*Dedicated to our mentor, Barry M. Brenner,
founding editor of* The Kidney,
pioneering investigator and visionary academic

Brenner & Rector's
The Kidney
9th Edition

Maarten W. Taal, MBChB, MMed, MD, FCP(SA), FRCP
Consultant Nephrologist and Honorary Associate Professor
Royal Derby Hospital and University of Nottingham
Derby, United Kingdom

Glenn M. Chertow, MD, MPH
Professor of Medicine
Chief, Division of Nephrology
Stanford University School of Medicine
Palo Alto, California

Philip A. Marsden, MD
Professor of Medicine
Keenan Chair in Medical Research at St. Michael's Hospital
Oreopoulos-Baxter Division Director of Nephrology
    at the University of Toronto
Department of Medicine, University of Toronto
Toronto, Ontario, Canada

Karl Skorecki, MD
Professor of Medicine
Division of Nephrology
Director, Rappaport Research Institute
Technion—Israel Institute of Technology
Director of Medical Research and Development
Rambam Health Care Campus
Haifa, Israel

Alan S. L. Yu, MB, B Chir
Harry Statland and Solon Summerfield Professor of Medicine
Director, Division of Nephrology and
    Hypertension and the Kidney Institute
University of Kansas Medical Center
Kansas City, Kansas

Barry M. Brenner, MD, AM(Hon), DSc(Hon), DMSc(Hon), MD(Hon), Dipl(Hon), FRCP(London, Hon)
Samuel A. Levine Distinguished Professor of Medicine
Harvard Medical School
Director Emeritus, Renal Division, and Senior Physician
Department of Medicine
Brigham and Women's Hospital
Boston, Massachusetts

Volume 1

ELSEVIER
SAUNDERS

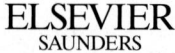
SAUNDERS

1600 John F. Kennedy Blvd.
Ste 1800
Philadelphia, PA 19103-2899

BRENNER & RECTOR'S THE KIDNEY   ISBN: 978-1-4160-6193-9

**Copyright © 2012, 2008, 2004, 2000, 1996, 1991, 1986, 1981, 1976 by Saunders,
an imprint of Elsevier Inc.**

Notice

Knowledge and best practice in this field are constantly changing. As new research and experience broaden our understanding, changes in research methods, professional practices, or medical treatment may become necessary.

Practitioners and researchers must always rely on their own experience and knowledge in evaluating and using any information, methods, compounds, or experiments described herein. In using such information or methods they should be mindful of their own safety and the safety of others, including parties for whom they have a professional responsibility.

With respect to any drug or pharmaceutical products identified, readers are advised to check the most current information provided (i) on procedures featured or (ii) by the manufacturer of each product to be administered, to verify the recommended dose or formula, the method and duration of administration, and contraindications. It is the responsibility of practitioners, relying on their own experience and knowledge of their patients, to make diagnoses, to determine dosages and the best treatment for each individual patient, and to take all appropriate safety precautions.

To the fullest extent of the law, neither the Publisher nor the authors, contributors, or editors, assume any liability for any injury and/or damage to persons or property as a matter of products liability, negligence or otherwise, or from any use or operation of any methods, products, instructions, or ideas contained in the material herein.

Library of Congress Cataloging-in-Publication Data

Brenner & Rector's the kidney / [edited by] Maarten W. Taal ... [et al.]. -- 9th ed.
    p. ; cm.
  Brenner and Rector's the kidney
  Kidney
  Includes bibliographical references and index.
  ISBN 978-1-4160-6193-9 (hardcover : alk. paper)
  I. Taal, Maarten W. II. Brenner, Barry M., 1937 - III. Rector, Floyd C. IV. Title: Brenner and Rector's the kidney. V. Title: Kidney.
  [DNLM: 1. Kidney Diseases. 2. Kidney--physiology. 3. Kidney--physiopathology. WJ 300]
  LC classification not assigned
  616.6'1--dc23
                                                                        2011032278

Acquisitions Editor: Kate Dimock
Developmental Editor: Joan Ryan
Publishing Services Manager: Jeff Patterson
Project Manager: Clay S. Broeker
Design Direction: Steven Stave

Printed in the United States of America

Last digit is the print number: 9 8 7 6 5 4 3 2 1

CONTRIBUTORS

Andrew Advani, BSc, MBChB(Hons), FRCP(UK), PhD
Assistant Professor
Clinician Scientist and Staff Endocrinologist
University of Toronto
St. Michael's Hospital
Toronto, Ontario, Canada
Vasoactive Molecules and the Kidney

Michael Allon, MD
Professor of Medicine, Division of Nephrology
University of Alabama at Birmingham
Birmingham, Alabama
Interventional Nephrology

Amanda Hyre Anderson, PhD, MPH
Research Associate
Center for Clinical Epidemiology and Biostatistics
University of Pennsylvania, Perelman
    School of Medicine
Philadelphia, Pennsylvania
Demographics of the Kidney

Gerald B. Appel, MD
Professor of Clinical Medicine
Columbia University, College of Physicians and Surgeons
The New York Presbyterian Hospital
New York, New York
Secondary Glomerular Disease

Suheir Assady, MD, PhD
Director, Department of Nephrology
Rambam Health Care Campus
Haifa, Israel
Near and Middle East

Anthony Atala, MD
Director, Institute for Regenerative Medicine
W.H. Boyce Professor and Chair, Department of Urology
Wake Forest University School of Medicine
Winston-Salem, North Carolina
Tissue Engineering, Stem Cells, and Cell Therapy in Nephrology

Colin Baigent
Professor of Epidemiology
Clinical Trial Service Unit and Epidemiological
    Studies Unit
University of Oxford
Oxford, United Kingdom
Cardiovascular Consequences of Kidney Disease

Sevcan A. Bakkaloglu, MD
Professor of Pediatrics, Faculty of Medicine
Department of Pediatric Nephrology
Gazi University
Ankara, Turkey
Diseases of the Kidney and Urinary Tract in Children

Gina-Marie Barletta, MD
Pediatric Nephrology
Phoenix Children's Hospital
Phoenix, Arizona
Dialysis in Children

Gavin J. Becker, MD, FRACP
Professor and Director of Nephrology
The Royal Melbourne Hospital and The University of
    Melbourne
Melbourne, Victoria, Australia
Renal Disease in the Oceania Region

Rinaldo Bellomo, MBBS, MD, FRACP, FCICM
Professor, Department of Medicine
University of Melbourne
Director of Intensive Care Research
Department of Intensive Care
Austin Health
Melbourne, Victoria, Australia
Critical Care Nephrology

Jeffrey S. Berns, MD
Professor of Medicine and Pediatrics
Renal-Electrolyte, and Hypertension Division
Perelman School of Medicine at the University of
    Pennsylvania
Hospital of the University of Pennsylvania
Philadelphia, Pennsylvania
Demographics of the Kidney

Vivek Bhalla, MD, FASN
Assistant Professor, Department of Medicine/Nephrology
Stanford University School of Medicine
Stanford University Hospitals and Clinics
Stanford, California
Aldosterone Regulation of Ion Transport

Jürg Biber, PhD
Institute of Physiology
University of Zurich
Zurich, Switzerland
Transport of Calcium, Magnesium, and Phosphate

Daniel G. Bichet, MD, MSc
Professor, Medicine and Physiology
Université de Montréal
Nephrologist
Hôpital du Sacré-Coeur de Montréal
Montreal, Quebec, Canada
Inherited Disorders of the Renal Tubule

René J.M. Bindels, PhD
Physiology
Radboud University Nijmegen Medical Centre
Nijmegen, The Netherlands
Transport of Calcium, Magnesium, and Phosphate

Melissa B. Bleicher, MD
Assistant Professor
Renal-Electrolyte and Hypertension Division
Department of Medicine
University of Pennsylvania
Philadelphia, Pennsylvania
Demographics of Kidney Disease

Jon D. Blumenfeld, MD
Professor of Clinical Medicine
Weill Medical College of Cornell University
Director
Hypertension and the Susan R. Knafel Polycystic Kidney
    Disease Center
The Rogosin Institute
Attending Physician, Medicine
New York Presbyterian Hospital
Attending Physician
The Rockefeller University Hospital
New York, New York
Primary and Secondary Hypertension

Alain Bonnardeaux, MD, PhD
Full Professor, Medicine
Université de Montréal
Staff Nephrologist
Hôpital Maisonneuve-Rosemont
Montreal, Quebec, Canada
Inherited Disorders of the Renal Tubule

Joseph V. Bonventre, MD, PhD
Samuel A. Levine Professor of Medicine
Harvard University
Cambridge, Massachusetts
Chief, Division of Renal Medicine
Chief, Biomedical Engineering Division, Medicine
Brigham and Women's Hospital
Boston, Massachusetts
Biomarkers in Acute and Chronic Kidney Diseases

William D. Boswell, Jr. MD, FACR
Professor Emeritus of Radiology and Urology
Keck School of Medicine
University of Southern California
Los Angeles, California
Professor and Chairman, Department of Diagnostic Radiology
City of Hope National Medical Center
Duarte, California
Diagnostic Kidney Imaging

Donald W. Bowden, PhD
Professor of Biochemistry and Internal Medicine
Center for Genomics and Personalized Medicine Research
Wake Forest University School of Medicine
Winston-Salem, North Carolina
Genetic Basis of Kidney Disease

Barry M. Brenner, MD, AM(Hon), DSc(Hon), DMSc(Hon), MD(Hon), Dipl(Hon), FRCP(London, Hon)
Samuel A. Levine Distinguished Professor of Medicine
Harvard Medical School
Director Emeritus, Renal Division, and Senior Physician
Department of Medicine
Brigham and Women's Hospital
Boston, Massachusetts
The Renal Circulations and Glomerular Ultrafiltration
Nephron Endowment
*Adaptation to Nephron Loss and Mechanisms of Progression in Chronic
    Kidney Disease*

Matthew D. Breyer, MD
Chief Scientific Officer, Lead Generation
Biotechnology Discovery Research
Eli Lilly and Company
Indianapolis, Indiana
Arachidonic Acid Metabolites and the Kidney

Richard M. Breyer, PhD
Professor, Medicine (Nephrology)
Vanderbilt University School of Medicine
Nashville, Tennessee
Arachidonic Acid Metabolites and the Kidney

Dennis Brown, PhD
Professor of Medicine
Harvard Medical School
Director, MGH Program in Membrane Biology
MGH Center for Systems Biology and Division of
    Nephrology
Massachusetts General Hospital
Simches Research Center
Boston, Massachusetts
The Cell Biology of Vasopressin Action

Carlo Brugnara, MD
Professor of Pathology, Department of Pathology
Harvard Medical School
Director of the Hematology Laboratory
Department of Laboratory Medicine
Children's Hospital Boston
Hematologic Aspects of Kidney Disease

Timothy E. Bunchman, MD
Professor and Director, Pediatric Nephrology
Children's Hospital of Richmond
Virginia Commonwealth University
Richmond, Virginia
Dialysis in Children

David A. Bushinsky, MD
Professor of Medicine and Pharmacology and Physiology
Department of Medicine
University of Rochester School of Medicine and Dentistry
Chief, Division of Nephrology
University of Rochester Medical Center
Rochester, New York
Nephrolithiaisis

Stéphan Busque, MD, MSc, FRCSC
Associate Professor, Surgery
Stanford University School of Medicine
Director, Adult Kidney and Pancreas Transplant Program
Stanford Hospital and Clinics
Stanford, California
Clinical Management

Juan Jesús Carrero, Pharm, PhD Pharm, PhD Med, MBA
Assistant Professor, Division of Renal Medicine
Department of Clinical Science, Intervention and Technology
Karolinska Institutet
Stockholm, Sweden
Endocrine Aspects of Chronic Kidney Disease

Daniel Cattran, MD, FRCP(c), FACP
Professor of Medicine
Medicine/Nephrology
University Health Network
Senior Scientist
Toronto General Research Institute
Toronto, Ontario, Canada
Overview of Therapy for Glomerular Disease

James C. Chan, MD
Professor of Pediatrics
Tufts University
Boston, Massachusetts
Director of Research, Department of Pediatrics
Barbara Bush Children's Hospital
Maine Medical Center
Portland, Maine
Fluid, Electrolyte, and Acid-Base Disorders in Children

Anil Chandraker, MB, ASN, FRCP
Associate Professor, Medicine
Harvard Medical School
Boston, Massachusetts
Transplantation Immunobiology

Ingrid J. Chang, MD
Partner and Clinical Physician
Western Nephrology
Denver, Colorado
Extracorporeal Treatment of Poisoning

Devasmita Choudhury, MD
Associate Professor of Medicine
University of Texas Southwestern Medical School
Director, In-Center and Home Dialysis
VA North Texas Health Care System
Dallas VA Medical Center
Dallas, Texas
Aging and Kidney Disease

Fredric L. Coe, MD
Professor of Medicine, Renal Section
University of Chicago
Chicago, Illinois
Nephrolithiaisis

John F. Collins, FRACP
Clinical Associate Professor, Medicine
University of Auckland
Doctor, Renal Medicine
Auckland City Hospital
Auckland, New Zealand
Renal Disease in the Oceania Region

H. Terence Cook, FRCPath, FMedSci
Professor of Renal Pathology
Department of Medicine
Imperial College
London, United Kingdom
The Renal Biopsy

Ricardo Correa-Rotter, MD
Head, Department of Nephrology and Mineral Metabolism
Instituto Nacional de Ciencias Médicas y Nutricion Salvador Zubirán
Professor of Nephrology
Universidad Nacional Autónoma de México
Mexico City, Mexico
Peritoneal Dialysis

Shawn E. Cowper, MD
Associate Professor of Dermatology and Pathology
Yale University School of Medicine
Yale New Haven Hospital
New Haven, Connecticut
Dermatologic Conditions in Kidney Disease

Paolo Cravedi, MD
Unit of Nephrology and Dialysis
Azienda Ospedaliera Ospedali Riuniti di Bergamo
Mario Negri Institute for Pharmacological Research
Bergamo, Italy
Microvascular and Macrovascular Diseases of the Kidney

Alfonso M. Cueto-Manzano, MD, MSc, PhD
Head, Medical Research Unit of Kidney Diseases
Hospital de Especialidades, CMNO, IMSS
Guadalajara, Jalisco, Mexico
Peritoneal Dialysis

Vivette D. D'Agati, MD
Professor of Pathology
Columbia University, College of Physicians and Surgeons
Director, Renal Pathology Laboratory
Department of Pathology
Columbia University Medical Center
New York, New York
Secondary Glomerular Disease

Mogomat Razeen Davids, MD
Associate Professor, Department of Medicine and Division
    of Nephrology
Stellenbosch University
Head, Division of Nephrology
Department of Medicine
Tygerberg Hospital
Cape Town, South Africa
*Interpretation of Electrolyte and Acid-Base Parameters in Blood
    and Urine*

Scott E. Delacroix, Jr., MD
Clinical Instructor, Department of Urology
Louisiana State University School of Medicine
New Orleans, Louisiana
Fellow, Urologic Oncology
Department of Urology
The University of Texas M.D. Anderson Cancer Center
Houston, Texas
Renal Neoplasia

Bradley M. Denker, MD
Associate Professor of Medicine
Harvard Medical School
Physician, Division of Nephrology
Beth Israel Deaconess Medical Center
Chief of Nephrology
Harvard Vanguard Medical Associates
Boston, Massachusetts
Plasmapheresis

Thomas A. Depner, MD
Professor of Medicine, Division of Nephrology
Director of Dialysis Services
University of California—Davis Health System
Sacramento, California
Hemodialysis

Thomas D. DuBose, Jr., MD
Tinsley R. Harrison Professor and Chair of Internal
    Medicine
Professor of Physiology and Pharmacology
Wake Forest School of Medicine
Winston-Salem, North Carolina
Disorders of Acid-Base Balance

Kai-Uwe Eckardt, MD
Professor of Medicine
Department of Nephrology and Hypertension
University of Erlangen-Nürnberg
Erlangen, Germany
University Clinic Erlangen
Erlangen, Germany
Community Hospital Nürnberg
Nürnberg, Germany
Hematologic Aspects of Kidney Disease

Mohamed T. Eldehni, MD, MSc, MRCP(UK)
Research Fellow in Renal Medicine
School of Graduate Entry Medicine and Health
University of Nottingham Medical School at Derby
Derby, United Kingdom
Prescribing Drugs in Kidney Disease

David H. Ellison, MD
Division Chief and Professor of Medicine and Physiology
    and Pharmacology
Division of Nephrology and Hypertension
School of Medicine, Department of Medicine
Oregon Health and Science University
Portland, Oregon
Diuretics

Michael Emmett, MD, MACP
Chairman, Department of Internal Medicine
Baylor University Medical Center
Dallas, Texas
Professor of Internal Medicine
Texas A&M Health Science Center, College of Medicine
Bryan, Texas
Approach to the Patient with Kidney Disease

Ronald J. Falk, MD
Allen Brewster Distinguished Professor
UNC Kidney Center
Chief, Division of Nephrology and Hypertension
Department of Medicine, School of Medicine
Director, UNC Kidney Center
University of North Carolina at Chapel Hill
University of North Carolina Hospitals
Chapel Hill, North Carolina
Primary Glomerular Disease

Harold I. Feldman, MD, MSCE
Professor of Medicine and Epidemiology
Director, Division of Epidemiology, and Director, Clinical
    Epidemiology Unit
Department of Biostatistics and Epidemiology
Center for Clinical Epidemiology and Biostatistics
Department of Medicine
Professor of Medicine and Epidemiology
Renal-Electrolyte and Hypertension Division
Department of Medicine
University of Pennsylvania
Philadelphia, Pennsylvania
Demographics of Kidney Disease

Robert A. Fenton, BSc(Hons), PhD
Professor of Molecular Cell Biology
Department of Biomedicine
Aarhus University
Aahrus, Denmark
Anatomy of the Kidney
Urine Concentration and Dilution
The Cell Biology of Vasopressin Action

Andrew Z. Fenves, MD, FACP
Director, Nephrology Division
Internal Medicine
Baylor University Medical Center
Dallas, Texas
Professor of Internal Medicine
Internal Medicine
Texas A&M Health Science Center, College of Medicine
Bryan, Texas
Approach to the Patient with Kidney Disease

Kevin W. Finkel, MD, FACP, FASN, FCCM
Professor of Medicine and Director
Division of Renal Diseases and Hypertension
Professor of Medicine
General Internal Medicine, Section of Nephrology
University of Texas Health Science Center at Houston
Chief of Nephrology
Memorial-Herman Hospital, Texas Medical Center
Houston, Texas
Renal Disease in Cancer Patients

Paola Fioretto, MD, PhD
Professor of Endocrinology
University of Padua Medical School
Padua, Italy
Diabetic Nephropathy

Damian G. Fogarty, BSc, MD, FRCP
Senior Lecturer in Renal Medicine
Centre for Public Health
Queen's University of Belfast
Consultant Nephrologist
Regional Nephrology and Transplant Unit
Belfast City Hospital at the Belfast Health and Social Care
    Trust
Belfast, Northern Ireland
Chairman, United Kingdom Renal Registry
A Stepped Care Approach to the Management of Chronic Kidney Disease

John R. Foringer, MD
Associate Professor of Medicine
Division of Renal Diseases and Hypertension
University of Texas Health Science Center at Houston
Chief of Medicine
LBJ General Hospital
Associate Professor of Medicine
General Internal Medicine, Section of Nephrology
The University of Texas Anderson Cancer Center
Houston, Texas
Renal Disease in Cancer Patients

Denis Fouque, MD, PhD
Professor of Nephrology
University Claude Bernard Lyon 1
Chief
Division of Nephrology
Hospital Edouard Herriot
Lyon, France
Dietary Approaches to Kidney Diseases

Barry I. Freedman, MD
John H. Felts, III Professor and Chief
Section on Nephrology
Professor, Urology
Wake Forest School of Medicine
Winston-Salem, North Carolina
Genetic Basis of Kidney Disease

Jørgen Frøkiaer, MD, PhD
Professor, Institute of Clinical Medicine
Aarhus University
Chief Physician
Department of Clinical Physiology
Aarhus University Hospital
Aarhus, Denmark
Urinary Tract Obstruction

John W. Funder, MD, PhD, FRACP, FRCP
Senior Fellow, Prince Henry's Institute
Monash Medical Centre
Clayton, Australia
Aldosterone Regulation of Ion Transport

**David S. Game, MA(Cantab), BMBCh(Oxon,) PhD,
    MRCP(UK)**
Consultant Nephrologist
Guy's Hospital
Kings Health Partners
London, United Kingdom
Vasoactive Molecules and the Kidney

Richard E. Gilbert, MBBS, PhD, FRCPC
Professor of Medicine and Canada Research Chair
University of Toronto
St. Michael's Hospital
Toronto, Ontario, Canada
Vasoactive Molecules and the Kidney

Jared J. Grantham, MD
University Distinguished Professor
Kidney Institute/Internal Medicine
Kansas University Medical Center
University Distinguished Professor
Internal Medicine
University of Kansas Hospital
Kansas City, Kansas
Cystic Diseases of the Kidney

Mitchell L. Halperin, MD, FRCPC, FRS
Emeritus Professor of Medicine
Medicine/Nephrology
Staff, Research Division
Keenan Research Building
Li Ka Shing Medical Knowledge Institute
Attending Staff, Nephrology
Medicine
St. Michaels Hospital
University of Toronto
Toronto, Ontario, Canada
*Interpretation of Electrolytes and Acid-Base Parameters in Blood
    and Urine*

Matthew Hand, DO
Division Director, Pediatric Nephrology
Tufts/Maine Medical Center School of Medicine
Division Director, Pediatric Nephrology
Pediatrics
The Barbara Bush Children's Hospital at Maine Medical
    Center
Portland, Maine
Fluid, Electrolyte, and Acid-Base Disorders in Children

Donna S. Hanes, MD, FACP
Associate Professor of Medicine
University of Maryland Medical Systems
Baltimore, Maryland
Antihypertensive Drugs

David C.H. Harris, MD, BS, FRACP
Associate Dean and Head of School
Sydney Medical School—Westmead
The University of Sydney
Sydney, New South Wales, Australia
Renal Disease in the Oceania Region

Raymond C. Harris, MD
Ann and Roscoe Robinson Professor of Medicine and Chief
Division of Nephrology
Medicine
Vanderbilt University School of Medicine
Nashville, Tennessee
Arachidonic Acid Metabolites and the Kidney

Richard Haynes, MA, BM, BCh, MRCP
Clinical Research Fellow
Clinical Trial Service Unit and Epidemiological Studies Unit
University of Oxford
Specialist Registrar
Oxford Kidney Unit
Oxford Radcliffe Hospitals NHS Trust
Oxford, Oxfordshire, United Kingdom
Cardiovascular Aspects of Kidney Disease

Joost G. J. Hoenderop, PhD
Physiology
Radboud University Nijmegen Medical Centre
Nijmegen, The Netherlands
Transport of Calcium, Magnesium, and Phosphate

Ewout J. Hoorn, MD, PhD
Renal Fellow
Department of Internal Medicine—Nephrology
Erasmus Medical Center
Rotterdam, Netherlands
Diuretics

Thomas H. Hostetter, MD
Professor of Medicine
Case Western Reserve University School of Medicine
Cleveland, Ohio
Pathophysiology of Uremia

Chi-yuan Hsu, MD, MSc
Professor and Chief, Division of Nephrology
University of California—San Francisco
San Francisco, California
Epidemiology of Kidney Disease

Shih Hua-Lin, MD
Professor, Department of Medicine
National Defense Medical Center
Chief, Division of Nephrology
Department of Medicine
Tri-Service General Hospital
Taipei, Taiwan
Interpretation of Electrolyte and Acid-Base Parameters in Blood and Urine

Hassan N. Ibrahim, MD, MS
Associate Professor of Medicine
Director, Division of Renal Diseases and Hypertension
Medicine
Nephrologist, Transplant Department
University of Minnesota Medical Center—Fairview
University of Minnesota
Minneapolis, Minnesota
Donor and Recipient Issues

Ajay K. Israni, MD, MS
Associate Professor, Medicine
University of Minnesota
Attending Physician, Medicine
Hennepin County Medical Center
Deputy Director
Scientific Registry of Transplant Recipients
Minneapolis Medical Research Foundation
Minneapolis, Minnesota
Laboratory Assessment of Kidney Disease: Glomerular Filtration Rate, Urinalysis, and Proteinuria

Jossein Jadvar, MD, PhD, MPH, MBA
Associate Professor of Radiology and Biomedical
    Engineering and Director of Research
Keck School of Medicine
University of Southern California
Attending Physician
Department of Radiology
Keck Medical Center of University of Southern California
Los Angeles, California
Diagnostic Kidney Imaging

J. Charles Jennette, MD
Kenneth M. Brinkhous Distinguished Professor and Chair
Department of Pathology and Laboratory Medicine
The University of North Carolina at Chapel Hill
Chapel Hill, North Carolina
Primary Glomerular Disease

Eric Jonasch, MD
Associate Professor
Department of Genitourinary Medical Oncology
The University of Texas M.D. Anderson Cancer Center
Houston, Texas
Renal Neoplasia

Kamel S. Kamel M.D, FRCP(c)
Professor of Medicine
University of Toronto
Head, Division of Nephrology
Medicine
St. Michael's Hospital
Toronto, Ontario, Canada
Interpretation of Electrolyte and Acid-Base Parameters in Blood and Urine

S. Ananth Karumanchi, MD
Associate Professor, Medicine
Harvard Medical School
Attending Nephrologist
Medicine
Beth Israel Deaconess Medical Center
Boston, Massachusetts
Hypertension and Kidney Disease in Pregnancy

Bertram L. Kasiske, MD
Department of Medicine
Hennepin County Medical Center
Minneapolis, Minnesota
*Laboratory Assessment of Kidney Disease: Glomerular Filtration Rate,
Urinalysis, and Proteinuria*
Donor and Recipient Issues

John A. Kellum, MD
Professor and Vice Chair
Critical Care Medicine
University of Pittsburgh
Pittsburgh, Pennsylvania
Critical Care Nephrology

Carolyn J. Kelly, MD
Professor and Associate Dean
Department of Medicine
University of Calfornia at San Diego
San Diego, California
Tubulointerstitial Diseases

Ramesh Khanna, MD
Karl D. Nolph, M.D. Chair in Nephrology and Professor of
Medicine
Department of Internal Medicine, Division of Nephrology
University of Missouri
Columbia, Missouri
Peritoneal Dialysis

David K. Klassen, MD
Professor of Medicine
Division of Nephrology, Department of Medicine
University of Maryland School of Medicine
Baltimore, Maryland
Antihypertensive Drugs

Christine J. Ko, MD
Associate Professor of Dermatology and Pathology
Yale University
New Haven, Connecticut
Dermatologic Conditions in Kidney Disease

Harbir Singh Kohli, MD, DM
Professor, Nephrology
Post Graduate Institute of Medical Education and Research
Chandigarh, India
Indian Subcontinent

Curtis K. Kost, Jr., RPh, PhD
Associate Professor of Physiology and Pharmacology
Division of Basic Biomedical Sciences
Sanford School of Medicine
University of South Dakota
Vermillion, South Dakota
The Renal Circulations and Glomerular Ultrafiltration

L. Spencer Krane, MD
Department of Urology
Wake Forest University
Winston-Salem, North Carolina
Tissue Engineering, Stem Cells, and Cell Therapy in Nephrology

Jordan Kreidberg, MD, PhD
Associate Professor, Pediatrics
Harvard Medical School
Boston, Massachusetts
Embryology of the Kidney

Tae-Hwan Kwon, MD, PhD
Department of Biochemistry and Cell Biology
School of Medicine
Kyungpook National University
Daegu, Korea
Anatomy of the Kidney

Amit Lahoti, MD
Assistant Professor
General Internal Medicine, Section of Nephrology
The University of Texas M. D. Anderson Cancer Center
Houston, Texas
Renal Disease in Cancer Patients

Martin J. Landray, PhD, FRCP, FASN
Reader in Epidemiology
Clinical Trial Service Unit and Epidemiological Studies Unit
Honorary Consultant Physician
Oxford Radcliffe Hospitals NHS Trust
University of Oxford
Oxford, Oxfordshire, United Kingdom
Cardiovascular Consequences of Kidney Disease

John H. Laragh, MD
Cardiothoracic Surgery
Weill Cornell Medical College
Attending Physician
New York Presbyterian Hospital
New York, New York
Primary and Secondary Hypertension

Harold E. Layton, PhD
Professor of Mathematics
Duke University
Durham, North Carolina
Urine Concentration and Dilution

Moshe Levi, MD
Professor of Medicine and Physiology and Biophysics
and Bioengineering
Division of Renal Diseases and Hypertension
University of Colorado at Denver
Aurora, Colorado
Aging and Kidney Disease

Bengt Lindholm, MD, PhD
Adjunct Professor
Divisions of Baxter Novum and Renal Medicine
Department of Clinical Science, Intervention and
Technology
Karolinska Institute
Stockholm, Sweden
Endocrine Aspects of Chronic Kidney Disease

Frank Liu, MD
Assistant Professor of Medicine
Department of Medicine
Weill Cornell Medical College
Nephrologist
The Rogosin Institute
Assistant Attending Physician
Department of Medicine
New York Presbyterian Hospital, Weill Cornell Center
New York, New York
Primary and Secondary Hypertension

Valerie A. Luyckx, MBBCh
Associate Professor
Division of Nephrology, Department of Medicine
University of Alberta
Division of Nephrology, Department of Medicine
University of Alberta Hospital
Edmonton, Alberta, Canada
Nephron Endowment

David A. Maddox, PhD, FASN
Professor, Internal Medicine and Basic Biomedical Sciences
Sanford School of Medicine
University of South Dakota
Coordinator, Research and Development
Sioux Falls VA Healthcare System
Senior Research Scientist (WOC)
Avera Research Institute
Avera McKennan Hospital
Sioux Falls, South Dakota
The Renal Circulations and Glomerular Ultrafiltration

Yoshiro Maezawa, MD
Samuel Lunenfeld Research Institute
Mount Sinai Hospital
Toronto, Ontario, Canada
Embryology of the Kidney

Arthur J. Matas, MD
Professor, Surgery
University of Minnesota
Minneapolis, Minnesota
Donor and Recipient Issues

Michael Mauer, MD
Professor, Pediatrics and Medicine
Amplatz Children's Hospital
Pediatrics
University of Minnesota
Minneapolis, Minnesota
Diabetic Nephropathy

Ivan D. Maya, MD, FACP
Associate Professor of Medicine and Radiology Medicine
University of Central Florida
Staff Nephrology Attending Medicine
Florida Hospital
Orlando, Florida
Interventional Nephrology

Sharon E. Maynard, MD
Adjunct Associate Professor of Medicine
George Washington University School of Medicine
Washington, DC
Physician, Division of Nephrology
Lehigh Valley Health Network
Allentown, Pennsylvania
Hypertension and Kidney Disease in Pregnancy

Alicia A. McDonough, PhD
Professor, Cell and Neurobiology
Keck School of Medicine
University of Southern California
Los Angeles, California
Metabolic Basis of Solute Transport

Christopher W. McIntyre, MD, DM
Associate Professor and Reader in Vascular Medicine
School of Graduate Entry Medicine and Health
University of Nottingham
Nottingham, United Kingdom
Honorary Consultant Nephrologist
Department of Renal Medicine
Royal Derby Hospital
Derby, United Kingdom
Prescribing Drugs in Kidney Disease

Timothy W. Meyer, MD
Professor of Medicine
Stanford University
Stanford, California
VA Palo Alto Health Care System
Palo Alto, California
Pathophysiology of Uremia

William E. Mitch, MD
Gordon A. Cain Chair in Nephrology
Department of Medicine, Division of Nephrology
Baylor College of Medicine
Houston, Texas
Dietary Approaches to Kidney Diseases

Orson W. Moe, MD
Professor of Internal Medicine and Physiology
Internal Medicine
University of Texas Southwestern Medical Center
Director
Charles and Jane Pak Center of Mineral Metabolism
University of Texas Southwestern Medical Center
Dallas, Texas
Renal Handling of Organic Solutes Nephrolithiasis

Sharon M. Moe, MD
Professor of Medicine and Anatomy and Cell Biology
Director, Division of Nephrology, Department of Medicine
Indiana University School of Medicine
Indiana University Health
Indianapolis, Indiana
Chronic Kidney Disease–Mineral Bone Disorder

Bruce A. Molitoris, MD
Professor of Medicine
Department of Medicine
Indiana University School of Medicine
Professor of Medicine
Roudebush VA Medical Center
Indianapolis, Indiana
Biomarkers in Acute Kidney Injury

Alvin H. Moss, MD, FACP, FAAHPM
Professor of Medicine
Section of Nephrology, Department of Medicine
Director, Center for Health Ethics and Law
West Virginia University
Morgantown, West Virginia
Ethical Dilemmas Facing Nephrology: Past, Present, and Future

David B. Mount, MD, FRCPC
Assistant Professor of Medicine
Harvard Medical School
Physician, Renal Division
Brigham and Women's Hospital and VA Boston Healthcare
    System
Boston, Massachusetts
Transport of Sodium, Chloride, and Potassium
Disorders of Potassium Balance

Karen A. Munger, PhD
Associate Professor of Medicine
Internal Medicine
Sanford School of Medicine
University of South Dakota
Director, Basic and Applied Research
Avera Research Institute
Avera McKennan Hospital and University Health Center
Research Physiologist
Research and Development
Sioux Falls VA Healthcare System
Sioux Falls, South Dakota
The Renal Circulations and Glomerular Ultrafiltration

Patrick H. Nachman, MD
Professor of Medicine
Division of Nephrology and Hypertension
Department of Medicine
University of North Carolina at Chapel Hill
Attending Physician, Department of Medicine
University of North Carolina Hospitals
Chapel Hill, North Carolina
Primary Glomerular Disease

Saraladevi Naicker, MB ChB, MRCP, FRCP, PhD
Professor of Nephrology and Academic Head, Internal
    Medicine
Faculty of Health Sciences
University of the Witwatersrand
Professor of Nephrology
Division of Nephrology
Charlotte Maxeke Johannesburg Academic Hospital
Johannesburg, South Africa
Africa

Søren Nielsen, MD, PhD
Professor of Cell Biology and Pathophysiology
Institute of Anatomy
Aarhus University
Aarhus, Denmark
Anatomy of the Kidney

Eric G. Neilson, MD
Vice President for Medical Affairs and Dean
Feinberg School of Medicine
Northwestern University
Chicago, Illinois
Tubulointerstitial Diseases

Lindsay E. Nicolle, MD FRCPC
Professor of Internal Medicine and Medical Microbiology
University of Manitoba
Winnipeg, Manitoba, Canada
Urinary Tract Infection in Adults

Daniel B. Ornt, MD, FACP
Vice Dean for Education and Academic Affairs and Interim
    Chair of Anatomy
Director, Center for Medical Education, and Professor of
    Medicine
Case Western Reserve University School of Medicine
Cleveland, Ohio
Hemodialysis

Manuel Palacín, PhD
Full Professor, Biochemistry and Molecular Biology
Universitat de Barcelona
Group Leader
Unit 731
CIBERER (The Spanish Network Center for Rare Diseases)
Group Leader
Molecular Medicine Program
Institute for Research in Biomedicine of Barcelona
Barcelona, Spain
Renal Handling of Organic Solutes

Paul M. Palevsky, MD
Chief, Renal Section
VA Pittsburgh Healthcare System
Professor of Medicine and Clinical and Translational Science
Renal-Electrolyte Division, Department of Medicine
University of Pittsburgh School of Medicine
Pittsburgh, Pennsylvania
Acute Kidney Injury

Suzanne L. Palmer, MD
Associate Professor of Clinical Radiology and Internal
    Medicine
Division Chief, Body Imaging
Attending Physician
Department of Radiology
Keck School of Medicine, University of Southern California
Los Angeles, California
Diagnostic Kidney Imaging

Hans-Henrik Parving, MD, DMSc
Professor and Chief Physician
University of Copenhagen
Professor and Chief Physician
Medical Endocrinology
Rigshospitalet
Copenhagen, Denmark
Diabetic Nephropathy

Jaakko Patrakka, MD, PhD
Assistant Professor
Department of Medical Biochemistry and Biophysics
Karolinska Institute
Nephrology Fellow
Division of Nephrology
Karolinska University Hospital
Stockholm, Sweden
Inherited Disorders of the Glomerulus

David Pearce, MD
Professor of Medicine and Cellular and Molecular
    Pharmacology
University of California at San Francisco
Chief, Division of Nephrology
San Francisco General Hospital
San Francisco, California
Aldosterone Regulation of Ion Transport

Roberto Pecoits-Filho, MD, PhD
Professor, Nephrology
Pontificia Universidade Católica do Paraná
Head, Internal Medicine
Cajurú University Hospital
Curitiba, Paraná, Brazil
Latin America

Carmen A. Peralta, MD
Assistant Professor of Medicine
University of California at San Francisco
Medicine
University of California—San Francisco Medical Center
Health Disparities in Nephrology

Norberto Perico, MD
Mario Negri Institute for Pharmacological Research
Bergamo, Italy
Mechanisms and Consequences of Proteinuria

Neil R. Powe, MD
Constance B. Wofsy Distinguished Professor of Medicine
University of California at San Francisco
Chief of Medicine
San Francisco General Hospital
San Francisco, California
Health Disparities in Nephrology

Kearkiat Praditpornsilpa, MD, MS
Associated Professor
Division of Nephrology
Chulalongkorn University
Nephrologist, Division of Nephrology
King Chulalongkorn Memorial Hospital
Bangkok, Thailand
Far East

Jeppe Prætorius, MD
Department of Anatomy
Aarhus University
Aarhus, Denmark
Anatomy of the Kidney

Susan E. Quaggin, MD
Professor, Medicine
University of Toronto
Senior Scientist
Samuel Lunenfeld Research Institute
Mount Sinai Hospital
Staff Nephrologist
St. Michael's Hospital
Toronto, Ontario, Canada
Embryology of the Kidney

L. Darryl Quarles, MD
Professor, Medicine—Nephrology
The University of Tennessee Health Science Center
Memphis, Tennessee
Vitamin D, Calcimimetic Agents, and Phosphate Binders

Jai Radhakrishnan, MD, MS
Associate Professor of Clinical Medicine
Department of Medicine, Division of Nephrology
Columbia University College of Physicians and Surgeons
Director, Nephrology Fellowship
New York, Presbyterian Hospital,
New York, New York
Secondary Glomerular Disease

Rawi Ramadan, MD
Adjunct Senior Lecturer, Faculty of Medicine
Technion—Israel Institute of Technology
Director of Kidney Transplantation Follow-Up Unit
Department of Nephrology
Rambam Health Care Campus
Haifa, Israel
Near and Middle East

Piero Reggenenti, MD
Unit of Nephrology and Dialysis
Azienda Ospedaliera Ospedali Riuniti di Bergamo
Mario Negri Institute for Pharmacological Research
Bergamo, Italy
Microvascular and Macrovascular Diseases of the Kidney

Heather N. Reich, MD CM, PhD, FRCP(C)
Assistant Professor, Medicine
University of Toronto
Clinician Scientist and Staff Nephrologist
Medicine
University Health Network
Toronto, Ontario, Canada
Overview of Therapy for Glomerular Disease

Andrea Remuzzi, EngD
University of Bergamo
Mario Negri Institute for Pharmacological Research
Bergamo, Italy
Mechanisms and Consequences of Proteinuria

Giuseppe Remuzzi, MD
Unit of Nephrology and Dialysis
Azienda Ospedaliera Ospedali Riuniti di Bergamo
Mario Negri Institute for Pharmacological Research
Bergamo, Italy
Microvascular and Macrovascular Diseases of the Kidney
Mechanisms and Consequences of Proteinuria

Stephen S. Rich, PhD
Harrison Professor and Vice-Chair
Department of Public Health Sciences
Director, Center for Public Health Genomics
University of Virginia
Charlottesville, Virginia
Genetic Basis of Kidney Disease

Miguel C. Riella, MD, PhD, FACP
Professor of Medicine
Catholic University of Parana
Chief, Nephrology and Transplant Division
Evangelic University Hospital
Chief, Nephrology and Transplant Division
Cajuru University Hospital, Catholic University of Parana
Curitiba, Brazil
Latin America

Eberhard Ritz, MD
Professor Emeritus
Department of Internal Medicine
Ruperto Carola University
Heidelberg, Germany
Diabetic Nephropathy

Claudio Ronco, MD
Director, Department of Nephrology, Dialysis, and
 Transplantation
International Renal Research Institute—Vicenza
San Bortolo Hospital
Vicenza, Italy
Critical Care Nephrology

Norman D. Rosenblum, MD
Professor of Paediatrics, Physiology, and Laboratory
 Medicine and Pathobiology
University of Toronto
Staff Nephrologist and Senior Scientist
Paediatrics and Research Institute
The Hospital for Sick Children
Toronto, Ontario, Canada
Malformation of the Kidney: Structural and Functional Consequences

Peter Rossing, MD, DMSc
Director of Research and Chief Physician
Steno Diabetes Center
Gentofte-Denmark
Diabetic Nephropathy

Dvora Rubinger, MD
Associate Professor of Medicine
Nephrology and Hypertensive Services, Department of
 Medicine
Hadassah Hebrew University Medical Center
Jerusalem, Israel
Near and Middle East

Robert K. Rude, MD*
Professor of Medicine
Division of Endocrinology, Diabetes and Metabolism
Keck School of Medicine
University of Southern California, Los Angeles County
University of Southern California Medical Center
Los Angeles, California
Disorders of Calcium, Magnesium, and Phosphate Balance

Ernesto Sabath, MD, PhD
Chief, Nephrology, Hemodialysis Unit
Hospital General de Queretaro
Queretaro, Mexico
Plasmapheresis

Venkata Sabbisetti, PhD
Instructor in Medicine
Harvard Medical School
Associate Biologist
Renal Division, Department of Medicine
Brigham and Women's Hospital
Boston, Massachusetts
Biomarkers in Acute and Chronic Kidney Diseases

Vinay Sakhuja, MD, DM, FAMS
Professor and Head
Department of Nephrology
Post Graduate Institute of Medical Education and Research
Chandigarh, India
Indian Subcontinent

*Deceased

Alan D. Salama, MBBS, MA, PhD, FRCP
Reader and Honorary Consultant in Nephrology
Centre for Nephrology
University College London, Royal Free Hospital
London, United Kingdom
The Renal Biopsy

Jeff M. Sands, MD
Juha P. Kokko Professor of Medicine and Physiology
Director, Renal Division
Executive Vice-Chair, Department of Medicine
Emory University
Atlanta, Georgia
Urine Concentration and Dilution

Fernando Santos, MD
Professor of Pediatrics
Medicine
University of Oviedo
Chairman of Pediatrics
Hospital Universitario Central de Asturias
Oviedo Asturias, Spain
Fluid, Electrolyte, and Acid-Base Disorders in Children

Mohamed H. Sayegh, MD, FAHA, FASN, ASCI, AAP
Director, Schuster Family Transplantation Research Center
Brigham and Women's Hospital and Children's Hospital
  Boston
Visiting Professor of Pediatrics and Medicine
Harvard Medical School
Boston, Massachusetts
Raja N. Khuri Dean, Faculty of Medicine
Professor of Medicine and Immunology
Vice President of Medical Affairs
American University of Beirut
New York, New York
Transplantation Immunobiology

John D. Scandling, MD
Professor of Medicine
Department of Medicine
Stanford University School of Medicine
Medical Director, Kidney and Pancreas Transplantation
Stanford Hospital and Clinics
Stanford, California
Clinical Management

Franz Schaefer, MD
Professor of Pediatrics, Faculty of Medicine
Ruprecht-Karls University
Head, Division of Pediatric Nephrology
Pediatrics I
Center for Pediatrics and Adolescent Medicine
Heidelberg, Germany
Diseases of the Kidney and Urinary Tract in Children

Jon I. Scheinman, MD
Fairway, Kansas
Pediatric Transplantation

John C. Schwartz, MD
Program Director, Nephrology Fellowship
Internal Medicine
Baylor University Medical Center
Dallas, Texas
Approach to the Patient with Kidney Disease

Asif A. Sharfuddin, MD
Assistant Professor of Clinical Medicine
Medicine/Nephrology
Indiana University School of Medicine
Staff Nephrologist/Transplant Nephrologist
Medicine/Nephrology
RLR VA Medical Center
Indianapolis, Indiana
Acute Kidney Injury

Susan Shaw, MRPharmS, DPharm
Renal Pharmacist
Renal Services
Royal Derby Hospital
Derby, United Kingdom
Prescribing Drugs in Kidney Disease

Visith Sitprija, MD, PhD
Emeritus Professor of Medicine
Department of Medicine
Chulalongkorn University Medical School
Department of Medicine
King Chulalongkorn Memorial Hospital
Director
Queen Saovabha Memorial Institute
Bangkok, Thailand
Far East

Karl L. Skorecki, MD
Professor of Medicine
Division of Nephrology
Director, Rappaport Research Institute
Technion—Israel Institute of Technology
Director of Medical Research and Development
Rambam Health Care Campus
Haifa, Israel
Disorders of Sodium Balance

Itzchak N. Slotki, MD
Senior Lecturer, Faculty of Medicine
Hebrew University, Hadassah Medical School
Head, Division of Adult Nephrology
Shaare Zedek Medical Center
Jerusalem, Israel
Disorders of Sodium Balance

James P. Smith, MD, MS
Clinical Lecturer
Internal Medicine, Division of Nephrology
University of Michigan
Ann Arbor, Michigan
Extracorporeal Treatment of Poisoning

Miroslaw J. Smogorzewski, MD, PhD
Associate Professor of Medicine
Division of Nephrology, Department of Medicine
Keck School of Medicine
University of Southern California
Attending Physician
Nephrology and Kidney Transplantation Services
Department of Medicine
USC University Hospital
Attending Physician
Nephrology Service
Division of Nephrology, Department of Medicine
LAC & USC Medical Center
Los Angeles, California
Disorders of Calcium, Magnesium, and Phosphate Balance

Stuart M. Sprague, DO
Professor, Medicine
University of Chicago Pritzker School of Medicine
Chicago, Illinois
Division Chief
Division of Nephrology and Hypertension
NorthShore University HealthSystem
Evanston, Illinois
Chronic Kidney Disease–Mineral Bone Disorder

Peter Stenvinkel, MD, PhD
Professor
Department of Nephrology
CLINTEC
Karolinska Institutet
Senior Consultant
Department of Nephrology
Karolinska University Hospital at Huddinge
Stockholm, Sweden
Endocrine Aspects of Chronic Kidney Disease

John B. Stokes, MD
Professor and Director
Division of Nephrology
Executive Vice-Chair
Department of Internal Medicine
University of Iowa
Staff Physician
Veteran's Affairs Medical Center
Iowa City, Iowa
Aldosterone Regulation of Ion Transport

Maarten W. Taal, MBChB, MMed, MD, FCP(SA), FRCP
Consultant Nephrologist and Honorary Associate Professor
Royal Derby Hospital and University of Nottingham
Derby, United Kingdom
Risk Factors and Chronic Kidney Disease
Adaptation to Nephron Loss and Mechanisms of Progression in Chronic Kidney Disease
A Stepped Care Approach to the Management of Chronic Kidney Disease

Manjula Kurella Tamura, MD, MPH
Assistant Professor
Department of Medicine, Division of Nephrology
Stanford University
Palo Alto, California
Neurologic Aspects of Kidney Disease

Jane C. Tan, MD, PhD
Associate Professor of Medicine
Department of Medicine
Stanford University School of Medicine
Kidney and Pancreas Transplantation
Stanford Hospital and Clinics
Stanford, California
Clinical Management

Stephen C. Textor, MD
Professor of Medicine
Division of Nephrology and Hypertension
Mayo Clinic College of Medicine
Rochester, Minnesota
Renovascular Hypertension and Ischemic Nephropathy

Ravi Thadhani, MD, MPH
Associate Professor of Medicine
Division of Nephrology
Senior Scientist in Obstetrics and Gynecology
Massachusetts General Hospital
Harvard Medical School
Boston, Massachusetts
Hypertension and Kidney Disease in Pregnancy

Scott C. Thomson, MD
Professor of Medicine
Division of Nephrology—Hypertension
University of California at San Diego
Chief of Nephrology Section
VA San Diego Healthcare System
Metabolic Basis of Solute Transport

Vincente E. Torres, MD, PhD
Professor of Medicine
Department of Nephrology and Hypertension
Mayo Clinic
Mayo Clinic Transplant Center
Rochester, Minnesota
Cystic Diseases of the Kidney

Karl Tryggvason, MD, PhD
Professor of Medical Chemistry
Department of Medical Biochemistry and Biophysics
Karlinska Institute
Stockholm, Sweden
Inherited Disorders of the Glomerulus

Meryem Tuncel, MD, FACP, FASN
Associate Professor of Medicine
Division of Nephrology and Hypertension
Texas Tech University Health Sciences Center
Lubbock, Texas
Aging and Kidney Disease

Kriang Tungsanga, MD
Professor of Medicine
Faculty of Medicine, Chulalongkorn University
Bangkok, Thailand
Far East

Joseph G. Verbalis, MD
Professor of Medicine and Chief
Division of Endocrinology and Metabolism
Director
Georgetown-Howard Universities Center for Clinical and
    Translational Science
Georgetown University
Washington, DC
Disorders of Water Balance

Jill W. Verlander, DVM
Associate Scientist and Director
College of Medicine Electron Microscopy Core Facility
Division of Nephrology, Hypertension, and Renal
    Transplantation
Department of Medicine
University of Florida College of Medicine
Gainesville, Florida
Renal Acidification Mechanisms

**Shoyab Wadee, MBBCh(Wits), FCP(SA), MMed(Wits),
    Cert Neph**
Doctor
Division of Nephrology, Department of Medicine
University of the Witwatersrand
Doctor
Wits Kidney and Dialysis Centre
Wits Donald Gordon Medical Centre
Johannesburg, Gauteng, South Africa
Africa

I. David Weiner, MD
C. Craig and Audrae Tisher Chair in Nephrology and Professor
    of Medicine, Physiology and Functional Genomics
Medicine
University of Florida College of Medicine
Attending Physician
Division of Nephrology
Shands Hospital at the University of Florida
Chief Nephrology and Hypertension Section
Medical Service
North Florida/South Georgia Veterans Health System
Gainesville, Florida
Renal Acidification Mechanisms

Matthew R. Weir, MD
Professor of Medicine
Director, Division of Nephrology
Department of Medicine
University of Maryland School of Medicine
Baltimore, Maryland
Antihypertensive Drugs

Steven D. Weisbord, MD, MSc
Assistant Professor of Medicine and Clinical and
    Translational Science
Department of Medicine
University of Pittsburgh School of Medicine
Staff Physician, Renal Section
Core Investigator, Center for Health Equity Research and
    Promotion
VA Pittsburgh Healthcare System
Pittsburgh, Pennsylvania
Acute Kidney Injury

David C. Wheeler, MD
Reader in Nephrology
UCL Centre for Nephrology
University College London
Consultant Nephrologist
Department of Nephrology
Royal Free (Hampstead) NHS Trust
London, United Kingdom
Cardiovascular Aspects of Kidney Disease

Christopher S. Wilcox, MD, PhD, FASN
Georgetown University Medical Center
Washington, DC
Diuretics

Christopher G. Wood, MD
Professor
Department of Urology
The University of Texas M.D. Anderson Cancer Center
Houston, Texas
Renal Neoplasia

Stephen H. Wright, PhD
Professor, Physiology
University of Arizona
Tucson, Arizona
Renal Handling of Organic Solutes

Jane Y. Yeun, MD, FACP
Professor of Clinical Medicine
Internal Medicine, Division of Nephrology
University of California, Davis, Health Sciences
Staff Physician
Medical Service, Nephrology Section
Sacramento Veterans Administration Medical Center
Mather, California
Hemodialysis

Alan S.L. Yu, MB, B Chir
Harry Statland and Solon Summerfield Professor of
    Medicine
Director, Division of Nephrology and Hypertension and the
    Kidney Institute
University of Kansas Medical Center
Kansas City, Kansas
Disorders of Calcium, Magnesium, and Phosphate Balance

Kambiz Zandi-Nejad, MD
Instructor in Medicine
Harvard Medical School
Staff Physician
Division of Nephrology
Beth Israel Deaconess Medical Center
Staff Physician
Division of Nephrology
Harvard Vanguard Medical Associates
Renal Division
Brigham and Women's Hospital
Boston, Massachusetts
Disorders of Potassium Balance

Mark L. Zeidel, MD
Herrman L. Blumgart Professor of Medicine
Harvard Medical School
Chair, Department of Medicine, and Physician-in-Chief
Beth Israel Deaconess Medical Center
Boston, Massachusetts
Urinary Tract Obstruction

FOREWORD

The book you, the reader, now hold in your hands (or are viewing electronically) has a very distinguished pedigree. Comprehensive treatises on diseases of organs, organ systems and organisms have an illustrious history. The ninth edition of *The Kidney* cannot only be directly traced to its origins in 1976 but also to its distinguished predecessors, such as *Nephrologie* by Jean Hamburger and Colleagues (1966), *Diseases of the Kidney* by Maurice Strauss and Louis Welt (1963), *The Kidney* by Hugh de Wardener (1958), *The Kidney; Structure and Function in Health and Disease* by Homer W. Smith (1951), *Renal Disease* by ET Bell (1950), *Die Bright'sche Nierenkrankheit, Klinik, Patholgie und Atlas* by Franz Volhard and Karl Theodor Fahr (1914); and even to the *Principles and Practice of Medicine* by Sir William Osler (1892) or *Reports on Medical Cases* by Richard Bright (1827). In many respects the first edition of *The Kidney,* then co-edited by Barry Brenner and Floyd Rector, was a landmark publication, and it unequivocally had a profound impact on the newly minted discipline of Nephrology. As with its predecessors, this multi-authored book encapsulated the great advances in renal physiology, pathology, cellular chemistry, and clinical diagnosis and treatment in a comprehensive and integrative manner. The book quickly established itself as the prime source of definitive information on the kidney in health and disease, just as Homer Smith's book accomplished a quarter century earlier and Volhard and Fahr's work did more than 7 decades previously. With the passage of time, it has become a prime tutorial for novices and a respected refresher of knowledge for advanced practitioners of the art. It has many mimics but few peers.

In the Foreword to the first edition in 1976, the late Robert Berliner, an early mentor of Brenner, drew attention to the importance of methodological innovations on the emergence of Nephrology as a distinct discipline, including renal biopsy and the application of immunofluorescence and electron microscopy as well as the development of the techniques of extracorporeal dialysis and renal transplantation. He also speculated that research on the fundamental mechanisms of kidney damage would eventually relegate dialysis to "iron lung" status. Now, more than 3 decades later, curing chronic kidney disease still largely remains an unanswered challenge, but untold lives have enjoyed prolonged dialysis-free intervals. Ever more magnificent new methodologies have appeared since 1976, and many of these exhibit great promise for fulfillment of the ultimate goal—eradication of kidney disease. Indeed, the methods of molecular biology and genetics as well as cellular and structural biology have already transformed diagnosis, prognosis, and treatment of kidney disease in spectacular ways. The emergence of Nephrology (from the perspective of renal physiology) as a "scientific discipline of formidable sophistication" was highlighted by Donald Seldin in his Foreword to the second edition of *The Kidney* in 1981. The breadth and depth of the eventual domain of Nephrology could only be glimpsed at this early juncture.

We now seem to be rapidly approaching an era of "personalized medicine" guided by the deciphering of the genome, with a virtually limitless potential for modifying diseased organs by genetic engineering and replacement of damaged tissues by cellular transplantation. *The Kidney* has kept pace with this steady and remarkable progress of science and its application to human disease by evolving its content and embracing the ever expanding realm of Nephrology. The ninth edition of *The Kidney* is no exception to this remarkable record of transformation, coherence, and excellence. The reader has new sections/chapters to explore on pediatric nephrology, biomarkers of renal injury, interventional nephrology, and extensions to global aspects of kidney disease to name a few. This latter new feature responds to the global reach of Nephrology, an aspect compellingly advanced in the Foreword to the seventh edition of *The Kidney* by John Dirks in 2004.

Perhaps the most significant change in the ninth edition of *The Kidney* is the editorship. For the first four editions (1976-1991), Barry Brenner and Floyd Rector served as co-editors. For the next four editions (1996-2008), Barry Brenner served as the sole editor. The ninth edition of *The Kidney* will be published with a new masthead and with Maarten W. Taal as the lead editor and five additional editors, including Barry Brenner. Thus, after 36 years, Barry Brenner's prodigious editorial efforts and manifest accomplishments will transition to a new generation. Nephrology owes a great debt to the foresight of the founding editors of *The Kidney* for crafting such a vital and comprehensive source of knowledge in Nephrology.

It is fitting to reflect on how this monumental task has chronicled the evolution of Nephrology over these more than 3 decades. In 1976, Nephrology was a teenager, the term having been coined by Jean Hamburger in 1960. Physiological inquiry stood at its pinnacle, while immunology and pathology of the kidney were gaining ascendency. Molecular biology, molecular genetics, and cellular chemistry were barely visible. For example, adult polycystic kidney disease, the monogenic kidney disease *par excellence,* was covered in approximately one page without mentioning a gene in the first edition of *The Kidney.* In the ninth edition, this topic has its own greatly expanded chapter, with diagrams describing the genes that determine the disease. The revolution of molecular biology, pervading all of medicine, has impacted Nephrology enormously as well. The sea change brought about by this new understanding of life and the origins of disease offers much hope and many challenges for the future, some of them of an ethical nature. Newer imaging techniques, such as magnetic resonance and computer assisted tomography, unheard of 1976, have also transformed diagnosis in polycystic kidney disease and in many other areas of Nephrology. Many new, heretofore unrecognized diseases entities have been described—HIV nephropathy, nephrogenic systemic fibrosis, and BK virus nephropathy in renal transplants, for example. Treatment approaches have also evolved. Continuous ambulatory peritoneal dialysis was not an option for treatment of ESRD in 1976. Cyclosporine, tacrolimus, mycophenolic acid salts, sirolimus, everolimus, and immunomodulatory biological products (anti-T cell and anti-B cell monoclonal antibodies) were still in an early phase of laboratory study or not even imagined. The concept of "reno-protection" by inhibition of the renin-angiotensin-aldosterone system was in its infancy; the maladaptive glomerular capillary hypertension seen in response to glomerular inquiry was already well described, but its significance was not yet well appreciated. The therapeutic armamentarium available to clinical nephrology practice in 1976 was quite limited; today, the pharmacopeia is dauntingly complex. End-stage renal disease (ESRD) is still with us, and its treatment has burgeoned to "epidemic" status brought about in part by unprecedented governmental action in 1972 to create the Medicare ESRD program. Chronic renal failure or renal insufficiency (or Bright's disease if you are a history buff) has a new name (chronic kidney disease, or CKD), a new way of estimating the degree of loss of kidney function (eGFR), and a myriad of guidelines for how to detect and manage the conditions associated with loss of renal function. The prospects for extension of survival and a better quality of life for the unfortunates with ESRD have greatly increased, but much still needs to be done. The use of randomized clinical trials to assess the safety and efficacy of new approaches to the treatment of kidney disease has increased greatly, but not nearly to the extent needed nor to the level approached by other disciplines (e.g., Cardiology). These are but a few of the evolutionary changes that have been well documented in the pages of *The Kidney* over the past 36 years.

What can we expect in the future? If the Shakespearian adage "past is prologue" remains correct and some catastrophic disaster does not befall society, we can with some confidence expect that creative scholarship (research) will provide a richness and variety of new knowledge for the editors of *The Kidney* to contemplate and describe. The sources of this new knowledge can be dimly perceived even now, driven by the next generation of methodological advances—namely, proteomics, metabolomics, genomics, transcriptomics, bio-informatics, and structural biology. But surprises from unexpected sources may also appear. Translating these expected and unanticipated advances in basic knowledge into practical and safe tools for recognizing, classifying, and treating human kidney disease will be difficult, expensive, time-consuming, and unpredictable. Clearly a more complete understanding of the mechanisms initiating and driving disease and its progression lies at the heart of reaching the ever elusive goals of attenuating or eradicating kidney disease and making future editions of *The Kidney* obsolete. Yet, hope springs eternal; Berliner drew similar conclusions in the first foreword to *The Kidney* in 1976.

We can only imagine what is on the horizon, but we can be sure that whatever comes to pass, this treasure of a book will capture its essence and communicate it to the next generation of readers in the gold-standard fashion to which we have become accustomed.

Richard J. Glassock, MD, MACP
Emeritus Professor
The David Geffen School of Medicine at UCLA

PREFACE

We are pleased to present the ninth edition of Brenner and Rector's *The Kidney*. This edition marks the planned change in editorship from Barry M. Brenner, who has undertaken the Herculean task of editing the book on his own for the past six editions, to a group of editors who I have been privileged to lead. It is only as we have engaged in this task that we have fully appreciated the enormous effort and determination it has taken for Dr. Brenner to achieve and maintain the highest possible standards of writing and scholarly investigation that have made *The Kidney* the most authoritative text in Nephrology over 4 decades. We have been privileged to have Dr. Brenner serve as one of the editors for this edition and have all gained enormously from his experience and wisdom as he has handed over his editorial responsibilities. There can be no doubt that Dr. Brenner deserves our thanks and recognition for the major contribution he has made through *The Kidney* to education and research in Nephrology. It was therefore fitting that he was honored with the Robert G. Narins Award for teaching by the American Society of Nephrology in November of 2010. Furthermore, in recognition of the founding editors and Dr. Brenner's career-long dedication to the book, we have decided to preserve the title *Brenner and Rector's The Kidney* in perpetuity.

In keeping with *The Kidney's* commitment to remaining comprehensive and current, we have introduced several changes for this edition. The reader will be impressed by ongoing development with respect to the appearance of the book. The cover and layout have been redesigned to make information more accessible and figures have been redrawn to ensure clarity and ease of interpretation. All chapters have been extensively updated or entirely rewritten. In order to keep the text dynamic, new authors have been invited to completely rewrite approximately one third of established chapters. These changes in authorship should not be interpreted to imply any dissatisfaction with the contributions of previous authors, to whom we remain indebted, but rather a desire to keep *The Kidney* vibrant and current by asking new authors to re-examine established topics. Additionally, we have sought to reflect recent developments in Nephrology by adding new sections and chapters. Consequently the number of chapters has been substantially expanded from 70 to 86. To reflect and promote the welcome growth in the development of Nephrology care and research worldwide, we have for the first time added Section XIII, "Global Considerations in Nephrology." In this section, leading nephrologists from each major geographical region outside Europe and North America (Latin America, Africa, Near and Middle East, Indian Subcontinent, Far East, Oceania, and Australia) present their expert insights into specific conditions that may affect the kidney as well as progress and challenges in the development of Nephrology. Globalization implies that it is increasingly likely that nephrologists working in Europe and North America will encounter patients whose renal pathology may have originated in a different part of the globe. Furthermore, it is hoped that giving prominence to the opportunities and challenges faced by nephrologists in other regions will promote collaborative efforts to improve Nephrology care worldwide, as well as continue research to further investigate renal pathologies unique to specific regions. As improvements in our understanding of pediatric renal disease translate into improved therapy and outcomes for children with renal disease who consequently can now expect to survive into adulthood, it is increasingly relevant for adult nephrologists to have some knowledge of renal pathologies that are usually present in childhood. We have therefore added Section XII, "Pediatric Nephrology," including chapters on "Malformation of the Kidney; Structural and Functional Consequences," "Fluid, Electrolyte, and Acid-Base Disorders in Children," "Diseases of the Kidney and Urinary Tract in Children," "Dialysis in Children," and "Pediatric Transplantation," to address this need. To reflect the very latest developments in Nephrology, we have added exciting new chapters including "Aldosterone Regulation of Ion Transport," "Demographics of Kidney Disease," "Biomarkers in Acute and Chronic Kidney Diseases," "Overview of Therapy for Glomerular Disease," "Renal Disease in Cancer Patients," "Genetic Basis of Kidney Disease," "Dermatologic Conditions in Kidney Disease," "A Stepped Care Approach to the Management of Chronic Kidney Disease," "Ethical Dilemmas Facing Nephrology: Past, Present, and Future," and "Health Disparities in Nephrology."

Many have argued that the rapid growth in information technology will portend the demise of traditional textbooks, and sadly, several celebrated texts are already no longer published. We hope that the reader will agree that the excellence of writing and scholarly rigor displayed by the authors in *The Kidney* make a strong argument for its endurance as an outstanding resource for education, teaching, and research in Nephrology. As in previous editions, authors were asked to emphasize references since 2000 and have gone to great lengths to report the very latest research developments; recent references have been added to the text until the last possible stage of production. To make the content of *The Kidney* readily accessible, portable, and available to as large a readership as possible, the full text and figures will again be available as an online version. We will continue to provide electronic updates on relevant articles that are published between editions to keep information as current as possible and maintain *The Kidney* as a "living textbook."

Publishing *The Kidney* is in every way a collaborative effort. I am deeply indebted to our team of editors—Barry M. Brenner, Glenn M. Chertow, Philip A. Marsden, Karl L. Skorecki and Alan S. L. Yu—who have each made major contributions in editing and writing chapters as well as being generous with their support and wisdom. Together we salute and thank our authors, who have shown extraordinary commitment to maintaining the excellent standard for which *The Kidney* is renowned. Many are leading academics with great demands on their time, and their willingness to devote many hours to writing reflects their unselfish dedication to promoting scholarship and research in Nephrology. Our thanks go also to Dick Glassock, a long-time supporter of *The Kidney* and friend to many of the editors and authors, for his scholarly and thoughtful foreword. We owe a great debt of thanks to the publishing team: Adrianne Brigido and Kate Dimock for their excellent leadership as Acquisitions Editors for the ninth edition; Joan Ryan for her tireless support and hard work as Senior Developmental Editor; Clay Broeker, Senior Project Manager, who ably led final production; and the rest of the dedicated team at Elsevier. Finally, as a team of editors, we would each like to express our heartfelt thanks to our families, friends, and colleagues for their support during times when our work on *The Kidney* has meant less time for them.

When the current editors were assembled, it was agreed that the lead editorship would in future rotate with each edition. It is therefore likely that this will be my single opportunity to act in that role, and I count it to have been an enormous privilege.

Maarten W. Taal, FRCP
Derby, United Kingdom, 2011

CONTENTS

C20051765

Section I

Normal Structure
and Function

Embryology of the Kidney

Yoshiro Maezawa, Jordan Kreidberg, and Susan E. Quaggin

Over the past several decades, the genes and molecular pathways required for normal renal development have been identified, and this information has provided insight into the understanding of well-known developmental disorders such as renal agenesis and renal dysplasia. However, many of the genes identified have also been shown to play roles in adult-onset and acquired renal diseases, such as focal segmental glomerulosclerosis. The number of nephrons present in the kidney at birth, which is determined during fetal life, is predictive of the risk of renal disease and hypertension later in life; a reduced number is associated with greater risk.[1-3] Discovery of novel therapeutic targets and strategies to slow and reverse kidney disease requires an understanding of the molecular mechanisms that underlie kidney development.

Mammalian Kidney Development: Embryology

Development of the Urogenital System

The vertebrate kidney derives from the intermediate mesoderm of the urogenital ridge, a structure found along the posterior wall of the abdomen in the developing fetus.[4] It develops in three successive stages, known as the *pronephros, the mesonephros,* and the *metanephros* (Figure 1-1). Only the metanephros gives rise to the definitive adult kidney; however, earlier stages are required for development of other organs, such as the adrenal gland and gonad, which also develop within the urogenital ridge. Furthermore, many of the signaling pathways and genes that play important roles in the metanephric kidney appear to play parallel roles during earlier stages of renal development, in the pronephros and mesonephros.

The pronephros consists of pronephric tubules and the pronephric duct (also known as the precursor to the wolffian duct) and develops from the rostralmost region of the urogenital ridge at 22 days of gestation in humans and 8 days post coitum (d.p.c.) in mice. It functions in the larval stages of amphibians and fish but not in mammals. The mesonephros develops caudal to the pronephric tubules in the midsection of the urogenital ridge. The mesonephros becomes the functional excretory apparatus in lower vertebrates and may perform a filtering function during embryonic life in mammals. However, it largely degenerates before birth. Before its degeneration, endothelial, peritubular myoid, and steroidogenic cells from the mesonephros migrate into the adjacent adrenogonadal primordia, which ultimately form the adrenal gland and gonads.[5] Abnormal mesonephric migration leads to gonadal dysgenesis, a fact that emphasizes the intricate association between these organ systems during development and underlies the common association of gonadal and renal defects in congenital syndromes.[6,7] In male vertebrates, production of

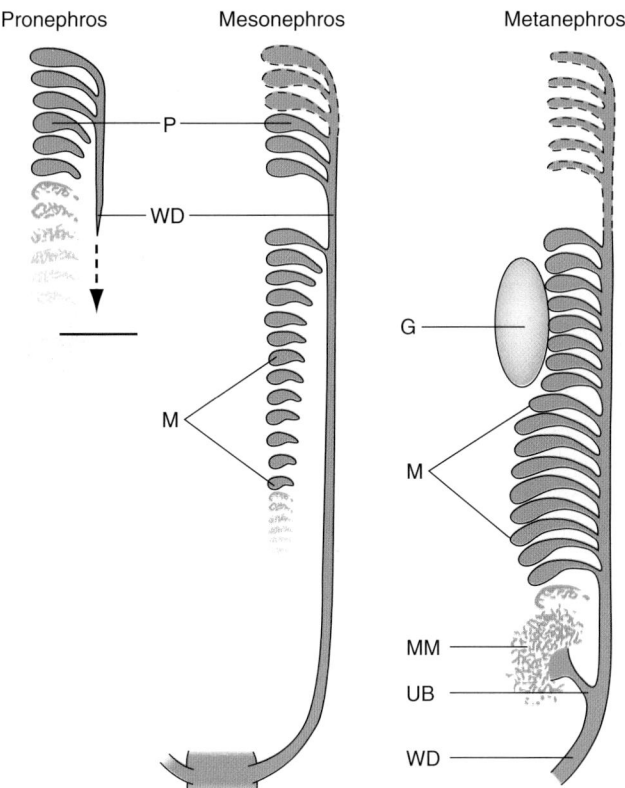

Pronephros Mesonephros Metanephros

P

WD

M

G

M

MM

UB

WD

FIGURE 1-1 Three stages of mammalian kidney development. The pronephros (P) and mesonephros (M) develop in a rostral-to-caudal direction, and the tubules are aligned adjacent to the wolffian, or nephric, duct (WD). The metanephros develops from an outgrowth of the distal end of the wolffian duct known as the ureteric bud epithelium (UB) and a cluster of cells known as the metanephric mesenchyme (MM). Cells migrate from the mesonephros (M) into the developing gonad (G), which develop in close association with one another. (Adapted from Saxen L: *Organogenesis of the kidney,* Cambridge, UK, 1987, Cambridge University Press.)

testosterone also induces the formation of seminal vesicles, tubules of the epididymis, and portions of the vas deferens from the wolffian duct.

Development of the Metanephros

The metanephros, the third and final stage of kidney development, gives rise to the definitive adult kidney in higher vertebrates; it results from a series of inductive interactions that occur between the metanephric mesenchyme and the epithelial ureteric bud at the caudal end of the urogenital ridge. The ureteric bud (UB) is first visible as an outgrowth at the distal end of the wolffian duct at approximately 5 weeks of gestation in humans and at 10.5 d.p.c. in mice. The metanephric mesenchyme (MM) becomes histologically distinct from the surrounding mesenchyme and is found adjacent to the UB. Upon invasion of UB into the MM at 11.5 d.p.c. in mice and 5 weeks in humans, signals from the MM cause the UB to branch into a T-tubule and then to undergo dichotomous branching, which gives rise to the urinary collecting system and all of the collecting ducts (Figure 1-2). Simultaneously, the UB sends reciprocal signals to the MM, which is induced to condense along the surface of the UB. After condensation, a subset of MM aggregates adjacent and inferior to the tips of the branching

ureteric bud. These collections of cells are known as *pretubular aggregates,* which undergo mesenchymal-to-epithelial conversion to become the renal vesicle (Figure 1-3).

Development of the Nephron

The renal vesicle segments and proceeds through a series of morphologic changes to form the glomerulus and components of the tubular nephron from the proximal convoluted tubule to the distal nephron. These stages are known as *comma shape, S-shape, capillary loop,* and *mature stages* and require precise proximal-to-distal patterning and structural transformation (see Figure 1-3). This process is, remarkably, repeated 600,000 to 1 million times in each developing human kidney as new nephrons are sequentially "born" at the tips of the UB throughout fetal life.

The glomerulus develops from the most proximal end of the renal vesicle that is farthest from the UB tip.[8,9] Distinct cell types of the glomerulus can first be identified in the S-shape stage, in which presumptive podocytes appear as a columnar-shaped epithelial cell layer. A vascular cleft develops and separates the presumptive podocyte layer from more distal cells that will form the proximal tubule. Parietal epithelial cells differentiate and flatten, becoming Bowman's capsule, a structure that surrounds the urinary space and is continuous with the proximal tubular epithelium. Concurrently, endothelial cells migrate into the vascular cleft. Together with the glomerular visceral epithelial cells, the endothelial cells produce the glomerular basement membrane (GBM), a major component of the mature filtration barrier.

Initially, the podocytes are connected by intercellular tight junctions at their apical surface.[10] As glomerulogenesis proceeds, the podocytes revert to a mesenchymal-type phenotype, flatten, and spread out to cover the increased surface area of the growing glomerular capillary bed. They develop microtubule-based primary processes and actin-based secondary foot processes. During this time, the intercellular junctions become restricted to the basal aspect of the podocyte and eventually are replaced by a modified adherens-like structure known as the slit diaphragm (SD).[10] At the same time, the podocyte foot processes of adjacent cells become highly interdigitated. The slit diaphragms function as signaling centers and as structural components of the renal filtration apparatus that connect foot processes of adjacent podocytes and link the SD to the specialized cytoskeleton that supports foot process structure.[11-13] Mesangial cell ingrowth follows the migration of endothelial cells and is required for development and patterning of the capillary loops that are found in normal glomeruli. The endothelial cells also flatten considerably, and capillary lumens are formed as a result of apoptosis of a subset of endothelial cells.[14] At the capillary loop stage, glomerular endothelial cells develop fenestrae, which are transmembrane pores found in semipermeable capillary beds exposed to high flux. Positioning of the foot processes on the GBM and spreading of podocyte cell bodies are still incompletely understood, but many of their features are similar to those of synapse formation and neuronal migration.[15-17]

In the mature stage glomerulus, the podocytes, fenestrated endothelial cells, and intervening GBM constitute the filtration barrier that separates the urinary space from the blood space. Together, these components provide a size- and

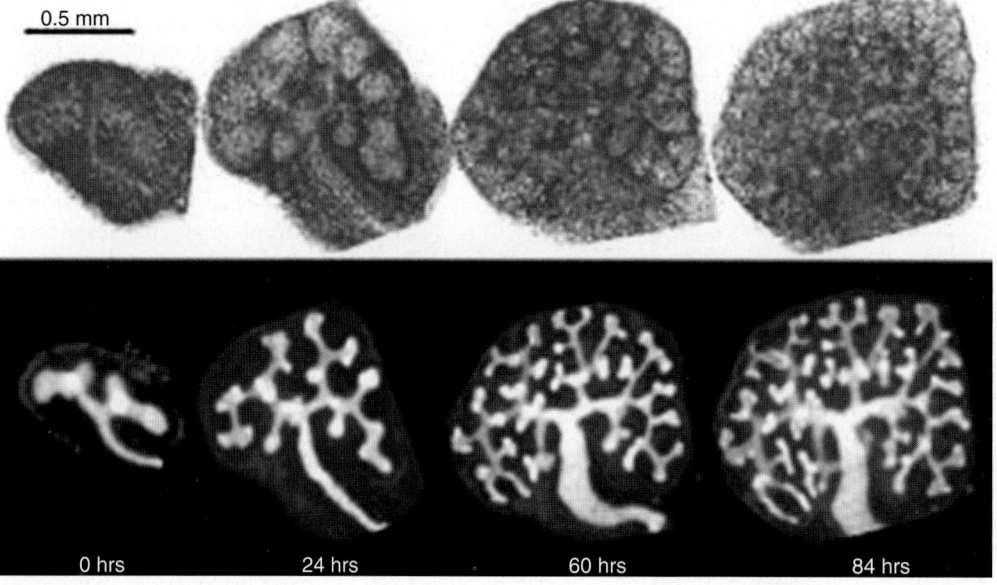

FIGURE 1-2 Organ culture of rat metanephroi dissected at T-tubule stage. Within 84 hours, dichotomous branching of the ureteric bud has occurred to provide basic architecture of the kidney. *Bottom panel* is stained with dolichos biflorus agglutinin—a lectin specific for the ureteric bud. (Adapted from Saxen L: *Organogenesis of the kidney,* Cambridge, UK, 1987, Cambridge University Press.)

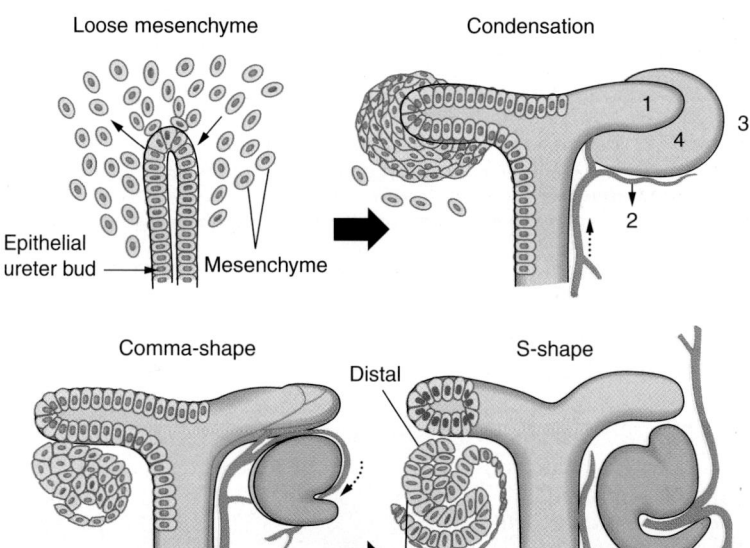

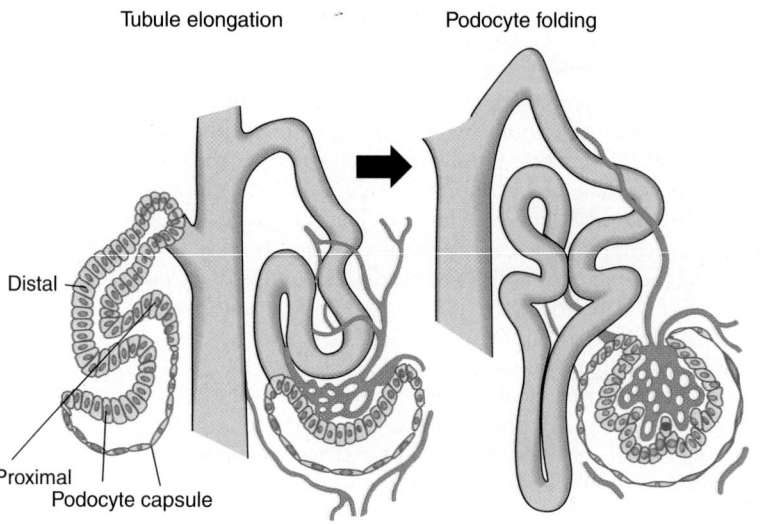

FIGURE 1-3 Schematic diagram of nephron development. Reciprocal interaction between the ureteric bud and metanephric mesenchyme results in a series of well-defined morphologic stages leading to formation of the nephron. (From Mugrauer G, Alt FW, Ekblom P: *N-myc* proto-oncogene expression during organogenesis in the developing mouse as revealed by in situ hybridization, *J Cell Biol* 1988;107:1325-1335. Copyright 1988, The Rockefeller University Press.)

charge-selective barrier that allows free passage of small solutes and water but prevents the loss of larger molecules such as proteins. The mesangial cells are found between the capillary loops (approximately three per loop); they provide ongoing structural support to the capillaries and possess smooth-muscle cell–like characteristics that have the capacity to contract, which may account for the dynamic properties of the glomerulus.

The tubular portion of the nephron becomes segmented in a proximal-distal order, into the proximal convoluted tubule, the descending and ascending loops of Henle, and the distal convoluted tubule. The latter portion connects to the collecting ducts, which are derived from the ureteric bud derivatives and not from the original mesenchymal component of the metanephric rudiment. Fusion events between the MM- and UB-derived portions of the nephron are required, but they are poorly understood at present.

Although all segments of the nephron are present at birth and filtration occurs before birth, maturation of the tubule continues in the postnatal period. Increased levels of transporters, switches in transporter isoforms, alterations in paracellular transport mechanisms, and the development of permeability and biophysical properties of tubular membranes have all been observed to occur postnatally.[18] Although additional studies are needed, these observations emphasize the importance of considering the developmental stage of the nephron in interpretation of renal transport and may explain the age at onset of symptoms in inherited transport disorders; some of these issues may be recapitulated in acute renal injury.

The Nephrogenic Zone

After the first few rounds of branching of the ureteric bud derivatives and the concomitant induction of nephrons from the mesenchyme, the kidney begins to become divided into an outer cortical region where nephrons are being induced and an inner medullary region where the collecting system will form. As growth continues, successive groups of nephrons are induced at the peripheral regions of the kidney, known as the *nephrogenic zone* (Figure 1-4). Thus, within the developing kidney, the most mature nephrons are found in the innermost

layers of the cortex, and the most immature nephrons are found in the most peripheral regions. At the extreme peripheral lining, under the renal capsule, a process that appears to recapitulate the induction of the original nephrons nearly exactly can be observed, in which numerous ureteric bud–like structures are inducing areas of condensed mesenchyme. Indeed, whether there are significant molecular differences between the induction of the original nephrons and these subsequent inductive events is not known. Certain mesenchymal cells found immediately adjacent and inferior to the tips of the ureteric buds in the nephrogenic zone appear to function as epithelial progenitors. They undergo self-renewal and give rise to every epithelial cell lineage of the nephron, including parietal epithelial cells, podocytes, and all tubular epithelial cells down to the distal nephron.[19,20]

Branching Morphogenesis: Development of the Collecting System

The collecting system is composed of hundreds of tubules through which the filtrate produced by the nephrons is conducted out of the kidney and to the ureter and then the bladder. Water and salt absorption and excretion, NH_3 transport, and $H^{\pm}$ ion secretion required for acid-base homeostasis also occur in the collecting ducts, under regulatory mechanisms and through transporters and channels different from those that are active in the tubular portions of the nephron. The collecting ducts are all derived from the original ureteric bud. Thus, whereas each nephron is an individual unit separately induced and originating from a distinct pretubular aggregate, the collecting ducts are the product of branching morphogenesis from the ureteric bud. Considerable remodeling is involved in forming collecting ducts from branches of ureteric bud, and how this occurs remains incompletely understood.[21] The branching is highly patterned: The first several rounds of branching are somewhat symmetric, followed by additional rounds of asymmetric branching in which a main trunk of the collecting duct continues to extend toward the nephrogenic zone, and smaller ureteric buds branch as they induce new nephrons within the nephrogenic zone. Originally, the ureteric bud derivatives are branching within a surrounding mesenchyme. Ultimately, they form a funnel-shaped structure in which a cone-shaped grouping of ducts or papillae sits within a funnel or calyx that drains into the ureter. The mouse kidney has a single papilla and calyx, whereas a human kidney has 8 to 10 papillae, each of which drains into a minor calyx, and several minor calyces drain into a smaller number of major calyces.

Renal Stroma and Interstitial Populations

For decades in classic embryologic studies of kidney development, emphasis has been placed on the reciprocal inductive signals between MM and UB. However, in recent years, investigators have become interested in the stromal cell as a key regulator of nephrogenesis.[9,22-24] Stromal cells also derive from the metanephric mesenchyme but are not induced to condense by the UB. Two distinct populations of stromal cells have been described: cortical stromal cells, which exist as a thin layer beneath the renal capsule, and medullary stromal cells, which

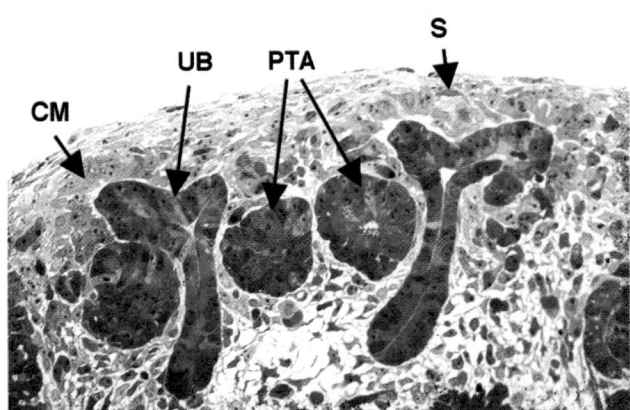

FIGURE 1-4 The nephrogenic zone. Nephrons are continually produced in the nephrogenic zone throughout fetal life. *CM,* condensing mesenchyme; *PTA,* pretubular aggregate; *S,* stromal cell lineage (spindle-shaped cells); *UB,* ureteric bud.

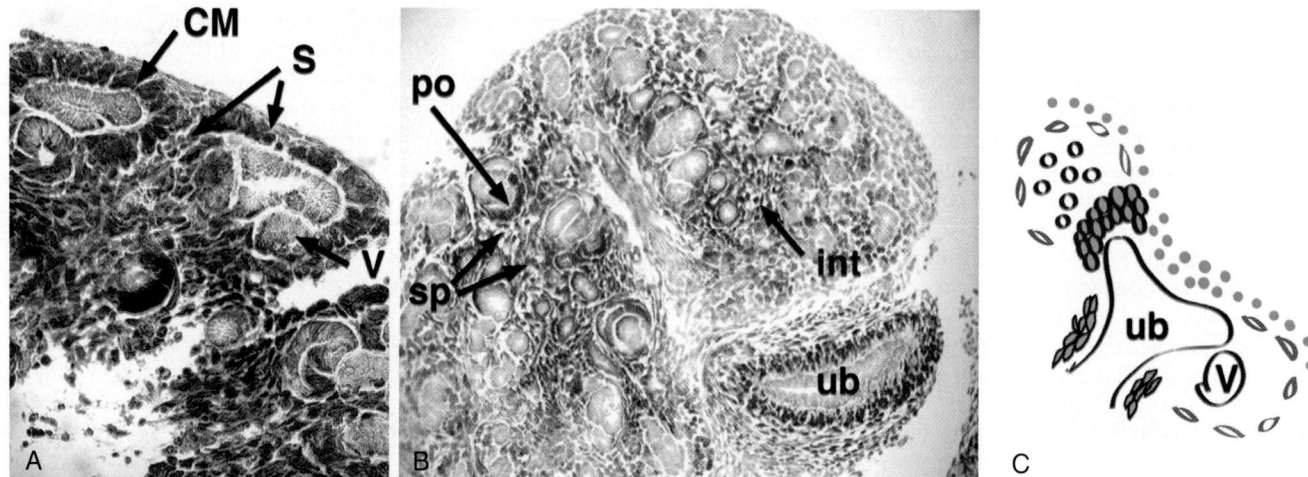

FIGURE 1-5 Populations of cells within the metanephric mesenchyme. As described in the text, these populations are defined by morphologic and molecular characteristics. Metanephroi from a Pod1/lacZ mouse, 14.5 days post coitum (**A**) and 15.5 days post coitum (**B**), are stained with X-gal. Pod1-expressing cells turn blue with this stain. Stromal cells (S; *pink* in C) are seen surrounding condensing mesenchyme (CM). Metanephrogenic population (*green* in C) remain unstained. By 15.5 days post coitum, an interstitial compartment is well developed and consists of peritubular fibroblasts, medullary fibroblasts, and pericytes. Loose and condensed mesenchymal cells are also observed around the stalk of the ureteric bud (**B**). v, renal vesicle; po, podocyte precursors; sp, stromal pericytes; int, interstitium. **C,** Schematic diagram of mesenchymal populations include the metanephrogenic precursors (*green*), uninduced mesenchyme (*white*), condensing mesenchyme around the ureteric bud tips and stalk (*blue*), and stromal cell lineage (*pink*). (Reproduced with permission from Developmental Dynamics.)

populate the interstitial space between the collecting ducts and tubules (Figure 1-5). Cortical stromal cells also surround the condensates and provide signals required for ureteric bud branching and patterning of the developing kidney. Disruption or loss of these stromal cells leads to failure of UB branching, a reduction in nephron number, and disrupted patterning of nephric units with failure of cortical-medullary boundary formation.

A reciprocal signaling loop from the UB exists to properly pattern stromal cell populations. Loss of these UB-derived signals leads to a buildup of stromal cells beneath the capsule that are several layers thick. As nephrogenesis proceeds, stromal cells differentiate into peritubular interstitial cells and pericytes that are required for vascular remodeling and for production of the extracellular matrix responsible for proper nephric formation.[24] These cells migrate from their position around the condensates to areas between the developing nephrons within the medulla. Although stromal cells derive from MM, it is not yet clear whether MM that gives rise to stromal cell and nephric lineages derives from the same progenitor cell or a different cell.

Development of the Vasculature

The microcirculations of the kidney include the specialized glomerular capillary system responsible for production of the ultrafiltrate and the vasa rectae, peritubular capillaries involved in the countercurrent mechanism. In the adult, each kidney receives 10% of the cardiac output.

Vasculogenesis and angiogenesis have been described as two distinct processes in blood vessel formation. *Vasculogenesis* is the *de novo* differentiation of previously nonvascular cells into structures that resemble capillary beds, whereas *angiogenesis* refers to the sprouting of the cells from these early beds to form mature vessel structures, including arteries, veins, and capillaries. Both processes are involved in development of the renal vasculature. At the time of UB invasion in mice

(11 d.p.c.), the MM is avascular, but by 12 d.p.c. a rich capillary network is present, and by 14 d.p.c. vascularized glomeruli are present. Transplantation experiments have shown that endothelial progenitors within the MM give rise to renal vessels in situ,[25] although the origin of large blood vessels is still debated. At 13 d.p.c., capillaries form networks around the developing nephric tubules and by 14 d.p.c., the hilar artery and first-order interlobar renal artery branches can be identified. These branches will form the corticomedullary arcades and interlobular arteries that branch from these arcades. Further branching produces the glomerular afferent arterioles.

From 13.5 d.p.c. onward, endothelial cells migrate into the vascular cleft of developing glomeruli, where they undergo differentiation to form the glomerular capillary loops. The efferent arterioles carry blood away from the glomerulus to a system of fenestrated peritubular capillaries that are in close contact with the adjacent tubules and receive filtered water and solutes reabsorbed from the filtrate. These capillaries have few pericytes. In comparison, the vasa rectae, which surround the medullary tubules and are involved in urinary concentration, are also fenestrated but have more pericytes. They arise from the efferent arterioles of deep glomeruli. The peritubular capillary system surrounding the proximal tubules is well developed in the late fetal period, whereas the vasa rectae mature 1 to 3 weeks postnatally.

Model Systems to Study Kidney Development

Organ Culture

The Kidney Organ Culture System: Classical Studies

Metanephric kidney organ culture (Figure 1-6) formed the basis for extensive classical studies of embryonic induction. Parameters of induction such as the temporal and physical

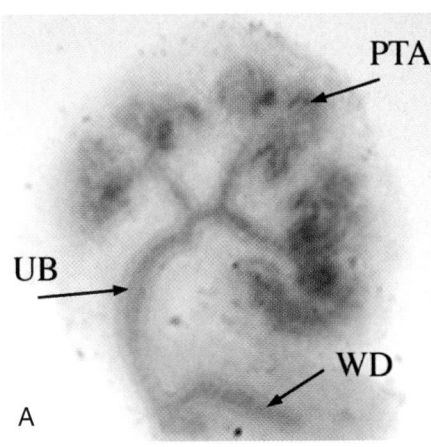 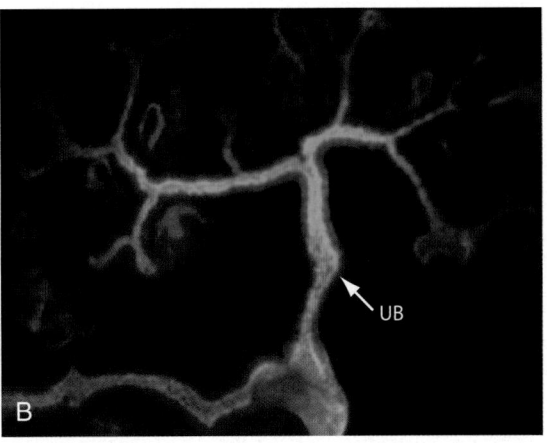

FIGURE 1-6 Metanephric organ explants. **A,** In situ analysis for Pax2 that marks pretubular aggregates (PTA) and the ureteric bud (UB) and wolffian duct (WD). **B,** Immunohistochemical stain for proximal tubular cell brush border (*red*) and pan cytokeratin (*green*) marks the developing nephrons and ureteric bud, respectively.

constraints on exposure of the inductive tissue to the mesenchyme were determined, as were the time periods during which various tubular elements of the nephron were first observed in culture.

Mutant Phenotypic Analyses

As originally shown by Grobstein,[26] Saxen,[4] and their colleagues in classical studies of embryonic induction, the two major components of the metanephric kidney, the mesenchyme and the ureteric bud, could be separated from each other, and the isolated mesenchyme could be induced to form nephron-like tubules by a selected set of other embryonic tissues, the best example of which is embryonic neural tube. This phenomenon can be observed by placing the whole metanephric rudiment, including the ureteric bud, in culture: When the whole rudiment is placed in culture, induction of nephrons, branching of the ureteric bud, and continued growth of the rudiment occur. In contrast, when neural tube is used to induce the separated mesenchyme, there is terminal differentiation of the mesenchyme into tubules but not significant tissue expansion.

The isolated mesenchyme experiment has proved useful in the analysis of phenotypes of renal agenesis, in which no outgrowth of the ureteric bud occurs. In these cases, the mesenchyme can be placed in contact with the neural tube to determine whether it has the intrinsic ability to differentiate. Most often, when renal agenesis results from the mutation of a transcription factor, tubular induction is not rescued by the neural tube, as could be predicted for transcription factors, which would be expected to act in a cell-autonomous manner.[27] In the converse situation, in which renal agenesis is caused by loss of function of a gene in the ureteric bud, such as *Emx2*, it is usually possible for the embryonic neural tube to induce tubule formation in isolated mesenchymes.[28] Therefore, the organ culture induction assay can be used to test hypotheses concerning whether a particular gene is required in the mesenchyme or ureteric bud. As chemical inhibitors specific for various signal transduction pathways have been synthesized and become available, it has been possible to add these to organ cultures and observe effects that are informative about the roles of specific pathways in development of the kidney. Examples are the use of mitogen-activated protein (MAP) kinase inhibitors and inhibitors of the Notch signaling pathway.

Antisense Oligonucleotides and Small Interfering RNA in Organ Culture

Several studies have described the use of antisense oligonucleotides and more recently, small interfering RNA (siRNA) molecules, to inhibit gene expression in kidney organ culture. Among the earliest of these was the inhibition of the low-affinity nerve growth factor receptor p75, or NGFR, by antisense oligonucleotides,[29] a treatment that decreased the growth of the organ culture. A subsequent study could not duplicate this phenotype,[30] although there may have been differences in experimental techniques.[31] An additional study in which antisense oligonucleotides to Pax2 were used also showed this gene to be crucial in the mesenchymal-to-epithelial transformation.[32,33] More recently, siRNA to the wt1 and Pax2 genes was demonstrated to inhibit early nephron differentiation.[34]

Organ Culture Microinjection

A novel approach to the organ culture system has also yielded insights as to a possible function of the wt1 gene in early kidney development. A system was established to microinject and electroporate DNA plasmid expression constructs into the condensed mesenchyme of organ cultures.[35]

Transgenic and Knockout Mouse Models

Over the past two decades, the generation and analysis of knockout (KO) and transgenic mice have provided tremendous insight into kidney development (Table 1-1).[36,37] Homologous recombination to delete genes within the germline, also known as standard KO technology, has provided information about the biologic functions of many genes in kidney development; however, several disadvantages exist. Disruption of gene function in embryonic stem (ES) cells may result in embryonic or perinatal death, which precludes the functional analysis of the gene in the kidney that develops relatively late in fetal life. In addition, many genes are expressed in multiple cell types, and the resulting KO phenotypes can be complex and difficult or impossible to dissect. The ability to limit gene targeting to specific renal cell types overcomes some of these problems, and the temporal control of gene expression allows more precise dissection of a gene's function. A number of existing mouse lines may be used to target

TABLE 1-1 Summary of Knockout and Transgenic Models for Kidney Development			
KIDNEY PHENOTYPE	**MOUSE (KNOCKOUT OR MUTATION): DISORDERS AND OTHER AFFECTED ORGANS**	**HUMAN (NATURALLY OCCURRING MUTATION): DISORDERS**	**REFERENCES**
Aplasia (Variable)			
Wt1	Gonad, mesothelium, heart, lung	Wilms' tumor, WAGR, Denys-Drash syndrome	27,93,211
Pax2	Genital tract, gonad	Renal hypoplasia, VUR, and optic nerve colobomas	32,33
Pax2/Pax8	Defect in intermediate mesoderm transition, failure of pronephric duct formation		236
Emx2	Genital tract, gonad		28
Lim1	Genital tract, gonads, anterior head		70
HoxA11/HoxD11	Distal limbs, vas deferens		237
Retinoic acid receptor $\alpha\gamma/\alpha\beta_2$	Skeleton; many visceral abnormalities, including renal hypoplasia and dysplasia		7,9,238
GDNF, c-Ret, GRFα1	Ureteric bud failure, enteric neurons	Hirschsprung's disease Multiple endocrine neoplasm type IIA (ret)	71,72,73,86,239, 240,241,242
Integrin-α_8	Reduced ureteric bud branching		107
Danforth Short Tail	Short tail, ureteric bud failure		243
KAL mutation		Kallman's syndrome (olfactory bulb agenesis)	308
Integrin-β_1	Disrupted ureteric bud branching, bilateral renal agenesis, hypoplastic collecting duct system (UB selective) Podocyte dedifferentiation (podocyte selective)		125,212,213
Heparan sulfate 2–sulfotransferase	Lack of ureteric bud branching and mesenchymal condensation		244
Eya1 (eyes absent–1)	Lack of metanephric mesenchyme, absence of UB outgrowth, defects of inner ear	Branchio-oto-renal syndrome (branchial fistulae, deafness)	65,79
Six1	UB failure; defects of inner ear, skeletal muscle, and skeleton	Branchio-oto-renal syndrome	67
Gremlin	UB failure, lung defects, distal limb defects		75
Sall1	Severe renal dysplasia/renal agenesis	Townes-Brock syndrome (anal, renal, limb, ear anomalies)	69,245
Odd1 (Osr1)	Lack of metanephric mesenchyme; adrenal gland, gonads; defects in formation of pericardium and atrial septum		66,78
Gdf11	Ureteric bud failure, skeletal defects		74,246
Fras1	Ureteric bud failure, defect of GDNF expression	Fraser syndrome (eyeball covered by skin, fused digits, and kidney malformation)	247
Nephronectin	Delay of ureteric bud invasion into metanephric mesenchyme		109
Dysplasia/Hypoplasia/Low Nephron Mass			
FoxD1 (BF-2)	Reduced ureteric bud branching/stromal patterning defects		23,248
Bmp7	Reduced metanephric mesenchyme survival		105
Wnt4	Failure of metanephric mesenchyme induction		101,249
Wnt9b	Vestigial kidney, failure of metanephric mesenchyme induction, cystic kidney (hypomorphic collecting duct stalk selective)		100,145
Ap2	Metanephric mesenchyme failure, craniofacial and skeletal defects		250
Cyclooxygenase-2	Oligonephronia		251

TABLE 1-1 Summary of Knockout and Transgenic Models for Kidney Development—cont'd

KIDNEY PHENOTYPE	MOUSE (KNOCKOUT OR MUTATION): DISORDERS AND OTHER AFFECTED ORGANS	HUMAN (NATURALLY OCCURRING MUTATION): DISORDERS	REFERENCES
Lmx1β	Renal dysplasia, skeletal abnormalities	Nail-patella syndrome	207,252
Fgf7	Small kidneys, reduction in nephron number		113
Fgf8	Renal dysplasia, arrested nephrogenesis at pretubular aggregate stage (mesenchyme selective)	Hypogonadotropic hypogonadism, Kallmann's syndrome	97,98
Pbx1	Reduced ureteric bud branching, delayed mesenchyme-to-epithelial transformation, dysgenesis of adrenal gland and gonads		253,254
GATA3	Ectopic ureteric budding, kidney agenesis/dysplasia, hydroureter, gonad dysgenesis	HDR syndrome (hypoparathyroidism, sensorineural deafness, renal disease)	255
β-Catenin	Severely hypoplastic kidney, lack of nephrogenic zone, and S-shaped body (cap mesenchyme selective)	Colorectal cancer, hepatoblastoma, hepatocellular cancer	103
Wnt7b	Complete absence of medulla		110
ALK3	Hypoplasia of medulla, fewer ureteric bud branches (UB selective)	Juvenile polyposis syndrome	118
Increased Branching			
Slit2/Robo2	Increased branching of ureteric bud		127
Sprouty1	Supernumerary ureteric buds, multiple ureters		130,256
Cysts			
Kif3A	Polycystic kidney disease (tubular and collecting duct selective)		257
HNF1β	Polycystic kidney disease (tubular and collecting duct selective, systemic inducible)	Renal cysts, MODY5	146,147
Von Hippel–Lindau	Renal cysts (tubular selective)		258
Peroxisomal assembly factor–1	Renal tubular ectasia	Zellweger's syndrome	309
Bcl2	Renal hypoplasia and cysts		310
Mks1	Renal hypoplasia and cysts	Meckel's syndrome (multicystic dysplasia, neural tube defect)	259
Pkd1, Pkd2	Renal cysts	Autosomal dominant PKD	260
Fat4	Renal cysts, disrupted hair cell organization in inner ear		148
MafB	Decreased glomeruli, cysts and tubular dysgenesis		261
Glis3	Polycystic kidney, neonatal diabetes	Congenital hypothyroidism, diabetes mellitus	262
Xylosyltransferase 2	Polycystic liver, kidneys		263
PTEN	Abnormal ureteric bud branching, cysts (UB selective)	Cowden's disease, Bannayan-Riley-Ruval syndrome, various tumors	95
Later Phenotypes (Glomerular, Vascular, Glomerular Basement Membrane)			
PDGF-B/PDGFR-β	Lack of mesangial cells, ballooned glomerular capillary loop		204,205
Mpv17	Nephrotic syndrome		264
Integrin-α₃	Reduced ureteric bud branching, glomerular defects, poor foot process formation, lung		121,124
CD151	Focal segmental glomerulosclerosis, massive proteinuria, disorganized GBM, tubular cystic dilation	End-stage kidney failure, regional skin blistering, sensorineural deafness	265
Col4a3 Col4a3/Col4a4 Col4a5 Col4a1	Alport's syndrome	Alport's syndrome; intracerebral hemorrhage and strokes (a1)	266-270

Continued

KIDNEY PHENOTYPE	MOUSE (KNOCKOUT OR MUTATION): DISORDERS AND OTHER AFFECTED ORGANS	HUMAN (NATURALLY OCCURRING MUTATION): DISORDERS	REFERENCES
	TABLE 1-1 Summary of Knockout and Transgenic Models for Kidney Development—cont'd		
Lamb2	Proteinuria before the onset of foot process effacement		271,272
Lama5	Defective glomerulogenesis, abnormal GBM, poor podocyte adhesion, loss of mesangial cells		273
Lama5; Mr51	Ballooned capillary loop, proteinuria		274
Lama5; Mr5G2	Nephrotic syndrome		275
Agrin	No glomerular permeability defect (podocyte selective)		276
Perlecan heparan sulfated sites	No baseline defects; proteinuria with albumin loading		277
Agrin (podocyte specific) and perlecan	Normal, no measurable proteinuria		278
Entactin-1	Abnormal GBM		279
Angiotensin II type 2 receptor	Various collecting system defects	CAKUT syndrome	189,190,192
Bmp4 (heterozygous)	Renal hypoplasia/dysplasia, hydroureter, ectopic uterovesical junction		111
FoxC1 (Mf1)	Renal duplication, multiple ureters, hydroureter/hydronephrosis		126
Mf2	Small kidneys with few nephrons		280
Glypican-3	Disorganized tubules and medullary cysts	Simpson-Golabi-Behmel syndrome	281-283
Notch2	Lack of glomerular endothelial and mesangial cells (standard knockout) Lack of podocytes and proximal tubular cells (metanephric mesenchyme selective) Decreased number of glomeruli (cap mesenchyme selective)	Alagille's syndrome (cholestatic liver disease, cardiac disease, kidney dysplasia, renal cysts, renal tubular acidosis)	133,134,139
Notch1 and Notch2	Severely compromised nephron formation (cap mesenchyme selective)		284
Pod1/Tcf21	Lung and cardiac defects, sex reversal and gonadal dysgenesis, vascular defects, disruption in ureteric bud branching, impaired podocyte differentiation, dilated glomerular capillary, poor mesangial migration		6,151
FoxC2	Impaired podocyte differentiation, dilated glomerular capillary loop, poor mesangial migration		50
Kreisler (maf-1)	Abnormal podocyte differentiation		208
Nephrin	Absence of slit diaphragms, congenital nephritic syndrome	Congenital nephrosis of the Finnish type, childhood-onset steroid-resistant nephritic syndrome, childhood- and adult-onset FSGS	214
Neph 1	Abnormal slit diaphragm function, FSGS		48
Podocin	Congenital nephrosis, FSGS, vascular defects	Steroid-resistant FSGS, congenital nephrotic syndrome	222,285
PLCE1		Diffuse mesangial sclerosis; FSGS	286
GNE/MNK (M712T)	Hyposialation defect, foot process effacement, GBM splitting, proteinuria and hematuria	Hereditary inclusion body myopathy	287
Fat1	Foot process fusion, failure of foot process formation		288
Nck1/Nck2	Failure of foot process formation (podocyte selective)		11
CD2AP	FSGS, immunotactoid nephropathy		225
α-Actinin 4	Glomerular developmental defects, FSGS	Autosomal dominant FSGS	223,224

TABLE 1-1 Summary of Knockout and Transgenic Models for Kidney Development—cont'd

KIDNEY PHENOTYPE	MOUSE (KNOCKOUT OR MUTATION): DISORDERS AND OTHER AFFECTED ORGANS	HUMAN (NATURALLY OCCURRING MUTATION): DISORDERS	REFERENCES
VEGF-A	Endotheliosis, disruption of glomerular filtration barrier formation, nephrotic syndrome (podocyte selective)		159,160,289
VEGFR-2	No proteinuria, no histologic/ultrastructural abnormality (podocyte selective)		311
Angiopoietin-2	Cortical peritubular capillary abnormalities		173
ILK1	Nephrotic syndrome (podocyte selective)		290
Von Hippel–Lindau	RPGN (podocyte selective)		182
Pax transactivation domain–interacting protein	Defects in urine concentration and osmotolerance (tubular and collecting duct selective)		291
β1 integrin	Podocyte loss, capillary and mesangial degeneration, glomerulosclerosis (podocyte selective)		212,213
aPKC	Defect of podocyte foot processes, nephrotic syndrome (podocyte selective)		219,220
Bmp7	Hypoplastic kidney, impaired maturation of nephron, reduced proximal tubules (podocyte selective)		180
Dicer and Rab3A	Podocyte damage, albuminuria, end-stage renal failure (podocyte selective)	Pleuropulmonary blastoma	232-234
	Reduced renin production, renal vascular abnormalities, striped fibrosis (juxtaglomerular cells selective)		203
	Albuminuria, disorganization of podocyte foot process structure		17

CAKUT, Congenital anomalies of kidney and urinary tract; *FSGS,* focal segmental glomerulosclerosis; *GBM,* glomerular basement membrane; *GDNF,* glial cell line–derived neurotrophic factor; *HDR,* hypoparathyroidism, sensorineural deafness, and renal dysplasia; *HNF1β,* hepatocyte nuclear factor 1β; *ILK1,* integrin-linked kinase 1; *MODY5,* maturity-onset diabetes of youth type 5; *PDGF-B,* platelet-derived growth factor type B; *PDGFR-β,* platelet-derived growth factor receptor β; *PKD,* polycystic kidney disease; *PLCE1,* phosphylipase epsilon 1; *PTEN,* phosphatase and tensin homolog; *RPGN,* rapidly progressive glomerulonephritis; *UB,* ureteric bud; *VEGF-A,* vascular epidermal growth factor type A; *VEGFR-2,* vascular epidermal growth factor receptor 2; *VUR,* vesicoureteral reflux; *WAGR,* Wilms' tumor, aniridia, genitourinary abnormalities, and mental retardation.

specific kidney cell lineages (Table 1-2; Figure 1-7). As with any experimental procedure, the investigator must take into account numerous caveats in interpretation of data (reviewed by Gawlik and Quaggin[38,39]); these include determining the completeness of excision at the locus of interest, the timing and extrarenal expression of the promoters, and general toxicity of expressed proteins to the cell of interest. In spite of these caveats, these mouse lines remain a powerful tool. The next generation of targeting includes improved efficiency with bacterial artificial chromosome (BAC) targeting approaches, siRNA and microRNA approaches, and large genomewide targeting efforts already under way at many academic and pharmaceutical institutions.

In contrast to gene targeting experiments, in which the gene is known at the beginning of the experiment (reverse genetics), random mutagenesis represents a complimentary phenotype-driven approach (forward genetics). Random mutations are introduced into the genome at high efficiency by chemical or "gene-trap" mutagenesis. Consecutively, large numbers of animals are screened systematically for specific phenotypes of interest. As soon as a phenotype is identified, test breeding is used to confirm the genetic nature of the trait. The mutated gene is then identified by chromosomal mapping and positional cloning. Genomewide-based approaches have two major advantages over reverse genetics: (1) Most KOs lead to major gene disruptions, which may

not be relevant to the subtle gene alterations that underlie human renal disease, and (2) many of the complex traits underlying congenital anomalies and acquired diseases of the kidney are unknown, which makes predictions about the nature of the genes that are involved in these diseases difficult.

One of the most powerful and well-characterized mutagens in the mouse is the chemical mutagen N-ethyl-N-nitrosourea (ENU). It acts through random alkylation of nucleic acids, inducing point mutations in spermatogonial stem cells of injected male mice.[40,41] This results in multiple point mutations within the spermatogonia of the male, which is then bred to a female mouse of different genetic background. Resulting F1 offspring are screened for renal phenotypes of interest (e.g., dysplastic, cystic) and heritability. Mutations may be manifested as complete or partial loss of function, gain of function, or altered function and can be dominant or recessive. The specific locus mutation frequency of ENU is 1 per 1000. If the total number of genes in the mouse genome is 25,000 to 40,000, a single treated male mouse should have between 25 and 40 different heterozygous mutagenized genes. In the case of multigenic phenotypes, segregation of the mutations in the next generation enables the researcher to focus on monogenic traits. In each generation, 50% of the mutations are lost, and only the mutation underlying the selected phenotype is maintained in the colony. A breeding strategy that includes

TABLE 1-2 Conditional Mouse Cell Lines for the Kidney			
PROMOTER	**RENAL EXPRESSION**	**EXTRARENAL EXPRESSION**	**REFERENCE**
Kidney androgen promoter 2	Proximal tubules	Brain	92
γ-Glutamyl transpeptidase	Cortical tubules	None	293
Na/glucose cotransporter (SGLT-2)	Proximal tubules	None	294
PEPCK	Proximal tubules	Liver	258
Aquaporin-2	Principal cells of collecting duct	Testis, vas deferens	295
Hox-B7	Collecting ducts, ureteric bud, wolffian bud, ureter	Spinal cord, dorsal root ganglia	296
Ksp-cadherin	Renal tubules, collecting ducts, ureteric bud, wolffian duct, mesonephros	Müllerian duct	297
Tamm-Horsfall protein	Thick ascending limbs of loops of Henle	Testis, brain	298
Nephrin	Podocytes	Brain	299,300
Podocin	Podocytes		301
Renin	Juxtaglomerular cells, afferent arterioles	Adrenal gland, testis, sympathetic ganglia, etc.	187
Fox-D1/BF-2	Stromal cells	Unknown	302
Six-2	Cap mesenchyme	Unknown	20
Pax3	Metanephric mesenchyme	Neural tube, neural crest	303,304
Pax2	Metanephric mesenchyme, ureteric bud	Inner ear, midbrain, cerebellum, olfactory bulb	305
Cited1	Cap mesenchyme	Unknown	19
Pax8	Proximal and distal tubule and collecting duct (tet-on system)		306
Pod1/Tcf21	Metanephric mesenchyme, cap mesenchyme, podocytes, stromal cells	Epicardium, lung mesenchyme, gonad, spleen, adrenal gland	Maezawa and Quaggin, unpublished

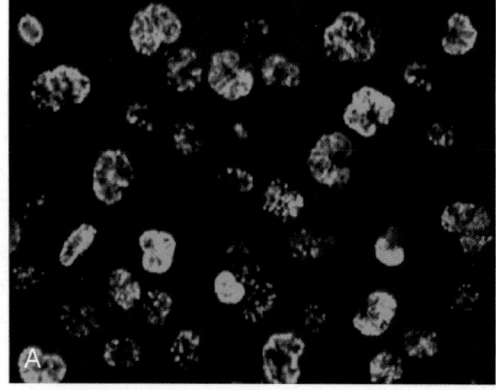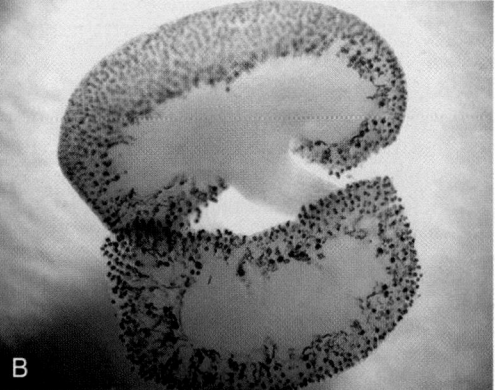

FIGURE 1-7 Glomeruli expressing cyan fluorescent protein (**A**) or β-galactosidase (**B**). Transgenic mice were generated through the use of the nephrin promoter to direct expression of either cyan fluorescent protein or β-galactosidase specifically to developing and mature podocytes.

backcrossing to the female genetic strain enables rapid mapping of the ENU mutation that occurred on the male genetic background.

The screening in experiments with ENU mutagenesis can focus on dominant or recessive renal mutations. Screening for dominant phenotypes is popular inasmuch as breeding schemes are simple and many mutants can be recovered through this approach. About 2% of all F1 mice display a heritable phenotypic abnormality.[42,43] A number of large ENU mutagenesis projects are now under way, with mutant strains available to interested researchers. One of the fruitful results obtained by this approach is the identification of a mutation in the aquaporin-11 gene, which causes severe proximal tubule

injury and giant vacuoles in renal cortex and results in perinatal death from renal failure.[44] It is possible to design "sensitized screens" on a smaller scale, which increases the ability to identify genes in a pathway of interest. For example, in renal glomerular development, the phenotype of a genetic mouse strain with a tendency to develop congenital nephrosis (e.g., CD2AP haploinsufficiency[45]) may be enhanced or suppressed by breeding to a mutagenized male. The modifier gene may then be mapped by means of the approach outlined earlier. This approach has been used successfully to identify genes involved in neural development.[46,47]

Other genomewide-based approaches that have led to the discovery of novel genes in kidney development and disease include gene trap consortia[48,49] and transcriptome/proteome projects.[50-52] The interested reader is referred to the websites of the Centre for Modeling Human Disease (www.cmhd.ca), the International Gene Trap Consortium (www.genetrap.org), Knockout Resources to Conquer Human Disease (www.tigm.org), and the Human Kidney & Urine Proteome Project (www.hkupp.org).

Nonmammalian Model Systems for Kidney Development

Organisms that differ from humans by millions of years of evolution are nonetheless useful models for studying the genetic basis and function of mammalian kidney development. This is because all these organisms possess excretory organs designed to remove metabolic wastes from the body, and genetic pathways involved in other aspects of invertebrate development may serve as templates to dissect pathways in mammalian kidney development. In support of the latter argument, the elucidation of the genetic interactions and molecular mechanism of the Neph1 ortholog (Syg1) and nephrin-like molecule (Syg2) in synapse formation in *Caenorhabditis elegans* is providing major clues to the function of these genes in glomerular and slit diaphragm formation and function in mammals.[53]

The excretory organs of invertebrates range in size from a few cells in the soil nematode *C. elegans* to several hundred cells in the malpighian tubules of *Drosophila* flies, and their structure and complexity differ greatly from those of the more recognizable kidneys in amphibians, birds, and mammals. In *C. elegans,* the excretory system consists of a single large H-shaped excretory cell, a pore cell, a duct cell, and a gland cell.[54,55] *C. elegans* provides many benefits as a model system: the availability of powerful genetic tools, a short life and reproductive cycle, a publicly available genome sequence and resource database (www.wormbase.org), the ease of performing genetic enhancer-suppressor screens in worms, and the fact that they share many genetic pathways with mammals. Studies of *C. elegans* have yielded major contributions to the understanding of the function of polycystic and cilia-related genes. The Pkd1 and Pkd2 homologs, Lov1 and Lov2, are involved in cilia development and function of the mating organ required for mating behavior.[56,57] Progress in understanding the function of the slit diaphragm has also been made as a result of studies of *C. elegans.*

In *Drosophila* flies, the "kidney" consists of malpighian tubules that develop from the hindgut and perform a secretion reabsorption filtering function.[58] These flies express a number of mammalian gene homologs (e.g., Cut, members of the Wingless pathway) that have been shown to play major roles in mammalian kidney development. Furthermore, studies on myoblast fusion and neural development in *Drosophila* species—two processes that may not appear to be related to kidney development at first glance—have provided major clues into development and function of slit diaphragms.[59] Mutations in the irregular chiasm C-roughest (irreC-rst) locus, a Neph ortholog, are associated with neuronal defects and abnormal patterning of the eye.[60,61] Recently, nephpocytes that are similar to podocytes in mammalians have been characterized, providing additional insights.[312]

The pronephros, which is only the first of three stages of kidney development in mammals, is the final and only kidney of jawless fish, whereas the mesonephros is the definitive kidney in amphibians. The pronephros found in larval-stage zebrafish consists of two tubules connected to a fused, single, midline glomerulus. The zebrafish pronephric glomerulus expresses many of the same genes found in mammalian glomeruli, including that for vascular endothelial growth factor–A (VEGF-A), Nphs1, Nphs2, and Wt1, and it contains podocytes and fenestrated endothelial cells.[62] Advantages of using the zebrafish as a model system include its short reproductive cycle, transparency of the larvae with easy visualization of defects in pronephric development without the need to sacrifice the organism, availability of the genome sequence, the ability to rapidly knock down gene function by using morpholino oligonucleotides, and the ability to perform functional studies of filtration by using fluorescently tagged labels of varying sizes.[63] These features enable investigators to use both forward and reverse genetic screens in zebrafish, and several laboratories are currently performing knockdown screens of mammalian homologs in zebrafish and genomewide mutagenesis screens to study renal function.

The pronephros of *Xenopus* frogs has also been used as a simple model to study early events in nephrogenesis. As in the fish, the pronephros in these frogs consists of a single glomus, paired tubules, and a duct. The fact that *Xenopus* embryos develop rapidly (all major organ systems are formed by 6 days of age); the ease of injecting DNA, messenger RNA, and protein; and the ability to perform grafting and in vitro culture experiments establish the frog as a valuable model system with which to dissect early inductive and patterning cues.[64]

Genetic Analysis of Mammalian Kidney Development

Much has been learned about the molecular genetic basis of kidney development since the mid-1990s. This understanding has been gained primarily through the phenotypic analysis of mice carrying targeted mutations that affect kidney development. Additional information has been gained from identification and study of genes that are expressed in the developing kidney, even though the targeted mutation, or KO, either has not yet been achieved or has not affected kidney development or function. In this section, the genetic defects are categorized on the basis of the major phenotype and stage of disrupted development. It must be emphasized that many genes are expressed at multiple time stages of renal development and may play pleiotropic roles that are not yet entirely clear.

Interaction of the Ureteric Bud and Metanephric Mesenchyme

The molecular analysis of the initiation of metanephric kidney development has included a series of classical experiments with organ culture systems that allow separation of the ureteric bud and metanephric mesenchyme and, more recently, the analysis of many gene-targeted mice whose phenotypes have included various degrees of renal agenesis. The organ culture system has been in use since the seminal experiments, beginning in the 1950s, of Grobstein,[26] Saxen,[4] and their colleagues. These experiments showed that the induction of the mesenchymal-to-epithelial transformation within the mesenchyme required the presence of an inducing agent, provided by the ureteric bud. The embryonic neural tube was able to substitute for the epithelial bud, and experiments involving the placement of the inducing agent on the opposite side of a porous filter from the mesenchyme provided information about the degree of contact required between them. A large series of experiments with the organ culture provided information about the timing of appearance of different proteins normally observed during the induction of nephrons, as well as the time intervals that were crucial in maintaining contact between the inducing agent and the mesenchyme to obtain induction of tubules.

The work with the organ culture system provided an extensive framework on which to base further studies of organ development, and this framework remains in extensive use. However, the modern era of studies on the early development of the kidney began with the observation of renal agenesis phenotypes in gene-targeted or KO mice; the earliest among these was the KO of several transcription factors, including the Wilms' tumor–1 gene (also known as Wt1),[27] Pax2,[33] Eya1,[65] Odd1,[66] Six1,[67,68] Sall1,[69] Lim1,[70] and Emx2.[28] The KO of several secreted signaling molecules such as glial cell line–derived neurotrophic factor (GDNF),[71-73] Gdf11,[74] Gremlin,[75] or their receptors, including c-Ret[76] and GFRα1,[77] also resulted in renal agenesis, at least in the majority of embryos.

Early Lineage Determination of Metanephric Mesenchyme

In embryos with the phenotype of renal agenesis, the most common observation is the presence of a histologically distinct patch of mesenchyme in the normal location of the metanephric mesenchyme, but no outgrowth of the ureteric bud. Two exceptions are the Odd1 and Eya1 mutant embryos, in which this distinct patch of mesenchyme is not found, which suggests that Odd1 and Eya1 represent the earliest determinants of the metanephric mesenchyme yet identified (Figure 1-8). Together, the phenotypes of these KO mice have provided an initial molecular hierarchy of early kidney development.[65,78] Odd1 is localized to mesenchymal cells within the mesonephric and metanephric kidney and is subsequently downregulated upon epithelial differentiation. Mice lacking Odd1 do not form the distinct patch of metanephric mesenchyme and do not express several other factors required for metanephric kidney formation, including Eya1, Six2, Pax2, Sall1, and GDNF.[78]

Another factor implicated in the earliest stages of the determination of metanephric mesenchyme cell fate is the Eya1/Six1 pathway. Eya1 and Six1 mutations are found in humans with branchio-oto-renal syndrome.[79] It is now known, as a result of in vitro experiments, that Eya1 and Six1 form a regulatory complex that appears to be involved in transcriptional regulation.[80,81] Of interest is that a phosphatase activity is associated with this complex.[81] Moreover, Eya and Six family genes are coexpressed in several tissues in mammals, *Xenopus* frogs, and *Drosophila* flies, which is further evidence of a functional interaction of these genes.[65,67,68,82,83] Direct transcriptional targets of this complex appear to include the pro-proliferative factor c-Myc.[81] In the urogenital ridge of the Eya1-deficient phenotype, unlike that of some other renal agenesis phenotypes, it has been demonstrated that there is no histologically distinct group of cells in the normal location of the metanephric

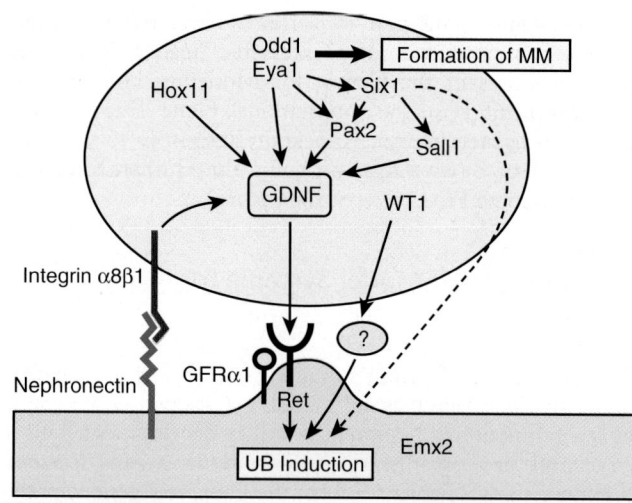

FIGURE 1-8 Early lineage determination of metanephric mesenchyme and transcriptional regulation of glial cell line–derived neurotrophic factor (GDNF). Odd1 and Eya1 seem to be the earliest determinants of the metanephric mesenchyme. Various factors whose deletions result in renal agenesis are involved in transactivation of GDNF. Secreted GDNF binds to the Ret-GFRα1 receptor complex and activates ureteric budding and branching. A GDNF-independent pathway mediated by Wt1 also exists, but the precise mechanism remains to be clarified. (Modified from Bouchard M: Transcriptional control of kidney development, *Differentiation* 2004;72[7]:295-306.)

mesenchyme.[84] Consistent with this finding is the observation that Six1 is either not expressed or highly diminished in expression in the location of the metanephric mesenchyme of Eya1[-/-] embryos.[81-84] These findings may indicate that Eya1 is a gene involved in early commitment of this group of cells to the metanephric lineage. Although Six1 and Eya1 may act in a complex together, the Six1 phenotype is somewhat different, in that a histologically distinct mesenchyme is present at E11.5, without an invading ureteric bud, which is a similar feature in the other renal agenesis phenotypes.[67,68] Eya1 is expressed in the Six1[-/-] mesenchyme, which suggests that Eya1 is upstream of Six1. In addition, Sall1 and Pax2 are not expressed in the Six1 mutant mesenchyme, although Wt1 is expressed.[67,68,84] (The literature contains discrepancies about Pax2 expression in Six1 mutant embryos, which may reflect the exact position along the anterior-posterior axis of the urogenital ridge of Six1 mutant embryos from which sections are obtained.)

Ureteric Bud Induction: Transcriptional Regulation of GDNF

In many cases of renal agenesis in humans, a failure of the GDNF-Ret axis has been identified.[85,313] GDNF belongs to the transforming growth factor (TGF)–β superfamily and is secreted from metanephric mesenchymal cells activating the Ret-GFRα1 receptor complex that is expressed by cells of the ureteric bud. The key role of GDNF–Ret-GFRα1 signaling in ureteric bud induction was elucidated by dramatic phenotypes observed in mouse mutants. Disruption of each of these genes results in similar urinary tract defects, ranging from bilateral renal agenesis to small rudimentary metanephroi.[71-73,77,86] In addition, organ culture experiments with GDNF-soaked beads have shown that ectopic GDNF protein is sufficient for ureteric bud induction.

A number of transcription factors have been shown to be involved in the transcriptional regulation of GDNF. Among the most important of these factors are Eya1, Pax2, the Hox11 paralog group, and Sall1 (see Figure 1-8). Targeted deletion of any one of these genes results in renal agenesis, with a failure of GDNF expression. As mentioned previously, Eya1 mutants fail to form metanephric mesenchyme. Pax2 is a transcriptional regulator of the paired-box family and is expressed widely during the development of both ureteric bud and mesenchymal components of the urogenital system.[87] In Pax2$^{-/-}$ embryos, Eya1, Six1, and Sal1 are expressed,[67] which suggests that the Eya1/Six1 pathway is not downstream but may be upstream of Pax2. Through a combination of molecular and in vivo studies, it has been demonstrated that Pax2 appears to act as a transcriptional activator of GDNF[88] and also regulates the expression of Ret.[89] Pax2 also appears to regulate kidney formation through epigenetic control as it is involved in the assembly of a histone H3 lysine 4 methyltransferase complex through the ubiquitously expressed nuclear factor PTIP, which regulates the histone methylation.[90] The HOX genes are conserved in all metazoans and specify positional information along the body axis. Hox11 paralogs include HoxA11, HoxC11, and HoxD11. Mice carrying mutations in any one of these genes do not have kidney abnormalities; however, mice with triple mutations in these genes demonstrate a complete absence of metanephric kidney induction.[91] Of interest in these mutant mice is that the formation of condensing metanephric mesenchyme and the expression of Eya1, Pax2, and Wt1 remain unperturbed, which suggests that Hox11 is not upstream of these factors. Although there seems to be some hierarchy, Eya1, Pax2, and Hox11 appear to form a complex to coordinately regulate the expression of GDNF.[92]

Non-GDNF Pathway in Metanephric Mesenchyme

Another pathway in early development of the metanephric mesenchyme involves Wt1 and vascular endothelial growth factor–A (VEGF-A).[35] Induction of the ureteric bud does not occur in persons with the Wt1 mutations, although GDNF is expressed in the metanephric mesenchyme, which indicates the existence of a GDNF-independent UB-induction mechanism.[27] However, details of this pathway still remain to be clarified. A novel approach to the organ culture system involving microinjection and electroporation has also yielded insights as to a possible function of the Wt1 gene in early kidney development. Overexpression of Wt1 from an expression construct led to high-level expression of VEGF-A. The target of VEGF-A appeared to be Flk1 (vascular endothelial growth factor receptor 2 [VEGFR-2])–expressing angioblasts at the periphery of the mesenchyme. Blocking signaling through Flk1, if done when the metanephric rudiment was placed in culture, blocked expression of Pax2 and GDNF and, consequently, the continued branching of the ureteric bud and induction of nephrons by the ureteric bud. Addition of the Flk1 blockade after the organ had been in culture for 48 hours had no effect, which indicates that the angioblast-derived signal was necessary to initiate kidney development but not to maintain continued development.[35] The signal provided by the angioblasts is not yet known, nor is it known whether Wt1 is a direct transcriptional activator of VEGF-A. Flk1 signaling is also known to be necessary to initiate hepatocyte differentiation during liver development. More recently,

a comprehensive catalog of Wt1 target genes in nephron progenitors was reported, in which chromatin immunoprecipitation (ChIP) coupled to mouse promoter microarray (ChIP-chip) was analyzed with the use of chromatin prepared from embryonic mouse kidney tissues.[93]

Genes Required by the Ureteric Bud in Early Kidney Development

Genes expressed by the ureteric bud are also crucially involved in the inductive events of early kidney development. Examples include Emx2, a transcription factor, and c-Ret, the receptor for GDNF. c-Ret is a receptor tyrosine kinase and presumably transduces signals to the epithelial cells of the UB that result in continued branching and proliferation. The molecular events downstream of c-Ret require clarification but certainly involve the phosphatidylinositol-3-kinase (PI3K) pathway.[94] PI3K pathway can be suppressed by the phosphatase and tensin homolog (PTEN), and conditional PTEN inactivation in ureteric bud disrupts normal branching.[95] Of interest is that the failure of ureteric bud growth and branching of the GDNF homozygous mutant embryos can be "rescued" in situations in which the embryo also carries a transgene that specifically directs GDNF expression in the ureteric bud and not in the mesenchyme. This autocrine-like rescue of ureteric bud growth and branching indicates that the pattern of branching is not determined by a specific pattern of GDNF expression in the mesenchyme; rather, any local source of GDNF elicits the usual pattern of branching.

Signaling Factors in Early Kidney Development

The signaling pathways described in the metanephric mesenchyme were identified by mutation of transcription factors. Presumably these transcription factors direct the expression of genes that encode proteins that act within the cell, in addition to genes encoding secreted molecules that act to convey signals from one group of cells to an adjacent or nearby group of cells. As previously mentioned, it has been demonstrated that Pax2 regulates the expression of GDNF, and Wt1 regulates VEGF-A. In the case of other signaling molecules, the transcription factors that control their expression in different cell types within the early kidney have yet to be determined. Nevertheless, several groups of signaling molecules have been identified to be of great importance in early kidney development.

Fibroblast growth factors (FGFs) have been implicated in the very early stages of differentiation of the nephron. Conditional mutation of FGF receptors in the murine mesenchyme results in renal agenesis with a ureteric bud, with expression of early markers such as Eya1 and Six1 in the vicinity of the ureteric bud but without expression of slightly later markers such as Six2 or Pax2 and without branching of the UB or induction of nephrons.[96] Two groups have published conditional mutations in the Fgf8 gene, which eliminate expression of fibroblast growth factor–8 (Fgf8) in the mesenchyme of the early kidney.[97,98] Failure to properly express Fgf8 did not block formation of a Wt1- and Pax2-expressing condensed mesenchyme, but Wnt4-expressing pretubular aggregates were not present; consequently, S-shaped bodies, the precursor of the nephron, never developed.[97,98] Of interest was that these conditionally mutant kidneys were smaller with fewer branches of the collecting ducts, which suggests that nephron differentiation may have a role in driving continued branching morphogenesis of the collecting system (Figure 1-9).

Two members of the Wingless type MMTV (mouse mammary tumor virus) integration site (Wnt) family of signaling molecules are expressed by the ureteric bud: Wnt11 and Wnt9b. The Wnt family was originally discovered as the Wingless mutation in *Drosophila* species and as genes found at retroviral integration sites in mammary tumors in mice. Wnt11 is expressed at the tips of the buds, and decreased branching is observed in its absence, although there is no specific effect on the induction of the mesenchymal-to-epithelial transformation.[99] In contrast, Wnt9b, which is expressed in the entire ureteric bud except the very tips, appears to be the vital molecule expressed by the bud that induces the mesenchyme. In the absence of Wnt9b, the bud merges from the wolffian duct and invades the mesenchyme, which condenses around the bud, but pretubular aggregates do not form, and the mesenchymal-to-epithelial transformation does not occur. No further branching of the bud is observed. Thus, to date, Wnt9b is the molecule produced by the bud that appears to be most crucial in stimulating induction of the nephrons.[100]

A third member of the Wnt family, Wnt4, is expressed in the pretubular aggregate, and is required for the mesenchymal-to-epithelial transformation.[101] In Wnt4-mutant embryos, pretubular aggregates are present but fail to undergo the mesenchymal-to-epithelial transformation into the tubular precursor of the mature nephron; this is indicative of a role for Wnt4 in the formation of epithelial cells from mesenchyme.[101] The role of Wnt signaling has been studied in vitro by exposure of isolated metanephric mesenchyme to fibroblast cultures transfected with Wnt-expressing DNA vectors. Several Wnt proteins were found to be able to induce the mesenchymal-to-epithelial transformation, similar to that observed in studies with embryonic neural tube. In view of the more recently published Wnt9b phenotype, it is worth considering whether the neural tube induction experiment can be viewed as a recapitulation of either the Wnt4 or Wnt9b function, or both. As previously noted, a distinction between induction by the ureteric bud and induction by the neural tube is that the bud stimulates both proliferation and mesenchymal-to-epithelial transformation, whereas the neural tube, or Wnt4 expression by fibroblasts, stimulates only differentiation, without significant proliferation. On the other hand, both the classical neural tube experiment and the Wnt-expressing fibroblast experiment seemingly bypass a step normally observed in kidney development: formation of the pretubular aggregate inferior to the tips of the bud. Instead, aggregates form randomly within the isolated mesenchyme. Therefore, the neural tube rescue experiments are consistent more with a Wnt4 function than with a Wnt 9b function. Further experimentation is needed, however, to determine whether Wnt9b, in the absence of the bud, can stimulate proliferation in addition to differentiation, in order to determine whether the expression of Wnt 9b is the major criterion that distinguishes the induction by the bud from induction by neural tube.

Two major Wnt-signaling branches exist downstream of the Fz receptor: a canonical, or Wnt/β-catenin–dependent, pathway and a noncanonical, or β-catenin–independent, pathway.[102] In the canonical pathway, Wnt-mediated signaling suppresses a phosphorylation-triggered pathway of proteosomal degradation, enabling the stabilization of β-catenin, which results in the formation of an activation complex between β-catenin and the TCF/LEF family of DNA binding proteins that directly regulates transcriptional targets. Numerous studies demonstrate the importance of the canonical Wnt pathway for renal development: Conditional deletion of β-catenin from the cap mesenchyme completely blocks both renal vesicle formation and expression of markers of induction such as Wnt4, Fgf8, and Pax8.[103] In contrast, activation of stabilized β-catenin in the same cell population causes ectopic expression of mesenchymal induction markers in vitro and functionally prevents the defects observed in Wnt4- or Wnt9b-deficient mesenchyme. Inhibitors of GSK3, a member of the β-catenin degradation complex, results in the ectopic differentiation of metanephric mesenchyme (see Figure 1-9).[104]

The bone morphogenetic protein (BMP) family of proteins is an additional family of secreted signaling proteins that plays a crucial role in the developing kidney. BMP7 is expressed first in the ureteric bud and then in the condensed mesenchyme.[105,106] In the absence of BMP7, the first round of nephrons are induced, but there is no further kidney development.[105,106] It has been suggested that this first round of nephrons might result from maternal contribution of BMP7 across the placenta, and it is not known whether BMP7 is absolutely required for the induction of nephrons.

Adhesion Proteins in Early Kidney Development

A current theme in cell biology is that growth factor signaling often occurs coordinately with signals from the extracellular matrix transduced by adhesion receptors, such as members of the integrin family. α8β1 Integrin is expressed by cells of the metanephric mesenchyme,[107] which binds a molecule named nephronectin,[108] expressed on the ureteric bud. In most embryos with α8 integrin mutations, outgrowth of the UB is arrested upon contact with the metanephric mesenchyme.[107] In a small portion of such embryos, this block is overcome, and a single, usually hypoplastic, kidney develops. Mice with

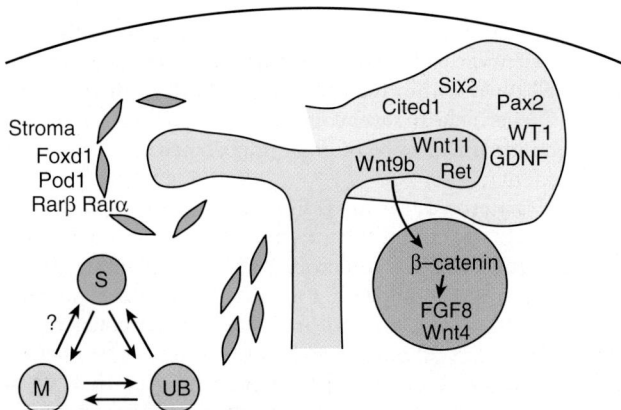

FIGURE 1-9 Six2 and Cited1 are expressed in cap mesenchyme that surrounds the ureteric bud, and they characterize the mesenchymal progenitor population that gives rise to every epithelial component of the nephron down to the distal tubules. Wnt9b from ureteric bud stimulates canonical pathway of WNT signaling with subsequent expression of Wnt4 and fibroblast growth factor-8 (FGF8), which results in formation of pretubular aggregates. Reciprocal interactions occur among all three major components of the metanephros (stroma [S], mesenchyme [M], and ureteric bud [UB]). (Modified from Schedl A: Renal abnormalities and their developmental origin, *Nat Rev Genet* 2007;8[10]:791-802.)

KO mutations for nephronectin exhibit renal agenesis or severe hypoplasia.[109] Thus, the interaction of α8β1 integrin with nephronectin must have an important role in the continued growth of the ureteric bud into the mesenchyme. Both α8 integrin and nephronectin-KO phenotypes appear to result from a reduction in GDNF expression.[109]

Formation of the Collecting System

Formation of the collecting system is the result of the branching morphogenesis of the ureteric bud and its derivative branches, followed by extensive remodeling of those initial branches, to finally form the papillary region of the medulla, as well as the collecting ducts within the cortex and outer medulla. The overall structure of the kidney is largely patterned by the collecting system, and an understanding of the pathways that drive the formation of the collecting system is essential for understanding how the overall structure of the kidney is derived.

The molecular events crucial to the development of the collecting system occur largely as interactions between the mesenchymal cells and the epithelial derivatives of the ureteric bud. This is especially true in the early phases of kidney development, when the epithelial branches of the bud are surrounded by mesenchyme. At later stages of development, when the cortex and medulla form distinct areas of the kidney and when nephrons and stromal cells compose much of the cortex, it is currently much less clear what the important cellular interactions are, even when specific molecules are known to be important.

Wnt7b is expressed in the ureteric bud epithelium that gives rise to the collecting duct system and ureter. In Wnt7b-mutant mice, cortical nephron development is normal, but the medullary zone and collecting duct system fails to form, which results in urinary concentrating defects. Interestingly, deletion of β-catenin from the interstitial cell population phenocopies the Wnt7b defects, which suggests that the canonical Wnt pathway is involved in the formation of both the collecting system and pretubular aggregates.[110]

Several families of secreted growth factors have been demonstrated to be important in the patterning of the collecting system, including members of the Wnt7b,[110] BMP,[111] sonic hedgehog,[112] and FGF families.[113] The role of GDNF, required for initial outgrowth of the ureteric bud and to drive continued branching, was previously discussed. Conditional gene targeting of FGF receptor 2 (but not of FGF receptor 1) in the ureteric bud results in greatly decreased branching of the bud.[114] Mice carrying a mutation of Fgf7 have smaller collecting systems,[113] although this phenotype is not as severe as the conditional mutation of FGF receptor 2, which implies that additional FGFs are probably involved in branching of the ureteric bud. The role of FGF8 in the mesenchyme, with regard to nephron development, was previously discussed. Whether FGF8 or another FGF is also driving development of the collecting system is not clear, but it is of interest that mutations that block induction of nephrons also tend to eliminate further branching and growth of the derivative branches of the ureteric bud.

The role of Bmp7 in early kidney development has been discussed in a previous section. Two other prominent members of the BMP family, Bmp2 and Bmp4, also have significant roles in formation of the collecting system,[111,115-116] which were more difficult to decipher because mouse embryos carrying mutations in these factors die too early to identify an effect on kidney development. In organ culture, Bmp7 stimulates branching, whereas Bmp2 was found to inhibit branching of the derivatives of the ureteric bud.[115,116] In further study of the role of Bmp2, researchers used a constitutively active form of the Bmp2 receptor, activin receptor–like kinase-3 (ALK3), specifically expressed in the derivatives of the ureteric bud. This resulted in medullary dysplasia, resembling medullary cystic disease observed in humans.[117] Furthermore, conditional deletion of ALK3 in the UB lineage results in renal malformation associated with a decreased number of collecting ducts and their progenitor UB branches. The embryonic mutant kidneys demonstrate a biphasic branching defect, which manifests in an early increase in the number of primary and secondary UB branches but a decrease in the number of subsequent branches that are formed, which results in an overall reduction in UB number. Together, these results suggest that Bmp2-ALK3 signaling functions to limit UB branching at the earliest stages of branching morphogenesis but is required for further branching of the ureteric bud. Of interest is that postnatal mice with ALK3 deficiency restricted to the UB lineage (Alk3UB$^{-/-}$) exhibit a dysplastic renal phenotype characterized by hypoplasia of the renal medulla, a decreased number of medullary collecting ducts, and abnormal expression of β-catenin. A similar phenotype has been observed in mutants of Wnt7b (see previous discussion), which suggests that there may be crosstalk between BMP signaling and the canonical Wnt pathway.[118] It appears that Bmp2 signaling normally acts to suppress a proliferation signal mediated by SMAD signaling and β-catenin, which acts to stimulate expression of the pro-proliferative transcription factor c-Myc.[119]

Diminished branching is also observed in kidneys of sonic hedgehog (Shh)–deficient embryos.[112] This phenotype bears resemblance to the renal dysplasia observed in humans with mutations of the Gli3 gene, which encodes an effector of the Shh signaling pathway.[120] Increased expression of Pax2 and Sal1, required for normal kidney development, as well as cell cycle regulatory genes MycN and cyclin D1, were observed in Shh-deficient kidneys.[120] Interestingly, the Shh-deficient kidney phenotype was rescued by inhibiting signaling through Gli3, which provided genetic confirmation that Gli3 is a regulator of the Shh pathway.[120]

Targeted mutation in mice of the α3 integrin gene, discussed later in regard to its role in glomerular development, also results in a poorly formed papilla, with fewer collecting ducts and increased interstitium.[121] α3β1 Integrin is expressed in the ureteric bud and collecting ducts.[122] in vitro, α3β1 integrin appears to have a role both in cell-matrix and cell-cell interaction,[123] but the latter role has not been verified in vivo, although α3β1 integrin is expressed basolaterally in developing tubules, which is consistent with both roles. Conditional deletion of the α3 integrin gene from ureteric bud epithelium results in malformation of the papilla with reduction of Wnt7b expression.[124] In accordance, conditional deletion of β1 integrin in ureteric bud also results in various degrees of phenotypes ranging from a hypoplastic medullary collecting duct system to bilateral renal agenesis caused by disrupted branching morphogenesis.[125] As integrins are known to signal in coordination with growth factor receptors, it is of interest to determine whether α3β1 integrin is involved in any of the signaling pathways discussed previously in this section.

Positioning of the Ureteric Bud

A final aspect of kidney development that is of great relevance to renal and urologic congenital defects in humans is related to the positioning of the ureteric bud. Incorrect position or duplication of the UB results in abnormally shaped kidneys, incorrect insertion of the ureter into the bladder, or both and in resultant ureteral reflux that can predispose to infection and scarring of the kidneys and urologic tract.

FoxC1 is a transcription factor of the Forkhead family, expressed in the intermediate mesoderm and the metanephric mesenchyme adjacent to the Wolffian duct. In the absence of FoxC1, the expression of GDNF adjacent to the wolffian duct is less restricted than in wild-type embryos, and the result is ectopic ureteric buds, giving rise to duplex ureters, one of which is a hydroureter, and to hypoplastic kidneys (Figure 1-10).[126,307] Additional molecules that regulate the location of ureteric bud outgrowth are Slit2 and Robo2, signaling molecules best known for their role in axon guidance in the developing nervous system. Slit is a secreted factor, and Roundabout (Robo) is its receptor. Slit2 is expressed mainly in the Wolffian duct, whereas Robo2 is expressed in the mesenchyme.[127] In embryos deficient in either Slit2 or Robo2, the UB are ectopic, as in the FoxC1 mutant. (Dissimilar to the FoxC1 phenotype was the observation that none of the ureters in Slit2/Robo2 mutants failed to undergo the normal remodeling that results in insertion in the bladder; instead,

the ureters remained connected to the nephric duct.[127]) The domain of GDNF expression is expanded anteriorly in the absence of either Slit2 or Robo2. Indeed, mutations in Robo2 have been identified in patients with vesicoureteral junction defects and vesicoureteral reflux.[128] The expression of Pax2, Eya1, and FoxC1, all thought to regulate GDNF expression, was not dramatically different in the absence of Slit2 or Robo2, which suggests that Slit/Robo signaling was not upstream of these genes. It is possible that Slit/Robo signaling is regulating the point of ureteric bud outgrowth by regulating the GDNF expression domain downstream of Pax2 or Eya1. An alternative explanation is that Slit/Robo are acting independently of GDNF and that the expanded GDNF domain is a response to, rather than a cause of, ectopic ureteric buds.

Since 2005, genetic studies have identified two additional negative regulators of UB branching: Sprouty1 and Bmp4. Sprouty1 is a negative regulator of Ras/Erk MAP kinase signaling (one of the signaling pathways activated by GDNF/Ret signaling)[129] that is expressed strongly in the posterior wolffian duct. Embryos lacking Sprouty1 develop supernumerary ureteric buds, but unlike FoxC1, Slit2, or Robo2 mutants, they do not display changes in GDNF expression.[130] The phenotype of Sprouty1 mutants can be rescued by reducing the GDNF expression dosage.[130] Sprouty 1 deletion also mitigates the renal agenesis defect in mice lacking the tyrosine phosphorylation residue of Ret that is the binding site for molecules such as Grb, Sos, and Ras.[131] Thus, Sprouty1 appears to regulate the response to GDNF by regulating post-receptor signaling functions of the Ret receptor.

Another negative regulator of branching is Bmp4, which is expressed in the mesenchyme surrounding the wolffian duct. Bmp4 heterozygous mutants have duplicated ureters, and in organ culture, Bmp4 blocks the induction of ectopic UBs by GDNF-soaked beads.[111] Furthermore, KO of Gremlin, a secreted BMP inhibitor, causes renal agenesis, a finding that supports a role for BMP in the suppression of UB formation.[132]

Molecular Biology of Nephron Development: Tubulogenesis

Whereas gene targeting and other analyses have identified many genes involved in the initial induction of the metanephric kidney and the formation of the pretubular aggregate, much less is currently known about how the pretubular aggregate develops into the mature nephron, a process through which a simple tubule elongates, convolutes, and differentiates into multiple distinct segments with different functions. The process by which this segmentation occurs may be similar to other aspects of development, such as the limb or neural tube, for which segmentation occurs along various axes.

The Notch group of signaling molecules has been implicated in directing segmentation of the nephron. Notch family members are transmembrane proteins whose cytoplasmic domains are cleared by the γ-secretase enzyme, upon the interaction of the extracellular domain with transmembrane ligand proteins of the Delta and Jagged families, found on adjacent cells.[133] Thus, Notch signaling occurs between adjacent cells, in contrast to signaling by secreted growth factors, which may occur at a distance from the growth factor–expressing cells. The cleaved portion of the Notch cytoplasmic domain translocates to the nucleus, where it has a role in directing gene expression.

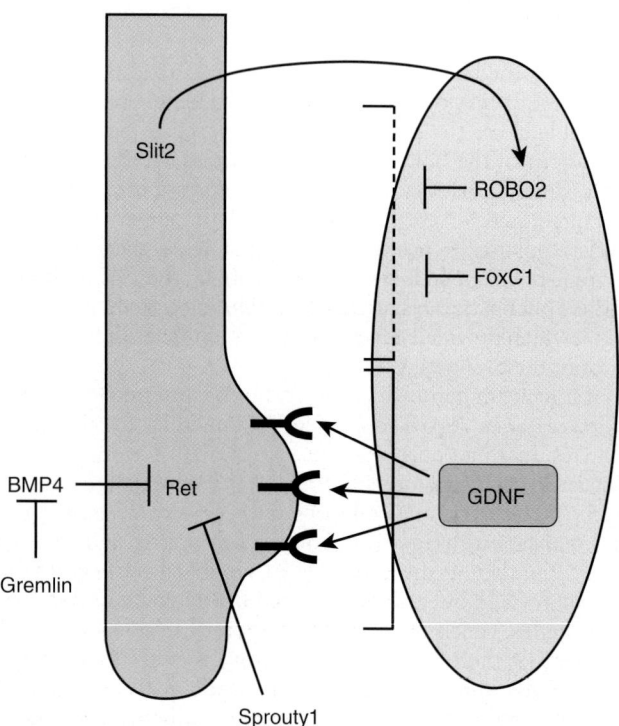

FIGURE 1-10 Positioning of the ureteric bud. The anterior part of glial cell line–derived neurotrophic factor (GDNF) expression is restricted by FoxC1 and Slit/Robo2 signaling. Sprouty1 suppresses the post-receptor activity of Ret. Bmp4 inhibits the response of GDNF and is suppressed by Gremlin. (Modified from Costantini F, Shakya R: GDNF/Ret signaling and the development of the kidney, *Bioessays* 2006;28(2):117-127.)

Mice homozygous for a hypomorphic allele of Notch2 have abnormal glomeruli, with a failure to form a mature capillary tuft.[134,135] Because null mutants of Notch family members usually result in early embryonic lethality, Notch family function in kidney development has been further analyzed with the organ culture model. When metanephric rudiments are cultured in the presence of a γ-secretase inhibitor,[136,137] expression of podocyte and proximal tubule markers is diminished, in comparison with distal tubule markers and branching of the ureteric bud. When the γ-secretase inhibitor is removed, recovery of expression of proximal tubule markers seems better, in comparison with markers of podocyte differentiation. Similar results were observed in mice carrying targeted mutation of the Psen1 and Psen2 genes that encode a component of the γ-secretase complex.[138] These observations are supported by results from conditional deletion of Notch2 in metanephric mesenchyme; these mice have hypoplastic kidneys that do not develop glomeruli or proximal tubules, despite the presence of distal tubules and collecting ducts. Of interest is that the condensed mesenchyme and pretubular aggregates initiate epithelialization expressing Pax2 and E-cadherin, but they do not proceed to form S-shaped bodies. In contrast, Notch1-deficient metanephroi are phenotypically wild-type, which suggests that Notch1 is not critical for determination of cell fate during early nephron formation. Local activation of Notch2 during tubule morphogenesis is thus critical in determining the proximal cell fate after the epithelialization of renal vesicle.[139]

There is one example so far of a transcription factor being involved in the differentiation of a specific cell type in the kidney. The phenotype is actually found in the collecting ducts, rather than in the nephron itself, but is discussed in this section because it is demonstrative of the types of phenotypes expected to be found as additional mutant mice are examined. Two cell types are normally found in the collecting ducts: principal cells, which mediate water and salt reabsorption, and intercalated cells, which mediate acid-base transport. In the absence of the FoxI1 transcription factor, only one cell type is present in collecting ducts, and many acid-base transport proteins normally expressed by intercalated cells are absent.[140]

In addition to cell differentiation, spatial orientation of cells is essential for tubule elongation and morphogenesis. In epithelia, cells are uniformly organized along an apical-basal plane of polarity. However, in addition, cells in most tissues require positional information in the plane perpendicular to the apical-basal axis. This type of polarization, referred to as *planar cell polarity* (PCP), is critical for morphogenesis of metazoans.[141,142] Using cell lineage analysis and close examination of the mitotic axis of dividing cells, investigators have shown that lengthening of renal tubules is associated with mitotic orientation of cells along the tubule axis, which demonstrates intrinsic planar cell polarity.[143] Dysregulation of oriented cell division results in the dysregulation of diameter and length of tubules, which results in multiple cyst formation.[144] To date, molecules implicated in PCP and tubule elongation include HNF1β-PKHD axis, the PCP ortholog Fat4, and Wnt9b.[143,145-150]

Molecular Analysis of the Nephrogenic Zone

Since the preceding publication of this chapter, molecular characterization of the nephrogenic zone has advanced tremendously, largely as a result of cell fate mapping studies in mice. As noted previously, the histologic features of this peripheral zone resemble the early developing kidney, with condensed mesenchyme expressing Six2, Cited1, Pax2, and low levels of Wt1 surrounding the tips of ureteric bud–like structures. Using various mouse strains that express Cre under the control of the Six2 or Cited1 promoters, investigators were able to demonstrate that this cell population replenishes and retains the potential to differentiate into all epithelial cell types of the nephron (from podocytes to distal tubules), exhibiting stem cell–like characteristics.[19,20] However, it is still not known whether there is a small subset of stem cells within those that express these markers or whether these stem cell–like properties apply to the whole population of Six2-positive condensed mesenchyme.

Molecular Genetics of the Stromal Cell Lineage

In recent years, a key role for the stromal cell lineage in kidney development was discovered largely through the analysis of KO mice. FoxD1 (formerly known as Bf2) is a winged helix transcription factor; in the kidney, it is expressed only in stromal cells that are found in a rim beneath the renal capsule and as a layer of cells surrounding the mesenchymal condensates.[23] Despite the restricted distribution of FoxD1-positive cells, major defects in the development of adjacent renal tubules and glomeruli were observed in FoxD1-KO mice. These results demonstrate that stromal cells are required for nephrogenesis and furthermore that the model of reciprocal signaling between the UB and condensates must be extended to include the stromal cell compartment (see Figure 1-5).[9]

Pod1 (Tcf21/capsulin/epicardin), a member of the basic-helix–loop-helix family of transcription factors, is also expressed in the stromal cell lineage, as well as in condensing MM.[151,152] Pod1 is also expressed in a number of differentiated renal cell types that derive from these mesenchymal cells and include developing and mature podocytes of the renal glomerulus, cortical and medullary peritubular interstitial cells, pericytes surrounding small renal vessels, and adventitial cells surrounding larger blood vessels. The defect in nephrogenesis observed in Pod1-KO mice is similar to the defect seen in Bf2-KO mice, with disruption of branching morphogenesis and an arrest and delay in glomerulogenesis and tubulogenesis. Analysis of chimeric mice that are derived from Pod1-KO ES cells and green fluorescent protein (GFP)–expressing embryos demonstrated both cell autonomous and non–cell-autonomous roles for Pod1 in nephrogenesis.[153] The most striking feature is that the glomerulogenesis defect is prevented by the presence of wild-type stromal cells (i.e., mutant cells epithelialize and form nephrons normally as long as they are surrounded by wild-type stromal cells, in keeping with the model outlined in Figures 1-5 and 1-9). In addition, there is a cell-autonomous requirement for Pod1 in stromal mesenchymal cells to allow differentiation into interstitial cell and pericyte cell lineages of the cortex and medulla as Pod1 null ES cells were unable to contribute to these populations.

Although many of the defects in the Pod1 mutant kidneys phenocopy those seen in the Bf2 mutant kidneys, there are important differences. The kidneys of Pod1-KO mice contain vascular anomalies and absence of pericyte differentiation that were not reported in FoxD1-mutant mice. These differences might result from the broader domain of Pod1 expression,

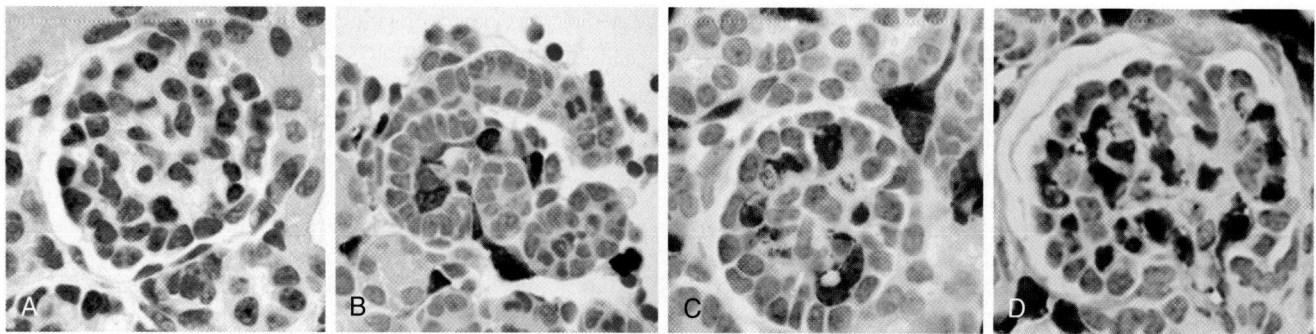

FIGURE 1-11 Developing glomeruli stained with an antibody to the green fluorescent protein (GFP). Control glomerulus from a wild-type mouse. Comma-shaped **(A)**, S-shaped **(B)**, capillary **(C)**, and mature **(D)** glomeruli in a metanephros from an Flk1-GFP mouse strain 18.5 days post coitum. All endothelial cells express the GFP protein that is expressed under control of the endogenous Flk1/VEGFR-2 promoter. (Reproduced with permission from the *Journal of American Society of Nephrology.*)

which also includes the condensing mesenchyme, podocytes, and medullary stromal cells, in addition to the stromal cells that surround the condensates. In contrast to FoxD1, Pod1 is not highly expressed in the thin rim of stromal cells found immediately beneath the capsule, which suggests that FoxD1 and Pod1 might mark early and late stromal cell lineages, respectively, with overlap in the stroma that surrounds the condensates.[24] However, definitive colabeling studies to address this issue have not been performed. Because both Pod1 and FoxD1 are transcription factors, it is possible that they interact or regulate the expression of a common stromal "inducing factor."

Vitamin A deficiency has been associated with a variety of birth defects, including renal dysplasia; vitamin A is the ligand for retinoic acid receptors (RARs), including RARA and RARB2, both of which are expressed in the stromal cell lineage. Mice that lack both of these receptors, and thus have decreased vitamin A signaling, demonstrate decreased branching of the UB, patterning defects in the stromal cell lineage with a buildup of stromal cell layers beneath the capsule and defects in nephron patterning.[9,24,154] Transgenic overexpression of the tyrosine kinase receptor c-Ret under the regulation of a ureteric bud–specific promoter from the Hoxb7 gene prevented the observed defects, although retinoic acid treatment alone could not. Together, these results show that a vitamin A–dependent signal is required in stromal cells for UB branching and that UB branching is necessary to pattern the stroma.

Molecular Genetics of Vascular Formation

Vasculogenesis and angiogenesis both contribute to vascular development within the kidney. Endothelial cells may be identified through the expression of the tyrosine kinase–signaling receptor VEGFR-2 (Flk1/KDR).[155] Reporter mouse strains that carry lacZ or GFP complementary DNA cassettes "knocked into" the VEGFR-2 locus enable precise snapshots of vessel development, inasmuch as all the vascular progenitor and differentiated cells in these organs express a blue or green color (Figure 1-11). Use of other knockin strains allows identification of endothelial cells lining arteriolar or venous vessels.[156]

Since 2000, a number of growth factors and their receptors that are required for vasculogenesis and angiogenesis have been identified. Gene deletion studies in mice have shown that VEGF-A and its cognate receptor VEGFR-2 are essential for vasculogenesis.[155,157] Mice that have a null VEGF-A genotype die at 9.5 days post coitum from a failure of vasculogenesis, whereas mice lacking a single VEGF-A allele (i.e., they are heterozygotes for the VEGF-A gene) die at 11.5 d.p.c. also from vascular defects.[157] These data demonstrate gene dosage sensitivity to VEGF-A during development. In the developing kidney, podocytes and renal tubular epithelial cells express VEGF-A[158] and continue to express it constitutively in the adult kidney, while the cognate tyrosine kinase receptors for VEGF-A, VEGFR-1 (Flt1), and VEGFR-2 (Flk1/KDR) are predominantly expressed by all endothelial cells. Which non-endothelial cells might also express the VEGF receptors in the kidney in vivo is still debated, although renal cell lines clearly do, and metanephric mesenchymal cells express VEGFR-2 in organ culture, as outlined earlier.

Conditional gene targeting experiments and cell-selective deletion of VEGF-A from podocytes demonstrate that VEGF-A signaling is required for formation and maintenance of the glomerular filtration barrier.[159,160] Glomerular endothelial cells express VEGFR-2 as they migrate into the vascular cleft. Although a few endothelia migrate into the developing glomeruli of VEGF^Lox/Lox/Pod-Cre mice (mice with selective deletion of VEGF from podocytes)—probably because a small amount of VEGF-A is produced by presumptive podocytes at the S-shaped stage of glomerular development before Cre-mediated genetic deletion—the endothelia failed to develop fenestrations and rapidly disappeared, leaving capillary "ghosts" (Figure 1-12). In a finding similar to the dosage sensitivity observed in the whole embryo, deletion of a single VEGF-A allele from podocytes also led to glomerular endothelial defects known as *endotheliosis* that progressed to end-stage kidney failure at 3 months of age; as the dose of VEGF-A decreased, the associated endothelial phenotypes became more severe (Figure 1-13). Upregulation of the major 164 angiogenic VEGF-A isoform in developing podocytes of transgenic mice led to massive proteinuria and collapse of the glomerular tuft by 5 days of age. Together, these results show a requirement for VEGF-A for development and maintenance of the specialized glomerular endothelia and demonstrate a major paracrine signaling function for VEGF-A in the glomerulus. Furthermore, tight regulation of the dose of VEGF-A is essential for proper formation of the glomerular capillary system; the molecular basis and mechanism of dosage sensitivity is unclear at present and is particularly intriguing in view of the documented inducible regulation of VEGF-A by hypoxia-inducible factors at a transcriptional level. Despite this, it is clear that in vivo, a single VEGF-A allele is unable to

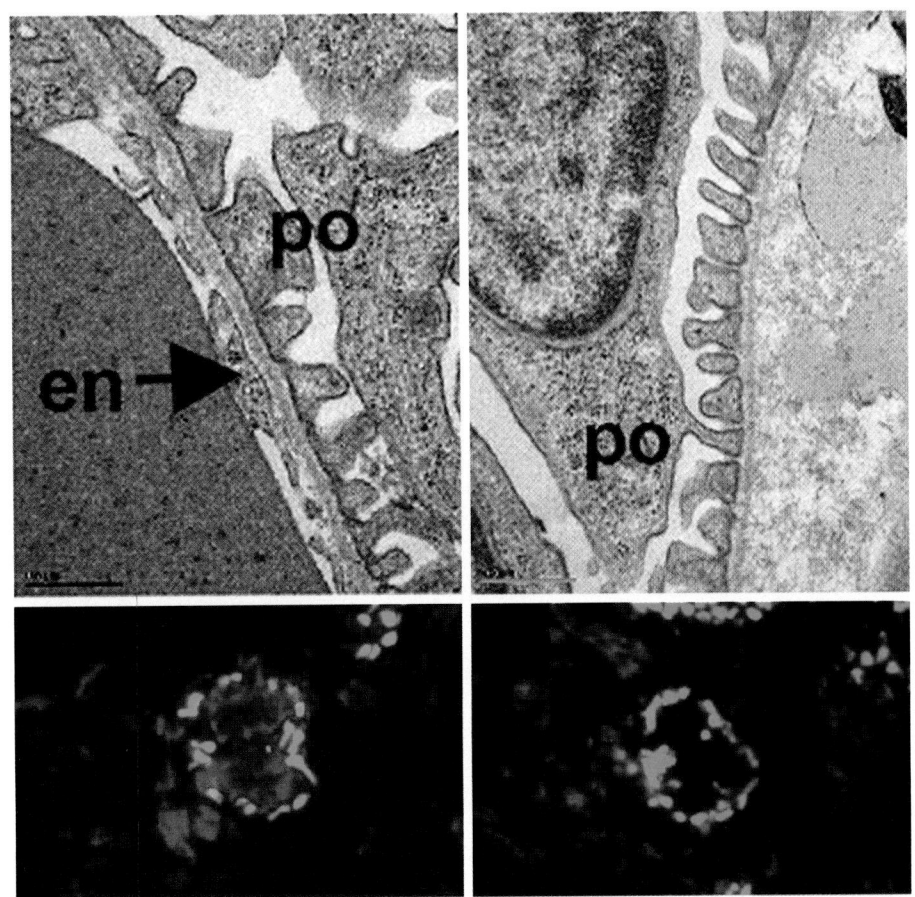

FIGURE 1-12 Transmission electron micrographs of the glomerular filtration barrier from a wild-type mouse (*left*) or transgenic mouse with selective knockout of vascular endothelial growth factor (VEGF) from the podocytes (*right*). Podocytes (po) are seen in both, but the endothelial layer (en) is entirely missing from the knockout mouse, leaving a "capillary ghost." Immunostaining for Wt1 (podocytes; green) and platelet-endothelial cell adhesion molecule (PECAM; red) confirms the absence of capillary wall in VEGF knockouts. (Adapted from Eremina V, Sood M, Haigh J, et al: Glomerular-specific alterations of VEGF-A expression lead to distinct congenital and acquired renal diseases, *J Clin Invest* 2003;111:707-716.)

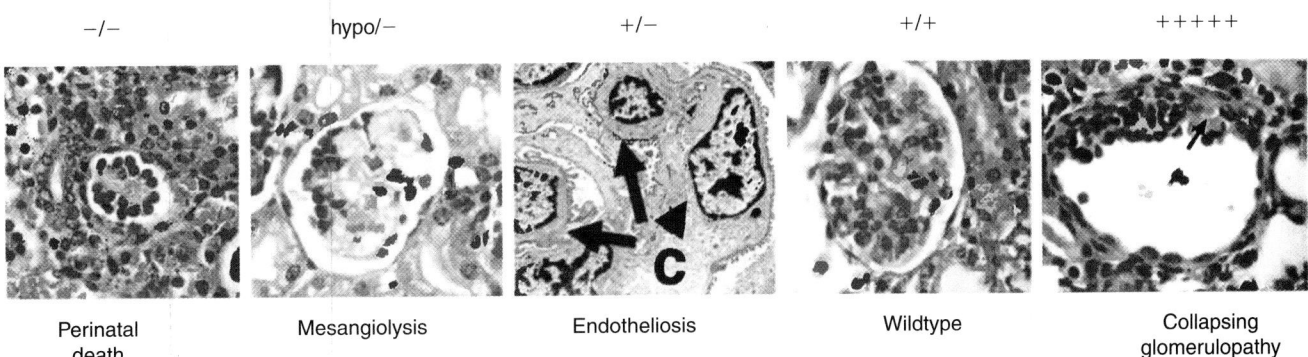

−/−	hypo/−	+/−	+/+	++++
Perinatal death	Mesangiolysis	Endotheliosis	Wildtype	Collapsing glomerulopathy

FIGURE 1-13 Vascular endothelial growth factor dose and glomerular development: Photomicrographs of glomeruli from mice carrying different copy numbers of the vascular endothelial growth factor (VEGF) gene within podocytes. A total knockout (loss of both alleles; −/−) results in failure of glomerular filtration barrier formation and perinatal death; a single hypomorphic allele (hypo/−) leads to massive mesangiolysis in the first weeks of life and death at 3 weeks of age; loss of one copy (+/−) results in endotheliosis (swelling of the endothelium) and death at 12 weeks of age. Overexpression (20-fold increase in VEGF;++++) results in collapsing glomerulopathy. (Adapted from Eremina V, Baeld HJ, Quaggin SE: Role of the VEGF-A signaling pathway in the glomerulus: evidence for crosstalk between components of the glomerular filtration barrier, *Nephron Physiol* 2007;106:32-37.)

compensate for loss of the other. Immortalized podocyte cell lines express a variety of VEGF receptors; however, deletion of VEGFR-2 from podocytes does not disrupt glomerular structure and function, which means that paracrine, not autocrine, VEGF signaling is important in the glomerular vasculature.[311]

A second major receptor tyrosine kinase (RTK)–signaling pathway required for maturation of developing blood vessels is the angiopoietin-Tie signaling system. Angiopoietin 1 (Ang1) stabilizes newly formed blood vessels and is associated with loss of vessel plasticity and concurrent recruitment of pericytes or vascular support cells to the vascular wall.[164] The molecular switch or pathway leading to vessel maturation through activation of Tie2 (previously known as Tek), the major receptor for Ang1, is not known and appears to be independent of the platelet-derived growth factor (PDGF)–signaling system that is also required for pericyte recruitment. Ang1-KO mice die at 12.5 d.p.c, which precludes analysis of its role in glomerular development, but exogenous recombinant Ang1 enhances the growth of interstitial capillaries in mouse metanephric organ culture[165]; thus, Ang1 may facilitate the capillary formation in glomeruli. In contrast, it is proposed that angiopoietin 2 (Ang2) functions as a natural antagonist of the Tie2 receptor, inasmuch as Ang2 can bind to this receptor but fails to phosphorylate it in endothelial cultures.[166,167] Consistent with this hypothesis is the fact that overexpression of Ang2 in transgenic mice results in a phenotype similar to the Ang1- or Tie2-KO mice. Ang1, Ang2, Tie2, and Tie1 (an orphan receptor for this system) are all expressed in the developing kidney.[168-172] Whereas Ang1 is quite broadly expressed in condensing mesenchyme, podocytes, and tubular epithelial cells, Ang2 is more restricted to pericytes and smooth muscle cells surrounding cortical and large vessels, as well as in the mesangium. Ang2-KO mice were viable but exhibited defects in peritubular cortical capillary development; they died before differentiation of vasa rectae, which precluded analysis of the role of Ang2 in these other capillary beds.[173] Podocyte-specific Ang2 overexpression causes proteinuria and increased apoptosis in formed glomerular capillaries.[174] Both angiopoietin ligands function in concert with VEGF, although the precise degree of crosstalk between these pathways is still under investigation. (VEGF and Ang2 work together to promote sprouting.) Chimeric studies demonstrated that the orphan receptor Tie1 is required for development of the glomerular capillary system because Tie1-null cells are not able to contribute to glomerular capillary endothelium.[175]

The Ephrin-Eph family is a third tyrosine kinase–dependent growth factor–signaling system that is expressed in the developing kidney; in the whole embryo, it is involved in neural sprouting and axon finding, as well as in arterial and venous specification of arterial and venous components of the vasculature.[176,177] Ephrins and their cognate receptors are expressed widely during renal development. Overexpression of Eph4 leads to defects in glomerular arteriolar formation, whereas conditional deletion of EphrinB2 from perivascular smooth muscle cells and mesangial cells leads to glomerular vascular abnormalities.[178,179] How this occurs is not entirely clear, inasmuch as EphrinB2 has a dynamic pattern of expression in the developing glomerulus, beginning in podocyte precursors and rapidly switching to glomerular endothelial cells and mesangial cells.[156]

Dysregulation of BMP within the podocyte compartment also results in glomerular vascular defects; overexpression of Bmp4 leads to defects in endothelial and mesangial recruitment, whereas overexpression of Noggin the antagonist for Bmp2/4/7, leads to collapse of the glomerular tuft. Interestingly, deletion of Bmp7 from podocytes results not in glomerular but tubular defects. Additional studies are needed to fully understand the role of this family of growth factors in glomeruli.[180,181]

An additional pathway that is likely to play a role in glomerular endothelial development and perhaps of the entire vasculature of the kidney is the CXCR4-SDF1 axis. CXCR4, a chemokine receptor, is expressed by bone marrow–derived cells, but it is also expressed in endothelial cells. SDF1 (Cxcl12), the only known ligand for CXCR4, is expressed in a dynamic segmental pattern in the podocyte-endothelial compartment and later in the mesangial cells of the glomerulus.[182]

Embryonic deletion of CXCR4 results in glomerular developmental defects with a dilated capillary network.[183]

Mice carrying a hypomorphic allele of Notch2, which is missing two epidermal growth factor (EGF) motifs, are born with a reduced number of glomeruli that lack both endothelial and mesangial cells, as discussed in the section on nephron segmentation ("Molecular Biology of Nephron Development: Tubulogenesis").[133,134]

There is evidence from other model systems that vascular development is required for patterning and terminal differentiation of adjacent tissues. For example, vascular signals and basement membrane produced by adjacent endothelial cells are required for differentiation of the islet cells of the pancreas.[184,185] In the kidney, it is possible that vascular signals are required for branching morphogenesis and patterning of the nephron; this requirement may explain some of the defects observed in mutants such as Pod1 (Tcf21)–KO mice. In view of the complex reciprocal interactions between tissue types, sorting out these signals will be a challenge but, with the increasing arsenal of genetic tools, should be possible.

The Juxtaglomerular Apparatus and the Renin-Angiotensin System

The juxtaglomerular (JG) apparatus consists of juxtaglomerular cells that line the afferent arteriole, the macula densa cells of the distal tubule, and the extraglomerular mesangial cells that are in contact with intraglomerular mesangium.[186] Renin-expressing cells may be seen in arterioles in early mesonephric kidneys in 5-week human fetuses and in metanephric kidney by week 8, at a stage before hemodynamic flow changes within the kidney. Sequeira López and colleagues[187] generated a renin-knockin mouse that expresses Cre recombinase in the renin locus. In the offspring of matings between the renin-Cre and a reporter strain that expresses β-galactosidase or GFP upon Cre-mediated DNA excision, renin-expressing cells may be found within MM and give rise not only to JG cells but also to mesangial cells, epithelial cells, and extrarenal cells, including interstitial Leydig cells of the XY gonad and cells within the adrenal gland. Although most of these cells cease to express renin in the adult, they appear to reexpress renin in stress conditions and are recruited to the afferent arteriole.

The only known substrate for renin, angiotensinogen, is converted to angiotensin I (AT1) and angiotensin II (AT2) by angiotensin-converting enzyme (ACE).[188] The renin-angiotensin-aldosterone system is required for normal renal development. In humans, the use of ACE inhibitors in early or late pregnancy has been associated with congenital defects that include renal anomalies.[189,190] Two subtypes of angiotensin receptors exist[191]: AT1 receptors, which are responsible for most of the classically recognized functions of the renin-angiotensin-aldosterone system, including pressor effects and aldosterone release mediated through angiotensin; and AT2 receptors, whose functions have been more difficult to characterize but generally seem to oppose the actions of the AT1 receptors. Genetic deletion of angiotensinogen[192,193] or the ACE[194,195] results in hypotension and defects in formation of the renal papilla and pelvis. Humans have one AT1 gene, whereas mice have two: At1a and At1b. Mice carrying a KO for either AT1 receptor alone exhibit no major defects,[196,197] but combined deficiency phenocopies the angiotensinogen and ACE phenotypes.[198,199] Although AT2 receptor expression is markedly upregulated in the embryonic kidney, genetic deletion of the AT2 receptor does not cause major impairment of renal development.[200,201] However, an association between AT2 receptor deficiency and malformations of the collecting system, including vesicoureteral reflux (VUR) and ureteropelvic junction obstruction, has been reported.[202]

Deletion of Dicer (an enzyme required for the production of functional microRNA) from renin-expressing cells results in severely reduced number of juxtaglomerular cells, reduced renin production, and lower blood pressure. The kidney develops severe vascular abnormalities and striped fibrosis along the affected blood vessels, which suggests that microRNAs are required for normal morphogenesis and function of the kidney.[203]

Nephron Development and Glomerulogenesis

Mesangial Cell Ingrowth

Mesangial cells grow into the developing glomerulus and come to sit between the capillary loops. Gene deletion studies have demonstrated a critical role for PDGF type B (PDGF-B)/PDGF receptor β signaling in this process. Deletion of PDGF-B, which is expressed by glomerular endothelia, or of the PDGF receptor β, which is expressed by mesangial cells, results in glomeruli with a single balloon-like capillary loop, instead of the intricately folded glomerular endothelial capillaries of wild-type kidneys. Furthermore, the glomeruli contain no mesangial cells.[204] Endothelial cell–specific deletion of PDGF-B results in the same glomerular phenotype and shows that production of PDGF-B by the endothelium is required for mesangial migration.[205] In turn, mesangial cells and the matrix that they produce are necessary to pattern the glomerular capillary system. Loss of podocyte-derived factors such as VEGF-A also lead to failure of mesangial cell ingrowth, probably through primary loss of endothelial cells and failure of PDGF-B signaling.[160]

A number of other KOs demonstrate defects in both vascular/capillary development and mesangial cell ingrowth. Transcription factors expressed by podocytes, including Pod1 and FoxC2, show defects in mesangial cell migration (Figure 1-14).[50,151] The factors that are disrupted in these mutant mice to result in the phenotype are not yet known, but their existence emphasizes the importance of "crosstalk" among cell compartments within the glomerulus.

Glomerular Epithelial Development

Presumptive podocytes are observed at the most proximal end of the *S*-shape body at the furthest point away from the ureteric bud tip. They form as columnar epithelial cells in opposition to the developing vascular cleft. A number of transcription factors have been identified that are expressed within developing and mature podocytes, including Wilms' tumor suppressor 1, Pod1 (Tcf21), Kreisler (Maf1), FoxC2, and Lmx1b (Figure 1-15).[27,50,151,152,207,208] Genetic deletion studies have shown that Pod1, FoxC2, Lmx1b, and Kreisler are all required for elaboration of podocyte foot processes and spreading of podocytes around the glomerular capillary beds. Pod1 appears to function upstream of Kreisler, inasmuch as the latter factor is downregulated in glomeruli from Pod1-KO mice.[208] Transcriptional programs regulated by these factors are incompletely known; however, Pod1-, FoxC2-, and Lmx1b-KO mice all display remarkably similar glomerular phenotypes with major podocyte developmental/maturation defects together with abnormalities in capillary loop, GBM, and mesangial ingrowth. It is believed that loss of podocyte-expressed factors regulated by these proteins leads to the dramatic arrest in development, resulting in abnormal capillary loop–stage glomeruli. Immunostaining and gene expression profiling performed in glomeruli from each of these mutant mice have identified reduced expression of some common downstream effector molecules, including collagen α4. In turn, a podocyte-specific protein, podocin (NPHS2) is reduced in the glomeruli of FoxC2-, Lmx1b-, and Pod1-KO mice.[50,209] Mutations in Lmx1b are associated with nail-patella syndrome in humans, a disease characterized by absence of patellae and nephrotic syndrome in a subset of patients. All these genes are expressed from the S-shape stage onward and remain constitutively expressed in adult glomeruli.

Wt1 is also expressed in presumptive and mature podocytes. Because Wt1-KO mice fail to develop any kidneys, the role of Wt1 in the developing and mature podocyte is not entirely clear. However, a series of experimental models support an important role for Wt1 in the podocyte. The null phenotype was largely rescued with a yeast artificial chromosome (YAC) containing the human Wt1 gene[5,210]; depending on the level of Wt1 expression, the affected mice developed crescentic glomerulonephritis or mesangial sclerosis. These defects in the glomerulus were reminiscent of some of the human phenotypes observed with Denys-Drash syndrome resulting from mutations in the KTS isoform (affecting amino acids lysine,

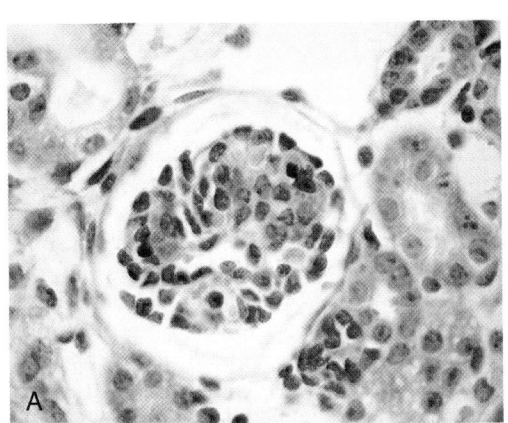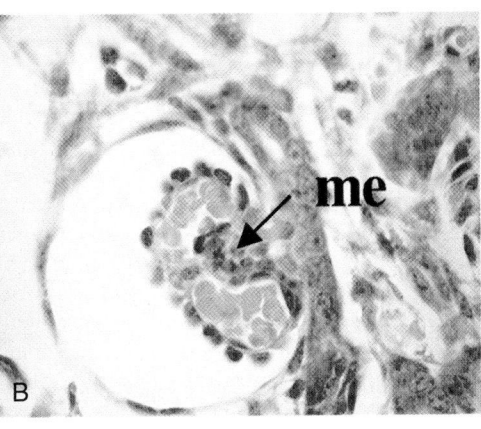

FIGURE 1-14 Glomeruli from wild-type (**A**) or Pod1-knockout mice (**B**). Note dilated capillary loop and poor ingrowth of mesangial cells (ME).

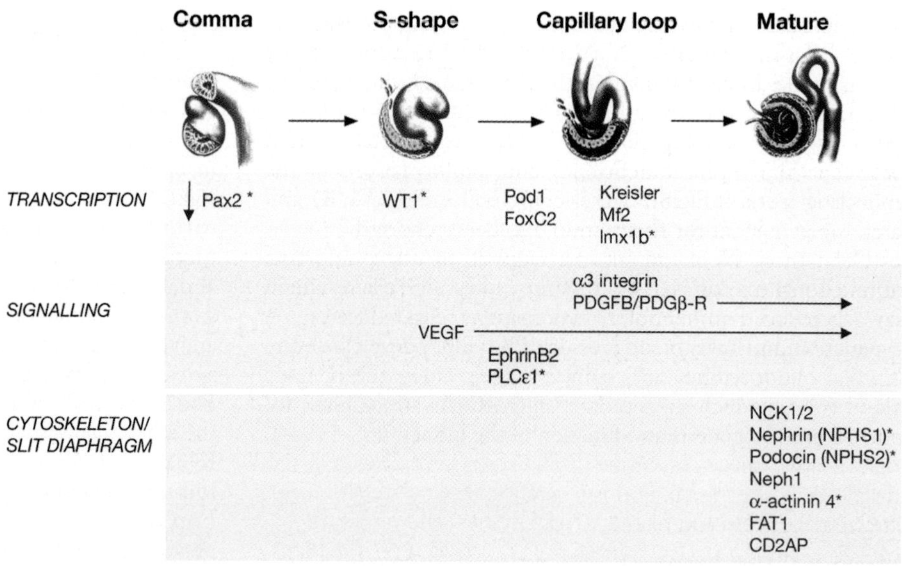

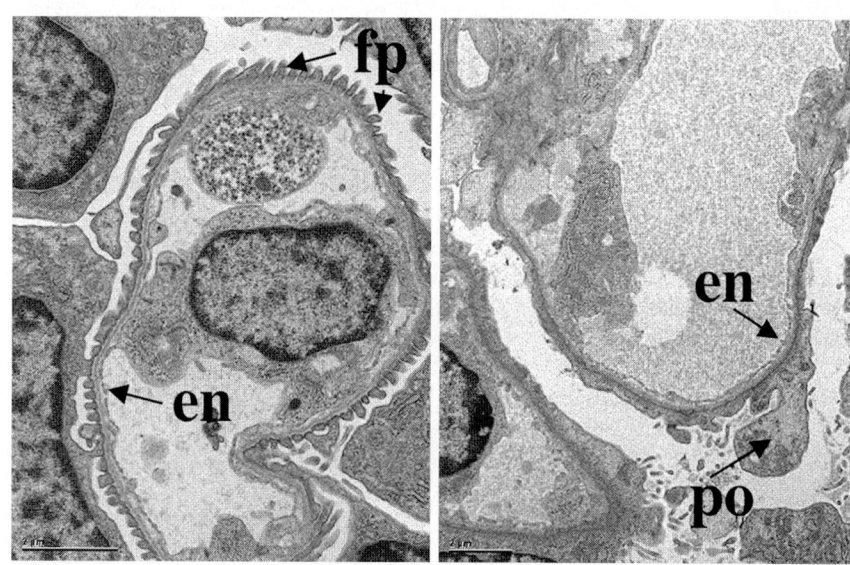

	Comma	S-shape	Capillary loop	Mature
TRANSCRIPTION	Pax2 *	WT1*	Pod1 FoxC2	Kreisler Mf2 lmx1b*
SIGNALLING		VEGF ———————————————→	α3 integrin PDGFB/PDGβ-R ———→ EphrinB2 PLCε1*	
CYTOSKELETON/ SLIT DIAPHRAGM				NCK1/2 Nephrin (NPHS1)* Podocin (NPHS2)* Neph1 α-actinin 4* FAT1 CD2AP

FIGURE 1-15 Molecular basis of glomerular development. Key factors are shown; time point of major effect observed in knockout or transgenic studies is identified. Many factors play roles at more than one time point. *Mutations identified in patients with glomerular disease. (Top panel adapted from Saxen L: *Organogenesis of the kidney,* Cambridge, UK, 1987, Cambridge University Press.)

FIGURE 1-16 Foot processes (fp) are seen surrounding a capillary loop of a newborn wild-type mouse. *Right,* A capillary loop from a Nck1/Nck2-knockout mouse shows complete lack of foot process formation. En, glomerular endothelial cell. (Adapted from Jones N, Blasutig IM, Eremina V, et al: Nck adaptor proteins link nephrin to the actin cytoskeleton of kidney podocytes, *Nature* 2006;440:818-823.)

threonine, and serine) of Wt1.[210] Transgenic mice expressing a Denys-Drash mutant Wt1 allele under the regulation of a podocyte-specific promoter also developed glomerular disease with abnormalities observed in the adjacent endothelium.[211]

α3 Integrin–KO mice also demonstrate defects in glomerular development with specific abnormalities in podocyte maturation.[121] α3 Integrin forms a heterodimer with β1 integrin and is expressed by podocytes. Loss of this integrin results in poorly formed foot processes and abnormalities in adjacent GBM. Podocyte-specific deletion of β1 integrin also manifests proteinuria at birth with podocyte foot process effacement and abnormal GBM.[212,213] Elaboration of foot processes during development requires the interaction of an adaptor signaling molecule, NCK, with slit diaphragm proteins. The slit diaphragm is a specialized intercellular junction that connects foot processes of adjacent podocytes. In mature glomeruli, the slit diaphragm appears as a dense band on transmission electron micrographs. In 1998, Karl Tryggvason's group[214] identified the nephrin (NphS1) gene and showed that mutations in this gene cause congenital nephrosis of the Finnish (CNF) variety. Glomeruli from infants with CNF

lack slit diaphragms, and the patients die from renal failure and nephrotic syndrome unless they receive renal replacement therapy. Nephrin is a member of the immunoglobulin superfamily and makes up a major structural component of the slit diaphragm. It has been shown that the nephrin molecule contains three intracellular tyrosine residues (1176, 1193, 1217) that can be phosphorylated leading to recruitment of the SH2 adaptor proteins, NCK1 and NCK2.[11,12] In vitro, this association leads to reorganization of the actin cytoskeleton, the backbone of foot process structure. Mice born with podocyte-selective deletion of the Nck1 and Nck2 genes exhibit congenital nephrosis and fail to form any foot processes (Figure 1-16), which emphasizes the biologic link between the slit diaphragm and cytoskeleton in vivo.

The phenotype observed in NCK-deficient mice is similar to that of Fat1-KO mice, with complete absence of foot process formation and podocyte effacement. Fat1 is a large protocadherin expressed in podocytes. In contrast, nephrin-KO mice exhibit narrowed slits with loss of the diaphragm, but the degree of foot process effacement or fusion varies and may be dependent on mouse strain. Additional proteins of the slit diaphragm and cytoskeleton have been identified that play major roles in glomerulogenesis and in human disease. Three nephrin-like molecules exist (Neph1 to Neph3) that are also expressed in podocytes and interact with other slit diaphragm proteins.[215,216] Mice generated through a gene-trap screen with loss of Neph1 function develop focal segmental glomerulosclerosis (FSGS), which suggests that these molecules are also important for function of the slit diaphragm.[48] Interestingly, these Neph-nephrin proteins bind the Par3-Par6–atypical protein kinase C (aPKC) complex. This is a widely conserved protein complex that regulates apical-basal cell polarity, cell migration, and asymmetric cell division in many tissues.[217] In epithelia, this complex is recruited to tight junctions.[218] In podocytes, the complex localizes at the insertion site of the slit diaphragm. Podocyte-specific aPKC-KO mice demonstrate severe proteinuria and nephrotic syndrome and die 5 weeks after birth. Podocytes in the mutant mice demonstrate mislocalization of the slit diaphragm and a disturbance of apical-basal polarity, indicating that the Par3-Par6-aPKC complex is required for cell polarity in podocytes.[219,220]

Nphs2 (podocin) is a homolog of the *C. elegans* mechanosensory channel (MEC) Mec2 and co-localizes with nephrin at the slit diaphragm. Mutations in Nphs2 have been identified in patients with steroid-resistant congenital autosomal recessive FSGS.[221] Although foot process effacement is a feature of the Nphs2-KO mice, vascular defects are also observed and suggest that podocin or the slit diaphragm (or both) may regulate components of the crosstalk between podocytes and endothelium.[222] Mutations in α-actinin 4, a component of the actin cytoskeleton, were identified in autosomal dominant FSGS, a disease with onset in adulthood.[223] Kos and colleagues[224] hypothesized that the mutant actinin functions in a dominant negative manner to cause the phenotype. Of interest is that Actn4-KO mice also develop glomerular disease, despite the protein's rather ubiquitous expression. Clearly, elucidation of the mechanism is important and will provide exciting insights into glomerular biology.

CD2AP (CD2-associated protein), is an Sh3 domain–containing protein in lymphoid cells and podocytes that interacts with the cytoplasmic tail of nephrin and with the actin cytoskeleton.[225] Mice with the null CD2AP genotype rapidly develop massive proteinuria and mesangial sclerosis, a finding that highlights the interplay of all of these molecules in the glomerulus. CD2AP heterozygous mice are susceptible to glomerular disease and exhibit glomerular lesions at 12 to 18 months that are similar to immunotactoid glomerulopathy in humans.[45,226] CD2AP has been implicated in endocytosis and lysosomal sorting and may be necessary to clear immunoglobulins that are normally filtered at the glomerulus. In accordance with this hypothesis, the investigators showed that a large proportion of CD2AP-heterozygous mice develop FSGS-like lesions when injected with a nephrotoxic antibody.[226] Mutations in the Trpc6 channel underlie another inherited form of autosomal dominant FSGS in patients. Some, but not all, of the identified mutations lead to activation of the channel and increased influx of calcium inside the cell.[227,228] Trpc6 is expressed in podocytes but also other glomerular cell types. Elucidation of the mechanism whereby Trpc6 leads to glomerular disease may yield a mechanism that is amenable to pharmacologic intervention. Inf2 is a formin protein that is involved in polymerization and depolymerization of actin filaments. This protein is expressed in podocytes

and other cell types in glomeruli, and its mutations have been identified in families with autosomal dominant FSGS.[229-231]

MicroRNAs are regulatory RNAs that act as antisense posttranscriptional repressors by binding the 3′-untranslated region of target messenger RNAs. Eukaryotes express hundreds of microRNAs that can regulate thousands of messenger RNAs, and they have been shown to play an important role in development and disease, including in differentiation, signaling pathways, proliferation, apoptosis, and tumorigenicity. Three research groups generated mice carrying a podocyte-specific deletion of Dicer.[232-234] Podocyte-specific Dicer-KO mice developed albuminuria by 3 weeks of age and rapidly deteriorated to end-stage renal failure by approximately 6 weeks. A number of potential microRNA targets were identified, but their functional significance in the podocyte in vivo are not yet known.

All these studies demonstrated that intrinsic proteins and functions of podocytes play a key role in the development and maintenance of the permselective properties of the glomerular filtration barrier; however, as outlined earlier in the section on vascular development, podocytes also function as vasculature supporting cells producing VEGF and other angiogenic growth factors. It is likely that endothelial cells also produce factors required for terminal differentiation of podocytes, although these factors are currently unknown.

Maturation of Glomerular Endothelial Cells and Glomerular Basement Membrane

After migration into the glomerular vascular cleft, endothelial cells are rounded, and capillaries do not possess a lumen. During glomerulogenesis, lumina form through apoptosis of a subset of endothelial cells, and the endothelial cells flatten considerably and develop fenestrations and a complex glycocalyx. This process is believed to be dependent on a TGFβ1-dependent signal.[14] Loss of these specialized features of the glomerular endothelium, as in endotheliosis, leads to disruption of the filtration barrier and protein loss, which emphasizes the major role that this layer of the GFB plays in permselectivity.

Another chapter in the book deals with properties and development of the GBM, although informative KOs are included in Table 1-1 for completeness. It is important to note that components are produced by both podocytes and glomerular endothelium and that a number of vital growth factors, such as VEGF-A, are stored and processed in the glomerular basement membrane.[235]

References

1. Zandi-Nejad K, Luyckx VA, Brenner BM. Adult hypertension and kidney disease: the role of fetal programming. *Hypertension.* 2006;47(3):502-558.
2. Luyckx VA, Brenner BM. Low birth weight, nephron number, and kidney disease. *Kidney Int Suppl.* 2005;(97):S68-S77.
3. Rossing P, et al. Low birth weight. A risk factor for development of diabetic nephropathy? *Diabetes.* 1995;44(12):1405-1407.
4. Saxen L. *Organogenesis of the kidney.* Cambridge, UK: Cambridge University Press; 1987.
5. Capel B, et al. Migration of mesonephric cells into the mammalian gonad depends on Sry. *Mech Dev.* 1999;84(1-2):127-131.
6. Cui S, et al. Disrupted gonadogenesis and male-to-female sex reversal in Pod1 knockout mice. *Development.* 2004;131(16):4095-4105.
7. Mendelsohn C, et al. Function of the retinoic acid receptors (RARs) during development (II). Multiple abnormalities at various stages of organogenesis in RAR double mutants. *Development.* 1994;120(10):2749-2771.

8. Kreidberg JA. Podocyte differentiation and glomerulogenesis. *J Am Soc Nephrol*. 2003;14(3):806-814.

9. Batourina E, et al. Vitamin A controls epithelial/mesenchymal interactions through Ret expression. *Nat Genet*. 2001;27(1):74-78.

10. Reeves W, Caulfield JP, Farquhar MG. Differentiation of epithelial foot processes and filtration slits: sequential appearance of occluding junctions, epithelial polyanion, and slit membranes in developing glomeruli. *Lab Invest*. 1978;39(2):90-100.

11. Jones N, et al. Nck adaptor proteins link nephrin to the actin cytoskeleton of kidney podocytes. *Nature*. 2006;440(7085):818-823.

12. Verma R, et al. Nephrin ectodomain engagement results in Src kinase activation, nephrin phosphorylation, Nck recruitment, and actin polymerization. *J Clin Invest*. 2006.

13. Tryggvason K, Pikkarainen T, Patrakka J. Nck links nephrin to actin in kidney podocytes. *Cell*. 2006;125(2):221-224.

14. Fierlbeck W, et al. Endothelial cell apoptosis during glomerular capillary lumen formation in vivo. *J Am Soc Nephrol*. 2003;14(5):1349-1354.

15. Rastaldi MP, et al. Glomerular podocytes possess the synaptic vesicle molecule Rab3A and its specific effector rabphilin-3a. *Am J Pathol*. 2003;163(3):889-899.

16. Kobayashi N, et al. Process formation of the renal glomerular podocyte: is there common molecular machinery for processes of podocytes and neurons? *Anat Sci Int*. 2004;79(1):1-10.

17. Giardino L, et al. Podocyte glutamatergic signaling contributes to the function of the glomerular filtration barrier. *J Am Soc Nephrol*. 2009;20(9):1929-1940.

18. Baum M, Quigley R, Satlin L. Maturational changes in renal tubular transport. *Curr Opin Nephrol Hypertens*. 2003;12(5):521-526.

19. Boyle S, et al. Fate mapping using Cited1-CreERT2 mice demonstrates that the cap mesenchyme contains self-renewing progenitor cells and gives rise exclusively to nephronic epithelia. *Dev Biol*. 2008;313(1):234-245.

20. Kobayashi A, et al. Six2 defines and regulates a multipotent self-renewing nephron progenitor population throughout mammalian kidney development. *Cell Stem Cell*. 2008;3(2):169-181.

21. Osathanondh V, Potter EL. Development of human kidney as shown by microdissection. III. Formation and interrelationship of collecting tubules and nephrons. *Arch Pathol*. 1963;76:290-302.

22. Bard J. A new role for the stromal cells in kidney development. *Bioessays*. 1996;18(9):705-707.

23. Hatini V, et al. Essential role of stromal mesenchyme in kidney morphogenesis revealed by targeted disruption of Winged Helix transcription factor BF-2. *Genes Dev*. 1996;10(12):1467-1478.

24. Levinson R, Mendelsohn C. Stromal progenitors are important for patterning epithelial and mesenchymal cell types in the embryonic kidney. *Semin Cell Dev Biol*. 2003;14(4):225-231.

25. Robert B, et al. Evidence that embryonic kidney cells expressing Flk-1 are intrinsic, vasculogenic angioblasts. *Am J Physiol*. 1996;271(3 Pt 2):F744-F753.

26. Grobstein C. Inductive epitheliomesenchymal interaction in cultured organ rudiments of the mouse. *Science*. 1953;118(3054):52-55.

27. Kreidberg JA, et al. Wt-1 is required for early kidney development. *Cell*. 1993;74(4):679-691.

28. Miyamoto N, et al. Defects of urogenital development in mice lacking Emx2. *Development*. 1997;124(9):1653-1664.

29. Sariola H, et al. Dependence of kidney morphogenesis on the expression of nerve growth factor receptor. *Science*. 1991;254(5031):571-573.

30. Durbeej M, et al. Differential expression of neurotrophin receptors during renal development. *Development*. 1993;119(4):977-989.

31. Sainio K, et al. Antisense inhibition of low-affinity nerve growth factor receptor in kidney cultures: power and pitfalls. *Cell Mol Neurobiol*. 1994;14(5):439-457.

32. Rothenpieler UW, Dressler GR. Pax-2 is required for mesenchyme-to-epithelium conversion during kidney development. *Development*. 1993;119(3):711-720.

33. Torres M, et al. Pax-2 controls multiple steps of urogenital development. *Development*. 1995;121(12):4057-4065.

34. Davies JA, et al. Development of an siRNA-based method for repressing specific genes in renal organ culture and its use to show that the Wt1 tumour suppressor is required for nephron differentiation. *Hum Mol Genet*. 2004;13(2):235-246.

35. Gao X, et al. Angioblast-mesenchyme induction of early kidney development is mediated by Wt1 and Vegfa. *Development*. 2005;132(24):5437-5449.

36. Vainio S, Lin Y. Coordinating early kidney development: lessons from gene targeting. *Nat Rev Genet*. 2002;3(7):533-543.

37. Dressler GR. Kidney development branches out. *Dev Genet*. 1999;24:189-193.

38. Gawlik A, Quaggin SE. Deciphering the renal code; advances in conditional gene targeting in the kidney. *Physiology (Bethesda)*. 2004;19:245-252.

39. Gawlik A, Quaggin SE. Conditional gene targeting in the kidney. *Curr Mol Med*. 2005;5(5):527-536.

40. Justice M. Capitalizing on large-scale mouse mutagenesis screens. *Nat Rev Genet*. 2000;2(1):109-115.

41. Justice M, et al. Effects of ENU dosage on mouse strains. *Mamm Genome*. 2000;11(7):484-488.

42. Hrabe de Angelis MH, et al. Genome-wide, large-scale production of mutant mice by ENU mutagenesis. *Nat Genet*. 2000;25(4):444-447.

43. Nolan PM, et al. A systematic, genome-wide, phenotype-driven mutagenesis programme for gene function studies in the mouse. *Nat Genet*. 2000;25(4):440-443.

44. Tchekneva EE, et al. Single amino acid substitution in aquaporin 11 causes renal failure. *J Am Soc Nephrol*. 2008;19(10):1955-1964.

45. Huber TB, et al. Bigenic mouse models of focal segmental glomerulosclerosis involving pairwise interaction of CD2AP, Fyn, and synaptopodin. *J Clin Invest*. 2006;116(5):1337-1345.

46. Beier DR, Herron BJ. Genetic mapping and ENU mutagenesis. *Genetica*. 2004;122(1):65-69.

47. Cordes SP. *N*-ethyl-*N*-nitrosourea mutagenesis: boarding the mouse mutant express. *Microbiol Mol Biol Rev*. 2005;69(3):426-439.

48. Donoviel DB, et al. Proteinuria and perinatal lethality in mice lacking Neph1, a novel protein with homology to nephrin. *Mol Cell Biol*. 2001;21(14):4829-4836.

49. Stanford WL, Cohn JB, Cordes SP. Gene-trap mutagenesis: past, present and beyond. *Nat Rev Genet*. 2001;2(10):756-768.

50. Takemoto M, et al. Large-scale identification of genes implicated in kidney glomerulus development and function. *EMBO J*. 2006;25(5):1160-1174.

51. Yoshida Y, et al. Overview of kidney and urine proteome databases. *Contrib Nephrol*. 2008;160:186-197.

52. Miyamoto M, et al. In-depth proteomic profiling of the normal human kidney glomerulus using two-dimensional protein prefractionation in combination with liquid chromatography–tandem mass spectrometry. *J Proteome Res*. 2007;6(9):3680-3690.

53. Shen K, Fetter RD, Bargmann CI. Synaptic specificity is generated by the synaptic guidepost protein SYG-2 and its receptor, SYG-1. *Cell*. 2004;116(6):868-881.

54. Nelson FK, Albert PS, Riddle DL. Fine structure of the *Caenorhabditis elegans* secretory-excretory system. *J Ultrastruct Res*. 1983;82(2):156-171.

55. Barr MM. *Caenorhabditis elegans* as a model to study renal development and disease: sexy cilia. *J Am Soc Nephrol*. 2005;16(2):305-312.

56. Barr MM, et al. The *Caenorhabditis elegans* autosomal dominant polycystic kidney disease gene homologs Lov-1 and Pkd-2 act in the same pathway. *Curr Biol*. 2001;11(17):1341-1346.

57. Simon JM, Sternberg PW. Evidence of a mate-finding cue in the hermaphrodite nematode *Caenorhabditis elegans*. *Proc Natl Acad Sci U S A*. 2002;99(3):1598-1603.

58. Jung AC, et al. Renal tubule development in *Drosophila*: a closer look at the cellular level. *J Am Soc Nephrol*. 2005;16(2):322-328.

59. Dworak HA, et al. Characterization of *Drosophila hibris*, a gene related to human nephrin. *Development*. 2001;128(21):4265-4276.

60. Schneider T, et al. Restricted expression of the irreC-rst protein is required for normal axonal projections of columnar visual neurons. *Neuron*. 1995;15(2):259-271.

61. Venugopala Reddy G, et al. Irregular chiasm-C-roughest, a member of the immunoglobulin superfamily, affects sense organ spacing on the *Drosophila* antenna by influencing the positioning of founder cells on the disc ectoderm. *Dev Genes Evol*. 1999;209(10):581-591.

62. Majumdar A, Drummond IA. Podocyte differentiation in the absence of endothelial cells as revealed in the zebrafish avascular mutant, cloche. *Developmental Genetics*. 1999;24(3-4):220-229.

63. Drummond IA. Kidney development and disease in the zebrafish. *J Am Soc Nephrol*. 2005;16(2):299-304.

64. Jones EA. *Xenopus*: a prince among models for pronephric kidney development. *J Am Soc Nephrol*. 2005;16(2):313-321.

65. Xu PX, et al. Eya1-deficient mice lack ears and kidneys and show abnormal apoptosis of organ primordia. *Nat Genet*. 1999;23(1):113-117.

66. Wang Q, et al. Odd-skipped related 1 (Odd 1) is an essential regulator of heart and urogenital development. *Dev Biol*. 2005;288(2):582-594.

67. Xu PX, et al. Six1 is required for the early organogenesis of mammalian kidney. *Development*. 2003;130(14):3085-3094.

68. Laclef C, et al. Thymus, kidney and craniofacial abnormalities in Six 1 deficient mice. *Mech Dev*. 2003;120(6):669-679.

69. Nishinakamura R, et al. Murine homolog of Sall1 is essential for ureteric bud invasion in kidney development. *Development*. 2001;128(16):3105-3115.

70. Shawlot W, Behringer RR. Requirement for Lim1 in head-organizer function. *Nature*. 1995;374(6521):425-430.

71. Moore MW, et al. Renal and neuronal abnormalities in mice lacking GDNF. *Nature*. 1996;382(6586):76-79.

72. Pichel JG, et al. Defects in enteric innervation and kidney development in mice lacking GDNF. *Nature*. 1996;382(6586):73-76.

73. Sanchez MP, et al. Renal agenesis and the absence of enteric neurons in mice lacking GDNF. *Nature*. 1996;382(6586):70-73.

74. Esquela AF, Lee SJ. Regulation of metanephric kidney development by growth/differentiation factor 11. *Dev Biol.* 2003;257(2):356-370.

75. Michos O, et al. Gremlin-mediated BMP antagonism induces the epithelial-mesenchymal feedback signaling controlling metanephric kidney and limb organogenesis. *Development.* 2004;131(14):3401-3410.

76. Schuchardt A, et al. RET-deficient mice: an animal model for Hirschsprung's disease and renal agenesis. *J Intern Med.* 1995;238(4):327-332.

77. Cacalano G, et al. GFRα1 is an essential receptor component for GDNF in the developing nervous system and kidney. *Neuron.* 1998;21(1):53-62.

78. James RG, et al. Odd-skipped related 1 is required for development of the metanephric kidney and regulates formation and differentiation of kidney precursor cells. *Development.* 2006;133(15):2995-3004.

79. Buller C, et al. Molecular effects of Eya1 domain mutations causing organ defects in BOR syndrome. *Hum Mol Genet.* 2001;10(24):2775-2781.

80. Ikeda K, et al. Molecular interaction and synergistic activation of a promoter by Six, Eya, and Dach proteins mediated through CREB binding protein. *Mol Cell Biol.* 2002;22(19):6759-6766.

81. Li X, et al. Eya protein phosphatase activity regulates Six1-Dach-Eya transcriptional effects in mammalian organogenesis. *Nature.* 2003; 426(6964):247-254.

82. Fougerousse F, et al. Six and Eya expression during human somitogenesis and MyoD gene family activation. *J Muscle Res Cell Motil.* 2002;23(3):255-264.

83. Pandur PD, Moody SA. *Xenopus* Six1 gene is expressed in neurogenic cranial placodes and maintained in the differentiating lateral lines. *Mech Dev.* 2000;96(2):253-257.

84. Sajithlal G, et al. Eya 1 acts as a critical regulator for specifying the metanephric mesenchyme. *Dev Biol.* 2005;284(2):323-336.

85. Bouchard M. Transcriptional control of kidney development. *Differentiation.* 2004;72(7):295-306.

86. Schuchardt A, et al. Defects in the kidney and enteric nervous system of mice lacking the tyrosine kinase receptor Ret. *Nature.* 1994;367(6461):380-383.

87. Dressler GR, et al. Pax2, a new murine paired-box-containing gene and its expression in the developing excretory system. *Development.* 1990;109(4): 787-795.

88. Brophy PD, et al. Regulation of ureteric bud outgrowth by Pax2-dependent activation of the glial derived neurotrophic factor gene. *Development.* 2001;128(23):4747-4756.

89. Clarke JC, et al. Regulation of c-Ret in the developing kidney is responsive to Pax2 gene dosage. *Hum Mol Genet.* 2006;15(23):3420-3428.

90. Patel SR, et al. The BRCT-domain containing protein PTIP links Pax2 to a histone H3, lysine 4 methyltransferase complex. *Dev Cell.* 2007;13(4):580-592.

91. Wellik DM, Hawkes PJ, Capecchi MR. Hox11 paralogous genes are essential for metanephric kidney induction. *Genes Dev.* 2002;16(11):1423-1432.

92. Gong KQ, et al. A Hox-Eya-Pax complex regulates early kidney developmental gene expression. *Mol Cell Biol.* 2007;27(21):7661-7668.

93. Hartwig S, et al. Genomic characterization of Wilms' tumor suppressor 1 targets in nephron progenitor cells during kidney development. *Development.* 2010;137(7):1189-1203.

94. Tang MJ, et al. Ureteric bud outgrowth in response to RET activation is mediated by phosphatidylinositol 3-kinase. *Dev Biol.* 2002;243(1):128-136.

95. Kim D, Dressler GR. PTEN modulates GDNF/RET mediated chemotaxis and branching morphogenesis in the developing kidney. *Dev Biol.* 2007;307(2):290-299.

96. Poladia DP, et al. Role of fibroblast growth factor receptors 1 and 2 in the metanephric mesenchyme. *Dev Biol.* 2006;291(2):325-339.

97. Perantoni AO, et al. Inactivation of FGF8 in early mesoderm reveals an essential role in kidney development. *Development.* 2005;132(17):3859-3871.

98. Grieshammer U, et al. FGF8 is required for cell survival at distinct stages of nephrogenesis and for regulation of gene expression in nascent nephrons. *Development.* 2005;132(17):3847-3857.

99. Majumdar A, et al. Wnt11 and Ret/Gdnf pathways cooperate in regulating ureteric branching during metanephric kidney development. *Development.* 2003;130(14):3175-3185.

100. Carroll TJ, et al. Wnt9b plays a central role in the regulation of mesenchymal to epithelial transitions underlying organogenesis of the mammalian urogenital system. *Dev Cell.* 2005;9(2):283-292.

101. Stark K, et al. Epithelial transformation of metanephric mesenchyme in the developing kidney regulated by Wnt-4. *Nature.* 1994;372(6507):679-683.

102. Merkel CE, Karner CM, Carroll TJ. Molecular regulation of kidney development: is the answer blowing in the Wnt? *Pediatr Nephrol.* 2007; 22(11):1825-1838.

103. Park JS, Valerius MT, McMahon AP. WNT/beta-catenin signaling regulates nephron induction during mouse kidney development. *Development.* 2007;134(13):2533-2539.

104. Kuure S, et al. Glycogen synthase kinase-3 inactivation and stabilization of beta-catenin induce nephron differentiation in isolated mouse and rat kidney mesenchymes. *J Am Soc Nephrol.* 2007;18(4):1130-1139.

105. Dudley AT, Lyons KM, Robertson EJ. A requirement for bone morphogenetic protein-7 during development of the mammalian kidney and eye. *Genes Dev.* 1995;9(22):2795-2807.

106. Luo G, et al. BMP-7 is an inducer of nephrogenesis, and is also required for eye development and skeletal patterning. *Genes Dev.* 1995;9(22):2808-2820.

107. Muller U, et al. Integrin α8β1 is critically important for epithelial-mesenchymal interactions during kidney morphogenesis. *Cell.* 1997;88(5):603-613.

108. Brandenberger R, et al. Identification and characterization of a novel extracellular matrix protein nephronectin that is associated with integrin α8β1 in the embryonic kidney. *J Cell Biol.* 2001;154(2):447-458.

109. Linton JM, Martin GR, Reichardt LF. The ECM protein nephronectin promotes kidney development via integrin α8β1-mediated stimulation of Gdnf expression. *Development.* 2007;134(13):2501-2509.

110. Yu J, et al. A Wnt7b-dependent pathway regulates the orientation of epithelial cell division and establishes the cortico-medullary axis of the mammalian kidney. *Development.* 2009;136(1):161-171.

111. Miyazaki Y, et al. Bone morphogenetic protein 4 regulates the budding site and elongation of the mouse ureter. *J Clin Invest.* 2000;105(7):863-873.

112. Chiang C, et al. Cyclopia and defective axial patterning in mice lacking Sonic hedgehog gene function. *Nature.* 1996;383(6599):407-413.

113. Qiao J, et al. FGF-7 modulates ureteric bud growth and nephron number in the developing kidney. *Development.* 1999;126(3):547-554.

114. Zhao H, et al. Role of fibroblast growth factor receptors 1 and 2 in the ureteric bud. *Dev Biol.* 2004;276(2):403-415.

115. Gupta IR, et al. BMP-2/ALK3 and HGF signal in parallel to regulate renal collecting duct morphogenesis. *J Cell Sci.* 2000;113(Pt 2):269-278.

116. Piscione TD, et al. BMP-2 and OP-1 exert direct and opposite effects on renal branching morphogenesis. *Am J Physiol.* 1997;273(6 Pt 2):F961-F975.

117. Hu MC, Piscione TD, Rosenblum ND. Elevated SMAD1/beta-catenin molecular complexes and renal medullary cystic dysplasia in ALK3 transgenic mice. *Development.* 2003;130(12):2753-2766.

118. Hartwig S, et al. BMP receptor ALK3 controls collecting system development. *J Am Soc Nephrol.* 2008;19(1):117-124.

119. Hu MC, Rosenblum ND. Smad1, beta-catenin and Tcf4 associate in a molecular complex with the Myc promoter in dysplastic renal tissue and cooperate to control Myc transcription. *Development.* 2005;132(1):215-225.

120. Hu MC, et al. GLI3-dependent transcriptional repression of Gli1, Gli2 and kidney patterning genes disrupts renal morphogenesis. *Development.* 2006;133(3):569-578.

121. Kreidberg JA, et al. α3β1 Integrin has a crucial role in kidney and lung organogenesis. *Development.* 1996;122(11):3537-3547.

122. Korhonen M, et al. The alpha 1-alpha 6 subunits of integrins are characteristically expressed in distinct segments of developing and adult human nephron. *J Cell Biol.* 1990;111(3):1245-1254.

123. Chattopadhyay N, et al. α3β1 integrin-CD151, a component of the cadherin-catenin complex, regulates PTPmu expression and cell-cell adhesion. *J Cell Biol.* 2003;163(6):1351-1362.

124. Liu Y, et al. Coordinate integrin and c-Met signaling regulate WNT gene expression during epithelial morphogenesis. *Development.* 2009;136(5):843-853.

125. Wu W, et al. Beta1-integrin is required for kidney collecting duct morphogenesis and maintenance of renal function. *Am J Physiol Renal Physiol.* 2009;297(1):F210-F217.

126. Kume T, Deng K, Hogan BL. Murine Forkhead/Winged Helix genes FoxC1 (Mf1) and FoxC2 (Mfh1) are required for the early organogenesis of the kidney and urinary tract. *Development.* 2000;127(7):1387-1395.

127. Grieshammer U, et al. SLIT2-mediated ROBO2 signaling restricts kidney induction to a single site. *Dev Cell.* 2004;6(5):709-717.

128. Lu W, et al. Disruption of ROBO2 is associated with urinary tract anomalies and confers risk of vesicoureteral reflux. *Am J Hum Genet.* 2007;80(4): 616-632.

129. Kim HJ, Bar-Sagi D. Modulation of signalling by Sprouty: a developing story. *Nat Rev Mol Cell Biol.* 2004;5(6):441-450.

130. Basson MA, et al. Sprouty1 is a critical regulator of GDNF/RET-mediated kidney induction. *Dev Cell.* 2005;8(2):229-239.

131. Rozen EJ, et al. Loss of Sprouty1 rescues renal agenesis caused by Ret mutation. *J Am Soc Nephrol.* 2009;20(2):255-259.

132. Michos O, et al. Reduction of BMP4 activity by Gremlin 1 enables ureteric bud outgrowth and GDNF/Wnt11 feedback signalling during kidney branching morphogenesis. *Development.* 2007;134(13):2397-2405.

133. McCright B. Notch signaling in kidney development. *Curr Opin Nephrol Hypertens.* 2003;12(1):5-10.

134. McCright B, et al. Defects in development of the kidney, heart and eye vasculature in mice homozygous for a hypomorphic Notch2 mutation. *Development.* 2001;128(4):491-502.

135. McCright B, Lozier J, Gridley T. A mouse model of Alagille syndrome: Notch2 as a genetic modifier of Jag1 haploinsufficiency. *Development.* 2002;129(4):1075-1082.

136. Cheng HT, Kopan R. The role of Notch signaling in specification of podocyte and proximal tubules within the developing mouse kidney. *Kidney Int.* 2005;68(5):1951-1952.

137. Cheng HT, et al. Gamma-secretase activity is dispensable for mesenchyme-to-epithelium transition but required for podocyte and proximal tubule formation in developing mouse kidney. *Development.* 2003;130(20):5031-5042.

138. Wang P, et al. Presenilins are required for the formation of comma- and S-shaped bodies during nephrogenesis. *Development*. 2003;130(20):5019-5029.

139. Cheng HT, et al. Notch2, but not Notch1, is required for proximal fate acquisition in the mammalian nephron. *Development*. 2007;134(4):801-811.

140. Blomqvist SR, et al. Distal renal tubular acidosis in mice that lack the Forkhead transcription factor FoxI1. *J Clin Invest*. 2004;113(11):1560-1570.

141. Seifert JR, Mlodzik M. Frizzled/PCP signalling: a conserved mechanism regulating cell polarity and directed motility. *Nat Rev Genet*. 2007;8(2): 126-138.

142. Zallen JA. Planar polarity and tissue morphogenesis. *Cell*. 2007;129(6): 1051-1063.

143. Fischer E, et al. Defective planar cell polarity in polycystic kidney disease. *Nat Genet*. 2006;38(1):21-23.

144. Bacallao RL, McNeill H. Cystic kidney diseases and planar cell polarity signaling. *Clin Genet*. 2009;75(2):107-117.

145. Karner CM, et al. Wnt9b signaling regulates planar cell polarity and kidney tubule morphogenesis. *Nat Genet*. 2009;41(7):793-799.

146. Gresh L, et al. A transcriptional network in polycystic kidney disease. *EMBO J*. 2004;23(7):1657-1668.

147. Verdeguer, F, et al. A mitotic transcriptional switch in polycystic kidney disease. *Nat Med*. 16(1):106-110.

148. Saburi S, et al. Loss of Fat4 disrupts PCP signaling and oriented cell division and leads to cystic kidney disease. *Nat Genet*. 2008;40(8):1010-1015.

149. Ma Z, et al. Mutations of HNF-1β inhibit epithelial morphogenesis through dysregulation of SOCS-3. *Proc Natl Acad Sci U S A*. 2007; 104(51):20386-20391.

150. Hiesberger T, et al. Role of the hepatocyte nuclear factor-1β (HNF-1β) C-terminal domain in Pkhd1 (ARPKD) gene transcription and renal cystogenesis. *J Biol Chem*. 2005;280(11):10578-10586.

151. Quaggin SE, et al. The basic-helix–loop-helix protein Pod-1 is critically important for kidney and lung organogenesis. *Development*. 1999;126: 5771-5783.

152. Quaggin SE, Vanden Heuvel GB, Igarashi P. Pod-1, a mesoderm-specific basic-helix–loop-helix protein expressed in mesenchymal and glomerular epithelial cells in the developing kidney. *Mech Dev*. 1998;71:37-48.

153. Cui S, Schwartz L, Quaggin SE. Pod1 is required in stromal cells for glomerulogenesis. *Dev Dyn*. 2003;226(3):512-522.

154. Mendelsohn C, et al. Stromal cells mediate retinoid-dependent functions essential for renal development. *Development*. 1999;126:1139-1148.

155. Shalaby F, et al. Failure of blood-island formation and vasculogenesis in Flk-1–deficient mice. *Nature*. 1995;376(6535):62-66.

156. Takahashi T, et al. Temporally compartmentalized expression of ephrin-B2 during renal glomerular development. *J Am Soc Nephrol*. 2001;12(12): 2673-2682.

157. Carmeliet P, et al. Abnormal blood vessel development and lethality in embryos lacking a single VEGF allele. *Nature*. 1996;380(6573):435-439.

158. Villegas G, Lange-Sperandio B, Tufro A. Autocrine and paracrine functions of vascular endothelial growth factor (VEGF) in renal tubular epithelial cells. *Kidney Int*. 2005;67(2):449-457.

159. Eremina V, et al. Glomerular-specific alterations of VEGF-A expression lead to distinct congenital and acquired renal diseases. *J Clin Invest*. 2003; 111(5):707-716.

160. Eremina V, Cui S, Gerber H, et al. Vascular endothelial growth factor A signaling in the podocyte-endothelial compartment is required for mesangial cell migration and survival. *J Am Soc Nephrol*. 2006;17(3):724-735.

161. Foster RR, et al. Functional evidence that vascular endothelial growth factor may act as an autocrine factor on human podocytes. *Am J Physiol Renal Physiol*. 2003;284(6):F1263-F1273.

162. Foster RR, et al. Vascular endothelial growth factor and nephrin interact and reduce apoptosis in human podocytes. *Am J Physiol Renal Physiol*. 2005;288(1):F48-F57.

163. Guan F, et al. Autocrine VEGF-A system in podocytes regulates podocin and its interaction with CD2AP. *Am J Physiol Renal Physiol*. 2006; 291(2):F422-F4228.

164. Suri C, et al. Requisite role of angiopoietin-1, a ligand for the TIE2 receptor, during embryonic angiogenesis [see comments]. *Cell*. 1996;87(7):1171-1180.

165. Kolatsi-Joannou M, et al. Expression and potential role of angiopoietins and Tie-2 in early development of the mouse metanephros. *Dev Dyn*. 2001;222(1):120-126.

166. Maisonpierre PC, et al. Angiopoietin-2, a natural antagonist for Tie2 that disrupts in vivo angiogenesis [see comments]. *Science*. 1997;277(5322): 55-60.

167. Augustin HG, Breier G. Angiogenesis: molecular mechanisms and functional interactions. *Thromb Haemost*. 2003;89(1):190-197.

168. Yuan HT, et al. Expression of angiopoietin-1, angiopoietin-2, and the Tie-2 receptor tyrosine kinase during mouse kidney maturation. *J Am Soc Nephrol*. 1999;10(8):1722-1736.

169. Woolf AS, Yuan HT. Angiopoietin growth factors and Tie receptor tyrosine kinases in renal vascular development. *Pediatr Nephrol*. 2001;16(2):177-184.

170. Yuan HT, et al. Angiopoietin-2 is a site-specific factor in differentiation of mouse renal vasculature. *J Am Soc Nephrol*. 2000;11(6):1055-1066.

171. Satchell SC, Harper SJ, Mathieson PW. Angiopoietin-1 is normally expressed by periendothelial cells. *Thromb Haemost*. 2001;86(6):1597-1598.

172. Satchell SC, et al. Human podocytes express angiopoietin 1, a potential regulator of glomerular vascular endothelial growth factor. *J Am Soc Nephrol*. 2002;13(2):544-550.

173. Pitera JE, et al. Dysmorphogenesis of kidney cortical peritubular capillaries in angiopoietin-2–deficient mice. *Am J Pathol*. 2004;165(6):1895-1906.

174. Davis B, et al. Podocyte-specific expression of angiopoietin-2 causes proteinuria and apoptosis of glomerular endothelia. *J Am Soc Nephrol*. 2007;18(8):2320-2329.

175. Partanen J, et al. Cell autonomous functions of the receptor tyrosine kinase TIE in a late phase of angiogenic capillary growth and endothelial cell survival during murine development. *Development*. 1996;122(10): 3013-3021.

176. Gerety SS, Anderson DJ. Cardiovascular EphrinB2 function is essential for embryonic angiogenesis. *Development*. 2002;129(6):1397-1410.

177. Wang HU, Anderson DJ. Eph family transmembrane ligands can mediate repulsive guidance of trunk neural crest migration and motor axon outgrowth. *Neuron*. 1997;18(3):383-396.

178. Andres AC, et al. EphB4 receptor tyrosine kinase transgenic mice develop glomerulopathies reminiscent of aglomerular vascular shunts. *Mech Dev*. 2003;120(4):511-516.

179. Foo SS, et al. Ephrin-B2 controls cell motility and adhesion during blood-vessel–wall assembly. *Cell*. 2006;124(1):161-173.

180. Kazama I, et al. Podocyte-derived BMP7 is critical for nephron development. *J Am Soc Nephrol*. 2008;19(11):2181-2191.

181. Ueda H, et al. Bmp in podocytes is essential for normal glomerular capillary formation. *J Am Soc Nephrol*. 2008;19(4):685-694.

182. Ding M, et al. Loss of the tumor suppressor Vhlh leads to upregulation of Cxcr4 and rapidly progressive glomerulonephritis in mice. *Nat Med*. 2006;12(9):1081-1087.

183. Takabatake Y, et al. The CXCL12 (SDF-1)/CXCR4 axis is essential for the development of renal vasculature. *J Am Soc Nephrol*. 2009;20(8):1714-1723.

184. Nikolova G, et al. The vascular basement membrane: a niche for insulin gene expression and beta cell proliferation. *Dev Cell*. 2006;10(3):397-405.

185. Lammert E, Cleaver O, Melton D. Induction of pancreatic differentiation by signals from blood vessels. *Science*. 2001;294(5542):564-567.

186. Schnermann J, Homer W. Smith Award lecture. The juxtaglomerular apparatus: from anatomical peculiarity to physiological relevance. *J Am Soc Nephrol*. 2003;14(6):1681-1694.

187. Sequeira López ML, et al. Renin cells are precursors for multiple cell types that switch to the renin phenotype when homeostasis is threatened. *Dev Cell*. 2004;6(5):719-728.

188. Husain A, Graham R. *Enzymes and receptors of the renin-angiotensin system: celebrating a century of discovery*. Sidney, Australia: Harwood Academic; 2000.

189. Cooper WO, et al. Major congenital malformations after first-trimester exposure to ACE inhibitors. *N Engl J Med*. 2006;354(23):2443-2451.

190. Friberg P, et al. Renin-angiotensin system in neonatal rats: induction of a renal abnormality in response to ACE inhibition or angiotensin II antagonism. *Kidney Int*. 1994;45(2):485-492.

191. Timmermans PB, et al. Angiotensin II receptors and angiotensin II receptor antagonists. *Pharmacol Rev*. 1993;45(2):205-251.

192. Niimura F, et al. Gene targeting in mice reveals a requirement for angiotensin in the development and maintenance of kidney morphology and growth factor regulation. *J Clin Invest*. 1995;96(6):2947-2954.

193. Kim HS, et al. Genetic control of blood pressure and the angiotensinogen locus. *Proc Natl Acad Sci U S A*. 1995;92(7):2735-2739.

194. Krege JH, et al. Male-female differences in fertility and blood pressure in ACE-deficient mice. *Nature*. 1995;375(6527):146-148.

195. Esther Jr CR, et al. Mice lacking angiotensin-converting enzyme have low blood pressure, renal pathology, and reduced male fertility. *Lab Invest*. 1996;74(5):953-965.

196. Ito M, et al. Regulation of blood pressure by the type 1A angiotensin II receptor gene. *Proc Natl Acad Sci U S A*. 1995;92(8):3521-3525.

197. Sugaya T, et al. Angiotensin II type 1a receptor–deficient mice with hypotension and hyperreninemia. *J Biol Chem*. 1995;270(32):18719-18722.

198. Tsuchida S, et al. Murine double nullizygotes of the angiotensin type 1A and 1B receptor genes duplicate severe abnormal phenotypes of angiotensinogen nullizygotes. *J Clin Invest*. 1998;101(4):755-760.

199. Oliverio MI, et al. Reduced growth, abnormal kidney structure, and type 2 (AT2) angiotensin receptor–mediated blood pressure regulation in mice lacking both AT1A and AT1B receptors for angiotensin II. *Proc Natl Acad Sci U S A*. 1998;95(26):15496-15501.

200. Ichiki T, et al. Effects on blood pressure and exploratory behaviour of mice lacking angiotensin II type-2 receptor. *Nature*. 1995;377(6551):748-750.

201. Hein L, et al. Behavioural and cardiovascular effects of disrupting the angiotensin II type-2 receptor in mice. *Nature*. 1995;377(6551):744-747.

202. Nishimura H, et al. Role of the angiotensin type 2 receptor gene in congenital anomalies of the kidney and urinary tract, CAKUT, of mice and men. *Mol Cell.* 1999;3(1):1-10.
203. Sequeira-López ML, Weatherford ET, Borges GR, et al. The microRNA-processing enzyme Dicer maintains juxtaglomerular cells. *J Am Soc Nephrol.* 2010;21(3):460-467.
204. Lindahl P, et al. Paracrine PDGF-B/PDGF-Rβ signaling controls mesangial cell development in kidney glomeruli. *Development.* 1998;125(17):3313-3322.
205. Bjarnegard M, et al. Endothelium-specific ablation of PDGFB leads to pericyte loss and glomerular, cardiac and placental abnormalities. *Development.* 2004;131(8):1847-1857.
206. Deleted in page proofs.
207. Chen H, et al. Limb and kidney defects in Lmx1b mutant mice suggest an involvement of LMX1B in human nail patella syndrome. *Nat Genet.* 1998;19(1):51-55.
208. Sadl V, et al. The mouse Kreisler (Krml1/MafB) segmentation gene is required for differentiation of glomerular visceral epithelial cells. *Dev Biol.* 2002;249(1):16-29.
209. Cui S, et al. Rapid isolation of glomeruli coupled with gene expression profiling identifies downstream targets in Pod1 knockout mice. *J Am Soc Nephrol.* 2005;16:3247-3255.
210. Moore AW, et al. YAC complementation shows a requirement for Wt1 in the development of epicardium, adrenal gland and throughout nephrogenesis. *Development.* 1999;126:1845-1857.
211. Natoli TA, et al. A mutant form of the Wilms' tumor suppressor gene Wt1 observed in Denys- Drash syndrome interferes with glomerular capillary development. *J Am Soc Nephrol.* 2002;13(8):2058-2067.
212. Kanasaki K, et al. Integrin β1-mediated matrix assembly and signaling are critical for the normal development and function of the kidney glomerulus. *Dev Biol.* 2008;313(2):584-593.
213. Pozzi A, Jarad G, Moeckel GW, et al. β1 Integrin expression by podocytes is required to maintain glomerular structural integrity. *Dev Biol.* 2008;316(2):288-301.
214. Kestilä M, Lenkkeri U, Männikkö M, et al. Positionally cloned gene for a novel glomerular protein—nephrin—is mutated in congenital nephrotic syndrome. *Mol Cell.* 1998;1(4):575-582.
215. Sellin L, et al. NEPH1 defines a novel family of podocin interacting proteins. *FASEB J.* 2003;17(1):115-117.
216. Huber TB, et al. Nephrin and CD2AP associate with phosphoinositide 3-OH kinase and stimulate AKT-dependent signaling. *Mol Cell Biol.* 2003;23(14):4917-4928.
217. Suzuki A, Ohno S. The PAR-aPKC system: lessons in polarity. *J Cell Sci.* 2006;119(Pt 6):979-987.
218. Hartleben B, et al. Neph-Nephrin proteins bind the Par3-Par6-atypical protein kinase C (aPKC) complex to regulate podocyte cell polarity. *J Biol Chem.* 2008;283(34):23033-23038.
219. Hirose T, et al. An essential role of the universal polarity protein, aPKCλ, on the maintenance of podocyte slit diaphragms. *PLoS One.* 2009;4(1):E4194.
220. Huber TB, et al. Loss of podocyte aPKCλ/ι causes polarity defects and nephrotic syndrome. *J Am Soc Nephrol.* 2009;20(4):798-806.
221. Lenkkeri U, et al. Structure of the gene for congenital nephrotic syndrome of the Finnish type (NPHS1) and characterization of mutations. *Am J Hum Genet.* 1999;64(1):51-61.
222. Roselli S, et al. Early glomerular filtration defect and severe renal disease in podocin-deficient mice. *Mol Cell Biol.* 2004;24(2):550-560.
223. Kaplan JM, et al. Mutations in ACTN4, encoding alpha-actinin-4, cause familial focal segmental glomerulosclerosis. *Nat Genet.* 2000;24(3):251-256.
224. Kos CH, Le TC, Sinha S, et al. Mice deficient in alpha-actinin-4 have severe glomerular disease. *J Clin Invest.* 2003;111(11):1683-1690.
225. Shih NY, et al. Congenital nephrotic syndrome in mice lacking CD2-associated protein [see comments]. *Science.* 1999;286(5438):312-315.
226. Kim JM, et al. CD2-associated protein haploinsufficiency is linked to glomerular disease susceptibility. *Science.* 2003;300(5623):1298-1300.
227. Winn MP, et al. A mutation in the TRPC6 cation channel causes familial focal segmental glomerulosclerosis. *Science.* 2005;308(5729):1801-1804.
228. Reiser J, et al. TRPC6 is a glomerular slit diaphragm–associated channel required for normal function. *Nat Genet.* 2005;37(7):739-744.
229. Brown EJ, et al. Mutations in the formin gene INF2 cause focal segmental glomerulosclerosis. *Nat Genet.* 2010;42(1):72-76.
230. Chhabra ES, Higgs HN. INF2 Is a WASP homology 2 motif–containing formin that severs actin filaments and accelerates both polymerization and depolymerization. *J Biol Chem.* 2006;281(36):26754-26767.
231. Chhabra ES, et al. INF2 is an endoplasmic reticulum-associated formin protein. *J Cell Sci.* 2009;122(Pt 9):1430-1440.
232. Shi S, et al. Podocyte-selective deletion of Dicer induces proteinuria and glomerulosclerosis. *J Am Soc Nephrol.* 2008;19(11):2159-2169.
233. Harvey SJ, et al. Podocyte-specific deletion of Dicer alters cytoskeletal dynamics and causes glomerular disease. *J Am Soc Nephrol.* 2008;19(11):2150-2158.
234. Ho J, et al. Podocyte-specific loss of functional microRNAs leads to rapid glomerular and tubular injury. *J Am Soc Nephrol.* 2008;19(11):2069-2075.
235. Schedl A. Renal abnormalities and their developmental origin. *Nat Rev Genet.* 2007;8(10):791-802.
236. Narlis M, et al. Pax2 and Pax8 regulate branching morphogenesis and nephron differentiation in the developing kidney. *J Am Soc Nephrol.* 2007;18(4):1121-1129.
237. Patterson LT, Pembaur M, Potter SS. Hoxa11 and Hoxd11 regulate branching morphogenesis of the ureteric bud in the developing kidney. *Development.* 2001;128(11):2153-2161.
238. Batourina E, et al. Apoptosis induced by vitamin A signaling is crucial for connecting the ureters to the bladder. *Nat Genet.* 2005;37(10):1082-1089.
239. Srinivas S, et al. Dominant effects of RET receptor misexpression and ligand-independent RET signaling on ureteric bud development. *Development.* 1999;126:1375-1386.
240. Vega QC, et al. Glial cell line–derived neurotrophic factor activates the receptor tyrosine kinase RET and promotes kidney morphogenesis. *Proc Natl Acad Sci U S A.* 1996;93(20):10657-10661.
241. Jing S, et al. GDNF-induced activation of the Ret protein tyrosine kinase is mediated by GDNFR-alpha, a novel receptor for GDNF. *Cell.* 1996;85 (June 28, 1996):1113–1124.
242. Schuchardt A, et al. Renal agenesis and hypodysplasia in Ret-k⁻ mutant mice result from defects in ureteric bud development. *Development.* 1996;122(6):1919-1929.
243. Mesrobian HG, Sulik KK. Characterization of the upper urinary tract anatomy in the Danforth spontaneous murine mutation. *J Urol.* 1992; 148(2 Pt 2):752-755.
244. Bullock SL, et al. Renal agenesis in mice homozygous for a gene trap mutation in the gene encoding heparan sulfate 2-sulfotransferase. *Genes Dev.* 1998;12(12):1894-1906.
245. Sato A, et al. Sall1, a causative gene for Townes-Brocks syndrome, enhances the canonical Wnt signaling by localizing to heterochromatin. *Biochem Biophys Res Commun.* 2004;319(1):103-113.
246. McPherron AC, Lawler AM, Lee SJ. Regulation of anterior/posterior patterning of the axial skeleton by growth/differentiation factor 11. *Nat Genet.* 1999;22(3):260-264.
247. Pitera JE, Scambler PJ, Woolf AS. Fras1, a basement membrane–associated protein mutated in Fraser syndrome, mediates both the initiation of the mammalian kidney and the integrity of renal glomeruli. *Hum Mol Genet.* 2008;17(24):3953-3964.
248. Levinson RS, et al. FoxD1-dependent signals control cellularity in the renal capsule, a structure required for normal renal development. *Development.* 2005;132(3):529-539.
249. Kispert A, Vainio S, McMahon AP. Wnt-4 is a mesenchymal signal for epithelial transformation of metanephric mesenchyme in the developing kidney. *Development.* 1998;125(Pt 21):4225-4234.
250. Moser M, et al. Enhanced apoptotic cell death of renal epithelial cells in mice lacking transcription factor AP-2β. *Genes Dev.* 1997;11(15):1938-1948.
251. Norwood VF, Morham SG, Smithies O. Postnatal development and progression of renal dysplasia in cyclooxygenase-2 null mice. *Kidney Int.* 2000;58(6):2291-2300.
252. Dreyer SD, et al. Mutations in LMX1B cause abnormal skeletal patterning and renal dysplasia in nail patella syndrome. *Nat Genet.* 1998;19(May 1998):47–50.
253. Schnabel CA, Godin RE, Cleary ML. Pbx1 regulates nephrogenesis and ureteric branching in the developing kidney. *Dev Biol.* 2003;254(2):262-276.
254. Schnabel CA, Selleri L, Cleary ML. Pbx1 is essential for adrenal development and urogenital differentiation. *Genesis.* 2003;37(3):123-130.
255. Grote D, et al. Gata3 acts downstream of beta-catenin signaling to prevent ectopic metanephric kidney induction. *PLoS Genet.* 2008;4(12):e1000316.
256. Basson MA, et al. Branching morphogenesis of the ureteric epithelium during kidney development is coordinated by the opposing functions of GDNF and Sprouty1. *Dev Biol.* 2006;299(2):466-477.
257. Lin F, et al. Kidney-specific inactivation of the KIF3A subunit of kinesin-II inhibits renal ciliogenesis and produces polycystic kidney disease. *Proc Natl Acad Sci U S A.* 2003;100(9):5286-5291.
258. Rankin EB, Tomaszewski JE, Haase VH. Renal cyst development in mice with conditional inactivation of the von Hippel–Lindau tumor suppressor. *Cancer Res.* 2006;66(5):2576-2583.
259. Kyttala M, et al. MKS1, encoding a component of the flagellar apparatus basal body proteome, is mutated in Meckel syndrome. *Nat Genet.* 2006;38(2):155-157.
260. Lu W, et al. Perinatal lethality with kidney and pancreas defects in mice with a targeted Pkd1 mutation. *Nat Genet.* 1997;17(2):179-181.
261. Moriguchi T, et al. MafB is essential for renal development and F4/80 expression in macrophages. *Mol Cell Biol.* 2006;26(15):5715-5727.
262. Kang HS, et al. Glis3 is associated with primary cilia and Wwtr1/TAZ and implicated in polycystic kidney disease. *Mol Cell Biol.* 2009;29(10):2556-2569.

263. Condac E, et al. Polycystic disease caused by deficiency in xylosyltransferase 2, an initiating enzyme of glycosaminoglycan biosynthesis. *Proc Natl Acad Sci U S A.* 2007;104(22):9416-9421.

264. Weiher H, et al. Transgenic mouse model of kidney disease: insertional inactivation of ubiquitously expressed gene leads to nephrotic syndrome. *Cell.* 1990;62(3):425-434.

265. Sachs N, et al. Kidney failure in mice lacking the tetraspanin CD151. *J Cell Biol.* 2006;175(1):33-39.

266. Miner JH, Sanes JR. Molecular and functional defects in kidneys of mice lacking collagen alpha 3(IV): implications for Alport syndrome. *J Cell Biol.* 1996;135(5):1403-1413.

267. Cosgrove D, et al. Collagen COL4A3 knockout: a mouse model for autosomal Alport syndrome. *Genes Dev.* 1996;10(23):2981-2992.

268. Lu W, et al. Insertional mutation of the collagen genes Col4a3 and Col4a4 in a mouse model of Alport syndrome. *Genomics.* 1999;61(2):113-124.

269. Rheault MN, et al. Mouse model of X-linked Alport syndrome. *J Am Soc Nephrol.* 2004;15(6):1466-1474.

270. Gould DB, et al. Role of Col4a1 in small-vessel disease and hemorrhagic stroke. *N Engl J Med.* 2006;354(14):1489-1496.

271. Noakes PG, et al. The renal glomerulus of mice lacking s-laminin/laminin β2: nephrosis despite molecular compensation by laminin β1. *Nat Genet.* 1995;10(4):400-406.

272. Jarad G, et al. Proteinuria precedes podocyte abnormalities in Lamb2$^{-/-}$ mice, implicating the glomerular basement membrane as an albumin barrier. *J Clin Invest.* 2006;116(8):2272-2279.

273. Miner JH, Li C. Defective glomerulogenesis in the absence of laminin α5 demonstrates a developmental role for the kidney glomerular basement membrane. *Dev Biol.* 2000;217(2):278-289.

274. Kikkawa Y, Virtanen I, Miner JH. Mesangial cells organize the glomerular capillaries by adhering to the G domain of laminin α5 in the glomerular basement membrane. *J Cell Biol.* 2003;161(1):187-196.

275. Kikkawa Y, Miner JH. Molecular dissection of laminin α5 in vivo reveals separable domain-specific roles in embryonic development and kidney function. *Dev Biol.* 2006;296(1):265-277.

276. Harvey SJ, et al. Disruption of glomerular basement membrane charge through podocyte-specific mutation of agrin does not alter glomerular permselectivity. *Am J Pathol.* 2007;171(1):139-152.

277. Morita H, et al. Heparan sulfate of perlecan is involved in glomerular filtration. *J Am Soc Nephrol.* 2005;16(6):1703-1710.

278. Goldberg S, et al. Glomerular filtration is normal in the absence of both agrin and perlecan-heparan sulfate from the glomerular basement membrane. *Nephrol Dial Transplant.* 2009;24(7):2044-2051.

279. Lebel SP, et al. Morphofunctional studies of the glomerular wall in mice lacking entactin-1. *J Histochem Cytochem.* 2003;51(11):1467-1478.

280. Kume T, Deng K, Hogan BL. Minimal phenotype of mice homozygous for a null mutation in the Forkhead/Winged Helix gene, Mf2. *Mol Cell Biol.* 2000;20(4):1419-1425.

281. Cano-Gauci DF, et al. Glypican-3–deficient mice exhibit developmental overgrowth and some of the abnormalities typical of Simpson-Golabi-Behmel syndrome. *J Cell Biol.* 1999;146(1):255-264.

282. Grisaru S, Rosenblum ND. Glypicans and the biology of renal malformations. *Pediatr Nephrol.* 2001;16(3):302-306.

283. Grisaru S, et al. Glypican-3 modulates BMP- and FGF-mediated effects during renal branching morphogenesis. *Dev Biol.* 2001;231(1):31-46.

284. Surendran K, Boyle S, Barak H, et al. The contribution of Notch1 to nephron segmentation in the developing kidney is revealed in a sensitized Notch2 background and can be augmented by reducing Mint dosage. *Dev Biol.* 2009;337(2):386-395.

285. Boute N, et al. NPHS2, encoding the glomerular protein podocin, is mutated in autosomal recessive steroid-resistant nephrotic syndrome [in process citation]. *Nat Genet.* 2000;24(4):349-354.

286. Hinkes B, et al. Positional cloning uncovers mutations in PLCE1 responsible for a nephrotic syndrome variant that may be reversible. *Nat Genet.* 2006;38(12):1397-1405.

287. Galeano B, et al. Mutation in the key enzyme of sialic acid biosynthesis causes severe glomerular proteinuria and is rescued by N-acetylmannosamine. *J Clin Invest.* 2007;117(6):1585-1594.

288. Ciani L, et al. Mice lacking the giant protocadherin Mfat1 exhibit renal slit junction abnormalities and a partially penetrant cyclopia and anophthalmia phenotype. *Mol Cell Biol.* 2003;23(10):3575-3582.

289. Eremina V, et al. VEGF inhibition and renal thrombotic microangiopathy. *N Engl J Med.* 2008;358(11):1129-1136.

290. El-Aouni C, et al. Podocyte-specific deletion of integrin-linked kinase results in severe glomerular basement membrane alterations and progressive glomerulosclerosis. *J Am Soc Nephrol.* 2006;17(5):1334-1344.

291. Kim D, et al. Pax transactivation-domain interacting protein is required for urine concentration and osmotolerance in collecting duct epithelia. *J Am Soc Nephrol.* 2007;18(5):1458-1465.

292. Lavoie JL, Lake-Bruse KD, Sigmund CD. Increased blood pressure in transgenic mice expressing both human renin and angiotensinogen in the renal proximal tubule. *Am J Physiol Renal Physiol.* 2004;286(5):F965-F971.

293. Sepulveda AR, et al. A 346–base pair region of the mouse gamma-glutamyl transpeptidase type II promoter contains sufficient *cis*-acting elements for kidney-restricted expression in transgenic mice. *J Biol Chem.* 1997;272(18):11959-11967.

294. Rubera I, et al. Specific Cre/Lox recombination in the mouse proximal tubule. *J Am Soc Nephrol.* 2004;15(8):2050-2056.

295. Nelson RD, et al. Expression of an AQP2 Cre recombinase transgene in kidney and male reproductive system of transgenic mice. *Am J Physiol.* 1998;275(1 Pt 1):C216-C226.

296. Srinivas S, et al. Expression of green fluorescent protein in the ureteric bud of transgenic mice: a new tool for the analysis of ureteric bud morphogenesis. *Dev Genet.* 1999;24(3-4):241-251.

297. Shao X, Somlo S, Igarashi P. Epithelial-specific Cre/Lox recombination in the developing kidney and genitourinary tract. *J Am Soc Nephrol.* 2002;13(7):1837-1846.

298. Zhu X, et al. Isolation of mouse THP gene promoter and demonstration of its kidney- specific activity in transgenic mice. *Am J Physiol Renal Physiol.* 2002;282(4):F608-F617.

299. Moeller MJ, Kovari IA, Holzman LB. Evaluation of a new tool for exploring podocyte biology: mouse Nphs1 5′ flanking region drives LacZ expression in podocytes. *J Am Soc Nephrol.* 2000;11(12):2306-2314.

300. Wong MA, Cui S, Quaggin SE. Identification and characterization of a glomerular-specific promoter from the human nephrin gene. *Am J Physiol Renal Physiology.* 2000;279(6):F1027-F1032.

301. Moeller MJ, et al. Two gene fragments that direct podocyte-specific expression in transgenic mice. *J Am Soc Nephrol.* 2002;13(6):1561-1567.

302. Humphreys, B.D., et al., Fate tracing reveals the pericyte and not epithelial origin of myofibroblasts in kidney fibrosis. Am J Pathol. 176(1):85-97.

303. Engleka KA, et al. Insertion of Cre into the Pax3 locus creates a new allele of Splotch and identifies unexpected Pax3 derivatives. *Dev Biol.* 2005;280(2):396-406.

304. Li J, Chen F, Epstein JA. Neural crest expression of Cre recombinase directed by the proximal Pax3 promoter in transgenic mice. *Genesis.* 2000;26(2):162-164.

305. Ohyama T, Groves AK. Generation of Pax2-Cre mice by modification of a Pax2 bacterial artificial chromosome. *Genesis.* 2004;38(4):195-199.

306. Traykova-Brauch M, et al. An efficient and versatile system for acute and chronic modulation of renal tubular function in transgenic mice. *Nat Med.* 2008;14(9):979-984.

307. Costantini F, Shakya R. GDNF/Ret signaling and the development of the kidney. *Bioessays.* 2006;28(2):117-127.

308. Sato N, Katsumata N, Kagami M, et al. Clinical assessment and mutation analysis of Kallmann syndrome 1 (KAL1) and fibroblast growth factor receptor 1 (FGFR1, or KAL2) in five families and 18 sporadic patients. *J Clin Endocrinol Metab.* 2004;89(3):1279-1288.

309. Faust P, Hatten M. Targeted deletion of the PEX2 peroxisome assembly gene in mice provides a model for Zellweger syndrome, a human neuronal migration disorder. *J Cell Biol.* 1997;139(5):1293-1305.

310. Nakayama K, Nakayama K, Negishi I, et al. Targeted disruption of Bcl-2 alpha beta in mice: occurrence of gray hair, polycystic kidney disease, and lymphocytopenia. *Proc Natl Acad Sci USA.* 1994;26;91(9):3700-3704.

311. Sison K, Eremina V, Baelde H, et al. Glomerular structure and function require paracrine, not autocrine, VEGF-VEGFR-2 signaling. *J Am Soc Nephrol.* 2010;21(10):1691-1701.

312. Weavers H, Prieto-Sanchez S, Grawe F, et al. The insect nephrocyte is a podocyte-like cell with a filtration slit diaphragm. *Nature.* 2009;457(7227):322-326.

313. Skinner M, Safford S, Reeves J, et al. Renal aplasia in humans is associated with RET mutations. *Am J Hum Genet.* 2008;82(2):344-351.

Chapter

2

Anatomy of the Kidney

Søren Nielsen, Tae-Hwan Kwon, Robert A. Fenton, and
Jeppe Prætorious

Knowledge of the complex structure of the mammalian kidney provides a basis for understanding the multitude of functional characteristics of this organ in both healthy and diseased states. In this chapter, an overview of the renal organization is presented through gross anatomic observations as well as light microscopic and ultrastructural information, including examples of immunohistochemical localization of selected channels, transporters, and regulatory proteins.

Gross Features

The kidneys are paired retroperitoneal organs situated one on each side of the vertebral column. In the human, the upper pole of each kidney lies opposite the twelfth thoracic vertebra, and the lower pole lies opposite the third lumbar vertebra. The right kidney is usually slightly more caudal in position. The weight of each kidney ranges from 125 to 170 g in the adult male and from 115 to 155 g in the adult female. The human kidney is approximately 11 to 12 cm in length, 5.0 to 7.5 cm in width, and 2.5 to 3.0 cm in thickness. Located on the medial or concave surface of each kidney is a slit, called the *hilum*, through which the renal pelvis, the renal artery and vein, the lymphatics, and a nerve plexus pass into the sinus of the kidney. The organ is surrounded by a thin tough fibrous capsule, which is smooth and easily removable under normal conditions.

In the human, as in most mammals, each kidney is normally supplied by a single renal artery, although the presence of one or more accessory renal arteries is not uncommon. The renal artery enters the hilar region and usually divides to form an anterior and a posterior branch. Three segmental or lobar arteries arise from the anterior branch and supply the upper, middle, and lower thirds of the anterior surface of the kidney (Figure 2-1). The posterior branch supplies more than half of the posterior surface and occasionally gives rise to a small apical segmental branch. However, the apical segmental or lobar branch arises most commonly from the anterior division. No collateral circulation has been demonstrated between individual segmental or lobar arteries or their subdivisions. The kidneys often receive aberrant arteries from the superior mesenteric, suprarenal, testicular, or ovarian arteries. True accessory arteries that arise from the abdominal aorta usually supply the lower pole of the kidney. The arterial and venous circulations in the kidney are described in detail in Chapter 3 and are not discussed further in this chapter.

Two distinct regions can be identified on the cut surface of a bisected kidney: a pale outer region, the cortex, and a darker inner region, the medulla (Figure 2-2). In humans, the medulla is divided into 8 to 18 striated conical masses, the renal pyramids. The base of each pyramid is positioned at the corticomedullary boundary, and the apex extends toward the renal pelvis to form a papilla. On the tip of each papilla are 10 to 25 small openings that represent the distal ends of the collecting ducts (ducts of Bellini). These openings form the area cribrosa (Figure 2-3). A renal pyramid and the corresponding cortex is referred to as a *renal lobus*. In contrast to the human kidney, the kidney of the rat and of many other laboratory animals has a single renal pyramid with its overlying cortex and is therefore termed *unipapillate*. Otherwise, these kidneys resemble the human kidney in their gross appearance.

In humans, the renal cortex is about 1 cm in thickness, forms a cap over the base of each renal pyramid, and extends downward between the individual pyramids to form the renal columns of Bertin (Figure 2-4; see also Figure 2-2). From the base of the renal pyramid, at the corticomedullary junction, longitudinal elements termed the *medullary rays of Ferrein* extend into the cortex. Despite their name, the medullary rays are actually considered a part of the cortex and are formed by the collecting ducts and the straight segments of the proximal and distal tubules. The renal pelvis is lined with transitional epithelium and represents the expanded portion of the upper urinary tract. In humans, two and sometimes three outpouchings, the major calyces, extend outward from the upper dilated end of the renal pelvis. From each of the major calyces, several minor calyces extend toward the papillae of the pyramids and drain the urine formed by each pyramidal unit. In mammals possessing a unipapillate kidney, the papilla is directly surrounded by the renal pelvis. The ureters originate from the lower portion of the renal pelvis at the ureteropelvic junction, and in humans they descend a distance of approximately 28 to 34 cm to open into the fundus of the bladder. The papilla, the walls of the calyces, pelvis, and ureters contain smooth muscle that contracts rhythmically to propel the urine to the bladder.

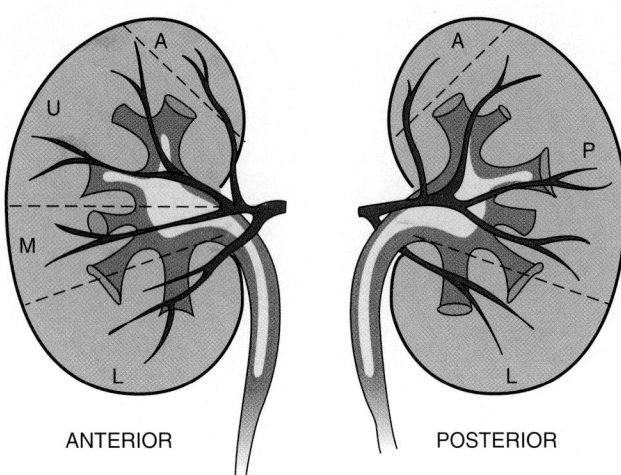

ANTERIOR   POSTERIOR

FIGURE 2-1 Diagram of the vascular supply of the human kidney. The anterior half of the kidney can be divided into upper (U), middle (M), and lower (L) segments, each supplied by a segmental branch of the anterior division of the renal artery. A small apical segment (A) is usually supplied by a division from the anterior segmental branch. The posterior half of the kidney is divided into apical (A), posterior (P), and lower (L) segments, each supplied by branches of the posterior division of the renal artery. (Modified from Graves FT: The anatomy of the intrarenal arteries and its application to segmental resection of the kidney, *Br J Surg* 42:132, 1954.)

Nephron

The nephron is often referred to as the *functional unit* of the kidney. Each human kidney contains about 0.6 to 1.4 × 10⁶ nephrons,[1-3] which contrasts with the approximately 30,000 nephrons in each adult rat kidney.[4-6] The essential components of the nephron include the renal or malpighian corpuscle (comprised of the glomerulus and Bowman's capsule), the proximal tubule, the thin limbs, the distal tubule, and the connecting tubule. The origin of the nephron is the metanephric blastema. Although there has not been universal agreement on the origin of the connecting tubule, it is now generally believed also to derive from the metanephric blastema.[7]

The collecting duct system, which includes the initial collecting tubule, the cortical collecting duct (CCD), the outer medullary collecting duct (OMCD), and the inner medullary

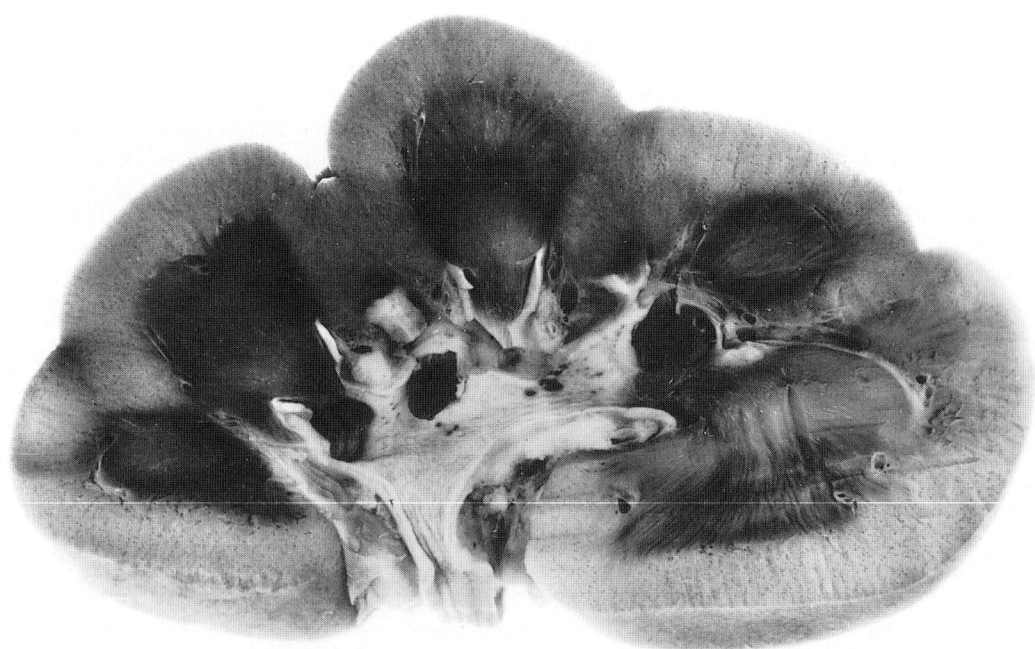

FIGURE 2-2 Bisected kidney from a 4-year-old child, demonstrating the difference in appearance between the light-staining cortex and the dark-staining outer medulla. The inner medulla and papillae are less dense than the outer medulla. The columns of Bertin can be seen extending downward to separate the papillae.

collecting duct (IMCD), is not considered to be an anatomical part of the nephron, because it embryologically arises from the ureteric bud. However, all of the components of the nephron and the collecting duct system are functionally interrelated.

Several populations of nephrons are recognizable in the kidney that have varying lengths of the loop of Henle (Figure 2-5). The loop of Henle is composed of the straight portion of the proximal tubule (pars recta), the thin limb segments, and the straight portion of the distal tubule (thick ascending limb,

or pars recta). The length of the loop of Henle is generally related to the position of its parent renal corpuscle in the cortex. Most nephrons originating from superficial and midcortical locations have shorter loops of Henle that bend within the inner stripe of the outer medulla close to the inner medulla. A few species, including humans, also possess cortical nephrons with extremely short loops that never enter the medulla but turn back within the cortex. Nephrons originating from the juxtamedullary region near the corticomedullary boundary

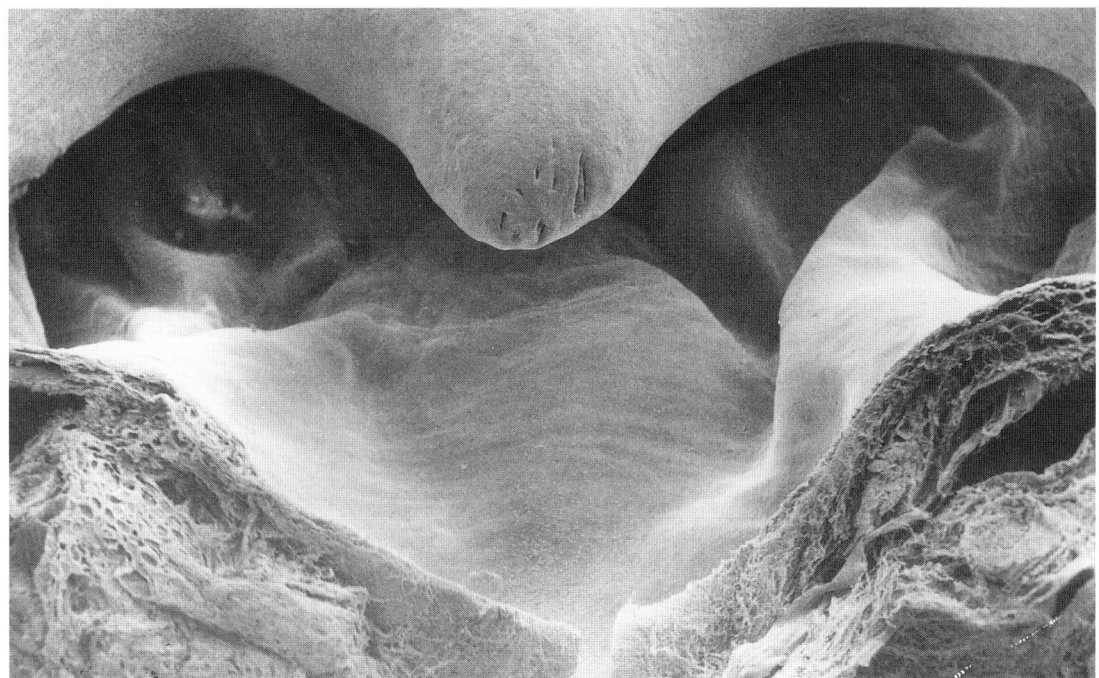

FIGURE 2-3 Scanning electron micrograph of a papilla from rat kidney (*upper center*), illustrating the area cribrosa formed by slitlike openings where the ducts of Bellini terminate. The renal pelvis (*below*) surrounds the papilla. (×24.)

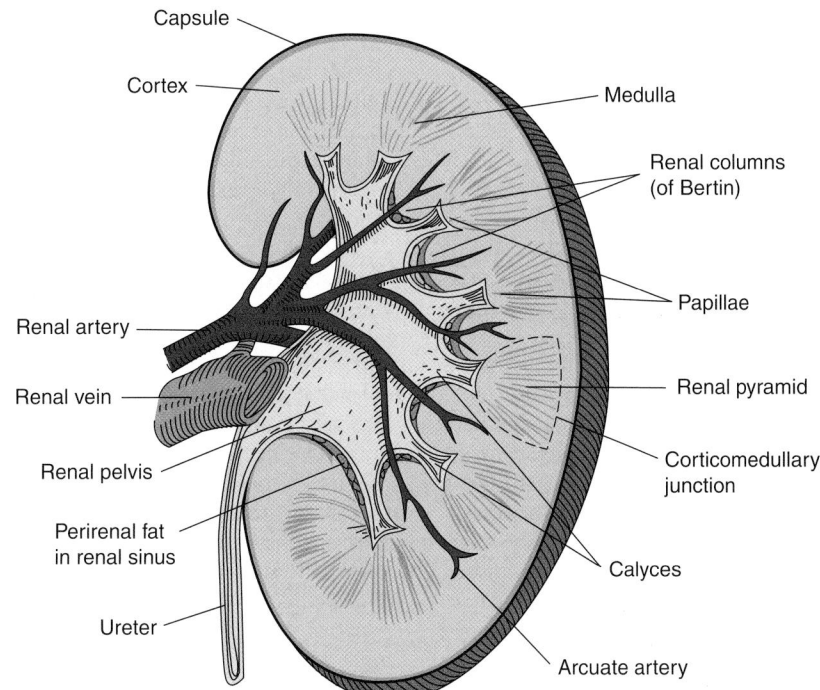

FIGURE 2-4 Diagram of the cut surface of a bisected kidney, depicting important anatomic structures.

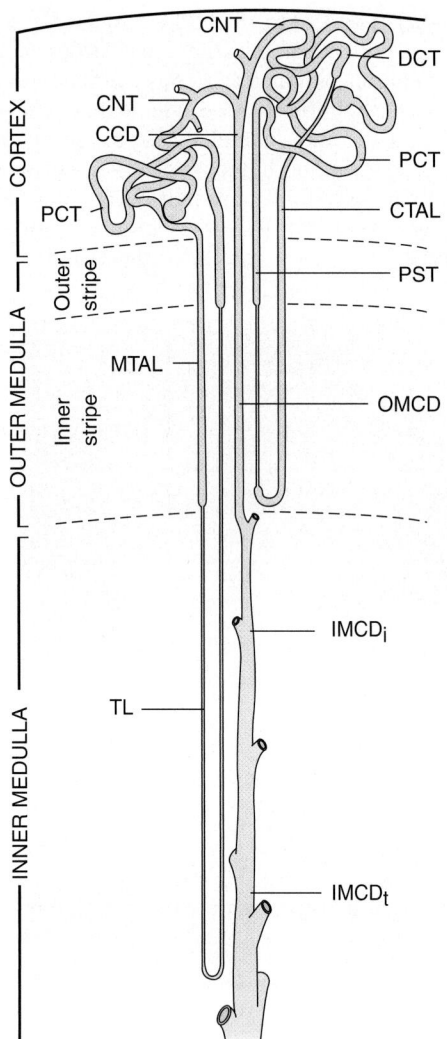

FIGURE 2-5 Diagram illustrating a superficial and juxtamedullary nephron. CCD, Cortical collecting duct; CNT, connecting tubule; CTAL, cortical thick ascending limb; DCT, distal convoluted tubule; IMCDi, initial inner medullary collecting duct; IMCDt, terminal inner medullary collecting duct; MTAL, medullary thick ascending limb; OMCD, outer medullary collecting duct; PCT, proximal convoluted tubule; PST, proximal straight tubule; TL, thin limb of loop of Henle. (Modified from Madsen KM, Tisher CC: Structural-functional relationship along the distal nephron, *Am J Physiol* 250:F1, 1986.)

have long loops of Henle with long descending and ascending thin limb segments that enter the inner medulla. Many variations exist, however, between the two basic types of nephrons, depending on their relative position in the cortex.

Recently, three-dimensional reconstruction studies of the rat and mouse kidney have provided insight into the anatomic distribution of various nephrons.[8-12] These studies have highlighted that the ratio of long- and short-looped nephrons varies among species, with humans and rodents having a larger number of short-looped than long-looped nephrons. Due to these anatomic differences, caution should be exercised in interpreting micropuncture data for understanding the urinary concentrating mechanism, because the majority of micropuncture data are obtained from studies of long-looped nephrons.

On the basis of the segmentation of the renal tubule, the medulla can be divided into an inner and an outer zone, with the outer zone further subdivided into an inner and an outer stripe (see Figure 2-5). The inner medulla contains both descending and ascending thin limbs and large collecting ducts, including the ducts of Bellini. In the inner stripe of the outer medulla, thick ascending limbs are present in addition to descending thin limbs and collecting ducts. The outer stripe of the outer medulla of human kidney contains the terminal segments of the pars recta of the proximal tubule, the thick ascending limbs (pars recta of the distal tubule), and collecting ducts. The division of the kidney into cortical and medullary zones and the further subdivision of the medulla into inner and outer zones are of considerable importance in relating renal structure to the ability of an animal to form a maximally concentrated urine.

Renal Corpuscle

The renal corpuscle is the initial part of the nephron and is composed of a capillary network lined by a thin layer of endothelial cells (glomerulus); a central mesangial region of mesangial cells with surrounding matrix material; the visceral epithelial layer of Bowman's capsule and the associated basement membrane; and the parietal layer of Bowman's capsule with its basement membrane (Figures 2-6 through 2-8). Between the two epithelial cell layers is a narrow cavity called *Bowman's space*, or the *urinary space*. Although the term *renal corpuscle* is more precise anatomically than the term *glomerulus* when referring to that portion of the nephron composed of the glomerular tuft and Bowman's capsule, the term *glomerulus* is employed throughout this chapter because of its common use.

The visceral epithelium is continuous with the parietal epithelium at the vascular pole, where the afferent arteriole enters and the efferent arteriole exits the glomerulus. The parietal layer of Bowman's capsule continues into the epithelium of the proximal tubule at the so-called urinary pole. The average diameter of the glomerulus is approximately 200 μm in the human kidney and 120 μm in the rat kidney. However, glomerular number and size vary significantly with age and gender as well as birth weight and renal health. The average glomerular volume has been reported to be 3 to 7 million μm^3 in humans[1-3] and 0.6 to 1 million μm^3 in the rat.[4,5] In the rat, juxtamedullary glomeruli are larger than glomeruli in the superficial cortex. However, this is not the case in the human kidney.[13]

The glomerulus is responsible for the production of an ultrafiltrate of plasma. The filtration barrier between the blood and the urinary space is composed of a fenestrated endothelium, the peripheral glomerular basement membrane (GBM), and the slit pores between the foot processes of the visceral epithelial cells (Figure 2-9). The mean area of filtration surface per glomerulus has been reported to be 0.203 mm^2 in the human kidney[14] and 0.184 mm^2 in the rat kidney.[15]

The glomerular capillary wall functions as a sieve or filter that allows the passage of small molecules, but almost completely restricts the passage of molecules the size of albumin or larger. Physiologic studies have established that the glomerular capillary wall possesses both size-selective and charge-selective properties.[16] To cross the capillary wall, a molecule must pass sequentially through the fenestrated endothelium, the GBM, and the epithelial slit diaphragm. The fenestrated endothelium, with its negatively charged glycocalyx, excludes

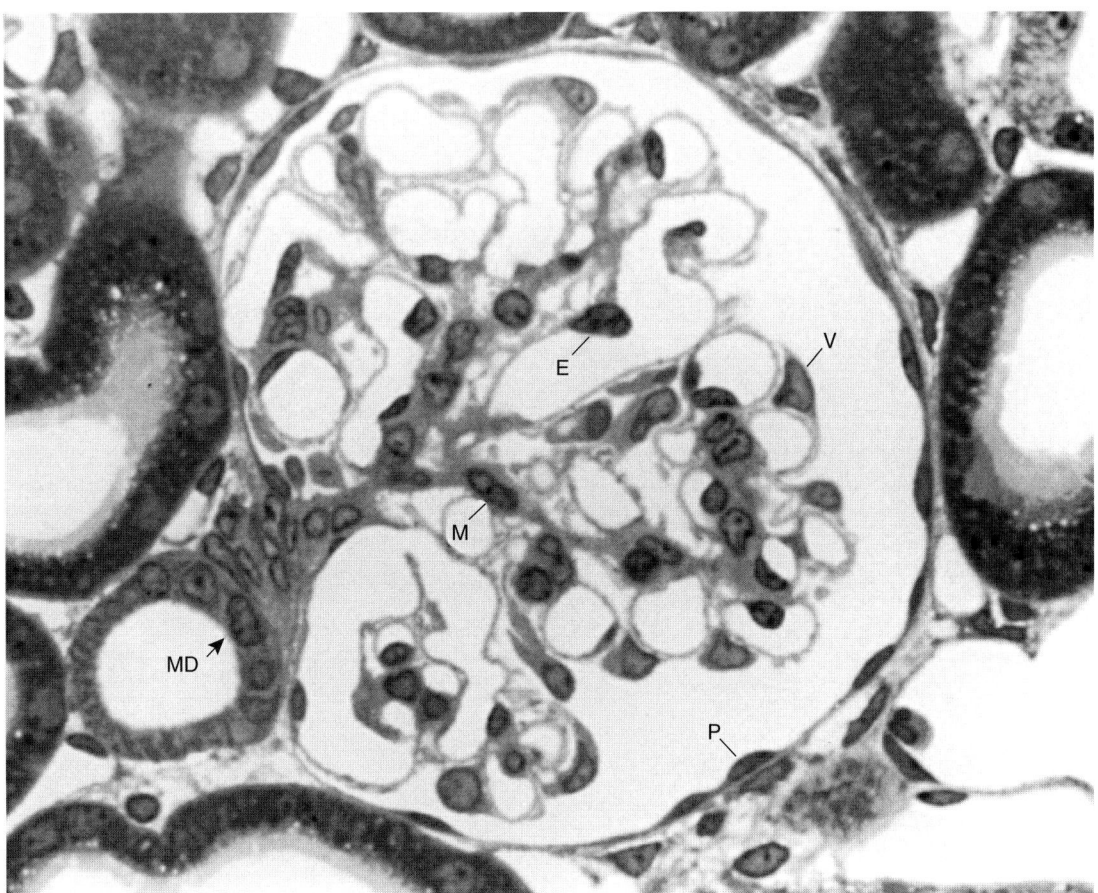

FIGURE 2-6 Light micrograph of a normal glomerulus from a rat, demonstrating the four major cellular components: mesangial cell (M), endothelial cell (E), visceral epithelial cell (V), and parietal epithelial cell (P). (×750.) MD, Macula densa.

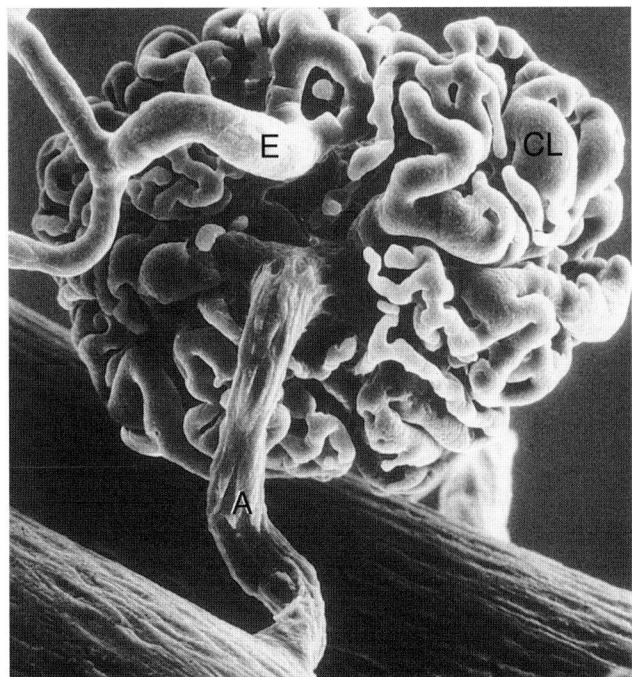

FIGURE 2-7 Scanning electron micrograph of a cast of a glomerulus with its many capillary loops (CL) and adjacent renal vessels. The afferent arteriole (A) takes its origin from an interlobular artery (*lower left*). The efferent arteriole (E) branches to form the peritubular capillary plexus (*upper left*). (×300.) (Courtesy of Waykin Nopanitaya, PhD.)

formed elements of the blood and probably plays a role in determining the access of proteins to the GBM.

Endothelial Cells

The glomerular capillaries are lined by a thin fenestrated endothelium (Figure 2-10; see also Figure 2-9). The endothelial cell nucleus usually lies adjacent to the mesangium, away from the urinary space, and the remainder of the cell is irregularly attenuated around the capillary lumen (see Figure 2-8). The endothelium is perforated by pores or fenestrae, which in the human kidney range from 70 to 100 nm in diameter (see Figure 2-10).[17] Thin protein diaphragms have been observed extending across these fenestrae, and electron microscopic studies using a modified fixation method reported the presence of filamentous sieve plugs in the fenestrae.[18] The function of these plugs remains to be established, and it is not known whether they represent a significant barrier to the passage of macromolecules. However, a recent study suggests that adult glomerular endothelial cells lack diaphragms, whereas these cells have diaphragmed fenestrae in the embryo, where they could compensate for the functional immaturity of the embryonic glomerular filtration barrier.[19] The presence of electron-dense filamentous material in the fenestrae and a thick filamentous surface layer on the endothelial cells have also been demonstrated.[20]

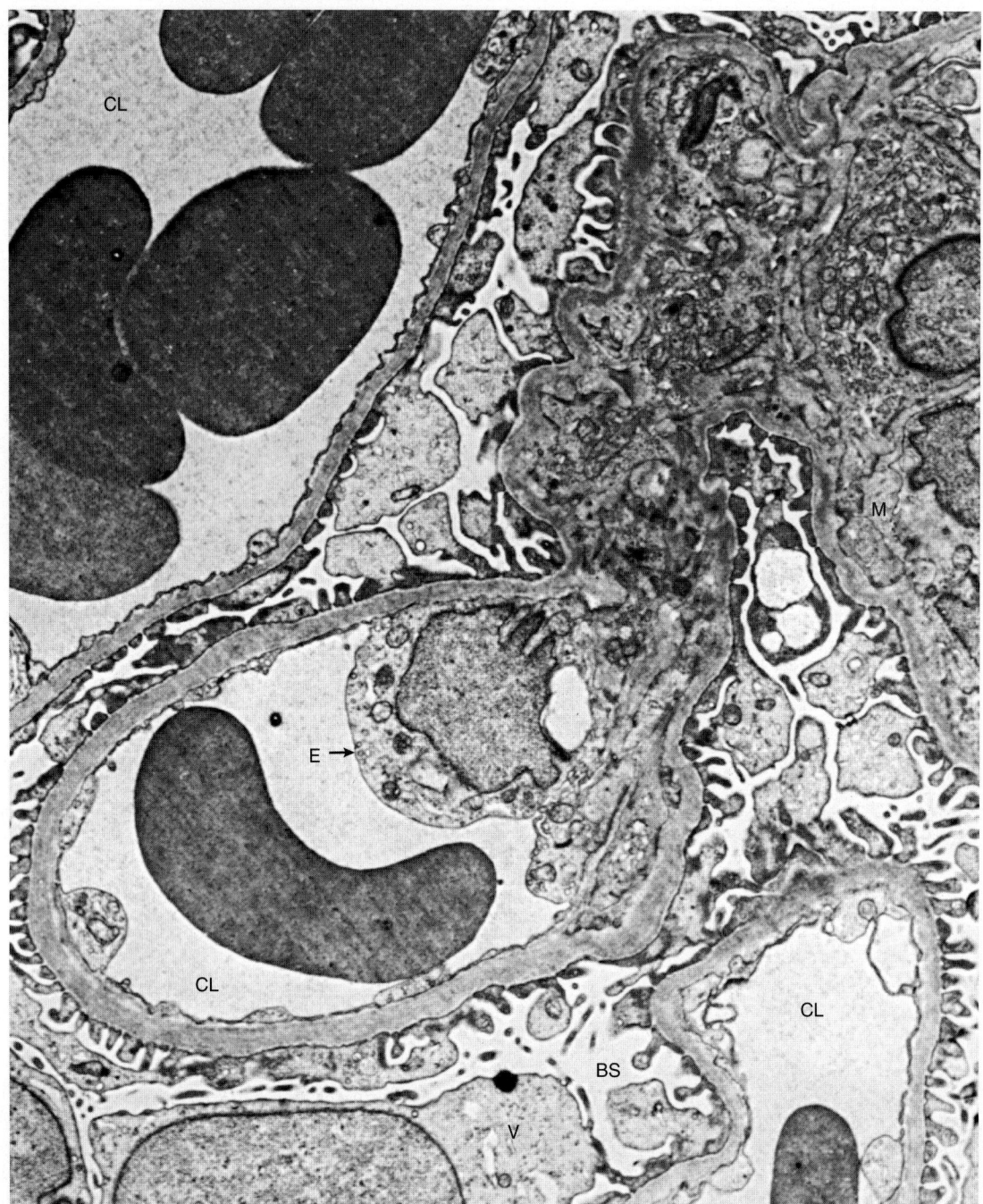

FIGURE 2-8 Electron micrograph of a portion of a glomerulus from normal human kidney in which segments of three capillary loops (CL) are evident. The relationship among mesangial cells (M), endothelial cells (E), and visceral epithelial cells (V) is demonstrated. Several electron-dense erythrocytes lie in the capillary lumens. (×6700.) BS, Bowman's space.

Nonfenestrated, ridgelike structures termed *cytofolds* are found near the cell borders. In both human and rat kidney, an extensive network of intermediate filaments and microtubules is present in the endothelial cells and microfilaments surround the endothelial fenestrations.[21] Knowledge of the exact functions of the cytoskeleton in these cells is incomplete.

The surface of the glomerular endothelial cells is negatively charged because of the presence of a surface coat or glycocalyx rich in polyanionic glycosaminoglycans and glycoproteins that are synthesized by the endothelial cells.[22] Studies have suggested that the endothelial cell glycocalyx contributes to

the charge-selective properties of the glomerular capillary wall and thus may constitute an important part of the filtration barrier.[23]

The glomerular endothelial cells synthesize both nitric oxide (NO), previously called endothelium-derived relaxing factor, and endothelin-1, a vasoconstrictor.[24] The synthesis of NO is catalyzed by endothelial nitric oxide synthase (eNOS), which is expressed in glomerular endothelial cells.[25]

Receptors for vascular endothelial growth factor (VEGF) are expressed on the surface of the glomerular endothelial cells.[26] VEGF is produced by the glomerular visceral epithelial

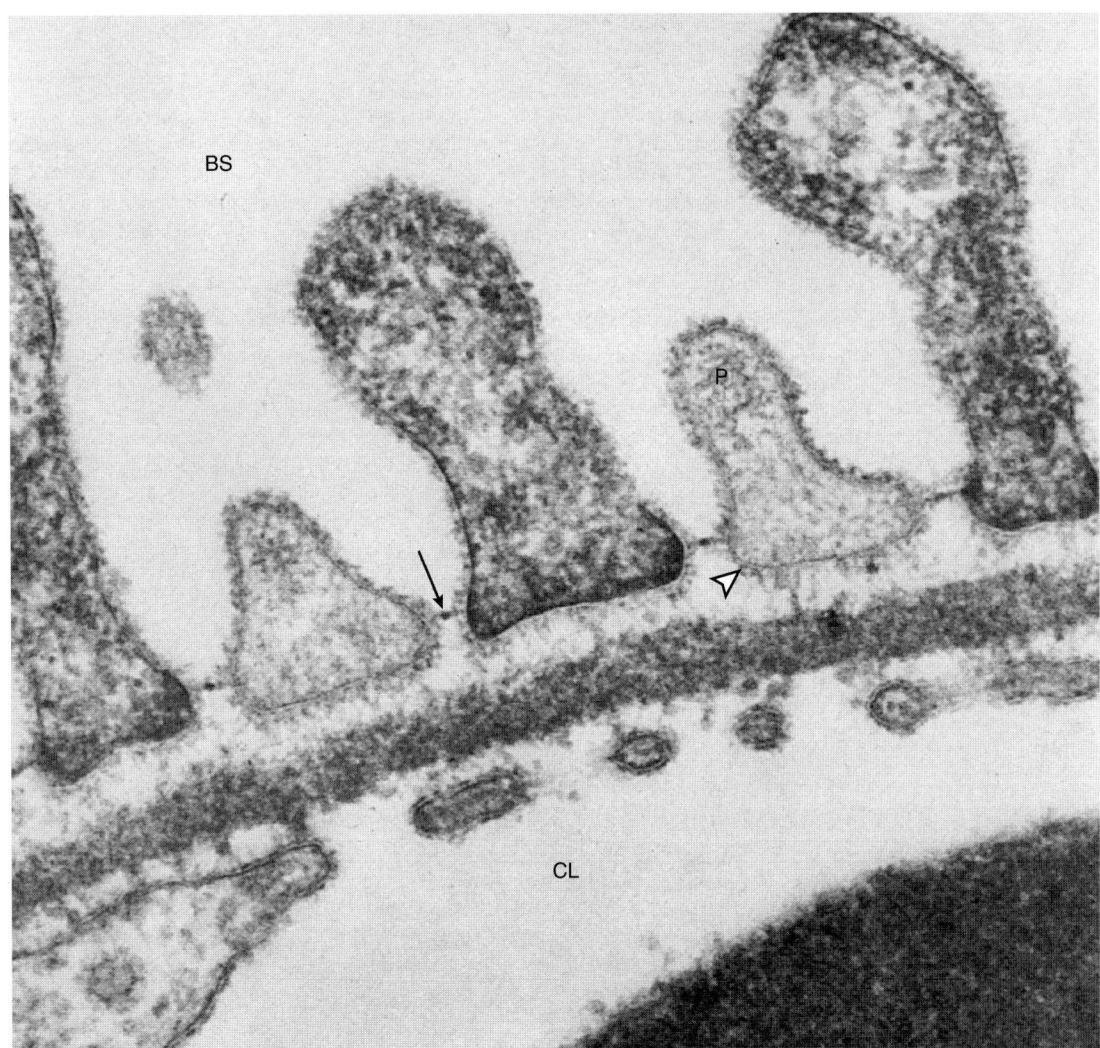

FIGURE 2-9 Electron micrograph of a normal rat glomerulus fixed in a 1% glutaraldehyde solution containing tannic acid. Note the relationship among the three layers of the glomerular basement membrane and the presence of the pedicels (P) embedded in the lamina rara externa (*thick arrow*). The filtration slit diaphragm with the central dense spot (*thin arrow*) is especially evident between the individual pedicels. The fenestrated endothelial lining of the capillary loop is shown below the basement membrane. A portion of an erythrocyte is located in the extreme lower right corner. (×120,000.) BS, Bowman's space; CL, capillary lumen.

cells and is an important regulator of microvascular permeability.[26,27] In vitro studies in endothelial cells of different origins have demonstrated that VEGF increases endothelial cell permeability and induces the formation of endothelial fenestrations.[28,29] VEGF-induced formation of fenestrae has also been demonstrated in renal microvascular endothelial cells.[30] Gene deletion studies in mice have demonstrated that VEGF is required for normal differentiation of glomerular endothelial cells,[31,32] and there is evidence that VEGF is important for endothelial cell survival and repair in glomerular diseases characterized by endothelial cell damage.[33] Thus, VEGF produced by the visceral epithelial cells plays a critical role in the differentiation and maintenance of glomerular endothelial cells and is an important regulator of endothelial cell permeability.

Endothelial cells form the initial barrier to the passage of blood constituents from the capillary lumen to Bowman's space, and they contribute to the charge-selective properties of the glomerular capillary wall through their negatively charged glycocalyx. Under normal conditions, the formed elements of

the blood, including erythrocytes, leukocytes, and platelets, do not gain access to the subendothelial space.

Glomerular Basement Membrane

The GBM is composed of a central dense layer, the lamina densa, and two thinner, more electron-lucent layers, the lamina rara externa and the lamina rara interna (see Figure 2-9). The latter two layers measure approximately 20 to 40 nm in thickness.[17] The layered configuration of the GBM results in part from the fusion of endothelial and epithelial basement membranes during development.[34] Several investigators have provided estimates of the width of the GBM of peripheral glomerular capillary loops. Jørgensen and Bentzon[35] reported a geometric mean of 329 nm in 24 patients who showed no clinical evidence of renal disease, and Østerby[36] calculated a mean width of 310 nm in five individuals. Steffes and colleagues[37] determined the GBM width in a large group of donor transplant kidneys and found a significantly thicker basement membrane in men (373 nm) than in women

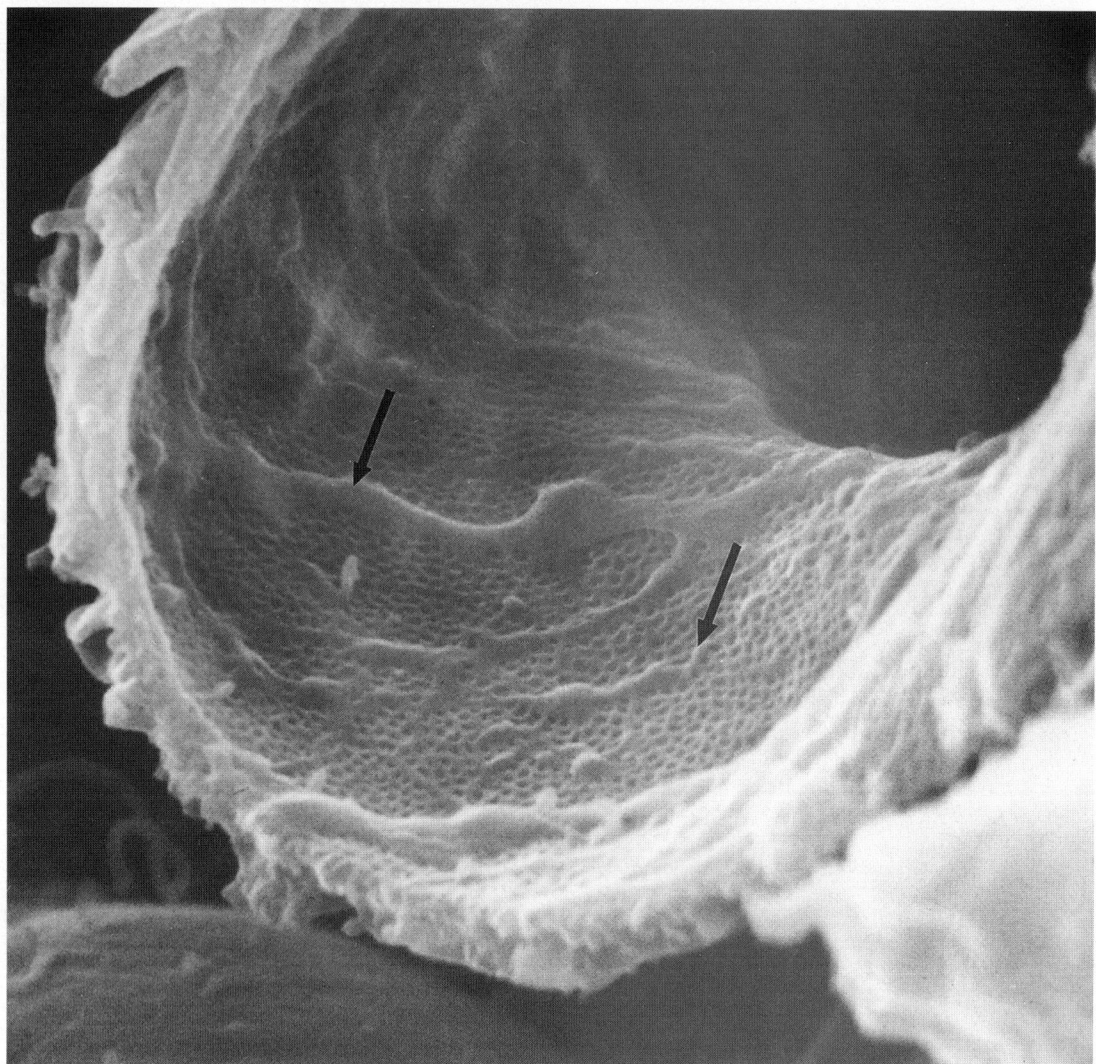

FIGURE 2-10 Scanning electron micrograph demonstrating the endothelial surface of a glomerular capillary from the kidney of a normal rat. Numerous endothelial pores, or fenestrae, are evident. The ridgelike structures (*arrows*) represent localized thickenings of the endothelial cells. (×21,400.)

(326 nm). For the purpose of comparison with the human, the thickness of the GBM in the rat was found to be 132 nm.[38]

Like other basement membranes in the body, the GBM is composed primarily of collagen IV, laminin, entactin (nidogen), and sulfated proteoglycans.[39-43] In addition, the GBM contains specific components such as laminin-11, distinct collagen IV α-chains, and the proteoglycans agrin and perlecan[43-45] that most likely reflect its specialized function as part of the glomerular filtration barrier. As reviewed by Kashtan,[46] six isomeric chains, designated α1 through α6 (IV), comprise the type IV collagen family of proteins.[47] Of these six chains, α1 through α5 have been identified in the normal GBM.[46] Mutations in the genes encoding α3, α4, and α5 (IV) chains are known to cause Alport's syndrome, a hereditary basement membrane disorder associated with progressive glomerulopathy.[46,48]

The exact role of the GBM in establishing the glomerular filtration barrier remains somewhat controversial. Ultrastructural tracer studies have provided evidence that the GBM constitutes both a size-selective and a charge-selective barrier. Caulfield and Farquhar[49] infused dextrans of different molecular weights into rats and demonstrated that filtration depended on the size of the molecule and that the GBM was the main barrier to filtration. Rennke and colleagues[50,51] used ultrastructural tracers such as ferritin and horseradish peroxidase with isoelectric points varying from 4.5 to 11.5 to examine the effect of molecular charge on the filtration of macromolecules. Their studies demonstrated that the clearance of cationic molecules greatly exceeded that of neutral and anionic molecules. Furthermore, the electrostatic barrier appeared to be located mainly in the GBM. However, the role of the GBM as the main determinant of charge selectivity was challenged subsequently, because studies in the isolated GBM failed to demonstrate charge selectivity in vitro.[52] The GBM possesses fixed, negatively charged sites that have been hypothesized to act as the putative charge barrier. Caulfield and Farquhar[53] demonstrated the existence of anionic sites in all three layers of the GBM with use of the cationic protein lysozyme. Additional studies revealed a lattice of anionic sites with a spacing of approximately 60 nm (Figure 2-11) throughout the lamina rara interna and lamina rara externa that might contribute to the formation of the charge barrier.[54]

Kanwar and Farquhar[55,56] demonstrated that the anionic sites in the GBM consist of glycosaminoglycans rich in

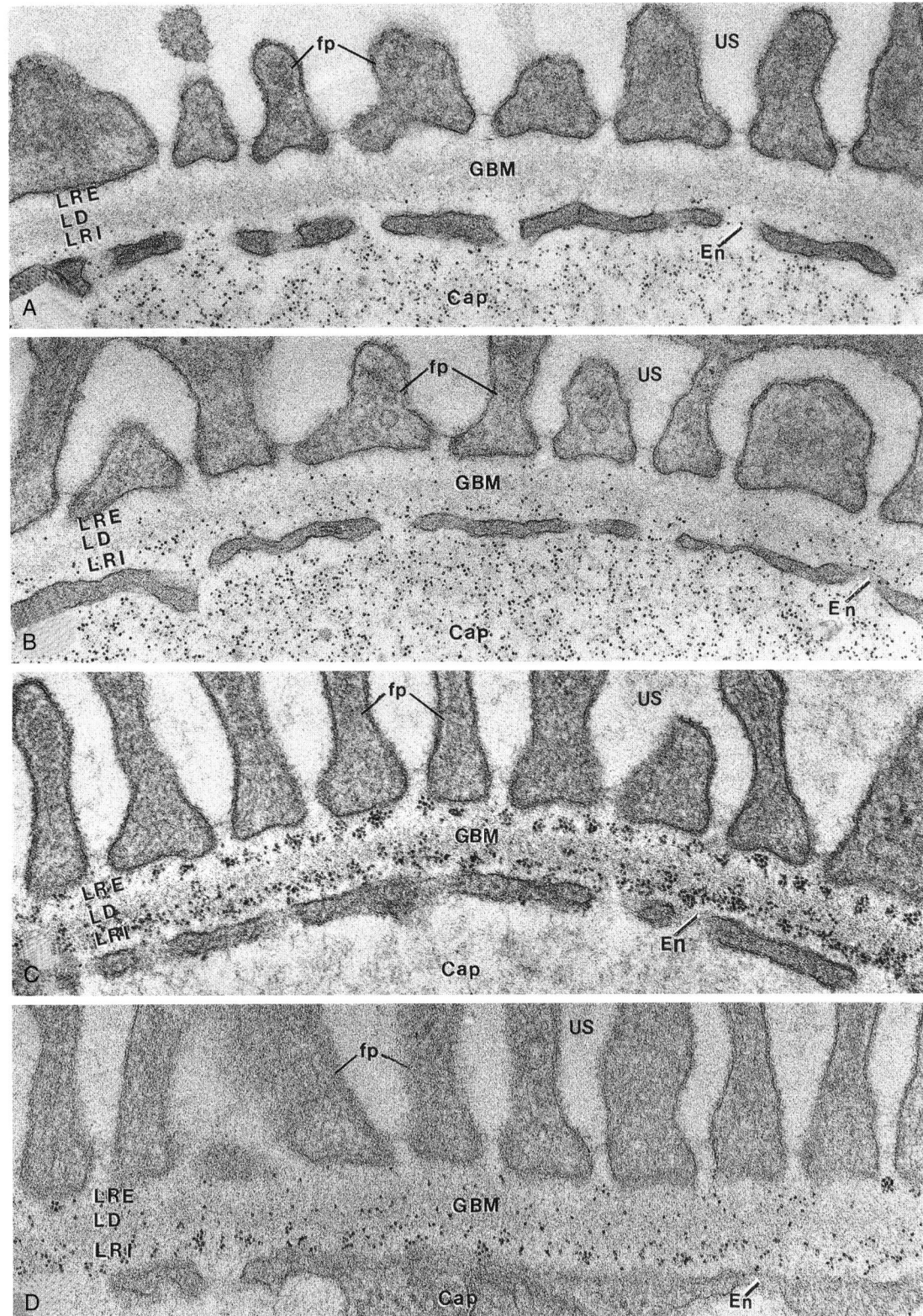

FIGURE 2-11 Transmission electron micrographs of glomerular filtration barrier in normal rats perfused with native anionic ferritin (**A**) or cationic ferritin (**C**) and in rats treated with heparitinase before perfusion with anionic (**B**) or cationic (**D**) ferritin. In normal animals, anionic ferritin is present in the capillary (Cap) but does not enter the glomerular basement membrane (GBM), as shown in **A.** In contrast, cationic ferritin binds to the negatively charged sites in the lamina rara interna (LRI) and lamina rara externa (LRE) of the GBM (see **C**). After treatment with heparitinase, both anionic (**B**) and cationic (**D**) ferritin penetrates into the GBM, but there is no labeling of negatively charged sites by cationic ferritin. En, Endothelial fenestrae; fp, foot processes; LD, lamina densa; US, urinary space. (×80,000.) (From Kanwar YS: Biophysiology of glomerular filtration and proteinuria, *Lab Invest* 51:7, 1984.)

heparan sulfate. Three distinct heparan sulfate proteoglycans are found in the GBM: perlecan, collagen XVIII, and agrin. Removal of their heparan sulfate side chains by enzymatic digestion resulted in an increase in the in vitro permeability of the GBM to ferritin[57] and to bovine serum albumin,[58] which suggests that glycosaminoglycans might play a role in establishing the permeability properties of the GBM to plasma proteins (see Figure 2-11). However, in vivo digestion of heparan sulfates with heparinase in rats did not result in proteinuria.[59] Furthermore, neither mice genetically engineered to lack agrin and perlecan heparin sulfate side chains[60,61] nor collagen XVIII–deficient mice[62] develop significant proteinuria. Thus, the role of electrostatic sites in the GBM as a charge-selective barrier has been largely refuted.

Due to the unique structure of the negatively charged filtration slit diaphragm of the podocyte and recent advances in its molecular characterization demonstrating that lack of distinct proteins associated with the slit diaphragm leads to massive proteinuria, it is now generally accepted that this structure plays a major role in establishing the ultrafiltration characteristics of the glomerular capillary wall (see later discussion). Most investigators, however, believe that the sequential existence of all three structural components of the filtration barrier is important for the normal permeability properties of the glomerulus. The strongest evidence for a specific role of the GBM in the filtration barrier is the finding that mice deficient in laminin-β2, a major component of the GBM, develop massive proteinuria,[63] as do patients with mutations in this gene.[64] Importantly, in laminin-β2 knockout mice, proteinuria is associated with increases in the permeability of the GBM that precede the onset of any abnormalities in the podocyte.[65]

Visceral Epithelial Cells

The visceral epithelial cells, also called *podocytes,* are the largest cells in the glomerulus (see Figure 2-6). They have long cytoplasmic processes, or trabeculae, that extend from the main cell body and divide into individual foot processes, or pedicels, that come into direct contact with the lamina rara externa of the GBM (see Figures 2-8 and 2-9). By scanning electron microscopy, it is apparent that adjacent foot processes are derived from different podocytes (Figure 2-12). The podocytes contain a well-developed Golgi complex, and lysosomes are often observed. Large numbers of microtubules, microfilaments, and intermediate filaments are present in the cytoplasm,[21] and actin filaments are especially abundant in the foot processes,[66] where they connect the slit membrane with the GBM.

In a healthy glomerulus, the distance between adjacent foot processes near the GBM varies from 25 to 60 nm (see Figure 2-9). This gap, referred to as the *filtration slit* or *slit pore,* is bridged by a thin membrane called the *filtration slit membrane*[67,68] or *slit diaphragm,*[69] which is located approximately 60 nm from the GBM. A continuous central filament with a diameter of approximately 11 nm can be seen in the filtration slit diaphragm.[67] Detailed studies of the slit diaphragm in the rat, mouse, and human glomerulus have revealed that the 11-nm-wide central filament is connected to the cell membrane of the adjacent foot processes by regularly spaced cross-bridges approximately 7 nm in diameter and 14 nm in length, which give the slit diaphragm a zipper-like configuration (Figure 2-13).[69,70] The dimensions of the pores between the cross-bridges are approximately 4 × 14 nm. The slit diaphragm has the morphologic features of an adherens junction,[71] and the ZO-1 protein that is specific to tight junctions has been localized to the sites where the slit diaphragm is connected to the plasma membrane of the foot processes.[72]

The molecular components of the slit diaphragm and their role in determining the permselective properties of the filtration barrier are now well established. The slit diaphragm is formed by a complex of the transmembrane proteins nephrin, NEPH1 through NEPH3, podocin, Fat1, VE-cadherin, and P-cadherin. Mutations in nephrin and podocin cause inherited nephrotic syndrome,[73-75] and knockout of nephrin, NEPH1, and podocin cause proteinuria in mice.[76] In addition, mutations in linker proteins that connect the slit diaphragm to the actin cytoskeleton, such as CD2-associated protein (CD2AP) and Nck, also cause proteinuria.[77,78] These observations establish the importance of the slit diaphragm in the glomerular filtration barrier (Figure 2-14).

In many diseases associated with proteinuria, the foot processes are replaced by a continuous cytoplasmic band along the GBM. This process is commonly referred to as *foot process fusion* or *effacement.* Similar ultrastructural changes have been described in the rat kidney after intraarterial infusion of protamine sulfate, a polycationic substance that interacts with anionic sites on the cell membrane.[79] Furthermore, perfusion of rat kidneys with neuraminidase, which removes sialic acid, causes a detachment of both endothelial and epithelial cells from the GBM,[80] a finding that suggests that negatively charged sites on these cells are important for the maintenance of normal structure and function of the filtration barrier. Therefore, anionic sites on the podocytes as well as the presence of an intact slit diaphragm are important in establishing the selective properties of the filtration barrier. The visceral epithelial cells are capable of endocytosis, and the heterogeneous content of their lysosomes most likely reflects the uptake of proteins and other components from the ultrafiltrate.

Mesangial Cells

The mesangial cells and their surrounding matrix constitute the mesangium, which is separated from the capillary lumen by the endothelium (see Figures 2-6 and 2-8). In 1933, Zimmermann provided the first detailed description of the mesangium by light microscopy and proposed the current nomenclature based on his theory of the development of the glomerulus by invagination.[17] It was not until the advent of the electron microscope, however, that the mesangial cell was distinguished clearly from the endothelial cell and described in detail.[81,82]

The mesangial cell is irregular in shape, with a dense nucleus and elongated cytoplasmic processes that can extend around the capillary lumen and insinuate themselves between the GBM and the overlying endothelium (see Figure 2-8). In addition to the usual complement of subcellular organelles, mesangial cells possess an extensive array of microfilaments composed at least in part of actin, α-actinin, and myosin.[83] The contractile mesangial cell processes appear to bridge the gap in the GBM encircling the capillary, and bundles of microfilaments interconnect opposing parts of the GBM, an

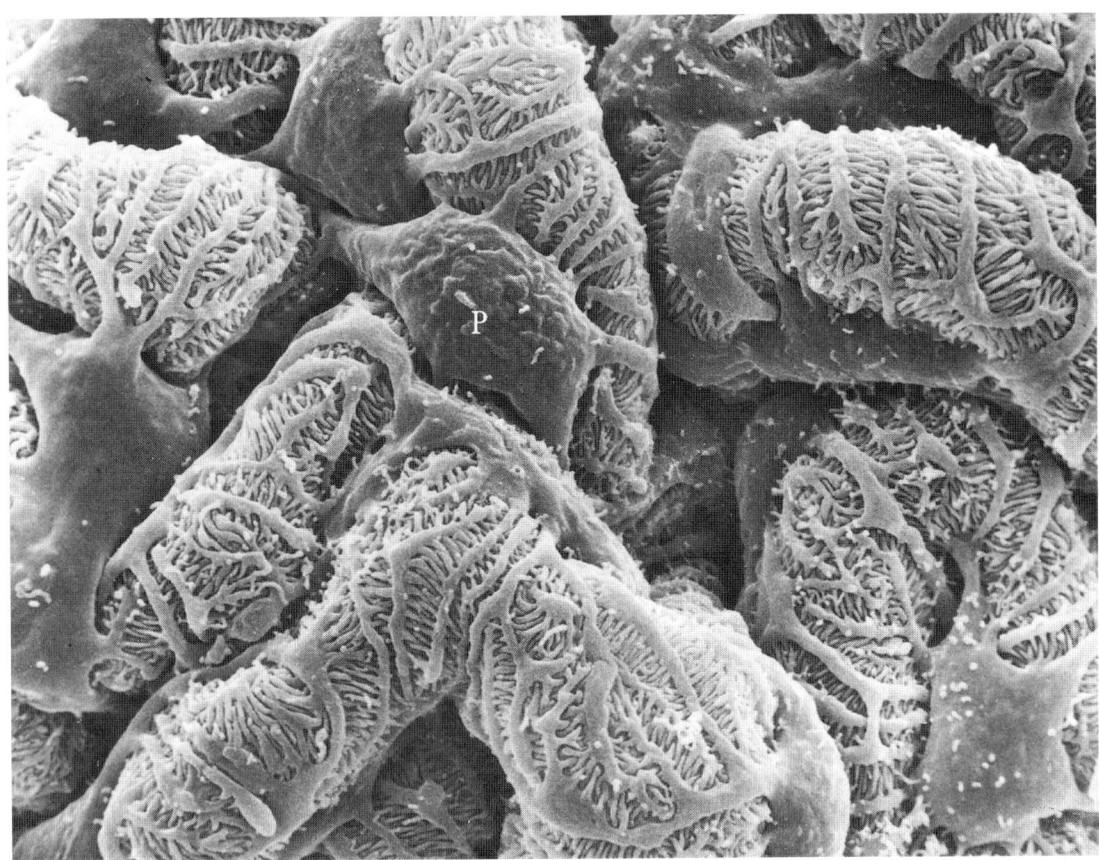

FIGURE 2-12 Scanning electron micrograph of a glomerulus from the kidney of a normal rat. The visceral epithelial cells, or podocytes (P), extend multiple processes outward from the main cell body to wrap around individual capillary loops. Immediately adjacent pedicels, or foot processes, arise from different podocytes. (×6000.)

arrangement that is believed to prevent capillary wall distension secondary to elevation of the intracapillary hydraulic pressure.[83,84]

The mesangial cell is surrounded by a matrix that is similar to but not identical with the GBM. The mesangial matrix is more coarsely fibrillar and slightly less electron dense. Several cell surface receptors of the β-integrin family have been identified on the mesangial cells, including α1β1, α3β1, and the fibronectin receptor, α5β1.[85-87] An additional α-chain, α8, has been identified on mesangial cells in human as well as rat and mouse kidneys.[88] The α8β1 integrin receptor can also serve as a receptor for fibronectin. The integrin receptors mediate attachment of the mesangial cells to specific molecules in the extracellular mesangial matrix and link the matrix to the cytoskeleton. The attachment to the mesangial matrix is important for cell anchorage, contraction, and migration, and ligand-integrin binding also serves as a signal transduction mechanism that regulates the production of extracellular matrix as well as the synthesis of various vasoactive mediators, growth factors, and cytokines.[89]

As reviewed by Schlondorff,[90] the mesangial cell in all likelihood represents a specialized pericyte and possesses many of the functional properties of smooth muscle cells. In addition to providing structural support for the glomerular capillary loops, the mesangial cell has contractile properties and is believed to play a role in the regulation of glomerular filtration. It is possible that mesangial cell contraction decreases glomerular filtration by reducing blood flow through selected capillary loops, thereby eliminating their contribution to the process of filtration.[90] The local generation of autocoids, such as prostaglandin E_2 (PGE_2), by the mesangial cell may provide a counterregulatory mechanism to oppose the effect of vasoconstrictors. Mesangial cells also exhibit phagocytic properties and participate in the clearance or disposal of macromolecules from the mesangium.[90,91] Finally, mesangial cells are involved in the generation and metabolism of the extracellular mesangial matrix and participate in various forms of glomerular injury.[89,90]

Morphologic aspects of the phagocytic properties of the mesangial cells are well documented.[91] Uptake of tracers such as ferritin,[81] colloidal carbon,[92] aggregated proteins,[93] and immune complexes has been described, and investigators have suggested that phagocytosed material may be cleared from the mesangium by cell-to-cell transport to the extraglomerular mesangial region at the vascular pole of the glomerular tuft.[92] Although some have reported that much of the phagocytic capability of the mesangium resides in the bone marrow–derived resident monocytes-macrophages, a population of cells possessing immune region–associated (Ia) antigens,[94,95] there is evidence that the mesangial cell is also capable of phagocytosis. The interaction among cytokines, mesangial cells, and prostaglandins may be important for understanding the mechanisms of the glomerular injury that is associated with mesangial cell proliferation and mesangial expansion in a host of kidney diseases.

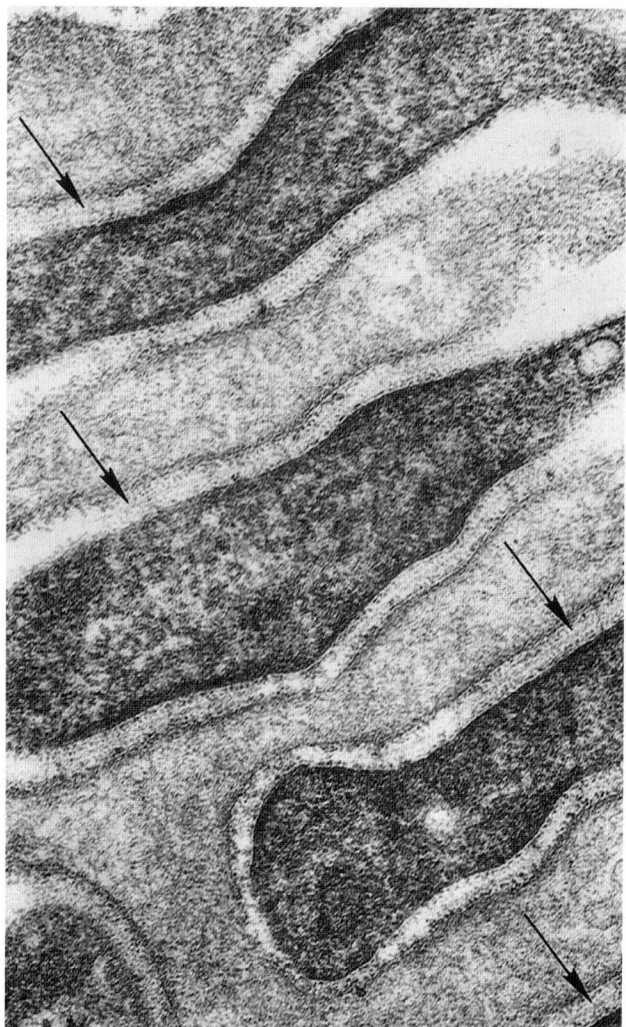

FIGURE 2-13 Electron micrograph showing the epithelial foot processes of normal rat glomerulus preserved in a 1% glutaraldehyde solution containing tannic acid. In several areas, the slit diaphragm has been sectioned parallel to the plane of the basement membrane, revealing a highly organized substructure. The thin central filament corresponding to the central dot observed on cross section (see Figure 2-9) is indicated by the *arrows.* (×52,000.)

Parietal Epithelial Cells

The parietal epithelium, which forms the outer wall of Bowman's capsule, is continuous with the visceral epithelium at the vascular pole. The parietal epithelial cells are squamous in character, but at the urinary pole there is an abrupt transition to the taller cuboidal cells of the proximal tubule, which have a well-developed brush border (Figures 2-15 and 2-16). The parietal epithelium of the capsule was described in detail by Jørgensen.[17] The cells are 0.1 to 0.3 μm in height except at the nucleus, where they increase to 2.0 to 3.5 μm. Each cell has a long cilium and occasional microvilli up to 600 nm in length. Cell organelles are generally sparse and include small mitochondria, numerous vesicles that are 40 to 90 nm in diameter, and the Golgi apparatus. Large vacuoles and multivesicular bodies are rare. The thickness of the basement membrane of Bowman's capsule varies from 1200 to 1500 nm.[17] The basement membrane is composed of multiple layers, or lamellae, that increase in thickness in many disease processes. At both the vascular pole and the urinary pole, the thickness of Bowman's capsule decreases markedly.

The parietal epithelial cell functions as the final permeability barrier for the urinary filtrate. In experimental glomerulonephritis, this barrier is compromised and macromolecules can leak into the space between the parietal cell and the basement membrane of Bowman's capsule, and into the periglomerular space.[96] There is also recent evidence that the parietal epithelial cell can transdifferentiate into podocytes and even repopulate the glomerular tuft.[97,98] In certain disease processes, such as rapidly progressive glomerulonephritis, the parietal epithelial cells proliferate, contributing to the formation of crescents.

Peripolar Cells

Ryan[99] and colleagues have described a peripolar cell that they believe is a component of the juxtaglomerular apparatus. It is located at the origin of the glomerular tuft in Bowman's space and is interposed between the visceral and parietal epithelial cells. The base of these cells rests on the basement membrane of Bowman's capsule, and the opposite surface is exposed

FIGURE 2-14 Diagram illustrating the hypothetical assembly of nephrin forming the filter of the podocyte slit diaphragm. Nephrin molecules from adjacent interdigitating foot processes are shown in different shades of gray. *X* indicates proteins interacting with nephrin and connecting with the plasma membrane. (From Tryggvason K: Unraveling the mechanisms of glomerular ultrafiltration: nephrin, a key component of the slit diaphragm, *J Am Soc Nephrol* 10:2440, 1999.)

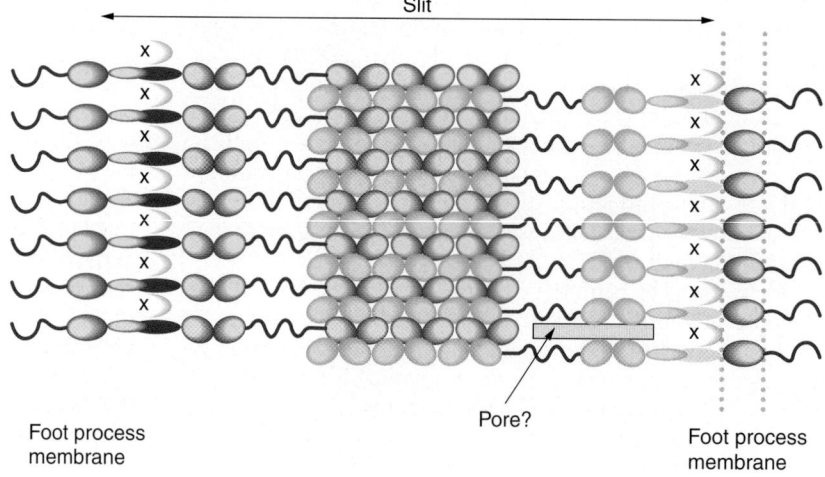

Slit

Foot process membrane

Pore?

Foot process membrane

to the urinary space. The cells contain multiple membrane-bound electron-dense granules and are separated from the afferent arteriole only by the basement membrane of Bowman's capsule.[99] The peripolar cells are especially prominent in sheep, but they have also been identified in other species, including humans, and have been localized predominantly in glomeruli in the outer cortex.[100]

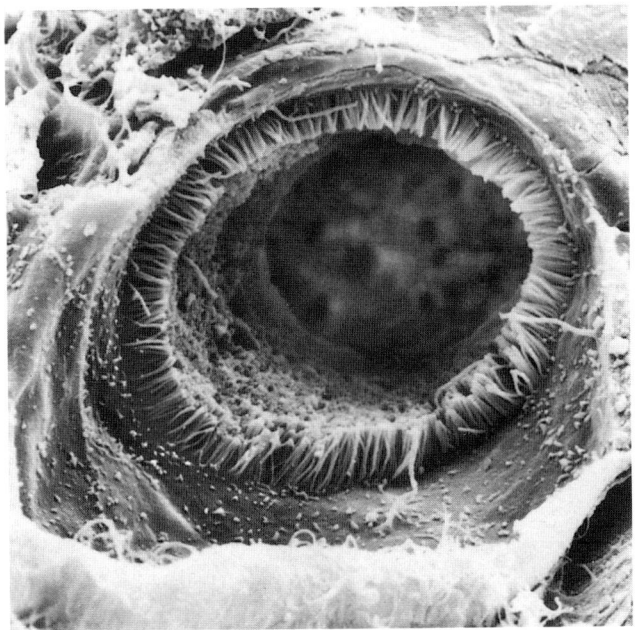

FIGURE 2-15 Scanning electron micrograph depicting the transition from the parietal epithelial cells of Bowman's capsule (*foreground*) to the proximal tubule cells, with their well-developed brush border, in the kidney of a rat. (×3200.)

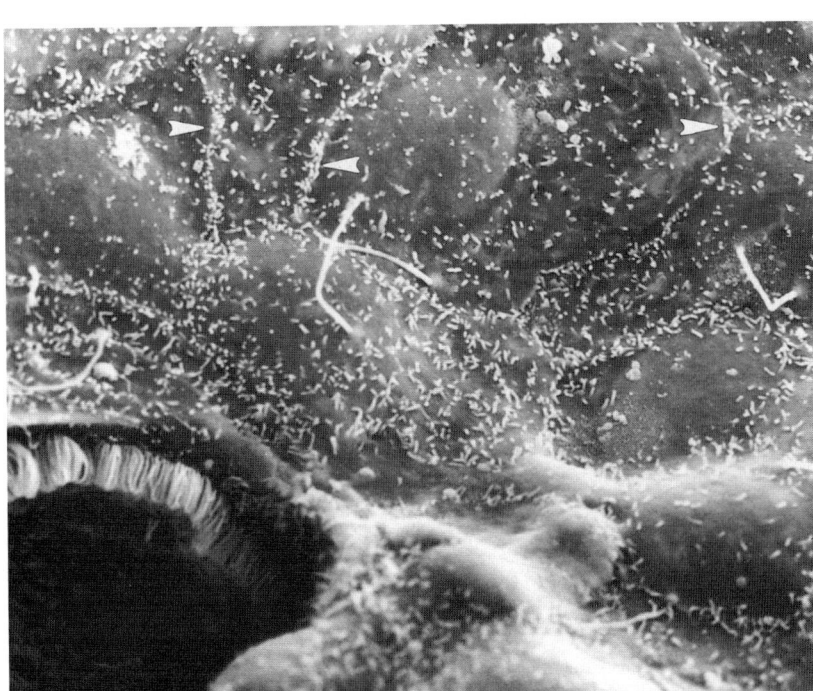

FIGURE 2-16 Scanning electron micrograph illustrating the appearance of the surface of the parietal epithelial cells adjacent to the early proximal tubule at the urinary pole (*lower left*). Parietal epithelial cells possess a single cilium, and their lateral cell margins are accentuated by short microvilli (*arrowheads*). (×12,500.) (Courtesy of Jill W. Verlander, DVM.)

Juxtaglomerular Apparatus

The juxtaglomerular apparatus is located at the vascular pole of the glomerulus, where a portion of the distal nephron comes into contact with its parent glomerulus. It has a vascular and a tubular component. The vascular component is composed of the terminal portion of the afferent arteriole, the initial portion of the efferent arteriole, and the extraglomerular mesangial region. The tubular component is the macula densa, which forms the transition between the thick ascending limb and the distal convoluted tubule (i.e., the transition between straight and convoluted segments of the distal tubule), which is in contact with the vascular component.[101-103] The extraglomerular mesangial region, which has also been referred to as the *polar cushion* (*polkissen*) or the *lacis*, is bounded by the cells of the macula densa, the specialized regions of the afferent and efferent glomerular arterioles, and the mesangial cells of the glomerular tuft (the intraglomerular mesangial cells). Within the vascular component of the juxtaglomerular apparatus, two distinct cell types can be distinguished: the juxtaglomerular granular cells, also called *epithelioid* or *myoepithelial cells*, and the agranular extraglomerular mesangial cells, which are also referred to as the *lacis cells*.

Juxtaglomerular Granular Cells

The granular cells are located primarily in the walls of the afferent and efferent arterioles.[101,103-105] They exhibit features of both smooth muscle cells and secretory epithelial cells and therefore have been called *myoepithelial cells*.[101] The juxtaglomerular granular cells are believed to represent modified smooth muscle cells. They contain myofilaments in the cytoplasm and, except for the presence of granules, are indistinguishable from the neighboring arteriolar smooth muscle cells. They also exhibit features suggestive of secretory activity, including a well-developed endoplasmic reticulum and a Golgi complex containing small granules with a crystalline substructure.[101,106]

The juxtaglomerular granular cells are characterized by the presence of numerous membrane-bound granules of variable size and shape (Figure 2-17).[105] Some of these granules, termed *protogranules,* have a crystalline substructure and are believed to represent precursors that fuse to form the larger mature granules.[105,107] In addition to these so-called specific granules, lipofuscin-like granules are commonly observed in the human kidney.[104,106]

As early as 1945, Goormaghtigh proposed that the granular cells were the source of renin, a hypothesis later proven correct by immunohistochemical and in situ hybridization studies as well as biochemical studies demonstrating renin enzyme activity in the juxtaglomerular apparatus.[103,105] Immunohistochemical studies demonstrated the presence of both renin and angiotensin II in the juxtaglomerular granular cells, with activities being highest in the afferent arteriole.[108] Through use of the immunogold technique in combination with electron microscopy, renin and angiotensin II were found to coexist in the same granules.[105] Studies using in situ hybridization techniques demonstrated renin messenger RNA (mRNA)

in the juxtaglomerular cells in normal kidneys, thus providing evidence that these cells produce renin.[109] Histochemical and immunocytochemical studies also have demonstrated the presence of lysosomal enzymes, including acid phosphatase and cathepsin B, in renin-containing granules of the juxtaglomerular epithelioid cells, which suggests that these granules may represent modified lysosomes.[105]

Extraglomerular Mesangium

Located between the afferent and efferent arterioles in close contact with the macula densa (see Figure 2-17), the extraglomerular mesangium is continuous with the intraglomerular mesangium and is composed of cells that are similar in ultrastructure to the mesangial cells.[101,103] The extraglomerular mesangial cells possess long, thin cytoplasmic processes that are separated by basement membrane material. Under normal conditions, these cells do not contain granules; however, juxtaglomerular granular cells are occasionally observed in the extraglomerular mesangium. The extraglomerular mesangial cells are in contact with the arterioles and the macula densa, and gap junctions are commonly observed between the various cells of the vascular portion of the juxtaglomerular apparatus.[110,111] Gap junctions have also been described between

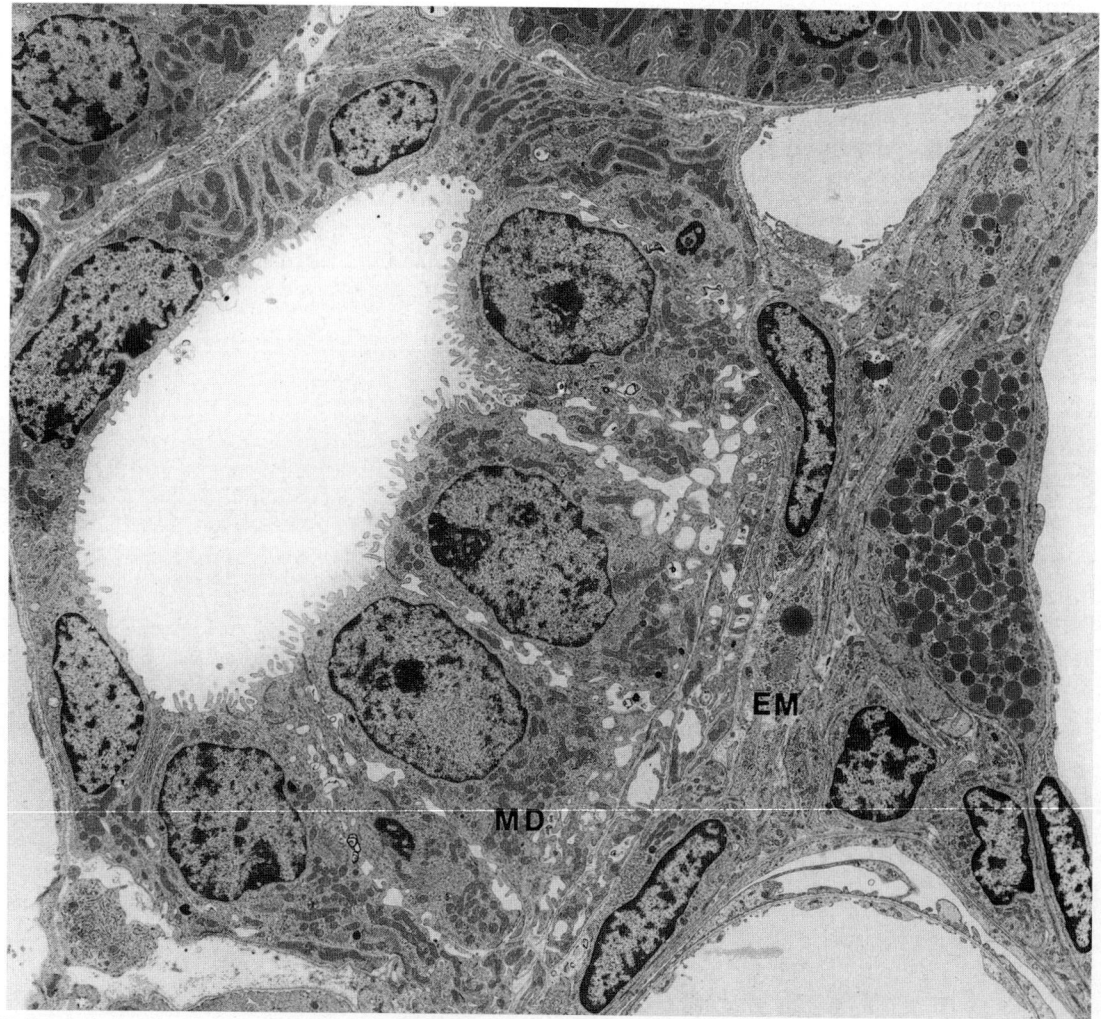

FIGURE 2-17 Transmission electron micrograph of the juxtaglomerular apparatus of rabbit kidney, illustrating macula densa (MD), extraglomerular mesangium (EM), and a portion of an arteriole (*on the right*) containing numerous electron-dense granules. (×3700.)

extraglomerular and intraglomerular mesangial cells, which suggests that the extraglomerular mesangium may serve as a functional link between the macula densa and the glomerular arterioles and mesangium.[111] Moreover, there is evidence that mesangial cell damage and selective disruption of gap junctions eliminate the tubuloglomerular feedback response.[112]

Macula Densa

The macula densa is a specialized region of the distal tubule adjacent to the hilum of the parent glomerulus (see Figure 2-17). Only those cells immediately adjacent to the hilum are morphologically distinctive from the surrounding cells of the thick ascending limb, forming the macula densa, and are columnar cells with an apically placed nucleus. With electron microscopy,[101,102] the cell base is seen to interdigitate with the adjacent extraglomerular mesangial cells. Although mitochondria are numerous, their orientation is not perpendicular to the base of the cell, and they are rarely enclosed within foldings of the basolateral plasma membrane. The position of the Golgi apparatus is lateral to and beneath the cell nucleus. In addition, other cell organelles, including lysosomes, autophagic vacuoles, ribosomes, and profiles of smooth and granular endoplasmic reticulum, are located principally beneath the cell nucleus.

The basement membrane of the macula densa is continuous with that surrounding the granular and agranular cells of the extraglomerular mesangial region, which in turn is continuous with the matrix material surrounding the mesangial cells within the glomerular tuft. Macula densa cells lack the lateral cell processes and interdigitations that are characteristic of the thick ascending limb. Ultrastructural studies have provided evidence that the width of the lateral intercellular spaces in the macula densa varies, depending on the physiologic status of the animal.[113] Furthermore, direct visualization of the isolated perfused macula densa by the use of differential interference contrast microscopy has revealed reversible dilatation of the lateral intercellular spaces between the macula densa cells with reduction of luminal osmolality.[114]

Morphologic evidence suggests that the autonomic nervous system is involved in the regulation of the function of the juxtaglomerular apparatus. Electron microscopic studies have demonstrated the existence of synapses between granular and agranular cells of the juxtaglomerular apparatus and autonomic nerve endings.[115] On serial sections of the rat juxtaglomerular apparatus, Barajas and Müller[116] analyzed the frequency of contacts between axons and the various cellular components of the juxtaglomerular apparatus. Nerve endings, principally adrenergic in type, were observed to be in contact with approximately one third of the cells of the efferent arteriole and with somewhat fewer than one third of the cells of the afferent arteriole in the region of the juxtaglomerular apparatus. The frequency of innervation of the tubule component of the juxtaglomerular apparatus was far less. Electron microscopic autoradiography demonstrated uptake of tritiated norepinephrine in axons in contact with afferent and efferent arterioles, which suggests that the nerves are adrenergic in character.[117]

Extensive studies by Kopp and DiBona[118] provided convincing evidence that renin secretion is modulated by renal sympathetic nerve activity, which is consistent with the existence of neuroeffector junctions on renin-positive granular cells of the juxtaglomerular apparatus. The juxtaglomerular apparatus (see earlier) represents a major structural component of the renin-angiotensin system. The role of the juxtaglomerular apparatus is to regulate glomerular arteriolar resistance and glomerular filtration and to control the synthesis and secretion of renin.[119,120]

The cells of the macula densa sense changes in the luminal concentrations of sodium and chloride, presumably via absorption of these ions across the luminal membrane by the Na^+-K^+-$2Cl^-$ cotransporter,[121,122] which is expressed in the macula densa.[123] This initiates the tubuloglomerular feedback response (see Chapter 3) by which signals generated by acute changes in sodium chloride concentration are transferred via the macula densa cells to the glomerular arterioles to control the glomerular filtration rate. Signals from the macula densa, in response to changes in luminal sodium and chloride, are also transmitted to the renin-secreting cells in the afferent arteriole.[120]

Renin synthesis and secretion by the juxtaglomerular granular cells are controlled by several factors, including neurotransmitters of the sympathetic nervous system, glomerular perfusion pressure (presumably through arteriolar baroreceptors), and mediators in the macula densa.[120,124,125] There is increasing evidence that the macula densa control of renin secretion is mediated by nitric oxide, cyclooxygenase products such as PGE_2, and adenosine.[120,125-127] There is both structural and functional evidence that both nitric oxide and cyclooxygenase-2 (COX-2)–generated prostaglandins participate in the signaling pathway between the macula densa and the renin-producing cells in the afferent arteriole. However, studies suggest that the increase in COX-2 expression in the macula densa in response to a low-salt diet is mediated by nitric oxide.[128,129] In addition to serving as a mediator of the tubuloglomerular feedback response, adenosine appears to be required for the inhibition of renin secretion that occurs in response to an increased sodium chloride concentration at the macula densa.[130]

Proximal Tubule

The proximal tubule begins abruptly at the urinary pole of the glomerulus (see Figure 2-15). It consists of an initial convoluted portion, the pars convoluta, which is a direct continuation of the parietal epithelium of Bowman's capsule, and a straight portion, the pars recta, which is located in the medullary ray (see Figure 2-5). The length of the proximal tubule is approximately 10 mm in the rabbit,[131] 8 mm in the rat, and 4 to 5 mm in the mouse,[11] compared with approximately 14 mm in the human. The outside diameter of the proximal tubule is about 40 μm. In the rat, three morphologically distinct segments—S1, S2, and S3— have been identified.[132] The S1 segment is the initial portion of the proximal tubule; it begins at the glomerulus and constitutes approximately two thirds of the pars convoluta. The S2 segment consists of the remainder of the pars convoluta and the initial portion of the pars recta. The S3 segment represents the remainder of the proximal tubule, located in the deep inner cortex and the outer stripe of the outer medulla.

The structural features that distinguish the cells in the three segments in the rat have been described in detail by Maunsbach[132] and are illustrated in Figures 2-18 through 2-20.

The S1 segment has a tall brush border and a well-developed vacuolar-lysosomal system. The basolateral plasma membrane forms extensive lateral invaginations, and lateral cell processes extending from the apical to the basal surface interdigitate with similar processes from adjacent cells. Elongated mitochondria are located in the lateral cell processes in proximity to the plasma membrane.

The ultrastructure of the S2 segment is similar to that of the S1 segment; however, the brush border is shorter, the basolateral invaginations are less prominent, and the mitochondria are smaller. Numerous small lateral processes are located close to the base of the cell. The endocytic compartment is less prominent than in the S1 segment. However, the number and size of the lysosomes vary among species and between males and females, and numerous large lysosomes are often observed in the S2 segment of the male rat.[131,132]

In the S3 segment, lateral cell processes and invaginations are essentially absent, and mitochondria are small and randomly distributed within the cell. The length of the brush border in the S3 segment varies among species. It is tall in the rat, fairly short in the rabbit, and intermediate in length in the human kidney. Considerable species variation is also observed in the vacuolar-lysosomal compartment in the S3 segment. In the rat[132] and the human,[133] endocytic vacuoles and lysosomes are small and sparse, whereas in the rabbit, large endocytic vacuoles and numerous small lysosomes are present in the S3 segment.[131] Peroxisomes are present throughout the proximal tubule. They increase in number along the length of the proximal tubule and are most prominent in the S3 segment.

Three segments have also been described in the proximal tubule of the rabbit[134,135] and the rhesus monkey.[136] According to Kaissling and Kriz,[134] however, in the rabbit the S2 segment is not clearly demarcated morphologically and represents a transition between the S1 and S3 segments. Interestingly, an ultrastructural study found no evidence of structural segmentation along the proximal tubule of the mouse.[11] Only the pars convoluta and the pars recta have been positively identified and described in the nondiseased human kidney.[133]

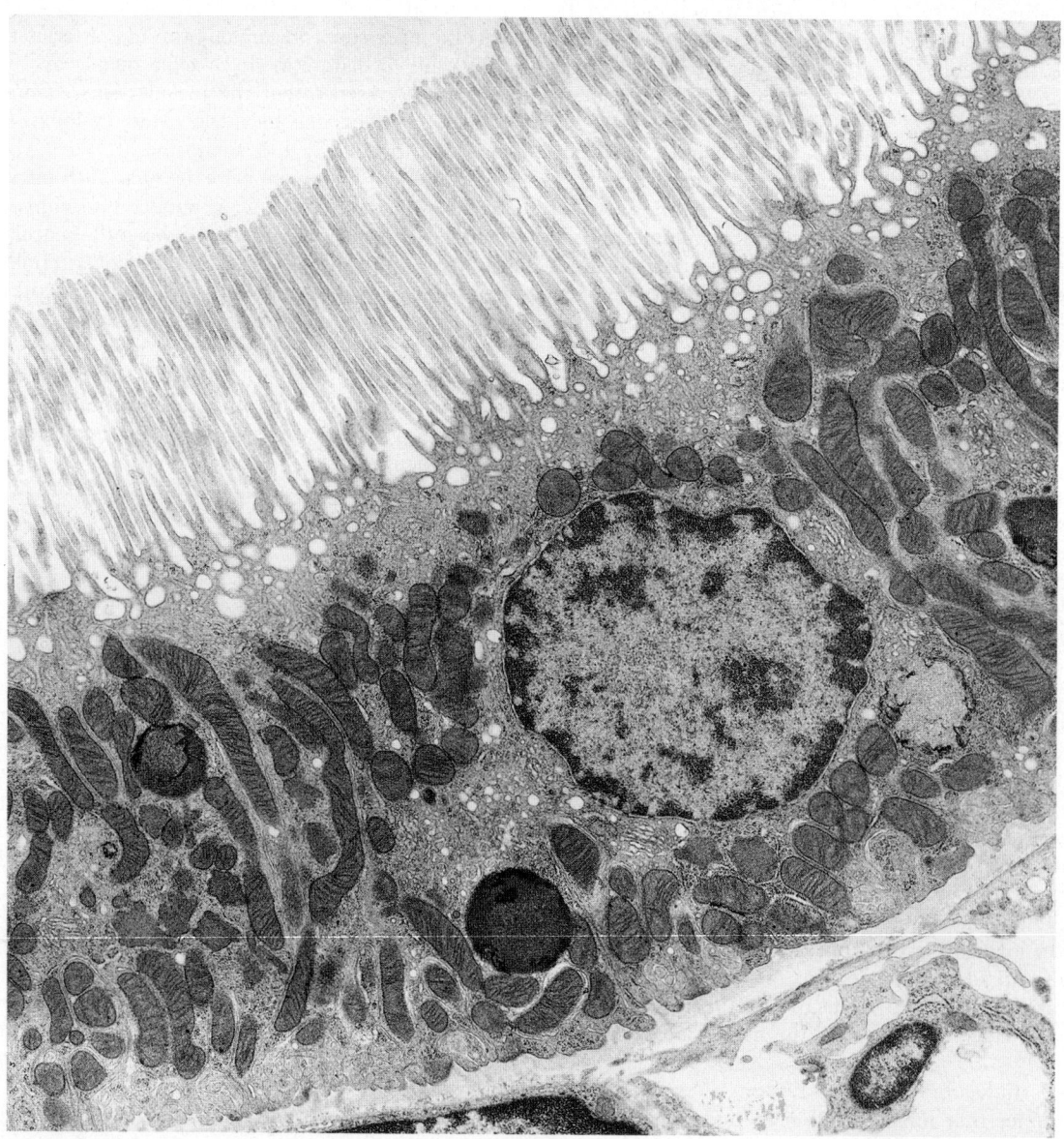

FIGURE 2-18 Transmission electron micrograph of the S1 segment of rat proximal tubule. The cells are characterized by a tall brush border, a prominent endocytic-lysosomal apparatus, and extensive invaginations of the basolateral plasma membrane. (×10,600.)

Since most functional studies have distinguished between the convoluted and the straight portions of the proximal tubule rather than the S1, S2, and S3 segments, the former distinction is used in the following description.

Pars Convoluta

The individual cells of the pars convoluta are extremely complex in shape as described for the S1 segment of the rat proximal tubule (Figure 2-21).[137] From the main cell body, large primary ridges extend laterally from the apical to the basal surface of the cells. Lateral processes large enough to contain mitochondria extend outward from the primary ridges and interdigitate with similar processes from adjacent cells. These lateral processes can be demonstrated by scanning electron microscopy (Figure 2-22). At the luminal surface of the cells, smaller lateral processes extend outward from the primary ridges to interdigitate with those of adjacent cells. Small basal villi that do not contain mitochondria are found along the basal cell surface (see Figure 2-21).

As a result of the extensive interdigitations of lateral and basal processes of adjacent cells, a complex extracellular compartment is formed. It is referred to as the *basolateral intercellular space* (Figure 2-23; see also Figure 2-22). This space

is separated from the tubule lumen by a specialization of the plasma membrane called the *zonula occludens*, or *tight junction*.[138] Physiologic and electrophysiologic studies have revealed the presence of a low-resistance shunt pathway in parallel with a high-resistance pathway across the apical and basal plasma membranes of the proximal tubule cell.[139-141] Claudins, a diverse family of tight junction proteins with various ion permeability properties, likely mediate the paracellular permeability properties of the tight junction.[142] In particular, claudin-2 is highly expressed in the tight junctions of the renal proximal tubules and constitutes leaky and cation (Na^+)-selective paracellular channels within these tight junctions.[143]

Immediately beneath the tight junction is a second specialized region of the plasma membrane, termed the *intermediate junction* or *zonula adherens*.[138] It is a seven-layered structure formed by the two adjacent triple-layered plasma membranes separated by a narrow upper extension of the intercellular space. Dense condensations of cytoplasm are located adjacent to the regions of the plasma membranes that form the intermediate junction. Desmosomes, also found in the proximal convoluted tubule, are distributed randomly at variable distances beneath the intermediate junction. These seven-layered structures are also formed by the two adjacent plasma membranes and the intervening intercellular space. However, they

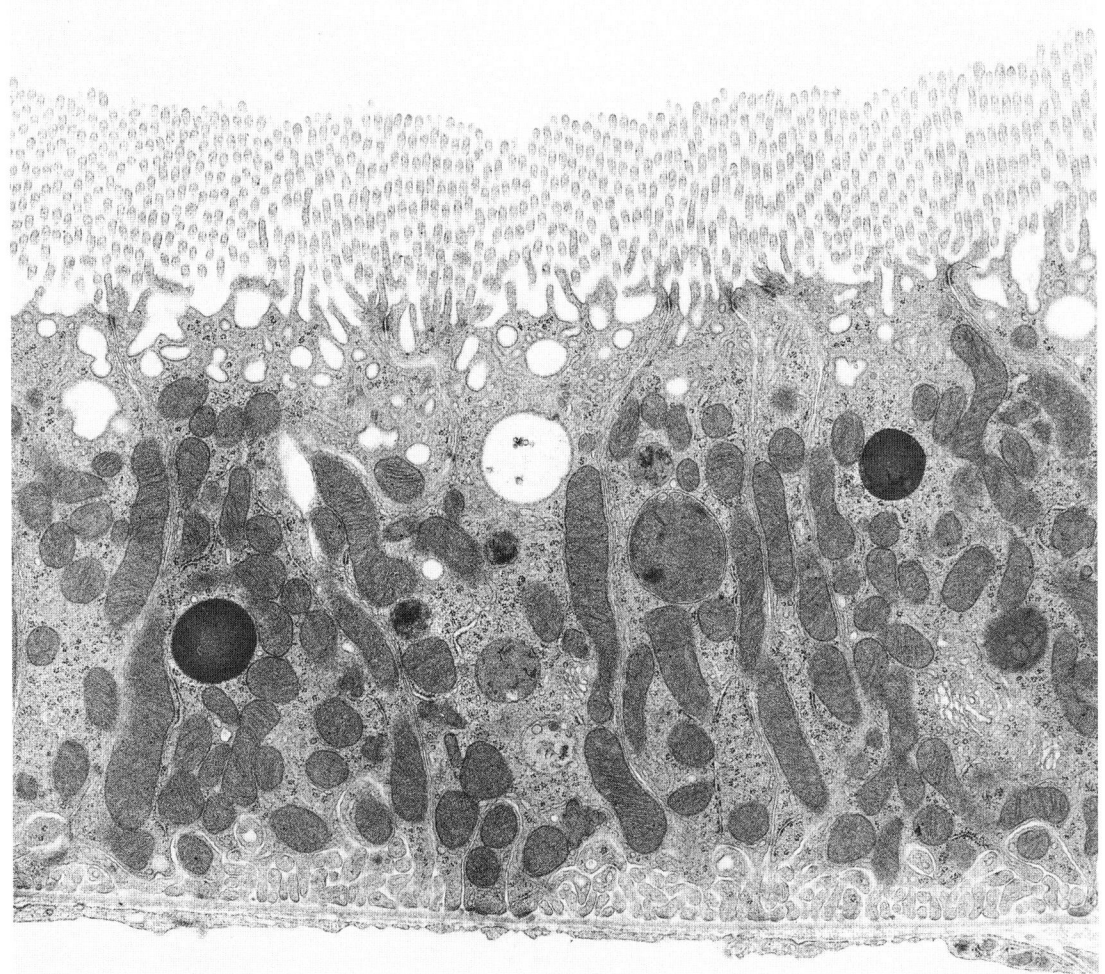

FIGURE 2-19 Transmission electron micrograph of the S2 segment of rat proximal tubule. The brush border is less prominent than in the S1 segment. Note numerous small lateral processes at the base of the cell. (×10,600.)

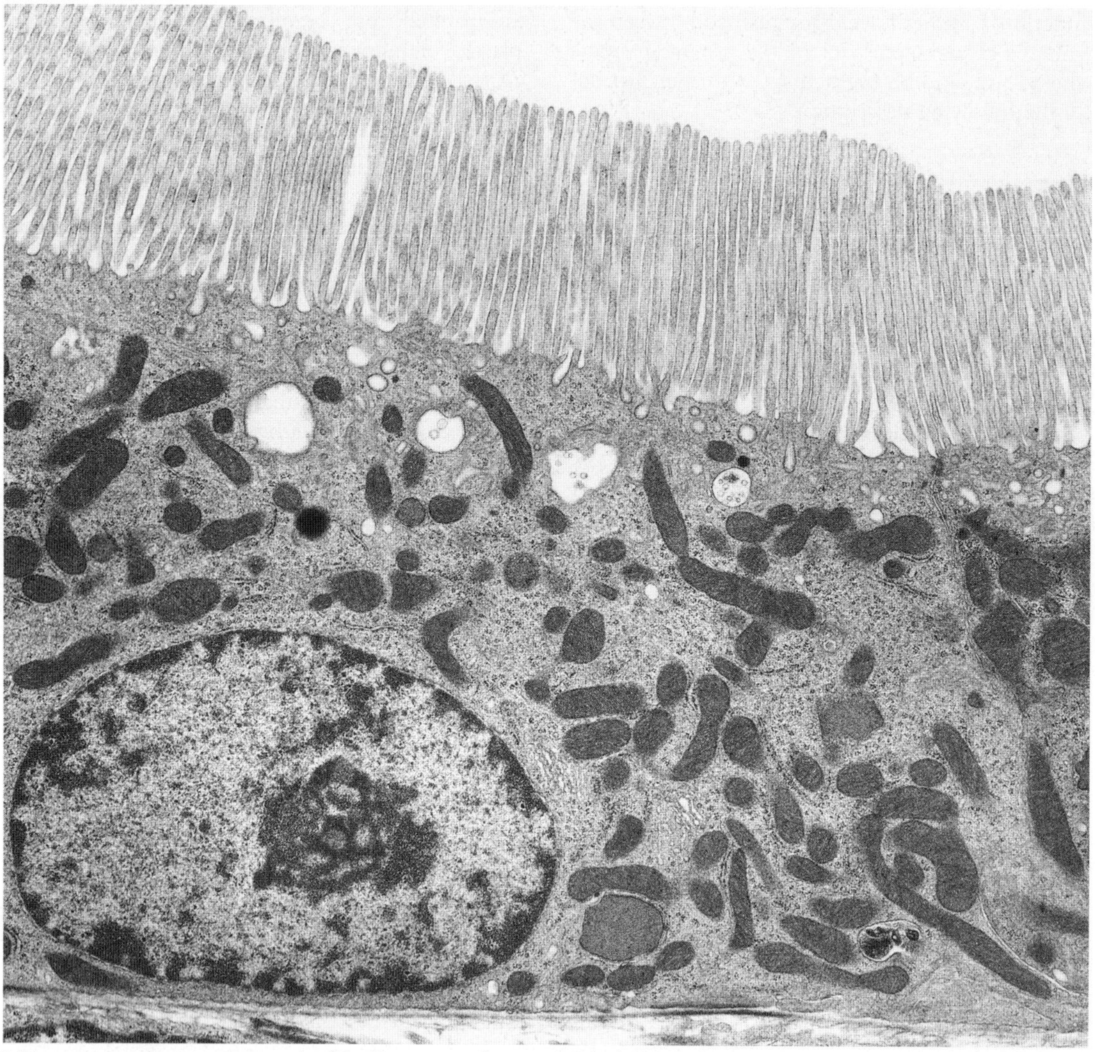

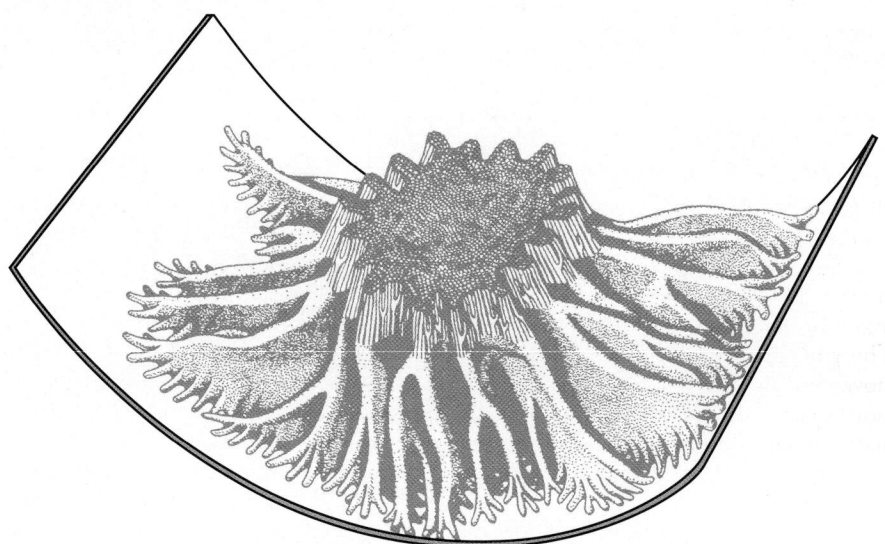

FIGURE 2-20 Transmission electron micrograph of the S3 segment of rat proximal tubule. The brush border is tall, but the endocytic-lysosomal apparatus is less prominent than in the S1 and S2 segments. Basolateral invaginations are sparse, and mitochondria are scattered randomly throughout the cytoplasm. (×10,600.)

FIGURE 2-21 Schematic drawing illustrating the three-dimensional configuration of a proximal convoluted tubule cell. (From Welling LW, Welling DJ: Shape of epithelial cells and intercellular channels in the rabbit proximal nephron, *Kidney Int* 9:385, 1976.)

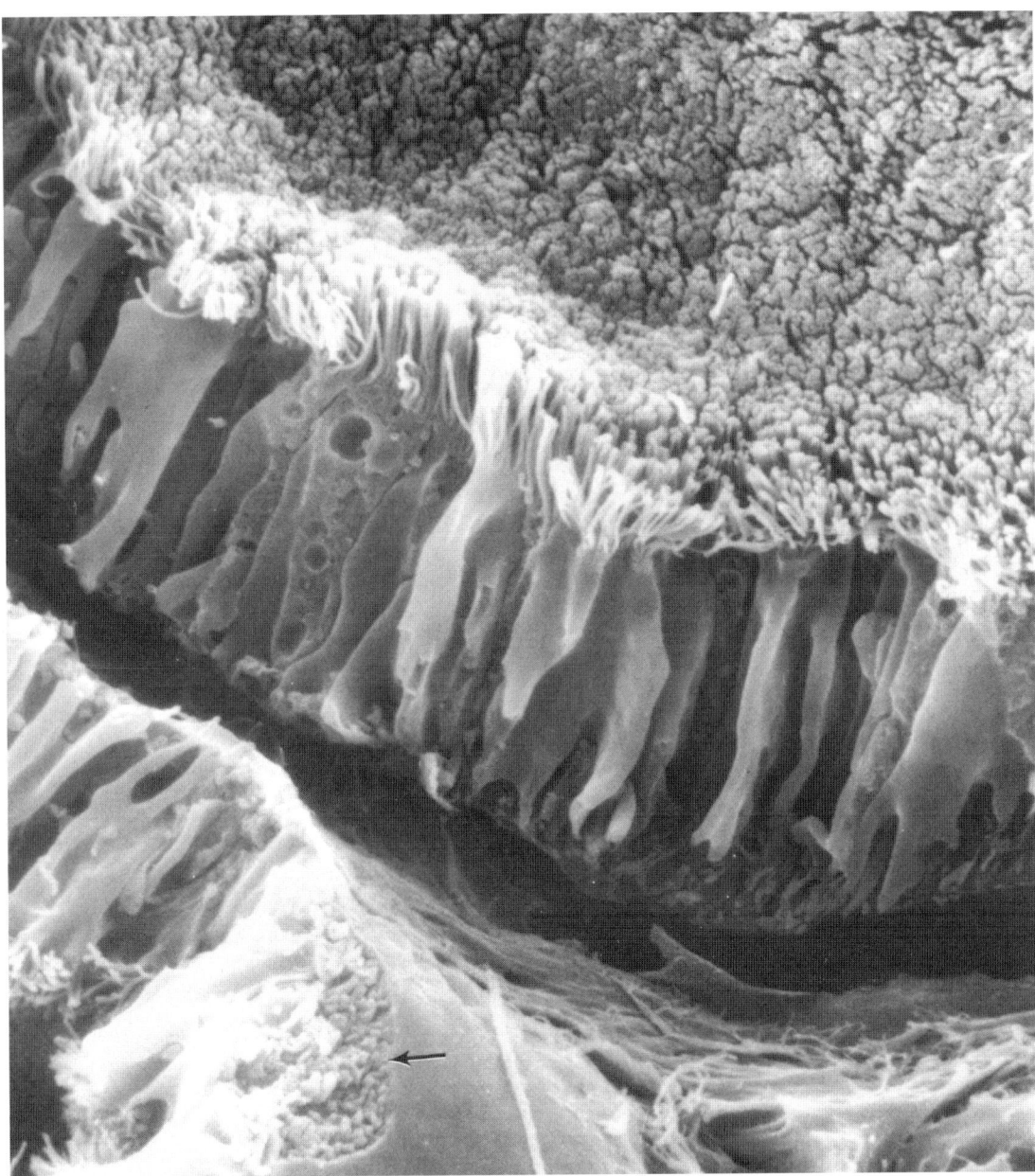

FIGURE 2-22 Scanning electron micrograph of a proximal convoluted tubule illustrating prominent lateral cell processes. *Arrow* on the adjacent proximal convoluted tubule denotes small basal processes. (×8200.) (From Madsen KM, Brenner BM: Structure and function of the renal tubule and interstitium, in Tisher CC, Brenner BM [editors]: *Renal pathology with clinical and functional correlations,* Philadelphia, 1989, JB Lippincott, p 606.)

are disk-shaped rather than beltlike in configuration, and they are responsible for cell-cell adhesion.

Gap junctions are present in small numbers in mammalian and invertebrate renal proximal tubules.[144] They are specialized connections between adjacent cells where the plasma membranes are separated by a 2-nm gap that contains characteristic subunits. The gap junction is believed to provide a pathway for the movement of ions between cells and for cell-cell communication. These functions of the gap junction are likely to be mediated by a family of proteins known as *connexins.*[145]

The intercellular space is open toward the basement membrane, which separates it from the peritubular interstitium and capillaries. The thickness of the basement membrane gradually decreases along the proximal tubule. In the rhesus monkey, it

decreases in thickness from approximately 250 nm in the S1 segment to 145 nm in the S2 segment and to only 70 nm in the S3 segment.[136] In the rat, the basement membrane of the proximal convoluted tubule was found to be 143 nm in thickness.[146] The lateral cell processes and invaginations of the plasma membrane serve to increase the intercellular space and the area of the basolateral plasma membrane, where the sodium–potassium–adenosine triphosphatase (Na^+–K^+–adenosine triphosphatase [ATPase]) or Na^+ pump is located.[147,148]

Morphometric studies of the proximal convoluted tubule in the rabbit have demonstrated that the area of the lateral surface equals that of the luminal surface and amounts to 2.9 mm^2/mm of tubule.[149] Elongated mitochondria are located in the lateral cell processes in close proximity to the plasma membrane (see Figure 2-23), an arrangement that is characteristic of epithelia involved in active ion transport. With standard transmission electron microscopy, these organelles appear rod-shaped and tortuous; however, studies using high-voltage electron microscopy have revealed that many mitochondria in the proximal tubule are branched and anastomose with one another.[150]

A system of smooth membranes, called the *paramembranous cisternal system,* is often observed between the plasma membrane and the mitochondria. The function of the paramembranous cisternal system is not known, but studies suggest that it is in continuity with the smooth endoplasmic reticulum.[151] The cells throughout the proximal tubule contain large quantities of smooth and rough endoplasmic reticulum, and free ribosomes are also abundant in the cytoplasm. A well-developed Golgi apparatus is located above and lateral to the nucleus in the midregion of the cell. It is composed of four basic elements: smooth-surfaced sacs or cisternae, coated vesicles, uncoated vesicles, and larger vacuoles. The cisternae form parallel stacks that possess a convex surface, the *cis* side, and a concave surface, the *trans* side, from which small coated vesicles appear to bud off (Figure 2-24).

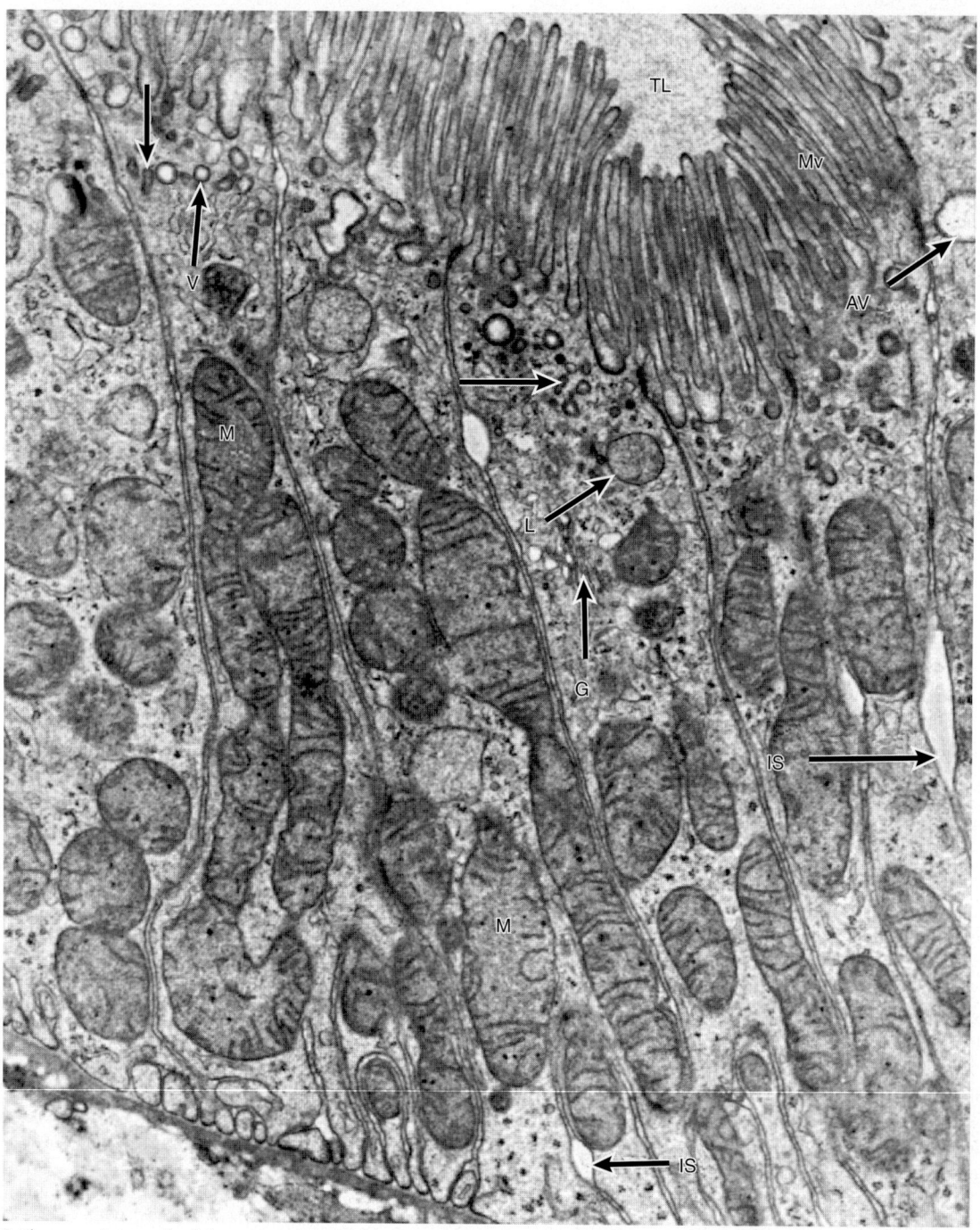

FIGURE 2-23 Electron micrograph of the pars convoluta of the proximal tubule from a normal human kidney. The mitochondria (M) are elongated and tortuous, occasionally doubling back on themselves. The endocytic apparatus, composed of apical vacuoles (AV), apical vesicles (V), and apical dense tubules (*arrows*), is well developed. (×15,000.) G, Golgi apparatus; IS, intercellular space; L, lysosome; Mv, microvilli forming the brush border; TL, tubule lumen.

An extensive system of microtubules is located throughout the cytoplasm of the proximal tubule cells. A well-developed brush border forms the apical or luminal surface of the proximal convoluted tubule. It is formed by numerous finger-like projections of the apical plasma membrane, the microvilli (see Figures 2-18 through 2-20). Morphometric studies performed on isolated segments of rabbit proximal convoluted tubules found that the brush border increases the apical cell surface 36-fold.[149] On cross section, 6 to 10 filaments, approximately 6 nm in diameter, can be seen within individual microvilli, often extending downward into the apical region of the cell for considerable distances. A network of filaments, called the *terminal web,* is located in the apical cytoplasm just beneath and perpendicular to the microvilli.[152] The filaments of the microvilli are actin filaments. Immunocytochemical studies have demonstrated the presence of the cytoskeletal proteins villin and fimbrin in the microvillar core, whereas myosin and spectrin are found in the terminal web.[153]

It is well established that the protein composition of the brush border membrane is different from that of the basolateral membrane.[154] Biochemical studies have reported the presence

of alkaline phosphatase, aminopeptidase, 5′-nucleotidase, and Mg^{2+}-ATPase activity within brush border membranes from the kidney cortex, whereas while Na^+-K^+-ATPase is present in the basolateral plasma membrane.[154] Furthermore, immunocytochemical studies have demonstrated microdomains with different glycoproteins in brush border membranes. The protein megalin (Heymann's nephritis antigen or gp330) is located mainly in the apical invaginations between the microvilli, whereas maltase, a disaccharidase, is concentrated on the microvilli.[155] Ecto-5′-nucleotidase, which is involved in the generation of adenosine, is also expressed in the brush border of the proximal tubule.[156]

The pars convoluta of the proximal tubule contains a well-developed endocytic-lysosomal apparatus that is involved in the reabsorption and degradation of macromolecules from the ultrafiltrate.[157] The endocytic compartment consists of an extensive system of coated pits, small coated vesicles, apical dense tubules, and larger endocytic vacuoles without a cytoplasmic coat (Figure 2-25). The coated pits are invaginations of the apical plasma membrane at the base of the microvilli that form the brush border. The cytoplasmic coat of the small

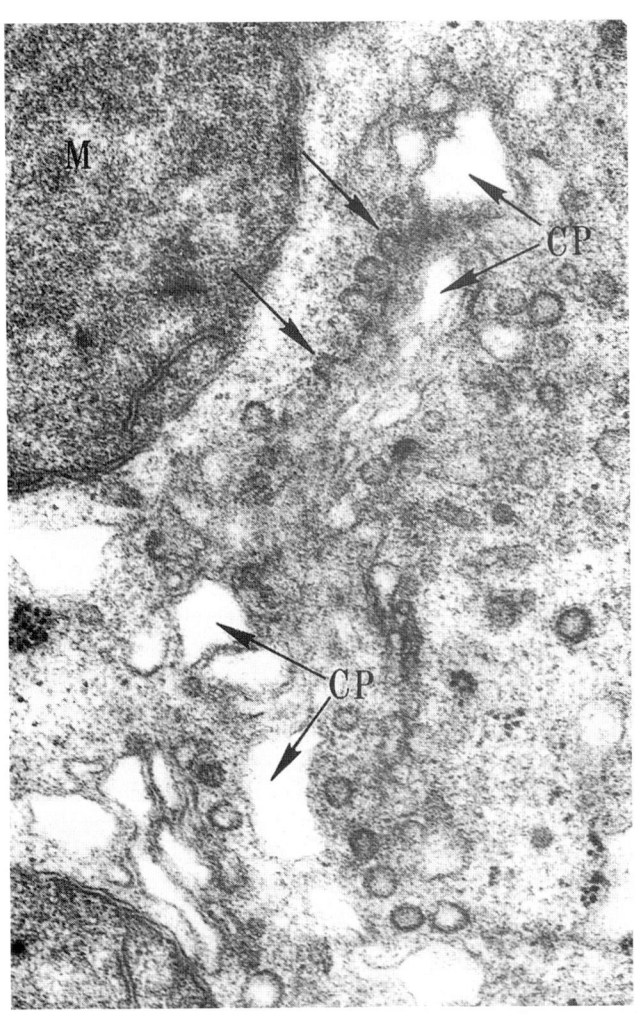

FIGURE 2-24 Electron micrograph of a Golgi apparatus from a normal human proximal tubule. Small vesicles (*arrows*) consistent with the appearance of primary lysosomes are seen budding from the larger cisternal profiles (CP). M, Mitochondrion. (×32,900.) (From Tisher CC, Bulger RE, Trump BF: Human renal ultrastructure. I. Proximal tubule of healthy individuals, *Lab Invest* 15:1357, 1966.)

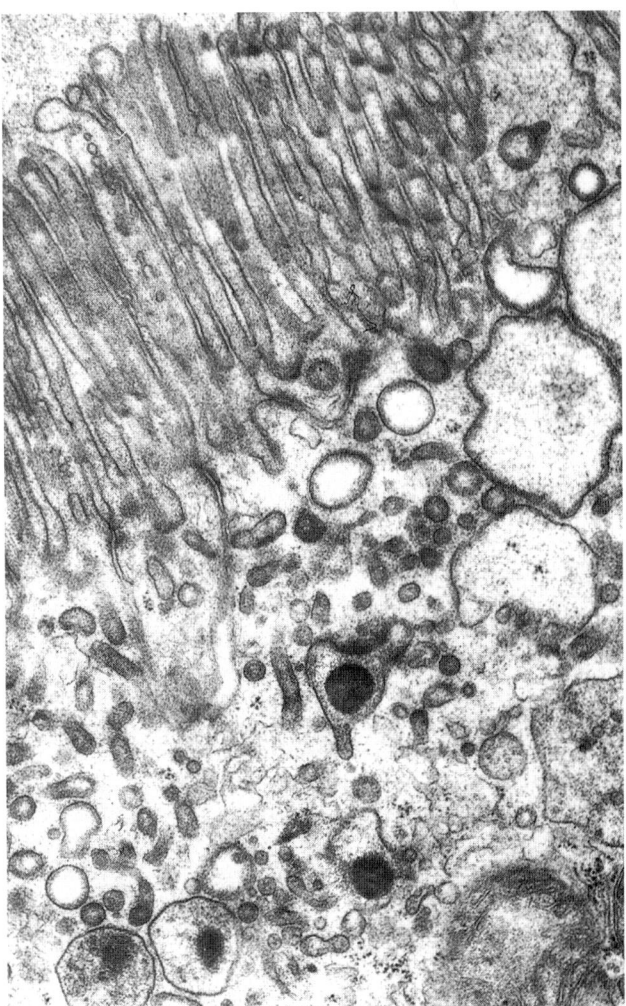

FIGURE 2-25 Transmission electron micrograph of the apical region of a human proximal tubule illustrating the endocytic apparatus, including coated pits, coated vesicles, apical dense tubules, and endosomes. (×18,500.)

vesicles is similar in ultrastructure to the coat that is present on the cytoplasmic side of the coated pits. Immunocytochemical studies have demonstrated that this coat contains clathrin[158] and megalin,[155,159] proteins involved in receptor-mediated endocytosis.

A large number of lysosomes are present in the proximal convoluted tubule. Lysosomes are membrane-bound, heterogeneous organelles that contain a variety of acid hydrolases, including acid phosphatase, and various proteases, lipases, and glycosidases (Figure 2-26).[157,160] They vary considerably in size, shape, and ultrastructural appearance. Lysosomes are involved in the degradation of material absorbed by endocytosis (heterophagocytosis), and they often contain multiple electron-dense deposits that are believed to represent reabsorbed substances such as proteins (see Figure 2-26). Lysosomes also play a role in the normal turnover of intracellular constituents by autophagocytosis, and autophagic vacuoles containing fragments of cell organelles are often seen in the proximal tubule (see Figure 2-26).[160] Lysosomes containing nondigestible residues are called *residual bodies,* and they can empty their contents into the tubule lumen by exocytosis. Multivesicular bodies that are part of the vacuolar-lysosomal system are often observed in the cytoplasm of the proximal convoluted tubule. They are believed to be involved in membrane retrieval and/or membrane disposal.

Biochemical studies in combination with immunohistochemical studies have demonstrated the presence of an electrogenic H^+ pump (H^+-ATPase) in endosomes and the apical plasma membrane of the proximal tubule.[161,162]

The vacuolar-lysosomal system plays an important role in the reabsorption and degradation of albumin and low-molecular-weight plasma proteins from the glomerular filtrate.[157,163,164] Proteins are absorbed from the tubule lumen by endocytosis or pinocytosis (Figure 2-27). By this process, the protein becomes located in invaginations of the apical plasma membrane—the so-called coated pits—which pinch off to form small coated vesicles. The coated vesicles fuse with endosomes, and the absorbed protein is transferred through the endosomal compartment to the lysosomes, where it is catabolized by proteolytic enzymes. The apical dense tubules are part of the vacuolar system and are believed to be involved in the recycling of membrane back to the luminal surface.[165]

Under normal conditions, the vacuolar-lysosomal system is most prominent in the S1 segment.[131,132] In proteinuric states, however, with large amounts of protein being presented to the proximal tubule cells, large vacuoles—so-called protein droplets—and lysosomes can be observed in the proximal tubule, especially in the S2 segment. In agreement with these ultrastructural observations, biochemical studies of individual tubule segments have demonstrated that under normal nonproteinuric conditions, the activity of the lysosomal proteolytic enzymes cathepsin B and cathepsin L is significantly higher in the S1 segment than in the S2 and S3 segments of the proximal tubule.[131,166] In proteinuric conditions, the activity of cathepsins B and L in the proximal tubule is increased, and activity is highest in the S2 segment.[166]

Studies in the isolated perfused rat kidney,[167] in vivo micropuncture studies,[168] and studies using isolated perfused rabbit proximal tubule[169,170] have provided evidence that the absorption of protein by the proximal tubule is a selective process

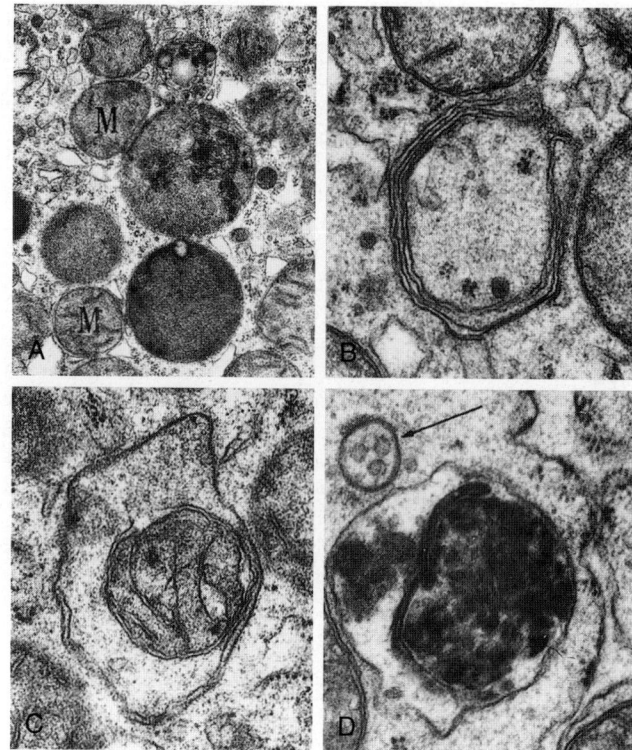

FIGURE 2-26 Electron micrographs illustrating the appearance of different types of lysosomes from human proximal tubules. **A,** Lysosomes. Several mitochondria (M) are also shown. (×15,500.) **B,** Early stage of formation of an autophagic vacuole. (×23,500.) **C,** Fully formed autolysosome containing a mitochondrion undergoing digestion. (×28,500.) **D,** Autolysosome containing a microbody undergoing digestion. A multivesicular body (*arrow*) is also shown. (×29,250.) (From Tisher CC, Bulger RE, Trump BF: Human renal ultrastructure. I. Proximal tubule of healthy individuals, *Lab Invest* 15:1357, 1966.)

determined by the net charge, size, and configuration of the protein molecule and possibly by the presence of preferential endocytic sites on the apical plasma membrane.

Based on studies by Farquhar and colleagues[171] and by Christensen and Birn,[172] it is now generally accepted that the reabsorption of numerous proteins and polypeptides by the proximal tubule is mediated by megalin, a multiligand endocytic receptor. Kerjaschki and Farquhar[159] purified megalin (gp330) from rat kidney brush border membrane and demonstrated that it represents the antigen for Heymann's nephritis in rats. Megalin was subsequently cloned and found to be a 600-kDa glycoprotein belonging to the low-density lipoprotein receptor gene family.[173] Immunocytochemical studies have demonstrated that megalin is located in the brush border, coated pits, endocytic vesicles, and apical dense tubules in the proximal tubule, particularly in the S2 segment (Figure 2-28).[155,174,175] As reviewed in detail by Christensen and Birn,[172] megalin serves as a receptor for numerous ligands, including low-molecular-weight proteins,[176] polypeptide hormones,[176] albumin,[177] vitamin-binding proteins,[178-180] and polybasic drugs such as aminoglycosides.[181] Orlando and colleagues[176] demonstrated that megalin binds and internalizes insulin, and evidence was also provided from ligand blotting assays that megalin serves as a receptor for various low-molecular-weight polypeptides, including β_2-microglobulin, lysozyme, prolactin, cytochrome C, and epidermal growth factor. Moestrup and colleagues[178-180] demonstrated that

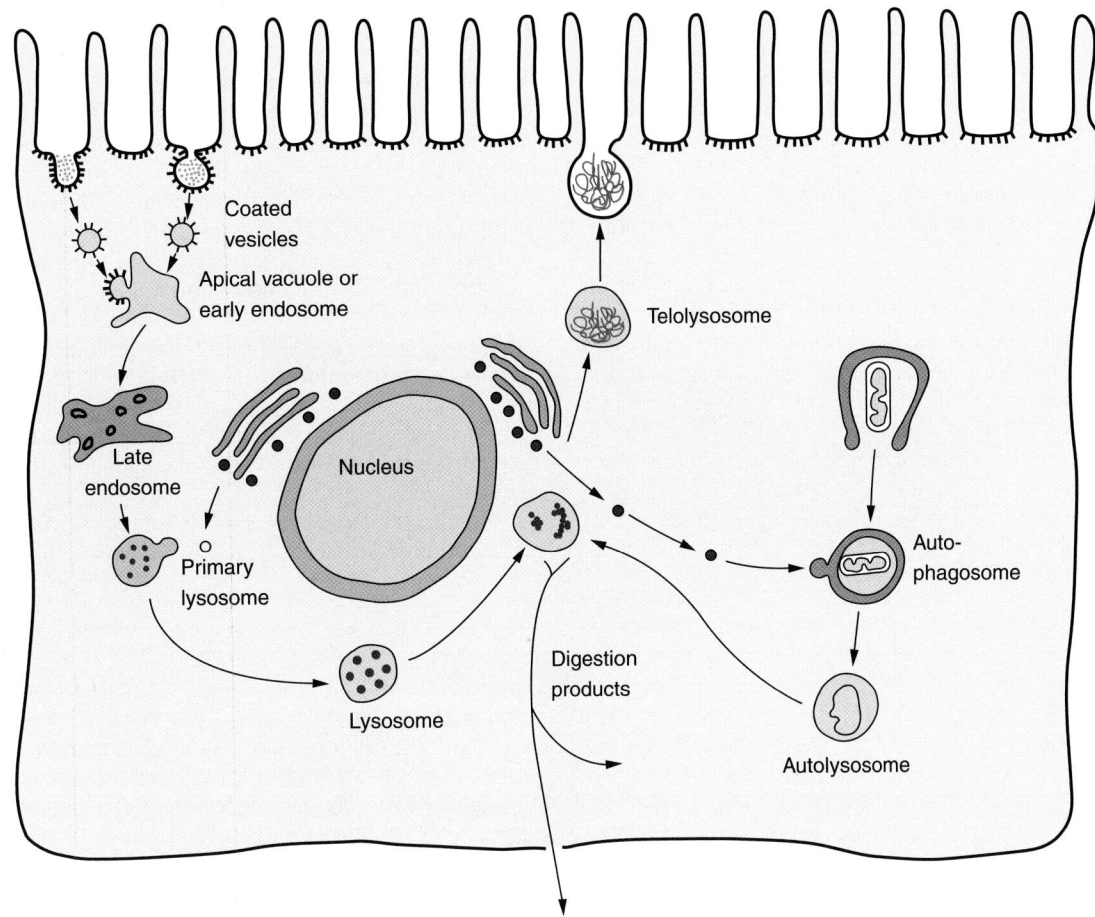

FIGURE 2-27 Schematic drawing of the endocytic-lysosomal system in a proximal tubule cell.

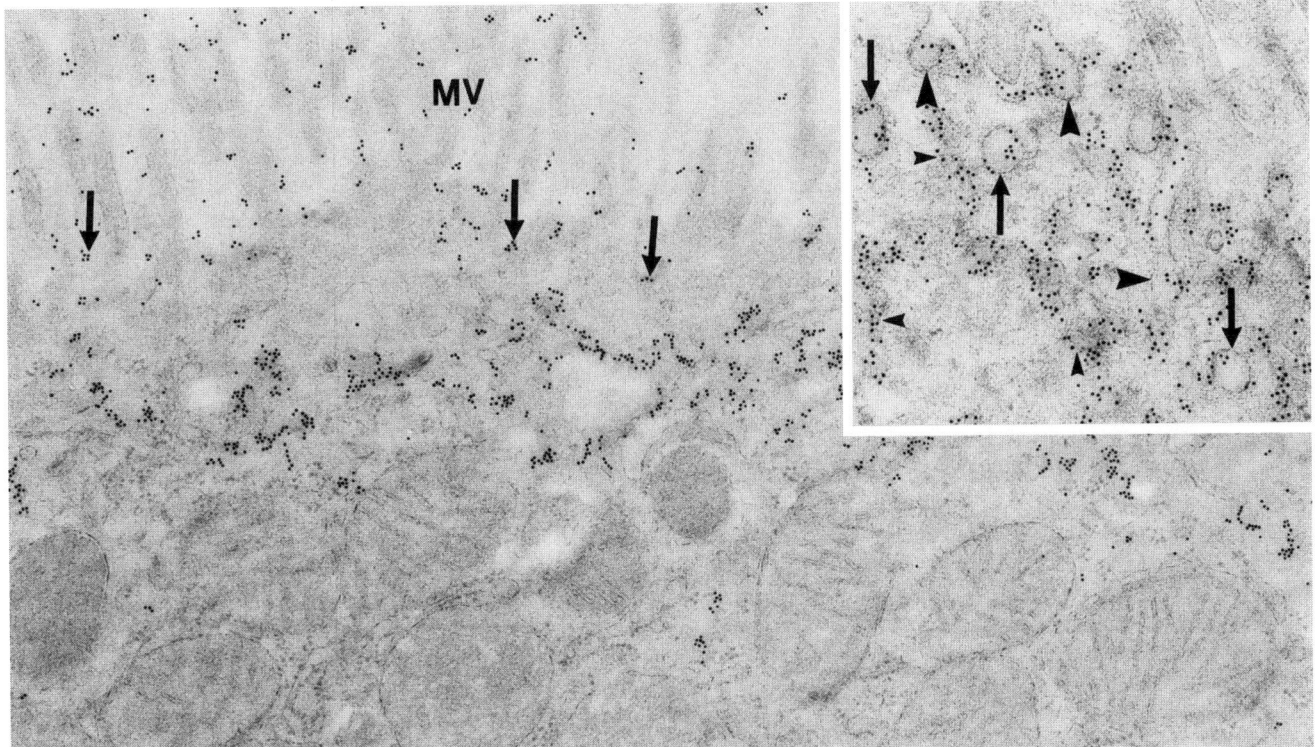

FIGURE 2-28 Transmission electron micrograph illustrating immunogold localization of megalin in a proximal tubule cell from normal mouse kidney. Labeling of megalin is seen on microvilli (MV), coated pits (*arrows*), and the apical endocytic apparatus. (×35,000.) *Inset* is a higher-magnification micrograph illustrating the labeling of coated pits (*large arrowheads*), apical endosomes (*arrows*), and apical dense tubules (*small arrowheads*). (×53,000.) (From Christensen EI, Willnow TE: Essential role of megalin in renal proximal tubule for vitamin homeostasis, *J Am Soc Nephrol* 10:2224, 1999.)

megalin serves as the principal receptor for the carrier proteins of various vitamins, including vitamin B_{12}, vitamin D, and retinol, which suggests that megalin may play a role in vitamin metabolism and homeostasis.[182] Other studies demonstrated a loss of components of the endocytic apparatus and increased excretion of low-molecular-weight proteins in the urine of megalin-deficient mice, findings that provide further support for the role of megalin in proximal tubule reabsorption of protein.[182,183]

A second multiligand endocytic receptor, cubilin, which is identical to the intestinal intrinsic factor–cobalamin receptor, has been identified in the proximal tubule.[172,184] Cubilin is a 460-kDa glycoprotein that binds to megalin. It is expressed in the brush border and in the endocytic compartment in a pattern similar to that of megalin.[172] Cubilin binds several ligands present in the glomerular ultrafiltrate, including albumin and various vitamin-binding proteins, and both megalin and cubilin are essential for the reabsorption of these proteins in the proximal tubule.[184,185]

Pars Recta

The pars recta of the proximal tubule consists of the terminal portion of the S2 segment and the entire S3 segment. The epithelium of the S3 segment is simpler than that of the S1 and S2 segments.[132,134] Basolateral invaginations of the plasma membrane are virtually absent, mitochondria are small and randomly scattered throughout the cytoplasm, and the intercellular spaces are smaller and less complex (Figure 2-29; see also Figure 2-20). These morphologic characteristics are in agreement with the results of biochemical studies demonstrating that Na$^+$-K$^+$-ATPase activity is significantly lower in the pars recta than in the pars convoluta.[186] In addition, studies examining transport parameters in individual segments of the proximal tubule have demonstrated that fluid reabsorption is significantly less in the S3 segment than in the S1 and S2 segments.[187]

The morphologic appearance of the pars recta varies considerably among species. In the rat, the microvilli of the brush

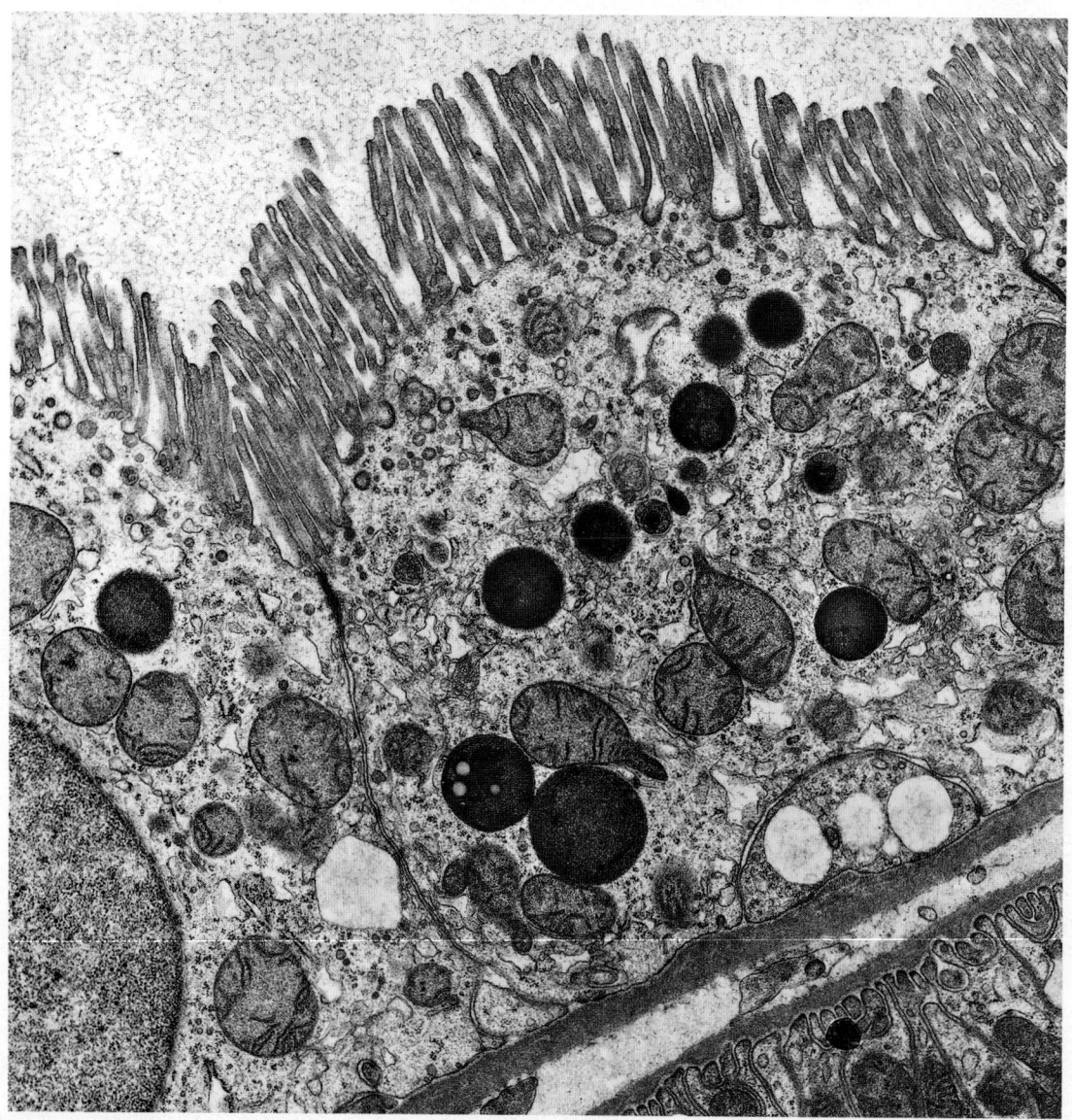

FIGURE 2-29 Low-magnification electron micrograph of a segment of the pars recta of a proximal tubule from human kidney. The microvilli on the convex apical cell surface are not as long as those in the pars recta of the rat. The lysosomes are extremely electron dense. The clear, single membrane–limited structures at the base of the cell to the right represent lipid droplets. (×10,400.) (Courtesy of R. E. Bulger, PhD.)

border measure up to 4 µm in length, whereas in the rabbit and human kidney they are much shorter. The vacuolar-lysosomal system is less prominent in the S3 segment of the proximal tubule. However, in both rabbit and human, many small lysosomes with electron-dense membrane-like material are common in the S3 segment.[131,133] The specific role of lysosomes in this segment is not known. Peroxisomes are common in the pars recta. In contrast to lysosomes, the peroxisomes are surrounded by a 6.5-nm-thick membrane and do not contain acid hydrolases.[160] Peroxisomes are irregular in shape and vary considerably in appearance among species. In the rat, small, circular profiles can be observed just inside the limiting membrane, and rod-shaped structures often project outward from the organelle. In addition, a small nucleoid is often present in peroxisomes in the rat proximal tubule. The functional significance of the peroxisomes in the kidney is not known with certainty; however, they are believed to be involved in lipid metabolism and to play a role in fatty acid oxidation. They have a high content of catalase, which is involved in the degradation of hydrogen peroxide, and of various oxidative enzymes, including L-α-hydroxy acid oxidase and D-amino acid oxidase.[188,189]

The proximal convoluted tubule plays a major role in the reabsorption of Na^+, HCO_3^-, Cl^-, K^+, Ca^{2+}, PO_4^{3-}, water, and organic solutes such as vitamins, glucose, and amino acids. Approximately 70% of the ultrafiltrate is reabsorbed in the proximal tubule. Fluid reabsorption is coupled to the active transport of Na^+, and little change occurs in the osmolality or in the Na^+ concentration of the tubule fluid along the proximal tubule, which indicates that fluid reabsorption in this segment is isosmotic.[190] The rate of fluid absorption from the proximal tubule to the peritubular capillaries is influenced by the hydraulic and oncotic pressures across the tubule and capillary wall. Changes in these parameters cause significant ultrastructural changes in the proximal tubule, especially in the configuration of the lateral intercellular spaces.[191,192]

In the early 1990s Preston and colleagues cloned a water channel protein, CHIP28 or aquaporin-1 (AQP1), from human erythrocytes.[193,194] AQP1 is believed to mediate osmotic water permeability in red blood cells as well as in some renal tubule cells. Immunocytochemical studies[195-197] using antibodies to AQP1 demonstrated the presence of this water channel protein in the proximal tubule (Figure 2-30), the descending thin limb, and the vasa recta. Recent studies demonstrated that AQP1 is not localized to descending limbs of short-looped nephrons, but is expressed in long-looped nephrons.[198] In these segments, labeling was observed in both the apical and the basolateral plasma membrane, which indicates that water is reabsorbed across the epithelium through these channels in response to the osmotic gradient generated by NaCl reabsorption (see Chapter 10). The importance of AQP1 in water reabsorption is highlighted by studies in knockout mice.[199,200]

Sodium reabsorption by the proximal tubule is an active process driven by the basolateral Na^+-K^+-ATPase. The active transport of Na^+ out of the cell across the basolateral membrane creates a lumen-to-cell concentration gradient for Na^+. The transport of various anions and organic solutes is coupled with the transport of Na^+ down its concentration gradient.[201] HCO_3^- reabsorption takes place primarily in the early proximal tubule. The mechanisms involve luminal conversion of secreted H^+ and filtered HCO_3^- to form CO_2 and H_2O.

The reverse reaction takes place in the cytosol of the proximal tubule cell aided by intracellular carbonic anhydrase II. HCO_3^- is extruded across the basolateral membrane and H^+ is recycled to the lumen. This H^+ secretion is mediated predominantly by an Na^+/H^+ exchange mechanism located in the brush border membrane.[202,203] Studies in several laboratories have demonstrated expression of the Na^+/H^+ exchanger isoform 3 (NHE3) in the brush border of the proximal tubule.[204,205] In addition, there is evidence that active H^+ secretion mediated by an H^+-ATPase occurs in the proximal tubule.[206] An H^+-ATPase has been demonstrated in brush border membrane vesicles[207] as well as in endosome vesicles isolated from the kidney cortex.[161] Studies in mice lacking NHE3 have confirmed the importance of NHE3 for bicarbonate and fluid reabsorption in the proximal convoluted tubule.[208,209] The expression and activity of NHE3 are regulated by various hormones, including parathyroid hormone, angiotensin II, and aldosterone.[210,211]

Basolateral bicarbonate extrusion is the final step in proximal tubule HCO_3^- reabsorption and is mediated by an electrogenic sodium-bicarbonate cotransporter, NBCe1, with a stoichiometry of 3 HCO_3^- ions for each Na^+ ion.[212,213] Sodium-bicarbonate cotransporter 1 (NBC1) belongs to a superfamily of bicarbonate transporters that includes the anion exchangers and the sodium-bicarbonate cotransporters.[214] NBCe1 in the proximal tubule was the first sodium-bicarbonate cotransporter to be identified. It was cloned initially from *Ambystoma*[215] and later from both human[216] and rat kidney.[217] In situ hybridization studies in the rabbit kidney demonstrated that NBCe1 mRNA was present only in the renal cortex, where it was localized to the proximal tubule.[218] Subsequent immunofluorescence studies in rat and rabbit[219] and high-resolution electron microscopic studies in the rat kidney[220] revealed that NBCe1 was expressed exclusively in the basolateral plasma membrane of the S1 and S2 segments of the proximal tubule (Figure 2-31). Humans with mutations in NBCe1 develop permanent proximal renal tubular acidosis with associated ocular abnormalities consistent with NBCe1's being the primary pathway for basolateral bicarbonate transport.[221]

The proximal tubule is a major site of ammonia production in the kidney.[222-224] Ammonia is produced in the mitochondria from the metabolism of glutamine. At the pH that exists in the proximal tubule cells, ammonia combines with H^+ to form NH_4^+, which is secreted into the tubule lumen.[225] The pars recta of the proximal tubule can also secrete organic anions and cations, and it is a portion of the nephron that is often damaged by nephrotoxic compounds, including various drugs and heavy metals. Woodhall and colleagues[135] examined the secretion of *p*-aminohippuric acid, an organic anion, in individual S1, S2, and S3 segments of superficial and juxtamedullary proximal tubules of the rabbit and found that secretion was significantly higher in the S2 segment of both nephron populations. In similar studies of organic cation transport, McKinney[226] demonstrated that the secretion of procainamide was greatest in S1 segments of superficial nephrons and in S1 and S2 segments of juxtamedullary nephrons.

Studies at several laboratories have identified a family of transporters involved in the uptake of organic anions and cations across the basolateral membrane into the cells of the proximal tubule.[227] The organic ion transporters play an important role in the excretion of numerous commonly used

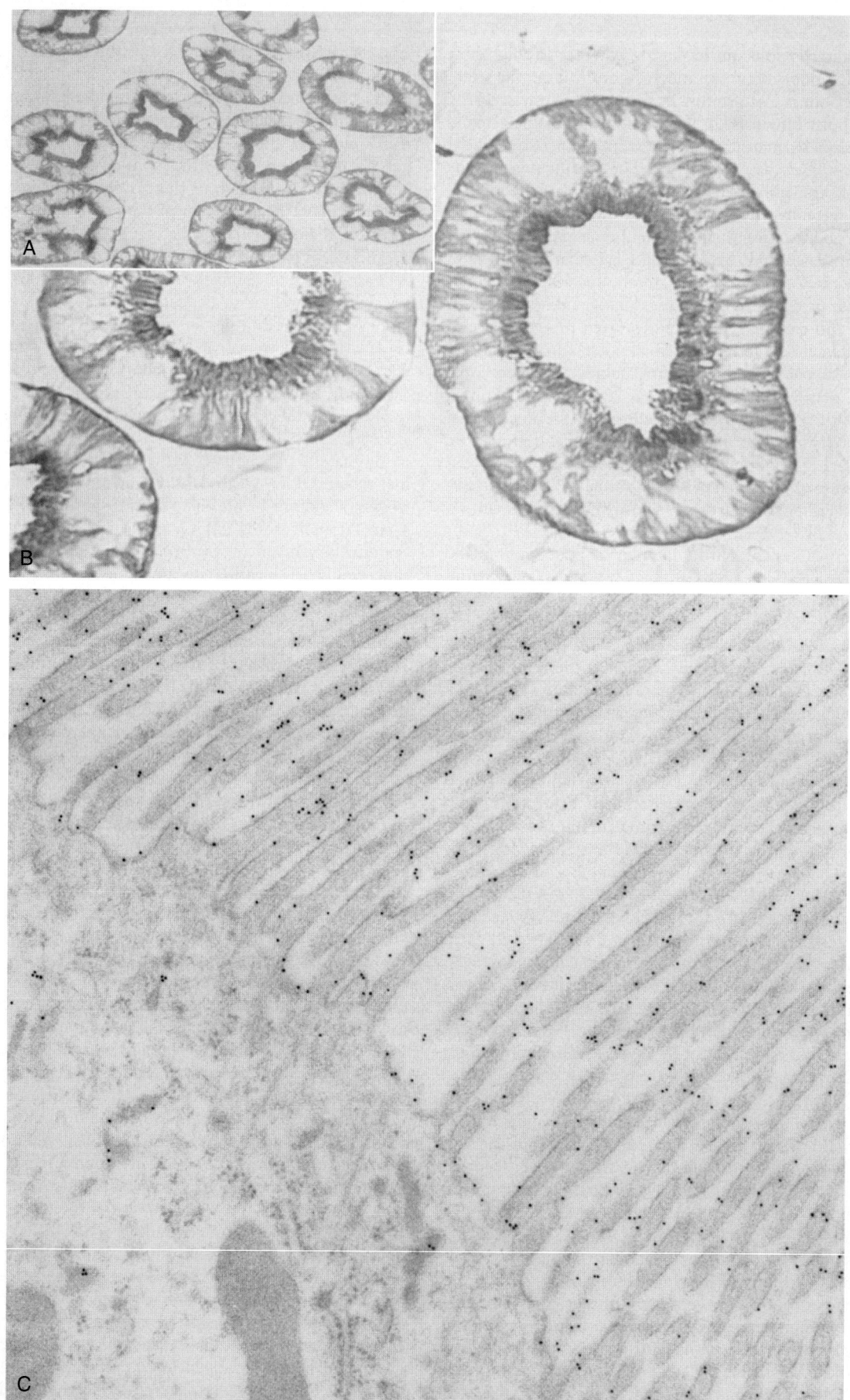

FIGURE 2-30 Immunolocalization of aquaporin-1 water channels in the rat proximal tubule. **A** and **B,** Light micrographs of cryosections, illustrating immunostaining of the apical and basolateral plasma membrane of the S3 segment of the proximal tubule with use of a horseradish peroxidase technique. (**A,** ×670; **B,** ×800.) **C,** Electron micrograph of cryosubstituted Lowicryl section, illustrating immunogold labeling of microvilli and apical invaginations of the S3 segment of the proximal tubule. (×48,000.)

drugs, including various antibiotics, nonsteroidal antiinflammatory drugs, loop diuretics, and the immunosuppressive drug cyclosporine.[227] The uptake of organic anions, including *p*-aminohippuric acid, from the blood into the proximal tubule cells is mediated by an organic anion transporter, OAT1.[228-230] In the kidney, OAT1 is present only in the basolateral plasma membrane of the proximal tubule, and in the rat, OAT1 is expressed predominantly in the S2 segment of the proximal tubule.[231] Organic cation transporters OCT1 and OCT2 have also been demonstrated in the proximal tubule of the rat.[232] By in situ hybridization, expression of both OCT1 and OCT2 was detected in all three segments of the proximal tubule. By immunohistochemical study, OCT1 was observed to be located mainly in S1 and S2 segments, whereas OCT2 was expressed in S2 and S3 segments.[232]

AQP11 is a channel protein with unusual pore-forming NPA (asparagine-proline-alanine) boxes.[233] Immunocytochemical studies have demonstrated intracellular expression of AQP11 in the proximal tubule.[234] A predominantly intracellular expression has also been reported in other cell types, including cells in the brain.[235] AQP11-null mice exhibit vacuolization and cyst formation of the proximal tubule.[234]

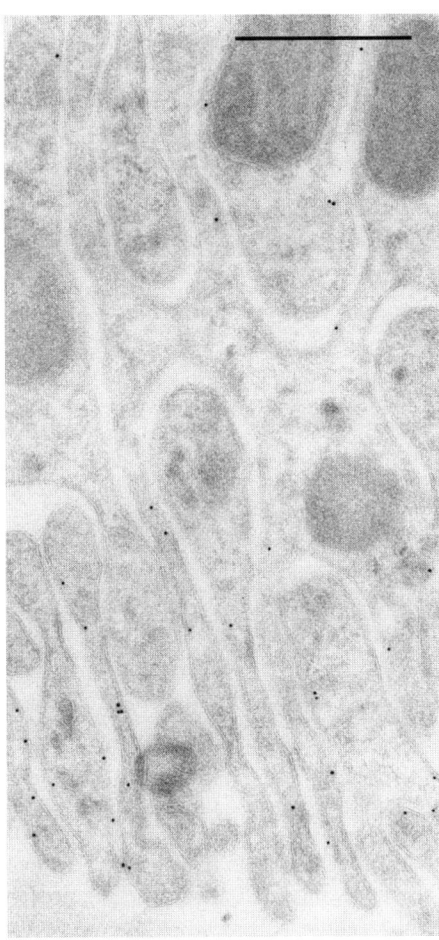

FIGURE 2-31 Transmission electron micrograph illustrating immunogold localization of sodium-bicarbonate cotransporter 1 (NBC1) in the basal part of a proximal convoluted tubule cell from normal rat kidney. Labeling of NBC1 is seen on the cytoplasmic side of the basolateral plasma membrane. (×68,000.) (From Maunsbach AB, Vorum H, Kwon TH, et al: Immunoelectron microscopic localization of the electrogenic Na/HCO₃ cotransporter in rat and *Ambystoma* kidney, *J Am Soc Nephrol* 11:2179, 2000.)

The mice appeared normal at birth, but developed polycystic kidneys and died before weaning due to advanced renal failure. Interestingly, primary cultured proximal tubule cells from AQP11-null mice exhibited an endosomal acidification defect. However, the physiologic role of AQP11 in the proximal tubule remains to be identified. AQP7, an aquaglyceroporin, is expressed exclusively in the pars recta brush border.[236,237] AQP7 knockout mice fail to reabsorb glycerol and exhibit marked glyceroluria,[238] which indicates a role for AQP7 in glycerol reabsorption.

Thin Limb of the Loop of Henle

The transition from the proximal tubule to the descending thin limb of the loop of Henle is abrupt (Figures 2-32 and 2-33) and marks the boundary between the outer and inner stripes of the outer medulla. Short-looped nephrons originating from superficial and midcortical glomeruli have a short descending thin limb located in the inner stripe of the outer medulla. Close to the hairpin turn of the short loops of Henle, the thin limb continues into the thick ascending limb. Long-looped nephrons originating from juxtamedullary glomeruli have a long descending thin limb that extends into the inner medulla and a long ascending thin limb that continues into the thick ascending limb. The transition from the thin to the thick ascending limb forms the boundary between the outer and inner medulla (see Figure 2-5). Nephrons arising in the extreme outer cortex may possess short cortical loops that do not extend into the medulla. Variations on this basic organization have been demonstrated; studies have also highlighted the interspecies variability in nephron organization.[9,12,198]

The histotopographic organization of the renal medulla has been studied in several laboratory animals, including recent three-dimensional reconstruction studies of the nephron.[9,12] These studies have highlighted the complexity of the organization of the medulla and are discussed in Chapter 10. Early ultrastructural studies demonstrated that the cells of the initial part of the descending thin limb of Henle were complex because of extensive interdigitation with one another, whereas the cells of the ascending thin limb near the transition with the thick ascending limb, and thin limb cells in the inner medulla, were less complex in configuration.

Dieterich and associates[239] later described the presence of four types of epithelia (types I through IV) in the thin limbs of the mouse kidney and devised a classification based on the ultrastructural characteristics of the cells and their location within the different regions of the medulla. Subsequent studies in other species, including rat,[240] rabbit,[134] hamster,[241] and *Psammomys obesus*,[242,243] confirmed the existence of four morphologically distinct segments in the thin limb of Henle (Figure 2-34). In these animals, type I epithelium is found exclusively in the descending thin limb of short-looped nephrons. Type II epithelium forms the descending thin limb of long-looped nephrons in the outer medulla. This epithelium gives way to type III epithelium in the inner medulla. Type IV epithelium forms the bends of the long loops and the entire ascending thin limb to the transition into the thick ascending limb at the boundary between the inner and outer medulla.

In all animals studied thus far, type I epithelium is extremely thin and has few basal or luminal surface specializations, the latter in the form of microvilli (see Figure 2-34).

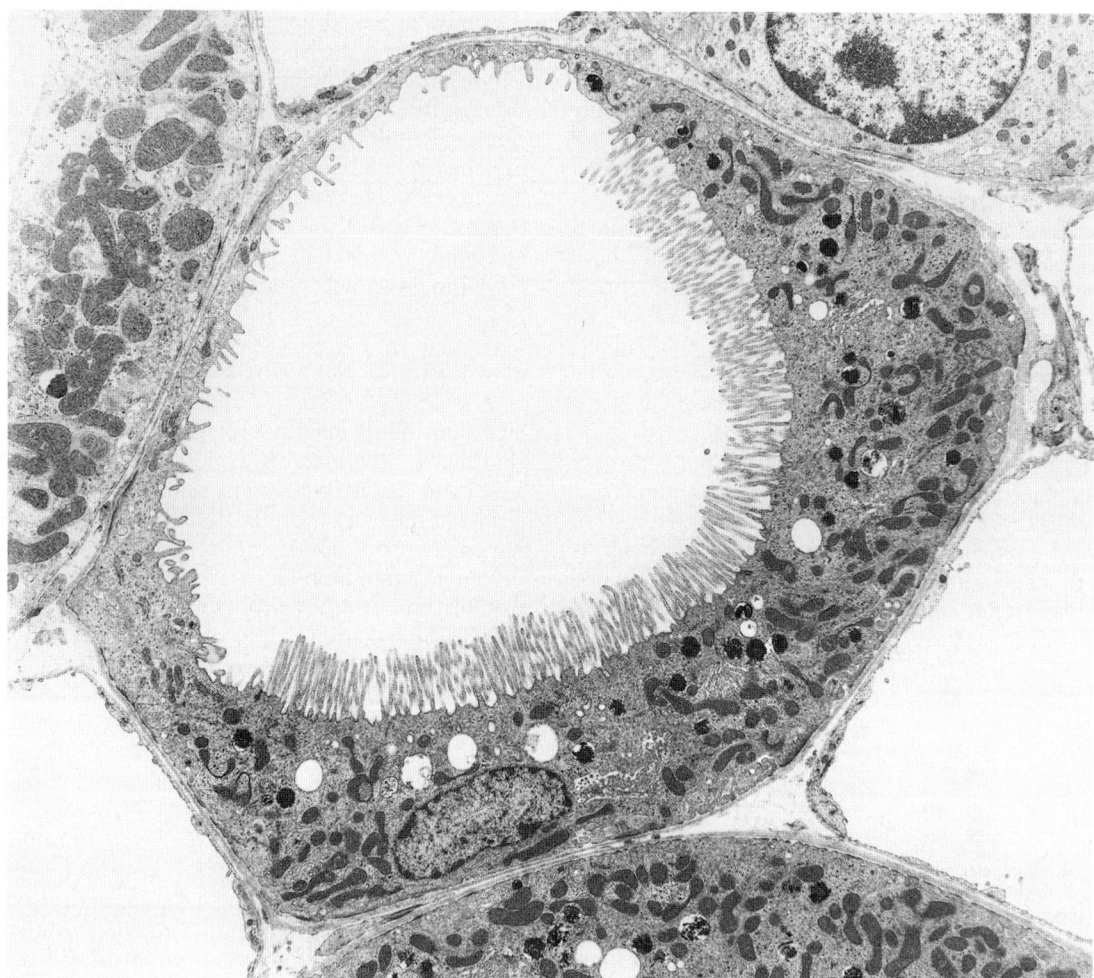

FIGURE 2-32 Transmission electron micrograph of rabbit kidney illustrating the transition from the pars recta of the proximal tubule to the descending thin limb of the loop of Henle. (×4500.) (From Madsen KM, Park CH: Lysosome distribution and cathepsin B and L activity along the rabbit proximal tubule, *Am J Physiol* 253:F1290-F1301, 1987.)

There is a virtual absence of lateral interdigitations with adjacent cells, and cellular organelles are relatively sparse. Microbodies have not been identified in the thin limbs of the loop of Henle. Tight junctions between cells are intermediate in depth with several junctional strands, which suggests a tight epithelium.[244-246]

Type II epithelium is taller and exhibits considerable species differences. In the rat,[247] mouse,[239] *P. obesus*,[242] and hamster,[241] the type II epithelium is complex and characterized by extensive lateral and basal interdigitations and a well-developed paracellular pathway (Figure 2-35). The tight junctions are extremely shallow and contain a single junctional strand, which is characteristic of a "leaky" epithelium. The luminal surface is covered by short blunt microvilli, and cell organelles, including mitochondria, are more prominent than in other segments of the thin limb. In the rabbit,[134] the type II epithelium is less complex. Lateral interdigitations and paracellular pathways are less prominent, and tight junctions are deeper.[245] As in the rat and mouse, the luminal surface is covered with short microvilli, and many small mitochondria are present in the cytoplasm.

In comparison with type II epithelium, type III epithelium is lower and has a simpler structure. The cells do not interdigitate, the tight junctions are intermediate in depth, and fewer microvilli cover the luminal surface.

Type IV epithelium (see Figure 2-34) is generally low and flattened and possesses relatively few organelles. It is characterized by an absence of surface microvilli but has an abundance of lateral cell processes and interdigitations as well as prominent paracellular pathways. The tight junctions are shallow and are characteristic of a leaky epithelium.

The basement membrane of the thin limb segments varies greatly in thickness from species to species and in many animals is multilayered. Freeze-fracture studies have confirmed the structural heterogeneity along the thin limb of the loop of Henle in the rat,[246] rabbit,[245] and *P. obesus*.[244] Segmental as well as species differences were found in the number of strands and the depth of the tight junctions. The most striking finding in these studies was an extremely high density of intramembrane particles in both the luminal and the basolateral membrane of type II epithelium in all animals studied. Biochemical studies in isolated nephron segments,[248] as well as histochemical studies,[249] demonstrated significant levels of Na^+-K^+-ATPase activity in type II epithelium of the thin limb in the rat. Little or no activity was present in other segments of the rat thin limb or in any segment of the rabbit thin limb.[250] The functional significance of these observations is not known. However, physiologic studies determining the permeability properties of isolated perfused segments of

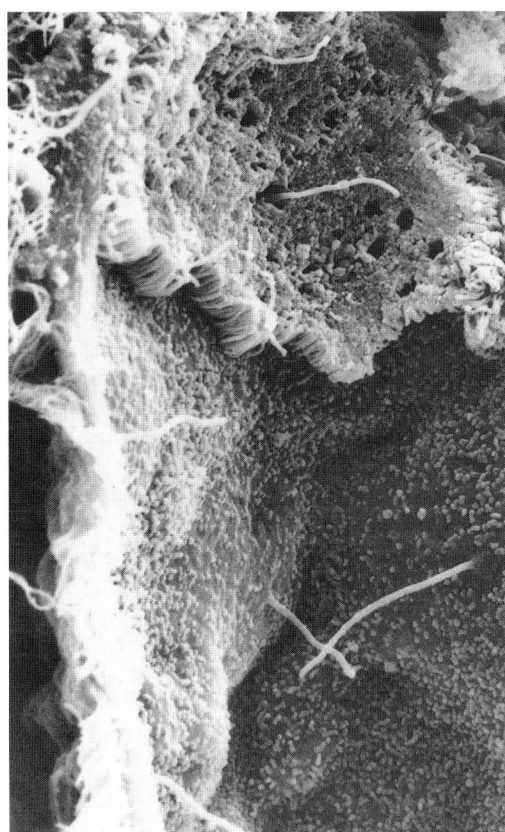

FIGURE 2-33 Scanning electron micrograph of normal rat kidney depicting the transition from the terminal S3 segment of the proximal tubule (*above*) to the early descending thin limb of Henle (*below*). Note the elongated cilia projecting into the lumen from cells of the proximal tubule and the thin limb of Henle. (×4500.)

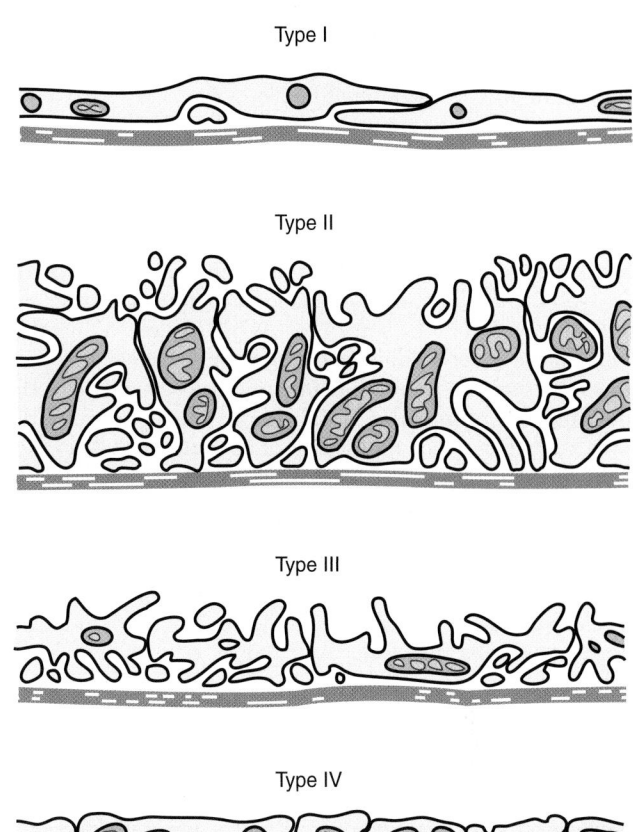

Type I

Type II

Type III

Type IV

FIGURE 2-34 Diagram depicting the appearance of the four types of thin limb segments in rat kidney. (See text for explanation.)

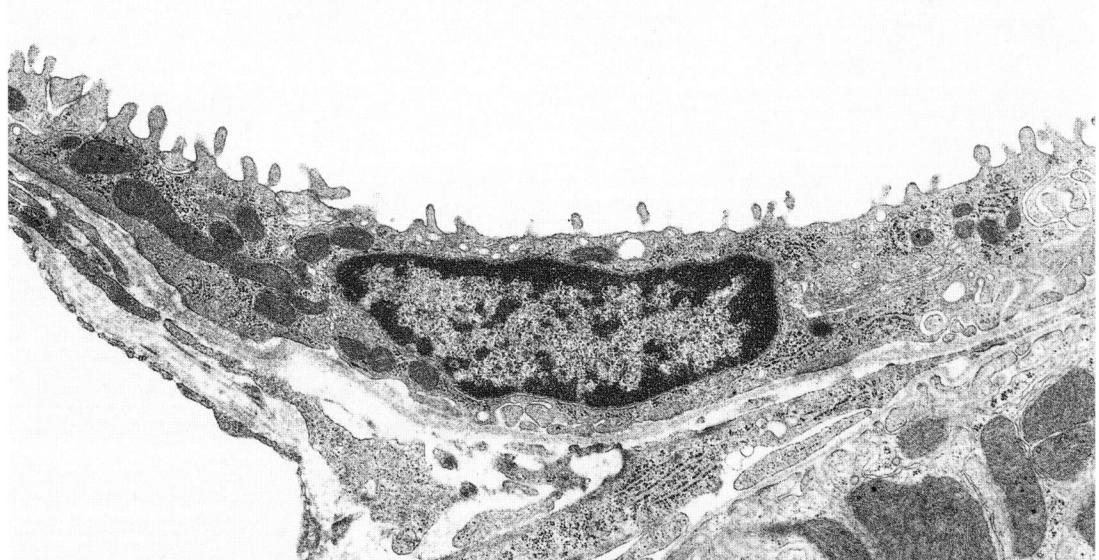

FIGURE 2-35 Transmission electron micrograph of type II epithelium of the thin limb of the loop of Henle in the inner stripe of the outer medulla of rat kidney. (×11,800.)

descending thin limbs from different species have demonstrated that the permeability of the type II epithelium to Na^+ and K^+ is higher in the rat and hamster than in the rabbit,[251] which supports the described ultrastructural and biochemical differences among species in this epithelium.

Studies of salt and water permeability in descending thin limb segments from the hamster have demonstrated that both type I and type II epithelia in this species are highly permeable to water, whereas the permeability to Na^+ and Cl^- is significantly higher in type II than in type I epithelium.[252] In contrast, urea permeability is higher in type I epithelium.[252] No evidence has been found for active transport of Na+ or Cl- in the thin limb of the loop of Henle.

In support of the reported permeability characteristics of the different thin limb segments, immunohistochemical studies have demonstrated high levels of expression of the water channel protein AQP1 in the type II epithelium of long-looped nephrons in the outer medulla (Figure 2-36).[195,253] There is no AQP1 immunoreactivity in the ascending thin limb and the type I epithelium of short-looped nephrons in mouse, rat, and human.[198] The expression of AQP1 in descending thin limbs in the inner medulla is heterogenous. Descending thin limbs that form loops more than 1 mm below the base of the inner medulla express AQP1 only in the initial portion of the segment, which leaves almost 60% of the inner medullary segment of long-looped thin descending limbs with no detectable AQP1 expression.[254] Moreover, AQP1 expression in the descending thin limbs and collecting ducts is separated into two distinct lateral compartments, which suggests that water transport may occur between these compartments.[255]

The innermost part of the thin descending limb of short-looped nephrons that lacks AQP1 does express high levels of the urea transporter UT-A2, as demonstrated at both the mRNA[256] and protein level (Figure 2-37).[257-261] There is also weak expression of UT-A2 mRNA and protein in the type III epithelium of the descending thin limb of long-looped nephrons in the outer portion of the inner medulla[256,257,259-261] upon vasopressin stimulation.[260,261] It is generally accepted that the permeability properties of the thin limb epithelium are important for the maintenance of a hypertonic interstitium. The role of the thin limb in the maintenance of a hypertonic medullary interstitium and in the dilution and concentration of the urine via countercurrent multiplication is discussed in detail in Chapter 10.

Distal Tubule

The distal tubule is composed of morphologically distinct segments: the thick ascending limb of the loop of Henle (pars recta), the macula densa, the distal convoluted tubule (pars convoluta), and the connecting tubules. Some studies[134,262] have revealed that the cortical thick ascending limb extends beyond the vicinity of the macula densa and forms an abrupt transition with the distal convoluted tubule. These data, combined with the observation that thick ascending limb proteins are not observed by immunohistochemical methods after the macula densa, suggest that the macula densa is a specialized region of the thick ascending limb.

Thick Ascending Limb

The thick ascending limb, or pars recta, represents the initial portion of the distal tubule and can be divided into a medullary and a cortical segment (see Figure 2-5). In long-looped nephrons, there is an abrupt transition from the thin ascending limb to the thick ascending limb, which marks the boundary between the inner medulla and the inner stripe of the outer medulla. In short-looped nephrons, the transition to the thick ascending limb can occur shortly before the hairpin turn, but this is not the case in all species.[12] From its transition with the thin limb, the thick ascending limb extends upward

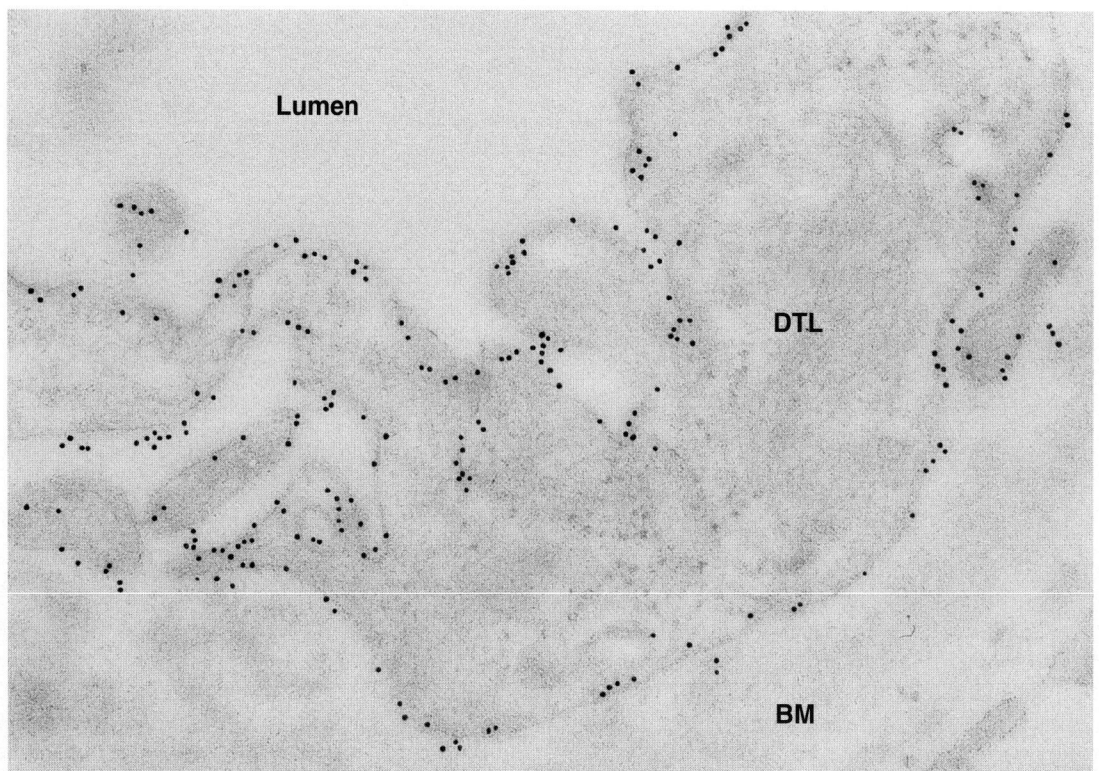

FIGURE 2-36 Transmission electron micrograph illustrating immunogold labeling of aquaporin-1 in the descending thin limb (DTL) of a long-looped nephron from rat kidney. Labeling of aquaporin-1 is seen in both the apical and basolateral plasma membrane. BM, Basement membrane. (×120,000.) (From Nielsen S, Kwon TH, Christensen BM, et al: Physiology and pathophysiology of renal aquaporins, *J Am Soc Nephrol* 10:647, 1999.)

through the outer medulla and the cortex to the glomerulus of the nephron of origin, where the macula densa is formed. At the point of contact with the extraglomerular mesangial region, only the immediately contiguous portion of the wall of the tubule actually forms the macula densa. The transition to the distal convoluted tubule occurs immediately after the macula densa.

The cells forming the medullary segment in the inner stripe of the outer medulla measure approximately 7 to 8 μm in height.[134,263] As the tubule ascends toward the cortex, cell height gradually decreases to approximately 5 μm in the cortical thick ascending limb of the rat[263] and to 2 μm in the terminal part of the cortical thick ascending limb of the rabbit. Welling and colleagues[264] reported an average cell height of 4.5 μm in the cortical thick ascending limb of the rabbit kidney.

The cells of the thick ascending limb are characterized by extensive invaginations of the basolateral plasma membrane and interdigitations between adjacent cells. The lateral invaginations often extend a distance of two thirds or more from the base to the luminal border of the cell. This arrangement is most prominent in the thick ascending limb of the

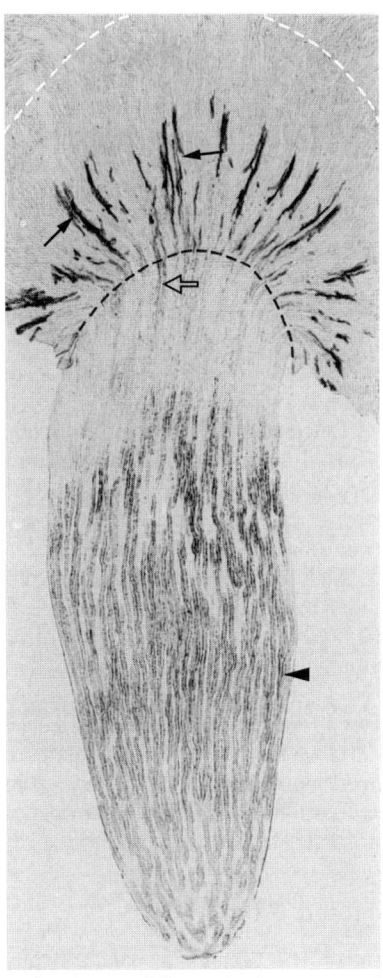

FIGURE 2-37 Light micrograph illustrating immunoperoxidase staining of the urea transporters UT-A2 in the descending thin limb of short-looped nephrons (*closed arrows*) and UT-A1 in the inner medullary collecting duct (*arrowhead*) in normal rat kidney. *Open arrow* indicates weak UT-A2 immunolabeling in descending thin limb segments of long-looped nephrons in the outer part of the inner medulla. (×20.) (Courtesy of Young-Hee Kim, PhD.)

inner stripe of the outer medulla (Figure 2-38). Numerous elongated mitochondria are located in lateral cell processes, and their orientation is perpendicular to the basement membrane. The mitochondria resemble those in the proximal tubule but contain very prominent granules in the matrix. Other subcellular organelles in this segment of the nephron include a well-developed Golgi complex, multivesicular bodies and lysosomes, and abundant quantities of smooth- and rough-surfaced endoplasmic reticulum. Numerous small vesicles are commonly observed in the apical portion of the cytoplasm.

The cells are attached to one another via tight junctions that are 0.1 to 0.2 μm in depth in the rat.[138] Intermediate junctions are also present, but desmosomes appear to be lacking. Scanning electron microscopy of the thick ascending limb of the rat kidney has revealed the existence of two distinct surface configurations of the luminal membrane.[262] Some cells have a rough surface because of the presence of numerous small microprojections, whereas others have a smooth surface that is largely devoid of microprojections except along the apical cell margins (Figure 2-39). Like all other cells from the parietal layer of Bowman's capsule to the terminal collecting duct (except intercalated cells), thick ascending limb cells possess a primary cilium. The rough-surfaced cells possess more extensive lateral processes radiating from the main cell body than do the smooth-surfaced cells. In contrast, small vesicles and tubulovesicular profiles are more numerous in the apical region of the smooth-surfaced cells. A predominance of cells with the smooth surface pattern is observed in the medullary segment. As the thick limb ascends toward the cortex, the number of cells with a rough surface pattern increases, and luminal microprojections and apical lateral invaginations become more prominent. Consequently, the surface area of the luminal plasma membrane is significantly greater in the cortical than in the medullary thick ascending limb.[263]

The thick ascending limb is involved in active transport of NaCl from the lumen to the surrounding interstitium. Since this epithelium is almost impermeable to water, the reabsorption of salt contributes to the formation of a hypertonic medullary interstitium and the delivery of a dilute tubule fluid to the distal convoluted tubule (see Chapter 5). The reabsorption of NaCl in both the medullary and the cortical segments of the thick ascending limb is mediated by a Na^+-K^+-$2Cl^-$ cotransport mechanism,[265-268] which is inhibited by loop diuretics such as furosemide and bumetanide.[268] The bumetanide-sensitive Na^+-K^+-$2Cl^-$ cotransporter (BSC1 or NKCC2) is expressed in the cortical and medullary thick ascending limb,[123,269,270] where it localizes to the apical plasma membrane domains.[269,271,272] Different splice variants of NKCC2 that possess different transport kinetics and affinity for Na^+, K^+, and Cl^- have a spatial distribution in the kidney, which indicates that they may play specialized roles.[273] Furthermore, phosphorylation of the amino-terminal of NKCC2 plays an important role in transporter function.[274,275]

The energy for the reabsorptive process is provided by the Na^+-K^+-ATPase that is located in the basolateral plasma membrane. Biochemical[276] and histochemical[249] studies have demonstrated that Na^+-K^+-ATPase activity is greatest in the segment of the thick ascending limb that is located in the inner stripe of the outer medulla, which also has a larger basolateral membrane area and more mitochondria than does the

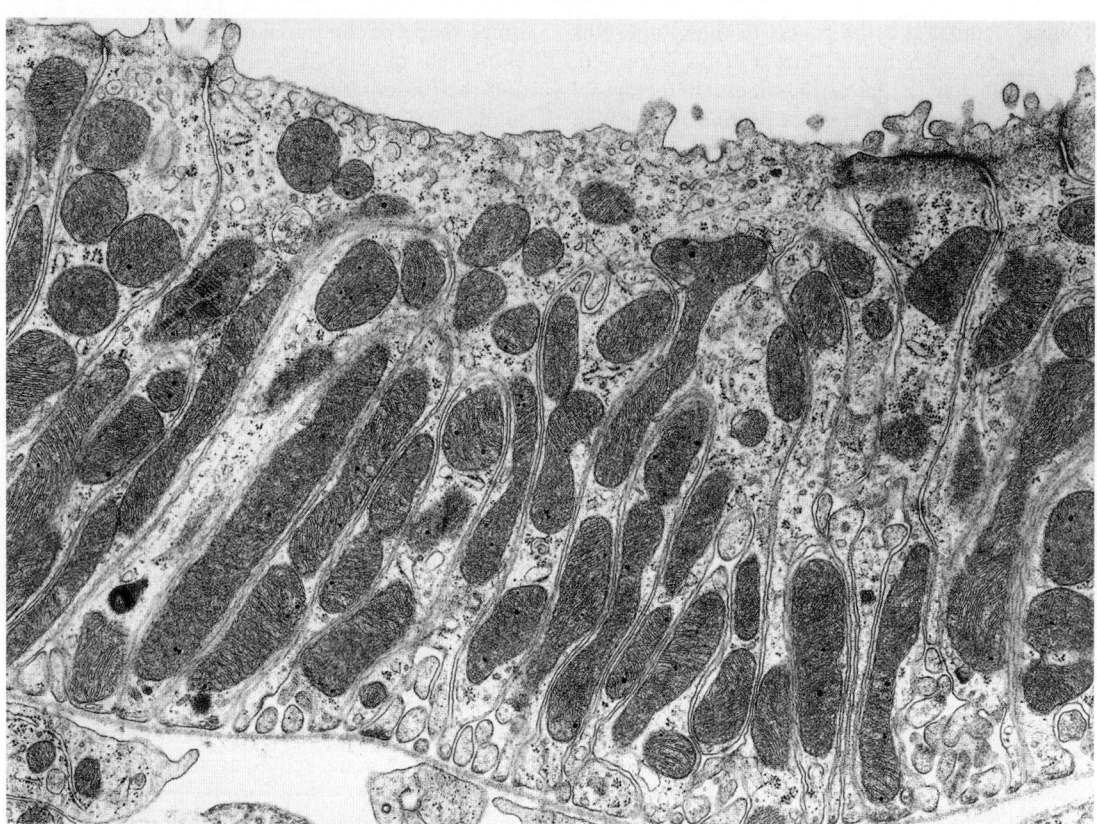

FIGURE 2-38 Transmission electron micrograph of a thick ascending limb in the outer stripe of the outer medulla of the rat. Note the deep, complex invaginations of the basal plasma membrane, which enclose elongated mitochondria and extend into the apical region of the cell. (×13,000.)

remainder of the thick ascending limb.[263] In agreement with these observations, physiologic studies using the isolated perfused tubule technique have demonstrated that NaCl transport is greater in the medullary segment than in the cortical segment of the thick ascending limb.[277] However, the cortical segment can create a steeper concentration gradient and therefore can achieve a lower NaCl concentration and a lower osmolality in the tubule fluid.[278] Thus, an excellent correlation exists between the structural and functional properties of the thick ascending limb.

Studies by Good and colleagues[279,280] provided evidence that the thick ascending limb is involved in HCO_3^- reabsorption in the rat. The reabsorption of $HCO3^-$ is Na^+ dependent and is inhibited by amiloride, which indicates that it is mediated by an Na^+/H^+ exchanger.[279] The identity of the Na^+/H^+ exchanger isoform responsible for HCO_3^- reabsorption in the thick ascending limb was established by immunohistochemical studies demonstrating strong expression of NHE3 in the apical plasma membrane.[205] Immunohistochemical studies[281] also demonstrated labeling for carbonic anhydrase IV in the rat thick ascending limb, thus providing additional support for a role of this part of the nephron in acid-base transport in the rat. Activation of adenylate cyclase by various peptide hormones was shown to inhibit HCO_3^- reabsorption in the thick ascending limb.[282] There is no evidence for HCO_3^- reabsorption or carbonic anhydrase activity in the thick ascending limb of the rabbit,[203] and NHE3 is not expressed in this segment in this species.[204] The mechanism of base exit across the basolateral plasma membrane is not known with certainty. However, studies in rat, mouse, nord human kidneys have demonstrated that a Cl^-/HCO_3^- exchanger, anion exchanger 2 (AE2), is

expressed in the thick ascending limb, which suggests that this transporter may be at least partly responsible for HCO_3^- exit from the cells.[283-285]

The medullary thick ascending limbs are also involved in the proposed medullary ammonium shortcut by which the tubules reabsorb ammonium for subsequent secretion into the medullary collecting duct lumen. Immunohistochemical study revealed that an electroneutral sodium bicarbonate cotransporter, NBCn1, is also expressed in the basolateral membrane of the medullary thick ascending limb in the rat.[286] NBCn1 was expressed only in the renal medulla, and there was no labeling of the cortical thick ascending limb.[286]

Finally, the thick ascending limb is involved in the paracellular transport of divalent cations such as Ca^{2+} ions[287] and Mg^{2+} ions.[288] The extracellular Ca^{2+}/polyvalent cation–sensing receptor, which was cloned originally from bovine parathyroid gland[289] and subsequently from rat kidney,[290] is strongly expressed in the distal tubule, particularly in the cortical thick ascending limb.[291,292] It modulates various cellular functions in response to changes in extracellular Ca^{2+} and other polyvalent cations and is believed to play a central role in mineral ion homeostasis.[293,294]

Distal Convoluted Tubule

The distal convoluted tubule, or pars convoluta, measures approximately 1 mm in length[134,295] and extends to the connecting tubule, which connects the nephron with the collecting duct. The cells of the distal convoluted tubule resemble those of the thick ascending limb but are considerably taller (Figure 2-40). By light microscopy, the cells appear tall and

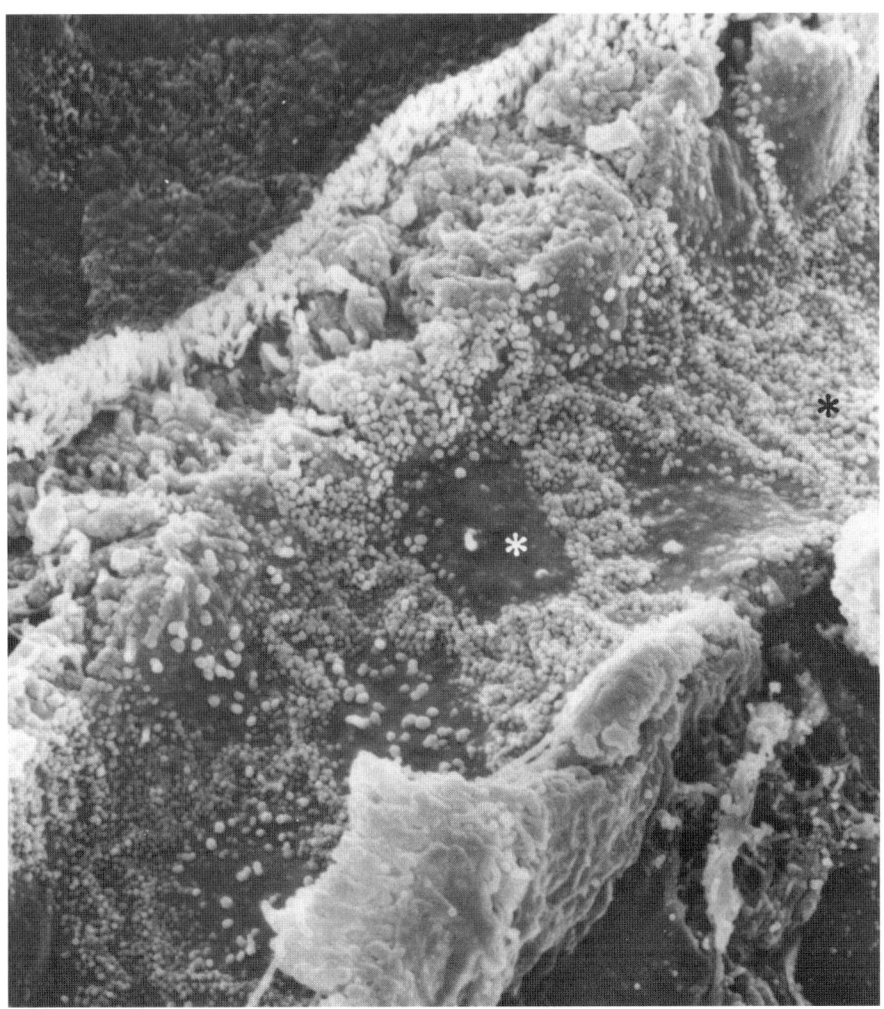

FIGURE 2-39 Scanning electron micrograph illustrating the luminal surface of rat medullary thick ascending limb. The *white asterisk* denotes smooth-surfaced cells; the *black asterisk* identifies rough-surfaced cells. (×4300.) (From Madsen KM, Verlander JW, Tisher CC: Relationship between structure and function in distal tubule and collecting duct, *J Electron Microsc Tech* 9:187, 1988.)

cuboid, and they contain numerous mitochondria. The cell nuclei occupy a central to apical position.

The distal convoluted tubule lacks the well-developed brush border and the extensive endocytic apparatus that are characteristic of the pars convoluta of the proximal tubule. Scanning electron microscopy has demonstrated that the luminal surface of the distal convoluted tubule differs substantially from that of the thick ascending limb (Figure 2-41; compare with Figure 2-39). The distal convoluted tubule is covered with numerous small microprojections or microplicae, and the lateral cell margins are straight, without the interdigitations between adjacent cells that are characteristic of the thick ascending limb. The individual cells possess one centrally placed primary cilium on the apical surface. The epithelium of the distal convoluted tubule is characterized by extensive invaginations of the basolateral plasma membrane and by interdigitations between adjacent cells similar to the arrangement in the thick ascending limb. Transmission electron microscopy reveals numerous elongated mitochondria that are located in lateral cell processes and are closely aligned with the plasma membrane. They are oriented perpendicular to the basement membrane and often extend from the basal to the apical cell surface (Figure 2-42). The junctional complex in this segment of the nephron is composed of a tight junction, which is approximately 0.3 μm in depth, and an intermediate junction.[138]

Lysosomes and multivesicular bodies are common in the cells of the distal convoluted tubule, but microbodies are absent. The Golgi complex is well developed, and its location is lateral to the cell nucleus. The cells contain numerous microtubules and abundant quantities of rough- and smooth-surfaced endoplasmic reticulum and free ribosomes. The basement membrane is complex, often multilayered, and frequently irregular in configuration. Numerous small vesicles are located in the apical region of the cells.

Investigators working with micropuncture techniques arbitrarily defined the distal tubule as that region of the nephron that begins just after the macula densa and extends to the first junction with another renal tubule. When that definition is used, however, the distal tubule can be formed by as many as four different types of epithelia. In general, the "early" distal tubule corresponds largely to the distal convoluted tubule and, in some species, the short segment of the thick ascending limb that extends beyond the macula densa, whereas the "late" distal tubule actually represents the connecting tubule and the first portion of the collecting duct, which is sometimes referred to as the *initial collecting tubule* (Figure 2-43).[295,296] (A more detailed discussion of the anatomy of this region of the renal tubule can be found in the next section, which describes the connecting tubule.)

Micropuncture studies in the rat have demonstrated net NaCl reabsorption and K⁺ secretion in the distal tubule,[297]

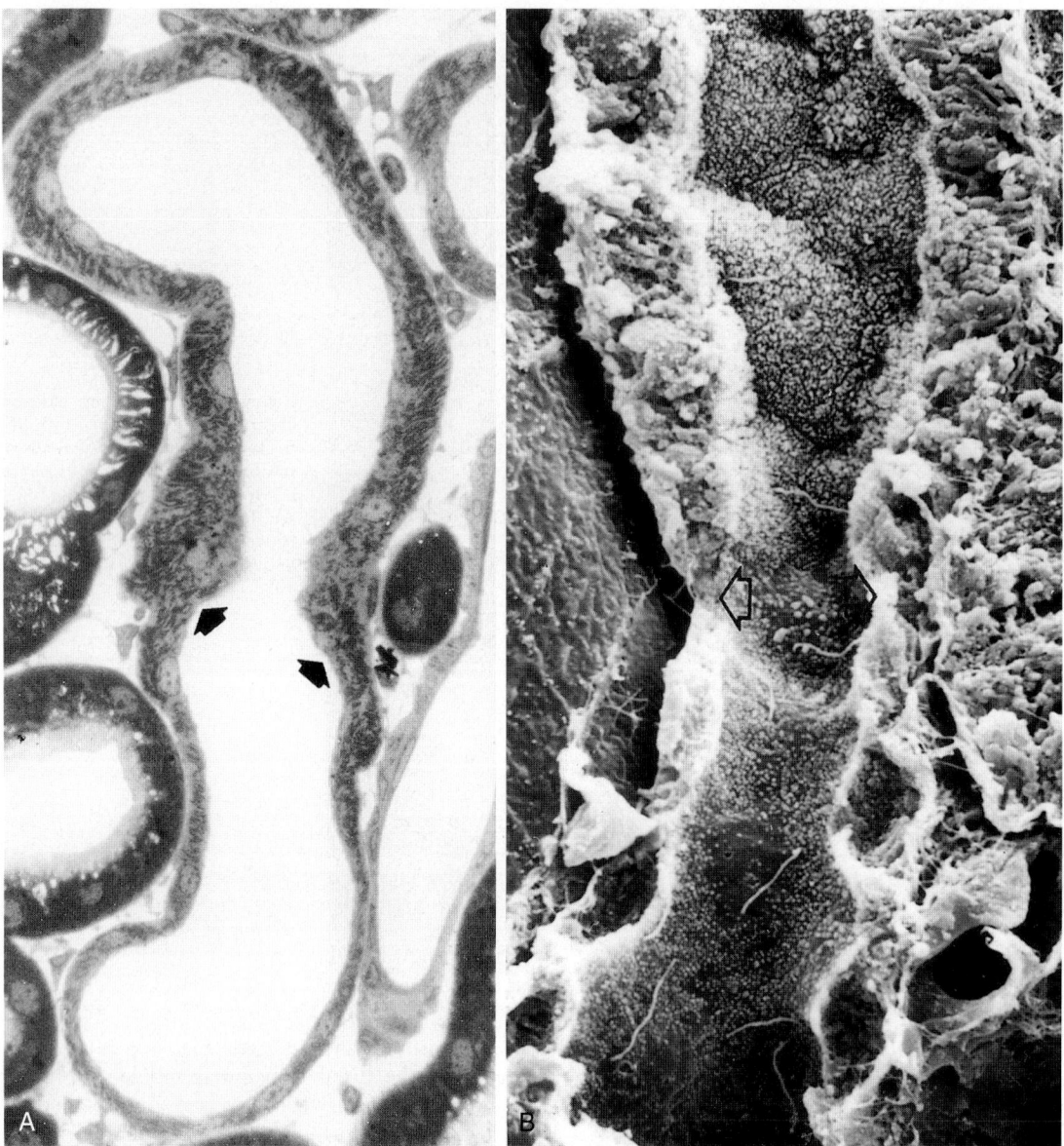

FIGURE 2-40 Micrographs depicting the abrupt transition (*arrows*) from the thick ascending limb of Henle (*below*) to the distal convoluted tubule (*above*). **A,** Light micrograph of normal rat kidney. (×775.) **B,** Scanning electron micrograph of normal rabbit kidney. (×2700.) (**B** courtesy of Ann LeFurgey, PhD.)

although it is not possible to state with certainty whether these functional properties are limited to the early distal tubule or whether they occurred along the entire "distal tubule." Stanton and Giebisch,[298] using in vivo microperfusion, succeeded in perfusing short segments of the rat distal tubule. They demonstrated that Na$^+$ is reabsorbed in both early and late segments, whereas K$^+$ is secreted only in the late segment of the distal tubule, corresponding to the connecting tubule and the initial collecting tubule. These findings agree with the results of a combined structural-functional study from the same laboratory that demonstrated significant morphologic changes in the connecting tubule and initial collecting tubule of the rat during K$^+$ loading but no changes in the distal convoluted tubule.[299] Ultrastructural changes were also seen in the connecting tubule and cortical collecting duct of the rabbit after ingestion of a high-potassium, low-sodium diet, whereas no changes occurred in the distal convoluted tubule.[300]

The distal convoluted tubule has a higher Na$^+$-K$^+$-ATPase activity than any other segment of the nephron[186,250] and provides the driving force for ion transport in this segment. Reabsorption of sodium and chloride is one function of the distal convoluted tubule. It is mediated by a thiazide-sensitive Na$^+$-Cl$^-$ cotransporter, NCC (originally called *TSC*), that is distinct from the Na$^+$-K$^+$-2Cl$^-$ cotransporter NKCC2 of the thick ascending limb.[297] NCC is expressed exclusively in the distal convoluted tubule, where it localizes to the apical plasma membrane and subapical vesicles.[301-304] The mineralocorticoid receptor and the enzyme that confers mineralocorticoid specificity, 11β-hydroxysteroid dehydrogenase, are detected in the distal convoluted tubule, and NCC abundance is increased by the mineralocorticoid.[305-307]

Studies in the rat have distinguished between the early segment, DCT1, and the late segment, DCT2, of the distal convoluted tubule.[305,306] NCC is expressed throughout the distal convoluted tubule, whereas the Na$^+$/Ca^{2+} exchanger NCX1,

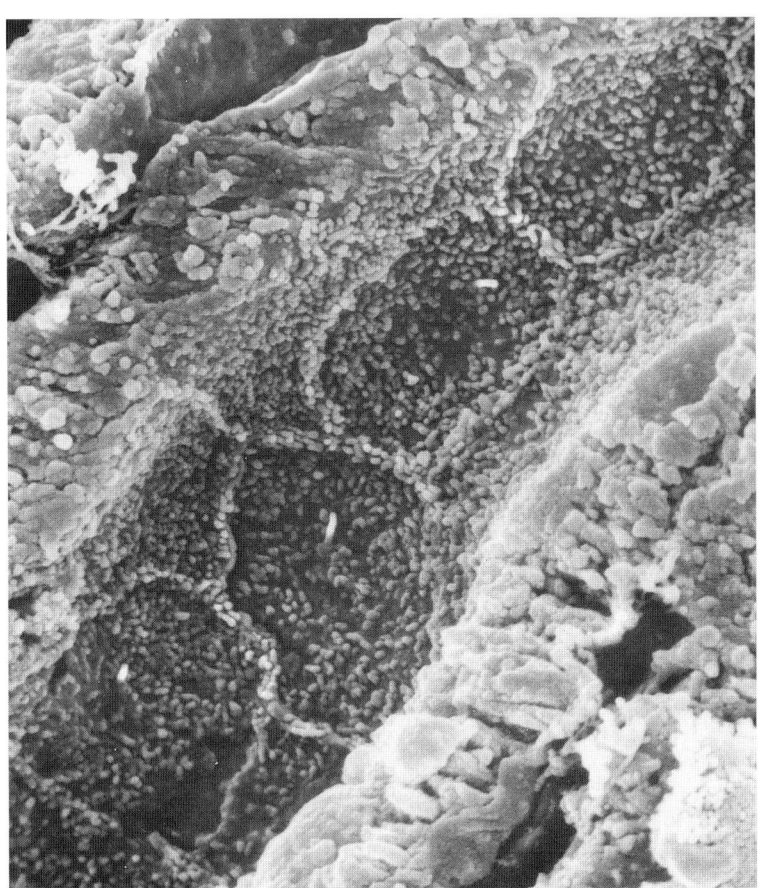

FIGURE 2-41 Scanning electron micrograph illustrating the appearance of the luminal surface of a distal convoluted tubule from rat kidney. Microvilli are prominent, but there is a marked absence of lateral interdigitations in the apical region of the cells. The cell boundaries are accentuated by taller microvilli. (×3000.) (Modified from Madsen KM, Verlander JW, Tisher CC: Relationship between structure and function in distal tubule and collecting duct, *J Electron Microsc Tech* 9:187, 1988.)

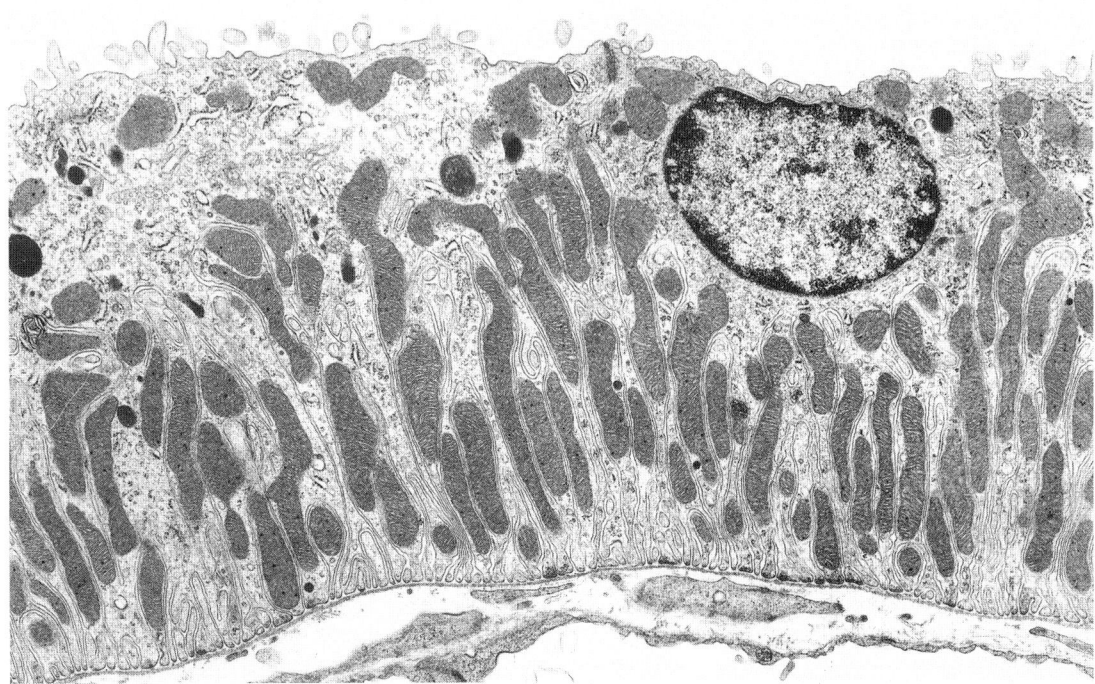

FIGURE 2-42 Transmission electron micrograph illustrating a typical portion of the pars convoluta segment of the distal tubule of a rat. The ultrastructural features closely resemble those of the pars recta of the distal tubule (see Figure 2-40). (×10,000.)

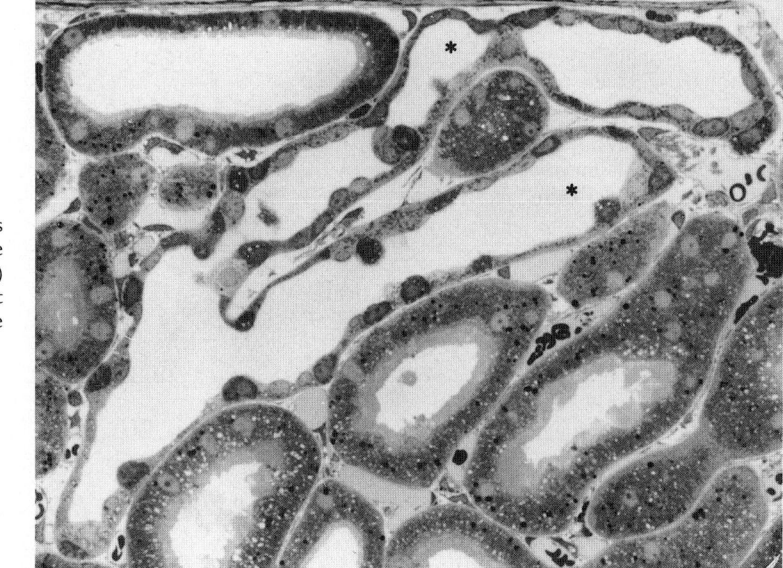

FIGURE 2-43 Light micrograph of initial collecting tubules (*asterisks*) of a cortical collecting duct in rat kidney. One tubule is situated just beneath the surface of the capsule (*top of picture*) and hence is easily accessible to micropuncture. This segment of the cortical collecting duct corresponds to the so-called late distal tubule as defined at the micropuncture table. (×360.)

the calcium-binding protein calbindin-D28K, and the Ca^{2+} channel TRPV5 (transient receptor potential cation channel subfamily V member 5), normally expressed in the connecting segment, have been found in DCT2 but not in DCT1. A similar distinction between DCT1 and DCT2 could not be established in the mouse kidney with respect to the Na^+/Ca^{2+} exchanger and calbindin that were expressed in most of the distal convoluted tubule.[308] However, the expression patterns are the same for NCC and TRPV5 in rat and mouse kidneys.[309,310]

As indicated by the many Ca^{2+} transporters and calbindin expression in DCT2, the distal convoluted tubule is also involved in the reabsorption of Ca^{2+} and has a higher Ca^{2+}-Mg^{2+}-ATPase activity than any other segment of the nephron.[311] Immunohistochemical studies using antibodies to the erythrocyte Ca^{2+}-Mg^{2+}-ATPase demonstrated labeling of the basolateral plasma membrane of the distal convoluted tubule cells,[312] and immunoreactivity for a vitamin D–dependent Ca^{2+}-binding protein has also been observed in this segment.[313]

Kaissling and colleagues[314-316] demonstrated that the ultrastructure and the functional capacity of the distal convoluted tubule and connecting tubule are highly dependent on the delivery and uptake of sodium. Animals treated with the loop diuretic furosemide and given sodium chloride in their drinking water exhibited a striking increase in epithelial cell volume and in basolateral membrane area in the distal convoluted tubule and connecting tubule, and in vivo microperfusion studies demonstrated increased rates of sodium reabsorption in these nephron segments. The observed structural and functional changes were independent of changes in extracellular fluid volume and levels of aldosterone and vasopressin.[314-316]

The consensus is that the distal convoluted tubule, like the thick ascending limb, is relatively impermeable to water. However, the distal convoluted tubule does express vasopressin receptors, and vasopressin positively regulates both Na^+ transport and NCC abundance and activity.[317-319]

The existence of several human diseases that result from abnormal distal tubule function, such as Gitelman's syndrome, nephrolithiasis, and autosomal recessive

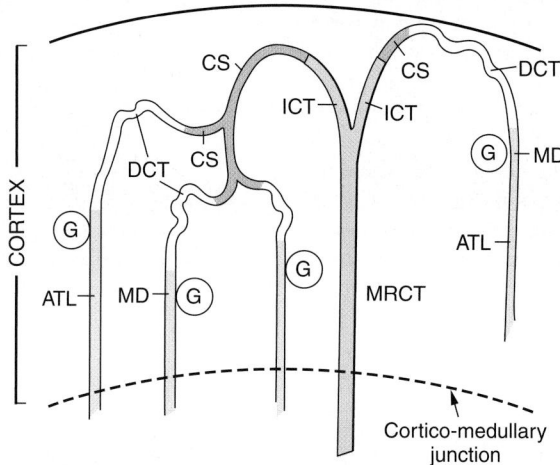

FIGURE 2-44 Diagram of the various anatomic arrangements of the distal tubule and cortical collecting duct in superficial and juxtamedullary nephrons. (See text for detailed explanation.) ATL, Ascending thick limb (of Henle); CS, connecting segment; DCT, distal convoluted tubule; G, glomerulus; ICT, initial collecting tubule; MD, macula densa; MRCT, medullary ray collecting tubule.

pseudohypoaldosteronism type 1, emphasize the importance of this relatively short nephron segment.[297]

Connecting Tubule

The connecting tubule (or connecting segment) represents a transitional region between the distal nephron and the collecting duct, and it constitutes the main portion of the late distal tubule as defined in the micropuncture literature. The connecting tubules of superficial nephrons continue directly into initial collecting tubules, whereas connecting tubules from midcortical and juxtamedullary nephrons join to form arcades that ascend in the cortex and continue into initial collecting tubules (Figure 2-44; see also Figure 2-43).[134,320]

In the rabbit, the connecting tubule is a well-defined segment composed of two cell types: the connecting tubule cell and the intercalated cell.[134,300] In most other species, however, including rat,[295,296] mouse,[300] and human,[321] there is a gradual transition from the distal convoluted tubule to the cortical collecting duct, and the connecting tubule is not clearly demarcated because of intermingling of cells from neighboring segments.

The connecting tubule in the rat measures 150 to 200 μm in length.[296] It is composed of four different cell types: connecting tubule cells, intercalated cells, distal convoluted tubule cells, and principal cells, which are similar to principal cells in the cortical collecting duct.

The connecting tubule cell is characteristic of this segment. It is intermediate in ultrastructure between the distal convoluted tubule cell and the principal cell and exhibits a mixture of lateral invaginations and basal infoldings of the plasma membrane.[322] Connecting tubule cells are taller than principal cells and have an apically located nucleus. Mitochondria are fewer and more randomly distributed than in the distal tubule.

In the rat, variations in the density of the cytoplasm of intercalated cells were reported in the connecting tubule.[295] Two configurations of intercalated cells, type A and type B, were described in both the connecting tubule and the cortical collecting duct of the rat.[323] In the connecting tubule, type A cells were more numerous than type B cells. A third type of intercalated cell was identified in the connecting tubule of both rat and mouse.[324,325] This cell has been referred to as the *non-A, non-B type* of intercalated cell. In the mouse, this is the most prevalent form of intercalated cell in the connecting tubule.[324]

The function of the intercalated cells in the connecting tubule is not known with certainty. However, ultrastructural changes have been demonstrated in the type A intercalated cells in both the connecting tubule and the cortical collecting duct of rats with acute respiratory acidosis, which indicates that these cells may be involved in acid secretion, as are the intercalated cells in the outer medullary collecting duct. The functional properties and immunohistochemical features of the intercalated cells have been studied extensively and are described later.

As are the thick ascending limbs and distal convoluted tubule, the connecting tubule is an important site for regulation of Na⁺ reabsorption, but in contrast with those segments, it is also capable of transporting large amounts of water. Subunits of the amiloride-sensitive epithelial sodium channel ENaC, which are also responsible for sodium absorption in the collecting duct, are highly expressed in the connecting tubule as well as in DCT2.[326] Studies in collecting duct–selective gene knockout mice generated by exploiting the Cre-loxP approach revealed that selective deletion of α-ENaC in the collecting duct system with retained expression in the DCT2 and connecting tubule failed to produce major phenotypic changes.[327] In contrast, global gene knockout of the α-subunit was postnatally lethal, although this phenotype is attributed to reduced fluid removal in the lungs.[328] Thus, the DCT2 and connecting tubule represent the major aldosterone-sensitive pathway for sodium reabsorption.

The vasopressin V_2 receptor and the vasopressin-regulated water channel AQP2 are also expressed in the connecting tubule.[324,329] In contrast to the ENaC knockout models, collecting duct–specific AQP2 gene knockout animals developed using the same Cre-loxP approach exhibited a dramatic phenotype with severe polyuria.[330] Mice with global AQP2 gene knockout died postnatally within 2 weeks with severe

hydronephrosis.[330] Thus, unlike the situation for ENaC (with regard to sodium reabsorption), expression of AQP2 in the entire connecting tubule and collecting duct is essential for water balance regulation.[330]

As described in the section on distal convoluted tubules, the connecting tubule is an important site of calcium reabsorption. Immunohistochemical studies have demonstrated the presence of an Na⁺/Ca²⁺ exchanger, NCX1,[302,331] as well as Ca²⁺-ATPase,[312,332] in the basolateral plasma membrane of the connecting tubule cells. Expression of the vitamin D–dependent calcium-binding protein calbindin D28K and the apical Ca²⁺ entry pathway TRPV5 has also been demonstrated in the connecting tubule cells.[313–334] Immunohistochemical studies in rats[306,331] revealed that a subpopulation of cells in the late part of the distal convoluted tubule, at the transition to the connecting tubule, expresses both the NaCl cotransporter, NCC, and the Na⁺/Ca²⁺ exchanger, which are traditionally considered specific for distal convoluted tubule cells and connecting tubule cells, respectively. In the rabbit, the connecting tubule constitutes a distinct segment with respect to both structure and function, and there is no coexpression of NCC and the Na⁺/Ca²⁺ exchanger in any cells in the distal convoluted tubule or connecting tubule.[301]

Morphologic and physiologic studies have provided evidence that the connecting tubule plays an important role in K⁺ secretion, which is at least in part regulated by mineralocorticoids.[297] Free-flow micropuncture studies in rats demonstrated high levels of K⁺ secretion in the superficial distal tubule.[335] In a combined structural-functional study, Stanton and colleagues[299] demonstrated that chronic K⁺ loading, which stimulates aldosterone secretion, caused an increase in K⁺ secretion by the late distal tubule and a simultaneous increase in the surface area of the basolateral plasma membrane of connecting tubule cells and principal cells in both the connecting tubule and the initial collecting tubule—results that indicate that these cells are responsible for K⁺ secretion. No changes were observed in the cells of the distal convoluted tubule. Studies in the rabbit revealed a similar increase in the basolateral membrane area of the connecting tubule cells after ingestion of a high-potassium, low-sodium diet.[300] Studies in adrenalectomized rats demonstrated a decrease in K⁺ secretion in the superficial distal tubule[336] as well as a decrease in the surface area of the basolateral membrane of the principal cells in the initial collecting tubule.[337] Both structural and functional changes could be prevented by aldosterone treatment, which indicates that K⁺ secretion in the connecting tubule and initial collecting tubule is regulated by mineralocorticoids.

Collecting Duct

The collecting duct extends from the connecting tubule in the cortex through the outer and inner medulla to the tip of the papilla. It can be divided into at least three regions, based primarily on their location in the kidney: the cortical collecting duct, the outer medullary collecting duct, and the IMCD. The inner medullary segments terminate as the ducts of Bellini, which open on the surface of the papilla to form the area cribrosa (see Figure 2-3). Traditionally, two types of cells have been described in the mammalian collecting duct: principal cells and intercalated cells. The principal cells are the major cell type; they were originally believed to be present in the entire collecting duct, whereas intercalated cells disappear at different lengths along the IMCD depending on the species. There is also both structural and functional evidence that the cells in the terminal portion of the IMCD constitute a distinct population of IMCD cells.[338] Furthermore, at least two, and in certain species three, configurations of intercalated cells have been described in the cortical collecting duct.[323] Therefore, significant structural axial heterogeneity exists along the collecting duct.

Cortical Collecting Duct

The cortical collecting duct can be further subdivided into two parts: the initial collecting tubule and the medullary ray portion (see Figure 2-5). The cells of the initial collecting tubule are taller than those of the medullary ray segment, but otherwise no major morphologic differences exist between the two subsegments. The cortical collecting duct is composed of principal cells and intercalated cells, the latter constituting approximately one third of the cells in this segment in the rat,[324,339] the mouse,[324,325] and the rabbit.[340] Principal cells have a light-staining cytoplasm and relatively few cell organelles (Figure 2-45). They are characterized by numerous infoldings of the basal plasma membrane below the nucleus. The infoldings do not enclose mitochondria or other cell organelles, which causes the basal region to appear as a light rim by light microscopy. Lateral cell processes and interdigitations are virtually absent.[341] Mitochondria are small and scattered randomly in the cytoplasm. A few lysosomes, autophagic vacuoles, and multivesicular bodies are also present, as are rough- and smooth-surfaced endoplasmic reticulum and free ribosomes. Scanning electron microscopy of the luminal surface of the principal cells reveals a relatively smooth membrane covered with short, stubby microvilli and a single primary cilium (Figure 2-46).

Intercalated cells in the cortical collecting duct have a densely staining cytoplasm and therefore are sometimes referred to as *dark cells* (Figure 2-47). They are characterized by the presence of various tubulovesicular membrane structures in the cytoplasm and prominent microprojections on the luminal surface. In addition, numerous mitochondria and polyribosomes are located throughout the cells, which also contain a well-developed Golgi apparatus. Previous studies have described two distinct populations of intercalated cells, type A and type B, in the cortical collecting duct of the rat,[323,342] each constituting approximately 50% of the intercalated cells in this segment (see Figure 2-47).

Type A intercalated cells are similar in ultrastructure to intercalated cells in the outer medullary collecting duct. They have a prominent tubulovesicular membrane compartment that includes both spherical and invaginated vesicles and flat saccules or cisternae that appear as tubular profiles on section (Figure 2-48). The cytoplasmic face of these membrane structures is coated with characteristic club-shaped particles or studs, similar to the coat that lines the cytoplasmic face of the apical plasma membrane.[343] The ultrastructural appearance of the apical region of type A intercalated cells can vary considerably, depending on the physiologic state. Some cells have numerous tubulovesicular structures and few microprojections on the luminal surface, whereas other cells have extensive microprojections on the surface but only a few tubulovesicular structures in the apical cytoplasm.

Type B intercalated cells have a denser cytoplasm and more mitochondria than type A cells, which gives them a darker appearance (see Figure 2-47). Numerous vesicles are present throughout the cytoplasm, but tubular profiles and studded membrane structures are rare in the cytoplasm of type B cells. The apical membrane exhibits small, blunt microprojections, and often a band of dense cytoplasm without organelles is present just beneath the apical membrane. Morphometric analysis in the rat has demonstrated that type B intercalated cells

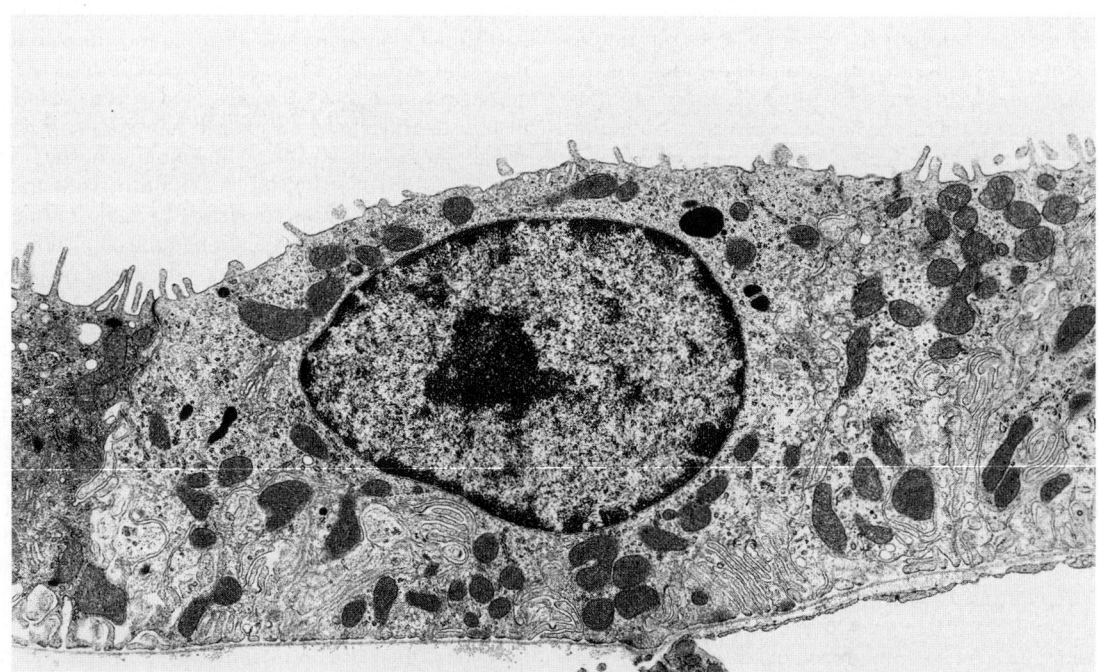

FIGURE 2-45 Transmission electron micrograph of a principal cell from the cortical collecting duct of normal rat kidney. Note the extensive infoldings of the basal plasma membrane. (×11,000.) (From Madsen KM, Tisher CC: Structural-functional relationship along the distal nephron, *Am J Physiol* 250:F1, 1986.)

have a smaller apical membrane area but a larger basolateral membrane area compared with type A cells.[323]

By scanning electron microscopy, two different surface configurations have been described in the rat.[323] Type A cells have a large luminal surface covered with microplicae or a mixture of microplicae and microvilli. Type B cells have a smaller, angular surface with a few microprojections, mostly in the form of small microvilli (see Figure 2-46). Both type A and type B intercalated cells are present in the cortical collecting duct of the mouse.[325] However, type B cells are less common than in the rat. More recent studies have identified and characterized a third type of intercalated cell in both rat[324] and mouse.[324,325] This so-called non-A, non-B type of intercalated cell constitutes approximately 40% to 50% percent of the intercalated cells in the connecting tubule and initial collecting duct of the mouse but is fairly rare in the rat.[324]

Kaissling and Kriz[134] described both light and dark manifestations of intercalated cells in the collecting duct of the rabbit. The light form was most commonly observed in the outer medulla, whereas the dark form was observed mainly in the cortex. Flat and invaginated vesicles were present in both cell configurations. The two manifestations of intercalated cells in the rabbit possibly correspond to type A and type B intercalated cells in the rat. Scanning electron microscopy has also revealed different surface configurations of intercalated cells in the collecting duct of the rabbit.[340] Cells with either microplicae or microvilli, or both, have been described, but their relationship to the two cell types has not been investigated. Cells with microvilli are prevalent in the cortex, however.

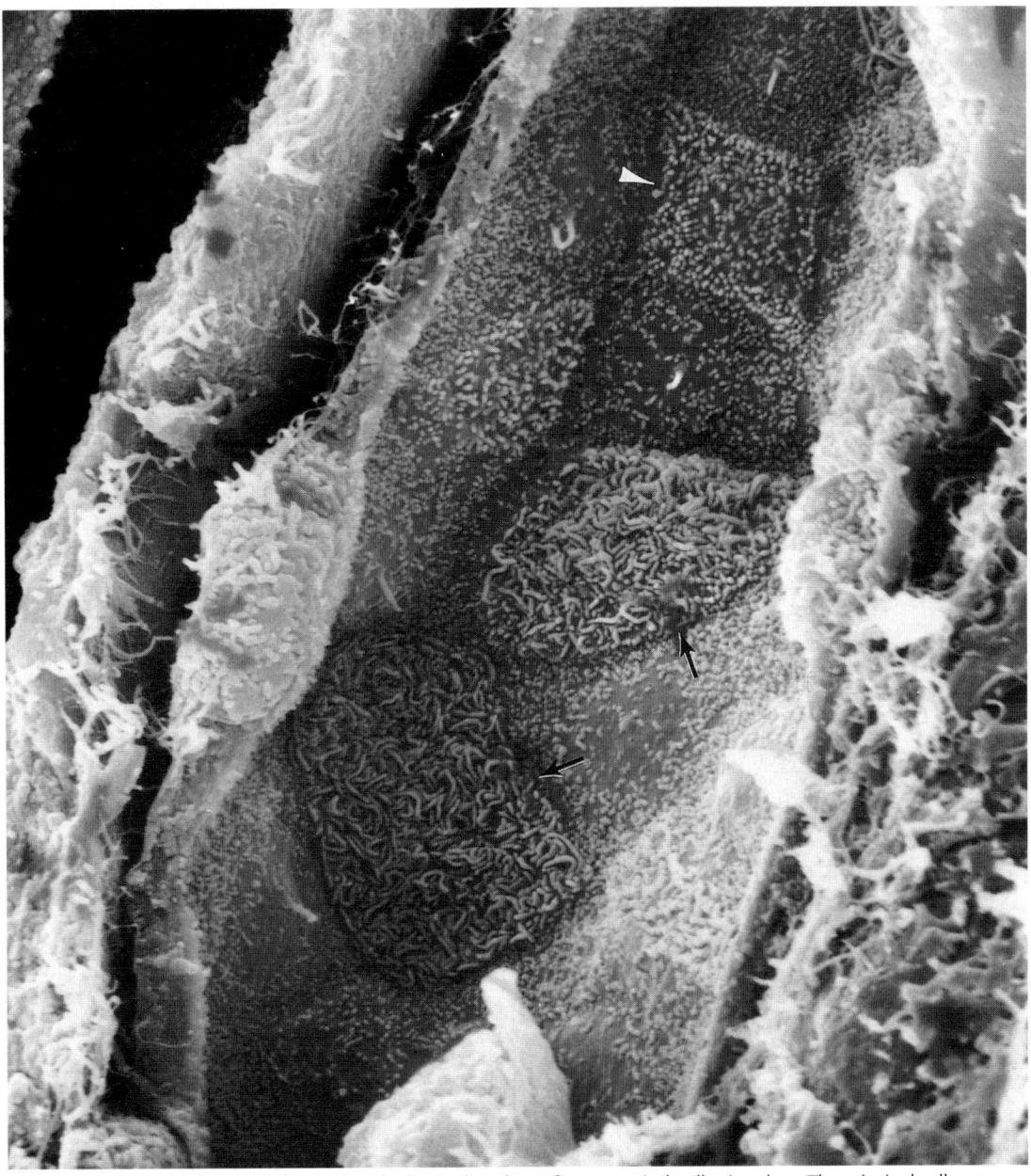

FIGURE 2-46 Scanning electron micrograph illustrating the luminal surface of a rat cortical collecting duct. The principal cells possess small, stubby microprojections and a single cilium. Two configurations of intercalated cells are present: type A (*arrows*), with a large luminal surface covered mostly with microplicae, and type B (*arrowhead*), with a more angular outline and a surface covered mostly with small microvilli. (×5900.) (From Madsen KM, Verlander JW, Tisher CC: Relationship between structure and function in distal tubule and collecting duct, *J Electron Microsc Tech* 9:187, 1988.)

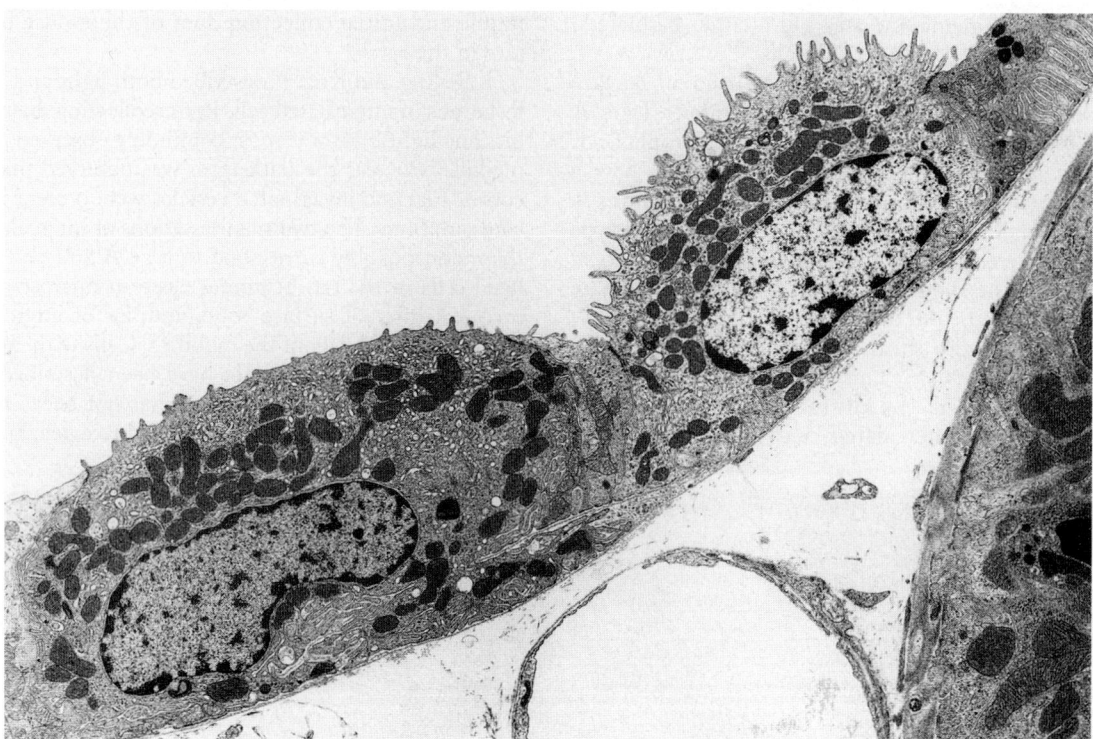

FIGURE 2-47 Transmission electron micrograph of a rat cortical collecting duct illustrating type A (*right*) and type B (*left*) intercalated cells. Note differences in the density of the cytoplasm and in apical microprojections. (×5300.) (From Madsen KM, Verlander JW, Tisher CC: Relationship between structure and function in distal tubule and collecting duct, *J Electron Microsc Tech* 9:187, 1988.)

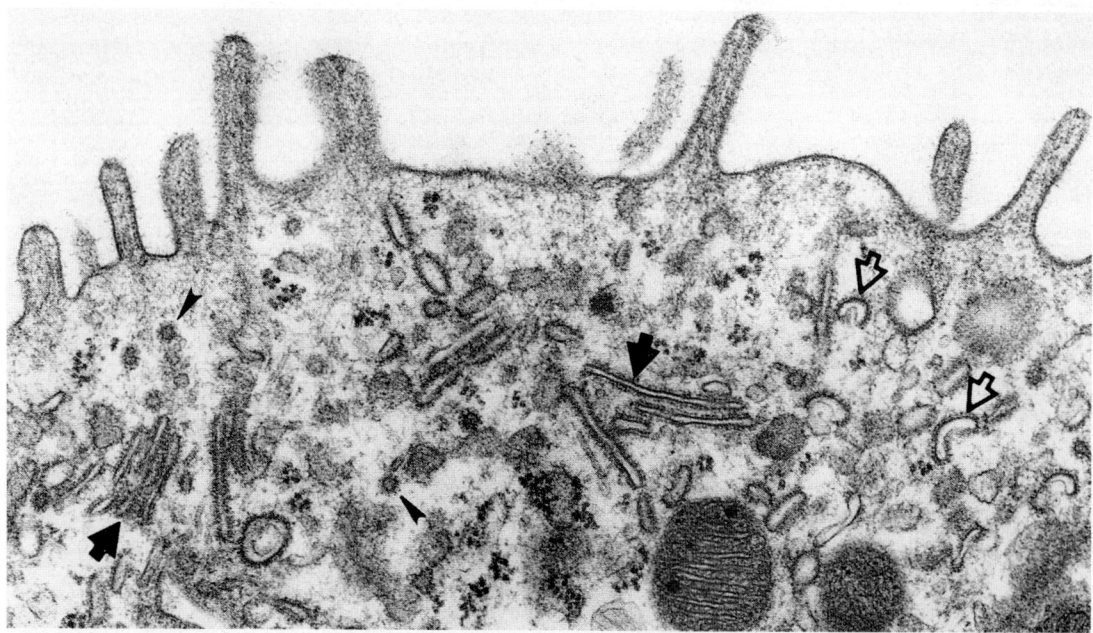

FIGURE 2-48 Higher-magnification transmission electron micrograph illustrating the apical region of an intercalated cell from rat kidney. Note especially the large number of tubulocisternal profiles (*solid arrows*), invaginated vesicles (*open arrows*), and small coated vesicles with the appearance of clathrin vesicles (*arrowheads*). (×38,000.)

High levels of carbonic anhydrase are detectable in intercalated cells,[344-346] which suggests that these cells are involved in tubule fluid acidification in the collecting duct. The cortical collecting duct is capable of both reabsorption and secretion of HCO_3^-. Studies using the isolated perfused tubule technique have demonstrated that cortical collecting tubules from acid-loaded rats[347] and rabbits[348,349] reabsorb HCO_3^- (i.e., secrete

H^+), whereas tubules from HCO_3^--loaded or deoxycorticosterone-treated rats[347,350] and rabbits[348,351,352] secrete HCO_3^-.

Both morphologic and immunocytochemical studies have provided evidence that the type A intercalated cells are involved in H^+ secretion in the cortical collecting duct of the rat.[353] In a study of the effect of acute respiratory acidosis on the cortical collecting duct of the rat, Verlander and

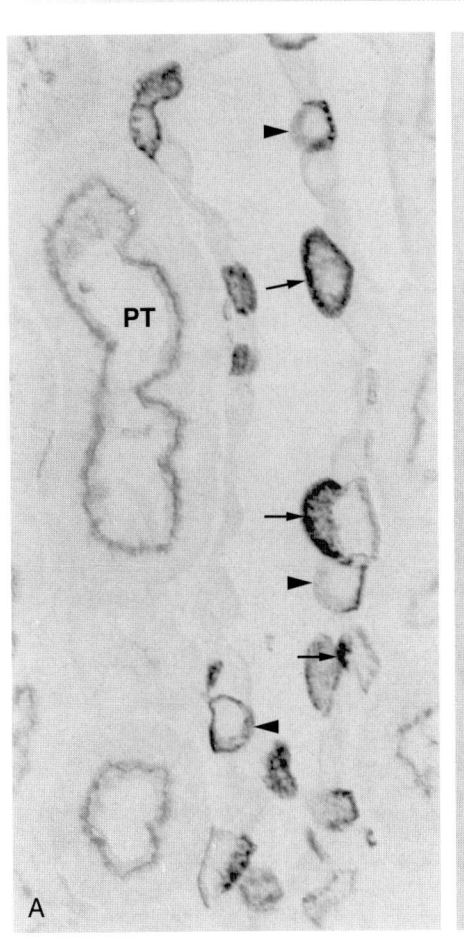
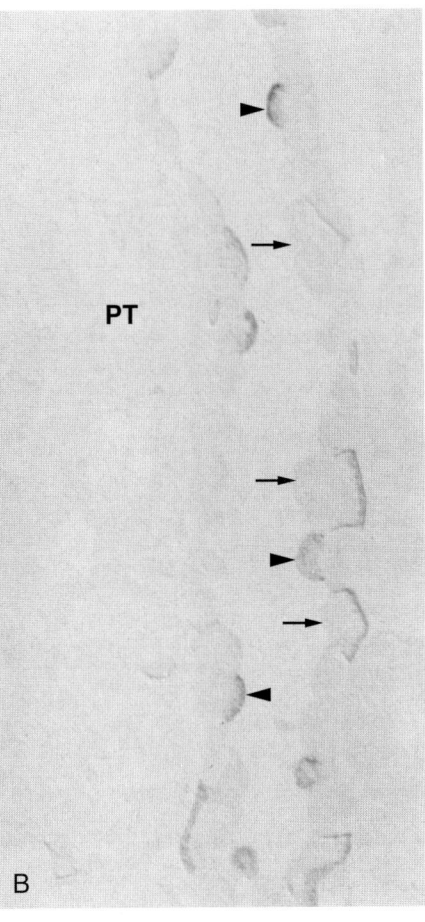

FIGURE 2-49 Light micrograph illustrating immunostaining for (**A**) the vacuolar H$^+$-ATPase and the anion exchanger, AE1, and (**B**) pendrin and AE1 in serial sections of the mouse cortical collecting duct with use of a horseradish peroxidase technique. In **A**, type A intercalated cells (*arrows*) have strong apical labeling for H$^+$-ATPase and basolateral labeling for AE1, whereas type B intercalated cells (*arrowheads*) have basolateral and diffuse labeling for H$^+$-ATPase and no AE1 labeling. In contrast, type B intercalated cells have apical labeling for pendrin (**B**). PT, Proximal tubule. (Differential interference microscopy; ×800.) (Courtesy of Jin Kim, MD, Catholic University, Seoul, Korea.)

colleagues[323] demonstrated a significant increase in the surface area of the apical plasma membrane of type A intercalated cells. No ultrastructural changes were observed in type B intercalated cells. Similar ultrastructural findings were reported in intercalated cells in the outer cortex of rats with acute metabolic acidosis; however, no distinction was made between type A and type B cells.[354]

Immunocytochemical studies using antibodies to the vacuolar H$^+$-ATPase and the erythrocyte anion exchanger band 3 protein (now known as *AE1*) have confirmed the presence of two types of intercalated cells in the cortical collecting duct of both mouse and rat. Type A intercalated cells have an apical H$^+$-ATPase (Figure 2-49)[324,325,355-359] and a basolateral band 3–like Cl$^-$/HCO$_3^-$ exchanger, AE1,[324,325,355,360,361] which indicates that they are involved in H$^+$ secretion. In contrast, type B intercalated cells have the H$^+$-ATPase in the basolateral plasma membrane and in cytoplasmic vesicles throughout the cell (see Figure 2-49*A*), and they do not express AE1.[324,325,355,361]

There is convincing evidence that type B cells secrete HCO$_3^-$ by an apical Cl$^-$/HCO$_3^-$ exchanger that is distinct from AE1, the anion exchanger in the type A cells. Studies have demonstrated that the anion exchanger pendrin is expressed in a subpopulation of cells in the renal cortex.[362,363] Mutations in the gene encoding pendrin causes Pendred's syndrome, a genetic disorder associated with deafness and goiter.[364] Immunohistochemical studies revealed that pendrin is restricted to the apical region of AE1–negative intercalated cells (see Figure 2-49*B*), which suggests that pendrin might

represent the long sought after apical Cl$^-$/HCO$_3^-$ exchanger of type B intercalated cells.[362,365] Immunogold electron microscopy confirmed that pendrin is located in the apical plasma membrane and subapical cytoplasmic vesicles of type B cells (Figure 2-50) as well as in non-A, non-B intercalated cells in the connecting tubule and cortical collecting duct of both mouse and rat.[365]

Microperfusion studies in isolated cortical collecting duct segments from alkali-loaded mice deficient in pendrin demonstrated a failure to secrete HCO$_3^-$, compared with tubules from wild-type mice,[362] which indicates that pendrin is important for HCO$_3^-$ secretion in the cortical collecting duct. This conclusion is also supported by studies in the rat demonstrating that the expression of pendrin in the renal cortex is significantly increased in chronic metabolic alkalosis and decreased in chronic metabolic acidosis.[366] In addition, ultrastructural studies have demonstrated changes in type B intercalated cells during experimental conditions designed to stimulate HCO$_3^-$ secretion in the collecting duct.[357,358]

Recent studies have focused on the possible role of pendrin in hypertension. Deoxycorticosterone induces hypertension and metabolic alkalosis in mice. However, pendrin-deficient mice appear resistant to deoxycorticosterone-induced hypertension and more sensitive to deoxycorticosterone-induced metabolic alkalosis.[367] In addition, Wall and colleagues found that during NaCl restriction, Cl$^-$ excretion and urinary volume were increased in pendrin-deficient mice compared with wild-type animals; this suggests that pendrin may play a role in renal Cl$^-$ conservation.[368] There is an inverse relationship

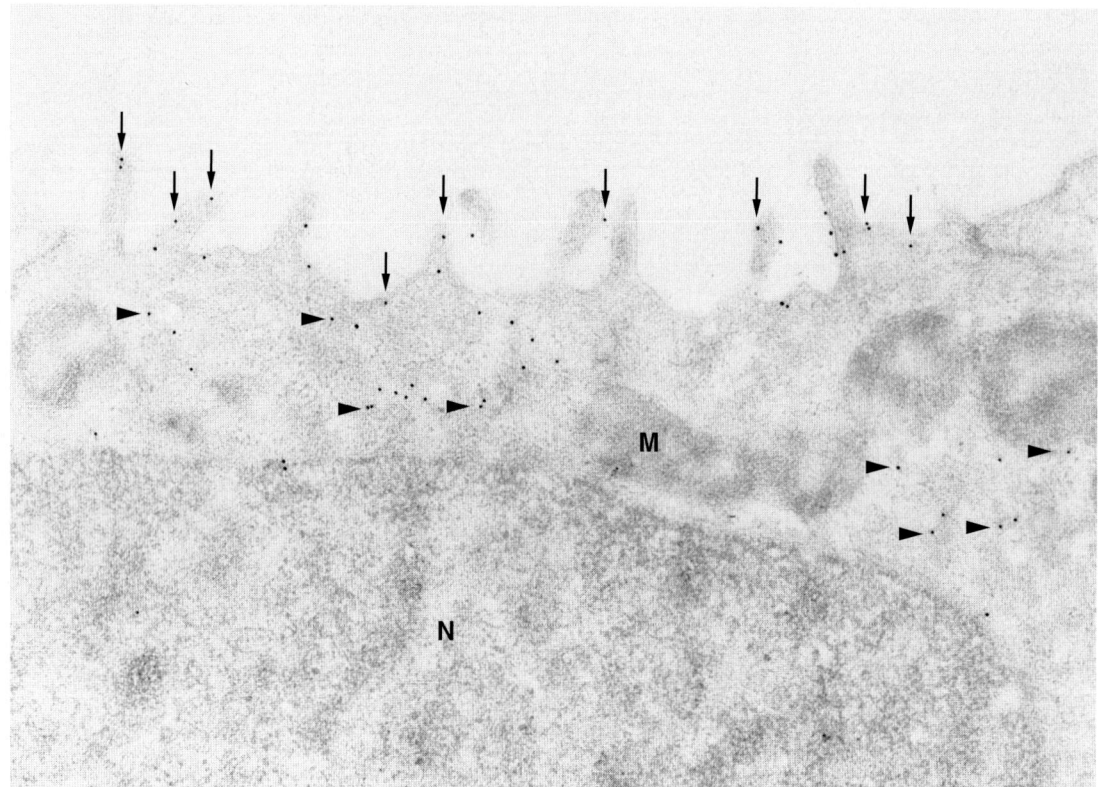

FIGURE 2-50 Transmission electron micrograph illustrating immunogold localization of pendrin in a type B intercalated cell from rat kidney. Labeling of pendrin is seen in the apical plasma membrane (*arrows*) and in small vesicles (*arrowheads*) in the apical cytoplasm. (×46,000.) M, Mitochondrion; N, nucleus. (Courtesy of Tae-Hwan Kwon, MD, University of Aarhus, Denmark.)

between pendrin expression and the level of dietary chloride loading, which provides evidence that distal chloride delivery may be the chief regulator of pendrin expression.[369,370]

In the cortical collecting duct of the rabbit, AE1 immunoreactivity is seen mainly in intracellular vesicles and multivesicular bodies in a subpopulation of intercalated cells, and there is little labeling of the basolateral plasma membrane.[371] Immunocytochemical studies have demonstrated that H+-ATPase is located in intracellular vesicles in most intercalated cells in the rabbit cortical collecting duct, and only a minority of intercalated cells have H+-ATPase immunoreactivity in the apical plasma membrane as is characteristic of type A intercalated cells.[372] These observations suggest that, under normal conditions, most type A intercalated cells in the rabbit cortical collecting duct are not functionally active. However, after long-term ammonium chloride loading there is increased AE1 immunolabeling in the basolateral plasma membrane and increased labeling for H+-ATPase in the apical plasma membrane of intercalated cells in the cortical collecting duct of the rabbit.[373] In addition, a subpopulation of intercalated cells in the rabbit cortical collecting duct exhibits H+-ATPase immunolabeling in the basolateral plasma membrane, which is characteristic of type B intercalated cells.[372]

It has been suggested that the type A and type B configurations of intercalated cells could represent different functional states of the same cell population and that these cells may change polarity in response to changes in the acid-base status of the animal.[374] Support for this hypothesis was provided by the presence of H+-ATPase in the apical membrane of the acid-secreting type A cell and in the basolateral membrane of the type B cell, which might suggest a reversed polarity.[356]

However, the observation that AE1 is expressed only in type A intercalated cells,[361] whereas pendrin is expressed only in type B and non-A, non-B intercalated cells,[365] is more consistent with the concept that type A and type B cells represent structurally and functionally distinct cell types. This concept is also supported by studies demonstrating that distinct members of the chloride channel gene family are expressed in the two types of intercalated cells. Chloride channel 3 (ClC-3) mRNA is present only in type B intercalated cells, whereas ClC-5 mRNA is expressed in type A intercalated cells.[375]

In the connecting tubule and collecting duct, sodium is absorbed through an amiloride-sensitive sodium channel, ENaC, that is located in the apical plasma membrane of connecting tubule cells and principal cells.[376,377] The amiloride-sensitive sodium channel is composed of three homologous ENaC subunits, α, β, and γ, that together constitute the functional channel.[378] All three subunits are expressed in connecting tubule cells and principal cells in the collecting duct.[376,377] However, high-resolution immunohistochemical studies and immunogold electron microscopy revealed that α-ENaC was expressed in both the apical plasma membrane and apical cytoplasmic vesicles, whereas β-ENaC and γ-ENaC appeared to be located in small vesicles throughout the cytoplasm.[377]

The activity of ENaC in the collecting duct is regulated by aldosterone and vasopressin as well as by other hormonal systems via mechanisms that involve complex signaling pathways and incorporate changes in expression and subcellular trafficking of ENaC subunits. In mice consuming a high-sodium diet, which is associated with a low plasma aldosterone level, α-ENaC was not detectable and β- and γ-ENaC were distributed throughout the cytoplasm.[379] In mice consuming a low-sodium diet, which is associated with high plasma aldosterone levels, all three subunits of ENaC were expressed in the apical and subapical region of the connecting tubule cells and in principal cells of the cortical collecting duct. In the medullary collecting duct, however, cytoplasmic staining for β- and γ-ENaC was still observed.[379] Vasopressin increases the abundance of all three ENaC subunits in the rat kidney,[380] and angiotensin II also plays a role in the regulation of ENaC.[381,382]

The regulation of epithelial Na^+ transport by ENaC is complex, involving multiple mechanisms that control ENaC abundance at the apical cell surface. These mechanisms involve regulated exocytosis, endocytosis, and degradation and are reviewed in detail.[383,384] The importance of ENaC in epithelial Na^+ transport is emphasized in conditions where regulation of ENaC is abnormal. This often results in salt retention or wasting by the collecting duct.[383,385] In addition, certain single-gene defects affecting ENaC or its regulation by aldosterone cause severe hypertension, whereas others cause sodium wasting and hypotension. Such gene defects underscore the role of the collecting duct in maintaining normal extracellular volume and blood pressure.

Another major function of the cortical collecting duct is the secretion of K^+. This process is regulated at least partly by mineralocorticoids, which stimulate K^+ secretion and Na^+ reabsorption in the isolated perfused cortical collecting duct of the rabbit.[386,387] Treatment with mineralocorticoids has also been shown to stimulate Na^+-K^+-ATPase activity in individual segments of the cortical collecting duct of both rat[388] and rabbit.[250,389]

Morphologic studies of the collecting duct of rabbits given a low-sodium, high-potassium diet[300] and of rabbits treated with deoxycorticosterone[390] demonstrated a significant increase in the surface area of the basolateral plasma membrane of the principal cells. The observed changes were similar to those reported in principal cells in the connecting segment and in the initial collecting duct of rats on a high-potassium diet,[299] which indicates that these cells are responsible for K^+ secretion in the connecting tubule and cortical collecting duct. This K^+ secretion is likely mediated by ROMK (regulation of Kir 1.1) and maxi-K channels.[391]

Outer Medullary Collecting Duct

In this chapter, the collecting duct segments in the outer and inner stripes of the outer medulla are abbreviated *OMCDo* and *OMCDi*, respectively. The outer medullary collecting duct is composed of principal cells and intercalated cells. In the rat[339] and mouse,[325] intercalated cells constitute approximately one third of the cells in both the OMCDo and the OMCDi, and a similar ratio between the two cell types is found in the OMCDo of the rabbit. In the rabbit OMCDi, however, the number of intercalated cells varies among animals. In some animals intercalated cells are present only in the outer half, where they represent 10% to 15% of the total cell population.

Principal cells in the outer medullary collecting duct are similar in ultrastructure to those in the cortical collecting duct. The cells become slightly taller, however, and the number of organelles and basal infoldings decreases as the collecting duct descends through the outer medulla. Whether principal cells in the outer medullary collecting duct are functionally similar to those in the cortical collecting duct is not known with certainty. They express Na^+-K^+-ATPase in the basolateral plasma membrane[148] and ENaC in the apical plasma membrane,[376,377] and they are believed to be involved in Na^+ reabsorption; however, there is no evidence that they secrete K^+ as in the cortical collecting duct. In fact, the OMCDi is a site of K^+ reabsorption, at least in the rabbit.[392] In the rat, intercalated cells in the outer medullary collecting duct are similar in ultrastructure to type A intercalated cells in the cortical collecting duct (Figure 2-51).

In the OMCDi, the cells become taller and less electron dense, and little or no difference in the density of the cytoplasm exists between intercalated cells and principal cells in this segment. The main characteristics of the intercalated cells in the outer medulla are numerous tubulovesicular structures in the apical cytoplasm and prominent microprojections on the luminal surface. Scanning electron microscopy has revealed that intercalated cells are covered with microplicae and often bulge into the tubule lumen.

The outer medullary collecting duct plays an important role in urine acidification,[349] which is believed to be a primary function of this segment. There is evidence that H^+ secretion in the OMCDi is an Na^+-independent electrogenic process.[393] Morphologic studies have demonstrated characteristic ultrastructural changes in intercalated cells in the collecting duct after stimulation of H^+ secretion. In rats with acute respiratory acidosis[343] or chronic metabolic acidosis,[394] the surface area of the apical plasma membrane increased concomitant with a decrease in the number of tubulovesicular structures in the apical cytoplasm. On the basis of these observations, it was suggested that membrane containing H^+-ATPase is transferred from the tubulovesicular structures to the luminal membrane in intercalated cells in response to stimulation of H^+ secretion.

Subsequent immunocytochemical studies using antibodies against the H^+-ATPase from bovine renal medulla confirmed the presence of an H^+-ATPase in the tubulovesicular structures and apical membrane of intercalated cells.[395] These studies, together with the demonstration that antibodies against AE1 label the basolateral membrane of intercalated cells, provided convincing evidence that these cells are involved in acid secretion in the collecting duct. Finally, there is now convincing evidence that mutations in the human H^+-ATPase gene lead to renal tubular acidosis (extensively reviewed by Wagner and colleagues[396]).

There is evidence that an H^+-K^+-ATPase is present in the collecting duct, where it plays an important role in K^+ reabsorption as well as H^+ secretion.[397] Biochemical studies have demonstrated H^+-K^+-ATPase activity in individual segments of both the cortical collecting duct and the outer medullary collecting duct of the rat[398] and the rabbit[398,399] that increases after consumption of a potassium-deficient diet,[398] which suggests that the transporter may be involved in K^+ reabsorption. Transport studies in the isolated perfused OMCDi of rabbits receiving a potassium-deficient diet also demonstrated K^+ reabsorption and H^+ secretion that were inhibited by omeprazole.[400] Furthermore, immunohistochemical studies revealed that antibodies to the gastric H^+-K^+-ATPase label the intercalated cells in the collecting duct of both the rat and the rabbit.[401] Subsequent in situ hybridization studies confirmed the expression of the gastric isoform of H^+-K^+-ATPase in intercalated cells of rat and rabbit collecting duct.[402,403]

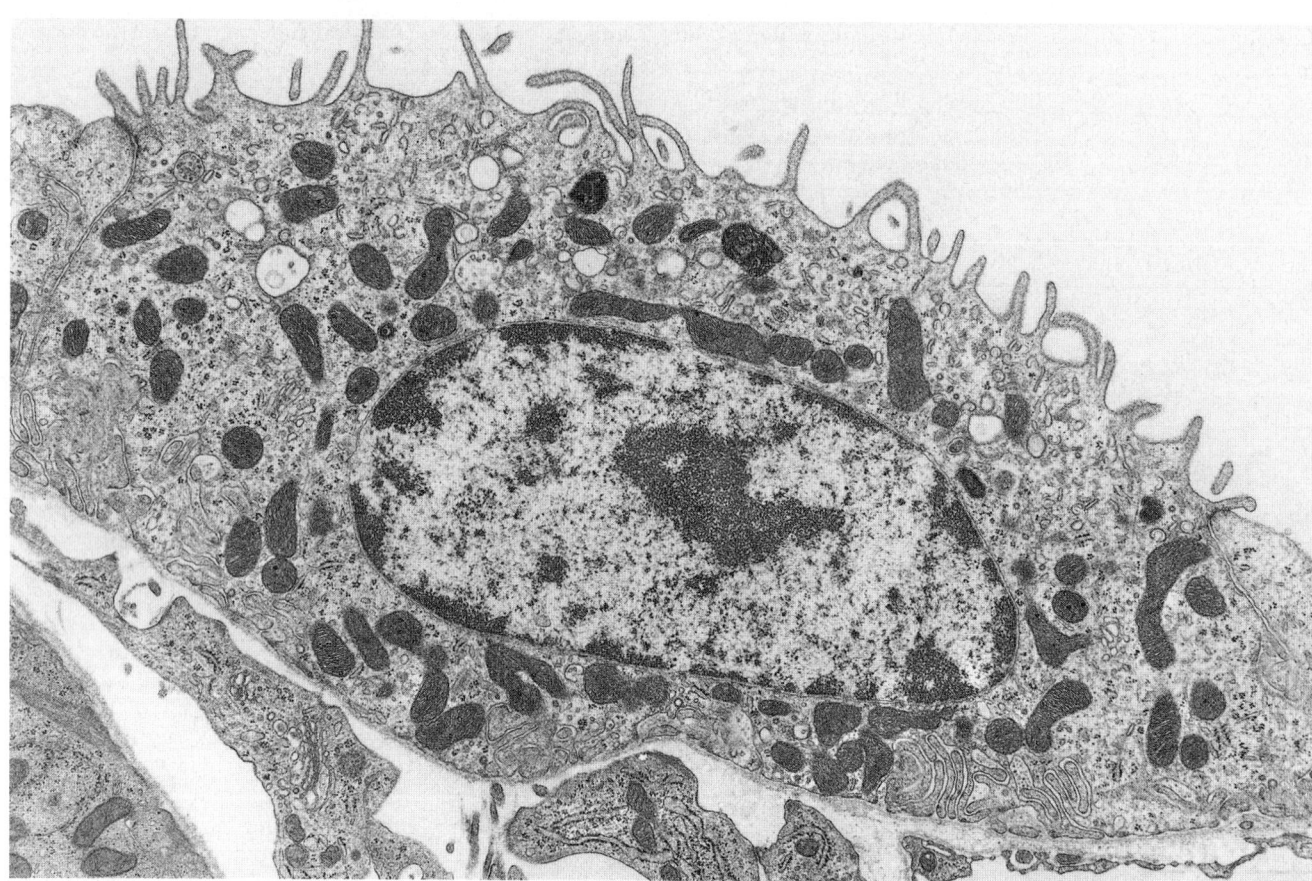

FIGURE 2-51 Transmission electron micrograph of an intercalated cell in the outer medullary collecting duct of normal rat kidney. The cell has a prominent tubulovesicular membrane compartment and many microprojections on the apical surface. (×10,000.) (From Madsen KM, Tisher CC: Response of intercalated cells of rat outer medullary collecting duct to chronic metabolic acidosis, *Lab Invest* 51:268, 1984.)

Therefore, intercalated cells are capable of both electrogenic H^+ secretion, mediated by a vacuolar-type H^+-ATPase, and electroneutral H^+ secretion in exchange for K^+, mediated by an H^+-K^+-ATPase. However, the two processes seem to be regulated differently. A study examining the role of aldosterone and dietary potassium in the regulation of ATPase activity in the collecting duct reported that H^+-ATPase activity is dependent on plasma aldosterone levels, whereas H^+-K^+-ATPase activity varies with changes in dietary potassium.[404] Moreover, an isoform of the α-subunit of the colonic H^+-K^+-ATPase, encoded by the H^+-K^+-α_2 gene, has been shown to be expressed in the kidney, where it mainly localizes to the outer medullary collecting duct principal cells.[405,406] In addition, transgenic mice expressing green fluorescent protein after exposure to the H^+-K^+-α_2 promoter show fluorescence in the collecting duct system.[407]

The colonic H^+-K^+-ATPase isoform has been shown to be regulated by long-term Na^+ and K^+ depletion,[405,406] and in cells of the inner third of the IMCD vasopressin and forskolin stimulate H^+-K^+-α_2 mRNA abundance, as does overexpression of cyclic adenosine monophosphate/Ca^{2+}–responsive element–binding protein.[408] Immunohistochemical studies have also demonstrated that a splice variant of the colonic isoform of H^+-K^+-ATPase is expressed in the apical domain of both intercalated cells and principal cells in the rabbit collecting duct.[409] Mice deficient in colonic H^+-K^+-ATPase showed no apparent renal phenotype either with or without K^+ depletion.[410]

Secretion of ammonia-ammonium by the collecting duct is an important component of net acid secretion. Members of the Rhesus protein superfamily have been proposed to function as NH_3/NH_4^+ transporters in the kidney.[411,412] Rh B and Rh G glycoproteins (RhBG and RhCG) are coexpressed in cells along the connecting tubule and collecting duct with strong immunoreactivity in intercalated cells and weaker expression in principal cells.[413-415] The RhCG protein is predominantly expressed in the apical plasma membrane, whereas RhBG is expressed in the basolateral membrane. Moreover, RhCG appears to be regulated in response to chronic metabolic acidosis, whereas RhBG remained unchanged.[416,417] RhBG-deficient mice did not exhibit any phenotypical changes, which suggests that RhBG may not contribute significantly to distal tubular ammonium excretion.[418] By contrast, global knockout of RhCG[419] or collecting duct-specific RhCG knockout[420] in mice decreased basal urinary ammonia excretion, whereas intercalated cell–specific knockout inhibited acidosis-stimulated but not basal ammonia excretion.[421] This suggests that RhCG in principal cells mediates basal ammonia excretion, whereas RhCG in intercalated cells is necessary for the normal renal response to metabolic acidosis.

Inner Medullary Collecting Duct

The IMCD extends from the boundary between the outer and inner medulla to the tip of the papilla. As the individual collecting ducts descend through the inner medulla, they

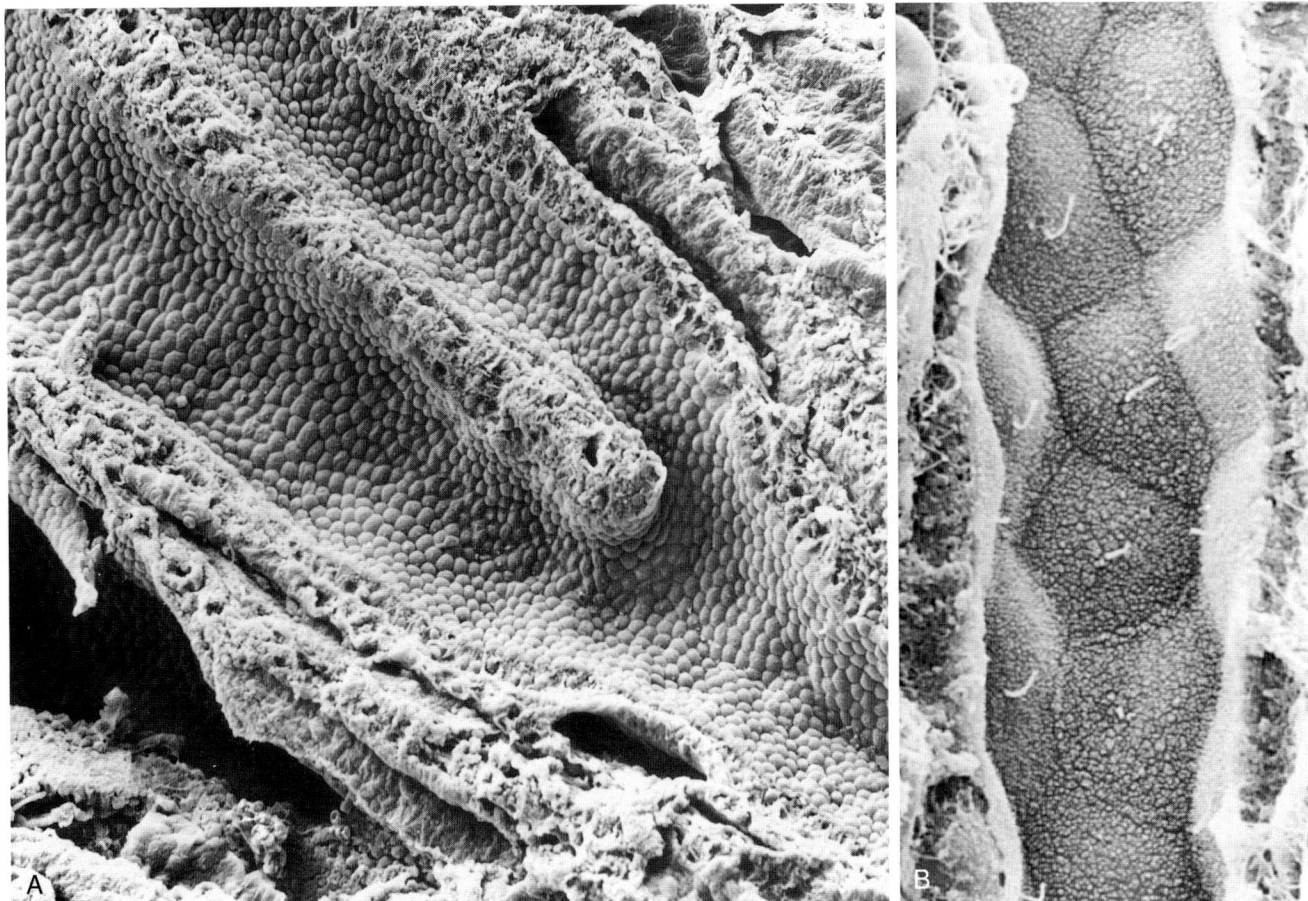

FIGURE 2-52 Scanning electron micrographs of a normal papillary collecting duct in rabbit kidney. **A,** The junction between two subdivisions at low magnification. (×600.) **B,** Higher-magnification view illustrating the luminal surface of individual cells with prominent microvilli and a single cilium. (×4250.) (**A** courtesy of Ann LeFurgey, PhD; **B** from LeFurgey A, Tisher CC: Morphology of rabbit collecting duct, *Am J Anat* 155:111, 1979.)

undergo successive fusions, which result in fewer tubules that have larger diameters (Figure 2-52). The final ducts, the ducts of Bellini, open on the tip of the papilla to form the area cribrosa (see Figure 2-3). The epithelium of the ducts of Bellini is tall, columnar, and similar to that covering the tip of the papilla.[134,422] There are considerable species differences in the length of the papilla, the number of fusions of the collecting ducts, and the height of the cells.[240,422] In the rabbit, the height of the cells gradually increases from approximately 10 μm in the initial portion to approximately 50 μm close to the papillary tip. In the rat the epithelium is considerably lower, and the increase in height occurs mainly in the inner half, from approximately 6 μm to 15 μm at the papillary tip.[338,422]

The IMCD has been subdivided arbitrarily into three portions: the outer third (IMCD1), middle third (IMCD2), and inner third (IMCD3).[338,423,424] The IMCD1 is similar in ultrastructure to the OMCDi, but most of the IMCD2 and the IMCD3 appear to represent a distinct segment.[424] The IMCD was originally believed to be a functionally homogeneous segment. However, transport studies have provided evidence that two functionally distinct segments exist in the inner medulla: an initial portion, the IMCDi, which corresponds to the IMCD1, and a terminal portion, the IMCDt, which includes most of the IMCD2 and the IMCD3. In the following text, the terms *IMCDi* and *IMCDt* are used to distinguish these two functionally distinct segments of the IMCD.

In both rat[423] and mouse,[325] the IMCDi consists of principal cells (Figure 2-53) and intercalated cells, the latter constituting approximately 10% of the total cell population.[423] Both cell types are similar in ultrastructure to the cells in the OMCDi and are believed to have the same functional properties. In the rabbit, the IMCDi is often composed of only one cell type, similar in ultrastructure to the predominant cell type in the OMCDi.[134] However, in some rabbits, intercalated cells can be found in this segment. In the rat, the transition from the IMCDi to the IMCDt is gradual and occurs in the outer part of the IMCD2.[338,424]

The IMCDt consists mainly of one cell type, the IMCD cell. It is cuboid to columnar with a light-staining cytoplasm and few cell organelles (Figure 2-54). It contains numerous ribosomes and many small, coated vesicles resembling clathrin-coated vesicles. Small electron-dense bodies representing lysosomes or lipid droplets are present in the cytoplasm, often located beneath the nucleus. The luminal membrane has short microvilli that are more numerous than those on principal cells, and they are covered with an extensive glycocalyx. Infoldings of the basal plasma membrane are sparse. By scanning electron microscopy, the luminal surface of IMCD cells is covered with numerous small microvilli (Figures 2-55 and 2-56). However, these cells lack the central cilium.[424]

The functional properties of the IMCD have been studied by in vivo micropuncture of the exposed rat papilla by microcatheterization through a duct of Bellini[240,338] and by the

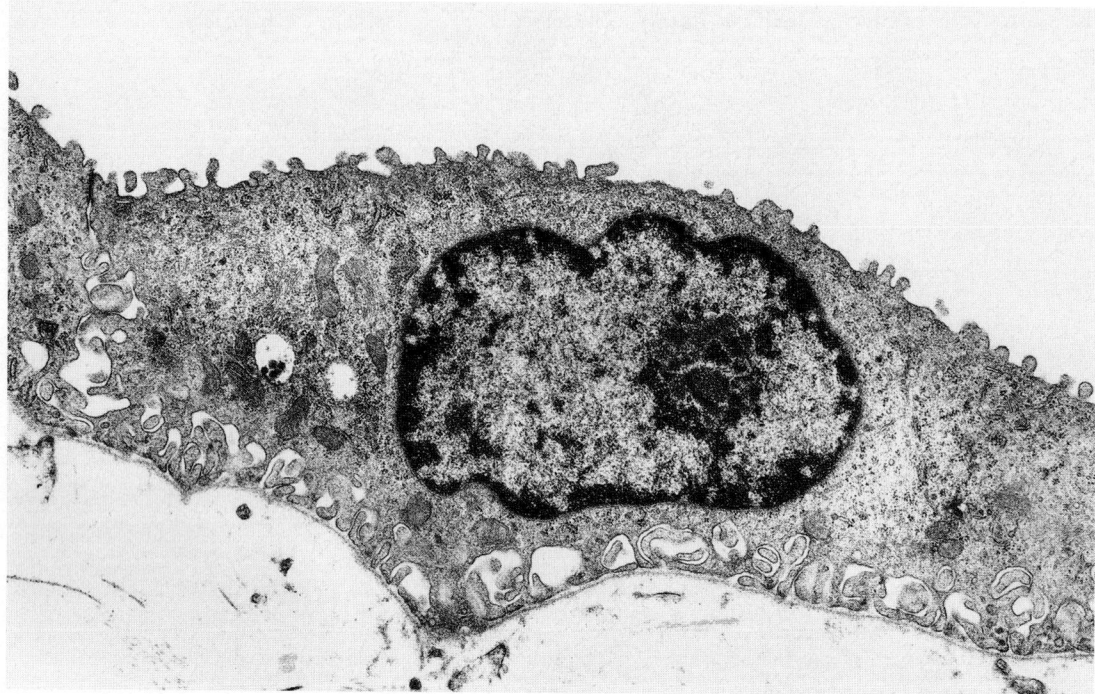

FIGURE 2-53 Transmission electron micrograph of a principal cell from the initial portion of the rat inner medullary collecting duct (IMCDi). Few organelles are present in the cytoplasm, and apical microprojections are sparse. (×11,750.) (From Madsen KM, Clapp WL, Verlander JW: Structure and function of the inner medullary collecting duct, *Kidney Int* 34:441, 1988.)

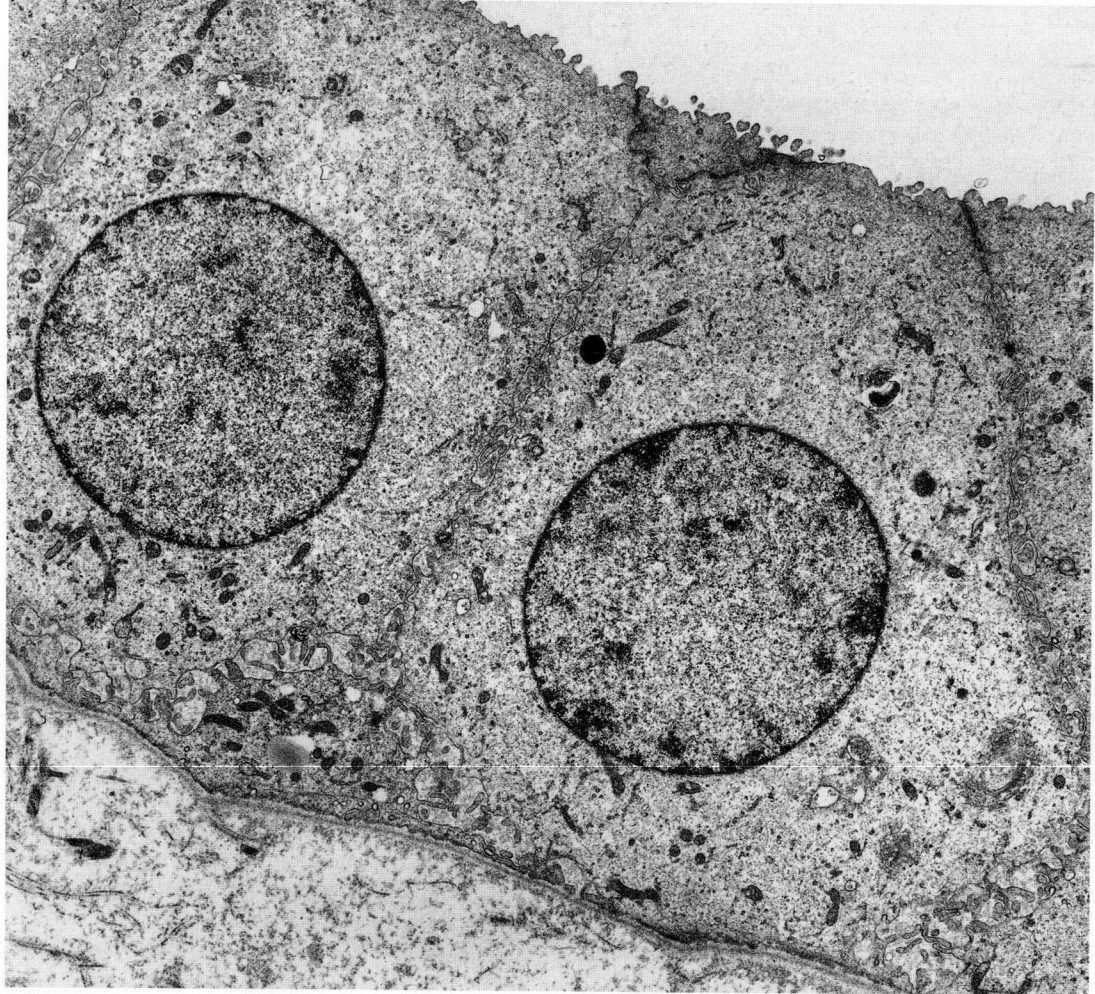

FIGURE 2-54 Transmission electron micrograph of cells from the terminal portion of the rabbit inner medullary collecting duct (IMCDt). The cells are tall, possess few organelles, and exhibit small microprojections on the apical surface. Ribosomes and small coated vesicles are scattered throughout the cytoplasm. (×7000.)

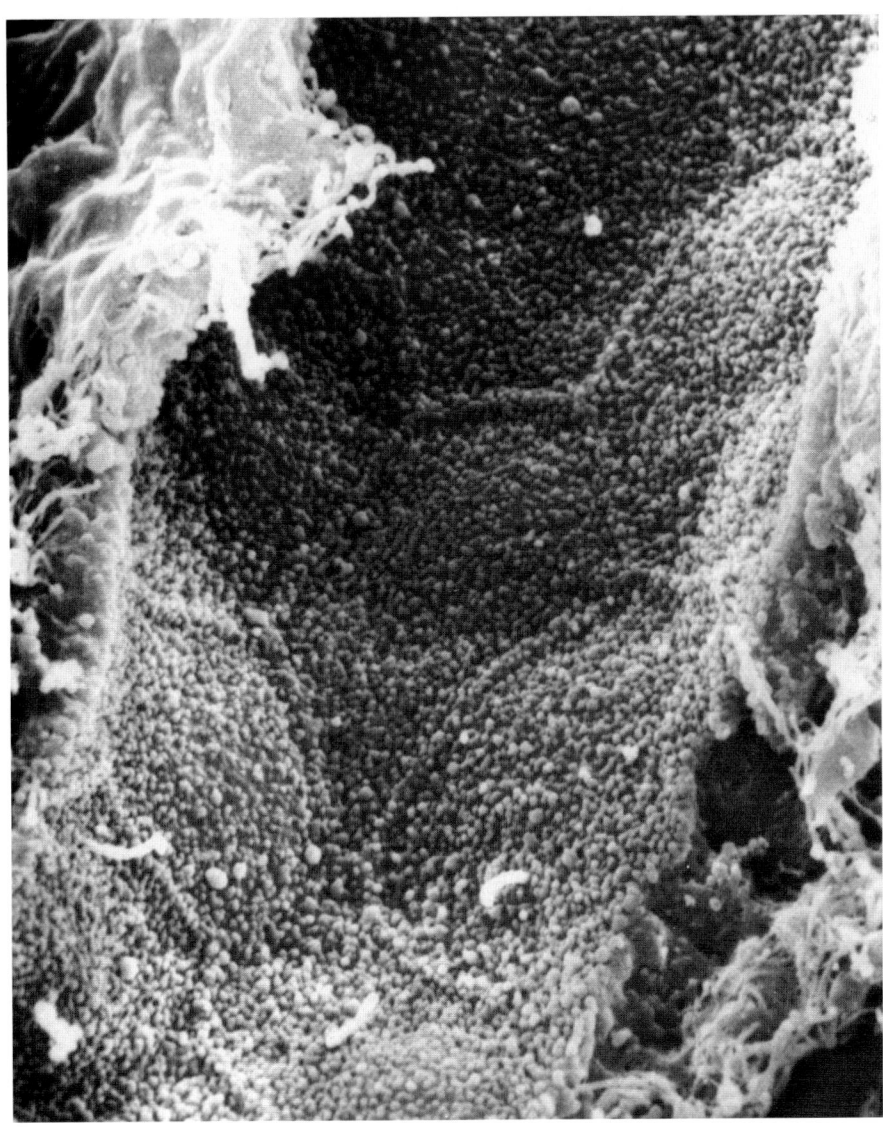

FIGURE 2-55 Scanning electron micrograph of the middle portion of the rat inner medullary collecting duct. The luminal surface is covered with small microvilli, and some cells possess a single cilium. (×10,500.) (From Madsen KM, Clapp WL, Verlander JW: Structure and function of the inner medullary collecting duct, *Kidney Int* 34:441, 1988.)

isolated perfused tubule technique. Use of these techniques has established that the IMCD is involved in the reabsorption of Na^+, Cl^-, K^+, urea, and water. Sands and Knepper,[425] using an improved method of microdissection and perfusion of segments of the IMCD from both rat and rabbit, demonstrated significant functional differences between the IMCDi and the IMCDt.[425,426] In the absence of vasopressin, the IMCDi is impermeable to both urea and water, whereas significant permeabilities for both urea and water were demonstrated in the IMCDt. Vasopressin stimulated water permeability in both segments of the IMCD, but urea permeability was stimulated only in the IMCDt.

Salt, water, and urea transport in the IMCD is regulated by other factors in addition to vasopressin, including atrial natriuretic peptides, ATP, glucagon, and glucocorticoids. In the following, a brief overview of the permeability of the collecting duct to water and urea is provided (see Chapter 10 for detailed discussion).

In the presence of vasopressin, all segments of the collecting duct are permeable to water. Morphologic changes, including cell swelling, dilatation of intercellular spaces, and an increased number of intracellular vacuoles, have been demonstrated along the entire collecting duct in association with vasopressin-induced osmotic water reabsorption (Figure 2-57).[296,427-429] Freeze-fracture studies have demonstrated characteristic intramembrane particle aggregates in the apical membrane of vasopressin-responsive cells in the collecting duct,[430,431] which are suggested to represent water channels.[432] Transmission electron microscopy has revealed the presence of coated pits in the luminal plasma membrane of principal cells. These coated pits correspond to the location of intramembrane particle clusters, which suggests that endocytosis plays a role in the regulation of water permeability.[433] Studies using horseradish peroxidase as a marker of endocytosis demonstrated that removal of vasopressin stimulates endocytosis in principal cells of the collecting duct in the rabbit[434]; these results suggest that water channels are internalized from the luminal membrane. Similar studies in Brattleboro rats with hereditary diabetes insipidus also indirectly suggested that insertion and retrieval of water channels in the principal cells are regulated by vasopressin.[435]

Nielsen and colleagues demonstrated that the water channel AQP2 was expressed in the principal cells and IMCD cells along the entire collecting duct of the rat (Figure 2-58).[436] AQP2 is detected at the apical plasma membrane and in small subapical vesicles.[437,438] Subsequent immunohistochemical

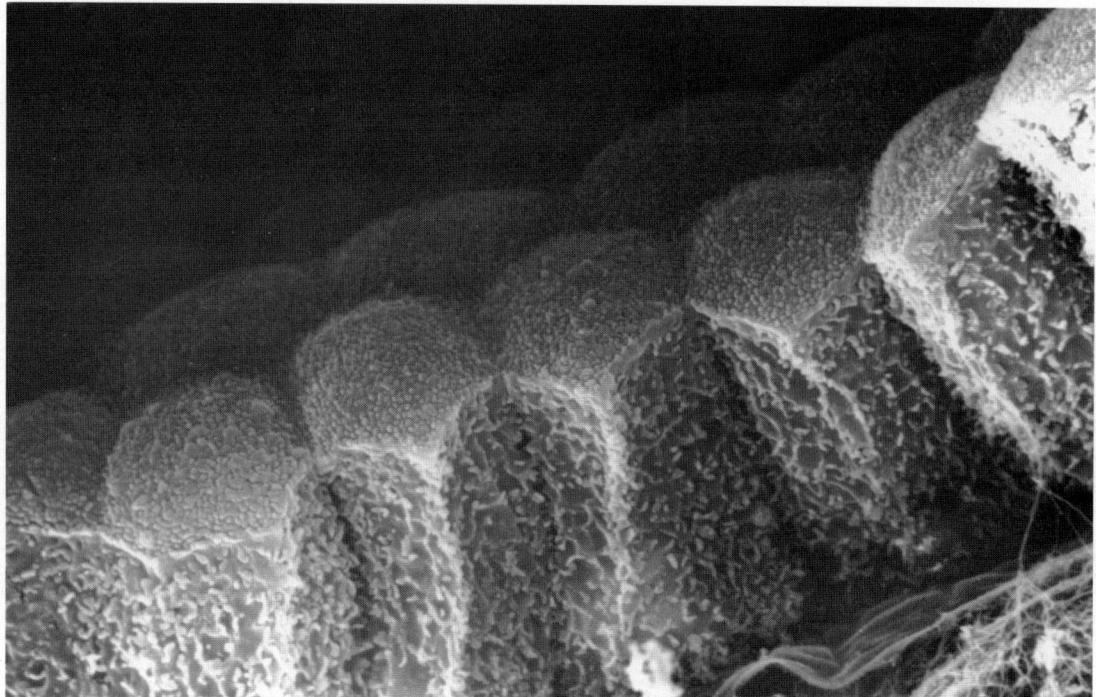

FIGURE 2-56 Scanning electron micrograph of the terminal portion of the rabbit inner medullary collecting duct (IMCDt). The cells are tall and covered with small microvilli on the luminal surface. Small lateral cell processes project into the lateral intercellular spaces. (×6000.) (From Madsen KM, Clapp WL, Verlander JW: Structure and function of the inner medullary collecting duct, *Kidney Int* 34:441, 1988.)

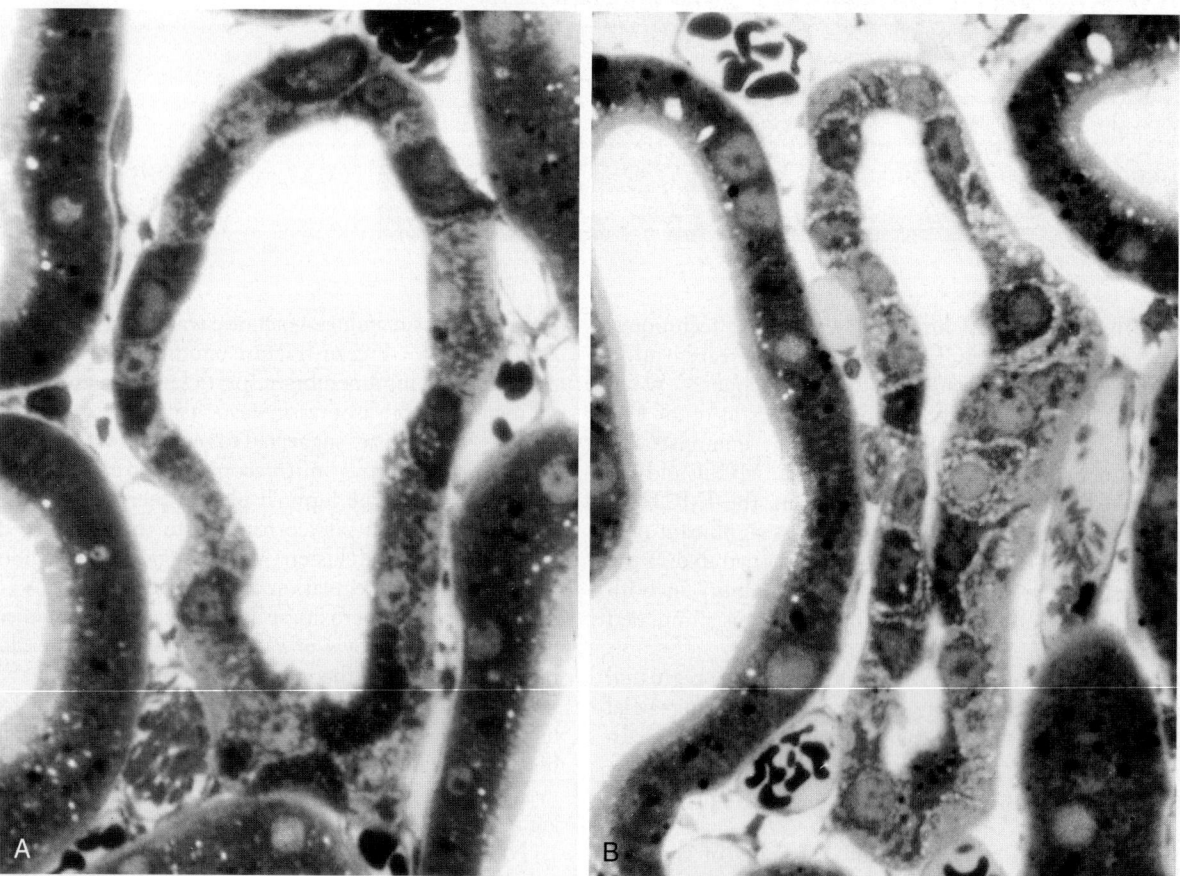

FIGURE 2-57 Light micrographs of cortical collecting ducts of rats with hypothalamic diabetes insipidus. **A,** Tissue preserved during water diuresis in the absence of exogenous vasopressin. (×960.) **B,** Tissue preserved after water diuresis was interrupted by intravenous administration of exogenous vasopressin. Note the presence of cell swelling and marked dilatation of the intercellular spaces. (×960.)

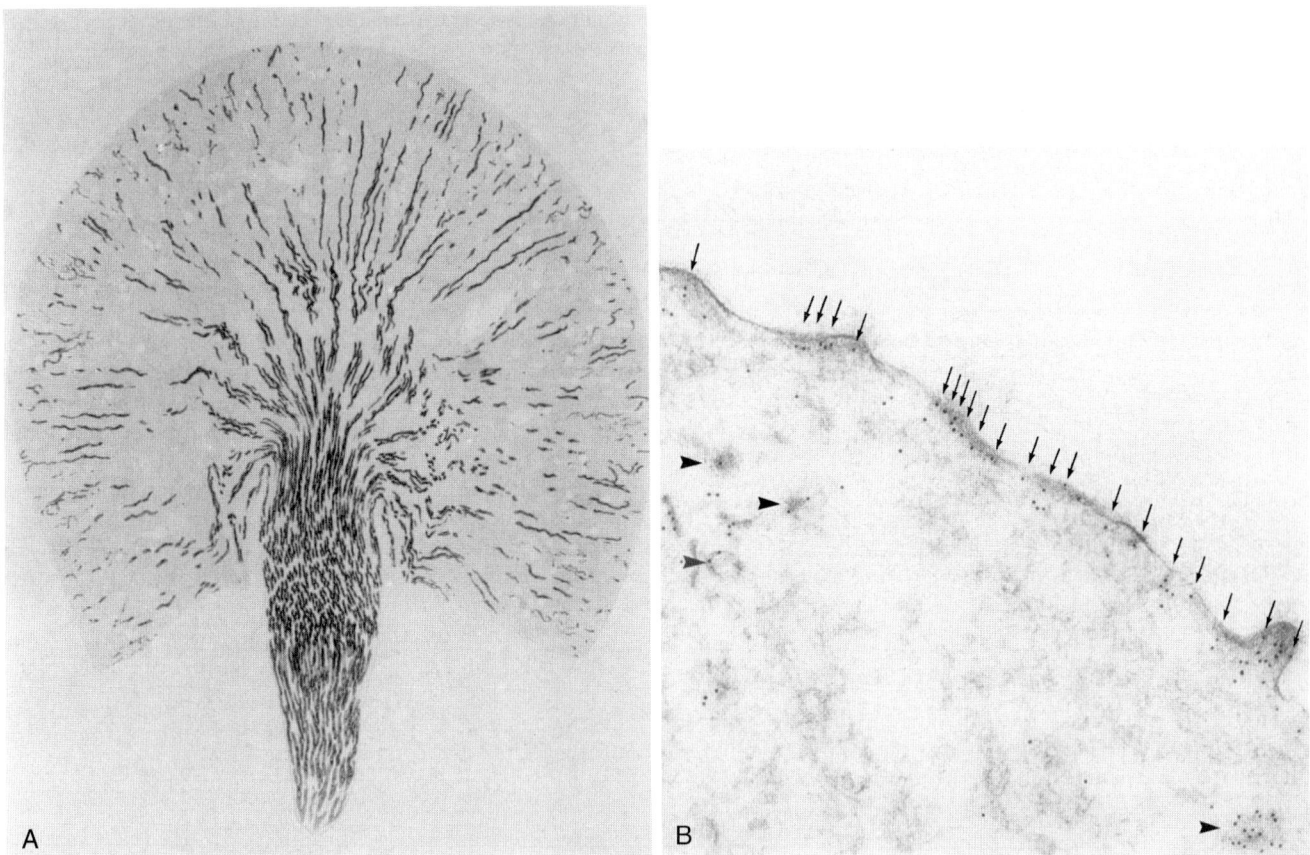

FIGURE 2-58 **A,** Light micrographs of 50-μm Vibratome sections of rat kidney, illustrating immunolocalization of the vasopressin-sensitive aquaporin-2 water channel in the collecting duct using a horseradish peroxidase procedure. Labeling of aquaporin-2 is seen in the connecting tubule and in principal cells throughout the collecting duct. **B,** Immunogold labeling of aquaporin-2 in the apical plasma membrane of principal cells in the cortical collecting duct showing expression at the apical plasma membrane (*arrows*) and in intracellular vesicles (*arrowheads*). (×20,000.) (**A** courtesy of Jin Kim, MD, Catholic University, Seoul, Korea.)

studies demonstrated that AQP3 and AQP4 are expressed in the basolateral plasma membrane, representing exit pathways for water reabsorbed through AQP2 channels.[439-442] AQP2 is also expressed in the basolateral membrane in the connecting tubule and the cortical collecting duct in response to aldosterone treatment.[443,444] The regulation of AQP2 is described in detail in Chapter 11.

Although the entire collecting duct is permeable to water, only the IMCD is permeable to urea.[445] Urea transport in the IMCDt is a facilitated process that is mediated by specific transport proteins located in the plasma membrane of the IMCD cells. The UT-A group of renal urea transporters belongs to a large family of urea transporters that also includes the erythrocyte urea transporter UT-B, which is expressed in the descending vasa recta. Studies of the segmental distribution of these transporters by in situ hybridization and immunohistochemical methods revealed that UT-A1 was expressed exclusively in the IMCDt, whereas UT-A2 was expressed in the descending thin limb of the loop of Henle (see Figure 2-37).[256-258] A third isoform, UT-A3, has also been identified in the IMCDt.[446] UT-A1 and UT-A3 are expressed exclusively in IMCD cells, and immunocytochemical studies have revealed that UT-A1 is present in the apical region of the IMCD,[258,447] whereas UT-A3 is localized both intracellularly and in the basolateral membrane.[446,448]

The role of urea transport in the inner medulla for the urinary concentrating mechanism was highlighted by Fenton and colleagues, who developed a mouse model by deleting both UT-A1 and UT-A3 using standard gene-targeting techniques.[449] These mice were found to have a severe urinary concentrating defect.[450]

The IMCD is also involved in urine acidification. Microcatheterization experiments estimating in situ pH demonstrated a decrease in pH along the IMCD,[451] and micropuncture of the papillary collecting duct revealed reabsorption of bicarbonate, which could be inhibited with acetazolamide.[452,453] In addition, microcatheterization studies demonstrated an increase in net acid secretion in the IMCD of rats with acute and chronic metabolic acidosis.[454,455]

The mechanism of H[+] secretion in this segment of the collecting duct is not known. In the rat, intercalated cells are present in the IMCDi. They are similar in ultrastructure to intercalated cells in the outer medullary collecting duct, and they exhibit immunostaining for both H[+]-ATPase and AE1, which suggests that they are involved in H[+] secretion.

Urine acidification has been demonstrated along the papillary portion of the collecting duct, where there are no intercalated cells, which indicates that the IMCD cells must also be involved in H[+] secretion; however, carbonic anhydrase has not been demonstrated in IMCD cells of adult animals, and these cells are also negative for AE1. An H[+]-ATPase has been isolated from both bovine[456] and rat[457] renal medulla, but the exact cellular origin of this ATPase is not known.

Although there is no immunoreactivity for either H⁺-ATPase or H⁺-K⁺-ATPase in IMCD cells, studies in cultured IMCD cells have demonstrated acid secretion mediated by H⁺-ATPase[458] as well as H⁺-K⁺-ATPase.[459] Moreover, acid secretion mediated by an H⁺-K⁺-ATPase was demonstrated in isolated perfused IMCDt segments from the rat kidney.[460] Interestingly, studies in AQP1-deficient mice revealed strong H⁺-ATPase immunoreactivity in the apical plasma membrane of IMCD cells and increased H⁺-ATPase protein expression in the inner medulla of AQP1-null mice compared with wild-type mice.[461]

Interstitium

The renal interstitium is composed of interstitial cells and a loose, flocculent extracellular matrix material consisting of sulfated and nonsulfated glucosaminoglycans.[462,463] The amount of interstitial tissue in the cortex is limited, and the tubules and capillaries are often directly apposed to each other. The interstitium constitutes 7% to 9% of the cortical volume in the rat.[464,465] Three percent of the 7% represents the interstitial cells, and the remaining 4% represents the extracellular space.[462] In the medulla, a gradual increase occurs in interstitial volume, from 10% to 20% in the outer medulla to approximately 30% to 40% at the papillary tip in both the rat and the rabbit.[422,465] In a study using the volume of distribution of inulin and similar extracellular markers, the interstitial volume in the rat kidney was found to constitute approximately 13% of the total kidney volume; in the rabbit kidney, the value was 17.5%.[466]

Cortical Interstitium

The cortical interstitium can be divided into a wide interstitial space, located between two or more adjacent renal tubules, and a narrow or slitlike interstitial space, located between the basement membrane of a single tubule and the adjacent peritubular capillary.[467,468] Whether such a division has any functional significance is unknown; however, it is of interest that approximately two thirds of the total peritubular capillary wall faces the narrow compartment and that this portion of the vessel wall is fenestrated.[464] This relationship might facilitate the control of fluid reabsorption across the basolateral membrane of the proximal tubule by Starling's forces.

There are two types of interstitial cells in the cortex: one that resembles a fibroblast (type 1 cortical interstitial cell) (Figure 2-59) and another, less common mononuclear or lymphocyte-like cell (type 2 cortical interstitial cell).[462,467] Type 1 cells are positioned between the basement membranes of adjacent tubules and peritubular capillaries. They have a stellate appearance and contain an irregularly shaped nucleus and a well-developed rough- and smooth-surfaced endoplasmic

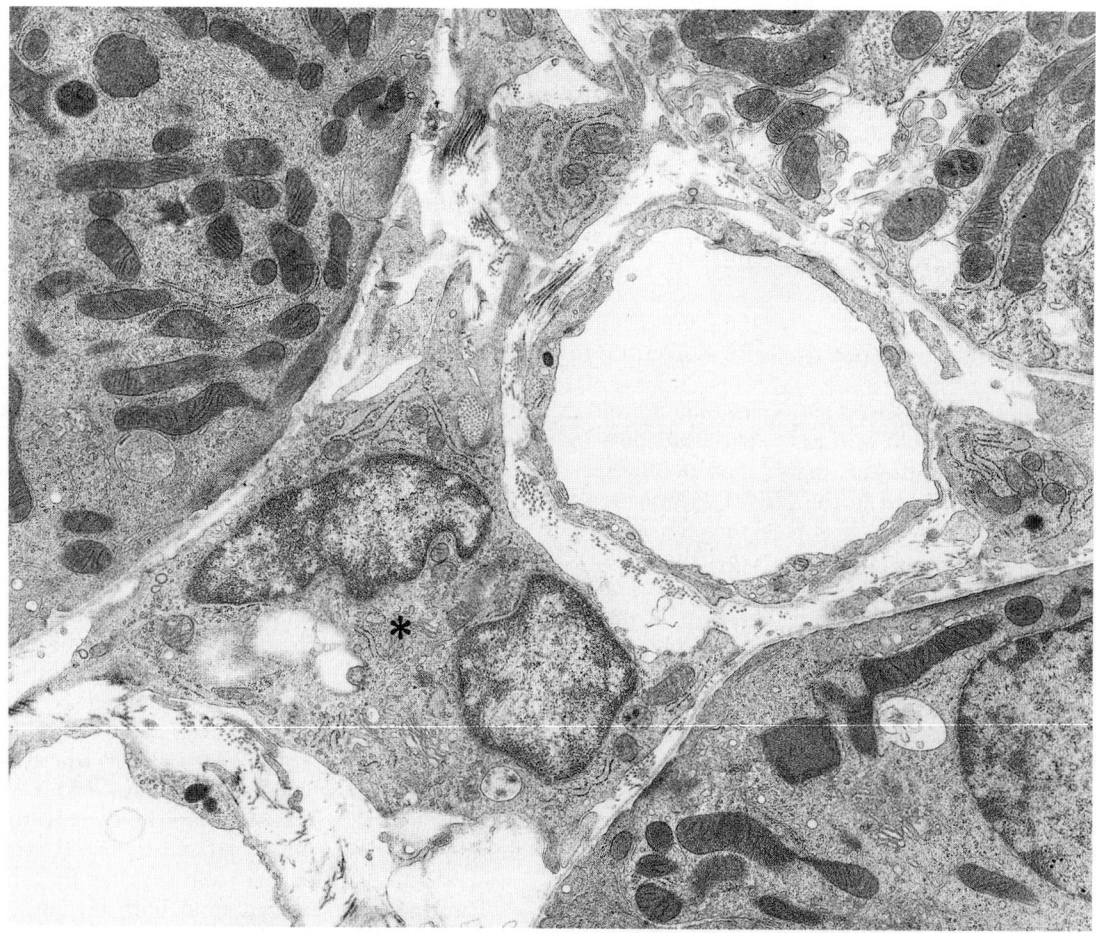

FIGURE 2-59 Transmission electron micrograph of a type 1 cortical interstitial cell (*asterisk*) from rat kidney. A peritubular capillary is located at *right center.* (×9300.)

reticulum. Type 2 cells are usually round, with sparse cytoplasm and few cell organelles. Studies by Kaissling and Le Hir[469] demonstrated antigen-presenting dendritic cells among the fibroblasts in the peritubular interstitium in both the cortex and outer medulla of the normal rat kidney. The interstitial space contains a loose, flocculent material of low density and small bundles of collagen fibrils. Immunocytochemical staining of immature and mature human kidney has revealed types I and III collagen and fibronectin in the interstitium of the cortex.[470] Type V collagen has been described in the cortical interstitium of the rat.[471]

There is evidence that the peritubular, fibroblast-like interstitial cells are the site of erythropoietin production in the kidney. In situ hybridization studies using sulfur 35–labeled probes detected erythropoietin mRNA in peritubular cells in the kidney cortex of anemic mice.[472] This localization was confirmed by Bachmann and colleagues,[473] who demonstrated co-localization of erythropoietin mRNA and immunoreactivity for ecto-5′-nucleotidase, a marker of the fibroblast-like interstitial cells in the renal cortex,[474] and thus identified the erythropoietin-producing cells in the renal cortex as being interstitial cells. The lymphocyte-like interstitial cells in the cortex are believed to represent bone marrow–derived cells.

Medullary Interstitium

Bohman[468] described three types of interstitial cells in the rat renal medulla. Type 1 cells are the prominent, lipid-containing interstitial cells and resemble the type 1 cells in the cortex. However, they do not express erythropoietin mRNA and do not contain ecto-5′-nucleotidase.[473,474] They are present throughout the inner medulla and are also found in the inner stripe of the outer medulla. The type 2 medullary interstitial cell is a lymphocyte-like cell that is virtually identical to the mononuclear cell (type 2 interstitial cell) described previously in the cortex. It is present in the outer medulla and in the outer part of the inner medulla. It is free of lipid droplets, but lysosome-like bodies are often observed. Type 2 cells are sometimes found together with type 1 cells. The type 3 cell is a pericyte that is located in the outer medulla and the outer portion of the inner medulla. It is closely related to the descending vasa recta, where it is found between two leaflets of the basement membrane. These three types of interstitial cells are also found in the rabbit.[467]

Most interstitial cells in the inner medulla are the lipid-containing type 1 interstitial cells,[475] which are often referred to as the *renomedullary interstitial cells.* They have long cytoplasmic projections that give them an irregular, star-shaped appearance. The cells are often arranged in rows between the loops of Henle and vasa recta, with their long axes perpendicular to those of adjacent tubules and vessels, so that they resemble the rungs of a ladder (Figure 2-60). The elongated cell processes are in close contact with the thin limbs of Henle and the vasa recta, but direct contact with collecting ducts is observed only rarely. Often, a single cell is in contact with several vessels and thin limbs.[468] The long cytoplasmic processes from different cells are often connected by specialized cell junctions that vary in both size and shape and contain elements of tight junctions, intermediate junctions, and gap junctions.[476,477]

Several investigators have described the ultrastructure of the type 1 medullary interstitial cells in rat,[468] rabbit,[467,475] and human kidney. These cells contain numerous lipid inclusions or droplets in the cytoplasm that vary considerably in both size and number (Figure 2-61). An average diameter of 0.4 to 0.5 μm has been reported in the rat, but profiles of up to 1 μm in diameter were also observed.[478] The droplets have a homogeneous content, but they have no limiting membrane; however, they are often surrounded by smooth cytomembranes with a thickness of 6 to 7 nm. The cells contain large amounts of rough endoplasmic reticulum that often is continuous with elements of the smooth cytoplasmic membranes. Mitochondria are sparse and scattered randomly in the cytoplasm. A small number of lysosomes are present, but endocytic vacuoles are sparse, although interstitial cells are capable of endocytosis of particulate material.

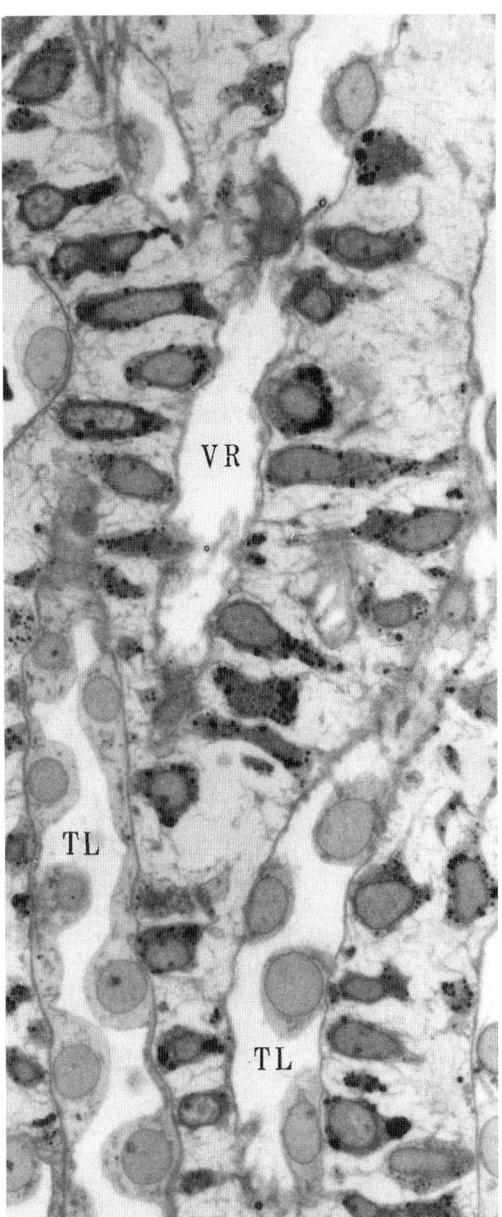

FIGURE 2-60 Light micrograph of the renal medullary interstitium from a normal rat. The lipid-laden type 1 interstitial cells bridge the interstitial space between adjacent thin limbs of Henle (TL) and vasa recta (VR). (×830.)

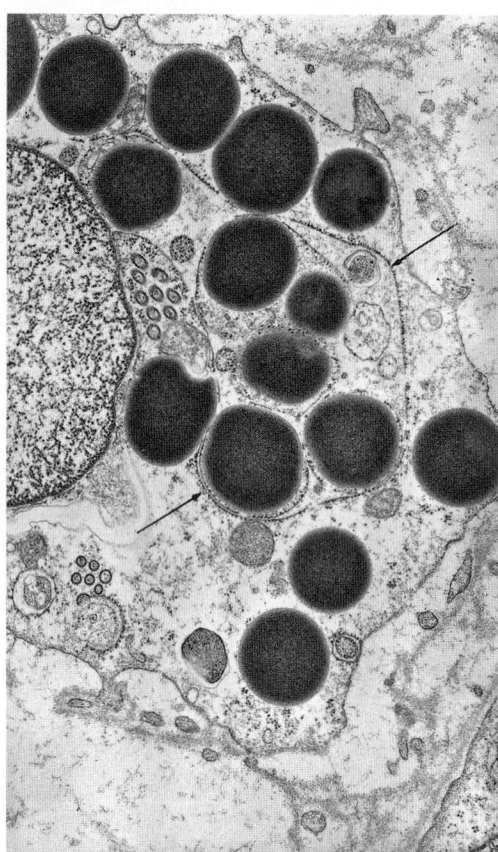

FIGURE 2-61 Higher-magnification electron micrograph illustrating the relationship between the electron-dense lipid droplets, which almost fill the type 1 medullary interstitial cells, and the granular endoplasmic reticulum (*arrows*). Wisps of basement membrane–like material adjacent to the surface of the cells are contiguous with the basement membrane of the adjacent tubules (*lower right*). (×12,000.)

An unusual type of cylindrical body, measuring 0.1 to 0.2 μm in diameter and up to 11 mm in length and believed to be derived from the endoplasmic reticulum, has been described in the type 1 interstitial cells.[462,479-481] These structures were observed originally in rats with dehydration and were believed to represent a response to severe dehydration,[479] but subsequent studies demonstrated their presence under normal conditions.[480] The wall of the cylinders consists of two triple-layered membranes, each measuring 6 nm in thickness, and connections between the walls and the membranes of the endoplasmic reticulum have been observed.[479] The functional significance of these cylindrical structures remains unknown.

The number and size of the lipid inclusions in type 1 medullary interstitial cells vary considerably, depending on the physiologic state of the animal[482,483] and the species.[475] In the rat, lipid droplets constitute 2% to 4% of the interstitial cell volume, and the volume depends largely on the physiologic state of the animal.[478] The lipid droplets were originally reported to decrease in both size and number after 24 hours of dehydration,[483] but in a later study Bohman and Jensen[478] were unable to confirm these findings.

The function of type 1 interstitial cells (renomedullary interstitial cells) is incompletely understood. They probably provide structural support in the medulla because of their special arrangement that is perpendicular to the tubules and vessels. The close relationship between these cells and the thin limbs and capillaries also suggests a possible interaction with these structures. Because of the presence of a well-developed endoplasmic reticulum and prominent lipid droplets, researchers have suggested that the type 1 interstitial cells may also be secretory.[484] The lipid droplets are not secretory granules in the usual sense, however, because they have no limiting membrane and there is no evidence that they are secreted by the cell. The droplets have been isolated from homogenates of the renal medulla of both rat[485,486] and rabbit.[487] They consist mainly of triglycerides and small amounts of cholesterol esters and phospholipids.[486] The triglycerides are rich in unsaturated fatty acids, including arachidonic acid.[485,487]

The renomedullary interstitial cells are a major site of prostaglandin synthesis, with the major product being PGE_2.[488] Prostaglandin synthesis in the renomedullary interstitial cells is mediated by COX-2.[489] The expression of COX-2 in these cells increases in response to water deprivation and hypertonicity.[128,489,490] Binding sites for several vasoactive peptides, including angiotensin II, are present in renomedullary interstitial cells,[491,492] and there is evidence that angiotensin may be involved in the regulation of prostaglandin production in the renal medulla.[493]

Using histochemical techniques, Kugler[494] demonstrated the presence of aminopeptidase A (EC 3.4.11.7), an angiotensinase that is capable of degrading angiotensin, in the type 1 renomedullary interstitial cells of rat, rabbit, golden hamster, and guinea pig. Therefore, another possible mechanism for control of angiotensin stimulation of prostaglandin production seems to be present in the medulla.

Finally, the interstitial cells are responsible for the synthesis of the glycosaminoglycans—in particular, hyaluronic acid—that are present in the matrix material of the interstitium.[495] Little is known about the function of the type 2 and type 3 medullary interstitial cells. Bohman[462] suggested that the type 2 cells are probably phagocytic, but the function of type 3 cells remains unknown.

Lymphatics

Interstitial fluid can leave the kidney by two different lymphatic networks, a superficial capsular system and a deeper hilar system.[496,497] Our knowledge of the distribution of lymphatics within the kidney, however, is limited. Intrarenal lymphatics are embedded in the periarterial loose connective tissue around the renal arteries and are distributed primarily along the interlobular and arcuate arteries in the cortex.[496-498] Kriz and Dieterich[498] believed that the cortical lymphatics begin as lymphatic capillaries in the area of the interlobular arteries and that these capillaries drain into the arcuate lymphatic vessels at the region of the corticomedullary junction (Figure 2-62). The arcuate lymphatic vessels drain to hilar lymphatic vessels through interlobar lymphatics. Numerous valves have been described within the interlobar and hilar lymphatic channels.[498]

Similar findings were reported by Bell and associates[497] in both calves and dogs. In the horse, glomeruli are often completely surrounded by lymphatic channels, whereas in the dog, only a portion of the glomerulus is surrounded by lymphatics.[497] Electron microscopic studies in the dog kidney after injection of India ink into capsular lymphatic vessels revealed the presence of small lymphatic channels in close apposition to both proximal and distal tubules, in addition to the interlobular

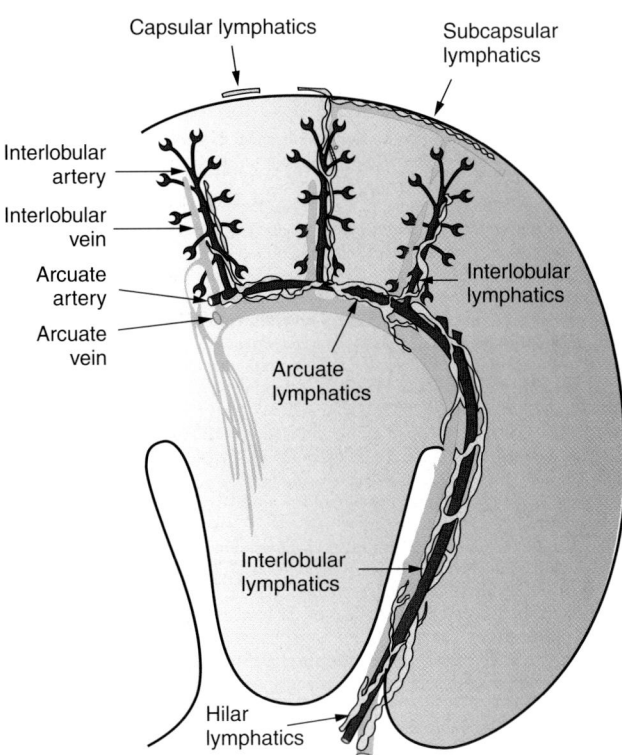

FIGURE 2-62 Diagram of the lymphatic circulation in the mammalian kidney. (Modified from Kriz W, Dieterich HJ: The lymphatic system of the kidney in some mammals. Light and electron microscopic investigations, *Z Anat Entwicklungsgesch* 131:111, 1970.)

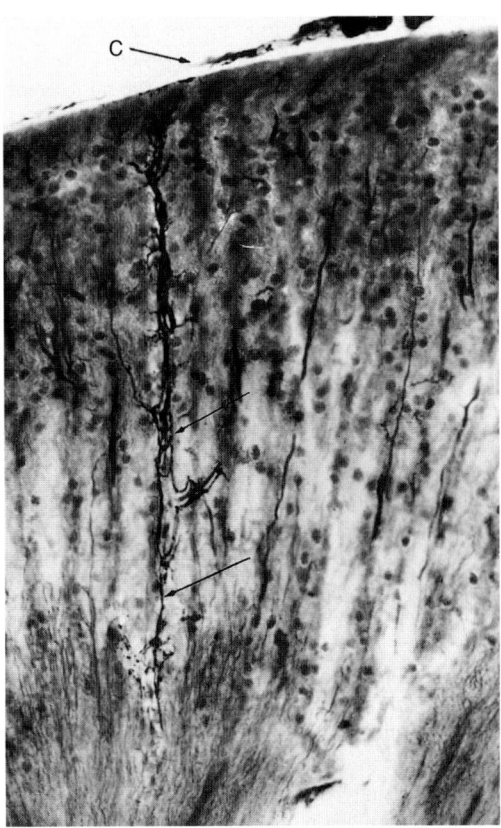

FIGURE 2-63 Light micrograph of a sagittal section through the cortex and outer medulla of dog kidney. A capsular lymphatic (C) was injected with India ink. Intrarenal lymphatics (*arrows*) follow the distribution of the interlobular arteries in the cortex. (×10.) (From Bell RD, Keyl MJ, Shrader FR, et al: Renal lymphatics: the internal distribution, *Nephron* 5:454, 1968.)

arteries.[499] An electron microscopic study of the lymphatic system in the dog kidney demonstrated the existence of cortical intralobular lymphatics closely associated with terminal arteries, arterioles, renal corpuscles, and tubule elements.[500]

Morphometric analysis revealed that the cross-sectional area of interlobular lymphatics was almost twice that of intralobular lymphatics in the cortex. The volume density of renal cortical lymphatics was 0.17%.[500] Similar morphometric studies in the rat, hamster, and rabbit revealed volume densities of cortical lymphatics of 0.11%, 0.37%, and 0.02%, respectively.[501]

A less extensive system of lymphatic vessels is present within and immediately beneath the renal capsule.[497,498] The lymphatic vessels of the renal capsule drain into subcapsular lymphatic channels that lie adjacent to interlobular arteries located just beneath the renal capsule. These lymphatic vessels appear to provide continuity between the major intrarenal lymphatic vessels within the cortex (interlobular and arcuate lymphatic vessels) and the capsular lymphatic vessels; thus, in some animals, a continuous system of lymphatic drainage has been observed from the renal capsule, through the cortex, and into the hilar region (Figure 2-63).

In the dog kidney, two types of tributaries have been described in association with the surface lymphatics.[502] So-called communicating lymphatic channels were found in small numbers, usually in association with an interlobular artery and vein; these lymphatics penetrated the capsule and appeared to represent a connection between the hilar and capsular systems. The second type of vessel, the so-called perforating lymphatic channel, penetrated the capsule alone or in association with a small vein; these channels appeared to represent a primary pathway for lymph drainage from the superficial cortex.

From a study in the dog kidney, investigators concluded that intramedullary lymphatics do not exist in this species, and they suggested that interstitial fluid from the medulla may drain to the arcuate or interlobar lymphatics.[503] It has also been suggested that plasma proteins are cleared from the medullary interstitium through the ascending vasa recta.[504-506] On microscopic examination, the wall of the interlobular lymphatic vessel is formed by a single endothelial layer and does not have the support of a basement membrane.[498] The arcuate and interlobar lymphatic vessels are similar in appearance, although the latter possess valves.

Innervation

The efferent nerve supply to the kidney arises largely from the celiac plexus, with additional contributions originating from the greater splanchnic nerve, the intermesenteric plexus, and the superior hypogastric plexus.[507] The postganglionic sympathetic nerve fiber distribution generally follows the arterial vessels throughout the cortex and outer stripe of the outer medulla.[508] Adrenergic fibers have been observed lying adjacent to smooth muscle cells of arcuate and interlobular arteries and afferent arterioles.[509-511] An extensive innervation of the efferent arteriolar vessels of the juxtamedullary glomeruli, which eventually divide to form the afferent vasa recta, has been described.[510,512] However, quantitation of monoaminergic innervation by autoradiography revealed a higher density of norepinephrine-containing nerves associated with the afferent rather than the efferent arteriole.[511] Newstead and Munkacsi[512] reported the existence of large bundles of unmyelinated nerve fibers that accompanied the efferent arterioles from the region of the juxtamedullary glomeruli to the level of the inner stripe of the outer medulla. Nerve fibers and nerve endings were no longer present at the site at which the smooth muscle layer of the efferent arterioles and arteriolae rectae gave way to the pericytes surrounding the arterial vasa recta, which begin in the deep inner stripe of the outer medulla. There is also evidence for the presence of transitory adrenergic fibers in the inner medulla of the cat kidney.[513]

For some time, controversy has existed regarding the presence of direct tubule innervation in the renal cortex. Nerve bundles arising from perivascular nerves have been described in proximity to both proximal and distal tubules.[514] Structures termed *varicosities*, which are believed to represent nerve endings, have been described as being in close contact with proximal and distal tubules, often in the vicinity of the hilum of the glomerulus and the juxtaglomerular apparatus,[116,514,515] and in the connecting segment and the cortical collecting duct.[516] Autoradiographic studies have also revealed that injected tritiated norepinephrine is taken up by both proximal and distal convoluted tubules, which indicates monoaminergic innervation of these tubules.[517] The thick ascending limb of Henle receives the largest nerve supply.[517] Both myelinated and unmyelinated nerve fibers have been demonstrated in the corticomedullary region and in perivascular connective tissue.[518] Electron microscopic autoradiography revealed that tritiated norepinephrine is concentrated mainly on unmyelinated fibers, which suggests that these fibers are adrenergic.[518] There is evidence that renal nerves possess fibers containing neuropeptide Y, a potent vasoconstrictor,[519,520] as well as immunoreactive somatostatin and neurotensin.[520] Vasoactive intestinal polypeptide–immunoreactive nerve fibers are also well documented in the kidney.[520] Earlier studies describing cholinergic nerve fibers within the renal parenchyma have fallen into disrepute because the conclusions were based largely on the presence of acetylcholinesterase.[509]

The afferent renal nerves are found principally in the pelvic region, the major vessels, and the corticomedullary connective tissue.[515] Most, although not all, afferent renal nerves are unmyelinated.[521] Largely on the basis of immunocytochemical localization of calcitonin gene–related peptide, a marker of afferent nerve fibers, Barajas and colleagues[515] suggested that these immunoreactive nerve fibers may be involved in baroreceptor and afferent nerve responses to changes in arterial, venous, interstitial, or intrapelvic pressure.

Acknowledgment

This chapter is a continuation of the chapter by Dr. C. Craig Tisher and Dr. Kirsten Madsen.

References

1. Hughson M, Farris III AB, Douglas-Denton R, et al. Glomerular number and size in autopsy kidneys: the relationship to birth weight. *Kidney Int.* 2003;63:2113.
2. Keller G, Zimmer G, Mall G, Ritz E, et al. Nephron number in patients with primary hypertension. *N Engl J Med.* 2003;348:101.
3. Nyengaard JR, Bendtsen TF. Glomerular number and size in relation to age, kidney weight, and body surface in normal man. *Anat Rec.* 1992;232:194.
4. Bertram JF, Soosaipillai MC, Ricardo SD, et al. Total numbers of glomeruli and individual glomerular cell types in the normal rat kidney. *Cell Tissue Res.* 1992;270:37.
5. Nyengaard JR. The quantitative development of glomerular capillaries in rats with special reference to unbiased stereological estimates of their number and sizes. *Microvasc Res.* 1993;45:243.
6. Baines AD, de Rouffignac C. Functional heterogeneity of nephrons. II. Filtration rates, intraluminal flow velocities and fractional water reabsorption. *Pflugers Arch.* 1969;308:260.
7. Neiss WF. Morphogenesis and histogenesis of the connecting tubule in the rat kidney. *Anat Embryol (Berl).* 1982;165:81.
8. Pannabecker TL, Dantzler WH. Three-dimensional architecture of inner medullary vasa recta. *Am J Physiol Renal Physiol.* 2006;290:F1355-F1366.
9. Pannabecker TL, Dantzler WH. Three-dimensional architecture of collecting ducts, loops of Henle, and blood vessels in the renal papilla. *Am J Physiol Renal Physiol.* 2007;293:F696-F704.
10. Pannabecker TL. Loop of Henle interaction with interstitial nodal spaces in the renal inner medulla. *Am J Physiol Renal Physiol.* 2008;295:F1744-F1751.
11. Zhai XY, Birn H, Jensen KB, et al. Digital three-dimensional reconstruction and ultrastructure of the mouse proximal tubule. *J Am Soc Nephrol.* 2003;14:611.
12. Zhai XY, Thomsen JS, Birn H, et al. Three-dimensional reconstruction of the mouse nephron. *J Am Soc Nephrol.* 2006;17:77.
13. Samuel T, Hoy WE, Douglas-Denton R, et al. Determinants of glomerular volume in different cortical zones of the human kidney. *J Am Soc Nephrol.* 2005;16:3102.
14. Guasch A, Myers BD. Determinants of glomerular hypofiltration in nephrotic patients with minimal change nephropathy. *J Am Soc Nephrol.* 1994;4:1571.
15. Shea SM, Morrison AB. A stereological study of the glomerular filter in the rat. Morphometry of the slit diaphragm and basement membrane. *J Cell Biol.* 1975;67:436.
16. Brenner BM, Bohrer MP, Baylis C, et al. Determinants of glomerular permselectivity: insights derived from observations in vivo. *Kidney Int.* 1977;12:229.
17. Jørgensen F. *The ultrastructure of the normal human glomerulus.* Copenhagen: Ejnar Munksgaard; 1966.
18. Rostgaard J, Thuneberg L. Electron microscopical observations on the brush border of proximal tubule cells of mammalian kidney. *Z Zellforsch Mikrosk Anat.* 1972;132:473.
19. Ichimura K, Stan RV, Kurihara H, et al. Glomerular endothelial cells form diaphragms during development and pathologic conditions. *J Am Soc Nephrol.* 2008;19:1463.
20. Hjalmarsson C, Johansson BR, Haraldsson B. Electron microscopic evaluation of the endothelial surface layer of glomerular capillaries. *Microvasc Res.* 2004;67:9.
21. Vasmant D, Maurice M, Feldmann G. Cytoskeleton ultrastructure of podocytes and glomerular endothelial cells in man and in the rat. *Anat Rec.* 1984;210:17.
22. Sorensson J, Bjornson A, Ohlson M, et al. Synthesis of sulfated proteoglycans by bovine glomerular endothelial cells in culture. *Am J Physiol Renal Physiol.* 2003;284:F373-F380.
23. Jeansson M, Haraldsson B. Morphological and functional evidence for an important role of the endothelial cell glycocalyx in the glomerular barrier. *Am J Physiol Renal Physiol.* 2006;290:F111-F116.
24. Ballermann BJ, Marsden PA. Endothelium-derived vasoactive mediators and renal glomerular function. *Clin Invest Med.* 1991;14:508.
25. Bachmann S, Bosse HM, Mundel P. Topography of nitric oxide synthesis by localizing constitutive NO synthases in mammalian kidney. *Am J Physiol.* 1995;268:F885-F898.
26. Simon M, Grone HJ, Johren O, et al. Expression of vascular endothelial growth factor and its receptors in human renal ontogenesis and in adult kidney. *Am J Physiol.* 1995;268:F240-F250.
27. Brown LF, Berse B, Tognazzi K, et al. Vascular permeability factor mRNA and protein expression in human kidney. *Kidney Int.* 1992;42:1457.
28. Esser S, Wolburg K, Wolburg H, et al. Vascular endothelial growth factor induces endothelial fenestrations in vitro. *J Cell Biol.* 1998;140:947.
29. Roberts WG, Palade GE. Increased microvascular permeability and endothelial fenestration induced by vascular endothelial growth factor. *J Cell Sci.* 1995;108(pt 6):2369.
30. Chen J, Braet F, Brodsky S, et al. VEGF-induced mobilization of caveolae and increase in permeability of endothelial cells. *Am J Physiol Cell Physiol.* 2002;282:C1053-C1063.
31. Ballermann BJ. Glomerular endothelial cell differentiation. *Kidney Int.* 2005;67:1668.
32. Eremina V, Sood M, Haigh J, et al. Glomerular-specific alterations of VEGF-A expression lead to distinct congenital and acquired renal diseases. *J Clin Invest.* 2003;111:707.

33. Ostendorf T, Kunter U, Eitner F, et al. VEGF(165) mediates glomerular endothelial repair. *J Clin Invest.* 1999;104:913.
34. Abrahamson DR. Structure and development of the glomerular capillary wall and basement membrane. *Am J Physiol.* 1987;253:F783-F794.
35. Jørgensen F, Bentzon MW. The ultrastructure of the normal human glomerulus. Thickness of glomerular basement membrane. *Lab Invest.* 1968;18:42.
36. Østerby R. Morphometric studies of the peripheral glomerular basement membrane in early juvenile diabetes. I. Development of initial basement membrane thickening. *Diabetologia.* 1972;8:84.
37. Steffes MW, Barbosa J, Basgen JM, et al. Quantitative glomerular morphology of the normal human kidney. *Lab Invest.* 1983;49:82.
38. Rasch R. Prevention of diabetic glomerulopathy in streptozotocin diabetic rats by insulin treatment. *Diabetologia.* 1979;16:319.
39. Courtoy PJ, Kanwar YS, Hynes RO, et al. Fibronectin localization in the rat glomerulus. *J Cell Biol.* 1980;87:691.
40. Courtoy PJ, Timpl R, Farquhar MG. Comparative distribution of laminin, type IV collagen, and fibronectin in the rat glomerulus. *J Histochem Cytochem.* 1982;30:874.
41. Dean DC, Barr JF, Freytag JW, et al. Isolation of type IV procollagen-like polypeptides from glomerular basement membrane. Characterization of pro-alpha 1(IV). *J Biol Chem.* 1983;258:590.
42. Katz A, Fish AJ, Kleppel MM, et al. Renal entactin (nidogen): isolation, characterization and tissue distribution. *Kidney Int.* 1991;40:643.
43. Miner JH. Renal basement membrane components. *Kidney Int.* 1999;56:2016.
44. Groffen AJ, Hop FW, Tryggvason K, et al. Evidence for the existence of multiple heparan sulfate proteoglycans in the human glomerular basement membrane and mesangial matrix. *Eur J Biochem.* 1997;247:175.
45. Groffen AJ, Ruegg MA, Dijkman H, et al. Agrin is a major heparan sulfate proteoglycan in the human glomerular basement membrane. *J Histochem Cytochem.* 1998;46:19.
46. Kashtan CE. Alport syndrome and thin glomerular basement membrane disease. *J Am Soc Nephrol.* 1998;9:1736.
47. Zhou J, Reeders ST. The alpha chains of type IV collagen. *Contrib Nephrol.* 1996;117:80.
48. Hudson BG, Tryggvason K, Sundaramoorthy M, et al. Alport's syndrome, Goodpasture's syndrome, and type IV collagen. *N Engl J Med.* 2003;348:2543.
49. Caulfield JP, Farquhar MG. The permeability of glomerular capillaries to graded dextrans. Identification of the basement membrane as the primary filtration barrier. *J Cell Biol.* 1974;63:883.
50. Rennke HG, Venkatachalam MA. Glomerular permeability: in vivo tracer studies with polyanionic and polycationic ferritins. *Kidney Int.* 1977;11:44.
51. Rennke HG, Patel Y, Venkatachalam MA. Glomerular filtration of proteins: clearance of anionic, neutral, and cationic horseradish peroxidase in the rat. *Kidney Int.* 1978;13:278.
52. Deen WM, Lazzara MJ, Myers BD. Structural determinants of glomerular permeability. *Am J Physiol Renal Physiol.* 2001;281:F579-F596.
53. Caulfield JP, Farquhar MG. Distribution of anionic sites in glomerular basement membranes: their possible role in filtration and attachment. *Proc Natl Acad Sci USA.* 1976;73:1646.
54. Kanwar YS, Farquhar MG. Anionic sites in the glomerular basement membrane. In vivo and in vitro localization to the laminae rarae by cationic probes. *J Cell Biol.* 1979;81:137.
55. Kanwar YS, Farquhar MG. Isolation of glycosaminoglycans (heparan sulfate) from glomerular basement membranes. *Proc Natl Acad Sci USA.* 1979;76:4493.
56. Kanwar YS, Farquhar MG. Presence of heparan sulfate in the glomerular basement membrane. *Proc Natl Acad Sci USA.* 1979;76:1303.
57. Kanwar YS, Linker A, Farquhar MG. Increased permeability of the glomerular basement membrane to ferritin after removal of glycosaminoglycans (heparan sulfate) by enzyme digestion. *J Cell Biol.* 1980;86:688.
58. Rosenzweig LJ, Kanwar YS. Removal of sulfated (heparan sulfate) or nonsulfated (hyaluronic acid) glycosaminoglycans results in increased permeability of the glomerular basement membrane to 125I-bovine serum albumin. *Lab Invest.* 1982;47:177.
59. Wijnhoven TJ, Lensen JF, Wismans RG, et al. Removal of heparan sulfate from the glomerular basement membrane blocks protein passage. *J Am Soc Nephrol.* 2007;18:3119.
60. Goldberg S, Harvey SJ, Cunningham J, et al. Glomerular filtration is normal in the absence of both agrin and perlecan-heparan sulfate from the glomerular basement membrane. *Nephrol Dial Transplant.* 2009;24:2044.
61. Harvey SJ, Jarad G, Cunningham J, et al. Disruption of glomerular basement membrane charge through podocyte-specific mutation of agrin does not alter glomerular permselectivity. *Am J Pathol.* 2007;171:139.
62. Utriainen A, Sormunen R, Kettunen M, et al. Structurally altered basement membranes and hydrocephalus in a type XVIII collagen deficient mouse line. *Hum Mol Genet.* 2004;13:2089.
63. Noakes PG, Miner JH, Gautam M, et al. The renal glomerulus of mice lacking s-laminin/laminin beta 2: nephrosis despite molecular compensation by laminin beta 1. *Nat Genet.* 1995;10:400.
64. Zenker M, Aigner T, Wendler O, et al. Human laminin beta2 deficiency causes congenital nephrosis with mesangial sclerosis and distinct eye abnormalities. *Hum Mol Genet.* 2004;13:2625.
65. Jarad G, Cunningham J, Shaw AS, et al. Proteinuria precedes podocyte abnormalities in Lamb2-/- mice, implicating the glomerular basement membrane as an albumin barrier. *J Clin Invest.* 2006;116:2272.
66. Andrews PM, Bates SB. Filamentous actin bundles in the kidney. *Anat Rec.* 1984;210:1.
67. Farquhar MG, Wissig SL, Palade GE. Glomerular permeability. I. Ferritin transfer across the normal glomerular capillary wall. *J Exp Med.* 1961;113:47.
68. Latta H. The glomerular capillary wall. *J Ultrastruct Res.* 1970;32:526.
69. Rodewald R, Karnovsky MJ. Porous substructure of the glomerular slit diaphragm in the rat and mouse. *J Cell Biol.* 1974;60:423.
70. Schneeberger EE, Levey RH, McCluskey RT, et al. The isoporous substructure of the human glomerular slit diaphragm. *Kidney Int.* 1975;8:48.
71. Reiser J, Kriz W, Kretzler M, et al. The glomerular slit diaphragm is a modified adherens junction. *J Am Soc Nephrol.* 2000;11:1.
72. Schnabel E, Anderson JM, Farquhar MG. The tight junction protein ZO-1 is concentrated along slit diaphragms of the glomerular epithelium. *J Cell Biol.* 1990;111:1255.
73. Kestila M, Lenkkeri U, Mannikko M, et al. Positionally cloned gene for a novel glomerular protein—nephrin—is mutated in congenital nephrotic syndrome. *Mol Cell.* 1998;1:575.
74. Lenkkeri U, Mannikko M, McCready P, et al. Structure of the gene for congenital nephrotic syndrome of the Finnish type (NPHS1) and characterization of mutations. *Am J Hum Genet.* 1999;64:51.
75. Boute N, Gribouval O, Roselli S, et al. NPHS2, encoding the glomerular protein podocin, is mutated in autosomal recessive steroid-resistant nephrotic syndrome. *Nat Genet.* 2000;24:349.
76. Patrakka J, Tryggvason K. New insights into the role of podocytes in proteinuria. *Nat Rev Nephrol.* 2009;5:463.
77. Jones N, Blasutig IM, Eremina V, et al. Nck adaptor proteins link nephrin to the actin cytoskeleton of kidney podocytes. *Nature.* 2006;440:818.
78. Shih NY, Li J, Cotran R, et al. CD2AP localizes to the slit diaphragm and binds nephrin via a novel C-terminal domain. *Am J Pathol.* 2001;159:2303.
79. Seiler MW, Venkatachalam MA, Cotran RS. Glomerular epithelium: structural alterations induced by polycations. *Science.* 1975;189:390.
80. Kanwar YS, Farquhar MG. Detachment of endothelium and epithelium from the glomerular basement membrane produced by kidney perfusion with neuraminidase. *Lab Invest.* 1980;42:375.
81. Farquhar MG, Palade GE. Functional evidence for the existence of a third cell type in the renal glomerulus. *J Cell Biol.* 1962;13:55.
82. Latta H, Maunsbach AB, Madden SC. The centrolobular region of the renal glomerulus studied by electron microscopy. *J Ultrastruct Res.* 1960;4:455.
83. Drenckhahn D, Schnittler H, Nobiling R, et al. Ultrastructural organization of contractile proteins in rat glomerular mesangial cells. *Am J Pathol.* 1990;137:1343.
84. Kriz W, Elger M, Mundel P, et al. Structure-stabilizing forces in the glomerular tuft. *J Am Soc Nephrol.* 1995;5:1731.
85. Kerjaschki D, Ojha PP, Susani M, et al. A beta 1-integrin receptor for fibronectin in human kidney glomeruli. *Am J Pathol.* 1989;134:481.
86. Cosio FG, Sedmak DD, Nahman Jr NS. Cellular receptors for matrix proteins in normal human kidney and human mesangial cells. *Kidney Int.* 1990;38:886.
87. Petermann A, Fees H, Grenz H, et al. Polymerase chain reaction and focal contact formation indicate integrin expression in mesangial cells. *Kidney Int.* 1993;44:997.
88. Hartner A, Schocklmann H, Prols F, et al. Alpha8 integrin in glomerular mesangial cells and in experimental glomerulonephritis. *Kidney Int.* 1999;56:1468.
89. Rupprecht HD, Schocklmann HO, Sterzel RB. Cell-matrix interactions in the glomerular mesangium. *Kidney Int.* 1996;49:1575.
90. Schlondorff D. The glomerular mesangial cell: an expanding role for a specialized pericyte. *FASEB J.* 1987;1:272.
91. Michael AF, Keane WF, Raij L, et al. The glomerular mesangium. *Kidney Int.* 1980;17:141.
92. Elema JD, Hoyer JR, Vernier RL. The glomerular mesangium: uptake and transport of intravenously injected colloidal carbon in rats. *Kidney Int.* 1976;9:395.
93. Mauer SM, Fish AJ, Blau EB, et al. The glomerular mesangium. I. Kinetic studies of macromolecular uptake in normal and nephrotic rats. *J Clin Invest.* 1972;51:1092.
94. Schreiner GF, Cotran RS. Localization of an Ia-bearing glomerular cell in the mesangium. *J Cell Biol.* 1982;94:483.

95. Schreiner GF, Kiely JM, Cotran RS, et al. Characterization of resident glomerular cells in the rat expressing Ia determinants and manifesting genetically restricted interactions with lymphocytes. *J Clin Invest.* 1981;68:920.

96. Ohse T, Chang AM, Pippin JW, et al. A new function for parietal epithelial cells: a second glomerular barrier. *Am J Physiol Renal Physiol.* 2009;297:F1566-F1574.

97. Appel D, Kershaw DB, Smeets B, et al. Recruitment of podocytes from glomerular parietal epithelial cells. *J Am Soc Nephrol.* 2009;20:333.

98. Ohse T, Vaughan MR, Kopp JB, et al. De novo expression of podocyte proteins in parietal epithelial cells during experimental glomerular disease. *Am J Physiol Renal Physiol.* 2010;298:F702-F711.

99. Ryan GB, Coghlan JP, Scoggins BA. The granulated peripolar epithelial cell: a potential secretory component of the renal juxtaglomerular complex. *Nature.* 1979;277:655.

100. Gall JA, Alcorn D, Butkus A, et al. Distribution of glomerular peripolar cells in different mammalian species. *Cell Tissue Res.* 1986;244:203.

101. Barajas L. Anatomy of the juxtaglomerular apparatus. *Am J Physiol.* 1979;237:F333-F343.

102. Barajas L. The ultrastructure of the juxtaglomerular apparatus as disclosed by three-dimensional reconstructions from serial sections. The anatomical relationship between the tubular and vascular components. *J Ultrastruct Res.* 1970;33:116.

103. Barajas L, Salido E. Pathology of the juxtaglomerular apparatus. In:Tisher CC, Brenner BM(eds). *Renal pathology with clinical and functional correlations.* Philadelphia: Lippincott, 1994, p 948.

104. Tisher CC, Bulger RE, Trump BF. Human renal ultrastructure. 3. The distal tubule in healthy individuals. *Lab Invest.* 1968;18:655.

105. Hackenthal E, Paul M, Ganten D, et al. Morphology, physiology, and molecular biology of renin secretion. *Physiol Rev.* 1990;70:1067.

106. Biava CG, West M. Fine structure of normal human juxtaglomerular cells. II. Specific and nonspecific cytoplasmic granules. *Am J Pathol.* 1966;49:955.

107. Barajas L. The development and ultrastructure of the juxtaglomerular cell granule. *J Ultrastruct Res.* 1966;15:400.

108. Celio MR, Inagami T. Angiotensin II immunoreactivity coexists with renin in the juxtaglomerular granular cells of the kidney. *Proc Natl Acad Sci USA.* 1981;78:3897.

109. Deschepper CF, Mellon SH, Cumin F, et al. Analysis by immunocytochemistry and in situ hybridization of renin and its mRNA in kidney, testis, adrenal, and pituitary of the rat. *Proc Natl Acad Sci USA.* 1986;83:7552.

110. Pricam C, Humbert F, Perrelet A, et al. Gap junctions in mesangial and lacis cells. *J Cell Biol.* 1974;63:349.

111. Taugner R, Schiller A, Kaissling B, et al. Gap junctional coupling between the JGA and the glomerular tuft. *Cell Tissue Res.* 1978;186:279.

112. Ren Y, Carretero OA, Garvin JL. Role of mesangial cells and gap junctions in tubuloglomerular feedback. *Kidney Int.* 2002;62:525.

113. Kaissling B, Kriz W. Variability of intercellular spaces between macula densa cells: a transmission electron microscopic study in rabbits and rats. *Kidney Int.* 1982;12(Suppl):S9.

114. Kirk KL, Bell PD, Barfuss DW, et al. Direct visualization of the isolated and perfused macula densa. *Am J Physiol.* 1985;248:F890-F894.

115. Barajas L. The innervation of the juxtaglomerular apparatus. An electron microscopic study of the innervation of the glomerular arterioles. *Lab Invest.* 1964;13:916.

116. Barajas L, Müller J. The innervation of the juxtaglomerular apparatus and surrounding tubules: a quantitative analysis by serial section electron microscopy. *J Ultrastruct Res.* 1973;43:107.

117. Barajas L, Wang P. Localization of tritiated norepinephrine in the renal arteriolar nerves. *Anat Rec.* 1979;195:525.

118. Kopp UC, DiBona GF. Neural regulation of renin secretion. *Semin Nephrol.* 1993;13:543.

119. Schnermann J, Briggs JP. The function of the juxtaglomerular apparatus: control of glomerular hemodynamics and renin secretion. In: Seldin DW, Giebisch G, eds. *The kidney: physiology and pathophysiology.* New York: Raven Press, 1992, p 1249.

120. Schnermann J. Juxtaglomerular cell complex in the regulation of renal salt excretion. *Am J Physiol.* 1998;274:R263-R279.

121. Schlatter E, Salomonsson M, Persson AE, et al. Macula densa cells sense luminal NaCl concentration via furosemide sensitive $Na^+2Cl^-K^+$ cotransport. *Pflugers Arch.* 1989;414:286.

122. Lapointe JY, Laamarti A, Hurst AM, et al. Activation of Na:2Cl:K cotransport by luminal chloride in macula densa cells. *Kidney Int.* 1995;47:752.

123. Obermuller N, Kunchaparty S, Ellison DH, et al. Expression of the Na-K-2Cl cotransporter by macula densa and thick ascending limb cells of rat and rabbit nephron. *J Clin Invest.* 1996;98:635.

124. Kurtz A, Wagner C. Cellular control of renin secretion. *J Exp Biol.* 1999;202:219.

125. Persson AE, Bachmann S. Constitutive nitric oxide synthesis in the kidney—functions at the juxtaglomerular apparatus. *Acta Physiol Scand.* 2000;169:317.

126. Kim SM, Mizel D, Huang YG, et al. Adenosine as a mediator of macula densa–dependent inhibition of renin secretion. *Am J Physiol Renal Physiol.* 2006;290:F1016-F1023.

127. Peti-Peterdi J, Harris RC. Macula densa sensing and signaling mechanisms of renin release. *J Am Soc Nephrol.* 2010.

128. Harris RC, Breyer MD. Physiological regulation of cyclooxygenase-2 in the kidney. *Am J Physiol Renal Physiol.* 2001;281:F1.

129. Cheng HF, Wang JL, Zhang MZ, et al. Nitric oxide regulates renal cortical cyclooxygenase-2 expression. *Am J Physiol Renal Physiol.* 2000;279:F122-F129.

130. Kim SM, Mizel D, Huang YG, et al. Adenosine as a mediator of macula densa–dependent inhibition of renin secretion. *Am J Physiol Renal Physiol.* 2006;290:F1016-F1023.

131. Madsen KM, Park CH. Lysosome distribution and cathepsin B and L activity along the rabbit proximal tubule. *Am J Physiol.* 1987;253:F1290-F1301.

132. Maunsbach AB. Observations on the segmentation of the proximal tubule in the rat kidney. Comparison of results from phase contrast, fluorescence and electron microscopy. *J Ultrastruct Res.* 1966;16:239.

133. Tisher CC, Bulger RE, Trump BF. Human renal ultrastructure. I. Proximal tubule of healthy individuals. *Lab Invest.* 1966;15:1357.

134. Kaissling B, Kriz W. Structural analysis of the rabbit kidney. *Adv Anat Embryol Cell Biol.* 1979;56:1.

135. Woodhall PB, Tisher CC, Simonton CA, et al. Relationship between para-aminohippurate secretion and cellular morphology in rabbit proximal tubules. *J Clin Invest.* 1978;61:1320.

136. Tisher CC, Rosen S, Osborne GB. Ultrastructure of the proximal tubule of the rhesus monkey kidney. *Am J Pathol.* 1969;56:469.

137. Welling LW, Welling DJ. Shape of epithelial cells and intercellular channels in the rabbit proximal nephron. *Kidney Int.* 1976;9:385.

138. Farquhar MG, Palade GE. Junctional complexes in various epithelia. *J Cell Biol.* 1963;17:375.

139. Grandchamp A, Boulpaep EL. Pressure control of sodium reabsorption and intercellular backflux across proximal kidney tubule. *J Clin Invest.* 1974;54:69.

140. Schultz SG. The role of paracellular pathways in isotonic fluid transport. *Yale J Biol Med.* 1977;50:99.

141. Lutz MD, Cardinal J, Burg MB. Electrical resistance of renal proximal tubule perfused in vitro. *Am J Physiol.* 1973;225:729.

142. Balkovetz DF. Tight junction claudins and the kidney in sickness and in health. *Biochim Biophys Acta.* 2009;1788:858.

143. Muto S, Hata M, Taniguchi J, et al. Claudin-2–deficient mice are defective in the leaky and cation-selective paracellular permeability properties of renal proximal tubules. *Proc Natl Acad Sci USA.* 2010;107:8011.

144. Silverblatt FJ, Bulger RE. Gap junctions occur in vertebrate renal proximal tubule cells. *J Cell Biol.* 1970;47:513.

145. Hanner F, Sorensen CM, Holstein-Rathlou NH, et al. Connexins and the kidney. *Am J Physiol Regul Integr Comp Physiol.* 2010;298:RR1143.

146. Christensen EI, Madsen KM. Renal age changes: observations of the rat kidney cortex with special reference to structure and function of the lysosomal system in the proximal tubule. *Lab Invest.* 1978;39:289.

147. Ernst SA. Transport ATPase cytochemistry: ultrastructural localization of potassium-dependent and potassium-independent phosphatase activities in rat kidney cortex. *J Cell Biol.* 1975;66:586.

148. Kashgarian M, Biemesderfer D, Caplan M, et al. Monoclonal antibody to Na, K-ATPase: immunocytochemical localization along nephron segments. *Kidney Int.* 1985;28:899.

149. Welling LW, Welling DJ. Surface areas of brush border and lateral cell walls in the rabbit proximal nephron. *Kidney Int.* 1975;8:343.

150. Bergeron M, Guerette D, Forget J, et al. Three-dimensional characteristics of the mitochondria of the rat nephron. *Kidney Int.* 1980;17:175.

151. Bergeron M, Thiery G. Three-dimensional characteristics of the endoplasmic reticulum of rat tubule cells, an electron microscopy study in thick sections. *Biol Cell.* 1981;42:43.

152. Coudrier E, Kerjaschki D, Louvard D. Cytoskeleton organization and submembranous interactions in intestinal and renal brush borders. *Kidney Int.* 1988;34:309.

153. Rodman JS, Mooseker M, Farquhar MG. Cytoskeletal proteins of the rat kidney proximal tubule brush border. *Eur J Cell Biol.* 1986;42:319.

154. Heidrich HG, Kinne R, Kinne-Saffran E, et al. The polarity of the proximal tubule cell in rat kidney. Different surface charges for the brush-border microvilli and plasma membranes from the basal infoldings. *J Cell Biol.* 1972;54:232.

155. Kerjaschki D, Noronha Blob L, Sacktor B, et al. Microdomains of distinctive glycoprotein composition in the kidney proximal tubule brush border. *J Cell Biol.* 1984;98:1505.

156. Le Hir M, Kaissling B. Distribution and regulation of renal ecto-5′-nucleotidase: implications for physiological functions of adenosine. *Am J Physiol*. 1993;264:F377-F387:(editorial).
157. Christensen EI, Nielsen S. Structural and functional features of protein handling in the kidney proximal tubule. *Semin Nephrol*. 1991;11:414.
158. Rodman JS, Kerjaschki D, Merisko E, et al. Presence of an extensive clathrin coat on the apical plasmalemma of the rat kidney proximal tubule cell. *J Cell Biol*. 1984;98:1630.
159. Kerjaschki D, Farquhar MG. The pathogenic antigen of Heymann nephritis is a membrane glycoprotein of the renal proximal tubule brush border. *Proc Natl Acad Sci USA*. 1982;79:5557.
160. Maunsbach AB. Observations on the ultrastructure and acid phosphatase activity of the cytoplasmic bodies in rat kidney proximal tubule cells. With a comment on their classification. *J Ultrastruct Res*. 1966;16:197.
161. Sabolic I, Burckhardt G. Characteristics of the proton pump in rat renal cortical endocytotic vesicles. *Am J Physiol*. 1986;250:F817-F826.
162. Brown D, Hirsch S, Gluck S. Localization of a proton-pumping ATPase in rat kidney. *J Clin Invest*. 1988;82:2114.
163. Maunsbach AB. Absorption of I^{125}-labeled homologous albumin by rat kidney proximal tubule cells. A study of microperfused single proximal tubules by electron microscopic autoradiography and histochemistry. 1966 [classic article]. *J Am Soc Nephrol*. 1997;8:323.
164. Maack T, Johnson V, Kau ST, et al. Renal filtration, transport, and metabolism of low-molecular-weight proteins: a review. *Kidney Int*. 1979;16:251.
165. Christensen EI. Rapid membrane recycling in renal proximal tubule cells. *Eur J Cell Biol*. 1982;29:43.
166. Olbricht CJ, Cannon JK, Garg LC, et al. Activities of cathepsins B and L in isolated nephron segments from proteinuric and nonproteinuric rats. *Am J Physiol*. 1986;250:F1055-F1062.
167. Sumpio BE, Maack T. Kinetics, competition, and selectivity of tubular absorption of proteins. *Am J Physiol*. 1982;243:F379-F392.
168. Christensen EI, Rennke HG, Carone FA. Renal tubular uptake of protein: effect of molecular charge. *Am J Physiol*. 1983;244:F436-F441.
169. Park CH, Maack T. Albumin absorption and catabolism by isolated perfused proximal convoluted tubules of the rabbit. *J Clin Invest*. 1984;73:767.
170. Park CH. Time course and vectorial nature of albumin metabolism in isolated perfused rabbit PCT. *Am J Physiol*. 1988;255:F520-F528.
171. Farquhar MG, Saito A, Kerjaschki D, et al. The Heymann nephritis antigenic complex: megalin (gp330) and RAP. *J Am Soc Nephrol*. 1995;6:35.
172. Christensen EI, Birn H. Megalin and cubilin: synergistic endocytic receptors in renal proximal tubule. *Am J Physiol Renal Physiol*. 2001;280:F562-F573.
173. Saito A, Pietromonaco S, Loo AK, et al. Complete cloning and sequencing of rat gp330/"megalin," a distinctive member of the low density lipoprotein receptor gene family. *Proc Natl Acad Sci USA*. 1994;91:9725.
174. Abbate M, Bachinsky D, Zheng G, et al. Location of gp330/a$_2$-m receptor–associated protein (a$_2$-MRAP) and its binding sites in kidney: distribution of endogenous a$_2$-MRAP is modified by tissue processing. *Eur J Cell Biol*. 1993;61:139.
175. Christensen EI, Nielsen S, Moestrup SK, et al. Segmental distribution of the endocytosis receptor gp330 in renal proximal tubules. *Eur J Cell Biol*. 1995;66:349.
176. Orlando RA, Rader K, Authier F, et al. Megalin is an endocytic receptor for insulin. *J Am Soc Nephrol*. 1998;9:1759.
177. Cui S, Verroust PJ, Moestrup SK, et al. Megalin/gp330 mediates uptake of albumin in renal proximal tubule. *Am J Physiol*. 1996;271:F900-F907.
178. Christensen EI, Moskaug JO, Vorum H, et al. Evidence for an essential role of megalin in transepithelial transport of retinol. *J Am Soc Nephrol*. 1999;10:685.
179. Moestrup SK, Birn H, Fischer PB, et al. Megalin-mediated endocytosis of transcobalamin-vitamin-B$_{12}$ complexes suggests a role of the receptor in vitamin-B$_{12}$ homeostasis. *Proc Natl Acad Sci USA*. 1996;93:8612.
180. Nykjaer A, Dragun D, Walther D, et al. An endocytic pathway essential for renal uptake and activation of the steroid 25-(OH) vitamin D$_3$. *Cell*. 1999;96:507.
181. Moestrup SK, Cui S, Vorum H, et al. Evidence that epithelial glycoprotein 330/megalin mediates uptake of polybasic drugs. *J Clin Invest*. 1995;96:1404.
182. Christensen EI, Willnow TE. Essential role of megalin in renal proximal tubule for vitamin homeostasis. *J Am Soc Nephrol*. 1999;10:2224.
183. Leheste JR, Rolinski B, Vorum H, et al. Megalin knockout mice as an animal model of low molecular weight proteinuria. *Am J Pathol*. 1999;155:1361.
184. Christensen EI, Birn H. Megalin and cubilin: multifunctional endocytic receptors. *Nat Rev Mol Cell Biol*. 2002;3:256.
185. Birn H, Fyfe JC, Jacobsen C, et al. Cubilin is an albumin binding protein important for renal tubular albumin reabsorption. *J Clin Invest*. 2000;105:1353.
186. Katz AI, Doucet A, Morel F. Na-K-ATPase activity along the rabbit, rat, and mouse nephron. *Am J Physiol*. 1979;237:F114-F120.
187. Clapp WL, Park CH, Madsen KM, et al. Axial heterogeneity in the handling of albumin by the rabbit proximal tubule. *Lab Invest*. 1988;58:549.
188. Ohno S. Peroxisomes of the kidney. *Int Rev Cytol*. 1985;95:131.
189. Angermuller S, Leupold C, Zaar K, et al. Electron microscopic cytochemical localization of alpha-hydroxyacid oxidase in rat kidney cortex. Heterogeneous staining of peroxisomes. *Histochemistry*. 1986;85:411.
190. Burg MB. Renal handling of sodium, chloride, water, amino acids and glucose. In: Brenner BM, Rector Jr FC, eds. *The kidney*. Philadelphia: WB Saunders; 1986:pp 145.
191. Maunsbach AB, Tripathi S, Boulpaep EL. Ultrastructural changes in isolated perfused proximal tubules during osmotic water flow. *Am J Physiol*. 1987;253:F1091-F1104.
192. Tripathi S, Boulpaep EL, Maunsbach AB. Isolated perfused *Ambystoma* proximal tubule: hydrodynamics modulates ultrastructure. *Am J Physiol*. 1987;252:F1129-F1147.
193. Agre P, Preston GM, Smith BL, et al. Aquaporin CHIP: the archetypal molecular water channel. *Am J Physiol*. 1993;265:F463-F476.
194. Preston GM, Agre P. Isolation of the cDNA for erythrocyte integral membrane protein of 28 kilodaltons: member of an ancient channel family. *Proc Natl Acad Sci USA*. 1991;88:11110.
195. Nielsen S, Smith B, Christensen EI, et al. CHIP28 water channels are localized in constitutively water-permeable segments of the nephron. *J Cell Biol*. 1993;120:371.
196. Sabolic I, Valenti G, Verbavatz JM, et al. Localization of the CHIP28 water channel in rat kidney. *Am J Physiol*. 1992;263:C1225-C1233.
197. Maunsbach AB, Marples D, Chin E, et al. Aquaporin-1 water channel expression in human kidney. *J Am Soc Nephrol*. 1997;8:1.
198. Zhai XY, Fenton RA, Andreasen A, et al. Aquaporin-1 is not expressed in descending thin limbs of short-loop nephrons. *J Am Soc Nephrol*. 2007;18:2937.
199. Ma T, Yang B, Gillespie A, et al. Severely impaired urinary concentrating ability in transgenic mice lacking aquaporin-1 water channels. *J Biol Chem*. 1998;273:4296.
200. Fenton RA, Knepper MA. Mouse models and the urinary concentrating mechanism in the new millennium. *Physiol Rev*. 2007;87:1083.
201. Rector Jr FC. Sodium, bicarbonate, and chloride absorption by the proximal tubule. *Am J Physiol*. 1983;244:F461-F471.
202. Aronson PS. Mechanisms of active H$^+$ secretion in the proximal tubule. *Am J Physiol*. 1983;245:F647-F659.
203. Alpern RJ, Stone DK, Rector Jr FC. Renal acidification mechanisms. In: Brenner BM, Rector Jr FC, eds. *The kidney*, 4th ed. vol. I. Philadelphia: Saunders; 1991:pp 318-379.
204. Biemesderfer D, Pizzonia J, Abu-Alfa A, et al. NHE3: a Na$^+$/H$^+$ exchanger isoform of renal brush border. *Am J Physiol*. 1993;265:F736-F742.
205. Amemiya M, Loffing J, Lotscher M, et al. Expression of NHE-3 in the apical membrane of rat renal proximal tubule and thick ascending limb. *Kidney Int*. 1995;48:1206.
206. Preisig PA, Ives HE, Cragoe Jr EJ, et al. Role of the Na$^+$/H$^+$ antiporter in rat proximal tubule bicarbonate absorption. *J Clin Invest*. 1987;80:970.
207. Kinne-Saffran E, Beauwens R, Kinne R. An ATP-driven proton pump in brush-border membranes from rat renal cortex. *J Membr Biol*. 1982;64:67.
208. Lorenz JN, Schultheis PJ, Traynor T, et al. Micropuncture analysis of single-nephron function in NHE3-deficient mice. *Am J Physiol*. 1999;277:F447-F453.
209. Schultheis PJ, Clarke LL, Meneton P, et al. Renal and intestinal absorptive defects in mice lacking the NHE3 Na$^+$/H$^+$ exchanger. *Nat Genet*. 1998;19:282.
210. Hayashi H, Szaszi K, Grinstein S. Multiple modes of regulation of Na$^+$/H$^+$ exchangers. *Ann N Y Acad Sci*. 2002;976:248.
211. Good DW, George T, Watts III BA. Nongenomic regulation by aldosterone of the epithelial NHE3 Na$^+$/H$^+$ exchanger. *Am J Physiol Cell Physiol*. 2006;290:C757-C763.
212. Alpern RJ. Mechanism of basolateral membrane H$^+$/OH$^-$/HCO$_3^-$ transport in the rat proximal convoluted tubule. A sodium-coupled electrogenic process. *J Gen Physiol*. 1985;86:613.
213. Soleimani M, Grassi SM, Aronson PS. Stoichiometry of Na$^+$-HCO$_3^-$ cotransport in basolateral membrane vesicles isolated from rabbit renal cortex. *J Clin Invest*. 1987;79:1276.
214. Soleimani M, Burnham CE. Na$^+$:HCO$_3^-$ cotransporters (NBC): cloning and characterization. *J Membr Biol*. 2001;183:71.
215. Romero MF, Hediger MA, Boulpaep EL, et al. Expression cloning and characterization of a renal electrogenic Na$^+$/HCO$_3^-$ cotransporter. *Nature*. 1997;387:409.
216. Burnham CE, Amlal H, Wang Z, et al. Cloning and functional expression of a human kidney Na$^+$:HCO$_3^-$ cotransporter. *J Biol Chem*. 1997;272:19111.
217. Romero MF, Fong P, Berger UV, et al. Cloning and functional expression of rNBC, an electrogenic Na$^+$-HCO$_3^-$ cotransporter from rat kidney. *Am J Physiol*. 1998;274:F425-F432.

218. Abuladze N, Lee I, Newman D, et al. Axial heterogeneity of sodium-bicarbonate cotransporter expression in the rabbit proximal tubule. *Am J Physiol Renal Physiol*. 1998;274:F628-F633.

219. Schmitt BM, Biemesderfer D, Romero MF, et al. Immunolocalization of the electrogenic Na⁺-HCO₃⁻ cotransporter in mammalian and amphibian kidney. *Am J Physiol*. 1999;276:F27-F38.

220. Maunsbach AB, Vorum H, Kwon TH, et al. Immunoelectron microscopic localization of the electrogenic Na/HCO(3) cotransporter in rat and *Ambystoma* kidney. *J Am Soc Nephrol*. 2000;11:2179.

221. Igarashi T, Inatomi J, Sekine T, et al. Mutations in SLC4A4 cause permanent isolated proximal renal tubular acidosis with ocular abnormalities. *Nat Genet*. 1999;23:264.

222. Good DW, Burg MB. Ammonia production by individual segments of the rat nephron. *J Clin Invest*. 1984;73:602.

223. Good DW, DuBose Jr TD. Ammonia transport by early and late proximal convoluted tubule of the rat. *J Clin Invest*. 1987;79:684.

224. Nagami GT, Kurokawa K. Regulation of ammonia production by mouse proximal tubules perfused in vitro. Effect of luminal perfusion. *J Clin Invest*. 1985;75:844.

225. Knepper MA, Packer R, Good DW. Ammonium transport in the kidney. *Physiol Rev*. 1989;69:179.

226. McKinney TD. Heterogeneity of organic base secretion by proximal tubules. *Am J Physiol*. 1982;243:F404-F407.

227. Burckhardt G, Wolff NA. Structure of renal organic anion and cation transporters. *Am J Physiol Renal Physiol*. 2000;278:F853-F866.

228. Lopez-Nieto CE, You G, Bush KT, et al. Molecular cloning and characterization of NKT, a gene product related to the organic cation transporter family that is almost exclusively expressed in the kidney. *J Biol Chem*. 1997;272:6471.

229. Sekine T, Watanabe N, Hosoyamada M, et al. Expression cloning and characterization of a novel multispecific organic anion transporter. *J Biol Chem*. 1997;272:18526.

230. Sweet DH, Wolff NA, Pritchard JB. Expression cloning and characterization of ROAT1. The basolateral organic anion transporter in rat kidney. *J Biol Chem*. 1997;272:30088.

231. Tojo A, Sekine T, Nakajima N, et al. Immunohistochemical localization of multispecific renal organic anion transporter 1 in rat kidney. *J Am Soc Nephrol*. 1999;10:464.

232. Karbach U, Kricke J, Meyer-Wentrup F, et al. Localization of organic cation transporters OCT1 and OCT2 in rat kidney. *Am J Physiol Renal Physiol*. 2000;279:F679-F687.

233. Ishibashi K, Kuwahara M, Kageyama Y, et al. Molecular cloning of a new aquaporin superfamily in mammals: AQPX1 and AQPX2. In: Hohmann S, Nielsen S, eds. *Molecular biology and physiology of water and solute transport*. New York: Kluwer Academic/Plenum; 2006:pp 123-126.

234. Morishita Y, Matsuzaki T, Hara-chikuma M, et al. Disruption of aquaporin-11 produces polycystic kidneys following vacuolization of the proximal tubule. *Mol Cell Biol*. 2005;25:7770.

235. Gorelick D, Praetorius J, Tsunenari T, et al. Aquaporin-11: a channel protein lacking apparent transport function expressed in brain. *BMC Biochem*. 2006;7:14.

236. Nejsum LN, Elkjaer M-L, Hager H, et al. Localization of aquaporin-7 in rat and mouse kidney using RT-PCR, immunoblotting, and immunocytochemistry. *Biochem Biophys Res Commun*. 2000;277:164.

237. Ishibashi K, Imai M, Sasaki S. Cellular localization of aquaporin 7 in the rat kidney. *Nephron Exp Nephrol*. 2000;8:252.

238. Sohara E, Rai T, Miyazaki JI, et al. Defective water and glycerol transport in the proximal tubules of AQP7 knockout mice. *Am J Physiol Renal Physiol*. 2005;289:F1195-F1200.

239. Dieterich HJ, Barrett JM, Kriz W, et al. The ultrastructure of the thin loop limbs of the mouse kidney. *Anat Embryol (Berl)*. 1975;147:1.

240. Jamison RL, Kriz W. *Urinary concentrating mechanism: structure and function*. New York: Oxford University Press; 1982.

241. Bachmann S, Kriz W. Histotopography and ultrastructure of the thin limbs of the loop of Henle in the hamster. *Cell Tissue Res*. 1982;225:111.

242. Barrett JM, Kriz W, Kaissling B, et al. The ultrastructure of the nephrons of the desert rodent (*Psammomys obesus*) kidney. II. Thin limbs of Henle of long-looped nephrons. *Am J Anat*. 1978;151:499.

243. Barrett JM, Kriz W, Kaissling B, et al. The ultrastructure of the nephrons of the desert rodent (*Psammomys obesus*) kidney. I. Thin limb of Henle of short-looped nephrons. *Am J Anat*. 1978;151:487.

244. Kriz W, Schiller A, Taugner R. Freeze-fracture studies on the thin limbs of Henle's loop in *Psammomys obesus*. *Am J Anat*. 1981;162:23.

245. Schiller A, Taugner R, Kriz W. The thin limbs of Henle's loop in the rabbit. A freeze fracture study. *Cell Tissue Res*. 1980;207:249.

246. Schwartz MM, Karnovsky MJ, Venkatachalam MA. Regional membrane specialization in the thin limbs of Henle's loops as seen by freeze-fracture electron microscopy. *Kidney Int*. 1979;16:577.

247. Schwartz MM, Venkatachalam MA. Structural differences in thin limbs of Henle: physiological implications. *Kidney Int*. 1974;6:193.

248. Garg LC, Tisher CC. Na-K-ATPase activity in thin limbs of rat nephron. *Kidney Int*. 1983;23:255:abstract.

249. Ernst SA, Schreiber JH. Ultrastructural localization of Na⁺, K⁺-ATPase in rat and rabbit kidney medulla. *J Cell Biol*. 1981;91:803.

250. Garg LC, Knepper MA, Burg MB. Mineralocorticoid effects on Na-K-ATPase in individual nephron segments. *Am J Physiol*. 1981;240:F536-F544.

251. Imai M. Functional heterogeneity of the descending limbs of Henle's loop. II. Interspecies differences among rabbits, rats, and hamsters. *Pflugers Arch*. 1984;402:393.

252. Imai M, Hayashi M, Araki M. Functional heterogeneity of the descending limbs of Henle's loop. I. Internephron heterogeneity in the hamster kidney. *Pflugers Arch*. 1984;402:385.

253. Nielsen S, Pallone TL, Smith BL, et al. Aquaporin-1 water channels in short and long loop descending thin limbs and in descending vasa recta in rat kidney. *Am J Physiol*. 1995;268:F1023-F1037.

254. Pannabecker TL, Abbott DE, Dantzler WH. Three-dimensional functional reconstruction of inner medullary thin limbs of Henle's loop. *Am J Physiol Renal Physiol*. 2004;286:F38-F45.

255. Pannabecker TL, Dantzler WH. Three-dimensional lateral and vertical relationships of inner medullary loops of Henle and collecting ducts. *Am J Physiol Renal Physiol*. 2004;287:F767-F774.

256. Shayakul C, Knepper MA, Smith CP, et al. Segmental localization of urea transporter mRNAs in rat kidney. *Am J Physiol*. 1997;272:F654-F660.

257. Kim YH, Kim DU, Han KH, et al. Expression of urea transporters in the developing rat kidney. *Am J Physiol Renal Physiol*. 2002;282:F530-F540.

258. Nielsen S, Terris J, Smith CP, et al. Cellular and subcellular localization of the vasopressin-regulated urea transporter in rat kidney. *Proc Natl Acad Sci USA*. 1996;93:5495.

259. Sands JM, Timmer RT, Gunn RB. Urea transporters in kidney and erythrocytes. *Am J Physiol*. 1997;273:F321-F339.

260. Shayakul C, Smith CP, Mackenzie HS, et al. Long-term regulation of urea transporter expression by vasopressin in Brattleboro rats. *Am J Physiol Renal Physiol*. 2000;278:F620-F627.

261. Wade JB, Lee AJ, Liu J, et al. UT-A2: a 55-kDa urea transporter in thin descending limb whose abundance is regulated by vasopressin. *Am J Physiol Renal Physiol*. 2000;278:F52-F62.

262. Allen F, Tisher CC. Morphology of the ascending thick limb of Henle. *Kidney Int*. 1976;9:8.

263. Kone BC, Madsen KM, Tisher CC. Ultrastructure of the thick ascending limb of Henle in the rat kidney. *Am J Anat*. 1984;171:217.

264. Welling LW, Welling DJ, Hill JJ. Shape of cells and intercellular channels in rabbit thick ascending limb of Henle. *Kidney Int*. 1978;13:144.

265. Greger R, Schlatter E. Presence of luminal K⁺, a prerequisite for active NaCl transport in the cortical thick ascending limb of Henle's loop of rabbit kidney. *Pflugers Arch*. 1981;392:92.

266. Hebert SC, Andreoli TE. Control of NaCl transport in the thick ascending limb. *Am J Physiol*. 1984;246:F745-F756.

267. Greger R, Schlatter E, Lang F. Evidence for electroneutral sodium chloride cotransport in the cortical thick ascending limb of Henle's loop of rabbit kidney. *Pflugers Arch*. 1983;396:308.

268. Schlatter E, Greger R, Weidtke C. Effect of "high ceiling" diuretics on active salt transport in the cortical thick ascending limb of Henle's loop of rabbit kidney. Correlation of chemical structure and inhibitory potency. *Pflugers Arch*. 1983;396:210.

269. Kaplan MR, Plotkin MD, Lee WS, et al. Apical localization of the Na-K-Cl cotransporter, rBSC1, on rat thick ascending limbs. *Kidney Int*. 1996;49:40.

270. Yang T, Huang YG, Singh I, et al. Localization of bumetanide- and thiazide-sensitive Na-K-Cl cotransporters along the rat nephron. *Am J Physiol Renal Physiol*. 1996;271:F931-F939.

271. Ecelbarger CA, Terris J, Hoyer JR, et al. Localization and regulation of the rat renal Na(+)-K(+)-2Cl⁻ cotransporter, BSC-1. *Am J Physiol*. 1996;271:F619-F628.

272. Nielsen S, Maunsbach AB, Ecelbarger CA, et al. Ultrastructural localization of Na-K-2Cl cotransporter in thick ascending limb and macula densa of rat kidney. *Am J Physiol*. 1998;275:F885-F893.

273. Castrop H, Schnermann J. Isoforms of renal Na-K-2Cl cotransporter NKCC2: expression and functional significance. *Am J Physiol Renal Physiol*. 2008;295:F859-F866.

274. Gimenez I, Forbush B. Regulatory phosphorylation sites in the NH2 terminus of the renal Na-K-Cl cotransporter (NKCC2). *Am J Physiol Renal Physiol*. 2005;289:F1341-F1345.

275. Richardson C, Alessi DR. The regulation of salt transport and blood pressure by the WNK-SPAK/OSR1 signalling pathway. *J Cell Sci*. 2008;121:3293.

276. Garg LC, Mackie S, Tisher CC. Effect of low potassium-diet on Na-K-ATPase in rat nephron segments. *Pflugers Arch*. 1982;394:113.

277. Rocha AS, Kokko JP. Sodium chloride and water transport in the medullary thick ascending limb of Henle. Evidence for active chloride transport. *J Clin Invest.* 1973;52:612.

278. Burg MB, Green N. Function of the thick ascending limb of Henle's loop. *Am J Physiol.* 1973;224:659.

279. Good DW. Sodium-dependent bicarbonate absorption by cortical thick ascending limb of rat kidney. *Am J Physiol.* 1985;248:F821-F829.

280. Good DW, Knepper MA, Burg MB. Ammonia and bicarbonate transport by thick ascending limb of rat kidney. *Am J Physiol.* 1984;247:F35-F44.

281. Brown D, Zhu XL, Sly WS. Localization of membrane-associated carbonic anhydrase type IV in kidney epithelial cells. *Proc Natl Acad Sci USA.* 1990;87:7457.

282. Good DW. Inhibition of bicarbonate absorption by peptide hormones and cyclic adenosine monophosphate in rat medullary thick ascending limb. *J Clin Invest.* 1990;85:1006.

283. Alper SL, Stuart-Tilley AK, Biemesderfer D, et al. Immunolocalization of AE2 anion exchanger in rat kidney. *Am J Physiol.* 1997;273:F601-F614:(published erratum in Am J Physiol 274[3 pt 2]:7433, 1998).

284. Stuart-Tilley AK, Shmukler BE, Brown D, et al. Immunolocalization and tissue-specific splicing of AE2 anion exchanger in mouse kidney. *J Am Soc Nephrol.* 1998;9:946.

285. Castillo JE, Martinez-Anso E, Malumbres R, et al. In situ localization of anion exchanger-2 in the human kidney. *Cell Tissue Res.* 2000;299:281.

286. Vorum H, Kwon TH, Fulton C, et al. Immunolocalization of electroneutral Na-HCO(3)(−) cotransporter in rat kidney. *Am J Physiol Renal Physiol.* 2000;279:F901-F909.

287. Suki WN, Rouse D, Ng RC, et al. Calcium transport in the thick ascending limb of Henle. Heterogeneity of function in the medullary and cortical segments. *J Clin Invest.* 1980;66:1004.

288. Shareghi GR, Agus ZS. Magnesium transport in the cortical thick ascending limb of Henle's loop of the rabbit. *J Clin Invest.* 1982;69:759.

289. Brown EM, Pollak M, Chou YH, et al. Cloning and functional characterization of extracellular Ca(2+)-sensing receptors from parathyroid and kidney. *Bone.* 1995;17:7S.

290. Riccardi D, Park J, Lee WS, et al. Cloning and functional expression of a rat kidney extracellular calcium/polyvalent cation–sensing receptor. *Proc Natl Acad Sci USA.* 1995;92:131.

291. Riccardi D, Lee WS, Lee K, et al. Localization of the extracellular Ca(2+)-sensing receptor and PTH/PTHrP receptor in rat kidney. *Am J Physiol.* 1996;271:F951-F956.

292. Riccardi D, Hall AE, Chattopadhyay N, et al. Localization of the extracellular Ca^{2+}/polyvalent cation–sensing protein in rat kidney. *Am J Physiol.* 1998;274:F611-F622.

293. Brown EM, Pollak M, Hebert SC. The extracellular calcium-sensing receptor: its role in health and disease. *Annu Rev Med.* 1998;49:15.

294. Brown EM, Hebert SC. A cloned Ca^{2+}-sensing receptor: a mediator of direct effects of extracellular Ca^{2+} on renal function? *J Am Soc Nephrol.* 1995;6:1530.

295. Crayen ML, Thoenes W. Architecture and cell structures in the distal nephron of the rat kidney. *Cytobiologie.* 1978;17:197.

296. Woodhall PB, Tisher CC. Response of the distal tubule and cortical collecting duct to vasopressin in the rat. *J Clin Invest.* 1973;52:3095.

297. Reilly RF, Ellison DH. Mammalian distal tubule: physiology, pathophysiology, and molecular anatomy. *Physiol Rev.* 2000;80:277.

298. Stanton BA, Giebisch GH. Potassium transport by the renal distal tubule: effects of potassium loading. *Am J Physiol.* 1982;243:F487-F493.

299. Stanton BA, Biemesderfer D, Wade JB, et al. Structural and functional study of the rat distal nephron: effects of potassium adaptation and depletion. *Kidney Int.* 1981;19:36.

300. Kaissling B. Structural aspects of adaptive changes in renal electrolyte excretion. *Am J Physiol.* 1982;243:F211-F226.

301. Bachmann S, Velazquez H, Obermuller N, et al. Expression of the thiazide-sensitive Na-Cl cotransporter by rabbit distal convoluted tubule cells. *J Clin Invest.* 1995;96:2510.

302. Obermuller N, Bernstein P, Velazquez H, et al. Expression of the thiazide-sensitive Na-Cl cotransporter in rat and human kidney. *Am J Physiol.* 1995;269:F900-F910.

303. Plotkin MD, Kaplan MR, Verlander JW, et al. Localization of the thiazide sensitive Na-Cl cotransporter, rTSC1 in the rat kidney. *Kidney Int.* 1996;50:174.

304. Sandberg MB, Maunsbach AB, McDonough AA. Redistribution of distal tubule Na$^+$-Cl$^-$ cotransporter (NCC) in response to a high-salt diet. *Am J Physiol Renal Physiol.* 2006;291:F503-F508.

305. Bachmann S, Bostanjoglo M, Schmitt R, et al. Sodium transport–related proteins in the mammalian distal nephron—distribution, ontogeny and functional aspects. *Anat Embryol (Berl).* 1999;200:447.

306. Bostanjoglo M, Reeves WB, Reilly RF, et al. 11Beta-hydroxysteroid dehydrogenase, mineralocorticoid receptor, and thiazide-sensitive Na-Cl cotransporter expression by distal tubules. *J Am Soc Nephrol.* 1998;9:1347.

307. Kim GH, Masilamani S, Turner R, et al. The thiazide-sensitive Na-Cl cotransporter is an aldosterone-induced protein. *Proc Natl Acad Sci USA.* 1998;95:14552.

308. Campean V, Kricke J, Ellison D, et al. Localization of thiazide-sensitive Na(+)-Cl(−) cotransport and associated gene products in mouse DCT. *Am J Physiol Renal Physiol.* 2001;281:F1028-F1035.

309. Hofmeister MV, Fenton RA, Praetorius J. Fluorescence isolation of mouse late distal convoluted tubules and connecting tubules: effects of vasopressin and vitamin D$_3$ on Ca^{2+} signaling. *Am J Physiol Renal Physiol.* 2009;296:F194-F203.

310. Loffing J, Vallon V, Loffing-Cueni D, et al. Altered renal distal tubule structure and renal Na(+) and Ca(2+) handling in a mouse model for Gitelman's syndrome. *J Am Soc Nephrol.* 2004;15:2276.

311. Doucet A, Katz AI. High-affinity Ca-Mg-ATPase along the rabbit nephron. *Am J Physiol.* 1982;242:F346-F352.

312. Borke JL, Minami J, Verma A, et al. Monoclonal antibodies to human erythrocyte membrane Ca^{++}-Mg^{++} adenosine triphosphatase pump recognize an epitope in the basolateral membrane of human kidney distal tubule cells. *J Clin Invest.* 1987;80:1225.

313. Roth J, Brown D, Norman AW, et al. Localization of the vitamin D–dependent calcium-binding protein in mammalian kidney. *Am J Physiol.* 1982;243:F243-F252.

314. Kaissling B, Bachmann S, Kriz W. Structural adaptation of the distal convoluted tubule to prolonged furosemide treatment. *Am J Physiol.* 1985;248:F374-F381.

315. Kaissling B, Stanton BA. Adaptation of distal tubule and collecting duct to increased sodium delivery. I. Ultrastructure. *Am J Physiol.* 1988;255: F1256-F1268.

316. Stanton BA, Kaissling B. Adaptation of distal tubule and collecting duct to increased Na delivery. II. Na$^+$ and K$^+$ transport. *Am J Physiol.* 1988;255:F1269-F1275.

317. Fenton RA, Brond L, Nielsen S, et al. Cellular and subcellular distribution of the type-2 vasopressin receptor in the kidney. *Am J Physiol Renal Physiol.* 2007;293:F748-F760.

318. Pedersen NB, Hofmeister MV, Rosenbaek LL, et al. Vasopressin induces phosphorylation of the thiazide-sensitive sodium chloride cotransporter in the distal convoluted tubule. *Kidney Int.* 2010.

319. Elalouf JM, Roinel N, de Rouffignac C. Effects of antidiuretic hormone on electrolyte reabsorption and secretion in distal tubules of rat kidney. *Pflugers Arch.* 1984;401:167.

320. Morel F, Chabardes D, Imbert M. Functional segmentation of the rabbit distal tubule by microdetermination of hormone-dependent adenylate cyclase activity. *Kidney Int.* 1976;9:264.

321. Myers CE, Bulger RE, Tisher CC, et al. Human renal ultrastructure. IV. Collecting duct of healthy individuals. *Lab Invest.* 1966;16:655.

322. Welling LW, Evan AP, Welling DJ, et al. Morphometric comparison of rabbit cortical connecting tubules and collecting ducts. *Kidney Int.* 1983;23:358.

323. Verlander JW, Madsen KM, Tisher CC. Effect of acute respiratory acidosis on two populations of intercalated cells in rat cortical collecting duct. *Am J Physiol.* 1987;253:F1142-F1156.

324. Kim J, Kim YH, Cha JH, et al. Intercalated cell subtypes in connecting tubule and cortical collecting duct of rat and mouse. *J Am Soc Nephrol.* 1999;10:1.

325. Teng-umnuay P, Verlander JW, Yuan W, et al. Identification of distinct subpopulations of intercalated cells in the mouse collecting duct. *J Am Soc Nephrol.* 1996;7:260.

326. Loffing J, Loffing-Cueni D, Valderrabano V, et al. Distribution of transcellular calcium and sodium transport pathways along mouse distal nephron. *Am J Physiol Renal Physiol.* 2001;281:F1021-F1027.

327. Rubera I, Loffing J, Palmer LG, et al. Collecting duct-specific gene inactivation of αENaC in the mouse kidney does not impair sodium and potassium balance. *J Clin Invest.* 2003;112:554.

328. Hummler E, Barker P, Gatzy J, et al. Early death due to defective neonatal lung liquid clearance in αENaC-deficient mice. *Nat Genet.* 1996;12:325.

329. Kishore BK, Mandon B, Oza NB, et al. Rat renal arcade segment expresses vasopressin-regulated water channel and vasopressin V2 receptor. *J Clin Invest.* 1996;97:2763.

330. Rojek A, Fuchtbauer EM, Kwon TH, et al. Severe urinary concentrating defect in renal collecting duct–selective AQP2 conditional-knockout mice. *Proc Natl Acad Sci U S A.* 2006;103(15):6037.

331. Reilly RF, Shugrue CA, Lattanzi D, et al. Immunolocalization of the Na$^+$/Ca^{2+} exchanger in rabbit kidney. *Am J Physiol.* 1993;265:F327-F332.

332. Borke JL, Caride A, Verma AK, et al. Plasma membrane calcium pump and 28-kDa calcium binding protein in cells of rat kidney distal tubules. *Am J Physiol.* 1989;257:F842-F849.

333. Yang CW, Kim J, Kim YH, et al. Inhibition of calbindin D28K expression by cyclosporin A in rat kidney: the possible pathogenesis of cyclosporin A–induced hypercalciuria. *J Am Soc Nephrol.* 1998;9:1416.

334. Boros S, Bindels RJ, Hoenderop JG. Active Ca(2+) reabsorption in the connecting tubule. *Pflugers Arch*. 2009;458:99.

335. Wright FS, Giebisch G. Renal potassium transport: contributions of individual nephron segments and populations. *Am J Physiol*. 1978;235:F515-F527.

336. Field MJ, Stanton BA, Giebisch GH. Differential acute effects of aldosterone, dexamethasone, and hyperkalemia on distal tubular potassium secretion in the rat kidney. *J Clin Invest*. 1984;74:1792.

337. Stanton B, Janzen A, Klein-Robbenhaar G, et al. Ultrastructure of rat initial collecting tubule. Effect of adrenal corticosteroid treatment. *J Clin Invest*. 1985;75:1327.

338. Madsen KM, Clapp WL, Verlander JW. Structure and function of the inner medullary collecting duct. *Kidney Int*. 1988;34:441.

339. Hansen GP, Tisher CC, Robinson RR. Response of the collecting duct to disturbances of acid-base and potassium balance. *Kidney Int*. 1980;17:326.

340. LeFurgey A, Tisher CC. Morphology of rabbit collecting duct. *Am J Anat*. 1979;155:111.

341. Welling LW, Evan AP, Welling DJ. Shape of cells and extracellular channels in rabbit cortical collecting ducts. *Kidney Int*. 1981;20:211.

342. Madsen KM, Tisher CC. Structural-functional relationship along the distal nephron. *Am J Physiol*. 1986;250:F1.

343. Madsen KM, Tisher CC. Cellular response to acute respiratory acidosis in rat medullary collecting duct. *Am J Physiol*. 1983;245:F670-F679.

344. Holthofer H, Schulte BA, Pasternack G, et al. Immunocytochemical characterization of carbonic anhydrase–rich cells in the rat kidney collecting duct. *Lab Invest*. 1987;57:150.

345. Kim J, Tisher CC, Linser PJ, et al. Ultrastructural localization of carbonic anhydrase II in subpopulations of intercalated cells of the rat kidney. *J Am Soc Nephrol*. 1990;1:245.

346. Lonnerholm G, Ridderstrale Y. Intracellular distribution of carbonic anhydrase in the rat kidney. *Kidney Int*. 1980;17:162.

347. Atkins JL, Burg MB. Bicarbonate transport by isolated perfused rat collecting ducts. *Am J Physiol*. 1985;249:F485-F489.

348. McKinney TD, Burg MB. Bicarbonate transport by rabbit cortical collecting tubules. Effect of acid and alkali loads in vivo on transport in vitro. *J Clin Invest*. 1977;60:766.

349. Lombard WE, Kokko JP, Jacobson HR. Bicarbonate transport in cortical and outer medullary collecting tubules. *Am J Physiol*. 1983;244:F289-F296.

350. Knepper MA, Good DW, Burg MB. Ammonia and bicarbonate transport by rat cortical collecting ducts perfused in vitro. *Am J Physiol*. 1985;249:F870-F877.

351. Garcia-Austt J, Good DW, Burg MB, et al. Deoxycorticosterone-stimulated bicarbonate secretion in rabbit cortical collecting ducts: effects of luminal chloride removal and in vivo acid loading. *Am J Physiol*. 1985;249:F205-F212.

352. Star RA, Burg MB, Knepper MA. Bicarbonate secretion and chloride absorption by rabbit cortical collecting ducts. Role of chloride/bicarbonate exchange. *J Clin Invest*. 1985;76:1123.

353. Verlander JW, Madsen KM, Tisher CC. Structural and functional features of proton and bicarbonate transport in the rat collecting duct. *Semin Nephrol*. 1991;11:465.

354. Dorup J. Structural adaptation of intercalated cells in rat renal cortex to acute metabolic acidosis and alkalosis. *J Ultrastruct Res*. 1985;92:119.

355. Alper SL, Natale J, Gluck S, et al. Subtypes of intercalated cells in rat kidney collecting duct defined by antibodies against erythroid band 3 and renal vacuolar H⁺-ATPase. *Proc Natl Acad Sci USA*. 1989;86:5429.

356. Brown D, Hirsch S, Gluck S. An H⁺-ATPase in opposite plasma membrane domains in kidney epithelial cell subpopulations. *Nature*. 1988;331:622.

357. Kim J, Welch WJ, Cannon JK, et al. Immunocytochemical response of type A and type B intercalated cells to increased sodium chloride delivery. *Am J Physiol*. 1992;262:F288-F302.

358. Verlander JW, Madsen KM, Galla JH, et al. Response of intercalated cells to chloride depletion metabolic alkalosis. *Am J Physiol*. 1992;262:F309-F319.

359. Bastani B, Purcell H, Hemken P, et al. Expression and distribution of renal vacuolar proton-translocating adenosine triphosphatase in response to chronic acid and alkali loads in the rat. *J Clin Invest*. 1991;88:126.

360. Drenckhahn D, Schluter K, Allen DP, et al. Colocalization of band 3 with ankyrin and spectrin at the basal membrane of intercalated cells in the rat kidney. *Science*. 1985;230:1287.

361. Verlander JW, Madsen KM, Low PS, et al. Immunocytochemical localization of band 3 protein in the rat collecting duct. *Am J Physiol*. 1988;255:F115-F125.

362. Royaux IE, Wall SM, Karniski LP, et al. Pendrin, encoded by the Pendred syndrome gene, resides in the apical region of renal intercalated cells and mediates bicarbonate secretion. *Proc Natl Acad Sci USA*. 2001;98:4221.

363. Soleimani M, Greeley T, Petrovic S, et al. Pendrin: an apical Cl⁻OH⁻/HCO₃⁻ exchanger in the kidney cortex. *Am J Physiol Renal Physiol*. 2001;280:F356-F364.

364. Everett LA, Glaser B, Beck JC, et al. Pendred syndrome is caused by mutations in a putative sulphate transporter gene (PDS). *Nat Genet*. 1997;17:411.

365. Kim YH, Kwon TH, Frische S, et al. Immunocytochemical localization of pendrin in intercalated cell subtypes in rat and mouse kidney. *Am J Physiol Renal Physiol*. 2002;283:F744-F754.

366. Frische S, Kwon TH, Frokiaer J, et al. Regulated expression of pendrin in rat kidney in response to chronic NH₄Cl or NaHCO₃ loading. *Am J Physiol Renal Physiol*. 2003;284:F584-F593.

367. Verlander JW, Hassell KA, Royaux IE, et al. Deoxycorticosterone upregulates PDS (Slc26a4) in mouse kidney: role of pendrin in mineralocorticoid-induced hypertension. *Hypertension*. 2003;42:356.

368. Wall SM, Kim YH, Stanley L, et al. NaCl restriction upregulates renal Slc26a4 through subcellular redistribution: role in Cl⁻ conservation. *Hypertension*. 2004;44:982.

369. Vallet M, Picard N, Loffing-Cueni D, et al. Pendrin regulation in mouse kidney primarily is chloride-dependent. *J Am Soc Nephrol*. 2006;17:2153.

370. Quentin F, Chambrey R, Trinh-Trang-Tan MM, et al. The Cl⁻/HCO₃⁻ exchanger pendrin in the rat kidney is regulated in response to chronic alterations in chloride balance. *Am J Physiol Renal Physiol*. 2004;287:F1179-F1188.

371. Madsen KM, Kim J, Tisher CC. Intracellular band 3 immunostaining in type A intercalated cells of rabbit kidney. *Am J Physiol*. 1992;262:F1015-F1022.

372. Verlander JW, Madsen KM, Stone DK, et al. Ultrastructural localization of H⁺ATPase in rabbit cortical collecting duct. *J Am Soc Nephrol*. 1994;4:1546.

373. Verlander JW, Madsen KM, Cannon JK, et al. Activation of acid-secreting intercalated cells in rabbit collecting duct with ammonium chloride loading. *Am J Physiol*. 1994;266:F633-F645.

374. Schwartz GJ, Barasch J, Al-Awqati Q. Plasticity of functional epithelial polarity. *Nature*. 1985;318:368.

375. Obermuller N, Gretz N, Kriz W, et al. The swelling-activated chloride channel ClC-2, the chloride channel ClC-3, and ClC-5, a chloride channel mutated in kidney stone disease, are expressed in distinct subpopulations of renal epithelial cells. *J Clin Invest*. 1998;101:635.

376. Duc C, Farman N, Canessa CM, et al. Cell-specific expression of epithelial sodium channel alpha, beta, and gamma subunits in aldosterone-responsive epithelia from the rat: localization by in situ hybridization and immunocytochemistry. *J Cell Biol*. 1907;127:1994.

377. Hager H, Kwon TH, Vinnikova AK, et al. Immunocytochemical and immunoelectron microscopic localization of alpha-, beta-, and gamma-ENaC in rat kidney. *Am J Physiol Renal Physiol*. 2001;280:F1093-F1106.

378. Canessa CM, Schild L, Buell G, et al. Amiloride-sensitive epithelial Na⁺ channel is made of three homologous subunits. *Nature*. 1994;367:463.

379. Loffing J, Pietri L, Aregger F, et al. Differential subcellular localization of ENaC subunits in mouse kidney in response to high- and low-Na diets. *Am J Physiol Renal Physiol*. 2000;279:F252-F258.

380. Ecelbarger CA, Kim GH, Terris J, et al. Vasopressin-mediated regulation of epithelial sodium channel abundance in rat kidney. *Am J Physiol Renal Physiol*. 2000;279:F46-F53.

381. Peti-Peterdi J, Warnock DG, Bell PD. Angiotensin II directly stimulates ENaC Activity in the cortical collecting duct via AT1 receptors. *J Am Soc Nephrol*. 2002;13:1131.

382. Beutler KT, Masilamani S, Turban S, et al. Long-term regulation of ENaC expression in kidney by angiotensin II. *Hypertension*. 2003;41:1143.

383. Hamm LL, Feng Z, Hering-Smith KS. Regulation of sodium transport by ENaC in the kidney. *Curr Opin Nephrol Hypertens*. 2010;19:98.

384. Loffing J, Korbmacher C. Regulated sodium transport in the renal connecting tubule (CNT) via the epithelial sodium channel (ENaC). *Pflugers Arch*. 2009;458:111.

385. Bhalla V, Hallows KR. Mechanisms of ENaC regulation and clinical implications. *J Am Soc Nephrol*. 1845;19:2008.

386. O'Neil RG, Helman SI. Transport characteristics of renal collecting tubules: influences of DOCA and diet. *Am J Physiol*. 1977;233:F544-F558.

387. Schwartz GJ, Burg MB. Mineralocorticoid effects on cation transport by cortical collecting tubules in vitro. *Am J Physiol*. 1978;235:F576-F585.

388. Mujais SK, Chekal MA, Jones WJ, et al. Regulation of renal Na-K-ATPase in the rat. Role of the natural mineralo- and glucocorticoid hormones. *J Clin Invest*. 1984;73:13.

389. Petty KJ, Kokko JP, Marver D. Secondary effect of aldosterone on Na-K ATPase activity in the rabbit cortical collecting tubule. *J Clin Invest*. 1981;68:1514.

390. Wade JB, O'Neil RG, Pryor JL, et al. Modulation of cell membrane area in renal collecting tubules by corticosteroid hormones. *J Cell Biol*. 1979;81:439.

391. Rodan AR, Huang CL. Distal potassium handling based on flow modulation of maxi-K channel activity. *Curr Opin Nephrol Hypertens*. 2009;18:350.

392. Wingo CS. Potassium transport by medullary collecting tubule of rabbit: effects of variation in K intake. *Am J Physiol*. 1987;253:F1136-F1141.

393. Stone DK, Seldin DW, Kokko JP, et al. Mineralocorticoid modulation of rabbit medullary collecting duct acidification. A sodium-independent effect. *J Clin Invest.* 1983;72:77.

394. Madsen KM, Tisher CC. Response of intercalated cells of rat outer medullary collecting duct to chronic metabolic acidosis. *Lab Invest.* 1984;51:268.

395. Brown D, Gluck S, Hartwig J. Structure of the novel membrane-coating material in proton-secreting epithelial cells and identification as an H+ATPase. *J Cell Biol.* 1987;105:1637.

396. Wagner CA, Finberg KE, Breton S, et al. Renal vacuolar H+-ATPase. *Physiol Rev.* 2004;84:1263.

397. Wingo CS, Cain BD. The renal H-K-ATPase: physiological significance and role in potassium homeostasis. *Annu Rev Physiol.* 1993;55:323.

398. Doucet A, Marsy S. Characterization of K-ATPase activity in distal nephron: stimulation by potassium depletion. *Am J Physiol.* 1987;253:F418-F423.

399. Garg LC, Narang N. Ouabain-insensitive K-adenosine triphosphatase in distal nephron segments of the rabbit. *J Clin Invest.* 1988;81:1204.

400. Wingo CS. Active proton secretion and potassium absorption in the rabbit outer medullary collecting duct. Functional evidence for proton-potassium-activated adenosine triphosphatase. *J Clin Invest.* 1989;84:361.

401. Wingo CS, Madsen KM, Smolka A, et al. H-K-ATPase immunoreactivity in cortical and outer medullary collecting duct. *Kidney Int.* 1990;38:985.

402. Ahn KY, Kone BC. Expression and cellular localization of mRNA encoding the "gastric" isoform of H(+)-K(+)-ATPase alpha-subunit in rat kidney. *Am J Physiol Renal Physiol.* 1995;268:F99.

403. Campbell-Thompson ML, Verlander JW, Curran KA, et al. In situ hybridization of H-K-ATPase beta-subunit mRNA in rat and rabbit kidney. *Am J Physiol.* 1995;269:F345-F354.

404. Eiam-Ong S, Kurtzman NA, Sabatini S. Regulation of collecting tubule adenosine triphosphatases by aldosterone and potassium. *J Clin Invest.* 1993;91:2385.

405. Ahn KY, Park KY, Kim KK, et al. Chronic hypokalemia enhances expression of the H(+)-K(+)-ATPase alpha 2-subunit gene in renal medulla. *Am J Physiol.* 1996;271:F314-F321.

406. Sangan P, Rajendran VM, Mann AS, et al. Regulation of colonic H-K-ATPase in large intestine and kidney by dietary Na depletion and dietary K depletion. *Am J Physiol.* 1997;272:C685-C696.

407. Zhang W, Xia X, Zou L, et al. in vivo expression profile of a H+-K+-ATPase α2-subunit promoter-reporter transgene. *Am J Physiol Renal Physiol.* 2004;286:F1171-F1177.

408. Xu X, Zhang W, Kone BC. CREB trans-activates the murine H+-K+-ATPase α2-subunit gene. *Am J Physiol Cell Physiol.* 2004;287:C903-C911.

409. Verlander JW, Moudy RM, Campbell WG, et al. Immunohistochemical localization of H-K-ATPase alpha(2c)-subunit in rabbit kidney. *Am J Physiol Renal Physiol.* 2001;281:F357-F365.

410. Meneton P, Schultheis PJ, Greeb J, et al. Increased Sensitivity to K+ deprivation in colonic H, K-ATPase-deficient mice. *J Clin Invest.* 1998;101:536.

411. Nakhoul N, Hamm LL. Non-erythroid Rh glycoproteins: a putative new family of mammalian ammonium transporters. *Pflugers Archiv.* 2004;447:807.

412. Weiner ID. The Rh gene family and renal ammonium transport. *Curr Opin Nephrol Hypertens.* 2004;13:533.

413. Eladari D, Cheval L, Quentin F, et al. Expression of RhCG, a new putative NH(3)/NH(4)(+) transporter, along the rat nephron. *J Am Soc Nephrol.* 1999;13:2002.

414. Quentin F, Eladari D, Cheval L, et al. RhBG and RhCG, the putative ammonia transporters, are expressed in the same cells in the distal nephron. *J Am Soc Nephrol.* 2003;14:545.

415. Verlander JW, Miller RT, Frank AE, et al. Localization of the ammonium transporter proteins RhBG and RhCG in mouse kidney. *Am J Physiol Renal Physiol.* 2003;284:F323-F337.

416. Seshadri RM, Klein JD, Kozlowski S, et al. Renal expression of the ammonia transporters, Rhbg and Rhcg, in response to chronic metabolic acidosis. *Am J Physiol Renal Physiol.* 2006;290:F397-F408.

417. Seshadri RM, Klein JD, Smith T, et al. Changes in subcellular distribution of the ammonia transporter, Rhcg, in response to chronic metabolic acidosis. *Am J Physiol Renal Physiol.* 2006;290:F1443-F1452.

418. Chambrey R, Goossens D, Bourgeois S, et al. Genetic ablation of Rhbg in the mouse does not impair renal ammonium excretion. *Am J Physiol Renal Physiol.* 2005;289:F1281-F1290.

419. Biver S, Belge H, Bourgeois S, et al. A role for Rhesus factor Rhcg in renal ammonium excretion and male fertility. *Nature.* 2008;456:339.

420. Lee HW, Verlander JW, Bishop JM, et al. Collecting duct-specific Rh C glycoprotein deletion alters basal and acidosis-stimulated renal ammonia excretion. *Am J Physiol Renal Physiol.* 2009;296:F1364-F1375.

421. Lee HW, Verlander JW, Bishop JM, et al. Effect of intercalated cell-specific Rh C glycoprotein deletion on basal and metabolic acidosis-stimulated renal ammonia excretion. *Am J Physiol Renal Physiol.* 2010;299:F369-F379.

422. Knepper MA, Danielson RA, Saidel GM, et al. Quantitative analysis of renal medullary anatomy in rats and rabbits. *Kidney Int.* 1977;12:313.

423. Clapp WL, Madsen KM, Verlander JW, et al. Intercalated cells of the rat inner medullary collecting duct. *Kidney Int.* 1987;31:1080.

424. Clapp WL, Madsen KM, Verlander JW, et al. Morphologic heterogeneity along the rat inner medullary collecting duct. *Lab Invest.* 1989;60:219.

425. Sands JM, Knepper MA. Urea permeability of mammalian inner medullary collecting duct system and papillary surface epithelium. *J Clin Invest.* 1987;79:138.

426. Sands JM, Nonoguchi H, Knepper MA. Vasopressin effects on urea and H₂O transport in inner medullary collecting duct subsegments. *Am J Physiol.* 1987;253:F823-F832.

427. Ganote CE, Grantham JJ, Moses HL, et al. Ultrastructural studies of vasopressin effect on isolated perfused renal collecting tubules of the rabbit. *J Cell Biol.* 1968;36:355.

428. Grantham JJ, Ganote CE, Burg MB, et al. Paths of transtubular water flow in isolated renal collecting tubules. *J Cell Biol.* 1969;41:562.

429. Tisher CC, Bulger RE, Valtin H. Morphology of renal medulla in water diuresis and vasopressin-induced antidiuresis. *Am J Physiol.* 1971;220:87.

430. Harmanci MC, Kachadorian WA, Valtin H, et al. Antidiuretic hormone–induced intramembranous alterations in mammalian collecting ducts. *Am J Physiol.* 1978;235:440.

431. Harmanci MC, Stern P, Kachadorian WA, et al. Vasopressin and collecting duct intramembranous particle clusters: a dose-response relationship. *Am J Physiol.* 1980;239:F560-F564.

432. Wade JB, Stetson DL, Lewis SA. ADH action: evidence for a membrane shuttle mechanism. *Ann NY Acad Sci.* 1981;372:106.

433. Brown D, Orci L. Vasopressin stimulates formation of coated pits in rat kidney collecting ducts. *Nature.* 1983;302:253.

434. Strange K, Willingham MC, Handler JS, et al. Apical membrane endocytosis via coated pits is stimulated by removal of antidiuretic hormone from isolated, perfused rabbit cortical collecting tubule. *J Membr Biol.* 1988;103:17.

435. Brown D, Weyer P, Orci L. Vasopressin stimulates endocytosis in kidney collecting duct principal cells. *Eur J Cell Biol.* 1988;46:336.

436. Nielsen S, DiGiovanni SR, Christensen EI, et al. Cellular and subcellular immunolocalization of vasopressin-regulated water channel in rat kidney. *Proc Natl Acad Sci USA.* 1993;90:11663.

437. Kwon TH, Nielsen J, Moller HB, et al. Aquaporins in the kidney. *Handb Exp Pharmacol.* 2009;190:95.

438. Nielsen S, Frokiar J, Marples D, et al. Aquaporins in the kidney: from molecules to medicine. *Physiol Rev.* 2002;82:205.

439. Ecelbarger CA, Terris J, Frindt G, et al. Aquaporin-3 water channel localization and regulation in rat kidney. *Am J Physiol.* 1995;269:F663-F672.

440. Terris J, Ecelbarger CA, Marples D, et al. Distribution of aquaporin-4 water channel expression within rat kidney. *Am J Physiol.* 1995;269:F775-F785.

441. Frigeri A, Gropper MA, Turck CW, et al. Immunolocalization of the mercurial-insensitive water channel and glycerol intrinsic protein in epithelial cell plasma membranes. *Proc Natl Acad Sci USA.* 1995;92:4328.

442. Kwon TH, Nielsen J, Masilamani S, et al. Regulation of collecting duct AQP3 expression: response to mineralocorticoid. *Am J Physiol Renal Physiol.* 2002;283:F1403-F1421.

443. de Seigneux S, Nielsen J, Olesen ET, et al. Long-term aldosterone treatment induces decreased apical but increased basolateral expression of AQP2 in CCD of rat kidney. *Am J Physiol Renal Physiol.* 2007;293:F87-F99.

444. Nielsen J, Kwon TH, Praetorius J, et al. Aldosterone increases urine production and decreases apical AQP2 expression in rats with diabetes insipidus. *Am J Physiol Renal Physiol.* 2006;290:F438-F449.

445. Fenton RA. Essential role of vasopressin-regulated urea transport processes in the mammalian kidney. *Pflugers Arch.* 2009;458:169.

446. Terris JM, Knepper MA, Wade JB. UT-A3: localization and characterization of an additional urea transporter isoform in the IMCD. *Am J Physiol Renal Physiol.* 2001;280:F325-F332.

447. Fenton RA, Stewart GS, Carpenter B, et al. Characterization of mouse urea transporters UT-A1 and UT-A2. *Am J Physiol Renal Physiol.* 2002;283:F817-F825.

448. Stewart GS, Fenton RA, Wang W, et al. The basolateral expression of mUT-A3 in the mouse kidney. *Am J Physiol Renal Physiol.* 2004;286:F979.

449. Fenton RA, Chou CL, Stewart GS, et al. Urinary concentrating defect in mice with selective deletion of phloretin-sensitive urea transporters in the renal collecting duct. *Proc Natl Acad Sci USA.* 2004;101:7469.

450. Fenton RA. Urea transporters and renal function: lessons from knockout mice. *Curr Opin Nephrol Hypertens.* 2008;17:513.

451. Graber ML, Bengele HH, Schwartz JH, et al. pH and PCO₂ profiles of the rat inner medullary collecting duct. *Am J Physiol.* 1981;241:F659-F668.

452. Richardson RM, Kunau Jr RT. Bicarbonate reabsorption in the papillary collecting duct: effect of acetazolamide. *Am J Physiol.* 1982;243:F74-F80.

453. Ullrich KJ, Papavassiliou F. Bicarbonate reabsorption in the papillary collecting duct of rats. *Pflugers Arch.* 1981;389:271.

454. Bengele HH, Schwartz JH, McNamara ER, et al. Chronic metabolic acidosis augments acidification along the inner medullary collecting duct. *Am J Physiol.* 1986;250:F690-F694.

455. Graber ML, Bengele HH, Mroz E, et al. Acute metabolic acidosis augments collecting duct acidification rate in the rat. *Am J Physiol.* 1981;241:F669-F676.

456. Gluck S, Al-Awqati Q. An electrogenic proton-translocating adenosine triphosphatase from bovine kidney medulla. *J Clin Invest.* 1984;73:1704.

457. Kaunitz JD, Gunther RD, Sachs G. Characterization of an electrogenic ATP and chloride-dependent proton translocating pump from rat renal medulla. *J Biol Chem.* 1985;260:11567.

458. Schwartz JH, Masino SA, Nichols RD, et al. Intracellular modulation of acid secretion in rat inner medullary collecting duct cells. *Am J Physiol.* 1994;266:F94.

459. Ono S, Guntupalli J, DuBose Jr TD. Role of H(+)-K(+)-ATPase in pHi regulation in inner medullary collecting duct cells in culture. *Am J Physiol.* 1996;270:F852-F861.

460. Wall SM, Truong AV, DuBose Jr TD. H(+)-K(+)-ATPase mediates net acid secretion in rat terminal inner medullary collecting duct. *Am J Physiol.* 1996;271:F1037-F1044.

461. Kim YH, Kim J, Verkman AS, et al. Increased expression of H⁺-ATPase in inner medullary collecting duct of aquaporin-1–deficient mice. *Am J Physiol Renal Physiol.* 2003;285:F550-F557.

462. Bohman SO. The ultrastructure of the renal medulla and the interstitial cells. In: Mandal AK, Bohman SO, eds. *The renal papilla and hypertension.* New York: Plenum; 1980, p 7.

463. Lemley KV, Kriz W. Anatomy of the renal interstitium. *Kidney Int.* 1991;39:370.

464. Pedersen JC, Persson AE, Maunsbach AB. Ultrastructure and quantitative characterization of the cortical interstitium in the rat kidney. In: Maunsbach AB, Olsen TS, Christensen EI, eds. *Functional ultrastructure of the kidney.* London: Academic Press; 1980, p 443.

465. Pfaller W. *Structure function correlation on rat kidney: quantitative correlation of structure and function in the normal and injured rat kidney.* Berlin: Springer-Verlag; 1982.

466. Wolgast M, Larson M, Nygren K. Functional characteristics of the renal interstitium. *Am J Physiol.* 1981;241:F105-F111.

467. Bulger RE, Nagle RB. Ultrastructure of the interstitium in the rabbit kidney. *Am J Anat.* 1973;136:183.

468. Bohman SO. The ultrastructure of the rat renal medulla as observed after improved fixation methods. *J Ultrastruct Res.* 1974;47:329.

469. Kaissling B, Le Hir M. Characterization and distribution of interstitial cell types in the renal cortex of rats. *Kidney Int.* 1994;45:709.

470. Mounier F, Foidart JM, Gubler MC. Distribution of extracellular matrix glycoproteins during normal development of human kidney. An immunohistochemical study. *Lab Invest.* 1986;54:394.

471. Martinez-Hernandez A, Gay S, Miller EJ. Ultrastructural localization of type V collagen in rat kidney. *J Cell Biol.* 1982;92:343.

472. Lacombe C, Da Silva JL, Bruneval P, et al. Peritubular cells are the site of erythropoietin synthesis in the murine hypoxic kidney. *J Clin Invest.* 1988;81:620.

473. Bachmann S, Le HM, Eckardt KU. Co-localization of erythropoietin mRNA and ecto-5′-nucleotidase immunoreactivity in peritubular cells of rat renal cortex indicates that fibroblasts produce erythropoietin. *J Histochem Cytochem.* 1993;41:335.

474. Le Hir M, Kaissling B. Distribution of 5′-nucleotidase in the renal interstitium of the rat. *Cell Tissue Res.* 1989;258:177.

475. Bohman SO, Jensen PK. The interstitial cells in the renal medulla of rat, rabbit, and gerbil in different states of diuresis. *Cell Tissue Res.* 1978;189:1.

476. Schiller A, Taugner R. Junctions between interstitial cells of the renal medulla: a freeze-fracture study. *Cell Tissue Res.* 1979;203:231.

477. Majack RA, Larsen WJ. The bicellular and reflexive membrane junctions of renomedullary interstitial cells: functional implications of reflexive gap junctions. *Am J Anat.* 1980;157:181.

478. Bohman SO, Jensen PK. Morphometric studies on the lipid droplets of the interstitial cells of the renal medulla in different states of diuresis. *J Ultrastruct Res.* 1976;55:182.

479. Bulger RE, Griffith LD, Trump BF. Endoplasmic reticulum in rat renal interstitial cells: molecular rearrangement after water deprivation. *Science.* 1966;151:83.

480. Ledingham JM, Simpson FO. Bundles of intracellular tubules in renal medullary interstitial cells. *J Cell Biol.* 1973;57:594.

481. Moffat DB. A new type of cell inclusion in the interstitial cells of the medulla of the rat kidney. *J Microsc.* 1967;6:1073.

482. Nissen HM. On lipid droplets in renal interstitial cells. II. A histological study on the number of droplets in salt depletion and acute salt repletion. *Z Zellforsch Mikrosk Anat.* 1968;85:483.

483. Nissen HM. On lipid droplets in renal interstitial cells. 3. A histological study on the number of droplets during hydration and dehydration. *Z Zellforsch Mikrosk Anat.* 1968;92:52.

484. Mandal AK, Frolich ED, Claude P. A morphologic study of the renal papillary granule: analysis in the interstitial cell and in the interstitium. *J Lab Clin Med.* 1975;85:120.

485. Nissen HM, Bojesen I. On lipid droplets in renal interstitial cells. IV. Isolation and identification. *Z Zellforsch Mikrosk Anat.* 1969;97:274.

486. Bohman SO, Maunsbach AB. Ultrastructure and biochemical properties of subcellular fractions from rat renal medulla. *J Ultrastruct Res.* 1972;38:225.

487. Anggard E, Bohman SO, Griffin JE, et al. Subcellular localization of the prostaglandin system in the rabbit renal papilla. *Acta Physiol Scand.* 1972;84:231.

488. Zusman RM, Keiser HR. Prostaglandin biosynthesis by rabbit renomedullary interstitial cells in tissue culture. Stimulation by angiotensin II, bradykinin, and arginine vasopressin. *J Clin Invest.* 1977;60:215.

489. Guan Y, Chang M, Cho W, et al. Cloning, expression, and regulation of rabbit cyclooxygenase-2 in renal medullary interstitial cells. *Am J Physiol.* 1997;273:F18-F26.

490. Kotnik P, Nielsen J, Kwon TH, et al. Altered expression of COX-1, COX-2, and mPGES in rats with nephrogenic and central diabetes insipidus. *Am J Physiol Renal Physiol.* 2005;288:F1053-F1068.

491. Maric C, Aldred GP, Antoine AM, et al. Effects of angiotensin II on cultured rat renomedullary interstitial cells are mediated by AT1A receptors. *Am J Physiol.* 1996;271:F1020-F1028.

492. Zhuo J, Dean R, Maric C, et al. Localization and interactions of vasoactive peptide receptors in renomedullary interstitial cells of the kidney. *Kidney Int.* 1998;(Suppl 67):S22-S28.

493. Brown CA, Zusman RM, Haber E. Identification of an angiotensin receptor in rabbit renomedullary interstitial cells in tissue culture. Correlation with prostaglandin biosynthesis. *Circ Res.* 1980;46:802.

494. Kugler P. Angiotensinase A in the renomedullary interstitial cells. *Histochemistry.* 1983;77:105.

495. Pitcock JA, Lyons H, Brown PS, et al. Glycosaminoglycans of the rat renomedullary interstitium: ultrastructural and biochemical observations. *Exp Mol Pathol.* 1988;49:373.

496. Peirce EC. Renal lymphatics. *Anat Rec.* 1944;90:315.

497. Bell RD, Keyl MJ, Shrader FR, et al. Renal lymphatics: the internal distribution. *Nephron.* 1968;5:454.

498. Kriz W, Dieterich HJ. The lymphatic system of the kidney in some mammals. Light and electron microscopic investigations. *Z Anat Entwicklungsgesch.* 1970;131:111.

499. Nordquist RE, Bell RD, Sinclair RJ, et al. The distribution and ultrastructural morphology of lymphatic vessels in the canine renal cortex. *Lymphology.* 1973;6:13.

500. Albertine KH, O'Morchoe CC. Distribution and density of the canine renal cortical lymphatic system. *Kidney Int.* 1979;16:470.

501. Niiro GK, Jarosz HM, O'Morchoe PJ, et al. The renal cortical lymphatic system in the rat, hamster, and rabbit. *Am J Anat.* 1986;177:21.

502. Holmes MJ, O'Morchoe PJ, O'Morchoe CC. Morphology of the intrarenal lymphatic system. Capsular and hilar communications. *Am J Anat.* 1977;149:333.

503. Albertine KH, O'Morchoe CC. An integrated light and electron microscopic study on the existence of intramedullary lymphatics in the dog kidney. *Lymphology.* 1980;13:100.

504. Michel CC. Renal medullary microcirculation: architecture and exchange. *Microcirculation.* 1995;2:125.

505. Tenstad O, Heyeraas KJ, Wiig H, et al. Drainage of plasma proteins from the renal medullary interstitium in rats. *J Physiol.* 2001;536:533.

506. Wang W, Michel CC. Modeling exchange of plasma proteins between microcirculation and interstitium of the renal medulla. *Am J Physiol Renal Physiol.* 2000;279:F334-F344.

507. Mitchell GA. The nerve supply of the kidneys. *Acta Anat (Basel).* 1950;10:1.

508. Gosling JA. Observations on the distribution of intrarenal nervous tissue. *Anat Rec.* 1969;163:81.

509. McKenna OC, Angelakos ET. Acetylcholinesterase-containing nerve fibers in the canine kidney. *Circ Res.* 1968;23:645.

510. McKenna OC, Angelakos ET. Adrenergic innervation of the canine kidney. *Circ Res.* 1968;22:345.

511. Barajas L, Powers K. Monoaminergic innervation of the rat kidney: a quantitative study. *Am J Physiol.* 1990;259:F503-F511.

512. Newstead J, Munkacsi I. Electron microscopic observations on the juxtamedullary efferent arterioles and *Arteriolae rectae* in kidneys of rats. *Z Zellforsch Mikrosk Anat.* 1969;97:465.

513. Knight DS, Russell HW, Cicero SR, et al. Transitory inner medullary nerve terminals in the cat kidney. *Neurosci Lett.* 1990;114:173.

514. Barajas L. Innervation of the renal cortex. *Fed Proc.* 1978;37:1192.

515. Barajas L, Liu L, Powers K. Anatomy of the renal innervation: intrarenal aspects and ganglia of origin. *Can J Physiol Pharmacol.* 1992;70:735.

516. Barajas L, Powers K, Wang P. Innervation of the late distal nephron: an autoradiographic and ultrastructural study. *J Ultrastruct Res.* 1985;92:146.

517. Barajas L, Powers K, Wang P. Innervation of the renal cortical tubules: a quantitative study. *Am J Physiol.* 1984;247:F50-F60.

518. Barajas L, Wang P. Myelinated nerves of the rat kidney. A light and electron microscopic autoradiographic study. *J Ultrastruct Res*. 1978; 65:148.
519. Ballesta J, Polak JM, Allen JM, et al. The nerves of the juxtaglomerular apparatus of man and other mammals contain the potent peptide NPY. *Histochemistry*. 1984;80:483.
520. Reinecke M, Forssmann WG. Neuropeptide (neuropeptide Y, neurotensin, vasoactive intestinal polypeptide, substance P, calcitonin gene-related peptide, somatostatin) immunohistochemistry and ultrastructure of renal nerves. *Histochemistry*. 1988;89:1.
521. Knuepfer MM, Schramm LP. The conduction velocities and spinal projections of single renal afferent fibers in the rat. *Brain Res*. 1987;435:167.

The Renal Circulations and Glomerular Ultrafiltration

Karen A. Munger, Curtis K. Kost Jr., Barry M. Brenner,
and David A. Maddox

Under resting conditions, blood flow to the kidneys represents approximately 20% of cardiac output in humans, even though these organs constitute less than 1% of body mass. This rate of blood flow, approximately 400 mL/100 g of tissue per minute, is significantly greater than that observed in other vascular beds considered to be well perfused, such as those of the heart, liver, and brain.[1] From this enormous blood flow (1.0 to 1.2 L/minute), only a small quantity of urine is formed (1 mL/minute). Although the metabolic energy requirement of urine production is relatively high (approximately 10% of basal O_2 consumption), the renal arteriovenous O_2 difference reveals that blood flow far exceeds metabolic demands. In fact, the high rate of blood flow is essential to the process of urine formation, as described later.

The kidney contains several distinct microvascular networks, including the glomerular microcirculation, the cortical peritubular microcirculation, and the unique microcirculations that nourish and drain the inner and outer medulla. In Chapter 2, the gross anatomy of the kidney and arrangement

of tubular segments are described. The first portion of this chapter is a consideration of (1) the intrarenal organization of the discrete microcirculatory networks and (2) the total and regional renal blood flows (RBFs). Later, the physiologic factors that regulate RBF and glomerular filtration rate (GFR) are discussed.

Major Arteries and Veins

Blood supply for each kidney is provided by a renal artery that branches directly from the abdominal aorta. The human renal artery typically branches into multiple segmental vessels at a point just before entry into the renal parenchyma (Figure 3-1). Therefore, complete obstruction of an arterial segmental vessel results in ischemia and infarction of the tissue in the vessel's area of distribution. In fact, ligation of individual segmental arteries has frequently been performed in the rat to reduce renal mass and produce the remnant kidney model of

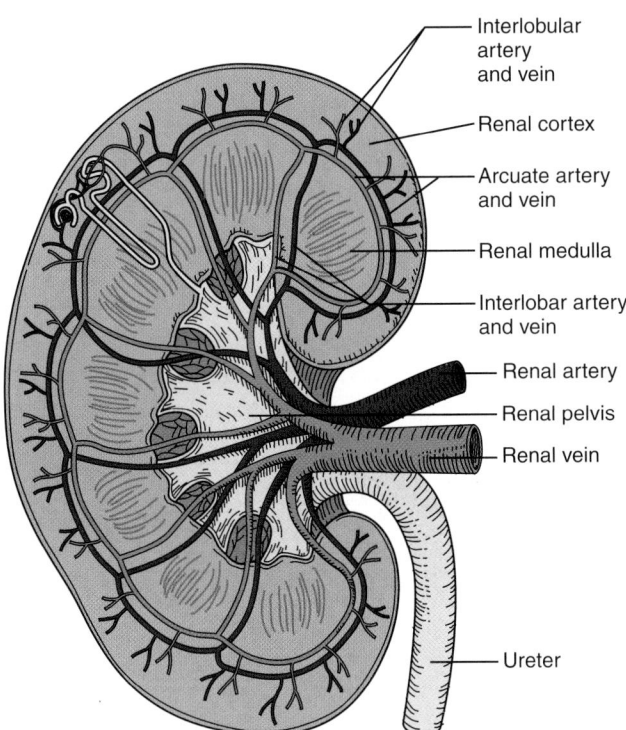

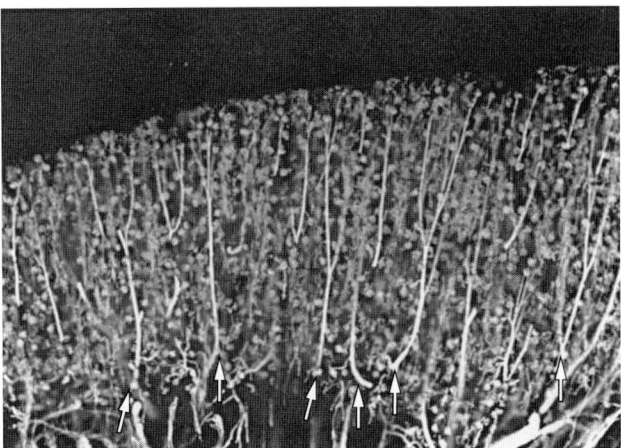

FIGURE 3-2 Low-power photomicrograph of silicone-injected vascular structures in human renal cortex. The tissue has been made transparent by dehydration and clearing procedures after injection. Interlobular arteries (some indicated by *arrows*) arise from arcuate arteries (not seen) and extend toward the kidney surface. The glomeruli, visible as small round objects, arise from the interlobular vessels at all cortical levels. (Magnification ×5.) (Courtesy of R. Beeuwkes, Ph.D.)

FIGURE 3-1 Simplified drawing of the human kidney in cross-section, illustrating the organization of vasculature. A single nephron is also drawn to show the interlobular artery entering into the glomerular capillary network. (From Fox SI: *Human physiology,* ed 6, New York, 1999, McGraw-Hilll, p 529. Reproduced with permission of The McGraw-Hill Companies.)

chronic renal failure. Morphologic studies in this model reveal the presence of ischemic zones adjacent to the totally infarcted areas. These regions contain viable glomeruli that appear shrunken and crowded together, demonstrating that some portions of the renal cortex may have partial dual perfusion.[2]

The anatomic distribution just described is most common; however, other patterns may occur.[3,4] "Accessory" renal arteries frequently result from division of the renal artery at the aorta. These vessels, which most often supply the lower pole,[5] are not in fact accessory, because each is the sole arterial supply of some part of the organ.[6] Such additional arteries are found in 20% to 30% of normal people.

Within the renal sinus of the human kidney, division of the segmental arteries gives rise to the interlobar arteries. These vessels, in turn, give rise to the arcuate arteries, whose several divisions lie at the border between the cortex and medulla (see Figure 3-1). From the arcuate arteries, the interlobular arteries branch more or less sharply, most often as a common trunk that divides two to five times as it extends toward the kidney surface[7,8] (Figure 3-2). Afferent arterioles leading to glomeruli arise from the smaller branches of the interlobular arteries (Figure 3-3). Glomeruli are classified according to their position within the cortex as superficial (i.e., near the kidney surface), midcortical, or juxtamedullary (near the corticomedullary border). The capillary network of each glomerulus is connected to the postglomerular (peritubular) capillary circulation by way of the efferent arterioles. Both the nomenclature and pattern of the renal arterial system are similar in most of the mammals commonly used experimentally. For example, the main arterial branches that lie beside the medullary

pyramid are called *interlobar,* even in animals such as rodents that have only a single lobe.

Organization and Function of the Intrarenal Microcirculations

Hydraulic Pressure Profile of the Renal Circulation

The pressure drop between the systemic vasculature and the end of the interlobular artery in both the superficial and juxtamedullary microvasculature can be as much as 25 mm Hg at normal perfusion pressures; the majority of that pressure drop occurs along the interlobular arteries (Figure 3-4). However, according to studies of the vasculature of a unique set of juxtamedullary nephrons,[9,10] most of the preglomerular pressure drop between the arcuate artery and the glomerulus occurs along the afferent arterioles. Approximately 70% of the postglomerular hydraulic pressure drop takes place along the efferent arterioles; approximately 40% of the total postglomerular resistance is accounted for by the early efferent arterioles (see Figure 3-4). Of note, results of studies of juxtamedullary nephrons perfused via the arcuate artery indicate that the very late portion of the afferent arterioles (the last 50 to 150 μm) and the very early portion of the efferent arterioles (the first 50 to 150 μm) provide a large portion of the total preglomerular and postglomerular resistance.[9,10] In fact, elegant work by Peti-Peterdi and associates,[11,12] who used multiphoton imaging, indicated the presence of an intraglomular precapillary sphincter (Figure 3-5).

Structure of the Glomerular Microcirculation

The glomerulus and glomerular filtration are discussed in detail later in this chapter. Figure 2-7 in Chapter 2 is a scanning electron micrograph of a resin-filled cast of a glomerulus with the afferent arterioles branching from the interlobular

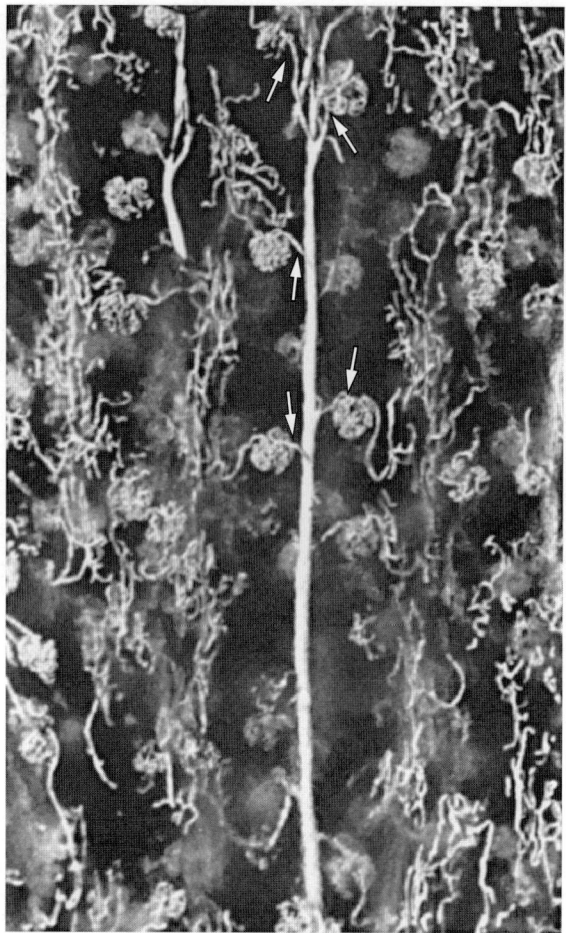

FIGURE 3-3 Photomicrograph of a single interlobular artery and glomeruli arising from it, as seen in a cleared section of a silicone rubber–injected human kidney. Afferent arterioles (*arrows*) extend to glomeruli. Efferent vessels emerging from glomeruli branch to form the cortical postglomerular capillary network. The photomicrograph is oriented so that the outer cortex is at the top and the inner cortex is at the bottom. (Magnification ×25.) (Courtesy of R. Beeuwkes, Ph.D.)

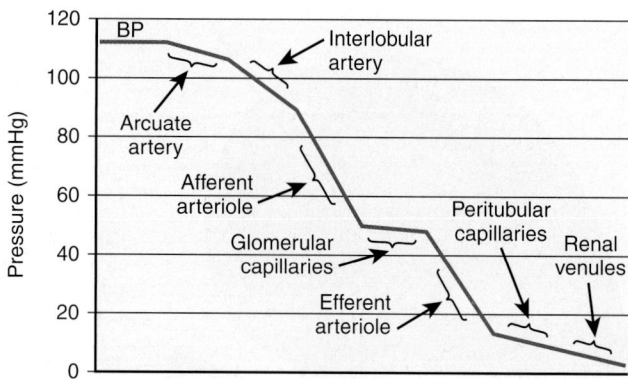

FIGURE 3-4 Hydraulic pressure profile in the renal vasculature, based on findings from various micropuncture studies in superficial nephrons of the rat and squirrel monkey and on values obtained by micropuncture of juxtamedullary nephrons in the rat. In the latter studies, the arcuate artery was perfused with whole blood at normal arterial pressures (BP) and at hydraulic pressures measured at downstream sites, including the interlobular artery, the proximal and distal portions of the afferent arterioles, the glomerular capillaries, the proximal and late segments of the efferent arterioles, the peritubular capillaries, and the renal vein. (Profile generated from data from Maddox et al.[76] and Maddox and Brenner.[87])

artery, the many loops of the glomerular capillaries, and the efferent arterioles emerging from the glomerular tuft. Elger and colleagues[13] provided a detailed ultrastructural analysis of the vascular pole of the renal glomerulus. They described significant differences in the structure and branching patterns of the afferent and efferent arterioles as they enter and exit the tuft. Afferent arterioles lose their internal elastic layer and smooth muscle cell layer before entering the glomerular tuft. Smooth muscle cells are replaced by renin-positive, myosin-negative granular cells that are in close contact with the extraglomerular mesangium.[14] As described by Elger and colleagues,[13] afferent arterioles, upon entering Bowman's space, branch immediately and are distributed along the surface of the glomerular tuft. These primary branches have wide lumens and immediately acquire features of glomerular capillaries, including a fenestrated endothelium, characteristic glomerular basement membrane, and epithelial foot processes.

In contrast, the efferent arterioles arise deep within the tuft, from the convergence of capillaries arising from multiple lobules. Additional tributaries join the arterioles as they travel toward the vascular pole. The structure of the capillary wall begins to change even before the vessels coalesce

to form the efferent arterioles, losing fenestrae progressively until a smooth epithelial lining is formed. At its terminal portion within the tuft, endothelial cells may bulge into the lumen, reducing its internal diameter. Typically, the diameter of the efferent arterioles within the tuft is significantly less than that of the afferent arterioles in the outer cortex. Efferent arterioles of the juxtamedullary nephrons, however, may be larger in diameter than the afferent arterioles and have a thicker wall.[15] Moreover, both the efferent and afferent arterioles of the juxtamedullary nephrons appear to be larger in diameter than those of more superficial nephrons[15] (Figure 3-6). Efferent arterioles acquire a smooth muscle cell layer, which is observed distal to the entry point of the final capillary. The efferent arterioles are also in close contact with the glomerular mesangium as it forms inside the tuft and with the extraglomerular mesangium as it exits the tuft. This precise and close anatomic relationship between the afferent and efferent arterioles and the mesangium is of uncertain physiologic significance, but it is consistent with the presence of an intraglomerular signaling system that may participate in the regulation of blood flow and filtration rate.

The appearance of the vascular pathways within the glomerulus may change under different physiologic conditions. Some insight into the mechanism by which intraglomerular flow patterns might be changed has been obtained. The glomerular mesangium has been shown to contain contractile elements[13,16] (Figure 3-7) and exhibits contractile activity when exposed to angiotensin II.[17] Mesangial cells, which possess specific receptors for angiotensin II, undergo contraction when exposed to this peptide in vitro.[18] Three-dimensional reconstruction of the entire mesangium in the rat suggests that approximately 15% of capillary loops may be entirely enclosed within armlike extensions of mesangial cells that, together with the body of the mesangial cell, are anchored to the extracellular matrix.[19] Contraction of these cells might alter local blood flow and filtration rate, as well as the intraglomerular distribution of blood flow and total filtration surface area. Many hormones and other vasoactive substances capable of

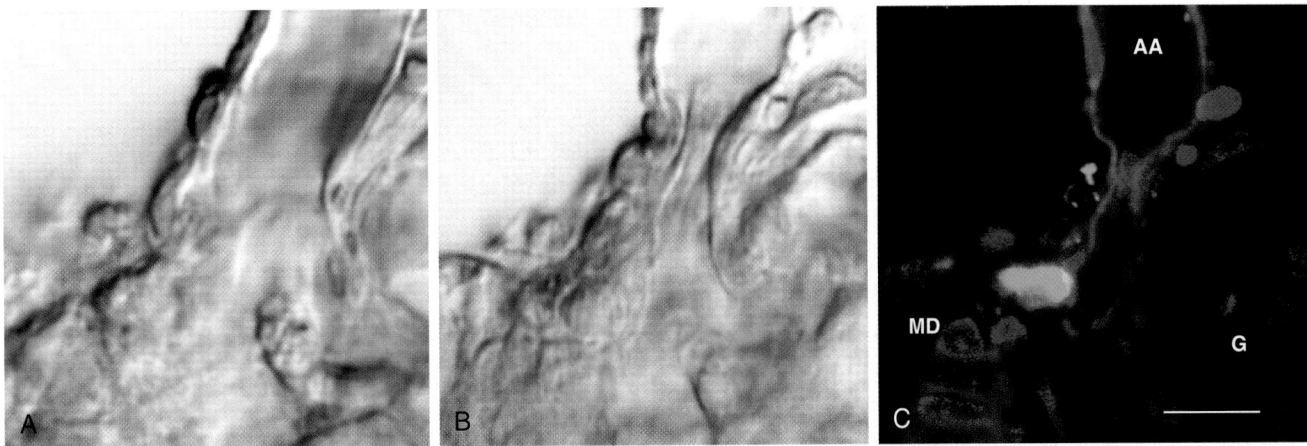

FIGURE 3-5 Constriction of the terminal afferent arterioles (AA), an intraglomerular precapillary sphincter, in response to elevations in distal tubular salt content. **A,** Control (NaCl concentration at the macula densa is 10 mM). **B,** NaCl concentration is increased to 60 mM, which results in an almost complete closure of AA. Transmitted light–differential interference contrast (DIC) images. **C,** Fluorescence image of same preparation as shown in **B.** Vascular endothelium and tubular epithelium are labeled with R18 (*red*), renin granules with quinacrine (*green*), and cell nuclei with Hoechst 33342 (*blue*). Note that renin-positive granular cells constitute the sphincter. Scale bar represents 10 μm. *AA,* Afferent arteriole; *G,* glomerulus; *MD,* macula densa. (From Peti-Peterdi J: Multiphoton imaging of renal tissues in vitro, *Am J Physiol Renal Physiol* 2005;288:F1079-F1083.)

altering glomerular filtration may bring about this adjustment, partly by altering the state of contraction of mesangial cells.

In the outermost, or subcapsular, region of the cortex, the efferent arterioles give rise to a dense capillary network that surrounds the convoluted tubule segments arising from the superficial glomeruli (Figure 3-8). There is evidence that this arrangement is of great importance for reabsorption of water and electrolytes in proximal tubule segments of superficial nephrons. In contrast, the efferent arterioles originating from the comparatively fewer juxtamedullary glomeruli extend into the medulla and give rise to the medullary microcirculatory patterns: an intricate capillary network in the outer medulla and long, unbranched capillary loops (the vasa recta) in the inner medulla. More localized, inner cortical capillary networks may also arise from juxtamedullary glomeruli. The arrangement of the medullary microcirculation plays an important role in the process of concentration of urine.

Venous drainage of the most superficial cortex is by way of superficial cortical veins.[7,20] In middle and inner cortex, venous drainage is achieved mainly by the interlobular veins. The dense peritubular capillary network surrounding the interlobular vessels drains directly into the interlobular veins through multiple connections, whereas the less dense, long-meshed network of the medullary rays appears to anastomose with the interlobular network and thus drain laterally. The medullary circulation also shows two different types of drainage: The outer medullary networks typically extend into the medullary rays before joining interlobular veins, whereas the long vascular bundles of the inner medulla (vasa recta) converge abruptly and join the arcuate veins (see discussion of medullary circulation in the later section Renal Autoregulation).

Vascular-Tubule Relations

Cortical vascular-tubule relations have been described most completely in the canine kidney.[7,21,22] These studies show that, except for convoluted tubule segments in the outermost region of the cortex, the efferent peritubular capillary network and the nephron arising from each glomerulus are often dissociated. In addition, even though the blood supply of many superficial proximal and distal convoluted tubules is derived from peritubular capillaries arising from the parent glomerulus of the same nephron (see Figure 3-8), the loops of Henle of such nephrons, descending in the medullary ray, are surrounded by blood vessels emerging from many midcortical glomeruli through efferent arterioles that extend directly into the medullary ray. Nephrons originating from midcortical glomeruli have proximal and distal convoluted tubule segments lying close to the interlobular axis in the region above the glomerulus of origin. This region is perfused by capillary networks arising from the efferent vessels of more superficial glomeruli. It is in the inner cortex, however, that this dissociation between individual tubules and the corresponding postglomerular capillary network is most apparent. The convoluted tubule segments of these nephrons lie above the glomeruli, surrounded either by the dense network close to the interlobular vessels or by capillary networks arising from other inner cortical glomeruli.

Efferent vessel patterns and vascular-tubule relationships in the human kidney are similar to those in the dog.[22,23] Vascular-tubule relationships in the superficial cortex of the rat have also been defined in micropuncture studies. In general, a close association between the initial portions of peritubular capillaries and early and late proximal tubule segments of the same glomerulus has been shown.[24-26] However, this close association does not mean that each vessel adjacent to a given tubule necessarily arises from the same glomerulus. In fact, Briggs and Wright[27] found that although superficial nephron segments and vessels arising from the same glomerulus are closely associated, each vessel may serve segments of more than one nephron.

Peritubular Capillary Dynamics

The same Starling forces that control fluid movement across all capillary beds govern the rate of fluid movement across peritubular capillary walls. Because the resistance along the afferent and efferent arterioles is relatively high, a large drop in hydraulic pressure occurs before blood enters the peritubular capillaries. In addition, as protein-free fluid is filtered

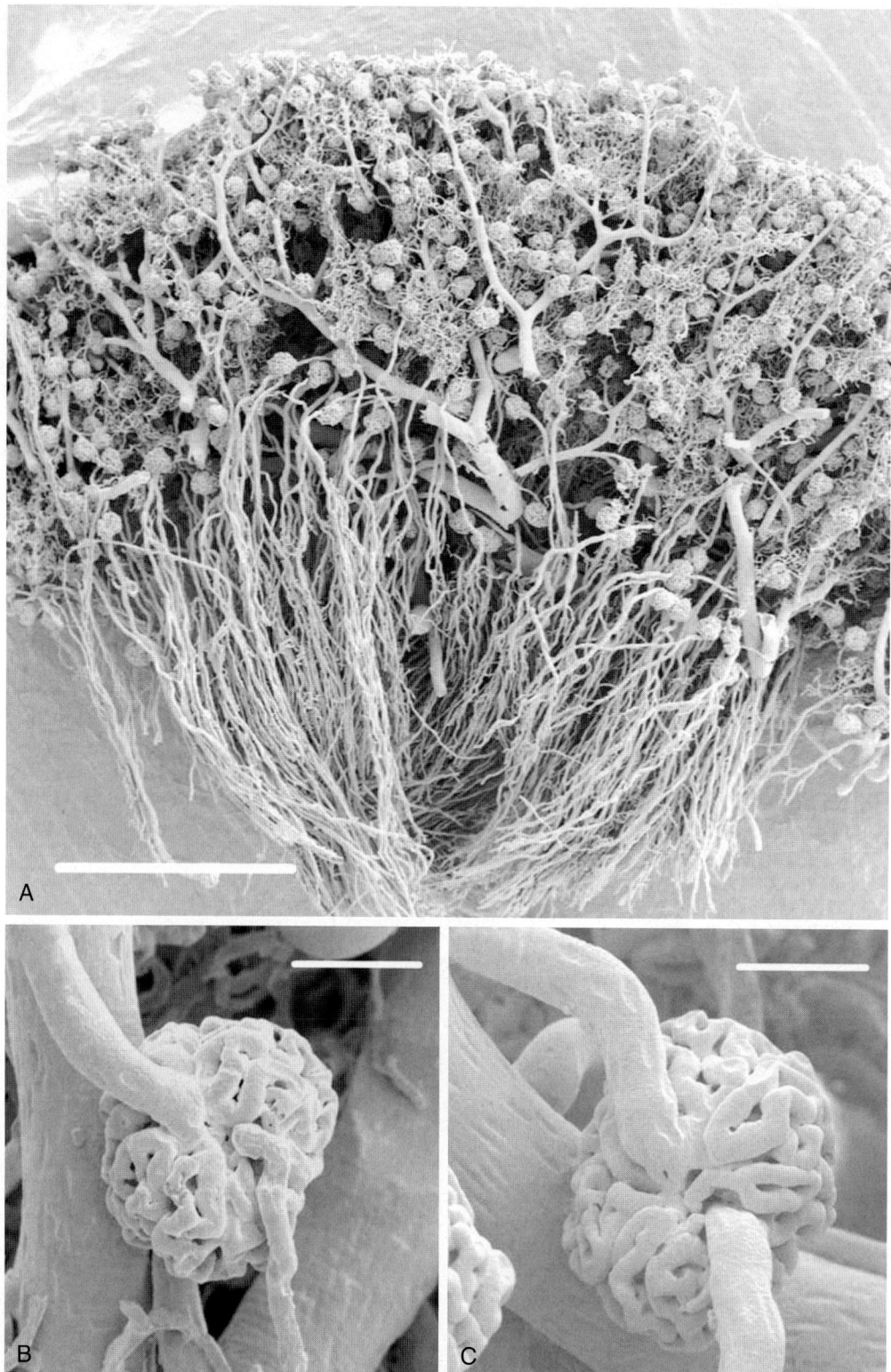

FIGURE 3-6 The renal vasculature of a rabbit. **A,** Resin cast of the vasculature, depicting both cortical and medullary vessels (scale bar represents 1 mm). Note that the diameters of cortical peritubular capillaries are considerably less than those of medullary vasa recta. **B,** Cortical glomeruli showing afferent (upper vessel) and efferent arterioles and the capillary tuft (scale bar represents 60 μm). **C,** Juxtamedullary glomeruli showing afferent (upper vessel) and efferent arterioles and the capillary tuft (scale bar represents 60 μm). Note that the diameters of the juxtamedullary arterioles are larger than those of the cortical glomerular arterioles, particularly the efferent arterioles. (From Evans RG, Eppel GA, Anderson WP, et al: Mechanisms underlying the differential control of blood flow in the renal medulla and cortex, *J Hypertens* 2004;22:1439-1451.)

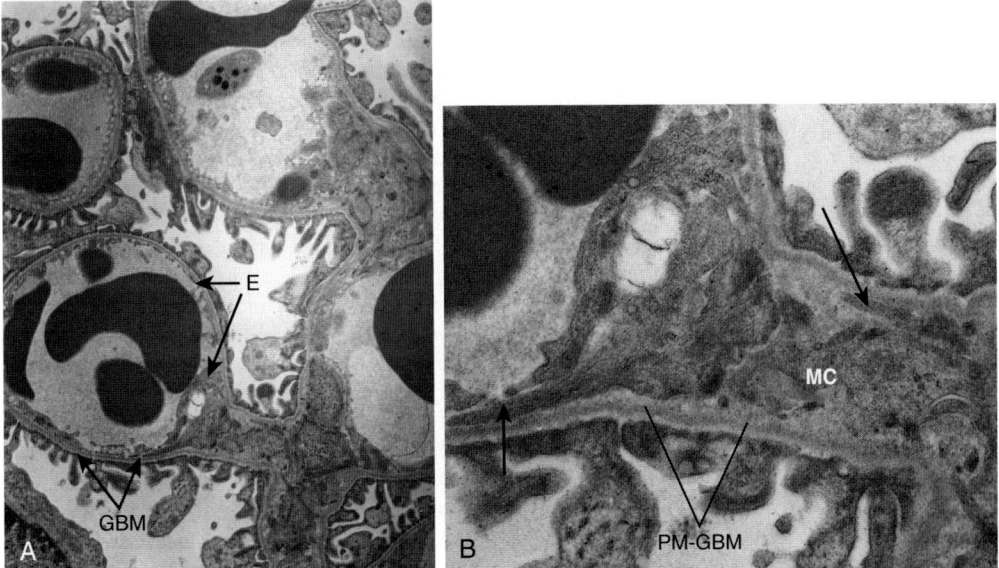

FIGURE 3-7 Electron micrographs of glomerular capillaries of a Munich-Wistar rat. **A,** Overview of several capillaries (magnification ≈×14,500). The majority of the glomerular capillary endothelium (E) is in contact with the glomerular basement membrane (GBM); only a small portion is in contact with the mesangium. At its outer aspect, the GBM is covered by podocyte foot processes. Note that there is no basement membrane separating the endothelium from the mesangium at their interface. **B,** The mesangial cell (MC) extends outward to meet the glomerular capillary (magnification ≈×42,000). Kriz and colleagues[16,41] suggested that within these cylinder-like stalks are contractile filament bundles (*thin arrow*) that attach to the perimesangial glomerular basement membranes (PM-GBM) and extend to the GBM at the mesangial angles (*thick arrow*). For this preparation, the nephron was perfusion-fixed by micropuncture (D. A. Maddox) with 1.25% glutaraldehyde through Bowman's space, thereby yielding the fixation of glomerular structures as well as the red blood cells in the capillaries.

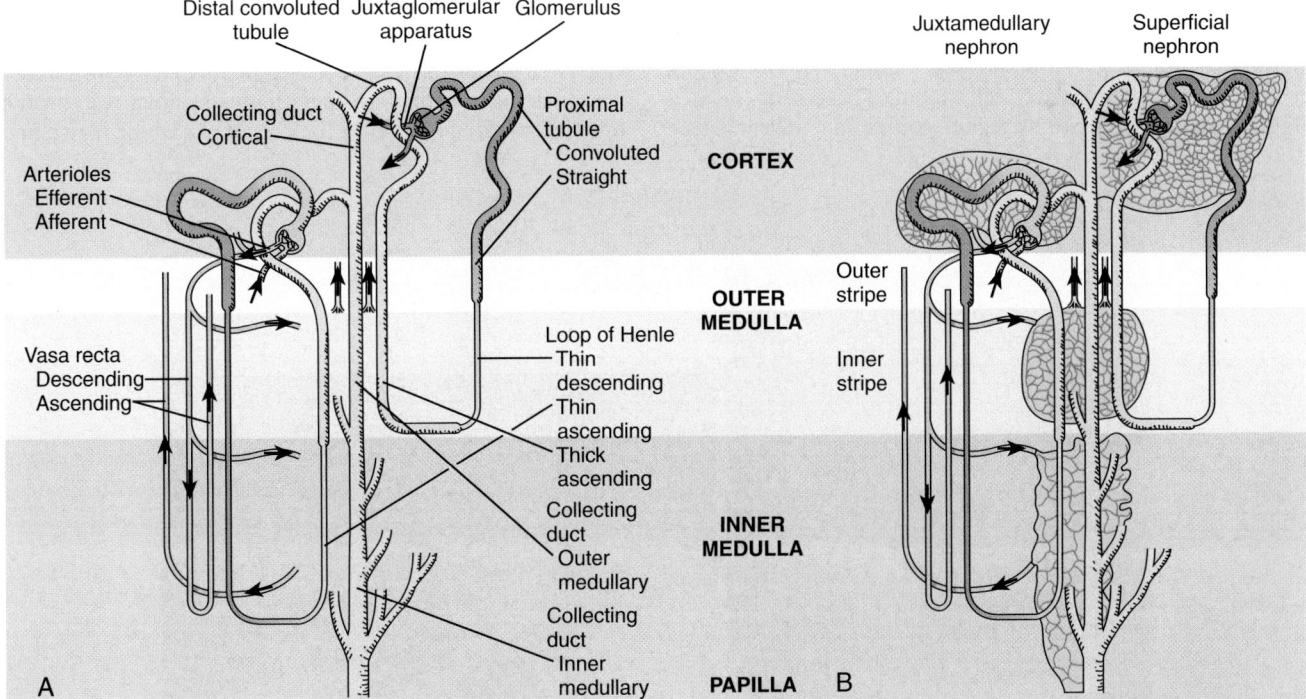

FIGURE 3-8 A, Superficial and juxtamedullary nephrons and their vasculature. The glomerulus plus the surrounding Bowman's capsule constitute the renal corpuscle. The beginning of the proximal tubule (the urinary pole) lies opposite the vascular pole, where the afferent and efferent arterioles enter and leave the glomerulus. The early distal tubule is always opposed to the vascular pole belonging to the same nephron; the juxtaglomerular apparatus is located at the point of contact. **B,** Capillary networks have been superimposed on the nephrons illustrated in **A.** Both diagrams are highly schematic (for a more accurate portrayal, see Beeuwkes and Bonventre[22]), and they do not accurately reflect some relationships that probably have functional meanings. In the rat, for example, long, thin descending limbs of Henle are located next to collecting ducts, and short, thin descending limbs are closely associated with the vascular bundles made up of descending and ascending vasa recta in the outer medulla. (Drawings based on Kriz and Bankir,[525] from Valtin H, Schafer JA: *Renal function,* ed 3, Philadelphia,1995, Lippincott Williams & Wilkins.)

out of the glomerular capillaries and into Bowman's space, the oncotic pressure of blood flowing into the peritubular capillaries increases as a result of "trapped" plasma proteins. Accordingly, the sum of these forces favors fluid movement into the peritubular capillaries. In fact, alterations in the net driving force for reabsorption (i.e., the balance between the transcapillary oncotic and hydraulic pressure gradients) have significant effects on net proximal reabsorption.[28] The absolute amount of movement resulting from this driving force also depends on the peritubular capillary surface area available for fluid uptake and the hydraulic conductivity of the capillary wall. Values for the hydraulic conductivity of the peritubular capillaries are not as high as those for the glomerular capillaries, but this difference is offset by the much larger total surface area of the peritubular capillary network.

In the rat, it has been estimated that approximately 50% of the peritubular capillary surface is composed of fenestrated areas.[29] Unlike the glomerular capillaries, peritubular capillary fenestrations are bridged by a thin diaphragm[29] that is negatively charged.[30] Beneath the fenestrae of the endothelial cells lies a basement membrane that completely surrounds the capillary. For the most part, peritubular capillaries are closely opposed to cortical tubules (Figure 3-9) so that the extracellular space between the tubules and capillaries constitutes only about 5% of the cortical volume.[31] The tubular epithelial cells are surrounded by the tubular basement membrane, which is distinct from and wider than the capillary basement membrane (see Figure 3-9). Numerous microfibrils connect the tubular and capillary basement membranes, which may help limit expansion of the interstitium and maintain close contact between tubular epithelial cells and the peritubular capillaries during periods of high fluid flux.[32] Thus, the pathway for fluid reabsorption from the tubular lumen to the peritubular capillary is composed, in series, of the epithelial cell, tubular basement membrane, a narrow interstitial region containing microfibrils,

the capillary basement membrane, and the thin membrane bridging the endothelial fenestrae.[32]

Like the endothelial cells, the basement membrane of the peritubular capillaries possesses anionic sites.[30] The electronegative charge density of the peritubular capillary basement membrane is significantly greater than that observed in the unfenestrated capillaries of skeletal muscle and similar to that observed in the glomerular capillary bed. The function of the anionic sites in the peritubular capillaries is uncertain; however, by analogy to the glomerulus, it is likely that they are an adaptation to compensate for the greater permeability of fenestrated capillaries, allowing free exchange of water and small molecules while restricting anionic plasma proteins to the circulation. In fact, some researchers have reported that the renal peritubular capillaries are more permeable to both small and large molecules than are other beds.[33] This conclusion is based on results of tracer studies in which the renal artery was clamped or the kidney removed before fixation. However, because normal plasma flow conditions appear necessary for the maintenance of the glomerular permeability barrier,[34] it is possible that these high stop-flow peritubular permeabilities occur as an artifact of the unfavorable experimental conditions employed. In fact, findings of studies by Deen and associates[35] indicate that, at least under free-flow conditions, the permeability of these vessels to dextrans and albumin is extremely low.

Inasmuch as the peritubular capillaries that surround a given nephron are derived from many efferent vessels, regulatory processes related to capillary factors need not be viewed as a mechanism only for balancing filtration and reabsorption in a single nephron. Instead, if capillary dynamics throughout the cortex are the same as has thus far been defined for the microcirculation of the superficial cortex, then within broad regions of the cortex, all tubule segments may be surrounded by capillary vessels that are operating in a similar reabsorptive mode. Thus, the function of the cortex as a whole may reflect

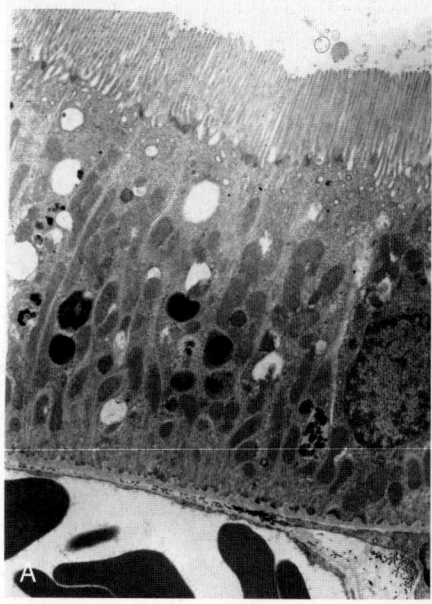
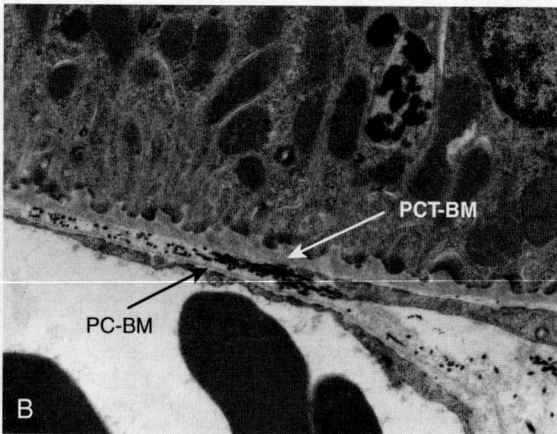

FIGURE 3-9 Electron micrograph (by D. A. Maddox) of a proximal tubule of a Munich Wistar rat. Tubule was perfusion fixed with 1.25% glutaraldehyde, which thereby also fixed red blood cells in adjacent capillaries. **A,** The apposition of the basolateral surface of the tubule cells with the adjacent peritubular capillaries is close, leaving little interstitial space where the two come in contact (magnification ≈×13,000). **B,** The proximal tubule basement membrane (PCT-BM) is thick in comparison with the peritubular capillary endothelial basement membrane (PC-BM) (magnification ≈×25,000).

the average reabsorptive capacity of all cortical peritubular vessels.

Medullary Microcirculation

Vascular Patterns

The precise location of the boundary between the renal cortex and medulla is difficult to discern because the medullary rays of the cortex merge imperceptibly with the medulla. In general, the arcuate arteries or the sites at which the interlobar arteries branch into arcuate arteries mark this boundary. When considering the medullary circulation, most investigators focus on its relation to the countercurrent mechanism as facilitated by the parallel array of descending and ascending vasa recta. However, although this configuration is characteristic of the inner medulla, the medulla also contains an outer zone, which consists of two morphologically distinct regions: the outer and inner stripes of the outer medulla (see Figure 3-8). The boundary between the outer and inner medullae is defined by the beginning of the thick ascending limbs of Henle (see Figure 3-8). In addition to the thick ascending limbs, the outer medulla contains descending straight segments of proximal tubules (pars recta), descending thin limbs, and collecting ducts. The nephron segments of the inner stripe of the outer medulla include thick ascending limbs, thin descending limbs, and collecting ducts. Each of these morphologically distinct medullary regions is supplied and drained by an independent, specific vascular system.

The blood supply of the medulla is entirely derived from the efferent arterioles of the juxtamedullary glomeruli (see Figure 3-8).[20,22,36,37] Depending on the species and the method of evaluation, it has been estimated that from 7% to 18% of glomeruli give rise to efferent vessels that ultimately supply the medulla.[20,38] Efferent arterioles of juxtamedullary nephrons are larger in diameter and possess a thicker endothelium and more prominent smooth muscle layer than do arterioles originating from superficial glomeruli.[15,39]

Although the vasculature of the outer medulla displays both vertical and lateral heterogeneity, both the outer and inner stripes generally contain two distinct circulatory regions. These are the vascular bundles, formed by the coalescence of the descending and ascending vasa recta, and the interbundle capillary plexus. Vascular bundles of descending and ascending vasa recta arise from the efferent arterioles of juxtamedullary glomeruli and descend through the outer stripe of the outer medulla to supply the inner stripe of the outer medulla and the inner medulla (Figure 3-10). Within the outer stripe, the descending vasa recta also give rise, via small side branches, to a complex capillary plexus. Results of early studies suggested that this capillary network was limited and, therefore, not the main blood supply to this region. Instead, it was thought that nutrient flow was provided by the ascending vasa recta rising from the inner stripe. This was further suggested by the large area of contact between ascending vasa recta and the descending proximal straight tubules within this zone (Figure 3-11).[29,38,40]

The outer medulla includes the metabolically active thick ascending limbs. Nutrients and O₂ to this energy-demanding tissue to the inner stripe are delivered by a dense capillary plexus arising from a few descending vasa recta at the periphery of the bundles. Approximately 10% to 15% of total RBF is directed to the medulla, and of this amount, probably the largest portion perfuses this inner stripe capillary plexus. The smooth muscle cells of the descending vasa recta are replaced by pericytes surrounding the endothelium with subsequent loss of the pericytes and transformation into medullary capillaries accompanied by endothelial fenestrations (Figure 3-12).[41,42]

The rich capillary network of the inner stripe drains into numerous veins that, for the most part, do not join the vascular bundles but ascend directly to the outer stripe. These veins subsequently rise to the cortical-medullary junction, and the majority join with cortical veins at the level of the inner cortex.[41] A minority of the veins may extend within the medullary rays to regions near the kidney surface.[7,36,41] Thus, the capillary network of the inner stripe makes no contact with the vessels draining the inner medulla.

The inner medulla contains thin descending and thin ascending limbs of Henle, together with collecting ducts

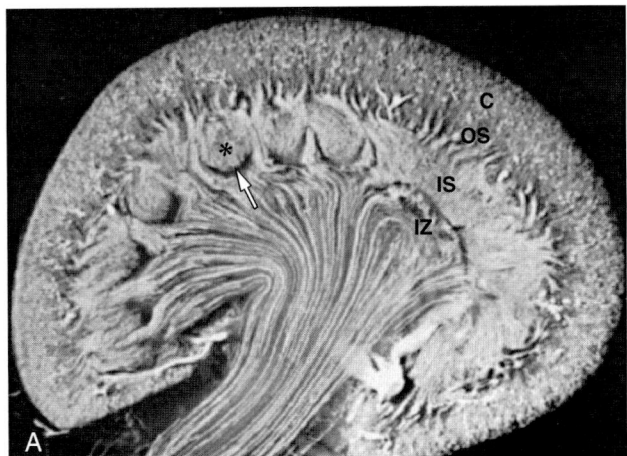

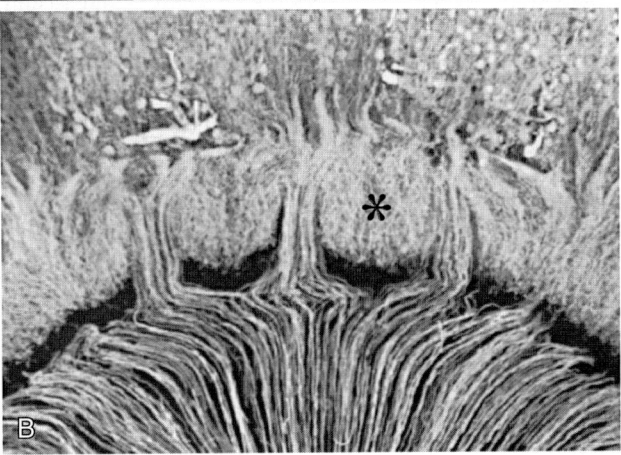

FIGURE 3-10 Longitudinal section of kidney of the sand rat (*Psammomys obesus*) after arterial injection of Microfil silicone rubber and clearing. **A,** The low-power magnification reveals distinct zonation of the kidney (*C*, cortex; *OS* and *IS*, outer and inner stripes of the outer medulla, respectively; *IZ*, inner medulla). The inner medulla is long and extends a short distance below the bottom of the picture. Giant vascular bundles, including a mixture of descending and ascending vasa recta, traverse the outer medulla to supply blood to the inner medulla. **B,** The outer medulla at a higher magnification. Between the vascular bundles (three are visible), a rich capillary plexus (*asterisk*) supplies the tubule segments present in this zone. (From Bankir L, Kaissling B, de Rouffignac C, et al: The vascular organization of the kidney of *Psammomys obesus, Anat Embryol* 1979;155:149.)

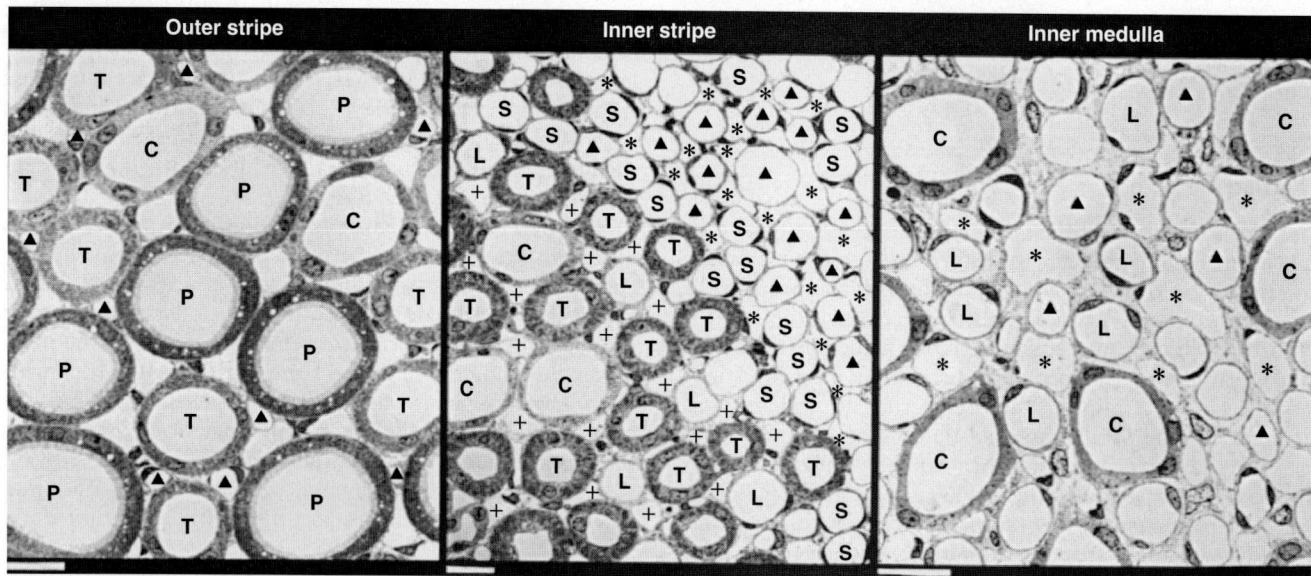

FIGURE 3-11 Electron micrograph showing cross-sections of both outer stripe and inner stripe of outer medulla and a cross-section of inner medulla. C, collecting duct; P, pars recta; S and L, thin descending limbs of short and long loops, respectively; T, thick ascending limb. *Triangles* indicate arterial descending vasa recta; *asterisks* indicate venous ascending vasa recta. In the outer stripe, note the large area of contact between ascending vasa recta and pars recta and the paucity of interstitial space. In the inner stripe, part of a vascular bundle is shown in the upper right half of the photograph, and the interbundle region is shown in the lower half. Note that the thin descending limbs of short loops are surrounded by venous vasa recta ascending from the inner medulla. The wall of these vessels adapts to available space between the descending vasa recta and the thin limbs, offering a large area of contact with these descending structures. Thin limbs of long loops lie in the interbundle region and are surrounded by vessels belonging to the interbundle capillary plexus. In the inner medulla, abundant interstitium surrounds all tubule and vascular structures. Walls of tubules and vessels are not in direct contact. (Outer stripe is from rabbit kidney; inner stripe and inner medulla are from rat kidney.) Bar represents approximately 30 μm. (Adapted from Bankir L, de Rouffignac C: Urinary concentration ability: insights derived from comparative anatomy, *Am J Physiol* 1985;249:R643.)

(see Figure 3-8). Within this region, the straight, unbranching vasa recta descend in bundles, with individual vessels leaving at every level to divide into a simple capillary network characterized by elongated links (see Figure 3-12 and also Figure 3-8).[38,41,42] These capillaries converge to form the venous vasa recta. Within the inner medulla, the descending and ascending vascular pathways remain in close apposition, although distinct vascular regions can no longer be clearly discerned. The venous vasa recta rise toward the outer medulla in parallel with the supply vessels to join the vascular bundles. Thus, the outer medullary vascular bundles include both supplying and draining vessels of the inner medulla. Within the outer stripe of the outer medulla, the vascular bundles spread out and traverse the outer stripe as wide, tortuous channels that lie in close opposition to the tubules, eventually emptying into arcuate or deep interlobular veins.[38] The venous pathways within the bundles are both larger and more numerous than the arterial vessels, which suggests that flow velocities are lower in the ascending (venous) direction than in the descending (arterial) direction.[43] The close apposition of the arterial and venous pathways within the vascular bundles is important for maintaining the hypertonicity of the inner medulla.

Morphologists have recognized important differences in the structure of the ascending and descending vasa recta. The descending vasa recta possess a contractile layer composed of smooth muscle cells in the early segments that evolve into pericytes by the more distal portions of the vessels. Immunohistochemical studies demonstrate that these pericytes contain smooth muscle α-actin, which suggests that they may serve as contractile elements and participate in the regulation of medullary blood flow.[44] These vessels also have a continuous endothelium that persists until the hairpin turn is reached

and the vessels divide to form the medullary capillaries. In contrast, ascending vasa recta, like true capillaries, lack a contractile layer and are characterized by a highly fenestrated endothelium.[45,46]

Vascular-Tubule Relations

The mechanism of urine concentration requires coordinated function of the vascular and tubule components of the medulla. In species capable of marked concentrating ability, medullary vascular-tubule relations show a high degree of organization favoring particular exchange processes by the juxtaposition of specific tubule segments and blood vessels.[41] In addition to anatomic proximity, the absolute magnitude of these exchanges is greatly influenced by the permeability characteristics of the structures involved, which may vary significantly among species.[47] The anatomic relations and permeability characteristics of the various medullary structures play an important role in urine concentration.

Most of the detailed knowledge of vascular-tubule relations within the medulla is based on histologic studies of rodent species.[37,40,41,44,48,49] As already discussed, the inner stripe of the outer medulla contains two distinct territories: the vascular bundles and the interbundle regions (see Figures 3-10 and 3-12). In most mammals, the vascular bundles contain only closely juxtaposed descending and ascending vasa recta running in parallel. The tubule structures of the inner stripe, including thin descending limbs, thick ascending limbs, and collecting ducts, are found in the interbundle regions and are supplied by the dense capillary bed described earlier.[41] The interbundle territory is commonly organized with the long loops of the juxtamedullary nephrons lying closest to the

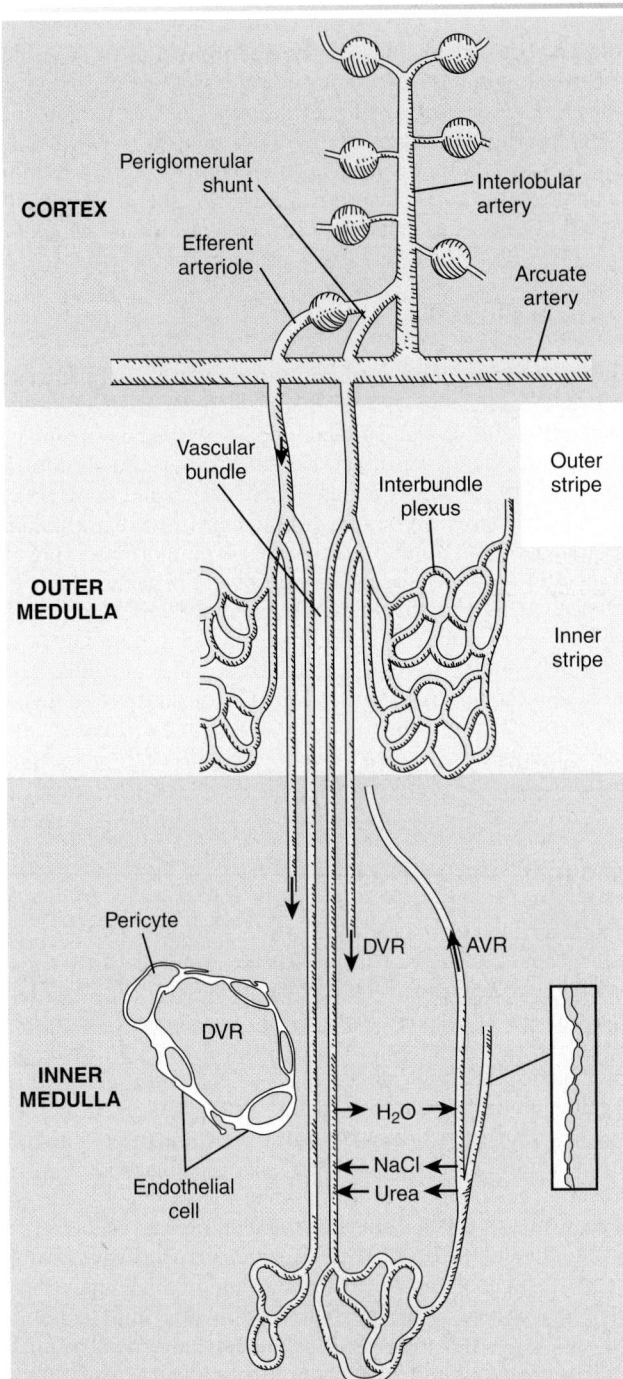

FIGURE 3-12 Anatomy of the medullary microcirculation. In the cortex, interlobular arteries arise from the arcuate artery and ascend toward the cortical surface. Cortical and juxtamedullary glomeruli branch from the interlobular artery. The majority of blood flow reaches the medulla through juxtamedullary efferent arterioles; however, there is evidence that some flow may also be from periglomerular shunt pathways. In the outer medulla, juxtamedullary efferent arterioles in the outer stripe give rise to descending vasa recta (DVR) that coalesce to form vascular bundles in the inner stripe. DVR on the periphery of vascular bundles give rise to the interbundle capillary plexus that surrounds nephron segments (thick ascending limb, collecting duct, long looped thin descending limbs; not shown). DVR in the center continue across the inner-outer medullary junction to perfuse the inner medulla. Thin descending limbs of short looped nephrons may also associate with the vascular bundles in a manner that is species dependent (not shown). Vascular bundles disappear in the inner medulla, and vasa recta become dispersed with nephron segments. Ascending vasa recta (AVR) that arise from the sparse capillary plexus of inner medulla return to the cortex by passing through outer medullary vascular bundles. DVR have a continuous endothelium (**inset**). (From Pallone TL, Zhang Z, Rhinehart K: Physiology of the renal medullary microcirculation, *Am J Physiol* 2003;284: F253-F266.)

vascular bundles. The shorter loops arising from superficial glomeruli are more peripheral and, therefore, closer to the collecting ducts. The vascular bundles themselves contain no tubule structures.

Medullary Capillary Dynamics

The functional role of the medullary peritubular vasculature is basically the same as that of cortical peritubular vessels. These capillaries supply the metabolic needs of nearby tissues and are responsible for the uptake and removal of water extracted from collecting ducts during the process of urine concentration. However, because the urinary concentration process is based on the maintenance of a hypertonic interstitium, the countercurrent arrangement of medullary blood flow plays a vital role in maintaining the medullary solute gradient through passive countercurrent exchange.

Total Renal Blood Flow

Total RBF in humans typically exceeds 20% of the cardiac output, or about 1 to 1.2 L/min for a man. The classic method of calculating total renal blood flow is first to determine renal plasma flow rate (RPF) by measuring from the time of disappearance of an indicator substance from blood passing through the kidney to its subsequent appearance in the urine. If the substance is neither metabolized nor synthesized in the kidney, then its rate of appearance in the urine equals its rate of extraction from the blood. The blood extraction rate is equal to the RPF multiplied by the difference between the arterial and renal venous plasma concentrations. This can be expressed mathematically as

$$U_x V = (Art_x - Vein_x) \times (RPF), \qquad (1)$$

where U_x = urine concentration of the indicator; V = urine flow rate; and Art_x and $Vein_x$ = arterial and renal venous concentrations of the indicator, respectively. This equation can be rearranged as

$$RPF = U_x V / (Art_x - Vein_x). \qquad (2)$$

RBF can then be calculated by dividing RPF by the plasma fraction of whole blood (from the hematocrit):

$$RBF = RPF / (1 - Hematocrit) \qquad (3)$$

Historically, investigators have estimated RBF from determinations of RPF by using *p*-aminohippuric acid (PAH) as the indicator. This substance is both filtered at the glomerulus and actively secreted by the tubules, which result in the renal extraction of 70% to 90% of PAH from the blood. Not all the PAH is removed from the kidney circulation because some flow is through regions of the kidney (e.g., medulla) that do not perfuse proximal tubule segments where secretion occurs, because of incomplete removal of PAH in (some) cortical regions, and because of the presence of periglomerular shunts (see Figure 3-12). If the extraction is assumed to be equal to 100% (renal venous concentration = 0), then the clearance of PAH (($U_{PAH} \times V$)/Art_{PAH}) provides a simple, noninvasive approximation of RPF. This is often termed "effective" renal plasma flow (ERPF) and provides an estimate of RPF without the need to obtain a renal venous blood sample. However, this estimate of RPF is much less accurate in the presence of renal disease because extraction is further reduced by damage

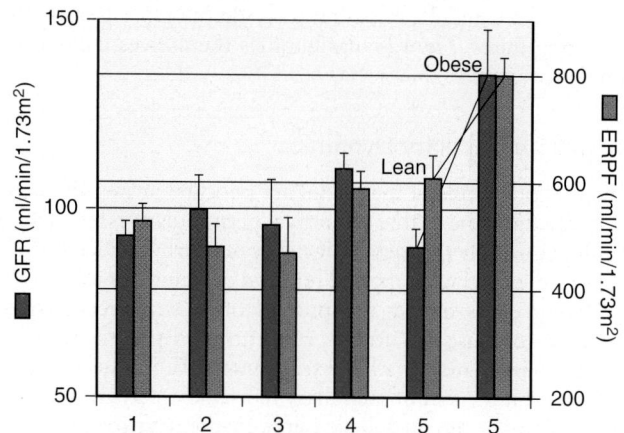

FIGURE 3-13 Typical values for glomerular filtration rate (GFR) and effective renal plasma flow (ERPF) in adult humans. Values from men and women were pooled. The numbers under each set of bars refer to data obtained from Giordano and DeFronzo[438] (1); Winetz et al[526] (2); Hostetter[527] (3); Deen et al[528] (4); and Chagnac et al[472] (5). For studies 1, 2, 3, and 5, values were obtained after approximately 12 hours of fasting; subjects in study 4 were allowed food ad libitum. For study 5, values from lean subjects (average body mass index = 22) were compared with those from obese nondiabetic individuals (body mass index > 38) after a 10-hour fast, and those values were not corrected for body surface area.

to proximal tubule segments involved in PAH secretion.[50] Figure 3-13 shows some typical values for ERPF and GFR in adult humans from a number of studies.

Micropuncture studies performed in vivo in experimental animals have provided more accurate and detailed information about cortical blood flow, but the medulla is less accessible to micropuncture, and thus the medullary blood flow has been less studied. For detailed discussion of historical methods of RBF measurements, the reader is referred to Dworkin and Brenner.[50] More recently, improved methods of RBF measurement have been introduced with laser Doppler flowmetry, video microscopy, and imaging techniques such as positron emission tomography (PET), high-speed computed tomography (CT), and magnetic resonance imaging (MRI).[50-54] These methods have been especially useful in determining regional blood flow as discussed next.

Intrarenal Blood Flow Distribution

The cortex accounts for filtration and the majority of reabsorption, whereas the medulla's primary function is maintenance of a hypertonic gradient and urine concentration. Therefore, RBF to these regions is differentially regulated in response to the differing demands of these two kidney regions.[15] Structural differences between the vascular components of the cortex and those of the medulla may account for differences in RBF: namely, the organization of the afferent and efferent arterioles of the cortical and juxtamedullary glomeruli. Studies conducted in rabbits demonstrated that cortical afferent arterioles have larger internal diameters than do the efferent arterioles, whereas juxtamedullary afferent and efferent arterioles are significantly larger and the efferent arterioles are more muscular than are the cortical arterioles.[15,55] In addition, the

cortical peritubular capillaries, derived from efferent arterioles of cortical glomeruli, are about half the size of the medullary vasa recta derived from efferent arterioles of the juxtamedullary glomeruli (see Figure 3-6).[15] These features may partially explain the differential control of medullary versus cortical blood flow. Additional factors include sympathetic nerve activity and hormonal influences, described later in this chapter.

Cortical Blood Flow

The majority of RBF perfuses the cortex. Vasoconstrictors such as angiotensin II, endothelin, and noradrenaline have much greater effects on cortical blood flow than on medullary blood flow, whereas vasodilators such as bradykinin and nitric oxide tend to selectively increase medullary blood flow.[15] As a result, blood flow can be redistributed extensively in the kidney under various conditions that may be important in physiologic and pathophysiologic conditions.[56] In fact, studies by Trueta[57] of RBF distribution after hemorrhage were among the first performed. His findings indicated that in shock states, RBF appeared to be shunted through the medulla. This phenomenon, observed in the 1950s in qualitative studies of the distribution of India ink and radiographic contrast media, was subsequently termed *cortical ischemia with maintained blood flow through the medulla*.[58]

Medullary Blood Flow

Medullary blood flow constitutes about 10% to 15% of total RBF[50,59] and is derived from efferent arterioles of the juxtamedullary nephrons.[42,55] Although these medullary flow rates are less than one fourth as high as cortical flow rates, medullary flow is still substantial. Thus, per gram of tissue, outer medullary flow exceeds that of liver, and inner medullary flow is comparable with that of resting muscle or brain.[60] The fact that such large flow rates are compatible with the existence and maintenance of the inner medullary solute concentration gradient attests to the efficiency of countercurrent mechanisms in this region. The descending vasa recta have a continuous endothelium with water movement across water channels and urea movement through endothelial carriers.[61,62] The ascending vasa recta are fenestrated with a high hydraulic conductivity; water movement is probably governed by transcapillary hydraulic and oncotic pressure gradients.[62] Medullary blood flow is highest under conditions of water diuresis and declines during antidiuresis.[59] This decrease depends, at least in part, on a direct vasoconstrictive action of vasopressin on the medullary microcirculation.[63] Vasodilatory factors act to preserve medullary blood flow and prevent ischemia. Acetylcholine,[64] vasodilator prostaglandins,[65] kinins,[66] adenosine,[67] atrial peptides,[68] bradykinin,[52] and nitric oxide[69] increase medullary RBF. In contrast to their vasoconstrictor effects in the renal cortex, angiotensin II[70-72] and endothelin[70] increase medullary blood flow, effects mediated in part by vasodilatory prostaglandins,[71,72] whereas vasopressin decreases medullary blood flow.[63,73] Alterations in medullary blood flow may be a key determinant of medullary tonicity and, therefore, of solute transport in the loops of Henle. In addition, the medullary circulation may play an important role in the control of sodium excretion and blood pressure.[74]

Determinants of Glomerular Ultrafiltration

Urine formation begins with filtration of a nearly protein-free fluid from the glomerular capillaries into Bowman's space. The barrier to filtration includes the fenestrated endothelial surface of the glomerular capillaries, the three layers of the glomerular basement membrane, the filtration slits between adjacent pedicels or foot processes of the visceral epithelial cells (podocytes) that surround the capillaries, and the filtration slit diaphragm that extends along the filtration slits and connects adjacent foot processes to form the ultimate barrier to filtration (see Chapter 2 and Figure 3-7). Water, electrolytes, amino acids, glucose, and other endogenous or exogenous compounds with molecular radii smaller than 20 Å are freely filtered from the blood into Bowman's space while molecules larger than approximately 50 Å are virtually excluded from filtration.[75-80] At any given point of a glomerular capillary wall, the process of ultrafiltration of fluid (J_v) is governed by the net balance between the transcapillary hydraulic pressure gradient (ΔP), the transcapillary colloid osmotic pressure gradient ($\Delta \pi$), and the hydraulic permeability of the filtration barrier (k) based on the expression

$$J_v = k(\Delta P - \Delta \pi)$$
$$= k[(P_{GC} - P_{BS}) - (\pi_{GC} - \pi_{BS})], \quad (4)$$

where P_{GC} and P_{BS} are the hydraulic pressures in the glomerular capillaries and Bowman's space, respectively, and π_{GC} and π_{BS} are the corresponding colloid osmotic pressures. Because the protein concentration of the fluid in Bowman's space is essentially zero, π_{BS} is also zero. Total GFR of fluid for a single nephron (SNGFR) is equal to the product of the surface area for filtration (S), the hydraulic permeability of the filtration barrier (k), and average values along the length of the glomerular capillaries of the right-sided terms in equation 4, which yields the expression

$$SNGFR = kS(\overline{\Delta P} - \overline{\Delta \pi})$$
$$= K_f \overline{P}_{UF}, \quad (5)$$

where K_f, the glomerular capillary ultrafiltration coefficient, is the product of S and k, and $\overline{P}_{UF}$, the mean net ultrafiltration pressure, is the difference between the mean transcapillary and colloid osmotic pressure differences, $\overline{\Delta P}$ and $\overline{\Delta \pi}$, respectively.

On the basis of known ultrastructural detail and the hydrodynamic properties of the individual components of the filtration barrier, mathematical modeling suggests that only approximately 2% of the total hydraulic resistance is accounted for by the fenestrated capillary endothelium, whereas the basement membrane accounts for nearly 50%.[81-83] The remaining hydraulic resistance resides in the filtration slit diaphragm of the filtration slits.[82,83] A reduction in the frequency of intact filtration slits is an important factor in the deterioration of filtration in some disease states.[82,84]

Hydraulic Pressures in the Glomerular Capillaries and Bowman's Space

Direct measurements of glomerular capillary hydraulic pressure (P_{GC}) were first obtained in the Munich Wistar rat in 1971 by Brenner and colleagues,[75] who found that $\overline{P}_{GC}$ (representing the average value for the mean pulsatile glomerular capillary hydraulic pressure as measured along the whole glomerulus) averaged 46 mm Hg. Subsequent studies confirmed the original observations, demonstrating that $\overline{P}_{GC}$ values averaged 43

to 49 mm Hg (Figure 3-14) with similar values found in the squirrel monkey.[85] $\overline{P}_{GC}$ is nearly constant along the length of the capillary bed, which results in a transcapillary hydraulic pressure difference that averages 34 mm Hg in the hydropenic Munich-Wistar rat (see Figure 3-14). These hydraulic pressure measurements are coupled with determinations of systemic plasma protein concentration and efferent arteriolar protein concentrations of superficial nephrons in order to determine the hydraulic and oncotic pressures that govern glomerular ultrafiltration at the beginning and end of the capillary network.

The early direct measurements of $\overline{P}_{GC}$ were obtained in the hydropenic rats, which exhibited a surgically induced reduction in plasma volume and GFR.[86] In subsequent studies in which plasma volume was restored to the "euvolemic" state, equal to that of the awake animal,[86] by infusion of isooncotic plasma, SNGFR was substantially higher in euvolemic animals than in hydropenic rats, primarily as a consequence of a marked increase in glomerular plasma flow (Q_A) associated with a fall in preglomerular arteriolar resistance (R_A) and efferent arteriolar resistance (R_E) values (see Figure 3-14). The use of the Munich-Wistar rat with surface glomeruli allows direct determinations of hydraulic pressure drops, preglomerular blood flow, and postglomerular blood flow and hence of R_A and R_E. Because surface glomeruli are not available in most experimental animals, the stop-flow technique has been used by a number of investigators to estimate $\overline{P}_{GC}$. With this technique, fluid movement in the early proximal tubule is blocked, which results in an increase in intratubular pressure until filtration at the glomerulus is stopped. At that point, the sum of this hydrostatic pressure in the early proximal tubule and the systemic colloid oncotic pressure is equal to the pressure in the glomerular capillaries (P_{GCSF}). P_{GCSF} calculated with this stop-flow technique enables a reasonable estimate of $\overline{P}_{GC}$: P_{GCSF} is, in general, approximately 2 mm Hg greater than $\overline{P}_{GC}$ measured directly.[87]

Glomerular Capillary Hydraulic and Colloid Osmotic Pressure Profiles

Glomerular capillary hydraulic and oncotic pressure profiles for hydropenic and euvolemic Munich-Wistar rats are shown in Figure 3-15; the profiles are based on the mean values determined from the studies shown in Figure 3-14. By the time the blood reaches the efferent end of the glomerular capillaries, plasma oncotic pressure (π_E) rises to a value that, on average, equals $\overline{\Delta P}$. As a consequence, the net local ultrafiltration pressure, $P_{UF}[P_{GC} - (P_T + \pi_{GC})]$, where P_T represent the proximal tubule hydraulic pressure, is reduced from approximately 17 mm Hg at the afferent end of the glomerular capillary network to essentially 0 by the efferent end in hydropenic animals. The equality between π_E and $\overline{\Delta P}$ is referred to as *filtration pressure equilibrium.* As seen in Figure 3-15, filtration pressure equilibrium ($\pi_E / \overline{\Delta P} \cong 1.00$) is almost always observed in the hydropenic Munich-Wistar rat but is present in only approximately 40% of the studies in the euvolemic rat, which suggests that the normal condition in the glomerulus is to be on the verge of disequilibrium.

The decline in P_{UF} between the afferent and efferent ends of the glomerular capillary network in the hydropenic animal is primarily a result of the rise in π_{GC}, inasmuch as ΔP remains nearly constant along the glomerular capillaries (see Figure 3-15). Curve A in Figure 3-15 shows that the decline in P_{UF} (the difference between ΔP and $\Delta \pi$ curves) is nonlinear. This occurs because

(1) filtration is more rapid at the afferent end of the capillary, where P_{UF} is greatest, and (2) the relationship between plasma protein concentration and colloid osmotic pressure is nonlinear (see Maddox et al[76] and Maddox and Brenner[87]). Under conditions of filtration pressure equilibrium, the exact profile of $\Delta\pi$ along the capillary network cannot be determined, and curves A and B in Figure 3-15 are only two of many possibilities.

Determination of the Ultrafiltration Coefficient

As was shown in equation 5, SNGFR equals the glomerular capillary ultrafiltration coefficient (K_f) multiplied by the net driving force for ultrafiltration averaged over the length of the glomerular capillaries ($\overline{P}_{UF}$). Under conditions of filtration pressure equilibrium, a unique value of $\overline{P}_{UF}$ cannot be

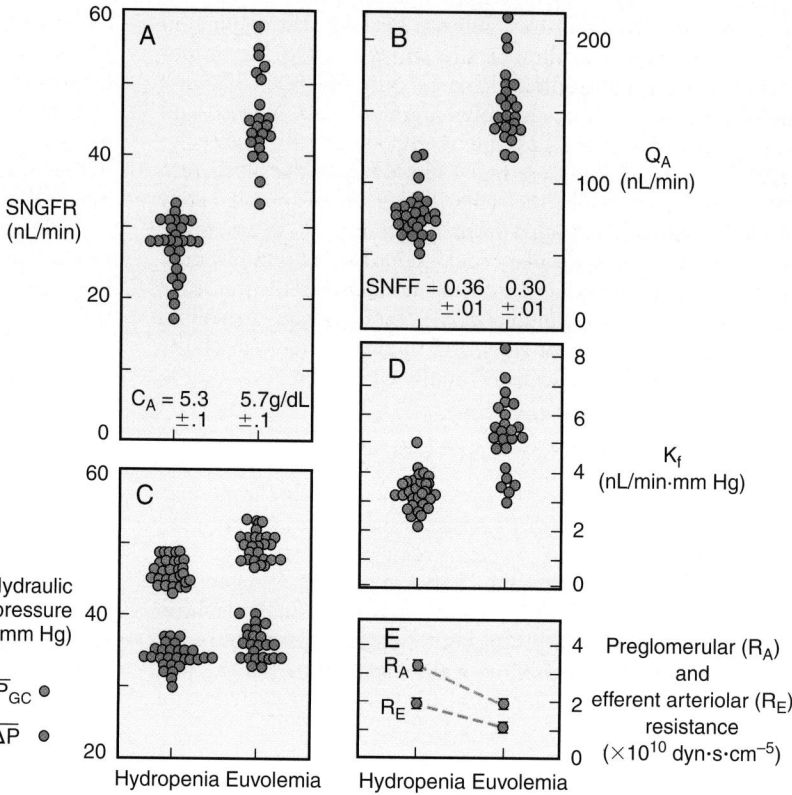

FIGURE 3-14 Glomerular ultrafiltration in the Munich-Wistar rat. Each point represents the mean value reported for studies in hydropenic and euvolemic rats, which were provided food and water ad libitum until the time of study. Results shown are from only studies in which male rats or a mix of male and female rats were used. Values of the ultrafiltration coefficient, K_f (*red circles* in **D**), denote minimum values, inasmuch as the animals were in filtration pressure equilibrium. *Blue circles* represent unique values of K_f calculated under conditions of filtration pressure disequilibrium ($\pi_E/\overline{\Delta P}$ ≤ 0.95). (Data from Maddox et al[76,479] and Maddox and Brenner.[87])

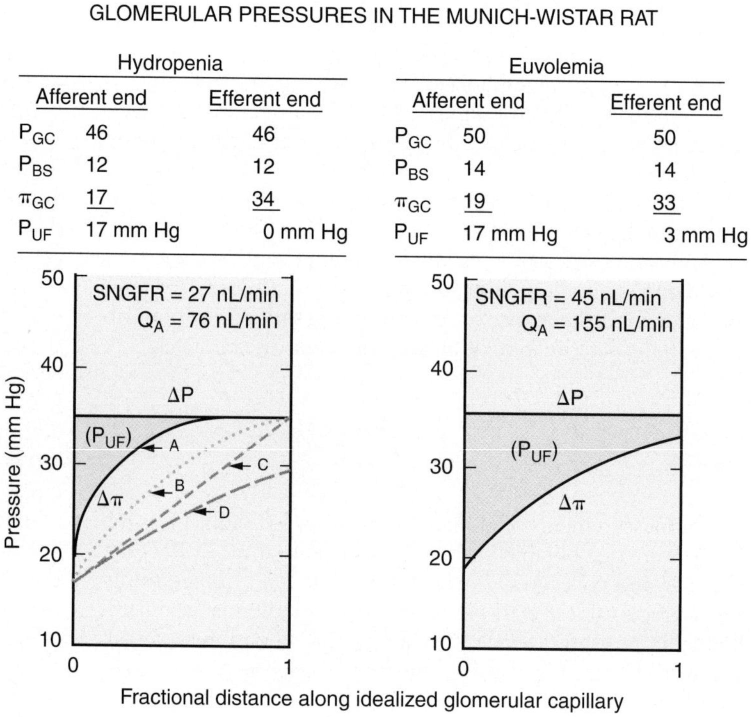

FIGURE 3-15 Hydraulic and colloid osmotic pressure profiles along idealized glomerular capillaries in hydropenic and euvolemic rats. Values shown are mean values derived from the studies shown in Figure 3-14. The transcapillary hydraulic pressure gradient, ΔP, is equal to $P_{GC} - P_T$, and the transcapillary colloid osmotic pressure gradient, $\Delta\pi$, is equal to $\pi_{GC} - \pi_T$, where P_{GC} and P_{BS} are the hydraulic pressures in the glomerular capillary and Bowman's space, respectively, and π_{GC} and π_T are the corresponding colloid osmotic pressures. Because the value of π_T is negligible, $\Delta\pi$ essentially equals π_{GC}. P_{UF} is the ultrafiltration pressure at any point. The area between the ΔP and $\Delta\pi$ curves represents the net ultrafiltration pressure, $\overline{P}_{UF}$. *Left*, Curves A and B represent two of the many possible profiles under conditions of filtration pressure equilibrium; line D represents disequilibrium. Line C represents the hypothetical linear $\Delta\pi$ profile.

GLOMERULAR PRESSURES IN THE MUNICH-WISTAR RAT

	Hydropenia		Euvolemia	
	Afferent end	Efferent end	Afferent end	Efferent end
P_{GC}	46	46	50	50
P_{BS}	12	12	14	14
π_{GC}	17	34	19	33
P_{UF}	17 mm Hg	0 mm Hg	17 mm Hg	3 mm Hg

Fractional distance along idealized glomerular capillary

determined because an exact $\Delta\pi$ profile cannot be defined. If, however, a linear rise in $\Delta\pi$ between the afferent and efferent ends of the glomerular capillaries is assumed, then a maximum value for $\overline{P}_{UF}$ can be determined (curve C, dashed line in Figure 3-15). With this maximum value for P_{UF} and measured values of SNGFR, a minimum estimate of K_f can be obtained. This minimum estimate of K_f in the hydropenic Munich-Wistar rat averages 3.5 ± 0.2 nL/(min • mm Hg) (see Figure 3-14D). In the euvolemic Munich-Wistar rat, K_f increases with age, and few differences are noted between sexes when body mass is taken into account (see Figure 3-16).

Changes in glomerular plasma flow rate (Q_A) (in the absence of changes in any other determinants of SNGFR) are predicted to result in proportional changes in SNGFR under conditions of filtration pressure equilibrium.[88] This occurs because an increase in Q_A slows the rate of increase of plasma protein concentration, and therefore $\Delta\pi$, along the glomerular capillary network, shifting the point at which filtration equilibrium is achieved toward the efferent end of the glomerular capillary network. As a result, the total capillary surface area exposed to a positive net ultrafiltration pressure is effectively increased, as is the magnitude of the local P_{UF} at any point along the glomerular capillary network. This is illustrated in Figure 3-15, which shows that even in the absence of changes in ΔP or plasma protein concentration, an increase in Q_A can result in a change in the profile from that seen with curve A to that of curve B while filtration pressure equilibrium is

still achieved. For curve B, however, P_{UF} (the area under the curve) is significantly greater than that for curve A, and hence SNGFR increases proportionately.

Filtration pressure disequilibrium is obtained if Q_A increases enough so that $\Delta\pi$ no longer rises to an extent that efferent arteriolar oncotic pressure (π_E) equals $\overline{\Delta P}$.[88] A unique profile of $\Delta\pi$ can then be derived, $\overline{P}_{UF}$ can be accurately determined, and a unique value of K_f can be calculated.[88] Deen and colleagues[88] expanded iso-oncotic plasma volume to increase Q_A sufficiently to produce filtration pressure disequilibrium; they thereby obtained the first unique determinations of K_f in the Munich-Wistar rat. Under these conditions, they observed that K_f exceeded the minimum estimate obtained in hydropenic rats by 37%, averaging 4.8 nL/(min • mm Hg). Because this value remained essentially unchanged over a twofold range of changes in Q_A, the data suggested that changes in Q_A per se did not affect K_f.[88]

The values of K_f for a large number of studies in euvolemic Munich-Wistar rats (shown in Figure 3-14) averaged 5.0 ± 0.3 nL/(min • mm Hg) and are similar to those obtained in plasma-expanded Munich Wistar rats in which only unique values of K_f were obtained (4.8 ± 0.3 nL/(min • mm Hg)).[76,88] Although measured values of $\overline{\Delta P}$ are slightly higher in euvolemic rats than in hydropenic animals (see Figure 3-14), this is offset by higher plasma protein concentrations in the afferent arterioles (C_A and hence the colloid osmotic pressure, π_A), so that P_{UF} at the afferent end of the glomerular capillary network is nearly

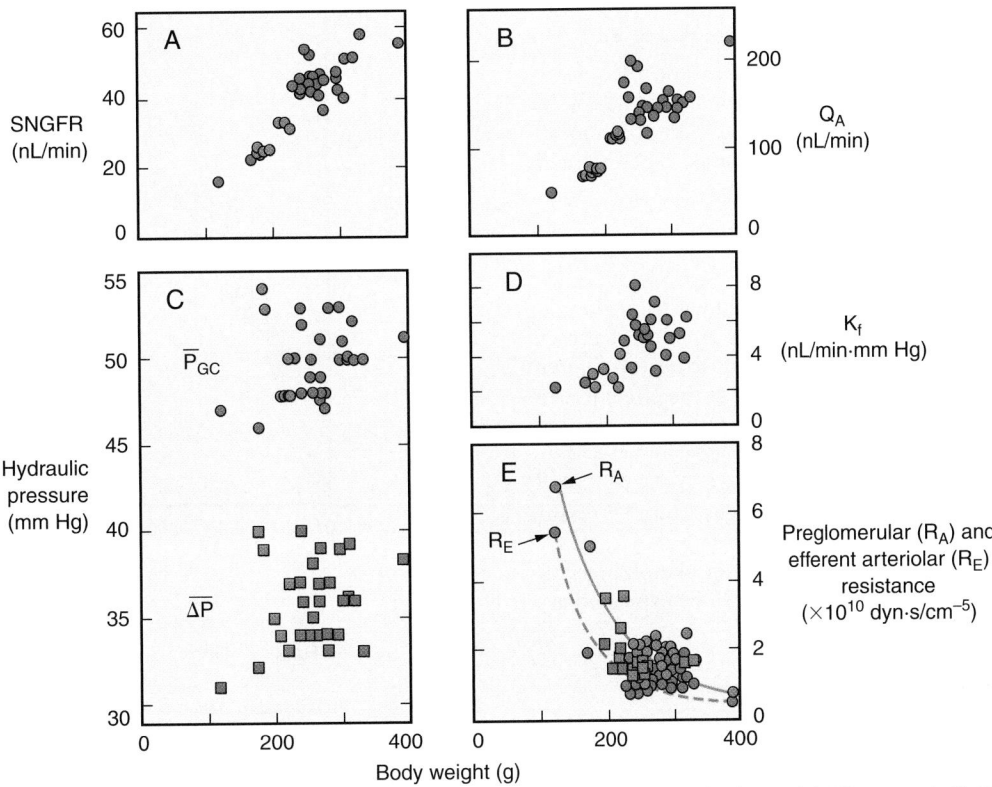

FIGURE 3-16 Maturational alterations in the determinants of glomerular ultrafiltration in the euvolemic Munich-Wister rat. **A, B, C,** and **D,** *Red symbols* denote values obtained from female rats; *blue symbols* denote values from studies of male rats or both male and female rats. **E,** *Red symbols* denote values of preglomerular arteriolar resistance (R_A); *blue symbols* denote values of efferent arteriolar resistance (R_E); *circles* represent values from studies of male rats or both male and female rats; and *squares* represent values from studies of female animals. Each point represents the mean value for a given study. (Data from Maddox et al[76,479] and Maddox and Brenner.[87])

identical in states of euvolemia and hydropenia (see Figure 3-15). Thus the higher SNGFR observed in euvolemic rats is a result primarily of increases in Q_A (see Figure 3-14), which yield a higher value of $\overline{P}_{UF}$ (see Figure 3-15).

K_f is the product of the total surface area available for filtration (S) and the hydraulic conductivity of the filtration barrier (k). In the rat, total capillary basement membrane surface area per glomerulus (A_s) is approximately 0.003 cm² in superficial nephrons and 0.004 cm² in the deep nephrons.[89] Only the peripheral area of the capillaries surrounded by podocytes participates in filtration, inasmuch as a large portion faces the mesangium. This peripheral area available for filtration (A_p) is only about half that of A_s (≈0.0016 to 0.0018 cm² and 0.0019 to 0.0022 cm² in the superficial and deep glomeruli, respectively).[89] Using a value of K_f of approximately 5 nL/min • mm Hg, as determined by micropuncture techniques with these estimates of A_p, yields a hydraulic conductivity (k) of 45 to 48 nL/(s • mm Hg • cm²). These estimates of k for the rat glomerulus are all one to two orders in magnitude higher than those reported for capillary networks in mesentery, skeletal muscle, and omentum and those for peritubular capillaries of the kidney.[76,87] As a consequence of this very high glomerular hydraulic permeability, filtration across glomerular capillaries occurs at very rapid rates despite mean net ultrafiltration pressures (P_{UF}) of only 5 to 6 mm Hg in hydropenia and 8 to 9 mm Hg in euvolemia.

Selective Alterations in the Primary Determinants of Glomerular Ultrafiltration

The four primary determinants of ultrafiltration are Q_A, $\overline{\Delta P}$, K_f, and π_A, and alterations in each of these affect GFR. The degree to which such alterations modify SNGFR has been examined in mathematical modeling,[88] and the modifications have been compared to values obtained experimentally (see Maddox and Brenner[87]).

Glomerular Plasma Flow Rate (Q_A)

Under normal conditions, protein is excluded from the glomerular ultrafiltrate; as a result, the total amount of protein entering the glomerular capillary network from the afferent arterioles equals the total amount leaving at the efferent arterioles, as dictated by the conservation of mass:

$$Q_A C_A = Q_E C_E, \tag{6}$$

where Q_A is, in this equation, the afferent arteriolar plasma flow rate; Q_E is the efferent arteriolar plasma flow rate; and C_A and C_E are the afferent and efferent arteriolar plasma concentrations of protein, respectively. This can be expressed as

$$Q_A C_A = (Q_A - \text{SNGFR}) C_E. \tag{7}$$

Equation 7 can be rearranged as

$$\text{SNGFR} = (1 - [C_A / C_E]) \times Q_A \tag{8}$$

with

$$\text{SNFF} = 1 - (C_A / C_E), \tag{9}$$

where SNFF is the single nephron filtration fraction. Although the relationship between colloid osmotic pressure

(π_A) and protein concentration deviates from linearity,[90] equation 8 can be approximated as

$$\text{SNGFR} \cong (1 - [\pi_A / \pi_E]) \times Q_A. \tag{10}$$

At filtration pressure equilibrium, $\pi_E = \overline{\Delta P}$, so that

$$\text{SNGFR} \cong (1 - (\pi_A / \pi_P)) \times Q_A. \tag{11}$$

Under conditions of filtration pressure equilibrium, filtration fraction, approximately $1 - (\pi_A / \overline{\Delta P})$, is constant if π_A and ΔP are unchanged. SNGFR then varies directly with changes in Q_A (equation 11). If Q_A increases enough to produce disequilibrium ($\pi_E < \overline{\Delta P}$), then C_E will fall, SNFF will decrease (equation 8), and SNGFR will no longer vary linearly with Q_A. Brenner and colleagues[91] first demonstrated the plasma flow dependence of GFR. As shown in Figure 3-17, increases in glomerular plasma flow are associated with increases in SNGFR, according to a number of studies of rats, dogs, nonhuman primates, and humans. Filtration pressure equilibrium was obtained in most studies at plasma flow rates less than 100 to 150 nL/min. As a consequence, increases in Q_A result in proportional increases in SNGFR, and SNFF remains constant. Further increases in Q_A are associated with proportionately lower increases in SNGFR, which result in decreased SNFF as filtration pressure disequilibrium is achieved.

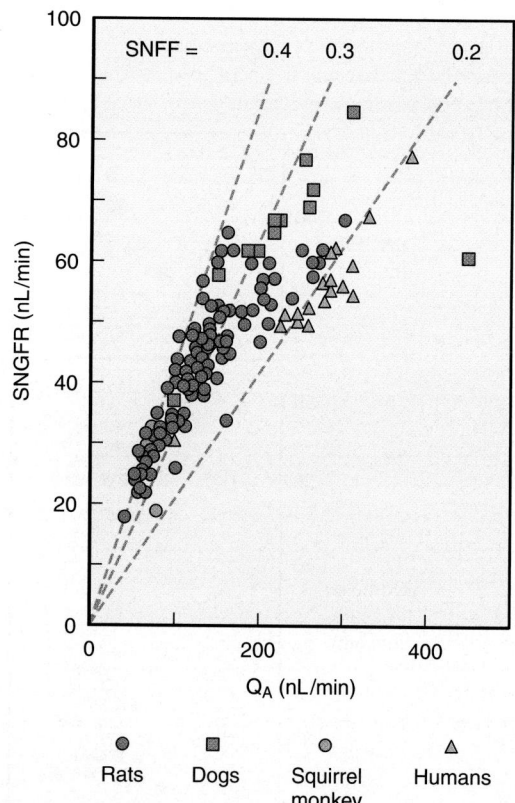

FIGURE 3-17 Relationship between single-nephron glomerular filtration rate (SNGFR) and glomerular plasma flow rate. Values from studies in rats are denoted by *blue circles*; data from dogs are represented by *red squares*. Also shown are values from primates, including the squirrel monkey (*orange circles*) and humans (*green triangles*). The values for SNGFR and Q_A for humans were calculated by dividing whole kidney glomerular filtration rate (GFR) and renal plasma flow by the estimated total number of nephrons/kidney (1 million). Each point represents the mean value for a given study. (Data from Maddox and Brenner[87] and Maddox et al.[479])

Transcapillary Hydraulic Pressure Difference (ΔP)

Mathematical modeling also suggests that isolated changes in the glomerular transcapillary hydraulic pressure gradient affect SNGFR.[88] No filtration can take place until ΔP exceeds the colloid osmotic pressure (π_A) at the afferent end of the glomerular capillary. Once that point is reached, SNGFR increases as ΔP increases. The rate of increase is nonlinear, however, because the rise in SNGFR at any given fixed value of Q_A results in a concurrent (but smaller) increase in $\Delta\pi$. Because $\overline{\Delta P}$ is normally 30 to 40 mm Hg (see Figure 3-14), changes in $\overline{\Delta P}$ generally result in relatively minor variations in SNGFR.

The Glomerular Capillary Ultrafiltration Coefficient (K_f)

Glomerular damage from a variety of kidney diseases can result in a reduction in K_f, partly as a consequence of a reduction in surface area available for filtration as glomerulosclerosis progresses. Studies of the hydraulic permeability of the glomerular basement membrane have demonstrated an inverse relationship to $\overline{\Delta P}$, which indicates that K_f, the product of surface area and hydraulic conductivity, may be directly affected by $\overline{\Delta P}$.[92] The hydraulic conductivity of the glomerular basement membrane, and thus of K_f, is also affected by the plasma protein concentration (see the next section). Because filtration pressure equilibrium is generally observed at low values of Q_A, reductions in K_f do not affect SNGFR until K_f is reduced enough to produce filtration pressure disequilibrium. At low Q_A values, increases in K_f above normal values move the point of equilibrium closer to the afferent end of the capillaries but have little effect on SNGFR.[87,88] For high Q_A values, filtration pressure disequilibrium occurs, and the relationship between K_f and SNGFR is more direct.[87,88]

Colloid Osmotic Pressure (π_A)

SNGFR and SNFF are each predicted to vary reciprocally as a function of π_A (see equations 8 and 9).[88] When Q_A, ΔP, and K_f are held constant, reductions in π_A will increase P_{UF}, which leads to an increase in SNGFR. An increase in π_A should produce a decrease in SNGFR until π_A equals $\overline{\Delta P}$ (normally ≈ 35 mm Hg), at which point filtration stops and SNFF is zero. In contrast to theoretical predictions, experimentally induced reductions in π_A do not lead to a rise in SNGFR. Studies in rats have revealed a direct relationship between π_A and K_f when plasma protein concentrations were varied between 3.4 and 5.9 g/dL (see Maddox and Brenner[87]) so that a reduction in π_A results in a reduction in K_f, thereby offsetting variations in P_{UF} that occur with changes in a (see Maddox and Brenner[87]). Studies in isolated glomeruli, however, indicated that extremely low concentrations of albumin produce an increase in K_f, whereas extremely high concentrations of albumin result in a decrease in K_f.[87] These divergent results of the effect of protein concentration on K_f can be explained partly by the results from studies of isolated glomerular basement membranes by Daniels and associates,[92] who observed a biphasic relationship between albumin concentration and hydraulic permeability. They observed lower values of hydraulic permeability at albumin concentrations of 4 g/dL than at either 0 or 8 g/dL, but they did not study the effects of extremely high protein concentrations. Their findings are suggestive of a primary effect of protein on hydraulic conductivity,[92] but the mechanism is unknown.

Regulation of Renal Hemodynamics and Glomerular Filtration

Vasomotor Properties of the Renal Microcirculations

A variety of hormonal, neural, and vasoactive substances influence RBF and glomerular ultrafiltration. The arcuate arteries, interlobular arteries, and both afferent and efferent arterioles are all influenced by such substances; thus the tone of preglomerular and postglomerular resistance vessels is regulated to control RBF, glomerular hydraulic pressure, and the transcapillary hydraulic pressure gradient. The glomerular mesangium is also the site of action and production of many such substances. Various growth factors can affect renal hemodynamics and promote mesangial cell proliferation and expansion of the extracellular matrix, which lead to obliteration of capillary loops and a reduction in the glomerular capillary ultrafiltration coefficient (K_f). A number of vasoactive compounds may also affect K_f by changing the effective surface area for filtration through contraction of mesangial cells, which causes shunting of blood to fewer capillary loops.[93,94] In addition, contraction of glomerular epithelial cells (podocytes), which contain filamentous actin molecules, may decrease the size of the filtration slit pores, thereby altering hydraulic conductivity of the filtration pathway and reducing K_f.[95]

Information about afferent and efferent vascular reactivity to neural, hormonal, and vasoactive substances has, to a large part, come from micropuncture studies of glomerular hemodynamics. Other methods have included grafting renal tissue from neonatal hamsters into the cheek pouch of adult hamsters[96]; this method provided access to afferent and efferent arterioles and enabled the examination of the effects of local application of vasoactive agents. Several other models have been developed to study functional responses of the preglomerular and postglomerular vasculature. Steinhausen and colleagues[97] applied epiillumination and transillumination microscopic techniques to the split hydronephrotic rat kidney. This preparation enables the arcuate arteries, interlobular arteries, afferent arterioles, and efferent arterioles to be visualized and studied in situ during perfusion with systemic blood, independent of tubular influences (e.g., tubuloglomerular feedback, as described later). Changes in the diameter of these vessels have been documented in response to systemically or locally applied vasoactive substances.

Loutzenhiser and associates[98-100] used a modification of the hydronephrotic kidney technique in which the kidney is mounted and perfused in vitro to examine the response of the afferent arterioles to various stimuli. in vitro perfusion of rat kidney has also been performed to assess segmental vascular reactivity directly in the juxtamedullary nephrons that lie in opposition to the pelvic cavity.[101] Edwards[102] developed an in vitro technique to study the reactivity of isolated segments of interlobular arteries and superficial afferent and efferent arterioles dissected from rabbit kidneys. Ito and colleagues[103] further developed the in vitro approach to study changes in preglomerular resistance by using the isolated perfused afferent arterioles with attached glomeruli. Thus, various techniques have been used to provide insight into the vasoactive properties of the preglomerular and postglomerular vasculature that control renal hemodynamics and GFR.

The renal vasculature and glomerular mesangium respond to a number of endogenous hormones and vasoactive peptides by vasoconstriction, reductions in RBF and GFR, and reductions in the glomerular capillary ultrafiltration coefficient (K_f). Among the vasoconstrictors are angiotensin II, norepinephrine, leukotriences C_4 and D_4 (LTC4 and LTD4), platelet-activating factor (PAF), adenosine 5'-triphosphate (ATP), endothelin, vasopressin, serotonin, and epidermal growth factor. Similarly, vasodilatory substances such as endothelium-derived relaxing factor (now known to be nitric oxide), prostaglandins E_2 and I_2 (PGE_2 and PGI_2), histamine, bradykinin, acetylcholine, insulin, insulin-like growth factor (IGF), calcitonin gene–related peptide (CGRP), cyclic adenosine monophosphate (cAMP), and relaxin can increase RBF and GFR. However, in addition to having their own direct effects on blood flow and GFR, a number of these vasodilator substances stimulate angiotensin II production, which masks their primary effect. In addition, vasoconstrictor substances

such as angiotensin II can result in a feedback stimulation of renal vasodilator production, which increases the complexity of the interaction for the control of renal hemodynamics. Cellular mechanisms of action of some of these compounds are covered in detail in other chapters.

Role of the Renin-Angiotensin System in the Control of Renal Blood Flow and Glomerular Filtration Rate

The renin-angiotensin system plays an important role in modulating RBF and filtration rate. Results of numerous studies indicate that preglomerular vessels—including the arcuate arteries, interlobular arteries, and afferent arterioles—and the postglomerular efferent arterioles constrict in response to exogenous and endogenous angiotensin II.[103-108] Figure 3-18 shows the effects of angiotensin II on diameters and estimated changes in resistance in these vessels. The efferent arterioles, however, have a 10- to 100-fold greater sensitivity to angiotensin II.[103,106-108] The vasoconstrictor effects of angiotensin II are blunted by the endogenous production of

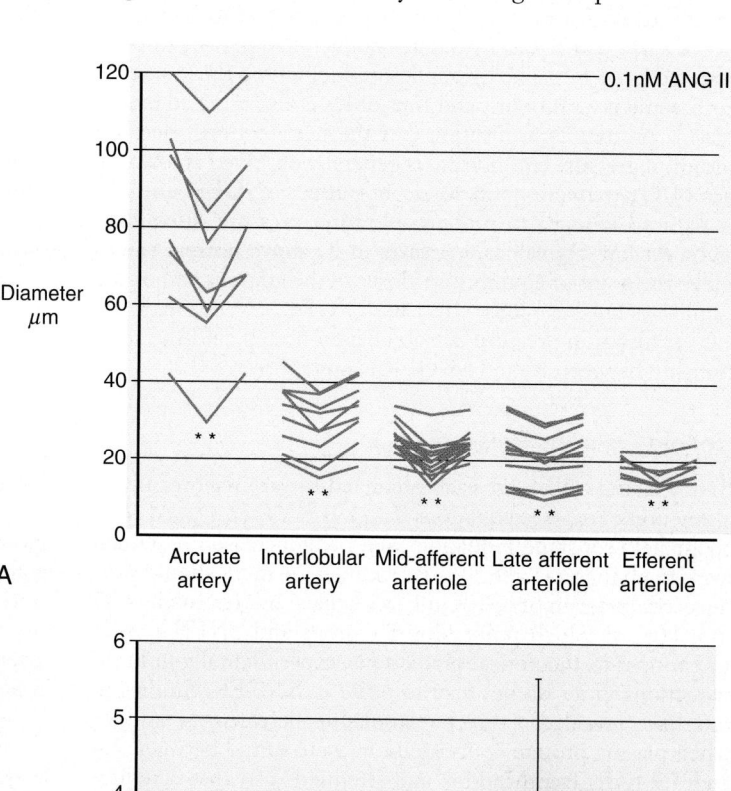

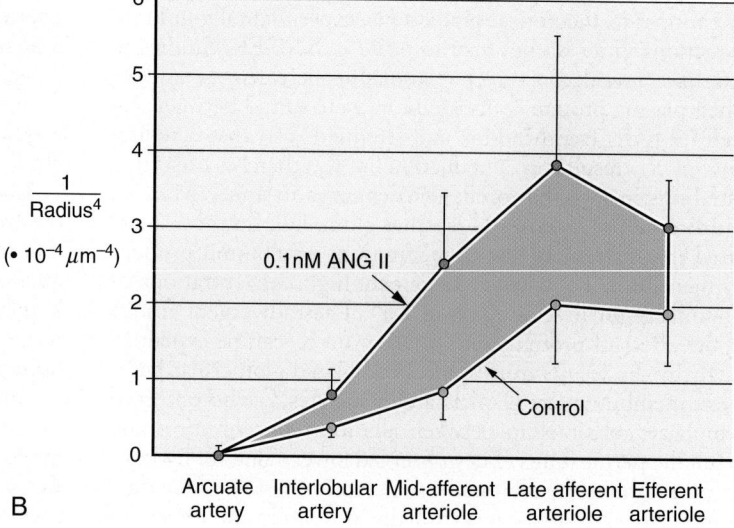

FIGURE 3-18 Effect of angiotensin II on the blood-perfused juxtamedullary nephron microvasculature. **A,** Vessel inside-diameter responses to angiotensin II (ANG II). Each line denotes observations of a single vessel segment during control, angiotensin II, and recovery periods. **B,** Estimation of angiotensin II–induced changes in segmental vascular resistance, calculated from data in the top panel. **$P < .01$. (From Navar LG, Gilmore JP, Joyner WL, et al: Direct assessment of renal microcirculatory dynamics, *Fed Proc* 1986;45:2851.)

vasodilators, including nitric oxide, as well as cyclooxygenase and cytochrome P450 epoxygenase metabolites in afferent but not efferent arterioles.[99,103,108-113] Angiotensin II–simulated release of nitric oxide in the afferent arterioles occurs through activation of the angiotensin II type 1 (AT_1) receptors.[114,115] Angiotensin II increases the production of prostaglandins in afferent arteriolar smooth muscle cells (both PGE_2 and PGI_2) and PGE_2, PGI_2, and cAMP all blunt angiotensin II–induced calcium entry into these cells,[110] which potentially explains, at least in part, the different effects of angiotensin II on vasoconstriction of the afferent and efferent arterioles.[109,110] PGE_2 had no effect on angiotensin II–induced vasoconstriction of the efferent arterioles.[99] The effects of PGE_2 on angiotensin II–induced vasoconstriction of the afferent arterioles are concentration dependent; low concentrations act as a vasodilator through interaction with prostaglandin EP_4 receptors, whereas high concentrations of PGE_2 act on prostaglandin EP_3 receptors to restore the angiotensin II effects in that segment.[99] Although angiotensin II infusion alone has little effect on SNGFR, angiotensin II when combined with cyclooxygenase inhibition causes marked reductions in both SNGFR and glomerular plasma flow rate (Q_A) when combined with cyclooxygenase inhibition; thus, endogenous vasodilatory prostaglandins may have an important role in ameliorating the vasoconstrictor effects of angiotensin II.[116] Because angiotensin II increases renal production of vasodilatory prostaglandins, a feedback loop may exist to modulate the vasoconstrictor effects on angiotensin II under chronic conditions when the renin-angiotensin system is stimulated.[87]

In addition to causing renal vasoconstriction, reduced blood flow, and glomerular capillary hypertension, angiotensin II causes a decrease in the glomerular ultrafiltration coefficient (K_f).[116] As discussed in the earlier section "Determinants of Glomerular Ultrafiltration," K_f is the product of the surface area available for filtration (S) and hydraulic conductivity of the filtration barrier (k) and is one of the primary determinants of SNGFR. A decrease in K_f induced by angiotensin II could be the result of a decrease in either S or k. As noted earlier, glomerular angiotensin II receptors are found on the mesangial cells, glomerular capillary endothelial cells, and podocytes. Because angiotensin II causes contraction of mesangial cells,[117] one possibility is that contraction of the mesangial cells reduces effective filtration area by blocking flow through some glomerular capillaries, but no direct evidence that would support this hypothesis has been obtained. Alternatively, the angiotensin II–induced decrease in K_f could be the result of a decrease in hydraulic conductivity rather than a reduction in the surface area available for filtration.[118] A role for glomerular epithelial cells in the effects of angiotensin II on K_f is suggested by the fact that they possess both AT_1 and angiotensin II type 2 (AT_2) receptors and respond to angiotensin II by increasing cAMP production.[119] Alterations in epithelial structure or the size of the filtration slits have not been detected after infusion of angiotensin II at a dose sufficient to decrease GFR and K_f.[120] Thus the mechanisms by which angiotensin II causes a reduction in K_f have not yet been determined.

Just as the renal vascular effects of angiotensin II are moderated by production of vasodilator prostaglandins and nitric oxide, angiotensin II–induced changes in K_f are also be affected by such substances. Endogenous prostaglandins help to prevent the reduction in K_f caused by angiotensin II.[116] The vasoconstrictive effect of angiotensin II on glomerular mesangial cells is markedly reduced by nitric oxide.[121] Mesangial cells co-incubated with endothelial cells have increased cyclic guanosine monophosphate (cGMP) production induced by nitric oxide release from the endothelial cells, which resulted in decreased vasoconstrictive effects of angiotensin II; this finding indicates that local nitric oxide production can modify the effects of agents such as angiotensin II.[121] Whether a similar effect would be observed for glomerular epithelial cells co-incubated with endothelial cells and whether either would translate into protection from angiotensin II–induced alterations on glomerular capillary surface area or hydraulic conductivity is not known, but inhibition of nitric oxide production in the normal rat does produce a marked decrease in K_f.[121-123]

Arima and associates[124] examined AT_2 receptor–mediated effects on afferent arteriolar tone. When the AT_1 receptor was blocked, angiotensin II caused a dose-dependent dilation of the afferent arterioles that could be blocked by disruption of the endothelium or by simultaneous inhibition of the cytochrome P450 pathway. These data suggest that AT_2 receptor–mediated vasodilation in afferent arterioles is endothelium dependent, possibly through the synthesis of epoxyeicosatrienoic acids via a cytochrome P450 pathway, and thus counteracts the vasoconstrictor effects of angiotensin II at AT_1 receptors.[124,125]

Since 1990, the classical renin-angiotensin-aldosterone system (RAAS) has become better understood. For example, the octapeptide angiotensin II produces prohypertensive and renal vasoconstrictor effects via activation of AT_1 receptors, whereas activation of AT_2 receptors results in vasodilation, as described previously.[124] Furthermore, fragments of angiotensin II that were once believed to be inactive have been shown to have physiologic effects within the kidney, often opposing the actions of angiotensin II. Although findings from multiple laboratories and in various preparations have not always been consistent, angiotensin-(1-7) has been shown to induce vasodilation of preconstricted renal arterioles.[126] These effects of angiotensin-(1-7) occur independently of binding to AT_1 or AT_2 receptors and appear to involve activation of the G protein–coupled Mas receptor,[127] which has been shown to be expressed in the afferent arterioles.[128] In addition, an isoform of angiotensin-converting enzyme (ACE) known as ACE_2 was recently identified[129,130] and appears to be involved in the formation of angiotensin-(1-7).[131] Angiotensin-(1-7), ACE_2, and the Mas receptor have all been detected within the kidney. The balance between opposing actions of the vasoconstrictor peptide, angiotensin II, and the vasodilator peptide angiotensin-(1-7) may be influenced by the ratio of ACE to ACE_2 content and the ratio of AT_1 to Mas receptor content within specific vascular regions (as well as tubular segments) of the kidney. In fact, cardiovascular and renal disease may involve an imbalance of these peptides, enzymes, or receptors.[128]

The hormone aldosterone has become a subject of interest. Once believed to be involved solely in salt and water balance manifest through tubular effects, aldosterone has more recently been studied for direct renovascular effects, possibly through activation of rapid nongenomic mechanisms. In one study, aldosterone induced a rapid vasoconstriction that was not blocked by spironolactone in perfused arterioles isolated from rabbit kidneys.[132] Data are somewhat controversial, but other studies have shown either no effect or a vasodilator effect in vasculature with intact endothelium, whereas a vasoconstrictor effect of aldosterone is consistently observed when endothelial function is impaired by inhibition of nitric oxide production (for review, see Arima[133] and Schmidt[134]). Finally, the peptide apelin has been found to serve as an endogenous ligand for the orphan G protein–coupled receptor APJ, which shares significant homology with the AT_1 receptor.[135] Apelin immunoreactivity and APJ receptor messenger RNA have been detected in the kidney and are believed to play a counterregulatory role with regard to renovascular and tubular effects of the RAAS.[136,137]

Endothelial Factors in the Control of Renal Hemodynamics and Glomerular Filtration

Endothelial cells were once considered "vascular cellophane," simple metabolically inactive cells that passively lined the vascular tree, providing a nonstick surface for blood cells. The pioneering work of Robert Furchgott, Louis Ignarro, Ferid Murad, and Masashi Yanigasawa revealed that these cells produce a number of substances that can profoundly alter vascular tone, including vasodilators, such as nitric oxide, and vasoconstrictors, such as the endothelins. These factors play an important role in the minute-to-minute regulation of renal vascular flow and resistance.

Nitric Oxide

In 1980, Furchgott and Zawadzki[138] demonstrated that the vasodilatory action of acetylcholine required the presence of an intact endothelium. The binding of acetylcholine and many other vasodilator substances to receptors on endothelial cells leads to the formation and release of nitric oxide.[139,140] Nitric oxide is formed from L-arginine[141] by a family of enzymes that are encoded by separate genes called nitric oxide synthases (NOSs) that are present in many cells, including vascular endothelial cells, macrophages, neurons,[142] glomerular mesangial cells,[143] the beginning of the distal convoluted tubule (known as the macula densa),[144] and renal tubular cells. Once released by the endothelium, nitric oxide diffuses into adjacent and downstream vascular smooth muscle cells,[145] where it activates soluble guanylate cyclase and thus leads to accumulation of cGMP.[121,146-150] cGMP modulates intracellular calcium concentration, in part, through a cGMP-dependent protein kinase–mediated phosphorylation of targets believed to include inositol 1,4,5-trisphosphate (IP_3) receptors, calcium channels, and phospholipase A_2,[151] thereby reducing the amount of calcium available for contraction and hence promoting relaxation.[152] The breakdown of cGMP is catalyzed by a family of phosphodiesterases (PDEs) that are either selective for cGMP (e.g., PDE_5 and PDE_6) or that are capable of metabolizing both cGMP and cAMP (e.g., PDE_1, PDE_2, PDE_{10}, and PDE_{11}).[153] Inhibitors of the PDEs as potential therapeutic agents in kidney disease are currently under investigation.

In addition to stimulation by acetylcholine, nitric oxide formation in the vascular endothelium increases in response to bradykinin,[121,154-157] thrombin,[158] PAF,[159] endothelin,[160] and CGRP.[155,161-164] Increased flow through blood vessels with intact endothelium or across cultured endothelial cells, resulting in increased shear stress, also increases nitric oxide release,[147,154,156,165-169] and elevated perfusion pressure/shear stress increases nitric oxide release from afferent arterioles.[170]

Both pulse frequency and amplitude modulate flow-induced nitric oxide release.[165]

In the kidney, nitric oxide has numerous important functions, including the regulation of renal hemodynamics, maintenance of medullary perfusion, blunting of tubuloglomerular feedback, inhibition of tubular sodium reabsorption, modulation of renal sympathetic neural activity, and mediation of pressure natriuresis.[171] The net effect of nitric oxide in the kidney is to promote natriuresis and diuresis.[172] In fact, in experimental models in which both renal perfusion pressure and medullary blood flow were increased in a stepwise manner, pressure natriuresis involved increased medullary nitric oxide release[173] that could exert direct tubular effects to promote sodium and water excretion. Although tubular epithelial cells are capable of releasing nitric oxide, the vasa recta may be a primary source of the nitric oxide produced during increased medullary flow, inasmuch as Zhang and Pallone[174] observed flow-dependent increases of nitric oxide during microperfusion of isolated outer medullary vasa recta.

Experimental studies also support the presence of an important interaction among nitric oxide, angiotensin II, and renal nerves in the control of renal function.[175] Renal hemodynamics are continuously affected by endogenous nitric oxide production, as evidenced by the fact that nonselective NOS inhibition results in marked decreases in RPF, an increase in mean arterial blood pressure, and, in general, a reduction in GFR.[176-178] These effects are largely prevented by the simultaneous administration of excess L-arginine, the NOS substrate.[176] Selective inhibition of neuronal NOS (nNOS, or type I NOS)—which is found in the thick ascending limb of the loop of Henle, the macula densa, and efferent arterioles[144,179]—decreases GFR without affecting blood pressure or RBF.[180] Because endothelial NOS (eNOS, or type II NOS) is found in the endothelium of renal blood vessels, including the afferent and efferent arterioles and glomerular capillary endothelial cells,[144] differences in the effects of inhibition of nitric oxide formation on RBF between generalized NOS inhibition and specific inhibition of nNOS appear to be related to the distinct distribution of eNOS versus nNOS in the kidney. Both acute and chronic inhibition of nitric oxide production results in systemic and glomerular capillary hypertension, an increase in R_A and R_E, a decrease in K_f, and decreases in both Q_A and SNGFR.[122,123,181-183] As shown in Figure 3-19, acute administration of pressor doses of a blocker of nitric oxide production resulted in declines in SNGFR, Q_A, and K_f and increases in both R_A and R_E. Administration of nonpressor doses of the inhibitor of nitric oxide formation through the renal artery yielded an increase in R_A and a decrease in SNGFR and K_f but no effect on R_E (see Figure 3-19).[123] These results suggested that the cortical afferent, but not efferent, arterioles were under tonic control by nitric oxide. However, in other research, the renal artery, arcuate and interlobular arteries, and afferent and efferent arterioles have all been shown to produce nitric oxide and to constrict in response to inhibition of endogenous nitric oxide production.[103,108,145,184-187] In agreement with this finding, other investigators[10,187] have reported that nitric oxide dilates both efferent and afferent arterioles in the perfused juxtamedullary nephron.

The role of the renin-angiotensin system in the genesis of the increase in vascular resistance that follows blockade of NOS is controversial. According to studies of in vitro perfused

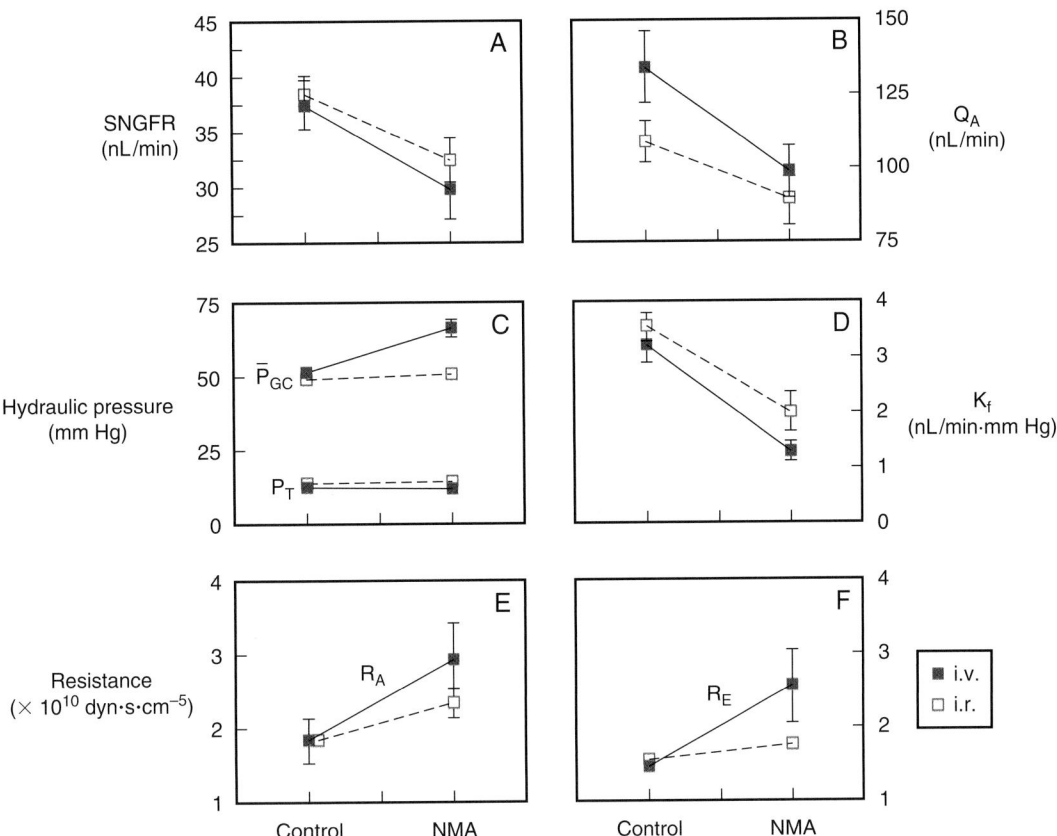

FIGURE 3-19 Role of endothelium-derived relaxing factor (EDRF; now known to be nitric oxide) in the control of glomerular ultrafiltration. Studies were performed in euvolemic Munich-Wistar rats either receiving intravenous pressor doses of the EDRF blocker *N*-monomethyl-L-arginine (NMA) (i.v., denoted by *filled squares*) or nonpressor doses of NMA at the origin of the renal artery (i.r., denoted by *open square*). (Data [mean ± standard error] from Deng and Baylis.[123])

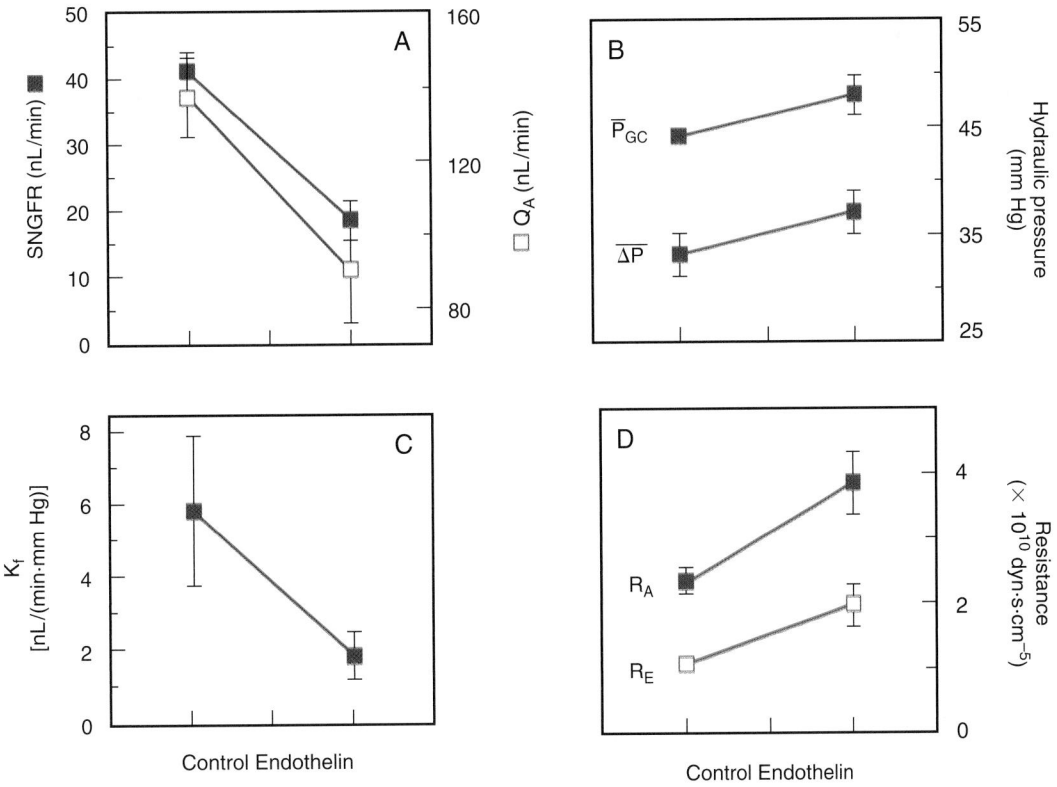

FIGURE 3-20 Effects of intravenous administration of endothelin (subpressor dose) on glomerular ultrafiltration. (Data [mean ± standard error] obtained in euvolemic Munich-Wistar rats from Badr et al.[226])

nephrons[187] and of anesthetized rats in vivo,[188] the increase in renal vascular resistance that follows NOS blockade may be blunted when angiotensin II formation or binding is blocked. Nitric oxide inhibits renin release, whereas acute angiotensin II infusion increases cortical NOS activity and protein expression, and chronic angiotensin II infusion increases messenger RNA levels for both eNOS and nNOS.[188,189] Angiotensin II increases nitric oxide production in isolated perfused afferent arterioles through activation of the AT_1 receptors.[114] On the other hand, Deng and colleagues[190] reported that nonselective NOS inhibition increased renal oxygen consumption, which was independent of angiotensin II. In addition, Baylis and colleagues[191] reported that inhibition of NOS in conscious rats had similar effects on renal hemodynamics in the intact and angiotensin II–blocked state. This suggests that the vasoconstrictor response of NOS blockade is not mediated by angiotensin II. In the same laboratory, Baylis and colleagues[192] later showed that when the angiotensin II level was acutely raised by infusion of exogenous peptide, acute nitric oxide blockade amplified the renal vasoconstrictor actions of angiotensin II. In agreement with this finding, Ito and colleagues[103] showed that intrarenal inhibition of nitric oxide enhanced angiotensin II–induced afferent, but not efferent, arteriolar vasoconstriction in rabbits. Similar results have also been obtained in dogs.[111] Although no clear consensus exists, these data suggest that nitric oxide modulates the vasoconstrictor effects of angiotensin II on glomerular arterioles in vivo, perhaps blunting its vasoconstrictor response in the afferent arterioles but not in the efferent arterioles. This may provide a mechanism for the proposed preferential vasoconstrictor response to angiotensin II in the efferent arterioles that is observed in settings in which angiotensin II levels are elevated.

Endothelin

Endothelin, a potent vasoconstrictor derived primarily from vascular endothelial cells, was first described by Yanagisawa and colleagues.[193] There are three distinct genes for endothelin, each encoding a distinct 21–amino acid isopeptide (ET-1, ET-2, and ET-3).[193-195] Endothelin is produced after cleavage by endothelin-converting enzyme of proendothelin (38 to 40 amino acids), which, in turn, is produced from proteolytic cleavage of prepro-endothelin (≈212 amino acids) by furin.[196,197] ET-1 is the primary endothelin produced in the kidney—including arcuate arteries and veins, interlobular arteries, afferent and efferent arterioles, glomerular capillary endothelial cells, glomerular epithelial cells, and glomerular mesangial cells of both rats and humans[198-209]—and acts in an autocrine or paracrine manner or both[210] to alter a variety of biologic processes in these cells. Endothelins are extremely potent vasoconstrictors, and the renal vasculature is highly sensitive to these agents.[211] Once released from endothelial cells, both ET-1 and ET-2 bind to specific receptors on vascular smooth muscle, the endothelin type A (ET_A) receptors.[210,212-215] Endothelin type B (ET_B) receptors are expressed in the glomerulus on mesangial cells and podocytes with equal affinity for ET-1, ET-2, and ET-3.[214,215] There are two subtypes of ET_B receptors: ET_{B1}, which is linked to vasodilation, and ET_{B2}, which is linked to vasoconstriction.[216] An endothelin-specific protease modulates endothelin levels in the kidney.[217]

Endothelin production is stimulated by physical factors, including increased shear stress and vascular stretch.[218,219] In addition, a variety of hormones, growth factors, and vasoactive peptides increase endothelin production; these substances include transforming growth factor–β, platelet-derived growth factor, tumor necrosis factor–α, angiotensin II, arginine vasopressin, insulin, bradykinin, thromboxane A_2, and thrombin.[198,202,204,208,220-223] Endothelin production is inhibited by atrial and brain natriuretic peptides acting through a cGMP-dependent process[217,224] and by factors that increase intracellular cAMP and protein kinase A activation, such as β-adrenergic agonists.[204]

Typically, intravenous infusion of ET-1 induces a marked, prolonged pressor response,[193,225] accompanied by increases in R_A and R_E and decreases in RBF and GFR.[225] As shown in Figure 3-20, infusion of subpressor doses of ET-1 also decreases SNGFR, Q_A, and whole kidney RBF and GFR,[226-230] again accompanied by increases in both R_A and R_E and filtration fraction.[226,228,231] Vasoconstriction of afferent and efferent arterioles by endothelin has been confirmed in the split hydronephrotic rat kidney preparation[232,233] and in isolated perfused arterioles.[106,185,234] In both micropuncture studies[226] and isolated arteriole studies,[106] the sensitivity and response of the efferent arterioles exceeded those of the afferent vessels. Endothelin also causes mesangial cell contraction.[195,235] Finally, results of other studies have suggested that the vasoconstrictor effects of the endothelins can be modulated by a number of factors,[213,236] including nitric oxide,[185,237] bradykinin,[238] PGE_2,[239] and prostacyclin.[239,240]

There are multiple endothelin receptors; most is known about the ET_A and ET_B receptors, which have been cloned and characterized.[215,241,242] According to the traditional view, ET_A receptors, abundant on vascular smooth muscle, have a high affinity for ET-1 and play a prominent role in the pressor response to endothelin.[243] ET_B receptors are present on endothelial cells, where they may mediate nitric oxide release and endothelial-dependent relaxation.[242] However, the distribution and function of ET_A and ET_B receptors vary greatly among species and, in the rat, even among strains. In the normal rat, both ET_A and ET_B receptors are expressed in the media of interlobular arteries, afferent arterioles, and efferent arterioles. In interlobar and arcuate arteries, only ET_A receptors were found to be present on vascular smooth muscle cells.[244] ET_B receptor immunoreactivity is sparse on endothelial cells of renal arteries, whereas there is strong labeling of peritubular and glomerular capillaries and of vasa recta endothelium.[244] ET_A receptors are evident on glomerular mesangial cells and pericytes of descending vasa recta bundles.[244] In the rat, endogenous endothelin may actually tonically dilate the afferent arterioles and lower K_f through ET_B receptors.[245] However, ET_B receptors on vascular smooth muscle also mediate vasoconstriction in the rat, and this is potentiated in hypertensive animals.[246]

Endothelin stimulates the production of vasodilatory prostaglandins,[229,237,240,247,248] which effects a feedback loop to modify the vasoconstrictor effects of endothelin. ET-1, ET-2, and ET-3 also stimulate nitric oxide production in the arterioles and glomerular mesangium through activation of the ET_B receptor.[158,160,185,237,249] Resistance in the renal and systemic vasculature are markedly increased during inhibition of nitric oxide production, and these effects can be partially reversed by ET_A blockade or inhibition of endothelin-converting enzyme;

this fact highlights the dynamic interrelationship between nitric oxide and endothelin effects.[250,251] The vasoconstrictive effects of angiotensin II may be mediated, in part, by a stimulation of ET-1 production that acts on ET_A receptors to produce vasoconstriction.[220,223] In fact, chronic administration of angiotensin II reduces RBF, an effect prevented by administration of a mixed ET_A/ET_B receptor antagonist, which suggests that endothelin makes an important contribution to the renal vasoconstrictive effects of angiotensin II.[220]

Renal Autoregulation

Many organs are capable of maintaining relative constancy of blood flow in the presence of major changes in perfusion pressure. Although the efficiency with which blood flow is maintained differs from organ to organ (being highest in brain and kidney), virtually all organs and tissues, including skeletal muscle and intestine, exhibit this property, termed *autoregulation*. As shown in Figure 3-21, the kidney autoregulates RBF and GFR over a wide range of renal perfusion pressures.

Autoregulation of blood flow requires changes in resistance that parallel changes in perfusion pressure. However, if efferent arteriolar resistance declined significantly when perfusion pressure was reduced, glomerular capillary pressure and GFR would also fall. Therefore, the finding that both RBF and GFR are autoregulated suggests that the principal resistance change is in the preglomerular vasculature. Studies of the Munich-Wistar rat, which has glomeruli on the renal cortical surface that are readily accessible to micropuncture, afforded an opportunity to observe the renal cortical microvascular adjustments that take place in response to variations in renal arterial perfusion pressure. Figure 3-22 summarizes the effects in the normal hydropenic rat of graded reductions in renal perfusion pressure on glomerular capillary blood flow rate, mean glomerular capillary hydraulic pressure (P_{GC}), and preglomerular (R_A) and efferent arteriolar (R_E) resistance.[252] As shown in Figure 3-22, graded reduction in renal perfusion pressure from 120 to 80 mm Hg resulted in only a modest decline in glomerular capillary blood flow, whereas further

reduction in perfusion pressure to 60 mm Hg led to a more pronounced decline. Despite the decline in perfusion pressure from 120 to 80 mm Hg, values of $\overline{P}_{GC}$ fell only modestly on average, from 45 to 40 mm Hg. Further reduction in perfusion pressure, from 80 to 60 mm Hg, resulted in a further fall in $\overline{P}_{GC}$, from 40 to 35 mm Hg. Calculated values for R_A and R_E are shown in Figure 3-22. Autoregulation of glomerular capillary blood flow and $\overline{P}_{GC}$ as perfusion pressure decreased from 120 to 80 mm Hg resulted from a pronounced decrease in R_A with little change in R_E. Over the range of renal perfusion pressure from 120 to 60 mm Hg, R_E tended to increase slightly. In Robertson and associates' study,[252] when plasma volume was expanded, R_A declined, whereas R_E increased as renal perfusion pressure was lowered; thus $\overline{P}_{GC}$ and ΔP were virtually unchanged over the entire range of renal perfusion pressures. In plasma-expanded animals, the mean glomerular transcapillary hydraulic pressure difference ($\overline{\Delta P}$) exhibited nearly perfect autoregulation over the entire range of perfusion pressures because of concomitant increases in R_E as R_A fell.[252] These results indicate that autoregulation of GFR is the consequence of the autoregulation of both glomerular blood flow and glomerular capillary pressure.

The medullary circulation has also been shown to possess autoregulatory capacity.[253-255] The extent of autoregulation of the medullary circulation may be influenced by the volume status of the animal.[254] Preglomerular vessels, including the

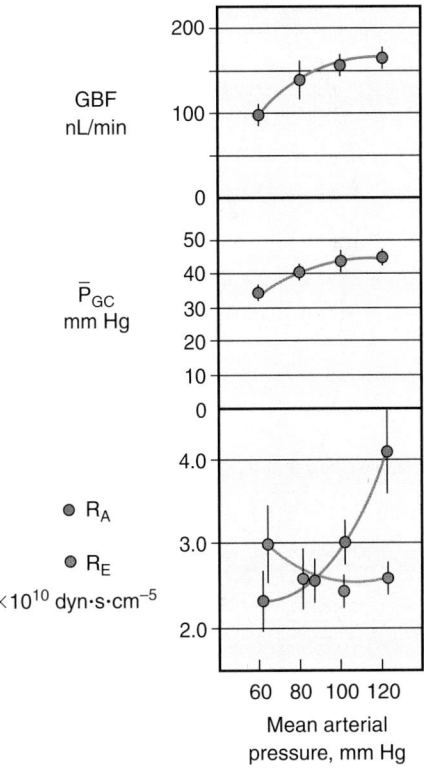

FIGURE 3-22 Glomerular dynamics in response to reduction of renal arterial perfusion pressure in the normal hydropenic rat. As can be seen, glomerular blood flow (GBF) and glomerular capillary hydraulic pressure ($\overline{P}_{GC}$) remained relatively constant as blood pressure was lowered from approximately 120 mm Hg to approximately 80 mm Hg, over the range of perfusion pressure examined, primarily as a result of a marked decrease in preglomerular arteriolar resistance (R_A). Efferent arteriolar resistance (R_E) was relatively constant. (Adapted from Robertson CR, Deen WM, Troy JL, et al: Dynamics of glomerular ultrafiltration in the rat. III. Hemodynamics and autoregulation, *Am J Physiol* 1972;223:1191.)

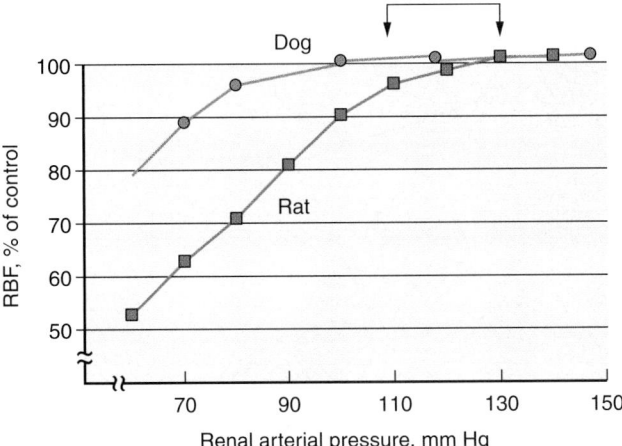

FIGURE 3-21 Autoregulatory response of total renal blood flow to changes in renal perfusion pressure in the dog and rat. In general, the normal anesthetized dog exhibits greater autoregulatory capability to lower arterial pressure than does the rat. (From Navar LG, Bell PD, Burke TJ: Role of a macula densa feedback mechanism as a mediator of renal autoregulation, *Kidney Int* 1982;22:S157.)

afferent arterioles and vessels as large as the arcuate and inter-lobular arteries, participate in the autoregulatory response. In the split hydronephrotic rat kidney preparation, Steinhausen and colleagues[256] observed dilation of all preglomerular vessels from the arcuate to interlobular arteries in response to reductions in perfusion pressure from 120 to 95 mm Hg. The proximal afferent arterioles did not respond to pressure changes in this range but did dilate when perfusion pressure was reduced to 70 mm Hg. The diameter of the distal afferent arterioles did not change at any pressure. Another finding consistent with an important role of large, preglomerular vessels in the autoregulatory response was that of Heyeraas and Aukland,[257] who reported that interlobular arterial pressure remained constant when renal perfusion pressure was reduced by 20 mm Hg, which again suggests that these vessels contribute importantly to the constancy of outer cortical blood flow in the upper autoregulatory range. A number of observations have provided evidence that the major preglomerular resistor is located close to the glomerulus, at the level of the afferent arterioles.[12,258-260] As in superficial nephrons, direct observations of perfused juxtamedullary nephrons revealed parallel reductions in the luminal diameters of arcuate, interlobular, and afferent arterioles in response to elevation in perfusion pressure. However, because quantitatively similar reductions in vessel diameter produce much greater elevations in resistance in small vessels than in large vessels, the predominant effect of these changes is an increase in afferent arteriolar resistance.[258]

Cellular Mechanisms Involved in Renal Autoregulation

Autoregulation of the afferent arterioles and interlobular artery is blocked by administration of L-type calcium channel blockers, inhibition of mechanosensitive cation channels, and a calcium-free perfusate.[261-264] The autoregulatory response thus involves gating of mechanosensitive channels, which

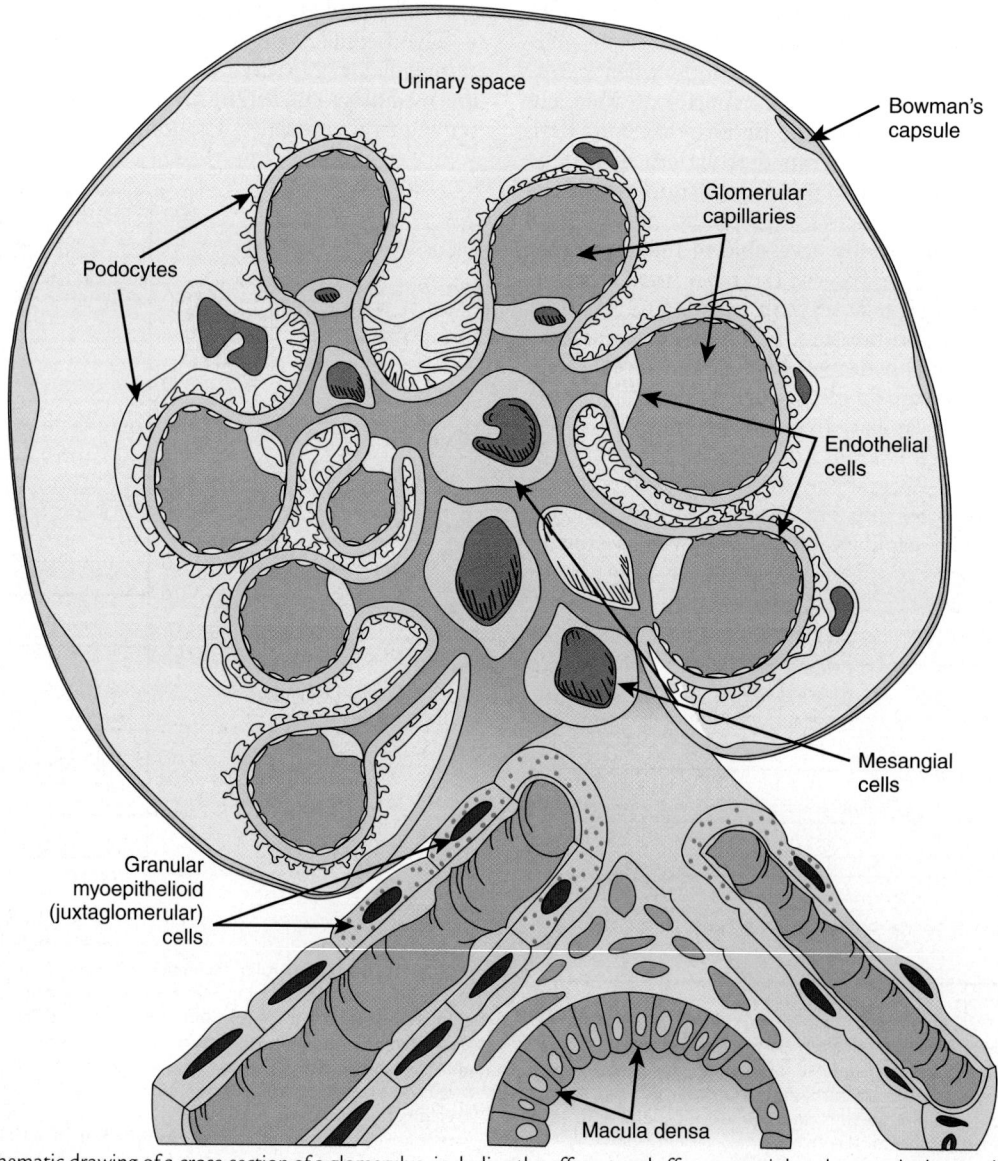

FIGURE 3-23 Schematic drawing of a cross-section of a glomerulus, including the afferent and efferent arterioles, the macula densa cells of the early distal tubule, the glomerular capillaries, mesangial cells, and podocytes. (Drawing by D. A. Maddox.)

produces membrane depolarization and activation of voltage-dependent calcium channels and leads to an increase in intracellular calcium concentration and vasoconstriction.[261,265,266] In fact, calcium channel blockade almost completely blocks autoregulation of RBF.[267,268] The autoregulatory capacity of the afferent arterioles is attenuated by intrinsic metabolites of the cytochrome P450 epoxygenase pathway, whereas metabolites of the cytochrome P450 hydroxylase pathway enhance autoregulatory responsiveness.[269]

Autoregulation of both GFR and RBF occur in the presence of inhibition of nitric oxide, but values for RBF were reduced at any given renal perfusion pressure, in comparison with control values.[177,270-272] In the isolated perfused juxtamedullary afferent arteriole, the initial vasodilation observed when pressure was increased was of shorter duration when endogenous nitric oxide formation was blocked but the autoregulatory response was unaffected.[266] Cortical and juxtamedullary preglomerular vessels in the split hydronephrotic rat kidney also autoregulate in the presence of nitric oxide inhibition.[184] The majority of evidence therefore suggests that nitric oxide is not essential at least for the myogenic component of renal autoregulation, although nitric oxide may play a role in tubuloglomerular feedback (see later discussion).[273]

The Myogenic Mechanism for Autoregulation

According to the myogenic theory, arterial smooth muscle contracts and relaxes in response to increases and decreases in vascular wall tension.[274] Thus an increase in perfusion pressure, which initially distends the vascular wall, is followed by a contraction of resistance vessels, which results in a recovery of blood flow from an initial elevation to a value comparable with the control level. Fray and associates[275] and Lush and Fray[276] presented a model of myogenic control of RBF that was based on the assumption that flow remains constant when the distending force and the constricting forces, determined by the properties of the vessel wall, are equal. The constricting force is envisioned to have both a passive and an active component, the latter sensitive to stretch in the vessel. Myogenic control of renal vascular resistance had been estimated to contribute up to 50% of the total autoregulatory response.[277]

Several lines of evidence indicate that such a myogenic mechanism is important in renal autoregulation. Autoregulation of RBF is observed even when tubuloglomerular feedback is inhibited by furosemide; this fact is suggestive of an important role for a myogenic mechanism.[105] This myogenic mechanism of autoregulation occurs very rapidly, reaching a full response in 3 to 10 seconds.[105] Autoregulation occurs in all of the preglomerular resistance vessels of the in vitro blood-perfused juxtamedullary nephron preparation.[259,269,278-280] Of note, the afferent arterioles in this preparation were able to constrict in response to rapid changes in perfusion pressure even when all flow to the macula densa was stopped by resection of the papilla; this finding is further support of an important role for a myogenic mechanism in autoregulation.[280] Isolated perfused rabbit afferent arterioles respond to step increases of intraluminal pressure with a decrease in luminal diameter.[102] In contrast, efferent arteriolar segments showed vasodilation when submitted to the same procedure, which probably reflects simple passive physical properties. Autoregulation is also observed in the afferent arterioles and in the arcuate and interlobular arteries of the split hydronephrotic rat kidney,[184,261,263,264,281] but, again, the efferent arterioles were not autoregulated in this model.[184] Further evidence that the renal vasculature is indeed intrinsically responsive to variations in the transmural hydraulic pressure difference was obtained by Gilmore and associates,[282] who observed myogenic autoregulation in renal vessels transplanted into a cheek pouch of the hamster. In this nonfiltering system, contraction of afferent but not efferent arterioles was observed in response to increased interstitial pressure in the pouch. In vivo, however, efferent arteriolar resistance may increase in response to decreases in arterial pressure,[283,284] and this may result from increased activity of the renin-angiotensin system. These data may also explain why autoregulation of GFR is more efficient than autoregulation of RBF.

The autoregulatory threshold can be reset in response to a variety of perturbations. Autoregulation in the afferent arterioles is greatly attenuated in diabetic kidneys and may contribute to the hyperfiltration that occurs early in this disease.[281] Autoregulation is partially restored by insulin treatment or by inhibition of endogenous prostaglandin production, or by both.[281] Autoregulation in the remnant kidney is markedly attenuated 24 hours after the reduction in renal mass and is again restored by cyclooxygenase inhibition, which suggests that release of vasodilator prostaglandins may be involved in the initial response to increased SNGFR in the remaining nephrons after acute partial nephrectomy.[285] Pressures much higher than normal are necessary to evoke a vasoconstrictor response in the afferent arterioles during the development of spontaneous hypertension.[286] The intermediate portion of the interlobular artery of the spontaneously hypertensive rat exhibits an enhanced myogenic response, with a lower threshold pressure and a greater maximal response.[263] Both the afferent arterioles and the interlobular arteries of the Dahl salt-sensitive hypertensive rat exhibit a reduced myogenic responsiveness to increases in perfusion pressure in rats fed a high-salt diet.[287] Thus, in a variety of disease states, autoregulatory responses of the renal vasculature are altered for the control of RBF and glomerular ultrafiltration.

Autoregulation Mediated by Tubuloglomerular Feedback

The nephron is uniquely organized so that the same tubule that descends from the cortex into the medulla eventually returns to the originating glomerulus to provide a regulatory mechanism known as tubuloglomerular feedback. There is a specialized nephron segment lying between the end of the thick ascending limb of the loop of Henle and the beginning of the distal convoluted tubule known as the macula densa. The macula densa cells are adjacent to the cells of the extraglomerular mesangium, which fill the angle formed by the afferent and efferent arterioles of the glomerulus (Figure 3-23). This anatomic arrangement of macula densa cells, extraglomerular mesangial cells, arteriolar smooth muscle cells, and renin-secreting cells of the afferent arterioles is known as the *juxtaglomerular apparatus* (JGA). The JGA is ideally suited for a feedback system whereby a stimulus received at the macula densa may be transmitted to the arterioles of the same nephron to alter RBF and GFR. Changes in the delivery rate and composition of the fluid flowing past the macula densa have been shown to elicit rapid changes in glomerular filtration of the same nephron; increases in delivery of fluid result in decreases in SNGFR and glomerular capillary hydraulic pressure (P_{GC}) of the same nephron.[288,289] This tubuloglomerular feedback system senses delivery of fluid to the macula densa and "feeds back" to control filtration rate; thus it is a powerful mechanism to regulate the pressures and flows that govern GFR in response to acute perturbations in delivery of fluid to the JGA. The tubuloglomerular feedback mechanism has been suggested as a mechanism that, in addition to the myogenic response, explains the autoregulation of RBF and GFR. Increased RBF or glomerular capillary pressure would lead to increased GFR, and delivery of solute to the distal tubule would therefore rise. Increased distal delivery is sensed by the macula densa, which activates effector mechanisms that increase preglomerular resistance, thereby reducing RBF, glomerular pressure, and GFR. A number of observations support this hypothesis. Perfusion of the renal distal tubule at increasing flows causes reduction in glomerular blood flow and GFR.[290] Furthermore, as reviewed by Navar and colleagues,[273,291] a variety of experimental maneuvers that cause distal tubule fluid flow to decline or cease induce afferent arteriolar vasodilation and interfere with the normal autoregulatory response. In addition, infusion of furosemide into the macula densa segment of juxtamedullary nephrons significantly abrogated the normal constrictor response of afferent arterioles to increased perfusion pressure,[292] presumably by blocking the uptake of Na^+ and Cl^- from the tubule lumen.[293] A similar observation was made by Takenaka and associates.[259] These studies suggested that the autoregulatory response in juxtamedullary nephrons was dependent mainly on the tubuloglomerular feedback mechanism. Moreover, deletion of the A_1 adenosine receptor gene in mice to block tubuloglomerular feedback results in less efficient autoregulation; this finding, too, is indicative of the role of tubuloglomerular feedback in the autoregulatory response.[294]

To examine the role of tubuloglomerular feedback in autoregulation, investigators have studied spontaneous oscillations in proximal tubule pressure and RBF and the response of the renal circulation to high-frequency oscillations in tubule flow rates or renal perfusion pressure.[295] Oscillations in tubule pressure have been observed in anesthetized rats at a rate of about three cycles per minute that are sensitive to small changes in delivery of fluid to the macula densa.[296] These spontaneous oscillations are eliminated by loop diuretics[297]; such findings are consistent with the hypothesis that they are mediated by the tubuloglomerular feedback response. To examine this hypothesis, Holstein-Rathlou[295] induced sinusoidal oscillations in distal tubule flow in rats at a frequency similar to that of the spontaneous fluctuations in tubule pressure. Varying distal delivery at this rate caused parallel fluctuations in stop-flow pressure (an index of glomerular capillary pressure), probably mediated by alterations in afferent resistance, which, again, was consistent with dynamic regulation of glomerular blood flow by the tubuloglomerular feedback system. To investigate the role of this system in autoregulation, Holstein-Rathlou and colleagues[298] examined the effects of sinusoidal variations in arterial pressure at varying frequencies on RBF in rats. Two separate components of autoregulation were identified: one operating at about the same frequency as the spontaneous fluctuations in tubule pressure (the tubuloglomerular feedback component) and one operating at a much higher frequency, consistent with spontaneous fluctuations in vascular smooth muscle tone (the myogenic component). Subsequently, Flemming and associates[299] reported that renal vascular responses to alterations in renal perfusion pressure varied considerably, depending on the dynamics of the change, and that rapid and slow changes in perfusion pressure could have opposite effects. They suggested that slow pressure changes elicited a predominant tubuloglomerular feedback response, whereas rapid changes invoked the myogenic mechanism.

Despite these observations, the conclusion that the tubuloglomerular feedback system plays a central role in autoregulation is complicated by several factors. One is the process of glomerulotubular balance, by which proximal tubule reabsorption increases as GFR rises. This mechanism tends to blunt the effects of alterations in GFR on distal delivery. In addition, the persistence of autoregulatory behavior in nonfiltering kidneys[300] and in isolated blood vessels suggests that the delivery of filtrate to the distal tubule is not absolutely required for constancy of blood flow, at least in superficial nephrons. In accordance with this view, Just and colleagues[105,301] demonstrated in the conscious dog that although tubuloglomerular feedback contributes to maximum autoregulatory capacity of RBF, autoregulation is observed even when tubuloglomerular feedback is inhibited by furosemide, which is suggestive of an important role for a myogenic mechanism. However, Wang and colleagues[302] found that the myogenic responses of the afferent arterioles are affected by inhibition of the $Na^+/K^+/2Cl^-$ cotransporter with furosemide in the absence of tubuloglomerular feedback. The myogenic and tubuloglomerular feedback mechanisms are not mutually exclusive, and Aukland and Oien[303] proposed a model of renal autoregulation that incorporates both systems. Because the myogenic and tubuloglomerular feedback responses share the same effector site, the afferent arterioles; interactions between these two systems are unavoidable, and each response is capable of modulating the other. The prevailing view is that these two mechanisms act in concert to accomplish the same end, a stabilization of renal function when blood pressure is altered.[277,304] Just[277] suggested that the myogenic component of autoregulation requires less than 10 seconds for completion and normally follows first-order kinetics without rate-sensitive components. The response time for the tubuloglomerular feedback may occur as rapidly as 5 seconds,[260] although some authorities have suggested that it takes 30 to 60 seconds and spontaneous oscillations occur at 0.025 to 0.033 Hz.[277] The myogenic and tubuloglomerular feedback mechanisms account for the majority of the autoregulatory response.[277]

Mechanisms of Tubuloglomerular Feedback Control of Renal Blood Flow and Glomerular Filtration Rate

Several factors have been identified as possible tubular signals for tubuloglomerular feedback.[305] Changes in delivery of Na^+, K^+, and Cl^- are thought to be sensed by the macula densa through the $Na^+/K^+/2Cl^-$ cotransporter (also known as the NKCC2 or BSC1 cotransporter) on the luminal cell membrane of the macula densa cells.[306] Alterations in Na^+, K^+, and Cl^- reabsorption result in inverse changes in SNGFR and renal vascular resistance, primarily in the preglomerular vessels. For instance, when the salt delivery to the distal tubule increases, the feedback mechanism decreases glomerular filtration. Agents such as furosemide that interfere with the Na$^+$/K$^+$/2Cl$^-$ cotransporter in the macula densa cells[293] inhibit the feedback response.[307]

Adenosine, and possibly ATP, plays a central role in mediating the relationship between Na$^+$, K$^+$, and Cl$^-$ transport at the luminal cell membrane of the macula densa and the GFR of the same nephron. This role is illustrated in Figure 3-24.[289] According to this scheme, increased delivery of solute to the macula densa results in concentration-dependent increases in solute uptake by the Na$^+$/K$^+$/2Cl$^-$ cotransporter. This, in turn, stimulates Na$^+$/K$^+$--adenosine triphosphatase (ATPase) activity on the basolateral side of the cells, which leads to the formation of adenosine diphosphate (ADP) and subsequent formation of adenosine monophosphate (AMP). Dephosphorylation of AMP by cytosolic 5′ nucleotidase or endo-5′ nucleotidase bound to the cell membrane yields the formation of adenosine.[289] AMP is extruded into the interstitium, where it is converted to adenosine by ecto-5′ nucleotidases. Once adenosine leaves the macula densa cells, or is formed in the adjacent interstitium, it interacts with adenosine A$_1$ receptors on the extraglomerular mesangial cells, which results in an increase in intracellular calcium concentration ([Ca^{2+}]$_i$).[308] The increase in [Ca^{2+}]$_i$ may occur, in part, through basolateral membrane depolarization via the Cl$^-$ channel, followed by

Ca^{2+} entry into the cells via voltage-gated Ca^{2+} channels.[309] As indicated in Figure 3-25, gap junctions then transmit the calcium transient to the adjacent afferent arterioles, which leads to vasoconstriction.[289] In addition, adenosine can directly constrict the afferent arterioles through calcium release from the sarcoplasmic reticulum, activation of calcium-dependent chloride channels, and influx of calcium through voltage-dependent calcium channels.[310] Macula densa cells may also respond to an increase in luminal sodium chloride concentration ([NaCl]) by releasing ATP at the basolateral cell membrane through ATP-permeable large conductance anion channels, possibly providing a communication link between macula densa cells and adjacent mesangial cells through purinergic receptors on the latter.[311]

Several studies have yielded evidence of the role of adenosine in mediating tubuloglomerular feedback. Intraluminal administration of an adenosine A$_1$ receptor agonist enhances the tubuloglomerular feedback response.[312] In addition, tubuloglomerular feedback is completely absent in adenosine A$_1$ receptor–deficient mice.[313,314] Blocking adenosine A$_1$ receptors, or inhibition of adenosine synthesis through inhibition of 5′-nucleotidase, reduces tubuloglomerular feedback efficiency, and combining the two inhibitors almost completely blocks tubuloglomerular feedback.[315] Addition of adenosine to the afferent arterioles causes vasoconstriction through activation of the adenosine A$_1$ receptor, and addition of an adenosine A$_1$ receptor antagonist blocks both the effects of adenosine and those of high macula densa [NaCl].[316] Of note, these effects occur only when adenosine is added to the extravascular space and do not occur when adenosine is added to the lumen of the macula densa.[316] These results are consistent with the proposed scheme in Figure 3-24, which suggests that an increase in [NaCl] to the macula densa stimulates Na$^+$/K$^+$-ATPase activity, leading to increased adenosine synthesis and followed by constriction of the afferent arterioles via adenosine A$_1$ receptor activation.[316]

Efferent arterioles preconstricted with norepinephrine vasodilate in response to an increase in [NaCl] at the macula densa, an effect blocked with adenosine A$_2$ receptor antagonists but not the adenosine A$_1$ receptor antagonists.[317] The changes in efferent arteriolar resistance are the opposite of those of the afferent arterioles, which vasoconstrict in response to increased [NaCl] at the macula densa.[316,318] The net result is decreased glomerular blood flow, decreased glomerular hydraulic pressure, and a reduction in SNGFR.

Angiotensin appears to be another regulatory factor. Tubuloglomerular feedback is blunted by angiotensin II antagonists and angiotensin II synthesis inhibitors, and tubuloglomerular feedback is absent in mice lacking either the angiotensin II type 1A (AT$_{1A}$) receptor or ACE. Furthermore, systemic infusion of angiotensin II in ACE-knockout mice restores tubuloglomerular feedback.[319-324] Angiotensin II enhances tubuloglomerular feedback via activation of AT$_1$ receptors on the luminal membrane of the macula densa.[325] Acute inhibition of the AT$_1$ receptor in normal mice blocks tubuloglomerular feedback and reduces autoregulatory efficiency.[320] Other studies have demonstrated the interaction of adenosine and angiotensin in feedback mechanisms. In these studies, administration of adenosine A$_1$ receptor antagonist results in decreased afferent arteriolar resistance and increased transcapillary hydraulic pressure differences ($\overline{\Delta P}$), whereas pretreatment with an AT$_1$ receptor antagonist prevented these

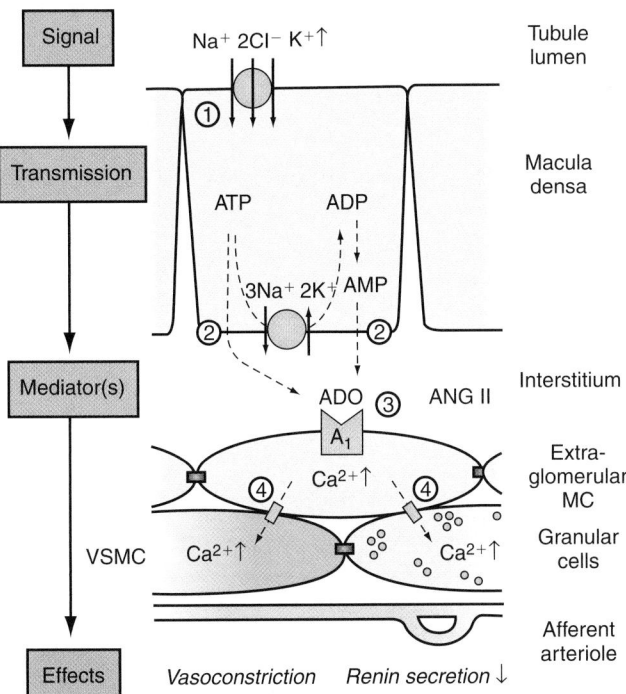

FIGURE 3-24 Proposed mechanism of tubuloglomerular feedback (TGF). The sequence of events (*numbers in circles*) are (1) uptake of Na$^+$, K$^+$, and Cl$^-$ by the Na$^+$/K$^+$/2Cl$^-$ cotransporter on the luminal cell membrane of the macula densa cells; (2) intracellular or extracellular production of adenosine (ADO); (3) ADO activation of adenosine A$_1$ receptors, which triggers an increase in cytosolic Ca^{2+} in extraglomerular mesangial cells (MC); and (4) coupling between extraglomerular MC and granular cells (containing renin) and smooth muscle cells of the afferent arterioles (VSMC) by gap junctions, which allows propagation of the increased intracellular calcium concentration ([Ca^{2+}]$_i$) and thereby results in afferent arteriolar vasoconstriction and inhibition of renin release. Local angiotensin II and neuronal nitric oxide synthase (nNOS) activity modulate the response. (From Vallon V: Tubuloglomerular feedback and the control of glomerular filtration rate, *News Physiol Sci* 2003;18:169-174.)

changes.[326] Although it is known that angiotensin II is not the primary regulator of tubuloglomerular feedback, these results indicate that angiotensin II plays a prominent role in modulating tubuloglomerular feedback and that this response is mediated through the AT_1 receptor, which may also link to the adenosine regulation.

Neuronal nitric oxide synthase (nNOS, or NOS 1) is present in the macula densa.[327] Nitric oxide derived from nNOS in the macula densa provides a vasodilatory influence on tubuloglomerular feedback, decreasing the amount of vasoconstriction of the afferent arterioles that otherwise would occur.[327,328] Increased distal NaCl delivery to the macula densa stimulates nNOS activity and also increases activity of the inducible form of cyclooxygenase-2 (COX-2), which counteracts tubuloglomerular feedback–mediated constriction of the afferent arterioles.[327,328] Macula densa cell pH increases in response to increased luminal sodium concentration and may be related to the stimulation of nNOS.[329] Inhibition of macula densa guanylate cyclase increases the tubuloglomerular feedback response to high luminal [NaCl], which is a further indication of the importance of nitric oxide in modulating tubuloglomerular feedback.[318] Ito and Ren,[186] using an isolated perfused complete JGA preparation, found that microperfusion of the macula densa with an inhibitor of nitric oxide production led to constriction of the adjacent afferent arterioles. When the macula densa was perfused with a low-sodium solution, however, the response was blocked, which indicates that solute reabsorption is required.[186] Microperfusion of the macula densa with the precursor of nitric oxide, L-arginine, blunts tubuloglomerular feedback, especially in salt-depleted animals.[330-332] Therefore, it appears that the afferent arterioles vasodilate acutely in response to nitric oxide, thus blunting tubuloglomerular feedback. An increase in nitric oxide production may also inhibit renin release by increasing cGMP in the granular cells of the afferent arterioles,[333] thereby accentuating its vasodilatory effects. Schnermann and associates,[321] however, reported that when nitric oxide production is chronically blocked in mice lacking nNOS, tubuloglomerular feedback in response to acute perturbations in distal sodium delivery is normal. They did observe that the presence of intact nNOS in the JGA is, nonetheless, required for sodium chloride–dependent renin secretion.[321] The tubuloglomerular feedback system, which elicits vasoconstriction and a reduction in SNGFR in response to acute increases in delivery to the macula densa, appears to secondarily activate a vasodilatory response. Stimulation of nitric oxide production in response to increased distal salt delivery under conditions of volume expansion would be advantageous by resetting tubuloglomerular feedback and limiting tubuloglomerular feedback–mediated vasoconstrictor responses.

Tubuloglomerular feedback responses might be temporally divided into two opposing events. The initial rapid (within seconds) tubuloglomerular feedback response would yield vasoconstriction and a decrease in GFR and $\overline{P}_{GC}$ when sodium delivery out of the proximal tubule is acutely increased. The same increase in delivery would be expected with time (in minutes) to decrease renin secretion, which, in the presence of a continued stimulus such as volume expansion, would reduce angiotensin II production and allow filtration rate to increase, thereby helping to increase urinary excretion rates. The rapid tubuloglomerular feedback system would prevent large changes in GFR under such conditions as spontaneous

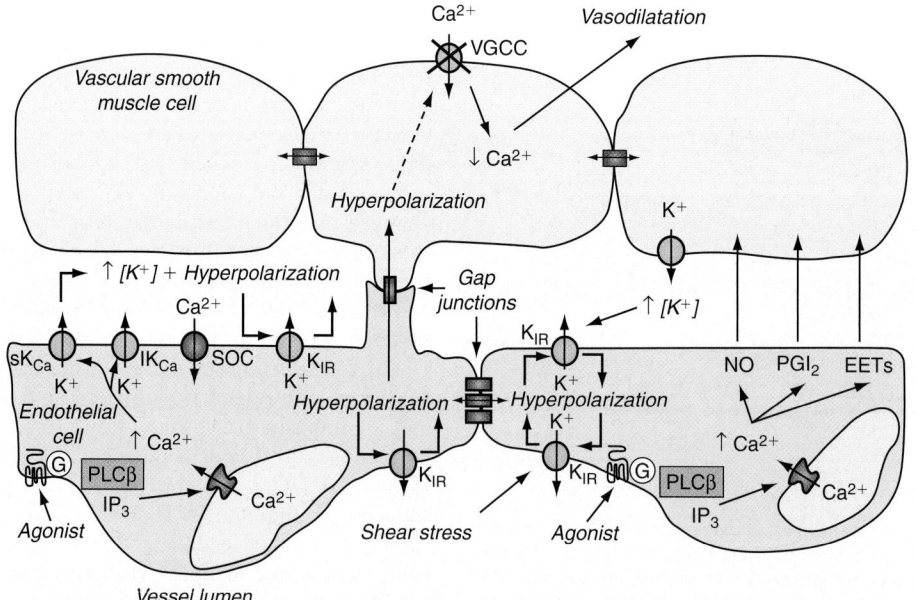

FIGURE 3-25 Potential mechanisms involved in endothelium-dependent vasodilation in response to agonists such as acetylcholine, bradykinin, and adenosine triphosphate (ATP). Coupling of agonists to G-protein–coupled receptors activates the β isoform of protein kinase C (PKC), leading to the production of inositol 1,4,5-trisphosphate (IP_3) with subsequent rapid release of intracellular calcium stores, followed by increased calcium influx through store-operated calcium channels (SOC). Increased intracellular calcium concentration ($[Ca^{2+}]_i$) opens intermediate (IKCa) or small (sKCa) Ca^{2+}-activated K^+ channels, which leads to endothelial cell membrane hyperpolarization. The hyperpolarization may activate inwardly rectifying potassium channels (K^+IR), contributing to the hyperpolarization. Endothelial shear stress may also active these channels. Coupling of endothelial cell hyperpolarization to adjacent vascular smooth muscle cells through gap junctions may then cause closure of voltage-gated calcium channels (VGCC), which leads to a fall in smooth muscle $[Ca^{2+}]_i$ concentration and vasodilation. Agonist-induced increases in endothelial cell $[Ca^{2+}]_i$ also increase production of nitric oxide and of cyclooxygenase- and epoxygenase-derived vasodilator compounds, which, when combined with hyperpolarization, effects smooth muscle vasodilation. (From Jackson WF: Silent inward rectifier K^+ channels in hypercholesterolemia, *Cir Res* 2006;98:982-984.)

fluctuations in blood pressure that might otherwise occur, thereby maintaining tight control of distal sodium delivery in the short term.[321] Schnermann and associates[321] hypothesized that the JGA functions to maintain tight control of distal sodium delivery only for the short term. Over the long term, renin secretion is controlled by the JGA in accordance with the requirements for sodium balance, and the tubuloglomerular feedback system is reset at a new sodium delivery rate.[321] The tubuloglomerular feedback system then continues to operate in accordance with this new set point. The resetting of the tubuloglomerular feedback system may thus be the result of sustained increases in GFR and distal delivery rather than the cause of the resetting.[321,334,335]

Autoregulation Mediated by Metabolic Mechanisms

The metabolic theory predicts that, in view of the relative constancy of tissue metabolism, a decrease in organ blood flow leads to local accumulation of a vasodilator metabolite, which maintains blood flow at or near its previous level, whether in tissues such as muscle or in kidney.[304,336,337] The tubuloglomerular feedback system is affected by compounds that are closely linked to cellular metabolism: ATP and its metabolites ADP and adenosine. These metabolites have important effects on renal vascular smooth muscle and thus may provide a metabolic link to autoregulation through the tubuloglomerular feedback mechanism.[271,338,339]

Other Factors Involved in Autoregulation

Studies have shown that endothelium-dependent factors might play a role in the myogenic response of renal arteries and arterioles to changes in perfusion pressure. For example, in 1992, Hishikawa and associates[340] reported that increased transmural pressure increased nitric oxide release by cultured endothelial cells. In addition, Tojo and colleagues[341] used histochemical techniques to demonstrate the presence of NOS in the macula densa, which suggests that nitric oxide also participates in the tubuloglomerular feedback response. Findings of more recent studies suggest that nitric oxide produced by the macula densa can dampen the tubuloglomerular feedback response.[330] In fact, investigators have examined the role of this endothelial factor in the autoregulatory response. In dogs, inhibition of production of nitric oxide leads to an increase in blood pressure and a decline in basal renal vascular resistance; however, autoregulatory ability is unimpaired.[177] On the other hand, Salom and associates[342] reported that inhibition of nitric oxide production causes a greater decline in RBF in the kidneys of rats perfused at hypertensive pressure than in those perfused with normotensive pressure. This suggests that increased nitric oxide production might modulate the vasoconstrictor response to an increase in perfusion pressure.

Elevations in transmural pressure also increase endothelin release by cultured endothelial cells, and this increase was not altered by the presence of either a calcium channel blocker, nifedipine, or a channel activator, gadolinium.[343] These findings suggest that endothelin, through a mechanism other than extracellular Ca^{2+} influx, may play a role in pressure-induced

control of RBF. Of note, endothelin production is also stimulated by a rise in sheer stress.[219] However, infusions of endothelin produce a prolonged constrictor response that is ill suited to an autoregulatory role,[344] and endothelin acting through ET_A receptors does not seem to play an important role in the autoregulation of RBF.[345]

Other Hormones and Vasoactive Substances Controlling Renal Blood Flow and Glomerular Filtration Rate

Adenosine Nucleotides

Navar[273] proposed that ATP may function as a metabolic regulator of tubuloglomerular feedback and autoregulation of RBF. ATP is present in, and required for the function of, all cells. ATP is released from vascular smooth muscle cells and endothelial cells,[346] as well as from ATP-releasing, or "purinergic," nerve fibers.[346-348] When ATP is released from the nerves or other types of cells into the extracellular space, it activates two types of purinoceptors, the P_{2X} and the P_{2Y} receptors, resulting in vasoconstriction.[349-353] Activation of P_{2X} receptors by ATP leads to increases in $[Ca^{2+}]_i$ through an initial rapid influx via nonselective ligand-gated cation channels, followed by sustained entry through opening of voltage-dependent L-type calcium channels.[351,354,355] ATP also activates P_{2Y} receptors, leading to activation of phospholipase C, formation of inositol 1,4,5-trisphosphate, and mobilization of intracellular calcium stores and thereby promoting vasoconstriction.[350,351,355,356] Superfusion with ATP leads to vasoconstriction of arcuate arteries, interlobular arteries, and the afferent arterioles; effects on the afferent arterioles are stronger and last longer than do those in the other vessels, but ATP does not constrict the efferent arterioles.[351-354,357] ATP promotes a transient vasoconstriction in the arcuate and interlobular arteries, which is followed by a gradual return to control diameter.[354] In the afferent arterioles, ATP induces a rapid initial vasoconstriction (vessel diameter ≈70% smaller than control diameter), which is followed by a gradual relaxation to a final diameter still at least 10% smaller than control diameter.[354] This suggests that the vasoconstrictor effects of ATP may be more prolonged in the afferent arterioles than in other preglomerular vessels. These results are indicative of a unique role for ATP in the selective control of preglomerular resistance.

Despite the ability of ATP to promote vasoconstriction when applied from the extravascular side of the blood vessel,[351-354,357] intrarenal infusion of ATP leads to renal vasodilation rather than vasoconstriction.[149,272] ATP from the luminal side of the blood vessel activates P_{2Y} receptors on vascular endothelial cells, which leads to increased synthesis and release of nitric oxide, as well as stimulation of the production of prostacyclin, and vasodilation results.[149,272] The net effect of ATP on renal vascular resistance in vivo may depend on whether the ATP is delivered from the blood side or the interstitial side, and nitric oxide and prostacyclin production stimulated by ATP in the endothelium may modulate any direct vasoconstrictive effects of this compound on the renal circulation.[351-354,357] Thus ATP serves as a metabolic regulator of RBF and GFR. Majid and associates[271] found that infusion of ATP in large enough amounts to saturate the P_2 receptors completely blocked autoregulation, which was then fully restored after discontinuation of the ATP infusion. Interstitial levels of ATP decrease with reductions in perfusion pressure, which would cause a decrease in ATP-induced preglomerular vasoconstriction.[358] These results thus suggest that ATP-mediated effects on autoregulation are significant.

ADP also may play a role in the control of RBF and GFR. ADP acts as a vasodilator by activating ATP-sensitive potassium (K_{ATP}) channels, which results in membrane hyperpolarization, whereas ATP closes the channel, which results in membrane depolarization.[359-361] When intracellular ATP levels are decreased and ADP concentrations are increased (as in the state of glycolysis inhibition), vasodilation occurs,[361,362] which suggests that either ADP concentration or the ATP/ADP ratio, or both, plays a significant role in regulating renal vascular tone. Exogenous ADP does not affect the renal vasculature,[361] but alterations in intracellular ADP concentrations may play an important role in modulating renal vascular resistance and glomerular ultrafiltration by its effects on the K_{ATP} channel. The vasodilation induced by ADP is, at least in part, endothelium dependent.[359] These data suggest that ADP has a potential role in the metabolic control of renal hemodynamics and autoregulation, but further studies are needed.

Adenosine

The metabolism of ATP or cAMP generates the purinergic agonist adenosine, which binds to the P_1 class of purinergic receptors that bind adenosine preferentially over ATP, ADP, or AMP.[346,363,364] Four subtypes of membrane bound G protein–coupled adenosine receptors of the P_1 class have been identified: A_1, A_{2a}, A_{2b}, and A_3.[346,365,366] Low levels of adenosine (nanomolar concentrations) activate adenosine A_1 receptors, which results in inhibition of adenylate cyclase activity, mobilization of intracellular Ca^{2+}, and vasoconstriction, whereas activation of either adenosine A_{2a} or A_{2b} receptor by higher adenosine levels (micromolar concentrations) stimulates adenylate cyclase activity and promotes vasorelaxation.[365,367-369] Intracellular adenosine formation is an important component in the macula densa cells for tubuloglomerular feedback control of GFR (see later discussion) and thus is involved in that component of autoregulation. Delivery of solute to the macula densa cells increases $Na^+/K^+/2Cl^-$ transport at the luminal cell membrane, which leads to increased basolateral Na^+/K^+-ATPase activity and the formation of ADP. Conversion of ADP to AMP by intracellular PDE and subsequently to adenosine by intracellular 5'-nucleotidase results in adenosine formation, with subsequent effects on vascular tone and renin production of the adjacent arterioles, as described in the earlier section "Autoregulation Mediated by Tubuloglomerular Feedback." An additional pathway leading to adenosine production is the transport of intracellular cAMP to the extracellular compartment, which leads to the production of adenosine by membrane-bound ectophosphodiesterase and ecto-5'-nucleotidase.[365,368,370] This extracellular adenosine may then directly regulate vascular tone through interaction with vascular adenosine receptors and indirectly affect tone by inhibition of renin release from juxtaglomerular cells through

activation of adenosine A_1 receptors[80,371] (the "adenosine brake" hypothesis) to block production of the vasoconstrictor angiotensin II.[326,365,370,372]

Intravenous infusion of adenosine results in a transient renal vasoconstriction followed by vasodilation and an increase in RBF.[373,374] The initial vasoconstriction is potentiated, and the duration of the contraction prolonged by nitric oxide inhibition, which suggests that at least a portion of the recovery from adenosine-induced renal vasoconstriction is mediated by increases in nitric oxide production,[374] and, indeed, adenosine stimulates nitric oxide production in vascular endothelial cells.[369] Both adenosine A_1 and A_{2b} receptors are present in afferent and efferent arterioles, and activation of the adenosine A_1 receptor by low concentrations of adenosine results in vasoconstriction of these vessels, whereas activation of the adenosine A_{2b} receptors by high concentrations of adenosine results in vasodilation.[100,357,375,376] Selective blockade of the adenosine A_{2a} receptors significantly augmented the vasoconstrictor response of the arterioles to adenosine, which indicates that adenosine-mediated vasoconstriction is modified by vasodilatory influences of adenosine A_{2a} receptor activation.[375]

Adenosine A_1 receptors in the afferent arterioles are selectively activated from the interstitial side; the result is vasoconstriction, which suggests that adenosine has a paracrine role in the control of GFR.[373] Vasoconstriction of the afferent and efferent arterioles in response to addition of adenosine to the bathing solution is prevented by adenosine receptor blockade.[377] Adenosine concentrations in cortical and medullary interstitial fluid averaged 23 and 55 nmol/L, respectively, in animals on a low-sodium (0.15%) diet and increased markedly to 418 and 1040 nmol/L in the cortex and medulla, respectively in rats on a high-salt (4%) diet.[378] High adenosine levels under conditions of a high-salt diet may contribute to a decrease in macula densa–mediated reductions in renin secretion.[379] Intravenous infusion of adenosine in conscious, healthy humans results in a decrease in GFR with only slight (nonsignificant) declines in RPF,[380] whereas administration of a selective adenosine A_1 antagonist produces increases in GFR[381]; under normal circumstances, adenosine concentrations may be low enough to activate the vasoconstrictor response through adenosine A_1 receptors, but activation of adenosine A_{2a} receptors provides counteracting vasodilation. Glomerular mesangial cells constrict in response to adenosine via adenosine A_1 receptors.[308] In view of the effects of adenosine on the mesangial cell, an adenosine-induced decrease in GFR may be related, in part, to a decrease in the glomerular capillary ultrafiltration coefficient (K_f). Specific adenosine A_1 receptor antagonists block tubuloglomerular feedback–mediated reductions in glomerular pressure in response to increases in delivery of fluid out of the proximal tubule; this suggests that at least part of the vasoconstrictor effect of adenosine is mediated through the tubuloglomerular feedback loop and thus might affect autoregulation.[382] Because of the link between local adenosine concentrations and the divergent hemodynamic responses that can result, adenosine plays an important role in the control of RBF and GFR. Data from genetically altered mice indicates that tubuloglomerular feedback control of GFR and RBF starts with the transcellular NaCl transport across the macula densa in association with the generation of adenosine through the dephosphorylation of ATP that, in conjunction with angiotensin II, elicits afferent arteriolar constriction.[306]

Arachidonic Acid Metabolites

Prostaglandins

Processing of linoleic acid (an essential polyunsaturated fatty acid in the diet) by the liver yields arachidonic acid, which is then stored in membrane phospholipids. After interaction of a variety of hormones and vasoactive substances with their membrane receptors, phospholipase A_2 is activated, which causes the release of arachidonic acid from the cell membranes, allowing the enzymatic action of cyclooxygenase to process arachidonic acid into prostaglandins G_2 (PGG_2) and, subsequently, H_2 (PGH_2). PGH_2 is then converted into a number of biologically active prostaglandins, including PGE_2 and PGI_2 (also known as prostacyclin); prostaglandins $F_2\alpha$ ($PGF_2\alpha$), E_1 (PGE_1), and D_2 (PGD_2); and thromboxane (see Chapter 13).

PGE_1, PGE_2, and PGI_2 are vasodilator prostaglandins that generally increase RPF and yet produce little or no increase in GFR and SNGFR, in part because of a large decline in K_f.[383-385] During blockade of endogenous prostaglandin production, infusion of PGE_2 or PGI_2 induces large declines in SNGFR and Q_A, which are accompanied by an increase in renal vascular resistance (particularly R_E), increases in $\overline{P}_{GC}$ and $\overline{\Delta P}$, and a decline in K_f.[386] Additional blockade of angiotensin II receptors during cyclooxygenase inhibition yields marked vasodilation in response to PGE_2 or PGI_2, which results in a return of SNGFR and Q_A to control values or higher, a fall in $\overline{P}_{GC}$ below control values, and a return of K_f to normal.[386] Thus, the renal vasoconstriction induced by exogenous PGE_2 or PGI_2 appears to be mediated by induction of renin and angiotensin II production. Vasodilation at the whole kidney level that results from PGI_2 infusion during cyclooxygenase and angiotensin II inhibition has not always been observed.[387] Topical (but not luminal) application of PGE_2 to the afferent arterioles increased the vasoconstrictive effect of angiotensin II and norepinephrine, whereas PGI_2 attenuated only norepinephrine-induced vasoconstriction.[388] PGE_2 also constricted interlobular arteries, but neither PGE_2 nor PGI_2 produced vasodilation of vessels preconstricted by angiotensin II.[388] Indomethacin alone induced vasoconstriction of all preglomerular and postglomerular resistance vessels of superficial and juxtamedullary nephrons, which suggests that vasodilatory prostaglandins normally modulate endogenous vasoconstrictors.[389] However, there appear to be gender-dependent differences in mechanisms, inasmuch as indomethacin treatment results in net renal vasodilation in female rats.[390] The combination of cyclooxygenase inhibition with an ACE inhibitor caused vasodilation of preglomerular but not postglomerular vessels of the cortical nephrons as a result of the effects of continued nitric oxide production on preglomerular vessels.[389] These data together indicate that there could indeed be differences between superficial and deep nephrons in their responses to vasoactive prostaglandins.

Leukotrienes and Lipoxins

Leukotrienes are a class of lipid products formed from arachidonic acid. Leukotrienes known to affect glomerular filtration and RBF are LTC_4, LTD_4, and leukotriene B_4 (LTB_4). LTC_4 and LTD_4 are potent vasoconstrictors,[391] whereas LTB_4 produces moderate renal vasodilation and an increase in RBF with no change in GFR in the normal rat.[392] Intravenous infusion of LTC_4 increases renal vascular resistance, thereby leading to a fall in RBF and GFR, as well as a decrease in plasma volume and cardiac output.[393,394] The decline in RBF is partially but not completely reversed by the peptide saralasin (an angiotensin II receptor antagonist) and indomethacin (an inhibitor of cyclooxygenase), which indicates that (1) angiotensin II and cyclooxygenase products are involved in the response to LTC_4 and (2) LTC_4 has an additional direct effect on the renal resistance vessels.[393] Similarly, LTD_4 induces a marked decrease in K_f; a rise in renal vascular resistance, particularly in R_E; a fall in Q_A and SNGFR; and a rise in $\overline{P}_{GC}$ and $\overline{\Delta P}$ during blockade of angiotensin II and control of renal perfusion pressure. These findings demonstrate a direct effect of this leukotriene on renal hemodynamics.[395]

Inflammatory injury also activates the 5-, 12-, and 15-lipoxygenase pathways in neutrophils and platelets to form acyclic eicosanoids called lipoxins, of which there are two main types: lipoxins A_4 and B_4 (LXA_4 and LXB_4).[396] The lipoxins produce diverse effects on renal hemodynamics. LXB_4 and 7-*cis*-11-*trans*-LXA_4 produce renal vasoconstriction.[397] In contrast, intrarenal infusion of LXA_4 induces a marked reduction in preglomerular arteriolar resistance (R_A) without affecting R_E, thereby resulting in increases in $\overline{P}_{GC}$ and $\overline{\Delta P}$.[395] The specific vasodilation of the preglomerular vessels by LXA_4 was blocked by cyclooxygenase inhibition, which indicates that vasodilatory prostaglandins were responsible for this effect.[395,397] A finding that was unique to this compound was that LXA_4 produced vasodilation while simultaneously causing a reduction in K_f.[397] Because $\overline{P}_{GC}$, $\overline{\Delta P}$, and Q_A were increased, however, SNGFR also increased.[395] Furthermore, transfection of rat kidney with the 15-lipoxygenase gene suppressed inflammation and preserved function in experimental glomerulonephritis.[398]

Miscellaneous Factors

Norepinephrine

Systemic infusion of norepinephrine increases arterial blood pressure and induces vasoconstriction of the preglomerular vessels and the efferent arterioles, which result in a decrease in Q_A, but the effects on K_f are unknown.[399] P_{GC} and ΔP increase with norepinephrine infusion, however, so that SNGFR is relatively unchanged.[399] Like angiotensin II, norepinephrine constricts the arcuate artery, the interlobular arteries, and the afferent and efferent arterioles, as well as mesangial cells.[107,108,266,388,399,400] Vasoconstriction of the afferent and efferent arterioles occurs through activation of α_1 receptors.[401] This is partially counterbalanced, however, by activation of COX-2 to increase production of the PGE_2 and $PGF_2\alpha$.[400]

Acetylcholine

Acetylcholine is a potent vasodilator that increases RBF without changing SNGFR.[342,383,402] The interlobular arteries and afferent and efferent arterioles vasodilate in response to acetylcholine, and the effects can be prevented by muscarinic receptor antagonists.[383,402,403] In one study, as a consequence of the decrease in renal vascular resistance, Q_A increased in response to acetylcholine in the rat, as did $\overline{\Delta P}$ (R_A decreased more than R_E, so that $\overline{P}_{GC}$ and $\overline{\Delta P}$ increased), and yet SNGFR remained unchanged because of a marked decline in K_f.[383]

Acetylcholine-induced renal and systemic vasodilation is mediated in part through the stimulation of nitric oxide production,[138,164,187,266,342,404-406] enhanced production of vasodilatory prostaglandins,[157,342,407] and production of a putative endothelium-derived hyperpolarizing factor (EDHF) that hyperpolarizes adjacent vascular smooth muscle.[148,370,407-411] Figure 3-25 summarizes the mechanisms by which a number of vasodilators, including acetylcholine and bradykinin, might lead to vasodilation. Acetylcholine acts on muscarinic receptors of the endothelium to increase endothelial $[Ca^{2+}]_i$, which causes Ca^{2+}-activated K^+ channels to open and hyperpolarization of endothelial membrane.[412] By way of myoendothelial gap junctions, hyperpolarization of adjacent smooth muscle cells results in closure of voltage-gated Ca^{2+} channels, a decrease in $[Ca^{2+}]_i$, and vasodilation.[409,412] The increase in endothelial $[Ca^{2+}]_i$ after stimulation of the muscarinic receptors also triggers the production of nitric oxide and prostanoids in the endothelium, which hyperpolarize the underlying smooth muscle by activation of ATP-sensitive K^+ channels.[148] Thus acetylcholine can stimulate three endothelium-dependent vasodilation pathways: the production of vasodilatory prostaglandins, the production of nitric oxide, and the production of EDHF.[413]

Bradykinin

Bradykinin is a potent vasodilator that produces large increases in RBF as a result of dilation of both the preglomerular blood vessels and the efferent arterioles, mediated through the bradykinin B_2 receptor.[383,414-416] Although in the rat bradykinin had no significant effects on $\overline{\Delta P}$, the increase in Q_A that might be expected to cause an increase SNGFR failed to do so because K_f fell to levels of half those seen in normal rats.[383] Figure 3-25 summarizes potential mechanisms of bradykinin-induced vasodilation. Bradykinin stimulates inositol 1,4,5-trisphosphate production and increased cytosolic free $[Ca^{2+}]$ in cultured mesangial cells, glomerular epithelial cells, and vascular endothelial cells.[265,389,417,418] Subsequent activation of Ca^{2+}-dependent potassium channels and activation of chloride channels leads to membrane depolarization and relaxation.[157,419-421] In the rat,[403] low concentrations of bradykinin induce vasodilation of isolated afferent and efferent arterioles that is mediated by bradykinin B_2 receptors.[389] In the rabbit, low concentrations of bradykinin (10^{-12} to 10^{-10} mol/L) dilate the afferent arterioles through B_2 receptor activation, whereas high concentrations (10^{-9} to 10^{-8} mol/L) result in vasoconstriction.[416] In contrast, high concentrations of bradykinin cause vasodilation of the efferent arterioles in the rabbit.[416] Vasoconstriction of the afferent arterioles to high concentrations of bradykinin appears to be mediated through vasoconstrictor prostanoids.[422] Bradykinin-induced vasodilation of the afferent arterioles is mediated by cyclooxygenase vasodilator products, including PGE_2 and epoxyeicosatrienoic acids (EETs), through increased epoxygenase activity.[423] Retrograde perfusion of the efferent arterioles with bradykinin, acting at B_2 receptors, results in a dose-dependent vasodilation that is independent of either nitric oxide or cyclooxygenase metabolites.[422] Thus the vasodilator effects in that segment under such conditions are mediated by cytochrome P450 metabolites, probably EETs.[422] In the absence of cyclooxygenase inhibitors, bradykinin infused in an orthograde manner through the afferent arterioles induces the glomerular release of a vasoconstrictor (20-hydroxyeicosatetraenoic acid [20-HETE]) that blunts the vasodilator effects of bradykinin-induced release of EETs from the efferent arterioles and glomerulus.[424]

Insulin

Insulin, necessary for tissue glucose metabolism, is also a vasoactive hormone important in the regulation of blood pressure and GFR.[425] Insulin is a vasodilator in the systemic and renal vasculature, acting in part through a stimulation of nitric oxide formation.[425-429] Glomerular hyperfiltration occurs in response to the infusion of L-arginine, and this response to L-arginine occurs in conjunction with an increase in both nitric oxide and insulin production.[430] When insulin release is blocked with octreotide, the increase in GFR in response to L-arginine is blocked. In the presence of octreotide plus an AT_1 receptor blocker, the response to L-arginine was restored, which suggested that the relationship between several hormonal systems was complex.[430] Vasodilation in response to insulin can still take place during inhibition of nitric oxide synthesis, however, and this effect is mediated in part through increased production of the metabolite adenosine.[431] In normal rats, acute insulin infusion (during euglycemic clamp) decreases preglomerular and efferent arteriolar resistance, causing increases in Q_A, SNGFR, and $\overline{\Delta P}$.[432]

Early insulin-dependent diabetes is characterized by high rates of RBF and glomerular filtration caused, in part, by elevations in levels of atrial natriuretic peptide and vasodilatory prostaglandins.[432,433] Insulin administration in diabetic animals produces preglomerular vasoconstriction rather than the vasodilation seen in normal animals; the results are decreases in Q_A, $\overline{P}_{GC}$, $\overline{\Delta P}$, and SNGFR.[432] The increase in preglomerular resistance observed after insulin infusion in diabetic animals could be related to a stimulation of vasoconstrictor prostaglandin (thromboxane A_2) and endothelin production, which might obviate any vasodilatory effects of insulin.[198,432]

Insulin-like Growth Factor

IGF is produced as two peptide hormones, IGF-I and IGF-II, which, upon secretion, are more than 99% bound to IGF-binding proteins that regulate the bioavailability of IGFs.[434] IGF-I is produced in several portions of the nephron, including mesangial cells, which also contain IGF-I receptors.[434,435] High dietary protein intake (which increases GFR) increases IGF-I production and increases the bioavailability of the peptide, whereas decreased protein intake or fasting decreases IGF-I production and increases binding protein levels.[434] The response to IGF-I overload is vasodilation of preglomerular blood vessels and the efferent arterioles, which leads to increases in GFR and RPF.[177,436-439] Administration of IGF-I to either nonstarved rats (after a 12-hour food restriction) or in rats with short-term starvation (after a 60- to 72-hour food restriction), which would have low levels of circulating IGF-I, resulted in increases in SNGFR and Q_A.[436] The increase in SNGFR was a consequence of the large increases in Q_A and a near doubling of K_f, inasmuch as $\overline{P}_{GC}$ and $\overline{\Delta P}$ were unaffected by IGF-I.[436] Increases in vasodilatory prostaglandin levels and nitric oxide production, combined with stimulation of the renal kalikrein-kinin system, are largely responsible for the renal vasodilation induced by IGF-I.[436,439,440] Inhibition of the effects of angiotensin II by IGF-I[125] may be responsible for the increase in K_f observed with IGF-I infusions.[436]

Natriuretic Peptides

Increased left atrial pressure, such as that induced by blood volume expansion, leads to natriuresis and diuresis[441,442] as a result of release of an atrial natriuretic peptide (ANP).[443] ANP is synthesized as part of a larger (151–amino acid) prepro-hormone (preproANP) and is stored in the atria as a high–molecular weight 126–amino acid precursor, proANP.[444] Upon release from the atria, proANP is cleaved into two polypeptides, including the 28–amino acid active form of the peptide ANP.[444] Other ANP-like natriuretic compounds include brain natriuretic peptide (BNP) and two ANP-like natriuretic peptides produced by the kidney, one a natriuretic peptide known as urodilatin that contains 32 amino acids[419,445] and the other a C-type natriuretic peptide (C-ANP).[446,447] Receptors for ANP have been identified in the glomerulus,[448] the arcuate and interlobular arteries, and the afferent and efferent arterioles.[449] ANP type A receptors mediate the vascular response to ANP in the afferent and efferent arterioles, but ANP binds to both ANP type A and ANP type C receptors.[449] The biologic effects of urodilatin are mediated by cGMP after interaction with an ANP type A receptor; C-ANP binds to both ANP types C and B receptors but exerts its effects only through the ANP type B receptor, located primarily in the glomerulus, the afferent arterioles, and distal portions of the nephron.[125,446,447,449] The C-ANP dilates afferent arterioles via a prostaglandin–nitric oxide pathway. A third type of ANP receptor, the ANP type C receptor, serves to clear natriuretic peptides with no vasoactive effects.[449] ANP stimulates secretion of urodilatin, which causes large increases in circulating urodilatin.[450] Glomerular ANP receptor density is downregulated in rats on a high-salt diet and upregulated in rats on a low-salt diet.[448,451] ANP stimulates nitric oxide production and increases guanylate cyclase activity and cGMP production in the kidney.[404]

As a result of acute and chronic blood volume expansion and increased atrial pressure, plasma levels of ANP and BNP increase.[452-455] In response to exogenous ANP, systemic blood pressure decreases, and GFR, filtration fraction, and salt and water excretion increase.[452,455,456] Studies in the hydronephrotic kidney preparation demonstrated increased glomerular blood flow in a dose-dependent manner in response to both ANP and urodilatin.[389] In the euvolemic rat, pretreatment with an ANP receptor antagonist resulted in a significantly lower GFR during subsequent ANP infusion than was observed in control rats receiving vehicle before the ANP infusion,[433,457] which again suggests that ANP has a role in the control of GFR in the normal rat. Renal hemodynamics are not altered by ANP antibody administration or ANP receptor antagonists in rats with myocardial infarction or congestive heart failure.[452,458] ANP receptor antagonists decreased GFR in deoxycorticosterone acetate (DOCA)–salt hypertension, a model associated with elevated ANP and BNP levels.[453] In diabetic animals that already had elevated baseline values of GFR and RPF, infusion of ANP antibodies reduced GFR toward normal levels, which indicates that high endogenous ANP contributes to hyperfiltration in early diabetes.[454,459] The effect of natriuretic peptide inhibition on GFR and RPF is greatest under conditions of high levels of endogenous natriuretic peptides such as chronic high sodium intake.[454,459] Elevated PGI_2 and PGE_2 production also contribute to the hyperfiltration seen in diabetes.[454,460]

As shown in Figure 3-26, ANP increases SNGFR without altering Q_A in the rat, which results in an increase in filtration fraction.[68] ANP has a property unique among vasoactive agents: it induces preglomerular vasodilation (arcuate arteries, interlobular arteries, and afferent arterioles) but efferent arteriolar vasoconstriction.[68,389,446,449] As a consequence, $\overline{P}_{GC}$ and $\overline{\Delta P}$ increased with little effect on K_f, which indicates that the increase in SNGFR was almost entirely the consequence of the increase in ΔP.[68] The preglomerular vasodilation and efferent arteriolar constriction occurred even when angiotensin II receptors were blocked or renal perfusion pressure was controlled.[68]

Urodilatin also produces effects similar to those of ANP: dose-dependent vasodilation of the arcuate and interlobular arteries and afferent arterioles, vasoconstriction of the efferent arterioles, and a net increase in glomerular blood flow in both cortical and juxtamedullary nephrons.[389] Low doses of urodilatin inhibit the renin-angiotensin system, whereas high concentrations activate it, leading to effects on RPF and GFR that vary depending on the dose used.[389,433,461,462] ACE inhibition, the combination of ACE inhibition with cyclooxygenase inhibition, or endothelin receptor blockade reduced the urodilatin-induced vasodilation of the preglomerular vessels.[389] Urodilatin-induced vasoconstriction of the efferent arterioles is exaggerated by nitric oxide blockade and is completely blocked by combined angiotensin II and cyclooxygenase inhibition, by bradykinin receptor blockade, and by endothelin blockade.[389] C-ANP induces dose-dependent vasodilation of both the preglomerular and postglomerular vessels and a large increase in RBF.[449]

In addition to the various hormones and vasoactive substances discussed in the preceding sections, many others also affect GFR and RBF. Some of these are summarized in Table 3-1.

Neural Regulation of Glomerular Filtration Rate

The renal vasculature, including the afferent and efferent arterioles, the macula densa cells of the distal tubule, and the glomerular mesangium, are richly innervated.[87,463] Innervation includes renal efferent sympathetic adrenergic nerves[463,464] and renal afferent sensory fibers containing peptides such as CGRP and substance P.[87,463] Acetylcholine is a potent vasodilator of the renal vasculature (discussed previously), and so circulating acetylcholine has a potential role in the control of the renal circulation. Sympathetic efferent nerves are found in all segments of the vascular tree from the main renal artery to the afferent arterioles (including the renin-containing juxtaglomerular cells) and the efferent arterioles[464,465] and play an important role in the regulation of renal hemodynamics, sodium transport, and renin secretion.[466] Afferent nerves containing CGRP and substance P are localized primarily in the main renal artery and interlobar arteries; some innervation is also observed in the arcuate arteries, the interlobular arteries, and the afferent arterioles, including the JGA.[464,465] Peptidergic nerve fibers immunoreactive for neuropeptide Y, neurotensin, vasoactive intestinal polypeptide, and somatostatin are also found in the kidney.[76] Neurons immunoreactive to nNOS have been identified in the kidney.[463,465] The

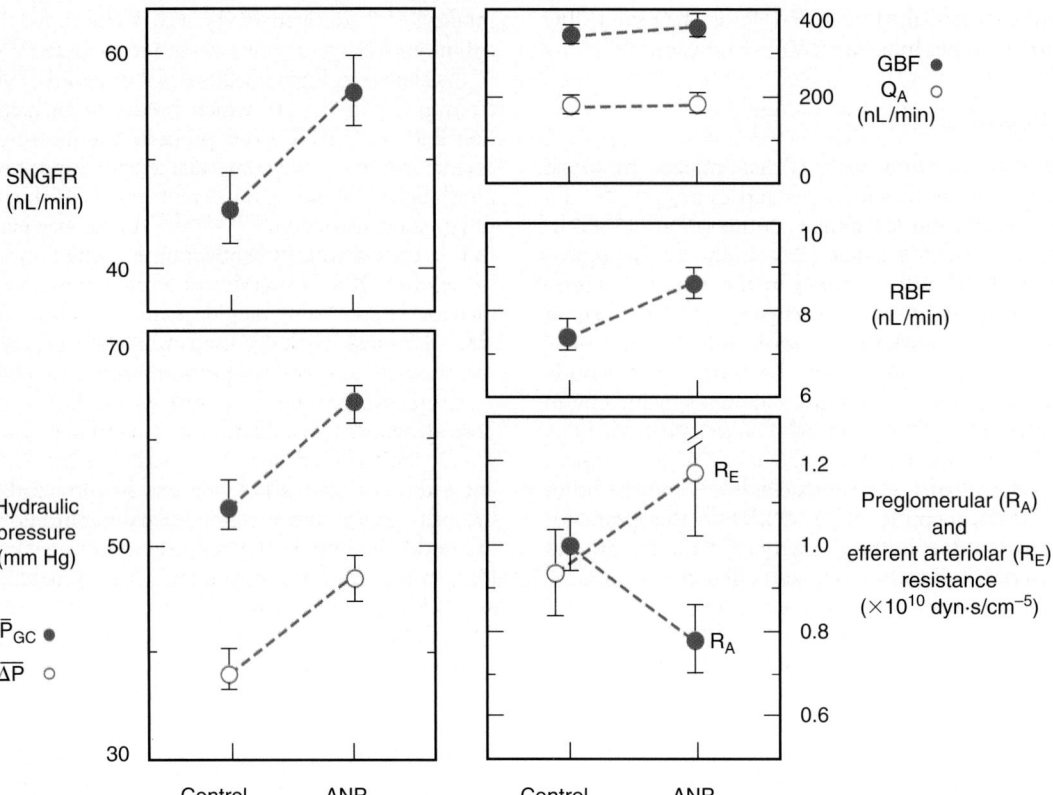

FIGURE 3-26 Effects of atrial natriuretic peptide (ANP) on glomerular hemodynamics in the euvolemic Munich-Wistar rat. During the control period, renal perfusion pressure was lowered slightly by aortic constriction to yield pressures observed after ANP infusion (95 to 100 mm Hg). GBF, glomerular blood flow; RBF, whole-kidney (renal) blood flow. (Data [mean ± standard error] from Dunn BR, Ichikawa I, Pfeffer JM, et al: Renal and systemic hemodynamic effects of synthetic atrial natriuretic peptide in the anesthetized rat, *Circ Res* 1986;59:237-246.)

TABLE 3-1   Additional Substances That Affect Renal Hemodynamics and Glomerular Ultrafiltration

VASOACTIVE SUBSTANCE	RENAL EFFECTS	REFERENCES
Adrenomedullin (ADM)	Intra-renal infusion increases RBF and GFR through interaction with CGRP receptors, ADM-specific binding sites, or both.	481-487
Calcitonin gene–related peptide (CGRP)	Infusion causes increase of RBF and GFR; effect is probably mediated through nitric oxide production and possibly increases of cAMP	488-492
Dopamine	Low dose increases GFR and RBF by stimulating cAMP production after activation of dopamine receptors Appears to dilate both afferent and efferent arterioles	493,494
Parathyroid hormone (PTH)	Intrarenal infusion increases RBF; effects on GFR vary as a result of secondary release of counteracting substances that yield dose-dependent effects on K_f and $\overline{\Delta P}$	386,495-501
Parathyroid hormone-related protein (PTHrP)	Intrarenal infusion at low doses increases RBF and GFR, with preferential vasodilator effect in preglomerular vessels	495,499,502-507
Platelet-activating factor (PAF)	Intrarenal infusion at low doses increases RBF through enhanced nitric oxide Infusion at higher doses decreases flow, K_f and SNGFR, possibly through increased thromboxane and angiotensin II production	159,344,508-511
Relaxin	May be involved in alterations of renal hemodynamics during pregnancy Infusion increases RBF and GFR, possibly through effects on endothelial factors	512-515
Vasopressin (also known as antidiuretic hormone [ADH])	Variable effects on renal hemodynamics Infusion may produce vasodilation of arterioles and increase of RBF mediated by V_2 receptors or constriction of arterioles mediated by V_1 receptors Complex effects on GFR, which typically increases during infusion as a result of increase of $\overline{\Delta P}$, despite decrease of K_f.	516-524

cAMP, Cyclic adenosine monophosphate; *GFR,* glomerular filtration rate; *K_f,* glomerular capillary ultrafiltration coefficient; $\overline{\Delta P}$, transcapillary hydraulic pressure gradient; *RBF,* renal blood flow; *SNGFR,* single-nephron glomerular filtration rate.

NOS-containing neuronal somata are seen in the wall of the renal pelvis, at the renal hilus close to the renal artery, along the interlobar arteries and the arcuate arteries, and extending to the afferent arterioles, which suggests that they have a role in the control of RBF.[463,465] They are also present in nerve bundles that have vasomotor and sensory fibers; therefore, they might modulate renal neural function.[463,465]

In micropuncture studies of the effects of renal nerve stimulation (RNS), RNS alone increased R_A and R_E, which resulted in a fall in Q_A and SNGFR without any effect on K_f.[467] When prostaglandin production was inhibited by indomethacin, however, the same level of RNS produced even greater increases in R_A and R_E, accompanied by very large declines in Q_A and SNGFR and decreases in K_f, $\overline{P}_{GC}$, and $\overline{\Delta P}$.[467] When saralasin was administered as a competitive inhibitor of endogenous angiotensin II in conjunction with indomethacin, RNS had no effect on K_f, but both R_A and R_E were still increased, and ΔP was slightly reduced.[467] Release of norepinephrine by RNS enhances angiotensin II production to yield arteriolar vasoconstriction and reduction in K_f. The increase in angiotensin II production may then enhance vasodilator prostaglandin production,[467,468] which partially ameliorates the constriction. Continued vasoconstriction by RNS during blockade of endogenous prostaglandins and angiotensin II suggests that norepinephrine has separate vasoconstrictive properties by itself. In agreement with this suggestion are the findings that norepinephrine causes constriction of preglomerular vessels.[109] Inhibition of NOS results in a decline in SNGFR in normal rats but not in rats with surgical renal denervation; this finding, in turn, suggests that nitric oxide normally modulates the effects of renal adrenergic activity.[469] This modulation does not appear, however, to be related to sympathetic modulation of renin secretion.[470]

Renal denervation in animals undergoing acute water deprivation (48-hour duration) or with congestive heart failure produces increases in SNGFR, Q_A, and K_f.[471] The natural activity of the renal nerves in these settings may thus play an important role in the constriction of the arterioles and reduction in K_f that were observed.[471] The vasoconstrictive effects of the renal nerves in both settings were mediated in part by a stimulatory effect on angiotensin II release, together with a direct vasoconstrictive effect on the preglomerular and postglomerular blood vessels.[471] These studies demonstrate the important role of the renal nerves in pathophysiologic settings.

Obesity-Linked Glomerular Hyperfiltration

Nondiabetic humans who were severely obese (body mass index > 38) were found to have increased values of GFR and RPF—51% and 31%, respectively, above that in normal body-weight subjects (body mass index ≈ 22; see Figure 3-13)—accompanied by an increase in filtration fraction, hypertension, and insulin resistance.[472] Both GFR and RPF are also increased in either normotensive or hypertensive nondiabetic patients with mild to moderate obesity,[473-475] in addition to increases in cardiac output and total blood volume.[474] The increase in GFR in the obese patients was correlated with increased protein intake, as estimated from the urinary excretion of urea.[475] Hall and colleagues[476] induced obesity in dogs through a diet supplemented with high fat, resulting in a 50% increase in body weight in 5 weeks. As in obese humans, GFR and RPF increased markedly and were accompanied by sodium retention, hypertension, increased cardiac output, and increased extracellular fluid volume.[476] Glomerular hemodynamics have been examined by micropuncture in the young obese Zucker rat (hydropenic), and no differences in P_{GC} (measured by the stop-flow technique) or $\overline{\Delta P}$ were observed in comparison with values in lean Zucker rats (Figure 3-27),

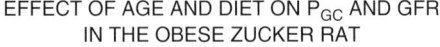

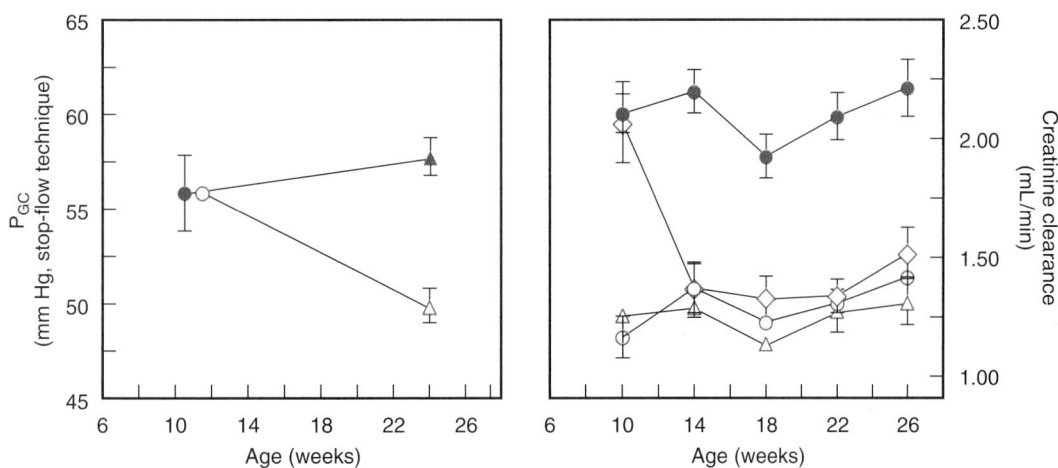

FIGURE 3-27 Glomerular capillary hydraulic pressure (by stop-flow technique) as a function of age in anesthetized obese and lean Zucker rats (*left*). Data from young lean rats are represented by *open circles,* and data from young obese rats are represented by *filled circles* (these data obtained from O'Donnell and colleagues[477]). Data from older lean rats are represented by *open triangles,* and data from older obese rats are represented by *filled triangles* (these data obtained from Schmitz and associates[478]). Glomerular filtration rate (GFR) (from 24-hour creatinine clearance) in conscious lean and obese Zucker rats is shown as a function of age (*right*). Data are from obese rats fed ad libitum, which hence ate approximately 28 g of food per day (*filled circles*); from lean animals fed 14 g/day (normal consumption) (*open circles*); and from obese rats whose food intake was restricted to 14 g/day beginning at either 6 weeks of age (*open triangles*) or at 12 weeks of age (*open diamonds*). (Data from Maddox DA, Alavi FK, Santella RN, et al: Prevention of obesity-linked renal disease: age-dependent effects of dietary food restriction, *Kidney Int* 2002;62:208-219.)

despite a higher GFR in the obese animals.[477] Glomerular pressures in both groups were elevated in comparison with those normally seen in hydropenic Munich-Wistar rats (see Figure 3-14). However, by the time the rats were 22 to 26 weeks of age, both Schmitz and associates[478] and Park and colleagues[44] observed significantly higher values of $\overline{P}_{GC}$ and ΔP in obese Zucker rats than in lean Zucker rats as values in the latter group declined toward those normally seen in lean Munich-Wistar rats (see Figure 3-27). Maddox and co-workers[479] examined the relationship between diet and GFR in conscious Zucker rats and observed that hyperphagic obese animals (which normally consume twice as much food as their lean littermates) had markedly elevated values of GFR (estimated from 24-hour creatinine clearance measurements) in comparison with lean animals (see Figure 3-27, *right*). This is in accord with observations in humans that protein intake in both normal and obese patients is correlated directly with GFR.[475,480] When food was restricted in obese Zucker rats to amounts consumed by lean littermates, the differences in GFR between lean and obese Zucker rats disappeared (see Figure 3-27, *right*). Of importance is that when food to obese Zucker rats was limited early in life (6 weeks of age), obesity-linked renal and tubulointerstitial disease did not appear at all in these animals, despite the fact that the animals eventually grew to more than 175% of the body weight of the lean animals.[479] Food restriction later in life (at 26 or 50 weeks of age) markedly reduced proteinuria in obese Zucker rats.[479] These data suggest that the development of proteinuria and renal disease in obese humans can be slowed or prevented by improved dietary habits at an early age and that limitation of food intake even after renal disease has begun can halt further damage to the kidneys.

References

1. Stein JH, Fadem SZ. The renal circulation. *JAMA*. 1978;239:1308-1312.
2. Correa-Rotter R, Hostetter TH, Manivel JC, et al. Renin expression in renal ablation. *Hypertension*. 1992;20:483-490.
3. Sykes D. The correlation between renal vascularisation and lobulation of the kidney. *Br J Urol*. 1964;36:549-555.
4. Sykes D. The arterial supply of the human kidney with special reference to accessory renal arteries. *Br J Surg*. 1963;50:368-374.
5. Boijsen E. Angiographic studies of the anatomy of single and multiple renal arteries. *Acta Radiol Suppl*. 1959;183:1-135.
6. Graves F. *The arterial anatomy of the kidney*. Baltimore: Williams & Wilkins; 1971.
7. Beeuwkes III R. Efferent vascular patterns and early vascular-tubular relations in the dog kidney. *Am J Physiol*. 1971;221:1361-1374.
8. Kosinski H. Variation of the structure and course of the interlobular arteries in human kidney. *Folia Morphol (Warsz)*. 1997;56:249-252.
9. Casellas D, Navar LG. In vitro perfusion of juxtamedullary nephrons in rats. *Am J Physiol*. 1984;246:F349-F358.
10. Imig JD, Roman RJ. Nitric oxide modulates vascular tone in preglomerular arterioles. *Hypertension*. 1992;19:770-774.
11. Peti-Peterdi J. Multiphoton imaging of renal tissues in vitro. *Am J Physiol Renal Physiol*. 2005;288:F1079-1083.
12. Peti-Peterdi J, Toma I, Sipos A, et al. Multiphoton imaging of renal regulatory mechanisms. *Physiology (Bethesda)*. 2009;24:88-96.
13. Elger M, Sakai T, Kriz W. The vascular pole of the renal glomerulus of rat. *Adv Anat Embryol Cell Biol*. 1998;139:1-98.
14. Rosivall L, Peti-Peterdi J. Heterogeneity of the afferent arteriole—correlations between morphology and function. *Nephrol Dial Transplant*. 2006;21:2703-2707.
15. Evans RG, Eppel GA, Anderson WP, et al. Mechanisms underlying the differential control of blood flow in the renal medulla and cortex. *J Hypertens*. 2004;22:1439-1451.
16. Kriz W, Elger M, Mundel P, et al. Structure-stabilizing forces in the glomerular tuft. *J Am Soc Nephrol*. 1995;5:1731-1739.
17. Sraer JD, Adida C, Peraldi MN, et al. Species-specific properties of the glomerular mesangium. *J Am Soc Nephrol*. 1993;3:1342-1350.
18. Feng Z, Wei C, Chen X, et al. Essential role of Ca^{2+} release channels in angiotensin II–induced Ca^{2+} oscillations and mesangial cell contraction. *Kidney Int*. 2006;70:130-138.
19. Inkyo-Hayasaka K, Sakai T, Kobayashi N, et al. Three-dimensional analysis of the whole mesangium in the rat. *Kidney Int*. 1996;50:672-683.
20. Moffat DB, Fourman J. A vascular pattern of the rat kidney. 1963. *J Am Soc Nephrol*. 2001;12:624-632.
21. Beeuwkes III R, Bonventre JV. The organization and vascular perfusion of canine renal tubules. *The Physiologist*. 1973;16:264.
22. Beeuwkes III R, Bonventre JV. Tubular organization and vascular-tubular relations in the dog kidney. *Am J Physiol*. 1975;229:695-713.
23. Beeuwkes III R. The vascular organization of the kidney. *Annu Rev Physiol*. 1980;42:531-542.
24. Steinhausen M. Further information on the cortical countercurrent system in rat kidney. *Yale J Biol Med*. 1972;45:451-456.
25. Steinhausen M, Eisenbach GM, Galaske R. Countercurrent system in the renal cortex of rats. *Science*. 1970;167:1631-1633.
26. Weinstein SW, Szyjewicz J. Superficial nephron tubular-vascular relationships in the rat kidney. *Am J Physiol*. 1978;234:F207-214.
27. Briggs JP, Wright FS. Feedback control of glomerular filtration rate: site of the effector mechanism. *Am J Physiol*. 1979;236:F40-F47.
28. Brenner BM, Troy JL. Postglomerular vascular protein concentration: evidence for a causal role in governing fluid reabsorption and glomerulotubular balance by the renal proximal tubule. *J Clin Invest*. 1971;50:336-349.
29. Edwards JG. Efferent arterioles of glomeruli in the juxtamedullary zone of the human kidney. *Anat Rec*. 1956;125:521-529.
30. Charonis AS, Wissig SL. Anionic sites in basement membranes. Differences in their electrostatic properties in continuous and fenestrated capillaries. *Microvasc Res*. 1983;25:265-285.
31. Kriz W, Napiwotzky P. Structural and functional aspects of the renal interstitium. *Contrib Nephrol*. 1979;16:104-108.
32. Aukland K, Bogusky RT, Renkin EM. Renal cortical interstitium and fluid absorption by peritubular capillaries. *Am J Physiol*. 1994;266:F175-F184.
33. Venkatachalam MA, Karnovsky MJ. Extravascular protein in the kidney. An ultrastructural study of its relation to renal peritubular capillary permeability using protein tracers. *Lab Invest*. 1972;27:435-444.
34. Ryan GB, Karnovsky MJ. Distribution of endogenous albumin in the rat glomerulus: role of hemodynamic factors in glomerular barrier function. *Kidney Int*. 1976;9:36-45.
35. Deen WM, Ueki IF, Brenner BM. Permeability of renal peritubular capillaries to neutral dextrans dextrans and endogenous albumin. *Am J Physiol*. 1976;231:283-291.
36. Fourman J. Structural aspects of the kidney. *J Endocrinol* 50: 4-5. 1971.
37. Kriz W, Koepsell H. The structural organization of the mouse kidney. *Z Anat Entwicklungsgesch*. 1974;144:137-163.
38. Kriz W. Structural organization of renal medullary circulation. *Nephron*. 1982;31:290-295.
39. Dieterich HJ. [Structure of blood vessels in the kidney]. *Norm Pathol Anat (Stuttg)*. 1978;35:1-108.
40. Kriz W, Schnermann J, Koepsell H. The position of short and long loops of Henle in the rat kidney. *Z Anat Entwicklungsgesch*. 1972;138:301-319.
41. Kriz W, Kaissling B. *Structural organization of the mammalian kidney*. Philadelphia: Lippincott Williams & Wilkins; 2000.
42. Pallone TL, Zhang Z, Rhinehart K. Physiology of the renal medullary microcirculation. *Am J Physiol Renal Physiol*. 2003;284:F253-F266.
43. Marsh DJ, Segel LA. Analysis of countercurrent diffusion exchange in blood vessels of the renal medulla. *Am J Physiol*. 1971;221:817-828.
44. Park F, Mattson DL, Roberts LA, et al. Evidence for the presence of smooth muscle alpha-actin within pericytes of the renal medulla. *Am J Physiol*. 1997;273:R1742-R1748.
45. Kriz W, Barrett JM, Peter S. The renal vasculature: anatomical-functional aspects. *Int Rev Physiol*. 1976;11:1-21.
46. Schwartz MM, Karnovsky MJ. Ultrastructural differences between rat inner medullary descending and ascending vasa recta. *Lab Invest*. 1976;35:161-170.
47. Imai M. Functional heterogeneity of the descending limbs of Henle's loop. II. Interspecies differences among rabbits, rats, and hamsters. *Pflugers Arch*. 1984;402:393-401.
48. Valtin H. Structural and functional heterogeneity of mammalian nephrons. *Am J Physiol*. 1977;233:F491-F501.
49. Yamamoto K, Wilson DR, Baumal R. Blood supply and drainage of the outer medulla of the rat kidney: scanning electron microscopy of microvascular casts. *Anat Rec*. 1984;210:273-277.
50. Dworkin LD, Brenner BM. *The kidney*. Philadelphia: WB Saunders; 2004.

51. Kost Jr CK, Li P, Williams DS, et al. Renal vascular responses to angiotensin II in conscious spontaneously hypertensive and normotensive rats. *J Cardiovasc Pharmacol.* 1998;31:854-861.
52. Matsuda H, Hayashi K, Arakawa K, et al. Zonal heterogeneity in action of angiotensin-converting enzyme inhibitor on renal microcirculation: role of intrarenal bradykinin. *J Am Soc Nephrol.* 1999;10:2272-2282.
53. Sommer G, Corrigan G, Fredrickson J, et al. Renal blood flow: measurement in vivo with rapid spiral MR imaging. *Radiology.* 1998;208:729-734.
54. Sommer G, Noorbehesht B, Pelc N, et al. Normal renal blood flow measurement using phase-contrast cine magnetic resonance imaging. *Invest Radiol.* 1992;27:465-470.
55. Pallone TL, Robertson CR, Jamison RL. Renal medullary microcirculation. *Physiol Rev.* 1990;70:885-920.
56. Cowley Jr AW. Renal medullary oxidative stress, pressure-natriuresis, and hypertension. *Hypertension.* 2008;52:777-786.
57. Perez FL. [Studies on the kidney and the renal circulation, by Josep Trueta i Raspall (1897–1977)]. *Actas Urol Esp.* 2008;32:276-280.
58. Daniel PM, Peabody CN, Prichard MM. Cortical ischaemia of the kidney with maintained blood flow through the medulla. *Q J Exp Physiol Cogn Med Sci.* 1952;37:11-18.
59. Zimmerhackl B, Robertson CR, Jamison RL. The microcirculation of the renal medulla. *Circ Res.* 1985;57:657-667.
60. Inoue M, Maeda M, Takao S. Regional differentiation of blood flow responses to microinjection of sodium nitroprusside into the nucleus tractus solitarius of anesthetized rats. *J Auton Nerv Syst.* 1997;63:172-178.
61. Lim SW, Han KH, Jung JY, et al. Ultrastructural localization of UT-A and UT-B in rat kidneys with different hydration status. *Am J Physiol Regul Integr Comp Physiol.* 2006;290:R479-R492.
62. Edwards A, Silldforff EP, Pallone TL. The renal medullary microcirculation. *Front Biosci.* 2000;5:E36-E52.
63. Zimmerhackl B, Robertson CR, Jamison RL. Effect of arginine vasopressin on renal medullary blood flow. A videomicroscopic study in the rat. *J Clin Invest.* 1985;76:770-778.
64. Fadem SZ, Hernandez-Llamas G, Patak RV, et al. Studies on the mechanism of sodium excretion during drug-induced vasodilatation in the dog. *J Clin Invest.* 1982;69:604-610.
65. Ganguli M, Tobian L, Ferris T, et al. Acute prostaglandin reduction with indomethacin and chronic prostaglandin reduction with an essential fatty acid deficient diet both decrease plasma flow to the renal papilla in the rat. *Prostaglandins.* 1989;38:3-19.
66. Nafz B, Berger K, Rosler C, et al. Kinins modulate the sodium-dependent autoregulation of renal medullary blood flow. *Cardiovasc Res.* 1998;40:573-579.
67. Zou AP, Nithipatikom K, Li PL, et al. Role of renal medullary adenosine in the control of blood flow and sodium excretion. *Am J Physiol.* 1999;276:R790-R798.
68. Dunn BR, Ichikawa I, Pfeffer JM, et al. Renal and systemic hemodynamic effects of synthetic atrial natriuretic peptide in the anesthetized rat. *Circ Res.* 1986;59:237-246.
69. Pallone TL, Mattson DL. Role of nitric oxide in regulation of the renal medulla in normal and hypertensive kidneys. *Curr Opin Nephrol Hypertens.* 2002;11:93-98.
70. Oliver JJ, Rajapakse NW, Evans RG. Effects of indomethacin on responses of regional kidney perfusion to vasoactive agents in rabbits. *Clin Exp Pharmacol Physiol.* 2002;29:873-879.
71. Badzynska B, Grzelec-Mojzesowicz M, Dobrowolski L, et al. Differential effect of angiotensin II on blood circulation in the renal medulla and cortex of anaesthetised rats. *J Physiol.* 2002;538:159-166.
72. Sarkis A, Liu KL, Lo M, et al. Angiotensin II and renal medullary blood flow in Lyon rats. *Am J Physiol Renal Physiol.* 2003;284:F365-F372.
73. Kiberd B, Robertson CR, Larson T, et al. Effect of V2-receptor–mediated changes on inner medullary blood flow induced by AVP. *Am J Physiol.* 1987;253:F576-F581.
74. Mattson DL. Importance of the renal medullary circulation in the control of sodium excretion and blood pressure. *Am J Physiol Regul Integr Comp Physiol.* 2003;284:R13-R27.
75. Brenner BM, Troy JL, Daugharty TM. The dynamics of glomerular ultrafiltration in the rat. *J Clin Invest.* 1971;50:1776-1780.
76. Maddox DA, Deen WM, Brenner BM. *Handbook of physiology: section 8; renal physiology.* New York: Oxford University Press; 1992.
77. Oliver III JD, Anderson S, Troy JL, et al. Determination of glomerular size-selectivity in the normal rat with Ficoll. *J Am Soc Nephrol.* 1992;3:214-228.
78. Scandling JD, Myers BD. Glomerular size-selectivity and microalbuminuria in early diabetic glomerular disease. *Kidney Int.* 1992;41:840-846.
79. Walker AM, Bott PA, Oliver JJ, et al. The collection and analysis of fluid from single nephrons of the mammalian kidney. *Am J Physiol.* 1941;134:580-595.
80. Wearn JT, Richards AN. Observations on the composition of glomerular urine, with particular reference to the problem of reabsorption in the renal tubule. *Am J Physiol.* 1924;71:209-227.
81. Deen WM. What determines glomerular capillary permeability? *J Clin Invest.* 2004;114:1412-1414.
82. Deen WM, Lazzara MJ, Myers BD. Structural determinants of glomerular permeability. *Am J Physiol Renal Physiol.* 2001;281:F579-F596.
83. Drumond MC, Deen WM. Structural determinants of glomerular hydraulic permeability. *Am J Physiol.* 1994;266:F1-F12.
84. Drumond MC, Kristal B, Myers BD, et al. Structural basis for reduced glomerular filtration capacity in nephrotic humans. *J Clin Invest.* 1994;94:1187-1195.
85. Maddox DA, Deen WM, Brenner BM. Dynamics of glomerular ultrafiltration: VI. Studies in the primate. *Kidney Int.* 1974;5:271-278.
86. Maddox DA, Price DC, Rector Jr FC. Effect of surgery on plasma volume and salt and water excretion in rats. *Am J Physiol.* 1977;233:F600-F606.
87. Maddox DA, Brenner BM. *The kidney.* Philadelphia: WB Saunders; 2004.
88. Deen WM, Robertson CR, Brenner BM. A model of glomerular ultrafiltration in the rat. *Am J Physiol.* 1972;223:1178-1183.
89. Pinnick RV, Savin VJ. Filtration by superficial and deep glomeruli of normovolemic and volume-depleted rats. *Am J Physiol.* 1986;250:F86-F91.
90. Brenner BM, Ueki IF, Daugharty TM. On estimating colloid osmotic pressure in pre- and postglomerular plasma in the rat. *Kidney Int.* 1972;2:51-53.
91. Brenner BM, Troy JL, Daugharty TM, et al. Dynamics of glomerular ultrafiltration in the rat. II. Plasma-flow dependence of GFR. *Am J Physiol.* 1972;223:1184-1190.
92. Daniels BS, Hauser EB, Deen WM, et al. Glomerular basement membrane: in vitro studies of water and protein permeability. *Am J Physiol.* 1992;262:F919-F926.
93. Haley DP, Sarrafian M, Bulger RE, et al. Structural and functional correlates of effects of angiotensin-induced changes in rat glomerulus. *Am J Physiol.* 1987;253:F111-F119.
94. Zimmerhackl B, Parekh N, Kücherer H, Steinhausen M. Influence of systemically applied angiotensin II on the microcirculation of glomerular capillaries in the rat. *Kidney Int.* 1985;27:17-24.
95. Andrews PM, Coffey AK. Cytoplasmic contractile elements in glomerular cells. *Fed Proc.* 1983;42:3046-3052.
96. Click RL, Joyner WL, Gilmore JP. Reactivity of gomerular afferent and efferent arterioles in renal hypertension. *Kidney Int.* 1979;15:109-115.
97. Steinhausen M, Sterzel RB, Fleming JT, et al. Acute and chronic effects of angiotensin II on the vessels of the split hydronephrotic kidney. *Kidney Int Suppl.* 1987;20:S64-S73.
98. Loutzenhiser R, Bidani A, Chilton L. Renal myogenic response: kinetic attributes and physiological role. *Circ Res.* 2002;90:1316-1324.
99. Tang L, Loutzenhiser K, Loutzenhiser R. Biphasic actions of prostaglandin E(2) on the renal afferent arteriole: role of EP(3) and EP(4) receptors. *Circ Res.* 2000;86:663-670.
100. Tang L, Parker M, Fei Q, et al. Afferent arteriolar adenosine A_{2a} receptors are coupled to K_{ATP} in in vitro perfused hydronephrotic rat kidney. *Am J Physiol.* 1999;277:F926-F933.
101. Carmines PK, Morrison TK, Navar LG. Angiotensin II effects on microvascular diameters of in vitro blood-perfused juxtamedullary nephrons. *Am J Physiol.* 1986;251:F610-F618.
102. Edwards RM. Segmental effects of norepinephrine and angiotensin II on isolated renal microvessels. *Am J Physiol.* 1983;244:F526-F534.
103. Ito S, Johnson CS, Carretero OA. Modulation of angiotensin II–induced vasoconstriction by endothelium-derived relaxing factor in the isolated microperfused rabbit afferent arteriole. *J Clin Invest.* 1991;87:1656-1663.
104. Denton KM, Anderson WP, Sinniah R. Effects of angiotensin II on regional afferent and efferent arteriole dimensions and the glomerular pole. *Am J Physiol Regul Integr Comp Physiol.* 2000;279:R629-R638.
105. Just A, Ehmke H, Toktomambetova L, et al. Dynamic characteristics and underlying mechanisms of renal blood flow autoregulation in the conscious dog. *Am J Physiol Renal Physiol.* 2001;280:F1062-F1071.
106. Lanese DM, Yuan BH, McMurtry IF, et al. Comparative sensitivities of isolated rat renal arterioles to endothelin. *Am J Physiol.* 1992;263:F894-F899.
107. Yuan BH, Robinette JB, Conger JD. Effect of angiotensin II and norepinephrine on isolated rat afferent and efferent arterioles. *Am J Physiol.* 1990;258:F741-F750.
108. Ito S, Arima S, Ren YL, et al. Endothelium-derived relaxing factor/nitric oxide modulates angiotensin II action in the isolated microperfused rabbit afferent but not efferent arteriole. *J Clin Invest.* 1993;91:2012-2019.
109. Juncos LA, Ren Y, Arima S, et al. Angiotensin II action in isolated microperfused rabbit afferent arterioles is modulated by flow. *Kidney Int.* 1996;49:374-381.
110. Purdy KE, Arendshorst WJ. Prostaglandins buffer ANG II–mediated increases in cytosolic calcium in preglomerular VSMC. *Am J Physiol.* 1999;277:F850-F858.

111. Schnackenberg CG, Wilkins FC, Granger JP. Role of nitric oxide in modulating the vasoconstrictor actions of angiotensin II in preglomerular and postglomerular vessels in dogs. *Hypertension*. 1995;26:1024-1029.

112. Kohagura K, Endo Y, Ito O, et al. Endogenous nitric oxide and epoxyeicosatrienoic acids modulate angiotensin II–induced constriction in the rabbit afferent arteriole. *Acta Physiol Scand*. 2000;168:107-112.

113. Patzak A, Kleinmann F, Lai EY, et al. Nitric oxide counteracts angiotensin II induced contraction in efferent arterioles in mice. *Acta Physiol Scand*. 2004;181:439-444.

114. Patzak A, Lai EY, Mrowka R, et al. AT₁ receptors mediate angiotensin II–induced release of nitric oxide in afferent arterioles. *Kidney Int*. 2004;66:1949-1958.

115. Patzak A, Lai E, Persson PB, et al. Angiotensin II–nitric oxide interaction in glomerular arterioles. *Clin Exp Pharmacol Physiol*. 2005;32:410-414.

116. Baylis C, Brenner BM. Modulation by prostaglandin synthesis inhibitors of the action of exogenous angiotensin II on glomerular ultrafiltration in the rat. *Circ Res*. 1978;43:889-898.

117. Takeda K, Meyer-Lehnert H, Kim JK, et al. Effect of angiotensin II on Ca²⁺ kinetics and contraction in cultured rat glomerular mesangial cells. *Am J Physiol*. 1988;254:F254-F266.

118. Wiegmann TB, MacDougall ML, Savin VJ. Glomerular effects of angiotensin II require intrarenal factors. *Am J Physiol*. 1990;258:F717-F721.

119. Sharma M, Sharma R, Greene AS, et al. Documentation of angiotensin II receptors in glomerular epithelial cells. *Am J Physiol*. 1998;274:F623-F627.

120. Pagtalunan ME, Rasch R, Rennke HG, et al. Morphometric analysis of effects of angiotensin II on glomerular structure in rats. *Am J Physiol*. 1995;268:F82-F88.

121. Shultz PJ, Schorer AE, Raij L. Effects of endothelium-derived relaxing factor and nitric oxide on rat mesangial cells. *Am J Physiol*. 1990;258:F162-F167.

122. Baylis C, Mitruka B, Deng A. Chronic blockade of nitric oxide synthesis in the rat produces systemic hypertension and glomerular damage. *J Clin Invest*. 1992;90:278-281.

123. Deng A, Baylis C. Locally produced EDRF controls preglomerular resistance and ultrafiltration coefficient. *Am J Physiol*. 1993;264:F212-F215.

124. Arima S, Endo Y, Yaoita H, et al. Possible role of P-450 metabolite of arachidonic acid in vasodilator mechanism of angiotensin II type 2 receptor in the isolated microperfused rabbit afferent arteriole. *J Clin Invest*. 1997;100:2816-2823.

125. Inishi Y, Okuda T, Arakawa T, et al. Insulin attenuates intracellular calcium responses and cell contraction caused by vasoactive agents. *Kidney Int*. 1994;45:1318-1325.

126. Ren Y, Garvin JL, Carretero OA. Vasodilator action of angiotensin–(1-7) on isolated rabbit afferent arterioles. *Hypertension*. 2002;39:799-802.

127. Santos RA, Simoes e Silva AC, et al. Angiotensin–(1-7) is an endogenous ligand for the G protein-coupled receptor Mas. *Proc Natl Acad Sci U S A*. 2003;100:8258-8263.

128. Chappell MC. Emerging evidence for a functional angiotensin-converting enzyme 2-angiotensin–(1-7)–MAS receptor axis: more than regulation of blood pressure? *Hypertension*. 2007;50:596-599.

129. Tipnis SR, Hooper NM, Hyde R, Karran E, Christie G, Turner AJ. A human homolog of angiotensin-converting enzyme. Cloning and functional expression as a captopril-insensitive carboxypeptidase. *J Biol Chem*. 2000;275:33238-33243.

130. Turner AJ, Tipnis SR, Guy JL, et al. ACEH/ACE₂ is a novel mammalian metallocarboxypeptidase and a homologue of angiotensin-converting enzyme insensitive to ACE inhibitors. *Can J Physiol Pharmacol*. 2002;80:346-353.

131. Zisman LS, Meixell GE, Bristow MR, et al. Angiotensin–(1-7) formation in the intact human heart: in vivo dependence on angiotensin II as substrate. *Circulation*. 2003;108:1679-1681.

132. Arima S, Kohagura K, Xu HL, et al. Nongenomic vascular action of aldosterone in the glomerular microcirculation. *J Am Soc Nephrol*. 2003;14:2255-2263.

133. Arima S. Aldosterone and the kidney: rapid regulation of renal microcirculation. *Steroids*. 2006;71:281-285.

134. Schmidt BM. Rapid non-genomic effects of aldosterone on the renal vasculature. *Steroids*. 2008;73:961-965.

135. Tatemoto K, Hosoya M, Habata Y, et al. Isolation and characterization of a novel endogenous peptide ligand for the human APJ receptor. *Biochem Biophys Res Commun*. 1998;251:471-476.

136. O'Carroll AM, Selby TL, Palkovits M, et al. Distribution of mRNA encoding B78/apj, the rat homologue of the human APJ receptor, and its endogenous ligand apelin in brain and peripheral tissues. *Biochim Biophys Acta*. 2000;1492:72-80.

137. Hus-Citharel A, Bouby N, Frugiere A, et al. Effect of apelin on glomerular hemodynamic function in the rat kidney. *Kidney Int*. 2008;74:486-494.

138. Furchgott RF, Zawadzki JV. The obligatory role of endothelial cells in the relaxation of arterial smooth muscle by acetylcholine. *Nature*. 1980;288:373-376.

139. Ignarro LJ, Buga GM, Wood KS, et al. Endothelium-derived relaxing factor produced and released from artery and vein is nitric oxide. *Proc Natl Acad Sci U S A*. 1987;84:9265-9269.

140. Palmer RM, Ferrige AG, Moncada S. Nitric oxide release accounts for the biological activity of endothelium-derived relaxing factor. *Nature*. 1987;327:524-526.

141. Ignarro LJ. Nitric oxide. A novel signal transduction mechanism for transcellular communication. *Hypertension*. 1990;16:477-483.

142. Romero JC, Lahera V, Salom MG, et al. Role of the endothelium-dependent relaxing factor nitric oxide on renal function. *J Am Soc Nephrol*. 1992;2:1371-1387.

143. Shultz PJ, Tayeh MA, Marletta MA, et al. Synthesis and action of nitric oxide in rat glomerular mesangial cells. *Am J Physiol*. 1991;261:F600-F606.

144. Bachmann S, Bosse HM, Mundel P. Topography of nitric oxide synthesis by localizing constitutive NO synthases in mammalian kidney. *Am J Physiol*. 1995;268:F885-F898.

145. Kon V, Harris RC, Ichikawa I. A regulatory role for large vessels in organ circulation. Endothelial cells of the main renal artery modulate intrarenal hemodynamics in the rat. *J Clin Invest*. 1990;85:1728-1733.

146. Greenberg SG, He XR, Schnermann JB, et al. Effect of nitric oxide on renin secretion. I. Studies in isolated juxtaglomerular granular cells. *Am J Physiol*. 1995;268:F948-F952.

147. Lamontagne D, Pohl U, Busse R. Mechanical deformation of vessel wall and shear stress determine the basal release of endothelium-derived relaxing factor in the intact rabbit coronary vascular bed. *Circ Res*. 1992;70:123-130.

148. Murphy ME, Brayden JE. Apamin-sensitive K⁺ channels mediate an endothelium-dependent hyperpolarization in rabbit mesenteric arteries. *J Physiol*. 1995;489(Pt 3):723-734.

149. Radermacher J, Forstermann U, Frolich JC. Endothelium-derived relaxing factor influences renal vascular resistance. *Am J Physiol*. 1990;259:F9-F17.

150. Tolins JP, Palmer RM, Moncada S, et al. Role of endothelium-derived relaxing factor in regulation of renal hemodynamic responses. *Am J Physiol*. 1990;258:H655-H662.

151. Lucas KA, Pitari GM, Kazerounian S, et al. Guanylyl cyclases and signaling by cyclic GMP. *Pharmacol Rev*. 2000;52:375-414.

152. Rapoport RM. Cyclic guanosine monophosphate inhibition of contraction may be mediated through inhibition of phosphatidylinositol hydrolysis in rat aorta. *Circ Res*. 1986;58:407-410.

153. Cheng J, Grande JP. Cyclic nucleotide phosphodiesterase (PDE) inhibitors: novel therapeutic agents for progressive renal disease. *Exp Biol Med (Maywood)*. 2007;232:38-51.

154. Buga GM, Gold ME, Fukuto JM, et al. Shear stress-induced release of nitric oxide from endothelial cells grown on beads. *Hypertension*. 1991;17:187-193.

155. Chin JH, Azhar S, Hoffman BB. Inactivation of endothelial derived relaxing factor by oxidized lipoproteins. *J Clin Invest*. 1992;89:10-18.

156. Cooke JP, Rossitch Jr E, Andon NA, et al. Flow activates an endothelial potassium channel to release an endogenous nitrovasodilator. *J Clin Invest*. 1991;88:1663-1671.

157. Luckhoff A, Busse R. Calcium influx into endothelial cells and formation of endothelium-derived relaxing factor is controlled by the membrane potential. *Pflugers Arch*. 1990;416:305-311.

158. Marsden PA, Brock TA, Ballermann BJ. Glomerular endothelial cells respond to calcium-mobilizing agonists with release of EDRF. *Am J Physiol*. 1990;258:F1295-F1303.

159. Handa RK, Strandhoy JW. Nitric oxide mediates the inhibitory action of platelet-activating factor on angiotensin II–induced renal vasoconstriction, in vivo. *J Pharmacol Exp Ther*. 1996;277:1486-1491.

160. Edwards RM, Pullen M, Nambi P. Activation of endothelin ET_B receptors increases glomerular cGMP via an l-arginine–dependent pathway. *Am J Physiol*. 1992;263:F1020-1025.

161. Fiscus RR, Zhou HL, Wang X, et al. Calcitonin gene–related peptide (CGRP)–induced cyclic AMP, cyclic GMP and vasorelaxant responses in rat thoracic aorta are antagonized by blockers of endothelium-derived relaxant factor (EDRF). *Neuropeptides*. 1991;20:133-143.

162. Samuelson UE, Jernbeck J. Calcitonin gene–related peptide relaxes porcine arteries via one endothelium-dependent and one endothelium-independent mechanism. *Acta Physiol Scand*. 1991;141:281-282.

163. Gray DW, Marshall I. Nitric oxide synthesis inhibitors attenuate calcitonin gene–related peptide endothelium–dependent vasorelaxation in rat aorta. *Eur J Pharmacol*. 1992;212:37-42.

164. Gray DW, Marshall I. Human alpha-calcitonin gene–related peptide stimulates adenylate cyclase and guanylate cyclase and relaxes rat thoracic aorta by releasing nitric oxide. *Br J Pharmacol*. 1992;107:691-696.

165. Hutcheson IR, Griffith TM. Release of endothelium-derived relaxing factor is modulated both by frequency and amplitude of pulsatile flow. *Am J Physiol*. 1991;261:H257-H262.

166. Koller A, Kaley G. Endothelial regulation of wall shear stress and blood flow in skeletal muscle microcirculation. *Am J Physiol*. 1991;260:H862-H868.

167. Nollert MU, Eskin SG, McIntire LV. Shear stress increases inositol trisphosphate levels in human endothelial cells. *Biochem Biophys Res Commun*. 1990;170:281-287.

168. O'Neill WC. Flow-mediated NO release from endothelial cells is independent of K^+ channel activation or intracellular Ca^{2+}. *Am J Physiol*. 1995;269:C863-C869.

169. Pohl U, Herlan K, Huang A, et al. EDRF-mediated shear-induced dilation opposes myogenic vasoconstriction in small rabbit arteries. *Am J Physiol*. 1991;261:H2016-H2023.

170. Pittner J, Wolgast M, Casellas D, et al. Increased shear stress–released NO and decreased endothelial calcium in rat isolated perfused juxtamedullary nephrons. *Kidney Int*. 2005;67:227-236.

171. Blantz RC, Deng A, Lortie M, et al. The complex role of nitric oxide in the regulation of glomerular ultrafiltration. *Kidney Int*. 2002;61:782-785.

172. Mount PF, Power DA. Nitric oxide in the kidney: functions and regulation of synthesis. *Acta Physiol (Oxf)*. 2006;187:433-446.

173. Jin C, Hu C, Polichnowski A, et al. Effects of renal perfusion pressure on renal medullary hydrogen peroxide and nitric oxide production. *Hypertension*. 2009;53:1048-1053.

174. Zhang Z, Pallone TL. Response of descending vasa recta to luminal pressure. *Am J Physiol Renal Physiol*. 2004;287:F535-F542.

175. Gabbai FB, Blantz RC. Role of nitric oxide in renal hemodynamics. *Semin Nephrol*. 1999;19:242-250.

176. Baylis C, Harton P, Engels K. Endothelial derived relaxing factor controls renal hemodynamics in the normal rat kidney. *J Am Soc Nephrol*. 1990;1:875-881.

177. Baumann JE, Persson PB, Ehmke H, et al. Role of endothelium-derived relaxing factor in renal autoregulation in conscious dogs. *Am J Physiol*. 1992;263:F208-F213.

178. Treeck B, Aukland K. Effect of L-NAME on glomerular filtration rate in deep and superficial layers of rat kidneys. *Am J Physiol*. 1997;272: F312-F318.

179. Welch WJ, Tojo A, Lee JU, et al. Nitric oxide synthase in the JGA of the SHR: expression and role in tubuloglomerular feedback. *Am J Physiol*. 1999;277:F130-F138.

180. Sigmon DH, Beierwaltes WH. Influence of nitric oxide derived from neuronal nitric oxide synthase on glomerular filtration. *Gen Pharmacol*. 2000;34:95-100.

181. Gonzalez JD, Llinas MT, Nava E, et al. Role of nitric oxide and prostaglandins in the long-term control of renal function. *Hypertension*. 1998;32:33-38.

182. Qiu C, Baylis C. Endothelin and angiotensin mediate most glomerular responses to nitric oxide inhibition. *Kidney Int*. 1999;55:2390-2396.

183. Zatz R, de Nucci G. Effects of acute nitric oxide inhibition on rat glomerular microcirculation. *Am J Physiol*. 1991;261:F360-F363.

184. Hoffend J, Cavarape A, Endlich K, Steinhausen M. Influence of endothelium-derived relaxing factor on renal microvessels and pressure-dependent vasodilation. *Am J Physiol*. 1993;265:F285-F292.

185. Ito S, Juncos LA, Nushiro N, et al. Endothelium-derived relaxing factor modulates endothelin action in afferent arterioles. *Hypertension*. 1991;17:1052-1056.

186. Ito S, Ren Y. Evidence for the role of nitric oxide in macula densa control of glomerular hemodynamics. *J Clin Invest*. 1993;92:1093-1098.

187. Ohishi K, Carmines PK, Inscho EW, et al. EDRF–angiotensin II interactions in rat juxtamedullary afferent and efferent arterioles. *Am J Physiol*. 1992;263:F900-F906.

188. Sigmon DH, Carretero OA, Beierwaltes WH. Endothelium-derived relaxing factor regulates renin release in vivo. *Am J Physiol*. 1992;263:F256-F261.

189. Moreno C, Lopez A, Llinas MT, et al. Changes in NOS activity and protein expression during acute and prolonged ANG II administration. *Am J Physiol Regul Integr Comp Physiol*. 2002;282:R31-R37.

190. Deng A, Miracle CM, Suarez JM, et al. Oxygen consumption in the kidney: effects of nitric oxide synthase isoforms and angiotensin II. *Kidney Int*. 2005;68:723-730.

191. Baylis C, Engels K, Samsell L, et al. Renal effects of acute endothelial-derived relaxing factor blockade are not mediated by angiotensin II. *Am J Physiol*. 1993;264:F74-F78.

192. Baylis C, Harvey J, Engels K. Acute nitric oxide blockade amplifies the renal vasoconstrictor actions of angiotension II. *J Am Soc Nephrol*. 1994;5:211-214.

193. Yanagisawa M, Kurihara H, Kimura S, et al. A novel potent vasoconstrictor peptide produced by vascular endothelial cells. *Nature*. 1988;332:411-415.

194. Goraca A. New views on the role of endothelin (minireview). *Endocr Regul*. 2002;36:161-167.

195. Simonson MS, Dunn MJ. Endothelin-1 stimulates contraction of rat glomerular mesangial cells and potentiates beta-adrenergic–mediated cyclic adenosine monophosphate accumulation. *J Clin Invest*. 1990;85: 790-797.

196. Barnes K, Brown C, Turner AJ. Endothelin-converting enzyme: ultrastructural localization and its recycling from the cell surface. *Hypertension*. 1998;31:3-9.

197. Barnes K, Murphy LJ, Takahashi M, et al. Localization and biochemical characterization of endothelin-converting enzyme. *J Cardiovasc Pharmacol*. 1995;26(Suppl 3):S37-S39.

198. Bakris GL, Fairbanks R, Traish AM. Arginine vasopressin stimulates human mesangial cell production of endothelin. *J Clin Invest*. 1991;87:1158-1164.

199. Herman WH, Emancipator SN, Rhoten RL, et al. Vascular and glomerular expression of endothelin-1 in normal human kidney. *Am J Physiol*. 1998;275:F8-F17.

200. Karet FE, Davenport AP. Localization of endothelin peptides in human kidney. *Kidney Int*. 1996;49:382-387.

201. Kasinath BS, Fried TA, Davalath S, et al. Glomerular epithelial cells synthesize endothelin peptides. *Am J Pathol*. 1992;141:279-283.

202. Kohan DE. Production of endothelin-1 by rat mesangial cells: regulation by tumor necrosis factor. *J Lab Clin Med*. 1992;119:477-484.

203. Marsden PA, Dorfman DM, Collins T, et al. Regulated expression of endothelin 1 in glomerular capillary endothelial cells. *Am J Physiol*. 1991;261:F117-F125.

204. Sakamoto H, Sasaki S, Nakamura Y, et al. Regulation of endothelin-1 production in cultured rat mesangial cells. *Kidney Int*. 1992;41:350-355.

205. Sakamoto H, Sasaki S, Hirata Y, et al. Production of endothelin-1 by rat cultured mesangial cells. *Biochem Biophys Res Commun*. 1990;169:462-468.

206. Ujiie K, Terada Y, Nonoguchi H, et al. Messenger RNA expression and synthesis of endothelin-1 along rat nephron segments. *J Clin Invest*. 1992;90:1043-1048.

207. Wilkes BM, Susin M, Mento PF, et al. Localization of endothelin-like immunoreactivity in rat kidneys. *Am J Physiol*. 1991;260:F913-F920.

208. Zoja C, Orisio S, Perico N, et al. Constitutive expression of endothelin gene in cultured human mesangial cells and its modulation by transforming growth factor-beta, thrombin, and a thromboxane A2 analogue. *Lab Invest*. 1991;64:16-20.

209. Badr KF, Munger KA, Sugiura M, et al. High and low affinity binding sites for endothelin in cultured rat glomerular mesangial cells. *Biochem Biophys Res Commun*. 1989;161:776-781.

210. Kohan DE. Endothelins in the normal and diseased kidney. *Am J Kidney Dis*. 1997;29:2-26.

211. Madeddu P, Troffa C, Glorioso N, et al. Effect of endothelin on regional hemodynamics and renal function in awake normotensive rats. *J Cardiovasc Pharmacol*. 1989;14:818-825.

212. Clozel M, Fischli W. Human cultured endothelial cells do secrete endothelin-1. *J Cardiovasc Pharmacol*. 1989;13(Suppl 5):S229-231.

213. Marsden PA, Danthuluri NR, Brenner BM, et al. Endothelin action on vascular smooth muscle involves inositol trisphosphate and calcium mobilization. *Biochem Biophys Res Commun*. 1989;158:86-93.

214. Martin ER, Brenner BM, Ballermann BJ. Heterogeneity of cell surface endothelin receptors. *J Biol Chem*. 1990;265:14044-14049.

215. Sakurai T, Yanagisawa M, Masaki T. Molecular characterization of endothelin receptors. *Trends Pharmacol Sci*. 1992;13:103-108.

216. Pollock DM, Keith TL, Highsmith RF. Endothelin receptors and calcium signaling. *Faseb J*. 1995;9:1196-1204.

217. Deng Y, Martin LL, DelGrande D, et al. A soluble protease identified from rat kidney degrades endothelin-1 but not proendothelin-1. *J Biochem*. 1992;112:168-172.

218. Katusic ZS, Shepherd JT, Vanhoutte PM. Endothelium-dependent contraction to stretch in canine basilar arteries. *Am J Physiol*. 1987;252:H671-H673.

219. Yoshizumi M, Kurihara H, Sugiyama, et al. Hemodynamic shear stress stimulates endothelin production by cultured endothelial cells. *Biochem Biophys Res Commun*. 1989;161:859-864.

220. Herizi A, Jover B, Bouriquet N, et al. Prevention of the cardiovascular and renal effects of angiotensin II by endothelin blockade. *Hypertension*. 1998;31:10-14.

221. Kohno M, Horio T, Ikeda M, et al. Angiotensin II stimulates endothelin-1 secretion in cultured rat mesangial cells. *Kidney Int*. 1992;42:860-866.

222. Marsden PA, Brenner BM. Transcriptional regulation of the endothelin-1 gene by TNF-alpha. *Am J Physiol*. 1992;262:C854-861.

223. Rajagopalan S, Laursen JB, Borthayre A, et al. Role for endothelin-1 in angiotensin II–mediated hypertension. *Hypertension*. 1997;30:29-34.

224. Munger KA, Sugiura M, Takahashi K, et al. A role for atrial natriuretic peptide in endothelin-induced natriuresis. *J Am Soc Nephrol*. 1991;1:1278-1283.

225. King AJ, Brenner BM, Anderson S. Endothelin: a potent renal and systemic vasoconstrictor peptide. *Am J Physiol*. 1989;256:F1051-1058.

226. Badr KF, Murray JJ, Breyer MD, et al. Mesangial cell, glomerular and renal vascular responses to endothelin in the rat kidney. Elucidation of signal transduction pathways. *J Clin Invest*. 1989;83:336-342.

227. Clavell AL, Stingo AJ, Margulies KB, et al. Role of endothelin receptor subtypes in the in vivo regulation of renal function. *Am J Physiol.* 1995;268:F455-F460.

228. Heller J, Kramer HJ, Horacek V. Action of endothelin-1 on glomerular haemodynamics in the dog: lack of direct effects on glomerular ultrafiltration coefficient. *Clin Sci (Lond).* 1996;90:385-391.

229. Perico N, Dadan J, Gabanelli M, et al. Cyclooxygenase products and atrial natriuretic peptide modulate renal response to endothelin. *J Pharmacol Exp Ther.* 1990;252:1213-1220.

230. Stacy DL, Scott JW, Granger JP. Control of renal function during intrarenal infusion of endothelin. *Am J Physiol.* 1990;258:F1232-F1236.

231. Kon V, Yoshioka T, Fogo A, Ichikawa I. Glomerular actions of endothelin in vivo. *J Clin Invest.* 1989;83:1762-1767.

232. Fretschner M, Endlich K, Gulbins E, et al. Effects of endothelin on the renal microcirculation of the split hydronephrotic rat kidney. *Ren Physiol Biochem.* 1991;14:112-127.

233. Loutzenhiser R, Epstein M, Hayashi K, et al. Direct visualization of effects of endothelin on the renal microvasculature. *Am J Physiol.* 1990;258:F61-F68.

234. Edwards RM, Trizna W, Ohlstein EH. Renal microvascular effects of endothelin. *Am J Physiol.* 1990;259:F217-F221.

235. Dlugosz JA, Munk S, Zhou X, et al. Endothelin-1–induced mesangial cell contraction involves activation of protein kinase C-alpha, -delta, and -epsilon. *Am J Physiol.* 1998;275:F423-F432.

236. Noll G, Wenzel RR, Luscher TF. Endothelin and endothelin antagonists: potential role in cardiovascular and renal disease. *Mol Cell Biochem.* 1996;157:259-267.

237. Lin H, Smith Jr MJ, Young DB. Roles of prostaglandins and nitric oxide in the effect of endothelin-1 on renal hemodynamics. *Hypertension.* 1996;28:372-378.

238. Momose N, Fukuo K, Morimoto S, et al. Captopril inhibits endothelin-1 secretion from endothelial cells through bradykinin. *Hypertension.* 1993;21:921-924.

239. Prins BA, Hu RM, Nazario B, et al. Prostaglandin E_2 and prostacyclin inhibit the production and secretion of endothelin from cultured endothelial cells. *J Biol Chem.* 1994;269:11938-11944.

240. Chou SY, Dahhan A, Porush JG. Renal actions of endothelin: interaction with prostacyclin. *Am J Physiol.* 1990;259:F645-F652.

241. Arai H, Hori S, Aramori I, et al. Cloning and expression of a cDNA encoding an endothelin receptor. *Nature.* 1990;348:730-732.

242. Sakurai T, Yanagisawa M, Takuwa Y, et al. Cloning of a cDNA encoding a non–isopeptide-selective subtype of the endothelin receptor. *Nature.* 1990;348:732-735.

243. Ihara M, Noguchi K, Saeki T, et al. Biological profiles of highly potent novel endothelin antagonists selective for the ET_A receptor. *Life Sci.* 1992;50:247-255.

244. Wendel M, Knels L, Kummer W, et al. Distribution of endothelin receptor subtypes ET_A and ET_B in the rat kidney. *J Histochem Cytochem.* 2006;54:1193-1203.

245. Qiu C, Engels K, Baylis C. Endothelin modulates the pressor actions of acute systemic nitric oxide blockade. *J Am Soc Nephrol.* 1995;6:1476-1481.

246. Gellai M, DeWolf R, Pullen M, et al. Distribution and functional role of renal ET receptor subtypes in normotensive and hypertensive rats. *Kidney Int.* 1994;46:1287-1294.

247. Oyekan A, Balazy M, McGiff JC. Renal oxygenases: differential contribution to vasoconstriction induced by ET-1 and ANG II. *Am J Physiol.* 1997;273:R293-R300.

248. Stier Jr CT, Quilley CP, McGiff JC. Endothelin-3 effects on renal function and prostanoid release in the rat isolated kidney. *J Pharmacol Exp Ther.* 1992;262:252-256.

249. Owada A, Tomita K, Terada Y, et al. Endothelin (ET)–3 stimulates cyclic guanosine 3′,5′-monophosphate production via ET_B receptor by producing nitric oxide in isolated rat glomerulus, and in cultured rat mesangial cells. *J Clin Invest.* 1994;93:556-563.

250. Filep JG. Endogenous endothelin modulates blood pressure, plasma volume, and albumin escape after systemic nitric oxide blockade. *Hypertension.* 1997;30:22-28.

251. Thompson A, Valeri CR, Lieberthal W. Endothelin receptor A blockade alters hemodynamic response to nitric oxide inhibition in rats. *Am J Physiol.* 1995;269:H743-H748.

252. Robertson CR, Deen WM, Troy JL, et al. Dynamics of glomerular ultrafiltration in the rat. 3. Hemodynamics and autoregulation. *Am J Physiol.* 1972;223:1191-1200.

253. Eppel GA, Bergstrom G, Anderson WP, et al. Autoregulation of renal medullary blood flow in rabbits. *Am J Physiol Regul Integr Comp Physiol.* 2003;284:R233-R244.

254. Pallone TL, Silldorff EP, Turner MR. Intrarenal blood flow: microvascular anatomy and the regulation of medullary perfusion. *Clin Exp Pharmacol Physiol.* 1998;25:383-392.

255. Majid DS, Navar LG. Medullary blood flow responses to changes in arterial pressure in canine kidney. *Am J Physiol.* 1996;270:F833-F838.

256. Steinhausen M, Blum M, Fleming JT, et al. Visualization of renal autoregulation in the split hydronephrotic kidney of rats. *Kidney Int.* 1989;35:1151-1160.

257. Heyeraas KJ, Aukland K. Interlobular arterial resistance: influence of renal arterial pressure and angiotensin II. *Kidney Int.* 1987;31:1291-1298.

258. Carmines PK, Inscho EW, Gensure RC. Arterial pressure effects on preglomerular microvasculature of juxtamedullary nephrons. *Am J Physiol.* 1990;258:F94-F102.

259. Takenaka T, Harrison-Bernard LM, Inscho EW, et al. Autoregulation of afferent arteriolar blood flow in juxtamedullary nephrons. *Am J Physiol.* 1994;267:F879-F887.

260. Peti-Peterdi J, Morishima S, Bell PD, et al. Two-photon excitation fluorescence imaging of the living juxtaglomerular apparatus. *Am J Physiol Renal Physiol.* 2002;283:F197-F201.

261. Takenaka T, Suzuki H, Okada H, et al. Mechanosensitive cation channels mediate afferent arteriolar myogenic constriction in the isolated rat kidney. *J Physiol.* 1998;511(Pt 1):245-253.

262. Davis MJ, Hill MA. Signaling mechanisms underlying the vascular myogenic response. *Physiol Rev.* 1999;79:387-423.

263. Hayashi K, Epstein M, Loutzenhiser R. Enhanced myogenic responsiveness of renal interlobular arteries in spontaneously hypertensive rats. *Hypertension.* 1992;19:153-160.

264. Hayashi K, Epstein M, Loutzenhiser R. Determinants of renal actions of atrial natriuretic peptide. Lack of effect of atrial natriuretic peptide on pressure-induced vasoconstriction. *Circ Res.* 1990;67:1-10.

265. Wagner AJ, Holstein-Rathlou NH, Marsh DJ. Endothelial Ca^{2+} in afferent arterioles during myogenic activity. *Am J Physiol.* 1996;270:F170-F178.

266. Yip KP, Marsh DJ. $[Ca^{2+}]_i$ in rat afferent arteriole during constriction measured with confocal fluorescence microscopy. *Am J Physiol.* 1996; 271:F1004-F1011.

267. Navar LG, Inscho EW, Imig JD, et al. Heterogeneous activation mechanisms in the renal microvasculature. *Kidney Int.* 1998;67(Suppl):S17-S21.

268. Griffin KA, Hacioglu R, Abu-Amarah I, et al. Effects of calcium channel blockers on "dynamic" and "steady-state step" renal autoregulation. *Am J Physiol Renal Physiol.* 2004;286:F1136-F1143.

269. Imig JD, Falck JR, Inscho EW. Contribution of cytochrome P450 epoxygenase and hydroxylase pathways to afferent arteriolar autoregulatory responsiveness. *Br J Pharmacol.* 1999;127:1399-1405.

270. Beierwaltes WH, Sigmon DH, Carretero OA. Endothelium modulates renal blood flow but not autoregulation. *Am J Physiol.* 1992;262:F943-F949.

271. Majid DS, Inscho EW, Navar LG. P_2 purinoceptor saturation by adenosine triphosphate impairs renal autoregulation in dogs. *J Am Soc Nephrol.* 1999;10:492-498.

272. Majid DS, Navar LG. Suppression of blood flow autoregulation plateau during nitric oxide blockade in canine kidney. *Am J Physiol.* 1992;262:F40-F46.

273. Navar LG. Integrating multiple paracrine regulators of renal microvascular dynamics. *Am J Physiol.* 1998;274:F433-F444.

274. Bayliss W. On the local reactions of the arterial wall to changes in internal pressure. *J Physiol.* 1902;28:220.

275. Fray JC, Lush DJ, Park CS. Interrelationship of blood flow, juxtaglomerular cells, and hypertension: role of physical equilibrium and Ca. *Am J Physiol.* 1986;251:R643-R662.

276. Lush DJ, Fray JC. Steady-state autoregulation of renal blood flow: a myogenic model. *Am J Physiol.* 1984;247:R89-R99.

277. Just A. Mechanisms of renal blood flow autoregulation: dynamics and contributions. *Am J Physiol Regul Integr Comp Physiol.* 2007;292:R1-R17.

278. Casellas D, Moore LC. Autoregulation of intravascular pressure in preglomerular juxtamedullary vessels. *Am J Physiol.* 1993;264:F315-F321.

279. Casellas D, Bouriquet N, Moore LC. Branching patterns and autoregulatory responses of juxtamedullary afferent arterioles. *Am J Physiol.* 1997;272:F416-F421.

280. Walker MR, Harrison-Bernard LM, Cook AK, et al. Dynamic interaction between myogenic and TGF mechanisms in afferent arteriolar blood flow regulation. *Am J Physiol.* 2000;279:F858-F865.

281. Hayashi K, Epstein M, Loutzenhiser R, et al. Impaired myogenic responsiveness of the afferent arteriole in streptozotocin-induced diabetic rats: role of eicosanoid derangements. *J Am Soc Nephrol.* 1992;2:1578-1586.

282. Gilmore JP, Cornish KG, Rogers SD, et al. Direct evidence for myogenic autoregulation of the renal microcirculation in the hamster. *Circ Res.* 1980;47:226-230.

283. Heller J, Horacek V. Autoregulation of superficial nephron function in the alloperfused dog kidney. *Pflugers Arch.* 1979;382:99-104.

284. Robertson CR, Deen WM, Troy JL, et al. Dynamics of glomerular ultrafiltration in the rat. III. Hemodynamics and autoregulation. *Am J Physiol.* 1972;223:1191-1200.

285. Pelayo JC, Westcott JY. Impaired autoregulation of glomerular capillary hydrostatic pressure in the rat remnant nephron. *J Clin Invest.* 1991;88:101-105.

286. Hayashi K, Epstein M, Loutzenhiser R. Pressure-induced vasoconstriction of renal microvessels in normotensive and hypertensive rats. *Circ Res.* 1989;65:1475-1484.

287. Takenaka T, Forster H, De Micheli A, et al. Impaired myogenic responsiveness of renal microvessels in Dahl salt-sensitive rats. *Circ Res.* 1992;71:471-480.

288. Schnermann J, Wright FS, Davis JM, et al. Regulation of superficial nephron filtration rate by tubulo-glomerular feedback. *Pflugers Arch.* 1970;318:147-175.

289. Vallon V. Tubuloglomerular feedback and the control of glomerular filtration rate. *News Physiol Sci.* 2003;18:169-174.

290. Schnermann J. Localization, mediation and function of the glomerular vascular response to alterations of distal fluid delivery. *Fed Proc.* 1981;40:109-115.

291. Navar LG, Bell PD, Burke TJ. Role of a macula densa feedback mechanism as a mediator of renal autoregulation. *Kidney Int.* 1982;12(Suppl):S157-S164.

292. Moore LC, Casellas D. Tubuloglomerular feedback dependence of autoregulation in rat juxtamedullary afferent arterioles. *Kidney Int.* 1990;37:1402-1408.

293. Schlatter E, Salomonsson M, Persson AE, et al. Macula densa cells sense luminal NaCl concentration via furosemide sensitive Na$^+$2Cl$^-$K$^+$ cotransport. *Pflügers Arch.* 1989;414:286-290.

294. Hashimoto S, Huang Y, Briggs J, Schnermann J. Reduced autoregulatory effectiveness in adenosine 1 receptor–deficient mice. *Am J Physiol Renal Physiol.* 2006;290:F888-F891.

295. Holstein-Rathlou NH. Oscillations and chaos in renal blood flow control. *J Am Soc Nephrol.* 1993;4:1275-1287.

296. Leyssac PP, Baumbach L. An oscillating intratubular pressure response to alterations in Henle loop flow in the rat kidney. *Acta Physiol Scand.* 1983;117:415-419.

297. Leyssac PP, Holstein-Rathlou NH. Effects of various transport inhibitors on oscillating TGF pressure responses in the rat. *Pflugers Arch.* 1986;407:285-291.

298. Holstein-Rathlou NH, Wagner AJ, Marsh DJ. Tubuloglomerular feedback dynamics and renal blood flow autoregulation in rats. *Am J Physiol.* 1991;260:F53-F68.

299. Flemming B, Arenz N, Seeliger E, et al. Time-dependent autoregulation of renal blood flow in conscious rats. *J Am Soc Nephrol.* 2001;12:2253-2262.

300. Gotshall R, Hess T, Mills T. Efficiency of canine renal blood flow autoregulation in kidneys with or without glomerular filtration. *Blood Vessels.* 1985;22:25-31.

301. Just A, Wittmann U, Ehmke H, et al. Autoregulation of renal blood flow in the conscious dog and the contribution of the tubuloglomerular feedback. *J Physiol.* 1998;506(Pt 1):275-290.

302. Wang X, Breaks J, Loutzenhiser K, et al. Effects of inhibition of the Na$^+$/K$^+$/2Cl$^-$ cotransporter on myogenic and angiotensin II responses of the rat afferent arteriole. *Am J Physiol Renal Physiol.* 2007;292:F999-F1006.

303. Aukland K, Oien AH. Renal autoregulation: models combining tubuloglomerular feedback and myogenic response. *Am J Physiol.* 1987;252:F768-F783.

304. Loutzenhiser R, Griffin K, Williamson G, et al. Renal autoregulation: new perspectives regarding the protective and regulatory roles of the underlying mechanisms. *Am J Physiol Regul Integr Comp Physiol.* 2006;290:R1153-R1167.

305. Singh P, Thomson SC. Renal homeostasis and tubuloglomerular feedback. *Curr Opin Nephrol Hypertens.* 2010;19:59-64.

306. Schnermann J, Briggs JP. Tubuloglomerular feedback: mechanistic insights from gene-manipulated mice. *Kidney Int.* 2008;74:418-426.

307. Gutsche HU, Brunkhorst R, Muller-Ott K, et al. Effect of diuretics on the tubuloglomerular feedback response. *Can J Physiol Pharmacol.* 1984;62:412-417.

308. Olivera A, Lamas S, Rodriguez-Puyol D, et al. Adenosine induces mesangial cell contraction by an A$_1$-type receptor. *Kidney Int.* 1989;35:1300-1305.

309. Peti-Peterdi J, Bell PD. Cytosolic [Ca^{2+}] signaling pathway in macula densa cells. *Am J Physiol.* 1999;277:F472-F476.

310. Hansen PB, Friis UG, Uhrenholt TR, et al. Intracellular signalling pathways in the vasoconstrictor response of mouse afferent arterioles to adenosine. *Acta Physiol (Oxf).* 2007;191:89-97.

311. Bell PD, Lapointe JY, Sabirov R, et al. Macula densa cell signaling involves ATP release through a maxi anion channel. *Proc Natl Acad Sci U S A.* 2003;100:4322-4327.

312. Franco M, Bell PD, Navar LG. Effect of adenosine A$_1$ analogue on tubuloglomerular feedback mechanism. *Am J Physiol.* 1989;257:F231-F236.

313. Brown R, Ollerstam A, Johansson B, et al. Abolished tubuloglomerular feedback and increased plasma renin in adenosine A$_1$ receptor–deficient mice. *Am J Physiol Regul Integr Comp Physiol.* 2001;281:R1362-R1367.

314. Sun D, Samuelson LC, Yang T, et al. Mediation of tubuloglomerular feedback by adenosine: evidence from mice lacking adenosine 1 receptors. *Proc Natl Acad Sci U S A.* 2001;98:9983-9988.

315. Thomson S, Bao D, Deng A, et al. Adenosine formed by 5′-nucleotidase mediates tubuloglomerular feedback. *J Clin Invest.* 2000;106:289-298.

316. Ren Y, Arima S, Carretero OA, et al. Possible role of adenosine in macula densa control of glomerular hemodynamics. *Kidney Int.* 2002;61:169-176.

317. Ren Y, Garvin JL, Carretero OA. Efferent arteriole tubuloglomerular feedback in the renal nephron. *Kidney Int.* 2001;59:222-229.

318. Ren YL, Garvin JL, Carretero OA. Role of macula densa nitric oxide and cGMP in the regulation of tubuloglomerular feedback. *Kidney Int.* 2000;58:2053-2060.

319. Traynor T, Yang T, Huang YG, et al. Tubuloglomerular feedback in ACE-deficient mice. *Am J Physiol.* 1999;276:F751-F757.

320. Traynor TR, Schnermann J. Renin-angiotensin system dependence of renal hemodynamics in mice. *J Am Soc Nephrol.* 1999;10(Suppl 11):S184-S188.

321. Schnermann J, Traynor T, Yang T, et al. Tubuloglomerular feedback: new concepts and developments. *Kidney Int.* 1998;67(Suppl):S40-S45.

322. Schnermann JB, Traynor T, Yang T, et al. Absence of tubuloglomerular feedback responses in AT$_{1A}$ receptor–deficient mice. *Am J Physiol.* 1997;273:F315-F320.

323. Welch WJ, Wilcox CS. Feedback responses during sequential inhibition of angiotensin and thromboxane. *Am J Physiol.* 1990;258:F457-F466.

324. Vallon V. Tubuloglomerular feedback in the kidney: insights from gene-targeted mice. *Pflügers Arch.* 2003;445:470-476.

325. Wang H, Garvin JL, Carretero OA. Angiotensin II enhances tubuloglomerular feedback via luminal AT(1) receptors on the macula densa. *Kidney Int.* 2001;60:1851-1857.

326. Munger KA, Jackson EK. Effects of selective A$_1$ receptor blockade on glomerular hemodynamics: involvement of renin-angiotensin system. *Am J Physiol.* 1994;267:F783-F790.

327. Wilcox CS, Welch WJ, Murad F, et al. Nitric oxide synthase in macula densa regulates glomerular capillary pressure. *Proc Natl Acad Sci U S A.* 1992;89:11993-11997.

328. Ichihara A, Imig JD, Inscho EW, et al. Cyclooxygenase-2 participates in tubular flow-dependent afferent arteriolar tone: interaction with neuronal NOS. *Am J Physiol.* 1998;275:F605-F612.

329. Liu R, Carretero OA, Ren Y, et al. Increased intracellular pH at the macula densa activates nNOS during tubuloglomerular feedback. *Kidney Int.* 2005;67:1837-1843.

330. Thorup C, Erik A, Persson G. Macula densa derived nitric oxide in regulation of glomerular capillary pressure. *Kidney Int.* 1996;49:430-436.

331. Welch WJ, Wilcox CS. Macula densa arginine delivery and uptake in the rat regulates glomerular capillary pressure. Effects of salt intake. *J Clin Invest.* 1997;100:2235-2242.

332. Wilcox CS, Welch WJ. Macula densa nitric oxide synthase: expression, regulation, and function. *Kidney Int.* 1998;67(Suppl):S53-S57.

333. Vidal MJ, Romero JC, Vanhoutte PM. Endothelium-derived relaxing factor inhibits renin release. *Eur J Pharmacol.* 1988;149:401-402.

334. Thomson SC, Blantz RC, Vallon V. Increased tubular flow induces resetting of tubuloglomerular feedback in euvolemic rats. *Am J Physiol.* 1996;270:F461-F468.

335. Thomson SC, Vallon V, Blantz RC. Resetting protects efficiency of tubuloglomerular feedback. *Kidney Int.* 1998;67(Suppl):S65-S70.

336. Haddy FJ, Scott JB. Metabolically linked vasoactive chemicals in local regulation of blood flow. *Physiol Rev.* 1968;48:688-707.

337. Jones RD, Berne RM. Evidence for a metabolic mechanism in autoregulation of blood flow in skeletal muscle. *Circ Res.* 1965;17:540-554.

338. Spielman WS, Thompson CI. A proposed role for adenosine in the regulation of renal hemodynamics and renin release. *Am J Physiol.* 1982;242:F423-F435.

339. Blantz RC, Deng A. Coordination of kidney filtration and tubular reabsorption: considerations on the regulation of metabolic demand for tubular reabsorption. *Acta Physiol Hung.* 2007;94:83-94.

340. Hishikawa K, Nakaki T, Suzuki H, et al. Transmural pressure inhibits nitric oxide release from human endothelial cells. *Eur J Pharmacol.* 1992;215:329-331.

341. Tojo A, Gross SS, Zhang L, et al. Immunocytochemical localization of distinct isoforms of nitric oxide synthase in the juxtaglomerular apparatus of normal rat kidney. *J Am Soc Nephrol.* 1994;4:1438-1447.

342. Salom MG, Lahera V, Romero JC. Role of prostaglandins and endothelium-derived relaxing factor on the renal response to acetylcholine. *Am J Physiol.* 1991;260:F145-F149.

343. Hishikawa K, Nakaki T, Marumo T, et al. Pressure enhances endothelin-1 release from cultured human endothelial cells. *Hypertension.* 1995;25:449-452.

344. Badr KF, DeBoer DK, Takahashi K, et al. Glomerular responses to platelet-activating factor in the rat: role of thromboxane A$_2$. *Am J Physiol.* 1989;256:F35-F43.

345. Braun C, Lang C, Hocher B, et al. Influence of the renal endothelin A system on the autoregulation of renal hemodynamics in SHRs and WKY rats. *J Cardiovasc Pharmacol.* 1998;31:643-648.
346. Olsson RA, Pearson JD. Cardiovascular purinoceptors. *Physiol Rev.* 1990;70:761-845.
347. Inscho EW, Mitchell KD, Navar LG. Extracellular ATP in the regulation of renal microvascular function. *FASEB J.* 1994;8:319-328.
348. Katsuragi T, Tokunaga T, Ogawa S, et al. Existence of ATP-evoked ATP release system in smooth muscles. *J Pharmacol Exp Ther.* 1991;259:513-518.
349. Navar LG, Inscho EW, Majid SA, et al. Paracrine regulation of the renal microcirculation. *Physiol Rev.* 1996;76:425-536.
350. Inscho EW. P₂ receptors in regulation of renal microvascular function. *Am J Physiol.* 2001;280:927-944.
351. Inscho EW, Cook AK. P₂ receptor–mediated afferent arteriolar vasoconstriction during calcium blockade. *Am J Physiol Renal Physiol.* 2002;282:F245-F255.
352. Inscho EW, Cook AK, Mui V, et al. Direct assessment of renal microvascular responses to P₂-purinoceptor agonists. *Am J Physiol.* 1998;274:F718-F727.
353. Inscho EW, Ohishi K, Navar LG. Effects of ATP on pre- and postglomerular juxtamedullary microvasculature. *Am J Physiol.* 1992;263:F886-F893.
354. Inscho EW, Ohishi K, Cook, et al. Calcium activation mechanisms in the renal microvascular response to extracellular ATP. *Am J Physiol.* 1995;268:F876-F884.
355. Inscho EW, Schroeder AC, Deichmann PC, et al. ATP-mediated Ca²⁺ signaling in preglomerular smooth muscle cells. *Am J Physiol.* 1999;276:F450-F456.
356. Pfeilschifter J. Extracellular ATP stimulates polyphosphoinositide hydrolysis and prostaglandin synthesis in rat renal mesangial cells. Involvement of a pertussis toxin-sensitive guanine nucleotide binding protein and feedback inhibition by protein kinase C. *Cell Signal.* 1990;2:129-138.
357. Inscho EW, Carmines PK, Navar LG. Juxtamedullary afferent arteriolar responses to P₁ and P₂ purinergic stimulation. *Hypertension.* 1991;17:1033-1037.
358. Nishiyama A, Majid DS, Walker 3rd M, et al. Renal interstitial ATP responses to changes in arterial pressure during alterations in tubuloglomerular feedback activity. *Hypertension.* 2001;37:753-759.
359. Brayden JE. Hyperpolarization and relaxation of resistance arteries in response to adenosine phosphate. *Circ Res.* 1991;69:1415-1420.
360. Brayden JE, Nelson MT. Regulation of arterial tone by activation of calcium-dependent potassium channels. *Science.* 1992;256:532-535.
361. Lorenz JN, Schnermann J, Brosius FC, et al. Intracellular ATP can regulate afferent arteriolar tone via ATP-sensitive K⁺ channels in the rabbit. *J Clin Invest.* 1992;90:733-740.
362. Gaposchkin CG, Tornheim K, Sussman I, et al. Glucose is required to maintain ATP/ADP ratio of isolated bovine cerebral microvessels. *Am J Physiol.* 1990;258:E543-E547.
363. Jackson EK, Ren J, Mi Z. Extracellular 2′,3′-cAMP is a source of adenosine. *J Biol Chem.* 2009;284:33097-33106.
364. Le Hir M, Kaissling B. Distribution and regulation of renal ecto-5′-nucleotidase: implications for physiological functions of adenosine. *Am J Physiol.* 1993;264:F377-F387.
365. Jackson EK, Dubey RK. Role of the extracellular cAMP-adenosine pathway in renal physiology. *Am J Physiol Renal Physiol.* 2001;281:F597-F612.
366. Stehle JH, Rivkees SA, Lee JJ, et al. Molecular cloning and expression of the cDNA for a novel A₂-adenosine receptor subtype. *Mol Endocrinol.* 1992;6:384-393.
367. Spielman WS, Arend LJ. Adenosine receptors and signaling in the kidney. *Hypertension.* 1991;17:117-130.
368. Lai EY, Patzak A, Steege A, et al. Contribution of adenosine receptors in the control of arteriolar tone and adenosine–angiotensin II interaction. *Kidney Int.* 2006;70:690-698.
369. Li JM, Fenton RA, Cutler BS, et al. Adenosine enhances nitric oxide production by vascular endothelial cells. *Am J Physiol.* 1995;269:C519-C523.
370. Jackson EK, Mi Z. Preglomerular microcirculation expresses the cAMP-adenosine pathway. *J Pharmacol Exp Ther.* 2000;295:23-28.
371. Weaver DR, Reppert SM. Adenosine receptor gene expression in rat kidney. *Am J Physiol.* 1992;263:F991-F995.
372. Jackson EK. A physiological brake on renin release. *Annu Rev Pharmacol Toxicol.* 1991;31:1-35.
373. Hansen PB, Schnermann J. Vasoconstrictor and vasodilator effects of adenosine in the kidney. *Am J Physiol Renal Physiol.* 2003;285:F590-F599.
374. Okumura M, Miura K, Yamashita Y, et al. Role of endothelium-derived relaxing factor in the in vivo renal vascular action of adenosine in dogs. *J Pharmacol Exp Ther.* 1992;260:1262-1267.
375. Nishiyama A, Inscho EW, Navar LG. Interactions of adenosine A₁ and A₂ₐ receptors on renal microvascular reactivity. *Am J Physiol Renal Physiol.* 2001;280:F406-F414.
376. Weihprecht H, Lorenz JN, Briggs JP, et al. Vasomotor effects of purinergic agonists in isolated rabbit afferent arterioles. *Am J Physiol.* 1992;263:F1026-F1033.
377. Carmines PK, Inscho EW. Renal arteriolar angiotensin responses during varied adenosine receptor blockade. *Hypertension.* 1994;23(Suppl I):I-114-I-119.
378. Siragy HM, Linden J. Sodium intake markedly alters renal interstitial fluid adenosine. *Hypertension.* 1996;27:404-407.
379. Lorenz JN, Weihprecht H, He XR, et al. Effects of adenosine and angiotensin on macula densa-stimulated renin secretion. *Am J Physiol.* 1993;265:F187-F194.
380. Balakrishnan VS, Coles GA, Williams JD. Effects of intravenous adenosine on renal function in healthy human subjects. *Am J Physiol.* 1996;271:F374-F381.
381. Balakrishnan VS, Coles GA, Williams JD. A potential role for endogenous adenosine in control of human glomerular and tubular function. *Am J Physiol.* 1993;265:F504-F510.
382. Kawabata M, Ogawa T, Takabatake T. Control of rat glomerular microcirculation by juxtaglomerular adenosine A₁ receptors. *Kidney Int.* 1998;67(Suppl):S228-S230.
383. Baylis C, Deen WM, Myers BD, et al. Effects of some vasodilator drugs on transcapillary fluid exchange in renal cortex. *Am J Physiol.* 1976;230:1148-1158.
384. Nielsen CB, Bech JN, Pedersen EB. Effects of prostacyclin on renal haemodynamics, renal tubular function and vasoactive hormones in healthy humans. A placebo-controlled dose-response study. *Br J Clin Pharmacol.* 1997;44:471-476.
385. Villa E, Garcia-Robles R, Haas J, et al. Comparative effect of PGE₂ and PGI₂ on renal function. *Hypertension.* 1997;30:664-666.
386. Schor N, Ichikawa I, Brenner B. Mechanisms of action of various hormones and vasoactive substances on glomerular ultrafiltration in the rat. *Kidney Int.* 1981;20:442-451.
387. Yoshioka T, Yared A, Miyazawa H, et al. In vivo influence of prostaglandin I₂ on systemic and renal circulation in the rat. *Hypertension.* 1985;7:867-872.
388. Inscho EW, Carmines PK, Navar LG. Prostaglandin influences on afferent arteriolar responses to vasoconstrictor agonists. *Am J Physiol.* 1990;259:F157-F163.
389. Endlich K, Forssmann WG, Steinhausen M. Effects of urodilatin in the rat kidney: comparison with ANF and interaction with vasoactive substances. *Kidney Int.* 1995;47:1558-1568.
390. Munger KA, Blantz RC. Cyclooxygenase-dependent mediators of renal hemodynamic function in female rats. *Am J Physiol.* 1990;258:F1211-F1217.
391. Dahlen SE, Bjork J, Hedqvist P, et al. Leukotrienes promote plasma leakage and leukocyte adhesion in postcapillary venules: in vivo effects with relevance to the acute inflammatory response. *Proc Natl Acad Sci U S A.* 1981;78:3887-3891.
392. Yared A, Albrightson-Winslow C, Griswold D, et al. Functional significance of leukotriene B₄ in normal and glomerulonephritic kidneys. *J Am Soc Nephrol.* 1991;2:45-56.
393. Badr KF, Baylis C, Pfeffer JM, et al. Renal and systemic hemodynamic responses to intravenous infusion of leukotriene C₄ in the rat. *Circ Res.* 1984;54:492-499.
394. Filep J, Rigter B, Frolich JC. Vascular and renal effects of leukotriene C₄ in conscious rats. *Am J Physiol.* 1985;249:F739-F744.
395. Badr KF, Serhan CN, Nicolaou KC, et al. The action of lipoxin-A on glomerular microcirculatory dynamics in the rat. *Biochem Biophys Res Commun.* 1987;145:408-414.
396. Serhan CN, Sheppard KA. Lipoxin formation during human neutrophil-platelet interactions. Evidence for the transformation of leukotriene A₄ by platelet 12-lipoxygenase in vitro. *J Clin Invest.* 1990;85:772-780.
397. Katoh T, Takahashi K, DeBoer DK, et al. Renal hemodynamic actions of lipoxins in rats: a comparative physiological study. *Am J Physiol.* 1992;263:F436-F442.
398. Munger KA, Montero A, Fukunaga M, et al. Transfection of rat kidney with human 15-lipoxygenase suppresses inflammation and preserves function in experimental glomerulonephritis. *Proc Natl Acad Sci U S A.* 1999;96:13375-13380.
399. Myers BD, Deen WM, Brenner B. Effects of norepinephrine and angiotensin II on the determinants of glomerular ultrafiltration and proximal tubule fluid reabsorption in the rat. *Circ Res.* 1975;37:101-110.
400. Llinas MT, Lopez R, Rodriguez F, et al. Role of COX-2–derived metabolites in regulation of the renal hemodynamic response to norepinephrine. *Am J Physiol Renal Physiol.* 2001;281:F975-F982.
401. Edwards RM, Trizna W. Characterization of α-adrenoceptors on isolated rabbit renal arterioles. *Am J Physiol.* 1988;254:F178-F183.
402. Thomas CE, Ott CE, Bell PD, et al. Glomerular filtration dynamics during renal vasodilatation with acetylcholine in the dog. *Am J Physiol.* 1983;244:F606-F611.

403. Edwards RM. Response of isolated renal arterioles to acetylcholine, dopamine, and bradykinin. *Am J Physiol*. 1985;248:F183-F189.

404. Burton GA, MacNeil S, de Jonge A, et al. Cyclic GMP release and vasodilatation induced by EDRF and atrial natriuretic factor in the isolated perfused kidney of the rat. *Br J Pharmacol*. 1990;99:364-368.

405. Jacobs M, Plane F, Bruckdorfer KR. Native and oxidized low-density lipoproteins have different inhibitory effects on endothelium-derived relaxing factor in the rabbit aorta. *Br J Pharmacol*. 1990;100:21-26.

406. Mugge A, Elwell JH, Peterson TE, et al. Release of intact endothelium-derived relaxing factor depends on endothelial superoxide dismutase activity. *Am J Physiol*. 1991;260:C219-C225.

407. Urakami-Harasawa L, Shimokawa H, Nakashima M, et al. Importance of endothelium-derived hyperpolarizing factor in human arteries. *J Clin Invest*. 1997;100:2793-2799.

408. Brayden JE. Membrane hyperpolarization is a mechanism of endothelium-dependent cerebral vasodilation. *Am J Physiol*. 1990;259:H668-H673.

409. Jackson WF. Potassium channels in the peripheral microcirculation. *Microcirculation*. 2005;12:113-127.

410. Komori K, Vanhoutte PM. Endothelium-derived hyperpolarizing factor. *Blood Vessels*. 1990;27:238-245.

411. Najibi S, Cowan CL, Palacino JJ, et al. Enhanced role of potassium channels in relaxations to acetylcholine in hypercholesterolemic rabbit carotid artery. *Am J Physiol*. 1994;266:H2061-H2067.

412. Jackson WF. Silent inward rectifier K$^+$ channels in hypercholesterolemia. *Circ Res*. 2006;98:982-984.

413. Hayashi K, Loutzenhiser R, Epstein M, et al. Multiple factors contribute to acetylcholine-induced renal afferent arteriolar vasodilation during myogenic and norepinephrine- and KCl-induced vasoconstriction. Studies in the isolated perfused hydronephrotic kidney. *Circ Res*. 1994;75:821-828.

414. Hoagland KM, Maddox DA, Martin DS. Bradykinin B$_2$-receptors mediate the pressor and renal hemodynamic effects of intravenous bradykinin in conscious rats. *J Auton Nerv Syst*. 1999;75:7-15.

415. Siragy HM, Jaffa AA, Margolius HS. Bradykinin B$_2$ receptor modulates renal prostaglandin E$_2$ and nitric oxide. *Hypertension*. 1997;29:757-762.

416. Yu H, Carretero OA, Juncos LA, et al. Biphasic effect of bradykinin on rabbit afferent arterioles. *Hypertension*. 1998;32:287-292.

417. Bascands JL, Emond C, Pecher C, et al. Bradykinin stimulates production of inositol (1,4,5) trisphosphate in cultured mesangial cells of the rat via a BK2-kinin receptor. *Br J Pharmacol*. 1991;102:962-966.

418. Pavenstadt H, Spath M, Fiedler C, et al. Effect of bradykinin on the cytosolic free calcium activity and phosphoinositol turnover in human glomerular epithelial cells. *Ren Physiol Biochem*. 1992;15:277-288.

419. Greenwald JE, Needleman P, Wilkins MR, et al. Renal synthesis of atriopeptin-like protein in physiology and pathophysiology. *Am J Physiol*. 1991;260:F602-F607.

420. Mehrke G, Pohl U, Daut J. Effects of vasoactive agonists on the membrane potential of cultured bovine aortic and guinea-pig coronary endothelium. *J Physiol*. 1991;439:277-299.

421. Pavenstadt H, Bengen F, Spath M, et al. Effect of bradykinin and histamine on the membrane voltage, ion conductances and ion channels of human glomerular epithelial cells (hGEC) in culture. *Pflugers Arch*. 1993;424:137-144.

422. Ren Y, Garvin J, Carretero OA. Mechanism involved in bradykinin-induced efferent arteriole dilation. *Kidney Int*. 2002;62:544-549.

423. Imig JD, Falck JR, Wei S, et al. Epoxygenase metabolites contribute to nitric oxide–independent afferent arteriolar vasodilation in response to bradykinin. *J Vasc Res*. 2001;38:247-255.

424. Wang H, Garvin JL, Falck JR, et al. Glomerular cytochrome P-450 and cyclooxygenase metabolites regulate efferent arteriole resistance. *Hypertension*. 2005;46:1175-1179.

425. Kotchen TA. Attenuation of hypertension by insulin-sensitizing agents. *Hypertension*. 1996;28:219-223.

426. Hayashi K, Fujiwara K, Oka K, et al. Effects of insulin on rat renal microvessels: studies in the isolated perfused hydronephrotic kidney. *Kidney Int*. 1997;51:1507-1513.

427. Scherrer U, Randin D, Vollenweider P, et al. Nitric oxide release accounts for insulin's vascular effects in humans. *J Clin Invest*. 1994;94:2511-2515.

428. Schroeder Jr CA, Chen YL, Messina EJ. Inhibition of NO synthesis or endothelium removal reveals a vasoconstrictor effect of insulin on isolated arterioles. *Am J Physiol*. 1999;276:H815-H820.

429. Steinberg HO, Brechtel G, Johnson A, et al. Insulin-mediated skeletal muscle vasodilation is nitric oxide dependent. A novel action of insulin to increase nitric oxide release. *J Clin Invest*. 1994;94:1172-1179.

430. Ruiz M, Singh P, Thomson SC, et al. L-Arginine–induced glomerular hyperfiltration response: the roles of insulin and ANG II. *Am J Physiol Regul Integr Comp Physiol*. 2008;294:R1744-R1751.

431. McKay MK, Hester RL. Role of nitric oxide, adenosine, and ATP-sensitive potassium channels in insulin-induced vasodilation. *Hypertension*. 1996;28:202-208.

432. Tucker BJ, Anderson CM, Thies RS, et al. Glomerular hemodynamic alterations during acute hyperinsulinemia in normal and diabetic rats. *Kidney Int*. 1992;42:1160-1168.

433. Zhang PL, Jimenez W, Mackenzie HS, et al. HS-142-1, a potent antagonist of natriuretic peptides in vitro and in vivo. *J Am Soc Nephrol*. 1994;5:1099-1105.

434. Hirschberg R, Adler S. Insulin-like growth factor system and the kidney: physiology, pathophysiology, and therapeutic implications. *Am J Kidney Dis*. 1998;31:901-919.

435. Aron DC, Rosenzweig JL, Abboud HE. Synthesis and binding of insulin-like growth factor I by human glomerular mesangial cells. *J Clin Endocrinol Metab*. 1989;68:585-591.

436. Hirschberg R, Kopple JD, Blantz RC, et al. Effects of recombinant human insulin-like growth factor I on glomerular dynamics in the rat. *J Clin Invest*. 1991;87:1200-1206.

437. Hirschberg R, Brunori G, Kopple JD, et al. Effects of insulin-like growth factor I on renal function in normal men. *Kidney Int*. 1993;43:387-397.

438. Giordano M, DeFronzo RA. Acute effect of human recombinant insulin-like growth factor I on renal function in humans. *Nephron*. 1995;71:10-15.

439. Jaffa AA, LeRoith D, Roberts Jr CT, et al. Insulin-like growth factor I produces renal hyperfiltration by a kinin-mediated mechanism. *Am J Physiol*. 1994;266:F102-F107.

440. Tsukahara H, Gordienko DV, Tonshoff B, et al. Direct demonstration of insulin-like growth factor-I–induced nitric oxide production by endothelial cells. *Kidney Int*. 1994;45:598-604.

441. Henry JP, Gauer OH, Reeves JL. Evidence of the atrial location of receptors influencing urine flow. *Circ Res*. 1956;4:85-90.

442. Henry JP, Gauer OH, Sieker HO. The effect of moderate changes in blood volume on left and right atrial pressures. *Circ Res*. 1956;4:91-94.

443. DeBold A, Borenstain HB, Veress AT, et al. A rapid and potent natriuretic response to intravenous injection of atrial myocardial extracts in rats. *Life Sci*. 1981;28:89-94.

444. Brenner BM, Ballermann BJ, Gunning ME, et al. Diverse biological actions of atrial natriuretic peptide. *Physiol Rev*. 1990;70:665-699.

445. Saxenhofer H, Raselli A, Weidmann P, et al. Urodilatin, a natriuretic factor from kidneys, can modify renal and cardiovascular function in men. *Am J Physiol*. 1990;259:F832-F838.

446. Amin J, Carretero OA, Ito S. Mechanisms of action of atrial natriuretic factor and C-type natriuretic peptide. *Hypertension*. 1996;27:684-687.

447. Lohe A, Yeh I, Hyver T, et al. Natriuretic peptide B receptor and C-type natriuretic peptide in the rat kidney. *J Am Soc Nephrol*. 1995;6:1552-1558.

448. Michel H, Meyer-Lehnert H, Backer A, et al. Regulation of atrial natriuretic peptide receptors in glomeruli during chronic salt loading. *Kidney Int*. 1990;38:73-79.

449. Endlich K, Steinhausen M. Natriuretic peptide receptors mediate different responses in rat renal microvessels. *Kidney Int*. 1997;52:202-207.

450. Maack T. Role of atrial natriuretic factor in volume control. *Kidney Int*. 1996;49:1732-1737.

451. Ballermann BJ, Hoover RL, Karnovsky MJ, et al. Physiologic regulation of atrial natriuretic peptide receptors in rat renal glomeruli. *J Clin Invest*. 1985;76:2049-2056.

452. Abassi Z, Haramati A, Hoffman A, et al. Effect of converting-enzyme inhibition on renal response to ANF in rats with experimental heart failure. *Am J Physiol*. 1990;259:R84-R89.

453. Hirata Y, Matsuoka H, Suzuki E, et al. Role of endogenous atrial natriuretic peptide in DOCA-salt hypertensive rats. Effects of a novel nonpeptide antagonist for atrial natriuretic peptide receptor. *Circulation*. 1993;87:554-561.

454. Perico N, Benigni A, Gabanelli M, et al. Atrial natriuretic peptide and prostacyclin synergistically mediate hyperfiltration and hyperperfusion of diabetic rats. *Diabetes*. 1992;41:533-538.

455. Lee RW, Raya TE, Michael U, et al. Captopril and ANP: changes in renal hemodynamics, glomerular-ANP receptors and guanylate cyclase activity in rats with heart failure. *J Pharmacol Exp Ther*. 1992;260:349-354.

456. Genovesi S, Protasoni G, Assi C, et al. Interactions between the sympathetic nervous system and atrial natriuretic factor in the control of renal functions. *J Hypertens*. 1990;8:703-710.

457. Zhang PL, Mackenzie HS, Troy JL, et al. Effects of an atrial natriuretic peptide receptor antagonist on glomerular hyperfiltration in diabetic rats. *J Am Soc Nephrol*. 1994;4:1564-1570.

458. Nishikimi T, Miura K, Minamino N, et al. Role of endogenous atrial natriuretic peptide on systemic and renal hemodynamics in heart failure rats. *Am J Physiol*. 1994;267:H182-H186.

459. Zhang PL, MacKenzie HS, Troy JL, et al. Effects of natriuretic peptide receptor inhibition on remnant kidney function in rats. *Kidney Int*. 1994;46:414-420.

460. Pomeranz A, Podjarny E, Rathaus M, et al. Atrial natriuretic peptide–induced increase of glomerular filtration rate, but not of natriuresis, is mediated by prostaglandins in the rat. *Miner Electrolyte Metab*. 1990;16:30-33.

461. Bestle MH, Olsen NV, Christensen P, et al. Cardiovascular, endocrine, and renal effects of urodilatin in normal humans. *Am J Physiol.* 1999;276:R684-R695.

462. Carstens J, Jensen KT, Pedersen EB. Effect of urodilatin infusion on renal hemodynamics, tubular function and vasoactive hormones. *Clin Sci.* 1997;92:397-407.

463. Liu GL, Liu L, Barajas L. Development of NOS-containing neuronal somata in the rat kidney. *J Auton Nerv Syst.* 1996;58:81-88.

464. Barajas L, Liu L, Powers K. Anatomy of the renal innervation: intrarenal aspects and ganglia of origin. *Can J Physiol Pharmacol.* 1992;70:735-749.

465. Liu L, Liu GL, Barajas L. Distribution of nitric oxide synthase–containing ganglionic neuronal somata and postganglionic fibers in the rat kidney. *J Comp Neurol.* 1996;369:16-30.

466. DiBona GF. Neural control of renal function in health and disease. *Clin Auton Res.* 1994;4:69-74.

467. Pelayo JC, Westcott JY. Renal adrenergic effector mechanisms: glomerular sites for prostaglandin interaction. *Am J Physiol.* 1988;254:F184-F190.

468. Pelayo JC, Ziegler MG, Blantz RC. Angiotensin II in adrenergic-induced alterations in glomerular hemodynamics. *Am J Physiol.* 1984;247:F799-F807.

469. Gabbai FB, Thomson SC, Peterson O, et al. Glomerular and tubular interactions between renal adrenergic activity and nitric oxide. *Am J Physiol.* 1995;268:F1004-F1008.

470. Beierwaltes WH. Sympathetic stimulation of renin is independent of direct regulation by renal nitric oxide. *Vascul Pharmacol.* 2003;40:43-49.

471. Kon V, Yared A, Ichikawa I. Role of sympathetic nerves in mediating hypoperfusion of renal cortical microcirculation in experimental congestive heart failure and acute extracellular volume depletion. *J Clin Invest.* 1985;76:1913-1920.

472. Chagnac A, Weinstein T, Korzets A, et al. Glomerular hemodynamics in severe obesity. *Am J Physiol Renal Physiol.* 2000;278:F817-822.

473. Porter LE, Hollenberg NK. Obesity, salt intake, and renal perfusion in healthy humans. *Hypertension.* 1998;32:144-148.

474. Reisin E, Messerli FG, Ventura HO, et al. Renal haemodynamic studies in obesity hypertension. *J Hypertens.* 1987;5:397-400.

475. Ribstein J, du Cailar G, Mimran A. Combined renal effects of overweight and hypertension. *Hypertension.* 1995;26:610-615.

476. Hall JE, Brands MW, Dixon WN, et al. Obesity-induced hypertension. Renal function and systemic hemodynamics. *Hypertension.* 1993;22:292-299.

477. O'Donnell MP, Kasiske BL, Cleary MP, et al. Effects of genetic obesity on renal structure and function in the Zucker rat. II. Micropuncture studies. *J Lab Clin Med.* 1985;106:605-610.

478. Schmitz PG, O'Donnell MP, Kasiske BL, et al. Renal injury in obese Zucker rats: glomerular hemodynamic alterations and effects of enalapril. *Am J Physiol.* 1992;263:F496-F502.

479. Maddox DA, Alavi FK, Santella RN, et al. Prevention of obesity-linked renal disease: age-dependent effects of dietary food restriction. *Kidney Int.* 2002;62:208-219.

480. Lew SW, Bosch JP. Effect of diet on creatinine clearance and excretion in young and elderly healthy subjects and in patients with renal disease. *J Am Soc Nephrol.* 1991;2:856-865.

481. Kitamura K, Kangawa K, Kawamoto M, et al. Adrenomedullin: a novel hypotensive peptide isolated from human pheochromocytoma. *Biochem Biophys Res Commun.* 1993;192:553-560.

482. Kohno M, Yasunari K, Yokokawa K, et al. Interaction of adrenomedullin and platelet-derived growth factor on rat mesangial cell production of endothelin. *Hypertension.* 1996;27:663-667.

483. Edwards RM, Trizna W, Stack E, et al. Effect of adrenomedullin on cAMP levels along the rat nephron: comparison with CGRP. *Am J Physiol.* 1996;271:F895-F899.

484. Hjelmqvist H, Keil R, Mathai M, et al. Vasodilation and glomerular binding of adrenomedullin in rabbit kidney are not CGRP receptor mediated. *Am J Physiol.* 1997;273:R716-R724.

485. Jougasaki M, Wei CM, Aarhus LL, et al. Renal localization and actions of adrenomedullin: a natriuretic peptide. *Am J Physiol.* 1995;268:F657-F663.

486. Vari RC, Adkins SD, Samson WK. Renal effects of adrenomedullin in the rat. *Proc Soc Exp Biol Med.* 1996;211:178-183.

487. Ebara T, Miura K, Okumura M, et al. Effect of adrenomedullin on renal hemodynamics and functions in dogs. *Eur J Pharmacol.* 1994;263:69-73.

488. Amuchastegui CS, Remuzzi G, Perico N. Calcitonin gene–related peptide reduces renal vascular resistance and modulates ET-1–induced vasoconstriction. *Am J Physiol.* 1994;267:F839-F844.

489. Edwards RM, Trizna W. Calcitonin gene-related peptide: effects on renal arteriolar tone and tubular cAMP levels. *Am J Physiol.* 1990;258:F121-F125.

490. Bankir L, Martin H, Dechaux M, et al. Plasma cAMP: a hepatorenal link influencing proximal reabsorption and renal hemodynamics? *Kidney Int.* 1997;59(Suppl):S50-S56.

491. Reslerova M, Loutzenhiser R. Renal microvascular actions of calcitonin gene–related peptide. *Am J Physiol.* 1998;274:F1078-F1085.

492. Castellucci A, Maggi CA, Evangelista S. Calcitonin gene–related peptide (CGRP)1 receptor mediates vasodilation in the rat isolated and perfused kidney. *Life Sci.* 1993;53:PL153-PL158.

493. McDonald Jr RH, Goldberg LI, McNay JL, et al. Effect of dopamine in man: augmentation of sodium excretion, glomerular filtration rate, and renal plasma flow. *J Clin Invest.* 1964;43:1116-1124.

494. Sasser JM, Baylis C. The natriuretic and diuretic response to dopamine is maintained during rat pregnancy. *Am J Physiol Renal Physiol.* 2008;294:F1342-F1344.

495. Massfelder T, Parekh N, Endlich K, et al. Effect of intrarenally infused parathyroid hormone-related protein on renal blood flow and glomerular filtration rate in the anaesthetized rat. *Br J Pharmacol.* 1996;118:1995-2000.

496. Ichikawa I, Humes HD, Dousa TJ, et al. Influence of parathyroid hormone on glomerular ultrafiltration in the rat. *Am J Physiol.* 1978;234:F393-F401.

497. Marchand GR. Effect of parathyroid hormone on the determinants of glomerular filtration in dogs. *Am J Physiol.* 1985;248:F482-F486.

498. Pang PKT, Janssen HF, Yee JA. Effects of synthetic parathyroid hormone on vascular beds of dogs. *Pharmacology.* 1980;21:213-222.

499. Trizna W, Edwards RM. Relaxation of renal arterioles by parathyroid hormone and parathyroid hormone-related protein. *Pharmacology.* 1991;42:91-96.

500. Saussine C, Massfelder T, Parnin F, et al. Renin stimulating properties of parathyroid hormone-related peptide in the isolated perfused rat kidney. *Kidney Int.* 1993;44:764-773.

501. Bosch RJ, Rojo-Linares P, Torrecillas-Casamayor G, et al. Effects of parathyroid hormone-related protein on human mesangial cells in culture. *Am J Physiol.* 1999;277:E990-E995.

502. Massfelder T, Stewart AF, Endlich K, et al. Parathyroid hormone-related protein detection and interaction with NO and cyclic AMP in the renovascular system. *Kidney Int.* 1996;50:1591-1603.

503. Endlich K, Massfelder T, Helwig JJ, et al. Vascular effects of parathyroid hormone and parathyroid hormone-related protein in the split hydronephrotic rat kidney. *J Physiol.* 1995;483:481-490.

504. Musso MJ, Plante M, Judes C, et al. Renal vasodilatation and microvessel adenylate cyclase stimulation by synthetic parathyroid hormone-like protein fragments. *Eur J Pharmacol.* 1989;174:139-151.

505. Kalinowski L, Dobrucki LW, Malinski T. Nitric oxide is the second messenger in parathyroid hormone–related protein signaling. *J Endocrinol.* 2001;170:433-440.

506. Simeoni U, Massfelder T, Saussine C, et al. Involvement of nitric oxide in the vasodilatory response to parathyroid hormone–related peptide in the isolated rabbit kidney. *Clin Sci (Lond).* 1994;86:245-249.

507. Jiang B, Morimoto S, Fukuo K, et al. Parathyroid hormone–related protein inhibits endothelin-1 production. *Hypertension.* 1996;27:360-363.

508. Handa RK, Strandhoy JW, Buckalew Jr VM. Platelet-activating factor is a renal vasodilator in the anesthetized rat. *Am J Physiol.* 1990;258:F1504-F1509.

509. Lianos EA, Zanglis A. Biosynthesis and metabolism of 1- *O*-alkyl-2-acetyl-*sn*-glycero-3-phosphocholine in rat glomerular mesangial cells. *J Biol Chem.* 1987;262:8990-8993.

510. Juncos LA, Ren YL, Arima S, et al. Vasodilator and constrictor actions of platelet-activating factor in the isolated microperfused afferent arteriole of the rabbit kidney. Role of endothelium-derived relaxing factor/nitric oxide and cyclooxygenase products. *J Clin Invest.* 1993;91:1374-1379.

511. Lopez-Farre A, Gomez-Garre D, Bernabeu F, et al. Renal effects and mesangial cell contraction induced by endothelin are mediated by PAF. *Kidney Int.* 1991;39:624-630.

512. Danielson LA, Kercher LJ, Conrad KP. Impact of gender and endothelin on renal vasodilation and hyperfiltration induced by relaxin in conscious rats. *Am J Physiol Regul Integr Comp Physiol.* 2000;279:R1298-R1304.

513. Danielson LA, Sherwood OD, Conrad KP. Relaxin is a potent renal vasodilator in conscious rats. *J Clin Invest.* 1999;103:525-533.

514. Novak J, Danielson LA, Kerchner LJ, et al. Relaxin is essential for renal vasodilation during pregnancy in conscious rats. *J Clin Invest.* 2001;107:1469-1475.

515. Novak J, Ramirez RJ, Gandley RE, et al. Myogenic reactivity is reduced in small renal arteries isolated from relaxin-treated rats. *Am J Physiol Regul Integr Comp Physiol.* 2002;283:R349-R355.

516. Naitoh M, Suzuki H, Murakami M, et al. Arginine vasopressin produces renal vasodilation via V_2 receptors in conscious dogs. *Am J Physiol.* 1993;265:R934-R942.

517. Ichikawa I, Brenner BM. Evidence for glomerular action of ADH and dibutyryl cyclic AMP in the rat. *Am J Physiol.* 1977;233:F102-F117.

518. Bouby N, Ahloulay M, Nsegbe E, et al. Vasopressin increases glomerular filtration rate in conscious rats through its antidiuretic action. *J Am Soc Nephrol.* 1996;7:842-851.

519. Aki Y, Tamaki T, Kiyomoto H, et al. Nitric oxide may participate in V$_2$ vasopressin-receptor–mediated renal vasodilation. *J Cardiovasc Pharmacol*. 1994;23:331-336.

520. Rudichenko VM, Beierwaltes WH. Arginine vasopressin–induced renal vasodilation mediated by nitric oxide. *J Vasc Res*. 1995;32:100-105.

521. Yared A, Kon V, Ichikawa I. Mechanism of preservation of glomerular perfusion and filtration during acute extracellular fluid volume depletion. Importance of intrarenal vasopressin-prostaglandin interaction for protecting kidneys from constrictor action of vasopressin. *J Clin Invest*. 1985;75:1477-1487.

522. Briner VA, Tsai P, Choong HL, et al. Comparative effects of arginine vasopressin and oxytocin in cell culture systems. *Am J Physiol*. 1992;263:F222-F227.

523. Tamaki T, Kiyomoto K, He H, et al. Vasodilation induced by vasopressin V$_2$ receptor stimulation in afferent arterioles. *Kidney Int*. 1996;49:722-729.

524. Weihprecht H, Lorenz JN, Briggs JP, et al. Vaoconstrictor effect of angiotensin and vasopressin in isolated rabbit afferent arterioles. *Am J Physiol*. 1991;261:F273-F282.

525. Kriz W, Bankir L. A standard nomenclature for structures of the kidney. The Renal Commission of the International Union of Physiological Sciences (IUPS). *Kidney Int*. 1988;33:1-7.

526. Winetz JA, Golbetz HV, Spencer RJ, et al. Glomerular function in advanced human diabetic nephropathy. *Kidney Int*. 1982;21:750-756.

527. Hostetter TH. Human renal response to meat meal. *Am J Physiol*. 1986;250:F613-F618.

528. Deen WM, Bridges CR, Brenner BM, et al. Heteroporous model of glomerular size selectivity: application to normal and nephrotic humans. *Am J Physiol*. 1985;249:F374-F389.

Metabolic Basis of Solute Transport

Alicia A. McDonough and Scott C. Thomson

How much energy is required to make the urine? Of the major body organs, the kidney consumes the second highest amount of oxygen per gram of tissue (2.7 mmol/kg/min vs. 4.3 mmol/kg/min for the heart).[1] Most of the potential energy developed by renal oxidative metabolism is committed to epithelial transport, which determines the volume and composition of the urine. It has been asserted that, because the kidney reabsorbs 99% of the glomerular filtrate, it must use a lot of energy. But this logic is incorrect. The minimum net energy required for reabsorption does not depend on the amount of fluid that is reabsorbed. Forming a volume of urine with a solute composition equal to that of the body fluid from which it is formed is the thermodynamic equivalent of partitioning a bucket into two compartments by the use of a divider. No net energy is required for this. On the other hand, energy is required to form a urine that differs in solute composition from that of the body fluids. The minimum amount of energy required for this is equal to the temperature multiplied by the decrease in mixing entropy represented by the differential solute composition of urine versus plasma.

Interest in kidney metabolism antedates most knowledge of the kidney's inner workings or of biochemistry. The theoretical minimum amount of energy required to make the urine was determined from the laws of thermodynamics nearly a century ago. Specifically, the cost of converting filtrate into urine by an idealized process that is 100% efficient, infinitely slow, completely reversible, involves no backleak, and generates no heat is about 0.5 cal/min/1.73 m² for a human in balance consuming a typical diet.[2] In real life, the kidney consumes more than 50-fold this amount of energy. On this basis alone, one might argue that the kidney is horribly inefficient, even after one subtracts the cost of the kidney's keeping itself alive. On the other hand, the requirement to make urine in a finite time, the need for flexibility to rapidly alter the volume and composition of the urine, the stoichiometric constraints of biochemistry, a 50% limit on the thermodynamic efficiency of oxidative phosphorylation, and the intrinsic permeabilities of tissues to electrolytes, gases, and urea impose added costs.

The thermodynamic requirement may be a small fraction of the actual expenditure, but before one concludes that the body is unconcerned with thermodynamics, it may be noted that the thermodynamic energy required of the kidney to maintain salt and nitrogen balance with consumption of a typical diet is minimized when the water intake is 1 to 2 L, which is what most people choose to drink. Also, the thermodynamic cost of excreting urea declines as blood urea nitrogen (BUN) concentration increases. Thus by allowing BUN to rise in kidney failure, the kidney lowers the thermodynamic cost associated with its role in nitrogen balance. These features were deduced in a mathematical model by Newburgh in 1943.[3]

This chapter provides an overview of the interdependence of renal solute transport and renal metabolism, including (1) the role of the sodium pump, Na^+–K^+–adenosine triphosphatase (ATPase), in epithelial transport; (2) the role of renal blood flow, the glomerular filtration rate, and tubuloglomerular feedback in controlling fluid and electrolyte filtration and tissue oxygenation; (3) the metabolic efficiency of sodium reabsorption (oxygen consumption/sodium reabsorption rate, or Qo_2/T_{Na}); (4) the metabolic substrates fueling active transport along the nephron; and (5) the regulation of the metabolic efficiency of transport during normal perturbations and disease.

Energy and the Sodium Pump

Na^+-K^+-ATPase, also referred to as the *sodium pump*, is an ubiquitous plasma membrane protein that transports intracellular sodium out of the cell and extracellular potassium into the cell, thereby generating opposite concentration gradients for sodium and potassium ions across the cell membrane. This process of separating sodium from potassium across the cell membrane is fueled by the hydrolysis of adenosine triphosphate (ATP).[4,5] Each cycle of the pump consumes 1 ATP molecule while transporting 3 Na^+ and 2 K^+ ions across the cell membrane. The hydrolysis of ATP and the associated transport of ions are mutually dependent[4,5] and constitute an example of *primary active transport*. Given the intrinsic free energy of ATP hydrolysis, the pump can generate gradients that store up to approximately 0.6 eV of electrochemical potential per 3 Na^+ plus 2 K^+ ions. For a typical cell in a typical environment, about 0.4 eV is required to cycle the pump, which means that cells tend to operate with some reserve to further reduce their sodium or increase their potassium concentrations.

Structure of the Sodium Pump

The sodium pump is composed of an α catalytic subunit that transports Na^+ and K^+ across the membrane and hydrolyzes the ATP, a β-subunit that is critical for functional maturation and delivery of Na^+-K^+-ATPase to the plasma membrane, and an FXYD protein that can modulate the kinetics of Na^+-K^+-ATPase in a tissue-specific manner[6] (Figure 4-1). There are multiple isoforms of each subunit. The α1β1 heterodimer is likely the exclusive Na^+-K^+-ATPase in renal epithelia,[7] whereas several FXYD protein subunits are expressed differentially along the nephron.[6-9] Biophysical models describing the turnover of the sodium pump through its functional cycle are described in a review by Horisberger.[4]

Other Adenosine Triphosphatases

Besides Na^+-K^+-ATPase, additional ion-translocating ATPases are expressed in renal epithelia along the nephron[10] including H^+-K^+-ATPase,[11,12] Ca^{2+}-ATPases[13] and H^+-ATPases.[14,15] These transport ATPases play important roles in maintaining acid-base and ion homeostasis as discussed in Chapters 5, 7, and 9. These ATPases do not contribute significantly to the reabsorption of the bulk of the filtrate.

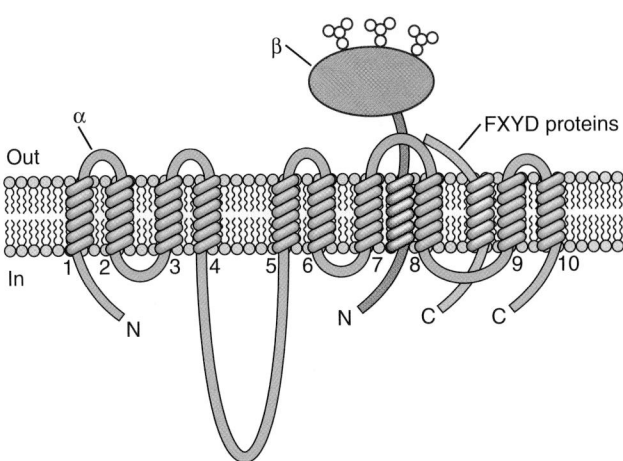

FIGURE 4-1 Na^+-K^+-ATPase is composed of a catalytic α-subunit (*teal*), an obligatory β-subunit (*pink*), and tissue-specific FXYD proteins (*green*). The α-submit has 10 transmembrane segments. It hydrolyzes ATP, is phosphorylated in the large cytoplasmic loop, and transports sodium and potassium. The β-subunit is a type II glycoprotein that is located close to M7/M10 and interacts with the extracellular loop between transmembrane segments M7 and M8 and with intracellular regions of the α-subunit.[3] FXYD proteins are type I membrane proteins that interact with M9 with the β-subunit,[4] and in the case of FXYD1 with the intracellular lipid surface and the cytoplasmic domain of the α-subunit [5•]. (From Geering K: Functional roles of Na,K-ATPase subunits, *Curr Opin Nephrol Hypertens* 17[5]:526-532, 2008.)

Pump-Leak Process and the Sodium Potential

For a cell in steady state, sodium and potassium must leak in and out across the cell membrane at the same rate that they are pumped out and in by the sodium pump. The back-leak of ions is an example of electrodiffusion. Electrodiffusion is a passive process that generates an electric field to retard diffusion of the most mobile charged species. Since cell membranes are generally more permeable to potassium than to sodium, potassium diffusion contributes more to the cell voltage than sodium diffusion, even though three sodium ions leak into the cell for every two potassium ions that leak out. Thus diffusion of potassium out of the cell dominates the cell voltage, making it negative. The negative cell voltage, in turn, neutralizes the net driving force for further potassium egress and augments the net driving force for sodium entry. Since cell membranes are poor capacitors, an imperceptible charge imbalance suffices to form the entire membrane voltage. This allows the transmembrane concentration differences for sodium and potassium to remain nearly equal and opposite in spite of the much greater leakiness to potassium. The net outcome of this pump-leak process is that electrochemical potential, which originates with ATP hydrolysis, becomes concentrated in the transmembrane sodium gradient, whereas potassium resides near to electrochemical equilibrium.

Harnessing the Sodium Potential for Work

The difference in electrochemical potential for sodium across the cell membrane is available to drive the unfavorable passage of other solutes across the membrane by a variety of exchangers and cotransporters. Examples include

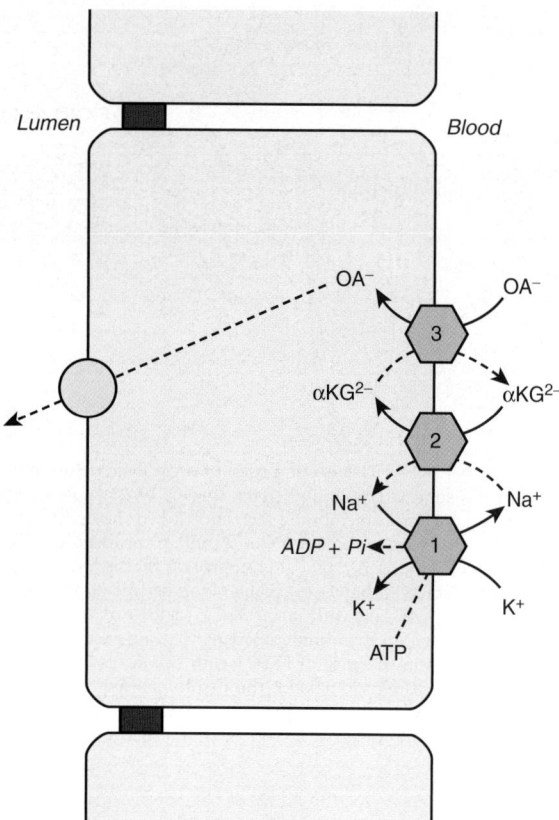

FIGURE 4-2 Different modes of active uphill transport as exemplified by organic acid (OA) secretion in proximal tubule epithelial cells. Transport across the basolateral membrane involves three steps functioning in parallel: *Primary active transport* (①) of Na and K by Na⁺-K⁺-ATPase coupled to the hydrolysis of ATP establishes the inwardly directed Na gradient. *Secondary active transport* (②) of α-ketoglutarate (α-KG) with Na on an Na/α-KG cotransporter uses the inwardly directed Na gradient to drive α-KG into the cell. *Tertiary active transport* (③) of OA with α-KG on an OA/α-KG antiporter uses the outward downhill transport of α-KG to drive the inward uphill transport of OA. The α-KG is recycled through the Na/α-KG cotransporter, which thus links the uphill transport of OA to the generation of the Na gradient by the Na⁺-K⁺-ATPase. Ultimately OAs are secreted down the OA concentration gradient into the tubular lumen. (From Dantzler WH, Wright SH: The molecular and cellular physiology of basolateral organic anion transport in mammalian renal tubules, *Biochim Biophys Acta* 1618[2]:185-193, 2003.)

the proximal tubule Na⁺/H⁺ exchanger, sodium-glucose cotransporters (SGLTs), the basolateral Na/α-ketoglutarate (α-KG) cotransporter, the furosemide-sensitive Na-K-2Cl cotransporter, (NKCC2) and the thiazide-sensitive Na-Cl cotransporter (NCC). Generically, transport that directly uses free energy from the sodium gradient to drive uphill flux of another solute is referred to as *secondary active transport*[16] (α-KG cotransport in Figure 4-2). *Tertiary active transport* refers to the net flux of a solute against its electrochemical potential gradient coupled indirectly to the Na⁺ gradient (three transport processes working in parallel). An example of tertiary active transport is the uptake of various organic anions from the peritubular blood into the proximal tubular cell by the so-called organic anion transporters (OATs). Energy from the sodium gradient is converted into a gradient for α-KG to diffuse out of the cell by Na/α-KG cotransport. OATs use this potential difference to exchange α-KG for another organic anion[17] (see Figure 4-2).

Cell Polarity and Vectorial Transport

The polar arrangement of transporters in renal cells is essential for vectorial transport. Wherever it is expressed along the nephron, the sodium pump, which removes sodium from the cell, is restricted to the basolateral membrane. Meanwhile, the variety of exchangers, cotransporters, and sodium channels through which sodium enters the tubular cell are restricted to the apical membrane. These include the principal Na⁺/H⁺ exchanger (NHE3) and SGLTs in the proximal tubule, the NKCC2 in the thick ascending limb (TAL) of the loop of Henle, the NCC in the distal convoluted tubule, and epithelial sodium channels in the connecting tubule and collecting duct (see Chapter 5). These apical sodium transporters effect secondary active transport coupled to the primary active transporter, Na⁺-K⁺-ATPase.

Close coordination of sodium uptake across the apical membrane with sodium extrusion across the basolateral membrane is required to avoid osmotic swelling and shrinking of the cell. Assuming ATP is not limiting for basolateral exit, the magnitude of transepithelial transport is a function of both the number of transporters in the plasma membrane, which can be varied by changes in synthesis or degradation rates and/or trafficking between intracellular and plasma membranes, and the activity per transporter, which can be varied by covalent modification (e.g., phosphorylation or proteolysis) or protein-protein interaction (e.g., Na⁺-K⁺-ATPase kinetics are influenced by FXYD subunit association[6]). The rate of apical sodium entry is also subject to influence by the availability of substrates for cotransport. For example, the amount of sodium-glucose cotransport depends on the availability of glucose in proximal tubular fluid, and the sodium entry at a given point along the TAL is subject to variations in the local chloride concentration, because the NKCC has a relatively low affinity for chloride.

Many factors and hormones known to regulate renal sodium reabsorption (including angiotensin II, aldosterone, dopamine, parathyroid hormone, and blood pressure) act in parallel to affect the activity, distribution, or abundance of apical transporters and basolateral sodium pumps.[7,18] The molecular basis of this apical-basolateral crosstalk is not clearly understood, especially in the light of close cell volume control; however, there is evidence for a role of elevated cellular calcium level in response to depressed sodium transport,[19] recent evidence for a salt-inducible kinase that responds to slight elevations in cell Na and Ca,[20] as well as evidence for coupling of Na⁺-K⁺-ATPase to apical channel activity.[21]

Control of Renal Oxygenation: Role of Renal Blood Flow, Glomerular Filtration Rate, and Tubuloglomerular Feedback

The kidneys are faced with the challenge of maintaining intrarenal oxygen levels so as to avoid both hypoxia, which leads to energy failure, and hyperoxia, which promotes oxidant damage.[22] In organs where blood flow is not a principal determinant of O₂ demand, tissue oxygen can be stabilized by simple negative feedback. In such an arrangement, increased utilization of oxygen produces a signal that results in more blood flow to that organ. But the kidney cannot rely on this simple mode of metabolic autoregulation because, unlike other organs that receive blood for their own benefit, the kidney receives blood to regulate blood volume and composition; that is, to benefit the blood itself.

Renal blood flow (RBF) creates its own demand, because RBF determines glomerular filtration rate (GFR), which in turn determines the rate of sodium reabsorption (T_{Na}), which is the main determinant of O_2 consumption (Q_{O_2}).[23,24] If the kidneys were to modulate RBF as a means of stabilizing renal O_2 content, this would create a vicious cycle of positive feedback in which increased O_2 delivery increases O_2 consumption, which calls for more O_2 delivery. Positive feedback is inherently destabilizing, so this arrangement alone could not work to stabilize either RBF or renal O_2 content. Hence, the kidney is compelled to invoke mechanisms that are more complex.

There are two generic routes for the kidney to stabilize its O_2 content. One is to dissociate RBF from GFR. The other is to alter the metabolic efficiency of Na^+ transport (Q_{O_2}/T_{Na}) (Table 4-1). Further details are discussed shortly. The amount of oxygen available to a given cell in the kidney depends on the amount of oxygen delivered in the arterial blood, on the amount consumed by other cells, and on the vascular anatomy of the kidney, which facilitates diffusion of oxygen directly from preglomerular arteries to postcapillary veins (arteriovenous [AV] O_2 shunting)[25] (Figure 4-3).

The phenomenon of O_2 shunting from descending to ascending vasa recta in the medulla has been accepted for decades. Evidence for AV O_2 shunting in the kidney cortex was provided more recently when it was shown, by the use of oxygen-sensing microelectrodes, that the oxygen tension is substantially higher in the renal vein (50 mm Hg) than in efferent arterioles (45 mm Hg) or tubules (40 mm Hg).[26] The fraction of incident oxygen subject to AV O_2 shunting is estimated at 50%. This causes tissue oxygen pressure (Po_2) in the kidney cortex to be lower than otherwise expected and similar to that of other organs with lower venous Po_2 in which perfusion is matched more closely to metabolic demand.

Noting the similarity of tissue Po_2 in the kidney and in other organs, some have argued that the renal AV O_2 shunt is an adaptive mechanism for preventing the exposure of cortical tubules to toxic levels of oxygen while permitting a high RBF, which is needed for clearance[27] (see Figure 4-3). As mentioned earlier, there is substantial shunting of oxygen from descending to ascending vasa recta in the renal medulla due to countercurrent flow in these vessels. Countercurrent flow in "hairpin loops" formed by the vasa recta facilitates the recycling of solutes to the inner medulla, where a high osmolarity is essential to the formation of concentrated urine (see Chapter 10). As an inherent consequence of this countercurrent mechanism for maintaining a medullary osmotic gradient, there arises a negative oxygen gradient from cortex to inner medulla, where Po_2 falls to 10 mm Hg.[28] This results from the combination of slow blood flow through the vasa recta, O_2 consumption by active transport in the outer medullary TAL, and diffusion of O_2 from descending to ascending vasa recta.[28]

Consideration of O_2 transport was recently incorporated into a mathematical model of the rat outer medulla by Chen and colleagues.[29,30] The model takes into account fine details of the medullary anatomy, which includes positioning of the long descending vasa recta in the center of vascular bundles and the positioning of the TAL and collecting ducts at some distance from those vascular bundles (see Figure 3-11

TABLE 4-1 Mechanisms for Changing the Amount of Oxygen Consumed per Work Performed
Dissociate glomerular filtration rate from renal blood flow.
Alter the amount of O_2 consumed per Na^+ reabsorbed.
Shift transport between tubular segments that make more or less use of passive reabsorption.
Alter backleak permeability of the tubule.
Change the coupling ratio of adenosine triphosphate generated to O_2 consumed by mitochondria.

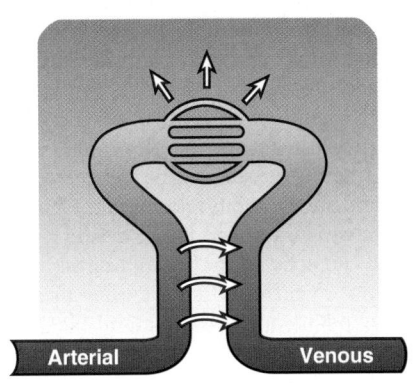

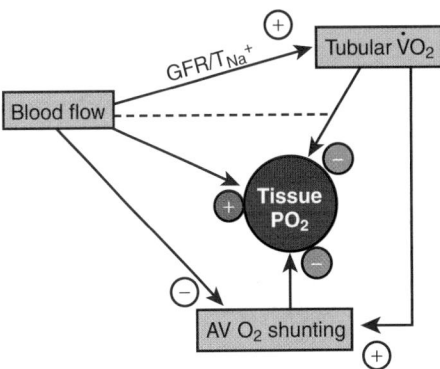

FIGURE 4-3 Control of intrarenal oxygenation. Renal arteriovenous (AV) oxygen shunting is a structural antioxidant mechanism that contributes to dynamic regulation of intrarenal oxygenation. Because of AV oxygen shunting, much of the oxygen entering the kidney never enters the renal microcirculation, instead diffusing from arterial blood to the closely associated veins. This mechanism helps maintain stable renal tissue oxygen tension. A model of the control of renal tissue oxygen tension (Po_2) is shown. In this model blood flow affects tissue Po_2. (Modified from Evans RG, et al: Intrarenal oxygenation: unique challenges and the biophysical basis of homeostasis. *Am J Physiol Renal Physiol* 295:F1259-F1270, 2008.)

in Chapter 3). The model predicts negative transverse O_2 gradients from vascular bundles to corresponding TALs and a compromise between the TAL and inner medulla with respect to the provision of oxygen.[31]

Ultimately, the rate at which the kidney consumes oxygen must be linked to the GFR. This is true because the main use of oxygen is to reabsorb sodium, which is linked to GFR by glomerulotubular balance (GTB). GTB is defined as the direct effect of the filtered load on tubular reabsorption, and it operates in all nephron segments, although the mechanism differs between segments. In the proximal tubule, shear strain tied to tubular flow exerts torque on the apical microvilli, which leads to upregulation of apical sodium transporters.[32] In cases in which filtration fraction increases, the parallel increase in peritubular capillary oncotic pressure will increase the Starling's force driving fluid reabsorption. In the TAL, flux through NKCC2 is limited by chloride concentration, which declines more slowly along the TAL at high flow rates. But although GTB applies to net reabsorption, increased flow rate in the tubule also shortens the time that a given sodium ion is exposed to the reabsorptive machinery. This leads to the prediction that GTB can do no better than maintain constant fractional reabsorption.[23]

Significant fluctuations in RBF, GFR, and filtered Na+ load would overwhelm the kidney's ability to accurately match Na+ and volume output to input and compromise homeostasis of extracellular fluid volume. This does not normally occur because RBF and GFR are tightly controlled by the tubuloglomerular feedback mechanism (described in detail in Chapter 3): In short, if RBF and/or GFR increases and GTB maintains a constant fractional reabsorption along the proximal tubule, an increasing amount of salt will be delivered to the macula densa, which sets off the tubuloglomerular feedback response. Specifically, increases in apical NaCl delivery or flow to this region provoke the cells of the macula densa to release ATP into the interstitium surrounding the afferent arterioles. This response is dependent on the basolateral Na+-K+-ATPase to maintain the inward-directed Na+ gradient.[33] ATP release is via maxi-anion channels.[34] Some fraction of the released ATP is converted to adenosine by local ecto–nucleoside triphosphate diphosphohydrolase 1 (ecto-NTPDase1) and ecto-5′-nucleotidase.[35] This adenosine activates A1 adenosine receptors on the afferent arteriole, causing vasoconstriction. The arteriolar constriction reduces RBF and GFR in concert until Na+ delivery to the macula densa is realigned. Thus, an inverse relationship is established between tubular NaCl load and the GFR of the same nephron.[24]

Due to the time it takes for information to pass through the tubuloglomerular feedback system, the system is prone to oscillate with a period of around 30 seconds. Rhythmic oscillations of kidney P_{O_2} occur at the same frequency as tubuloglomerular feedback–mediated oscillations in tubular flow. This illustrates the simultaneous influence of tubuloglomerular feedback over minute-to-minute tubular flow rate and oxygen levels in the kidney.[36]

Adenosine mediates tubuloglomerular feedback as a vasoconstrictor. Adenosine-mediated vasoconstriction is unique to the afferent arteriole. In all other beds where adenosine is vasoactive, it exerts a vasodilatory effect mediated by A2 receptors. In addition to adenosine receptors, the afferent arteriole expresses P_{2X} purinergic receptors that also mediate a vasoconstrictor response, in this case to interstitial ATP. These P_{2X} receptors are essential to pressure-mediated RBF autoregulation,[37] but adenosine A1 receptors are sufficient to explain the tubuloglomerular feedback response.[35]

tubuloglomerular feedback adjusts the renal workload by affecting GFR. A number of other autocrine and paracrine factors stabilize the medullary energy balance through local adjustments in blood flow and transport.[38] Examples include vasodilatory prostaglandins, nitric oxide, and adenosine, which increase medullary blood flow while inhibiting sodium transport in the TAL.[39,40] Adenosine, in particular, is a case study in local metabolic regulation by negative feedback in the medulla. When ATP levels decline, adenosine is released from TAL cells into the renal interstitium, where it binds to adenosine A1 receptors and inhibits Na+ reabsorption in the

TAL and inner medullary collecting duct (IMCD). This has the effect of increasing P_{O_2} by reducing Q_{O_2}. The same pool of adenosine also activates vascular adenosine A2 receptors in the deep cortex and medullary vasa recta to increase blood flow.[41,42]

By these mechanisms, the TAL looks after its own interest. But since TAL sodium reabsorption normally exceeds the urinary sodium excretion by 40-fold, any significant decline in TAL reabsorption must be compensated for by increasing active transport somewhere else or by reducing GFR through tubuloglomerular feedback. Activation of A1 receptors in the glomerulus, proximal tubule, or TAL each contributes to lessening the amount of work imposed on the hypoxic outer medulla, whereas activating A2 receptors in the vasa recta supports O2 delivery to the medulla (summarized in Figure 4-4).

The cost of renal sodium transport can be estimated from the sodium pump stoichiometry and the amount of oxygen required to produce ATP. Sodium pump stoichiometry dictates that hydrolysis of one ATP molecule is coupled to the transport of 3 Na+ ions out of the cell and 2 K+ ions into the cell,[4] and oxidative metabolism generates approximately 6 ATP molecules per O2 molecule consumed (Table 4-1 and Figure 4-5).

In the 1960s, several investigators undertook to measure the metabolic cost of tubular reabsorption in various species of mammal. Each adopted a similar standard, which was to express suprabasal renal oxygen consumption (Q_{O_2}) as a function of sodium reabsorption (T_{Na}). Suprabasal O2 consumption was obtained by subtracting from total O2 consumption the amount required for basal metabolism. The latter was determined by various methods. One method was to plot Q_{O_2} against T_{Na} and then extrapolate to the y-intercept to obtain basal Q_{O_2}. Another approach was to reduce renal perfusion pressure to the point that glomerular filtration ceased, then ascribe the residual measured Q_{O_2} to basal metabolism.

These approaches for obtaining basal O2 consumption have their unique limitations, and both require the dubious assumption that basal metabolism is unaffected by T_{Na} per se. Nonetheless, there is fair consensus among four oft-cited studies published between 1961 and 1966 that the relationship between Q_{O_2} and T_{Na} is fairly linear and that the kidney reabsorbs 25 to 29 Na+ ions per molecule of O2 consumed in the process.[43-46] A representative figure from one of these studies is shown in Figure 4-6.

If one assumes that kidney mitochondria make 6 molecules of ATP per molecule of O2, the kidney must then reabsorb 4 to 5 Na+ per ATP molecule. This exceeds the 3:1 stoichiometry of the Na+-K+-ATPase, which was known at the time (reviewed in Burg and Good[47]). Since there are thermodynamic difficulties with the idea of an undiscovered basolateral sodium pump capable of forcing 5 Na+ from a tubular cell with energy from a single ATP molecule, it was surmised that a considerable fraction of overall sodium reabsorption must be passive and paracellular, as is now accepted.

It was later suggested, by Cohen[48] and others, that these calculated ratios of Q_{O_2}/T_{Na} actually underestimate the true efficiency of sodium reabsorption because a fraction of the oxygen consumed during Na+ transport is also spent metabolizing organic substrates that enter the cell by Na cotransport. The most important example of this is lactate, which is converted to glucose in the proximal tubule via the Cori cycle. The capacity for renal gluconeogenesis from lactate is large,

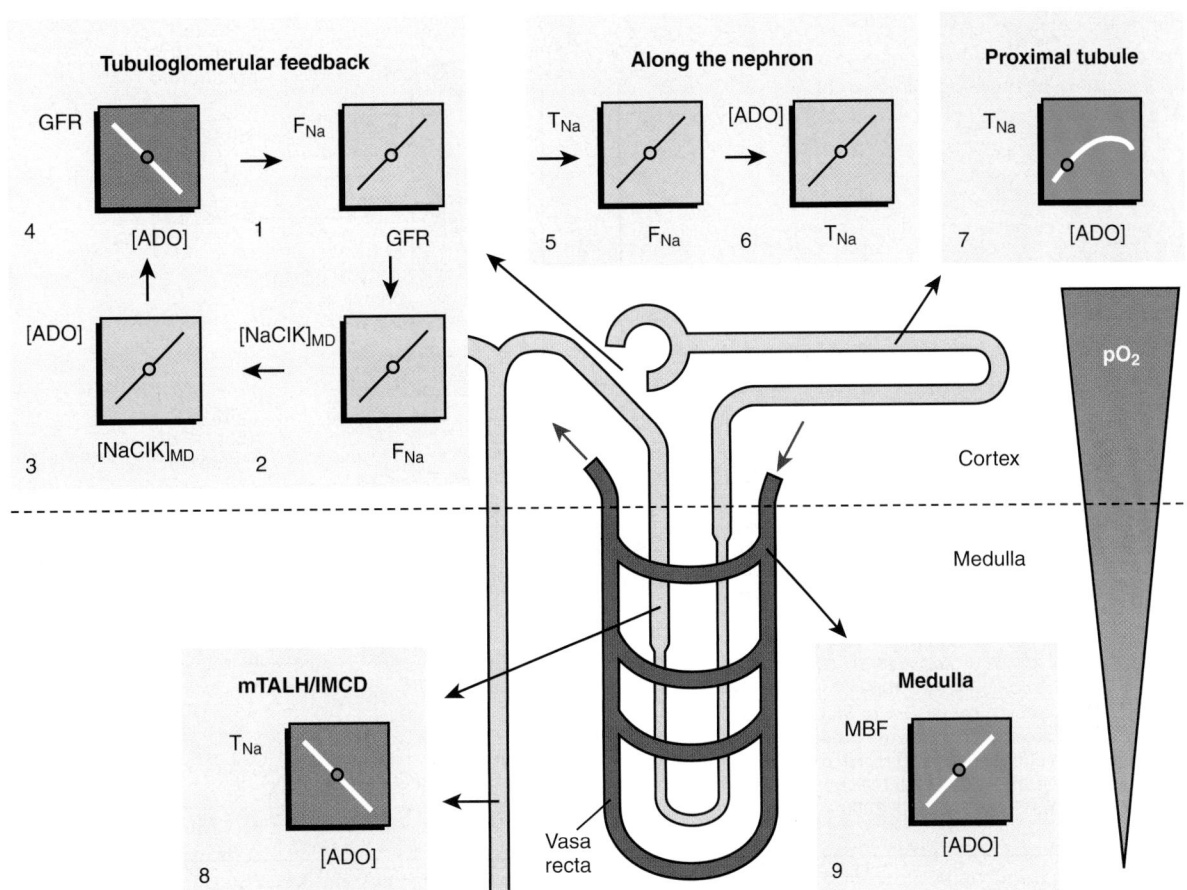

FIGURE 4-4 Role of extracellular adenosine (ADO) in protecting the renal medulla from hypoxia. The line plots illustrate the relationships between the given parameters. *Small circles* on these lines indicate ambient physiologic conditions. *1,* A rise in glomerular filtration rate (GFR) increases the Na$^+$ load (F$_{Na}$) to the tubular system in cortex and medulla. *2,* This rise in F$_{Na}$ increases the salt concentration sensed by the macula densa ([Na-Cl-K]$_{MD}$). *3,* The increase in [Na-Cl-K]$_{MD}$, in turn, enhances local ADO. *4,* ADO lowers GFR and thus F$_{Na}$, which closes a negative feedback loop and thus provides a basis for an oscillating system. *5,* F$_{Na}$ determines Na$^+$ transport work (T$_{Na}$) and O$_2$ consumption in every nephron segment, and thus oscillations in F$_{Na}$ may help protect the medulla. *6,* A rise in T$_{Na}$ increases ADO along the nephron. *7,* In the cortical proximal tubule, ADO stimulates T$_{Na}$ and thus lowers the Na$^+$ load to segments residing in the medulla. *8,* In contrast, ADO inhibits transport work in the medulla, including medullary thick ascending limb (mTAL) and inner medullary collecting duct (IMCD). *9,* In addition, ADO enhances medullary blood flow (MBF), which increases O$_2$ delivery and further limits O$_2$-consuming transport in the medulla. (Modified from Vallon V, et al: Adenosine and kidney function. *Physiol Rev* 86:901-940, 2006. © 2006 American Physiological Society.)

and it has been estimated that the kidney can consume up to 25% as much energy converting lactate to glucose as it spends reabsorbing sodium.[48] Proximal tubular gluconeogenesis will appear invisible from outside the kidney when the substrate is lactate made by glycolysis in the TAL and processed back into glucose without leaving the kidney.

The specific factors contributing to this Qo$_2$/T$_{Na}$ stoichiometry as well as to the basal metabolic rate in the kidney have been the subject of numerous reviews.[49,50] It is theoretically possible to alter Qo$_2$/T$_{Na}$ in a number of ways: First, Qo$_2$/T$_{Na}$ should increase if overall transport is made less efficient by shifting more of the burden for overall sodium transport from the efficient proximal tubule to the less efficient distal nephron, where all reabsorbed Na must pass through the sodium pump (discussed later). Second, O$_2$ might be diverted to some other purpose, such as gluconeogenesis. Finally, ATP production might be uncoupled from oxygen consumption (discussed later in the section on regulation of metabolic efficiency).

The metabolic cost of active sodium transport should vary along the nephron. As reviewed earlier, the overall stoichiometry of Na$^+$ reabsorbed to O$_2$ consumed is estimated at 25 to 30 (microequivalents Na$^+$/micromoles O$_2$).[43,44] This ratio

translates to 5 Na$^+$ reabsorbed for every ATP molecule consumed, which is much higher than the ratio of 3 Na$^+$ to every ATP molecule predicted by sodium pump stoichiometry. In fact, one might expect a ratio lower than 3 because of the basal metabolic functions of the kidney that are independent of sodium transport (i.e., insensitive to the Na$^+$-K$^+$-ATPase inhibitor ouabain) (Figure 4-7) and because of tubular backleak.

One reason for this higher than expected efficiency of sodium reabsorption is that the kidney can leverage excess free energy in the gradients created by primary and secondary active transport to drive passive paracellular reabsorption of sodium chloride. Free energy for paracellular reabsorption is available in the midproximal tubule and early ascending limb.[47] In the proximal tubule, the driving force for the passive transport develops as a result of the preferential absorption of bicarbonate over chloride earlier in the tubule.[51,52]

The decline in tubular bicarbonate concentration is paralleled by a rise in chloride concentration as water follows HCO$_3^-$ osmoles across the leaky proximal tubule (see Figure 5-3). This favorable lumen-to-blood Cl$^-$ gradient drives passive paracellular chloride reabsorption. The transepithelial

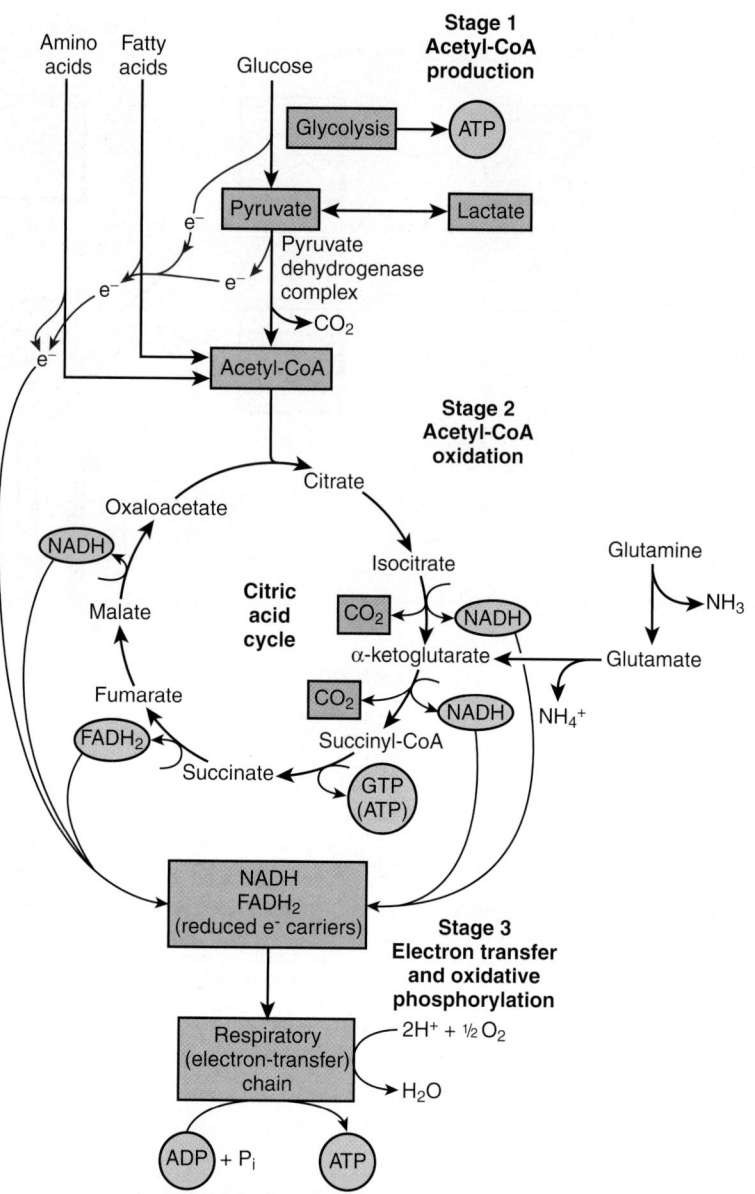

FIGURE 4-5 Catabolism of proteins, fats, and carbohydrates in three stages of cellular respiration. *Stage 1:* Oxidation of fatty acids, glucose, and some amino acids yields acetyl–coenzyme A (CoA). *Stage 2:* Oxidation of acetyl groups in the citric acid cycle includes four steps in which electrons are abstracted. *Stage 3:* Electrons carried by reduced nicotinamide adenine dinucleotide (NADH) and reduced flavin adenine dinucleotide (FADH$_2$) are funneled into a chain of mitochondrial (or, in bacteria, plasma membrane-bounds) electron carriers—the respiratory chain—that ultimately reduces O$_2$ to H$_2$O. This electron flow drives the production of ATP. Also indicated are two proximal tubule pathways: (1) oxidation of lactate through pyruvate and acetyl-CoA, and (2) glutamine conversion to glutamate and α-ketoglutarate in the mitochondria with the production of 2 mol NH$_3$, which is the main source of NH$_3$ secreted during acidosis. (Modified from Nelson DL, Cox MM. *Lehninger principles of biochemistry* [ed 5]. New York: WH Freeman; 2008.)

voltage that arises from electrodiffusion of chloride, in turn, drives passive sodium reabsorption. Since the NaCl reflection coefficient is less than that for NaHCO$_3$ in this region,[52] coupled sodium chloride reabsorption also occurs secondary to solvent drag.[53] Although estimates vary, this passive reabsorption may increase the number of Na$^+$ ions reabsorbed to O$_2$ molecules consumed in the proximal tubule from 18 to 48.[54]

Simultaneously blocking both cytosolic and membrane carbonic anhydrase with acetazolamide reduces bicarbonate reabsorption and Q$_{O_2}$ in a 16:1 molar ratio as expected for simple coupling to the sodium pump.[55] But inhibiting bicarbonate reabsorption with a membrane-specific carbonic anhydrase inhibitor, which acidifies the tubular lumen, paradoxically increases Q$_{O_2}$ both in vivo and in isolated proximal tubules, an effect that is prevented by also blocking the apical Na$^+$/H$^+$ exchanger NHE3.[56] A simple explanation is lacking for why increasing the cell-to-lumen proton gradient should increase Q$_{O_2}$ in the proximal tubule, but these results establish the phenomenon in vitro and in vivo.

The early portion of the TAL is also capable of paracellular Na$^+$ reabsorption. In this region, Na$^+$ can be transported transcellularly by the apical Na-K-2Cl cotransporter or apical Na$^+$/H$^+$ exchanger, secondary to a high density of Na$^+$-K$^+$-ATPase extruding Na$^+$ across the basolateral membranes. In addition, Na$^+$ can be reabsorbed paracellularly as long as there is a lumen positive transepithelial voltage sufficient to overcome the force for back diffusion associated with an unfavorable concentration difference. A lumen positive voltage develops in the TAL because the apical membrane has a high concentration of K$^+$ channels, whereas the basolateral membrane has both K$^+$ and Cl$^-$ channels. As predicted by the Goldman-Hodgkin-Katz voltage equation, the chloride conductance causes the basolateral membrane potential to be less negative than the apical membrane potential, which results in a positive transepithelial gradient.[57,58]

Further along the nephron in the distal tubule and collecting duct the tubular fluid sodium concentration is too low to allow paracellular reabsorption of sodium. In those segments, a lower

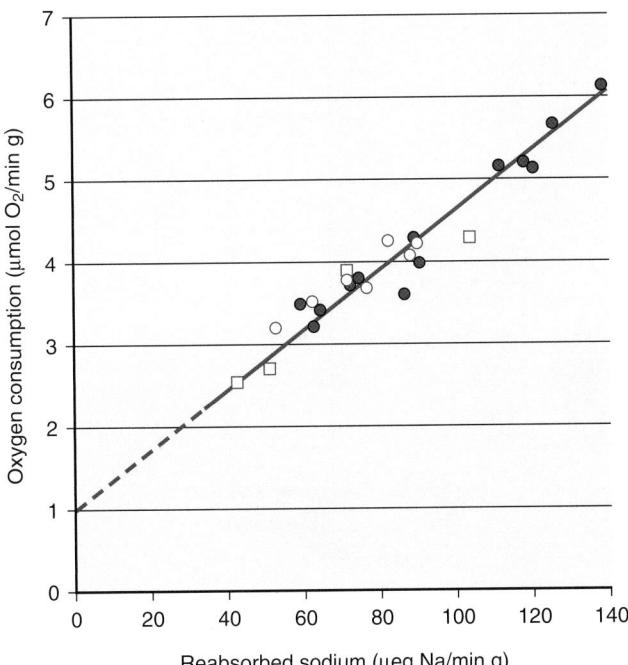

FIGURE 4-6 Oxygen consumption as a function of net sodium reabsorption in whole dog kidney. •, Control; o, hypoxia; □, hydrochlorothiazide. (Modified from Thurau K: Renal Na-reabsorption and O_2-uptake in dogs during hypoxia and hydrochlorothiazide infusion, *Proc Soc Exp Biol Med* 106:714-717, 1961; and Mandel LJ, Balaban RS: Stoichiometry and coupling of active transport to oxidative metabolism in epithelial tissues, *Am J Physiol* 240[5]:F357-F371, 1981.)

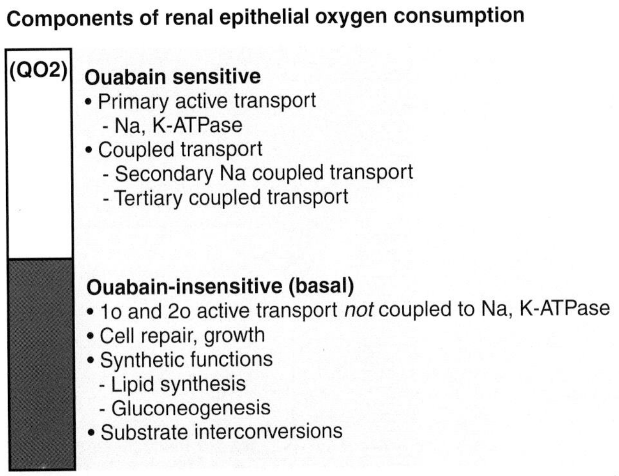

Components of renal epithelial oxygen consumption

(QO2)

Ouabain sensitive
- Primary active transport
  - Na, K-ATPase
- Coupled transport
  - Secondary Na coupled transport
  - Tertiary coupled transport

Ouabain-insensitive (basal)
- 1o and 2o active transport *not* coupled to Na, K-ATPase
- Cell repair, growth
- Synthetic functions
  - Lipid synthesis
  - Gluconeogenesis
- Substrate interconversions

FIGURE 4-7 A large fraction of renal epithelial oxygen consumption (Q_{O_2}) in renal cells is sensitive to the Na^+-K^+-ATPase–specific inhibitor ouabain, and this Q_{O_2} drives primary active transport and transport coupled to sodium pump activity. The fraction of renal oxygen consumption that does not change in the presence of ouabain is, by definition, independent of Na^+-K^+-ATPase activity in the cell and is roughly equivalent to the basal Q_{O_2}, which fuels transport not coupled to sodium gradients, cell repair and growth, biosynthesis, and substrate interconversions.

limit on the cost of Na^+ reabsorption is set by the 3 Na^+/1 ATP ratio of the sodium pump. Although active transport of sodium is a pacemaker for renal respiration, there are ways to reset the relationship of Q_{O_2} to sodium pump activity. Examples of this were provided by Silva and Epstein, who measured both O_2 consumption and Na^+-K^+-ATPase activity in rat kidney slices in which an increase in the latter had been induced by prior treatment of the animals with triiodothyronine (T_3), methylprednisolone, potassium loading, or subtotal nephrectomy. Although each of these maneuvers increased ex vivo sodium pump activity, only T_3 and methylprednisolone increased Q_{O_2}.[59]

It has also been shown that the thermogenic effect of catecholamines, normally associated with brown fat and striated muscle, also occurs in the kidney, which responds to dopamine infusion with a near doubling of overall metabolic rate, but minimal change in sodium reabsorption.[60] Dopamine inhibits Na^+ reabsorption in the proximal tubule,[61,62] thereby shifting the reabsorptive burden to less-efficient downstream segments. However, heat accumulates in both cortex and medulla during dopamine infusion, which suggests that the mechanism is not as simple as a shift in transport and that a direct effect of catecholamines on renal metabolism should be considered when interpreting the relationship between sodium reabsorption and energy consumption.

Weinstein and Szyjewicz[63,64] also examined Q_{O_2}/T_{Na} using 10% body weight short-term saline expansion as another way to inhibit proximal Na^+ reabsorption in rats. Using this maneuver, they were able to reduce fractional Na^+ reabsorption by 30% in the proximal tubule leading to a GTB-mediated increase in net reabsorption downstream of the proximal

tubule. Yet overall Q_{O_2} did not increase but actually fell. It was conjectured that energy for this increase in downstream reabsorption was derived anaerobically, but the full details of this remain to be clarified. It appears that the energy cost of transport in the proximal versus distal nephron during inhibition of proximal tubule transport depends on the stimulus provoking the change in transport as well as the metabolic environment.

Metabolic Substrates Fueling Active Transport along the Nephron

Mitchell has noted that "biochemists generally accept the idea that metabolism is the cause of membrane transport. The underlying thesis of the hypothesis put forward here is that if the processes that we call metabolism and transport represent events in a sequence, not only can metabolism be the cause of transport, but also transport can be the cause of metabolism. Thus, we might be inclined to recognize that transport and metabolism, as usually understood by biochemists, may be conceived advantageously as different aspects of one and the same process of vectorial metabolism."[65]

Metabolism Basics

Detailed accounts of cellular metabolism are provided in many excellent texts[66]; nonetheless, an abbreviated overview relevant to renal metabolism is warranted. Substrates enter the kidney by RBF and GFR and enter renal epithelial cells by substrate transporters, often facilitated by the inward-directed Na^+ gradient created by the sodium pump (see Figure 4-2), as discussed thoroughly in Chapter 8. Oxygen is likewise delivered by RBF to the epithelial cells. Once in the cell, substrates face one of three fates: (1) transport across the epithelium back into the blood (reabsorption), (2) conversion into another substrate (e.g., lactate to pyruvate), or (3) oxidization

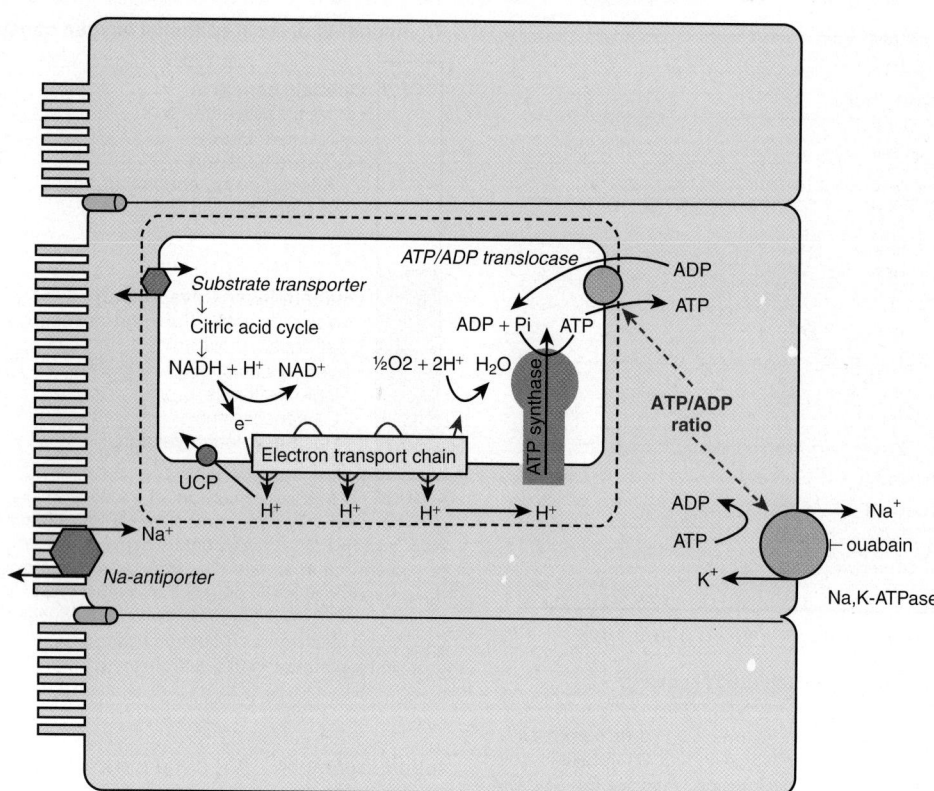

FIGURE 4-8 Whittam model. Coupling of ATP utilization by Na⁺-K⁺-ATPase to ATP production by mitochondrial oxygen consumption (Qo_2). Hydrolysis of ATP produces ADP plus inorganic phosphate (Pi), which lowers the ATP/ADP ratio, a signal to increase ADP uptake into the mitochondria and increase ATP synthesis.

to CO_2 in the process of cellular ATP production.[67] This section traces the roadmap that connects substrates to production of ATP in the mitochondrion and to ATP utilization by the sodium pump, and the feedback connections between production and utilization.

Renal epithelia, except in the descending and thin ascending limbs of the loop of Henle, are packed with mitochondria (see Chapter 2). All of the pathways of fuel oxidation take place in the mitochondrial matrix except for glycolysis, which occurs in the cytosol. Substrates in the cytosol can freely cross the outer mitochondrial membrane through integral membrane porins. These substrates, as well as adenosine diphosphate (ADP) and phosphate (the building blocks of ATP), cross the inner mitochondrial membrane into the mitochondrial matrix via specific substrate transporters driven by their respective concentration gradients or by the H⁺ gradient created by the electron transport chain (Figure 4-8).

As illustrated in Figure 4-5, amino acids, fatty acids, and pyruvate are metabolized to acetyl–coenzyme A and enter the citric acid cycle. With each turn of the cycle, 3 molecules of reduced nicotinamide adenine dinucleotide (NADH), 1 molecule of reduced flavin adenine dinucleotide (FADH₂), 1 molecule of guanosine triphosphate (GTP) or ATP, and 2 molecules of CO_2 are released in oxidative decarboxylation reactions (Table 4-2). Electrons carried by NADH and FADH₂ are transferred into the mitochondrial electron transport chain, a series of integral membrane complexes located within the inner mitochondrial membrane, where the electrons are sequentially transferred, ultimately to oxygen, which is reduced to H_2O. NADH and FADH₂ oxidization provoke

TABLE 4-2 Adenosine Triphosphate (ATP) Yield		
PROCESS	**DIRECT PRODUCT**	**FINAL ATP**
ATP Yield from Complete Oxidation of Glucose		
Glycolysis	2 NADH (cytosol)	5*
	2 ATP	2
Pyruvate oxidation (two per glucose)	2 NADH (mitochondrial matrix)	5
Acetyl–coenzyme A oxidation in citric acid cycle (two per glucose)	6 NADH (mitochondrial matrix) 2 FADH2	
Total yield per glucose		30
ATP Yield from Glycolysis of Glucose		
Glycolysis	2 ATP, 2 NADH	2

*Malate-aspartate shuttle in kidney.
FADH₂, Reduced flavin adenine dinucleotide; *NADH*, reduced nicotinamide adenine dinucleotide.

the transport of H⁺ from the matrix to the inner mitochondrial space.

The release of the potential energy stored in the H⁺ gradient across the inner mitochondrial membrane provides the driving force for ATP synthesis from ADP by the ATP synthase: H⁺ is transported into the matrix coupled to the production of ATP from ADP and inorganic phosphate (Pi) (see Figure 4-8). These are the fundamental pieces of the chemiosmotic mechanism of oxidative phosphorylation proposed by Peter Mitchell in 1961.[65] The newly synthesized ATP is extruded from the matrix into the intermembrane space via the ADP-ATP countertransporter known as *adenine nucleotide translocase* and then exits the mitochondria across the permeable outer membrane. In the cytosol, ATP is available to bind to ATPases such as plasma membrane Na$^+$-K$^+$-ATPase.

In summary, the flow of electrons through the electron transport chain generates a proton gradient across the inner mitochondrial membrane that provides the energy to drive ATP synthesis from ADP + Pi by ATP synthase and is also sufficient to extrude the ATP across the mitochondrial membrane.[66] The coupling between oxygen consumption and ATP production is one of the mechanisms that can change Qo$_2$/ T$_{Na}$. This coupling can be influenced by uncoupling protein isoforms (UCPs) located in the mitochondrial inner membrane and expressed in a tissue-specific manner. Simply stated, UCPs create a proton leak that dissipates the proton gradient available to drive oxidative phosphorylation (see Figure 4-8). It has been reported that UCP-2 is expressed in renal proximal tubule and TAL (not in glomerulus or the distal nephron) and that its expression is elevated in kidneys of diabetic rats.[68] However, the physiologic consequences of the expression and regulation of UCP in kidneys has not been explored experimentally.

Whittam Model

In the early 1960s, the coupling between active transport, respiration, and Na$^+$-K$^+$-ATPase activity was recognized by Whittam and Blond,[69,70] who tested the idea that inhibition of active ion transport at the plasma membrane would cause a fall in oxygen consumption (Qo$_2$) in the mitochondria. Using brain or kidney samples studied in vitro, they demonstrated that inhibition of Na$^+$-K$^+$-ATPase activity by removal of sodium or addition of the sodium pump–specific inhibitor ouabain (neither of which directly inhibits mitochondrial respiration) markedly reduced Qo$_2$, which led the investigators to conclude that an extramitochondrial ATPase, sensitive to Na$^+$ and ouabain, as well as to K$^+$ and Ca^{++}, is one of the pacemakers of respiration of kidney cortex.[69,70]

A careful study by Balaban and colleagues two decades later[71] used a suspension of renal cortical tubules to reexamine this Whittam model (see Figure 4-8) in more detail by measuring the redox state of mitochondrial nicotinamide adenine dinucleotide (NAD), cellular ATP and ADP concentrations, ATP/ ADP ratio, and oxygen consumption rate (Qo$_2$) in the same samples. If transport and respiration are assumed to be coupled, inhibition of transport is predicted to provoke a mitochondrial transition to a resting state[72] accompanied by an increase in NADH/NAD$^+$ (reduced to oxidized NAD), increase in [ATP], decrease in [ADP] and [Pi], increase in ATP/ADP ratio, and decrease in Qo$_2$. Stimulation of active transport would provoke the opposite pattern: decreased NADH, ATP, and ATP/ADP ratio, and increased Qo$_2$. Predictably, incubating the renal cortical tubule suspension with the Na$^+$-K$^+$-ATPase inhibitor ouabain caused a 50% decline in Qo$_2$, reduction of NAD to NADH, and a 30% increase in the ATP/ADP ratio, all evidence for coupling of mitochondrial ATP production to ATP consumption via Na$^+$-K$^+$-ATPase. Similarly, in tubules deprived of K$^+$ (which is required for Na$^+$-K$^+$-ATPase turnover), adding 5 mmol/L K$^+$ increased Qo$_2$ by more than 50%, oxidized NADH to NAD$^+$, and decreased the cellular ATP/ADP ratio by 50%. These results provide evidence for the coupling of both

Na$^+$-K$^+$-ATPase and ATP production via ATP synthase to the cellular ATP/ADP ratio (see Figure 4-8).

Energy Requirements and Substrate Use along the Nephron

In all renal epithelial cells from the proximal convoluted tubule to the IMCD, the basolateral sodium pump uses the hydrolysis of ATP to drive primary active transport of Na$^+$ out of and K$^+$ into the cell, and the gradients created are used to drive coupled transport of ions and substrates across both the apical and basolateral membranes.

In spite of consistent distribution and function, the relative abundance of Na,K-ATPase as a function of tubular location along the nephron is highly variable. Na,K-ATPase activity, ouabain binding, and Na,K-ATPase subunit abundance have been studied in dissected tubules and with imaging techniques. Na,K-ATPase and ouabain binding patterns along the nephron are very similar.[10,73] The pronounced differences in activity can largely be accounted for by differences in sodium pump number measured either by ouabain binding or by immunoblot of subunits in dissected nephron segments (Figure 4-9).[74]

The patterns of Na$^+$-K$^+$-ATPase protein expression and activity as a function of tubule length are what is to be expected from what is understood of the physiology of the nephron segments: moderate levels are expressed in the proximal tubule where two thirds of the sodium is reabsorbed across a leaky epithelium, and lower levels are expressed in the straight than in the convoluted segments reflecting the amount of sodium transported in these two regions. Very low levels are detected in the thin limbs of the loop of Henle, whereas high levels are expressed in the medullary and cortical TAL ("diluting segments") that must reabsorb a significant fraction of NaCl without water against an increasingly steep transepithelial gradient. The Na$^+$-K$^+$-ATPase activity and expression in the distal convoluted tubule (DCT), which is responsible for reabsorbing another 5% to 7% of the filtered load against a very steep transepithelial gradient, is very high. In the collecting duct, which reabsorbs a smaller fraction of Na$^+$ via channels electrically coupled to the secretion of K$^+$ or H$^+$ and has variable H$_2$O permeability, the Na$^+$-K$^+$-ATPase is quite low, albeit sufficient to drive sodium reabsorption in this region. The distribution of the ATP-producing mitochondria along the nephron, reported as percent of cytoplasmic volume,[75] parallels the distribution of the ATP-consuming sodium pumps but is somewhat less variable, ranging from 10% or less of the cell volume in the thin loop of Henle and medullary collecting duct to 20% in the cortical collecting duct and proximal straight tubule to 30% to 40% of cell volume in the proximal tubule and TAL[75] (Figure 4-9C).

Determining which substrates support ATP production and Na$^+$-K$^+$-ATPase activity along the nephron has been the subject of many studies and reviews.[67,76,77] To obtain nephron-specific information, investigators have dissected nephron segments and assayed for either metabolic pathway enzyme distribution or examined how specific substrates affected ATP levels. Although these in vitro approaches lack the in vivo realities of blood flow, tubular flow, and autocrine-paracrine, hormonal, and nervous system inputs that are evident in the whole kidney, the studies do provide information about the metabolic potential of each segment under defined conditions.

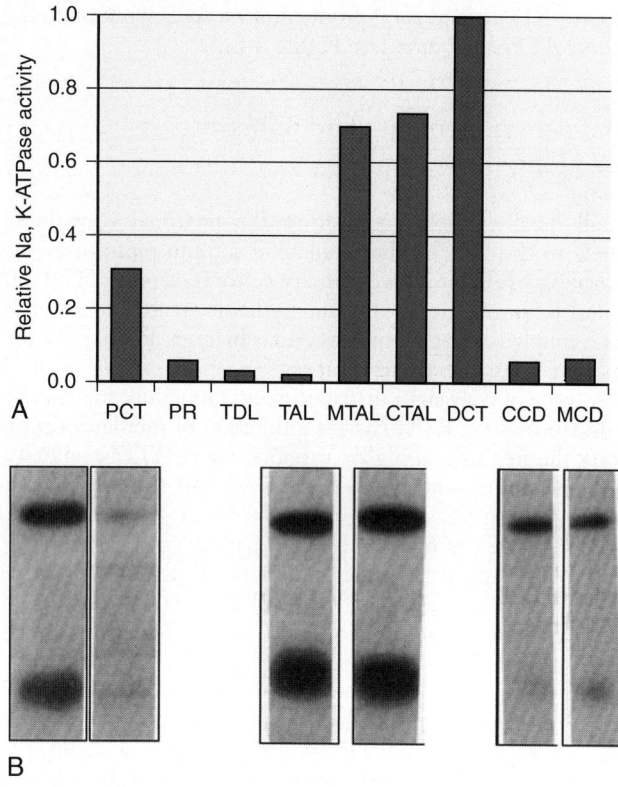

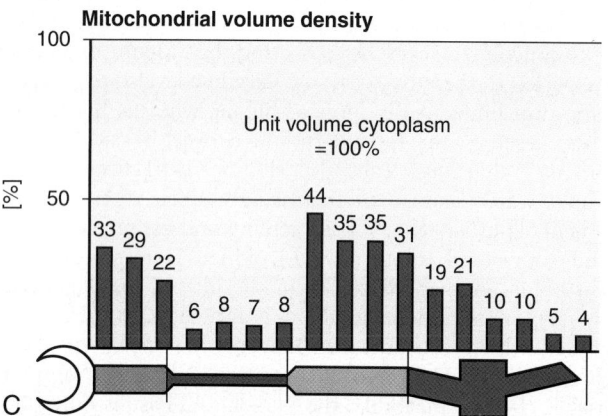

FIGURE 4-9 A, Relative levels of Na+-K+ATPase activity measured in individual segments of the rat nephron. (Data are normalized to that of the distal convoluted tubule.) **B,** Detection of Na+-K+-ATPase α1- and β1-subunits along the nephron. Tubule segments 40 mm long were resolved by sodium dodecyl sulfate–polyacrylamide gel electrophoresis (SDS-PAGE) and subjected to immunoblotting with subunit-specific antisera. Blots placed below corresponding tubule label indicated in **A. C,** Morphologic analysis of mitochondrial density relative to a unit of cytoplasm. *CCD,* Cortical collecting duct; *CTAL,* cortical thick ascending limb of the loop of Henle; *DCT,* distal convoluted tubule; *MCD,* outer medullary collecting duct; *MTAL,* medullary thick ascending limb of the loop of Henle; *PCT,* proximal convoluted tubule; *PR,* pars recta (proximal straight tubule); *TAL,* thin ascending limb of the loop of Henle; *TDL,* thin descending limb of the loop of Henle. (**A** redrawn from Katz AI, Doucet A, Morel F: Na+-K+-ATPase activity along the rabbit, rat, and mouse nephron, *Am J Physiol* 237:F114-F120, 1979; **B** based on data from McDonough AA, Magyar CE, Komatsu Y: Expression of Na[+]-K[+]-ATPase alpha- and beta-subunits along rat nephron: isoform specificity and response to hypokalemia, *Am J Physiol* 267:C901-C908, 1994; **C** based on data from Pfaller W, Rittinger M: Quantitative morphology of the rat kidney, *Int J Biochem* 12[1-2]:17-22, 1980.)

Isolated nephron segments had been reported to have low levels of cellular ATP, so Uchida and Endou[78] reasoned that if the segments were incubated with fuels that could be utilized by the segment, their ATP levels should increase toward physiologic levels. They examined a range of substrates for their ability to maintain cellular ATP levels in microdissected glomeruli and nephron segments (excluding thin sections of loop of Henle and papillary duct). The substrates studied (all at 2 mmol/L) included L-glutamine, D-glucose, β-hydroxybutyrate (HBA), and DL-lactate. Because the preincubation did not fully deplete the TAL and distal nephron segments of ATP, the ionophore monensin was included in the incubation with the substrate to dissipate the Na+ gradient and promote ATP consumption.

The change in ATP per millimeter of tubule (or glomerulus) as a function of substrate addition, shown in Figure 4-10, illustrates that each segment had a distinct ability to utilize these substrates. Lactate was very effective at maintaining ATP levels in all nephron segments tested, notably in the proximal tubule. The S1, S2, and S3 segments of the proximal tubule all utilized glutamine effectively as a fuel, which is consistent with the role of the proximal tubule in ammoniagenesis. Glutamine is the main amino acid oxidized by the proximal tubule, where it is deaminated and converted to α-KG, yielding 2 NH_3 molecules that are secreted during acidosis, as illustrated in Figure 4-5 and discussed in Chapter 9. Glutamine was not a preferred fuel in the more distal nephron segments. Glucose is completely reabsorbed along the proximal tubule yet, glucose is not an effective metabolic fuel for the S1 or S2 regions of the proximal tubule. In contrast, all the more distal segments tested readily used glucose to maintain cellular ATP. The ketone HBA was utilized effectively in all nephron segments tested; however, in S1 and S2 of the proximal tubule the capacity of HBA to support ATP production was far less than that provided by glutamine or lactate.

The distribution along the nephron of numerous enzymes involved in metabolic pathways, collated from many studies, has been summarized by Guder and Ross.[77] Their description of glycolytic (Figure 4-11*A*) and gluconeogenic (Figure 4-11*B*) enzymes along the rat nephron[79-81] demonstrate very low glycolytic potential in the proximal tubule and high glycolytic potential from medullary ascending limb to medullary collecting tubule. In contrast, gluconeogenic enzymes are found almost exclusively in the proximal tubule.

In summary, the proximal tubule reabsorbs glucose and can synthesize glucose biosynthetically, but does not metabolize glucose. There are both practical and theoretical explanations for the lack of glucose metabolism in this segment. The proximal tubule is specialized to reabsorb the filtered load of glucose from the tubular fluid back into the blood. Because of the enormous load of glucose moving through these cells, a proximal tubule hexokinase would need to have exceedingly low affinity for glucose, which would be difficult to regulate. In contrast, more distal regions of the nephron such as the loop of Henle and distal nephron normally have little or no glucose in their tubular fluid, have no Na-glucose cotransporters in their apical membranes, and cannot synthesize glucose, but these regions use glucose delivered via RBF as a metabolic fuel (which could be provided by gluconeogenesis in the proximal tubule during fasting). A summary of substrate preferences along the nephron is provided in Figure 4-12.[76]

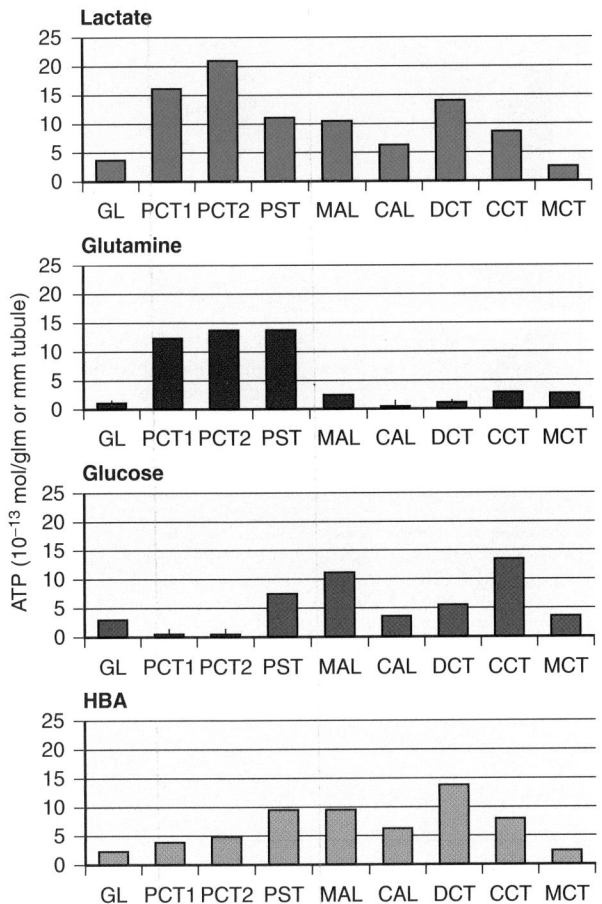

FIGURE 4-10 ATP production in glomeruli and dissected nephron segments as a function of substrates. In glomeruli and PCT1, PCT2, and PST segments, the values equal the differences in ATP content between samples incubated with and without each substrate for 30 minutes. **B,** In MAL, CAL, DCT, CCT, and MCT, the values equal the differences in ATP content between samples incubated with and without each substrate in the presence of monensin (10 pg/mL) for 15 minutes. (Data from Uchida S, Endou H: Substrate specificity to maintain cellular ATP along the mouse nephron, *Am J Physiol* 255[5 pt 2]:F977-F983, 1988.)

Renal Gluconeogenesis and Lactate Handling

In a review of renal gluconeogenesis, Gerich and colleagues[82] comment that the kidney can be considered two separate organs, because the proximal tubule makes and releases glucose from noncarbohydrate precursors, whereas glucose utilization occurs primarily in the medulla. Since the kidney is both a consumer and a producer of glucose, net arteriovenous glucose differences across the kidney can be uninformative, because glucose consumption in the medulla can mask glucose release by the cortex.

Gerich and colleagues[82] also make the case that the kidney is a significant gluconeogenic organ in normal humans based on the following: (1) In humans fasted overnight, proximal tubule gluconeogenesis can be as much as 40% of whole-body gluconeogenesis.[82] (2) During liver transplantation, endogenous glucose release falls to only 50% of control levels by 1 hour after liver removal.[83] (3) Pathologically in type 2 diabetes, renal glucose release is increased by about the same fraction as hepatic glucose release.[84] Zucker diabetic fatty rats also exhibit marked stimulation of gluconeogenesis compared with their lean litter mate controls.[85]

As discussed earlier, oxygen consumption by the kidney has been described as a linear function of sodium reabsorption.[86] Yet the kidney performs other functions that also require energy. For example, the proximal tubule can devote considerable energy to gluconeogenesis, especially in the postabsorptive or fasting states, and in diabetes.[84,87,88] In these states it becomes plausible for renal gluconeogenesis to consume oxygen on a par with sodium reabsorption, as discussed earlier. Hence, Q_{O_2}/T_{Na} can increase due to energy consumption by nontransport functions. The literature discussed in this chapter often refers to Q_{O_2}/T_{Na} as an index of transport efficiency. But in light of the fact that oxygen can be diverted to do other work, an increase in Q_{O_2}/T_{Na} is not necessarily due to "decreased transport efficiency."

Lactate can reach the nephron by filtration or blood flow and can also be produced along the nephron. Within the kidney, lactate can be (1) oxidized to produce energy with generation of CO_2, a process that consumes oxygen but generates ATP; or (2) converted to glucose via gluconeogenesis in the proximal tubule, a process that consumes oxygen and ATP. This is shown in Figure 4-13. Studies by Cohen[48] in isolated whole kidney perfused with just lactate as substrate demonstrated a change in carbon 14–lactate utilization as a function of its concentration in the perfusate: at low concentrations, all the lactate was oxidized (detected as CO_2) in order to fuel transport and basal metabolism; when [lactate] in perfusate was raised above 2 mmol/L some of the lactate was used for synthesis of glucose (gluconeogenesis); and at high [lactate] in perfusate the metabolic and synthetic rates approach maximum, and some lactate is conserved (reabsorbed). However, it is not the normal circumstance that lactate is the sole substrate, and it is now appreciated that the metabolism of lactate is affected by the presence of other substrates; for example, lactate uptake and oxidation are inhibited in the presence of fatty acids.[67,89]

The kidney's ability to convert lactate to glucose provides evidence that it can participate in cell-cell lactate shuttle, also known as the *Cori cycle*.[90] This cycle is important when oxidative phosphorylation is inhibited in vigorously exercising muscle, which becomes hypoxic. In the muscle, pyruvate is reduced to lactate to regenerate NAD^+ from NADH, which is necessary for ATP production by glycolysis to continue. Lactate is released into the blood and can be taken up by tissues capable of gluconeogenesis, such as liver and kidney. In the proximal tubule, the lactate that is not oxidized can be converted to glucose, and since this substrate is not used by the proximal tubule, glucose will be reabsorbed back into the blood, where it will be available for metabolism by the exercising muscle. Overall, this cycle is metabolically costly: glycolysis produces 2 ATP molecules at a cost of 6 ATP molecules consumed in the gluconeogenesis. Thus, the Cori cycle is an energy-requiring process that shifts the metabolic burden away from the exercising muscle during hypoxia. This cell-cell lactate shuttle could also operate within the kidney between nephron segments that produce lactate anaerobically and the proximal tubule.

Renal medullary lactate concentration was explored in a 1965 study in rats by Scaglione and colleagues[91] to test the idea that the medulla utilized glycolysis in the low-oxygen environment. Medullary lactate concentration is a function of delivery via the blood flow, production in the medulla, and removal by the blood flow, because there is no gluconeogenesis

GUDER AND ROSS

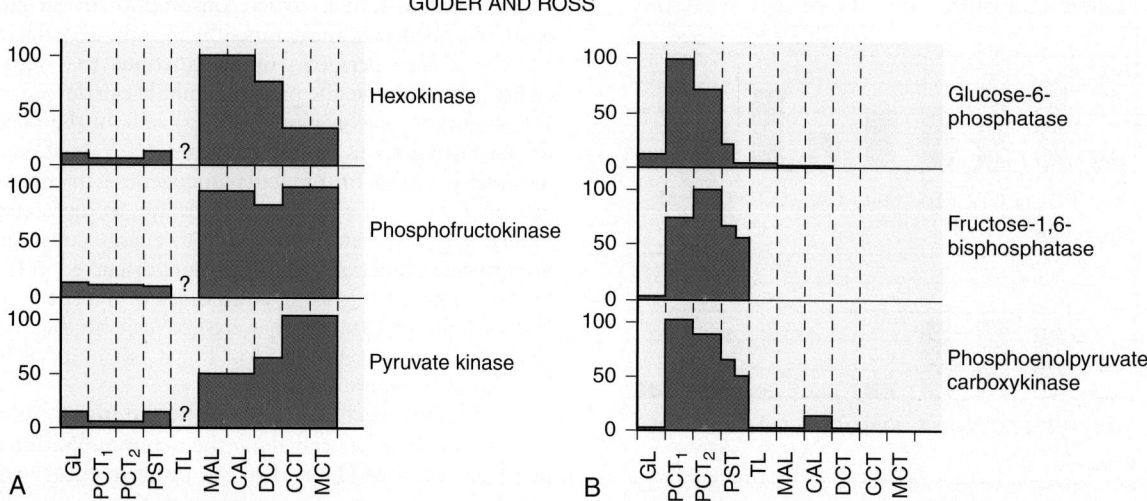

FIGURE 4-11 Distribution of glycolytic and gluconeogenic enzymes along the rat nephron. Nephron segments were dissected from fed (**A**) and starved (**B**) rats, respectively. The activity of hexokinase, phosphofructokinase, pyruvate kinase, glucose-6-phosphatase, fructose 1,6-bisphosphatase, and phospho*enol*-pyruvate carboxykinase. Were determined in individual segments. Enzyme activities are expressed as a percentage of the maximal value observed, based on the original activity per gram of dry weight. *CAL,* Cortical ascending limb; *DCT,* distal convoluted tubule; *CCT,* cortical collecting tubule; *GL,* glomerulus; *MAL,* medullary thick ascending limb; *MCT,* medullary collecting tubule; *PCT₁,* early proximal convoluted tubule; *PCT₂,* late proximal convoluted tubule; *PST,* proximal straight tubule; *TL,* loop of Henle, thin limbs. (Modified from Guder WG, Ross BD: Enzyme distribution along the nephron, *Kidney Int* 26[2]:101-111, 1984.)

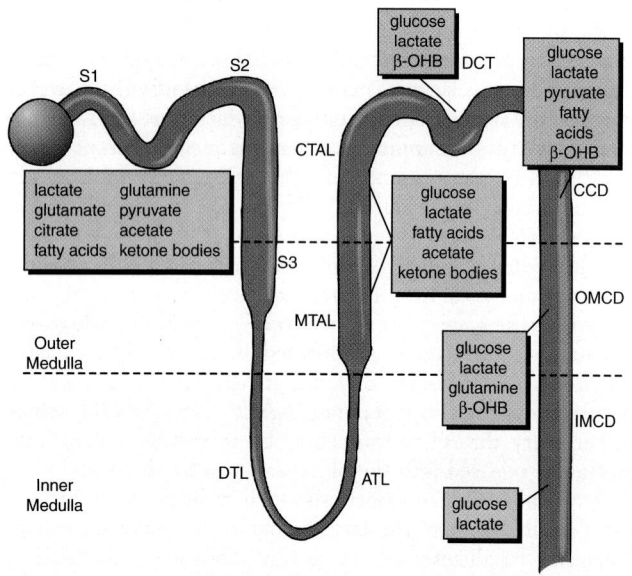

FIGURE 4-12 Substrate preferences along the nephron. Summary of preferred substrates to fuel active transport in nephron segments as gleaned primarily from studies using oxygen consumption (Qo₂), ion fluxes, radioactive carbon (¹⁴C)-labeled carbon dioxide generation from ¹⁴C-labeled substrates, ATP contents, and reduced nicotinamide adenine dinucleotide (NADH) fluorescence. *β-OHB,* β-Hydroxybutyrate. (Taken from Kone BC. Metabolic basis of solute transport. In *Brenner and Rector's the kidney* [ed 5]. Saunders; 2008.)

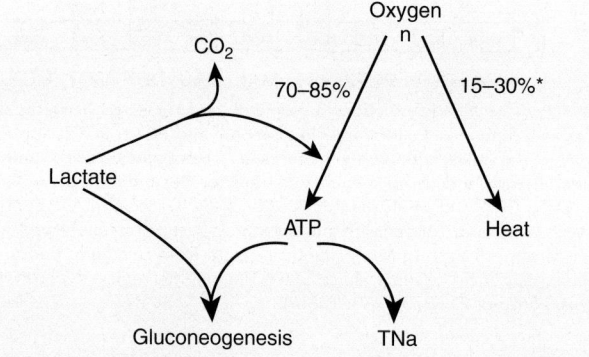

FIGURE 4-13 Fate of lactate and oxygen in renal metabolism. Oxygen can be utilized to generate ATP via oxidative phosphorylation or heat if uncoupling occurs. Lactate can act as a substrate for gluconeogenesis (GNG), which consumes energy, or enter into the citric acid cycle to generate energy.

in this region to consume lactate. Because of the countercurrent arrangement of the vasa recta, lactate would be expected to concentrate in the medulla somewhat. The study results indicated that lactate concentration was twice as high in the inner medulla as in the cortex and that during osmotic diuresis the medullary [lactate] doubled, whereas cortical lactate

remained unchanged. The authors postulated that increased medullary lactate was evidence for increased glycolysis during osmotic diuresis because the diuresis and increased flow through the vasa recta would be expected to decrease [lactate] if synthesis rates were unchanged. Sodium delivery to the distal nephron would also increase during osmotic diuresis and the accompanying increased Na⁺ reabsorption could drive the increased glycolysis.

Twenty years later, Bagnasco and colleagues[92] studied lactate production along the nephron in dissected rat nephron segments incubated in vitro with glucose with or without an inhibitor of oxidative metabolism, antimycin A. The only pathway for lactate production in the kidney is from pyruvate via lactate dehydrogenase. Proximal tubules produced no lactate with or without antimycin A. The distal segments

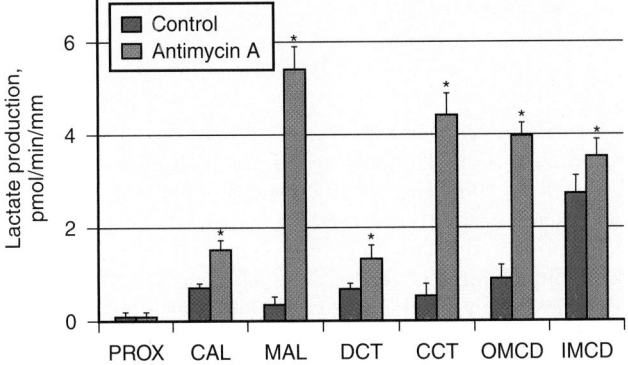

LACTATE PRODUCTION IN NEPHRON SEGMENTS

FIGURE 4-14 Lactate production by rat nephron segments under control conditions and in the presence of antimycin A. (From Bagnasco S, Good D, Balaban R, et al: Lactate production in isolated segments of the rat nephron, *Am J Physiol* 248:F522-F526, 1985.)

all produced lactate, and the production was significantly increased (approximately 10-fold in TAL) during antimycin A incubation (Figure 4-14), which led the authors to conclude that significant amounts of lactate can be produced by anaerobic glycolysis during anoxia in the distal segments. The IMCD, a region with low oxygen tension under control conditions, had high levels of lactate production even without antimycin A, which indicates that it is primed for anaerobic glycolysis.

Nephron Region–Specific Metabolic Considerations

Proximal Tubule

Studies carried out in a number of laboratories provide evidence that sodium transport and gluconeogenesis compete for ATP in the proximal convoluted tubule.[38,93,94] Friedrichs and Schoner[93] studied both processes in rat renal tubules and slices and found that ouabain inhibition of Na^+-K^+-ATPase increased renal gluconeogenesis by 10% to 40% depending on the substrate, and that stimulating Na^+-K^+-ATPase activity with high extracellular K^+- inhibited gluconeogenesis. The authors concluded that inhibition of the sodium pump induced a higher energy state of the cell, which would favor energy-requiring synthetic processes.

Nagami and Lee[94] used an isolated perfused mouse proximal tubule preparation to address this issue. When tubules were perfused at higher rates, delivering more sodium to the proximal tubule, glucose production rate was decreased by 50%; when tubules were incubated with ouabain in the bath or perfused with amiloride (to inhibit apical transport) glucose production rate increased above that seen in unperfused tubules. These authors also verified that the reduction in glucose production seen at elevated perfusion rates does not result from increased glucose utilization and is not dependent on the presence of specific substrates.

Because gluconeogenesis requires ATP, this relationship between sodium transport and glucose production can mask an effect of transport inhibitors or stimulators on the Q_{O_2}/T_{Na} ratio. Gluconeogenesis is localized to the proximal tubule,

so this effect will be most marked when transport is altered in the proximal tubule alone. Gullans and colleagues reevaluated these relationships in rabbit proximal tubule suspensions and perfused tubules.[89] They found that adding fatty acids to incubation fluid could increase gluconeogenesis twofold to threefold without affecting cellular ATP levels or fluid reabsorption. They concluded that the relationship between gluconeogenesis and active transport in the proximal tubule cannot be ascribed to competition for ATP and that under normal circumstances, with mixed substrates including fatty acids, the proximal tubule can meet the energetic needs of both processes.[89]

Thick Ascending Limb

The TAL has a very high rate of Na^+ transport against a steep concentration gradient, very high levels of Na^+-K^+-ATPase activity and expression, and, perhaps not unexpectedly, 40% of its cytosolic volume occupied by mitochondria (see Figure 4-9). Although the TALs have a far greater capacity for anaerobic metabolism than the proximal tubules, this region still requires oxidative metabolism to maintain cellular ATP levels and active Na^+ reabsorption.[78,95]

Cortical Collecting Duct

Cortical collecting duct (CCD) metabolism has been studied by Hering-Smith and Hamm.[96] This region is particularly interesting because it is made up of distinctly different cell types: principal cells that reabsorb sodium and intercalated cells that can secrete bicarbonate. Rabbit CCDs were microperfused, Na^+ reabsorption was measured by sodium 22 ion flux from lumen to bath, and bicarbonate transport was assayed by microcalorimetry in the presence of substrates with and without inhibitors. Both Na^+ reabsorption and HCO_3^- secretion were inhibited by antimycin A, which provides evidence for dependence on oxidative phosphorylation. However, neither was dependent on either glycolysis or the hexose-monophosphate shunt pathways. A small component of sodium transport was supported by endogenous substrates. Na^+ reabsorption was supported best by a mixture of basolateral glucose and acetate, whereas HCO_3^- secretion was fully supported by either glucose or acetate. HCO_3^- secretion (but not sodium transport) was supported to some extent by luminal glucose. In sum, this study indicates that principal cells and intercalated cells have distinct metabolic phenotypes.

Medullary Collecting Duct

Medullary collecting ducts contribute to final urinary acidification. Comparing the outer medullary collecting duct (OMCD) with the CCD, Hering-Smith and Hamm[96] found that HCO_3^- secretion in the OMCD could be fully supported by endogenous substrates. This region has far less sodium transport and few mitochondria (see Figure 4-9). Stokes and colleagues[97] isolated IMCDs and examined their metabolic characteristics. In the absence of exogenous substrate, IMCD can maintain cellular ATP and respire normally, which is evidence for the presence of significant endogenous substrate. In the presence of rotenone, an inhibitor of oxidative phosphorylation, glycolysis increased 56%, which provides evidence for anaerobic metabolism, as supported by enzymatic profiles. Inhibition of sodium pump activity reduced Q_{O_2} by 25% to 35%, which provides evidence for a requirement for a linkage between sodium pump activity and oxidative metabolism.

In studies that examined the metabolic determinants of K^+ transport in isolated IMCD,[12] glucose increased both Q_{O_2} and cell K^+ content by more than 10%, whereas an inhibitor of glycolysis promoted a release of cell K^+. Nor could cell K^+ content be maintained during inhibition of mitochondrial oxidative phosphorylation. Thus, in the IMCD, both glycolysis and oxidative phosphorylation are required to maintain optimal Na^+-K^+-ATPase activity to preserve cellular K^+ gradients. Given the low P_{O_2} and low density of mitochondria in this region, the collecting ducts have a higher reliance on anaerobic metabolism, but still take advantage of oxidative metabolism to fully support transport.

Regulation of the Metabolic Efficiency of Transport during Normal Perturbations and Disease

The kidneys have developed multiple mechanisms to minimize changes in oxygen delivery and to cope with falls in P_{O_2}. Some of these are specific to the kidney and some are present in many tissues. Diseases of mitochondria can also affect renal function.

Physiologic Regulation: Filtration Fraction and Q_{O_2}/T_{Na}

As reviewed earlier, there are two generic routes for the kidney to achieve a stable content of O_2: dissociation of RBF from GFR, and alteration of Q_{O_2}/T_{Na}. Both routes are subject to regulation. Dissociating RBF from GFR equates to changing the glomerular filtration fraction. This can work to stabilize kidney O_2 because lowering filtration fraction increases the ratio of supply to demand for O_2. For nephrons in filtration equilibrium, this requires independent control of the afferent and efferent arterioles, which can be achieved by modulating relative activities of purinergic, angiotensin, nitric oxide, and other signaling systems in the glomerulus. A full discussion of glomerular hemodynamics is available in Chapter 3, but a few features are noted here.

To begin, filtration fraction can be lowered by constricting the afferent arteriole (which reduces net O_2 delivery) or dilating the efferent arteriole (which increases net O_2 delivery). Constricting the afferent arteriole confers initial energy savings by reducing GFR faster than RBF, but there is diminishing return as O_2 delivery declines toward the basal requirement. Dilating the efferent arteriole only reduces GFR when glomerular capillary pressure is low to begin with, such as during hypotension or with high afferent resistance.[98] When angiotensin II acts on the afferent and efferent arterioles to stabilize GFR in the face of low blood pressure or high upstream resistance by preferentially constricting efferent arterioles, the kidney is accepting a decrease in the ratio of O_2 supply to O_2 demand. Conversely, adenosine signaling in the glomerulus decreases filtration fraction and so manages to stabilize nephron function without compromising the O_2 supply-demand balance. Adenosine in the nanomolar range constricts the afferent arteriole via high-affinity A_1 adenosine receptors. Higher adenosine concentration dilates the efferent arteriole via low-affinity A_2 adenosine receptors. Interstitial adenosine concentration rises as more NaCl is delivered into the nephron. The prototype for this is tubuloglomerular feedback signaling through the macula densa, although other sources are not precluded (see Figure 4-4). When the kidney is operating in the domain of modest distal delivery, increasing the tubuloglomerular feedback signal constricts the afferent arteriole. When the kidney is operating in the domain of high distal delivery, further increase causes the efferent arteriole to dilate,[99] which can be viewed as a shift in priority toward maintaining the O_2 supply as the supply diminishes.

The second generic means for stabilizing kidney O_2 is to alter Q_{O_2}/T_{Na}. Mechanisms to alter this ratio include the following: (1) Transport could be shifted from the proximal tubule, where efficient use of energy from the Na^+-K^+-ATPase drives passive transport, to other segments where all Na^+ reabsorbed passes through the Na^+-K^+-ATPase. (2) Tubular backleak permeability could change, which would affect the number of times that a given Na^+ ion must be reabsorbed to escape excretion into the urine. (3) The ratio of ATP produced per O_2 consumed could be altered by the regulated activity of UCPs (see Figure 4-8).[68] (4) ATP could be diverted to gluconeogenesis, such as during fasting.

The same neurohumoral factors that exert well-known effects on glomerular hemodynamics and O_2 supply, including nitric oxide, angiotensin II, adenosine, and catecholamines, also appear to participate in the regulation of kidney metabolism and oxygen consumption (Q_{O_2}/T_{Na}) by the tubule. Traditionally it has been argued that the oxygen consumed and ATP produced in the kidney are mainly used to support Na^+ transport and that the relationship between Q_{O_2} and T_{Na} is linear[43,86,99,100] (see Figure 4-6).

The bulk of sodium transport occurs in the proximal tubule, which relies on aerobic metabolism to generate ATP. Therefore, Q_{O_2}/T_{Na} has been used as a measure of metabolic efficiency. It has been shown[101,102] that administration of nonselective nitric oxide synthase (NOS) inhibitors increases Q_{O_2}/T_{Na}, essentially decreasing the efficiency of sodium reabsorption. Other experiments suggested that NOS-1 is the specific isoform that regulates this action in vivo. The changes in Q_{O_2} with NOS inhibition may occur due to (1) a shift in the site of sodium reabsorption to a less efficient nephron segment; (2) decreased efficiency of transport in the proximal tubule (i.e., decrease in the passive component of reabsorption); (3) less efficient use of O_2 by mitochondria; or (4) increased oxygen consumption by nontransport functions in the kidney (e.g., gluconeogenesis). For example, nitric oxide given directly to a proximal tubular cell is both a proximal diuretic[103] and a competitive inhibitor of O_2 flux through the electron transport chain in mitochondria.[104]

Most effects of nitric oxide are mediated by cyclic guanosine monophosphate, but the mitochondrial effect is presumed to occur through the competitive inhibition of cytochrome c oxidase.[104-106] Studies in normal rats,[107] in rats with experimental diabetes,[108] and in rats with untreated hypertension[109,110] have found an antagonistic relationship between nitric oxide and angiotensin II in terms of both glomerular hemodynamics and tubular reabsorption. Specifically, systemic NOS blockade causes renal vasoconstriction and activation of tubuloglomerular feedback, which can be prevented by angiotensin II blockers.

A parallel antagonistic relationship appears to exist in control of kidney metabolism as well. Angiotensin II was recently shown capable of increasing Q_{O_2} in spite of lowering T_{Na},[111] and studies in spontaneous hypertensive rats have suggested opposing effects of angiotensin II and nitric oxide on the Q_{O_2}/T_{Na} ratio in the kidney.[112] Rats with angiotensin-induced hypertension demonstrated an increased Q_{O_2}/T_{Na} that was reversed by a mimetic of superoxide dismutase, which is consistent with the theory that many angiotensin II effects are mediated by upregulating the activity of reduced nicotinamide adenine dinucleotide phosphate (NADPH) oxidase.[111] In addition there is evidence that angiotensin II contributes to mitochondrial dysfunction and oxygen consumption in aging rats.[113]

There is also known to exist a self-contained tubular angiotensin system that operates independently of the systemic renin-angiotensin system (RAS),[114-116] and it is possible to dissociate tubular and whole-kidney angiotensin II in the regulation of proximal reabsorption and salt homeostasis.[117] For example, a high-salt diet has a predictable inhibitory effect on plasma and whole-kidney angiotensin II but, surprisingly, leads to increased angiotensin II content of proximal tubular fluid. This finding explains why the tonic influence of endogenous angiotensin II over proximal reabsorption fails to decline with consumption of a high-salt diet. Thus, whereas the systemic RAS is oriented toward salt homeostasis, it appears that the tubular angiotensin II system is oriented toward a stable delivery beyond the proximal tubule.

By analogy to transport, it becomes reasonable to postulate that there may also be a different set of rules governing the effects of endogenously produced tubular angiotensin II compared with systemic RAS on kidney oxygen consumption. The role of angiotensin II in kidney metabolism is amplified in the ablation/infarction remnant kidney model of chronic kidney disease (CKD). Tissue pO2 is reduced in this model,[118] and local hypoxia has been proposed as a final common pathway to progression of CKD.[119] Rarefaction of capillaries leading to a decrease in blood supply may develop in late stages but does not explain the hypoxia observed in the early stages of CKD in which inefficient transport elevates Q_{O_2}/T_{na},[120, 121] which can be normalized by blocking angiotensin II.[122]

A connection has been established recently between local accumulation of the Krebs cycle intermediate succinate and activation of the RAS.[123] Succinate can accumulate extracellularly when oxygen supply does not match demand. In the extracellular fluid it can bind to its G protein–coupled receptor, GPR91. P_{O_2} in the juxtaglomerular region is reduced in the hyperglycemia of diabetes, and succinate levels are very high in urine and renal tissue of diabetic animals. Inhibition of the Krebs cycle's succinate dehydrogenase complex causes robust renin release. This effect is amplified in high-glucose conditions or with added succinate. In summary, GPR91-mediated signaling in the juxtaglomerular apparatus could modulate glomerular filtration rate and RAS activity in response to changes in metabolism (especially after a meal when glucose level is elevated). Pathologically, GPR91-mediated signaling could link metabolic diseases (such as diabetes) with RAS activation, systemic hypertension, and organ injury.

Hypoxia and Ischemia

Evans and colleagues[124] recently examined tissue oxygen tension (P_{O_2}) during moderate renal ischemia, when changes in renal oxygen delivery and consumption (Q_{O_2}) are mismatched. When renal artery pressure was reduced from 80 to 40 mm Hg, Q_{O_2} was reduced almost 40%, even though delivery was reduced only 26%. Renal angiotensin II infusion reduced O_2 delivery nearly 40%, and increased fractional oxygen extraction (renal venous P_{O_2} fell). When renal arterial pressure was higher than 40 mm Hg, renal P_{O_2} remained remarkably stable. With these protocols, reductions in Q_{O_2} were proportionally less than reductions in T_{Na}. Thus, reducing renal Q_{O_2} can help prevent tissue hypoxia during mild ischemia, and other mechanisms, not including increased efficiency of renal oxygen utilization for sodium reabsorption, apparently come into play to prevent a fall in renal P_{O_2} when renal Q_{O_2} is reduced less than O_2 delivery.

Recently, blood oxygen level–dependent magnetic resonance imaging (BOLD MRI) has been used to measure blood flow, oxygen tension, and regional tissue oxygenation in kidney cortex and medulla in humans with hypertension. The following were compared: kidneys with atherosclerotic renal artery stenosis, the kidneys contralateral to the stenotic kidneys, and kidneys in individuals with essential hypertension with no accompanying stenosis.[125,126] In the stenotic kidneys, as expected, tissue volume was decreased and blood flow was compromised; however, there was no significant decrease in P_{O_2} in the cortex or deep medulla compared with the contralateral kidney in the same person or compared with kidneys in individuals with essential hypertension. This led the authors to postulate that there was reduced oxygen consumption in the stenotic kidneys. Consistent with this interpretation, furosemide-suppressible Q_{O_2} in the medulla was significantly less in the stenotic kidney than in the contralateral kidney or kidneys in individuals with essential hypertension.[126]

BOLD MRI appears to be a useful technique for assessing whether renal artery stenosis is associated with tissue hypoxia and renal damage in a particular case.[127] BOLD MRI was also used recently to investigate the effect of sodium intake on renal tissue oxygenation.[128] In brief, 1 week of low Na^+ intake increased renal medullary oxygenation in both normotensive and hypertensive subjects, whereas a high-Na^+ diet reduced medullary oxygenation.

During hypoxia the cellular interior becomes acidic and the low cellular pH causes a small protein inhibitor called *inhibitory factor 1* (IF_1) to dimerize. In the dimeric state the IF_1 binds to two ATPase synthase molecules and inhibits their activity. This is an important adaptation, because during low-energy states ATPase synthase can actually operate in reverse (as an ATPase), which would cause further deterioration in the energy status of the cell. IF_1 inhibits the ATPase activity of ATP synthase, thereby preventing wasteful hydrolysis of ATP that could occur if there is insufficient oxygen to drive the electron transport chain. When oxygen delivery is normalized and cellular pH increases, the IF_1 dimer disassembles, and ATP synthase begins to operate in the ATP synthesis mode.[66]

In addition to the IF_1-mediated rapid posttranscriptional adaptation to hypoxia, there is an adaptive response to hypoxia mediated by hypoxia-inducible factor 1 (HIF-1).[129] Overall, HIF-1 is a transcription factor that accumulates in hypoxic cells, where it acts to regulate gene expression. HIF-1 regulates the expression of many genes during hypoxia, and the changes in gene expression culminate in a rise in erythropoiesis and tissue vascularization, which increases oxygen delivery, as well as a set of responses that conserve energy by decreasing substrate movement into the tricarboxylic acid cycle and increasing cellular glucose uptake and glycolytic enzymes to increase anaerobic ATP production; in addition, mitochondrial autophagy is stimulated.[129,130]

This last response is important in the context of renal physiology. During hypoxia there can be a buildup of reactive oxygen species (ROS) in the mitochondria that can provoke oxidative damage. For this reason, elimination of pathways leading to ROS production is adaptive during hypoxia. Recently, a study has suggested that dietary salt intake can also regulate HIF-1 expression: high salt intake leads to an increase in HIF-1 expression in the renal medulla of normotensive rats but not in that of Dahl salt-sensitive rats, which may represent a pathogenic mechanism producing salt-sensitive hypertension.[129] Whether this is mediated by hypoxia directly or indirectly remains to be determined.

Enzymes that regulate degradation of HIF-1 during normoxia (HIF-prolyl hydroxylases) are found predominantly in DCT, collecting duct, and podocytes, and levels are depressed during ischemia and reperfusion.[129,130] Although a tremendous amount of progress has been made in understanding how HIF-1 helps to maintain O_2 homeostasis, the study of this factor in the kidney under normal physiologic and pathophysiologic conditions is just in its infancy.

Adenosine Monophosphate–Activated Protein Kinase

The energy status of the cell can be detected by the ultrasensitive adenosine monophosphate (AMP)–activated protein kinase (AMPK). Cellular energy stress is detected as a rising concentration of AMP and an increase in the AMP/ATP ratio. AMP binding to one of the regulatory subunits of AMPK increases its activity in three ways: (1) AMP has a direct allosteric effect on activity. (2) The AMPK catalytic subunit becomes a better substrate for upstream kinases; phosphorylation of the catalytic subunit increases AMPK activity. (3) AMP binding inhibits dephosphorylation of the catalytic subunit. These three effects, working in concert, render the system exquisitely sensitive to changes in AMP, and all are antagonized by ATP—thus the importance of the AMP/ATP ratio.

The role of the energy sensor AMPK in renal physiology was recently reviewed.[131] Overall, AMPK becomes activated when ATP is limiting—that is, when the AMP/ATP ratio increases—and once activated it decreases ATP consumption and increases ATP synthesis. In the kidney, sodium transport is the major energy-consuming process, and AMPK can couple ion transport and energy metabolism. Hallows and colleagues[131] have determined that AMPK activation depresses transport mediated by the cystic fibrosis transmembrane conductance regulator, the epithelial sodium channel, the vacuolar H^+-ATPase, and NKCC (Figure 4-15). These effects are expected to decrease both renal Qo_2 and T_{Na}. in vivo, rats receiving a high-salt diet exhibited both increases in AMPK activity and phosphorylation.[132] Whether this effect is driven

by a change in cellular metabolism that results in an increase in AMP/ATP levels is not clear. Consumption of a high-salt diet does decrease the fraction of the filtered load of Na^+ that is absorbed, and given the effect of AMPK activation in inhibiting transporters, the findings suggest that AMPK participates in salt and water homeostasis.

The AMPK pathway provides another important layer of regulation between ATP production by mitochondria and ATP consumption by transporters. In the Whittam model illustrated in Figure 4-8, increased active transport provokes a decrease in the ATP/ADP ratio, which drives increased ATP production by the mitochondria. When ATP production by the mitochondria becomes limiting, however, AMPK will be activated, which will drive a reduction in ATP consumption by active membrane transporters.

AMPK was first characterized as a cellular fuel gauge that, once activated, would switch on ATP-generating processes such as cellular glucose uptake and glucose and fatty acid oxidation and switch off ATP-consuming processes such as lipid, glycogen, and protein synthesis as well as gluconeogenesis (see Figure 4-15). Although acute renal ischemia provokes a rapid and powerful activation of AMPK, its functional role in the response to ischemia remains unclear, because the role of AMPK in renal metabolism has not been explored. Whether AMPK abundance or its phosphorylation is higher in the hypoxia-prone medulla than in the cortex has not yet been investigated, nor have studies been conducted examining the effect of AMPK activation on renal gluconeogenesis or glycolysis. A key question is whether renal AMPK

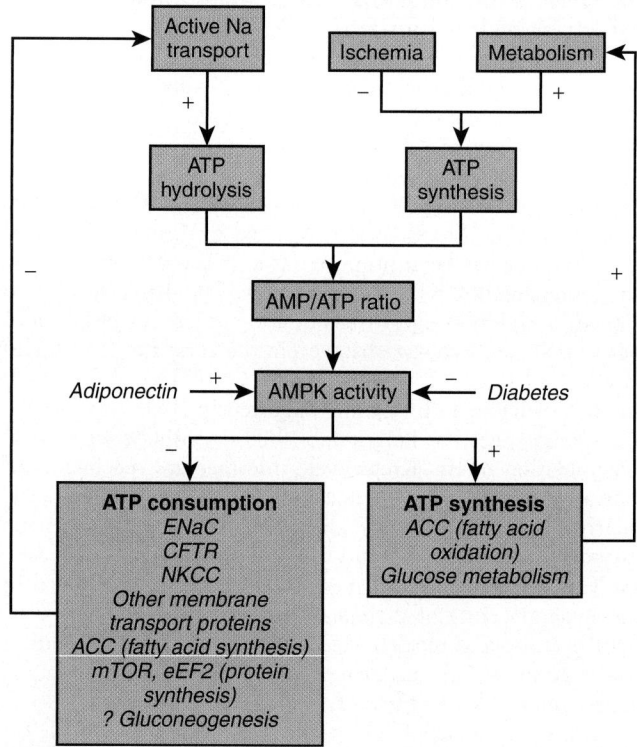

FIGURE 4-15 Proposed role of adenosine monophosphate–activated protein kinase (AMPK) in the kidney in coupling catabolic pathways requiring ATP hydrolysis (primarily sodium transport) with metabolic pathways leading to ATP synthesis (primarily fatty acid and glucose oxidation). +, Activating pathway; −, inhibitory pathway. (From Hallows KR, et al: Role of the energy sensor AMP-activated kinase in renal physiology and disease. *Am J Physiol Renal Physiol* 298:F1067-F1077, 2010.)

activation suppresses Na⁺-K⁺-ATPase activity along the nephron. AMPK activation has been reported to inhibit lung cell Na⁺-K⁺-ATPase transport activity mediated by endocytosis,[133] but AMPK activation had no apparent effect on skeletal muscle Na⁺-K⁺-ATPase activity or distribution,[134] which leaves the question open for the kidney.

Mitochondrial Diseases

Given the central role of mitochondria in producing ATP via oxidative phosphorylation, it is not surprising that genetic mutations affecting mitochondrial function have renal manifestations. The mitochondrial genome is distinct from the nuclear genome, and it encodes 13 of the 88 protein subunits of electron transport chain complexes I through V as well as 22 mitochondrial-specific transfer RNAs (tRNAs) and two RNA components of the translational apparatus. The nuclear genome encodes the remaining respiratory chain subunits as well as most of the mitochondrial DNA replication and expression components.

Disorders affecting mitochondrial oxidative phosphorylation can arise from mutations in either mitochondrial genes or nuclear genes encoding respiratory chain components or ancillary factors involved in maintenance of electron transport chain function or the overall number of mitochondria.[135] The incidence of genetic mitochondrial disorders is estimated at about 1 in 5000 births, with the most common affecting the sequence of a mitochondrial tRNA for leucine. Such mutations affect mitochondrial function in all tissues. Symptoms are evident before 2 months of age, and the number of organ systems affected increases with age.

Impairment of mitochondrial oxidative phosphorylation results in increased levels of reducing equivalents (NADH, FADH), which in the mitochondria transform acetoacetate to 3-hydroxybutyrate and in the cytosol transform pyruvate to lactate. Thus, elevated levels of lactic acid, ketone bodies, and impaired redox status are suggestive of a mitochondrial defect disorder.[136] If the genetic cause of the impairment can be pinpointed, then an appropriate therapy, if available, can be implemented to treat these life-threatening disorders; for example, coenzyme Q_{10} enzyme defects can be treated with coenzyme Q_{10} supplementation.[135]

Myopathies and cardiomyopathies are the most common manifestations of mitochondrial disease, and central nervous system symptoms, including encephalopathies, are very common. Renal system impairment can be present, but is not seen without other system deficiencies and is usually reported in children. Although glomerular disease and tubulointerstitial nephropathy have both been reported, the most frequently observed is impairment of proximal tubule reabsorption, known as *de Toni–Debré–Fanconi syndrome,* in which there are urinary losses of bicarbonate, amino acids, glucose, phosphate, uric acid, potassium, and water. All of these symptoms can be explained by lack of ATP to fuel Na⁺-K⁺-ATPase sufficiently to drive transepithelial transport. The symptoms can range from mild to more severe, and present in the neonatal period in most patients. Biopsy specimens show tubular dilations, casts, dedifferentiation, and cellular vacuolization. At the cellular level there are enlarged mitochondria. Supplements of sodium bicarbonate, potassium, vitamin D, phosphorus, and water are called for if these symptoms are evident.[135,136]

Summary

Most of the energy consumed by the kidney is traceable to the energy requirements for sodium reabsorption. Although all sodium reabsorption is linked to Na⁺-K⁺-ATPase, efficiency is achieved by leveraging Na⁺-K⁺-ATPase into transepithelial chloride or voltage gradients that allow some sodium to be reabsorbed without passing through the Na⁺-K⁺-ATPase itself. ATP production in the proximal tubule is solely by aerobic metabolism, whereas the medullary segments have additional capacity to produce energy by glycolysis. Transport activity regulates metabolism, metabolism may be rate limiting for transport, and the efficiency of transport can be made to vary at multiple levels from backleak permeability to the efficiency of mitochondrial respiration. With regard to metabolic autoregulation, the kidney faces a particular challenge because the usual mechanism for delivering more oxygen to the kidney also increases the demand for that oxygen. Several intermediaries have been identified as parts of the complex network of interactions between transport and metabolism that allow the kidney to meet this challenge while balancing the risk of hypoxia against the risk of oxygen toxicity. A partial list of these is adenosine, nitric oxide, prostaglandins, angiotensin II, succinate, uncoupling proteins, HIF, and AMPK. A multiscale systems model that incorporates these elements along with renal anatomy to recapitulate renal metabolism is expected in the future.

References

1. Cohen JJ, Kamm DE. Renal metabolism: relation to renal function. In: Brenner BM, Rector BA, eds. *The kidney.* Philadelphia: Saunders; 1981, p 147.
2. Rapoport S, Brodsky WA. West: Excretion of solutes and osmotic work of the resting kidney of hydropenic man. *Am J Physiol.* 1949;157(3):357-362.
3. Newburgh JD. The changes which alter renal osmotic work. *J Clin Invest.* 1943;22(3):439-446.
4. Horisberger JD. Recent insights into the structure and mechanism of the sodium pump. *Physiology (Bethesda).* 2004;19:377-387.
5. Skou JC. The identification of the sodium pump. *Biosci Rep.* 2004;24 (4-5):436-451.
6. Geering K. FXYD proteins: new regulators of Na-K-ATPase. *Am J Physiol Renal Physiol.* 2006;290(2):F241-F250.
7. Feraille E, Doucet A. Sodium-potassium-adenosinetriphosphatase-dependent sodium transport in the kidney: hormonal control. *Physiol Rev.* 2001;81(1):345-418.
8. Arystarkhova E, et al. Multiplicity of expression of FXYD proteins in mammalian cells: dynamic exchange of phospholemman and gamma-subunit in response to stress. *Am J Physiol Cell Physiol.* 2007;292(3):C1179-C1191.
9. Geering K. Functional roles of Na, K-ATPase subunits. *Curr Opin Nephrol Hypertens.* 2008;17(5):526-532.
10. Katz AI. Distribution and function of classes of ATPases along the nephron. *Kidney Int.* 1986;29(1):21-31.
11. Gumz ML, et al. The renal H⁺-K⁺-ATPases: physiology, regulation, and structure. *Am J Physiol Renal Physiol.* 2010;298(1):F12-F21.
12. Kone BC, et al. Cellular pathways of potassium transport in renal inner medullary collecting duct. *Am J Physiol.* 1989;256(4 pt 1):C823-C830.
13. Magyar CE, et al. Plasma membrane Ca²⁺-ATPase and NCX1 Na⁺/Ca²⁺ exchanger expression in distal convoluted tubule cells. *Am J Physiol Renal Physiol.* 2002;283(1):F29-F40.
14. Valles P, et al. Kidney vacuolar H⁺-ATPase: physiology and regulation. *Semin Nephrol.* 2006;26(5):361-374.
15. Wagner CA, et al. Renal vacuolar H⁺-ATPase. *Physiol Rev.* 2004;84(4):1263-1314.
16. Aronson PS. Identifying secondary active solute transport in epithelia. *Am J Physiol.* 1981;240(1):F1-F11.
17. Dantzler WH, Wright SH. The molecular and cellular physiology of basolateral organic anion transport in mammalian renal tubules. *Biochim Biophys Acta.* 2003;1618(2):185-193.

18. McDonough AA. Mechanisms of proximal tubule sodium transport regulation that link extracellular fluid volume and blood pressure. *Am J Physiol Regul Integr Comp Physiol.* 2010;298(4):R851-R861.

19. Lapointe JY, et al. Membrane crosstalk in the mammalian proximal tubule during alterations in transepithelial sodium transport. *Am J Physiol.* 1990;258(2 pt 2):F339-F345.

20. Sjostrom M, et al. SIK1 is part of a cell sodium-sensing network that regulates active sodium transport through a calcium-dependent process. *Proc Natl Acad Sci U S A.* 2007;104(43):16922-16927.

21. Muto S, et al. Basolateral Na^+ pump modulates apical Na^+ and K^+ conductances in rabbit cortical collecting ducts. *Am J Physiol.* 1999;276(1 pt 2):F143-F158.

22. O'Connor PM, et al. Renal preglomerular arterial-venous O_2 shunting is a structural anti-oxidant defence mechanism of the renal cortex. *Clin Exp Pharmacol Physiol.* 2006;33(7):637-641.

23. Thomson SC, Blantz RC. Glomerulotubular balance, tubuloglomerular feedback, and salt homeostasis. *J Am Soc Nephrol.* 2008;19(12):2272-2275.

24. Blantz RC, et al. Regulation of kidney function and metabolism: a question of supply and demand. *Trans Am Clin Climatol Assoc.* 2007;118:23-43.

25. Schurek HJ, et al. Evidence for a preglomerular oxygen diffusion shunt in rat renal cortex. *Am J Physiol.* 1990;259(6 pt 2):F910-F915.

26. Welch WJ, et al. Nephron pO2 and renal oxygen usage in the hypertensive rat kidney. *Kidney Int.* 2001;59(1):230-237.

27. Evans RG, et al. Intrarenal oxygenation: unique challenges and the biophysical basis of homeostasis. *Am J Physiol Renal Physiol.* 2008;295(5):F1259-F1270.

28. Neuhofer W, Beck FX. Cell survival in the hostile environment of the renal medulla. *Annu Rev Physiol.* 2005;67:531-555.

29. Chen J, Edwards A, Layton AT. A mathematical model of O_2 transport in the rat outer medulla. II. Impact of outer medullary architecture. *Am J Physiol Renal Physiol.* 2009;297(2):F537-F548.

30. Chen J, Layton AT, Edwards A. A mathematical model of O_2 transport in the rat outer medulla. I. Model formulation and baseline results. *Am J Physiol Renal Physiol.* 2009;297(2):F517-F536.

31. Edwards A. Modeling transport in the kidney: investigating function and dysfunction. *Am J Physiol Renal Physiol.* 2010;298(3):F475-F484.

32. Du Z, et al. Mechanosensory function of microvilli of the kidney proximal tubule. *Proc Natl Acad Sci U S A.* 2004;101(35):13068-13073.

33. Lorenz JN, et al. Ouabain inhibits tubuloglomerular feedback in mutant mice with ouabain-sensitive alpha1 Na, K-ATPase. *J Am Soc Nephrol.* 2006;17(9):2457-2463.

34. Bell PD, et al. Macula densa cell signaling involves ATP release through a maxi anion channel. *Proc Natl Acad Sci U S A.* 2003;100(7):4322-4327.

35. Schnermann J, Briggs JP. Tubuloglomerular feedback: mechanistic insights from gene-manipulated mice. *Kidney Int.* 2008;74(4):418-426.

36. Schurek HJ, Johns O. Is tubuloglomerular feedback a tool to prevent nephron oxygen deficiency? *Kidney Int.* 1997;51(2):386-392.

37. Nishiyama A, et al. Relation between renal interstitial ATP concentrations and autoregulation-mediated changes in renal vascular resistance. *Circ Res.* 2000;86(6):656-662.

38. Epstein FH. Oxygen and renal metabolism. *Kidney Int.* 1997;51(2):381-385.

39. Lear S, et al. Prostaglandin E2 inhibits oxygen consumption in rabbit medullary thick ascending limb. *Am J Physiol.* 1990;258(5 pt 2):F1372-F1378.

40. Herrera M, Ortiz PA, Garvin JL. Regulation of thick ascending limb transport: role of nitric oxide. *Am J Physiol Renal Physiol.* 2006;290(6):F1279-F1284.

41. Vallon V. P2 receptors in the regulation of renal transport mechanisms. *Am J Physiol Renal Physiol.* 2008;294(1):F10-F27.

42. Vallon V, Muhlbauer B, Osswald H. Adenosine and kidney function. *Physiol Rev.* 2006;86(3):901-940.

43. Thurau K. Renal Na-reabsorption and O2-uptake in dogs during hypoxia and hydrochlorothiazide infusion. *Proc Soc Exp Biol Med.* 1961;106:714-717.

44. Kiil F, Aukland K, Refsum HE. Renal sodium transport and oxygen consumption. *Am J Physiol.* 1961;201:511-516.

45. Torelli G, et al. Energy requirement for sodium reabsorption in the in vivo rabbit kidney. *Am J Physiol.* 1966;211(3):576-580.

46. Knox FG, Fleming JS, Rennie DW. Effects of osmotic diuresis on sodium reabsorption and oxygen consumption of kidney. *Am J Physiol.* 1966;210(4):751-759.

47. Burg M, Good D. Sodium chloride coupled transport in mammalian nephrons. *Annu Rev Physiol.* 1983;45:533-547.

48. Cohen JJ. Relationship between energy requirements for Na^+ reabsorption and other renal functions. *Kidney Int.* 1986;29(1):32-40.

49. Mandel LJ, Balaban RS. Stoichiometry and coupling of active transport to oxidative metabolism in epithelial tissues. *Am J Physiol.* 1981;240(5):F357-F371.

50. Soltoff SP. ATP and the regulation of renal cell function. *Annu Rev Physiol.* 1986;48:9-31.

51. Neumann KH, Rector Jr FC. Mechanism of NaCl and water reabsorption in the proximal convoluted tubule of rat kidney. *J Clin Invest.* 1976;58(5):1110-1118.

52. Fromter E, Rumrich G, Ullrich KJ. Phenomenologic description of Na^+, Cl^- and HCO_3^- absorption from proximal tubules of rat kidney. *Pflugers Arch.* 1973;343(3):189-220.

53. Andreoli TE, et al. Solvent drag component of Cl^- flux in superficial proximal straight tubules: evidence for a paracellular component of isotonic fluid absorption. *Am J Physiol.* 1979;237(6):F455-F462.

54. Mathisen O, Monclair T, Kiil F. Oxygen requirement of bicarbonate-dependent sodium reabsorption in the dog kidney. *Am J Physiol.* 1980;238(3):F175-F180.

55. Ostensen J, et al. Low oxygen cost of carbonic anhydrase–dependent sodium reabsorption in the dog kidney. *Acta Physiol Scand.* 1989;137(2):189-198.

56. Deng A, et al. Kidney oxygen consumption, carbonic anhydrase, and proton secretion. *Am J Physiol Renal Physiol.* 2006;290(5):F1009-F1015.

57. Hebert SC. Roles of Na-K-2Cl and Na-Cl cotransporters and ROMK potassium channels in urinary concentrating mechanism. *Am J Physiol.* 1998;275(3 pt 2):F325-F327.

58. Hebert SC, Andreoli TE. Ionic conductance pathways in the mouse medullary thick ascending limb of Henle. The paracellular pathway and electrogenic Cl^- absorption. *J Gen Physiol.* 1986;87(4):567-590.

59. Silva P, et al. Relation between Na-K-ATPase activity and respiratory rate in the rat kidney. *Am J Physiol.* 1976;230(5):1432-1438.

60. Johannesen J, et al. Dopamine-induced dissociation between renal metabolic rate and sodium reabsorption. *Am J Physiol.* 1976;230(4):1126-1131.

61. Aperia A, Bertorello A, Seri I. Dopamine causes inhibition of Na^+-K^+-ATPase activity in rat proximal convoluted tubule segments. *Am J Physiol.* 1987;252(1 pt 2):F39-F45.

62. Aperia AC. Intrarenal dopamine: a key signal in the interactive regulation of sodium metabolism. *Annu Rev Physiol.* 2000;62:621-647.

63. Weinstein SW, Szyjewicz J. Individual nephron function and renal oxygen consumption in the rat. *Am J Physiol.* 1974;227(1):171-177.

64. Weinstein SW, Szyjewicz J. Single-nephron function and renal oxygen consumption during rapid volume expansion. *Am J Physiol.* 1976;231(4):1166-1172.

65. Mitchell P. Coupling of phosphorylation to electron and hydrogen transfer by a chemi-osmotic type of mechanism. *Nature.* 1961;191:144-148.

66. Nelson DL, Cox MM. *Lehninger principles of biochemistry.* ed 5, New York: WH Freeman; 2008.

67. Mandel LJ. Metabolic substrates, cellular energy production, and the regulation of proximal tubular transport. *Annu Rev Physiol.* 1985;47:85-101.

68. Friederich M, et al. Identification and distribution of uncoupling protein isoforms in the normal and diabetic rat kidney. *Adv Exp Med Biol.* 2009;645:205-212.

69. Whittam R. Active cation transport as a pace-maker of respiration. *Nature.* 1961;191:603-604.

70. Blond DM, Whittam R. The regulation of kidney respiration by sodium and potassium ions. *Biochem J.* 1964;92(1):158-167.

71. Balaban RS, et al. Coupling of active ion transport and aerobic respiratory rate in isolated renal tubules. *Proc Natl Acad Sci U S A.* 1980;77(1):447-451.

72. Chance B, Williams GR. The respiratory chain and oxidative phosphorylation. *Adv Enzymol Relat Subj Biochem.* 1956;17:65-134.

73. Katz AI, Doucet A, Morel F. Na-K-ATPase activity along the rabbit, rat, and mouse nephron. *Am J Physiol.* 1979;237(2):F114-F120.

74. McDonough AA, Magyar CE, Komatsu Y. Expression of Na(+)-K(+)-ATPase alpha- and beta-subunits along rat nephron: isoform specificity and response to hypokalemia. *Am J Physiol.* 1994;267(4 pt 1):C901-C908.

75. Pfaller W, Rittinger M. Quantitative morphology of the rat kidney. *Int J Biochem.* 1980;12(1-2):17-22.

76. Kone BC, Metabolic basis of solute transport. In *Brenner and Rector's the kidney.* Saunders; 2008.

77. Guder WG, Ross BD. Enzyme distribution along the nephron. *Kidney Int.* 1984;26(2):101-111.

78. Uchida S, Endou H. Substrate specificity to maintain cellular ATP along the mouse nephron. *Am J Physiol.* 1988;255(5 P t 2):F977-F983.

79. Schmidt U, Marosvari I, Dubach UC. Renal metabolism of glucose: anatomical sites of hexokinase activity in the rat nephron. *FEBS Lett.* 1975;53(1):26-28.

80. Schmid H, et al. Unchanged glycolytic capacity in rat kidney under conditions of stimulated gluconeogenesis. Determination of phosphofructokinase and pyruvate kinase in microdissected nephron segments of fasted and acidotic animals. *Hoppe Seylers Z Physiol Chem.* 1980;361(6):819-827.

81. Burch HB, et al. Distribution along the rat nephron of three enzymes of gluconeogenesis in acidosis and starvation. *Am J Physiol.* 1978;235(3):F246-F253.

82. Gerich JE, et al. Renal gluconeogenesis: its importance in human glucose homeostasis. *Diabetes Care.* 2001;24(2):382-391.

83. Joseph SE, et al. Renal glucose production compensates for the liver during the anhepatic phase of liver transplantation. *Diabetes.* 2000;49(3):450-456.
84. Meyer C, et al. Abnormal renal and hepatic glucose metabolism in type 2 diabetes mellitus. *J Clin Invest.* 1998;102(3):619-624.
85. Eid A, et al. Intrinsic gluconeogenesis is enhanced in renal proximal tubules of Zucker diabetic fatty rats. *J Am Soc Nephrol.* 2006;17(2):398-405.
86. Deetjen P, Kramer K. [The relation of O_2 consumption by the kidney to Na re-resorption]. *Pflugers Arch Gesamte Physiol Menschen Tiere.* 1961;273:636-650.
87. Ekberg K, et al. Contributions by kidney and liver to glucose production in the postabsorptive state and after 60 h of fasting. *Diabetes.* 1999;48(2):292-298.
88. Mithieux G, et al. Contribution of intestine and kidney to glucose fluxes in different nutritional states in rat. *Comp Biochem Physiol B Biochem Mol Biol.* 2006;143(2):195-200.
89. Gullans SR, et al. Interactions between gluconeogenesis and sodium transport in rabbit proximal tubule. *Am J Physiol.* 1984;246(6 pt 2):F859-F869.
90. Brooks GA. Cell-cell and intracellular lactate shuttles. *J Physiol.* 2009;587(pt 23):5591-5600.
91. Scaglione PR, Dell RB, Winters RW. Lactate concentration in the medulla of rat kidney. *Am J Physiol.* 1965;209(6):1193-1198.
92. Bagnasco S, et al. Lactate production in isolated segments of the rat nephron. *Am J Physiol.* 1985;248(4 pt 2):F522-F526.
93. Friedrichs D, Schoner W. Stimulation of renal gluconeogenesis by inhibition of the sodium pump. *Biochim Biophys Acta.* 1973;304(1):142-160.
94. Nagami GT, Lee P. Effect of luminal perfusion on glucose production by isolated proximal tubules. *Am J Physiol.* 1989;256(1 pt 2):F120-F127.
95. Chamberlin ME, Mandel LJ. Na$^+$-K$^+$-ATPase activity in medullary thick ascending limb during short-term anoxia. *Am J Physiol.* 1987;252(5 pt 2):F838-F843.
96. Hering-Smith KS, Hamm LL. Metabolic support of collecting duct transport. *Kidney Int.* 1998;53(2):408-415.
97. Stokes JB, Grupp C, Kinne RK. Purification of rat papillary collecting duct cells: functional and metabolic assessment. *Am J Physiol.* 1987;253(2 pt 2):F251-F262.
98. Thomson SC, Blantz RC. Biophysical basis of glomerular filtration. In: Alpern R, Hebert S, eds. *Seldin and Giebisch's the kidney: physiology and pathophysiology.* Boston: Elsevier/Academic Press; 2007.
99. Ren Y, Garvin JL, Carretero OA. Efferent arteriole tubuloglomerular feedback in the renal nephron. *Kidney Int.* 2001;59(1):222-229.
100. Deetjen P, Kramer K. The relation of O_2 consumption by the kidney to Na re-resorption. *Pflugers Arch Gesamte Physiol Menschen Tiere.* 1961;273:636-650.
101. Deng A, et al. Oxygen consumption in the kidney: effects of nitric oxide synthase isoforms and angiotensin II. *Kidney Int.* 2005;68(2):723-730.
102. Laycock SK, et al. Role of nitric oxide in the control of renal oxygen consumption and the regulation of chemical work in the kidney. *Circ Res.* 1998;82(12):1263-1271.
103. Yip KP. Flash photolysis of caged nitric oxide inhibits proximal tubular fluid reabsorption in free-flow nephron. *Am J Physiol Regul Integr Comp Physiol.* 2005;289(2):R620-R626.
104. Beltran B, et al. The effect of nitric oxide on cell respiration: a key to understanding its role in cell survival or death. *Proc Natl Acad Sci U S A.* 2000;97(26):14602-14607.
105. Borutaite V, Brown GC. Rapid reduction of nitric oxide by mitochondria, and reversible inhibition of mitochondrial respiration by nitric oxide. *Biochem J.* 1996;315(pt 1):295-299.
106. Koivisto A, et al. Oxygen-dependent inhibition of respiration in isolated renal tubules by nitric oxide. *Kidney Int.* 1999;55(6):2368-2375.
107. De Nicola L, Blantz RC, Gabbai FB. Nitric oxide and angiotensin II. Glomerular and tubular interaction in the rat. *J Clin Invest.* 1992;89(4):1248-1256.
108. De Nicola L, Blantz RC, Gabbai FB. Renal functional reserve in the early stage of experimental diabetes. *Diabetes.* 1992;41(3):267-273.
109. De Nicola L, Blantz RC, Gabbai FB. Renal functional reserve in treated and untreated hypertensive rats. *Kidney Int.* 1991;40(3):406-412.
110. De Nicola L, et al. Angiotensin II and renal functional reserve in rats with Goldblatt hypertension. *Hypertension.* 1992;19(6 pt 2):790-794.
111. Welch WJ, et al. Angiotensin-induced defects in renal oxygenation: role of oxidative stress. *Am J Physiol Heart Circ Physiol.* 2005;288(1):H22-H28.
112. Welch WJ, et al. Renal oxygenation defects in the spontaneously hypertensive rat: role of AT1 receptors. *Kidney Int.* 2003;63(1):202-208.
113. Adler S, et al. Oxidant stress leads to impaired regulation of renal cortical oxygen consumption by nitric oxide in the aging kidney. *J Am Soc Nephrol.* 2004;15(1):52-60.
114. Navar LG, Harrison-Bernard LM, Imig JD, et al. Intrarenal angiotensin II generation and renal effects of AT1 receptor blockade. *J Am Soc Nephrol.* 1999;10(suppl 12):S266-S272.
115. Kobori H, et al. The intrarenal renin-angiotensin system: from physiology to the pathobiology of hypertension and kidney disease. *Pharmacol Rev.* 2007;59(3):251-287.
116. Rohrwasser A, et al. Elements of a paracrine tubular renin-angiotensin system along the entire nephron. *Hypertension.* 1999;34(6):1265-1274.
117. Thomson SC, et al. An unexpected role for angiotensin II in the link between dietary salt and proximal reabsorption. *J Clin Invest.* 2006;116(4):1110-1116.
118. Manotham K, et al. Evidence of tubular hypoxia in the early phase in the remnant kidney model. *J Am Soc Nephrol.* 2004;15(5):1277-1288.
119. Nangaku M. Chronic hypoxia and tubulointerstitial injury: a final common pathway to end-stage renal failure. *J Am Soc Nephrol.* 2006;17(1):17-25.
120. Harris DC, Chan L, Schrier RW. Remnant kidney hypermetabolism and progression of chronic renal failure. *Am J Physiol.* 1988;254(2 pt 2):F267-F276.
121. Nath KA, Croatt AJ, Hostetter TH. Oxygen consumption and oxidant stress in surviving nephrons. *Am J Physiol.* 1990;258(5 pt 2):F1354-F1362.
122. Deng A, et al. Regulation of oxygen utilization by angiotensin II in chronic kidney disease. *Kidney Int.* 2009;75(2):197-204.
123. Toma I, et al. Succinate receptor GPR91 provides a direct link between high glucose levels and renin release in murine and rabbit kidney. *J Clin Invest.* 2008;118(7):2526-2534.
124. Evans RG, et al. Multiple mechanisms act to maintain kidney oxygenation during renal ischemia in anesthetized rabbits. *Am J Physiol Renal Physiol.* 2010;298:F1235-F1243.
125. Gloviczki ML, et al. Comparison of 1.5 and 3 T BOLD MR to study oxygenation of kidney cortex and medulla in human renovascular disease. *Invest Radiol.* 2009;44(9):566-571.
126. Gloviczki ML, et al. Preserved oxygenation despite reduced blood flow in poststenotic kidneys in human atherosclerotic renal artery stenosis. *Hypertension.* 2010;55:961-966.
127. Carey RM. Are kidneys not ischemic in human renal vascular disease? *Hypertension.* 2010;55:838-839.
128. Pruijm M, et al. Effect of sodium loading/depletion on renal oxygenation in young normotensive and hypertensive men. *Hypertension.* 2010;55(5):1116-1122.
129. Semenza GL. Regulation of oxygen homeostasis by hypoxia-inducible factor 1. *Physiology (Bethesda).* 2009;24:97-106.
130. Gunaratnam L, Bonventre JV. HIF in kidney disease and development. *J Am Soc Nephrol.* 2009;20(9):1877-1887.
131. Hallows KR, et al. Role of the energy sensor AMP-activated protein kinase in renal physiology and disease. *Am J Physiol Renal Physiol.* 2010;298:F1067-1077.
132. Fraser S, et al. Regulation of the energy sensor AMP-activated protein kinase in the kidney by dietary salt intake and osmolality. *Am J Physiol Renal Physiol.* 2005;288(3):F578-F586.
133. Vadasz I, et al. AMP-activated protein kinase regulates CO_2-induced alveolar epithelial dysfunction in rats and human cells by promoting Na, K-ATPase endocytosis. *J Clin Invest.* 2008;118(2):752-762.
134. Zheng D, et al. AMPK activation with AICAR provokes an acute fall in plasma [K$^+$]. *Am J Physiol Cell Physiol.* 2008;294(1):C126-C135.
135. Di Donato S. Multisystem manifestations of mitochondrial disorders. *J Neurol.* 2009;256(5):693-710.
136. Niaudet P, Rotig A. The kidney in mitochondrial cytopathies. *Kidney Int.* 1997;51(4):1000-1007.

Transport of Sodium, Chloride, and Potassium

David B. Mount

Sodium and Chloride Transport

Na^+ is the principal osmole in extracellular fluid. Because of this, the total body content of Na^+ and Cl^-, its primary anion, determine the extracellular fluid volume. Renal excretion or retention of salt (Na^+-Cl^-) is thus the major determinant of extracellular fluid volume, so that genetic losses or gains in function in renal Na^+-Cl^- transport can be associated with relative hypotension or hypertension, respectively.

On a quantitative level, at a glomerular filtration rate (GFR) of 180 L/day and serum Na^+ of approximately 140 mmol/L, the kidney filters some 25,200 mmol/day of Na^+. This is equivalent to approximately 1.5 kg of salt, which would occupy roughly 10 times the extracellular space.[1] Minute changes in renal Na^+-Cl^- excretion can thus have massive effects on the extracellular fluid volume. In addition, 99.6% of filtered Na^+-Cl^- must be reabsorbed to excrete 100 mmol/L per day.

Energetically, this renal absorption of Na^+ consumes 1 molecule of adenosine triphosphate (ATP) per 5 molecules of Na^+.[1] This is gratifyingly economical, given that the absorption of Na^+-Cl^- is driven by basolateral Na^+–K^+–adenosine triphosphatase (Na^+-K^+-ATPase), which has a stoichiometry of 3 molecules of transported Na^+ per molecule of ATP. This estimate reflects a net expenditure, however, because the cost of transepithelial Na^+-Cl^- transport varies considerably along the nephron, from a predominance of passive transport by thin ascending limbs to the purely active transport mediated by the aldosterone-sensitive distal nephron (distal convoluted tubule [DCT], connecting tubule, and collecting duct). The bulk of filtered Na^+-Cl^- transport is reabsorbed by the proximal tubule and thick ascending limb (Figure 5-1), nephron segments that

utilize their own peculiar combinations of paracellular and transcellular Na^+-Cl^- transport. Although the proximal tubule can theoretically absorb as many as 9 Na^+ molecules for each hydrolyzed ATP molecule,[1] paracellular Na^+ transport by the thick ascending limb doubles the efficiency of transepithelial Na^+-Cl^- transport (6 Na^+ per ATP).[2]

Finally, the "fine tuning" of renal Na^+-Cl^- absorption occurs at full cost[1] (3 Na^+ per ATP) in the aldosterone-sensitive distal nephron, while affording the generation of considerable transepithelial gradients. The nephron thus constitutes a serial arrangement of tubule segments with considerable heterogeneity in the physiologic consequences, mechanisms, and regulation of transepithelial Na^+-Cl^- transport. These issues are reviewed in this section, in anatomic order of the involved structures, with an emphasis on particularly recent developments.

Proximal Tubule

A primary function of the renal proximal tubule is the near-isosmotic reabsorption of two thirds to three quarters of the glomerular ultrafiltrate. This encompasses the reabsorption of approximately 60% of filtered Na^+-Cl^- (see Figure 5-1), so that this nephron segment plays a critical role in the maintenance of extracellular fluid volume. Although all segments of the proximal tubule share the ability to transport a variety of inorganic and organic solutes, there are considerable differences in the transport characteristics and capacity of early, middle, and late segments of the proximal tubule. There is thus a gradual reduction in the volume of transported fluid and solutes as one proceeds along the proximal nephron. This corresponds

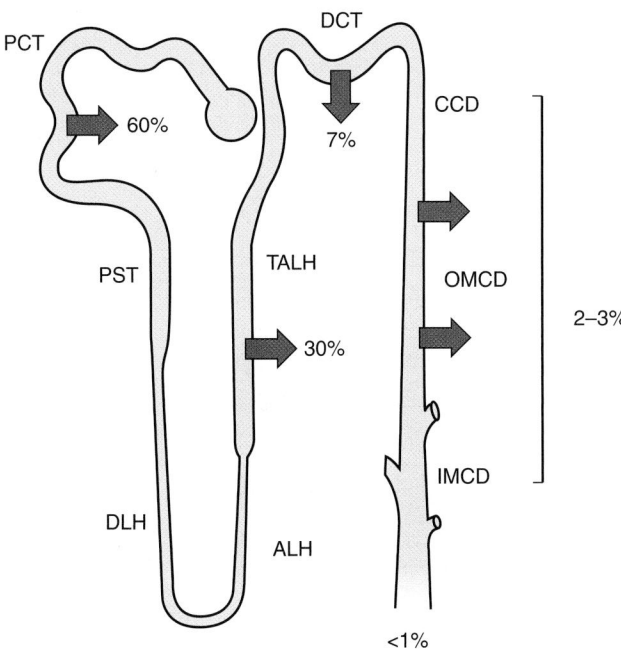

FIGURE 5-1 Percentage reabsorption of filtered Na⁺-Cl⁻ along the euvolemic nephron. *ALH,* Thin ascending limb of the loop of Henle; *CCD,* cortical collecting duct; *DCT,* distal convoluted tubule; *DLH,* thin descending limb of the loop of Henle; *IMCD,* inner medullary collecting duct; *OMCD,* outer medullary collecting duct; *PCT,* proximal convoluted tubule; *PST,* proximal straight tubule; *TAL,* thick ascending limb. (From Moe OW, Baum M, Berry CA, et al: Renal transport of glucose, amino acids, sodium, chloride, and water, in Brenner BM [editor]: *Brenner and Rector's the kidney,* ed 7, Philadelphia, 2004, Saunders, pp 413-452.)

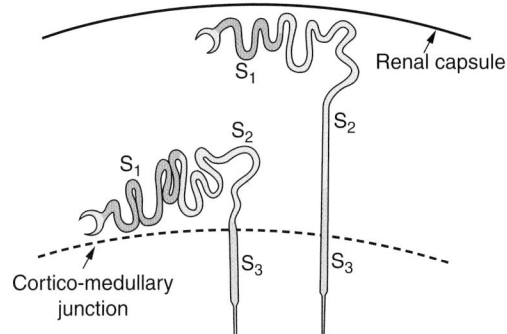

FIGURE 5-2 Schematic representation of the distribution of S1, S2, and S3 segments in the proximal tubules of superficial (SF) and juxtamedullary (JM) nephrons. (From Woodhall PB, Tisher CC, Simonton CA, et al: Relationship between para-aminohippurate secretion and cellular morphology in rabbit proximal tubules, *J Clin Invest* 61:1320-1329, 1978.)

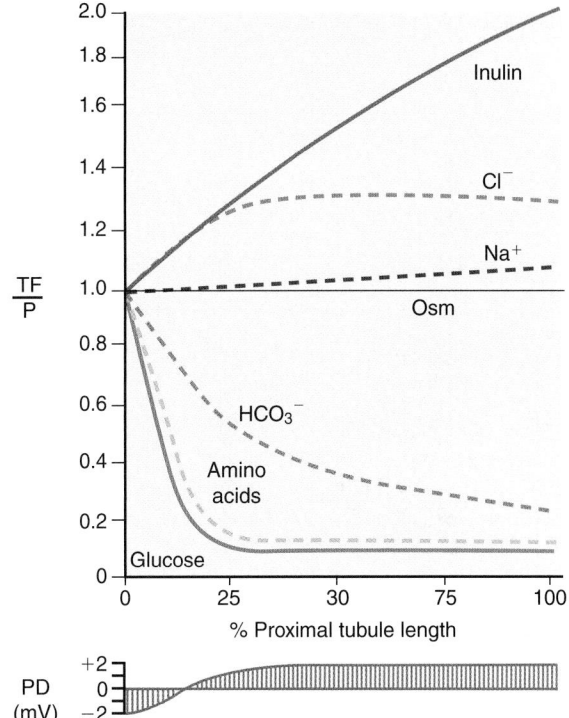

FIGURE 5-3 Reabsorption of solutes along the proximal tubule in relation to transepithelial potential difference (PD). TF/P represents the ratio of tubule fluid to plasma concentration. *Osm,* Osmolality. (From Rector FC Jr: Sodium, bicarbonate, and chloride absorption by the proximal tubule, *Am J Physiol* 244:F461-F471, 1983.)

to distinct ultrastructural characteristics in the tubular epithelium, moving from the S1 segment (early proximal convoluted tubule), to the S2 segment (late proximal convoluted tubule and beginning of the proximal straight tubule), and the S3 segment (remainder of the proximal straight tubule) (Figure 5-2).

Cells of the S1 segment are characterized by a tall brush border, with extensive lateral invaginations of the basolateral membrane.[3] Numerous elongated mitochondria are located in lateral cell processes, with a proximity to the plasma membrane that is characteristic of epithelial cells involved in active transport. The ultrastructure of the S2 segment is similar, albeit with a shorter brush border, fewer lateral invaginations, and less prominent mitochondria. In epithelial cells of the S3 segment, lateral cell processes and invaginations are essentially absent, and small mitochondria are randomly distributed within the cell.[3]

The extensive brush border of proximal tubular cells serves to amplify the apical cell surface that is available for reabsorption; again, this amplification is axially distributed, increasing the apical area 36-fold in S1 and 15-fold in S3.[4] At the functional level, there is a rapid drop in the absorption of bicarbonate (HCO_3^-) and Cl^- after the first millimeter of perfused proximal tubule, consistent with a much greater reabsorptive capacity in S1 segments.[5] There is also considerable axial heterogeneity in the quantitative capacity of the proximal nephron for organic solutes such as glucose and amino acids, with predominant reabsorption of these substrates in S1 segments.[6]

The Na⁺-dependent reabsorption of glucose, amino acids, and other solutes in S1 segments results in a transepithelial potential difference (PD) that is initially lumen negative, due

to electrogenic removal of Na⁺ from the lumen[7] (Figure 5-3). This is classically considered the first phase of volume reabsorption by the proximal tubule.[8] The lumen-negative PD serves to drive both paracellular Cl⁻ absorption and a backleak of Na⁺ from the peritubular space to the lumen. Paracellular Cl⁻ absorption in this setting accomplishes the net transepithelial absorption of a solute such as glucose, along with equal amounts of Na⁺ and Cl⁻. In contrast, backleak of Na⁺ leads only to reabsorption of the organic solute, with no net transepithelial transport of Na⁺ or Cl⁻.

The amount of Cl⁻ reabsorption that is driven by this lumen-negative PD depends on the relative permeability of the paracellular pathway to Na⁺ and Cl⁻. There appears to be

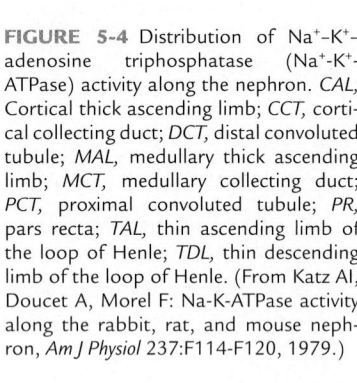

FIGURE 5-4 Distribution of Na+-K+-adenosine triphosphatase (Na+-K+-ATPase) activity along the nephron. *CAL,* Cortical thick ascending limb; *CCT,* cortical collecting duct; *DCT,* distal convoluted tubule; *MAL,* medullary thick ascending limb; *MCT,* medullary collecting duct; *PCT,* proximal convoluted tubule; *PR,* pars recta; *TAL,* thin ascending limb of the loop of Henle; *TDL,* thin descending limb of the loop of Henle. (From Katz AI, Doucet A, Morel F: Na-K-ATPase activity along the rabbit, rat, and mouse nephron, *Am J Physiol* 237:F114-F120, 1979.)

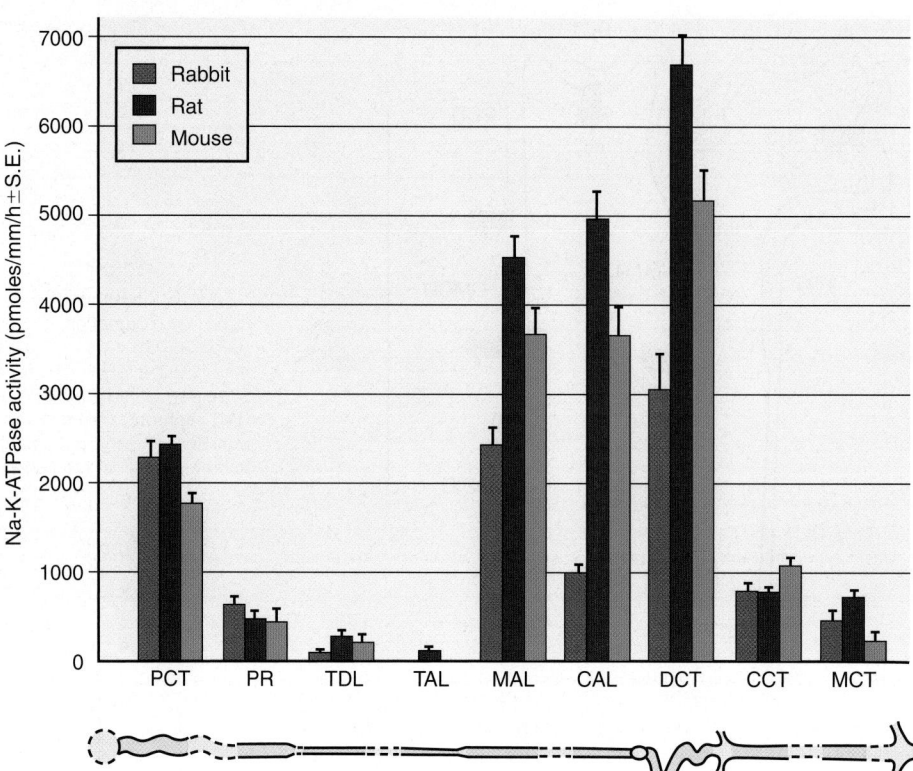

considerable heterogeneity in the relative paracellular permeability to Na+ and Cl−. For example, whereas superficial proximal convoluted tubules and proximal straight tubules in the rabbit are Cl− selective, juxtamedullary proximal tubules in this species are reportedly Na+ selective.[9,10] Regardless, the component of paracellular Cl− transport that is driven by this lumen-negative PD is restricted to the very early proximal tubule.

The second phase of volume reabsorption by the proximal tubule is dominated by Na+-Cl− reabsorption, via both paracellular and transcellular pathways.[8] Not only does Na+-dependent reabsorption of organic solutes occur in the early proximal tubule, but this portion of the proximal tubule also has a much higher capacity for HCO3− absorption,[6] via the coupling of apical Na+/H+ exchange, carbonic anhydrase, and basolateral Na+-HCO3− cotransport. As the luminal concentrations of HCO3− and other solutes begin to drop, the concentration of Na+-Cl− rises to a value greater than that of the peritubular space.[11] This is accompanied by a reversal of the lumen-negative PD to a lumen-*positive* value generated by passive Cl− diffusion[12] (see Figure 5-3). This lumen-positive PD serves to drive paracellular Na+ transport, whereas the *chemical* gradient between the lumen and peritubular space provides the driving force for paracellular reabsorption of Cl−.

This passive, paracellular pathway is thought to mediate approximately 40% of transepithelial Na+-Cl− reabsorption by the mid to late proximal tubule.[10] Of note, however, heterogeneity may be seen in the relative importance of this paracellular pathway, and there is evidence that active (i.e., transcellular) reabsorption predominates in proximal convoluted tubules from juxtamedullary nephrons but not in those from superficial nephrons.[13] Regardless, the combination of both passive and active transport of Na+-Cl− explains how

the proximal tubule is able to reabsorb approximately 60% of filtered Na+-Cl− despite Na+-K+-ATPase activity that is considerably lower than that of distal segments of the nephron[14] (Figure 5-4).

The transcellular component of Na+-Cl− reabsorption was initially recognized in studies of the effect of cyanide, ouabain, luminal anion transport inhibitors, cooling, and luminal-peritubular K+ removal.[8] For example, the luminal addition of SITS (4-acetamido-4′-isothiocyanostilbene-2,2′-disulfonic acid), an inhibitor of anion transporters, reduces volume reabsorption by proximal convoluted tubules perfused with a high-Cl−, low-HCO3− solution that mimics the luminal composition of the late proximal tubule; this occurs in the absence of an effect on carbonic anhydrase.[11] This transcellular component of Na+-Cl− reabsorption is clearly electroneutral. For example, in the absence of anion gradients across the perfused proximal tubule there is no change in transepithelial PD after the inhibition of active transport by ouabain, despite a marked reduction in volume reabsorption.[15] Transcellular Na+-Cl− reabsorption is accomplished by the coupling of luminal Na+/H+ exchange or Na+-SO4²− cotransport with a heterogeneous population of anion exchangers, as reviewed later.

Paracellular Na+-Cl− Transport

A number of factors serve to optimize the conditions for paracellular Na+-Cl− transport by the mid to late proximal tubule. First, the proximal tubule is a low-resistance, "leaky" epithelium[10] with tight junctions that are highly permeable to both Na+ and Cl−.[9] Second, these tight junctions are preferentially permeable to Cl− over HCO3− ions,[11] a feature that helps generate the lumen-positive PD in the mid to late proximal tubule. Third, the increase in luminal Na+-Cl− concentrations in the mid to late proximal tubule generates the electrical and chemical driving forces for paracellular transport.

Diffusion of Cl⁻ thus generates a lumen-positive PD,[12] which drives paracellular Na⁺ transport. The *chemical* gradient between the lumen and peritubular space provides the driving force for paracellular reabsorption of Cl⁻. This rise in luminal Na⁺-Cl⁻ is the direct result of the robust reabsorption of HCO_3^- and other solutes by the early S1 segment,[6] combined with the isosmotic reabsorption of filtered water.[16]

A highly permeable paracellular pathway is a consistent feature of epithelia that function in the near-isosmolar reabsorption of Na⁺-Cl⁻, including small intestine, proximal tubule, and gallbladder. Morphologically, the apical tight junction of proximal tubular cells and other leaky epithelia is considerably less complex than that of tight epithelia. Freeze-fracture microscopy thus reveals that the tight junction of proximal tubular cells is comparatively shallow, with as few as one junctional strand (Figure 5-5); in contrast, high-resistance epithelia have deeper tight junctions with a complex, extensive network of junctional strands.[17]

At the functional level, tight junctions of epithelia function as charge- and size-selective paracellular tight junction channels,[11] physiologic characteristics that are thought to be conferred by integral membrane proteins that cluster together at the tight junction.[18] Changes in the expression of these proteins can have marked effects on permeability without affecting the number of junctional strands.[19] In particular, the charge[20] and size[21] selectivity of tight junctions appears to be conferred in large part by the claudins, a large (>20-member) gene family of tetraspan transmembrane proteins. The repertoire of claudins expressed by proximal tubular epithelial cells may thus determine the high paracellular permeability of this nephron segment. At a minimum, proximal tubular cells coexpress claudin-2, claudin-10, and claudin-11.[11,22]

The robust expression of claudin-2 in proximal tubule is of particular interest, since this claudin can dramatically decrease the resistance of transfected epithelial cells.[19] Overexpression of claudin-2, but not of claudin-10, also increases Na⁺-dependent water flux in epithelial cell lines, which suggests that claudin-2 directly modulates paracellular water permeability.[23] Consistent with this cellular phenotype, targeted deletion of claudin-2 in knockout mice generates a tight epithelium in the proximal tubule, with a reduction in Na⁺, Cl⁻, and fluid absorption.[24] Loss of claudin-2 expression does not affect the ultrastructure of tight junctions, but leads to a reduction in paracellular cation permeability and secondary reduction in transepithelial Cl⁻ transport.[24]

The reabsorption of HCO_3^- and other solutes from the glomerular ultrafiltrate would be expected to generate an osmotic gradient across the epithelium, resulting in a hypotonic lumen. This appears to be the case, although the absolute difference in osmolality between lumen and peritubular space has been a source of considerable controversy.[16] Another controversial issue has been the relative importance of paracellular versus transcellular water transport from this hypotonic lumen.

These issues have both been elegantly addressed through characterization of knockout mice with a targeted deletion of aquaporin-1, a water channel protein expressed at the apical and basolateral membranes of the proximal tubule. Mice deficient in aquaporin-1 have an 80% reduction in water permeability in perfused S2 segments, with a 50% reduction in

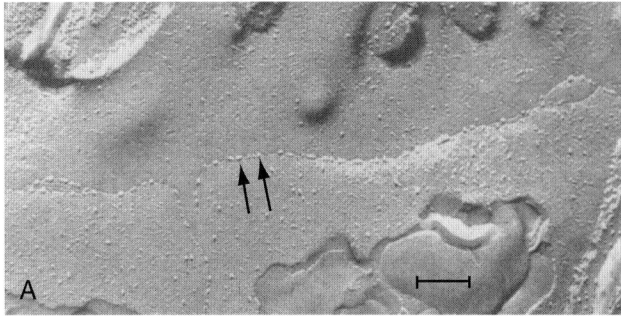

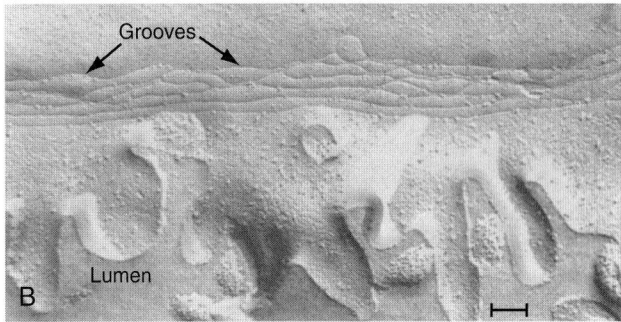

FIGURE 5-5 Freeze-fracture electron micrographs of tight junctions in mouse proximal and distal nephron. **A,** Proximal convoluted tubule, a "leaky" epithelium. The tight junction contains only one junctional strand, seen as a groove in the fracture face (*arrows*). **B,** Distal convoluted tubule, a "tight" epithelium. The tight junction is deeper and contains several anastamosing strands, seen as grooves in the fracture face. (From Claude P, Goodenough DA: Fracture faces of zonulae occludentes from "tight" and "leaky" epithelia, *J Cell Biol* 58:390-400, 1973.)

transepithelial fluid transport.[25] Aquaporin-1 deficiency also results in a marked increase in luminal hypotonicity, which provides definitive proof that near-isosmotic reabsorption by the proximal tubule requires transepithelial water transport via aquaporin-1.[16] The residual water transport in the proximal tubules of aquaporin-1 knockout mice is mediated in part by the aquaporin-7 water channel[26] and/or by claudin-2–dependent paracellular water transport.[24]

Alternative pathways for water reabsorption may include "cotransport" of H_2O via the multiple Na⁺-dependent solute transporters in the early proximal tubule[27]; however, this novel hypothesis is a source of considerable controversy.[28] A related issue is the relative importance of diffusional versus convective ("solvent drag") transport of Na⁺-Cl⁻ across the paracellular tight junction.[10] Convective transport of Na⁺-Cl⁻ with water would seem to play a lesser role than diffusion, given the evidence that the transcellular pathway is the dominant transepithelial pathway for water in the proximal tubule.[16,25,26]

Transcellular Na⁺-Cl⁻ Transport

APICAL MECHANISMS

Apical Na⁺/H⁺ exchange plays a critical role in both transcellular and paracellular reabsorption of Na⁺-Cl⁻ by the proximal tubule. In addition to providing an entry site in the transcellular transport of Na⁺, Na⁺/H⁺ exchange plays a dominant role in the robust absorption of HCO_3^- by the early proximal tubule.[29] This absorption of HCO_3^- serves to increase the luminal concentration of Cl⁻, which in turn increases the driving forces for the passive paracellular transport of both Na⁺ and Cl⁻. Increases in luminal Cl⁻ also help

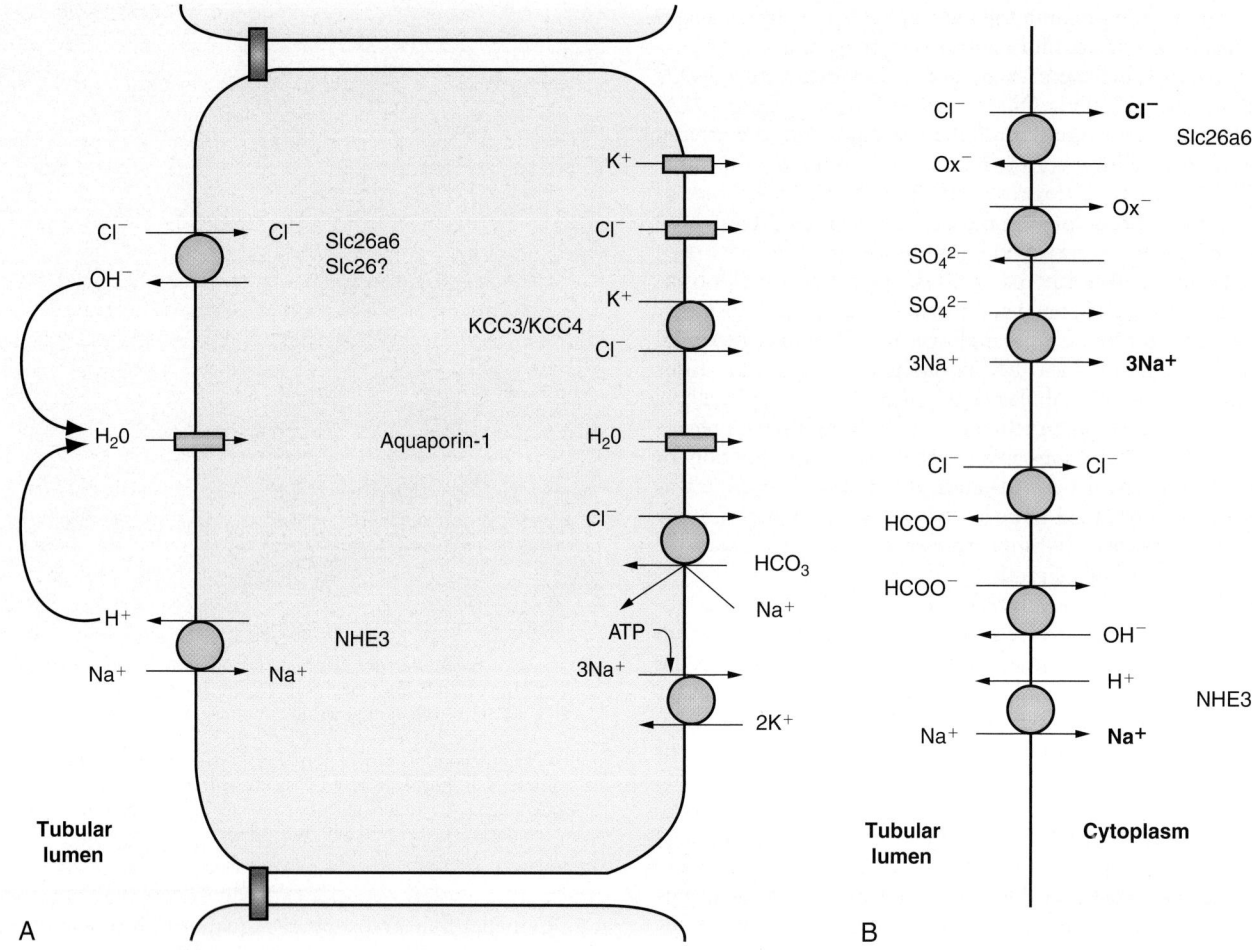

FIGURE 5-6 Transepithelial Na$^+$-Cl$^-$ transport in the proximal tubule. **A,** In the simplest scheme, Cl$^-$ enters the apical membrane via a Cl$^-$/OH$^-$ exchanger, coupled to Na$^+$ entry via Na$^+$/H$^+$ exchanger isoform 3 (NHE3). **B,** Alternative apical anion exchange activities couple to Na$^+$/H$^+$ exchange and Na$^+$-SO$_4^{2-}$ cotransport. See text for details.

drive the apical uptake of Cl$^-$ during transcellular transport. Not surprisingly, there is a considerable reduction in fluid transport of perfused proximal tubules exposed to concentrations of amiloride that are sufficient to inhibit proximal tubular Na$^+$/H$^+$ exchange.[11]

Na$^+$/H$^+$ exchange is predominantly mediated by the NHE proteins, encoded by the nine members of the SLC9 (solute carrier 9) gene family. NHE3, in particular, plays an important role in proximal tubular physiology.[30] The NH3 protein is expressed at the apical membrane of S1, S2, and S3 segments.[31] The apical membrane of the proximal tubule also expresses alternative Na$^+$-dependent H$^+$ transporters,[32] including NHE8.[30] NHE8 predominates over NHE3 in neonatal proximal tubule, with subsequent induction of NHE3 and downregulation of NHE8 in mature, adult nephrons.[30] The primacy of NHE3 in mature proximal tubules is illustrated by the renal phenotype of *NHE3*-null knockout mice, which have a 62% reduction in proximal fluid absorption[33] and a 54% reduction in baseline chloride absorption.[34]

Much as amiloride and other inhibitors of Na$^+$/H$^+$ exchange revealed an important role for this transporter in transepithelial salt transport by the proximal tubule,[11] evidence for the involvement of an apical anion exchanger first came from the use of anion transport inhibitors. DIDS (4,4′-diisothiocyanostilbene-2,2′-disulfonic acid), furosemide,

and SITS all reduce fluid absorption from the lumen of proximal tubule segments perfused with solutions containing Na$^+$-Cl$^-$.[11]

In the simplest arrangement for the coupling of Na$^+$/H$^+$ exchange to Cl$^-$ exchange, Cl$^-$ would be exchanged with the OH$^-$ ion during Na$^+$-Cl$^-$ transport (Figure 5-6). Evidence for such a Cl$^-$/OH$^-$ exchanger was reported by a number of groups in the early 1980s using membrane vesicles isolated from the proximal tubule (reviewed in Kurtz and colleagues[35]). These findings could not be replicated, however, in similar studies performed by other groups.[35,36]

Moreover, experimental evidence was provided for the existence of a dominant Cl$^-$/formate exchange activity in brush border vesicles, in the absence of significant Cl$^-$/OH$^-$ exchange.[36] It was postulated that recycling of formate by the back diffusion of formic acid would sustain the net transport of Na$^+$-Cl$^-$ across the apical membrane. Vesicle formate transport stimulated by a pH gradient (H$^+$-formate cotransport or formate/OH$^-$ exchange) is saturable, which is consistent with a carrier-mediated process rather than diffusion of formic acid across the apical membrane of the proximal tubule.[37] Transport studies using brush border vesicles have also detected the presence of Cl$^-$/oxalate exchange mechanisms in the apical membrane of the proximal tubule,[38] in addition to SO$_4^{2-}$/oxalate exchange.[39]

Based on differences in the affinities and inhibitor sensitivity of the Cl⁻/oxalate and Cl⁻/formate exchange activities, it was suggested that there are two separate apical exchangers in the proximal nephron, a Cl⁻/formate exchanger and a Cl⁻/formate/oxalate exchanger capable of transporting both formate and oxalate (see Figure 5-6). The physiologic relevance of apical Cl/formate and Cl/oxalate exchange has been addressed by perfusing individual proximal tubule segments with solutions containing Na⁺-Cl⁻ and either formate or oxalate. Both formate and oxalate significantly increased fluid transport under these conditions in rabbit, rat, and mouse proximal tubule.[34] This increase in fluid transport was inhibited by DIDS, which suggests involvement of the DIDS-sensitive anion exchanger(s) detected in brush border vesicle studies. A similar mechanism for Na⁺-Cl⁻ transport in the DCT has also been detected, independent of thiazide-sensitive Na⁺-Cl⁻ cotransport.[40]

Further experiments indicated that the oxalate- and formate-dependent anion transporters in the proximal tubule are coupled to distinct Na⁺ entry pathways: Na⁺-SO₄²⁻ cotransport and Na⁺/H⁺ exchange, respectively.[41] The coupling of Cl⁻-oxalate transport to Na⁺-SO₄²⁻ cotransport requires the additional presence of SO₄²⁻/oxalate exchange, which has been demonstrated in brush border membrane vesicle studies.[39] The obligatory role of NHE3 in formate-stimulated Cl⁻ transport was illustrated using *NHE3*-null mice, in which the formate effect is abolished[34]; as expected, oxalate stimulation of Cl⁻ transport is preserved in the *NHE3*-null mice. Finally, tubular perfusion data from superficial and juxtamedullary proximal convoluted tubules suggest that there is heterogeneity in the dominant mode of anion exchange along the proximal tubule, so that Cl⁻/formate exchange is absent in juxtamedullary proximal convoluted tubules, in which Cl⁻/OH⁻ exchange may instead be dominant.[11]

The molecular identity of the apical anion exchanger(s) involved in transepithelial Na⁺-Cl⁻ transport by the proximal tubule has been the object of almost three decades of investigation. A key breakthrough was the observation that the SLC26A4 (SLC family 26, subfamily A, isoform 4) anion exchanger, also known as *pendrin*, is capable of Cl⁻/formate exchange when expressed in *Xenopus laevis* oocytes.[42] However, expression of SLC26A4 in the proximal tubule is minimal or absent in several species, and formate-stimulated Na⁺-Cl⁻ transport in this nephron segment is unimpaired in SLC26A4-null mice.[11] Nevertheless, there is robust expression of SLC26A4 in distal type B intercalated cells.[43] The role of this exchanger in Cl⁻ transport by the distal nephron is reviewed elsewhere in this chapter (see the section "Cl⁻ Transport" under "Connecting Tubules and Cortical Collecting Duct").

These data for SLC26A4 led to the identification and characterization of SLC26A6, a widely occurring member the SLC26 family that is expressed at the apical membrane of proximal tubular cells. Murine Slc26a6, when expressed in *Xenopus* oocytes, mediates the multiple modes of anion exchange that have been implicated in transepithelial Na⁺-Cl⁻ transport by the proximal tubule, including Cl⁻/formate exchange, Cl⁻/OH⁻ exchange, Cl⁻/SO₄²⁻ exchange, and SO₄²⁻/oxalate exchange.[44] However, tubule perfusion experiments in mice deficient in Slc26a6 do not reveal a reduction in baseline Cl⁻ or fluid transport, which is indicative of considerable heterogeneity in apical Cl⁻ transport by the proximal tubule.[45]

Candidates for the residual Cl⁻ transport in Slc26a6-deficient mice include Slc26a7, which is expressed at the apical membrane of proximal tubule[46]; however, this member of the SLC26 family appears to function as a Cl⁻ channel rather than as an exchanger.[47] SLC26A2 may also contribute to apical anion exchange in the proximal tubule.[48] It does appear, however, that Slc26a6 is the dominant Cl⁻/oxalate exchanger of the proximal brush border; the usual increase in tubular fluid transport induced by oxalate is abolished in Slc26a6-knockout mice,[45] with an attendant loss of Cl⁻/oxalate exchange in brush border membrane vesicles.[49]

Somewhat surprisingly, Slc26a6 mediates electrogenic Cl⁻/OH⁻ and Cl⁻/HCO₃⁻ exchange,[44] and most if not all the members of this family are electrogenic in at least one mode of anion transport.[11,44,47,50,51] This begs the question of how the electroneutrality of transcellular Na⁺-Cl⁻ transport is preserved. Notably, however, the stoichiometry and electrophysiology of Cl⁻-base exchange differ for individual members of the family; for example, Slc26a6 exchanges one Cl⁻ for two HCO₃⁻ anions, whereas SLC26A3 exchanges two Cl⁻ anions for one HCO₃⁻ anion.[11,50] Coexpression of two or more electrogenic SLC26 exchangers in the same membrane may thus yield a net electroneutrality of apical Cl⁻ exchange. Alternatively, apical K⁺ channels in the proximal tubule may function to stabilize membrane potential during Na⁺-Cl⁻ absorption.[52]

Another puzzle is why Cl⁻/formate exchange preferentially couples to Na⁺/H⁺ exchange mediated by the NHE3 exchanger[34] (see Figure 5-6), without evident coupling of Cl⁻/oxalate exchange to Na⁺/H⁺ exchange or Cl⁻/formate exchange to Na⁺-SO₄²⁻ cotransport. It is evident that Slc26a6 is capable of mediating SO₄²⁻/formate exchange,[44] which would be necessary to support coupling between Na⁺-SO₄²⁻ cotransport and formate. Scaffolding proteins may serve to cluster these different transporters together in separate "microdomains," which would lead to preferential coupling. Notably, whereas both Slc26a6 and NHE have been reported to bind to the scaffolding protein PDZK1 (PDZ domain–containing 1), distribution of Slc26a6 is selectively impaired in PDZK1 knockout mice.[53] Petrovic and colleagues have also reported a novel activation of proximal Na⁺/H⁺ exchange by luminal formate, which suggests a direct effect of formate itself on NHE3.[54] This may in part explain the preferential coupling of Cl⁻/formate exchange to NHE3.

BASOLATERAL MECHANISMS

As in other absorptive epithelia, basolateral Na⁺-K⁺-ATPase activity establishes the Na⁺ gradient for transcellular Na⁺-Cl⁻ transport by the proximal tubule and provides a major exit pathway for Na⁺. To preserve the electroneutrality of transcellular Na⁺-Cl⁻ transport,[15] this exit of Na⁺ across the basolateral membrane must be balanced by an equal exit of Cl⁻. Several exit pathways for Cl⁻ have been identified in proximal tubular cells, including K⁺-Cl⁻ cotransport, Cl⁻ channels, and various modalities of Cl⁻/HCO₃⁻ exchange (see Figure 5-6).

Several lines of evidence support the existence of a swelling-activated basolateral K⁺-Cl⁻ cotransporter (KCC) in the proximal tubule.[55] The KCC proteins are encoded by four members of the cation-chloride cotransporter gene family. KCC1, KCC3, and KCC4 are all expressed in kidney. In particular, there is very heavy coexpression of KCC3 and KCC4 at the basolateral membrane of the proximal tubule, from S1 to S3.[56]

At the functional level, basolateral membrane vesicles from the renal cortex reportedly contain K⁺-Cl⁻ cotransport activity.[55] The use of ion-sensitive microelectrodes, combined with luminal charge injection and manipulation of bath K^+ and Cl^-, suggest the presence of an electroneutral KCC at the basolateral membrane proximal straight tubules. Increases or decreases in basolateral K^+ increase or decrease intracellular Cl^- activity, respectively, with reciprocal effects of basolateral Cl^- on K^+ activity; these data are consistent with coupled K^+-Cl^- transport.[57,58]

Notably, a 1 mmol/L concentration of furosemide, sufficient to inhibit all four of the KCCs, does not inhibit this K^+-Cl^- cotransport under baseline conditions.[57] However, only 10% of baseline K^+ efflux in the proximal tubule is mediated by furosemide-sensitive K^+-Cl^- cotransport, which is likely quiescent in the absence of cell swelling. Thus the activation of apical Na^+-glucose transport in proximal tubular cells strongly activates a barium-resistant (Ba^{2+}) K^+ efflux pathway that is 75% inhibited by 1 mmol/L furosemide.[59] In addition, volume-regulatory decrease in Ba^{2+}-blocked proximal tubules swollen by hypotonic conditions is blocked by 1 mmol/L furosemide.[55]

Cell swelling in response to apical Na^+ absorption[11] is postulated to activate a volume-sensitive basolateral KCC that participates in transepithelial absorption of Na^+-Cl^-. Notably, targeted deletion of KCC3 and KCC4 in the respective knockout mice reduces volume-regulatory decrease in the proximal tubule.[60] Furthermore, perfused proximal tubules from KCC3-deficient mice have a considerable reduction in transepithelial fluid transport,[61] which suggests an important role for basolateral K^+-Cl^- cotransport in transcellular Na^+-Cl^- reabsorption. The basolateral chloride conductance of mammalian proximal tubular cells is relatively low, which indicates a lesser role for Cl^- channels in transepithelial Na^+-Cl^- transport. Basolateral anion substitutions have minimal effect on the membrane potential, despite considerable effects on intracellular Cl^- activity[62]; for that matter, changes in basolateral membrane potential also have no affect on intracellular Cl^-.[57,58] However, as with basolateral K^+-Cl^- cotransport, basolateral Cl^- channels in the proximal tubule may be relatively inactive in the absence of cell swelling. Cell swelling thus activates both K^+ and Cl^- channels at the basolateral membranes of proximal tubular cells.[11,63,64]

Seki and colleagues have reported the presence of a basolateral Cl^- channel within S3 segments of the rabbit nephron, in which they did not see an affect of the KCC inhibitor H74 on intracellular Cl^- activity.[65] The molecular identity of these and other basolateral Cl^- channels in the proximal nephron is not known with certainty, although S3 segments have been shown to exclusively express messenger RNA (mRNA) for the swelling-activated ClC-2 Cl^- channel.[66] The role of this channel in transcellular Na^+-Cl^- reabsorption is not yet clear.

Finally, there is functional evidence for both Na^+-dependent and Na^+-independent Cl^-/HCO_3^- exchange at the basolateral membrane of proximal tubular cells.[9,62,67] The impact of Na^+-independent Cl^-/HCO_3^- exchange on basolateral exit is thought to be minimal.[62] For one thing, this exchanger is expected to mediate Cl^- *entry* under physiologic conditions.[67] Second, there is only a modest difference between the rate of decrease in intracellular Cl^- activity with combined removal of Na^+ and Cl^- and the rate of decrease with Cl^- and HCO_3^- removal, which suggests that pure Cl^-/HCO_3^- exchange does not contribute significantly to Cl^- exit. In contrast, there is a 75% decrease in intracellular Cl^- activity after the removal of

basolateral Na^+.[62] The Na^+-dependent Cl^-/HCO_3^- exchanger may thus play a considerable role in basolateral Cl^- exit, with recycled exit of Na^+ and HCO_3^- via the basolateral Na^+-HCO_3^- cotransporter NBC1 (see Figure 5-6). The molecular identity of this proximal tubular Na^+-dependent Cl^-/HCO_3^- exchanger is not yet known.

Regulation of Proximal Tubular Na⁺-Cl⁻ Transport

GLOMERULOTUBULAR BALANCE

A fundamental property of the kidney is the phenomenon of glomerulotubular balance, whereby changes in GFR are balanced by equivalent changes in tubular reabsorption so that a constant *fractional* reabsorption of fluid and Na^+-Cl^- is maintained (Figure 5-7). Although the distal nephron is capable of adjusting reabsorption in response to changes in tubular flow,[68] the impact of GFR on Na^+-Cl^- reabsorption by the proximal tubule is particularly pronounced (Figure 5-8).

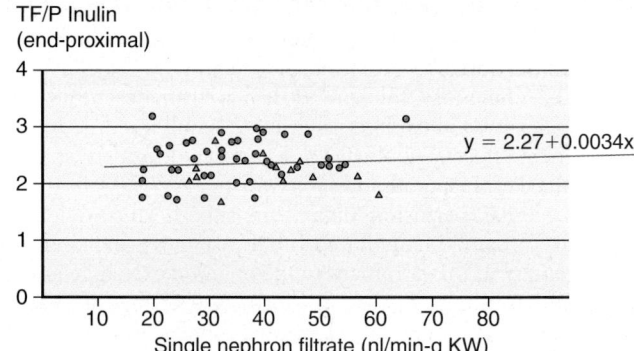

FIGURE 5-7 Glomerulotubular balance. The tubule fluid/plasma ratio of the nonreabsorbable marker inulin (TF/P Inulin) at the end of the proximal tubule, which is used as a measure of fractional water absorption by the proximal tubule, does not change as a function of single-nephron glomerular filtration rate (GFR). (From Schnermann J, Wahl M, Liebau G, et al: Balance between tubular flow rate and net fluid reabsorption in the proximal convolution of the rat kidney. I. Dependency of reabsorptive net fluid flux upon proximal tubular surface area at spontaneous variations of filtration rate, *Pflugers Arch* 304:90-103, 1968.)

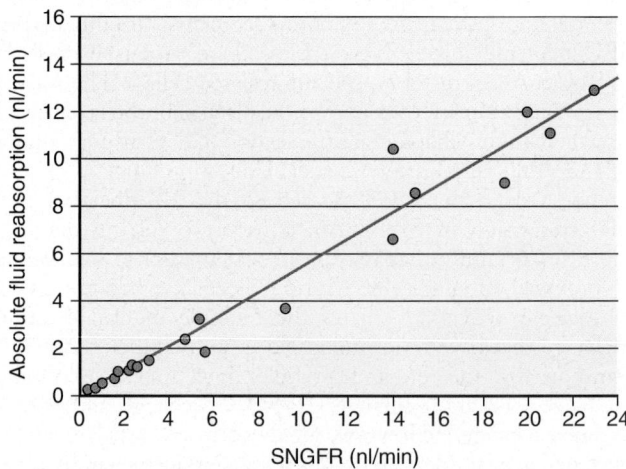

FIGURE 5-8 Glomerulotubular balance. Linear increase in absolute fluid reabsorption by the late proximal tubule as a function of single-nephron glomerular filtration rate (SNGFR). (From Spitzer A, Brandis M: Functional and morphologic maturation of the superficial nephrons. Relationship to total kidney function, *J Clin Invest* 53:279-287, 1974.)

Glomerulotubular balance is independent of direct neurohumoral control and is thought to be mediated by the additive effects of luminal and peritubular factors.[69] At the luminal side, changes in GFR increase the filtered load of HCO_3^-, glucose, and other solutes, which increases their reabsorption by the load-responsive proximal tubule[6] and thus preserves a constant fractional reabsorption. Changes in tubular flow rate have additional stimulatory effects on luminal transport in both the proximal and distal nephron.[68] In the proximal tubule, increases in tubular perfusion clearly increase the rate of both Na^+ and HCO_3^- absorption, due to increases in luminal Na^+/H^+ exchange.[68] Increases in GFR during volume expansion are also accompanied by a modest increase in the capacity of Na^+/H^+ exchange, as measured in brush border membrane vesicles, with the opposite effect in volume contraction.[68]

Notably, influential experiments from almost four decades ago, performed in rabbit proximal tubules, failed to demonstrate a significant effect of tubular flow on fluid absorption.[70] This issue has been revisited by Du and colleagues, who recently reported a considerable flow dependence of fluid and HCO_3^- transport in perfused murine proximal tubules[69,71] (Figure 5-9). These data were analyzed using a mathematical model that estimated microvillus torque as a function of tubular flow.[71] When increases in tubular diameter, which reduce torque, are taken into account, there is a linear relationship between calculated torque and both fluid and HCO_3^- absorption.[69,71] Consistent with an effect of torque rather than of flow per se, increasing the viscosity of the perfusate by adding dextran increases the effect on fluid transport; the extra viscosity increases the hydrodynamic effect of flow and thus increases torque.

The mathematical analysis of Du and colleagues provides an excellent explanation of the discrepancy between their results and those of Burg and Orloff.[70] Whereas Burg and Orloff performed their experiments in rabbit,[70] the more recent report utilized mice.[69,71] Other studies that had found an effect of flow used perfused rat proximal tubules, presumably more similar to those of mouse than of rabbit.[68] Increased flow has a considerably greater effect on tubular diameter in rabbit proximal tubule, which reduces the increase in torque. Mathematical analysis of the rabbit data[70] thus predicts a 43% increase in torque, due to a 41% increase in tubule diameter at a threefold increase in flow; this corresponds to the statistically insignificant 36% increase in volume reabsorption reported by Burg and Orloff (Table 2 in their article[70]).

Pharmacologic inhibition reveals that tubular flow activates proximal HCO_3^- reabsorption mediated by both NHE3 and apical H^+-ATPase.[69] The flow-dependent increase in proximal fluid and HCO_3^- reabsorption is also attenuated in NHE3-deficient knockout mice.[69,71] Inhibition of the actin cytoskeleton with cytochalasin D reduces the effect of flow on fluid and HCO_3^- transport, which suggests that flow-dependent movement of microvilli serves to activate NHE3 and H^+-ATPase via their linkage to the cytoskeleton (see Figure 5-13 for NHE3 activation). Fluid shear stress induces dense distribution of peripheral actin bands and increases the formation of tight junctions and adherens junctions in cultured tubule cells. This "junctional buttressing" is hypothesized to maximize flow-activated transcellular salt and water absorption.[72]

Peritubular factors also play an important, additive role in glomerulotubular balance. Specifically, increases in GFR result in an increase in filtration fraction and an attendant increase in postglomerular protein and peritubular oncotic pressure. It has long been appreciated that changes in peritubular protein concentration have important effects on proximal tubular Na^+-Cl^- reabsorption.[73] These effects are also seen in combined capillary and tubular perfusion experiments (reviewed in Du and colleagues[69]). Peritubular protein also has an effect in isolated perfused proximal tubule segments, where the effect of hydrostatic pressure is abolished.[69] Increases in peritubular protein concentration have an additive effect on flow-dependent activation of proximal fluid and HCO_3^- absorption (see Figure 5-9). The effect of peritubular protein on HCO_3^- absorption, which is a predominantly transcellular phenomenon,[11] suggests that changes in peritubular oncotic pressure do not affect transport via the paracellular pathway. However, the mechanism of the stimulatory effect of peritubular protein on transcellular transport is still not completely clear.[69]

NEUROHUMORAL INFLUENCES

Fluid and Na^+-Cl^- reabsorption by the proximal tubule is affected by a number of hormones and neurotransmitters. The major hormonal influences on renal Na^+-Cl^- transport are shown in Figure 5-10. Renal sympathetic tone exerts a particularly important stimulatory influence, as does angiotensin II. Dopamine is a major inhibitor of proximal tubular Na^+-Cl^- reabsorption.

Unilateral denervation of the rat kidney causes marked natriuresis and a 40% reduction in proximal Na^+-Cl^- reabsorption, without effects on single-nephron GFR or on the

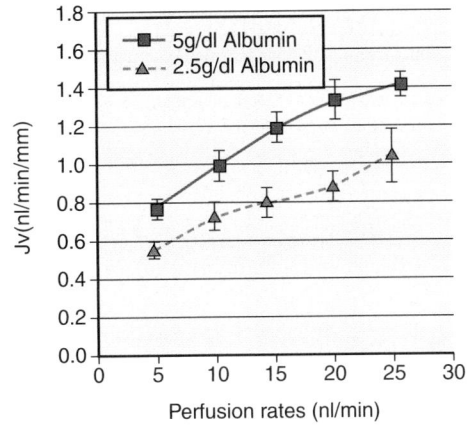

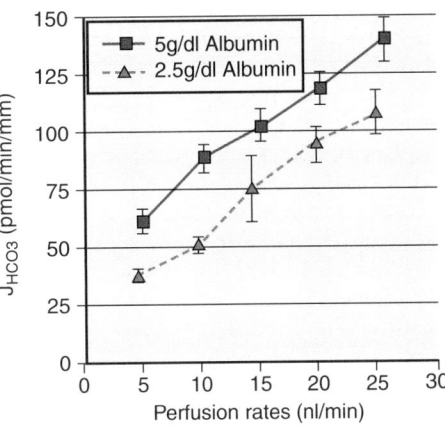

FIGURE 5-9 Glomerulotubular balance. Flow-dependent increases in absorption of fluid (J_v) and HCO_3^- (J_{HCO3}) by perfused mouse proximal tubules. Absorption increases when bath albumin concentration increases from 2.5 to 5 g/dL. (From Du Z, Yan Q, Duan Y, et al: Axial flow modulates proximal tubule NHE3 and H-ATPase activities by changing microvillus bending moments, *Am J Physiol Renal Physiol* 290:F289-F296, 2006.)

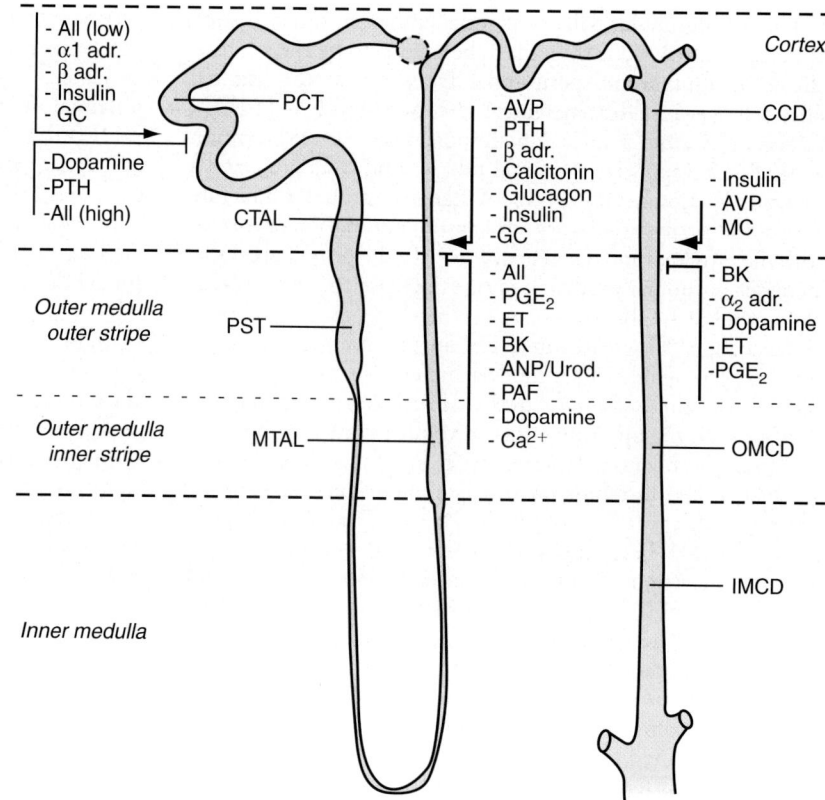

FIGURE 5-10 Neurohumoral influences on Na⁺-Cl⁻ absorption by the proximal tubule, thick ascending limb, and collecting duct. Factors that stimulate (→) and inhibit (⊣) sodium reabsorption are as follows: angiotensin II (ANG II; "low" and "high" refer to picomolar and micromolar concentrations, respectively), adrenergic agonists (adr), arginine vasopressin (AVP), parathyroid hormone (PTH), glucocorticoids (GC), mineralocorticoids (MC), prostaglandin E_2 (PGE_2), endothelin (ET), atrial natriuretic peptide and urodilatin (ANP/Urod), platelet-activating factor (PAF), and bradykinin (BK). CCD, Cortical collecting duct; CTAL, cortical thick ascending limb; IMCD, inner medullary collecting duct; MTAL, medullary thick ascending limb; OMCD, outer medullary collecting duct; PCT, proximal convoluted tubule; PST, proximal straight tubule. (From Feraille E, Doucet A: Sodium-potassium-adenosinetriphosphatase-dependent sodium transport in the kidney: hormonal control, *Physiol Rev* 81:345-418, 2001.)

contralateral innervated kidney.[74] In contrast, low-frequency electrical stimulation of renal sympathetic nerves reduces proximal tubular fluid absorption, with a 32% drop in natriuresis and no change in GFR.[75]

Basolateral epinephrine and/or norepinephrine stimulates proximal Na⁺-Cl⁻ reabsorption via both α- and β-adrenergic receptors. Several lines of evidence suggest that α_1-adrenergic receptors exert a stimulatory effect on proximal Na⁺-Cl⁻ transport, via activation of basolateral Na⁺-K⁺-ATPase and apical Na⁺/H⁺ exchange; the role of α_2-adrenergic receptors is more controversial.[76] Ligand-dependent recruitment of the scaffolding protein NHE regulatory factor 1 (NHERF-1) by β_2-adrenergic receptors results in direct activation of apical NHE3,[77] which bypasses the otherwise negative effect of downstream cyclic adenosine monophosphate (cAMP; see later).

Angiotensin II has potent, complex effects on proximal Na⁺-Cl⁻ reabsorption. Several issues unique to angiotensin II deserve emphasis. First, it has been appreciated for three decades that this hormone has a biphasic effect on the proximal tubule[78]; stimulation of Na⁺-Cl⁻ reabsorption occurs at low doses (10^{-12} to 10^{-10} mol/L), whereas concentrations higher than 10^{-7} mol/L are inhibitory (Figure 5-11).

Further complexity arises from the presence of AT_1 receptors for angiotensin II at both luminal and basolateral membranes in the proximal tubule.[79] Angiotensin II application to either the luminal or peritubular side of perfused tubules has a similar biphasic effect on fluid transport, albeit with more potent effects at the luminal side.[80] Experiments using both receptor antagonists and knockout mice have indicated that the stimulatory and inhibitory effects of angiotensin II are both mediated via AT_1 receptors, due to signaling at both the luminal and basolateral membrane.[81]

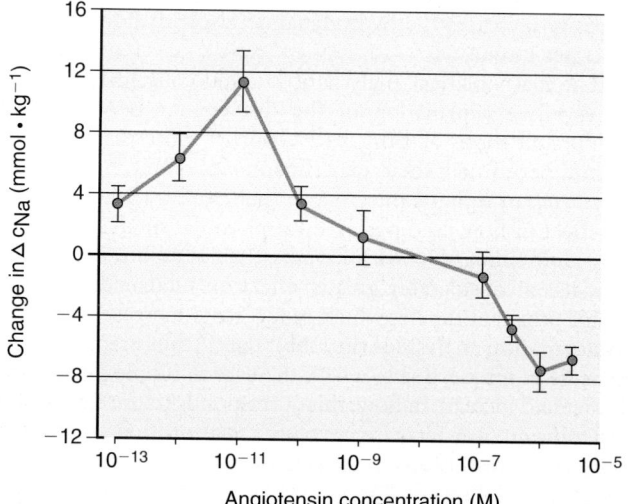

FIGURE 5-11 Biphasic effect of angiotensin II (ANG II) on proximal tubular Na⁺-Cl⁻ absorption. The steady-state Na⁺ concentration gradient (ΔC_{Na}) across the proximal tubular epithelium is plotted as a function of peritubular ANG II concentration. Low concentrations activate Na⁺-Cl⁻ absorption by the proximal tubule, whereas higher concentrations inhibit absorption. (From Harris PJ, Navar LG: Tubular transport responses to angiotensin, *Am J Physiol* 248:F621-F630, 1985.)

Finally, angiotensin II is also synthesized and secreted by the proximal tubule, exerting a potent autocrine effect on proximal tubular Na⁺-Cl⁻ reabsorption.[82] Proximal tubular cells express mRNA for angiotensinogen, renin, and angiotensin converting enzyme,[76] which allows for autocrine generation of angiotensin II. Indeed, luminal concentrations of angiotensin II can be 100- to 1000-fold higher than circulating

Vehicle   Luminal DA, 10⁻⁵mol/L   Bath DA, 10⁻⁵ mol/L

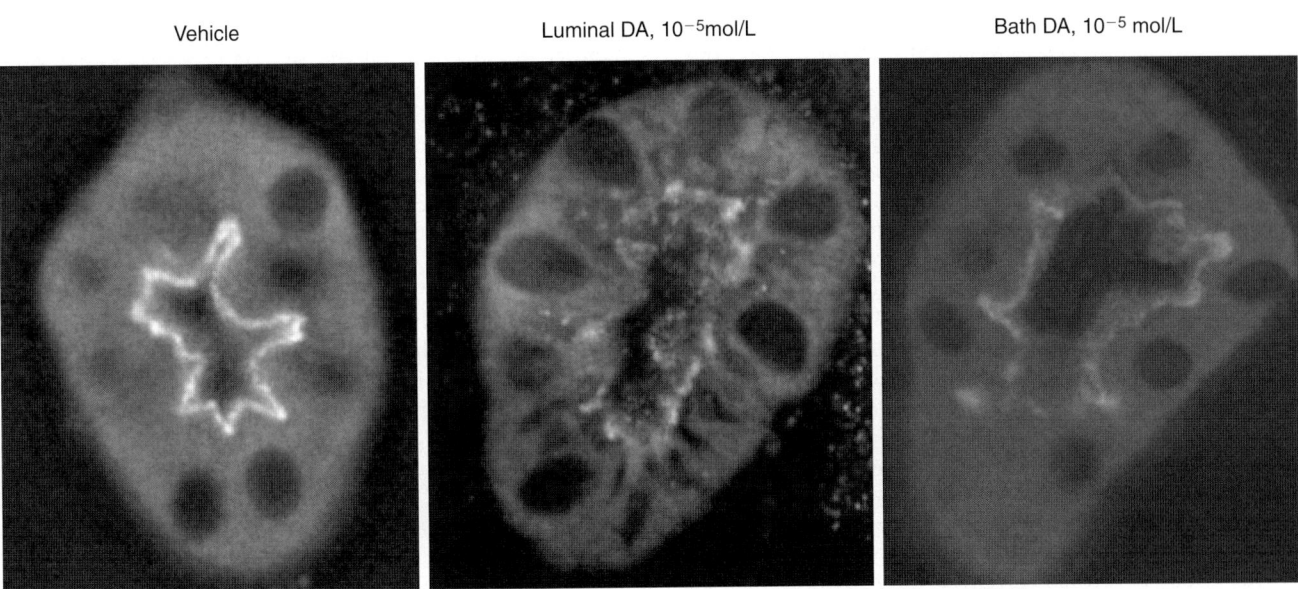

FIGURE 5-12 Effect of dopamine (DA) on trafficking of the Na⁺/H⁺ exchanger NHE3 in the proximal tubule. Microdissected proximal convoluted tubules were perfused for 30 minutes with 10⁻⁵ mol/L DA in the lumen or the bath, which induced a retraction of immunoreactive NHE3 protein from the apical membrane. (From Bacic D, Kaissling B, McLeroy P, et al: Dopamine acutely decreases apical membrane Na/H exchanger NHE3 protein in mouse renal proximal tubule, *Kidney Int* 64:2133-2141, 2003.)

levels of the hormone.[76] Proximal tubular and systemic synthesis of angiotensin II may be subject to different control. Androgens increase proximal tubular Na⁺-Cl⁻ reabsorption via marked induction of renal angiotensinogen, presumptively within the proximal tubule.[83] Thomson and colleagues have demonstrated that proximal tubular angiotensin II is increased considerably after consumption of a high-salt diet, with a preserved inhibitory effect of losartan on proximal fluid reabsorption.[84] These authors have argued that the increase in proximal tubular angiotensin II after a high-salt diet contributes to a more stable distal salt delivery.[84]

The proximal tubule is also a target for natriuretic hormones. In particular, dopamine synthesized in the proximal tubule has negative autocrine effects on proximal Na⁺-Cl⁻ reabsorption.[76] Proximal tubular cells have the requisite enzymatic machinery for the synthesis of dopamine, using L-dopa reabsorbed from the glomerular ultrafiltrate. Dopamine synthesis by proximal tubular cells and release into the tubular lumen is increased after volume expansion or consumption of a high-salt diet, which results in a considerable natriuresis.[85,86] Luminal dopamine antagonizes the stimulatory effect of epinephrine on volume absorption in perfused proximal convoluted tubules,[87] which is consistent with an autocrine effect of dopamine released into the tubular lumen.[85]

Dopamine primarily exerts its natriuretic effect via D_1-like dopamine receptors (D_1 and D_5 in human). As is the case for the AT_1 receptors for angiotensin II,[79] D_1 receptors are expressed at both the apical and luminal membranes of proximal tubule.[88] Targeted deletion of the D_{1A}[89] and D_5 receptors[90] in mice leads to hypertension, by mechanisms that include reduced proximal tubular natriuresis.[89]

The natriuretic effect of dopamine in the proximal tubule is modulated by atrial natriuretic peptide (ANP), which inhibits apical Na⁺/H⁺ exchange via a dopamine-dependent mechanism.[11] ANP appears to induce recruitment of the D_1 dopamine receptor to the plasma membrane of proximal tubular cells, thus sensitizing the tubule to the effect of dopamine.[91]

The inhibitory effect of ANP on basolateral Na⁺-K⁺-ATPase occurs via a D_1-dependent mechanism, with a synergistic inhibition of Na⁺-K⁺-ATPase by the two hormones.[91] Furthermore, dopamine and D_1 receptors appear to play critical permissive roles in the in vivo natriuretic effect of ANP.[11]

Finally, there is considerable crosstalk between the major antinatriuretic and natriuretic influences on the proximal tubule. For example, ANP inhibits angiotensin II–dependent stimulation of proximal tubular fluid absorption,[92] presumably via the dopamine-dependent mechanisms discussed earlier.[11] Dopamine also decreases the expression of AT_1 receptors for angiotensin II in cultured proximal tubular cells.[93] Furthermore, the provision of L-dopa in the drinking water of rats decreases AT_1 receptor expression in the proximal tubule, which suggests that dopamine synthesis in the proximal tubule "resets" the sensitivity to angiotensin II.[93] Angiotensin II signaling through AT_1 receptors decreases expression of the D_5 dopamine receptor, whereas renal cortical expression of AT_1 receptors is, in turn, increased in knockout mice deficient in the D_5 receptor.[94] Similar interactions have been found between proximal tubular AT_1 receptors and the D_2-like D_3 receptor.[95]

REGULATION OF PROXIMAL TUBULAR TRANSPORTERS

The apical Na⁺/H⁺ exchanger NHE3 and the basolateral Na⁺-K⁺-ATPase are primary targets for signaling pathways elicited by the various antinatriuretic and natriuretic stimuli discussed earlier. NHE3 mediates the rate-limiting step in transepithelial Na⁺-Cl⁻ absorption[71] and for this reason is the dominant target for regulatory pathways. NHE3 is regulated by the combined effects of direct phosphorylation and dynamic C-terminal interaction with scaffolding proteins and signal transduction proteins, which primarily regulate transport via changes in trafficking of the exchanger protein to and from the brush border membrane (Figure 5-12).[30,96] Basal activity of the exchanger is also dependent on C-terminal binding of casein kinase 2 (CK2). Phosphorylation of the serine at residue 719 (S719) by CK2 contributes significantly to the transport activity of NHE3 by modulating membrane trafficking of the transport protein.[97]

Increases in cAMP have a profound inhibitory effect on apical Na^+/H^+ exchange in the proximal tubule. Intracellular cAMP is increased in response to dopamine signaling via D_1-like receptors and/or parathyroid hormone (PTH)–dependent signaling via the PTH receptor, whereas angiotensin II–dependent activation of NHE3 is associated with a reduction in cAMP.[98] PTH is a potent inhibitor of NHE3, presumably so as to promote distal delivery of Na^+-HCO_3^- and an attendant stimulation of distal calcium reabsorption.[99]

The activation of protein kinase A (PKA) by increased cAMP results in direct phosphorylation of NHE3. Although several sites in NHE3 are phosphorylated by PKA, the phosphorylation of S552 and S605 have been specifically implicated in the inhibitory effect of cAMP on Na^+/H^+ exchange.[100] "Phosphospecific" antibodies that specifically recognize the phosphorylated forms of S552 and S605 demonstrate dopamine-dependent increases in the phosphorylation of both these serines.[101] Moreover, immunostaining of rat kidney revealed that S552-phosphorylated NHE3 localizes at the coated pit region of the brush border membrane,[101] where the oligomerized inactive form of NHE3 predominates.[102] The cAMP-stimulated phosphorylation of NHE3 by PKA thus results in a redistribution of the transporter from the microvillar membrane to an inactive, submicrovillar population (see Figure 5-12).

Notably, however, phosphorylation of these residues appears to be necessary but not sufficient for regulation of NHE3.[30] The regulation of NHE3 by cAMP also requires the participation of homologous scaffolding proteins that contain protein-protein interaction motifs known as *PDZ domains* (named for the PSD95, discs large [*Drosophila*], and ZO-1 proteins in which these domains were first discovered) (Figure 5-13). The first of these proteins, the NHE regulatory factor NHERF-1, was purified as a cellular factor required for the inhibition of NHE3 by PKA.[103] NHERF-2 was in turn cloned by yeast two-hybrid screens as a protein that interacts with the C terminus of NHE3. NHERF-1 and NHERF-2 have very similar effects on the regulation of NHE3 in cultured cells. The related protein PDZK1 interacts with NHE3 and a number of other epithelial transporters, and is required for expression of the anion exchanger Slc26a6 at brush border membranes of the proximal tubule.[53]

NHERF-1 and NHERF-2 are both expressed in human and mouse proximal tubule cells. NHERF-1 co-localizes with NHE3 in microvilli of the brush border, whereas NHERF-2 is predominantly expressed at the base of microvilli in the vesicle-rich domain.[103] The NHERFs assemble a multiprotein, dynamically regulated signaling complex that includes NHE3 and several other transport proteins. In addition to NHE3 they bind to the actin-associated protein ezrin, thus linking NHE3 to the cytoskeleton.[103] This linkage to the cytoskeleton may be particularly important for the mechanical activation of NHE3 by microvillar bending, as has been implicated in glomerulotubular balance (see earlier).[69,71] Ezrin also interacts directly with NHE3, binding to a separate binding site within the C terminus of the transport protein.[96] Ezrin functions as an anchoring protein for PKA, bringing PKA into close proximity with NHE3 and facilitating its phosphorylation[103] (see Figure 5-13). Characterization

of knockout mice for NHERF-1 has revealed that it is not required for baseline activity of NHE3; as expected, however, it is required for cAMP-dependent regulation of the exchanger by PTH.[103]

One longstanding paradox has been that β-adrenergic receptors, which increase cAMP in the proximal tubule, cause an activation of apical Na^+/H^+ exchange.[76] This was resolved by the observation that the first PDZ domain of NHERF-1 interacts with the $β_2$-adrenergic receptor in an agonist-dependent fashion; this interaction serves to disrupt the interaction between the second PDZ domain and NHE3, which results in stimulation of the exchanger despite the catecholamine-dependent increase in cAMP.[103]

As discussed earlier, at concentrations higher than 10^{-7} mol/L (see Figure 5-11) angiotensin II has an inhibitory effect on proximal tubular Na^+-Cl^- absorption.[78] This inhibition is dependent on the activation of brush border phospholipase A_2, which results in the liberation of arachidonic acid.[80] Metabolism of arachidonic acid by cytochrome P450 monooxygenases in turn generates 20-hydroxyeicosatetraenoic acid (20-HETE) and epoxyeicosatrienoic acids (EETs), compounds that inhibit NHE3 and basolateral Na^+-K^+-ATPase.[76,104] EETs and 20-HETE have also been implicated in the reduction in proximal Na^+-Cl^- absorption that occurs during pressure natriuresis, inhibiting Na^+-K^+-ATPase and retracting NHE3 from the brush border membrane.[105]

Antinatriuretic stimuli such as angiotensin II acutely increase expression of NHE3 at the apical membrane, at least in part by inhibiting the generation of cAMP.[98] Low-dose angiotensin II (10^{-10} mol/L) also increases exocytic insertion of NHE3 into the plasma membrane via a mechanism that is dependent on phosphatidylinositol-3-kinase (PI3K).[106]

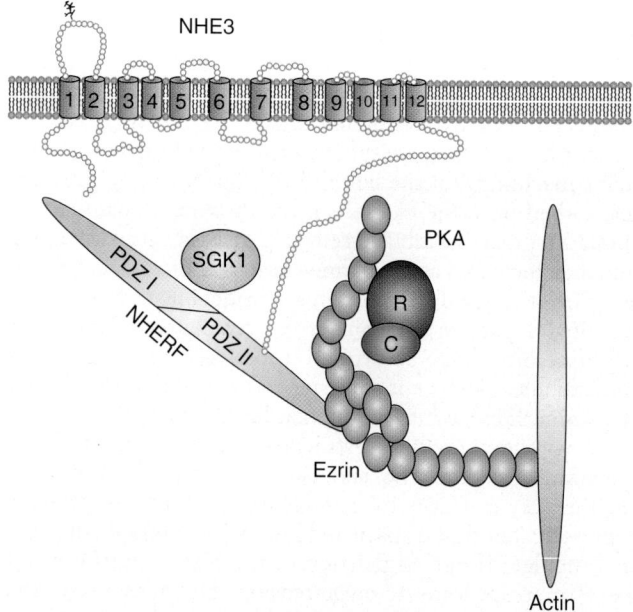

FIGURE 5-13 Scaffolding protein NHERF (Na^+/H^+ exchanger regulatory factor) links the Na^+/H^+ exchanger NHE3 to the cytoskeleton and signaling proteins. NHERF binds to ezrin, which in turn links to protein kinase A (PKA) and the actin cytoskeleton. NHERF also binds to SGK1 (serum- and glucocorticoid-regulated kinase 1), which activates NHE3. *PDZ*, Domain named for the PSD95, discs large (*Drosophila*), and ZO-1 proteins. (From Weinman EJ, Cunningham R, Shenolikar S: NHERF and regulation of the renal sodium-hydrogen exchanger NHE3, *Pflugers Arch* 450:137-144, 2005.)

Treatment of rats with captopril thus results in a retraction of NHE3 and associated proteins from the brush border of proximal tubule cells.[107]

Glucocorticoids also increase NHE3 activity, due to both transcriptional induction of the NHE3 gene and acute stimulation of exocytosis of the exchanger to the plasma membrane.[30] Glucocorticoid-dependent exocytosis of NHE3 appears to require NHERF-2, which acts in this context as a scaffolding protein for the glucocorticoid-induced serine-threonine kinase SGK1 (see also the section "Aldosterone" under "Regulation of Na^+-Cl^- Transport in the Connecting Tubule and Cortical Collecting Duct").[108] The acute effect of dexamethasone has thus been shown to require direct phosphorylation of S663 in the NHE3 protein by SGK1.[109]

Finally, many of the natriuretic and antinatriuretic pathways that influence NHE3 have parallel effects on basolateral Na^+-K^+-ATPase (see Feraille and Doucet[76] for a detailed review). The molecular mechanisms underlying inhibition of Na^+-K^+-ATPase by dopamine have been particularly well characterized. Inhibition by dopamine is associated with removal of active Na^+-K^+-ATPase units from the basolateral membrane,[110] analogous somewhat to the effect on NHE3 expression at the apical membrane. This inhibitory effect is primarily mediated by protein kinase C (PKC), which directly phosphorylates the α_1-subunit of Na^+-K^+-ATPase, the predominant α-subunit in the kidney.[76] The effect of dopamine requires phosphorylation of S18 of the α_1-subunit by PKC. This phosphorylation event does not affect enzymatic activity of the Na^+-K^+-ATPase, but rather induces a conformational change that enhances the binding of PI3K to an adjacent proline-rich domain. The PI3K recruited by this phosphorylated α_1-subunit then stimulates the dyamin-dependent endocytosis of the Na^+-K^+-ATPase complex via clathrin-coated pits.[110]

Loop of Henle and Thick Ascending Limb

The loop of Henle encompasses the thin descending limb, the thin ascending limb, and the thick ascending limb (TAL). The descending and ascending thin limbs function in passive absorption of water[111] and Na^+-Cl^-,[112] respectively, whereas the TAL reabsorbs approximately 30% of filtered Na^+-Cl^- via active transport. There is considerable cellular and functional heterogeneity along the entire length of the loop of Henle, with consequences for the transport of water, Na^+-Cl^-, and other solutes. The thin descending limb begins in the outer medulla after an abrupt transition from S3 segments of the proximal tubule, marking the boundary between the outer and inner stripes of the outer medulla. Thin descending limbs end at a hairpin turn at the end of the loop of Henle. Short-looped nephrons that originate from superficial and midcortical nephrons have a short descending limb within the inner stripe of the outer medulla; close to the hairpin turn of the loop these tubules merge abruptly into the TAL (see also later). Long-looped nephrons originating from juxtamedullary glomeruli have a long ascending thin limb that then merges with the TAL. The TALs of long-looped nephrons begin at the boundary between the inner and outer medulla, whereas the TALs of short-looped nephrons may be entirely cortical. The ratio of medullary to cortical TAL for a given nephron is a function of the depth of its origin; superficial nephrons are primarily composed of cortical TALs, whereas juxtamedullary nephrons primarily possess medullary TALs.

Transport Characteristics of the Thin Descending Limb

It has long been appreciated that the osmolality of tubular fluid increases progressively between the corticomedullary junction and the papillary tip, due to either active secretion of solutes or passive absorption of water along the thin descending limb.[113] Subsequent reports revealed a very high water permeability of perfused outer medullary thin descending limbs in the absence of significant permeability to Na^+-Cl^-.[114] Notably, however, the permeability properties of thin descending limbs vary as a function of depth in the inner medulla and inclusion in short- versus long-looped nephrons.[115,116]

Thin descending limbs from short-looped nephrons contain type I cells—very flat, endothelium-like cells with intermediate-depth tight junctions suggesting a relative tight epithelium (reviewed in Imai and colleagues[115] and Chou and Knepper[116]). The epithelium of descending limbs from long-looped nephrons is initially more complex, with taller type II cells possessing more elaborate apical microvilli and more prominent mitochondria. In the lower medullary portion of long-looped nephrons these cells change into a type III morphology, endothelium-like cells similar to the type I cells from short-looped nephrons.[115]

The permeability properties appear to change as a function of cell type, with a progressive axial drop in water permeability of long-looped descending limbs; the water permeability of thin descending limbs in the middle part of the inner medulla is thus approximately 42% that of outer medullary thin descending limbs.[117] Furthermore, the distal 20% of thin descending limbs have a very low water permeability.[117] These changes in water permeability along the thin descending limb are accompanied by a progressive increase in Na^+-Cl^- permeability, although the ionic permeability remains considerably less than that of the thin ascending limb.[116]

Consistent with a primary role in passive water and solute absorption, Na^+-K^+-ATPase activity in the thin descending limb is almost undetectable,[14] which suggests that these cells do not actively transport Na^+-Cl^-. Those ion transport pathways that have been identified in thin descending limb cells are thought to contribute primarily to cellular volume regulation.[118]

In contrast to the relative lack of Na^+-Cl^- transport, transcellular water reabsorption by the thin descending limb is a critical component of the renal countercurrent concentrating mechanism.[111,114] Consistent with this role, epithelial cells of the thin descending limbs express very high levels of the aquaporin-1 water channel at both apical and basolateral membranes.[119] The expression is highest in type II cells of thin descending limbs in the outer medulla,[119] which have the highest aquaporin-1 content of all the tubule segments along the nephron.[120] Aquaporin-1 is also expressed in type I cells of short-looped nephrons.[119] Notably, however, aquaporin-1–expressing cells in descending limbs from short-looped nephrons extend into segments that do not express aquaporin-1, just prior to the juncture with TALs.[119] In addition, the terminal sections of deep descending limbs of long-looped nephrons, which do not exhibit appreciable water permeability,[117] do not express aquaporin-1.[121]

Characterization of knockout mice with targeted deletion of aquaporin-1 has dramatically proven the primary role of water absorption, as opposed to solute secretion, in the progressive increase in osmolality along the thin descending limb.[113] Homozygous aquaporin-1 knockout mice have a marked reduction in water permeability of perfused thin descending limbs, which results in a vasopressin-resistant concentrating defect.[111]

Na⁺-Cl⁻ Transport in the Thin Ascending Limb

Fluid entering the thin ascending limb has a very high concentration of Na⁺-Cl⁻, due to osmotic equilibration by the water-permeable descending limbs. The passive reabsorption of this delivered Na⁺-Cl⁻ by the thin ascending limb is a critical component of the passive equilibration model of the renal countercurrent multiplication system. Consistent with this role, the permeability properties of the thin ascending limb are dramatically different from those of the thin descending limb, with a much higher permeability to Na⁺-Cl⁻[116] and vanishingly low water permeability.[122]

Passive Na⁺-Cl⁻ reabsorption by thin ascending limbs occurs via a combination of paracellular Na⁺ transport[112,123,124] and transcellular Cl⁻ transport.[125-127] The inhibition of paracellular conductance by protamine thus selectively inhibits Na⁺ transport across perfused thin ascending limbs, consistent with paracellular transport of Na⁺.[123] As in the descending limb, thin ascending limbs have a modest Na⁺-K⁺-ATPase activity (see Figure 5-4); however, the active transport of Na⁺ across thin ascending limbs accounts for only an estimated 2% of Na⁺ reabsorption by this nephron segment.[128]

Chloride channel blockers[126] reduce Cl⁻ permeability of the thin ascending limb, consistent with passive transcellular Cl⁻ transport. Direct measurement of the membrane potential of impaled hamster thin ascending limbs has also yielded evidence for apical and basolateral Cl⁻ channel activity.[127] This transepithelial transport of Cl⁻, but not Na⁺, is activated by vasopressin, with a pharmacology that is consistent with direct activation of thin ascending limb Cl⁻ channels.[129]

Both apical and basolateral Cl⁻ transport in the thin ascending limb appear to be mediated by the ClC-K1 chloride channel, in cooperation with the barttin subunit (see also the section "Basolateral Mechanisms" under "Na⁺-Cl⁻ Transport in the Thick Ascending Limb"). Immunofluorescence[130] and in situ hybridization[131] studies indicate a selective expression of ClC-K1 in thin ascending limbs, although single-tubule reverse transcriptase polymerase chain reaction (RT-PCR) studies have suggested additional expression in the TAL, DCT, and cortical collecting duct.[132] Notably, immunofluorescence and immunogold labeling indicate that ClC-K1 is expressed exclusively at both the apical and basolateral membrane of thin ascending limbs,[130] so that both the luminal and basolateral Cl⁻ channels of this nephron segment[127] are encoded by the same gene. Homozygous knockout mice with a targeted deletion of ClC-K1 have a vasopressin-resistant nephrogenic diabetes insipidus,[133] reminiscent of the phenotype of aquaporin-1 knockout mice.[111]

Given that ClC-K1 is potentially expressed in the TAL,[132] dysfunction of this nephron segment might also contribute to the renal phenotype of ClC-K1 knockout mice; however, the closely homologous channel ClC-K2 (CLC-NKB) is clearly expressed in TAL,[132] where it can likely substitute for ClC-K1.

Furthermore, loss-of-function mutations in ClC-NKB are an important cause of Bartter's syndrome,[134] which indicates that ClC-K2, rather than ClC-K1, is critical for transport function of the TAL.

Detailed characterization of ClC-K1 knockout mice has revealed a selective impairment in Cl⁻ transport by the thin ascending limb.[112] Although Cl⁻ absorption is profoundly reduced, Na⁺ absorption by thin ascending limbs is not significantly impaired (Figure 5-14). The diffusion voltage induced by a transepithelial Na⁺-Cl⁻ gradient is reversed by the absence of ClC-K1, from +15.5 mV in homozygous wild-type controls (+/+) to −7.6 mV in homozygous knockout mice (−/−). This change in diffusion voltage is due to the dominance of paracellular Na⁺ transport in the ClC-K1–deficient (−/−) mice, which leads to a lumen-negative potential; this corresponds to a marked reduction in the permeability of Cl⁻ relative to that of Na⁺ (P_{Cl}/P_{Na}), from 4.02 to 0.63 (see Figure 5-14).

The inhibition of paracellular transport by protamine has a comparable effect on the diffusion voltage in −/− mice compared with +/− and +/+ mice that have been treated with NPPB (5-nitro-2-[3-phenylpropylamino]-benzoate) to inhibit ClC-K1; the respective diffusion voltages are 7.9 mV (−/− plus protamine), 8.6 mV (+/− plus protamine and NPPB), and 9.8 (+/+ plus protamine and NPPB). Therefore, the paracellular Na⁺ conductance is unimpaired and essentially the same in ClC-K1 mice compared with littermate controls. This study thus provides elegant proof of the relative independence of paracellular and transcellular conductances of Na⁺ and Cl⁻, respectively, in thin ascending limbs.

Finally, ClC-K1 associates with barttin, a novel accessory subunit identified via positional cloning of the gene for Bartter's syndrome with sensorineural deafness[135] (see also the section "Basolateral Mechanisms" under "Na⁺-Cl⁻ Transport in the Thin Ascending Limb"). Barttin is expressed with ClC-K1 in thin ascending limbs, in addition to TAL, DCT, and α-intercalated cells.[132,135] Rat ClC-K1 is unique among the ClC-K orthologs and paralogs (ClC-K1/2 in rodent, CLC-NKB/NKA in humans) in that it can generate Cl⁻ channel activity in the absence of coexpression with barttin[130,136]; however, its human ortholog CLC-NKA is nonfunctional in the absence of barttin.[135] Regardless, barttin coimmunoprecipitates with ClC-K1[132] and increases expression of the channel protein at the cell membrane.[132,136] This chaperone function seems to involve the transmembrane core of barttin, whereas domains within the cytoplasmic C terminus modulate channel properties (open probability and unitary conductance).[136]

Na⁺-Cl⁻ Transport in the Thick Ascending Limb

Apical Na⁺-Cl⁻ Transport

The TAL reabsorbs approximately 30% of filtered Na⁺-Cl⁻ (see Figure 5-1). Not only does the TAL play an important role in the defense of the extracellular fluid volume, but Na⁺-Cl⁻ reabsorption by the water-impermeable TAL is a critical component of the renal countercurrent multiplication system. The separation of Na⁺-Cl⁻ and water in the TAL is thus responsible for the capacity of the kidney to either dilute or concentrate the urine. In collaboration with the countercurrent mechanism, Na⁺-Cl⁻ reabsorption by the thin and thick ascending limb increases medullary tonicity, facilitating water absorption by the collecting duct.

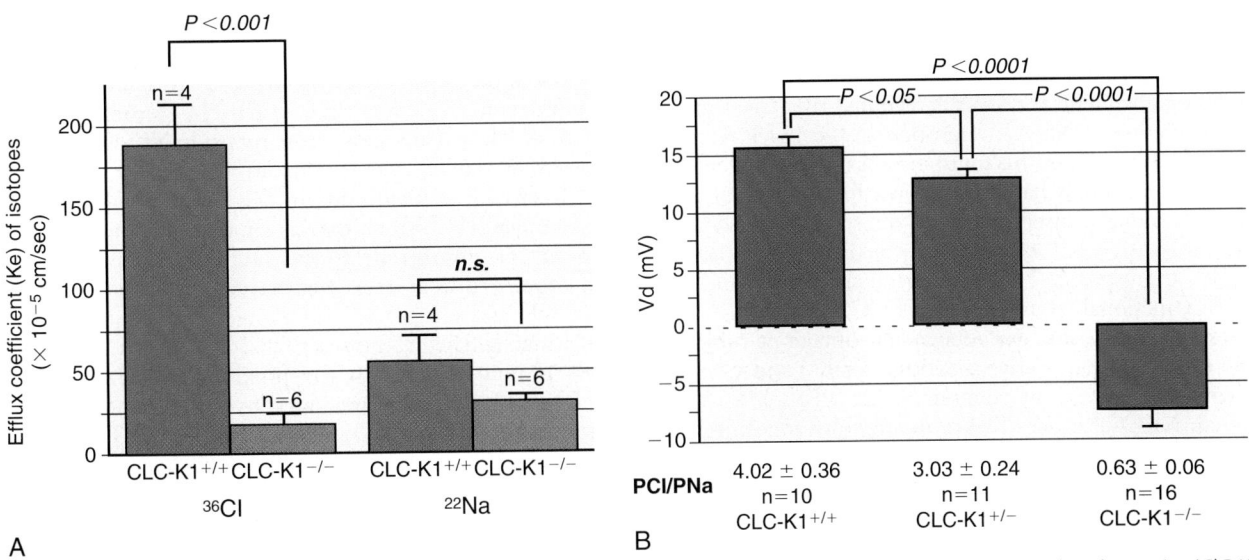

FIGURE 5-14 Role of the ClC-K1 chloride channel in Na⁺ and Cl⁻ transport by thin ascending limbs. Data for homozygous knockout mice (ClC-K1⁻/⁻) are compared with those for their littermate controls (ClC-K1⁺/⁺). **A,** Efflux coefficients for chloride Cl 36 (³⁶Cl⁻) and sodium Na 22 (²²Na⁺) in the thin ascending limbs are shown. Cl⁻ absorption is essentially abolished in the knockout mice, whereas there is no significant effect of ClC-K1 deficiency on Na⁺ transport. **B,** The diffusion voltage induced by a transepithelial Na⁺-Cl⁻ gradient is reversed by the absence of ClC-K1, from +15.5 mV in controls to −7.6 mV in homozygous knockout mice. This change in diffusion voltage is due to the dominance of paracellular Na⁺ transport in the ClC-K1–deficient (−/−) mice, which leads to a lumen-negative potential. This corresponds to a marked reduction in the permeability of Cl⁻ relative to that of Na⁺ (P_{Cl}/P_{Na} ratio), from 4.02 to 0.63. (From Liu W, Morimoto T, Kondo Y, et al: Analysis of NaCl transport in thin ascending limb of Henle's loop in ClC-K1 null mice, *Am J Physiol Renal Physiol* 282:F451-F457, 2002.)

The TAL begins abruptly after the thin ascending limb of long-looped nephrons and after the aquaporin-negative segment of short-limbed nephrons.[119] The TAL extends into the renal cortex, where it meets its parent glomerulus at the vascular pole. The plaque of cells at this junction forms the macula densa, which functions as the tubular sensor for both tubuloglomerular feedback and tubular regulation of renin release by the juxtaglomerular apparatus.

Cells in the medullary TAL are 7 to 8 μm in height, with extensive invaginations of the basolateral plasma membrane and interdigitations between adjacent cells.[3] As in the proximal tubule, these lateral cell processes contain numerous elongated mitochondria, perpendicular to the basement membrane. Cells in the cortical TAL are considerably shorter, 2 μm in height at the end of the cortical TAL in rabbit, with fewer mitochondria and a simpler basolateral membrane.[3]

Macula densa cells also lack the lateral cell processes and interdigitations that are characteristic of medullar TAL cells.[3] However, scanning electron microscopy has revealed that the TAL of both rat[137] and hamster[138] contains two morphologic subtypes, a rough-surfaced cell type (R cells) with prominent apical microvilli and a smooth-surfaced cell type (S cells) with an abundance of subapical vesicles.[3,139] In the hamster TAL, cells can also be separated into those with high apical and low basolateral K⁺ conductance and a weak basolateral Cl⁻ conductance (LBC cells), versus a second population with low apical and high basolateral K⁺ conductance, combined with high basolateral Cl⁻ conductance (HBC cells).[127,138] The relative frequency of the morphologic and functional subtypes in the cortical and medullary TAL suggests that HBC cells correspond to S cells and LBC cells to R cells.[138]

Morphologic heterogeneity notwithstanding, the cells of the medullary TAL, cortical TAL, and macula densa share the same basic transport mechanisms (Figure 5-15).

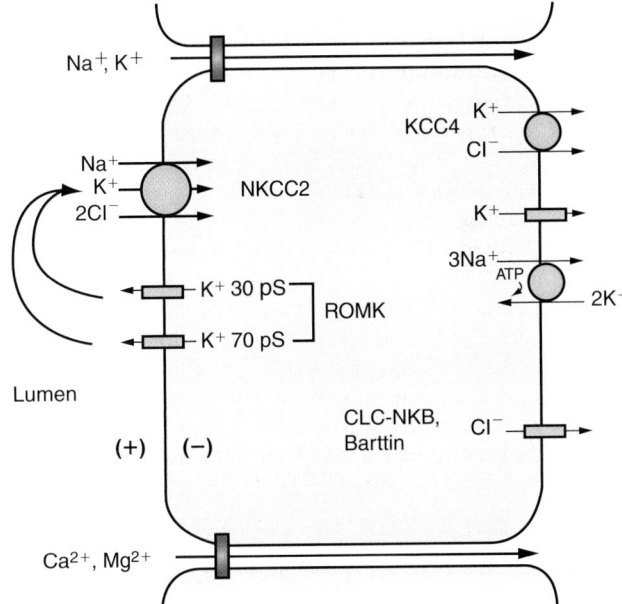

FIGURE 5-15 Transepithelial Na⁺-Cl⁻ transport pathways in the thick ascending limb (TAL). barttin, Cl⁻ channel subunit; CLC-NKB, human chloride channel; KCC4, K⁺-Cl⁻ cotransporter 4; NKCC2, Na⁺-K⁺-2Cl⁻ cotransporter 2; ROMK, renal outer medullary K⁺ channel (Kir 1.1).

Na⁺-Cl⁻ reabsorption by the TAL is thus a secondarily active process, driven by the favorable electrochemical gradient for Na⁺ established by the basolateral Na⁺-K⁺-ATPase.[11,140] Na⁺, K⁺, and Cl⁻ are cotransported across by the apical membrane by an electroneutral Na⁺-K⁺-2Cl⁻ cotransporter (NKCC). This transporter generally requires the simultaneous presence of all three ions, so that the transport of Na⁺ and the transport of Cl⁻ across the epithelium are codependent as well as dependent on the luminal presence of K⁺.[11] Of note, under certain circumstances apical Na⁺-Cl⁻ transport in the TAL appears to be K⁺ independent; this issue is reviewed later (see the section "Regulation of Na⁺-Cl⁻ Transport in the Thick Ascending Limb"). Regardless, this transporter is universally sensitive to furosemide, which has been known for more than three decades to inhibit transepithelial Cl⁻ transport by the TAL.[141]

Apical Na⁺-K⁺-2Cl⁻ cotransport is mediated by the cation-chloride cotransporter NKCC2, encoded by the *SLC12A1* gene.[142] Functional expression of NKCC2 in *Xenopus laevis* oocytes yields Cl⁻- and Na⁺-dependent uptake of rubidium Rb 86 (⁸⁶Rb⁺) (a radioactive substitute for K⁺) and Cl⁻- and K⁺-dependent uptake of sodium Na 22 (²²Na⁺).[142-144] As expected, NKCC2 is sensitive to micromolar concentrations of furosemide, bumetanide, and other loop diuretics.[142] Immunofluorescence testing indicates expression of NKCC2 protein along the entire length of the TAL.[142] In particular, immunoelectron microscopy reveals expression in both rough (R) and smooth (S) cells of the TAL (see above).[139] NKCC2 expression in subapical vesicles is particularly prominent in smooth cells,[139] which suggests a role for vesicular trafficking in the regulation of NKCC2 (see the section "Regulation of Na⁺-Cl⁻ Transport in the Thick Ascending Limb").

NKCC2 is also expressed in macula densa cells,[139] which have been shown to possess apical Na⁺-K⁺-2Cl⁻ cotransport activity.[145] This latter observation is of considerable significance, given the role of the macula densa in tubuloglomerular feedback and renal renin secretion. Luminal loop diuretics block both tubuloglomerular feedback[11] and the suppression of renin release by luminal Cl⁻.[11]

Alternative splicing of exon 4 of the *SLC12A1* gene yields NKCC2 proteins that differ within transmembrane domain 2 and the adjacent intracellular loop. There are three different variants of exon 4, denoted *A, B,* and *F;* the variable inclusion of these cassette exons yields the NKCC2A, NKCC2B, and NKCC2F proteins.[142,144] Kinetic characterization reveals that these isoforms differ dramatically in ion affinities.[142,144] In particular, NKCC2F has a very low affinity for Cl⁻ (K_m of 113 mmol/L), and NKCC2B has a very high affinity (K_m of 8.9 mmol/L); NKCC2A has an intermediate affinity for Cl⁻ (K_m of 44.7 mmol/L).[144] These isoforms differ in axial distribution along the tubule, with the F cassette expressed in the inner stripe of the outer medulla, the A cassette in the outer stripe, and the B cassette in cortical TAL.[11] There is thus an axial distribution of the anion affinity of NKCC2 along the TAL, from a low-affinity, high-capacity transporter (NKCC2F) to a high-affinity, low-capacity transporter (NKCC2B).

Although technically compromised by the considerable homology between the 3′ end of these 96-base-pair exons, in situ hybridization has suggested that rabbit macula densa exclusively expresses the NKCC2B isoform.[11] Notably, however, selective knockout of the B cassette exon 4 does not eliminate NKCC2 expression in the murine macula densa, which also seems to express NKCC2A as determined by in situ hybridization.[146]

The comparative phenotypes of NKCC2A and NKCC2B knockout mice are consistent with the relative Cl⁻ affinity of each isoform, with NKCC2B functioning as a high affinity/low capacity isoform and NKCC2A functioning as a low affinity/high capacity isoform. Thus targeted deletion of NKCC2A selectively reduces tubuloglomerular feedback responses at the higher range of tubular flow rates (a low affinity/high capacity situation), whereas NKCC2B deletion reduces responses at low flow rates.[147] Loss of NKCC2A virtually abolishes the suppression of plasma renin activity by isotonic saline infusion, which is, if anything, more robust in NKCC2B knockout mice than in wild-type littermates.[147]

It should be mentioned in this context that the Na⁺/H⁺ exchanger NHE3 functions as an alternative mechanism for apical Na⁺ absorption by the TAL. There is also evidence in mouse cortical TAL for Na⁺-Cl⁻ transport via parallel Na⁺/H⁺ and Cl⁻/HCO₃⁻ exchange,[11] although the role of this mechanism in transepithelial Na⁺-Cl⁻ transport seems less prominent than in the proximal tubule. Indeed, apical Na⁺/H⁺ exchange mediated by NHE3 appears to function primarily in HCO₃⁻ absorption by the TAL.[148] There is thus a considerable upregulation of both apical Na⁺/H⁺ exchange and NHE3 protein in the TAL of acidotic animals,[149] paired with an induction of AE2, a basolateral Cl⁻/HCO₃⁻ exchanger.[150]

APICAL K⁺ CHANNELS

Microperfused TALs develop a lumen-positive PD during perfusion with Na⁺-Cl⁻.[151,152] This lumen-negative PD plays a critical role in the physiology of the TAL, driving the paracellular transport of Na⁺, Ca²⁺, and Mg²⁺ (see Figure 5-15). Originally attributed to electrogenic Cl⁻ transport,[152] the lumen-positive, transepithelial PD in the TAL is generated by the combination of apical K⁺ channels and basolateral Cl⁻ channels.[11,140] The conductivity of the apical membrane of TAL cells is predominantly, if not exclusively, K⁺ selective. Luminal recycling of K⁺ via Na⁺-K⁺-2Cl⁻ cotransport and apical K⁺ channels, along with basolateral depolarization due to Cl⁻ exit through Cl⁻ channels, results in the lumen-negative transepithelial PD.[11,140]

Several lines of evidence indicate that apical K⁺ channels are required for transepithelial Na⁺-Cl⁻ transport by the TAL.[11,140] First, the removal of K⁺ from luminal perfusate results in a marked decrease in Na⁺-Cl⁻ reabsorption by the TAL, as measured by short-circuit current. The residual Na⁺-Cl⁻ transport in the absence of luminal K⁺ is sustained by the exit of K⁺ via apical K⁺ channels, since the combination of K⁺ removal and a luminal K⁺ channel inhibitor (barium) almost abolishes the short-circuit current.[11] Apical K⁺ channels are thus required for continued functioning of NKCC2, the apical Na⁺-K⁺-2Cl⁻ cotransporter; the low luminal concentration of K⁺ in this nephron segment would otherwise become limiting for transepithelial Na⁺-Cl⁻ transport.

Second, the net transport of K⁺ across perfused TAL is less than 10% that of Na⁺ and Cl⁻[153]; approximately 90% of the K⁺ transported by NKCC2 is recycled across the apical membrane via K⁺ channels, which results in minimal net K⁺ absorption by the TAL.[11]

Third, the intracellular K⁺ activity of perfused TAL cells is approximately 15 to 20 mV above equilibrium, due to furosemide-sensitive entry of K⁺ via NKCC2.[154] Given an estimated apical K⁺ conductivity of approximately 12 m/cm², this intracellular K⁺ activity yields a calculated K⁺ current of approximately 200 μA/cm²; this corresponds quantitatively to the uptake of K⁺ by the apical NKCC.[140]

Finally, the observation that Bartter's syndrome can be caused by mutations in ROMK (renal outer medullary K⁺ channel; also known as *Kir 1.1*)[155] provides genetic proof for the importance of K[+] channels in Na[+]-Cl[−] absorption by the TAL (see later).

Three types of apical K[+] channels have been identified in the TAL, a 30-picosiemen channel, a 70-picosiemen channel, and a high-conductance, calcium-activated maxi-K[+] channel[156-158] (see Figure 5-15). The higher open probability and greater density of the 30-picosiemen and 70-picosiemen channels compared with the maxi-K[+] channel suggest that these are the primary route for K[+] recycling across the apical membrane; the 70-picosiemen channel, in turn, appears to mediate approximately 80% of the apical K[+] conductance of TAL cells.[159]

The low-conductance 30-picosiemen channel shares several electrophysiologic and regulatory characteristics with ROMK, the cardinal inward-rectifying K[+] channel that was initially cloned from renal outer medulla.[11] ROMK protein has been identified at the apical membrane of medullary TAL, cortical TAL, and macula densa.[160] Furthermore, the 30-picosiemen channel is also absent from the apical membrane of mice with homozygous deletion of the gene encoding ROMK.[161] Notably, not all cells in the TAL are labeled with ROMK antibody, which suggests that ROMK might be absent in the so-called HBC cells with high basolateral Cl[−] conductance and low apical/high basolateral K[+] conductance (see also earlier).[127,138] HBC cells are thought to correspond to the smooth-surfaced morphologic subtype of TAL cells (S cells)[138]; however, data showing the distribution of ROMK protein by immunoelectron microscopy have not yet been published.

ROMK clearly plays a critical role in Na[+]-Cl[−] absorption by the TAL, given that loss-of-function mutations in this gene are associated with Bartter's syndrome.[155] The role of ROMK in Bartter's syndrome was initially discordant with the data, which suggested that the 70-picosiemen K[+] channel has the dominant conductance at the apical membrane of TAL cells.[159] Heterologous expression of the ROMK protein in *Xenopus* oocytes had yielded a channel with a conductance of approximately 30 picosiemens,[11] a finding implying that the 70-picosiemen channel is distinct from ROMK. This paradox has been resolved by the observation that the 70-picosiemen channel is absent from the TAL of ROMK knockout mice, which indicates that ROMK proteins form a subunit of the 70-picosiemen channel.[162]

ROMK activity in the TAL is clearly modulated by association with other proteins, so coassociation with other subunits to generate the 70-picosiemen channel is perfectly compatible with the known physiology of this protein. ROMK associates with scaffolding proteins NHERF-1 and NHERF-2 (see the section "Neurohumoral Influences" under "Regulation of Proximal Tubular Na[+]-Cl[−] Transport") via the C-terminal PDZ-binding motif of ROMK; NHERF-2 is coexpressed with ROMK in the TAL.[163] The association of ROMK with NHERFs serves to bring ROMK into closer proximity to the cystic fibrosis transmembrane regulator (CFTR) protein.[163] This ROMK-CFTR interaction is, in turn, required for the native ATP and glibenclamide sensitivity of apical K[+] channels in the TAL.[164]

PARACELLULAR TRANSPORT

TALs microperfused with Na[+]-Cl[−] develop a lumen-positive transepithelial PD,[151,152] generated by the combination of apical K[+] secretion and basolateral Cl[−] efflux.[11,140,154] This lumen-positive PD plays a critical role in the paracellular reabsorption of Na[+], Ca[2+], and Mg[2+] by the TAL (see Figure 5-15). In the transepithelial transport of Na[+], the stoichiometry of NKCC2 (1 Na[+] to 1 K[+] to 2Cl[−]) is such that other mechanisms are necessary to balance the exit of Cl[−] at the basolateral membrane. Consistent with this requirement, data from mouse TAL indicate that approximately 50% of transepithelial Na[+] transport occurs via the paracellular pathway.[2,165] For example, the ratio of net Cl[−] transepithelial absorption to net Na[+] absorption through the paracellular pathway is 2.4 ± 0.3 in microperfused mouse medullary TAL segments,[165] the expected ratio if 50% of Na[+] transport occurs via the paracellular pathway.

In the absence of vasopressin, apical Na[+]-Cl[−] cotransport is not K[+] dependent (see the section "Regulation of Na[+]-Cl[−] Transport in the Thick Ascending Limb"), which reduces the lumen-positive PD. Switching to K[+]-dependent Na[+]-K[+]-2Cl[−] cotransport in the presence of vasopressin results in a doubling of Na[+]-Cl[−] reabsorption, without affecting oxygen consumption.[2] Therefore, the combination of a cation-permeable paracellular pathway and an active transport lumen-positive PD,[140] generated indirectly by the basolateral Na[+]-K[+]-ATPase,[166] results in a doubling of active Na[+]-Cl[−] transport for a given level of oxygen consumption.[2]

Unlike in the proximal tubule,[12] the voltage-positive PD in the TAL is generated almost entirely by transcellular transport, rather than diffusion across the lateral tight junction. In vasopressin-stimulated mouse TAL segments, with a lumen-positive PD of 10 mV, the maximal increase in Na[+]-Cl[−] in the lateral interspace is approximately 10 mmol/L.[165] Tight junctions in the TAL are cation selective, with P_{Na}/P_{Cl} ratios of 2 to 5.[140,165] Notably, however, P_{Na}/P_{Cl} ratios can be highly variable in individual tubules, ranging from 2 to 5 in a single study of perfused mouse TAL.[165] Regardless, if one assumes a P_{Na}/P_{Cl} ratio of approximately 3, the maximal dilution potential in the mouse TAL is between 0.7 and 1.1 mV, consistent with a dominant effect of transcellular processes on the lumen-positive PD.[165]

The reported transepithelial resistance in the TAL is between 10 and 50 $\Omega \cdot cm^2$. Although this resistance is higher than that of the proximal tubule, the TAL is not considered a tight epithelium.[11,140] Notably, however, the water permeability of the TAL is extremely low, less than 1% that of the proximal tubule.[140] These "hybrid" characteristics[11]—relatively low resistance and very low water permeability—allow the TAL to generate and sustain Na[+]-Cl[−] gradients of up to 120 mmol/L.[140]

Not unexpectedly, given its lack of water permeability, the TAL does not express aquaporin water channels; as in the proximal tubule, the particular repertoire of claudins expressed in the TAL determines the resistance and ion selectivity of this nephron segment. Mouse TAL segments coexpress claudins 3, 10, 11, 16, and 19.[11,167,168] Notably, the expression of claudin-19 in TAL cells is heterogeneous,[168] analogous perhaps to the heterogeneity of ROMK expression (see earlier). Mutations in human claudin-16 (paracellin-1)[11] and claudin-19[167] are associated with hereditary hypomagnesemia, which suggests that these claudins are particularly critical for the cation selectivity of TAL tight junctions.

Heterologous expression of claudin-16 (paracellin-1) in the anion-selective LLC-PK$_1$ cell line (a strain of epithelium-like pig kidney cells) markedly increases Na[+] permeability without affecting Cl[−] permeability; this generates a significant increase in the P_{Na}/P_{Cl} ratio (Figure 5-16).[169] LLC-PK$_1$ cells expressing claudin-16 also have increased permeability to other monovalent cations. There is, however, only a modest

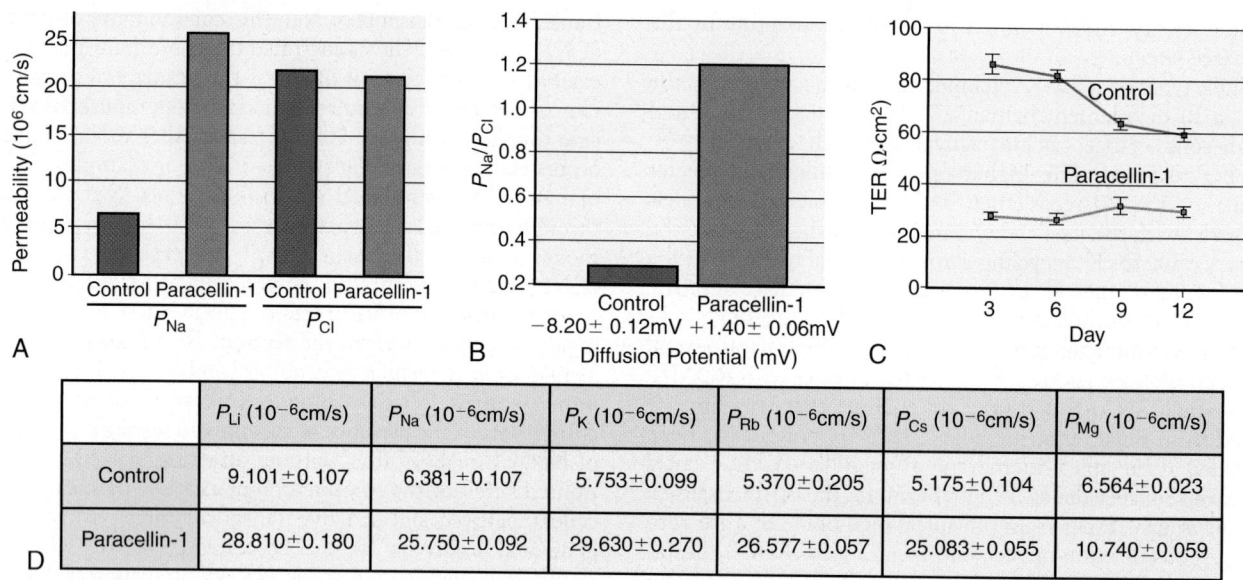

FIGURE 5-16 Effect of claudin-16 (paracellin-1) overexpression in LLC-PK$_1$ cells. **A,** Effects of paracellin-1 on the permeability of Na$^+$ and Cl$^-$ in LLC-PK$_1$ cells. **B,** Ratio of Na$^+$ permeability (P_{Na}) to Cl$^-$ permeability (P_{Cl}) and diffusion potential (*bottom*) across an LLC-PK$_1$ cell monolayer. **C,** Transepithelial resistance across an LLC-PK$_1$ cell monolayer over a period of 12 days in cells expressing paracellin-1 and in control cells. **D,** Summary of the effects of paracellin-1 on permeability of various cations in LLC-PK$_1$ cells. (From Hou J, Paul DL, Goodenough DA: Paracellin-1 and the modulation of ion selectivity of tight junctions, *J Cell Sci* 118:5109-5118, 2005.)

increase in Mg^{2+} permeability, which suggests that claudin-16 does not form a Mg^{2+}-specific pathway in the tight junction; rather, it may serve to increase the overall cation selectivity of the tight junction. Claudin-19, in turn, appears to reduce P$_{Cl}$ in LLC-PK$_1$ cells without having much effect on Mg^{2+} or Na$^+$ permeability.[170]

The claudin-16 and claudin-19 proteins interact in multiple systems,[170,171] and coexpression of claudin-16 and claudin-19 synergistically increases the P$_{Na}$/P$_{Cl}$ ratio in LLC-PK$_1$ cells.[170] Knockdown of claudin-16 in transgenic mice increases Na$^+$ absorption in the downstream collecting duct, with the development of hypovolemic hyponatremia after treatment with amiloride.[172] Claudin-19 knockdown mice exhibit an increase in fractional excretion of Na$^+$ and a doubling in serum aldosterone level.[171] In summary, claudin-16 and claudin-19 interact to confer the cation selectivity of tight junctions in the TAL, contributing significantly to the transepithelial absorption of Na$^+$ in this nephron segment.

BASOLATERAL MECHANISMS

Basolateral Na$^+$-K$^+$-ATPase is the primary exit pathway for Na$^+$ at the basolateral membrane of TAL cells. The Na$^+$ gradient generated by Na$^+$-K$^+$-ATPase activity is also thought to drive the apical entry of Na$^+$, K$^+$, and Cl$^-$ via NKCC2, the furosemide-sensitive Na$^+$-K$^+$-2Cl$^-$ cotransporter.[11] Inhibition of Na$^+$-K$^+$-ATPase with ouabain thus collapses the lumen-positive PD and abolishes transepithelial Na$^+$-Cl$^-$ transport in the TAL.[151,152,166]

Basolateral exit of Cl$^-$ from TAL cells is primarily but not exclusively[173] electrogenic, mediated by Cl$^-$ channel activity.[11,140] Reductions in basolateral Cl$^-$ depolarize the basolateral membrane, whereas increases in intracellular Cl$^-$ induced by luminal furosemide have a hyperpolarizing effect.[11] Intracellular Cl$^-$ activity during transepithelial Na$^+$-Cl$^-$ transport is above its electrochemical equilibrium,[11] with an intracellular negative voltage of −40 to −70 mV that drives basolateral Cl$^-$ exit.[11,140]

At least two ClC chloride channels, ClC-K1 and ClC-K2 (CLC-NKA and CLC-NKB in humans), are coexpressed in this nephron segment.[132,135] However, an increasing body of evidence indicates that the dominant Cl$^-$ channel in the TAL is encoded by ClC-K2. First, ClC-K1 is heavily expressed at both apical and basolateral membranes of the thin ascending limb,[130] and the phenotype of the corresponding knockout mouse is consistent with primary dysfunction of the thin ascending limbs, rather than the TAL[112,133] (see the section "Na$^+$-Cl$^-$ Transport in the Thin Ascending Limb"). Second, loss-of-function mutations in CLC-NKB are associated with Bartter's syndrome,[134] genetic evidence for a dominant role of this channel in Na$^+$-Cl$^-$ transport in the TAL. More recently, a very common polymorphism in human CLC-NKB in which threonine at residue 481 is replaced by serine (T481S) was shown to increase channel activity by a factor of 20.[11] Preliminary data indicate an association with hypertension,[174] which suggests that this gain-of-function in CLC-NKB increases Na$^+$-Cl$^-$ transport by the TAL and/or other segments of the distal nephron. Finally, ClC-K2 protein is heavily expressed at the basolateral membrane of the mouse TAL, with additional expression in the DCT, CNT, and α-intercalated cells.[175]

A key advance was the characterization of the barttin subunit of ClC-K channels, which is coexpressed with ClC-K1 and ClC-K2 in several nephron segments, including TAL[132,135] (see also the section "Na$^+$-Cl$^-$ Transport in the Thin Ascending Limb"). Unlike rat ClC-K1, rat ClC-K2, human CLC-NKA, and human CLC-NKB paralogs are not functional in the absence of barttin coexpression.[135,136] CLC-NKB coexpressed with barttin is highly selective for Cl$^-$, with a permeability series of Cl$^-$ >> Br$^-$ = NO$_3^-$ > I$^-$.[11,132,135]

CLC-NKB/barttin channels are activated by increases in extracellular Ca^{2+} and are pH sensitive, with activation at alkaline extracellular pH and marked inhibition at acidic pH.[135] CLC-NKA/barttin channels have similar pH and calcium sensitivities, but exhibit higher permeability to Br⁻.[135] Strikingly, despite the considerable homology between the CLC-NKA and CLC-NKB proteins, these channels also differ considerably in pharmacologic sensitivity to various Cl⁻ channel blockers, potential lead compounds for the development of paralog-specific inhibitors.[176]

Correlation between functional characteristics of ClC-K proteins and native Cl⁻ channels in TAL has been problematic. In particular, a wide variation in single-channel conductance has been reported for basolateral Cl⁻ channels in this nephron segment (reviewed in Palmer and Frindt[177]). This is perhaps due to the use of collagenase and other conditions associated with the preparation of tubule fragments and/or basolateral vesicles, manipulations that potentially affect channel characteristics.[177] There may also be considerable molecular heterogeneity of Cl⁻ channels in the TAL, although the genetic evidence would seem to suggest a functional dominance of CLC-NKB.[134]

Single-channel conductance has not been reported for CLC-NKB/barttin channels, due to the difficulty in expressing the channel in heterologous systems. This complicates the comparison of CLC-NKB/barttin with native Cl⁻ channels. Single-channel conductance has been reported, however, for the V166E mutant of rat ClC-K1, which alters gating of the channel without expected effects on single-channel amplitude; notably, coexpression with barttin increases the single-channel conductance of V166E ClC-K1 from approximately 7 picosiemens to approximately 20 picosiemens.[136] Therefore, part of the reported variability in native single-channel conductance may reflect heterogeneity in the interaction between CLC-NKB and/or CLC-NKA with barttin.

Regardless, a recent study using whole-cell recording techniques suggests that ClC-K2 (CLC-NKB in humans) is the dominant Cl⁻ channel in TAL and other segments of the rat distal nephron.[177] Like CLC-NKB/barttin,[11,132,135] this native channel is highly Cl⁻-selective, with considerably weaker conductance for Br⁻ and I⁻[177]; CLC-NKA/barttin channels exhibit higher permeability to Br⁻.[135] This renal channel is also inhibited by acidic extracellular pH,[177] but seems to lack the activation by alkaline pH seen in CLC-NKB/barttin-expressing cells.[135]

Electroneutral K⁺-Cl⁻ cotransport has also been implicated in transepithelial Na⁺-Cl⁻ transport in the TAL (see Figure 5-15), functioning in K⁺-dependent Cl⁻ exit at the basolateral membrane.[11] The K⁺-Cl⁻ cotransporter KCC4 is expressed at the basolateral membrane of medullary and cortical TAL, in addition to macula densa.[178,179] There is also functional evidence for K⁺-Cl⁻ cotransport at the basolateral membrane of this section of the nephron.

First, TAL cells contain a Cl⁻-dependent NH₄⁺ transport mechanism that is sensitive to 1.5 mmol/L furosemide and 10 mmol/L barium (Ba²⁺).[180] NH₄⁺ ions have the same ionic radius as K⁺ and are transported by KCC4 and other K⁺-Cl⁻ cotransporters.[181] KCC4 is also sensitive to Ba²⁺ and millimolar furosemide,[182] which is consistent with the pharmacology of NH₄⁺-Cl⁻ cotransport in the TAL.[180]

Second, to account for the effects on transmembrane PD of basolateral Ba²⁺ and/or increased K⁺, it has been suggested that the basolateral membrane of TAL contains a Ba²⁺-sensitive K⁺-Cl⁻ transporter[11]; this is also consistent with the known expression of Ba²⁺-sensitive[182] KCC4 at the basolateral membrane.[178,179]

Third, increases in basolateral K⁺ cause Cl⁻-dependent cell swelling in *Amphiuma* early distal tubule, an analog of the mammalian TAL. In *Amphiuma* LBC cells with low basolateral conductance, which are analogous to mammalian LBC cells[127,138] (see the section "Apical Na⁺-Cl⁻ Transport" under "Na⁺-Cl⁻ Transport in the Thick Ascending Limb"), this cell swelling was not accompanied by changes in basolateral membrane voltage or resistance,[183] which is consistent with K⁺-Cl⁻ transport.

There is thus considerable evidence for basolateral K⁺-Cl⁻ cotransport in the TAL, mediated by KCC4.[178,179] However, direct confirmation of a role for basolateral K⁺-Cl⁻ cotransport in transepithelial Na⁺-Cl⁻ transport is lacking. Indeed, KCC4-deficient mice do not have a prominent defect in the function of the TAL, but instead exhibit a renal tubular acidosis.[179] The renal tubular acidosis in these mice has been attributed to defects in acid extrusion by H⁺-ATPase in α-intercalated cells[179]; however, this phenotype is conceivably caused by reduction in medullary NH₄⁺ reabsorption by the TAL,[184] due to the loss of basolateral NH₄⁺ exit mediated by KCC4.[181]

Finally, there is also evidence for the existence of Ba²⁺-sensitive K⁺ channel activity at the basolateral membrane of the TAL,[185-187] which provides an alternative exit pathway for K⁺ to that mediated by KCC4. These channels may function in transepithelial transport of K⁺; however, such K⁺ transport is less than 10% that of Na⁺ and Cl⁻ transport by the TAL.[153] Basolateral K⁺ channels may also attenuate the increases in intracellular K⁺ that are generated by the basolateral Na⁺-K⁺-ATPase, thus maintaining transepithelial Na⁺-Cl⁻ transport.[185-187] In addition, basolateral K⁺ channel activity may help stabilize the basolateral membrane potential above the equilibrium potential for Cl⁻,[187] thus maintaining a continuous driving force for Cl⁻ exit via CLC-NKB/barttin Cl⁻ channels.

REGULATION OF NA⁺-CL⁻ TRANSPORT IN THE THICK ASCENDING LIMB

Activating Influences. Transepithelial Na⁺-Cl⁻ transport by the TAL is regulated by a complex blend of competing neurohumoral influences. In particular, increases in intracellular cAMP tonically stimulate ion transport in the TAL. The list of stimulatory hormones and mediators that increase cAMP in this nephron segment includes vasopressin, PTH, glucagon, calcitonin, and β-adrenergic activation (see Figure 5-10). These overlapping cAMP-dependent stimuli are thought to result in maximal baseline stimulation of transepithelial Na⁺-Cl⁻ transport.[76] For example, characterization of the in vivo effect of these hormones requires the prior simultaneous suppression or absence of circulating vasopressin, PTH, calcitonin, and glucagon.[76] This baseline activation is in turn modulated by a number of negative influences, most prominently prostaglandin E₂ (PGE₂) and extracellular Ca²⁺ (see Figure 5-10).

Vasopressin is perhaps the most extensively studied positive modulator of transepithelial Na⁺-Cl⁻ transport in the TAL. The TAL expresses V₂ vasopressin receptors at both the mRNA and protein level, and microdissected TALs respond to the hormone with an increase in intracellular cAMP.[188] Vasopressin activates apical Na⁺-K⁺-2Cl⁻ cotransport within minutes in perfused mouse TAL segments and also exerts longer term influence on NKCC2 expression and function. The acute activation of apical Na^+-K^+-$2Cl^-$ cotransport is achieved at least in part by the stimulated exocytosis of NKCC2 proteins from subapical vesicles to the plasma membrane.[189] This trafficking-dependent activation is abrogated by treatment of perfused tubules with tetanus toxin, which cleaves the vesicle-associated membrane proteins VAMP-2 and VAMP-3.[189]

Activation of NKCC2 is also associated with the phosphorylation of a cluster of N-terminal threonines in the transporter protein. Treatment of rats with the V_2 agonist desmopressin (DDAVP) induces phosphorylation of these residues in vivo, as measured with a potent phosphospecific antibody.[189] These threonine residues are substrates for the SPAK (STE20/SPS1-related proline/alanine-rich kinase) and OSR1 (oxidative stress–responsive kinase 1) kinases, recently identified by Delpire's group as key regulatory kinases for NKCC1 and other cation-chloride cotransporters.[190]

SPAK and OSR1, in turn, are activated by upstream WNK (*with no lysine* [*K*]) kinases (see also the section "Regulation of Na^+-Cl^- Transport" under "Distal Convoluted Tubule"), so that SPAK or OSR1 requires coexpression with WNK4 to fully activate NKCC1.[190] WNK kinases can, however, influence transport when coexpressed alone in *Xenopus* oocytes with cation-chloride cotransporters, in the absence of exogenous SPAK/OSR1, which is reflective perhaps of the activation of endogenous *Xenopus laevis* orthologs of SPAK and/or OSR1. Regardless, coexpression with WNK3 in *Xenopus* oocytes results in activating phosphorylation of the N-terminal threonines in NKCC2 that are phosphorylated in TAL cells after treatment with DDAVP.[189,191]

The WNK3 protein is also expressed in TAL cells,[191] although the links between activation of the V_2 receptor and this particular kinase are as yet uncharacterized. The N-terminal phosphorylation of NKCC2 by SPAK kinase appears to be critical for the activity of the transporter in the native TAL. The N terminus of NKCC2 contains a predicted binding site for the SPAK kinase,[192] proximal to the sites of regulatory phosphorylation; the analogous binding site is required for activation of the NKCC1 cotransporter.[193] SPAK also requires the sorting receptor SORLA (sorting protein–related receptor with A-type repeats) for proper trafficking within TAL cells, so that targeted deletion of SORLA results in marked reduction in N-terminal NKCC2 phosphorylation.[194]

The role of the upstream WNK kinases is illustrated by the phenotype of a knock-in mouse strain in which mutant SPAK cannot be activated by upstream WNK kinases.[195] These mice have a marked reduction in N-terminal phosphorylation of both NKCC2 and the thiazide-sensitive Na^+-Cl^- cotransporter NCC, with associated salt-sensitive hypotension. The upstream WNK kinases appear to regulate SPAK and NKCC2 in chloride-dependent fashion, phosphorylating and activating SPAK and the transporter in response to a reduction in intracellular chloride concentration.[196]

Vasopressin has also been shown to alter the stoichiometry of furosemide-sensitive apical Cl^- transport in the TAL, from a K^+-independent Na^+-Cl^- mode to the classical Na^+-K^+-$2Cl^-$ cotransport stoichiometry.[2] In the absence of vasopressin, $^{22}Na^+$ uptake by mouse medullary TAL cells is not dependent on the presence of extracellular K^+, whereas the addition of the hormone induces a switch to K^+-dependent $^{22}Na^+$ uptake. In a process that underscores the metabolic advantages of paracellular Na^+ transport, which is critically dependent on

the apical entry of K^+ via Na^+-K^+-$2Cl^-$ cotransport (see earlier), vasopressin accomplishes a doubling of transepithelial Na^+-Cl^- transport without affecting $^{22}Na^+$ uptake (an indicator of transcellular Na^+-Cl^- transport); this doubling in transepithelial absorption occurs without an increase in oxygen consumption,[2] which highlights the energy efficiency of ion transport by the TAL.

The mechanism of this shift in the apparent stoichiometry of NKCC2 is not completely clear. However, splice variants of mouse NKCC2 with a novel, shorter C terminus have been found to confer sensitivity to cAMP when coexpressed with full-length NKCC2.[197] Notably, these shorter splice variants appear to encode furosemide-sensitive, K^+-independent Na^+-Cl^- cotransporters when expressed alone in *Xenopus* oocytes.[198] The in vivo relevance of these phenomena is not clear, however, nor is it known whether similar splice variants exist in species other than mouse.

In addition to its acute effects on NKCC2, the apical Na^+-K^+-$2Cl^-$ cotransporter, vasopressin increases transepithelial Na^+-Cl^- transport by activating apical K^+ channels and basolateral Cl^- channels in the TAL.[76,188] Details have yet to emerge of the regulation of the basolateral CLC-NKB/barttin Cl^- channel complex by vasopressin, cAMP, and related pathways. However, the apical K^+ channel ROMK is directly phosphorylated by PKA on three serine residues (S25, S200, and S294 in the ROMK2 isoform). Phosphorylation of at least two of these three serines is required for detectable K^+ channel activity in *Xenopus* oocytes; mutation of all three serines to alanine abolishes phosphorylation and transport activity, and all three serines are required for full channel activity.[199]

These three phosphoacceptor sites have distinct effects on ROMK activity and expression.[200] Phosphorylation of the N-terminal S25 residue appears to regulate trafficking of the channel to the cell membrane, without affecting channel gating; this serine is also a substrate for the SGK1 kinase, which activates the channel via an increase in expression at the membrane.[200] In contrast, phosphorylation of the two C-terminal serines modulates open channel probability via effects on pH-dependent gating[201] and on activation by the binding of phosphatidylinositol bisphosphate (PIP_2) to the C-terminal domain of the channel.[202]

Vasopressin also has considerable long-term effects on transepithelial Na^+-Cl^- transport by the TAL. Sustained increases in circulating vasopressin result in marked hypertrophy of medullary TAL cells, accompanied by a doubling in baseline active Na^+-Cl^- transport.[188] Water restriction or treatment with DDAVP also results in an increase in abundance of the NKCC2 protein in rat TAL cells. Consistent with a direct effect of vasopressin-dependent signaling, expression of NKCC2 is reduced in mice with a heterozygous deletion of the G_s (stimulatory) G protein, through which the V_2 receptor activates cAMP generation.[188] Increases in cAMP are thought to directly induce transcription of the *SLC12A1* gene that encodes NKCC2, given the presence of a cAMP-response element in the 5′ promoter.[188,189] Abrogation of the tonic negative effect of PGE_2 on cAMP generation with indomethacin also results in a considerable increase in abundance of the NKCC2 protein.[188] Finally, in addition to these effects on NKCC2 expression, water restriction or DDAVP treatment increases abundance of the ROMK protein at the apical membrane of TAL cells.[203]

Inhibitory Influences. The tonic stimulation of transepithelial Na^+-Cl^- transport by cAMP-generating hormones (vasopressin, PTH, etc.) is modulated by a number of negative neurohumoral influences (see Figure 5-10 and Feraille and Doucet[76]). In particular, extracellular Ca^{2+} and PGE_2 exert dramatic inhibitory effects on ion transport by this and other segments of the distal nephron, through a plethora of synergistic mechanisms. Both extracellular Ca^{2+} and PGE_2 activate the G_i (inhibitory) G protein in TAL cells, opposing the stimulatory, G_s-dependent effects of vasopressin on intracellular levels of cAMP.[204,205] Extracellular Ca^{2+} exerts its effect through the calcium-sensing receptor (CaSR), which is heavily expressed at the basolateral membrane of TAL cells.[205,206] PGE_2 primarily signals through EP3 prostaglandin receptors.[76]

The increases in intracellular Ca^{2+} caused by the activation of the CaSR and other receptors directly inhibits cAMP generation by a Ca^{2+}-inhibitable adenylate cyclase that is expressed in the TAL, accompanied by an increase in phosphodiesterase-dependent degradation of cAMP[205,207] (Figure 5-17). Activation of the CaSR and other receptors in the TAL also results in the downstream generation of arachidonic acid metabolites with potent negative effects on Na^+-Cl^- transport (see Figure 5-17). For instance, extracellular Ca^{2+} activates phospholipase A_2 in TAL cells, which leads to the liberation of arachidonic acid. This arachidonic acid is in turn metabolized by P450 ω-hydroxylase to 20-HETE or by cyclooxygenase-2 (COX-2) to PGE_2. P450 ω-hydroxylation generally predominates in response to activation of the CaSR in TAL.[205] 20-HETE has very potent negative effects on apical Na^+-K^+-$2Cl^-$ cotransport, apical K^+ channels, and the basolateral Na^+-K^+-ATPase.[76,205] Phospholipase A_2–dependent generation of 20-HETE also underlies in part the negative effect of bradykinin and angiotensin II on Na^+-Cl^- transport.[76,205] Activation of the CaSR also induces tumor necrosis factor-α expression in the TAL, which activates COX-2 and thus generation of PGE_2 (see Figure 5-17); this PGE_2 in turn results in additional inhibition of Na^+-Cl^- transport.[205]

The relative importance of the CaSR in the regulation of Na^+-Cl^- transport by the TAL is dramatically illustrated by the phenotype of a handful of patients with gain-of-function mutations in this receptor. In addition to suppressed PTH and hypocalcemia, the usual phenotype caused by gain-of-function mutations in the CaSR (autosomal dominant hypoparathyroidism), these patients manifest a hypokalemic alkalosis, polyuria, and increases in circulating renin and aldosterone.[208,209] Therefore, the persistent inhibition of Na^+-Cl^- transport in the TAL by these overactive mutants of the CaSR causes a rare subtype of Bartter's syndrome, type 5 in the genetic classification of this disease.[205]

Distal Convoluted Tubule, Connecting Tubule, and Collecting Duct

The distal nephron that extends beyond the TAL is the final determiner of urinary Na^+-Cl^- excretion and a critical target for both natriuretic and antinatriuretic stimuli. The understanding of the cellular organization and molecular phenotype of the distal nephron continues to evolve and merits a brief review here.

The DCT begins at a variable distance after the macula densa, with an abrupt transition between NKCC2-positive cortical TAL cells and DCT cells that express the thiazide-sensitive Na^+-Cl^- cotransporter NCC. Considerable progress has been made in the phenotypic classification of cell types in the DCT and adjacent nephron segments, based on the

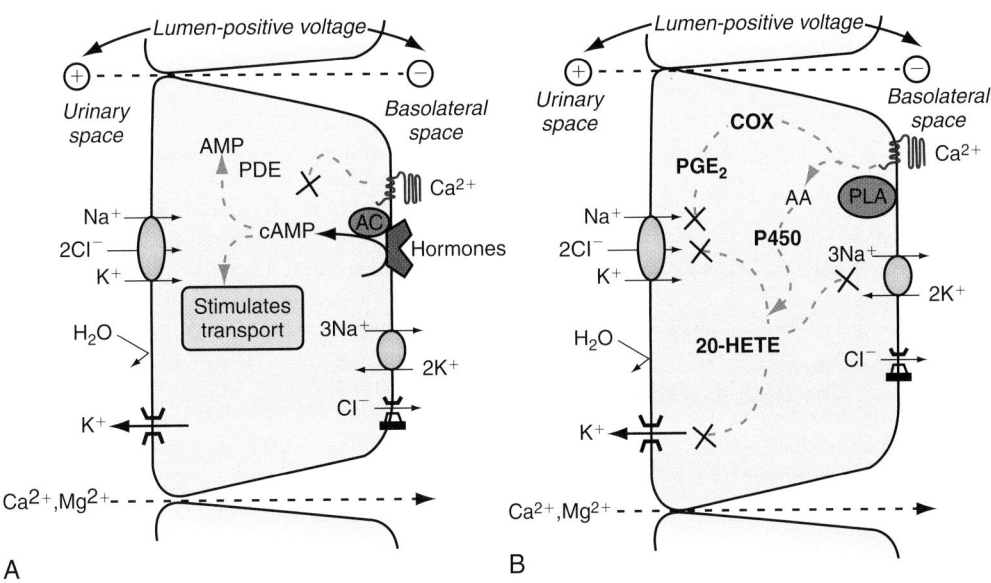

FIGURE 5-17 Inhibitory effects of the calcium-sensing receptor (CaSR) on transepithelial Na^+-Cl^- transport in the thick ascending limb (TAL). **A,** Activation of the basolateral CaSR inhibits the generation of cyclic adenosine monophosphate (cAMP) in response to vasopressin and other hormones (see text for details). **B,** Stimulation of phospholipase A_2 by the CaSR leads to liberation of arachidonic acid, which in turn is metabolized by P450 ω-hydroxylase to 20-hydroxyeicosatetraenoic acid (20-HETE), or by cyclooxygenase-2 (COX-2) to prostaglandin E_2 (PGE_2). 20-HETE is a potent natriuretic factor, inhibiting apical Na^+-K^+-$2Cl^-$ cotransport, apical K^+ channels, and basolateral Na^+-K^+-adenosine triphosphatase (Na^+-K^+-ATPase). Activation of the CaSR also induces tumor necrosis factor-α (TNF-α) expression in the TAL, which activates COX-2 and thus generation of PGE_2; this leads to additional inhibition of Na^+-Cl^- transport. (From Hebert SC: Calcium and salinity sensing by the thick ascending limb: a journey from mammals to fish and back again, *Kidney Int Suppl* [91]:S28-S33, 2004.)

expression of an expanding list of transport proteins and other markers.[210] This analysis has revealed considerable differences in the organization of the DCT, connecting tubule (CNT), and cortical collecting duct (CCD) in rodent, rabbit, and human kidneys. In general, rabbit kidneys are unique in the axial demarcation of DCT, CNT, and CCD segments, at both a molecular and morphologic level; the organization of the DCT to CCD is considerably more complex in other species, with boundaries that are much less absolute.[210] Notably, however, the overall set of transport proteins expressed does not vary among these species; what differs is the specific cellular and molecular organization of this segment of the nephron.

The early DCT (DCT1) of mouse kidney expresses NCC and a specific marker, parvalbumin, that also distinguishes the DCT1 from the adjacent cortical TAL[211] (Figure 5-18). Targeted deletion of parvalbumin in mice reveals that this intracellular Ca^{2+}-binding protein is required for full activity of NCC in the DCT.[212] Mouse DCT2 cells coexpress NCC with proteins involved in transcellular Ca^{2+} transport, including the apical epithelial calcium channel ECaC1, the cytosolic calcium-binding protein calbindin-D28K, and the basolateral Na^+/Ca^{2+} exchanger NCX.[211] NCC is coexpressed with the amiloride-sensitive epithelial Na^+ channel (ENaC) in the late DCT2 of mouse, with robust expression of ENaC continuing in the downstream CNT and CCD.[211] In contrast, rabbit kidney does not have a DCT1 or DCT2 and exhibits abrupt transitions between NCC- and ENaC-positive DCT and CNT segments, respectively.[210]

Human kidneys that have been studied thus far exhibit expression of calbindin-D28K all along the DCT and CNT, extending into the CCD; however, the intensity of expression varies at these sites. Approximately 30% of cells in the distal convolution of human kidney express NCC, with 70% expressing ENaC (CNT cells). ENaC and NCC overlap in expression at the end of the human DCT segment. Finally, cells of the early CNT of human kidneys express ENaC in the absence of aquaporin-2, the apical vasopressin-sensitive water channel.[210]

Although primarily contiguous with the DCT, CNT cells share several traits with principal cells of the CCD, including apical expression of ENaC and ROMK, the K^+-secretory channel. The capacity for Na^+-Cl^- reabsorption and K^+ secretion in this nephron segment is as much as 10 times higher than that in the CCD[213] (see also the section "Apical Na^+ Transport" under "Connecting Tubules and Cortical Collecting Duct").

Intercalated cells are the minority cell type within the distal nephron, emerging within the DCT and CNT and extending into the early inner medullary collecting duct (IMCD).[214] Three subtypes of intercalated cells have been defined, based on differences in the subcellular distribution of the H^+-ATPase and the presence or absence of the basolateral AE1 Cl^-/HCO_3^- exchanger. Type A intercalated cells extrude protons via an apical H^+-ATPase in series with basolateral AE1. Type B intercalated cells secrete HCO_3^- and OH^- via an apical anion exchanger (SLC26A4 or pendrin) in series with basolateral H^+-ATPase.[214] In rodents, the most prevalent subtype of intercalated cells in the CNT is the non-A, non-B intercalated cell, which possesses an apical Cl^-/HCO_3^- exchanger (SLC26A4 or pendrin) along with apical H^+-ATPase.[214] Although intercalated cells play a dominant role in acid-base homeostasis, Cl^- transport by type B intercalated cells performs an increasingly appreciated role in distal nephron Na^+-Cl^- transport (see the section "Cl^- Transport" under "Connecting Tubules and Cortical Collecting Duct").

The outer medullary collecting duct (OMCD) encompasses two separate subsegments, corresponding to the outer and inner stripes of the outer medulla, or OMCDo and OMCDi, respectively. The OMCDo and OMCDi contain principal cells with apical amiloride-sensitive Na^+ channels (ENaC)[215]; however, the primary role of this nephron segment is renal acidification, with a particular dominance of type A intercalated cells in the OMCDi.[3] The OMCD also plays a critical role in K^+ reabsorption via the activity of apical H^+-K^+-ATPase pumps.[216-218]

Finally, the IMCD begins at the boundary between the outer and inner medulla, and extends to the tip of the papilla. The IMCD is arbitrarily separated into three equal zones, denoted IMCD1, IMCD2, and IMCD3. At the functional level, an early IMCD (IMCDi) and a terminal portion (IMCDt) can be appreciated.[3] The IMCD plays particularly prominent roles in vasopressin-sensitive water and urea transport.[3] The early IMCD contains both principal cells and intercalated cells; all three subsegments (IMCD1 to IMCD3) express apical ENaC protein, albeit this expression is considerably weaker than in the CNT and CCD.[219]

The roles of the IMCD and OMCD in Na^+-Cl^- homeostasis have been more elusive than those of the CNT and CCD; however, to the extent that ENaC is expressed in the IMCD and OMCD, homologous mechanisms are expected to function in Na^+-Cl^- reabsorption by CNT, CCD, OMCD, and IMCD segments.

Distal Convoluted Tubule

MECHANISMS OF NA⁺-CL⁻ TRANSPORT

Earlier micropuncture studies that did not distinguish between early and late DCT indicate that this nephron segment reabsorbs approximately 10% of filtered Na^+-Cl^-.[220,221] The apical absorption of Na^+ and of Cl^- by the DCT are mutually dependent; ion substitution does not affect transepithelial voltage, which suggests electroneutral transport.[222] The absorption of Na^+ by perfused DCT segments is also inhibited by

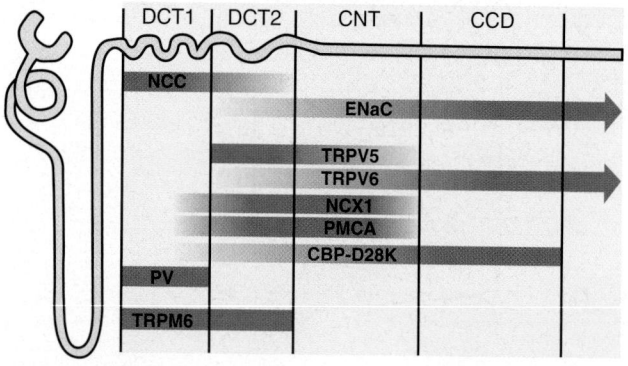

FIGURE 5-18 Schematic representation of the segmentation of the mouse distal nephron and of the distribution and abundance of Na^+-, Ca^{2+}- and Mg^{2+}-transporting proteins. *CBP-D28K,* Calbindin-D28K; *ENaC,* epithelial Na^+ channel; *NCC,* thiazide-sensitive Na^+-Cl^- cotransporter; *NCX1,* Na^+/Ca^{2+} exchanger 1; *PMCA,* plasma membrane Ca^{2+}-adenosine triphosphatase; *PV,* parvalbumin; *TRPM6,* apical Mg^{2+} entry channel; *TRPV5* and *TRPV6,* apical Ca^{2+} entry channels. (Data from Loffing et al,[211] Nijenhuis et al,[441] and Voets et al.[442])

chlorothiazide, localized proof that this nephron segment is the target for thiazide diuretics.[223] Similar thiazide-sensitive Na$^+$-Cl$^-$ cotransport exists in the urinary bladder of winter flounder, the species in which the thiazide-sensitive Na$^+$-Cl$^-$ cotransporter NCC was first identified by expression cloning.[224]

Functional characterization of rat NCC indicates very high affinities for both Na$^+$ and Cl$^-$ (Michaelis-Menten constants of 7.6 ± 1.6 and 6.3 ± 1.1 mmol/L, respectively).[225] Equally high affinities had previously been obtained by Velazquez and colleagues in perfused rat DCT.[222] The measured Hill coefficients of rat NCC are approximately 1 for each ion, which is consistent with electroneutral cotransport.[225]

NCC expression is the defining characteristic of the DCT[210] (Figure 5-19). There is also evidence for expression of this transporter in osteoblasts, peripheral blood mononuclear cells, and intestinal epithelium[226]; however, kidney is the dominant expression site.[142] Loss-of-function mutations in the *SLC12A2* gene encoding human NCC cause Gitelman's syndrome, familial hypokalemic alkalosis with hypomagnesemia and hypocalciuria (see also Chapter 15). Mice with homozygous deletion of the *Slc12a2* gene encoding NCC exhibit marked morphologic defects in the early DCT,[227,228] with both a reduction in the absolute number of DCT cells and changes in ultrastructural appearance. Similarly, thiazide treatment promotes marked apoptosis of the DCT,[229] which suggests that thiazide-sensitive Na$^+$-Cl$^-$ cotransport plays an important role in modulating growth and regression of this nephron segment (see also the section "Regulation of Na$^+$-Cl$^-$ Transport" under "Distal Convoluted Tubule").

Coexpression of NCC and the amiloride-sensitive Na$^+$ channel ENaC occurs in the late DCT and CNT segments of many species, either in the same cells or in adjacent cells in the same tubule.[210] Notably, ENaC is the primary Na$^+$ transport pathway of CNT and CCD cells, rather than DCT cells. There is, however, evidence for other Na$^+$ and Cl$^-$ entry pathways in DCT cells. In particular, the Na$^+$/H$^+$ exchanger NHE2 is coexpressed with NCC at the apical membrane of rat DCT cells.[230]

As in the proximal tubule, perfusion of DCT with formate and oxalate stimulates DIDS-sensitive Na$^+$-Cl$^-$ transport that is distinct from the thiazide-sensitive transport mediated by NCC.[40] Therefore, a parallel arrangement of Na$^+$/H$^+$ exchange and Cl$^-$/anion exchangers may play an important role in electroneutral Na$^+$-Cl$^-$ absorption by the DCT (see Figure 5-19). Of note, the anion exchanger SLC26A6 is evidently expressed in the human distal nephron, including perhaps in DCT cells.[231] NHE2[230] and SLC26A6 are thus candidates mechanisms for this alternative pathway of DCT Na$^+$-Cl$^-$ absorption.

At the basolateral membrane, as in other nephron segments, Na$^+$ exits via Na$^+$-K$^+$-ATPase. Although one must bear in mind the considerable caveats in morphologic identification of the DCT,[210] this nephron segment appears to have the highest Na$^+$-K$^+$-ATPase activity of the entire nephron[14] (see Figure 5-4). Basolateral membranes of DCT cells in both rabbit[232] and mouse[178] express the K$^+$-Cl$^-$ cotransporter KCC4, a potential exit pathway for Cl$^-$. However, several lines of evidence indicate that Cl$^-$ primarily exits DCT cells via basolateral Cl$^-$ channels. First, the basolateral membrane of rabbit DCT contains Cl$^-$ channel activity, with functional characteristics that are similar to those of ClC-K2.[177,233] Second, ClC-K2 protein is expressed at the basolateral membrane of DCT and CNT cells[175]; mRNA for ClC-K1 can also be detected by RT-PCR of microdissected DCT segments.[132]

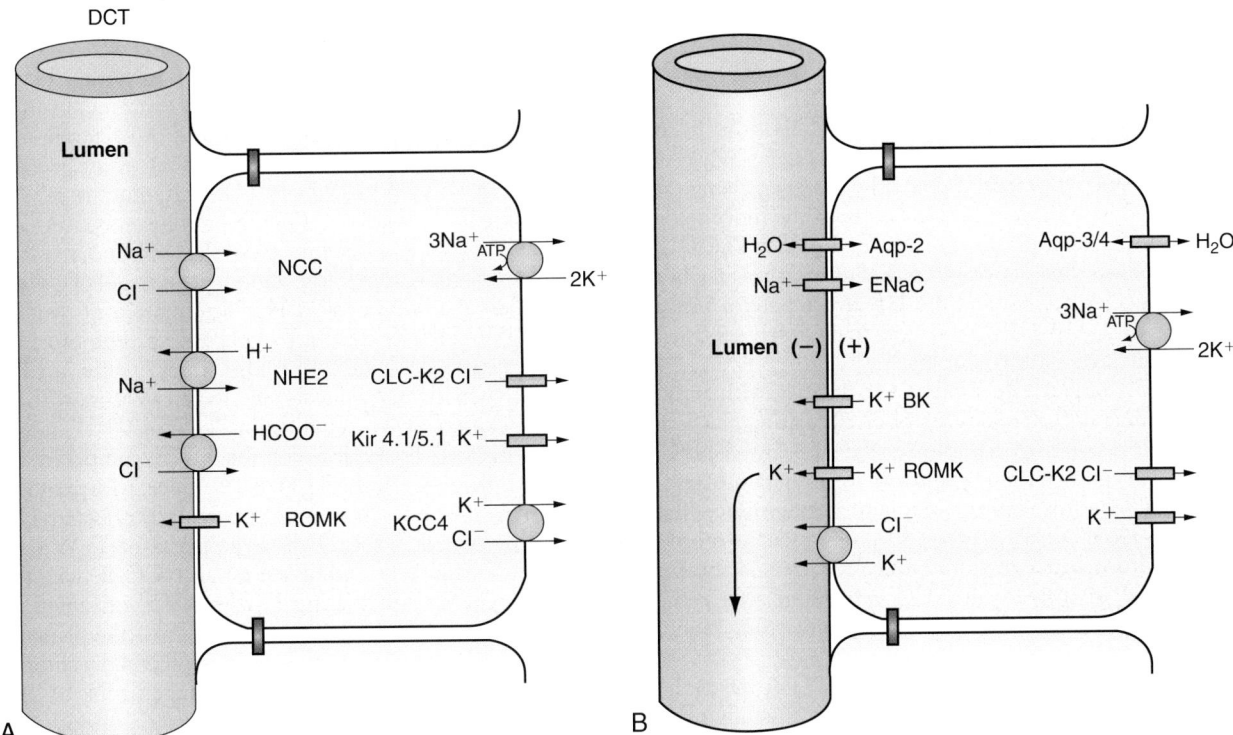

A

B

FIGURE 5-19 Transport pathways for Na$^+$-Cl$^-$ and K$^+$. **A,** Distal convoluted tubule (DCT) cells. *Kir 4.1/5.1,* basolateral inwardly rectifying K$^+$ channels 4.1 and 5.1; *KCC4,* K$^+$-Cl$^-$ cotransporter 4. **B,** Principal cells of the connecting tubule (CNT) and cortical collecting duct (CCD). *ENaC,* Epithelial Na$^+$ channel; *NCC,* thiazide-sensitive Na$^+$-Cl$^-$ cotransporter; *NHE2,* Na$^+$/H$^+$ exchanger 2; *ROMK,* renal outer medullary K$^+$ channel (Kir 1.1).

Third, loss-of-function mutations in CLC-NKB, the human ortholog of ClC-K2, typically cause Bartter's syndrome (dysfunction of the TAL)[134]; however, in some of these patients, mutations in CLC-NKB lead to more of a Gitelman's syndrome phenotype, consistent with loss-of-function of DCT segments.[234]

K$^+$ channels at the basolateral membrane of DCT cells play a critical role in the function of this nephron segment. Cell-attached patches in basolateral membranes of microdissected DCTs detect an inwardly rectifying K$^+$ channel with characteristics similar to those of heteromeric Kir 4.1/Kir 5.1 and Kir 4.2/Kir 5.1 channels.[235] Basolateral membranes of the DCT express immunoreactive Kir 4.1[236,237] and Kir 5.1[238] protein, and DCT cells express Kir 4.2 mRNA.[235]

Patients with loss-of-function mutations in the *KCNJ10* gene that encodes KIR4.1 develop a syndrome that includes epilepsy, ataxia, sensorineural deafness, and tubulopathy (EAST or SeSAME syndrome).[237,239] The associated tubulopathy includes hypokalemia, metabolic alkalosis, hypocalciuria, and hypomagnesemia.[237,239] Kir 4.1 knockout mice demonstrate a greater natriuresis than littermate controls, in addition to hypocalciuria.[237]

The Kir 4.1/Kir 5.1 and Kir 4.2/Kir 5.1 channels at the basolateral membrane of DCT cells are hypothesized to function in basolateral K$^+$ recycling, maintenance of adequate Na$^+$-K$^+$-ATPase activity for Na$^+$-Cl$^-$ absorption, and other aspects of DCT function. Notably, the calcium-sensing receptor coassociates with Kir 4.1 and Kir 4.2 proteins and inhibits their activity, which provides a mechanism for dynamic modulation of Na$^+$-Cl$^-$, calcium, and magnesium transport by the DCT.[236]

REGULATION OF NA$^+$-CL$^-$ TRANSPORT

Considerable hypertrophy of the DCT occurs in response to long-term increases in delivery of Na$^+$-Cl$^-$ to the DCT, typically induced by furosemide treatment with dietary Na$^+$-Cl$^-$ supplementation.[210,220] These morphologic changes are reportedly independent of changes in aldosterone or glucocorticoid levels, which suggests that increased Na$^+$-Cl$^-$ entry via NCC promotes hypertrophy of the DCT.[210] This is the inverse of the hypomorphic changes seen in NCC deficiency[227,228] and with thiazide treatment.[210] Notably, however, changes in aldosterone do have dramatic effects on both the morphology of the DCT[240] and expression of NCC.[210,241,242] The DCT is thus an aldosterone-sensitive epithelium, expressing both mineralocorticoid receptor and the 11β-hydroxysteroid dehydrogenase type 2 (11β-HSD2) enzyme that confers specificity for aldosterone over glucocorticoids.[210]

Mice with a targeted deletion of 11β-HSD2, with activation of the mineralocorticoid receptor by circulating glucocorticoid, exhibit massive hypertrophy of what appear to be DCT cells[240]; this suggests an important role for mineralocorticoid activity in shaping this nephron segment. Furthermore, NCC expression is dramatically increased by treatment of normal rats with fludrocortisone or aldosterone.[241] Adrenalectomized rats also show an increase in NCC expression after rescue with aldosterone, and treatment with spironolactone reduces expression of NCC in salt-restricted rats.[242]

Considerable insight into the role of NCC in the pathobiology of the DCT has recently emerged from study of the WNK1 and WNK4 kinases.[243] *WNK1* and *WNK4* were initially identified as causative genes for familial hyperkalemic hypertension (FHHt, also known as *pseudohypoaldosteronism type 2* and *Gordon's syndrome*). FHHt is in every respect the mirror image of Gitelman's syndrome, encompassing hypertension, hyperkalemia, hyperchloremic metabolic acidosis, suppressed plasma renin activity and aldosterone, and hypercalciuria.[244] Furthermore, FHHt behaves like a gain-of-function in NCC and/or the DCT, in that treatment with thiazides typically results in resolution of the entire syndrome.[244]

Intronic mutations in WNK1 have been detected in patients with FHHt, leading to increased abundance of WNK1 mRNA in patient leukocytes; WNK4-associated disease is due to clustered point mutations in an acidic-rich, conserved region of the protein.[245] The WNK1 and WNK4 proteins are coexpressed within the distal nephron, in both DCT and CCD cells. Whereas WNK1 localizes to the cytoplasm and basolateral membrane, WNK4 protein is found at the apical tight junctions.[245]

Consistent with the physiologic gain-of-function in NCC associated with FHHt,[244] WNK4 coexpression with NCC in *Xenopus* oocytes inhibits transport, and both kinase-dead and disease-associated mutations abolish the effect.[246,247] WNK1 has no effect on NCC, but abrogates the inhibitory effect of WNK4.[248] WNK4 coexpression with NCC reduces transporter expression at the membrane of both *Xenopus* oocytes and mammalian cells, which suggests a prominent effect on membrane trafficking.[249-251]

The WNK4 kinase activates lysosomal degradation of the transporter protein, rather than inducing dynamin- and clathrin-dependent endocytosis.[252,253] This occurs through effects of WNK4 on the interaction of NCC with both the lysosomal targeting receptor sortilin[253] and the AP-3 adaptor complex.[252] Dynamin-dependent endocytosis of NCC is induced by phosphorylation of ERK1/2 (extracellular signal–regulated kinases 1 and 2) via activation of H-Ras, Raf, and MEK1/2 (mitogen-activated protein kinase kinase 1 and 2), which results in ubiquitination of NCC and endocytosis of the transporter.[254,255]

To develop in vivo models relevant to both FHHt and the physiologic role of WNK4 in the distal nephron, Lalioti and colleagues generated two strains of bacterial artificial chromosome (BAC) transgenic mice that overexpress wild-type WNK4 (TgWnk4^{WT}) or a FHHt mutant of WNK4 (TgWnk4^{PHAII}, bearing a Q562E mutation associated with the disease).[243] Consistent with the inhibitory effect of WNK4 on NCC,[246,247] the blood pressure of TgWnk4^{WT} mice is less than that of wild-type littermate controls; in contrast, TgWnk4^{PHAII} mice are hypertensive. The biochemical phenotype of TgWnk4^{PHAII} is also similar to that of FHHt, that is, hyperkalemia, acidosis, and hypercalciuria, with a suppressed expression of renal renin. TgWnk4^{PHAII} mice also exhibit marked hyperplasia of the DCT, compared with a relative hypoplasia in the TgWnk4^{WT} mice. Morphology and phenotype of the CCD was not particularly affected. Of particular significance, the DCT hyperplasia of TgWnk4^{PHAII} mice was completely suppressed on an NCC-deficient background, generated by mating TgWnk4^{PHAII} mice with NCC knockout mice.[227,228] Therefore, the DCT is the primary target for FHHt-associated mutations in WNK4. In addition, as suggested by prior studies,[210,227,228] changes in Na$^+$-Cl$^-$ entry via NCC can evidently modulate hyperplasia or regression of the DCT.[243]

The results obtained with transgenic mice[243] provide a dramatic validation of the selective use of *Xenopus* oocytes for the analysis of regulatory interactions with ion transport proteins such as NCC.[246-248] Under certain conditions, a *stimulatory* effect of the WNK kinases appears to dominate. The WNK kinases seem to exert their effect on NCC and other cation-chloride cotransporters via the phosphorylation and activation of the SPAK and OSR1 serine/threonine kinases, which in turn phosphorylate the transporter proteins.[190,256,257] Specifically, in NCC, WNK-dependent phosphorylation and activation of SPAK or OSR1 lead to phosphorylation of a cluster of N-terminal threonines, which results in the activation of Na+-Cl- cotransport.[195,258]

The various mechanistic models for the regulation of NCC by upstream WNK1, WNK4, and the SPAK/OSR1 kinases have recently been reviewed.[249] Interactions between WNK4 and both WNK3[259] and SGK1[260] also contribute to the complexity. Competing divergent mechanisms can be reconciled by the likelihood that the physiologic context determines whether WNK4 will have an activating or inhibitory effect on NCC. For example, the *activation* of NCC by the AT$_1$ angiotensin II receptor appears to require the downstream activation of SPAK by WNK4.[251,261] Changes in circulating and local levels of angiotensin II,[251,261] aldosterone,[262] vasopressin,[263,264] and K$^+$[265] are thus expected to have different and often opposing effects on the activity of NCC in the DCT[249-251] (see also the section "Integrated Na+-Cl- and K+ transport in the Distal Nephron" and Figure 5-26).

Connecting Tubules and Cortical Collecting Duct

Apical Na+ Transport

The apical membrane of CNT cells and principal cells contain prominent Na+ and K+ conductances,[213,266,267] without a measurable apical conductance for Cl-.[177] The entry of Na+ occurs via the highly selective ENaC, which is sensitive to micromolar concentrations of amiloride[268] (see Figure 5-19). This selective absorption of positive charge generates a lumen-negative PD, the magnitude of which varies considerably as a function of mineralocorticoid status and other factors (see also the section "Regulation of Na+-Cl- Transport in the Connecting Tubule and Cortical Collecting Duct"). This lumen-negative PD serves to drive the following critical processes: (1) K+ secretion via apical K+ channels, (2) paracellular Cl- transport through the adjacent tight junctions, and/or (3) electrogenic H+ secretion via adjacent type A intercalated cells.[269]

ENaC is a heteromeric channel complex formed by the assembly of separate homologous subunits, denoted α-, β-, and γ-ENaC.[11] These channel subunits share a common structure, with intracellular N- and C-terminal domains, two transmembrane segments, and a large glycosylated extracellular loop.[11] *Xenopus* oocytes expressing α-ENaC alone have detectable Na+ channel activity (Figure 5-20), which facilitated the initial identification of this subunit by expression cloning; functional complementation of this modest activity was then used to clone the other two subunits by expression cloning.[11] Full channel activity requires the coexpression of all three subunits, which causes a dramatic increase in expression of the channel complex at the plasma membrane[270] (see Figure 5-20). The subunit stoichiometry has been a source of considerable controversy, with some reports favoring a tetramer with ratios of two α-ENaC proteins to one each of β- and γ-ENaC (2α:1β:1γ), and others favoring a higher-order assembly with a stoichiometry of 3α:3β:3γ.[271]

Regardless, the single-channel characteristics of heterologously expressed ENaC are essentially identical to those of the amiloride-sensitive channel detectable at the apical membrane of CCD cells.[11] ENaC plays a critical role in renal Na+-Cl- reabsorption and maintenance of the extracellular fluid volume (see also the section "Regulation of Na+-Cl- Transport in the Connecting Tubule and Cortical Collecting Duct"). In particular, recessive loss-of-function mutations in the three

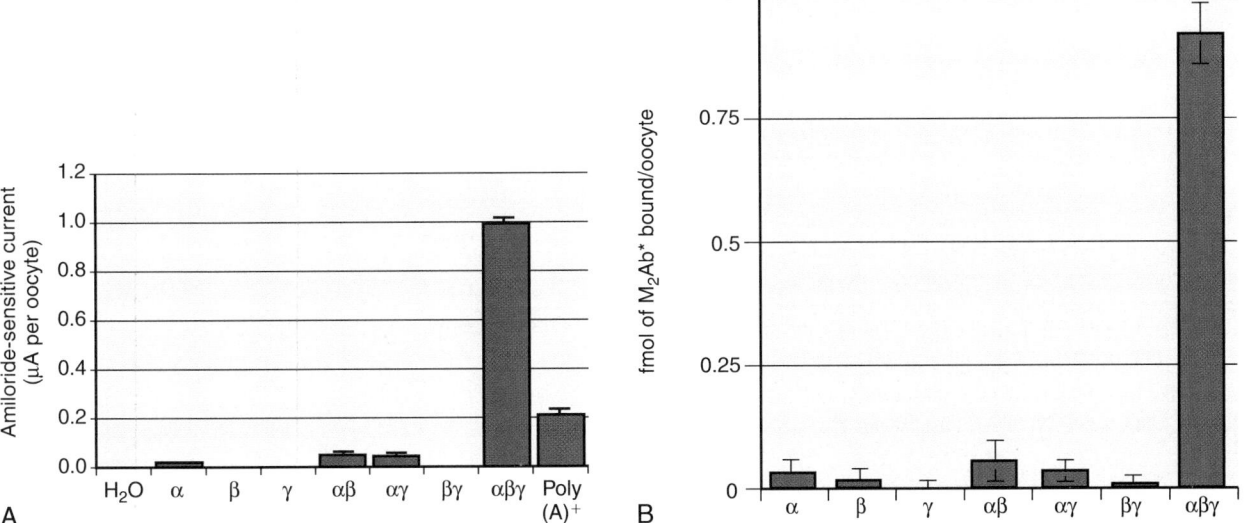

FIGURE 5-20 Maximal expression of the amiloride-sensitive epithelial Na+ channel (ENaC) at the plasma membrane requires the coexpression of all three subunits (α-, β-, and γ-ENaC). **A,** Amiloride-sensitive current in *Xenopus* oocytes expressing the individual subunits and various combinations thereof. **B,** Marked enhancement of surface expression in *Xenopus* oocytes that coexpress all three subunits. The individual complementary DNAs (cDNAs) were engineered with an external epitope tag; expression of the channel proteins at the cell surface was measured by binding of a monoclonal antibody (M$_2$Ab*) to the tag. (**A** from Canessa CM, Schild L, Buell G, et al: Amiloride-sensitive epithelial Na+ channel is made of three homologous subunits, *Nature* 367:463-467, 1994; **B** from Firsov D, Schild L, Gautschi I, et al: Cell surface expression of the epithelial Na channel and a mutant causing Liddle syndrome: a quantitative approach, *Proc Natl Acad Sci U S A* 93:15370-15375, 1996.)

subunits of ENaC are a cause of pseudohypoaldosteronism type 1.[11] Patients with this syndrome typically present with severe neonatal salt wasting, hypotension, acidosis, and hyperkalemia. This dramatic phenotype underscores the critical roles of ENaC activity in renal Na^+-Cl^- reabsorption, K^+ secretion, and H^+ secretion. Gain-of-function mutations in the β- and γ-ENaC subunits are, in turn, a cause of Liddle's syndrome, an autosomal dominant hypertensive syndrome accompanied by suppressed aldosterone and variable hypokalemia.[272] With one exception,[273] ENaC mutations associated with Liddle's syndrome disrupt interactions between a PPxY motif in the C terminus of channel subunits and the Nedd4-2 (neural developmentally downregulated isoform 4-2) ubiquitin ligase (see also the section "Regulation of Na^+-Cl^- Transport in the Connecting Tubule and Cortical Collecting Duct").

The ENaC protein is detectable at the apical membrane of CNT cells and principal cells in the CCD, OMCD, and IMCD.[215,219] Notably, however, several lines of evidence support the hypothesis that the CNT makes the dominant contribution to amiloride-sensitive Na^+ reabsorption by the distal nephron. First, amiloride-sensitive Na^+ currents in the CNT are twofold to fourfold higher than in the CCD. The maximal capacity of the CNT for Na^+ reabsorption is estimated to be approximately 10 times higher than that of the CCD.[213] Second, targeted deletion of α-ENaC in the collecting duct abolishes amiloride-sensitive currents in CCD principal cells, but does not affect Na^+ or K^+ homeostasis. The residual ENaC expression in the late DCT and CNT of these knockout mice easily compensates for the loss of the channel in CCD cells.[274] Third, Na^+-K^+-ATPase activity in the CCD is considerably less than that in the DCT[14] (see also Figure 5-4). This speaks to a greater capacity for transepithelial Na^+-Cl^- absorption by the DCT and CNT. Fourth, the apical recruitment of ENaC subunits in response to dietary Na^+ restriction begins in the CNT, with progressive recruitment of subunits in the downstream CCD at lower levels of dietary Na^+.[275] Under conditions of high Na^+-Cl^- and low K^+ intake, the bulk of aldosterone-stimulated Na^+ transport likely occurs prior to the entry of tubular fluid into the CCD.[276]

Cl^- Transport

There are two major pathways for Cl^- absorption in the CNT and CCD: paracellular transport across the tight junction, and transcellular transport across type B intercalated cells (Figure 5-21).[214,277] The CNT and CCD are tight epithelia, with comparatively low paracellular permeability that is not selective for Cl^- over Na^+; however, voltage-driven paracellular Cl^- transport in the CCD may play a considerable role in transepithelial Na^+-Cl^- absorption.[278] The CNT, DCT, and collecting duct coexpress claudins 3, 4, and 8.[11,279] Claudin-8 in particular may function as a paracellular cation barrier that prevents backleak of Na^+, K^+, and H^+ in this segment of the nephron.[279]

Regulated changes in paracellular permeability may also contribute to Cl^- absorption by the CNT and CCD. In particular, wild-type WNK4 appears to increase paracellular Cl^- permeability in transfected Madin-Darby canine kidney II (MDCK II) cell lines. A WNK4 FHHt mutant has a much larger effect, with no effect seen in cells expressing kinase-dead WNK4 constructs.[280] Yamauchi and colleagues have also reported that FHHt-associated WNK4 increases paracellular

permeability, due perhaps to an associated hyperphosphorylation of claudin proteins.[281]

Transcellular Cl^- absorption across intercalated cells is thought to play a quantitatively greater role in the CNT and CCD than that of paracellular transport.[277] In the simplest scheme, this process requires the concerted function of both type A and type B intercalated cells, achieving net electrogenic Cl^- absorption without affecting HCO_3^- or H^+ excretion[277] (see also Figure 5-21). Chloride thus enters type B intercalated cells via apical Cl^-/HCO_3^- exchange, followed by exit from the cell via basolateral Cl^- channels. Recycling of Cl^- at the basolateral membrane of adjacent type A intercalated cells results in HCO_3^- absorption and extrusion of H^+ at the apical membrane. The net effect of apical Cl^-/HCO_3^- exchange in type B intercalated cells, which leads to apical secretion of HCO_3^-, and recycling of Cl^- at the basolateral membrane of type A intercalated cells, which leads to apical secretion of H^+, is electrogenic Cl^- absorption across type B intercalated cells (see Figure 5-21).

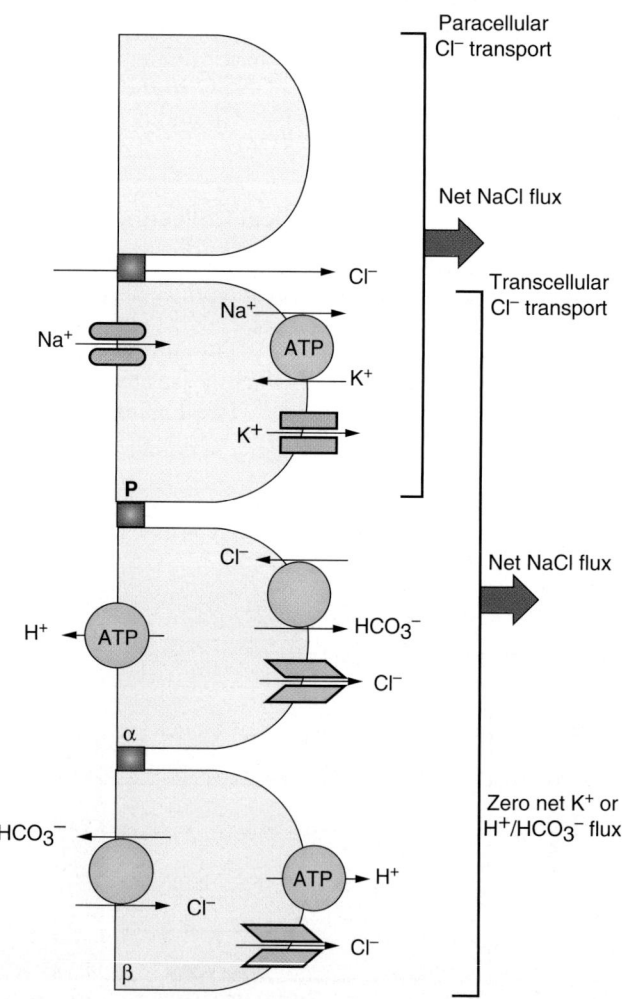

FIGURE 5-21 Transepithelial Cl^- transport by principal and intercalated cells. The lumen-negative potential difference (PD) generated by principal cells drives paracellular Cl^- absorption. Alternatively, transepithelial transport occurs in type B intercalated cells via apical Cl^-/HCO_3^- exchange (SLC26A4/pendrin) and basolateral Cl^- exit via the chloride channel ClC-K2. (Modified from Moe OW, Baum M, Berry CA, e al: Renal transport of glucose, amino acids, sodium, chloride, and water, in Brenner BM [editor]: *Brenner and Rector's the kidney*, ed 7, Philadelphia, 2004, Saunders, pp 413-452.)

At the basolateral membrane, intercalated cells have a very robust Cl^- conductance with transport characteristics similar to those of ClC-K2/barttin.[177] ClC-K2 protein has also been detected at the basolateral membrane of type A intercalated cells, although expression in type B cells was not clarified.[175]

At the apical membrane, the SLC26A4 exchanger (also known as *pendrin*), has been conclusively identified as the elusive Cl^-/HCO_3^- exchanger of type B and non-A, non-B intercalated cells.[214] This exchanger functions as the apical entry site during transepithelial Cl^- transport by the distal nephron. Human SLC26A4 is mutated in Pendred's syndrome, which encompasses sensorineural hearing loss and goiter; these patients do not have an appreciable renal phenotype.[214] However, Slc26a4-deficient knockout mice are sensitive to restriction of dietary Na^+-Cl^-, developing hypotension during severe restriction.[282] Slc26a4 knockout mice are also resistant to mineralocorticoid-induced hypertension.[283] Finally, dietary Cl^- restriction with provision of Na^+-HCO_3^- results in Cl^- wasting in Slc26a4 knockout mice and increased apical expression of Slc26a4 protein in the type B intercalated cells of normal littermate controls.[284]

Several groups have reported that Slc26a4 expression is exquisitely responsive to changes in distal chloride delivery.[285] Therefore, Slc26a4 plays a critical role in distal nephron Cl^- absorption, which underlined the particular importance of transcellular Cl^- transport in this process. Of broader relevance, these studies have served to emphasize the important role of Cl^- homeostasis in the maintenance of extracellular volume and the pathogenesis of hypertension.[285]

ELECTRONEUTRAL Na^+-Cl^- COTRANSPORT

Thiazide-sensitive Na^+-Cl^- cotransport is considered the exclusive provenance of the DCT, which expresses the canonical thiazide-sensitive transporter NCC (see the section "Mechanisms of Na^+-Cl^- Transport" under "Distal Convoluted Tubule"). However, Knepper and colleagues demonstrated many years ago that approximately 50% of Na^+-Cl^- transport in rat CCD is electroneutral, amiloride resistant, and thiazide sensitive.[286,287] Thiazide-sensitive electroneutral Na^+-Cl^- transport has also been demonstrated in mouse CCD.[288] This transport activity is preserved in CCDs from mice with genetic disruption of NCC and ENaC, which indicates independence from the dominant apical Na^+ transport pathways in the distal nephron.

This thiazide-sensitive electroneutral Na^+-Cl^- transport appears to be mediated by the parallel activity of the Na^+-driven SLC4A8 Cl^-/HCO_3^- exchanger and the SLC26A4 Cl^-/HCO_3^- exchanger (pendrin, see earlier).[288] In particular, amiloride-resistant Na^+-Cl^- absorption is abolished in CCDs from Slc4a8-null knockout mice. Notably, however, heterologously expressed recombinant Slc4a8 and Slc26a4 are resistant to and partially sensitive to thiazide, respectively, so the in vivo pharmacology of this electroneutral Na^+-Cl^- absorption is not completely explained. Furthermore, localization of Slc4a8 within the CCD has not yet been reported; hence, it is unknown whether Slc4a8 and Slc26a4 are coexpressed in type B intercalated cells. Regardless, the combined activity of Slc4a8 and Slc26a4 appears to play a major role in Na^+-Cl^- transport within the CCD, with significant implications for both Na^+-Cl^- and K^+ homeostasis (see also the section "Integrated Na^+-Cl^- and K^+ Transport in the Distal Nephron").

REGULATION OF Na^+-Cl^- TRANSPORT IN THE CONNECTING TUBULE AND CORTICAL COLLECTING DUCT

Aldosterone. The DCT, CNT, and collecting ducts collectively constitute the aldosterone-sensitive distal nephron, expressing both the mineralocorticoid receptor and the 11β-HSD2 enzyme that protects against unwanted activation by glucocorticoids.[210] Aldosterone plays a dominant positive role in the regulation of distal nephron Na^+-Cl^- transport, with a plethora of mechanisms and transcriptional targets[289] (see also Chapter 6). For example, aldosterone increases expression of the Na^+-K^+-ATPase α_1- and β_1-subunits in the CCD,[290] in addition to inducing Slc26a4, the apical Cl^-/HCO_3^- exchanger in intercalated cells.[283] Aldosterone may also affect paracellular permeability of the distal nephron via posttranscriptional modification of claudins and other components of the tight junction.[291] Particularly impressive progress has been made, however, in the understanding of the downstream effects of aldosterone on synthesis, trafficking, and membrane-associated activity of ENaC subunits.

Aldosterone increases the abundance of α-ENaC via a glucocorticoid response element in the promoter of the *SCNN1A* gene that encodes this subunit.[292] Aldosterone also relieves a tonic inhibition of the *SCNN1A* gene by a complex that includes the Dot1a (disruptor of telomere silencing splicing variant *a*) and the AF9 and AF17 transcription factors.[293] This transcriptional activation results in an increased abundance of α-ENaC protein in response to either exogenous aldosterone or dietary Na^+-Cl^- restriction[294,295] (Figure 5-22). The response to Na^+-Cl^- restriction is blunted by spironolactone, which indicates involvement of the mineralocorticoid receptor.[242]

At baseline, α-ENaC transcripts in the kidney are less abundant than those encoding β- and γ-ENaC[296] (see Figure 5-22). All three subunits are required for efficient processing of heteromeric channels in the endoplasmic reticulum and trafficking to the plasma membrane (see Figure 5-20), so that the induction of α-ENaC is thought to relieve a major "bottleneck" in the processing and trafficking of active ENaC complexes.[296]

Aldosterone also plays an indirect role in the regulated trafficking of ENaC subunits to the plasma membrane via the regulation of accessory proteins that interact with preexisting ENaC subunits (see also Chapter 6). Aldosterone rapidly induces expression of a serine-threonine kinase denoted *SGK1* (serum- and glucocorticoid-regulated kinase 1)[297,298]; coexpression of SGK1 with ENaC subunits in *Xenopus* oocytes results in a dramatic activation of the channel, due to increased expression at the plasma membrane.[295] Notably, an analogous redistribution of ENaC subunits occurs in the CNT and early CCD, from a largely cytoplasmic location during dietary Na^+-Cl^- excess to a purely apical distribution after aldosterone or Na^+-Cl^- restriction (see Figure 5-22).[242,275,295] Furthermore, there is a temporal correlation between the appearance of induced SGK1 protein in the CNT and the redistribution of ENaC protein to the plasma membrane.[295]

SGK1 modulates membrane expression of ENaC by interfering with regulated endocytosis of its channel subunits (see also Chapter 6). Specifically, the kinase interferes with interactions between ENaC subunits and the ubiquitin ligase Nedd4-2.[296] PPxY domains in the C termini of all three ENaC subunits bind to WW domains of Nedd4-2.[299] These

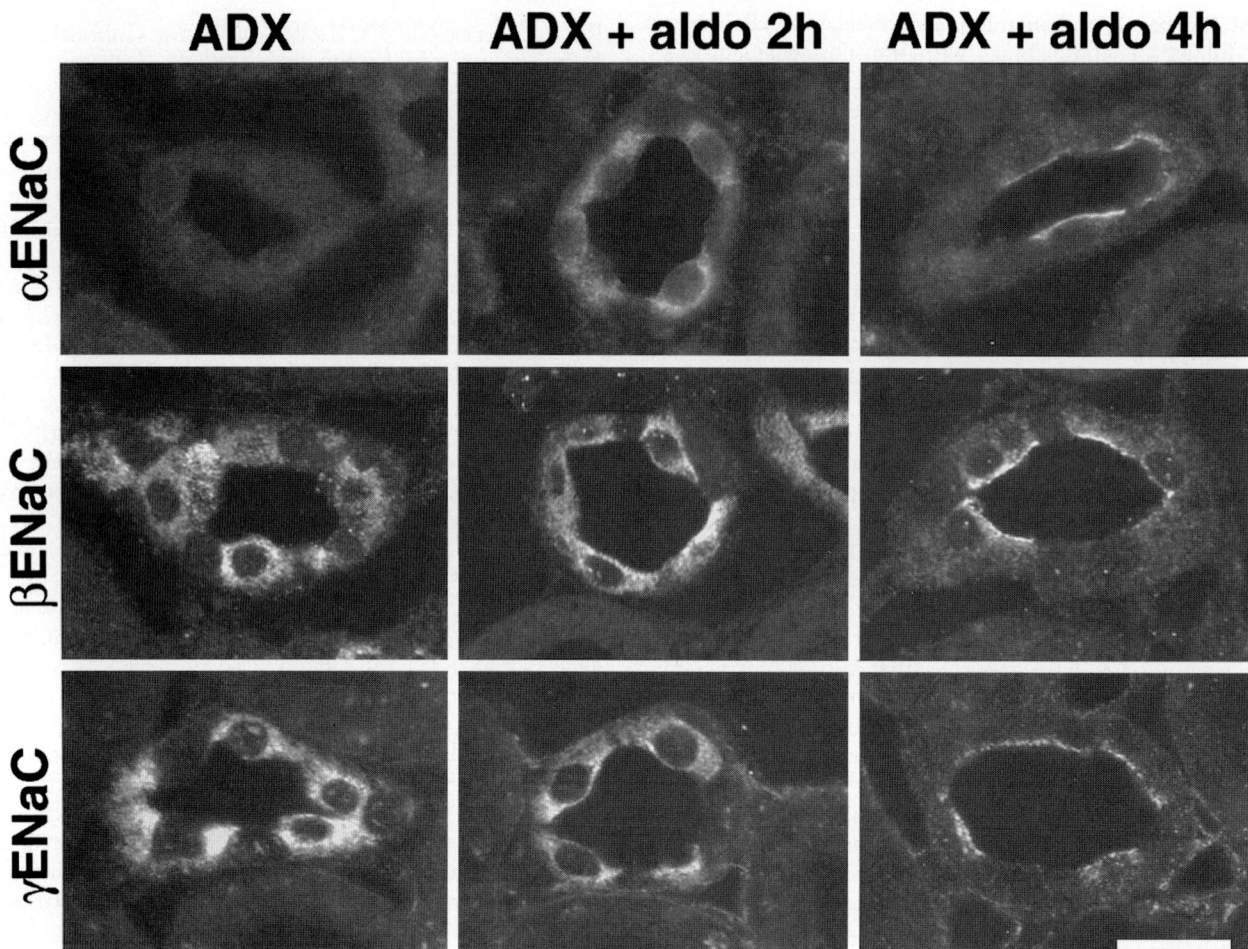

FIGURE 5-22 Immunofluorescence images of connecting tubule (CNT) profiles in kidneys from adrenalectomized (ADX) rats and from ADX rats 2 and 4 hours after aldosterone injection. Antibodies against the α-, β-, and γ-subunits of the epithelial Na⁺ channel (ENaC) reveal absent expression of the α-subunit in ADX rats, with progressive induction by aldosterone. All three subunits traffic to the apical membrane in response to aldosterone. This coincides with rapid aldosterone induction of serum- and glucocorticoid-regulated kinase (SGK) in the same cells. SGK is known to increase the expression of ENaC at the plasma membrane (see text for details). Bar equals 15 μm. (From Loffing J, Zecevic M, Féraille E, et al: Aldosterone induces rapid apical translocation of ENaC in early portion of renal collecting system: possible role of SGK, *Am J Physiol Renal Physiol* 280:F675-F682, 2001.)

PPxY domains are deleted, truncated, or mutated in patients with Liddle's syndrome,[272] which leads to a gain of function in channel activity.[270] Coexpression of Nedd4-2 with wild-type ENaC channel results in a marked inhibition of channel activity due to retrieval from the cell membrane, whereas channels bearing Liddle's syndrome mutations are resistant. Nedd4-2 is thought to ubiquitinate ENaC subunits, which result in the removal of channel subunits from the cell membrane and degradation in lysosomes and the proteosome.[296]

A PPxY domain in SGK1 also binds to Nedd4-2, which is a phosphorylation substrate for the kinase. Phosphorylation of Nedd4-2 by SGK1 abrogates its inhibitory effect on ENaC subunits.[300,301] Aldosterone also stimulates Nedd4-2 phosphorylation in vivo.[302] Nedd4-2 phosphorylation in turn results in ubiquitin-mediated degradation of SGK1,[303] which suggests that there is considerable feedback regulation in this system. Furthermore, the hormone reduces Nedd4-2 protein expression in cultured CCD cells,[304] a finding that indicates additional levels of in vivo regulation.

The induction of SGK1 by aldosterone thus appears to stimulate the redistribution of ENaC subunits from the cytoplasm to the apical membrane of CNT and CCD cells. This

phenomenon involves SGK1-dependent phosphorylation of the Nedd4-2 ubiquitin ligase, which is coexpressed with ENaC and SGK1 in the distal nephron.[304] Of note, there is considerable axial heterogeneity in the recruitment and redistribution of ENaC to the plasma membrane, which begins in the CNT and only extends into the CCD and OMCD in Na⁺-Cl⁻ restricted or aldosterone-treated animals.[210,295] The underlying causes of this progressive axial recruitment are not yet clear.[210] However, Nedd4-2 expression is inversely related to the apical distribution of ENaC, with low expression in the CNT and increased expression levels in the CCD.[304] In all likelihood, the relative balance between SGK1, ENaC, and Nedd4-2 figures prominently in the recruitment of the channel subunits to the apical membrane.

Finally, aldosterone indirectly activates ENaC channels through the induction of channel-activating proteases, which increase open channel probability by cleavage of the extracellular domain of α- and γ-ENaC. Western blotting of renal tissue from rats subjected to Na⁺-Cl⁻ restriction or treatment with aldosterone reveals α- and γ-ENaC subunits of lower molecular mass than those detected in control animals, which indicates that aldosterone induces proteolytic cleavage.[294,305]

Proteases that have been implicated in the processing of ENaC include furin, elastase, and three novel membrane-associated proteases denoted *channel-activating proteases 1, 2, and 3* (CAP1, CAP2, and CAP3).[306-308] Filtered proteases such as plasmin may also contribute to ENaC activation in nephrotic syndrome.[308]

CAP1 was initially identified from *Xenopus* A6 cells as an ENaC-activating protease.[309] The mammalian ortholog is an aldosterone-induced protein in principal cells.[310] Urinary excretion of CAP1, also known as *prostasin*, is increased in hyperaldosteronism, with a reduction after adrenalectomy.[310] CAP1 is tethered to the plasma membrane by a glycosylphosphatidylinositol (GPI) linkage,[309] whereas CAP2 and CAP3 are transmembrane proteases.[307] All three of these proteases activate ENaC by increasing the open probability of the channel without increasing expression at the cell surface.[307]

Proteolytic cleavage of ENaC appears to activate the channel by removing the self-inhibitory effect of external Na^+.[306] In the case of furin-mediated proteolysis of α-ENaC, this appears to involve the removal of an inhibitory domain from within the extracellular loop.[311] The structures of the extracellular domains of ENaC and related channels resemble an outstretched hand holding a ball, with defined subdomains termed the *wrist, finger, thumb, palm, β-ball,* and *knuckle.* Functionally relevant proteolytic events target the finger domains of ENaC subunits.[308] Unprocessed channels at the plasma membrane are thought to function as a reserve pool, capable of rapid activation by membrane-associated luminal proteases.[306]

Vasopressin and Other Factors. Although not classically considered an antinatriuretic hormone, vasopressin has well-characterized stimulatory effects on Na^+-Cl^- transport by the CCD.[76,312] Vasopressin directly activates ENaC in murine CCD, increasing the open probability of the channel.[313] In perfused rat CCD segments, vasopressin and aldosterone can have synergistic effects on Na^+ transport, with a combined effect that exceeds that of the individual hormones.[312] In addition, water and Na^+ restriction synergistically increase the open probability of ENaC in murine CCDs.[313]

Prostaglandins inhibit this effect of vasopressin, particularly in the rabbit CCD; this inhibition occurs at least in part through reductions in vasopressin-generated cAMP.[76,312] There are, however, considerable species-dependent differences in the interactions between vasopressin and negative modulators of Na^+-Cl^- transport in the CCD, which include prostaglandins, bradykinin, endothelin, and α_2-adrenergic tone.[76,312] Regardless, cAMP causes a rapid increase in the Na^+ conductance of apical membranes in the CCD. This appears to be due to increases in surface expression of ENaC subunits at the plasma membrane,[314] in addition to effects on open channel probability.[313,315] Notably, cAMP inhibits retrieval of ENaC subunits from the plasma membrane, via PKA-dependent phosphorylation of the phosphoacceptor sites in Nedd4-2 that are targeted by SGK1.[316] Therefore, both aldosterone and vasopressin converge on Nedd4-2 in the regulation of ENaC activity in the distal nephron. Analogous to the effect on trafficking of aquaporin-2 in principal cells, cAMP also seems to stimulate exocytosis of ENaC subunits to the plasma membrane.[315] Finally, similar to the long-term effects of vasopressin on aquaporin-2 expression and NKCC2 expression,[188] long-term treatment with DDAVP results in an increase in abundance of the α- and γ-ENaC subunits.[317]

Systemic generation of circulating angiotensin II induces aldosterone release by the adrenal gland, with downstream activation of ENaC. However, angiotensin II also directly activates amiloride-sensitive Na^+ transport in perfused CCDs. Blockade by losartan or candesartan suggests that this activation is mediated by AT_1 receptors.[318] Of particular significance, the effect of luminal angiotensin II (10^{-9} mol/L) was greater than that of angiotensin II in the bath, which suggests that intratubular angiotensin II may regulate ENaC in the distal nephron. Angiotensin II also activates chloride absorption across intercalated cells, via a pendrin (SLC26A4)- and H^+-ATPase–dependent mechanism.[319]

Stimulation of ENaC is seen when tubules are perfused with angiotensin I. This effect is blocked by angiotensin converting enzyme inhibition with captopril, which suggests that intraluminal conversion of angiotensin I to angiotensin II can occur in the CCD.[320] Notably, CNT cells express considerable amounts of immunoreactive renin, versus the vanishingly low expression of renin mRNA in the proximal tubule.[321] Angiotensinogen secreted into the tubule by proximal tubule cells[321] may thus be converted to angiotensin II in the CNT via locally generated renin and angiotensin converting enzyme, and/or related proteases.

Luminal perfusion with adenosine trisphosphate (ATP) or uridine triphosphate (UTP) inhibits amiloride-sensitive Na^+ transport and reduces ENaC open probability in the CCD, via activation of luminal $P2Y_2$ purinergic receptors.[322,323] Targeted deletion of the murine $P2Y_2$ receptor results in salt-resistant hypertension, due in part to an upregulation of NKCC2 activity in the TAL. Resting ENaC activity is also increased,[323] but suppression of aldosterone and downregulation of the α-subunit of ENaC blunts the role of amiloride-sensitive transport.[324]

Clamping mineralocorticoid activity at higher levels via the administration of exogenous mineralocorticoid reveals that $P2Y_2$ receptor activation may be a major mechanism for modulation of ENaC open probability in response to changes in dietary Na^+-Cl^-.[325] Increased dietary Na^+-Cl^- thus leads to increased urinary ATP and UTP excretion in mice,[323] endogenous ATP from principal cells inhibits ENaC,[323] and ENaC activity is not responsive to increased dietary Na^+-Cl^- in $P2Y_2$ receptor knockout mice.[325] In addition, the activation of apical ionotropic purinergic receptors, likely $P2X_4$ and/or $P2X_4$/$P2X_6$, can inhibit or activate ENaC, depending on luminal Na^+ concentration. These receptors may also participate in fine tuning of ENaC activity in response to dietary Na^+-Cl^-.[326]

As in other segments of the nephron, Na^+-Cl^- transport by the CNT and CCD is modulated by metabolites of arachidonic acid generated by cytochrome P450 monooxygenases. In particular, arachidonic acid inhibits ENaC channel activity in the rat CCD via generation of the epoxygenase product 11,12-EET by the CYP2C23 enzyme expressed in principal cells.[327] Targeted deletion of the murine Cyp4a10 enzyme, another P450 monooxygenase, results in salt-sensitive hypertension. Urinary excretion of 11,12-EET is reduced in these knockout mice, with a blunted effect of arachidonic acid on ENaC channel activity in the CCD.[328] These mice also became normotensive after treatment with amiloride, which is indicative of in vivo activation of ENaC. It appears that deletion of Cyp4a10 reduces activity of the murine ortholog of rat CYP2C23 (Cyp2c44 in mouse), and/or related epoxygenases, via reduced generation of a ligand for peroxisome proliferator–activated receptor α (PPARα) that induces epoxygenase activity.[328] The mechanism by which 11,12-EET inhibits ENaC is not yet known. However, renal 11,12-EET production is known to be salt sensitive, which suggests that generation of this mediator may serve to reduce ENaC activity during high dietary Na^+-Cl^- intake.[327] Finally, activation of PPARγ by thiazolidinediones (TZDs) results in amiloride-sensitive hypertension, which indicates in vivo activation of ENaC.[329,330]

The TZDs (rosiglitazone, pioglitazone, and troglitazone) are insulin-sensitizing drugs used for the treatment of type 2 diabetes. Treatment with these agents is frequently associated with fluid retention, which suggests an effect on renal Na^+-Cl^- transport. Given robust expression of PPARγ in the collecting duct, activation of ENaC was an attractive hypothesis for this TZD-associated edema syndrome.[329,330] This appears to be the case, because selective deletion of the murine PPARγ gene in principal cells abrogates the increase in amiloride-sensitive transport seen in response to TZDs.[329,330] TZDs appear to induce transcription of the *Sccn1g* gene encoding γ-ENaC,[329] in addition to inducing SGK1.[331] Targeted deletion of SGK1 in knockout mice attenuates but does not abolish TZD-associated edema.[332] Notably, however, other studies have failed to detect an effect of TZDs on ENaC activity,[333] which indicates that these drugs may instead activate a nonspecific cation channel within the IMCD.[334] Regardless, the beneficial effect of spironolactone in type 2 diabetic patients with TZD-associated volume expansion is consistent with in vivo activation of Na^+-Cl^- absorption in the aldosterone-responsive distal nephron.[335] In addition, the risk of peripheral edema is increased considerably in patients treated with both TZDs and insulin therapy. Notably, insulin appears to activate ENaC via SGK1-dependent mechanisms,[336,337] and PPARγ is required for the full activating effect of insulin on ENaC,[333] so that this clinical observation may reflect synergistic activation of ENaC by insulin and TZDs.

Potassium Transport

Maintenance of K^+ balance is important for a multitude of physiologic processes. Changes in intracellular K^+ impact cell volume regulation, regulation of intracellular pH, enzymatic function, protein synthesis, DNA synthesis, and apoptosis.[11] Changes in the ratio of intracellular to extracellular K^+ affect the resting membrane potential, leading to depolarization in hyperkalemia and hyperpolarization in hypokalemia. As a consequence, disorders of extracellular K^+ have a dominant effect on excitable tissues, chiefly heart and muscle. In addition, a growing body of evidence implicates hypokalemia and/or reduced dietary K^+ in the pathobiology of hypertension, heart failure, and stroke. These and other clinical consequences of K^+ disorders are reviewed in Chapter 17.

Potassium is predominantly an intracellular cation, with only 2% of total body K^+ residing in the extracellular fluid. Extracellular K^+ is maintained within a very narrow range by three primary mechanisms. First, the distribution of K^+ between the intracellular and extracellular space is determined by the activity of a number of transport pathways, namely Na^+-K^+-ATPase, the Na^+-K^+-$2Cl^-$ cotransporter NKCC1, the four K^+-Cl^- cotransporters, and a large number of K^+ channels. Skeletal muscle contains as much as 75% of body

potassium (see Figure 17-1), and exerts considerable influence on extracellular K^+. Short-term and long-term regulation of muscle Na^+-K^+-ATPase plays a dominant role in determining the distribution of K^+ between the intracellular and extracellular space. The various hormones and physiologic conditions that affect the uptake of K^+ by skeletal muscle are reviewed in Chapter 17 (see Table 17-1).

Second, the colon has the ability to absorb and secrete K^+, and considerable mechanistic[338] and regulatory[11] similarities are seen with renal K^+ secretion. K^+ secretion in the distal colon is increased after dietary loading[11] and in end-stage renal disease.[339] However, the colon has a relatively limited capacity for K^+ excretion, so that changes in renal K^+ excretion play the dominant role in responding to changes in K^+ intake. In particular, regulated K^+ secretion by the CNT and CCD play a critical role in the response to hyperkalemia and K^+ loading; increases in the reabsorption of K^+ by the CCD and OMCD function in the response to hypokalemia or K^+ deprivation.

This section reviews the mechanisms and regulation of transepithelial K^+ transport along the nephron. As in other sections of this chapter, the emphasis is on particularly recent developments in elucidating the molecular physiology of renal K^+ transport. Of note, transport pathways for K^+ play important roles in renal Na^+-Cl^- transport, particularly within the TAL. Furthermore, Na^+ absorption via ENaC in the aldosterone-sensitive distal nephron generates a lumen-negative PD that drives distal K^+ excretion. These pathways are discussed primarily in the section on renal Na^+-Cl^- transport; related issues relevant to K^+ homeostasis per se are specifically addressed in this section.

Proximal Tubule

The proximal tubule reabsorbs some 50% to 70% of filtered K^+ (Figure 5-23). Proximal tubules generate minimal transepithelial K^+ gradients, and fractional reabsorption of K^+ is similar to that of Na^+.[216] K^+ absorption follows that of fluid, Na^+, and other solutes,[340,341] so that this nephron segment does not play a direct role in regulated renal excretion. Notably, however, changes in Na^+-Cl^- reabsorption by the proximal tubule have considerable effects on distal tubular flow and distal tubular Na^+ delivery, with attendant effects on the excretory capacity for K^+ (see the section "K^+ Secretion by the Distal Convoluted Tubule, Collecting Tubule, and Cortical Collecting Duct").

The mechanisms involved in transepithelial K^+ transport by the proximal tubule are not completely clear, although active transport does not appear to play a major role.[341,342] Luminal barium has modest effects on transepithelial K^+ transport by the proximal tubule, which suggests a component of transcellular transport via barium-sensitive K^+ channels.[343] However, the bulk of K^+ transport is thought to occur via the paracellular pathway,[343,344] driven by the lumen-positive PD in the middle to late proximal tubule (see Figure 5-3). The total K^+ permeability of the proximal tubule is thus rather high, apparently due to characteristics of the paracellular pathway.[343,344] The combination of luminal K^+ concentrations that are approximately 10% higher than that of plasma, a lumen-positive PD of approximately 2 mV (see Figure 5-3), and high paracellular permeability leads to considerable paracellular absorption in

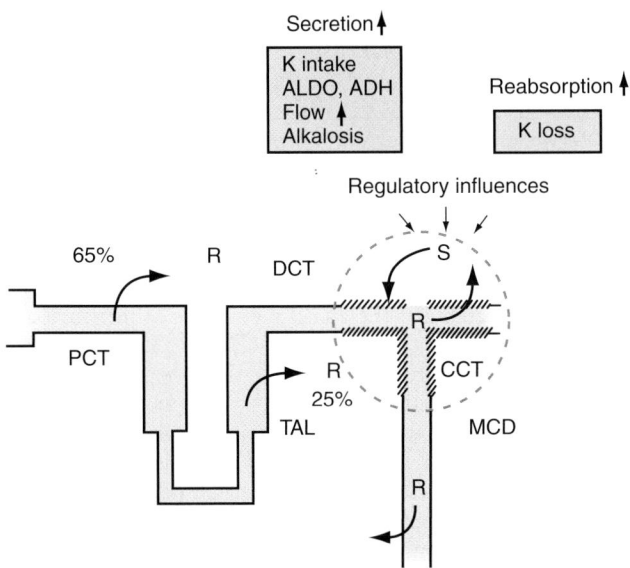

FIGURE 5-23 K+ transport along the nephron. Approximately 90% of filtered K+ is reabsorbed by the proximal tubule and the loop of Henle. K+ is secreted along the initial and cortical collecting tubule. Net reabsorption occurs in response to K+ depletion, primarily within the medullary collecting duct. ADH, Antidiuretic hormone; ALDO, aldosterone; CCT, cortical collecting tubule; DCT, distal convoluted tubule; ICT, initial connecting tubule; MCD, medullary collecting duct; PCT, proximal tubule; R, reabsorption; S, secretion; TAL, thick ascending limb.

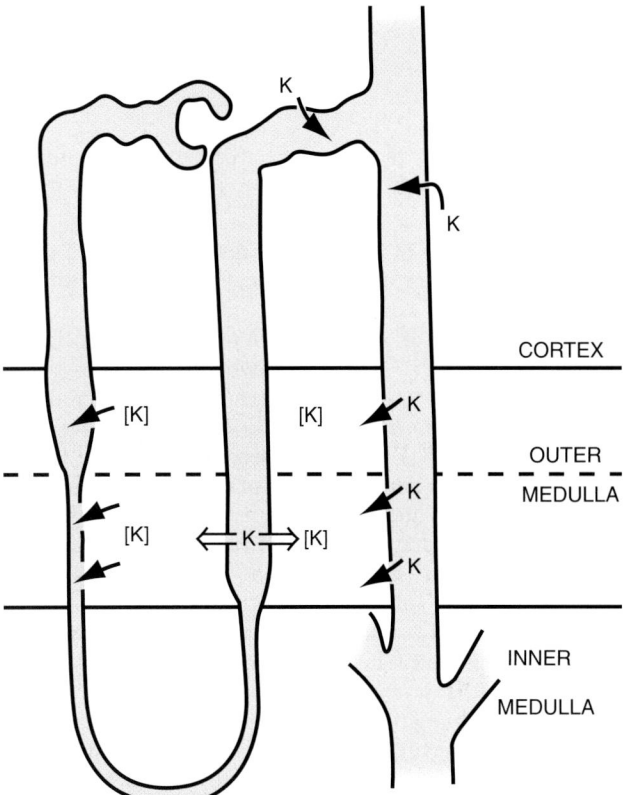

FIGURE 5-24 Schematic representation of medullary K+ recycling. Medullary interstitial K+ increases considerably after dietary K+ loading due to the combined effects of secretion in the cortical collecting duct (CCD); absorption in the outer medullary collecting duct (OMCD), thick ascending limb (TAL), and inner medullary collecting duct (IMCD); and secretion in the thin descending limb (see text for details). (From Stokes JB: Consequences of potassium recycling in the renal medulla. Effects of ion transport by the medullary thick ascending limb of Henle's loop, *J Clin Invest* 70:219-229, 1982.)

the proximal tubule. This absorption is thought to primarily proceed via convective transport—"solvent drag" due to frictional interactions between water and K+—rather than diffusional transport.[345] Notably, however, the primary pathway for water movement in the proximal tubule is quite conclusively transcellular, via aquaporin-1 and aquaporin-7 water channels in the apical and basolateral membrane.[16,25,26] Therefore, the apparent convective transport of K+ would have to constitute "pseudo–solvent drag," with hypothetical uncharacterized interactions between water traversing the transcellular route and diffusion of K+ along the paracellular pathway.[345]

Loop of Henle and Medullary K+ Recycling

Transport by the loop of Henle plays a critical role in medullary K+ recycling (Figure 5-24). Several lines of evidence indicate that a considerable fraction of K+ secreted by the CCD is reabsorbed by the medullary collecting ducts and then secreted into the late proximal tubule and/or thin descending limbs of long-looped nephrons.[346] In potassium-loaded rats there is thus a doubling of luminal K+ in terminal thin descending limbs, with a sharp drop after inhibition of CCD K+ secretion by amiloride.[347] Enhancement of CCD K+ secretion by treatment with DDAVP also results in an increase in luminal K+ in thin descending limbs.[348] This recycling pathway (secretion in CCD, absorption in OMCD and IMCD, secretion in thin descending limb) is associated with a marked increase in medullary interstitial K+. Passive transepithelial K+ absorption by the thin ascending limb and active absorption by the TAL[153] also contribute to this increase in interstitial K+ (see Figure 5-24). Specifically, the absorption of K+ by thin ascending limb, TAL, and OMCD exceeds the secretion by thin descending limbs, thus trapping K+ in the interstitium.

The physiologic significance of medullary K+ recycling is not completely clear. However, an increase in interstitial K+ from 5 to 25 mmol/L dramatically inhibits Cl− transport by perfused TALs.[153] By inhibiting Na+-Cl− absorption by the TAL, increases in interstitial K+ would increase Na+ delivery to the CNT and CCD, thus enhancing the lumen-negative PD in these tubules and increasing K+ secretion.[153] Alternatively, the marked increase in medullary interstitial K+ after dietary K+ loading could serve to limit the difference between luminal and peritubular K+ in the collecting duct, thus minimizing passive K+ loss from the collecting duct.

K+ is secreted into thin descending limbs by passive diffusion, driven by the high medullary interstitial K+ concentration. Thin descending limbs thus have a very high K+ permeability, without evidence for active transepithelial K+ transport.[349] Transepithelial K+ transport by thin ascending limbs has not to the authors' knowledge been measured; however, as is the case for Na+-Cl− transport (see the section "Na+-Cl− Transport in the Thin Ascending Limb"), the absorption of K+ by thin ascending limbs is presumably passive. Active transepithelial K+ transport across the TAL includes both a transcellular component, via apical Na+-K+-2Cl− cotransport mediated by NKCC2, and a paracellular pathway (see Figure 5-15). Luminal K+ channels play a critical role in generating the lumen-positive PD in the TAL, as summarized in the section on Na$^+$-Cl$^-$ transport (see the section "Apical K$^+$ Channels" under "Na$^+$-Cl$^-$ Transport in the Thick Ascending Limb").

K$^+$ Secretion by the Distal Convoluted Tubule, Connecting Tubule, and Cortical Collecting Duct

Approximately 90% of filtered K$^+$ is reabsorbed by the proximal tubule and loop of Henle (see Figure 5-23); the fine tuning of renal K$^+$ excretion occurs in the remaining distal nephron. The bulk of regulated secretion occurs in principal cells within the CNT and CCD, whereas K$^+$ reabsorption primarily occurs in the OMCD (see later). K$^+$ secretion is initially detectable in the early DCT,[350] where NCC-positive cells express ROMK, the apical K$^+$ secretory channel.[160] Classically, the CCD is considered the primary site for distal K$^+$ secretion, partially due to the greater ease with which this segment is perfused and studied. However, as is the case for Na$^+$-Cl$^-$ absorption (see the section "Apical Na$^+$ Transport" under "Collecting Tubules and Cortical Collecting Duct"), the bulk of distal K$^+$ secretion appears to occur prior to the CCD,[216] within the CNT.[267] In principal cells, apical Na$^+$ entry via ENaC generates a lumen-negative PD, which drives passive K$^+$ exit through apical K$^+$ channels. Distal K$^+$ secretion is therefore dependent on delivery of adequate luminal Na$^+$ to the CNT and CCD[351,352] and essentially ceases when luminal Na$^+$ drops below 8 mmol/L.[353] Dietary Na$^+$ intake also influences K$^+$ excretion. Excretion is enhanced by excess Na$^+$ intake and reduced by Na$^+$ restriction.[351,352]

Secreted K$^+$ enters principal cells via the basolateral Na$^+$-K$^+$-ATPase, which also generates the gradient that drives apical Na$^+$ entry via ENaC (see Figure 5-23). Two major subtypes of apical K$^+$ channels function in secretion by the CNT and CCD, and possibly the DCT: a small-conductance 30-picosiemen (SK) channel[161,267] and a large-conductance, Ca^{2+}-activated 150-picosiemen (maxi-K or BK) channel.[267,354] The density and high open probability of the SK channel indicate that this pathway alone is sufficient to mediate the bulk of K$^+$ secretion in the CCD under baseline conditions[355]; hence its designation as the "secretory" K$^+$ channel. Notably, SK channel density is considerably higher in the CNT than in the CCD,[267] consistent with the greater capacity for Na$^+$ absorption and K$^+$ secretion in the CNT.

The characteristics of the SK channel are similar to those of the ROMK K$^+$ channel,[356] and ROMK protein has been localized at the apical membrane of principal cells.[160] SK channel activity is absent from apical membranes of the CCD in homozygous knockout mice with a targeted deletion of the *Kcnj1* gene that encodes ROMK, definitive proof that ROMK is the SK channel.[161] The observation that these knockout mice are normokalemic with an *increased* excretion of K$^+$ illustrates the considerable redundancy in distal K$^+$ secretory pathways[161]; distal K$^+$ secretion in these mice is mediated by apical BK channels[357] (see later).

Of interest, loss-of-function mutations in human *KCNJ1* are associated with Bartter's syndrome; ROMK expression is critical for the 30-picosiemen and 70-picosiemen channels that generate the lumen-positive PD in the TAL[161,162] (see Figure 5-15). These patients typically have slightly higher serum K$^+$ levels than patients with the other genetic forms of Bartter's syndrome.[155] Affected patients with severe neonatal

hyperkalemia have also been described[11]; this neonatal hyperkalemia is presumably the result of a transient developmental deficit in apical BK channel activity.

The apical Ca^{2+}-activated BK channel plays a critical role in *flow*-dependent K$^+$ secretion by the CNT and CCD.[354] BK channels have a heteromeric structure, with α-subunits that form the ion channel pore and modulatory β-subunits that affect the biophysical, regulatory, and pharmacologic characteristics of the channel complex.[354] BK α-subunit transcripts are expressed in multiple nephron segments, and channel protein is detectable at the apical membrane of principal and intercalated cells in the CCD and CNT.[354] The β-subunits are differentially expressed within the distal nephron. Thus β$_1$ subunits are restricted to the CNT,[354] with no expression in intercalated cells,[358] whereas β$_4$ subunits are detectable at the apical membranes of TAL, DCT, and intercalated cells.[358]

Increased distal flow has a well-established stimulatory effect on K$^+$ secretion, due in part both to enhanced delivery and absorption of Na$^+$ and to increased removal of secreted K$^+$.[351,352] The pharmacology of flow-dependent K$^+$ secretion in the CCD is consistent with dominant involvement of BK channels,[359] and flow-dependent K$^+$ secretion is reduced in mice with targeted deletion of the α$_1$- and β$_1$-subunits.[354,360,361] Both mice strains develop hyperaldosteronism that is exacerbated by a high-K$^+$ diet,[361] which leads to hypertension in the α$_1$-subunit knockout.[361]

One persistent puzzle has been the greater density of BK channels in intercalated cells than in principal cells in both the CCD[362] and the CNT.[363] This suggested a role for intercalated cells in K$^+$ secretion; however, the much lower density of Na$^+$-K$^+$-ATPase activity in intercalated cells was considered inadequate to support K$^+$ secretion across the apical membrane.[364] The role of BK channels has recently been addressed through characterization of knockout mice deficient in β$_4$ subunits,[364] the BK subunit expressed in intercalated cells.[358] Intercalated cell volume drops dramatically in tubules from wild-type but not β$_4$-deficient mice, which indicates a role for BK channels in volume regulation of intercalated cells.[364] Intercalated cells thus function as "speed bumps" that protrude into the lumen of distal tubules; flow-activated BK channels decrease the cell volume of intercalated cells, which reduces tubular resistance and increases tubular flow rates.[364]

The physiologic rationale for the presence of two apical secretory K$^+$ channels—ROMK/SK and BK channels—is not completely clear. However, the high density and higher open probability of SK/ROMK channels perhaps makes them better suited for a role in basal K$^+$ secretion, with additional recruitment of the higher-capacity, flow-activated BK channels when additional K$^+$ secretion is required.[354] The two K$^+$ channels can substitute for one another, with BK-dependent K$^+$ secretion in ROMK knockout mice[357] and an upregulation of ROMK in the distal nephron of α$_1$-subunit BK knockouts.[360]

Other K$^+$ channels reportedly expressed at the luminal membranes of the CNT and CCD include voltage-sensitive channels such as Kv 1.3,[365,366] double-pore K$^+$ channels such as TWIK-1 (tandem of P domains in weak inward rectifier K$^+$ channel 1),[367] and KCNQ1 (voltage-gated potassium channel, KQT-like subfamily, member 1).[368] KCNQ1 mediates K$^+$ secretion in the inner ear and is expressed at the apical membrane of principal cells in the CCD,[368] whereas TWIK-1 is expressed at the apical membrane of intercalated cells.[367] The roles of these channels in renal K^+ secretion or absorption have not been fully characterized. However, Kv 1.3 may play a role in distal K^+ secretion, because luminal margatoxin, a specific blocker of this channel, reduces K^+ secretion in CCDs of rat kidneys from animals consuming a high-K^+ diet.[369]

Other apical K^+ channels in the distal nephron may subserve other physiologic functions. For example, the apical Kv 1.1 channel is critically involved in Mg^{2+} transport by the DCT, likely by hyperpolarizing the apical membrane and increasing the driving force for Mg^{2+} influx via TRPM6 (transient receptor potential cation channel 6). Missense mutations in Kv 1.1 are a cause of genetic hypomagnesemia.[370]

K^+ channels present at the *basolateral* membrane of principal cells appear to set the resting potential of the basolateral membrane and function in K^+ secretion and Na^+ absorption at the apical membrane, the latter via K^+ recycling at the basolateral membrane to maintain the activity of Na^+-K^+-ATPase. A variety of different K^+ channels have been described in the electrophysiologic characterization of the basolateral membrane of principal cells, which has a number of technical barriers to overcome (reviewed in Gray and colleagues[371]). However, a single predominant activity can be identified in principal cells from the rat CCD, using whole-cell recording techniques under conditions in which ROMK is inhibited (low intracellular pH or presence of the ROMK inhibitor tertiapin-Q).[371] This basolateral current is tetraethylammonium insensitive, barium sensitive, and acid sensitive (pK_a of approximately 6.5), with a conductance of approximately 17 picosiemens and weak inward rectification.

These properties do not correspond exactly to specific characterized K^+ channels or combinations thereof. However, candidate inwardly rectifying K^+ channel subunits that have been localized at the basolateral membrane of the CCD include Kir 4.1, Kir 5.1, Kir 7.1, and Kir 2.3.[371] A more recent report suggests that Kir 4.1/Kir 5.1 channels generate a predominant 40-picosiemen basolateral K^+ channel in murine principal cells.[372] Notably, basolateral K^+ channel activity increases when a high-K^+ diet is consumed, which suggests a role in transepithelial K^+ secretion.[371]

In addition to apical K^+ channels, considerable evidence implicates apical K^+-Cl^- cotransport (or functionally equivalent pathways[373]) in distal K^+ secretion.[55,351,374] Thus in rat distal tubules, a reduction in luminal Cl^- markedly increases K^+ secretion[375]; the replacement of luminal Cl^- with SO_4^- or gluconate has an equivalent stimulatory effect on K^+ secretion. This anion-dependent component of K^+ secretion is not influenced by luminal Ba^{2+},[375] which suggests that it does not involve apical K^+ channel activity. Perfused surface distal tubules are a mixture of DCT, CNT, and initial collecting duct; however, Cl^--coupled K^+ secretion is detectable in both the DCT and in early CNT.[376] In addition, similar pathways are detectable in rabbit CCD, where a decrease in luminal Cl^- from 112 mmol/L to 5 mmol/L increases K^+ secretion by 48%.[377] A reduction in basolateral Cl^- also decreases K^+ secretion without an effect on transepithelial voltage or Na^+ transport, and the direction of K^+ flux can be reversed by a lumen-to-bath Cl^- gradient, which results in K^+ absorption.[377]

In perfused CCDs from rats treated with mineralocorticoid, vasopressin increases K^+ secretion.[378] Because this increase in K^+ secretion is resistant to luminal Ba^{2+} (2 mmol/L), vasopressin may stimulate Cl^--dependent K^+ secretion.[11] Pharmacologic studies of perfused tubules are consistent with

K^+-Cl^- cotransport mediated by the KCCs[55,374]; however, of the three renal KCCs, only KCC1 is apically expressed along the nephron (D. Mount, unpublished observations). Other functional possibilities for Cl^--dependent K^+ secretion include parallel operation of apical H^+/K^+ exchange and Cl^-/HCO_3^- exchange in type B intercalated cells.[373]

A recent provocative study by Frindt and Palmer serves to underline the importance of ENaC-independent K^+ excretion, be it mediated by apical K^+-Cl^- cotransport and/or by other mechanisms[379] (see also the section "Integrated Na^+-Cl^- and K^+ Transport in the Distal Nephron"). Rats were infused with amiloride via osmotic minipumps to generate urinary concentrations considered sufficient to inhibit more than 98% of ENaC activity. Whereas amiloride almost abolished K^+ excretion in rats with a normal K^+ intake, consumption of short-term and long-term high-K^+ diets led to an increasing fraction of K^+ excretion that was independent of ENaC activity (approximately 50% after 7 to 9 days on a high-K^+ diet).

K^+ Reabsorption by the Collecting Duct

In addition to K^+ secretion, the distal nephron is capable of considerable reabsorption, primarily during restriction of dietary K^+.[216-218] This reabsorption is accomplished in large part by intercalated cells in the OMCD via the activity of apical H^+-K^+-ATPase pumps. Under K^+-replete conditions, apical H^+-K^+-ATPase activity recycles K^+ with an apical K^+ channel, with no effect on transepithelial K^+ absorption. Under K^+-restricted conditions, K^+ absorbed via apical H^+-K^+-ATPase appears to exit intercalated cells via a *basolateral* K^+ channel, which thus achieves the transepithelial transport of K^+.[380]

H^+-K^+-ATPase holoenzymes are members of the P-type family of ion transport ATPases, which also includes subunits of the basolateral Na^+-K^+-ATPase.[381] $HK\alpha_1$ and $HK\alpha_2$ are also referred to as the *gastric* and *colonic* subunits, respectively. Humans also have an $HK\alpha_4$ subunit.[381,382] A specific $HK\beta$ subunit interacts with the $HK\alpha$ subunits to ensure delivery to the cell surface and complete expression of H^+-K^+-ATPase activity.[383] $HK\alpha_2$ and $HK\alpha_4$ subunits are also capable of interaction with Na^+-K^+-ATPase β-subunits.[11]

The pharmacology of H^+-K^+-ATPase holoenzymes differs considerably: the gastric $HK\alpha_1$ is classically sensitive to the H^+-K^+-ATPase inhibitors Schering 28080 (SCH-28080) and omeprazole and resistant to ouabain; the colonic $HK\alpha_2$ subunit is usually sensitive to ouabain and resistant to SCH-28080.[383]

Within the kidney, the $HK\alpha_1$ subunit is expressed at the apical membrane of at least a subset of type A intercalated cells in the distal nephron.[382] $HK\alpha_2$ distribution in the distal nephron is more diffuse,[384] with robust expression at the apical membrane of type A and B intercalated cells and CNT cells and lesser expression in principal cells.[385,386] The human $HK\alpha_4$ subunit is reportedly expressed in intercalated cells.[382] $HK\alpha_1$ and $HK\alpha_2$ are both constitutively expressed in the distal nephron. However, tubule perfusion of K^+-replete animals suggests a functional dominance of omeprazole/SCH-28080–sensitive, ouabain-resistant H^+-K^+-ATPase activity, which is consistent with holoenzymes containing $HK\alpha_1$.[387] K^+ deprivation increases the overall activity of H^+-K^+-ATPase in the collecting duct, with the emergence of a ouabain-sensitive H^+-K^+-ATPase activity[11]; this is consistent with a relative dominance of HKα$_2$ during K$^+$-restricted conditions. K$^+$-restriction also induces a dramatic upregulation of HKα$_2$ transcript and protein in the outer and inner medulla during K$^+$ depletion; HKα$_1$ expression is unaffected.[11]

Mice with a targeted deletion of HKα$_2$ exhibit lower plasma and muscle K$^+$ than wild-type littermates when maintained on a K$^+$-deficient diet. However, this appears to be due to marked loss of K$^+$ in the colon rather than the kidney, because renal K$^+$ excretion is appropriately reduced in the K$^+$-depleted knockout mice.[388] Presumably the lack of an obvious renal phenotype in either HKα$_1$[389] or HKα$_2$[388] knockout mice reflects the marked redundancy in the expression of HKα subunits in the distal nephron. Indeed, collecting ducts from the HKα$_1$ knockout mice have significant residual ouabain-resistant and SCH-28080-sensitive H$^+$-K$^+$-ATPase activities, consistent with the expression of other HKα subunits that confer characteristics similar to that of gastric H$^+$-K$^+$-ATPase.[390] However, data from HKα$_1$ and HKα$_2$ knockout mice suggest that compensatory mechanisms in these mice are not accounted for by ATPase-type mechanisms.[391]

The importance of K$^+$ reabsorption mediated by the collecting duct is dramatically illustrated by the phenotype of transgenic mice with generalized overexpression of a gain-of-function mutation in H$^+$-K$^+$-ATPase, which effectively bypasses the redundancy and complexity of this reabsorptive pathway. This transgene expresses a mutant form of the HKβ subunit in which a tyrosine to alanine mutation within the C-terminal tail abrogates regulated endocytosis from the plasma membrane. These mice have higher plasma K$^+$ levels than their wild-type littermates, with approximately half the fractional excretion of K$^+$.[392]

Regulation of Distal K$^+$ Transport

Aldosterone and K$^+$ Loading

Aldosterone has a potent kaliuretic effect,[393] with important interrelationships between circulating K$^+$ and aldosterone. Aldosterone release by the adrenal glands is induced by hyperkalemia and/or a high-K$^+$ diet, which suggests an important feedback effect of aldosterone on K$^+$ homeostasis.[394] Aldosterone also has clinically relevant effects on K$^+$ homeostasis, with a clear relationship at all levels of serum K$^+$ between circulating levels of the hormone and the ability to excrete K$^+$ (see Chapter 17).

Aldosterone has no effect on the density of apical SK channels in the CCD.[395] It does, however, induce a marked increase in the density of apical Na$^+$ channels in the CNT and CCD.[395] This hormone activates ENaC via interrelated effects on the synthesis, trafficking, and membrane-associated activity of the subunits encoding the channel (see the section "Regulation of Na$^+$-Cl$^-$ Transport in the Collecting Tubule and Cortical Collecting Duct"). Aldosterone is thus induced by consumption of a high-K$^+$ diet and strongly stimulates apical ENaC activity, which provides the lumen-negative PD that stimulates K$^+$ secretion by principal cells.

The important relationships between K$^+$ and aldosterone notwithstanding, it is increasingly clear that much of the adaptation to high K$^+$ intake is aldosterone independent. For example, a high-K$^+$ diet in adrenalectomized animals increases apical Na$^+$ reabsorption and K$^+$ secretion in the CCD.[396] At the tubular level, when basolateral K$^+$ is increased there is a

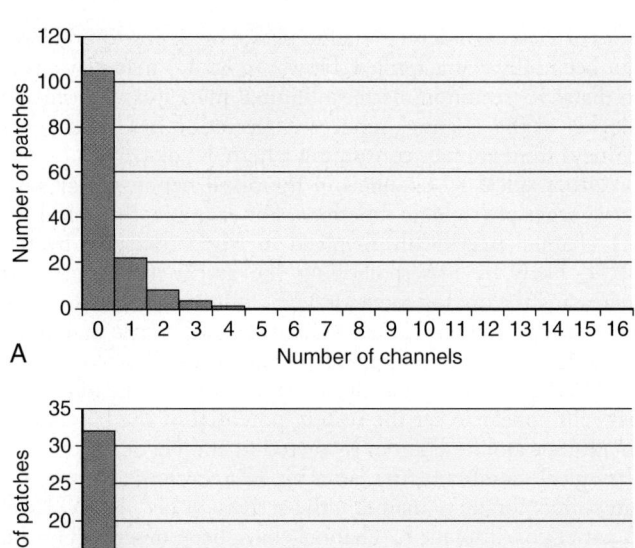

A

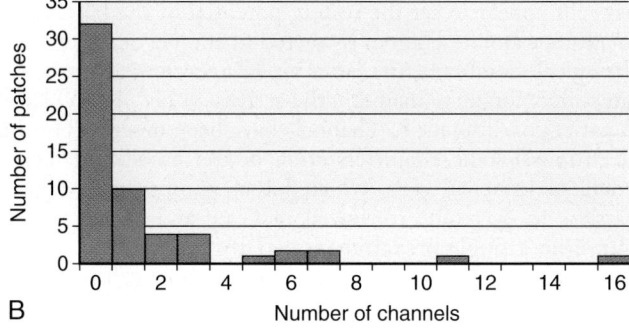

B

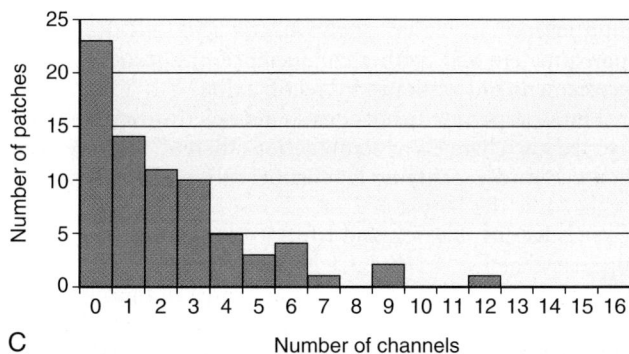

C

FIGURE 5-25 Rapid activation of small-conductance (SK) channels in the cortical collecting duct (CCD), mediated by the renal outer medullary K$^+$ channel (ROMK/Kir 1.1), in response to K$^+$ intake. Histograms of N (number of channels per patch) are shown for rats consuming a control diet (**A**), a high-K$^+$ diet for 6 hours (**B**), and a high-K$^+$ diet for 48 hours (**C**). Each determination of N represents a single cell-attached patch. Consumption of a high-K$^+$ diet results in a progressive recruitment of SK channels at the apical membrane. (From Palmer LG, Frindt G: Regulation of apical K channels in rat cortical collecting tubule during changes in dietary K intake, *Am J Physiol* 277:F805-F812, 1999.)

significant activation of Na$^+$-K$^+$-ATPase, accompanied by a secondary activation of apical Na$^+$ and K$^+$ channels.[397]

Increased dietary K$^+$ also leads to a marked increase in the density of SK channels in the CCD, along with a modest increase in Na$^+$ channel (ENaC) density.[395] This is associated with changes in the subcellular distribution of the ROMK protein, with an increase in apical expression.[398] Notably, this increase in ENaC and SK density in the CCD occurs within hours of consuming a high-K$^+$ diet, with a minimal associated increase in circulating aldosterone[399] (Figure 5-25). In contrast, a week of low–Na$^+$-Cl$^-$ intake, with almost a 1000-fold increase in aldosterone level, has no effect on SK channel density, nor for that matter does 2 days of aldosterone infusion, despite the development of hypokalemia[399] (Table 5-1).

TABLE 5-1 Effects of a High-K+ Diet, Aldosterone Level, and/or Na+-Cl− Restriction on SK Channel Density in the Rat Cortical Collecting Duct			
CONDITION	**K+ CHANNEL DENSITY (per µm²)**	**PLASMA ALDO (ng/dL)**	**PLASMA K+ (mmol/L)**
Control	0.41	15	3.68
High-K+ diet, 6 hr	1.51	36	NM
High-K+ diet, 48 hr	2.13	98	4.37
Low-Na+ diet, 7 days	0.48	1260	NM
Aldo infusion, 48 hr	0.44	550	2.44
Aldo + high-K+ diet	0.32	521	3.80

Aldo, Aldosterone; *NM*, not measured; *SK channel*, small-conductance K+ channel.
Modified from Palmer LG, Frindt G: Regulation of apical K channels in rat cortical collecting tubule during changes in dietary K intake, *Am J Physiol* 277:F805-F812, 1999.

Of note, unlike the marked increase seen in the CCD,[395,399] the density of SK channels in the CNT has not been found to be increased by high dietary K+.[267] This appears to be due to difficulties in estimating channel densities in small membrane patches, however, because measurement of whole-cell currents using the ROMK inhibitor tertiapin-Q indicates an upregulation of ROMK activity in the CNT in response to a high-K+ diet.[400]

BK channels in the CNT and CCD play an important role in the flow-activated component of distal K+ excretion.[354] These channels are also activated by dietary K+ loading. Flow-stimulated K+ secretion by the CCD of both mice[357] and rats[401] is enhanced by consumption of a high-K+ diet, with an absence of flow-dependent K+ secretion in rats consuming a low-K+ diet.[401] This is accompanied by the appropriate changes in transcript levels for the α-subunit and β₂- through β₄-subunits of the BK channel proteins in microdissected CCDs (β₁-subunits are restricted to the CNT[354]).

Trafficking of BK subunits is also affected by dietary K+, with largely intracellular distribution of α-subunits in K+-restricted rabbits and prominent apical expression in K+-loaded rabbits.[401] Aldosterone does not contribute to the regulation of BK channel activity or expression in response to a high-K+ diet.[402] The changes in trafficking and/or activity of the ROMK channel that are induced by dietary K+ appear in large part to involve tyrosine phosphorylation and dephosphorylation of the ROMK protein (see later). However, a recent series of reports have linked changes in expression of WNK1 kinase subunits to the response to a high-K+ diet.

WNK1 and WNK4 were initially identified as causative genes for FHHt (see also the section "Regulation of Na+-Cl− Transport" under "Distal Convoluted Tubule"). ROMK expression at the membrane of *Xenopus* oocytes is significantly reduced by coexpression of WNK4. FHHt-associated mutations dramatically increase this effect, which suggests a direction inhibition of SK channels in FHHt.[403]

The study of WNK1 is further complicated by the transcriptional complexity of its gene, which has at least three separate promoters and a number of alternative splice forms

(Figure 5-26). In particular, the predominant intrarenal WNK1 isoform is generated by a distal nephron transcriptional site that bypasses the N-terminal exons that encode the kinase domain, which yields a kinase-deficient short form of the protein[404] (WNK1-S). Full-length WNK1 (WNK1-L) inhibits ROMK activity by inducing endocytosis of the channel protein.[405-407] Kinase activity and/or the N-terminal kinase domain of WNK1 appear to be required for this effect,[406,407] although Cope and colleagues have reported that a kinase-dead mutant of WNK1 is unimpaired.[405]

WNK1 and WNK4 induce endocytosis of ROMK via interaction with intersectin, a multimodular endocytic scaffold protein.[408] Additional binding of ROMK to the clathrin adaptor protein known as *autosomal recessive hypercholesterolemia* (ARH) is required for basal and WNK1-stimulated endocytosis of the channel protein.[409] Ubiquitination of ROMK protein is also involved in clathrin-dependent endocytosis, which requires interaction between the channel and the U3 ubiquitin ligase POSH (plenty of SH₃ domains).[410]

The shorter WNK1-S isoform, which lacks the kinase domain, appears to inhibit the effect of WNK1-L.[406,407] The ratio of WNK1-S to WNK1-L transcripts is reduced by K+ restriction (greater endocytosis of ROMK)[407,411] and increased by K+ loading (reduced endocytosis of ROMK),[406,411] which suggests that this ratio between WNK1-S and WNK1-L functions as a switch to regulate distal K+ secretion (see also Figure 5-26). The inhibitory effect of WNK1-S tracks to the first 253 amino acids of the protein, encompassing the initial 30 amino acids unique to this isoform and an adjacent auto-inhibitory domain.[412] Transgenic mice that overexpress this inhibitory domain of WNK1-S have lower serum K+ concentrations, higher fractional excretion of K+, and increased expression of ROMK protein at the apical membrane of CNT and CCD cells—all consistent with an important inhibitory effect of WNK1-S.[412]

K+ Deprivation

A reduction in dietary K+ leads within 24 hours to a dramatic drop in urinary K+ excretion.[411,413] This drop in excretion is due to both an induction of reabsorption by intercalated cells in the OMCD[217,218] and a reduction in SK channel activity in principal cells.[11] The mechanisms involved in K+ reabsorption by intercalated cells were discussed earlier; notably, H+-K+-ATPase activity in the collecting duct does not appear to be regulated by aldosterone.[414] Considerable progress has recently been made in defining the signaling pathways that regulate the activity of the SK channel (ROMK) in response to changes in dietary K+. Dietary K+ intake modulates trafficking of the ROMK channel protein to the plasma membrane of principal cells, with a marked increase in the relative proportion of intracellular channel protein in K+-depleted animals[398,415] and clearly defined expression at the plasma membrane of CCD cells from animals consuming a high-K+ diet.[398]

The membrane insertion and activity of ROMK is modulated by tyrosine phosphorylation of the channel protein: phosphorylation of tyrosine residue 337 stimulates endocytosis, and dephosphorylation induces exocytosis.[416,417] This tyrosine phosphorylation appears to play a key role in the regulation of ROMK by dietary K+.[418] Although the levels of protein tyrosine phosphatase 1D do not vary with K+

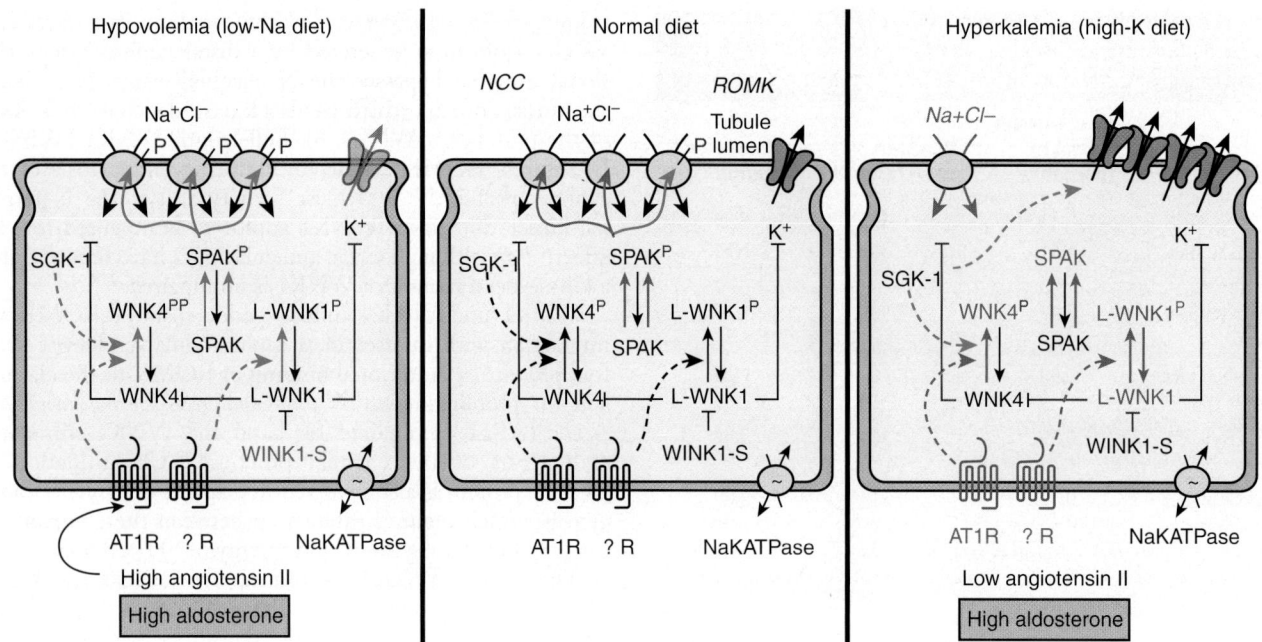

FIGURE 5-26 Simplified models of the effect of high and low K⁺ intake on the activity of the epithelial Na⁺ channel (ENaC) and renal outer medullary K⁺ channel (ROMK/Kir 1.1) in principal cells. These models omit the effects of K⁺ intake on large-conductance (BK) channels, which are also activated by high K⁺ intake and inhibited by low K⁺ intake. Also not shown is the effect of K⁺ intake on Na⁺-Cl⁻ cotransporter (NCC)–mediated Na⁺-Cl⁻ in the upstream distal convoluted tubule (DCT), which is inhibited by high K⁺ intake and activated by low K⁺ intake (see text). Negative effects are denoted by a *blunted line,* whereas predominantly positive effects are denoted by *arrows. Black circles with an X* denote inhibition of a particular pathway. **A,** Effect of low K⁺ intake. Low K⁺ intake reduces ROMK expression and ROMK activity at the plasma membrane of principal cells. A decrease in the ratio of kinase-deficient WNK1 (WINK1-S) to full-length WNK1 (with no lysine kinase 1) results in predominant inhibition of ROMK trafficking to the plasma membrane. Low K⁺ intake also increases circulating renin and angiotensin II, which affect ROMK activity via several pathways. Activation of src-like protein tyrosine kinases (PTKs) blocks the negative effects of WNK4 phosphorylation by serum- and glucocorticoid-regulated kinase 1 (SGK1), so that WNK4-dependent inhibition of ROMK trafficking is unopposed. WNK4-dependent inhibition of ENaC is also unmasked, which reduces the lumen-negative potential difference that stimulates K⁺ secretion. Direct tyrosine phosphorylation of ROMK by src-like PTKs also reduces expression and thus activity of ROMK at the plasma membrane. Finally, angiotensin II–dependent activation of mitogen-activated protein kinases (MAPKs) results in inhibition of ROMK. **B,** Effect of high K⁺ intake. High K⁺ intake reduces renin and angiotensin II, which abrogates the negative downstream effects of angiotensin II on ROMK trafficking and activity. The ratio of WINK1-S to full-length WNK1 is increased; this abolishes the negative effects of full-length WNK1 on ROMK trafficking and activity. High K⁺ intake also stimulates aldosterone release from the adrenal gland, which activates ENaC via SGK1. SGK1-dependent phosphorylation of WNK4 abolishes the inhibitory effect of WNK4 on ROMK, thus enhancing ROMK-dependent K⁺ secretion. (Adapted from Wang WH, Giebisch G: Regulation of potassium [K] handling in the renal collecting duct, *Pflugers Arch* 458:157-168, 2009.)

intake, intrarenal activity of the cytoplasmic tyrosine kinases c-src and c-yes are inversely related to dietary K⁺ intake, with a decrease under high-K⁺ conditions and a marked increase after several days of K⁺ restriction.[11,419] Localization studies indicate coexpression of c-src with ROMK in the TAL and principal cells of the CCD.[398] Moreover, inhibition of protein tyrosine phosphatase activity, which leads to a dominance of tyrosine phosphorylation, dramatically increases the proportion of intracellular ROMK in the CCDs of animals consuming a high-K⁺ diet.[398]

The neurohumoral factors that induce the K⁺-dependent trafficking and expression of apical ROMK[398,415] and BK channels[401] have only recently come into focus. Several studies have implicated the intrarenal generation of superoxide anions in the activation of cytoplasmic tyrosine kinases and downstream phosphorylation of the ROMK channel protein by K⁺ depletion.[420-422] Potential candidates for the upstream kaliuretic factor include angiotensin II and growth factors such as insulin-like growth factor-1.[420] Angiotensin II inhibits ROMK activity in K⁺-restricted rats, but not in rats consuming a normal K⁺ diet.[423] This inhibition involves downstream activation of superoxide production and c-src activity; thus the well-known induction of angiotensin II by consumption of a low-K⁺ diet appears to play a major role in reducing distal

tubular K⁺ secretion[424] (see also Figure 5-26). Mitogen-activated protein kinases (MAPKs) are also activated by angiotensin II in K⁺-restricted rats.[422,424] MAPK activation inhibits both ROMK[425] and BK[426] channels in the CCD. Finally, within principal cells, increases in aldosterone induce the SGK1 kinase, which phosphorylates WNK4 and attenuates the inhibitory effect of WNK4 on ROMK.[427] When dietary K⁺ intake is reduced, however, the increase in c-src tyrosine kinase activity abrogates the effect of SGK1 on WNK4,[428] so that inhibition of ROMK by WNK4 is unopposed (see also Figure 5-26).

Reports of a marked postprandial kaliuresis in sheep, independent of changes in plasma K⁺ or aldosterone levels, have led to the suggestion that an enteric or hepatoportal K⁺ "sensor" controls kaliuresis via a sympathetic reflex.[429] Changes in dietary K⁺ absorption may thus have a direct anticipatory effect on K⁺ homeostasis in the absence of changes in plasma K⁺ concentration. Such a feed-forward control has the theoretical advantage of greater stability, since it operates prior to changes in plasma K⁺ concentration.[430] Notably, changes in ROMK phosphorylation status and insulin-sensitive muscle uptake can be seen in K⁺-deficient animals in the absence of a change in plasma K⁺ level,[431] which suggests that upstream activation of the major mechanisms that serve to reduce

K+ excretion (reduced K+ secretion in the CNT and CCD, decreased peripheral uptake, and increased K+ reabsorption in the OMCD) does not require changes in plasma K+ concentration. Consistent with this hypothesis, moderate K+ restriction—without an associated drop in plasma K+ level—is sufficient to induce angiotensin II–dependent superoxide generation and c-src activation, which leads to inhibition of ROMK channel activity.[424]

The serine protease tissue kallikrein has recently emerged as a potential mediator for aldosterone-independent postprandial kaliuresis.[432] Mice trained to eat their daily ration of food within a 4-hour window demonstrate a marked postprandial kaliuresis, accompanied by an increase in urinary kallikrein. Mice with a targeted deletion of the kallikrein gene demonstrate a marked postprandial increase in plasma K+ concentration. Kallikrein is secreted by CNT cells, activating ENaC channels in principal cells and inhibiting downstream H+-K+-ATPase in intercalated cells. Postprandial, K+-stimulated kallikrein secretion thus results in an aldosterone-independent activation of K+ secretion and a concomitant inhibition of K+ reabsorption, with a net increase in K+ excretion.[432]

Vasopressin

Vasopressin has a well-characterized stimulatory effect on K+ secretion by the distal nephron.[348,433] Teleologically, this vasopressin-dependent activation serves to preserve K+ secretion during dehydration and extracellular volume depletion, when circulating levels of vasopressin are high and tubular delivery of Na+ and fluid is reduced. The stimulation of basolateral V_2 receptors results in an activation of ENaC, which increases the driving force for K+ secretion by principal cells. The relevant mechanisms were discussed earlier in this chapter (see the section "Vasopressin and Other Factors" under "Regulation of Na+-Cl− Transport in the Connecting Tubule and Cortical Collecting Duct"). In addition, vasopressin activates SK channels directly in the CCD,[434] as does cAMP.[355] ROMK is directly phosphorylated by PKA on three serine residues (S25, S200, and S294 in the ROMK2 isoform), with phosphorylation of all three sites required for full activity in *Xenopus* oocytes (see the section "Activating Influences" under "Regulation of Na+-Cl− Transport in the Thick Ascending Limb"). Finally, the stimulation of luminal V_1 receptors also stimulates K+ secretion in the CCD, apparently via activation of BK channels.[435]

Integrated Na+-Cl− and K+ Transport in the Distal Nephron

In the classical model of renal K+ secretion, the lumen-negative PD generated by Na+ entry via ENaC induces the exit of K+ via apical K+-selective channels. This general scheme explains much of the known physiology and pathophysiology of renal K+ secretion, yet has several key consequences that bear emphasis. First, enhanced Na+-Cl− reabsorption upstream of the CNT and CCD will reduce the delivery of luminal Na+ to the CNT and CCD,[351,352] decrease the lumen-negative PD, and thus decrease K+ secretion. K+ secretion by the CCD essentially stops when luminal Na+ drops below 8 mmol/L.[353] In this respect, the increasingly refined phenotypic understanding of FHHt, caused by kinase-induced gain

of function of the DCT (see also the section "Regulation of Na+-Cl− Transport" under "Distal Convoluted Tubule"), has served to underline that variation in NCC-dependent Na+-Cl− absorption just upstream of the CNT has truly profound effects on the ability to excrete dietary K+.[243]

Second, aldosterone is a kaliuretic hormone, induced by hyperkalemia. However, under certain circumstances associated with marked induction of aldosterone, such as dietary sodium restriction, sodium balance is maintained without effects on K+ homeostasis. This "aldosterone paradox"—how does the kidney independently regulate Na+-Cl− and K+ handling by the aldosterone-sensitive distal nephron?—is only recently beginning to yield to investigative efforts.

The major factors in the integrated control of Na+-Cl− and K+ transport appear to include electroneutral thiazide-sensitive Na+-Cl− transport within the CCD[286-288] (see the section "Electroneutral Na+-Cl− Transport" under "Connecting Tubules and Cortical Collecting Duct"), ENaC-independent K+ excretion within the distal nephron,[379] and the differential regulation of various signaling pathways by aldosterone, angiotensin II, dietary K+, and kallikrein.[428,432,436] Electroneutral thiazide-sensitive Na+-Cl− transport within the CCD is evidently mediated by the parallel activity of the Na+-driven SLC4A8 Cl−/HCO3− exchanger and the SLC26A4 Cl−/HCO3− exchanger (see also the section "Electroneutral Na+-Cl− Transport" under "Connecting Tubules and Cortical Collecting Duct").[288]

The molecular identity of this transport mechanism has only recently emerged[288]; hence, regulatory influences are not fully characterized. However, electroneutral Na+-Cl− transport within the CCD is evidently induced by both volume depletion and mineralocorticoid treatment.[286-288] This mechanism appears to mediate approximately 50% of Na+ transport in the CCD under these conditions, all without affecting the lumen PD and thus without direct effect on K+ excretion. Therefore, electroneutral thiazide-sensitive Na+-Cl− transport affords the ability to increase the reabsorption of Na+ within the CCD without affecting K+ excretion. The converse occurs after several days' accommodation to a high-K+ diet, which increases the fraction of ENaC-independent, amiloride-resistant K+ excretion to approximately 50%. Again, this presumptively electroneutral, aldosterone-independent pathway for K+ excretion serves to uncouple distal tubular Na+ and K+ excretion.[379]

In a landmark study in 2003, Kahle and colleagues established that the WNK4 kinase, encoded by a disease gene for FHHt, causes inhibition of ROMK activity in *Xenopus* oocytes; FHHt-associated mutations potentiated this effect.[403] This finding identified WNK-dependent signaling as a major pathway for integrating Na+-Cl− and K+ transport within the distal nephron. Details of the relevant effects of WNK kinases on NCC and ROMK were discussed earlier (see Figure 5-26, the section "Regulation of Distal K+ Transport," and the section "Regulation of Na+-Cl− Transport" under "Distal Convoluted Tubule"). However, key elements include the differential influence of K+ intake on circulating angiotensin II, ROMK activity (i.e., K+ secretory capacity), the ratio of WNK1 isoforms, and the activity of NCC in the DCT.

Angiotensin II activates NCC via the WNK4-SPAK pathway,[261,437,438] reducing delivery of Na+ to the CNT and limiting K+ secretion. In contrast, angiotensin II inhibits ROMK activity via several mechanisms, including downstream activation of c-src tyrosine kinases.[422-424] Whereas K+ restriction induces renin and circulating angiotensin II, increases in dietary K$^+$ are suppressive.[424,439] A decrease in circulating and local angiotensin II presumably explains why NCC phosphorylation and activity is downregulated by high-K$^+$ diet.[265] Teleologically, this serves to *increase* delivery of Na$^+$ to the CNT, which increases K$^+$ secretion.

Finally, within principal cells, increases in aldosterone induce the SGK1 kinase, which phosphorylates WNK4 and attenuates the effect of WNK4 on ROMK,[427] while activating ENaC via Nedd4-2–dependent effects (see the section "Regulation of Na$^+$-Cl$^-$ Transport in the Connecting Tubule and Cortical Collecting Duct"). When dietary K$^+$ intake is reduced, however, c-src tyrosine kinase activity increases under the influence of increased angiotensin II, causing direction inhibition of ROMK activity via tyrosine phosphorylation of the channel[416,418,440] (see the section "Regulation of Distal K$^+$ Transport"). The increase in c-src tyrosine kinase activity also abrogates the effect of SGK1 on WNK4[428] (see also Figure 5-26).

References

1. Greger R. Physiology of renal sodium transport. *Am J Med Sci.* 2000;319:51-62.
2. Sun A, Grossman EB, Lombardi M, et al. Vasopressin alters the mechanism of apical Cl$^-$ entry from Na$^+$:Cl$^-$ to Na$^+$:K$^+$:2Cl$^-$ cotransport in mouse medullary thick ascending limb. *J Membr Biol.* 1991;120:83-94.
3. Madsen KM, Tisher CC. Anatomy of the kidney. In: Brenner BM, ed. *Brenner and Rector's the kidney.* Philadelphia: Saunders; 2004:3-72.
4. Welling LW, Welling DJ. Surface areas of brush border and lateral cell walls in the rabbit proximal nephron. *Kidney Int.* 1975;8:343-348.
5. Liu FY, Cogan MG. Axial heterogeneity of bicarbonate, chloride, and water transport in the rat proximal convoluted tubule. Effects of change in luminal flow rate and of alkalemia. *J Clin Invest.* 1986;78:1547-1557.
6. Maddox DA, Gennari FJ. The early proximal tubule: a high-capacity delivery-responsive reabsorptive site. *Am J Physiol.* 1987;252:F573-F584.
7. Kokko JP. Proximal tubule potential difference. Dependence on glucose on glucose, HCO$_3$, and amino acids. *J Clin Invest.* 1973;52:1362-1367.
8. Alpern RJ, Howlin KJ, Preisig PA. Active and passive components of chloride transport in the rat proximal convoluted tubule. *J Clin Invest.* 1985;76:1360-1366.
9. Moe OW, Baum M, Berry CA, et al. Renal transport of glucose, amino acids, sodium, chloride, and water. In: Brenner BM, ed. *Brenner and Rector's the kidney.* Philadelphia: Saunders; 2004:413-452.
10. Schild L, Giebisch G, Green R. Chloride transport in the proximal renal tubule. *Annu Rev Physiol.* 1988;50:97-110.
11. Mount DB, Yu AS. Transport of inorganic solutes: sodium, potassium, calcium, magnesium, and phosphate. In: Brenner BM, ed. *Brenner and Rector's the kidney.* Philadelphia: Saunders; 2007:156-213.
12. Barratt LJ, Rector Jr FC, Kokko JP, et al. Factors governing the transepithelial potential difference across the proximal tubule of the rat kidney. *J Clin Invest.* 1974;53:454-464.
13. Jacobson HR. Characteristics of volume reabsorption in rabbit superficial and juxtamedullary proximal convoluted tubules. *J Clin Invest.* 1979;63:410-418.
14. Katz AI, Doucet A, Morel F. Na-K-ATPase activity along the rabbit, rat, and mouse nephron. *Am J Physiol.* 1979;237:F114-F120.
15. Baum M, Berry CA. Evidence for neutral transcellular NaCl transport and neutral basolateral chloride exit in the rabbit proximal convoluted tubule. *J Clin Invest.* 1984;74:205-211.
16. Vallon V, Verkman AS, Schnermann J. Luminal hypotonicity in proximal tubules of aquaporin-1-knockout mice. *Am J Physiol Renal Physiol.* 2000;278:F1030-F1033.
17. Claude P, Goodenough DA. Fracture faces of zonulae occludentes from "tight" and "leaky" epithelia. *J Cell Biol.* 1973;58:390-400.
18. Yu AS. Paracellular solute transport: more than just a leak? *Curr Opin Nephrol Hypertens.* 2000;9:513-515.
19. Furuse M, Furuse K, Sasaki H, et al. Conversion of zonulae occludentes from tight to leaky strand type by introducing claudin-2 into Madin-Darby canine kidney I cells. *J Cell Biol.* 2001;153:263-272.
20. Yu AS, Enck AH, Lencer WI, et al. Claudin-8 expression in Madin-Darby canine kidney cells augments the paracellular barrier to cation permeation. *J Biol Chem.* 2003;278:17350-17359.
21. Nitta T, et al. Size-selective loosening of the blood-brain barrier in claudin-5–deficient mice. *J Cell Biol.* 2003;161:653-660.
22. Enck AH, Berger UV, Yu AS. Claudin-2 is selectively expressed in proximal nephron in mouse kidney. *Am J Physiol Renal Physiol.* 2001;281:F966-F974.
23. Rosenthal R, et al. Claudin-2, a component of the tight junction, forms a paracellular water channel. *J Cell Sci.* 2010;123:1913-1921.
24. Muto S, et al. Claudin-2-deficient mice are defective in the leaky and cation-selective paracellular permeability properties of renal proximal tubules. *Proc Natl Acad Sci U S A.* 2010;107:8011-8016.
25. Schnermann J, et al. Defective proximal tubular fluid reabsorption in transgenic aquaporin-1 null mice. *Proc Natl Acad Sci U S A.* 1998;95:9660-9664.
26. Sohara E, et al. Defective water and glycerol transport in the proximal tubules of AQP7 knockout mice. *Am J Physiol Renal Physiol.* 2005;289:F1195-F1200.
27. Zeuthen T, Meinild AK, Loo DD, et al. Isotonic transport by the Na$^+$-glucose cotransporter SGLT1 from humans and rabbit. *J Physiol.* 2001;531:631-644.
28. Charron FM, Blanchard MG, Lapointe JY. Intracellular hypertonicity is responsible for water flux associated with Na$^+$/glucose cotransport. *Biophys J.* 2006;90:3546-3554.
29. Maddox DA, Gennari FJ. Load dependence of HCO$_3$ and H$_2$O reabsorption in the early proximal tubule of the Munich-Wistar rat. *Am J Physiol.* 1985;248:F113-F121.
30. Bobulescu IA, Moe OW. Luminal Na(+)/H(+) exchange in the proximal tubule. *Pflugers Arch.* 2009;458:5-21.
31. Bacic D, et al. Dopamine acutely decreases apical membrane Na/H exchanger NHE3 protein in mouse renal proximal tubule. *Kidney Int.* 2003;64:2133-2141.
32. Choi JY, et al. Novel amiloride-sensitive sodium-dependent proton secretion in the mouse proximal convoluted tubule. *J Clin Invest.* 2000;105:1141-1146.
33. Schultheis PJ, et al. Renal and intestinal absorptive defects in mice lacking the NHE3 Na$^+$/H$^+$ exchanger. *Nat Genet.* 1998;19:282-285.
34. Wang T, et al. Essential role of NHE3 in facilitating formate-dependent NaCl absorption in the proximal tubule. *Am J Physiol Renal Physiol.* 2001;281:F288-F292.
35. Kurtz I, et al. Mechanism of apical and basolateral Na(+)-independent Cl$^-$/base exchange in the rabbit superficial proximal straight tubule. *J Clin Invest.* 1994;94:173-183.
36. Karniski LP, Aronson PS. Chloride/formate exchange with formic acid recycling: a mechanism of active chloride transport across epithelial membranes. *Proc Natl Acad Sci U S A.* 1985;82:6362-6365.
37. Saleh AM, Rudnick H, Aronson PS. Mechanism of H(+)-coupled formate transport in rabbit renal microvillus membranes. *Am J Physiol.* 1996;271:F401-F407.
38. Karniski LP, Aronson PS. Anion exchange pathways for Cl$^-$ transport in rabbit renal microvillus membranes. *Am J Physiol.* 1987;253:F513-F521.
39. Kuo SM, Aronson PS. Pathways for oxalate transport in rabbit renal microvillus membrane vesicles. *J Biol Chem.* 1996;271:15491-15497.
40. Wang T, Agulian SK, Giebisch G, et al. Effects of formate and oxalate on chloride absorption in rat distal tubule. *Am J Physiol.* 1993;264:F730-F736.
41. Wang T, Egbert Jr AL, Abbiati T, et al. Mechanisms of stimulation of proximal tubule chloride transport by formate and oxalate. *Am J Physiol.* 1996;271:F446-F450.
42. Scott DA, Karniski LP. Human pendrin expressed in *Xenopus laevis* oocytes mediates chloride/formate exchange. *Am J Physiol Cell Physiol.* 2000;278:C207-C211.
43. Royaux IE, et al. Pendrin, encoded by the Pendred syndrome gene, resides in the apical region of renal intercalated cells and mediates bicarbonate secretion. *Proc Natl Acad Sci U S A.* 2001;98:4221-4226.
44. Xie Q, Welch R, Mercado A, et al. Molecular characterization of the murine Slc26a6 anion exchanger, functional comparison to Slc26a1. *Am J Physiol.* 2002;283:F826-F838.
45. Wang Z, et al. Renal and intestinal transport defects in Slc26a6-null mice. *Am J Physiol Cell Physiol.* 2005;288:C957-C965.
46. Dudas PL, Greineder CF, Mentone SA, et al. Immunolocalization of anion exchanger Slc26a7 in mouse kidney. *J Am Soc Nephrol.* 2003;14:313A.
47. Kim KH, Shcheynikov N, Wang Y, et al. SLC26A7 is a Cl$^-$ channel regulated by intracellular pH. *J Biol Chem.* 2005;280:6463-6470.
48. Chapman JM, Karniski LP. Protein localization of SLC26A2 (DTDST) in rat kidney. *Histochem Cell Biol.* 2010;133:541-547.
49. Jiang Z, et al. Calcium oxalate urolithiasis in mice lacking anion transporter Slc26a6. *Nat Genet.* 2006;38(4):474-478.
50. Ohana E, Yang D, Shcheynikov N, et al. Diverse transport modes by the solute carrier 26 family of anion transporters. *J Physiol.* 2009;587:2179-2185.
51. Chang MH, et al. Slc26a9-anion exchanger, channel and Na(+) transporter. *J Membr Biol.* 2009;228:125-140.
52. Vallon V, et al. KCNQ1-dependent transport in renal and gastrointestinal epithelia. *Proc Natl Acad Sci U S A.* 2005;102:17864-17869.

53. Thomson RB, et al. Role of PDZK1 in membrane expression of renal brush border ion exchangers. *Proc Natl Acad Sci U S A*. 2005;102:13331-13336.

54. Petrovic S, Barone S, Weinstein AM, et al. Activation of the apical Na^+/H^+ exchanger NHE3 by formate: a basis of enhanced fluid and electrolyte reabsorption by formate in the kidney. *Am J Physiol Renal Physiol*. 2004;287:F336-F346.

55. Mount DB, Gamba G. Renal K-Cl cotransporters. *Curr Opin Nephrol Hypertens*. 2001;10:685-692.

56. Mercado A, et al. NH2-terminal heterogeneity in the KCC3 K^+-Cl^- cotransporter. *Am J Physiol Renal Physiol*. 2005;289:F1246-F12461.

57. Ishibashi K, Rector Jr FC, Berry CA. Chloride transport across the basolateral membrane of rabbit proximal convoluted tubules. *Am J Physiol*. 1990;258:F1569-F15678.

58. Sasaki S, Ishibashi K, Yoshiyama N, et al. KCl co-transport across the basolateral membrane of rabbit renal proximal straight tubules. *J Clin Invest*. 1988;81:194-199.

59. Avison MJ, Gullans SR, Ogino T, et al. Na^+ and K^+ fluxes stimulated by Na^+-coupled glucose transport: evidence for a Ba^{2+}-insensitive K^+ efflux pathway in rabbit proximal tubules. *J Membr Biol*. 1988;105:197-205.

60. Boettger T, et al. Loss of K-Cl co-transporter KCC3 causes deafness, neurodegeneration and reduced seizure threshold. *EMBO J*. 2003;22:5422-5434.

61. Wang T, Delpire E, Giebisch G, et al. Impaired fluid and bicarbonate absorption in proximal tubules (PT) of KCC3 knockout mice. *FASEB J*. 2003;17:A464.

62. Ishibashi K, Rector Jr FC, Berry CA. Role of Na-dependent Cl/HCO_3 exchange in basolateral Cl transport of rabbit proximal tubules. *Am J Physiol*. 1993;264:F251-F258.

63. Macri P, Breton S, Beck JS, et al. Basolateral K^+, Cl^-, and HCO_3^- conductances and cell volume regulation in rabbit PCT. *Am J Physiol*. 1993;264:F365-F3676.

64. Welling PA, O'Neil RG. Cell swelling activates basolateral membrane Cl and K conductances in rabbit proximal tubule. *Am J Physiol*. 1990;258:F951-F962.

65. Seki G, Taniguchi S, Uwatoko S, et al. Evidence for conductive Cl^- pathway in the basolateral membrane of rabbit renal proximal tubule S3 segment. *J Clin Invest*. 1993;92:1229-1235.

66. Obermuller N, Gretz N, Kriz W, et al. The swelling-activated chloride channel ClC-2, the chloride channel ClC-3, and ClC-5, a chloride channel mutated in kidney stone disease, are expressed in distinct subpopulations of renal epithelial cells. *J Clin Invest*. 1998;101:635-642.

67. Alpern RJ, Chambers M. Basolateral membrane Cl/HCO_3 exchange in the rat proximal convoluted tubule. Na-dependent and -independent modes. *J Gen Physiol*. 1987;89:581-598.

68. Wang T. Flow-activated transport events along the nephron. *Curr Opin Nephrol Hypertens*. 2006;15:530-536.

69. Du Z, et al. Axial flow modulates proximal tubule NHE3 and H-ATPase activities by changing microvillus bending moments. *Am J Physiol Renal Physiol*. 2006;290:F289-F296.

70. Burg MB, Orloff J. Control of fluid absorption in the renal proximal tubule. *J Clin Invest*. 1968;47:2016-2024.

71. Du Z, et al. Mechanosensory function of microvilli of the kidney proximal tubule. *Proc Natl Acad Sci U S A*. 2004;101:13068-13073.

72. Duan Y, et al. Shear-induced reorganization of renal proximal tubule cell actin cytoskeleton and apical junctional complexes. *Proc Natl Acad Sci U S A*. 2008;105:11418-11423.

73. Brenner BM, Troy JL. Postglomerular vascular protein concentration: evidence for a causal role in governing fluid reabsorption and glomerulotubular balance by the renal proximal tubule. *J Clin Invest*. 1971;50:336-349.

74. Bello-Reuss E, Colindres RE, Pastoriza-Munoz E, et al. Effects of acute unilateral renal denervation in the rat. *J Clin Invest*. 1975;56:208-217.

75. Bell-Reuss E, Trevino DL, Gottschalk CW. Effect of renal sympathetic nerve stimulation on proximal water and sodium reabsorption. *J Clin Invest*. 1976;57:1104-1107.

76. Feraille E, Doucet A. Sodium-potassium-adenosinetriphosphatase-dependent sodium transport in the kidney: hormonal control. *Physiol Rev*. 2001;81:345-418.

77. Hall RA, et al. The beta$_2$-adrenergic receptor interacts with the Na^+/H^+-exchanger regulatory factor to control Na^+/H^+ exchange. *Nature*. 1998;392:626-630.

78. Harris PJ, Young JA. Dose-dependent stimulation and inhibition of proximal tubular sodium reabsorption by angiotensin II in the rat kidney. *Pflugers Arch*. 1977;367:295-297.

79. Harrison-Bernard LM, Navar LG, Ho MM, et al. Immunohistochemical localization of ANG II AT1 receptor in adult rat kidney using a monoclonal antibody. *Am J Physiol*. 1997;273:F170-F177.

80. Li L, Wang YP, Capparelli AW, et al. Effect of luminal angiotensin II on proximal tubule fluid transport: role of apical phospholipase A2. *Am J Physiol*. 1994;266:F202-F209.

81. Zheng Y, et al. Biphasic regulation of renal proximal bicarbonate absorption by luminal AT(1A) receptor. *J Am Soc Nephrol*. 2003;14:1116-1122.

82. Quan A, Baum M. Endogenous production of angiotensin II modulates rat proximal tubule transport. *J Clin Invest*. 1996;97:2878-2882.

83. Quan A, et al. Androgens augment proximal tubule transport. *Am J Physiol Renal Physiol*. 2004;287:F452-F459.

84. Thomson SC, et al. An unexpected role for angiotensin II in the link between dietary salt and proximal reabsorption. *J Clin Invest*. 2006;116:1110-1116.

85. Wang ZQ, Siragy HM, Felder RA, et al. Intrarenal dopamine production and distribution in the rat. Physiological control of sodium excretion. *Hypertension*. 1997;29:228-234.

86. Hegde SS, Jadhav AL, Lokhandwala MF. Role of kidney dopamine in the natriuretic response to volume expansion in rats. *Hypertension*. 1989;13:828-834.

87. Baum M, Quigley R. Inhibition of proximal convoluted tubule transport by dopamine. *Kidney Int*. 1998;54:1593-1600.

88. Yu P, et al. D1 dopamine receptor hyperphosphorylation in renal proximal tubules in hypertension. *Kidney Int*. 2006;70:1072-1029.

89. Albrecht FE, et al. Role of the D1A dopamine receptor in the pathogenesis of genetic hypertension. *J Clin Invest*. 1996;97:2283-2288.

90. Hollon TR, et al. Mice lacking D5 dopamine receptors have increased sympathetic tone and are hypertensive. *J Neurosci*. 2002;22:10801-10810.

91. Holtback U, et al. Receptor recruitment: a mechanism for interactions between G protein–coupled receptors. *Proc Natl Acad Sci U S A*. 1999;96:7271-7275.

92. Harris PJ, Thomas D, Morgan TO. Atrial natriuretic peptide inhibits angiotensin-stimulated proximal tubular sodium and water reabsorption. *Nature*. 1987;326:697-698.

93. Cheng HF, Becker BN, Harris RC. Dopamine decreases expression of type-1 angiotensin II receptors in renal proximal tubule. *J Clin Invest*. 1996;97:2745-2752.

94. Zeng C, et al. Interaction of angiotensin II type 1 and D5 dopamine receptors in renal proximal tubule cells. *Hypertension*. 2005;45:804-810.

95. Zeng C, et al. Activation of D3 dopamine receptor decreases angiotensin II type 1 receptor expression in rat renal proximal tubule cells. *Circ Res*. 2006;99:494-500.

96. Donowitz M, et al. NHE3 regulatory complexes. *J Exp Biol*. 2009;212:1638-1646.

97. Sarker R, et al. Casein kinase 2 binds to the C terminus of Na^+/H^+ exchanger 3 (NHE3) and stimulates NHE3 basal activity by phosphorylating a separate site in NHE3. *Mol Biol Cell*. 2008;19:3859-3870.

98. Liu FY, Cogan MG. Angiotensin II stimulates early proximal bicarbonate absorption in the rat by decreasing cyclic adenosine monophosphate. *J Clin Invest*. 1989;84:83-91.

99. Collazo R, et al. Acute regulation of Na^+/H^+ exchanger NHE3 by parathyroid hormone via NHE3 phosphorylation and dynamin-dependent endocytosis. *J Biol Chem*. 2000;275:31601-31608.

100. Zhao H, et al. Acute inhibition of Na/H exchanger NHE-3 by cAMP. Role of protein kinase a and NHE-3 phosphoserines 552 and 605. *J Biol Chem*. 1999;274:3978-3987.

101. Kocinsky HS, et al. Use of phospho-specific antibodies to determine the phosphorylation of endogenous Na^+/H^+ exchanger NHE3 at PKA consensus sites. *Am J Physiol Renal Physiol*. 2005;289:F249-F258.

102. Biemesderfer D, DeGray B, Aronson PS. Active (9.6 s) and inactive (21 s) oligomers of NHE3 in microdomains of the renal brush border. *J Biol Chem*. 2001;276:10161-10167.

103. Weinman EJ, Cunningham R, Shenolikar S. NHERF and regulation of the renal sodium-hydrogen exchanger NHE3. *Pflugers Arch*. 2005;450:137-144.

104. Sanchez-Mendoza A, et al. Angiotensin II modulates ion transport in rat proximal tubules through CYP metabolites. *Biochem Biophys Res Commun*. 2000;272:423-430.

105. Dos Santos EA, Dahly-Vernon AJ, Hoagland KM, et al. Inhibition of the formation of EETs and 20-HETE with 1-aminobenzotriazole attenuates pressure natriuresis. *Am J Physiol Regul Integr Comp Physiol*. 2004;287:R58-R68.

106. du Cheyron D, et al. Angiotensin II stimulates NHE3 activity by exocytic insertion of the transporter: role of PI 3-kinase. *Kidney Int*. 2003;64:939-949.

107. Leong PK, et al. Effects of ACE inhibition on proximal tubule sodium transport. *Am J Physiol Renal Physiol*. 2006;290:F854-F863.

108. Yun CC, Chen Y, Lang F. Glucocorticoid activation of Na(+)/H(+) exchanger isoform 3 revisited. The roles of SGK1 and NHERF2. *J Biol Chem*. 2002;277:7676-7683.

109. Wang D, Sun H, Lang F, et al. Activation of NHE3 by dexamethasone requires phosphorylation of NHE3 at Ser663 by SGK1. *Am J Physiol Cell Physiol*. 2005;289:C802-C810.

110. Pedemonte CH, Efendiev R, Bertorello AM. Inhibition of Na, K-ATPase by dopamine in proximal tubule epithelial cells. *Semin Nephrol*. 2005;25:322-327.

111. Chou CL, et al. Reduced water permeability and altered ultrastructure in thin descending limb of Henle in aquaporin-1 null mice. *J Clin Invest.* 1999;103:491-496.

112. Liu W, et al. Analysis of NaCl transport in thin ascending limb of Henle's loop in CLC-K1 null mice. *Am J Physiol Renal Physiol.* 2002;282:F451-F457.

113. Gottschalk CW, et al. Micropuncture study of composition of loop of Henle fluid in desert rodents. *Am J Physiol.* 1963;204:532-535.

114. Kokko JP. Sodium chloride and water transport in the descending limb of Henle. *J Clin Invest.* 1970;49:1838-1846.

115. Imai M, Taniguchi J, Yoshitomi K. Transition of permeability properties along the descending limb of long-loop nephron. *Am J Physiol.* 1988;254:F323-F328.

116. Chou CL, Knepper MA. in vitro perfusion of chinchilla thin limb segments: urea and NaCl permeabilities. *Am J Physiol.* 1993;264:F337-F343.

117. Chou CL, Knepper MA. in vitro perfusion of chinchilla thin limb segments: segmentation and osmotic water permeability. *Am J Physiol.* 1992;263:F417-F426.

118. Lopes AG, Amzel LM, Markakis D, et al. Cell volume regulation by the thin descending limb of Henle's loop. *Proc Natl Acad Sci U S A.* 1988;85:2873-2877.

119. Nielsen S, et al. Aquaporin-1 water channels in short and long loop descending thin limbs and in descending vasa recta in rat kidney. *Am J Physiol.* 1995;268:F1023-F1037.

120. Maeda Y, Smith BL, Agre P, et al. Quantification of aquaporin-CHIP water channel protein in microdissected renal tubules by fluorescence-based ELISA. *J Clin Invest.* 1995;95:422-428.

121. Chou CL, Nielsen S, Knepper MA. Structural-functional correlation in chinchilla long loop of Henle thin limbs: a novel papillary subsegment. *Am J Physiol.* 1993;265:F863-F874.

122. Imai M. Function of the thin ascending limb of Henle of rats and hamsters perfused in vitro. *Am J Physiol.* 1977;232:F201-F209.

123. Koyama S, Yoshitomi K, Imai M. Effect of protamine on ion conductance of ascending thin limb of Henle's loop from hamsters. *Am J Physiol.* 1991;261:F593-F599.

124. Takahashi N, et al. Characterization of Na^+ transport across the cell membranes of the ascending thin limb of Henle's loop. *Kidney Int.* 1995;47:789-794.

125. Kondo Y, Yoshitomi K, Imai M. Effects of anion transport inhibitors and ion substitution on Cl^- transport in TAL of Henle's loop. *Am J Physiol.* 1987;253:F1206-F1215.

126. Isozaki T, Yoshitomi K, Imai M. Effects of Cl^- transport inhibitors on Cl^- permeability across hamster ascending thin limb. *Am J Physiol.* 1989;257:F92-F98.

127. Yoshitomi K, Kondo Y, Imai M. Evidence for conductive Cl^- pathways across the cell membranes of the thin ascending limb of Henle's loop. *J Clin Invest.* 1988;82:866-871.

128. Kondo Y, et al. Direct evidence for the absence of active Na^+ reabsorption in hamster ascending thin limb of Henle's loop. *J Clin Invest.* 1993;91:5-11.

129. Takahashi N, et al. Vasopressin stimulates Cl^- transport in ascending thin limb of Henle's loop in hamster. *J Clin Invest.* 1995;95:1623-1627.

130. Uchida S, et al. Localization and functional characterization of rat kidney-specific chloride channel, ClC-K1. *J Clin Invest.* 1995;95:104-113.

131. Wolf K, et al. Parallel down-regulation of chloride channel CLC-K1 and barttin mRNA in the thin ascending limb of the rat nephron by furosemide. *Pflugers Arch.* 2003;446:665-671.

132. Waldegger S, et al. Barttin increases surface expression and changes current properties of ClC-K channels. *Pflugers Arch.* 2002;444:411-418.

133. Matsumura Y, et al. Overt nephrogenic diabetes insipidus in mice lacking the CLC-K1 chloride channel. *Nat Genet.* 1999;21:95-98.

134. Simon DB, et al. Mutations in the chloride channel gene, CLCNKB, cause Bartter's syndrome type III. *Nat Genet.* 1997;17:171-178.

135. Estevez R, et al. Barttin is a Cl^- channel beta-subunit crucial for renal Cl^- reabsorption and inner ear K^+ secretion. *Nature.* 2001;414:558-561.

136. Scholl U, et al. Barttin modulates trafficking and function of ClC-K channels. *Proc Natl Acad Sci U S A.* 2006;103:11411-11416.

137. Allen F, Tisher CC. Morphology of the ascending thick limb of Henle. *Kidney International.* 1976;9:8-22.

138. Tsuruoka S, Koseki C, Muto S, et al. Axial heterogeneity of potassium transport across hamster thick ascending limb of Henle's loop. *Am J Physiol.* 1994;267:F121-F129.

139. Nielsen S, Maunsbach AB, Ecelbarger CA, et al. Ultrastructural localization of Na-K-2Cl cotransporter in thick ascending limb and macula densa of rat kidney. *Am J Physiol.* 1998;275:F885-F893.

140. Greger R. Ion transport mechanisms in thick ascending limb of Henle's loop of mammalian nephron. *Physiol Rev.* 1985;65:760-797.

141. Burg M, Stoner L, Cardinal J, et al. Furosemide effect on isolated perfused tubules. *Am J Physiol.* 1973;225:119-124.

142. Hebert SC, Mount DB, Gamba G. Molecular physiology of cation-coupled Cl^- cotransport: the SLC12 family. *Pflugers Arch.* 2004;447:580-593.

143. Plata C, Mount DB, Rubio V, et al. Isoforms of the apical Na-K-2Cl transporter in murine thick ascending limb. II: Functional characterization and mechanism of activation by cyclic-AMP. *Am J Physiol.* 1999;276:F359-F366.

144. Gimenez I, Isenring P, Forbush B. Spatially distributed alternative splice variants of the renal Na-K-Cl cotransporter exhibit dramatically different affinities for the transported ions. *J Biol Chem.* 2002;277:8767-8770.

145. Lapointe JY, Laamarti A, Bell PD. Ionic transport in macula densa cells. *Kidney Int Suppl.* 1998;67:S58-S64.

146. Oppermann M, et al. Macula densa control of renin secretion and preglomerular resistance in mice with selective deletion of the B isoform of the Na, K,2Cl co-transporter. *J Am Soc Nephrol.* 2006;17:2143-2152.

147. Castrop H, Schnermann J. Isoforms of renal Na-K-2Cl cotransporter NKCC2: expression and functional significance. *Am J Physiol Renal Physiol.* 2008;295:F859-F866.

148. Good DW, Watts 3rd BA. Functional roles of apical membrane Na^+/H^+ exchange in rat medullary thick ascending limb. *Am J Physiol.* 1996;270:F691-F699.

149. Laghmani K, et al. Chronic metabolic acidosis enhances NHE-3 protein abundance and transport activity in the rat thick ascending limb by increasing NHE-3 mRNA. *J Clin Invest.* 1997;99:24-30.

150. Quentin F, et al. Regulation of the Cl^-/HCO_3^- exchanger AE2 in rat thick ascending limb of Henle's loop in response to changes in acid-base and sodium balance. *J Am Soc Nephrol.* 2004;15:2988-2997.

151. Burg MB, Green N. Function of the thick ascending limb of Henle's loop. *Am J Physiol.* 1973;224:659-668.

152. Rocha AS, Kokko JP. Sodium chloride and water transport in the medullary thick ascending limb of Henle. Evidence for active chloride transport. *J Clin Invest.* 1973;52:612-623.

153. Stokes JB. Consequences of potassium recycling in the renal medulla. Effects of ion transport by the medullary thick ascending limb of Henle's loop. *J Clin Invest.* 1982;70:219-229.

154. Greger R, Weidtke C, Schlatter E, et al. Potassium activity in cells of isolated perfused cortical thick ascending limbs of rabbit kidney. *Pflugers Arch.* 1984;401:52-57.

155. Simon DB, et al. Genetic heterogeneity of Bartter's syndrome revealed by mutations in the K^+ channel, ROMK. *Nat Genet.* 1996;14:152-156.

156. Taniguchi J, Guggino WB. Membrane stretch: a physiological stimulator of Ca^{2+}-activated K^+ channels in thick ascending limb. *Am J Physiol.* 1989;257:F347-F352.

157. Bleich M, Schlatter E, Greger R. The luminal K^+ channel of the thick ascending limb of Henle's loop. *Pflugers Arch.* 1990;415:449-460.

158. Wang WH. Two types of K^+ channel in thick ascending limb of rat kidney. *Am J Physiol.* 1994;267:F599-F605.

159. Wang W, Lu M. Effect of arachidonic acid on activity of the apical K^+ channel in the thick ascending limb of the rat kidney. *J Gen Physiol.* 1995;106:727-743.

160. Xu JZ, et al. Localization of the ROMK protein on apical membranes of rat kidney nephron segments. *Am J Physiol.* 1997;F739-F748.

161. Lu M, et al. Absence of small conductance K^+ channel (SK) activity in apical membranes of thick ascending limb and cortical collecting duct in ROMK (Bartter's) knockout mice. *J Biol Chem.* 2002;277:37881-37887.

162. Lu M, et al. ROMK is required for expression of the 70-pS K channel in the thick ascending limb. *Am J Physiol Renal Physiol.* 2004;286:F490-F495.

163. Yoo D, et al. Assembly and trafficking of a multiprotein ROMK (Kir 1.1) channel complex by PDZ interactions. *J Biol Chem.* 2004;279:6863-6873.

164. Lu M, et al. CFTR is required for PKA-regulated ATP sensitivity of Kir1.1 potassium channels in mouse kidney. *J Clin Invest.* 2006;116:797-807.

165. Hebert SC, Andreoli TE. Ionic conductance pathways in the mouse medullary thick ascending limb of Henle. The paracellular pathway and electrogenic Cl^- absorption. *J Gen Physiol.* 1986;87:567-590.

166. Hebert SC, Culpepper RM, Andreoli TE. NaCl transport in mouse medullary thick ascending limbs. II. ADH enhancement of transcellular NaCl cotransport; origin of transepithelial voltage. *Am J Physiol.* 1981;241:F432-F442.

167. Konrad M, et al. Mutations in the tight-junction gene claudin 19 (CLDN19) are associated with renal magnesium wasting, renal failure, and severe ocular involvement. *Am J Hum Genet.* 2006;79:949-957.

168. Angelow S, El-Husseini R, Kanzawa SA, et al. Renal localization and function of the tight junction protein, claudin-19. *Am J Physiol Renal Physiol.* 2007;293:F166-F177.

169. Hou J, Paul DL, Goodenough DA. Paracellin-1 and the modulation of ion selectivity of tight junctions. *J Cell Sci.* 2005;118:5109-5118.

170. Hou J, et al. Claudin-16 and claudin-19 interact and form a cation-selective tight junction complex. *J Clin Invest.* 2008;118:619-628.

171. Hou J, et al. Claudin-16 and claudin-19 interaction is required for their assembly into tight junctions and for renal reabsorption of magnesium. *Proc Natl Acad Sci U S A.* 2009;106:15350-15355.

172. Himmerkus N, et al. Salt and acid-base metabolism in claudin-16 knockdown mice: impact for the pathophysiology of FHHNC patients. *Am J Physiol Renal Physiol.* 2008;295:F1641-F1647.

173. Greger R, Schlatter E. Properties of the basolateral membrane of the cortical thick ascending limb of Henle's loop of rabbit kidney. A model for secondary active chloride transport. *Pflugers Arch.* 1983;396:325-334.

174. Geller DS. A genetic predisposition to hypertension? *Hypertension.* 2004;44:27-28.

175. Kobayashi K, Uchida S, Mizutani S, et al. Intrarenal and cellular localization of clc-k2 protein in the mouse kidney. *J Am Soc Nephrol.* 2001;12:1327-1334.

176. Picollo A, et al. Molecular determinants of differential pore blocking of kidney CLC-K chloride channels. *EMBO Rep.* 2004;5:584-589.

177. Palmer LG, Frindt G. Cl⁻ channels of the distal nephron. *Am J Physiol Renal Physiol.* 2006;291(6):F1157-1168.

178. Song L, Delpire E, Gamba G, et al. Localization of the K-Cl cotransporters KCC3 and KCC4 in mouse kidney. *FASEB J.* 2000;A341.

179. Boettger T, et al. Deafness and renal tubular acidosis in mice lacking the K-Cl co-transporter Kcc4. *Nature.* 2002;416:874-878.

180. Amlal H, Paillard M, Bichara M. Cl⁻-dependent NH4⁺ transport mechanisms in medullary thick ascending limb cells. *Am J Physiol.* 1994;267:C1607-C1615.

181. Bergeron MJ, Gagnon E, Wallendorff B, et al. Ammonium transport and pH regulation by K(+)-Cl(−) cotransporters. *Am J Physiol Renal Physiol.* 2003;285:F68-F78.

182. Mercado A, Song L, Vazquez N, et al. Functional comparison of the K⁺-Cl⁻ cotransporters KCC1 and KCC4. *J Biol Chem.* 2000;275:30326-30334.

183. Guggino WB. Functional heterogeneity in the early distal tubule of the *Amphiuma* kidney: evidence for two modes of Cl⁻ and K⁺ transport across the basolateral cell membrane. *Am J Physiol.* 1986;250:F430-F440.

184. Good DW. Ammonium transport by the thick ascending limb of Henle's loop. *Annu Rev Physiol.* 1994;56:623-647.

185. Hurst AM, Duplain M, Lapointe JY. Basolateral membrane potassium channels in rabbit cortical thick ascending limb. *Am J Physiol.* 1992;263:F262-F267.

186. Paulais M, Lachheb S, Teulon J. A Na⁺- and Cl⁻-activated K⁺ channel in the thick ascending limb of mouse kidney. *J Gen Physiol.* 2006;127:205-215.

187. Paulais M, Lourdel S, Teulon J. Properties of an inwardly rectifying K(+) channel in the basolateral membrane of mouse TAL. *Am J Physiol Renal Physiol.* 2002;282:F866-FF876.

188. Knepper MA, Kim GH, Fernandez-Llama P, et al. Regulation of thick ascending limb transport by vasopressin. *J Am Soc Nephrol.* 1999;10:628-634.

189. Mount DB. Membrane trafficking and the regulation of NKCC2. *Am J Physiol Renal Physiol.* 2006;290:F606-F607.

190. Gagnon KB, England R, Delpire E. Volume sensitivity of cation-chloride cotransporters is modulated by the interaction of two kinases: SPAK and WNK4. *Am J Physiol Cell Physiol.* 2006;290:C134-C142.

191. Rinehart J, et al. WNK3 kinase is a positive regulator of NKCC2 and NCC, renal cation-Cl⁻ cotransporters required for normal blood pressure homeostasis. *Proc Natl Acad Sci U S A.* 2005;102:16777-16782.

192. Delpire E, Gagnon KB. Genome-wide analysis of SPAK/OSR1 binding motifs. *Physiol Genomics.* 2007;28:223-231.

193. Gagnon KB, England R, Delpire E. A single binding motif is required for SPAK activation of the Na-K-2Cl cotransporter. *Cell Physiol Biochem.* 2007;20:131-142.

194. Reiche J, et al. SORLA/SORL1 functionally interacts with SPAK to control renal activation of Na(+)-K(+)-Cl(−) cotransporter 2. *Mol Cell Biol.* 2010;30:3027-3037.

195. Rafiqi FH, et al. Role of the WNK-activated SPAK kinase in regulating blood pressure. *EMBO Mol Med.* 2010;2:63-75.

196. Ponce-Coria J, et al. Regulation of NKCC2 by a chloride-sensing mechanism involving the WNK3 and SPAK kinases. *Proc Natl Acad Sci U S A.* 2008;105:8458-8463.

197. Mount DB, et al. Isoforms of the Na-K-2Cl cotransporter in murine TAL I. Molecular characterization and intrarenal localization. *Am J Physiol.* 1999;276:F347-F358.

198. Plata C, et al. Alternatively spliced isoform of apical Na(+)-K(+)-Cl(−) cotransporter gene encodes a furosemide-sensitive Na(+)-Cl(−) cotransporter. *Am J Physiol Renal Physiol.* 2001;280:F574-F582.

199. Xu ZC, Yang Y, Hebert SC. Phosphorylation of the ATP-sensitive, inwardly rectifying K⁺ channel, ROMK, by cyclic AMP-dependent protein kinase. *J Biol Chem.* 1996;271:9313-9319.

200. Yoo D, et al. Cell surface expression of the ROMK (Kir 1.1) channel is regulated by the aldosterone-induced kinase, SGK-1, and protein kinase A. *J Biol Chem.* 2003;278:23066-23075.

201. Leipziger J, et al. PKA site mutations of ROMK2 channels shift the pH dependence to more alkaline values. *Am J Physiol Renal Physiol.* 2000;279:F919-F926.

202. Liou HH, Zhou SS, Huang CL. Regulation of ROMK1 channel by protein kinase A via a phosphatidylinositol 4,5-bisphosphate-dependent mechanism. *Proc Natl Acad Sci U S A.* 1999;96:5820-5825.

203. Ecelbarger CA, et al. Regulation of potassium channel Kir 1.1 (ROMK) abundance in the thick ascending limb of Henle's loop. *J Am Soc Nephrol.* 2001;12:10-18.

204. Takaichi K, Kurokawa K. Inhibitory guanosine triphosphate-binding protein-mediated regulation of vasopressin action in isolated single medullary tubules of mouse kidney. *J Clin Invest.* 1988;82:1437-1444.

205. Hebert SC. Calcium and salinity sensing by the thick ascending limb: a journey from mammals to fish and back again. *Kidney Int Suppl.* 2004;S28-S33.

206. Riccardi D, et al. Localization of the extracellular Ca²⁺/polyvalent cation-sensing protein in rat kidney. *Am J Physiol.* 1998;274:F611-F622.

207. de Jesus Ferreira MC, et al. Co-expression of a Ca²⁺-inhibitable adenylyl cyclase and of a Ca²⁺-sensing receptor in the cortical thick ascending limb cell of the rat kidney. Inhibition of hormone-dependent cAMP accumulation by extracellular Ca²⁺. *J Biol Chem.* 1998;273:15192-15202.

208. Watanabe S, et al. Association between activating mutations of calcium-sensing receptor and Bartter's syndrome. *Lancet.* 2002;360:692-694.

209. Vargas-Poussou R, et al. Functional characterization of a calcium-sensing receptor mutation in severe autosomal dominant hypocalcemia with a Bartter-like syndrome. *J Am Soc Nephrol.* 2002;13:2259-2266.

210. Loffing J, Kaissling B. Sodium and calcium transport pathways along the mammalian distal nephron: from rabbit to human. *Am J Physiol Renal Physiol.* 2003;284:F628-F643.

211. Loffing J, et al. Distribution of transcellular calcium and sodium transport pathways along mouse distal nephron. *Am J Physiol Renal Physiol.* 2001;281:F1021-F1027.

212. Belge H, et al. Renal expression of parvalbumin is critical for NaCl handling and response to diuretics. *Proc Natl Acad Sci U S A.* 2007;104:14849-14854.

213. Frindt G, Palmer LG. Na channels in the rat connecting tubule. *Am J Physiol Renal Physiol.* 2004;286:F669-F674.

214. Wall SM. Recent advances in our understanding of intercalated cells. *Curr Opin Nephrol Hypertens.* 2005;14:480-484.

215. Duc C, Farman N, Canessa CM, et al. Cell-specific expression of epithelial sodium channel alpha, beta, and gamma subunits in aldosterone-responsive epithelia from the rat: localization by in situ hybridization and immunocytochemistry. *J Cell Biol.* 1994;127:1907-1921.

216. Malnic G, Klose RM, Giebisch G. Micropuncture study of renal potassium excretion in the rat. *Am J Physiol.* 1964;206:674-686.

217. Wingo CS, Armitage FE. Rubidium absorption and proton secretion by rabbit outer medullary collecting duct via H-K-ATPase. *Am J Physiol.* 1992;263:F849-F857.

218. Okusa MD, Unwin RJ, Velazquez H, et al. Active potassium absorption by the renal distal tubule. *Am J Physiol.* 1992;262:F488-F493.

219. Hager H, et al. Immunocytochemical and immunoelectron microscopic localization of alpha-, beta-, and gamma-ENaC in rat kidney. *Am J Physiol Renal Physiol.* 2001;280:F1093-F1106.

220. Ellison DH, Velazquez H, Wright FS. Adaptation of the distal convoluted tubule of the rat. Structural and functional effects of dietary salt intake and chronic diuretic infusion. *J Clin Invest.* 1989;83:113-126.

221. Khuri RN, Strieder N, Wiederholt M, et al. Effects of graded solute diuresis on renal tubular sodium transport in the rat. *Am J Physiol.* 1975;228:1262-1268.

222. Velazquez H, Good DW, Wright FS. Mutual dependence of sodium and chloride absorption by renal distal tubule. *Am J Physiol.* 1984;247:F904-F911.

223. Costanzo LS. Localization of diuretic action in microperfused rat distal tubules: Ca and Na transport. *Am J Physiol.* 1985;248:F527-F535.

224. Gamba G, et al. Primary structure and functional expression of a cDNA encoding the thiazide-sensitive, electroneutral sodium-chloride cotransporter. *Proc Natl Acad Sci U S A.* 1993;90:2749-2753.

225. Monroy A, Plata C, Hebert SC, et al. Characterization of the thiazide-sensitive Na(+)-Cl(−) cotransporter: a new model for ions and diuretics interaction. *Am J Physiol Renal Physiol.* 2000;279:F161-F169.

226. Bazzini C, et al. Thiazide-sensitive NaCl-cotransporter in the intestine: possible role of hydrochlorothiazide in the intestinal Ca²⁺ uptake. *J Biol Chem.* 2005;280:19902-19910.

227. Schultheis PJ, et al. Phenotype resembling Gitelman's syndrome in mice lacking the apical Na⁺-Cl⁻ cotransporter of the distal convoluted tubule. *J Biol Chem.* 1998;273:29150-29155.

228. Loffing J, et al. Altered renal distal tubule structure and renal Na(+) and Ca(2+) handling in a mouse model for Gitelman's syndrome. *J Am Soc Nephrol.* 2004;15:2276-2288.

229. Loffing J, et al. Thiazide treatment of rats provokes apoptosis in distal tubule cells. *Kidney Int.* 1996;50:1180-1190.

230. Chambrey R, et al. Immunolocalization of the Na⁺/H⁺ exchanger isoform NHE2 in rat kidney. *Am J Physiol.* 1998;275:F379-F386.

231. Kujala M, et al. SLC26A6 and SLC26A7 anion exchangers have a distinct distribution in human kidney. *Nephron Exp Nephrol.* 2005;101:e50-e58.

232. Velazquez H, Silva T. Cloning and localization of KCC4 in rabbit kidney: expression in distal convoluted tubule. *Am J Physiol Renal Physiol.* 2003;285:F49-F58.

233. Lourdel S, Paulais M, Marvao P, et al. A chloride channel at the basolateral membrane of the distal-convoluted tubule: a candidate ClC-K channel. *J Gen Physiol*. 2003;121:287-300.

234. Jeck N, et al. Mutations in the chloride channel gene, CLCNKB, leading to a mixed Bartter-Gitelman phenotype. *Pediatr Res*. 2000;48:754-758.

235. Lourdel S, et al. An inward rectifier K(+) channel at the basolateral membrane of the mouse distal convoluted tubule: similarities with Kir4-Kir5.1 heteromeric channels. *J Physiol*. 2002;538:391-404.

236. Huang C, et al. Interaction of the Ca²⁺-sensing receptor with the inwardly rectifying potassium channels Kir4.1 and Kir4.2 results in inhibition of channel function. *Am J Physiol Renal Physiol*. 2007;292:F1073-F1081.

237. Bockenhauer D, et al. Epilepsy, ataxia, sensorineural deafness, tubulopathy, and KCNJ10 mutations. *N Engl J Med*. 2009;360:1960-1970.

238. Tanemoto M, Abe T, Onogawa T, et al. PDZ binding motif-dependent localization of K⁺ channel on the basolateral side in distal tubules. *Am J Physiol Renal Physiol*. 2004;287:F1148-F1153.

239. Scholl UI, et al. Seizures, sensorineural deafness, ataxia, mental retardation, and electrolyte imbalance (SeSAME syndrome) caused by mutations in KCNJ10. *Proc Natl Acad Sci U S A*. 2009;106:5842-5847.

240. Kotelevtsev Y, et al. Hypertension in mice lacking 11beta-hydroxysteroid dehydrogenase type 2. *J Clin Invest*. 1999;103:683-689.

241. Kim GH, et al. The thiazide-sensitive Na-Cl cotransporter is an aldosterone-induced protein. *Proc Natl Acad Sci U S A*. 1998;95:14552-14557.

242. Nielsen J, et al. Sodium transporter abundance profiling in kidney: effect of spironolactone. *Am J Physiol Renal Physiol*. 2002;283:F923-F933.

243. Lalioti MD, et al. Wnk4 controls blood pressure and potassium homeostasis via regulation of mass and activity of the distal convoluted tubule. *Nat Genet*. 2006;38:1124-1132.

244. Mayan H, et al. Pseudohypoaldosteronism type II: marked sensitivity to thiazides, hypercalciuria, normomagnesemia, and low bone mineral density. *J Clin Endocrinol Metab*. 2002;87:3248-3254.

245. Wilson FH, et al. Human hypertension caused by mutations in WNK kinases. *Science*. 2001;293:1107-1112.

246. Wilson FH, et al. Molecular pathogenesis of inherited hypertension with hyperkalemia: the Na-Cl cotransporter is inhibited by wild-type but not mutant WNK4. *Proc Natl Acad Sci U S A*. 2003;100:680-684.

247. Golbang AP, et al. Regulation of the expression of the Na/Cl cotransporter (NCCT) by WNK4 and WNK1: evidence that accelerated dynamin-dependent endocytosis is not involved. *Am J Physiol Renal Physiol*. 2006;291(6):F1369-1376.

248. Yang CL, Angell J, Mitchell R, et al. WNK kinases regulate thiazide-sensitive Na-Cl cotransport. *J Clin Invest*. 2003;111:1039-1045.

249. Ko B, Hoover RS. Molecular physiology of the thiazide-sensitive sodium-chloride cotransporter. *Curr Opin Nephrol Hypertens*. 2009;18:421-427.

250. Welling PA, Chang YP, Delpire E, et al. Multigene kinase network, kidney transport, and salt in essential hypertension. *Kidney Int*. 2010;77(12):1063-1069.

251. Gamba G. The thiazide-sensitive Na⁺-Cl⁻ cotransporter: molecular biology, functional properties, and regulation by WNKs. *Am J Physiol Renal Physiol*. 2009;297:F838-F848.

252. Subramanya AR, Liu J, Ellison DH, et al. WNK4 diverts the thiazide-sensitive NaCl cotransporter to the lysosome and stimulates AP-3 interaction. *J Biol Chem*. 2009;284:18471-18480.

253. Zhou B, et al. WNK4 enhances the degradation of NCC through a sortilin-mediated lysosomal pathway. *J Am Soc Nephrol*. 2010;21(1):82-92.

254. Ko B, et al. RasGRP1 stimulation enhances ubiquitination and endocytosis of the sodium chloride cotransporter. *Am J Physiol Renal Physiol*. 2010;299(2):F300-309.

255. Ko B, et al. Phorbol ester stimulation of RasGRP1 regulates the sodium-chloride cotransporter by a PKC-independent pathway. *Proc Natl Acad Sci U S A*. 2007;104:20120-20125.

256. Vitari AC, Deak M, Morrice NA, et al. The WNK1 and WNK4 protein kinases that are mutated in Gordon's hypertension syndrome phosphorylate and activate SPAK and OSR1 protein kinases. *Biochem J*. 2005;391:17-24.

257. Moriguchi T, et al. WNK1 regulates phosphorylation of cation-chloride-coupled cotransporters via the STE20-related kinases, SPAK and OSR1. *J Biol Chem*. 2005;280:42685-42693.

258. Richardson C, et al. Activation of the thiazide-sensitive Na⁺-Cl⁻ cotransporter by the WNK-regulated kinases SPAK and OSR1. *J Cell Sci*. 2008;121:675-684.

259. Yang CL, Zhu X, Ellison DH. The thiazide-sensitive Na-Cl cotransporter is regulated by a WNK kinase signaling complex. *J Clin Invest*. 2007;117:3403-3411.

260. Rozansky DJ, et al. Aldosterone mediates activation of the thiazide-sensitive Na-Cl cotransporter through an SGK1 and WNK4 signaling pathway. *J Clin Invest*. 2009;119:2601-2612.

261. San-Cristobal P, et al. Angiotensin II signaling increases activity of the renal Na-Cl cotransporter through a WNK4-SPAK-dependent pathway. *Proc Natl Acad Sci U S A*. 2009;106:4384-4389.

262. Chiga M, et al. Dietary salt regulates the phosphorylation of OSR1/SPAK kinases and the sodium chloride cotransporter through aldosterone. *Kidney Int*. 2008;74:1403-1409.

263. Pedersen NB, Hofmeister MV, Rosenbaek LL, et al. Vasopressin induces phosphorylation of the thiazide-sensitive sodium chloride cotransporter in the distal convoluted tubule. *Kidney Int*. 2010;78(2):160-169.

264. Mutig K, et al. Short-term stimulation of the thiazide-sensitive Na⁺-Cl⁻ cotransporter by vasopressin involves phosphorylation and membrane translocation. *Am J Physiol Renal Physiol*. 2010;298(3):F502-509.

265. Vallon V, Schroth J, Lang F, et al. Expression and phosphorylation of the Na⁺-Cl⁻ cotransporter NCC in vivo is regulated by dietary salt, potassium, and SGK1. *Am J Physiol Renal Physiol*. 2009;297:F704-F712.

266. Frindt G, Palmer LG. Low-conductance K channels in apical membrane of rat cortical collecting tubule. *Am J Physiol*. 1989;256:F143-F151.

267. Frindt G, Palmer LG. Apical potassium channels in the rat connecting tubule. *Am J Physiol Renal Physiol*. 2004;287:F1030-F1037.

268. Palmer LG, Frindt G. Amiloride-sensitive Na channels from the apical membrane of the rat cortical collecting tubule. *Proc Natl Acad Sci U S A*. 1986;83:2767-2770.

269. Wagner CA, Devuyst O, Bourgeois S, et al. Regulated acid-base transport in the collecting duct. *Pflugers Arch*. 2009;458:137-156.

270. Firsov D, et al. Cell surface expression of the epithelial Na channel and a mutant causing Liddle syndrome: a quantitative approach. *Proc Natl Acad Sci U S A*. 1996;93:15370-15375.

271. Staruschenko A, Adams E, Booth RE, et al. Epithelial Na⁺ channel subunit stoichiometry. *Biophys J*. 2005;88:3966-3975.

272. Findling JW, Raff H, Hansson JH, et al. Liddle's syndrome: prospective genetic screening and suppressed aldosterone secretion in an extended kindred. *J Clin Endocrinol Metab*. 1997;82:1071-1074.

273. Hiltunen TP, et al. Liddle's syndrome associated with a point mutation in the extracellular domain of the epithelial sodium channel gamma subunit. *J Hypertens*. 2002;20:2383-2390.

274. Rubera I, et al. Collecting duct-specific gene inactivation of αENaC in the mouse kidney does not impair sodium and potassium balance. *J Clin Invest*. 2003;112:554-565.

275. Loffing J, et al. Differential subcellular localization of ENaC subunits in mouse kidney in response to high- and low-Na diets. *Am J Physiol Renal Physiol*. 2000;279:F252-F258.

276. Meneton P, Loffing J, Warnock DG. Sodium and potassium handling by the aldosterone-sensitive distal nephron: the pivotal role of the distal and connecting tubule. *Am J Physiol Renal Physiol*. 2004;287:F593-F601.

277. Schuster VL, Stokes JB. Chloride transport by the cortical and outer medullary collecting duct. *Am J Physiol*. 1987;253:F203-F212.

278. Warden DH, Schuster VL, Stokes JB. Characteristics of the paracellular pathway of rabbit cortical collecting duct. *Am J Physiol*. 1988;255:F720-F727.

279. Li WY, Huey CL, Yu AS. Expression of claudin-7 and -8 along the mouse nephron. *Am J Physiol Renal Physiol*. 2004;286:F1063-F10671.

280. Kahle KT, et al. Paracellular Cl⁻ permeability is regulated by WNK4 kinase: insight into normal physiology and hypertension. *Proc Natl Acad Sci U S A*. 2004;101:14877-14882.

281. Yamauchi K, et al. Disease-causing mutant WNK4 increases paracellular chloride permeability and phosphorylates claudins. *Proc Natl Acad Sci U S A*. 2004;101:4690-4694.

282. Wall SM, et al. NaCl restriction upregulates renal Slc26a4 through subcellular redistribution. Role in Cl⁻ conservation. *Hypertension*. 2004;44(6):982-987.

283. Verlander JW, et al. Deoxycorticosterone upregulates PDS (Slc26a4) in mouse kidney: role of pendrin in mineralocorticoid-induced hypertension. *Hypertension*. 2003;42:356-362.

284. Verlander JW, et al. Dietary Cl(−) restriction upregulates pendrin expression within the apical plasma membrane of type B intercalated cells. *Am J Physiol Renal Physiol*. 2006;291:F833-F839.

285. Eladari D, Chambrey R, Frische S, et al. Pendrin as a regulator of ECF and blood pressure. *Curr Opin Nephrol Hypertens*. 2009;18:356-362.

286. Tomita K, Pisano JJ, Burg MB, et al. Effects of vasopressin and bradykinin on anion transport by the rat cortical collecting duct. Evidence for an electroneutral sodium chloride transport pathway. *J Clin Invest*. 1986;77:136-141.

287. Terada Y, Knepper MA. Thiazide-sensitive NaCl absorption in rat cortical collecting duct. *Am J Physiol*. 1990;259:F519-F528.

288. Leviel F, et al. The Na⁺-dependent chloride-bicarbonate exchanger SLC4A8 mediates an electroneutral Na⁺ reabsorption process in the renal cortical collecting ducts of mice. *J Clin Invest*. 2010;120:1627-1635.

289. Fuller PJ, Young MJ. Mechanisms of mineralocorticoid action. *Hypertension*. 2005;46:1227-1235.

290. Welling PA, Caplan M, Sutters M, et al. Aldosterone-mediated Na/K-ATPase expression is alpha 1 isoform specific in the renal cortical collecting duct. *J Biol Chem*. 1993;268:23469-23476.

291. Le Moellic C, et al. Aldosterone and tight junctions: modulation of claudin-4 phosphorylation in renal collecting duct cells. *Am J Physiol Cell Physiol*. 2005;289:C1513-C1521.

292. Mick VE, et al. The alpha-subunit of the epithelial sodium channel is an aldosterone-induced transcript in mammalian collecting ducts, and this transcriptional response is mediated via distinct cis-elements in the 5'-flanking region of the gene. *Mol Endocrinol*. 2001;15:575-588.
293. Reisenauer MR, et al. AF17 competes with AF9 for binding to Dot1a to up-regulate transcription of epithelial Na+ channel alpha. *J Biol Chem*. 2009;284:35659-35669.
294. Masilamani S, Kim GH, Mitchell C, et al. Aldosterone-mediated regulation of ENaC alpha, beta, and gamma subunit proteins in rat kidney. *J Clin Invest*. 1999;104:R19-R23.
295. Loffing J, et al. Aldosterone induces rapid apical translocation of ENaC in early portion of renal collecting system: possible role of SGK. *Am J Physiol Renal Physiol*. 2001;280:F675-F682.
296. Snyder PM. Minireview: regulation of epithelial Na+ channel trafficking. *Endocrinology*. 2005;146:5079-5085.
297. Chen SY, et al. Epithelial sodium channel regulated by aldosterone-induced protein sgk. *Proc Natl Acad Sci U S A*. 1999;96:2514-2519.
298. Naray-Fejes-Toth A, Canessa C, Cleaveland ES, et al. sgk is an aldosterone-induced kinase in the renal collecting duct. Effects on epithelial Na+ channels. *J Biol Chem*. 1999;274:16973-16978.
299. Kamynina E, Tauxe C, Staub O. Distinct characteristics of two human Nedd4 proteins with respect to epithelial Na(+) channel regulation. *Am J Physiol Renal Physiol*. 2001;281:F469-F477.
300. Snyder PM, Olson DR, Thomas BC. Serum and glucocorticoid-regulated kinase modulates Nedd4-2-mediated inhibition of the epithelial Na+ channel. *J Biol Chem*. 2002;277:5-8.
301. Debonneville C, et al. Phosphorylation of Nedd4-2 by Sgk1 regulates epithelial Na(+) channel cell surface expression. *EMBO J*. 2001;20:7052-7059.
302. Flores SY, et al. Aldosterone-induced serum and glucocorticoid-induced kinase 1 expression is accompanied by Nedd4-2 phosphorylation and increased Na+ transport in cortical collecting duct cells. *J Am Soc Nephrol*. 2005;16:2279-2287.
303. Zhou R, Snyder PM. Nedd4-2 phosphorylation induces serum and glucocorticoid-regulated kinase (SGK) ubiquitination and degradation. *J Biol Chem*. 2005;280:4518-4523.
304. Loffing-Cueni D, et al. Dietary sodium intake regulates the ubiquitin-protein ligase nedd4-2 in the renal collecting system. *J Am Soc Nephrol*. 2006;17:1264-1274.
305. Ergonul Z, Frindt G, Palmer LG. Regulation of maturation and processing of ENaC subunits in the rat kidney. *Am J Physiol Renal Physiol*. 2006;291:F683-F693.
306. Kleyman TR, Myerburg MM, Hughey RP. Regulation of ENaCs by proteases: an increasingly complex story. *Kidney Int*. 2006;70:1391-1392.
307. Vuagniaux G, Vallet V, Jaeger NF, et al. Synergistic activation of ENaC by three membrane-bound channel-activating serine proteases (mCAP1, mCAP2, and mCAP3) and serum- and glucocorticoid-regulated kinase (Sgk1) in *Xenopus* oocytes. *J Gen Physiol*. 2002;120:191-201.
308. Kleyman TR, Carattino MD, Hughey RP. ENaC at the cutting edge: regulation of epithelial sodium channels by proteases. *J Biol Chem*. 2009;284:20447-20451.
309. Vallet V, Chraibi A, Gaeggeler HP, et al. An epithelial serine protease activates the amiloride-sensitive sodium channel. *Nature*. 1997;389:607-610.
310. Narikiyo T, et al. Regulation of prostasin by aldosterone in the kidney. *J Clin Invest*. 2002;109:401-408.
311. Carattino MD, et al. The epithelial Na+ channel is inhibited by a peptide derived from proteolytic processing of its alpha subunit. *J Biol Chem*. 2006;281:18901-18907.
312. Schafer JA. Abnormal regulation of ENaC: syndromes of salt retention and salt wasting by the collecting duct. *Am J Physiol Renal Physiol*. 2002;283:F221-F235.
313. Bugaj V, Pochynyuk O, Stockand JD. Activation of the epithelial Na+ channel in the collecting duct by vasopressin contributes to water reabsorption. *Am J Physiol Renal Physiol*. 2009;297:F1411-F1418.
314. Morris RG, Schafer JA. cAMP increases density of ENaC subunits in the apical membrane of MDCK cells in direct proportion to amiloride-sensitive Na(+) transport. *J Gen Physiol*. 2002;120:71-85.
315. Butterworth MB, Edinger RS, Johnson JP, et al. Acute ENaC stimulation by cAMP in a kidney cell line is mediated by exocytic insertion from a recycling channel pool. *J Gen Physiol*. 2005;125:81-101.
316. Snyder PM, Olson DR, Kabra R, et al. cAMP and serum and glucocorticoid-inducible kinase (SGK) regulate the epithelial Na(+) channel through convergent phosphorylation of Nedd4-2. *J Biol Chem*. 2004;279:45753-45758.
317. Ecelbarger CA, et al. Vasopressin-mediated regulation of epithelial sodium channel abundance in rat kidney. *Am J Physiol Renal Physiol*. 2000;279:F46-F53.
318. Peti-Peterdi J, Warnock DG, Bell PD. Angiotensin II directly stimulates ENaC activity in the cortical collecting duct via AT(1) receptors. *J Am Soc Nephrol*. 2002;13:1131-1135.
319. Pech V, et al. Angiotensin II increases chloride absorption in the cortical collecting duct in mice through a pendrin-dependent mechanism. *Am J Physiol Renal Physiol*. 2007;292:F914-F920.
320. Komlosi P, et al. Angiotensin I conversion to angiotensin II stimulates cortical collecting duct sodium transport. *Hypertension*. 2003;42:195-199.
321. Rohrwasser A, et al. Elements of a paracrine tubular renin-angiotensin system along the entire nephron. *Hypertension*. 1999;34:1265-1274.
322. Lehrmann H, Thomas J, Kim SJ, et al. Luminal P2Y2 receptor-mediated inhibition of Na+ absorption in isolated perfused mouse CCD. *J Am Soc Nephrol*. 2002;13:10-18.
323. Pochynyuk O, et al. Paracrine regulation of the epithelial Na+ channel in the mammalian collecting duct by purinergic P2Y2 receptor tone. *J Biol Chem*. 2008;283:36599-36607.
324. Rieg T, et al. Mice lacking P2Y2 receptors have salt-resistant hypertension and facilitated renal Na+ and water reabsorption. *FASEB J*. 2007;21(13):3717-3726.
325. Pochynyuk O, et al. Dietary Na+ inhibits the open probability of the epithelial sodium channel in the kidney by enhancing apical P2Y2-receptor tone. *FASEB J*. 2010;24:2056-2065.
326. Wildman SS, et al. Sodium-dependent regulation of renal amiloride-sensitive currents by apical P2 receptors. *J Am Soc Nephrol*. 2008;19:731-742.
327. Wei Y, et al. Arachidonic acid inhibits epithelial Na channel via cytochrome P450 (CYP) epoxygenase-dependent metabolic pathways. *J Gen Physiol*. 2004;124:719-727.
328. Nakagawa K, et al. Salt-sensitive hypertension is associated with dysfunctional Cyp4a10 gene and kidney epithelial sodium channel. *J Clin Invest*. 2006;116:1696-1702.
329. Guan Y, et al. Thiazolidinediones expand body fluid volume through PPARγ stimulation of ENaC-mediated renal salt absorption. *Nat Med*. 2005;11:861-866.
330. Zhang H, et al. Collecting duct–specific deletion of peroxisome proliferator–activated receptor gamma blocks thiazolidinedione-induced fluid retention. *Proc Natl Acad Sci U S A*. 2005;102:9406-9411.
331. Hong G, et al. PPARγ activation enhances cell surface ENaCα via up-regulation of SGK1 in human collecting duct cells. *FASEB J*. 2003;17:1966-1968.
332. Artunc F, et al. Lack of the serum and glucocorticoid-inducible kinase SGK1 attenuates the volume retention after treatment with the PPARγ agonist pioglitazone. *Pflugers Arch*. 2008;456:425-436.
333. Pavlov TS, Levchenko V, Karpushev AV, et al. Peroxisome proliferator-activated receptor gamma antagonists decrease Na+ transport via the epithelial Na+ channel. *Mol Pharmacol*. 2009;76:1333-1340.
334. Vallon V, et al. Thiazolidinedione-induced fluid retention is independent of collecting duct αENaC activity. *J Am Soc Nephrol*. 2009;20:721-729.
335. Karalliedde J, et al. Effect of various diuretic treatments on rosiglitazone-induced fluid retention. *J Am Soc Nephrol*. 2006;17(12):3482-3490.
336. Alvarez de la Rosa D, Canessa CM. Role of SGK in hormonal regulation of epithelial sodium channel in A6 cells. *Am J Physiol Cell Physiol*. 2003;284:C404-C414.
337. Wang J, et al. SGK integrates insulin and mineralocorticoid regulation of epithelial sodium transport. *Am J Physiol Renal Physiol*. 2001;280:F303-F313.
338. Sausbier M, et al. Distal colonic K(+) secretion occurs via BK channels. *J Am Soc Nephrol*. 2006;17:1275-1282.
339. Bastl C, Hayslett JP, Binder HJ. Increased large intestinal secretion of potassium in renal insufficiency. *Kidney Int*. 1977;12:9-16.
340. Bomsztyk K, Wright FS. Dependence of ion fluxes on fluid transport by rat proximal tubule. *Am J Physiol*. 1986;250:F680-F689.
341. Kaufman JS, Hamburger RJ. Passive potassium transport in the proximal convoluted tubule. *Am J Physiol*. 1985;248:F228-F232.
342. Wilson RW, Wareing M, Green R. The role of active transport in potassium reabsorption in the proximal convoluted tubule of the anaesthetized rat. *J Physiol*. 1997;500(pt 1):155-164.
343. Kibble JD, Wareing M, Wilson RW, et al. Effect of barium on potassium diffusion across the proximal convoluted tubule of the anesthetized rat. *Am J Physiol*. 1995;268:F778-F783.
344. Wilson RW, Wareing M, Kibble J, et al. Potassium permeability in the absence of fluid reabsorption in proximal tubule of the anesthetized rat. *Am J Physiol*. 1998;274:F1109-F1112.
345. Wareing M, Wilson RW, Kibble JD, et al. Estimated potassium reflection coefficient in perfused proximal convoluted tubules of the anaesthetized rat in vivo. *J Physiol*. 1995;488(pt 1):153-161.
346. Johnston PA, Battilana CA, Lacy FB, et al. Evidence for a concentration gradient favoring outward movement of sodium from the thin loop of Henle. *J Clin Invest*. 1977;59:234-240.
347. Battilana CA, et al. Effect of chronic potassium loading on potassium secretion by the pars recta or descending limb of the juxtamedullary nephron in the rat. *J Clin Invest*. 1978;62:1093-1103.
348. Elalouf JM, Roinel N, de Rouffignac C. Effects of dDAVP on rat juxtamedullary nephrons: stimulation of medullary K recycling. *Am J Physiol*. 1985;249:F291-F298.

349. Tabei K, Imai M. K transport in upper portion of descending limbs of long-loop nephron from hamster. *Am J Physiol.* 1987;252:F387-F392.

350. Schnermann J, Weihprecht H, Briggs JP. Inhibition of tubuloglomerular feedback during adenosine1 receptor blockade. *Am J Physiol.* 1990;258:F553-F561.

351. Giebisch G. Renal potassium transport: mechanisms and regulation. *Am J Physiol.* 1998;274:F817-F833.

352. Muto S. Potassium transport in the mammalian collecting duct. *Physiol Rev.* 2001;81:85-116.

353. Stokes JB. Potassium secretion by cortical collecting tubule: relation to sodium absorption, luminal sodium concentration, and transepithelial voltage. *Am J Physiol.* 1981;241:F395-F402.

354. Pluznick JL, Sansom SC. BK channels in the kidney: role in K(+) secretion and localization of molecular components. *Am J Physiol Renal Physiol.* 2006;291:F517-F529.

355. Gray DA, Frindt G, Palmer LG. Quantification of K^+ secretion through apical low-conductance K channels in the CCD. *Am J Physiol Renal Physiol.* 2005;289:F117-F126.

356. Palmer LG, Choe H, Frindt G. Is the secretory K channel in the rat CCT ROMK? *Am J Physiol.* 1997;273:F404-F410.

357. Bailey MA, et al. Maxi-K channels contribute to urinary potassium excretion in the ROMK-deficient mouse model of type II Bartter's syndrome and in adaptation to a high-K diet. *Kidney Int.* 2006;70:51-59.

358. Grimm PR, Foutz RM, Brenner R, et al. Identification and localization of BK-beta subunits in the distal nephron of the mouse kidney. *Am J Physiol Renal Physiol.* 2007;293:F350-F359.

359. Woda CB, Bragin A, Kleyman TR, et al. Flow-dependent K^+ secretion in the cortical collecting duct is mediated by a maxi-K channel. *Am J Physiol Renal Physiol.* 2001;280:F786-F793.

360. Rieg T, et al. The role of the BK channel in potassium homeostasis and flow-induced renal potassium excretion. *Kidney Int.* 2007;72(5):566-573.

361. Grimm PR, Irsik DL, Settles DC, et al. Hypertension of Kcnmb1$^{-/-}$ is linked to deficient K secretion and aldosteronism. *Proc Natl Acad Sci U S A.* 2009;106:11800-11805.

362. Pacha J, Frindt G, Sackin H, et al. Apical maxi K channels in intercalated cells of CCT. *Am J Physiol.* 1991;261:F696-F705.

363. Palmer LG, Frindt G. High-conductance K channels in intercalated cells of the rat distal nephron. *Am J Physiol Renal Physiol.* 2007;292:F966-F973.

364. Holtzclaw JD, Grimm PR, Sansom SC. Intercalated cell BK-alpha/beta4 channels modulate sodium and potassium handling during potassium adaptation. *J Am Soc Nephrol.* 2010;21:634-645.

365. Giebisch GH. A trail of research on potassium. *Kidney Int.* 2002;62:1498-1512.

366. Giebisch G. Renal potassium channels: function, regulation, and structure. *Kidney Int.* 2001;60:436-445.

367. Lesage F, Lazdunski M. Molecular and functional properties of two-pore-domain potassium channels. *Am J Physiol Renal Physiol.* 2000;279:F793-F801.

368. Zheng W, et al. Cellular distribution of the potassium channel KCNQ1 in normal mouse kidney. *Am J Physiol Renal Physiol.* 2007;292(1):F456-466.

369. Carrisoza-Gaytan R, et al. Potassium secretion by voltage-gated potassium channel Kv1.3 in the rat kidney. *Am J Physiol Renal Physiol.* 2010;299:F255-F264.

370. Glaudemans B, et al. A missense mutation in the Kv1.1 voltage-gated potassium channel-encoding gene KCNA1 is linked to human autosomal dominant hypomagnesemia. *J Clin Invest.* 2009;119:936-942.

371. Gray DA, Frindt G, Zhang YY, et al. Basolateral K^+ conductance in principal cells of rat CCD. *Am J Physiol Renal Physiol.* 2005;288:F493-F504.

372. Lachheb S, et al. Kir4.1/Kir5.1 channel forms the major K^+ channel in the basolateral membrane of mouse renal collecting duct principal cells. *Am J Physiol Renal Physiol.* 2008;294:F1398-F1407.

373. Zhou X, Xia SL, Wingo CS. Chloride transport by the rabbit cortical collecting duct: dependence on H, K-ATPase. *J Am Soc Nephrol.* 1998;9:2194-2202.

374. Amorim JB, Bailey MA, Musa-Aziz R, et al. Role of luminal anion and pH in distal tubule potassium secretion. *Am J Physiol Renal Physiol.* 2003;284:F381-F388.

375. Ellison DH, Velazquez H, Wright FS. Unidirectional potassium fluxes in renal distal tubule: effects of chloride and barium. *Am J Physiol.* 1986;250:F885-F894.

376. Velazquez H, Ellison DH, Wright FS. Chloride-dependent potassium secretion in early and late renal distal tubules. *Am J Physiol.* 1987;253:F555-F562.

377. Wingo CS. Potassium secretion by the cortical collecting tubule: effect of C1 gradients and ouabain. *Am J Physiol.* 1989;256:F306-F313.

378. Schafer JA, Troutman SL. Potassium transport in cortical collecting tubules from mineralocorticoid-treated rat. *Am J Physiol.* 1987;253:F76-F88.

379. Frindt G, Palmer LG. K^+ secretion in the rat kidney: Na^+ channel-dependent and -independent mechanisms. *Am J Physiol Renal Physiol.* 2009;297:F389-F396.

380. Zhou X, Lynch IJ, Xia SL, et al. Activation of H^+-K^+-ATPase by CO_2 requires a basolateral Ba^{2+}-sensitive pathway during K restriction. *Am J Physiol Renal Physiol.* 2000;279:F153-F160.

381. Jaisser F, Beggah AT. The nongastric H^+-K^+-ATPases: molecular and functional properties. *Am J Physiol.* 1999;276:F812-F824.

382. Kraut JA, et al. Detection and localization of H^+-K^+-ATPase isoforms in human kidney. *Am J Physiol Renal Physiol.* 2001;281:F763-F768.

383. Sangan P, Thevananther S, Sangan S, et al. Colonic H-K-ATPase alpha- and beta-subunits express ouabain-insensitive H-K-ATPase. *Am J Physiol Cell Physiol.* 2000;278:C182-C189.

384. Fejes-Toth G, Naray-Fejes-Toth A, Velazquez H. Intrarenal distribution of the colonic H, K-ATPase mRNA in rabbit. *Kidney Int.* 1999;56:1029-1036.

385. Verlander JW, Moudy RM, Campbell WG, et al. Immunohistochemical localization of H-K-ATPase alpha(2c)-subunit in rabbit kidney. *Am J Physiol Renal Physiol.* 2001;281:F357-F365.

386. Fejes-Toth G, Naray-Fejes-Toth A. Immunohistochemical localization of colonic H-K-ATPase to the apical membrane of connecting tubule cells. *Am J Physiol Renal Physiol.* 2001;281:F318-F325.

387. Silver RB, Soleimani M. H^+-K^+-ATPases: regulation and role in pathophysiological states. *Am J Physiol.* 1999;276:F799-F811.

388. Meneton P, et al. Increased sensitivity to K^+ deprivation in colonic H, K-ATPase-deficient mice. *J Clin Invest.* 1998;101:536-542.

389. Spicer Z, et al. Stomachs of mice lacking the gastric H, K-ATPase alpha-subunit have achlorhydria, abnormal parietal cells, and ciliated metaplasia. *J Biol Chem.* 2000;275:21555-21565.

390. Petrovic S, Spicer Z, Greeley T, et al. Novel Schering and ouabain-insensitive potassium-dependent proton secretion in the mouse cortical collecting duct. *Am J Physiol Renal Physiol.* 2002;282:F133-F143.

391. Dherbecourt O, Cheval L, Bloch-Faure M, et al. Molecular identification of Sch28080-sensitive K-ATPase activities in the mouse kidney. *Pflugers Arch.* 2006;451:769-775.

392. Abuladze N, et al. Axial heterogeneity of sodium-bicarbonate cotransporter expression in the rabbit proximal tubule. *Am J Physiol.* 1998;274:F628-F633.

393. August JT, Nelson DH, Thorn GW. Response of normal subjects to large amounts of aldosterone. *J Clin Invest.* 1958;37:1549-1555.

394. Palmer LG, Frindt G. Aldosterone and potassium secretion by the cortical collecting duct. *Kidney Int.* 2000;57:1324-1328.

395. Palmer LG, Antonian L, Frindt G. Regulation of apical K and Na channels and Na/K pumps in rat cortical collecting tubule by dietary K. *J Gen Physiol.* 1994;104:693-710.

396. Muto S, Sansom S, Giebisch G. Effects of a high potassium diet on electrical properties of cortical collecting ducts from adrenalectomized rabbits. *J Clin Invest.* 1988;81:376-380.

397. Muto S, Asano Y, Seldin D, et al. Basolateral Na^+ pump modulates apical Na^+ and K^+ conductances in rabbit cortical collecting ducts. *Am J Physiol.* 1999;276:F143-F158.

398. Lin DH, et al. Protein tyrosine kinase is expressed and regulates ROMK1 location in the cortical collecting duct. *Am J Physiol Renal Physiol.* 2004;286:F881-F892.

399. Palmer LG, Frindt G. Regulation of apical K channels in rat cortical collecting tubule during changes in dietary K intake. *Am J Physiol.* 1999;277:F805-F812.

400. Frindt G, Shah A, Edvinsson J, et al. Dietary K regulates ROMK channels in connecting tubule and cortical collecting duct of rat kidney. *Am J Physiol Renal Physiol.* 2009;296:F347-F354.

401. Najjar F, et al. Dietary K^+ regulates apical membrane expression of maxi-K channels in rabbit cortical collecting duct. *Am J Physiol Renal Physiol.* 2005;289:F922-F932.

402. Estilo G, et al. Effect of aldosterone on BK channel expression in mammalian cortical collecting duct. *Am J Physiol Renal Physiol.* 2008;295:F780-F788.

403. Kahle KT, et al. WNK4 regulates the balance between renal NaCl reabsorption and K^+ secretion. *Nat Genet.* 2003;35:372-376.

404. Delaloy C, et al. Multiple promoters in the WNK1 gene: one controls expression of a kidney-specific kinase-defective isoform. *Mol Cell Biol.* 2003;23:9208-9221.

405. Cope G, et al. WNK1 affects surface expression of the ROMK potassium channel independent of WNK4. *J Am Soc Nephrol.* 2006;17:1867-1874.

406. Wade JB, et al. WNK1 kinase isoform switch regulates renal potassium excretion. *Proc Natl Acad Sci U S A.* 2006;103:8558-8563.

407. Lazrak A, Liu Z, Huang CL. Antagonistic regulation of ROMK by long and kidney-specific WNK1 isoforms. *Proc Natl Acad Sci U S A.* 2006;103:1615-1620.

408. He G, Wang HR, Huang SK, et al. Intersectin links WNK kinases to endocytosis of ROMK1. *J Clin Invest.* 2007;117:1078-1087.

409. Fang L, Garuti R, Kim BY, et al. The ARH adaptor protein regulates endocytosis of the ROMK potassium secretory channel in mouse kidney. *J Clin Invest.* 2009;119:3278-3789.

410. Lin DH, et al. POSH stimulates the ubiquitination and the clathrin-independent endocytosis of ROMK1 channels. *J Biol Chem*. 2009;284:29614-29624.

411. O'Reilly M, et al. Dietary electrolyte-driven responses in the renal WNK kinase pathway in vivo. *J Am Soc Nephrol*. 2006;17:2402-2413.

412. Liu Z, Wang HR, Huang CL. Regulation of ROMK channel and K⁺ homeostasis by kidney-specific WNK1 kinase. *J Biol Chem*. 2009;284:12198-12206.

413. Ornt DB, Tannen RL. Demonstration of an intrinsic renal adaptation for K⁺ conservation in short-term K⁺ depletion. *Am J Physiol*. 1983;245:F329-F338.

414. Eiam-Ong S, Kurtzman NA, Sabatini S. Regulation of collecting tubule adenosine triphosphatases by aldosterone and potassium. *J Clin Invest*. 1993;91:2385-2392.

415. Mennitt PA, Frindt G, Silver RB, et al. Potassium restriction downregulates ROMK expression in rat kidney. *Am J Physiol Renal Physiol*. 2000;278:F916-F924.

416. Lin DH, et al. K depletion increases protein tyrosine kinase-mediated phosphorylation of ROMK. *Am J Physiol Renal Physiol*. 2002;283:F671-F677.

417. Sterling H, et al. Inhibition of protein-tyrosine phosphatase stimulates the dynamin-dependent endocytosis of ROMK1. *J Biol Chem*. 2002;277:4317-4323.

418. Lin DH, Sterling H, Wang WH. The protein tyrosine kinase-dependent pathway mediates the effect of K intake on renal K secretion. *Physiology (Bethesda)*. 2005;20:140-146.

419. Wei Y, Bloom P, Lin D, et al. Effect of dietary K intake on apical small-conductance K channel in CCD: role of protein tyrosine kinase. *Am J Physiol Renal Physiol*. 2001;281:F206-F212.

420. Babilonia E, et al. Superoxide anions are involved in mediating the effect of low K intake on c-Src expression and renal K secretion in the cortical collecting duct. *J Biol Chem*. 2005;280:10790-10796.

421. Babilonia E, et al. Role of gp91phox -containing NADPH oxidase in mediating the effect of K restriction on ROMK channels and renal K excretion. *J Am Soc Nephrol*. 2007;18:2037-2045.

422. Wang ZJ, et al. Decrease in dietary K intake stimulates the generation of superoxide anions in the kidney and inhibits K secretory channels in the CCD. *Am J Physiol Renal Physiol*. 2010;298:F1515-F1522.

423. Wei Y, Zavilowitz B, Satlin LM, et al. Angiotensin II inhibits the ROMK-like small conductance K channel in renal cortical collecting duct during dietary potassium restriction. *J Biol Chem*. 2007;282:6455-6462.

424. Jin Y, Wang Y, Wang ZJ, et al. Inhibition of angiotensin type 1 receptor impairs renal ability of K conservation in response to K restriction. *Am J Physiol Renal Physiol*. 2009;296:F1179-F1184.

425. Babilonia E, et al. Mitogen-activated protein kinases inhibit the ROMK (Kir 1.1)–like small conductance K channels in the cortical collecting duct. *J Am Soc Nephrol*. 2006;17:2687-2696.

426. Li D, et al. Inhibition of MAPK stimulates the Ca²⁺-dependent big-conductance K channels in cortical collecting duct. *Proc Natl Acad Sci U S A*. 2006;103:19569-19574.

427. Ring AM, et al. An SGK1 site in WNK4 regulates Na⁺ channel and K⁺ channel activity and has implications for aldosterone signaling and K⁺ homeostasis. *Proc Natl Acad Sci U S A*. 2007;104:4025-4029.

428. Yue P, et al. Src family protein tyrosine kinase (PTK) modulates the effect of SGK1 and WNK4 on ROMK channels. *Proc Natl Acad Sci U S A*. 2009;106:15061-15066.

429. Rabinowitz L. Aldosterone and potassium homeostasis. *Kidney Int*. 1996;49:1738-1742.

430. McDonough AA, Youn JH. Role of muscle in regulating extracellular [K+]. *Semin Nephrol*. 2005;25:335-342.

431. Chen P, et al. Modest dietary K⁺ restriction provokes insulin resistance of cellular K⁺ uptake and phosphorylation of renal outer medulla K⁺ channel without fall in plasma K⁺ concentration. *Am J Physiol Cell Physiol*. 2006;290:C1355-C1363.

432. El Moghrabi S, et al. Tissue kallikrein permits early renal adaptation to potassium load. *Proc Natl Acad Sci U S A*. 2010;107:13526-13531.

433. Field MJ, Stanton BA, Giebisch GH. Influence of ADH on renal potassium handling: a micropuncture and microperfusion study. *Kidney Int*. 1984;25:502-511.

434. Cassola AC, Giebisch G, Wang W. Vasopressin increases density of apical low-conductance K⁺ channels in rat CCD. *Am J Physiol*. 1993;264:F502-F509.

435. Amorim JB, Musa-Aziz R, Mello-Aires M, et al. Signaling path of the action of AVP on distal K⁺ secretion. *Kidney Int*. 2004;66:696-704.

436. Welling PA, Chang YP, Delpire E, et al. Multigene kinase network, kidney transport, and salt in essential hypertension. *Kidney Int*. 2010;77:1063-1069.

437. Sandberg MB, Riquier AD, Pihakaski-Maunsbach K, et al. ANG II provokes acute trafficking of distal tubule Na⁺-Cl⁻ cotransporter to apical membrane. *Am J Physiol Renal Physiol*. 2007;293:F662-F669.

438. Yang LE, Sandberg MB, Can AD, et al. Effects of dietary salt on renal Na⁺ transporter subcellular distribution, abundance, and phosphorylation status. *Am J Physiol Renal Physiol*. 2008;295:F1003-F1016.

439. Sealey JE, Clark I, Bull MB, et al. Potassium balance and the control of renin secretion. *J Clin Invest*. 1970;49:2119-2127.

440. Sterling D, Brown NJ, Supuran CT, et al. The functional and physical relationship between the DRA bicarbonate transporter and carbonic anhydrase II. *Am J Physiol Cell Physiol*. 2002;283:C1522-C1529.

441. Nijenhuis T, Hoenderop JG, van der Kemp AW, et al. Localization and regulation of the epithelial Ca²⁺ channel TRPV6 in the kidney. *J Am Soc Nephrol*. 2003;14:2731-2740.

442. Voets T, et al. TRPM6 forms the Mg²⁺ influx channel involved in intestinal and renal Mg²⁺ absorption. *J Biol Chem*. 2004;279:19-25.

Aldosterone Regulation of Ion Transport

David Pearce, Vivek Bhalla, John W. Funder, and John B. Stokes

In mammals, the control of extracellular fluid volume and blood pressure is intimately intertwined with the regulation of epithelial ion transport. Aldosterone, which is essential for survival, is the central hormone regulating the relevant epithelial transport processes, particularly of ions such as Na^+, K^+, and Cl^-. Virtually all circulating aldosterone is generated in the adrenal glomerulosa, where its synthesis and secretion are under the control of angiotensin II and potassium, and its major epithelial actions occur in the distal nephron and colon. The former extends from the late distal convoluted tubule (DCT) through the connecting segment and the entire cortical and medullary collecting ducts. These segments, rich in the mineralocorticoid receptor (MR), are often referred to as the *aldosterone-sensitive distal nephron* (ASDN).[1] Most if not all effects of aldosterone are mediated by MR, a hormone-regulated transcription factor related closely to the glucocorticoid receptor and more distantly to other members of the nuclear receptor superfamily. The physiologic effects of aldosterone on epithelia entail direct gene regulatory actions of MR. Thus, a sound foundation for understanding aldosterone's physiologic effects on the extracellular fluid, blood pressure, and electrolyte concentrations can be had through familiarity with MR-dependent effects on the transcription of various genes, which in turn alter epithelial ion transport. Aldosterone actions in certain disease states involve both genomic and nongenomic effects in both epithelial and nonepithelial tissues. This chapter addresses the cellular and molecular mechanisms underlying aldosterone action, focusing primarily on its effects on ion transport in epithelia, but also highlighting key aspects of nonepithelial actions, which are of particular importance to its pathophysiologic effect.

General Introduction to Aldosterone and Mineralocorticoid Receptors

Steroid hormones are derived from cholesterol and produced in systemically relevant amounts in a relatively narrow range of tissues (adrenal glands, gonads, placenta, skin).

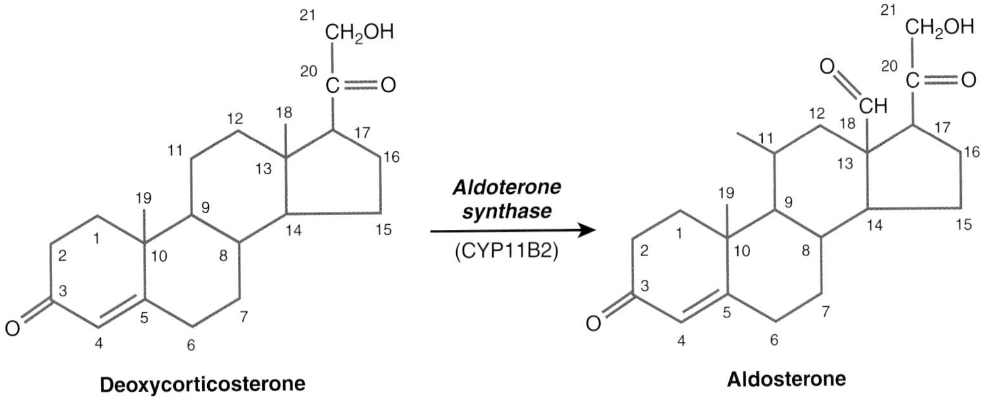

Deoxycorticosterone

Aldoterone synthase

(CYP11B2)

Aldosterone

FIGURE 6-1 Final step in aldosterone synthesis. Note that the hemiacetal form of aldosterone is shown. Most aldosterone (>99%) exists as the hemiketal form, which is cyclized and does not allow access of 11β-hydroxysteroid dehydrogenase type 2 (11β-HSD2) to the 11-hydroxyl. See text for details.

In mammalian physiology six classes of steroid hormones are commonly recognized: mineralocorticoid, glucocorticoid, androgen, estrogen, progestin, and the secosteroid vitamin D_3. This classification was based on their observed effects and has proven robust despite our current appreciation of a much more diverse physiology of steroid hormones over and above their classical roles. In further support of this original classification is the characterization of six intracellular receptors (mineralocorticoid, MR; glucocorticoid, GR; androgen, AR; estrogen, ER; progestin, PR; vitamin D_3, VDR). As addressed further later, it is now appreciated that a one-to-one relationship between receptor and hormone does not hold, and this is particularly the case for MR. Aldosterone was isolated and characterized in 1953. Crucial for its isolation was the application of radioisotopic techniques to measure $[Na^+]$ and $[K^+]$ flux across epithelia in the laboratory of Sylvia Simpson, a biologist, and Jim Tait, a physicist.[2,3] Because of this, the active principle was initially called *electrocortin*; the name was soon changed to *aldosterone* when its unique aldehyde (rather than methyl) group at carbon 18 was discovered in collaborative studies between investigators in London and Basel.[4] Aldosterone is commonly depicted so as to highlight this aldehyde group (Figure 6-1, *left*). In vivo, the very reactive aldehyde group cyclizes with the β-hydroxyl group at carbon 11 to form the 11,18 hemiacetal (see Figure 6-1, *right*) and in addition may exist in an 11,18 hemiketal form. This cyclization of the 11β-hydroxyl group protects aldosterone from dehydrogenation by the enzyme 11β-hydroxysteroid dehydrogenase in epithelial tissue, which enables it to activate epithelial MR and thus regulate ion transport at very low (subnanomolar) circulating levels.[5,6] There is broad evidence that aldosterone is not the only cognate ligand for MR, its essential effects via MR on epithelial ion transport notwithstanding. MRs are found in high abundance in the hippocampus and cardiomyocytes, and in such nonepithelial tissues—which lack 11β-hydroxysteroid dehydrogenase type 2 (11β-HSD2; see "11β-Hydroxysteroid Dehydrogenase Type 2" section later)—are essentially constitutively occupied by glucocorticoids (cortisol in humans, corticosterone in rodents). This is due to the comparable affinity and markedly higher plasma free levels (≥100-fold) of glucocorticoids compared with those of aldosterone. In terms of evolution, MR appeared well before aldosterone synthase (e.g., in fish).[7] It is commonly assumed that MR and GR share a common immediate evolutionary precursor,[8] although this has recently been challenged on sequence grounds,[9] and MR may have been the first of the MR/GR/AR/PR subfamily to branch off the ancestral receptor. A final reason not to equate MR and aldosterone action derives from a comparison of the MR knockout and aldosterone synthase knockout ($AS^{-/-}$) phenotypes. MR knockout mice (which lack all functional MR) cannot survive sodium restriction; $AS^{-/-}$ mice (which have no detectable aldosterone) survive even stringent sodium restriction, but die when their fluid intake is restricted to that of wild-type animals.[10] This suggests an as yet poorly defined dependence upon aldosterone for vasopressin action, mediated via mechanisms other than classical MR.[11]

Aldosterone Synthesis

Aldosterone is synthesized in the adrenal cortex, which has three functional zones. The outermost layer of cells represents the zona glomerulosa, which is the unique site of aldosterone biosynthesis. Cortisol is synthesized in the middle zone, the zona fasciculata, and the innermost zona reticularis secretes adrenal androgens in many species, including humans, but not in rats or mice. Normally the glomerulosa secretes aldosterone at the rate of 50 to 200 µg/day, to give plasma levels of 4 to 21 µg/dL; in contrast, secretion of cortisol is at levels 200- to 500-fold higher. Underlying the separate synthesis of cortisol and aldosterone is expression of the enzyme 17α-hydroxylase uniquely in the zona fasciculata, and that of aldosterone synthase uniquely in the glomerulosa.

In most species, aldosterone synthase, or cytochrome P450 (CYP) enzyme 11B2, is responsible for the conversion of deoxycortisterone to aldosterone in a three-step process of sequential 11β-hydroxylation, 18-hydroxylation, and 18-methyl oxidation, to produce the characteristic C18-aldehyde from which aldosterone derives its name (Figure 6-2, *left*). Although CYP11B2 is distinct from CYP11B1 (11β-hydroxylase) in most species,[12,13] in some (e.g., bovine) only a single CYP11B is expressed. How this enzyme is responsible for the three-step process of aldosterone synthesis in the glomerulosa but not the fasciculata is yet to be determined.

Figure 6-2 also shows key steps in biosynthesis of cortisol to illustrate the overlap and similarities with that of aldosterone. The genes encoding CYP11B1 and CYP11B2 lie close to one another on human chromosome band 8q24.3, so that an unequal crossing over at meiosis has been shown to be responsible for the syndrome of glucocorticoid remediable aldosteronism, in which the 3′ end of the CYP11B1 is fused to the 5′ end of CYP11B2. The chimeric gene product[14] is expressed in the fasciculata and responds to adrenocorticotrophic hormone (ACTH) with aldosterone synthesis, producing a syndrome of

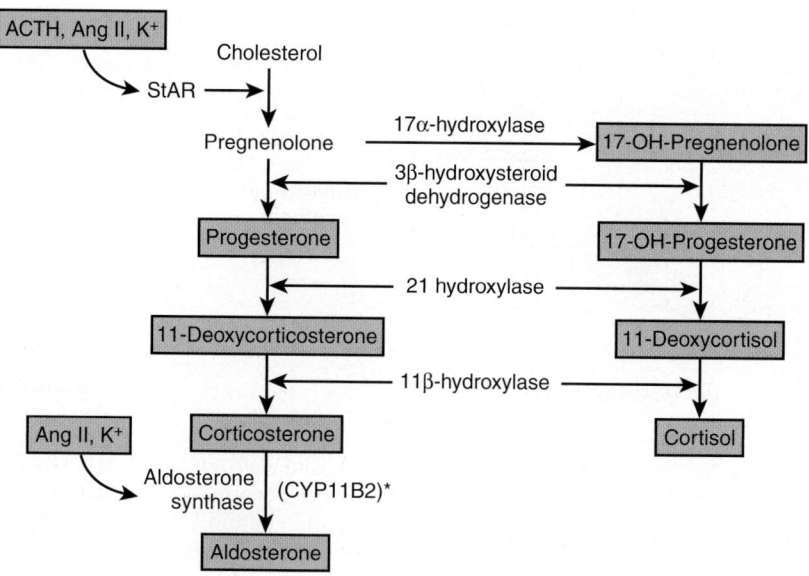

FIGURE 6-2 Overview of aldosterone synthetic pathway showing key regulatory nodes. Note that adrenocorticotropic hormone (ACTH), angiotensin II (Ang II), and K^+ regulate steroidogenic acute regulatory protein (StAR), which stimulates cholesterol uptake by mitochondria and thus substrate availability for synthesis of all of the steroid hormones. Aldosterone synthase (AS; gene name CYP11B2), which is selectively expressed in the adrenal glomerulosa, mediates the final step in aldosterone synthesis. It is also regulated by Ang II and K^+. Aldosterone synthesis is shown on the *left*. Cortisol synthesis is also shown (*right*) to emphasize the interconnections and similarities between these pathways.

*Aldosterone synthase = CYP11B2

juvenile-onset hyperaldosteronism and hypertension. The final step in synthesizing aldosterone involves 11β-hydroxylation, 18-hydroxylation, and 18-methyl oxidation, all of which can be catalyzed by aldosterone synthase, or CYP11B2, present in the cells of the zona glomerulosa (see Figure 6-1).

Normal glomerulosa secretion of aldosterone is primarily regulated by angiotensin II in response to posture and acute lowering of circulating volume, to plasma $[K^+]$ in response to chronic Na^+ deficiency or potassium loading, and to ACTH to the extent of entrainment of the circadian fluctuation in plasma aldosterone levels with those of cortisol. Aldosterone secretion is lowered by high levels of atrial natriuretic peptide and by the administration of heparin, somatostatin, and dopamine. As yet incompletely characterized molecules of adipocyte origin have been shown to stimulate aldosterone secretion in vitro, and roles in the metabolic syndrome have been proposed on this basis.[15]

Angiotensin and plasma $[K^+]$ stimulate aldosterone secretion primarily by increasing the expression and activity of key steroidogenic enzymes as well as the steroidogenic acute regulatory protein (StAR).[16] StAR is required for cholesterol transport into mitochondria and hence is available for steroid synthesis.[17] Regulated steroidogenic enzymes include side-chain cleavage enzyme, 3β-hydroxysteroid dehydrogenase, and, most notably, aldosterone synthase, which mediates the final step in aldosterone synthesis. Common to the mechanism of stimulation by angiotensin II and $[K^+]$ is elevation of intracellular $[Ca^{2+}]$; angiotensin activates angiotensin type I receptors in the glomerulosa cell membrane, which in turn activate phospholipase C, and elevated $[K^+]$ increases intracellular $[Ca^{2+}]$ by depolarizing the cell membrane and activating voltage-sensitive Ca^{2+} channels.[18,19] Subsequently, the pathways diverge, with the $[K^+]$ effect but not the angiotensin effect dependent on Ca^{2+} calmodulin kinase. Patients taking angiotensin converting enzyme inhibitors or angiotensin receptor blockers usually show a degree of suppression of aldosterone secretion, reflected in a modest (0.2 to 0.3 μg/L) elevation in plasma $[K^+]$. This is often sufficient to establish a new steady state, with plasma aldosterone levels rising into the

normal range, a process best termed *breakthrough* rather than *escape*, given the time-honored usage of the latter for escape from progression of the salt and water effect of mineralocorticoid excess in the medium and long term.[20]

Recent data have shed new light on the regulation of aldosterone production by the adrenal glomerulosa in health and disease. Choi and associates found recurrent somatic mutations in the K^+ channel Kir3.4 (encoded by the gene KCNJ5), which were present in more than a third of human aldosterone-producing adenomas studied.[351] These mutations increased Na^+ conductance through Kir3.4 and resulted in increased Ca^{2+} entry and enhanced aldosterone production and glomerulosa cell proliferation. Interestingly, an inherited mutation in KCNJ5 is associated with hypertension associated with marked bilateral adrenal hyperplasia.[352] These findings suggest that KCNJ5 may provide tonic inhibition of aldosterone production and glomerulosa cell proliferation. In glomerulosa cells harboring mutant channel, both proliferation rate and aldosterone synthesis are increased.

Mechanisms of MR Function and Gene Regulation

Mammals cannot survive without MR, except with massive NaCl supplementation. This member of the nuclear receptor superfamily appears to have both genomic and nongenomic actions; however, the latter are not essential to the control of epithelial ion transport. This section focuses exclusively on the function of MR as a hormone-regulated transcription factor.

MR Function as a Hormone-Regulated Transcription: General Features and Subcellular Localization

In the presence of specific agonists, MR binds to specific genomic sites and alters the transcription rate of a subset of genes. Figure 6-3 shows the fundamental paradigm of

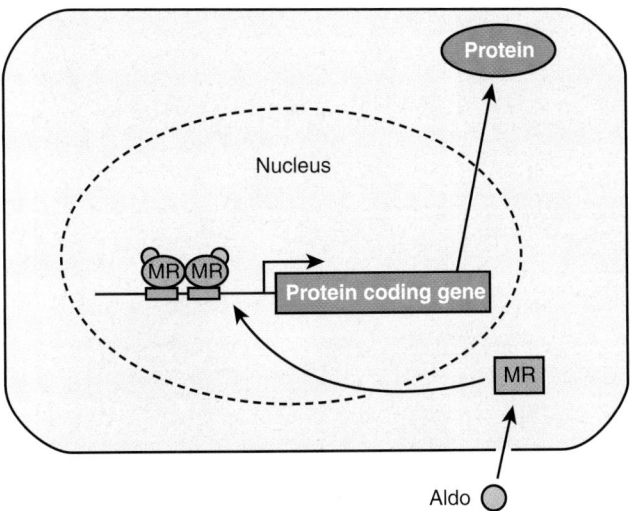

FIGURE 6-3 General mechanism of aldosterone action through the mineralocorticoid receptor (MR). This simple schematic shows the general features of MR regulation of a "simple" hormone response element (HRE), common to a large subset (but not all) of aldosterone-stimulated genes. Note that in the absence of hormone, MR is found in both nucleus and cytoplasm (see Figure 6-6). Aldosterone triggers nuclear translocation of cytoplasmic MR, binding as a dimer to HREs, and stimulation of transcription initiation complex formation (*arrow* upstream of "protein coding gene" defines the site of transcription initiation). See text for further details.

MR function. All nuclear receptors shuttle in and out of the nucleus; however, in the absence of hormone some, such as the estrogen and the vitamin D receptors* are predominantly nuclear, whereas others, like GR, are almost exclusively cytoplasmic. In the absence of hormone, MR is distributed fairly evenly between nuclear and cytoplasmic compartments, but in the presence of hormone, like all steroid-nuclear receptors it is highly concentrated in the nucleus (Figure 6-4).[21,22] It is also notable that in addition to this marked change in MR cellular distribution, its subnuclear organization and protein-protein interactions are also changed.[22] Like its close cousin the GR, the unliganded MR (in the absence of hormone) is complexed with a set of chaperone proteins, which include the heat shock proteins, hsp90, hsp70, and hsp56, and immunophilins.[23,24] This chaperone complex is essential for several aspects of MR function, notably high-affinity hormone binding and trafficking to the nucleus.[24] It was thought for many years that after binding hormone, the hsp90-containing chaperone complex is jettisoned. However, recently it has become clear that this complex remains associated with the receptor and plays an important role in nuclear trafficking.[23] Several members of the immunophilin family—including FKBP52, FKBP51, and CyP40—are present in the chaperone complex, and provide a bridge between hsp90 and the cytoplasmic motor protein dynein, which moves the receptor-hsp90 complex retrograde along microtubules to the nuclear envelope.[24] Here, the receptor is handed off to the nuclear pore

protein, importin-α, and translocated into the nucleus, where it functions as a transcription factor, stimulating transcription of certain genes and repressing the transcriptional activity of others. In the regulation of ion transport, stimulation of key target genes is paramount. Transcriptional repression may be essential for effects in nonepithelial cells, including neurons, cardiomyocytes, smooth muscle cells, and macrophages.[25]

Domain Structure of MR

The MR of all vertebrates is highly conserved. There are only minor differences between MR in rodents and humans.[25] In general, the steroid and nuclear receptors have been divided into three major domains (Figure 6-5): (1) an N-terminal transcriptional regulatory domain; (2) a central DNA-binding domain; and (3) a C-terminal ligand/hormone–binding domain (LBD). Each of these broadly defined domains has more than one function, and not all of the functions can be neatly assigned to separate distinct domains; however, much of what MR does can be understood from this point of view. In the following sections, the domains are described roughly in the historical order in which they were characterized, which also parallels the clarity of functional and structural knowledge about them.

DNA-Binding Domain

The sine qua non of MR function as a transcription factor is its ability to bind specifically to DNA. This protein-DNA interaction is mediated by the receptor's compact modular "DNA-binding domain" (DBD) (amino acids 603 to 688 of human MR; Figure 6-6 shows a strip diagram and two-dimensional structure), which forms a variety of contacts with a specific 15-nucleotide DNA sequence termed a *hormone response element* (HRE). Receptor binding to the HRE in the vicinity of regulated genes promotes the recruitment of coactivators and components of the general transcription machinery, such as the TATA-binding protein (TBP), which binds to the thymidine (T) and adenosine (A)-rich DNA sequence found upstream of many genes and is required for correct transcription initiation. These types of HREs have been identified near or in many of the key MR-regulated genes, such as SGK1 (serum- and glucocorticoid-regulated kinase 1), GILZ (glucocorticoid-induced leucine zipper), and α ENaC (epithelial Na channel, α-subunit) Although in many cases, differential binding to HREs is a key determinant of the specificity of many transcription factors, it should be noted that some steroid receptors (notably MR and GR) have only minor differences within this domain and have identical DNA-binding properties.[26] Specificity in these cases is determined through other mechanisms.[25,27]

The canonical MR HRE is a 15-nucleotide sequence that forms a partial palindrome (inverted repeat), which is bound by a receptor homodimer. A dimer interface embedded within the DBD is essential for MR to form these requisite homodimers, as well as to form heterodimers with GR.[28,29] Mutations that disrupt this interface have complex effects on receptor activity in animals[30] and cultured cells,[31] and similar mutations in other receptors (AR in particular) result in disease

---

*The steroid receptors are members of a large class of "nuclear receptors" that share a common structural layout. The nonsteroid nuclear receptors such as vitamin D, retinoic acid, and thyroid receptors are often referred to simply as *nuclear receptors* to distinguish them from the closely related steroid receptors.

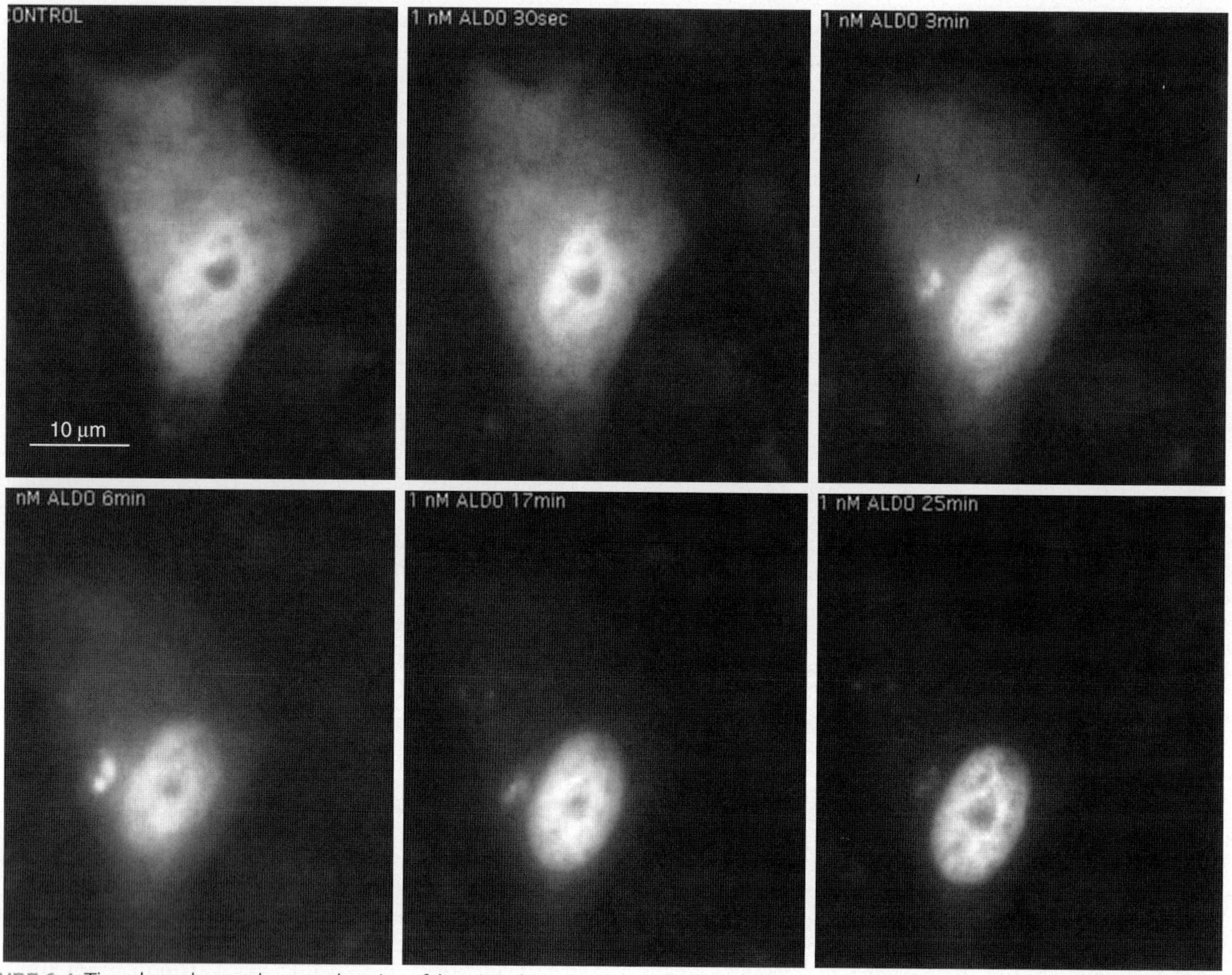

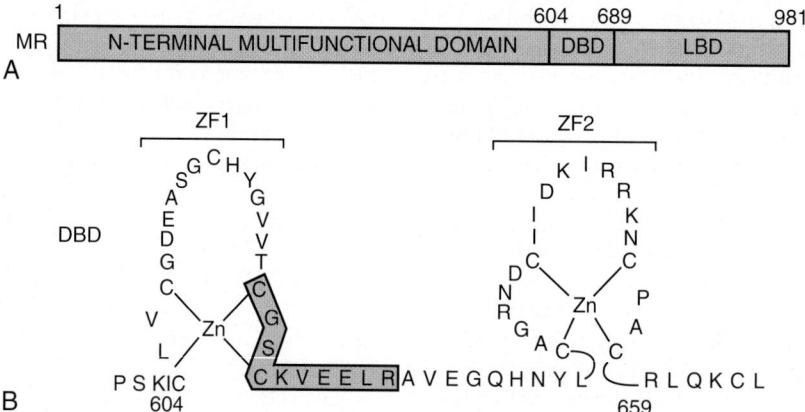

FIGURE 6-4 Time-dependent nuclear translocation of the mineralocorticoid receptor (MR) in the presence of aldosterone. Cultured cells expressing green fluorescent protein-MR fusion protein (GFP-MR) were grown in a steroid-free medium and treated with 1 nmol/L aldosterone. Translocation of GFP-MR was followed in real time, and images were captured at indicated times. It is notable that nuclear accumulation of GFP-MR started within 30 sec, was half-maximal at 7.5 min, and was complete by 10 min. Control: MR distribution prior to addition of aldosterone. (From Fejes-Toth G, Pearce D, Naray-Fejes-Toth A: Subcellular localization of mineralocorticoid receptors in living cells: effects of receptor agonists and antagonists, *Proc Natl Acad Sci U S A* 95(6):2973-2978, 1998, Figure 3.)

FIGURE 6-5 Mineralocorticoid receptor (MR) ligand/hormone-binding domain (LBD) crystal structure. Structure of the MR LBD bound to corticosterone and coactivator peptides (SRC1-4). **A** and **B,** Two views of the complex (rotated by 90 degrees about the vertical axis) are shown in ribbon representation. MR is colored in *gold* and SRC1-4 peptide in *yellow.* Corticosterone, which binds MR with an affinity comparable to that of aldosterone, is shown in *ball and stick* representation. Note that hormone is located in a deep pocket formed by helices 3, 5, and 7, which explains the slow off rate and high affinity. **C,** Sequence alignment of the human MR LBD with other steroid hormone receptors (GR, glucocorticoid; AR, androgen; PR, progesterone; and ER, estrogen). Residues that form the steroid-binding pockets are shaded in *gray.* Key structural features for the binding of SRC peptides are noted with *stars,* and the residues that determine MR/GR hormone specificity are labeled by *arrowheads.* See Li and others[25a] for further details. (From Li Y, et al: Structural and biochemical mechanisms for the specificity of hormone binding and coactivator assembly by mineralocorticoid receptor. *Mol Cell* 19:367-380, 2005.)

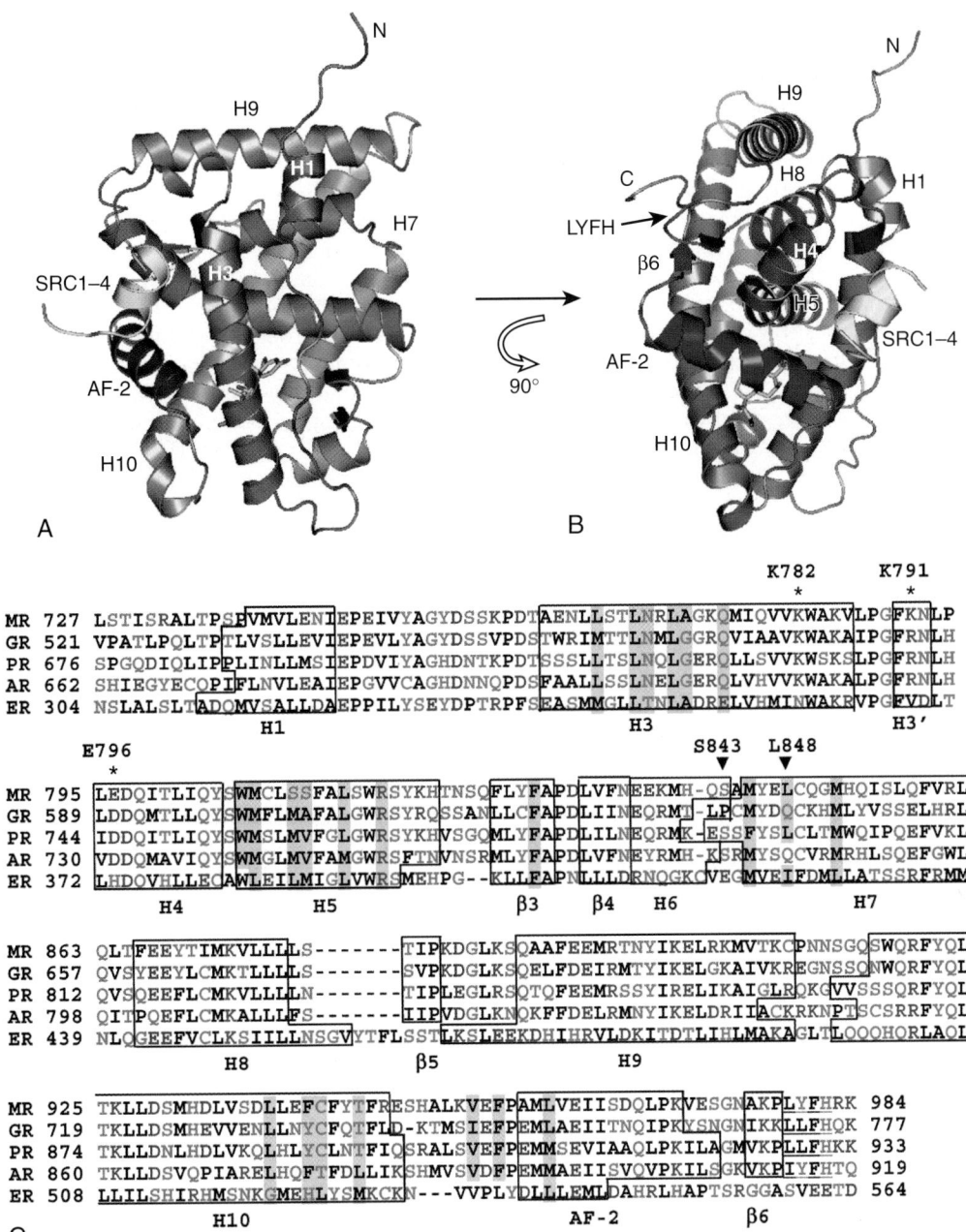

FIGURE 6-6 Domain structure of the mineralocorticoid receptor (MR). Three major domains have been defined, which are common to all steroid/nuclear receptors. Further refinements have led some to use a six-letter system, which is shown; however, this adds little to the understanding of receptor structure or function, and the authors prefer the three global domain system. These large receptor sections should not be confused with the many small functional domains that have been identified, as discussed in the text. The size and amino acid designations used here are for rat MR (981 amino acids total); they apply with minor variations to human MR (984 amino acids total). **A,** Strip diagram of MR. N-terminus is to the *left,* C-terminus to the *right.* **B,** Schematic of MR DNA-binding domain (DBD), showing the two zinc fingers, and the positions of the coordinating Zn ions. *Boxed region* is the α-helix, which intercalates into the major groove of the DNA and provides the major protein-DNA interaction contacts. The dimerization interface is comprised of amino acids within the second zinc finger, which form van der Waals and salt bridge interactions. *LBD,* Ligand-binding domain.

states.[32] Also, in at least one kindred of the autosomal dominant form of type 1 pseudohypoaldosteronism, an MR DBD mutation appears to be causative, although the mechanistic basis has not elucidated.[33]

In addition to supporting DNA binding and dimerization, the DBD also harbors a nuclear localization signal,[34,35] as well as surfaces that contact distant parts of the receptor and that mediate interactions with other proteins, as has been shown for GR and in some cases MR.[36-38]

Ligand/Hormone-Binding Domain

The MR LBD is comprised of amino acids 689 to 981 (see Figure 6-6*A*). Like the DBD, the LBD has multiple functions: In addition to binding with high affinity to various MR agonists and antagonists, it also harbors interaction surfaces for coactivators, dimerization, and N-C interactions.[39-41] MR is distinct from GR in that it binds with high affinity to both corticosterone and cortisol (the physiologic glucocorticoids in rodents and primates, respectively) and aldosterone. Indeed, as discussed later, MR likely functions purely as a high-affinity glucocorticoid receptor in some tissues, including brain and heart. High-resolution representations of the crystal structures of wild-type and mutant MR have identified the structural features of the LBD and specific amino acid contacts involved in binding to the mineralocorticoid desoxycorticosterone (DOC) (see Figure 6-5).[42,43] Key features include the following: (1) The LBD of MR, like that of other nuclear receptors, is arranged into 11 α-helices and four small β-strands. (2) The C-terminal α-helix, H12, contains the activation function AF2. (3) Hormone is deeply embedded into a pocket comprised of α-helices H3, H4, H5, H7, and H10, and two β-strands; numerous contacts are made between amino acids of the pocket and the hormone. This accounts for the slow off rate and high affinity of mineralocorticoids for their receptor.[42] The crystal structure of the constitutively active mutant S810L, implicated in a form of pseudohyperaldosteronism,[44] reveals that H12 is stabilized with AF2 in the active conformation.[43] The crystal structure of wild-type MR LBD also provides insight into the mechanisms underlying some forms of type 1 pseudohypoaldosteronism. Notably, MR/S818L is an LBD mutation in helix 5, which is predicted to disrupt interaction with the steroid ring structure,[45] whereas Q776R and L979P have been demonstrated to have markedly reduced aldosterone binding.[33] Structural analysis reveals that Q776 is located in helix H3 at the extremity of the hydrophobic ligand-binding pocket and anchors the steroid C3-ketone group.

MR binds cortisol and corticosterone with affinities similar to that of aldosterone. 11β-HSD2 is an essential determinant of aldosterone specificity, through its effect in limiting concentrations of the glucocorticoids in collecting duct principal cells, as discussed later. MR binding to glucocorticoids is physiologically relevant, and it acts as a glucocorticoid receptor in many tissues.[46-48]

N-Terminal Domain

As its noncommittal name implies, the N-terminal region of MR has diverse functions, which appear to revolve primarily around protein-protein interactions and recruitment of coactivators and corepressors. It has two potent transcriptional regulatory motifs, usually termed *AF1a* and *AF1b*.[39,49] This domain bears some functional and sequence similarity to the homologous region of GR and is capable of stimulating gene transcription when fused to an unrelated DBD.[39] Overall, however, MR and GR differ markedly in the N-terminal domain, and this region of the receptor is a central determinant of specificity.[50] Recent evidence supports the idea that this domain has functional sequences that limit receptor activity through recruitment of corepressors, in addition to transcriptional activation functions.[38,51] Its role in coactivator and corepressor recruitment is addressed further in the following section.

MR Regulation of Transcription Initiation: Coactivators and Corepressors

The major mechanism of MR action is its effects on transcription initiation; however, there may also be effects on transcript elongation.[52,53] Much has been learned over the last decade about the generation of an initiation complex and the particular roles that steroid receptors play in this process. For reviews of the biochemistry of the general transcription machinery, transcription initiation, promoter escape, and processive elongation, there are several review articles and book chapters that address these issues in depth.[54-56] Most of the coactivators identified so far interact with the C-terminal AF2 domain and include the prototypical GRIP1/TIF2 and SRC,[57,58] which sequentially recruit a series of different components of the transcriptional machinery and result in the formation of a preinitiation complex (PIC). This PIC includes all of the key components of the transcription machinery, including RNA polymerase II. A detailed picture of MR-dependent PIC formation has not been obtained. However, the general features are likely similar to those for ER[59] and involve the sequential recruitment by the receptor of (1) chromatin-remodeling SWI/SNF and CARM1/PRTM1 proteins, which promote chromatin remodeling and initiation of complex formation; (2) histone acetylase CBP/P300 (cyclic adenosine monophosphate [cAMP] response element–binding protein), which promotes an active chromatin conformation[55]; and (3) direct or indirect recruitment of the TATA-binding protein and other components of the general transcription machinery.[59]

The aforementioned mechanisms are generic and are used by many transcription factors, including all steroid receptors, through interactions with the C-terminal AF2 domain. The N-terminal region of MR, which harbors the AF1 domain, diverges from the other steroid receptors, and recent evidence has identified coregulators that interact selectively with this receptor domain. ELL (eleven-nineteen lysine-rich leukemia factor) is a coactivator for MR that specifically interacts with AF1b and assists in PIC formation.[52] It was originally identified as an elongation factor, and it may also affect transcript elongation. Other specific coregulators include the synergy inhibitory protein PIAS1,[51] Ubc9,[60] and p68 RNA helicase.[61]

Regulation of Sodium Absorption and Potassium Secretion

General Model of Aldosterone Action

Aldosterone enters the cell passively, binds to the MR, and triggers changes in gene transcription (as addressed in "Mechanisms of MR Function and Gene Regulation"), and potentially has nongenomic effects. Aldosterone effects in the ASDN have been divided into three major phases: latent, early, and late.[1] This designation goes back to the early observations by Ganong and Mulrow that after aldosterone infusion into experimental animals, no effect was observed for at least 15 to 20 minutes.[62] A similar delay was observed in isolated epithelia.[63] The early phase, which is now known to involve primarily MR-dependent regulation of signaling mediators such as SGK1, culminates in increased apical localization—and possibly increased probability of the open state—of ENaC. In the late phase, aldosterone stimulates transcription of a variety of effector genes, including those that encode components of the ion transport machinery, notably the ENaC and Na⁺-K⁺–adenosine triphosphatase (ATPase) subunits. The major direct effect is to increase Na⁺ reabsorption, which is accompanied variably by Cl⁻ reabsorption and/or K⁺ secretion, and ultimately water reabsorption. Aldosterone's actions in the principal cells of the connecting segment and collecting duct (Figure 6-7) are of primary significance; however, it also has been shown to influence fluid and electrolyte transport in other tubule segments, as well as in other organs. These actions of aldosterone can be surmised from the clinical features of individuals with aldosterone-secreting tumors; they have volume expansion with high blood pressure and are hypokalemic (usually).[64,65] In general, the effects of aldosterone on Na^+ absorption and K^+ secretion work together. However, there are ways that these actions can be separated, as is discussed later.

The two basic cell processes that aldosterone regulates—Na^+ absorption and K^+ secretion—are depicted in Figure 6-7. Most aspects of this mechanism are relevant to the various aldosterone target tissues.

Na^+-K^+-ATPase, located on the basolateral membrane (blood side), establishes the essential electrochemical gradients that drive ion transport (see Chapters 4 and 5). The most important, rate-limiting step is that of Na^+ entry into the cell via the epithelial Na^+ channel, ENaC. The discovery of the molecular composition of ENaC in 1993[66,67] opened the door to understanding how aldosterone functions to regulate this critically important ion channel. Most Na^+ transporters are encoded by a single gene product. In contrast, ENaC is composed of three similar but distinct subunits, each encoded by a unique gene. All three subunits come together (the stoichiometry is controversial) to form an ion channel with unique biophysical characteristics, the most striking of which is the relatively long time it stays open or closed.[68] The complete loss of any one of these subunits in mice is incompatible with life.[69-71]

The entry of Na^+ into the cell via ENaC in the apical membrane is the rate-limiting step in both Na^+ absorption and K^+ secretion.[72] Na^+ enters the cell down a steep electrochemical gradient; intracellular [Na^+] is approximately 10 mmol/L, and the membrane voltage is strongly negative inside the cell. The Na inside the cell is pumped out across the basolateral membrane by Na^+-K^+-ATPase, as addressed in detail in Chapter 5. Most epithelial cells have a greater density of K^+ channels on the basolateral membrane and thus recycle K^+ back into the blood. The distal nephron is unique in that it has an unusually high density of K channels on the apical membrane (primarily regulation of Kir 1.1 [ROMK] and BK channels).[73,74] This distribution of K^+ channels permits a large amount of K^+ that enters the cell via Na^+-K^+-ATPase to exit the cell into the lumen and be excreted into the urine. The vast majority of K^+ that appears in the urine is secreted by the distal nephron.

Much attention has been focused on the early phase of aldosterone action because it appears to be more tractable to dissection and the majority of change in Na^+ current occurs during this phase. This separation is probably somewhat artificial, however, and there is considerable overlap in events that define the early and late phases. Moreover, many efforts to manipulate mediators of the early phase (through overexpression and knockdown experiments) have been evaluated after prolonged alteration. Nevertheless, there is some heuristic value in considering early and late phases of aldosterone action separately.

In cultured collecting duct cells deprived of corticosteroids and then exposed to high concentrations of aldosterone, an increase in ENaC-mediated Na^+ transport can be observed in well under an hour, which is consistent with animal studies.[62,75] Na^+ transport continues to increase for 2 to 3 hours, then plateaus for a few hours, and then gradually increases over the next several hours. After 12 hours of exposure to saturating aldosterone concentrations, the increase in

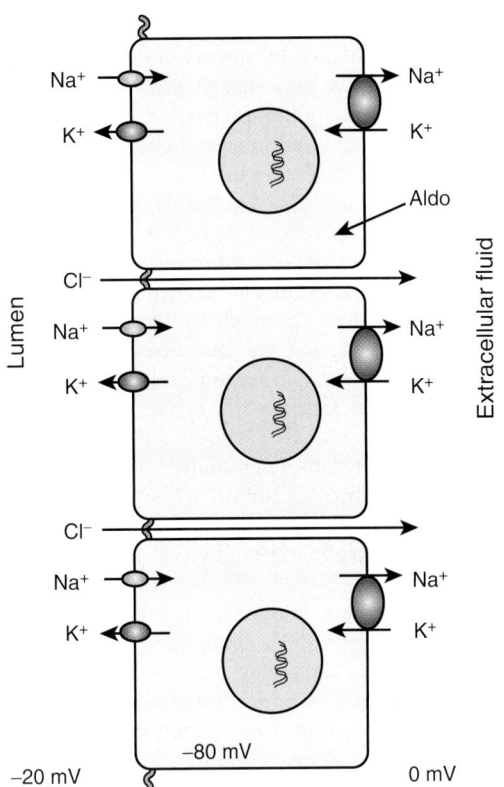

FIGURE 6-7 Schematic of principal cells in the aldosterone-sensitive distal nephron (ASDN). The ASDN includes the distal third of the distal convoluted tubule (DCT), the connecting tubule (CNT), and the collecting duct. The Na^+-K^+-adenosine triphosphatase (ATPase) establishes the gradients for passive apical entry of sodium through the epithelial sodium channel (ENaC). Transport of sodium through the ENaC creates a negative lumen potential that drives potassium secretion into the lumen. Potassium is also recycled at the basolateral surface, which facilitates potassium exchange across the Na^+-K^+-ATPase. Chloride (Cl^-) moves via paracellular and transcellular pathways. There is evidence to support aldosterone actions in other segments, particularly the sodium-chloride cotransporter (NCC)-expressing portions of the DCT (DCT1 and DCT2).

ENaC activity is near maximal. The molecular basis for this increase in ENaC activity has been intensively investigated, and several key events are now apparent.

For aldosterone to increase ENaC activity, a change in gene transcription must occur. One of the earliest response genes is SGK1.[76-78] This discovery has had a major impact on the direction of research on aldosterone action, and this gene is addressed separately—together with its major target, Nedd4-2—later in this chapter. SGK1 is particularly important for the early actions of aldosterone.[79,80] An important consideration in evaluating our understanding of this molecular pathway is that the genetic disease Liddle's syndrome provided the first clues that the C-terminal portions of the ENaC subunits were essential in regulating ENaC surface expression[81,82] (see Chapter 44).

Aldosterone and Epithelial Sodium Channel Trafficking

The major action of aldosterone is to increase the number of functional ENaC units on the apical membrane. This process can involve either an increase in the number of channel complexes on the surface or activation of existing complexes, or both. There is evidence to support both, although the bulk of evidence favors the idea that changes in the number of ENaC complexes (*N*) predominates.[83-85] The redistribution of ENaC to the apical membrane can be detected in less than 2 hours after aldosterone exposure.[75]

It is less well established whether *N* is increased through increased insertion, decreased removal, or both. Aldosterone probably contributes to both processes. Rapid insertion of ENaC complexes is best understood with regard to the actions of cAMP.[86] The extent to which the molecules involved in cAMP-mediated insertion are also involved in aldosterone action is uncertain, but some common mechanisms probably are used. Trafficking to the apical membrane appears to involve hsp70,[87] SNARE (soluble NEM-sensitive factor attachment protein receptor) proteins,[88] and the aldosterone-induced protein melanophilin.[89] The mitogen-activated protein kinase pathway may also be involved, because interruption of ERK phosphorylation by GILZ[90] increases ENaC surface expression.

Considerably more is known about how ENaC complexes are retrieved from the apical membrane. This understanding is the direct result of dissecting the molecular consequences of Liddle's syndrome, in which mutations in the C terminus of ENaC lead to increased residence time in the apical membrane.[81,82] The missing or mutated domains in the β- or γ-subunit of ENaC in this syndrome normally bind to Nedd4-2, a ubiquitin ligase, which ultimately is responsible for initiating endocytosis and degradation.[91,92] The interactions of Sgk1 and Nedd4-2 in the actions of aldosterone is discussed later. ENaC is internalized via clathrin-coated vesicles and processed into early endosomes, then further processed into recycling endosomes and late endosomes.[93,94] Degradation is via lysosomes or proteasomes.[95,96] The processing of ENaC by vesicular trafficking and its regulation by aldosterone has recently been reviewed.[97]

Phosphatidylinositol-3-kinase (PI3K)–dependent signaling is essential for epithelial Na+ transport. It controls SGK1 activity (addressed later) and also appears to have independent effects on ENaC open probability through direct actions of 3-phosphorylated phosphoinositides, particularly phosphatidylinositol (3,4,5) trisphosphate.[98,99] Ras-dependent signaling may also regulate ENaC and the pump in complex ways that depend both on downstream signaling through Raf, MEK and ERK, as well as through PI3K.[100-105]

The late phase of ENaC activation by aldosterone is less well understood than the early phase. A simple evaluation of the late phase is that aldosterone increases the transcription and protein abundance of the ENaC subunits. This idea comes from the fact that aldosterone increases the mRNA and protein abundance of the α ENaC subunit in kidney[84,106] after a lag of several hours.[107] However, whereas aldosterone produces an increase in α-subunit expression in kidney, it produces an increase of β- and γ-subunits in colon.[107,108] Dietary Na restriction, one of two major physiologically relevant maneuvers that increase aldosterone secretion, clearly increases ENaC surface expression in the renal distal nephron.[85] However, there appear to be some important differences between chronic aldosterone administration to an Na-replete animal and chronic dietary Na restriction.[106,109] The role of increased expression of the α ENaC subunit in the long-term actions of aldosterone has recently been questioned, because overexpression of this subunit does not increase ENaC activity in models of collecting duct and lung epithelia.[110] It appears that increased expression of the α ENaC subunit may be important for the consolidation of the increase, but it is not sufficient to reproduce the steroid-mediated increase in ENaC activity.

Basolateral Membrane Effects of Aldosterone

Over the years, research on aldosterone action has focused with varying degrees of intensity on apical effects,[111,112] basolateral effects,[113-115] and effects on metabolism.[63] There is general agreement now that the early effects of aldosterone are on apical events, primarily on ENaC, and that basolateral and metabolic effects come later. In addition, although it is somewhat less settled whether the basolateral effects are direct or result indirectly from the enhanced entry of Na+ into cells, the bulk of evidence favors the latter view. Notably, increased Na+ entry has been found to control more than 80% of increased Na+-K+-ATPase activity and basolateral membrane density in the rat[116] and rabbit[117] cortical collecting tubule. Furthermore, striking increases in basolateral membrane folding and surface area occur in aldosterone-treated animals,[118] an effect that is markedly attenuated in animals fed a low-Na diet. This result strongly suggests that apical Na+ entry is required for basolateral changes to occur. However, it is important to note that there is good evidence for direct transcriptional stimulation of Na+-K+-ATPase subunit expression,[119,120] as well as reports supporting some direct effects of aldosterone in increasing basolateral pump activity[113,121] or at least in constituting the pool of latent pumps, which are then recruited to the basolateral membrane in response to a rise in intracellular [Na+].[122]

Activation of the Epithelial Sodium Channel by Proteolytic Cleavage

There is now clear evidence that when ENaC is delivered to the apical membrane it can be activated by proteolytic cleavage. The first hint of this process was the demonstration that rats fed a low-Na diet or given aldosterone over the long term showed the appearance of a proteolytic fragment of the γ ENaC subunit.[84] Subsequently, investigators have shown that both the α and the γ (but not the β) ENaC subunits can be cleaved. Furthermore, cleavage at each site apparently initiates a degree of activation of the channel complex. ENaC complexes are activated by cleavage because specific regions of the large extracellular domain (26 residues in the α ENaC and 46 residues in the γ ENaC) are excised. These regions contain inhibitory sequences that, when applied exogenously, can inhibit ENaC function. Removing these regions by proteolytic cleavage releases this inhibition.[123]

Several proteases can cleave either the α or γ ENaC subunits. Among them are furin, prostasin, CAP2, kallikrein, elastase, matriptase, plasmin, and trypsin. It is not clear whether activation of ENaC by proteolytic cleavage can be regulated by aldosterone, but the idea certainly has attractive features. Were aldosterone able to regulate expression of one or more rate-limiting proteases, it would be able to regulate both the number of complexes in the apical membrane and the ability of the channel complex to be active. It appears that aldosterone may regulate the expression of prostasin.[124] Aldosterone may also regulate the expression of the protease nexin-1, an inhibitor of prostasin and other proteases.[125]

The discovery of ENaC activation by cleavage helps to explain how aldosterone might increase ENaC activity by increasing both surface expression and the activity of a single ENaC complex. By phosphorylating Nedd4-2 via SGK1 and reducing its ability to bind to the PY domains of the ENaC subunits, aldosterone increases ENaC residence time on the apical membrane. This additional time permits proteolytic activation by one or more endogenous proteases.[126]

Potassium Secretion and Aldosterone

One of the major effects of aldosterone is to increase K^+ secretion (and thus excretion). This phenomenon has been demonstrated in countless patients with aldosterone-secreting tumors and in hundreds of studies in animals given excess amounts of aldosterone. The general mechanism whereby aldosterone increases K^+ secretion is depicted in Figure 6-8. The key feature of this process involves the increased absorption of Na^+ via ENaC. The dependency of K^+ secretion on Na^+ absorption is the basis of the action of the "K-sparing" diuretics amiloride and triamterene, both of which inhibit ENaC. These drugs have no direct effect on the apical K^+ channels.

Increasing ENaC activity produces two major secondary effects that in turn enhance K^+ secretion. First, the enhanced Na^+ conductance of the apical membrane produces depolarization of that membrane and hence a more favorable electrical driving force for K^+ efflux into the lumen. The second effect relates to the activity of the Na^+-K^+ pump on the basolateral membrane. The more Na^+ that enters across the apical membrane, the more that must be extruded by the pump. Since the stoichiometry of the pump is constant (3Na and 2K), more K^+ enters the cell. In isolated, perfused cortical collecting ducts, the amount of secreted K^+ is highly related to the amount of absorbed Na^+ when the stimulus for Na^+ absorption is mineralocorticoid hormone.[127]

Two kinds of K channels are found in the apical membrane of the ASDN: small conductance (SK, 30 to 40 picosiemens) channels created by the ROMK gene, and large conductance (BK, 100 to 200 picosiemens) found in many kinds of cells, including the apical membrane of the colon. The majority of the K channels on the apical membrane of the principal cells appear to be SK, at least as far as can be assessed by patch clamp analysis. The activity of these channels is not increased by aldosterone.[128]

A feature of K^+ secretion is that although apical K^+ channels are abundant in the proximal portion of the ASDN (connecting tubule and cortical collecting duct), they are strikingly less abundant in the medullary collecting duct.[129-131] Because apical K channels are not regulated by aldosterone, their absence in the medullary collecting duct might uncouple aldosterone-regulated Na^+ reabsorption from K^+ secretion in this segment.

Recent advances in understanding genetic forms of hypertension have uncovered an important role for a family of kinases that lack an otherwise conserved lysine residue in the catalytic domain. These kinases, called *WNK* (*with no lysine*; *K* is also the abbreviation for lysine), have potent effects on pathways regulating Na^+ and K^+ transport in the distal nephron. An important feature of one member of this family,

WNK4, is its ability to modulate the activity of ROMK.[132,133] The activity of ROMK can be regulated via WNK4 by signaling events activated by aldosterone but modulated by serum $[K^+]$, Na balance via angiotensin II, and SGK1 activity. The importance of this information is that it provides a molecular mechanism for the collecting duct separately to regulate Na^+ absorption via ENaC and K^+ secretion via ROMK.

Separation of Sodium Absorption and Potassium Secretion by the Aldosterone-Sensitive Distal Nephron

One of the challenging features of understanding how aldosterone acts is to rationalize its Na^+-retaining effects and its K^+-secretory effects. Is aldosterone an Na-regulatory hormone or a K-regulatory hormone? Of course, the answer is that it is both, but the organism does not ingest a fixed amount of Na^+ and K^+, so inexorable linkage between Na^+ absorption and K^+ secretion by the ASDN cannot possibly occur all the time. Investigators have proposed several possibilities to explain how these processes can be separated.

The most attractive possibility involves separate regulation of ENaC and ROMK by specific stimuli depending on the state of Na and K intake. With a constant Na intake, one could envision that a high-K diet could enhance the activity of ROMK, while a low-K diet would reduce its activity. Such an effect would cause more or less of the K entering the cell via the Na-K pump to be recycled across the basolateral membrane. This mechanism, although probably very complex in its execution, is appealing in its teleologic simplicity. The actions of WNK4 may be central to the regulation of ROMK.

There are several other possibilities, however. One set involves the differing nature of Na^+ and K^+ transport along the distal nephron. The DCT absorbs Na^+ and Cl^- primarily (via the Na-Cl cotransporter), and enhanced activity in this segment would favor more electroneutral NaCl absorption and less K^+ secretion. Such a situation occurs in Gordon's syndrome (also referred to as *pseudohypoaldosteronism type 2* or *familial hyperkalemic hypertension*).[134] Another possibility involves modulation of Na^+ absorption by the medullary collecting duct, a segment that has little capacity to secrete K^+. The environment of the renal medulla is very different from that of the cortex, and endogenous paracrine factors such as prostaglandins E_2 and transforming growth factor-β, both of which have potent inhibitory effects on Na^+ transport, are increased in response to a high-NaCl diet.[135,136]

A third possibility involves the independent regulation of Cl^- transport by the collecting duct. Cl^- can be absorbed by the paracellular pathway (i.e., between cells) driven by the lumen-negative voltage across the epithelium. This pathway can be influenced by aldosterone.[137] Cl^- can also be absorbed through the cells by specific transporters. One example of a Cl^- transporter in the collecting duct is pendrin, an anion exchanger present on the apical membrane of intercalated cells. Mice that lack this transporter do not tolerate NaCl restriction as well as normal mice.[138] This transporter seems not to be upregulated by aldosterone, but is dependent on Cl^- delivery to the distal nephron and is upregulated by angiotensin II.[139,140] Results of intense investigation into the signaling systems activated by aldosterone and its modulating systems will continue to provide us with a rich understanding of the

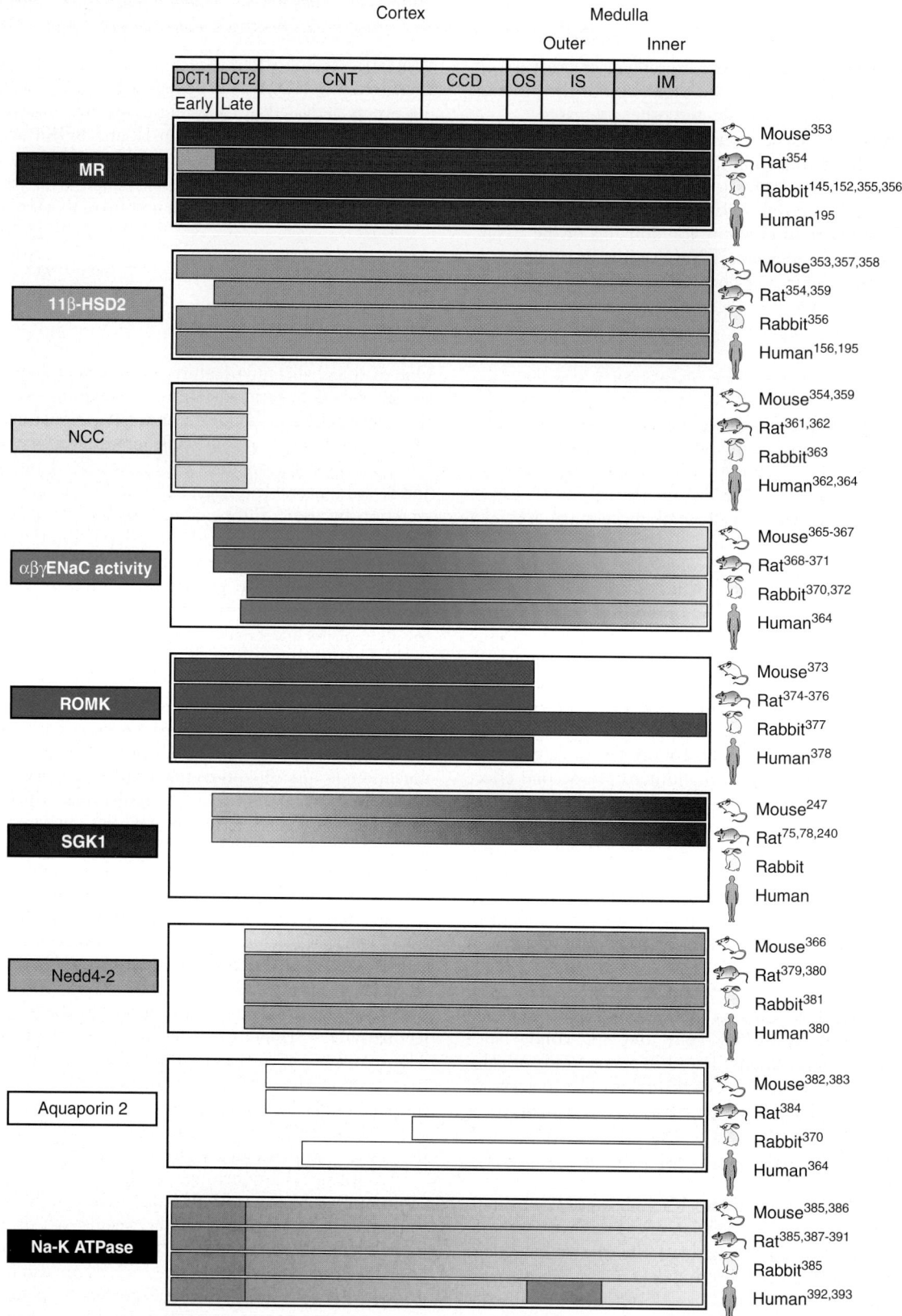

FIGURE 6-8 Expression and/or activity of the mineralocorticoid-dependent transport machinery in principal cells along the aldosterone-sensitive distal nephron (ASDN). Aldosterone specificity is conferred by the presence of the mineralocorticoid receptor (MR) and 11β-hydroxysteroid dehydrogenase 2 (11β-HSD2) beginning primarily from the latter part of the distal convoluted tubule (DCT). The thiazide-sensitive sodium-chloride cotransporter (NCC) is expressed exclusively in the DCT, but after the transition from the DCT to the connecting tubule (CNT), sodium reabsorption is distinctly determined by epithelial sodium channel (ENaC) activity. ENaC activity is strongest in the CNT and decreases down to the inner medulla (IMCD). Variation in gene expression or activity along the nephron is indicated by the intensity of shading. Note that there is some variation gene expression from mouse to human. However, the machinery for sodium reabsorption in the ASDN is predominantly conserved across species. Each nephron segment is drawn to scale, but expression of channels and transporters in intercalated cells is omitted. Expression and/or activity is based on messenger RNA, protein, and biochemical studies. (Adapted from Loffing J, Korbmacher C: Regulated sodium transport in the renal connecting tubule [CNT] via the epithelial sodium channel [ENaC], *Pflugers Archiv* 458[1]:111-135, 2009.)

complexities of how aldosterone acts and how other signaling systems modulate Na$^+$, K$^+$, and Cl$^-$ transport.

Sites of MR Expression and Locus of Action along the Nephron

Aldosterone-Sensitive Distal Nephron

In the kidney, MR is expressed at the highest levels in distal nephron cells extending from the last third of the DCT through the medullary collecting duct,[141] which is frequently referred to as the *aldosterone-sensitive distal nephron* (ASDN) (see Figure 6-8).[1] This pattern of expression was first demonstrated using labeled hormone–binding studies performed before the cloning of MR[142] and has been confirmed since by several methods, including polymerase chain reaction,[143] in situ hybridization,[144] and immunohistochemical analysis.[145] Effects of aldosterone on electrogenic Na$^+$ and K$^+$ transport in principal cells have been found consistently in these nephron segments,[141] which also express ENaC, and 11β-HSD2, as addressed in detail earlier. Collecting duct intercalated cells also express MR and respond specifically to aldosterone and alter proton secretion. Aldosterone directly increases the activity of the H$^+$-ATPase in the collecting duct, and its absence results in decreased proton secretion.[146-148] Interestingly, nongenomic stimulation of H$^+$-ATPase activity in type A intercalated cells has been demonstrated in isolated murine collecting ducts.[149] Consistent with these effects, aldosterone deficiency results in distal renal tubular acidosis type 4, and excess aldosterone results in metabolic alkalosis.[150] It should be noted that aldosterone also impacts H$^+$ secretion due to effects on principal cell Na$^+$ transport, which alter the electrical gradient.

Other Sites of Expression

MR has been identified at some level in all parts of the nephron examined, including the glomerulus.[143,151-156] Its effects, at least at some of these sites, are likely to be physiologically relevant in states of volume depletion and acid-base disturbances; however, the data are not as robust and consistent as those for the ASDN.

Glomerulus

MR is expressed in glomerular mesangial cells, where it is thought to affect proliferation and production of reactive oxygen species[157,158] and to have profibrotic effects through SGK1.[159] These effects have been suggested to be important in the progression of renal damage, particularly in diabetic nephropathy,[160] but the physiologic role of mesangial cell MR is uncertain.

Proximal Convoluted Tubule

Hierholzer and Stolte showed through elegant microperfusion studies that the sodium reabsorptive capacity of the proximal convolution was decreased in adrenalectomized animals and restored with administration of aldosterone.[161] Chronic volume depletion increases sodium reabsorption in the proximal convoluted tubule, which is in part mediated by aldosterone. The mechanisms of action in this nephron segment are controversial. Recent studies indicate an MR-dependent increase in the activity of Na$^+$/H$^+$ exchanger isoform 3, possibly through an increase in trafficking of the transporter to the membrane.[162-165] This transporter contributes to sodium

and bicarbonate reabsorption. Aldosterone may also activate the Na$^+$-K$^+$-ATPase in the basolateral membrane of the proximal convoluted tubule to maintain a gradient for sodium reabsorption.[166-169]

Medullary Thick Ascending Limb

In the medullary thick ascending limb, mineralocorticoids but not glucocorticoids increase sodium and chloride reabsorption. In rodents, adrenalectomy impairs reabsorption of NaCl in the medullary thick ascending limb, and aldosterone restores this process.[170,171] This reabsorptive defect may contribute to the urinary concentrating and diluting abnormality measured in patients with Addison's disease and in mice lacking aldosterone synthase.[147,161,172] The medullary thick ascending limb also participates in the regulation of acid-base balance by reabsorbing most of the filtered HCO$_3$ that is not reabsorbed by the proximal tubule. In this context, aldosterone has been shown to stimulate the Na$^+$/H$^+$ exchanger in amphibian thick ascending limb, possibly through a rapid nongenomic effect.[173] Recent evidence has also implicated regulation of the Na-K-2Cl cotransporter type 2 in the thick ascending limb—as well as the Na-Cl cotransporter (NCC) in the DCT (see later)—by oxidative stress response kinase 1 (OSR1), and STE20/SPS1-related proline/alanine–rich kinase (SPAK) (OSR1/SPAK).[174]

Distal Convoluted Tubule

The DCT is also capable of mineralocorticoid specificity.[175,176] Hormone studies in rodents demonstrate that aldosterone increases expression of the NCC and its apical membrane abundance[177-179] without changes in mRNA expression.[179,180] The recently described family of WNK kinases may play a pivotal role in mediating this effect. Aldosterone acts through MR to increase NCC phosphorylation, which appears to be important for the changes in its expression and apical targeting.[181,182] Recent evidence supports the idea that aldosterone-induced NCC phosphorylation occurs through a signaling cascade in which SGK1 phosphorylates WNK4,[183,184] which in turn phosphorylates OSR1 and SPAK.[181,185] OSR1/SPAK then directly phosphorylates NCC at three serine/threonine sites,[186] which results in increased expression. It is interesting to note that SGK1 may also be a target of WNK1.[187]

Nonrenal Aldosterone-Responsive Tight Epithelia

The mineralocorticoid effects of aldosterone have predominantly been studied in the distal nephron, but do influence other—mostly ENaC-expressing—tight epithelia. ENaC is present in visceral epithelial cells of the distal colon, distal lung, salivary glands, sweat glands, and taste buds.

Colon

Under physiologic conditions, approximately 1.3 to 1.8 L of electrolyte-rich fluid is reabsorbed per day from the colonic epithelium, which accounts for about 90% of the salt and water that enter the proximal colon from the terminal ileum. In nonmammalian vertebrates, sodium conservation by the colon plays an even more significant role.[188] This transport is regulated by several transporters and channels, including ENaC. Like the nephron, the proximal colon reabsorbs sodium via an electroneutral, ENaC-independent process. In the distal colon, electrogenic Na⁺ absorption via ENaC channels is the predominate mode of sodium transport.[189-192] In disease states such as inflammatory bowel disease, ENaC-mediated sodium reabsorption can be reduced,[193] although in diarrheal states, elevated aldosterone levels may attenuate sodium and water loss from the colon.[194] It should be noted that in the colon, as in the distal nephron, aldosterone signaling is enhanced over that of glucocorticoids by 11β-HSD2.[195] Aldosterone increases electrogenic sodium absorption and potassium secretion, and inhibits electroneutral absorption.[196] This is in contrast to glucocorticoids, which activate GR to stimulate electroneutral absorption in the proximal and distal colon.[72,197] As in the distal nephron, the aldosterone response can be characterized by an early and late response. The early response gene, SGK1, is upregulated by aldosterone via MR.[198] However, opposite to aldosterone's effects in kidney, aldosterone and a low-salt diet have been shown to stimulate transcription of β but not α ENaC in rat models.[199,200]

Aldosterone stimulates electrogenic potassium secretion from colonic epithelia. The significance of this secretion is evident in anuric patients. Potassium secretion from the colon is much higher in patients undergoing long-term hemodialysis than in patients not undergoing dialysis.[201-203] Indeed, administration of fludrocortisone, a mineralocorticoid agonist, to dialysis patients has been showed to reduce hyperkalemia in small clinical trials.[204] However, use of the common MR antagonist spironolactone does not result in significant hyperkalemia.[205-207]

Lung

Vectorial transport of salt and water across the distal airway epithelium (ciliated Clara cells, nonciliated cuboidal cells) and alveoli (type I and type II alveoli) primarily determine fluid clearance from the lung. ENaC is the rate-limiting step in sodium transport in the lung and plays a primary role in several physiologic and pathophysiologic conditions that are determined by fluid clearance.[208] At birth, the lung must assume a resorptive phenotype, and lack of functional ENaC channels leads to neonatal respiratory distress syndrome in mouse knockout models.[209] In children, lack of functional ENaC (e.g., autosomal recessive pseudohypoaldosteronism type 1)[210-212] results in increased rates of recurrent infection due to increased airway liquid.[211] In the mature lung, defective ENaC channels can lead to pulmonary edema and pathologic conditions (e.g., acute respiratory distress syndrome[213] and high-altitude pulmonary edema[214]). Conversely, hyperabsorption through ENaC is emerging as an important mechanism of decreased mucus clearance in cystic fibrosis.[215]

The molecular apparatus for mineralocorticoid-stimulated liquid reabsorption via ENaC (concomitant MR and 11β-HSD2) is present in late gestational and mature adult lung in humans[195,216,217] and rats,[218] and there is some evidence for a significant physiologic role of aldosterone in ENaC-mediated sodium transport in the lung.[218] However, glucocorticoids acting through GR are likely to play the predominant role in lung.[106,198,219-222] Importantly, not only do glucocorticoids—but not mineralocorticoids—play a critical clinical role in lung maturation in humans, but GR knockout mice, like ENaC-α knockout mice, die of respiratory insufficiency within hours of birth. In contrast, MR knockout mice demonstrate a severe salt-wasting phenotype but no significant lung phenotype.[146,223]

Exocrine Glands and Sensors

ENaC-mediated sodium reabsorption is also measurable in salivary and sweat glands.[224] The importance of these tissues for sodium and water homeostasis is underscored by rare genetic mutations that confer elevated plasma aldosterone levels and pseudohypoaldosteronism with normal renal tubular function but significant sodium loss from salivary or sweat glands.[225,226] ENaC channels also play an important role in transduction of sodium salt taste in the anterior papillae of the tongue.[227,228] The appropriate molecular machinery for mineralocorticoid-responsive sodium reabsorption is expressed in these organs,[195,229,230] and these epithelia are model systems for the study of ENaC regulation.[224,231] As in colonic epithelia, aldosterone stimulates expression of β and γ ENaC and sodium transport in glands and taste buds in animal models.[228,232] Moreover, in humans, changes in dietary sodium are inversely proportional to sodium transport across salivary epithelia.[233] As in the aldosterone-responsive distal nephron and distal colon, sodium uptake is coupled with potassium secretion in salivary epithelia. This effect is evident in humans with hyperaldosteronism. Such patients have a salivary [Na⁺]/[K⁺] ratio significantly lower than that of subjects without the disorder[234,235]; however, this has not been accepted as a valid means to screen for hyperaldosteronism.

Role of Serum- and Glucocorticoid-Regulated Kinase in Mediating Aldosterone Effects

Induction of SGK1 by Aldosterone

In the early to mid 1960s, primarily from the work of Izzy Edelman and colleagues, it became clear that aldosterone, like cortisol, exerted most—if not all—of its key physiologic effects by altering transcription rates of a specific subset of genes.[236] In particular, hormone-induced changes in gene transcription were shown to be essential for its effects on epithelial Na⁺ transport.[63] Attention focused first on enzymes of intermediary metabolism, particularly citrate synthase,[237,238] and after the cloning of the transporters involved in Na⁺ translocation (Na⁺-K⁺-ATPase and ENaC), these were also found to be regulated by aldosterone at the transcriptional level. However, these effects are manifest several hours after most of the change in Na⁺ transport has already occurred and hence could not explain the early—and greatest proportion of—the effects of aldosterone.[1] Considerable effort by many groups went into unbiased screening for aldosterone-regulated proteins[239] and later aldosterone-regulated mRNAs (reviewed in Verrey[1]). In 1999, SGK1 was identified as the first early-onset aldosterone-induced gene product, which clearly stimulates ENaC-mediated sodium reabsorption in the distal nephron[198,240,241] without pleiotropic effects on other cellular processes. The physiologic relevance of SGK1 is now firmly established, and investigations by numerous laboratories into its mechanism of action have revealed critical general features of the mechanism underlying hormone-regulated ion transport. Hence, it is addressed in some detail here. SGK1 mRNA levels are increased within 15 minutes—and protein levels within 30 minutes—in cultured cells upon stimulation by aldosterone[240,242,243] and in the collecting duct by aldosterone or a low-salt diet (a physiologic stimulus for aldosterone secretion) in vivo.[75,198,244] Notably, SGK1 is increased more abundantly in kidney cortex (connecting tubule and cortical collecting duct) than in medulla, which corresponds to the potency of ENaC activation in these nephron segments.[245,246] SGK1 is expressed in other nephron segments, including glomeruli, proximal tubule, and papilla[75,198,247]; however, its rapid induction specifically in the ASDN appears to provide most of the basis for its role in aldosterone-regulated sodium and potassium transport. It is of interest that SGK1 is highly expressed in glomeruli and inner medulla and papilla in the absence of aldosterone[248]; recent data are consistent with the idea that its inner medullary induction is related to its role in osmotic responses.[249]

Molecular Mechanisms of SGK1 Action in the Aldosterone-Sensitive Distal Nephron

SGK1 is a serine/threonine kinase of the AGC protein kinase superfamily,[250] and its kinase activity appears to be essential for Na⁺ transport regulation. Although it does have mild effects on proliferation and apoptosis in kidney cells, these effects appear to be minor, and the control of ENaC[248] and other transporters[251] predominates. SGK1 transcription is induced by a variety of stimuli in addition to aldosterone. As its name implies, these include serum and glucocorticoids, but also follicle-stimulating hormone, transforming growth factor–β, and hypotonic and hypertonic stress.[252-255] Of these, osmotic regulation is of the clearest physiologic relevance.[256] SGK1 is interesting as a signaling kinase in that both its expression level and its activity are highly regulated. Regulation of the former occurs primarily through effects on gene transcription, although protein stability is also regulated, whereas regulation of the latter occurs through phosphorylation.[257,259] Like that of its close relative Akt, SGK1 phosphorylation is stimulated by a variety of growth factors including insulin and insulin-like growth factor–1,[257,259-261] which act through PI3K to trigger phosphorylation at two key residues, an activation loop (residue T256), and hydrophobic motif (S422). Both of these phosphorylation events appear to be PI3K dependent. Specifically, the α isoform of the p110 subunit of PI3K stimulates PI3K-dependent kinase 1 and mTORC2 (PDK2) repectively.[259,261-264,349] (Recent evidence has established that PDK2 is in fact the mammalian target of rapamycin [mTOR] in its complex 2 variant.[349-350]) In turn, these upstream kinases phosphorylate and hence activate SGK1 kinase, which is required for its stimulation of ENaC.[264-266] Thus, SGK1 serves as a convergence point for different classes of stimuli, which act on the one hand to control its expression (aldosterone) and the other to control its activity (insulin), which results in the coordinate regulation of ENaC. In the study of the physiologic and pathophysiologic role of SGK1 in the ASDN, mice lacking SGK1 have provided considerable insight. Unlike MR knockout mice,[146] mice lacking SGK1 survive the neonatal period and appear normal when consuming a diet with normal salt levels, although their aldosterone levels are markedly elevated. When subjected to a low-salt diet, these mice have a profound sodium-wasting phenotype (pseudohypoaldosteronism type 1).[267,268] Notably, this is a significantly milder phenotype than in the MR knockout. This comparison suggests that disruption of SGK1 signaling may be insufficient to eliminate aldosterone-mediated sodium transport due to additional aldosterone-induced and aldosterone-repressed proteins that could compensate for the lack of SGK1. Other early aldosterone-induced genes, including K-ras, GILZ, kidney-specific WNK1, Usp45, melanophilin, and promyocytic leukemia zinc finger,[269-274] have also been implicated in the stimulation of ENaC. Their distinct mechanisms of action have not been studied in vivo and are beyond the scope of this chapter. Alternatively, SGK1 may play a more significant role in states of aldosterone excess or upregulation of hormonal activators of SGK1 (e.g., insulin). Indeed, SGK1 knockout mice are protected from the development of salt-sensitive hypertension, which accompanies the hyperinsulinemia of the metabolic syndrome.[275,276] Despite its accepted role as a mediator of aldosterone-stimulated sodium reabsorption, the mechanisms by which SGK1 stimulates ENaC are not fully characterized. Several mechanistic studies have demonstrated that SGK1 is rapidly induced but also rapidly degraded.[198,240,277,278] The N terminus of the kinase, which distinguishes SGK1 from other kinase family members (e.g., Akt), is important for stimulation of sodium transport, but is also the target for rapid degradation of the kinase via the ubiquitin-proteasome system.[279-282] In addition, several naturally occurring variants of SGK1 possess distinct N termini that modify the ability to stimulate ENaC and to be degraded.[283-285] The pathophysiologic implications of the N terminus for sodium transport are unclear, but may involve a negative feedback loop to limit sodium reabsorption in states of hypertension.

The molecular mechanisms of ENaC stimulation by SGK1 can be divided into three known categories: (1) posttranslational effects on the E3 ubiquitin ligase Nedd4-2; (2) posttranslational Nedd4-2–independent effects; and (3) transcription of gene products such as α ENaC (Figure 6-9).

SGK1 Inhibits the Ubiquitin Ligase Nedd4-2

Before the discovery of SGK1 as an aldosterone-induced early gene product, the E3 ubiquitin ligase known as *neural developmentally downregulated isoform 4-2* (Nedd4-2) was shown to interact with the C-terminal tails of β ENaC and γ ENaC[286] and decrease surface expression of the channel via channel ubiquitination, and hence to inhibit sodium current.[96,287,288] The genetic defect in Liddle's syndrome (ENaC-mediated hypertension, hypokalemia, and metabolic alkalosis) consists of a gain-of-function mutation in the C-terminal tail of these subunits, which results in decreased inhibition by Nedd4-2 and hence increased ENaC activity.[289] Lack of Nedd4-2 in vivo results in increased ENaC activity and salt-sensitive hypertension,[290,291] recapitulating a Liddle's syndrome–like phenotype. SGK1 interacts with and phosphorylates Nedd4-2[243,265] in an ENaC signaling complex[101] and enhances cell surface expression of ENaC,[242,292] a surrogate for ENaC activity. This interaction coordinates phosphorylation-dependent binding of 14-3-3 proteins to inhibit Nedd4-2 and prevent ubiquitination of ENaC.[293-295] This disinhibition of ENaC parallels a recurring theme in the regulation of ion transport in the kidney seen with the WNK kinases and the Na-Cl cotransporter,

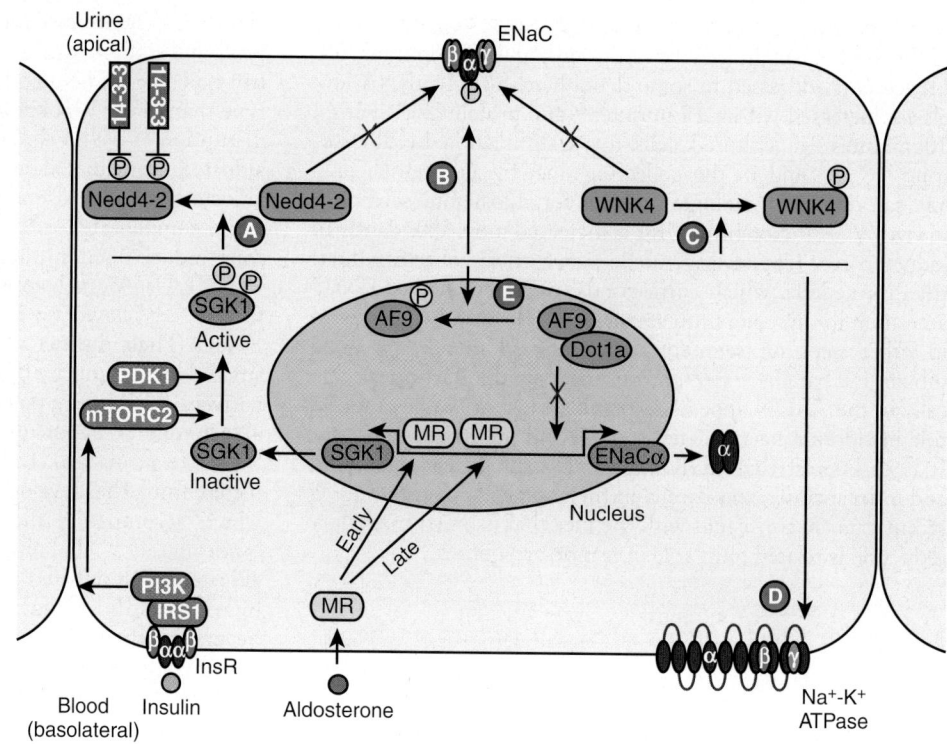

FIGURE 6-9 Mechanisms of serum- and glucocorticoid-regulated kinase 1 (SGK1)–mediated stimulation of the epithelial sodium channel (ENaC). Within principal cells of the mammalian kidney, SGK1 is transcriptionally upregulated as an early aldosterone-induced gene product. SGK1 is then phosphorylated twice via a phosphatidylinositol-3-kinase (PI3K)–dependent cascade of upstream kinases leading to active SGK1. Active SGK1 has multiple effects: it increases apical plasma membrane ENaC by inhibiting Nedd4-2 and Raf-1, and it induces transcription of the ENaC-α subunit (thereby influencing late effects of aldosterone). **A** to **E** (clockwise), The individual mechanisms that have been elucidated in principal cells. See text for details.

other aldosterone-regulated gene products (e.g., GILZ) and ENaC, and NHERF2 and ROMK.[250,296]

SGK1 Enhances Epithelial Sodium Channel Activity Independently of Nedd4-2

In cell culture systems, mutation of SGK1 phosphorylation sites on Nedd4-2 does not completely abolish the ability of SGK1 to stimulate ENaC.[265] Furthermore, SGK1 has been shown to stimulate ENaC channels with Liddle's syndrome mutations, which are unable to bind Nedd4-2.[198,242] Consequently, other Nedd4-2–independent mechanisms of SGK1 stimulation have been proposed. SGK1 directly phosphorylates a serine residue in the intracellular C-terminal tail of α ENaC, which directly activates channels at the cell surface.[297] Recently, SGK1 has been implicated in the stimulation of ENaC via phosphorylation of WNK4, a kinase mutated in pseudohypoaldosteronism type 2.[183] SGK1 may also have a small effect on modulation of the open probability of the channel.[298] In addition to showing effects on ENaC, SGK1 has been found to stimulate the activity of basolateral Na$^+$-K$^+$-ATPase, which separately increases ENaC-mediated sodium transport.[299,300] The time course of these effects and their relative importance compared with Nedd4-2–dependent inhibition have not been explored.[297] The next generation of molecular studies of SGK1 will elucidate the relative importance of each of these pathways.

SGK1 Stimulates the Components of Sodium Transport Machinery

SGK1 also regulates the expression of late aldosterone-responsive genes, primarily ENaC-α.[301,302] Active SGK1 is an important mediator of aldosterone-sensitive ENaC-α

transcription in vivo via inhibition of a transcriptional repression element, the disruptor of telomeric silencing alternative splice variant a (Dot1a)–ALL1–fused gene from chromosome 9 (Af9) complex.[302] SGK1 phosphorylates Af9 and reduces interaction between Dot1a and Af9. This releases suppression of ENaC transcription by this complex. Thus, SGK1 not only acts on ENaC channels to rapidly enhance sodium channel activity through the increase of active channels at the apical surface and increase of the Na$^+$-K$^+$-ATPase at the basolateral surface, but also stimulates transcription of elements of the machinery for sodium transport to promote a sustained response to aldosterone. SGK1 is an early-onset gene, but its effects influence both immediate and long-term aldosterone-stimulated sodium reabsorption.

SGK1 Stimulates Potassium Secretion in the Aldosterone-Sensitive Distal Nephron

Further evidence of a role for SGK1 in the regulation of sodium transport in the ASDN is revealed by the study of potassium secretion. As outlined earlier, sodium reabsorption through ENaC increases the negative charge on the luminal surface of the apical membrane of principal cells, thereby providing an electrical driving force for potassium secretion through the ROMK channel. If SGK1 enhances ENaC-mediated sodium transport, the potential difference across the apical-to-basolateral surface of principal cells should be higher (more negative) and thus should indirectly stimulate potassium secretion. SGK1 knockout mice are unable to adequately secrete potassium in both the short and long term when challenged with a high-potassium diet. Moreover, the potential difference across collecting duct epithelia from these knockout mice indicates that the effect of SGK1 on potassium secretion occurs via ENaC, not through direct regulation of ROMK.[303]

11β-Hydroxysteroid Dehydrogenase Type 2

11β-HSD2: An Essential Determinant of Mineralocorticoid Specificity

Central to the ability of aldosterone to selectively regulate epithelial ion transport is the coexpression with MR of the enzyme 11β-HSD2 at very high levels.[5,6] The physiologic glucocorticoid cortisol (corticosterone in rats and mice) have a high affinity for MR equivalent to that of aldosterone and, as noted earlier, circulates at plasma free concentrations that are 100-fold or more those of aldosterone. 11β-HSD2 converts cortisol/corticosterone to receptor-inactive 11-keto steroids (cortisone in humans, 11-dehydrocorticosterone in rats and mice), using nicotinamide adenine dinucleotide (NAD) as a cosubstrate and generating sufficient amounts of the reduced form of NAD (NADH) to alter the redox potential of the cell. This dependence sets it in contrast to 11β-HSD1, which uses the reduced form of nicotinamide adenine dinucleotide phosphate (NADPH), preferentially catalyzes the conversion of the oxidized to the reduced form, and has received substantial attention recently as a target for treatment of metabolic syndrome.[304] Aldosterone has a very reactive aldehyde group at carbon 18 (see Figure 6-1), which forms an 11,18-hemiacetal (see Figure 6-1, *right*) and is protected from dehydrogenation by 11β-HSD2.[5,6] 11β-HSD2 is localized predominantly to nonnuclear subcellular locations, which is consistent with its role in excluding glucocorticoids from MR.

Sites of 11β-HSD2 Expression

In the kidney, 11β-HSD2 is expressed at high levels throughout the ASDN,[144,155,305] where it is coexpressed with MR and ENaC.[306] Consistent with aldosterone regulation of the NCC, it is also coexpressed in DCT with this transporter as well.[307,308] Interestingly, expression has also been found in the thick ascending limb,[155] although expression levels appear to be substantially lower, and increase progressively in DCT. Expression is by far highest in the connecting tubule and cortical collecting duct.[305,308] It is also expressed in the aldosterone-sensitive segments of the colon, particularly the distal colon, as is the case for MR, although there is species variability.[309] 11β-HSD2 expression has also been described in several nonepithelial tissues, including placenta,[310] the nucleus tractus solitarius in the brain,[311] and the vessel wall,[47] which makes all of these tissues potential aldosterone target tissues.

Impact of 11β-HSD2 on MR Activity

The initial[5,6] and still widely held interpretation of the role of 11β-HSD2 was that of excluding active glucocorticoids from epithelial MR, which allowed aldosterone unfettered access. This is only part of the picture, however; to reduce the signal-to-noise ratio from 100-fold to 10% would require that 999 of every 1000 cortisol molecules entering the cell be metabolized to cortisone, a very tall order in an organ such as the kidney that commands 20% to 25% of cardiac output. 11β-HSD2 in epithelia (and in other tissues in which it is expressed) clearly

does reduce glucocorticoid levels by an order of magnitude,[312] but may still leave them at intracellular levels above those of aldosterone. At the same time, although it is clear that when 11β-HSD2 is operative glucocorticoid-occupied MR are not transcriptionally active, it is also clear that when the enzyme is deficient (as in apparent mineralocorticoid excess) or blocked (as in licorice abuse), cortisol can activate MR and ion transport. Although the subcellular mechanisms involved are yet to be established, it appears that glucocorticoid-MR complexes are conformationally distinct from aldosterone-MR, and one intriguing possibility is that these hormone-receptor complexes—in contrast to aldosterone-MR complexes—are held inactive by the obligate generation of NADH from the cosubstrate NAD, required for the operation of 11β-HSD2.[313] There is direct evidence to support the idea that redox potential affects the activity of the glucocorticoid receptor through effects on thioredoxin.[314]

Apparent Mineralocorticoid Excess: A Disease of Defective 11β-HSD2

Apparent mineralocorticoid excess was first described by Maria New, and the molecular mechanisms responsible were established after an intense but fruitless search for a novel mineralocorticoid.[315] The condition reflects partial or complete deficiency of 11β-HSD2 activity, is more common in consanguinity, and manifests as severe juvenile hypertension.[316] Confectionery licorice (or that added to chewing tobacco) contains glycyrrhizic and glycyrrhetinic acid suicide substrate for 11β-HSD2, which acts as a competitive inhibitor of the enzyme. Lack of functional 11β-HSD2 results in high levels of MR occupancy by cortisol and inappropriate mineralocorticoid-like stimulation of ENaC-mediated Na$^+$ reabsorption. This causes severe hypertension, often accompanied by hypokalemia. Plasma renin, angiotensin II, and aldosterone are suppressed. Treatment of apparent mineralocorticoid excess is the use of MR antagonists and additional antihypertensives as required. Treatment of licorice abuse is moderation.

Role of 11β-HSD2 in Blood Vessels

Studies of 11β-HSD2 in the human vascular wall[317] defined the activity of aldosterone and cortisol in this physiologic aldosterone target tissue. Aldosterone at nanomolar concentrations caused a rapid rise in intracellular pH, reflecting nongenomic activation of the Na$^+$/H$^+$ exchanger. Cortisol alone over a range of doses produced no effect, but when carbenoxolone was added to inhibit 11β-HSD2 cortisol mimicked aldosterone. Inhibitor studies revealed that the effects of both aldosterone and cortisol were mediated by classical MR. In other studies involving tissue damage, mineralocorticoid antagonists were protective, whereas aldosterone or cortisol worsened injury. The inference from these results was that cortisol becomes an MR agonist in the context of tissue damage (or when 11β-HSD2 is pharmacologically inhibited), with alteration of reactive oxygen species generation and redox potential.[318] It is further notable that aldosterone has been shown to have both vasodilatory and vasoconstricting effects in animals and humans.[319] These contradictory results have not been fully reconciled[320] but likely reflect a combination of direct effects on vascular smooth muscle to stimulate myosin light-chain phosphorylation through ERK activation,[321,322] on the one hand, and stimulatory effects on endothelial cell nitric oxide synthase,[319] on the other. Finally, it is of considerable interest that vascular smooth muscle cells express ENaC, in addition to MR, and that the channel might play a role in vascular tone.[323]

Summary

In summary, the enzyme 11β-HSD2 is crucial for aldosterone-selective activation of epithelial MR and possibly of MR in other tissues, including blood vessel, nucleus of the solitary tract, and placenta. It does this in part by debulking intracellular glucocorticoids by an order of magnitude, which is not sufficient to account for its blockade of cortisol agonist activity. Current evidence supports the possibility that 11β-HSD2–mediated generation of NADH renders glucocorticoid-occupied MR inactive. Partial or complete deficiency of 11β-HSD2 results in the syndrome of apparent mineralocorticoid excess, which is mimicked by licorice abuse.

Nongenomic Effects

The classical effects of aldosterone on ion transport are genomic, with MR acting at the nuclear level to regulate DNA-directed, RNA-mediated protein synthesis and thereby sodium transport. Such genomic effects are characterized by a lag period of 45 to 60 minutes before changes in ion transport can be measured, commensurate with a homeostatic role for aldosterone action in regulating sodium and potassium status in response to dietary intake. In other circumstances (e.g., orthostasis, acute blood volume depletion), aldosterone secretion rises rapidly, and acute nongenomic effects are an understandable response. Such rapid effects were first demonstrated 25 years ago in the laboratory[324]; in human vascular tissues they have been amply demonstrated both in vitro[317] and in vivo.[325] Although most of these rapid nongenomic effects appear to be mediated via activation of classical MR,[317,324] there is recent evidence from atomic force microscopy studies for non-MR membrane sites binding aldosterone with high affinity on cultured endothelial cells.[326] Such nongenomic effects are not unique to aldosterone, having been shown for the other recognized classes of steroid hormones[327] and reported for dehydroepiandrosterone (DHEA).[319] Genomic effects commonly have a lag period of 20 minutes or longer and are abrogated by inhibitors of transcription such as actinomycin D. Most nongenomic effects of steroids have time courses from onset to plateau of 5 to 10 minutes and are mediated by a variety of pathways. MR does not have a myristoylation site (unlike, for example, estrogen receptors[328]), and there is little evidence for membrane-associated classical MR. Most rapid nongenomic effects of aldosterone appear to be mediated by classical MR, in that they are inhibited by the MR antagonist RU 28318. In some instances[317] spironolactone is ineffective as an inhibitor: exclusive reliance on blockade by spironolactone led to the assumption of a widely distributed aldosterone receptor distinct from classical MR, and a long and unsuccessful search for such a membrane-bound species.[329] The physiology of nongenomic aldosterone actions has been slow to be accepted, which in part reflects the major emphasis on the

clearly genomic actions of aldosterone in the kidney. The most obvious example is the conjunction of rapid secretion of aldosterone in response to orthostasis and its demonstrated rapid vascular effects.[320,330] With the recent interest in the pathophysiologic effects of MR activation, particularly in nonclassical aldosterone target tissues, there has been renewed interest in rapid nongenomic effects of aldosterone (and the physiologic glucocorticoids) via classical MR. Further details of the nongenomic actions of aldosterone can be found in Funder[330] and other sources.[331,332]

Disease States

Primary Aldosteronism

Clinically, by far the most prevalent disorder directly involving aldosterone is Conn's syndrome, or primary aldosteronism.[333] In this syndrome aldosterone secretion is elevated and (relatively) autonomous as a result of an adrenal adenoma or, more frequently, bilateral adrenal hyperplasia, and very rarely adrenal carcinoma or the inherited disorder glucocorticoid remediable aldosteronism.[334] Once considered rare (<1% of all cases of hypertension), necessarily characterized by hypokalemia and relatively benign, primary aldosteronism is now thought to account for approximately 8% to 13% of all hypertension, which reflects improved case detection and diagnosis. In contrast with previous teaching, frank hypokalemia is relatively uncommon, and the incidence of cardiovascular pathology (fibrosis, fibrillation, infarct, stroke) is substantially higher than in age-, sex-, and blood pressure–matched individuals with essential hypertension.[335,336] Guidelines for the case detection, diagnosis, and management of primary aldosteronism have been published[337] as a first step in addressing what is increasingly recognized as a major public health issue. It has long been thought, and taught, that the role of aldosterone in blood pressure regulation reflects its epithelial effects leading to retention of sodium, and with it water, which thus increases circulating volume. This increase, in turn, is reflected in an increased cardiac output, which is reflexively normalized by vasoconstriction and thus elevation of blood pressure (in keeping with the Guyton hypothesis[338]). Although the epithelial effects of aldosterone on vascular volume are indisputably homeostatically important, there are compelling experimental and clinical studies to suggest a role for nonepithelial effects in mineralocorticoid-induced hypertension.[339,340] Very recently, in addition to MR-mediated central nervous system and vascular effects in hypertension, roles for macrophages have been demonstrated by two groups using distinct and complementary experimental approaches.[341,342]

Recent data have suggested a role for a mutated K+ channel (KCNJ5) in the pathogenesis of both aldosterone-producing adrenal adenomas and bilateral adrenal hyperplasia.[351,352] See section "Aldosterone Synthesis" for additional details.

Congestive Heart Failure

Aldosterone has been implicated in the pathophysiology of congestive heart failure since soon after its discovery in the mid-1950s.[343,344] Until fairly recently, most of the focus has been on the counterproductive effects of aldosterone in epithelia. More recently, the beneficial effects of MR antagonists in congestive heart failure have suggested an additional effect in myocardium itself.[345] In the Randomized Aldactone Evaluation Study (RALES) trial,[345] addition of low-dose (mean 26 mg/day) spironolactone to standard-of-care treatment in patients with progressive heart failure produced a 30% reduction in mortality and 35% fewer hospitalizations. This result is often attributed to spironolactone's antagonizing the effect of aldosterone on cardiomyocyte MR, but may actually reflect its antagonizing of cortisol acting as an MR agonist under ischemic conditions. Subsequently, the Eplerenone's Neurohormonal Efficacy and Survival Study (EPHESUS) trial examined the effect of eplerenone, an MR antagonist with improved specificity relative to spironolactone, on heart failure due to systolic dysfunction complicating acute myocardial infarction. The study showed that adding eplerenone (25 mg/day) on top of conventional therapy significantly decreased mortality due to all causes (31%) and cardiovascular mortality (13%).[346] Potassium concentration was only slightly higher in the eplerenone-treated group than in the placebo-treated group (4.47 mmol/L and 4.54 mmol/L, respectively). Coupled with the recent literature on direct cardiac and vascular effects of aldosterone addressed earlier, these data suggest that MR antagonists have a beneficial effect that cannot be accounted for by diuretic actions in the kidney alone.[347] It is also notable that a recent trial (Eplerenone in Mild Patients Hospitalization And Survival Study in Heart Failure [EMPHASIS-HF]) examining the effect of eplerenone in class II heart failure (milder than previously examined) was stopped early because a significant benefit was found in the treated group.[348] In summary, the pathophysiologic effects of aldosterone on the cardiovascular system in primary aldosteronism are well documented, and MR also plays an important role in essential hypertension and heart failure. Importantly, MR expressed in cardiac and vascular cells likely plays an important role. In this latter setting, MR may actually be activated not only by aldosterone but also by cortisol, which is calculated to be present in serum at levels that are higher by 100-fold or more and mimics aldosterone in the context of tissue damage.

References

1. Verrey F. Early aldosterone action: toward filling the gap between transcription and transport. *Am J Physiol*. 1999;277(3 pt 2):F319-F327.
2. Simpson SA, Tait JF. A quantitative method for the bioassay of the effect of adrenal cortical steroids on mineral metabolism. *Endocrinology*. 1952;50(2):150-161.
3. Simpson SA, Tait JF. Physiochemical methods of detection of a previously unidentified adrenal hormone. *Mem Soc Endocrinol*. 1953;2:9-24.
4. Simpson SA, et al. [Constitution of aldosterone, a new mineralocorticoid]. *Experientia*. 1954;10(3):132-133.
5. Funder JW, et al. Mineralocorticoid action: target tissue specificity is enzyme, not receptor, mediated. *Science*. 1988;242(4878):583-585.
6. Edwards CR, et al. Localisation of 11 beta-hydroxysteroid dehydrogenase—tissue specific protector of the mineralocorticoid receptor. *Lancet*. 1988;2(8618):986-989.
7. Colombe L, et al. A mineralocorticoid-like receptor in the rainbow trout, *Oncorhynchus mykiss*: cloning and characterization of its steroid binding domain. *Steroids*. 2000;65(6):319-328.
8. Nuclear Receptors Nomenclature Committee. A unified nomenclature system for the nuclear receptor superfamily. *Cell*. 1999;97(2):161-163.
9. Hu X, Funder JW. The evolution of mineralocorticoid receptors. *Mol Endocrinol*. 2006;20(7):1471-1478.
10. Makhanova N, et al. Disturbed homeostasis in sodium-restricted mice heterozygous and homozygous for aldosterone synthase gene disruption. *Hypertension*. 2006;48(6):1151-1159.
11. Funder JW. Aldosterone and mineralocorticoid receptors: lessons from gene deletion studies. *Hypertension*. 2006;48(6):1018-1019.
12. Mornet E, et al. Characterization of two genes encoding human steroid 11β-hydroxylase (P-450 11β). *J Biol Chem*. 1989;264:20961-20967.
13. Curnow KM, et al. The product of the CYP11B2 gene is required for aldosterone biosynthesis in the human adrenal cortex. *Mol Endocrinol*. 1991;5:1513-1522.
14. Lifton RP, et al. A chimaeric 11β-hydroxylase/aldosterone synthase gene causes glucocorticoid-remediable aldosteronism and human hypertension. *Nature*. 1992;355:262-265.
15. Ehrhart-Bornstein M, et al. Human adipocytes secrete mineralocorticoid-releasing factors. *Proc Natl Acad Sci U S A*. 2003;100(24):14211-14216.
16. Nogueira EF, Bollag WB, Rainey WE. Angiotensin II regulation of adrenocortical gene transcription. *Mol Cell Endocrinol*. 2009;302(2):230-236.
17. Miller WL. StAR search—what we know about how the steroidogenic acute regulatory protein mediates mitochondrial cholesterol import. *Mol Endocrinol*. 2007;21(3):589-601.
18. Ganguly A, Davis JS. Role of calcium and other mediators in aldosterone secretion from the adrenal glomerulosa cells. *Pharmacol Rev*. 1994;46(4):417-447.
19. Foster RH, MacFarlane CH, Bustamante MO. Recent progress in understanding aldosterone secretion. *Gen Pharmacol*. 1997;28(5):647-651.
20. Schrier RW. Aldosterone "escape" vs. "breakthrough." *Nat Rev Nephrol*. 6(2):61.
21. DeFranco DB. Navigating steroid hormone receptors through the nuclear compartment. *Mol Endocrinol*. 2002;16(7):1449-1455.
22. Fejes-Toth G, Pearce D, Naray-Fejes-Toth A. Subcellular localization of mineralocorticoid receptors in living cells: effects of receptor agonists and antagonists. *Proc Natl Acad Sci U S A*. 1998;95(6):2973-2978.
23. Pratt WB, et al. Role of hsp90 and the hsp90-binding immunophilins in signalling protein movement. *Cell Signal*. 2004;16(8):857-872.
24. Gallo LI, et al. Differential recruitment of tetratricopeptide repeat domain immunophilins to the mineralocorticoid receptor influences both heat-shock protein 90-dependent retrotransport and hormone-dependent transcriptional activity. *Biochemistry*. 2007;46(49):14044-14057.
25. Viengchareun S, et al. The mineralocorticoid receptor: insights into its molecular and (patho)physiological biology. *Nucl Recept Signal*. 2007;5:e012.
25a. Li Y, et al. Structural and biochemical mechanisms for the specificity of hormone binding and coactivator assembly by mineral corticoid receptor. *Mol Cell*. 2005;19:367-380.
26. Arriza JL, et al. The neuronal mineralocorticoid receptor as a mediator of glucocorticoid response. *Neuron*. 1988;1(9):887-900.
27. Bhargava A, Pearce D. Mechanisms of mineralocorticoid action: determinants of receptor specificity and actions of regulated gene products. *Trends Endocrinol Metab*. 2004;15(4):147-153.
28. Liu W, et al. Steroid receptor heterodimerization demonstrated in vitro and in vivo. *Proc Natl Acad Sci U S A*. 1995;92(26):12480-12484.
29. Trapp T, et al. Heterodimerization between mineralocorticoid and glucocorticoid receptor: a new principle of glucocorticoid action in the CNS. *Neuron*. 1994;13(6):1457-1462.
30. Reichardt HM, et al. DNA binding of the glucocorticoid receptor is not essential for survival. *Cell*. 1998;93(4):531-541.
31. Liu W, et al. Steroid receptor transcriptional synergy is potentiated by disruption of the DNA-binding domain dimer interface. *Mol Endocrinol*. 1996;10(11):1399-1406.
32. Kaspar F, et al. A mutant androgen receptor from patients with Reifenstein syndrome: identification of the function of a conserved alanine residue in the D box of steroid receptors. *Mol Cell Biol*. 1993;13(12):7850-7858.
33. Sartorato P, et al. Different inactivating mutations of the mineralocorticoid receptor in fourteen families affected by type I pseudohypoaldosteronism. *J Clin Endocrinol Metab*. 2003;88(6):2508-2517.
34. Picard D, Yamamoto KR. Two signals mediate hormone-dependent nuclear localization of the glucocorticoid receptor. *EMBO J*. 1987;6(3333):3333-3340.
35. Walther RF, et al. A serine/threonine-rich motif is one of three nuclear localization signals that determine unidirectional transport of the mineralocorticoid receptor to the nucleus. *J Biol Chem*. 2005;280(17):17549-17561.
36. Starr DB, et al. Intracellular receptors use a common mechanism to interpret signaling information at response elements. *Genes Dev*. 1996;10(10):1271-1283.
37. Prefontaine GG, et al. Recruitment of octamer transcription factors to DNA by glucocorticoid receptor. *Mol Cell Biol*. 1998;18(6):3416-3430.
38. Iniguez-Lluhi JA, Pearce D. A common motif within the negative regulatory regions of multiple factors inhibits their transcriptional synergy. *Mol Cell Biol*. 2000;20(16):6040-6050.
39. Fuse H, Kitagawa H, Kato S. Characterization of transactivational property and coactivator mediation of rat mineralocorticoid receptor activation function-1 (AF-1). *Mol Endocrinol*. 2000;14(6):889-899.
40. Savory JG, et al. Glucocorticoid receptor homodimers and glucocorticoid-mineralocorticoid receptor heterodimers form in the cytoplasm through alternative dimerization interfaces. *Mol Cell Biol*. 2001;21(3):781-793.

41. Rogerson FM, Fuller PJ. Interdomain interactions in the mineralocorticoid receptor. *Mol Cell Endocrinol.* 2003;200(1-2):45-55.

42. Li Y, et al. Structural and biochemical mechanisms for the specificity of hormone binding and coactivator assembly by mineralocorticoid receptor. *Mol Cell.* 2005;19(3):367-380.

43. Fagart J, et al. Crystal structure of a mutant mineralocorticoid receptor responsible for hypertension. *Nat Struct Mol Biol.* 2005;12(6):554-555.

44. Geller DS, et al. Activating mineralocorticoid receptor mutation in hypertension exacerbated by pregnancy. *Science.* 2000;289(5476):119-123.

45. Geller DS, et al. Autosomal dominant pseudohypoaldosteronism type 1: mechanisms, evidence for neonatal lethality, and phenotypic expression in adults. *J Am Soc Nephrol.* 2006;17(5):1429-1436.

46. Krozowski ZS, Funder JW. Renal mineralocorticoid receptors and hippocampal corticosterone-binding species have identical intrinsic steroid specificity. *Proc Natl Acad Sci U S A.* 1983;80(19):6056-6060.

47. Funder JW, et al. Vascular type I aldosterone binding sites are physiological mineralocorticoid receptors. *Endocrinology.* 1989;125(4):2224-2226.

48. De Kloet ER. Hormones and the stressed brain. *Ann N Y Acad Sci.* 2004;1018:1-15.

49. Kitagawa H, et al. Ligand-selective potentiation of rat mineralocorticoid receptor activation function 1 by a CBP-containing histone acetyltransferase complex. *Mol Cell Biol.* 2002;22(11):3698-3706.

50. Pearce D, Yamamoto KR. Mineralocorticoid and glucocorticoid receptor activities distinguished by nonreceptor factors at a composite response element. *Science.* 1993;259(5098):1161-1165.

51. Tallec LP, et al. Protein inhibitor of activated signal transducer and activator of transcription 1 interacts with the N-terminal domain of mineralocorticoid receptor and represses its transcriptional activity: implication of small ubiquitin-related modifier 1 modification. *Mol Endocrinol.* 2003;17(12):2529-2542.

52. Pascual-Le Tallec L, et al. The elongation factor ELL (eleven-nineteen lysine-rich leukemia) is a selective coregulator for steroid receptor functions. *Mol Endocrinol.* 2005;19(5):1158-1169.

53. Choudhry MA, Ball A, McEwan IJ. The role of the general transcription factor IIF in androgen receptor-dependent transcription. *Mol Endocrinol.* 2006;20(9):2052-2061.

54. Roeder RG. Transcriptional regulation and the role of diverse coactivators in animal cells. *FEBS Lett.* 2005;579(4):909-915.

55. Lee DY, et al. Role of protein methylation in regulation of transcription. *Endocr Rev.* 2005;26(2):147-170.

56. Watson JD. *Molecular biology of the gene,* ed 6. Benjamin Cummings, 2007.

57. Hong H, et al. GRIP1, a novel mouse protein that serves as a transcriptional coactivator in yeast for the hormone binding domains of steroid receptors. *Proc Natl Acad Sci U S A.* 1996;93(10):4948-4952.

58. Onate SA, et al. Sequence and characterization of a coactivator for the steroid hormone receptor superfamily. *Science.* 1995;270(5240):1354-1357.

59. Metivier R, et al. Estrogen receptor-alpha directs ordered, cyclical, and combinatorial recruitment of cofactors on a natural target promoter. *Cell.* 2003;115(6):751-763.

60. Yokota K, et al. Coactivation of the N-terminal transactivation of mineralocorticoid receptor by Ubc9. *J Biol Chem.* 2007;282(3):1998-2010.

61. Endoh H, et al. Purification and identification of p68 RNA helicase acting as a transcriptional coactivator specific for the activation function 1 of human estrogen receptor alpha. *Mol Cell Biol.* 1999;19(8):5363-5372.

62. Ganong WF, Mulrow PJ. Rate of change in sodium and potassium excretion after injection of aldosterone into the aorta and renal artery of the dog. *Am J Physiol.* 1958;195(2):337-342.

63. Edelman IS, Fimognari GM. On the biochemical mechanism of action of aldosterone. *Recent Prog Horm Res.* 1968;24(1):1-44.

64. Ganguly A. Primary aldosteronism. *N Engl J Med.* 1998;339:1828-1834.

65. Conn JW, Knopf RF, Nesbit RM. Clinical characteristics of primary aldosteronism from an analysis of 145 cases. *Am J Surg.* 1964;107:159-172.

66. Canessa CM, et al. Amiloride-sensitive epithelial Na+ channel is made of three homologous subunits. *Nature.* 1994;367(6462):463-467.

67. Canessa CM, Horisberger JD, Rossier BC. Epithelial sodium channel related to proteins involved in neurodegeneration. *Nature.* 1993;361(6411):467-470.

68. Garty H, Palmer LG. Epithelial sodium channels: function, structure, and regulation. *Physiol Rev.* 1997;77:359-396.

69. Hummler E, et al. Early death due to defective neonatal lung liquid clearance in αENaC-deficient mice. *Nat Genet.* 1996;12:325-328.

70. Barker PM, et al. Role of γENaC subunit in lung liquid clearance and electrolyte balance in newborn mice. Insights into perinatal adaptation and pseudohypoaldosteronism. *J Clin Invest.* 1998;102:1634-1640.

71. McDonald FJ, et al. Disruption of the β subunit of the epithelial Na+ channel in mice: hyperkalemia and neonatal death associated with a pseudohypoaldosteronism phenotype. *Proc Natl Acad Sci U S A.* 1999;96:1727-1731.

72. Kunzelmann K, Mall M. Electrolyte transport in the mammalian colon: mechanisms and implications for disease. *Physiol Rev.* 2002;82(1):245-289.

73. Giebisch G. Renal potassium transport: mechanisms and regulation. *Am J Physiol.* 1998;274(5 pt 2):F817-F833.

74. Palmer LG. Potassium secretion and the regulation of distal nephron K channels. *Am J Physiol.* 1999;277(6 pt 2):F821-F825.

75. Loffing J, et al. Aldosterone induces rapid apical translocation of ENaC in early portion of renal collecting system: possible role of SGK. *Am J Physiol Renal Physiol.* 2001;280(4):F675-F682.

76. Chen S, et al. Epithelial sodium channel regulated by aldosterone-induced protein sgk. *Proc Natl Acad Sci U S A.* 1999;96:2514-2519.

77. Naray-Fejes-Toth A, et al. sgk is an aldosterone-induced kinase in the renal collecting duct. Effects on epithelial Na+ channels. *J Biol Chem.* 1999;274:16973-16978.

78. Shigaev A, et al. Regulation of sgk by aldosterone and its effects on the epithelial Na(+) channel. *Am J Physiol.* 2000;278(4):F613-F619.

79. McCormick JA, et al. SGK1: a rapid aldosterone-induced regulator of renal sodium reabsorption. *Physiology.* 2005;20(2):134-139.

80. Vallon V, et al. Role of Sgk1 in salt and potassium homeostasis. *Am J Physiol Regul Integr Comp Physiol.* 2005;288(1):R4-10.

81. Schild L, et al. A mutation in the epithelial sodium channel causing Liddle disease increases channel activity in the *Xenopus laevis* oocyte expression system. *Proc Natl Acad Sci U S A.* 1995;92:5699-5703.

82. Snyder PM, et al. Mechanism by which Liddle's syndrome mutations increase activity of a human epithelial Na+ channel. *Cell.* 1995;83:969-978.

83. Loffing J, et al. Aldosterone induces rapid apical translocation of ENaC in early portion of renal collecting system: possible role of SGK. *Am J Physiol Renal Physiol.* 2001;280(4):F675-F682.

84. Masilamani S, et al. Aldosterone-mediated regulation of ENaC alpha, beta, and gamma subunit proteins in rat kidney. *J Clin Invest.* 1999;104:R19-R23.

85. Frindt G, Ergonul Z, Palmer LG. Surface expression of epithelial Na channel protein in rat kidney. *J Gen Physiol.* 2008;131(6):617-627.

86. Butterworth MB, et al. Acute ENaC stimulation by cAMP in a kidney cell line is mediated by exocytic insertion from a recycling channel pool. *J Gen Physiol.* 2004;125(1):81-101.

87. Goldfarb SB, et al. Differential effects of Hsc70 and Hsp70 on the intracellular trafficking and functional expression of epithelial sodium channels. *Proc Natl Acad Sci U S A.* 2006;103(15):5817-5822.

88. Butterworth MB, et al. PKA-dependent ENaC trafficking requires the SNARE-binding protein complexin. *Am J Physiol Renal Physiol.* 2005;289(5):F969-F977.

89. Martel JA, et al. Melanophilin, a novel aldosterone-induced gene in mouse cortical collecting duct cells. *Am J Physiol Renal Physiol.* 2007;293(3):F904-F913.

90. Soundararajan R, et al. A novel role for glucocorticoid-induced leucine zipper protein in epithelial sodium channel-mediated sodium transport. *J Biol Chem.* 2005;280(48):39970-39981.

91. Goulet CC, et al. Inhibition of the epithelial Na+ channel by interaction of Nedd4 with a PY motif deleted in Liddle's syndrome. *J Biol Chem.* 1998;273:30012-30017.

92. Schild L, et al. Identification of PY motif in the epithelial Na channel subunits as a target sequence for mutations causing channel activation found in Liddle syndrome. *EMBO J.* 1996;15:2381-2387.

93. Wang H, et al. Clathrin-mediated endocytosis of the epithelial sodium channel: role of epsin. *J Biol Chem.* 2006;281(20):14129-14135.

94. Shimkets RA, Lifton RP, Canessa CM. The activity of the epithelial sodium channel is regulated by clathrin-mediated endocytosis. *J Biol Chem.* 1997;272:25537-25541.

95. Malik B, et al. Regulation of epithelial sodium channels by the ubiquitin-proteasome proteolytic pathway. *Am J Physiol Renal Physiol.* 2006;290(6):F1285-F1294.

96. Staub O, et al. Regulation of stability and function of the epithelial Na+ channel (ENaC) by ubiquitination. *EMBO J.* 1997;16(21):6325-6336.

97. Butterworth MB, et al. Regulation of the epithelial sodium channel by membrane trafficking. *Am J Physiol Renal Physiol.* 2009;296(1):F10-F24.

98. Pochynyuk O, et al. Regulation of the epithelial Na+ channel (ENaC) by phosphatidylinositides. *Am J Physiol Renal Physiol.* 2006;290(5):F949-F957.

99. Tong Q, et al. Direct activation of the epithelial Na(+) channel by phosphatidylinositol 3,4,5-trisphosphate and phosphatidylinositol 3,4-bisphosphate produced by phosphoinositide 3-OH kinase. *J Biol Chem.* 2004;279(21):22654-22663.

100. Stockand JD, et al. Regulation of Na(+) reabsorption by the aldosterone-induced small G protein K-Ras2A. *J Biol Chem.* 1999;274(50):35449-35454.

101. Soundararajan R, et al. Epithelial sodium channel regulated by differential composition of a signaling complex. *Proc Natl Acad Sci U S A.* 2009;106(19):7804-7809.

102. Staruschenko A, et al. Ras activates the epithelial Na+ channel through phosphoinositide 3-OH kinase signaling. *J Biol Chem.* 2004;279(36):37771-37778.

103. Falin RA, Cotton CU. Acute downregulation of ENaC by EGF involves the PY motif and putative ERK phosphorylation site. *J Gen Physiol.* 2007;130(3):313-328.

104. Shi H, et al. Interactions of beta and gamma ENaC with Nedd4 can be facilitated by an ERK-mediated phosphorylation. *J Biol Chem.* 2002;277(16):13539-13547.

105. Staruschenko A, Pochynyuk O, Stockand JD. Regulation of epithelial Na^+ channel activity by conserved serine/threonine switches within sorting signals. *J Biol Chem.* 2005;280(47):39161-39167.

106. Stokes JB, Sigmund RD. Regulation of rENaC mRNA by dietary NaCl and steroids: organ, tissue, and steroid heterogeneity. *Am J Physiol Cell Physiol.* 1998;274:C1699-C1707.

107. Masilamani S, et al. Time course of renal Na-K-ATPase, NHE3, NKCC2, NCC, and ENaC abundance changes with dietary NaCl restriction. *Am J Physiol Renal Physiol.* 2002;283(4):F648-F657.

108. Johnson DW, et al. TGF-β1 dissociates human proximal tubule cell growth and Na^+-H^+ exchange activity. *Kidney Int.* 1998;53:1601-1607.

109. Ergonul Z, Frindt G, Palmer LG. Regulation of maturation and processing of ENaC subunits in the rat kidney. *Am J Physiol Renal Physiol.* 2006;291(3):F683-F693.

110. Husted RF, et al. Discordant effects of corticosteroids and expression of subunits on ENaC activity. *Am J Physiol Renal Physiol.* 2007;293(3):F813-F820.

111. Crabbe J. Site of action of aldosterone on the toad bladder. *Nature.* 1963;200(4908):787-788.

112. Sharp GW, et al. Evidence for a mucosal effect of aldosterone on sodium transport in the toad bladder. *J Clin Invest.* 1966;45(10):1640-1647.

113. Pellanda AM, et al. Sodium-independent effect of aldosterone on initial rate of ouabain binding in A6 cells. *Am J Physiol.* 1992:C899-C906.

114. Verrey F, et al. Regulation by aldosterone of Na^+, K^+-ATPase mRNAs, protein synthesis, and sodium transport in cultured kidney cells. *J Cell Biol.* 1987;104(5):1231-1237.

115. Park CS, Edelman IS. Dual action of aldosterone on toad bladder: Na^+ permeability and Na^+ pump modulation. *Am J Physiol.* 1984:F517-F525.

116. Palmer LG, Antonian L, Frindt G. Regulation of the Na-K pump of the rat cortical collecting tubule by aldosterone. *J Gen Physiol.* 1993;102(1):43-57.

117. Coutry N, et al. Time course of sodium-induced Na^+-K^+-ATPase recruitment in rabbit cortical collecting tubule. *Am J Physiol Cell Physiol.* 1992;263:C61-C68.

118. Wade JB, et al. Morphological and physiological responses to aldosterone: time course and sodium dependence. *Am J Physiol.* 1990;259(1 pt 2):F88-F94.

119. Verrey F, Kraehenbuhl JP, Rossier BC. Aldosterone induces a rapid increase in the rate of Na, K-ATPase gene transcription in cultured kidney cells. *Mol Endocrinol.* 1989;3(9):1369-1376.

120. Kolla V, Robertson NM, Litwack G. Identification of a mineralocorticoid/glucocorticoid response element in the human Na/K ATPase alpha1 gene promoter. *Biochem Biophys Res Commun.* 1999;266(1):5-14.

121. Nagel W. Rheogenic sodium transport in a tight epithelium, the amphibian skin. *J Physiol.* 1980;302:281-295.

122. Blot-Chabaud M, et al. Cell sodium-induced recruitment of Na^+-K^+-ATPase pumps in rabbit cortical collecting tubules is aldosterone-dependent. *J Biol Chem.* 1990;265:11676-11681.

123. Kleyman TR, Carattino MD, Hughey RP. ENaC at the cutting edge: regulation of epithelial sodium channels by proteases. *J Biol Chem.* 2009.

124. Narikiyo T, et al. Regulation of prostasin by aldosterone in the kidney. *J Clin Invest.* 2002;109(3):401-408.

125. Wakida N, et al. Inhibition of prostasin-induced ENaC activities by PN-1 and regulation of PN-1 expression by TGF-beta1 and aldosterone. *Kidney Int.* 2006;70(8):1432-1438.

126. Knight KK, et al. Liddle's syndrome mutations increase Na^+ transport through dual effects on epithelial Na^+ channel surface expression and proteolytic cleavage. *Proc Natl Acad Sci U S A.* 2006;103(8):2805-2808.

127. Stokes JB. Potassium secretion by cortical collecting tubule: relation to sodium absorption, luminal sodium concentration, and transepithelial voltage. *Am J Physiol Renal Fluid Electrolyte Physiol.* 1981;241:F395-F402.

128. Palmer LG, Antonian L, Frindt G. Regulation of apical K and Na channels and Na/K pumps in rat cortical collecting tubule by dietary K. *J Gen Physiol.* 1994;104:693-710.

129. Diezi J, et al. Micropuncture study of electrolyte transport across papillary collecting duct of the rat. *Am J Physiol.* 1973;224:623-634.

130. Stokes JB. Ion transport by the cortical and outer medullary collecting tubule. *Kidney Int.* 1982;22:473-484.

131. Koeppen BM. Conductive properties of the rabbit outer medullary collecting duct: inner stripe. *Am J Physiol Renal Physiol.* 1985;248(4):F500-F506.

132. Lazrak A, Liu Z, Huang CL. Antagonistic regulation of ROMK by long and kidney-specific WNK1 isoforms. *Proc Natl Acad Sci U S A.* 2006;103(5):1615-1620.

133. Kahle KT, Ring AM, Lifton RP. Molecular physiology of the WNK kinases. *Annu Rev Physiol.* 2008;70(1):329-355.

134. McCormick JA, Yang CL, Ellison DH. WNK kinases and renal sodium transport in health and disease: an integrated view. *Hypertension.* 2008;51(3):588-596.

135. Stokes JB. Physiologic resistance to the action of aldosterone. *Kidney Int.* 2000;57:1319-1323.

136. Harris RC, Breyer MD. Physiological regulation of cyclooxygenase-2 in the kidney. *Am J Physiol Renal Physiol.* 2001;281(1):F1-11.

137. Le Moellic C, et al. Aldosterone and tight junctions: modulation of claudin-4 phosphorylation in renal collecting duct cells. *Am J Physiol Cell Physiol.* 2005;289(6):C1513-C1521.

138. Wall SM, et al. NaCl restriction upregulates renal Slc26a4 through subcellular redistribution: role in Cl^- conservation. *Hypertension.* 2004;44(6):982-987.

139. Pech V, et al. Angiotensin II increases chloride absorption in the cortical collecting duct in mice through a pendrin-dependent mechanism. *Am J Physiol Renal Physiol.* 2007;292(3):F914-F920.

140. Vallet M, et al. Pendrin regulation in mouse kidney primarily is chloride-dependent. *J Am Soc Nephrol.* 2006;17(8):2153-2163.

141. Marver D, Kokko JP. Renal target sites and the mechanism of action of aldosterone. *Miner Electrolyte Metab.* 1983;9(1):1-18.

142. Bonvalet JP. Binding and action of aldosterone, dexamethasone, 1-25(OH)₂D₃, and estradiol along the nephron. *J Steroid Biochem.* 1987;27(4-6):953-961.

143. Todd-Turla KM, et al. Distribution of mineralocorticoid and glucocorticoid receptor mRNA along the nephron. *Am J Physiol.* 1993:F781-F791.

144. Roland BL, Krozowski ZS, Funder JW. Glucocorticoid receptor, mineralocorticoid receptors, 11 beta-hydroxysteroid dehydrogenase-1 and -2 expression in rat brain and kidney: in situ studies. *Mol Cell Endocrinol.* 1995;111(1):R1-R7.

145. Farman N, et al. Immunolocalization of gluco- and mineralocorticoid receptors in rabbit kidney. *Am J Physiol.* 1991;260(2 pt 1):C226-C233.

146. Berger S, et al. Mineralocorticoid receptor knockout mice: pathophysiology of Na^+ metabolism. *Proc Natl Acad Sci U S A.* 1998;95(16):9424-9429.

147. Makhanova N, et al. Kidney function in mice lacking aldosterone. *Am J Physiol Renal Physiol.* 2006;290(1):F61-F69.

148. Stone DK, et al. Mineralocorticoid modulation of rabbit medullary collecting duct acidification. A sodium-independent effect. *J Clin Invest.* 1983;72(1):77-83.

149. Winter C, et al. Nongenomic stimulation of vacuolar H^+-ATPases in intercalated renal tubule cells by aldosterone. *Proc Natl Acad Sci U S A.* 2004;101(8):2636-2641.

150. Wagner CA, et al. Regulated acid-base transport in the collecting duct. *Pflugers Arch.* 2009;458(1):137-156.

151. Marver D, Schwartz MJ. Identification of mineralocorticoid target sites in the isolated rabbit cortical nephron. *Proc Natl Acad Sci U S A.* 1980;77(6):3672-3676.

152. Doucet A, Katz AI. Mineralcorticoid receptors along the nephron: [3H] aldosterone binding in rabbit tubules. *Am J Physiol.* 1981;241(6):F605-F611.

153. Vandewalle A, et al. Aldosterone binding along the rabbit nephron: an autoradiographic study on isolated tubules. *Am J Physiol.* 1981;240(3):F172-F179.

154. Gnionsahe A, et al. Aldosterone binding sites along nephron of *Xenopus* and rabbit. *Am J Physiol.* 1989;257(1 pt 2):R87-R95.

155. Krozowski Z, et al. Immunohistochemical localization of the 11 beta-hydroxysteroid dehydrogenase type II enzyme in human kidney and placenta. *J Clin Endocrinol Metab.* 1995;80(7):2203-2209.

156. Kyossev Z, Walker PD, Reeves WB. Immunolocalization of NAD-dependent 11 beta-hydroxysteroid dehydrogenase in human kidney and colon. *Kidney Int.* 1996;49(1):271-281.

157. Miyata K, et al. Aldosterone stimulates reactive oxygen species production through activation of NADPH oxidase in rat mesangial cells. *J Am Soc Nephrol.* 2005;16(10):2906-2912.

158. Nishiyama A, et al. Involvement of aldosterone and mineralocorticoid receptors in rat mesangial cell proliferation and deformability. *Hypertension.* 2005;45(4):710-716.

159. Terada Y, et al. Aldosterone-stimulated SGK1 activity mediates profibrotic signaling in the mesangium. *J Am Soc Nephrol.* 2008;19(2):298-309.

160. Cha DR, et al. Role of aldosterone in diabetic nephropathy. *Nephrology (Carlton).* 2005;10(suppl):S37-S39.

161. Hierholzer K, Stolte H. The proximal and distal tubular action of adrenal steroids on Na reabsorption. *Nephron.* 1969;6(3):188-204.

162. Wiederholt M, et al. Sodium conductance changes by aldosterone in the rat kidney. *Pflugers Arch.* 1974;348(2):155-165.

163. Pergher PS, Leite-Dellova D, de Mello-Aires M. Direct action of aldosterone on bicarbonate reabsorption in in vivo cortical proximal tubule. *Am J Physiol Renal Physiol.* 2009;296(5):F1185-F1193.

164. Leite-Dellova DC, et al. Genomic and nongenomic dose-dependent biphasic effect of aldosterone on Na$^+$/H$^+$ exchanger in proximal S3 segment: role of cytosolic calcium. *Am J Physiol Renal Physiol*. 2008;295(5):F1342-F1352.

165. Krug AW, et al. Aldosterone stimulates surface expression of NHE3 in renal proximal brush borders. *Pflugers Arch*. 2003;446(4):492-496.

166. ElMernissi G, Doucet A. Short-term effects of aldosterone and dexamethasone on Na-K-ATPase along the rabbit nephron. *Pflugers Arch*. 1983;399:147-151.

167. Garg LC, Knepper MA, Burg MB. Mineralocorticoid effects on Na-K-ATPase in individual nephron segments. *Am J Physiol*. 1981;240(6):F536-F544.

168. Schmidt U, et al. Sodium- and potassium-activated ATPase: a possible target of aldosterone. *J Clin Invest*. 1975;55(3):655-660.

169. Schmid H, et al. Hormonal effects on Na-K-ATPase of various parts of the rat nephron. *Curr Probl Clin Biochem*. 1975;4:214-217.

170. Stanton BA. Regulation by adrenal corticosteroids of sodium and potassium transport in loop of Henle and distal tubule of rat kidney. *J Clin Invest*. 1986;78(6):1612-1620.

171. Work J, Jamison RL. Effect of adrenalectomy on transport in the rat medullary thick ascending limb. *J Clin Invest*. 1987;80(4):1160-1164.

172. Crabbe J. The role of aldosterone in the renal concentration mechanism in man. *Clin Sci*. 1962;23:39-46.

173. Oberleithner H, et al. Aldosterone activates Na$^+$/H$^+$ exchange and raises cytoplasmic pH in target cells of the amphibian kidney. *Proc Natl Acad Sci U S A*. 1987;84:1464-1468.

174. Ponce-Coria J, et al. Regulation of NKCC2 by a chloride-sensing mechanism involving the WNK3 and SPAK kinases. *Proc Natl Acad Sci U S A*. 2008;105(24):8458-8463.

175. Rundle SE, et al. Immunocytochemical demonstration of mineralocorticoid receptors in rat and human kidney. *J Steroid Biochem*. 1989;33(6):1235-1242.

176. Gonzalez-Nunez D, et al. In vitro characterization of aldosterone and cAMP effects in mouse distal convoluted tubule cells. *Am J Physiol Renal Physiol*. 2004;286(5):F936-F944.

177. Nielsen J, et al. Sodium transporter abundance profiling in kidney: effect of spironolactone. *Am J Physiol Renal Physiol*. 2002;283(5):F923-F933.

178. Abdallah JG, et al. Loop diuretic infusion increases thiazide-sensitive Na(+)/Cl(−)-cotransporter abundance: role of aldosterone. *J Am Soc Nephrol*. 2001;12(7):1335-1341.

179. Masilamani S, et al. Time course of renal Na-K-ATPase, NHE3, NKCC2, NCC, and ENaC abundance changes with dietary NaCl restriction. *Am J Physiol Renal Physiol*. 2002;283(4):F648-F657.

180. Wang XY, et al. The renal thiazide-sensitive Na-Cl cotransporter as mediator of the aldosterone-escape phenomenon. *J Clin Invest*. 2001;108(2):215-222.

181. Yang SS, et al. Molecular pathogenesis of pseudohypoaldosteronism type II: generation and analysis of a Wnk4(D561A/$^+$) knockin mouse model. *Cell Metab*. 2007;5(5):331-344.

182. Kim GH, et al. The thiazide-sensitive Na-Cl cotransporter is an aldosterone-induced protein. *Proc Natl Acad Sci U S A*. 1998;95(24):14552-14557.

183. Ring AM, et al. An SGK1 site in WNK4 regulates Na$^+$ channel and K$^+$ channel activity and has implications for aldosterone signaling and K$^+$ homeostasis. *Proc Natl Acad Sci U S A*. 2007;104(10):4025-4029.

184. Rozansky DJ, et al. Aldosterone mediates activation of the thiazide-sensitive Na-Cl cotransporter through an SGK1 and WNK4 signaling pathway. *J Clin Invest*. 2009;119(9):2601-2612.

185. Chiga M, et al. Dietary salt regulates the phosphorylation of OSR1/SPAK kinases and the sodium chloride cotransporter through aldosterone. *Kidney Int*. 2008;74(11):1403-1409.

186. Richardson C, et al. Activation of the thiazide-sensitive Na$^+$-Cl$^-$-cotransporter by the WNK-regulated kinases SPAK and OSR1. *J Cell Sci*. 2008;121(pt 5):675-684.

187. Xu BE, et al. WNK1 activates SGK1 by a phosphatidylinositol 3-kinase–dependent and non-catalytic mechanism. *J Biol Chem*. 2005;280(40):34218-34223.

188. Braun EJ. Regulation of renal and lower gastrointestinal function: role in fluid and electrolyte balance. *Comp Biochem Physiol A Mol Integr Physiol*. 2003;136(3):499-505.

189. Levitan R, et al. Water and salt absorption in the human colon. *J Clin Invest*. 1962;41:1754-1759.

190. Clauss W, et al. Ion transport and electrophysiology of the early proximal colon of rabbit. *Pflugers Arch*. 1987;408(6):592-599.

191. Sandle GI, et al. Electrophysiology of the human colon: evidence of segmental heterogeneity. *Gut*. 1986;27(9):999-1005.

192. Yau WM, Makhlouf GM. Comparison of transport mechanisms in isolated ascending and descending rat colon. *Am J Physiol*. 1975;228(1):191-195.

193. Greig ER, et al. Decreased expression of apical Na$^+$ channels and basolateral Na$^+$, K$^+$-ATPase in ulcerative colitis. *J Pathol*. 2004;204(1):84-92.

194. Levitan R, Ingelfinger FJ. Effect of d-aldosterone on salt and water absorption from the intact human colon. *J Clin Invest*. 1965;44:801-808.

195. Hirasawa G, et al. Colocalization of 11 beta-hydroxysteroid dehydrogenase type II and mineralocorticoid receptor in human epithelia. *J Clin Endocrinol Metab*. 1997;82(11):3859-3863.

196. Turnamian SG, Binder HJ. Regulation of active sodium and potassium transport in the distal colon of the rat: role of the aldosterone and glucocorticoid receptors. *J Clin Invest*. 1989;84(6):1924-1929.

197. Fromm M, Schulzke JD, Hegel U. Control of electrogenic Na$^+$ absorption in rat late distal colon by nanomolar aldosterone added in vitro. *Am J Physiol*. 1993;264(1 pt 1):E68-E73.

198. Shigaev A, et al. Regulation of sgk by aldosterone and its effects on the epithelial Na(+) channel. *Am J Physiol Renal Physiol*. 2000;278(4):F613-F619.

199. Asher C, et al. Aldosterone-induced increase in the abundance of Na$^+$ channel subunits. *Am J Physiol*. 1996;271(2 pt 1):C605-C611.

200. Epple HJ, et al. Early aldosterone effect in distal colon by transcriptional regulation of ENaC subunits. *Am J Physiol Gastrointest Liver Physiol*. 2000;278(5):G718-G724.

201. Gifford JD, et al. Control of serum potassium during fasting in patients with end-stage renal disease. *Kidney Int*. 1989;35(1):90-94.

202. Hayes Jr CP, McLeod ME, Robinson RR. An extrarenal mechanism for the maintenance of potassium balance in severe chronic renal failure. *Trans Assoc Am Physicians*. 1967;80:207-216.

203. Sandle GI, et al. Enhanced rectal potassium secretion in chronic renal insufficiency: evidence for large intestinal potassium adaptation in man. *Clin Sci*. 1986;71(4):393-401.

204. Imbriano LJ, Durham JH, Maesaka JK. Treating interdialytic hyperkalemia with fludrocortisone. *Semin Dial*. 2003;16(1):5-7.

205. Hussain S, et al. Is spironolactone safe for dialysis patients? *Nephrol Dial Transplant*. 2003;18(11):2364-2368.

206. Saudan P, et al. Safety of low-dose spironolactone administration in chronic haemodialysis patients. *Nephrol Dial Transplant*. 2003;18(11):2359-2363.

207. Gross E, et al. Effect of spironolactone on blood pressure and the renin-angiotensin-aldosterone system in oligo-anuric hemodialysis patients. *Am J Kidney Dis*. 2005;46(1):94-101.

208. Eaton DC, et al. The contribution of epithelial sodium channels to alveolar function in health and disease. *Annu Rev Physiol*. 2009;71:403-423.

209. Hummler E, et al. Early death due to defective neonatal lung liquid clearance in alpha-ENaC-deficient mice. *Nat Genet*. 1996;12(3):325-328.

210. Malagon-Rogers M. A patient with pseudohypoaldosteronism type 1 and respiratory distress syndrome. *Pediatr Nephrol*. 1999;13(6):484-486.

211. Kerem E, et al. Pulmonary epithelial sodium-channel dysfunction and excess airway liquid in pseudohypoaldosteronism. *N Engl J Med*. 1999;341:156-162.

212. Sheridan MB, et al. Mutations in the beta-subunit of the epithelial Na$^+$ channel in patients with a cystic fibrosis-like syndrome. *Hum Mol Genet*. 2005;14(22):3493-3498.

213. Matthay MA, Robriquet L, Fang X. Alveolar epithelium: role in lung fluid balance and acute lung injury. *Proc Am Thorac Soc*. 2005;2(3):206-213.

214. Scherrer U, et al. High-altitude pulmonary edema: from exaggerated pulmonary hypertension to a defect in transepithelial sodium transport. *Adv Exp Med Biol*. 1999;474:93-107.

215. Myerburg MM, et al. Airway surface liquid volume regulates ENaC by altering the serine protease-protease inhibitor balance: a mechanism for sodium hyperabsorption in cystic fibrosis. *J Biol Chem*. 2006;281(38):27942-27949.

216. Hirasawa G, et al. 11Beta-hydroxysteroid dehydrogenase type 2 and mineralocorticoid receptor in human fetal development. *J Clin Endocrinol Metab*. 1999;84(4):1453-1458.

217. Suzuki T, et al. 11Beta-hydroxysteroid dehydrogenase type 2 in human lung: possible regulator of mineralocorticoid action. *J Clin Endocrinol Metab*. 1998;83(11):4022-4025.

218. Suzuki S, et al. Modulation of transalveolar fluid absorption by endogenous aldosterone in adult rats. *Experimental lung research*. 2001;27(2):143-155.

219. Champigny G, et al. Regulation of expression of the lung amiloride-sensitive Na$^+$ channel by steroid hormones. *EMBO J*. 1994;13(9):2177-2181.

220. Renard S, et al. Localization and regulation by steroids of the alpha, beta and gamma subunits of the amiloride-sensitive Na$^+$ channel in colon, lung and kidney. *Pflugers Arch*. 1995;430(3):299-307.

221. Illek B, Fischer H, Clauss W. Aldosterone regulation of basolateral potassium channels in alveolar epithelium. *Am J Physiol*. 1990;259(4 pt 1):L230-L237.

222. Keller-Wood M, von Reitzenstein M, McCartney J. Is the fetal lung a mineralocorticoid receptor target organ? Induction of cortisol-regulated genes in the ovine fetal lung, kidney and small intestine. *Neonatology*. 2009;95(1):47-60.

223. Berger SA. Molecular genetic analysis of glucocorticoid and mineralocorticoid signaling in development and physiological processes. *Steroids*. 1996;61(4):236-239.

224. Cook DI, et al. Patch-clamp studies on epithelial sodium channels in salivary duct cells. *Cell Biochem Biophys.* 2002;36(2-3):105-113.

225. Anand SK, et al. Pseudohypoaldosteronism due to sweat gland dysfunction. *Pediatric research.* 1976;10(7):677-682.

226. Sanderson IR, et al. Familial salivary gland insensitivity to aldosterone: a variant of pseudohypoaldosteronism. *Horm Res.* 1989;32(4):145-147.

227. Kretz O, et al. Differential expression of RNA and protein of the three pore-forming subunits of the amiloride-sensitive epithelial sodium channel in taste buds of the rat. *J Histochem Cytochem.* 1999;47(1):51-64.

228. Lin W, et al. Epithelial Na⁺ channel subunits in rat taste cells: localization and regulation by aldosterone. *J Comp Neurol.* 1999;405(3):406-420.

229. Sasano H, et al. Immunolocalization of mineralocorticoid receptor in human kidney, pancreas, salivary, mammary and sweat glands: a light and electron microscopic immunohistochemical study. *J Endocrinol.* 1992;132(2):305-310.

230. Duc C, et al. Cell-specific expression of epithelial sodium channel alpha, beta, and gamma subunits in aldosterone-responsive epithelia from the rat: localization by in situ hybridization and immunocytochemistry. *J Cell Biol.* 1994;127(6):1907-1921.

231. Rauh R, et al. Stimulation of the epithelial sodium channel (ENaC) by the serum- and glucocorticoid-inducible kinase (Sgk) involves the PY motifs of the channel but is independent of sodium feedback inhibition. *Pflugers Arch.* 2006;452(3):290-299.

232. Riad F, et al. Aldosterone regulates salivary sodium secretion in cattle. *J Endocrinol.* 1986;108(3):405-411.

233. Wotman S, et al. Salivary electrolytes, renin, and aldosterone during sodium loading and depletion. *J Appl Physiol.* 1973;35(3):322-324.

234. McVie R, Levine LS, New MI. The biologic significance of the aldosterone concentration in saliva. *Pediatr Res.* 1979;13(6):755-759.

235. Adlin EV, Marks AD, Channick BJ. Racial difference in salivary sodium-potassium ratio in low renin essential hypertension. *Arch Intern Med.* 1982;142(4):703-706.

236. Porter GA, Bogoroch R, Edelman IS. On the mechanism of action of aldosterone on sodium transport: the role of RNA synthesis. *Proc Natl Acad Sci U S A.* 1964;52:1326-1333.

237. Kirsten E, et al. Increased activity of enzymes of the tricarboxylic acid cycle in response to aldosterone in the toad bladder. *Pflugers Arch Gesamte Physiol Menschen Tiere.* 1968;300(4):213-225.

238. Law PY, Edelman IS. Induction of citrate synthase by aldosterone in the rat kidney. *J Membr Biol.* 1978;41:41-64.

239. Blazer-Yost B, Cox M. Aldosterone-induced proteins: characterization using lectin-affinity chromatography. *Am J Physiol.* 1985:C215-C225.

240. Chen SY, et al. Epithelial sodium channel regulated by aldosterone-induced protein sgk. *Proc Natl Acad Sci U S A.* 1999;96(5):2514-2519.

241. Naray-Fejes-Toth A, et al. sgk is an aldosterone-induced kinase in the renal collecting duct: effects on epithelial Na⁺ channels. *J Biol Chem.* 1999;274(24):16973-16978.

242. Alvarez de la Rosa D, et al. The serum and glucocorticoid kinase sgk increases the abundance of epithelial sodium channels in the plasma membrane of *Xenopus* oocytes. *J Biol Chem.* 1999;274(53):37834-37839.

243. Flores SY, et al. Aldosterone-induced serum and glucocorticoid-induced kinase 1 expression is accompanied by Nedd4-2 phosphorylation and increased Na⁺ transport in cortical collecting duct cells. *J Am Soc Nephrol.* 2005;16(8):2279-2287.

244. Bhargava A, et al. The serum- and glucocorticoid-induced kinase is a physiological mediator of aldosterone action. *Endocrinology.* 2001;142(4):1587-1594.

245. Loffing J, Korbmacher C. Regulated sodium transport in the renal connecting tubule (CNT) via the epithelial sodium channel (ENaC). *Pflugers Archiv.* 2009;458(1):111-135.

246. Rubera I, et al. Collecting duct-specific gene inactivation of αENaC in the mouse kidney does not impair sodium and potassium balance. *J Clin Invest.* 2003;112(4):554-565.

247. Hou J, et al. Sgk1 gene expression in kidney and its regulation by aldosterone: spatio-temporal heterogeneity and quantitative analysis. *J Am Soc Nephrol.* 2002;13(5):1190-1198.

248. Chen S-Y, et al. Epithelial sodium channel regulated by aldosterone-induced protein sgk. *Proc Natl Acad Sci U S A.* 1999;96(5):2514-2519.

249. Chen WS, et al. Leptin deficiency and beta-cell dysfunction underlie type 2 diabetes in compound Akt knockout mice. *Mol Cell Biol.* 2009;29(11):3151-3162.

250. Bhalla V, et al. Disinhibitory pathways for control of sodium transport: regulation of ENaC by SGK1 and GILZ. *Am J Physiol Renal Physiol.* 2006;291(4):F714-F721.

251. Lang F, et al. (Patho)physiological significance of the serum- and glucocorticoid-inducible kinase isoforms. *Physiol Rev.* 2006;86(4):1151-1178.

252. Waldegger S, et al. h-sgk serine-threonine protein kinase gene as transcriptional target of transforming growth factor beta in human intestine. *Gastroenterology.* 1999;116:1081-1088.

253. Gonzalez-Robayna IJ, et al. Follicle-stimulating hormone (FSH) stimulates phosphorylation and activation of protein kinase B (PKB/Akt) and serum and glucocorticoid-Induced kinase (Sgk): evidence for A kinase-independent signaling by FSH in granulosa cells. *Mol Endocrinol.* 2000;14(8):1283-1300.

254. Webster MK, et al. Characterization of sgk, a novel member of the serine/threonine protein kinase gene family which is transcriptionally induced by glucocorticoids and serum. *Mol Cell Biol.* 1993;13(4):2031-2040.

255. Rozansky DJ, et al. Hypotonic induction of SGK1 and Na⁺ transport in A6 cells. *Am J Physiol Renal Physiol.* 2002;283(1):F105-F113.

256. Pearce D. The role of SGK1 in hormone-regulated sodium transport. *Trends Endocrinol Metab.* 2001;12(8):341-347.

257. Wang J, et al. SGK integrates insulin and mineralocorticoid regulation of epithelial sodium transport. *Am J Physiol Renal Physiol.* 2001;280(2):F303-F313.

258. Deleted in page proofs.

259. Park J, et al. Serum- and glucocorticoid-inducible kinase (SGK) is a target of the PI 3-kinase-stimulated signaling pathway. *EMBO J.* 1999;18(11):3024-3033.

260. Kobayashi T, et al. Characterization of the structure and regulation of two novel isoforms of serum- and glucocorticoid-induced protein kinase. *Biochem J.* 1999;344(pt 1):189-197.

261. Kobayashi T, Cohen P. Activation of serum- and glucocorticoid-regulated protein kinase by agonists that activate phosphatidylinositol 3-kinase is mediated by 3-phosphoinositide-dependent protein kinase-1 (PDK1) and PDK2. *Biochem J.* 1999;339(pt 2):319-328.

262. Garcia-Martinez JM, Alessi DR. mTOR complex 2 (mTORC2) controls hydrophobic motif phosphorylation and activation of serum- and glucocorticoid-induced protein kinase 1 (SGK1). *Biochem J.* 2008;416(3):375-385.

263. Jones KT, et al. Rictor/TORC2 regulates *Caenorhabditis elegans* fat storage, body size, and development through sgk-1. *PLoS Biol.* 2009;7(3):e60.

264. Wang J, et al. Activity of the p110-alpha subunit of phosphatidylinositol-3-kinase is required for activation of epithelial sodium transport. *Am J Physiol Renal Physiol.* 2008;295(3):F843-F850.

265. Debonneville C, et al. Phosphorylation of Nedd4-2 by Sgk1 regulates epithelial Na(+) channel cell surface expression. *EMBO J.* 2001;20(24):7052-7059.

266. Snyder PM, Olson DR, Thomas BC. Serum- and glucocorticoid-regulated kinase modulates Nedd4-2-mediated inhibition of the epithelial Na⁺ channel. *J Biol Chem.* 2002;277(1):5-8.

267. Wulff P, et al. Impaired renal Na(+) retention in the sgk1-knockout mouse. *J Clin Invest.* 2002;110(9):1263-1268.

268. Fejes-Toth G, et al. Epithelial Na⁺ channel activation and processing in mice lacking SGK1. *Am J Physiol Renal Physiol.* 2008;294(6):F1298-F1305.

269. Fakitsas P, et al. Early aldosterone-induced gene product regulates the epithelial sodium channel by deubiquitylation. *J Am Soc Nephrol.* 2007;18(4):1084-1092.

270. Martel JA, et al. Melanophilin, a novel aldosterone-induced gene in mouse cortical collecting duct cells. *Am J Physiol Renal Physiol.* 2007;293(3):F904-F913.

271. Mastroberardino L, et al. Ras pathway activates epithelial Na⁺ channel and decreases its surface expression in *Xenopus* oocytes. *Mol Biol Cell.* 1998;9(12):3417-3427.

272. Naray-Fejes-Toth A, Boyd C, Fejes-Toth G. Regulation of epithelial sodium transport by promyelocytic leukemia zinc finger protein. *Am J Physiol Renal Physiol.* 2008;295(1):F18-F26.

273. Naray-Fejes-Toth A, Snyder PM, Fejes-Toth G. The kidney-specific WNK1 isoform is induced by aldosterone and stimulates epithelial sodium channel-mediated Na⁺ transport. *Proc Natl Acad Sci U S A.* 2004;101(50):17434-17439.

274. Soundararajan R, et al. A novel role for glucocorticoid-induced leucine zipper protein in epithelial sodium channel-mediated sodium transport. *J Biol Chem.* 2005;280(48):39970-39981.

275. Huang DY, et al. Blunted hypertensive effect of combined fructose and high-salt diet in gene-targeted mice lacking functional serum- and glucocorticoid-inducible kinase SGK1. *Am J Physiol Regul Integr Comp Physiol.* 2006;290(4):R935-R944.

276. Huang DY, et al. Resistance of mice lacking the serum- and glucocorticoid-inducible kinase SGK1 against salt-sensitive hypertension induced by a high-fat diet. *Am J Physiol Renal Physiol.* 2006;291(6):F1264-F1273.

277. Bhargava A, Wang J, Pearce D. Regulation of epithelial ion transport by aldosterone through changes in gene expression. *Mol Cell Endocrinol.* 2004;217(1-2):189-196.

278. Webster MK, Goya L, Firestone GL. Immediate-early transcriptional regulation and rapid mRNA turnover of a putative serine/threonine protein kinase. *J Biol Chem.* 1993;268(16):11482-11485.

279. Brickley DR, et al. Ubiquitin modification of serum and glucocorticoid-induced protein kinase-1 (SGK-1). *J Biol Chem.* 2002;277(45):43064-43070.

280. Naray-Fejes-Toth A, et al. Regulation of sodium transport in mammalian collecting duct cells by aldosterone-induced kinase, SGK1: structure/function studies. *Mol Cell Endocrinol.* 2004;217(1-2):197-202.

281. Pao AC, et al. NH2 terminus of serum and glucocorticoid-regulated kinase 1 binds to phosphoinositides and is essential for isoform-specific physiological functions. *Am J Physiol Renal Physiol.* 2007;292(6):F1741-F1750.

282. Zhou R, Snyder PM. Nedd4-2 phosphorylation induces serum- and glucocorticoid-regulated kinase (SGK) ubiquitination and degradation. *J Biol Chem.* 2005;280(6):4518-4523.

283. Arteaga MF, et al. Multiple translational isoforms give functional specificity to serum- and glucocorticoid-induced kinase 1. *Mol Biol Cell.* 2007;18(6):2072-2080.

284. Arteaga MF, et al. A brain-specific SGK1 splice isoform regulates expression of ASIC1 in neurons. *Proc Natl Acad Sci U S A.* 2008;105(11):4459-4464.

285. Raikwar NS, Snyder PM, Thomas CP. An evolutionarily conserved N-terminal Sgk1 variant with enhanced stability and improved function. *Am J Physiol Renal Physiol.* 2008;295(5):F1440-F1448.

286. Staub O, et al. WW domains of Nedd4 bind to the proline-rich PY motifs in the epithelial Na⁺ channel deleted in Liddle's syndrome. *EMBO J.* 1996;15(10):2371-2380.

287. Abriel H, et al. Defective regulation of the epithelial Na⁺ channel by Nedd4 in Liddle's syndrome. *J Clin Invest.* 1999;103(5):667-673.

288. Knight KK, et al. Liddle's syndrome mutations increase Na⁺ transport through dual effects on epithelial Na⁺ channel surface expression and proteolytic cleavage. *Proc Natl Acad Sci U S A.* 2006;103(8):2805-2808.

289. Kamynina E, et al. A novel mouse Nedd4 protein suppresses the activity of the epithelial Na⁺ channel. *FASEB J.* 2001;15(1):204-214.

290. Shi PP, et al. Salt-sensitive hypertension and cardiac hypertrophy in mice deficient in the ubiquitin ligase Nedd4-2. *Am J Physiol Renal Physiol.* 2008;295:F462-F470.

291. Snyder PM, Steines JC, Olson DR. Relative contribution of Nedd4 and Nedd4-2 to ENaC regulation in epithelia determined by RNA interference. *J Biol Chem.* 2004;279(6):5042-5046.

292. Alvarez de la Rosa D, Canessa CM. Role of SGK in hormonal regulation of epithelial sodium channel in A6 cells. *Am J Physiol Cell Physiol.* 2003;284(2):C404-C414.

293. Bhalla V, et al. Serum- and glucocorticoid-regulated kinase 1 regulates ubiquitin ligase neural precursor cell-expressed, developmentally down-regulated protein 4-2 by inducing interaction with 14-3-3. *Mol Endocrinol.* 2005;19(12):3073-3084.

294. Liang X, et al. 14-3-3 isoforms are induced by aldosterone and participate in its regulation of epithelial sodium channels. *J Biol Chem.* 2006;281(24):16323-16332.

295. Ichimura T, et al. 14-3-3 proteins modulate the expression of epithelial Na⁺ channels by phosphorylation-dependent interaction with Nedd4-2 ubiquitin ligase. *J Biol Chem.* 2005;280(13):13187-13194.

296. Rossier BC. Negative regulators of sodium transport in the kidney: key factors in understanding salt-sensitive hypertension? *J Clin Invest.* 2003;111(7):947-950.

297. Diakov A, Korbmacher C. A novel pathway of epithelial sodium channel activation involves a serum- and glucocorticoid-inducible kinase consensus motif in the C terminus of the channel's alpha-subunit. *J Biol Chem.* 2004;279(37):38134-38142.

298. Vuagniaux G, et al. Synergistic activation of ENaC by three membrane-bound channel-activating serine proteases (mCAP1, mCAP2, and mCAP3) and serum- and glucocorticoid-regulated kinase (Sgk1) in *Xenopus* oocytes. *J Gen Physiol.* 2002;120(2):191-201.

299. Alvarez de la Rosa D, et al. SGK1 activates Na⁺-K⁺-ATPase in amphibian renal epithelial cells. *Am J Physiol Cell Physiol.* 2006;290(2):C492-C498.

300. Zecevic M, et al. SGK1 increases Na, K-ATP cell-surface expression and function in *Xenopus laevis* oocytes. *Pflugers Arch.* 2004;448(1):29-35.

301. Boyd C, Naray-Fejes-Toth A. Gene regulation of ENaC subunits by serum- and glucocorticoid-inducible kinase-1. *Am J Physiol Renal Physiol.* 2005;288(3):F505-F512.

302. Zhang W, et al. Aldosterone-induced Sgk1 relieves Dot1a-Af9-mediated transcriptional repression of epithelial Na⁺ channel alpha. *J Clin Invest.* 2007;117(3):773-783.

303. Huang DY, et al. Impaired regulation of renal K⁺ elimination in the sgk1-knockout mouse. *J Am Soc Nephrol.* 2004;15(4):885-891.

304. Tomlinson JW, Stewart PM. Mechanisms of disease: selective inhibition of 11beta-hydroxysteroid dehydrogenase type 1 as a novel treatment for the metabolic syndrome. *Nat Clin Pract Endocrinol Metab.* 2005;1(2):92-99.

305. Naray-Fejes-Toth A, Fejes-Toth G. Extranuclear localization of endogenous 11beta-hydroxysteroid dehydrogenase-2 in aldosterone target cells. *Endocrinology.* 1998;139(6):2955-2959.

306. Bachmann S, et al. Sodium transport–related proteins in the mammalian distal nephron—distribution, ontogeny and functional aspects. *Anat Embryol (Berl).* 1999;200(5):447-468.

307. Velazquez H, et al. Rabbit distal convoluted tubule coexpresses NaCl cotransporter and 11 beta-hydroxysteroid dehydrogenase II mRNA. *Kidney Int.* 1998;54(2):464-472.

308. Bostanjoglo M, et al. 11Beta-hydroxysteroid dehydrogenase, mineralocorticoid receptor, and thiazide-sensitive Na-Cl cotransporter expression by distal tubules. *J Am Soc Nephrol.* 1998;9(8):1347-1358.

309. Whorwood CB, et al. 11 Beta-hydroxysteroid dehydrogenase and corticosteroid hormone receptors in the rat colon. *Am J Physiol.* 1993;264(6 pt 1):E951-E957.

310. Challis JR, Connor K. Glucocorticoids, 11beta-hydroxysteroid dehydrogenase: mother, fetus, or both? *Endocrinology.* 2009;150(3):1073-1074.

311. Geerling JC, Loewy AD. Aldosterone in the brain. *Am J Physiol Renal Physiol.* 2009;297(3):F559-F576.

312. Funder J, Myles K. Exclusion of corticosterone from epithelial mineralocorticoid receptors is insufficient for selectivity of aldosterone action: in vivo binding studies. *Endocrinology.* 1996;137(12):5264-5268.

313. Funder JW. Is aldosterone bad for the heart? *Trends Endocrinol Metab.* 2004;15(4):139-142.

314. Makino Y, et al. Direct association with thioredoxin allows redox regulation of glucocorticoid receptor function. *J Biol Chem.* 1999;274(5):3182-3188.

315. Wilson RC, et al. Steroid 21-hydroxylase deficiency: genotype may not predict phenotype. *J Clin Endocrinol Metab.* 1995;80(8):2322-2329.

316. Wilson RC, Nimkarn S, New MI. Apparent mineralocorticoid excess. *Trends Endocrinol Metab.* 2001;12(3):104-111.

317. Alzamora R, Michea L, Marusic ET. Role of 11beta-hydroxysteroid dehydrogenase in nongenomic aldosterone effects in human arteries. *Hypertension.* 2000;35(5):1099-1104.

318. Mihailidou KS, et al. Glucocorticoids activate cardiac mineralocorticoid receptors during experimental myocardiac infarction. *Hypertension.* 2009;54(6):1306-1312.

319. Liu SL, et al. Aldosterone regulates vascular reactivity: short-term effects mediated by phosphatidylinositol 3-kinase-dependent nitric oxide synthase activation. *Circulation.* 2003;108(19):2400-2406.

320. Oberleithner H. Is the vascular endothelium under the control of aldosterone? Facts and hypothesis. *Pflugers Arch.* 2007;454(2):187-193.

321. Molnar GA, et al. Glucocorticoid-related signaling effects in vascular smooth muscle cells. *Hypertension.* 2008;51(5):1372-1378.

322. Gros R, et al. Rapid effects of aldosterone on clonal human vascular smooth muscle cells. *Am J Physiol Cell Physiol.* 2007;292(2):C788-C794.

323. Kusche-Vihrog K, et al. The epithelial sodium channel (ENaC): mediator of the aldosterone response in the vascular endothelium? *Steroids.* 2009;75(8-9):544-549.

324. Moura AM, Worcel M. Direct action of aldosterone on transmembrane 22Na efflux from arterial smooth muscle: rapid and delayed effects. *Hypertension.* 1984;6(3):425-430.

325. Romagni P, et al. Aldosterone induces contraction of the resistance arteries in man. *Atherosclerosis.* 2003;166(2):345-349.

326. Wildling L, et al. Aldosterone receptor sites on plasma membrane of human vascular endothelium detected by a mechanical nanosensor. *Pflugers Arch.* 2009;458(2):223-230.

327. Kelly MJ, Levin ER. Rapid actions of plasma membrane estrogen receptors. *Trends Endocrinol Metab.* 2001;12(4):152-156.

328. Wang Z, et al. A variant of estrogen receptor-α, hER-α36: transduction of estrogen- and antiestrogen-dependent membrane-initiated mitogenic signaling. *Proc Natl Acad Sci U S A.* 2006;103(24):9063-9068.

329. Boldyreff B, Wehling M. Rapid aldosterone actions: from the membrane to signaling cascades to gene transcription and physiological effects. *J Steroid Biochem Mol Biol.* 2003;85(2-5):375-381.

330. Funder JW. The nongenomic actions of aldosterone. *Endocr Rev.* 2005;26(3):313-321.

331. Chun TY, Pratt JH. Nongenomic renal effects of aldosterone: dependency on NO and genomic actions. *Hypertension.* 2006;47(4):636-637.

332. Good DW. Nongenomic actions of aldosterone on the renal tubule. *Hypertension.* 2007;49(4):728-739.

333. Young WF. Primary aldosteronism: renaissance of a syndrome. *Clin Endocrinol (Oxf).* 2007;66(5):607-618.

334. Lifton RP, et al. A chimaeric 11 beta-hydroxylase/aldosterone synthase gene causes glucocorticoid-remediable aldosteronism and human hypertension. *Nature.* 1992;355(6357):262-265.

335. Stowasser M, et al. Evidence for abnormal left ventricular structure and function in normotensive individuals with familial hyperaldosteronism type I. *J Clin Endocrinol Metab.* 2005;90(9):5070-5076.

336. Milliez P, et al. Evidence for an increased rate of cardiovascular events in patients with primary aldosteronism. *J Am Coll Cardiol.* 2005;45(8):1243-1248.

337. Funder JW, et al. Case detection, diagnosis, and treatment of patients with primary aldosteronism: an Endocrine Society clinical practice guideline. *J Clin Endocrinol Metab.* 2008;93(9):3266-3281.

338. Guyton AC, et al. Salt balance and long-term blood pressure control. *Annu Rev Med.* 1980;31:15-27.

339. Gomez-Sanchez EP, Fort CM, Gomez-Sanchez CE. Intracerebroventricular infusion of RU28318 blocks aldosterone-salt hypertension. *Am J Physiol*. 1990;258(3 pt 1):E482-E484.

340. Levy DG, Rocha R, Funder JW. Distinguishing the antihypertensive and electrolyte effects of eplerenone. *J Clin Endocrinol Metab*. 2004;89(6): 2736-2740.

341. Machnik A, et al. Macrophages regulate salt-dependent volume and blood pressure by a vascular endothelial growth factor-C–dependent buffering mechanism. *Nat Med*. 2009;15(5):545-552.

342. Rickard AJ, et al. Deletion of mineralocorticoid receptors from macrophages protects against deoxycorticosterone/salt-induced cardiac fibrosis and increased blood pressure. *Hypertension*. 2009;54(3):537-543.

343. Ball Jr WC, et al. Increased excretion of aldosterone in urine from dogs with right-sided congestive heart failure and from dogs with thoracic inferior vena cava constriction. *Am J Physiol*. 1956;187(1):45-50.

344. Luetscher Jr JA, Neher R, Wettstein A. Isolation of crystalline aldosterone from the urine of patients with congestive heart failure. *Experientia*. 1956;12(1):22-23.

345. Pitt B, et al. The effect of spironolactone on morbidity and mortality in patients with severe heart failure. Randomized Aldactone Evaluation Study Investigators. *N Engl J Med*. 1999;341(10):709-717.

346. Pitt B, et al. Eplerenone reduces mortality 30 days after randomization following acute myocardial infarction in patients with left ventricular systolic dysfunction and heart failure. *J Am Coll Cardiol*. 2005;46(3): 425-431.

347. Rossi G, et al. Aldosterone as a cardiovascular risk factor. *Trends Endocrinol Metab*. 2005;16(3):104-107.

348. Zannad F, et al. Rationale and design of the Eplerenone in Mild Patients Hospitalization And SurvIval Study in Heart Failure (EMPHASIS-HF). *Eur J Heart Fail*. 12(6):617-622.

349. Lu M, et al. mTOR complex-2 activates ENaC by phosphorylating SGK1. *J Am Soc Nephrol*. 2010;21:811-818.

350. Garcia-Martinez JM, Alessi DR. mTOR complex 2 (mTORC2) controls hydrophobic motif phosphorylation and activation of serum- and glucocorticoid-induced protein kinase 1 (SGK1). *Biochem J*. 2008;416: 375-385.

351. Choi M, et al. K+ channel mutations in adrenal aldosterone-producing adenomas and hereditary hypertension. *Science*. 2011;331:768-772.

352. Geller DS, et al. A novel form of human mendelian hypertension featuring nonglucocorticoid-remediable aldosteronism. *J Clin Endocrinol Metab*. 2008;93:3117-3123.

353. Kenouch S, et al. Multiple patterns of 11 beta-hydroxysteroid dehydrogenase catalytic activity along the mammalian nephron. *Kidney Int*. 1992;42:56-60.

354. Bostanjoglo M, et al. 11Beta-hydroxysteroid dehydrogenase, mineralocorticoid receptor, and thiazide-sensitive Na-Cl cotransporter expression by distal tubules. *J Am Soc Nephrol*. 1998;9:1347-1358.

355. Lombes M, et al. Immunohistochemical localization of renal mineralocorticoid receptor by using an anti-idiotypic antibody that is an internal image of aldosterone. *Proc Natl Acad Sci U S A*. 1990;87:1086-1088.

356. Bonvalet JP, et al. Distribution of 11 beta-hydroxysteroid dehydrogenase along the rabbit nephron. *J Clin Invest*. 1990;86:832-837.

357. Naray-Fejes-Toth A, Fejes-Toth G. Novel mouse strain with Cre recombinase in 11beta-hydroxysteroid dehydrogenase-2-expressing cells. *Am J Physiol Renal Physiol*. 2007;292:F486-F494.

358. Cole TJ. Cloning of the mouse 11 beta-hydroxysteroid dehydrogenase type 2 gene: tissue specific expression and localization in distal convoluted tubules and collecting ducts of the kidney. *Endocrinology*. 1995;136: 4693-4696.

359. Smith RE, et al. Immunohistochemical and molecular characterization of the rat 11 beta-hydroxysteroid dehydrogenase type II enzyme. *Endocrinology*. 1997;138:540-547.

360. Campean V, et al. Localization of thiazide-sensitive Na(+)-Cl(-) cotransport and associated gene products in mouse DCT. *Am J Physiol Renal Physiol*. 2001;281:F1028-F1035.

361. Plotkin MD, et al. Localization of the thiazide sensitive Na-Cl cotransporter, rTSC1 in the rat kidney. *Kidney Int*. 1996;50:174-183.

362. Obermuller N, Bernstein P, Velazquez H, Reilly R, Moser D, Ellison DH, Bachmann S. Expression of the thiazide-sensitive Na-Cl cotransporter in rat and human kidney. *Am J Physiol*. 1995;269:F900-F910.

363. Bachmann S, et al. Expression of the thiazide-sensitive Na-Cl cotransporter by rabbit distal convoluted tubule cells. *J Clin Invest*. 1995;96:2510-2514.

364. Biner HL, et al. Human cortical distal nephron: distribution of electrolyte and water transport pathways. *J Am Soc Nephrol*. 2002;13:836-847.

365. Ciampolillo F, et al. Cell-specific expression of amiloride-sensitive, Na(+)-conducting ion channels in the kidney. *Am J Physiol*. 1996;271:C1303-C1315.

366. Loffing-Cueni D, et al. Dietary sodium intake regulates the ubiquitin-protein ligase nedd4-2 in the renal collecting system. *J Am Soc Nephrol*. 2006;17:1264-1274.

367. Loffing J, et al. Distribution of transcellular calcium and sodium transport pathways along mouse distal nephron. *Am J Physiol Renal Physiol*. 2001;281:F1021-F1027.

368. Duc C, et al. Cell-specific expression of epithelial sodium channel alpha, beta, and gamma subunits in aldosterone-responsive epithelia from the rat: localization by in situ hybridization and immunocytochemistry. *Journal Cell Biol*. 1994;127:1907-1921.

369. Palmer LG, Frindt G. Amiloride-sensitive Na channels from the apical membrane of the rat cortical collecting tubule. *Proc Natl Acad Sci U S A*. 1986;83:2767-2770.

370. Loffing J, et al. Localization of epithelial sodium channel and aquaporin-2 in rabbit kidney cortex. *Am J Physiol Renal Physiol*. 2000;278:F530-F539.

371. Schmitt R, et al. Developmental expression of sodium entry pathways in rat nephron. *Am J Physiol*. 1999;276:F367-F381.

372. Dijkink L, et al. Time-dependent regulation by aldosterone of the amiloride-sensitive Na+ channel in rabbit kidney. *Pflugers Arch*. 1999;438:354-360.

373. Lu M, et al. Absence of small conductance K+ channel (SK) activity in apical membranes of thick ascending limb and cortical collecting duct in ROMK (Bartter's) knockout mice. *J Biol Chem*. 2002;277:37881-37887.

374. Xu JZ, et al. Localization of the ROMK protein on apical membranes of rat kidney nephron segments. *Am J Physiol*. 1997;273:F739-F748.

375. Mennitt PA, et al. Localization of ROMK channels in the rat kidney. *J Am Soc Nephrol*. 1997;8:1823-1830.

376. Kohda Y, et al. Localization of the ROMK potassium channel to the apical membrane of distal nephron in rat kidney. *Kidney Int*. 1998;54:1214-1223.

377. Benchimol C, Zavilowitz B, Satlin LM. Developmental expression of ROMK mRNA in rabbit cortical collecting duct. *Pediatr Res*. 2000;47:46-52.

378. Nusing RM, et al. Expression of the potassium channel ROMK in adult and fetal human kidney. *Histochem Cell Biol*. 2005;123:553-559.

379. Staub O, et al. Immunolocalization of the ubiquitin-protein ligase Nedd4 in tissues expressing the epithelial Na+ channel (ENaC). *Am J Physiol*. 1997;272:C1871-C1880.

380. Umemura M, et al. Transcriptional diversity and expression of NEDD4L gene in distal nephron. *Biochem Biophys Res Commun*. 2006;339:1129-1137.

381. Velazquez H, et al. The distal convoluted tubule of rabbit kidney does not express a functional sodium channel. *Am J Physiol Renal Physiol*. 2001;280:F530-F539.

382. Breton S, et al. Depletion of intercalated cells from collecting ducts of carbonic anhydrase II-deficient (CAR2 null) mice. *Am J Physiol*. 1995;269:F761-F774.

383. Nelson RD, et al. Expression of an AQP2 Cre recombinase transgene in kidney and male reproductive system of transgenic mice. *Am J Physiol*. 1998;275:C216-C226.

384. Coleman RA, et al. Expression of aquaporins in the renal connecting tubule. *Am J Physiol Renal Physiol*. 2000;279:F874-F883.

385. Katz AI, Doucet A, Morel F. Na-K-ATPase activity along the rabbit, rat, and mouse nephron. *Am J Physiol*. 1979;237:F114-F120.

386. Piepenhagen PA, et al. Differential expression of Na(+)-K(+)-ATPase, ankyrin, fodrin, and E-cadherin along the kidney nephron. *Am J Physiol*. 1995;269:C1417-C1432.

387. Baskin DG, Stahl WL. Immunocytochemical localization of Na+, K+-ATPase in the rat kidney. *Histochemistry*. 1982;73:535-548.

388. Charles PG, Dowling JP, Fuller PJ. Characterization of renal Na-K-ATPase gene expression by in situ hybridization. *Ren Physiol Biochem*. 1992;15:10-15.

389. McDonough AA, Magyar CE, Komatsu Y. Expression of Na(+)-K(+)-ATPase alpha- and beta-subunits along rat nephron: isoform specificity and response to hypokalemia. *Am J Physiol*. 1994;267:C901-C908.

390. Wetzel RK, Sweadner KJ. Immunocytochemical localization of Na-K-ATPase alpha- and gamma-subunits in rat kidney. *Am J Physiol Renal Physiol*. 2001;281:F531-F545.

391. Kashgarian M, et al. Monoclonal antibody to Na, K-ATPase: immunocytochemical localization along nephron segments. *Kidney Int*. 1985;28:899-913.

392. Beeuwkes 3rd R, Rosen S. Renal sodium-potassium adenosine triphosphatase. Optical localization and x-ray microanalysis. *J Histochem Cytochem*. 1975;23:828-839.

393. Kwon O, et al. Distribution of cell membrane-associated proteins along the human nephron. *J Histochem Cytochem*. 1998;46:1423-1434.

Transport of Calcium, Magnesium, and Phosphate

René J.M. Bindels, Joost G.J. Hoenderop, and Jürg Biber

The maintenance of calcium, magnesium, and phosphate homeostasis involves the concerted action of intestine, bone, and kidney. These minerals play an essential role in various biologic processes in the body. The kidney determines the final excretion of these ions and therefore performs an important step in homeostatic control. This chapter discusses the normal regulation of renal calcium, magnesium, and phosphate handling to provide scientists with an understanding of molecular transport mechanisms and clinicians with a basis for diagnosis and management of the common disorders that involve this homeostatic system.

Calcium Transport

Ca²⁺ Homeostasis

The tight control of blood calcium (Ca²⁺) levels within a narrow range is essential to the performance of many vital physiologic functions. Muscle contraction, intracellular signaling events, neuronal excitation, and bone formation all require Ca²⁺.[1,2] Disturbances in the Ca²⁺ balance result in serious symptoms, which include seizures, rickets, and heart failure. It is the collaborative action of intestine, bone, and kidney that controls the Ca²⁺ balance through the regulation of intestinal absorption, bone metabolism, and renal excretion of Ca²⁺, respectively. The majority of whole-body Ca²⁺ is stored in the

skeleton. In blood 45% of Ca²⁺ is present as the free, ionized form, whereas approximately 45% is bound to plasma proteins. The remaining fraction, 10%, forms complexes with anions like citrate, sulfate, and phosphate. Intestinal Ca²⁺ absorption occurs largely in the duodenum, but also takes place along the other more distal intestinal parts like the colon.[3] Fine tuning of Ca²⁺ excretion from the body via the urine takes place in the kidney, which preserves a constant Ca²⁺ concentration in the blood.

Renal Handling of Ca²⁺

In the kidney, approximately 8 g of Ca²⁺ is filtered at the glomerulus daily, of which less than 2% is excreted into the urine. Ca²⁺ can pass through the tubular system and reach the blood compartment via passive paracellular and active transcellular reabsorption through the epithelial cell layers.

Proximal Tubule

The proximal tubules (PTs), including the proximal convoluted tubule (PCT) and proximal straight tubule (PST), are responsible for the absorption of the bulk of the Ca²⁺ from the filtrate. Approximately 65% of the filtered Ca²⁺ is reabsorbed here, as has been demonstrated using micropuncture experiments.[4-7] This transport is passive and follows the local Na⁺

and water reabsorption. Therefore, this nephron site does not provide an independent regulation of Ca^{2+} reabsorption.[8]

Thick Ascending Limb of the Loop of Henle

In the subsequent nephron segment—that is, the thin descending and thin ascending limbs of the loop of Henle—virtually no Ca^{2+} is reabsorbed.[9] However, the thick ascending limb of the loop of Henle (TAL) is again permeable to Ca^{2+}, and this segment accounts for approximately 20% of the total Ca^{2+} reabsorption.[10-16] Several studies suggest that Ca^{2+} mainly follows the paracellular pathway in this diluting segment.[17-19] This was further confirmed when mutations in paracellin-1 (claudin-16), localized in the tight junctions of TAL, were found to be associated with renal Ca^{2+} wasting due to impaired paracellular reabsorption.[20] Recent work has shown that claudin-16 and claudin-19 together form paracellular pores and determine the Ca^{2+} and Mg^{2+} selectivity of the paracellular junctions.[21]

Distal Convoluted Tubule and Connecting Tubule

In the distal convoluted tubule (DCT) and connecting tubule (CNT) Ca^{2+} reabsorption takes place against its electrochemical gradient, which indicates that the transport is active.[22]

Tight junctions in the DCT and CNT are nearly impermeable to Ca^{2+}, consistent with a predominant role for an active transcellular Ca^{2+} transport pathway. The relative contribution of the initial (DCT1) and later (DCT2) segments of the DCT and of the CNT to active Ca^{2+} reabsorption is not entirely clear. Microperfusion studies in the past showed active Ca^{2+} transport in both the DCT and CNT,[23] whereas other studies indicated a predominant role for the CNT.[24]

In addition to the ubiquitously expressed Na^+–K^+–adenosine triphosphatase (Na^+-K^+-ATPase), Na^+/Ca^{2+} exchanger 1 (NCX1) and plasma membrane Ca^{2+}-ATPase isoform 1b (PMCA1b) have been found along the basolateral site of the DCT2 and CNT region. The DCT2 shares similarities with the CNT segment, because both segments express transient receptor potential cation channel, vanilloid subfamily, member 5 (TRPV5) and the Ca^{2+}-binding protein calbindin-D28K. Transepithelial transport of Ca^{2+} is a three-step procedure as outlined in more detail later (Figure 7-1). Ca^{2+} influx across the apical membrane is mediated by TRPV5. Subsequently, entered Ca^{2+} is sequestered by the specialized intracellular carrier protein calbindin-D28K, and this complex diffuses toward the basolateral membrane. Finally, transporter proteins such as NCX1 and PMCA1b extrude Ca^{2+} from the epithelial cell back into the circulation.

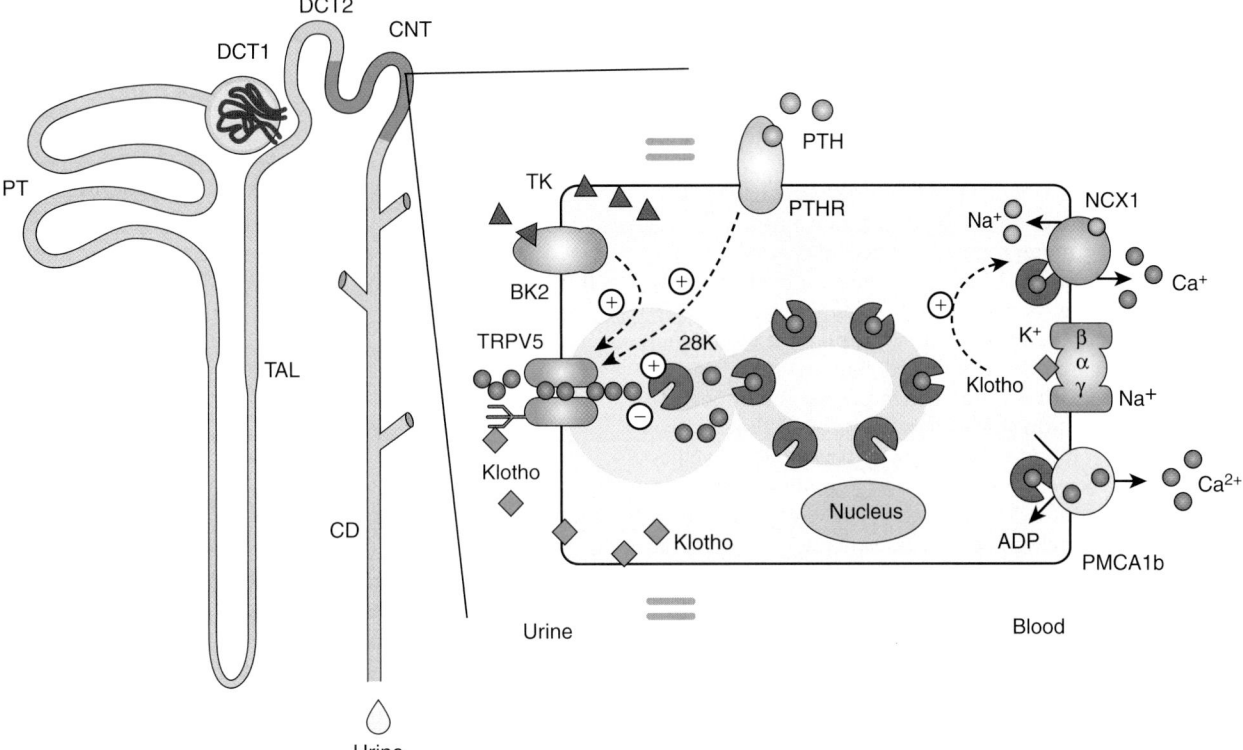

FIGURE 7-1 Model of active Ca^{2+} reabsorption in the late segment of the distal convoluted tubule (DCT2) and the connecting tubule (CNT). The distal part of the nephron comprises anatomically discrete segments, including the thick ascending limb of the loop of Henle (TAL) and the DCT, which ends in the CNT. The DCT2 and CNT play an important role in fine tuning the excretion of Ca^{2+}. The epithelial Ca^{2+} channel (TRPV5) is primarily expressed apically in these segments and co-localizes with calbindin-D28K (28K), the Na^+/Ca^{2+} exchanger (NCX1), and the plasma membrane ATPase (PMCA1b). Upon entry via TRPV5, Ca^{2+} is buffered by calbindin-D28K and diffuses to the basolateral membrane, where it is released and extruded by a concerted action of NCX1 and PMCA1b. In addition, the basolateral membrane exposes a parathyroid hormone receptor (PTHR) and Na^+-K^+-ATPase. PTHR activation by PTH stimulates TRPV5 activity, and entered Ca^{2+} can subsequently control the expression level of the Ca^{2+} transporters. At the apical membrane, there is a bradykinin receptor (BK2) that is activated by urinary tissue kallikrein (TK) to stimulate TRPV5-mediated Ca^{2+} influx. In the cell, entered Ca^{2+} acts as a negative feedback on channel activity, and calbindin-D28K plays a regulatory role by association with TRPV5 under low intracellular Ca^{2+} concentrations. Extracellular urinary Klotho directly stimulates TRPV5 at the apical membrane by modification of the *N*-glycan, whereas intracellular Klotho enhances Na^+-K^+-ATPase surface expression, which in turn activates NCX1-mediated Ca^{2+} efflux. (Adapted from Boros S, Bindels RJ, Hoenderop JG: Active Ca^{2+} reabsorption in the connecting tubule, *Pflugers Arch* 458[1]:99-109, 2009.)

Collecting Duct

Studies carried out before 1970 suggested that the cortical part of the collecting duct (CCD) accounts for small amount (3%) of Ca^{2+} reabsorption. Because net transport occurs against the electrochemical gradient for Ca^{2+}, Ca^{2+} reabsorption must be active here as well, but so far data regarding the mechanism are lacking. It is not always clear whether the CNT can be fully excluded in the analysis of studied isolated CCD segments.

Passive and Active Ca^{2+} Reabsorption

The paracellular component of epithelial Ca^{2+} transport is passive and directly connects the luminal compartment with the blood compartment, whereas the transcellular component is active and involves the passage of at least two membrane barriers. Importantly, the transcellular pathway is the main target site for specific regulation of Ca^{2+} (re)absorption by various calciotropic hormones. Passive Ca^{2+} reabsorption takes place in the PTs and TAL, whereas active transport is confined to the DCT and CNT by Ca^{2+} transporters like TRPV5, calbindin-D28K, the Na^+/Ca^{2+} exchanger, and ATP-driven Ca^{2+}-ATPase identified in the following sections.

Apical Entry of Ca^{2+} via TRPV5

The epithelial Ca^{2+} channel known as *TRPV5* is a member of the TRP channel superfamily.[3] This channel consists of large and flexible intracellular amino- and carboxy-terminal tails flanking six transmembrane segments, and an additional hydrophobic stretch between segments 5 and 6, predicted to be the pore-forming region. The amino-terminal tail contains multiple ankyrin repeats[25,26] that are important structural elements for both channel assembly and protein-protein interactions.[25,27] Furthermore, the first extracellular loop between transmembrane segments 1 and 2 contains an evolutionarily conserved asparagine at residue 358 (N358) crucial for its complex glycosylation and, in turn, for regulation of channel activity.[27-29] The carboxy-terminal tail contains three potential protein kinase C (PKC) sites, which suggests an important role for phosphorylation in the regulation of channel activity. Moreover, in cultured mammalian cell systems, as well as in oocytes, TRPV5 is assembled into large homotetramers to acquire an active conformation state.[28,30] Facing each other, the hydrophobic stretches between transmembrane segments 5 and 6 in each subunit are postulated to form the aqueous pore centered at the fourfold-symmetric axis (Figure 7-2).

Generation of a TRPV5-null mouse strain (TRPV5$^{-/-}$) provided compelling evidence for the physiologic function of this channel. Active Ca^{2+} reabsorption in DCT2 and the CNT is severely impaired in these transgenic animals, because TRPV5$^{-/-}$ mice excrete approximately 10-fold more Ca^{2+} than their wild-type littermates; that is in line with the postulated gatekeeper function of TRPV5 in active Ca^{2+} reabsorption.[1]

Shortly after the identification of TRPV5, a homologous channel, sharing a high protein sequence identity (75%), was cloned from the proximal intestine and named *TRPV6*.[31] Although there are some functional differences between these channels, TRPV6 exhibits the same high Ca^{2+} selectively and channel characteristics.[32-34] Moreover, this latter channel has been postulated to play an important role in intestinal Ca^{2+} absorption.

Intracellular Carrier Calbindin-D28K

The principal cells of the DCT2 and CNT segments are continuously challenged by a substantial Ca^{2+} influx through TRPV5, yet the cells manage to maintain a low intracellular Ca^{2+} concentration ($[Ca^{2+}]_i$). Importantly, an increased $[Ca^{2+}]_i$ has been shown to inhibit the activity of TRPV5.[35] Intracellular diffusion of Ca^{2+} is facilitated by the vitamin D_3–dependent Ca^{2+}-binding protein calbindin-D28K in the principal cells of this Ca^{2+}-transporting segment[36,37] (see Figure 7-1). Calbindin-D28K has three pairs of EF hands that form the structural basis of its high Ca^{2+} affinity binding capacity.[38] It has also recently been shown that calbindin-D28K translocates to the TRPV5-containing plasma membranes upon a decrease in $[Ca^{2+}]_i$ to directly associate with this Ca^{2+} channel.[39] Importantly, due to the relatively slow Ca^{2+}-binding kinetics of calbindin-D28K, hormone-induced Ca^{2+} signaling can occur independently of the transcellular Ca^{2+} transport rate.[40] Bound to calbindin-D28K, Ca^{2+} is shuttled toward the basolateral membrane, where Ca^{2+} is discharged into the blood compartment by the basolateral Ca^{2+} extrusion systems. Some studies have reported that calbindin-D28K$^{-/-}$ mice fed a high-Ca^{2+} diet have impaired renal Ca^{2+} handling, because they excrete more Ca^{2+} in their urine than their wild-type control littermates[41]; other studies have not observed a difference, however, probably due to the compensatory increase of renal calbindin-D9K expression.[42] These data suggest that calbindin-D28K facilitates the intracellular diffusion of Ca^{2+} in DCT2 and the CNT.

Basolateral Extrusion Systems: NCX1 and PMCA1b

The energy-consuming step of transepithelial Ca^{2+} transport is formed by the Ca^{2+} efflux process. Here, intracellular Ca^{2+} is transported across the basolateral membrane against its electrochemical gradient, and the ions are extruded back into the blood compartment. Two transporters have been implicated in this mechanism, PMCA1b and NCX1. Plasma membrane

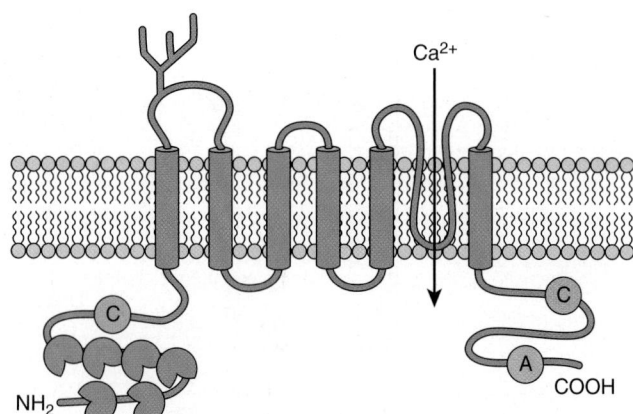

FIGURE 7-2 Epithelial Ca^{2+} channel TRPV5. The proposed topology of TRPV5 includes six transmembrane (TM)-spanning domains and a pore-forming region between TM5 and TM6. Ankyrin repeats are present in the amino-terminal of TRPV5. TRPV5 contains protein kinase C (C) and protein kinase A (A) phosphorylation sites that are important for tissue kallikrein and parathyroid hormone (PTH)-stimulated channel activity, respectively. In addition, the channel is N-glycosylated at asparagine position 358 (N358; numbering in rabbit species) between TM1 and TM2. The functional channel is based on the formation of a homotetramer exposing the pore-forming domain to the inner part of the tetramer to create a selective Ca^{2+} pore.

ATPases are high-affinity Ca^{2+} efflux pumps that maintain the resting Ca^{2+} concentration in virtually all cells.[43] The highest Ca^{2+}-ATPase activity in kidney was reported in the DCT segment. However, earlier studies have also suggested that the capacity of this Ca^{2+} pump in the CNT seems to be insufficient to keep pace with the absorptive flux of Ca^{2+}, because it can transport only approximately 30% of the total Ca^{2+} efflux.[44,45]

In contrast to PMCA1b, Na^+/Ca^{2+} exchange has been shown to be a prerequisite for transepithelial Ca^{2+} transport.[44,45] Moreover, NCX1 is a widely expressed protein that can be found in several tissues, including heart, brain, and skeletal muscle.[46] In the kidney, the expression of NCX1 is restricted to the distal part of the nephron, particularly the CNT segment, where it predominantly localizes along the basolateral membrane[47-49] and accounts for the remaining 70% of Ca^{2+} efflux.[44,45]

Characteristics of TRPV5

Electrophysiologic studies have demonstrated a constitutive activity of TRPV5 at low intracellular Ca^{2+} concentrations and physiologic membrane potentials.[35] The current-voltage relationship of TRPV5 shows strong inward rectification.[3,35,50] Another important functional feature of TRPV5 is its 100 times larger selectivity for Ca^{2+} than for Na^+, which makes the epithelial Ca^{2+} channel the most Ca^{2+}-selective member of the TRP superfamily.[35] The pore residue D542 appears to be crucial for high-affinity Ca^{2+} binding and selectivity. Patch clamp studies revealed a constitutively open channel, because no stimulus or ligand was required for TRPV5-mediated Ca^{2+} entry.[51]

The subcellular localization of TRPV5 was studied using fluorescence microscopy and enhanced green fluorescent protein (eGFP)–tagged TRPV5. Although not visible and mainly localized in intracellular vesicles, cell surface expression of eGFP-TRPV5 was confirmed using biochemical and functional studies.[52] Thus, TRPV5 expression at the plasma membrane is limited, providing a mechanism allowing controlled Ca^{2+} influx. TRPV5 presence at the plasma membrane was found to be to be highly dynamic.[52] After an irreversible chemical block of TRPV5 channels present at the cell surface, TRPV5 activity was restored for approximately 50% of channels within a 10-minute recovery phase.[52] After reaching the cell surface, the TRPV5 channel is reinternalized via dynamin- and clathrin-dependent processes. While in contact with the extracellular environment, TRPV5 channels exhibit closed and open states, during which Ca^{2+} enters the cell. The probability of a channel's being open is termed *open probability*, whereas conductance is the amount of current transmitted during the open state. Together, conductance and open probability determine TRPV5 single-channel activity, which is under the control of various factors such as intracellular Ca^{2+}, hormones, and other intracellular cascade messengers.

Protein-Protein Interactions of TRPV5

Several regulatory proteins of TRPV5 have been described in detail (for an overview see Table 7-1 and the review in Hoenderop and colleagues[3]). These regulators modify the trafficking of the channel, in particular. A few examples are described in the following sections.

S100A10-Annexin 2

S100A10 (S100 calcium-binding protein A10) has been identified as a protein linked with TRPV5 that specifically associates with the carboxy-terminals of TRPV5.[53] Several members of the S100 protein family form heteromeric complexes with annexins, and S100A10 is often found tightly associated with annexin 2 to form a tetrameric complex. The association of S100A10 with TRPV5 is restricted to a short conserved peptide sequence VATTV located in the carboxy-terminals of this channel. Mutation of this motif has been found to be accompanied by a major disturbance in TRPV5 subcellular localization, which indicates that the S100A10–annexin 2 heterotetramer facilitates the translocation of TRPV5 toward the plasma membrane. These findings show that the S100A10–annexin 2 complex is a significant component in the trafficking of TRPV5 and, therefore, in Ca^{2+} homeostasis.

80K-H

80K-H has been identified as a protein involved in Ca^{2+}-dependent regulation of TRPV5.[54] A specific interaction between 80K-H and TRPV5, co-localization of both proteins in the DCT, and similar transcriptional regulation by 1,25-dihydroxyvitamin D_3 and dietary Ca^{2+} has been demonstrated. 80K-H directly binds Ca^{2+} via its two EF-hand structures. Electrophysiologic studies using 80K-H mutants showed that three domains of 80K-H (two EF-hand structures, the highly acidic glutamic stretch, and the HDEL sequence) are critical determinants of TRPV5 activity. 80K-H did not alter the plasma membrane localization of TRPV5, which suggests that this associated protein has a direct effect on channel activity. In summary, 80K-H acts as novel Ca^{2+} sensor controlling TRPV5 channel activity.

Rab11a

The small guanosine triphosphatase (GTPase) Rab11a, involved in trafficking via recycling endosomes, was identified as a novel TRPV5 binding partner.[55] Rab11a co-localized with TRPV5 in the DCT and CNT. Importantly, the Ca^{2+} channel and Rab11a were both present in vesicular structures underlying the apical plasma membrane. It was demonstrated that TRPV5 preferentially interacts with Rab11a in its guanosine diphosphate (GDP)–bound conformation. Expression of a mutant Rab11a protein locked in the GDP-bound state resulted in a marked decrease of channels at the cell surface, which indicates a direct role of Rab11a in the trafficking of the Ca^{2+} channel toward the plasma membrane. Interestingly, Zobiack and colleagues have demonstrated that the S100A10–annexin 2 complex controls the distribution of Rab11-positive endosomes.[56] This suggests that two crucial pathways controlling the cell surface expression of TRPV5 are closely linked.

Regulation of Active Ca^{2+} Reabsorption by Calciotropic Factors

Vitamin D

The vitamin D_3 endocrine system is essential for proper development and maintenance of Ca^{2+} balance.[57] The active form of vitamin D, 1,25-dihydroxyvitamin D_3 (1,25[OH]$_2D_3$),

TABLE 7-1 Overview of the Regulation of Active Ca²⁺ Reabsorption

	Apical Membrane	Cytoplasm	Basolateral Membrane		
	TRANSPORTER TRPV5 / ACTION	TRANSPORTER CALBINDIN-D28K / ACTION	TRANSPORTER NCX1 PMCA1B	ACTION	REFERENCES
Hormones					
1,25-dihydroxyvitamin D₃	Gene expression ↑	Gene expression ↑	NCX1 PMCA1b	Gene expression ↑, =	85
Estrogen	Gene expression ↑	Gene expression ↑	NCX1 PMCA1b	Gene expression ↑	83
Insulin	Gene expression ↓	Gene expression ↓			311
Parathyroid hormone	Gene expression ↑ Activity ↑	Gene expression ↑	NCX1	Gene expression ↑	78, 80
Transporter Trafficking Regulators					
S100A10–annexin 2	Plasma membrane abundance ↑				53
Clathrin	Plasma membrane abundance ↑				312
Caveolin	Plasma membrane abundance ↑				313
Rab11a	Plasma membrane abundance ↑				55
Transporter Activity Regulators					
[Ca²⁺]ᵢ	Activity ↓				49
[Mg²⁺]ᵢ	Activity ↓				32
PIP₂	Activity ↑				314
80K-H	Activity ↑				54
Extracellular Factors					
Alkaline pH	Plasma membrane retention ↑ Activity ↑				95, 315
[Mg²⁺]pro-urine	Activity ↓				316
Tissue kallikrein/bradykinin	Plasma membrane retention ↑				317
Klotho	Plasma membrane retention ↑		Na⁺-K⁺-ATPase, NCX1	Plasma membrane abundance ↑ Indirect increase in NCX activity	122, 123

↑, Increased gene expression, increased channel activity, or increased plasma membrane abundance; ↓, downregulation of gene expression or inhibition of channel activity; =, no effect; $ATPase$, adenosine triphosphatase; $[Ca^{2+}]_i$, intracellular Ca²⁺ concentration; $[Mg^{2+}]_i$, intracellular Mg²⁺ concentration; $[Mg^{2+}]_{pro-urine}$, Mg²⁺ concentration of pro-urine; NCX, Na⁺/Ca²⁺ exchanger; $NCX1$, Na⁺/Ca²⁺ exchanger 1; PIP_2, phosphatidylinositol 4,5-bisphosphate; $PMCA1b$, plasma membrane Ca²⁺-ATPase isoform 1b; $TRPV5$, transient receptor potential cation channel, vanilloid subfamily, member 5.

is synthesized in the PTs by the renal cytochrome P450 enzyme 25-hydroxyvitamin D_3–1α-hydroxylase.[57,58] The biologic effects of $1,25(OH)_2D_3$ on target organs are mediated by genomic transcriptional mechanisms.[57] $1,25(OH)_2D_3$ transcriptionally controls the expression of a particular set of target genes. The genomic mechanism involves the specific interaction of $1,25(OH)_2D_3$ with a nuclear vitamin D receptor (VDR). Upon binding of $1,25(OH)_2D_3$, the VDR undergoes a conformational change and forms a complex with a retinoid X receptor (RXR). This VDR-RXR complex binds to DNA elements in the promoter region of target genes described as vitamin D response elements (VDREs). Binding to these VDREs controls the rate of gene transcription. Importantly, VDR is expressed in epithelia that play a role in Ca^{2+} (re) absorption. The intestine and kidney are the main target organs for the calciotropic action of this hormone, although vitamin D affects many other processes, notably in the skin and immune system but also directly in bone and parathyroid gland.[59]

Direct evidence for a role of vitamin D in the positive regulation of TRPV5 comes from two distinct double-knockout models. First, it was shown that the increased vitamin D levels observed in TRPV5$^{-/-}$ mice are critical for the compensatory intestinal hyperabsorption seen in these mice. This was demonstrated using TRPV5$^{-/-}$ and 1α-hydroxylase$^{-/-}$ double-knockout mice.[60] Second, 1α-hydroxylase$^{-/-}$ and parathyroid hormone (PTH) double-knockout mice were created to eliminate a possible role of PTH during vitamin D administration. Administration of $1,25(OH)_2D_3$ upregulated messenger RNA (mRNA) and protein levels of renal TRPV5, calbindin-D28K, calbindin-D9K, and NCX1; increased serum Ca^{2+} concentration; and stimulated bone formation.[61]

The correlation between vitamin D and the expression level of the Ca^{2+} transport proteins has also been addressed in several cell models. Wood and colleagues observed the correlation between the $1,25(OH)_2D_3$-induced expression of TRPV6, calbindin-D9K, and PMCA1b, and transcellular Ca^{2+} transport in Caco-2 cells, a model duodenal cell line.[62,63] Furthermore, in controlled tissue culture conditions using primary cultures from the distal part of the nephron including the DCT and CNT, a direct relationship between $1,25(OH)_2D_3$-induced expression of Ca^{2+} transport proteins and transcellular Ca^{2+} transport also was shown.[45,64]

TRPV5 and TRPV6 promoter analysis indicated that there are functional VDREs located upstream of the start codon.[65-68] Mutation of the VDREs within the −2.1 kilobase (kb) and −4.3 kb region and the VDRE at −1.2 kb abolished all response to $1,25(OH)_2D_3$ when examined within the TRPV6 promoter.[65] Taken together, findings from vitamin D–deficient animal models and epithelial cell lines demonstrate a consistent $1,25(OH)_2D_3$ sensitivity of TRPV5, TRPV6, and the calbindins and, to a lesser extent, the basolateral extrusion systems NCX1 and PMCA1b.

Parathyroid Hormone

The parathyroid glands play a key role in maintaining the extracellular Ca^{2+} concentration ($[Ca^{2+}]_e$) through their secretion of PTH.[69] PTH controls the extracellular Ca^{2+} balance by activation of the PTH receptor, regulating predominantly Ca^{2+} transport in bone and kidney. Parathyroid cells sense decreases in $[Ca^{2+}]_e$ by means of the Ca^{2+}-sensing receptor (CaSR) to increase PTH secretion. In addition to parathyroid tissue, the receptor is also expressed in regions of the kidney involved in regulated Ca^{2+} and Mg^{2+} reabsorption.[70,71]

PTH itself acts primarily on kidney and bone, where it activates the PTH receptor.[72,73] PTH stimulates the activity of 1α-hydroxylase in the PT.[74] Thereby, PTH increases the $1,25(OH)_2D_3$-dependent (re)absorption of Ca^{2+}. Activation of the PTH receptor directly enhances Ca^{2+} (re)absorption in kidney. Several groups localized PTH receptor mRNA in rat kidney to glomerular podocytes, PCTs, PSTs, cortical TAL, and DCT, but the receptor was not detected in the thin limb of the loop of Henle or in the collecting duct (CD).[70,71] PTH directly stimulates active Ca^{2+} reabsorption in the distal part of the nephron.[24] In the TAL, it was shown that PTH increases the transepithelial driving force for Ca^{2+} reabsorption, enhancing paracellular Ca^{2+} transport.[19]

Various mechanisms of PTH action have been proposed for the effect in the DCT, including membrane insertion of apical Ca^{2+} channels,[75] opening of basolateral chloride channels resulting in cellular hyperpolarization,[76] and modulation of PMCA activity.[77] Van Abel and colleagues reported that PTH stimulates renal Ca^{2+} reabsorption through the coordinated expression of renal transcellular Ca^{2+} transport proteins. They showed that parathyroidectomy in rats resulted in decreased serum PTH levels and hypocalcemia, which was accompanied by reduced levels of TRPV5, calbindin-D28K, and NCX1.[78] Supplementation with PTH restored serum Ca^{2+} concentrations and abundance of the Ca^{2+} transport proteins.

Similarly, infusion of a calcimimetic compound (a chemical that activates CaSR at low serum Ca^{2+} concentrations) decreased PTH levels and resulted in reduced expression of TRPV5, calbindin, and NCX1, which is consistent with diminished Ca^{2+} reabsorption and in line with the observed hypocalcemia in these mice.[78] Importantly, serum $1,25(OH)_2D_3$ levels and renal VDR or CaSR mRNA abundance did not significantly change during these treatments.[78] Furthermore, PTH injection in mice increased both TRPV5 and TRPV6 mRNA expression in kidney.[79] Recently, de Groot and colleagues demonstrated a short-term effect of PTH in which a threonine residue in the carboxy-terminal of TRPV5 is phosphorylated to increase the open probability of the channel and, therefore, TRPV5 activity.[80] Together, all these findings demonstrate the important role of PTH in renal Ca^{2+} reabsorption (see Figure 7-1, and Table 7-1).

Estrogens

Estrogen deficiency after menopause results in bone loss, which is associated with an increase in plasma and urinary Ca^{2+}. In vivo studies have demonstrated that estrogen deficiency is associated with increased renal Ca^{2+} loss, which can be corrected by estrogen replacement therapy.[81,82] Furthermore, estrogen receptors also reside in proximal and distal tubules within the nephron. It was demonstrated that estrogen upregulates the expression of TRPV5 in kidney in a $1,25$-$(OH)_2D_3$-independent manner.[83] In ovariectomized 1α-hydroxylase knockout mice estradiol-17β replacement therapy resulted in upregulation of renal TRPV5 mRNA and protein levels, leading to normalization of plasma Ca^{2+} levels. Van Cromphaut and colleagues reported that renal TRPV5 expression is reduced in estrogen receptor-α knockout mice and upregulated by estrogen treatment.[84] The mechanism of estrogen-controlled upregulation of TRPV5 mRNA remains to be elucidated.

Dietary Ca^{2+} Intake

To investigate the mechanisms underlying the effect of dietary Ca^{2+} intake, the expression level of several Ca^{2+} transport proteins was studied in various mice models. Importantly, high dietary Ca^{2+} intake restored the reduced expression level of renal TRPV5, calbindin-D28K, and NCX1 in 1α-hydroxylase$^{-/-}$ mice and normalized the serum Ca^{2+} concentration.[85] Likewise, the expression of the intestinal Ca^{2+} transport proteins TRPV6, calbindin-D9K, and PMCA1b was normalized by this rescue Ca^{2+} diet.[86] Comparable observations were made in VDR knockout mice in which duodenal TRPV5 and TRPV6 mRNA levels were upregulated by dietary Ca^{2+}.[87] These findings suggest that dietary Ca^{2+} can affect active Ca^{2+} (re)absorption via vitamin D–independent modulation of the expression of Ca^{2+} transport proteins. However, the molecular mechanism of this vitamin D–independent Ca^{2+}-sensitive pathway remains to be further elucidated.

A high dietary Ca^{2+} intake can eventually result in hypercalciuria, which is an important risk factor for Ca^{2+} complex formation, including kidney stones. In an alkaline environment, inorganic phosphate (Pi) is present in divalent form and can conjugate with Ca^{2+} to form Ca^{2+}-Pi precipitations. To prevent the tubular lumen from hypercalciuria in this alkaline state, TRPV5 channels are more abundantly expressed at the plasma membrane to allow the reabsorption of Ca^{2+} from the pro-urine.[52] Likewise, extracellular acidification induces TRPV5 retrieval from the luminal membrane and consequently less Ca^{2+} reabsorption.

Recently, Renkema and colleagues demonstrated that hypercalciuria enhances H$^+$-ATPase–mediated acid secretion and also downregulation of aquaporin-2 via activation of the CaSR in the CD.[88] TRPV5 knockout (TRPV5$^{-/-}$) mice manifest hypercalciuria, because the DCT and CNT of these mice lack the ability to reabsorb Ca^{2+} into the blood compartment.[1] Consequently, activation of the CaSR by increased luminal Ca^{2+} leads to urinary acidification and polyuria. These beneficial adaptations facilitate the excretion of large amounts of soluble Ca^{2+} and are crucial to prevent the formation of kidney stones.

Another regulatory role of Ca^{2+} is initiated by increased plasma Ca^{2+} concentrations. Hypercalcemia also activates the CaSR in the TAL, which subsequently inhibits the activity of Na$^+$-K$^+$-2Cl$^-$ cotransporter 2 (NKCC2) and therefore passive paracellular Ca^{2+} transport.[21]

Finally, it was demonstrated that the CaSR and TRPV5 co-localize at the luminal membrane of the DCT and CNT. In these segments activation of the CaSR may lead to elevated TRPV5-mediated Ca^{2+} reabsorption and increases intracellular Ca^{2+} levels in cells coexpressing TRPV5 and CaSR.[89] These data suggest that activation of the CaSR stimulates TRPV5-mediated Ca^{2+} influx via a PKC-dependent pathway.

Acidosis and Alkalosis

Acid-base homeostasis is known to affect renal Ca^{2+} handling.[90,91] For instance, chronic metabolic acidosis is associated with increased renal Ca^{2+} excretion. Long-standing metabolic acidosis can lead to Ca^{2+} loss from bone and ultimately result in metabolic bone disorders, including osteomalacia and osteoporosis.[92] It has been shown by several groups that extracellular protons inhibit TRPV5 channel activity.[93-96] Furthermore, earlier studies, including micropuncture experiments, suggested that systemic acid-base disturbances specifically affect Ca^{2+} reabsorption in the DCT and CNT.[90,97]

Nijenhuis and colleagues addressed the mechanisms underlying acid-base balance on renal Ca^{2+} handling in more detail. Metabolic alkalosis was induced by oral NaHCO$_3$ loading and metabolic acidosis by NH$_4$Cl loading as well as by acetazolamide administration in wild-type and TRPV5$^{-/-}$ mice.[98] Acetazolamide specifically inhibits proximal tubular bicarbonate reabsorption, which results in a self-limiting metabolic acidosis and, in contrast to NH$_4$Cl loading, an alkaline urine pH.[99-101]

Chronic metabolic acidosis, induced by NH$_4$Cl loading or administration of acetazolamide, enhanced the calciuresis and was accompanied by decreased renal TRPV5 and calbindin-D28K mRNA and protein abundance in mice. In contrast, metabolic acidosis did not affect Ca^{2+} excretion in TRPV5$^{-/-}$ mice, in which active Ca^{2+} reabsorption is effectively abolished.[98] This demonstrates that downregulation of renal Ca^{2+} transport proteins is responsible for the hypercalciuria. Conversely, chronic metabolic alkalosis, induced by NaHCO$_3$ administration, increased the expression of Ca^{2+} transport proteins and was accompanied by diminished urine Ca^{2+} excretion in mice. However, this Ca^{2+}-sparing action persisted in TRPV5$^{-/-}$ mice, which suggests that additional mechanisms apart from upregulation of active Ca^{2+} reabsorption contributed to the hypocalciuria. These data indicate that renal Ca^{2+} transport proteins play an instrumental role in the effect of acid-base status on renal Ca^{2+} handling.

Regulation by Immunosuppressives and Diuretics

Calcineurin Inhibitors

The use of calcineurin inhibitors such as tacrolimus (FK506) and cyclosporine has led to major advances in the field of transplantation and made possible an excellent short-term outcome. However, the long-term nephrotoxicity of these drugs is a significant problem. Tacrolimus is a widely prescribed immunosuppressant drug and is known to induce significant adverse effects on mineral homeostasis, including increased bone turnover, a negative Ca^{2+} balance, and hypercalciuria.[102,103]

In theory, downregulation of Ca^{2+} transporter proteins in the distal part of the nephron may be involved in the pathogenesis of hypercalciuria during drug treatment. Previous reports showed reduced calbindin-D28K levels during tacrolimus treatment, which suggests that tacrolimus can affect active Ca^{2+} transport.[104] In addition, it was demonstrated that tacrolimus treatment significantly increased urinary Ca^{2+} excretion, accompanied by a downregulation of the renal mRNA and protein expression of TRPV5.[105] The fact that serum Ca^{2+} concentrations and the glomerular filtration rate (GFR) in drug-treated animals did not differ from those in control animals confirmed that impaired Ca^{2+} reabsorption rather than an increased filtered load caused the hypercalciuria. This data supported the hypothesis that tacrolimus induces a primary defect of renal active Ca^{2+} reabsorption by specifically downregulating the proteins involved in active Ca^{2+} transport.

The molecular mechanism underlying the downregulation of the epithelial Ca^{2+} channel by tacrolimus remains elusive. In previous studies, plasma $1,25-(OH)_2D_3$ levels were either unaltered or moderately increased by similar doses of tacrolimus, whereas plasma PTH levels were not affected, which excludes the possibility that the reduced Ca^{2+} transport protein expression levels are secondary to decreased circulating levels of calciotropic hormones.

In addition, cyclosporine treatment induces high bone turnover, osteopenia, and hypercalciuria.[106] Cyclosporine administration suppresses the expression of calbindin-D28K in mice, but has no effect on TRPV5 gene expression. The pathogenesis of cyclosporine-induced hypercalciuria involves both downregulation of calbindin-D28K and subsequent impaired renal Ca^{2+} reabsorption.

Furosemide

Furosemide is known to inhibit renal Ca^{2+} reabsorption, which leads to various effects including alterations in the structure and stability of bone. The molecular mechanism underlying its action on Ca^{2+} reabsorption includes the following events. Furosemide inhibits the NKCC2 transporter of the TAL, which results in a reduction in NaCl reabsorption and K^+ recycling across the apical membrane. This action diminishes the lumen-positive potential that drives the paracellular reabsorption of Ca^{2+}, which explains the hypercalciuric effect of furosemide. As a consequence, there is enhanced delivery of Ca^{2+} to the DCT and CNT, which are the primary sites of active Ca^{2+} reabsorption.[3] Studies by Lee and colleagues have shown that these latter nephron segments partly compensate for the hypercalciuric effect of the loop diuretics. In this respect, it is interesting to note that furosemide was found to increase the expression level of TRPV5 and calbindin-D28K.[107]

Thiazide

Thiazide diuretics, in contrast to loop diuretics, have the unique characteristic of decreasing Na^+ reabsorption while increasing Ca^{2+} reabsorption. In addition, mutations in the thiazide-sensitive Na^+-Cl^- cotransporter (NCC) have been shown to cause Gitelman's syndrome. Patients with this syndrome have hypovolemia, hypokalemic alkalosis, hypomagnesemia, and hypocalciuria.[108]

Intriguingly, the molecular mechanisms responsible for the hypocalciuria and hypomagnesemia of thiazide administration and Gitelman's syndrome remain elusive. Two hypotheses exist with respect to the Ca^{2+}-sparing effect of thiazides.[3] According to the first hypothesis, renal salt and water loss due to thiazide treatment results in contraction of the extracellular volume (ECV), which triggers a compensatory increase in proximal Na^+ reabsorption. This would in turn enhance the electrochemical gradient, driving passive Ca^{2+} transport in proximal tubular segments.[108-110] Early studies by Weinman and Eknoyan had already demonstrated that the escape from the long-term effects of chlorothiazide is due to a decrease in the GFR and to an increase in fractional reabsorption in the PT.[111] Subsequently, Nijenhuis and colleagues showed that hydrochlorothiazide-induced hypocalciuria in rats was accompanied by a significant decrease in body weight compared with controls, which illustrates that ECV contraction occurred.[112] Because Na^+ depletion resulted in a similar hypocalciuria, it is likely that the ECV contraction by itself is responsible for the thiazide-induced hypocalciuria. This is further supported by the finding that Na^+ repletion during hydrochlorothiazide treatment, which prevented the ECV contraction, normalized the calciuresis.

The second hypothesis draws on microperfusion experiments suggesting that acute administration of thiazides in the tubular lumen stimulates Ca^{2+} reabsorption in the DCT.[23] Subsequently, several molecular mechanisms were postulated to explain this latter stimulatory effect. These included hyperpolarization of the plasma membrane resulting in increased apical Ca^{2+} entry through TRPV5 and, alternatively, enhanced basolateral Na^+/Ca^{2+} exchange due to a decreased intracellular Na^+ concentration.[109] This last proposal was based on substantial co-localization in the DCT of NCC and the proteins involved in active Ca^{2+} transport. However, immunohistochemical studies demonstrated only minor overlap, whereas the Ca^{2+} transporters (i.e., TRPV5, calbindin-D28K, NCX1, and PMCA1b) completely co-localized.[3] Interestingly, it was demonstrated that in the DCT epithelium the Ca^{2+} transport proteins, including TRPV5, calbindin-D28K, and PMCA1b, were decreased in animals treated with high thiazide doses. In addition, the localization of the NCC protein was shifted from the luminal membrane to the basal membrane.

Schultheis and colleagues generated NCC knockout mice exhibiting hypocalciuria and hypomagnesemia, representing a valuable animal model explaining Gitelman's syndrome.[113] In these mice Ca^{2+} reabsorption was unaltered in the DCT and CNT as indicated by real-time reverse transcriptase polymerase chain reaction, Western blotting, and immunohistochemical analysis for TRPV5 and NCX1 as well as micropuncture experiments.[114] Micropuncture data indicated that reduced glomerular filtration and enhanced fractional reabsorption of Na^+ and Ca^{2+} upstream of the DCT provide compensation for the Na^+ transport defect in the DCT and contribute to the hypocalciuria.[114]

Taken together, these data support the hypothesis that enhanced proximal tubular Na^+ transport as a consequence of ECV contraction stimulates paracellular Ca^{2+} transport and comprises the molecular mechanism explaining thiazide-induced hypocalciuria.

Extracellular Regulation of TRPV5 by Novel Calciotropic Hormones

Klotho

Mice lacking the antiaging hormone Klotho show a phenotype resembling those of patients with premature aging syndromes: arteriosclerosis, osteoporosis, age-related skin changes, and ectopic calcifications, together with short lifespan and infertility.[115] Klotho is secreted and activated by cleavage of the amino-terminal extracellular domain, and this secreted form of Klotho exhibits β-glucuronidase activity.[116,117]

Several observations connect Klotho with Ca^{2+} metabolism. First, Klotho-deficient mice have a slight hypercalcemia that is associated with high levels of $1,25(OH)_2D_3$, caused by increased expression of renal 1α-hydroxylase.[118] Furthermore, administration of $1,25(OH)_2D_3$ induces Klotho expression in the kidney.[119] Second, Klotho$^{-/-}$ mice show bone abnormalities, including an approximately 20% lower bone mineral density than control mice.[115] In humans, allelic variants of Klotho are associated with osteoporosis, which confirms this phenotype.[120,121] Third, Klotho is strongly expressed in the DCT/CNT and the parathyroid gland, which further supports a role in epithelial Ca^{2+} handling.[115,122] Fourth, Chang and colleagues demonstrated a novel mechanism employed by Klotho to directly stimulate active Ca^{2+} reabsorption. Mutation of the conserved *N*-glycosylation site of TRPV5 (asparagine at residue 358 replaced by glutamine [N358Q]) abolished both Klotho- and β-glucuronidase–mediated activation of TRPV5, a finding indicating that Klotho may work by affecting the extracellular glycosylation status of the channel.[122]

Membrane protein biotinylation studies indicated a significant increase in plasma membrane localization of TRPV5 after Klotho or β-glucuronidase stimulation. Galectin-1 has been postulated as an anchoring molecule binding to TRPV5.[29] Together, these findings indicate that Klotho entraps the channels in the plasma membrane, which thereby increases TRPV5-mediated Ca^{2+} influx activity. Recently a molecular association of Klotho and Na^+-K^+-ATPase also was demonstrated that results in increased expression of the pump at the plasma membrane. The increased Na^+ gradient created by Na^+-K^+-ATPase activity might drive transepithelial Ca^{2+} transport in cooperation with Ca^{2+} influx mechanisms in the choroid plexus and the kidney.[123]

Tissue Kallikrein

Tissue kallikrein (TK) is a serine protease that is expressed mainly in the DCT and CNT. TK has been shown to be involved in the regulation of water, sodium, and potassium metabolism. The role of TK in the regulation of Ca^{2+} balance was not well studied until the discovery of a marked hypercalciuria in TK-deficient mice.[138] Gkika and colleagues further explored the molecular mechanism of TK involved in renal Ca^{2+} handling in vitro. Using TRPV5-expressing primary cultures of renal Ca^{2+}-transporting epithelial cells, they showed that TK activates Ca^{2+} reabsorption.[139] The stimulatory effect of TK was mimicked by bradykinin and could be inhibited by application of a bradykinin (BK) receptor blocker. The cell surface biotinylation studies revealed that TK increased the number of wild-type TRPV5 channels. Taken together, these data indicate that TK enhances active Ca^{2+} reabsorption through an increased TRPV5 plasma membrane expression via the BK-activated phospholipase/diacylglycerol/PKC pathway.

Concluding Remarks

Ca^{2+} reabsorption in the kidney, and particularly in the distal DCT2/CNT segments, is critical in the maintenance of Ca^{2+} balance. The identification and characterization of the proteins mediating this active Ca^{2+} transport have provided novel insight and a means to study the molecular aspects. In these segments, TRPV5 functions as the gatekeeper of Ca^{2+} entry, and therefore tight control of its activity enables the organism to adjust Ca^{2+} reabsorption according to the demands of the body. The control of cell surface expression of this TRPV5 channel, with modification of its *N*-linked glycosylation and phosphorylation of the channel induced by extracellular TK or PTH, is a newly discovered mechanism for regulation of active Ca^{2+} reabsorption. The molecular mechanism of Ca^{2+} shuttling between calbindin-D28K on one site and NCX1 and PMCA1b on the other site is not clear. Whether there is

a crosstalk between the apical Ca^{2+} entry and the basolateral Ca^{2+} extrusion regulatory systems is not known.

Magnesium Transport

Mg^{2+} Homeostasis

Mg^{2+} is the second most abundant intracellular cation in the body. Approximately 50% of the total body Mg^{2+} is mineralized in bone, whereas almost all of the other half is localized intracellularly; only 1% of the total body Mg^{2+} is present extracellularly.[124] Of the intracellular Mg^{2+}, only up to 10% exists as the metabolically active ionized form, but it plays a crucial role as a cofactor in many biochemical and physiologic processes such as activation of ATPases, regulation of many plasma membrane ion channels, and translational processes.[125-127] In plasma, 60% of the Mg^{2+} exists as the physiologically active ionized form; 30% is protein bound, mainly to albumin[128]; and the remaining 10% forms complexes with plasma anions such as phosphates and citrates.[129]

Disturbances of plasma Mg^{2+} levels can result in serious symptoms such as seizures and coma.[124,130] Therefore, an adequate homeostasis of Mg^{2+} resulting in tight regulation of plasma Mg^{2+} levels within a narrow range of 0.7 to 1.1 mmol/L is essential.[131] The extracellular Mg^{2+} concentration is controlled by the concerted action of renal Mg^{2+} reabsorption, intestinal absorption, and exchange of Mg^{2+} from bone. The principal organ responsible for the regulation of the body Mg^{2+} balance is the kidney, which tightly matches the intestinal absorption of Mg^{2+}.

Renal Handling of Mg^{2+}

About 80% of the total plasma Mg^{2+} is filtered in the glomerules. At a GFR of 125 mL/min, approximately 140 mmol Mg^{2+} per day is filtered, of which the majority is reabsorbed along the nephron. In the presence of hypermagnesemia the fractional excretion of Mg^{2+} can raise to nearly 100%. In contrast, with hypomagnesemia or reduced Mg^{2+} intake, the kidney minimizes urinary losses by increasing reabsorption and as a consequence can lower the fractional excretion to less than 1%.[124,132]

Proximal Tubule

In the PT approximately 20% of the filtered Mg^{2+} is reabsorbed. Although Mg^{2+} reabsorption in this segment is not well understood it appears to be paracellular and dependent on the filtered load as well as net salt and water reabsorption.[133]

Thick Ascending Loop of Henle

The major site of Mg^{2+} transport (70%) is the TAL, where paracellular Mg^{2+} transport is driven by a favorable lumen-positive electrochemical gradient, which is generated by the transcellular reabsorption of NaCl. The latter is dependent on the concerted activity of the Na^+-K^+-$2Cl^-$ cotransporter NKCC2, the renal outer medullary K^+ channel (ROMK, also known as *Kir 1.1*), Na^+-K^+-ATPase, and the renal Cl^- channel ClC-Kb.[134] The lumen-positive electrochemical gradient allows Mg^{2+} to be transported into the blood compartment via the tight junction proteins claudin-16 and claudin-19.[20,135]

Reabsorption of Na^+ along the length of the TAL reduces the intraluminal Na^+ concentration. Under these conditions, backflux of Na^+ from the interstitium to the tubular lumen may further augment the membrane voltage.[136] The calciotropic hormone PTH stimulates NaCl transport in the TAL, probably by modulating the activity of NKCC2. Interestingly, after application of PTH, changes in net Mg^{2+} transport appear much higher than the associated alterations observed in response to the transepithelial voltage. These data suggest that changes in the permeability of the paracellular pathway can modulate transepithelial Mg^{2+} transport via the claudins.

In addition, the CaSR receptor is expressed in the basolateral membrane of the TAL where it regulates transport in response to changes in extracellular Ca^{2+} and Mg^{2+} concentrations. Stimulation of the receptor is likely to reduce NKCC2 abundance. The reason why 60% of filtered Mg^{2+} and only 20% of the filtered Ca^{2+} is reabsorbed in the TAL is not entirely clear, but this disparity may represent differences in either delivery of divalent cations to the bend of the loop of Henle or permeability differences for divalent cations within the TAL.

Distal Convoluted Tubule

The DCT actively reabsorbs 5% to 10% of the filtered Mg^{2+} and the transport rate in this segment defines the final urinary Mg^{2+} concentration, as no reabsorption takes place beyond this segment.[127] In kidney, the function of DCT in active ion transport is underlined by the fact that cells of this nephron segment have the highest energy consumption of the nephron.[110] In addition to the proteins described in detail below the functioning of NCC, which is exclusively present in DCT, the CaSR and ClC-Kb are also important for active Mg^{2+} reabsorption in DCT.[137,140]

Collecting Duct

There are no data suggesting Mg^{2+} reabsorption in the CD segments. Approximately 3% of the filtered Mg^{2+} is excreted in the urine.

Active Mg^{2+} Reabsorption

Cellular Transport and Extrusion

Basically, the process of active transcellular Mg^{2+} transport in kidney can be envisioned as the following sequential steps (Figure 7-3). Driven by a favorable transmembrane potential, Mg^{2+} enters the DCT cell through an apical epithelial Mg^{2+} channel. The chemical driving force for Mg^{2+} is negligible, because the extracellular and intracellular Mg^{2+} concentrations are comparable. Importantly, Mg^{2+} entry into the cells appears to be the rate-limiting step and the site of regulation. Subsequently, Mg^{2+} diffuses through the cytosol to be extruded actively against an electrochemical gradient across the basolateral membrane.[141]

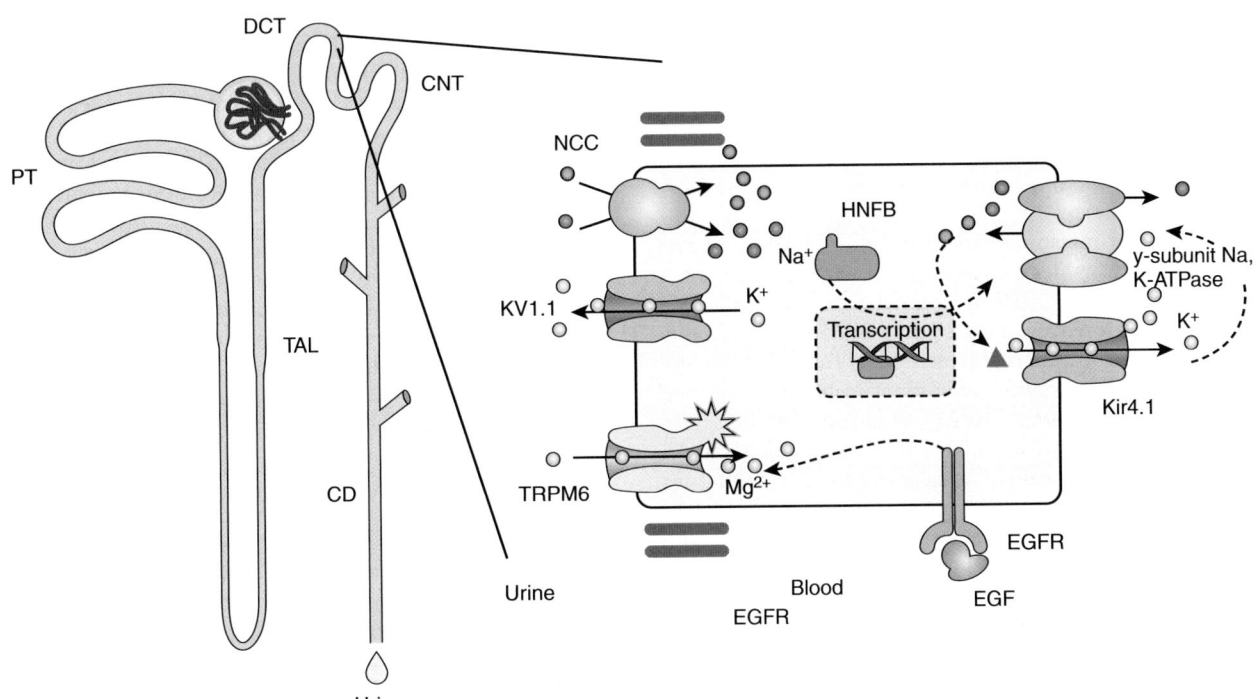

FIGURE 7-3 Model of active Mg^{2+} reabsorption. The distal tubule in the nephron comprises anatomically discrete segments, including the thick ascending limb of the loop of Henle (TAL) and the distal convoluted tubule (DCT), which ends in the connecting tubule (CNT). The DCT plays an important role in fine tuning renal excretion of Mg^{2+}. The epithelial Mg^{2+} channel (TRPM6) is predominantly expressed in the initial segment of the DCT (DCT1) with a lower abundance in the late segment (DCT2). TRPM6 co-localizes with the Na^+-Cl^- cotransporter (NCC) and parvalbumin in DCT1 and with calbindin-D28K in DCT2. Mg^{2+} influx via TRPM6 is controlled by the luminal and intracellular free Mg^{2+}. The basolateral membrane harbors the epidermal growth factor receptor (EGFR), Na^+-K^+-ATPase, the Kir 4.1 potassium channel, and possibly an Na^+/Mg^{2+} exchanger and Mg^{2+}-ATPase. The molecular identities of the Na^+/Mg^{2+} exchanger and Mg^{2+}-ATPase are still elusive. EGFR activation by EGF can enhance Mg^{2+} influx by increasing TRPM6 membrane expression. The protein encoded by *FXYD2* may bind as a γ-subunit with the α- and β-subunit of Na^+-K^+-ATPase. (Adapted from Xi Q, Hoenderop JG, Bindels RJ: Regulation of magnesium reabsorption in DCT, *Pflugers Arch* 458[1]:89-98, 2009.)

The key molecules that represent the cytosolic Mg^{2+}-binding proteins (if present) and the mechanism of basolateral Mg^{2+} extrusion in the process of transcellular Mg^{2+} transport are still elusive. As of now, specific Mg^{2+}-binding proteins have not been identified, but it is interesting to note that the Ca^{2+}-binding proteins parvalbumin and the calbindins, which are present in the DCT, also bind Mg^{2+}.[141,142] For the basolateral Mg^{2+} extrusion mechanism, most physiologic studies favor an Na^+-dependent exchange mechanism.[126] Other candidate mechanisms include an ATP-dependent Mg^{2+} pump.

TRPM6—The Apical Gate

Mg^{2+} enters the epithelial cell through the apical epithelial Mg^{2+} channel known as *transient receptor potential cation channel, subfamily M, member 6* (TRPM6). TRPM6 is a cation channel composed of six transmembrane-spanning domains and a conserved pore-forming region that assemble in a tetrameric configuration. Investigations of families who have autosomal recessive hypomagnesemia with secondary hypocalcemia (HSH) have identified mutations in TRPM6.[143,144] Through these and other studies, TRPM6 was discovered as an essential molecular determinant in transcellular Mg^{2+} transport in renal and intestinal epithelia.[141,143,144]

TRPM6 is one of the eight members of the identified TRPM cation channel subfamily and is composed of 2022 amino acids encoded by a large gene that contains 39 exons.[143-145] The TRPM6 protein shows 52% homology with its closest homolog TRPM7. TRPM6 displays a restricted expression pattern and is predominantly present in (re)absorbing epithelia.[141,143,144] In kidney, TRPM6 is localized along the apical membrane of the DCT, known to be the main site of active transcellular Mg^{2+} reabsorption along the nephron.[141] This localization is in line with the expected function of TRPM6 as the gatekeeper of Mg^{2+} influx. In the small intestine, TRPM6 is detected along the brush border membrane of the absorptive epithelial cells.[141,143]

The renal and intestinal expression of TRPM6, in addition to the renal Mg^{2+} leak in patients with HSH, emphasizes the important role of TRPM6 in renal and intestinal Mg^{2+} (re)absorption. Moreover, the role of TRPM6 in total-body Mg^{2+} homeostasis is underlined by the fact that TRPM6 and TRPM7 are not functionally redundant in humans, because the ubiquitously expressed TRPM7 cannot rescue the severe phenotype of HSH patients.[146] Interestingly, deletion of TRPM6 or TRPM7 in mice revealed that it is essential for embryonic development.[147,148]

TRPM6 is a unique bifunctional protein that has both Mg^{2+}-permeable cation channel properties and protein kinase activity and is therefore referred to as a *chanzyme*.[149] Electrophysiologic characterization of TRPM6 demonstrated that TRPM6-transfected human embryonic kidney 293 (HEK293) cells exhibited outwardly rectifying currents upon establishment of the whole-cell configuration as demonstrated for TRPM7.

It has been shown that the fused α-kinase domain is not a prerequisite for channel activity. However, studies have revealed an indirect regulatory role in the modulation of channel functioning.[146,150,151] Along this line, a receptor for activated C-kinase 1 (RACK1) has been identified as the first TRPM6-associated partner. This protein is expressed in the DCT and interacts with the α-kinase domain, thereby inhibiting TRPM6 channel activity. The inhibitory effect of RACK1 was shown to be dependent on autophosphorylation of a threonine residue (T1851) in the α-kinase domain. These data suggest a novel feedback mechanism of TRPM6-mediated Mg^{2+} influx via autophosphorylation, which activates the inhibitory effect of RACK1 and thereby prevents Mg^{2+} overload during active Mg^{2+} reabsorption.

Recently, a new TRPM6-interacting protein, repressor of estrogen receptor activity (REA), has been described.[152] REA inhibits TRPM6 channel activity in an α-kinase activity–dependent manner, because REA has no functional effect on the TRPM6 phosphotransferase-deficient mutant (K1804R).[152] These data suggest another indirect regulation of TRPM6 activity that is independent of autophosphorylation, but reliant on TRPM6 α-kinase activity. REA thus appears to act as another negative modulator involved in renal Mg^{2+} handling via regulation of TRPM6-mediated Mg^{2+}-influx.

Kv 1.1

Another protein assumed to regulate Mg^{2+} reabsorption via TRPM6 is the voltage-gated K^+ channel Kv 1.1. Recently, a mutation in the *KCNA1* gene coding for the Kv 1.1 was shown to be causative for autosomal dominant hypomagnesemia. The phenotype, detectable from infancy, consists of recurrent muscle cramps, tetany, tremor, muscle weakness, cerebellar atrophy, and myokymia. The K^+ channel co-localizes with TRPM6 along the luminal membrane of the DCT. Functional characterization showed that the mutation results in a nonfunctional channel with a dominant negative effect on wild-type channel function.

The Mg^{2+} influx via TRPM6 is energized by the local electrochemical gradient. Importantly, the DCT cell lacks a substantial chemical gradient for Mg^{2+}. The luminal membrane potential in the DCT is approximately -70 mV, which favors Mg^{2+} influx. Thus, the movement of Mg^{2+} into the DCT cell seems driven mainly by the electrical gradient. Kv 1.1 is postulated to hyperpolarize the luminal membrane of the DCT, which thus promotes TRPM6-mediated Mg^{2+} reabsorption. Consequently, loss-of-function mutation of Kv 1.1 leads to impairment of renal Mg^{2+} handling.

γ-Subunit of Na^+-K^+-ATPase

Another identified gene involved in hypomagnesemia is *FXYD2*. *FXYD2* encodes the γ-subunit of basolateral Na^+-K^+-ATPase and is mutated in patients with autosomal dominant renal hypomagnesemia associated with hypocalciuria. The *FXYD2* gene encodes two splice variants, γa and γb, which locate to different segments of the nephron. Splice variant γa is specifically expressed in the macula densa and the CD, whereas γb localizes along the basolateral membrane of the DCT and CNT. Currently, the exact molecular mechanism by which the γ-subunit controls Mg^{2+} handling in the DCT remains elusive. It has been postulated that the γ-subunit facilitates the basolateral extrusion of Mg^{2+} in renal epithelial cells.[153] Others suggest a role for the γ-subunit in the regulation of other transport mechanisms that localize to the basolateral membrane, such as Na^+-K^+-ATPase, Kir 4.1/5.1, and the unidentified basolateral Mg^{2+} extrusion mechanism.

HNF1B

Additional evidence for an active role of the γ-subunit in Mg^{2+} reabsorption was provided by a study demonstrating that the transcription factor known as *hepatocyte nuclear factor 1 homeobox B* (HNF1B) is linked to the regulation of the *FXYD2* gene.[154] Hypomagnesemia, hypermagnesuria, and hypocalciuria were observed in 44% of the *HNF1B* mutation carriers. Analysis of the *FXYD2* promoter region resulted in the identification of a highly conserved HNF1B recognition site. Future studies should confirm the role of HNF1B in the regulation of *FXYD2* and possibly other components of the molecular machinery involved in renal Mg^{2+} handling.

Kir 4.1

A new syndrome with a phenotype closely resembling that of Gitelman's syndrome was recently identified.[155,156] One study reporting on this syndrome described two nonrelated consanguineous families with a disorder characterized by epilepsy, ataxia, sensorineural deafness, and tubulopathy (referred to as *EAST syndrome*).[156] A second study described four kindreds with similar clinical manifestations.[155] Both studies revealed a mutation in the *KCNJ10* gene as the underlying cause of the syndrome in these patients. The *KCNJ10* gene encodes the inwardly rectifying K^+ channel Kir 4.1, which is expressed in brain, ear, and kidney, in line with the phenotype observed in these patients.

The renal phenotype of EAST syndrome is similar to that of Gitelman's syndrome and consists of polyuria, hypokalemic metabolic alkalosis, hypomagnesemia, and hypocalciuria. In the kidney, Kir 4.1 is expressed at the basolateral membrane of distal tubular epithelia, together with Na^+-K^+-ATPase. Kir 4.1 is suggested to recycle K^+ into the interstitium to allow a sufficient supply of K^+ for optimal Na^+-K^+-ATPase activity, which may be necessary to support the substantial transport of NaCl and Mg^{2+}.

Regulation of Epithelial Mg^{2+} Transport

Several hormones, including PTH, calcitonin, $1,25(OH)_2D_3$, insulin, glucagon, antidiuretic hormone, aldosterone, and sex steroids (estrogens) have been implicated in Mg^{2+} transport in vitro.[157-159] Moreover, it was demonstrated that Mg^{2+} transport in the DCT is influenced by dietary Mg^{2+} restriction and various hormones, and that PTH in vivo stimulates Mg^{2+} reabsorption in the TAL and DCT.[160-162] In addition, it was shown that Mg^{2+} transport in rat colon is not responsive to $1,25(OH)_2D_3$.[163,164] In spite of these reports, hormonal regulation of active transcellular Mg^{2+} reabsorption remains largely undefined.[127,133,161,165] Moreover, it has been suggested that the hormones influencing the Mg^{2+} balance are only indirect regulators of Mg^{2+} homeostasis, because Mg^{2+} lacks a specific endocrine control similar to that existing for Ca^{2+}, Na^+, and K^+.[158]

Until recently there was no evidence of specific physiologic hormonal control of Mg^{2+} (re)absorption. Apical Mg^{2+} influx is the initial step of transcellular Mg^{2+} transport. Therefore, this step is an ideal target for hormonal regulation of active Mg^{2+} (re)absorption. Potentially, the regulation of TRPM6 channel activity can be controlled at discrete processing levels, including transcription, translation, posttranslational modification, trafficking to the plasma membrane, channel gating, and ultimately protein degradation; however, it remains elusive whether these regulatory processes all apply to TRPM6. The following sections summarize the recent discoveries regarding the molecular mechanisms controlling TRPM6 activity, including the role of novel magnesiotropic hormones (Table 7-2).

Calcineurin Inhibitors

Hypomagnesemia occurs frequently in tacrolimus- and cyclosporine-treated patients. Navaneethan and colleagues studied the correlation between renal Mg^{2+} wasting and tacrolimus blood levels in renal transplant patients.[166] Based on these studies it was concluded that hypomagnesemia in renal transplant recipients results from renal Mg^{2+} wasting. Studies of longer duration are needed to assess the long-term effects of this early posttransplant hypomagnesemia. Administration of tacrolimus to rats by daily oral gavage significantly enhanced the urinary excretion of Mg^{2+} and induced a significant hypomagnesemia. Renal wasting was explained by decreased expression of TRPM6 in kidney during tacrolimus treatment.[167] Similarly, cyclosporine causes hypomagnesemia by decreasing the expression of TRPM6.[168]

TABLE 7-2 Genes and Hormones Involved in Active Mg^{2+} Reabsorption

	(POTENTIAL) MECHANISM	REFERENCES
Major Factors		
Estrogen	Transport in DCT ↑, TRPM6 expression ↑	173
Epidermal growth factor	Transport in DCT ↑, TRPM6 activation ↑	174
Insulin	Transport in DCT ↓, TRPM6 expression ↓	311
Thiazide	Transport in DCT ↓, TRPM6 expression ↓	177
Tacrolimus	Transport in DCT ↓, TRPM6 expression ↓	167
Hypovolemic status	Transport in DCT ↓, TRPM6 expression ↓	177
Mutated Genes		
TRPM6	Transport in DCT ↓	143, 144
NCC	Transport in DCT ↓, TRPM6 expression ↓	177
KCNA1	Transport in DCT ↓, TRPM6-mediated Mg^{2+} influx ↓	318
HNF1B	Unknown	154
FXYD2	Unknown	319
KCNJ10	Transport in DCT ↓, Na^+-K^+-ATPase activity ↓	155, 156

NOTE: Increased or decreased active Mg^{2+} reabsorption in the DCT does not necessarily mean that total renal Mg^{2+} reabsorption is increased or reduced.

↑, Increased gene expression, increased channel activity; ↓, downregulation of gene expression or inhibition of channel activity; *ATPase*, adenosine triphosphatase; *DCT*, distal convoluted tubule; *TRPM6*, transient receptor potential, subfamily M, member 6.

Estrogen

It has been previously shown that estrogen influences whole-body Mg^{2+} balance, which may explain the hypermagnesuria seen in postmenopausal women.[169-172] Recently, Groenestege and colleagues demonstrated that the renal TRPM6 mRNA level in ovariectomized rats is significantly reduced, whereas supplementation with 17β-estradiol normalizes TRPM6 mRNA levels in these rats.[173] Of note, the renal mRNA abundance of TRPM7 remained unaltered under these conditions.[173] This finding provides insight into the molecular mechanism of estrogen deficiency–induced hypermagnesuria.

Epidermal Growth Factor

Epidermal growth factor (EGF) has been identified as a magnesiotropic hormone directly stimulating TRPM6 activity.[174] Genetic analysis and a positional cloning strategy revealed that a point mutation in the *pro-EGF* gene causes a rare inherited autosomal recessive form of renal hypomagnesemia. Previous studies demonstrated that EGF acts as an autocrine-paracrine magnesiotropic hormone, specifically increasing TRPM6 activity via engagement of its receptor on the basolateral membrane of DCT cells. This effect is specific for TRPM6, because the stimulatory effect of EGF is not observed on the homologous TRPM7 channel.[174] These findings provide the first insight into the molecular regulation of TRPM6 by extracellular EGF. Moreover, it demonstrates the molecular basis for the magnesium wasting that is a side effect of cetuximab treatment of colorectal cancer and identifies TRPM6 as a potential pharmacologic target during cetuximab therapy.[174,175]

Diuretics

It has been known for a long time that diuretics can affect the Mg^{2+} balance. Thiazide diuretics are among the most commonly prescribed drugs, particularly in the treatment of hypertension. These compounds inhibit NCC present in the apical membrane of the DCT to enhance renal Na^+ excretion.[176] Besides having this diuretic effect, thiazides are known to cause hypomagnesemia.

Several features of long-term thiazide treatment are mimicked in NCC knockout mice, which are an animal model for Gitelman's syndrome.[113,114] Intriguingly, the molecular mechanisms responsible for hypomagnesemia during thiazide administration and Gitelman's syndrome have remained elusive. The level of renal expression of TRPM6 in NCC knockout mice and in mice receiving thiazides long term was analyzed. Renal TRPM6 mRNA expression was significantly reduced in NCC knockout mice compared with control littermates. Immunohistochemical analysis revealed that TRPM6 protein abundance along the apical membrane of the DCT is profoundly decreased in these mice. Similarly, renal TRPM6 expression was diminished in thiazide-treated animals. NCC expression was enhanced in these animals, which illustrates that TRPM6 downregulation is a specific nondeleterious effect.[177] Together, these findings demonstrate that long-term administration of thiazide diuretics results in specific downregulation of renal TRPM6, leading to inappropriately high renal Mg^{2+} excretion and hypomagnesemia.

Concluding Remarks

The identification of TRPM6 and its regulatory factors has advanced our knowledge of the control of renal Mg^{2+} handling. Moreover, understanding of the regulation of TRPM6 channel activity in a short time scale has been improved by unraveling of the signaling pathway of EGF receptor activation and the finding of estrogen stimulation of epithelial Mg^{2+} transport. Further investigation into the hormonal control of TRPM6 trafficking and activity will provide more detail to aid our understanding of the body Mg^{2+} balance. Currently, limited experimental evidence is available on the cellular diffusion and basolateral extrusion of Mg^{2+} in the DCT. Future studies of families with rare inherited forms of renal hypomagnesemia will be instrumental to elucidate novel genes and the molecular mechanisms in active Mg^{2+} handling.

Phosphate Transport

Phosphate Homeostasis

Total Body Phosphate

Phosphate has multiple functions in the body. Phosphate is a key component of the bony skeleton and is an important limiting factor for metabolic processes, including the formation of high-energy phosphate bonds such as those in ATP. It is also an important component of nucleic acids and phospholipids. Phosphorylation of cellular proteins is an important mechanism for regulation of cellular function. Finally, phosphate is an important blood and urinary pH buffer.

The total body phosphorus content is 700 g in an average adult, of which 85% is in bone and teeth, 14% is in soft tissues, and only 1% is present in extracellular fluid. In plasma, phosphorus is present primarily as HPO_4^{2-} and $H_2PO_4^-$ (phosphate ions) that exist in a pH-dependent equilibrium ($pK_a = 6.8$). Thus, at pH 7.4, the ratio of HPO_4^{2-} to $H_2PO_4^-$ is 4:1. The normal mean concentration of phosphate in human plasma is 3 to 4.5 mg/dL, corresponding to 1.0 to 1.5 mmol/L.

Plasma phosphate exists in ionized, complexed, and protein-bound forms. If phosphate were totally filterable in the glomerulus, its concentration in the ultrafiltrate would be 1.18 times that of plasma (corrected for plasma water and the Gibbs-Donnan factor). Measured ratios of ultrafilterable phosphate to plasma phosphate have been found to range from 0.89 to 0.96, which indicates that a small portion of plasma phosphate is nonfilterable (e.g., protein bound). Nevertheless, independent of plasma concentration, the concentration of phosphate in the ultrafiltrate is approximately the same as in plasma. Due to complex formation with Ca^{2+} ions the fraction of ultrafilterable phosphate may decline under certain conditions, for example, hypercalcemia.

Intracellular phosphate is primarily present as free phosphate and may be sequestered to some extent in intracellular organelles. Phosphate is also incorporated into organic compounds such as creatine phosphate, adenosine phosphates, nucleic acids, phospholipids, and, in erythrocytes, 2,3-diphosphoglycerate. In steady state, the cytosolic free inorganic phosphate concentration in soft tissues has been estimated to be around 1 mmol/L. This value is above its electrochemical equilibrium value as predicted from the membrane potential, which suggests that there must be active transport of phosphate into cells.

The regulation of intracellular phosphate levels is closely linked to cellular metabolic activity. Inhibition of phosphate uptake impairs cellular metabolic function, whereas increasing extracellular phosphate concentration stimulates mitochondrial respiration.

Intake and Output

The daily dietary intake of phosphate is 800 mg to 1500 mg (Figure 7-4). Phosphate is found in many foods, including dairy products, meat, and cereal grains, so that dietary deficiency is rare. Approximately 65% of ingested phosphate is absorbed in the small intestine. Dietary polyvalent cations such as Ca^{2+}, Mg^{2+}, and Al^{3+} bind to intestinal luminal phosphate and decrease its absorption. Secreted digestive juices contain about 3 mg/kg/day of phosphate. Once absorbed, phosphate in the extracellular fluid may exchange with the pool in bone, with 200 mg of phosphate typically entering and leaving the skeleton daily as it is continuously remodeled.

Ultimately, the kidneys are responsible for the excretion of a substantial excess of phosphate, about 900 mg/day. During periods of growth, a greater proportion of phosphate is retained for bone deposition, but this still constitutes a small percentage of dietary intake. Thus, renal phosphate excretion is the principal mechanism by which the body regulates extracellular phosphate balance.

Overview of Regulation of Phosphate Homeostasis

The plasma concentration of phosphate is maintained by numerous humoral and local factors. The predominant humoral factors are PTH and the phosphatonins (Figure 7-5). Both PTH and phosphatonins inhibit renal tubular phosphate reabsorption and hence increase phosphate excretion.[178] The term *phosphatonins* refers to a group of humoral phosphaturic factors, of which the most well characterized is fibroblast growth factor 23 (FGF-23),[179] that were first isolated from tumors of patients with tumor-induced osteomalacia and are produced primarily in bone.[180,181]

Orchestration of plasma concentration of PTH and FGF-23 is achieved by serum calcium, serum phosphate, and $1,25(OH)_2D_3$, which inhibits PTH secretion and stimulates FGF-23 secretion.[182,183] A rise in serum phosphate level causes a fall in serum free Ca^{2+}, which acutely stimulates PTH release via activation of the CaSR.[184] Hyperphosphatemia also stimulates FGF-23 expression and release in bone.[185,186] In addition, hyperphosphatemia inhibits expression of the enzyme 25-hydroxyvitamin D_3–1α-hydroxylase in the PT, likely mediated by FGF-23.[185,187] A decreased level of $1,25(OH)_2D_3$ reduces its inhibition of PTH secretion[188] and results in decreased intestinal phosphate absorption. The concerted actions of these factors contribute to the restoration of normal plasma phosphate levels. A fall in plasma phosphate level triggers the opposite effects.

Renal Handling of Phosphate

Phosphate concentration of fluid in Bowman's space is approximately equal to the total plasma free phosphate concentration. Renal clearance studies have demonstrated that 80% to 97% of the filtered load of phosphate is reabsorbed by the renal tubules, so that only 3% to 20% is ultimately

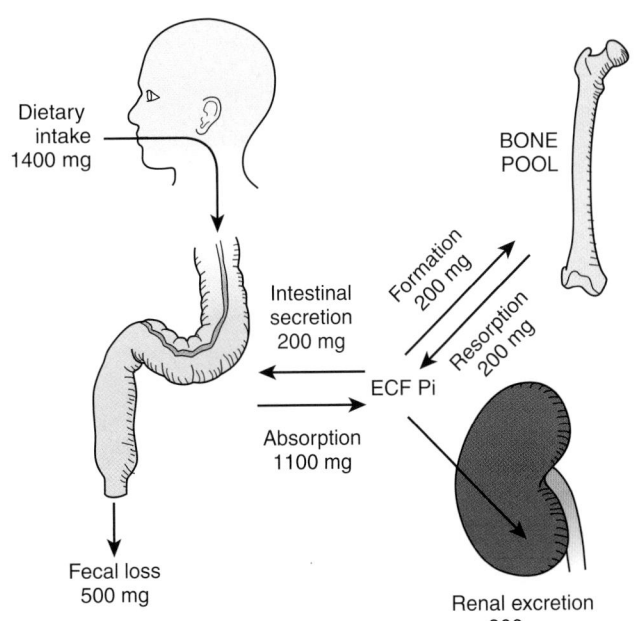

FIGURE 7-4 Daily phosphate intake and output for a normal adult in neutral phosphate balance.

excreted. The relationship between plasma phosphate level and phosphate excretion is shown in Figure 7-6. Initially, as the plasma phosphate concentration, and hence filtered load, increases, there is a commensurate increase in the reabsorption of phosphate, so that minimal phosphate appears in the urine. When the plasma phosphate concentration exceeds a certain level, the renal threshold, phosphate begins to appear in the urine, increasing in proportion to the filtered load. This indicates that tubular reabsorption of phosphate is saturable. In humans, at a GFR above 40 mL/min, the maximal tubular reabsorption rate of phosphate (TmP) varies proportionately with GFR. Thus, TmP/GFR, which is the theoretical renal threshold, is kept constant and is a reliable index of tubule reabsorptive capacity. With advanced renal insufficiency (GFR of <40 mL/min), TmP is further decreased (in part due to secondary hyperparathyroidism) and the fractional excretion of phosphate further increased. However, the decrease in TmP is less than the decrease in GFR, so that TmP/GFR rises and hyperphosphatemia ensues.

Phosphate Handling by Different Nephron Segments

About 80% of filtered phosphate is reabsorbed in the PT. There is likely no reabsorption of phosphate in the loop of Henle and the CD. Some evidence has been provided that in distal nephron segments approximately 5% of filtered phosphate may be reabsorbed (see later).

PROXIMAL TUBULE

In PTs there is marked axial heterogeneity in reabsorptive activity. Micropuncture studies showed that 60% to 70% of filtered phosphate is reabsorbed within the proximal convoluted tubules itself. Of this, most is reabsorbed in the S1 segment.[189,190] In agreement with the functional studies mentioned, the abundance of Na/Pi cotransporters under normal dietary conditions, as estimated by immunofluorescence, was higher in the proximal convoluted tubule segments.[178,191] Altogether, these findings indicated that the earliest convolutions

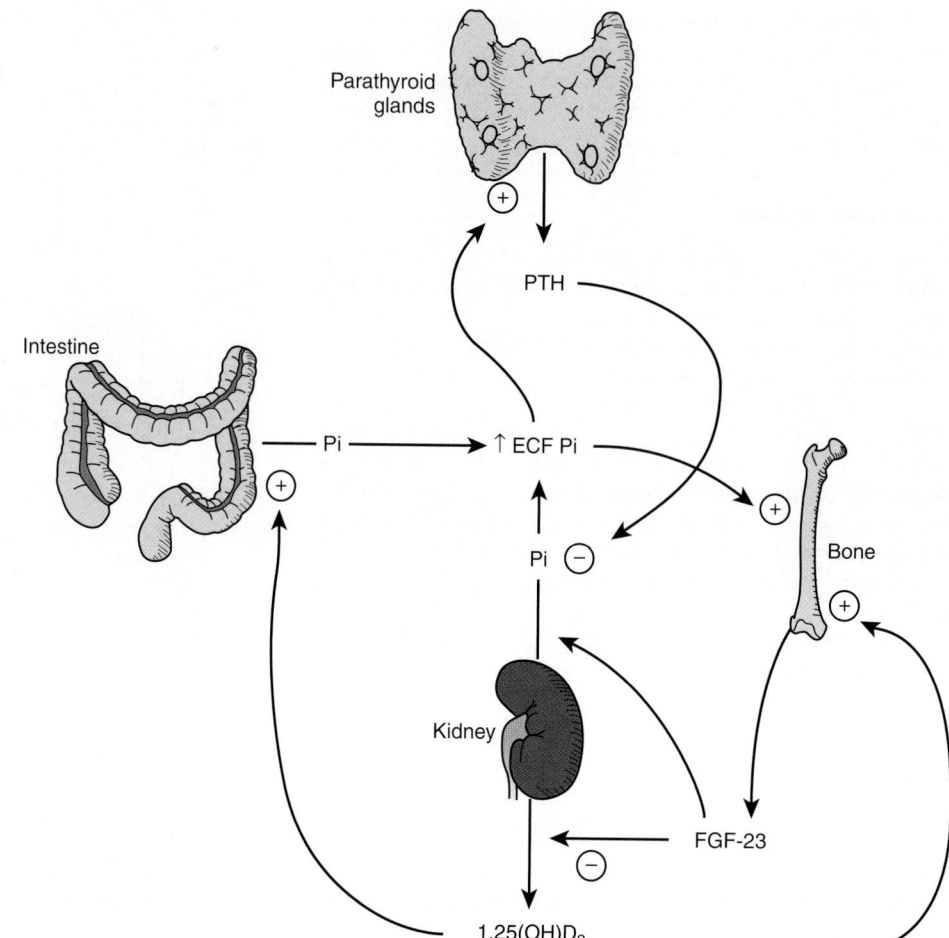

FIGURE 7-5 Schematic view of overall phosphate homeostasis. Several endocrine feedback loops that involve parathyroid hormone (PTH), fibroblast growth factor 23 (FGF-23), and 1,25-dihydroxyvitamin D regulate serum phosphate concentrations.

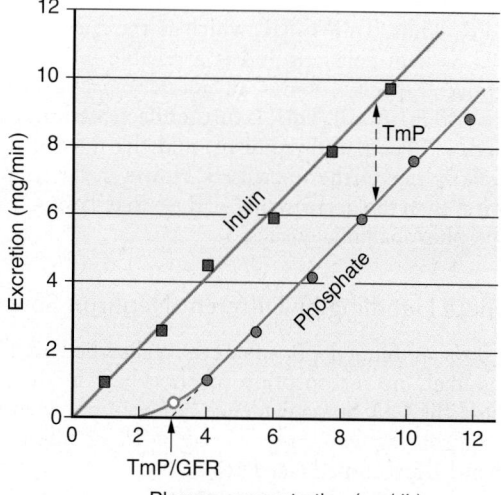

FIGURE 7-6 Effect of fasting and phosphate infusion on phosphate balance. Relationship between urinary excretion rate and plasma concentration of phosphate is shown for a normal human subject during fasting (*open circle*) and phosphate infusion (*solid circles*). Also shown is the excretion-concentration relationship for inulin (*squares*). The slope of both lines is the same and equal to the glomerular filtration rate (GFR). The vertical distance between the two lines represents the maximal tubular reabsorption rate of phosphate (TmP). The *x*-intercept, extrapolated from the line connecting the solid circles, represents the theoretical renal phosphate threshold (TmP/GFR). (From Bijvoet OL: Relation of plasma phosphate concentration to renal tubular reabsorption of phosphate, *Clin Sci* 37[1]:23-36, 1969.)

of the proximal convoluted tubule have the highest density of Na/Pi cotransporters and the highest capacity to reabsorb phosphate. There is also some evidence for internephron heterogeneity in reabsorptive activity. The fractional delivery of phosphate to the micropuncture-accessible DCT, which is derived from superficial nephrons, is consistently greater than that delivered to the bend of the loop of Henle of juxtamedullary nephrons. This suggests that the proximal reabsorptive capacity of juxtamedullary nephrons is greater than that of superficial nephrons.

DISTAL CONVOLUTED TUBULE
Whether phosphate is reabsorbed in distal nephron segments remains controversial. Several studies have failed to find phosphate transport in the distal tubules from animals consuming a normal diet. However, several lines of evidence suggested that under conditions of phosphate deprivation there may be true distal tubule phosphate reabsorption. If it does occur, the cellular mechanism of this phosphate reabsorption in the DCT is unknown.

Molecular Mechanisms of Proximal Tubular Phosphate Reabsorption

Phosphate reabsorption along the PTs is a unidirectional, transcellular process that has been studied in detail (see Figure 7-7 and Biber and colleagues[178]). Intracellular phosphate levels

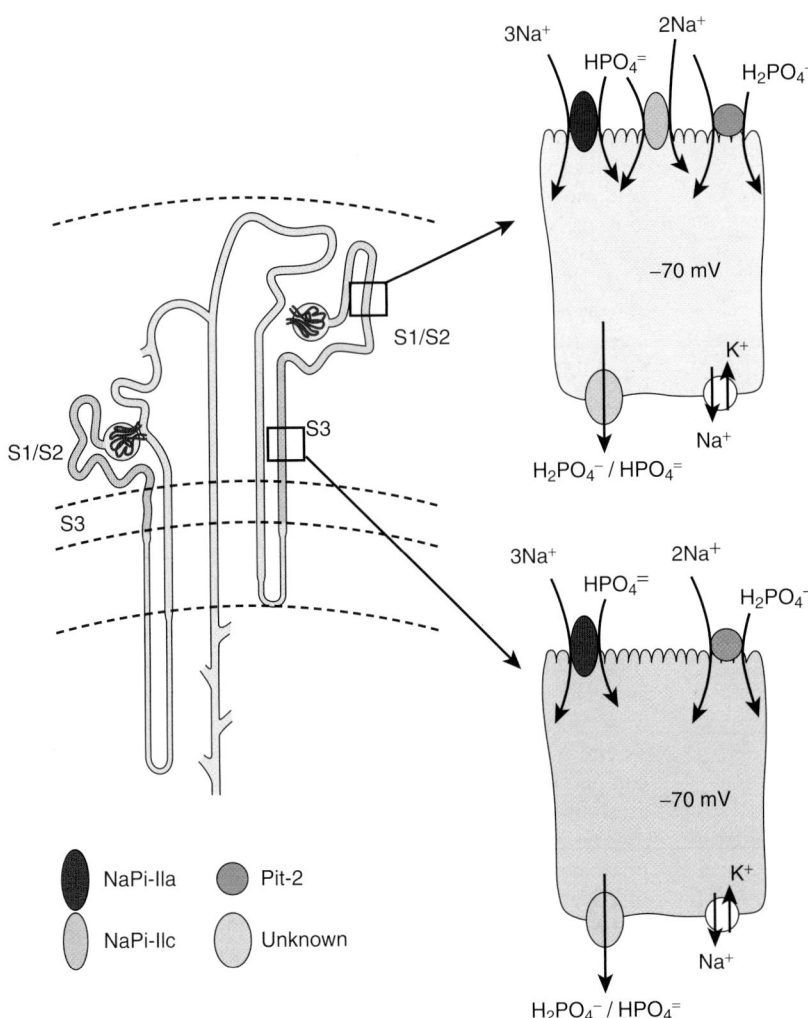

FIGURE 7-7 Apically localized Na/Pi cotransporters involved in the reabsorption of phosphate in proximal tubular segments S1/S2 and S3. (Adapted from Biber J, Hernando N, Forster I, et al: Regulation of phosphate transport in proximal tubules, *Pflugers Arch* 458[1]:39-52, 2009.)

have been estimated to be in the range of 1 mmol/L and thus are higher than the level expected for electrochemical equilibrium with luminal fluid. Therefore, apical entry must occur by active transport, whereas basolateral exit may occur by passive diffusion. At the brush border membrane phosphate entry is dependent on Na^+ ions and is mediated by several sodium-dependent phosphate cotransporters that, depending on the coupling ratio of Na^+ to phosphate ions, theoretically could give rise to a 100- to 10,000-fold concentration of intracellular phosphate. Thus, the capacity of phosphate reabsorption is determined not by the driving force, but by the abundance of Na/Pi cotransporters residing in the brush border membrane. Therefore, regulation of proximal tubular reabsorption of phosphate is mostly achieved by changes in the number of Na/Pi cotransporters.

Apical Na/Pi Cotransporters

The entry of phosphate at the apical site of proximal tubular cells is the rate-limiting step in transcellular phosphate transport and the target for virtually all physiologic mechanisms that alter proximal tubular reabsorption of phosphate. Initially some of the key features of the apical Na^+-phosphate cotransporter emerged from studies using isolated brush border membrane vesicles.[192] The coupling ratio of Na^+ to phosphate

ions is greater than unity, and, depending on the transporter protein, Na/Pi cotransport is electrogenic (movement of net positive charge with phosphate entry) or electroneutral (Table 7-3). There is normally a steep inward concentration gradient for Na^+ ions across the plasma membrane, which is maintained by the basolaterally localized Na^+-K^+-ATPase, and an inside-negative membrane potential. Thus, the high coupling ratio and electrogenicity are both thermodynamically important for the secondary active transport of phosphate against its steep electrochemical gradient at the apical membrane.[193]

Na/Pi cotransporters identified so far belong to the solute carrier families SLC17, SLC20, and SLC34.[194] Members of the latter two SLC families were shown to be involved in proximal tubular Pi reabsorption and thus in phosphate homeostasis (see Figure 7-5). The type I Na/Pi cotransporter (SLC17A1) has been cloned based on Na/Pi cotransport activity and was localized at the brush border of PTs.[195] However, the transport characteristics of the type I Na/Pi cotransporter do not resemble the characteristics of renal brush border Na/phosphate cotransport,[196] which makes it unlikely that SLC17A1 plays an important role in the transcellular phosphate transport.

SLC family 20 consists of two members, PiT-1 and PiT-2 (type III Na/Pi cotransporters).[197] In rat kidney PiT-2 was localized at the brush border membrane in PTs[198] (Figure 7-7).

TABLE 7-3   Characterization of Na/Pi Cotransporters Involved in Renal Reabsorption of Phosphate

	TYPE II			TYPE III
Protein name	NaPi-IIa	NaPi-IIb	NaPi-IIc	PiT-1 (Glvr-1) PiT-2 (Ram-1)
Gene name	*SLC34A1*	*SLC34A2*	*SLC34A3*	*SLC20A1/2*
Tissue expression	Kidney cortex/PT	Intestine, lung, etc.	Kidney cortex/PT	Ubiquitous PiT-2 in PT
Substrates	HPO_4^-	HPO_4^-	HPO_4^-	$H_2PO_4^-$
K_m (Pi)	0.1-0.2 mmol/L	0.05 mmol/L	0.07 mmol/L	0.025 mmol/L
K_m (Na^+)	~60 mmol/L	~30 mmol/L	~50 mmol/L	~50 mmol/L
Coupling ratio (Na:Pi)	3:1	3:1	2:1	2:1
Transport	Electro-genic	Electro-genic	Electro-neutral	Electrogenic
Dependence on pH	Stimulated at high pH	Inhibited at high pH	Stimulated at high pH	Inhibited at high pH
Inhibited by	PFA	PFA	PFA	

PFA, Phosphonoformic acid; *PT,* proximal tubules.

Na/Pi cotransport by PiT-2 is electrogenic and, in contrast to the type II Na/Pi cotransporter family SLC34, PiT-2 prefers monovalent phosphate.[194,199] The relative importance of Pit-2 in overall renal reabsorption of phosphate has not been established.

The solute carrier family SLC34 includes three homologous isoforms of type II Na/Pi cotransporters.[200] Isoforms IIa (SLC34A1) and IIc (SLC34A3) are located at the proximal tubular brush border membrane. Isoform IIb (SLC34A2) is expressed in the small intestine and other tissues, such as lung and testis. NaPi-IIa and NaPi-IIc are regarded as the major players in renal handling of phosphate, yet their relative importance varies in different species.

In rodents, the NaPi-IIa cotransporter appears to be the predominant one. Mice with targeted inactivation of the Na/Pi cotransporter gene *Npt2a* exhibited phosphaturia, hypophosphatemia, and an appropriate elevation in the serum concentration of $1,25(OH)_2D_3$ with attendant hypercalcemia, hypercalciuria, and decreased serum PTH levels.[201] Na/Pi cotransport in brush border membrane vesicles (BBMVs) derived from the *Npt2* knockout mice was reduced by 70% compared with that in BBMVs from wild-type controls, which indicates that the cause of the phosphaturia was loss of the major brush border Na^+-phosphate transport system, namely NaPi-IIa (SLC34A1).

In humans, the relative contribution of the NaPi-IIa cotransporter is controversial. Two patients have been described who have heterozygous inactivating mutations in NaPi-IIa cotransporter. Both have idiopathic hypophosphatemia with renal Pi wasting, associated in one case with recurrent nephrolithiasis and in the other with osteoporosis.[202] However, a detailed analysis of described NaPi-IIa variants showed no differences in function or expression compared with the wild-type transporters.[203] Furthermore, it was demonstrated

that several NaPi-IIa mutants that were reported in patients with hypercalciuria and increased excretion of phosphate do not represent a major cause of phosphaturia in humans.[204]

The NaPi-IIc cotransporter is expressed primarily in the kidney at the apical membrane of the PT and at significantly higher levels in weaning animals than in adults.[205] In PTs of rat and mouse kidneys, NaPi-IIc is absent in S3 segments. Deletion of NaPi-IIc in mice does not result in hyperphosphaturia or hypophosphatemia.[206,207] The physiologic importance of NaPi-IIc appears to be different in humans than in mice. Analysis of patients with hereditary hypophosphatemic rickets with hypercalciuria revealed missense mutations and large deletions of the *SLC34A3* gene, which indicates that, in humans, NaPi-IIc contributes significantly to renal phosphate excretion.[208-210]

Transport Characteristics of Type IIa and IIc Na/Pi Cotransporters

Na/Pi cotransport by the NaPi-IIa cotransporter is electrogenic and has been investigated in detail after expression in *Xenopus laevis* oocytes.[194,211] The general kinetic characteristics derived from these studies are depicted in Table 7-3. By simultaneous measurement of substrate flux and charge movement under voltage-clamp conditions, the stoichiometry was determined to be 3 Na^+ ions to 1 (divalent) phosphate ion.[212] Na/Pi cotransport by NaPi-IIa is higher at more alkaline pH values due to both a competitive interaction of H^+ ions with the Na^+ binding site and an additional effect on reorientation of the empty transporter.[213]

The NaPi-IIc cotransporter exhibits Na^+-dependent phosphate cotransport that is electroneutral, with a stoichiometry of 2 Na^+ ions to 1 (divalent) phosphate ion, and is stimulated by an alkaline extracellular pH.[205,214] The 2:1 stoichiometry, and thus the lack of coupled movement of net charge, would be expected to reduce the thermodynamic ability of the transporter to concentrate phosphate within the PT epithelial cell.

Protein-Protein Interactions of Type IIa and IIc Na/Pi Cotransporters

The NaPi-IIa cotransporter participates in multiple protein interactions via a PDZ-binding motif (TRL) located on its C-terminal tail.[215,216] This peptide motif binds to PDZ (PSD95, discs large [*Drosophila*], and ZO-1 proteins) domains of the Na^+/H^+ exchanger regulatory factor (NHERF) protein family,[217] which includes NHERF-1, NHERF-2, NHERF-3 (PDZK1, or "PDZ domain–containing 1") and NHERF-4 (PDZK2). All NHERF proteins are located at the apical site of proximal tubular cells.[216,218] Disruption of these interactions by competition with PDZ domain peptides or by deletion mutations prevents normal trafficking of the NaPi-IIa cotransporter to the apical membrane.[219]

The importance of NHERF-1 for proper apical localization of NaPi-IIa was demonstrated by using knockout mice lacking NHERF-1.[220] In these mice, the apical abundance of NaPi-IIa proteins is reduced and the proteins are aberrantly localized intracellularly. Consistent with this, NHERF-1 null mice are phosphaturic. By contrast, and despite robust in vitro interactions of the NaPi-IIa cotransporter with NHERF-3, NHERF-3 knockout mice show very few phenotypic characteristics related to renal handling of phosphate.[221] Interaction of the NaPi-IIa cotransporter with the PDZ proteins NHERF-1 and NHERF-3 has been described,[222] but the physiologic significance of these interactions remains to be elucidated.

Basolateral Phosphate Exit

Transport of phosphate through the basolateral membrane in the PT must be sufficiently flexible to support two different functions. First, to mediate transcellular phosphate reabsorption it must be able to efflux some or all of the phosphate that enters from the luminal membrane. Second, it must be able to mediate influx of phosphate for intracellular metabolic processes if apical phosphate entry is insufficient to meet cellular requirements.

The mechanisms for basolateral phosphate exit and the identity of the molecules involved are poorly understood. Several studies have found evidence for Na^+-independent phosphate uptake in basolateral membrane vesicles that is driven by an intravesicular-positive membrane potential or trans-stimulated by intravesicular loading with phosphate or other inorganic anions. Thus, there may be support for the existence of an electrogenic phosphate-anion exchanger as the probable basolateral phosphate efflux system. In addition, Na^+-phosphate cotransport has been found in basolateral membranes from dog kidney, but not in those from the rat. It has been suggested that such conflicting results may be caused by variable contamination of basolateral vesicle preparations with brush border membranes. If basolateral Na/Pi cotransport does occur, it would likely serve as a "housekeeping" phosphate influx system.[192]

Regulation of Renal Phosphate Handling

Renal phosphate handling is influenced by a myriad of hormones, phosphatonins, and metabolic factors (summarized in Table 7-4) that are either of renal or extrarenal origin.[223] Orchestration of the activity of many of these factors is achieved by complex endocrine networks that involve several organs, such as kidneys, small intestine, bones, and parathyroid gland.[180,182,183,224,225] Several pathophysiologic states have been described that interfere at singles nodes of these regulatory networks. Regulation of proximal tubular phosphate reabsorption occurs by alterations in the numbers of apical Na/Pi cotransporters.[178]

Parathyroid Hormone

PTH is an important hormonal regulator of renal phosphate handling. It inhibits tubule phosphate reabsorption along the entire PT of both deep and superficial nephrons.[226,227] In mice and rats, the acute effect of PTH on phosphate reabsorption in PTs is primarily mediated by its effect on the NaPi-IIa cotransporter. In knockout mice that lack NaPi-IIa, PTH has no effect on serum phosphate concentration, fractional excretion of phosphate, or Na^+-dependent phosphate transport in the BBMV.[228] The effect of PTH on the NaPi-IIc cotransporter is less pronounced and is observed only several hours after PTH infusion, and internalized NaPi-IIc cotransporters do not traffic to the lysosomes.[229] It remains to be determined if PTH affects the SLC20a1 (PiT-2) transporter.

PTH causes endocytosis of type IIa proteins from the apical surface at the intermicrovillar clefts. At this site the

TABLE 7-4 Hormonal and Nonhormonal Factors Affecting Reabsorption of Phosphate

PHOSPHATE EXCRETION INCREASED BY	PHOSPHATE EXCRETION DECREASED BY
Parathyroid hormone	Parathyroidectomy
Atrial natriuretic peptide	Insulin
Glucocorticoids	Growth hormone
Dopamine	Stanniocalcin 1
Phosphatonins:	Metabolic alkalosis
Fibroblast growth factor 23 (FGF-23)	Phosphate depletion
Secreted frizzled-related protein 4 (sFRP-4)	Volume contraction
Matrix extracellular phosphoglycoprotein (MEPE)	Hypocalcemia
Metabolic acidosis	
Phosphate loading	
Volume expansion	
Diuretics	
Estrogen	
Hypercalcemia	
Hypokalemia	

transporter is internalized into clathrin- and adapter protein 2–coated vesicles and is transiently trafficked to early endosomes in the subapical region.[226] Unlike other membrane transport proteins, NaPi-IIa cotransporters are not routed to a recycling compartment from which they can be recruited back to the surface. Instead, they are trafficked directly to the lysosomes and irreversibly degraded.[226,230] A recognition signal for PTH-mediated endocytosis was identified as a dibasic peptide KR motif located in the last intracellular loop of the NaPi-IIa protein.[231] This KR motif was reported to interact with PEX19, a protein normally involved in the binding and trafficking of peroxisomal proteins.[232]

Withdrawal of PTH, or parathyroidectomy, reverses these changes and upregulates brush border NaPi-IIa cotransporters. The cellular mechanisms involved in the recovery after PTH inhibition of phosphate reabsorption are not well understood. After PTH infusion, restoration of the amount of NaPi-IIa abundance apparently is a slow process.[233]

Different signaling pathways are involved in the signaling of the PTH receptor in PTs. These include the classical adenylate cyclase–protein kinase A (PKA) pathway, phospholipase C–PKC pathway, and extracellular signal–regulated kinase (ERK) pathway.[178] PTH receptors are localized at both the brush border and the basolateral membrane, and depending on the localization, PTH decreases the amount of NaPi-IIa via activation of either the PKA or PKC pathway. By perfusion of either luminal or peritubular compartments of PTs with PTH analogs, it was demonstrated that activation of PTH receptors at either surface was sufficient to cause internalization of NaPi-IIa.[234] Because PTH is a small polypeptide that is probably freely filtered at the glomerulus, a sufficiently high concentration is likely to be present normally in the lumen of the PT to be sensed by brush border receptors.

The importance of luminal signaling is indicated by studies in mice with targeted inactivation of *CLC5*, the Dent's disease gene.[235] These mice, which have defective endocytosis of luminal PTH and therefore high concentrations of PTH in PT luminal fluid, exhibit abnormal internalization of the NaPi-IIa cotransporter, and hence phosphaturia. The luminal receptors signal preferentially via PKC, whereas the basolateral receptors activate both PKA and PKC pathways.[234]

Apical PTH receptors interact with NHERF-1,[217] and in NHERF-1–deficient mice inhibition of phosphate reabsorption by stimulation of apical PTH receptors is impaired.[236] Activation of PTH receptors results in phosphorylation of a serine residue within the PDZ domain of NHERF-1 that interacts with the NaPi-IIa protein.[237] Phosphorylation of NHERF-1 thus may explain the increased rate of endocytic retrieval of NaPi-IIa upon PTH stimulation due to a decrease in the affinity of NaPi-IIa for NHERF 1.

In addition to affecting NaPi-IIa cotransporter abundance, PTH inhibits phosphate reabsorption by several other mechanisms. PTH inhibits basolateral Na^+-K^+-ATPase and thereby indirectly prevents secondary active Na^+ gradient–dependent phosphate transport at the apical membrane. The signal transduction pathways for this are complex and involve an early phase and late phase, both dependent on PKC, PKA, phospholipase A_2, and ERK.[238] PTH-stimulated cyclic adenosine monophosphate (cAMP) generation may also inhibit phosphate transport via another pathway rather than by directly activating the PKA pathway. It has been postulated that the cAMP generated can be exported to the tubule lumen, where it is metabolized by 5′-ectonucleotidase to adenosine, which reenters the cell and inhibits phosphate transport.[239]

Dopamine

Dopamine is a phosphaturic hormone. Renal dopamine is produced in the PT from its precursor L-dopa. A small amount is also released from nerve endings. Dopamine production is stimulated by a high-phosphate diet and suppressed by a low-phosphate diet.[240] Inhibition of endogenous dopamine production with carbidopa decreased renal phosphate excretion and increased Na/Pi cotransport in BBMV.[241] A synthetic L-dopa analog that is selectively activated in the PTs was shown to inhibit BBMV Na/Pi cotransport and to cause phosphaturia.[242] Dopamine provokes internalization of the NaPi-IIa protein.[243] This effect is mediated by D_{A1} receptors and can be completely blocked by inhibition of the PKA pathway.[243,244] In addition, dopamine inhibits basolateral Na^+-K^+-ATPase, a process dependent on both PKA and PKC.[238]

Phosphatonins

Phosphatonins are humoral factors secreted by tumors of patients with tumor-induced osteomalacia that have phosphaturic activity. Phosphatonins inhibit phosphate reabsorption as well as the synthesis of $1,25(OH)_2D_3$. Several proteins have now been found to be overexpressed by such tumors: fibroblast growth factors FGF-23 and FGF-7, matrix extracellular phosphoglycoprotein (MEPE), and secreted frizzled-related protein 4 (sFRP-4).[180]

The evidence for a role in regulating renal phosphate excretion is strongest for FGF-23. FGF-23 is expressed in osteoblasts and osteocytes.[181] Its secretion is increased by hyperphosphatemia and by $1,25(OH)_2D_3$.[186,245-247] Changes in serum concentrations of FGF-23 occur more slowly than changes in PTH concentrations. In a feedback loop, FGF-23 inhibits the production of $1,25(OH)_2D_3$ by inhibition of 1α-hydroxylase. Targeted ablation of FGF-23 in mice causes hyperphosphatemia.[248] Mutations in FGF-23 that prevent its cleavage (and presumably increase functional levels) cause autosomal dominant hypophosphatemic rickets-osteomalacia,[249-251] and missense mutations in FGF-23 that presumably abolish its function have been identified in patients with familial tumoral calcinosis, which is characterized by decreased urinary excretion of phosphorus, hyperphosphatemia, and ectopic calcification.[252,253]

FGF-23 inhibits Na^+-dependent phosphate transport in kidneys and in isolated PTs.[254,255] In FGF-23 transgenic mice, reduction in mRNA expression of both NaPi-IIa and NaPi-IIc is the cause of phosphaturia.[256] Of the four different FGF receptors (FGFR-1 through FGFR-4) only FGFR-1 is responsible for the phosphaturic action of FGF-23.[257,258] Regulation of phosphate reabsorption by FGF-23 requires Klotho as a cofactor (see later) and involves mitogen-activated protein kinase (MAPK)–dependent mechanisms or production of prostaglandin E_2.[259,260] An intrarenal signaling axis has been proposed, because both FGFR-1 and Klotho were found to be localized in the DCT.[261] sFRP-4 increases renal phosphate excretion by inducing internalization of NaPi-IIa from the brush border of the PT.[262] Similarly, infusion of MEPE resulted in phosphaturia, most likely due to inhibition of PT reabsorption of phosphate.[263]

Klotho

As discussed earlier, accumulated evidence suggests that the Klotho protein plays an important role in mineral homeostasis.[264] Klotho is a type I membrane protein. The extracellular domain of Klotho is anchored by a single transmembrane segment and shows approximately 40% homology with β-glycosidase family 1 enzymes and thus may enzymatically alter sugar moieties of membrane proteins.[117] The extracellular domain of Klotho can be shed from the cell surface and detected in the plasma.[264] Thus the soluble extracellular domain can circulate and act as an endocrine, paracrine, or autocrine factor.

In kidney, Klotho is predominantly expressed in DCTs.[265] Homozygous Klotho mutant (kl/kl) mice show hyperphosphatemia that is correlated with increased amounts of NaPi-IIa and NaPi-IIc cotransporters,[266] which suggests that Klotho acts on proximal tubular phosphate reabsorption. In humans, missense mutations and overproduction of Klotho cause hyperphosphatemia and hypophosphatemia, respectively.[267,268]

The action of Klotho on proximal tubular Pi handling can be explained in two ways. On the one hand, Klotho is required for conversion of canonical FGF receptors into FGF-23 receptors.[269] In kl/kl mice, this requirement of Klotho for FGF-23 action can explain the lack of downregulation of proximal tubular Na/Pi cotransporters despite the high plasma concentration of FGF-23. On the other hand, Klotho may exert a direct effect on proximal tubular Na/Pi cotransporters. As shown in isolated tubules and isolated BBMV, the enzymatic activity of the extracellular domain of Klotho may alter the degree of glycosylation of NaPi-IIa and thereby may affect its membrane expression or activity. The origin of the Klotho that acts on PT cells is not clear. Although Klotho is expressed mainly in distal tubules, proximal tubular expression of Klotho cannot be ruled out.

Vitamin D

The effects of vitamin D metabolites on renal phosphate handling are complex. The action of $1,25(OH)_2D_3$ on renal handling of phosphate has to be considered in the context of regulatory networks that affect serum levels of PTH and FGF-23.[182,183,270] In addition, because $1,25(OH)_2D_3$ stimulates intestinal absorption of phosphate,[270] $1,25(OH)_2D_3$ action on proximal phosphate reabsorption can be indirect via a phosphate overload. Production of $1,25(OH)_2D_3$ in PTs is stimulated by low serum levels of phosphate and PTH[270] and inhibited by FGF-23.[182,185] Long-term administration of vitamin D causes phosphaturia, a reduction in renal cortical BBMV phosphate transport, and reduced renal cortical expression of NaPi-IIa mRNA and protein.[271] Acute administration of vitamin D metabolites reduces renal phosphate excretion. This effect requires the presence of PTH, is associated with a decrease in urinary cAMP and renal tubular adenylate cyclase activity, and can be inhibited by cycloheximide, which blocks de novo protein synthesis.[272] In vitamin D–deficient rats, NaPi-IIa mRNA and protein is downregulated.[273]

Insulin and Glucagon

Insulin reduces renal phosphate excretion and has been shown to stimulate phosphate uptake.[274] Insulin treatment of isolated PTs increased Na/Pi cotransport in isolated BBMV, which indicates that insulin acts on proximal tubular cells directly. Glucagon is phosphaturic.[275] The effects of both insulin and glucagon may be explained by altered metabolic pathways, because insulin inhibits and glucagon stimulates gluconeogenesis.

Stanniocalcin 1

The mammalian stanniocalcins, STC1 and STC2, are homologs of a fish anticalcemic hormone. Both STC1 and STC2 are ubiquitously expressed.[276] The intrarenal sites of STC1 expression are controversial, and renal expression of STC2 is negligible. In humans, STC1 protein appears to be expressed in the distal tubule and CD.[277] In rodents, STC1 mRNA has been detected in CDs only, whereas STC1 protein is found in almost all tubule segments,[278] which suggests a paracrine function. The highest amounts of STC1 mRNA are found in neonates, and level is regulated by dietary phosphate intake.[279] STC1 is an antiphosphaturic hormone. Recombinant human STC1, when injected into rats, caused a decrease in fractional excretion of phosphate, and an increase in Na/Pi cotransport in the BBMV.[280] However, STC1 knockout mice have normal serum Ca^{2+} and phosphate levels, which raises doubt as to the physiologic significance of STC1.[281] Whether or not STC2 plays a role in renal phosphate excretion remains undetermined.

Dietary Phosphate

Clearance studies have demonstrated that phosphate excretion is remarkably responsive to antecedent dietary phosphate intake. The phosphate reabsorption capacity adapts to altered intake of phosphate within hours (acute adaptation) and remains changed during prolonged intake of altered amount of dietary phosphate.[282,283] Fractional excretion of phosphate increases with a high-phosphate diet and decreases with a low-phosphate diet. Micropuncture studies show that the major site of adaptation is the PT. Superficial nephrons demonstrate a greater suppression of phosphate reabsorption on a high-phosphate diet than do juxtamedullary nephrons.

BBMV transport studies demonstrate that this adaptation is due to changes in the maximum velocity (V_{max}) of apical Na/Pi cotransport.[282]

The short-term adaptive changes in response to dietary phosphate are due to altered trafficking of the NaPi-IIa, NaPi-IIc, or PiT-2 cotransporters, whereas long-term adaptive changes may also include changes in transcription and translation. Adaptive changes in the abundance of NaPi-IIa, NaPi-IIc, and PiT-2 proteins differ in terms of both time course and trafficking.[198] In rats fed a high-phosphate diet over the long term, NaPi-IIa protein abundance is low. Immunofluorescence analysis shows that the transporter is found mostly in juxtamedullary nephrons.[284] After a short-term switch to a low-phosphate diet, brush border membrane transporter protein is increased. This redistribution is dependent on microtubules[285] and is not inhibited by cycloheximide,[283] which indicates that protein synthesis is not required.

In weaning mice, under long-term low-phosphate conditions, the amount of NaPi-IIa mRNA was increased.[286] The basis of transcriptional activation of the *Npt2* gene in response to long-term low-phosphate diet has been investigated by DNA footprinting analysis. A putative phosphate response element in the Npt2 promoter that binds to mouse transcription factor μE3 (TFE3) was identified. TFE3 was found to be upregulated by a low-phosphate diet, and stimulated transcription from the Npt2 promoter. However, in adult mice, increase of NaPi-IIc but not of NaPi-IIa mRNA was detected.[287]

In the short term, after a switch to a high-phosphate diet, the NaPi-IIa protein is internalized by membrane retrieval from the apical surface and sequestrated in the subapical vacuolar network. The endocytosed protein is subsequently trafficked to lysosomes for degradation.[230] Similarly, a high-phosphate diet causes internalization of NaPi-IIc protein but, unlike NaPi-IIa protein, NaPi-IIc cotransporters are not trafficked to the lysosomes.[288]

The upstream signals that mediate the short-term and long-term effects of dietary phosphate intake are not well understood. On the one hand, altered serum phosphate concentration affects levels of free Ca^{2+}-concentration, PTH $1,25(OH)_2D_3$, and FGF-23[180,183,186]; on the other hand, however, adaptation to dietary phosphate intake also occurs independently of PTH, $1,25(OH)_2D_3$, and growth factors.[283,289] Because dietary phosphate affects the concentrations of phosphate in plasma and in tubular fluid, it is possible that that PT cells sense phosphate directly. Alternatively, short-term regulation of renal excretion of phosphate may be explained by an intestinal-renal axis that may involve endocrine factors.[290] Studies showed that insertion of a phosphate bolus into the duodenum provokes a rapid change in phosphate excretion independent of PTH, FGF-23, and plasma phosphate levels.

Calcium and Magnesium

Acute hypercalcemia, especially when severe, decreases phosphate excretion by several mechanisms. Hypercalcemia decreases the plasma concentration of ultrafilterable phosphate because of the formation Ca^{2+}-phosphate-proteinate complexes. Hypercalcemia also decreases renal blood flow and GFR. As a consequence, filtered load of phosphate falls. Furthermore, phosphate reabsorption can be increased due to a reduction in circulating PTH. Whether acute hypercalcemia directly affects tubule phosphate reabsorption is controversial. in vitro microperfused PT S2 segments showed increased phosphate reabsorption in response to increased luminal Ca^{2+}, whereas S3 segments did not. Because the CaSR is expressed at the brush border of the PT, predominantly in S1 and S2 segments,[291] this raises the possibility that the CaSR might mediate the effects of proximal luminal Ca^{2+} on phosphate transport. In contrast to acute hypercalcemia, chronic hypercalcemia decreases tubule phosphate reabsorption, whereas chronic hypocalcemia increases phosphate reabsorption, independent of the effects of PTH, vitamin D, or serum Ca^{2+}.[292] The mechanisms are unknown.

Like Ca^{2+}, Mg^{2+} activates the CaSR.[293] High serum Mg^{2+} concentration decreases phosphate excretion due to an increased abundance of NaPi-IIa and NaPi-IIc cotransporters. This effect was shown to be dependent on PTH.[294]

Acid-Base Status

Metabolic acidosis increases and metabolic alkalosis decreases phosphate excretion. Increased excretion of phosphate under conditions of metabolic acidosis is explained mainly by the release of phosphate from bone.[92] In rats, after a few hours of metabolic acidosis the number of NaPi-IIa cotransporters at the brush border is decreased, but the abundance of the protein in total cortical homogenate as well as mRNA abundance remain unchanged, which suggests that there is retrieval of transporters from the apical membrane.[295] After several days of metabolic acidosis the abundance of NaPi-IIa cotransporter mRNA decreases progressively. Similarly, in mice metabolic acidosis decreases the amount of NaPi-IIa and NaPi-IIc mRNA; however, the numbers of NaPi-IIa and NaPi-IIc cotransporters in brush border membranes were not reduced.[296]

Respiratory acidosis and alkalosis are associated with an increase and decrease in phosphate excretion, respectively. Acute respiratory alkalosis causes a redistribution of phosphate into cells, resulting in hypophosphatemia, so the effects on renal excretion may be attributable to alterations in filtered load. Indeed, in rats fed a high-phosphate diet, which would be expected to induce saturating phosphate concentrations, the effect of acute respiratory alkalosis on fractional excretion of phosphate was abolished. In opossum kidney (OK) cells, decreasing the HCO_3^-/CO_2 concentration of the medium without changing the pH caused an increase in NaPi-IIa expression due to transcriptional activation.[297] This suggests that the effects of respiratory acid-base status may be mediated by a direct effect of CO_2 on PT cells.

Potassium

Hypokalemia is associated with hypophosphatemia and increased renal excretion of phosphate,[298] whereas potassium loading decreases the fractional excretion of phosphate.[299] Dietary potassium deficiency reduced Na/Pi cotransport in brush border membranes despite an increase of NaPi-IIa protein abundance.[300] The discrepancy with regard to phosphaturia observed in potassium deficiency can be explained by altered lipid composition of the brush border membrane[300] or by downregulation of the Na/Pi cotransporters NaPi-IIc and PiT-2.[301]

Diuretics

Most diuretics are somewhat phosphaturic.[292] Mannitol modestly increases phosphate excretion by decreasing Na^+ and water reabsorption in the PT, and hence diluting luminal phosphate. Acetazolamide, which inhibits carbonic anhydrase, is quite phosphaturic, probably because it sets up an acidic disequilibrium pH in the PT lumen that inhibits the NaPi-IIa cotransporter. Thiazides and furosemide in high dosages have a small phosphaturic effect.

Extracellular Volume

Extracellular volume expansion increases (and volume contraction decreases) phosphate excretion by several mechanisms.[215,292] First, volume expansion increases GFR and the filtered load of phosphate. Second, volume expansion inhibits PT Na^+ and water reabsorption, which dilutes the concentration of luminal phosphate available for reabsorption. Third, volume expansion decreases plasma Ca^{2+} and increases PTH, which inhibits PT phosphate reabsorption. Finally, volume expansion probably has a direct inhibitory effect on tubule phosphate reabsorption that is independent of filtered load, plasma Ca^{2+}, or PTH.

Ontogeny

In contrast to other tubule transport processes, phosphate reabsorption is highest in infants and declines with age.[302] This is important to maintain positive phosphate balance in the immature animal during active growth and development. BBMVs from neonates show a greater V_{max} for Na/Pi cotransport than those of adults.[302,303] NaPi-IIa cotransporter protein is concomitantly increased.[303-305] Early in development, NaPi-IIa is expressed in the brush borders of all PTs, whereas in adulthood it is primarily expressed in the brush borders of juxtamedullary nephrons.[305] Furthermore, the NaPi-IIc cotransporter is expressed in weaning animals but not in adults, which suggests that it may supply added capacity for phosphate reabsorption just during development.[205] The mechanisms for regulating these developmental changes are unknown, but growth hormone[306] and triiodothyronine appear to play a role.[307]

References

1. Hoenderop JG, et al. Renal Ca^{2+} wasting, hyperabsorption, and reduced bone thickness in mice lacking TRPV5. *J Clin Invest.* 2003;112(12):1906-1914.
2. Takeda E, et al. Inorganic phosphate homeostasis and the role of dietary phosphorus. *J Cell Mol Med.* 2004;8(2):191-200.
3. Hoenderop JG, Nilius B, Bindels RJ. Calcium absorption across epithelia. *Physiol Rev.* 2005;85(1):373-422.
4. Edwards BR, et al. Micropuncture study of diuretic effects on sodium and calcium reabsorption in the dog nephron. *J Clin Invest.* 1973;52(10):2418-2427.
5. Friedman PA. Calcium transport in the kidney. *Curr Opin Nephrol Hypertens.* 1999;8(5):589-595.
6. Sutton RA, Dirks JH. The renal excretion of calcium: a review of micropuncture data. *Can J Physiol Pharmacol.* 1975;53(6):979-988.
7. Ullrich KJ, et al. Micropuncture study of composition of proximal and distal tubular fluid in rat kidney. *Am J Physiol.* 1963;204:527-531.
8. Suki WN. Calcium transport in the nephron. *Am J Physiol.* 1979;237(1):F1-F6.
9. Rocha AS, Magaldi JB, Kokko JP. Calcium and phosphate transport in isolated segments of rabbit Henle's loop. *J Clin Invest.* 1977;59(5):975-983.

10. Bailly C, et al. Isoproterenol increases Ca, Mg, and NaCl reabsorption in mouse thick ascending limb. *Am J Physiol*. 1990;258(5 pt 2):F1224-F1231.

11. Bourdeau JE, Burg MB. Effect of PTH on calcium transport across the cortical thick ascending limb of Henle's loop. *Am J Physiol*. 1980;239(2):F121-F126.

12. Bourdeau JE, Langman CB, Bouillon R. Parathyroid hormone-stimulated calcium absorption in cTAL from vitamin D–deficient rabbits. *Kidney Int*. 1987;31(4):913-917.

13. Di Stefano A, et al. Effects of parathyroid hormone and calcitonin on Na$^+$, Cl$^-$, K$^+$, Mg^{2+} and Ca^{2+} transport in cortical and medullary thick ascending limbs of mouse kidney. *Pflugers Arch*. 1990;417(2):161-167.

14. Friedman PA. Basal and hormone-activated calcium absorption in mouse renal thick ascending limbs. *Am J Physiol*. 1988;254(1 pt 2):F62-F70.

15. Imai M. Calcium transport across the rabbit thick ascending limb of Henle's loop perfused in vitro. *Pflugers Arch*. 1978;374(3):255-263.

16. Ng RC, Peraino RA, Suki WN. Divalent cation transport in isolated tubules. *Kidney Int*. 1982;22(5):492-497.

17. Bourdeau JE, Burg MB. Voltage dependence of calcium transport in the thick ascending limb of Henle's loop. *Am J Physiol*. 1979;236(4):F357-F364.

18. Shareghi GR, Agus ZS. Magnesium transport in the cortical thick ascending limb of Henle's loop of the rabbit. *J Clin Invest*. 1982;69(4):759-769.

19. Wittner M, et al. Hormonal stimulation of Ca^{2+} and Mg^{2+} transport in the cortical thick ascending limb of Henle's loop of the mouse: evidence for a change in the paracellular pathway permeability. *Pflugers Arch*. 1993;423(5-6):387-396.

20. Simon DB, et al. Paracellin-1, a renal tight junction protein required for paracellular Mg^{2+} resorption. *Science*. 1999;285(5424):103-106.

21. Gunzel D, Yu AS. Function and regulation of claudins in the thick ascending limb of Henle. *Pflugers Arch*. 2009;458(1):77-88.

22. Costanzo LS, Windhager EE, Ellison DH. Calcium and sodium transport by the distal convoluted tubule of the rat. *J Am Soc Nephrol*. 2000;11(8):1562-1580.

23. Costanzo LS, Windhager EE. Calcium and sodium transport by the distal convoluted tubule of the rat. *Am J Physiol*. 1978;235(5):F492-F506.

24. Greger R, Lang F, Oberleithner H. Distal site of calcium reabsorption in the rat nephron. *Pflugers Arch*. 1978;374(2):153-157.

25. Erler I, et al. Ca^{2+}-selective transient receptor potential V channel architecture and function require a specific ankyrin repeat. *J Biol Chem*. 2004;279(33):34456-34463.

26. Phelps CB, et al. Structural analyses of the ankyrin repeat domain of TRPV6 and related TRPV ion channels. *Biochemistry*. 2008;47(8):2476-2484.

27. Chang Q, et al. Molecular determinants in TRPV5 channel assembly. *J Biol Chem*. 2004;279(52):54304-54311.

28. Hoenderop JG, et al. Homo- and heterotetrameric architecture of the epithelial Ca^{2+} channels TRPV5 and TRPV6. *EMBO J*. 2003;22(4):776-785.

29. Cha SK, et al. Removal of sialic acid involving Klotho causes cell-surface retention of TRPV5 channel via binding to galectin-1. *Proc Natl Acad Sci U S A*. 2008;105(28):9805-9810.

30. Hellwig N, et al. Homo- and heteromeric assembly of TRPV channel subunits. *J Cell Sci*. 2005;118(pt 5):917-928.

31. Peng JB, et al. Molecular cloning and characterization of a channel-like transporter mediating intestinal calcium absorption. *J Biol Chem*. 1999;274(32):22739-22746.

32. Hoenderop JG, et al. Function and expression of the epithelial Ca(2+) channel family: comparison of mammalian ECaC1 and 2. *J Physiol*. 2001;537(pt 3):747-761.

33. Yue L, et al. CaT1 manifests the pore properties of the calcium-release-activated calcium channel. *Nature*. 2001;410(6829):705-709.

34. Niemeyer BA, et al. Competitive regulation of CaT-like-mediated Ca^{2+} entry by protein kinase C and calmodulin. *Proc Natl Acad Sci U S A*. 2001;98(6):3600-3605.

35. Vennekens R, et al. Permeation and gating properties of the novel epithelial Ca(2+) channel. *J Biol Chem*. 2000;275(6):3963-3969.

36. Feher JJ. Facilitated calcium diffusion by intestinal calcium-binding protein. *Am J Physiol*. 1983;244(3):C303-C307.

37. Bronner F. Renal calcium transport: mechanisms and regulation—an overview. *Am J Physiol*. 1989;257(5 pt 2):F707-F711.

38. Bouhtiauy I, et al. Two vitamin D$_3$-dependent calcium binding proteins increase calcium reabsorption by different mechanisms. I. Effect of CaBP 28K. *Kidney Int*. 1994;45(2):461-468.

39. Lambers TT, et al. Calbindin-D28K dynamically controls TRPV5-mediated Ca^{2+} transport. *EMBO J*. 2006;25(13):2978-2988.

40. Koster HP, et al. Calbindin-D28K facilitates cytosolic calcium diffusion without interfering with calcium signaling. *Cell Calcium*. 1995;18(3):187-196.

41. Sooy K, et al. Calbindin-D(28k) controls [Ca^{2+}]$_i$ and insulin release. Evidence obtained from calbindin-D(28k) knockout mice and beta cell lines. *J Biol Chem*. 1999;274(48):34343-34349.

42. Gkika D, et al. Critical role of the epithelial Ca^{2+} channel TRPV5 in active Ca^{2+} reabsorption as revealed by TRPV5/calbindin-D28K knockout mice. *J Am Soc Nephrol*. 2006;17(11):3020-3027.

43. Blaustein MP, et al. Na/Ca exchanger and PMCA localization in neurons and astrocytes: functional implications. *Ann N Y Acad Sci*. 2002;976:356-366.

44. Bindels RJ, et al. Role of Na$^+$/Ca^{2+} exchange in transcellular Ca^{2+} transport across primary cultures of rabbit kidney collecting system. *Pflugers Arch*. 1992;420(5-6):566-572.

45. Van Baal J, et al. Localization and regulation by vitamin D of calcium transport proteins in rabbit cortical collecting system. *Am J Physiol*. 1996;271(5 pt 2):F985-F993.

46. Lytton J. Na$^+$/Ca^{2+} exchangers: three mammalian gene families control Ca^{2+} transport. *Biochem J*. 2007;406(3):365-382.

47. Loffing J, et al. Distribution of transcellular calcium and sodium transport pathways along mouse distal nephron. *Am J Physiol Renal Physiol*. 2001;281(6):F1021-F1027.

48. Biner HL, et al. Human cortical distal nephron: distribution of electrolyte and water transport pathways. *J Am Soc Nephrol*. 2002;13(4):836-847.

49. Vennekens R, et al. Permeation and gating properties of the novel epithelial Ca^{2+} channel. *J Biol Chem*. 2000;275(6):3963-3969.

50. Vassilev PM, et al. Single-channel activities of the human epithelial Ca^{2+} transport proteins CaT1 and CaT2. *J Membr Biol*. 2001;184(2):113-120.

51. Nilius B, et al. The single pore residue Asp542 determines Ca^{2+} permeation and Mg^{2+} block of the epithelial Ca^{2+} channel. *J Biol Chem*. 2001;276(2):1020-1025.

52. Lambers TT, et al. Extracellular pH dynamically controls cell surface delivery of functional TRPV5 channels. *Mol Cell Biol*. 2007;27(4):1486-1494.

53. Van de Graaf SF, et al. Functional expression of the epithelial Ca^{2+} channels (TRPV5 and TRPV6) requires association of the S100A10–annexin 2 complex. *EMBO J*. 2003;22(7):1478-1487.

54. Gkika D, et al. 80K-H as a new Ca^{2+} sensor regulating the activity of the epithelial Ca^{2+} channel transient receptor potential cation channel V5 (TRPV5). *J Biol Chem*. 2004;279(25):26351-26357.

55. Van de Graaf SF, et al. Direct interaction with Rab11a targets the epithelial Ca^{2+} channels TRPV5 and TRPV6 towards the plasma membrane. *Mol Cell Biol*. 2006;26(1):303-312.

56. Zobiack N, et al. The annexin 2/S100A10 complex controls the distribution of transferrin receptor–containing recycling endosomes. *Mol Biol Cell*. 2003;14(12):4896-4908.

57. Jones G, Strugnell SA, DeLuca HF. Current understanding of the molecular actions of vitamin D. *Physiol Rev*. 1998;78(4):1193-1231.

58. Fraser DR, Kodicek E. Unique biosynthesis by kidney of a biological active vitamin D metabolite. *Nature*. 1970;228(273):764-766.

59. DeLuca HF. Overview of general physiologic features and functions of vitamin D. *Am J Clin Nutr*. 2004;80(suppl 6):1689S-1696S.

60. Renkema KY, et al. Hypervitaminosis D mediates compensatory Ca^{2+} hyperabsorption in TRPV5 knockout mice. *J Am Soc Nephrol*. 2005;16(11):3188-3195.

61. Xue Y, et al. Exogenous 1,25-dihydroxyvitamin D$_3$ exerts a skeletal anabolic effect and improves mineral ion homeostasis in mice which are homozygous for both the 1α-hydroxylase and parathyroid hormone null alleles. *Endocrinology*. 2006;147(10):4801-4810.

62. Wood RJ, Tchack L, Taparia S. 1,25-dihydroxyvitamin D$_3$ increases the expression of the CaT1 epithelial calcium channel in the Caco-2 human intestinal cell line. *BMC Physiol*. 2004;1(1):11.

63. Fleet JC, et al. Vitamin D–inducible calcium transport and gene expression in three Caco-2 cell lines. *Am J Physiol Gastrointest Liver Physiol*. 2002;283(3):G618-G625.

64. Bindels RJ, et al. Active Ca^{2+} transport in primary cultures of rabbit kidney CCD: stimulation by 1,25-dihydroxyvitamin D$_3$ and PTH. *Am J Physiol*. 1991;261(5 pt 2):F799-807.

65. Meyer MB, et al. The human Trpv6 distal promoter contains multiple vitamin D Receptor binding sites that mediate activation by 1,25-dihydroxyvitamin D$_3$ in intestinal cells. *Mol Endocrinol*. 2006;20(6):1447-1461.

66. Weber K, et al. Gene structure and regulation of the murine epithelial calcium channels ECaC1 and 2. *Biochem Biophys Res Commun*. 2001;289(5):1287-1294.

67. Hoenderop JG, et al. Calcitriol controls the epithelial calcium channel in kidney. *J Am Soc Nephrol*. 2001;12(7):1342-1349.

68. Peng JB, et al. Human calcium transport protein CaT1. *Biochem Biophys Res Commun*. 2000;278(2):326-332.

69. Potts JT. Parathyroid hormone: past and present. *J Endocrinol*. 2005;187(3):311-325.

70. Lee K, et al. Localization of parathyroid hormone/parathyroid hormone–related peptide receptor mRNA in kidney. *Am J Physiol*. 1996;270(1 pt 2):F186-F191.

71. Yang T, et al. Expression of PTHrP, PTH/PTHrP receptor, and Ca^{2+}-sensing receptor mRNAs along the rat nephron. *Am J Physiol*. 1997;272(6 pt 2):F751-F758.

72. Mannstadt M, Juppner H, Gardella TJ. Receptors for PTH and PTHrP: their biological importance and functional properties. *Am J Physiol.* 1999;277(5 pt 2):F665-F675.

73. Juppner H, et al. A G protein–linked receptor for parathyroid hormone and parathyroid hormone–related peptide. *Science.* 1991;254(5034):1024-1026.

74. Fraser DR, Kodicek E. Regulation of 25-hydroxycholecalciferol-1-hydroxylase activity in kidney by parathyroid hormone. *Nat New Biol.* 1973;241(110):163-166.

75. Bacskai BJ, Friedman PA. Activation of latent Ca^{2+} channels in renal epithelial cells by parathyroid hormone. *Nature.* 1990;347(6291):388-391.

76. Friedman PA, Gesek FA. Hormone-responsive Ca^{2+} entry in distal convoluted tubules. *J Am Soc Nephrol.* 1994;4(7):1396-1404.

77. Tsukamoto Y, Saka S, Saitoh M. Parathyroid hormone stimulates ATP-dependent calcium pump activity by a different mode in proximal and distal tubules of the rat. *Biochim Biophys Acta.* 1992;1103(1):163-171.

78. Van Abel M, et al. Coordinated control of renal Ca^{2+} transport proteins by parathyroid hormone. *Kidney Int.* 2005;68(4):1708-1721.

79. Okano T, et al. Regulation of gene expression of epithelial calcium channels in intestine and kidney of mice by $1\alpha,25$-dihydroxyvitamin D_3. *J Steroid Biochem Mol Biol.* 2004;89-90(1-5):335-338.

80. de Groot T, et al. Parathyroid hormone activates TRPV5 via PKA-dependent phosphorylation. *J Am Soc Nephrol.* 2009;20(8):1693-1704.

81. Nordin BE, et al. Evidence for a renal calcium leak in postmenopausal women. *J Clin Endocrinol Metab.* 1991;72(2):401-407.

82. Prince RL, et al. Prevention of postmenopausal osteoporosis. A comparative study of exercise, calcium supplementation, and hormone-replacement therapy. *N Engl J Med.* 1991;325(17):1189-1195.

83. Van Abel M, et al. 1,25-dihydroxyvitamin D_3–independent stimulatory effect of estrogen on the expression of ECaC1 in the kidney. *J Am Soc Nephrol.* 2002;13(8):2102-2109.

84. Van Cromphaut SJ, et al. Intestinal calcium transporter genes are upregulated by estrogens and the reproductive cycle through vitamin D receptor–independent mechanisms. *J Bone Miner Res.* 2003;18(10):1725-1736.

85. Hoenderop JG, et al. Modulation of renal Ca^{2+} transport protein genes by dietary Ca^{2+} and 1,25-dihydroxyvitamin D_3 in 25-hydroxyvitamin D_3–1α-hydroxylase knockout mice. *FASEB J.* 2002;16(11):1398-1406.

86. Van Abel M, et al. Regulation of the epithelial Ca^{2+} channels in small intestine as studied by quantitative mRNA detection. *Am J Physiol.* 2003;285(1):G78-G85.

87. Van Cromphaut SJ, et al. Duodenal calcium absorption in vitamin D receptor-knockout mice: functional and molecular aspects. *Proc Natl Acad Sci U S A.* 2001;98(23):13324-13329.

88. Renkema KY, et al. The calcium-sensing receptor promotes urinary acidification to prevent nephrolithiasis. *J Am Soc Nephrol.* 2009;20(8):1705-1713.

89. Topala CN, et al. Activation of the Ca^{2+}-sensing receptor stimulates the activity of the epithelial Ca^{2+} channel TRPV5. *Cell Calcium.* 2009;45(4):331-339.

90. Sutton RA, Wong NL, Dirks JH. Effects of metabolic acidosis and alkalosis on sodium and calcium transport in the dog kidney. *Kidney Int.* 1979;15(5):520-533.

91. Canzanello VJ, et al. Effect of chronic respiratory acidosis on urinary calcium excretion in the dog. *Kidney Int.* 1990;38(3):409-416.

92. Lemann Jr J, Bushinsky DA, Hamm LL. Bone buffering of acid and base in humans. *Am J Physiol Renal Physiol.* 2003;285(5):F811-F832.

93. Yeh BI, et al. Conformational changes of pore helix coupled to gating of TRPV5 by protons. *EMBO J.* 2005;24(18):3224-3234.

94. Yeh BI, et al. Mechanism and molecular determinant for regulation of rabbit transient receptor potential type 5 (TRPV5) channel by extracellular pH. *J Biol Chem.* 2003;278(51):51044-51052.

95. Vennekens R, et al. Modulation of the epithelial Ca^{2+} channel ECaC by extracellular pH. *Pflugers Arch.* 2001;442(2):237-242.

96. Peng JB, et al. A rat kidney-specific calcium transporter in the distal nephron. *J Biol Chem.* 2000;275(36):28186-28194.

97. Wong NL, Quamme GA, Dirks JH. Effects of acid-base disturbances on renal handling of magnesium in the dog. *Clin Sci (Lond).* 1986;70(3):277-284.

98. Nijenhuis T, et al. Acid-base status determines the renal expression of Ca^{2+} and Mg^{2+} transport proteins. *J Am Soc Nephrol.* 2006;17(3):617-626.

99. Soleimani M. Na^+:HCO_3^- cotransporters (NBC): expression and regulation in the kidney. *J Nephrol.* 2002;15(suppl 5):S32-S40.

100. Soleimani M, Aronson PS. Effects of acetazolamide on Na^+-HCO_3^- cotransport in basolateral membrane vesicles isolated from rabbit renal cortex. *J Clin Invest.* 1989;83(3):945-951.

101. Dirks JH, Cirksena WJ, Berliner RW. Micropuncture study of the effect of various diuretics on sodium reabsorption by the proximal tubules of the dog. *J Clin Invest.* 1966;45(12):1875-1885.

102. Reid IR. Glucocorticoid osteoporosis—mechanisms and management. *Eur J Endocrinol.* 1997;137(3):209-217.

103. Rodino MA, Shane E. Osteoporosis after organ transplantation. *Am J Med.* 1998;104(5):459-469.

104. Aicher L, et al. Decrease in kidney calbindin-D 28kDa as a possible mechanism mediating cyclosporine A– and FK-506–induced calciuria and tubular mineralization. *Biochem Pharmacol.* 1997;53(5):723-731.

105. Nijenhuis T, Hoenderop JG, Bindels RJ. Downregulation of Ca^{2+} and Mg^{2+} transport proteins in the kidney explains tacrolimus (FK506)–induced hypercalciuria and hypomagnesemia. *J Am Soc Nephrol.* 2004;15(3):549-557.

106. Lee CT, et al. Cyclosporine A–induced hypercalciuria in calbindin-D28k knockout and wild-type mice. *Kidney Int.* 2002;62(6):2055-2061.

107. Lee CT, et al. Effects of furosemide on renal calcium handling. *Am J Physiol Renal Physiol.* 2007;293(4):F1231-F1237.

108. Ellison DH. Divalent cation transport by the distal nephron: insights from Bartter's and Gitelman's syndromes. *Am J Physiol Renal Physiol.* 2000;279(4):F616-F625.

109. Friedman PA. Codependence of renal calcium and sodium transport. *Annu Rev Physiol.* 1998;60:179-197.

110. Reilly RF, Ellison DH. Mammalian distal tubule: physiology, pathophysiology, and molecular anatomy. *Physiol Rev.* 2000;80(1):277-313.

111. Weinman EJ, Eknoyan G. Chronic effects of chlorothiazide on reabsorption by the proximal tubule of the rat. *Clin Sci Mol Med.* 1975;49(2):107-113.

112. Nijenhuis T, et al. Thiazide-induced hypocalciuria is accompanied by a decreased expression of Ca^{2+} transporting proteins in the distal tubule. *Kidney Int.* 2003;64(2):555-564.

113. Schultheis PJ, et al. Phenotype resembling Gitelman's syndrome in mice lacking the apical Na^+-Cl^- cotransporter of the distal convoluted tubule. *J Biol Chem.* 1998;273(44):29150-29155.

114. Loffing J, et al. Altered renal distal tubule structure and renal Na^+ and Ca^{2+} handling in a mouse model for Gitelman's syndrome. *J Am Soc Nephrol.* 2004;15(9):2276-2288.

115. Kuro-o M, et al. Mutation of the mouse klotho gene leads to a syndrome resembling ageing. *Nature.* 1997;390(6655):45-51.

116. Imura A, et al. Secreted Klotho protein in sera and CSF: implication for post-translational cleavage in release of Klotho protein from cell membrane. *FEBS Lett.* 2004;565(1-3):143-147.

117. Tohyama O, et al. Klotho is a novel beta-glucuronidase capable of hydrolyzing steroid beta-glucuronides. *J Biol Chem.* 2004;279(11):9777-9784.

118. Yoshida T, Fujimori T, Nabeshima Y. Mediation of unusually high concentrations of 1,25-dihydroxyvitamin D in homozygous klotho mutant mice by increased expression of renal 1α-hydroxylase gene. *Endocrinology.* 2002;143(2):683-689.

119. Tsujikawa H, et al. Klotho, a gene related to a syndrome resembling human premature aging, functions in a negative regulatory circuit of vitamin D endocrine system. *Mol Endocrinol.* 2003;17(12):2393-2403.

120. Kawano K, et al. Klotho gene polymorphisms associated with bone density of aged postmenopausal women. *J Bone Miner Res.* 2002;17(10):1744-1751.

121. Ogata N, et al. Association of klotho gene polymorphism with bone density and spondylosis of the lumbar spine in postmenopausal women. *Bone.* 2002;31(1):37-42.

122. Chang Q, et al. The beta-glucuronidase klotho hydrolyzes and activates the TRPV5 channel. *Science.* 2005;310(5747):490-493.

123. Imura A, et al. α-Klotho as a regulator of calcium homeostasis. *Science.* 2007;316(5831):1615-1618.

124. Topf JM, Murray PT. Hypomagnesemia and hypermagnesemia. *Rev Endocr Metab Disord.* 2003;4(2):195-206.

125. Flatman PW. Magnesium transport across cell membranes. *J Membr Biol.* 1984;80(1):1-14.

126. Flatman PW. Mechanisms of magnesium transport. *Annu Rev Physiol.* 1991;53:259-271.

127. Dai LJ, et al. Magnesium transport in the renal distal convoluted tubule. *Physiol Rev.* 2001;81(1):51-84.

128. Kulpmann WR, Gerlach M. Relationship between ionized and total magnesium in serum. *Scand J Clin Lab Invest Suppl.* 1996;224:251-258.

129. Thienpont LM, Dewitte K, Stockl D. Serum complexed magnesium—a cautionary note on its estimation and its relevance for standardizing serum ionized magnesium. *Clin Chem.* 1999;45(1):154-155.

130. Agus ZS. Hypomagnesemia. *J Am Soc Nephrol.* 1999;10(7):1616-1622.

131. Hoenderop JG, Bindels RJ. Epithelial Ca^{2+} and Mg^{2+} channels in health and disease. *J Am Soc Nephrol.* 2005;16(1):15-26.

132. Sutton RA, Domrongkitchaiporn S. Abnormal renal magnesium handling. *Miner Electrolyte Metab.* 1993;19(4-5):232-240.

133. Quamme GA, Dirks JH. Magnesium transport in the nephron. *Am J Physiol.* 1980;239(5):F393-F401.

134. Quamme GA. Renal magnesium handling: new insights in understanding old problems. *Kidney Int.* 1997;52(5):1180-1195.

135. Konrad M, et al. Mutations in the tight-junction gene claudin 19 (CLDN19) are associated with renal magnesium wasting, renal failure, and severe ocular involvement. *Am J Hum Genet.* 2006;79(5):949-957.

136. Hou J, Paul DL, Goodenough DA. Paracellin-1 and the modulation of ion selectivity of tight junctions. *J Cell Sci.* 2005;118(pt 21):5109-5118.

137. Simon DB, et al. Gitelman's variant of Bartter's syndrome, inherited hypokalaemic alkalosis, is caused by mutations in the thiazide-sensitive Na-Cl cotransporter. *Nat Genet.* 1996;12(1):24-30.

138. Picard N, Van Abel M, Campone C, et al. Tissue kallikrein-deficient mice display a defect in renal tubular calcium absorption. *J Am Soc Nephrol.* 2005;16(12):3602-3610.

139. Gkika D, Topala CN, Chang Q, et al. Tissue kallikrein stimulates Ca^{2+} reabsorption via PKC-dependent plasma membrane accumulation of TRPV5. *EMBO J.* 2006;25(20):4707-4716.

140. Chattopadhyay N, Vassilev PM, Brown EM. Calcium-sensing receptor: roles in and beyond systemic calcium homeostasis. *Biol Chem.* 1997;378(8):759-768.

141. Voets T, et al. TRPM6 forms the Mg^{2+} influx channel involved in intestinal and renal Mg^{2+} absorption. *J Biol Chem.* 2004;279(1):19-25.

142. Yang W, et al. Structural analysis, identification, and design of calcium-binding sites in proteins. *Proteins.* 2002;47(3):344-356.

143. Schlingmann KP, et al. Hypomagnesemia with secondary hypocalcemia is caused by mutations in TRPM6, a new member of the TRPM gene family. *Nat Genet.* 2002;31(2):166-170.

144. Walder RY, et al. Mutation of TRPM6 causes familial hypomagnesemia with secondary hypocalcemia. *Nat Genet.* 2002;31(2):171-174.

145. Clapham DE, Runnels LW, Strubing C. The TRP ion channel family. *Nat Rev Neurosci.* 2001;2(6):387-396.

146. Schmitz C, et al. The channel kinases TRPM6 and TRPM7 are functionally nonredundant. *J Biol Chem.* 2005;280(45):37763-37771.

147. Walder RY, et al. Mice defective in Trpm6 show embryonic mortality and neural tube defects. *Hum Mol Genet.* 2009;18(22):4367-4375.

148. Jin J, et al. Deletion of Trpm7 disrupts embryonic development and thymopoiesis without altering Mg^{2+} homeostasis. *Science.* 2008;322(5902):756-760.

149. Montell C. Mg^{2+} homeostasis: the Mg^{2+}nificent TRPM chanzymes. *Curr Biol.* 2003;13(20):R799-R801.

150. Cao G, et al. RACK1 inhibits TRPM6 activity via phosphorylation of the fused alpha-kinase domain. *Curr Biol.* 2008;18(3):168-176.

151. Schmitz C, et al. Regulation of vertebrate cellular Mg^{2+} homeostasis by TRPM7. *Cell.* 2003;114(2):191-200.

152. Cao G, et al. Regulation of the epithelial Mg^{2+} channel TRPM6 by estrogen and the associated repressor protein of estrogen receptor activity (REA). *J Biol Chem.* 2009;284(22):14788-14795.

153. Sha Q, et al. Human FXYD2 G41R mutation responsible for renal hypomagnesemia behaves as an inward-rectifying cation channel. *Am J Physiol Renal Physiol.* 2008;295(1):F91-F99.

154. Adalat S, et al. HNF1B mutations associate with hypomagnesemia and renal magnesium wasting. *J Am Soc Nephrol.* 2009;20(5):1123-1131.

155. Scholl UI, et al. Seizures, sensorineural deafness, ataxia, mental retardation, and electrolyte imbalance (SeSAME syndrome) caused by mutations in KCNJ10. *Proc Natl Acad Sci U S A.* 2009;106(14):5842-5847.

156. Bockenhauer D, et al. Epilepsy, ataxia, sensorineural deafness, tubulopathy, and KCNJ10 mutations. *N Engl J Med.* 2009;360(19):1960-1970.

157. Quamme GA. Renal handling of magnesium: drug and hormone interactions. *Magnesium.* 1986;5(5-6):248-272.

158. Kelepouris E, Agus ZS. Hypomagnesemia: renal magnesium handling. *Semin Nephrol.* 1998;18(1):58-73.

159. de Rouffignac C, et al. Hormonal control of renal magnesium handling. *Miner Electrolyte Metab.* 1993;19(4-5):226-231.

160. Bailly C, Roinel N, Amiel C. Stimulation by glucagon and PTH of Ca^{2+} and Mg^{2+} reabsorption in the superficial distal tubule of the rat kidney. *Pflugers Arch.* 1985;403(1):28-34.

161. de Rouffignac C, Quamme G. Renal magnesium handling and its hormonal control. *Physiol Rev.* 1994;74(2):305-322.

162. Shafik IM, Quamme GA. Early adaptation of renal magnesium reabsorption in response to magnesium restriction. *Am J Physiol.* 1989;257(6 pt 2):F974-F977.

163. Karbach U. Magnesium transport across colon ascendens of the rat. *Dig Dis Sci.* 1989;34(12):1825-1831.

164. Karbach U. Cellular-mediated and diffusive magnesium transport across the descending colon of the rat. *Gastroenterology.* 1989;96(5 pt 1):1282-1289.

165. Quamme GA, Dirks JH. Intraluminal and contraluminal magnesium on magnesium and calcium transfer in the rat nephron. *Am J Physiol.* 1980;238(3):F187-F198.

166. Navaneethan SD, et al. Tacrolimus-associated hypomagnesemia in renal transplant recipients. *Transplant Proc.* 2006;38(5):1320-1322.

167. Nijenhuis T, Hoenderop JG, Bindels RJ. Downregulation of Ca^{2+} and Mg^{2+} transport proteins in the kidney explains tacrolimus (FK506)–induced hypercalciuria and hypomagnesemia. *J Am Soc Nephrol.* 2004;15(3):549-557.

168. Ikari A, et al. Down-regulation of TRPM6-mediated magnesium influx by cyclosporin A. *Naunyn Schmiedebergs Arch Pharmacol.* 2008;377(4-6):333-343.

169. Bogoroch R, Belanger LF. Skeletal effects of magnesium deficiency in normal, ovariectomized, and estrogen-treated rats. *Anat Rec.* 1975;183(3):437-447.

170. McNair P, Christiansen C, Transbol I. Effect of menopause and estrogen substitution therapy on magnesium metabolism. *Miner Electrolyte Metab.* 1984;10(2):84-87.

171. Muneyyirci-Delale O, et al. Serum ionized magnesium and calcium in women after menopause: inverse relation of estrogen with ionized magnesium. *Fertil Steril.* 1999;71(5):869-872.

172. Seelig MS. Consequences of magnesium deficiency on the enhancement of stress reactions; preventive and therapeutic implications (a review). *J Am Coll Nutr.* 1994;13(5):429-446.

173. Groenestege WM, et al. The epithelial Mg^{2+} channel transient receptor potential melastatin 6 is regulated by dietary Mg^{2+} content and estrogens. *J Am Soc Nephrol.* 2006;17(4):1035-1043.

174. Groenestege WM, et al. Impaired basolateral sorting of pro-EGF causes isolated recessive renal hypomagnesemia. *J Clin Invest.* 2007;117(8):2260-2267.

175. Tejpar S, et al. Magnesium wasting associated with epidermal-growth-factor receptor-targeting antibodies in colorectal cancer: a prospective study. *Lancet Oncol.* 2007;8(5):387-394.

176. Gamba G, et al. Primary structure and functional expression of a cDNA encoding the thiazide-sensitive, electroneutral sodium-chloride cotransporter. *Proc Natl Acad Sci U S A.* 1993;90(7):2749-2753.

177. Nijenhuis T, et al. Enhanced passive Ca^{2+} reabsorption and reduced Mg^{2+} channel abundance explains thiazide-induced hypocalciuria and hypomagnesemia. *J Clin Invest.* 2005;115(6):1651-1658.

178. Biber J, et al. Regulation of phosphate transport in proximal tubules. *Pflugers Arch.* 2009;458(1):39-52.

179. Fukumoto S. Physiological regulation and disorders of phosphate metabolism—pivotal role of fibroblast growth factor 23. *Intern Med.* 2008;47(5):337-343.

180. Berndt T, Kumar R. Phosphatonins and the regulation of phosphate homeostasis. *Annu Rev Physiol.* 2007;69:341-359.

181. Feng JQ, Ye L, Schiavi S. Do osteocytes contribute to phosphate homeostasis? *Curr Opin Nephrol Hypertens.* 2009;18(4):285-291.

182. Quarles LD. Endocrine functions of bone in mineral metabolism regulation. *J Clin Invest.* 2008;118(12):3820-3828.

183. Silver J, Naveh-Many T. Phosphate and the parathyroid. *Kidney Int.* 2009;75(9):898-905.

184. Brown EM, et al. Cloning and characterization of an extracellular Ca(2+)-sensing receptor from bovine parathyroid. *Nature.* 1993;366(6455):575-580.

185. Perwad F, et al. Dietary and serum phosphorus regulate fibroblast growth factor 23 expression and 1,25-dihydroxyvitamin D metabolism in mice. *Endocrinology.* 2005;146(12):5358-5364.

186. Weber TJ, et al. Serum FGF23 levels in normal and disordered phosphorus homeostasis. *J Bone Miner Res.* 2003;18(7):1227-1234.

187. Perwad F, et al. Fibroblast growth factor 23 impairs phosphorus and vitamin D metabolism in vivo and suppresses 25-hydroxyvitamin D–1α-hydroxylase expression in vitro. *Am J Physiol Renal Physiol.* 2007;293(5):F1577-F1583.

188. Naveh-Many T, et al. Parathyroid cell proliferation in normal and chronic renal failure rats. The effects of calcium, phosphate, and vitamin D. *J Clin Invest.* 1995;96(4):1786-1793.

189. Ullrich KJ, Rumrich G, Kloss S. Phosphate transport in the proximal convolution of the rat kidney. I. Tubular heterogeneity, effect of parathyroid hormone in acute and chronic parathyroidectomized animals and effect of phosphate diet. *Pflugers Arch.* 1977;372(3):269-274.

190. Levi M. Heterogeneity of Pi transport by BBM from superficial and juxtamedullary cortex of rat. *Am J Physiol.* 1990;258(6 pt 2):F1616-F1624.

191. Custer M, et al. Expression of Na-P(i) cotransport in rat kidney: localization by RT-PCR and immunohistochemistry. *Am J Physiol.* 1994;266(5 pt 2):F767-F774.

192. Gmaj P, Murer H. Cellular mechanisms of inorganic phosphate transport in kidney. *Physiol Rev.* 1986;66(1):36-70.

193. Forster IC, et al. Proximal tubular handling of phosphate: a molecular perspective. *Kidney Int.* 2006;70(9):1548-1559.

194. Virkki LV, et al. Phosphate transporters: a tale of two solute carrier families. *Am J Physiol Renal Physiol.* 2007;293(3):F643-F654.

195. Biber J, et al. Localization of NaPi-1, a Na/Pi cotransporter, in rabbit kidney proximal tubules. II. Localization by immunohistochemistry. *Pflugers Arch.* 1993;424(3-4):210-215.

196. Broer S, et al. Chloride conductance and Pi transport are separate functions induced by the expression of NaPi-1 in *Xenopus* oocytes. *J Membr Biol.* 1998;164(1):71-77.

197. Collins JF, Bai L, Ghishan FK. The SLC20 family of proteins: dual functions as sodium-phosphate cotransporters and viral receptors. *Pflugers Arch.* 2004;447(5):647-652.

198. Villa-Bellosta R, et al. The Na⁺-Pi cotransporter PiT-2 (SLC20A2) is expressed in the apical membrane of rat renal proximal tubules and regulated by dietary Pi. *Am J Physiol Renal Physiol.* 2009;296(4):F691-F699.

199. Ravera S, et al. Deciphering PiT transport kinetics and substrate specificity using electrophysiology and flux measurements. *Am J Physiol Cell Physiol.* 2007;293(2):C606-G620.

200. Murer H, Forster I, Biber J. The sodium phosphate cotransporter family SLC34. *Pflugers Arch.* 2004;447(5):763-767.

201. Beck L, et al. Targeted inactivation of Npt2 in mice leads to severe renal phosphate wasting, hypercalciuria, and skeletal abnormalities. *Proc Natl Acad Sci U S A.* 1998;95(9):5372-5377.

202. Prie D, et al. Nephrolithiasis and osteoporosis associated with hypophosphatemia caused by mutations in the type 2a sodium-phosphate cotransporter. *N Engl J Med.* 2002;347(13):983-991.

203. Virkki LV, et al. Functional characterization of two naturally occurring mutations in the human sodium-phosphate cotransporter type IIa. *J Bone Miner Res.* 2003;18(12):2135-2141.

204. Lapointe JY, et al. NPT2a gene variation in calcium nephrolithiasis with renal phosphate leak. *Kidney Int.* 2006;69(12):2261-2267.

205. Segawa H, et al. Growth-related renal type II Na/Pi cotransporter. *J Biol Chem.* 2002;277(22):19665-19672.

206. Segawa H, et al. Npt2a and Npt2c in mice play distinct and synergistic roles in inorganic phosphate metabolism and skeletal development. *Am J Physiol Renal Physiol.* 2009;297(3):F671-F678.

207. Segawa H, et al. Type IIc sodium-dependent phosphate transporter regulates calcium metabolism. *J Am Soc Nephrol.* 2009;20(1):104-113.

208. Bergwitz C, et al. SLC34A3 mutations in patients with hereditary hypophosphatemic rickets with hypercalciuria predict a key role for the sodium-phosphate cotransporter NaPi-IIc in maintaining phosphate homeostasis. *Am J Hum Genet.* 2006;78(2):179-192.

209. Lorenz-Depiereux B, et al. Hereditary hypophosphatemic rickets with hypercalciuria is caused by mutations in the sodium-phosphate cotransporter gene SLC34A3. *Am J Hum Genet.* 2006;78(2):193-201.

210. Jaureguiberry G, et al. A novel missense mutation in SLC34A3 that causes hereditary hypophosphatemic rickets with hypercalciuria in humans identifies threonine 137 as an important determinant of sodium-phosphate cotransport in NaPi-IIc. *Am J Physiol Renal Physiol.* 2008;295(2):F371-F379.

211. Andrini O, et al. The leak mode of type II Na(+)-P(i) cotransporters. *Channels (Austin).* 2008;2(5):Epub September 20, 2008.

212. Forster IC, Loo DD, Eskandari S. Stoichiometry and Na$^+$ binding cooperativity of rat and flounder renal type II Na$^+$-Pi cotransporters. *Am J Physiol.* 1999;276(4 Pt 2):F644-F649.

213. Forster IC, Biber J, Murer H. Proton-sensitive transitions of renal type II Na(+)-coupled phosphate cotransporter kinetics. *Biophys J.* 2000;79(1):215-230.

214. Bacconi A, et al. Renouncing electroneutrality is not free of charge: switching on electrogenicity in a Na$^+$-coupled phosphate cotransporter. *Proc Natl Acad Sci U S A.* 2005;102(35):12606-12611.

215. Gisler SM, et al. Monitoring protein-protein interactions between the mammalian integral membrane transporters and PDZ-interacting partners using a modified split-ubiquitin membrane yeast two-hybrid system. *Mol Cell Proteomics.* 2008;7(7):1362-1377.

216. Biber J, et al. Protein/protein interactions (PDZ) in proximal tubules. *J Membr Biol.* 2005;203(3):111-118.

217. Shenolikar S, et al. Regulation of ion transport by the NHERF family of PDZ proteins. *Physiology (Bethesda).* 2004;19:362-369.

218. Wade JB, et al. Differential renal distribution of NHERF isoforms and their colocalization with NHE3, ezrin, and ROMK. *Am J Physiol Cell Physiol.* 2001;280(1):C192-C198.

219. Hernando N, et al. PDZ-domain interactions and apical expression of type IIa Na/P(i) cotransporters. *Proc Natl Acad Sci U S A.* 2002;99(18):11957-11962.

220. Shenolikar S, et al. Targeted disruption of the mouse NHERF-1 gene promotes internalization of proximal tubule sodium-phosphate cotransporter type IIa and renal phosphate wasting. *Proc Natl Acad Sci U S A.* 2002;99(17):11470-11475.

221. Capuano P, et al. Expression and regulation of the renal Na/phosphate cotransporter NaPi-IIa in a mouse model deficient for the PDZ protein PDZK1. *Pflugers Arch.* 2005;449(4):392-402.

222. Villa-Bellosta R, et al. Interactions of the growth-related, type IIc renal sodium/phosphate cotransporter with PDZ proteins. *Kidney Int.* 2008;73(4):456-464.

223. Murer H, et al. Proximal tubular phosphate reabsorption: molecular mechanisms. *Physiol Rev.* 2000;80(4):1373-1409.

224. Kiela PR, Ghishan FK. Recent advances in the renal-skeletal-gut axis that controls phosphate homeostasis. *Lab Invest.* 2009;89(1):7-14.

225. Prie D, Urena Torres P, Friedlander G. Latest findings in phosphate homeostasis. *Kidney Int.* 2009;75(9):882-889.

226. Bacic D, et al. The renal Na$^+$/phosphate cotransporter NaPi-IIa is internalized via the receptor-mediated endocytic route in response to parathyroid hormone. *Kidney Int.* 2006;69(3):495-503.

227. Berndt T, Knox FG. The Kidney. In: Seldom DW, Giebisch GH, eds. *Renal regulation of phosphate excretion.* Philadelphia: Lippincott Williams & Wilkins; 1992:pp 2511-2532.

228. Zhao N, Tenenhouse HS. Npt2 gene disruption confers resistance to the inhibitory action of parathyroid hormone on renal sodium-phosphate cotransport. *Endocrinology.* 2000;141(6):2159-2165.

229. Segawa H, et al. Parathyroid hormone–dependent endocytosis of renal type IIc Na-Pi cotransporter. *Am J Physiol Renal Physiol.* 2007;292(1):F395-F403.

230. Keusch I, et al. Parathyroid hormone and dietary phosphate provoke a lysosomal routing of the proximal tubular Na/Pi-cotransporter type II. *Kidney Int.* 1998;54(4):1224-1232.

231. Karim-Jimenez Z, et al. A dibasic motif involved in parathyroid hormone–induced down-regulation of the type IIa NaPi cotransporter. *Proc Natl Acad Sci U S A.* 2000;97(23):12896-12901.

232. Ito M, et al. Interaction of a farnesylated protein with renal type IIa Na/Pi co-transporter in response to parathyroid hormone and dietary phosphate. *Biochem J.* 2004;377(pt 3):607-616.

233. Friedlaender MM, et al. Recovery of renal tubule phosphate reabsorption despite reduced levels of sodium-phosphate transporter. *Eur J Endocrinol.* 2004;151(6):797-801.

234. Traebert M, et al. Luminal and contraluminal action of 1-34 and 3-34 PTH peptides on renal type IIa Na-P(i) cotransporter. *Am J Physiol Renal Physiol.* 2000;278(5):F792-F798.

235. Piwon N, et al. ClC-5 Cl$^-$ -channel disruption impairs endocytosis in a mouse model for Dent's disease. *Nature.* 2000;408(6810):369-373.

236. Capuano P, et al. Defective coupling of apical PTH receptors to phospholipase C prevents internalization of the Na$^+$-phosphate cotransporter NaPi-IIa in Nherf1-deficient mice. *Am J Physiol Cell Physiol.* 2007;292(2):C927-C934.

237. Weinman EJ, et al. Parathyroid hormone inhibits renal phosphate transport by phosphorylation of serine 77 of sodium-hydrogen exchanger regulatory factor-1. *J Clin Invest.* 2007;117(11):3412-3420.

238. Khundmiri SJ, Lederer E. PTH and DA regulate Na-K ATPase through divergent pathways. *Am J Physiol Renal Physiol.* 2002;282(3):F512-F522.

239. Siegfried G, et al. Parathyroid hormone stimulates ecto-5′-nucleotidase activity in renal epithelial cells: role of protein kinase-C. *Endocrinology.* 1995;136(3):1267-1275.

240. Friedlander G. Autocrine/paracrine control of renal phosphate transport. *Kidney Int.* 1998;65 (Suppl):S18-S23.

241. Debska-Slizien A, et al. Endogenous renal dopamine production regulates phosphate excretion. *Am J Physiol.* 1994;266(6 pt 2):F858-F867.

242. de Toledo FG, et al. γ-L-glutamyl-L-DOPA inhibits Na$^+$-phosphate cotransport across renal brush border membranes and increases renal excretion of phosphate. *Kidney Int.* 1999;55(5):1832-1842.

243. Bacic D, et al. Activation of dopamine D$_1$-like receptors induces acute internalization of the renal Na$^+$/phosphate cotransporter NaPi-IIa in mouse kidney and OK cells. *Am J Physiol Renal Physiol.* 2005;288(4):F740-F747.

244. Cunningham R, et al. Signaling pathways utilized by PTH and dopamine to inhibit phosphate transport in mouse renal proximal tubule cells. *Am J Physiol Renal Physiol.* 2009;296(2):F355-F361.

245. Liu S, Quarles LD. How fibroblast growth factor 23 works. *J Am Soc Nephrol.* 2007;18(6):1637-1647.

246. Mirams M, et al. Bone as a source of FGF23: regulation by phosphate? *Bone.* 2004;35(5):1192-1199.

247. Collins MT, et al. Fibroblast growth factor-23 is regulated by 1α,25-dihydroxyvitamin D. *J Bone Miner Res.* 2005;20(11):1944-1950.

248. Shimada T, et al. Targeted ablation of Fgf23 demonstrates an essential physiological role of FGF23 in phosphate and vitamin D metabolism. *J Clin Invest.* 2004;113(4):561-568.

249. Shimada T, et al. Mutant FGF-23 responsible for autosomal dominant hypophosphatemic rickets is resistant to proteolytic cleavage and causes hypophosphatemia in vivo. *Endocrinology.* 2002;143(8):3179-3182.

250. White KE, et al. Autosomal-dominant hypophosphatemic rickets (ADHR) mutations stabilize FGF-23. *Kidney Int.* 2001;60(6):2079-2086.

251. Autosomal dominant hypophosphataemic rickets is associated with mutations in FGF23. *Nat Genet.* 2000;26(3):345-348.

252. Larsson T, et al. A novel recessive mutation in fibroblast growth factor-23 causes familial tumoral calcinosis. *J Clin Endocrinol Metab.* 2005;90(4):2424-2427.

253. Benet-Pages A, et al. An FGF23 missense mutation causes familial tumoral calcinosis with hyperphosphatemia. *Hum Mol Genet.* 2005;14(3):385-390.

254. Saito H, et al. Human fibroblast growth factor-23 mutants suppress Na$^+$-dependent phosphate co-transport activity and 1α,25-dihydroxyvitamin D$_3$ production. *J Biol Chem.* 2003;278(4):2206-2211.

255. Baum M, et al. Effect of fibroblast growth factor-23 on phosphate transport in proximal tubules. *Kidney Int.* 2005;68(3):1148-1153.

256. Larsson T, et al. Transgenic mice expressing fibroblast growth factor 23 under the control of the alpha1(I) collagen promoter exhibit growth retardation, osteomalacia, and disturbed phosphate homeostasis. *Endocrinology.* 2004;145(7):3087-3094.

257. Gattineni J, et al. FGF23 decreases renal NaPi-2a and NaPi-2c expression and induces hypophosphatemia in vivo predominantly via FGF receptor 1. *Am J Physiol Renal Physiol.* 2009;297(2):F282-F291.

258. Liu S, et al. FGFR3 and FGFR4 do not mediate renal effects of FGF23. *J Am Soc Nephrol.* 2008;19(12):2342-2350.

259. Syal A, et al. Fibroblast growth factor-23 increases mouse PGE_2 production in vivo and in vitro. *Am J Physiol Renal Physiol*. 2006;290(2):F450-F455.

260. Yamashita T, et al. Fibroblast growth factor (FGF)-23 inhibits renal phosphate reabsorption by activation of the mitogen-activated protein kinase pathway. *J Biol Chem*. 2002;277(31):28265-28270.

261. Farrow EG, et al. Initial FGF23-mediated signaling occurs in the distal convoluted tubule. *J Am Soc Nephrol*. 2009;20(5):955-960.

262. Berndt TJ, et al. Secreted frizzled-related protein-4 reduces sodium-phosphate co-transporter abundance and activity in proximal tubule cells. *Pflugers Arch*. 2006;451(4):579-587.

263. Dobbie H, et al. Matrix extracellular phosphoglycoprotein causes phosphaturia in rats by inhibiting tubular phosphate reabsorption. *Nephrol Dial Transplant*. 2008;23(2):730-733.

264. Kuro-o M. Endocrine FGFs and Klothos: emerging concepts. *Trends Endocrinol Metab*. 2008;19(7):239-245.

265. Li SA, et al. Immunohistochemical localization of Klotho protein in brain, kidney, and reproductive organs of mice. *Cell Struct Funct*. 2004;29(4):91-99.

266. Segawa H, et al. Correlation between hyperphosphatemia and type II Na-Pi cotransporter activity in klotho mice. *Am J Physiol Renal Physiol*. 2007;292(2):F769-F779.

267. Ichikawa S, et al. A homozygous missense mutation in human KLOTHO causes severe tumoral calcinosis. *J Musculoskelet Neuronal Interact*. 2007;7(4):318-319.

268. Brownstein CA, et al. A translocation causing increased alpha-klotho level results in hypophosphatemic rickets and hyperparathyroidism. *Proc Natl Acad Sci U S A*. 2008;105(9):3455-3460.

269. Urakawa I, et al. Klotho converts canonical FGF receptor into a specific receptor for FGF23. *Nature*. 2006;444(7120):770-774.

270. Dusso AS, Brown AJ, Slatopolsky E. Vitamin D. *Am J Physiol Renal Physiol*. 2005;289(1):F8-F28.

271. Friedlaender MM, et al. Vitamin D reduces renal NaPi-2 in PTH-infused rats: complexity of vitamin D action on renal P(i) handling. *Am J Physiol Renal Physiol*. 2001;281(3):F428-F433.

272. Brezis M, et al. Blockade of the renal tubular effects of vitamin D by cycloheximide in the rat. *Pflugers Arch*. 1983;398(3):247-252.

273. Taketani Y, et al. Regulation of type II renal Na^+-dependent inorganic phosphate transporters by 1,25-dihydroxyvitamin D_3. Identification of a vitamin D–responsive element in the human NAPi-3 gene. *J Biol Chem*. 1998;273(23):14575-14581.

274. Hammerman MR. Interaction of insulin with the renal proximal tubular cell. *Am J Physiol*. 1985;249(1 pt 2):F1-F11.

275. Rubinger D, et al. Effect of intravenous glucagon on the urinary excretion of adenosine 3′,5′-monophosphate in man and in rats. Evidence for activation of renal adenylate cyclase and formation of nephrogenous cAMP. *Miner Electrolyte Metab*. 1988;14(4):211-220.

276. Ishibashi K, Imai M. Prospect of a stanniocalcin endocrine/paracrine system in mammals. *Am J Physiol Renal Physiol*. 2002;282(3):F367-F375.

277. De Niu P, et al. Immunolocalization of stanniocalcin in human kidney. *Mol Cell Endocrinol*. 1998;137(2):155-159.

278. Wong CK, Ho MA, Wagner GF. The co-localization of stanniocalcin protein, mRNA and kidney cell markers in the rat kidney. *J Endocrinol*. 1998;158(2):183-189.

279. Deol H, et al. Post-natal ontogeny of stanniocalcin gene expression in rodent kidney and regulation by dietary calcium and phosphate. *Kidney Int*. 2001;60(6):2142-2152.

280. Wagner GF, et al. Human stanniocalcin inhibits renal phosphate excretion in the rat. *J Bone Miner Res*. 1997;12(2):165-171.

281. Chang AC, et al. The murine stanniocalcin 1 gene is not essential for growth and development. *Mol Cell Biol*. 2005;25(23):10604-10610.

282. Levi M, et al. Molecular regulation of renal phosphate transport. *J Membr Biol*. 1996;154(1):1-9.

283. Levine BS, et al. Renal adaptation to phosphorus deprivation: characterization of early events. *J Bone Miner Res*. 1986;1(1):33-40.

284. Ritthaler T, et al. Effects of phosphate intake on distribution of type II Na/Pi cotransporter mRNA in rat kidney. *Kidney Int*. 1999;55(3):976-983.

285. Lotscher M, et al. Role of microtubules in the rapid regulation of renal phosphate transport in response to acute alterations in dietary phosphate content. *J Clin Invest*. 1997;99(6):1302-1312.

286. Kido S, et al. Identification of regulatory sequences and binding proteins in the type II sodium/phosphate cotransporter NPT2 gene responsive to dietary phosphate. *J Biol Chem*. 1999;274(40):28256-28263.

287. Madjdpour C, et al. Segment-specific expression of sodium-phosphate cotransporters NaPi-IIa and -IIc and interacting proteins in mouse renal proximal tubules. *Pflugers Arch*. 2004;448(4):402-410.

288. Segawa H, et al. Internalization of renal type IIc Na-Pi cotransporter in response to a high-phosphate diet. *Am J Physiol Renal Physiol*. 2005;288(3):F587-F596.

289. Capuano P, et al. Intestinal and renal adaptation to a low-Pi diet of type II NaPi cotransporters in vitamin D receptor- and 1αOHase-deficient mice. *Am J Physiol Cell Physiol*. 2005;288(2):C429-434.

290. Berndt T, et al. Evidence for a signaling axis by which intestinal phosphate rapidly modulates renal phosphate reabsorption. *Proc Natl Acad Sci U S A*. 2007;104(26):11085-11090.

291. Riccardi D, et al. Localization of the extracellular Ca^{2+}/polyvalent cation-sensing protein in rat kidney. *Am J Physiol*. 1998;274(3 pt 2):F611-F622.

292. Yu AS. Renal transport of calcium, magnesium and phosphate. In: Brenner BM, ed. *Brenner and Rector's the kidney*. 7th ed. Philadelphia: Saunders; 2004:pp 535-572.

293. Ba J, Friedman PA. Calcium-sensing receptor regulation of renal mineral ion transport. *Cell Calcium*. 2004;35(3):229-237.

294. Thumfart J, et al. Magnesium stimulates renal phosphate reabsorption. *Am J Physiol Renal Physiol*. 2008;295(4):F1126-F1133.

295. Ambuhl PM, et al. Regulation of renal phosphate transport by acute and chronic metabolic acidosis in the rat. *Kidney Int*. 1998;53(5):1288-1298.

296. Nowik M, et al. Renal phosphaturia during metabolic acidosis revisited: molecular mechanisms for decreased renal phosphate reabsorption. *Pflugers Arch*. 2008;457(2):539-549.

297. Jehle AW, et al. Type II Na-Pi cotransport is regulated transcriptionally by ambient bicarbonate/carbon dioxide tension in OK cells. *Am J Physiol*. 1999;276(1 pt 2):F46-F53.

298. Sebastian A, et al. Dietary potassium influences kidney maintenance of serum phosphorus concentration. *Kidney Int*. 1990;37(5):1341-1349.

299. Jaeger P, et al. Influence of acute potassium loading on renal phosphate transport in the rat kidney. *Am J Physiol*. 1983;245(5 pt 1):F601-F605.

300. Zajicek HK, et al. Glycosphingolipids modulate renal phosphate transport in potassium deficiency. *Kidney Int*. 2001;60(2):694-704.

301. Breusegem SY, et al. Differential regulation of the renal sodium-phosphate cotransporters NaPi-IIa, NaPi-IIc, and PiT-2 in dietary potassium deficiency. *Am J Physiol Renal Physiol*. 2009;297(2):F350-F361.

302. Spitzer A, Barac-Nieto M. Ontogeny of renal phosphate transport and the process of growth. *Pediatr Nephrol*. 2001;16(9):763-771.

303. Taufiq S, Collins JF, Ghishan FK. Posttranscriptional mechanisms regulate ontogenic changes in rat renal sodium-phosphate transporter. *Am J Physiol*. 1997;272(1 pt 2):R134-R141.

304. Woda C, et al. Renal tubular sites of increased phosphate transport and NaPi-2 expression in the juvenile rat. *Am J Physiol Regul Integr Comp Physiol*. 2001;280(5):R1524-R1533.

305. Traebert M, et al. Distribution of the sodium/phosphate transporter during postnatal ontogeny of the rat kidney. *J Am Soc Nephrol*. 1999;10(7):1407-1415.

306. Haramati A, Mulroney SE, Lumpkin MD. Regulation of renal phosphate reabsorption during development: implications from a new model of growth hormone deficiency. *Pediatr Nephrol*. 1990;4(4):387-391.

307. Euzet S, Lelievre-Pegorier M, Merlet-Benichou C. Effect of 3,5,3′-triiodothyronine on maturation of rat renal phosphate transport: kinetic characteristics and phosphate transporter messenger ribonucleic acid and protein abundance. *Endocrinology*. 1996;137(8):3522-3530.

308. Boros S, Bindels RJ, Hoenderop JG. Active Ca(2+) reabsorption in the connecting tubule. *Pflugers Arch*. 2009;458(1):99-109.

309. Xi Q, Hoenderop JG, Bindels RJ. Regulation of magnesium reabsorption in DCT. *Pflugers Arch*. 2009;458(1):89-98.

310. Bijvoet OL. Relation of plasma phosphate concentration to renal tubular reabsorption of phosphate. *Clin Sci*. 1969;37(1):23-36.

311. Lee CT, et al. Increased renal calcium and magnesium transporter abundance in streptozotocin-induced diabetes mellitus. *Kidney Int*. 2006;69(10):1786-1791.

312. van de Graaf SF, et al. TRPV5 is internalized via clathrin-dependent endocytosis to enter a Ca^{2+}-controlled recycling pathway. *J Biol Chem*. 2008;283(7):4077-4086.

313. Cha SK, Wu T, Huang CL. Protein kinase C inhibits caveolae-mediated endocytosis of TRPV5. *Am J Physiol Renal Physiol*. 2008;294(5):F1212-F12121.

314. Lee J, et al. PIP2 activates TRPV5 and releases its inhibition by intracellular Mg^{2+}. *J Gen Physiol*. 2005;126(5):439-451.

315. Lambers TT, et al. Recruitment of the epithelial Ca^{2+} channel TRPV5 to the plasma membrane is dependent on extracellular pH. *Abstracts: The American Society for Cell Biology 45th Annual Meeting*. Bethesda, Md: American Society for Cell Biology; 2005:p 112a, abstract 400.

316. Bonny O, et al. Mechanism of urinary calcium regulation by urinary magnesium and pH. *J Am Soc Nephrol*. 2008;19(8):1530-1537.

317. Gkika D, et al. Tissue kallikrein stimulates Ca(2+) reabsorption via PKC-dependent plasma membrane accumulation of TRPV5. *EMBO J*. 2006;25(20):4707-4716.

318. Glaudemans B, et al. A missense mutation in the Kv1.1 voltage-gated potassium channel-encoding gene KCNA1 is linked to human autosomal dominant hypomagnesemia. *J Clin Invest*. 2009;119(4):936-942.

319. Meij IC, et al. Dominant isolated renal magnesium loss is caused by misrouting of the Na^+, K^+-ATPase gamma-subunit. *Nat Genet*. 2000;26(3):265-266.

Renal Handling of Organic Solutes

Orson W. Moe, Stephen H. Wright, and Manuel Palacín

Archaic nephrons are largely secretory in nature. Kidneys in higher vertebrates handle solutes through the processes of filtration, reabsorption, and secretion. The handling of organic solutes involves all three of these means. The renal tubules reabsorb a large volume of glomerular filtrate to conserve the essential nutrients (glucose, amino acids, Krebs cycle intermediates, vitamins), to eliminate potentially toxic substances (organic acids and bases), and to reduce the quantity of valuable solute and water excreted in the final urine. The handling of organic solutes spans a wide range: from a clearance that exceeds glomerular filtration rate (GFR) in the form of filtration followed by secretion (fractional excretion >1) to filtration followed by complete reabsorption (fractional excretion = 0) (Figure 8-1).

The kidney adjusts the body fluid content, as well as concentration of specific solutes, usually in the plasma or extracellular fluid volume. To achieve these regulatory functions, there must be sensing mechanisms for both the pool size and the concentration of the solute. In contrast to inorganic solutes such as sodium or potassium, the total pool for organic solutes is difficult to define because these solutes are constantly being absorbed, excreted, synthesized, and metabolized. For glucose, the maintenance of a discrete plasma concentration is clearly important. For amino acids, organic cations (OCs), and organic anions, it is less clear whether plasma levels are as tightly regulated. The renal regulation of these three types of organic solutes is more concerned with external balance.

A filtration-reabsorption design is absolutely crucial for maintaining a high GFR, which is required for the complex metabolism and homeothermy of terrestrial mammals, inasmuch as tubular reabsorption salvages all the valuable solutes

(e.g., sodium, bicarbonate, glucose) that would have otherwise be lost in the urine (see Figure 8-1). In addition to maintaining a high GFR, the filtration-reabsorption process commences by disposing everything and then selectively reclaiming and retaining substances that the organism needs to keep in the appropriate amount. This mechanism economizes on gene products necessary to identify and excrete the myriad of undesirable substances. In the secretion mode, the burden is on the kidneys to recognize the substrates to be secreted. Therefore, in contrast to glucose reabsorption, which is highly specific to certain hexose structures, organic anion and cation secretion can engage hundreds of structurally distinct substrates.

Unlike the handling of many other solutes, the reabsorption and secretion of organic solutes are performed primarily by the proximal tubule with little or no contribution past the pars recta. This chapter summarizes the physiologic and molecular biologic characteristics of organic solute transport in the kidney. Although only renal mechanisms are covered in this chapter, it is important to note that homeostasis of organic solutes involves the concerted action of multiple organs.

Glucose

Physiology of Renal Glucose Transport

Plasma glucose concentration is regulated at about 5 mmol, with actions of glucose ingestion, glycogenolysis, and gluconeogenesis balanced against those of glucose utilization and, in some circumstances, renal glucose excretion. Although transient increments and decrements of plasma glucose are

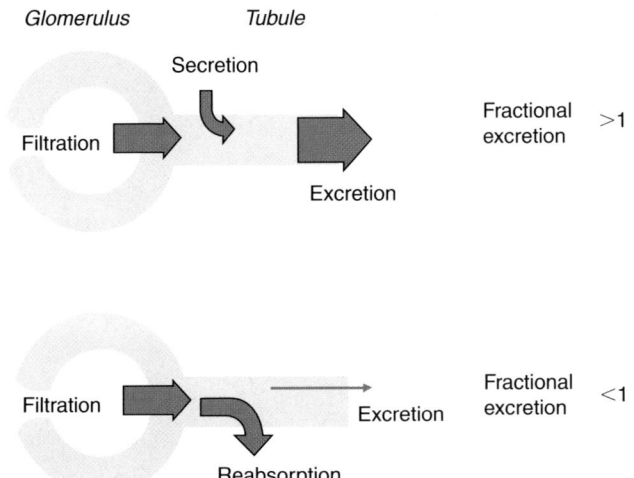

FIGURE 8-1 Secretory and reabsorptive modes of the mammalian nephron.

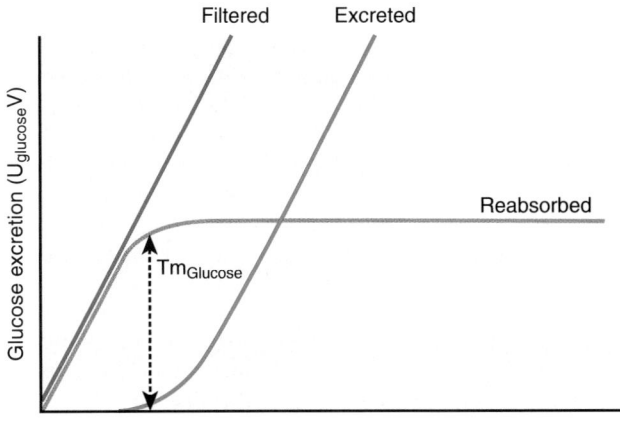

FIGURE 8-2 Urinary glucose excretion and tubular reabsorption as a function of filtered load. Tubular reabsorption increases linearly with filtered load as a part of glomerulotubular balance. When reabsorption reaches the tubular maximum ($Tm_{glucose}$), glucose starts appearing in the urine. Excretion is indicated by the *green line*. The plasma glucose concentration for the given glomerular filtration rate (GFR) is the glycosuric threshold.

tolerated in postprandial and fasting states, neither hypoglycemia nor hyperglycemia is desirable for the organism. The robust metabolic rate of mammals mandates a high GFR, and so the amount of glucose lost through the ultrafiltrate is colossal if it is not reclaimed. Therefore, the main physiologic task of the kidneys is to retrieve as much glucose as possible so that the normal urine is glucose free. This was described by Cushny as early as 1917.[1]

Renal Glucose Handling

Plasma glucose is neither protein bound nor complexed with macromolecules; thus it is filtered freely at the glomerulus. Glucose reabsorption by the proximal tubule increases as the filtered load increases (plasma [glucose] × GFR) until it reaches a threshold, the tubular maximum ($Tm_{Glucose}$), which represents the maximal reabsorptive capacity of the proximal tubule, beyond which glycosuria ensues (Figure 8-2).

With normal GFR, the threshold of plasma glucose for glycosuria to occur is about 11 mmol, or 200 mg/dL. Glycosuria occurs at lower plasma glucose concentrations in physiologic states of hyperfiltration such as pregnancy or the presence of a unilateral kidney (e.g., because of nephrectomy or transplant allograft); in these conditions, glycosuria may not be indicative of significant hyperglycemia. Conversely, in patients with reduced GFR, plasma glucose concentration may have to be higher for glycosuria to occur if $Tm_{Glucose}$ is relatively preserved. Some of the whole organism values for humans can be summarized as follows:

Excretion rate: 3.4 mmol/day
Urine concentration: 0.50 to 0.65 mmol
Reabsorptive capacity: 1.85 to 2.17 mmol/min
$Tm_{Glucose}$: 2664 to 3125 mmol/day

The maximal rate of glucose transport slows as one progresses from the early (S1) to late (S3) segments of the proximal tubule (Figure 8-3).[2] However, the affinity for glucose rises, with a Michaelis constant (K_m; concentration of substrate in which half the maximal rate of transport is attained) of approximately 2 mmol in the S1 segment to 0.4 mmol in the S3 segment.[2] The result is that the S1 segment reabsorbs glucose with higher capacity, but the S3 segment can decrease the tubule fluid glucose concentration to a much lower level.

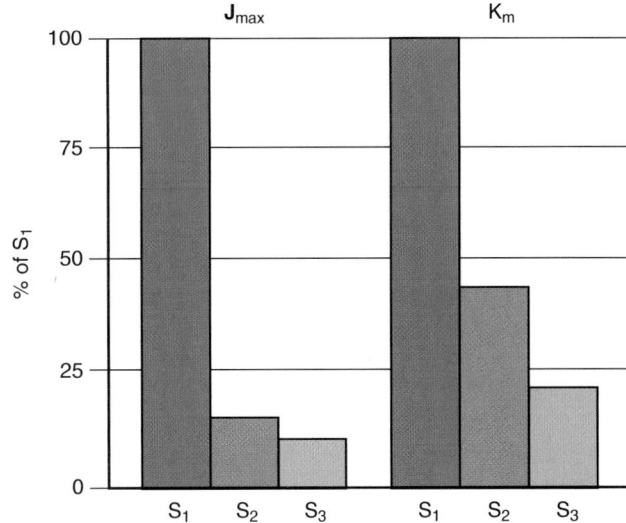

FIGURE 8-3 Relative magnitude of glucose transport characteristics in different segments of the proximal tubule. J_{max}, Maximal glucose transport rate; K_m, affinity (Michaelis) constant for glucose. (Data from Barfuss DW, Schafer JA: Differences in active and passive glucose transport along the proximal nephron, *Am J Physiol* 241:F322-F332, 1981.)

Clearly, a single uniform segment cannot perform both high-capacity and high-gradient glucose absorption. Results of transport studies with brush border membrane vesicles (BBMVs) and molecular cloning methods have demonstrated the existence of two transport systems with kinetic characteristics consistent with earlier microperfusion findings. When Na^+ and glucose move as a net positive charge into the negatively charged cell interior, they partially depolarize the cell interior.[3] Elimination of Na^+-glucose cotransport results in 14 mV of hyperpolarization in the S1 and early S2 segments of the proximal tubule and about 4 mV in the late S2 segment.[3] Na^+-glucose transport accounts for approximately 15% of the apical membrane current and for about half of the luminal negative potential difference in the early proximal convoluted tubule.

Aronson and Sacktor[4,5] described Na^+-dependent glucose transport in renal brush border vesicles. The two major

Na$^+$-glucose transporters are distinguished by their glucose transport capacity; their affinities for glucose, Na$^+$, and phlorhizin; and their location within the kidney. In the outer cortex, where the S1 and S2 segments of the proximal tubule are located, there is predominantly a high-capacity, low-affinity glucose transport system.[6-8] The low-affinity system has a Michaelis constant for glucose of approximately 6 mmol and carries one Na$^+$ molecule per glucose molecule, with a Michaelis constant for Na$^+$ of 228 mmol.[8] Phlorhizin binds and inhibits the transporter with a dissociation constant (K_d) of 1 mmol to 2 mmol.[8] In the outer medulla, where the S3 segment is located, there is a high-affinity system with a Michaelis constant for glucose of approximately 0.3 mmol, carrying two Na$^+$ molecules per glucose molecule.[7,8] The coupling of two Na$^+$ molecules to one glucose molecule allows the cotransporter to amplify the electrochemical driving force of Na$^+$ to energize glucose uptake. For the transporter in the S3, $K_m \approx 50$ mmol for Na$^+$. This transporter binds phlorhizin ($K_d = 1$ mmol to 2 mmol), and glucose transport is inhibited ($K_d = 50$ mmol). The transporter in the S3 segment has an affinity for D-galactose that is more than 10-fold higher than that of the transporter in the S1 segment.[7]

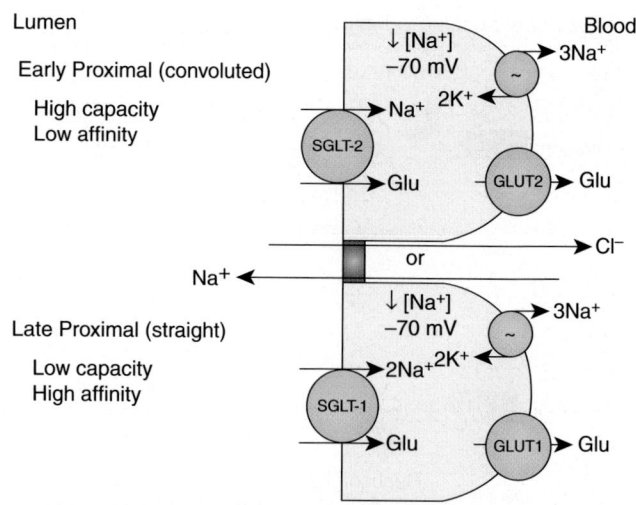

FIGURE 8-4 Model of proximal tubule glucose absorption. Na$^+$-K$^+$-ATPase lowers cell [Na$^+$] and generates a negative interior voltage. This drives the uphill Na$^+$-coupled glucose entry from the apical membrane via the sodium-glucose–linked cotransporters 1 and 2 (SGLT1 and SGLT2). Glucose leaves the basolateral membrane via the facilitative glucose transporters 1 and 2 (GLUT1 and GLUT2) down its electrochemical gradient.

Molecular Biology of Renal Glucose Transport Proteins

Cell Model of Proximal Tubule Glucose Transport

Glucose reabsorption in the proximal tubule cell occurs in two steps: (1) carrier-mediated Na$^+$-glucose cotransport across the apical membrane and (2) facilitated glucose transport and active Na$^+$ extrusion across the basolateral membrane (Figure 8-4). Electroneutrality is maintained by either paracellular Cl$^-$ diffusion or Na$^+$ back diffusion, depending on the relative permeabilities of the intercellular tight junction to Na$^+$ and Cl$^-$ (see Figure 8-4). Two Na$^+$-coupled carriers—sodium-glucose–linked cotransporters 1 and 2 (SGLT1 and SGLT2)—have been identified in the apical membrane of the proximal tubule cell. A third sodium-glucose–linked transporter (SGLT3) has been cloned from a porcine kidney cell line and is expressed in the kidneys. SGLT3 has been studied in a heterologously expressed system, but its localization and functional role in the kidneys is undetermined; thus, the current paradigm still concerns only SGLT1 and SGLT2 (see Figure 8-4).

The translocation of Na$^+$ and glucose across the apical cell membrane is driven by the electrochemical driving force for Na$^+$ from tubule fluid to cell and is therefore termed *secondary active transport*. Exit of glucose across the basolateral membrane does not consume energy but is mediated by specific carriers belonging to the glucose transporter (*GLUT*) gene family (see Figure 8-4). SGLT1 and SGLT2 belongs to SLC5, a broader group of solute carriers that currently encompasses 11 members in the human genome, of which 6 are Na$^+$-glucose cotransporters.[9]

Apical Entry: Transporter Proteins

Molecular studies have confirmed with striking fidelity the physiologic data obtained in perfused tubules and membrane vesicles. It is known that patients with congenital disorder of glucose-galactose malabsorption have a partial defect in renal

and intestinal absorption of glucose,[10-13] but patients with renal glycosuria have normal intestinal glucose transport.[10] This finding led to the conjecture that one of the two renal glucose transporters may also be found in the intestine. Hediger and colleagues[11] and Ikeda and associates[12] cloned the first intestinal Na$^+$-glucose transporter and found expression in both the intestines and the kidneys. Within the kidneys, it is expressed almost exclusively in the S3 segment of the proximal tubule.[14] This transporter, SGLT1, has a Michaelis constant for glucose of 0.4 mmol, is inhibited by 5 to 10 mmol of phlorhizin, and binds two Na$^+$ molecules, with a Michaelis constant for Na$^+$ of 32 mmol.[12] The high affinity allows SGLT1 to reclaim low concentrations glucose from the late proximal urinary lumen. The stoichiometry of two Na$^+$ molecules to one glucose molecule amplifies the electrochemical driving force. These properties are virtually identical to those of the glucose transport system in the S3 segment, determined from earlier microperfusion studies and transport studies in membrane vesicles.

Kanai and colleagues[15] and Wells and Hediger[16] cloned a second glucose transporter termed SGLT2, which is 59% homologous to SGLT1 and is expressed in the kidneys but not in the intestines.[16] SGLT2 confers phlorhizin-sensitive (1- to 5-mmol) glucose transport, with a Michaelis constant for glucose of approximately 1.6 mmol. One Na$^+$ molecule is bound per glucose molecule, with a Michaelis constant for Na$^+$ of 200 to 300 mmol (Table 8-1). Through in situ hybridization, researchers localized SGLT2 to the cortex in the S1 segment of the proximal tubule. SGLT2 is probably the "low-affinity" glucose transporter previously described.

SGLT1 and SGLT2 are responsible for bringing glucose into the proximal tubule cell via secondary active transport, but a different system is clearly needed to return this glucose from the cell to the blood. The transporter was found to be inhibited by phloretin and cytochalasin B but not by phlorhizin.[17,18] Although stereospecific for D-glucose, it also transports 2-deoxy-D-glucose and 3-O-methyl-D-glucose, but not α-methyl-D-glucoside.[17] These characteristics are similar to

TABLE 8-1 Sodium-Glucose–Linked Transporter (SGLT) Family			
FEATURE	SGLT1	SGLT2	SGLT3
Gene name	*SLC5A1*	*SLC5A2*	*SLC5A4*
Human chromosome	22p13.1	16p11.2	22p12.1
OMIM code	182380	233100	—
Genetic disease	Intestinal glucose-galactose malabsorption	Familial renal glycosuria	—
Amino acids (number)	664	672	659
Tissue distribution	Kidney, intestine, liver, spleen	Kidney	Kidney, intestine, muscle
Renal expression	Proximal straight tubule	Proximal convoluted tubule	Unknown
K_m, glucose (mmol)	0.4	2	6
Hexose selectivity	Glucose = galactose	Glucose >> galactose	Glucose >> galactose
K_m, sodium (mmol)	32	100	1.5
Substrate stoichiometry	2 Na^+ molecules to 1 glucose molecule	1 Na^+ molecule to 1 glucose molecule	2 Na^+ molecules to 1 glucose molecule

K_m, Michaelis constant; OMIM, Online Mendelian Inheritance in Man (database).

those of proteins found in polarized intestinal and liver cells and to those of the insulin-sensitive D-glucose transporters in red blood cells, muscle cells, and adipocytes.

Another complementary DNA from the SGLT family was cloned and is now termed SGLT3.[19] SGLT3 resembles SGLT2 in terms of its low affinity for glucose and high specificity for glucose over other hexose substrates, but it functions more like SGLT1 in terms of its tissue distribution and 2:1 stoichiometry for Na^+ and glucose (see Table 8-1).[20,21] SGLT3 transcript is present in the kidneys but in low levels; its distribution in the nephron segment is not yet known. At present, SGLT3 has been characterized in expression systems, but its role in the kidneys is unclear. Differences in substrate specificity and affinity exist among species.[19,21] SGLT3 has been proposed to function as a glucose sensor in enteric neurons and at the neuromuscular junction in skeletal muscle.[22,23]

A seminal achievement in this field was attained when Faham and colleagues[24] solved the structure of the *Vibrio* sodium-galactose transporter (vSGLT), which has 32% identity and 60% similarity to SGLT1 in the presence of Na^+ and galactose to approximately 3 Å resolution.

The predicted structure of the protein is shown in Figure 8-5. This structure was not predictable from the amino acid sequence of vSGLT, but it has striking similarity to the structure of the leucine transporter LeuT, which shares almost no primary sequence similarity with vSGLT. The galactose binding site is interposed between hydrophobic residues that form intracellular and extracellular portals of entry. This "5+5" motif is discussed in more detail later in the "Structural Information of Amino Acid Transporters" section. An alternative access model was proposed to account to the translocation of the galactose and Na^+ ions (see Figure 8-5). This knowledge should provide clues to the structure of the human SGLTs and guide further studies in transporter function and drug design.

Basolateral Exit: Transporter Proteins

In the basolateral membrane of the proximal tubule, glucose transport has been clarified with the discovery of a large gene family termed the *GLUT* genes. There are now 18 known genes of the *GLUT* family, of which 14 have known gene products (Table 8-2).[25] A thorough discussion is beyond the scope of this book; several excellent reviews are available.[25,26] The two isoforms believed to be important for transepithelial glucose transport are GLUT1 and GLUT2 (see Figure 8-4). GLUT1 was the first member of the GLUT family discovered in red blood cells with high affinity for glucose ($K_m s$ = 1 to 2 mmol) and is found at variable levels in virtually all nephron segments.[27,28] Its expression may be correlated with nutritive requirements of the cell,[28] and it is probably also the main mechanism for glucose exit in the S3 segment.[29] GLUT2 is a high-capacity, low-affinity ($K_m s$ = 15 to 20 mmol) basolateral transporter found in tissues with large glucose fluxes, such as intestine, liver, and pancreas, and the S1 segment of the proximal convoluted tubule.[28,29] GLUT4 is the insulin-responsive glucose transporter found almost exclusively in fat and muscle.[30,31] This transporter has been found in glomeruli and renal microvessels, but its role in tubular absorption is probably minimal.[32,33]

The role of GLUT2 in renal glucose transport has been demonstrated by the presence of renal glycosuria in mice with the GLUT2 deletion,[34] as well as in humans with GLUT2 mutations who present with Fanconi's syndrome, which is glycosuria with generalized proximal tubule dysfunction.[35,36] Transcripts of some of the other GLUT transporters have been detected in the kidneys (see Table 8-2), but the location of their protein and their roles are unclear.

Renal Glucose Transport in Disease States

Monogenic Defects of Glucose Transport

SGLT1

The best characterized monogenic disease in the SGLT family is glucose-galactose malabsorption caused by inactivating mutation of *SGLT1* (Online Mendelian Inheritance in Man database [OMIM] code 182380).[33,37-40] This rare autosomal recessive disease manifests in infancy with osmotic diarrhea, which resolves upon cessation of dietary glucose, galactose, and lactose, which are substrates of SGLT1. The diarrhea returns when the patient is rechallenged with one or more these substrates. The disease is readily diagnosed through oral administration of glucose or galactose, followed by a breath test for the presence of lactic acid. Patients with inactivating

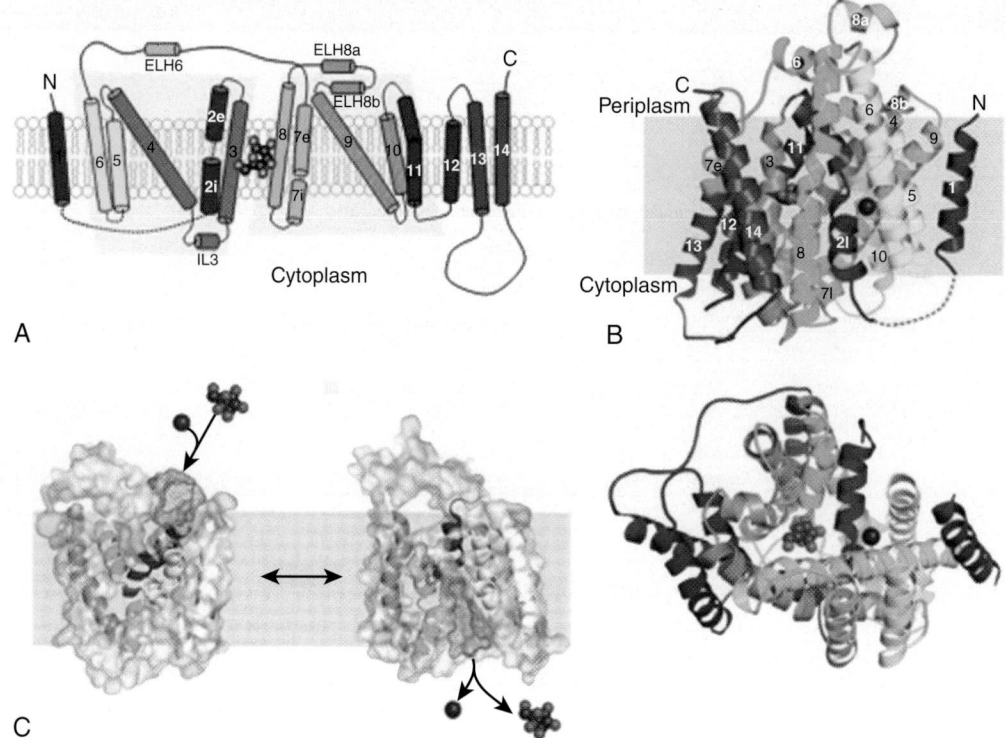

FIGURE 8-5 Structure of *Vibrio* sodium-galactose transporter (vSGLT). **A,** Topology. The protein has 14 transmembrane helices (TMHs) with both termini in the extracellular space. A structural core is formed from inverted repeats of two five-transmembrane helices (TMH2 to TMH6 and TMH7 to TMH11). Galactose is at the central heart of the core seven helices (TMH2, TMH3, TMH4, TMH7, TMH8, TMH9, TMH11). The two *gray trapezoids* represent the inverted topology of TMH2 to TMH6 and TMH7 to TMH11. Galactose traversing the central core is shown as *black spheres* (carbon atoms) and *red spheres* (oxygen atoms). **B,** *Top,* The structure as viewed in the membrane plane. The coloring scheme matches that of **A.** Bound galactose is shown as *black and red spheres* as in **A.** Na$^+$ ion is shown as a *blue sphere*. **B,** *Bottom,* The view from the intracellular side. **C,** Alternating accessibility. The depiction of the protein on the left is a slice through the surface of the outward-facing model viewed from the membrane plane. An externally facing cavity is depicted by the *blue mesh*. The depiction of the protein on the right is a slice through the surface of the inward-facing structure of vSGLT in the membrane plane, showing the internally facing cavity. Helices showing structural rearrangement during the transport cycle are colored *orange* (for TMH3), *green* (for TMH7), and *blue* (for TMH11). Helices with little movement during transport are *white*. The surface is shown in *beige*. Galactose is shown as *black and red spheres* as in **A.** Na$^+$ ion is shown as *blue spheres*. (Adated from Faham S, Watanabe A, Besserer GM, et al: The crystal structure of a sodium galactose transporter reveals mechanistic insights into Na$^+$/sugar symport, *Science* 321:810-814, 2008.)

TABLE 8-2 Facilitative Glucose Transporters (GLUTs)				
PROTEIN	**GENE NAME**	**TRANSPORTER CLASS**	**RENAL EXPRESSION**	**EXTRARENAL EXPRESSION**
GLUT1	*SLC2A1*	I	All nephron segments Proximal tubule, basolateral S2 segment	Erythrocytes, brain
GLUT2	*SLC2A2*	I	Proximal tubule, basolateral S1 segment	Liver, islet cells, intestine
GLUT3	*SLC2A3*	I	None	Brain, testis
GLUT4	*SLC2A4*	I	Messenger RNA in situ in thick ascending limb	Adipocyte, muscle
GLUT5	*SLC2A5*	II	Messenger RNA in situ in proximal straight tubule	Testis, intestine, muscle
GLUT6	*SLC2A6*	III	None	Brain, spleen, leukocyte
GLUT7	*SLC2A7*	II	Unknown	Intestine, prostate, testis
GLUT8	*SLC2A8*	III	None	Testis, brain, adipocyte
GLUT9	*SLC2A9*	II	Messenger RNA present	Liver
GLUT10	*SLC2A10*	III	Messenger RNA present	Liver, pancreas
GLUT11	*SLC2A11*	II	None	Pancreas, placenta, muscle
GLUT12	*SLC2A12*	III	Unknown	Heart, prostate
GLUT14	*SLC2A14*	I	None	Testis
HMIT	*SLC2A13*	III	Unknown	Brain
No gene product	*SLC2A3P1*	—		

Continued

		TRANSPORTER		
PROTEIN	**GENE NAME**	**CLASS**	**RENAL EXPRESSION**	**EXTRARENAL EXPRESSION**
No gene product	*SLC2A3P2*	—		
No gene product	*SLC2A3P3*	—		
No gene product	*SLC2AXP1*	—		

TABLE 8-2 Facilitative Glucose Transporters (GLUTs)—cont'd

HMIT, H+-myo-inositol transporter.

mutations of SGLT1 exhibit some degree of renal glycos-uria.[13] Because of redundancy in SGLT2, glycosuria is mild, and reduction of $Tm_{glucose}$ is not always demonstrable. This is in keeping, however, with the low capacity of the SGLT1 transport system in the late proximal tubule.

RENAL GLYCOSURIA

Because of the lack of intestinal defect and the renal restricted distribution of SGLT2, *SGLT2* is expected to be the gene responsible for congenital renal glycosuria. There is considerable controversy as to the inheritance pattern (auto-somal dominant vs. recessive), clinical classification of the reabsorptive defect (glucose threshold, maximal absorptive capacity, or both), and associated overlapping defects with aminoaciduria in this syndrome.[41,42] To date, the strongest evidence that SGLT2 is the major transporter involved in the reabsorption of glucose from the glomerular filtrate comes from the analysis of a patient with autosomal recessive renal glycosuria with a homozygous nonsense mutation in exon 11 of *SGLT2* and a heterozygous mutation in both parents and a younger brother.[43] In contrast, the linkage of the autoso-mal dominant form of renal glycosuria to the HLA complex on chromosome 6 has not yielded evidence that the SGLT transporters are causative.[44] On the basis of circumstantial evidence, an autoimmune mechanism has been proposed for this disease.[45] This entity probably represents a heteroge-neous group of disorders.

DISEASES OF GLUCOSE TRANSPORTERS

The first patient reported with Fanconi-Bickel syndrome[46] had hepatorenal glycogenosis and renal manifestations of Fanconi's syndrome[47] and presented at age 6 months with failure to thrive, polydipsia, and constipation, followed by osteopenia, short stature, hepatomegaly, and a proximal tubulopathy consisting of glycosuria, phosphaturia, amino-aciduria, proteinuria, and hyperuricemia. The liver was infiltrated with glycogen and fat. Disturbance of glucose homeostasis included fasting hypoglycemia, ketosis, and postprandial hyperglycemia. A mutation in the *GLUT2* gene was demonstrated.[36] Most patients with the Fanconi-Bickel syndrome are homozygous for the disease-related muta-tions, but some patients have been shown to be compound heterozygotes.[48] The mechanism by which *GLUT2* muta-tion cause the proximal tubulopathy is unclear. It is conceiv-able that impaired basolateral exit of glucose in the proximal convoluted tubule can lead to glucose accumulation and gly-cotoxicity.[49] Deletion of the *GLUT2* gene in rodents leads to glucose-insensitive islet cells, but proximal tubulopathy has not been described.[34] *GLUT1* mutations manifest pri-marily as a neurologic syndrome with no documented renal involvement.[46,50,51]

PHARMACOLOGIC MANIPULATION OF SODIUM-GLUCOSE–LINKED COTRANSPORTER

Antidiabetic therapy traditionally targets several broad pro-cesses: gut glucose absorption, insulin release, and insulin sensitivity. One additional strategy is providing a glucose sink to alleviate hyperglycemia and the ravages of glycose toxicity without actual direct manipulation of insulin secre-tion or sensitivity.[52] If the capacity of proximal absorption is decreased, the same filtered load leads to more severe glycos-uria, resulting in lower plasma glucose concentration (Figure 8-6). In addition to providing a glucose sink, the proximal osmotic diuresis can potentially act through tubuloglomeru-lar feedback to reduce GFR, especially in the setting of dia-betic hyperfiltration. One advantage of this approach is the self-limiting effect. In the presence of reduced proximal reab-sorption, increased filtered load from hyperglycemia increases glycosuria (see Figure 8-6). Once hyperglycemia is corrected and filtered load is reduced, the renal glucose leak ceases, even if the drug is still in the patient's body (see Figure 8-6). This approach is receiving increasing attention[52,53] with new technical advances in high-throughput screening.[54,55] Various compounds with widely divergent structures have been shown to inhibit SGLT function.[56-66] Glycemic control with these agents has been demonstrated in animal models.[53,55,67-70] The long-term consequence of escalated glycosylation of epithelial proteins exposed to the urinary lumen has not been examined. Because hyperglycemia fluctuates, so does osmotic diuresis. The staccato natriuresis may present a challenge in control of extracellular fluid volume.

Organic Cations

Physiology of Renal Organic Cation Transport

The kidneys have the astonishing capability to clear the plasma of organic solutes that share little in common other than possessing a net positive charge at physiologic pH. These OCs include a structurally diverse array of primary, second-ary, tertiary, or quaternary amines, although compounds that have nonnitrogen cationic moieties (e.g., phosphoniums)[66] can also interact effectively with what is frequently referred to as the *classical organic cation secretory pathway.*[9,64] Studies with stop-flow techniques, micropuncture, and microperfusion have identified the renal proximal tubule as the principal site of renal secretion of OCs.[9,64] Although a number of endog-enous OCs are actively secreted by the proximal tubule—such as N^1-methylnicotinamide, choline, epinephrine, and dopamine—an equally (if not more) important function is clearing of xenobiotic compounds,[9,64] including a wide range of alkaloids and other positively charged, heterocyclic dietary

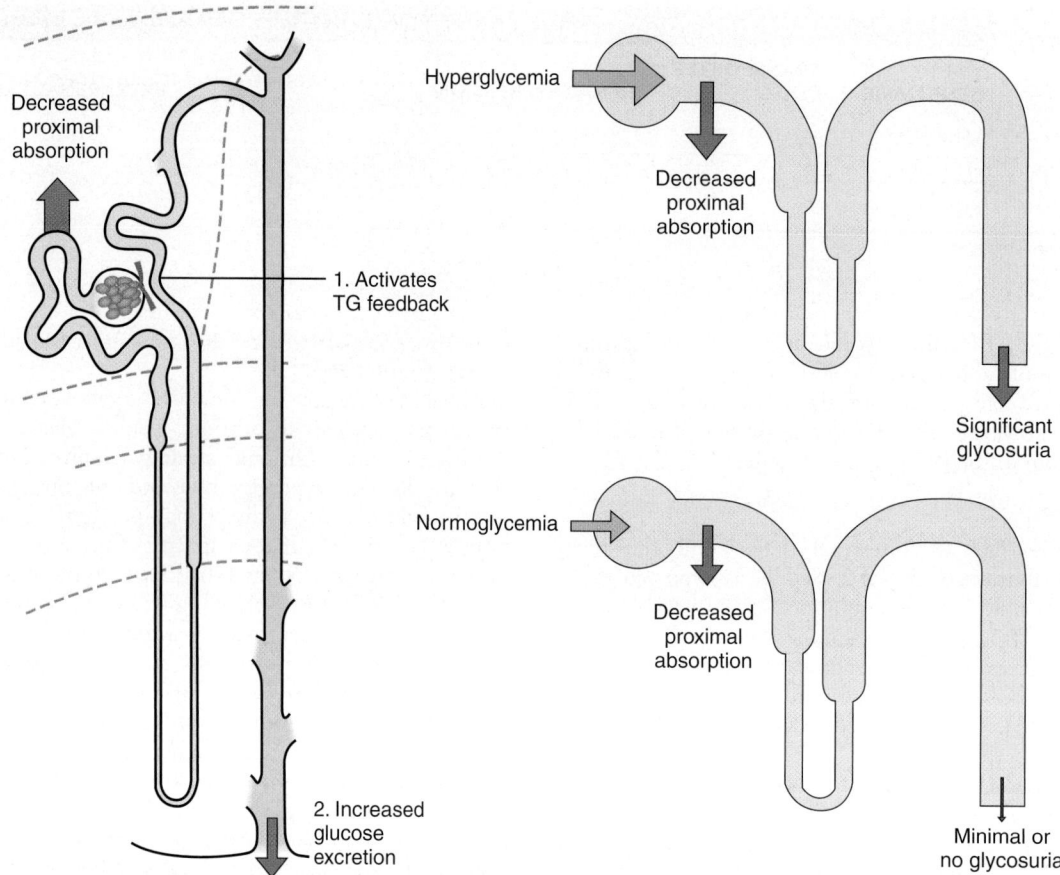

FIGURE 8-6 Effect of sodium-glucose–linked transporter (SGLT) inhibition. Inhibition of proximal absorption leads to increased glucose excretion. Proximal osmotic diuresis activates tubuloglomerular (TG) feedback and reduces hyperfiltration. The renal glucose sink has self-adjusting features (*right*). As plasma glucose level falls, so does filtered load, and glycosuria ceases; even proximal absorption is still inhibited.

constituents; cationic drugs of therapeutic or recreational use; or other cationic toxins of environmental origin (e.g., nicotine). Of importance is that OC secretion is also of clinical significance in humans. For example, therapeutic doses of cimetidine retard the renal elimination of procainamide[65] and nicotine.[62]

Renal Secretion of Organic Cations

Renal secretion of OCs involves the concerted activity of a suite of distinct transport processes arranged either in series in the basolateral (peritubular) and apical (luminal) poles of proximal tubule cells or in parallel within the same pole. In developing a functional model of this complexity, it is useful to consider the "type I" and "type II" classifications for different structural classes of OCs originally developed to describe OC secretion in the liver.[63] Type I OCs are relatively small (generally <400 Da) monovalent compounds, such as tetraethylammonium (TEA), tributylmethylammonium, and procainamide ethobromide. The majority of cationic drugs from many clinical classes, including antihistamines, skeletal muscle relaxants, antiarrhythmics, and β-adrenoceptor–blocking agents, are adequately described as type I OCs.

Type II OCs are usually bulkier (generally >500 Da) and frequently polyvalent; they include *d*-tubocurarine, vecuronium, and hexafluorenium. Although the kidneys play a quantitatively significant role in the secretion of selected type II OCs,

the liver plays a predominant role in excretion (into the bile) of large hydrophobic cations.[70] In contrast, renal excretion is the prime avenue for clearance of type I OCs. Whereas renal handling of type II OCs is only briefly described as they are currently understood, the renal transport of type I OCs of substrates is the focus of this discussion. Reviews of the molecular biologic and physiologic properties of multidrug-resistant transporter 1 (MDR1) provide more depth on the handling of type II OCs.[67,69,71]

Basolateral Entry of Organic Cations

Figure 8-7 depicts a model of transcellular OC transport by the proximal tubule that is consistent with results of studies in isolated renal plasma membranes and intact proximal tubules[64,72] and supported by molecular data. For type I OCs, the entry step involves either an electrogenic uniport (facilitated diffusion), driven by the inside negative electrical potential,[73] or an electroneutral antiport (exchange) of OCs.[73,74] It is likely that these two mechanisms represent alternative modes of action of the same transporter(s).[75] The potential difference across the basolateral membrane of is on the order of 60 mV (inside negative),[76,77] which is sufficient to account for an accumulation of OCs within proximal cells to levels approximately 10 times that in the blood. A hallmark of peritubular OC uptake is its broad selectivity, frequently termed *multispecificity*.[78] Ullrich and colleagues[78,79]

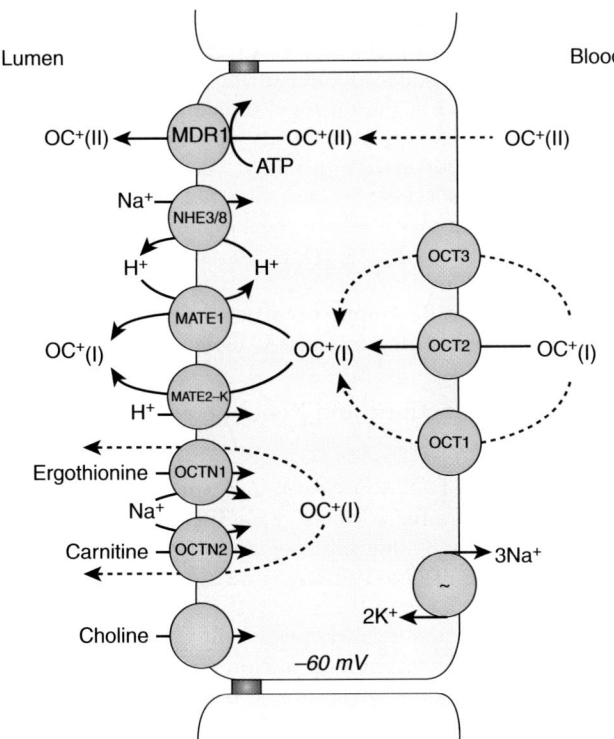

Lumen   Blood

OC⁺(II) ← MDR1 — OC⁺(II) ← - - - - - OC⁺(II)

FIGURE 8-7 Schematic model of the transport processes associated with the secretion of organic cations (OCs) by renal proximal tubule cells. *Circles* represent carrier-mediated transport processes. *Arrows* indicate the direction of net substrate transport. *Solid lines* represent what are believed to be principal pathways of substrate transport; *dotted lines* represent pathways that are believed to be of secondary importance; the *dashed line* represents diffusive movement. Each of the numbered processes is currently believed to play a role, direct or indirect, in transepithelial organic cation (OC) secretion. Principal basolateral processes include (1) Na⁺–K–adenosine triphosphatase (ATPase), which maintains the K⁺ gradient associated with the inside negative membrane potential and the inwardly directed Na⁺ gradient, both of which represent driving forces associated with active OC secretion; (2) organic cation transporters (OCT1, OCT2, and OCT3), which support electrogenic uniport (facilitated diffusion) of type I OCs from the blood (these processes are also believed to support electroneutral OC/OC exchange); and (3) diffusive flux of type II OCs. Principal apical transport processes include (4) multidrug-resistant transporter 1 (MDR1), which supports the adenosine triphosphate (ATP)-dependent, active luminal export of type II OCs; (5) Na⁺/H⁺ exchanger isoforms 3 and 8 (NHE3 and NHE8), which support the Na⁺/H⁺ exchange activity that sustains the inwardly directed hydrogen electrochemical gradient that, in turn, supports activity of multidrug and toxin extrusion (MATE) transporters; (6) MATE1 and MATE2-K, which support the mediated electroneutral exchange of luminal H⁺ for intracellular type I OCs; (7) novel organic cation transporters 1 and 2 (OCTN1 and OCTN2), which principally support electrogenic Na⁺-dependent reabsorptive fluxes of ergothioneine and carnitine, respectively; and (8) physiologically characterized electrogenic choline reabsorption pathway (possibly choline transporter-like protein 1 [CTL1]).

showed that the structural specificity of peritubular transport of OCs in microperfused rat proximal tubules in vivo exhibits a correlation between an increase in substrate hydrophobicity and an increase in interaction with basolateral OC transporters, although it is also clear that steric factors influence this interaction.[80-82] As discussed later, basolateral OC entry in human renal proximal tubules is probably dominated by the organic cation transporter 2 (OCT2).

The mechanisms for basolateral entry of type II OCs are less clear. The bulky ring structures that characterize type II OCs generally render them substantially more hydrophobic than type I OCs and, in the liver, type II OCs (e.g., rocuronium) tend to be substrates for the organic anion transporting polypeptide (OATP) superfamily of transporters (SLCO; also called SLC21, as described later).[83] In the rat, however, as discussed later, renal OATP expression is typically low in comparison with that in the liver (the sole exception is Oatp5, whose function and location in rat kidney is unknown and for which no human ortholog has been identified).[84] It is possible that the marked hydrophobicity of most type II OCs results in a substantial diffusive flux across the peritubular membrane that provides type II OCs with a passive, electrically conductive avenue for entry into proximal cells.

Apical Exit of Organic Cations

Exit of type I OCs across the luminal membrane involves carrier-mediated antiport of OC for H⁺ (see Figure 8-7), described in BBMVs in multiple species.[64] Luminal OC efflux is considered to be the rate-limiting step in transtubular OC secretion.[85] Of importance is that net OC secretion probably does not require a transluminal H⁺-gradient. In fact, in the early proximal tubule, where the pH of the tubular filtrate is about 7.4, tubular secretion exceeds that of later segments,[85] even though these latter regions are where an inwardly directed (lumen into cell) H⁺ gradient is present.[86] The electrically silent nature of the exchanger (which involves the obligatory 1:1 exchange of monovalent cations),[87] even in the absence of an inwardly directed H⁺ gradient, allows OCs to exit the electrically negative cytoplasm of cells in the renal proximal tubule and to develop a luminal concentration as large as (or larger than, if there is an inwardly directed H⁺ gradient) that in the cytoplasm. Net transepithelial secretion is therefore a consequence of combining electrically driven flux of OCs across the basolateral membrane with luminal OC/H⁺ exchange.

From an energetic perspective, OC/H⁺ antiport depends on the displacement of H⁺ away from electrochemical equilibrium, a state maintained through the activity in the luminal membrane of the Na⁺/H⁺ exchanger[88] and, to a lesser extent, that of the V (vacuolar)-type H⁺–adenosine triphosphatase (ATPase).[89] The basolateral Na⁺-K⁺-ATPase ultimately drives OC secretion by (1) maintaining the inside negative membrane potential that supports concentrative uptake of OCs across the basolateral membrane (result of the K⁺ gradient) and (2) sustaining the inwardly directed Na⁺ gradient that drives the aforementioned luminal Na⁺/H⁺ exchange. Evidence on the structural specificity of luminal transport of OCs indicates that, as with peritubular transport, binding of substrate to the OC/H⁺ exchanger is profoundly influenced by substrate hydrophobicity and, to a lesser extent, the three-dimensional structure of the substrate.[90]

At least two distinct OC/H⁺ exchangers, distinguished by their substrate selectivities, have been described in the BBMVs of the renal cortex. One, which is regarded as being the principal avenue for luminal secretion of OCs, displays a very broad selectivity and accepts TEA as a substrate.[90] The second displays mechanistically similar characteristics[91] but narrower selectivity and accepts guanidine (but not TEA) as a substrate.[92] The molecular identity of the principal (i.e., TEA-accepting) route of apical OC/H⁺ exchange activity probably includes two novel members of the multidrug and toxin extrusion (MATE) family of drug resistance transporters, MATE1 and MATE2-K.[93]

The apical export of type II OCs probably involves MDR1, which is expressed in the apical membrane and has been implicated in the apical efflux of type II OCs (and other bulky hydrophobic substrates) in in vitro studies.[94-96] However, whereas the influence of MDR1 in biliary excretion of type II OCs is evident (e.g., in studies employing *Mdr1*-knockout mice),[97] the quantitative influence of MDR1 on renal secretion is less clear. Whereas biliary excretion of doxorubicin is markedly decreased in *Mdr1*-knockout mice, urinary clearance increases.[98] Similarly, elimination of MDR1 by gene deletion is associated with marked changes in the distribution of type II OCs across brain, intestinal, and hepatic barriers, whereas the renal phenotype is modest.[97]

Axial Distribution of Organic Cation Transport in the Renal Proximal Tubule

Renal secretion of TEA and procainamide by isolated perfused renal proximal tubule in rabbits shows marked axial heterogeneity that differs from that for secretion of *p*-aminohippuric acid (PAH)[99,100]; its profile is of TEA secretion in the S1 segment (highest), S2 segment, and S3 segment (lowest)[85] and procainamide secretion in the S1 and S2 segments (higher) and in the S3 segment.[101] This axial heterogeneity is correlated (in rats and rabbits) with differences in the distribution of basolateral transporters, wherein expression of organic cation transporter 1 (OCT1) dominates in the early proximal tubule and OCT2 in the middle and later portions of the proximal tubule.[9,102] Despite these differences, the kinetics of basolateral TEA uptake, as determined in isolated nonperfused tubules, is effectively the same in all three segments[9]; thus, apical exit for OCs may be both rate limiting and the source of the axial heterogeneity observed for TEA secretion.[85] Consistent with this conclusion is the observation that the maximal rate of TEA/H[+] exchange is significantly higher in the BBMVs isolated from the outer renal cortex in rabbits (enriched in membranes from the S1 and S2 segments) than in those isolated from the outer medulla (enriched in membranes from S3 segments).[103]

MATE1 and MATE2-K are expressed in the luminal membrane of cells in the renal proximal tubule, including those in humans,[93,104] although it is not known whether they are distributed heterogeneously along the length of the tubule. MATE1, at least, is also expressed in the luminal membrane of distal tubules in human kidneys[93]; it is not yet clear whether MATE2-K has a similarly broad distribution in the kidneys. The role of these apical OC exporters in the distal tubule is also not clear.

Reabsorption of Organic Cations

Whereas secretion dominates the net flux of OCs transported by the proximal tubule, net reabsorption has been reported for a few cationic substrates, most notably choline.[64,105,106] The proximal apical membrane has an electrogenic uniporter that accepts choline and structurally similar compounds with relatively high affinity.[107,108] In contrast, the apical OC/H[+] exchanger has a low affinity (but high capacity) for choline.[108] Consequently, choline is effectively reabsorbed when plasma concentration do not exceed low physiologic concentrations (10 to 20 μmol) and is secreted when concentrations are raised to levels exceeding 100 μmol.[105] The molecular identity of the apical choline transporter is unclear, but the rat renal tubule epithelial cell line, NRK-52E, displays functional plasma membrane expression of choline transporter–like protein 1 (CTL1); this demonstration led to speculation that this pH-sensitive choline transporter could play a role in renal maintenance of plasma choline homeostasis.[109] However, the absence of information on the site and level of CTL1 expression in native renal cells complicates development of a model of the cellular handling of choline that includes CTL1.

Substrate Interactions and Renal Clearance of Organic Cations

Renal secretion of OCs possesses sufficient transport capacity to extract more than 90% of many OCs, when present in low physiologic and clinically relevant concentrations, during a single passage of blood through the kidneys.[110] The presence of multiple OCs in the blood can result in competition between these compounds for one or more OC secretory pathways, leading to decreased rates of elimination of one or more of these compounds and elevations in blood levels. A well-studied example was demonstrated from the coadministration of the antiarrhythmic procainamide with either cimetidine or ranitidine[65,111] (Figure 8-8).

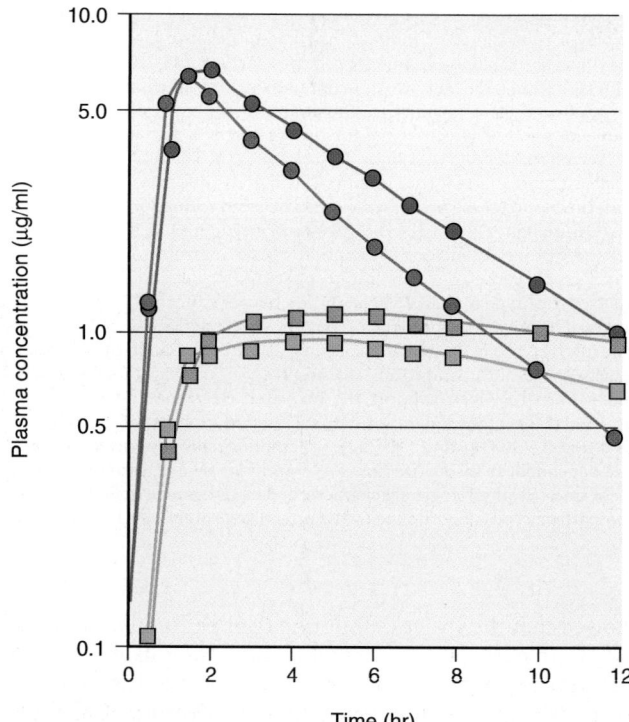

FIGURE 8-8 Effect of drug-drug competition at the level of renal organic cation secretion on mean plasma concentration-time profiles of procainamide (denoted by *circles*) and *N*-acetylprocainamide (denoted by *squares*) in six subjects who received (denoted by *blue* or *orange symbols*) or did not receive (denoted by *red* or *green symbols*) coadministration of cimetidine. (Data from Somogyi A, McLean A, Heinzow B: Cimetidine-procainamide pharmacokinetic interaction in man: evidence of competition for tubular secretion of basic drugs, *Eur J Clin Pharmacol* 25:339-345, 1983.)

Molecular Biology of Renal Organic Cation Transport

The cloning of OCT1[112] in 1994 resulted in a rapid increase in understanding of the molecular and cellular basis of renal transport of OCs. Strong evidence supports the conclusions that (1) basolateral entry of type I OCs occurs through a combination of the activities of OCT1, OCT2, and organic cation transporter 3 (OCT3) and (2) that apical exit of type I OCs includes a combination of the activities of MATE1 and MATE2-K (Table 8-3). Among different species, however, the levels of expression of these transporters differ markedly. For example, whereas both OCT1 and OCT2 have major roles in basolateral transport of OCs in rabbits[113] and rodents,[114] human kidney expresses very low levels of OCT1 (and OCT3); thus, OCT2 appears to dominate basolateral transport of OCs. Also, whereas human kidneys express similar levels of messenger RNA for MATE1 and MATE2-K, rodent kidneys express only MATE1.[115]

OCTs belong to the SLC22A family of solute carriers, and because they share a common set of structural features, they also belong to the major facilitator superfamily of transport proteins.[116] The MATEs are members of the multidrug/oligosaccharidyl-lipid/polysaccharide superfamily of transporters[93] and of the SLC47A family of solute carriers.[117] Renal secretion of type II OCs involves MDR1 in the luminal membrane, although its role in clearance of these compounds from the body is still a subject of speculation. The molecular characteristics of the these transport proteins are described as follows.

Basolateral Transporters of Organic Cations

OCT Family

Basolateral transport of OCs is dominated by the combined activity of three members of the SLC22A family of transport proteins: OCT1 (SLC22A1), OCT2 (SLC22A2), and OCT3 (SLC22A3).[9] As transporters in the major facilitator superfamily, they share several structural characteristics, including 12 transmembrane-spanning helices (TMHs), cytoplasmic N- and C-termini, a long cytoplasmic loop between TMH6 and TMH7, and several conserved sequence motifs.[9] Several additional features are unique to the OCT members of SLC22A, including a long ($\approx$110–amino acid–residue) extracellular loop between TMH1 and TMH2, as well as a distinguishing sequence motif.[118] The human orthologs of OCT1, OCT2, and OCT3 contain 554, 555, and 556 amino acid residues, respectively, and several consensus sites for phosphorylation mediated by protein kinase C, protein kinase A, protein kinase G, casein kinase II (CKII), and/or calcium/calmodulin-dependent protein kinase II (CaMII) located within or near the long cytoplasmic loop between TMH6 and TMH7 or in the cytoplasmic C-terminal sequence.[119] The long extracellular loop between TMH1 and TMH2 contains three *N*-linked glycosylation sites in all three homologs. In OCT2, all three sites are glycosylated, and their elimination is associated with both decreased trafficking of protein to the membrane and changes in apparent affinity for substrate.[120] The latter observation suggests that the configuration of the long extracellular loop influences the position of TMH1 and TMH2, which are elements of the hydrophilic "binding cleft" common to the OCTs and in which substrate is suspected to bind (see later discussion).[121,122]

TABLE 8-3 Renal Transporters of Organic Cations					
NAME	GENE NAME	HUMAN CHROMOSOME	PROXIMAL TUBULE LOCALIZATION	PRINCIPAL TRANSPORT MODE	SUBSTRATE
OCT Family					
OCT1	*SLC22A1*	6q26	Basolateral (low in human kidney)	Electrogenic uniport	Type I organic cations (e.g., TEA, MPP, clonidine)
OCT2	*SLC22A2*	6q26	Basolateral	Electrogenic uniport	Type I organic cations (e.g., TEA, MPP, metformin, cimetidine)
OCT3	*SLC22A3*	6q26-27	Basolateral (modest in human kidney)	Electrogenic uniport	Type I organic cations (e.g., MPP, catecholamines)
OCTN1	*SLC22A4*	5q31.1	Apical	Na cotransport	Ergothioneine
OCTN2	*SLC22A5*	5q31	Apical	Na cotransport	Carnitine
MATE Family					
MATE1	*SLC47A1*	17p11.2	Apical	H+-driven exchange	Type I organic cations (e.g., TEA, MPP, metformin, cimetidine)
MATE2-K	*SLC47A2*	17p11.2	Apical	H+-driven exchange	Type I organic cations (e.g., TEA, MPP, metformin, cimetidine)
MDR Family					
MDR1	*ABCB1*	7q21.1	Apical	ATP-dependent	Type II organic cations, neutral steroids, cardiac glycosides (e.g., doxorubicin, dexamethasone, digoxin)

ATP, Adenosine triphosphate; *MATE,* multidrug and toxin extrusion; *MDR,* multidrug-resistant transporter; *MPP,* 1-methyl-4-phenylpyridinium; *OCT,* organic cation transporter; *OCTN,* carnitine/organic cation transporters; *TEA,* tetraethylammonium.

The human genes for OCT1, OCT2, and OCT3 have 11 coding exons,[123] but several alternatively spliced variants of OCT1 have been described. In rats, OCT1A lacks putative TMH1 and TMH2 and the large extracellular loop that separates those two TMHs, and yet it supports mediated transport of TEA.[124] In the human, four alternatively spliced isoforms of OCT1 are present in human glioma cells[125]: a long (full-length) form and three shorter forms. Only the long form (hOCT1G/L554) supports transport when expressed in human embryonic kidney 293 cells.[125] Human kidneys express at least one splice variant of OCT2, designated hOCT2-A; it is characterized by the insertion of 1169 base pairs arising from the intron between exons 7 and 8 of hOCT2,[126] which results in a truncated protein that is missing the last three putative TMHs (i.e., TMH10, TMH11, and TMH12). Despite the absence of these last three helices, hOCT2-A retains the capacity to transport TEA and cimetidine, but not guanidine.

In rats and rabbits, OCT1 appears to dominate basolateral OC entry in the S1 segment of the renal proximal tubule, whereas OCT2 expression appears to dominate in the S2 and S3 segments.[9,102] However, in the human kidneys, basolateral OC transport is probably dominated by activity of OCT2. The level of OCT2 messenger RNA is in the top quartile of all messenger RNAs expressed in human kidneys,[127] and the relative expression profile of messenger RNAs coding for OCT1, OCT2, and OCT3 in the human renal cortex is 1:100:10.[128] Because OCT1 activity dominates OC transport in the early proximal tubule in rabbits, despite the fact that OCT2 messenger RNA expression is more than 10 times larger,[113] OCT1 and OCT3 actually may influence renal clearance of selected compounds by human kidneys.

The relative role of OCTs in the proximal tubule may also be influenced by the site of their expression. In rodents and rabbits, the early proximal tubule is dominated by OCT1 expression, whereas OCT2 expression is restricted to the later portions of the proximal tubule.[102] Jonker and associates[114] found that targeted elimination of OCT1 actually resulted in an increase in renal clearance of TEA (which presumably reflects the increase in plasma TEA levels that resulted from the elimination of OCT1-mediated hepatic clearance of TEA), and elimination of OCT2 had no effect on renal clearance of TEA. In other words, the level of *functional* expression of each transporter was sufficient to maintain fractional clearance of TEA at control levels in the absence of the other. Of importance is that the elimination of both OCT1 and OCT2 completely eliminated active secretion of TEA (Figure 8-9),[114] which indicates that in mice, OCT3 plays no significant role in renal clearance of TEA. In fact, mice with OCT3 deletion display no apparent renal phenotype,[129] although OCT3 may still play a role in the renal elimination of substrates for which it displays a particularly high affinity.[9] Thus, under normal conditions, transporters restricted to later portions of the proximal tubule may encounter little or no substrate if that compound is effectively cleared by transporters in upstream portions of the tubule. Transport capacity in later portions of the tubule may come into play only when the activity in the early segment is saturated or inhibited, as may occur in a drug-drug interaction.

All the OCTs share a common transport mechanism: electrogenic uniport. Transport is independent of extracellular Na^+ and H^+; membrane potential provides the driving force for concentrative uptake of cationic substrates.[75,130] The transport of positively charged substrates is electrogenic, as shown directly in studies in which investigators characterized the saturable inward currents that result from exposing *Xenopus* oocytes injected with the complementary RNA for OCT1,[75] OCT2,[130] or OCT3[131] to increasing concentrations of substrate. Busch and colleagues[75] showed that membrane potential provides the driving force for OCT1-mediated TEA, N^1-methylnicotinamide, and choline uptake and that OCT1 can also support the electrogenic efflux of substrate in the presence of energetically favorable outwardly directed substrate gradients, as well as electroneutral OC/OC exchange. In rats, simultaneous measurement of rat OCT2-mediated flux of current versus radiolabeled OC revealed charge-to-substrate ratios that vary between 1.5 and 4.0, depending on the substrate and membrane potential.[132] The excess charge flux appears to involve a nonselective "cotransport" (which does not involve energetic coupling) of OC substrates with small cations, which could include molecules as distinct as Na^+ or lysine$^+$. Modeling of the outwardly directed binding surface of rat OCT2 revealed a binding surface with more anionic residues than those accessible in the inward-facing mode of the transporter, thereby facilitating the parallel net influx of small charged cations with each cycle of conformational changes associated with the transport process. Of importance is that mutation of one of the anionic glutamate residue at position 448 to the neutral glutamine reduced the charge-to-TEA ratio at 0 mV from 3.5 to unity.[132] The observed charge excess associated with OC uptake into depolarized cells was suggested to contribute to tubular damage in renal failure.

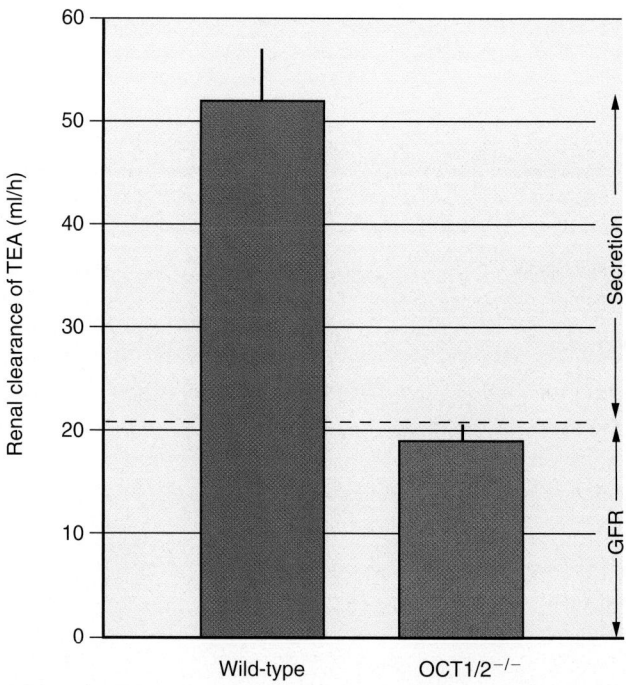

FIGURE 8-9 Renal clearance of tetraethylammonium (TEA) in wild-type and *Oct1*- and *Oct2*-knockout mice. Renal clearance was calculated by dividing the amount of TEA excreted in the urine over 60 minutes by the plasma area under the curve (AUC) (0 to 60). The estimated glomerular filtration rate (GFR) was approximately 21 mL/hour for both genotypes and is represented by a *dashed line*. (Data from Jonker JW, Wagenaar E, Van Eijl S, et al: Deficiency in the organic cation transporters 1 and 2 (Oct1/Oct2 [Slc22A1/Slc22A2]) in mice abolishes renal secretion of organic cations, *Mol Cell Biol* 23:7902-7908, 2003.)

Although the three OCTs display marked overlap in substrate selectivity, they are also distinguished by their selectivities for specific compounds. For example, OCT1 and OCT2 generally have a similar affinity for TEA (20 to 200 μmol),[9] whereas OCT3 has a very low affinity for TEA (≈2 mmol).[133] Cimetidine has a much higher (50-fold) affinity for OCT2 than for OCT1,[134] whereas tyramine has a higher (20-fold) affinity for OCT1 than for OCT2,[134] and all three homologs display a similar, comparatively high affinity for 1-methyl-4-phenylpyridinium (MPP).[135] In general, the three homologs all support transport of a structurally diverse array of type I OCs[9] and interact with a limited number of neutral and even anionic substrates.[136] With regard to the latter observation that OCTs can interact with selected neutral or anionic substrates, Ullrich and colleagues[137] observed "crossover" interactions of a number of what they referred to as "bisubstrates" with both cation and anion transport pathways in rat kidneys. Nevertheless, despite the generally weak interaction of neutral and anionic substrates with OCTs, the presence of a charged moiety clearly enhances interaction with these transporters, as shown in studies demonstrating more efficient interaction of the weak base cimetidine (pK_a = 6.9) with OCT2 when the substrate is protonated.[138] OCTs also typically interact with type II OCs, although this interaction appears to be restricted to binding with modest or no translocation of substrate.[83]

The molecular determinants that influence the interaction of substrates and inhibitors with OCTs have been assessed in several studies with computational methods. Through the use of several three-dimensional quantitative structure/activity relationship methods, a number of common structural elements have been identified for substrates and inhibitors of OCT1, including a positive ion interaction site, one or more hydrophobic surface interaction sites, and hydrogen bond acceptor sites.[80,139] Computational assessment of ligand binding to OCT2 has also clarified the influence of the distance between hydrophobic (i.e., aromatic) elements and the center of positive charge,[81,140] as well as the importance of topologic polar surface area as a criterion in the prediction of substrate interaction with transporter binding region.[140]

The binding kinetics of OCTs with many, if not most, substrates is probably asymmetric; that is, the activity differs when the interaction occurs at the extracellular versus cytoplasmic aspect of the membrane. Volk and colleagues,[141] using giant excised patches of *Xenopus* oocyte membrane, determined that the IC50 values for interaction of corticosterone and tetrabutylammonium with the extracellular aspect of rat OCT2 are 20-fold higher and 4-fold lower, respectively, than those measured for interaction with the intracellular aspect of the transporter. This is not a surprising observation in view of information concerning the probable three-dimensional structure of OCTs and the likelihood that binding regions will have (at least) modestly different three-dimensional configurations when exposed to the inside versus the outside of cells. As noted earlier, modeling of the outward- versus inward-facing conformations of rat OCT2 revealed functional differences in the physicochemical characteristics of the postulated binding surfaces.[132] This is discussed in more detail in later sections.

In addition to operating as electrogenic uniporters, the OCTs also support OC/OC exchange.[75,142-145] *Xenopus* oocytes loaded with unlabeled TEA stimulates the uptake of [3H]MPP by OCT1.[142] The symmetry of this type of *trans*-effect is apparent in observations of accelerated efflux

of preloaded [3H]MPP from rat OCT1–expressing oocytes in the presence of inwardly directed gradients of unlabeled TEA[75] or MPP.[143] Human OCT1 also supports *trans*-stimulation of both influx and efflux (of TEA), but quantitative differences in the extent of these fluxes produced by some substrates (e.g., tributylmethylammonium) support the notion of asymmetric binding properties on the extracellular versus intracellular aspect of the transporter.[144]

OCT Structure. The elucidation of the crystal structure of two transporters in the major facilitator superfamily, LacY[146] and GlpT,[147] and the discovery that these two proteins are markedly homologous in structure, including a common helical fold, despite having low homology (<15%) with regard to sequence, paved the way for efforts to use homology modeling as a means of developing structural models for other transporters in the major facilitator superfamily.[148] LacY and GlpT served as "templates" for the modeling of OCT1[121] and OCT2,[122] respectively, and the resulting models share a number of common structural features (as a result, in part, of shared structural features of the templates), including a large hydrophilic "cleft" formed by the juxtaposition of the N- and C-terminal halves of the proteins composed of the amino acid residues of the "pore-forming" helices: TMH1, TMH2, TMH4, TMH5, TMH7, TMH8, TMH10, and TMH11 (Figure 8-10).

Amino acid residues that were shown in site-directed studies to influence substrate binding are found, in both OCT models, at locations consistent with roles in stabilizing substrate-transporter interactions. In particular, an aspartate in TMH11 conserved in all OCT homologs (i.e., D475 in human OCT2) markedly influences substrate binding in rat OCT1[149] (and in rat OCT2[150]) and is directed toward the hydrophilic pore at a position within the protein that coincides closely with the binding site identified both in GlpT[147] and in LacY[146] (see Figure 8-10). Similarly, residues within TMH4 and TMH10 that influence substrate binding are also directed toward the pore region of OCT1[121] and OCT2,[122] including three residues in TMH10 that play a key role in defining the selectivity differences that distinguish OCT1 and OCT2.[121,122,151] The comparatively large extent of the pore or cleft region of OCTs (20Å × 60Å × 80Å)[121] is consistent with the suggestion that the broad substrate selectivity of these proteins reflects binding interactions over a large surface that contains several distinct sites or regions.[122,151] In OCT1 and OCT2, the native cysteine residues that are accessible to impermeable thiol-reactive reagents are found in the pore-lining helices, TMH10 and TMH11, in positions clearly exposed to the water-filled cleft.[121,122] In addition, increasing evidence suggests that OCTs (and organic anion transporters [OATs]) may form multimeric complexes,[152,153] although the influence of such interactions on transport activity is not known.

As noted earlier, the charge-to-substrate ratio for OCT2-mediated transport generally exceeds 1 and varies according to membrane potential and the identity of the OC substrate.[132] A nonspecific "cotransport" (i.e., one not involving energetic coupling between cotransported substrates) of small cations (e.g., Na^+ ions) that is larger in the influx direction than in the efflux direction appears to be responsible for the excess charge translocated with OC substrate. Computational modeling of the outward-facing binding site revealed a more markedly negative surface charge than that of the inward-facing binding

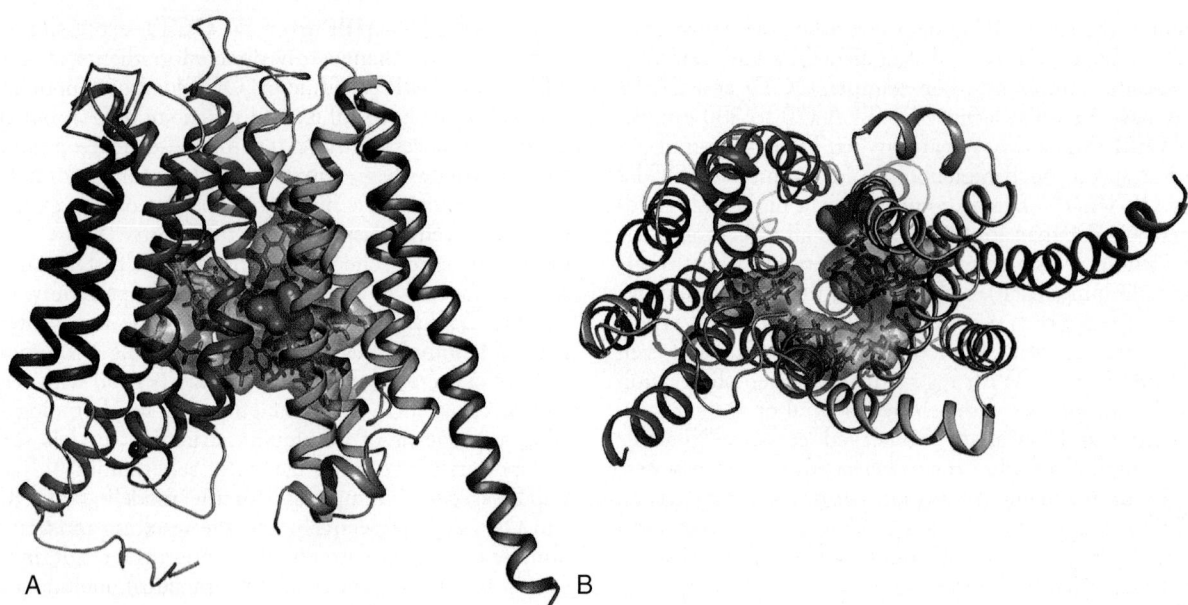

FIGURE 8-10 Model of the three-dimensional structure of the rabbit ortholog of organic cation 2 (OCT2), based on structural homology with the major facilitator superfamily (MFS) transporter GlpT. **A,** Side view of OCT2, with the cytoplasmic aspect directed downward. The transmembrane-spanning helices (TMHs) 1 to 6, which constitute the N-terminal half of the protein, are *blue;* the helices that constitute the C-terminal half of the protein are *cyan.* The lighter colored helices (TMH1, TMH2, TMH4, TMH5, TMH7, TMH8, TMH10, and TMH11) border the hydrophilic cleft region formed by the juxtaposition of the N- and C-terminal halves of the protein. The amino acid residues that constitute the postulated substrate-binding region within the cleft are rendered as sticks with a *pink* van der Waals surface. D475 is rendered as a space-filling residue in *orange.* Note that residues from the long extracellular loop (between TMH1 and TMH2) and the cytoplasmic loop (between TMH6 and TMH7) were eliminated to facilitate homology modeling with the GlpT template. **B,** An end-on view of the cleft and postulated binding region from the cytoplasmic aspect of the protein. (Adapted from Zhang X, Shirahatti NV, Mahadevan D, et al: A conserved glutamate residue in transmembrane helix 10 influences substrate specificity of rabbit OCT2 (Slc22A2), *J Biol Chem* 280:34813-34822, 2005.)

site, which may account for the increased tendency of cations to occupy the cleft when exposed to the external solution. The external aspect of the binding cleft in rat OCT1 also appears to include one or more binding sites capable of interacting with selected OCs (including MPP and tetrabutylammonium) with K_d values lower than 1 nmol, in addition to the lower affinity sites that appear to play predominant roles in substrate translocation (i.e., K_t values >1 μmol). The influence of the very high-affinity sites on OCT transport is not clear, although the presence of "high-affinity" ligands could influence the binding and translocation of other substrates.

The discovery of altered transport function of human OCT1 and OCT2 in which the genes contain single-nucleotide polymorphisms, present in different ethnic populations,[154-156] has underscored the importance of understanding structure-activity relationships. For example, 28 variable sites in the human *OCT2* gene were discovered in a collection of 247 ethnically diverse DNA samples (white American, African American, Asian American, Mexican American, and Pacific Islander). Eight of these polymorphisms caused nonsynonymous amino acid changes, of which four were present in at least 1% of an ethnic population. These four displayed altered transporter function, including up to a threefold change in K_t values for MPP and tetrabutylammonium, changes that could result in differences in the pharmacokinetics of renal drug excretion between individuals expressing different variants of human *OCT2*. However, population-genetic analysis suggests that selection has acted against amino acid changes to human *OCT2*, which may reflect a necessary role of OCT2 in the renal elimination of endogenous amines or xenobiotics.[154]

Substantial effort has been directed toward understanding the impact of the nonsynonomous polymorphism of human

OCT2, G808T, which results in A270S in the protein. This variant is present in approximately 16% of white Americans, 11% of African Americans, 17% of native Japanese, and 13% of native Chinese.[157,158] The A270S variant displays only a modest decrease in the apparent affinity for MPP and tetrabutylammonium when expressed in *Xenopus* oocytes,[155] and transport of metformin is profoundly depressed, principally because of a large decrease in maximum velocity (V_{max}) (despite expression of the protein at the plasma membrane). However, subjects expressing the reference or A270S variant of *OCT2* showed no differences in either maximal clearance or area under the curve for metformin, although the marked inhibition of metformin clearance produced by coadminstration of cimetidine typically seen in affected patients was not observed in subjects with the A270S variant.[158] Of importance is that other *OCT2* single-nucleotide polymorphisms have, however, been shown to influence renal clearance of metformin.[159]

According to the current structural models of OCT proteins, A270 lies within the small extracellular loop between TMH5 and TMH6[122] or, alternatively, in the middle of TMH6.[121] Interestingly, neither position is in or near the putative binding region within the hydrophilic cleft between the N- and C-terminal halves of OCT transporters. In fact, in major facilitator proteins, TMH6 is postulated to play a structural role in stabilizing the protein within the lipid bilayer.[146] These data suggest that mutations in regions far from actual sites of direct substrate interaction can exert a marked effect on transporter function.

Regulation of OCT-Mediated Transport. OCT activity responds to both short- and long-term regulation, although there appear to be significant species differences in the extent of such responses.[119] For example, when expressed heterologously, activation of protein kinase A acutely upregulates rat OCT1–mediated transport[160] but downregulates human OCT1–mediated transport.[161] Of particular significance to the issue of short-term regulation of renal OC transport in humans is the observation that basolateral uptake of the fluorescent cation 4-[4-(dimethylamino)-styryl]-*N*-methylpyridinium into isolated single nonperfused proximal tubules from human kidneys is acutely downregulated after activation of protein kinase C.[162] This event presumably reflects acute regulation of OCT2 activity. In fact, human OCT2 (expressed heterologously) is acutely downregulated after activation of protein kinase A, protein kinase C, Ca^{2+}–calcium/calmodulin-dependent protein kinase (CaM), or phosphatidylinositol-3-kinase (PI3).[163]

The inhibition of human OCT2 in association with acute activation of these kinases appears to reflect a decrease in the maximal rate of transport (i.e., K_t is not affected),[164] which is consistent with the hypothesis that acute downregulation of OCT2 activity reflects the rapid sequestration of transporters into a cytoplasmic vesicular compartment, a mechanism that has been shown to account for the acute downregulation of the closely related OAT transporters.[165] Activity of rat OCT2 is also downregulated by activation of Ca^{2+}/CaM, although that regulation appears to involve changes in apparent affinity of the transporter for substrate, rather than a change in V$_{max}$.[166] Interestingly, the acute inhibition of OCT2 in rat kidneys is gender dependent: It is evident in renal proximal tubules (S3 segment) only from male rats.[166]

Sex steroids have been shown to regulate the long-term activity of OCT2. TEA uptake is greater, and expression of messenger RNA and protein is higher, in renal cortical slices from male rats than in those from female rats and is correlated with a higher level of expression of OCT2; no sex-linked differences occur in either OCT1 or OCT3.[167] Moreover, treatment of male and female rats with testosterone significantly increases OCT2 expression in the kidney,[168] through the androgen receptor–mediated transcriptional pathway,[169] which suggests that testosterone plays a significant role in the transcriptional regulation of the OCT2 gene in rats.

A similar profile is not, however, evident in all species. Although levels of OCT2 messenger RNA are higher in kidneys from male rabbits than in those from female rabbits, this difference does not extend to differences in either protein expression or in rates of TEA transport in renal tubules isolated from male and female rabbit kidneys.[170] Also, treating opossum kidney cells with estrogen for 6 days caused a 30% to 40% reduction in basolateral TEA transport that was correlated with a 40% to 50% reduction in OCT1 protein expression, with no effect on OCT2 expression.[171] Humans, like rats, exhibit a significant sex difference in the renal excretion of the OC substrate amantadine, which is a substrate for OCT1, OCT2, and OCT3.[172,173] It is noteworthy that renal clearance involves transport across both basolateral and apical membranes. Thus, sex differences in renal clearance may involve apical transporters either in addition to or rather than basolateral transporters.

Apical Organic Cation Transporters

Although the physiologic characteristics of apical OC transport have been studied extensively in isolated BBMVs,[9,64] the molecular identity of the principal transporters that mediate the exit step in renal secretion of type I OCs—that is, the OC/H$^+$ exchanger—has only more recently been clarified. Whereas the carnitine/OC transporters (OCTNs; i.e., OCTN1 and OCTN2) were once thought to play a role in the mediating transport of at least some OCs (e.g., as suggested by Yabuuchi and associates[91]), it is more likely that the transporters MATE1 and MATE2-K are the major elements in apical OC secretion.

OCTN Family

OCTN1 (SLC22A4) and OCTN2 (SLC22A5) are peptides, 551 to 557 amino acids in length, approximately 30% to 33% identical in sequence to human OCT1. Like other members of the OCT family, the OCTNs have 12 putative TMHs and, consistent with the OCTs, three *N*-linked glycosylation sites and a number of consensus sites for phosphorylation mediated by protein kinase A, protein kinase C, and CKII. OCTN1, although widely expressed in human tissues, is weakly expressed in the kidneys.[128] OCTN2, in contrast, is most heavily expressed in the kidneys, heart, placenta, skeletal muscle, and pancreas.[174]

OCTN1 supports electroneutral transport of TEA. TEA uptake in *Xenopus* oocyte is *trans*-stimulated by oppositely oriented H$^+$ gradients[91]; thus, researchers have speculated that OCTN1 may play a role in the OC/H$^+$ exchange in isolated preparations of the renal BBMVs. However, TEA/H$^+$ exchange has been noted in very few tissues, most notably in isolated membranes from apical BBMVs in the kidneys[9] and canalicular BBMVs in the liver.[175] OCTN1, however, is expressed in many tissues, including the placenta and intestines,[176] neither of which supports TEA/H$^+$ exchange. The comparatively low level of expression of OCTN1 in human kidneys[128] also appears to be inconsistent with the observation that OC/H$^+$ exchange is the dominant mechanism for OC flux across isolated BBMVs in human kidneys.[177] In addition, the kinetic/selectivity characteristics of OCTN1 are inconsistent with this process, playing a major role in luminal OC transport. Grundemann and associates[178] showed that OCTN1, like its congener OCTN2 (see next paragraph), supports the narrowly selective Na$^+$-coupled cotransport of the fungal metabolite and antioxidant ergothionine, and it is suggested that this is the principal role of its excretion.[178]

OCTN2 supports both Na$^+$-independent electrogenic facilitated diffusion of selected type I OCs and the Na$^+$-dependent transport of the zwitterion carnitine (and related compounds). Of importance is that lesions in OCTN2 result in primary carnitine deficiency in humans[179,180] and in mice[181]; the Na$^+$-dependent interaction of OCTN2 with carnitine and its role in supporting the reabsorption of this important metabolite is discussed elsewhere.[182] The Na$^+$-independent transport of TEA, MPP, and a wide range of other type I OCs occurs electrogenically.[174,183] In view of its apical location, operation of OCTN2 in this mode is expected to support OC reabsorption, rather than secretion. There is evidence that OCTN2 can support electroneutral exchange of selected OCs (including TEA) for Na$^+$-carnitine interaction.[184] However, other than for selected zwitterions (e.g., carnitine), OC transport mediated by OCTN2 displays extremely low transport efficiencies (the ratio of V$_{max}$/K$_t$),[185] a finding that strongly supports the contention that, like OCTN1, OCTN2 does not play a quantitatively significant role in general renal OC secretion.[178,186]

MATE FAMILY

Two members of the multidrug/oligosaccharidyl-lipid/polysaccharide superfamily of transport proteins, MATE1 and MATE2, have been cloned in humans and mice.[93,187] In humans, MATE1 is expressed in the kidneys and liver (less so in the heart), where it is found in the apical and canalicular membranes of renal proximal tubules and hepatocytes, respectively.[93] MATE2 appears to be more broadly expressed; however, whereas MATE1 clearly supports OC transport (see later discussion), the function of MATE2 has yet to be demonstrated. However, a sequence variant (in which 36 amino acids are missing from the putative intracellular loop between TMH4 and TMH5) that is highly expressed in the kidney, MATE2-K,[104] has transport function that closely parallels that of its homolog, MATE1.[104,188] The human ortholog of MATE1 is a protein with 570 amino acids and 13 putative TMHs, no N-linked glycosylation sites (in extracellular loops), and three consensus phosphorylation sites for protein kinase G (and none for protein kinase C, protein kinase A, CKII, or CaMII). Of importance is that MATE1-mediated transport of TEA is electroneutral, pH-sensitive, and markedly $trans$-stimulated by oppositely oriented H[+] gradients. TEA transport is cis-inhibited by type I OCs, including cimetidine, quinidine, and MPP; only weakly inhibited by N^1-methylnicotinamide and choline; and refractory to guanidine, PAH, and probenecid.[187] Thus, the expression profile, energetic mechanism, and selectivity characteristics of MATE1 are quite comparable with those of the apical OC/H[+] exchanger in renal BBMVs, and MATE1 (and MATE2-K) is therefore a strong candidate for apical OC/H[+] exchange.

The role of MATEs in the apical secretion of OCs in the renal proximal tubule is thought to be significant, on the basis of the observation that $Mate1$-null mice display an 82% reduction of total renal clearance, and 86% reduction in renal secretion, of the cationic drug metformin.[189] Mice do not express MATE2 in the kidneys (its expression is highest in the testes),[115] and this complicates the estimation of the fractional contribution of MATE1 to renal secretion of OCs in the humans who express both MATE1 and MATE2-K. Nevertheless, these data strongly implicate MATE transporters as being quantitatively significant contributors to the renal handling of OCs.

MDR FAMILY

MDR1 (also known as ABCB1, P-glycoprotein, or p-GP) was first characterized for its role in the development of cross-resistance of cancer cells to a structurally diverse range of chemotherapeutic agents. The human ortholog of MDR1 is a protein of 1279 amino acids (141 kDa) composed of two homologous halves, each containing six transmembrane-spanning domains and an adenosine triphosphate (ATP)–binding domain, separated by a linker polypeptide. The normal expression of MDR1 in barrier epithelia, including those of the intestines, liver, and kidneys, supports the conclusion that it plays a role in limiting absorption (in the intestines) and facilitating excretion (in the liver and kidneys) of xenobiotic compounds. In the kidneys, MDR1 is expressed in the apical membrane of proximal tubule cells in humans[190] and in mice.[191] MDR1 is also expressed, albeit at lower levels, in the mesangium, thick ascending limb, and collecting tubule of normal human kidneys.[192]

MDR1 supports ATP-dependent export of a structurally diverse range of comparatively bulky, hydrophobic cationic substrates that, in general, are classified as type II OCs. These traditional MDR1 substrates include the vinca alkaloids (e.g., vinblastine, vincristine), cyclosporine, anthracyclines (e.g., daunorubicin, doxorubicin), and verapamil. In addition, MDR1 mediates the transport of a number of relatively hydrophobic compounds that are either completely uncharged or are titrated to neutral charge at physiologic pH, including digoxin, colchicine, propafenone, and selected corticosteroids. Although MDR1 is probably involved in the luminal secretion of at least type II OCs, its quantitative significance is not known.

Clinical Diseases of Organic Cation Transporters

Lesions in OCTN2 have been clearly linked to systemic carnitine deficiency, because of the central role of this transporter in reabsorption of carnitine from the tubular filtrate.[181,193,194] In addition, single-nucleotide polymorphisms in the genes coding for OCTN1 and OCTN2 have been linked to increased incidence of inflammatory bowel diseases, including Crohn's disease.[195] A clear disease phenotype is not, however, associated with the failure of renal secretion of OCs, as shown by the normal phenotypes of mice in which OCT1, OCT2, OCT3, or MATE1 (or a combination of these) has been eliminated.[9,114,189] Instead, the focus has been more on the influence of naturally occurring genetic variations in OCTs and OCTNs within human populations and the influence that such variation may have on the pharmacokinetics of drug elimination.[154]

A study of six pairs of monozygotic twins showed that genetic factors contribute substantially to the renal clearance of metformin, a drug that is a substrate of OCT2 and eliminated exclusively by the kidneys. In fact, the genetic contribution to variation in renal clearance of metformin, which undergoes transporter-mediated secretion, is suspected to be particularly high (>90%).[156] Genetic variation in OCT2 may explain a large part of this pharmacokinetic variability. Common variants of OCT2—as well as genetic variants of OCT1, OCTN1, OCTN2, and MATE1—may alter protein function and could cause interindividual differences in the renal handling of OC drugs. Genetic variants of all these transporters have been identified in human populations,[154-156,196-199] and studies in heterologous expressions systems have confirmed that common single-nucleotide polymorphisms (typically, those that occur in specific population groups at a rate of >1%), can result in substantial changes in transporter activity. Further examinations of the pharmacokinetic phenotypes of individuals harboring genetic variants that change transport function should help to define the roles of each transporter in renal elimination. Such studies may also help identify particular genetic variants that lead to susceptibility to toxic effects that result from drug-drug interactions.

Organic Anions

Physiology of Organic Anion Transport

Organic anions represent an immensely broad group of solutes transported by the kidneys; thus, a single section seems inadequate for discussing them. This chapter provides a general overview, followed by discussion of specific topics, without attempting to be exhaustive.

An organic anion is loosely defined as any organic compound that bears a net negative charge at the pH of the fluid in which the compound resides. These compounds can be endogenous substances or exogenously acquired toxins or drugs. The physiologic processes can potentially include conservation with extremely low fractional excretion. Such is the case with metabolic intermediates such as monocarboxylates and dicarboxylates (see Figure 8-1; fractional excretion ≈ 0). In contrast, the system can also gear itself for elimination through combined glomerular filtration and secretion (see Figure 8-1; fractional excretion > 1). In addition to the large range of fractional excretion rates, this group of transporters also has the broadest array of substrates, which spans compounds with completely disparate chemical structures. Multispecificity in substrate recognition is a prevalent feature within each gene family and across different families of organic anion transporters.

The precise analysis of the field of renal anion excretion was initiated in 1923 by the seminal work of Marshall and Vickers,[200] who studied the elimination of dyes and concluded that mammalian renal tubules possess high-capacity secretory function. This observation was followed in 1945 by the classical studies of Smith and colleagues,[201] who described the tubular secretion of PAH and provided a marker for estimating renal plasma flow by PAH clearance for decades that followed. Reabsorptive physiology was illustrated in the "Glucose" section. Figure 8-11 illustrates the secretory nature of the proximal tubule, in which PAH is used as a surrogate. In low plasma concentrations, PAH has a fractional excretion rate of >1, and the rate of PAH clearance approaches that of renal plasma flow, inasmuch as most (albeit not all) of the PAH is removed from the plasma in a single pass. As plasma levels of PAH increase, both filtered and secreted PAH levels increase, and PAH clearance rate remains a good estimate of renal plasma flow rate. When the secretory maximum is reached and subsequently exceeded, the increment in excretion is contributed solely by increasing filtered load. At this stage, PAH clearance rate starts to gradually lag behind renal plasma flow rate, toward the value of GFR (see Figure 8-11).

Classic studies with stop-flow techniques, micropuncture, and microperfusion[202-204] demonstrated organic anion secretion in the proximal tubule. As in the case for OCs, the secretory mode mandates uphill energetic and broad substrate recognition, and the organism simply cannot afford to devote one gene per compound that must be excreted. Table 8-4 is an illustrative but incomplete inventory of the extremely broad spectrum of organic anions handled by the kidneys. It is impossible to fathom any structural similarities among these compounds. In addition, the number of substances transported far exceeds the number of proteins necessary to excrete these substances. This situation is classical for proteins such as the OCTs, MATEs, MDR1, or the multiligand receptor megalin, for which the ability to engage with multiple compounds is intrinsic to their biologic function.[205,206] Fritzsch and colleagues proposed that at minimum, a hydrophobic region in the anion must be a substrate.[207] The protein structure that allows this broad range of substrate to be bound and transported is unknown but will undoubtedly be fascinating.

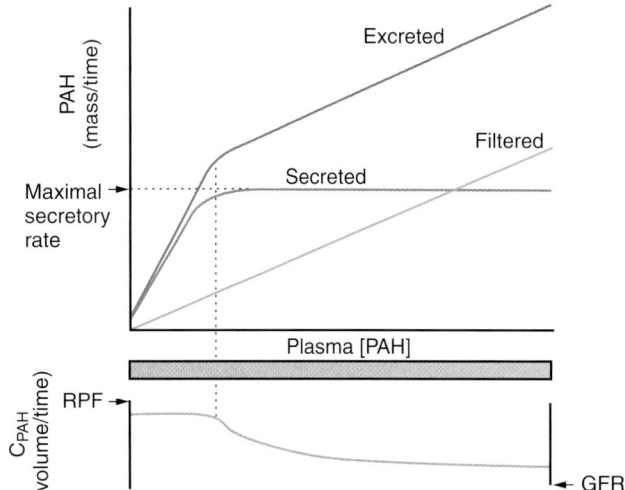

FIGURE 8-11 Illustration of filtration-secretion through the use of *p*-aminohippuric acid (PAH) clearance. When plasma [PAH] is low, the rate of PAH clearance approximates that of renal plasma flow (RPF). When plasma [PAH] is high, the rate of PAH clearance is lower than that of RPF and higher than glomerular filtration rate (GFR).

TABLE 8-4 Classes of Organic Anions Transported by the Proximal Tubule

TYPE OF AGENT	EXAMPLE
Endogenous	
Metabolic intermediates	α-Ketoglutarate, succinate, citrate
Eicosanoids	Prostaglandins E_1, E_2, D_2, $F_2\alpha$, I_2
Thromboxane B_2 cyclic nucleotides	cAMP, cGMP
Others	Urate, folate, bile acids, oxalate, 5-HIA, homovanillic acid
Metabolic Conjugates	
Sulfate	Estrone sulfate, DHEAS
Glucuronide	Estradiol glucuronide, salicyl glucuronide
Acetyl	Acetylated sulfonamide
Glycine	PAH, *o*-hydroxyhippurate
Cysteine	CTFC, DCVC, *N*-acetyl-*S*-farnesyl–cysteine
Drugs	
Antibiotic	β-Lactam, cephem, tetracycline, sulfonamide
Antiviral	Acyclovir, amantadine, adefovir
Antiinflammatory	Salicylates, indomethacin
Diuretic	Loop diuretics, thiazides, acetazolamide
Antihypertensive	ACE inhibitors, ARBs
Chemotherapeutic	Methotrexate, azathioprine, cyclophosphamide, 5-fluorouracil
Antiepileptic	Valproate
Uricosuric	Probenecid
Environmental Toxins	
Fungal product	Ochratoxins A and B, aflatoxin G1, patulin
Herbicide	2,4-Dichlorophenoxyacetic acid

ACE, angiotensin converting enzyme; *ARB*, angiotensin receptor blockers; *cAMP*, cyclic adenosine monophosphate; *cGMP*, cyclic guanidine monophosphate; *CTFC*, S-(2-chloro-1,1,2-trifluoroethyl)-L-cysteine; *DCVC*, S-(1,2-dichlorovinyl)-L-cysteine; *DHEAS*, dihydroxyepiandrosterone sulfate; *5-HIA*, 5-hydroxyindoleacetate; *PAH*, *p*-aminohippuric acid.

Molecular Biology of Organic Anion Transporters

In contrast to other organic ions, the segregation into apical and basolateral classes of tandem transporters are not that distinct for organic anions because of the assorted secretory and absorptive functions and the widespread use of anion-exchange mechanisms; hence, the same family of transporters can be found on both membranes. Three families of solute transporters are described here: the Na⁺ dicarboxylate (NaDC)–sulfate transporters (NaDC family; SLC13A family; both apical and basolateral), the organic anion transporters (OAT family; SLC22A family; both apical and basolateral), and the OATPs (SLCO family; basolateral). In addition, uric acid transport is given some attention. A detailed account is beyond the scope of this chapter, but a review is available.[208]

NaDC (*SLC13A*) Family

These transporters mainly reclaim filtered solutes, and their functions are opposite those of the secretory transporter proteins. This family is related by similarities in primary sequences, but the isoforms have quite distinct function. The nomenclature is still evolving, and five genes have been identified to date (Table 8-5). NaS1 is a low-affinity sulfate transporter expressed at the proximal tubule apical membrane (see Table 8-5). Although NaS1 is crucial for sulfate homeostasis, it is not an organic anion transporter and hence is not discussed here. NaS2 and NaCT are not expressed in the kidney (see Table 8-5). NaDC1 and NaDC3 are the main transporters of interest.

NaDC1

NaDC1 was first cloned by Bai and Pajor[209] and Pajor.[210,211] NaDC1 is on the apical membranes of both the renal proximal tubule and the small intestine, where it mediates absorption of tricarboxylic acid cycle intermediates from the glomerular filtrate or the intestinal lumen. The preferred substrates are 4-carbon dicarboxylates such as succinate, fumarate, and α-ketoglutarate. Citrate exists mostly as a tricarboxylate at plasma pH, but in the proximal tubule lumen, because of apical H⁺ transport, $citrate^{3-}$ is titrated ($citrate^{3-}/citrate^{2-}$ pK, 5.7 to 6.0) and is taken up as $citrate^{2-}$. The Michaelis constant for dicarboxylates ranges between 0.3 and 1.0 mmol. Transport of one divalent anion substrate is coupled to three Na⁺ ions. Once across the apical membrane, cytosolic citrate is either metabolized through ATP citrate lyase, which cleaves citrate to oxaloacetate and acetyl coenzyme A, or transported into the mitochondria, where it can be metabolized in the tricarboxylic acid cycle to neutral end products such as carbon dioxide (Figure 8-12).[212,213] When a divalent organic anion is converted to neutral products, two H⁺ molecules

TABLE 8-5 Organic Anion Transporters				
TRANSPORTER NAME	**GENE NAME**	**HUMAN CHROMOSOME**	**RENAL TUBULE LOCALIZATION**	**TRANSPORT MODE OR SUBSTRATE (NA⁺-INDEPENDENT)**
NaDC Family				
NaS1	*SLC13A1*	7q31-32	Apical	Sulfate, thiosulfate, selenate
NaDC1	*SLC13A2*	17p11.1-q11.1	Apical	Succinate, citrate, α-ketoglutarate
NaDC3	*SLC13A3*	20q12-13.1	Basolateral	Succinate, citrate, α-ketoglutarate
NaS2	*SLC13A4*	7q33	Absent	Sulfate
NaCT	*SLC13A5*	12q12-13	Absent	Citrate, succinate, pyruvate
OAT Family				
OAT1	*SLC22A6*	11q12.3	Basolateral	OA dicarboxylate exchange
OAT2	*SLC22A7*	6q21.1-2	Basolateral	OA dicarboxylate exchange
OAT3	*SLC22A8*	11q12.3	Basolateral	OA dicarboxylate exchange
OAT4	*SLC22A11*	11q13.1	Apical	OA dicarboxylate exchange
URAT1	*SLC22A12*	11q13.1	Apical	Urate OA exchange
OAT5	*Slc22A19*	(murine)	—	—
OATP Family				
OATP4C1	*SLCO4C1*	5q21	Proximal tubule: basolateral	Digoxin, ouabain, T_3
OATP1A2	*SLCO1A2*	12p12	Cortical collecting duct: basolateral	Bile salts, estrogen conjugates prostaglandins, T_3, T_4, antibiotics, ouabain, ochratoxin A
OATP2A1	*SLCO2A1*	3q21	Messenger RNA	Prostaglandins
OATP2B1	*SLCO2B1*	11q13	Messenger RNA	Estrogen conjugates, antibiotics
OATP3A1	*SLCO3A1*	15q26	Messenger RNA	Estrogen conjugates, antibiotics
OATP4A1	*SLCO4A1*	20q13.1	Messenger RNA	Bile salts, estrogen conjugates, prostaglandins, T_3, T_4, antibiotics

NaDC, Na⁺-dicarboxylate cotransporter; *OA*, organic anion (broad substrate specificity); *OAT*, organic anion transporter; *OATP*, organic anion transport polypeptide; *T_3*, triiodothyronine; *T_4*, thyroxine; *URAT1*, uric acid transporter 1.

are consumed, which renders citrate^{2+} an important urinary base.[214] Deletion of the gene for NaDC1 in rodents was found to lead to increased excretion of dicarboxylic acids in the urine, but the phenotype was not examined from the viewpoint of acid-base balance.[215]

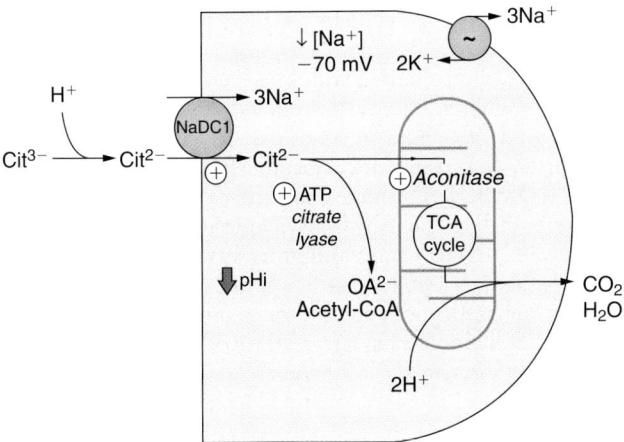

FIGURE 8-12 Absorption and metabolism of citrate in the proximal tubule. Na$^+$-K$^+$-ATPase activity generates the low cell [Na$^+$]. As a secondary active transporter, Na$^+$-dicarboxylate cotransporter 1 (NaDC1) uses the electrochemical gradient to pick up filtered citrate, which is metabolized in the cytoplasm or the mitochondria. Ambient and cytoplasmic pH increase citrate uptake and metabolism. Acidification of urinary lumen titrates citrate to the divalent transported species. NaDC1 activity is directly activated by pH, and chronic low pH increases expression of NaDC1 (*circled arrow*). Intracellular acidification increases the expression of adenosine triphosphate (ATP) citrate lyase and aconitase (*circled arrows*).

NaDC3

NaDC3 has a wider tissue distribution and much broader substrate specificity than does NaDC1. NaDC3 is expressed on basolateral membranes in renal proximal tubule cells,[216] as well as in liver, brain, and placenta tissue. The basolateral localization signal of NaDC3 was mapped to a motif in its N-terminal cytoplasmic domain.[217] The Michaelis constant for succinate in NaDC3 is lower than that for NaDC1 (10 vs. 100 μmol).[217] Similarly, NaDC3 displays a much higher affinity for α-ketoglutarate than does NaDC1.[218] Like NaDC1, NaDC3 is Na$^+$-coupled and electrogenic, and so NaDC3 probably does not mediate citrate efflux from the proximal tubule into the peritubular space. It is more likely that the NaDC3 supports the outwardly directed α-ketoglutarate gradient required for OATs to perform organic anion exchange (see later discussion). NaDC3 has been shown to support approximately 50% of the OAT-mediated uptake of the organic anion across the basolateral membrane in isolated renal tubules of rabbits[219]; half of this effect reflects the accumulation of exogenous α-ketoglutarate from the blood, and the other half is attributable to "recycling" of endogenous α-ketoglutarate that exited the cell in OAT-mediated exchange for the organic anion substrate.

OAT (*SLC22A*) Family

A few features of these transporters should again be emphasized: their role as anion exchangers, their high capacity, their tremendously diverse substrate selectivity (see Table 8-5), and their presence on both membranes. These proteins are vital in rescuing the organism from succumbing to toxins. The uptake of substrates from the basolateral membrane of the proximal tubule is a thermodynamically uphill process

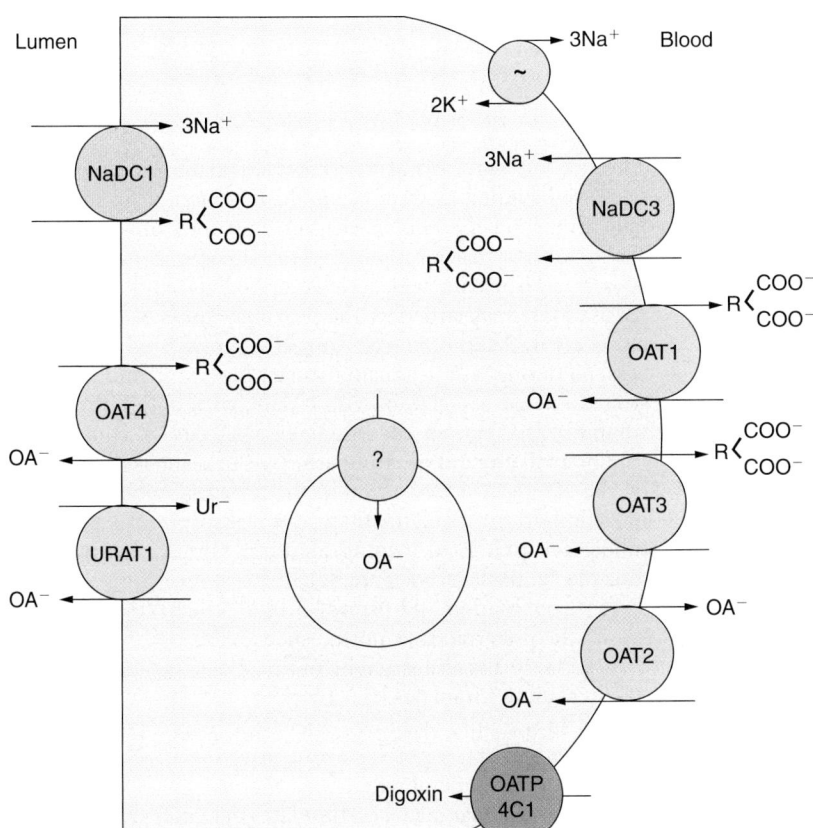

FIGURE 8-13 Families of anionic transporters in the proximal tubule: Na$^+$-dicarboxylate cotransporter (NaDC; *green*), organic anion transporter (OAT; *blue*), and organic anion transporting polypeptide (OATP; *purple*). The intracellular transport and sequestration of organic anions are not understood. OA, organic anion; Ur, urate.

involving tertiary active transport (Figure 8-13). The Na^+ and voltage gradient generated by Na^+-K^+-ATPase activity drives the accumulation of the dicarboxylate α-ketoglutarate in the proximal tubule via NaDC3 transport, which in a tertiary manner (thrice removed from ATP hydrolysis) energizes uptake of other organic anions into the proximal tubule (see Figure 8-13). Endogenously produced α-ketoglutarate from deamination and deamidation of glutamine (ammonia genesis) may also participate in the exchange. Some of the organic anions transported may be endogenous or relatively innocuous exogenous compounds, but many of the substrates (see Table 8-4) are toxins.

Although its function is in defending the body, the proximal tubule cells cannot afford a self-sacrificial approach because the end result can be destruction of the very mechanism that secretes these toxins. There exists a detoxifying mechanism in the proximal tubule cell that protects the cell while the toxins are en route to the apical membrane to be disposed. The details of these mechanisms are still elusive, but current data from studies in isolated tubules and cell culture models is suggestive of compartmentalization that may serve to sequester the toxins from imparting their harmful effects.[220]

BASOLATERAL ORGANIC ANION TRANSPORTERS

More than half a century after Smith and colleagues[201] described PAH secretion into the urine, the PAH transporter was cloned by several laboratories almost contemporaneously.[221-223] OAT1 and OAT3 are present in the basolateral membrane of the proximal tubule (see Figure 8-13, Table 8-5). OAT1-mediated uptake of PAH is stimulated by an outwardly directed gradient of dicarboxylates such as α-ketoglutarate, which indicates that OAT1 is an organic anion/dicarboxylate exchanger.[224] The substrate selectivity of OAT1 is extremely broad, with affinities for substrate that are comparable with those reported for the functional PAH transport system. OAT3 is localized in the basolateral membrane of the kidneys and, like OAT1, has broad extrarenal expression.[225] OAT3 also has a promiscuous list of substrates comparable with that of OAT1. The purpose for the OAT1 and OAT3 redundancy in the kidneys is unclear. OAT2 was originally identified from the liver, and its expression in the kidneys appears to be weaker than that of OAT1 and OAT3.[226] It transports PAH, dicarboxylates, prostaglandins, salicylate, acetylsalicylate, and tetracycline.

APICAL ORGANIC ANION TRANSPORTERS

There is no overlap of polarized expression of OATs in the proximal tubule. OAT4 was cloned from the kidneys and is expressed in the apical membrane of the proximal tubule.[227] In oocytes, it transports PAH, conjugated sex hormones, prostaglandins, and mycotoxins in an organic anion/dicarboxylate exchange mode and is capable of bidirectional movement of organic anions.[228] It is not known whether OAT4 represents an exceptional OAT-mediated luminal uptake, although it is hard to fathom from the list of candidate substrates why OAT would participate in absorption of some rather noxious substances. The other apical transporter is uric acid transporter 1 (URAT1), which is renal specific in its expression.[229] Human URAT1 appears to be quite specific for urate transport,[229] which is discussed later. The role of URAT1 as a urate transporter was proved at the whole-organism level from an experiment of nature in humans with renal hypouricemia.

OATP (*SLCO*) Family

The OATPs constitute a superfamily of transporters, designated SLCO (*solute carrier OATP*).[208] One noteworthy point is that considerable interspecies differences between rodents and humans engender difficulties in extrapolating rodent data to humans. This family of OATPs consists of 11 members in humans[208] that are expressed widely in the brain, choroid plexus, liver, heart, intestines, kidneys, placenta, and testes and, like the OATs, also have a wide spectrum of substrates.[230,231] The first member, *Oatp1*, was cloned from rat liver by Jacquemin and associates[232] as a Na^+-independent bile acid transporter. Substrates are enormously diverse in structure, including multiple hormones and their conjugates, bile salts, and drugs such as the 3-hydroxy-3-methylglutaryl–coenzyme A (HMG-CoA) reductase inhibitors, cardiac glycosides, antimicrobial agents, and anticancer agents. They play important roles in drug absorption, distribution, and excretion. The presence and functional characterization of naturally occurring variations in human OATP genes render this class of transporters a focus of intensive pharmacogenomic research.

Among human OATPs, only OATP4C1 is definitively expressed in the kidney. In rodents, there exist myriad isoforms whose presence has not been confirmed in humans.[208] One important compound carried by OATP4C1 is the cardiac glycoside digoxin.[233] OATP4C1 is expressed exclusively in the basolateral membrane of proximal tubular cells and mediates the high-affinity transport of digoxin (K_m = 7.8 μmol) and ouabain (K_m = 0.38 μmol), as well as thyroid hormones such as triiodothyronine (K_m = 5.9 μmol). The apical pathway for digoxin has been presumed, although not proven, to be an ATP-dependent efflux pump, such as MDR1.

Clinical Relevance of Organic Anion Transporters

Disorders of Citrate Transport

The role of NaDC1 in physiology and pathophysiology has been well studied. Citrate has multiple functions in mammalian urine, and the two most important ones are as a chelator for urinary calcium and as a physiologic urinary base.[214] It is a tricarboxylic acid cycle intermediate, and the majority of citrate reabsorbed by the proximal tubule is oxidized to electroneutral end products; thus, H^+ is consumed in the process, rendering citrate a major urinary base. Calcium has a 1:1 stoichiometric association with citrate, with high affinity and solubility as a monovalent anionic ($Ca^{2+}citrate^{3-}$)$^-$ complex.[214]

The final amount of citrate excreted in urine is determined by the extent of reabsorption in the proximal tubule, and the most important regulator of citrate reabsorption is proximal tubule cell pH. Acid loading increases citrate absorption by four mechanisms (see Figure 8-12):

(1) Low luminal pH titrates citrate^{3-} to citrate^{2-}, which is the preferred transported species.[234]
(2) NaDC1 is also gated by pH in such a way that low pH acutely stimulates its activity.[235]
(3) Intracellular acidosis increases expression of the NaDC1 transporter[236] and insertion of NaDC1 into the apical membrane.
(4) Intracellular acidosis stimulates enzymes that metabolize citrate in the cytoplasm and mitochondria.[237,238]

This is a well-concerted process, and an appropriate response of the proximal tubule to cellular acidification is hypocitraturia. Although perfectly adaptive from an acid-base point of view, this response is detrimental to prevention of calcium precipitation. All conditions that lead to proximal tubular cellular acidification (e.g., distal renal tubular acidosis, high-protein diet, potassium deficiency) are clinical risk factors for calcareous nephrolithiasis. Hypocitraturia can cause kidney stones by itself or by acting with other risk factors such as hypercalciuria. Therapy with potassium citrate reverses the biochemical defect and reduces the rate of stone recurrence.

Uric Acid

COMPLEXITY OF URIC ACID HANDLING BY THE PROXIMAL TUBULE

Before a discussion of disorders of uric acid and the role of the kidney, the current knowledge base about uric acid handling must be reviewed. At present, renal handling of uric acid still remains poorly understood. Although there is some merit to the classical multicomponent, quadruple-tandem model of filtration-reabsorption-secretion-reabsorption, much debate has been generated as to the accuracy of this model, mainly because of its heavy dependence on inhibitors for interpreting results and the lack of direct measurements of axial differences in uric acid secretion and reabsorption. For example, the assumption that pyrazinamide, probenecid, benzbromarone, and sulfinpyrazone are pure inhibitors of uric acid secretion or absorption is rather unfounded,[239] and the existence of postsecretory absorption is conjectural at best. In addition, ambiguous molecular identity of the transporters and their locale, as well as the disparity between rodents and humans, renders the construction of a full model very difficult.

Molecular identification and functional evidence of the proteins involved are just beginning to emerge. If researchers compile a list of anion transporters that accept uric acid as a substrate in expression systems and confirm their location in the proximal tubule, it is possible to conjure a model such as that shown in Figure 8-14. It is premature to place these transporters in the same cell of a model and definitely not appropriate to try to assign them to the four-component model.

APICAL TRANSPORTERS

The apical membrane hosts numerous urate transporters from diverse transporter families. URAT1 (SLC22A12), which is a member of the OAT family, exchanges urate for an array of anions[229] (see Figure 8-14). The best evidence of the role of URAT1 as an apical urate absorber is that homozygous or compound heterozygous inactivating mutations of URAT1 in humans lead to hypouricemia from renal leakage.[240] Likewise, in *Urat*-null mice (rodent equivalent of URAT1 is RST), reabsorption of uric acid is defective.[241] Inhibition of URAT1 by drugs such as probenecid, losartan, benzbromarone, and high-dose salicylates probably explains the uricosuric effects of these agents.[229] OAT4 on the apical membrane also exchanges urate for various anions, including monocarboxylates[228] (see Figure 8-14). The Na+-coupled sodium

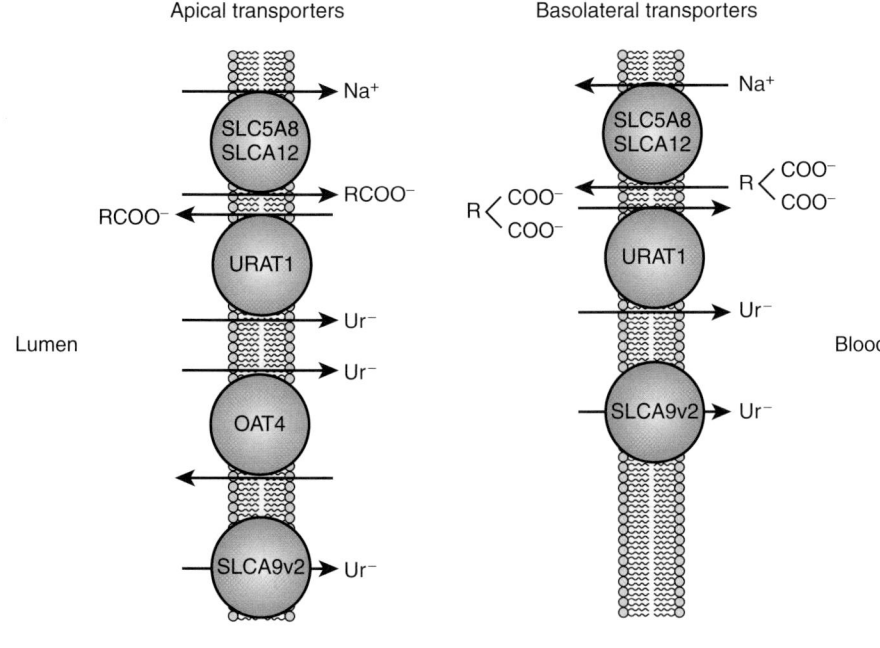

FIGURE 8-14 Potential uric acid transporters in the two membranes of the proximal tubule. A cell model is not presented because there is no evidence yet to suggest that all these transporters are expressed in the same cell. Modes that sustain urate (Ur⁻) absorption are represented by *black arrows*. Modes that sustain Ur⁻ secretion are represented by *red arrows*. GLUT, glucose transporter; MRP, multidrug resistance–related protein; NaDC, Na+ dicarboxylate cotransporter; NPT, sodium inorganic phosphate transporter; OAT, organic anion transporter; SMCT, sodium monocarboxylate transporter; UAT, uric acid transporter; URAT, uric acid anion transporter.

monocarboxylate transporters 1 and 2 (SMCT1 and SMCT2; SLC5A8 and SLC5A12) provides the monocarboxylate for URAT1 in a tertiary active transport mode. In support of this model is the observation that double deletion of SMCT1 and SMCT2 in the kidneys leads to hyperuricosuria without a decrease in URAT1. OAT4 also supports urate/organic dicarboxylate exchange and can theoretically couple with NaDC1, but there is currently no evidence of what role OAT4 plays in urate absorption.

Uric acid transporter/channel (UAT; galectin 9) is a ubiquitous protein belonging to family of glycan-binding proteins that also sustains uric acid transport in vitro and can potentially function as a "channel" that facilitates diffusion.[242] If UAT mediates uric acid transport in vivo, it is difficult to predict whether UAT will transport urate into the lumen or cell. NPT1 (OATv1) was originally cloned functionally as a Na^+-dependent inorganic phosphate cotransporter, but it was subsequently shown to be a voltage-gated OAT that could transport urate.[243] Multidrug resistance–related protein 4 (MRP4), which belongs to the ATP-binding cassette family of proteins, resides on the apical membrane and may secrete urate energized by ATP.[244,245] The association between plasma levels of uric acid and one member of the facilitative glucose transporter 9 (GLUT9) led to the examination and discovery of this protein as a urate transporter ($K_m \approx 1$ mmol) and interest in it as a possible hexose/urate exchanger.[246] Quite distinct from the other candidates, GLUT9 is not coupled to other organic anions. A triple coupling of SMCT, URAT1, and GLUT9 has been proposed to represent net Na^+-glucose cotransport with urate and monocarboxylate recycling.[247] Figure 8-14 summarizes these transporters and depicts them in the predicted mode of transport.

BASOLATERAL TRANSPORTERS

The basolateral transporters are equally diverse, and their proven function is similarly uncertain. OAT1 and OAT3 are located in the basolateral side, and both transport urate; OAT1 has higher affinity.[240] Urate transport is *trans*-stimulated by dicarboxylic anions such as α-ketoglutarate and PAH.[248] Basolateral NaDC3 provides influx of dicarboxylate anions to facilitate urate efflux.[216,217] Conversely, OAT1 and OAT3 can sustain urate uptake from the blood into the cell and participate in tubular urate secretion. Compatible with this notion is the fact that in *Oat1*- and *Oat3*-null mice, secretion and not absorption is decreased.[241] Like UAT, GLUT9 is also expressed in both apical and basolateral membranes and can potentially function in an opposing manner. The interior negative voltage would be greatly conducive to negative electrogenic urate efflux, but the movement of glucose from cell to plasma is conducive to urate uptake. The basolateral efflux mode is supported by the finding that inactivating mutations lead to hypouricemia.[249]

CLINICAL IMPLICATIONS

Clinical disorders of uric acid have reached new levels of significance beyond that of gouty arthritis, uric acid nephrolithiasis, and acute urate nephropathy. The effect of hyperuricemia on cardiovascular morbidity has been controversial, but new experimental and human data continue to emerge to support this connection.[250] The existence of chronic urate nephropathy and whether uric acid is an independent risk factor for renal disease from all causes continues to be a topic of intense debate.[251] From studies of population genetics, a large number of genes have been either shown to be or implicated as determinants of plasma uric acid levels (e.g., *SLC2A9, SLC5A8, SLC13A3, SLC16A9, SLC17A1, SLC22A6, SLC22A8, SLC22A11, SLC22A12, ABCC4, ABCG2, GCKR, LRRC16A, PDZK1*). Included among these are 11 proteins that are either proven or putative uric acid transporters. Some of the candidate genes such as that for GLUT9 (*SLC2A9*) were demonstrated to transport urate[252,253] and, in several population-based studies, to contribute to plasma uric acid levels.[254-256]

A host of uricosuric substances such as probenecid, phenylbutazone, sulfinpyrazone, benzbromarone, and some nonsteroidal antiinflammatory agents inhibit URAT1 from the luminal aspect.[257] The angiotensin II receptor losartan, which lowers blood uric acid through its uricosuric actions, also inhibits URAT1.[258]

Mutations involving URAT1 (*SLC22A12*) cause idiopathic renal hypouricemia,[229,240] a rare autosomal recessive disorder observed in Japanese persons and Iraqi Jews. The lack of functional URAT1 transporter leads to hypouricemia and hyperuricosuria, resulting in crystalluria and kidney stones. Some patients can experience exercise-induced acute renal failure, probably from a combination of rhabdomyolysis and acute urate nephropathy.[259] Sequencing of *SLC22A12* in Japanese cohorts with idiopathic renal hypouricemia revealed two patients who did not have missense mutations in this gene.[240] This suggests that noncoding sequences or additional loci related to urate transport or metabolism could be involved in renal hypouricemia.

Uremic Toxins

Many substances that are collectively referred to as "uremic toxins" are retained in renal failure, and their accumulation contributes to the uremic state. The expanding group of proven and putative uremic toxins is estimated to exceed 110 substances. These highly diverse compounds have chemical properties as expansive as their identities. No single transporter possesses the ability to handle their excretion, but a variety of organic anion and cation transporters participate in uremic toxin clearance.[260] Transporters in the SLCO family accept an extremely broad range of substrates. SLCO4C1 expression is reduced in 5/6 nephrectomized rats with chronic kidney disease,[233] and genetic overexpression of SLCO4C1 in mice reduces plasma levels of specific potential uremic toxins, such as asymmetric dimethyl arginine, guanidine succinate, and *trans*-aconitate,[261] and in amelioration of hypertension and histologic indices of renal inflammation. The role of transporters in uremic toxin elimination is still being studied and holds promise for therapeutic potential.[251]

Amino Acids

Physiology of Renal Amino Acid Transport

The amount of free amino acids in the plasma total approximately 2.5 mmol,[262] and the daily filtered load amounts to approximately 400 mmol. Studies involving stop-flow techniques, micropuncture, and microperfusion identified the renal proximal tubule as the principal site of renal amino acid reabsorption.[262] Although net transepithelial reabsorption typically predominates, there is also a physiologically important influx of many amino acids from the blood into renal cells across the basolateral membrane. The situation is further complicated by tubular amino acid metabolism. Renal glutamine breakdown plays a key role in acid-base balance, and renal conversion of citrulline to arginine is the most important source of this dibasic amino acid in the whole body.[263]

In contrast to the other transport processes highlighted in this chapter that are generally restricted to the proximal tubule, all cells of the renal nephron express an array of distinct amino acid transporters that play some role in the metabolic needs of the cells. In addition, amino acid transporters in Henle's loop contribute to high concentrations of amino acids that serve a protective role against the high ionic strength associated with the urine-concentrating mechanism.[264] The tubular and organ physiology of renal amino acid transport deduced from classical studies was discussed in detail by Silbernagl.[265] In this chapter, attention is focused on the molecular and cellular physiology of amino acid transport in the proximal tubule.

Molecular Biology of Amino Acid Transport

Renal reabsorption of amino acids occurs mainly in the proximal convoluted tubule (S1 and S2 segments) and, to a lesser extent, in the proximal straight tubule (S3 segment).[265] Findings in physiologic studies defined transport systems of amino

acids in renal and intestinal epithelium, and results of cloning of mammalian amino acid transporters established the molecular correlates and showed that the epithelial cells in the gut and kidneys have a similar set of amino acid transporters on their plasma membrane.[266] Amino acid transport in the kidneys is more complex than in the intestines because for some amino acids, low-affinity and high-affinity transporters are differentially distributed along the convoluted and straight tubules, respectively.

Transepithelial flux of amino acids from the lumen to the interstitial space requires transport through apical and basolateral plasma membranes (Figure 8-15). The easier accessibility to apical membranes allowed researchers to obtain faster and deeper knowledge of the transporters in the apical membranes in the past. This situation still stands in the age of genome research.

Neutral Amino Acids

APICAL TRANSPORTERS
In the mouse genome region homologous to the human Hartnup locus, Bioinformatic screen for membrane proteins identified the Na+-dependent neutral amino acid transporter B0AT1.[267] Through sequence comparison, this transporter was designated as a new member of the "orphan transporter" branch of the neurotransmitter sodium symporter family, which prompted functional screening of other members with no neurotransmitter transport function. As a result, IMINO,[267a,267b] B0AT2,[268,269] XT2,[269a] and taurine

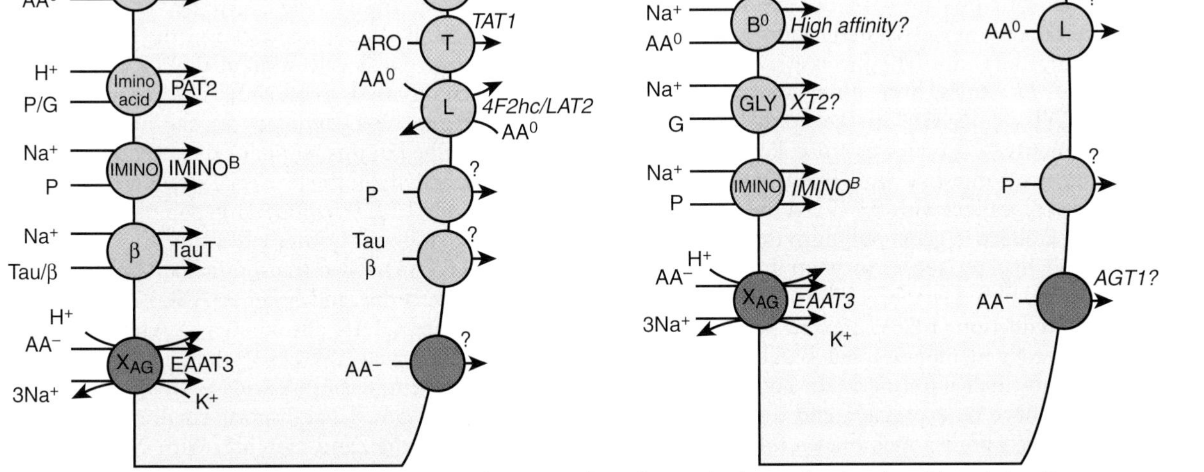

FIGURE 8-15 Transporters involved in renal reabsorption of amino acids in the proximal convoluted and straight tubules. Transporters are colored depending on the substrates: dibasic (*blue*), neutral (*beige*), and anionic (*red*). Letters *inside the spheres* refer to the amino acid transport systems, and letters in *italics* refer to the molecular identity of the transporter (see text for details). Efflux system L and efflux systems for proline (P), taurine (Tau), β-alanine (β), and anionic amino acids (AA−) have been detected in the basolateral membrane, but their molecular entity (indicated by *question marks*) has not been identified (see text for details; by Bröer[341]). Not depicted are basolateral Na+-dependent transporters with no clear function in renal reabsorption, such as EAAT2 for anionic amino acids in the proximal convoluted and straight tubules; system N amino acid transporter 3 [SNAT3] for glutamine, histidine, and asparagine in the proximal straight tubule; glycine transporter in the proximal straight tubule; and system β for taurine and β-alanine. *AA0*, Neutral amino acids; *AA+*, dibasic amino acids; *ARO*, aromatic amino acids; *CSSC*, cystine; *CSH*, cysteine; *G*, glycine.

transporter (TauT)[269b,269c,269d] were identified. Proton amino acid transporters 1 and 2 (PAT1 and PAT2; SLC36 family) were cloned by sequence homology to plant members of the H$^+$-coupled amino acid auxin permease (AAAP) superfamily. **B^{0}AT1 (SLC6A19).** B^{0}AT1 corresponds to the major apical neutral amino acid transport system B^0 (or neutral brush border).[270] An additional B^0-like activity in the proximal straight tubule (S3 segment) has unknown molecular identity.[341] Main characteristics of B^{0}AT1 are as follows: (1) It is an amino acid symporter of low affinity (Michaelis constant in the low millimolar range for L-leucine) with Na$^+$ with 1:1 stoichiometry; (2) it is different from other neurotransmitter transporters of SLC6 family in that it is chloride independent; (3) it transports all neutral amino acids with preference for large aliphatic amino acids; and (4) Michaelis constants for amino acid substrate and Na$^+$ are highly dependent on the concentration of the cotransported molecule.[272] B^{0}AT1 is expressed in the apical membranes of epithelial cells from glomerulus to S1 and S2 (and even S3) segments and in the small intestine.[267,273,274]

Major data concerning the functional role of B^{0}AT1 came from studies of Hartnup's disorder (OMIM code 234500)[273,275] (Table 8-6), an inherited aminoaciduria with hyperexcretion of all neutral amino acids except proline. Twenty-one B^{0}AT1 mutations have been identified (missense, nonsense, frameshift, and splice-site).[276,277] Hartnup's disorder has been linked to B^{0}AT1 mutations in all affected families that have been studied[276] except one.[273] Clearly, B^{0}AT1 is the predominant transporter for neutral amino acid reabsorption in the renal tubule. Most clinical symptoms could be explained by tryptophan deficiency, resulting from defective intestinal and renal absorption, which is a relevant precursor of serotonin and niacin biosynthesis.

Auxiliary Proteins for B^{0}AT1. Collectrin and angiotensin converting enzyme 2 (ACE2) are two type 1 membrane proteins needed for cell surface expression of B^{0}AT1 and proper transport function.[277-279] The transmembrane segment and flanking regions of collectrin and ACE2 are homologous, but collectrin lacks the extracellular HEMGH carboxypeptidase domain (a single catalytic domain with zinc-binding motif). Murine collectrin is mainly expressed in the kidneys (proximal tubule and collecting duct), in the pancreas, and, to a lesser extent, in the small intestines, liver, heart, and stomach.[278] Collectrin and B^{0}AT1 colocalize in the apical membrane in S1 and S2 segments.[278] In contrast to collectrin, ACE2 is expressed in the small intestine with B^{0}AT1 in the apical membrane and also colocalizes with B^{0}AT1 in the S1, S2, and S3 segments.[277,279] Collectrin gene–null mice exhibited tyrosine crystalluria and hyperexcretion of neutral amino acids, a syndrome that resembled Hartnup's disorder.[278,279a] These mice also exhibited reduction of B^{0}AT1 expression and activity in renal brush border membranes, but B^{0}AT1 expression was unaffected in the small intestine.[277] In contrast, ACE2 gene knockout mice have no expression and transport function of B^{0}AT1 in brush border membranes form the small intestine, whereas expression of B^{0}AT1 in renal brush borders is not affected.[277] The different behavior of some missense B^{0}AT1 mutations with collectrin and ACE2 also explains the different involvement of the kidneys and intestines in cases of Hartnup's disorder. B^{0}AT1 mutations involving D173N and P265L are activated by ACE2 but not by collectrin, correlating with cases with affected kidney, but not intestinal,

phenotype.[277] Mutations that disrupt ACE2 interaction with B^{0}AT1 cause intestinal malabsorption of neutral amino acids without renal aminoaciduria.[280]

The mechanism by which collectrin and ACE2 promote B^{0}AT1 expression and function is not well understood. In the absence of collectrin (and ACE2), B^{0}AT1 is not expressed in the plasma membrane. Ablation of collectrin in mice also depletes other renal brush border transporters of the SLC6 transporter family, such as IMINO and XT2.[278,279a] In this sense, hyperexcretion of amino acids in urine in the B^{0}AT1 gene–knockout mice also include acid and basic amino acids,[278] which suggests that collectrin may also have a role in other amino acid transporters. Collectrin has been linked with function of the exocytotic machinery.[281] How the collectrin-exocytotic pathway is connected to apical expression of transporters in the proximal tubule remains to be established.

Once in the membrane, collectrin and ACE2 interact noncovalently with SLC6 transporters (B^{0}AT1 and XT2 for collectrin and B^{0}AT1 for ACE2).[277,278] The auxiliary proteins may also affect the activity of the associated transporters. The transport activity of B^{0}AT1 is increased 6- to 10-fold by coexpression of ACE2, whereas surface expression of the transporters is increased only twofold to threefold.[277] ACE2 may have an additional mechanism of activation of B^{0}AT1. ACE2 is a carboxypeptidase, which removes the terminal amino acid from peptides and thus converts angiotensins I and II to angiotensins 1-9 and 1-7, respectively; as a result, its homolog ACE is antagonized (reviewed by Camargo et al[277]). The ACE2-B^{0}AT1 connection fosters the idea that ACE2 might channel amino acid substrates from peptide degradation in the intestinal lumen to B^{0}AT1. In fact, this has been demonstrated in *Xenopus* oocytes that coexpress both proteins.[279]

B^{0}AT2 (SLC6A15). Functional studies demonstrated that B^{0}AT2 (also known as v7-3 and SBAT1) is a Na$^+$-dependent high-affinity (K$_m$ ≈ 200 μmol) transporter of neutral branched amino acids (leucine, isoleucine, and valine), methionine, and proline, similar to B^{0}AT1.[268,269] B^{0}AT2 transports other neutral amino acids with low affinity (Michaelis constant in the millimolar range) and does not transport aromatic amino acids, β-amino acids, glycine, and γ-aminobutyric acid (GABA). B^{0}AT2 is expressed in the kidneys, but to the authors' knowledge, localization of B^{0}AT2 along the nephron has not been reported. Because B^{0}AT2 is expressed in the S3 segment, it may be a candidate for the high-affinity B^0-like activity described in this region of the proximal tubule. A system B^0-like activity in the proximal straight tubule (putatively B^{0}AT2 in the 12q21 region) is a potential explanation for unexplained cases of Hartnup's disorder.

ASCT2 (SLC1A5). Two transporters are isoforms of the system for alanine, serine, and cysteine (ASC): ASCT1 (SLC1A4) and ASCT2 (SLC1A5; also known as ATB^0). ASCT2 is the correlate of intestinal ASC.[282,283] ASCT2 is a Na$^+$-dependent exchanger of neutral amino acids with variable stoichiometry for Na$^+$.[283a] ASCT2 transports small neutral amino acids (e.g., alanine, serine, and cysteine) with Michaelis constants of approximately 20 μmol and transports other neutral amino acids (e.g., glycine, leucine, and methionine) with affinity of an order of magnitude lower.[283] ASCT2 is expressed in the proximal tubule apical membrane.[284]

Beside the location of ASCT2, there is limited evidence that this transporter has a role in renal reabsorption. Because ASCT2 is an antiporter, its participation in active amino

TABLE 8-6 Primary Inherited Aminoacidurias

DISORDER	OMIM CODE	PREVALENCE	INHERITANCE	GENE	CHROMOSOME	MUTATIONS	TRANSPORT SYSTEM	PROTEIN	LOCALE
Cystinuria*	220100	1:7000	AR/ADIP	*SLC3A1*	2p16.3	133	$b^{0,+}$	rBAT	apical
				SLC7A9	19q13.1	95	$b^{0,+}$	$B^{0,+}AT$	apical
LPI	222700	≈200 cases	AR	*SLC7A7*	14q11	49	$y^{+}L$	$y^{+}LAT1$	baso-lateral
Hyperdibasic aminoaciduria type I	222690	very rare	AD	?	?	?	?	?	?
Hartnup's disorder	234500	1:26000	AR	*SLC6A19*	5p15	21	B^{0}	$B^{0}AT1$	apical
Renal familial iminoglycinuria	242600	1:15000	Complex	*SLC36A2*	5q33	2	Imino acid	PAT2	apical
				(*SLC6A20*)	3921	1	IMINO	IMINO	apical
				(*SLC6A19*)	5p15	1 Poly$	B^{0}	$B^{0}AT1$	apical
(Glycinuria)	138500	1:15000	Complex	(*SLC6A18*)	5p15	2 and 2 Poly$	?	XT2	apical
Dicarboxylic aminoaciduria	222730	very rare	AR?	*SLC1A1*	9p24	KO null	X_{AG}^{-}	EAAT3	apical

AR, autosomal recessive; *ADIP*, autosomal dominant with incomplete penetrance; *AD*, autosomal dominant; *AR?*, unclear but familial studies in the very few cases described for these diseases suggest an autosomal recessive mode of inheritance; *LPI*, lysinuric protein intolerance; *PAT2*, proton amino acid transporter 2. Complex inheritance refers to autosomal recessive mode on inheritance of a major gene (*SLC36A2*) with other genes (*SLC6A20, SLC6A19, SLC6A18*) acting as modifiers indicated in parenthesis. * , Four phenotypes of cystinuria, depending on the obligate heterozygotes, are considered: type I (with AR inheritance), type non-I (ADIP inheritance), mixed type (combination of both) and isolated cystinuria. $, Poly, polymorphism. See text for details and references.

acid reabsorption could be envisaged only in terms of cooperation with a secondary active transporter (i.e., analogous to the cooperation of the heterodimer rBAT/b$^{0,+}$AT and B^{0}AT1 for reabsorption of cationic amino acids and cystine). In this sense, ASCT2 at low pH interacts with anionic amino acids (apparent K$_m$ ≈ 1.6 mmol for L-glutamate).[283a] Thus, uptake of glutamate in exchange with neutral amino acids through ASCT2, followed by recapture of neutral amino acids by B^{0}AT1, might represent a tertiary active reabsorption system for glutamate. This mechanism could be the basis of the moderate hyperexcretion of glutamate in patients with Hartnup's disorder caused by B^{0}AT1 mutations.

IMINO (SLC6A20). There are three transport systems for proline, hydroxyproline, and glycine in the brush border membranes of the proximal tubule[285]: (1) a low-affinity system shared by the three amino acids (reminiscent of the intestinal IMINO system); (2) a high-affinity system specific for proline and hidroxyproline (system IMINO); and (3) a high-affinity system specific for glycine (system Gly). The transporter IMINO (also known as SIT, XT3, STRP3, and rB21A) is the molecular correlate of system IMINO. IMINO transports proline, hydroxyproline, and N-methylated amino acids and analogs in a Na$^+$- and Cl$^-$-dependent manner, characteristic of the SLC6 family. Broer and colleagues[341] proposed naming the human transporter SLC6A20, the rat transporter XT3 (also known as rB21A), and the mouse XT3s1 transporter as *IMINO^B*, to distinguish from *IMINO^K*, a highly homologous gene with syntenic locations in rat (XT3s1) and mouse (XT3) genomes and with no ascribed transport function. *IMINO^B* is expressed in brain and in the apical membrane of the small intestine and kidney,[274] particularly in the S2 and S3 segments.[269] Mutations in this transporter, in combination with mutations in PAT2, resulted in iminoglycinuria,[271] characterized by hyperexcretion of proline, hydroxyproline, and glycine (see upcoming "PAT2 (SLC36A2)" section and Table 8-6).

XT2 (SLC6A18). XT2 is expressed only in the kidneys and localizes in the apical membrane of the S3 segment.[286] Expression of XT2 (also known as XTRP2 and Rosit) in a heterologous system showed no transport function with the substrates tested.[287] However, XT2 gene–knockout mice do have moderate glycinuria (values threefold higher than those of controls).[286] Brush border membranes prepared from the renal medullae of these mice lacked a high-affinity component of glycine transport. In humans, mutation G496R and polymorphisms Y319X and L478P of XT2 showed some correlation with iminoglyvinuria and hyperglycinuria caused by mutations in PAT2.[271] XT2 with Y319X is expected to obliterate function but is highly prevalent and in Hardy-Weinberg equilibrium in human populations (around 0.4:1 in French-Canadian, Australian, and Japanese populations).[288] Thus, about 16% of humans would be devoid of XT2 transport activity. This suggests that there is very little evolutionary pressure on this human gene. An interesting feature in XT2 gene–knockout mice is systolic hypertension,[286] which is perhaps indicative of a potential role of glycine in blood pressure control. In the only human study, there was no association between the Y319X polymorphism and hypertension in 1000 individuals from a region in Japan.[288] As a whole, functional differences between humans and rodents are expected for XT2, and the exact role of human XT2 is unclear at present.

PAT1 (SLC36A1). PAT1 is the molecular correlate of the intestinal imino acid system.[289] Main characteristics of PAT1

are as follows: (1) It is a low-affinity (Michaelis constant in the low millimolar range for preferred substrates) amino acid symporter with H$^+$ with 1:1 stoichiometry; (2) glycine, proline, and alanine are preferred substrates, and PAT1 also transports GABA, β-alanine, and N-methyl amino acids (e.g., 2-[methylamino]-isobutyrate [MeAIB], sarcosine) with similar affinity; and (3) it is not stereospecific for L- and D-isomers.[289,289a] PAT1 has a steep pH dependence. The intestinal imino acid system was initially defined as Na$^+$ dependent. Functional coupling between PAT1 (H$^+$–amino acid transporter) and Na$^+$/H$^+$ exchanger isoform 3 in intact intestinal epithelia explains the apparent Na$^+$ dependence of the imino acid carrier in mammalian intestine.[289] PAT1 is highly expressed in the kidneys, but its location along the nephron is not yet known. Despite the biochemical evidence of a role of PAT1 in renal reabsorption of glycine and proline, individuals with iminoglycinuria and hyperglycinuria do not have mutations in the gene for this transporter.[271]

PAT2 (SLC36A2). PAT2 is considered to be the high-affinity isoform of the Imino acid system. PAT2 has a transport mechanism similar to that of PAT1 (H$^+$ symport with 1:1 stoichiometry), with small differences: (1) less steep pH dependence, (2) higher apparent affinity for the preferred substrates, (3) among the preferred substrates, a higher maximum velocity of glycine than of proline and alanine, and (4) lower affinity for GABA and β-alanine.[289b] PAT2 is expressed in the apical membrane of the S1 segment, close to the glomerulus.[271]

The role of PAT2 in reabsorption of renal imino acids (proline and hydroxyproline) and glycine has been elegantly demonstrated by data from studies of renal familial iminoglycinuria (OMIM code 242600) and glycinuria (OMIM code 138500)[271] (see Table 8-6). Autosomal recessive iminoglycinuria is characterized by hyperexcretion of imino acids and glycine, and heterozygotes were considered to present isolated hyperglycinuria.[290] Mutations of known imino acid and glycine transporters revealed a more complex situation.[271]

Mutations in one or two alleles of PAT2 segregate with iminoglycinuria and hyperglycinuria. In addition, mutations and polymorphisms in the genes for three other transporters (IMINO^B, B^{0}AT1, and XT2) act as modifier genes. In patients with the PAT2 missense mutation G87V, activity for proline and glycine is decreased as a result of decreased substrate affinity. Splice-site mutations in the first intron (IVs1+1G→A) in donor genes alter normal splicing and yield a nonfunctional truncated protein. One missense mutation (T199M) in IMINO^B also cosegregates with iminoglycinuria and has normal expression at the cell surface but loses 90% of proline transport. These three mutations explain six of the seven cases of iminoglycinuria studied and 12 of the 14 cases of hyperglycinuria studied. The authors identified a B^{0}AT1 polymorphism (IVS7-4G→A; present in >20% in the general population) that exists in the homozygous state in the unexplained case of iminoglycinuria and in the heterozygous state in the two other cases of hyperglycinuria. This polymorphism is not sufficient explanation alone, inasmuch as individuals with neither iminoglycinuria nor hyperglycinuria in the study are homozygous for IVS7-4G→A. The two unexplained cases of hyperglycinuria were in patients in the same family, and so it is possible that a missing mutation (e.g., in intronic regions) in PAT2 may finally explain these cases.

Two mutations (G79S and G496R) and two polymorphisms (Y319X and L478P) in XT2 are correlated weakly with the presence of iminoglycinuria and hyperglycinuria. The role of XT2 in renal reabsorption of imino acids and glycine is not clear because XT2 has not been functionally expressed. In summary, PAT2 and IMINO^B are the major players in the apical reabsorption of imino acids and glycine.

TauT (SLC6A6). TauT is the molecular correlate of the amino acid transport system β, a Na$^+$- and Cl$^-$-dependent, high-affinity transporter for taurine, β-alanine, and GABA in renal brush border membranes of the proximal tubule.[291,292] In contrast, a basolateral efflux pathway for taurine has not been described in the renal proximal tubule. TauT mediates highly concentrative (three orders of magnitude) taurine transport ($K_m \approx 20$ μmol); the stoichiometric relationships are expressed as >2Na$^+$:1Cl$^-$:taurine.[269b,269c,269d] TauT may play two major roles in the kidneys. Upregulation of TauT in Madin-Darby canine kidney cells after hyperosmotic stress suggests that TauT has a role in osmotic regulation. In fact, TauT gene-knockout mice show impaired ability to lower urine osmolality and increase water excretion.[293] These animals have a fractional excretion of taurine similar to the GFR, which suggests that TauT is the major system for renal taurine reabsorption.

BASOLATERAL TRANSPORTERS

The light subunit LAT2 were cloned through methods involving homology[294,295] and TAT1 by expression cloning from rat intestine.[295a] Absorption requires net efflux of neutral amino acids across the basolateral membrane. Beside the TAT1 system for aromatic amino acids (described next), no other uniports for neutral amino acids have been identified in the basolateral membrane of the small intestine and the renal proximal tubule. Orphan transporters from the monocarboxylate transporter family (SLC16)[296] and from the glycoprotein independent L-type transporters (SLC43)[297,298] are candidates for such activities.

TAT1 (SLC16A10). TAT1 is the molecular correlate of system T (Na$^+$-independent uniport system for aromatic amino acids), in which substrate affinity is low ($K_m \approx$ mmol), and it also transports L-dopa and *N*-methylated aromatic amino acids.[295a] TAT1 belongs to the H$^+$-monocarboxylate cotransporter family (SLC16).[296] TAT1, in contrast to other SLC16 members,[300] neither cotransports H$^+$ nor needs ancillary proteins (e.g., basigin and embigin) to reach the plasma membrane and maintain the catalytic activity. TAT1 is highly expressed in the small intestine and kidneys in humans and mice, but it is strangely absent from rat kidneys.[299] Mouse TAT1 is expressed in the basolateral membrane of renal proximal convoluted tubules (S1 and S2 segments).[299] Expression in this location suggests that TAT1 has a direct role in the basolateral efflux of aromatic amino acids or a cooperative role with the 4F2hc/LAT2 exchanger in the basolateral efflux of all neutral amino acids during renal reabsorption.[299] Proof of this notion awaits the study of TAT1-deficient mice. TAT1 is a potential candidate for blue diaper syndrome (OMIM code 211000), an inherited disease characterized by tryptophan malabsorption that results from defective transport in the intestines.

4F2hc/LAT2 (SLC3A2/SLC7A8). This a heterodimer with a heavy subunit (4F2hc) and a light subunit (LAT2) linked by a disulfide bridge, characteristic of the heteromeric amino acid transporters (HATs). No larger oligomeric state has been detected in kidneys or expression in cultured cells.[301] 4F2hc/LAT2 mediates high-affinity (Michaelis constant values in the micromolar range) obligatory exchange of all neutral amino acids except proline with 1:1 stoichiometry.[294,295,302] This activity resembles the classical system L in nonepithelial cells,[302] but with broader substrate specificity, and it resembles the Na$^+$-independent neutral amino acid transport defined in the renal basolateral membrane.[303] LAT2 is highly expressed in the kidneys and small intestine.[294,295] LAT2 localizes to the basolateral membrane in the proximal convoluted tubule (most highly in the S1 segment, less so in the S2 segment, and far less in the S3 segment).[294] This distribution parallels the reabsorption capacity for neutral amino acids along the nephron.[265]

4F2hc/LAT2 is an antiporter and thus cannot mediate net basolateral efflux of neutral amino acids during reabsorption. The transporter, with similar substrate selectivity at both sides of the membrane, has higher affinity for substrates (K_ms $\approx$ 40 to 200 μmol) on the outside[295] than in the cytosolic aspect (Michaelis constants two orders of magnitude higher, in the millimolar range).[304] This asymmetry suggests that the extracellular concentration of neutral amino acids controls the activity of the transporter, but the species of amino acid exchanged depends on the relative concentration of each amino acid on both sides of the basolateral membrane. Knockdown of LAT2 in the proximal tubule–like opossum kidney epithelial (OK) cells resulted in increased intracellular cysteine content; decreased alanine, serine, and threonine content; and lower transepithelial flux of cystine.[305] This suggests that 4F2hc/LAT2 plays a role in cysteine efflux, which is generated after reduction of cystine by glutathione in the cytosol.[306] Whether the transporter has a role in the basolateral uptake of alanine, serine and threonine in the proximal tubule in vivo is unknown.

It is speculated that 4F2hc/LAT2 (with broad substrate specificity), in cooperation with a uniport with highly specific neutral amino acids, can mediate basolateral efflux of any neutral amino acid by recycling common substrates. TAT1, the aromatic amino acid uniport (described previously), colocalizes with 4F2hc/LAT2 in the basolateral membrane of the human proximal convoluted tubule.[307] Coexpression of 4F2hc/LAT2 and TAT1 in oocytes resulted in net efflux of alanine, serine, glutamine, and asparagine, which are not TAT1 substrates.[307] This coupling does not require physical interaction between the transporters and is not specific, inasmuch as 4F2hc/LAT1 (system L exchanger) and LAT4 (SLC43A1; system L uniport) have similar functional cooperation.

Cationic Amino Acids

APICAL TRANSPORTERS

Only one transporter with molecular identity for dibasic amino acids has been identified in the proximal apical membrane: the heterodimer rBAT/b$^{0,+}$AT (related to b$^{0,+}$ amino acid transporter).[16,308,309] The homologous protein 4F2hc also demonstrated amino acid transport in oocytes.[308,310] 4F2hc needs the activity of accompanying proteins for full transport activity.[311] Coexpression with 4F2hc was used to identify LAT1 (system L exchanger)[312,313] and xCT (system x$_c^-$)[314] The rest of the subunits associated with 4F2hc and rBAT, like b$^{0,+}$AT and y$^+$LAT1 were identified by homology.[315,316]

Results of transport studies in proximal tubule suggest that transport for cationic amino acids in the apical membrane is Na$^+$ dependent or Na$^+$ modulated. A defect in such a transport activity may cause hyperdibasic aminoaciduria type I (OMIM code 222690), which differs from cystinuria because of the absence of cystine hyperexcretion and from lysinuric protein intolerance (LPI) because of the absence of hyperammonemia and protein intolerance. The candidate gene is unknown.

rBAT/b[0,+]AT (SLC3A1/SLC7A9). This is the molecular correlate of the renal and intestinal cationic amino acid transport system b[0,+] in brush border membranes from the small intestine and kidneys.[317,318] The heavy subunit (rBAT) and the light subunit (b[0,+]AT) are linked by a disulfide bridge, forming a heterodimer, characteristic of the HATs.[319-321] rBAT/b[0,+]AT mediates obligatory exchange of cationic amino acids, cystine (i.e., two cysteines bound by a disulfide bridge), and neutral amino acids (except imino acids) with 1:1 stoichiometry. Functional characteristics include the following: (1) high affinity for cationic amino acids (lysine, arginine, and ornithine) and for cystine ($K_m \approx 100\ \mu mol$); (2) affinity that is apparently three orders of magnitude higher in the extracellular site than in the intracellular site; and (3) reversible electrogenic exchange of cationic and neutral amino acids.[322-325] The heterodimer rBAT/b[0,+]AT is expressed in the apical membrane of the S1 and S2 segments,[326] in which more than 90% of cystine reabsorption occurs.[265]

Under physiologic conditions, only cationic amino acids are reabsorbed by system b[0,+], in exchange with neutral amino acids (efflux),[344] probably driven by the membrane potential (i.e., negative inside). Similarly, system b[0,+] mediates uptake of cystine from the lumen because once in the epithelial cell, the amino acid is reduced to cysteine. This exchange of system b[0,+] was verified by the fact that mutations in system b[0,+] cause cystinuria,[315,328] characterized by hyperexcretion in urine and intestinal malabsorption of cationic amino acids (lysine, arginine, and ornithine) and cystine but not of other neutral amino acids.[329] Cystine has low solubility and forms cystine crystals and calculi. Moreover, mice with defective rBAT (D140G mutation)[330] or b[0,+]AT (knockout)[331] and Newfoundland dogs with defective rBAT (natural nonsense mutation)[331a] have cystinuria and cystine stones similar to those in humans.

Cystinuria (OMIM code 220100) is recessively inherited; homozygotes hyperexcrete cationic amino acids (mainly lysine) and cystine[332] (Table 8-7; see also Table 8-6). A total of 133 mutations in the rBAT gene (*SLC3A1;* cystinuria type A) and 95 mutations in the b[0,+]AT gene (*SLC7A9;* cystinuria type B) have been identified in humans.[333] In a small proportion of patients ($\approx$3%), no mutations have been identified in exons. These patients may have mutations in promoter genes, regulatory genes, or introns that were not studied. Alternatively, haplotypes with several b[0,+]AT gene polymorphisms may contribute to the cystinuria phenotype, as it has been shown for the group of b[0,+]AT heterozygotes who are cystine stone formers.[335] Brodehl and associates[336] reported a family transmitting isolated cystinuria (i.e., hyperexcretion of cystine without cationic aminoaciduria) with a heterozygous b[0,+]AT gene mutation (T123M) that explained the isolated cystinuria.[337] It is believed that all cases of classic and isolated cystinuria are caused by mutations in system b[0,+]. The rate of cystine clearance is close to the GFR in classic cystinuria[326] (see Table 8-7); thus, system b[0,+] is the major transporter for cystine reabsorption. In contrast, clearance of cationic amino acids is only partially affected in cystinuria,[338] which suggests that other apical transport systems participate in the reabsorption of these amino acids. In fact, a lysine transport activity has been reported in the human kidneys, which was also present in patients with cystinuria.[339] The molecular identity of this transporter is currently unknown.

All b[0,+]AT subunits are linked by a disulfide bridge to rBAT, but not all renal rBAT subunits form heterodimers with b[0,+]AT.[326] rBAT has the higher expression in the S3 segment,[340] where it forms disulfide-linked heterodimers ($\approx$140 kDa) with an unidentified light subunit.[326] This heterodimer (rBAT-X) is in renal brush border membranes from b[0,+]AT gene–knockout mice.[331] It is speculated that this rBAT heterodimer is the Na[+]-stimulated cationic amino acid transporter.[341] However, the mean and range (i.e., fifth to ninety-fifth percentile limits) of cystine, lysine, arginine, and ornithine in the urine of patients with mutations in rBAT and b[0,+]AT genes are almost identical (see Table 8-7).[332] This result is expected because all b[0,+]AT forms heterodimers with rBAT (system b[0,+]) in renal brush border membranes, and it rules out the role of rBAT-X heterodimer in cystine and cationic amino acid reabsorption.

Oligomeric Structure and Biogenesis of rBAT/b[0,+]AT. The native oligomeric state of system b[0,+] is a heterotetramer

TABLE 8-7 Urine Amino Acid Excretion Classified by Genotype and Type of Cystinuria

GENOTYPE	CYSTINURIA TYPE	n	CYSTINE	LYSINE	ARGININE	ORNITHINE
			URINE AMINO ACID EXCRETED (mmol/g CREATININE)			
AA	I	34	1.66 [0.65-3.40]	6.58 [2.65-11.6]	3.14 [0.23-8.37]	1.74 [0.59-3.44]
AA	Mixed	3	0.78, 2.12, 5.56	3.31, 5.72, 11.4	1.23, 2.82, 7.03	0.72, 1.64, 1.92
AA(B)	Mixed	1	2.57	9.84	2.95	5.17
BB	I	1	2.69	2.28	111	0.30
BB	non-I	37	1.62 [0.50-3.30]	6.51 [1.72-14.7]	3.45 [0.50-6.15]	2.20 [0.30-4.77]
B+	non-I carriers	3	0.26*, 0.44*, 0.80	1.64*, 2.45, 3.88	0.02*, 0.12*, 0.15*	0.04*, 0.27*, 0.29*
BB	Mixed	11	1.82 [0.43- 3.18]	4.58 [1.57-8.72]	1.54 [0.21-3.51]	1.33 [0.47-2.45]
BB(A)	Mixed	1	0.43	3.27	489	603

The mean of the amino acid levels for each group is indicated, with the exception of categories with less than 11 patients, for which individual data are shown. When applicable, the fifth and ninety-fifth percentile limits are shown in square brackets. For genotype, A represents one mutated allele in rBAT (SLC3A1); B, one mutated allele in B[0,+]AT (SLC7A9); and +, nonmutated allele in B[0,+]AT. *n*, number of patients.

*Arginine and ornithine excretion values are below fifth percentile of those for homozygotes of cystinuria type non-I (BB) in carriers of cystinuria type non-I.

From Font-Llitjos M, Jimenez-Vidal M, Bisceglia L, et al: New insights into cystinuria: 40 new mutations, genotype-phenotype correlation, and digenic inheritance causing partial phenotype, *J Med Genet* 42:58-68, 2005.

(dimer of heterodimers), in which two dimers catalyze transport independently.[301] Both subunits rBAT and b[0,+]AT need to be coexpressed to reach the plasma membrane. Reconstitution of b[0,+]AT alone revealed full transport activity, which demonstrated that this is the catalytic subunit.[325] Mutations in the rBAT gene cause trafficking defects,[342-344] whereas mutations in the b[0,+]AT gene cause either trafficking defects or inactivation of the transporter, or both.[325,334] The only exception to this rule is the rBAT mutation R365W, which affects both trafficking and transport.[344] The effect of cystinuria-specific rBAT mutations on system b[0,+] trafficking in mammalian cells has been studied in detail, and investigators have developed a minimal working model for the biogenesis of the transporter.[342] Fast interactions of the transmembrane segment of rBAT with folded b[0,+]AT determine formation of the heterodimer within the endoplasmic reticulum. Assembly with b[0,+]AT blocks rBAT degradation via the endoplasmic reticulum–associated degradation (ERAD) pathway. These early steps do not require the calnexin chaperone system, but after assembly, the rBAT extracellular domain folds within that chaperone system. Heterotetramerization proceeds immediately after rBAT folding or is interspersed within the final folding steps. Only the heterotetramers exit the endoplasmic reticulum and proceed to the Golgi complex. Mutations of the extracellular domain of rBAT (T216M, R365W, M467T, and M467K) disrupt or delay the postassembly folding of rBAT, hindering stable oligomerization, and lead to degradation.

BASOLATERAL TRANSPORTERS

Only one transporter for dibasic amino acids has been identified at the molecular level in the basolateral membranes of renal epithelial cells: 4F2hc/y[+]LAT1.[316,345]

4F2hc/y[+]LAT1 (SLC3A2/SLC7A7). This is one of the two molecular correlates of system y[+]L and is the mediator of cationic amino acid efflux in epithelial cells. The heavy subunit (4F2hc) and the light subunit (y[+]LAT1) are linked by a disulfide bridge and form a heterodimer, characteristic of the HATs.[316] 4F2hc/y[+]LAT1 mediates electroneutral high-affinity ($K_m \approx 20$ μmol) exchange of cationic amino acids with neutral amino acids plus Na[+] with 1:1:1 stoichiometry.[316,345] The affinity of neutral, but not cationic, amino acids increases by two orders of magnitude in the presence of Na[+]. 4F2hc/y[+]LAT1 is highly expressed in the kidneys, small intestine, placenta, spleen, and macrophages.[347] In epithelial cells, the transporter has a basolateral location.[348] The other system y[+]L isoform (4F2hc/y[+]LAT2) is widely expressed, but less in the kidneys and small intestine than is 4F2hc/y[+]LAT1.[347]

Under physiologic conditions, the high extracellular Na[+] concentration drives the efflux of cationic amino acids in exchange for neutral amino acids. This electroneutral transporter mediates the efflux of cationic amino acids against the membrane potential (negative inside). Proof for this exchange mode is supported by the fact that mutations in y[+]LAT1 cause LPI[349,350] (Table 8-8), which is characterized by increased renal clearance excretion and intestinal malabsorption of only cationic amino acids.[351] Lysinuria is the most prominent aminoaciduria in patients with LPI, with renal clearance values of approximately 25 mL · min[-1] · 1.73 m[-2].

LPI (OMIM code 222700) is a very rare disease (≈200 patients known), probably as a result in part of misdiagnosis, and its mode of inheritance is recessive. Impairment of both intestinal and renal reabsorption of cationic amino acids in homozygotes causes a metabolic derangement characterized by low plasma concentration of cationic amino acids, which causes dysfunction of the urea cycle and thereby leads

TABLE 8-8 Plasma and Urine Amino Acids in LPI and Cystinuria

Plasma Amino Acids

AMINO ACID	NORMAL CHILDREN	PATIENTS WITH LPI MEAN (μmol)	RANGE (μmol)	CONTROLS WITHOUT CYSTINURIA (μmol: MEAN ± SD)	PATIENTS WITH CYSTINURIA (μmol: MEAN ± SD)
Lysine	71-151	70	32-179	171 ± 26	121 ± 30
Arginine	23-86	27	12-58	82 ± 16	46 ± 12
Ornithine	27-86	21	2-83	58 ± 11	36 ± 11
Cystine	48-140	80	57-105	79 ± 12	43 ± 12
Glutamine	57-467	5583	3644-7161	n.d.	n.d.
Alanine	173-305	772	417-1017	n.d.	n.d.

Amino Acids in Urine

AMINO ACID	CONTROLS (n = 83) (mmol/g CREATININE) MEAN	RANGE*	PATIENTS (n = 4) WITH LPI (mmol/1.73 m²/24 h) MEAN	RANGE	PATIENTS (n = 37) WITH CYSTINURIA TYPE B (mmol/g CREATININE) MEAN	RANGE*
Lysine	0.18	0.04-0.50	4.13	1.02-7.00	6.51	1.72-14.7
Arginine	0.02	0.00-0.05	0.36	0.08-0.69	3.45	0.50-6.15
Ornithine	0.03	0.01-0.07	0.11	0.09-0.13	2.20	0.30-4.77
Cystine	0.05	0.02-0.11	0.12	0.06-0.21	1.62	0.50- 3.30

Data for normal children and pediatric patients with lysinuric protein intolerance (LPI) are from Simell.[140a] Plasma glutamine data also include asparagine concentration. Data concerning plasma amino acids from 12 controls and 8 patients with cystinuria are from Morin et al.[193a] Cystinuria type B is the disease caused by mutations in *SLC7A9*; data extracted from Table 8-7.

n.d., Not determined; *SD,* standard deviation.
*Fifth to ninety-fifth percentiles.

to hyperammonemia and protein aversion. In contrast to disorders of apical amino acid transporters (Hartnup's disorder and cystinuria), the basolateral location of the LPI transporter cannot be bypassed by the apical intestinal absorption of peptides containing dibasic amino acids.[352] Thus, affected patients fail to thrive normally. Similarly, the few y$^+$LAT1-null mice that survive the neonatal period display metabolic derangement similar to that of humans with LPI.[353]

Forty-nine mutations (missense, nonsense, and splice-site mutations; frameshift deletions and insertions; and large rearrangements) have been described in y$^+$LAT1.[354,355] Beside aminoaciduria, other symptoms vary widely among patients, even those with the same mutation, which precludes meaningful genotype-phenotype correlations.[351] Four mutations (E36del, G54V, F152L, L334R) are characterized by defective system y$^+$L transport activity despite normal trafficking in heterologous systems, which indicates that transporter activity is defective.[356] Interestingly, mutation E36del causes a dominant negative effect when coexpressed in *Xenopus* oocytes with wild-type y$^+$LAT1 or even y$^+$LAT2.[356] This suggests that 4F2hc/y$^+$LAT1 has a multiheteromeric structure that includes y$^+$LAT2, but biochemical evidence for multiheterodimerization is missing.

As for other HATs, 4F2hc is needed to bring the heterodimer 4F2hc/y$^+$LAT1 to the plasma membrane and specifically to the basolateral membrane in epithelial cells.[352] No LPI mutations have been identified in 4F2hc, which suggests that they may be lethal. In fact, 4F2hc knockout is lethal.[357] 4F2hc serves for six amino acid transporter subunits (LAT1, LAT2, y$^+$LAT1, y$^+$LAT2, xCT, and asc1)[346]; in addition, 4F2hc is necessary for proper function of β1 integrin.[358,359] Thus, defective 4F2hc is probably incompatible with life.

Anionic Amino Acids

The glutamate transporters EAAT3 (also known as EAAC1)[360] and EAAT2 (also known as GLT1) (Pines et al., 1992), from the SLC1 family,[362] were cloned from kidney and brain respectively. The glutamate transporter AGT1 was identified by its homology to b$^{0,+}$AT (SLC7 family) from the kidneys.[362a] Transporters EAAT3 and AGT1 might have a role in renal reabsorption of amino acids in humans. EAAT2 transporter is expressed in the kidneys,[364] but its location in the proximal tubule has not yet been studied. Na$^+$-dependent transport of anionic amino acids has been reported in the basolateral membrane of renal epithelial cells.[365]

APICAL TRANSPORTERS

EAAT3 (SLC1A1). EAAT3 is the molecular correlate of system X$^-_{AG}$. Its activity fits all properties of the high-affinity (K$_m$ < 20 μmol) L-glutamate transporter described in the kidneys and intestines.[341] EAAT3 cotransports three Na$^+$ molecules, one glutamate molecule, and one H$^+$ molecule, and the return of the transporters is facilitated by the binding of one K$^+$ molecule.[363,366] The transporter shows preference for D-aspartate over L-glutamate and transports cystine with a Michaelis constant of approximately 100 μmol. EAAT3 is expressed in the apical membrane of the S2 and S3 segments, with weaker signals in the S1 segment, descending thin limbs of long-loop nephrons, medullary thick ascending limbs, and distal convoluted tubules.[367] This distribution is only partially consistent with reabsorption of glutamate along the nephron[368]: More

than 90% occurs in the S1 segment, where EAAT3 expression is low, and reabsorption remains significant until the process reaches the distal convoluted tubules, which also express EAAT3.

The strongest support for EAAT3 in renal reabsorption is the fact that EAAT3 gene–knockout mice develop dicarboxylic aminoaciduria (values 1400- and 10-fold higher than control values for glutamate and aspartate, respectively).[369] Human dicarboxylic aminoaciduria (OMIM code 222730) is characterized by urinary hyperexcretion of glutamate and aspartate[370] (see Table 8-6). Loss-of-function mutations in human EAAT3 cause dicarboxylic aminoaciduria.[370a]

BASOLATERAL TRANSPORTERS

AGT1 (SLC7A13). AGT1 is one of the light subunits of HATs. Thus, AGT1 forms a disulfide bond between light chain and heavy chain subunits of these transporters. In contrast, none of the two heavy subunits identified (4F2hc and rBAT) resulted in functional coexpression of AGT1 in *Xenopus* oocytes. It is possible that an unknown heavy subunit may form a heterodimer with AGT1.[362a] AGT1 showed Na$^+$-independent transport for acidic amino acids (for L-aspartate and L-glutamate, K$_m$ ≈ 20 μmol). In contrast to the Na$^+$-independent cystine/glutamate transporter xCT, AGT1 does not accept cystine, homocysteate, and l-α-aminoadipate. AGT1 is expressed predominantly in the basolateral membrane of the proximal straight tubules and distal convoluted tubules. No experimental data on human AGT1 are available. The role of AGT1 in renal reabsorption of anionic amino acids is not clear. HATs, with the exception of system ASC isoforms (4F2hc/asc1 and asc2), are tightly coupled amino acid antiporters.[320] If AGT1 is a uniport, the transporter could mediate basolateral net efflux of anionic amino acids in renal reabsorption.

Structural Information of Amino Acid Transporters

Since 2000, the atomic resolution structures of some prokaryotic models of several mammalian amino acids transporters have been reported: (1) the glycerol-3-phosphate/phosphate exchanger GlpT of the major facilitator superfamily, a model for the SLC16 family of transporters (e.g., TAT1)[147]; (2) the Na$^+$-dependent aspartate transporter GltPh of the family of dicarboxylate/amino acid:cation symporters (DAACS), a model for the SLC1 family of transporters (e.g., ASCT2 and EAAT3);[371] (3) the Na$^+$-dependent leucine transporter LeuT, a model for SLC6 (neurotransmitter:sodium symporter) family of transporters (e.g., B^{0}AT1, B^{0}AT2, IMINO, XT2, and TauT)[372]; and the arginine/agmatine exchanger AdiC of the amino acid, polyamine, and organocation (APC) family of transporters, a model for SLC7 family of transporters (light subunits of HATs; e.g., AGT1, b$^{0,+}$AT, LAT2, and y$^+$LAT1).[373,376]

These structures shed light on transport mechanisms and will eventually help explain the basis of the defects associated with human mutations that cause aminoacidurias. In this section, the focus is on transporters with the so-called 5+5 inverted repeat fold of LeuT shared by SLC6 and SLC7 transporters, which are involved in primary inherited aminoacidurias.

Transporters with 5⁺5 Inverted Repeat Fold

The fold of LeuT revealed an internal twofold pseudosymmetric axis, running parallel to the membrane plane through the center of the transporter, which relates the first five transmembrane-spanning helices (TMH1 to TMH5) to the second five helices (TMH6 to TMH10)[372] (Figure 8-16). The LeuT fold has also been observed in other structures such as the galactose transporter vSGLT (solute:sodium symporter family),[24] the benzyl-hydantoin transporter Mhp1 (nucleobase:cation symporter family),[374] the betaine transporter BetP (betaine/choline/carnitine transporter family),[375] and the arginine/agmatine exchanger AdiC (amino acids, polyamines, and organoCations [APC] super family of transporters).[373,376] Amino acid sequences have limited identity (≈10%) among these members, and the members do not even have the same number of transmembrane segments; however, all these new structures contain the 5⁺5 inverted repeat fold defined by TMH1 to TMH10 of LeuT.

The 5⁺5 transmembrane motif consist of two interior pairs of symmetry related helices (TMH1 and TMH6; TMH3 and TMH8), which are surrounded by an arch of outer helices (also related by the two-fold axis of symmetry; TMH2 and TMH7, TMH4 and TMH9, and TMH5 and TMH10, numbered according to LeuT) (see Figure 8-16). In the outer arch of helices, TMH2 and TMH7 link TMH1 and TMH6 with the intracellular and extracellular helix-loop-helix structures IL1 and EL4. The two interior pairs largely define the central translocation pathway that contains the binding sites for substrate and ions, which is consistent with findings in mutagenesis and functional studies.[377] LeuT has a principal substrate-binding site at its center, surrounded by the interior helices, which is similarly but not identically located in vSGLT, Mhp1, and BetP. In transporters with 5⁺5 inverted repeat fold TMH1 and TMH6 (according to LeuT numbering) have a central interruption in their helical conformations, which divides these helices in two parts (TMH1a and TMH1b, and TMH6a and TMH6b). These central interruptions expose main-chain hydrogen-bonding partners and orients the helical dipoles to create a polar environment for coordination of substrate and ions within the lipid bilayer.

These electrostatic elements, together with side-chain atoms, sculpt the steric, chemical, and electric properties of the binding pocket, conferring on a given transporter its particular substrate selectivity.[377] In LeuT, a second substrate binding site lies between the primary site and the external medium, which is suggestive of an allosteric mechanism or a transiently occupied site in the way to the primary binding site from the extracellular vestibule.[378]

LeuT cotransports two Na⁺ molecules per leucine molecule, and the atomic structure of LeuT revealed two Na⁺ binding sites (Na1 and Na2).[372] Na⁺ at the Na1 site is coordinated by five ligands in TMH1, TMH6, and TMH7, and the carboxylate of the substrate leucine reveals direct coupling of the binding of Na⁺ and leucine. The Na2 site is located approximately 6Å away from the Na1 site. Na⁺ binds this site by coordinating with five lateral chains from residues in TMH1 and TMH8. Functional and molecular dynamic studies suggest that Na2 corresponds to the low-affinity Na⁺ site that first dissociates to promote release of leucine. The Na2 site, but not the Na1 site, seems to be conserved in vSGLT and Mhp1 with substrate:Na⁺ stoichiometry of 1:1.[24,374]

Beside intrinsic differences between the different transporter families sharing the 5⁺5 inverted repeat fold, some common themes emerge from the comparisons of the structures of LeuT, Mhp1, vSGLT, BetP, and AdiC providing evidence for the conformation changes of these transporters through the transport cycle.[377,378a] The primary substrate- and ion-binding sites are flanked by two gates, one controlling access to the outside of the cell, the other controlling access to the inside. Only one of these gates is open at a time, allowing substrates and ions to reach the primary binding sites without opening up a continuous transmembrane pore. This is consistent with the alternating access mechanisms depicted in the 1950s[379,380]: an open-to-out conformation of the transporter (Tᵒᵘᵗ) binds substrate and ions (TᴹSᵒᵘᵗ) and then isomerizes to an open-to-in conformation (TᴹSⁱⁿ) before the substrate is released in the cytoplasm (Tⁱⁿ) (Figure 8-17). The main gate closing access to the binding site from the other side of the membrane is a thick (≈20 Å) barrier. Thus, five transmembrane segments, along with the N terminus and IL1, block access to the cytosol in the outward-facing LeuT-leucine structure, whereas

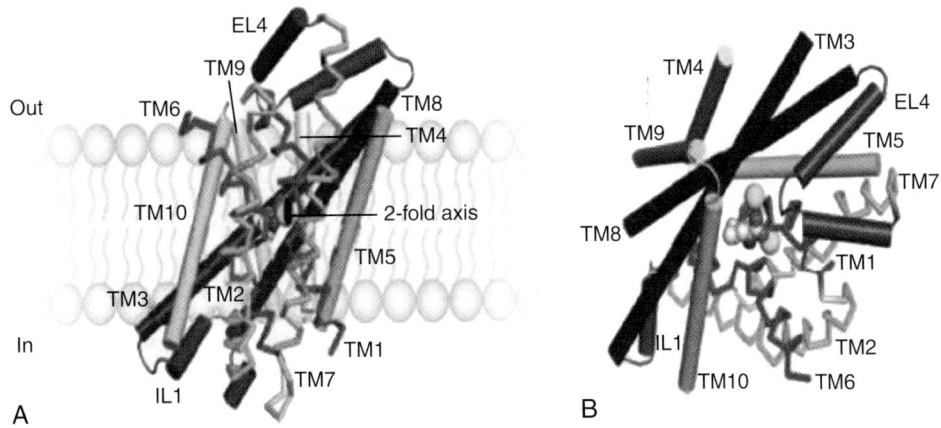

FIGURE 8-16 Architecture of the LeuT fold (5⁺5 inverted repeat fold). Views parallel (**A**) and perpendicular (**B**) to the membrane views of the core 5⁺5 repeat structure of LeuT show the inverted scaffold of TMH4, TMH5, TMH9, and TMH10 holding the two interior pair of helices: the long-tilted helices (TMH3 and TMH8) and the centrally unwounded helices (TMH1 and TMH6; *red*). TMH2 and TMH7 (*green*) embrace TMH1 and TMH6. Reentrant pseudo–two-fold related loops IL1 and EL4 are shown in *brown*. Bound-leucine (carbon, *gray*; oxygen, *red*; nitrogen, *blue*) and two sodium ions (*yellow*) are shown. *TMH*, Transmembrane-spanning helix. (From Krishnamurthy H, Piscitelli CL, Gouaux E: Unlocking the molecular secrets of sodium-coupled transporters, *Nature* 459:347-355, 2009.)

almost the same transmembrane segments, along with EL4, block access to the extracellular medium in the inward-facing vSGLT-galactose structure (see Figure 8-17). The thick gate of each transporter is related to the extracellular or intracellular pathway by the internal two-fold symmetry: the structural elements of the solvent-filled pathway are reciprocal (with regard to the axis of the two-fold symmetry) to those of the thick gates.

According to the findings in studies of crystal structures and functional and molecular dynamics,[381] two major classes of transition occur during the transport cycle.[377] First, substrate binding closes, and unbinding opens, the thin gates to occlude or expose the substrate in the primary binding site, and this involves local conformational changes. Second, the opening and closing of the thick gates switch the transporter between outward-facing and inward-facing states. The thick-gate transition reorients the occluded substrate-transporter complex by rotating a set of membrane-spanning

helices (the "bundle" composed of TMH1, 2, 6 and 7, or the "hash" composed of TMH3, 4, 8 and 9, depending on the transporter) about a central axis approximately perpendicular to the axis of internal two-fold symmetry. The most relevant changes in the LeuT transporter involve rotation of TMH1 and TMH6 (see Figure 8-17). In this scheme, the totally occluded betaine-bound BetP structure[375] may represent an intermediate state between the open-to-out and open-to-in states.

Harnessing Structural Knowledge to Understand Function and Dysfunction

SLC6 Family
The structure of the prokaryotic homolog LeuT from *Aquifex aeolicus* crystallized by Yamashita and associates[372] is approximately 30% identical in amino acid to the mammalian

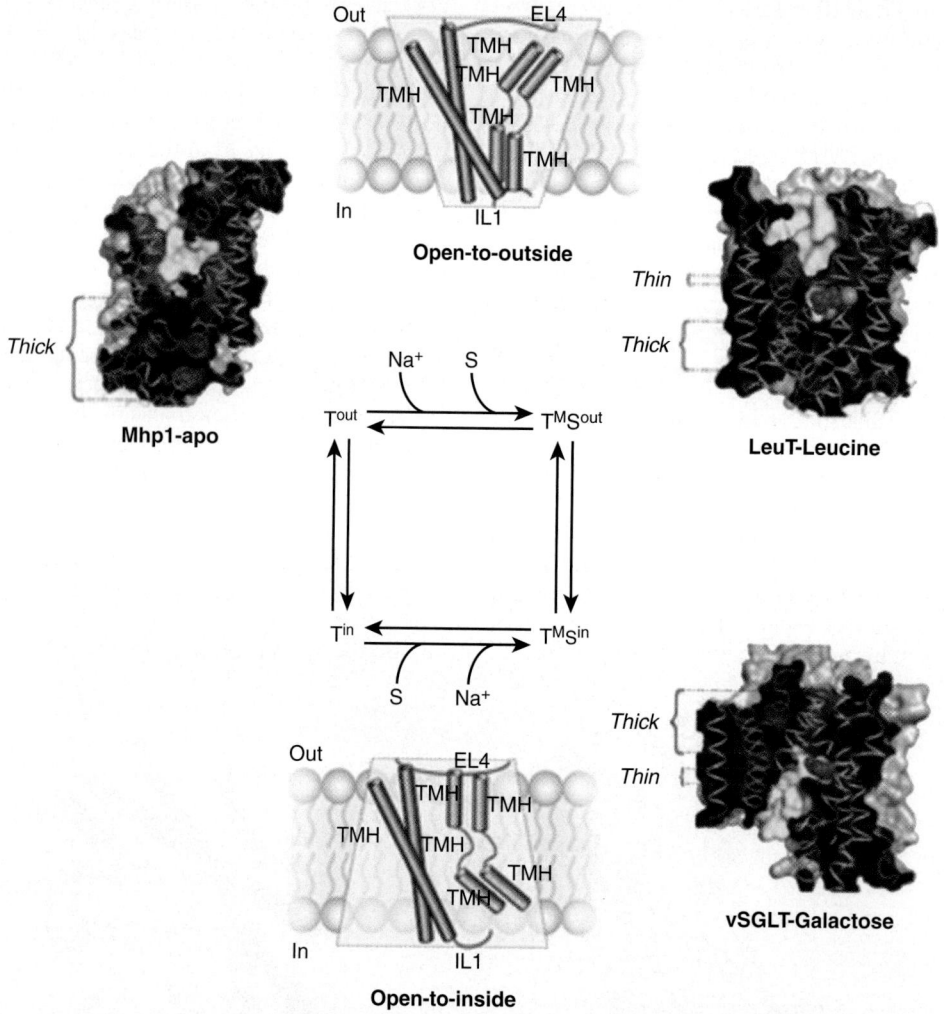

FIGURE 8-17 Crystal structures of transport intermediates of transporters with the LeuT fold. Transport cycle based on an alternating-access type of mechanism together with insights from atomic structures (Mhp1-apo, Protein Data Bank code 2JLN; LeuT-leucine, Protein Data Bank code 2A65; vSGLT-galactose, Protein Data Bank code 3DH4). Cross-sectional illustrations of the crystal structures of each transporter show associations with the states of the cycle that they represent. The positions of the "thin" and "thick" gates are indicated by *red dashed lines* (see text for details). The solvent-accessible solvent areas are shown in *light blue*. Surfaces of the substrate binding site and associated cavities are shown in *yellow*. Van der Waals spheres represent the substrates (*magenta*) and sodium ions (*orange*). The transition between outward-facing states (top) and inward-facing states (bottom) is illustrated in the middle. Transmembrane segments TMH1, TMH3, TMH6, and TMH8 line the central translocation pathway, with EL4 and IL1 acting as lids that seal the extracellular and intracellular gates, respectively, in their closed states. TMH1 and TMH6 rotate approximately 37 degrees in relation to TMH3 and TMH8 in transitioning from the outward-facing state adopted by LeuT (top) to the inward-facing state adopted by vSGLT (bottom). *TMH,* Transmembrane-spanning helix; *vSGLT, Vibrio* sodium-galactose transporter. (From Krishnamurthy H, Piscitelli CL, Gouaux E: Unlocking the molecular secrets of sodium-coupled transporters, *Nature* 459:347-355, 2009.)

transporters of the SLC6 family. Thus, good structural models have been made on the basis of this structure for human B⁰AT1.[277,279] Because the carboxyl group of leucine forms part of the Na1 site in LeuT, these models explain the mutual influence of substrate and Na⁺ on each other's Michaelis constant, which has been observed in B⁰AT1, B⁰AT2, and IMINO[B].[341] Similarly, the Cl⁻-binding site identified in GABA transporter 1 (GAT1) after LeuT structure[381a,382] is conserved in the SLC6 Cl⁻-dependent transporters (e.g., IMINO[B] and TauT) but also in B⁰AT1 and B⁰AT2, which are not Cl⁻-dependent. Therefore, it is possible that a static Cl⁻ ion stabilizes the structure of B⁰AT1 and B⁰AT2.[341]

LeuT-based models of B⁰AT1 structure help investigators understand the molecular bases of mutations that cause Hartnup's disorder. At present, 11 missense mutations have been described, and 9 have been studied for expression at the cell surface and transport function.[277,279] As a result, three categories of mutations for Hartnup's disorder have been proposed.[277] In the first group (R57C, G93R, L242P, E501K, and P579L), the mutations are not active in foreign expression systems either in the absence or in the presence of the auxiliary proteins collectrin and ACE2, probably because of folding defects, with the exception of G93R and E501K. These two mutations affect the intrinsic activity of the transporter. Interestingly, G93 in TMH2 interacts with the intracellular part of TMH6b, and E501 in TMH10 interacts with one of two water molecules that hold the structure of the unwound residues between TMH6a and TMH6b, which interact with the amino acid substrate and Na⁺ at the Na1 site (Figure 8-18). Thus, mutations E501K and G93R most probably affect the folding and position of this unwound region, thereby compromising binding and eventually substrate translocation.

In another group of B⁰AT1 mutations (A69T and R240Q), neither collectrin nor ACE2 stimulates transport. R240Q

co-immunoprecipitates with collectrin and ACE2, but there is no increase in cell surface expression of B⁰AT1, whereas the A69T mutant shows increased surface expression with the auxiliary proteins, but transport function is abolished. This situation suggests that, in addition to increasing B⁰AT1 cell surface expression, collectrin and ACE2 stimulate transport, and this mechanism is affected in the A69T mutation, which results in complete inactivation of B⁰AT1. Of interest is that both residues are related to the extracellular TMH5-TMH6 loop: Ala69 is located in the beginning of TMH2, interacting with the TMH5-TMH6 loop, and R240Q is located at the end of TMH5 (see Figure 8-18). This suggests that the TMH5-TMH6 loop is involved in B⁰AT1 activation by collectrin and ACE2.

The third group of mutations causing Hartnup's disorder (D173N, P265L) abolish functional interaction with collectrin but not with ACE2. ACE2 increases P265L cell surface expression, and transport is activated only partially (in <10% of wild-type organisms). Thus, P265L resembles A69T (a group 2 mutation) but with less inactivation upon ACE2 interaction. Of interest is that Pro265 is located at the beginning of TMH6a, a location similar to that of group 2 mutations (see Figure 8-18). D173N is a hypomorphic polymorphism (frequency of >1:100 in healthy individuals) with 20% of transport function upon activation with ACE2. Asp173 is located in the extracellular EL2 loop (between TMH3 and TMH4), opposite the TMH5-TMH6 loop (see Figure 8-18). This suggests that activation of B⁰AT1 by collectrin and ACE2 involves overall conformational changes in the extracellular loops and not restricted only to the TMH5-TMH6 loop.

Heteromeric Amino Acid Transporters. With the exception of 4F2hc/asc1, HATs are tightly coupled amino acid antiporters[327] composed of a heavy chain (rBAT or 4F2hc) linked by a disulfide bridge to a light subunit (in mammals,

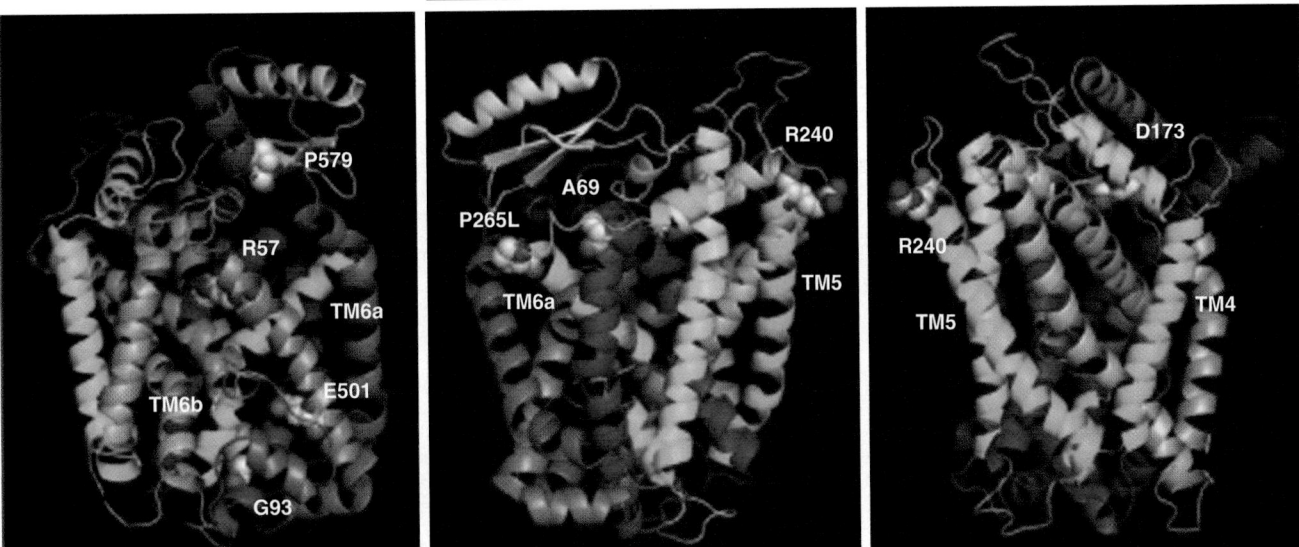

Group 1   Group 2 and 3

FIGURE 8-18 Location of mutated B⁰AT1 residues in Hartnup disorder. Secondary structure illustration of a homology model generated using the atomic structure of the related transporters LeuT[372] and kindly provided by S. Broer[279] Van der Waals spheres (carbon, *gray;* oxygen, *red;* nitrogen, *blue*) representing the residues involved in missense mutations in Hartnup disease are indicated, and distributed by their group of phenotype (see text for details). Transmembrane-spanning helix 12 has been omitted for clarity.

$b^{0,+}AT$ for rBAT; LAT1, LAT2, y^+LAT1, y^+LAT2, asc1, and xCT for 4F2hc; asc2, AGT1, and arpAT for an unidentified heavy subunit). The amino acids of rBAT and 4F2hc (also known as CD98 and FRP1) are less than 30% identical. The heavy subunits (molecular masses ≈ 90 kDa for rBAT and ≈ 80 kDa for 4F2hc) are type II membrane N-glycoproteins with a single transmembrane segment, an intracellular N-terminus, and an extracellular C-terminus domain significantly homologous to insect and bacterial α-amylases (Figure 8-19). The conserved cysteine residue responsible for the intersubunit disulfide bridge is located between the transmembrane segment and the ectodomain. X-ray diffraction of the extracellular domain of human 4F2hc revealed a three-dimensional structure similar to that of bacterial glucosidases: domain A, a triose phosphate isomerase barrel [(αβ)8] and domain C, eight antiparallel β-strands at the C-terminal part (see Figure 8-19).[383] The 4F2hc ectodomain is highly soluble with positively charged residues in the surface connected with the transmembrane segment, which is suggestive of an electrostatic interaction with the plasma membrane.

In contrast to rBAT, for which only the function is as a component of system $b^{0,+}$, 4F2hc has a dual role: as a component of six amino acid transporters and as a necessary component for β1 integrin signaling.[359] Domain swapping and analysis of cystinuria-related point mutations revealed that the rBAT transmembrane segment and the cytoplasmic N-terminus are essential for amino acid transport function.[342,384] In contrast, the 4F2hc ectodomain might be necessary for amino acid transport function,[385] whereas the transmembrane segment and the cytoplasmic N-terminus are essential for stimulation of β1 integrin signaling.[386]

Reconstitution experiments have revealed that a given light subunit is the catalytic component and confers specificity to the holotransporter.[325] Light subunits (≈50 kDa) are highly hydrophobic, not glycosylated, and belong to the family of L–amino acid transporters within the APC superfamily.[387] The atomic structure of AdiC,[373,376,378a] a prokaryotic member of the APA family within the APC superfamily, is currently the best structural model available for the light subunits of HATs. The amino acids of AdiC are approximately 20% identical to those of the eukaryotic L–amino acid transporters, and its atomic structure is fully consistent with the findings of previous low-resolution structural studies of the light subunits of HATs. Thus, results of cysteine-scanning mutagenesis studies of xCT are indicative of 12–transmembrane-domain topology, with the N- and C-terminals located inside the cell and with the intracellular TMH2-TMH3 loop (IL1) accessible to the external medium[388] (see Figure 8-19). The conserved cysteine residue responsible for the intersubunit disulfide bridge is located in the extracellular TMH3-TMH4 loop. Moreover, structural models of $b^{0,+}AT$ and y^+LAT1 based on AdiC structure show that almost half of the more than 60 reported missense mutations causing cystinuria and LPI are located in the two interior pairs of symmetry-related helices (TMH1 and TMH6, and TMH3 and TMH8). This highlights the relevance of the inner helices for transport function of HATs.

The reported structures of AdiC bound to its substrate correspond to the outward-facing states. The open-to-out

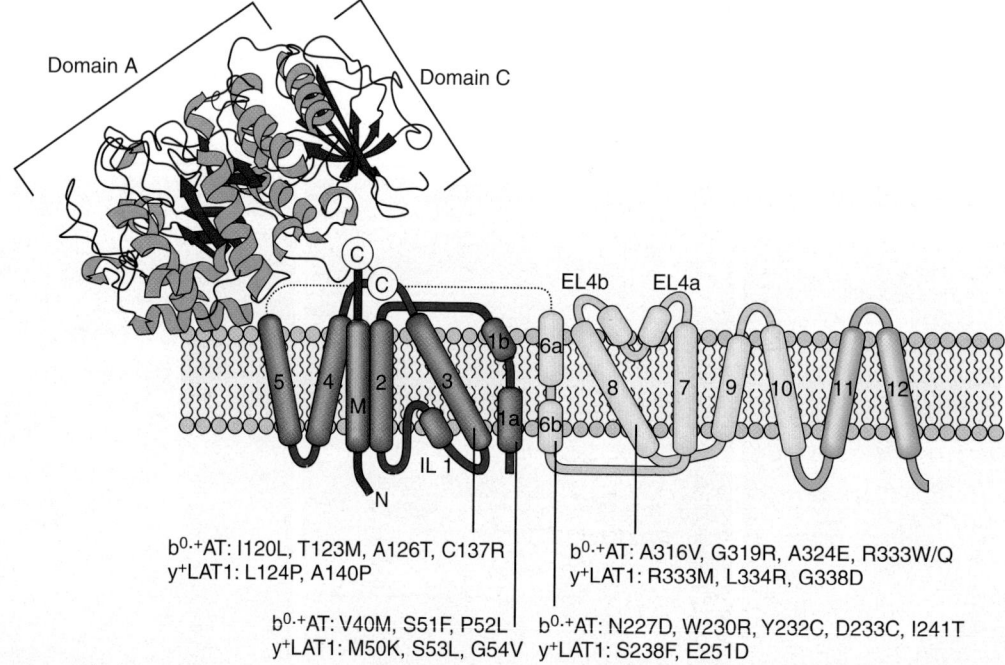

b[0,+]AT: I120L, T123M, A126T, C137R
y[+]LAT1: L124P, A140P

b[0,+]AT: A316V, G319R, A324E, R333W/Q
y[+]LAT1: R333M, L334R, G338D

b[0,+]AT: V40M, S51F, P52L
y[+]LAT1: M50K, S53L, G54V

b[0,+]AT: N227D, W230R, Y232C, D233C, I241T
y[+]LAT1: S238F, E251D

FIGURE 8-19 Structure of the heteromeric amino acid transporters (HATs). The heavy subunit (4F2hc) is represented by a secondary structure illustration of the ectodomain (Protein Data Bank code 2DH2)[383] connected by a short stretch of amino acids to the putative transmembrane domain and the structurally undefined cytosolic N-terminus (*pink*). The position of the ectodomain on the plasma membrane is a subject of speculation based on the distribution of positive charges in the protein surface and in the atomic structure of 4F2hc-ectodomain homodimers (Protein Data Bank code 2DH3). The light subunit is represented by a topologic diagram based on the atomic structure of the homologous protein AdiC (Protein Data Bank code 3HQK).[373] Repeat 1 and repeat 2, related by the pseudo–two-fold axis of symmetry, are colored in *red* and *yellow*, respectively. The conserved cysteine residues that link both subunits are shown in the "neck" interconnecting the ectodomain and the transmembrane segment of 4F2hc and in the TMH3-TMH4 loop of the light subunit. Missense mutations for cystinuria (B[0,+]AT) and lysinuric protein intolerance (LPI; y[+]LAT1) located in the two inner pair of transmembrane-spanning helices (TMHs; TMH1 and TMH6; TMH3 and TMH8) are shown (see text for details).

arginine-bound structure shows the initial substrate recognition.[378a] The outward-facing arginine-occluded structure corresponds to the substrate-bound occluded state.[389] These structures delineate a substrate binding site similar to that of LeuT. Thus, the alpha-amino carboxy moiety of the substrate interacts with the unwound regions of TMH1 and TMH6, and the lateral chain of the substyrate interacts with residues in TMH8 and TMH3. This model of substrate binding site seems to be conserved in LAT transporters (i.e. light subunits of HATs),[390] but the low amino acid sequence identity of AdiC precludes generation of robust structural models of the light subunits of HATs. Thus, crystal structures of LAT transporters are necessary to unravel the molecular transport mechanisms of HAT and the defects associated with amino-aciduria-causing mutations.

References

1. Cushny AR. The excretion of urea and sugar by the kidney. *J Physiol.* 1917;51:36-44.
2. Barfuss DW, Schafer JA. Differences in active and passive glucose transport along the proximal nephron. *Am J Physiol.* 1981;241:F322-F332.
3. Biagi B, Kubota T, Sohtell M, et al. Intracellular potentials in rabbit proximal tubules perfused in vitro. *Am J Physiol.* 1981;240:F200-F210.
4. Aronson PS, Sacktor B. Transport of D-glucose by brush border membranes isolated from the renal cortex. *Biochim Biophys Acta.* 1974;356:231-243.
5. Aronson PS, Sacktor B. The Na$^+$ gradient–dependent transport of D-glucose in renal brush border membranes. *J Biol Chem.* 1975;250:6032-6039.
6. Quamme GA, Freeman HJ. Evidence for a high-affinity sodium-dependent D-glucose transport system in the kidney. *Am J Physiol.* 1987;253:F151-F157.
7. Turner RJ, Moran A. Heterogeneity of sodium-dependent D-glucose transport sites along the proximal tubule: evidence from vesicle studies. *Am J Physiol.* 1982;242:F406-F414.
8. Turner RJ, Moran A. Further studies of proximal tubular brush border membrane D-glucose transport heterogeneity. *J Membr Biol.* 1982;70:37-45.
9. Wright SH, Dantzler WH. Molecular and cellular physiology of renal organic cation and anion transport. *Physiol Rev.* 2004;84:987-1049.
10. Elsas LJ, Rosenberg LE. Familial renal glycosuria: a genetic reappraisal of hexose transport by kidney and intestine. *J Clin Invest.* 1969;48:1845-1854.
11. Hediger MA, Coady MJ, Ikeda TS, et al. Expression cloning and cDNA sequencing of the Na$^+$/glucose co-transporter. *Nature.* 1987;330:379-381.
12. Ikeda TS, Hwang ES, Coady MJ, et al. Characterization of a Na$^+$/glucose cotransporter cloned from rabbit small intestine. *J Membr Biol.* 1989;110:87-95.
13. Lindquist B, Meeuwisse GW, Melin K. Glucose-glactose malabsorption. *Lancet.* 1962;2:666.
14. Lee WS, Kanai Y, Wells RG, et al. The high affinity Na$^+$/glucose cotransporter. Re-evaluation of function and distribution of expression. *J Biol Chem.* 1994;269:12032-12039.
15. Kanai Y, Lee WS, You G, et al. The human kidney low affinity Na$^+$/glucose cotransporter SGLT2. Delineation of the major renal reabsorptive mechanism for D-glucose. *J Clin Invest.* 1994;93:397-404.
16. Wells RG, Pajor AM, Kanai Y, et al. Cloning of a human kidney cDNA with similarity to the sodium-glucose cotransporter. *Am J Physiol.* 1992;263(3 pt 2):F459-F465.
17. Cheung PT, Hammerman MR. Na$^+$-independent D-glucose transport in rabbit renal basolateral membranes. *Am J Physiol.* 1988;254:F711-F718.
18. Ling KY, Im WB, Faust RG. Na$^+$-independent sugar uptake by rat intestinal and renal brush border and basolateral membrane vesicles. *Int J Biochem.* 1981;13:693-700.
19. Diez-Sampedro A, Lostao MP, Wright EM, et al. Glycoside binding and translocation in Na(+)-dependent glucose cotransporters: comparison of SGLT1 and SGLT3. *J Membr Biol.* 2000;176:111-117.
20. Diez-Sampedro A, Eskandari S, Wright EM, et al. Na$^+$-to-sugar stoichiometry of SGLT3. *Am J Physiol Renal Physiol.* 2001;280:F278-F282.
21. Mackenzie B, Loo DD, Panayotova-Heiermann M, Wright EM. Biophysical characteristics of the pig kidney Na$^+$/glucose cotransporter SGLT2 reveal a common mechanism for SGLT1 and SGLT2. *J Biol Chem.* 1996;271:32678-32683.
22. Diez-Sampedro A, Hirayama BA, Osswald C, et al. A glucose sensor hiding in a family of transporters. *Proc Natl Acad Sci U S A.* 2003;100:11753-11758.
23. Freeman SL, Bohan D, Darcel N, et al. Luminal glucose sensing in the rat intestine has characteristics of a sodium-glucose cotransporter. *Am J Physiol Gastrointest Liver Physiol.* 2006;291:G439-G445.
24. Faham S, Watanabe A, Besserer GM, et al. The crystal structure of a sodium galactose transporter reveals mechanistic insights into Na$^+$/sugar symport. *Science.* 2008;321:810-814.
25. Joost HG, Thorens B. The extended GLUT-family of sugar/polyol transport facilitators: nomenclature, sequence characteristics, and potential function of its novel members (review). *Mol Membr Biol.* 2001;18:247-256.
26. Uldry M, Thorens B. The SLC2 family of facilitated hexose and polyol transporters. *Pflugers Arch.* 2004;447:480-489.
27. Takata K, Kasahara T, Kasahara M, et al. Localization of Na(+)-dependent active type and erythrocyte/HepG2-type glucose transporters in rat kidney: immunofluorescence and immunogold study. *J Histochem Cytochem.* 1991;39:287-298.
28. Thorens B, Lodish HF, Brown D. Differential localization of two glucose transporter isoforms in rat kidney. *Am J Physiol.* 1990;259:C286-C294.
29. Dominguez JH, Camp K, Maianu L, et al. Glucose transporters of rat proximal tubule: differential expression and subcellular distribution. *Am J Physiol.* 1992;262:F807-F812.
30. Birnbaum MJ. Identification of a novel gene encoding an insulin-responsive glucose transporter protein. *Cell.* 1989;57:305-315.
31. James DE, Strube M, Mueckler M. Molecular cloning and characterization of an insulin-regulatable glucose transporter. *Nature.* 1989;338:83-87.
32. Brosius 3rd FC, Briggs JP, Marcus RG, et al. Insulin-responsive glucose transporter expression in renal microvessels and glomeruli. *Kidney Int.* 1992;42:1086-1092.
33. Lam JT, Martin MG, Turk E, et al. Missense mutations in SGLT1 cause glucose-galactose malabsorption by trafficking defects. *Biochim Biophys Acta.* 1999;1453:297-303.
34. Guillam MT, Hummler E, Schaerer E, et al. Early diabetes and abnormal postnatal pancreatic islet development in mice lacking *Glut-2. Nat Genet.* 1997;17:327-330.
35. Sakamoto O, Ogawa E, Ohura T, et al. Mutation analysis of the *GLUT2* gene in patients with Fanconi-Bickel syndrome. *Pediatr Res.* 2000;48:586-589.
36. Santer R, Schneppenheim R, Dombrowski A, et al. Mutations in *GLUT2,* the gene for the liver-type glucose transporter, in patients with Fanconi-Bickel syndrome. *Nat Genet.* 1997;17:324-326.
37. Kasahara M, Maeda M, Hayashi S, et al. A missense mutation in the Na(+)/glucose cotransporter gene SGLT1 in a patient with congenital glucose-galactose malabsorption: normal trafficking but inactivation of the mutant protein. *Biochim Biophys Acta.* 2001;1536:141-147.
38. Martin MG, Lostao MP, Turk E, et al. Compound missense mutations in the sodium/D-glucose cotransporter result in trafficking defects. *Gastroenterology.* 1997;112:1206-1212.
39. Martin MG, Turk E, Lostao MP, et al. Defects in Na$^+$/glucose cotransporter (SGLT1) trafficking and function cause glucose-galactose malabsorption. *Nat Genet.* 1996;12:216-220.
40. Turk E, Zabel B, Mundlos S, et al. Glucose/galactose malabsorption caused by a defect in the Na$^+$/glucose cotransporter. *Nature.* 1991;350:354-356.
41. Brodehl J, Oemar BS, Hoyer PF. Renal glucosuria. *Pediatr Nephrol.* 1987;1:502-508.
42. Desjeux JF, Turk E, Wright E. Congenital selective Na D-glucose cotransport defects leading to renal glycosuria and congenital intestinal malabsorption of glucose and galactose. In: Scriver CR, Beaudet AL, Sly WS, et al, eds. *The Metabolic and Molecular Basis of Inherited Diseases.* New York: McGraw-Hill: 1995: p 3563.
43. van den Heuvel LP, Assink K, Willemsen M, et al. Autosomal recessive renal glucosuria attributable to a mutation in the sodium glucose cotransporter (SGLT2). *Hum Genet.* 2002;111:544-547.
44. De Marchi S, Cecchin E, Basile A, et al. Close linkage between HLA and renal glycosuria. *Am J Nephrol.* 1984;4:280-286.
45. De Paoli P, Battistin S, Jus A, et al. Immunological characterization of renal glycosuria patients. *Clin Exp Immunol.* 1984;56:289-294.
46. Pascual JM, Wang D, Lecumberri B, et al. GLUT1 deficiency and other glucose transporter diseases. *Eur J Endocrinol.* 2004;150:627-633.
47. Fanconi G, Bickel H. [Die chronische aminoacidurie (aminosaeurediabetes oder nephrotischglukosurisscher zwergwuchs) ber der glykogenose und cystinkrankheit]. *Helv Paediatr Acta.* 1949;4:359-396.
48. Santer R, Groth S, Kinner M, et al. The mutation spectrum of the facilitative glucose transporter gene SLC2A2 (GLUT2) in patients with Fanconi-Bickel syndrome. *Hum Genet.* 2002;110:21-29.
49. Moe OW, Seldin DW, Baum M. The Fanconi syndrome. In: Lifton RP, Somlo S, Giebisch G, et al, eds. *Genetic diseases of the kidney.* Burlington, Mass: Academic Press; 2009:171-197.
50. De Vivo DC, Trifiletti RR, Jacobson RI, et al. Defective glucose transport across the blood-brain barrier as a cause of persistent hypoglycorrhachia, seizures, and developmental delay. *N Engl J Med.* 1991;325:703-709.

51. Seidner G, Alvarez MG, Yeh JI, et al. GLUT-1 deficiency syndrome caused by haploinsufficiency of the blood-brain barrier hexose carrier. *Nat Genet.* 1998;18:188-191.
52. Asano T, Ogihara T, Katagiri H, et al. Glucose transporter and Na$^+$/glucose cotransporter as molecular targets of anti-diabetic drugs. *Curr Med Chem.* 2004;11:2717-2724.
53. Ueta K, Ishihara T, Matsumoto Y, et al. Long-term treatment with the Na$^+$-glucose cotransporter inhibitor T-1095 causes sustained improvement in hyperglycemia and prevents diabetic neuropathy in Goto-Kakizaki rats. *Life Sci.* 2005;76:2655-2668.
54. Castaneda F, Kinne RK. A 96-well automated method to study inhibitors of human sodium-dependent D-glucose transport. *Mol Cell Biochem.* 2005;280:91-98.
55. Ueta K, Yoneda H, Oku A, et al. Reduction of renal transport maximum for glucose by inhibition of Na(+)-glucose cotransporter suppresses blood glucose elevation in dogs. *Biol Pharm Bull.* 2006;29:114-118.
56. Ader P, Block M, Pietzsch S, et al. Interaction of quercetin glucosides with the intestinal sodium/glucose co-transporter (SGLT-1). *Cancer Lett.* 2001;162:175-180.
57. Ohsumi K, Matsueda H, Hatanaka T, et al. Pyrazole-O-glucosides as novel Na(+)-glucose cotransporter (SGLT) inhibitors. *Bioorg Med Chem Lett.* 2003;13:2269-2272.
58. Tsujihara K, Hongu M, Saito K, et al. Na(+)-glucose cotransporter inhibitors as antidiabetics. I. Synthesis and pharmacological properties of 4'-dehydroxyphlorizin derivatives based on a new concept. *Chem Pharm Bull (Tokyo).* 1996;44:1174-1180.
59. Tsujihara K, Hongu M, Saito K, et al. Na(+)-glucose cotransporter (SGLT) inhibitors as antidiabetic agents. 4. Synthesis and pharmacological properties of 4'-dehydroxyphlorizin derivatives substituted on the B ring. *J Med Chem.* 1999;42:5311-5324.
60. Yoo O, Lee DH. Inhibition of sodium glucose cotransporter-I expressed in *Xenopus laevis* oocytes by 4-acetoxyscirpendiol from *Cordyceps takaomantana* (anamorph = *Paecilomyces tenuipes*). *Med Mycol.* 2006;44:79-85.
61. Yoo O, Son JH, Lee DH. 4-Acetoxyscirpendiol of *Paecilomyces tenuipes* inhibits Na(+)/D-glucose cotransporter expressed in *Xenopus laevis* oocytes. *J Biochem Mol Biol.* 2005;38:211-217.
62. Bendayan R, Sullivan JT, Shaw C, et al. Effect of cimetidine and ranitidine on the hepatic and renal elimination of nicotine in humans. *Eur J Clin Pharmacol.* 1990;38:165-169.
63. Meijer DK, Mol WE, Muller M, et al. Carrier-mediated transport in the hepatic distribution and elimination of drugs, with special reference to the category of organic cations. *J Pharmacokinet Biopharm.* 1990;18:35-70.
64. Pritchard JB, Miller DS. Mechanisms mediating renal secretion of organic anions and cations. *Physiol Rev.* 1993;73:765-796.
65. Somogyi A, McLean A, Heinzow B. Cimetidine-procainamide pharmacokinetic interaction in man: evidence of competition for tubular secretion of basic drugs. *Eur J Clin Pharmacol.* 1983;25:339-345.
66. Wright SH, Wunz TM. Influence of substrate structure on turnover of the organic cation/H$^+$ exchanger of the renal luminal membrane. *Pflugers Arch.* 1998;436:469-477.
67. Ambudkar SV, Dey S, Hrycyna CA, et al. Biochemical, cellular, and pharmacological aspects of the multidrug transporter. *Annu Rev Pharmacol Toxicol.* 1999;39:361-398.
68. Arakawa K, Ishihara T, Oku A, et al. Improved diabetic syndrome in C57BL/KsJ-db/db mice by oral administration of the Na(+)-glucose cotransporter inhibitor T-1095. *Br J Pharmacol.* 2001;132:578-586.
69. Blackmore CG, McNaughton PA, van Veen HW. Multidrug transporters in prokaryotic and eukaryotic cells: physiological functions and transport mechanisms. *Mol Membr Biol.* 2001;18:97-103.
70. Chandra P, Brouwer KL. The complexities of hepatic drug transport: current knowledge and emerging concepts. *Pharm Res.* 2004;21:719-735.
71. Higgins CF, Callaghan R, Linton KJ, et al. Structure of the multidrug resistance P-glycoprotein. *Semin Cancer Biol.* 1997;8:135-142.
72. Pritchard JB, Miller DS. Renal secretion of organic anions and cations. *Kidney Int.* 1996;49:1649-1654.
73. Sokol PP, McKinney TD. Mechanism of organic cation transport in rabbit renal basolateral membrane vesicles. *Am J Physiol.* 1990;258:F1599-F1607.
74. Dantzler WH, Wright SH, Chatsudthipong V, et al. Basolateral tetraethylammonium transport in intact tubules: specificity and *trans*-stimulation. *Am J Physiol.* 1991;261:F386-F392.
75. Busch AE, Quester S, Ulzheimer JC, et al. Electrogenic properties and substrate specificity of the polyspecific rat cation transporter rOCT1. *J Biol Chem.* 1996;271:32599-32604.
76. Bello-Reuss E. Electrical properties of the basolateral membrane of the straight portion of the rabbit proximal renal tubule. *J Physiol.* 1982;326:49-63.
77. Cardinal J, Lapointe JY, Laprade R. Luminal and peritubular ionic substitutions and intracellular potential of the rabbit proximal convoluted tubule. *Am J Physiol.* 1984;247:F352-F364.
78. Ullrich KJ, Rumrich G, Neiteler K, et al. Contraluminal transport of organic cations in the proximal tubule of the rat kidney. II. Specificity: anilines, phenylalkylamines (catecholamines), heterocyclic compounds (pyridines, quinolines, acridines). *Pflugers Arch.* 1992;420:29-38.
79. Ullrich KJ, Papavassiliou F, David C, et al. Contraluminal transport of organic cations in the proximal tubule of the rat kidney. I. Kinetics of N^1-methylnicotinamide and tetraethylammonium, influence of K$^+$, HCO$_3^-$, pH; inhibition by aliphatic primary, secondary and tertiary amines and mono- and bisquaternary compounds. *Pflugers Arch.* 1991;419:84-92.
80. Bednarczyk D, Ekins S, Wikel JH, et al. Influence of molecular structure on substrate binding to the human organic cation transporter, hOCT1. *Mol Pharmacol.* 2003;63:489-498.
81. Suhre WM, Ekins S, Chang C, et al. Molecular determinants of substrate/inhibitor binding to the human and rabbit renal organic cation transporters hOCT2 and rbOCT2. *Mol Pharmacol.* 2005;67:1067-1077.
82. Ullrich KJ, Rumrich G. Morphine analogues: relationship between chemical structure and interaction with proximal tubular transporters—contraluminal organic cation and anion transporter, luminal H$^+$/organic cation exchanger, and luminal choline transporter. *Cell Physiol Biochem.* 1995;5:290.
83. van Montfoort JE, Muller M, Groothuis GM, et al. Comparison of "type I" and "type II" organic cation transport by organic cation transporters and organic anion–transporting polypeptides. *J Pharmacol Exp Ther.* 2001;298:110-115.
84. Li N, Hartley DP, Cherrington NJ, et al. Tissue expression, ontogeny, and inducibility of rat organic anion transporting polypeptide 4. *J Pharmacol Exp Ther.* 2002;301:551-560.
85. Schali C, Schild L, Overney J, et al. Secretion of tetraethylammonium by proximal tubules of rabbit kidneys. *Am J Physiol.* 1983;245:F238-F246.
86. Yoshitomi K, Fromter E. Cell pH of rat renal proximal tubule in vivo and the conductive nature of peritubular HCO$_3^-$ (OH$^-$) exit. *Pflugers Arch.* 1984;402:300-305.
87. Wright SH, Wunz TM. Transport of tetraethylammonium by rabbit renal brush-border and basolateral membrane vesicles. *Am J Physiol.* 1987;253:F1040-F1050.
88. Wright SH. Transport of N^1-methylnicotinamide across brush border membrane vesicles from rabbit kidney. *Am J Physiol.* 1985;249:F903-F911.
89. Gluck S, Nelson R. The role of the V-ATPase in renal epithelial H$^+$ transport. *J Exp Biol.* 1992;172:205-218.
90. Wright SH, Wunz TM, Wunz TP. Structure and interaction of inhibitors with the TEA/H$^+$ exchanger of rabbit renal brush border membranes. *Pflugers Arch.* 1995;429:313-324.
91. Yabuuchi H, Tamai I, Nezu J, et al. Novel membrane transporter OCTN1 mediates multispecific, bidirectional, and pH-dependent transport of organic cations. *J Pharmacol Exp Ther.* 1999;289:768-773.
92. Miyamoto Y, Tiruppathi C, Ganapathy V, et al. Multiple transport systems for organic cations in renal brush-border membrane vesicles. *Am J Physiol.* 1989;256:F540-F548.
93. Otsuka M, Matsumoto T, Morimoto R, et al. A human transporter protein that mediates the final excretion step for toxic organic cations. *Proc Natl Acad Sci U S A.* 2005;102:17923-17928.
94. Gutmann H, Miller DS, Droulle A, et al. P-glycoprotein– and mrp2-mediated octreotide transport in renal proximal tubule. *Br J Pharmacol.* 2000;129:251-256.
95. Miller DS, Fricker G, Drewe J. P-glycoprotein–mediated transport of a fluorescent rapamycin derivative in renal proximal tubule. *J Pharmacol Exp Ther.* 1997;282:440-444.
96. Miller DS, Sussman CR, Renfro JL. Protein kinase C regulation of P-glycoprotein–mediated xenobiotic secretion in renal proximal tubule. *Am J Physiol.* 1998;275:F785-F795.
97. Chen C, Liu X, Smith BJ. Utility of *Mdr1*-gene deficient mice in assessing the impact of P-glycoprotein on pharmacokinetics and pharmacodynamics in drug discovery and development. *Curr Drug Metab.* 2003;4:272-291.
98. Hartmann G, Vassileva V, Piquette-Miller M. Impact of endotoxin-induced changes in P-glycoprotein expression on disposition of doxorubicin in mice. *Drug Metab Dispos.* 2005;33:820-828.
99. Shimomura A, Chonko AM, Grantham JJ. Basis for heterogeneity of para-aminohippurate secretion in rabbit proximal tubules. *Am J Physiol.* 1981;240:F430-F436.
100. Woodhall PB, Tisher CC, Simonton CA, et al. Relationship between para-aminohippurate secretion and cellular morphology in rabbit proximal tubules. *J Clin Invest.* 1978;61:1320-1329.
101. McKinney TD. Heterogeneity of organic base secretion by proximal tubules. *Am J Physiol.* 1982;243:F404-F407.
102. Karbach U, Kricke J, Meyer-Wentrup F, et al. Localization of organic cation transporters OCT1 and OCT2 in rat kidney. *Am J Physiol Renal Physiol.* 2000;279:F679-F687.
103. Montrose-Rafizadeh C, Roch-Ramel F, Schali C. Axial heterogeneity of organic cation transport along the rabbit renal proximal tubule: studies with brush-border membrane vesicles. *Biochim Biophys Acta.* 1987;904:175-177.

104. Masuda S, Terada T, Yonezawa A, et al. Identification and functional characterization of a new human kidney-specific H⁺/organic cation antiporter, kidney-specific multidrug and toxin extrusion 2. *J Am Soc Nephrol.* 2006;17:2127-2135.

105. Acara M, Rennick B. Regulation of plasma choline by the renal tubule: bidirectional transport of choline. *Am J Physiol.* 1973;225:1123-1128.

106. Acara M, Roch-Ramel F, Rennick B. Bidirectional renal tubular transport of free choline: a micropuncture study. *Am J Physiol.* 1979;236:F112-F118.

107. Ullrich KJ, Rumrich G. Luminal transport system for choline⁺ in relation to the other organic cation transport systems in the rat proximal tubule. Kinetics, specificity: alkyl/arylamines, alkylamines with OH, O, SH, NH₂, ROCO, RSCO and H₂PO₄-groups, methylaminostyryl, rhodamine, acridine, phenanthrene and cyanine compounds. *Pflugers Arch.* 1996;432:471-485.

108. Wright SH, Wunz TM, Wunz TP. A choline transporter in renal brush-border membrane vesicles: energetics and structural specificity. *J Membr Biol.* 1992;126:51-65.

109. Yabuki M, Inazu M, Yamada T, et al. Molecular and functional characterization of choline transporter in rat renal tubule epithelial NRK-52E cells. *Arch Biochem Biophys.* 2009;485:88-96.

110. Besseghir K, Pearce LB, Rennick B. Renal tubular transport and metabolism of organic cations by the rabbit. *Am J Physiol.* 1981;241:F308-F314.

111. Christian Jr CD, Meredith CG, Speeg Jr KV. Cimetidine inhibits renal procainamide clearance. *Clin Pharmacol Ther.* 1984;36:221-227.

112. Grundemann D, Gorboulev V, Gambaryan S, et al. Drug excretion mediated by a new prototype of polyspecific transporter. *Nature.* 1994;372:549-552.

113. Wright SH, Evans KK, Zhang X, et al. Functional map of TEA transport activity in isolated rabbit renal proximal tubules. *Am J Physiol Renal Physiol.* 2004;287:F442-F451.

114. Jonker JW, Wagenaar E, Van Eijl S, et al. Deficiency in the organic cation transporters 1 and 2 (Oct1/Oct2 [Slc22A1/Slc22A2]) in mice abolishes renal secretion of organic cations. *Mol Cell Biol.* 2003;23:7902-7908.

115. Lickteig AJ, Cheng X, Augustine LM, et al. Tissue distribution, ontogeny and induction of the transporters multidrug and toxin extrusion (MATE) 1 and MATE2 mRNA expression levels in mice. *Life Sci.* 2008;83:59-64.

116. Pao SS, Paulsen IT, Saier Jr MH. Major facilitator superfamily. *Microbiol Mol Biol Rev.* 1998;62:1-34.

117. Terada T, Inui K. Physiological and pharmacokinetic roles of H⁺/organic cation antiporters (MATE/SLC47A). *Biochem Pharmacol.* 2008;75:1689-1696.

118. Schomig E, Spitzenberger F, Engelhardt M, et al. Molecular cloning and characterization of two novel transport proteins from rat kidney. *FEBS Lett.* 1998;425:79-86.

119. Ciarimboli G, Schlatter E. Regulation of organic cation transport. *Pflugers Arch.* 2005;449:423-441.

120. Pelis RM, Suhre WM, Wright SH. Functional influence of *N*-glycosylation in OCT2-mediated tetraethylammonium transport. *Am J Physiol Renal Physiol.* 2006;290:F1118-F1126.

121. Popp C, Gorboulev V, Muller TD, et al. Amino acids critical for substrate affinity of rat organic cation transporter 1 line the substrate binding region in a model derived from the tertiary structure of lactose permease. *Mol Pharmacol.* 2005;67:1600-1611.

122. Zhang X, Shirahatti NV, Mahadevan D, et al. A conserved glutamate residue in transmembrane helix 10 influences substrate specificity of rabbit OCT2 (Slc22A2). *J Biol Chem.* 2005;280:34813-34822.

123. Eraly SA, Monte JC, Nigam SK. Novel Slc22 transporter homologs in fly, worm, and human clarify the phylogeny of organic anion and cation transporters. *Physiol Genomics.* 2004;18:12-24.

124. Zhang J, Bobulescu IA, Goyal S, et al. Characterization of Na⁺/H⁺ exchanger NHE8 in cultured renal epithelial cells. *Am J Physiol Renal Physiol.* 2007;293:F761-F766.

125. Hayer M, Bonisch H, Bruss M. Molecular cloning, functional characterization and genomic organization of four alternatively spliced isoforms of the human organic cation transporter 1 (hOCT1/SLC22A1). *Ann Hum Genet.* 1999;63:473-482.

126. Urakami Y, Akazawa M, Saito H, et al. cDNA cloning, functional characterization, and tissue distribution of an alternatively spliced variant of organic cation transporter hOCT2 predominantly expressed in the human kidney. *J Am Soc Nephrol.* 2002;13:1703-1710.

127. Bleasby K, Castle JC, Roberts CJ, et al. Expression profiles of 50 xenobiotic transporter genes in humans and pre-clinical species: a resource for investigations into drug disposition. *Xenobiotica.* 2006;36:963-988.

128. Motohashi H, Sakurai Y, Saito H, et al. Gene expression levels and immunolocalization of organic ion transporters in the human kidney. *J Am Soc Nephrol.* 2002;13:866-874.

129. Zwart R, Verhaagh S, Buitelaar M, et al. Impaired activity of the extraneuronal monoamine transporter system known as uptake-2 in Orct3/Slc22A3-deficient mice. *Mol Cell Biol.* 2001;21:4188-4196.

130. Budiman T, Bamberg E, Koepsell H, et al. Mechanism of electrogenic cation transport by the cloned organic cation transporter 2 from rat. *J Biol Chem.* 2000;275:29413-29420.

131. Kekuda R, Prasad PD, Wu X, et al. Cloning and functional characterization of a potential-sensitive, polyspecific organic cation transporter (OCT3) most abundantly expressed in placenta. *J Biol Chem.* 1998;273:15971-15979.

132. Schmitt BM, Gorbunov D, Schlachtbauer P, et al. Charge-to-substrate ratio during organic cation uptake by rat OCT2 is voltage dependent and altered by exchange of glutamate 448 with glutamine. *Am J Physiol Renal Physiol.* 2009;296:F709-F722.

133. Wu X, Huang W, Ganapathy ME, et al. Structure, function, and regional distribution of the organic cation transporter OCT3 in the kidney. *Am J Physiol Renal Physiol.* 2000;279:F449-F458.

134. Kaewmokul S, Chatsudthipong V, Evans KK, et al. Functional mapping of rbOCT1 and rbOCT2 activity in the S2 segment of rabbit proximal tubule. *Am J Physiol Renal Physiol.* 2003;285:F1149-F1159.

135. Sata R, Ohtani H, Tsujimoto M, et al. Functional analysis of organic cation transporter 3 expressed in human placenta. *J Pharmacol Exp Ther.* 2005;315:888-895.

136. Arndt P, Volk C, Gorboulev V, et al. Interaction of cations, anions, and weak base quinine with rat renal cation transporter rOCT2 compared with rOCT1. *Am J Physiol Renal Physiol.* 2001;281:F454-F468.

137. Ullrich KJ, Rumrich G, David C, et al. Bisubstrates: substances that interact with renal contraluminal organic anion and organic cation transport systems. I. Amines, piperidines, piperazines, azepines, pyridines, quinolines, imidazoles, thiazoles, guanidines and hydrazines. *Pflugers Arch.* 1993;425:280-299.

138. Barendt WM, Wright SH. The human organic cation transporter (hOCT2) recognizes the degree of substrate ionization. *J Biol Chem.* 2002;277:22491-22496.

139. Moaddel R, Ravichandran S, Bighi F, et al. Pharmacophore modelling of stereoselective binding to the human organic cation transporter (hOCT1). *Br J Pharmacol.* 2007;151:1305-1314.

140. Zolk O, Solbach TF, Konig J, et al. Structural determinants of inhibitor interaction with the human organic cation transporter OCT2 (SLC22A2). *Naunyn Schmiedebergs Arch Pharmacol.* 2009;379:337-348.

140a. Simell O. Lysinuric protein intolerance and other cationic aminoacidurias. In: Scriver CR, Beaudet AL, Sly WS, et al, eds. *The metabolic and molecular bases of inherited disease.* New York: McGraw-Hill; 2001:4933-4956.

141. Volk C, Gorboulev V, Budiman T, et al. Different affinities of inhibitors to the outwardly and inwardly directed substrate binding site of organic cation transporter 2. *Mol Pharmacol.* 2003;64:1037-1047.

142. Dresser MJ, Gray AT, Giacomini KM. Kinetic and selectivity differences between rodent, rabbit, and human organic cation transporters (OCT1). *J Pharmacol Exp Ther.* 2000;292:1146-1152.

143. Nagel G, Volk C, Friedrich T, et al. A reevaluation of substrate specificity of the rat cation transporter rOCT1. *J Biol Chem.* 1997;272:31953-31956.

144. Zhang L, Gorset W, Dresser MJ, et al. The interaction of *N*-tetraalkylammonium compounds with a human organic cation transporter, hOCT1. *J Pharmacol Exp Ther.* 1999;288:1192-1198.

145. Zhang L, Schaner ME, Giacomini KM. Functional characterization of an organic cation transporter (hOCT1) in a transiently transfected human cell line (HeLa). *J Pharmacol Exp Ther.* 1998;286:354-361.

146. Abramson J, Smirnova I, Kasho V, et al. Structure and mechanism of the lactose permease of *Escherichia coli. Science.* 2003;301:610-615.

147. Huang Y, Lemieux MJ, Song J, et al. Structure and mechanism of the glycerol-3-phosphate transporter from *Escherichia coli. Science.* 2003;301:616-620.

148. Vardy E, Arkin IT, Gottschalk KE, et al. Structural conservation in the major facilitator superfamily as revealed by comparative modeling. *Protein Sci.* 2004;13:1832-1840.

149. Gorboulev V, Volk C, Arndt P, et al. Selectivity of the polyspecific cation transporter rOCT1 is changed by mutation of aspartate 475 to glutamate. *Mol Pharmacol.* 1999;56:1254-1261.

150. Bahn A, Hagos Y, Rudolph T, et al. Mutation of amino acid 475 of rat organic cation transporter 2 (rOCT2) impairs organic cation transport. *Biochimie.* 2004;86:133-136.

151. Gorboulev V, Shatskaya N, Volk C, et al. Subtype-specific affinity for corticosterone of rat organic cation transporters rOCT1 and rOCT2 depends on three amino acids within the substrate binding region. *Mol Pharmacol.* 2005;67:1612-1619.

152. Hong M, Xu W, Yoshida T, et al. Human organic anion transporter hOAT1 forms homooligomers. *J Biol Chem.* 2005;280:32285-32290.

153. Keller T, Schwarz D, Bernhard F, et al. Cell free expression and functional reconstitution of eukaryotic drug transporters. *Biochemistry.* 2008;47:4552-4564.

154. Leabman MK, Huang CC, DeYoung J, et al. Natural variation in human membrane transporter genes reveals evolutionary and functional constraints. *Proc Natl Acad Sci U S A.* 2003;100:5896-5901.

155. Leabman MK, Huang CC, Kawamoto M, et al. Polymorphisms in a human kidney xenobiotic transporter, OCT2, exhibit altered function. *Pharmacogenetics*. 2002;12:395-405.

156. Shu Y, Leabman MK, Feng B, et al. Evolutionary conservation predicts function of variants of the human organic cation transporter, OCT1. *Proc Natl Acad Sci U S A*. 2003;100:5902-5907.

157. Takane H, Shikata E, Otsubo K, et al. Polymorphism in human organic cation transporters and metformin action. *Pharmacogenomics*. 2008;9:415-422.

158. Wang ZJ, Yin OQ, Tomlinson B, et al. OCT2 polymorphisms and in-vivo renal functional consequence: studies with metformin and cimetidine. *Pharmacogenet Genomics*. 2008;18:637-645.

159. Song IS, Shin HJ, Shim EJ, et al. Genetic variants of the organic cation transporter 2 influence the disposition of metformin. *Clin Pharmacol Ther*. 2008;84:559-562.

160. Mehrens T, Lelleck S, Cetinkaya I, et al. The affinity of the organic cation transporter rOCT1 is increased by protein kinase C–dependent phosphorylation. *J Am Soc Nephrol*. 2000;11:1216-1224.

161. Ciarimboli G, Struwe K, Arndt P, et al. Regulation of the human organic cation transporter hOCT1. *J Cell Physiol*. 2004;201:420-428.

162. Pietig G, Mehrens T, Hirsch JR, et al. Properties and regulation of organic cation transport in freshly isolated human proximal tubules. *J Biol Chem*. 2001;276:33741-33746.

163. Cetinkaya I, Ciarimboli G, Yalcinkaya G, et al. Regulation of human organic cation transporter hOCT2 by PKA, PI3K, and calmodulin-dependent kinases. *Am J Physiol Renal Physiol*. 2003;284:F293-F302.

164. Biermann J, Lang D, Gorboulev V, et al. Characterization of regulatory mechanisms and states of human organic cation transporter 2. *Am J Physiol Cell Physiol*. 2006;290:C1521-1531.

165. Wolff NA, Thies K, Kuhnke N, et al. Protein kinase C activation downregulates human organic anion transporter 1–mediated transport through carrier internalization. *J Am Soc Nephrol*. 2003;14:1959-1968.

166. Wilde S, Schlatter E, Koepsell H, et al. Calmodulin-associated post-translational regulation of rat organic cation transporter 2 in the kidney is gender dependent. *Cell Mol Life Sci*. 2009;66:1729-1740.

167. Urakami Y, Nakamura N, Takahashi K, et al. Gender differences in expression of organic cation transporter OCT2 in rat kidney. *FEBS Lett*. 1999;461:339-342.

168. Urakami Y, Okuda M, Saito H, et al. Hormonal regulation of organic cation transporter OCT2 expression in rat kidney. *FEBS Lett*. 2000;473:173-176.

169. Asaka J, Terada T, Okuda M, et al. Androgen receptor is responsible for rat organic cation transporter 2 gene regulation but not for rOCT1 and rOCT3. *Pharm Res*. 2006;23:697-704.

170. Groves CE, Suhre WB, Cherrington NJ, et al. Sex differences in the mRNA, protein, and functional expression of organic anion transporter (Oat) 1, Oat3, and organic cation transporter (Oct) 2 in rabbit renal proximal tubules. *J Pharmacol Exp Ther*. 2006;316:743-752.

171. Pelis RM, Hartman RC, Wright SH, et al. Influence of estrogen and xenoestrogens on basolateral uptake of tetraethylammonium by opossum kidney cells in culture. *J Pharmacol Exp Ther*. 2007;323:555-561.

172. Goralski KB, Lou G, Prowse MT, et al. The cation transporters rOCT1 and rOCT2 interact with bicarbonate but play only a minor role for amantadine uptake into rat renal proximal tubules. *J Pharmacol Exp Ther*. 2002;303:959-968.

173. Kristufek D, Rudorfer W, Pifl C, et al. Organic cation transporter mRNA and function in the rat superior cervical ganglion. *J Physiol*. 2002;543:117-134.

174. Wu X, Prasad PD, Leibach FH, et al. cDNA sequence, transport function, and genomic organization of human OCTN2, a new member of the organic cation transporter family. *Biochem Biophys Res Commun*. 1998;246:589-595.

175. Moseley RH, Jarose SM, Permoad P. Organic cation transport by rat liver plasma membrane vesicles: studies with tetraethylammonium. *Am J Physiol*. 1992;263:G775-G785.

176. Wu X, George RL, Huang W, et al. Structural and functional characteristics and tissue distribution pattern of rat Octn1, an organic cation transporter, cloned from placenta. *Biochim Biophys Acta*. 2000;1466:315-327.

177. Ott RJ, Hui AC, Yuan G, Giacomini KM. Organic cation transport in human renal brush-border membrane vesicles. *Am J Physiol*. 1991;261:F443-F451.

178. Grundemann D, Harlfinger S, Golz S, et al. Discovery of the ergothioneine transporter. *Proc Natl Acad Sci U S A*. 2005;102:5256-5261.

179. Tang NL, Ganapathy V, Wu X, et al. Mutations of *OCTN2*, an organic cation/carnitine transporter, lead to deficient cellular carnitine uptake in primary carnitine deficiency. *Hum Mol Genet*. 1999;8:655-660.

180. Wang Y, Ye J, Ganapathy V, et al. Mutations in the organic cation/carnitine transporter OCTN2 in primary carnitine deficiency. *Proc Natl Acad Sci U S A*. 1999;96:2356-2360.

181. Lu K, Nishimori H, Nakamura Y, et al. A missense mutation of mouse *Octn2*, a sodium-dependent carnitine cotransporter, in the juvenile visceral steatosis mouse. *Biochem Biophys Res Commun*. 1998;252:590-594.

182. Tein I. Carnitine transport: pathophysiology and metabolism of known molecular defects. *J Inherit Metab Dis*. 2003;26:147-169.

183. Wagner CA, Lukewille U, Kaltenbach S, et al. Functional and pharmacological characterization of human Na(+)-carnitine cotransporter hOCTN2. *Am J Physiol Renal Physiol*. 2000;279:F584-F591.

184. Ohashi R, Tamai I, Nezu Ji J, et al. Molecular and physiological evidence for multifunctionality of carnitine/organic cation transporter OCTN2. *Mol Pharmacol*. 2001;59:358-366.

185. Schomig E, Lazar A, Grundemann D. Extraneuronal monoamine transporter and organic cation transporters 1 and 2: a review of transport efficiency. *Handb Exp Pharmacol*. 2006:151-180.

186. Grigat S, Fork C, Bach M, et al. The carnitine transporter SLC22A5 is not a general drug transporter, but it efficiently translocates mildronate. *Drug Metab Dispos*. 2009;37:330-337.

187. Hiasa M, Matsumoto T, Komatsu T, et al. Wide variety of locations for rodent Mate1, a transporter protein that mediates the final excretion step for toxic organic cations. *Am J Physiol Cell Physiol*. 2006;291:C678-C686.

188. Zhang X, Wright SH. MATE1 has an external COOH terminus, consistent with a 13-helix topology. *Am J Physiol Renal Physiol*. 2009;297:F263-F271.

189. Tsuda M, Terada T, Mizuno T, et al. Targeted disruption of the multidrug and toxin extrusion 1 (*Mate1*) gene in mice reduces renal secretion of metformin. *Mol Pharmacol*. 2009;75:1280-1286.

190. Thiebaut F, Tsuruo T, Hamada H, et al. Cellular localization of the multidrug-resistance gene product P-glycoprotein in normal human tissues. *Proc Natl Acad Sci U S A*. 1987;84:7735-7738.

191. Ernest S, Bello-Reuss E. Expression and function of P-glycoprotein in a mouse kidney cell line. *Am J Physiol*. 1995;269:C323-C333.

192. Ernest S, Rajaraman S, Megyesi J, et al. Expression of MDR1 (multidrug resistance) gene and its protein in normal human kidney. *Nephron*. 1997;77:284-289.

193. Lahjouji K, Mitchell GA, Qureshi IA. Carnitine transport by organic cation transporters and systemic carnitine deficiency. *Mol Genet Metab*. 2001;73:287-297.

193a. Morin CL, Thompson MW, Jackson SH, et al. Biochemical and genetic studies in cystinuria: observations on double heterozygotes of genotype I-II. *J Clin Invest*. 1971;50:1961.

194. Tamai I, Ohashi R, Nezu J, et al. Molecular and functional identification of sodium ion–dependent, high affinity human carnitine transporter OCTN2. *J Biol Chem*. 1998;273:20378-20382.

195. Peltekova VD, Wintle RF, Rubin LA, et al. Functional variants of OCTN cation transporter genes are associated with Crohn disease. *Nat Genet*. 2004;36:471-475.

196. Becker ML, Visser LE, van Schaik RH, et al. Genetic variation in the multidrug and toxin extrusion 1 transporter protein influences the glucose-lowering effect of metformin in patients with diabetes: a preliminary study. *Diabetes*. 2009;58:745-749.

197. Fukushima-Uesaka H, Maekawa K, Ozawa S, et al. Fourteen novel single nucleotide polymorphisms in the *SLC22A2* gene encoding human organic cation transporter (OCT2). *Drug Metab Pharmacokinet*. 2004;19:239-244.

198. Itoda M, Saito Y, Maekawa K, et al. Seven novel single nucleotide polymorphisms in the human *SLC22A1* gene encoding organic cation transporter 1 (OCT1). *Drug Metab Pharmacokinet*. 2004;19:308-312.

199. Kajiwara M, Terada T, Ogasawara K, et al. Identification of multidrug and toxin extrusion (MATE1 and MATE2-K) variants with complete loss of transport activity. *J Hum Genet*. 2009;54:40-46.

200. Marshall Jr EK, Vickers JL. The mechanism of elimination of phenolsulphonphthalein by the kidney—a proof of secretion by the convoluted tubules. *Johns Hopkins Hosp (Bull)*. 1923;34:1.

201. Smith HW, Finkelstein N, Aliminosa L, et al. The renal clearances of substituted hippuric acid derivatives and other aromatic acids in dog and man. *J Clin Invest*. 1945;24:388-404.

202. Cortney MA, Mylle M, Lassiter WE, et al. Renal tubular transport of water, solute, and PAH in rats loaded with isotonic saline. *Am J Physiol*. 1965;209:1199-1205.

203. Malvin RL, Wilde WS, Sullivan LP. Localization of nephron transport by stop flow analysis. *Am J Physiol*. 1958;194:135-142.

204. Tune BM, Burg MB, Patlak CS. Characteristics of *p*-aminohippurate transport in proximal renal tubules. *Am J Physiol*. 1969;217:1057-1063.

205. Christensen EI, Birn H. Megalin and cubilin: multifunctional endocytic receptors. *Nat Rev Mol Cell Biol*. 2002;3:256-266.

206. Deeley RG, Cole SP. Substrate recognition and transport by multidrug resistance protein 1 (ABCC1). *FEBS Lett*. 2006;580:1103-1111.

207. Fritzsch G, Rumrich G, Ullrich KJ. Anion transport through the contraluminal cell membrane of renal proximal tubule. The influence of hydrophobicity and molecular charge distribution on the inhibitory activity of organic anions. *Biochim Biophys Acta*. 1989;978:249-256.

208. Hagenbuch B, Meier PJ. Organic anion transporting polypeptides of the OATP/SLC21 family: phylogenetic classification as OATP/SLCO superfamily, new nomenclature and molecular/functional properties. *Pflugers Arch*. 2004;447:653-665.

209. Bai L, Pajor AM. Expression cloning of NaDC-2, an intestinal Na(+)- or Li(+)-dependent dicarboxylate transporter. *Am J Physiol.* 1997;273:G267-G274.

210. Pajor AM. Sequence and functional characterization of a renal sodium/dicarboxylate cotransporter. *J Biol Chem.* 1995;270:5779-5785.

211. Pajor AM. Molecular cloning and functional expression of a sodium-dicarboxylate cotransporter from human kidney. *Am J Physiol.* 1996;270:F642-F648.

212. Simpson DP. Citrate excretion: a window on renal metabolism. *Am J Physiol.* 1983;244:F223-F234.

213. Srere PA. The molecular physiology of citrate. *Curr Top Cell Regul.* 1992;33:261-275.

214. Moe OW, Preisig PA. Dual role of citrate in mammalian urine. *Curr Opin Nephrol Hypertens.* 2006;15:419-424.

215. Ho HT, Ko BC, Cheung AK, et al. Generation and characterization of sodium-dicarboxylate cotransporter–deficient mice. *Kidney Int.* 2007;72:63-71.

216. Hentschel H, Burckhardt BC, Scholermann B, et al. Basolateral localization of flounder Na⁺-dicarboxylate transporter (fNaDC-3) in the kidney of *Pleuronectes americanus. Pflugers Arch.* 2003;446:578-584.

217. Pajor AM, Gangula R, Yao X. Cloning and functional characterization of a high-affinity Na(+)/dicarboxylate cotransporter from mouse brain. *Am J Physiol Cell Physiol.* 2001;280:C1215-C1223.

218. Pajor AM, Sun N. Functional differences between rabbit and human Na(+)-dicarboxylate cotransporters, NaDC-1 and hNaDC-1. *Am J Physiol.* 1996;271:F1093-F1099.

219. Welborn JR, Shpun S, Dantzler WH, et al. Effect of alpha-ketoglutarate on organic anion transport in single rabbit renal proximal tubules. *Am J Physiol.* 1998;274:F165-F174.

220. Miller DS, Stewart DE, Pritchard JB. Intracellular compartmentation of organic anions within renal cells. *Am J Physiol.* 1993;264:R882-R890.

221. Sekine T, Watanabe N, Hosoyamada M, et al. Expression cloning and characterization of a novel multispecific organic anion transporter. *J Biol Chem.* 1997;272:18526-18529.

222. Sweet DH, Wolff NA, Pritchard JB. Expression cloning and characterization of rOAT1. The basolateral organic anion transporter in rat kidney. *J Biol Chem.* 1997;272:30088-30095.

223. Wolff NA, Werner A, Burkhardt S, et al. Expression cloning and characterization of a renal organic anion transporter from winter flounder. *FEBS Lett.* 1997;417:287-291.

224. Shimada H, Moewes B, Burckhardt G. Indirect coupling to Na⁺ of *p*-aminohippuric acid uptake into rat renal basolateral membrane vesicles. *Am J Physiol.* 1987;253:F795-F801.

225. Kusuhara H, Sekine T, Utsunomiya-Tate N, et al. Molecular cloning and characterization of a new multispecific organic anion transporter from rat brain. *J Biol Chem.* 1999;274:13675-13680.

226. Sekine T, Cha SH, Tsuda M, et al. Identification of multispecific organic anion transporter 2 expressed predominantly in the liver. *FEBS Lett.* 1998;429:179-182.

227. Cha SH, Sekine T, Kusuhara H, et al. Molecular cloning and characterization of multispecific organic anion transporter 4 expressed in the placenta. *J Biol Chem.* 2000;275:4507-4512.

228. Ekaratanawong S, Anzai N, Jutabha P, et al. Human organic anion transporter 4 is a renal apical organic anion/dicarboxylate exchanger in the proximal tubules. *J Pharmacol Sci.* 2004;94:297-304.

229. Enomoto A, Kimura H, Chairoungdua A, et al. Molecular identification of a renal urate anion exchanger that regulates blood urate levels. *Nature.* 2002;417:447-452.

230. Meier PJ, Eckhardt U, Schroeder A, et al. Substrate specificity of sinusoidal bile acid and organic anion uptake systems in rat and human liver. *Hepatology.* 1997;26:1667-1677.

231. Tamai I, Nezu J, Uchino H, et al. Molecular identification and characterization of novel members of the human organic anion transporter (OATP) family. *Biochem Biophys Res Commun.* 2000;273:251-260.

232. Jacquemin E, Hagenbuch B, Stieger B, et al. Expression cloning of a rat liver Na(+)-independent organic anion transporter. *Proc Natl Acad Sci U S A.* 1994;91:133-137.

233. Mikkaichi T, Suzuki T, Onogawa T, et al. Isolation and characterization of a digoxin transporter and its rat homologue expressed in the kidney. *Proc Natl Acad Sci U S A.* 2004;101:3569-3574.

234. Brennan S, Hering-Smith K, Hamm LL. Effect of pH on citrate reabsorption in the proximal convoluted tubule. *Am J Physiol.* 1988;255:F301-F306.

235. Wright SH, Kippen I, Wright EM. Effect of pH on the transport of Krebs cycle intermediates in renal brush border membranes. *Biochim Biophys Acta.* 1982;684:287-290.

236. Aruga S, Wehrli S, Kaissling B, et al. Chronic metabolic acidosis increases NaDC-1 mRNA and protein abundance in rat kidney. *Kidney Int.* 2000;58:206-215.

237. Melnick JZ, Preisig PA, Moe OW, et al. Renal cortical mitochondrial aconitase is regulated in hypo- and hypercitraturia. *Kidney Int.* 1998;54:160-165.

238. Melnick JZ, Srere PA, Elshourbagy NA, et al. Adenosine triphosphate citrate lyase mediates hypocitraturia in rats. *J Clin Invest.* 1996;98:2381-2387.

239. Roch-Ramel F, Guisan B. Renal transport of urate in humans. *News Physiol Sci.* 1999;14:80-84.

240. Ichida K, Hosoyamada M, Hisatome I, et al. Clinical and molecular analysis of patients with renal hypouricemia in Japan—influence of URAT1 gene on urinary urate excretion. *J Am Soc Nephrol.* 2004;15:164-173.

241. Eraly SA, Vallon V, Rieg T, et al. Multiple organic anion transporters contribute to net renal excretion of uric acid. *Physiol Genomics.* 2008;33:180-192.

242. Leal-Pinto E, Tao W, Rappaport J, et al. Molecular cloning and functional reconstitution of a urate transporter/channel. *J Biol Chem.* 1997;272:617-625.

243. Jutabha P, Kanai Y, Hosoyamada M, et al. Identification of a novel voltage-driven organic anion transporter present at apical membrane of renal proximal tubule. *J Biol Chem.* 2003;278:27930-27938.

244. Van Aubel RA, Smeets PH, van den Heuvel JJ, et al. Human organic anion transporter MRP4 (ABCC4) is an efflux pump for the purine end metabolite urate with multiple allosteric substrate binding sites. *Am J Physiol Renal Physiol.* 2005;288:F327-F333.

245. El-Sheikh AA, van den Heuvel JJ, Koenderink JB, et al. Effect of hypouricaemic and hyperuricaemic drugs on the renal urate efflux transporter, multidrug resistance protein 4. *Br J Pharmacol.* 2008;155:1066-1075.

246. Vitart V, Rudan I, Hayward C, et al. SLC2A9 is a newly identified urate transporter influencing serum uric acid concentration, urate excretion and gout. *Nat Genet.* 2008;40:437-442.

247. Cheeseman C. Solute carrier family 2, member 9 and uric acid homeostasis. *Curr Opin Nephrol Hypertens.* 2009;18:428-432.

248. Bakhiya A, Bahn A, Burckhardt G, et al. Human organic anion transporter 3 (hOAT3) can operate as an exchanger and mediate secretory urate flux. *Cell Physiol Biochem.* 2003;13:249-256.

249. Anzai N, Ichida K, Jutabha P, et al. Plasma urate level is directly regulated by a voltage-driven urate efflux transporter URATv1 (SLC2A9) in humans. *J Biol Chem.* 2008;283:26834-26838.

250. Heinig M, Johnson RJ. Role of uric acid in hypertension, renal disease, and metabolic syndrome. *Cleve Clin J Med.* 2006;73:1059-1064.

251. Moe OW. Posing the question again: does chronic uric acid nephropathy exist? *J Am Soc Nephrol.* 2010;21:395-397.

252. Bibert S, Hess SK, Firsov D, et al. Mouse GLUT9: evidences for a urate uniporter. *Am J Physiol Renal Physiol.* 2009;297:F612-F619.

253. Doblado MA, Moley KH. Facilitative glucose transporter 9, a unique hexose and urate transporter. *Am J Physiol Endocrinol Metab.* 2009;297(4):E831-835.

254. Li S, Sanna S, Maschio A, et al. The *GLUT9* gene is associated with serum uric acid levels in Sardinia and Chianti cohorts. *PLoS Genet.* 2007;3:e194.

255. McArdle PF, Parsa A, Chang YP, et al. Association of a common nonsynonymous variant in *GLUT9* with serum uric acid levels in Old Order Amish. *Arthritis Rheum.* 2008;58:2874-2881.

256. Stark K, Reinhard W, Neureuther K, et al. Association of common polymorphisms in *GLUT9* gene with gout but not with coronary artery disease in a large case-control study. *PLoS One.* 2008;3:e1948.

257. Sekine T, Cha SH, Endou H. The multispecific organic anion transporter (OAT) family. *Pflugers Arch.* 2000;440:337-350.

258. Nakashima M, Uematsu T, Kosuge K, et al. Pilot study of the uricosuric effect of DuP-753, a new angiotensin II receptor antagonist, in healthy subjects. *Eur J Clin Pharmacol.* 1992;42:333-335.

259. Kikuchi Y, Koga H, Yasutomo Y, et al. Patients with renal hypouricemia with exercise-induced acute renal failure and chronic renal dysfunction. *Clin Nephrol.* 2000;53:467-472.

260. Enomoto A, Niwa T. Roles of organic anion transporters in the progression of chronic renal failure. *Ther Apher Dial.* 2007;11(suppl 1):S27-S31.

261. Toyohara T, Suzuki T, Morimoto R, et al. SLCO4C1 transporter eliminates uremic toxins and attenuates hypertension and renal inflammation. *J Am Soc Nephrol.* 2009;20:2546-2555.

262. Silbernagl S, Volkl H. Molecular specificity of the tubular resorption of "acidic" amino acids. A continuous microperfusion study in rat kidney in vivo. *Pflugers Arch.* 1983;396:225-230.

263. Windmueller HG, Spaeth AE. Source and fate of circulating citrulline. *Am J Physiol.* 1981;241:E473-E480.

264. Handler JS, Kwon HM. Kidney cell survival in high tonicity. *Comp Biochem Physiol A Physiol.* 1997;117:301-306.

265. Silbernagl S. The renal handling of amino acids and oligopeptides. *Physiol Rev.* 1988;68:911-1007.

266. Palacín M, Estevez R, Bertran J, et al. Molecular biology of mammalian plasma membrane amino acid transporters. *Physiol Rev.* 1998;78:969-1054.

267. Broer A, Klingel K, Kowalczuk S, et al. Molecular cloning of mouse amino acid transport system B⁰, a neutral amino acid transporter related to Hartnup disorder. *J Biol Chem.* 2004;279:24467-24476.

267a. Böhmer C, Bröer A, Munzinger M, et al. Characterization of mouse amino acid transporter B0AT1 (slc6a19). *Biochem J.* 2005;389(pt 3): 745-751.

267b. Takanaga H, Mackenzie B, Suzuki Y, et al. Identification of mammalian proline transporter SIT1 (SLC6A20) with characteristics of classical system imino. *J Biol Chem.* 2005;280(10):8974-8984.

268. Bröer A, Tietze N, Kowalczuk S, et al. The orphan transporter v7-3 (slc6a15) is a Na+-dependent neutral amino acid transporter (B0AT2). *Biochem J.* 2006;393(pt 1):421-430.

269. Takanaga H, Mackenzie B, Peng JB, et al. Characterization of a branched-chain amino-acid transporter SBAT1 (SLC6A15) that is expressed in human brain. *Biochem Biophys Res Commun.* 2005;337:892-900.

269a. Wasserman JC, Delpire E, Tonidandel W, et al. Molecular characterization of ROSIT, a renal osmotic stress-induced Na(+)-Cl(-)-organic solute cotransporter. *Am J Physiol.* 1994;267(4 pt 2):F688-F694.

269b. Liu QR, López-Corcuera B, Nelson H, et al. Cloning and expression of a cDNA encoding the transporter of taurine and beta-alanine in mouse brain. *Proc Natl Acad Sci USA.* 1992;89(24):12145-12149.

269c. Smith KE, Borden LA, Wang CH, et al. Cloning and expression of a high affinity taurine transporter from rat brain. *Mol Pharmacol.* 1992;42(4): 563-569.

269d. Uchida S, Kwon HM, Yamauchi A, et al. Molecular cloning of the cDNA for an MDCK cell Na(+)- and Cl(-)-dependent taurine transporter that is regulated by hypertonicity. *Proc Natl Acad Sci USA.* 1992;89(17):8230-8234.

270. Doyle FA, McGivan JD. The bovine renal epithelial cell line NBL-1 expresses a broad specificity Na(+)-dependent neutral amino acid transport system (system Bo) similar to that in bovine renal brush border membrane vesicles. *Biochim Biophys Acta.* 1992;1104:55-62.

271. Broer S, Bailey CG, Kowalczuk S, et al. Iminoglycinuria and hyperglycinuria are discrete human phenotypes resulting from complex mutations in proline and glycine transporters. *J Clin Invest.* 2008;118:3881-3892.

272. Bohmer C, Broer A, Munzinger M, et al. Characterization of mouse amino acid transporter B⁰AT1 (Slc6A19). *Biochem J.* 2005;389:745-751.

273. Kleta R, Romeo E, Ristic Z, et al. Mutations in SLC6A19, encoding B⁰AT1, cause Hartnup disorder. *Nat Genet.* 2004;36:999-1002.

274. Romeo E, Dave MH, Bacic D, et al. Luminal kidney and intestine SLC6 amino acid transporters of B0AT-cluster and their tissue distribution in *Mus musculus. Am J Physiol Renal Physiol.* 2006;290:F376-F383.

275. Seow HF, Broer S, Broer A, et al. Hartnup disorder is caused by mutations in the gene encoding the neutral amino acid transporter SLC6A19. *Nat Genet.* 2004;36:1003-1007.

276. Azmanov DN, Kowalczuk S, Rodgers H, et al. Further evidence for allelic heterogeneity in Hartnup disorder. *Hum Mutat.* 2008;29:1217-1221.

277. Camargo SM, Singer D, Makrides V, et al. Tissue-specific amino acid transporter partners ACE2 and collectrin differentially interact with hartnup mutations. *Gastroenterology.* 2009;136:872-882.

278. Danilczyk U, Sarao R, Remy C, et al. Essential role for collectrin in renal amino acid transport. *Nature.* 2006;444:1088-1091.

279. Kowalczuk S, Broer A, Tietze N, et al. A protein complex in the brush-border membrane explains a Hartnup disorder allele. *FASEB J.* 2008;22:2880-2887.

279a. Malakauskas SM, Quan H, Fields TA, et al. Aminoaciduria and altered renal expression of luminal amino acid transporters in mice lacking novel gene collectrin. *Am J Physiol Renal Physiol.* 2007;292(2):F533-F544.

280. Hillman RE. Amino-acid transport defect in intestine not affecting kidney. *Pediatric Res.* 1986;20:A265.

281. Fukui K, Yang Q, Cao Y, et al. The HNF-1 target collectrin controls insulin exocytosis by SNARE complex formation. *Cell Metab.* 2005;2:373-384.

282. Kekuda R, Prasad PD, Fei YJ, et al. Cloning of the sodium-dependent, broad-scope, neutral amino acid transporter B⁰ from a human placental choriocarcinoma cell line. *J Biol Chem.* 1996;271:18657-18661.

283. Utsunomiya-Tate N, Endou H, Kanai Y. Cloning and functional characterization of a system ASC-like Na⁺-dependent neutral amino acid transporter. *J Biol Chem.* 1996;271:14883-14890.

283a. Bröer A, Wagner C, Lang F, et al. Neutral amino acid transporter ASCT2 displays substrate-induced Na+ exchange and a substrate-gated anion conductance. *Biochem J.* 2000;346(pt 3):705-710.

284. Avissar NE, Ryan CK, Ganapathy V, et al. Na(+)-dependent neutral amino acid transporter ATB(0) is a rabbit epithelial cell brush-border protein. *Am J Physiol Cell Physiol.* 2001;281:C963-C971.

285. Scriver CR, Schafer IA, Efron ML. New renal tubular amino-acid transport system and a new hereditary disorder of amino-acid metabolism. *Nature.* 1961;192:672-673.

286. Quan H, Athirakul K, Wetsel WC, et al. Hypertension and impaired glycine handling in mice lacking the orphan transporter XT2. *Mol Cell Biol.* 2004;24:4166-4173.

287. Nash SR, Giros B, Kingsmore SF, et al. Cloning, gene structure and genomic localization of an orphan transporter from mouse kidney with six alternatively-spliced isoforms. *Receptors Channels.* 1998;6:113-128.

288. Eslami B, Kinboshi M, Inoue S, et al. A nonsense polymorphism (Y319X) of the solute carrier family 6 member 18 (*SLC6A18*) gene is not associated with hypertension and blood pressure in Japanese. *Tohoku J Exp Med.* 2006;208:25-31.

289. Anderson CM, Grenade DS, Boll M, et al. H⁺/amino acid transporter 1 (PAT1) is the imino acid carrier: an intestinal nutrient/drug transporter in human and rat. *Gastroenterology.* 2004;127:1410-1422.

289a. Boll M, Foltz M, Anderson CM, et al. Substrate recognition by the mammalian proton-dependent amino acid transporter PAT1. *Mol Membr Biol.* 2003;20(3):261-269.

289b. Foltz M, Oechsler C, Boll M, et al. Substrate specificity and transport mode of the proton-dependent amino acid transporter mPAT2. *Eur J Biochem.* 2004;271(16):3340-3347.

290. Scriver CR, Efron ML, Schafer IA. Renal tubular transport of proline, hydroxyproline, and glycine in health and in familial hyperprolinemia. *J Clin Invest.* 1964;43:374-385.

291. Dantzler WH, Silbernagl S. Renal tubular reabsorption of taurine, gamma-aminobutyric acid (GABA) and beta-alanine studied by continuous microperfusion. *Pflugers Arch.* 1976;367:123-128.

292. Turner RJ. Beta-amino acid transport across the renal brush-border membrane is coupled to both Na and Cl. *J Biol Chem.* 1986;261:16060-16066.

293. Huang DY, Boini KM, Lang PA, et al. Impaired ability to increase water excretion in mice lacking the taurine transporter gene *TauT. Pflugers Arch.* 2006;451:668-677.

294. Pineda M, Fernandez E, Torrents D, et al. Identification of a membrane protein, LAT-2, that co-expresses with 4F2 heavy chain, an L-type amino acid transport activity with broad specificity for small and large zwitterionic amino acids. *J Biol Chem.* 1999;274:19738-19744.

295. Rajan DP, Kekuda R, Huang W, et al. Cloning and functional characterization of a Na(+)-independent, broad-specific neutral amino acid transporter from mammalian intestine. *Biochim Biophys Acta.* 2000;1463: 6-14.

295a. Kim DK, Kanai Y, Chairoungdua A, et al. Expression cloning of a Na+-independent aromatic amino acid transporter with structural similarity to H+/monocarboxylate transporters. *J Biol Chem.* 2001;276(20):17221-17228.

296. Halestrap AP, Meredith D. The *SLC16* gene family—from monocarboxylate transporters (MCTs) to aromatic amino acid transporters and beyond. *Pflugers Arch.* 2004;447:619-628.

297. Babu E, Kanai Y, Chairoungdua A, et al. Identification of a novel system L amino acid transporter structurally distinct from heterodimeric amino acid transporters. *J Biol Chem.* 2003;278:43838-43845.

298. Bodoy S, Martin L, Zorzano A, et al. Identification of LAT4, a novel amino acid transporter with system L activity. *J Biol Chem.* 2005;280:12002-12011.

299. Ramadan T, Camargo SM, Summa V, et al. Basolateral aromatic amino acid transporter TAT1 (Slc16A10) functions as an efflux pathway. *J Cell Physiol.* 2006;206:771-779.

300. Wilson MC, Meredith D, Fox JE, et al. Basigin (CD147) is the target for organomercurial inhibition of monocarboxylate transporter isoforms 1 and 4: the ancillary protein for the insensitive MCT2 is EMBIGIN (gp70). *J Biol Chem.* 2005;280:27213-27221.

301. Fernandez E, Jimenez-Vidal M, Calvo M, et al. The structural and functional units of heteromeric amino acid transporters. The heavy subunit rBAT dictates oligomerization of the heteromeric amino acid transporters. *J Biol Chem.* 2006;281:26552-26561.

302. Oxender DL, Christensen HN. Distinct mediating systems for the transport of neutral amino acids by the Ehrlich cell. *J Biol Chem.* 1963;238:3686-3699.

303. Hopfer U, Sigrist-Nelson K, Ammann E, et al. Differences in neutral amino acid and glucose transport between brush border and basolateral plasma membrane of intestinal epithelial cells. *J Cell Physiol.* 1976;89:805-810.

304. Meier C, Ristic Z, Klauser S, et al. Activation of system L heterodimeric amino acid exchangers by intracellular substrates. *Embo J.* 2002;21:580-589.

305. Fernandez E, Torrents D, Chillaron J, et al. Basolateral LAT-2 has a major role in the transepithelial flux of L-cystine in the renal proximal tubule cell line OK. *J Am Soc Nephrol.* 2003;14:837-847.

306. Crawhall JC, Segal S. The intracellular cysteine-cystine ratio in kidney cortex. *Biochem J.* 1966;99:19C-20C.

307. Ramadan T, Camargo SM, Herzog B, et al. Recycling of aromatic amino acids via TAT1 allows efflux of neutral amino acids via LAT2-4F2hc exchanger. *Pflugers Arch.* 2007;454:507-516.

308. Bertran J, Werner A, Moore ML, et al. Expression cloning of a cDNA from rabbit kidney cortex that induces a single transport system for cystine and dibasic and neutral amino acids. *Proc Natl Acad Sci USA.* 1992;89(12): 5601-5605.

309. Tate SS, Yan N, Udenfriend S. Expression cloning of a Na(+)-independent neutral amino acid transporter from rat kidney. *Proc Natl Acad Sci U S A.* 1992;89:1-5.

310. Wells RG, Lee WS, Kanai Y, et al. The 4F2 antigen heavy chain induces uptake of neutral and dibasic amino acids in *Xenopus* oocytes. *J Biol Chem.* 1992;267:15285-15288.

311. Estevez R, Camps M, Rojas AM, et al. The amino acid transport system y⁺L/4F2hc is a heteromultimeric complex. *FASEB J.* 1998;12:1319-1329.

312. Kanai Y, Segawa H, Miyamoto K, et al. Expression cloning and characterization of a transporter for large neutral amino acids activated by the heavy chain of 4F2 antigen (CD98). *J Biol Chem.* 1998;273:23629-23632.

313. Mastroberardino L, Spindler B, Pfeiffer R, et al. Amino-acid transport by heterodimers of 4F2hc/CD98 and members of a permease family. *Nature.* 1998;395:288-291.

314. Sato H, Tamba M, Ishii T, et al. Cloning and expression of a plasma membrane cystine/glutamate exchange transporter composed of two distinct proteins. *J Biol Chem.* 1999;274:11455-11458.

315. Feliubadalo L, Font M, Purroy J, et al. Non–type I cystinuria caused by mutations in SLC7A9, encoding a subunit (b⁰,⁺AT) of rBAT. *Nat Genet.* 1999;23:52-57.

316. Torrents D, Estevez R, Pineda M, et al. Identification and characterization of a membrane protein (y⁺L amino acid transporter-1) that associates with 4F2hc to encode the amino acid transport activity y⁺L. A candidate gene for lysinuric protein intolerance. *J Biol Chem.* 1998;273:32437-32445.

317. Munck BG. Lysine transport across the small intestine. Stimulating and inhibitory effects of neutral amino acids. *J Membr Biol.* 1980;53:45-53.

318. Munck BG. Transport of neutral and cationic amino acids across the brush-border membrane of the rabbit ileum. *J Membr Biol.* 1985;83:1-13.

319. Palacín M, Bertran J, Chillaron J, et al. Lysinuric protein intolerance: mechanisms of pathophysiology. *Mol Genet Metab.* 2004;81(suppl 1):S27-S37.

320. Palacín M, Nunes V, Font-Llitjos M, et al. The genetics of heteromeric amino acid transporters. *Physiology (Bethesda).* 2005;20:112-124.

321. Verrey F, Closs EI, Wagner CA, et al. CATs and HATs: the SLC7 family of amino acid transporters. *Pflugers Arch.* 2004;447:532-542.

322. Busch AE, Herzer T, Waldegger S, et al. Opposite directed currents induced by the transport of dibasic and neutral amino acids in *Xenopus* oocytes expressing the protein rBAT. *J Biol Chem.* 1994;269:25581-25586.

323. Chillaron J, Estevez R, Mora C, et al. Obligatory amino acid exchange via systems b⁰,⁺-like and y⁺L-like. A tertiary active transport mechanism for renal reabsorption of cystine and dibasic amino acids. *J Biol Chem.* 1996;271:17761-17770.

324. Mora C, Chillaron J, Calonge MJ, et al. The rBAT gene is responsible for L-cystine uptake via the b⁰,(+)-like amino acid transport system in a "renal proximal tubular" cell line (OK cell). *J Biol Chem.* 1996;271:10569-10576.

325. Reig N, Chillaron J, Bartoccioni P, et al. The light subunit of system b(0,+) is fully functional in the absence of the heavy subunit. *Embo J.* 2002;21:4906-4914.

326. Fernandez E, Carrascal M, Rousaud F, et al. rBAT-b(0,+)AT heterodimer is the main apical reabsorption system for cystine in the kidney. *Am J Physiol Renal Physiol.* 2002;283:F540-F548.

327. Deleted in page proofs.

328. Calonge MJ, Gasparini P, Chillaron J, et al. Cystinuria caused by mutations in rBAT, a gene involved in the transport of cystine. *Nat Genet.* 1994;6:420-425.

329. Palacín M, Goodyer P, Nunes V, et al, eds. *Cystinuria.* New York: McGraw-Hill; 2001.

330. Peters T, Thaete C, Wolf S, et al. A mouse model for cystinuria type I. *Hum Mol Genet.* 2003;12:2109-2120.

331. Feliubadalo L, Arbones ML, Manas S, et al. *Slc7a9*-deficient mice develop cystinuria non-I and cystine urolithiasis. *Hum Mol Genet.* 2003;12:2097-2108.

331a. Henthorn PS, Liu J, Gidalevich T, et al. Canine cystinuria: polymorphism in the canine SLC3A1 gene and identification of a nonsense mutation in cystinuric Newfoundland dogs. *Hum Genet.* 2000;107(4):295-303.

332. Font-Llitjos M, Jimenez-Vidal M, Bisceglia L, et al. New insights into cystinuria: 40 new mutations, genotype-phenotype correlation, and digenic inheritance causing partial phenotype. *J Med Genet.* 2005;42:58-68.

333. Chillarón J, Font-Llitjós M, Fort J, et al. Pathophysiology and treatment of cystinuria. *Nat Rev Nephrol.* 2010;6(7):424-434.

334. Shigeta Y, Kanai Y, Chairoungdua A, et al. A novel missense mutation of SLC7A9 frequent in Japanese cystinuria cases affecting the C-terminus of the transporter. *Kidney Int.* 2006;69:1198-1206.

335. Chatzikyriakidou A, Sofikitis N, Kalfakakou V, et al. Evidence for association of SLC7A9 gene haplotypes with cystinuria manifestation in SLC7A9 mutation carriers. *Urol Res.* 2006;34:299-303.

336. Brodehl J, Gellissen K, Kowalewski S. Isolated cystinuria (without lysin-, ornithinand argininuria) in a family with hypocalcemic tetany. *Monatsschr Kinderheilkd.* 1967;115:317-320.

337. Eggermann T, Elbracht M, Haverkamp F, et al. Isolated cystinuria (OMIM 238200) is not a separate entity but is caused by a mutation in the cystinuria gene *SLC7A9. Clin Genet.* 2007;71:597-598.

338. Crawhall JC, Scowen EF, Thompson CJ, et al. The renal clearance of amino acids in cystinuria. *J Clin Invest.* 1967;46:1162-1171.

339. Rosenberg LE, Albrecht I, Segal S. Lysine transport in human kidney: evidence for two systems. *Science.* 1967;155:1426-1428.

340. Furriols M, Chillaron J, Mora C, et al. rBAT, related to L-cysteine transport, is localized to the microvilli of proximal straight tubules, and its expression is regulated in kidney by development. *J Biol Chem.* 1993;268:27060-27068.

341. Bröer S. Amino acid transport across mammalian intestinal and renal epithelia. *Physiol Rev.* 2008;88:249-286.

342. Bartoccioni P, Rius M, Zorzano A, et al. Distinct classes of trafficking rBAT mutants cause the type I cystinuria phenotype. *Hum Mol Genet.* 2008;17:1845-1854.

343. Chillaron J, Estevez R, Samarzija I, et al. An intracellular trafficking defect in type I cystinuria rBAT mutants M467T and M467K. *J Biol Chem.* 1997;272:9543-9549.

344. Pineda M, Wagner CA, Broer A, et al. Cystinuria-specific rBAT (R365W) mutation reveals two translocation pathways in the amino acid transporter rBAT-b⁰,⁺AT. *Biochem J.* 2004;377:665-674.

345. Pfeiffer R, Rossier G, Spindler B, et al. Amino acid transport of y⁺L-type by heterodimers of 4F2hc/CD98 and members of the glycoprotein-associated amino acid transporter family. *Embo J.* 1999;18:49-57.

346. Palacín M, Kanai Y. The ancillary proteins of HATs: SLC3 family of amino acid transporters. *Pflugers Arch.* 2004;447:490-494.

347. Shoji Y, Noguchi A, Shoji Y, et al. Five novel SLC7A7 variants and y⁺L gene-expression pattern in cultured lymphoblasts from Japanese patients with lysinuric protein intolerance. *Hum Mutat.* 2002;20:375-381.

348. Bauch C, Forster N, Loffing-Cueni D, et al. Functional cooperation of epithelial heteromeric amino acid transporters expressed in Madin-Darby canine kidney cells. *J Biol Chem.* 2003;278:1316-1322.

349. Borsani G, Bassi MT, Sperandeo MP, et al. SLC7A7, encoding a putative permease-related protein, is mutated in patients with lysinuric protein intolerance. *Nat Genet.* 1999;21:297-301.

350. Torrents D, Mykkanen J, Pineda M, et al. Identification of SLC7A7, encoding y⁺LAT-1, as the lysinuric protein intolerance gene. *Nat Genet.* 1999;21:293-296.

351. Palacín M, Borsani G, Sebastio G. The molecular bases of cystinuria and lysinuric protein intolerance. *Curr Opin Genet Dev.* 2001;11:328-335.

352. Rajantie J, Simell O, Perheentupa J. Basolateral-membrane transport defect for lysine in lysinuric protein intolerance. *Lancet.* 1980;1:1219-1221.

353. Sperandeo MP, Annunziata P, Bozzato A, et al. Slc7a7 disruption causes fetal growth retardation by downregulating Igf1 in the mouse model of lysinuric protein intolerance. *Am J Physiol Cell Physiol.* 2007;293:C191-C198.

354. Font-Llitjos M, Rodriguez-Santiago B, Espino M, et al. Novel SLC7A7 large rearrangements in lysinuric protein intolerance patients involving the same AluY repeat. *Eur J Hum Genet.* 2009;17:71-79.

355. Sperandeo MP, Andria G, Sebastio G. Lysinuric protein intolerance: update and extended mutation analysis of the SLC7A7 gene. *Hum Mutat.* 2008;29:14-21.

356. Sperandeo MP, Paladino S, Maiuri L, et al. A y(+)LAT-1 mutant protein interferes with y(+)LAT-2 activity: implications for the molecular pathogenesis of lysinuric protein intolerance. *Eur J Hum Genet.* 2005;13:628-634.

357. Tsumura H, Suzuki N, Saito H, et al. The targeted disruption of the CD98 gene results in embryonic lethality. *Biochem Biophys Res Commun.* 2003;308:847-851.

358. Cantor J, Browne CD, Ruppert R, et al. CD98hc facilitates B cell proliferation and adaptive humoral immunity. *Nat Immunol.* 2009;10:412-419.

359. Feral CC, Nishiya N, Fenczik CA, et al. CD98hc (SLC3A2) mediates integrin signaling. *Proc Natl Acad Sci U S A.* 2005;102:355-360.

360. Kanai Y, Hediger MA. Primary structure and functional characterization of a high-affinity glutamate transporter. *Nature.* 1992;360:467-471.

361. Pines G, Danbolt NC, Bjørås M, et al. Cloning and expression of a rat brain L-glutamate transporter. *Nature.* 1992;360(6403):464-467.

362. Kanai Y, Hediger MA. The glutamate/neutral amino acid transporter family SLC1: molecular, physiological and pharmacological aspects. *Pflugers Arch.* 2004;447:469-479.

362a. Matsuo H, Kanai Y, Kim JY, et al. Identification of a novel Na+-independent acidic amino acid transporter with structural similarity to the member of a heterodimeric amino acid transporter family associated with unknown heavy chains. *J Biol Chem.* 2002;277(23):21017-21026.

363. Zerangue N, Kavanaugh MP. Flux coupling in a neuronal glutamate transporter. *Nature.* 1996;383:634-637.

364. Welbourne TC, Matthews JC. Glutamate transport and renal function. *Am J Physiol.* 1999;277:F501-F505.

365. Sacktor B, Rosenbloom IL, Liang CT, et al. Sodium gradient– and sodium plus potassium gradient–dependent L-glutamate uptake in renal basolateral membrane vesicles. *J Membr Biol.* 1981;60:63-71.

366. Kanai Y, Stelzner M, Nussberger S, et al. The neuronal and epithelial human high affinity glutamate transporter. Insights into structure and mechanism of transport. *J Biol Chem.* 1994;269:20599-20606.

367. Shayakul C, Kanai Y, Lee WS, et al. Localization of the high-affinity glutamate transporter EAAC1 in rat kidney. *Am J Physiol.* 1997;273:F1023-F1029.

368. Dantzler WH, Silbernagl S. Amino acid transport by juxtamedullary nephrons: distal reabsorption and recycling. *Am J Physiol.* 1988;255:F397-F407.

369. Peghini P, Janzen J, Stoffel W. Glutamate transporter EAAC-1–deficient mice develop dicarboxylic aminoaciduria and behavioral abnormalities but no neurodegeneration. *Embo J.* 1997;16:3822-3832.

370. Swarna M, Rao DN, Reddy PP. Dicarboxylic aminoaciduria associated with mental retardation. *Hum Genet.* 1989;82:299-300.

370a. Bailey CG, Ryan RM, Thoeng AD, et al. Loss-of-function mutations in the glutamate transporter SLC1A1 cause human dicarboxylic aminoaciduria. *J Clin Invest.* 2011;121(1):446-453.

371. Yernool D, Boudker O, Jin Y, et al. Structure of a glutamate transporter homologue from *Pyrococcus horikoshii. Nature.* 2004;431:811-818.

372. Yamashita A, Singh SK, Kawate T, et al. Crystal structure of a bacterial homologue of Na⁺/Cl⁻-dependent neurotransmitter transporters. *Nature.* 2005;437:215-223.

373. Fang Y, Jayaram H, Shane T, et al. Structure of a prokaryotic virtual proton pump at 3.2 Å resolution. *Nature.* 2009;460:1040-1043.

374. Weyand S, Shimamura T, Yajima S, et al. Structure and molecular mechanism of a nucleobase-cation-symport-1 family transporter. *Science.* 2008;322:709-713.

375. Ressl S, Terwisscha van Scheltinga AC, et al. Molecular basis of transport and regulation in the Na(+)/betaine symporter BetP. *Nature.* 2009;458:47-52.

376. Gao X, Lu F, Zhou L, et al. Structure and mechanism of an amino acid antiporter. *Science.* 2009;324:1565-1568.

377. Krishnamurthy H, Piscitelli CL, Gouaux E. Unlocking the molecular secrets of sodium-coupled transporters. *Nature.* 2009;459:347-355.

378. Shi L, Quick M, Zhao Y, et al. The mechanism of a neurotransmitter:sodium symporter—inward release of Na⁺ and substrate is triggered by substrate in a second binding site. *Mol Cell.* 2008;30:667-677.

378a. Kowalczyk L, Ratera M, Paladino A, et al. Molecular basis of substrate-induced permeation by an amino acid antiporter. *Proc Natl Acad Sci USA.* 2011;108(10):3935-3940.

379. Mitchell P. A general theory of membrane transport from studies of bacteria. *Nature.* 1957;180:134-136.

380. Patlak CS. Contributions to the theory of active transport: II. The gate type non-carrier mechanism and generalizations concerning tracer flow, efficiency, and measurement of energy expenditure. *Bull Math Biophys.* 1957;19:209-235.

381. Forrest LR, Zhang YW, Jacobs MT, et al. Mechanism for alternating access in neurotransmitter transporters. *Proc Natl Acad Sci U S A.* 2008;105:10338-10343.

381a. Forrest LR, Tavoulari S, Zhang YW, et al. Identification of a chloride ion binding site in Na+/Cl -dependent transporters. *Proc Natl Acad Sci USA.* 2007;104(31):12761-12766.

382. Zomot E, Bendahan A, Quick M, et al. Mechanism of chloride interaction with neurotransmitter:sodium symporters. *Nature.* 2007;449(7163):726-730.

383. Fort J, de la Ballina LR, Burghardt HE, et al. The structure of human 4F2hc ectodomain provides a model for homodimerization and electrostatic interaction with plasma membrane. *J Biol Chem.* 2007;282:31444-31452.

384. Franca R, Veljkovic E, Walter S, et al. Heterodimeric amino acid transporter glycoprotein domains determining functional subunit association. *Biochem J.* 2005;388:435-443.

385. Broer A, Friedrich B, Wagner CA, et al. Association of 4F2hc with light chains LAT1, LAT2 or y⁺LAT2 requires different domains. *Biochem J.* 2001;355:725-731.

386. Fenczik CA, Zent R, Dellos M, et al. Distinct domains of CD98hc regulate integrins and amino acid transport. *J Biol Chem.* 2001;276:8746-8752.

387. Reig N, del Rio C, Casagrande F, et al. Functional and structural characterization of the first prokaryotic member of the L–amino acid transporter (LAT) family: a model for APC transporters. *J Biol Chem.* 2007;282:13270-13281.

388. Gasol E, Jimenez-Vidal M, Chillaron J, et al. Membrane topology of system xc- light subunit reveals a re-entrant loop with substrate-restricted accessibility. *J Biol Chem.* 2004;279:31228-31236.

389. Gao X, Zhou L, Jiao X, et al. Mechanism of substrate recognition and transport by an amino acid antiporter. *Nature.* 2010;463(7282):828-832.

390. Bartoccioni P, Del Rio C, Ratera M, et al. Role of transmembrane domain 8 in substrate selectivity and translocation of SteT, a member of the L-amino acid transporter (LAT) family. *J Biol Chem.* 2010;285(37):28764-28776.

Renal Acidification Mechanisms

I. David Weiner and Jill W. Verlander

Acid-base homeostasis is critical for normal health, growth, and development. Acid-base disorders can lead to a wide variety of clinical problems, including growth retardation in neonates and children; nausea and vomiting; electrolyte disturbances; increased susceptibility to cardiac arrhythmias; decreased catecholamine sensitivity, particularly in the cardiovascular system; osteoporosis and osteomalacia; recurrent nephrolithiasis; skeletal muscle atrophy; paresthesias; and coma.

The kidneys have two major functions in acid-base homeostasis: reabsorption of filtered bicarbonate and generation of new bicarbonate. In the normal adult, daily filtered bicarbonate averages approximately 4200 mmol/day and is reabsorbed almost completely by renal epithelial cells. This process is termed *bicarbonate reabsorption*. Both intracellular and extracellular bicarbonate are used to buffer acids produced from cellular metabolism, oral ingestion, and gastrointestinal alkali losses, and must be continually replenished to maintain acid-base homoeostasis. The kidneys produce bicarbonate; this process is termed *bicarbonate generation*. In addition, the kidneys can excrete alkali, both in the form of bicarbonate and in the form of organic anions, which are necessary for multiple physiologic functions, including prevention of or recovery from respiratory and metabolic alkalosis and prevention of renal stone formation.

Bicarbonate Reabsorption

Bicarbonate reabsorption involves coordinated effects in multiple nephron segments. As shown in Figure 9-1, the majority of bicarbonate reabsorption occurs in the proximal tubule. Little to no reabsorption occurs in the thin descending limb of the loop of Henle, moderate amounts occur in the thick ascending limb of the loop of Henle (TAL), and the remaining filtered bicarbonate is reabsorbed in distal nephron sites, including the distal convoluted tubule (DCT), connecting tubule (CNT), initial collecting tubule (ICT), and collecting duct.

Proximal Tubule

General Transport Mechanisms

Proximal tubule bicarbonate reabsorption involves four distinct and interconnected processes (Figure 9-2). First, protons (H^+) are secreted into the luminal fluid. Two proteins mediate H^+ secretion, the apical Na^+/H^+ exchanger isoform 3 (NHE3), and an apical H^+–adenosine triphosphatase (ATPase). NHE3 is responsible for 60% to 70% of apical H^+ secretion and H^+-ATPase accounts for the remainder. Secreted H^+ combines with luminal HCO_3^- to form carbonic acid (H_2CO_3). Luminal carbonic acid dissociates to water (H_2O) and carbon dioxide (CO_2). Although this can occur spontaneously, the spontaneous dehydration rate is relatively slow and inadequate to support normal rates of proximal tubule bicarbonate reabsorption. The dehydration reaction is catalyzed by carbonic anhydrase IV (CA IV), a membrane-bound carbonic anhydrase isoform present in the proximal tubule brush border. Luminal CO_2 moves across the apical plasma membrane. Although this process has traditionally been thought to occur through lipid-phase diffusion, increasing evidence indicates that aquaporin-1 (AQP1) contributes to CO_2 transport across the apical plasma membrane as necessary for bicarbonate reabsorption.[41] Cytosolic CO_2 is then hydrated, forming carbonic acid. Similar to the luminal

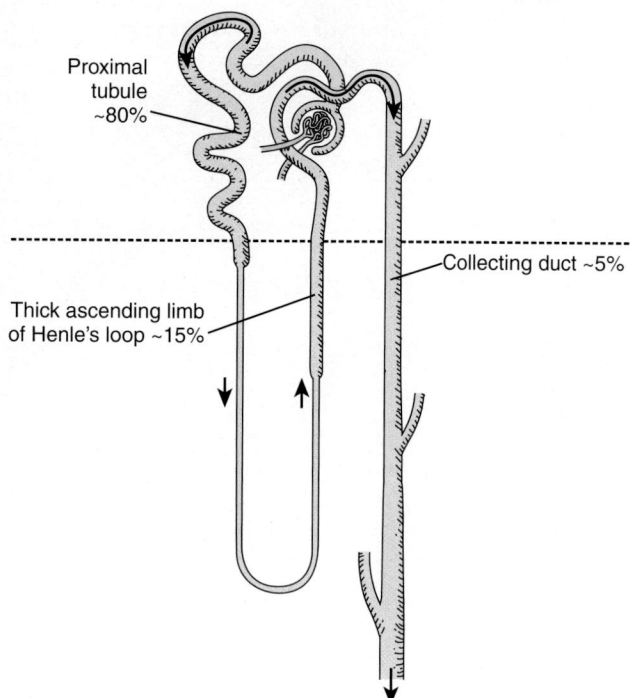

Proximal tubule ~80%

Collecting duct ~5%

Thick ascending limb of Henle's loop ~15%

FIGURE 9-1 Summary of sites of bicarbonate reabsorption. The proximal tubule is the primary site quantitatively for filtered bicarbonate reabsorption. Minimal reabsorption occurs in the thin limb of the loop of Henle, whereas in the thick ascending limb of the loop of Henle there is reabsorption of the majority of the bicarbonate not reabsorbed in the proximal tubule. The collecting duct is the primary site for reabsorption of the remaining filtered bicarbonate.

reaction, this process is accelerated by a cytosolic carbonic anhydrase, CA II. Cytosolic carbonic acid spontaneously dissociates to H^+ and HCO_3^-. This "replenishes" the H^+ secreted across the apical plasma membrane by apical NHE3 and H^+-ATPase. Cytosolic HCO_3^- is secreted across the basolateral plasma membrane. In the S1 and S2 segments of the proximal tubule the primary HCO_3^- transport mechanism is a sodium-coupled, electrogenic bicarbonate cotransporter, NBCe1.[1,223] In the S3 segment a basolateral Na^+-dependent Cl^-/HCO_3^- exchanger appears be the primary mechanism of basolateral HCO_3^- movement,[189] although NBCe1 may also contribute.[246] In addition to active H^+ secretion and luminal bicarbonate reabsorption, the proximal tubule also exhibits passive H^+ and bicarbonate transport. Because bicarbonate reabsorption decreases the luminal bicarbonate concentration and increases the luminal H^+ concentration relative to the peritubular space, passive H^+ and/or bicarbonate transport counteracts active bicarbonate reabsorption and thereby limits bicarbonate reabsorption. Backleak rates limit the net amount of bicarbonate reabsorbed.[11] There is both H^+ and bicarbonate permeability, but the bicarbonate permeability is greater than the H^+ permeability.[135] Accordingly, this process is generally referred to as *bicarbonate backleak*. The specific mechanisms of the peritubular bicarbonate permeability are unclear, but it is known to be both developmentally regulated (permeability is lower in newborn than in adult animals[277]) and hormonally regulated (angiotensin II decreases bicarbonate backleak[207]). H^+ permeability is at least in part transcellular and involves specific membrane proteins, but not NHE3.[135,270]

Regulation of Proximal Tubule Bicarbonate Reabsorption

EXTRACELLULAR pH

Multiple conditions alter proximal tubule bicarbonate transport. Perhaps the most extensively studied condition is altered extracellular pH. Metabolic and respiratory acidosis increase and alkalosis decreases bicarbonate reabsorption. These changes occur with both acute and chronic pH conditions, although the effects are substantially greater with chronic acidosis. Respiratory-induced changes in extracellular pH, that is, changes in CO_2 pressure (Pco_2), also alter proximal tubule transport.[73] However, the effects of acute CO_2 changes are substantially less than those observed with chronic changes.[71,72] Luminal bicarbonate also regulates proximal tubule bicarbonate reabsorption. However, the direction of the changes is opposite to the effects of systemic and peritubular bicarbonate: increased luminal bicarbonate concentration increases bicarbonate reabsorption, and decreased luminal bicarbonate decreases it. These parallel changes are a form of glomerular-tubular balance in which changes in filtered load regulate transport rates.

Mechanism by Which Extracellular pH Regulates Proximal Tubule Bicarbonate Reabsorption. Recent studies have begun to elucidate the mechanisms by which extracellular bicarbonate and CO_2 regulate proximal tubule bicarbonate reabsorption. Isohydric (constant pH) CO_2/HCO_3^- addition to the peritubular solution stimulated apical H^+ secretion, but luminal addition did not.[247] Because these studies were performed at constant pH, they show that extracellular pH is not a primary regulator of apical H^+ secretion; it is either CO_2 or HCO_3^- or both. Furthermore, because CO_2/HCO_3^- addition to the luminal or peritubular solutions had similar effects on intracellular pH, intracellular pH is not the primary mechanism through which extracellular CO_2/HCO_3^- regulates apical H^+ secretion. Finally, the observation that peritubular CO_2/HCO_3^- regulates transport suggests a role for one or more basolateral plasma membrane proteins that "sense" CO_2 and/or HCO_3^-. To differentiate the effects of CO_2 and HCO_3^- on transport, a method was needed to separately alter these without altering pH. Conventional studies examining the different roles of pH, CO_2, and HCO_3^- have been limited, because these three parameters are in equilibrium with each other through the following reaction:

$$CO_2 + H_2O \overset{1}{\Leftrightarrow} H_2CO_3 \overset{2}{\Leftrightarrow} H^+ + HCO_3^-$$

A technique to generate "out-of-equilibrium" solutions was developed and uses the knowledge that there are two major reactions in the preceding equation, reaction 1 in which CO_2 hydration forms carbonic acid (H_2CO_3), which occurs relatively slowly, and reaction 2 in which carbonic acid dissociates to H^+ and HCO_3^-, which occurs rapidly. Taking advantage of this, Boron and colleagues developed techniques to rapidly mix two solutions with different compositions and then use the resulting solution before it has come to equilibrium, thereby generating "out-of-equilibrium" solutions that enable study of the specific roles of extracellular CO_2, HCO_3^- and pH.[415] Use of this technique produced a series of remarkable results. First, increasing peritubular HCO_3^- concentration, at constant pH and Pco_2, decreased bicarbonate reabsorption.[421] Increasing peritubular Pco_2, at constant pH and HCO_3^-, increased bicarbonate reabsorption. And altering peritubular pH, at

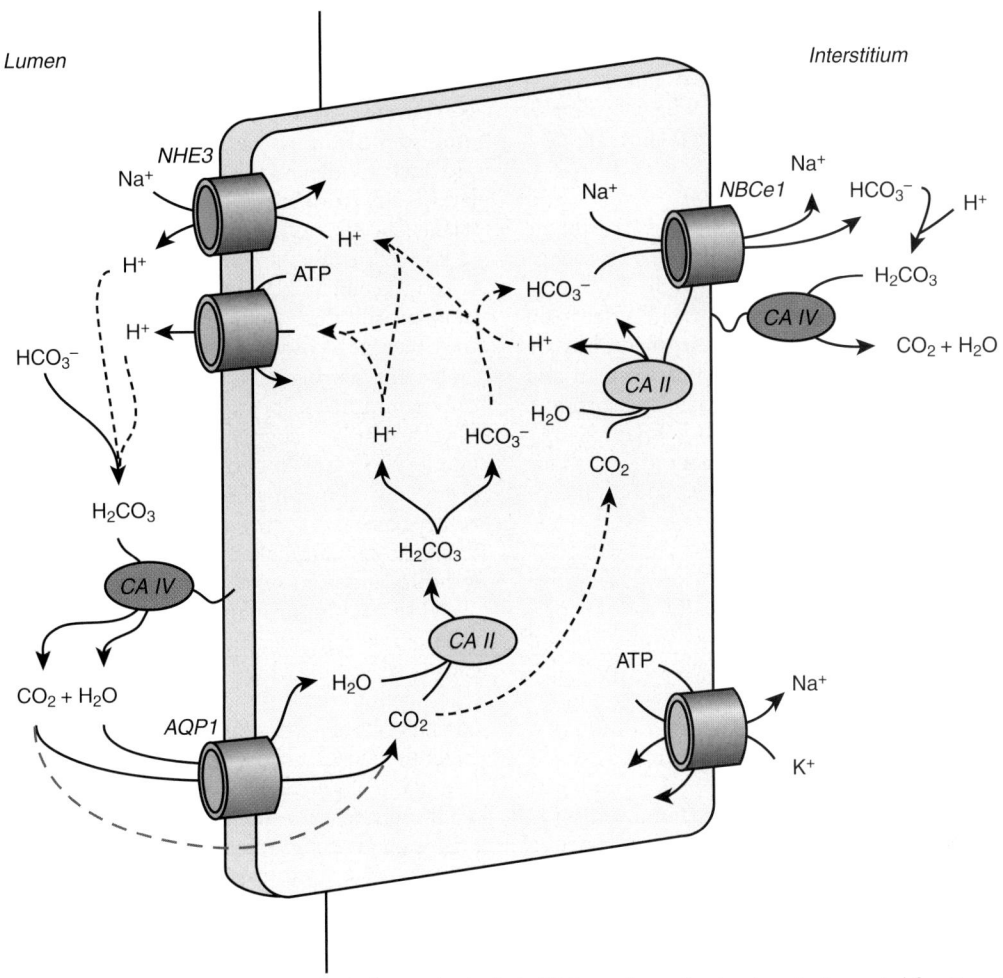

FIGURE 9-2 Bicarbonate reabsorption in the proximal tubule. Proximal tubule HCO_3^- reabsorption involves the integrated function of multiple proteins. H^+ ions are secreted by both the Na^+/H^+ exchanger NHE3 and H^+-ATPase, and titrate luminal HCO_3^- to H_2CO_3. Luminal H_2CO_3 dehydration to H_2O and CO_2 is accelerated by luminal carbonic anhydrase (CA) activity mediated by CA IV. CO_2 enters the cell via aquaporin-1 (AQP1) and, most likely, via diffusive movement, where its hydration to H_2CO_3 is accelerated by cytoplasmic CA II. H_2CO_3 rapidly dissociates to H^+ and HCO_3^-, thereby replenishing the secreted cytosolic H^+. Cytosolic HCO_3^- exits across the basolateral plasma membrane primarily by the $Na^+(HCO_3^-)_3$ cotransporter NBCe1. Basolateral CA II and CA IV facilitate HCO_3^- transport.

fixed HCO_3^- and PCO_2, did not alter bicarbonate reabsorption.[421] Thus, the proximal tubule has basolateral HCO_3^- and CO_2 "sensors," and peritubular pH does not independently regulate bicarbonate transport. These responses were specific to bicarbonate reabsorption, because fluid reabsorption did not parallel bicarbonate reabsorption. Active investigation is ongoing into the specific mechanisms through which peritubular HCO_3^- and CO_2 regulate proximal tubule bicarbonate reabsorption. These appear to involve members of the ErbB family of receptor tyrosine kinases.[419] These acute effects of peritubular HCO_3^- and CO_2 also appear to involve the intrarenal angiotensin system. Peritubular addition of CO_2 appears to stimulate intracellular angiotensin II production and luminal secretion, which acts through an apical AT_1 receptor to stimulate bicarbonate reabsorption.[418,420]

Long-Term Effects of Metabolic Acidosis. Chronic metabolic acidosis increases proximal tubule bicarbonate reabsorption to extents greater than observed with acute metabolic acidosis. This adaptive increase involves increased NHE3 expression and activity,[15,269] but not detectable changes in NBCe1 expression.[191] Enzymatic assays suggest that metabolic acidosis increases proximal tubule H^+-ATPase activity.[63]

Total renal H^+-ATPase expression does not change with chronic metabolic acidosis,[29] but H^+-ATPase is expressed in multiple sites other than the proximal tubule. Glucocorticoid levels increase with chronic metabolic acidosis,[397] and glucocorticoid receptor activation increases acidosis-induced increases in NHE3 expression and apical trafficking.[16]

LUMINAL FLOW RATE

Another important regulatory mechanism is luminal flow rate. Renal bicarbonate reabsorption changes in parallel with glomerular filtration rate,[264] mediated, at least in part, by flow-dependent changes in proximal tubule transport.[12] Multiple mechanisms likely contribute to flow-dependent bicarbonate reabsorption. First, increased luminal flow increases NHE3 insertion into the apical plasma membrane.[268] In addition, bicarbonate reabsorption decreases luminal bicarbonate concentration. Increased flow minimizes these changes, enabling higher mean luminal bicarbonate concentration, which, because bicarbonate reabsorption parallels luminal bicarbonate concentration, facilitates increased bicarbonate reabsorptive rates.[12] Second, proximal tubule brush border microvilli may function as flow sensors, with drag force mediated through the actin filament altering cytoskeletal elements and regulating transport.[88] Similarly, apical cilia in renal epithelial cells respond to luminal flow rates, regulating ion transport through changes in intracellular calcium.[266] The specific role of proximal tubule cilia remains incompletely identified.

Angiotensin II

Angiotensin II is an important regulator of proximal tubule ion transport, including bicarbonate reabsorption. Low concentrations of angiotensin II increase and high concentrations inhibit bicarbonate reabsorption.[67,378] The effects on bicarbonate transport are greatest in the S1 segment, but are also observed in the S2 and S3 segments. Both luminal and peritubular angiotensin II stimulate bicarbonate reabsorption, mediated predominantly through apical and basolateral AT_1 receptors. Increased bicarbonate reabsorption in metabolic acidosis may be mediated partly through increased AT_1 receptor expression.[242]

Potassium

Systemic potassium is another important modulator of proximal tubule bicarbonate transport; hypokalemia stimulates and hyperkalemia inhibits transport.[279] This occurs in part due to altered apical Na^+/H^+ exchange and basolateral sodium-bicarbonate cotransport activity[317] and also due to increased apical and basolateral plasma membrane AT_1 receptor expression.[110] Acute changes in extracellular potassium concentration do not alter proximal tubule bicarbonate transport,[66] however, probably because the response to hypokalemia requires new protein synthesis.

Endothelin

Endothelin has important and direct effects on ion transport in a variety of renal epithelial cells, including the proximal tubule. Endothelin can be produced in the proximal tubule and exhibits an autocrine effect to stimulate NHE3.[204] In particular, metabolic acidosis–induced increases in NHE3 expression may require endothelin receptor B (ET-B) activation.[193]

Parathyroid Hormone

Parathyroid hormone (PTH), acting through adenylyl cyclase and intracellular cyclic adenosine monophosphate (cAMP) production, inhibits proximal tubule bicarbonate reabsorption.[228] PTH also inhibits proximal tubule phosphate reabsorption, which increases distal phosphate delivery and may thereby increase luminal buffer available for titratable acid excretion.

Transporters Involved in Proximal Tubule Bicarbonate Reabsorption

Na⁺/H⁺ Exchangers

Na^+/H^+ exchangers are expressed widely in the kidney, where they function in intracellular pH regulation, transepithelial bicarbonate reabsorption, and vacuolar acidification. Mammalian Na^+/H^+ exchangers are members of an extended Na^+/H^+ exchanger family present in prokaryotes, lower eukaryotes, and higher eukaryotes, including fungi, plants, and animals. All members of this family utilize the extracellular-to-intracellular Na^+ gradient generated by the ubiquitous Na^+-K^+-ATPase to enable secondarily active electroneutral H^+ secretion with a stoichiometry of 1:1. Although the preferred binding ions are Na^+ and H^+, Li^+ can compete for the Na^+ binding site and NH_4^+ can substitute for H^+.[178] The latter process, which enables Na^+/NH_4^+ exchange, is important in proximal tubule NH_4^+ secretion.[236] Intracellular $[H^+]$ regulates Na^+/H^+ exchange activity more than expected from the change in electrochemical gradients, with a Hill coefficient of approximately 2.6.[230] This suggests the presence of at least two intracellular H^+-binding sites. One may be an allosteric modifier site that regulates sensitivity to intracellular pH, and the other is the binding site for H^+ translocation.

Na^+/H^+ exchangers are members of a large monovalent cation-proton antiporter (CPA) family.[45] NHE3 is one of nine currently recognized Na^+/H^+ exchangers in the CPA1 family. NHE1 is ubiquitous, with high levels of expression in essentially all mammalian cells. In the kidney, NHE1 is generally expressed in the basolateral plasma membrane. Table 9-1 lists the mammalian Na^+/H^+ exchangers, their subcellular location, and their renal expression.

NHE3 is the primary Na^+/H^+ exchanger in the proximal tubule apical membrane and mediates the majority of apical H^+ secretion, which is necessary for luminal bicarbonate reabsorption. In addition, coupling of NHE3 to Cl^-/base and Cl^-/anion exchangers enables NaCl reabsorption and thereby facilitates H_2O reabsorption. Genetic deletion of NHE3 results in volume depletion, metabolic acidosis, and decreased renal reabsorption of HCO_3^-, Na^+, Cl^-, and H_2O.[296] Both micropuncture and microperfusion studies show that NHE3 deletion decreases proximal tubule solute and bicarbonate reabsorption.[214,296]

NHE2 and NHE8 are other Na^+/H^+ exchanger isoforms expressed in the kidney. NHE2 appears to be expressed in the apical membrane in macula densa, cortical TALs, DCTs, and CNTs, with weaker expression in medullary TALs and in some thin limbs in the inner medulla.[64,260] Whether NHE2 is present in the proximal tubule is unclear. However, studies in mice with genetic deletion of NHE3 and NHE2 and inhibitor-based studies find no functional evidence for NHE2-mediated H^+ secretion in the proximal tubule.[380] NHE8 is expressed in apical plasma membrane in the proximal tubule,[127] which raises the possibility that it may mediate the NHE3-independent component of proximal tubule Na^+-dependent H^+ secretion.[127]

An ever-increasing list of mechanisms regulates NHE3 expression and activity. Agonists that regulate NHE3 are presented in Table 9-2. In addition, NHE3 activity is regulated through a wide variety of mechanisms, including transcription, protein synthesis, phosphorylation, trafficking, and protein-protein interactions.

The best-studied hormonal regulation involves PTH, dopamine, and angiotensin II. Both PTH and dopamine inhibit NHE3 activity, whereas angiotensin II has a biphasic effect, stimulatory at low concentrations and inhibitory at high concentrations. Both PTH and dopamine increase intracellular cAMP levels, which leads to decreased NHE3 activity.[74] Dopamine is also protein kinase C (PKC) dependent.[116] Angiotensin II decreases cAMP levels and activates PKC, tyrosine kinase, and phosphatidylinositol-3-kinase.[151]

The NHE3 5′-promoter region contains multiple transcriptional regulatory elements. These include glucocorticoid and thyroid response elements and multiple transcription factor consensus binding sites (Sp1, AP-2, MZF-1, CdxA,

TABLE 9-1 Mammalian Na$^+$/H$^+$ Exchangers (NHEs)		
PROTEIN	**SUBCELLULAR LOCATION**	**RENAL EXPRESSION**
NHE1	Plasma membrane, basolateral in epithelial cells	Basolateral; present in essentially all cells with exception of macula densa
NHE2	Plasma membrane, apical in epithelial cells	Thick ascending limb of loop of Henle and DCT
NHE3	Apical plasma membrane and recycling endosomes	Proximal tubule and thick ascending limb
NHE4	Basolateral plasma membrane	Throughout nephron, greatest expression in thick ascending limb
NHE5	Plasma membrane	Very low level mRNA expression
NHE6	Recycling endosomes	mRNA present, protein expression unknown
NHE7	Trans-Golgi network	mRNA present, protein expression unknown
NHE8	Apical membrane and recycling endosomes of epithelial cells	Apical plasma membrane in proximal tubule
NHE9	Recycling endosomes	mRNA present, protein expression unknown
Sperm-NHE	Sperm flagellum	Absent
NHA1	Unknown	Absent
NHA2	Mitochondria, endosomes, plasma membrane	DCT

DCT, Distal convoluted tubule; NHA, Sodium-hydrogen antiporter; mRNA, messenger RNA.

TABLE 9-2 Immediate and Long-Term Regulation of Na$^+$/H$^+$ Exchanger Isoform 3		
AGONIST	**IMMEDIATE EFFECTS**	**LONG-TERM EFFECTS**
α-Adrenergic agonists	↓	?
Extracellular acidosis	↑	↑
Adenosine	↑	↓
Albumin	↓	↓
Aldosterone	↑	↑
Angiotensin II	↓/↑ (concentration dependent)	↑
Adenosine triphosphate depletion	↓	?
Atrial natriuretic peptide	↓	?
Cyclic adenosine monophosphate	↓	↑
Dopamine	↓	↓
Endothelin 1	↑	↑
Glucocorticoids	↑	↑
Hyperosmolarity	↓	↑
Insulin	↑	↑
Long-chain fatty acids	?	↓
Nitric oxide	↓	↑
Ouabain	?	↓
Parathyroid hormone	↓	↓
Thyroid hormone	?	↑

Cdx-2, steroid and nonsteroid hormone receptor binding sites, and a phorbol-12-myristate-13-acetate response element).[166] In general, increased NHE3 messenger RNA (mRNA) expression is associated with increased protein expression.

The NHE3 carboxy-terminal cytoplasmic domain contains multiple phosphorylation sites, many of which regulate transporter activity. Serine 552 is a consensus protein kinase A (PKA) phosphorylation site. NHE3 phosphorylated at serine 552 localizes to the coated pit region of the brush border membrane where NHE3 is inactive, which suggests that phosphorylation at this site regulates subcellular trafficking in vivo.[185] Similarly, phosphorylation of rabbit serine 719 regulates insertion into the plasma membrane.[291] Dephosphorylation, mediated by the serine/threonine phosphatase PP1, but not PP2, at serines 552 and 605 and at other novel phosphorylation sites stimulates NHE3 activity.[91] Alterations in the subcellular distribution commonly regulate transporter function. NHE3 exists in a variety of subcellular domains in proximal tubule cells, including microvilli, intermicrovillar clefts, endosomes, and a cytoplasmic "storage compartment." Only NHE3 in microvilli is functionally active in bicarbonate reabsorption.[6] Redistribution within these domains is regulated by a variety of factors, including renal sympathetic nerve activity, glucocorticoids and insulin,[35,225] angiotensin II,[285] dopamine,[24] and PTH.[74] This process of regulated changes in NHE3 subcellular distribution involves the complex interaction of a number of cellular elements, including PKA–mediated NHE3 phosphorylation, dynamin, NHERF-1, clathrin-coated vesicles, calcineurin homologous protein-1, ezrin phosphorylation, G protein α-subunits, and G protein β-γ dimers.[5,85,152] A major advance during the past several years has been the identification of a number of proteins that directly interact with NHE3. NHERF-1 is a major regulatory protein necessary for cAMP-mediated inhibition of NHE3.[413] NHERF-1 and NHERF-2 are members of the PDZ domain family of adapter proteins and appear to enable indirect association of PKA with NHE3.[6] A related protein, NHERF-2, also can bind NHE3 and mediate cAMP-dependent inhibition of NHE3,[194] and NHERF-3, also known as *PDZK1*, also interacts with NHE3.[115] However, genetic deletion of NHERF-1 or NHERF-3 does not alter either acid-base homeostasis or proximal tubule NHE3 expression.[308,335]

H$^+$-ATPASE

The second major mechanism of proximal tubule apical H$^+$ secretion is through the vacuolar H$^+$-ATPase. This is a multisubunit protein involved in both plasma membrane

H+ secretion and acidification of subcellular compartments, including Golgi apparatus, lysosomes, endosomes, and clathrin-coated vesicles. Proximal tubule H+-ATPase is expressed in the brush border microvilli, the base of the brush border, and apical invaginations between clathrin-coated domains.[48] It appears to mediate the approximately 40% of proton secretion that is not mediated by Na+/H+ exchange.[379] In addition, H+-ATPase acidifies proximal tubule endosomes and lysosomes, senses endosomal pH, and is involved in recruiting trafficking proteins to acidified vesicles, thereby assuring appropriate progression from early endosomes to lysosomes.[51] Proximal tubule H+-ATPase activity is increased by angiotensin II, increased axial flow, and chronic metabolic acidosis.[63,89,364]

ELECTROGENIC SODIUM-BICARBONATE COTRANSPORTER 1 (SLC4A4)

The electrogenic sodium-bicarbonate cotransporter NBCe1 is a member of the sodium-coupled bicarbonate transporter family. NBCe1 is thought to have large cytoplasmic amino- and carboxy-terminals tails and 10 to 14 transmembrane domains[40,286] and to function as a homodimer composed of functionally active subunits.[167] Three splice variants of the NBCe1 gene are known; they result from two alternative amino- and two alternative carboxy-tail gene products. Only NBCe1-A, also known as *kNBC1*, is expressed in the kidney in the basolateral plasma membrane in the proximal tubule.[56,223] The basolateral expression of NBCe1-A appears to be mediated through the carboxy 23 amino acids.[203] Metabolic acidosis increases proximal tubule HCO_3^- reabsorption and increases proximal tubule basolateral HCO_3^- transport, but does not alter NBCe1-A expression.[191] Instead, phosphorylation may regulate NBCe1-A activity.[99]

NBCe1-A in the proximal tubule mediates the coupled net movement of Na+ and HCO_3^- in a 1:3 ratio. This could reflect either transport of 3 HCO_3^- molecules or 1 HCO_3^- and 1 CO_3^{2-} molecule. In nonrenal mammalian tissues and in *Xenopus* oocytes, NBCe1-A transports Na+ and HCO_3^- in a 1:2 ratio.[128,147] These differences in the coupling ratio are physiologically relevant: 1:3 coupling mediates net HCO_3^- efflux, whereas a 1:2 ratio mediates net HCO_3^- influx under typical cellular Na+ and HCO_3^- concentrations and membrane potential. Intracellular calcium and transporter phosphorylation are known to alter this substrate coupling ratio.[129,234]

NBCe1-A also appears to facilitate transport through other basolateral proteins present in the proximal tubule. The carboxy-terminal may bind both CA II and CA IV, thereby facilitating HCO_3^- transport,[13,274] although some studies have failed to verify these interactions.[215] NBCe1-A also appears to be functionally coupled to the basolateral monocarboxylate cotransporter MCT1, enabling lactate uptake while minimizing intracellular pH changes,[31] and can couple functionally with the glutamine transporter SNAT3, facilitating glutamine transport while minimizing intracellular pH changes due to H+ transport by SNAT3.[398] Defects in NBCe1 are the most common cause of autosomal recessive proximal tubule renal tubular acidosis (RTA).[158] Ocular tissues also express NBCe1, and ocular abnormalities, including band keratopathy, cataracts, and glaucoma, which can lead to blindness, are common in patients with a genetic lack of NBCe1.[158]

CARBONIC ANHYDRASE II

Carbonic anhydrases are a family of zinc metalloenzymes that catalyze the reversible hydration of CO_2 to form carbonic acid (H_2CO_3), reaction 1 in the following equation:

$$CO_2 + H_2O \overset{1}{\Leftrightarrow} H_2CO_3 \overset{2}{\Leftrightarrow} H^+ + HCO_3^-$$

Dissociation of carbonic acid to H+ and HCO_3^- (reaction 2) is rapid. Consequently, carbonic anhydrases facilitate interconversion of CO_2 and H_2O with H+ and HCO_3^-. At least 15 carbonic anhydrase isoforms are known. CA II is the predominant carbonic anhydrase in the kidney, accounting for approximately 95% of total renal carbonic anhydrase activity, and is the predominant carbonic anhydrase in the proximal tubule. CA II is a 29-kDa protein expressed in the cytoplasm of the proximal tubule, in addition to multiple other sites in the kidney, including the thin descending limb, TAL, and intercalated cells. In the mouse kidney, CA II is also expressed in collecting duct principal cells.

CA II binds to a variety of bicarbonate transporters, further facilitating urine acidification and transepithelial bicarbonate transport. These interactions include those with NBCe1 in the proximal tubule basolateral membrane (detailed earlier); with anion exchanger 1 (AE1) in intercalated cells,[360] AE2, and AE3; and with NBC3, an apical anion exchanger present in intercalated cells in the outer medullary collecting duct (OMCD).[271] In the proximal tubule CA II interacts with SLC26A6, an anion exchanger present in the brush border, where it facilitates coupled Na+ and Cl− reabsorption.[14]

CARBONIC ANHYDRASE IV

CA IV is a membrane-associated carbonic anhydrase isoform expressed in the proximal tubule and in intercalated cells in the collecting duct.[299] CA IV is linked to the plasma membrane via a glycosylphosphatidylinositol (GPI) anchor, which makes it unique among carbonic anhydrase isoforms.[422] In the proximal tubule, CA IV is expressed in both apical and basolateral plasma membranes where, by facilitating HCO_3^- interconversion with CO_2, it contributes to transepithelial bicarbonate reabsorption.[50] In the collecting duct, CA IV expression is limited to the apical membrane.[271] CA IV interacts with multiple bicarbonate transporters, including AE1, AE2, and AE3,[324] and proximal tubule NBCe1,[13] which may facilitate proximal tubule bicarbonate reabsorption.

Loop of Henle

The TAL of the loop of Henle contributes to acid-base homeostasis through its roles in reabsorbing approximately 15% to 20% of the filtered bicarbonate load and in contributing to the development of the medullary interstitial ammonia gradient that is critical for collecting duct ammonia secretion. The mechanisms and regulation of bicarbonate reabsorption are described in the following sections.

The overall schema of TAL bicarbonate reabsorption is similar to that in the proximal tubule. Cytosolic H+ is secreted by apical Na+/H+ exchange activity and vacuolar H+-ATPase. Quantitatively, apical Na+/H+ exchange activity is the predominant apical H+ secretory mechanism; vacuolar H+-ATPase is also present, but has at most a minor role in TAL bicarbonate reabsorption.[59,126] Two Na+/H+ exchanger isoforms are present in the TAL, NHE2 and NHE3, and inhibitor sensitivity studies suggest that NHE3 is the predominant isoform involved in bicarbonate reabsorption.[348,380] Secreted H^+ reacts with luminal HCO_3^-, forming H_2CO_3, which dissociates to CO_2 and H_2O. Whether luminal CA IV is present is unclear; some studies[50] but not others[342] find CA IV in the TAL. Luminal CO_2 moves down its concentration gradient across the apical plasma membrane into the cell cytoplasm. Cytoplasmic CA II catalyzes CO_2 hydration to form H_2CO_3, which dissociates to H^+ and HCO_3^-, thereby recycling the H^+ secreted across the apical plasma membrane. Absence of CA II in the rabbit TAL correlates with diminished bicarbonate reabsorption rate.[86] Cytosolic HCO_3^- exits via a basolateral Cl^-/HCO_3^- exchanger, possibly AE2; via an electroneutral sodium-bicarbonate cotransporter (NBCn1); and possibly via basolateral Cl^- channels.[10,361,396] An apical K^+-dependent HCO_3^- transporter mediates coupled K^+ and HCO_3^- transport, functions in parallel with apical Na^+/H^+ exchange, and, because of a cytoplasmic to luminal K^+ gradient, may secrete HCO_3^-.[382] Several other plasma membrane ion transporters either directly or indirectly alter TAL bicarbonate reabsorption. Inhibition of the apical Na^+-K^+-$2Cl^-$ cotransporter NKCC2 increases bicarbonate reabsorption.[59] This likely results because inhibiting NKCC2 decreases apical Na^+ entry, which decreases intracellular Na^+; this raises the Na^+ uptake gradient by apical Na^+/H^+ exchange activity and thereby increases net bicarbonate reabsorption. TAL expresses a basolateral Na^+/H^+ exchange activity, likely NHE1, and inhibiting basolateral Na^+/H^+ exchange activity inhibits bicarbonate reabsorption by inhibiting apical NHE3–mediated H^+ secretion.[124] This effect appears to result from alterations in the organization of the actin cytoskeleton, which likely decreases apical plasma membrane NHE3 insertion.[381]

Regulation of Thick Ascending Limb Bicarbonate Reabsorption

TAL bicarbonate reabsorption is regulated by a variety of physiologic stimuli. Acute and chronic metabolic acidosis increase TAL bicarbonate reabsorption.[61,117] Whether the long-term effects are specific to metabolic acidosis or due to other mechanisms, possibly intravascular volume changes, is unclear. In in vivo studies, oral NH_4Cl (used to induce metabolic acidosis) and NaCl loading induce equivalent changes in medullary TAL bicarbonate reabsorption.[117] In other studies, TAL NHE3 abundance increases with NH_4Cl-induced metabolic acidosis, but not with NaCl loading.[173] Chloride-depletion metabolic alkalosis, a model in which plasma volume does not change, decreases TAL bicarbonate reabsorption.[120] This finding suggests that alkalosis directly regulates TAL bicarbonate transport. Several hormones regulate bicarbonate reabsorption, including angiotensin II, glucocorticoids, and mineralocorticoids. Angiotensin II stimulates TAL bicarbonate reabsorption, likely through activation of AT_1 receptors.[60,233] Glucocorticoid receptors are present in the TAL, and glucocorticoid availability is necessary for normal bicarbonate reabsorption.[347] At high concentrations mineralocorticoids stimulate bicarbonate reabsorption,[120] but their absence does not alter basal transport.[347] The relatively minor role of mineralocorticoids parallels relatively low mineralocorticoid receptor expression in the TAL.[336] Arginine vasopressin inhibits bicarbonate reabsorption through prostaglandin

E_2–mediated inhibition of apical Na^+/H^+ exchange activity.[39,118] Cytokines regulate bicarbonate transport in this segment. Lipopolysaccharide (LPS) inhibits transport; this effect involves the cytokine receptor TLR4, and involves separate pathways activated by luminal and by peritubular LPS. In particular, luminal LPS involves the mTOR pathway whereas peritubular LPS functions through the MEK/ERK pathway.[125] Another important regulatory factor is renal medullary tonicity. Increased tonicity inhibits and decreased tonicity stimulates bicarbonate reabsorption through changes in apical Na^+/H^+ exchange activity involving phosphatidylinositol-3-kinase.[119,123] This effect is additive to the inhibitory effect of antidiuretic hormone on bicarbonate reabsorption and may function to limit bicarbonate reabsorption in the medullary TAL and shift it to the cortical TAL, thereby minimizing medullary interstitial bicarbonate accumulation.

Paracellular Bicarbonate Transport

Unlike in the proximal tubule where substantial paracellular HCO_3^- transport limits bicarbonate reabsorption, in the TAL paracellular backleak is minimal. The paracellular permeability of HCO_3^- is approximately 10% of the permeability to Cl^- in the mouse and approximately 4% of the permeability to Cl^- in the rabbit TAL.[120] Consequently, changes in luminal voltage, which can result in response to altered rates of NaCl reabsorption, do not appear to alter TAL bicarbonate reabsorption significantly.[120]

Acid-Base Transporters in the Thick Ascending Limb

Many of the major H^+ and HCO_3^- transporters in the TAL were discussed earlier in relation to the proximal tubule and are not described again here.

ELECTRONEUTRAL SODIUM-BICARBONATE COTRANSPORTER 1 (SLC4A7)
NBCn1 facilitates the electroneutral coupled transport of Na^+ and HCO_3^-. In the kidney, NBCn1 is expressed in the basolateral membrane in the TAL and in the apical membranes of the outer and inner medullary collecting duct intercalated cells[191,273] Both metabolic acidosis and hypokalemia increase TAL NBCn1 expression.[160,191] Because these conditions increase TAL bicarbonate reabsorption, increased basolateral bicarbonate entry via increased NBCn1 is unlikely to contribute to transepithelial bicarbonate reabsorption. However, both metabolic acidosis and hypokalemia stimulate TAL ammonia reabsorption, and TAL apical ammonia entry causes acute intracellular acidification because the primary molecular form transported is NH_4^+.[172] Increased basolateral NBCn1 expression/activity in metabolic acidosis, in which there is increased apical NH_4^+ uptake, may buffer this intracellular acid load rather than contributing to bicarbonate reabsorption.

Distal Convoluted Tubule

The DCT is an important site for bicarbonate reabsorption.[395] The DCT consists of two cell types, DCT cells and intercalated cells, and the mechanisms of bicarbonate reabsorption appear to differ for DCT and intercalated cells. DCT

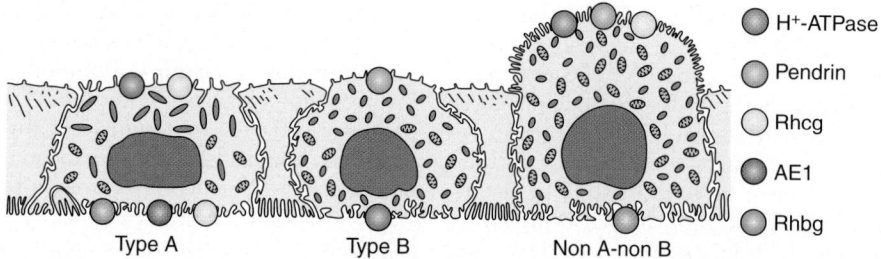

FIGURE 9-3 Intercalated cell subtypes in the distal nephron. The distal nephron—that is, the connecting segment, initial collecting tubule, cortical collecting duct (CCD), outer medullary collecting duct (OMCD), and inner medullary collecting duct (IMCD)—has multiple distinct cell types. Three intercalated cell types can be distinguished based on differential expression in different plasma membrane domains of several proteins involved in renal acid-base transport, including H⁺–adenosine triphosphatase (ATPase), anion exchanger 1 (AE1), pendrin, Rh B glycoprotein (Rhbg), and Rh C glycoprotein (Rhcg). (Modified from an original drawing by of Ki-Hwan Han, M.D., Ph.D., Ewha Womans University, Seoul, Korea.)

cells express apical NHE2,[64] and pharmacologic inhibitors of NHE2 decrease bicarbonate reabsorption.[380] A basolateral Cl^-/HCO_3^- exchange-mediated bicarbonate exit mechanism is postulated and is likely mediated by basolateral AE2.[10] A basolateral Cl^- channel that has partial HCO_3^- permeability may also mediate as much as 20% of basolateral HCO_3^- exit.[394] Cytosolic CA II is present, but not apical CA IV.[50] In the late DCT intercalated cells are present.[218] Quantitatively, intercalated cells comprise only a very small proportion of all cells in the DCT, approximately 4% and 7% in the mouse and rat kidneys, respectively.[176] The majority of intercalated cells in the DCT are type A and type C (non-A, non-B) intercalated cells.[176]

Collecting Duct

The renal collecting duct is the site of the final regulation of urinary acid excretion. It has several transport functions that contribute to acid-base homeostasis, including bicarbonate reabsorption and secretion, and ammonia secretion. These functions are regulated and performed by specific transporters in specific epithelial cell types, which vary in type and frequency in the different collecting duct segments.

Collecting Duct Segments

Technically, the collecting duct begins with the ICT, distal to the CNT, in the cortical labyrinth. The CNT arises from a different embryonic origin than the ICT and the more distal portions of the collecting duct. However, the CNT is included in the discussion of the role of the collecting duct in acid-base regulation because it has cell types and acid-base transport mechanisms similar to those of the collecting duct. The portions of the medullary collecting duct are identified by the region of the kidney in which they reside: outer medullary collecting duct in the outer stripe (OMCDo), outer medullary collecting duct in the inner stripe (OMCDi), and inner medullary collecting duct (IMCD). The IMCD subsegments in rodents are designated by various terms. The most proximal portion, located in the base of the inner medulla, is called either *IMCD1* or *initial IMCD* (IMCDi). The IMCD in the papilla in rodents is either called the *terminal IMCD* (IMCDt) or divided into IMCD2 and IMCD3, with IMCD3 being the most distal part. The cellular composition and function of the IMCD subsegments vary, so that differentiating these segments is important.

Cell Composition

Collecting ducts contain several distinct epithelial cell subtypes and exhibit axial heterogeneity in the cellular composition. From the ICT through the OMCD or IMCD (depending on species), two fundamentally distinct cell types, intercalated cells and principal cells, are present. Principal cells account for approximately 60% to 65% of cells, and intercalated cells account for the remaining cells through the OMCD. Current evidence suggests that there are at least three distinct intercalated cell subtypes: the type A intercalated cell, the type B intercalated cell, and a third, distinct intercalated cell type, the non-A, non-B intercalated cell (Figure 9-3). Distal to the OMCD, the percentage of intercalated cells decreases; they are absent from the terminal portion of the IMCD, where the epithelium is composed of IMCD cells, a unique cell type distinct from both intercalated cells and principal cells. The CNT contains intercalated cells; a cell type specific to the CNT, termed the *CNT cell;* and, in some species, principal cells similar to those in the ICT.

Type A Intercalated Cell

The type A intercalated cell is present in collecting ducts in the cortex (CNT through cortical collecting duct [CCD]), the OMCD, and the IMCD. Bicarbonate reabsorption involves integrated activity of multiple proteins, including H⁺ transporters, anion exchangers, and carbonic anhydrase (Figure 9-4). Immunocytochemical studies, both at the light microscopic and ultrastructural level, show that multiple vacuolar H⁺-ATPase subunits are abundant in the apical plasma membrane and in apical cytoplasmic tubulovesicles in intercalated cells. In response to physiologic perturbations, H⁺-ATPase is redistributed between the cytoplasmic compartment and the apical plasma membrane, which enables regulated apical H⁺ secretion. A second means of H⁺ secretion by intercalated cells is electroneutral and dependent on the presence of luminal potassium and is mediated by H⁺-K⁺-ATPase proteins.[131] At least two H⁺-K⁺-ATPase α-isoforms are present. One, $HK\alpha_1$, is similar to the α-isoform involved in gastric acid secretion and is sensitive to Schering 28080, whereas the other, $HK\alpha_2$, is similar to the α-isoform in the colon and is sensitive to low concentrations of ouabain. K⁺ reabsorbed via apical H⁺-K⁺-ATPase can either recycle across the apical plasma membrane or exit the cell across the basolateral plasma membrane. K⁺ movement across the apical versus basolateral plasma membrane appears to be regulated by dietary K⁺ intake.[417] A truncated isoform of the erythrocyte anion exchanger, kidney

Lumen

Interstitium

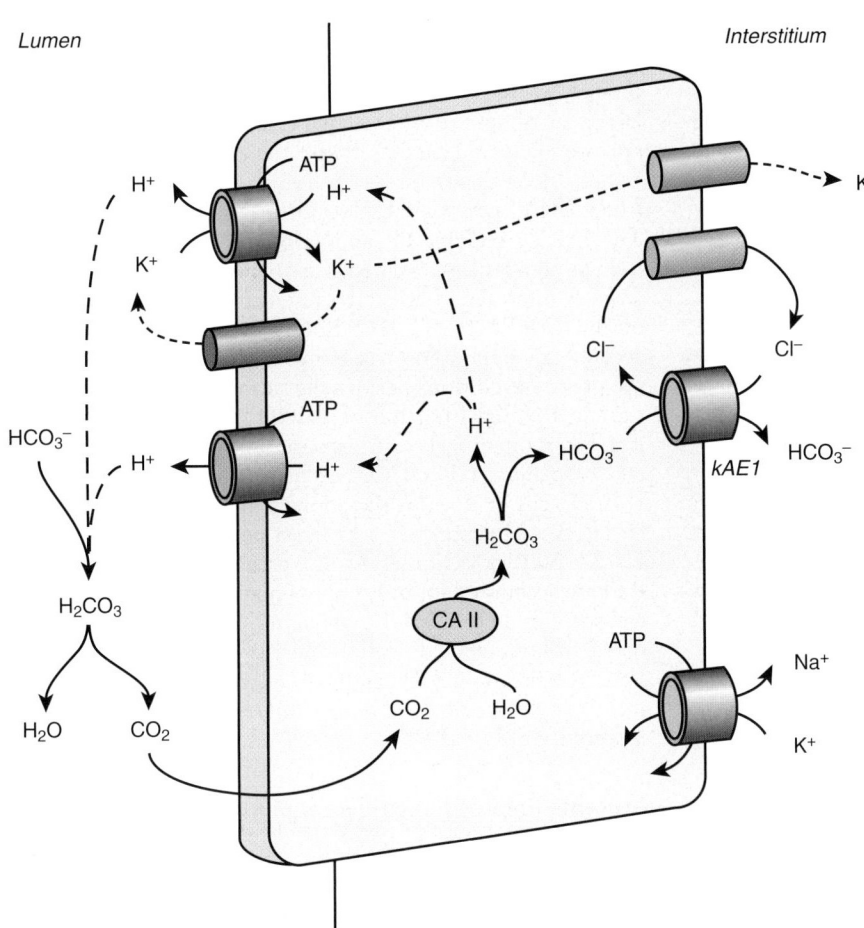

FIGURE 9-4 Bicarbonate reabsorption by the type A intercalated cell. The type A intercalated cell is present from the connecting segment through the initial inner medullary collecting duct (IMCD). Two families of H^+ transporters, H^+–adenosine triphosphatase (ATPase) and H^+-K^+-ATPase, are present in the apical plasma membrane. Secreted H^+ ions titrate luminal HCO_3^- to form H_2CO_3, which dehydrates to H_2O and CO_2. Luminal carbonic anhydrase activity, most likely mediated by carbonic anhydrase IV (CA IV), is variably present in the collecting duct (see text for details). Cytosolic H^+ and HCO_3^- are formed from CA II–accelerated hydration of CO_2 and rapid dissociation of H_2CO_3. Cytosolic HCO_3^- exits across the basolateral plasma membrane via the kidney isoform of anion exchanger 1, kAE1. Cl^- that enters via kAE1 recycles via a basolateral Cl^- channel. K^+ that enters via apical H^+-K^+-ATPase can either recycle via an apical Ba^+-sensitive K^+ channel or be reabsorbed via a basolateral Ba^+-sensitive K^+ channel. A basolateral Na^+/H^+ exchanger is present, but does not contribute to bicarbonate reabsorption and is not shown.

anion exchanger 1 (kAE1), is present in the basolateral plasma membrane and mediates basolateral bicarbonate exit.[8] Cl^- that enters the cell via basolateral Cl^-/HCO_3^- exchange exits via a basolateral Cl^- channel, presumably ClC-Kb in humans and ClC-K2 in rodents.[184] Cytoplasmic CA II is abundant in type A intercalated cells. In addition, membrane-associated carbonic anhydrases are present in the apical region (CA IV) and, at least in mouse and rabbit, in the basolateral region (CA XII) of intercalated cells.[271]

TYPE B INTERCALATED CELL
The type B intercalated cell, which is almost exclusively located in the CNT through CCD, contains basolateral H^+-ATPase and an apical Cl^-/HCO_3^- exchanger, pendrin.[9] H^+-ATPase is also present in vesicles throughout the cell, but ultrastructural studies using immunogold localization of H^+-ATPase show that it is not present in the apical plasma membrane. Both $HK\alpha_1$ and $HK\alpha_2$ are present in type B intercalated cells.[358,404] In the rabbit and mouse, functional studies suggest the presence of an apical Schering 28080–sensitive H^+-K^+-ATPase,[217,389] whereas in the rat Sch28080 inhibits bicarbonate secretion, which suggests basolateral rather than apical H^+-K^+-ATPase activity.[112] The type B cell also has cytoplasmic CA II, which facilitates intracellular H^+ and HCO_3^- production.

It is important to recognize that the apical Cl^-/HCO_3^- exchange activity present in the type B intercalated cell is distinct from kAE1, which is basolateral in the type A intercalated cell. Apical Cl^-/HCO_3^- exchange is relatively disulfonic

stilbene insensitive; this contrasts with kAE1, which is highly disulfonic stilbene sensitive.[386] Apical kAE1 has not been identified in any of many immunohistochemistry studies examining its localization, and studies using pendrin-null mice show that pendrin is responsible for the majority of apical bicarbonate secretion.[288]

Studies in the isolated perfused rabbit CCD suggest that type B, or β, intercalated cells also have basolateral anion exchange activity. Initial studies found that approximately 50% of CCD intercalated cells with apical Cl^-/HCO_3^- exchange activity also possessed basolateral Cl^-/HCO_3^- exchange activity.[98] However, subsequent studies showed that *all* CCD intercalated cells with apical Cl^-/HCO_3^- exchange have basolateral Cl^-/HCO_3^- exchange activity.[391] This basolateral exchanger has not been identified.

NON-A, NON-B (TYPE C) INTERCALATED CELL
A third intercalated cell subtype is present in the CNT and ICT.[176,334] This cell has distinct morphologic features, expresses both pendrin and H^+-ATPase in the apical plasma membrane and in apical cytoplasmic vesicles, does not express either basolateral plasma membrane H^+-ATPase or the anion exchanger AE1, and expresses basolateral Rh B glycoprotein (Rhbg) and apical Rh C glycoprotein (Rhcg) (see Figure 9-3). Thus, it does not have the phenotypic characteristics of either type A or type B intercalated cells. Studies of the developing mouse kidney indicate that the non-A, non-B intercalated cells in the CNT arise from separate foci than do type B intercalated cells.[142,318] This cell type was dubbed *non-A, non-B*

cell in early studies; alternative names include *non-A, non-B intercalated cell* and *type C intercalated cell.*

The function of the non-A, non-B intercalated cell remains to be defined. Treating mice with a mineralocorticoid analog increased pendrin-mediated CCD bicarbonate secretion and increased apical plasma membrane pendrin protein expression in type B intercalated cells as well as in non-A, non-B intercalated cells.[161] In other models of increased pendrin-mediated bicarbonate secretion there is increased apical plasma membrane pendrin expression in type B cells, but not in non-A, non-B cells.[351,370] Thus, it is likely that non-A, non-B intercalated cells have a role in bicarbonate secretion and chloride uptake, but their basal activity and regulation differ from those of type B intercalated cells.

PRINCIPAL CELL
Principal cells are widely recognized for their major role in transepithelial sodium, potassium, and water transport, but there also is evidence that they may play a role in acid secretion. In particular, functional studies have demonstrated both apical H^+ secretion and basolateral HCO_3^- transporters,[385,392] and, at least in the mouse and rat kidney, carbonic anhydrase activity in principal cells in the OMCDi and IMCDi.[87,179] Immunocytochemical studies have demonstrated that principal cells express H^+-ATPase,[49,362] at least two isoforms of H^+-K^+-ATPase,[131] and both ammonia transporters, Rhcg and Rhbg.[174] Increased principal cell Rhbg and Rhcg expression is a component of the renal response to metabolic acidosis.[197,198,306]

INNER MEDULLARY COLLECTING DUCT CELL
The terminal IMCD is composed primarily of the distinct IMCD cell, which exhibits carbonic anhydrase activity,[179] both H^+-ATPase and H^+-K^+-ATPase activity,[131,373] and basolateral Cl^-/HCO_3^- exchange.[383]

Functional Role of Different Collecting Duct Segments

CONNECTING TUBULE AND INITIAL COLLECTING TUBULE
Less information is available on the functional role of the CNT and ICT in acid-base homeostasis than on the role of other segments. Morphologic and immunolocalization studies suggest that the CNT and ICT contain type A and type B intercalated cell types similar to those in the CCD and that the type C (or non-A, non-B) intercalated cell is most prevalent here.[176,334,355] Under basal conditions, the CNT, at least in the rabbit, secretes bicarbonate through a luminal mechanism dependent on Cl^-, carbonic anhydrase, and H^+-ATPase[344] that likely involves apical pendrin, cytosolic CA II, and basolateral H^+-ATPase.

CORTICAL COLLECTING DUCT
Unlike the OMCD and IMCD, which can secrete only acid, the CCD both reabsorbs and secretes bicarbonate. The basal direction of bicarbonate transport varies among species, but both net bicarbonate absorption and secretion can be induced in response to systemic acid or alkali loading.[19,211,226] The ability to secrete bicarbonate, which is not found in the OMCD or IMCD, correlates with expression of the type B intercalated cell in the CCD, but not in more distal collecting duct segments.

OUTER MEDULLARY COLLECTING DUCT
The OMCD is responsible for approximately 40% to 50% of the net acid secretion in the collecting duct. Acid secretion is largely attributed to intercalated cells in this segment, which are essentially of a single subtype, the type A intercalated cell.

INNER MEDULLARY COLLECTING DUCT
The IMCD secretes H^+ and reabsorbs luminal bicarbonate even though few intercalated cells are present in the IMCD.[371] Type A intercalated cells are present in the proximal portion of the IMCD (IMCD1/IMCDi) in mouse and rat; they account for only 10% of cells in IMCD1 in rat kidney, and the prevalence diminishes distally so that no intercalated cells exist in the distal portion of IMCD (IMCD3).[70] Nonetheless, bicarbonate reabsorption occurs in the terminal IMCD, and basolateral Cl^-/HCO_3^- exchange is present in cultured IMCD cells.[383] Proton secretion is at least partly mediated by H^+-K^+-ATPase.[376] In rats fed a potassium-deficient diet, H^+-K^+-ATPase activities were upregulated,[373] but H^+-K^+-ATPase accounted for only approximately 50% of bicarbonate reabsorption in the IMCD, which indicates that other mechanisms of luminal acidification must exist in the IMCD. The IMCD expresses CA IV, and luminal, cytoplasmic, and lateral membrane-associated carbonic anhydrase activity has been reported.[179,369]

Proteins Involved in Collecting Duct H^+/Bicarbonate Transport

Transepithelial proton and bicarbonate transport in the collecting duct is mediated by the coordinated activity of specific proton and bicarbonate transporters located in the plasma membrane and carbonic anhydrase isoforms. Carbonic anhydrases and vacuolar H^+-ATPase are involved in both proton and bicarbonate secretion, but distinct Cl^-/HCO_3^- exchangers mediate bicarbonate reabsorption and secretion.

CARBONIC ANHYDRASE
At least three carbonic anhydrase isoforms, CA II, CA IV, and CA XII, are present in the collecting duct. CA II is a cytosolic form of carbonic anhydrase that is abundant both in the proximal tubule (discussed earlier), in intercalated cells in the collecting duct, and in principal cells in the mouse collecting duct.[357] Although not as abundant as in A cells, CA II is present in type B and C (non-A, non-B) intercalated cells as well.

CA IV is an extracellular, membrane-associated carbonic anhydrase tethered to the membrane through a GPI lipid-anchoring protein that is expressed apically in the majority of cells in rabbit OMCD and IMCD and in type A intercalated cells in the CCD.[302] In the OMCDi, luminal carbonic anhydrase inhibition decreases bicarbonate absorption, which suggests an important role for CA IV in acid-base homeostasis.[343]

CA XII is another extracellular, membrane-associated carbonic anhydrase in the collecting duct, but unlike CA IV, which is tethered to the plasma membrane, CA XII has a single transmembrane-spanning region.[271] CA XII is expressed in the collecting duct, although there may be significant species differences in cellular distribution.[271] Basolateral CA XII immunoreactivity has been reported in principal cells in human kidney, but in mouse collecting duct, CA XII immunoreactivity is reported to be basolateral in type A intercalated cells in cortical and medullary collecting ducts.[272]

Mutations in CA II lead to a mixed form of RTA because of the importance of CA II in both the proximal tubule and the collecting duct for generation of intracellular bicarbonate. Several mutations in CA II produce autosomal recessive RTA in humans, and in general the clinical syndromes resulting from CA II deficiencies are severe and include osteopetrosis and cerebral calcification along with RTA.[30,252] Mice with CA II deletion develop RTA and almost complete loss of intercalated cells in the medullary collecting duct and substantial decrease in both type A and type B intercalated cells in the CCD.[43]

H⁺-ATPASE

Electrogenic apical proton secretion in acid-secreting intercalated cells and basolateral proton transport by bicarbonate-secreting intercalated cells is mediated by the vacuolar H⁺-ATPase. In the collecting duct, H⁺-ATPase is most abundant in intercalated cells. Intercalated cells in the medullary collecting ducts and type A intercalated cells in the CCD contain H⁺-ATPase in the apical plasma membrane and in an apical cytoplasmic vesicle pool. Acid secretion is regulated in large part by redistribution of H⁺-ATPase between the cytoplasmic vesicle pool and the apical plasma membrane; changes in total H⁺-ATPase expression are not a major mechanism regulating H⁺ secretion.[29] H⁺-ATPase is also present in the apical region of principal cells and CNT cells, but the expression level is less than in intercalated cells. The role of apical H⁺-ATPase in nonintercalated cells has not been clearly defined; it may be involved in endosomal trafficking and fusion,[155] although in the OMCDi it can also mediate luminal proton secretion.[385]

Vacuolar H⁺-ATPase is an assembly of multiple subunits that form two main domains, the V_1 domain, which is extramembranous and hydrolyzes ATP, and the V_0 domain, which is a transmembranous portion and transports protons. The V_0 domain is composed of six subunits; the V_1 domain is composed of eight subunits and is linked to the V_0 domain via a stalk region comprised of subunits of both V_0 and V_1. Distinct isoforms and splice variants have been identified for many of these H⁺-ATPase subunits, and their cell-specific distribution may contribute to cell-specific regulation of proton and bicarbonate transport.

In the V_1 domain, two isoforms of the 56-kDa B subunit have been demonstrated in the collecting duct.[251] In the kidney, the B1 isoform is almost exclusively expressed in intercalated cells, in a polarized pattern specific to the intercalated cell subtype. In intercalated cells in the medullary collecting ducts and in type A intercalated cells in cortical segments, the B1 subunit is associated with both the apical plasma membrane and subapical cytoplasmic vesicles. In type B intercalated cells, the B1 subunit is present in both the apical and basolateral regions, although the apical H-ATPase in B cells has only been found in cytoplasmic vesicles and not in the apical plasma membrane by ultrastructural methods.[44] The B1 subunit in type B intercalated cells interacts with the scaffolding protein NHERF-1, whereas in type A intercalated cells it does not.[44] This cell-specific interaction with NHERF-1 likely plays a role in the basolateral H⁺-ATPase targeting essential for bicarbonate secretion.

The B2 isoform is widely distributed in the kidney and is primarily associated with intracellular organelles, such as endocytic vesicles and lysosomes, in proximal tubules, TALs, and collecting ducts. However, B2 immunoreactivity is intensified in the apical region of acid-secreting intercalated cells throughout the collecting duct and is expressed in the apical plasma membrane in these cells,[257] which suggests that B2 may have a role in H⁺ secretion by intercalated cells. B2 immunoreactivity is only weakly expressed in the basolateral membrane region of most type B intercalated cells.

In the V_0 domain, four isoforms of the a subunit and two isoforms of the d subunit have been identified in kidney. Intercalated cells express all four a subunit isoforms, but in specific cellular and subcellular locations in the different intercalated cell subtypes. In AE1-positive intercalated cells, a1 and a4 expression is exclusively apical. However, in the cortical segments, a1 and a4 expression varies in AE1-negative, pendrin-positive intercalated cells; a1 and a4 expression is either basolateral, diffuse, or bipolar. In the CNT, where the majority of the pendrin-positive intercalated cells are type C (non-A, non-B), a1 and a4 expression is exclusively apical.[297,323] Expression of the a3 isoform is strongest in the CCD, and it is apical in all intercalated cells. Expression of the a2 isoform is also apical in intercalated cells, but is restricted to type A intercalated cells and is strongest in the medullary collecting ducts.

Two d subunit isoforms are present in the kidney. The d1 isoform is ubiquitous, whereas d2 isoform expression is restricted to collecting duct intercalated cells. The d2 isoform colocalizes with the a4 subunit isoform in intercalated cells and can be immunoprecipitated with the B1 subunit, which suggests it may be involved in transepithelial proton transport.[316]

Genetic defects in several H⁺-ATPase subunit mutations have been shown to cause distal renal tubular acidosis (dRTA) in humans, often accompanied by sensorineural hearing loss and nephrocalcinosis. Defects in the B1 subunit in the ATP-hydrolytic V_1 domain resulting from recessive mutations in the ATP6V1B1 gene can produce early-onset hearing loss with severe dRTA.[168,169,326] Mice with B1 subunit deletion have incomplete distal RTA.[101] In these mice the B2 subunit appears to partially replace the B1 subunit, which allows partial compensation.[256] Mutations in the a4 subunit (ATP6V0A4) in the proton-translocating V_0 domain also produce recessive, severe, early-onset dRTA, with variable onset of hearing loss.[315,326,349]

KIDNEY ANION EXCHANGER 1 (SLC4A1)

The basolateral anion exchanger in intercalated cells in the medullary collecting duct and in type A intercalated cells in the cortex is a truncated splice variant of AE1, also known as *band 3 protein*, the anion exchanger found in erythrocytes. In the human, rat, and mouse kidney AE1 is expressed almost entirely in the basolateral plasma membrane. In the rabbit kidney under basal conditions, AE1 is present in intracytoplasmic multivesicular bodies, as well as in the basolateral plasma membrane; metabolic acidosis decreases intracellular AE1 and increases basolateral AE1, which suggests that regulated trafficking contributes to bicarbonate reabsorption.[352]

AE1 is an integral membrane protein with multiple membrane-spanning regions and cytoplasmic carboxy- and amino-terminals. The kidney AE1 (kAE1) carboxy-terminal lacks the initial 65 amino acids of the full-length erythrocyte AE1. The transmembrane portion mediates anion exchange. Basolateral targeting of AE1 requires sorting sequences in the carboxy terminus[84]; in cultured MDCK cells sorting sequences in both the amino- and carboxy- terminals are needed for polarized distribution of the transporter.[340] The AE1 carboxy-terminal may bind CA II, although perhaps not directly[263]; this physical proximity may facilitate bicarbonate transport by facilitating interconversion of HCO_3^- and CO_2.

Several mutations in AE1 have been identified as causes of both autosomal dominant and autosomal recessive dRTA. Even though AE1 is also expressed in erythrocytes, the majority of the genetic defects associated with autosomal dominant dRTA are not associated with altered erythrocyte AE1 expression. Instead, the defect that leads to dRTA development is most commonly a trafficking defect resulting in either mistargeting to the apical plasma membrane or failure of plasma membrane insertion.[278,307] Autosomal recessive dRTA caused by AE1 is most commonly associated with mutations that result in functionally inactive kAE1 due to intracellular protein retention.[332] Genetic defects in erythrocyte AE1 that lead to Southeast Asian ovalocytosis (SAO) result in nonfunctional kAE1 that has normal plasma membrane expression; expression of a single abnormal SAO allele decreases AE1 activity approximately 50% but is insufficient to cause dRTA.[130]

PENDRIN (SLC26A4)

Generation of pendrin-null mice and multiple studies employing whole-animal physiology, in vitro microperfusion, and evaluation of protein expression have demonstrated that pendrin is responsible for normal bicarbonate secretion in response to various physiologic stimuli. Pendrin protein is an integral membrane protein predicted to have 11 to 12 transmembrane domains and cytoplasmic amino- and carboxyterminals. In the kidney, pendrin protein is expressed exclusively in type B and C (non-A, non-B) intercalated cells in the apical plasma membrane and in apical cytoplasmic vesicles in type B and non-A, non-B intercalated cells in the CNT, ICT, and CCD. Under basal conditions, pendrin is predominantly expressed in the apical plasma membrane in non-A, non-B intercalated cells and in subapical cytoplasmic vesicles in type B intercalated cells.[377] Several conditions associated with increased pendrin expression, such as dietary Cl^- deficiency, increase apical plasma membrane pendrin expression in type B, but not type C, intercalated cells.[351]

Pendrin also appears to play an important role in extracellular fluid volume and blood pressure regulation. This seems to involve roles in both transcellular Cl^- reabsorption and, through luminal alkalinization due to HCO_3^- secretion, activation of the principal cell epithelial Na^+ transporter, ENaC.[94,374]

Pendrin-null mice have been used effectively to identify pendrin protein as the apical Cl^-/HCO_3^- exchanger responsible for bicarbonate secretion in the CCD and to characterize its importance in chloride uptake and blood pressure regulation in addition to bicarbonate secretion. However, patients with Pendred's syndrome typically have no apparent renal phenotype resulting from the loss of functional pendrin protein. Recently, a report described the development of severe hypokalemic metabolic alkalosis in a patient with Pendred's syndrome after treatment with hydrochlorothiazide.[259] The lack of pendrin-mediated bicarbonate secretion likely explains the increased severity of metabolic alkalosis in this patient.

H+-K+-ATPASE

Another mechanism of active H^+ secretion in the collecting duct is electroneutral H^+-K^+ exchange.[131] At least two main forms of H^+-K^+-ATPase, a P-type ATPase similar to the proton pump responsible for gastric parietal cell acid secretion,[131] exist in the kidney. The active pump is a heterodimer composed of α- and β-subunits. The α-subunit is an integral membrane protein with multiple membrane-spanning domains and contains the catalytic portion of the enzyme. The β-subunit has only a single membrane-spanning region and is necessary for targeting of the α-subunit to the plasma membrane and for transport function.[131]

Two isoforms of the α-subunit have been identified. HKα$_1$, the gastric isoform, is sensitive to omeprazole and Schering 28080. HKα$_1$ forms heterodimers with its specific β-subunit, HKβ. HKα$_2$, the colonic isoform, is sensitive to low concentrations of ouabain; three splice variants of HKα$_2$ have been identified in the kidney. HKα$_2$ forms heterodimers with the β$_1$-subunit of Na^+-K^+-ATPase.

Both the gastric and colonic H^+-K^+-ATPase isoforms are expressed throughout the collecting duct, with greater expression of HKα$_1$, HKα$_2$, and HKβ mRNA in intercalated cells than in principal cells.[3,4,58] Both the gastric and colonic H^+-K^+-ATPase isoforms are present in type A as well as type B intercalated cell subtypes.[217,229,389] Immunohistochemical studies have yielded variable results with respect to the precise cellular distribution of the HKα$_1$ and HKα$_2$ isoforms. HKα$_1$ immunoreactivity was found in both AE1-positive (type A) and AE1-negative intercalated cells in both rat and rabbit kidney,[404] but in human kidney, diffuse HKα$_1$ immunoreactivity was present in both intercalated and principal cells.[188] HKα$_2$ immunoreactivity was consistently apical, but in different cell types in different studies. It was found exclusively in the CNT cell in rabbit in one study[100] and exclusively in the OMCD principal cell in rat in another.[290] A third study found the splice variant HKα$_{2c}$ in intercalated cells, principal cells, and cells from the CNT through the IMCDi in rabbit kidney.[358]

Multiple physiologic conditions alter H^+-K^+-ATPase expression and activity. Metabolic acidosis increases expression of mRNA for HKα$_1$ and HKα$_2$ and H^+-K^+-ATPase activity in the CCD, which suggests that H^+-K^+-ATPase contributes to H^+ secretion.[131] In the rat, metabolic alkalosis increases Schering 28080–sensitive H^+-K^+-ATPase activity in the isolated perfused CCD, which suggests basolateral H^+-K^+-ATPase.[112] In contrast, other studies identified apical, but not basolateral, H^+-K^+-ATPase activity in the type B intercalated cells in both the mouse and rabbit kidney.[389,416] Extracellular ammonia, which increases in response to both metabolic acidosis and hypokalemia, increases H^+-K^+-ATPase–mediated H^+ secretion in both type A and type B intercalated cells in the CCD.[105,107] This effect is not due to changes in intracellular pH but involves changes in intracellular calcium and mechanisms dependent on microtubules and SNARE (soluble NEM-sensitive factor attachment protein receptor) proteins.[106]

OTHER ANION TRANSPORTERS

Cl^- entering via basolateral kAE1 recycles across the basolateral plasma membrane. The potassium-chloride cotransporter KCC4 is basolateral in acid-secreting intercalated cells and appears to facilitate chloride exit.[36] The Cl^- channel ClC-K2 is present in the basolateral plasma membrane of intercalated cells and, when expressed in heterologous expression systems, has functional characteristics similar to those observed in these cells.[255]

Several other anion transporters have been identified in the collecting duct, including anion exchangers and sodium bicarbonate cotransporters, but their roles in acid-base homeostasis have not been defined. AE2 (Slc4a2) is expressed in collecting ducts, particularly in the basolateral plasma membrane of IMCD cells in the terminal IMCD.[109] Slc26a7 has been reported to mediate basolateral Cl^-/HCO_3^- exchange in OMCD intercalated cells.[262] Slc26a7 mRNA and protein expression increases in the outer and inner medulla with acid loading in rats, which suggests that it may contribute to regulated bicarbonate reabsorption in the medullary collecting ducts.[328] AE4 (Slc4a9) has been reported in the collecting duct, but both its location and function are in question. One study reported that AE4 immunoreactivity is exclusively apical in type B intercalated cells in rabbit kidney,[341] whereas another found apical and lateral AE4 immunoreactivity in rabbit type A intercalated cells, and basolateral immunoreactivity in both type A and type B intercalated cells in the rat CCD.[183] In addition, sodium bicarbonate cotransporters are expressed in collecting duct. NBCn1 (Slc4a7), an electroneutral sodium-bicarbonate cotransporter, is expressed in rat inner medulla and is basolateral in IMCD cells in the distal IMCD, where it appears to contribute to stilbene-insensitive sodium- and bicarbonate-dependent intracellular pH correction after cell acidification.[267] In other studies, another product of the SLC4A7 gene, designated *NBC3* in these studies, was found in the apical region of OMCD intercalated cells and type A intercalated cells in the CCD and in the basolateral region of type B intercalated cells.[192] In intercalated cells in the OMCDi, it contributes to intracellular pH regulation, but not significantly to net bicarbonate flux.[411] NBCe2 (Slc4a5), an electrogenic sodium-bicarbonate cotransporter, is apical in intercalated cells in the medullary collecting duct.[81]

Finally, Oat8 (Slc22a9), a sodium-independent organic anion transporter, colocalizes with H^+-ATPase in intercalated cells (apical in type A cells, basolateral in B cells). Oat8 may be involved in endosomal acidification and vesicular trafficking, but the polar distribution and colocalization with H^+-ATPase in intercalated cells suggest that Oat8 may be involved in transepithelial transport.[412]

Regulation of Collecting Duct Acid-Base Transport

The collecting duct is the final site providing renal acid-base regulation. It responds quickly to physiologic conditions to increase acid or bicarbonate excretion as needed to maintain systemic acid-base homeostasis.

ACIDOSIS

The collecting duct response to the challenge of excreting an increased acid load includes immediate and long-term adaptations and involves all segments of the collecting duct and the CNT. The known mechanisms involved typically are alterations in the abundance, subcellular location, and activity of the major proteins connected with proton and bicarbonate transport. Increased acid secretion in the collecting duct during acidosis is primarily mediated by H^+-ATPase. Both metabolic and respiratory acidosis increase apical H^+-ATPase activity and apical plasma membrane H^+-ATPase in acid-secreting collecting duct intercalated cells. Redistribution of H^+-ATPase from a subapical vesicle pool to the apical plasma membrane is the primary means of activation of proton secretion and

involves vesicular trafficking that requires SNARE proteins and Rab guanosine triphosphatases.[49,362] In most models of metabolic acidosis, total renal H^+-ATPase mRNA and protein expression do not change,[323,362] but recent studies using serial analysis for gene expression in OMCDs isolated from mice subjected to metabolic acidosis found increased mRNA for several H^+-ATPase subunits, including the B1 and a4 subunits.[69] During metabolic acidosis, AE1 mRNA and AE1 protein expression in the basolateral plasma membrane in OMCD and CCD type A intercalated cells is increased. In rats and mice, AE1 is present in the basolateral membrane under basal conditions, and the subcellular distribution does not change with metabolic acidosis.[153,289] In rabbits fed a normal diet, AE1 is in both intracellular multivesicular bodies and the basolateral plasma membrane in type A intercalated cells. Metabolic acidosis increases the amount of AE1 immunoreactivity in the basolateral plasma membrane and reduces intracellular AE1.[352] During ammonium chloride loading, pendrin expression in type B and non-A, non-B intercalated cells decreases along with decreased apical Cl^-/HCO_3^- exchange in type B intercalated cells in the CCD.[108,261,363] Reduced bicarbonate secretion by B cells during acid loading thus may contribute to increased net bicarbonate reabsorption. Carbonic anhydrase activity and the expression of CA II and CA IV in the collecting duct are increased by metabolic acidosis.[271] CA IV expression is upregulated in the OMCD, whereas CA II expression is upregulated in the CNT, CCD, and OMCD.

The collecting duct response to respiratory acidosis appears to be similar to the response to metabolic acidosis. Respiratory acidosis stimulates structural changes in OMCD and CCD type A intercalated cells consistent with translocation of H^+-ATPase–bearing membrane from the apical vesicle pool to the apical plasma membrane.[354] Respiratory acidosis also stimulates NEM-sensitive ATPase activity[92,362] and bicarbonate reabsorption in isolated CCDs,[227] consistent with activation of H^+-ATPase–mediated proton secretion. In addition, chronic respiratory acidosis increases kAE1 mRNA.[80] Pendrin expression is downregulated during respiratory acidosis,[83] which likely mediates decreased bicarbonate secretion.

An important and ongoing issue is whether acidosis and alkalosis alter the cellular composition of the collecting duct. Some studies have suggested that there can be interconversion between different intercalated cell subtypes, particularly in the CCD, whereas other studies have found no evidence for interconversion. This issue is discussed in more detail later.

ALKALOSIS

Metabolic alkalosis induces coordinated changes in acid-base transport throughout the collecting duct. In the OMCD of bicarbonate-loaded animals, bicarbonate reabsorption persists, but is decreased compared with that in control animals,[211] and in the IMCD, bicarbonate loading abolishes acid secretion.[33] In the CCD, bicarbonate loading in animals produces net bicarbonate secretion.[226]

The cellular response to alkalosis in OMCD and CCD type A cells entails essentially the reverse of processes that occur to stimulate acid secretion. H^+-ATPase is redistributed from the apical plasma membrane into the apical vesicle pool, and basolateral AE1 immunoreactivity decreases.[28,289,353] Depending on the animal model, alkalosis increases pendrin expression and its apical distribution in type B and non-A, non-B intercalated cells,[108,363] and increases pendrin-mediated CCD bicarbonate secretion.[196] However, pendrin expression, subcellular location, and functional activity are regulated by other factors independent of acid-base status, particularly chloride balance and luminal chloride delivery.[275,351] The recognition of pendrin as the apical anion exchanger responsible for CCD bicarbonate secretion and its functional dependence on chloride provides a mechanistic explanation for the importance of chloride in the correction of metabolic alkalosis.[111]

HORMONAL REGULATION OF COLLECTING DUCT ACID-BASE TRANSPORT

In addition to extracellular pH, multiple other factors regulate collecting duct acid-base transport. Importantly, in vivo acid-base changes cause greater adaptations than equivalent in vitro changes, which suggests that in vivo regulatory mechanisms play a critical role in the response to acid-base disturbances.[113] Several hormones and receptors are known to regulate bicarbonate transport in the collecting duct, particularly aldosterone and its analogs, and angiotensin II.

Aldosterone is an important regulator of collecting duct bicarbonate transport.[325] Both in vivo and in vitro mineralocorticoids increase OMCD bicarbonate reabsorption.[325] This involves, at least in vitro, increased H^+-ATPase activity and apical translocation in OMCD intercalated cells, stimulated through a nongenomic pathway not inhibited by mineralocorticoid receptor blockade.[405] Long-term mineralocorticoid treatment also increases CCD bicarbonate secretion; this is dependent on luminal chloride, mediated by pendrin, and involves increased pendrin mRNA and protein expression and pendrin redistribution from cytoplasmic vesicles to the apical plasma membrane in type B intercalated cells.[288,350]

Angiotensin II is an important regulator of renal acid-base homeostasis and exerts effects on the proximal tubule, TAL, DCT, and collecting ducts. The collecting duct expresses apical AT_1 receptors in both principal cells and intercalated cells.[287] In mouse OMCD and CCD, angiotensin II in vitro increases H^+-ATPase activity in acid-secreting intercalated cells by trafficking H^+-ATPase to the apical plasma membrane.[258,287] In mouse OMCD, angiotensin II stimulation of H^+-ATPase activity is mediated through a G protein–coupled phosphokinase C pathway and requires the B1 H^+-ATPase subunit.[287] However, in other studies, angiotensin II decreased bicarbonate reabsorption in rat OMCD in vivo and in vitro, and angiotensin II decreased H^+-ATPase activity via AT_1 receptors in vitro.[337,367] The apparent discrepancy between these observations and the documentation of angiotensin II–stimulated H^+-ATPase activity and acid secretion by type A intercalated cells in mouse studies has not been resolved.

The role of angiotensin II–stimulated H^+-ATPase activity in the CCD may relate more to the regulation of chloride reabsorption and extracellular volume than to acid-base balance. In vitro angiotensin II stimulates pendrin-mediated chloride uptake in mouse CCD,[258] which is consistent with earlier reports that in vitro angiotensin II stimulates apical Cl^-/HCO_3^- exchange in rabbit type B intercalated cells.[390] The pendrin-mediated transport depends on the activation of H^+-ATPase and acid secretion by type A intercalated cells, presumably by providing a sink for secreted bicarbonate and a driving force for continued anion exchange.[258]

Endothelin has important effects on collecting duct acid-base transport that are mediated partly by nitric oxide. Dietary protein intake stimulates urinary acidification through a process involving H^+-ATPase activation, mediated by endothelin and nitric oxide.[399] Endothelin 1 (ET-1) is synthesized in native collecting duct and cultured collecting duct cells.[309,327] Endothelin receptors A and B (ET-A and ET-B) are present in the collecting duct, but ET-B predominates.[186] In vitro metabolic acidosis normally increases acid secretion by type A cells and decreases bicarbonate secretion by type B cells. ET-B, in conjunction with nitric oxide synthase, regulates the type B intercalated cell response to metabolic acidosis, whereas the ET-B receptor, but not nitric oxide synthase, regulates the type A cell response.[345]

The calcium-sensing receptor is apical in IMCD cells and in type A intercalated cells[282] and mediates luminal Ca^{2+} stimulation of H^+-ATPase.[281] Luminal acidification stimulated by this pathway may inhibit calcium precipitation and minimize development of nephrolithiasis.[281]

Other hormones affect acid-base transport in the collecting duct, but their effects have not been fully characterized. These include kallikrein, which inhibits bicarbonate secretion[220]; calcitonin, which stimulates H^+-ATPase–dependent bicarbonate reabsorption in the rabbit CCD[310]; and isoproterenol, which stimulates bicarbonate secretion by type B intercalated cells.[298]

It is well established that both type A and type B intercalated cells respond to physiologic conditions with remodeling of the apical region and subcellular redistribution of important acid-base transporters, including H^+-ATPase, pendrin, and Rhcg. Whether there is true interconversion of these two intercalated cell types, however, is unclear. Early papers examining the rabbit isolated perfused CCD equated apical endocytosis with acid-secreting type A (α) intercalated cells and used apical peanut lectin binding as an empirical marker of bicarbonate-secreting type B (β) intercalated cells. Stimuli that increased luminal acidification increased the number of intercalated cells exhibiting apical endocytosis and decreased the number of cells that bound peanut lectin; the interpretation was that intercalated cell subtypes in the CCD could interconvert, with β intercalated cells reversing polarity to meet the physiologic demand for increased acid secretion.[301] Subsequent cell culture experiments showed reversal of the polar distribution of AE1, the basolateral anion exchanger found in native medullary CD and CCD type A intercalated cells, an effect that is mediated by expression of an extracellular matrix protein, hensin.[300] However, apical expression of AE1 has never been reported in native intercalated cells in any animal model. In addition, despite several studies of animal models that suppress apical bicarbonate secretion, there are no reports of expression of basolateral pendrin, the apical anion exchanger of type B intercalated cells. More recent studies have suggested instead that there can be a functional reversal of the direction of bicarbonate and proton extrusion, particularly in type B intercalated cells, that allows B cells to secrete protons rather than bicarbonate. In support of this possibility, isolated perfused tubule studies have demonstrated that all intercalated cells in the rabbit CCD that express an apical Cl^-/HCO_3^- exchange activity have both apical H^+-K^+-ATPase and basolateral Cl^-/HCO_3^- exchange activity as well.[389,391] Thus, it is possible that the type B intercalated cell can secrete H^+ and reabsorb luminal HCO_3^- via apical H^+-K^+-ATPase and basolateral Cl^-/HCO_3^- exchange activity. It also has been proposed that under certain conditions in vivo, type B intercalated cells can convert to type A intercalated cells; that is, rather than reversing polarity, they can eliminate pendrin expression, express basolateral AE1, and reverse the plasma membrane location of H+-ATPase. Although some studies report changes in the percentage of type A and B intercalated cells under various physiologic perturbations,[25,29,301] others do not.[153,289,355] The explanation for the differences in the results of these studies remains to be determined, but could include differences in the experimental models, species examined, and intercalated cell identification and quantitation methods.

Bicarbonate Generation

Renal acid-base homeostasis requires new bicarbonate generation, in addition to reabsorption of filtered bicarbonate. There are two major components of bicarbonate generation: titratable acid excretion and ammonia excretion. In addition, bicarbonate generation also requires consideration of organic ion excretion, which because the metabolism of retained organic anions generates equimolar bicarbonate, is physiologically equivalent to bicarbonate excretion.

Titratable Acid Excretion

Titratable acids are solutes in the urine that buffer secreted protons, enabling H+ excretion without substantial changes in urine pH. Titratable acid excretion comprises approximately 30% to 40% of net acid excretion under basal conditions. Metabolic acidosis increases titratable acid excretion by as much as 50% above baseline, which contributes to recovery from this acid-base disorder (Figure 9-5).[136,292] Multiple solutes contribute to titratable acid excretion. Figure 9-6 shows the relative contributions of major urinary buffers, taking into account the amount excreted under basal conditions and the pK_a. Although ammonia is frequently considered a urinary buffer, because of its high pK_a it does not contribute substantially to titratable acid excretion. Phosphate is the predominant titratable acid, typically accounting for more than 50% of total titratable acid.[136,408] Citrate and creatinine also contribute to

titratable acid excretion, but to a lesser extent. Although sulfate is excreted in relatively large amounts, because of its low pK_a it does not effectively buffer secreted H+ and therefore does not contribute significantly to titratable acid excretion.

Phosphate as a Titratable Acid

The amount of phosphate excreted that functions as a titratable acid is determined by filtered load, renal tubular reabsorption, and urine pH. Plasma phosphate is not bound to proteins, and consequently it is almost completely filtered at the glomerulus. Renal tubular phosphate reabsorption and urine pH are the major factors regulating titratable acid excretion in the form of phosphate. Phosphate exists in serum in equilibrium between two molecular forms, $H_2PO_4^-$ and HPO_4^{2-}. The relative amount of these two forms is determined by the following formula:

$$10^{pH - 6.8} = \frac{[HPO_4^{2-}]}{[H_2PO_4^-]}$$

Accordingly, at a typical serum pH of 7.4, approximately 80% of filtered phosphate is HPO_4^{2-} and 20% is $H_2PO_4^-$. Because the pK_a of the buffer reaction $H_2PO_4^- + H^+ \rightleftharpoons H_3PO_4$ is approximately 2.2, essentially no phosphate is in the form, H_3PO_4. Titratable acid excretion in the form of phosphate thus reflects the amount of filtered HPO_4^{2-} that is not reabsorbed and that buffers H+ secreted in the proximal tubule, loop of Henle, distal tubule, and collecting duct. Regulation of renal tubular phosphate transport is a complex process and is discussed in more detail elsewhere in this text. Here, only the factors that regulate this process in response to acid-base disorders are reviewed. The proximal tubule is the primary site of phosphate reabsorption and the location where metabolic acidosis and other acid-base disorders regulate phosphate transport. Minimal phosphate reabsorption occurs distal to the proximal tubule, and distal sites do not appear to contribute to regulated titratable acid excretion. Acute and chronic metabolic acidosis

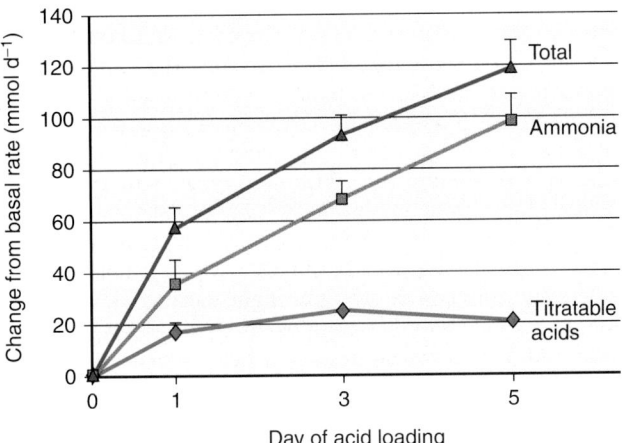

FIGURE 9-5 Relative responses of titratable acid and ammonia excretion in the response to metabolic acidosis. Healthy human volunteers were acid loaded with approximately 2 mmol/kg/day of ammonium chloride, and changes in urinary ammonia and titratable acid excretion were quantified. (Data recalculated from Elkinton and others.[95])

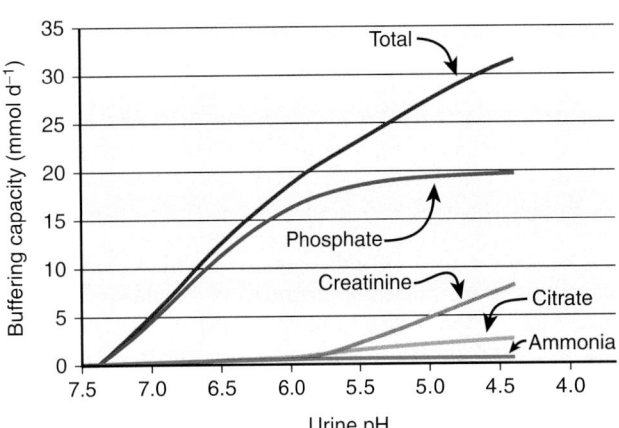

FIGURE 9-6 Relative contribution of various urinary buffers to titratable acid excretion. Ability of various urinary buffers to contribute to titratable acid excretion depends on their urinary excretion rate, pKa, and final urine pH. Figure shows buffering capacity of each of four major urinary buffers—phosphate, creatinine, citrate, and ammonia—at differing urine pH. Rates were calculated with the following daily excretion rates and pKa values, respectively: phosphate, 25 mmol/day and 6.8; creatinine, 11 mmol/day and 4.9; citrate, 3 mmol/day and 5.6; and ammonia, 40 mmol/day and 9.15.

decrease proximal tubule phosphate reabsorption through a variety of mechanisms. The decrease involves decreased apical plasma membrane Na^+-dependent phosphate transport and decreased NaPi-IIa protein and mRNA expression.[17,132] Metabolic acidosis decreases luminal pH by decreasing the filtered bicarbonate load and increasing luminal bicarbonate reabsorption, and luminal acidification independently inhibits proximal tubule phosphate uptake.[148,346] In acute metabolic acidosis, decreased phosphate transport may involve changes in the subcellular distribution of NaPi-IIa.[17] PTH likely contributes to the decreased phosphate reabsorption in response to metabolic acidosis. Metabolic acidosis increases PTH release, thereby inhibiting proximal tubule phosphate reabsorption and increasing luminal phosphate availability as a titratable acid. Multiple phosphate transporters, including NaPi-IIa, NaPi-IIc, and Pit-2 are present in the proximal tubule apical plasma membrane. The central role of NaPi-IIa was shown in studies in which NaPi-IIa deletion prevents changes in phosphate excretion with metabolic acidosis.[253] Whether NaPi-IIc changes with metabolic acidosis is unclear, because some studies find decreased expression[359] and others do not.[253] Pit-2 expression, although regulated by dietary phosphate availability, is not altered in metabolic acidosis in phosphate-replete conditions, but does increase in response to metabolic acidosis in conditions of phosphate depletion.[359] The specific signals that stimulate changes in NaPi-IIa phosphate transport are incompletely defined. In particular, acid loading can alter NaPi-IIa expression in the absence of steady-state changes in systemic pH.[359] Acidosis-induced changes in phosphate excretion depend on systemic phosphate availability. In the presence of dietary phosphate restriction, basal phosphate excretion is greatly reduced, and the normal increases in urinary phosphate excretion in response to metabolic acidosis are greatly blunted.[359] This lack of change in phosphate excretion parallels a lack of change in NaPi-IIa protein or mRNA abundance.[17] NaPi-IIc and Pit-2 expression actually increase in phosphate-restricted animals exposed to metabolic acidosis.[359] Changes in extrarenal phosphate transport contribute to increased phosphate availability for excretion as titratable acid. Metabolic acidosis increases small intestinal Na^+-dependent phosphate uptake, and this is associated with increased expression of both protein and mRNA for the primary small intestinal apical plasma membrane phosphate transporter NaPi-IIb.[322] There is also increased phosphate release from bone in response to both acute and chronic metabolic acidosis.[199] The net effect of these extrarenal effects is to enable changes in urinary phosphate excretion without resulting changes in systemic phosphate concentration.

Hypokalemia is a second common condition that increases phosphaturia by inhibiting proximal tubule phosphate transport. Increased phosphate excretion enables increased titratable acid excretion and can thereby contribute to the metabolic alkalosis that can occur with hypokalemia. This occurs through decreased NaPi-IIc and Pit-2 expression, through changes in the subcellular distribution of NaPi-IIc, and through altered activity, diffusion, and clustering of NaPi-IIa.[46,414]

Other Urinary Buffers

Creatinine, although typically used to assess glomerular filtration, has a pK_a of approximately 4.9 and is excreted in sufficient quantities, approximately 11 mmol/day, that it can contribute to titratable acid excretion. This is particularly true in conditions in which urinary pH is 5.5 or less, when creatinine can account for as much as 20% of titratable acid excretion.[136] Uric acid, although it has a pK_a of 5.6, which is ideal as a urinary buffer, is typically excreted in such small amounts, approximately 4 mmol/day, as to limit its role as a titratable acid. In ketoacidosis, β-hydroxybutyric acid and acetoacetic acid excretion increases, which increases titratable acid excretion. Because ketoacids can be metabolized to bicarbonate, however, their loss in the urine has no net effect on acid-base homeostasis.

Organic Anion Excretion

Multiple organic anions in the urine can contribute to acid-base homeostasis. At least 95 different urinary organic anions have been identified, and many, including hippuric, erythronic, threonic, tartaric, and uric acid, are excreted in substantial quantities.[62] In general, their role in acid-base homeostasis is not as titratable acids but as alkali equivalents, because their metabolism produces bicarbonate. Some, however, such as citrate and uric acid, can function both as titratable acids and as metabolizable organic anions. In this case, they contribute to acid-base homeostasis both as titratable acids and as alkali equivalents, with the specific role in part determined by urinary pH.

Citrate Excretion

Citrate plays an important role in both acid-base homeostasis and urinary calcium excretion. The latter function relates to citrate's ability to complex calcium and enables excretion of calcium at high urinary concentrations, and is discussed in other sections of this textbook. This chapter discusses citrate's role in acid-base homeostasis. Citrate is a tricarboxylic acid with four molecular forms: $citrate^{3-}$, $citrate^{2-}$, $citrate^-$, and citric acid. The pK_a values for the interconversion of these molecular forms are 5.6, 4.3, and 2.9, respectively. In plasma almost all citrate is in the form of $citrate^{3-}$. In urine, the two major molecular forms are $citrate^{3-}$ and $citrate^{2-}$, with the relative amounts of each determined by pH. Unless specified explicitly, the term *citrate* refers to the sum of all molecular forms in this chapter. Citrate has two roles in acid-base homeostasis: as a urinary buffer contributing to titratable acid excretion and as a substrate for the tricarboxylic acid cycle. Plasma citrate is approximately 99% in the molecular form of $citrate^{3-}$, and at a urine pH of 5.6 approximately 50% of urinary citrate is in the form $citrate^{2-}$, which enables citrate to function as titratable acid (see Figure 9-6). However, because the pK_a' is 5.6 for the $H^+ + citrate^{3-} \rightleftharpoons H\text{-}citrate^{2-}$ buffer reaction, at a urine pH of approximately 6.0, less than 30% of urinary citrate is in the molecular form of $H\text{-}citrate^{2-}$, which is able to buffer secreted protons and thereby contribute to titratable acid excretion. Citrate is also a key component of the tricarboxylic acid cycle, and its metabolism results in HCO_3^- generation. Thus, citrate excretion is functionally equivalent to HCO_3^- excretion. Because the majority of urinary citrate is in the molecular form of $citrate^{3-}$, not $citrate^{2-}$, the predominant effect of variations in citrate excretion is mediated through its role as a substrate in the tricarboxylic acid cycle and thereby as an alkali equivalent. Changes in renal citrate excretion appear to have a substantial impact on acid-base homeostasis, particularly in modest acid-base disorders.[52,171] Multiple factors regulate renal citrate excretion. Metabolic acidosis decreases citrate excretion, and both respiratory and metabolic alkalosis increase it.[27] Decreased citrate excretion with metabolic acidosis decreases its availability as a titratable acid, but because citrate is also a metabolic alkali equivalent, decreased citrate excretion results in decreased alkali equivalent excretion and a net beneficial effect on systemic acid-base homeostasis. Hypokalemia reduces citrate excretion.[2,104] This effect is likely independent of systemic pH, because hypokalemia normally induces metabolic alkalosis. Both the carbonic anhydrase inhibitor acetazolamide and high dietary intake of either NaCl or protein decrease citrate excretion.[133,187] Lithium chloride, even when administered at therapeutic dosages, increases citrate excretion, at least in animal models,[37] but studies in humans have not confirmed this finding.[38] Renal citrate handling determines renal citrate excretion and is limited to glomerular filtration and proximal tubule metabolism. In humans, plasma citrate levels average approximately 0.1 mmol/L, and changes in plasma levels are not an important regulatory mechanism. Plasma citrate is essentially completely filtered at the glomerulus and 10% to 35% of filtered citrate is excreted in the urine. The proximal tubule reabsorbs 65% to 90% of filtered citrate, and reabsorption rises in parallel with changes in the filtered load. In addition, there is basolateral citrate uptake, but no evidence for citrate secretion. Instead, citrate transported into proximal tubule epithelial cells, whether across apical or basolateral plasma membranes, is metabolized, which enables citrate to serve as a significant component of renal oxidative metabolism.[133] There does not appear to be a significant component of citrate transport in other renal sites. Proximal tubule apical citrate uptake is a secondarily active process, involving electrogenic cotransport of 3 Na^+ with citrate^{2-}, and is dependent on basolateral Na^+-K^+-ATPase activity.[133] Apical citrate transport is believed to be mediated by the sodium-dicarboxylate cotransporter NaDC-1, an 11 transmembrane segment, integral membrane protein highly expressed in apical plasma membrane in the proximal tubule and in the small intestine.[254,304] Multiple mechanisms regulate proximal tubule citrate transport. First, the transported citrate form is citrate^{2-}; luminal acidification, as present with metabolic acidosis, shifts the buffer reaction citrate^{3-} + H^+ ⇔ citrate^{2-} to the right, which increases luminal citrate^{2-} concentration and citrate uptake. Metabolic acidosis also increases apical citrate transport capacity when measured in brush border membrane vesicles,[162] most likely by increasing NaDC-1 expression.[18] Both hypokalemia and starvation, which decrease citrate excretion, increase citrate transport activity measured in brush border membrane vesicles.[202,403] Basolateral citrate transport in the proximal tubule has different characteristics than apical transport. Uptake is pH independent, Na^+ dependent, and electroneutral, involves 3 Na^+ transported with 1 citrate^{3-},[133,163] and appears to be mediated by NaDC-3.[55] Approximately 20% of proximal tubule citrate uptake appears to be mediated by basolateral uptake. However, because the proximal tubule does not secrete citrate, basolateral citrate uptake does not regulate renal citrate excretion.

Other Organic Anions

Humans excrete 26 to 52 mEq/day of organic anions other than citrate. Because organic anions can be metabolized to bicarbonate, organic anion excretion is functionally equivalent to alkali excretion and thus can contribute to acid-base regulation. The extent of change in organic anion excretion with acid-base disturbances is not clear. Some studies indicate that acid or alkali loading does not alter urinary organic anion excretion,[200] whereas other, more recent studies show that organic anion excretion is increased by alkali loading and decreased by a ketogenic, acid-producing diet.[150] Studies in experimental animal models indicate an important role for organic anions in acid-base homeostasis. In the rat, changes in organic anion excretion in response to acid-base loading can be as much as 40% of the total change in net acid excretion.[52,68,206] Quantitatively, there are important species-dependent differences in the magnitude of organic anion excretion. In humans, basal organic anion excretion averages 0.3 to 0.7 mEq/kg/day,[200] whereas in the rat organic anion excretion has been reported at between 2 and 8 mEq/kg/day.[52,283] Studies in the dog report 1 to 2 mEq/kg/day[250] and in the rabbit an average of 4 mEq/kg/day.[283] In part, this species-dependent variation reflects species-dependent differences in intestinal absorption of dietary organic anions.[283]

Ammonia Metabolism

Renal ammonia metabolism and transport is a predominant mechanism of the renal response to most acid-base disorders, and generally changes in renal ammonia excretion are quantitatively greater than changes in titratable acid excretion (see Figure 9-5). Ammonia metabolism involves the integrated function of multiple portions of the kidney. Only a minimal amount of urinary ammonia derives from glomerular filtration, which makes urinary ammonia unique among the major compounds present in the urine. Instead, ammonia is produced by the kidney and is then selectively transported either into the urine or into the renal vein. Ammonia's selective transport into the urine, where it can be excreted, or into the renal interstitium and then into the renal veins, which results in return to the systemic circulation, determines its effect on acid-base homeostasis. Ammonia excreted into the urine as NH_4^+ results in equimolar new bicarbonate formation. Ammonia returned to the systemic circulation is metabolized by the liver; this process uses equimolar amounts of bicarbonate and thereby consumes the bicarbonate produced during ammoniagenesis. Selective transport of ammonia into either the urine or the renal vein involves integrated transport in the proximal tubule, TAL of the loop of Henle, and collecting duct (Figure 9-7). Renal ammonia metabolism is subject to a number of known stimuli (Table 9-3).

Ammonia Chemistry

Ammonia exists in two molecular forms, NH_3 and NH_4^+. The relative amounts of each are governed by the buffer reaction NH_3 + H^+ ⇔ NH_4^+. This reaction occurs essentially instantaneously and has a pK_a' under biologically relevant conditions of approximately 9.15. Accordingly, the majority of ammonia is present as NH_4^+; at pH 7.4 only approximately 1.7% of total ammonia is present as NH_3. Because most biologic fluids exist at a pH substantially below the pK_a' of this buffer reaction, small changes in pH cause exponential changes in NH_3 concentration, but almost no change in NH_4^+ concentration.

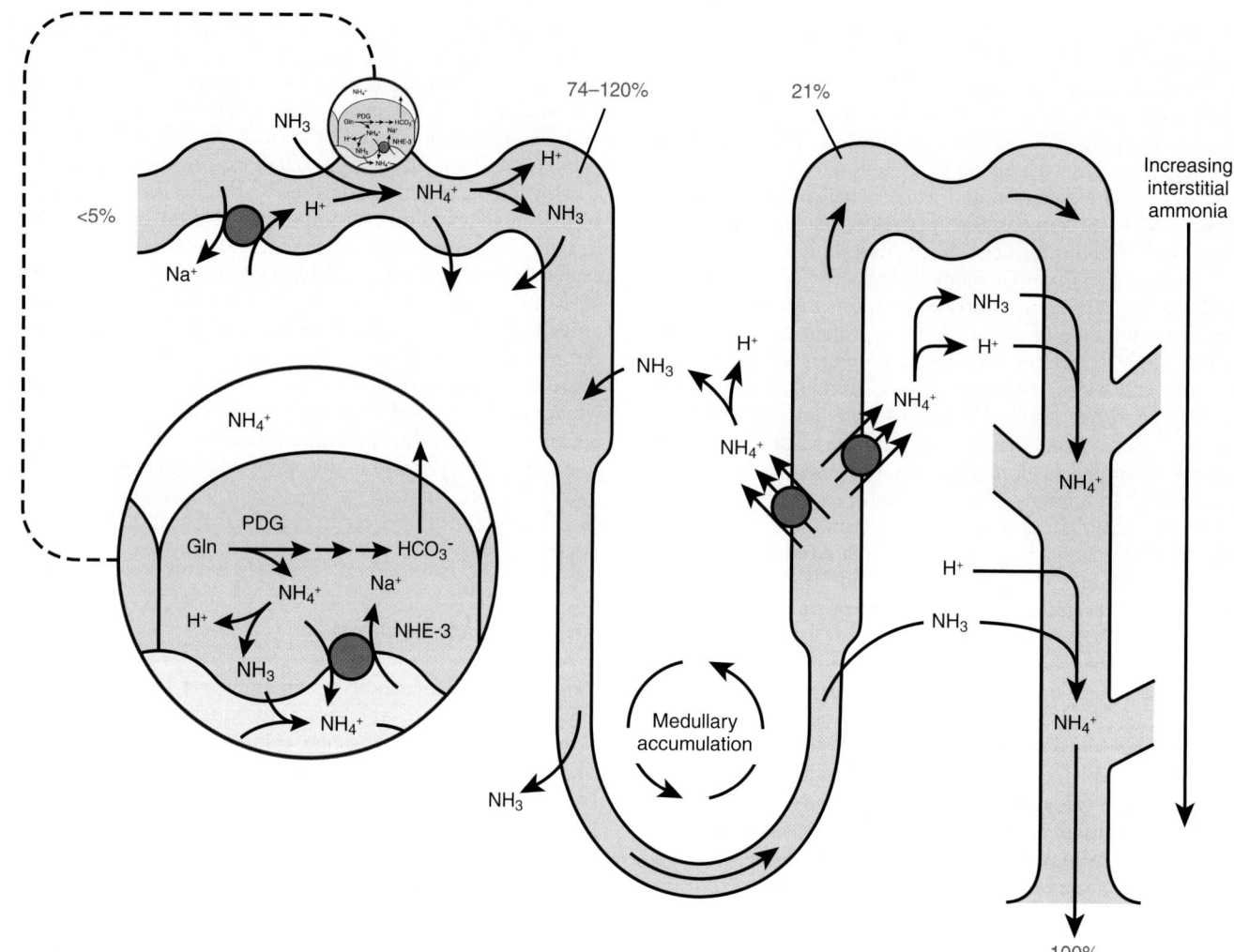

FIGURE 9-7 Summary of renal ammonia metabolism. The proximal tubule produces ammonia, as NH_4^+, from glutamine. NH_4^+ is then secreted preferentially into the luminal fluid, primarily by Na^+/H^+ exchanger isoform 3 (NHE3). It is then reabsorbed by the thick ascending limb of the loop of Henle (TAL), primarily by Na^+-K^+-$2Cl^-$ cotransporter type 2 (NKCC2). This results in delivery of ammonia to the distal nephron, which accounts for approximately 20% of final urinary ammonia; the remaining approximately 80% is secreted in the collecting duct through parallel NH_3 and H^+ transport. Numbers in red indicate the proportion of total urinary ammonia present at the indicated sites under baseline conditions.

NH_3, although uncharged, has an asymmetric arrangement of positively charged hydrogen nuclei surrounding a central nitrogen; as a result, NH_3 actually is a relatively polar molecule. This molecular polarity causes NH_3 to have limited lipid permeability and finite permeability across plasma membranes.[387]

NH_4^+ also has limited permeability across lipid bilayers in the absence of specific transport proteins. However, in aqueous solutions NH_4^+ and K^+ have nearly identical biophysical characteristics (Table 9-4), which enables NH_4^+ to be transported at the K^+ transport site of many proteins.[387]

Ammonia Production

Ammonia is produced by almost all renal epithelial cells, but the proximal tubule is the primary site for physiologically relevant ammoniagenesis. In particular, the glomeruli, S1, S2, S3, proximal tubule segments, descending thin limb of the loop of Henle, medullary and cortical TAL of the loop of Henle, DCT, CCD, OMCD, and IMCD all have the capability to synthesize ammonia, with glutamine being the primary metabolic substrate.[122] Phosphate-dependent glutaminase (PDG)

is involved in this process in each of these segments.[78] However, rates of ammoniagenesis increase in response to metabolic acidosis only in the S1 and S2 proximal tubule segments.[122,407] When the production rates per unit length and the relative lengths of the different nephron segments are taken into account, the proximal tubule accounts for 60% to 70% of total renal ammonia production under basal conditions and at least 70% to 80% of production in response to metabolic acidosis (Figure 9-8).[122]

Although multiple pathways for ammoniagenesis are present in the proximal tubule (Figure 9-9), the predominant ammoniagenic pathway involves PDG. PDG is an inner mitochondrial membrane-bound enzyme that metabolizes glutamine to glutamate, producing NH_4^+. Glutamine can also be metabolized by γ-glutamyl transpeptidase (γ-GT), also known as *phosphate-independent glutaminase*, although this is unlikely to be a major mechanism of renal ammoniagenesis. Another pathway involves sequential metabolism through glutamine ketoacid aminotransferase and ω-amidase, which forms α-ketoglutarate (α-KG) and releases NH_4^+. Quantitative assessments suggest that this pathway does not contribute substantially to net ammoniagenesis, either under

TABLE 9-3 Known Stimuli of Renal Ammonia Metabolism

Acidosis

Hypokalemia

Glucocorticoids

Mineralocorticoids

Cyclic adenosine monophosphate

Circulating non-dialyzable factor

TABLE 9-4 Biophysical Characteristics of Common Cations[387]

CATION	IONIC RADIUS (Å)	HYDRO-DYNAMIC RADIUS (Å)	MOBILITY IN H_2O (10^{-4} CM^2/SEC/V)	TRANS-FERENCE NUMBER IN H_2O ($T_i^{H_2O}$)
Li^+	0.060	1.73	4.01	0.33
Na^+	0.095	1.67	5.19	0.39
NH_4^+	0.133	1.14	7.60	0.49
K^+	0.143	1.14	7.62	0.49

Reprinted from Weiner ID, Hamm LL. Molecular mechanisms of renal ammonia transport. *Annu Rev Physiol.* 2007;69:317-340.

basal conditions or in response to acute or chronic metabolic acidosis.[331]

Glutamate then undergoes further metabolism through multiple pathways. The major pathways involve either glutamate dehydrogenase (GDH), which mediates conversion to α-KG with release of NH_4^+, or transamination via glutamic-oxaloacetic transaminase (GOT) to aspartate. GDH-mediated metabolism of glutamate to form α-KG is the quantitatively predominant mechanism and is regulated in parallel with changes in total renal ammoniagenesis. Although transamination of glutamate via GOT does not release NH_4^+, the aspartate produced can be metabolized through the purine nucleotide cycle (PNC), which forms fumarate and releases NH_4^+. Quantitatively, the PNC pathway plays only a minor role in overall ammoniagenesis.[331] Glutamate can also be metabolized through glutamate decarboxylase to form γ-aminobutyric acid (GABA), but this pathway does not alter net ammoniagenesis because GABA metabolism results in regeneration of glutamate. Glutamate can also be converted back to glutamine via the enzyme glutamine synthetase. Because this reaction utilizes NH_4^+ as a cosubstrate, it results in decreased net NH_4^+ formation. Glutamine synthetase is expressed in the proximal tubule of the rat and mouse, primarily in late proximal tubule segments. Metabolic acidosis decreases glutamine synthetase activity,[201] but not protein expression,[333] in the rat kidney and decreases both activity and expression in the mouse kidney.[75] α-KG can be metabolized through α-KG dehydrogenase and succinate dehydrogenase, forming oxaloacetic acid. Oxaloacetic acid can serve as a substrate for phospho*enol*pyruvate carboxykinase (PEPCK) to form phospho*enol*pyruvate, which can then be used for gluconeogenesis. Conditions that increase ammonia, such as metabolic acidosis, increase flux through this pathway and stimulate renal gluconeogenesis. Pyruvate can also be metabolized by pyruvate dehydrogenase, forming HCO_3^- and acetyl–coenzyme A.

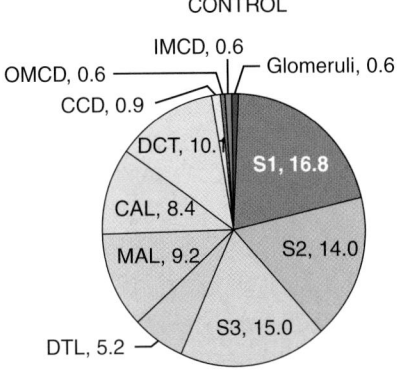

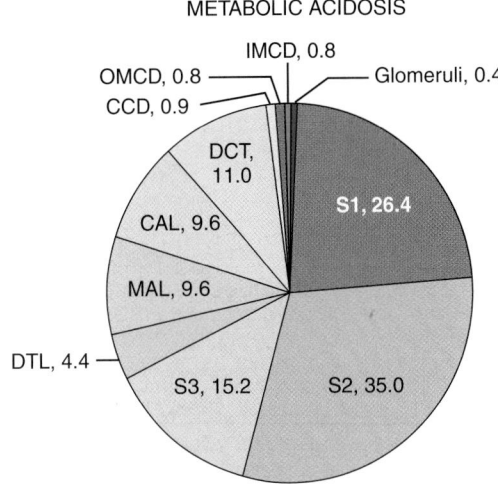

FIGURE 9-8 Ammonia production in various renal segments. Ammonia production rates in different renal components were measured in microdissected segments from rats on control diets and after induction of metabolic acidosis. All segments tested produce net ammonia. Metabolic acidosis increases total renal ammoniagenesis, but only through increased production in proximal tubule segments (S1, S2, and S3). Rates were calculated from measured ammonia production rates and mean length per segment as described in Good and Burg.[122] The size of the pie graph is proportional to total renal ammoniagenesis rates. *CAL,* Cortical thick ascending limb of the loop of Henle; *CCD,* cortical collecting duct; *DCT,* distal convoluted tubule; *DTL,* descending thin limb of the loop of Henle; *IMCD,* inner medullary collecting duct; *MAL,* medullary thick ascending limb of the loop of Henle; *OMCD,* outer medullary collecting duct.

Glutamine Transport in Ammoniagenesis

Glutamine is the primary metabolic source for renal ammoniagenesis. Under conditions of normal acid-base balance, the kidneys extract very little glutamine, less than 3% of delivered glutamine. However, acute metabolic acidosis induces a rapid, approximately twofold increase in plasma glutamine levels; this results primarily from increased skeletal muscle glutamine release.[333] In parallel, renal glutamine uptake increases to approximately 20% of delivered glutamine, which enables increased ammoniagenesis.[154,333] With chronic metabolic acidosis, renal extraction increases to as much as 50% of delivered glutamine, even though plasma glutamine levels actually decrease.[154] Increased renal glutamine utilization is balanced by increased skeletal muscle and liver glutamine release.[333] Filtered glutamine is almost completely reabsorbed in the proximal convoluted tubule.[311] Apical glutamine transport, assessed in brush border membrane vesicles, is Na^+ dependent and has inhibitor characteristics similar to those identified

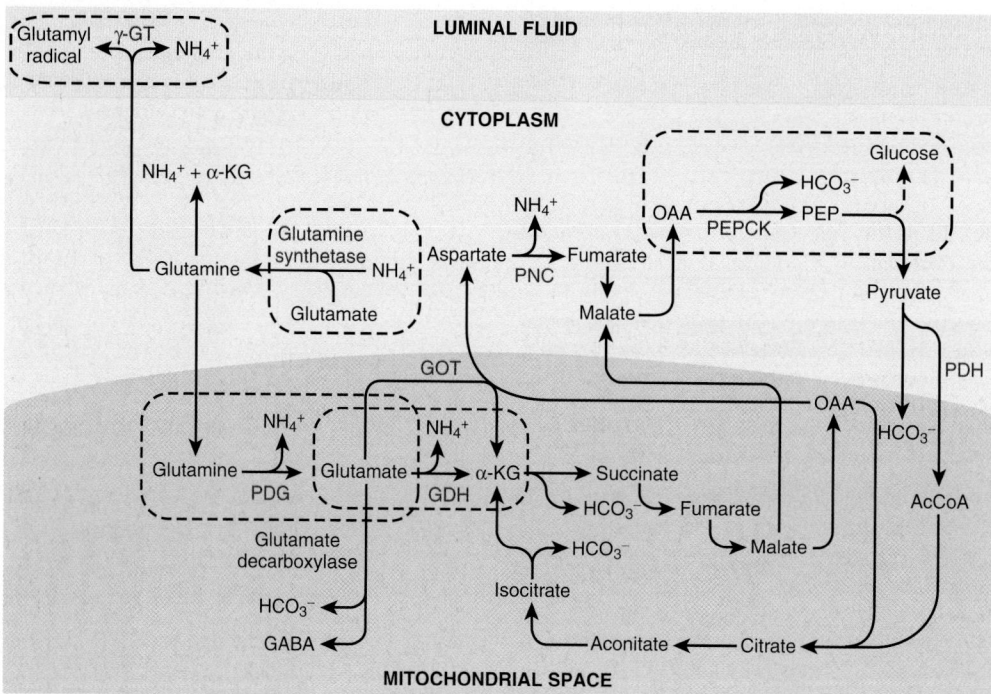

FIGURE 9-9 Mechanisms of ammoniagenesis. Multiple pathways for enzymatic ammonia production originating from glutamine metabolism are present in the proximal tubule. Glutamine metabolism through phosphate-dependent glutaminase (PDG) and glutamate dehydrogenase (GDH) and involving phospho*enol*pyruvate carboxykinase (PEPCK) is the quantitatively most significant component of renal ammoniagenesis and the primary pathway stimulated in response to metabolic acidosis.

for SNAT3/SN1 (SLC38A3).[170] SNAT3 has been identified by immunoblot analysis in brush border membrane vesicles under basal conditions,[170] but not by immunohistochemical analysis,[57] so that the role of SNAT3 in glutamine reabsorption in the proximal convoluted tubule is unclear. Multiple other glutamine transporters are expressed in the apical membrane in the proximal tubule, including the Na+-dependent neutral amino acid transporters B0AT1 (SLC6A19) and B0AT3 (SLC6A18). Under basal conditions, relatively little of the glutamine reabsorbed in the proximal tubule is metabolized but instead is transported across the basolateral membrane into the peritubular space, which results in net glutamine reabsorption. Chronic metabolic acidosis increases both apical glutamine transport and SNAT3 protein expression, at least as assessed in brush border membrane vesicles.[170] However, immunohistochemical studies have not identified apical SNAT3 expression in the proximal tubule.[57,231] Chronic metabolic acidosis does not alter expression of the other apical glutamine transporters, B0AT1 and B0AT3.[231] Chronic metabolic acidosis also increases basolateral glutamine transport, assessed in basolateral membrane vesicles, and it increases basolateral SNAT3 protein expression.[170] Immunohistochemical studies show basolateral SNAT3 immunolabel in the S3 proximal tubule segment under basal conditions, and multiple conditions that increase ammoniagenesis, such as chronic metabolic acidosis, hypokalemia, and high protein intake, increase SNAT3 protein expression. Moreover, not only is SNAT3 expression increased, but there is induction of detectable expression in the basolateral plasma membrane in the proximal tubule S2 segment and increased basolateral expression in the S3 segment.[57,231] Increased basolateral SNAT3 expression presumably mediates increased peritubular glutamine uptake, which enables increased ammoniagenesis

and explains the observation that renal glutamine extraction can exceed glutamine filtration. In addition, a system ASC glutamine transporter may also be present, at least in the renal cortex, and contribute to glutamine transport under basal conditions.[170] In the basolateral membrane, in addition to SNAT3, is the cationic amino acid/neutral amino acid exchanger y+-LAT1 (SLC7A7). During chronic metabolic acidosis y+-LAT1 expression decreases, which suggests that it does not contribute to increased glutamine uptake in this condition.[231] Mitochondrial glutamine uptake involves a specific transporter-mediated mechanism.[293] This uptake is *trans*-stimulated and *cis*-inhibited by alanine, demonstrates a positive cooperativity effect by glutamine, and is stimulated by metabolic acidosis.[293] The transporter appears to have a molecular weight of 41.5 kDa and may also transport asparagines.[159] The specific molecular identity of this protein has not been identified.

Regulation of Ammoniagenesis

Multiple conditions stimulate renal ammoniagenesis (see Table 3). Both acute and chronic metabolic acidosis stimulate ammoniagenesis[331] and appear to do so by stimulating the PDG pathway. Although acute respiratory acidosis stimulates ammoniagenesis, the effect of chronic respiratory acidosis is unclear, because different studies have either identified no change or an increase.[330] In metabolic acidosis, the majority of evidence suggests that changes in extracellular pH, which then alter cytoplasmic and mitochondrial pH, are a proximate stimuli.[243,294] However, metabolic acidosis can also stimulate ammoniagenesis through a pH-independent mechanism involving a small, nondialyzable factor.[7] Chronic metabolic acidosis is associated with increases in PDG, GDH, and PEPCK expression and activity.[331] Chronic hypokalemia increases ammoniagenesis through mechanisms involving increased enzyme expression and activity similar to those identified for chronic metabolic acidosis. Acute changes in extracellular K^+ also regulate proximal tubule ammoniagenesis. These effects are directly mediated by extracellular K^+ and, because they can be observed within 45 minutes of change in extracellular K^+, likely do not require changes in protein expression.[238] The observation that increased ammoniagenesis decreases renal potassium excretion,[329] and that this is associated with specific changes in collecting duct potassium secretion and reabsorption,[107,134] suggests that ammonia may also play a role as an intrarenal signaling molecule that regulates renal potassium excretion.

Ammoniagenesis can be modulated independently of acid-base status by a variety of factors, including tricarboxylic acid cycle intermediates, hormones that increase cAMP, prostaglandin $F_{2\alpha}$, insulin, growth hormone, angiotensin II, corticosteroids, aldosterone, and tubular flow rate.[331] Increasing evidence suggests an important role for angiotensin II in regulating ammoniagenesis. In particular, luminal angiotensin II stimulates and peritubular angiotensin II inhibits proximal tubule ammoniagenesis.[239]

Ammonia Transport

Ammonia produced in the proximal tubule is secreted preferentially into the tubule lumen, although there is some transport across the basolateral membrane. Preferential apical secretion results from multiple factors, including increased luminal acidification, which facilitates "trapping" of secreted NH_3 as NH_4^+; and NHE3-mediated Na^+/NH_4^+ exchange expression and activity.[237,313] An apical Ba^{2+}-sensitive K^+ channel and a diffusive NH_3 transport component also appear to be involved in ammonia secretion.[138,313] The proximal tubule also can reabsorb luminal ammonia; this appears to occur primarily in the late proximal tubule.[137] These portions of the proximal tubule express glutamine synthetase, which catalyzes the reaction of NH_4^+ with glutamate to form glutamine.[53] Metabolic acidosis converts late proximal tubule ammonia transport from net reabsorption to net secretion[137]; the molecular mechanisms that underlie this conversion involve decreased glutamine synthetase–mediated NH_4^+ metabolism.[75,280] The TAL reabsorbs luminal ammonia. The apical $Na^+-K^+-2Cl^-$ cotransporter NKCC2 mediates the majority of ammonium reabsorption. An apical K^+/NH_4^+ antiporter and amiloride-sensitive NH_4^+ conductance are also present.[20] Metabolic acidosis increases both TAL ammonia reabsorption and NKCC2 expression.[22] Intracellular NH_4^+ can dissociate into NH_3 and H^+, which results in intracellular acidification. Ammonia exit across the basolateral plasma membrane likely involves a component of diffusive NH_3 movement, although recent evidence suggests that NH_4^+ also exits via basolateral Na^+/NH_4^+ exchange mediated by NHE4.[42]

Some of the ammonia absorbed by the medullary TAL of the loop of Henle undergoes recycling into the thin descending limb of the loop of Henle, which results in countercurrent amplification of medullary interstitial ammonia concentration. Ammonia recycling predominantly involves NH_3 transport, with a smaller component of NH_4^+ transport.[102]

The net effect of ammonia absorption by the TAL of the loop of Henle and passive ammonia secretion into the thin descending limb of the loop of Henle is development of axial ammonia concentration in the medullary interstitium that parallels the hypertonicity gradient. Moreover, as a result of ammonia absorption by the medullary TAL, ammonia delivery to the distal tubule accounts for only approximately 20% to 40% of final urinary ammonia content.[90,136] There is likely to be a small component of ammonia secretion in the regions of the distal tubule prior to the collecting duct, that is, the DCT, CNT, and ICT. Micropuncture studies in the rat kidney have generally shown net ammonia secretion between the early and late portions of the micropuncturable distal tubule, which accounts for approximately 10% to 15% of total urinary ammonia excretion under basal conditions.[312,402] Ammonia secretion by the collecting duct accounts for the majority of urinary ammonia content. Several studies examining the CCD, OMCD, and IMCD have uniformly shown that collecting duct ammonia secretion involves parallel NH_3 and H^+ transport, with little to no pH-independent NH_4^+ permeability.[90,180] H^+ secretion likely involves both H^+-ATPase and H^+-K^+-ATPase, as detailed in previous sections discussing bicarbonate reabsorption. Carbonic anhydrase also contributes to ammonia secretion, probably through a role in supplying cytosolic H^+ for secretion.[366] The presence or absence of luminal carbonic anhydrase activity, mediated by apical CA IV, has an important impact on the rate of collecting duct ammonia secretion. In the absence of luminal carbonic anhydrase activity, the luminal $[H^+]$ increases above equilibrium levels due to delayed dissociation of H_2CO_3. This is termed a luminal *disequilibrium pH*. Because the $H^+ + NH_3 \rightleftharpoons NH_4^+$ reaction occurs rapidly, increased luminal H^+ concentration in the absence of luminal carbonic anhydrase activity shifts the ammonia buffer reaction toward NH_4^+, decreasing the luminal NH_3 concentration and thereby increasing the transepithelial gradient for NH_3 secretion. Detailed studies of the collecting duct have demonstrated the presence of a luminal disequilibrium pH in the OMCDi and the terminal IMCD of the rat kidney[103,369] and in the CCD[181,321] and OMCDo in the rabbit,[320] but not in the OMCDi in the rabbit.[320] NH_3 movement across collecting duct cell apical and basolateral membranes appears to involve both diffusive and transporter-mediated NH_3 transport. The transporter-mediated component is Na^+- and K^+-independent, electroneutral, facilitated NH_3 transport and is the predominant route at physiologically relevant ammonia concentrations.[143,144] Subsequent studies showed that the Rh glycoprotein Rhcg plays a critical role in renal ammonia excretion. Rhcg is an ammonia-specific transporter with no identifiable affinity for solutes other than ammonia and its methyl derivative, methyl ammonia.[26,219,224,232] Rhcg is expressed in the DCT, CNT, ICT, CCD, OMCD, and IMCD of the human, rat, and mouse kidney.[93,139,357] Rhcg is expressed both in intercalated cells and in principal cells, DCT cells and CNT cells in these regions, with the exception that it is not expressed in nonintercalated cells in the IMCD under basal conditions or in type B intercalated cells.[139,357] In the human kidney, Rhcg expression has the same distribution, except that principal cells do not express Rhcg.[139] Although Rhcg was identified initially only in the apical membrane, more recent studies have shown both apical and basolateral Rhcg expression in the mouse, rat, and human kidney.[47,139,174,305,306] Rhcg's essential role in renal ammonia excretion has been shown in gene deletion studies. Both global and collecting duct–specific Rhcg deletion decrease basal urinary ammonia excretion and impair the normal increase in urinary ammonia excretion in response to metabolic acidosis.[34,197] Intercalated cell–specific Rhcg deletion impairs the response to metabolic acidosis.[198] Global Rhcg deletion decreases apical NH_3 permeability in perfused collecting duct segments and decreases transepithelial collecting duct ammonia permeability.[34] Thus, collecting duct NH_3 transport involves, at least in part, Rhcg-mediated transport. Rhbg is a related member of the Rh glycoprotein family. Like Rhcg, Rhbg is an ammonia-specific transporter, with the majority of studies identifying facilitated NH_3 transport,[216,219,423] but one study identifying only NH_4^+ transport.[249] Rhbg is expressed in the same cells that express Rhcg, with the significant difference that that Rhbg has basolateral expression, in contrast to the apical and basolateral expression of Rhcg.[276,357] Another mechanism for basolateral ammonia uptake involves basolateral Na^+-K^+-ATPase. In particular, in the IMCD the basolateral Na^+-K^+-ATPase contributes to basolateral NH_4^+ uptake.[365,375] Intracellular NH_4^+ dissociates to H^+ and NH_3, which are then secreted across the apical membrane. In the CCD, however, basolateral Na^+-K^+-ATPase does not contribute to ammonia secretion,[181] and its role in the OMCD has not been reported. Overall, collecting duct ammonia secretion appears to involve the integrated function of a number of proteins (Figure 9-10).

Specific Proteins Involved in Renal Ammonia Metabolism

PHOSPHATE-DEPENDENT GLUTAMINASE
PDG catalyzes the reaction L-glutamine + H_2O → L-glutamate$^-$ + NH_4^+. PDG is present in many extrarenal tissues, including liver and brain. In humans, the gene for the kidney-type

isoform has 19 exons and gives rise to at least two transcripts, a KGA mRNA that results from joining exons 1 to 14 and 16 to 19, and a GAC mRNA product that uses only exons 1 to 15.[222] A separate gene gives rise to an LGA isoform. The KGA protein is ubiquitously expressed, including in the renal proximal tubule. The GAC isoform is expressed primarily in the kidney, at least at the level of mRNA expression. The LGA isoform is widely expressed, including in liver, brain, pancreas, and breast cancer.[222] The KGA isoform is increased in response to metabolic acidosis and appears to be the source of the majority of renal PDG. Metabolic acidosis increases proximal tubule PDG activity; these increases derive from increased protein synthesis and correlate with increased mRNA expression.[338,339] Interestingly, metabolic acidosis increases PDG mRNA via increased stability of the mRNA product, not via increased transcription.[156] A direct repeat of an 8-nt AU sequence functions as a pH-response element and is both necessary and sufficient to generate pH-response gene stabilization. This response element binds multiple RNA-binding proteins, including ς-crystallin, AU factor 1, and HuR. Acidosis also causes an endoplasmic reticulum–stress response that leads to formation of cytoplasmic stress granules; ς-crystallin undergoes transient movement to stress granules, and simultaneously HuR is translocated from the nucleus to the cytoplasm.[157]

GLUTAMATE DEHYDROGENASE
GDH is a mitochondrial enzyme that catalyzes the reaction L-glutamate$^-$ + H_2O + NAD^+ (or $NADP^+$) → α-KG^{2-} + NH_4^+ + NADH (or NADPH) + H^+ (where NAD and NADP are

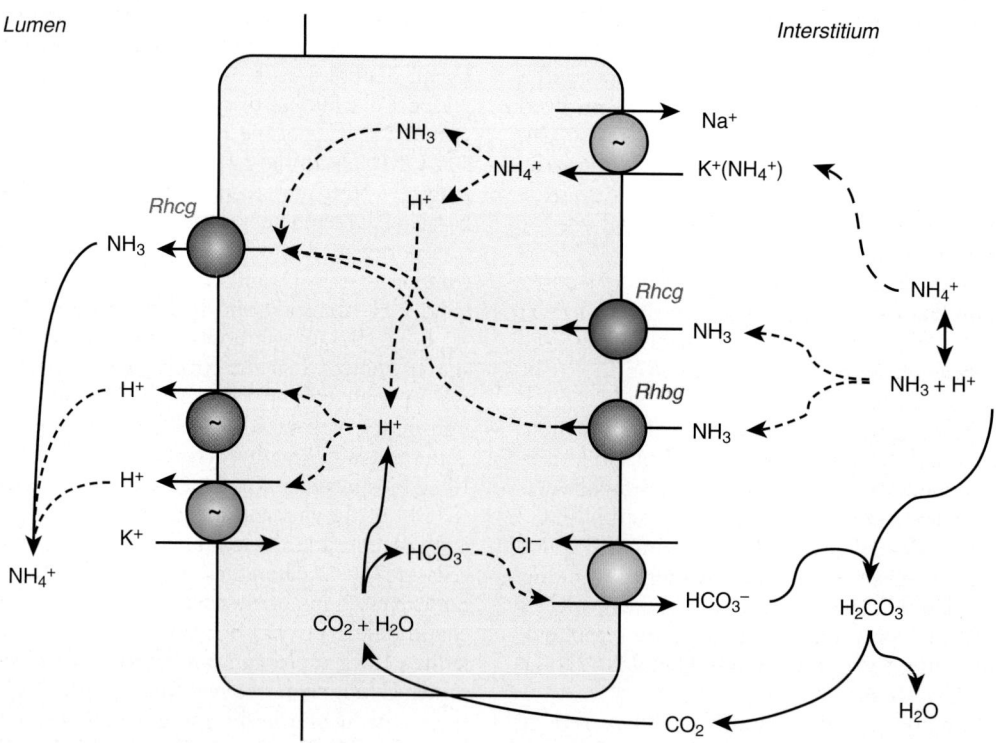

FIGURE 9-10 Detailed model of collecting duct ammonia transport. Interstitial NH_4^+ is in equilibrium with NH_3 and H^+. NH_3 is transported across the basolateral membrane, predominantly by Rh C glycoprotein (Rhcg), but also possibly partly by Rh B glycoprotein (Rhbg). In the inner medullary collecting duct (IMCD), basolateral Na^+-K^+-adenosine triphosphatase (ATPase) transports NH_4^+. Intracellular NH_3 is secreted across the apical membrane by apical Rh C glycoprotein (Rhcg). H^+-ATPase and H^+-K^+-ATPase secrete H^+, which combines with luminal NH_3 to form NH_4^+, which is "trapped" in the lumen. Intracellular H^+ is generated by carbonic anhydrase II (CA II)–accelerated CO_2 hydration that forms carbonic acid, which dissociates to H^+ and HCO_3^-. Basolateral Cl^-/HCO_3^- exchange transports HCO_3^- across the basolateral membrane. HCO_3^- combines with H^+ released from NH_4^+ to form carbonic acid, which dissociates to CO_2 and H_2O. This CO_2 can recycle into the cell, supplying the CO_2 used for cytosolic H^+ production. The net result is NH_4^+ transport from the peritubular space into the luminal fluid.

nicotinamide adenine dinucleotide and nicotinamide adenine dinucleotide phosphate, respectively, and NADH and NADPH are their reduced forms). There are two GDH isoforms that are products of two different genes: GLUD1, which is widely expressed, and GLUD2, which appears to be a nerve- and testicle-specific isoform.[265] High levels of GDH activity are found not only in kidney but also in mammalian liver, brain, heart, pancreas, ovaries, and testes. Brain and testicular GDH consists of products of GLUD1 and GLUD2, whereas in most other tissues, including the kidney, GDH is a product of GLUD1 mRNA.

Metabolic acidosis stimulates renal GDH activity,[406] protein,[79] and mRNA (GLUD1) expression.[77] The increased mRNA expression appears to be related to increased gene stability, not increased transcription.[165] Four AU-rich elements are present in the promoter region, bind ς-cystallin, and appear to confer pH-responsive stabilization of GDH mRNA.[295]

PHOSPHOENOLPYRUVATE CARBOXYKINASE

Renal PEPCK is a cytosolic enzyme that is the product of the PCK1 gene. In the kidney, as in extrarenal sites, including liver, adipose tissue, and small intestine, PEPCK is a key enzyme in gluconeogenesis through its role in conversion of oxaloacetate into phosphoenolpyruvate and CO_2. It also plays an important role in the renal response to metabolic acidosis[54] coincident with increased renal gluconeogenesis. The adaptive increase in PEPCK activity and protein expression results from increased protein synthesis and mRNA expression.[77] Unlike with PDG and GDH, the increased PEPCK mRNA expression appears to result from increased gene transcription.[146] Acidosis-induced increases in gene transcription appear to involve binding to the P3(II) and CRE-1 elements in the PCK1 promoter.[77] The 3′ nontranslated region of PEPCK mRNA contains an instability element that facilitates its rapid turnover and contributes to the regulation of PEPCK gene expression.[195] Metabolic acidosis also stimulates PEPCK gene expression through p38 mitogen-activated protein kinase phosphorylation of ATF-2, which binds to the CRE-1 element and either recruits or interacts with additional transcription factors that activate gene transcription.[77]

Γ-GLUTAMYL TRANSPEPTIDASE

γ-GT accounts for phosphate-independent glutaminase activity identified in many early enzymatic studies of renal ammoniagenesis. However, γ-GT is primarily expressed in the proximal straight tubule,[78] and micropuncture studies suggest that glutamine is completely reabsorbed by the proximal convoluted tubule, so that ammoniagenesis via γ-GT in the proximal straight tubule is unlikely to contribute significantly to renal ammoniagenesis. Studies examining the late proximal convoluted tubule have determined that γ-GT activity contributes only approximately 10% of total ammoniagenesis.[314] Finally, chronic metabolic acidosis does not alter γ-GT activity.[78] Thus, γ-GT is unlikely to play a significant role in either basal or acidosis-stimulated renal ammoniagenesis.

NA⁺/H⁺ EXCHANGER 3

Multiple lines of evidence suggest that the apical Na⁺/H⁺ exchanger NHE3 secretes NH_4^+ through binding of NH_4^+ at the H⁺ binding site. These data indicate that proximal tubule brush border membrane vesicles exhibit NH_4^+/Na^+ exchange

activity[178]; that combining a low luminal Na⁺ concentration with the Na⁺/H⁺ exchange inhibitor amiloride decreases ammonia secretion[236]; and that the Na⁺/H⁺ exchange inhibitor ethylisopropyl amiloride blunts ammonia secretion when alternative secretory pathways are blocked.[313] Apical NHE3 is also present in the TAL. However, since this transporter secretes NH_4^+ and the TAL reabsorbs NH_4^+, NHE3 is unlikely to play an important role in loop of Henle ammonia transport.

NHE3 appears to be important in the regulation of proximal tubule ammonia transport. In response to chronic metabolic acidosis, changes in extracellular potassium and angiotensin II and changes in NHE3 expression and activity parallel changes in ammonia secretion.[15,96,238,243] In both S2 and S3 segments, chronic metabolic acidosis increases AT₁ receptor–mediated stimulation of NHE3.[240,241,244] Other studies show that increased ET-1 expression with subsequent activation of the ET-B receptor plays an important role in increasing NHE3 expression and renal ammonia excretion in metabolic acidosis.[193]

POTASSIUM CHANNELS

At a molecular level, K⁺ and NH_4^+ have nearly identical biophysical characteristics. In general, the relative conductance for NH_4^+ is 10% to 20% of that observed for K⁺.[387] The primary evidence that K⁺ channels contribute to proximal tubule ammonia transport comes from in vitro microperfusion studies showing that barium, a nonspecific K⁺ channel inhibitor, can inhibit proximal tubule ammonia transport.[313] Multiple K⁺ channels are present in the apical membrane of the proximal tubule, including KCNA10, TWIK-1, and KCNQ1; which of these mediate ammonia transport is not currently known. In the TAL, K⁺ channels can contribute to luminal NH_4^+ uptake when apical Na⁺-K⁺-2Cl⁻ cotransport is inhibited.[20] However, NKCC2 inhibitors completely inhibit TAL ammonia transport, which suggests that apical K⁺ channels are unlikely to play a quantitatively important role in TAL ammonia transport.[121]

NA⁺-K⁺-2CL⁻ COTRANSPORT

NKCC1 is a widely expressed Na⁺-K⁺-2Cl⁻ cotransporter family isoform that in the kidney is present in the basolateral membrane of type A intercalated cells in the OMCD and IMCD cells.[114] Because peritubular bumetanide, an NKCC1/NKCC2 inhibitor, does not alter OMCD ammonia secretion, NKCC1 is unlikely to play a quantitatively important role in OMCD ammonia secretion.[366] In the IMCD, although NH_4^+ and K⁺ compete for a common binding site on NKCC1, inhibiting NKCC1 does not appear to significantly alter peritubular NH_4^+ uptake.[365] Thus, NKCC1 is unlikely to play a substantial role in renal ammonia secretion.

NKCC2 is a kidney-specific isoform expressed in the apical plasma membrane of the TAL and is the major mechanism for ammonia reabsorption in the TAL of the loop of Henle.[121] Luminal NH_4^+ competes with K⁺ for binding to the K⁺ transport site, which allows alterations in luminal K⁺ in hypokalemia and hyperkalemia to alter net NH_4^+ transport and lead to alterations in medullary interstitial ammonia concentration in conditions of altered potassium homeostasis. The ability of NH_4^+ to be transported at the K⁺ binding site of NKCC2 may also contribute to TAL Na Cl transport.[396] Changes in TAL ammonia transport contribute to the increase in renal ammonia excretion that is seen in chronic metabolic acidosis.[117] These changes involve transcriptionally mediated increases in NKCC2 expression,[22] which may be related to the elevation in systemic glucocorticoids that occurs with chronic metabolic acidosis.[23]

NA⁺-K⁺-ATPASE

Na⁺-K⁺-ATPase is present in the basolateral plasma membrane of renal epithelial cells, and its expression is greatest in the medullary TAL of the loop of Henle, with lesser expression in the cortical TAL, DCT, CCD, MCD, and proximal tubule.[164] NH_4^+ competes with K^+ at the K^+ binding site of Na⁺-K⁺-ATPase, which permits net Na⁺-NH_4^+ exchange.[190,372] However, the relative affinities of Na⁺-K⁺-ATPase for NH_4^+ (approximately 11 mmol/L) and for K^+ (approximately 1.9 mmol/L) have important effects on Na⁺-K⁺-ATPase–mediated NH_4^+ transport. In the cortex, interstitial ammonia concentrations are less than 1 mmol/L, which suggests that NH_4^+ is unlikely to be transported to a significant extent by basolateral Na⁺-K⁺-ATPase.[190] Moreover, even in the presence of high concentrations of peritubular ammonia, basolateral Na⁺-K⁺-ATPase does not appear to contribute to CCD ammonia secretion.[181] In contrast, interstitial ammonia concentrations in the inner medulla are high, and Na⁺-K⁺-ATPase–mediated basolateral NH_4^+ uptake is critical for IMCD ammonia and acid secretion.[190,372] In hypokalemia, decreased interstitial K^+ concentrations, by facilitating increased NH_4^+ uptake by Na⁺-K⁺-ATPase, allow increased rates of NH_4^+ secretion independent of changes in Na⁺-K⁺-ATPase expression.[368]

H⁺-K⁺-ATPASE

H⁺-K⁺-ATPase proteins are members of the P-type ATPase family and transport NH_4^+. The majority of evidence suggests that NH_4^+ binds to and is transported at the K^+ binding site. However, potassium deficiency increases expression of colonic H⁺-K⁺-ATPase, which has been postulated to mediate increased NH_4^+ secretion via binding of NH_4^+ to and transport at the H^+ binding site.[245]

K⁺/NH₄⁺ (H⁺) EXCHANGE

An electroneutral Ba^{2+}- and verapamil-inhibitable apical K^+/NH_4^+ (H^+) activity is present in the apical membrane of the TAL.[21] The gene product and the protein that correlate with this transport activity have not yet been identified. However, the observation that NKCC2 inhibitors almost completely inhibit the transcellular component of ammonia transport in the TAL suggests that K^+/NH_4^+ (H^+) exchange activity may not play a major role in TAL ammonia reabsorption.

AQUAPORINS

The aquaporin family is an extended family of proteins that facilitate water transport. Because both H_2O and NH_3 have similar molecular sizes and charge distribution, several studies have examined the role of aquaporins in NH_3 transport. Importantly, many but not all aquaporins transport ammonia.[235] AQP1 was the first aquaporin shown to transport ammonia. Studies involving AQP1 expression in *Xenopus* oocytes demonstrated that AQP1 expression increases NH_3 transport.[235,248] However, not all studies have confirmed NH_3 transport by AQP1.[149] AQP1 is present in the thin descending limb of the loop of Henle, which suggests that it may contribute to ammonia permeability in this segment.

AQP3 is present in the basolateral membrane of collecting duct principal cells and, when expressed in *Xenopus* oocytes, transports NH_3.[149] Whether AQP3 contributes to renal principal cell basolateral NH_3 transport has not been determined.

AQP8 is expressed in intracellular sites in the proximal tubule, CCD, and OMCD in the kidney, but not in the plasma membrane.[97] The specific intracellular site of AQP8 in mammalian cells has not been determined, but it localizes to the inner mitochondrial membrane when expressed in yeast.[319] The role of AQP8 in renal ammonia metabolism is unclear. Genetic deletion alters hepatic ammonia accumulation, renal excretion of infused ammonia, and intrarenal ammonia concentrations but does not alter serum chloride concentration, urine ammonia concentration, or urine pH either under basal conditions or in response to acid loading.[409,410] The molecular specificity of ammonia transport by aquaporins may relate to specific amino acids in the aromatic/arginine constriction region of these proteins. This region is located below the channel mouth and may be narrower than the NPA constriction.[82] Site-directed mutagenesis has shown that specific amino acids of AQP1—phenylalanine 56, histidine 180, and arginine 195—are necessary for ammonia permeability, but not for water permeability.[32] The central NPA constriction, while important for aquaporin water permeability, does not appear to be critical for aquaporin ammonia permeability.[32]

CARBONIC ANHYDRASE

Carbonic anhydrase, in addition to playing a role in bicarbonate reabsorption, also contributes to ammonia secretion. Direct studies have shown that carbonic anhydrase inhibition, presumably through effects on CA II, block OMCD ammonia secretion.[366] Figure 9-10 shows the putative role of cytoplasmic CA II in facilitating transepithelial ammonia secretion.

In contrast, collecting duct CA IV, although functioning to increase bicarbonate reabsorption, likely decreases collecting duct ammonia secretion through its effects to prevent a luminal disequilibrium pH. Apical CA IV expression has been demonstrated in the rabbit CCD type A intercalated cell, in the rabbit OMCD and IMCD,[303] and in the human CCD and OMCD,[212] but not in the rat collecting duct.[50] This pattern is inconsistent with evidence of luminal disequilibrium pH in the rat CCD and OMCD,[103,182] but is consistent with the evidence of luminal disequilibrium pH in the rabbit CCD and OMCDo segments.[320,321]

RH GLYCOPROTEINS

Rh glycoproteins are mammalian orthologs of Mep/AMT proteins, ammonia transporter family proteins present in yeast, plants, bacteria, and many other organisms. Three mammalian Rh glycoproteins have been identified to date, Rh A glycoprotein (RhAG/Rhag), Rh B glycoprotein (RhBG/Rhbg), and Rh C glycoprotein (RhCG/Rhcg). By convention, Rh A glycoprotein is termed *RhAG* in human tissues and *Rhag* in nonhuman organisms. Terminology is similar for RhBG/Rhbg and RhCG/Rhcg.

RhAG/Rhag. RhAG/Rhag is a component of the Rh complex, which consists of the nonglycosylated Rh proteins RhD and RhCE in humans and Rh30 in nonhuman mammals, in association with RhAG/Rhag. RhAG mediates electroneutral NH_3 transport.[221,284,400,401] However, RhAG/Rhag is an erythrocyte- and erythroid precursor–specific protein,[208] and studies of the human kidney have found no evidence of renal RhAG expression.[384] At present, RhAG/Rhag appears unlikely to contribute to renal ammonia metabolism.

RhBG/Rhbg. RhBG/Rhbg is expressed in a wide variety of organs involved in ammonia metabolism, including kidney, liver, skin, lung, stomach, and intestinal tract.[140,145,210,276,357,388] The kidneys express basolateral Rhbg immunoreactivity in the DCT, CNT, ICT, CCD, OMCD, and IMCD.[276,357] In general, both intercalated and principal cells express Rhbg, with greater expression in intercalated cells than in principal cells. The exceptions to this rule are the IMCD, where only intercalated cells express Rhbg, and the CCD type B intercalated cells, which do not express Rhbg detectable with immunohistochemical techniques.[357] The basolateral expression of Rhbg appears to be due to basolateral stabilization through specific interactions of its cytoplasmic carboxy-terminal with ankyrin-G.[213] The human kidney expresses high amounts of RhBG mRNA,[210] but a recent study using a variety of antibodies did not detect RhBG protein expression.[47]

RhBG/Rhbg transports ammonia and the ammonia analog methylammonia, but does not appear to have other known substrates. Different studies have reached different conclusions regarding the exact ammonia species transported, NH_3 or NH_4^+. Most studies show that Rhbg mediates electroneutral, Na^+- and K^+-independent NH_3 transport,[216,219,423] but one study identified only electrogenic NH_4^+ transport.[249] In all of these studies, the affinity for ammonia was approximately 2 to 4 mmol/L. The explanation for the seemingly differing molecular mechanisms in different studies has not been determined at present. Importantly, both electroneutral NH_3 transport and electrogenic NH_4^+ transport result in basolateral ammonia uptake in renal collecting duct cells. The specific role of Rhbg in renal ammonia metabolism is unclear. In the mouse, one study showed increased mRNA expression with metabolic acidosis, but the effect on Rhbg protein expression was not reported.[69] In another study, genetic deletion of pendrin, an apical Cl^-/HCO_3^- exchanger present in the type B intercalated cell and non-A, non-B cell, decreased Rhbg expression.[177] Since pendrin deletion increases urine acidification, the decreased Rhbg expression may have been a compensatory mechanism to maintain normal ammonia excretion. Genetic deletion of Rhcg from acid-loaded mice increased Rhbg expression, which suggests that increased Rhbg protein expression may contribute to ammonia excretion under these conditions.[197,198] In contrast, an Rhbg knockout mouse had normal basal acid-base parameter values, normal responses to acid loading, and normal basolateral NH_3 and NH_4^+ transport in microperfused CCD segments.[65]

RhCG/Rhcg. RhCG/Rhcg is expressed in multiple ammonia transporting and metabolizing structures, including kidney, central nervous system, testes, lung, liver, and gastrointestinal tract.[140,145,209,388] In the kidney, Rhcg expression parallels Rhbg expression; that is, it is found in the DCT, CNT, ICT, CCD, OMCD, and IMCD.[93,357] Intercalated cell expression exceeds principal cell expression in the DCT, CNT, ICT, CCD, and OMCD, and in the IMCD Rhcg is expressed only in intercalated cells.[93,357] However, the subcellular location of Rhcg differs from the exclusive basolateral location observed for Rhbg. In the human, rat, and mouse kidney, RhCG/Rhcg exhibits both apical and basolateral immunoreactivity.[47,139,174,305,306] Rhcg is also present in subapical sites, and changes in apical plasma membrane and subapical Rhcg expression suggest that trafficking between these two sites is an important regulatory

mechanism.[306] Basolateral Rhcg expression is approximately 20% of total cellular expression, at least in the rat OMCDi.[306] In the mouse there are significant strain-specific variations in the extent of basolateral Rhcg expression, and these differences correlate with the ability to excrete ammonia in response to acid loading.[174,393]

Multiple studies have addressed the molecular ammonia species transported by RhCG/Rhcg. Some studies suggest that RhCG/Rhcg mediates electroneutral NH_3 transport,[216,219,423] whereas others have reported both NH_3 and NH_4^+ transport.[26] The explanation for these differing observations is unclear at present.

Rhcg's expression parallels ammonia excretion in multiple models. Chronic metabolic acidosis significantly increases Rhcg protein expression in both the OMCD and the IMCD, but not in the cortex.[305] These changes appear to occur through posttranscriptional mechanism, since Rhcg steady-state mRNA expression is not detectably altered.[305] In response to reduced renal mass, where there is increased single-nephron ammonia secretion, apical Rhcg expression increases in CCD type A intercalated cells, CCD principal cells, OMCD intercalated cells, and OMCD principal cells, and basolateral expression increases in CCD principal cells, OMCD intercalated cells, and OMCD principal cells.[175] In ischemia-reperfusion injury, in which there is decreased renal ammonia excretion despite intact interstitial ammonia concentrations, there is selective damage to Rhcg-expressing OMCD intercalated cells, with induction of apoptosis and cellular extrusion.[141] Cyclosporine A nephropathy is associated with decreased Rhcg expression, which likely contributes to impaired ammonia excretion and to development of metabolic acidosis.[205]

At least two distinct mechanisms contribute to increased Rhcg expression in these models. First, there is increased Rhcg protein expression, which, because Rhcg mRNA expression does not change, suggests regulation through posttranscriptional mechanisms.[306] Second, there are changes in Rhcg's subcellular location. Under basal conditions, Rhcg is located in both the apical and basolateral plasma membrane and in subapical sites in both principal cells and intercalated cells. In response to chronic metabolic acidosis, particularly in the intercalated cells, apical plasma membrane expression increases and cytoplasmic expression decreases.[306] The relative roles of these two mechanisms differ in different cell types, with subcellular distribution changes being the predominant adaptive response in OMCD intercalated cells and increased protein expression being the predominant mechanism in OMCD principal cells.[306] Chronic metabolic acidosis also increases basolateral plasma membrane Rhcg expression.[175,306] This increase does not appear to involve redistribution from cytoplasmic sites to the basolateral plasma membrane.[306] Most recently, genetic deletion studies have confirmed the key role of Rhcg in renal ammonia excretion. Global Rhcg deletion decreases basal ammonia excretion and impairs urinary ammonia excretion in response to metabolic acidosis.[34] Collecting duct–specific Rhcg deletion produces identical findings, which indicates that these effects of Rhcg deletion reflect impaired collecting duct ammonia secretion and are not indirectly mediated through an extrarenal Rhcg-related mechanism.[197] Moreover, Rhcg deletion decreases transepithelial ammonia permeability in perfused collecting duct segments and decreases apical membrane NH_3 permeability.[34]

Nonglycosylated Rh Proteins. The nonglycosylated Rh proteins RhD and RhCE in humans and Rh30 in nonhumans are present in erythrocytes in a multimeric complex with RhAG. RhCE appears neither to transport ammonia or its analog, methylammonia, nor to alter transport by RhAG.[400] Structural models suggest that the arrangement of key amino acids is sufficiently different in RhCE and RhD that they either do not transport ammonia or that they do so by mechanisms different from those used by the glycosylated Rh glycoproteins and their bacterial orthologs.[76]

Acknowledgments

The authors thank the many talented investigators with whom we have been fortunate to work; the superb mentors who have supported, encouraged, and, in many cases, enabled our scientific endeavors; and our wonderful spouses and families who have supported all aspects of our lives. The preparation of this chapter was supported in part by funds from National Institutes of Health grant R01-DK-45788.

References

1. Abuladze N, Lee I, Newman D, et al. Axial heterogeneity of sodium-bicarbonate cotransporter expression in the rabbit proximal tubule. *Am J Physiol.* 1998;274:F628-F633.
2. Adler S, Zett B, Anderson B. Renal citrate in the potassium-deficient rat: role of potassium and chloride ions. *J Lab Clin Med.* 1974;84:307-316.
3. Ahn KY, Kone BC. Expression and cellular localization of mRNA encoding the "gastric" isoform of the H⁺-K⁺-ATPase alpha-subunit in rat kidney. *Am J Physiol.* 1995;268:F99-F109.
4. Ahn KY, Turner PB, Madsen KM, et al. Effects of chronic hypokalemia on renal expression of the "gastric" H⁺-K⁺-ATPase alpha-subunit gene. *Am J Physiol.* 1996;270:F557-F566.
5. Albrecht FE, Xu J, Moe OW, et al. Regulation of NHE3 activity by G protein subunits in renal brush-border membranes. *Am J Physiol Regul Integr Comp Physiol.* 2000;278:R1064-R1073.
6. Alexander RT, Grinstein S. Tethering, recycling and activation of the epithelial sodium-proton exchanger, NHE3. *J Exp Biol.* 2009;212:1630-1637.
7. Alleyne GA, Barnswell J, McFarlane-Anderson N, et al. Renal ammoniagenic factor in the plasma of rats with acute metabolic acidosis. *Am J Physiol.* 1981;241:F112-F116.
8. Alper SL. Molecular physiology and genetics of Na⁺-independent SLC4 anion exchangers. *J Exp Biol.* 2009;212:1672-1683.
9. Alper SL, Natale J, Gluck S, et al. Subtypes of intercalated cells in rat kidney collecting duct defined by antibodies against erythroid band 3 and renal vacuolar H⁺-ATPase. *Proc Natl Acad Sci U S A.* 1989;86:5429-5433.
10. Alper SL, Stuart-Tilley AK, Biemesderfer D, et al. Immunolocalization of AE2 anion exchanger in rat kidney. *Am J Physiol.* 1997;273:F601-F614.
11. Alpern RJ, Cogan MG, Rector Jr FC. Effect of luminal bicarbonate concentration on proximal acidification in the rat. *Am J Physiol.* 1982;243:F53-F59.
12. Alpern RJ, Cogan MG, Rector Jr FC. Flow dependence of proximal tubular bicarbonate absorption. *Am J Physiol.* 1983;245:F478-F484.
13. Alvarez BV, Loiselle FB, Supuran CT, et al. Direct extracellular interaction between carbonic anhydrase iv and the human NBC1 sodium/bicarbonate co-transporter. *Biochemistry.* 2003;42:12321-12329.
14. Alvarez BV, Vilas GL, Casey JR. Metabolon disruption: a mechanism that regulates bicarbonate transport. *EMBO J.* 2005;24:2499-2511.
15. Ambuhl PM, Amemiya M, Danczkay M, et al. Chronic metabolic acidosis increases NHE3 protein abundance in rat kidney. *Am J Physiol.* 1996;271:F917-F925.
16. Ambuhl PM, Yang X, Peng Y, et al. Glucocorticoids enhance acid activation of the Na⁺/H⁺ exchanger 3 (NHE3). *J Clin Invest.* 1999;103:429-435.
17. Ambuhl PM, Zajicek HK, Wang H, et al. Regulation of renal phosphate transport by acute and chronic metabolic acidosis in the rat. *Kidney Int.* 1998;53:1288-1298.
18. Aruga S, Wehrli S, Kaissling B, et al. Chronic metabolic acidosis increases NaDC-1 mRNA and protein abundance in rat kidney. *Kidney Int.* 2000;58:206-215.
19. Atkins JL, Burg MB. Bicarbonate transport by isolated perfused rat collecting ducts. *Am J Physiol.* 1985;249:F485-F489.
20. Attmane-Elakeb A, Amlal H, Bichara M. Ammonium carriers in medullary thick ascending limb. *Am J Physiol Renal Physiol.* 2001;280:F1-F9.
21. Attmane-Elakeb A, Boulanger H, Vernimmen C, et al. Apical location and inhibition by arginine vasopressin of K⁺/H⁺ antiport of the medullary thick ascending limb of rat kidney. *J Biol Chem.* 1997;272:25668-25677.
22. Attmane-Elakeb A, Mount DB, Sibella V, et al. Stimulation by in vivo and in vitro metabolic acidosis of expression of rBSC-1, the Na⁺-K⁺ (NH₄⁺)-2Cl⁻ cotransporter of the rat medullary thick ascending limb. *J Biol Chem.* 1998;273:33681-33691.
23. Attmane-Elakeb A, Sibella V, Vernimmen C, et al. Regulation by glucocorticoids of expression and activity of rBSC1, the Na⁺-K⁺(NH₄⁺)-2Cl⁻ cotransporter of medullary thick ascending limb. *J Biol Chem.* 2000;275:33548-33553.
24. Bacic D, Kaissling B, McLeroy P, et al. Dopamine acutely decreases apical membrane Na/H exchanger NHE3 protein in mouse renal proximal tubule. *Kidney Int.* 2003;64:2133-2141.
25. Bagnis C, Marshansky V, Breton S, et al. Remodeling the cellular profile of collecting ducts by chronic carbonic anhydrase inhibition. *Am J Physiol Renal Physiol.* 2001;280:F437-F448.
26. Bakouh N, Benjelloun F, Hulin P, et al. NH₃ is involved in the NH₄⁺ transport induced by the functional expression of the human Rh C glycoprotein. *J Biol Chem.* 2004;279:15975-15983.
27. Balagura-Baruch S, Burich RL, King VF. Effects of alkalosis on renal citrate metabolism in dogs infused with citrate. *Am J Physiol.* 1973;225:385-388.
28. Bastani B, McEnaney S, Yang L, et al. Adaptation of inner medullary collecting duct vacuolar H-adenosine triphosphatase to chronic acid or alkali loads in the rat. *Exp Nephrol.* 1994;2:171-175.
29. Bastani B, Purcell H, Hemken P, et al. Expression and distribution of renal vacuolar proton-translocating adenosine triphosphatase in response to chronic acid and alkali loads in the rat. *J Clin Invest.* 1991;88:126-136.
30. Batlle D, Ghanekar H, Jain S, et al. Hereditary distal renal tubular acidosis: new understandings. *Annu Rev Med.* 2001;52:471-484.
31. Becker HM, Deitmer JW. Voltage dependence of H⁺ buffering mediated by sodium bicarbonate cotransport expressed in *Xenopus* oocytes. *J Biol Chem.* 2004;279:28057-28062.
32. Beitz E, Wu B, Holm LM, et al. Point mutations in the aromatic/arginine region in aquaporin 1 allow passage of urea, glycerol, ammonia, and protons. *Proc Natl Acad Sci U S A.* 2006;103:269-274.
33. Bengele HH, McNamara ER, Schwartz JH, et al. Suppression of acidification along inner medullary collecting duct. *Am J Physiol.* 1988;255:F307-F312.
34. Biver S, Belge H, Bourgeois S, et al. A role for Rhesus factor Rhcg in renal ammonium excretion and male fertility. *Nature.* 2008;456:339-343.
35. Bobulescu IA, Dwarakanath V, Zou L, et al. Glucocorticoids acutely increase cell surface Na⁺/H⁺ exchanger-3 (NHE3) by activation of NHE3 exocytosis. *Am J Physiol Renal Physiol.* 2005;289:F685-F691.
36. Boettger T, Hubner CA, Maier H, et al. Deafness and renal tubular acidosis in mice lacking the K-Cl co-transporter Kcc4. *Nature.* 2002;416:874-878.
37. Bond PA, Jenner FA. The effect of lithium and related metal ions on the urinary excretion of 2-oxoglutarate and citrate in the rat. *Br J Pharmacol.* 1974;50:283-289.
38. Bond PA, Jenner FA, Lee CR, et al. The effect of lithium salts on the urinary excretion of α-oxoglutarate in man. *Br J Pharmacol.* 1972;46:116-123.
39. Borensztein P, Juvin P, Vernimmen C, et al. cAMP-dependent control of Na⁺/H⁺ antiport by AVP, PTH, and PGE2 in rat medullary thick ascending limb cells. *Am J Physiol Renal Physiol.* 1993;264:F354-F364.
40. Boron WF, Chen L, Parker MD. Modular structure of sodium-coupled bicarbonate transporters. *J Exp Biol.* 2009;212:1697-1706.
41. Boron WF. Acid-base transport by the renal proximal tubule. *J Am Soc Nephrol.* 2006;17:2368-2382.
42. Bourgeois S, Meer LV, Wootla B, et al. NHE4 is critical for the renal handling of ammonia in rodents. *J Clin Invest.* 2010;120:1895-1904.
43. Breton S, Alper SL, Gluck SL, et al. Depletion of intercalated cells from collecting ducts of carbonic anhydrase II-deficient (CAR2 null) mice. *Am J Physiol.* 1995;269:F761-F774.
44. Breton S, Wiederhold T, Marshansky V, et al. The B1 subunit of the H⁺ATPase is a PDZ domain-binding protein. Colocalization with NHE-RF in renal B-intercalated cells. *J Biol Chem.* 2000;275:18219-18224.
45. Brett CL, Donowitz M, Rao R. Evolutionary origins of eukaryotic sodium/proton exchangers. *Am J Physiol Cell Physiol.* 2005;288:C223-C239.
46. Breusegem SY, Takahashi H, Giral-Arnal H, et al. Differential regulation of the renal sodium-phosphate cotransporters NaPi-IIa, NaPi-IIc, and PiT-2 in dietary potassium deficiency. *Am J Physiol Renal Physiol.* 2009;297:F350-F361.
47. Brown ACN, Hallouane D, Mawby WJ, et al. RhCG is the major putative ammonia transporter expressed in human kidney and RhBG is not expressed at detectable levels. *Am J Physiol Renal Physiol.* 2009;296:F1279-F1290.

48. Brown D, Hirsch S, Gluck S. Localization of a proton-pumping ATPase in rat kidney. *J Clin Invest.* 1988;82:2114-2126.
49. Brown D, Paunescu TG, Breton S, et al. Regulation of the V-ATPase in kidney epithelial cells: dual role in acid-base homeostasis and vesicle trafficking. *J Exp Biol.* 2009;212:1762-1772.
50. Brown D, Zhu XL, Sly WS. Localization of membrane-associated carbonic anhydrase type IV in kidney epithelial cells. *Proc Natl Acad Sci U S A.* 1990;87:7457-7461.
51. Brown D, Paunescu TG, Breton S, et al. Regulation of the V-ATPase in kidney epithelial cells: dual role in acid-base homeostasis and vesicle trafficking. *J Exp Biol.* 2009;212:1762-1772.
52. Brown JC, Packer RK, Knepper MA. Role of organic anions in renal response to dietary acid and base loads. *Am J Physiol.* 1989;257:F170-F176.
53. Burch HB, Choi S, McCarthy WZ, et al. The location of glutamine synthetase within the rat and rabbit nephron. *Biochem Biophys Res Commun.* 1978;82:498-505.
54. Burch HB, Narins RG, Chu C, et al. Distribution along the rat nephron of three enzymes of gluconeogenesis in acidosis and starvation. *Am J Physiol.* 1978;235:F246-F253.
55. Burckhardt BC, Burckhardt G. Transport of organic anions across the basolateral membrane of proximal tubule cells. *Rev Physiol Biochem Pharmacol.* 2003;146:95-158.
56. Burnham CE, Amlal H, Wang Z, et al. Cloning and functional expression of a human kidney Na$^+$:HCO3$^-$ cotransporter. *J Biol Chem.* 1997;272:19111-19114.
57. Busque SM, Wagner CA. Potassium restriction, high protein intake, and metabolic acidosis increase expression of the glutamine transporter SNAT3 (Slc38a3) in mouse kidney. *Am J Physiol Renal Physiol.* 2009;297:F440-F450.
58. Campbell-Thompson ML, Verlander JW, Curran KA, et al. In situ hybridization of H-K-ATPase beta-subunit mRNA in rat and rabbit kidney. *Am J Physiol.* 1995;269:F345-F354.
59. Capasso G, Unwin R, Agulian S, et al. Bicarbonate transport along the loop of Henle. I. Microperfusion studies of load and inhibitor sensitivity. *J Clin Invest.* 1991;88:430-437.
60. Capasso G, Unwin R, Ciani F, et al. Bicarbonate transport along the loop of Henle. II. Effects of acid-base, dietary, and neurohumoral determinants. *J Clin Invest.* 1994;94:830-838.
61. Capasso G, Unwin R, Rizzo M, et al. Bicarbonate transport along the loop of Henle: molecular mechanisms and regulation. *J Nephrol.* 2002;15(suppl 5):S88-S96.
62. Chalmers RA, Lawson AM. *Organic acids in man.* London: Chapman and Hall; 1982: pp 163-208.
63. Chambrey R, Paillard M, Podevin RA. Enzymatic and functional evidence for adaptation of the vacuolar H(+)-ATPase in proximal tubule apical membranes from rats with chronic metabolic acidosis. *J Biol Chem.* 1994;269:3243-3250.
64. Chambrey R, Warnock DG, Podevin RA, et al. Immunolocalization of the Na$^+$/H$^+$ exchanger isoform NHE2 in rat kidney. *Am J Physiol.* 1998;275:F379-F386.
65. Chambrey R, Goossens D, Bourgeois S, et al. Genetic ablation of Rhbg in mouse does not impair renal ammonium excretion. *Am J Physiol Renal Physiol.* 2005;289:F1281-F1290.
66. Chan YL, Biagi B, Giebisch G. Control mechanisms of bicarbonate transport across the rat proximal convoluted tubule. *Am J Physiol Renal Physiol.* 1982;242:F532-F543.
67. Chatsudthipong V, Chan YL. Inhibitory effect of angiotensin II on renal tubular transport. *Am J Physiol Renal Physiol.* 1991;260:340-F346.
68. Cheema-Dhadli S, Lin SH, Halperin ML. Mechanisms used to dispose of progressively increasing alkali load in rats. *Am J Physiol Renal Physiol.* 2002;282:F1049-F1055.
69. Cheval L, Morla L, Elalouf JM, et al. Kidney collecting duct acid-base "regulon." *Physiol Genomics.* 2006;27:271-281.
70. Clapp WL, Madsen KM, Verlander JW, et al. Intercalated cells of the rat inner medullary collecting duct. *Kidney Int.* 1987;31:1080-1087.
71. Cogan MG. Chronic hypercapnia stimulates proximal bicarbonate reabsorption in the rat. *J Clin Invest.* 1984;74:1942-1947.
72. Cogan MG. Effects of acute alterations in Pco$_2$ on proximal HCO3$^-$, Cl$^-$, and H$_2$O reabsorption. *Am J Physiol.* 1984;246:F21-F26.
73. Cogan MG, Alpern RJ. Regulation of proximal bicarbonate reabsorption. *Am J Physiol Renal Physiol.* 1984;247:F387-F395.
74. Collazo R, Fan L, Hu MC, et al. Acute regulation of Na$^+$/H$^+$ Exchanger NHE3 by parathyroid hormone via NHE3 phosphorylation and dynamin-dependent endocytosis. *J Biol Chem.* 2000;275:31601-31608.
75. Conjard A, Komaty O, Delage H, et al. Inhibition of glutamine synthetase in the mouse kidney: a novel mechanism of adaptation to metabolic acidosis. *J Biol Chem.* 2003;278:38159-38166.
76. Conroy MJ, Bullough PA, Merrick M, et al. Modelling the human Rhesus proteins: implications for structure and function. *Br J Haematol.* 2005;131:543-551.
77. Curthoys NP, Gstraunthaler G. Mechanism of increased renal gene expression during metabolic acidosis. *Am J Physiol Renal Physiol.* 2001;281:F381-F390.
78. Curthoys NP, Lowry OH. The distribution of glutaminase isoenzymes in the various structures of the nephron in normal, acidotic, and alkalotic rat kidney. *J Biol Chem.* 1973;248:162-168.
79. Curthoys NP, Taylor L, Hoffert JD, et al. Proteomic analysis of the adaptive response of rat renal proximal tubules to metabolic acidosis. *Am J Physiol Renal Physiol.* 2007;292:F140-F147.
80. Da Silva Júnior JC, Perrone RD, Johns CA, et al. Rat kidney band 3 mRNA modulation in chronic respiratory acidosis. *Am J Physiol.* 1991;260:F204-F209.
81. Damkier HH, Nielsen S, Praetorius J. Molecular expression of SLC4-derived Na$^+$-dependent anion transporters in selected human tissues. *Am J Physiol Regul Integr Comp Physiol.* 2007;293:R2136-R2146.
82. de Groot BL, Grubmuller H. Water permeation across biological membranes: mechanism and dynamics of aquaporin-1 and GlpF. *Science.* 2001;294:2353-2357.
83. de Seigneux S, Malte H, Dimke H, et al. Renal compensation to chronic hypoxic hypercapnia: downregulation of pendrin and adaptation of the proximal tubule. *Am J Physiol Renal Physiol.* 2007;292:F1256-F1266.
84. Devonald MA, Smith AN, Poon JP, et al. Non-polarized targeting of AE1 causes autosomal dominant distal renal tubular acidosis. *Nat Genet.* 2003;33:125-127.
85. DiSole F, Babich V, Moe OW. The calcineurin homologous protein-1 increases Na(+)/H(+) -exchanger 3 trafficking via ezrin phosphorylation. *J Am Soc Nephrol.* 2009;20:1776-1786.
86. Dobyan DC, Bulger RE. Renal carbonic anhydrase. *Am J Physiol Renal Physiol.* 1982;243:F311-F324.
87. Dobyan DC, Magill LS, Friedman PA, et al. Carbonic anhydrase histochemistry in rabbit and mouse kidneys. *Anat Rec.* 1982;204:185-197.
88. Du Z, Duan Y, Yan QS, et al. Mechanosensory function of microvilli of the kidney proximal tubule. *Proc Natl Acad Sci U S A.* 2004;101:13068-13073.
89. Du Z, Yan Q, Duan Y, et al. Axial flow modulates proximal tubule NHE3 and H-ATPase activities by changing microvillus bending moments. *Am J Physiol Renal Physiol.* 2006;290:F289-F296.
90. DuBose TD, Good DW, Hamm LL, et al. Ammonium transport in the kidney: new physiological concepts and their clinical implications. *J Am Soc Nephrol.* 1991;1:1193-1203.
91. Dynia DW, Steinmetz AG, Kocinsky HS. NHE3 function and phosphorylation are regulated by a calyculin A–sensitive phosphatase. *Am J Physiol Renal Physiol.* 2009;298:F745-F753.
92. Eiam-ong S, Laski ME, Kurtzman NA, et al. Effect of respiratory acidosis and respiratory alkalosis on renal transport enzymes. *Am J Physiol.* 1994;267:F390-F399.
93. Eladari D, Cheval L, Quentin F, et al. Expression of RhCG, a new putative NH$_3$/NH$_4^+$ transporter, along the rat nephron. *J Am Soc Nephrol.* 2002;13:1999-2008.
94. Eladari D, Chambrey R, Frische S, et al. Pendrin as a regulator of ECF and blood pressure. *Curr Opin Nephrol Hypertens.* 2009;18:356-362.
95. Elkinton JR, Huth EJ, Webster Jr GD, et al. The renal excretion of hydrogen ion in renal tubular acidosis. *Am J Med.* 1960;36:554-575.
96. Elkjar ML, Kwon TH, Wang W, et al. Altered expression of renal NHE3, TSC, BSC-1, and ENaC subunits in potassium-depleted rats. *Am J Physiol Renal Physiol.* 2002;283:F1376-F1388.
97. Elkjar ML, Nejsum LN, Gresz V, et al. Immunolocalization of aquaporin-8 in rat kidney, gastrointestinal tract, testis, and airways. *Am J Physiol Renal Physiol.* 2001;281:F1047-F1057.
98. Emmons C, Kurtz I. Functional characterization of three intercalated cell subtypes in the rabbit outer cortical collecting duct. *J Clin Invest.* 1994;93:417-423.
99. Espiritu DJD, Yang VL, Bernardo AA, et al. Regulation of Renal Na$^+$/HCO$_3^-$ cotransporter stimulation by CO$_2$: role of phosphorylation, exocytosis and protein synthesis. *J Membrane Biol.* 2004;199:39-49.
100. Fejes-Toth G, Naray-Fejes-Toth A. Immunohistochemical localization of colonic H-K-ATPase to the apical membrane of connecting tubule cells. *Am J Physiol Renal Physiol.* 2001;281:F318-F325.
101. Finberg KE, Wagner CA, Bailey MA, et al. The B1-subunit of the H$^+$ ATPase is required for maximal urinary acidification. *Proc Natl Acad Sci U S A.* 2005;102:13616-13621.
102. Flessner MF, Mejia R, Knepper MA. Ammonium and bicarbonate transport in isolated perfused rodent long-loop thin descending limbs. *Am J Physiol.* 1993;264:F388-F396.
103. Flessner MF, Wall SM, Knepper MA. Ammonium and bicarbonate transport in rat outer medullary collecting ducts. *Am J Physiol.* 1992;262:F1-F7.
104. Fourman P, Robinson JR. Diminished urinary excretion of citrate during deficiencies of potassium in man. *Lancet.* 1953;265:656-657.

105. Frank AE, Weiner ID. Effects of ammonia on acid-base transport by the B-type intercalated cell. *J Am Soc Nephrol.* 2001;12:1607-1614.
106. Frank AE, Wingo CS, Andrews PM, et al. Mechanisms through which ammonia regulates cortical collecting duct net proton secretion. *Am J Physiol Renal Physiol.* 2002;282:F1120-F1128.
107. Frank AE, Wingo CS, Weiner ID. Effects of ammonia on bicarbonate transport in the cortical collecting duct. *Am J Physiol Renal Physiol.* 2000;278:F219-F226.
108. Frische S, Kwon TH, Frokiaer J, et al. Regulated expression of pendrin in rat kidney in response to chronic NH4Cl or NaHCO3 loading. *Am J Physiol Renal Physiol.* 2003;284:F584-F593.
109. Frische S, Zolotarev AS, Kim YH, et al. AE2 isoforms in rat kidney: immunohistochemical localization and regulation in response to chronic NH4Cl loading. *Am J Physiol Renal Physiol.* 2004;286:F1163-F1170.
110. Fryer JN, Burns KD, Ghorbani M, et al. Effect of potassium depletion on proximal tubule AT1 receptor localization in normal and remnant rat kidney. *Kidney Int.* 2001;60:1792-1799.
111. Galla JH, Gifford JD, Luke RG, et al. Adaptations to chloride-depletion alkalosis. *Am J Physiol.* 1991;261:R771-R781.
112. Gifford JD, Rome L, Galla JH. H+-K+-ATPase activity in rat collecting duct segments. *Am J Physiol.* 1992;262:F692-F695.
113. Gifford JD, Ware MW, Luke RG, et al. HCO3− transport in rat CCD: rapid adaptation by in vivo but not in vitro alkalosis. *Am J Physiol.* 1993;264:F435-F440.
114. Ginns SM, Knepper MA, Ecelbarger CA, et al. Immunolocalization of the secretory isoform of Na-K-Cl cotransporter in rat renal intercalated cells. *J Am Soc Nephrol.* 1996;7:2533-2542.
115. Gisler SM, Pribanic S, Bacic D, et al. PDZK1: I. A major scaffolder in brush borders of proximal tubular cells1. *Kidney Int.* 2003;64:1733-1745.
116. Gomes P, Soares-da-Silva P. Dopamine acutely decreases type 3 Na+H+ exchanger activity in renal OK cells through the activation of protein kinases A and C signalling cascades. *Eur J Pharmacol.* 2004;488:51-59.
117. Good DW. Adaptation of HCO3− and NH4+ transport in rat MTAL: effects of chronic metabolic acidosis and Na+ intake. *Am J Physiol.* 1990;258:F1345-F1353.
118. Good DW. Inhibition of bicarbonate absorption by peptide hormones and cyclic adenosine monophosphate in rat medullary thick ascending limb. *J Clin Invest.* 1990;85:1006-1013.
119. Good DW. Effects of osmolality on bicarbonate absorption by medullary thick ascending limb of the rat. *J Clin Invest.* 1992;89:184-190.
120. Good DW. The thick ascending limb as a site of renal bicarbonate reabsorption. *Semin Nephrol.* 1993;13:225-235.
121. Good DW. Ammonium transport by the thick ascending limb of Henle's loop. *Annu Rev Physiol.* 1994;56:623-647.
122. Good DW, Burg MB. Ammonia production by individual segments of the rat nephron. *J Clin Invest.* 1984;73:602-610.
123. Good DW, Di Mari JF, Watts III BA. Hyposmolality stimulates Na(+)/H(+) exchange and HCO(3)(−) absorption in thick ascending limb via PI 3-kinase. *Am J Physiol Cell Physiol.* 2000;279:C1443-C1454.
124. Good DW, George T, Watts III BA. Basolateral membrane Na+/H+ exchange enhances HCO3− absorption in rat medullary thick ascending limb: evidence for functional coupling between basolateral and apical membrane Na+/H+ exchangers. *Proc Natl Acad Sci U S A.* 1995;92:12525-12529.
125. Good DW, George T, Watts III BA. Lipopolysaccharide directly alters renal tubule transport through distinct TLR4-dependent pathways in basolateral and apical membranes. *Am J Physiol Renal Physiol.* 2009;297:F866-F874.
126. Good DW, Watts III BA. Functional roles of apical membrane Na+/H+ exchange in rat medullary thick ascending limb. *Am J Physiol Renal Physiol.* 1996;270:F691-F699.
127. Goyal S, Vanden Heuvel G, Aronson PS. Renal expression of novel Na+/H+ exchanger isoform NHE8. *Am J Physiol Renal Physiol.* 2003;284:F467-F473.
128. Gross E, Hawkins K, Abuladze N, et al. The stoichiometry of the electrogenic sodium bicarbonate cotransporter NBC1 is cell-type dependent. *J Physiol.* 2001;531:597-603.
129. Gross E, Hawkins K, Pushkin A, et al. Phosphorylation of Ser982 in the sodium bicarbonate cotransporter kNBC1 shifts the HCO3−:Na+ stoichiometry from 3:1 to 2:1 in murine proximal tubule cells. *J Physiol (Lond).* 2001;537:659-665.
130. Groves JD, Ring SM, Schofield AE, et al. The expression of the abnormal human red cell anion transporter from South-East Asian ovalocytes (band 3 SAO) in Xenopus oocytes. *FEBS Lett.* 1993;330:186-190.
131. Gumz ML, Lynch IJ, Greenlee MM, et al. The renal H+-K+-ATPases: physiology, regulation, and structure. *Am J Physiol Renal Physiol.* 2010;298:F12-F21.
132. Guntupalli J, Eby B, Lau K. Mechanism for the phosphaturia of NH4Cl: dependence on acidemia but not on diet PO4 or PTH. *Am J Physiol.* 1982;242:F552-F560.
133. Hamm LL. Renal handling of citrate. *Kidney Int.* 1990;38:728-735.
134. Hamm LL, Gillespie C, Klahr S. NH4Cl inhibition of transport in the rabbit cortical collecting tubule. *Am J Physiol.* 1985;248:F631-F637.
135. Hamm LL, Pucacco LR, Kokko JP, et al. Hydrogen ion permeability of the rabbit proximal convoluted tubule. *Am J Physiol.* 1984;246:F3-11.
136. Hamm LL, Simon EE. Roles and mechanisms of urinary buffer excretion. *Am J Physiol.* 1987;253:F595-F605.
137. Hamm LL, Simon EE. Ammonia transport in the proximal tubule in vivo. *Am J Kidney Dis.* 1989;14:253-257.
138. Hamm LL, Simon EE. Ammonia transport in the proximal tubule. *Miner Electrolyte Metab.* 1990;16:283-290.
139. Han KH, Croker BP, Clapp WL, et al. Expression of the ammonia transporter, Rh C glycoprotein, in normal and neoplastic human kidney. *J Am Soc Nephrol.* 2006;17:2670-2679.
140. Han KH, Mekala K, Babida V, et al. Expression of the gas transporting proteins, Rh B glycoprotein and Rh C glycoprotein, in the murine lung. *Am J Physiol Lung Cell Mol Physiol.* 2009;297:L153-L163.
141. Han KH, Kim HY, Croker BP, et al. Effects of ischemia-reperfusion injury on renal ammonia metabolism and the collecting duct. *Am J Physiol Renal Physiol.* 2007;293:F1342-F1354.
142. Han KH, SY Lee, WY Kim, et al. Expression of the ammonia transporter family members, Rh B glycoprotein and Rh C glycoprotein, in the developing rat kidney. *Am J Physiol Renal Physiol.* 2009;299:F187-F198.
143. Handlogten ME, Hong SP, Westhoff CM, et al. Basolateral ammonium transport by the mouse inner medullary collecting duct cell (mIMCD-3). *Am J Physiol Renal Physiol.* 2004;287:F628-F638.
144. Handlogten ME, Hong SP, Westhoff CM, et al. Apical ammonia transport by the mouse inner medullary collecting duct cell (mIMCD-3). *Am J Physiol Renal Physiol.* 2005;289:F347-F358.
145. Handlogten ME, Hong SP, Zhang L, et al. Expression of the ammonia transporter proteins, Rh B glycoprotein and Rh C glycoprotein, in the intestinal tract. *Am J Physiol Gastrointest.* 2005;288:G1036-G1047.
146. Hanson RW, Reshef L. Regulation of phosphoenolpyruvate carboxykinase (GTP) gene expression. *Annu Rev Biochem.* 1997;66:581-611.
147. Heyer M, Muller-Berger S, Romero MF, et al. Stoichiometry of the rat kidney Na+-HCO3− cotransporter expressed in Xenopus laevis oocytes. *Pflugers Arch.* 1999;438:322-329.
148. Hoffmann N, Thees M, Kinne R. Phosphate transport by isolated renal brush border vesicles. *Pflugers Archiv.* 1976;362:147-156.
149. Holm LM, Jahn TP, Moller AL, et al. NH3 and NH4+ permeability in aquaporin-expressing Xenopus oocytes. *Pflugers Arch.* 2005;450:415-428.
150. Hood VL. pH regulation of endogenous acid production in subjects with chronic ketoacidosis. *Am J Physiol Renal Physiol.* 1985;249:F220-F226.
151. Houillier P, Chambrey R, Achard JM, et al. Signaling pathways in the biphasic effect of angiotensin II on apical Na/H antiport activity in proximal tubule. *Kidney Int.* 1996;50:1496-1505.
152. Hu MC, Fan L, Crowder LA, et al. Dopamine acutely stimulates Na+/H+ exchanger (NHE3) endocytosis via clathrin-coated vesicles: dependence on protein kinase A–mediated NHE3 phosphorylation. *J Biol Chem.* 2001;276:26906-26915.
153. Huber S, Asan E, Jons T, et al. Expression of rat kidney anion exchanger 1 in type A intercalated cells in metabolic acidosis and alkalosis. *Am J Physiol.* 1999;277:F841-F849.
154. Hughey RP, Rankin BB, Curthoys NP. Acute acidosis and renal arteriovenous differences of glutamine in normal and adrenalectomized rats. *Am J Physiol Renal Physiol.* 1980;238:F199-F204.
155. Hurtado-Lorenzo A, Skinner M, Annan JE, et al. V-ATPase interacts with ARNO and Arf6 in early endosomes and regulates the protein degradative pathway. *Nat Cell Biol.* 2006;8:124-136.
156. Hwang JJ, Perera S, Shapiro RA, et al. Mechanism of altered renal glutaminase gene expression in response to chronic acidosis. *Biochemistry.* 1991;30:7522-7526.
157. Ibrahim H, Lee YJ, Curthoys NP. Renal response to metabolic acidosis: role of mRNA stabilization. *Kidney Int.* 2007;73:11-18.
158. Igarashi T, Inatomi J, Sekine T, et al. Mutations in SLC4A4 cause permanent isolated proximal renal tubular acidosis with ocular abnormalities. *Nat Genet.* 1999;23:264-266.
159. Indiveri C, Abruzzo G, Stipani I, et al. Identification and purification of the reconstitutively active glutamine carrier from rat kidney mitochondria. *Biochem J.* 1998;333:285-290.
160. Jakobsen JK, Odgaard E, Wang W, et al. Functional up-regulation of basolateral Na+-dependent HCO3− transporter NBCn1 in medullary thick ascending limb of K+-depleted rats. *Pflugers Arch.* 2004;448:571-578.
161. Janoshazi A, Ojcius DM, Kone B, et al. Relation between the anion exchange protein in kidney medullary collecting duct cells and red cell band 3. *J Membr Biol.* 1988;103:181-189.
162. Jenkins AD, Dousa TP, Smith LH. Transport of citrate across renal brush border membrane: effects of dietary acid and alkali loading. *Am J Physiol Renal Physiol.* 1985;249:F590-F595.

163. Jorgensen KE, Kragh-Hansen U, Roigaard-Petersen H, et al. Citrate uptake by basolateral and luminal membrane vesicles from rabbit kidney cortex. *Am J Physiol Renal Physiol.* 1983;244:F686-F695.
164. Jorgensen PL. Sodium and potassium ion pump in kidney tubules. *Physiol Rev.* 1980;60:864-917.
165. Kaiser S, Hwang JJ, Smith H, et al. Effect of altered acid-base balance and of various agonists on levels of renal glutamate dehydrogenase mRNA. *Am J Physiol Renal Physiol.* 1992;262:F507-F512.
166. Kandasamy RA, Orlowski J. Genomic organization and glucocorticoid transcriptional activation of the rat Na/H exchanger Nhe3 gene. *J Biol Chem.* 1996;271:10551-10559.
167. Kao L, Sassani P, Azimov R, et al. Oligomeric structure and minimal functional unit of the electrogenic sodium bicarbonate cotransporter NBCe1-A. *J Biol Chem.* 2008;283:26782-26794.
168. Karet FE, Finberg KE, Nayir A, et al. Localization of a gene for autosomal recessive distal renal tubular acidosis with normal hearing (rdRTA2) to 7q33-34. *Am J Hum Genet.* 1999;65:1656-1665.
169. Karet FE, Finberg KE, Nelson RD, et al. Mutations in the gene encoding B1 subunit of H$^+$-ATPase cause renal tubular acidosis with sensorineural deafness. *Nat Genet.* 1999;21:84-90.
170. Karinch AM, Lin CM, Wolfgang CL, et al. Regulation of expression of the SN1 transporter during renal adaptation to chronic metabolic acidosis in rats. *Am J Physiol Renal Physiol.* 2002;283:F1011-F1019.
171. Kaufman AM, Kahn T. Complementary role of citrate and bicarbonate excretion in acid-base balance in the rat. *Am J Physiol Renal Physiol.* 1988;255:F182-F187.
172. Kikeri D, Sun A, Zeidel ML, et al. Cell membranes impermeable to NH$_3$. *Nature.* 1989;339:478-480.
173. Kim GH, Ecelbarger C, Knepper MA, et al. Regulation of thick ascending limb ion transporter abundance in response to altered acid/base intake. *J Am Soc Nephrol.* 1999;10:935-942.
174. Kim HY, Verlander JW, Bishop JM, et al. Basolateral expression of the ammonia transporter family member, Rh C glycoprotein, in the mouse kidney. *Am J Physiol Renal Physiol.* 2009;296:F545-F555.
175. Kim HY, Baylis C, Verlander JW, et al. Effect of reduced renal mass on renal ammonia transporter family, Rh C glycoprotein and Rh B glycoprotein, expression. *Am J Physiol Renal Physiol.* 2007;293:F1238-F1247.
176. Kim J, Kim YH, Cha JH, et al. Intercalated cell subtypes in connecting tubule and cortical collecting duct of rat and mouse. *J Am Soc Nephrol.* 1999;10:1-12.
177. Kim YH, Verlander JW, Matthews SW, et al. Intercalated cell H$^+$/OH$^-$ transporter expression is reduced in *Slc26a4* null mice. *Am J Physiol Renal Physiol.* 2005;289:F1262-F1272.
178. Kinsella JL, Aronson PS. Interaction of NH$_4^+$ and Li$^+$ with the renal microvillus membrane Na$^+$-H$^+$ exchanger. *Am J Physiol.* 1981;241:C220-C226.
179. Kleinman JG, Bain JL, Fritsche C, et al. Histochemical carbonic anhydrase in rat inner medullary collecting duct. *J Histochem Cytochem.* 1992;40:1535-1545.
180. Knepper MA. NH$_4^+$ transport in the kidney. *Kidney Int.* 1991;40:S95-S102.
181. Knepper MA, Good DW, Burg MB. Mechanism of ammonia secretion by cortical collecting ducts of rabbits. *Am J Physiol.* 1984;247:F729-F738.
182. Knepper MA, Good DW, Burg MB. Ammonia and bicarbonate transport by rat cortical collecting ducts perfused in vitro. *Am J Physiol.* 1985;249:F870-F877.
183. Ko SB, Luo X, Hager H, et al. AE4 is a DIDS-sensitive Cl(−)/HCO(−)(3) exchanger in the basolateral membrane of the renal CCD and the SMG duct. *Am J Physiol Cell Physiol.* 2002;283:C1206-C1218.
184. Kobayashi K, Uchida S, Mizutani S, et al. Intrarenal and cellular localization of CLC-K2 protein in the mouse kidney. *J Am Soc Nephrol.* 2001;12:1327-1334.
185. Kocinsky HS, Girardi ACC, Biemesderfer D, et al. Use of phospho-specific antibodies to determine the phosphorylation of endogenous Na$^+$/H$^+$ exchanger NHE3 at PKA consensus sites. *Am J Physiol Renal Physiol.* 2005;289:F249-F258.
186. Kohan DE. Biology of endothelin receptors in the collecting duct. *Kidney Int.* 2009;76:481-486.
187. Kok DJ, Iestra JA, Doorenbos CJ, et al. The effects of dietary excesses in animal protein and sodium on the composition and the crystallization kinetics of calcium oxalate monohydrate in urines of healthy men. *J Clin Endocrinol Metab.* 1990;71:861-867.
188. Kraut JA, Helander KG, Helander HF, et al. Detection and localization of H$^+$-K$^+$-ATPase isoforms in human kidney. *Am J Physiol Renal Physiol.* 2001;281:F763-F768.
189. Kurtz I. Basolateral membrane Na$^+$/H$^+$ antiport, Na$^+$/base cotransport and Na$^+$-independent Cl$^-$/base exchange in the rabbit S$_3$ proximal tubule. *J Clin Invest.* 1989;83:616-622.
190. Kurtz I, Balaban RS. Ammonium as a substrate for Na$^+$-K$^+$-ATPase in rabbit proximal tubules. *Am J Physiol.* 1986;250:F497-F502.
191. Kwon TH, Fulton C, Wang W, et al. Chronic metabolic acidosis upregulates rat kidney Na-HCO cotransporters NBCn1 and NBC3 but not NBC1. *Am J Physiol Renal Physiol.* 2002;282:F341-F351.
192. Kwon TH, Pushkin A, Abuladze N, et al. Immunoelectron microscopic localization of NBC3 sodium-bicarbonate cotransporter in rat kidney. *Am J Physiol Renal Physiol.* 2000;278:F327-F336.
193. Laghmani K, Preisig PA, Moe OW, et al. Endothelin-1/endothelin-B receptor–mediated increases in NHE3 activity in chronic metabolic acidosis. *J Clin Invest.* 2001;107:1563-1569.
194. Lamprecht G, Weinman EJ, Yun C-HC. The role of NHERF and E3KARP in the cAMP-mediated inhibition of NHE3. *J Biol Chem.* 1998;273:29972-29978.
195. Laterza OF, Taylor L, Unnithan S, et al. Mapping and functional analysis of an instability element in phospho *eno*/pyruvate carboxykinase mRNA. *Am J Physiol Renal Physiol.* 2000;279:F866-F873.
196. Launonen V, Vierimaa O, Kiuru M, et al. Inherited susceptibility to uterine leiomyomas and renal cell cancer. *Proc Natl Acad Sci U S A.* 2001;98:3387-3392. 051633798.
197. Lee HW, Verlander JW, Bishop JM, et al. Collecting duct-specific Rh C glycoprotein deletion alters basal and acidosis-stimulated renal ammonia excretion. *Am J Physiol Renal Physiol.* 2009;296:F1364-F1375.
198. Lee HW, Verlander JW, JM Bishop, et al. Effect of intercalated cell-specific Rh C glycoprotein deletion on basal and metabolic acidosis–stimulated renal ammonia excretion. *Am J Physiol Renal Physiol.* 2010;299:F369-F379.
199. Lemann Jr J, Bushinsky DA, Hamm LL. Bone buffering of acid and base in humans. *Am J Physiol Renal Physiol.* 2003;285:F811-F832.
200. Lemann Jr J, Lennon EJ, Goodman AD, et al. The net balance of acid in subjects given large loads of acid or alkali. *J Clin Invest.* 1965;44:507-517.
201. Lemieux G, Baverel G, Vinay P, et al. Glutamine synthetase and glutamyltransferase in the kidney of man, dog, and rat. *Am J Physiol.* 1976;231:1068-1073.
202. Levi M, McDonald LA, Preisig PA, et al. Chronic K depletion stimulates rat renal brush-border membrane Na-citrate cotransporter. *Am J Physiol Renal Physiol.* 1991;261:F767-F773.
203. Li HC, Worrell RT, Matthews JB, et al. Identification of a carboxyl-terminal motif essential for the targeting of Na$^+$-cotransporter NBC1 to the basolateral membrane. *J Biol Chem.* 2004;279:43190-43197.
204. Licht C, Laghmani K, Yanagisawa M, et al. An autocrine role for endothelin-1 in the regulation of proximal tubule NHE3. *Kidney Int.* 2004;65:1320-1326.
205. Lim SW, Ahn KO, Kim WY, et al. Expression of ammonia transporters, Rhbg and Rhcg, in chronic cyclosporine nephropathy in rats. *Nephron Exp Nephrol.* 2008;110:e49-e58.
206. Lin SH, Cheema-Dhadli S, Chayaraks S, et al. Physiological disposal of the potential alkali load in diet of the rat: steps to achieve acid-base balance. *Am J Physiol.* 1998;274:F1037-F1044.
207. Liu FY, Cogan MG. Angiotensin II stimulation of hydrogen ion secretion in the rat early proximal tubule: modes of action, mechanism, and kinetics. *J Clin Invest.* 1988;82:601-607.
208. Liu Z, Huang CH. The mouse Rhl1 and Rhag genes: sequence, organization, expression, and chromosomal mapping. *Biochem Genet.* 1999;37:119-138.
209. Liu Z, Chen Y, Mo R, et al. Characterization of human RhCG and mouse Rhcg as novel nonerythroid Rh glycoprotein homologues predominantly expressed in kidney and testis. *J Biol Chem.* 2000;275:25641-25651.
210. Liu Z, Peng J, Mo R, et al. Rh type B glycoprotein is a new member of the Rh superfamily and a putative ammonia transporter in mammals. *J Biol Chem.* 2001;276:1424-1433.
211. Lombard WE, Kokko JP, Jacobson HR. Bicarbonate transport in cortical and outer medullary collecting tubules. *Am J Physiol.* 1983;244:F289-F296.
212. Lonnerholm G, Wistrand PJ. Membrane-bound carbonic anhydrase CA IV in the human kidney. *Acta Physiol Scand.* 2008;141:231-234.
213. Lopez C, Metral S, Eladari D, et al. The ammonium transporter RhBG: requirement of a tyrosine-based signal and ankyrin-G for basolateral targeting and membrane anchorage in polarized kidney epithelial cells. *J Biol Chem.* 2004;280:8221-8228.
214. Lorenz JN, Schultheis PJ, Traynor T, et al. Micropuncture analysis of single-nephron function in NHE3-deficient mice. *Am J Physiol Renal Physiol.* 1999;277:F447-F453.
215. Lu J, Daly CM, Parker MD, et al. Effect of human carbonic anhydrase II on the activity of the human electrogenic Na/HCO$_3$ cotransporter NBCe1-A in *Xenopus* oocytes. *J Biol Chem.* 2006;281:19241-19250.
216. Ludewig U. Electroneutral ammonium transport by basolateral Rhesus B glycoprotein. *J Physiol.* 2004;559:751-759.
217. Lynch IJ, Rudin A, Xia SL, et al. Impaired acid secretion in cortical collecting duct intercalated cells from H-K-ATPase-deficient mice: role of HKα isoforms. *Am J Physiol Renal Physiol.* 2008;294:F621-F627.

218. Madsen KM, Tisher CC. Structural-functional relationship along the distal nephron. *Am J Physiol.* 1986;250:F1-15.
219. Mak DO, Dang B, Weiner ID, et al. Characterization of transport by the kidney Rh glycoproteins, RhBG and RhCG. *Am J Physiol Renal Physiol.* 2006;290:F297-F305.
220. Manucha W, Valles P. Effect of glandular kallikrein on distal bicarbonate transport: role of basolateral Cl⁻/HCO₃⁻ exchanger and vacuolar H(+)-ATPase. *Biocell.* 1999;23:161-170.
221. Marini AM, Matassi G, Raynal V, et al. The human Rhesus-associated RhAG protein and a kidney homologue promote ammonium transport in yeast. *Nat Genet.* 2000;26:341-344.
222. Marquez J, Lopez de la Oliva A, Mates JM, et al. Glutaminase: a multifaceted protein not only involved in generating glutamate. *Neurochem Int.* 2005;48:465-471.
223. Maunsbach AB, Vorum H, Kwon TH, et al. Immunoelectron microscopic localization of the electrogenic Na/HCO₃ cotransporter in rat and ambystoma kidney. *J Am Soc Nephrol.* 2000;11:2179-2189.
224. Mayer M, Schaaf G, Mouro I, et al. Different transport mechanisms in plant and human AMT/Rh-type ammonium transporters. *J Gen Physiol.* 2006;127:133-144.
225. McDonough AA, Biemesderfer D. Does membrane trafficking play a role in regulating the sodium/hydrogen exchanger isoform 3 in the proximal tubule? *Curr Opin Nephrol Hypertens.* 2003;12:533-541.
226. McKinney TD, Burg MB. Bicarbonate transport by rabbit cortical collecting tubules: effect of acid and alkali loads in vivo on transport in vitro. *J Clin Invest.* 1977;60:766-768.
227. McKinney TD, Davidson KK. Effects of respiratory acidosis on HCO₃⁻ transport by rabbit collecting tubules. *Am J Physiol.* 1988;255:F656-F665.
228. McKinney TD, Myers P. Bicarbonate transport by proximal tubules: effect of parathyroid hormone and dibutyryl cyclic AMP. *Am J Physiol.* 1980;238:F166-F174.
229. Milton AE, Weiner ID. Intracellular pH regulation in the rabbit cortical collecting duct A-type intercalated cell. *Am J Physiol.* 1997;273:F340-F347.
230. Montrose MH, Donowitz M. Functional characteristics of a cloned epithelial Na⁺/H⁺ exchanger (NHE3): resistance to amiloride and inhibition by protein kinase C. *Proc Natl Acad Sci USA.* 1993;90:9110-9114.
231. Moret C, Dave MH, Schulz N, et al. Regulation of renal amino acid transporters during metabolic acidosis. *Am J Physiol Renal Physiol.* 2007;292:F555-F566.
232. Mouro-Chanteloup I, Cochet S, Chami M, et al. Functional reconstitution into liposomes of purified human RhCG ammonia channel. *PLoS One.* 2010;5:e8921.
233. Mujais SK, Kauffman S, Katz AI. Angiotensin II binding sites in individual segments of the rat nephron. *J Clin Invest.* 1986;77:315-318.
234. Muller-Berger S, Ducoudret O, Diakov A, et al. The renal Na-HCO₃⁻-cotransporter expressed in *Xenopus laevis* oocytes: change in stoichiometry in response to elevation of cytosolic Ca²⁺ concentration. *Pflugers Arch.* 2001;442:718-728.
235. Musa-Aziz R, Chen LM, Pelletier MF, et al. Relative CO₂/NH₃ selectivities of AQP1, AQP4, AQP5, AmtB, and RhAG. *Proc Natl Acad Sci U S A.* 2009;106:5406-5411.
236. Nagami GT. Luminal secretion of ammonia in the mouse proximal tubule perfused in vitro. *J Clin Invest.* 1988;81:159-164.
237. Nagami GT. Ammonia production and secretion by the proximal tubule. *Am J Kidney Dis.* 1989;14:258-261.
238. Nagami GT. Effect of bath and luminal potassium concentration on ammonia production and secretion by mouse proximal tubules perfused in vitro. *J Clin Invest.* 1990;86:32-39.
239. Nagami GT. Effect of angiotensin II on ammonia production and secretion by mouse proximal tubules perfused in vitro. *J Clin Invest.* 1992;89:925-931.
240. Nagami GT. Enhanced ammonia secretion by proximal tubules from mice receiving NH(4)Cl role of angiotensin II. *Am J Physiol Renal Physiol.* 2002;282:F472-F477.
241. Nagami GT. Ammonia production and secretion by S3 proximal tubule segments from acidotic mice role of ANG II. *Am J Physiol Renal Physiol.* 2004;287:F707-F712.
242. Nagami GT, Kraut JA. Acid-base regulation of angiotensin receptors in the kidney. *Curr Opin Nephrol Hypertens.* 2010;19:91-97.
243. Nagami GT, Sonu CM, Kurokawa K. Ammonia production by isolated mouse proximal tubules perfused in vitro: effect of metabolic acidosis. *J Clin Invest.* 1986;78:124-129.
244. Nagami GT. Role of angiotensin II in the enhancement of ammonia production and secretion by the proximal tubule in metabolic acidosis. *Am J Physiol Renal Physiol.* 2008;294:F874-F880.
245. Nakamura S, Amlal H, Galla JH, et al. NH₄⁺ secretion in inner medullary collecting duct in potassium deprivation: role of colonic H⁺-K⁺-ATPase. *Kidney Int.* 1999;56:2160-2167.
246. Nakhoul NL, Chen LK, Boron WF. Intracellular pH regulation in rabbit S3 proximal tubule: basolateral Cl-HCO₃ exchange and Na-HCO₃ cotransport. *Am J Physiol.* 1990;258:F371-F381.
247. Nakhoul NL, Chen LK, Boron WF. Effect of basolateral CO₂/HCO₃⁻ on intracellular pH regulation in the rabbit S3 proximal tubule. *J Gen Physiol.* 1993;102:1171-1205.
248. Nakhoul NL, Hering-Smith KS, Abdulnour-Nakhoul SM, et al. Transport of NH(3)/NH in oocytes expressing aquaporin-1. *Am J Physiol Renal Physiol.* 2001;281:F255-F263.
249. Nakhoul NL, DeJong H, Abdulnour-Nakhoul SM, et al. Characteristics of renal Rhbg as an NH₄⁺ transporter. *Am J Physiol Renal Physiol.* 2004;288:F170-F181.
250. Needle MA, Kaloyanides GJ, Schwartz WB. The effects of selective depletion of hydrochloric acid on acid-base and electrolyte equilibrium. *J Clin Invest.* 1964;43:1836-1846.
251. Nelson RD, Guo XL, Masood K, et al. Selectively amplified expression of an isoform of the vacuolar H(+)-ATPase 56-kilodalton subunit in renal intercalated cells. *Proc Natl Acad Sci U S A.* 1992;89:3541-3545.
252. Nicoletta JA, Schwartz GJ. Distal renal tubular acidosis. *Curr Opin Pediatr.* 2004;16:194-198.
253. Nowik M, Picard N, Stange G, et al. Renal phosphaturia during metabolic acidosis revisited: molecular mechanisms for decreased renal phosphate reabsorption. *Pflugers Arch.* 2008;457:539-549.
254. Pajor AM. Molecular cloning and functional expression of a sodium-dicarboxylate cotransporter from human kidney. *Am J Physiol.* 1996;270:F642-F648.
255. Palmer LG, Frindt G. Cl⁻ channels of the distal nephron. *Am J Physiol Renal Physiol.* 2006;291:F1157-F1168.
256. Paunescu TG, Russo LM, Da Silva N, et al. Compensatory membrane expression of the V-ATPase B2 subunit isoform in renal medullary intercalated cells of B1-deficient mice. *Am J Physiol Renal Physiol.* 2007;293:F1915-F1926.
257. Paunescu TG, Silva ND, Marshansky V, et al. Expression of the 56-kDa B2 subunit isoform of the vacuolar H⁺-ATPase in proton-secreting cells of the kidney and epididymis. *Am J Physiol Cell Physiol.* 2004;287:C149-C162.
258. Pech V, Zheng W, Pham TD, et al. Angiotensin II activates H⁺-ATPase in type A intercalated cells. *J Am Soc Nephrol.* 2008;19:84-91.
259. Pela I, Bigozzi M, Bianchi B. Profound hypokalemia and hypochloremic metabolic alkalosis during thiazide therapy in a child with Pendred syndrome. *Clin Nephrol.* 2008;69:450-453.
260. Peti-Peterdi J, Chambrey R, Bebok Z, et al. Macula densa Na⁺/H⁺ exchange activities mediated by apical NHE2 and basolateral NHE4 isoforms. *Am J Physiol Renal Physiol.* 2000;278:F452-F463.
261. Petrovic S, Wang Z, Ma L, et al. Regulation of the apical Cl⁻/HCO₃⁻ exchanger pendrin in rat cortical collecting duct in metabolic acidosis. *Am J Physiol Renal Physiol.* 2003;284:F103-F112.
262. Petrovic S, Barone S, Xu J, et al. SLC26A7: a basolateral Cl⁻/HCO₃⁻ exchanger specific to intercalated cells of the outer medullary collecting duct. *Am J Physiol Renal Physiol.* 2004;286:F161-F169.
263. Piermarini PM, Kim EY, Boron WF. Evidence against a direct interaction between intracellular carbonic anhydrase II and pure C-terminal domains of SLC4 bicarbonate transporters. *J Biol Chem.* 2007;282:1409-1421.
264. Pitts RF, Lotspeich WD. Bicarbonate and the renal regulation of acid base balance. *Am J Physiol.* 1946;147:138-154.
265. Plaitakis A, Metaxari M, Shashidharan P. Nerve tissue-specific (GLUD2) and housekeeping (GLUD1) human glutamate dehydrogenases are regulated by distinct allosteric mechanisms. *J Neurochem.* 2002;75:1862-1869.
266. Praetorius HA, Spring KR. The renal cell primary cilium functions as a flow sensor. *Curr Opin Nephrol Hypertens.* 2003;12:517-520.
267. Praetorius J, Kim YH, Bouzinova EV, et al. NBCn1 is a basolateral Na⁺-HCO₃⁻ cotransporter in rat kidney inner medullary collecting ducts. *Am J Physiol Renal Physiol.* 2004;286:F903-F912.
268. Preisig PA. Luminal flow rate regulates proximal tubule H-HCO₃ transporters. *Am J Physiol.* 1992;262:F47-F54.
269. Preisig PA, Alpern RJ. Chronic metabolic acidosis causes an adaptation in the apical membrane Na/H antiporter and basolateral membrane Na(HCO₃)₃ symporter in the rat proximal convoluted tubule. *J Clin Invest.* 1988;82:1445-1453.
270. Preisig PA, Alpern RJ. Contributions of cellular leak pathways to net NaHCO₃ and NaCl absorption. *J Clin Invest.* 1989;83:1859-1867.
271. Purkerson JM, Schwartz GJ. The role of carbonic anhydrases in renal physiology. *Kidney Int.* 2006;71:103-115.
272. Purkerson JM, Schwartz GJ. Expression of membrane-associated carbonic anhydrase isoforms IV, IX, XII, and XIV in the rabbit: induction of CA IV and IX during maturation. *Am J Physiol Regul Integr Comp Physiol.* 2005;288:R1256-R1263.

273. Pushkin A, Yip KP, Clark I, et al. NBC3 expression in rabbit collecting duct: colocalization with vacuolar H⁺-ATPase. *Am J Physiol.* 1999;277:F974-F981.

274. Pushkin A, Abuladze N, Gross E, et al. Molecular mechanism of kNBC1-carbonic anhydrase II interaction in proximal tubule cells. *J Physiol (Lond).* 2004;559:55-65.

275. Quentin F, Chambrey R, Trinh-Trang-Tan MM, et al. The Cl⁻/HCO₃⁻ exchanger pendrin in the rat kidney is regulated in response to chronic alterations in chloride balance. *Am J Physiol Renal Physiol.* 2004;287:F1179-F1188.

276. Quentin F, Eladari D, Cheval L, et al. RhBG and RhCG, the putative ammonia transporters, are expressed in the same cells in the distal nephron. *J Am Soc Nephrol.* 2003;14:545-554.

277. Quigley R, Baum M. Developmental changes in rabbit proximal straight tubule paracellular permeability. *Am J Physiol Renal Physiol.* 2002;283:F525-F531.

278. Quilty JA, Li J, Reithmeier RA. Impaired trafficking of distal renal tubular acidosis mutants of the human kidney anion exchanger kAE1. *Am J Physiol Renal Physiol.* 2002;282:F810-F820.

279. Rector Jr FC, Bloomer HA, Seldin DW. Effect of potassium deficiency on the reabsorption of bicarbonate in the proximal tubule of the rat kidney. *J Clin Invest* 1964;43:1976.

280. Rector Jr FC, Orloff J. The effect of the administration of sodium bicarbonate and ammonium chloride on the excretion and production of ammonia. The absence of alterations in the activity of renal ammonia-producing enzymes in the dog. *J Clin Invest.* 1959;38:366-372.

281. Renkema KY, Velic A, Dijkman HB, et al. The calcium-sensing receptor promotes urinary acidification to prevent nephrolithiasis. *J Am Soc Nephrol.* 2009;20:1705-1713.

282. Riccardi D, Brown EM. Physiology and pathophysiology of the calcium-sensing receptor in the kidney. *Am J Physiol Renal Physiol.* 2010;298:F485-F499.

283. Richardson RM, Goldstein MB, Stinebaugh BJ, et al. Influence of diet and metabolism on urinary acid excretion in the rat and the rabbit. *J Lab Clin Med.* 1979;94:510-518.

284. Ripoche P, Bertrand O, Gane P, et al. Human Rhesus-associated glycoprotein mediates facilitated transport of NH₃ into red blood cells. *Proc Natl Acad Sci U S A.* 2004;101:17222-17227.

285. Riquier-Brison ADM, Leong PKK, Pihakaski-Maunsbach K, et al. Angiotensin II stimulates trafficking of NHE3, NaPi2, and associated proteins into the proximal tubule microvilli. *Am J Physiol Renal Physiol.* 2010;298:F177-F186.

286. Romero MF. Molecular pathophysiology of SLC4 bicarbonate transporters. *Curr Opin Nephrol Hypertens.* 2005;14:495-501.

287. Rothenberger F, Velic A, Stehberger PA, et al. Angiotensin II stimulates vacuolar H⁺-ATPase activity in renal acid-secretory intercalated cells from the outer medullary collecting duct. *J Am Soc Nephrol.* 2007;18:2085-2093.

288. Royaux IE, Wall SM, Karniski LP, et al. Pendrin, encoded by the Pendred syndrome gene, resides in the apical region of renal intercalated cells and mediates bicarbonate secretion. *Proc Natl Acad Sci U S A.* 2001;98:4221-4226.

289. Sabolic I, Brown D, Gluck SL, et al. Regulation of AE1 anion exchanger and H(+)-ATPase in rat cortex by acute metabolic acidosis and alkalosis. *Kidney Int.* 1997;51:125-137.

290. Sangan P, Kolla SS, Rajendran VM, et al. Colonic H-K-ATPase beta-subunit: identification in apical membranes and regulation by dietary K depletion. *Am J Physiol.* 1999;276:C350-C360.

291. Sarker R, Gronborg M, Cha B, et al. Casein kinase 2 binds to the C terminus of Na⁺/H⁺ exchanger 3 (NHE3) and stimulates NHE3 basal activity by phosphorylating a separate site in NHE3. *Mol Biol Cell.* 2008;19:3859.

292. Sartorius OW, Roemmelt JC, Pitts RF, et al. The renal regulation of acid-base balance in man. IV. The nature of the renal compensations in ammonium chloride acidosis. *J Clin Invest.* 1949;28:423-439.

293. Sastrasinh S, Sastrasinh M. Glutamine transport in submitochondrial particles. *Am J Physiol Renal Physiol.* 1989;257:F1050-F1058.

294. Schoolwerth AC, Gesek FA. Intramitochondrial pH and ammonium production in rat and dog kidney cortex. *Miner Electrolyte Metab.* 1990;16:264-269.

295. Schroeder JM, Liu W, Curthoys NP. pH-responsive stabilization of glutamate dehydrogenase mRNA in LLC-PK1-F⁺ cells. *Am J Physiol Renal Physiol.* 2003;285:F258-F265.

296. Schultheis PJ, Clarke LL, Meneton P, et al. Renal and intestinal absorptive defects in mice lacking the NHE3 Na⁺/H⁺ exchanger. *Nat Genet.* 1998;19:282-285.

297. Schulz N, Dave MH, Stehberger PA, et al. Differential localization of vacuolar H⁺-ATPases containing a1, a2, a3, or a4 (ATP6V0A1-4) subunit isoforms along the nephron. *Cell Physiol Biochem.* 2007;20:109-120.

298. Schuster VL. Cyclic adenosine monophosphate-stimulated bicarbonate secretion in the rabbit cortical collecting tubule. *J Clin Invest.* 1985;75:2056-2064.

299. Schwartz GJ. Physiology and molecular biology of renal carbonic anhydrase. *J Nephrol.* 2002;15(suppl 5):S61-S74.

300. Schwartz GJ, Al-Awqati Q. Role of hensin in mediating the adaptation of the cortical collecting duct to metabolic acidosis. *Curr Opin Nephrol Hypertens.* 2005;14:383-388.

301. Schwartz GJ, Barasch J, Al-Awqati Q. Plasticity of functional epithelial polarity. *Nature.* 1985;318:368-371.

302. Schwartz GJ, Kittelberger AM, Barnhart DA, et al. Carbonic anhydrase IV is expressed in H(+)-secreting cells of rabbit kidney. *Am J Physiol Renal Physiol.* 2000;278:F894-F904.

303. Schwartz GJ, Kittelberger AM, Barnhart DA, et al. Carbonic anhydrase IV is expressed in H⁺-secreting cells of rabbit kidney. *Am J Physiol Renal Physiol.* 2000;278:F894-F904.

304. Sekine T, Cha SH, Hosoyamada M, et al. Cloning, functional characterization, and localization of a rat renal Na⁺-dicarboxylate transporter. *Am J Physiol.* 1998;275:F298-F305.

305. Seshadri RM, Klein JD, Kozlowski S, et al. Renal expression of the ammonia transporters, Rhbg and Rhcg, in response to chronic metabolic acidosis. *Am J Physiol Renal Physiol.* 2006;290:F397-F408.

306. Seshadri RM, Klein JD, Smith T, et al. Changes in the subcellular distribution of the ammonia transporter Rhcg, in response to chronic metabolic acidosis. *Am J Physiol Renal Physiol.* 2006;290:F1443-F1452.

307. Shayakul C, Alper SL. Defects in processing and trafficking of the AE1 Cl⁻/HCO₃⁻ exchanger associated with inherited distal renal tubular acidosis. *Clin Exp Nephrol.* 2004;8:1-11.

308. Shenolikar S, Voltz JW, Minkoff CM, et al. Targeted disruption of the mouse NHERF-1 gene promotes internalization of proximal tubule sodium-phosphate cotransporter type IIa and renal phosphate wasting. *Proc Natl Acad Sci U S A.* 2002;99:11470-11475.

309. Shiraishi N, Kitamura K, Kohda Y, et al. Increased endothelin-1 expression in the kidney in hypercalcemic rats. *Kidney Int.* 2003;63:845-852.

310. Siga E, Houillier P, Mandon B, et al. Calcitonin stimulates H⁺ secretion in rat kidney intercalated cells. *Am J Physiol.* 1996;40:F1217-F1223.

311. Silbernagl S. Tubular reabsorption of l-glutamine studied by free-flow micropuncture and microperfusion of rat kidney. *Int J Biochem.* 1980;12:9-16.

312. Simon E, Martin D, Buerkert J. Contribution of individual superficial nephron segments to ammonium handling in chronic metabolic acidosis in the rat. Evidence for ammonia disequilibrium in the renal cortex. *J Clin Invest.* 1985;76:855-864.

313. Simon EE, Merli C, Herndon J, et al. Effects of barium and 5-(*N*-ethyl-*N*-isopropyl)-amiloride on proximal tubule ammonia transport. *Am J Physiol.* 1992;262:F36-F39.

314. Simon EE, Merli C, Herndon J, et al. Contribution of luminal ammoniagenesis to proximal tubule ammonia appearance in the rat. *Am J Physiol.* 1990;259:F402-F407.

315. Smith AN, Skaug J, Choate KA, et al. Mutations in ATP6N1B, encoding a new kidney vacuolar proton pump 116-kD subunit, cause recessive distal renal tubular acidosis with preserved hearing. *Nat Genet.* 2000;26:71-75.

316. Smith AN, Jouret F, Bord S, et al. Vacuolar H⁺-ATPase d2 subunit: molecular characterization, developmental regulation, and localization to specialized proton pumps in kidney and bone. *J Am Soc Nephrol.* 2005;16:1245-1256.

317. Soleimani M, Bergman JA, Hosford MA, et al. Potassium depletion increases luminal Na⁺/H⁺ exchange and basolateral Na⁺:CO₃=:HCO₃⁻ cotransport in rat renal cortex. *J Clin Invest.* 1990;86:1076-1083.

318. Song HK, Kim WY, Lee HW, et al. Origin and fate of pendrin-positive intercalated cells in developing mouse kidney. *J Am Soc Nephrol.* 2007;18:2672-2682.

319. Soria LR, Fanelli E, Altamura N, et al. Aquaporin 8-facilitated mitochondrial ammonia transport. *Biochem Biophys Res Commun.* 2010;393:217-221.

320. Star RA, Burg MB, Knepper MA. Luminal disequilibrium pH and ammonia transport in outer medullary collecting duct. *Am J Physiol.* 1987;252:F1148-F1157.

321. Star RA, Kurtz I, Mejia R, et al. Disequilibrium pH and ammonia transport in isolated perfused cortical collecting ducts. *Am J Physiol.* 1987;253:F1232-F1242.

322. Stauber A, Radanovic T, Stange G, et al. Regulation of intestinal phosphate transport II. Metabolic acidosis stimulates Na⁺-dependent phosphate absorption and expression of the Na⁺-Pi cotransporter NaPi-IIb in small intestine. *Am J Physiol Gastrointest.* 2005;288:G501-G506.

323. Stehberger PA, Schulz N, Finberg KE, et al. Localization and regulation of the ATP6V0A4 (a4) vacuolar H⁺-ATPase subunit defective in an inherited form of distal renal tubular acidosis. *J Am Soc Nephrol.* 2003;14:3027-3038.

324. Sterling D, Alvarez BV, Casey JR. The extracellular component of a transport metabolon. *J Biol Chem.* 2002;277:25239-25246.
325. Stone DK, Seldin DW, Kokko JP, et al. Mineralocorticoid modulation of rabbit medullary collecting duct acidification: a sodium-independent effect. *J Clin Invest.* 1983;72:77-83.
326. Stover EH, Borthwick KJ, Bavalia C, et al. Novel ATP6V1B1 and ATP6V0A4 mutations in autosomal recessive distal renal tubular acidosis with new evidence for hearing loss. *J Med Genet.* 2002;39:796-803.
327. Strait KA, Stricklett PK, Kohan JL, et al. Calcium regulation of endothelin-1 synthesis in rat inner medullary collecting duct. *Am J Physiol Renal Physiol.* 2007;293:F601-F606.
328. Sun X, Petrovic S. Increased acid load and deletion of AE1 increase Slc26a7 expression. *Nephron Physiol.* 2008;109:29-35.
329. Tannen RL. Relationship of renal ammonia production and potassium homeostasis. *Kidney Int.* 1977;11:453-465.
330. Tannen RL. Ammonia metabolism. *Am J Physiol Renal Physiol.* 1978;235:F265-F277.
331. Tannen RL, Sahai A. Biochemical pathways and modulators of renal ammoniagenesis. *Miner Electrolyte Metab.* 1990;16:249-258.
332. Tanphaichitr VS, Sumboonnanonda A, Ideguchi H, et al. Novel AE1 mutations in recessive distal renal tubular acidosis: loss-of-function is rescued by glycophorin a. *J Clin Invest.* 1998;102:2173-2179.
333. Taylor L, Curthoys NP. Glutamine metabolism: role in acid-base balance. *Biochem Mol Biol Educ.* 2004;32:291-304.
334. Teng-umnuay P, Verlander JW, Yuan W, et al. Identification of distinct subpopulations of intercalated cells in the mouse collecting duct. *J Am Soc Nephrol.* 1996;7:260-274.
335. Thomson RB, Wang T, Thomson BR, et al. Role of PDZK1 in membrane expression of renal brush border ion exchangers. *Proc Natl Acad Sci U S A.* 2005;102:13331-13336.
336. Todd-Turla KM, Schnermann J, Fejes-Toth G, et al. Distribution of mineralocorticoid and glucocorticoid receptor mRNA along the nephron. *Am J Physiol Renal Physiol.* 1993;264:F781-F791.
337. Tojo A, Tisher CC, Madsen KM. Angiotensin II regulates H+-ATPase activity in rat cortical collecting duct. *Am J Physiol.* 1994;267:F1045-F1051.
338. Tong J, Harrison G, Curthoys NP. The effect of metabolic acidosis on the synthesis and turnover of rat renal phosphate-dependent glutaminase. *Biochem J.* 1986;233:139-144.
339. Tong J, Shapiro RA, Curthoys NP. Changes in the levels of translatable glutaminase mRNA during onset and recovery from metabolic acidosis. *Biochemistry.* 1987;26:2773-2777.
340. Toye AM, Banting G, Tanner MJA. Regions of human kidney anion exchanger 1 (kAE1) required for basolateral targeting of kAE1 in polarised kidney cells: mis-targeting explains dominant renal tubular acidosis (dRTA). *J Cell Sci.* 2004;117:1399-1410.
341. Tsuganezawa H, Kobayashi K, Iyori M, et al. A new member of the HCO3-transporter superfamily is an apical anion exchanger of beta-intercalated cells in the kidney. *J Biol Chem.* 2001;276:8180-8189.
342. Tsuruoka S, Kittelberger AM, Schwartz GJ. Carbonic anhydrase II and IV mRNA in rabbit nephron segments: stimulation during metabolic acidosis. *Am J Physiol.* 1998;274:F259-F267.
343. Tsuruoka S, Schwartz GJ. HCO3- absorption in rabbit outer medullary collecting duct: role of luminal carbonic anhydrase. *Am J Physiol.* 1998;274:F139-F147.
344. Tsuruoka S, Schwartz GJ. Mechanisms of HCO(-)(3) secretion in the rabbit connecting segment. *Am J Physiol.* 1999;277:F567-F574.
345. Tsuruoka S, Watanabe S, Purkerson JM, et al. Endothelin and nitric oxide mediate adaptation of the cortical collecting duct to metabolic acidosis. *Am J Physiol Renal Physiol.* 2006;291:F866-F873.
346. Ullrich KJ, Rumrich G, Klöss S. Phosphate transport in the proximal convolution of the rat kidney. *Pflugers Archiv.* 1978;377:33-42.
347. Unwin R, Capasso G, Giebisch G. Bicarbonate transport along the loop of Henle effects of adrenal steroids. *Am J Physiol.* 1995;268:F234-F239.
348. Vallon V, Schwark JR, Richter K, et al. Role of Na+/H+ exchanger NHE3 in nephron function: micropuncture studies with S3226, an inhibitor of NHE3. *Am J Physiol Renal Physiol.* 2000;278:F375-F379.
349. Vargas-Poussou R, Houillier P, Le Pottier N, et al. Genetic investigation of autosomal recessive distal renal tubular acidosis: evidence for early sensorineural hearing loss associated with mutations in the ATP6V0A4 gene. *J Am Soc Nephrol.* 2006;17:1437-1443.
350. Verlander JW, Hassell KA, Royaux IE, et al. Deoxycorticosterone upregulates PDS (Slc26a4) in mouse kidney: role of pendrin in mineralocorticoid-induced hypertension. *Hypertension.* 2003;42:356-362.
351. Verlander JW, Kim YH, Shin W, et al. Dietary Cl(−) restriction upregulates pendrin expression within the apical plasma membrane of type B intercalated cells. *Am J Physiol Renal Physiol.* 2006;291:F833-F839.
352. Verlander JW, Madsen KM, Cannon JK, et al. Activation of acid-secreting intercalated cells in rabbit collecting duct with ammonium chloride loading. *Am J Physiol.* 1994;266:F633-F645.
353. Verlander JW, Madsen KM, Galla JH, et al. Response of intercalated cells to chloride depletion metabolic alkalosis. *Am J Physiol.* 1992;262:F309-F319.
354. Verlander JW, Madsen KM, Tisher CC. Effect of acute respiratory acidosis on two populations of intercalated cells in rat cortical collecting duct. *Am J Physiol.* 1987;253:F1142-F1156.
355. Verlander JW, Madsen KM, Tisher CC. Axial distribution of band 3-positive intercalated cells in the collecting duct of control and ammonium chloride-loaded rabbits. *Kidney Int Suppl.* 1996;57:S137-S147.
356. Deleted in page proofs.
357. Verlander JW, Miller RT, Frank AE, et al. Localization of the ammonium transporter proteins, Rh B glycoprotein and Rh C glycoprotein, in the mouse kidney. *Am J Physiol Renal Physiol.* 2003;284:F323-F337.
358. Verlander JW, Moudy RM, Campbell WG, et al. Immunohistochemical localization of H-K-ATPase alpha$_{2C}$ subunit in rabbit kidney. *Am J Physiol Renal Physiol.* 2001;281:F357-F365.
359. Villa-Bellosta R and V Sorribas. Compensatory regulation of the sodium/phosphate cotransporters NaPi-IIc (SCL34A3) and Pit-2 (SLC20A2) during Pi deprivation and acidosis. *Pflugers Arch.* 2009;459:499-508.
360. Vince JW, Reithmeier RA. Carbonic anhydrase II binds to the carboxyl terminus of human band 3, the erythrocyte Cl-/HCO3- exchanger. *J Biol Chem.* 1998;273:28430-28437.
361. Vorum H, Kwon TH, Fulton C, et al. Immunolocalization of electroneutral Na-HCO3- cotransporter in rat kidney. *Am J Physiol Renal Physiol.* 2000;279:F901-F909.
362. Wagner CA, Finberg KE, Breton S, et al. Renal vacuolar H+-ATPase. *Physiol Rev.* 2004;84:1263-1314.
363. Wagner CA, Finberg KE, Stehberger PA, et al. Regulation of the expression of the Cl-/anion exchanger pendrin in mouse kidney by acid-base status. *Kidney Int.* 2002;62:2109-2117.
364. Wagner CA, Giebisch G, Lang F, et al. Angiotensin II stimulates vesicular H+-ATPase in rat proximal tubular cells. *Proc Natl Acad Sci U S A.* 1998;95:9665-9668.
365. Wall SM. Ouabain reduces net acid secretion and increases pHi by inhibiting NH4+ uptake on rat tIMCD Na(+)-K(+)-ATPase. *Am J Physiol.* 1997;273:F857-F868.
366. Wall SM, Fischer MP. Contribution of the Na+-K+-2Cl- cotransporter (NKCC1) to transepithelial transport of H+, NH4+, K+, and Na+ in rat outer medullary collecting duct. *J Am Soc Nephrol.* 2002;13:827-835.
367. Wall SM, Fischer MP, Glapion DM, et al. ANG II reduces net acid secretion in rat outer medullary collecting duct. *Am J Physiol Renal Physiol.* 2003;285:F930-F937.
368. Wall SM, Fischer MP, Kim GH, et al. In rat inner medullary collecting duct, NH4+ uptake by the Na, K-ATPase is increased during hypokalemia. *Am J Physiol Renal Physiol.* 2002;282:F91-102.
369. Wall SM, Flessner MF, Knepper MA. Distribution of luminal carbonic anhydrase activity along rat inner medullary collecting duct. *Am J Physiol.* 1991;260:F738-F748.
370. Wall SM, Kim YH, Stanley L, et al. NaCl restriction upregulates renal Slc26a4 through subcellular redistribution: role in Cl- conservation. *Hypertension.* 2004;44:982-987.
371. Wall SM, Knepper MA. Acid-base transport in the inner medullary collecting duct. *Semin Nephrol.* 1990;10:148-158.
372. Wall SM, Koger LM. NH4+ transport mediated by Na+-K+-ATPase in rat inner medullary collecting duct. *Am J Physiol.* 1994;267:F660-F670.
373. Wall SM, Mehta P, DuBose TD. Dietary K+ restriction upregulates total and Sch-28080–sensitive bicarbonate absorption in rat tIMCD. *Am J Physiol.* 1998;275:F543-F549.
374. Wall SM, Pech V. The interaction of pendrin and the epithelial sodium channel in blood pressure regulation. *Curr Opin Nephrol Hypertens.* 2008;17:18-24.
375. Wall SM, Trinh HN, Woodward KE. Heterogeneity of NH4+ transport in mouse inner medullary collecting duct cells. *Am J Physiol.* 1995;269:F536-F544.
376. Wall SM, Truong AV, DuBose TD. H(+)-K(+)-ATPase mediates net acid secretion in rat terminal inner medullary collecting duct. *Am J Physiol.* 1996;271:F1037-F1044.
377. Wall SM, Hassell KA, Royaux IE, et al. Localization of pendrin in mouse kidney. *Am J Physiol Renal Physiol.* 2003;284:F229-F241.
378. Wang T, Chan YL. Mechanism of angiotensin II action on proximal tubular transport. *J Pharmacol Exp Ther.* 1990;252:689-695.
379. Wang T, Yang CL, Abbiati T, et al. Mechanism of proximal tubule bicarbonate absorption in NHE3 null mice. *Am J Physiol.* 1999;277:F298-F302.
380. Wang T, Hropot M, Aronson PS, et al. Role of NHE isoforms in mediating bicarbonate reabsorption along the nephron. *Am J Physiol Renal Physiol.* 2001;281:F1117-F1122.

381. Watts III BA, George T, Good DW. The basolateral NHE1 Na⁺/H⁺ exchanger regulates transepithelial HCO₃⁻ absorption through actin cytoskeleton remodeling in renal thick ascending limb. *J Biol Chem.* 2005;280:11439-11447.

382. Watts III BA, Good DW. An apical K(+)-dependent HCO(3)(−) transport pathway opposes transepithelial HCO(3)(−) absorption in rat medullary thick ascending limb. *Am J Physiol Renal Physiol.* 2004;287:F57-F63.

383. Weill AE, Tisher CC, Conde MF, et al. Mechanisms of bicarbonate transport by cultured rabbit inner medullary collecting duct cells. *Am J Physiol.* 1994;266:F466-F476.

384. Weiner ID. The Rh gene family and renal ammonium transport. *Curr Opin Nephrol Hyper.* 2004;13:533-540.

385. Weiner ID, Frank AE, Wingo CS. Apical proton secretion by the inner stripe of the outer medullary collecting duct. *Am J Physiol Renal Physiol.* 1999;276:F606-F613.

386. Weiner ID, Hamm LL. Regulation of intracellular pH in the rabbit cortical collecting tubule. *J Clin Invest.* 1990;85:274-281.

387. Weiner ID, Hamm LL. Molecular mechanisms of renal ammonia transport. *Annu Rev Physiol.* 2007;69:317-340.

388. Weiner ID, Miller RT, Verlander JW. Localization of the ammonium transporters, Rh B glycoprotein and Rh C glycoprotein in the mouse liver. *Gastroenterology.* 2003;124:1432-1440.

389. Weiner ID, Milton AE. H⁺-K⁺-ATPase in rabbit cortical collecting duct B-type intercalated cell. *Am J Physiol.* 1996;270:F518-F530.

390. Weiner ID, New AR, Milton AE, et al. Regulation of luminal alkalinization and acidification in the cortical collecting duct by angiotensin II. *Am J Physiol.* 1995;269:F730-F738.

391. Weiner ID, Weill AE, New AR. Distribution of Cl⁻/HCO₃⁻ exchange and intercalated cells in the rabbit cortical collecting duct. *Am J Physiol.* 1994;267:F952-F964.

392. Weiner ID, Wingo CS, Hamm LL. Regulation of intracellular pH in two cell populations of the inner stripe of the rabbit outer medullary collecting duct. *Am J Physiol.* 1993;265:F406-F415.

393. Weiner ID and Jw Verlander. Molecular physiology of the Rh ammonia transport proteins.. *Curr Opin Nephrol Hypertens.* 2010;19:471-477

394. Weinstein AM. A mathematical model of rat distal convoluted tubule. I. Cotransporter function in early DCT. *Am J Physiol Renal Physiol.* 2005;289:F699-F720.

395. Weinstein AM. A mathematical model of distal nephron acidification: diuretic effects. *Am J Physiol Renal Physiol.* 2008;295:F1353-F1364.

396. Weinstein AM, Krahn TA. A mathematical model of rat ascending Henle limb. II. Epithelial function. *Am J Physiol Renal Physiol.* 2009;298:F525-F542.

397. Welbourne TC. Acidosis activation of the pituitary-adrenal-renal glutaminase I axis. *Endocrinology.* 1976;99:1071-1079.

398. Wendel C, Becker HM, Deitmer JW. The sodium-bicarbonate cotransporter NBCe1 supports glutamine efflux via SNAT3 (SLC38A3) co-expressed in *Xenopus* oocytes. *Pflugers Arch.* 2008;455:885-893.

399. Wesson DE. Regulation of kidney acid excretion by endothelins. *Kidney Int.* 2006;70:2066-2073.

400. Westhoff CM, Ferreri-Jacobia M, Mak DO, et al. Identification of the erythrocyte Rh-blood group glycoprotein as a mammalian ammonium transporter. *J Biol Chem.* 2002;277:12499-12502.

401. Westhoff CM, Siegel DL, Burd CG, et al. Mechanism of genetic complementation of ammonium transport in yeast by human erythrocyte Rh-associated glycoprotein (RhAG). *J Biol Chem.* 2004;279:17443-17448.

402. Wilcox CS, Granges F, Kirk G, et al. Effects of saline infusion on titratable acid generation and ammonia secretion. *Am J Physiol.* 1984;247:F506-F519.

403. Windus DW, Cohn DE, Heifets M. Effects of fasting on citrate transport by the brush-border membrane of rat kidney. *Am J Physiol Renal Physiol.* 1986;251:F678-F682.

404. Wingo CS, Madsen KM, Smolka A, et al. H-K-ATPase immunoreactivity in cortical and outer medullary collecting duct. *Kidney Int.* 1990;38:985-990.

405. Winter C, Schulz N, Giebisch G, et al. Nongenomic stimulation of vacuolar H⁺-ATPases in intercalated renal tubule cells by aldosterone. *Proc Natl Acad Sci U S A.* 2004;101:2636-2641.

406. Wright PA, Knepper MA. Glutamate dehydrogenase activities in microdissected rat nephron segments: effects of acid-base loading. *Am J Physiol.* 1990;259:F53-F59.

407. Wright PA, Knepper MA. Phosphate-dependent glutaminase activity in rat renal cortical and medullary tubule segments. *Am J Physiol.* 1990;259:F961-F970.

408. Wrong O, Davies HE. The excretion of acid in renal disease. *Q J Med.* 1959;28:259-313.

409. Yang B, Song Y, Zhao D, et al. Phenotype analysis of aquaporin-8 null mice. *Am J Physiol Cell Physiol.* 2005;288:C1161-C1170.

410. Yang B, Zhao D, Solenov E, et al. Evidence from knockout mice against physiologically significant aquaporin 8–facilitated ammonia transport. *Am J Physiol Cell Physiol.* 2006;291:C417-C423.

411. Yip KP, Tsuruoka S, Schwartz GJ, et al. Apical H(+)/base transporters mediating bicarbonate absorption and pH(i) regulation in the OMCD. *Am J Physiol Renal Physiol.* 2002;283:F1098-F1104.

412. Yokoyama H, Anzai N, Ljubojevic M, et al. Functional and immunochemical characterization of a novel organic anion transporter Oat8 (Slc22a9) in rat renal collecting duct. *Cell Physiol Biochem.* 2008;21:269-278.

413. Yun CH, Oh S, Zizak M, et al. cAMP-mediated inhibition of the epithelial brush border Na⁺/H⁺ exchanger, NHE3, requires an associated regulatory protein. *Proc Natl Acad Sci U S A.* 1997;94:3010-3015.

414. Zajicek HK, Wang H, Puttaparthi K, et al. Glycosphingolipids modulate renal phosphate transport in potassium deficiency. *Kidney Int.* 2001;60:694-704.

415. Zhao J, Hogan EM, Bevensee MO, et al. Out-of-equilibrium CO₂/HCO₃⁻ solutions and their use in characterizing a new K/HCO₃ cotransporter. *Nature.* 1995;374:636-639.

416. Zheng W, Verlander JW, Cash M, et al. Cellular distribution of the potassium channel, KCNQ1, in normal mouse kidney. *Am J Physiol Renal Physiol.* 2007;292:F456-F466.

417. Zhou X, Lynch IJ, Xia SL, et al. Activation of H(+)-K(+)-ATPase by CO(2) requires a basolateral Ba(2+)-sensitive pathway during K restriction. *Am J Physiol Renal Physiol.* 2000;279:F153-F160.

418. Zhou Y, Boron WF. Role of endogenously secreted angiotensin II in the CO₂-induced stimulation of HCO₃ reabsorption by renal proximal tubules. *Am J Physiol Renal Physiol.* 2008;294:F245-F252.

419. Zhou Y, Bouyer P, Boron WF. Role of a tyrosine kinase in the CO₂-induced stimulation of HCO₃⁻ reabsorption by rabbit S2 proximal tubules. *Am J Physiol Renal Physiol.* 2006;291:F358-F367.

420. Zhou Y, Bouyer P, Boron WF. Role of the AT1A receptor in the CO₂-induced stimulation of HCO₃⁻ reabsorption by renal proximal tubules. *Am J Physiol Renal Physiol.* 2007;293:F110-F120.

421. Zhou Y, Zhao J, Bouyer P, et al. Evidence from renal proximal tubules that HCO₃⁻ and solute reabsorption are acutely regulated not by pH but by basolateral HCO₃⁻ and CO₂. *Proc Natl Acad Sci U S A.* 2005;102:3875-3880.

422. Zhu XL, Sly WS. Carbonic anhydrase IV from human lung: purification, characterization, and comparison with membrane carbonic anhydrase from human kidney. *J Biol Chem.* 1990;265:8795-8801.

423. Zidi-Yahiaoui N, Mouro-Chanteloup I, D'Ambrosio AM, et al. Human Rhesus B and Rhesus C glycoproteins: properties of facilitated ammonium transport in recombinant kidney cells. *Biochem J.* 2005;391:33-40.

Urine Concentration and Dilution

Jeff M. Sands, Harold E. Layton, and Robert A. Fenton

Independent Regulation of Water and Salt Excretion

The kidney is responsible for numerous homeostatic functions. For example, body fluid tonicity is tightly controlled by regulation of renal water excretion; extracellular fluid volume is controlled by regulated NaCl excretion; systemic acid-base balance is regulated via control of net acid excretion; systemic K^+ balance is controlled via regulated K^+ excretion; and the body maintains nitrogen balance through regulated urea excretion. The independent regulation of water and solute excretion is essential for the homeostatic functions of the kidney to be performed simultaneously. Essentially, this means that in the absence of changes in solute intake or of changes in metabolic production of waste solutes, the kidney is able to excrete different volumes of water in response to changes in water intake. This ability to excrete the appropriate amount of water without marked perturbations in solute excretion (i.e., without disturbing the other homeostatic functions of the kidney) is dependent on renal concentrating and diluting mechanisms, and its discussion forms the basis of this chapter (Figure 10-1). Renal water excretion is tightly regulated by the peptide hormone arginine vasopressin (antidiuretic hormone). Under normal circumstances, the circulating vasopressin level is determined by osmoreceptors in the hypothalamus that trigger increases in vasopressin secretion (by the posterior pituitary gland) when the osmolality of the blood rises above a threshold value, about 292 mOsm/kg H_2O. This mechanism can be modulated when other inputs to the hypothalamus (e.g., arterial underfilling, severe fatigue, or physical stress) override the osmotic mechanism. Upon an increase in plasma osmolality, vasopressin is secreted from the posterior pituitary gland into the peripheral plasma. The kidney responds to the variable vasopressin levels by varying urine flow (i.e., water excretion). For example, during extreme antidiuresis (high vasopressin levels), water excretion is greater than 100-fold lower than during major water diuresis (low vasopressin levels). These major changes in water excretion are obtained without substantial changes in steady-state solute excretion. This phenomenon is dependent on the kidney's ability to concentrate and dilute the urine. During low circulating vasopressin levels, urine osmolality is less than that of plasma (290 mOsm/kg H_2O)—the diluting function of the kidney. In contrast, when the circulating vasopressin levels are high, urine osmolality is much higher than that of plasma—the concentrating function of the kidney.

Criticality of the Parallel Organization of Structures in the Renal Medulla to the Urinary Concentrating and Diluting Processes

The kidney's ability to vary water excretion over a wide physiologic range without altering steady-state solute excretion cannot be explained as simply a consequence of the sequential

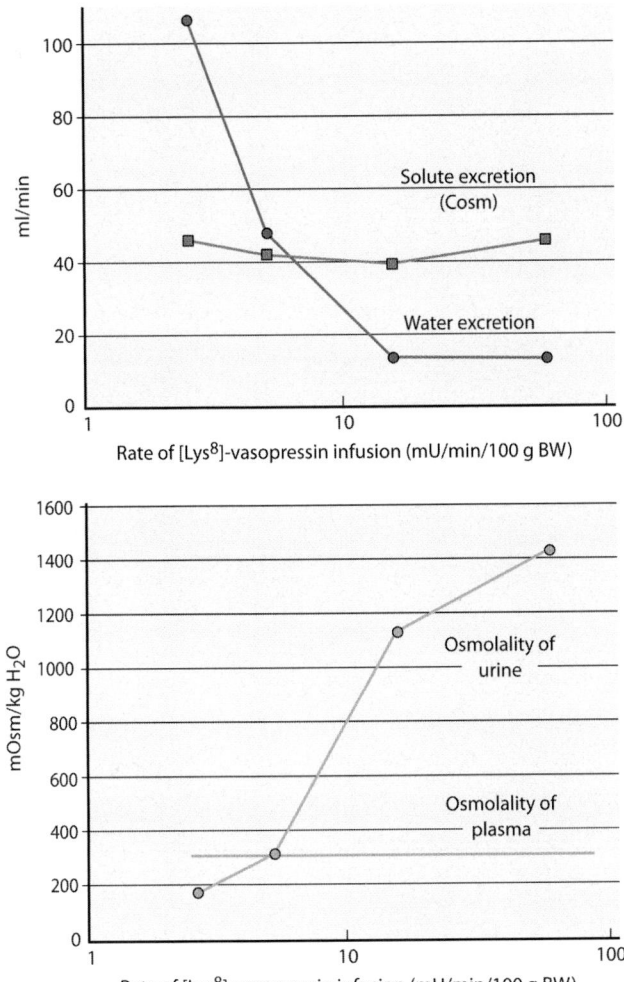

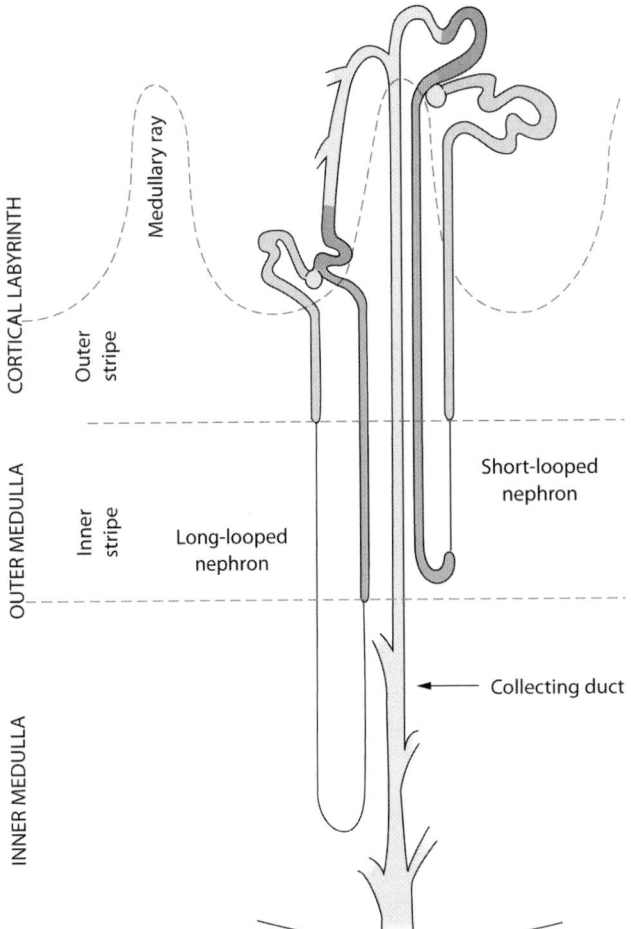

FIGURE 10-1 Steady-state renal response to varying rates of vasopressin infusion in conscious rats. A water load (4% of body weight) was maintained throughout the experiments to suppress endogenous vasopressin secretion. Although the urine flow rate was markedly reduced at higher vasopressin infusion rates, the osmolar clearance (solute excretion) changed little. In accordance with this, at higher vasopressin infusion rates, the osmolality of the urine increased significantly, whereas plasma osmolality remained constant. (Data from Atherton JC, Hai MA, Thomas S: The time course of changes in renal tissue composition during water diuresis in the rat, *J Physiol* 197:429-443, 1968.)

FIGURE 10-2 Mammalian renal structure. Major regions of the kidney are shown on the *left*. Configurations of a long-looped and a short-looped nephron are depicted. The major portions of the nephron are the proximal tubules (*medium blue*), thin limbs of the loops of Henle (*single line*), thick ascending limbs of the loops of Henle (*green*), distal convoluted tubules (*lavender*), and collecting duct system (*yellow*). (Modified from Knepper MA, Stephenson JL: Urinary concentrating and diluting processes. In Andreoli TE, Fanestil DD, Hoffman JF, et al, editors: *Physiology of membrane disorders,* ed 2, New York, 1986, Plenum, pp 713-726.)

transport processes along the nephron.[1] The independent regulation of water and sodium excretion occurs in the renal medulla, where the nephron segments and vasculature (vasa recta) are arranged in complex but specific anatomic relationships, both in terms of which segments connect to which segments and their three-dimensional configuration. Thus, it is necessary to consider the parallel interactions between nephron segments that occur as a result of the nephron's looped or hairpin structure. Figure 10-2 illustrates the regional architecture of the renal medulla and medullary rays.[2]

Renal Tubules

Loops of Henle

The kidney generally contains two populations of nephrons, long looped and short looped, which merge to form a common collecting duct system (see Figure 10-2). Both types of nephrons have loops of Henle that are arranged in a folded or hairpin configuration. Short-looped nephrons generally have glomeruli that are located more superficially in the cortex and have loops that bend in the outer medulla. Long-looped nephrons generally have glomeruli that are located more deeply within the cortex and have loops that bend at various levels of the inner medulla. Long-looped nephrons also contain a thin ascending limb, a segment that is not present in short-looped nephrons. Thin ascending limbs are found only in the inner medulla. The inner-outer medullary border is defined by the transition from thin to thick ascending limbs. Thus, the outer medulla contains only thick ascending limbs, regardless of the type of loop. The long-looped nephrons bend at various levels of the inner medulla from the inner-outer medullary border to the papillary tip. Thus, progressively fewer loops of Henle extend to deeper levels of the inner medulla. Some mammalian kidneys, such as human kidneys, also contain cortical nephrons, which are nephrons whose loops of Henle do not reach into the medulla.

The loops of Henle receive the tubular fluid from the proximal convoluted tubules. Tubular fluid exits the thick ascending limbs of both long- and short-looped nephrons, and from cortical nephrons in species that have them, and flows into distal convoluted tubules. Thus, the limbs of the loops of Henle have a countercurrent flow configuration and are composed of several different nephron segments (see Figure 10-2). The descending portion of the loop of Henle consists of the S2 proximal straight tubule in the medullary ray, the S3 proximal straight tubule (or pars recta) in the outer stripe of the outer medulla, and the thin descending limb in the inner stripe of the outer medulla and the inner medulla. The descending thin limb of short-looped nephrons differs structurally and functionally from the descending thin limb of long-looped nephrons.[3,4]

The location of the descending thin limb of short-looped nephrons within the outer medulla is illustrated in Figure 10-3 (labeled in green).[5] The descending thin limbs of short-looped nephrons surround the vascular bundles in the outer medulla and tend to be organized in a ring-like pattern (see Figure 10-3 *inset*). Thin descending limbs of long-looped nephrons in the outer medulla differ morphologically and functionally from thin descending limbs of long-looped nephrons in the inner medulla.[6-9] The histologic transition from the outer medullary to the inner medullary type of thin descending limbs of long-looped nephrons is gradual and often occurs at some distance into the inner medulla, rather than strictly at the inner-outer medullary border as is the case for the transition between thin and thick ascending limbs.

Pannabecker, Dantzler, and colleagues used immunohistochemical labeling and computer-assisted reconstruction to provide new detail about the functional architecture of the rat inner medulla (see recent review by Pannabecker and others.[10]). Figure 10-4 shows a computerized reconstruction of the inner medullary portion of several long-looped nephrons from rats that are labeled using antibodies to the water channel aquaporin-1 (AQP1, shown in red) and the kidney-specific chloride channel ClC-K1 (shown in green),[11] reviewed in Pannabecker and others.[10] AQP1 is a marker of the thin descending limb of a long-looped nephron in the outer medulla and is detected in the thin descending limb of a long-looped nephron in the inner medulla for a variable distance. However, AQP1 was not found in thin descending limbs of loops of Henle that turn within the upper first millimeter of the inner medulla. Correspondingly, Zhai and colleagues determined that AQP1 was not detectable along the entire length of thin descending limbs of short-looped nephrons.[12] In contrast, thin descending limbs of loops of Henle that turn below the first millimeter have three discernible functional subsegments: the upper 40% expresses AQP1, whereas the lower 60% do not. ClC-K1 is a marker of the thin ascending limb–type epithelium. It is first detected in the final approximately 165 μm of the thin descending limb, as well as the contiguous thin ascending limb. Thus, ClC-K1 is detected before the bend of the loops of Henle, which is consistent with several morphologic studies demonstrating that the descending limb to ascending limb transition occurs before the loop bend. A substantial portion of the inner medullary thin descending limb of long-looped nephrons do not express either AQP1 or ClC-K1, as indicated in gray.

Pannabecker and colleagues have also found evidence for mixed descending- and ascending-type thin limbs of the loops of Henle in the inner medulla.[13] The ascending portion of the loops of Henle consists of the thin ascending limbs (which are present only in long-looped nephrons), the medullary thick ascending limbs in the inner stripe of the outer medulla, and

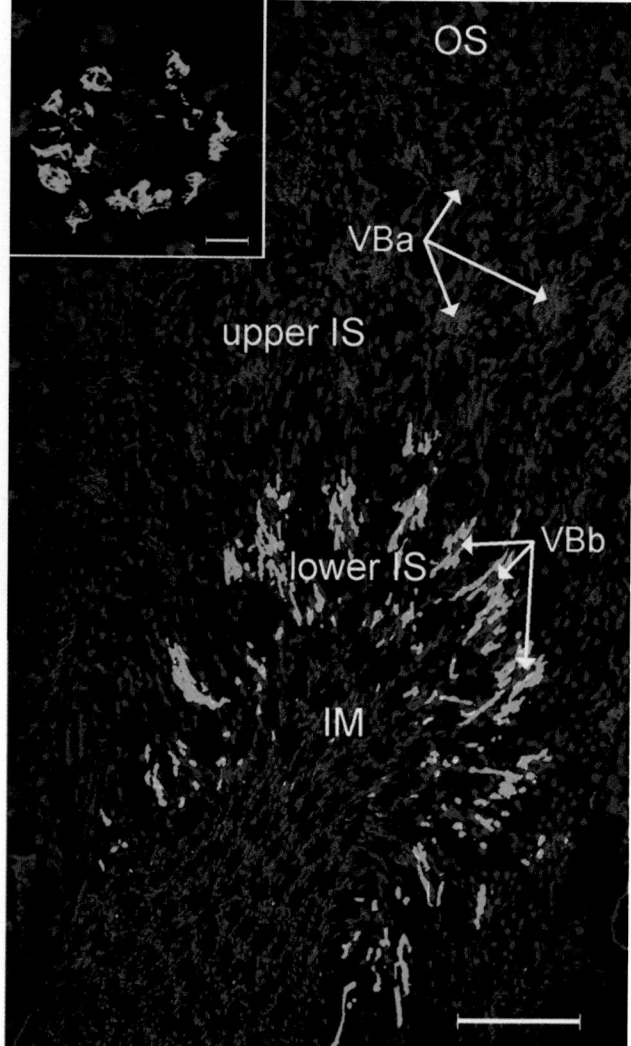

FIGURE 10-3 Triple immunolabeling of rat renal medulla showing localization of the urea transporter UT-A2 (*green*), marking the late thin descending limbs from short-looped nephrons; von Willebrand factor (*blue*), marking the endothelial cells of vasa recta; and aquaporin-1 (*red*), marking the thin descending limbs from outer medullary long-looped nephrons and early short-looped nephrons. *Inset* shows a cross section of a vascular bundle demonstrating that UT-A2-positive thin descending limbs from short-looped nephrons surround the vascular bundles in the deep part of the outer medulla. IM, Inner medulla; IS, inner stripe of outer medulla; OS, outer stripe of outer medulla; VBa, vascular bundles in outer part of inner stripe; VBb, vascular bundles in inner part of inner stripe. (From Wade JB, Lee AJ, Liu J, et al: UT-A2: a 55 kDa urea transporter protein in thin descending limb of Henle's loop whose abundance is regulated by vasopressin, *Am J Physiol Renal Physiol* 278:F52-F62, 2000.)

the cortical thick ascending limbs in the outer stripe of the outer medulla and medullary rays.

Distal Tubule Segments in the Cortical Labyrinth

After tubular fluid exits the loop of Henle through the cortical thick ascending limb, it enters the distal convoluted tubule within the cortical labyrinth. In most mammalian species, several distal tubules merge to form a connecting tubule arcade.[14] The connecting tubule cells express both the vasopressin-regulated water channel AQP2, and the type 2 vasopressin receptor (V_2R),[15] which suggests that the arcades are sites of vasopressin-regulated water reabsorption, similar to the

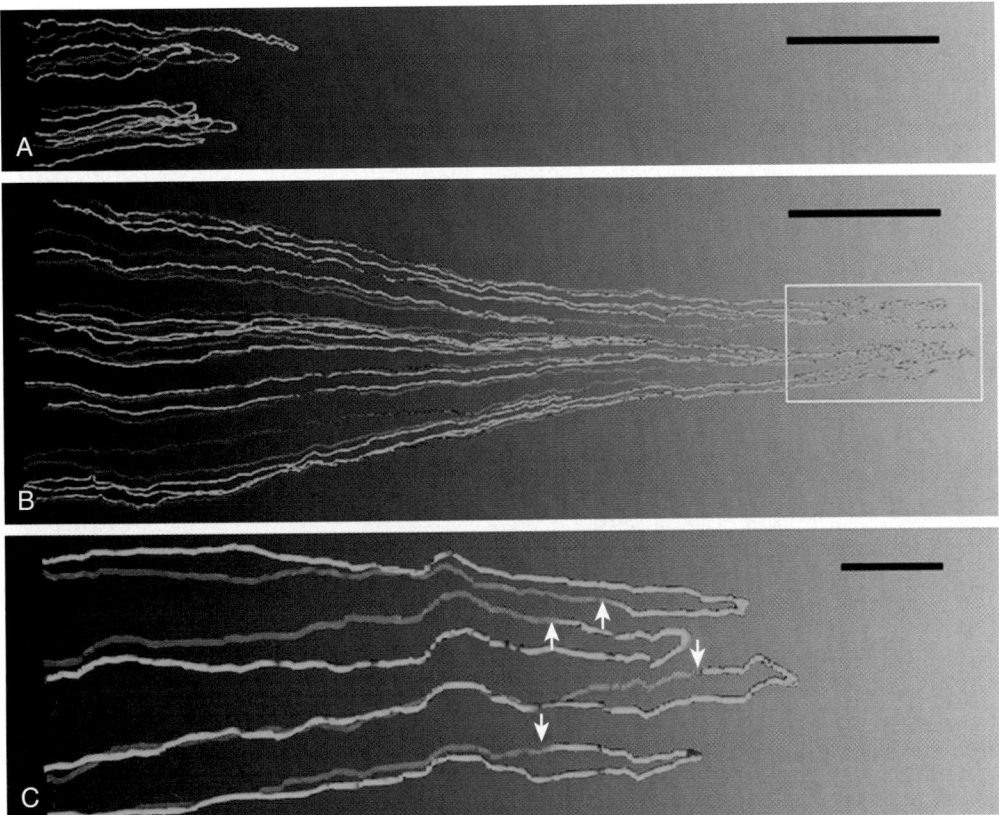

FIGURE 10-4 Computer-assisted reconstruction of loops of Henle from rat inner medulla showing expression of aquaporin-1 (AQP1; *red*) and the chloride channel ClC-K1 (*green*); gray regions (β-crystallin) express undetectable levels of AQP1 and ClC-K1. Loops are oriented along the corticopapillary axis, with the *left* edge of each image nearer the base of the inner medulla. **A,** Thin limbs that have their bends within the first millimeter beyond the outer-inner medullary boundary. Descending segments lack detectable AQP1. ClC-K1 is expressed continuously along the prebend segment and the thin ascending limb. **B,** Loops that have their bends beyond the first millimeter of the inner medulla. AQP1 is expressed along the initial 40% of each thin descending limb and is absent from the remainder of each loop. ClC-K1 is expressed continuously along the prebend segment and the thin ascending limb. **C,** Enlargement of near-bend regions of four thin limbs in box in **B.** ClC-K1 expression, corresponding to the thin descending limb prebend segment, begins, on average, 165 μm before the loop bend (*arrows*). Scale bars equal 500 μm in **A** and **B** and 100 μm in **C.** (From Pannabecker TL, Dantzler WH, Layton HE, et al: Role of three-dimensional architecture in the urine concentrating mechanism of the rat renal inner medulla, *Am J Physiol Renal Physiol* 295:F1271-F1285, 2008.)

collecting ducts (see later). Tubule fluid exits the connecting tubules within the arcades, enters the initial collecting tubules in the superficial cortex, and from thence flows into the cortical collecting ducts. In most rodent species studied, several nephrons merge to form a single cortical collecting duct.[3,16]

Collecting Duct System

The collecting duct system spans all regions of the kidney, starting in the cortex and running to the tip of the inner medulla (see Figure 10-2). The collecting ducts are arranged in parallel to the loops of Henle in the medullary rays, outer medulla, and inner medulla. Like the loops of Henle, the collecting duct system contains several morphologically and functionally discrete segments. In general, the collecting ducts descend straight through the medullary rays and outer medulla without joining with other collecting ducts. However, several collecting ducts merge as they descend within the inner medulla, which leads to a progressive reduction in the number of inner medullary collecting ducts (IMCDs) from the inner-outer medullary border to the papillary tip.[16] The tapered structure of the renal papilla results from the reduction in collecting duct number, accompanied by a progressive reduction in the number of loops of Henle, reaching the deepest levels of the inner medulla.

Detailed studies of inner medullary structure, both by Kriz and colleagues[17-20] and more recently by Pannabecker, Dantzler, and others,[11,21-23] find that the IMCDs in the inner medullary base (initial IMCDs), form clusters that coalesce along the corticomedullary axis. The thin descending limbs are predominantly present at the periphery of these clusters and appear to form an asymmetric ring around each collecting duct cluster, whereas the thin ascending limbs are distributed relatively uniformly among the collecting ducts and thin descending limbs.[22]

Pannabecker and Dantzler[21] identified three population groups of loops of Henle in Munich-Wistar rats, distinguished by the position of the thin ascending limb at the base of the inner medulla and by differing loop length (Figure 10-5). Group 1 loops have thin ascending limbs that are interposed between collecting ducts and reach a mean length of 700 μm into the inner medulla. Group 2 loops have thin ascending limbs that are adjacent to just one collecting duct and reach a mean length of 1500 μm. Group 3 loops have thin ascending limbs that lie more than 0.5 tubule diameters from a collecting duct and reach a mean length of 2200 μm. As the collecting ducts coalesce and the shorter loops of Henle disappear, the originating portions of the longer thin ascending limbs run alongside the collecting ducts for a substantial distance.[21]

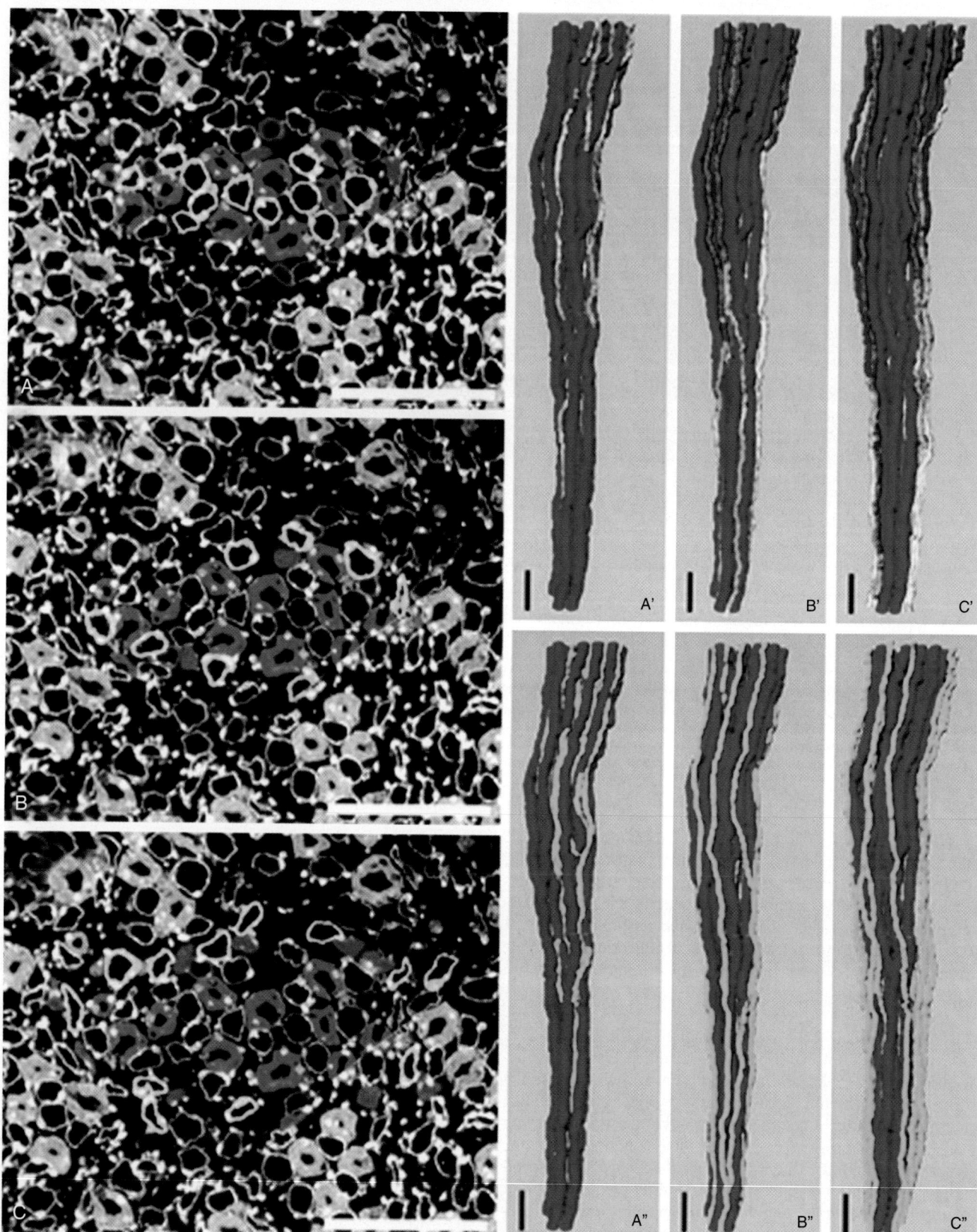

FIGURE 10-5 Spatial relationships between thin descending limbs (*red tubules*), thin ascending limbs (*green tubules*), and collecting ducts (*dark blue tubules*). Thin ascending limbs were categorized into three groups related to their lateral proximity to collecting ducts. Members of each group are shown in a transverse section located at the base of the inner medulla. **A,** Group 1. **B,** Group 2. **C,** Group 3. In panels **A** through **C,** *open red figures* represent aquaporin-1 (AQP1)–null thin descending limbs, *solid red figures* represent AQP1-expressing thin descending limbs, *white outlined figures* represent thin ascending limbs not associated with the collecting duct cluster, and *light blue figures* represent collecting ducts not associated with the collecting duct cluster. Two prebend segments from group 1 are included in **A.** One thin ascending limb from each of groups 2 and 3 (**B** and **C**) extends below the region of reconstruction, and their thin descending limbs were therefore not reconstructed. **A′, B′,** and **C′** show thin descending limbs and collecting ducts. **A″, B″,** and **C″** show thin ascending limbs and collecting ducts. *Gray tubules* in **A′, B′,** and **C′** represent AQP1-null thin descending limbs. Scale bars equal 100 µm. (From Pannabecker TL, Dantzler WH: Three-dimensional lateral and vertical relationships of inner medullary loops of Henle and collecting ducts, *Am J Physiol Renal Physiol* 287:F767-F774, 2004.)

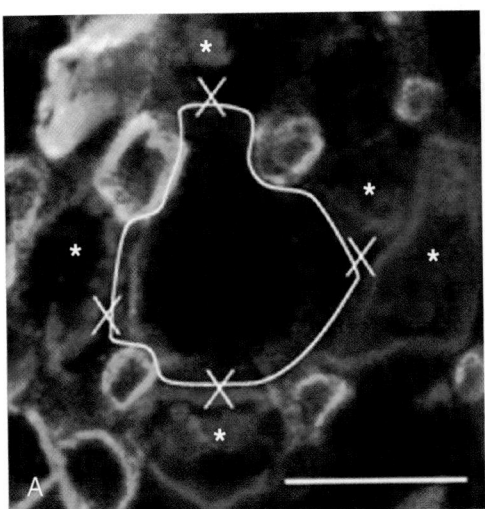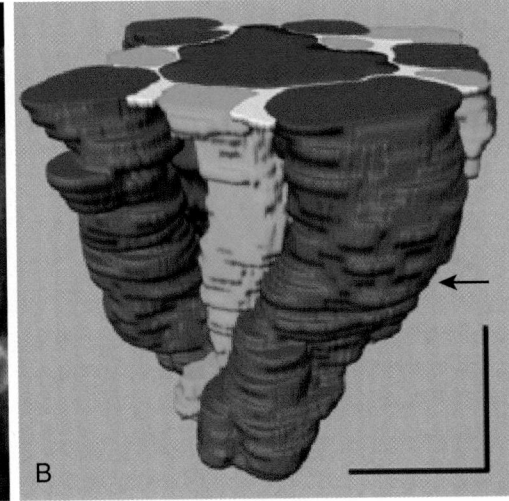

FIGURE 10-6 A, Interstitial nodal spaces (marked with *X*) surrounding one collecting duct in the outer zone of the inner medulla. *Red,* Thin ascending limb Cl channel (ClC-K1). *Green,* Ascending vasa recta/plasmalemmal vesicle protein 1 (PV-1). *Aqua,* Aquaporin-1 (AQP1)–positive thin descending limb. Approximate outer border of collecting duct, determined from autofluorescence and tubule dimensions, is outlined in *white. Asterisks* denote thin ascending limbs and prebend segments that make contact with interstitial nodal space. Confocal optical section from tissue slice dissected from approximately 1 mm below the outer-inner medullary boundary is shown. The image illustrates a configuration in which an AQP1-positive thin descending limb lies near thin ascending limbs associated with the nodal spaces. **B,** Three-dimensional reconstruction illustrating approximate interstitial nodal spaces (*white;* shown for the *top*most transverse section only) surrounding a single collecting duct in the outer zone of the inner medulla. Reconstruction was assembled from thirty-six 2-µm-thick confocal optical sections (same tissue as in **A**). *Black arrow* marks axial level of section shown in **A**. *Red,* ClC-K1; *green,* PV-1; *blue,* collecting duct estimated from autofluorescence and tubule dimensions. Scale bars equal 30 µm. (From Pannabecker TL: Loop of Henle interaction with interstitial nodal spaces in the renal inner medulla, *Am J Physiol Renal Physiol* 295:F1744-F1751, 2008.)

Vasculature

The major blood vessels that carry blood into and out of the renal medulla are named the *vasa recta*. Blood enters the descending vasa recta from the efferent arterioles of juxtamedullary nephrons and supplies it to the capillary plexuses at each level of the medulla. The outer medullary capillary plexus is considerably more dense and much better perfused than the plexus in the inner medulla.[24] Blood from the inner medullary capillary plexus feeds into ascending vasa recta (ascending vasa recta are never formed directly from descending vasa recta in a looplike structure.) Inner medullary ascending vasa recta traverse the inner stripe of the outer medulla in close physical association with the descending vasa recta in vascular bundles.[17] In many animal species, thin descending limbs of short-looped nephrons surround the vascular bundles, as shown in Figure 10-3. In the figure the thin descending limb segments are labeled with an antibody to the UT-A2 urea transporter,[5] which suggests a route for urea recycling from the vasa recta to the thin descending limbs of short-looped nephrons. The outer medullary capillary plexus is drained by vasa recta that ascend through the outer stripe of the outer medulla, separate from the descending vasa recta.[20]

The counterflow arrangement of vasa recta in the medulla promotes countercurrent exchange of solutes and water. This exchange is abetted by the presence of AQP1 water channels[25,26] and UT-B urea transporters[27,28] in the endothelial cells of the descending portion of the vasa recta. Countercurrent exchange provides a means of reducing the effective blood flow to the medulla while maintaining a high absolute perfusion rate.[29] The low effective blood flow that results from countercurrent exchange is thought to be important for the preservation of solute concentration gradients in the medullary tissue (see later).

In contrast to the medulla, the cortical labyrinth has a high effective blood flow. The rapid vascular perfusion to this region promotes the rapid return of solutes and water reabsorbed from the nephron to the general circulation. The rapid perfusion is thought to maintain the interstitial concentrations of most solutes at levels close to those in the peripheral plasma. The medullary rays of the cortex have a capillary plexus that is considerably sparser than that of the cortical labyrinth. Consequently, the effective blood flow to the medullary rays has been postulated to be lower than that of the cortical labyrinth.[1]

Medullary Interstitium

The renal medullary interstitium connects the tubules and vasculature (Figure 10-6).[30] It is a complex space that includes the medullary interstitial cells, microfibrils, extracellular matrix, and fluid.[30,31] The interstitium is relatively small in volume in the outer medulla and the outer portion of the inner medulla, which may be important in limiting the diffusion of solutes upward along the medullary axis.[1,22,30] In contrast, the interstitial space is much larger in the inner half of the inner medulla.[1,22,30] Within this region, it consists of a gelatinous matrix containing large amounts of highly polymerized hyaluronic acid, consisting of alternating *N*-acetyl-D-glucosamine and D-glucuronate moieties.[32] Recently, theories have been proposed in which the hyaluronic acid interstitial matrix plays a direct role in the generation of an inner medullary osmotic gradient through its ability to store and transduce energy from the smooth muscle contractions of the renal pelvis.[32]

Renal Pelvis

Urine exits the collecting duct system through the ducts of Bellini at the papillary tip and enters the renal pelvis (Figure 10-7). The renal pelvis (or calyx in multipapillate kidneys) is

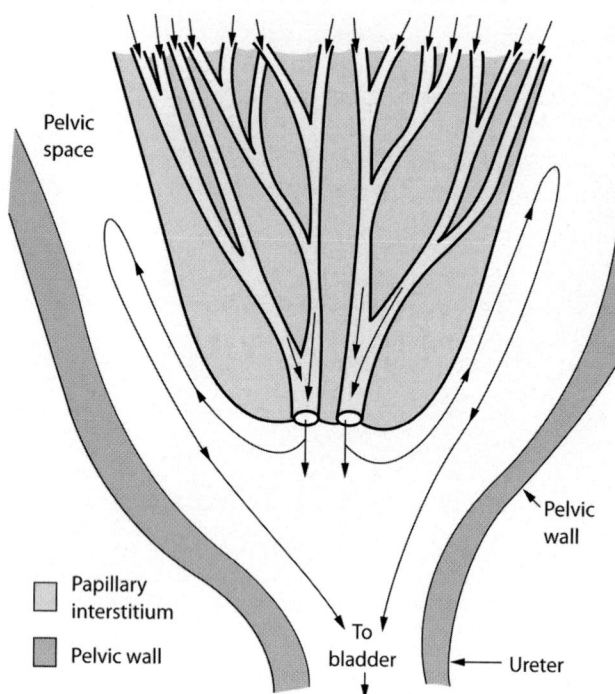

FIGURE 10-7 Pattern of urine flow in papillary collecting ducts and renal pelvis. Urine exits the papillary collecting ducts (ducts of Bellini) at the tip of the renal papilla and is carried to the urinary bladder by the ureter. (Compare with Figure 10-9.) Under some circumstances, a fraction of the urine may reflux backward in the pelvic space and contact the outer surface of the renal papilla. Solute and water exchange across the papillary surface epithelium has been postulated (see text).

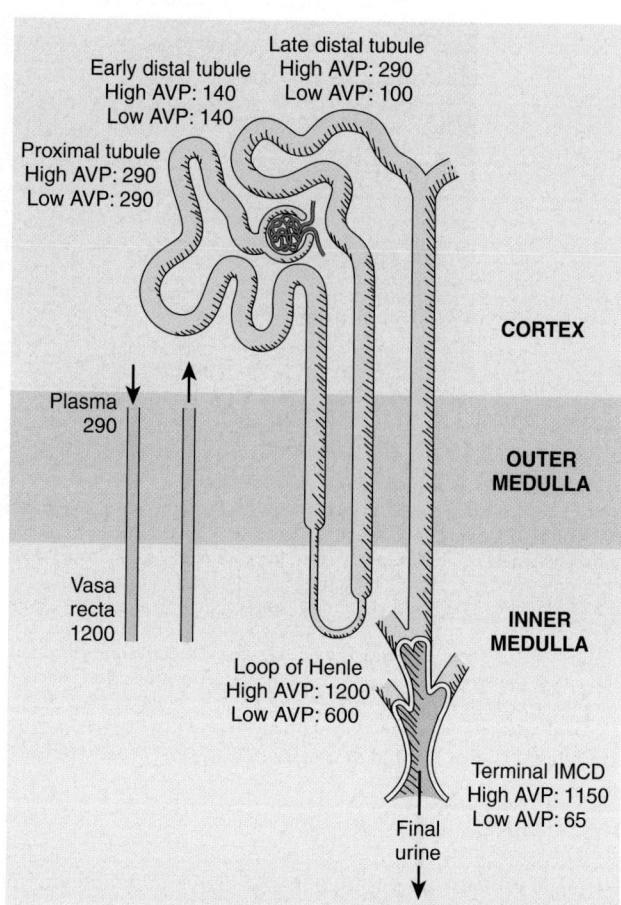

FIGURE 10-8 Typical osmolalities (in milliosmoles per kilogram H_2O) found in various vascular (**left**) and renal tubule (**right**) sites in rat kidneys. Fluid in the proximal tubule is always isosmotic with plasma (290 mOsm/kg H_2O). Fluid emerging from the loop of Henle (entering the early distal tubule) is always hypotonic. Osmolality in the late distal tubule increases to plasma levels only during antidiuresis. Final urine is hypertonic when the circulating vasopressin level is high and hypotonic when the vasopressin level is low. A high osmolality is always maintained in the loop of Henle and vasa recta. During antidiuresis, osmolalities in all inner medullary structures are nearly equal. Osmolalities are somewhat attenuated in the loop and vasa recta during water diuresis (not shown). (Based on results of micropuncture studies; see text.)

a complex intrarenal urinary space that surrounds the papilla. The renal pelvis (or calyx) has portions that extend into the outer medulla, which are called *fornices* and *secondary pouches*. Although a transitional epithelium lines most of the pelvic space, the renal parenchyma is separated from the pelvic space by a simple cuboidal epithelium.[33] It has been proposed that water and solute transport could occur across this epithelium, thereby modifying the composition of the renal medullary interstitial fluid.[34] There are two smooth muscle layers within the renal pelvic (calyceal) wall.[35] Contractions of these smooth muscle layers generate powerful peristaltic waves that appear to displace the renal papilla downward with a "milking" action.[36] These peristaltic waves may intermittently propel urine along the collecting ducts. The contractions compress all structures within the renal inner medulla, including the interstitium, loops of Henle, vasa recta, and collecting ducts.[37] According to some theories, these contractions furnish part of the energy for concentrating solutes, and hence concentrating urine, within the inner medulla,[32] as discussed later.

Urine Concentration and Dilution Processes along the Mammalian Nephron

Sites of Urine Concentration and Dilution

Micropuncture studies of the mammalian nephron have determined the major sites of tubule fluid concentration and dilution (Figure 10-8). Proximal tubule fluid is always isosmotic with plasma, regardless of whether the kidney is diluting or concentrating the urine.[38] In contrast, the fluid in the early distal convoluted tubule is always hypotonic, regardless of the final osmolality of the urine. Indeed, during antidiuresis and water diuresis the earliest tubule segment in which significant differences in tubule fluid osmolality can be detected is the late distal tubule. During antidiuresis, the tubule fluid of this segment becomes isosmotic with plasma. However, during water diuresis the tubule fluid remains hypotonic. During antidiuresis, the tubule fluid osmolality between the late distal tubule and the IMCDs rises to a level greater than that of plasma. However, during water diuresis it remains hypotonic. Thus, the conclusion from micropuncture studies is that the loop of Henle is the major site of dilution of tubule fluid and that dilution processes in the loop occur regardless of whether the final urine is dilute or concentrated. Further dilution of the tubule fluid can occur in the collecting ducts during water diuresis.[39] In contrast, the chief site of urine concentration is beyond the distal tubule (i.e., in the collecting duct system). The mechanisms of urinary dilution and of urinary concentration are discussed in the following sections.

Mechanism of Tubule Fluid Dilution

Micropuncture studies in rats have shown that the fluid in the early distal tubule is hypotonic, due chiefly to a reduction in luminal NaCl concentration relative to that in the proximal tubule.[40] The low luminal NaCl concentration could result either from active NaCl reabsorption from the loop of Henle or from water secretion into the loop of Henle. Micropuncture measurements in rats performed using inulin as a volume marker demonstrated net water reabsorption from the superficial loops of Henle during antidiuresis, which rules out water secretion as a potential mechanism of tubule fluid dilution.[41] Thus, one can conclude that luminal dilution occurs because of NaCl reabsorption from the loops of Henle in excess of water reabsorption. Classic studies of isolated perfused rabbit thick ascending limbs established the mechanism of tubule fluid dilution.[42,43] NaCl is rapidly reabsorbed by active transport, which lowers the luminal osmolality and NaCl concentration to levels below those in the peritubular fluid. The osmotic water permeability of the thick ascending limb is very low, which prevents dissipation of the transepithelial osmolality gradient by water flux.

The tubule fluid remains hypotonic throughout the distal tubule and collecting duct system during water diuresis, aided by the low osmotic water permeability of the collecting ducts when circulating levels of vasopressin are low. Even though the tubule fluid remains hypotonic in the collecting duct system, the solute composition of the tubule fluid is modified within the collecting duct, chiefly by Na+ absorption and K+ secretion. Active NaCl reabsorption from the collecting duct results in a further dilution of the collecting duct fluid beyond that achieved in the thick ascending limbs.[39]

Mechanism of Tubule Fluid Concentration

When circulating vasopressin levels are high, net water absorption occurs between the late distal tubule and the collecting ducts.[41] The reader is referred to Chapter 11 for a detailed discussion of the cell biology of vasopressin action. Since water is absorbed in excess of solutes, with a resulting rise in osmolality along the collecting ducts toward the papillary tip,[44] it can be concluded that collecting duct fluid is concentrated chiefly by water absorption, rather than by solute addition.

An axial osmolality gradient in the renal medullary tissue, with the highest degree of hypertonicity at the papillary tip, provides the osmotic driving force for water absorption along the collecting ducts. This osmolality gradient was initially reported by Wirz and colleagues.[45] In a classic study, they demonstrated, in rats in an antidiuretic state, the existence of a continuously increasing osmolality gradient along the outer and inner medulla, with the highest osmolality in the deepest part of the inner medulla, the papillary tip. In addition, within the medulla the osmolality of the collecting ducts was as high as that in the loops of Henle, and the osmolality of vasa recta blood, sampled from near the papillary tip, was virtually equal to that of the final urine.[45] Taken together these results demonstrated that the high tissue osmolality was not simply a manifestation of a high osmolality in a single structure, namely, the collecting duct. Micropuncture studies by Gottschalk and Mylle[38] confirmed that the osmolality of the fluid in the loops of Henle, the vasa recta, and the collecting ducts is approximately the same (see Figure 10-8), which supports

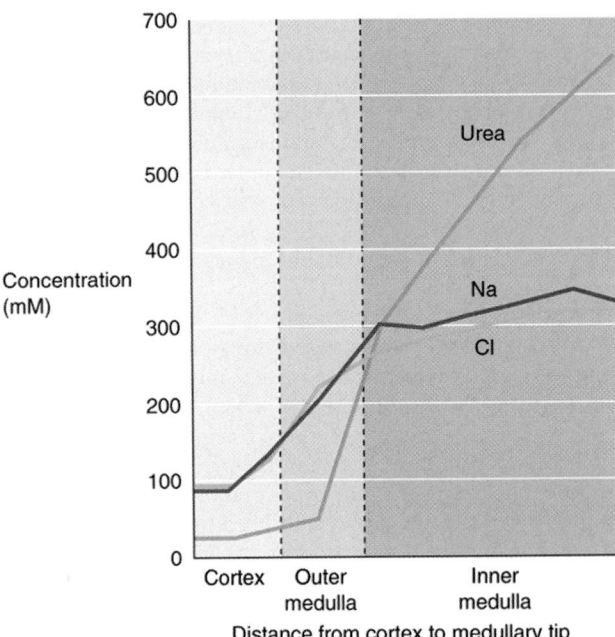

FIGURE 10-9 Corticomedullary gradients of urea, sodium, and chloride in kidneys of dogs in an antidiuretic state. Summary of data from Jarausch and Ullrich.[48] (From Giebisch G, Windhager EE: Urine concentration and dilution. In Boron WF, Boulpaep EL, editors: *Medical physiology,* Philadelphia, 2006, Saunders, pp 828-844.)

the hypothesis that the collecting duct fluid is concentrated by osmotic equilibration with a hypertonic medullary interstitium. Furthermore, in vitro studies demonstrated that collecting ducts have a high water permeability in the presence of vasopressin,[46,47] as is required for osmotic equilibration. The mechanism by which the corticomedullary osmolality gradient is generated is considered later.

Although the final axial osmolality gradient within the renal medulla is due to the combined gradients of several individual solutes, as initially demonstrated by Jarausch and Ullrich[48] using tissue slice analysis (Figure 10-9), the principal solutes responsible for the osmolality gradient are NaCl and urea. The increase in the NaCl concentration gradient along the corticomedullary axis occurs predominantly in the outer medulla, with only a small increase in the inner medulla. In contrast, the increase in urea concentration occurs predominantly in the inner medulla, with little or no increase in the initial outer medulla. The mechanisms for generating the NaCl gradient in the outer medulla and urea accumulation in the inner medulla are discussed in the following sections.

Generation of the Axial NaCl Gradient in the Renal Outer Medulla

A sustained osmolality gradient is maintained along the corticomedullary axis of the outer medulla (see Figure 10-9). That gradient, which is present in both diuresis and antidiuresis,[49] arises mostly from an accumulation of NaCl. The gradient is generated by the concentrating mechanism of the outer medulla. General considerations circumscribe the nature of that mechanism. Because the axial osmolality gradient is present in both diuresis and antidiuresis (in which the outer medullary collecting duct is water permeable to varying degrees), the accumulation of NaCl in the outer medulla cannot depend on a sustained osmolality difference across the collecting duct epithelium. Thus, the concentrating mechanism must depend on the loops of Henle, on the vasculature, and on their interactions within the outer medulla. Moreover, mass balance of water and NaCl must be maintained; thus, for example, concentrated fluid that flows into the inner medulla must be balanced by dilute fluid that flows into the cortex.

It has long been believed that the osmolality gradient of the outer medulla is generated by means of countercurrent multiplication of a single effect ("Vervielfältigung des Einzeleffektes"). In this paradigm, proposed by Kuhn and Ryffel in 1942,[50] osmotic pressure is raised along parallel but opposing flows in nearby tubes that are made contiguous by a hairpin turn (Figure 10-10): a transfer of solute from one tubule to another (i.e., a single effect) would augment (multiply), or reinforce, the osmotic pressure in the parallel flows. Thus, by means of the countercurrent configuration, a small transverse osmotic difference would be multiplied into a relatively large difference along the axes of flow. In support of this paradigm, Kuhn and Ryffel provided both a mathematical model and an apparatus that exemplified countercurrent multiplication.

As anatomic and physiologic understanding of the renal medulla increased, the countercurrent multiplication paradigm was reinterpreted and modified. In 1951, Hargitay and Kuhn[51] put the paradigm in the context of specific renal tubules. The loop of Henle was identified with the parallel tubes joined by a hairpin turn. Thus, the loops of Henle were proposed as the source of the outer medullary gradient, and that gradient was hypothesized to draw water out of water-permeable collecting ducts. In 1959, Kuhn and Ramel[52] used a mathematical model to show that active transport of NaCl from thick ascending limbs could serve as the single effect. Subsequent physiologic experiments confirmed the active NaCl transport and the osmotic absorption of water from collecting ducts.[41-44] Experiments indicating high water

permeability in hamster descending limbs of short loops[53] and in descending limbs of long loops[6,7,9] suggested that the accumulation of NaCl from thick limbs concentrated descending limb tubular fluid by osmotic water withdrawal, rather than by NaCl addition (see Figure 10-10).

In recent years doubts have arisen about whether the paradigm of countercurrent multiplication provides an accurate representation of the means by which the gradient is generated in the mammalian outer medulla. Several weaknesses have been noted:

1. The descending limbs of short loops are anatomically separated from ascending limbs, with inner stripe portions of short loops near (or within) the vascular bundles and thick limbs near the collecting ducts.[17,54] This configuration is not consistent with direct interactions between counterflowing limbs.

2. In short-looped rat nephrons, Wade and colleagues[5] found that AQP1 is not expressed in portions of descending limb segments in the distal inner stripe. Zhai and others[12] found that AQP1 is not expressed in descending limbs of short loops in the inner stripes of mice, rats, and humans. The absence of AQP1 suggests that the assumption of high water permeability in descending limbs of short loops merits further experimental study. (Dantzler and others[55] have found that the AQP1-null segments of descending limbs in the inner medulla are essentially impermeable to water.)

3. Using transport rates based on measured Na$^+$–K$^+$–adenosine triphosphatase (ATPase) activities, mathematical models predict substantial transepithelial NaCl gradients along the medullary portions of thick limbs.[56] This seems contrary to the notion of a small single effect.

4. It may well be that the concentrating mechanism of the outer medulla is placed under increased load, not less, if it has to concentrate water flowing in, and absorbed from, the descending limbs of short loops.[57]

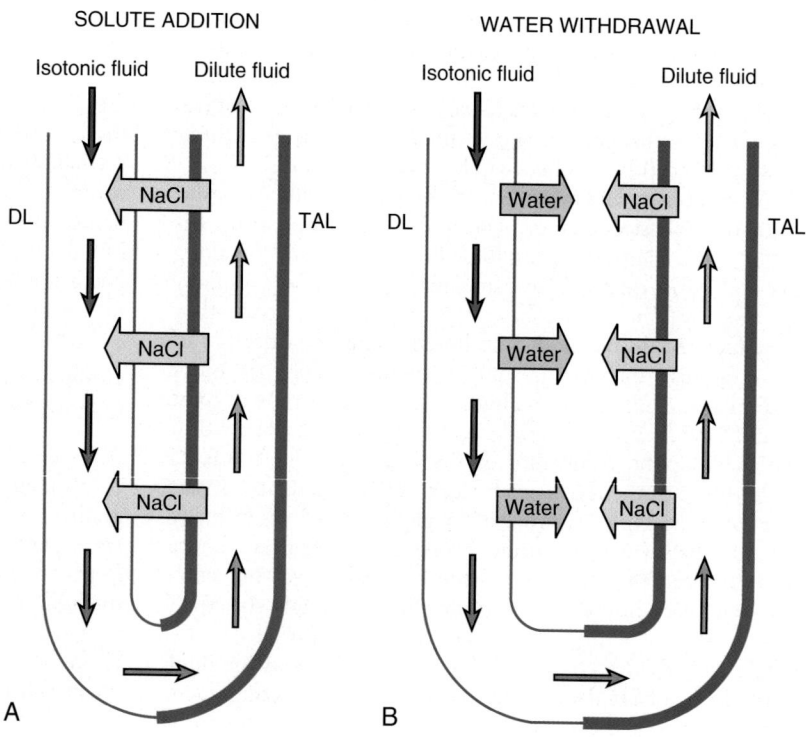

FIGURE 10-10 **A,** Countercurrent multiplication by means of NaCl transfer from an ascending flow to a descending flow. **B,** Countercurrent multiplication by means of water withdrawal from a descending flow. NaCl transport from the ascending flow into the interstitium raises interstitial osmolality; this results in passive water transport from the descending flow, which has lower osmolality than the interstitium. In both panels, tubular fluid flow direction is indicated by *blue arrows*; increasing osmolality is indicated by *darkening shades of blue*. Ascending flow may be considered to be in the thick ascending limb of the loop of Henle (TAL) and descending flow in the descending limb of Henle (DL). *Thick blue lines* indicate that a tubule is impermeable to water; *thin lines* indicate high permeability to water.

5. The absorption of water from the outer medullary portions of long loops has sometimes been considered to participate in a generalized form of countercurrent multiplication, and this may be the case for long loops that extend for sufficiently short distances into the inner medulla. In sufficiently long loops, however, tubular fluid is likely to be much altered by urea secretion and passive NaCl absorption within the inner medulla.

From these considerations, it seems reasonable, therefore, to hypothesize that the outer medullary osmolality gradient arises principally from vigorous active transport of NaCl, without accompanying water, from the thick ascending limbs of short- and long-looped nephrons. The tubular fluid of the thick limbs that enters the cortex is diluted well below plasma osmolality, and thus the requirement of mass balance is met. In rats and mice, the thick limbs are localized near the collecting ducts[58]; mathematical models suggest that at a given level of the outer medulla, the interstitial osmolality will be higher near the collecting ducts than near the vascular bundles.[56,57] This higher osmolality will facilitate water withdrawal from the descending limbs of long loops and from collecting ducts. Descending vasa recta are thought to be found only in the vascular bundles. Thus, the ascending vasa recta will collect water that is absorbed from the collecting ducts and from the descending limbs of long loops of Henle.

The countercurrent configuration of the ascending vasa recta, relative to the descending limbs and collecting ducts, is likely to aid in sustaining the axial gradient: as ascending vasa recta fluid rises toward the cortex, its osmolality will exceed that in the descending limbs of long loops and in the collecting ducts. Thus, ascending vasa recta fluid will be progressively diluted as that fluid contributes to the concentrating of fluid in descending limbs of long loops and in collecting ducts by giving up NaCl to, and absorbing water from, the interstitium (Figure 10-11).

The previous summary appears to account for the elevation of osmolality in the outer medulla without invoking a role for countercurrent multiplication. However, a question remains: Why does the osmolality gradient increase along the outer medulla as a function of increasing medullary depth? The answer likely lies in the local balance of NaCl absorption from thick limbs and water absorption from descending limbs of long loops and from collecting ducts. The rate of NaCl absorption from thick limbs may be higher at deeper medullary levels than at shallow levels, owing to a higher Na$^+$-K$^+$-ATPase activity at deeper levels[59] and to a saturation of transport proteins by the higher NaCl concentration in thick limb tubular fluid before dilution. Moreover, because of the water already absorbed in the upper outer medulla, the load of water presented to the thick limbs deep in the outer medulla by descending limbs of long loops and by the collecting ducts is much reduced.

Finally, a caveat is in order. Our understanding of the outer medulla is mostly based on information obtained from heavily studied laboratory animals, especially rats and mice. Outer medullary function and structure are likely to vary substantially in other species. For example, the human kidney has limited concentrating capability (relative to many other mammals) and only about one seventh of the loops of Henle are long[60]; the mountain beaver (*Aplodontia rufa*) has mostly cortical loops of Henle and essentially no inner medulla.[61] It seems likely that the outer medullary structure in these species differs substantially from that in rats and mice.

Accumulation of Urea in the Renal Inner Medulla

Urea accumulation within the inner medulla is dependent on variable urea permeabilities along the collecting duct system (Figure 10-12). Within the collecting duct system, only the terminal part of the IMCD possesses high urea permeability,[62] which can be further increased by acute vasopressin exposure.[47,63,64] This action of vasopressin is mediated (at least in part) by cyclic adenosine monophosphate (cAMP).[65] Specialized urea transporter proteins in the apical and basolateral

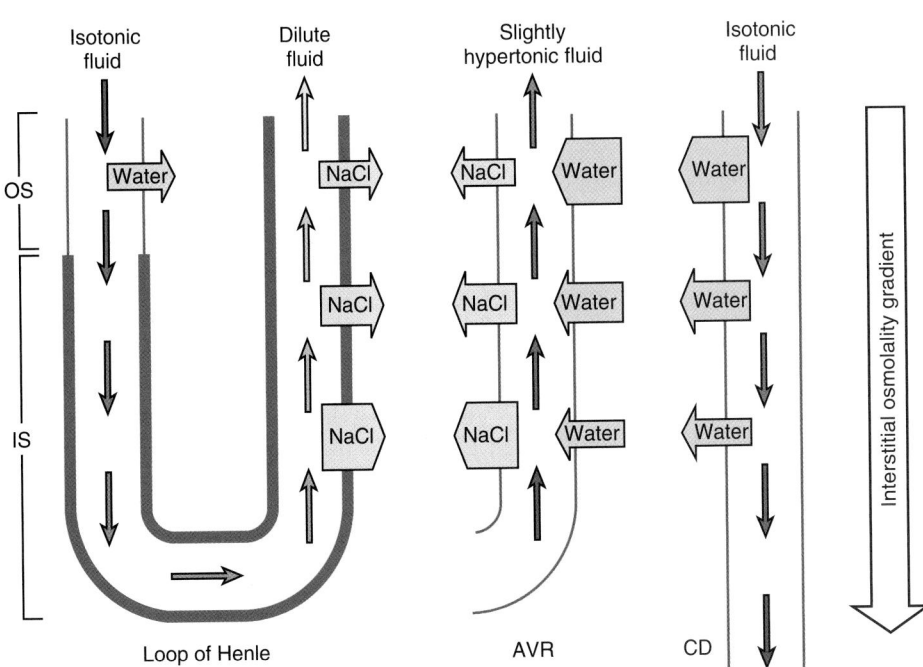

FIGURE 10-11 Outer medullary concentrating mechanism based on NaCl addition to the interstitium but without water absorption from descending limbs of short loops. *Arrows* indicate water (*cyan*) and NaCl (*yellow*) transepithelial transport; *arrow widths* suggest relative transport magnitudes. Isotonic fluid is considered to have the same osmolality as blood plasma. Flow entering the ascending vas rectum (AVR) is assumed to arise from a descending vas rectum that is in, or near, a vascular bundle. Out-flow from the collecting duct (CD) enters the inner medullary CD. Tubular fluid flow direction is indicated by *blue arrows;* increasing osmolality is indicated by *darkening shades of blue. Thick blue lines* indicate that a tubule is impermeable to water; *thin lines* indicate high permeability to water. *IS,* Inner stripe; *OS,* outer stripe.

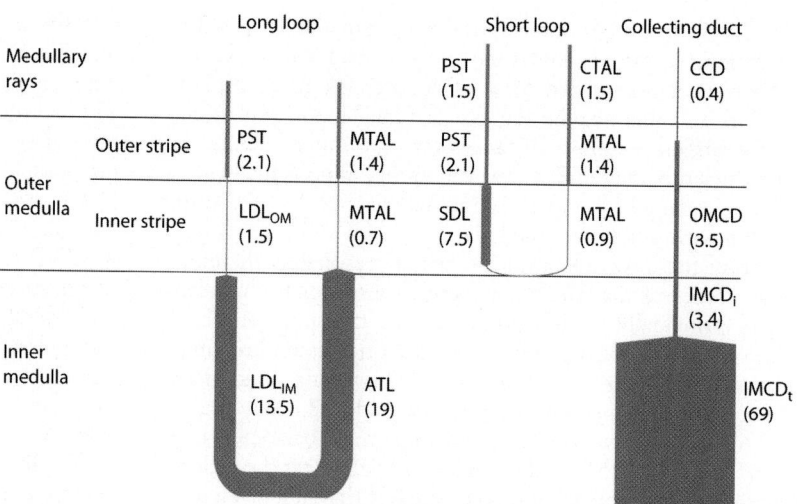

FIGURE 10-12 Urea permeabilities of mammalian renal tubule segments. The width of each segment in the diagram is distorted to be proportional to the urea permeability of that segment. Numbers in parentheses are measured values for the permeability coefficient ($\times 10^{-5}$ cm/sec). Values are from isolated perfused tubule studies.

plasma membranes of the IMCD cells are responsible for the high urea permeability of the terminal part of the IMCD. In contrast, the low urea permeability of the collecting duct system proximal to the terminal IMCD is due to a lack of urea transporter expression.

The mechanisms of urea accumulation in the renal medulla are depicted in Figure 10-13. Accumulation is predominantly a result of passive urea reabsorption from the IMCD. Tubular fluid entering the collecting duct system in the renal cortex has a relatively low urea concentration. During antidiuresis, water is osmotically reabsorbed from the urea-impermeable parts of the collecting duct system in the cortex and outer medulla, which causes a progressive increase in the luminal urea concentration along the connecting tubules, cortical collecting ducts, and outer medullary collecting ducts. Once the tubule fluid reaches the highly urea-permeable terminal IMCD, urea rapidly exits from the lumen to the inner medullary interstitium. This urea is "trapped" in the inner medulla by countercurrent urea exchange between descending and ascending flows in both vasa recta and loops of Henle. Under steady-state conditions, and in the continued presence of vasopressin, the urea permeability of the terminal IMCD is so high that urea nearly equilibrates across the IMCD epithelium. This allows urea in the interstitium to almost completely osmotically balance the urea in the collecting duct lumen. If the urea concentration in the collecting duct were higher transiently, then urea would diffuse from the collecting duct to restore the equilibrium between the urea concentration in the collecting duct and the concentration arising from the large store of urea in other inner medullary structures, thus buffering, as it were, possible instances of osmotic diuresis (Figure 10-14).

The descending and ascending vasa recta are in close association with each other in the inner medulla, which facilitates countercurrent exchange of urea between the two structures.[29] In the ascending vasa recta, aided by the extremely high ($>40 \times 10^{-5}$ cm/sec) permeability to urea, the concentration of urea exiting the inner medulla is similar to the concentration of urea in the descending vasa recta.[27,47] This minimizes the washout of urea from the inner medulla. Countercurrent exchange cannot completely eliminate loss of urea from the inner medullary interstitium, however, because the volume flow rate of blood in the ascending vasa recta exceeds that in the descending vasa recta.[66] During antidiuresis, water

is added to the vasa recta from both IMCDs and descending limbs, which results in a higher-volume flow rate and an increased mass flow rate of urea. This ensures that the inner medullary vasculature continually removes urea from the inner medulla. Quantitatively, the most important loss of urea from the inner medullary interstitium is thought to occur via the vasa recta,[67] but urea recycling pathways play a major role in limiting the loss of urea from the inner medulla. Three major urea recycling pathways are the following, and an overview of these is depicted in Figure 10-15.

1. *Recycling of urea through the ascending limbs, distal tubules, and collecting ducts.* Urea that escapes the inner medulla in the ascending limbs of the long loops of Henle is carried back through the thick ascending limbs, the distal convoluted tubules, and the early part of the collecting duct system by the flow of tubule fluid.[41] When it reaches the urea-permeable part of the inner medulla collecting ducts, it passively exits into the inner medullary interstitium.

2. *Recycling of urea through the vasa recta, short loops of Henle, and collecting ducts.* The delivery of urea to the superficial distal tubule exceeds the delivery out of the superficial proximal tubule.[41,68,69] This implies that net urea addition occurs somewhere along the short loops of Henle. One possible mechanism is that the urea leaving the inner medulla in the vasa recta is transferred to the descending limbs of the short loops of Henle[68] and is subsequently carried through the superficial distal tubules back to the urea-permeable part of the inner medulla collecting ducts, where it passively exits, completing the recycling pathway. The close physical association between the vasa recta and the descending limbs of the short loops in the vascular bundles of the inner stripe of the outer medulla would facilitate this transfer of urea from the vasa recta to the short loops of Henle.[20,70] Furthermore, the existence of a facilitative urea transporter, UT-A2, in the thin descending limb of the short loops of Henle[5,71] provides further support for this mechanism. However, results of recent studies involving UT-A2 knockout mice[72,73] have raised doubts about the importance of this pathway.

3. *Urea recycling between ascending and descending limbs of the loops of Henle.* Urea permeability measurements in isolated perfused thick ascending limbs from the inner stripe of the outer medulla show that urea permeability is too low to

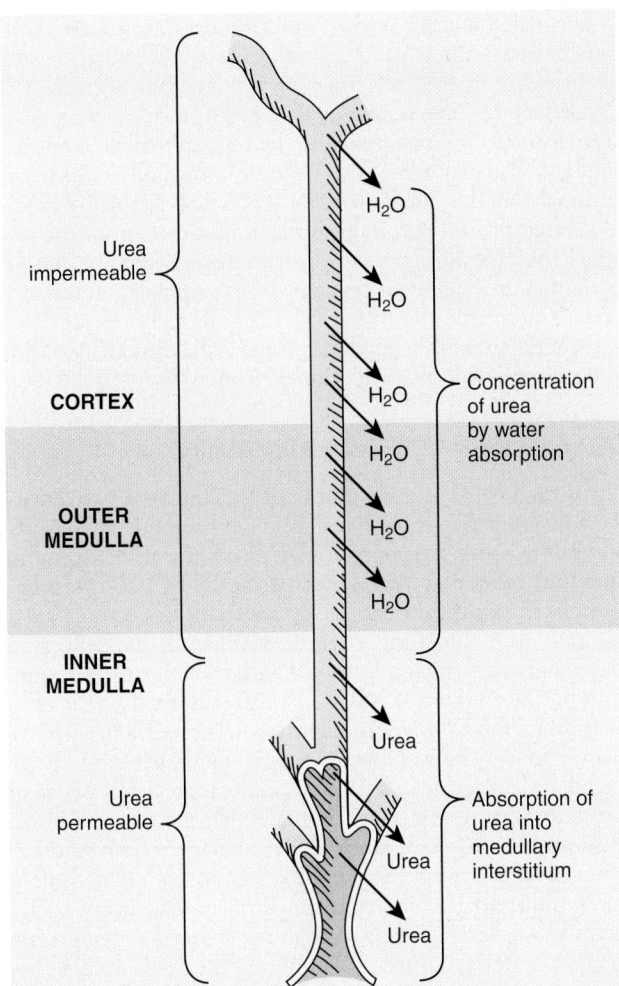

FIGURE 10-13 Schematic representation of the mammalian collecting duct system showing principal sites of water absorption and urea absorption. Water is absorbed in the early part of the collecting duct system, driven by an osmotic gradient. Since urea permeabilities of cortical collecting duct, outer medullary collecting duct, and initial inner medullary collecting duct (IMCD) are very low, the water absorption concentrates urea in the lumen of these segments. When the tubule fluid reaches the terminal IMCD, which is highly permeable to urea, urea rapidly exits from the lumen. This urea is trapped in the inner medulla as a result of countercurrent exchange.

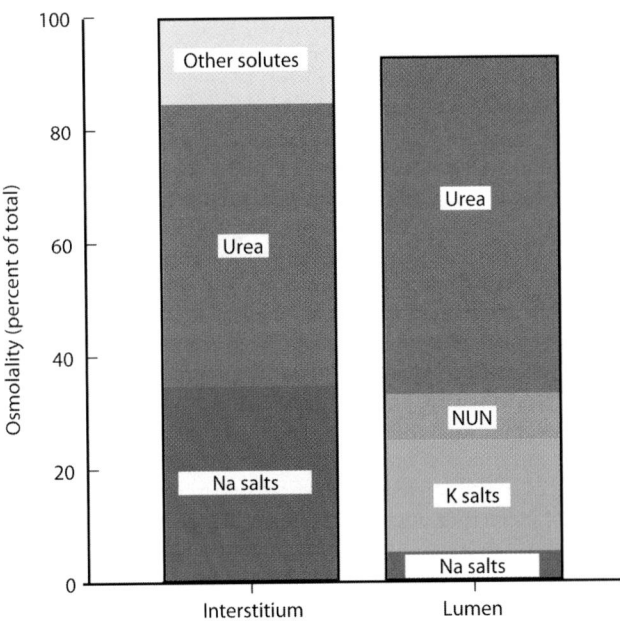

FIGURE 10-14 Solutes that account for osmolality of medullary interstitium and tubule fluid in the inner medullary collecting duct during antidiuresis in rats. Urea nearly equilibrates across the inner medullary collecting duct (IMCD) epithelium as a result of rapid facilitated urea transport. Although the osmolalities of the fluid in the two spaces are nearly equal, the nonurea solutes can differ considerably between the two compartments. Typical values in untreated rats are presented. Values can differ considerably in other species and in the same species with consumption of different diets. NUN, Nonurea nitrogen.

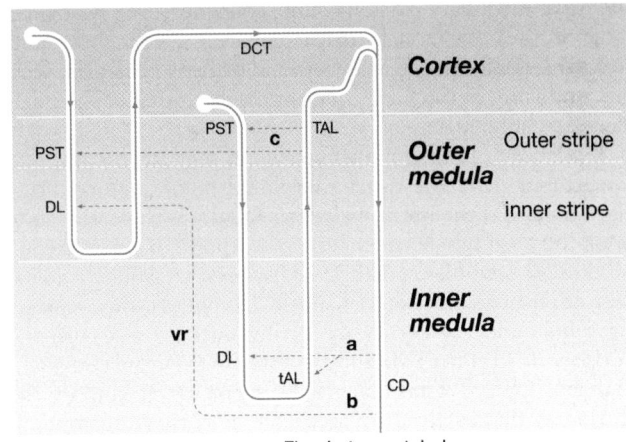

FIGURE 10-15 *Pathways of urea recycling in renal medulla. Solid blue lines represent a short-looped nephron (**left**) and a long-looped nephron (**right**). Transfer of urea between nephron segments is indicated by dashed red arrows labeled a, b, and c corresponding to recycling pathways described in the text. CD, Collecting duct; DCT, distal convoluted tubule; DL, descending limb; PST, proximal straight tubule; tAL, thin ascending limb; TAL, thick ascending limb; vr, vasa recta. (From Knepper MA, Roch-Ramel F: Pathways of urea transport in the mammalian kidney,* Kidney Int *31:629-633, 1987.)*

permit a substantial amount of urea absorption from this nephron segment.[74,75] However, higher urea permeability values are found when similar measurements are made in nephron segments located in the outer stripe of the outer medulla and the medullary rays.[74,76] A urea recycling pathway has been proposed in which urea is reabsorbed from thick ascending limbs and is secreted into neighboring proximal straight tubules, forming a recycling pathway between the ascending and descending limbs of the loop of Henle.[1,67] Urea recycling from the thick ascending limbs and the proximal straight tubules is facilitated by the parallel relationship of these two structures in the outer stripe of the outer medulla and in the medullary rays. The transfer of urea may also depend on a relatively attenuated effective blood flow in these regions of the kidney. Urea secretion into the proximal straight tubules can occur by passive diffusion,[76] active transport,[77] or a combination of both. Urea presumably enters the proximal straight tubules of both

short- and long-looped nephrons. The urea that enters the short-looped nephrons is carried back to the inner medulla by the flow of tubule fluid through the superficial distal tubules and cortical collecting ducts, reentering the inner medullary interstitium by reabsorption from the terminal IMCD. The urea that enters proximal straight tubules of long-looped nephrons returns to the inner medulla directly through the descending limbs of the loops of Henle.[67]

Collecting Duct Water Absorption and Osmotic Equilibration

The urinary concentrating mechanism is built on two independent processes: (1) generation of a hypertonic medullary interstitium by concentration of NaCl and urea via countercurrent processes, and (2) osmotic equilibration of the tubule fluid within the medullary collecting ducts with the hypertonic medullary interstitium, thus forming a final hypertonic urine. In reality these two processes are not truly separable, particularly with regard to urea, the major solute responsible for waste nitrogen elimination in mammals. The generation of the hypertonic medullary interstitium was described earlier, and in the following the mechanism of osmotic equilibration is discussed.

The antidiuretic hormone arginine vasopressin regulates the degree of water excretion, mainly due to its effects on regulation of collecting duct water permeability. When circulating vasopressin levels are low, for example during water diuresis, the water permeability of the collecting ducts is also extremely low, and relatively little water is reabsorbed. Thus, the dilute tubule fluid that exits from the loops of Henle (made dilute because of the removal of solute by the thick ascending limb) remains dilute as it passes through the collecting duct system, yielding a large volume of hypotonic urine. In contrast, high circulating levels of vasopressin increase the water permeability of the collecting ducts to very high levels. Due to the large osmolality gradient between the lumen and the peritubular interstitium (generated by active solute transport in the thick ascending limb), water is rapidly reabsorbed from the cortical and outer medullary portions of the collecting duct system via aquaporin water channels (discussed later). Under these conditions, a small volume of hypertonic urine is produced, with the osmolality of the final urine approaching that of the inner medullary interstitium.

Evidence from micropuncture studies suggests that the late distal tubule (the late distal convoluted tubule, the connecting tubule, and the initial collecting tubule) is the earliest site along the renal tubule where water absorption increases during antidiuresis (see Figure 10-8).[78] The distal convoluted tubule does not express any water channels. In contrast, the connecting tubule and the cortical collecting duct express both the vasopressin receptor V_2R and the vasopressin-regulated water channel AQP2.[79] Thus, among the segments making up the portion of the distal tubule accessible by cortical micropuncture, only the connecting tubule and the initial collecting tubule appear to exhibit vasopressin-regulated water transport. Therefore, these segments are presumably sites of the distal tubular osmotic equilibration observed in micropuncture studies.

The volume of water absorption in the connecting segment and initial collecting tubule required to raise tubule fluid to isotonicity is considerably greater than the additional amount required to concentrate the urine above the osmolality of plasma in the medullary portion of the collecting duct system.[1] Consequently, during antidiuresis, most of the water reabsorbed from the collecting duct system enters the cortical labyrinth, where the effective blood flow is high enough to return the reabsorbed water to the general circulation without diluting the interstitium. In contrast, if such a large volume of water were reabsorbed along the medullary collecting ducts, it would have a significant dilution effect on the medullary interstitium and thus impair concentrating ability.[80,81]

Surprisingly, even during water diuresis, a modest corticomedullary osmolality gradient persists,[82,83] and the water permeability of the collecting ducts is low but not zero.[64,84] Consequently, some water is reabsorbed by the collecting ducts during water diuresis, driven by the transepithelial osmolality gradient. The majority of this water reabsorption occurs in the terminal IMCDs, where the transepithelial osmolality gradient is highest. In fact, more water is absorbed from the terminal IMCDs during water diuresis than during antidiuresis owing to a much greater transepithelial osmolality gradient.[80] Water reabsorption from the IMCDs is thought to contribute to the reduction of the medullary interstitial osmolality during water diuresis due to its dilutional effect.[81,85]

Determinants of Concentrating Ability

The overall concentrating ability of the kidney is based upon the interaction between several different components. In addition to the active transport of NaCl from the thick ascending limb and collecting duct water permeability, two other factors play a significant role in determining the osmolality of the final urine. One important determinant is the delivery of NaCl and water to the loop of Henle, which sets the upper limit on the amount of NaCl actively reabsorbed by the thick ascending limb to drive the countercurrent multiplier mechanism. Finally, the volume of tubule fluid delivered to the medullary collecting duct has an underappreciated effect on the concentrating process. Too much delivery saturates water reabsorption processes along the medullary collecting ducts, which leads to interstitial dilution caused by rapid osmotic water transport. In contrast, too little fluid delivery to the medullary collecting ducts, even in the absence of vasopressin, results in sustained osmotic equilibration across the collecting duct epithelium owing to the nonzero osmotic water permeability of the IMCD.[64,80,84]

Unresolved Question: Concentration of NaCl in the Renal Inner Medulla

Tissue slice studies have demonstrated that the corticomedullary osmolality gradient is made up largely of an NaCl gradient in the outer medulla and a urea gradient in the inner medulla (see Figure 10-9). Accordingly, the previous sections emphasized the processes that concentrate NaCl in the outer medulla and the processes responsible for urea accumulation in the inner medulla (passive urea absorption from the inner medullary collecting duct plus countercurrent exchange of urea via diffusion). The concentrating mechanism described earlier functions only in the renal outer medulla and medullary rays of the cortex. The ascending limbs of the loops of Henle that reach into the inner medulla are thin walled and do not actively transport NaCl[47,86,87]; nonetheless, in antidiuresis a substantial axial osmolality gradient is generated in the inner medulla of many mammals. For nearly 50 years, controversy has persisted regarding the nature of the mechanism that generates the inner medullary osmolality gradient. Another unresolved question is the energy source for concentration of nonurea solutes in the inner medullary interstitium. General analysis of inner medullary concentrating processes indicates that, to satisfy mass balance requirements, either an ascending stream (thin ascending limbs or ascending vasa recta) must be diluted relative to the inner medullary interstitium, or a descending stream (descending thin limbs, descending vasa recta, or collecting ducts) must be concentrated locally relative to the inner medulla.[32,88]

Three major hypotheses have been proposed for the concentrating mechanism of the inner medulla:

1. The "passive" countercurrent mechanism of Kokko and Rector[89] and Stephenson,[90] in which the absorption of urea and accompanying water from the inner medullary collecting ducts results in a transepithelial NaCl gradient that promotes NaCl absorption from the water-impermeable ascending thin limbs without a significant compensatory secretion of urea into those limbs.
2. The external solute hypothesis, proposed by Jen and Stephenson[91] and extended by Thomas and colleagues,[92-94] in which a net generation of osmotically active particles raises the osmolality of the inner medulla.
3. The mechano-osmotic induction hypothesis,[32,95] in which energy from the peristaltic contractions of the renal pelvic wall is used to concentrate solutes in the descending limbs and collecting ducts by water withdrawal, or, alternatively, the peristaltic contractions reduce sodium activity in the hyaluronan matrix of the interstitium, which results in the reabsorption of hypotonic fluid from that matrix into ascending vasa recta.

These hypotheses are described in more detail in the following sections.

"Passive" Mechanism

Kokko and Rector[89] and Stephenson[90] simultaneously and independently proposed a model by which the osmolality in the ascending thin limb could be lowered below that of the interstitium entirely by passive transport processes in the inner medulla. This mechanism is generally referred to as the *passive model* or the *passive countercurrent multiplier mechanism.* The passive mechanism depends on the separation of urea and NaCl that is accomplished by NaCl absorption from the thick ascending limbs; indeed, this absorption is the energy source for the passive mechanism. In this model, rapid urea reabsorption from the IMCD generates and maintains a high urea concentration in the inner medullary interstitium, causing the osmotic withdrawal of water from the thin descending limb. This concentrates NaCl in the *descending* limb lumen and results in a transepithelial gradient favoring the passive reabsorption of NaCl from the thin *ascending* limb of the loop of Henle. In addition, if the ascending limbs have extremely low urea permeability, then any NaCl that has been reabsorbed from the ascending thin limb will not be replaced by urea. Thus, the ascending limb fluid will be dilute relative to the fluid in other nephron segments, which will generate a "single effect" analogous to active NaCl absorption from thick ascending limbs. This single effect can then be multiplied by the counterflow between the ascending and descending limbs of Henle's loops. This model requires that the thin descending limbs be highly permeable to water but not to NaCl or urea, whereas the thin ascending limb would have to be permeable to NaCl but not to water or urea. Several objections have been made to the passive mechanism, both because of the high urea permeabilities that have been measured in the thin descending limb and thin ascending limb (summarized in Gamba and Knepper[96]) and new studies in urea transporter knockout mice in which urea accumulation in the inner medulla was largely eliminated, but inner medullary NaCl accumulation was not

affected[79,97,98] (see "UT-A1/3 Urea Transporter Knockout Mice" section).

Layton and colleagues[99] reevaluated the passive mechanism in the context of the emerging information coming from the studies by Pannabecker and Dantzler. This study showed that water absorption from descending limbs was not a requirement for the passive mechanism to generate an osmolality gradient. That study also identified a second concentrating passive mode in which the loops of Henle are highly urea permeable and serve as a highly effective countercurrent urea exchanger. However, neither mode was able to account fully for the high urine osmolalities attained by some animals.

Concentrating Mechanism Driven by External Solute

Jen and Stephenson[91] proposed that the concentrating mechanism of the inner medulla depends on a solute other than NaCl and urea. By means of a mathematical model, they demonstrated, in principle, that the continuous addition of small amounts of an unspecified but osmotically active solute to the inner medullary interstitium could produce a substantial axial osmolality gradient. Such a solute would have to be generated in the inner medulla by a chemical reaction that produces more osmotically active particles than it consumes. The mechanism of concentration is similar to that driven by urea in the passive models proposed by Kokko and Rector[89] and by Stephenson[90]: the thin descending limbs of inner medulla are assumed impermeable to the solute (thus it is an "external" solute), and as a result, water is withdrawn from the descending limbs and the concentration of NaCl is raised in descending limb tubular fluid. Beginning at the loop bend, elevated NaCl concentration within the loop will result in a substantial NaCl efflux that will dilute the ascending flow and that is sufficient to generate the axial gradient.

The feasibility of this mechanism was subsequently confirmed by Thomas and Wexler[94] in the context of a more detailed mathematical model. In further modeling studies, Thomas[92] and Hervy and Thomas[93] proposed that lactate, generated by anaerobic glycolysis (the predominant means of adenosine triphosphate [ATP] generation in the inner medulla), could serve as the solute. Two lactate ions are generated per glucose consumed:

$$glucose \rightarrow 2\ lactate^- + 2\ H^+$$

However, as pointed out by Knepper and others,[32] the net generation of osmotically active particles depends on which buffering anions are titrated by the protons. If the protons titrate bicarbonate, there may be a net removal of osmotically active particles; if instead the protons titrate other buffers (e.g., phosphate or NH_3), there will be a net generation of osmotically active particles.

A mathematical model developed by Zhang and Edwards[101] predicted that vascular countercurrent exchange would tend to restrict significant availability of glucose to the outer medulla and the upper inner medulla and would thus limit the rate of lactate generation in the deep inner medulla where the highest osmolalities are found. Recent findings by Dantzler and colleagues[55] present an additional challenge to the external solute hypothesis: in a perfused tubule study, they found that the deepest 60% of inner medullary descending thin limbs (those limb portions that lack measurable AQP1) have essentially no osmotic water permeability.

Hyaluronan as a Mechano-osmotic Transducer

Hyaluronan (or hyaluronic acid) is a glycosaminoglycan (GAG). GAGs consist of unbranched polysaccharide chains composed of repeating disaccharide units. In addition to hyaluronan, the family of mammalian GAGs includes dermatan sulfate, chondroitin sulfates, keratan sulfate, heparan sulfate, and heparin. Hyaluronan differs from the other GAGs in that it is not covalently linked to proteins to form proteoglycans, and it is not sulfonated.[102] In contrast to other GAGs, which are produced in the Golgi apparatus, hyaluronan is synthesized at the plasma membrane by an integral membrane protein, hyaluronan synthase (HAS).[103,104] Three mammalian HAS genes have been identified: *HAS1*, *HAS2*, and *HAS3*. All three HAS proteins produce hyaluronan on the cytoplasmic side of the plasma membrane and transport it across the plasma membrane to the extracellular space. Therefore, hyaluronan secretion is not dependent on vesicular trafficking. Because of the importance of GAGs in the structure of connective tissues such as cartilage, tendon, bone, synovial fluid, intervertebral disks, and skin, the physiochemical properties of GAGs have been extensively investigated.[105]

Hyaluronan is abundant in the interstitium of the renal inner medulla.[106,107] Other GAGs are also present, but in much lower amounts. The hyaluronan in the inner medulla is produced by a specialized interstitial cell (the type 1 interstitial cell), which forms characteristic bridges between the thin limbs of Henle and the vasa recta.[108] (These bridges may delimit, above and below, the nodal compartments identified by Pannabecker and Dantzler.[23]) Thus, the inner medullary interstitium may be considered to be composed of a compressible, viscoelastic, hyaluronan matrix.

Several hypotheses have been advanced that depend on the peristalsis of the papilla as an integral component of the concentrating mechanism of the inner medulla.[109,110] Most recently, Knepper and colleagues[32] proposed that the periodic compression of the papilla, and the effects of that compression on the hyaluronan matrix, could explain the osmolality gradient along the inner medulla.

Two hypotheses were proposed. In the first hypothesis, which was suggested in part by Schmidt-Nielsen,[111] compression of the hyaluronan matrix stores some of the mechanical energy from the smooth muscle contraction that gives rise to the peristaltic wave. In the postwave decompression, the matrix exerts an elastic force that promotes water absorption from thin descending limbs and collecting ducts, and thereby increases tubular fluid osmolality. Water absorption from the descending limbs would raise tubular fluid NaCl concentration and thus promote a vigorous NaCl absorption from the loop bends and early ascending limbs. However, if, as is apparently the case in the rat, the lower 60% of inner medullary descending limbs are water impermeable,[55] water is unlikely to be absorbed from descending limbs in the deep portion of the inner medulla where the highest osmolalities are achieved.

The second hypothesis involves special properties of hyaluronan.[112] Hyaluronan is a large polyanion (1000 to 10,000 kDa). Its charge is due to the carboxylate (COO) groups of the glucuronic subunits. Hyaluronan is hydrophilic and assumes a highly expanded, random-coil confirmation that occupies a large volume of space relative to its mass. This extended state arises partly from electrostatic repulsion between carboxylate groups (which maximize the distances between neighboring negative charges) and partly from the extended conformations of the glycosidic bonds.

When hyaluronan is compressed, as occurs in the meniscus of the knee joint in response to load bearing, the repulsive forces of neighboring carboxylate groups are overcome, in part, by a condensation of cations (mainly Na^+), and a localized crystalloid structure is formed. Thus, compression of the hyaluronan gel results in a decrease of the local sodium ion activity in the gel.[32] In aqueous solutions that are in equilibrium with the gel, the NaCl concentration will decrease as a consequence of the compression-induced reduction in Na^+ activity within the gel. Therefore, the free fluid that is expressed from the hyaluronan matrix during the contraction phase will have a lower total solute concentration than that of the gel as a whole. The slightly hypotonic fluid expressed from the matrix is likely to escape the inner medulla via the ascending vasa recta, the only structure that remains open during the compressive phase of the contraction cycle.[111] As a consequence, the ascending fluid within ascending vasa recta would have a lower osmolality than the local interstitium, and therefore fluid in collecting ducts and descending vasa recta would be concentrated.

This mechanism is consistent with the nodal compartments found by Pannabecker and Dantzler.[23] These compartments, which are likely rich in hyaluronan, are in contact with collecting ducts, ascending thin limbs, and ascending vasa recta. Thus, they are well configured to be the sites of transduction; that is, the sites where the mechanical energy of peristalsis is harnessed to generate an ascending flow that is dilute relative to average local osmolality. However, no quantitative analyses or mathematical models have examined the mass balance consistency or the thermodynamic adequacy of hypotheses that depend on the peristaltic contractions.

The *HAS2* gene has been knocked out in mice, but the mice die in fetal development because of cardiac abnormalities.[113] Thus, the role of hyaluronan in the concentrating mechanism of the inner medulla cannot be evaluated in these mice.

Molecular Physiology of Urinary Concentrating and Diluting Processes

Transport Proteins Involved in Urinary Concentration and Dilution

Figure 10-16 presents a schematic representation of the mammalian nephron with the localization of major water channels (aquaporins), urea transporters, and ion transporters important to the urinary concentrating process. Figure 10-17 shows which of these transporters and channels are molecular targets for regulated vasopressin action, in terms of either abundance or activity. The function and regulation of several of these transporters are explained in detail elsewhere in this book. The following sections summarize the roles of these transport proteins in urinary concentrating and diluting mechanisms, with particular attention to their regulation via vasopressin. The reader is referred to Chapter 11 for a detailed discussion of the cell biology of vasopressin action.

Aquaporins

AQP1 in the mammalian kidney is responsible for water reabsorption along the proximal tubule. Abundant expression of AQP1 in the descending limbs of long-looped nephrons in

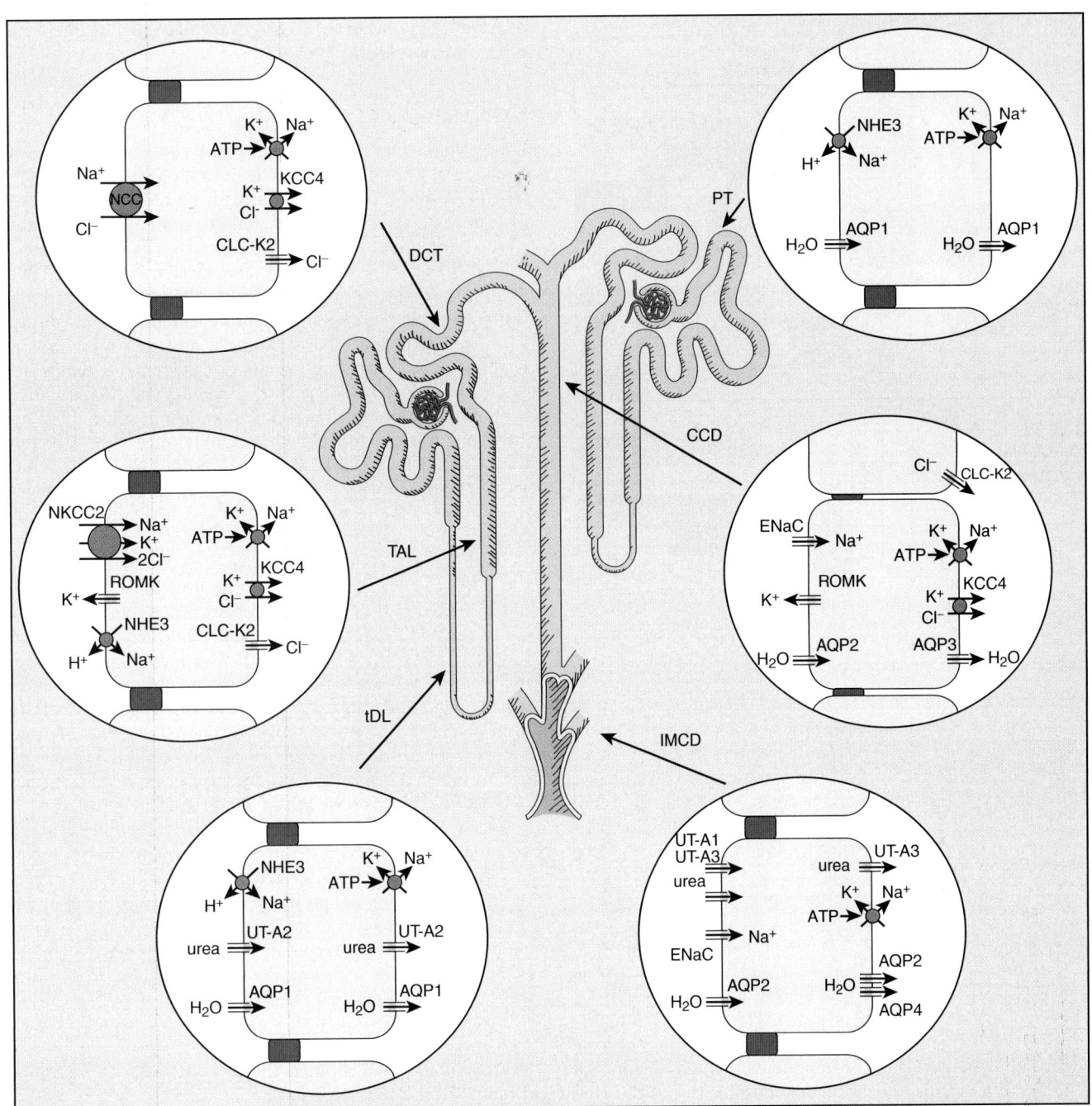

FIGURE 10-16 Major aquaporins, urea transporters, and ion transporters and channels that are important to the urinary concentrating and diluting process. Figure presents a schematic overview of a mammalian kidney tubule, showing the solute and water transport pathways in the proximal tubule (PT), thin descending limb of the loop of Henle (tDL), thick ascending limb (TAL), distal convoluted tubule (DCT), cortical collecting duct (CCD), and inner medullary collecting duct (IMCD). Tubule lumen side is always on the left-hand side of the cell, whereas the interstitium is on the right-hand side. *Arrows* represent direction of movement. (See text for details.) (Adapted from Fenton RA, Knepper MA: Mouse models and the urinary concentrating mechanism in the new millennium, *Physiol Rev* 87:1083-1112, 2007.)

the outer medulla accounts for the high water permeability in this segment.[7,114,115] In the inner medulla, AQP1-null segments of thin descending limbs have been detected.[13] In contrast, recent studies demonstrate that there is a complete absence of AQP1 along the entire length of descending thin limbs of 90% of short-looped nephrons in the outer medulla. Because the majority of nephrons are of the short-loop variety, the lack of AQP1 suggests that the mechanisms of water transport in the descending thin limbs of short-looped nephrons should be reevaluated. Likewise, the roles of AQP1 in

the countercurrent multiplier and in water conservation may need to be readdressed. In the ascending limb segments (thin ascending limb of the loop of Henle, medullary thick ascending limb, and cortical thick ascending limb), no known water channels are expressed, which accounts for the low osmotic water permeability measured in these segments.[42,63,75,86]

AQP2 is a major target for vasopressin action in the connecting tubule and throughout the collecting duct system (reviewed in Nielsen and colleagues[116]). Vasopressin regulates AQP2 via two independent mechanisms:

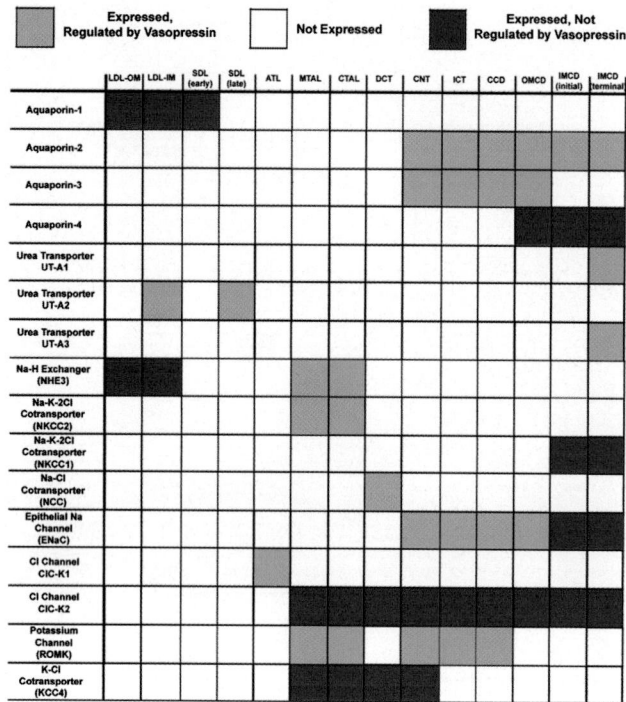

FIGURE 10-17 Grid showing sites of expression of water channels, urea transporters, and ion transporters important to the urinary concentrating process. (See text for details.)

1. *Short-term regulation of AQP2 trafficking to and from the apical plasma membrane.* Vasopressin regulates the abundance of AQP2 in the plasma membrane by triggering its redistribution from intracellular vesicles into the plasma membrane. This permits water entry. The translocation of AQP2 is initiated by an increase in cAMP following V_2R activation through vasopressin. The vasopressin-induced rise in cAMP activates protein kinase A (PKA) and potentially other kinases, which in turn phosphorylate AQP2 on at least four serine residues[117-121] and thereby trigger the redistribution of AQP2. Several proteins participating in the control of cAMP-dependent AQP2 trafficking have been identified (reviewed in Fenton and Moeller[122]); for example, A kinase anchoring proteins tethering PKA to cellular compartments; phosphodiesterases regulating the local cAMP level; cytoskeletal components such as F-actin and microtubules; small guanosine triphosphatases of the Rho family controlling cytoskeletal dynamics; motor proteins transporting AQP2-bearing vesicles to and from the plasma membrane for exocytic insertion and endocytic retrieval; soluble NEM-sensitive factor attachment protein receptor (SNARE) proteins inducing membrane fusion; and hsc70, a chaperone, important for endocytic retrieval. Recent mass spectrometry analysis has identified proteins that bind to AQP2 in a phosphorylation-dependent manner.[123]

2. *Long-term regulation of AQP2 protein abundance,* mainly through increased gene transcription (reviewed in Nielsen and colleagues[116]).

The basolateral component of water transport across connecting tubule cells and collecting duct principal cells is mediated by AQP3 and AQP4.[124,125] AQP3 is the dominant basolateral water channel in the connecting tubule and early parts of the collecting duct system, whereas AQP4 predominates in the inner medullary collecting ducts. The abundance of AQP3, but not that of AQP4, is regulated by the long-term effect of vasopressin.[124-126]

Urea Transporters

Urea plays a central role in the urinary concentrating mechanism. Urea's importance has been appreciated since 1934, when Gamble and colleagues initially described "an economy of water in renal function referable to urea,"[127] findings that were recently confirmed and advanced in knockout mice[128] (see also the "UT-A1/3 Urea Transporter Knockout Mice" section later). Many studies show that maximal urinary concentrating ability is decreased in protein-deprived or malnourished humans (and other mammals) and that urea infusion restores urine concentrating ability (reviewed in Sands and Layton[109]). Recently, urinary concentrating defects have been demonstrated in UT-A1/3[−/−] knockout mice,[97] UT-A2 knockout mice,[72] and UT-B knockout mice[129-131] (see also the "UT-A2 and UT-B Urea Transporter Knockout Mice" section later). Thus, an effect due to urea or urea transporters must be part of the mechanism by which the inner medulla concentrates urine.

Two urea transporter genes have been cloned in mammals: the UT-B (*Slc14A1*) gene encodes two protein isoforms,[132] and the UT-A (*Slc14A2*) gene encodes six protein and nine complementary DNA (cDNA) isoforms (reviewed in Sands and Layton[109]). UT-B, which is also the Kidd blood group antigen in humans, has been cloned from humans and rodents[133] and is reviewed in Sands and Layton.[109] The UT-A gene, which has been cloned from rat, human, and mouse, has two promoter elements: one upstream of exon 1 and a second that is located within intron 12 and drives the transcription of UT-A2 and UT-A2b[134-137]; it is reviewed in Sands and Layton.[109]

Analysis of UT-A promoter I shows that it contains a consensus tonicity enhancer (TonE) element and that hyperosmolality increases promoter activity.[135,138] This element may explain the finding that prolonged administration of vasopressin (12 days) is needed to increase UT-A1 protein abundance and inner medullary urea content in Brattleboro rats (which lack vasopressin and have central diabetes insipidus).[139-141] Vasopressin directly increases the transcription of the Na-K-2Cl cotransporter NKCC2/BSC1 in the thick ascending limb. The increase in NaCl reabsorption increases inner medullary osmolality, which then increases UT-A1 transcription through TonE.[142,143]

UT-A1 is expressed in the terminal IMCD and is detected in the apical plasma membrane (Figure 10-18).[71,136,144] UT-A3 is also expressed in the terminal IMCD; it is primarily detected in the basolateral plasma membrane but has also been identified in the apical plasma membrane in some studies.[145-147] UT-A2 is expressed in thin descending limbs.[5,71,144,148] UT-A4 messenger RNA (mRNA) is expressed in rat kidney medulla, although its protein has not been detected and UT-A4 mRNA has not been detected in mouse kidney.[131,137,149] UT-A5 and UT-A6 are not expressed in kidney but in testis and colon, respectively,[150,151] and thus do not play a role in urinary concentration. There are also three UT-A cDNA variants, UT-A1b, UT-A2b, and UT-A3b, which differ in their 3′ untranslated regions but not in their coding regions.[134] UT-B protein is expressed in descending vasa recta and red blood cells, as is phloretin-inhibitable urea transport (reviewed in Sands and Layton[109]).

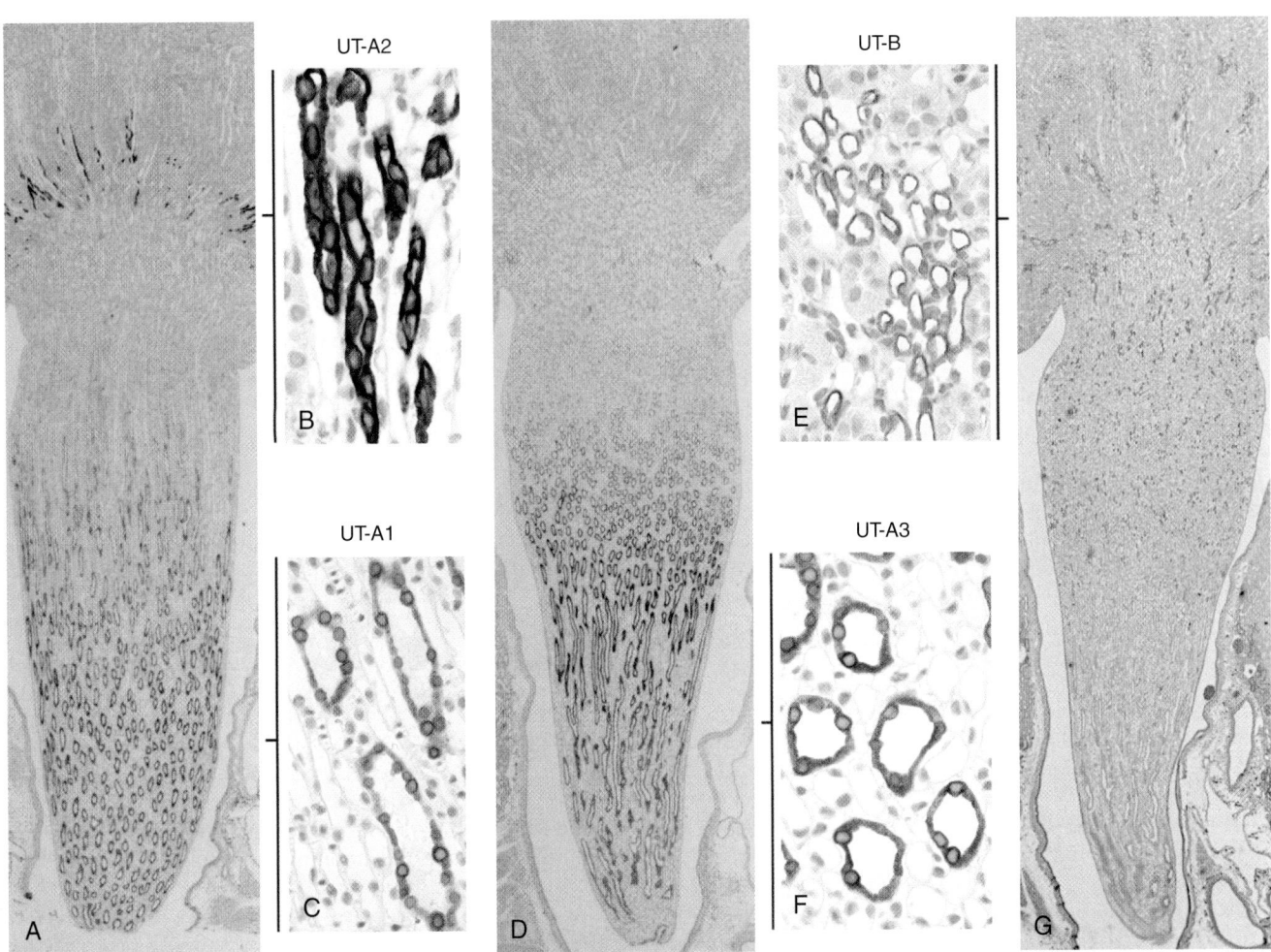

FIGURE 10-18 Localization of urea transporters. UT-A1 is localized to the terminal portion of the inner medullary collecting duct (IMCD), whereas UT-A2 is localized to the thin descending limbs of the loop of Henle in the inner stripe of the outer medulla (**A**). Higher magnification shows that both UT-A2 (**B**) and UT-A1 (**C**) are predominantly intracellular. UT-A3 is localized to the terminal portion of the IMCD (**D**) and is both intracellular and in the basolateral membrane domains (**F**). UT-B is expressed in the descending vasa recta (**G**), where it is localized to the basolateral and apical regions (**E**). (Adapted from Fenton RA, Knepper MA: Urea and renal function in the 21st century: insights from knockout mice, *J Am Soc Nephrol* 18:679-688, 2007.)

Vasopressin increases the phosphorylation and the apical plasma membrane accumulation of UT-A1 and of UT-A3 in freshly isolated suspensions of rat IMCDs.[147,152] UT-A1 is phosphorylated by vasopressin at serines 486 and 499.[153] Mutation of both serines, but not of either one alone, eliminates vasopressin stimulation of UT-A1 apical plasma membrane accumulation and urea transport.[153] The site in UT-A3 that is phosphorylated by vasopressin has not been determined, but neither of the two PKA consensus sites is involved.[151] Vasopressin stimulates urea transport and UT-A1 phosphorylation and apical plasma membrane accumulation through two cAMP-dependent pathways: PKA and Epac (exchange protein activated by cAMP).[154]

UT-A1 is linked to the SNARE machinery via snapin in rat IMCD, which suggests that the SNARE-SNAP vesicle trafficking mechanism may be functionally important for regulating urea transport.[155] UT-A1 can be ubiquitinated.[156,157] The ubiquitin ligase MDM2 mediates UT-A1 ubiquitination and degradation, which may contribute to the regulation of UT-A1.[157] UT-A1 also interacts with caveolin-1 in lipid rafts, which provides another mechanism for the regulation of UT-A1 activity within the plasma membrane.[158]

During antidiuresis, inner medullary osmolality is high. Hyperosmolality increases urea permeability in rat terminal IMCDs, even in the absence of vasopressin,[159-161] which suggests that it is an independent activator of urea transport. Both hyperosmolality and vasopressin increase urea permeability by increasing the V_{max} for urea transport, rather than by decreasing the K_m.[160,162] However, they do so through different second messenger pathways: hyperosmolality stimulates urea permeability via increases in activation of PKC and intracellular calcium,[163,164] whereas vasopressin stimulates urea permeability via increases in cAMP.[65] Hyperosmolality increases the phosphorylation and plasma membrane accumulation of both UT-A1 and UT-A3,[147,152,165,166] which is similar to the effects of vasopressin.

Sodium Transporters and Channels

Na⁺/H⁺ Exchanger 3

Na⁺/H⁺ exchanger isoform 3 (NHE3) plays a major role in sodium reabsorption in the proximal tubule. In addition, NHE3 is expressed in the thin descending limb of the loop of Henle and the medullary and cortical thick ascending limbs[167] (see Figure 10-9). Vasopressin (via cAMP production) inhibits

NHE3 activity in the thick ascending limb of the loop of Henle by reducing hypotonicity-induced, phosphatidylinositol-3-kinase–dependent NHE3 activation.[168]

Na-K-2Cl Cotransporters

Two Na-K-2Cl cotransporters are expressed in the kidney. The ubiquitous form, NKCC1, is expressed in the basolateral membrane of the inner medullary collecting duct, where it plays a role in NaCl secretion.[63,169] In addition, NKCC1 is expressed in the α intercalated cells of the outer medulla, where it localizes to the basolateral plasma membrane.[170] NKCC2 is expressed only in the kidney (see Figure 10-16). Three mRNA isoforms of NKCC2 are produced through differential splicing: NKCC2A, NKCC2B, and NKCC2F (reviewed in Castrop and Schnermann[171]). These splice variants differ in their localization along the thick ascending limb of the loop of Henle. NKCC2 protein is detected in the apical plasma membrane and subapical vesicles throughout the thick ascending limb of the loop of Henle and cortical thick ascending limb cells and in macula densa cells.[172-174] Of the isoforms, NKCC2F is detected in the medullary thick ascending limb, NKCC2A in both the medullary and cortical thick ascending limbs, and NKCC2B in the cortical thick ascending limb, including the macula densa.[171] Long-term vasopressin exposure increases NKCC2 protein abundance in the thick ascending limb,[56] which in turn is associated with an increase in maximal urinary concentrating capacity.[175,176] Vasopressin also acutely regulates NaCl reabsorption in the medullary thick ascending limb, in part by regulating trafficking of NKCC2 to the apical plasma membrane.[177-180] Vasopressin increases phosphorylation of the N-terminal tail of NKCC2 at threonine 184 and threonine 189, which increases apical targeting of the transporter.[177] This effect of vasopressin signaling may be mediated by the kinase WNK3.[181] Furthermore, recent studies suggest that vasopressin mediates apical insertion of NKCC2 by modulating its movement from nonraft to lipid raft fractions.[182]

Na-Cl Cotransporter and Epithelial Sodium Channel

Aldosterone partly regulates sodium excretion by regulating the function of both the thiazide-sensitive Na-Cl cotransporter NCC and the amiloride-sensitive sodium channel ENaC.[183,184] bNCC is expressed in the apical plasma membrane of distal convoluted tubule cells.[100,184-186] In contrast, ENaC is localized to the connecting tubule, initial collecting tubule, and throughout the collecting duct.[187,188] Long-term vasopressin treatment results in increased protein abundance of NCC and the β- and γ-subunits of ENaC.[189-191] Acute vasopressin exposure also increases Na reabsorption in the cortical collecting duct by increasing apical Na entry via ENaC,[192-194] possibly through vasopressin-induced trafficking of ENaC-containing vesicles from intracellular stores to the apical plasma membrane (reviewed in Snyder[195]).

Although evidence for a direct effect of NCC and ENaC in the urinary concentrating mechanism is not conclusive (see later), vasopressin-mediated increases in NaCl reabsorption in the distal convoluted tubule (via NCC) and connecting tubule and cortical collecting duct (via ENaC) could have a positive effect on urinary concentrating ability by reducing fluid delivery to the medullary collecting ducts.

Chloride Channels

The closely related chloride channels ClC-K1 and ClC-K2 are expressed in the mammalian kidney. ClC-K1 is localized to both the apical and basolateral plasma membrane of the thin ascending limb of Henle.[196] In addition, CLC-K1 mRNA has been detected in both the thick ascending limb and distal convoluted tubule.[197] In contrast ClC-K2 is localized to the basolateral membrane of the nephron from the thick ascending limb (see Figure 10-16) through the collecting ducts.[197-199] In isolated perfused tubules, chloride conductance of the thin ascending limb is increased by vasopressin exposure, as a result of either increased unit conductance or altered cellular localization of ClC-K1 chloride channels.[200]

ROMK Potassium Channel

The ROMK (regulation of Kir 1.1) potassium channel, an ATP-sensitive inwardly rectifier potassium channel, localizes to the thick ascending limb, distal convoluted tubule, connecting tubule, and collecting duct system, where it is predominantly associated with the apical plasma membrane[201-205] (see Figure 10-16). ROMK is essential for the urinary concentrating mechanism because of its critical role in active NaCl transport processes in the thick ascending limb of Henle. Long-term vasopressin treatment increases ROMK abundance in the thick ascending limb, thus contributing to vasopressin's long-term effect of increasing NaCl transport in this segment.[206,207] In addition, ROMK (alongside large-conductance Ca^{2+}-activated K^+ (BK) channels) is partially responsible for potassium secretion in the connecting tubule and collecting duct, and because of this helps regulate urinary potassium excretion and systemic potassium balance.[208] These processes are regulated by vasopressin; however, the secretory process may be an indirect consequence of vasopressin's action to increase sodium entry via ENaC, which results in depolarization and an increase in the electrochemical driving force for K movement through ROMK.[194,209] Alternatively, vasopressin may modulate the open probability of ROMK via its effects on CFTR.[210,211]

Use of Knockout Mice to Study the Urinary Concentrating Mechanism and Vasopressin Action

The function of several of the transporters and channels shown in Figure 10-16 have been evaluated using targeted gene deletion in mice (see Fenton and Knepper[73] for a comprehensive review). The phenotypes of these mice have been informative with regard to the role of these proteins in the urinary concentrating and diluting mechanism. An overview of the studies in these mice with respect to the urinary concentrating mechanism is provided here.

Aquaporin-1 Knockout Mice

AQP1 knockout mice have a drastically increased urine volume and reduced urinary osmolality that does not increase in response to water deprivation.[212] The concentrating defect is so severe that their average body weight decreases by 35% and serum osmolality increases to more than 500 mOsm/kg H_2O after 36 hours of water deprivation. Proximal tubule fluid absorption is markedly impaired in AQP1 knockout mice.

However, distal delivery of water and NaCl is not impaired, because of a reduction in glomerular filtration rate via the tubular-glomerular feedback mechanism.[213] The osmotic water permeability of isolated perfused thin descending limbs (from long loops of Henle) from AQP1 knockout mice was markedly reduced compared with control animals.[214] As previously discussed, rapid water absorption from the long-loop thin descending limbs is thought to be a major component of the countercurrent multiplication process in the outer medulla. Thus, the reduced water reabsorption of the thin descending limb from long loops of Henle is likely one factor responsible for the concentrating defect in AQP1 knockout mice. In addition, descending vasa recta, a second renal medullary site of AQP1 expression, also displayed a marked reduction in osmotic water permeability in AQP1 knockout mice.[25,26] Thus, countercurrent exchange processes involving the descending vasa recta are likely to be impaired in AQP1 knockout mice. Combined, the results of studies in these mice show that AQP1 is involved in the urine concentrating mechanism in the renal medulla.

Aquaporin-2 Gene Modified Mice

In 2001, a mouse knock-in model of AQP2-dependent nephrogenic diabetes insipidus (NDI), equivalent to humans with a form of autosomal NDI, was generated.[215] These mice failed to thrive and generally died within 1 week. Analysis of the urine and serum revealed serum hyperosmolality and low urine osmolality. Recently, several other mouse models have been developed that allow the role of AQP2 in the adult mouse to be examined. One model, developed by Rojek and colleagues, makes use of the Cre-loxP system of gene disruption to create a collecting duct–specific deletion of AQP2.[216] Another inducible mouse model for AQP2 deletion was developed by Yang and colleagues.[217] The major phenotype in both of these mouse lines is severe polyuria, with average basal urine volumes approximately equivalent to body weight. Despite the major polyuria, however, with free access to water, plasma concentrations of electrolytes, urea, and creatinine are no different in knockout mice than in controls. Thus, although they have relatively normal renal function, there is a major defect in the urinary concentrating mechanism in these mice. In addition, forward genetic screening of ethylnitrosourea-mutagenized mice isolated another mouse model of NDI with a F204V mutation in AQP2. These mice have a milder form of NDI.[218] Taken together, these mouse models confirm that AQP2 is responsible for the majority of transcellular water reabsorption in the collecting duct system.

Mouse models have been examined that indicate an essential role for AQP2 phosphorylation in transporter function.[219,220] One model has a single base change in codon 256 of AQP2, resulting in a serine to leucine amino acid substitution and loss of AQP2 phosphorylation at amino acid 256. This mutation results in an absence of AQP2 accumulation in the apical membrane. Another model has deletion of the distal COOH-terminal tail of AQP2 (from amino acid 230). Phenotypically, these phosphorylation-deficient mice produce large quantities of hypotonic urine and do not have a renal response to vasopressin, which is characteristic of NDI. These models provide direct genetic evidence that phosphorylation of AQP2 at serine 256 is essential for its apical membrane accumulation and maximal water reabsorption in the collecting duct.

Another mouse model has helped us to understand the molecular mechanisms behind AQP2-dependent autosomal dominant nephrogenic diabetes insipidus (AD-NDI).[221] These mice express 76 amino acids of the carboxy-terminal of a human AD-NDI mutant AQP2 (763-772del), fused to the wild-type 254 amino-terminus amino acids of mouse AQP2. Mice that are heterozygous for the mutation exhibited a severely impaired urinary concentrating ability, but after dehydration were able to moderately increase their urine osmolality.[222] Thus, this model is similar to the milder phenotype indicative of AD-NDI, rather than to autosomal recessive forms of NDI.[222] Additional studies in this mouse model determined that the phosphodiesterase 4 inhibitor rolipram was partially able to restore concentrating ability, which indicates that phosphodiesterase inhibitors may be useful drugs for the treatment of AD-NDI.

Finally, a conditional gene knock-in mouse model has been developed that has been used to screen for candidate protein folding correctors to address autosomal recessive NDI.[222a]

Aquaporin-3 Knockout Mice

The osmotic water permeability of the cortical collecting duct basolateral membrane of AQP3 knockout mice is reduced by greater that threefold compared with that of wild-type control mice.[223] The deletion of AQP3 and the reduced osmotic water permeability of the basolateral membrane would subsequently result in a decrease in transepithelial water transport in the connecting tubule, initial collecting tubule, and cortical collecting duct. This is emphasized by the finding that AQP3 knockout mice are markedly polyuric (10-fold greater daily urine volume than controls), with an average urine osmolality of less than 300 mOsm/kg H_2O. However, in contrast to AQP1 or AQP2 knockout mice, AQP3 knockout mice can slightly increase their urine osmolality after either water deprivation or vasopressin treatment. The relatively severe polyuria in AQP3 knockout mice is consistent with the view based on micropuncture data that the majority of post–macula densa fluid reabsorption is from the cortical portion of the collecting duct system, where AQP3 is normally the predominant basolateral water channel.[1]

Aquaporin-4 Knockout Mice

Isolated perfused tubule studies have demonstrated a fourfold decrease in IMCD osmotic water permeability in AQP4 knockout mice, which indicates that AQP4 is responsible for the majority of water movement across the basolateral membrane in this segment.[224,225] Despite this reduced IMCD water permeability, however, AQP4 knockout mice have relatively normal serum electrolyte concentrations and, compared with wild-type controls, have no difference in urine osmolality. AQP4 knockout mice have a significantly reduced maximal urine osmolality after 36 hours of water deprivation, and this reduced urine osmolality could not be further increased by vasopressin administration. The relatively modest decrease in urinary concentrating ability in AQP4 knockout mice, compared with the profound concentrating defect in AQP3 knockout mice, is likely due to the normal distribution of water transport along the collecting duct,[1] with much greater osmotic reabsorption of water in the cortical portion of the collecting duct system (where AQP3 is predominant), than in the medullary collecting ducts (where AQP4 is the predominant basolateral water channel).

UT-A1/3 Urea Transporter Knockout Mice

In 2004, a mouse model in which the two collecting duct urea transporters UT-A1 and UT-A3 were deleted (UT-A1/3$^{-/-}$ mice) was generated (extensively reviewed by Fenton[226,227] and Fenton and Knepper[228]). Perfused IMCD tubules from these mice had a complete absence of phloretin-sensitive and vasopressin-regulated urea transport.[97] On a normal protein (20% protein by weight) or high-protein (40% protein) diet, UT-A1/3$^{-/-}$ mice had a significantly greater fluid intake and urine flow, which resulted in decreased urine osmolality compared with wild-type mice.[97,98] In contrast, on a low-protein (4%) diet, UT-A1/3$^{-/-}$ mice did not show a substantial degree of polyuria. In the latter condition, hepatic urea production is low, and urea delivery to the IMCD is predicted to be low, which thus renders collecting duct urea transport largely immaterial to water balance. After 18 hours of water restriction, UT-A1/3$^{-/-}$ mice on a 20% or 40% protein diet are unable to reduce their urine flow to levels below those observed under basal conditions, which results in volume depletion and loss of body weight. In contrast, UT-A1/3$^{-/-}$ mice on a 4% protein diet are able to reduce their urine output to a level similar to that of control mice. Thus, the concentrating defect in UT-A1/3$^{-/-}$ mice is due to a urea-dependent osmotic diuresis; greater urea delivery to the IMCD results in greater levels of water excretion. These results are compatible with a model proposed in the 1950s by Berliner and colleagues, which predicted that luminal urea in the IMCD is normally osmotically ineffective because of the high concentrations of urea in the inner medullary interstitium, which balance osmotically the luminal urea and thus prevent the osmotic diuresis that would otherwise occur.[29]

UT-A1/3$^{-/-}$ mice have been exploited to study the mechanism responsible for Na$^+$ and Cl$^-$ accumulation in the inner medulla. A model independently proposed in 1972 by Stephenson[90] and by Kokko and Rector[89] has been the most widely accepted as the mechanism for concentration of Na$^+$ and Cl$^-$ in the inner medulla (see earlier). In this mechanism, generally referred to as the *passive model* or the *passive countercurrent multiplier mechanism*, the generation of a passive electrochemical gradient that drives the exit of Na$^+$ and Cl$^-$ from the thin ascending limb is indirectly dependent on rapid reabsorption of urea from the IMCD (see earlier for a full description). Based on this model, it would be predicted that UT-A1/3$^{-/-}$ mice would be unable to accumulate Na$^+$ and Cl$^-$ to a normal degree. However, three independent studies in UT-A1/3$^{-/-}$ mice failed to demonstrate in all regions of the inner medulla the predicted decline in Na$^+$ and Cl$^-$ concentrations, despite a profound decrease in urea accumulation.[97,127,227,228] Based on these results alone, the passive concentrating model in the form originally proposed by Stephenson and by Kokko and Rector, in which NaCl reabsorption from the loop of Henle depends on a high IMCD urea permeability, does not appear to be the only mechanism by which NaCl is concentrated in the inner medulla. However, a recent mathematical modeling analysis of these same data concluded that the results found in the UT-A1/3$^{-/-}$ mice are consistent with what one would predict for the passive mechanism.[10] Thus, the issue remains unresolved at present.

Another hypothesis regarding urea and the urinary concentrating mechanism was described nearly 75 years ago as "an economy of water in renal function referable to urea" and is affectionately known as the *Gamble phenomenon*.[127] Gamble described that (1) the water requirement for excretion of urea is less than that for excretion of an osmotically equivalent amount of NaCl, and (2) less water is required for the excretion of urea and NaCl together than is needed for excretion of an osmotically equivalent amount of either urea or NaCl alone. In UT-A1/3$^{-/-}$ mice both elements of the Gamble phenomenon were absent, which indicates that IMCD urea transporters play an essential role.[128] When wild-type mice were given progressively increasing amounts of urea or NaCl in the diet, both substances induced osmotic diuresis, but at different excretion levels (6000 micro-osmole/day for urea; 3500 micro-osmole/day for NaCl). Mice were unable to increase urinary NaCl concentrations above 420 mmol/L. Thus, the second component of the Gamble phenomenon derives from the fact that both urea and NaCl excretion are saturable, which presumably results from an ability to exceed the respective reabsorptive capacities for urea and NaCl, rather than a specific interaction of urea transport and NaCl transport at an epithelial level.

UT-A2 and UT-B Urea Transporter Knockout Mice

Mouse models with selective deletion of either UT-A2 or UT-B have been developed.[72,129,229] The role of these two urea transporters in the urinary concentrating mechanism is proposed to be predominantly in the process of urea recycling (see earlier), which helps maintain a high level of urea in the renal inner medulla. Recycling occurs when urea reabsorbed from the IMCD is resecreted into the loop of Henle, which causes it to be returned to the collecting duct lumen with the flow of tubule fluid. A major factor in urea secretion into the loop of Henle is believed to be transfer from the vasa recta to the thin descending limb of short-loop nephrons in the vascular bundles of the outer medulla where these two structures are in close proximity.[3] The urea transporter in the thin descending limb is UT-A2, whereas in the vasa recta UT-B is the major urea transporter. Deletion of either of these transporters is predicted to impair urea accumulation in the inner medulla, resulting in increased water excretion via urea-induced osmotic diuresis. However, UT-A2 knockout mice did not have a reduced concentrating ability or increased water excretion with a normal level of protein intake.[72] Thus, urea secretion into the thin descending limb does not appear to be as important in medullary urea accumulation as previously believed.

In contrast, UT-B knockout mice have a significantly higher daily urine output and lower urine osmolality than wild-type mice.[129] Their phenotype is very similar to that of humans with genetic loss of UT-B (Kidd antigen), who are unable to concentrate their urine above 800 mOsm/kg H$_2$O, even following overnight water deprivation and exogenous vasopressin administration.[230] UT-B–null mice have a "urea-selective" urinary concentrating defect, with a significantly higher plasma urea level and a severely reduced urine–to–plasma urea ratio.[229] UT-B is potentially important for both countercurrent exchange of urea between ascending and descending vasa recta and for transfer of urea from the vasa recta to the thin descending limb.

The concentrating defect observed in UT-B knockout mice is greater than that observed in UT-A2 knockout mice, which suggests that countercurrent exchange of urea between ascending and descending vasa recta is more important than the transfer of urea from the vasa recta to the thin descending limb for trapping urea in the inner medullary interstitium. However, UT-B is also present in red blood cells and contributes to their high urea permeability, and because of this erythrocytes from UT-B knockout mice have an approximately 45-fold lower urea permeability than do those from control mice.[231] Therefore, the concentrating defects observed in the UT-B knockout mice could be due to the loss of urea transport in the vasa recta, in red blood cells, or in both, and this may help to explain the apparent difference in concentrating ability between the UT-A2 knockout mice and UT-B knockout mice.

Na⁺/H⁺ Exchanger 3 and Na-K-2Cl Cotransporter 2 Knockout Mice

The major apical transporters mediating Na entry in the thick ascending limb, namely NHE3 and NKCC2/BSC1, have been knocked out in mice, but the effect on the urinary concentrating mechanism is drastically different in the two models.[232,233] NHE3 knockout mice have a marked reduction in proximal tubule fluid absorption, which confirms that NHE3 is the major Na entry pathway in proximal tubule cells. NHE3 knockout mice exhibit a compensatory decrease in glomerular filtration rate owing to an intact tubuloglomerular feedback mechanism.[234] On ad libitum water intake, NHE3 knockouts manifest a moderate increase in water intake associated with lower urinary osmolalities.[235] NHE3 knockout mice have a marked decrease in renal NKCC2 expression despite elevated circulating levels of vasopressin.[235,236] Overall, despite drastically reduced proximal tubule fluid reabsorption, NHE3 knockout mice have a very mild urinary concentrating defect that may be associated with reduced NKCC2 expression. In contrast, NKCC2 knockout mice die before weaning due to renal fluid wasting and dehydration.[233] Although these mice could be induced to survive by treatment with indomethacin and fluid administration, extreme polyuria, hydronephrosis, and growth retardation could not be abrogated. Why does deletion of NKCC2 result in such a severe phenotype, when deletion of NHE3, a transporter responsible for reabsorption of far more Na, results in a viable mouse capable of maintaining extracellular fluid volume? The answer appears to lie in the special role that NKCC2 plays in the macula densa in the mediation of tubuloglomerular feedback. Tubuloglomerular feedback allows NHE3 knockout mice to maintain a relatively normal distal delivery through a decrease in glomerular filtration rate, whereas NKCC2 mice cannot compensate in this manner because the transporter is necessary for the feedback to occur. Indeed, mice with isoform-specific deletion of NKCC2 have been generated that may be useful for examining the tubular versus tubuloglomerular feedback role of NKCC2 in the urinary concentrating mechanism.[237,238]

Na-K-2Cl Cotransporter 1 Knockout Mice

NKCC1-null mice have a reduced capacity to excrete free water relative to wild-type mice and also have a blunted increase in urinary osmolality after vasopressin administration.[239] These results suggest abnormalities in vasopressin signaling in the collecting duct, but may also be attributable to the NKCC1-dependent increase in IMCD cell swelling that results from vasopressin treatment.[240,241]

Na-Cl Cotransporter and Epithelial Sodium Channel Knockout Mice

The two major apical Na transporters mediating Na entry beyond the macula densa, namely NCC and ENaC, have been knocked out in mice. NCC knockout mice appear to have an essentially normal phenotype, with only a mild decrease in blood pressure and no difference in urine output.[242] Upon dietary potassium restriction, however, NCC knockout mice develop hypokalemia and polyuria, which seem to be associated with a central defect in the regulation of vasopressin secretion and suppressed AQP2 expression.[243] In contrast to the NCC knockout, deletion of any of the ENaC subunits results in a severe phenotype with neonatal death.[244-247] In α-ENaC knockout mice, early death appears to be due to failure to adequately clear fluid from the pulmonary alveoli after birth, whereas the β- and γ-ENaC knockout mice appear to die of hyperkalemia and sodium chloride wasting.[244,245,247] α-ENaC deletion from the collecting ducts alone, with ENaC expression left intact in the connecting tubule and nonrenal tissues, resulted in viable mice that had little or no difficulty in maintaining salt and fluid homeostasis.[248] Thus, Na absorption from the renal collecting duct via ENaC does not appear to be necessary for urinary concentration, or else connecting tubule ENaC plays an underestimated role in urinary concentration. Taken together, NCC deleted only from the distal convoluted tubule or ENaC deleted only from the collecting duct results in a very mild phenotype, possibly because one can compensate for the other with regard to sodium balance.

ClC-K1 Chloride Channel Knockout Mice

Microperfusion studies of ClC-K1–null mice (*Clcnk1⁻/⁻*) determined that there was drastically reduced transepithelial chloride transport in the thin ascending limb of these knockout mice.[249] Physiologic studies revealed that *Clcnk1⁻/⁻* mice had significantly greater urine volume and lower urine osmolality compared with controls, and even after water deprivation knockout mice were unable to concentrate their urine. This observed polyuria was insensitive to vasopressin administration and was due to water diuresis and not osmotic diuresis. Inner medulla concentrations of Na^+ and Cl^- in *Clcnk1⁻/⁻* mice were approximately half those in controls, which resulted in a significantly reduced osmolality of the papilla. These studies demonstrate that the ClC-K1 chloride channel is necessary for maintenance of a maximal osmolality in the inner medullary tissue. The findings in the *Clcnk1⁻/⁻* mice emphasize the importance of rapid chloride exit (and presumably Na^+ exit) from the thin ascending limb in the inner medullary concentrating process.

ROMK Potassium Channel Knockout Mice

The majority of ROMK potassium channel (Kir1.1) knockout mice die before weaning due to hydronephrosis and severe dehydration.[250] Approximately 5% of these mice survive the perinatal period, but surviving adults manifest polydipsia, polyuria, impaired urinary concentrating ability, hypernatremia, and reduced blood pressure, which is consistent with the known role of ROMK in active NaCl absorption in the thick ascending limb. From these animals, a line of mice has been derived that has a greater survival rate and no hydronephrosis in adult animals, but the concentrating defect still persists. Interestingly, more male mice survive than female mice, and this is associated with lower glomerular filtration rate, higher fractional Na excretion, and higher prostaglandin E_2 levels in the female mice.[251] Surprisingly, adult ROMK knockout mice do not exhibit hyperkalemia, which indicates that the connecting tubule and/or collecting duct principal cells must be capable of secreting K^+ via some other pathway, presumably flow-dependent, Ca^{2+}-activated K channels referred to as *Maxi-K channels*.[252,253]

Vasopressin V_2 Receptor Knockout Mice

A mouse model of X-linked NDI has provided insight into the role of V_2R in the urinary concentrating mechanism.[254] All male V_2R mutant mice ($V_2R^{-/y}$) died within 7 days after birth. Analysis of 3-day old pups revealed a severe state of hypernatremia, with drastically increased serum Na^+ and Cl^- levels, and significantly lower urine osmolality. The V_2R agonist desmopressin (DDAVP) had no effect in $V_2R^{-/y}$ mice, but increased urine osmolality significantly in control mice. Adult female $V_2R^{+/-}$ mice had an approximate 50% decrease in total vasopressin binding capacity and a 50% decrease in DDAVP-induced intracellular cAMP levels. This resulted in polyuria, polydipsia, and a reduced urinary concentrating ability, consistent with NDI. In addition, the expression of multiple other gene products, including those of the renin-angiotensin-aldosterone system, was altered in V_2R-deficient mice.[255] Taken together, these results are consistent with the general view that the antidiuretic effects of vasopressin are due to an initial interaction between vasopressin and the V_2R, which results in increased intracellular cAMP and eventually promotes water reabsorption in the kidney collecting duct via aquaporins. Furthermore, they demonstrate that there is no other significant compensatory event that can generate cAMP and increase water permeability in the renal collecting duct.

Acknowledgments

Drs. Mark A. Knepper, Jason D. Hoffert, and Randall K. Packer were coauthors of this chapter in the eighth edition, and some of the material in that chapter is carried forward to the present edition. This work was supported by National Institutes of Health grants R01-DK41707 and P01-DK61521 to Jeff Sands and R01-DK42091 to Harold Layton. Robert Fenton is supported by a Marie Curie Intra-European Fellowship, the Danish Medical Research Council, the Novo Nordisk Fund, the Carlsberg Foundation (Carlsbergfondet), and the Danish National Research Foundation (Danmarks Grundforskningsfond).

References

1. Knepper MA, Burg MB. Organization of nephron function. *Am J Physiol Renal Physiol.* 1983;244:F579-F589.
2. Knepper MA, Stephenson JL. Urinary concentrating and diluting processes. In: Andreoli TE, Hoffman JF, Fanestil DD, et al. eds. *Physiology of Membrane Disorders*. New York: Plenum; 1986.
3. Zhai XY, Thomsen JS, Birn H, et al. Three-dimensional reconstruction of the mouse kidney. *J Am Soc Nephrol.* 2006;17:77-88.
4. Imai M, Taniguchi J, Tabei K. Function of thin loops of Henle. *Kidney Int.* 1987;31:565-579.
5. Wade JB, Lee AJ, Liu J, et al. UT-A2: a 55 kDa urea transporter protein in thin descending limb of Henle's loop whose abundance is regulated by vasopressin. *Am J Physiol.* 2000;278:F52-F62.
6. Imai M, Taniguchi J, Yoshitomi K. Transition of permeability properties along the descending limb of long-loop nephron. *Am J Physiol.* 1988;254:F323-F328.
7. Chou C-L, Knepper MA. in vitro perfusion of chinchilla thin limb segments: segmentation and osmotic water permeability. *Am J Physiol Renal Physiol.* 1992;263:F417-F426.
8. Chou C-L, Knepper MA. in vitro perfusion of chinchilla thin limb segments: urea and NaCl permeabilities. *Am J Physiol Renal Physiol.* 1993;264:F337-F343.
9. Chou C-L, Nielsen S, Knepper MA. Structural-functional correlation in chinchilla long loop of Henle thin limbs: a novel papillary subsegment. *Am J Physiol Renal Fluid Electrolyte Physiol.* 1993;265:F863-F874.
10. Pannabecker TL, Dantzler WH, Layton HE, et al. Role of three-dimensional architecture in the urine concentrating mechanism of the rat renal inner medulla. *Am J Physiol Renal Physiol.* 2008;295:F1271-F1285.
11. Pannabecker TL, Abbott DE, Dantzler WH. Three-dimensional functional reconstruction of inner medullary thin limbs of Henle's loop. *Am J Physiol Renal Physiol.* 2004;286:F38-F45.
12. Zhai XY, Fenton RA, Andreasen A, et al. Aquaporin-1 is not expressed in descending thin limbs of short-loop nephrons. *J Am Soc Nephrol.* 2007;18:2937-2944.
13. Pannabecker TL, Dahlmann A, Brokl OH, et al. Mixed descending- and ascending-type thin limbs of Henle's loop in mammalian renal inner medulla. *Am J Physiol Renal Physiol.* 2000;278:F202-F208.
14. Kaissling B, Kriz W. Structural analysis of the rabbit kidney. In: Brodal A, Hild W, VanLimborgh J, et al. eds. *Advances in anatomy: embryology and cell biology*. vol. 56. Berlin: Springer Verlag; 1979.
15. Kishore BK, Mandon B, Oza NB, et al. Rat renal arcade segment expresses vasopressin-regulated water channel and vasopressin V_2 receptor. *J Clin Invest.* 1996;97:2763-2771.
16. Knepper MA, Danielson RA, Saidel GM, et al. Quantitative analysis of renal medullary anatomy in rats and rabbits. *Kidney Int.* 1977;12:313-323.
17. Kriz W. Der architektonische und funktionelle Aufbau der Rattenniere. *Z Zellforsch.* 1967;82:495-535.
18. Kriz W, Bankir L. Structural organization of the renal medullary counterflow system. *Fed Proc.* 1983;42:2379-2385.
19. Kriz W, Schnermann J, Koepsell H. The position of short and long loops of Henle in the rat kidney. *Z Anat Entwicklungsgesch.* 1972;138:301-319.
20. Lemley KV, Kriz W. Cycles and separations: the histotopography of the urinary concentrating process. *Kidney Int.* 1987;31:538-548.
21. Pannabecker TL, Dantzler WH. Three-dimensional lateral and vertical relationships of inner medullary loops of Henle and collecting ducts. *Am J Physiol Renal Physiol.* 2004;287:F767-F774.
22. Pannabecker TL, Henderson CS, Dantzler WH. Quantitative analysis of functional reconstructions reveals lateral and axial zonation in the renal inner medulla. *Am J Physiol Renal Physiol.* 2008;294:F1306-F1314.
23. Pannabecker TL, Dantzler WH. Three-dimensional architecture of collecting ducts, loops of Henle, and blood vessels in the renal papilla. *Am J Physiol Renal Physiol.* 2007;293:F696-F704.
24. Rolhuser H, Kriz W, Heinke W. Das Gefs system der Rattenniere. *Z Zellforsch.* 1964;64:381-403.
25. Nielsen S, Pallone T, Smith BL, et al. Aquaporin-1 water channels in short and long loop descending thin limbs and in descending vasa recta in rat kidney. *Am J Physiol Renal Fluid Electrolyte Physiol.* 1995;268:F1023-F1037.
26. Pallone TL, Kishore BK, Nielsen S, et al. Evidence that aquaporin-1 mediates NaCl-induced water flux across descending vasa recta. *Am J Physiol Renal Physiol.* 1997;272:F587-F596.
27. Pallone TL. Characterization of the urea transporter in outer medullary descending vasa recta. *Am J Physiol.* 1994;267:R260-R267.
28. Xu Y, Olives B, Bailly P, et al. Endothelial cells of the kidney vasa recta express the urea transporter HUT11. *Kidney Int.* 1997;51:138-146.
29. Berliner RW, Levinsky NG, Davidson DG, et al. Dilution and concentration of the urine and the action of antidiuretic hormone. *Am J Med.* 1958;24:730-744.
30. Pannabecker TL. Loop of Henle interaction with interstitial nodal spaces in the renal inner medulla. *Am J Physiol Renal Physiol.* 2008;295:F1744-F1751.
31. Bulger RE, Nagle RB. Ultrastructure of the interstitium in the rabbit kidney. *Am J Anat.* 1973;136:183-204.
32. Knepper MA, Saidel GM, Hascall VC, et al. Concentration of solutes in the renal inner medulla: interstitial hyaluronan as a mechano-osmotic transducer. *Am J Physiol Renal Physiol.* 2003;284:F433-F446.
33. Lacy ER, Schmidt-Nielsen B. Ultrastructural organization of the hamster renal pelvis. *Am J Anat.* 1979;155:403-424.

34. Schmidt-Nielsen B. Excretion in mammals: role of the renal pelvis in the modification of the urinary concentration and composition. *Fed Proc.* 1977;36:2493-2503.

35. Sheehan HL, Davis JC. Anatomy of the pelvis in the rabbit kidney. *J Anat.* 1959;93:499-502.

36. Reinking LN, Schmidt-Nielsen B. Peristaltic flow of urine in the renal papillary collecting ducts of hamsters. *Kidney Int.* 1981;20:55-60.

37. Schmidt-Nielsen B, Graves B. Changes in fluid compartments in hamster renal papilla due to peristalsis in the pelvic wall. *Kidney Int.* 1982;22:613-625.

38. Gottschalk CW, Mylle M. Micropuncture study of the mammalian urinary concentrating mechanism: evidence for the countercurrent hypothesis. *Am J Physiol.* 1959;196:927-936.

39. Jamison RL, Lacy ER. Evidence for urinary dilution by the collecting tubule. *Am J Physiol.* 1972;223:898-902.

40. Giebisch G, Windhager EE. Renal tubular transfer of sodium chloride and potassium. *Am J Med.* 1964;36:643-669.

41. Lassiter WE, Gottschalk CW, Mylle M. Micropuncture study of net transtubular movement of water and urea in nondiuretic mammalian kidney. *Am J Physiol.* 1961;200:1139-1146.

42. Burg MB, Green N. Function of the thick ascending limb of Henle's loop. *Am J Physiol.* 1973;224:659-668.

43. Rocha AS, Kokko JP. Sodium chloride and water transport in the medullary thick ascending limb of Henle: evidence for active chloride transport. *J Clin Invest.* 1973;52:612-623.

44. Ullrich KJ. Function of the collecting ducts. *Circulation.* 1960;21:869-874.

45. Wirz H, Hargitay B, Kuhn W. Lokalisation des Konzentrierungsprozesses in der Niere durch direkte Kryoskopie. *Helv Physiol Pharmacol Acta.* 1951;9:196-207.

46. Grantham JJ, Burg MB. Effect of vasopressin and cyclic AMP on permeability of isolated collecting tubules. *Am J Physiol.* 1966;211:255-259.

47. Morgan T, Berliner RW. Permeability of the loop of Henle, vasa recta, and collecting duct to water, urea, and sodium. *Am J Physiol.* 1968;215:108-115.

48. Jarausch KH, Ullrich KJ. Untersuchungen zum Problem der Harnkonzentrierung und Harnverdünnung; Über die Verteilung von Elektrolyten (Na, K, Ca, Mg, Cl, anorganischem Phosphat), Harnstoff, Aminosäuren und exogenem Kreatinin in Rinde und Mark der Hundeniere bei verschiedenen Diuresezustanden. *Pflugers Arch.* 1956;262:537-550.

49. Hai MA, Thomas S. The time-course of changes in renal tissue composition during lysine vasopressin infusion in the rat. *Pflugers Arch.* 1969;310:297-319.

50. Kuhn W, Ryffel K. Herstellung konzentrierter Lösungen aus verdünnten durch blosse Membranwirkung: Ein Modellversuch zur Funktion der Niere. *Hoppe-Seylers Z Physiol Chem.* 1942;276:145-178.

51. Hargitay B, Kuhn W. Das Multiplikationsprinzip als Grundlage der Harnkonzentrierung in der Niere. *Z Elektrochem.* 1951;55:539-558.

52. Kuhn W, Ramel A. Aktiver Salztransport als möglicher (und wahrscheinlicher) Einzeleffekt bei der Harnkonzentrierung in der Niere. *Helv Chim Acta.* 1959;42:628-660.

53. Imai M, Hayashi M, Araki M. Functional heterogeneity of the descending limbs of Henle's loop. I. Internephron heterogeneity in the hamster kidney. *Pflugers Arch.* 1984;402:385-392.

54. Rasch R, Grann BL, Andreasen A. 3D reconstruction of the bend of short loops from the loop of Henle. *J Am Soc Nephrol.* 2002;13: SA VP0017:(abstract).

55. Dantzler WH, Evans KE, Pannabecker TL. Osmotic water permeabilities in specific segments of rat inner medullary thin limbs of Henle's loops. *FASEB J.* 2009;23:970.3: (abstract).

56. Layton AT, Layton HE. A region-based mathematical model of the urine concentrating mechanism in the rat outer medulla. I. Formulation and base-case results. *Am J Physiol Renal Physiol.* 2005;289:F1346-F1366.

57. Layton AT, Layton HE. A region-based mathematical model of the urine concentrating mechanism in the rat outer medulla. II. Parameter sensitivity and tubular inhomogeneity. *Am J Physiol Renal Physiol.* 2005;289: F1367-F1381.

58. Kriz W, Koepsell H. The structural organization of the mouse kidney. *Z Anat Entwicklungsgesch.* 1974;144:137-163.

59. Garg LC, Mackie S, Tisher CC. Effect of low potassium-diet on Na-K-ATPase in rat nephron segments. *Pflugers Arch.* 1982;394:113-117.

60. Oliver J. *Nephrons and kidneys: a quantitative study of developmental and evolutionary mammalian renal architectonics.* New York: Harper & Row; 1968.

61. Pfeiffer EW, Nungesser WC, Iverson DA, et al. The renal anatomy of the primitive rodent, *Aplodontia rufa,* and a consideration of its functional significance. *Anat Rec.* 1960;137:227-235.

62. Sands JM, Knepper MA. Urea permeability of mammalian inner medullary collecting duct system and papillary surface epithelium. *J Clin Invest.* 1987;79:138-147.

63. Rocha AS, Kudo LH. Water, urea, sodium, chloride, and potassium transport in the in vitro perfused papillary collecting duct. *Kidney Int.* 1982;22:485-491.

64. Sands JM, Nonoguchi H, Knepper MA. Vasopressin effects on urea and H_2O transport in inner medullary collecting duct subsegments. *Am J Physiol.* 1987;253:F823-F832.

65. Star RA, Nonoguchi H, Balaban R, et al. Calcium and cyclic adenosine monophosphate as second messengers for vasopressin in the rat inner medullary collecting duct. *J Clin Invest.* 1988;81:1879-1888.

66. Zimmerhackl BL, Robertson CR, Jamison RL. The medullary microcirculation. *Kidney Int.* 1987;31:641-647.

67. Knepper MA, Roch-Ramel F. Pathways of urea transport in the mammalian kidney. *Kidney Int.* 1987;31:629-633.

68. de Rouffignac C, Morel F. Micropuncture study of water, electrolytes and urea movements along the loop of Henle in. *Psammomys. J Clin Invest.* 1969;48:474-486.

69. de Rouffignac C, Bankir L, Roinel N. Renal function and concentrating ability in a desert rodent: the gundi (*Ctenodactylus vali. Pflugers Arch.* 1981;390:138-144.

70. Kriz W. Structural organization of the renal medulla: comparative and functional aspects. *Am J Physiol Regul Integr Comp Physiol.* 1981;241:R3-R16.

71. Nielsen S, Terris J, Smith CP, et al. Cellular and subcellular localization of the vasopressin-regulated urea transporter in rat kidney. *Proc Natl Acad Sci U S A.* 1996;93:5495-5500.

72. Uchida S, Sohara E, Rai T, et al. Impaired urea accumulation in the inner medulla of mice lacking the urea transporter UT-A2. *Mol Cell Biol.* 2005;25:7357-7363.

73. Fenton RA, Knepper MA. Mouse models and the urinary concentrating mechanism in the new millennium. *Physiol Rev.* 2007;87:1083-1112.

74. Knepper MA. Urea transport in isolated thick ascending limbs and collecting ducts from rats. *Am J Physiol.* 1983;245:F634-F639.

75. Rocha AS, Kokko JP. Permeability of medullary nephron segments to urea and water: effect of vasopressin. *Kidney Int.* 1974;6:379-387.

76. Knepper MA. Urea transport in nephron segments from medullary rays of rabbits. *Am J Physiol.* 1983;244:F622-F627.

77. Kawamura S, Kokko JP. Urea secretion by the straight segment of the proximal tubule. *J Clin Invest.* 1976;58:604-612.

78. Wirz H. Der osmotische Druck in den corticolin Tubuli der rattenniere. *Helv Physiol Acta.* 1956;14:353-362.

79. Fenton RA, Brond L, Nielsen S, et al. Cellular and subcellular distribution of the type II vasopressin receptor in kidney. *Am J Physiol Renal Physiol.* 2007;293:F748-F760.

80. Jamison RL, Buerkert J, Lacy FB. A micropuncture study of collecting tubule function in rats with hereditary diabetes insipidus. *J Clin Invest.* 1971;50:2444-2452.

81. Schmidt-Nielsen B, Graves B, Roth J. Water removal and solute additions determining increases in renal medullary osmolality. *Am J Physiol.* 1983;244:F472-F482.

82. Hai MA, Thomas S. Acute effects of lysine-vasopressin infusion on rat renal tissue osmolality. *J Physiol.* 1969;202:117P+.

83. Saikia TC. Composition of the renal cortex and medulla of rats during water diuresis and antidiuresis. *Q J Exp Physiol Cogn Med Sci.* 1965;50: 146-157.

84. Lankford SP, Chou C-L, Terada Y, et al. Regulation of collecting duct water permeability independent of cAMP-mediated AVP response. *Am J Physiol Renal Fluid Electrolyte Physiol.* 1991;261:F554-F566.

85. Atherton JC, Hai MA, Thomas S. The time course of changes in renal tissue composition during water diuresis in the rat. *J Physiol.* 1968;197:429-443.

86. Imai M, Kokko JP. Sodium, chloride, urea, and water transport in the thin ascending limb of Henle. *J Clin Invest.* 1974;53:393-402.

87. Kondo Y, Abe K, Igarashi Y, et al. Direct evidence for the absence of active Na^+ reabsorption in hamster ascending thin limb of Henle's loop. *J Clin Invest.* 1993;91:5-11.

88. Knepper MA, Chou C-L, Layton HE. How is urine concentrated by the renal inner medulla? *Contrib Nephrol.* 1993;102:144-160.

89. Kokko JP, Rector FC. Countercurrent multiplication system without active transport in inner medulla. *Kidney Int.* 1972;2:214-223.

90. Stephenson JL. Concentration of urine in a central core model of the renal counterflow system. *Kidney Int.* 1972;2:85-94.

91. Jen JF, Stephenson JL. Externally driven countercurrent multiplication in a mathematical model of the urinary concentrating mechanism of the renal inner medulla. *Bull Math Biol.* 1994;56:491-514.

92. Thomas SR. Inner medullary lactate production and accumulation: a vasa recta model. *Am J Physiol Renal Physiol.* 2000;279:F468-F481.

93. Hervy S, Thomas SR. Inner medullary lactate production and urine-concentrating mechanism: a flat medullary model. *Am J Physiol Renal Physiol.* 2003;284:F65-F81.

94. Thomas SR, Wexler AS. Inner medullary external osmotic driving force in a 3D model of the renal concentrating mechanism. *Am J Physiol.* 1995;269:F159-F171.

95. Pruitt ME, Knepper MA, Graves B, et al. Effect of peristaltic contractions of the renal pelvic wall on solute concentrations of the renal inner medulla in the hamster. *Am J Physiol Renal Physiol.* 2006;290:F892-F896.

96. Gamba G, Knepper MA. Urinary concentration and dilution. In: Brenner BM, ed. *Brenner and Rector's the kidney*. Philadelphia: Saunders; 2004.

97. Fenton RA, Chou C-L, Stewart GS, et al. Urinary concentrating defect in mice with selective deletion of phloretin-sensitive urea transporters in the renal collecting duct. *Proc Natl Acad Sci U S A*. 2004;101:7469-7474.

98. Fenton RA, Flynn A, Shodeinde A, et al. Renal phenotype of UT-A urea transporter knockout mice. *J Am Soc Nephrol*. 2005;16:1583-1592.

99. Layton AT, Pannabecker TL, Dantzler WH, et al. Two modes for concentrating urine in rat inner medulla. *Am J Physiol Renal Physiol*. 2004;287:F816-F839.

100. Yang T, Huang YA, Singh I, et al. Localization of bumetanide- and thiazide-sensitive Na-K-Cl cotransporters along the rat nephron. *Am J Physiol*. 1996;271:F931-F939.

101. Zhang W, Edwards A. A model of glucose transport and conversion to lactate in the renal medullary microcirculation. *Am J Physiol Renal Physiol*. 2006;290:F87-F102.

102. Hascall VC, Heinegaard DK, Wight TN. Proteoglycans: metabolism and pathology. In: Hay ED, ed. *Cell biology of extracellular matrix*. New York: Plenum; 1991.

103. Weigel PH, Hascall VC, Tammi M. Hyaluronan synthases. *J Biol Chem*. 1997;272:13997-14000.

104. Toole BP. Hyaluronan is not just goo! *J Clin Invest*. 2000;106:335-336.

105. Comper WD, Laurent TC. Physiological function of connective tissue polysaccharides. *Physiol Rev*. 1978;58:255-315.

106. Castor CW, Greene JA. Regional distribution of acid mucopolysaccharides in the kidney. *J Clin Invest*. 1968;47:2125-2132.

107. Dwyer TM, Banks SA, Alonso-Calicia M, et al. Distribution of renal medullary hyaluronan in lean and obese rabbits. *Kidney Int*. 2000;58:721-729.

108. Pitcock JA, Lyons H, Brown PS, et al. Glycosaminoglycans of the rat renomedullary interstitium: ultrastructural and biochemical observations. *Exp Mol Pathol*. 1988;49:373-387.

109. Sands JM, Layton HE. The urine concentrating mechanism and urea transporters. In: Alpern RJ, Hebert SC, eds. *The kidney: physiology and pathophysiology*. San Diego: Academic Press; 2008.

110. Sands JM, Layton HE. The physiology of urinary concentration: an update. *Semin Nephrol*. 2009;29:178-195.

111. Schmidt-Nielsen B. The renal concentrating mechanism in insects and mammals: a new hypothesis involving hydrostatic pressures. *Am J Physiol*. 1995;268:R1087-R1100.

112. Laurent TC. *The chemistry, biology and medical applications of hyaluronan and its derivatives*. London: Portland Press; 1988.

113. Camenisch TD, Spicer AP, Brohm-Gibson T, et al. Disruption of hyaluronan synthase-2 abrogates normal cardiac morphogenesis and hyaluronan-mediated transformation of epithelium to mesenchyme. *J Clin Invest*. 2000;106:349-360.

114. Sabolic I, Valenti G, Verbavatz J-M, et al. Localization of the CHIP28 water channel in rat kidney. *Am J Physiol Cell Physiol*. 1992;263:C1225-C1233.

115. Nielsen S, Smith BL, Christensen EI, et al. CHIP28 water channels are localized in constitutively water-permeable segments of the nephron. *J Cell Biol*. 1993;120:371-383.

116. Nielsen S, Frokiaer J, Marples D, et al. Aquaporins in the kidney: from molecules to medicine. *Physiol Rev*. 2002;82:205-244.

117. Fenton RA, Moeller HB, Hoffert JD, et al. Acute regulation of aquaporin-2 phosphorylation at Ser-264 by vasopressin. *Proc Natl Acad Sci U S A*. 2008;105:3134-3139.

118. Hoffert JD, Fenton RA, Moeller HB, et al. Vasopressin-stimulated increase in phosphorylation at Ser269 potentiates plasma membrane retention of aquaporin-2. *J Biol Chem*. 2008;283:24617-24627.

119. Hoffert JD, Pisitkun T, Wang G, et al. Quantitative phosphoproteomics of vasopressin-sensitive renal cells: regulation of aquaporin-2 phosphorylation at two sites. *Proc Natl Acad Sci U S A*. 2006;103:7159-7164.

120. Moeller HB, Knepper MA, Fenton RA. Serine 269 phosphorylated aquaporin-2 is targeted to the apical membrane of collecting duct principal cells. *Kidney Int*. 2009;75:295-303.

121. Moeller HB, MacAulay N, Knepper MA, et al. Role of multiple phosphorylation sites in the COOH-terminal tail of aquaporin-2 for water transport: evidence against channel gating. *Am J Physiol Renal Physiol*. 2009;296:F649-F657.

122. Fenton RA, Moeller HB. Recent discoveries in vasopressin-regulated aquaporin-2 trafficking. *Prog Brain Res*. 2008;170:571-579.

123. Zwang NA, Hoffert JD, Pisitkun T, et al. Identification of phosphorylation-dependent binding partners of aquaporin-2 using protein mass spectrometry. *J Proteome Res*. 2009;8:1540-1554.

124. Ecelbarger CA, Terris J, Frindt G, et al. Aquaporin-3 water channel localization and regulation in rat kidney. *Am J Physiol*. 1995;269:F663-F672.

125. Terris J, Ecelbarger CA, Marples D, et al. Distribution of aquaporin-4 water channel expression within rat kidney. *Am J Physiol*. 1995;269:F775-F785.

126. Terris J, Ecelbarger CA, Nielsen S, et al. Long-term regulation of four renal aquaporins in rats. *Am J Physiol*. 1996;271:F414-F422.

127. Gamble JL, McKhann CF, Butler AM, et al. An economy of water in renal function referable to urea. *Am J Physiol*. 1934;109:139-154.

128. Fenton RA, Chou CL, Sowersby H, et al. Gamble's "economy of water" revisited: studies in urea transporter knockout mice. *Am J Physiol Renal Physiol*. 2006;291:F148-F154.

129. Yang B, Bankir L, Gillespie A, et al. Urea-selective concentrating defect in transgenic mice lacking urea transporter UT-B. *J Biol Chem*. 2002;277:10633-10637.

130. Yang B, Verkman AS. Analysis of double knockout mice lacking aquaporin-1 and urea transporter UT-B. *J Biol Chem*. 2002;277:36782-36786.

131. Klein JD, Sands JM, Qian L, et al. Upregulation of urea transporter UT-A2 and water channels AQP2 and AQP3 in mice lacking urea transporter UT-B. *J Am Soc Nephrol*. 2004;15:1161-1167.

132. Stewart GS, Graham C, Cattell S, et al. UT-B is expressed in bovine rumen: potential role in ruminal urea transport. *Am J Physiol Regul Integr Comp Physiol*. 2005;289:R605-R612.

133. Olives B, Neau P, Bailly P, et al. Cloning and functional expression of a urea transporter from human bone marrow cells. *J Biol Chem*. 1994;269:31649-31652.

134. Bagnasco SM, Peng T, Nakayama Y, et al. Differential expression of individual UT-A urea transporter isoforms in rat kidney. *J Am Soc Nephrol*. 2000;11:1980-1986.

135. Nakayama Y, Naruse M, Karakashian A, et al. Cloning of the rat Slc14a2 gene and genomic organization of the UT-A urea transporter. *Biochim Biophys Acta*. 2001;1518:19-26.

136. Bagnasco SM, Peng T, Janech MG, et al. Cloning and characterization of the human urea transporter UT-A1 and mapping of the human *Slc14a2* gene. *Am J Physiol Renal Physiol*. 2001;281:F400-F406.

137. Fenton RA, Cottingham CA, Stewart GS, et al. Structure and characterization of the mouse UT-A gene (*Slc14a2*). *Am J Physiol Renal Physiol*. 2002;282:F630-F638.

138. Nakayama Y, Peng T, Sands JM, et al. The TonE/TonEBP pathway mediates tonicity-responsive regulation of UT-A urea transporter expression. *J Biol Chem*. 2000;275:38275-38280.

139. Terris J, Ecelbarger CA, Sands JM, et al. Long-term regulation of collecting duct urea transporter proteins in rat. *J Am Soc Nephrol*. 1998;9:729-736.

140. Kim D-U, Sands JM, Klein JD. Role of vasopressin in diabetes mellitus–induced changes in medullary transport proteins involved in urine concentration in Brattleboro rats. *Am J Physiol Renal Physiol*. 2004;286:F760-F766.

141. Harrington AR, Valtin H. Impaired urinary concentration after vasopressin and its gradual correction in hypothalamic diabetes insipidus. *J Clin Invest*. 1968;47:502-510.

142. Yasui M, Zelenin SM, Celsi G, et al. Adenylate cyclase-coupled vasopressin receptor activates AQP2 promoter via a dual effect on CRE and AP1 elements. *Am J Physiol Renal Physiol*. 1997;272:F443-F450.

143. Igarashi P, Whyte DA, Nagami GT. Cloning and kidney cell-specific activity of the promoter of the murine renal Na-K-Cl cotransporter gene. *J Biol Chem*. 1996;271:9666-9674.

144. Kim Y-H, Kim D-U, Han K-H, et al. Expression of urea transporters in the developing rat kidney. *Am J Physiol Renal Physiol*. 2002;282:F530-F540.

145. Terris JM, Knepper MA, Wade JB. UT-A3: localization and characterization of an additional urea transporter isoform in the IMCD. *Am J Physiol Renal Physiol*. 2001;280:F325-F332.

146. Stewart GS, Fenton RA, Wang W, et al. The basolateral expression of mUT-A3 in the mouse kidney. *Am J Physiol Renal Physiol*. 2004;286:F979-F987.

147. Blount MA, Klein JD, Martin CF, et al. Forskolin stimulates phosphorylation and membrane accumulation of UT-A3. *Am J Physiol Renal Physiol*. 2007;293:F1308-F1313.

148. You G, Smith CP, Kanai Y, et al. Cloning and characterization of the vasopressin-regulated urea transporter. *Nature*. 1993;365:844-847.

149. Fenton RA, Stewart GS, Carpenter B, et al. Characterization of the mouse urea transporters UT-A1 and UT-A2. *Am J Physiol Renal Physiol*. 2002;283:F817-F825.

150. Fenton RA, Howorth A, Cooper GJ, et al. Molecular characterization of a novel UT-A urea transporter isoform (UT-A5) in testis. *Am J Physiol Cell Physiol*. 2000;279:C1425-C1431.

151. Smith CP, Potter EA, Fenton RA, et al. Characterization of a human colonic cDNA encoding a structurally novel urea transporter, UT-A6. *Am J Physiol Cell Physiol*. 2004;287:C1087-C1093.

152. Zhang C, Sands JM, Klein JD. Vasopressin rapidly increases the phosphorylation of the UT-A1 urea transporter activity in rat IMCDs through PKA. *Am J Physiol Renal Physiol*. 2002;282:F85-F90.

153. Blount MA, Mistry AC, Froehlich O, et al. Phosphorylation of UT-A1 urea transporter at serines 486 and 499 is important for vasopressin-regulated activity and membrane accumulation. *Am J Physiol Renal Physiol*. 2008;295:F295-F299.

154. Wang Y, Klein JD, Blount MA, et al. Epac regulation of the UT-A1 urea transporter in rat IMCDs. *J Am Soc Nephrol*. 2009;20:2018-2024.

155. Mistry AC, Mallick R, Froehlich O, et al. The UT-A1 urea transporter interacts with snapin, a SNARE-associated protein. *J Biol Chem.* 2007;282:30097-30106.

156. Stewart GS, O'Brien JH, Smith CP. Ubiquitination regulates the plasma membrane expression of renal UT-A urea transporters. *Am J Physiol Cell Physiol.* 2008;295:C121-C129.

157. Chen G, Huang H, Froehlich O, et al. MDM2 E3 ubiquitin ligase mediates UT-A1 urea transporter ubiquitination and degradation. *Am J Physiol Renal Physiol.* 2008;295:F1528-F1534.

158. Feng X, Huang H, Yang Y, et al. Caveolin-1 directly interacts with UT-A1 urea transporter: the role of caveolae/lipid rafts in UT-A1 regulation at the cell membrane. *Am J Physiol Renal Physiol.* 2009;296:F1514-F1520.

159. Sands JM, Schrader DC. An independent effect of osmolality on urea transport in rat terminal IMCDs. *J Clin Invest.* 1991;88:137-142.

160. Gillin AG, Sands JM. Characteristics of osmolarity-stimulated urea transport in rat IMCD. *Am J Physiol.* 1992;262:F1061-F1067.

161. Kudo LH, César KR, Ping WC, et al. Effect of peritubular hypertonicity on water and urea transport of inner medullary collecting duct. *Am J Physiol Renal Fluid Electrolyte Physiol.* 1992;262:F338-F347.

162. Chou C-L, Sands JM, Nonoguchi H, et al. Concentration dependence of urea and thiourea transport pathway in rat inner medullary collecting duct. *Am J Physiol.* 1990;258:F486-F494.

163. Gillin AG, Star RA, Sands JM. Osmolarity-stimulated urea transport in rat terminal IMCD: role of intracellular calcium. *Am J Physiol.* 1993;265:F272-F277.

164. Kato A, Klein JD, Zhang C, et al. Angiotensin II increases vasopressin-stimulated facilitated urea permeability in rat terminal IMCDs. *Am J Physiol Renal Physiol.* 2000;279:F835-F840.

165. Blessing NW, Blount MA, Sands JM, et al. Urea transporters UT-A1 and UT-A3 accumulate in the plasma membrane in response to increased hypertonicity. *Am J Physiol Renal Physiol.* 2008;295:F1336-F1341.

166. Klein JD, Froehlich O, Blount MA, et al. Vasopressin increases plasma membrane accumulation of urea transporter UT-A1 in rat inner medullary collecting ducts. *J Am Soc Nephrol.* 2006;17:2680-2686.

167. Biemesderfer D, Rutherford PA, Nagy T, et al. Monoclonal antibodies for high-resolution localization of NHE3 in adult and neonatal rat kidney. *Am J Physiol Renal Physiol.* 1997;273:F289-F299.

168. Good DW, Di Mari JF, Watts BA, III: Hyposmolality stimulates Na⁺/H⁺ exchange and HCO₃⁻ absorption in thick ascending limb via PI 3-kinase. *Am J Physiol Cell Physiol.* 2000;279:C1443-C1454.

169. Kaplan MR, Plotkin MD, Brown D, et al. Expression of the mouse Na-K-2Cl cotransporter, mBSC2, in the terminal inner medullary collecting duct, the glomerular and extraglomerular mesangium, and the glomerular afferent arteriole. *J Clin Invest.* 1996;98:723-730.

170. Ginns SM, Knepper MA, Ecelbarger CA, et al. Immunolocalization of the secretory isoform of Na-K-Cl cotransporter in rat renal intercalated cells. *J Am Soc Nephrol.* 1996;7:2533-2542.

171. Castrop H, Schnermann J. Isoforms of renal Na-K-2Cl cotransporter NKCC2: expression and functional significance. *Am J Physiol Renal Physiol.* 2008;295:FF859-F866.

172. Ecelbarger CA, Terris J, Hoyer JR, et al. Localization and regulation of the rat renal Na⁺-K⁺-2Cl⁻ cotransporter, BSC-1. *Am J Physiol Renal Physiol.* 1996;271:F619-F628.

173. Kaplan MR, Plotkin MD, Lee WS, et al. Apical localization of the Na-K-Cl cotransporter, rBSC1, on rat thick ascending limbs. *Kidney Int.* 1996;49:40-47.

174. Nielsen S, Maunsbach AB, Ecelbarger CA, et al. Ultrastructural localization of Na-K-2Cl cotransporter in thick ascending limb and macula densa of rat kidney. *Am J Physiol Renal Physiol.* 1998;275:F885-F893.

175. Kim GH, Ecelbarger CA, Mitchell C, et al. Vasopressin increases Na-K-2Cl cotransporter expression in thick ascending limb of Henle's loop. *Am J Physiol.* 1999;276:F96-F103.

176. Kim JK, Summer SN, Erickson AE, et al. Role of arginine vasopressin in medullary thick ascending limb on maximal urinary concentration. *Am J Physiol Renal Physiol.* 1986;251:F266-F270.

177. Giménez I, Forbush B. Short-term stimulation of the renal Na-K-Cl cotransporter (NKCC2) by vasopressin involves phosphorylation and membrane translocation of the protein. *J Biol Chem.* 2003;278:26946-26951.

178. Hall DA, Varney DM. Effect of vasopressin on electrical potential differences and chloride transport in mouse medullary thick ascending limb of Henle's loop. *J Clin Invest.* 1980;66:792-802.

179. Ortiz PA. cAMP increases surface expression of NKCC2 in rat thick ascending limbs: role of VAMP. *Am J Physiol Renal Physiol.* 2006;290:F608-F616.

180. Sasaki S, Imai M. Effects of vasopressin on water and NaCl transport across the in vitro perfused medullary thick ascending limb of Henle's loop of mouse, rat, and rabbit kidney. *Pflugers Arch.* 1980;383:215-221.

181. Rinehart J, Kahle KT, de Los Heros P, et al. WNK3 kinase is a positive regulator of NKCC2 and NCC, renal cation–Cl⁻ cotransporters required for normal blood pressure homeostasis. *Proc Natl Acad Sci U S A.* 2005;102:16777-16782.

182. Welker P, Bohlick A, Mutig K, et al. Renal Na⁺-K⁺-Cl⁻ cotransporter activity and vasopressin-induced trafficking are lipid raft–dependent. *Am J Physiol Renal Physiol.* 2008;295:F789-F802.

183. Masilamani S, Kim G-H, Mitchell C, et al. Aldosterone-mediated regulation of ENaC alpha, beta, and gamma subunit proteins in rat kidney. *J Clin Invest.* 1999;104:R19-R23.

184. Kim GH, Masilamani S, Turner R, et al. The thiazide-sensitive Na-Cl cotransporter is an aldosterone-induced protein. *Proc Natl Acad Sci U S A.* 1998;95:14552-14557.

185. Ellison DH, Biemesderfer D, Morrisey J, et al. Immunocytochemical characterization of the high-affinity thiazide diuretic receptor in rabbit renal cortex. *Am J Physiol Renal Physiol.* 1993;264:F141-F148.

186. Plotkin MD, Kaplan MR, Verlander JW, et al. Localization of the thiazide sensitive Na-Cl cotransporter, rTSC1, in the rat kidney. *Kidney Int.* 1996;50:174-183.

187. Hager H, Kwon TH, Vinnikova AK, et al. Immunocytochemical and immunoelectron microscopic localization of alpha-, beta-, and gamma-ENaC in rat kidney. *Am J Physiol Renal Physiol.* 2001;280:F1093-F1106.

188. Loffing J, Loffing-Cueni D, Macher A, et al. Localization of epithelial sodium channel and aquaporin-2 in rabbit kidney cortex. *Am J Physiol Renal Physiol.* 2000;278:F530-F539.

189. Ecelbarger CA, Kim GH, Terris J, et al. Vasopressin-mediated regulation of epithelial sodium channel abundance in rat kidney. *Am J Physiol Renal Physiol.* 2000;279:F46-F53.

190. Nicco C, Wittner M, DiStefano A, et al. Chronic exposure to vasopressin upregulates ENaC and sodium transport in the rat renal collecting duct and lung. *Hypertension.* 2001;38:1143-1149.

191. Sauter D, Fernandes S, Goncalves-Mendes N, et al. Long-term effects of vasopressin on the subcellular localization of ENaC in the renal collecting system. *Kidney Int.* 2006;69:1024-1032.

192. Schlatter E, Schafer JA. Electrophysiological studies in principal cells of rat cortical collecting tubules. ADH increases the apical membrane Na⁺-conductance. *Pflugers Arch.* 1987;409:81-92.

193. Reif MC, Troutman SL, Schafer JA. Sodium transport by rat cortical collecting tubule: effects of vasopressin and desoxycorticosterone. *J Clin Invest.* 1986;77:1291-1298.

194. Tomita K, Pisano JJ, Knepper MA. Control of sodium and potassium transport in the cortical collecting duct of the rat: effects of bradykinin, vasopressin, and deoxycorticosterone. *J Clin Invest.* 1985;76:132-136.

195. Snyder PM. Minireview: regulation of epithelial Na⁺ channel trafficking. *Endocrinology.* 2005;146:5079-5085.

196. Uchida S, Sasaki S, Nitta K, et al. Localization and functional characterization of rat kidney-specific chloride channel, ClC-K1. *J Clin Invest.* 1995;95:104-113.

197. Vandewalle A, Cluzeaud F, Bens M, et al. Localization and induction by dehydration of ClC-K chloride channels in the rat kidney. *Am J Physiol Renal Physiol.* 1997;272:F678-F688.

198. Yoshikawa M, Uchida S, Yamauchi A, et al. Localization of rat CLC-K2 chloride channel mRNA in the kidney. *Am J Physiol Renal Physiol.* 1999;276:F552-F558.

199. Kobayashi K, Uchida S, Mizutani S, et al. Intrarenal and cellular localization of CLC-K2 protein in the mouse kidney. *J Am Soc Nephrol.* 2001;12:1327-1334.

200. Takahashi N, Kondo Y, Ito O, et al. Vasopressin stimulates Cl⁻ transport in ascending thin limb of Henle's loop in hamster. *J Clin Invest.* 1995;95:1623-1627.

201. Boim MA, Ho K, Shuck ME, et al. ROMK inwardly rectifying ATP-sensitive K⁺ channel. II. Cloning and distribution of alternative forms. *Am J Physiol Renal Physiol.* 1995;268:F1132-F1140.

202. Lee W-S, Hebert SC. ROMK inwardly rectifying ATP-sensitive K⁺ channel. I. Expression in rat distal nephron segments. *Am J Physiol Renal Fluid Electrolyte Physiol.* 1995;268:F1124-F1131.

203. Kohda Y, Ding W, Phan E, et al. Localization of the ROMK potassium channel to the apical membrane of distal nephron in rat kidney. *Kidney Int.* 1998;54:1214-1223.

204. Mennitt PA, Wade JB, Ecelbarger CA, et al. Localization of ROMK channels in the rat kidney. *J Am Soc Nephrol.* 1997;8:1823-1830.

205. Xu JZ, Hall AE, Peterson LN, et al. Localization of the ROMK protein on apical membranes of rat kidney nephron segments. *Am J Physiol Renal Physiol.* 1997;273:F739-F748.

206. Besseghir K, Trimble ME, Stoner L. Action of ADH on isolated medullary thick ascending limb of the Brattleboro rat. *Am J Physiol.* 1986;251:F271-F277.

207. Ecelbarger CA, Kim GH, Knepper MA, et al. Regulation of potassium channel Kir 1.1 (ROMK) abundance in the thick ascending limb of Henle's loop. *J Am Soc Nephrol.* 2001;12:10-18.

208. Rieg T, Vallon V, Sausbier M, et al. The role of the BK channel in potassium homeostasis and flow-induced renal potassium excretion. *Kidney Int.* 2007;72:566-573.

209. Schafer JA, Troutman SL, Schlatter E. Vasopressin and mineralocorticoid increase apical membrane driving force for K⁺ secretion in rat CCD. *Am J Physiol.* 1990;258:F199-F210.

210. Konstas AA, Koch JP, Tucker SJ, et al. Cystic fibrosis transmembrane conductance regulator–dependent up-regulation of Kir1.1 (ROMK) renal K+ channels by the epithelial sodium channel. *J Biol Chem.* 2002;277: 25377-25384.

211. Lu M, Leng Q, Egan ME, et al. CFTR is required for PKA-regulated ATP sensitivity of Kir1.1 potassium channels in mouse kidney. *J Clin Invest.* 2006;116:797-807.

212. Ma TH, Yang BX, Gillespie A, et al. Severely impaired urinary concentrating ability in transgenic mice lacking aquaporin-1 water channels. *J Biol Chem.* 1998;273:4296-4299.

213. Schnermann J, Chou CL, Ma TH, et al. Defective proximal tubular fluid reabsorption in transgenic aquaporin-1 null mice. *Proc Natl Acad Sci U S A.* 1998;95:9660-9664.

214. Chou CL, Knepper MA, Van Hoek AN, et al. Reduced water permeability and altered ultrastructure in thin descending limb of Henle in aquaporin-1 null mice. *J Clin Invest.* 1999;103:491-496.

215. Yang B, Gillespie A, Carlson EJ, et al. Neonatal mortality in an aquaporin-2 knock-in mouse model of recessive nephrogenic diabetes insipidus. *J Biol Chem.* 2001;276:2775-2779.

216. Rojek A, Fuechtbauer EM, Kwon TH, et al. Severe urinary concentrating defect in renal collecting duct–selective AQP2 conditional-knockout mice. *Proc Natl Acad Sci U S A.* 2006;103:6037-6042.

217. Yang BX, Zhao D, Qian LM, et al. Mouse model of inducible nephrogenic diabetes insipidus produced by floxed aquaporin-2 gene deletion. *Am J Physiol Renal Physiol.* 2006;291:F465-F472.

218. Lloyd DJ, Hall FW, Tarantino LM, et al. Diabetes insipidus in mice with a mutation in aquaporin-2. *PLoS Genet.* 2005;1:E20.

219. McDill BW, Li SZ, Kovach PA, et al. Congenital progressive hydronephrosis (cph) is caused by an S256L mutation in aquaporin-2 that affects its phosphorylation and apical membrane accumulation. *Proc Natl Acad Sci U S A.* 2006;103:6952-6957.

220. Shi PP, Cao XR, Qu J, et al. Nephrogenic diabetes insipidus in mice caused by deleting COOH-terminal tail of aquaporin-2. *Am J Physiol Renal Physiol.* 2007;292:F1344.

221. Kuwahara M, Iwai K, Ooeda T, et al. Three families with autosomal dominant nephrogenic diabetes insipidus caused by aquaporin-2 mutations in the C-terminus. *Am J Hum Genet.* 2001;69:738-748.

222. Sohara E, Rai T, Yang SS, et al. Pathogenesis and treatment of autosomal-dominant nephrogenic diabetes insipidus caused by an aquaporin 2 mutation. *Proc Natl Acad Sci U S A.* 2006;103:14217-14222.

222a. Yang B, Zhao D, Verkman AS. Hsp90 inhibitor partially corrects nephrogenic diabetes insipidus in a conditional knock-in mouse model of aquaporin-2 mutation. *FASEB J.* 2009;23:503-512.

223. Ma TH, Song YL, Yang BX, et al. Nephrogenic diabetes insipidus in mice lacking aquaporin-3 water channels. *Proc Natl Acad Sci U S A.* 2000;97:4386-4391.

224. Ma TH, Yang BX, Gillespie A, et al. Generation and phenotype of a transgenic knockout mouse lacking the mercurial-insensitive water channel aquaporin-4. *J Clin Invest.* 1997;100:957-962.

225. Chou C-L, Ma TH, Yang BX, et al. Fourfold reduction of water permeability in inner medullary collecting duct of aquaporin-4 knockout mice. *Am J Physiol Cell Physiol.* 1998;274:C549-C554.

226. Fenton RA. Urea transporters and renal function: lessons from knockout mice. *Curr Opin Nephrol Hypertens.* 2008;17:513-518.

227. Fenton RA. Essential role of vasopressin-regulated urea transport processes in the mammalian kidney. *Pflugers Arch.* 2009;458:169-177.

228. Fenton RA, Knepper MA. Urea and renal function in the 21st century: insights from knockout mice. *J Am Soc Nephrol.* 2007;18:679-688.

229. Bankir L, Chen K, Yang B. Lack of UT-B in vasa recta and red blood cells prevents urea-induced improvement of urinary concentrating ability. *Am J Physiol Renal Physiol.* 2004;286:F144-F151.

230. Sands JM, Gargus JJ, Fröhlich O, et al. Urinary concentrating ability in patients with Jk(a–b–) blood type who lack carrier-mediated urea transport. *J Am Soc Nephrol.* 1992;2:1689-1696.

231. Timmer RT, Klein JD, Bagnasco SM, et al. Localization of the urea transporter UT-B protein in human and rat erythrocytes and tissues. *Am J Physiol Cell Physiol.* 2001;281:C1318-C1325.

232. Schultheis PJ, Clarke LL, Meneton P, et al. Renal and intestinal absorptive defects in mice lacking the NHE3 Na+/H+ exchanger. *Nat Genet.* 1998;19:282-285.

233. Cho CS, Elkahwaji J, Chang Z, et al. Modulation of the electrophoretic mobility of the linker for activation of T cells (LAT) by calcineurin inhibitors CsA and FK506: LAT is a potential substrate for PK and calcineurin signaling pathways. *Cell Signal.* 2003;15:85-93.

234. Lorenz JN, Schultheis PJ, Traynor T, et al. Micropuncture analysis of single-nephron function in NHE3-deficient mice. *Am J Physiol Renal Physiol.* 1999;277:F447-F453.

235. Amlal H, Ledoussal C, Sheriff S, et al. Downregulation of renal AQP2 water channel and NKCC2 in mice lacking the apical Na+-H+ exchanger NHE3. *J Physiol (Lond).* 2003;553:511-522.

236. Brooks HL, Sorensen AM, Terris J, et al. Profiling of renal tubule Na+ transporter abundances in NHE3 and NCC null mice using targeted proteomics. *J Physiol.* 2001;530:359-366.

237. Oppermann M, Mizel D, Kim SM, et al. Renal function in mice with targeted disruption of the A isoform of the Na-K-2Cl co-transporter. *J Am Soc Nephrol.* 2007;18:440-448.

238. Oppermann M, Mizel D, Huang G, et al. Macula densa control of renin secretion and preglomerular resistance in mice with selective deletion of the B isoform of the Na,K,2Cl co-transporter. *J Am Soc Nephrol.* 2006;17: 2143-2153.

239. Flagella M, Clarke LL, Miller ML, et al. Mice lacking the basolateral Na-K-2Cl cotransporter have impaired epithelial chloride secretion and are profoundly deaf. *J Biol Chem.* 1999;274:26946-26955.

240. Chou C-L, Yu MJ, Kassai EM, et al. Roles of basolateral solute uptake via NKCC1 and of myosin II in vasopressin-induced cell swelling in inner medullary collecting duct. *Am J Physiol Renal Physiol.* 2008;295: F192-F210.

241. Wall SM, Knepper MA, Hassell KA, et al. Hypotension in NKCC1 null mice: role of the kidneys. *Am J Physiol Renal Physiol.* 2006;290:F416.

242. Schultheis PJ, Lorenz JN, Meneton P, et al. Phenotype resembling Gitelman's syndrome in mice lacking the apical Na+-Cl− cotransporter of the distal convoluted tubule. *J Biol Chem.* 1998;273:29150-29455.

243. Morris RG, Hoorn EJ, Knepper MA. Hypokalemia in a mouse model of Gitelman syndrome. *Am J Physiol Renal Physiol.* 2006;290: F1416-F1420.

244. McDonald FJ, Yang B, Hrstka RF, et al. Disruption of the beta subunit of the epithelial Na+ channel in mice: hyperkalemia and neonatal death associated with a pseudohypoaldosteronism phenotype. *Proc Natl Acad Sci U S A.* 1999;96:1727-1731.

245. Hummler E, Barker P, Gatzy J, et al. Early death due to defective neonatal lung liquid clearance in alpha-ENaC–deficient mice. *Nat Genet.* 1996;12:325-328.

246. Hummler E, Barker P, Talbot C, et al. A mouse model for the renal salt-wasting syndrome pseudohypoaldosteronism. *Proc Natl Acad Sci U S A.* 1997;94:11710-11715.

247. Barker PM, Nguyen MS, Gatzy JT, et al. Role of gammaENaC subunit in lung liquid clearance and electrolyte balance in newborn mice: insights into perinatal adaptation and pseudohypoaldosteronism. *J Clin Invest.* 1998;102:1634-1640.

248. Rubera I, Loffing J, Palmer LG, et al. Collecting duct-specific gene inactivation of αENaC in the mouse kidney does not impair sodium and potassium balance. *J Clin Invest.* 2003;112:554-565.

249. Matsumura Y, Uchida S, Kondo Y, et al. Overt nephrogenic diabetes insipidus in mice lacking the CLC-K1 chloride channel. *Nat Genet.* 1999;21:95-98.

250. Lorenz JN, Baird NR, Judd LM, et al. Impaired renal NaCl absorption in mice lacking the ROMK potassium channel, a model for type II Bartter's syndrome. *J Biol Chem.* 2002;277:37871-37880.

251. Yan Q, Yang X, Cantone A, et al. Female ROMK null mice manifest more severe Bartter II phenotype on renal function and higher PGE2 production. *Am J Physiol Regul Integr Comp Physiol.* 2008;295:R997-R1004.

252. Woda CB, Bragin A, Kleyman TR, et al. Flow-dependent K+ secretion in the cortical collecting duct is mediated by a maxi-K channel. *Am J Physiol Renal Physiol.* 2001;280:F786-F793.

253. Bailey MA, Cantone A, Yan Q, et al. Maxi-K channels contribute to urinary potassium excretion in the ROMK-deficient mouse model of type II Bartter's syndrome and in adaptation to a high-K diet. *Kidney Int.* 2006;70:51-59.

254. Yun J, Schöneberg T, Liu J, et al. Generation and phenotype of mice harboring a nonsense mutation in the *V2 vasopressin receptor* gene. *J Clin Invest.* 2000;106:1361-1371.

255. Schliebe N, Strotmann R, Busse K, et al. V2 vasopressin receptor deficiency causes changes in expression and function of renal and hypothalamic components involved in electrolyte and water homeostasis. *Am J Physiol Renal Physiol.* 2008;295:F1177-F1190.

The Cell Biology of Vasopressin Action

Dennis Brown and Robert A. Fenton

In humans, the glomerulus can filter 180 L/day of fluid from plasma, of which 90% (about 162 L) is returned to the circulation by reabsorption in the proximal tubule and descending limb of the loop of Henle. Most of the remaining 18 L is reabsorbed under the regulation of vasopressin (VP) in the cortical and medullary collecting ducts. Failure of this regulated pathway for water reabsorption in the collecting ducts results in the production of copious amounts of dilute urine—a disease known as *diabetes insipidus* (DI). VP—the antidiuretic hormone—plays a multifaceted role in the urinary concentrating process in mammals by activating the type 2 VP receptor (V_2R), a G protein–coupled receptor (GPCR). VP increases collecting duct water permeability by increasing the plasma membrane accumulation of a water channel, aquaporin-2 (AQP2), in principal cells. It acts on thick ascending limbs of Henle to stimulate NaCl reabsorption, which increases the osmolality of the medullary interstitium. It facilitates the transepithelial movement of urea along its concentration gradient in terminal portions of the collecting duct, which allows high levels of urea to be excreted without reducing urinary concentrating ability.

Overall, the urinary concentration mechanism requires the tight coordination of cellular and molecular events within the context of the renal architecture and fluid dynamics in the vasculature. Several of these issues are dealt with in depth in other chapters of this book. This chapter focuses on the VP-activated renal concentrating mechanism and addresses the way in which the V_2R and the AQP2 water channel interact via intracellular signaling pathways to regulate collecting duct water reabsorption and urine concentration. Our understanding of how the V_2R signaling pathway is regulated so as to lead to an increase in epithelial water permeability and urinary concentration continues to evolve rapidly as the powerful new tools of genomics and proteomics are applied to renal physiology. With the exponential increase in the amount of raw data generated by these and other high-throughput screening technologies, it becomes increasingly important to process this emerging information in the context of whole-organ and whole-animal "systems" physiology.

Vasopressin—The Antidiuretic Hormone

The antidiuretic hormone of most mammals is a nine–amino acid peptide, arginine vasopressin (VP). A slightly different peptide known as *lysine VP*, in which a lysine replaces the arginine in position 8 of the molecule, is present in members of the pig family. Secretion of VP from the posterior pituitary is stimulated most notably by an increase in plasma osmolality, but also by a decrease in plasma volume.[295] A change in osmolality as small as 1% can cause a significant rise in plasma VP levels. VP then activates regulatory systems necessary to retain water and restore osmolality to normal. In contrast, a 5% to 10% decrease in volume is required to stimulate VP secretion, but VP nevertheless has important clinical applications in the control of vasodilatory shock.[184] One study indicates that VP gene transcription is activated by decreased plasma volume, but not by increased plasma osmolality,[117] whereas another shows increased VP heteronuclear RNA levels in the hypothalamus after acute salt loading of rats.[389] V_2R promoter activity is increased by hypertonicity in LLC-PK$_1$ cells (an epithelial pig kidney cell strain), but this effect is suppressed by $V_{1a}R$ activation.[148]

The effects of VP occur through the stimulation of receptors that are located on different cell types. The V_1 receptor activates a Ca^{++} pathway and is involved in the pressor effect of VP, whereas the V_2R activates a cyclic adenosine monophosphate (cAMP) pathway that regulates transepithelial water transport in kidney.[233,333] However, some cell types may express both V_1 and V_2 receptors. Indeed, the release of von Willebrand factor by some endothelial cells is V_2R mediated and depends on cAMP elevation.[166,196] Furthermore, VP also increases nitric oxide production by human umbilical vein endothelial cells via a V_2R-mediated pathway.[165] Other studies have suggested that the oxytocin receptor[348] or a receptor with mixed V_1 and V_2 characteristics[224] is expressed in endothelial cells. In situations in which it is critical to distinguish V_1 from V_2 receptor effects, a modified form of VP, known as *desamino-8-d-arginine VP* (dDAVP) is used, which is specific for the V_2R and has little or no V_1-related pressor effect. The remainder of this discussion focuses on the V_2R in renal epithelial cells.

Type 2 Vasopressin Receptor—A G Protein–Coupled Receptor

The V_2R is a member of the family of seven membrane-spanning domain receptors that couple to heterotrimeric G proteins (GPCRs).[14,198] In the kidney, it is expressed in collecting duct principal cells and the thick ascending limb of Henle.[83,107,171,234,379] Although some reports have used antibodies to detect the V_2R in situ with variable results,[84,257,311] most studies of V_2R recycling, downregulation, and desensitization have been performed on cell cultures, often using epitope-tagged V_2R constructs. LLC-PK$_1$ cells from porcine kidney expressing endogenous V_2R have also played an important role in the evaluation of ligand receptor interactions and signal transduction mechanisms via heterotrimeric guanosine triphosphate–binding proteins.[5]

When VP binds to the V_2R, adenylyl cyclase activity is stimulated and cytosolic cAMP levels increase.[322] This activates protein kinase A (PKA) and leads to the phosphorylation of several proteins, including AQP2. This water channel then accumulates in the apical plasma membrane of collecting duct principal cells, which increases transepithelial water permeability and facilitates osmotically driven water reabsorption (Figure 11-1). AQP2 contains several C-terminal residues whose phosphorylation status changes upon VP treatment of V_2R-expressing cells. Finally, intracellular calcium is also increased by VP via a mechanism involving interaction with calmodulin[243]; this is also involved in the regulated trafficking of AQP2.[53,125]

Structure of the V_2R

The V_2R has been cloned from several mammalian species, and the sequences are more than 90% identical. Several important features of the V_2R include the following: (1) an extracellular N terminus with a consensus site for N-linked glycosylation (N22); (2) two conserved cysteine residues in the second and third extracellular loops, which may form a disulfide bridge that is important for correct folding of the molecule and stabilization of the ligand binding site; (3) conserved sites for fatty acylation (palmitoylation), which may serve as an additional membrane anchor in the C-terminal tail and be involved in membrane accumulation or in endocytosis and mitogen-activated protein kinase (MAPK) signaling[47,306]; (4) hydrophobic residues at the C terminus, including a dileucine motif, that are involved in endoplasmic reticulum (ER) to Golgi transfer and in the receptor folding that is required for receptor transport from the ER[349]; (5) a cytoplasmic C terminus and large intracellular loop that contain multiple sites for serine and threonine phosphorylation and that probably play a role in receptor desensitization, internalization, sequestration, and recycling.[136-139]

Interaction of V_2R with Heterotrimeric G proteins and β-Arrestin

Upon ligand binding, the V_2R assumes an active configuration and the bound heterotrimeric G protein G_s dissociates into G_α and $G_{\beta\gamma}$ subunits.[322] This G protein is localized on the basolateral plasma membrane of thick ascending limb and principal cells.[41,330] Adenylyl cyclase is stimulated by activated $G_{\alpha s}$, and cAMP levels are increased. The predominant adenylyl cyclase isoform in the adult rat kidney is AC-6, but several other isoforms are expressed at lower levels, including AC-4, AC-5, AC-9, and calmodulin-sensitive AC-3.[318] Liganded V_2R interacts with G_s via its cytosolic domain, and a peptide corresponding to the third intracellular loop of the V_2R inhibits signaling through G_s.[106] The VP-V_2R association increases cellular cAMP, which initiates a cascade of events that increases collecting duct water permeability by changing the phosphorylation pattern of AQP2 and causing its accumulation at the cell surface (see later). Termination of this response depends on the internalization of the V_2R after VP binding and its delivery to and degradation in lysosomes (Figure 11-2).

Many accessory proteins are involved in V_2R downregulation, including inhibitory G_i proteins[322,367,378] and proteins involved in clathrin-mediated endocytosis.[25,262] Not only is there less receptor at the cell surface, the level of V_2R messenger RNA (mRNA) also decreases rapidly after elevation of plasma VP.[345] Additional mechanisms that downregulate the VP response include destruction of cAMP by cytosolic phosphodiesterases[74] and inhibition by prostaglandins,[329] dopamine,[193,239] adenosine receptor stimulation,[79] adrenergic agonists,[116] endothelin-1,[263] and bradykinin.[341] Changes in receptor conformation after VP binding are followed by receptor phosphorylation, desensitization, internalization, and sequestration.

One critical step in this process is the binding of β-arrestin to the V_2R,[71] which is triggered by phosphorylation of the V_2R by kinases, including G protein–coupled receptor kinases (GRKs). There are several phosphorylation sites in the V_2R C terminus,[136-138] but their specific roles remain unclear. For example, a point mutation in any one element of the serine cluster at residues 362 to 364 (S362-364) impedes V_2R

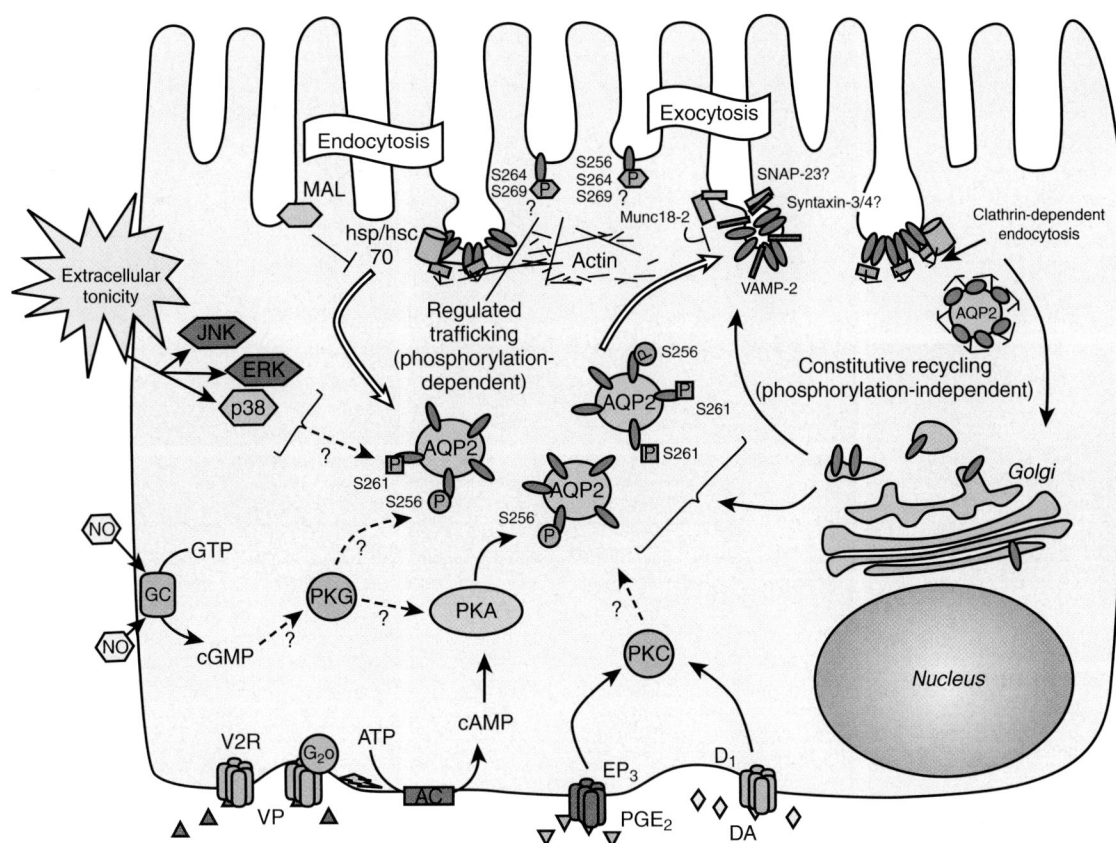

FIGURE 11-1 Diagram showing key events that contribute to the regulation of aquaporin-2 (AQP2) trafficking. The canonical pathway involves interaction of vasopressin (VP) with the type 2 VP receptor (V_2R) on the basolateral surface of the principal cell. This increases cyclic adenosine monophosphate (cAMP) formation after $G_{\alpha s}$ protein stimulation of adenylyl cyclase (AC). Phosphorylation of AQP2 occurs initially on residue S256, via protein kinase A (PKA) activation. After VP stimulation, residue S261 on AQP2 is dephosphorylated, and phosphorylation of residues S264 and S269 is increased. During exocytosis, AQP2 interacts with SNARE (soluble *N*-ethylmaleimide–sensitive factor attachment protein receptor) proteins and their regulatory proteins such as Munc18-2 (mammalian uncoordinated 18-2 protein), and these interactions may be regulated by phosphorylation. At the cell surface, phosphorylated AQP2 is present in endocytosis-resistant domains, and its interaction with heat shock cognate protein 70 (hsc70), which is required for clathrin-mediated endocytosis, is inhibited. The myelin and lymphocyte protein (MAL) also is involved in AQP2 endocytosis by an as yet unknown mechanism. Endocytosis of AQP2 is also facilitated by protein kinase C (PKC) activation (but possibly not by direct phosphorylation of AQP2), as well as by activation of receptors for dopamine (DA, D_1) and prostaglandin E_2 (PGE_2, EP_3). However, constitutive exocytosis of AQP2 occurs without VP stimulation and does not require AQP2 phosphorylation on residue S256. Accumulation of AQP2 at the plasma membrane is increased by inhibiting clathrin-mediated endocytosis. AQP2 phosphorylation can also be increased by stimulating the cyclic guanosine monophosphate/protein kinase G (cGMP/PKG) pathways using, for example, nitric oxide (NO). Extracellular hypertonicity activates the mitogen-activated protein (MAP) kinase pathway, and c-Jun N-terminal kinase (JNK), extracellular signal–regulated kinase (ERK), and p38 activities are all required for AQP2 surface accumulation after acute hypertonic shock. Finally, AQP2 trafficking involves the actin cytoskeleton, and actin depolymerization results in cell surface accumulation of AQP2 without the need for VP stimulation.

recycling by an as yet unknown mechanism. Recently, a novel phosphorylation site (of unknown function) in the third intracellular loop was identified at S255 and is phosphorylated by PKA in vitro.[380] Interestingly, different cellular responses to receptor phosphorylation can be dissected depending on the kinase involved in the phosphorylation process. Thus, phosphorylation of V_2R with GRK2 and GRK3 results in VP-dependent desensitization and recruitment of β-arrestins. In contrast, GRK5 and GRK6 phosphorylation is involved in extracellular signal–regulated kinase activation.[284]

Arrestin-receptor complexes recruit the clathrin adaptor protein 2, an important component of the endocytotic mechanism,[378] and the complex is then internalized via clathrin-mediated endocytosis.[25,261,267] Arrestins also uncouple GPCRs from heterotrimeric G proteins, producing a desensitized receptor.[266] After downregulation, restoration of prestimulation levels of V_2R at the cell surface requires several hours.[26,136,137] In contrast, prestimulation levels of the β_2-adrenergic receptor (β_2AR) are restored on the cell

surface within an hour of internalization.[136] This difference has been correlated with the association characteristics of the receptor/β-arrestin complex. The V_2R is a class B GPCR, which forms a more stable interaction with β-arrestin than GPCRs of the class A type, such as β_2AR.

The persistence of a tightly associated V_2R/β-arrestin complex throughout the internalization pathway is responsible for the intracellular retention of the V_2R[136,261] but does not dictate the final cellular destination of the receptor.[139] Upon binding to a liganded receptor, a change in conformation of β-arrestin takes place that could modify its function, for example by increasing its clathrin-binding affinity.[381] This is consistent with the biologic effect of β-arrestin-2 in vivo to stimulate clathrin-mediated endocytosis of the V_2R. A further effect of a V_2R-induced conformation change in β-arrestin-2 is to promote disassociation of the deubiquitinating enzyme USP33 from the complex, which prolongs the ubiquinated state of β-arrestin2 compared with that of more rapidly recycling receptors such as β_2AR.[319]

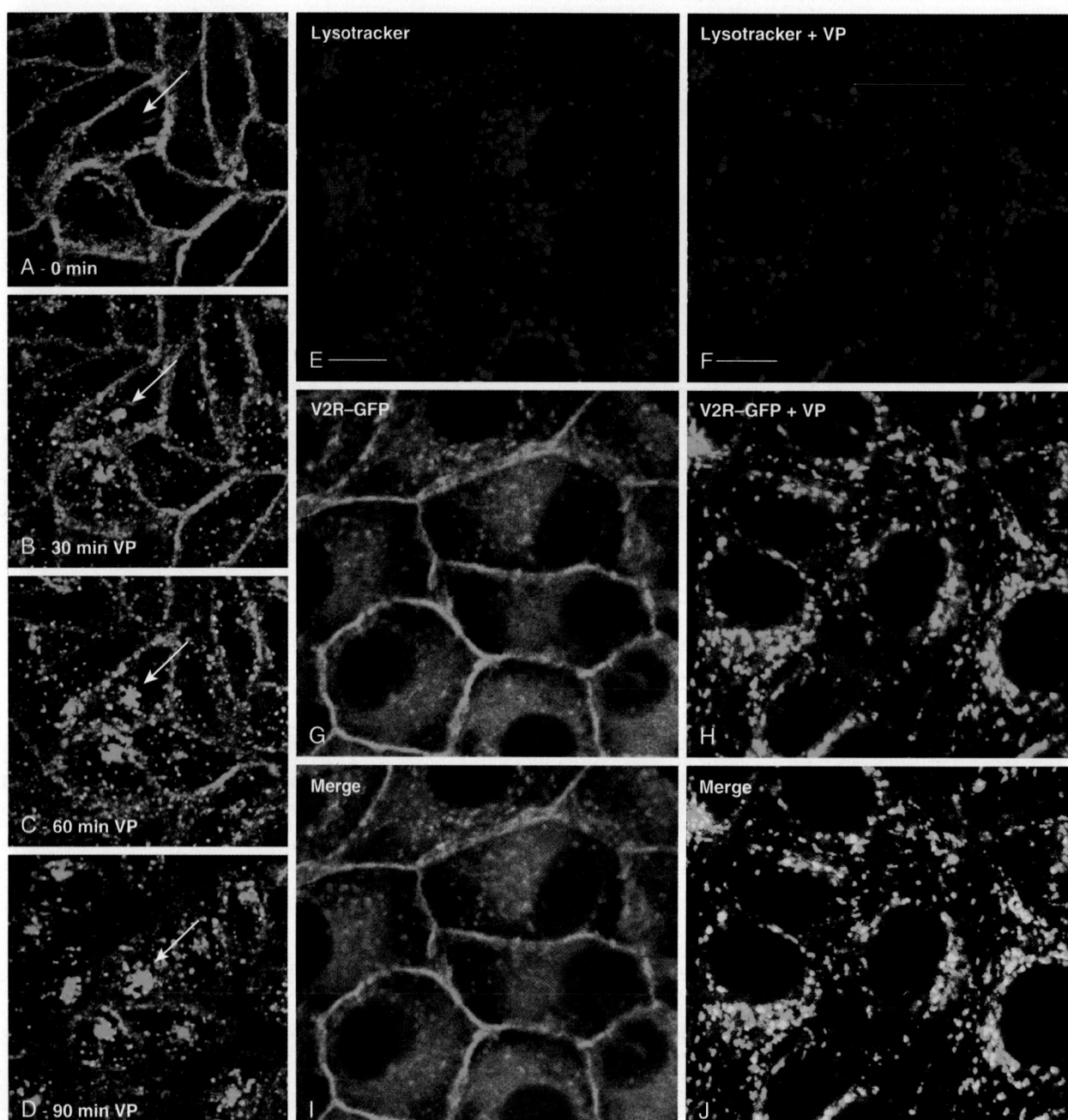

FIGURE 11-2 Internalized type 2 vasopressin receptor (V_2R) is mainly trafficked to lysosomes for degradation. Imaging of V_2R–green fluorescent protein (GFP) trafficking in LLC-PK$_1$ cells demonstrates internalization of V_2R into lysosomes. **A** through **D** show spinning disk confocal microscopy (live imaging of the same cells over time) of LLC-PK$_1$ cells stably expressing V_2R-GFP seen at various times (0 to 90 minutes) after addition of vasopressin (VP). Initially, most of the V_2R-GFP is located on the plasma membrane (**A**). After VP treatment, the V_2R-GFP is downregulated from the cell surface and is progressively internalized (**B, C,** and **D**) into a perinuclear compartment that is seen as a bright fluorescent patch (indicated by an *arrow* in each panel). **E** through **J** show localization of V_2R in lysosomes after VP treatment. In nonstimulated LLC-PK$_1$ cells, the patterns of staining for Lysotracker (**E**)—a marker of acidic lysosomes and late endosomes—and the V_2R-GFP (**G**) are distinct, with most of the V_2R-GFP at the plasma membrane, although some intracellular V_2R is also present (**I,** merged panel). After VP-induced downregulation, the V_2R-GFP is internalized (**H**) and accumulates in vesicles, many of which are also stained with Lysotracker (**F, J**). (Adapted from Brown D: Imaging protein trafficking, *Nephron Exp Nephrol* 103:e55-61, 2006; and from Bouley R, Lin HY, Raychowdhury MK, et al: Downregulation of the vasopressin type 2 receptor after vasopressin-induced internalization: involvement of a lysosomal degradation pathway, *Am J Physiol Cell Physiol* 288:C1390-C1401, 2005.)

Fate of V_2R after Internalization—Delivery to Lysosomes

VP stimulation leads to rapid, β-arrestin–dependent ubiquitination of the V_2R, internalization, and increased degradation.[221] Much of the V_2R that is internalized enters a lysosomal degradation compartment,[22,289] along with the VP ligand.[204] In transfected LLC-PK$_1$ cells, real-time microscopy[30] shows that after ligand binding, V_2R–green fluorescent protein moves to a perinuclear vesicular compartment that is composed predominantly of late endosomes and lysosomes (see Figure 11-2), where it is degraded.[21,22] Importantly, restoration of prestimulation levels of V_2R at the cell surface is greatly inhibited by cycloheximide, which shows that new protein synthesis is involved in the resensitization process.[22] In summary, the V_2R—classified as a "slow-recycling" GPCR—is mainly degraded in lysosomes after internalization. This pathway may allow the V_2R to function in the harsh environment of the renal medulla, which can be acidic and of high osmolality.[168,391] Receptors and ligand pairs often separate in the acidic environment of endosomes, but VP must actually associate with the V_2R in the acidic renal medulla, which indicates that it is at least partially resistant to pH-induced dissociation. Delivery of both the ligand and receptor to lysosomes may be required to terminate the physiologic response to VP.[391] Whether the continued association of the V_2R with VP during its intracellular transit also prolongs its signaling capacity within the cell is an interesting question that remains to be examined.

Diabetes Insipidus (Central and Nephrogenic)

Nephrogenic diabetes insipidus (NDI) is characterized by excessive water loss (up to 20 L of dilute urine per day) via the kidneys.[12,308] It can be either acquired or inherited. Failure of water reabsorption in the collecting duct is associated with most cases of DI. If not corrected, DI can result in severe dehydration, hypernatremia, bladder enlargement, and damage to the central nervous system. The most common manifestation of NDI is in bipolar patients treated with lithium, about 20% of whom develop NDI.[169] Both acquired and congenital forms of NDI have been linked to defects in VP signaling and AQP2 trafficking. Although the inherited forms of DI are much rarer, their molecular basis has been largely elucidated thanks to the cloning and sequencing of the key proteins involved: the V_2R,[14,198] the VP-sensitive collecting duct water channel AQP2,[100] and the gene coding for the VP-neurophysin-glycopeptide precursor protein from which active VP is generated.[170,315] Chapters 15 and 44 provide more extensive discussion of the pathophysiology of these diseases.

Central (Neurohypophyseal) Diabetes Insipidus

The central (neurohypophyseal) form of DI results from a defect in the production and release of functional VP.[57,97] Acquired forms of the disease have multiple causes, including damage to the neurohypophysis, or may be idiopathic. Hereditary forms of familial DI have been linked to over 40 different mutations of the gene encoding the VP–neurophysin II (VP-NPII) precursor.[57]

The congenital (or acquired) absence of functional VP generally can be treated by administration of VP or dDAVP, usually via nasal aerosol, because the V_2R and the AQP2 genes and proteins are unaffected in central diabetes insipidus (CDI).[209] However, VP is also involved in stimulating AQP2 transcription; AQP2 levels are significantly lower than normal in Brattleboro rats—a valuable animal model of CDI that does not produce functional VP due to a single amino acid mutation in the neurophysin domain of the VP gene.[170,358] It is likely, therefore, that the beneficial effect of VP in CDI results from not only increased AQP2 trafficking (see later) but also increased AQP2 protein levels following transcriptional activation of the AQP2 gene.

Nephrogenic Diabetes Insipidus

The loss of an appropriate renal response to VP that characterizes NDI is most often due to a functional defect in either the V_2R or AQP2 protein. Therefore, administration of VP is not usually sufficient to rectify the concentrating defect. However, some patients in whom the mutated V_2R has a reduced affinity for VP may respond if circulating VP levels are increased sufficiently. NDI also can be a congenital-hereditary or an acquired disease.[169] Acquired NDI is much more common than all hereditary forms, and the most prevalent of the acquired forms is lithium-induced NDI resulting from the use of this element in the treatment of bipolar disorder.[102] Exposure of rats to dietary lithium results in a dramatic reduction in AQP2 expression in the kidney,[215] but its mechanism of action remains unclear.

A variety of gene mutations that result in defective targeting and/or function of the V_2R or the AQP2 water channel result in several distinct forms of NDI. The predominant form (type 1) affecting the V_2R is an X-linked recessive trait resulting from mutations in the V_2R.[13,298] Mutations in the V_2R represent about 90% of hereditary NDI cases. Type 2 congenital NDI is a much less common autosomal recessive disease caused by mutations in AQP2,[288,308] representing about 10% of NDI cases. However, an autosomal dominant form of congenital NDI has also been described that results when the product of the mutated allele in heterozygous patients interacts with wild-type AQP2 to block normal trafficking and/or function of the AQP2 tetramer.[220]

Mutations in V_2R

As described in more detail in Chapter 44, over 200 mutations that result in NDI have been identified in the V_2R protein.[13,325] The mutation sites are distributed throughout all regions of the V_2R. Some introduce premature stop codons, and frameshifts can produce nonsense protein sequences. Some single-point mutations cause an amino acid replacement at critical locations in the V_2R,[81,176] whereas others allow the production of a full-length or near full-length protein but interfere with different aspects of the receptor-ligand signal transduction cascade.[13] Mutated receptors are often incorrectly folded and are retained and degraded in the rough ER, never reaching the plasma membrane. In other cases, the V_2R appears to be expressed normally at the cell surface, but either does not bind VP or shows a reduction in VP binding. Alternatively, the mutated receptor may bind VP normally at the cell surface, but fail to couple to $G_{\alpha s}$, so that adenylyl cyclase is not activated and the intracellular concentration of cAMP is not elevated.

Some defects in V_2R function result from changes in the ability of the receptor to be phosphorylated, which may affect V_2R trafficking and desensitization. One interesting mutation that results in substitution of arginine at position 137 by histidine (R137H) produces NDI because the V_2R is constitutively phosphorylated and sequestered in arrestin-containing vesicles even in the absence of VP.[7] This mutation can result in either severe or mild NDI, which indicates that genetic and/or environmental modifiers may affect the final phenotype within affected members of the same family.[158]

Some V_2R mutations are associated with specific functional defects that are believed to explain the loss of receptor function.

For example, some of the missense mutations (R181C, G185C, and Y205C) add cysteine residues that are believed to interfere with disulfide bond formation in the wild-type receptor. However, a Y205H substitution also abolishes receptor function and leads to NDI, which suggests that loss of the tyrosine is the cause of the dysfunction, rather than the addition of a cysteine, at least at residue 205.[310]

Many folding mutations are recognized by cellular quality control mechanisms, which leads to degradation. Different mutations are handled in various ways, and some mutated receptors temporarily escape from the ER before being rerouted back to this compartment for degradation. Although the L62P, L62-R64, del (deletion of residues 62-64), and S167L mutants are trapped in the ER, the R143P, Y205C, Q292ins (insertion of glutamine at position 292), V226E, and R337X mutant receptors actually reach the ER-Golgi intermediate compartment before being rerouted to the ER. Differences in the folding characteristics of these receptors that allow interactions with different sets of accessory proteins are thought to explain these differences.[123]

Correction of the Defect: Approaches to Treatment of Nephrogenic Diabetes Insipidus Involving the V₂R

Our increased understanding of V_2R cell biology and signaling pathways have led to the consideration and development of several potential therapeutic strategies for X-linked NDI. For example, inducing the cell surface delivery of mutated (often misfolded) receptors that are trapped in intracellular compartments would be beneficial. A variety of approaches, including the use of chemical- or drug-induced rescue of cell surface expression, have been attempted.

Among the first chemical chaperones to be tested were substances such as glycerol and dimethylsulfoxide. Additional drugs (thapsigargin/curcumin and ionomycin) that modify calcium levels in cellular compartments were also tested. However, of nine V_2R mutants used, the surface expression of only one of them—V_2R with the V206D mutation—was increased using these reagents.[292]

The use of V_2R antagonists to increase cell surface expression and functionality of mutant V_2R protein seems more promising.[235,287,347] Small, cell-permeant nonpeptidic antagonists were shown to rescue the cell surface appearance of eight mutant receptors.[291] Importantly, the antagonist SR49059, which was shown to be effective in three patients harboring the R137H V_2R mutation, acts by improving the maturation and cell surface targeting of the mutant receptor.[10] Furthermore, the pharmacologic V_2R antagonist SR121463B resulted in greater maturation and surface expression of the V_2R mutations V206D and S167T than did chemical chaperones.[292] When clinically relevant drug concentrations are considered, however, high-affinity nonpeptide antagonists such as OPC31260 and OPC41061 are the best potential candidates to treat NDI, based on results from cell culture studies.[291] Other membrane-permeant peptides, penetratin and its synthetic analog (an amino acid peptide known as KLAL), result in surface expression of the Y205C mutant, which has a post-ER defect, whereas plasma membrane delivery of the L62P mutant is not influenced by either peptide, probably because the peptides are unable to enter the ER.[265]

More recently, the use of small nonpeptide compounds that also act as agonists has also been proposed.[149] Aminoglycoside antibiotics are known to suppress premature stop codons in some instances. In the case of the V_2R, an E242X mutation produces a premature stop codon in humans, and when introduced into mice, this mutation causes NDI. Urine concentrating ability can be restored by administering the antibiotic G418 (Geneticin) to mice, and the VP-mediated cAMP response is increased by G418 in cultured cells expressing this V_2R mutation.[310] This provides a potential means of suppressing NDI that is caused by a premature stop codon in the V_2R.

Finally, although much attention has been focused on increasing the delivery of misfolded V_2R to the cell surface where interaction with VP can take place, a recent study has shown that cAMP can be generated by activation of some intracellular (i.e., mistrafficked) V_2R mutants using nonpeptide chemical agonists.[290] The generation of cAMP was sufficient to cause cell surface accumulation of AQP2 in the systems examined. These results require that the V_2R–G protein–adenylyl cyclase cascade be functional in intracellular compartments. The data represent a novel and exciting development in this area.

The Aquaporins—A Family of Water Channel Proteins

The first water channel (AQP1) was identified and characterized in a Nobel Prize–winning discovery by Peter Agre and his associates in 1988.[69,175,272,273] AQP1 is expressed not only in erythrocytes but also in many cells and tissues with high constitutive water permeability, including proximal tubules and thin descending limbs of Henle in the kidney,[251,304] the choroid plexus,[250] reabsorptive portions of the male reproductive tract that are embryologically related to renal tubules,[39] parts of the inner ear,[327] bile canaliculi cholangiocytes,[294,350] and many others.[18,366] Soon after the discovery of AQP1, the collecting duct VP-sensitive water channel, now called *AQP2*, was identified by homology cloning from the renal medulla,[100] and a variety of studies confirmed that it is the principal cell water channel that is involved in distal urinary concentration in the kidney.[2,31,95,146,312,357] A total of 12 mammalian aquaporin homologs are known, and dozens more have been identified in virtually all organisms, including invertebrates, plants, and microbes.

Aquaporins share structural similarities in their overall transmembrane organization, but important differences in the actual pore structure that help to explain some of the permeability differences among aquaporins have been revealed by X-ray crystallography. The membrane topography and some key features (e.g., phosphorylation sites) of AQP2 are illustrated in Figure 11-3. Many functional studies on aquaporins have relied on the use of mercurial compounds such as $HgCl_2$ as inhibitors that react with an exposed cysteine in the neck of the aqueous pore.[3,313] This cysteine residue is absent from AQP4, which is not inhibited by the addition of external mercurial compounds.[320]

Other Permeability Properties of Aquaporins

The single-channel water permeability of different aquaporins varies greatly. AQP1, AQP2, and AQP4 have high permeabilities, whereas AQP0 and AQP3 have much lower permeabilities.[385] Interestingly, some aquaporins, including AQP3,

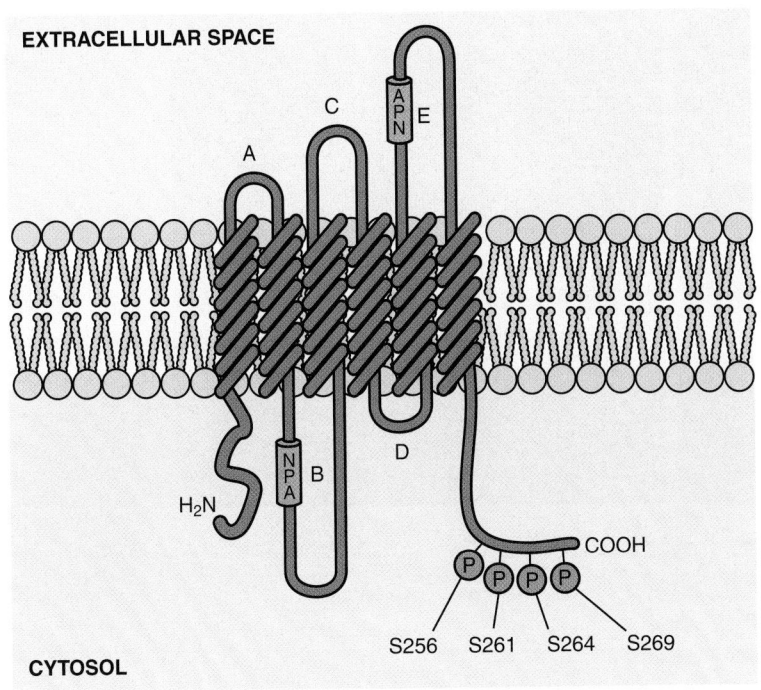

EXTRACELLULAR SPACE

CYTOSOL

FIGURE 11-3 Membrane topology of the aquaporin-2 (AQP2) water channel. This 271–amino acid protein spans the lipid bilayer six times. Both N and C termini are in the cytoplasm. Four important phosphorylation sites in the C-terminal region are shown, S256, S261, S264 and S269. The S256 site is a protein kinase A (PKA) target that was originally shown to be required for AQP2 membrane accumulation after vasopressin (VP) stimulation. It is now believed to be a "master regulator" for the other adjacent phosphorylation sites in the C terminus, but the precise function of these sites remains under investigation. (From Pisitkun T, Hoffert JD, Yu MJ, et al: Tandem mass spectrometry in physiology, *Physiology [Bethesda]* 22:390-400, 2007.)

AQP8, and AQP9—referred to as *aquaglyceroporins*—allow the passage of other molecules, including urea, glycerol, ammonia, and other small solutes.[1,129,141,143,353,385] Distinct physiologic functions for aquaporins in the transport of non-water molecules, including glycerol, have emerged and continue to evolve.[111] Furthermore, AQP6 seems to be located exclusively on intracellular membranes in some renal epithelial cells, including intercalated cells. Although it was originally believed to function as a Cl⁻ and/or Na⁺ channel that is activated by low pH or $HgCl_2$,[121,387] with a potential role in acid-base homeostasis,[280] its precise function remains unclear. Indeed other studies have suggested that it has a high specificity for nitrate,[135] and it is permeable to urea and glycerol.[130] Most recently AQP6 was shown to be a calcium-dependent calmodulin-binding protein.[281]

Unexpectedly, all aquaporins are impermeable to protons, a property that was first shown using isolated apical endosomes from rat kidney papilla.[187,305] Crystallographic evidence from several groups has shown that the central region of the aqueous channel with charged residues lining a constricted region renders the passage of protons energetically unfavorable.[48,227,238,334] Physiologically, the impermeability of aquaporins to protons is important. For example, the collecting duct luminal fluid is acidic due to proton secretion and can reach a pH of close to 5.5. It would presumably be disadvantageous if the cytosol of the principal cells equilibrated with the low pH of the tubule lumen simultaneously with an increase in membrane water permeability.

Several other unexpected permeabilities have also been reported for various members of the aquaporin family. Perhaps most controversially, AQP1 has been proposed to serve as a CO_2 channel,[59] although whole-animal studies using AQP1-deficient mice have refuted this claim.[82] Other groups examining the potential role of erythrocyte AQP1 in CO_2 transport have produced data in favor of[15] or against[286,336] a role for AQP1 in this process. Some data have shown that in erythrocytes, AQP1 is the major

pathway for CO_2 permeation, but that about 30% of the CO_2 crosses the membrane via an alternative mechanism.[80] One group has provided evidence that the permeation of CO_2 across lipid bilayers is always limited by the unstirred layer and is the same whether or not AQP1 is present.[225] Thus, although the central pore of some aquaporins may be permeant to gases, including CO_2, the physiologic relevance of this process remains in doubt, and it may be functionally important only in membranes with a low intrinsic gas permeability and/or in membranes that contain a very high amount of AQP1.[375]

AQP2—The Vasopressin-Sensitive Collecting Duct Water Channel

AQP2 is the VP-regulated water channel in kidney collecting duct principal cells.[100] VP stimulation of the kidney collecting duct results in the accumulation of AQP2 on the plasma membrane of principal cells (Figure 11-4) via a membrane trafficking mechanism that involves the recycling of AQP2 between intracellular vesicles and the cell surface.[2,31,68,95,142,241,248,357] However, both AQP3 and AQP4, which are found in the basolateral membrane of principal cells,[90,144] are also regulated at the expression level and possibly the functional level by VP and/or dehydration.[144,228,362]

What is the specific role of AQP2 in the urinary concentrating mechanism? The VP-induced low-to-high permeability state of collecting duct principal cells involves the redistribution of AQP2 from cytoplasmic vesicles to the apical plasma membrane. Because the basolateral membrane of these cells has a high constitutive water permeability due to the presence of AQP3 and/or AQP4, the luminal fluid can then equilibrate osmotically with the surrounding interstitium. The osmolality in the renal inner medulla reaches about 1200 mOsm/kg in humans, and the urine can reach the same concentration in the presence of VP.

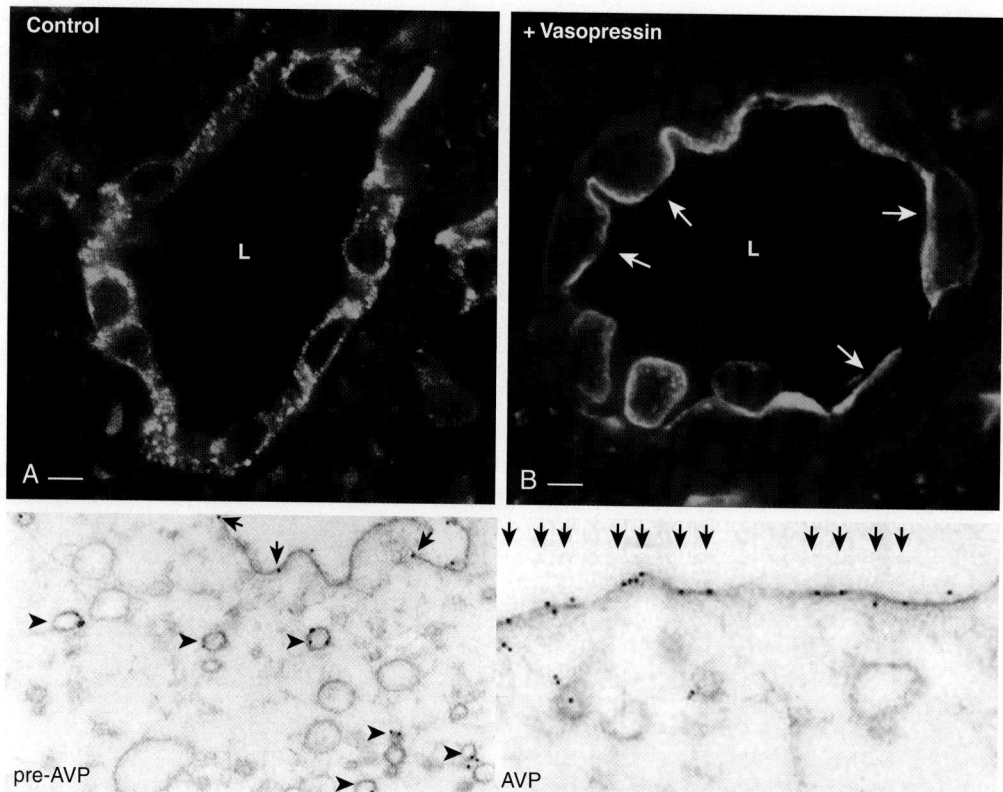

FIGURE 11-4 Increased plasma membrane expression of aquaporin-2 (AQP2) in principal cells of vasopressin (VP)–deficient Brattleboro rat kidney inner medullary collecting duct perfused with 4 nmol/L desamino-8-d-arginine VP (dDAVP) for 60 minutes. After perfusion kidneys were fixed, sectioned, and immunostained using anti-AQP2 antibodies. Under control conditions (**A**), AQP2 has a cytosolic distribution in principal cells. After perfusion with VP (**B**), AQP2 shows an increased apical localization in principal cells (*arrows*). A weaker basolateral localization of AQP2 in principal cells is also visible in this section (*L* indicates the tubule lumen). The lower two panels show the effect of VP on AQP2 distribution by immunogold electron microscopy. The left panel (pre-VP) shows the apical region of a principal cell, with gold particles (detecting AQP2) distributed on cytoplasmic vesicles, as well as a few on the apical plasma membrane (*arrows*). After VP treatment (right panel), the number of gold particles on the apical plasma membrane is greatly increased (*arrows*), and the number of labeled cytoplasmic vesicles is decreased. Bar equals 5 µm. (Lower panels adapted from Nielsen S, Chou CL, Marples D, et al: Vasopressin increases water permeability of kidney collecting duct by inducing translocation of aquaporin-CD water channels to plasma membrane, *Proc Natl Acad Sci USA* 92:1013-1017, 1995.)

AQP2 Recycling: The Shuttle Hypothesis of Vasopressin Action

The so-called shuttle hypothesis of VP action was proposed in 1981 by Wade and associates.[371] This elegant idea was based largely on studies using VP-sensitive amphibian epithelia, in which a large increase in water permeability is induced by the addition of VP or similar antidiuretic hormones (e.g., the amphibian equivalent, called *vasotocin*). Studies using amphibian urinary bladder and skin suggested that "water channels" are located on intracellular vesicles that fuse with the apical plasma membrane upon VP stimulation, and then are retrieved back into the cell by endocytosis after VP washout. In these early studies, water channels were recognized morphologically as characteristic aggregates of intramembraneous particles that were revealed by the specialized technique of freeze-fracture electron microscopy.[34,35,50,157,369] Following the identification of aquaporins, new tools and assays became available that allowed direct testing of the mechanism by which membrane water permeability is increased in VP target cells. Importantly, the availability of cell culture models expressing AQP2 allowed a correlation to be made between the freeze-fracture intramembranous particle (IMP) aggregates that were used initially to track the cellular itinerary of water channels in older studies, and the presence of AQP2 within the aggregates.[335]

Overview of Vasopressin-Regulated AQP2 Trafficking in Collecting Duct Principal Cells

Following the identification of AQP2,[100] specific antibodies were used to show that this water channel is expressed in the apical plasma membrane of collecting duct principal cells, as well as in intracellular vesicles.[100,247,303] In vitro and in vivo studies correlated the VP-stimulated increase in collecting duct water permeability and urinary concentration with relocalization of AQP2 from intracellular vesicles to the plasma membrane of principal cells (see Figure 11-4).[217,246,303,383] The reversibility of this membrane accumulation was demonstrated upon VP washout in isolated perfused collecting ducts and in whole animals infused with a V_2R antagonist or subjected to water loading.[54,118,307]

Taken together, these data indicated that VP acutely regulates the osmotic water permeability of collecting duct principal cells by inducing a shift in the steady-state distribution of AQP2 from its baseline location mainly in intracellular vesicles to the apical plasma membrane. Removal of the stimulus results in a return of AQP2 to its intracellular location, which restores the low baseline water permeability of the apical plasma membrane of principal cells.

One unexpected observation from these initial studies was that significant amounts of AQP2 were present on principal cell basolateral membranes in some kidney regions, and that this staining tended to increase after VP treatment. This issue is addressed in more detail later in this chapter. The internalized AQP2 that accumulates in endosomes after VP withdrawal follows a complex intracellular pathway prior to reinsertion into the plasma membrane.[20,109,241,339] Recycling of the existing cohort of AQP2 can occur in conditions in which protein synthesis is inhibited, which indicates that de novo protein synthesis is not required for sequential responses to VP stimulation.[163]

Not all AQP2 is recycled, however. A significant amount of AQP2 also accumulates in larger cellular structures, including multivesicular bodies (MVBs), in response to treatment of rats with a VP antagonist.[54] Proteins targeted for delivery to this compartment following endocytosis could then either be directed to lysosomes for degradation, be transferred to a recycling compartment via vesicular carriers that bud from the MVB, or be directly transported to the cell surface via other distinct transport vesicles that derive from the MVBs. The fate of internalized AQP2 seems to be at least in part regulated by ubiquitinylation, and this pathway is discussed later.

At least some of the MVBs approach the apical membrane of principal cells, and upon fusion, small vesicles that were inside the MVB are released into the tubule lumen, where they exist as structures known as *exosomes*. These exosomes contain AQP2 on their limiting membranes,[271,377] and it has been shown recently that they also contain AQP2 mRNA.[302] AQP2 can be detected in the urine, and the amount increases in conditions of antidiuresis when more AQP2 is present in the apical membrane of principal cells. The physiologic relevance of this urinary excretion of AQP2 remains unknown, but urinary exosomes also contain a host of proteins that are expressed in renal epithelial cells from all tubule segments. Interestingly, urinary AQP2 level correlates with the severity of nocturnal enuresis in children, and lowering urinary calcium levels (through consumption of a low-calcium diet) has a beneficial effect in reducing the severity of the enuresis and reducing AQP2 secretion in hypercalcemic children treated with dDVP.[279]

Exogenous Aquaporin Expression in Nonpolarized Cell Systems

Expression of Aquaporins in *Xenopus* Oocytes

Xenopus oocytes were the first model protein expression system that allowed the identification of AQP1 as a functional water channel using an oocyte swelling assay.[273,395] This system has also been valuable in assessing the function and regulation of mutated aquaporins[67] and in examining the role played by oligomerization and phosphorylation of AQP2 in its function.[162] Many of the mutant AQP2 proteins are not expressed or have different levels of expression at the cell surface of oocytes, probably due to folding defects that cause retention and ultimate degradation in the rough ER and/or retention in the Golgi apparatus.[46,237]

Expression of Aquaporins in Nonepithelial Cells

Chinese hamster ovary (CHO) and other nonpolarized cells are, of course, not appropriate models for studying the polarized expression of aquaporins in renal epithelia, but they can be used to monitor the functional and physical properties of aquaporins. For example, freeze-fracture studies of CHO cells revealed that the AQP1 protein assembles as a tetramer in the lipid bilayer,[364,392] in agreement with biochemical cross-linking data[323] and findings of cryo-electron and atomic force microscopy.[61,232,372] Transfection of CHO cells with AQP4 complementary DNA showed that this protein forms a characteristic pattern of orthogonal intramembranous particle arrays (OAPs) that are found in several cell types, including collecting duct principal cells.[264,384] A comparison of membrane organization in CHO cells expressing AQP1 to AQP5 showed that only AQP4 forms OAPs, that AQP2 does not spontaneously form IMP aggregates, and that AQP3 has a limited tendency to form small, densely packed clusters of IMPs.[361] Important information was gathered concerning the abnormal intracellular location and defective functional activity of AQP2 mutations,[46] and CHO cells were also used to demonstrate that chemical chaperones could increase the delivery of misfolded AQP2 protein to the cell surface.[340]

Expression of AQP2 in Polarized Epithelial Cells

Transfected Cells Expressing Exogenous AQP2

Because principal cells from the inner medullary collecting duct (IMCD) showed a progressive loss of AQP2 mRNA expression in culture,[98] several laboratories developed stably transfected cells with which to analyze AQP2 trafficking and V_2R signaling. These include LLC-PK$_1$ cells (Figure 11-5),[163] rabbit collecting duct epithelial cells,[355] Madin-Darby canine kidney (MDCK) cells,[66] and primary cultures of IMCD cells.[211] Transfected LLC-PK$_1$ and MDCK cells showed constitutive plasma membrane expression of AQP1, as predicted from its pattern of expression in vivo, whereas AQP2 accumulated at the cell surface only upon cAMP elevation by VP or forskolin.[65,163] Similar data were obtained using transformed rabbit collecting duct epithelial cells.[355] Since their initial development, AQP2-expressing cultured cell lines have proven to be reliable cell models that in most cases predict the in vivo behavior of the VP-stimulated AQP2 trafficking pathway.

Cells Expressing Endogenous AQP2

Some cell lines, including mpkCCD(cl4) cells (a highly differentiated mouse clonal cortical collecting duct principal cell line), do express endogenous AQP2[293] and can be used to examine factors regulating AQP2 transcription, for example, the involvement of the tonicity-responsive enhancer–binding protein and the nuclear factor-κB pathway in regulating AQP2 expression in response to hypertonicity and lipopolysaccharide.[114] They were also used to show that the effect of lithium on AQP2 downregulation was unrelated to adenylyl cyclase activity.[195] Other studies using mpkCCD cells to address issues of AQP2 expression and trafficking have also used this cell line.[43,115]

Use of Kidney Tissue Slices and Isolated Collecting Duct to Examine AQP2 Trafficking

Kidney slices and isolated tubules more closely mimic the in situ situation than cell culture monolayers and have been extremely valuable tools.[19,24,27,317] Tissue slices (150 to 200 μm thick) are useful for morphologic and biochemical studies because of the larger amount of material that is available. Although

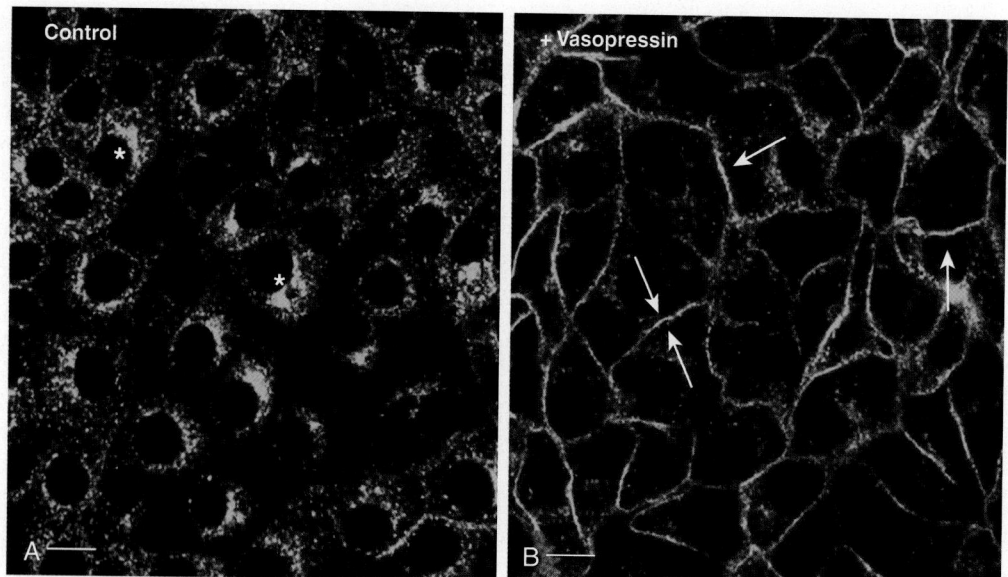

FIGURE 11-5 Immunofluorescence staining showing aquaporin-2 (AQP2) expressed in LLC-PK₁ cells. Under control conditions (**A**), AQP2 is located on perinuclear vesicles (*asterisks*) and more diffusely distributed intracellular vesicles, with very little plasma membrane staining. After vasopressin (VP) treatment for 10 minutes, AQP2 accumulates on the plasma membrane (**B**, *arrows*). Bar equals 5 μm.

there may be potential issues of oxygen, nutrient, and drug diffusion into the slices, dozens of slices can be prepared from the same kidney and treated simultaneously in paired studies. Isolated perfused tubules have been extensively used in kidney physiologic studies. They provide invaluable data, but the procedure is technically demanding and is accessible to only a few laboratories. Finally, isolated, microdissected collecting ducts in suspension have been exploited to provide, for example, a pure IMCD cell population for detailed proteomic analysis of IMCD cells before and after exposure to VP.[132]

Expression of Multiple Basolateral Aquaporins (AQP2, AQP3, and/or AQP4) in Principal Cells

The basolateral plasma membranes of collecting duct principal cells are constitutively permeable to water due to the presence of AQP3 and/or AQP4. AQP3 expression is predominant in the cortex and decreases toward the inner medulla. The reverse pattern is seen for AQP4, which is most abundant in the inner medulla.[144,346] This being the case, it is perhaps surprising that AQP2 is also localized in the basolateral plasma membrane of these cells in some regions of the collecting duct.[247] The bipolar expression of AQP2 is most evident in the cortical connecting segment (Figure 11-6*A*) and the inner medulla (Figure 11-6*B*),[56,58,217] although it is also detectable in other regions, including the outer medullary collecting duct (Figure 11-7). An example of AQP2 and AQP4 staining in the same principal cells from an outer medullary collecting duct is shown in Figure 11-7.

In the inner medulla, basolateral expression of AQP2 is greatly increased by VP (see Figure 11-6*B*) and oxytocin,[152,360] with hypertonicity in the medulla playing a modulating role.[360] Basolateral AQP2 expression in the cortical collecting duct is increased by long-term (6-day) aldosterone treatment in rats.[64] Importantly, basolateral membrane water permeability in this region is increased in a mercurial-sensitive manner by VP treatment, which rules out the contribution of

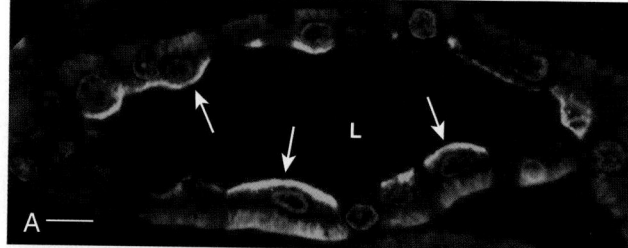

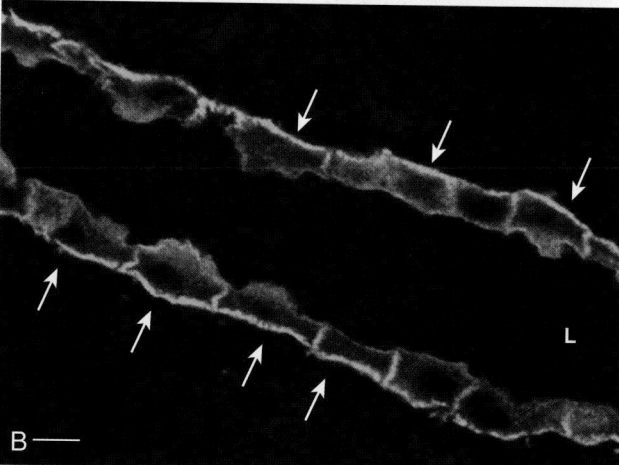

FIGURE 11-6 Immunofluorescence localization of aquaporin-2 (AQP2) in apical and basolateral plasma membranes of epithelial cells in the cortical connecting segment (CNS) (**A**) and the inner medullary collecting duct (IMCD) (**B**) of rat kidney. In the CNS, cells positive for AQP2 show a sharp apical band of staining (*arrows*). The basolateral staining appears broader, due to the relatively deep basolateral infoldings present in these CNS cells. The IMCD segment shown here is from the central portion of the papilla and is from a tubule that was exposed to vasopressin (VP) for approximately 15 minutes prior to fixation and staining. In this region, VP induces a marked basolateral accumulation of AQP2 (*arrows*). Nuclei are stained blue with DAPI (4,6-diamidino-2-phenylindole-2-HCl) in **A**. Bar equals 5 μm.

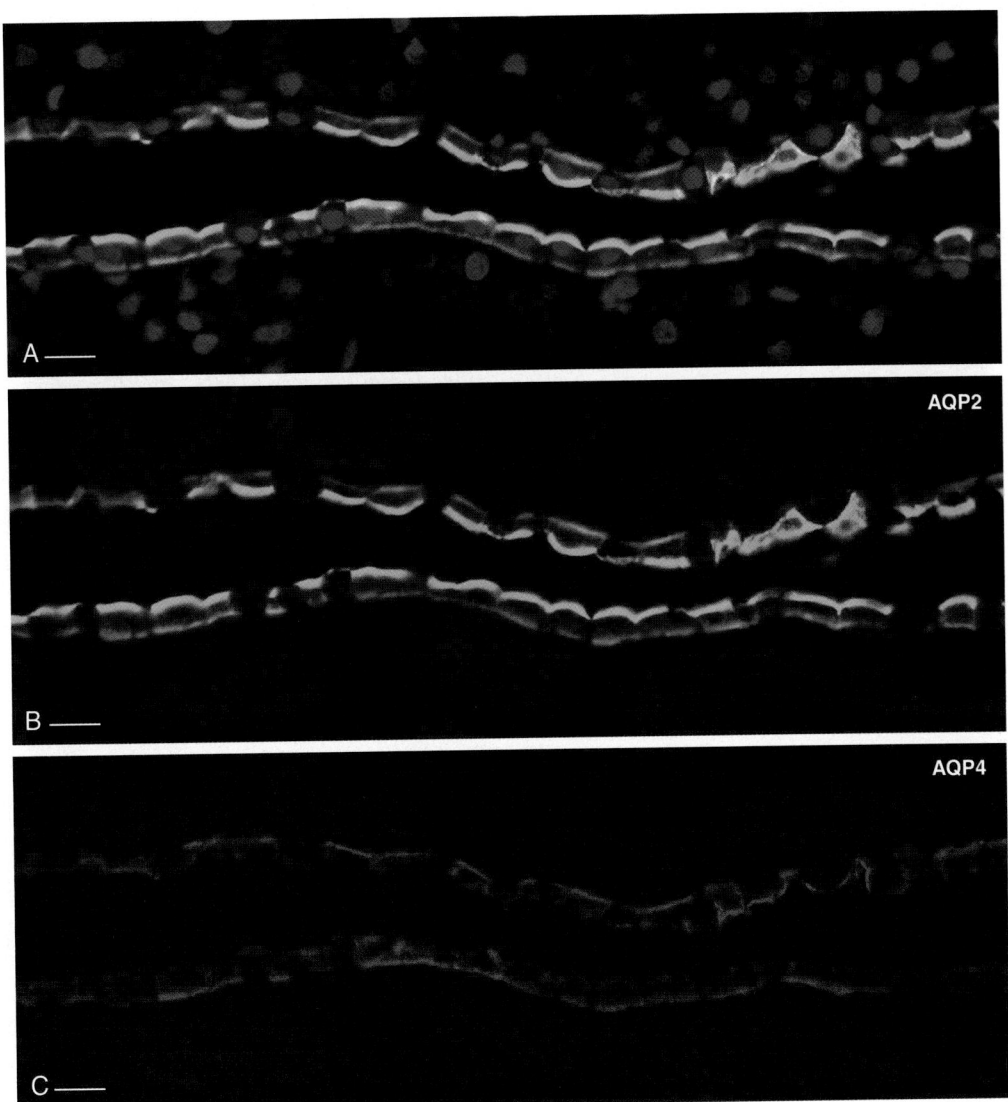

FIGURE 11-7 Example of a collecting duct from the outer medulla (outer stripe) of a rat kidney, immunostained for aquaporin-2 (AQP2) (*green*) and AQP4 (*red*). The merged image in **A** shows that AQP2 is largely apical in this region, but both AQP2 and AQP4 are present on basolateral membranes. This is best seen in the individual images in **B** (AQP2) and **C** (AQP4). All principal cells have some basolateral AQP2 staining at about the same intensity, whereas the basolateral staining for AQP4 varies somewhat among different, even adjacent, principal cells in this segment. Intercalated cells are not stained with either antibody and appear as darker gaps among the other cells. Nuclei are stained with DAPI (4,6-diamidino-2-phenylindole-2-HCl) in **A**. Bar equals 10 μm.

the mercurial-insensitive AQP4 to this process.[9] Nevertheless, the role of basolateral AQP2 remains unclear.

AQP3 may also function as a solute channel under normal circumstances, although AQP3 knockout mice have a significant concentrating defect.[205] AQP4, on the other hand, has much greater single-channel water permeability than AQP2 and AQP3,[385] but interestingly, AQP4 knockout mice have only a minor concentrating defect,[206] although the water permeability of isolated collecting ducts from these animals is reduced to about 25% of that measured in wild-type tubules.[52] Unexpectedly, kangaroo rats, which can concentrate their urine to more than 5000 mOsm/kg, do not express AQP4 in their kidneys. This indicates that AQP4 is not necessary for the extreme concentrating ability of these rodents.[133]

The apical to basolateral distribution of AQP2 in connecting segments and cortical collecting ducts is modified by aldosterone in rats with two types of DI, as well as in normal rats exposed to aldosterone for 6 days.[64] In lithium-treated rats,

aldosterone increases urine output even more than lithium alone and causes a significant redistribution of AQP2 to the basolateral plasma membrane.[245] A similar effect is seen in aldosterone-treated Brattleboro rats that lack endogenous VP, which indicates that this profound effect on AQP2 polarity is independent of VP action. However, a frameshift mutation in AQP2 that results in NDI in humans also results in basolateral targeting when expressed in polarized MDCK cells.[159] This shows that an increased basolateral expression of AQP2 is not sufficient to increase transepithelial water permeability in the collecting duct. Whether basolateral AQP2 represents a mechanism to further increase the water permeability of the basolateral membrane under some conditions or whether it represents a transient step in an indirect apical targeting pathway for the AQP2 protein remains uncertain. Finally, it is possible that basolateral AQP2 has an as yet undetermined effect on renal tubule biology that may or may not be related to its water channel function.

Intracellular Pathways of AQP2 Trafficking

It is now clear that rather than being "stored" in intracellular vesicles prior to the induction of membrane insertion by VP, AQP2 is in fact continually recycling between intracellular vesicles and the cell surface, even in the absence of VP stimulation. Membrane accumulation of AQP2 can then be achieved by a combination of stimulation of exocytosis and inhibition of endocytosis.[31,174] This pattern of trafficking has been described for some other membrane transporters, including the insulin-regulated glucose transporter GLUT4.[42]

Role of Clathrin-Coated Pits in AQP2 Recycling

Clathrin-coated pits concentrate and internalize selected populations of many plasma membrane proteins, including receptors,[378] transporters, and channels.[32] The role of clathrin-coated pits in V_2R internalization has been shown previously.[25,261] Based on early morphologic studies of collecting duct principal cells in situ, it was proposed that coated pits were also involved in the endocytotic step of water channel recycling long before aquaporins were identified.[37,40,331] These studies were subsequently confirmed by direct visualization of AQP2 in clathrin-coated pits by immunogold electron microscopy (Figure 11-8).[335]

A relationship between the water channel–containing IMP clusters first described two decades earlier[38,112] and AQP2 endocytosis was also shown using a technique known as *fracture labeling* in transfected LLC-PK$_1$ cells[335] (see Figure 11-8). Thus, the IMP clusters seen in principal cells are markers of endocytotic, but probably not exocytotic, events. It is now believed that they result from a concentration of AQP2 protein into clathrin-coated membrane domains during the internalization phase of AQP2 recycling. Whether exocytosis of AQP2 from intracellular stores results in the immediate formation of detectable membrane IMP clusters (representing concentrated patches of AQP2) at the sites of vesicle fusion with the plasma membrane remains uncertain.

When clathrin-mediated endocytosis was inhibited by the expression of a dominant negative form of the protein dynamin in LLC-PK$_1$ cells, AQP2 accumulated on the plasma membrane and was depleted from cytoplasmic vesicles.[335] Dynamin is a guanosine triphosphatase (GTPase) that is involved in the formation and pinching off of clathrin-coated pits to form clathrin-coated vesicles.[124] The dominant negative form has a single point mutation, K44A, that renders the protein GTPase deficient and arrests clathrin-mediated endocytosis. The cholesterol-depleting drug methyl-β-cyclodextrin (MBCD) also blocks clathrin-mediated endocytosis, and exposure to MBCD of both AQP2-expressing cell cultures and intact kidneys (using an isolated perfused kidney preparation) results in AQP2 accumulation on the plasma membrane within 15 minutes (Figure 11-9).[200,301] Taken together, these data demonstrate the critical role of clathrin-coated pits in AQP2 endocytosis.

AQP2 Localization in Intracellular Compartments during Recycling

Recycling of AQP2 was directly demonstrated in cycloheximide-treated, AQP2-transfected LLC-PK$_1$ cells, in which several rounds of exocytosis and endocytosis of AQP2 could be followed despite the complete inhibition of de novo AQP2

synthesis.[163] Several studies have been carried out to identify the intracellular compartments in which AQP2 resides during this recycling process, but the intracellular itinerary of AQP2 remains incompletely understood.

After internalization from the plasma membrane via clathrin-coated pits, AQP2 enters an early endosomal antigen 1 (EEA1)–positive compartment.[338] After forskolin washout from transfected MDCK cells, AQP2 enters an apical storage compartment that is sensitive to the phosphatidylinositol-3-kinase inhibitors wortmannin and LY294002. In the same cells, AQP2 is localized in a subapical recycling compartment that is distinct from organelles such as the Golgi apparatus, the trans-Golgi network (TGN), and lysosomes.[338] Furthermore, this AQP2 compartment does not contain transferrin receptor, and it is distinct from vesicles that contain GLUT4 (another recycling protein) in adipocytes that coexpress AQP2 and GLUT4.[276] Stimulation of these coexpressing cells with forskolin results in the membrane accumulation of AQP2, but not of GLUT4. Similarly, stimulation of cells with insulin causes membrane accumulation of GLUT4 but not of AQP2.[276]

Together, these data suggest that prior to insertion into the cell surface, AQP2—like GLUT4 in smooth muscle cells and adipocytes—is located in specialized vesicles that are not easily identified using markers of known intracellular compartments, although in the adipocyte system AQP2 showed significant overlap with the distribution of vesicle-associated membrane protein 2 (VAMP-2). Whether these vesicles represent a novel organelle that appears in cells transfected with AQP2 or whether AQP2 usurps an already existing pathway and modifies it based on intrinsic signals within the AQP2 sequence remains unclear.

It is likely that as newly synthesized AQP2 is loaded into transporting vesicles as it exits the TGN, the fate of the vesicles is indeed determined by signals on the AQP2 protein itself. However, when the recycling of AQP2 is interrupted by lowering the incubation temperature of the cells to 20° C or by incubating cells with bafilomycin, an inhibitor of the vacuolar hydrogen–adenosine triphosphatase (H$^+$-ATPase), AQP2 can be concentrated in a clathrin-positive, Golgi-associated compartment.[109] This accumulation occurs even in the presence of cycloheximide, an inhibitor of protein synthesis, which indicates that recycling AQP2 is also accumulating in this juxtanuclear compartment. The 20° C block prevents exit of proteins from the TGN,[222] and clathrin-coated vesicles are enriched in this cellular compartment.[108] However, some portions of the so-called recycling endosome, which is located in a similar juxtanuclear region of some cells, also have clathrin-coated domains.[101] Therefore, the AQP2 could be recycling either via the TGN, via a specialized clathrin-coated recycling endosome, or via both. Indeed recycling AQP2 is partially co-localized with rab11, a marker of the recycling endosomal compartment, in subapical vesicles.[240,337]

AQP2 as a Constitutively Recycling Membrane Protein

It is now clear that AQP2 recycles continually between intracellular vesicles and the cell surface, both in transfected cells in culture and in principal cells in situ.[20,31] This provides the opportunity to modulate the plasma membrane content of AQP2 by increasing the rate of exocytosis, decreasing endocytosis, or both. Such a dual action of VP was predicted by

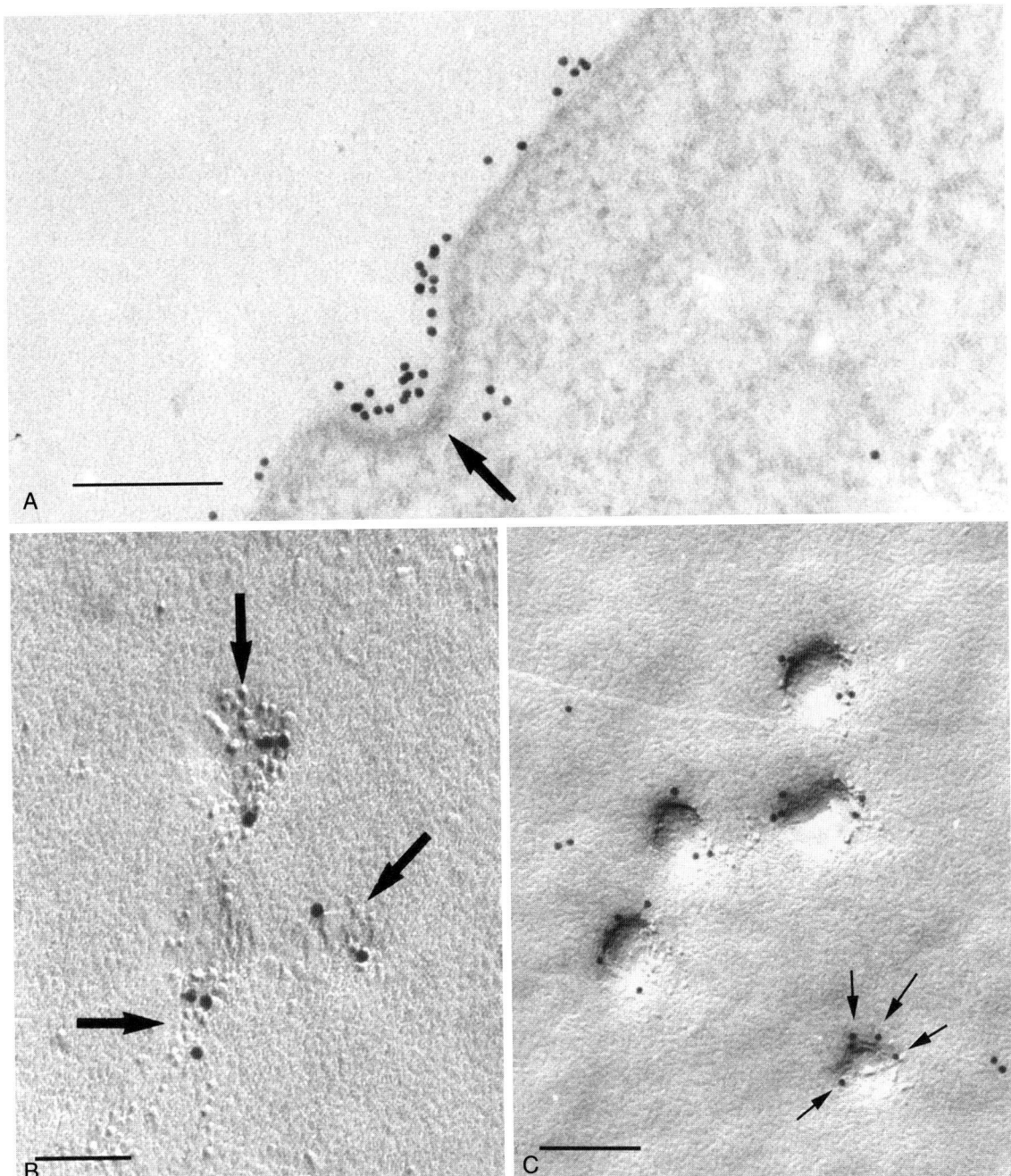

FIGURE 11-8 Internalization of aquaporin-2 (AQP2) by clathrin-coated pits. **A,** Immunogold labeling of AQP2 in clathrin-coated pit (*arrow*) at the apical plasma membrane of collecting duct principal cells. An antibody against an external epitope of AQP2 was used. **B** and **C,** Label-fracture images of LLC-PK₁ cells expressing AQP2. Immunogold label for AQP2 is located in intramembranous particle (IMP) clusters on the membrane (**B,** *arrows*) and is associated with membrane invaginations that resemble clathrin-coated pits (**C,** *arrows*). Bars equal 0.25 μm.

Knepper and Nielsen,[174] who compared mathematical models of VP-induced permeability changes to actual experimental data from isolated perfused collecting ducts.

Data showing that AQP2 recycles constitutively have been obtained by blocking the AQP2 recycling pathway, either in an intracellular perinuclear compartment identified as the TGN, as discussed earlier,[109] or at the cell surface.[200,335] When cells are infected with a dynamin K44A virus, clathrin-mediated endocytosis is arrested, and in parallel, AQP2 accumulates at the plasma membrane in a VP-independent manner.[335] This process takes several hours as the mutant dynamin is expressed in cultured cells and the endogenous wild-type dynamin is overwhelmed.

A more rapid means of preventing clathrin-mediated endocytosis is to treat cells with the cholesterol-depleting drug MBCD.[296,332] When this was done in LLC-PK₁ cells expressing AQP2, the water channel accumulated at the plasma membrane in a matter of minutes, which indicates that it is recycling rapidly through the plasma membrane and that inhibition of endocytosis is sufficient to cause membrane accumulation of AQP2 (see Figure 11-9).[200] Importantly, this drug also causes a significant accumulation of AQP2 in the apical membrane of collecting duct principal cells in situ (Figure 11-9*G, H*).[301] This observation raises the possibility that inhibition of endocytosis is a potential pathway by which AQP2 can be accumulated at

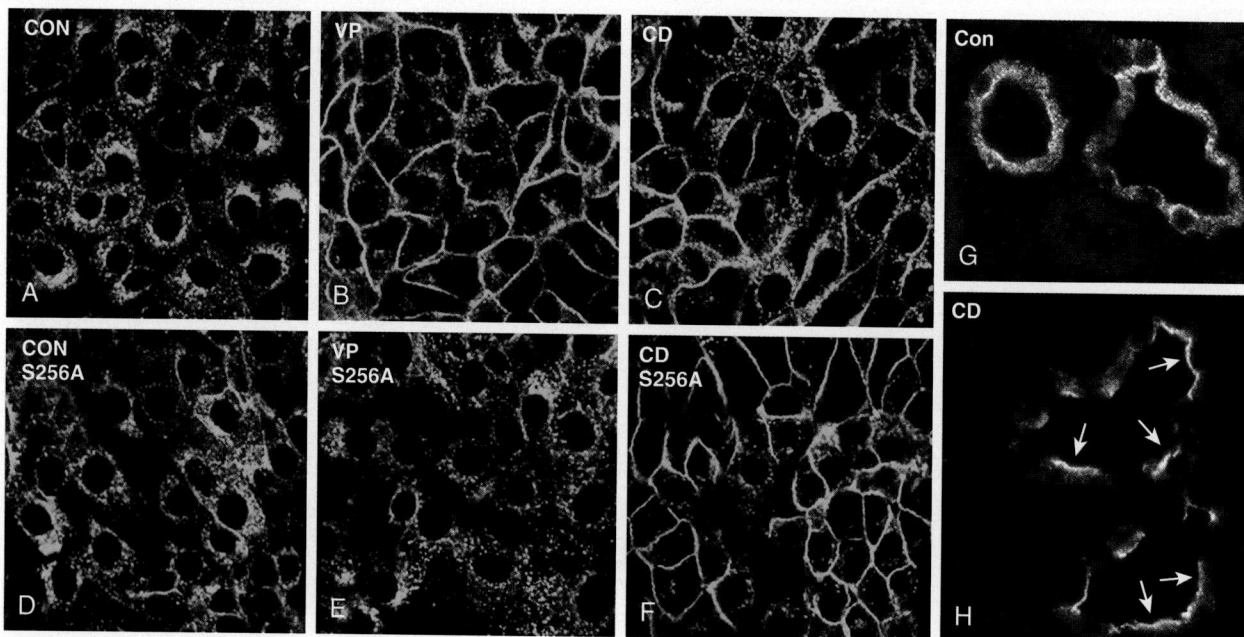

FIGURE 11-9 Stimulation of aquaporin-2 (AQP2) membrane accumulation by methyl-β-cyclodextrin (MBCD) in LLC-PK₁ cells (**A** through **F**) and collecting duct principal cells in situ (**G, H**). Immunofluorescence staining is shown for AQP2 in LLC-PK₁ cells expressing either wild-type AQP2 (**A** through **C**) or a mutant in which the serine at residue 256 has been replaced by alanine (S256A) (**D** through **F**). Under baseline conditions, both the wild-type (**A**) and the S256A mutation (**D**) are located mainly on intracellular vesicles, with very little plasma membrane staining. After vasopressin (VP) treatment, the wild-type AQP2 relocates to the plasma membrane (**B**), whereas the S256A mutation remains on intracellular vesicles (**E**). However, when endocytosis is inhibited in these cells by application of the cholesterol-depleting drug MBCD, both wild-type AQP2 and S256A-AQP2 accumulate at the cell surface (**C, F**). This result shows that both wild-type AQP2 and S256A-AQP2 are constitutively recycling between intracellular vesicles and the plasma membrane and that inhibiting endocytosis with MBCD (CD in the images) is sufficient to cause membrane accumulation, even in the absence of S256 phosphorylation of AQP2. In collecting duct principal cells (inner stripe of outer medulla) in situ, AQP2 is located on vesicles scattered throughout the cytoplasm after perfusion of intact kidneys in vitro (**G**). However, after perfusion of kidneys for 60 minutes with 5 mmol/L MBCD, increased apical plasma membrane expression of AQP2 is seen (**H,** *arrows*). This finding indicates that AQP2 is constitutively recycling through the apical plasma membrane in principal cells in situ and that membrane accumulation can be induced by blocking endocytosis (with MBCD) even in the absence of VP.

the cell surface of collecting duct principal cells in patients with X-linked NDI. Recently, the therapeutic use of cholesterol-depleting statins to increase AQP2 accumulation at the cell surface by blocking endocytosis has also been proposed.[20,193a,274] How these and other recent insights into AQP2 trafficking and signaling might provide novel strategies to alleviate the symptoms of NDI is discussed in more detail later.

Regulation of AQP2 Trafficking

Our understanding of AQP2 recycling continues to evolve in parallel with new discoveries related to the targeting and trafficking of membrane proteins in general. These discoveries include the presence of alternative signaling pathways for AQP2 trafficking in addition to the "conventional" cAMP pathway, the role of phosphorylation by various kinases, and the involvement of the actin cytoskeleton, as well as the gradual identification of accessory interacting proteins, including phosphorylation-dependent AQP2-binding proteins. However, several fundamental questions related to the cell biology of VP action remain unanswered, including how phosphorylation of AQP2 induces membrane accumulation of this water channel.

Role of Phosphorylation in AQP2 Trafficking

Phosphorylation of the C-terminal tail of AQP2 plays a complex regulatory role in trafficking and compartmentalization of the protein. AQP2 contains several putative phosphorylation

sites for kinases (see Figure 11-3), including protein kinase A (PKA), protein kinase G (PKG), protein kinase C (PKC), Golgi casein kinase, and casein kinase 2. The majority of work has focused on the role of PKA-induced phosphorylation of S256 in the VP-induced signaling cascade, because this site appears to be critical to the VP-induced membrane accumulation of AQP2.[99,164] However, S256 is part of a polyphosphorylated region at the C terminus of AQP2, which contains three further VP-regulated phosphorylation sites: S261, S264, and S269 (threonine in humans).[126,128]

The rise in intracellular cAMP following activation of G-coupled proteins by VP results in recruitment of PKA to AQP2-containing vesicles by PKA-anchoring proteins (AKAPs).[172] The co-localization of vesicular AQP2 with AKAP18δ makes this the most likely isoform to mediate this event.[122] Inhibition of the cAMP-specific phosphodiesterase 4D (PDE₄D) by rolipram increases AKAP-tethered PKA activity in AQP2-bearing vesicles and enhances AQP2 trafficking,[328] which indicates that a novel, compartmentalized cAMP-dependent signal transduction pathway consisting of anchored PDE₄D, AKAP18δ, and PKA plays an essential role in AQP2 translocation. Furthermore, the AKAP Ht31 directly interacts with the actin-modifying GTPase RhoA, which plays a crucial role in modulating AQP2 trafficking (see later).

In theory, phosphorylation could modulate the water permeability of AQP2 already in the plasma membrane, as previously discussed,[178] or it could be involved in the regulated trafficking of vesicles containing AQP2 and insertion of AQP2 into the plasma membrane. The permeability of AQP4 is inhibited by PKC-induced phosphorylation,[110,394] and phosphorylation-mediated gating of aquaporins has been described in plants.[154,352] However, several lines of evidence suggest that AQP2 is not gated by phosphorylation. Kamsteeg and colleagues showed that oocytes expressing S256D-AQP2 (mimicking the charge state of phosphorylation on this residue) have water permeability similar to that of wild-type AQP2.[161] In addition, PKA-dependent phosphorylation of AQP2 in purified endosomes had no effect on single-channel water permeability.[183] Most recently, a comprehensive study in oocytes demonstrated that phosphorylation of the C-terminal tail of AQP2 does not directly affect its water transport function.[230]

In contrast, regulation of membrane permeability by AQP2 trafficking has been established in a variety of experimental systems. Following PKA recruitment, phosphorylation of AQP2 on S256 is critical for VP-induced cell surface accumulation of AQP2 (Figure 11-9*B, E*).[99,164] In oocytes, S256 phosphorylation is required for AQP2 trafficking to the plasma membrane.[161] A mouse strain with an amino acid substitution at S256 (S256L) that prevents phosphorylation of this residue and inhibits AQP2 accumulation on the plasma membrane has polyuria and congenital progressive hydronephrosis.[223] The importance of S256 phosphorylation was shown in humans by the identification of a mutation in AQP2 (S254L) that destroys the PKA phosphorylation site at S256 and results in NDI.[62] The role of the three other phosphorylation sites, S261, S264, and S269 is still uncertain. Downstream phosphorylation of S264 and S269 requires prior PKA-mediated phosphorylation of S256,[126] whereas S261 phosphorylation is independent of that of any of the other sites.[230]

Acute VP exposure regulates the abundance of all three phosphorylated forms of AQP2, but whereas phosphorylated S261 (pS261) decreases in abundance, both pS264 and pS269 increase in abundance. All three phosphorylated forms are localized to some degree in the plasma membrane in vivo,[86,127,229] but cell culture studies have demonstrated that S261 phosphorylation is not required for either VP-stimulated AQP2 trafficking or constitutive recycling.[202] Interestingly, the pS269 form of AQP2 is exclusively detected in the apical plasma membrane, which suggests a regulatory role for this phosphorylation site directly in the plasma membrane.[229] Acute VP exposure for 15 minutes causes an increase in the abundance of pS264-AQP2 in the basolateral plasma membrane; whether this is due to trafficking or direct phosphorylation of AQP2 that is already in the basolateral membrane (see earlier) remains unknown.[86] As for other proteins with multiple kinase target sites, dissecting their individual contributions to AQP2 trafficking is likely to be a complex and difficult process.

Although phosphorylation of AQP2 at S256 plays a role in AQP2 accumulation at the cell surface, it is not (alone) necessary for its exocytotic insertion into the plasma membrane. As detailed earlier, AQP2 follows a constitutive recycling pathway, and the S256A mutant, from which the PKA phosphorylation site is absent, also accumulates on the plasma membrane upon inhibition of endocytosis with either K44A dynamin or MBCD (see Figure 11-9),[200] which suggests that the rate of AQP2 endocytosis also plays a major role in membrane AQP2 accumulation.

In line with this hypothesis, Nunes and colleagues[260] suggested that S256 phosphorylation plays a more significant role in the reduction of AQP2 endocytosis in response to VP, rather than acting as an on-switch for exocytosis. Thus, although VP-induced *accumulation* of AQP2 at the cell surface requires S256 phosphorylation, exocytotic *insertion* of AQP2 into the plasma membrane is independent of this phosphorylation event.

Although phosphorylation of AQP2 is usually required for cell surface expression, the internalization of AQP2 may not be dependent on its phosphorylation state at S256. Prostaglandin E_2 (PGE_2) stimulates removal of AQP2 from the surface of principal cells when added after VP treatment,[393] but was not reported to alter the S256 phosphorylation state of AQP2. PKC-mediated endocytosis of AQP2 is also independent of the S256 phosphorylation state. Furthermore, although the S256D-AQP2 mutant—which mimics a phosphorylated S256 residue—is constitutively expressed predominantly at the cell surface,[359] S256D-AQP2 internalization can be induced by either PGE_2 or dopamine, but only after preexposing cells to forskolin. This suggests that PGE_2 and dopamine induce internalization of AQP2 independently of AQP2 dephosphorylation,[242] and that preceding activation of cAMP production is necessary for PGE_2 and dopamine to cause AQP2 internalization.

These data imply that phosphorylation of another intracellular target or targets (presumably by forskolin-stimulated elevation of cAMP) is necessary for AQP2 endocytosis to occur (see later). However, recent data suggest that the effect of PGE_2 on AQP2 recycling depends on which PGE_2 receptor (EP receptor) it acts upon, because EP4 receptor stimulation is able to increase intracellular cAMP levels and presumably AQP2 membrane insertion.[192] Preventing dephosphorylation of AQP2 with the phosphatase inhibitor okadaic acid also has the expected effect of increasing cell surface accumulation of AQP2 in cultured cells, but surprisingly, the same effect of okadaic acid was observed in the presence of the PKA inhibitor H-89. The authors of that study concluded that okadaic acid stimulates the membrane translocation of AQP2 in a phosphorylation-independent manner.[356]

The transduction mechanism responsible for this effect remains to be determined, but these data support the idea that AQP2 can accumulate on the plasma membrane in an S256 phosphorylation–independent manner. Although there is clear evidence that AQP2 exocytosis and endocytosis can occur independently of S256 phosphorylation, the role of the downstream phosphorylation sites S261, S264, and S269 in either of these processes currently remains unknown.

The mechanism by which phosphorylation of AQP2 affects the steady-state redistribution of AQP2 is slowly unraveling. One report has suggested that a Golgi casein kinase–mediated phosphorylation of S256 is involved in the passage of AQP2 through the Golgi apparatus in its biosynthetic pathway.[277] Furthermore, accumulating evidence suggests that phosphorylation of AQP2 mediates its interaction with other proteins. These interactions may influence AQP2 exocytosis, for example by modification of interactions between AQP2-containing vesicles and the cytoskeleton, via microtubules and/or microtubule motors (see later), or the endocytotic step of AQP2 recycling.[201]

AQP2 forms a complex with proteins of the endocytotic machinery and phosphorylation modifies AQP2 interaction with key proteins that are involved in this process, including heat shock cognate/heat shock protein 70 (hsc/hsp70).[201] AQP2 is present in "endocytosis-resistant" membrane domains after VP treatment,[21] probably because the interaction of AQP2 with hsc/hsp70, a key protein required for clathrin-mediated endocytosis, is greatly reduced by phosphorylation of AQP2 at residue S256.[201] In support of this idea, AQP2 membrane accumulation was increased in cells expressing a dominant negative mutation of hsc70, presumably because of a decrease in clathrin-mediated endocytosis of AQP2. Subsequent studies have shown that the ability of AQP2 to coimmunoprecipitate not only with hsc70 but also with clathrin and dynamin is reduced significantly by S256 phosphorylation.[231] Recently, a comparative proteomic approach[270] has also been used to determine that several proteins, including Hsp70 isoforms 1, 2, and 5 (hsp70-1, hsp70-2, hsp70-5), and annexin 2, differentially interact with AQP2 depending on its phosphorylation status.[396]

The myelin and lymphocyte protein, MAL, is an AQP2-interacting protein that enhances AQP2 cell surface accumulation by reducing AQP2 internalization. As predicted from this hypothesis, MAL associates less with AQP256A that with wild-type AQP2.[160] However, it remains unclear whether this effect is due to AQP2 phosphorylation at S256 itself, because the association of MAL with both wild-type AQP2 and S256D-AQP2 seemed to be similar in coimmunoprecipitation experiments. It should also be noted that the reported association of MAL with AQP2 could not be confirmed by another group using MDCK cells expressing AQP2.[231]

Actin, Actin-Associated Proteins, and AQP2 Trafficking

The literature examining the involvement of actin in water channel trafficking dates back over three decades, but actin's role in this process still remains unclear. Actin has been shown to associate directly with AQP2,[33,256] which implies a functional relationship. Furthermore, both β- and γ-actin have been identified in kidney inner medulla in association with AQP2-containing vesicles.[8] Most recently, G-actin has been shown to be associated directly with non–S256-phosphorylated AQP2.[254]

Early studies conducted in rat inner medulla and toad urinary bladder demonstrated that VP induces a reduction in F-actin in apical regions of cells,[73,120] which presumably allows water channel–containing vesicles to break through the "actin barrier" and fuse with the plasma membrane. However, actin depolymerization resulting from the inactivation of RhoA, a GTPase that regulates the actin cytoskeleton, increases the membrane accumulation of AQP2 and membrane water permeability in cultured cells, even in the absence of VP.[173,342] F-actin depolymerizing agents, such as cytochalasins, inhibit responses to VP[70,147,370] but also increase AQP2 membrane accumulation in cultured renal epithelial cells.[173,342] Importantly, the pool of actin depolymerized by VP appears to overlap with the pool depolymerized by cytochalasin. Although these results appear conflicting (VP increases water permeability by depolymerization of actin, whereas cytochalasin decreases osmotic water permeability), they do suggest a dual role for actin: one to serve as a vesicle-holding network that allows membrane fusion upon VP stimulation, and another in transporting AQP2 vesicles to and from the apical membrane.[88]

Role of Actin Polymerization in AQP2 Trafficking

The potential role of actin in AQP2 trafficking was directly examined in transfected CD8 cells (a rabbit collecting duct cell line) in culture. Exposure of these cells to *Clostridium* toxin B, which inhibits Rho GTPases that are involved in regulating the actin cytoskeleton,[285] resulted in actin depolymerization and accumulation of AQP2 in the plasma membrane.[342] A similar AQP2 translocation was seen in cells treated with the downstream Rho kinase inhibitor Y-27632,[173] without detectable changes in intracellular cAMP levels. Conversely, expression of constitutively active RhoA in these cells induced stress fiber formation, indicating actin polymerization, and inhibited the normal AQP2 translocation response to forskolin.

It remains unclear whether the net accumulation of AQP2 under these conditions is due to increased exocytosis or decreased endocytosis. There is a considerable body of evidence showing that actin depolymerization inhibits endocytosis, although whether apical and/or basolateral endocytosis is most affected remains a matter of debate.[104,134,188] Interestingly, actin depolymerization was sufficient to provoke membrane accumulation of AQP2 in either the apical or the basolateral plasma membrane, depending upon the transfected cell type that was examined.[173,342]

Recently, a new hypothesis regarding the role of actin depolymerization in AQP2 trafficking has been proposed.[254] According to this hypothesis, AQP2 phosphorylation results in the release of AQP2 from G-actin and an increased affinity of AQP2 to α-tropomyosin 5b (TM5b). This causes a reduction in the amount of TM5b bound to F-actin, which induces F-actin destabilization and subsequent AQP2 trafficking to the plasma membrane. These findings also suggest a novel mechanism of protein trafficking, in which the channel protein itself critically regulates local actin reorganization to initiate its movement. This idea is supported by recent data from Nunes and colleagues[260] showing that VP induces a burst of exocytosis only in cells expressing AQP2 and not in cells that are AQP2 null. Thus, the presence of AQP2 influences the cellular effect of VP on target cells, despite the fact that cAMP levels are similarly increased under all conditions.

In contrast to the data discussed earlier showing membrane accumulation of AQP2 after actin depolymerization, a study using transfected MDCK cells reported that AQP2 was concentrated in an EEA1-positive early endosomal compartment upon actin filament disruption by either cytochalasin D or latrunculin.[337] These contrasting effects may reflect the use of different model systems. The physiologic role played by actin on AQP2 trafficking in renal principal cells in situ is still a matter of debate.

Identification of Actin-Associated Proteins Potentially Involved in AQP2 Trafficking

Many studies have implicated actin and associated proteins such as the myosins, as well as microtubules (see later), in sequential transport steps of vesicle trafficking.[11,297] Immunogold electron microscopy demonstrated that myosin I, an actin-associated motor protein, is associated with AQP2-containing vesicles.[219] In addition, various other myosin isoforms, including myosin IC, nonmuscle myosins IIA and IIB, myosin VI, and myosin IXB, were identified by mass spectrometry in immunoisolated AQP2-containing vesicles.[8] However, the profile of other identified proteins indicates that virtually all compartments in the secretory and recycling pathways were represented in the immunoprecipitated material, which makes a hypothesis regarding the role of myosin difficult.

Coupling of motor proteins to vesicles requires multiple Rab proteins, and recently myosin VB has been suggested to play a role in the AQP2 shuttle by Rab11 family–interacting protein 2–dependent recycling through a perinuclear Rab11 compartment.[240] Myosin light-chain kinase, the myosin regulatory light chain, and nonmuscle myosin IIA and IIB isoforms have also been detected in rat IMCD cells and implicated in a calcium/calmodulin-regulated pathway leading to AQP2 membrane accumulation.[51] These results support previous data showing that Ca²⁺ release from ryanodine-sensitive stores plays an essential role in VP-mediated AQP2 trafficking via a calmodulin-dependent mechanism.[53] A role for Epac (exchange protein directly activated by cAMP), which is expressed in the collecting duct,[194] in VP-induced calcium mobilization and AQP2 exocytosis in perfused collecting ducts has also been shown.[388] However, the role of calcium in the VP response was questioned by another group, who provided capacitance data in support of a cAMP-dependent but calcium-independent exocytotic process after VP stimulation.[199]

Immunoaffinity isolation of AQP2 followed by protein mass spectrometry has been used[270] to identify a "multiprotein complex" containing ionized calcium–binding adapter molecule 2, myosin regulatory light-chain smooth muscle isoforms 2A and 2B, TM5b, annexin A2 and A6, scinderin, gelsolin, α-actinin 4, αII-spectrin, and myosin heavy-chain nonmuscle type A.[255] Interestingly, the gelsolin-like protein adseverin is much more highly expressed in collecting duct principal cells than is gelsolin (which is abundant in intercalated cells); this indicates that it might be a physiologically important player in calcium-activated actin remodeling.[203]

In addition to myosins, moesin, a member of the ERM (ezrin-radixin-moesin) family of scaffolding proteins, has also been implicated in the apical trafficking process.[343] The GTPase Rap1 and signal-induced proliferation–associated gene 1 (SPA-1) may also have a role in regulating AQP2 trafficking.[253] Activation of Rap1 was found to inhibit AQP2 plasma membrane targeting, possibly by increasing actin polymerization mediated by SPA-1.

Based on these studies, it is clear that actin and its complex array of regulatory proteins play critical roles in the membrane accumulation and recycling of AQP2. However, what the precise steps in the pathway are and how these processes are regulated by VP have not been established in any detail, other than to show that disruption of the cytoskeleton has end results compatible with a perturbation of the physiologically regulated process.

Microtubules and AQP2 Trafficking

Intracellular vesicles can move along microtubules, driven by microtubule "mechanoenzymes" or motors.[4,316,354] It is, therefore, not surprising that microtubule-depolymerizing agents such as colchicine and nocodazole partially inhibit the VP-induced water permeability increase in target epithelia (e.g., Dousa and Barnes,[75] Phillips and Taylor,[269] Taylor and colleagues[344]). Colchicine treatment disrupts the apical localization of AQP2 in rat kidney principal cells, which results in AQP2 scattering in vesicles throughout the cytoplasm.[303] Furthermore, cold treatment, which depolymerizes microtubules,

also inhibits the VP response.[27] This indicates that caution must be exercised in the interpretation of data from cell or tissue preparations that involve a cold incubation step as part of the experimental procedure.

Two large protein families are of particular importance for microtubule-based vesicle movement. These are ATPases known as *motor proteins*, the dyneins[268] and the kinesins.[365] Minus end–directed motors, such as dynein, transport vesicles toward the microtubule-organizing center, whereas plus end–directed motors, such as kinesin, transport vesicles in the opposite direction.[29,283]

Dynein and dynactin, a protein complex thought to link dynein to microtubules and vesicles, are associated with AQP2-bearing vesicles.[218] An inhibitor of the dynein ATPase, erythro-9-[3-(2-hydroxynonyl)]adenine (EHNA), significantly reduces the effect of VP on water permeability in the amphibian urinary bladder.[213] However, although treatment of cells with nocodazole or colchicine to depolymerize microtubules resulted in dispersion of AQP2 vesicles throughout the cytoplasm, forskolin-induced AQP2 membrane accumulation was not inhibited.[337] Earlier work using toad bladder and collecting duct epithelia demonstrated that the effect of VP on transepithelial water flow was only partially inhibited by microtubule disruption (about 65% in collecting ducts).[269] Taken together, these data support the idea that microtubules are involved in the long-range trafficking of vesicles toward the plasma membrane, but that the final step of approach and fusion involves a cooperative interaction between the microtubule and actin-based cytoskeleton.

Furthermore, whether microtubules affect endocytic retrieval or the exocytic pathway of AQP2 remains unclear. Recently it has been shown that upon VP exposure, the microtubule network that is usually densely formed around the cell nucleus is reversibly reorganized with increased formation of microtubules in the cell periphery.[368] In the same study, depolymerization of microtubules prevented the perinuclear positioning of AQP2 in resting cells, and after internalization of AQP2 following VP washout, forskolin stimulation still caused a redistribution of AQP2 to the plasma membrane.[368] These results suggest that the microtubule-dependent translocation of AQP2 is predominantly responsible for trafficking and localization of AQP2 inside the cell after internalization, but not for its exocytic translocation.

In conclusion, the delivery of AQP2-containing vesicles to the sub–plasma membrane region probably involves both microtubules and the actin cytoskeleton, as well as their respective cohorts of accessory and motor proteins, which are also involved in membrane trafficking processes in most cell types. In addition, microtubules are probably involved in redistribution of AQP2 following endocytic retrieval. Most of the specific protein-protein interactions that render these processes VP sensitive in the collecting duct, as well as their regulation, remain to be elucidated.

SNARE Proteins and AQP2 Trafficking

As for the majority of membrane fusion events, it has been postulated that the docking step for VP-induced exocytosis of AQP2-containing vesicles could be mediated by vesicle-targeting proteins. The final accomplishment of vesicle tethering, docking, and fusion involves a complex series of protein-protein interactions that are combined under the name the *SNARE hypothesis*.[299,300,314,376] This process requires a complex interaction among integral membrane proteins, the SNAREs (soluble *N*-ethylmaleimide–sensitive factor attachment protein receptors), present in the vesicle (v-SNAREs) and the target membrane (t-SNAREs), as has been suggested for docking of synaptic vesicles to the presynaptic plasma membrane in the central nervous system.

In the collecting duct principal cell, several proteins of the SNARE complex are associated with AQP2-containing vesicles and/or the apical plasma membrane of principal cells. The SNARE protein VAMP-2 (vesicle-associated membrane protein 2, also known as *synaptobrevin 2*) has been found associated with AQP2 vesicles,[153,249] and disruption of VAMP-2 with tetanus toxin diminishes cAMP-dependent AQP2 trafficking.[105] Other SNARES that co-localize with AQP2 include VAMP-3 (cellubrevin), SNAP23 (synaptosomal-associated protein 23), and the ATPase Hrs-2 (hepatocyte growth factor–regulated tyrosine kinase substrate 2), which may regulate exocytosis via interaction with SNAP25.[89,140,321] The t-SNARE syntaxin 4 is present in the apical plasma membrane of collecting duct principal cells,[210] and SNAP23 has been found associated with syntaxin 4 and VAMP-2.[282]

The interaction of AQP2 and the t-SNARE complex may be mediated by the protein snapin.[226] Furthermore, other proteins that are involved in exocytotic processes in other cell types, such as members of the Rab GTPase family Rab3 and Rab5a,[197] have been identified in AQP2-containing vesicles and may also play a role in vesicle docking and fusion. Several additional SNARE proteins, including syntaxin 7, syntaxin 12, and syntaxin 13, were identified in a proteomic screen using vesicles immunoisolated with anti-AQP2 antibodies.[8] As mentioned previously, however, such isolated vesicles represent a mixed population that contain AQP2, but are not all in the exocytotic pathway.

A recent study utilizing small interfering siRNA has shown functionally that VAMP-2, VAMP-3, syntaxin 3, and SNAP23 are a complementary set of SNAREs responsible for AQP2 vesicle fusion into the apical plasma membrane, and Munc18b (mammalian uncoordinated 18b protein) is a negative regulator of the SNARE complex.[275] However, the functions of the other SNARE proteins in AQP2 trafficking have not been formally examined.

V₂R-Independent Membrane Insertion of AQP2: Potential Strategies for Treating Nephrogenic Diabetes Insipidus

Important progress has been made in the last few years in our understanding of intracellular signaling and alternative trafficking pathways that bypass the V_2R-cAMP-PKA cascade, allowing membrane accumulation of AQP2 even in the absence of a functional V_2R. This is especially important for the generation of novel strategies to alleviate the symptoms of X-linked NDI, in which a mutated V_2R is defective for any of a number of reasons (see earlier). Renal principal cells in these patients may still produce AQP2, but the defective V_2R signaling mechanism means that it does not accumulate at the cell surface to increase urine concentration upon an increase in circulating VP levels. Recent developments in understanding the cell biology of AQP2 trafficking have provided some hope that AQP2 can in fact accumulate at the cell surface independently of VP signaling in the collecting ducts of these patients. Four promising approaches are discussed here.

STIMULATION OF THE CAMP PATHWAY WITH ALTERNATIVE GPCR LIGANDS

Principal cells in different regions of the kidney express other adenylyl cyclase–coupled GPCRs in addition to the V_2R. Examples are the calcitonin receptor, mainly in the cortex, and the glucagon receptor. It has been shown recently that calcitonin treatment results in membrane accumulation of AQP2 in vitro and in vivo, and that this is dependent on the presence of S256 within the AQP2 C terminus.[23] In vivo, calcitonin increased apical membrane accumulation of AQP2 in principal cells of the cortex and outer stripe, but not in the inner medulla where calcitonin receptors are not expressed. Finally, and importantly, calcitonin infusion via osmotic minipump in VP-deficient Brattleboro rats resulted in a threefold reduction in urine output and a twofold increase in urine osmolality during the first 12 hours of treatment. These data confirm and extend the earlier findings of de Rouffignac and Elalouf that calcitonin has antidiuretic effects in hormonally deprived rats.[63]

Early studies reported that another GPCR ligand, glucagon, increased cAMP levels in microdissected cortical and medullary collecting ducts.[6] Glucagon receptors were also detected at various locations along the renal tubule, including in the collecting duct, by reverse transcriptase polymerase chain reaction[212] and radioligand binding.[45] Glucagon administration was reported to increase cAMP levels and water permeability in perfused IMCDs, and it also increased the expression of AQP2.[386] However, an earlier study could detect no increase in cAMP induced by glucagon in microdissected rat IMCD segments.[208] This discrepancy remains to be clarified.

ACTIVATION OF A CGMP SIGNALING PATHWAY

Both in cell cultures and principal cells of kidney slices in vitro, several hormones and drugs that increase levels of cyclic guanosine monophosphate (cGMP) also induce AQP2 accumulation at the cell surface. These include sodium nitroprusside (a nitric oxide donor), L-arginine (which stimulates nitric oxide synthase), and atrial natriuretic peptide.[19] Similar data showing that AQP2 surface expression can be increased in vivo following 90 minutes of atrial natriuretic peptide infusion have also been reported.[374] Elevation of intracellular cGMP using the PDE5 inhibitor sildenafil citrate (Viagra) also increases cell surface (plasma membrane) expression of AQP2 both in vitro and in vivo[24] (Figure 11-10). Although no significant increase in urinary concentration was detectable in rats treated with sildenafil for 90 minutes, possibly due to increased renal blood flow as a result of vasodilatation, this observation nevertheless provides a strategy to induce VP-independent cell surface accumulation of AQP2. Adaptation of this approach to the treatment of human disease requires further dose-response studies, as well as the potential development of PDE5 inhibitors that are more selective for tubular epithelial cells or that may be delivered more specifically to these cells at an appropriate concentration to elicit the required response.

INHIBITION OF AQP2 ENDOCYTOSIS

It is now evident that AQP2 recycles constitutively between the cell surface and intracellular vesicles. Thus, an attractive possibility is to modulate the endocytotic pathway in X-linked NDI as a means of increasing its cell surface expression. Use of a discovery approach to screen small chemical libraries for specific inhibitors of endocytosis that might be applied in vivo could be informative. Such a strategy was used to identify a

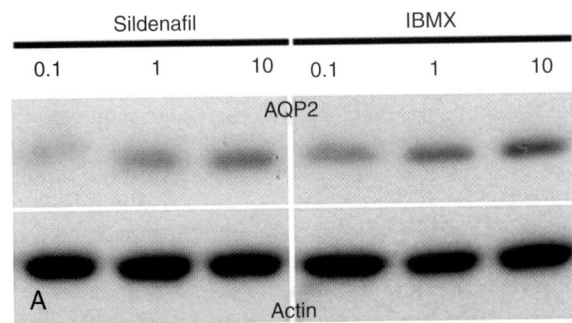

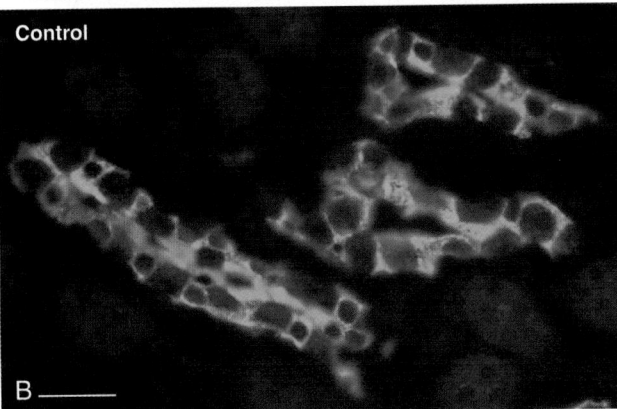

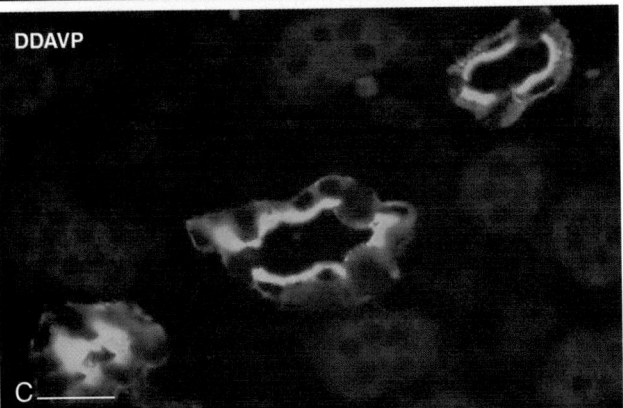

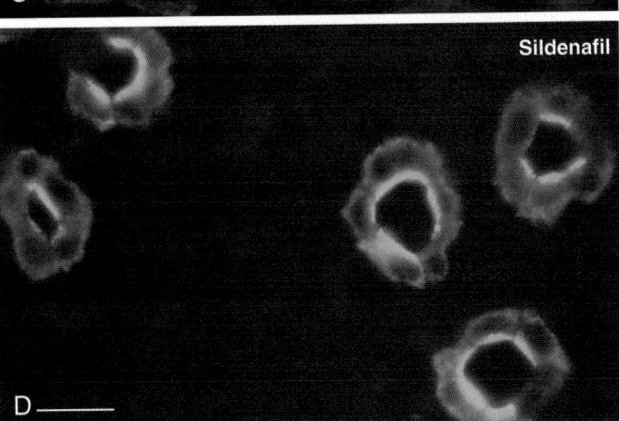

FIGURE 11-10 Stimulation of membrane accumulation of aquaporin-2 (AQP2) in kidney inner stripe collecting duct principal cells of Brattleboro rats after acute in vivo treatment with sildenafil citrate (Viagra). Animals were injected with saline, desamino-8-d-arginine VP (dDAVP), or sildenafil through the jugular vein. Injection of saline was used as a control (**A**) and compared with 25 mg/kg dADVP (**B**) and 4 mg/kg of sildenafil (**C**). In controls (**A**), AQP2 is diffusely located throughout the subapical cytoplasm of principal cells. The dDAVP (**B**) and sildenafil (**C**) both induce a marked redistribution of AQP2, which appears as a narrow, brightly stained band at the apical pole of principal cells, consistent with plasma membrane staining (*arrows*). Bar equals 10 μm.

small chemical named *dynasore* that is a specific inhibitor of the dynein GTPase, a protein critically involved in clathrin- and caveolin-mediated endocytosis.[207] Recently, the use of cholesterol-lowering statins has also been proposed as a means of increasing cell surface expression of AQP2.[20,193a,274]

STIMULATION OF RENAL EP4 PROSTANOID RECEPTORS

There is evidence that PGE_2 treatment results in internalization of AQP2,[242,393] and PGE_2 infusion can promote diuresis. However, a recent study suggests that treating a mouse model of X-linked NDI with a selective EP4 agonist bypasses the V_2R, resulting in increased levels of cAMP, enhanced collecting duct water permeability, and increased AQP2 levels.[192] Thus, the effect of PGE_2 in promoting diuresis seems to be dependent on activation of other PGE_2 receptor subtypes mediating inhibition of salt and water absorption along the nephron.[28] Selective activation of EP4 receptors, combined with inhibition of local PGE_2 effects, such as by use of indomethacin, could represent a new strategy for the treatment of X-linked NDI.

Long-Term Regulation of Water Balance

The actions of VP on the kidney collecting duct are mediated by two different but convergent mechanisms. As described earlier, VP-mediated short-term regulation of collecting duct water permeability is highly dependent on AQP2 trafficking events. Of equal importance are the long-term effects of prolonged VP exposure. Prolonged dehydration increases urinary concentrating ability to about the same extent as acute VP treatment,[156] whereas long-term water loading reduces urinary concentrating capacity.

The consequences of long-term dehydration are complex and probably result from numerous adaptational changes. For example, in addition to causing changes in circulating VP levels, dehydration alters circulating levels of glucocorticoids and prostaglandins and leads to adaptational changes in the kidney, such as reduction in glomerular filtration rate. However, one aspect of long-term regulation can be ascribed to changes in collecting duct water permeability. Lankford and colleagues demonstrated that perfused collecting ducts isolated from water-restricted rats displayed a much higher osmotic water permeability than tubules from water-loaded rats,[185] which suggests an adaptation in collecting duct principal cells.

One such adaptation is that AQP2 expression markedly increases in response to dehydration, with a greater abundance of AQP2 in the apical plasma membrane,[247] and recent studies have shown that long-term VP exposure results in increased abundance of several forms of phosphorylated AQP2.[85,86,231] Of course it is likely that both VP and VP-independent pathways are responsible for these changes,[72,77,119,214,217] with evidence suggesting that both secretin and oxytocin are important for VP-independent AQP2 translocation and expression.[186,191] Also, the long-term effects of VP on medullary hyperosmolality should not be underestimated, because extracellular tonicity, through activation of the tonicity-responsive enhancer–binding protein, increases VP-induced AQP2 transcription and subsequent whole-cell AQP2 abundance.[113]

AQP2 and Nephrogenic Diabetes Insipidus

Hereditary NDI, characterized by the inability of the kidney to respond to VP and produce a concentrated urine, can result from mutations in the V_2R or, more rarely, mutations in the AQP2 water channel. In addition to hereditary NDI, multiple forms of acquired NDI exist, and many of these disorders are associated with alterations in AQP2 expression or targeting.

Autosomal Recessive Nephrogenic Diabetes Insipidus and Mutations in AQP2

The role of AQP2 in non–X-linked NDI was discovered almost 15 years ago.[363] Currently, over 40 different mutations in AQP2 have been reported that result in NDI of varying degrees (see Nedvetsky and collegues[241] for a review). Of these mutations, 80% cause autosomal recessive NDI. AQP2 gene mutations producing full-length proteins could have at least two consequences that would result in a loss of principal cell VP-sensitivity: (1) an AQP2 channel that is inserted into the plasma membrane after VP stimulation but no longer functions as a water channel, and (2) AQP2 that is still functional, but is not targeted to the apical plasma membrane after VP stimulation.

All recessive mutations associated with NDI reported to date lead to AQP2 misfolding, retention in the ER, and subsequent degradation. The rarer autosomal dominant form of NDI is caused by mutations that affect intracellular sorting of the channel, in which AQP2 is either retained in the Golgi apparatus or sorted to late endosomes, to lysosomes, or to the basolateral plasma membrane.[16] Thus far, all dominant mutations have been found to be located within the C terminus of AQP2. It is likely that dominant NDI mutations effect AQP2 phosphorylation to some degree and therefore its trafficking.[36,85] In the majority of cases, mutant AQP2 monomers form heterotetramers with wild-type AQP2 and prevent wild-type AQP2 from reaching the cell surface.[16]

Although specific treatments for non–X-linked NDI are not available, numerous therapeutic guidelines have been recommended. These include consumption of a low-salt diet, combined with hydrochlorothiazide and amiloride treatment. In addition, inhibitors of cyclooxygenases, such as indomethacin, are often prescribed, despite their association with gastrointestinal disturbances. Recent studies in mice suggest that phosphodiesterase inhibitors might be useful drugs for the treatment of autosomal dominant NDI.[324]

Acquired Water Balance Disorders

Acquired forms of NDI are much more common than hereditary forms and arise as a consequence of drug treatments, electrolyte disturbances, and urinary tract obstruction (Table 11-1). In most manifestations of acquired NDI, dysregulation of AQP2, either in terms of protein abundance or in AQP2 membrane targeting, plays a fundamental role in the development of polyuria.[16,17,182] Quantitative data on AQP2 levels in various experimental conditions resulting in acquired NDI are summarized in Figure 11-11.

The downregulation of AQP2 observed in acquired NDI is most likely the primary cause of the NDI, rather than being a secondary event (e.g., as a consequence of the increased urine production or reduction in interstitial osmolality). For example, in models of hypokalemic and lithium-induced NDI, the changes in AQP2 expression in kidney cortex are identical to those seen in the inner medulla,[181,215,216] which indicates that interstitial tonicity is not a major factor. Moreover, washout of the medullary osmotic gradient for 1 or 5 days using the loop diuretic furosemide has no effect on AQP2 expression.[214,216] This also indicates that high urine flow in itself is not responsible for the reduced AQP2 expression in experimental NDI.

In the following sections, we focus on new developments in the field, and readers are directed to Chapters 15 and 44 or to the extensive review articles by Frokiaer and colleagues,[93] Kwon and colleagues,[182] and Nielsen and colleagues[248] for further information.

Lithium Treatment

Lithium is commonly used to treat bipolar affective mood disorders,[351] and 20% to 30% of lithium-treated patients develop VP-resistant polyuria (NDI). However, approximately 75% of filtered lithium is reabsorbed before the distal convoluted tubule by mechanisms similar to those for sodium reabsorption. Dietary sodium restriction results in lithium reabsorption in the connecting tubule and collecting duct. This process is probably mediated by the amiloride-sensitive epithelial sodium channel ENaC,[177] which provides a molecular rationale for treating patients with lithium-induced NDI with thiazide and amiloride.[60,167]

A major cause of lithium-induced NDI is decreased AQP2 and AQP3 expression and membrane localization in the kidney collecting duct (Figure 11-12A, B).[55,181,215,244,245] The mechanism responsible for the reduction in AQP2 expression was originally thought to involve interference with the normal intracellular signaling of VP, with impaired activity of adenylate cyclase and reduced cAMP production.[182] This hypothesis is consistent with the presence of a cAMP-responsive element in the AQP2 gene promoter and with the finding that mice with inherently low cAMP levels have decreased AQP2 expression.[94] However, recent in vitro studies using collecting duct–derived mpkCCD(c14) cells demonstrated that lithium-induced decreases in AQP2 gene transcription can occur without changes in intracellular cAMP levels.[195] In addition, both PGE_2, cyclooxygenase-2 (COX-2), and non–VP mediated effects, as well as collecting duct cellular reorganization resulting from lithium treatment (an increase in the number of intercalated cells and a corresponding decrease in principal cells), may be involved in the onset of polyuria (Figure 11-12C through E).[55,182]

A proteomic study identified numerous proteins involved in cell death, apoptosis, cell proliferation, and morphology that are affected by lithium treatment.[244] In the same study, members of several signaling pathways were found to be activated by lithium, including PKB/Akt kinase and the MAPKs.

TABLE 11-1 Physiologic and Pathophysiologic Conditions Associated with Altered Abundance and/or Targeting of Aquaporin-2 (AQP2)

REDUCED ABUNDANCE OF AQP2	INCREASED ABUNDANCE OF AQP2
With Polyuria	**With Expansion of Extracellular Fluid Volume**
Genetic defects	Vasopressin infusion (syndrome of inappropriate antidiuretic hormone secretion)
Brattleboro rats (central DI)	Congestive heart failure
DI +/+ severe mice (low cAMP)	Hepatic cirrhosis (carbon tetrachloride-induced noncompensated)?
Aquaporin-2 mutants (human)	Pregnancy
Vasopressin type 2 receptor variants (human)*	**With Polyuria**
Acquired NDI (rat models)	Osmotic diuresis (diabetes mellitus model in rat)
Lithium treatment	
Hypokalemia	
Hypercalcemia	
Postobstructive NDI	
Bilateral	
Unilateral	
Low-protein diet (urinary concentrating defect without polyuria)	
Water loading (compulsive water drinking)	
Chronic renal failure (5/6 nephrectomy model)	
Ischemia-induced acute renal failure (polyuric phase in rat model)	
Cisplatin-induced acute renal failure	
Calcium channel blocker (nifedipine) treatment (rat model)	
Age-induced NDI	
With Altered Urinary Concentration without Polyuria	
Nephrotic syndrome models (rat models)	
Puromycin aminonucleoside induced	
Doxorubicin (Adriamycin) induced	
Hepatic cirrhosis (common bile duct ligation, compensated)	
Ischemia-induced acute renal failure (oliguric phase in rat model)	

*Reduced vasopressin type 2 receptor density has a profound effect on aquaporin-2 targeting and expression.

cAMP, Cyclic adenosine monophosphate; *DI,* diabetes insipidus; *NDI,* nephrogenic diabetes insipidus.

Lithium treatment also increased the intracellular accumulation of β-catenin in association with increased levels of phosphorylated glycogen synthase kinase type 3β.[182]

Electrolyte Abnormalities: Hypokalemia and Hypercalcemia

Hypokalemia and hypercalcemia are both associated with significant VP-resistant polyuria and reduced expression of AQP2.[216,309] The polyuria associated with these conditions is less severe than that seen in lithium-induced NDI, and consistent with this, a less marked reduction in AQP2 is observed. In a mouse model of Gitelman's syndrome with hypokalemia, the mice also display drastically reduced AQP2 levels and severe polyuria.[236] In hypercalcemia, in addition to downregulation of AQP2, the expression levels of AQP1 and AQP3 protein are reduced, as are levels of the VP-regulated Na-K-2Cl cotransporter type 2 (NKCC2) and regulation of the Kir 1.1 (ROMK) potassium channel.[373] These changes are likely to result in reduced sodium reabsorption in the thick ascending limb, which would affect the countercurrent multiplication system and, subsequently, urine concentration. Hypercalciuria, commonly seen during hypercalcemia, could also result in impaired AQP2 expression and apical targeting. This has been proposed to result from altered signal transduction pathways via the actions of the extracellular calcium-sensing receptor (CaSR),[44,278,279] but further studies are required to fully understand the underlying pathogenic mechanisms.

Ureteral Obstruction

Chronic urinary outflow obstruction with impaired ability of the kidney to concentrate the urine is a common condition among elderly men. Moreover, acute obstruction in all age groups results in a similar concentrating defect. Several experimental animal models have been developed to study the physiology of this disorder and are discussed in detail in Chapter 37. Experimental bilateral ureteral obstruction (BUO) for 24 hours results in dramatically reduced expression of AQP1 through AQP4, key sodium transporters/channels and urea transporters.[91,92,189] The polyuria remains for up to 2 weeks following release of the obstruction, concurrent with a continued downregulation of AQP2 and AQP3 expression.

BUO is associated with COX-2 induction and cellular infiltration of the renal medulla.[49,258] Indeed, treatment with a specific COX-2 inhibitor prevents downregulation of AQP2 and reduces postobstructive polyuria.[258] The renin-angiotensin system is also involved in the pathophysiologic changes of BUO,[150] and blockade of the angiotensin II type 1 receptor prevents downregulation of the Na+/PO4 3− exchanger NaPi-2, NKCC2, and AQP2 following BUO release.[151]

In contrast to BUO, unilateral ureteral obstruction does not result in changes in the absolute excretion of water and solute, because the nonobstructed kidney is able to compensate.[91,189] Despite this, there is still a pronounced reduction in AQP1 through AQP4 and in phosphorylated AQP2 levels in the obstructed kidney, which suggests that local factors such as prostaglandins may play a role.[258,259] Inflammatory cytokines have also been implicated in ureteral obstruction,[390] and α-melanocyte–stimulating hormone (α-MSH) treatment of rats with ureteral obstruction or release of obstruction

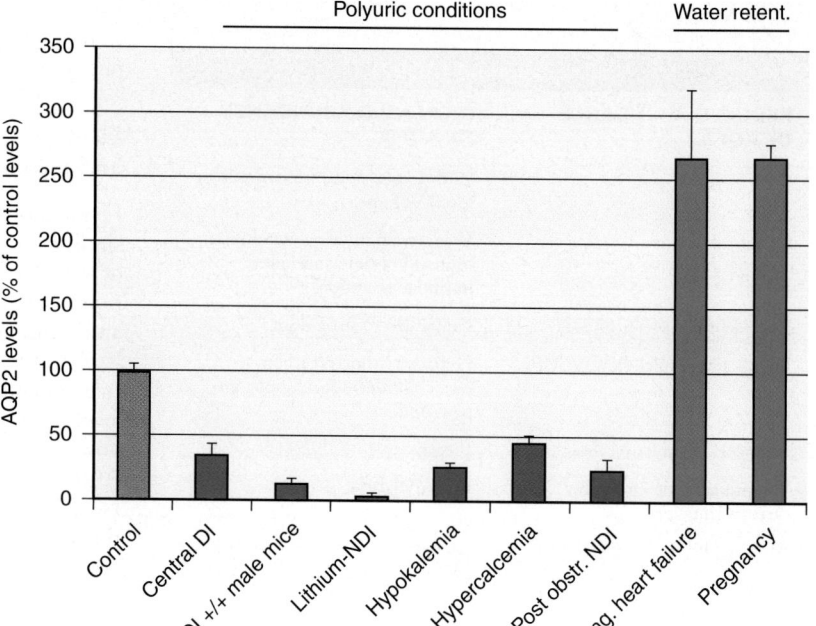

FIGURE 11-11 Quantitation of aquaporin-2 (AQP2) levels in various conditions of fluid and electrolyte imbalance, including acquired nephrogenic diabetes insipidus. *DI*, Diabetes insipidus.

markedly prevents the downregulation of several key aquaporins and sodium transporters.[190] Administration of α-MSH, an antiinflammatory cytokine that inhibits both neutrophil and nitric oxide pathways, attenuates the reduced expression of AQP1, AQP2, and AQP3 and impaired urinary concentration ability.[179]

Acute and Chronic Renal Failure

Acute renal failure (ARF) and chronic renal failure (CRF) associated with polyuria and impaired urinary concentration are discussed in detail in later chapters. In both conditions, a broad range of glomerulotubular abnormalities contribute to the overall renal dysfunction. In experimentally induced ARF, expression of both AQP2 and AQP3 in the collecting duct, as well as AQP1 expression in the proximal tubule, are significantly decreased.[87,179] Hemorrhagic shock–induced ARF also results in decreased expression of AQP2 and AQP3.[103] In CRF, V_2R mRNA in the inner medulla is virtually absent, which provides an explanation for the significant defects in collecting duct water reabsorption in response to VP in this condition. Consistent with these observations, the reduced levels of AQP2 and AQP3 resulting from experimentally induced CRF were not attenuated following long-term dDAVP infusion.[180]

Cirrhosis and Congestive Heart Failure

Hepatic cirrhosis and congestive heart failure (CHF) are just two conditions resulting in extracellular fluid expansion and hyponatremia due to sodium and water retention. Although no changes in AQP2 levels were observed in a model of compensatory heart failure, in experimentally induced CHF, a marked increase in AQP2 expression and apical targeting was observed.[252,382] Administration of the V_2R antagonist OPC 31260 in the latter case significantly increased diuresis, decreased urine osmolality, and reduced the observed increase in AQP2 levels. These observations support the view

that dysregulation of AQP2 may play a significant role in the development of water retention and hyponatremia in CHF, possibly due to a baroreceptor-mediated increase in circulating VP levels. It remains to be established why VP escape does not take place in rats with CHF.[78]

It should be emphasized that other mechanisms, including changes in NaCl transporter expression, are also likely to play a major role in the development of sodium and water retention in CHF.[326] Treatment of CHF rats with losartan normalized the levels of NKCC2 and AQP2, resulting in normalization of daily sodium excretion, and partially improved renal function.

In experimental models of severe hepatic cirrhosis, AQP2 protein abundance is greatly increased,[96,145] whereas in models of compensated biliary hepatic cirrhosis AQP2 expression is reduced.[155] Thus it appears that, unlike in CHF, the changes in AQP2 levels vary considerably between different experimental models of hepatic cirrhosis. Although an explanation for these differences remains to be determined, it is well known that the dysregulation of body water balance depends on the severity of cirrhosis.[182] Thus, the downregulation of AQP2 observed in milder forms of cirrhosis may represent a compensatory mechanism to prevent development of water retention. In contrast, the increased levels of VP seen in severe noncompensated cirrhosis with ascites may induce an inappropriate upregulation of AQP2 that would in turn participate in the development of water retention.

Vasopressin Escape and the Syndrome of Inappropriate Antidiuretic Hormone Secretion

Hyponatremia (serum Na < 135 mmol/L) is most commonly caused by the inappropriate secretion of VP relative to serum osmolality (syndrome of inappropriate antidiuretic hormone secretion, or SIADH). Vascular, infectious, or neoplastic abnormalities in the lung or central nervous system commonly result in SIADH. In a rat model

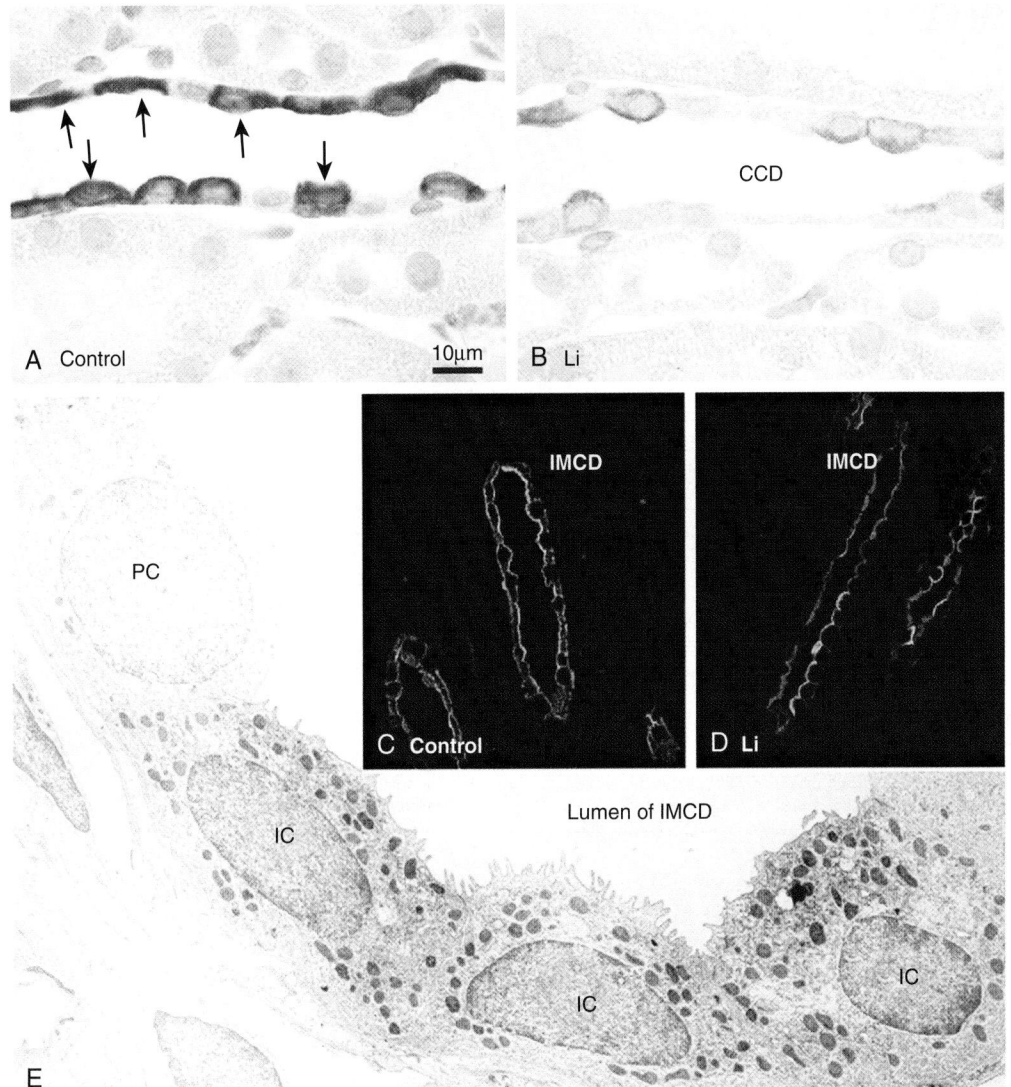

FIGURE 11-12 Effect of lithium treatment on aquaporin-2 (AQP2) expression and cellular composition of rat medullary collecting ducts. AQP2 levels in control rat kidneys (**A,** *arrows*) are considerably greater than those after treatment with lithium for 2 weeks (**B**), when levels of AQP2 fall dramatically, and some principal cells (PCs) show little or no immunoperoxidase staining. In parallel, the number of PCs is reduced in the collecting ducts of lithium-treated rats, and the number of intercalated cells (ICs) is increased. **C** shows the inner medulla of a kidney from a control rat stained for AQP2 (*green,* a PC marker; note as well the significant amount of basolateral AQP2 staining, as also seen in Figure 11-8) and vacuolar proton pumping adenosine triphosphatase (V-ATPase) (*red,* an IC marker). ICs are normally rare in this part of the kidney. However, after treatment with lithium many more ICs (*red*) appear, and the number of AQP2-stained (*green*) PCs is correspondingly lower (**D**). This striking increase in the number of ICs can also be seen with electron microscopy as in **E,** in which several adjacent ICs can be detected, in contrast to the very scattered population of ICs seen in the inner medullary collecting duct of control rats (not shown).

of SIADH, AQP2 levels were increased, which provides a molecular mechanism for the associated water retention and hyponatremia.[96]

VP escape is a physiologic process that limits the degree of hyponatremia after prolonged VP exposure and is characterized by a sudden increase in urine volume with a decrease in urine osmolality independent of high circulating VP levels. In a rat model of VP escape, the onset of escape coincided temporally with a marked decrease in AQP2 levels, but no changes in renal expression of AQP1, AQP3, and AQP4.[76,78] These results suggest that escape from VP-induced antidiuresis is attributable, at least in part, to a selective VP-independent decrease in AQP2 expression.

Recent proteomic studies have attempted to provide a rationale for the altered AQP2 abundance.[131] Thus, dysregulation

of aquaporin expression, targeting, and function is a major factor associated with a variety of water balance disorders in common kidney, liver, and heart diseases. In some cases, AQP2 dysfunction is a primary cause of the osmoregulatory defect, whereas in others it may be a secondary consequence that contributes to the pathophysiology. Further analysis of aquaporin expression and function in these and other conditions is underway in many laboratories.

Given our growing understanding of ion channel and transporter expression in the kidney, as well as new insights into renal development, signal transduction, and epithelial polarity, significant new advances to further illuminate the molecular nature of normal water balance and its disorders can be expected to emerge with increasing regularity over the next few years.

Acknowledgments

The work of Dennis Brown was supported by National Institutes of Health grant P01-DK38452. The work of Robert Fenton was supported by a grant from the Danish National Research Foundation (Danmarks Grundforskningsfonden) and the Danish Medical Research Council, Novo Nordisk Foundation, and the Lundbeck Foundation. The authors thank their many excellent colleagues for their invaluable contributions to the authors' research endeavors over the past several years.

References

1. Agre P, Bonhivers M, Borgnia MJ. The aquaporins, blueprints for cellular plumbing systems. *J Biol Chem.* 1998;273:14659-14662.
2. Agre P, Kozono D. Aquaporin water channels: molecular mechanisms for human diseases. *FEBS Lett.* 2003;555:72-78.
3. Agre P, Preston GM, Smith BL, et al. Aquaporin CHIP: the archetypal molecular water channel. *Am J Physiol.* 1993;265:F463-F476.
4. Allan VJ, Schroer TA. Membrane motors. *Curr Opin Cell Biol.* 1999;11:476-482.
5. Ausiello DA, Holtzman EJ, Gronich JH, et al. Cell signalling. In: Seldin DW, Giebisch G, eds. *The kidney: physiology and pathophysiology.* New York: Raven Press; 1992:pp 645-692.
6. Bailly C, Imbert-Teboul M, Chabardes D, et al. The distal nephron of rat kidney: a target site for glucagon. *Proc Natl Acad Sci U S A.* 1980;77:3422-3424.
7. Barak LS, Oakley RH, Laporte SA, et al. Constitutive arrestin-mediated desensitization of a human vasopressin receptor mutant associated with nephrogenic diabetes insipidus. *Proc Natl Acad Sci U S A.* 2001;98:93-98.
8. Barile M, Pisitkun T, Yu MJ, et al. Large scale protein identification in intracellular aquaporin-2 vesicles from renal inner medullary collecting duct. *Mol Cell Proteomics.* 2005;4:1095-1106.
9. Baturina GS, Isaeva LE, Khodus GR, et al. [Water permeability of the OMCD and IMCD cells' basolateral membrane under the conditions of dehydration and dDAVP action]. *Ross Fiziol Zh Im I M Sechenova.* 2004;90:865-873.
10. Bernier V, Lagace M, Lonergan M, et al. Functional rescue of the constitutively internalized V2 vasopressin receptor mutant R137H by the pharmacological chaperone action of SR49059. *Mol Endocrinol.* 2004;18:2074-2084.
11. Bi GQ, Morris RL, Liao G, et al. Kinesin- and myosin-driven steps of vesicle recruitment for Ca^{2+}-regulated exocytosis. *J Cell Biol.* 1997;138:999-1008.
12. Bichet DG. Nephrogenic diabetes insipidus. *Adv Chronic Kidney Dis.* 2006;13:96-104.
13. Bichet DG. Vasopressin receptor mutations in nephrogenic diabetes insipidus. *Semin Nephrol.* 2008;28:245-251.
14. Birnbaumer M, Seibold A, Gilbert S. Molecular cloning of the receptor for human antidiuretic hormone. *Nature.* 1992;357:333-335.
15. Blank ME, Ehmke H. Aquaporin-1 and HCO$_3^-$-Cl$^-$ transporter-mediated transport of CO$_2$ across the human erythrocyte membrane. *J Physiol.* 2003;550:419-429.
16. Boone M, Deen PM. Congenital nephrogenic diabetes insipidus: what can we learn from mouse models? *Exp Physiol.* 2009;94:186-190.
17. Boone M, Deen PM. Physiology and pathophysiology of the vasopressin-regulated renal water reabsorption. *Pflugers Arch.* 2008;456:1005-1024.
18. Borgnia M, Nielsen S, Engel A, et al. Cellular and molecular biology of the aquaporin water channels. *Annu Rev Biochem.* 1999;68:425-458.
19. Bouley R, Breton S, Sun T, et al. Nitric oxide and atrial natriuretic factor stimulate cGMP-dependent membrane insertion of aquaporin 2 in renal epithelial cells. *J Clin Invest.* 2000;106:1115-1126.
20. Bouley R, Hasler U, Lu HA, et al. Bypassing vasopressin receptor signaling pathways in nephrogenic diabetes insipidus. *Semin Nephrol.* 2008;28:266-278.
21. Bouley R, Hawthorn G, Russo LM, et al. Aquaporin 2 (AQP2) and vasopressin type 2 receptor (V2R) endocytosis in kidney epithelial cells: AQP2 is located in "endocytosis-resistant" membrane domains after vasopressin treatment. *Biol Cell.* 2006;98:215-232.
22. Bouley R, Lin HY, Raychowdhury MK, et al. Downregulation of the vasopressin type 2 receptor after vasopressin-induced internalization: involvement of a lysosomal degradation pathway. *Am J Physiol Cell Physiol.* 2005;288:C1390-C1401.
23. Bouley R, Lu HAJ, Nunes P, et al. Vasopressin-like effect of calcitonin on urinary concentration and aquaporin 2 trafficking. *J Am Soc Nephrol.* 2010;22:59-72.
24. Bouley R, Pastor-Soler N, Cohen O, et al. Stimulation of AQP2 membrane insertion in renal epithelial cells in vitro and in vivo by the cGMP phosphodiesterase inhibitor sildenafil citrate (Viagra). *Am J Physiol Renal Physiol.* 2005;288:F1103-F1112.
25. Bouley R, Sun TX, Chenard M, et al. Functional role of the NPxxY motif in internalization of the type 2 vasopressin receptor in LLC-PK$_1$ cells. *Am J Physiol Cell Physiol.* 2003;285:C750-C762.
26. Bowen-Pidgeon D, Innamorati G, Sadeghi HM, et al. Arrestin effects on internalization of vasopressin receptors. *Mol Pharmacol.* 2001;59:1395-1401.
27. Breton S, Brown D. Cold-induced microtubule disruption and relocalization of membrane proteins in kidney epithelial cells. *J Am Soc Nephrol.* 1998;9:155-166.
28. Breyer RM, Bagdassarian CK, Myers SA, et al. Prostanoid receptors: subtypes and signaling. *Annu Rev Pharmacol Toxicol.* 2001;41:661-690.
29. Brown CL, Maier KC, Stauber T, et al. Kinesin-2 is a motor for late endosomes and lysosomes. *Traffic.* 2005;6:1114-1124.
30. Brown D. Imaging protein trafficking. *Nephron Exp Nephrol.* 2006;103:e55-61.
31. Brown D. The ins and outs of aquaporin-2 trafficking. *Am J Physiol Renal Physiol.* 2003;284:F893-F901.
32. Brown D, Breton S, Ausiello DA, et al. Sensing, signaling and sorting events in kidney epithelial cell physiology. *Traffic.* 2009;10:275-284.
33. Brown D, Cunningham C, Hartwig J, et al. Association of AQP2 with actin in transfected LLC-PK$_1$ cells and rat papilla. *J Am Soc Nephrol.* 1996;7:1265a.
34. Brown D, Grosso A, DeSousa RC. Correlation between water flow and intramembrane particle aggregates in toad epidermis. *Am J Physiol.* 1983;245:C334-C342.
35. Brown D, Grosso A, DeSousa RC. Membrane architecture and water transport in epithelial cell membranes. In: Aloia RC, ed. *Advances in membrane fluidity, membrane transport and information storage.* vol. 4. New York: Alan Liss; 1990:pp 103-132.
36. Brown D, Hasler U, Nunes P, et al. Phosphorylation events and the modulation of aquaporin 2 cell surface expression. *Curr Opin Nephrol Hypertens.* 2008;17:491-498.
37. Brown D, Orci L. Vasopressin stimulates formation of coated pits in rat kidney collecting ducts. *Nature.* 1983;302:253-255.
38. Brown D, Shields GI, Valtin H, et al. Lack of intramembranous particle clusters in collecting ducts of mice with nephrogenic diabetes insipidus. *Am J Physiol.* 1985;249:F582-F589.
39. Brown D, Verbavatz JM, Valenti G, et al. Localization of the CHIP28 water channel in reabsorptive segments of the rat male reproductive tract. *Eur J Cell Biol.* 1993;61:264-273.
40. Brown D, Weyer P, Orci L. Vasopressin stimulates endocytosis in kidney collecting duct epithelial cells. *Eur J Cell Biol.* 1988;46:336-340.
41. Brunskill N, Bastani B, Hayes C, et al. Localization and polar distribution of several G-protein subunits along nephron segments. *Kidney Int.* 1991;40:997-1006.
42. Bryant NJ, Govers R, James DE. Regulated transport of the glucose transporter GLUT4. *Nat Rev Mol Cell Biol.* 2002;3:267-277.
43. Bustamante M, Hasler U, Kotova O, et al. Insulin potentiates AVP-induced AQP2 expression in cultured renal collecting duct principal cells. *Am J Physiol Renal Physiol.* 2005;288:F334-F344.
44. Bustamante M, Hasler U, Leroy V, et al. Calcium-sensing receptor attenuates AVP-induced aquaporin-2 expression via a calmodulin-dependent mechanism. *J Am Soc Nephrol.* 2008;19:109-116.
45. Butlen D, Morel F. Glucagon receptors along the nephron: [125I]glucagon binding in rat tubules. *Pflugers Arch.* 1985;404:348-353.
46. Canfield MC, Tamarappoo BK, Moses AM, et al. Identification and characterization of aquaporin-2 water channel mutations causing nephrogenic diabetes insipidus with partial vasopressin response. *Hum Mol Genet.* 1997;6:1865-1871.
47. Charest PG, Bouvier M. Palmitoylation of the V2 vasopressin receptor carboxyl tail enhances beta-arrestin recruitment leading to efficient receptor endocytosis and ERK1/2 activation. *J Biol Chem.* 2003;278:41541-41551.
48. Cheng A, van Hoek AN, Yeager M, et al. Three-dimensional organization of a human water channel. *Nature.* 1997;387:627-630.
49. Cheng X, Zhang H, Lee HL, et al. Cyclooxygenase-2 inhibitor preserves medullary aquaporin-2 expression and prevents polyuria after ureteral obstruction. *J Urol.* 2004;172:2387-2390.
50. Chevalier J, Bourguet J, Hugon JS. Membrane-associated particles: distribution in frog urinary bladder epithelium at rest and after oxytocin treatment. *Cell Tissue Res.* 1974;152:129-140.
51. Chou CL, Christensen BM, Frische S, et al. Non-muscle myosin II and myosin light chain kinase are downstream targets for vasopressin signaling in the renal collecting duct. *J Biol Chem.* 2004;279:49026-49035.
52. Chou CL, Ma T, Yang B, et al. Fourfold reduction of water permeability in inner medullary collecting duct of aquaporin-4 knockout mice. *Am J Physiol.* 1998;274:C549-C554.

53. Chou CL, Yip KP, Michea L, et al. Regulation of aquaporin-2 trafficking by vasopressin in the renal collecting duct. Roles of ryanodine-sensitive Ca²⁺ stores and calmodulin. *J Biol Chem.* 2000;275:36839-36846.
54. Christensen BM, Marples D, Jensen UB, et al. Acute effects of vasopressin V2-receptor antagonist on kidney AQP2 expression and subcellular distribution. *Am J Physiol.* 1998;275:F285-F297.
55. Christensen BM, Marples D, Wang W, et al. Decreased fraction of principal cells in parallel with increased fraction of intercalated cells in rats with lithium-induced NDI. *J Am Soc Nephrol.* 2002;13:270A.
56. Christensen BM, Wang W, Frokiaer J, et al. Axial heterogeneity in basolateral AQP2 localization in rat kidney: effect of vasopressin V2-receptor activation and deactivation. *Am J Physiol Renal Physiol.* 2003;284(4):F701-F717:Epub November 26, 2002.
57. Christensen JH, Siggaard C, Rittig S. Autosomal dominant familial neurohypophyseal diabetes insipidus. *APMIS Suppl.* 2003(109):92-95.
58. Coleman RA, Wu DC, Liu J, et al. Expression of aquaporins in the renal connecting tubule. *Am J Physiol Renal Physiol.* 2000;279:F874-F883.
59. Cooper GJ, Zhou Y, Bouyer P, et al. Transport of volatile solutes through AQP1. *J Physiol.* 2002;542:17-29.
60. Crawford JD, Kennedy GC. Chlorothiazide in diabetes insipidus. *Nature.* 1959;183:891-892.
61. de Groot BL, Heymann JB, Engel A, et al. The fold of human aquaporin 1. *J Mol Biol.* 2000;300:987-994.
62. de Mattia F, Savelkoul PJ, Kamsteeg EJ, et al. Lack of arginine vasopressin-induced phosphorylation of aquaporin-2 mutant AQP2-R254L explains dominant nephrogenic diabetes insipidus. *J Am Soc Nephrol.* 2005;16:2872-2880.
63. de Rouffignac C, Elalouf JM. Effects of calcitonin on the renal concentrating mechanism. *Am J Physiol.* 1983;245:F506-F511.
64. de Seigneux S, Nielsen J, Olesen ET, et al. Long-term aldosterone treatment induces decreased apical but increased basolateral expression of AQP2 in CCD of rat kidney. *Am J Physiol Renal Physiol.* 2007;293:F87-F99.
65. Deen PM, Nielsen S, Bindels RJ, et al. Apical and basolateral expression of aquaporin-1 in transfected MDCK and LLC-PK cells and functional evaluation of their transcellular osmotic water permeabilities. *Pflugers Arch.* 1997;433:780-787.
66. Deen PM, Rijss JP, Mulders SM, et al. Aquaporin-2 transfection of Madin-Darby canine kidney cells reconstitutes vasopressin-regulated transcellular osmotic water transport. *J Am Soc Nephrol.* 1997;8:1493-1501.
67. Deen PM, Verdijk MA, Knoers NV, et al. Requirement of human renal water channel aquaporin-2 for vasopressin-dependent concentration of urine. *Science.* 1994;264:92-95.
68. Deen PMT, Brown D. Trafficking of native and mutant mammalian MIP proteins. In: Hohmann S, Nielsen S, Agre P, eds. *Aquaporins*, vol 51 *of Current topics in membranes.* New York: Academic Press; 2001:pp 235-276.
69. Denker BM, Smith BL, Kuhajda FP, et al. Identification, purification and partial characterization of a novel Mr 28,000 integral membrane protein from erythrocytes and renal tubules. *J Biol Chem.* 1988;263:15634-15642.
70. DeSousa RC, Grosso A, Rufener C. Blockade of the hydroosmotic effect of vasopressin by cytochalasin B. *Experientia.* 1974;30:175-177.
71. DeWire SM, Ahn S, Lefkowitz RJ, et al. Beta-arrestins and cell signaling. *Annu Rev Physiol.* 2007;69:483-510.
72. DiGiovanni SR, Nielsen S, Christensen EI, et al. Regulation of collecting duct water channel expression by vasopressin in Brattleboro rat. *Proc Natl Acad Sci U S A.* 1994;91:8984-8988.
73. Ding GH, Franki N, Condeelis J, et al. Vasopressin depolymerizes F-actin in toad bladder epithelial cells. *Am J Physiol.* 1991;260:C9-C16.
74. Dousa TP. Cyclic-3′, 5′-nucleotide phosphodiesterases in the cyclic adenosine monophosphate (cAMP)–mediated actions of vasopressin. *Semin Nephrol.* 1994;14:333-340.
75. Dousa TP, Barnes LD. Effects of colchicine and vinblastine on the cellular action of vasopressin in mammalian kidney. A possible role of microtubules. *J Clin Invest.* 1974;54:252-262.
76. Ecelbarger CA, Chou CL, Lee AJ, et al. Escape from vasopressin-induced antidiuresis: role of vasopressin resistance of the collecting duct. *Am J Physiol.* 1998;274:F1161-F1166.
77. Ecelbarger CA, Chou CL, Lolait SJ, et al. Evidence for dual signaling pathways for V2 vasopressin receptor in rat inner medullary collecting duct. *Am J Physiol.* 1996;270:F623-F633.
78. Ecelbarger CA, Nielsen S, Olson BR, et al. Role of renal aquaporins in escape from vasopressin-induced antidiuresis in rat. *J Clin Invest.* 1997;99:1852-1863.
79. Edwards RM, Spielman WS. Adenosine A1 receptor–mediated inhibition of vasopressin action in inner medullary collecting duct. *Am J Physiol.* 1994;266:F791-F796.
80. Endeward V, Musa-Aziz R, Cooper GJ, et al. Evidence that aquaporin 1 is a major pathway for CO₂ transport across the human erythrocyte membrane. *FASEB J.* 2006;20:1974-1981.
81. Faerch M, Christensen JH, Rittig S, et al. Diverse vasopressin V2 receptor functionality underlying partial congenital nephrogenic diabetes insipidus. *Am J Physiol Renal Physiol.* 2009;297(6):F1518-F1525:Epub October 7, 2009.
82. Fang X, Yang B, Matthay MA, et al. Evidence against aquaporin-1–dependent CO₂ permeability in lung and kidney. *J Physiol.* 2002;542:63-69.
83. Fejes-Toth G, Naray-Fejes-Toth A. Isolated principal and intercalated cells: hormone responsiveness and Na⁺-K⁺-ATPase activity. *Am J Physiol.* 1989;256:F742-F750.
84. Fenton RA, Brond L, Nielsen S, et al. Cellular and subcellular distribution of the type-2 vasopressin receptor in the kidney. *Am J Physiol Renal Physiol.* 2007;293:F748-F760.
85. Fenton RA, Moeller HB. Recent discoveries in vasopressin-regulated aquaporin-2 trafficking. *Prog Brain Res.* 2008;170:571-579.
86. Fenton RA, Moeller HB, Hoffert JD, et al. Acute regulation of aquaporin-2 phosphorylation at Ser-264 by vasopressin. *Proc Natl Acad Sci U S A.* 2008;105:3134-3139.
87. Fernandez-Llama P, Andrews P, Turner R, et al. Decreased abundance of collecting duct aquaporins in post-ischemic renal failure in rats. *J Am Soc Nephrol.* 1999;10:1658-1668.
88. Franki N, Ding G, Gao Y, et al. Effect of cytochalasin D on the actin cytoskeleton of the toad bladder epithelial cell. *Am J Physiol.* 1992;263:C995-C1000.
89. Franki N, Macaluso F, Schubert W, et al. Water channel-carrying vesicles in the rat IMCD contain cellubrevin. *Am J Physiol.* 1995;269:C797-C801.
90. Frigeri A, Gropper MA, Umenishi F, et al. Localization of MIWC and GLIP water channel homologs in neuromuscular, epithelial and glandular tissues. *J Cell Sci.* 1995;108:2993-3002.
91. Frokiaer J, Christensen BM, Marples D, et al. Downregulation of aquaporin-2 parallels changes in renal water excretion in unilateral ureteral obstruction. *Am J Physiol.* 1997;273:F213-F223.
92. Frokiaer J, Marples D, Knepper MA, et al. Bilateral ureteral obstruction downregulates expression of vasopressin-sensitive AQP-2 water channel in rat kidney. *Am J Physiol.* 1996;270:F657-F668.
93. Frokiaer J, Marples D, Knepper MA, et al. Pathophysiology of aquaporin-2 in water balance disorders. *Am J Med Sci.* 1998;316:291-299.
94. Frokiaer J, Marples D, Valtin H, et al. Low aquaporin-2 levels in polyuric DI +/+ severe mice with constitutively high cAMP-phosphodiesterase activity. *Am J Physiol.* 1999;276:F179-F190.
95. Frokiaer J, Nielsen S, Knepper MA. Molecular physiology of renal aquaporins and sodium transporters: exciting approaches to understand regulation of renal water handling. *J Am Soc Nephrol.* 2005;16:2827-2829.
96. Fujita N, Ishikawa SE, Sasaki S, et al. Role of water channel AQP-CD in water retention in SIADH and cirrhotic rats. *Am J Physiol.* 1995;269:F926-F931.
97. Fujiwara TM, Bichet DG. Molecular biology of hereditary diabetes insipidus. *J Am Soc Nephrol.* 2005;16:2836-2846.
98. Furuno M, Uchida S, Marumo F, et al. Repressive regulation of the aquaporin-2 gene. *Am J Physiol.* 1996;271:F854-F860.
99. Fushimi K, Sasaki S, Marumo F. Phosphorylation of serine 256 is required for cAMP-dependent regulatory exocytosis of the aquaporin-2 water channel. *J Biol Chem.* 1997;272:14800-14804.
100. Fushimi K, Uchida S, Hara Y, et al. Cloning and expression of apical membrane water channel of rat kidney collecting tubule. *Nature.* 1993;361:549-552.
101. Futter CE, Gibson A, Allchin EH, et al. In polarized MDCK cells basolateral vesicles arise from clathrin-gamma-adaptin–coated domains on endosomal tubules. *J Cell Biol.* 1998;141:611-623.
102. Garofeanu CG, Weir M, Rosas-Arellano MP, et al. Causes of reversible nephrogenic diabetes insipidus: a systematic review. *Am J Kidney Dis.* 2005;45:626-637.
103. Gong H, Wang W, Kwon TH, et al. Reduced renal expression of AQP2, p-AQP2 and AQP3 in haemorrhagic shock–induced acute renal failure. *Nephrol Dial Transplant.* 2003;18:2551-2559.
104. Gottlieb TA, Ivanov IE, Adesnik M, et al. Actin microfilaments play a critical role in endocytosis at the apical but not the basolateral surface of polarized epithelial cells. *J Cell Biol.* 1993;120:695-710.
105. Gouraud S, Laera A, Calamita G, et al. Functional involvement of VAMP/synaptobrevin-2 in cAMP-stimulated aquaporin 2 translocation in renal collecting duct cells. *J Cell Sci.* 2002;115:3667-3674.
106. Granier S, Terrillon S, Pascal R, et al. A cyclic peptide mimicking the third intracellular loop of the V2 vasopressin receptor inhibits signaling through its interaction with receptor dimer and G protein. *J Biol Chem.* 2004;279:50904-50914.
107. Grantham JJ, Burg MB. Effect of vasopressin and cyclic AMP on permeability of isolated collecting tubules. *Am J Physiol.* 1966;211:255-259.
108. Griffiths G, Pfeiffer S, Simons K, et al. Exit of newly synthesized membrane proteins from the trans cisterna of the Golgi complex to the plasma membrane. *J Cell Biol.* 1985;101:949-964.

109. Gustafson CE, Katsura T, McKee M, et al. Recycling of aquaporin 2 occurs through a temperature- and bafilomycin-sensitive trans-Golgi–associated compartment in LLC-PK1 cells. *Am J Physiol Renal Physiol.* 1999;278:F317-F326.

110. Han Z, Wax MB, Patil RV. Regulation of aquaporin-4 water channels by phorbol ester-dependent protein phosphorylation. *J Biol Chem.* 1998;273:6001-6004.

111. Hara-Chikuma M, Verkman AS. Physiological roles of glycerol-transporting aquaporins: the aquaglyceroporins. *Cell Mol Life Sci.* 2006;63:1386-1392.

112. Harmanci MC, Stern P, Kachadorian WA, et al. Vasopressin and collecting duct intramembranous particle clusters: a dose-response relationship. *Am J Physiol.* 1980;239:F560-F564.

113. Hasler U, Jeon US, Kim JA, et al. Tonicity-responsive enhancer binding protein is an essential regulator of aquaporin-2 expression in renal collecting duct principal cells. *J Am Soc Nephrol.* 2006;17:1521-1531.

114. Hasler U, Leroy V, Martin PY, et al. Aquaporin-2 abundance in the renal collecting duct: new insights from cultured cell models. *Am J Physiol Renal Physiol.* 2009;297:F10-F18.

115. Hasler U, Nunes P, Bouley R, et al. Acute hypertonicity alters aquaporin-2 trafficking and induces a MAPK-dependent accumulation at the plasma membrane of renal epithelial cells. *J Biol Chem.* 2008;283:26643-26661.

116. Hawk CT, Kudo LH, Rouch AJ, et al. Inhibition by epinephrine of AVP- and cAMP-stimulated Na^+ and water transport in Dahl rat CCD. *Am J Physiol.* 1993;265:F449-F460.

117. Hayashi M, Arima H, Goto M, et al. Vasopressin gene transcription increases in response to decreases in plasma volume, but not to increases in plasma osmolality, in chronically dehydrated rats. *Am J Physiol Endocrinol Metab.* 2006;290:E213-E217.

118. Hayashi M, Sasaki S, Tsuganezawa H, et al. Expression and distribution of aquaporin of collecting duct are regulated by vasopressin V2 receptor in rat kidney. *J Clin Invest.* 1994;94:1778-1783.

119. Hayashi M, Sasaki S, Tsuganezawa H, et al. Role of vasopressin V2 receptor in acute regulation of aquaporin-2. *Kidney Blood Press Res.* 1996;19:32-37.

120. Hays RM, Condeelis J, Gao Y, et al. The effect of vasopressin on the cytoskeleton of the epithelial cell. *Pediatr Nephrol.* 1993;7:672-679.

121. Hazama A, Kozono D, Guggino WB, et al. Ion permeation of AQP6 water channel protein. Single channel recordings after Hg^{2+} activation. *J Biol Chem.* 2002;277:29224-29230.

122. Henn V, Edemir B, Stefan E, et al. Identification of a novel A-kinase anchoring protein 18 isoform and evidence for its role in the vasopressin-induced aquaporin-2 shuttle in renal principal cells. *J Biol Chem.* 2004;279:26654-26665.

123. Hermosilla R, Oueslati M, Donalies U, et al. Disease-causing V(2) vasopressin receptors are retained in different compartments of the early secretory pathway. *Traffic.* 2004;5:993-1005.

124. Hinshaw JE. Dynamin and its role in membrane fission. *Annu Rev Cell Dev Biol.* 2000;16:483-519.

125. Hoffert JD, Chou CL, Fenton RA, et al. Calmodulin is required for vasopressin-stimulated increase in cyclic AMP production in inner medullary collecting duct. *J Biol Chem.* 2005;280:13624-13630.

126. Hoffert JD, Fenton RA, Moeller HB, et al. Vasopressin-stimulated increase in phosphorylation at Ser269 potentiates plasma membrane retention of aquaporin-2. *J Biol Chem.* 2008;283:24617-24627.

127. Hoffert JD, Nielsen J, Yu MJ, et al. Dynamics of aquaporin-2 serine-261 phosphorylation in response to short-term vasopressin treatment in collecting duct. *Am J Physiol Renal Physiol.* 2007;292:F691-F700.

128. Hoffert JD, Pisitkun T, Wang G, et al. Quantitative phosphoproteomics of vasopressin-sensitive renal cells: regulation of aquaporin-2 phosphorylation at two sites. *Proc Natl Acad Sci U S A.* 2006;103:7159-7164.

129. Holm LM, Jahn TP, Moller AL, et al. NH3 and NH4+ permeability in aquaporin-expressing *Xenopus* oocytes. *Pflugers Arch.* 2005;450:415-428.

130. Holm LM, Klaerke DA, Zeuthen T. Aquaporin 6 is permeable to glycerol and urea. *Pflugers Arch.* 2004;448:181-186.

131. Hoorn EJ, Hoffert JD, Knepper MA. Combined proteomics and pathways analysis of collecting duct reveals a protein regulatory network activated in vasopressin escape. *J Am Soc Nephrol.* 2005;16:2852-2863.

132. Hoorn EJ, Pisitkun T, Yu MJ, et al. Proteomic approaches for the study of cell signaling in the renal collecting duct. *Contrib Nephrol.* 2008;160:172-185.

133. Huang Y, Tracy R, Walsberg GE, et al. Absence of aquaporin-4 water channels from kidneys of the desert rodent *Dipodomys merriami merriami. Am J Physiol Renal Physiol.* 2001;280:F794-F802.

134. Hyman T, Shmuel M, Altschuler Y. Actin is required for endocytosis at the apical surface of Madin-Darby canine kidney cells where ARF6 and clathrin regulate the actin cytoskeleton. *Mol Biol Cell.* 2006;17:427-437.

135. Ikeda M, Beitz E, Kozono D, et al. Characterization of aquaporin-6 as a nitrate channel in mammalian cells. Requirement of pore-lining residue threonine 63. *J Biol Chem.* 2002;277:39873-39879.

136. Innamorati G, Le Gouill C, Balamotis M, et al. The long and the short cycle. Alternative intracellular routes for trafficking of G-protein–coupled receptors. *J Biol Chem.* 2001;276:13096-13103.

137. Innamorati G, Sadeghi H, Birnbaumer M. Phosphorylation and recycling kinetics of G protein–coupled receptors. *J Recept Signal Transduct Res.* 1999;19:315-326.

138. Innamorati G, Sadeghi H, Eberle AN, et al. Phosphorylation of the V2 vasopressin receptor. *J Biol Chem.* 1997;272:2486-2492.

139. Innamorati G, Sadeghi HM, Tran NT, et al. A serine cluster prevents recycling of the V2 vasopressin receptor. *Proc Natl Acad Sci U S A.* 1998;95:2222-2226.

140. Inoue T, Nielsen S, Mandon B, et al. SNAP-23 in rat kidney: colocalization with aquaporin-2 in collecting duct vesicles. *Am J Physiol.* 1998;275:F752-F760.

141. Ishibashi K, Kuwahara M, Gu Y, et al. Cloning and functional expression of a new aquaporin (AQP9) abundantly expressed in the peripheral leukocytes permeable to water and urea but not to glycerol. *Biochem Biophys Res Commun.* 1998;244:268-274.

142. Ishibashi K, Kuwahara M, Sasaki S. Molecular biology of aquaporins. *Rev Physiol Biochem Pharmacol.* 2000;141:1-32.

143. Ishibashi K, Sasaki S, Fushimi K, et al. Molecular cloning and expression of a member of the aquaporin family with permeability to glycerol and urea in addition to water expressed at the basolateral membrane of kidney collecting duct cells. *Proc Natl Acad Sci U S A.* 1994;91:6269-6273:[see comments].

144. Ishibashi K, Sasaki S, Fushimi K, et al. Immunolocalization and effect of dehydration on AQP3, a basolateral water channel of kidney collecting ducts. *Am J Physiol.* 1997;272:F235-F241.

145. Ishikawa S, Saito T, Fujita N, et al. Expression and subcellular localization of water channel aquaporin-2 in conscious rats. *Kidney Int.* 1997;61(Suppl):S6-S9.

146. Ishikawa SE, Schrier RW. Pathophysiological roles of arginine vasopressin and aquaporin-2 in impaired water excretion. *Clin Endocrinol (Oxf).* 2003;58:1-17.

147. Iyengar R, Lepper KG, Mailman DS. Involvement of microtubules and microfilaments in the action of vasopressin in canine renal medulla. *J Supramol Struct.* 1976;5:521(373)-530(382).

148. Izumi Y, Nakayama Y, Memetimin H, et al. Regulation of V2R transcription by hypertonicity and V1aR-V2R signal interaction. *Am J Physiol Renal Physiol.* 2008;295:F1170-F1176.

149. Jean-Alphonse F, Perkovska S, Frantz MC, et al. Biased agonist pharmacochaperones of the AVP V2 receptor may treat congenital nephrogenic diabetes insipidus. *J Am Soc Nephrol.* 2009;20:2190-2203.

150. Jensen AM, Bae EH, Fenton RA, et al. Angiotensin II regulates V2 receptor and pAQP2 during ureteral obstruction. *Am J Physiol Renal Physiol.* 2009;296:F127-F134.

151. Jensen AM, Li C, Praetorius HA, et al. Angiotensin II mediates downregulation of aquaporin water channels and key renal sodium transporters in response to urinary tract obstruction. *Am J Physiol Renal Physiol.* 2006;291:F1021-F1032.

152. Jeon US, Joo KW, Na KY, et al. Oxytocin induces apical and basolateral redistribution of aquaporin-2 in rat kidney. *Nephron.* 2003;93:E36-E45.

153. Jo I, Harris HW, Amendt-Raduege AM, et al. Rat kidney papilla contains abundant synaptobrevin protein that participates in the fusion of antidiuretic hormone–regulated water channel–containing endosomes in vitro. *Proc Natl Acad Sci U S A.* 1995;92:1876-1880.

154. Johansson I, Karlsson M, Shukla VK, et al. Water transport activity of the plasma membrane aquaporin PM28A is regulated by phosphorylation. *Plant Cell.* 1998;10:451-459.

155. Jonassen TE, Nielsen S, Christensen S, et al. Decreased vasopressin-mediated renal water reabsorption in rats with compensated liver cirrhosis. *Am J Physiol.* 1998;275:F216-F225.

156. Jones RVH, DeWardener HF. Urine concentration after fluid deprivation or pitressin tannate in oil. *Br Med J.* 1956;1:271-274.

157. Kachadorian WA, Wade JB, Uiterwyk CC, et al. Membrane structural and functional responses to vasopressin in toad bladder. *J Membrane Biol.* 1977;30:381-401.

158. Kalenga K, Persu A, Goffin E, et al. Intrafamilial phenotype variability in nephrogenic diabetes insipidus. *Am J Kidney Dis.* 2002;39:737-743.

159. Kamsteeg EJ, Bichet DG, Konings IB, et al. Reversed polarized delivery of an aquaporin-2 mutant causes dominant nephrogenic diabetes insipidus. *J Cell Biol.* 2003;163:1099-1109.

160. Kamsteeg EJ, Duffield AS, Konings IB, et al. MAL decreases the internalization of the aquaporin-2 water channel. *Proc Natl Acad Sci U S A.* 2007;104:16696-16701.

161. Kamsteeg EJ, Heijnen I, van Os CH, et al. The subcellular localization of an aquaporin-2 tetramer depends on the stoichiometry of phosphorylated and nonphosphorylated monomers. *J Cell Biol.* 2000;151:919-930.

162. Kamsteeg EJ, Wormhoudt TA, Rijss JP, et al. An impaired routing of wild-type aquaporin-2 after tetramerization with an aquaporin-2 mutant explains dominant nephrogenic diabetes insipidus. *EMBO J.* 1999;18:2394-2400.
163. Katsura T, Ausiello DA, Brown D. Direct demonstration of aquaporin-2 water channel recycling in stably transfected LLC-PK1 epithelial cells. *Am J Physiol.* 1996;270:F548-F553.
164. Katsura T, Gustafson CE, Ausiello DA, et al. Protein kinase A phosphorylation is involved in regulated exocytosis of aquaporin-2 in transfected LLC-PK1 cells. *Am J Physiol.* 1997;272:F817-F822.
165. Kaufmann JE, Iezzi M, Vischer UM. Desmopressin (DDAVP) induces NO production in human endothelial cells via V2 receptor- and cAMP-mediated signaling. *J Thromb Haemost.* 2003;1:821-828.
166. Kaufmann JE, Oksche A, Wollheim CB, et al. Vasopressin-induced von Willebrand factor secretion from endothelial cells involves V2 receptors and cAMP. *J Clin Invest.* 2000;106:107-116.
167. Kennedy GC, Crawford JD. Treatment of diabetes insipidus with hydrochlorothiazide. *Lancet.* 1959;1:866-867.
168. Kersting U, Dantzler DW, Oberleithner H, et al. Evidence for an acid pH in rat renal inner medulla: paired measurements with liquid ion-exchange microelectrodes on collecting ducts and vasa recta. *Pflugers Arch.* 1994;426:354-356.
169. Khanna A. Acquired nephrogenic diabetes insipidus. *Semin Nephrol.* 2006;26:244-248.
170. Kim JK, Summer SN, Wood WM, et al. Arginine vasopressin secretion with mutants of wild-type and Brattleboro rats AVP gene. *J Am Soc Nephrol.* 1997;8:1863-1869.
171. Kirk K. Binding and internalization of a fluorescent vasopressin analogue by collecting duct cells. *Am J Physiol.* 1988;255:C622-C632.
172. Klussmann E, Maric K, Wiesner B, et al. Protein kinase A anchoring proteins are required for vasopressin-mediated translocation of aquaporin-2 into cell membranes of renal principal cells. *J Biol Chem.* 1999;274:4934-4938.
173. Klussmann E, Tamma G, Lorenz D, et al. An inhibitory role of Rho in the vasopressin-mediated translocation of aquaporin-2 into cell membranes of renal principal cells. *J Biol Chem.* 2001;276:20451-20457.
174. Knepper MA, Nielsen S. Kinetic model of water and urea permeability regulation by vasopressin in collecting duct. *Am J Physiol.* 1993;265:F214-F224.
175. Knepper MA, Nielsen S, Peter Agre. 2003 Nobel Prize winner in chemistry. *J Am Soc Nephrol.* 2004;15:1093-1095.
176. Knoers NV, Deen PM. Molecular and cellular defects in nephrogenic diabetes insipidus. *Pediatr Nephrol.* 2001;16:1146-1152.
177. Kortenoeven ML, Li Y, Shaw S, et al. Amiloride blocks lithium entry through the sodium channel thereby attenuating the resultant nephrogenic diabetes insipidus. *Kidney Int.* 2009;76:44-53.
178. Kuwahara M, Fushimi K, Terada Y, et al. cAMP-dependent phosphorylation stimulates water permeability of aquaporin-collecting duct water channel protein expressed in *Xenopus* oocytes. *J Biol Chem.* 1995;270:10384-10387.
179. Kwon TH, Frokiaer J, Fernandez-Llama P, et al. Reduced abundance of aquaporins in rats with ischemia-induced acute renal failure: prevention by alpha-MSH. *Am J Physiol.* 1999;277:F413-F427.
180. Kwon TH, Frokiaer J, Knepper MA, et al. Reduced AQP1, -2, and -3 levels in kidneys of rats with CRF induced by surgical reduction in renal mass. *Am J Physiol.* 1998;275:F724-F741.
181. Kwon TH, Laursen UH, Marples D, et al. Altered expression of renal AQPs and Na(+) transporters in rats with lithium-induced NDI. *Am J Physiol Renal Physiol.* 2000;279:F552-F564.
182. Kwon TH, Nielsen J, Moller HB, et al. Aquaporins in the kidney. *Handb Exp Pharmacol.* 2009:95-132.
183. Lande MB, Jo I, Zeidel ML, et al. Phosphorylation of aquaporin-2 does not alter the membrane water permeability of rat papillary water channel-containing vesicles. *J Biol Chem.* 1996;271:5552-5557.
184. Landry DW, Oliver JA. The pathogenesis of vasodilatory shock. *N Engl J Med.* 2001;345:588-595.
185. Lankford SP, Chou CL, Terada Y, et al. Regulation of collecting duct water permeability independent of cAMP-mediated AVP response. *Am J Physiol.* 1991;261:F554-F566.
186. Lencer WI, Brown D, Ausiello DA, et al. Endocytosis of water channels in rat kidney: cell specificity and correlation with in vivo antidiuresis. *Am J Physiol.* 1990;259:C920-C932.
187. Lencer WI, Verkman AS, Arnaout MA, et al. Endocytic vesicles from renal papilla which retrieve the vasopressin-sensitive water channel do not contain a functional H+ ATPase. *J Cell Biol.* 1990;111:379-389.
188. Leung SM, Rojas R, Maples C, et al. Modulation of endocytic traffic in polarized Madin-Darby canine kidney cells by the small GTPase RhoA. *Mol Biol Cell.* 1999;10:4369-4384.
189. Li C, Wang W, Kwon TH, et al. Downregulation of AQP1, -2, and -3 after ureteral obstruction is associated with a long-term urine-concentrating defect. *Am J Physiol Renal Physiol.* 2001;281:F163-F171.
190. Li C, Wang W, Kwon TH, et al. Alpha-MSH treatment prevents downregulation of AQP1, AQP2 and AQP3 expression in rats with bilateral ureteral obstruction. *J Am Soc Nephrol.* 2002;13:272A.
191. Li C, Wang W, Summer SN, et al. Molecular mechanisms of antidiuretic effect of oxytocin. *J Am Soc Nephrol.* 2008;19:225-232.
192. Li JH, Chou CL, Li B, et al. A selective EP4 PGE2 receptor agonist alleviates disease in a new mouse model of X-linked nephrogenic diabetes insipidus. *J Clin Invest.* 2009;119(10):3115-3126.
193. Li L, Schafer JA. Dopamine inhibits vasopressin-dependent cAMP production in the rat cortical collecting duct. *Am J Physiol.* 1998;275:F62-F67.
193a. Li W, Zhang Y, Bouley R, et al. Simvastatin enhances aquaporin 2 surface expression and urinary concentration in vasopressin deficient Brattleboro rats through modulation of Rho GTPase. *Am J Physiol Renal Physiol.* Epub ahead of print, April 20, 2011.
194. Li Y, Konings IB, Zhao J, et al. Renal expression of exchange protein directly activated by cAMP (Epac) 1 and 2. *Am J Physiol Renal Physiol.* 2008;295:F525-F533.
195. Li Y, Shaw S, Kamsteeg EJ, et al. Development of lithium-induced nephrogenic diabetes insipidus is dissociated from adenylyl cyclase activity. *J Am Soc Nephrol.* 2006;17:1063-1072.
196. Liard JF. L-NAME antagonizes vasopressin V2-induced vasodilatation in dogs. *Am J Physiol.* 1994;266:H99-H106.
197. Liebenhoff U, Rosenthal W. Identification of Rab3-, Rab5a- and synaptobrevin II–like proteins in a preparation of rat kidney vesicles containing the vasopressin-regulated water channel. *FEBS Lett.* 1995;365:209-213.
198. Lolait SJ, O'Carroll AM, Konig M, et al. Cloning and characterization of a vasopressin V2 receptor and possible link to nephrogenic diabetes insipidus. *Nature.* 1992;357:336-339.
199. Lorenz D, Krylov A, Hahm D, et al. Cyclic AMP is sufficient for triggering the exocytic recruitment of aquaporin-2 in renal epithelial cells. *EMBO Rep.* 2003;4:88-93.
200. Lu H, Sun TX, Bouley R, et al. Inhibition of endocytosis causes phosphorylation (S256)-independent plasma membrane accumulation of AQP2. *Am J Physiol Renal Physiol.* 2004;286:F233-F243.
201. Lu HA, Sun TX, Matsuzaki T, et al. Heat shock protein 70 interacts with aquaporin-2 and regulates its trafficking. *J Biol Chem.* 2007;282:28721-28732.
202. Lu HJ, Matsuzaki T, Bouley R, et al. The phosphorylation state of serine 256 is dominant over that of serine 261 in the regulation of AQP2 trafficking in renal epithelial cells. *Am J Physiol Renal Physiol.* 2008;295:F290-F294.
203. Lueck A, Brown D, Kwiatkowski DJ. The actin-binding proteins adseverin and gelsolin are both highly expressed but differentially localized in kidney and intestine. *J Cell Sci.* 1998;111:3633-3643.
204. Lutz W, Sanders M, Salisbury J, et al. Internalization of vasopressin analogs in kidney and smooth muscle cells: evidence for receptor-mediated endocytosis in cells with V2 or V1 receptors. *Proc Natl Acad Sci U S A.* 1990;87:6507-6511.
205. Ma T, Song Y, Yang B, et al. Nephrogenic diabetes insipidus in mice lacking aquaporin-3 water channels. *Proc Natl Acad Sci U S A.* 2000;97:4386-4391.
206. Ma T, Yang B, Gillespie A, et al. Generation and phenotype of a transgenic knockout mouse lacking the mercurial-insensitive water channel aquaporin-4. *J Clin Invest.* 1997;100:957-962.
207. Macia E, Ehrlich M, Massol R, et al. Dynasore, a cell-permeable inhibitor of dynamin. *Dev Cell.* 2006;10:839-850.
208. Maeda Y, Terada Y, Nonoguchi H, et al. Hormone and autacoid regulation of cAMP production in rat IMCD subsegments. *Am J Physiol.* 1992;263:F319-F327.
209. Makaryus AN, McFarlane SI. Diabetes insipidus: diagnosis and treatment of a complex disease. *Cleve Clin J Med.* 2006;73:65-71.
210. Mandon B, Chou CL, Nielsen S, et al. Syntaxin-4 is localized to the apical plasma membrane of rat renal collecting duct cells: possible role in aquaporin-2 trafficking. *J Clin Invest.* 1996;98:906-913.
211. Maric K, Oksche A, Rosenthal W. Aquaporin-2 expression in primary cultured rat inner medullary collecting duct cells. *Am J Physiol.* 1998;275:F796-F801.
212. Marks J, Debnam ES, Dashwood MR, et al. Detection of glucagon receptor mRNA in the rat proximal tubule: potential role for glucagon in the control of renal glucose transport. *Clin Sci (Lond).* 2003;104:253-258.
213. Marples D, Barber B, Taylor A. Effect of a dynein inhibitor on vasopressin action in toad urinary bladder. *J Physiol.* 1996;490(pt 3):767-774.
214. Marples D, Christensen BM, Frokiaer J, et al. Dehydration reverses vasopressin antagonist-induced diuresis and aquaporin-2 downregulation in rats. *Am J Physiol.* 1998;275:F400-F409.
215. Marples D, Christensen S, Christensen EI, et al. Lithium-induced downregulation of aquaporin-2 water channel expression in rat kidney medulla. *J Clin Invest.* 1995;95:1838-1845.

216. Marples D, Frokiaer J, Dorup J, et al. Hypokalemia-induced downregulation of aquaporin-2 water channel expression in rat kidney medulla and cortex. *J Clin Invest.* 1996;97:1960-1968.
217. Marples D, Knepper MA, Christensen EI, et al. Redistribution of aquaporin-2 water channels induced by vasopressin in rat kidney inner medullary collecting duct. *Am J Physiol.* 1995;269:C655-C664.
218. Marples D, Schroer TA, Ahrens N, et al. Dynein and dynactin colocalize with AQP2 water channels in intracellular vesicles from kidney collecting duct. *Am J Physiol.* 1998;274:F384-F394.
219. Marples D, Smith J, Nielsen S. Myosin-I is associated with AQP-2 water channel bearing vesicles in rat kidney and may be involved in the antidiuretic response to vasopressin. *J Am Soc Nephrol.* 1997;8:62a.
220. Marr N, Bichet DG, Lonergan M, et al. Heteroligomerization of an aquaporin-2 mutant with wild-type aquaporin-2 and their misrouting to late endosomes/lysosomes explains dominant nephrogenic diabetes insipidus. *Hum Mol Genet.* 2002;11:779-789.
221. Martin NP, Lefkowitz RJ, Shenoy SK. Regulation of V2 vasopressin receptor degradation by agonist-promoted ubiquitination. *J Biol Chem.* 2003;278:45954-45959.
222. Matlin KS, Simons K. Reduced temperature prevents transfer of a membrane glycoprotein to the cell surface but does not prevent terminal glycosylation. *Cell.* 1983;34:233-243.
223. McDill BW, Li SZ, Kovach PA, et al. Congenital progressive hydronephrosis (cph) is caused by an S256L mutation in aquaporin-2 that affects its phosphorylation and apical membrane accumulation. *Proc Natl Acad Sci U S A.* 2006;103:6952-6957.
224. Mechaly I, Laurent F, Portet K, et al. Vasopressin V2 (SR121463A) and V1a (SR49059) receptor antagonists both inhibit desmopressin vasorelaxing activity. *Eur J Pharmacol.* 1999;383:287-290.
225. Missner A, Kugler P, Saparov SM, et al. Carbon dioxide transport through membranes. *J Biol Chem.* 2008;283:25340-25347.
226. Mistry AC, Mallick R, Klein JD, et al. Syntaxin specificity of aquaporins in the inner medullary collecting duct. *Am J Physiol Renal Physiol.* 2009;297:F292-F300.
227. Mitra AK, Ren G, Reddy VS, et al. The architecture of a water-selective pore in the lipid bilayer visualized by electron crystallography in vitreous ice. *Novartis Found Symp.* 2002;245:33-46:discussion 46-50, 165–168.
228. Moeller HB, Fenton RA, Zeuthen T, et al. Vasopressin-dependent short-term regulation of aquaporin 4 expressed in *Xenopus* oocytes. *Neuroscience.* 2009;164:1674-1684.
229. Moeller HB, Knepper MA, Fenton RA. Serine 269 phosphorylated aquaporin-2 is targeted to the apical membrane of collecting duct principal cells. *Kidney Int.* 2009;75:295-303.
230. Moeller HB, MacAulay N, Knepper MA, et al. Role of multiple phosphorylation sites in the COOH-terminal tail of aquaporin-2 for water transport: evidence against channel gating. *Am J Physiol Renal Physiol.* 2009;296:F649-F657.
231. Moeller HB, Praetorius J, Rutzler MR, et al. Phosphorylation of aquaporin-2 regulates its endocytosis and protein-protein interactions. *Proc Natl Acad Sci U S A.* 2010;107(1):424-429:Epub December 4, 2009.
232. Moller C, Fotiadis D, Suda K, et al. Determining molecular forces that stabilize human aquaporin-1. *J Struct Biol.* 2003;142:369-378.
233. Morel A, O'Carroll AM, Brownstein MJ, et al. Molecular cloning and expression of a rat V1a arginine vasopressin receptor. *Nature.* 1992;356:523-526.
234. Morel F, Imbert-Teboul M, Chabardes D. Distribution of hormone-dependent adenylate cyclase in the nephron and its physiological significance. *Ann Rev Physiol.* 1981;43:569-581.
235. Morello JP, Salahpour A, Laperriere A, et al. Pharmacological chaperones rescue cell-surface expression and function of misfolded V2 vasopressin receptor mutants. *J Clin Invest.* 2000;105:887-895.
236. Morris RG, Hoorn EJ, Knepper MA. Hypokalemia in a mouse model of Gitelman's syndrome. *Am J Physiol Renal Physiol.* 2006;290:F1416-F1420.
237. Mulders SM, Bichet DG, Rijss JP, et al. An aquaporin-2 water channel mutant which causes autosomal dominant nephrogenic diabetes insipidus is retained in the Golgi complex. *J Clin Invest.* 1998;102:57-66.
238. Murata K, Mitsuoka K, Hirai T, et al. Structural determinants of water permeation through aquaporin-1. *Nature.* 2000;407:599-605.
239. Muto S, Tabei K, Asano Y, et al. Dopaminergic inhibition of the action of vasopressin on the cortical collecting tubule. *Eur J Pharmacol.* 1985;114:393-397.
240. Nedvetsky PI, Stefan E, Frische S, et al. A Role of myosin Vb and Rab11-FIP2 in the aquaporin-2 shuttle. *Traffic.* 2007;8:110-123.
241. Nedvetsky PI, Tamma G, Beulshausen S, et al. Regulation of aquaporin-2 trafficking. *Handb Exp Pharmacol.* 2009;(190):133-157.
242. Nejsum LN, Zelenina M, Aperia A, et al. Bidirectional regulation of AQP2 trafficking and recycling: involvement of AQP2-S256 phosphorylation. *Am J Physiol Renal Physiol.* 2005;288:F930-F938.
243. Nickols HH, Shah VN, Chazin WJ, et al. Calmodulin interacts with the V2 vasopressin receptor: elimination of binding to the C terminus also eliminates arginine vasopressin-stimulated elevation of intracellular calcium. *J Biol Chem.* 2004;279:46969-46980.
244. Nielsen J, Hoffert JD, Knepper MA, et al. Proteomic analysis of lithium-induced nephrogenic diabetes insipidus: mechanisms for aquaporin 2 down-regulation and cellular proliferation. *Proc Natl Acad Sci U S A.* 2008;105:3634-3639.
245. Nielsen J, Kwon TH, Praetorius J, et al. Aldosterone increases urine production and decreases apical AQP2 expression in rats with diabetes insipidus. *Am J Physiol Renal Physiol.* 2006;290:F438-F449.
246. Nielsen S, Chou CL, Marples D, et al. Vasopressin increases water permeability of kidney collecting duct by inducing translocation of aquaporin-CD water channels to plasma membrane. *Proc Natl Acad Sci USA.* 1995;92:1013-1017.
247. Nielsen S, DiGiovanni SR, Christensen EI, et al. Cellular and subcellular immunolocalization of vasopressin-regulated water channel in rat kidney. *Proc Natl Acad Sci U S A.* 1993;90:11663-11667.
248. Nielsen S, Frokiaer J, Marples D, et al. Aquaporins in the kidney: from molecules to medicine. *Physiol Rev.* 2002;82:205-244.
249. Nielsen S, Marples D, Birn H, et al. Expression of VAMP-2-like protein in kidney collecting duct intracellular vesicles. Colocalization with Aquaporin-2 water channels. *J Clin Invest.* 1995;96:1834-1844.
250. Nielsen S, Smith BL, Christensen EI, et al. Distribution of the aquaporin CHIP in secretory and resorptive epithelia and capillary endothelia. *Proc Natl Acad Sci U S A.* 1993;90:7275-7279.
251. Nielsen S, Smith BL, Christensen EI, et al. CHIP28 water channels are localized in constitutively water-permeable segments of the nephron. *J Cell Biol.* 1993;120:371-383.
252. Nielsen S, Terris J, Andersen D, et al. Congestive heart failure in rats is associated with increased expression and targeting of aquaporin-2 water channel in collecting duct. *Proc Natl Acad Sci U S A.* 1997;94:5450-5455.
253. Noda Y, Horikawa S, Furukawa T, et al. Aquaporin-2 trafficking is regulated by PDZ-domain containing protein SPA-1. *FEBS Lett.* 2004;568:139-145.
254. Noda Y, Horikawa S, Kanda E, et al. Reciprocal interaction with G-actin and tropomyosin is essential for aquaporin-2 trafficking. *J Cell Biol.* 2008;182:587-601.
255. Noda Y, Horikawa S, Katayama Y, et al. Identification of a multiprotein "motor" complex binding to water channel aquaporin-2. *Biochem Biophys Res Commun.* 2005;330:1041-1047.
256. Noda Y, Horikawa S, Katayama Y, et al. Water channel aquaporin-2 directly binds to actin. *Biochem Biophys Res Commun.* 2004;322:740-745.
257. Nonoguchi H, Owada A, Kobayashi N, et al. Immunohistochemical localization of V2 vasopressin receptor along the nephron and functional role of luminal V2 receptor in terminal inner medullary collecting ducts. *J Clin Invest.* 1995;96:1768-1778.
258. Norregaard R, Jensen BL, Li C, et al. COX-2 inhibition prevents downregulation of key renal water and sodium transport proteins in response to bilateral ureteral obstruction. *Am J Physiol Renal Physiol.* 2005;289:F322-F333.
259. Norregaard R, Jensen BL, Topcu SO, et al. Cyclooxygenase type 2 is increased in obstructed rat and human ureter and contributes to pelvic pressure increase after obstruction. *Kidney Int.* 2006;70:872-881.
260. Nunes P, Hasler U, McKee M, et al. A fluorimetry-based ssYFP secretion assay to monitor vasopressin-induced exocytosis in LLC-PK1 cells expressing aquaporin-2. *Am J Physiol Cell Physiol.* 2008;295:C1476-C1487.
261. Oakley RH, Laporte SA, Holt JA, et al. Association of beta-arrestin with G protein–coupled receptors during clathrin-mediated endocytosis dictates the profile of receptor resensitization. *J Biol Chem.* 1999;274:32248-32257.
262. Oakley RH, Laporte SA, Holt JA, et al. Differential affinities of visual arrestin, beta arrestin1, and beta arrestin2 for G protein–coupled receptors delineate two major classes of receptors. *J Biol Chem.* 2000;275:17201-17210.
263. Oishi R, Nonoguchi H, Tomita K, et al. Endothelin-1 inhibits AVP-stimulated osmotic water permeability in rat inner medullary collecting duct. *Am J Physiol.* 1991;261:F951-F956.
264. Orci L, Humbert F, Brown D, et al. Membrane ultrastructure in urinary tubules. *Int Rev Cytol.* 1981;73:183-242.
265. Oueslati M, Hermosilla R, Schonenberger E, et al. Rescue of a nephrogenic diabetes insipidus-causing vasopressin V2 receptor mutant by cell-penetrating peptides. *J Biol Chem.* 2007;282:20676-20685.
266. Perry SJ, Lefkowitz RJ. Arresting developments in heptahelical receptor signaling and regulation. *Trends Cell Biol.* 2002;12:130-138.
267. Pfeiffer R, Kirsch J, Fahrenholz F. Agonist and antagonist-dependent internalization of the human vasopressin V2 receptor. *Exp Cell Res.* 1998;244:327-339.
268. Pfister KK, Fisher EM, Gibbons IR, et al. Cytoplasmic dynein nomenclature. *J Cell Biol.* 2005;171:411-413.

269. Phillips ME, Taylor A. Effect of nocodazole on the water permeability response to vasopressin in rabbit collecting tubules perfused in vitro. *J Physiol (Lond)*. 1989;411:529-544.
270. Pisitkun T, Hoffert JD, Yu MJ, et al. Tandem mass spectrometry in physiology. *Physiology (Bethesda)*. 2007;22:390-400.
271. Pisitkun T, Shen RF, Knepper MA. Identification and proteomic profiling of exosomes in human urine. *Proc Natl Acad Sci U S A*. 2004;101:13368-13373.
272. Preston GM, Agre P. Isolation of the cDNA for erythrocyte integral membrane protein of 28 kilodaltons: member of an ancient channel family. *Proc Natl Acad Sci U S A*. 1991;88:11110-11114.
273. Preston GM, Carroll TP, Guggino WB, et al. Appearance of water channels in *Xenopus* oocytes expressing red cell CHIP28 protein. *Science*. 1992;256:385-387.
274. Procino G, Barbieri C, Carmosino M, et al. Lovastatin-induced cholesterol depletion affects both apical sorting and endocytosis of aquaporin 2 in renal cells. *Am J Physiol Renal Physiol*. 2010;298(2):F266-F278:Epub November 18, 2009.
275. Procino G, Barbieri C, Tamma G, et al. AQP2 exocytosis in the renal collecting duct—involvement of SNARE isoforms and the regulatory role of Munc18b. *J Cell Sci*. 2008;121:2097-2106.
276. Procino G, Caces DB, Valenti G, et al. Adipocytes support cAMP-dependent translocation of aquaporin-2 from intracellular sites distinct from the insulin-responsive GLUT4 storage compartment. *Am J Physiol Renal Physiol*. 2006;290:F985-F994.
277. Procino G, Carmosino M, Marin O, et al. Ser-256 phosphorylation dynamics of aquaporin 2 during maturation from the ER to the vesicular compartment in renal cells. *FASEB J*. 2003;17:1886-1888.
278. Procino G, Carmosino M, Tamma G, et al. Extracellular calcium antagonizes forskolin-induced aquaporin 2 trafficking in collecting duct cells. *Kidney Int*. 2004;66:2245-2255.
279. Procino G, Mastrofrancesco L, Mira A, et al. Aquaporin 2 and apical calcium-sensing receptor: new players in polyuric disorders associated with hypercalciuria. *Semin Nephrol*. 2008;28:297-305.
280. Promeneur D, Kwon TH, Yasui M, et al. Regulation of AQP6 mRNA and protein expression in rats in response to altered acid-base or water balance. *Am J Physiol Renal Physiol*. 2000;279:F1014-F1026.
281. Rabaud NE, Song L, Wang Y, et al. Aquaporin 6 binds calmodulin in a calcium-dependent manner. *Biochem Biophys Res Commun*. 2009;383:54-57.
282. Ravichandran V, Chawla A, Roche PA. Identification of a novel syntaxin- and synaptobrevin/VAMP-binding protein, SNAP-23, expressed in non-neuronal tissues. *J Biol Chem*. 1996;271:13300-13303.
283. Reilein AR, Rogers SL, Tuma MC, et al. Regulation of molecular motor proteins. *Int Rev Cytol*. 2001;204:179-238.
284. Ren XR, Reiter E, Ahn S, et al. Different G protein–coupled receptor kinases govern G protein and beta-arrestin–mediated signaling of V2 vasopressin receptor. *Proc Natl Acad Sci U S A*. 2005;102:1448-1453.
285. Ridley AJ. Rho proteins: linking signaling with membrane trafficking. *Traffic*. 2001;2:303-310.
286. Ripoche P, Goossens D, Devuyst O, et al. Role of RhAG and AQP1 in NH3 and CO_2 gas transport in red cell ghosts: a stopped-flow analysis. *Transfus Clin Biol*. 2006;13:117-122.
287. Robben JH, Deen PM. Pharmacological chaperones in nephrogenic diabetes insipidus: possibilities for clinical application. *BioDrugs*. 2007;21:157-166.
288. Robben JH, Knoers NV, Deen PM. Cell biological aspects of the vasopressin type-2 receptor and aquaporin 2 water channel in nephrogenic diabetes insipidus. *Am J Physiol Renal Physiol*. 2006;291:F257-F270.
289. Robben JH, Knoers NV, Deen PM. Regulation of the vasopressin V2 receptor by vasopressin in polarized renal collecting duct cells. *Mol Biol Cell*. 2004;15:5693-5699.
290. Robben JH, Kortenoeven ML, Sze M, et al. Intracellular activation of vasopressin V2 receptor mutants in nephrogenic diabetes insipidus by nonpeptide agonists. *Proc Natl Acad Sci U S A*. 2009;106:12195-12200.
291. Robben JH, Sze M, Knoers NV, et al. Functional rescue of vasopressin V2 receptor mutants in MDCK cells by pharmacochaperones: relevance to therapy of nephrogenic diabetes insipidus. *Am J Physiol Renal Physiol*. 2007;292:F253-F260.
292. Robben JH, Sze M, Knoers NV, et al. Rescue of vasopressin V2 receptor mutants by chemical chaperones: specificity and mechanism. *Mol Biol Cell*. 2006;17:379-386.
293. Robert-Nicoud M, Flahaut M, Elalouf JM, et al. Transcriptome of a mouse kidney cortical collecting duct cell line: effects of aldosterone and vasopressin. *Proc Natl Acad Sci U S A*. 2001;98:2712-2716.
294. Roberts SK, Yano M, Ueno Y, et al. Cholangiocytes express the aquaporin CHIP and transport water via a channel-mediated mechanism. *Proc Natl Acad Sci U S A*. 1994;91:13009-13013.
295. Robertson GL. Vasopressin. In: Seldin DW, Giebisch G, eds. *The kidney: physiology and pathophysiology*. Philadelphia: Lippincott Williams & Wilkins; 2000:pp 1133-1151.
296. Rodal SK, Skretting G, Garred O, et al. Extraction of cholesterol with methyl-beta-cyclodextrin perturbs formation of clathrin-coated endocytic vesicles. *Mol Biol Cell*. 1999;10:961-974.
297. Rogers SL, Gelfand VI. Myosin cooperates with microtubule motors during organelle transport in melanophores. *Curr Biol*. 1998;8:161-164.
298. Rosenthal WA, Seibold A, Antaramian A, et al. Molecular identification of the gene responsible for congenital nephrogenic diabetes insipidus. *Nature*. 1992;359:233-235.
299. Rothman JE, Sollner TH. Throttles and dampers: controlling the engine of membrane fusion. *Science*. 1997;276:1212-1213.
300. Rothman JE, Warren G. Implications of the SNARE hypothesis for intracellular membrane topology and dynamics. *Curr Biol*. 1994;4:220-233.
301. Russo LM, McKee M, Brown D. Methyl-beta-cyclodextrin induces vasopressin-independent apical accumulation of aquaporin-2 in the isolated, perfused rat kidney. *Am J Physiol Renal Physiol*. 2006;291:F246-F253.
302. Russo LM, Miranda KC, Bond DT, et al. Massively parallel sequencing of urinary exosomes for renal disease biomarker discovery. *J Am Soc Nephrol*. 2009:abstract: SA-FC372, 2009. American Society of Nephrology, San Diego, October 21–November 1, 2009.
303. Sabolic I, Katsura T, Verbavatz JM, et al. The AQP2 water channel: effect of vasopressin treatment, microtubule disruption, and distribution in neonatal rats. *J Membr Biol*. 1995;143:165-175.
304. Sabolic I, Valenti G, Verbavatz J-M, et al. Localization of the CHIP28 water channel in rat kidney. *Am J Physiol*. 1992;263:C1225-C1233.
305. Sabolic I, Wuarin F, Shi LB, et al. Apical endosomes isolated from kidney collecting duct principal cells lack subunits of the proton pumping ATPase. *J Cell Biol*. 1992;119:111-122.
306. Sadeghi HM, Innamorati G, Dagarag M, et al. Palmitoylation of the V2 vasopressin receptor. *Mol Pharmacol*. 1997;52:21-29.
307. Saito T, Ishikawa SE, Sasaki S, et al. Alteration in water channel AQP-2 by removal of AVP stimulation in collecting duct cells of dehydrated rats. *Am J Physiol*. 1997;272:F183-F191.
308. Sands JM, Bichet DG. Nephrogenic diabetes insipidus. *Ann Intern Med*. 2006;144:186-194.
309. Sands JM, Flores FX, Kato A, et al. Vasopressin-elicited water and urea permeabilities are altered in IMCD in hypercalcemic rats. *Am J Physiol*. 1998;274:F978-F985.
310. Sangkuhl K, Rompler H, Busch W, et al. Nephrogenic diabetes insipidus caused by mutation of Tyr205: a key residue of V2 vasopressin receptor function. *Hum Mutat*. 2005;25:505.
311. Sarmiento JM, Ehrenfeld P, Anazco CC, et al. Differential distribution of the vasopressin V receptor along the rat nephron during renal ontogeny and maturation. *Kidney Int*. 2005;68:487-496.
312. Sasaki S, Fushimi K, Ishibashi K, et al. Water channels in the kidney collecting duct. *Kidney Int*. 1995;48:1082-1087.
313. Savage DF, Stroud RM. Structural basis of aquaporin inhibition by mercury. *J Mol Biol*. 2007;368:607-617.
314. Scheller RH. Membrane trafficking in the presynaptic nerve terminal. *Neuron*. 1995;14:893-897.
315. Schmale H, Heinsohn S, Richter D. Structural organization of the rat gene for the arginine vasopressin-neurophysin precursor. *EMBO J*. 1983;2:763-767.
316. Schroer TA. Microtubules don and doff their caps: dynamic attachments at plus and minus ends. *Curr Opin Cell Biol*. 2001;13:92-96.
317. Shaw S, Marples D. A rat kidney tubule suspension for the study of vasopressin-induced shuttling of AQP2 water channels. *Am J Physiol Renal Physiol*. 2002;283:F1160-F1166.
318. Shen T, Suzuki Y, Poyard M, et al. Expression of adenylyl cyclase mRNAs in the adult, in developing, and in the Brattleboro rat kidney. *Am J Physiol*. 1997;273:C323-330.
319. Shenoy SK, Modi AS, Shukla AK, et al. Beta-arrestin–dependent signaling and trafficking of 7-transmembrane receptors is reciprocally regulated by the deubiquitinase USP33 and the E3 ligase Mdm2. *Proc Natl Acad Sci U S A*. 2009;106:6650-6655.
320. Shi LB, Verkman AS. Selected cysteine point mutations confer mercurial sensitivity to the mercurial-insensitive water channel MIWC/AQP-4. *Biochemistry*. 1996;35:538-544.
321. Shukla A, Hager H, Corydon TJ, et al. SNAP-25-associated Hrs-2 protein colocalizes with AQP2 in rat kidney collecting duct principal cells. *Am J Physiol Renal Physiol*. 2001;281:F546-F556.
322. Skorecki KL, Brown D, Ercolani L, et al. Molecular mechanisms of vasopressin action in the kidney. In: Windhager EE, ed. *Handbook of physiology*. New York: Oxford University Press; 1992:pp 1185-1218.
323. Smith BL, Agre P. Erythrocyte Mr 28,000 transmembrane protein exists as a multisubunit oligomer similar to channel proteins. *J Biol Chem*. 1991;266:6407-6415.
324. Sohara E, Rai T, Yang SS, et al. Pathogenesis and treatment of autosomal-dominant nephrogenic diabetes insipidus caused by an aquaporin 2 mutation. *Proc Natl Acad Sci U S A*. 2006;103:14217-14222.

325. Spanakis E, Milord E, Gragnoli C. AVPR2 variants and mutations in nephrogenic diabetes insipidus: review and missense mutation significance. *J Cell Physiol*. 2008;217:605-617.

326. Staahltoft D, Nielsen S, Janjua NR, et al. Losartan treatment normalizes renal sodium and water handling in rats with mild congestive heart failure. *Am J Physiol Renal Physiol*. 2002;282:F307-F315.

327. Stankovic KM, Adams JC, Brown D. Immunolocalization of aquaporin CHIP in the guinea pig inner ear. *Am J Physiol*. 1995;269:C1450-C1456.

328. Stefan E, Wiesner B, Baillie GS, et al. Compartmentalization of cAMP-dependent signaling by phosphodiesterase-4D is involved in the regulation of vasopressin-mediated water reabsorption in renal principal cells. *J Am Soc Nephrol*. 2007;18:199-212.

329. Stokes JB. Modulation of vasopressin-induced water permeability of the cortical collecting tubule by endogenous and exogenous prostaglandins. *Miner Electrolyte Metab*. 1985;11:240-248.

330. Stow JL, Sabolic I, Brown D. Heterogenous localization of G protein α-subunits in rat kidney. *Am J Physiol*. 1991;261:F831-F840.

331. Strange K, Willingham MC, Handler JS, et al. Apical membrane endocytosis via coated pits is stimulated by removal of antidiuretic hormone from isolated, perfused rabbit cortical collecting tubule. *J Membr Biol*. 1988;103:17-28.

332. Subtil A, Gaidarov I, Kobylarz K, et al. Acute cholesterol depletion inhibits clathrin-coated pit budding. *Proc Natl Acad Sci U S A*. 1999;96:6775-6780.

333. Sugimoto T, Saito M, Mochizuki S, et al. Molecular cloning and functional expression of a cDNA encoding the human V1b vasopressin receptor. *J Biol Chem*. 1994;269:27088-27092.

334. Sui H, Han BG, Lee JK, et al. Structural basis of water-specific transport through the AQP1 water channel. *Nature*. 2001;414:872-878.

335. Sun TX, Van Hoek A, Huang Y, et al. Aquaporin-2 localization in clathrin-coated pits: inhibition of endocytosis by dominant-negative dynamin. *Am J Physiol Renal Physiol*. 2002;282:F998-F1011.

336. Swenson ER, Deem S, Kerr ME, et al. Inhibition of aquaporin-mediated CO_2 diffusion and voltage-gated H^+ channels by zinc does not alter rabbit lung CO_2 and NO excretion. *Clin Sci (Lond)*. 2002;103:567-575.

337. Tajika Y, Matsuzaki T, Suzuki T, et al. Differential regulation of AQP2 trafficking in endosomes by microtubules and actin filaments. *Histochem Cell Biol*. 2005;124:1-12.

338. Tajika Y, Matsuzaki T, Suzuki T, et al. Aquaporin-2 is retrieved to the apical storage compartment via early endosomes and phosphatidylinositol 3-kinase-dependent pathway. *Endocrinology*. 2004;145:4375-4383.

339. Takata K. Aquaporin-2 (AQP2): its intracellular compartment and trafficking. *Cell Mol Biol (Noisy-le-grand)*. 2006;52:34-39.

340. Tamarappoo BK, Yang B, Verkman AS. Misfolding of mutant aquaporin-2 water channels in nephrogenic diabetes insipidus. *J Biol Chem*. 1999;274:34825-34831.

341. Tamma G, Carmosino M, Svelto M, et al. Bradykinin signaling counteracts cAMP-elicited aquaporin 2 translocation in renal cells. *J Am Soc Nephrol*. 2005;16:2881-2889.

342. Tamma G, Klussmann E, Maric K, et al. Rho inhibits cAMP-induced translocation of aquaporin-2 into the apical membrane of renal cells. *Am J Physiol Renal Physiol*. 2001;281:F1092-F1101.

343. Tamma G, Klussmann E, Oehlke J, et al. Actin remodeling requires ERM function to facilitate AQP2 apical targeting. *J Cell Sci*. 2005;118:3623-3630.

344. Taylor A, Mamelak M, Golbetz H, et al. Evidence for involvement of microtubules in the action of vasopressin in toad urinary bladder. I. Functional studies on the effects of antimitotic agents on the response to vasopressin. *J Membr Biol*. 1978;40:213-235.

345. Terashima Y, Kondo K, Mizuno Y, et al. Influence of acute elevation of plasma AVP level on rat vasopressin V2 receptor and aquaporin-2 mRNA expression. *J Mol Endocrinol*. 1998;20:281-285.

346. Terris J, Ecelbarger CA, Marples D, et al. Distribution of aquaporin-4 water channel expression within rat kidney. *Am J Physiol*. 1995;269:F775-F785.

347. Thibonnier M. Genetics of vasopressin receptors. *Curr Hypertens Rep*. 2004;6:21-26.

348. Thibonnier M, Conarty DM, Preston JA, et al. Human vascular endothelial cells express oxytocin receptors. *Endocrinology*. 1999;140:1301-1309.

349. Thielen A, Oueslati M, Hermosilla R, et al. The hydrophobic amino acid residues in the membrane-proximal C tail of the G protein–coupled vasopressin V2 receptor are necessary for transport-competent receptor folding. *FEBS Lett*. 2005;579:5227-5235.

350. Tietz PS, McNiven MA, Splinter PL, et al. Cytoskeletal and motor proteins facilitate trafficking of AQP1-containing vesicles in cholangiocytes. *Biol Cell*. 2006;98:43-52.

351. Timmer RT, Sands JM. Lithium intoxication. *J Am Soc Nephrol*. 1999;10:666-674.

352. Tornroth-Horsefield S, Wang Y, Hedfalk K, et al. Structural mechanism of plant aquaporin gating. *Nature*. 2006;439:688-694.

353. Tsukaguchi H, Shayakul C, Berger UV, et al. Molecular characterization of a broad selectivity neutral solute channel. *J Biol Chem*. 1998;273:24737-24743.

354. Vale RD, Milligan RA. The way things move: looking under the hood of molecular motor proteins. *Science*. 2000;288:88-95.

355. Valenti G, Frigeri A, Ronco PM, et al. Expression and functional analysis of water channels in a stably AQP2- transfected human collecting duct cell line. *J Biol Chem*. 1996;271:24365-24370.

356. Valenti G, Procino G, Carmosino M, et al. The phosphatase inhibitor okadaic acid induces AQP2 translocation independently from AQP2 phosphorylation in renal collecting duct cells. *J Cell Sci*. 2000;113:1985-1992.

357. Valenti G, Procino G, Tamma G, et al. Minireview: aquaporin 2 trafficking. *Endocrinology*. 2005;146:5063-5070.

358. Valtin H. The discovery of the Brattleboro rat, recommended nomenclature and the question of proper controls. *Ann N Y Acad Sci*. 1982;394:1-9.

359. Van Balkom BW, Savelkoul PJ, Markovich D, et al. The role of putative phosphorylation sites in the targeting and shuttling of the aquaporin-2 water channel. *J Biol Chem*. 2002;277:41473-41479.

360. van Balkom BW, van Raak M, Breton S, et al. Hypertonicity is involved in redirecting the aquaporin-2 water channel into the basolateral, instead of the apical, plasma membrane of renal epithelial cells. *J Biol Chem*. 2003;278:1101-1107.

361. Van Hoek A, Yang B, Kirmiz S, et al. Freeze-fracture analysis of plasma membranes of CHO cells stably expressing aquaporins 1-5. *J Membr Biol*. 1998;165:243-254.

362. Van Hoek AN, Bouley R, Lu Y, et al. Vasopressin-induced differential stimulation of AQP4 splice variants regulates the in-membrane assembly of orthogonal arrays. *Am J Physiol Renal Physiol*. 2009;296:F1396-F1404.

363. van Lieburg AF, Verdijk MA, Knoers VV, et al. Patients with autosomal nephrogenic diabetes insipidus homozygous for mutations in the aquaporin 2 water-channel gene. *Am J Hum Genet*. 1994;55:648-652.

364. Verbavatz J-M, Brown D, Sabolic I, et al. Tetrameric assembly of CHIP28 water channels in liposomes and cell membranes: a freeze-fracture study. *J Cell Biol*. 1993;123:605-618.

365. Verhey KJ, Hammond JW. Traffic control: regulation of kinesin motors. *Nat Rev Mol Cell Biol*. 2009;10:765-777.

366. Verkman AS. Novel roles of aquaporins revealed by phenotype analysis of knockout mice. *Rev Physiol Biochem Pharmacol*. 2005;155:31-55.

367. von Zastrow M. Mechanisms regulating membrane trafficking of G protein–coupled receptors in the endocytic pathway. *Life Sci*. 2003;74:217-224.

368. Vossenkamper A, Nedvetsky PI, Wiesner B, et al. Microtubules are needed for the perinuclear positioning of aquaporin-2 after its endocytic retrieval in renal principal cells. *Am J Physiol Cell Physiol*. 2007;293:C1129-C1138.

369. Wade JB. Membrane structural specialization of the toad urinary bladder revealed by the freeze-fracture technique. III. Location, structure and vasopressin dependence of intramembranous particle arrays. *J Membr Biol*. 1978;40(special issue):281-296.

370. Wade JB, Kachadorian WA. Cytochalasin B inhibition of toad bladder apical membrane responses to ADH. *Am J Physiol*. 1988;255:C526-C530.

371. Wade JB, Stetson DL, Lewis SA. ADH action: evidence for a membrane shuttle mechanism. *Ann N Y Acad Sci*. 1981;372:106-117.

372. Walz T, Tittmann P, Fuchs KH, et al. Surface topographies at subnanometer-resolution reveal asymmetry and sidedness of aquaporin-1. *J Mol Biol*. 1996;264:907-918.

373. Wang W, Li C, Kwon TH, et al. AQP3, p-AQP2, and AQP2 expression is reduced in polyuric rats with hypercalcemia: prevention by cAMP-PDE inhibitors. *Am J Physiol Renal Physiol*. 2002;283:F1313-F1325.

374. Wang W, Li C, Nejsum LN, et al. Biphasic effects of ANP infusion in conscious, euvolumic rats: roles of AQP2 and ENaC trafficking. *Am J Physiol Renal Physiol*. 2006;290:F530-F541.

375. Wang Y, Cohen J, Boron WF, et al. Exploring gas permeability of cellular membranes and membrane channels with molecular dynamics. *J Struct Biol*. 2007;157:534-544.

376. Weber T, Zemelman BV, McNew JA, et al. SNAREpins: minimal machinery for membrane fusion. *Cell*. 1998;92:759-772.

377. Wen H, Frokiaer J, Kwon TH, et al. Urinary excretion of aquaporin-2 in rat is mediated by a vasopressin-dependent apical pathway. *J Am Soc Nephrol*. 1999;10:1416-1429.

378. Wolfe BL, Trejo J. Clathrin-dependent mechanisms of G protein–coupled receptor endocytosis. *Traffic*. 2007;8:462-470.

379. Woodhall PB, Tisher CC. Response of the distal tubule and cortical collecting duct to vasopressin in the rat. *J Clin Invest*. 1973;52:3095-3108.

380. Wu S, Birnbaumer M, Guan Z. Phosphorylation analysis of G protein–coupled receptor by mass spectrometry: identification of a phosphorylation site in V2 vasopressin receptor. *Anal Chem*. 2008;80:6034-6037.

381. Xiao K, Shenoy SK, Nobles K, et al. Activation-dependent conformational changes in β-arrestin 2. *J Biol Chem*. 2004;279:55744-55753.

382. Xu DL, Martin PY, Ohara M, et al. Upregulation of aquaporin-2 water channel expression in chronic heart failure rat. *J Clin Invest*. 1997;99:1500-1505.

383. Yamamoto T, Sasaki S, Fushimi K, et al. Localization and expression of a collecting duct water channel, aquaporin, in hydrated and dehydrated rats. *Exp Nephrol*. 1995;3:193-201.
384. Yang B, Brown D, Verkman AS. The mercurial insensitive water channel (AQP-4) forms orthogonal arrays in stably transfected Chinese hamster ovary cells. *J Biol Chem*. 1996;271:4577-4580.
385. Yang B, Verkman AS. Water and glycerol permeabilities of aquaporins 1-5 and MIP determined quantitatively by expression of epitope-tagged constructs in *Xenopus* oocytes. *J Biol Chem*. 1997;272:16140-16146.
386. Yano Y, Cesar KR, Araujo M, et al. Aquaporin 2 expression increased by glucagon in normal rat inner medullary collecting ducts. *Am J Physiol Renal Physiol*. 2009;296:F54-F59.
387. Yasui M, Hazama A, Kwon TH, et al. Rapid gating and anion permeability of an intracellular aquaporin. *Nature*. 1999;402:184-187.
388. Yip KP. Epac mediated Ca^{2+} mobilization and exocytosis in inner medullary collecting duct. *Am J Physiol Renal Physiol*. 2006;291(4):F882-F890:Epub May 9, 2006.
389. Yue C, Mutsuga N, Scordalakes EM, et al. Studies of oxytocin and vasopressin gene expression in the rat hypothalamus using exon- and intron-specific probes. *Am J Physiol Regul Integr Comp Physiol*. 2006;290:R1233-R1241.
390. Zager RA, Johnson AC, Lund S. Uremia impacts renal inflammatory cytokine gene expression in the setting of experimental acute kidney injury. *Am J Physiol Renal Physiol*. 2009;297(4):F961-F970:Epub August 5, 2009.
391. Zalyapin EA, Bouley R, Hasler U, et al. Effects of the renal medullary pH and ionic environment on vasopressin binding and signaling. *Kidney Int*. 2008;74:1557-1567.
392. Zeidel ML, Nielsen S, Smith BL, et al. Ultrastructure, pharmacologic inhibition, and transport selectivity of aquaporin channel-forming integral protein in proteoliposomes. *Biochemistry*. 1994;33:1606-1615.
393. Zelenina M, Christensen BM, Palmer J, et al. Prostaglandin E(2) interaction with AVP: effects on AQP2 phosphorylation and distribution. *Am J Physiol Renal Physiol*. 2000;278:F388-F394.
394. Zelenina M, Zelenin S, Bondar AA, et al. Water permeability of aquaporin-4 is decreased by protein kinase C and dopamine. *Am J Physiol Renal Physiol*. 2002;283:F309-F318.
395. Zhang R, Logee K, Verkman AS. Expression of mRNA coding for kidney and red cell water channels in *Xenopus* oocytes. *J Biol Chem*. 1990;265:15375-15378.
396. Zwang NA, Hoffert JD, Pisitkun T, et al. Identification of phosphorylation-dependent binding partners of aquaporin-2 using protein mass spectrometry. *J Proteome Res*. 2009;8:1540-1554.

Vasoactive Molecules and the Kidney

Richard E. Gilbert, David S. Game, and Andrew Advani

Vasoactive peptides, arising both from the systemic circulation and from local tissue-based generation, play important roles in renal physiology, not only in the regulation of renal blood flow but also in electrolyte exchange, acid-base balance, and body fluid homeostasis. Please see Chapter 15 for a detailed discussion of this latter concept. More recent interest has focused on the role of these peptide systems in kidney development and in the pathogenesis of organ injury.

Renin-Angiotensin System

In their now seminal 1898 report, *Niere und Kreislauf,* Robert Tigerstedt and Per Bergman, who were working at the Karolinska Institute in Sweden, described the prolonged vasopressor effects of crude kidney extracts.[1] Although recognizing the impurity of the extract, Tigerstedt named the unidentified active substance "renin" on the basis of its organ of origin. More than 110 years later, the understanding of the renin-angiotensin system (RAS) continues to evolve with insights

into its pivotal role in both pathophysiologic and physiologic processes. Underlying this effort to fully understand the RAS is not only a desire for knowledge but also a profound appreciation of the therapeutic importance of its blockade. Much of this insight is derived from work by Anderson and colleagues[2] in 1985, who defined the renoprotective effects of angiotensin-converting enzyme (ACE) inhibition in a rodent model of progressive renal disease.

Classical Renin-Angiotensin System

The classical view of the RAS focuses on the endocrine aspects of this peptidergic system. Angiotensinogen synthesized by the liver enters the circulation, in which it is cleaved by renin to form angiotensin I, a peptidase that is secreted from the juxtaglomerular apparatus (JGA) of the kidneys. The terminal two amino acids of angiotensin I are then removed to form angiotensin II, as it traverses through the circulation and is exposed to ACE, a peptidase expressed on endothelial cells, particularly in the pulmonary vasculature. Angiotensin II, the principal effector molecule of the RAS, then binds to its type 1 receptor, which results in vasoconstriction, sodium retention, thirst, and aldosterone secretion. This traditional view of the RAS is still valid but has been augmented considerably, not only by the discovery of new enzymes, peptides, and receptors but also by an appreciation that, in addition to its endocrine paradigm, the RAS also has an independently functioning local tissue-based component that acts through paracrine, autocrine, and possibly intracrine mechanisms (Figure 12-1).

Angiotensinogen

Angiotensinogen is primarily, but by no means exclusively, synthesized in the liver, particularly the pericentral zone of the hepatic lobules.[3] In humans, it is coded by a single gene, composed of five exons and four introns, that spans approximately 13 kb of genomic sequence on chromosome 1 (1q42-q43). It is translated to a 453–amino acid globular glycoprotein with a molecular weight of between 45 and 65 kDa, depending on the extent of its glycosylation, that then undergoes posttranslational cleavage of a 24– or 33–amino acid signal peptide,[4] giving rise to the mature circulating form of angiotensinogen.[5] Structurally, angiotensinogen is substantially homologous to the serpin superfamily of protease inhibitors and, like many members of its family, behaves as an acute-phase reactant in the inflammatory setting,[6] which reflects the presence of an acute-phase response element that binds the transcription factor, nuclear factor κ–light-chain enhancer of activated B cells (NF-κB), in the promoter regulatory regions of the genomic DNA.[7]

Renin

Like angiotensinogen, the gene that encodes renin is also located on the long arm of chromosome 1 (1q32) and contains 10 exons and 9 introns, a feature similar to that of other aspartyl proteases.[8] Unlike humans and rats, which have only a single renin gene, the mouse has two genes, Ren-1 and Ren-2, expressed primarily in the kidneys and submandibular glands, respectively.

After its synthesis as a 406–amino acid preprohormone, the 23–amino acid leader sequence of preprorenin is cleaved in the rough endoplasmic reticulum, which gives rise to prorenin (also called *inactive renin* and *"big" renin*), which may then be rapidly secreted directly from the Golgi apparatus or from protogranules.[4] Alternatively, and virtually exclusively in the JGA, prorenin may be packaged into mature, dense granules that, instead of being immediately secreted, undergo further processing to the active enzyme renin (active renin). In contrast to the more constitutive secretion of prorenin, release of renin-containing granules is tightly regulated.[8]

Mature, active renin is a variably glycosylated 37- to 40-kDa aspartyl protease that is active at neutral pH and, in contrast to the more promiscuous activities of most other proteases in this class, has only a single known substrate, which cleaves the decapeptide angiotensin I from the amino terminal of angiotensinogen. Whereas the kidneys produce both renin and prorenin, a range of extrarenal tissues—including the adrenal glands, gonads, and placenta—produce prorenin and contribute to its presence in plasma. However, as evidenced by the near-total absence of active renin in anephric

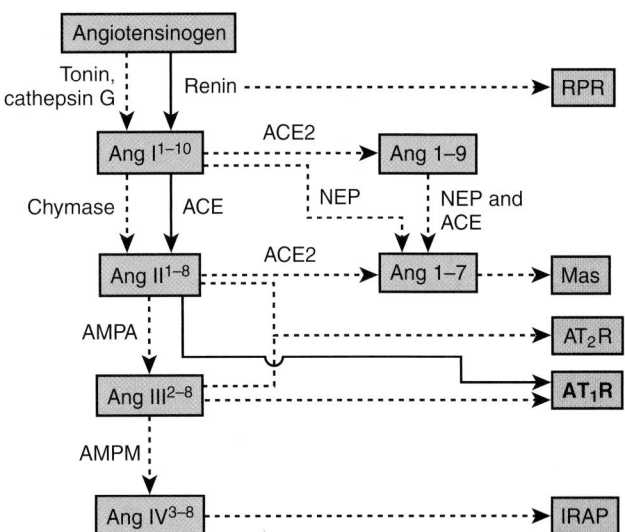

FIGURE 12-1 Current view of the expanded renin-angiotensin system. *ACE,* Angiotensin-converting enzyme; *ACE2,* angiotensin-converting enzyme 2; *AMPA,* aminopeptidase A; *AMPM,* aminopeptidase M; *AT₁R,* angiotensin type 1 receptor; *AT₂R,* angiotensin type 2 receptor; *IRAP,* insulin-regulated aminopeptidase; *Mas,* Mas oncogene, receptor for angiotensin-(1-7); *NEP,* neutral endopeptidase; *RPR,* renin/prorenin receptor. (Adapted from Fyhrquist F, Saijonmaa O: Renin-angiotensin system revisited. *J Intern Med* 2008;264:224-236.)

patients, the kidneys, and the JGA in particular, appear to be the only source of circulating renin in humans, at least in healthy tissues.

Factors that chronically stimulate renin secretion, such as a low-sodium diet and ACE inhibition, lead to an increase in the number of renin-secreting cells rather than an increase in cell size or in the number of granules that each JGA cell contains. This expansion of the renin-secreting mass occurs proximally by metaplastic transformation of vascular smooth muscle cells within the walls of the afferent arteriole. Ectopic renin expression within the extraglomerular mesangium, although sometimes mentioned, appears to be an extraordinarily rare event.[9]

Prorenin Activation

Prorenin is maintained as an inactive zymogen through the occupation of its catalytic cleft by its prosegment. The removal of this prosegment by either proteolytic or nonproteolytic means yields active renin; the term *active renin* refers to its enzymatic activity rather than its amino acid sequence (Figure 12-2). Within the dense core secretory granules of the JGA, acidification by vacuolar adenosine triphosphatases (ATPases) provides the optimal pH for the prosegment-cleaving enzymes proconvertase 1 and cathepsin B and may also assist the pH-dependent, nonenzymatic activation of prorenin.[9-11] Although various peptidases such as trypsin, plasmin, and kallikrein can also cleave the prosegment of prorenin in vitro, these do not appear to contribute to the generation of renin in the in vivo setting. Proteolytic activation of renin—although traditionally viewed as occurring only in the JGA—can also occur in cardiac and vascular smooth muscle cells by as-yet-unidentified serine proteases, according to cell culture–based studies.[12-14] The significance of these findings

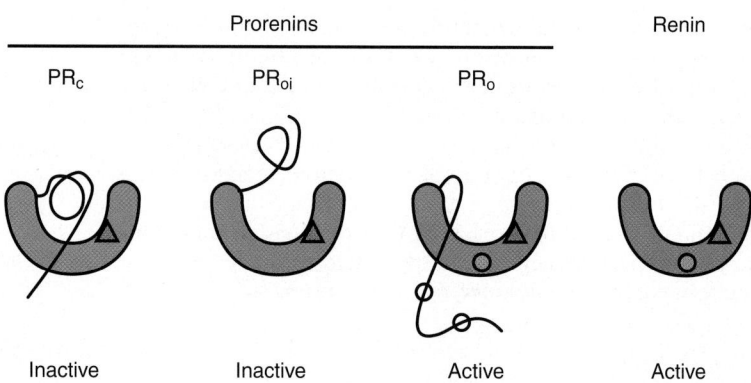

FIGURE   12-2 Prorenin activation. The conformational changes and the expression of immunoreactive epitopes associated with the activation of prorenin are depicted. The main body of the molecule, the substrate-binding cleft, and the prosegment are shown. The *closed triangle* represents the epitope of the main body expressed by PR_c (prorenin in the inactive closed conformation), PR_{oi} (prorenin in the inactive intermediary open conformation), PR_o (prorenin in the active open conformation), and renin. The *closed circle* represents the epitope of the main body, expressed by PR_o and renin, but not by PR_c and PR_{oi}. The *open circles* represent epitopes of the prosegment expressed by PR_o but not by PR_c and PR_{oi}. (Adapted from Schalekamp MADH, Derkx FHM, Deinum J, et al: Newly developed renin and prorenin assays and the clinical evaluation of renin inhibitors, *J Hypertens* 2008;26:928-937.)

in the intact organism, however, remains to be established. In addition to proteolytic cleavage of its prosegment, prorenin can also be reversibly activated nonenzymatically by a conformational change, so that the prosegment no longer occupies the enzymatic cleft. Under usual circumstances, less than 2% of prorenin is in this open active conformation. This process can, however, be induced by acid (pH < 4.0)[15,16] and, to a lesser extent, by cold.[17] More recently, the putative (pro)renin receptor (see later discussion) has also been shown to nonproteolytically activate prorenin.[18]

Regulation of Renin Secretion

Mechanical, neurologic, and chemical factors regulate the activity of the RAS by modulating renin secretion.

RENAL BARORECEPTOR

The existence of a renal baroreceptor mechanism was first conceptualized by Skinner and associates[19] to explain how renin secretion increases when afferent arteriolar perfusion pressure falls. Studies in conscious dogs have revealed that changes in renal perfusion pressure have only a small effect on renin secretion until a threshold of approximately 90 mm Hg is reached, below which renin secretion abruptly increases, doubling with every 2– to 3–mm Hg fall in pressure.[20] Accordingly, reduction in pressure below this level profoundly stimulates renin secretion, thereby acutely activating the RAS; as a result, a range of angiotensin II–dependent phenomena occur in an attempt to restore systemic pressure. Because of the location of the baroreceptor, the perfusion pressure can reflect aortic systemic pressure or, as in the case of renal artery stenosis, a perceived local pressure that is distinct from the aortic pressure. Despite the importance of the baroreceptor function, several decades of research have not identified precisely how the pressure signal is transduced into renin release, although postulated mediators include stretch-activated calcium channels, endothelins, and prostaglandins.

NEURAL CONTROL

The JGA is endowed with a rich network of noradrenergic nerve endings and their β_1 receptors. Stimulation of the renal sympathetic nerve activity leads to renin secretion that is independent of changes in renal blood flow, glomerular filtration rate (GFR), or Na^+ resorption. Moreover, this effect can be blocked surgically (by denervation) and pharmacologically (by the administration of β-adrenoreceptor blockers).[20] The role of cholinergic, dopaminergic, and adrenergic activation is controversial, although these agents have also been shown to modulate renin release under certain circumstances.

TUBULAR CONTROL

Chronic diminution in luminal NaCl delivery to the macula densa is a potent stimulus for renin secretion, reflecting a coordinate interaction among a range of mediators (including adenosine, nitric oxide, and prostaglandins) that affect not only renin release but also its transcription.[21] This mechanism is thought to account for the chronically high plasma renin activity (PRA) in subjects who adhere to a low-salt diet.[22]

METABOLIC CONTROL

The tricarboxylic acid cycle provides a final common pathway by which carbohydrates, fatty acids, and amino acids converge in the process of adenosine triphosphate (ATP) generation by aerobic electron transfer. Although the tricarboxylic acid cycle operates within mitochondria, its intermediates can be detected within the extracellular space, and they increase in abundance when local energy supply and demand are mismatched or when cells are exposed to hypoxia, toxins, or injury.[23] Succinate, for instance, has been shown to stimulate renin release, and its intravenous administration leads to hypertension, although the mechanisms underlying this effect remained unknown for a long time. In 2004, He and colleagues[24] reported that α-ketoglutarate and succinate are ligands for the G protein–coupled receptors GPR90 and GPR91 (previously orphaned), respectively, and that succinate-induced hypertension is abolished in GPR91-deficient mice. Indeed, in follow-up studies from this group, the location of GPR91 was pinpointed to the apical plasma membrane of macula densa cells, where succinate stimulation was shown to activate p38 and extracellular signal-regulated kinases 1 and 2 (ERK1/2) mitogen-activated protein (MAP) kinases, inducing cyclooxygenase-2–dependent synthesis of prostaglandin E_2, a well-established paracrine mediator of renin release.[25] Moreover, the ability of tubular succinate to induce juxtaglomerular renin secretion suggests that this phenomenon is probably an important determinant of JGA function in both physiologic and pathophysiologic settings. Elevated succinate levels have been detected in both plasma and urine of diabetic rats.[25]

OTHER LOCAL FACTORS

In addition to the factors just discussed, numerous locally active factors have also been shown to alter renin secretion. These include peptides (atrial natriuretic peptide [NP], kinins, vasoactive intestinal polypeptide, endothelin, calcitonin gene–related peptide), proinflammatory cytokines (tumor necrosis factor-α [TNF-α]), amines (dopamine and histamine), and arachidonic acid derivatives.[20]

Plasma Prorenin and Renin

Under usual circumstances, the plasma concentration of prorenin is approximately 10 times higher than that of renin. In some diabetic patients, however, plasma prorenin is disproportionately increased; such levels are predictive of the development of diabetic nephropathy (including microalbuminuria) and retinopathy.[26,27] In addition to its role in the research setting, measurement of plasma renin is an important clinical assay, providing important information, for example, in the evaluation of patients with possible hyperaldosteronism, in assessing volume status, and in predicting the response to, or monitoring adherence to, a regimen of an ACE inhibitor or an angiotensin receptor blocker. In broad terms, plasma renin is determined by either activity or immunologic assay methods.[28] The method most commonly used involves the measurement of PRA: The rate at which angiotensin I is produced from plasma angiotensinogen is assayed. To prevent degradation of angiotensin I or its conversion to angiotensin II, inhibitors of angiotensinase and ACE are added to the assay. Accordingly, PRA not only is dependent on renin and endogenous angiotensinogen concentrations but also is an overestimate of the extent of inhibition by renin inhibitors as a result of the displacement of protein-bound drug by the peptidase inhibitors. The probability of the latter scenario may be diminished by the use of an antibody capture method in which anti–angiotensin I antibody, instead of peptidase inhibitors, is used to prevent further catabolism of angiotensin I.[28] The nomenclature of renin assays can be quite confusing in that plasma renin concentration (PRC) may be measured by both activity and immunologic assays. With the activity method (PRCa), exogenous angiotensinogen is added to the assay, thereby preventing the influence of endogenous levels of the substrate. However, PRCa may also be affected by the presence of renin inhibitors. This can be circumvented with antibody capture method.[28] In the immunologic assay for renin (PRCi), the concentrations of renin and prorenin in their active, open conformation are assessed, so that the PRCi assay, like PRA and PRCa, is time and temperature dependent, inasmuch as lower temperatures increase the proportion of prorenin in its active conformation. Moreover, renin inhibitors, by binding to the active site of prorenin in its open conformation, prevent the refolding of the prosegment and may therefore lead to an overestimation of PRCi.[28,29]

Angiotensin-Converting Enzyme

ACE is a zinc-containing dipeptidyl carboxypeptidase that cleaves the terminal histidyl-leucine from angiotensin I to form the octapeptide angiotensin II. In contrast to the single substrate specificity of renin, ACE is not specific, cleaving the two terminal acids from peptides with the C′-terminal sequence R_1-R_2-R_3-OH, in which R_1 is the protected (non-cleaved) amino acid, R_2 is any nonproline L-amino acid, and R_3 is any nondicarboxylic (cysteine, ornithine, lysine, arginine) L-amino acid with a free carboxy-terminal.[4] Of importance, therefore, is that ACE also catalyzes the inactivation of bradykinin. Although encoded by a single ACE gene, two distinct tissue-specific messenger RNAs (mRNAs) are transcribed, each with different sites of transcription initiation and mRNA alternative splice sites.[30] The somatic form is present in almost all tissues and is a 1306–amino acid, 140- to 160-kDa glycoprotein with two active sites. In contrast, the 90- to 100-kDa testicular or germinal form is found exclusively in postmeiotic male germ cells, contains a single active site, and appears to be involved with spermatogenesis.[4,31,32] The somatic form of ACE is widely distributed and is active not only in tissues but also in most biologic fluids. In human kidneys, ACE is present to the greatest extent within proximal and distal tubules; however, both the magnitude of expression and its site-specific distribution may be altered by disease.[33]

AT₁ Receptor

The angiotensin type 1 (AT_1) receptor mediates most of the known physiologic effects of angiotensin II. The gene for this widely distributed 359–amino acid, 40-kDa, seven-transmembrane G protein–coupled receptor is located on chromosome 3 in humans.[34]

Within the kidneys, AT_1 receptors are widely expressed. In the glomerulus, they are found in both afferent and efferent arterioles, as well as in the mesangium, in endothelium, and on podocytes.[35] In accordance with the role of angiotensin II in Na^+ resorption, AT_1 receptors are highly abundant on the brush borders of proximal tubular epithelial cells.[36] Prominent expression has also been found in renal medullary interstitial cells, located between the renal tubules and vasa recta, where angiotensin II is purported to have a potential role in the regulation of medullary blood flow.[37]

Angiotensin II binding to the AT_1 receptor initiates cell signaling by several different mechanisms that have been studied mostly in vascular smooth muscle cells.[38] These include G protein–mediated pathways and the activation of tyrosine kinases, reduced nicotinamide adenine dinucleotide (NADH)/reduced nicotinamide adenine dinucleotide phosphate (NADPH) oxidases, and serine/threonine kinases.[34]

G Protein–Mediated Signaling

In the classical G protein–mediated pathway, AT_1 receptor ligand binding leads to activation of phospholipases C, D, and A_2. Phospholipase C rapidly hydrolyses phosphatidylinositol bisphosphate (PIP_2) to inositol trisphosphate (IP_3) and diacylglycerol (DAG), initiating intracellular calcium release and protein kinase C activation, respectively. Phospholipase D similarly generates DAG and activates protein kinase C, while phospholipase A_2 leads to the formation of various vasoactive and proinflammatory arachidonic acid derivatives.

Reactive Oxygen Species

Although reactive oxygen species were previously regarded as toxic waste products, emerging evidence indicates that they may also act as second messengers in AT_1 receptor signaling, activating not only other cell-signaling cascades such as p38 MAP kinase but also a number of transcription pathways implicated in the pathogeneses of inflammatory and degenerative disease.[34] Although the mechanisms by which the AT_1 receptor stimulates NADH/NADPH are not well understood, angiotensin II binding to this receptor results in the generation of both superoxide and hydrogen peroxide.

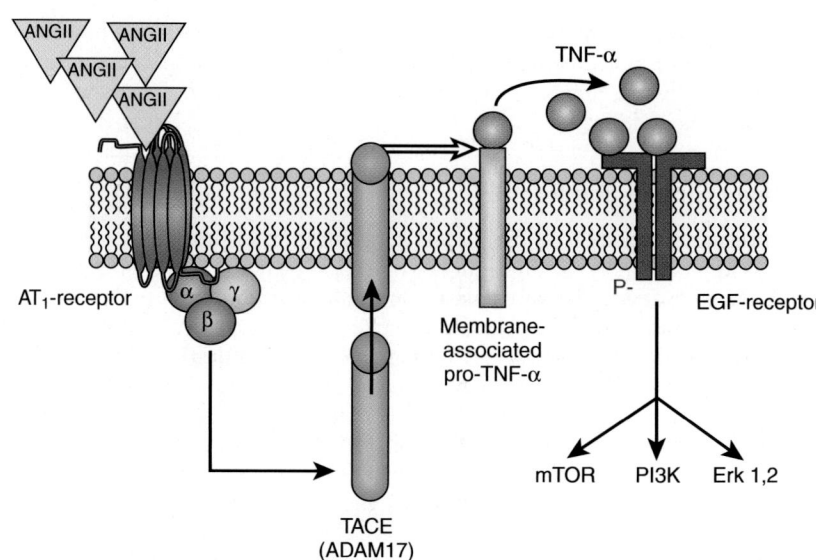

FIGURE 12-3 Angiotensin II–mediated transactivation of the epidermal growth factor (EGF) receptor. Angiotensin II binds to its angiotensin II type 1 (AT_1) receptor, a G protein–coupled receptor lacking intrinsic tyrosine kinase activity. Through as-yet-undescribed mechanisms, this interaction leads to the translocation of the metalloprotease tumor necrosis factor-α (TNF-α)–activating enzyme (TACE) from the cytosol to the cell surface, where it cleaves TNF-α from its membrane-associated promolecule, allowing it to bind and activate the epidermal growth factor (EGF) receptor. (Adapted from Wolf G: "As time goes by": angiotensin II–mediated transactivation of the EGF receptor comes of age, *Nephrol Dial Transplant* 2005;20:2050-2053.)

TYROSINE KINASES

Angiotensin II binding to the AT_1 receptor "transactivates" a number of nonreceptor tyrosine kinases (Src, Pyk2, FAK, JAK, and MAP kinase), as well as the growth factor receptor tyrosine kinases, including epidermal growth factor (EGF)[39,40] and platelet-derived growth factor (PDGF).[41,42] By binding to the AT_1 receptor, angiotensin II initiates the translocation of TNF-α–converting enzyme (TACE) to the cell surface. TACE then cleaves TNF-α from its membrane associated precursor (pro–TNF-α), allowing it to bind to EGF receptor on the cell surface. This ligand-receptor interaction then induces EGF receptor autophosphorylation and activates its downstream signaling pathways, which include those of the Akt family, ERK1/2, and mammalian target of rapamycin (mTOR) (Figure 12-3). Lautrette and colleagues[43] confirmed the in vivo relevance of this transactivation pathway: Using mice that express a dominant negative form of EGF receptor, they showed that despite similar blood pressures, mutant mice infused with angiotensin II had less proteinuria and renal fibrosis than did their wild-type counterparts. In accordance with these findings and with the pivotal role of the RAS in diabetic nephropathy, researchers using the specific EGF receptor tyrosine kinase inhibitor PKI 166 have also shown a reduction in early structural injury in a rat model of diabetic nephropathy.[44] The transactivation of the PDGF receptor by AT_1 receptor is also complex, involving the adaptor protein Shc.[41,42] In addition to studies in which the angiotensin II–PDGF receptor interaction has been explored in cell culture or organ baths,[45] a more recent report has shown that despite continued hypertension, inhibition of the PDGF receptor kinase in vivo can also dramatically attenuate angiotensin II–induced vascular remodeling.[46]

AT_1 RECEPTOR INTERNALIZATION

In addition to the conventional ligand-receptor–mediated pathways, a range of other signaling mechanisms that involve the AT_1 receptor have been described. These include receptor-interacting proteins, heterologous receptor dimerization, and ligand-independent activation[47] (Figure 12-4). These new insights, although adding greater complexity to the understanding of the RAS, provide the potential for new therapeutic targets in disease prevention and management.

After ligand binding and the initiation of signal transduction, AT_1 receptors are rapidly internalized, which is followed by either lysosomal degradation or recycling back to the plasma membrane. Several mechanisms account for AT_1 receptor internalization, including interaction with caveolae, phosphorylation of its carboxy-terminal by G protein receptor kinases[34] and association with the more recently described AT_1 receptor–interacting proteins.[47] To date, two such interacting proteins have been described: AT_1 receptor–associated protein (ATRAP),[48] which interacts with the C-terminal of AT_1 receptor, downregulates cell surface AT_1 receptor expression, and attenuates angiotensin II–mediated effects[47]; and AT_1 receptor–associated protein 1 (ARAP1),[49] which, although somewhat similar to ATRAP, promotes AT_1 receptor recycling to the plasma membrane in such a way that its kidney-specific overexpression induces hypertension and renal hypertrophy.[49]

AT_1 RECEPTOR DIMERIZATION

In addition to their ability to induce cell signaling in their monomeric state, G protein–coupled receptors such as AT_1 receptor, may also associate to form both homodimers and heterodimers.[50] Beyond its constitutive homodimerization,[51] AT_1 receptors may dimerize with angiotensin type 2 (AT_2) receptors and also form hetero-oligomers with receptors for bradykinin (B_2), epinephrine (β_2), dopamine (D1, D3, and D5), endothelin type B, Mas, and EGF that modulate their function.[52-55]

LIGAND-INDEPENDENT AT_1 RECEPTOR ACTIVATION

Without involvement of angiotensin II, cell stretch induces a conformational switch that initiates the AT_1 receptor's intracellular signaling pathways.[56,57] As might be expected from an understanding of this mechanism, an AT_1 receptor blocker, acting as an inverse agonist, will abrogate these effects, as described in both cardiac cells[57] and mesangial cells.[58] A similar means of ligand-independent activation has also been shown to result from the binding of agonist antibodies to AT_1 receptors in some women with preeclampsia[59] and in certain cases of renal allograft rejection.[60] The clinical relevance of the latter remains to be defined.

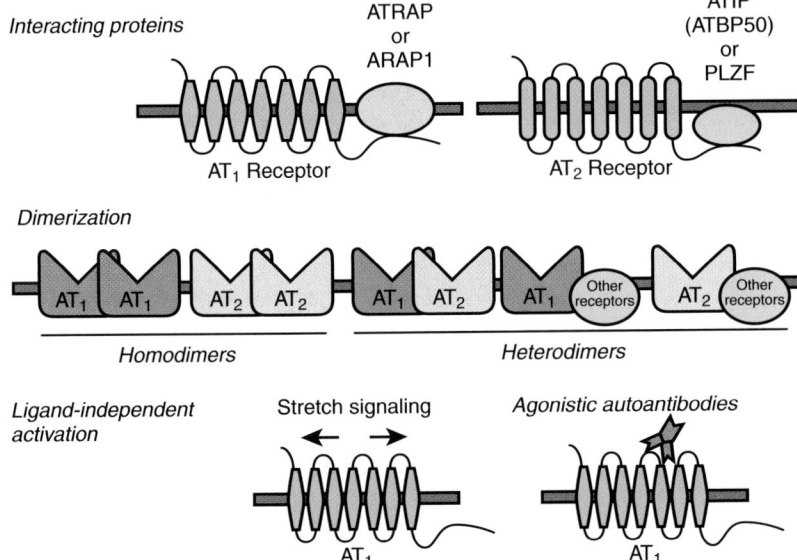

Interacting proteins

ATRAP or ARAP1

AT₁ Receptor

ATIP (ATBP50) or PLZF

AT₂ Receptor

Dimerization

AT₁ AT₁   AT₂ AT₂   AT₁ AT₂   AT₁ Other receptors   AT₂ Other receptors

Homodimers   Heterodimers

Ligand-independent activation

Stretch signaling

AT₁

Agonistic autoantibodies

AT₁

FIGURE 12-4 Developments in knowledge about the regulation of angiotensin receptors. (Adapted from Mogi M, Iwai M, Horiuchi M: New insights into the regulation of angiotensin receptors, *Curr Opin Nephrol Hypertens* 2009;18:138-143.)

Physiologic Effects of Angiotensin II in the Kidneys

The traditional actions of angiotensin II are related primarily to its effects on vascular tone and fluid balance that are mediated by its actions on AT_1 receptors in the vasculature, heart, kidneys, brain, and adrenal glands. In vascular smooth muscle, stimulation of AT_1 receptors by angiotensin II induces cell contraction and consequent vasoconstriction. In the adrenal cortex, this ligand-receptor interaction stimulates aldosterone release, thereby promoting sodium resorption in the distal nephron. Moreover, angiotensin II directly enhances sodium retention by the proximal tubule, and in the brain it stimulates thirst and salt craving. Additional effects include sympathoadrenal stimulation and the augmentation of cardiac contractility. Together these effects serve to maintain extracellular fluid volume and systemic blood pressure. In view of the central role of the kidneys in the regulation of these key aspects of mammalian homeostasis, it is not surprising that angiotensin II should have profound effects on renal physiology.

Hemodynamic Actions

The effects of exogenously administered angiotensin II are dose dependent. At low doses, angiotensin II infusion increases renal vascular resistance and lowers renal blood flow, without affecting GFR so that the filtration fraction is increased. At higher doses of angiotensin II, renal vascular resistance is further increased, which leads to an augmented reduction in renal blood flow and a fall in GFR.[61] However, because GFR is reduced to a lesser extent than is renal plasma flow, the filtration fraction remains elevated. Such findings are consistent with the view that limited stimulation of the RAS would serve mostly to enhance tubular sodium levels, as is seen, for instance, in populations unaccustomed to contemporary diets.[22] Greater activation of the RAS, on the other hand, as might be found in the setting of severe volume depletion, would result in angiotensin II–dependent reduction in renal blood flow that would aid in sustaining systemic blood pressure while further stimulating sodium resorption. Kidney micropuncture studies have been used extensively to explore the intrarenal sites of the effects of angiotensin II on vascular resistance. These studies

have demonstrated that although angiotensin II increases both afferent and efferent arteriolar resistance, intraglomerular capillary pressure (P_{GC}) is consistently elevated,[62] and the ultrafiltration coefficient (K_f) is reduced.[61] Moreover, as predicted by mathematical modeling, the glomerular hypertension induced by angiotensin II does not lead to acute proteinuria, because the structural barriers to macromolecular passage remain intact.[61] Chronic angiotensin II infusion with sustained intraglomerular hypertension, in contrast, leads to glomerular capillary damage and substantial proteinuria.

Tubular Transport

SODIUM

In accordance with its importance in the regulation of volume status, angiotensin II has profound effects on renal Na^+ handling. The proximal tubule is responsible for the resorption of approximately two thirds of the sodium from the glomerular filtrate, and binding sites for angiotensin II are particularly abundant in the proximal tubule with immunohistochemical localization of the AT_1 receptor to both apical and basolateral surfaces.[63] At picomolar concentrations, angiotensin II stimulates the luminal Na^+-H^+ exchanger, the basolateral Na^+-HCO_3^- cotransporter, and the basolateral Na^+-K^+-ATPase. However, at concentrations higher than 10^{-9} mol, angiotensin II inhibits the very same transporters. The mechanisms underlying this dose-dependent effect of angiotensin II on Na^+ transport, which also seem to occur in the loop of Henle,[63] are incompletely understood. In the distal tubule, the effects of angiotensin II on Na^+ transport are site dependent. In the early distal tubule, for instance, angiotensin II stimulates apical Na^+-H^+ exchange, whereas in the late distal tubule, it stimulates the amiloride-sensitive sodium channel.[63]

ACID-BASE REGULATION

The kidneys have a key role in the maintenance of physiologic pH by regulating the secretion and resorption of acids and bases. As for Na^+, angiotensin II also has substantial effects on acid-base transport in the proximal tubule, distal tubule, and collecting duct. Of particular interest is its actions in the collecting duct. In the collecting duct, angiotensin II not only stimulates Na^+-H^+ exchangers and Na^+-HCO_3^- cotransporters but has also been shown to stimulate the vacuolar H^+-ATPase in intercalated A cells through its AT_1 receptor.[64] Moreover, elegant and detailed electron microscopic studies have helped to unravel the mechanisms by which angiotensin II exerts its effects at this site, revealing translocation of the H^+-ATPase from the cytoplasm to the apical surface in response to ligand stimulation.[65]

Expanded Renin-Angiotensin System: Enzymes, Angiotensin Peptides, and Receptors

AT_2 Receptor

In humans, the AT_2 receptor is a 363–amino acid protein that maps to the X chromosome and is highly homologous to its rat and mouse counterparts.[66] Like the AT_1 receptor, the AT_2 receptor is a seven-transmembrane G protein–coupled receptor, although it is homologous to only 34% of the amino acids.

Despite substantial research, the actions of the AT_2 receptor are still not well understood and remain somewhat controversial.[67] In general, however, the actions of AT_2 receptor stimulation oppose those of AT_1 receptor stimulation. For instance, whereas the AT_1 receptor causes vasoconstriction and promotes Na^+ retention, AT_2 receptor stimulation leads to vasodilation[68] and natriuresis,[69] which are consistent with its abundance on the epithelium of the proximal tubule.[70] The vasodilatory effects of AT_2 receptor stimulation are mediated by increasing nitric oxide synthesis and cyclic guanosine monophosphate (cGMP) synthesis by bradykinin-dependent and -independent mechanisms.[71] Its natriuretic effects, however, seem to be dependent on the conversion of angiotensin II to angiotensin III by aminopeptidase N.[72] Like the activity of the AT_1 receptor, the activity of AT_2 receptor may be modulated by oligomerization, association with various interacting proteins, and ligand-independent effects.[71]

(Pro)renin Receptor

In 2002, an apparently novel, 350–amino acid, single-transmembrane protein that binds both renin and prorenin with high affinity was identified.[18] Ligand binding to this protein was shown to induce a fourfold increase in the catalytic cleavage of angiotensinogen, as well as stimulating intracellular signaling with activation of MAP kinases ERK1/2[18]; it was therefore named the (pro)renin receptor. The designation *(pro)renin* refers to its ability to interact with both renin and prorenin. Because of its localization to the mesangium in initial studies, its actions in augmenting local angiotensin II production, and its ability to increase mesangial transforming growth factor-β (TGF-β) production,[73] the (pro)renin receptor has been implicated in the pathogenesis of renal disease.[74] However, despite the conceptual appeal, it has been difficult to reconcile this view of the (pro)renin receptor with a number of other experimental findings, regarding not only its potentially pathogenetic role but also its pattern of distribution within the kidneys and its homology to other proteins. For instance, in view of the purported pathogenetic role of the (pro)renin receptor, the increase in the abundance of renin that follows the use of ACE inhibitors and angiotensin receptor blockers would be expected to have adverse effects, but these classes

of drugs have been repeatedly shown to be renoprotective. Second, although the (pro)renin receptor was initially localized to the glomerular mesangium, more recent and highly detailed studies have shown that it is expressed primarily in the collecting duct.[75] Third, although the (pro)renin receptor was initially reported to have no homology with any known membrane protein,[18] database interrogation has demonstrated that it is identical to two other proteins: endoplasmic reticulum–localized type 1 transmembrane adaptor precursor (CAPER) and ATPase-H^+–transporting, lysosomal accessory protein 2 (ATP6ap2),[76-80] a protein that associates with the vacuolar H^+-ATPase.[81] Although ATP6ap2 is expressed on the membranes of intracellular organelles, it is also found in striking abundance at the apical surface of collecting duct A-type intercalated cells, where it functions to expel protons into the tubular lumen and thereby regulates final urinary acidification.[82] Thus, the predominant expression of the (pro)renin receptor at the apex of acid-secreting cells in the collecting duct, in conjunction with its colocalization and homology with an accessory subunit of the vacuolar H^+-ATPase, suggests that the (pro)renin receptor may function primarily in urinary acidification.[75] However, its true function in either renal physiology or renal pathophysiology is, at present, unclear.

Angiotensin-Converting Enzyme 2

In 2000, two groups independently reported the existence of an ACE homolog, termed ACE2, an apparently novel zinc metalloprotease but considerably homologous (40% identity and 61% similarity) to ACE.[83,84] The gene encoding ACE2 is located on the X chromosome (Xp22) and contains 18 exons, several of which bear considerable similarity to the first 17 exons of human ACE. Its mRNA transcript size is 3.4 kb, and it generates an 805–amino acid peptide that is expressed most highly in the kidneys, heart, and testes but is also present in plasma and urine.[85,86] In contrast to ACE, ACE2 functions as a carboxypeptidase, removing the terminal C-terminal phenylalanine from angiotensin II to yield the vasodilatory heptapeptide angiotensin-(1-7). ACE2 may also indirectly lead to the formation of angiotensin-(1-7) by cleaving the C-terminal leucine from angiotensin I, thereby generating angiotensin-(1-9), which may then give rise to angiotensin-(1-7) under the influence of ACE or neutral endopeptidase (NEP).[86] Thus ACE2 contributes to both angiotensin II degradation and angiotensin-(1-7) synthesis. Accordingly, ACE and ACE2 were initially viewed as having opposing actions with regard to vascular tone and tissue injury. However, emerging data suggest that the situation is far from clear. For instance, although lentivirus-induced overexpression of ACE2 in the heart exerted a protective influence after experimental myocardial infarction,[87] a more recent study showed cardiac ACE2 overexpression led to cardiac dysfunction and fibrosis, despite lowering systemic blood pressure.[88]

In the kidneys, ACE2 colocalizes with ACE and angiotensin receptors in the proximal tubule, whereas in the glomerulus, it is expressed predominantly within podocytes and, to a lesser extent, in mesangial cells, in contrast to the endothelial predilection of ACE at that site.[89] In experimental diabetic nephropathy, pharmacologic ACE2 inhibition with MLN-4760 led to worsening albuminuria and glomerular injury[89]; similar findings were obtained in ACE2-knockout mice that were crossed with the Akita model of type 1 diabetes.[90] ACE2 has been shown to be the receptor for the severe adult respiratory syndrome (SARS) coronavirus.[91] Together, these findings suggest that the role of ACE2 and its purported mechanisms of action, although of future importance, are far from well understood.

Angiotensin Peptides

ANGIOTENSIN III, OR ANGIOTENSIN-(2-8)
Formed by the actions of aminopeptidase A, the heptapeptide angiotensin III—also known as angiotensin-(2-8)—like angiotensin II, exerts its effects by binding to AT_1 receptors and AT_2 receptors.[92] Initially, angiotensin III was thought to have a predominant role in regulating vasopressin release.[93] However, more recent studies indicate that although angiotensin III is equipotent to angiotensin II with regard to its effects on blood pressure, aldosterone secretion, and renal function, its metabolic clearance rate is approximately five times as rapid.[94]

ANGIOTENSIN IV, OR ANGIOTENSIN-(3-8)
Angiotensin IV is generated from angiotensin III by the actions of aminopeptidase M. Although some of its actions are mediated by the AT_1 receptor, the majority of angiotensin IV's biologic effects are thought to result from its binding to insulin-regulated aminopeptidase.[95]

Previously viewed as inactive, angiotensin IV does have actions in the central nervous system (CNS), where it not only enhances learning and memory but also possesses anticonvulsant properties and protects the brain from ischemic injury.[95] In addition to its CNS effects, angiotensin IV has also been implicated in atherogenesis, principally in relation to its ability to activate NF-κB and upregulate several proinflammatory factors that include monocyte chemoattractant protein-1, intercellular adhesion molecule-1, interleukin-6, and TNF-α, as well as enhancing the synthesis of prothrombotic factor plasminogen activator inhibitor-1.[96,97] In the kidneys, angiotensin IV is reported to have variable effects on blood flow and natriuresis.[95]

ANGIOTENSIN-(1-7)
The ostensibly vasodilatory and antitrophic angiotensin-(1-7) may be formed by the actions of several endopeptidases that include removal of the terminal tripeptide of angiotensin I by NEP, cleavage of the C-terminal phenylalanine of angiotensin II by ACE2, and excision of the dipeptidyl group from the C-terminal of angiotensin-(1-9) by ACE. Evolving evidence indicates that the actions of this heptapeptide are mediated by its binding to the previously orphaned G protein–coupled receptor MAS1.[98] Angiotensin-(1-7) induces vasodilation by a number of mechanisms that include the amplification of bradykinin's effects, stimulating cGMP synthesis, and inhibiting the release of norepinephrine.[99] In addition, angiotensin-(1-7) inhibits vascular smooth muscle proliferation and prevents neo-intima formation after balloon injury to the carotid arteries.[100] In contrast to these findings, however, is a demonstration that exogenous angiotensin-(1-7), rather than ameliorating diabetic nephropathy, as might have been predicted on basis of the prevailing paradigm, actually accelerated the progression of the disease.[90]

ANGIOTENSIN-(2-10)
In addition to angiotensin II and the other C-terminal cleavage products just discussed, angiotensin-(1-10) may also give rise to a number of other potentially biologically active peptides that result from removal of amino acids from its N terminus. Of these, angiotensin-(2-10), produced by the actions of aminopeptidase A, has been found to modulate the pressor activity of angiotensin II in rodents.[101]

PRO-ANGIOTENSIN-12
The latest addition to the angiotensin peptide family is pro-angiotensin-12, a dodecapeptide formed from angiotensinogen cleavage that has been identified in the intestines, spleen, liver, heart, and kidneys, where its abundance is increased in hypertensive rats. It can be cleaved to angiotensin II by chymase but only variably by ACE, which induces vasoconstriction in rat coronary arteries.[102] Whether it may also interact with its own non–AT_1 receptor is at present unknown.

Intrarenal Renin-Angiotensin System

In the traditional view of the RAS, angiotensin II functions as a hormone that, in a classical endocrine manner, circulates systemically to act at sites distant from those where it was formed. However, since the cloning of its components, it has become increasingly clear that an additional local, tissue-based RAS functions quasi-independently from its systemic counterpart, acting in paracrine, autocrine, and possibly even intracrine modes.[103] This is seen most clearly in the kidneys; pioneering work of several groups[104-106] has shown not only that the kidneys possess all the necessary molecular machinery to synthesize angiotensin II and other bioactive angiotensin peptides but also that their concentrations in glomerular filtrate, tubular fluid, and the interstitium are frequently between 10 and 1000 times higher than those in plasma.[36,107] Within the kidneys, renin-expressing cells have traditionally been considered to be terminally differentiated and confined to the JGA. In a series of elegant studies, however, Sequeira Lopez and colleagues,[108] using a fate-mapping Cre-loxP system, showed that renin-expressing cells are precursors to a range of other cell types in the kidneys, including those of the arteriolar media, mesangium, Bowman's capsule, and proximal tubule. Although normally quiescent, these cells may undergo metaplastic transformation to synthesize renin when homeostasis is challenged.[108] Such threats include not only those related to volume depletion but also those related to tissue injury. For instance, in the setting of single-nephron hyperfiltration and consequent progressive dysfunction that follows renal mass reduction, Gilbert and associates[109] noted the de novo expression of renin mRNA and angiotensin II peptide in tubular epithelial cells.

In addition to resident kidney cells, infiltrating mast cells may also contribute to activation of the local RAS in disease. Traditionally associated with allergic reactions and host responses to parasite infestation, mast cells have been increasingly recognized for their role in inflammation, immunomodulation, and chronic disease. In the kidneys, interstitial mast cell infiltration accompanies most forms of chronic kidney disease (CKD), in which their abundance is correlated with the extent of tubulointerstitial fibrosis and declining GFR, although not that of proteinuria.[110] Mast cells have been shown to synthesize renin,[111] in such a way that their degranulation releases large quantities of both renin and chymase, accelerating angiotensin II formation in the local environment.

INTRACRINE RENIN-ANGIOTENSIN SYSTEM
Peptide hormones traditionally bind to their cognate receptors on the plasma membrane and produce their effects

through the generation of secondary intermediates. However, emerging evidence suggests that certain peptides may also act directly within the cell's interior, having arrived there by either internalization or intracellular synthesis. For instance, not only has angiotensin II been localized within the cytoplasm and nucleus but also its introduction into the cytoplasm was shown as early as 1996 to have major effects on intracellular calcium currents.[112] Uptake of angiotensin II from the extracellular space probably contributes to its intracellular activity; more recently, however, investigators have focused predominantly on its endogenous synthesis. To date, much of the work on the intracrine RAS has been undertaken in cardiac cells,[113] and whether the same phenomena also apply to the kidneys remains to be established.

Renin-Angiotensin System in Renal Pathophysiology

In a critical series of experiments in the 1980s, Hostetter, Olson, and Rennke studied the hemodynamic effects of renal mass ablation in 5/6 nephrectomized rats, a well-established model of progressive renal disease.[114] In the setting of nephron loss, the glomeruli that remain undergo compensatory enlargement with increased single-nephron GFR (SNGFR) and elevations in P_{GC}, which ultimately leads to glomerulosclerosis and loss of function. That this phenomenon might be related to angiotensin II was suggested by previous work in which angiotensin II infusion was also demonstrated to result in elevated P_{GC}.[115] Together, these studies suggested that intraglomerular hypertension, as a consequence of the action of angiotensin II, was a pivotal factor underlying the inexorable progression of CKD and that strategies that reduce P_{GC} should lead to amelioration of CKD. Indeed, in proof-of-concept studies, blockade of angiotensin II formation with the ACE inhibitor enalapril was shown to result in dilation of the glomerular efferent arteriole, reduction in P_{GC}, and reduction in disease progression in 5/6 nephrectomized rats.[116] In contrast, combination therapy with hydralazine, reserpine, and hydrochlorothiazide, although equally effective in lowering systemic blood pressure, failed to ameliorate intraglomerular hypertension and disease progression.[116] These studies were soon followed by similar ones in other disease models, particularly diabetes, which, like the 5/6 nephrectomy in rats, is characterized by increased SNGFR and elevated P_{GC}.[117]

FIBROSIS
Since 1990, considerable research has focused on many of the nonhemodynamic effects of angiotensin II. For instance, in addition to their effects on P_{GC}, ACE inhibitors and angiotensin receptor blockers are highly effective in reducing interstitial fibrosis and tubular atrophy, each of which is closely correlated to progressive renal dysfunction. Underlying these effects is the ability of angiotensin II to potently induce expression of the profibrotic and proapoptotic growth factor TGF-β in a range of kidney cell types.[118,119] In accordance with these in vitro findings, TGF-β overexpression is seen in both the glomerular and tubulointerstitial compartments in the 5/6 nephrectomized and diabetic rats, in which studies also showed that both ACE inhibitors and angiotensin receptor blockers were effective at reducing TGF-β levels and disease progression.[120,121] Similarly, in human diabetic nephropathy,

the ACE inhibitor perindopril was found to reduce TGF-β mRNA in a sequential renal biopsy study,[122] and losartan was shown to lower urinary TGF-β excretion.[123]

PROTEINURIA
The development of proteinuria is both a cardinal manifestation of glomerular injury and a pathogenetic factor in the progression of renal dysfunction. Although P_{GC} remains an important factor in determining the transglomerular passage of albumin, podocytes are potential contributors. Indeed, podocyte injury is a cardinal manifestation of proteinuric renal disease, in which foot process effacement is prevented by both ACE inhibition and angiotensin receptor blockade.[124] In consideration of its crucial role in the development and function of the glomerular filtration barrier, other studies have focused on nephrin, a podocyte slit pore membrane protein. Of note, podocytes express the AT_1 receptor and respond to the addition of angiotensin II to the cell culture medium by dramatically decreasing their expression of nephrin.[125] In accordance with these findings, the reduction in nephrin expression in patients with diabetic nephropathy was shown to be ameliorated by 2 years' treatment with an ACE inhibitor.[126]

INFLAMMATION, IMMUNITY, AND THE RENIN-ANGIOTENSIN SYSTEM
Inflammatory cell infiltration is a long-recognized feature of CKD that is attenuated in rodent models by agents that block the RAS.[127] In the in vitro setting, angiotensin II activates NF-κB by both AT_1 receptor– and AT_2 receptor–dependent pathways, stimulating the expression of a number of potent chemokines such as macrophage chemotactic protein-1 and RANTES (regulated on activation, normal T expressed, and secreted), as well as cytokines, such as interleukin-6.[128] In addition to angiotensin II, angiotensin-(1-7), acting through the Mas receptor (MAS1), activates NF-κB, inducing proinflammatory effects in the kidneys under both basal and disease settings.[129] In addition to macrophages, mast cells, and other components of the innate immune system, the adaptive immune system also appears to be involved in the pathogenesis of angiotensin II–mediated organ injury. Of note, suppression of the adaptive immune system prevents the development of angiotensin II–dependent hypertension in experimental models,[130] and adoptive transfer of CD4+/CD25+ regulatory T cells is able to ameliorate angiotensin II–dependent injury.[131]

DIABETES PARADOX
Despite the fact that patients with long-standing diabetes characteristically have low plasma renin,[132-134] which suggests that the RAS is not activated by the disease, agents that block the RAS are the mainstay of therapy in diabetic nephropathy. Compounding this apparent paradox is the fact that although PRA is normal or low in diabetes, plasma prorenin levels are characteristically elevated. This dichotomy suggests a difference in cell-specific responses to diabetes, inasmuch as the JGA is the primary source of renin secretion, whereas prorenin is secreted by a much wider range of cell types. Peti-Peterdi and associates[135] explained the (pro)renin paradox of diabetes thus: Whereas the early stages of diabetes would lead to augmented succinate and enhanced JGA renin release, elevated angiotensin II levels would thereafter suppress JGA renin secretion. In contrast to this negative feedback at the JGA, angiotensin II has been shown to have the opposite effect

in the tubule, whereby diabetes causes a 3.5-fold increase in collecting duct renin that could be reduced by AT_1 receptor blockade.[136]

Endothelin

Endothelins (ETs) are potent vasoconstrictors that, although expressed primarily in the vascular endothelium, are also notably present within the renal medulla. The biologic effects of the ET system are mediated by two receptors: endothelin types A (ET-A) and B (ET-B). In the kidneys, these receptors contribute to the regulation of renal blood flow, salt and water balance, and acid-base homeostasis, as well as potentially mediating tissue inflammation and fibrosis. ET receptor blockade as a therapeutic strategy has been investigated in a range of renal diseases. In this regard, antagonist effects are determined largely by the relative specificity for each receptor isoform; nonselective ET receptor antagonists and specific ET-A receptor blockers have shown the most promise in preclinical and clinical studies of renal disease. An important therapeutic role has emerged for ET receptor antagonism in the treatment of pulmonary hypertension[137-140]; ET receptor antagonists have been granted regulatory authority approval for this indication in the United States and in Europe.[141]

Structure, Synthesis, and Secretion of the Endothelins

ETs consist of three 21–amino acid isoforms that are structurally and pharmacologically distinct: ET-1, ET-2, and ET-3. The dominant isoform in the cardiovascular system is ET-1. Differences in the amino acid sequence among the isopeptides are minor. All three isoforms share a common structure, with a typical hairpin loop configuration that results from two disulfide bonds at the amino terminus and a hydrophobic carboxy terminus that contains an aromatic indol side chain at Trp_{21} (Figure 12-5). Both the carboxy

terminus and the two disulfide bonds are responsible for the biologic activity of the peptide. ETs are synthesized from preprohormones by posttranslational proteolytic cleavage; this synthesis is mediated by furin and other enzymes. Dibasic pair–specific processing endopeptidases, which recognize Arg-Arg or Lys-Arg paired amino acids, cleave preproETs, reducing their size from approximately 203 to 39 amino acids. Subsequent proteolytic cleavage of the largely biologically inactive big ETs is mediated by endothelin-converting enzymes (ECEs), the key enzymes in the ET biosynthetic pathway. They are type II membrane-bound metalloproteases whose amino acid sequence is significantly homologous to that of NEP 24.11, so that most ECE inhibitors are also active against NEP.

Secretion of ET-1 is dependent on de novo protein synthesis, which is constitutive. However, a range of stimuli may also increase ET synthesis through both transcriptional and posttranscriptional regulation (Table 12-1). Once it is synthesized, ET-1 is secreted by endothelial cells into the basolateral compartment, toward the adjacent smooth muscle cells.

Within the kidneys, ET-1 expression is most abundant in the inner medulla. In fact, this region possesses the highest

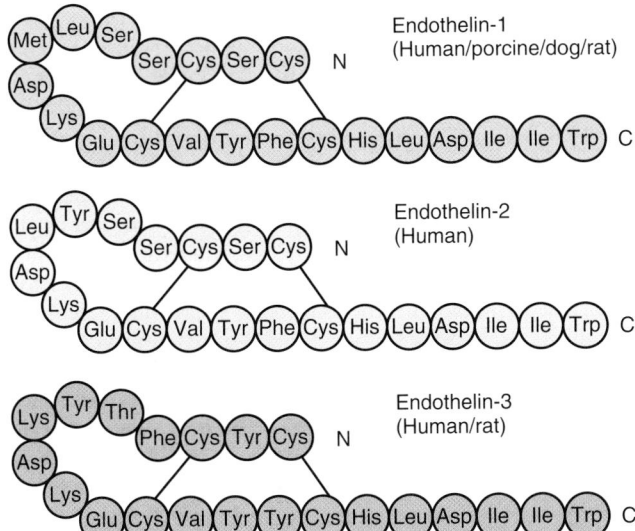

FIGURE 12-5 Molecular structure of the three endothelin isoforms. (Adapted from Schiffrin EL: Vascular endothelin in hypertension, *Vascul Pharmacol* 2005;43:19-29.)

TABLE 12-1 Regulation of Endothelin Gene and Protein Expression
Stimulation
Vasoactive peptides
Angiotensin II
Bradykinin
Vasopressin
Endothelin-1 (ET-1)
Epinephrine
Insulin
Glucocorticoids
Prolactin
Inflammatory mediators
Endotoxin
Interleukin-1
Tumor necrosis factor-α (TNF-α)
Interferon-β
Growth factors
Epidermal growth factor
Insulin-like growth factor
Transforming growth factor-β (TGF-β)
Coagulation factors
Thromboxane A_2
Tissue plasminogen activator
Other
Calcium
Hypoxia
Shear stress
Verotoxins (Shiga-like toxins)
Oxidized low-density lipoproteins
Heat shock
Inhibition
Atrial natriuretic peptide (ANP)
Brain natriuretic peptide (BNP)
Bradykinin
Heparin
Prostacyclin
Protein kinase A activators
Nitric oxide
Angiotensin-converting enzyme (ACE) inhibitors

concentration of ET-1 of any tissue bed.[142] In addition to their presence in the inner medullary collecting ducts (IMCDs), ETs have also been described in glomerular endothelial cells,[143] glomerular epithelial cells,[144] mesangial cells,[145] vasa recta,[146] and tubular epithelial cells.[147] The kidneys also synthesize ET-2 and ET-3, although at much lower levels than they do ET-1.[148] As with ET-1, endothelin-converting enzyme 1 (ECE) mRNA is also more abundant in the renal medulla than in the cortex under normal conditions. However, in disease states such as chronic heart failure, ECE1 mRNA is upregulated primarily within the cortex.[149] In human kidneys, ECE1 has been localized to endothelial and tubular epithelial cells in the cortex and medulla.[150]

Endothelin Receptors

ETs bind to two seven-transmembrane–domain G protein–coupled receptors, ET-A and ET-B. Within the vasculature, ET-A receptors are found on smooth muscle cells, where they mediate vasoconstriction. Although ET-B receptors localized on vascular smooth muscle cells can also mediate vasoconstriction, they are also expressed on endothelial cells, where their activation results in vasodilation through the production of nitric oxide and prostacyclin.[151] In addition to their role in mediating vascular tone, ET-B receptors act as clearance receptors for ET-1,[151] particularly in the lung, where ET-B receptor–binding accounts for approximately 80% of clearance.[152] In the kidneys, the ET-B receptor has predominantly renoprotective effects, including natriuresis and vasodilation.

In the kidneys, expression of both ET-A and ET-B receptors is most prominent within the IMCDs, although binding of ET-1 also occurs in smooth muscle cells, endothelial cells, renomedullary interstitial cells, thin descending limbs, and medullary thick ascending limbs.[146] ET-A receptors are localized to several renovascular structures, including vascular smooth muscle cells, arcuate arteries, and pericytes of descending vasa recta, as well as glomeruli. ET-B receptors, although prominently represented within the medullary collecting system, have also been demonstrated in proximal convoluted tubules, collecting ducts of the inner cortex, medullary thick ascending limbs, and podocytes.[153]

Physiologic Actions of Endothelin in the Kidneys

The ETs have several effects on normal renal function, including regulation of renal blood flow, sodium and water balance, and acid-base homeostasis. Although ET-1 has hemodynamic effects in almost all vessels, the sensitivity of different vascular beds varies. The renal vasculature, along with the mesenteric vessels, is the most sensitive: Vasoconstriction occurs at picomolar concentrations of ET-1,[154,155] increasing renal vascular resistance and decreasing renal blood flow. Mesangial cells are also important targets for ETs. ET-1 induces mesangial cell contraction,[156] which, together with arteriolar vasoconstriction,[157] results in an overall decline in GFR. However, long-lasting vasoconstriction that is mediated by the ET-A receptor may be preceded by a transient ET-B receptor–mediated vasodilation through release of nitric oxide from vascular endothelium; this vasodilation probably also involves

prostaglandin E$_2$ synthesis.[158] The latter effect plays an important role in the brief vasodepressor response observed immediately after bolus systemic administration of ET-1. Because of the site-specific distribution of ET receptors, ET-1 may exert different vasoconstrictive and vasodilatory effects in different regions of the kidneys. For example, by inducing nitric oxide release from adjacent tubular epithelial cells, ET-1 may actually increase blood flow in the renal medulla, where ET-B receptors predominate.[159]

In addition to effects on renal blood flow, the ET system also plays a direct role in renal sodium and water handling. In the renal medulla, ET is regulated by sodium intake and exerts its natriuretic and diuretic effects through the ET-B receptor.[160-162] Downstream signaling events for ET-B receptor–mediated increases in sodium and water excretion involve the enzyme neuronal nitric oxide synthase (NOS1), with subsequent generation of cGMP and stimulation of protein kinase G.[163] In addition to natriuretic and diuretic effects, the ET-B receptor may also contribute to acid-base homeostasis by stimulating proximal tubular sodium/proton exchanger isoform 3 (NHE3).[164] Although the role of ET-B receptor activation in urinary sodium excretion has been appreciated for some time, more recent evidence suggests that renal medullary ET-A receptors may also mediate natriuresis.[165] This may partly explain the edema that can occur as a side effect of ET-A or dual ET receptor antagonism.

Role of Endothelin in Essential Hypertension

In view of its potent vasoconstrictive properties, it is not surprising that ET-1 has been implicated in the pathogenesis of hypertension. In preclinical models of hypertension, ET antagonism may ameliorate heart failure, vascular injury, and renal failure, as well as reduce the incidence of stroke.[166,167] ET-A receptor antagonism has also been shown to normalize blood pressure in rats exposed to eucapnic intermittent hypoxia, which is analogous to sleep apnea in humans.[168] However, despite compelling preclinical evidence, it is not yet established whether the same beneficial effects can be extrapolated to a hypertensive patient population. PreproET-1 mRNA is increased in the endothelium of subcutaneous resistance arteries in patients with moderate to severe hypertension.[169] However, plasma ET-1 levels are not universally elevated[170]; an increase is found more commonly in the presence of end-organ damage or in salt-depleted, salt-sensitive patients with a blunted renin response.[171] A major component of this increase in disease is often decreased clearance by the kidneys. These findings suggest that certain patient subgroups may be more responsive than others to ET receptor blockade. Clinical experience with the long-term effects of ET receptor antagonism in hypertension is limited. In patients with essential hypertension, the nonselective ET receptor antagonist bosentan decreased blood pressure as effectively as did enalapril, without reflex neurohumoral activation, over a 4-week period.[172] Similarly, in 115 patients with resistant hypertension who were taking three or more agents, the selective ET-A receptor antagonist darusentan significantly reduced blood pressure at 10 weeks.[173] Currently, however, no ET receptor antagonists have a licensed indication for the treatment of essential hypertension.

Role of Endothelin in Renal Injury

Increasing evidence indicates that, beyond its effects on vascular tone, the ET system is also directly involved in the pathogenesis of fibrotic injury in CKD.[174] In patients with CKD, plasma ET-1 concentrations are elevated, as a result of both increased production and decreased renal clearance,[175,176] and urinary levels of ET-1 are also increased, which is indicative of increased renal ET-1 expression.[175,177]

One mechanism for increased renal ET-1 in CKD is a direct effect of urinary protein on ET-1 expression in tubular epithelial cells. In nephrotic patients, for instance, de novo expression of ET-1 occurs in tubular cells, and urinary ET-1 excretion declines in patients in whom proteinuria remits.[178] In support of this clinical observation, results of experimental studies suggest that protein overload of renal tubular cells leads to increased synthesis and secretion of ET-1 in a dose-dependent manner.[179,180] Beyond direct effects of urine protein, a number of proinflammatory factors induce ET-1 expression in the kidneys, including hypoxia, angiotensin II, thrombin, thromboxane A_2, TGF-β, and shear stress (see Table 12-1). Several distinct mechanisms may account for the injurious effects of ET-1 on the kidneys. Locally derived ET-1 has direct hemodynamic effects, increasing P_{GC} at high doses and causing vasoconstriction of the vasa recta and peritubular capillaries, with a resultant reduction in tissue oxygen tension. ET-1 also acts as a chemoattractant for inflammatory cells, which may express the peptide themselves, stimulating interstitial fibroblast and mesangial cell proliferation and mediating the production of a number of factors associated with collagenous matrix deposition, including TGF-β, matrix metalloproteinase-1, and tissue inhibitors of metalloproteinases-1 and -2. These profibrotic effects may be antagonized by ET-A receptor blockade[181] and are augmented by TGF-β.[182] Finally, ET-1 can induce cytoskeletal remodeling in both mesangial cells and podocytes. In mesangial cells and in response to injury, the ET system may induce transformation from a quiescent to an activated state. In podocytes, increased passage of protein across the filtration barrier causes cytoskeletal rearrangements and coincident upregulation of ET-1, which may act in an autocrine manner to further propagate ultrastructural injury in the same cells.[183]

The Endothelin System in Chronic Kidney Disease

ET receptor antagonists have been employed to study the role of ETs in renal pathophysiology in a range of experimental models, including the rat remnant kidney, lupus nephritis, and diabetes. In the remnant kidney model of progressive renal disease, although beneficial effects have been reported with nonselective ET receptor antagonists,[184] selective ET-A receptor inhibition appears to yield superior outcomes[185,186]; concomitant inhibition of ET-B receptors potentially abrogates any beneficial effects.[187] However, even taking receptor isoform specificity into account, it is unclear whether, in the remnant kidney model (which is exquisitely sensitive to RAS blockade), any approach to ET receptor antagonism offers added renal protection when used in combination with either an ACE inhibitor or an angiotensin II receptor blocker.[188]

Both plasma and urinary ET-1 levels are increased in patients with CKD[176,189,190]; plasma ET-1 levels are inversely correlated with estimated GFR. In a study of hypertensive patients with CKD, both selective ET-A receptor blockade and nonselective ET receptor inhibition lowered blood pressure.[191] However, whereas ET-A receptor blockade increased both renal blood flow and effective filtration fraction and decreased renal vascular resistance, dual blockade had no effect.[191] These observations suggest that although activation of the ET-B receptor does contribute to systemic vascular tone, its predominant role is probably in mediating renal vasodilation. Plasma ET-1 concentrations are also increased in patients who undergo chronic hemodialysis, falling after hemodialysis and correlating with systolic blood pressure, which suggests that ET-1 may play a role in blood pressure changes during dialysis.[192]

The Endothelin System in Diabetic Nephropathy

The ET system may contribute to the pathogenesis of diabetic nephropathy through both renal hemodynamic and trophic effects, which lead to regional tissue hypoxia and accumulation of extracellular matrix. However, as is the case in the remnant kidney, the role of ET regulation, in comparison with the pathogenetic importance of RAS activation, is slight.

Plasma levels of ET-1 are generally not elevated in individuals with uncomplicated type 1 and type 2 diabetes, although they may be increased in the setting of albuminuria, which is indicative of generalized endothelial dysfunction, and are correlated with the degree of albuminuria, as well as with the severity and duration of diabetes.[193,194] In diabetic patients with macrovascular disease, increased plasma ET-1 level is a consistent finding. Data with regard to an effect of glucose itself on ET synthesis and secretion are conflicting. Mesangial cell p38 MAP kinase activation in response to ET-1, angiotensin II, and PDGF is enhanced in the presence of high glucose levels.[195] In contrast, mesangial contraction in response to ET-1 is diminished under high-glucose conditions.[196,197] Insulin itself may also stimulate ET-1 secretion and ET receptor expression. Correspondingly, plasma ET-1 concentrations are increased in insulin-resistant patients. Circulating ET-1 concentrations are elevated in animal models of both type 1 and type 2 diabetes, although receptor levels are usually not affected. In experimental diabetic nephropathy, increased expression of ET-1 and its receptors has been found in glomeruli and in tubular epithelial cells,[179,198] although increased expression of ET receptors has not been a universal finding.[199] Diabetes also causes an increase in renal ECE1 expression, the effect being synergistic with that of radiocontrast media.[200]

A number of researchers have investigated the effect of both nonselective and selective ET-A receptor inhibitors in experimental diabetic nephropathy. In streptozotocin-diabetic rats, the nonselective ET receptor antagonist bosentan has yielded conflicting results,[198,201,202] whereas another nonselective ET receptor inhibitor, PD142893, improved renal function when administered to streptozotocin-diabetic rats that were already proteinuric.[179] The Otsuka Long Evans Tokushima Fatty (OLETF) rat is a useful animal model of type II diabetes with obesity. In OLETF rats, selective ET-A receptor blockade attenuated albuminuria, without affecting blood pressure, whereas ET-B receptor inhibition had no effect.[203] Diabetic ET-B receptor–deficient rats developed severe hypertension and progressive renal failure[204]; this finding supports a protective role for the ET-B receptor in diabetic nephropathy.

Accumulation of reactive oxygen species plays a major role in the pathogenesis of diabetic complications, particularly diabetic nephropathy,[205,206] and several observations suggest that the ET system may contribute to oxidative stress. In low-renin hypertension, ET-1 increases superoxide in carotid arteries,[207] and ET-A receptor blockade decreases vascular superoxide generation.[208,209] Similarly, ET-1 infusion increases urinary excretion of 8-isoprostane prostaglandin $F_2\alpha$ in rats, which is indicative of increased generation of reactive oxygen species.[210] In rats made diabetic with streptozotocin, the selective ET-A receptor antagonist ABT-627 prevented the development of albuminuria.[211] This effect occurred without an improvement in markers of oxidative stress but with a reduction in macrophage infiltration and urinary excretion of TGF-β and prostaglandin E_2 metabolites.[211] These observations suggest, at least in this model, that the renoprotective effect of ET-A receptor antagonism is more likely to be mediated through anti-inflammatory properties than through attenuation of oxidative damage. The effect of the ET-A receptor antagonist avosentan was examined, in addition to standard treatment with an ACE inhibitor or angiotensin II receptor blocker, in a placebo-controlled trial of 286 patients with diabetic nephropathy and macroalbuminuria.[212] At 12 weeks, avosentan was found to decrease urine albumin excretion rate without affecting blood pressure. In this study, treatment with avosentan, administered in a once-daily oral dosage for 12 weeks, was generally well tolerated with the main side effect being peripheral edema.[212] Accordingly, although a large, outcome-based trial is still lacking, selective ET-A receptor blockade may be a suitable adjunctive therapy with RAS-blockade in diabetic patients with macroalbuminuria.

The Endothelin System and Other Renal Diseases

In addition to diabetic and nondiabetic CKD, the role of the ET system has also been investigated in a number of other experimental models, including acute renal ischemia, cyclosporine-induced nephrotoxicity, and renal allograft rejection. Overall, these studies have suggested some degree of renoprotection with either selective ET-A or nonselective ET receptor inhibitors.

Endotoxemia

ET-1 may play a role in sepsis-mediated acute renal failure,[213] although, again, experimental findings have been conflicting, dependent to some extent on the ET receptor antagonist employed. For example, in a rat model of early normotensive endotoxemia, neither an ET-A receptor antagonist nor combined ET-A/ET-B receptor blockade improved GFR,[214] whereas ET-B receptor blockade alone resulted in a marked reduction in renal blood flow.[214] In contrast, in a porcine model of endotoxemic shock, the dual ET receptor antagonist, tezosentan attenuated the decrease in renal blood flow and increase in plasma creatinine.[215]

Systemic Lupus Erythematosus

Urinary ET-1 excretion is correlated with disease activity in patients with systemic lupus erythematosus (SLE),[216] and serum from such patients has been shown to stimulate ET-1 release from endothelial cells in culture.[217] In accordance with a pathogenetic role for the ET system in SLE, the ET-A receptor antagonist FR139317 attenuated renal injury in a murine model of lupus nephritis.[218] In one experimental study of the same mouse model, the peroxisome proliferator activator receptor γ (PPARγ) agonist rosiglitazone decreased blood pressure, urinary albumin excretion, glomerulosclerosis, and macrophage infiltration.[219] In these experiments, mice with SLE also demonstrated an increase in urinary ET-1 excretion that was attenuated with rosiglitazone.[219]

Hepatorenal Syndrome

Plasma ET-1 concentrations are increased in individuals with cirrhosis and ascites and in patients with type 2 hepatorenal syndrome (diuretic-resistant or refractory ascites with slowly progressive renal decline) in whom systemic vasodilation accompanies paradoxical renal vasoconstriction.[220] To investigate the therapeutic potential of ET receptor antagonism in this setting, the combined ET-A/ET-B receptor blocker tezosentan was administered to six patients in an early-phase clinical trial.[221] In this study, treatment was discontinued early in five patients, in one case because of systemic hypotension and in four because of concerns about worsening renal function.[221] These adverse effects are consistent with a dose-dependent decline in renal function in patients with acute heart failure treated with tezosentan, and they highlight the need for caution with the use of ET receptor antagonists in certain patient populations.

Endothelin Receptor Antagonists in Combination Therapy

The most likely role of ET receptor antagonists in the treatment of diabetic and nondiabetic renal disease is in combination with agents that block the RAS. Accordingly, a number of researchers have investigated the role of ET receptor antagonism in combination with RAS blockade in attenuating the progression of nephropathy, generally concluding that the combination of blockade of the RAS and the ET system is superior to antagonism of either system in isolation,[222,223] although this has not always been the case.[188]

Natriuretic Peptides

The NPs are a family of vasoactive hormones that play a role in salt and water homeostasis. The family consists of at least five structurally related but genetically distinct peptides: atrial natriuretic peptide (ANP), brain natriuretic peptide (BNP), C-type natriuretic peptide (CNP), *Dendroaspis* natriuretic peptide (DNP), and urodilatin. ANP was originally isolated from human and rat atrial tissues in 1984.[224] Since then, the NP family has been found to include several other members, all of which share a common 17–amino acid ring structure that is stabilized by a cysteine bridge and that contains several invariant amino acids.[225] Both BNP[226] and CNP[227] were originally identified in porcine brain tissue, and DNP was first isolated from the venom of the green mamba snake, *Dendroaspis angusticeps*.[228] Urodilatin is an NH_2-terminally extended form of ANP that was initially described in human urine.[229]

NP inactivation occurs through at least two distinct pathways: binding to a clearance receptor (natriuretic peptide receptor [NPR]–C) and enzymatic degradation. Other peptides also involved in salt and water balance include guanylin, uroguanylin, and adrenomedullin.

ANP and BNP act as endogenous antagonists of the RAS-mediating natriuresis, diuresis, vasodilation, and suppression of sympathetic activity, as well as inhibiting cell growth and decreasing secretion of aldosterone and renin.[230] The role of NPs in cardiovascular and renal disease, particularly BNP, has led to their adoption into clinical practice both as indicators of disease states and as novel therapeutic agents. NPs are important in cardiovascular, renal, and endocrine physiology and pathophysiology; however, their therapeutic potential is limited by their peptide nature and the need for intravenous administration. An alternative treatment strategy is to increase endogenous NP levels through inhibition of their enzymatic degradation by NEP EC 24.11 (neprilysin).

Structure and Synthesis of the Natriuretic Peptides

Atrial Natriuretic Peptide

ANP is a 28–amino acid peptide comprising a 17–amino acid ring linked by a disulfide bond between two cysteine residues and a COOH-terminal extension that confers its biologic activity (Figure 12-6). The gene for ANP, NP precursor type

A, is found on chromosome 1p36 and encodes the precursor preproANP, which is between 149 and 153 amino acids in length according to the species of origin. Human preproANP consists of 151–amino acids and is rapidly processed to the 126–amino acid proANP. ANP is identical in mammalian species except for a single amino acid substitution at residue 110, which is isoleucine in the rat, rabbit, and mouse and methionine in the human, pig, dog, sheep, and cow.

ANP synthesis occurs primarily within atrial cardiomyocytes, in which it is stored as proANP, the main constituent of the atrial secretory granules. The major stimulus to ANP release is mechanical stretch of the atria that is secondary to increased wall tension. A clinical correlate of this physiologic process is the observed natriuresis that accompanies paroxysmal atrial tachycardia. The atrial stretch observed with this supraventricular tachyarrhythmia is accompanied by increased plasma levels of ANP. In addition to atrial stretch, ANP synthesis and release may also be stimulated by neurohumoral factors such as glucocorticoids, ET, vasopressin, and angiotensin II, partly through changes in atrial pressure and partly through direct cellular effects. Although ANP mRNA levels are approximately 30- to 50-fold higher in the cardiac atria than in the ventricles, ventricular expression is dramatically increased in the developing heart and in conditions of hemodynamic overload such as heart failure and hypertension. Beyond the heart, the peptide has also been demonstrated in the kidneys, brain, lungs, adrenal glands, and liver. In the kidneys, alternate processing of proANP adds four amino acids

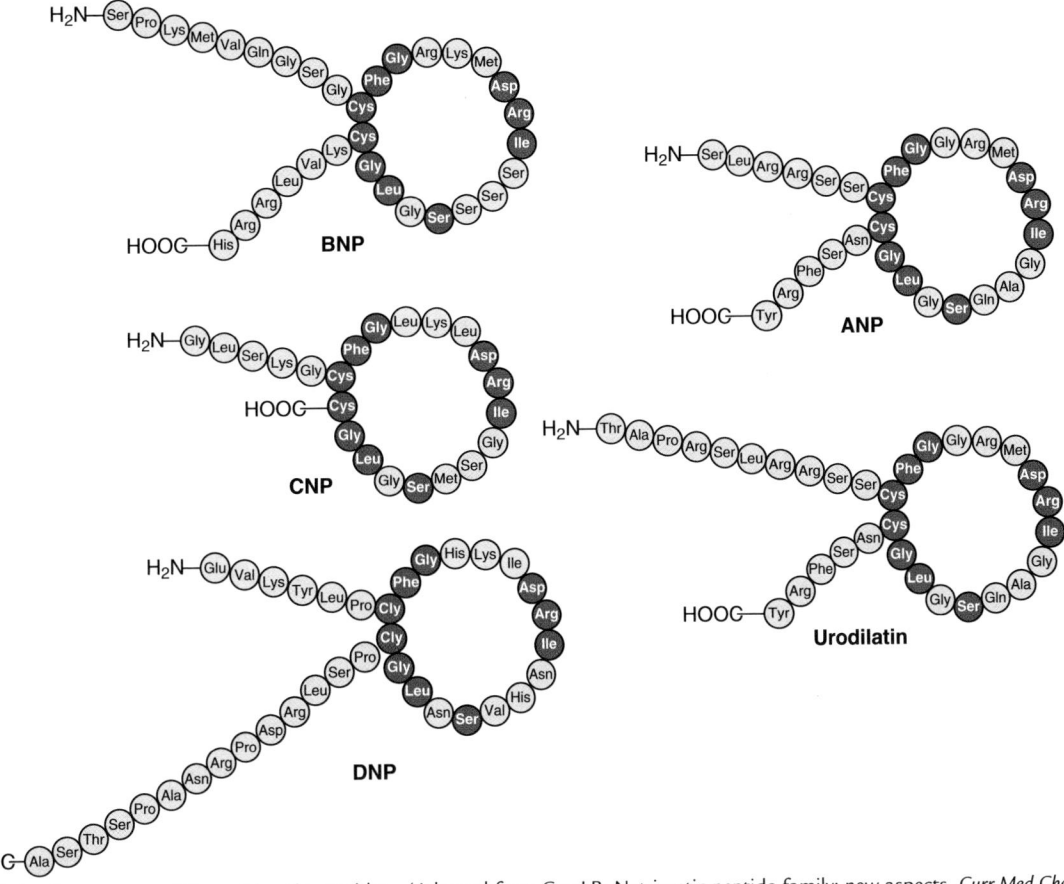

FIGURE 12-6 Molecular structure of the natriuretic peptides. (Adapted from Cea LB: Natriuretic peptide family: new aspects, *Curr Med Chem Cardiovasc Hematol Agents* 2005;3:87-98.)

to the NH_2-terminus of the ANP peptide to generate a 32–amino acid peptide: proANP 95-126, or urodilatin.

ANP is stored, primarily as proANP, in the secretory granules of the atrial cardiomyocytes and is released by fusion of the granules with the cell surface. During this process, proANP is cleaved to an NH_2-terminal 98–amino acid peptide (ANP 1-98) and the COOH-terminal 28–amino acid biologically active fragment (ANP 99-126). Both fragments circulate in the plasma; further processing of the NH_2-terminal fragment leads to the generation of peptides ANP 1-30 (long-acting NP), ANP 31-67 (vessel dilator), and ANP 79-98 (kaliuretic peptide), all of whose biologic actions may be similar to those of ANP.[231]

Brain Natriuretic Peptide

The BNP gene is located approximately only 8 kb upstream of the ANP gene on the short arm of chromosome 1 in humans, which suggests that the two genes may share both evolutionary origin and transcriptional regulation. In contrast, CNP is found separately, on chromosome 2. CNP is highly conserved across species; thus, it may represent the evolutionary ancestor of ANP and BNP. BNP, like ANP, is synthesized as a preprohormone, between 121 and 134 amino acids in length, according to species of origin. Human preproBNP (134 amino acids) is cleaved to produce the 108–amino acid precursor proBNP. Further processing leads to the production of the 32–amino acid, biologically active BNP (which corresponds to the C-terminal of the precursor), as well as a 76–amino acid N-terminal fragment (NT-proBNP).[232] Active BNP, NT-proBNP, and pro-BNP all circulate in the plasma. Circulating BNP contains the characteristic 17–amino acid ring structure closed by a disulfide bond between two cysteine residues, along with a 9–amino acid N-terminal tail and a 6–amino acid C-terminal tail (see Figure 12-6).[233]

The term *brain natriuretic peptide* is somewhat misleading, inasmuch as the primary sites of synthesis of BNP are the cardiac ventricles, and expression also occurs, to a lesser extent, in atrial cardiomyocytes. Like ANP, expression of BNP is regulated by changes in intracardiac pressure and stretch. However, unlike ANP, which is stored and released from secretory granules, BNP is regulated at the gene expression level and is synthesized and secreted in bursts. BNP expression is increased in heart failure, hypertension, and renal failure. Its plasma half-life is approximately 22 minutes; in contrast, the half-life of circulating ANP is 3 to 5 minutes, and the half-life of the biologically inactive NT-proBNP is 120 minutes. This difference is relevant to the utility of NP measurement as a biologic marker of cardiorenal disease. Changes in pulmonary capillary wedge pressure may be reflected by plasma BNP concentrations every 2 hours and by NT-proBNP levels every 12 hours.[234,235] The physiologic actions of BNP are similar to those of ANP, including effects on the kidneys (natriuresis and diuresis), vasculature (hypotension), endocrine systems (inhibition of plasma renin and aldosterone secretion), and the brain (central vasodepressor activity).

C-Type Natriuretic Peptide

As is the case for ANP and BNP, CNP is derived from a prepropeptide that undergoes posttranslational proteolytic cleavage. The initial translation product preproCNP is 126 amino acids in length and is cleaved to produce the 103–amino acid prohormone. Cleavage of proCNP yields two mature peptides made up of 22 and 53 amino acids: CNP and NH_2-terminally extended form of CNP, respectively. Of the 17 amino acids within the CNP ring structure, 11 are identical to those in the other NPs, although, uniquely, CNP lacks an amino tail at the carboxy-terminus (see Figure 12-6). CNP functions in an autocrine/paracrine manner with effects on vascular tone and muscle cell growth.[236] Accordingly, plasma concentrations of CNP are very low, although they are increased in the conditions of heart failure and renal failure. CNP is present in the heart, kidneys, and endothelium, and its receptor is also expressed in abundance in the hypothalamus and pituitary gland, which suggests that the peptide may also play a role as a neuromodulator or neurotransmitter. Because CNP is present in primarily noncardiac tissues, regulation of its expression is distinct from that of ANP and BNP and is controlled by a number of vasoactive mediators, including insulin, vascular endothelial growth factor, TGF-β, TNF-α and interleukin-1β.[225]

Dendroaspis Natriuretic Peptide

The physiologic role of DNP has been controversial since its original identification in the venom of the Green Mamba snake, *D. angusticeps*, in 1992.[228,237] DNP is a 38–amino acid peptide that shares the 17–amino acid ring structure common to all NPs, except that it has unique N- and C-terminal regions (see Figure 12-6).[235] Immunoreactivity for DNP has been reported in human plasma and atrial myocardium, and DNP has also been described in rat kidneys,[238] the rat colon,[239] and rat aortic vascular smooth muscle cells,[240] as well as pig ovarian granulosa cells.[241] DNP binds to natriuretic peptide receptor A (NPR-A)[242] and the clearance receptor NPR-C,[243] which may be of particular relevance in view of the peptide's apparent resistance to enzymatic degradation.[244] In dogs, either under normal conditions or in a pacing-induced heart failure model, administration of synthetic DNP decreased cardiac filling pressures; increased GFR, natriuresis, and diuresis; and lowered blood pressure, suppressing renin release and increasing plasma and urine cGMP levels.[245,246] Despite these propitious findings, several aspects of the biologic role of DNP remain contentious. In particular, the gene for the peptide has not been identified in mammals, nor has it yet been identified in the Green Mamba snake. Immunoreactivity experiments can be subject to artifact, and the fractionation of DNP from human samples has not been reported.[237] These uncertainties have led some authors to question whether DNP is, in fact, expressed at all in humans.[237]

Urodilatin

Urodilatin is a structural homolog of ANP, synthesized in renal distal tubular cells and differentially processed to a 32–amino acid NH_2-terminally extended form of ANP, and it shares the same 17–amino acid ring structure and COOH-terminal tail.[247] Urodilatin is not found in plasma; instead, it acts in a paracrine manner within the kidneys on receptors in the glomeruli and IMCDs to promote natriuresis and diuresis. Urodilatin is upregulated in diabetic animals[248] and in the remnant kidney[249] and is relatively resistant to enzymatic degradation, which may explain its more potent renal effects.

Natriuretic Peptide Receptors

NPs mediate their biologic effects by binding to three distinct guanylyl cyclase NPRs. The terminology can be somewhat confusing: NPR-A binds ANP and BNP, and natriuretic peptide receptor-B (NPR-B) binds CNP, whereas NPR-C acts as a clearance receptor for all three peptides.

NPR-A and NPR-B are structurally similar but share only 44% homology in the extracellular ligand-binding segment; this difference is probably responsible for the differences in ligand specificity. Both NPR-A and NPR-B have a molecular weight of approximately 120 kDa and consist of a ligand-binding extracellular domain, a single transmembrane segment, an intracellular kinase domain, and an enzymatically active guanylyl cyclase domain.[225] The kinase homology domain of NPR-A and NPR-B shares 30% homology with protein kinases but has no kinase activity. Ligand binding of NPR-A and NPR-B prevents the normal inhibitory action exerted by the kinase homology domain on the guanylyl cyclase domain, allowing the generation of cGMP, which acts as a second messenger responsible for most of the biologic effects of the NPs. NPR-C, in contrast to NPR-A and -B, lacks both the kinase homology domain and the catalytic guanylyl cyclase domain and therefore does not signal through a second-messenger system. Instead, the receptor contains the extracellular ligand-binding segment, a transmembrane domain, and a 37–amino acid cytoplasmic domain containing a G protein–activating sequence.[250] In NPR-C–knockout mice, blood pressure is reduced and the plasma half-life of ANP is increased; this finding supports the role of NPR-C as a clearance receptor.[251]

NPR-C binds all members of the NP family with high affinity and is the most abundantly expressed of the NPRs—present in the kidneys, vascular endothelium, smooth muscle cells, and heart—and represents approximately 95% of the total receptor population. Preferential binding of NPR-C to ANP over BNP may explain the relatively increased plasma half-life of BNP.[235] NPR-C clears NPs from the circulation through a process of receptor-mediated endocytosis and lysosomal degradation before rapid recycling of the internalized receptor to the cell surface. Although the primary function of NPR-C is as a clearance receptor, ligand binding may exert biologic effects on the cell through G protein–mediated inhibition of cyclic adenosine monophosphate.[252] The biologic effects of NPs are largely dependent on the distribution of their receptors. NPR-A mRNA is present mainly in the kidneys, especially in the IMCD cells (in which its expression is upregulated by 1,25-dihydroxyvitamin D_3[253]), although the receptor is also notably present within the glomeruli, renal vasculature, and proximal tubules. The distribution of NPR-B overlaps with that of NPR-A; the receptor is found in the kidneys, vasculature, and brain. However, in accordance with the paracrine effects of CNP on vascular tone, mitogenesis, and cell migration, NPR-B is expressed in greater abundance than is NPR-A within the vascular endothelium and smooth muscle, whereas expression levels are relatively lower within the kidneys.

Neutral Endopeptidase

Receptor-mediated endocytosis probably accounts for about 50% of clearance of the NPs from the circulation; catalytic degradation by the enzyme NEP is responsible for the majority of the rest, and direct renal excretion accounts for only a minor contribution.[235] Receptor clearance probably plays an even smaller role in conditions associated with chronically elevated NP levels, because of increased receptor occupancy and downregulation of NPR-C expression.

NEP is a membrane-bound zinc metalloproteinase, originally termed *enkephalinase* because of its ability to degrade opioid receptors in the brain. The enzyme has structural and catalytic similarity to other metallopeptidases, including aminopeptidase; ACE; ECE; and carboxypeptidases A, B, and E. ANP, BNP, and CNP are therefore not the only substrates for NEP; enzymatic activity has been demonstrated against a number of other vasoactive peptides, including ET-1, angiotensin II, substance P, bradykinin, neurotensin, insulin B chain, calcitonin gene–related peptide, and adrenomedullin. The primary mechanism of action of NEP is to hydrolyze peptide bonds on the NH_2 side of hydrophobic amino acid residues. In the case of ANP, NEP cleaves the Cys^{105}-Phe^{106} bond to disrupt the ring structure and inactivate the peptide. The Cys-Phe bond of BNP is relatively insensitive to enzymatic cleavage. NEP has a nearly ubiquitous tissue distribution; expression has been demonstrated in the kidneys, liver, heart, brain, lungs, gut, and adrenal glands. The metallopeptidase is present not only on the surface of endothelial cells but also on smooth muscle cells, fibroblasts, and cardiac myocytes[254]; it is most abundant in the brush border of the proximal tubules of the kidneys, where it rapidly degrades filtered ANP, preventing the peptide from reaching more distal luminal receptors.

Actions of the Natriuretic Peptides

In several respects, the NPs can be considered as endogenous antagonists of the RAS. In response to pressure overload and volume expansion, circulating levels of ANP and BNP increase, countering the effects of angiotensin II on blood pressure, vascular tone, renal tubular reabsorption, and aldosterone secretion.

Renal Effects of the Natriuretic Peptides

The natriuretic and diuretic actions of the NPs are consequences of both vasomotor and direct tubular effects. Both ANP and BNP cause an increase in glomerular capillary hydrostatic pressure and a rise in GFR by inducing afferent arteriolar vasodilation and efferent arteriolar vasoconstriction. These contrasting effects of the NPs on the afferent and efferent arterioles differ from the actions of classical vasodilators such as bradykinin. In addition to direct effects on vascular tone, ANP can also increase GFR through cGMP-mediated mesangial cell relaxation and consequent changes in the ultrafiltration coefficient. Plasma levels of ANP that do not increase GFR can induce natriuresis; this fact illustrates the potential for direct tubular effects, which may involve either locally produced NPs acting in a paracrine manner, such as urodilatin, or circulating NPs. A number of mechanisms may be responsible for the natriuresis, including direct effects on sodium transport in tubular epithelial cells and indirect effects through inhibition of renin secretion after increased sodium delivery to the macula densa.

NPs also antagonize vasopressin in the cortical collecting ducts. Similar mechanisms probably underlie the response to

ANP, BNP, and urodilatin. In contrast, CNP has little natriuretic or diuretic effect, which may indicate a requirement for the presence of the C-terminal extension of the peptide for renal effects. The NPs may have antifibrotic effects within the kidneys, as evidenced by an increase in renal fibrosis in NPR-A–knockout mice after unilateral ureteral obstruction.[255] In cultured proximal tubular cells, ANP attenuates high glucose–induced activation of TGF-β_1, Smad, and collagen synthesis, which illustrates the potentially antifibrotic properties of the peptide in the context of diabetic nephropathy.[256] In the same cell line, transfection of cells with ANP[257] highlighted potential autocrine effects, with attenuation of high glucose–activated TGF-β_1, collagen, and NF-κB.

Cardiovascular Effects

All NPs have vasodilatory and hypotensive properties. Heterozygous mutant mice with a disrupted proANP gene display evidence of salt-sensitive hypertension,[258] whereas hypotension is a feature of transgenic mice overexpressing ANP.[259] In a human patient population, a variant in the ANP promoter was associated with both lower levels of plasma ANP and increased susceptibility to early development of hypertension.[260] However, infusion of high concentrations of ANP can actually induce a rise in blood pressure, which suggests that counterregulatory baroreceptors may be activated.[261]

ANP lowers blood pressure through two major direct mechanisms. First, it increases vascular permeability with a shift of fluid from the intravascular to extravascular compartments by capillary hydraulic pressure. Second, ANP increases venous capacitance and lowering preload.[262] In addition, ANP and BNP also antagonize the vasoconstrictive effects of the RAS, ET, and the sympathetic nervous system[230] by decreasing sympathetic peripheral vascular tone, thereby suppressing the release of catecholamines and reducing central sympathetic outflow.[232] By lowering the activation threshold of vagal afferents, ANP prevents the vasoconstriction and tachycardia that normally follows a reduction in preload and thereby produces a sustained drop in blood pressure. CNP is a more potent vasodilator than either ANP or BNP. In fact, CNP relaxes human subcutaneous resistance arteries, whereas ANP and BNP have no effect.[263]

The endothelium-dependent effects of CNP on vasodilation in small resistance vessels has led some investigators to suggest that the peptide acts mainly as an endothelium-derived hyperpolarizing factor (EDHF).[264] However, intracellular microelectrode studies in the carotid arteries of guinea pigs have caused other investigators to question this role.[265,266] NPs have a number of other effects on the cardiovascular system distinct from their action on vasomotor tone. For example, NPs play a major role in cardiac remodeling. Mice with genetic deficiencies of ANP exhibit an increase in cardiac mass,[258] whereas heart size is diminished in mice transgenically overexpressing ANP.[259] The antimitogenic and antitrophic effects of NPs, which appear to be mediated by cGMP, have also been demonstrated in a range of cultured cell types, including cultured vascular cells, fibroblasts, and myocytes, and in vivo in response to balloon angioplasty. Further evidence for the role of ANP in mediating cardiac hypertrophy was obtained from population studies, in which variants in either the ANP promoter (associated with reduced circulating ANP) or in the NPR-A gene have been associated

with left ventricular hypertrophy.[267,268] BNP has been shown to have antifibrotic properties within the heart. In vitro, BNP antagonizes TGF-β induced fibrosis in cultured cardiac fibroblasts,[269] and in vivo, targeted genetic disruption of BNP in mice is associated with an increase in cardiac fibrosis, in the absence of either hypertension or ventricular hypertrophy.[270]

Other Effects of the Natriuretic Peptides

Even though they do not cross the blood-brain barrier, NPs exert important CNS effects that may augment their peripheral actions. ANP, BNP, and particularly CNP are all expressed within the brain. Circulating NPs may also exert central effects through actions at sites that are outside the blood-brain barrier. The NPR-B receptor is expressed throughout the CNS, which reflects the wide distribution of CNP, whereas the NPR-A receptor is expressed in areas adjacent to the third ventricle, which is indicative of a role of peripherally circulating ANP and BNP, as well as centrally expressed peptides. Complementing their natriuretic and diuretic effects, NPs inhibit both salt appetite and water drinking. ANP also prevents release of vasopressin and possibly adrenocorticotropic hormone (ACTH) from the pituitary gland, whereas sympathetic tone is increased by the actions of the NPs on the brainstem.

Recent clinical and experimental evidence suggests that NPs play a role in mediating metabolism. Circulating levels of NPs are decreased in obese individuals[271] and among patients with the metabolic syndrome,[272,273] correlating inversely with both plasma glucose and fasting insulin levels.[274] In accordance with these epidemiologic observations, infusion of ANP activates hormone-sensitive lipase from fat cells, which is indicative of lipolysis.[275] In vitro, ANP inhibits preadipocyte proliferation[276]; the lipolytic properties of the peptide are mediated by cGMP phosphorylation.[277,278]

Knockout mouse studies have revealed that although CNP is widely expressed, its primary role is likely to be in regulation of skeletal growth. CNP is an important regulator of cartilage homeostasis and endochondral bone formation.[279] Mice with genetic deficiencies of either CNP or its receptor NPR-B lack growth of longitudinal bones and vertebrae and have a shortened life span as a consequence of respiratory insufficiency secondary to abnormal ossification of the skull and vertebrae.[280,281] Mutations in the NPR-B gene have also been reported in patients with the autosomal recessive skeletal dysplasia, acromesomelic dysplasia type Maroteaux, and obligate carriers of the mutations have heights that are below predicted levels.[282]

Natriuretic Peptides as Biomarkers of Disease

Both ANP and BNP have been studied as clinical biomarkers of heart failure and renal failure. The short half-life of ANP (2 to 5 minutes) restricts its applicability.[283] However, the biologically inactive NH_2-terminal 98–amino acid peptide ANP 1-98 does not bind to NPR-A or NPR-C and so remains in the circulation longer than does ANP. In heart failure, ANP 1-98 levels closely reflect the degree of renal function.[284] Plasma concentrations of the midregional epitopes of the stable prohormones of both ANP and adrenomedullin are predictive of the progression of renal decline in patients with nondiabetic CKD.[285] Although this observation offers promise, measurement of ANP or one of its prohormone derivatives is currently not part of routine clinical care. Commercial assays are widely available for measurement of either BNP or the biologically inactive peptide fragment NT-proBNP. Correspondingly, since 2000, measurement of circulating BNP and NT-proBNP levels has been incorporated into several clinical practice guidelines for the management of heart failure. Important differences distinguish BNP and NT-proBNP from each other as clinical biomarkers. NT-proBNP is not removed from the circulation by binding to the clearance receptor NPR-C, and hence its circulating half-life of approximately 2 hours is significantly longer than that for BNP (approximately 20 minutes). In addition, both BNP and NT-proBNP are affected by renal impairment,[286] but the magnitude of the effect is greater for NT-proBNP.[287]

BNP and NT-proBNP as Biomarkers of Heart Failure

Measurement of circulating levels of either BNP or NT-proBNP has effectively helped guide clinical practice in several aspects of the management of heart failure, including diagnosis, screening, prognosis, and monitoring of therapy.[225] The primary role of BNP measurement in the assessment of dyspnea is as a "ruling out" test: A plasma BNP level lower than 100 pg/mL has a negative predictive value for heart failure of 90%.[288] In the ProBNP Investigation of Dyspnea in the Emergency Department (PRIDE), an NT-proBNP level lower than 300 pg/mL was optimal in ruling out heart failure, with a negative predictive value of 99%.[289] In the interpretation of plasma levels of BNP and NT-proBNP, a number of other biologic variables should be taken into account. NP levels rise with age and are higher in women, the latter effect possibly secondary to estrogen regulation, inasmuch as hormone replacement therapy increases BNP levels.[290] Conversely, NP levels fall with increasing obesity.

Role of BNP and NT-proBNP as Biomarkers in Renal Disease

The interpretation of NP concentrations in patients with renal disease merits special consideration. NP levels are increased in individuals with impaired renal function. This increase is probably multifactorial in origin and not solely the consequence of increased intravascular volume. Other factors that contribute to increased NP levels include decreased NP responsiveness, subclinical ventricular dysfunction, hypertension, left ventricular hypertrophy, subclinical ischemia, myocardial fibrosis, and RAS-activation,[291] as well as decreased filtration and reduced clearance by NPR-C and NEP.[292] Although, on the basis of observational studies, it has been widely considered that renal clearance plays a greater role in the removal of NT-proBNP from the circulation than removal of BNP, one study has challenged this view. By measuring both NT-proBNP and BNP in the renal arteries and veins of 165 subjects undergoing renal arteriography, investigators found that both NT-proBNP and BNP are equally dependent on renal clearance.[293] However, the NT-proBNP/BNP ratio did increase with declining GFR, which suggests that the two peptides may be differentially cleared at GFRs lower than 30 mL/min/1.73 m^2.[293]

Even though both BNP and NT-proBNP are affected by renal impairment, their clinical utility for the prediction of heart failure persists in CKD patients, in the context of appropriately adjusted reference ranges. For example in the

Breathing Not Properly study, BNP cutpoint values were approximately threefold higher to diagnose heart failure in patients with an estimated GFR lower than 60 mL/min relative to the conventional cutpoint value of 100 pg/mL.[294] In a cohort of 831 patients with dyspnea and a GFR <60ml/min, both BNP and NT-proBNP were effective predictors of heart failure, although NT-proBNP was superior in predicting mortality.[295] In asymptomatic patients with CKD, both BNP and NT-proBNP were equivalent and effective in indicating the presence of left ventricular hypertrophy or coronary artery disease.[296] In patients with CKD, BNP and NT-proBNP may be predictive of the progression of renal decline[297] and cardiovascular disease and of mortality. In a nondialysis CKD population, NT-proBNP, but not BNP, was an independent predictor of death[298]; in 994 black patients with hypertensive renal disease (GFR = 20 to 65 mL/min/1.73 m^2), NT-proBNP was predictive of cardiovascular disease and mortality, particularly among individuals with proteinuria.[299]

BNP and NT-proBNP have been studied extensively in dialysis recipients both as prognostic indicators and as markers of volume status. The molecular weights of BNP (3.5 kDa) and NT-proBNP (8.35 kDa) are low enough that both peptides may be cleared by high-flux dialysis.[300,301] Nevertheless, in contrast to ANP, which falls sharply after either hemodialysis or peritoneal dialysis, levels of BNP and NT-proBNP are less affected.[300,302] Overall, NP levels have not been shown to be good indicators of volume status in either hemodialysis or peritoneal dialysis recipients, which reflects not only extracellular water but also left ventricular mass and function.[286,294,303,304] Both BNP and NT-proBNP levels are predictive of mortality, heart failure, and coronary artery disease in the population undergoing dialysis.[305-309] Although levels of NT-proBNP are lower after than before hemodialysis, both are predictive of mortality.[310] Although measurement of BNP and NT-proBNP seems likely to offer prognostic advantage in hemodialysis recipients, no definite cutpoint values for diagnosing heart failure in these patients have been defined.[294]

Therapeutic Uses of Natriuretic Peptides

Even though NP levels are increased in heart failure, their biologic effects are blunted. Intravenous administration of recombinant NPs increases their circulating levels several-fold, overcoming this resistance. As such, two recombinant NPs are currently available as therapeutic agents for the treatment of heart failure. Recombinant ANP (carperitide) is available in Japan for the treatment of pulmonary edema. Recombinant BNP (nesiritide) is licensed in several countries, including the United States, for the treatment of acute decompensated heart failure.

Recombinant Atrial Natriuretic Peptide

ANP has a short half-life and a high total body clearance. Its intravenous administration causes a reduction in blood pressure, diuresis, and natriuresis in healthy individuals; this response is reduced in the setting of acute heart failure. In a 6-year open-label study of 3777 patients with acute heart failure treated with carperitide, clinical improvement was reported in 82%.[311] Results of early experimental studies were also suggestive of a potential benefit of exogenous ANP in acute renal failure; however, results in patients have generally been disappointing. Results of some small studies have suggested that the peptide may have a limited role in selected patient populations. For example, low-dose carperitide preserved renal function in patients undergoing repair of abdominal aortic aneurysm[312] and reduced the incidence of contrast-induced nephropathy in patients after coronary angiography.[313] However, a meta-analysis suggested that recombinant ANP has no effect on mortality in patients with acute renal injury, although a trend toward a reduction in the need for renal replacement therapy was shown.[314]

Recombinant Brain Natriuretic Peptide

Nesiritide is recombinant human BNP, manufactured from *Escherichia coli* and identical in structure to native human BNP, with a mean terminal half-life of 18 minutes in patients with heart failure.[315] Intravenous administration of nesiritide lowers pulmonary and systemic vascular resistance, decreases right atrial pressure, and increases cardiac output (presumably through effects on ventricular afterload) in a dose-dependent manner.[316] In contrast to nitroglycerin, nesiritide is associated with neither a reflex tachycardia nor tachyphylaxis and, unlike inotropes, such as dobutamine, it does not affect myocardial oxygen consumption or contractility and is not arrhythmogenic.

In the kidneys, nesiritide increases renal blood flow and GFR through both direct vasodilatory effects and indirect effects on cardiac output and norepinephrine inhibition.[317] Diuresis and natriuresis may also occur, although these effects are modest and may not be seen at the approved doses. Additional effects of nesiritide may also include inhibition of renin secretion in the kidneys and aldosterone production in the heart and adrenal glands. The recommended dose of nesiritide is a 2-μg/kg bolus, followed by a continuous infusion at a rate of 0.01 μg/kg/min; adjustment is not required in patients with renal dysfunction.[316,318] The main side effects of nesiritide are asymptomatic and symptomatic hypotension, which do not occur at more significant rates than with nitroglycerin.

Effects of Recombinant BNP on Renal Function

Findings of meta-analyses have raised safety concerns regarding the effects of nesiritide on both renal function and mortality. In a meta-analysis of five randomized clinical trials in which nesiritide was compared with either placebo or active control in patients with acute decompensated heart failure, nesiritide treatment was associated with a significant worsening of renal function.[319] However, this effect may have been weighted by nonstandard higher doses, infusion time, and use of large doses of diuretics.[320,321] In contrast, in the Nesiritide Administered Peri-Anesthesia in Patients Undergoing Cardiac Surgery (NAPA) study of patients with left ventricular dysfunction, nesiritide (0.01 μg/kg/min), in comparison with placebo, was associated with a lower peak rise in serum creatinine, smaller fall in GFR, and greater urine output in the immediate postoperative period.[322] This observation is supported by favorable results for preservation of renal function in a second population of patients undergoing cardiopulmonary bypass surgery, in whom nesiritide was administered at a rate of 5 ng/kg/min.[323] Similarly, in patients with acute decompensated heart failure, individuals receiving low-dose nesiritide (5 ng/kg/min) experienced an improvement in renal function, whereas those receiving the standard dose (2-μg/kg bolus, followed by 10 ng/kg/min) did not.[324]

With regard to the effect of nesiritide on mortality, a second meta-analysis revealed a trend toward an increase in death in nesiritide-treated patients in comparison with control subjects (hazard ratio = 1.80; 95% confidence interval = 0.98 to 3.31) in three trials in which inotrope-based control therapy was not used.[325] In contrast, an analysis of 15,230 patients as part of the Acute Decompensated Heart Failure National Registry (ADHERE) revealed that the mortality rate with nesiritide was equivalent to that with nitroglycerin and was reduced in comparison with the mortality rate with inotropes.[326] A subsequent meta-analysis also failed to identify an increase in 30- or 180-day mortality rate with nesiritide.[327] The controversies surrounding the potential adverse effects of nesiritide on renal function and mortality will, it is hoped, be resolved with the results of the ongoing 7000-patient Acute Study of Clinical Effectiveness of Nesiritide in Decompensated Heart Failure (ASCEND-HF).[328]

One approach aimed at optimizing the effect of recombinant BNP on the kidneys is direct delivery. In a canine pacing model of heart failure, local renal delivery of BNP was superior to systemic delivery of BNP with regard to natriuresis, diuresis, increase in GFR, and increase in urinary BNP excretion, without causing a significant reduction in mean arterial pressure.[329] Because there exist devices that enable the direct infusion of therapeutic agents into the renal arteries,[330] the potential exists, at least theoretically, to enhance the effects of BNP in patients with heart failure.

Therapeutic Uses of Other Natriuretic Peptides

The effects of urodilatin (ularitide) have been assessed in both heart failure and acute renal failure. However, the diuretic effect of urodilatin appears to be attenuated in heart failure patients, which reflects a blunted response, as observed for ANP and BNP.[331,332] Similarly, as with ANP and BNP, hypotension appears to be a dose-limiting side effect of uralatide therapy.[331,333] In the Safety and Efficacy of an Intravenous Placebo-Controlled Randomized Infusion of Ularitide in a Prospective Double-blind Study in Patients with Symptomatic, Decompensated Chronic Heart Failure (SIRIUS II) study, a phase II trial of 221 patients hospitalized for decompensated heart failure, a single 24-hour infusion of uralatide preserved short-term renal function.[334] The NP vessel dilator may offer theoretical advantages for the treatment of acute decompensated heart failure in comparison with current NP-based therapies.[335,336] In particular, vessel dilator may produce a greater and more sustained natriuresis than does ANP or BNP, without a blunted response in patients with heart failure, and may also improve renal function in the setting of experimental acute renal injury.[337] An alternative therapeutic approach is the development of novel chimeric peptides. For example, researchers have synthesized a peptide (CD-NP) that represents fusion of the 22–amino acid peptide CNP together with the 15–amino acid linear C terminus of DNP.[338] In vitro, this peptide activates cGMP and attenuates cardiac fibroblast proliferation. In vivo, CD-NP is both natriuretic and diuretic and increases GFR with less hypotension than does BNP.[338]

Neutral Endopeptidase Inhibition

Notwithstanding the recent concerns regarding the safety, efficacy, and cost effectiveness of recombinant NP therapy, a major limitation is the requirement for systemic administration, which is unsuitable for chronic treatment. Alternative methods to increase the biologic activity of NPs may offer a more feasible approach for chronic therapy. In particular, inhibition of the enzymatic degradation of NPs by NEP has been the focus of drug discovery efforts for a number of years. NEP is a zinc metallopeptidase with catalytic similarity to ACE and with a wide tissue distribution, although abundant at the proximal tubule brush border. The enzyme has activity against a number of substrates, including the vasodilating peptides ANP, BNP, and CNP; substance P; bradykinin; adrenomedullin; and the vasoconstrictors angiotensin II and ET-1. Several pharmacologic NEP inhibitors have been investigated (e.g., candoxatril, thiorphan, and phosphoramidon). Although these agents, in general, lead to an increase in plasma levels of the NPs and, under some experimental conditions, induce natriuresis and diuresis with peripheral vasodilation, results of clinical trials in hypertension and heart failure have generally been disappointing. Specifically, sustained antihypertensive effects have not been demonstrated, and some researchers have reported a paradoxical rise in blood pressure. The biologic actions of the NPs are, however, restored in the presence of an inhibited RAS, and this has led to the development of compounds that simultaneously inhibit both NEP and ACE, termed *vasopeptidase inhibitors* (VPIs).

Vasopeptidase Inhibitors

The rational design of metallopeptidase inhibitors—such as mixanpril (S21402), CGS30440, aladotril, MDL 100173, sampatrilat, and omapatrilat—is possible because of the similar structural characteristics of the catalytic sites of both ACE and NEP.[254] These VPIs have theoretical advantages over antagonists of either enzyme in isolation, and a number of preclinical studies have demonstrated their efficacy in experimental models of cardiovascular and renal disease. However, phase III clinical studies have not been able to demonstrate superiority of vasopeptidase inhibition over ACE inhibition, and an increase in the incidence of angioedema has raised safety concerns. As a result, development and clinical application of these compounds have been limited.

Although effective against both ACE and NEP, VPIs have different relative potencies for each enzyme. For example, the most extensively studied VPI, omapatrilat, has broadly equivalent potency for NEP (affinity constant $[K_i]$ = 8.9 nmol) and for ACE (K_i = 6.0 nmol) whereas the VPI gemopatrilat has an efficacy almost 100 times greater for ACE (K_i = 3.6 nmol) than for NEP (K_i = 305 nmol).[339] The broad substrate specificities of VPIs can also be expected to result in an increase in ET, adrenomedullin, and bradykinin and a reduction in the synthesis of angiotensin-(1-7). Omapatrilat lowers blood pressure and attenuates heart failure in experimental models, in association with dose-dependent increases in ANP and cGMP excretion, diuresis, and natriuresis and a decrease in PRA (although a paradoxical increase in PRA has also been reported).[339] In the subtotal (5/6) nephrectomy model of progressive renal disease, VPIs have consistently been found to be as effective as or better than ACE inhibitors[340-342]; similar benefits have been reported in diabetic apolipoprotein E–knockout mice.[343] In diabetic spontaneously hypertensive rats, the VPI S21402 was more effective than either ACE or NEP inhibition alone at lowering blood pressure and urinary albumin excretion.[344]

In contrast to the promising findings in preclinical models, trials of VPIs in human disease have, on the whole,

yielded disappointing results. In the Inhibition of Metalloproteinase in a Randomized Exercise and Symptoms Study in Heart Failure (IMPRESS) study of patients with New York Heart Association (NYHA) classes II to IV congestive heart failure, there was no difference between omapatrilat and lisinopril in outcome of the primary endpoint of maximum exercise tolerance at 12 weeks.[345] The Omapatrilat Cardiovascular Treatment vs. Enalapril (OCTAVE) trial randomly assigned 25,302 hypertensive patients to receive omapatrilat or enalapril.[346] Omapatrilat treatment was associated with a 3.6–mm Hg greater reduction in systolic blood pressure than was enalapril. However, angioedema occurred in 2.17% of omapatrilat-treated patients, in comparison with 0.68% of the enalapril-treated group.[346] This concerning side effect was even more common among black patients.[346] In the Omapatrilat Versus Enalapril Randomized Trial of Utility in Reducing Events (OVERTURE), there was no difference between enalapril and omapatrilat in outcome in the primary endpoint of combined risk of death or hospitalization for heart failure necessitating intravenous treatment, although a post hoc analysis revealed a significant 9% reduction in cardiovascular death or hospitalization.[347] In this trial, the incidence of angioedema was, again, increased among subjects receiving omapatrilat in comparison with those receiving enalapril (0.8% vs. 0.5%).[347]

SIDE EFFECTS OF VASOPEPTIDASE INHIBITORS

Limited data indicate that omapatrilat is not cleared by hemodialysis, and the dose need not be altered in the presence of renal dysfunction.[348,349] In general, the side effects of VPIs are qualitatively similar to those of ACE inhibitors, including cough (in approximately 10% of patients), dizziness, and postural hypotension.[347,350] Flushing appears more commonly with VPIs than with ACE inhibitors, which may be a consequence of increased circulating adrenomedullin concentrations.[351] The increased incidence of angioedema with omapatrilat has limited its clinical development, although it is currently unclear whether this effect is typical of its drug class or specific to this particular agent.[352] No angioedema was reported in a small study of the effect of the VPI GW660511X in 123 hypertensive individuals.[353]

TRIPLE VASOPEPTIDASE INHIBITORS

In addition to dual metallopeptidase inhibitors, agents that offer the potential for triple VPI action have been developed. For example, the compound CGS 35601 antagonizes the action of ECE, which normally converts big ET-1 to ET-1, and it has NEP and ACE inhibitory properties. This compound has been shown to reduce blood pressure in rodent models of hypertension and type 2 diabetes in a concentration-dependent manner.[354,355] Clinical studies of the safety and efficacy of triple VPIs are needed.

Other Natriuretic Peptides

Guanylin and Uroguanylin

The existence of intestinal NPs is suggested by the observation that sodium excretion is greater after an oral salt load than after an intravenous salt load. These intestinal peptides include guanylin and uroguanylin, both of which inhibit sodium absorption and increase anion secretion in response to a high-salt meal. Intestinal NPs may also act directly on the kidneys to promote natriuresis and diuresis, although they have no effect on vascular tone or GFR. It is currently unclear whether uroguanylin is a true intestinal NP or whether its actions in the kidneys and intestines are independent of each other.[356]

Adrenomedullin

Adrenomedullin is a 52–amino acid peptide originally isolated from human pheochromocytoma cells,[357] although it is synthesized mainly by vascular smooth muscle cells, endothelial cells, and macrophages[358] and is present in the plasma, vasculature, lungs, heart, and adipose tissue. The peptide is upregulated in patients with cardiovascular disease and has positive inotropic and vasodilatory properties. Systemic administration of adrenomedullin induces a nitric oxide–dependent natriuresis and an increase in GFR both under normal conditions and in patients with congestive heart failure; it also decreases plasma aldosterone levels without affecting renin activity.

Kallikrein-Kinin System

The kallikrein-kinin system (KKS) is a complex network of peptide hormones, receptors, and peptidases that is evolutionarily conserved with homologues in nonmammalian species.[359] Discovery of the KKS is attributed to J. E. Abelous and E. Bardier, who reported in 1909 that experimental injection of urine resulted in an acute fall in systemic blood pressure.[359a] Since that time, investigators have recognized that the physiologic actions of the KKS also include regulation of tissue blood flow, transepithelial water and electrolyte transport, cellular growth, capillary permeability, and inflammatory responses. The main components of the KKS are the enzyme kallikrein, its substrate kininogen, effector hormones known as *kinins* (especially bradykinin and kallidin [also termed lys-bradykinin]) and their inactivating enzymes, which include kininases I and II (ACE) and NEP EC 24.11 (neprilysin).

Kinins exert their biologic effects through binding to two receptors: the bradykinin B1 receptor (B1R) and bradykinin B2 receptor (B2R). The B2R is widely expressed and mediates all the physiologic actions of the kinins under physiologic conditions. The B1R is activated predominantly by des-Arg-bradykinin, a natural degradation product of bradykinin, generated by cleavage of the peptide by kininase I. The KKS may be subdivided into a circulatory (plasma) KKS and a tissue (including renal) KKS, which may be distinguished by their principal effector molecules, bradykinin and kallidin, respectively. In the kidneys, the kinins play a significant role in the modulation of renal hemodynamics, salt homeostasis, and water homeostasis. Although agents that specifically antagonize or augment the KKS are not currently available in clinics, the KKS is enhanced by ACE inhibition, which may account for some of the effects of this class of agents, independent of blood pressure lowering and distinct from those observed with AT_1 receptor blockers.

Components of the Kallikrein-Kinin System

Kininogen

Humans possess a single kininogen gene, which is localized to chromosome 3q26 and encodes both high–molecular weight (HMW) kininogens (626 amino acids, 88 to 120 kDa) and low–molecular weight (LMW) kininogens (409 amino acids, 50-68 kDa) through alternate splicing from 11 exons spread over a 27-kb genomic region. A second kininogen gene has been identified in mice.[360] In humans, kininogen deficiency may be relatively asymptomatic[361]; the kininogen-deficient Brown-Norway Katholiek rat strain, however, shows increased sensitivity to the pressor effects of salt, angiotensin II, and mineralocorticoid.[362,363]

Kallikrein

HMW and LMW kininogen are cleaved by the serine protease kallikrein. The name *kallikrein* is derived from the Greek term *kallikreas,* meaning "pancreas," after the work of E. K. Frey and others, in the 1930s, who extracted a kinin-producing enzyme from the pancreas of dogs.[363a] Since then, 15 tissue kallikreins have been identified, although, in humans, only one (KLK1) is involved in local kinin production. The human kallikrein genes are clustered on chromosome 19 at loci q13.3-13.4. Plasma kallikrein is found in the circulation and is involved largely with the coagulation cascade and activation of neutrophils. The tissue kallikreins are acid glycoproteins that are variably and extensively glycosylated. Human renal kallikrein is synthesized as a zymogen (prekallikrein) with a 17–amino acid signal peptide and a 7–amino acid activation sequence, which must be cleaved in order to activate the enzyme. In most mammals, including humans, tissue kallikrein cleaves kallidin (lys-bradykinin) from kininogens, whereas plasma kallikrein releases bradykinin.

Although the physiologic effects of kallikrein have been attributed to increased kinin generation, the enzyme may also have direct effects on the B2R, as well as actions independent of the kinin receptors.[364,365] For example, in kininogen-deficient Brown-Norway Katholiek rats, local injection of kallikrein into the myocardium after coronary artery ligation had a cardioprotective effect that was abolished by the nitric oxide synthase inhibitor Nω-nitro-L-arginine methyl ester and the selective B2R inhibitor, icatibant (Hoe 140).[364] As a serine protease, kallikrein may also elicit kinin receptor–independent effects on endothelial cell migration and survival through cleavage of growth factors and matrix metalloproteinases.[366] Transgenic mice overexpressing human kallikrein exhibit a sustained reduction in systemic blood pressure throughout their lifespan, which is indicative of the lack of sufficient compensatory mechanisms to reverse the hypotensive effect of kallikrein.[367] In humans, polymorphisms of the kallikrein gene KLK1 or its promoter can impair enzymatic activity, potentially influencing both kinin-dependent and kinin-independent effects. Among normotensive men with a common loss-of-function KLK1 polymorphism (R53H), an increase in wall shear stress and a paradoxical reduction in artery diameter and lumen were noted, although flow-mediated and endothelium-independent vasodilation were unaffected.[368]

Kinins

The kinins are bradykinin and kallidin in humans and bradykinin and kallidin-like peptide in rodents.[369] Plasma aminopeptidase can convert kallidin (10 amino acids: Lys-Arg-Pro-Pro-Gly-Phe-Ser-Pro-Phe-Arg) to bradykinin (9 amino acids: Arg-Pro-Pro-Gly-Phe-Ser-Pro-Phe-Arg) by cleavage of the first N-terminal lysine residue. Cleavage of the carboxy terminal arginine residue by kininase I (carboxy-peptidase-N) and carboxypeptidase-M generates their des-Arg derivatives, which are agonists of the B1R.[369] Removal of two C-terminal amino acids (Phe and Arg) by ACE (kininase II), NEP, or ECE is responsible for inactivation of the peptides.[369]

Bradykinin Receptors

B1R and B2R share 36% homology, and both are G protein-coupled receptors with seven-transmembrane domains. The genes for the two receptors are in tandem on a compact locus (14q23) separated by only 12 kb.[370] The B2R is the principal receptor mediating the actions of both of the kinins, is expressed in abundance by vascular endothelial cells, and is present in most tissues, including those of the kidneys, heart, skeletal muscle, CNS, vas deferens, trachea, intestines, uterus, and bladder. In general, the distribution and action of B1Rs are similar to those of the B2Rs. The B1R, on the other hand, is expressed at low levels under normal conditions but is upregulated in response to inflammatory stimuli (e.g., lipopolysaccharide, endotoxins, and cytokines such as interleukin-1β and TNF-α)[371] and in the setting of diabetes[372] and ischemia-reperfusion injury.[373] B2R binds both bradykinin and kallidin, whereas bradykinin has almost no effect at the B1R. The carboxypeptidase required to generate the des-Arg B1R-active kinin fragments is closely associated with the B1R on the cell surface.[374] This association would enable B2R agonists to rapidly activate B1Rs, particularly in response to inflammation.[374]

Ligand binding of both receptor subtypes induces activation of phospholipase C, which results in intracellular calcium mobilization through production of inositol 1,4,5-triphosphate and diacylglycerol via activation of G proteins, including Ga_q and Ga_i. The physiologic effects of bradykinin receptor activation are mediated through generation of both endothelial nitric oxide synthase (eNOS)–derived nitric oxide and prostaglandins. B2R activation leads to a rise in intracellular calcium concentrations in vascular endothelial cells.[369] However, bradykinin-induced vasodilation is not abolished by coadministration of nitric oxide synthase and cyclooxygenase inhibitors, which indicates that additional effectors are also likely to be involved, possibly an EDHF, inasmuch as vasodilation is abolished by inhibitors of calcium-activated potassium channels or high external potassium concentrations.[375] In addition, through binding to both B1R[376] and B2R,[377] bradykinin also increases the expression of inducible nitric oxide synthase (iNOS), at least in rodents. It is very difficult to induce the iNOS gene in human tissues, especially the vascular endothelium. Mice that have genetic deficiencies of B2R,[378] B1R[379] or both receptors[380] have been generated; the reported phenotypes of the different knockout strains have been varied, which may be a result of different genetic backgrounds, or, in the case of the single knockouts, differing compensatory effects of the remaining receptor. For example, some studies of B2R-deficient mice revealed an increase in resting systemic blood pressure, an exaggerated pressor response to angiotensin II[381] and salt sensitivity,[382] whereas others revealed no difference in resting blood pressure between B2R- or B1R-deficient mice and wild-type animals.[379,383] Double B2R-/B1R-knockout mice were also reported to have resting blood pressure identical to that in

wild-type mice and were resistant to lipopolysaccharide-induced hypotension.[380,384] In contrast, transgenic mice expressing the human B2R had a lower resting blood pressure than did wild-type controls [385] Transgenic mice expressing the rat B1R (as well as their native murine B2R) were normotensive but showed an exaggerated hypotensive response to lipopolysaccharide and, unexpectedly, a hypertensive response to des-Arg bradykinin.[386]

Kallistatin

Kallistatin is an endogenous serpin inhibitor of kallikrein that acts by forming a heat-stable complex with the enzyme. Surprisingly, administration of human kallistatin to rodents induced vasodilation and a decline in systemic blood pressure, which was unaltered by either a nitric oxide synthase inhibitor or the B2R antagonist icatibant; this suggests that the vasodilatory properties of kallistatin may be mediated through a smooth muscle mechanism independent of bradykinin receptor activation.[387]

Kininases

With the exception of the metabolites des-Arg-bradykinin and des-Arg-kallidin, kinin-cleavage products are biologically inactive. Kinins are cleaved by a number of enzymes, including carboxypeptidases, ACE, and NEP. ACE also truncates its own reaction product, bradykinin-(1-7), further to form bradykinin-(1-5). NEP, like ACE, cleaves bradykinin at the 7-8 position and has a broad substrate specificity that includes not only the kinins but also the NPs, substance P, angiotensin II, big-ET, enkephalins, oxytocin, and gastrin. The amino-terminal of bradykinin possesses two proline residues and is susceptible to cleavage by the proline-specific exopeptidase aminopeptidase P. The resultant peptide, bradykinin-(2-9), may be further cleaved by proteases that include the endothelial enzyme dipeptidyl-aminopeptidase IV, which reduces this metabolite to bradykinin-(4-9).

Plasma and Tissue Kallikrein-Kinin System

The two independent KKSs in humans (plasma and tissue) can be distinguished by the specific subtypes of kallikreins, kininogens, and kinins involved. The circulating plasma KKS includes HMW kininogen and plasma prekallikrein, both of which are synthesized in the liver and secreted in the plasma, in which kallikrein is generated by the cell matrix–associated prekallikrein activator prolylcarboxypeptidase.[388] Of importance is that bradykinin is the main effector molecule of the plasma KKS. The tissue-specific KKS, whose involvement includes the kidneys, consists of locally synthesized or liver-derived kininogen (HMW and LMW), tissue kallikrein, and the effector molecules kallidin in humans and kallidin-like peptide in rodents. The half-life of kinins is 10 to 30 seconds, but in tissues with high kallikrein content, such as those of the kidneys, local and plasma-derived LMW kininogen can be continuously cleaved to produce kallidin.

Figure 12-7 illustrates the enzymatic cascades of the plasma and tissue KKSs.

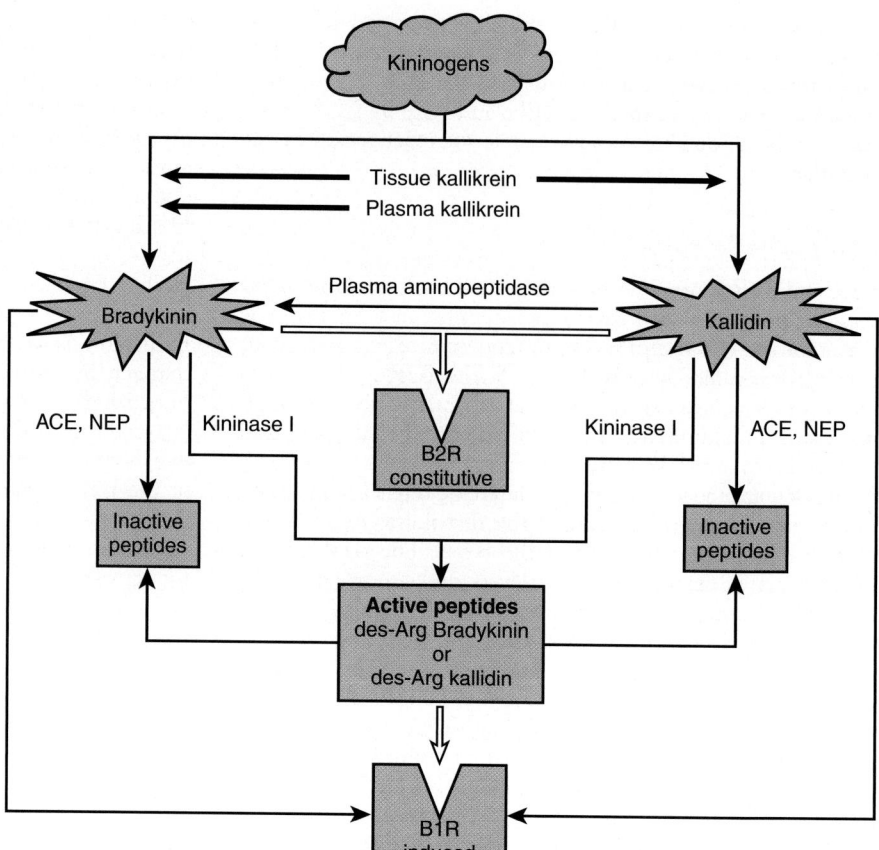

FIGURE 12-7 Enzymatic cascade of the kallikrein-kinin system. ACE, angiotensin converting enzyme; B1R, bradykinin B1 receptor; B2R, bradykinin B2 receptor; NEP, neutral endopeptidase.

Renal Kallikrein-Kinin System

The tissue KKS contributes to the physiologic functions of the kidneys with effects on renal vascular resistance, natriuresis, diuresis, and other vasoactive mediators, such as renin and angiotensin, eicosanoids, catecholamines, nitric oxide, vasopressin, and ET. In the kidneys, large quantities of kininogen and kallikrein are synthesized by the tubular epithelium and are excreted in the urine. Locally formed kinin is also detectable in the urine, renal interstitial fluid, and renal venous blood. In the human kidneys, kallikrein is localized to the connecting tubules with close anatomic association between the kallikrein-expressing tubules and the afferent arterioles of the JGA. Results of some studies suggest that renal kallikrein mRNA is also detectable by in situ hybridization at the glomerular vascular pole. This anatomic association highlights the physiologic relationship between the KKS and the RAS and is consistent with a paracrine function for the KKS in the regulation of renal blood flow, GFR, and renin release. In this regard, it has been suggested that, through effects on prostaglandin production, kinins may lower tubuloglomerular feedback sensitivity.

Expression of kallikrein within the kidneys is altered during development and is regulated by estrogen and progesterone, salt intake, thyroid hormone, and glucocorticoid.[389-392] The enzyme is not normally filtered at the glomerulus in the absence of glomerular injury. However, in the remnant kidney, kallikrein may be observed as absorption droplets within the proximal tubules, which is indicative of altered glomerular permeability.[393] Kininogens are localized mostly to connecting tubule principal cells near kallikrein, which can be found

in the connecting tubules of the same nephron. Once activated, renal kallikrein cleaves both HMW and LMW kininogens to release kallidin. The majority of the physiologic effects of kinins are mediated through activation of constitutively expressed B2Rs, with little or no B1R mRNA detectable in normal kidneys. In rats, administration of lipopolysaccharide, however, induces expression of B1R throughout the nephron (except the outer medullary collecting ducts), with strong expression in the efferent arteriole, medullary limb, and distal tubule.[394]

Activity of the renal KKS is usually assessed by measurement of urinary kallikrein concentrations. However, a number of factors may influence urinary kallikrein excretion: not only synthesis and secretion of the enzyme by tubular epithelial cells but also the presence of kallikrein inhibitors and kininases, as well as the pH and ionic concentration of the tubular fluid. Kinins may also be measured in the urine and vascular compartment. However, these peptides are rapidly degraded, and urinary or renal vein kinin concentrations may not reflect activity of the renal KKS. High-performance liquid chromatography–based radioimmunoassays have been developed for the specific measurement of hydroxylated and nonhydroxylated bradykinin and kallidin peptides and their metabolites.[395] With this technique, kallidin peptides were found to be more abundant than bradykinin peptides in the urine, and peptide levels in the urine were several orders of magnitude higher than those found in the plasma or tissue.[395,396]

The KKS is involved in the regulation of renal hemodynamics and tubular function; diuretic and natriuretic effects play a pivotal role in the contribution of the renal KKS to fluid and electrolyte balance. Kinins have been reported to increase renal blood flow and papillary blood flow and to mediate the hyperfiltration induced by a high-protein diet. These vasodilatory effects in the kidneys are mediated primarily by endothelium-derived nitric oxide, prostacyclin, and EDHF. Kinins also inhibit conductive sodium entry in the IMCDs,[397] and B2R-deficient mice demonstrate increased urinary concentration in response to vasopressin, which indicates that, through the B2R, endogenous kinins oppose the antidiuretic effect of vasopressin.[398] Kinins may therefore affect sodium reabsorption through direct effects on sodium transport along the nephron, through vasodilatory effects, and through changes in the osmotic gradient of the renal medulla. In addition to the effects on renal vascular tone, salt homeostasis, and water homeostasis, experiments with the B2R antagonist icatibant have yielded evidence that kinins may also have antihypertrophic and antiproliferative properties in mesangial cells, fibroblasts, and renomedullary interstitial cells. The antiproliferative effect of bradykinin in mesangial cells may be mediated through interaction of the B2R with the protein-tyrosine phosphatase SH2 domain–containing phosphatase-2 (SHP-2).[399] Finally, tissue kallikrein may play a role in renal tubular calcium transport. Tissue kallikrein–deficient mice, but not B2R-deficient mice, treated with a B1R antagonist showed impaired renal tubular calcium absorption, which is suggestive of a kinin-independent mechanism.[400] A distal tubular defect in calcium handling has also been reported in humans with the loss-of-function R53H polymorphism in the tissue kallikrein gene.[401]

Interactions of the Kallikrein-Kinin System and the Renin-Angiotensin System

The KKS and the RAS interact during growth, development, inflammation, blood pressure control, and regulation of renal function.[402] The central link between the KKS and the RAS is ACE, which regulates circulating levels of kinins and angiotensin II. Although increased bradykinin levels as a consequence of ACE inhibition are widely considered to mediate some of the blood pressure–independent effects of this class of agents[369] (including the side effect of cough), the RAS and KKS are linked at a number of additional levels. For example, there is an anatomic proximity of kallikrein- and renin-producing cells in the kidneys; B2R agonists stimulate renin release from isolated rat glomeruli[403]; and renal renin mRNA is reduced in B2R-knockout mice.[404] B2R activity is also potentiated by ACE inhibition independently of the effect on reduced kinin degradation, through angiotensin derivatives such as angiotensin-(1-7).[405] Kallikrein probably also acts as a prorenin-activating enzyme.[371] Both the AT_1 receptor and the B2R are seven transmembrane G protein–coupled receptors and are coexpressed in several renal cell types. The AT_1 receptor and B2R are capable of forming stable heterodimers, which leads to increased activation of Ga_q and Ga_i proteins and enhances signaling through both receptors.[52] Interestingly, preeclamptic women have been found to have increased levels of AT_1-B2R heterodimerization, which may contribute to the enhanced responsiveness to angiotensin II in these patients.[406] In addition to this physical association, the AT_1 receptor and B2R are also linked at the gene level, at which angiotensin II induces B2R expression through the AT_1 receptor.[407]

The Kallikrein-Kinin System in Renal Disease

Hypertension

Although it has been known for many years that kinin infusion results in an acute drop in systemic blood pressure by reducing peripheral resistance, the role of the KKS in mediating primary or secondary hypertension has yet to be fully established. Decreased activity of kallikrein has been reported in the urine of hypertensive patients and hypertensive rats. An inverse relationship between urinary kallikrein excretion and blood pressure in humans may be suggestive of a role for the renal KKS in protecting against hypertension.[408] However, an alternative interpretation may be that preexisting or hypertension-induced renal disease may itself lead to a reduction in renal kallikrein excretion. In the Dahl salt-sensitive rat model of hypertension, ACE inhibitors attenuate the progression of proteinuria and hypertensive nephrosclerosis better than do angiotensin II receptor blockers.[409] That this difference may be mediated by enhanced kinin activity with ACE inhibition is supported by the observations that infusion of either kallikrein[410] or bradykinin[411] in this model attenuated glomerulosclerosis without affecting blood pressure. Studies in two-kidney, one-clip hypertension have yielded conflicting results. The incidence of two-kidney, one-clip hypertension was increased in B2R-deficient mice, in comparison with wild-type animals.[412] In contrast, with regard to the response between tissue kallikrein–deficient mice and wild-type animals, there was no difference with regard to kidney size, renin release, systemic blood pressure increase, and cardiac remodeling.[413]

Despite the uncertainty about the role of the KKS in mediating the pathogenesis of hypertension, a variety of genetic mutations of the KKS have been associated with hypertension in animal models and in humans.[414] Inactivating mutations in the kallikrein gene have been identified in spontaneously hypertensive rats,[415] and an association between mutations in the regulatory region of the kallikrein gene KLK1 and hypertension has also been described in African Americans[416] and Chinese Han people.[417] A common loss-of-function polymorphism in humans, found in 5% to 7% of the white population, is the KLK1 R53H mutation.[418] However, this one single-nucleotide polymorphism (SNP) has not in itself been found to markedly alter blood pressure.[419] ACE polymorphisms, responsible for different plasma levels of the enzyme and, accordingly, altered kinin levels, have been identified as independent risk factors for progression of various diseases, including diabetic nephropathy, but they do not affect blood pressure. Finally, a number of SNPs in both the B2R and B1R genes have been associated with hypertension[420,421] and coronary risk in hypertensive individuals.[422]

Diabetic Nephropathy

Observations in both experimental animal models and in humans indicate a role for altered KKS activity in the pathogenesis of diabetic nephropathy. The KKS is markedly altered in rats with streptozotocin-induced diabetes; changes are correlated with those in renal plasma flow and GFR.[423] Renal and urinary levels of active kallikrein are increased in such rats with moderate hyperglycemia in association with reduced renal vascular resistance, increased GFR, and increased renal plasma flow.[423] Treatment of such animals with the kallikrein inhibitor aprotinin or with a B2R antagonist reduced renal blood flow and GFR.[423] In contrast, in non–insulin-treated streptozotocin-treated rats with severe hyperglycemia and hypofiltration, kallikrein excretion and expression were reduced.[423,424] In addition to its hemodynamic effects, the KKS may also play a renoprotective role in diabetic nephropathy through its antiinflammatory and antiproliferative properties.[371] Although the kinins induce proliferation of quiescent renal cells through activation of the B2R, mesangial cell proliferation induced through insulin-like growth factor-1–induced ERK1/2 activation is inhibited by bradykinin through calcium-dependent tyrosine phosphatase activation.[425]

Results of receptor antagonist studies initially suggested that the KKS had a limited role in preserving renal structure and function in diabetic nephropathy: Treatment of diabetic rats with icatibant had no effect on glomerular structure or on albuminuria, nor did it alter the attenuating effect of ACE inhibition on either of these parameters.[426] In contrast to this finding, however, the results of more contemporary work suggest that the beneficial effects of ACE inhibitors in experimental diabetic nephropathy may be attenuated by coadministration of a B2R antagonist.[427-429] For instance, in Akita diabetic mice lacking the B2R, there was a marked increase in mesangial sclerosis and a worsening of albuminuria,[430] in association with an increase in oxidative stress and mitochondrial damage[431]; however, another study revealed that B2R-knockout mice were relatively protected from the renal injury caused by streptozotocin-induced diabetes.[432] In support of a renoprotective effect of the KKS in diabetic nephropathy, one study showed that induction of diabetes by streptozotocin in mice caused a twofold increase in mRNA for kininogen, tissue kallikrein, kinins, and kinin receptors, with a doubling in albumin excretion in kallikrein-knockout mice in comparison with wild-type animals.[433] In another study, gene delivery of human tissue kallikrein with an adeno-associated virus vector attenuated renal injury in diabetes and decreased urinary albumin excretion.[434] Urinary kallikrein excretion in patients with type 1 diabetes demonstrates a similar association with GFR as observed in rats with streptozotocin-induced diabetes.[435] Active kallikrein excretion is increased in hyperfiltering individuals in comparison both with patients with type 1 diabetes who have a normal GFR and with normal controls, and it is correlated with both GFR and distal tubular sodium reabsorption.[435] Results of genetic association studies in diabetic patients have, however, been conflicting: One study demonstrated an association between B2R polymorphisms and albuminuria in 49 patients with type 1 diabetes and 112 patients with type 2 diabetes,[436] whereas another revealed no association between either B1R or B2R polymorphisms and incipient or overt nephropathy in 285 patients with type 2 diabetes.[437]

Ischemic Renal Injury

In models of ischemia-reperfusion injury, ACE inhibitors appear to be superior to angiotensin II receptor blockers in protecting against tubular necrosis, loss of endothelial function, and excretory dysfunction.[438] This superiority may be attributed to enhanced kinin activity with ACE inhibition, inasmuch as the effect is negated by B2R antagonists and inhibitors of nitric oxide synthase.[439,440] Bradykinin suppresses the opening of mitochondrial pores,[441] and nitric oxide suppresses oxidative metabolism; both observations indicate that the KKS may exert its protective effects in

ischemia-reperfusion injury through attenuation of oxidative damage. In mice with genetic deficiencies in either the B2R alone or both B1R and B2R, ischemic damage was enhanced in comparison with wild-type mice; injury was most severe in mice that lacked both receptors.[384] In contrast, tissue kallikrein infusion aggravated renal ischemia-reperfusion injury in rats.[442] Thus, although physiologic kinin levels may be protective in this setting, higher levels may be detrimental, possibly through pathologic reperfusion.[369]

Chronic Kidney Disease

In the remnant kidney model of progressive renal disease, adenovirus-mediated or adeno-associated virus–mediated gene delivery of kallikrein attenuated the decline in renal function.[443] In the model of unilateral ureteric obstruction, both genetic ablation of the B2R and pharmacologic blockade of the B2R increase tubulointerstitial fibrosis.[444] In contrast, expression of the B1R is increased after unilateral ureteric obstruction,[445] and treatment with a nonpeptide B1R antagonist reduced macrophage infiltration and fibrosis.[445] In the same model, B1R-deficient mice similarly showed less upregulation of inflammatory cytokines, reduced albumin excretion, and diminished fibrosis in comparison with wild-type mice.[446] Together, these observations suggest that although the B2R is renoprotective, B1R upregulation may contribute to the pathogenesis of renal fibrosis. In humans, polymorphisms in both the B1R gene[447,448] and B2R gene[447,449] have been associated with the development of end-stage renal disease.

Lupus Nephritis/Anti–Glomerular Basement Membrane Disease

Recent evidence has linked the KKS to the pathogenesis of the immune-mediated nephritides SLE, Goodpasture's syndrome (anti–glomerular basement membrane [GBM] disease), and spontaneous lupus nephritis. Mice strains differ in their susceptibility to anti-GBM antibody–induced nephritis. Comparison of disease-sensitive and control strains, by microarray analysis of renal cortical tissue, revealed that 360 gene transcripts were differentially expressed.[450] Of the underexpressed genes, one fifth belonged to the kallikrein gene family.[450] Furthermore, in disease-sensitive mice, B2R antagonism augmented proteinuria after anti-GBM challenge, whereas bradykinin administration attenuated disease.[450] In the same study, SNPs in the KLK1 and KLK3 promoters were also described in patients with SLE and lupus nephritis.[450] Extending their work further, the same investigators showed that adenoviral delivery of the KLK1 gene attenuated renal injury in congenic mice possessing a lupus-susceptibility interval on chromosome 7.[451]

Antineutrophil Cytoplasmic Antibody–Associated Vasculitis

Wegener's-type antineutrophil cytoplasmic antibody–associated vasculitis (AAV) may be associated with a necrotizing glomerulonephritis. The major antigenic target in Wegener's-type AAV is neutrophil-derived proteinase 3 (PR3). Incubation of PR3 with HMW kininogen resulted in the generation of a novel tridecapeptide kinin, termed *PR3-kinin*.[452] PR3-kinin binds to B1R directly and can also activate B2R after further processing to form bradykinin.[452] These observations suggest that, in Wegener's-type AAV, PR3 may activate the kinin pathway in a kallikrein-independent manner.

Cell Therapy

Both mesenchymal stem cells[453-457] and endothelial progenitor cells[458] have been shown to attenuate renal injury, particularly in the setting of acute injury. Ex vivo modulation of mesenchymal stem cells or endothelial progenitor cells has the potential to enhance their reparative capacity. In this regard, transfection of mesenchymal stem cells with human KLK1 increased the ability of mesenchymal stem cells to protect against renal injury after ischemia and reperfusion.[459] Bradykinin can act as a chemoattractant to endothelial progenitor cells through the B2R,[460] and KLK1-transfected endothelial progenitor cells may enhance blood flow recovery of ischemic hindlimbs.[366] Whether these properties can be translated to an improvement in renal ischemia remains to be determined.

Urotensin II

Urotensin II (U-II) is a potent vasoactive cyclic undecapeptide originally isolated from the caudal neurosecretory organ of teleost fish. The two principal regulatory peptides derived from this organ are urotensin I (U-I), which is homologous to mammalian corticotropin-releasing factor, and U-II, which bears sequence similarity to somatostatin[461] and has notable hemodynamic, gastrointestinal, reproductive, osmoregulatory, and metabolic functions in fish. Homologs of U-II have been identified in many species, including humans.

Synthesis, Structure, and Secretion of Urotensin II

Human U-II is derived from two prepropeptide alternate splice variants of 124 and 139 amino acids, differing only in the N-terminal sequence.[462,463] The C terminus is cleaved by

prohormone convertases to yield the mature 11–amino acid U-II peptide. U-II contains a cyclic Cys-Phe-Trp-Lys-Tyr-Cys hexapeptide sequence that is conserved across species and is essential for its biologic activity (Figure 12-8).[464] The N-terminal region of the precursor is highly variable across species. Prepro–U-II mRNA has been described in a range of cell types, including vascular smooth muscle cells, endothelial cells, neuronal cells, and cardiac fibroblasts. Multiple monobasic and polybasic amino acid sequences have been identified as posttranslational cleavage sites of the prohormone. However, a specific U-II converting enzyme has not yet been described. It is also currently unclear whether U-II is processed within the cells in which it is expressed or whether the prohormone is secreted and cleaved either at a remote site or within the circulation.[465,466] With regard to its tissue distribution, immunohistochemical staining has identified U-II protein in the blood vessels of various organs and also within the tubular epithelial cells of the kidneys.[461,467,468] A significant arteriovenous gradient exists across the heart, liver, and kidneys, which indicates that these organs are important sites of U-II production.[469]

In 1999, Ames and colleagues[463] identified U-II as the ligand for the previously orphan rat receptor GPR14/SENR. The U-II receptor (commonly referred to as the UT receptor) is a seven-transmembrane, G protein–coupled receptor encoded on chromosome 17q25.3 in humans.[470] The UT receptor bears structural similarity to both somatostatin receptor subtype 4 and the opioid receptors. Ligand binding of the receptor results in G protein–mediated activation of protein kinase C, calmodulin, and phospholipase C; evidence also links MAP kinases ERK1/2 and the Rho kinase pathway in the intracellular signaling cascade.[471-473]

The relationship between U-II and the UT receptor is not exclusive; the receptor also binds alternative U-II fragments such as U-II(4-11) and U-II(5-11), as well as urotensin-related peptide (URP).[466,474] URP was originally isolated from rat brain and binds with high affinity to the UT receptor.[474] Although this 8–amino acid peptide retains the cyclic hexapeptide sequence, it is derived from a different precursor to U-II and may have different physiologic properties.[465]

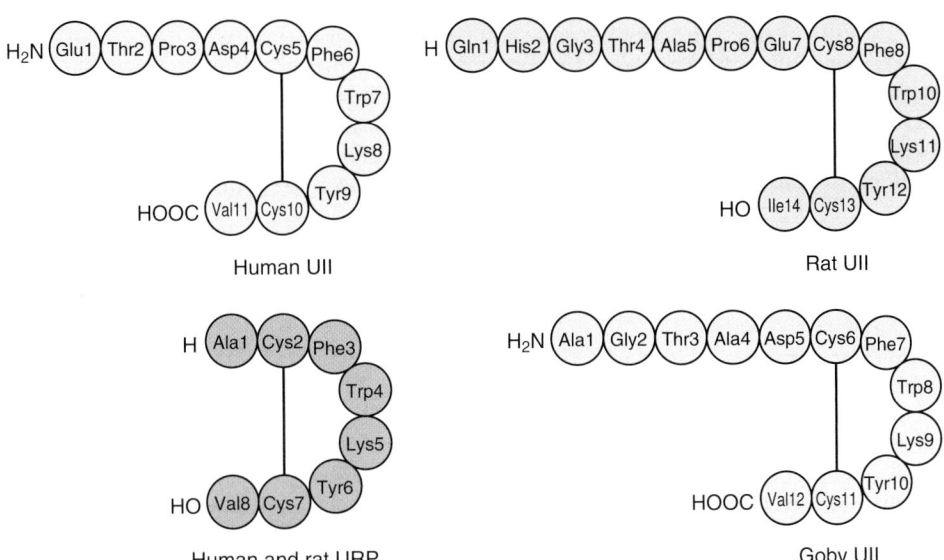

Human UII

Rat UII

Human and rat URP

Goby UII

FIGURE 12-8 Molecular structure of human, rat, and goby urotensin II. (Adapted from Ashton N: Renal and vascular actions of urotensin II, *Kidney Int* 2006;70:624-629.)

Physiologic Role of Urotensin II

U-II is the most potent vasoconstrictor known, being 16 times more potent than ET-1 in the isolated rat thoracic aorta.[463] However, its vasoconstrictive properties are not universal, varying between species and between vascular beds. For example, U-II has little or no effect on venous tone, and it does not cause constriction of rat abdominal aorta, femoral arteries, or renal arteries.[475] It also lacks systemic pressor activity when administered intravenously to anesthetized rats.[463,476] In cynomolgus monkeys, bolus intravenous injection of U-II induced myocardial depression, circulatory collapse, and death.[463] In contrast to the vasoconstrictive properties of vascular smooth muscle UT receptor, endothelial UT receptor may mediate vasodilation in pulmonary and mesenteric vessels.[477] The response to U-II may be dependent on the caliber of the artery; a small-vessel response is more endothelium mediated, and a large-vessel response is more dependent on vascular smooth muscle.[461] These disparities are among many examples of how the role of U-II may be influenced by a number of factors, including animal model, vascular bed, method of exogenous U-II administration, and the presence of comorbid conditions.

Urotensin II in the Kidneys

The kidney is a major site of U-II production; this is indicated by both the arteriovenous gradient of plasma U-II across the kidneys and the observation that urinary U-II clearance exceeds urinary creatinine clearance.[461,469] In fact, in humans, urinary concentrations of U-II are approximately three orders of magnitude higher than plasma concentrations.[478] U-II is present in a number of kidney cell types, including the smooth muscle cells and endothelium of arteries, proximal convoluted tubules, and particularly the distal tubules and collecting ducts.[468] UT receptor mRNA is also present in the kidneys, particularly within the renal medulla,[478-480] which suggests that the peptide may have autocrine or paracrine functions at this site. In addition, URP mRNA has also been described in both rat and human kidneys,[474,479,480] and its expression is increased in the kidneys of subtotally nephrectomized rats,[481] which potentially implicates this peptide in the pathogenesis of progressive renal disease. Studies of the role of U-II in normal renal physiology have yielded conflicting findings. In one report, continuous infusion of U-II into the renal artery of anesthetized rats caused nitric oxide–dependent increases in GFR, urinary water excretion, and urinary sodium excretion.[482] In contrast, another study showed that bolus injection of picomolar concentrations of U-II produced a dose-dependent decrease in GFR and a reduction in urine flow and urinary sodium excretion.[480] Furthermore, a third group of researchers reported that intravenous bolus injection of U-II in nanomolar amounts induced only a minor reduction in GFR and had no effect on sodium excretion.[483] These researchers also investigated the effect of U-II administration in the context of experimental congestive heart failure, in which the peptide induced an almost 30% increase in GFR.[483] Although these discrepancies may be explained partly by a difference in experimental models and method of administration, the variable results may also reflect differences in receptor reserve.[484]

Observational Studies of Urotensin II in Renal Disease

Increased concentrations of U-II in the plasma and urine have been found in a number of diseases. U-II levels in plasma may be increased in hypertensive individuals in comparison with normotensive controls and are correlated with systolic blood pressure.[485] U-II concentrations in plasma are also increased twofold in patients with renal disease not on hemodialysis and threefold in patients on hemodialysis.[486] Higher U-II levels in urine have been described in patients with essential hypertension, in patients with glomerular disease and hypertension, and in patients with renal tubular disorders, but not in normotensive patients with glomerular disease.[478] U-II levels in both plasma and urine have been reported to be higher in patients with type 2 diabetes and renal disease than in such patients with normal renal function.[487] Increased expression of both U-II and the UT receptor have also been demonstrated in biopsy samples of patients with diabetic nephropathy[488]; increased U-II levels have also been described in glomerulonephritis[489] and in minimal change disease.[490]

Epidemiologic Evidence for a Protective Role of Urotensin II in End-Stage Renal Disease

Initial observations of increased plasma levels of U-II in renal disease were interpreted as implicating the peptide in the pathogenesis of either renal disease or its associated cardiovascular complications; however, subsequent epidemiologic observations have challenged this view. In patients with end-stage renal disease, elevated plasma levels of U-II were correlated inversely with levels of sympathetic activity and BNP.[491] This finding suggests that either U-II downregulation is a counterregulatory response or, in this population at least, U-II may act as a protective factor. In accordance with this latter scenario, the same group of investigators[492] subsequently reported that in patients with end-stage renal disease, plasma levels of U-II were correlated inversely with rates of both fatal and nonfatal cardiovascular events and that higher U-II levels were associated with preserved left ventricular systolic function.[493] These observations have been extended to patients with stages 2 to 5 CKD, which again highlights an inverse correlation between plasma levels of U-II and rates of all-cause and cardiovascular mortality.[494] Because U-II is a potent nitric oxide–dependent vasodilator in pulmonary and mesenteric vessels, it is possible that increased U-II level in end-stage renal disease is an adaptive response to increased neurohumoral activation and nitric oxide inhibition.[466] Thus, in at least some circumstances, U-II may exert a protective effect in cardiorenal disease. Because of this possibility, results of interventional studies aimed at mitigating an activated urotensin system should be interpreted with caution.

Interventional Studies of Urotensin II in the Kidneys

In view of the elevation of U-II levels in a range of disease states, there has been a concerted effort to develop agents that antagonize the system. Both peptide and nonpeptide UT receptor antagonists are currently being studied. Urantide is a derivative of human U-II.[495] Continuous infusion of urantide into rats induces an increase in GFR and natriuresis,[480] although it is not clear whether the natriuresis is a consequence of altered renal vascular tone or a direct effect of U-II on the tubular epithelium. Although urantide is a potent antagonist of the rat UT receptor,[495] it has been found to have agonist properties in cells expressing the human UT receptor.[496] An alternative U-II peptide antagonist, UFP-803, also has partial agonist properties in human UT receptor–expressing cells,[497] which complicates the interpretation of a peptide-based approach to U-II inhibition. Two compounds in the nonpeptide group of U-II antagonists have been studied in experimental models: palosuran (ACT-058362) and SB-611812. Intravenous administration of palosuran protected against renal ischemia in a rat model.[498] The same compound was also studied in rats with streptozotocin-induced diabetes, in which it was found to significantly reduce the severity of albuminuria.[499] Actelion Pharmaceuticals, the developer of palosuran, initiated phase II studies of the agent in diabetic patients; however, the studies were terminated early because of a lack of efficacy. Although limited data are available from these studies, no safety issues were identified.[461] SB-611812 decreased the carotid intima/media ratio in a rat model of balloon angioplasty–induced stenosis.[500] The same compound attenuated myocardial remodeling and was associated with a reduced rate of mortality in a rat model of ischemic cardiomyopathy.[501,502] At present, there are no reports of the effect of SB-611812 in experimental models of renal disease.

References

1. Tigerstedt R, Bergman P. Niere und Kreislauf. *Skandinävisches Archiev für Physiologie.* 1898;8:223-271.
2. Anderson S, Meyer TW, Rennke HG, et al. Control of glomerular hypertension limits glomerular injury in rats with reduced renal mass. *J Clin Invest.* 1985;76:612-619.
3. Morris BJ, Iwamoto HS, Reid IA. Localization of angiotensinogen in rat liver by immunocytochemistry. *Endocrinology.* 1979;105:796-800.
4. Griendling KK, Murphy TJ, Alexander RW. Molecular biology of the renin-angiotensin system. *Circulation.* 1993;87:1816-1828.
5. Clauser E, Gaillard I, Wei L, et al. Regulation of angiotensinogen gene. *Am J Hypertens.* 1989;2:403-410.
6. Hoj Nielsen A, Knudsen F. Angiotensinogen is an acute-phase protein in man. *Scand J Clin Lab Invest.* 1987;47:175-178.
7. Ron D, Brasier AR, Habener JF. Angiotensinogen gene-inducible enhancer-binding protein 1, a member of a new family of large nuclear proteins that recognize nuclear factor kappa B-binding sites through a zinc finger motif. *Mol Cell Biol.* 1991;11:2887-2895.
8. Dzau VJ, Burt DW, Pratt RE. Molecular biology of the renin-angiotensin system. *Am J Physiol.* 1988;255:F563-F573.
9. Schweda F, Friis U, Wagner C, et al. Renin release. *Physiology (Bethesda).* 2007;22:310-319.
10. Neves FA, Duncan KG, Baxter JD. Cathepsin B is a prorenin processing enzyme. *Hypertension.* 1996;27:514-517.
11. Reudelhuber TL, Ramla D, Chiu L, et al. Proteolytic processing of human prorenin in renal and non-renal tissues. *Kidney Int.* 1994;46:1522-1524.
12. Saris JJ, Derkx FH, De Bruin RJ, et al. High-affinity prorenin binding to cardiac man-6-P/IGF-II receptors precedes proteolytic activation to renin. *Am J Physiol Heart Circ Physiol.* 2001;280:H1706-H1715.
13. van den Eijnden MM, Saris JJ, de Bruin RJ, et al. Prorenin accumulation and activation in human endothelial cells: importance of mannose 6-phosphate receptors. *Arterioscler Thromb Vasc Biol.* 2001;21:911-916.
14. Danser AH, Deinum J. Renin, prorenin and the putative (pro)renin receptor. *Hypertension.* 2005;46:1069-1076.
15. Lumbers ER. Activation of renin in human amniotic fluid by low pH. *Enzymologia.* 1971;40:329-336.
16. Skinner SL, Cran EJ, Gibson R, et al. Angiotensins I and II, active and inactive renin, renin substrate, renin activity, and angiotensinase in human liquor amnii and plasma. *Am J Obstet Gynecol.* 1975;121:626-630.
17. Pitarresi TM, Rubattu S, Heinrikson R, et al. Reversible cryoactivation of recombinant human prorenin. *J Biol Chem.* 1992;267:11753-11759.
18. Nguyen G, Delarue F, Burckle C, et al. Pivotal role of the renin/prorenin receptor in angiotensin II production and cellular responses to renin. *J Clin Invest.* 2002;109:1417-1427.
19. Skinner SL, McCubbin JW, Page IH. Control of renin secretion. *Circ Res.* 1964;15:64-76.
20. Hackenthal E, Paul M, Ganten D, et al. Morphology, physiology, and molecular biology of renin secretion. *Physiol Rev.* 1990;70:1067-1116.
21. Schnermann J. Juxtaglomerular cell complex in the regulation of renal salt excretion. *Am J Physiol.* 1998;274:R263-R279.
22. Oliver WJ, Cohen EL, Neel JV. Blood pressure, sodium intake, and sodium related hormones in the Yanomamo Indians, a "no-salt" culture. *Circulation.* 1975;52:146-151.
23. Hebert SC. Physiology: orphan detectors of metabolism. *Nature.* 2004;429:143-145.
24. He W, Miao FJ, Lin DC, et al. Citric acid cycle intermediates as ligands for orphan G-protein–coupled receptors. *Nature.* 2004;429:188-193.
25. Vargas SL, Toma I, Kang JJ, et al. Activation of the succinate receptor GPR91 in macula densa cells causes renin release. *J Am Soc Nephrol.* 2009;20:1002-1011.
26. Luetscher LA, Kraemer FB, Wilson DM, et al. Increased plasma inactive renin in diabetes mellitus. A marker of microvascular complications. *New Engl J Med.* 1985;312:1412.
27. Allen TJ, Cooper ME, Gilbert RE, et al. Serum total renin is increased before microalbuminuria in diabetes. *Kidney Int.* 1996;50:902-907.
28. Campbell DJ, Nussberger J, Stowasser M, et al. Activity assays and immunoassays for plasma renin and prorenin: information provided and precautions necessary for accurate measurement. *Clin Chem.* 2009;55:867-877.
29. Menard J, Guyene TT, Peyrard S, et al. Conformational changes in prorenin during renin inhibition in vitro and in vivo. *J Hypertens.* 2006;24:529-534.
30. Kumar RS, Thekkumkara TJ, Sen GC. The mRNAs encoding the two angiotensin-converting isozymes are transcribed from the same gene by a tissue-specific choice of alternative transcription initiation sites. *J Biol Chem.* 1991;266:3854-3862.
31. Atanassova N, Lakova E, Bratchkova Y, et al. Expression of testicular angiotensin-converting enzyme in adult spontaneously hypertensive rats. *Folia Histochem Cytobiol.* 2009;47:117-122.
32. Perich RB, Jackson B, Rogerson F, et al. Two binding sites on angiotensin-converting enzyme: evidence from radioligand binding studies. *Mol Pharmacol.* 1992;42:286-293.
33. Lai KN, Leung JC, Lai KB, et al. Gene expression of the renin-angiotensin system in human kidney. *J Hypertens.* 1998;16:91-102.
34. Mehta PK, Griendling KK. Angiotensin II cell signaling: physiological and pathological effects in the cardiovascular system. *Am J Physiol Cell Physiol.* 2007;292:C82-C97.
35. Gloy J, Henger A, Fischer KG, et al. Angiotensin II modulates cellular functions of podocytes. *Kidney Int.* 1998;54:S168-S170.
36. Velez JC. The importance of the intrarenal renin-angiotensin system. *Nat Clin Pract Nephrol.* 2009;5:89-100.
37. Zhuo J, Alcorn D, Allen AM, et al. High resolution localization of angiotensin II receptors in rat renal medulla. *Kidney Int.* 1992;42:1372-1380.
38. Touyz RM, Schiffrin EL. Signal transduction mechanisms mediating the physiological and pathophysiological actions of angiotensin II in vascular smooth muscle cells. *Pharmacol Rev.* 2000;52:639-672.
39. Murasawa S, Mori Y, Nozawa Y, et al. Angiotensin II type 1 receptor–induced extracellular signal-regulated protein kinase activation is mediated by Ca2+/calmodulin-dependent transactivation of epidermal growth factor receptor. *Circ Res.* 1998;82:1338-1348.
40. Eguchi S, Numaguchi K, Iwasaki H, et al. Calcium-dependent epidermal growth factor receptor transactivation mediates the angiotensin II–induced mitogen-activated protein kinase activation in vascular smooth muscle cells. *J Biol Chem.* 1998;273:8890-8896.
41. Heeneman S, Haendeler J, Saito Y, et al. Angiotensin II induces transactivation of two different populations of the platelet-derived growth factor beta receptor. Key role for the adaptor protein Shc. *J Biol Chem.* 2000;275:15926-15932.
42. Linseman DA, Benjamin CW, Jones DA. Convergence of angiotensin II and platelet-derived growth factor receptor signaling cascades in vascular smooth muscle cells. *J Biol Chem.* 1995;270:12563-12568.
43. Lautrette A, Li S, Alili R, et al. Angiotensin II and EGF receptor cross-talk in chronic kidney diseases: a new therapeutic approach. *Nat Med.* 2005;11:867-874.
44. Wassef L, Kelly DJ, Gilbert RE. Epidermal growth factor receptor inhibition attenuates early kidney enlargement in experimental diabetes. *Kidney Int.* 2004;66:1805-1814.
45. Eskildsen-Helmond YE, Mulvany MJ. Pressure-induced activation of extracellular signal-regulated kinase 1/2 in small arteries. *Hypertension.* 2003;41:891-897.
46. Kelly DJ, Cox AJ, Gow RM, et al. Platelet-derived growth factor receptor transactivation mediates the trophic effects of angiotensin II in vivo. *Hypertension.* 2004;44:195-202.

47. Mogi M, Iwai M, Horiuchi M. New insights into the regulation of angiotensin receptors. *Curr Opin Nephrol Hypertens*. 2009;18:138-143.

48. Daviet L, Lehtonen JY, Tamura K, et al. Cloning and characterization of ATRAP, a novel protein that interacts with the angiotensin II type 1 receptor. *J Biol Chem*. 1999;274:17058-17062.

49. Guo DF, Chenier I, Lavoie JL, et al. Development of hypertension and kidney hypertrophy in transgenic mice overexpressing ARAP1 gene in the kidney. *Hypertension*. 2006;48:453-459.

50. Prinster SC, Hague C, Hall RA. Heterodimerization of G protein–coupled receptors: specificity and functional significance. *Pharmacol Rev*. 2005;57:289-298.

51. Hansen JL, Theilade J, Haunso S, et al. Oligomerization of wild type and nonfunctional mutant angiotensin II type I receptors inhibits gαq protein signaling but not ERK activation. *J Biol Chem*. 2004;279:24108-24115.

52. AbdAlla S, Lother H, Quitterer U. AT_1-receptor heterodimers show enhanced G-protein activation and altered receptor sequestration. *Nature*. 2000;407:94-98.

53. Zeng C, Wang Z, Asico LD, et al. Aberrant ETB receptor regulation of AT receptors in immortalized renal proximal tubule cells of spontaneously hypertensive rats. *Kidney Int*. 2005;68:623-631.

54. Zeng C, Liu Y, Wang Z, et al. Activation of D_3 dopamine receptor decreases angiotensin II type 1 receptor expression in rat renal proximal tubule cells. *Circ Res*. 2006;99:494-500.

55. Mogi M, Iwai M, Horiuchi M. Emerging concepts of regulation of angiotensin II receptors: new players and targets for traditional receptors. *Arterioscler Thromb Vasc Biol*. 2007;27:2532-2539.

56. Yasuda N, Miura S, Akazawa H, et al. I: Conformational switch of angiotensin II type 1 receptor underlying mechanical stress–induced activation. *EMBO Rep*. 2008;9:179-186.

57. Zou Y, Akazawa H, Qin Y, et al. Mechanical stress activates angiotensin II type 1 receptor without the involvement of angiotensin II. *Nat Cell Biol*. 2004;6:499-506.

58. Yatabe J, Sanada H, Yatabe MS, et al. Angiotensin II type 1 receptor blocker attenuates the activation of ERK and NADPH oxidase by mechanical strain in mesangial cells in the absence of angiotensin II. *Am J Physiol Renal Physiol*. 2009;296:F1052-F1060.

59. Wallukat G, Homuth V, Fischer T, et al. Patients with preeclampsia develop agonistic autoantibodies against the angiotensin AT_1 receptor. *J Clin Invest*. 1999;103:945-952.

60. Dragun D, Muller DN, Brasen JH, et al. Angiotensin II type 1–receptor activating antibodies in renal-allograft rejection. *N Engl J Med*. 2005;352:558-569.

61. Toke A, Meyer TW. Hemodynamic effects of angiotensin II in the kidney. *Contrib Nephrol*. 2001;135:34-46.

62. Navar LG, Inscho EW, Majid SA, et al. Paracrine regulation of the renal microcirculation. *Physiol Rev*. 1996;76:425-536.

63. Kennedy CR, Burns KD. Angiotensin II as a mediator of renal tubular transport. *Contrib Nephrol*. 2001;135:47-62.

64. Rothenberger F, Velic A, Stehberger PA, et al. Angiotensin II stimulates vacuolar H^+-ATPase activity in renal acid-secretory intercalated cells from the outer medullary collecting duct. *J Am Soc Nephrol*. 2007;18:2085-2093.

65. Pech V, Zheng W, Pham TD, et al. Angiotensin II activates H^+-ATPase in type A intercalated cells. *J Am Soc Nephrol*. 2008;19:84-91.

66. Koike G, Horiuchi M, Yamada T, et al. Human type 2 angiotensin II receptor gene: cloned, mapped to the X chromosome, and its mRNA is expressed in the human lung. *Biochem Biophys Res Commun*. 1994;203:1842-1850.

67. Reudelhuber TL. The continuing saga of the AT_2 receptor: a case of the good, the bad, and the innocuous. *Hypertension*. 2005;46:1261-1262.

68. Savoia C, Touyz RM, Volpe M, et al. Angiotensin type 2 receptor in resistance arteries of type 2 diabetic hypertensive patients. *Hypertension*. 2007;49:341-346.

69. Padia SH, Howell NL, Siragy HM, et al. Renal angiotensin type 2 receptors mediate natriuresis via angiotensin III in the angiotensin II type 1 receptor–blocked rat. *Hypertension*. 2006;47:537-544.

70. Miyata N, Park F, Li XF, et al. Distribution of angiotensin AT_1 and AT_2 receptor subtypes in the rat kidney. *Am J Physiol*. 1999;277:F437-F446.

71. Carey RM, Padia SH. Angiotensin AT_2 receptors: control of renal sodium excretion and blood pressure. *Trends Endocrinol Metab*. 2008;19:84-87.

72. Padia SH, Kemp BA, Howell NL, et al. Intrarenal aminopeptidase N inhibition augments natriuretic responses to angiotensin III in angiotensin type 1 receptor–blocked rats. *Hypertension*. 2007;49:625-630.

73. Huang Y, Wongamorntham S, Kasting J, et al. Renin increases mesangial cell transforming growth factor–beta1 and matrix proteins through receptor-mediated, angiotensin II–independent mechanisms. *Kidney Int*. 2006;69:105-113.

74. van den Heuvel M, Batenburg WW, Danser AH. Diabetic complications: a role for the prorenin–(pro)renin receptor–TGF-beta(1) axis?. *Mol Cell Endocrinol*. 2009;302:213-218.

75. Advani A, Kelly DJ, Cox AJ, et al. The (pro)renin receptor: site-specific and functional linkage to the vacuolar H^+-ATPase in the kidney. *Hypertension*. 2009;54:261-269.

76. Burckle C, Bader M. Prorenin and its ancient receptor. *Hypertension*. 2006;48:549-551.

77. Ichihara A, Hayashi M, Kaneshiro Y, et al. Inhibition of diabetic nephropathy by a decoy peptide corresponding to the "handle" region for nonproteolytic activation of prorenin. *J Clin Invest*. 2004;114:1128-1135.

78. Strausberg RL, Feingold EA, Grouse LH, et al. Generation and initial analysis of more than 15,000 full-length human and mouse cDNA sequences. *Proc Natl Acad Sci U S A*. 2002;99:16899-16903.

79. Campbell DJ. Critical review of prorenin and (pro)renin receptor research. *Hypertension*. 2008;51:1259-1264.

80. Bader M. The second life of the (pro)renin receptor. *J Renin Angiotensin Aldosterone Syst*. 2007;8:205-208.

81. Ludwig J, Kerscher S, Brandt U, et al. Identification and characterization of a novel 9.2-kDa membrane sector–associated protein of vacuolar proton-ATPase from chromaffin granules. *J Biol Chem*. 1998;273:10939-10947.

82. Wagner CA, Finberg KE, Breton S, et al. Renal vacuolar H^+-ATPase. *Physiol Rev*. 2004;84:1263-1314.

83. Tipnis SR, Hooper NM, Hyde R, et al. A human homolog of angiotensin-converting enzyme. Cloning and functional expression as a captopril-insensitive carboxypeptidase. *J Biol Chem*. 2000;275:33238-33243.

84. Donoghue M, Hsieh F, Baronas E, et al. A novel angiotensin-converting enzyme–related carboxypeptidase (ACE2) converts angiotensin I to angiotensin 1-9. *Circ Res*. 2000;87:E1-E9.

85. Turner AJ, Tipnis SR, Guy JL, et al. ACEH/ACE2 is a novel mammalian metallocarboxypeptidase and a homologue of angiotensin-converting enzyme insensitive to ACE inhibitors. *Can J Physiol Pharmacol*. 2002;80:346-353.

86. Ingelfinger JR. Angiotensin-converting enzyme 2: implications for blood pressure and kidney disease. *Curr Opin Nephrol Hypertens*. 2009;18:79-84.

87. Der Sarkissian S, Grobe JL, Yuan L, et al. Cardiac overexpression of angiotensin converting enzyme 2 protects the heart from ischemia-induced pathophysiology. *Hypertension*. 2008;51:712-718.

88. Masson R, Nicklin SA, Craig MA, et al. Onset of experimental severe cardiac fibrosis is mediated by overexpression of angiotensin-converting enzyme 2. *Hypertension*. 2009;53:694-700.

89. Soler MJ, Wysocki J, Batlle D. Angiotensin-converting enzyme 2 and the kidney. *Exp Physiol*. 2008;93:549-556.

90. Wong DW, Oudit GY, Reich H, et al. Loss of angiotensin-converting enzyme–2 (ACE2) accelerates diabetic kidney injury. *Am J Pathol*. 2007;171:438-451.

91. Li W, Moore MJ, Vasilieva N, et al. Angiotensin-converting enzyme 2 is a functional receptor for the SARS coronavirus. *Nature*. 2003;426:450-454.

92. Fyhrquist F, Saijonmaa O. Renin-angiotensin system revisited. *J Intern Med*. 2008;264:224-236.

93. Zini S, Fournie-Zaluski MC, Chauvel E, et al. Identification of metabolic pathways of brain angiotensin II and III using specific aminopeptidase inhibitors: predominant role of angiotensin III in the control of vasopressin release. *Proc Natl Acad Sci U S A*. 1996;93:11968-11973.

94. Gammelgaard I, Wamberg S, Bie P. Systemic effects of angiotensin III in conscious dogs during acute double blockade of the renin-angiotensin-aldosterone system. *Acta Physiol (Oxf)*. 2006;188:129-138.

95. Stragier B, De Bundel D, Sarre S, et al. Involvement of insulin-regulated aminopeptidase in the effects of the renin-angiotensin fragment angiotensin IV: a review. *Heart Fail Rev*. 2008;13:321-337.

96. Esteban V, Ruperez M, Sanchez-Lopez E, et al. Angiotensin IV activates the nuclear transcription factor–κB and related proinflammatory genes in vascular smooth muscle cells. *Circ Res*. 2005;96:965-973.

97. Kerins DM, Hao Q, Vaughan DE. Angiotensin induction of PAI-1 expression in endothelial cells is mediated by the hexapeptide angiotensin IV. *J Clin Invest*. 1995;96:2515-2520.

98. Tallant EA, Ferrario CM, Gallagher PE. Angiotensin-(1-7) inhibits growth of cardiac myocytes through activation of the Mas receptor. *Am J Physiol Heart Circ Physiol*. 2005;289:H1560-H1566.

99. Ferrario CM. Angiotensin-converting enzyme 2 and angiotensin-(1-7): an evolving story in cardiovascular regulation. *Hypertension*. 2006;47:515-521.

100. Strawn WB, Ferrario CM, Tallant EA. Angiotensin-(1-7) reduces smooth muscle growth after vascular injury. *Hypertension*. 1999;33:207-211.

101. Dharmani M, Mustafa MR, Achike FI, et al. Effect of des-aspartate–angiotensin I on the actions of angiotensin II in the isolated renal and mesenteric vasculature of hypertensive and STZ-induced diabetic rats. *Regul Pept*. 2005;129:213-219.

102. Cummins PM. A new addition to the renin-angiotensin peptide family: proAngiotensin-12 (PA12). *Cardiovasc Res*. 2009;82:7-8.

103. Paul M, Poyan Mehr A, Kreutz R. Physiology of local renin-angiotensin systems. *Physiol Rev*. 2006;86:747-803.

104. Kobori H, Nangaku M, Navar LG, et al. The intrarenal renin-angiotensin system: from physiology to the pathobiology of hypertension and kidney disease. *Pharmacol Rev.* 2007;59:251-287.
105. Braam B, Mitchell KD, Fox J, et al. Proximal tubular secretion of angiotensin II in rats. *Am J Physiol.* 1993;264:F891-F898.
106. Ingelfinger JR, Zuo WM, Fon EA, et al. In situ hybridization evidence for angiotensinogen messenger RNA in rat proximal tubule. *J Clin Invest.* 1990;85:417-423.
107. Nishiyama A, Seth DM, Navar LG. Renal interstitial fluid concentrations of angiotensins I and II in anesthetized rats. *Hypertension.* 2002;39:129-134.
108. Sequeira Lopez ML, Pentz ES, Nomasa T, et al. Renin cells are precursors for multiple cell types that switch to the renin phenotype when homeostasis is threatened. *Dev Cell.* 2004;6:719-728.
109. Gilbert RE, Wu LL, Kelly DJ, et al. Pathological expression of renin and angiotensin II in the renal tubule after subtotal nephrectomy—implications for the pathogenesis of tubulointerstitial fibrosis. *Am J Pathol.* 1999;155:429-440.
110. Holdsworth SR, Summers SA. Role of mast cells in progressive renal diseases. *J Am Soc Nephrol.* 2008;19:2254-2261.
111. Silver RB, Reid AC, Mackins CJ, et al. Mast cells: a unique source of renin. *Proc Natl Acad Sci U S A.* 2004;101:13607-13612.
112. Haller H, Lindschau C, Erdmann B, et al. Effects of intracellular angiotensin II in vascular smooth muscle cells. *Circ Res.* 1996;79:765-772.
113. Re R. Intracellular renin-angiotensin system: the tip of the intracrine physiology iceberg. *Am J Physiol Heart Circ Physiol.* 2007;293:H905-H906.
114. Hostetter TH, Olson JL, Rennke HG. Hyperfiltration in remnant nephrons: a potentially adverse response to renal ablation. *Am J Physiol.* 1981;241:F85-F93.
115. Blantz RC, Konnen KS, Tucker BJ. Angiotensin II effects upon the glomerular microcirculation and ultrafiltration coefficient of the rat. *J Clin Invest.* 1976;57:419-434.
116. Anderson S, Rennke HG, Brenner BM. Therapeutic advantage of converting enzyme inhibitors in arresting progressive renal disease associated with systemic hypertension in the rat. *J Clin Invest.* 1986;77:1993-2000.
117. Zatz R, Dunn BR, Meyer TW, et al. Prevention of diabetic glomerulopathy by pharmacological amelioration of glomerular capillary hypertension. *J Clin Invest.* 1986;77:1925-1930.
118. Kagami S, Border WA, Miller DE, et al. Angiotensin II stimulates extracellular matrix protein synthesis through induction of transforming growth factor–beta expression in rat glomerular mesangial cells. *J Clin Invest.* 1994;93:2431-2437.
119. Wolf G, Mueller E, Stahl RAK, et al. Angiotensin II–induced hypertrophy of cultured murine proximal tubular cells is mediated by endogenous transforming growth factor–β. *J Clin Invest.* 1993;92:1366-1372.
120. Wu L, Cox A, Roe C, et al. Transforming growth factor β1 and renal injury following subtotal nephrectomy in the rat: role of the renin-angiotensin system. *Kidney Int.* 1997;51:1553-1567.
121. Gilbert RE, Cox A, Wu LL, et al. Expression of transforming growth factor–β1 and type IV collagen in the renal tubulointerstitium in experimental diabetes: effects of angiotensin converting enzyme inhibition. *Diabetes.* 1998;47:414-422.
122. Langham RG, Kelly DJ, Gow RM, et al. Transforming growth factor–beta in human diabetic nephropathy: effects of ACE inhibition. *Diabetes Care.* 2006;29:2670-2675.
123. Houlihan CA, Akdeniz A, Tsalamandris C, et al. Urinary transforming growth factor–beta excretion in patients with hypertension, type 2 diabetes, and elevated albumin excretion rate: effects of angiotensin receptor blockade and sodium restriction. *Diabetes Care.* 2002;25:1072-1077.
124. Mifsud SA, Allen TJ, Bertram JF, et al. Podocyte foot process broadening in experimental diabetic nephropathy: amelioration with renin-angiotensin blockade. *Diabetologia.* 2001;44:870-873.
125. Suzuki K, Han GD, Miyauchi N, et al. Angiotensin II type 1 and type 2 receptors play opposite roles in regulating the barrier function of kidney glomerular capillary wall. *Am J Pathol.* 2007;170:1841-1853.
126. Langham RG, Kelly DJ, Cox AJ, et al. Proteinuria and the expression of the podocyte slit diaphragm protein, nephrin, in diabetic nephropathy: effects of angiotensin converting enzyme inhibition. *Diabetologia.* 2002;45:1572-1576.
127. Wu LL, Yang N, Roe CJ, et al. Macrophage and myofibroblast proliferation in remnant kidney: role of angiotensin II. *Kidney Int.* 1997;52(Suppl 63):S221-S225.
128. Ruiz-Ortega M, Lorenzo O, Ruperez M, et al. Renin-angiotensin system and renal damage: emerging data on angiotensin II as a proinflammatory mediator. *Contrib Nephrol.* 2001:123-137.
129. Esteban V, Heringer-Walther S, Sterner-Kock A, et al. Angiotensin-(1-7) and the G protein–coupled receptor MAS are key players in renal inflammation. *PLoS One.* 2009;4:e5406.
130. Guzik TJ, Hoch NE, Brown KA, et al. Role of the T cell in the genesis of angiotensin II induced hypertension and vascular dysfunction. *J Exp Med.* 2007;204:2449-2460.
131. Kvakan H, Kleinewietfeld M, Qadri F, et al. Regulatory T cells ameliorate angiotensin II–induced cardiac damage. *Circulation.* 2009;119:2904-2912.
132. Lush DJ, King JA, Fray JC. Pathophysiology of low renin syndromes: sites of renal renin secretory impairment and prorenin overexpression. *Kidney Int.* 1993;43:983-999.
133. Paulsen EP, Seip RL, Ayers CR, et al. Plasma renin activity and albumin excretion in teenage type I diabetic subjects. A prospective study. *Hypertension.* 1989;13:781-788.
134. Levy SB, Lilley JJ, Frigon RP, et al. Urinary kallikrein and plasma renin activity as determinants of renal blood flow. The influence of race and dietary sodium intake. *J Clin Invest.* 1977;60:129-138.
135. Peti-Peterdi J, Kang JJ, Toma I. Activation of the renal renin-angiotensin system in diabetes—new concepts. *Nephrol Dial Transplant.* 2008;23:3047-3049.
136. Kang JJ, Toma I, Sipos A, et al. The collecting duct is the major source of prorenin in diabetes. *Hypertension.* 2008;51:1597-1604.
137. Jais X, D'Armini AM, Jansa P, et al. Bosentan for treatment of inoperable chronic thromboembolic pulmonary hypertension: BENEFiT (Bosentan Effects in iNopErable Forms of chronIc Thromboembolic pulmonary hypertension), a randomized, placebo-controlled trial. *J Am Coll Cardiol.* 2008;52:2127-2134.
138. Galie N, Manes A, Negro L, et al. A meta-analysis of randomized controlled trials in pulmonary arterial hypertension. *Eur Heart J.* 2009;30:394-403.
139. Barst RJ, Langleben D, Badesch D, et al. Treatment of pulmonary arterial hypertension with the selective endothelin-A receptor antagonist sitaxsentan. *J Am Coll Cardiol.* 2006;47:2049-2056.
140. Galie N, Rubin L, Hoeper M, et al. Treatment of patients with mildly symptomatic pulmonary arterial hypertension with bosentan (EARLY study): a double-blind, randomised controlled trial. *Lancet.* 2008;371:2093-2100.
141. Olsson KM, Hoeper MM. Novel approaches to the pharmacotherapy of pulmonary arterial hypertension. *Drug Discov Today.* 2009;14:284-290.
142. Morita S, Kitamura K, Yamamoto Y, et al. Immunoreactive endothelin in human kidney. *Ann Clin Biochem.* 1991;28(Pt 3):267-271.
143. Marsden PA, Dorfman DM, Collins T, et al. Regulated expression of endothelin 1 in glomerular capillary endothelial cells. *Am J Physiol.* 1991;261:F117-F125.
144. Ohta K, Hirata Y, Imai T, et al. Cytokine-induced release of endothelin-1 from porcine renal epithelial cell line. *Biochem Biophys Res Commun.* 1990;169:578-584.
145. Sakamoto H, Sasaki S, Hirata Y, et al. Production of endothelin-1 by rat cultured mesangial cells. *Biochem Biophys Res Commun.* 1990;169:462-468.
146. Kohan DE. The renal medullary endothelin system in control of sodium and water excretion and systemic blood pressure. *Curr Opin Nephrol Hypertens.* 2006;15:34-40.
147. Kohan DE. Endothelin synthesis by rabbit renal tubule cells. *Am J Physiol.* 1991;261:F221-F226.
148. Kohan DE. Endothelins in the normal and diseased kidney. *Am J Kidney Dis.* 1997;29:2-26.
149. Abassi Z, Winaver J, Rubinstein I, et al. Renal endothelin-converting enzyme in rats with congestive heart failure. *J Cardiovasc Pharmacol.* 1998;31(Suppl 1):S31-S34.
150. Pupilli C, Romagnani P, Lasagni L, et al. Localization of endothelin-converting enzyme–1 in human kidney. *Am J Physiol.* 1997;273:F749-F756.
151. Dhaun N, Goddard J, Webb DJ. The endothelin system and its antagonism in chronic kidney disease. *J Am Soc Nephrol.* 2006;17:943-955.
152. Luscher TF, Barton M. Endothelins and endothelin receptor antagonists: therapeutic considerations for a novel class of cardiovascular drugs. *Circulation.* 2000;102:2434-2440.
153. Yamamoto T, Hirohama T, Uemura H. Endothelin B receptor–like immunoreactivity in podocytes of the rat kidney. *Arch Histol Cytol.* 2002;65:245-250.
154. Katoh T, Chang H, Uchida S, et al. Direct effects of endothelin in the rat kidney. *Am J Physiol.* 1990;258:F397-F402.
155. Tomobe Y, Miyauchi T, Saito A, et al. Effects of endothelin on the renal artery from spontaneously hypertensive and Wistar Kyoto rats. *Eur J Pharmacol.* 1988;152:373-374.
156. Sorokin A, Kohan DE. Physiology and pathology of endothelin-1 in renal mesangium. *Am J Physiol Renal Physiol.* 2003;285:F579-F589.
157. Inscho EW, Imig JD, Cook AK, et al. ETA and ETB receptors differentially modulate afferent and efferent arteriolar responses to endothelin. *Br J Pharmacol.* 2005;146:1019-1026.
158. Hirata Y, Emori T, Eguchi S, et al. Endothelin receptor subtype B mediates synthesis of nitric oxide by cultured bovine endothelial cells. *J Clin Invest.* 1993;91:1367-1373.
159. Konishi F, Okada Y, Takaoka M, et al. Role of endothelin ET(B) receptors in the renal hemodynamic and excretory responses to big endothelin-1. *Eur J Pharmacol.* 2002;451:177-184.

160. Vanni S, Polidori G, Cecioni I, et al. ET(B) receptor in renal medulla is enhanced by local sodium during low salt intake. *Hypertension.* 2002;40:179-185.
161. Ge Y, Bagnall A, Stricklett PK, et al. Collecting duct–specific knockout of the endothelin B receptor causes hypertension and sodium retention. *Am J Physiol Renal Physiol.* 2006;291:F1274-F1280.
162. Ahn D, Ge Y, Stricklett PK, et al. Collecting duct–specific knockout of endothelin-1 causes hypertension and sodium retention. *J Clin Invest.* 2004;114:504-511.
163. Nakano D, Pollock JS, Pollock DM. Renal medullary ETB receptors produce diuresis and natriuresis via NOS1. *Am J Physiol Renal Physiol.* 2008;294:F1205-1211.
164. Chu TS, Peng Y, Cano A, et al. Endothelin(B) receptor activates NHE-3 by a Ca²⁺-dependent pathway in OKP cells. *J Clin Invest.* 1996;97:1454-1462.
165. Nakano D, Pollock DM. Contribution of endothelin A receptors in endothelin 1–dependent natriuresis in female rats. *Hypertension.* 2009;53:324-330.
166. Schiffrin EL. Endothelin: role in experimental hypertension. *J Cardiovasc Pharmacol.* 2000;35:S33-S35.
167. Touyz RM, Turgeon A, Schiffrin EL. Endothelin-A–receptor blockade improves renal function and doubles the lifespan of stroke-prone spontaneously hypertensive rats. *J Cardiovasc Pharmacol.* 2000;36:S300-S304.
168. Allahdadi KJ, Cherng TW, Pai H, et al. Endothelin type A receptor antagonist normalizes blood pressure in rats exposed to eucapnic intermittent hypoxia. *Am J Physiol Heart Circ Physiol.* 2008;295:H434-H440.
169. Schiffrin EL, Deng LY, Sventek P, et al. Enhanced expression of endothelin-1 gene in resistance arteries in severe human essential hypertension. *J Hypertens.* 1997;15:57-63.
170. Schiffrin EL. Role of endothelin-1 in hypertension and vascular disease. *Am J Hypertens.* 2001;14:83S-89S.
171. Elijovich F, Laffer CL, Amador E, et al. Regulation of plasma endothelin by salt in salt-sensitive hypertension. *Circulation.* 2001;103:263-268.
172. Krum H, Viskoper RJ, Lacourciere Y, et al. The effect of an endothelin-receptor antagonist, bosentan, on blood pressure in patients with essential hypertension. Bosentan Hypertension Investigators. *N Engl J Med.* 1998;338:784-790.
173. Black HR, Bakris GL, Weber MA, et al. Efficacy and safety of darusentan in patients with resistant hypertension: results from a randomized, double-blind, placebo-controlled dose-ranging study. *J Clin Hypertens (Greenwich).* 2007;9:760-769.
174. Gerstung M, Roth T, Dienes HP, et al. Endothelin-1 induces NF-κB via two independent pathways in human renal tubular epithelial cells. *Am J Nephrol.* 2007;27:294-300.
175. Orisio S, Benigni A, Bruzzi I, et al. Renal endothelin gene expression is increased in remnant kidney and correlates with disease progression. *Kidney Int.* 1993;43:354-358.
176. Koyama H, Tabata T, Nishzawa Y, et al. Plasma endothelin levels in patients with uraemia. *Lancet.* 1989;1:991-992.
177. Zoccali C, Leonardis D, Parlongo S, et al. Urinary and plasma endothelin 1 in essential hypertension and in hypertension secondary to renoparenchymal disease. *Nephrol Dial Transplant.* 1995;10:1320-1323.
178. Vlachojannis JG, Tsakas S, Petropoulou C, et al. Endothelin-1 in the kidney and urine of patients with glomerular disease and proteinuria. *Clin Nephrol.* 2002;58:337-343.
179. Benigni A, Colosio V, Brena C, et al. Unselective inhibition of endothelin receptors reduces renal dysfunction in experimental diabetes. *Diabetes.* 1998;47:450-456.
180. Benigni A, Zoja C, Corna D, et al. A specific endothelin subtype A receptor antagonist protects against injury in renal disease progression. *Kidney Int.* 1993;44:440-444.
181. Tian X, Tang G, Chen Y. [The effects of endothelin-1 and selective endothelin receptor–type A antagonist on human renal interstitial fibroblasts in vitro]. *Zhonghua Yi Xue Za Zhi.* 2002;82:5-9.
182. Dube J, Chakir J, Dube C, et al. Synergistic action of endothelin (ET)–1 on the activation of bronchial fibroblast isolated from normal and asthmatic subjects. *Int J Exp Pathol.* 2000;81:429-437.
183. Morigi M, Buelli S, Angioletti S, et al. In response to protein load podocytes reorganize cytoskeleton and modulate endothelin-1 gene: implication for permselective dysfunction of chronic nephropathies. *Am J Pathol.* 2005;166:1309-1320.
184. Nabokov A, Amann K, Wagner J, et al. Influence of specific and non-specific endothelin receptor antagonists on renal morphology in rats with surgical renal ablation. *Nephrol Dial Transplant.* 1996;11:514-520.
185. Opocensky M, Kramer HJ, Backer A, et al. Late-onset endothelin-A receptor blockade reduces podocyte injury in homozygous Ren-2 rats despite severe hypertension. *Hypertension.* 2006;48:965-971.
186. Vaneckova I, Kramer HJ, Backer A, et al. Early endothelin-A receptor blockade decreases blood pressure and ameliorates end-organ damage in homozygous Ren-2 rats. *Hypertension.* 2005;46:969-974.
187. Shimizu T, Hata S, Kuroda T, et al. Different roles of two types of endothelin receptors in partial ablation-induced chronic renal failure in rats. *Eur J Pharmacol.* 1999;381:39-49.
188. Cao Z, Cooper ME, Wu LL, et al. Blockade of the renin-angiotensin and endothelin systems on progressive renal injury. *Hypertension.* 2000;36:561-568.
189. Grenda R, Wuhl E, Litwin M, et al. Urinary excretion of endothelin-1 (ET-1), transforming growth factor-β₁ (TGF-β₁) and vascular endothelial growth factor (VEGF165) in paediatric chronic kidney diseases: results of the ESCAPE trial. *Nephrol Dial Transplant.* 2007;22:3487-3494.
190. Goddard J, Johnston NR, Cumming AD, et al. Fractional urinary excretion of endothelin-1 is reduced by acute ETB receptor blockade. *Am J Physiol Renal Physiol.* 2007;293:F1433-F1438.
191. Goddard J, Johnston NR, Hand MF, et al. Endothelin-A receptor antagonism reduces blood pressure and increases renal blood flow in hypertensive patients with chronic renal failure: a comparison of selective and combined endothelin receptor blockade. *Circulation.* 2004;109:1186-1193.
192. Tomic M, Galesic K, Markota I. Endothelin-1 and nitric oxide in patients on chronic hemodialysis. *Ren Fail.* 2008;30:836-842.
193. Letizia C, Iannaccone A, Cerci S, et al. Circulating endothelin-1 in non–insulin-dependent diabetic patients with retinopathy. *Horm Metab Res.* 1997;29:247-251.
194. Peppa-Patrikiou M, Dracopoulou M, Dacou-Voutetakis C. Urinary endothelin in adolescents and young adults with insulin-dependent diabetes mellitus: relation to urinary albumin, blood pressure, and other factors. *Metabolism.* 1998;47:1408-1412.
195. Tsiani E, Lekas P, Fantus IG, et al. High glucose–enhanced activation of mesangial cell p38 MAPK by ET-1, ANG II, and platelet-derived growth factor. *Am J Physiol Endocrinol Metab.* 2002;282:E161-169.
196. Dlugosz JA, Munk S, Ispanovic E, et al. Mesangial cell filamentous actin disassembly and hypocontractility in high glucose are mediated by PKC-zeta. *Am J Physiol Renal Physiol.* 2002;282:F151-F163.
197. Whiteside CI, Dlugosz JA. Mesangial cell protein kinase C isozyme activation in the diabetic milieu. *Am J Physiol Renal Physiol.* 2002;282:F975-F980.
198. Chen S, Evans T, Deng D, et al. Hyperhexosemia induced functional and structural changes in the kidneys: role of endothelins. *Nephron.* 2002;90:86-94.
199. Jandeleit-Dahm K, Allen TJ, Youssef S, et al. Is there a role for endothelin antagonists in diabetic renal disease?. *Diabetes Obes Metab.* 2000;2:15-24.
200. Khamaisi M, Raz I, Shilo V, et al. Diabetes and radiocontrast media increase endothelin converting enzyme–1 in the kidney. *Kidney Int.* 2008;74:91-100.
201. Kelly DJ, Skinner SL, Gilbert RE, et al. Effects of endothelin or angiotensin II receptor blockade on diabetes in the transgenic (mRen-2)27 rat. *Kidney Int.* 2000;57:1882-1894.
202. Cosenzi A, Bernobich E, Trevisan R, et al. Nephroprotective effect of bosentan in diabetic rats. *J Cardiovasc Pharmacol.* 2003;42:752-756.
203. Sugimoto K, Fujimori A, Yuyama H, et al. Renal protective effect of YM598, a selective endothelin type A receptor antagonist. *J Cardiovasc Pharmacol.* 2004;44(Suppl 1):S451-S454.
204. Pfab T, Thone-Reineke C, Theilig F, et al. Diabetic endothelin B receptor–deficient rats develop severe hypertension and progressive renal failure. *J Am Soc Nephrol.* 2006;17:1082-1089.
205. Brownlee M. Biochemistry and molecular cell biology of diabetic complications. *Nature.* 2001;414:813-820.
206. Advani A, Gilbert RE, Thai K, et al. Expression, localization, and function of the thioredoxin system in diabetic nephropathy. *J Am Soc Nephrol.* 2009;20:730-741.
207. Li L, Fink GD, Watts SW, et al. Endothelin-1 increases vascular superoxide via endothelin(A)–NADPH oxidase pathway in low-renin hypertension. *Circulation.* 2003;107:1053-1058.
208. Elmarakby AA, Dabbs Loomis E, et al. ETA receptor blockade attenuates hypertension and decreases reactive oxygen species in ETB receptor–deficient rats. *J Cardiovasc Pharmacol.* 2004;44(Suppl 1):S7-S10.
209. Callera GE, Touyz RM, Teixeira SA, et al. ETA receptor blockade decreases vascular superoxide generation in DOCA-salt hypertension. *Hypertension.* 2003;42:811-817.
210. Sedeek MH, Llinas MT, Drummond H, et al. Role of reactive oxygen species in endothelin-induced hypertension. *Hypertension.* 2003;42:806-810.
211. Sasser JM, Sullivan JC, Hobbs JL, et al. Endothelin A receptor blockade reduces diabetic renal injury via an anti-inflammatory mechanism. *J Am Soc Nephrol.* 2007;18:143-154.
212. Wenzel RR, Littke T, Kuranoff S, et al. Avosentan reduces albumin excretion in diabetics with macroalbuminuria. *J Am Soc Nephrol.* 2009;20:655-664.

213. Tschaikowsky K, Sagner S, Lehnert N, et al. Endothelin in septic patients: effects on cardiovascular and renal function and its relationship to proinflammatory cytokines. *Crit Care Med.* 2000;28:1854-1860.
214. Nitescu N, Grimberg E, Ricksten SE, et al. Endothelin B receptors preserve renal blood flow in a normotensive model of endotoxin-induced acute kidney dysfunction. *Shock.* 2008;29:402-409.
215. Fenhammar J, Andersson A, Frithiof R, et al. The endothelin receptor antagonist tezosentan improves renal microcirculation in a porcine model of endotoxemic shock. *Acta Anaesthesiol Scand.* 2008;52:1385-1393.
216. Dhaun N, Lilitkarntakul P, Macintyre IM, et al. Urinary endothelin-1 in chronic kidney disease and as a marker of disease activity in lupus nephritis. *Am J Physiol Renal Physiol.* 2009;296:F1477-F1483.
217. Yoshio T, Masuyama J, Mimori A, et al. Endothelin-1 release from cultured endothelial cells induced by sera from patients with systemic lupus erythematosus. *Ann Rheum Dis.* 1995;54:361-365.
218. Nakamura T, Ebihara I, Tomino Y, et al. Effect of a specific endothelin A receptor antagonist on murine lupus nephritis. *Kidney Int.* 1995;47:481-489.
219. Venegas-Pont M, Sartori-Valinotti JC, Maric C, et al. Rosiglitazone decreases blood pressure and renal injury in a female mouse model of systemic lupus erythematosus. *Am J Physiol Regul Integr Comp Physiol.* 2009;296:R1282-R1289.
220. Cardenas A, Gines P. Hepatorenal syndrome. *Clin Liver Dis.* 2006;10:371-385;ix-x.
221. Wong F, Moore K, Dingemanse J, et al. Lack of renal improvement with nonselective endothelin antagonism with tezosentan in type 2 hepatorenal syndrome. *Hepatology.* 2008;47:160-168.
222. Bauersachs J, Fraccarollo D, Schafer A, et al. Angiotensin-converting enzyme inhibition and endothelin antagonism for endothelial dysfunction in heart failure: mono- or combination therapy. *J Cardiovasc Pharmacol.* 2002;40:594-600.
223. Amann K, Simonaviciene A, Medwedewa T, et al. Blood pressure–independent additive effects of pharmacologic blockade of the renin-angiotensin and endothelin systems on progression in a low-renin model of renal damage. *J Am Soc Nephrol.* 2001;12:2572-2584.
224. Kangawa K, Tawaragi Y, Oikawa S, et al. Identification of rat gamma atrial natriuretic polypeptide and characterization of the cDNA encoding its precursor. *Nature.* 1984;312:152-155.
225. Woodard GE, Rosado JA. Recent advances in natriuretic peptide research. *J Cell Mol Med.* 2007;11:1263-1271.
226. Sudoh T, Kangawa K, Minamino N, et al. A new natriuretic peptide in porcine brain. *Nature.* 1988;332:78-81.
227. Sudoh T, Minamino N, Kangawa K, et al. C-type natriuretic peptide (CNP): a new member of natriuretic peptide family identified in porcine brain. *Biochem Biophys Res Commun.* 1990;168:863-870.
228. Schweitz H, Vigne P, Moinier D, et al. A new member of the natriuretic peptide family is present in the venom of the green mamba (*Dendroaspis angusticeps*). *J Biol Chem.* 1992;267:13928-13932.
229. Schulz-Knappe P, Forssmann K, et al. Isolation and structural analysis of "urodilatin," a new peptide of the cardiodilatin-(ANP)–family, extracted from human urine. *Klin Wochenschr.* 1988;66:752-759.
230. Silver MA. The natriuretic peptide system: kidney and cardiovascular effects. *Curr Opin Nephrol Hypertens.* 2006;15:14-21.
231. Vesely DL, Perez-Lamboy GI, Schocken DD. Long-acting natriuretic peptide, vessel dilator, and kaliuretic peptide enhance urinary excretion rate of albumin, total protein, and beta(2)-microglobulin in patients with congestive heart failure. *J Card Fail.* 2001;7:55-63.
232. de Lemos JA, McGuire DK, Drazner MH. B-type natriuretic peptide in cardiovascular disease. *Lancet.* 2003;362:316-322.
233. Valli N, Gobinet A, Bordenave L. Review of 10 years of the clinical use of brain natriuretic peptide in cardiology. *J Lab Clin Med.* 1999;134:437-444.
234. McCullough PA, Omland T, Maisel AS. B-type natriuretic peptides: a diagnostic breakthrough for clinicians. *Rev Cardiovasc Med.* 2003;4:72-80.
235. Vanderheyden M, Bartunek J, Goethals M. Brain and other natriuretic peptides: molecular aspects. *Eur J Heart Fail.* 2004;6:261-268.
236. Woodard GE, Rosado JA, Brown J. Expression and control of C-type natriuretic peptide in rat vascular smooth muscle cells. *Am J Physiol Regul Integr Comp Physiol.* 2002;282:R156-R165.
237. Richards AM, Lainchbury JG, Nicholls MG, et al. *Dendroaspis* natriuretic peptide: endogenous or dubious? *Lancet.* 2002;359:5-6.
238. Kim SW, Lee JU, Kim SZ, et al. Enhanced *Dendroaspis* natriuretic peptide immunoreactivity in experimental ureteral obstruction. *Nephron.* 2002;92:369-372.
239. Kim JH, Yang SH, Yu MY, et al. *Dendroaspis* natriuretic peptide system and its paracrine function in rat colon. *Regul Pept.* 2004;120:93-98.
240. Woodard GE, Rosado JA, Brown J. *Dendroaspis* natriuretic peptide–like immunoreactivity and its regulation in rat aortic vascular smooth muscle. *Peptides.* 2002;23:23-29.
241. Piao FL, Park SH, Han JH, et al. *Dendroaspis* natriuretic peptide and its functions in pig ovarian granulosa cells. *Regul Pept.* 2004;118:193-198.
242. Singh G, Maguire JJ, Kuc RE, et al. Characterization of the snake venom ligand [125I]–DNP binding to natriuretic peptide receptor–A in human artery and potent DNP mediated vasodilatation. *Br J Pharmacol.* 2006;149:838-844.
243. Johns DG, Ao Z, Heidrich BJ, et al. *Dendroaspis* natriuretic peptide binds to the natriuretic peptide clearance receptor. *Biochem Biophys Res Commun.* 2007;358:145-149.
244. Chen HH, Lainchbury JG, Burnett Jr JC. Natriuretic peptide receptors and neutral endopeptidase in mediating the renal actions of a new therapeutic synthetic natriuretic peptide *Dendroaspis* natriuretic peptide. *J Am Coll Cardiol.* 2002;40:1186-1191.
245. Lisy O, Jougasaki M, Heublein DM, et al. Renal actions of synthetic *Dendroaspis* natriuretic peptide. *Kidney Int.* 1999;56:502-508.
246. Lisy O, Lainchbury JG, Leskinen H, et al. Therapeutic actions of a new synthetic vasoactive and natriuretic peptide, dendroaspis natriuretic peptide, in experimental severe congestive heart failure. *Hypertension.* 2001;37:1089-1094.
247. Forssmann W, Meyer M, Forssmann K. The renal urodilatin system: clinical implications. *Cardiovasc Res.* 2001;51:450-462.
248. Shin SJ, Lee YJ, Tan MS, et al. Increased atrial natriuretic peptide mRNA expression in the kidney of diabetic rats. *Kidney Int.* 1997;51:1100-1105.
249. Totsune K, Mackenzie HS, Totsune H, et al. Upregulation of atrial natriuretic peptide gene expression in remnant kidney of rats with reduced renal mass. *J Am Soc Nephrol.* 1998;9:1613-1619.
250. Kone BC. Molecular biology of natriuretic peptides and nitric oxide synthases. *Cardiovasc Res.* 2001;51:429-441.
251. Matsukawa N, Grzesik WJ, Takahashi N, et al. The natriuretic peptide clearance receptor locally modulates the physiological effects of the natriuretic peptide system. *Proc Natl Acad Sci U S A.* 1999;96:7403-7408.
252. Murthy KS, Teng BQ, Zhou H, et al. G(i-1)/G(i-2)–dependent signaling by single-transmembrane natriuretic peptide clearance receptor. *Am J Physiol Gastrointest Liver Physiol.* 2000;278:G974-G980.
253. Chen S, Olsen K, Grigsby C, et al. Vitamin D activates type A natriuretic peptide receptor gene transcription in inner medullary collecting duct cells. *Kidney Int.* 2007;72:300-306.
254. Corti R, Burnett Jr JC, Rouleau JL, et al. Vasopeptidase inhibitors: a new therapeutic concept in cardiovascular disease? *Circulation.* 2001;104:1856-1862.
255. Nishikimi T, Inaba-Iemura C, Ishimura K, et al. Natriuretic peptide/natriuretic peptide receptor–A (NPR-A) system has inhibitory effects in renal fibrosis in mice. *Regul Pept.* 2009;154:44-53.
256. Lo CS, Chen ZH, Hsieh TJ, et al. Atrial natriuretic peptide attenuates high glucose–activated transforming growth factor–beta, Smad and collagen synthesis in renal proximal tubular cells. *J Cell Biochem.* 2008;103:1999-2009.
257. Lo CS, Chen CH, Hsieh TJ, et al. Local action of endogenous renal tubular atrial natriuretic peptide. *J Cell Physiol.* 2009;219:776-786.
258. John SW, Krege JH, Oliver PM, et al. Genetic decreases in atrial natriuretic peptide and salt-sensitive hypertension. *Science.* 1995;267:679-681.
259. Steinhelper ME, Cochrane KL, Field LJ. Hypotension in transgenic mice expressing atrial natriuretic factor fusion genes. *Hypertension.* 1990;16:301-307.
260. Rubattu S, Evangelista A, Barbato D, et al. Atrial natriuretic peptide (ANP) gene promoter variant and increased susceptibility to early development of hypertension in humans. *J Hum Hypertens.* 2007;21:822-824.
261. Levin ER, Gardner DG, Samson WK. Natriuretic peptides. *N Engl J Med.* 1998;339:321-328.
262. Vesely DL. Natriuretic peptides and acute renal failure. *Am J Physiol Renal Physiol.* 2003;285:F167-F177.
263. Garcha RS, Hughes AD. CNP, but not ANP or BNP, relax human isolated subcutaneous resistance arteries by an action involving cyclic GMP and BKCa channels. *J Renin Angiotensin Aldosterone Syst.* 2006;7:87-91.
264. Chauhan SD, Nilsson H, Ahluwalia A, et al. Release of C-type natriuretic peptide accounts for the biological activity of endothelium-derived hyperpolarizing factor. *Proc Natl Acad Sci U S A.* 2003;100:1426-1431.
265. Garland CJ, Dora KA. Evidence against C-type natriuretic peptide as an arterial "EDHF." *Br J Pharmacol.* 2008;153:4-5.
266. Leuranguer V, Vanhoutte PM, Verbeuren T, et al. C-type natriuretic peptide and endothelium-dependent hyperpolarization in the guinea-pig carotid artery. *Br J Pharmacol.* 2008;153:57-65.
267. Nakayama T, Soma M, Takahashi Y, et al. Functional deletion mutation of the 5′-flanking region of type A human natriuretic peptide receptor gene and its association with essential hypertension and left ventricular hypertrophy in the Japanese. *Circ Res.* 2000;86:841-845.
268. Rubattu S, Bigatti G, Evangelista A, et al. Association of atrial natriuretic peptide and type a natriuretic peptide receptor gene polymorphisms with left ventricular mass in human essential hypertension. *J Am Coll Cardiol.* 2006;48:499-505.
269. Kapoun AM, Liang F, O'Young G, et al. B-type natriuretic peptide exerts broad functional opposition to transforming growth factor–beta in primary human cardiac fibroblasts: fibrosis, myofibroblast conversion, proliferation, and inflammation. *Circ Res.* 2004;94:453-461.

270. Tamura N, Ogawa Y, Chusho H, et al. Cardiac fibrosis in mice lacking brain natriuretic peptide. *Proc Natl Acad Sci U S A.* 2000;97:4239-4244.
271. Wang TJ, Larson MG, Levy D, et al. Impact of obesity on plasma natriuretic peptide levels. *Circulation.* 2004;109:594-600.
272. Olsen MH, Hansen TW, Christensen MK, et al. N-terminal pro brain natriuretic peptide is inversely related to metabolic cardiovascular risk factors and the metabolic syndrome. *Hypertension.* 2005;46:660-666.
273. Rubattu S, Sciarretta S, Ciavarella GM, et al. Reduced levels of N-terminal–proatrial natriuretic peptide in hypertensive patients with metabolic syndrome and their relationship with left ventricular mass. *J Hypertens.* 2007;25:833-839.
274. Wang TJ, Larson MG, Keyes MJ, et al. Association of plasma natriuretic peptide levels with metabolic risk factors in ambulatory individuals. *Circulation.* 2007;115:1345-1353.
275. Birkenfeld AL, Boschmann M, Moro C, et al. Lipid mobilization with physiological atrial natriuretic peptide concentrations in humans. *J Clin Endocrinol Metab.* 2005;90:3622-3628.
276. Sarzani R, Marcucci P, Salvi F, et al. Angiotensin II stimulates and atrial natriuretic peptide inhibits human visceral adipocyte growth. *Int J Obes (Lond).* 2008;32:259-267.
277. Galitzky J, Sengenes C, Thalamas C, et al. The lipid-mobilizing effect of atrial natriuretic peptide is unrelated to sympathetic nervous system activation or obesity in young men. *J Lipid Res.* 2001;42:536-544.
278. Sengenes C, Bouloumie A, Hauner H, et al. Involvement of a cGMP-dependent pathway in the natriuretic peptide–mediated hormone-sensitive lipase phosphorylation in human adipocytes. *J Biol Chem.* 2003;278:48617-48626.
279. Pejchalova K, Krejci P, Wilcox WR. C-natriuretic peptide: an important regulator of cartilage. *Mol Genet Metab.* 2007;92:210-215.
280. Tamura N, Doolittle LK, Hammer RE, et al. Critical roles of the guanylyl cyclase B receptor in endochondral ossification and development of female reproductive organs. *Proc Natl Acad Sci U S A.* 2004;101:17300-17305.
281. Chusho H, Tamura N, Ogawa Y, et al. Dwarfism and early death in mice lacking C-type natriuretic peptide. *Proc Natl Acad Sci U S A.* 2001;98:4016-4021.
282. Bartels CF, Bukulmez H, Padayatti P, et al. Mutations in the transmembrane natriuretic peptide receptor NPR-B impair skeletal growth and cause acromesomelic dysplasia, type Maroteaux. *Am J Hum Genet.* 2004;75:27-34.
283. Doust JA, Glasziou PP, Pietrzak E, et al. A systematic review of the diagnostic accuracy of natriuretic peptides for heart failure. *Arch Intern Med.* 2004;164:1978-1984.
284. Trof RJ, Di Maggio F, Leemreis J, et al. Biomarkers of acute renal injury and renal failure. *Shock.* 2006;26:245-253.
285. Dieplinger B, Mueller T, Kollerits B, et al. Pro-A-type natriuretic peptide and pro-adrenomedullin predict progression of chronic kidney disease: the MMKD study. *Kidney Int.* 2009;75:408-414.
286. Khalifeh N, Haider D, Horl WH. Natriuretic peptides in chronic kidney disease and during renal replacement therapy: an update. *J Investig Med.* 2009;57:33-39.
287. Lee DS, Vasan RS. Novel markers for heart failure diagnosis and prognosis. *Curr Opin Cardiol.* 2005;20:201-210.
288. Silver MA, Maisel A, Yancy CW, et al. BNP Consensus Panel 2004: a clinical approach for the diagnostic, prognostic, screening, treatment monitoring, and therapeutic roles of natriuretic peptides in cardiovascular diseases. *Congest Heart Fail.* 2004;10:1-30.
289. Januzzi Jr JL, Camargo CA, Anwaruddin S, et al. The N-terminal Pro-BNP Investigation of Dyspnea in the Emergency department (PRIDE) study. *Am J Cardiol.* 2005;95:948-954.
290. McKie PM, Burnett Jr JC. B-type natriuretic peptide as a biomarker beyond heart failure: speculations and opportunities. *Mayo Clin Proc.* 2005;80:1029-1036.
291. Munagala VK, Burnett Jr JC, Redfield MM. The natriuretic peptides in cardiovascular medicine. *Curr Probl Cardiol.* 2004;29:707-769.
292. McDonald K, Dahlstrom U, Aspromonte N, et al. B-type natriuretic peptide: application in the community. *Congest Heart Fail.* 2008;14:12-16.
293. van Kimmenade RR, Januzzi Jr JL, Bakker JA, et al. Renal clearance of B-type natriuretic peptide and amino terminal pro–B-type natriuretic peptide a mechanistic study in hypertensive subjects. *J Am Coll Cardiol.* 2009;53:884-890.
294. Vanderheyden M, Bartunek J, Filippatos G, et al. Cardiovascular disease in patients with chronic renal impairment: role of natriuretic peptides. *Congest Heart Fail.* 2008;14:38-42.
295. deFilippi CR, Seliger SL, Maynard S, et al. Impact of renal disease on natriuretic peptide testing for diagnosing decompensated heart failure and predicting mortality. *Clin Chem.* 2007;53:1511-1519.
296. Khan IA, Fink J, Nass C, et al. N-terminal pro–B-type natriuretic peptide and B-type natriuretic peptide for identifying coronary artery disease and left ventricular hypertrophy in ambulatory chronic kidney disease patients. *Am J Cardiol.* 2006;97:1530-1534.
297. Spanaus KS, Kronenberg F, Ritz E, et al. B-type natriuretic peptide concentrations predict the progression of nondiabetic chronic kidney disease: the Mild-to-Moderate Kidney Disease Study. *Clin Chem.* 2007;53:1264-1272.
298. Vickery S, Webb MC, Price CP, et al. Prognostic value of cardiac biomarkers for death in a non-dialysis chronic kidney disease population. *Nephrol Dial Transplant.* 2008;23:3546-3553.
299. Astor BC, Yi S, Hiremath L, et al. N-terminal prohormone brain natriuretic peptide as a predictor of cardiovascular disease and mortality in blacks with hypertensive kidney disease: the African American Study of Kidney Disease and Hypertension (AASK). *Circulation.* 2008;117:1685-1692.
300. Wahl HG, Graf S, Renz H, Fassbinder W. Elimination of the cardiac natriuretic peptides B-type natriuretic peptide (BNP) and N-terminal proBNP by hemodialysis. *Clin Chem.* 2004;50:1071-1074.
301. Mehta RL. Continuous renal replacement therapy in the critically ill patient. *Kidney Int.* 2005;67:781-795.
302. Obineche EN, Pathan JY, Fisher S, et al. Natriuretic peptide and adrenomedullin levels in chronic renal failure and effects of peritoneal dialysis. *Kidney Int.* 2006;69:152-156.
303. Lee JA, Kim DH, Yoo SJ, et al. Association between serum N-terminal pro–brain natriuretic peptide concentration and left ventricular dysfunction and extracellular water in continuous ambulatory peritoneal dialysis patients. *Perit Dial Int.* 2006;26:360-365.
304. Wang AY, Lam CW, Yu CM, et al. N-terminal pro–brain natriuretic peptide: an independent risk predictor of cardiovascular congestion, mortality, and adverse cardiovascular outcomes in chronic peritoneal dialysis patients. *J Am Soc Nephrol.* 2007;18:321-330.
305. Zoccali C, Mallamaci F, Benedetto FA, et al. Cardiac natriuretic peptides are related to left ventricular mass and function and predict mortality in dialysis patients. *J Am Soc Nephrol.* 2001;12:1508-1515.
306. Guo Q, Barany P, Qureshi AR, et al. N-terminal pro–brain natriuretic peptide independently predicts protein energy wasting and is associated with all-cause mortality in prevalent HD patients. *Am J Nephrol.* 2009;29:516-523.
307. Roberts MA, Srivastava PM, Macmillan N, et al. B-type natriuretic peptides strongly predict mortality in patients who are treated with long-term dialysis. *Clin J Am Soc Nephrol.* 2008;3:1057-1065.
308. Gutierrez OM, Tamez H, Bhan I, et al. N-terminal pro–B-type natriuretic peptide (NT-proBNP) concentrations in hemodialysis patients: prognostic value of baseline and follow-up measurements. *Clin Chem.* 2008;54:1339-1348.
309. Niizuma S, Iwanaga Y, Yahata T, et al. Plasma B-type natriuretic peptide levels reflect the presence and severity of stable coronary artery disease in chronic haemodialysis patients. *Nephrol Dial Transplant.* 2009;24:597-603.
310. Madsen LH, Ladefoged S, Corell P, et al. N-terminal pro brain natriuretic peptide predicts mortality in patients with end-stage renal disease in hemodialysis. *Kidney Int.* 2007;71:548-554.
311. Suwa M, Seino Y, Nomachi Y, et al. Multicenter prospective investigation on efficacy and safety of carperitide for acute heart failure in the "real world" of therapy. *Circ J.* 2005;69:283-290.
312. Mitaka C, Kudo T, Jibiki M, et al. Effects of human atrial natriuretic peptide on renal function in patients undergoing abdominal aortic aneurysm repair. *Crit Care Med.* 2008;36:745-751.
313. Morikawa S, Sone T, Tsuboi H, et al. Renal protective effects and the prevention of contrast-induced nephropathy by atrial natriuretic peptide. *J Am Coll Cardiol.* 2009;53:1040-1046.
314. Nigwekar SU, Navaneethan SD, Parikh CR, et al. Atrial natriuretic peptide for management of acute kidney injury: a systematic review and meta-analysis. *Clin J Am Soc Nephrol.* 2009;4:261-272.
315. Elkayam U, Akhter MW, Tummala P, et al. Nesiritide: a new drug for the treatment of decompensated heart failure. *J Cardiovasc Pharmacol Ther.* 2002;7:181-194.
316. Lee CY, Burnett Jr JC. Natriuretic peptides and therapeutic applications. *Heart Fail Rev.* 2007;12:131-142.
317. Burger AJ. A review of the renal and neurohormonal effects of B-type natriuretic peptide. *Congest Heart Fail.* 2005;11:30-38.
318. Keating GM, Goa KL. Nesiritide: a review of its use in acute decompensated heart failure. *Drugs.* 2003;63:47-70.
319. Sackner-Bernstein JD, Skopicki HA, Aaronson KD. Risk of worsening renal function with nesiritide in patients with acutely decompensated heart failure. *Circulation.* 2005;111:1487-1491.
320. Elkayam U, Janmohamed M, Habib M, et al. Vasodilators in the management of acute heart failure. *Crit Care Med.* 2008;36:S95-S105.
321. Chow SL, Peng JT, Okamoto MP, et al. Effect of nesiritide infusion duration on renal function in acutely decompensated heart failure patients. *Ann Pharmacother.* 2007;41:556-561.
322. Mentzer Jr RM, Oz MC, Sladen RN, et al. Effects of perioperative nesiritide in patients with left ventricular dysfunction undergoing cardiac surgery: the NAPA Trial. *J Am Coll Cardiol.* 2007;49:716-726.

323. Chen HH, Sundt TM, Cook DJ, et al. Low dose nesiritide and the preservation of renal function in patients with renal dysfunction undergoing cardiopulmonary-bypass surgery: a double-blind placebo-controlled pilot study. *Circulation.* 2007;116:I134-I138.
324. Riter HG, Redfield MM, Burnett JC, et al. Nonhypotensive low-dose nesiritide has differential renal effects compared with standard-dose nesiritide in patients with acute decompensated heart failure and renal dysfunction. *J Am Coll Cardiol.* 2006;47:2334-2335.
325. Sackner-Bernstein JD, Kowalski M, Fox M, et al. Short-term risk of death after treatment with nesiritide for decompensated heart failure: a pooled analysis of randomized controlled trials. *JAMA.* 2005;293:1900-1905.
326. Abraham WT, Adams KF, Fonarow GC, et al. In-hospital mortality in patients with acute decompensated heart failure requiring intravenous vasoactive medications: an analysis from the Acute Decompensated Heart Failure National Registry (ADHERE). *J Am Coll Cardiol.* 2005;46:57-64.
327. Arora RR, Venkatesh PK, Molnar J. Short and long-term mortality with nesiritide. *Am Heart J.* 2006;152:1084-1090.
328. Hernandez AF, O'Connor CM, Starling RC, et al. Rationale and design of the Acute Study of Clinical Effectiveness of Nesiritide in Decompensated Heart Failure Trial (ASCEND-HF). *Am Heart J.* 2009;157:271-277.
329. Chen HH, Cataliotti A, Schirger JA, et al. Local renal delivery of a natriuretic peptide a renal-enhancing strategy for B-type natriuretic peptide in overt experimental heart failure. *J Am Coll Cardiol.* 2009;53:1302-1308.
330. Allie DE, Lirtzman MD, Wyatt CH, et al. Targeted renal therapy and contrast-induced nephropathy during endovascular abdominal aortic aneurysm repair: results of a feasibility pilot trial. *J Endovasc Ther.* 2007;14:520-527.
331. Mitrovic V, Seferovic PM, Simeunovic D, et al. Haemodynamic and clinical effects of ularitide in decompensated heart failure. *Eur Heart J.* 2006;27:2823-2832.
332. Mitrovic V, Luss H, Nitsche K, et al. Effects of the renal natriuretic peptide urodilatin (ularitide) in patients with decompensated chronic heart failure: a double-blind, placebo-controlled, ascending-dose trial. *Am Heart J.* 2005;150:1239.
333. Dorner GT, Selenko N, Kral T, et al. Hemodynamic effects of continuous urodilatin infusion: a dose-finding study. *Clin Pharmacol Ther.* 1998;64:322-330.
334. Luss H, Mitrovic V, Seferovic PM, et al. Renal effects of ularitide in patients with decompensated heart failure. *Am Heart J.* 2008;155:1012:e1011-e1018.
335. Vesely DL. Urodilatin: a better natriuretic peptide? *Curr Heart Fail Rep.* 2007;4:147-152.
336. Vesely DL. Which of the cardiac natriuretic peptides is most effective for the treatment of congestive heart failure, renal failure and cancer? *Clin Exp Pharmacol Physiol.* 2006;33:169-176.
337. Clark LC, Farghaly H, Saba SR, et al. Amelioration with vessel dilator of acute tubular necrosis and renal failure established for 2 days. *Am J Physiol Heart Circ Physiol.* 2000;278:H1155-H1564.
338. Lisy O, Huntley BK, McCormick DJ, et al. Design, synthesis, and actions of a novel chimeric natriuretic peptide: CD-NP. *J Am Coll Cardiol.* 2008;52:60-68.
339. Molinaro G, Rouleau JL, Adam A. Vasopeptidase inhibitors: a new class of dual zinc metallopeptidase inhibitors for cardiorenal therapeutics. *Curr Opin Pharmacol.* 2002;2:131-141.
340. Cao Z, Burrell LM, Tikkanen I, et al. Vasopeptidase inhibition attenuates the progression of renal injury in subtotal nephrectomized rats. *Kidney Int.* 2001;60:715-721.
341. Cohen DS, Mathis JE, Dotson RA, et al. Protective effects of CGS 30440, a combined angiotensin-converting enzyme inhibitor and neutral endopeptidase inhibitor, in a model of chronic renal failure. *J Cardiovasc Pharmacol.* 1998;32:87-95.
342. Taal MW, Nenov VD, Wong W, et al. Vasopeptidase inhibition affords greater renoprotection than angiotensin-converting enzyme inhibition alone. *J Am Soc Nephrol.* 2001;12:2051-2059.
343. Jandeleit-Dahm K, Lassila M, Davis BJ, et al. Anti-atherosclerotic and renoprotective effects of combined angiotensin-converting enzyme and neutral endopeptidase inhibition in diabetic apolipoprotein E–knockout mice. *J Hypertens.* 2005;23:2071-2082.
344. Tikkanen T, Tikkanen I, Rockell MD, et al. Dual inhibition of neutral endopeptidase and angiotensin-converting enzyme in rats with hypertension and diabetes mellitus. *Hypertension.* 1998;32:778-785.
345. Rouleau JL, Pfeffer MA, Stewart DJ, et al. Comparison of vasopeptidase inhibitor, omapatrilat, and lisinopril on exercise tolerance and morbidity in patients with heart failure: IMPRESS randomised trial. *Lancet.* 2000;356:615-620.
346. Kostis JB, Packer M, Black HR, et al. Omapatrilat and enalapril in patients with hypertension: the Omapatrilat Cardiovascular Treatment vs. Enalapril (OCTAVE) trial. *Am J Hypertens.* 2004;17:103-111.
347. Packer M, Califf RM, Konstam MA, et al. Comparison of omapatrilat and enalapril in patients with chronic heart failure: the Omapatrilat Versus Enalapril Randomized Trial of Utility in Reducing Events (OVERTURE). *Circulation.* 2002;106:920-926.
348. Ruschitzka F, Corti R, Quaschning T, et al. Vasopeptidase inhibitors—concepts and evidence. *Nephrol Dial Transplant.* 2001;16:1532-1535.
349. Sica DA, Liao W, Gehr TW, et al. Disposition and safety of omapatrilat in subjects with renal impairment. *Clin Pharmacol Ther.* 2000;68:261-269.
350. Weber MA. Vasopeptidase inhibitors. *Lancet.* 2001;358:1525-1532.
351. Troughton RW, Lewis LK, Yandle TG, et al. Hemodynamic, hormone, and urinary effects of adrenomedullin infusion in essential hypertension. *Hypertension.* 2000;36:588-593.
352. Jandeleit-Dahm KA. Dual ACE/NEP inhibitors—more than playing the ACE card. *J Hum Hypertens.* 2006;20:478-481.
353. Johnson AG, Pearce GL, Danoff TM. A randomized, double-blind, placebo-controlled, parallel-group study to assess the efficacy and safety of dual ACE/NEP inhibitor GW660511X in mild-to-moderate hypertensive patients. *J Hum Hypertens.* 2006;20:496-503.
354. Battistini B, Daull P, Jeng AY. CGS 35601, a triple inhibitor of angiotensin converting enzyme, neutral endopeptidase and endothelin converting enzyme. *Cardiovasc Drug Rev.* 2005;23:317-330.
355. Daull P, Benrezzak O, Arsenault D, et al. Triple vasopeptidase inhibition normalizes blood pressure in conscious, unrestrained, and spontaneously hypertensive rats. *Am J Hypertens.* 2005;18:1606-1613.
356. Sindic A, Schlatter E. Renal electrolyte effects of guanylin and uroguanylin. *Curr Opin Nephrol Hypertens.* 2007;16:10-15.
357. Kitamura K, Kangawa K, Kawamoto M, et al. Adrenomedullin: a novel hypotensive peptide isolated from human pheochromocytoma. *Biochem Biophys Res Commun.* 1993;192:553-560.
358. Yanagawa B, Nagaya N. Adrenomedullin: molecular mechanisms and its role in cardiac disease. *Amino Acids.* 2007;32:157-164.
359. Leeb-Lundberg LM, Marceau F, Muller-Esterl W, et al. International union of pharmacology. XLV. Classification of the kinin receptor family: from molecular mechanisms to pathophysiological consequences. *Pharmacol Rev.* 2005;57:27-77.
359a. Abelous JE, Bardier E. Les substances hypotensives de l'urine humaine normale. *CR Sco Boil.* 1909;66:511-520
360. Shesely EG, Hu CB, Alhenc-Gelas F, et al. A second expressed kininogen gene in mice. *Physiol Genomics.* 2006;26:152-157.
361. Colman RW, Bagdasarian A, Talamo RC, et al. Williams trait. Human kininogen deficiency with diminished levels of plasminogen proactivator and prekallikrein associated with abnormalities of the Hageman factor–dependent pathways. *J Clin Invest.* 1975;56:1650-1662.
362. Campbell DJ. The kallikrein-kinin system in humans. *Clin Exp Pharmacol Physiol.* 2001;28:1060-1065.
363. Damas J. The brown Norway rats and the kinin system. *Peptides.* 1996;17:859-872
363a. Kraut H, Frey EK, Werle E. Der Nachweis eines Kreislaufhormon in der Pankreasdrüse. *Hoppe-Seylers Z Physiol Chem.* 1930;189:97-106.
364. Chao J, Yin H, Gao L, et al. Tissue kallikrein elicits cardioprotection by direct kinin B_2 receptor activation independent of kinin formation. *Hypertension.* 2008;52:715-720.
365. Biyashev D, Tan F, Chen Z, et al. Kallikrein activates bradykinin B_2 receptors in absence of kininogen. *Am J Physiol Heart Circ Physiol.* 2006;290:H1244-H1250.
366. Krankel N, Madeddu P. Helping the circulatory system heal itself: manipulating kinin signaling to promote neovascularization. *Expert Rev Cardiovasc Ther.* 2009;7:215-219.
367. Chao J, Chao L. Functional analysis of human tissue kallikrein in transgenic mouse models. *Hypertension.* 1996;27:491-494.
368. Azizi M, Boutouyrie P, Bissery A, et al. Arterial and renal consequences of partial genetic deficiency in tissue kallikrein activity in humans. *J Clin Invest.* 2005;115:780-787.
369. Kakoki M, Smithies O. The kallikrein-kinin system in health and in diseases of the kidney. *Kidney Int.* 2009;75:1019-1030.
370. Cayla C, Merino VF, Cabrini DA, et al. Structure of the mammalian kinin receptor gene locus. *Int Immunopharmacol.* 2002;2:1721-1727.
371. Riad A, Zhuo JL, Schultheiss HP, et al. The role of the renal kallikrein-kinin system in diabetic nephropathy. *Curr Opin Nephrol Hypertens.* 2007;16:22-26.
372. Spillmann F, Altmann C, Scheeler M, et al. Regulation of cardiac bradykinin B_1– and B_2–receptor mRNA in experimental ischemic, diabetic, and pressure-overload–induced cardiomyopathy. *Int Immunopharmacol.* 2002;2:1823-1832.
373. Griol-Charhbili V, Messadi-Laribi E, Bascands JL, et al. Role of tissue kallikrein in the cardioprotective effects of ischemic and pharmacological preconditioning in myocardial ischemia. *FASEB J.* 2005;19:1172-1174.
374. Zhang X, Tan F, Zhang Y, et al. Carboxypeptidase M and kinin B_1 receptors interact to facilitate efficient B_1 signaling from B_2 agonists. *J Biol Chem.* 2008;283:7994-8004.
375. Hecker M, Bara AT, Bauersachs J, et al. Characterization of endothelium-derived hyperpolarizing factor as a cytochrome P450–derived arachidonic acid metabolite in mammals. *J Physiol.* 1994;481(Pt 2):407-414.

376. Ignjatovic T, Stanisavljevic S, Brovkovych V, et al. Kinin B_1 receptors stimulate nitric oxide production in endothelial cells: signaling pathways activated by angiotensin I–converting enzyme inhibitors and peptide ligands. *Mol Pharmacol.* 2004;66:1310-1316.

377. Savard M, Barbaz D, Belanger S, et al. Expression of endogenous nuclear bradykinin B_2 receptors mediating signaling in immediate early gene activation. *J Cell Physiol.* 2008;216:234-244.

378. Borkowski JA, Ransom RW, Seabrook GR, et al. Targeted disruption of a B_2 bradykinin receptor gene in mice eliminates bradykinin action in smooth muscle and neurons. *J Biol Chem.* 1995;270:13706-13710.

379. Pesquero JB, Araujo RC, Heppenstall PA, et al. Hypoalgesia and altered inflammatory responses in mice lacking kinin B_1 receptors. *Proc Natl Acad Sci U S A.* 2000;97:8140-8145.

380. Cayla C, Todiras M, Iliescu R, et al. Mice deficient for both kinin receptors are normotensive and protected from endotoxin-induced hypotension. *FASEB J.* 2007;21:1689-1698.

381. Madeddu P, Varoni MV, Palomba D, et al. Cardiovascular phenotype of a mouse strain with disruption of bradykinin B_2–receptor gene. *Circulation.* 1997;96:3570-3578.

382. Alfie ME, Yang XP, Hess F, et al. Salt-sensitive hypertension in bradykinin B_2 receptor knockout mice. *Biochem Biophys Res Commun.* 1996;224:625-630.

383. Milia AF, Gross V, Plehm R, et al. Normal blood pressure and renal function in mice lacking the bradykinin B(2) receptor. *Hypertension.* 2001;37:1473-1479.

384. Kakoki M, McGarrah RW, Kim HS, et al. Bradykinin B_1 and B_2 receptors both have protective roles in renal ischemia/reperfusion injury. *Proc Natl Acad Sci U S A.* 2007;104:7576-7581.

385. Wang DZ, Chao L, Chao J. Hypotension in transgenic mice overexpressing human bradykinin B_2 receptor. *Hypertension.* 1997;29:488-493.

386. Ni A, Yin H, Agata J, et al. Overexpression of kinin B_1 receptors induces hypertensive response to des-Arg9-bradykinin and susceptibility to inflammation. *J Biol Chem.* 2003;278:219-225.

387. Chao J, Stallone JN, Liang YM, et al. Kallistatin is a potent new vasodilator. *J Clin Invest.* 1997;100:11-17.

388. Moreira CR, Schmaier AH, Mahdi F, et al. Identification of prolylcarboxypeptidase as the cell matrix-associated prekallikrein activator. *FEBS Lett.* 2002;523:167-170.

389. el-Dahr SS, Chao J. Spatial and temporal expression of kallikrein and its mRNA during nephron maturation. *Am J Physiol.* 1992;262:F705-F711.

390. el-Dahr S, Yosipiv IV, Muchant DG, et al. Salt intake modulates the developmental expression of renal kallikrein and bradykinin B_2 receptors. *Am J Physiol.* 1996;270:F425-F431.

391. el-Dahr SS, Yosipiv I. Developmentally regulated kallikrein enzymatic activity and gene transcription rate in maturing rat kidneys. *Am J Physiol.* 1993;265:F146-F150.

392. Madeddu P, Glorioso N, Maioli M, et al. Regulation of rat renal kallikrein expression by estrogen and progesterone. *J Hypertens Suppl.* 1991;9:S244-S245.

393. Vio CP, Loyola S, Velarde V. Localization of components of the kallikrein-kinin system in the kidney: relation to renal function. State of the art lecture. *Hypertension.* 1992;19:II10-II16.

394. Marin-Castano ME, Schanstra JP, Praddaude F, et al. Differential induction of functional B_1-bradykinin receptors along the rat nephron in endotoxin induced inflammation. *Kidney Int.* 1998;54:1888-1898.

395. Duncan AM, Kladis A, Jennings GL, et al. Kinins in humans. *Am J Physiol Regul Integr Comp Physiol.* 2000;278:R897-R904.

396. Rosamilia A, Clements JA, Dwyer PL, et al. Activation of the kallikrein kinin system in interstitial cystitis. *J Urol.* 1999;162:129-134.

397. Zeidel ML, Jabs K, Kikeri D, et al. Kinins inhibit conductive Na^+ uptake by rabbit inner medullary collecting duct cells. *Am J Physiol.* 1990;258:F1584-F1591.

398. Alfie ME, Alim S, Mehta D, et al. An enhanced effect of arginine vasopressin in bradykinin B_2 receptor null mutant mice. *Hypertension.* 1999;33:1436-1440.

399. Duchene J, Schanstra JP, Pecher C, et al. A novel protein-protein interaction between a G protein–coupled receptor and the phosphatase SHP-2 is involved in bradykinin-induced inhibition of cell proliferation. *J Biol Chem.* 2002;277:40375-40383.

400. Picard N, Van Abel M, Campone C, et al. Tissue kallikrein–deficient mice display a defect in renal tubular calcium absorption. *J Am Soc Nephrol.* 2005;16:3602-3610.

401. Blanchard A, Azizi M, Peyrard S, et al. Partial human genetic deficiency in tissue kallikrein activity and renal calcium handling. *Clin J Am Soc Nephrol.* 2007;2:320-325.

402. Shen B, El-Dahr SS. Cross-talk of the renin-angiotensin and kallikrein-kinin systems. *Biol Chem.* 2006;387:145-150.

403. Madeddu P, Oppes M, Soro A, et al. The effects of aprotinin, a kallikrein inhibitor, on renin release and urinary sodium excretion in mild essential hypertensives. *J Hypertens.* 1987;5:581-586.

404. Yosipiv IV, Dipp S, El-Dahr SS. Targeted disruption of the bradykinin B(2) receptor gene in mice alters the ontogeny of the renin-angiotensin system. *Am J Physiol Renal Physiol.* 2001;281:F795-F801.

405. Tschope C, Schultheiss HP, Walther T. Multiple interactions between the renin-angiotensin and the kallikrein-kinin systems: role of ACE inhibition and AT_1 receptor blockade. *J Cardiovasc Pharmacol.* 2002;39:478-487.

406. AbdAlla S, Lother H, el Massiery A, et al. Increased AT(1) receptor heterodimers in preeclampsia mediate enhanced angiotensin II responsiveness. *Nat Med.* 2001;7:1003-1009.

407. Kintsurashvili E, Duka I, Gavras I, et al. Effects of ANG II on bradykinin receptor gene expression in cardiomyocytes and vascular smooth muscle cells. *Am J Physiol Heart Circ Physiol.* 2001;281:H1778-H1783.

408. Margolius HS, Horwitz D, Geller RG, et al. Urinary kallikrein excretion in normal man. Relationships to sodium intake and sodium-retaining steroids. *Circ Res.* 1974;35:812-819.

409. Hirawa N, Uehara Y, Kawabata Y, et al. Mechanistic analysis of renal protection by angiotensin converting enzyme inhibitor in Dahl salt-sensitive rats. *J Hypertens.* 1994;12:909-918.

410. Uehara Y, Hirawa N, Kawabata Y, et al. Long-term infusion of kallikrein attenuates renal injury in Dahl salt-sensitive rats. *Hypertension.* 1994;24:770-778.

411. Chao J, Li HJ, Yao YY, et al. Kinin infusion prevents renal inflammation, apoptosis, and fibrosis via inhibition of oxidative stress and mitogen-activated protein kinase activity. *Hypertension.* 2007;49:490-497.

412. Cervenka L, Vaneckova I, Maly J, et al. Genetic inactivation of the B_2 receptor in mice worsens two-kidney, one-clip hypertension: role of NO and the AT_2 receptor. *J Hypertens.* 2003;21:1531-1538.

413. Griol-Charhbili V, Sabbah L, Colucci J, et al. Tissue kallikrein deficiency and renovascular hypertension in the mouse. *Am J Physiol Regul Integr Comp Physiol.* 2009;296:R1385-R1391.

414. Madeddu P, Emanueli C, El-Dahr S. Mechanisms of disease: the tissue kallikrein-kinin system in hypertension and vascular remodeling. *Nat Clin Pract Nephrol.* 2007;3:208-221.

415. Woodley-Miller C, Chao J, Chao L. Restriction fragment length polymorphisms mapped in spontaneously hypertensive rats using kallikrein probes. *J Hypertens.* 1989;7:865-871.

416. Yu H, Bowden DW, Spray BJ, et al. Identification of human plasma kallikrein gene polymorphisms and evaluation of their role in end-stage renal disease. *Hypertension.* 1998;31:906-911.

417. Hua H, Zhou S, Liu Y, et al. Relationship between the regulatory region polymorphism of human tissue kallikrein gene and essential hypertension. *J Hum Hypertens.* 2005;19:715-721.

418. Slim R, Torremocha F, Moreau T, et al. Loss-of-function polymorphism of the human kallikrein gene with reduced urinary kallikrein activity. *J Am Soc Nephrol.* 2002;13:968-976.

419. Rossi GP, Taddei S, Ghiadoni L, et al. Tissue kallikrein gene polymorphisms induce no change in endothelium-dependent or independent vasodilation in hypertensive and normotensive subjects. *J Hypertens.* 2006;24:1955-1963.

420. Cui J, Melista E, Chazaro I, et al. Sequence variation of bradykinin receptors B_1 and B_2 and association with hypertension. *J Hypertens.* 2005;23:55-62.

421. Brull D, Dhamrait S, Myerson S, et al. Bradykinin B_2BKR receptor polymorphism and left-ventricular growth response. *Lancet.* 2001;358:1155-1156.

422. Dhamrait SS, Payne JR, Li P, et al. Variation in bradykinin receptor genes increases the cardiovascular risk associated with hypertension. *Eur Heart J.* 2003;24:1672-1680.

423. Harvey JN, Jaffa AA, Margolius HS, et al. Renal kallikrein and hemodynamic abnormalities of diabetic kidney. *Diabetes.* 1990;39:299-304.

424. Tschope C, Reinecke A, Seidl U, et al. Functional, biochemical, and molecular investigations of renal kallikrein-kinin system in diabetic rats. *Am J Physiol.* 1999;277:H2333-H2340.

425. Alric C, Pecher C, Cellier E, et al. Inhibition of IGF-I–induced Erk 1 and 2 activation and mitogenesis in mesangial cells by bradykinin. *Kidney Int.* 2002;62:412-421.

426. Allen TJ, Cao Z, Youssef S, et al. Role of angiotensin II and bradykinin in experimental diabetic nephropathy. Functional and structural studies. *Diabetes.* 1997;46:1612-1618.

427. Buleon M, Allard J, Jaafar A, et al. Pharmacological blockade of B_2-kinin receptor reduces renal protective effect of angiotensin-converting enzyme inhibition in db/db mice model. *Am J Physiol Renal Physiol.* 2008;294:F1249-F1256.

428. Tschope C, Seidl U, Reinecke A, et al. Kinins are involved in the antiproteinuric effect of angiotensin-converting enzyme inhibition in experimental diabetic nephropathy. *Int Immunopharmacol.* 2003;3:335-344.

429. Schafer S, Schmidts HL, Bleich M, et al. Nephroprotection in Zucker diabetic fatty rats by vasopeptidase inhibition is partly bradykinin B_2 receptor dependent. *Br J Pharmacol.* 2004;143:27-32.

430. Kakoki M, Takahashi N, Jennette JC, et al. Diabetic nephropathy is markedly enhanced in mice lacking the bradykinin B$_2$ receptor. *Proc Natl Acad Sci U S A.* 2004;101:13302-13305.
431. Kakoki M, Kizer CM, Yi X, et al. Senescence-associated phenotypes in Akita diabetic mice are enhanced by absence of bradykinin B$_2$ receptors. *J Clin Invest.* 2006;116:1302-1309.
432. Tan Y, Keum JS, Wang B, et al. Targeted deletion of B$_2$-kinin receptors protects against the development of diabetic nephropathy. *Am J Physiol Renal Physiol.* 2007;293:F1026-F1035.
433. Bodin S, Chollet C, Goncalves-Mendes N, et al. Kallikrein protects against microalbuminuria in experimental type I diabetes. *Kidney Int.* 2009;76:395-403.
434. Yuan G, Deng J, Wang T, et al. Tissue kallikrein reverses insulin resistance and attenuates nephropathy in diabetic rats by activation of phosphatidylinositol 3–kinase/protein kinase B and adenosine 5'-monophosphate–activated protein kinase signaling pathways. *Endocrinology.* 2007;148:2016-2026.
435. Harvey JN, Edmundson AW, Jaffa AA, et al. Renal excretion of kallikrein and eicosanoids in patients with type 1 (insulin-dependent) diabetes mellitus. Relationship to glomerular and tubular function. *Diabetologia.* 1992;35:857-862.
436. Maltais I, Bachvarova M, Maheux P, et al. Bradykinin B$_2$ receptor gene polymorphism is associated with altered urinary albumin/creatinine values in diabetic patients. *Can J Physiol Pharmacol.* 2002;80:323-327.
437. Zychma MJ, Gumprecht J, Trautsolt W, et al. Polymorphic genes for kinin receptors, nephropathy and blood pressure in type 2 diabetic patients. *Am J Nephrol.* 2003;23:112-116.
438. Pazoki-Toroudi HR, Hesami A, Vahidi S, et al. The preventive effect of captopril or enalapril on reperfusion injury of the kidney of rats is independent of angiotensin II AT$_1$ receptors. *Fundam Clin Pharmacol.* 2003;17:595-598.
439. Kitakaze M, Minamino T, Node K, et al. Beneficial effects of inhibition of angiotensin-converting enzyme on ischemic myocardium during coronary hypoperfusion in dogs. *Circulation.* 1995;92:950-961.
440. Liu YH, Yang XP, Sharov VG, et al. Paracrine systems in the cardioprotective effect of angiotensin-converting enzyme inhibitors on myocardial ischemia/reperfusion injury in rats. *Hypertension.* 1996;27:7-13.
441. Park SS, Zhao H, Mueller RA, et al. Bradykinin prevents reperfusion injury by targeting mitochondrial permeability transition pore through glycogen synthase kinase 3β. *J Mol Cell Cardiol.* 2006;40:708-716.
442. Chiang WC, Chien CT, Lin WW, et al. Early activation of bradykinin B$_2$ receptor aggravates reactive oxygen species generation and renal damage in ischemia/reperfusion injury. *Free Radic Biol Med.* 2006;41:1304-1314.
443. Wolf WC, Yoshida H, Agata J, et al. Human tissue kallikrein gene delivery attenuates hypertension, renal injury, and cardiac remodeling in chronic renal failure. *Kidney Int.* 2000;58:730-739.
444. Schanstra JP, Neau E, Drogoz P, et al. In vivo bradykinin B$_2$ receptor activation reduces renal fibrosis. *J Clin Invest.* 2002;110:371-379.
445. Klein J, Gonzalez J, Duchene J, et al. Delayed blockade of the kinin B$_1$ receptor reduces renal inflammation and fibrosis in obstructive nephropathy. *FASEB J.* 2009;23:134-142.
446. Wang PH, Cenedeze MA, Campanholle G, et al. Deletion of bradykinin B$_1$ receptor reduces renal fibrosis. *Int Immunopharmacol.* 2009;9:653-657.
447. Zychma MJ, Gumprecht J, Zukowska-Szczechowska E, et al. Polymorphisms in the genes encoding for human kinin receptors and the risk of end-stage renal failure: results of transmission/disequilibrium test. The End-Stage Renal Disease Study Group. *J Am Soc Nephrol.* 1999;10:2120-2124.
448. Bachvarov DR, Landry M, Pelletier I, et al. Characterization of two polymorphic sites in the human kinin B$_1$ receptor gene: altered frequency of an allele in patients with a history of end-stage renal failure. *J Am Soc Nephrol.* 1998;9:598-604.
449. Jozwiak L, Drop A, Buraczynska K, et al. Association of the human bradykinin B$_2$ receptor gene with chronic renal failure. *Mol Diagn.* 2004;8:157-161.
450. Liu K, Li QZ, Delgado-Vega AM, et al. Kallikrein genes are associated with lupus and glomerular basement membrane–specific antibody–induced nephritis in mice and humans. *J Clin Invest.* 2009;119:911-923.
451. Li QZ, Zhou J, Yang R, et al. The lupus-susceptibility gene kallikrein downmodulates antibody-mediated glomerulonephritis. *Genes Immun.* 2009;10:503-508.
452. Kahn R, Hellmark T, Leeb-Lundberg LM, et al. Neutrophil-derived proteinase 3 induces kallikrein-independent release of a novel vasoactive kinin. *J Immunol.* 2009;182:7906-7915.
453. Semedo P, Wang PM, Andreucci TH, et al. Mesenchymal stem cells ameliorate tissue damages triggered by renal ischemia and reperfusion injury. *Transplant Proc.* 2007;39:421-423.
454. Morigi M, Introna M, Imberti B, et al. Human bone marrow mesenchymal stem cells accelerate recovery of acute renal injury and prolong survival in mice. *Stem Cells.* 2008;26:2075-2082.
455. Togel F, Cohen A, Zhang P, et al. Autologous and allogeneic marrow stromal cells are safe and effective for the treatment of acute kidney injury. *Stem Cells Dev.* 2009;18:475-485.
456. Qian H, Yang H, Xu W, et al. Bone marrow mesenchymal stem cells ameliorate rat acute renal failure by differentiation into renal tubular epithelial-like cells. *Int J Mol Med.* 2008;22:325-332.
457. Semedo P, Palasio CG, Oliveira CD, et al. Early modulation of inflammation by mesenchymal stem cell after acute kidney injury. *Int Immunopharmacol.* 2009;9:677-682.
458. Patschan D, Krupincza K, Patschan S, et al. Dynamics of mobilization and homing of endothelial progenitor cells after acute renal ischemia: modulation by ischemic preconditioning. *Am J Physiol Renal Physiol.* 2006;291:F176-F185.
459. Hagiwara M, Shen B, Chao L, et al. Kallikrein-modified mesenchymal stem cell implantation provides enhanced protection against acute ischemic kidney injury by inhibiting apoptosis and inflammation. *Hum Gene Ther.* 2008;19:807-819.
460. Krankel N, Katare RG, Siragusa M, et al. Role of kinin B$_2$ receptor signaling in the recruitment of circulating progenitor cells with neovascularization potential. *Circ Res.* 2008;103:1335-1343.
461. Desai N, Sajjad J, Frishman WH. Urotensin II: a new pharmacologic target in the treatment of cardiovascular disease. *Cardiol Rev.* 2008;16:142-153.
462. Coulouarn Y, Lihrmann I, Jegou S, et al. Cloning of the cDNA encoding the urotensin II precursor in frog and human reveals intense expression of the urotensin II gene in motoneurons of the spinal cord. *Proc Natl Acad Sci U S A.* 1998;95:15803-15808.
463. Ames RS, Sarau HM, Chambers JK, et al. Human urotensin-II is a potent vasoconstrictor and agonist for the orphan receptor GPR14. *Nature.* 1999;401:282-286.
464. Davenport AP, Maguire JJ. Urotensin II: fish neuropeptide catches orphan receptor. *Trends Pharmacol Sci.* 2000;21:80-82.
465. Tolle M, van der Giet M. Cardiorenovascular effects of urotensin II and the relevance of the UT receptor. *Peptides.* 2008;29:743-763.
466. Carmine Z, Mallamaci F. Urotensin II: a cardiovascular and renal update. *Curr Opin Nephrol Hypertens.* 2008;17:199-204.
467. Zhu YC, Zhu YZ, Moore PK. The role of urotensin II in cardiovascular and renal physiology and diseases. *Br J Pharmacol.* 2006;148:884-901.
468. Shenouda A, Douglas SA, Ohlstein EH, et al. Localization of urotensin-II immunoreactivity in normal human kidneys and renal carcinoma. *J Histochem Cytochem.* 2002;50:885-889.
469. Charles CJ, Rademaker MT, Richards AM, et al. Urotensin II: evidence for cardiac, hepatic, and renal production. *Peptides.* 2005;26:2211-2214.
470. Protopopov A, Kashuba V, Podowski R, et al. Assignment of the GPR14 gene coding for the G-protein–coupled receptor 14 to human chromosome 17q25.3 by fluorescent in situ hybridization. *Cytogenet Cell Genet.* 2000;88:312-313.
471. Lin Y, Matsumura K, Tsuchihashi T, et al. Role of ERK and Rho kinase pathways in central pressor action of urotensin II. *J Hypertens.* 2004;22:983-988.
472. Sauzeau V, Le Mellionnec E, Bertoglio J, et al. Human urotensin II–induced contraction and arterial smooth muscle cell proliferation are mediated by RhoA and Rho-kinase. *Circ Res.* 2001;88:1102-1104.
473. Tamura K, Okazaki M, Tamura M, et al. Urotensin II–induced activation of extracellular signal-regulated kinase in cultured vascular smooth muscle cells: involvement of cell adhesion–mediated integrin signaling. *Life Sci.* 2003;72:1049-1060.
474. Sugo T, Murakami Y, Shimomura Y, et al. Identification of urotensin II–related peptide as the urotensin II–immunoreactive molecule in the rat brain. *Biochem Biophys Res Commun.* 2003;310:860-868.
475. Itoh H, McMaster D, Lederis K. Functional receptors for fish neuropeptide urotensin II in major rat arteries. *Eur J Pharmacol.* 1988;149:61-66.
476. Gibson A, Wallace P, Bern HA. Cardiovascular effects of urotensin II in anesthetized and pithed rats. *Gen Comp Endocrinol.* 1986;64:435-439.
477. Stirrat A, Gallagher M, Douglas SA, et al. Potent vasodilator responses to human urotensin-II in human pulmonary and abdominal resistance arteries. *Am J Physiol Heart Circ Physiol.* 2001;280:H925-H928.
478. Matsushita M, Shichiri M, Imai T, et al. Co-expression of urotensin II and its receptor (GPR14) in human cardiovascular and renal tissues. *J Hypertens.* 2001;19:2185-2190.
479. Ashton N. Renal and vascular actions of urotensin II. *Kidney Int.* 2006;70:624-629.
480. Song W, Abdel-Razik AE, Lu W, et al. Urotensin II and renal function in the rat. *Kidney Int.* 2006;69:1360-1368.
481. Mori N, Hirose T, Nakayama T, et al. Increased expression of urotensin II–related peptide and its receptor in kidney with hypertension or renal failure. *Peptides.* 2009;30:400-408.
482. Zhang AY, Chen YF, Zhang DX, et al. Urotensin II is a nitric oxide–dependent vasodilator and natriuretic peptide in the rat kidney. *Am J Physiol Renal Physiol.* 2003;285:F792-F798.

483. Ovcharenko E, Abassi Z, Rubinstein I, et al. Renal effects of human urotensin-II in rats with experimental congestive heart failure. *Nephrol Dial Transplant*. 2006;21:1205-1211.

484. Douglas SA, Dhanak D, Johns DG. From "gills to pills": urotensin-II as a regulator of mammalian cardiorenal function. *Trends Pharmacol Sci*. 2004;25:76-85.

485. Cheung BM, Leung R, Man YB, et al. Plasma concentration of urotensin II is raised in hypertension. *J Hypertens*. 2004;22:1341-1344.

486. Totsune K, Takahashi K, Arihara Z, et al. Role of urotensin II in patients on dialysis. *Lancet*. 2001;358:810-811.

487. Totsune K, Takahashi K, Arihara Z, et al. Elevated plasma levels of immunoreactive urotensin II and its increased urinary excretion in patients with type 2 diabetes mellitus: association with progress of diabetic nephropathy. *Peptides*. 2004;25:1809-1814.

488. Langham RG, Kelly DJ, Gow RM, et al. Increased expression of urotensin II and urotensin II receptor in human diabetic nephropathy. *Am J Kidney Dis*. 2004;44:826-831.

489. Balat A, Karakok M, Yilmaz K, et al. Urotensin-II immunoreactivity in children with chronic glomerulonephritis. *Ren Fail*. 2007;29:573-578.

490. Balat A, Pakir IH, Gok F, et al. Urotensin-II levels in children with minimal change nephrotic syndrome. *Pediatr Nephrol*. 2005;20:42-45.

491. Mallamaci F, Cutrupi S, Pizzini P, et al. Urotensin II in end-stage renal disease: an inverse correlate of sympathetic function and cardiac natriuretic peptides. *J Nephrol*. 2005;18:727-732.

492. Zoccali C, Mallamaci F, Tripepi G, et al. Urotensin II is an inverse predictor of incident cardiovascular events in end-stage renal disease. *Kidney Int*. 2006;69:1253-1258.

493. Zoccali C, Mallamaci F, Benedetto FA, et al. Urotensin II and cardiomyopathy in end-stage renal disease. *Hypertension*. 2008;51:326-333.

494. Ravani P, Tripepi G, Pecchini P, et al. Urotensin II is an inverse predictor of death and fatal cardiovascular events in chronic kidney disease. *Kidney Int*. 2008;73:95-101.

495. Patacchini R, Santicioli P, Giuliani S, et al. Urantide: an ultrapotent urotensin II antagonist peptide in the rat aorta. *Br J Pharmacol*. 2003;140:1155-1158.

496. Camarda V, Song W, Marzola E, et al. Urantide mimics urotensin-II induced calcium release in cells expressing recombinant UT receptors. *Eur J Pharmacol*. 2004;498:83-86.

497. Camarda V, Spagnol M, Song W, et al. in vitro and in vivo pharmacological characterization of the novel UT receptor ligand [Pen5, DTrp7, Dab8] urotensin II(4-11) (UFP-803). *Br J Pharmacol*. 2006;147:92-100.

498. Clozel M, Binkert C, Birker-Robaczewska M, et al. Pharmacology of the urotensin-II receptor antagonist palosuran (ACT-058362; 1-[2-(4-benzyl-4-hydroxy-piperidin-1-yl)-ethyl]-3-(2-methyl-quinolin-4-yl)-urea sulfate salt): first demonstration of a pathophysiological role of the urotensin system. *J Pharmacol Exp Ther*. 2004;311:204-212.

499. Clozel M, Hess P, Qiu C, et al. The urotensin-II receptor antagonist palosuran improves pancreatic and renal function in diabetic rats. *J Pharmacol Exp Ther*. 2006;316:1115-1121.

500. Rakowski E, Hassan GS, Dhanak D, et al. A role for urotensin II in restenosis following balloon angioplasty: use of a selective UT receptor blocker. *J Mol Cell Cardiol*. 2005;39:785-791.

501. Bousette N, Pottinger J, Ramli W, et al. Urotensin-II receptor blockade with SB-611812 attenuates cardiac remodeling in experimental ischemic heart disease. *Peptides*. 2006;27:2919-2926.

502. Bousette N, Hu F, Ohlstein EH, et al. Urotensin-II blockade with SB-611812 attenuates cardiac dysfunction in a rat model of coronary artery ligation. *J Mol Cell Cardiol*. 2006;41:285-295.

Arachidonic Acid Metabolites and the Kidney

Raymond C. Harris, Matthew D. Breyer, and Richard M. Breyer

Cellular Origin of Eicosanoids

Eicosanoids comprise a family of biologically active, oxygenated arachidonic acid (AA) metabolites. AA is a polyunsaturated fatty acid possessing 20 carbon atoms and four double bonds (C20:4) and is formed from linoleic acid (C18:2) by the addition of two carbon atoms to the chain and further desaturation. In mammals, linoleic acid is derived strictly from dietary sources. Essential fatty acid deficiency occurs when dietary fatty acid precursors, including linoleic acid, are omitted, which depletes the hormone-responsive pool of AA. Essential fatty acid deficiency thus reduces the intracellular availability of AA in response to hormonal stimulation and abrogates many biologic actions of hormone-induced eicosanoid release.[1]

Of the approximately 10 g of linoleic acid ingested per day, only about 1 mg/day is eliminated as end products of AA metabolism. Following its formation, AA is esterified into cell membrane phospholipids, principally at the 2 position of the phosphatidylinositol fraction (i.e., sn-2 esterified AA), the major hormone-sensitive pool of AA that is susceptible to release by phospholipases.

Multiple stimuli lead to release of membrane-bound AA via activation of cellular phospholipases, principally in the phospholipase A_2 (PLA_2) class.[2] This cleavage step is rate limiting in the production of biologically relevant arachidonate metabolites. In the case of PLA_2 activation, membrane receptors activate guanine nucleotide-binding (G) proteins, which leads to release of AA directly from membrane phospholipids. Activation of phospholipase C or D, on the other hand, releases AA via the sequential action of the phospholipase-mediated production of diacylglycerol (DAG) with subsequent release of AA from DAG by DAG lipase.[3] When eicosanoid formation is considered, the physiologic significance of AA release by these other phospholipases remains uncertain, because at least in the setting of inflammation, PLA_2 action appears essential for the generation of biologically active AA metabolites.[4]

More than 15 proteins with PLA_2 activity are known to exist, including secreted PLA_2 ($sPLA_2$) and cytoplasmic PLA_2 ($cPLA_2$) isoforms.[5,6] A mitogen-activated $cPLA_2$ has been found to mediate AA release in a calcium/calmodulin-dependent manner. Other hormones and growth factors, including epidermal growth factor (EGF) and platelet-derived growth factors, activate PLA_2 directly through tyrosine residue kinase activity, which allows the recruitment of coactivators to the enzyme without an absolute requirement for the intermediate action of calcium/calmodulin or other cellular kinases.

Following de-esterification, AA is rapidly re-esterified into membrane lipids or avidly bound by intracellular proteins, in which case it becomes unavailable to further metabolism. Should it escape re-esterification and protein binding, free AA becomes available as a substrate for one of three major enzymatic transformations, the common result of which is the incorporation of oxygen atoms at various sites of the fatty acid backbone, with accompanying changes in its molecular structure (such as ring formation).[7,8] This results in the formation of biologically active molecules, referred to as *eicosanoids*. The specific nature of the products generated is a function of the initial stimuli for AA release, as well as the metabolic

enzyme available, which is determined in part by the cell type involved.[8,9]

These products, in turn, either *mediate* or *modulate* the biologic actions of the agonist in question. AA release may also result from nonspecific stimuli such as cellular trauma, including ischemia and hypoxia,[10] oxygen free radicals,[11] and osmotic stress.[12] The identity of the specific AA metabolite generated in a particular cell system depends on both the proximate stimulus and the availability of the downstream AA metabolizing enzymes present in that cell.

Three major enzymatic pathways of AA metabolism are present in the kidney: cyclooxygenases, lipoxygenases, and cytochrome P450 enzymes (Figure 13-1). The cyclooxygenase pathway mediates the formation of prostaglandins and thromboxanes; the lipoxygenase pathway mediates the formation of mono-, di-, and trihydroxyeicosatetraenoic acids (HETEs), leukotrienes, and lipoxins; and the cytochrome P450–dependent oxygenation of AA mediates the formation of epoxyeicosatrienoic acids (EETs), their corresponding diols, HETEs, and monooxygenated AA derivatives. Fish oil diets are rich in ω-3 polyunsaturated fatty acids. The ω-3 fatty acids are those in which the double bond is three carbons from the terminal (ω) carbon, that is, the one furthest from the carboxy-group atom. AA is thus an ω-6 fatty acid. One can interfere with metabolism via all three pathways by competing with AA oxygenation, which results in the formation of biologically inactive end products.[14] Interference with the production of proinflammatory lipids has been hypothesized to underlie the beneficial effects of fish oil in immunoglobulin A nephropathy and other cardiovascular diseases.[15] The following sections describe the current understanding of the chemistry, biosynthesis, renal metabolism, mechanisms of release, receptor biology, signal transduction pathways, biologic activities, and functional significance of each of the metabolites generated by the three major routes of AA metabolism in the kidney.

Cyclooxygenase Pathway

Molecular Biology

The cyclooxygenase enzyme system is the major pathway for AA metabolism in the kidney (Figure 13-2). Cyclooxygenase (prostaglandin synthase G_2/H_2) is the enzyme responsible

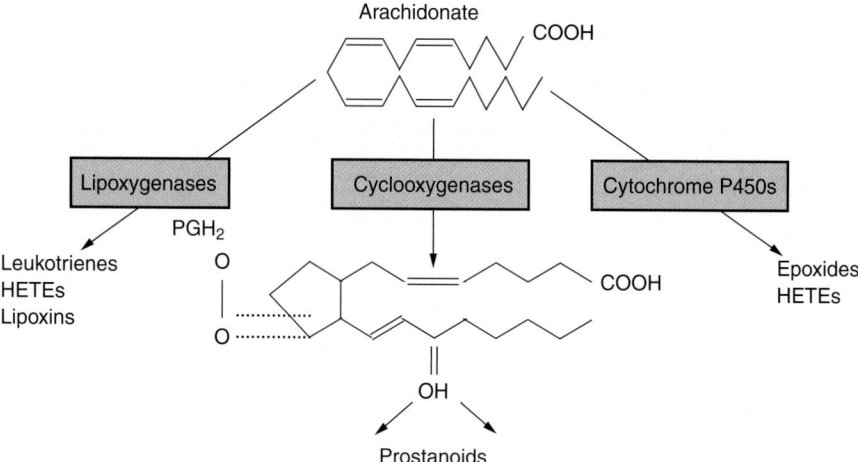

FIGURE 13-1 Pathways of enzymatically mediated arachidonic acid metabolism. Arachidonic acid can be converted into biologically active compounds through metabolism mediated by cyclooxygenase (COX), lipoxygenase (LO), or cytochrome P450 (CYP450).

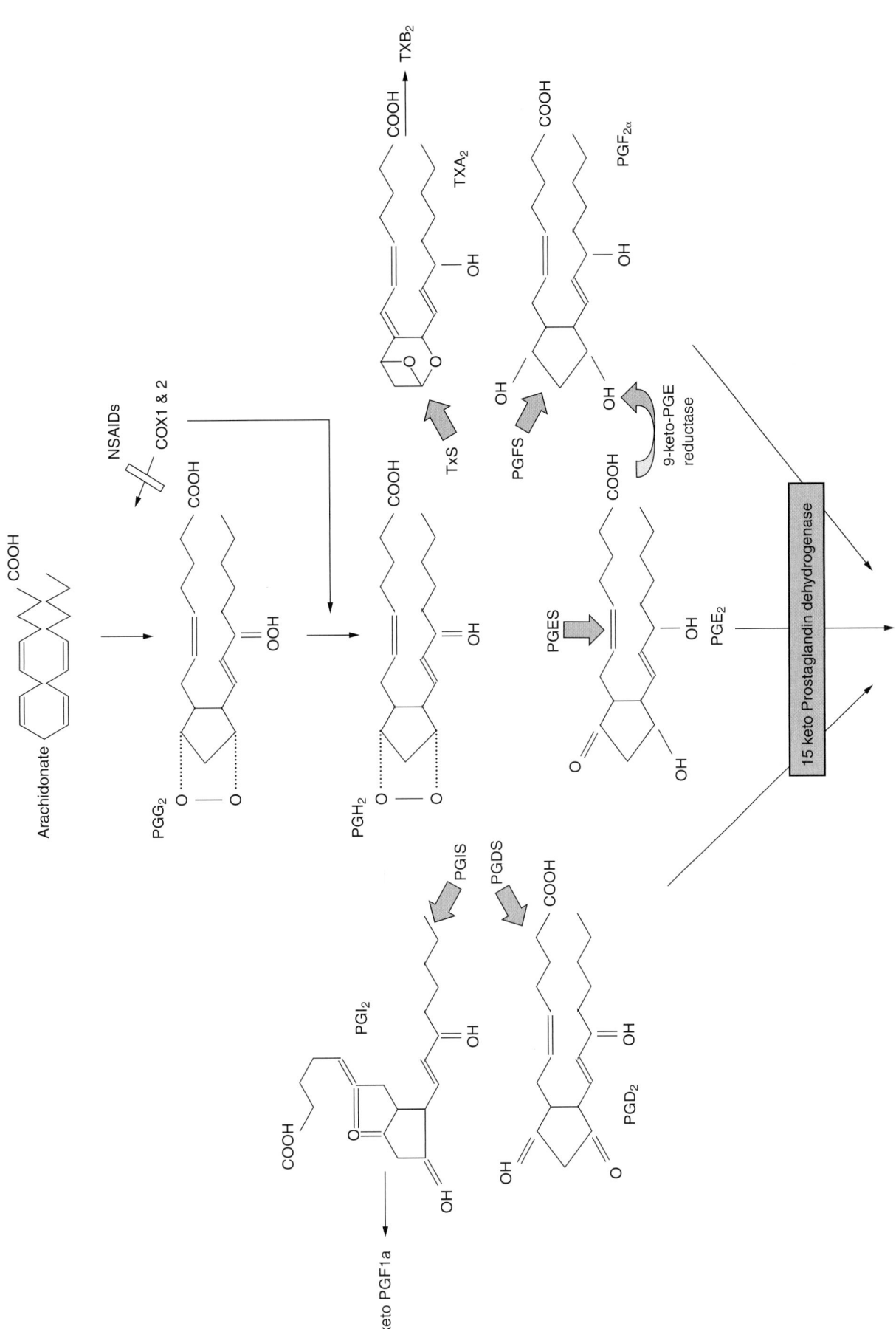

FIGURE 13-2 Cyclooxygenase (COX) metabolism of arachidonic acid (AA). Both COX-1 and COX-2 convert AA to prostaglandin H₂ (PGH₂). PGH₂ is then acted upon by specific synthases to produce prostanoids that act at G protein–coupled receptors which either increase or decrease cyclic adenosine monophosphate (cAMP) or increase intracellular calcium level.

for the initial conversion of AA to prostaglandin G_2 (PGG_2) and subsequently to PGH_2. Cyclooxygenase was first purified from ram seminal vesicles and cloned in 1988. The protein is widely expressed, and the level of activity is not dynamically regulated. Other studies supported the presence of a cyclooxygenase that was dynamically regulated and responsible for increased prostanoid production in inflammation. This second, inducible cyclooxygenase isoform was identified shortly after the cloning of the initial enzyme and designated cyclooxygenase-2 (COX-2), and the initially isolated isoform is now designated COX-1.[7,16,17] COX-1 and COX-2 are encoded by distinct genes located on different chromosomes. The human COX-1 gene (*PTGS1,* or prostaglandin synthase 1) is distributed over 40 kilobases (kb) on 11 exons on chromosome 9, whereas COX-2 is localized on chromosome 1 and spans approximately 9 kb. The genes are also subject to dramatically different regulatory signals.

Regulation of Cyclooxygenase Gene Expression

At the cellular level, COX-2 expression is highly regulated by several processes that alter its transcription rate, message export from the nucleus, message stability, and efficiency of message translation.[18,19] These processes tightly control the expression of COX-2 in response to many of the same cellular stresses that activate arachidonate release (e.g., cell volume changes, shear stress, hypoxia)[10,20] as well as to variety of cytokines and growth factors, including tumor necrosis factor, interleukin-1β, EGF, and platelet-derived growth factor. Activation of COX-2 gene transcription is mediated via the coordinated activation of several transcription factors that bind to and activate consensus sequences in the 5′ flanking region of the COX-2 gene for NF-κB (nuclear factor-κB), NF-IL6 (interleukin-6–regulated nuclear factor, also known as *C/EBP*-β [CCAAT/enhancer-binding protein-β]), and a cyclic adenosine monophosphate response element (CRE).[21] Induction of COX-2 messenger RNA (mRNA) transcription by endotoxin (lipopolysaccharide) may also involve CRE sites[22] and NF-κB sites.[23]

Regulation of Cyclooxygenase Expression by Antiinflammatory Steroids

A molecular basis linking the antiinflammatory effects of cyclooxygenase-inhibiting nonsteroidal antiinflammatory drugs (NSAIDs) and antiinflammatory glucocorticoids has long been sought. A novel mechanism for the suppression of arachidonate metabolism by corticosteroids involving translational inhibition of cyclooxygenase formation had been suggested prior to the molecular recognition of COX-2. With the cloning of COX-2 it became well established that glucocorticoids suppress COX-2 expression and prostaglandin synthesis, an effect now viewed as central to the antiinflammatory effects of glucocorticoids. Posttranscriptional control of COX-2 expression represents another robust mechanism by which adrenal steroids regulate COX-2 expression.[24] Accumulating evidence suggests that COX-2 is modulated at multiple steps in addition to transcription rate, including stabilization of the mRNA and enhanced translation.[18,25] Glucocorticoids, including dexamethasone, downregulate

COX-2 mRNA in part by destabilizing the mRNA.[25] The 3′-untranslated region of COX-2 mRNA contains 22 copies of an AUUUA motif, which are important in destabilizing COX-2 message in response to dexamethasone, where other 3′ sequences appear important for COX-2 mRNA stabilization in response to interleukin-1β.[25] Effects of the 3′-untranslated region as well as other factors regulating efficiency of COX-2 translation have also been suggested.[18] The factors determining the expression of COX-1 are more obscure.

Enzymatic Chemistry

Despite these differences, both prostaglandin synthases catalyze a similar reaction, which results in cyclization of carbons 8 to 12 of the AA backbone forming cyclic endoperoxide, accompanied by the concomitant insertion of two oxygen atoms at carbon 15 to form PGG_2 (a 15-hydroperoxide). In the presence of a reduced glutathione-dependent peroxidase, PGG_2 is converted to the 15-hydroxy derivative, PGH_2. The endoperoxides (PGG_2 and PGH_2) have very short half-lives of about 5 minutes and are biologically active in inducing aortic contraction and platelet aggregation.[26] However, under some circumstances, the formation of these endoperoxides may be strictly limited via the self-deactivating properties of the enzyme.

Expression of recombinant enzymes and determination of the crystal structure of COX-2 have provided further insight into the observed physiologic and pharmacologic similarities to, and differences from, COX-1. It is now clear that cyclooxygenase-inhibiting NSAIDs work by sterically blocking access of AA to the heme-containing active enzymatic site.[27] Particularly well conserved are sequences surrounding the aspirin-sensitive serine residues, at which acetylation by aspirin irreversibly inhibits activity.[28] More recent evidence has developed showing that COX-1 and COX-2 are capable of forming heterodimers and sterically modulating each other's function.[29] The substrate-binding pocket of COX-2 is larger and therefore accepting of bulkier inhibitors and substrates. This difference has allowed the development and marketing of both relatively and highly selective COX-2 inhibitors for clinical use as analgesics,[30] antipyretics,[31] and antiinflammatory agents.[30] Not only does COX-2 play central role in inflammation, but aberrantly upregulated COX-2 expression has been implicated in the pathogenesis of a number of epithelial cell carcinomas[32] and in Alzheimer's disease and other degenerative neurologic conditions.[33]

Renal COX-1 and COX-2 Expression

COX-2 Expression in the Kidney

There is now definitive evidence for significant COX-2 expression in the mammalian kidney (Figure 13-3). COX-2 mRNA and immunoreactive COX-2 are present at low but detectable levels in normal adult mammalian kidney, where in situ hybridization and immunolocalization have demonstrated localized expression of COX-2 mRNA and immunoreactive protein in the cells of the macula densa and a few cells in the cortical thick ascending limb cells immediately adjacent to the macula densa.[34] COX-2 expression is also

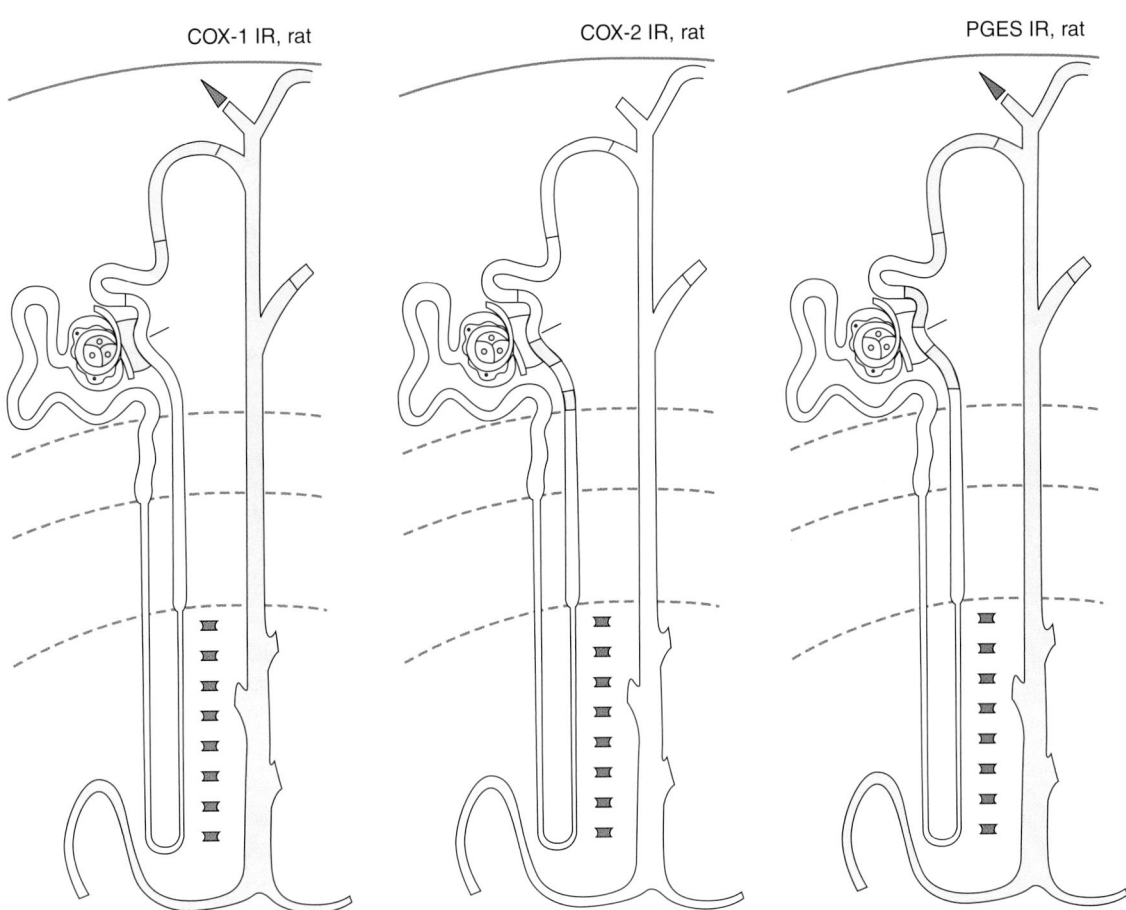

COX-1 IR, rat   COX-2 IR, rat   PGES IR, rat

FIGURE 13-3 Localization (indicated in *shaded areas*) of immunoreactive cyclooxygenases 1 and 2 (COX-1, COX-2) and microsomal prostaglandin E synthase along the rat nephron. (Courtesy of S. Bachmann.)

abundant in the lipid-laden medullary interstitial cells in the tip of the papilla.[34,35] Some investigators have reported that COX-2 may be expressed in inner medullary collecting duct cells or intercalated cells in the renal cortex.[36] Nevertheless COX-1 expression is constitutive, and COX-1 is clearly the most abundant isoform in the collecting duct, so the potential existence and physiologic significance of COX-2 coexpression in this segment remains uncertain.

COX-2 Expression in the Renal Cortex

It is now well documented that COX-2 is expressed in the macula densa/cortical thick ascending limb of the loop of Henle and in kidney of mouse, rat, rabbit, and dog.[1] Furthermore, despite initial controversy regarding COX-2 localization in primate and human kidney, more recent studies confirm a similar distribution of COX-2 in macula densa (as well as medullary interstitial cells), especially in kidneys of the elderly[37,38] and patients with diabetes mellitus, congestive heart failure,[39] and Bartter-like syndrome.[40]

The presence of COX-2 in the unique group of cells comprising the macula densa points to a potential role for COX-2–derived prostanoids in regulating glomerular function.[41] Studies of the prostanoid-dependent control of glomerular filtration rate (GFR) by the macula densa suggest influences via both dilator and constrictor effects of prostanoids contributing to tubuloglomerular feedback.[42,43] Some studies suggest

that COX-2–derived prostanoids are predominantly vasodilators.[44,45] By inhibiting production of dilator prostanoids contributing to the patency of adjacent afferent arterioles, COX-2 inhibition may contribute to the decline in GFR observed in patients taking NSAIDs or selective COX-2 inhibitors[46] (see later). The identity of the specific prostanoids elaborated by the COX-2–expressing macula densa cells remains uncertain.

The volume-depleted state is typified by low sodium chloride (NaCl) delivery to the macula densa, and COX-2 expression in the macula densa is also increased in states associated with volume depletion (Figure 13-4).[34] Of note, COX-2 expression in cultured macula densa cells and cells of the cortical thick ascending limb is also increased in vitro by reducing extracellular chloride (Cl^-) concentration. Perfusion studies of cortical thick limbs and associated glomeruli removed from rabbits pretreated with a low-salt diet to upregulate macula densa COX-2 demonstrated COX-2–dependent release of PGE_2 from the maculae densae in response to decreased Cl^- perfusate.[47] Furthermore the induction of COX-2 by low Cl^- can be blocked by a specific p38 mitogen-activated protein (MAP) kinase inhibitor.[48,49] Finally, in vivo, renal cortical expression of immunoreactive pp38 (the active form of p38) predominantly localized to the macula densa and cortical thick ascending limb, and increased in response to a low-salt diet.[48] These findings point to a molecular pathway whereby enhanced COX-2 expression occurring in circumstances associated with intracellular volume depletion could result from decreased luminal Cl^- delivery. Studies have also

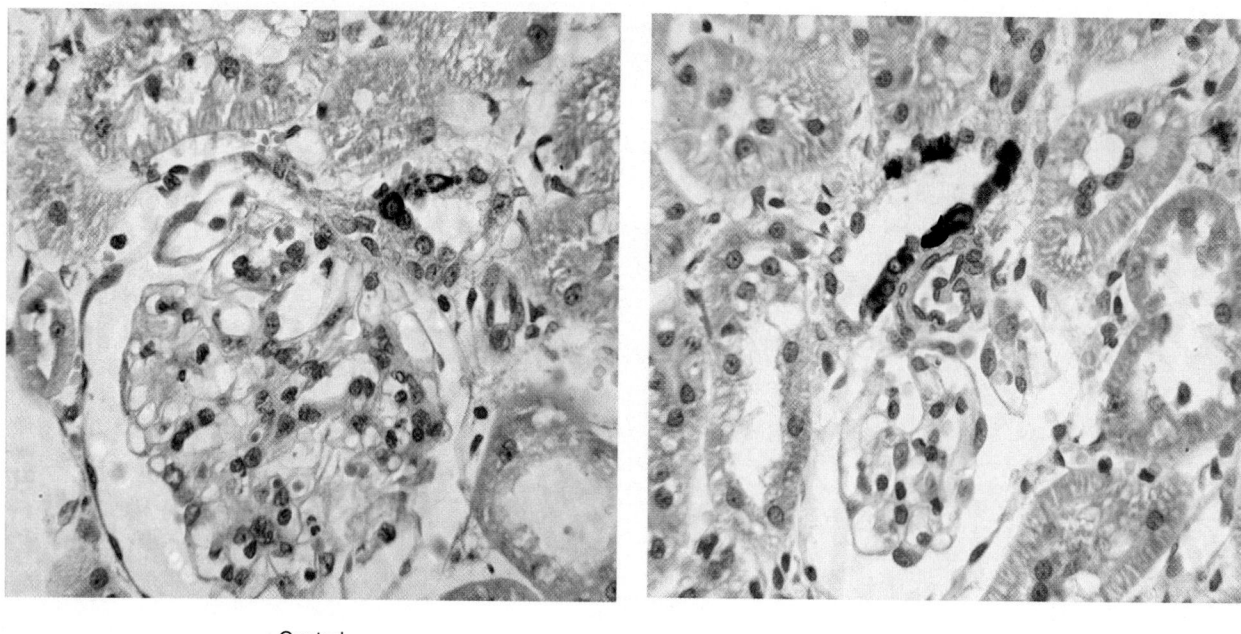

Control   Low salt

FIGURE 13-4 Cyclooxygenase-2 (COX-2) expression is regulated in renal cortex in rats. Under basal conditions, sparse immunoreactive COX-2 is localized to the macula densa and surrounding cortical thick ascending limb (CTAL). After long-term consumption of a sodium-deficient diet, COX-2 expression in the macula densa/CTAL increases markedly.

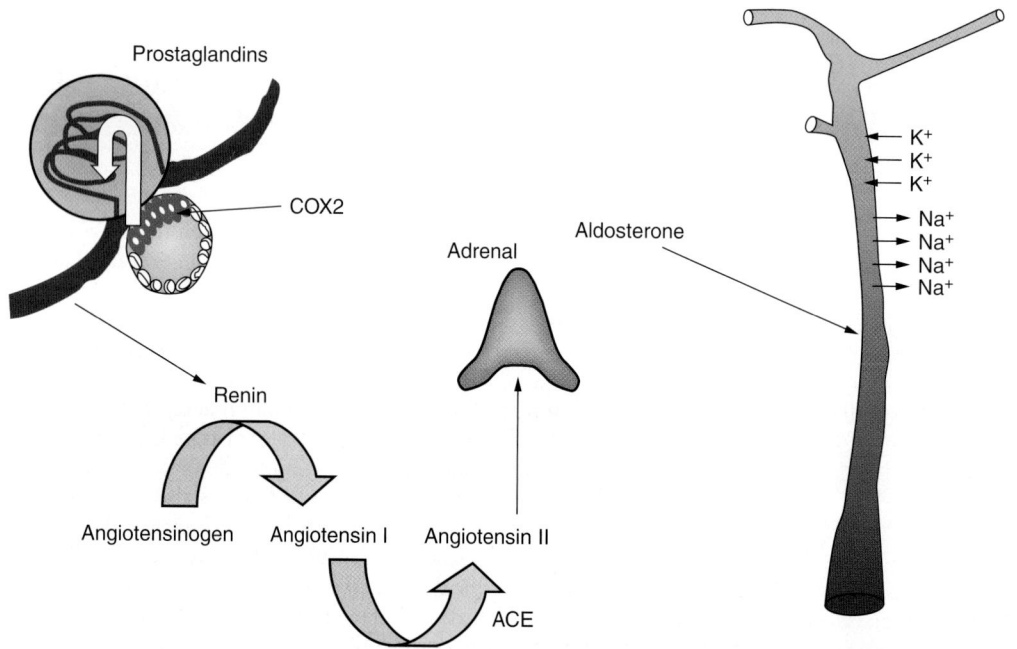

FIGURE 13-5 Proposed intrarenal roles for vasodilatory prostaglandins in the regulation of renal function and blood pressure control. Prostaglandins released from the macula densa and/or the afferent arteriole can both vasodilate the afferent arteriole and modulate renin release from juxtaglomerular cells.

indicated that dopamine and the carbonic anhydrase inhibitor acetazolamide may both indirectly regulate macula densa COX-2 expression by inhibiting proximal reabsorption and thereby increasing luminal macula densa Cl⁻ delivery.[50] In mice deficient in the Na^+/H^+ exchanger subtype 2 (NHE2), the macula densa is shrunken and expression of COX-2 and juxtaglomerular renin is increased, which suggests that NHE2 is the major isoform associated with macula densa cell volume regulation.[51]

In the mammalian kidney, the macula densa is involved in regulating renin release by sensing alterations in luminal Cl⁻ via changes in the rate of $Na^+/K^+/2Cl^-$ cotransport[42] (Figure 13-5). Measurements in vivo in isolated perfused kidney and in isolated perfused juxtaglomerular preparation all indicated that administration of nonspecific cyclooxygenase inhibitors prevented the increases in renin release mediated by macula densa sensing of decreases in luminal NaCl.[42] Induction of a high-renin state by imposition of a salt-deficient diet,

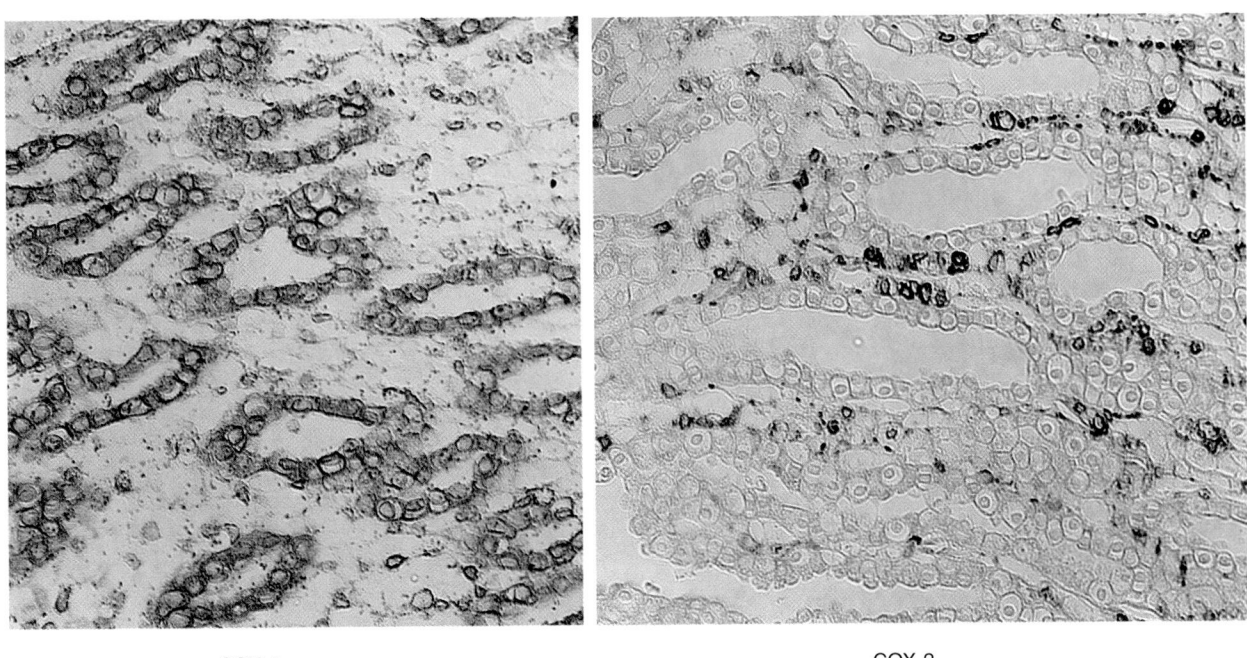

COX-1   COX-2

FIGURE 13-6 Differential immunolocalization of cyclooxygenases 1 and 2 (COX-1, COX-2) in the renal medulla of rodents. COX-1 is predominantly localized to the collecting duct and is also found in a subset of medullary interstitial cells, whereas COX-2 is predominantly localized to a subset of interstitial cells.

angiotensin converting enzyme (ACE) inhibition, diuretic administration, or experimental induction of renovascular hypertension all significantly increase macula densa/cortical thick ascending limb COX-2 mRNA and immunoreactive protein.[41] Administration of COX-2–selective inhibitors blocked elevations in plasma renin activity, renal renin activity, and renal cortical renin mRNA in response to loop diuretics, ACE inhibitors, or a low-salt diet,[41,52-54] and in an isolated perfused juxtaglomerular preparation, increased renin release in response to lowering of the perfusate NaCl concentration was blocked by COX-2 inhibition.[55] Increases in renin in response to a low-salt diet or ACE inhibition were significantly blunted in COX-2 knockout mice[56,57] but were unaffected in COX-1 knockout mice.[58,59] Macula densa COX-2–derived prostanoids appear to be predominantly involved in setting tonic levels of juxtaglomerular renin expression rather than necessarily mediating short-term renin release.[60,61] There is evidence that the effect of ACE inhibitors and angiotensin II receptor blockers in increasing macula densa COX-2 expression is mediated by feedback of angiotensin II on the macula densa, with angiotensin II type 1 (AT_1) receptor activation inhibiting and AT_2 receptor stimulating COX-2 expression.[52] In addition, prorenin and/or renin may stimulate macula densa COX-2 expression through activation of the prorenin receptor.[62]

COX-2 inhibitors have also been shown to decrease renin production in models of renovascular hypertension,[63,64] and studies of mice with targeted deletion of the prostacyclin receptor suggest a predominant role for prostacyclin in mediating renin production and release in these models.[64] In a model of sepsis, COX-2 expression increased in macula densa and both cortical and medullary thick ascending limb. This increased COX-2 expression was mediated by Toll-like receptor 4 (TLR4), and in TLR4$^{-/-}$ mice, juxtaglomerular apparatus renin expression was absent.[65]

In addition to mediating juxtaglomerular renin expression, COX-2 metabolites may also modulate tubuloglomerular feedback. However, investigators using different methodologies have reported that COX-2 metabolites predominantly modulate tubuloglomerular feedback by production of vasodilatory prostanoids[45,66] or mediate afferent arteriolar vasoconstriction by activating thromboxane receptors through generation of thromboxane A_2 (TXA_2) and/or PGH_2.[67] Further studies will be required to reconcile these divergent results.

There is recent evidence that macula densa COX-2 expression is sensitive not only to alterations in intravascular volume but also to alterations in renal metabolism. Specifically, the G protein–coupled receptor GPR91 has been shown to be a receptor for succinate, an intermediate of the citric acid cycle (the Krebs cycle).[68] GPR91 is expressed in macula densa, and both GPR91 and intrarenal production of succinate are increased in diabetes. Studies suggest that succinate activation of GPR91 leads to increased macula densa COX-2 expression.[69,70]

COX-2 Expression in the Renal Medulla

The renal medulla is a major site of prostaglandin synthesis and abundant COX-1 and COX-2 expression (Figure 13-6).[71] COX-1 and COX-2 exhibit differential compartmentalization within the medulla, with COX-1 predominating in the medullary collecting ducts and COX-2 predominating in medullary interstitial cells.[41] COX-2 may also be expressed in endothelial cells of the vasa recta supplying the inner medulla.

The factors determining this differential tissue expression of COX-2 remain uncertain but likely include distinct upstream promoter elements and gene organization. In the collecting duct or human ureter and bladder epithelium, which are also derived from ureteric bud, COX-2 expression is only detected in the setting of malignant transformation.[72] Because of the potential chemopreventive and therapeutic effects of NSAIDs in epithelial cancers,[73] the factors contributing to the aberrant expression of COX-2 in malignant epithelia is an area of intense investigation.[32] Aberrant methylation of COX-2 promoter DNA sequences has been associated with silencing of COX-2 mRNA expression in some colon cancers,[74] but whether differential DNA methylation contributes to the cellular compartmentalization of COX-2 in the normal kidney is unknown.

In those cells normally expressing COX-2, dynamic regulation of its expression appears to be an important adaptive response to physiologic stresses, including water deprivation and exposure to endotoxin.[36,71,75] After dehydration, renal medullary COX-2 mRNA and protein expression are significantly induced,[36,71] primarily in medullary interstitial cells.[71] In contrast, COX-1 expression is unaffected by water deprivation. Although hormonal factors could also contribute to COX-2 induction, shifting cultured renal medullary interstitial cells to hypertonic media (using either NaCl or mannitol) is sufficient to induce COX-2 expression directly. Since prostaglandins play an important role in maintaining renal function during volume depletion or water deprivation, induction of COX-2 by hypertonicity provides an important adaptive response.

As is the case for the macula densa, medullary interstitial cell COX-2 expression is transcriptionally regulated in response to renal extracellular salt and tonicity. Water deprivation activates COX-2 expression in medullary interstitial cells by activating the NF-κB pathway.[71] Other studies suggest roles for MAP kinase/c-Jun N-terminal kinase (JNK) in COX-2 induction following hypertonicity.[76] There is also evidence that nitric oxide (NO) may modulate medullary

COX-2 expression through MAP kinase–dependent pathways.[77] The mechanisms underlying upregulation of medullary COX-2 expression in response to volume expansion are probably multifactorial. There is clear evidence that increased medullary tonicity increases medullary COX-2 expression. Different studies have indicated a role for either NF-κB,[71] epidermal growth factor receptor (EGFR) transactivation,[78] or mitochondrial-generated reactive oxygen species (ROS).[79] Whether these represent parallel pathways or are all interrelated is not yet clear. However, it should be noted that the described EGFR transactivation is mediated by cleavage of the EGFR ligand TGF-α (transforming growth factor-α) by ADAM17 (a disintegrin and metalloproteinase domain 17, also called *TACE* [tumor necrosis factor-α–converting enzyme]), which is known to be activated by src; src, in turn, can be activated by ROS. In addition to medullary COX-2, cortical COX-2 expression increases in salt-sensitive hypertension, especially in the glomerulus, and is inhibited by either the superoxide dismutase mimetic tempol or an angiotensin II receptor blocker.[80]

COX-1 Expression in the Kidney

Although well-defined factors regulating COX-2 and factors determining the expression of COX-2 expression in the kidney are coming to light, the role of renal COX-1 remains more obscure. COX-1 is constitutively expressed in platelets,[81] in the renal microvasculature, and in glomerular parietal epithelial cells (Figure 13-7). In addition COX-1 is abundantly expressed in the collecting duct, but there is little COX-1 expressed in the proximal tubule or thick ascending limb.[44] COX-1 expression levels do not appear to be dynamically regulated. The factors accounting for the tissue-specific expression of COX-1 are uncertain but may involve histone

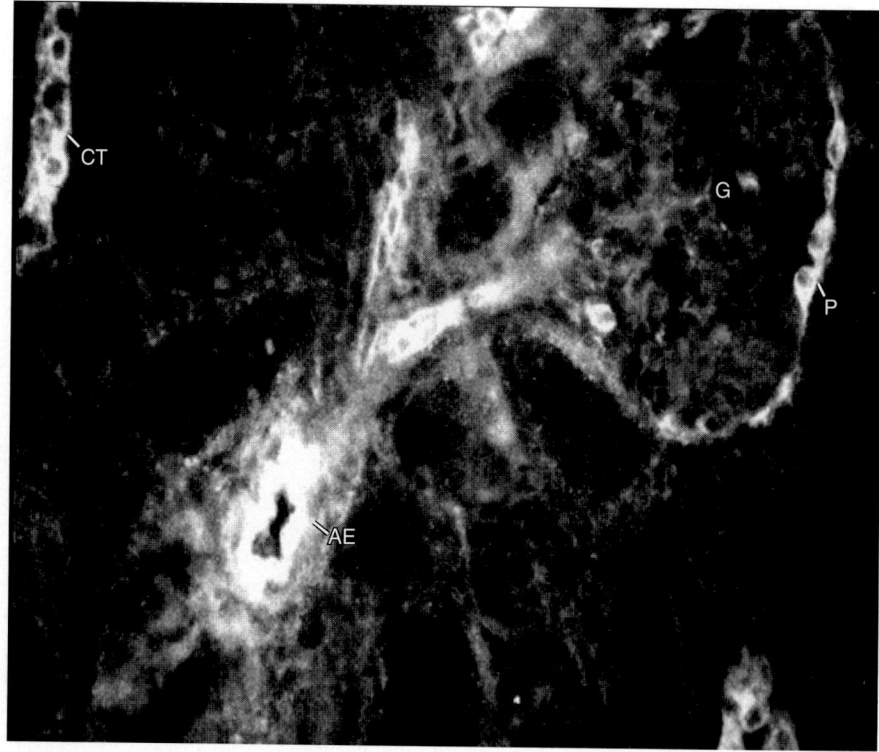

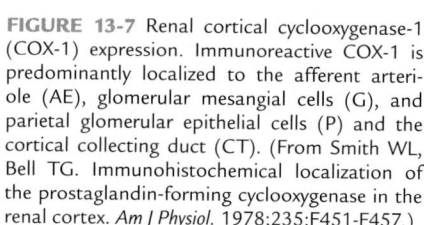

FIGURE 13-7 Renal cortical cyclooxygenase-1 (COX-1) expression. Immunoreactive COX-1 is predominantly localized to the afferent arteriole (AE), glomerular mesangial cells (G), and parietal glomerular epithelial cells (P) and the cortical collecting duct (CT). (From Smith WL, Bell TG. Immunohistochemical localization of the prostaglandin-forming cyclooxygenase in the renal cortex. *Am J Physiol.* 1978;235:F451-F457.)

acetylation and the presence of two tandem Sp1 sites in the upstream region of the gene.[82]

Renal Complications of the Use of Nonsteroidal Antiinflammatory Drugs

Sodium Retention, Edema, Hypertension

Use of nonselective NSAIDs may be complicated by the development of significant Na^+ retention, edema, congestive heart failure, and hypertension.[83] These complications are also apparent in patients using COX-2–selective NSAIDs. Studies with celecoxib and rofecoxib demonstrate that, like nonselective NSAIDs, these COX-2–selective NSAIDs reduce urinary Na^+ excretion and are associated with modest Na^+ retention in otherwise healthy individuals.[84,85]

COX-2 inhibition likely promotes salt retention via multiple mechanisms (Figure 13-8). Reduced GFR may limit the filtered Na^+ load and salt excretion.[86,87] In addition, PGE_2 directly inhibits Na^+ absorption in the thick ascending limb and collecting duct.[88] The relative abundance of COX-2 in medullary interstitial cells places this enzyme adjacent to both these nephron segments, which allows COX-2–derived PGE_2 to modulate salt absorption. COX-2 inhibitors decrease renal PGE_2 production[84,89] and thereby may enhance renal sodium retention. Finally, reduction in renal medullary blood flow by inhibition of vasodilator prostanoids may significantly reduce

renal salt excretion and promote the development of edema and hypertension. COX-2–selective NSAIDs have been demonstrated to exacerbate salt-dependent hypertension in rats.[90] Similarly, patients with preexisting treated hypertension commonly experience hypertensive exacerbations with COX-2–selective NSAIDs.[85] Taken together these data suggest that COX-2–selective NSAIDs have effects similar to those of nonselective NSAIDs with respect to salt excretion.

Hyperkalemia

Nonselective NSAIDs cause hyperkalemia due to suppression of the renin-aldosterone axis. Both decreased GFR and inhibition of renal renin release may compromise renal K^+ excretion. Two recent studies of patients consuming a salt-restricted diet demonstrated that a COX-2–selective inhibitor (either rofecoxib or celecoxib) decreased urinary K^+ excretion.[86,87] In subpopulations of patients at risk, development of overt hyperkalemia with the use of COX-2–selective inhibitors seems likely.

Papillary Necrosis

Both acute and subacute forms of papillary necrosis have been observed with NSAID use.[91-93] Acute NSAID-associated renal papillary injury is more likely to occur in the setting of

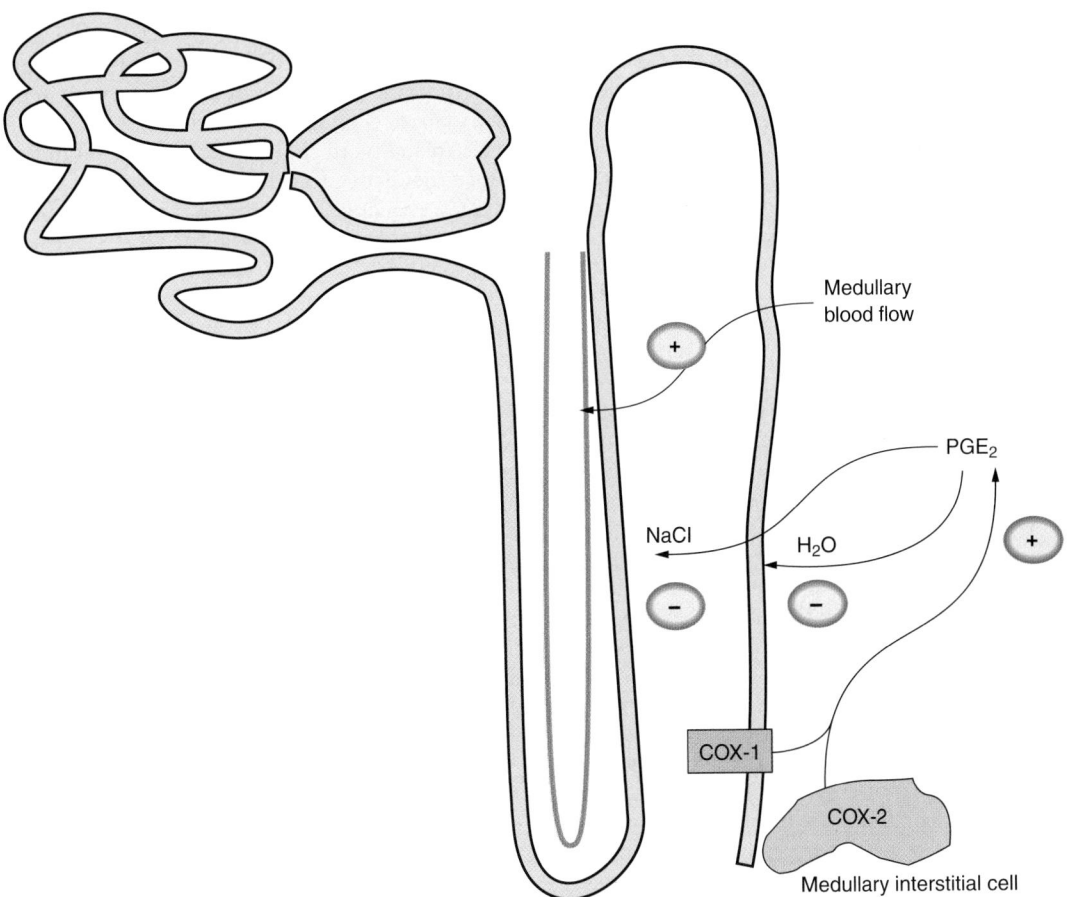

FIGURE 13-8 Integrated role of prostaglandin E_2 (PGE_2) in the regulation of salt and water excretion. PGE_2 can both increase medullary blood flow and directly inhibit NaCl reabsorption in the medullary thick ascending limb and water reabsorption in the collecting duct.

dehydration, which suggests a critical dependence of renal function on cyclooxygenase metabolism in this setting.[71] Long-term use of NSAIDs has been associated with papillary necrosis and progressive renal structural and functional deterioration, much as in the syndrome of analgesic nephropathy observed with the use of acetaminophen, aspirin, and caffeine combinations.[92]

Experimental studies suggest that renal medullary interstitial cells are an early target of injury in analgesic nephropathy.[94] COX-2 has been shown to be an important survival factor for cells exposed to a hypertonic medium.[35,71,95] The coincident localized expression of COX-2 in these interstitial cells[35,71] raises the possibility that, as with the use of nonselective NSAIDs, long-term use of COX-2–selective NSAIDs may contribute to the development of papillary necrosis and analgesic nephropathy.[96] Since the development of analgesic nephropathy requires the regular ingestion of NSAIDs or analgesics over a period of years, this possibility remains to be verified.

Acute Renal Insufficiency

Acute renal failure is a well-described complication of NSAID use.[83] It is generally considered to be a result of altered intrarenal microcirculation and glomerular filtration secondary to the inability to produce beneficial endogenous prostanoids when the kidney is dependent on them for normal function. Reports suggest that like the traditional nonselective NSAIDs, COX-2–selective NSAIDs will also reduce glomerular filtration in susceptible patients.[83] Although rare overall, NSAID-associated renal insufficiency occurs in a significant proportion of patients with underlying volume depletion, renal insufficiency, congestive heart failure, diabetes, and advanced age.[83] These risk factors are additive and rarely are present in patients included in study cohorts used for safety assessment of these drugs. It is therefore relevant that both celecoxib and rofecoxib caused a slight but significant fall in GFR in salt-depleted but otherwise healthy subjects.[86,87] More than 200 cases of acute renal insufficiency due to COX-2–selective NSAIDs have now been reported.[46,97]

Preclinical studies support the concept that inhibition of COX-2–derived prostanoids generated in the macula densa contributes to a fall in GFR by reducing the diameter of the afferent arteriole. In vivo video microscopy studies document reduced afferent arteriolar diameter after administration of a COX-2 inhibitor.[45] Taken together these animal data not only support the concept that COX-2 plays an important role regulating GFR but also the clinical observations that COX-2–selective inhibitors can cause renal insufficiency similar to that reported with nonselective NSAIDs.

Interstitial Nephritis

The gradual development of renal insufficiency characterized by a subacute inflammatory interstitial infiltrate may occur after several months of continuous NSAID ingestion. Less commonly, the interstitial nephritis and renal failure may be fulminant. The infiltrate is typically accompanied by eosinophils; however, the clinical picture is typically much less dramatic than the allergic interstitial nephritis associated with

β-lactam antibiotics, lacking fever or rash.[98] This syndrome has also been reported with the COX-2–selective drug celecoxib.[99,100] Dysregulation of the immune system is thought to play an important role in the syndrome, which typically abates rapidly following discontinuation of the NSAID or COX-2 inhibitor.

Nephrotic Syndrome

Like interstitial nephritis, nephrotic syndrome typically occurs in patients ingesting any one of a myriad of NSAIDs over a course of months.[98,101] The renal pathology is usually consistent with that of minimal change disease with foot process fusion of glomerular podocytes observed on electron microscopy, but membranous nephropathy has also been reported.[102] Typically, nephrotic syndrome occurs together with interstitial nephritis.[98] Nephrotic syndrome without interstitial nephritis, as well as immune complex glomerulopathy, may occur in a small subset of patients receiving NSAIDs. It remains uncertain whether this syndrome results from mechanism-based cyclooxygenase inhibition by these drugs, an idiosyncratic immune drug reaction, or a combination of both.

Renal Dysgenesis

Reports of renal dysgenesis and oligohydramnios in offspring of women administered nonselective NSAIDs during the third trimester of pregnancy[103] have implicated prostaglandins in the process of normal renal development. A similar syndrome of renal dysgenesis has been reported in mice with targeted disruption of the COX-2 gene, as well as in mice treated with the specific COX-2 inhibitor SC58236.[104] Since neither COX-1$^{-/-}$ mice or mice treated with the COX-1–selective inhibitor SC58560 exhibited altered renal development, a specific role for COX-2 in nephrogenesis is suggested.[105-107] A report of renal dysgenesis in the infant of a woman exposed to the COX-2–selective inhibitor nimesulide suggests that COX-2 also plays a role in renal development in humans.[103]

The intrarenal expression of COX-2 in the developing kidney peaks in mouse at postnatal day 4 and in the rat in the second postnatal week.[104,108] It has not yet been determined if a similar pattern of COX-2 expression is seen in humans. Although the most intense staining is observed in a small subset of cells in the nascent macula densa and cortical thick ascending limb, expression in the papilla is also observed.[104,108] Considering the similar glomerular developmental defects observed in rodents treated with a COX-2 inhibitor and in mice with targeted disruption of the COX-2 gene, it seems likely that prostanoids or other products resulting from COX-2 activity in cortical thick limb (and macula densa) act in a paracrine manner to influence glomerular development. The identity of the COX-2–derived prostanoids that promote glomerulogenesis remains uncertain. In vitro studies show that exogenous PGE_1 promotes renal metanephric development[109] and is a critical growth factor for renal epithelia cells. Nevertheless, none of the prostaglandin receptor knockout mice recapitulate the phenotype of the COX-2 knockout mouse.[110]

Cardiovascular Effects of COX-2 Inhibitors

Effects of COX-2 Inhibition on Vascular Tone

In addition to their propensity to reduce renal salt excretion and decrease medullary blood flow, NSAIDs and selective COX-2 inhibitors have been shown to exert direct effects on systemic resistance vessels. The acute pressor effect of angiotensin infusion in human subjects was significantly increased by pretreatment with the nonselective NSAID indomethacin at all angiotensin II doses studied. More recently, administration of selective COX-2 inhibitors or COX-2 gene knockout has been shown to accentuate the pressor effects of angiotensin II in mice.[44] These studies also demonstrated that angiotensin II–mediated blood pressure increases were markedly reduced by administration of a selective COX-1 inhibitor or in COX-1 gene knockout mice.[44] These findings support the conclusion that COX-1–derived prostaglandins participate in, and are integral to, the pressor activity of angiotensin II, whereas COX-2–derived prostaglandins are vasodilators that oppose and mitigate the pressor activity of angiotensin II. Other animal studies more directly show that both NSAIDs and COX-2 inhibitors blunt arteriolar dilation and decrease flow through resistance vessels.[111]

Increased Cardiovascular Thrombotic Events

COX-2 is known to be induced in vascular endothelial cells in response to shear stress,[112] and selective COX-2 inhibition reduces circulating prostacyclin levels in normal human subjects.[113] Therefore, increasing evidence indicates that COX-2–selective antagonism may carry increased thrombogenic risks due to selective inhibition of the endothelial-derived antithrombogenic prostacyclin without any inhibition of the prothrombotic platelet-derived thromboxane generated by COX-1.[114] Although animal studies have provided conflicting results about the role of COX-2 inhibition on the development of atherosclerosis[115-119] there are indications that COX-2 inhibition may destabilize atherosclerotic plaques,[120] as suggested by studies indicating increased COX-2 expression and co-localization with microsomal PGE synthase 1 and metalloproteinases 2 and 9 in carotid plaques from individuals with symptomatic disease before endarterectomy.[121] Because of the concerns about increased cardiovascular risk, two selective COX-2 inhibitors, rofecoxib and valdecoxib, have been withdrawn from the market, and remaining coxibs and other NSAIDs have been relabeled to highlight the increased risk of cardiovascular events.

Prostanoid Synthases

Once PGH_2 is formed in the cell, it can undergo a number of possible transformations, yielding biologically active prostaglandins and TXA_2. As seen in Figure 13-9, in the presence of isomerase and reductase enzymes, PGH_2 is converted to PGE_2 and $PGF_{2\alpha}$, respectively. Thromboxane synthase converts PGH_2 into a bicyclic oxetane-oxane ring metabolite, TXA_2, a prominent reaction product in the platelet and an established synthetic pathway in the glomerulus. Prostacyclin synthase, a 50-kDa protein located in plasma and nuclear membranes and found mostly in vascular endothelial cells,

catalyzes the biosynthesis of prostacyclin (PGI_2). PGD_2, the major prostaglandin product in mast cells, is also derived directly from PGH_2, but its role in the kidney is uncertain. The enzymatic machinery and their localization in the kidney are discussed in detail later.

Sources and Nephronal Distribution of Cyclooxygenase Products

Cyclooxygenase activity is present in arterial and arteriolar endothelial cells, including glomerular afferent and efferent arterioles.[41] The predominant metabolite from these vascular endothelial cells is PGI_2.[122,123] Whole glomeruli generate PGE_2, PGI_2, $PGF_{2\alpha}$, and TXA_2.[1] The predominant products in rat and rabbit glomeruli are PGE_2, followed by PGI_2 and $PGF_{2\alpha}$ and finally TXA_2.

Analysis of individual cultured glomerular cell subpopulations has also provided insight into the localization of prostanoid synthesis. Cultured mesangial cells are capable of generating PGE_2, and in some cases $PGF_{2\alpha}$ and PGI_2 have also been detected.[124] Other studies suggest that mesangial cells may produce the endoperoxide PGH_2 as a major cyclooxygenase product.[125] Glomerular epithelial cells also appear to participate in prostaglandin synthesis, but the profile of cyclooxygenase products generated in these cells remains controversial. Immunocytochemical studies of rabbit kidney demonstrate intense staining for COX-1 predominantly in the parietal epithelial cells. Glomerular capillary endothelial cell prostaglandin generation profiles remain undefined but may well include prostacyclin.

The predominant synthetic site of prostaglandin synthesis along the nephron is the collecting duct, particularly its medullary portion.[126] In the presence of exogenous AA, PGE_2 is the predominant prostaglandin formed in collecting duct, the variations among the other products being insignificant.[1] PGE_2 is also the major cyclooxygenase metabolite generated in medullary interstitial cells.[127] The role that specific prostanoid synthases may play in the generation of these products is outlined later.

Thromboxane Synthase

TXA_2 is produced from PGH_2 by thromboxane synthase, a microsomal protein of 533 amino acids with a predicted molecular weight of approximately 60 kDa. The amino acid sequence of the enzyme exhibits homology to the cytochrome P450s and is now classified as CYP5A1.[128] The human gene is localized on chromosome arm 7q and spans 180 kb. Thromboxane synthase mRNA is highly expressed in hematopoietic cells, including platelets, macrophages, and leukocytes. Thromboxane synthase mRNA is expressed in the thymus, kidney, lung, spleen, prostate, and placenta. Immunolocalization of thromboxane synthase demonstrates high expression in the dendritic cells of the interstitium, with lower expression in glomerular podocytes of human kidney.[129] TXA_2 synthase expression is regulated by dietary salt intake.[130] Furthermore, experimental use of ridogrel, a specific thromboxane synthase inhibitor, reduced blood pressure in spontaneously hypertensive rats.[131] The clinical use of TXA_2 synthase inhibitors is complicated by the fact that the endoperoxide precursors of TXA_2 synthase (PGG_2 and PGH_2) are also capable of activating its downstream target, the TP (TXA_2) receptor.[26]

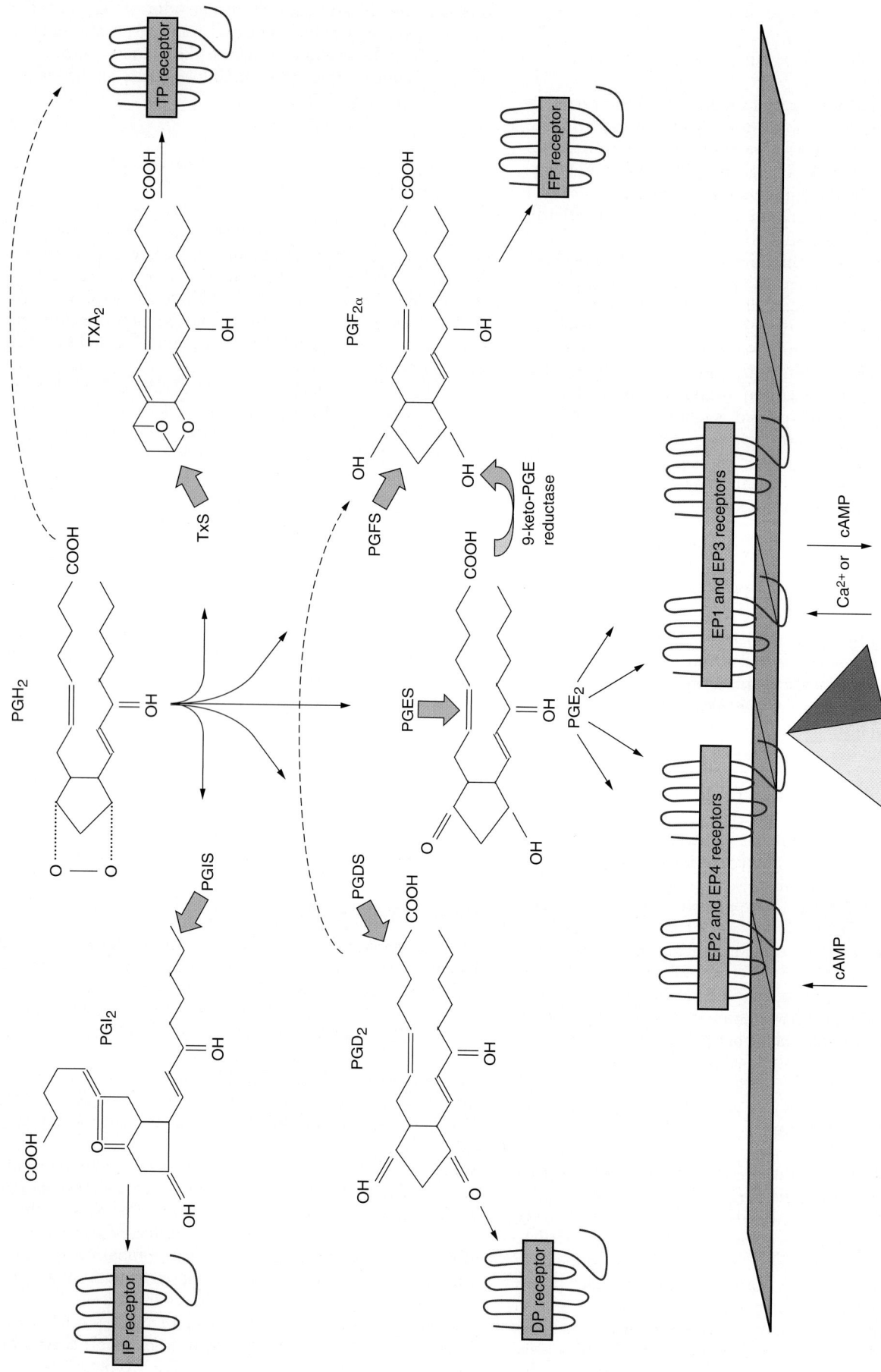

FIGURE 13-9 Prostaglandin synthases.

Prostacyclin Synthase

The biologic effects of prostacyclin are numerous and include nociception, antithrombosis, and vasodilator actions, which have been targeted therapeutically to treat pulmonary hypertension.

PGI_2 is derived by the enzymatic conversion of PGH_2 via prostacyclin synthase. The cloned complementary DNA (cDNA) contains a 1500–base pair open reading frame that encodes a 500–amino acid protein of approximately 56 kDa. The human prostacyclin synthase gene is present as a single copy per haploid genome and is localized on chromosome arm 20q. Northern blot analysis shows that prostacyclin synthase mRNA is widely expressed in human tissues and is particularly abundant in ovary, heart, skeletal muscle, lung, and prostate. PGI synthase exhibits segmental expression in the kidney, especially in kidney inner medulla tubules and interstitial cells.

PGI_2 synthase–null mice were generated.[132] PGI_2 levels in the plasma, kidneys, and lungs of these mice were reduced, which documents the role of this enzyme as an in vivo source of PGI_2. Blood pressure as well as blood urea nitrogen and creatinine levels in the prostacyclin synthase knockout mice were significantly increased, and renal pathologic findings included surface irregularity, fibrosis, cysts, arterial sclerosis, and hypertrophy of vessel walls. Thickening of the thoracic aortic media and adventitia were observed in aged PGI-null mice.[132] Interestingly, this is a phenotype different from that reported for the IP (prostacyclin) receptor knockout mouse.[133] These differences point to the presence of additional prostacyclin-independent PGI_2-activated signaling pathways. Regardless, these findings demonstrate the importance of PGI_2 to the maintenance of blood vessels and to the kidney.

Prostaglandin D Synthases

PGD_2 is derived from PGH_2 via the action of specific enzymes designated PGD synthases. Two major enzymes are capable of transforming PGH_2 to PGD_2, including a lipocalin-type PGD synthase and a hematopoietic-type PGD synthase.[134,135] Mice lacking the lipocalin D synthase gene exhibit altered sleep and pain sensation.[136] PGD_2 is the major prostanoid released from mast cells following challenge with immunoglobulin E. The kidney also appears capable of synthesizing PGD_2. RNA for the lipocalin-type PGD synthase has been reported to be widely expressed along the rat nephron, whereas the hematopoietic-type PGD synthase is restricted to the collecting duct.[137] Urinary excretion of lipocalin D synthase has recently been proposed as a biomarker predictive of renal injury,[138] and lipocalin D synthase knockout mice appear to be more prone to diabetic nephropathy.[139] However, the physiologic roles of these enzymes in the kidney remain less certain. Once synthesized, PGD_2 is available either to interact with the DP1 or DP2 (PGD_2) receptors (see later) or to undergo further metabolism to a PGF_2-like compound.

Prostaglandin F Synthesis

Prostaglandin $F_{2\alpha}$ is a major urinary cyclooxygenase product. Its synthesis may derive either directly from PGH_2 via a PGF synthase[140] or indirectly by metabolism of PGE_2 via a 9-keto-reductase.[140] Another more obscure pathway for PGF formation is by the action of a PGD_2 ketoreductase, which yields a stereoisomer of PGF_2, $9a,11\beta$-PGF_2 (11-epi-$PGF_{2\alpha}$).[140] This reaction and the conversion of PGD_2 into an apparently biologically active metabolite ($9a,11\beta$-$PGF_{2\alpha}$) have been documented in vivo.[141] Interestingly, this isomer can also ligate and activate the FP ($PGF_{2\alpha}$) receptor.[142] The physiologically relevant enzymes responsible for renal $PGF_{2\alpha}$ formation remain incompletely characterized.

Prostaglandin 9-Ketoreductase

Physiologically relevant transformations of cyclooxygenase products occur in the kidney via a reduced nicotinamide adenine dinucleotide phosphate (NADPH)–dependent 9-ketoreductase, which converts PGE_2 into $PGF_{2\alpha}$. This enzymatic activity is typically cytosolic[140] and may be detected in homogenates from renal cortex, medulla, or papilla. The activity appears to be particularly robust in suspensions from the thick ascending limb of the loop of Henle. Renal PGE_2 9-ketoreductase also exhibits 20α-hydroxysteroid reductase activity that could affect steroid metabolism.[140] This enzyme appears to be a member of aldo-keto reductase family 1C.[143]

Interestingly, some studies suggest that the activity of a 9-ketoreductase may be modulated by salt intake and AT_2 receptor activation and may play an important role in hypertension.[144] Mice deficient in the AT_2 receptor exhibit salt-sensitive hypertension, increased PGE_2 production, and reduced production of $PGF_{2\alpha}$,[145] consistent with reduced 9-ketoreductase activity. Other studies suggest that dietary potassium intake may also enhance the activity of conversion from PGE_2 to $PGF_{2\alpha}$.[146] The intrarenal sites of expression of this enzymatic activity remain to be characterized.

Prostaglandin E Synthases

PGE_2 is the other major product of cyclooxygenase-initiated AA metabolism in the kidney and is synthesized at high rates along the nephron, particularly in the collecting duct. Two membrane-associated PGE_2 synthases have been identified: a 33-kDa and a 16-kDa membrane-associated enzyme.[147,148] The initial report describing the cloning of a glutathione-dependent microsomal enzyme (the 16-kDa form) that specifically converts PGH_2 to PGE_2[148] showed that mRNA for this enzyme is highly expressed in reproductive tissues as well as in kidney. Genetic disruption studies confirm that microsomal PGE synthase 1 (mPGES-1)$^{-/-}$ mice exhibit a marked reduction in inflammatory responses compared with mPGES-1$^{+/+}$ mice[149] and indicate that mPGES-1 is also critical for the induction of inflammatory fever.[150]

Intrarenal expression of mPGES-1 has been demonstrated and mapped to collecting duct with lower expression in the medullary interstitial cells and macula densa[126,151] (see Figure 13-3). Thus in the kidney this isoform co-localizes with both COX-1 and COX-2. In contrast, in inflammatory cells, this PGE synthase is co-induced with COX-2 and appears to be functionally coupled to it.[152] Notably, the kidneys of mPGES-1$^{-/-}$ mice are normal and do not exhibit the renal dysgenesis observed in COX-2$^{-/-}$ mice.[106,153] Nor do these mice exhibit the perinatal death from patent ductus arteriosus observed in the EP4 (prostaglandin E_2 type 4) receptor knockout mouse.[154]

More recently another membrane-associated PGE synthase with a relative mass of approximately 33 kDa was purified

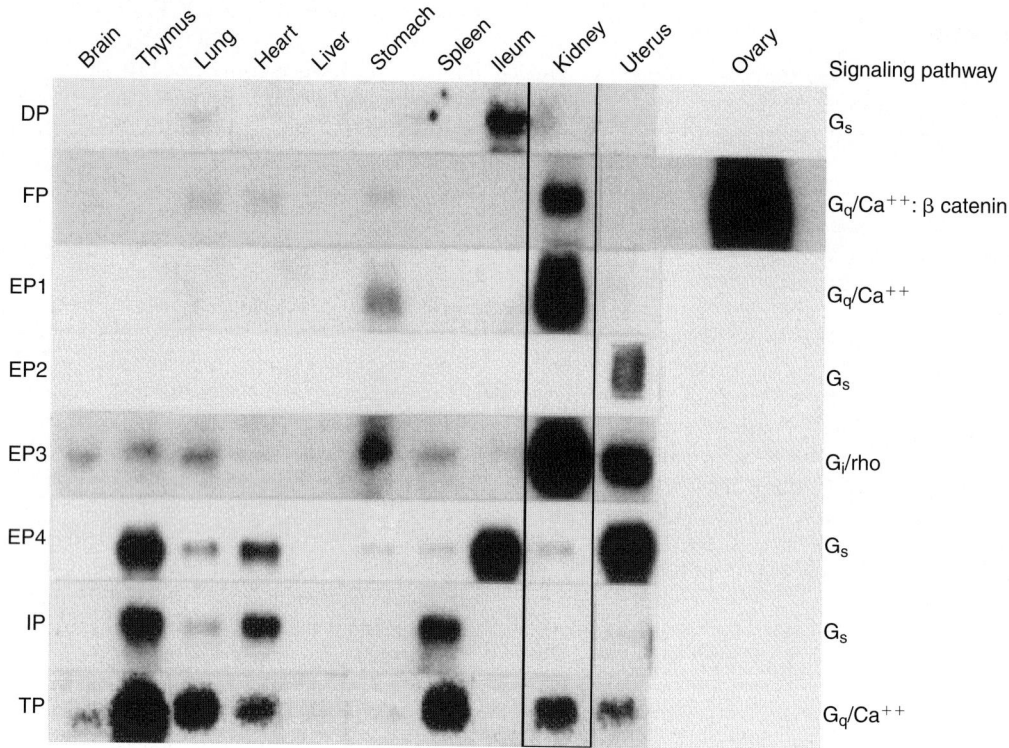

FIGURE 13-10 Tissue distribution of prostanoid receptor messenger RNA (mRNA). (Adapted from Sugimoto Y, Narumiya S, Ichikawa A. Distribution and function of prostanoid receptors: studies from knockout mice. *Prog Lip Res.* 2000;39:289-314.)

from heart. The recombinant enzyme was activated by several sulfhydral (SH)-reducing reagents, including dithiothreitol, glutathione, and β-mercaptoethanol. Moreover, the mRNA distribution was high in the heart and brain, and the mRNA was also expressed in the kidney, but it was not expressed in the seminal vesicles. The intrarenal distribution of this enzyme is, at present, uncharacterized.[147]

Other cytosolic proteins exhibit lower PGE synthase activity, including a 23-kDa glutathione S-transferase requiring cytoplasmic PGE synthase[155] that is expressed in the kidney and lower genitourinary tract.[156] Some evidence suggests that this isozyme may constitutively couple to COX-1 in inflammatory cells. In addition several cytosolic glutathione *S*-transferases have the ability to convert PGH_2 to PGE_2; however, their physiologic role in this process remains uncertain.[157]

Prostanoid Receptors (Figures 13-10 and 13-11)

TP Receptors

The TP receptor was originally purified by chromatography using a high-affinity ligand to capture the receptor.[158] This was the first eicosanoid receptor cloned and is a G protein–coupled transmembrane receptor capable of activating a calcium-coupled signaling mechanism (Figure 13-12). The cloning of other prostanoid receptors was achieved by finding cDNAs homologous to this TP receptor cDNA. Two alternatively spliced variants of the human thromboxane receptor have been described[159] that differ in their carboxy-terminal tail distal to the arginine at position 238. Similar patterns of alternative splicing have been described for both the EP3

receptor and the FP receptor.[160] Heterologous cyclic adenosine monophosphate (cAMP)–mediated signaling of the thromboxane receptor may occur via its heterodimerization with the prostacyclin (IP) receptor.[161]

Either the endoperoxide PGH_2 or its metabolite, TXA_2, can activate the TP receptor.[26] Competition radioligand binding studies have shown these radioligands to have the following rank order of potency on human platelet TP receptor: I-BOP and S-145 > SQ 29,548 > STA_2 > U 46619.[162,163] Whereas I-BOP, STA_2, and U 46619 are agonists, SQ 29,548 and S-145 are high-affinity TP receptor antagonists.[164] Studies have suggested that the TP receptor may mediate some of the biologic effects of the nonenzymatically derived isoprostanes,[165] including modulation of tubuloglomerular feedback.[166] This latter finding may have significance in pathophysiologic conditions associated with increased oxidative stress.[167] Signal transduction studies show that the TP receptor activates phosphatidylinositol hydrolysis (phosphatidylinositol bisphosphate [PIP_2])–dependent Ca^{2+} influx.[158,168] Northern blot analysis of mouse tissues revealed that the highest level of TP mRNA expression is in the thymus, followed by the spleen, lung, and kidney, with lower levels of expression in the heart, uterus, and brain.[169]

Thromboxane is a potent modulator of platelet shape change and aggregation as well as smooth muscle contraction and proliferation. Moreover, a point mutation (arginine to leucine at position 60) in the first cytoplasmic loop of the TXA_2 receptor was identified in a dominantly inherited bleeding disorder in humans, characterized by defective platelet response to TXA_2.[170] Targeted gene disruption of the murine TP receptor also resulted in prolonged bleeding times and reduction in collagen-stimulated platelet aggregation (Figure 13-13). Conversely, overexpression of the TP receptor in vascular tissue increases the severity of vascular pathology

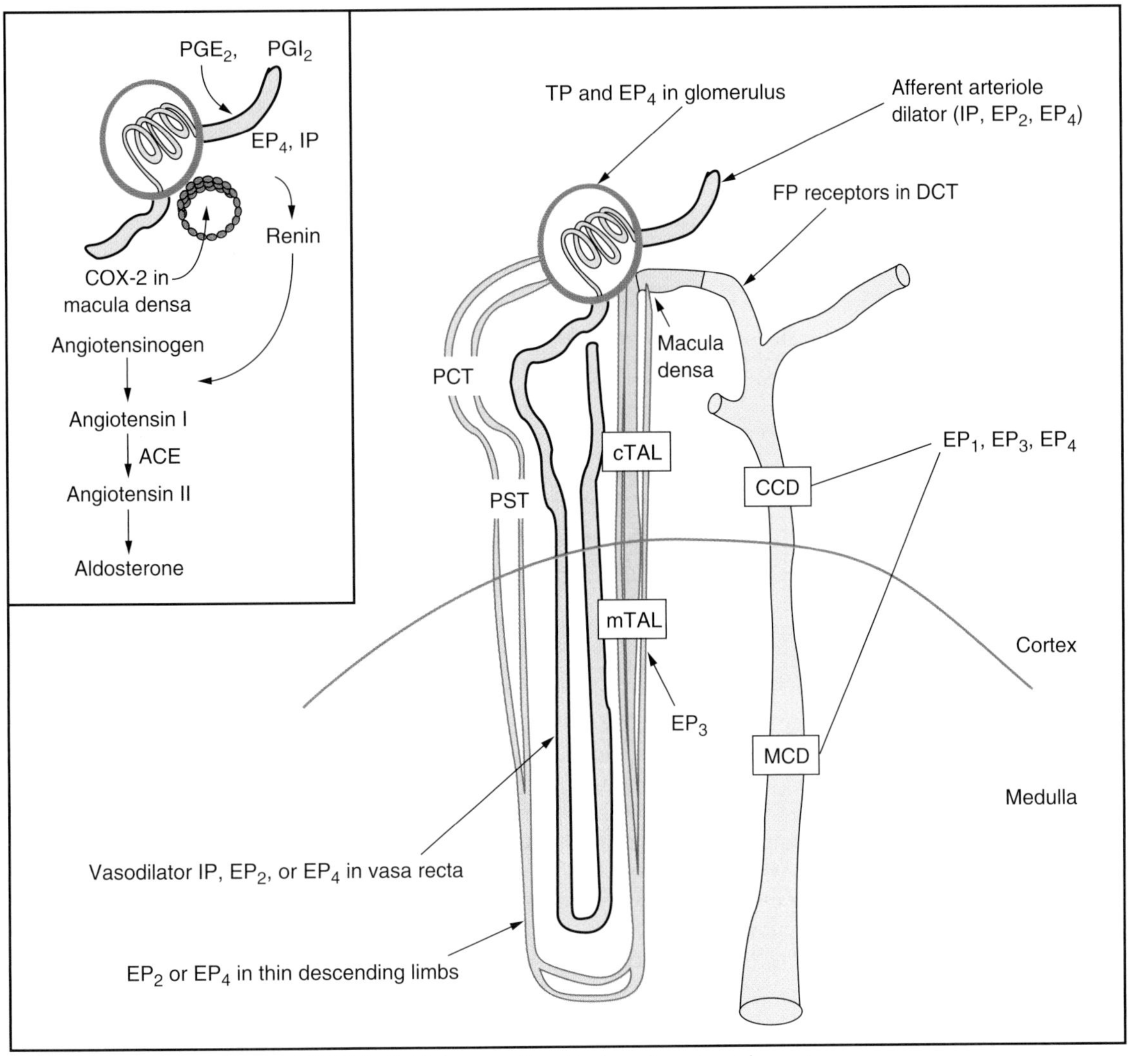

FIGURE 13-11 Intrarenal localization of prostanoid receptors.

following injury.[1] Increased thromboxane synthesis has been linked to cardiovascular diseases, including acute myocardial ischemia and heart failure, and inflammatory renal diseases.[1]

In the kidney, TP receptor mRNA has been reported in glomeruli and vasculature. Radioligand autoradiography using ^{125}I-BOP suggests a similar distribution of binding sites in mouse renal cortex, but additional renal medullary binding sites were observed.[171] These medullary TXA_2 binding sites are absent following disruption of the TP receptor gene, which suggests that they also represent authentic TP receptors.[172] Glomerular TP receptors may participate in potent vasoconstrictor effects of TXA_2 analogs on the glomerular microcirculation associated with reduced GFR.[1] Mesangial TP receptors coupled to phosphatidylinositol hydrolysis, protein kinase C activation and glomerular mesangial cell contraction may contribute to these effects.[173]

An important role for TP receptors in regulating renal hemodynamics and systemic blood pressure has also been suggested. Administration of a TP receptor antagonist reduces blood pressure in spontaneous hypertension in rats[131] and in angiotensin-dependent hypertension.[174] The TP receptor also appears to modulate renal blood flow in angiotensin II–dependent hypertension[175] and in endotoxemia-induced renal failure.[176] Modulation of renal TP receptor mRNA expression

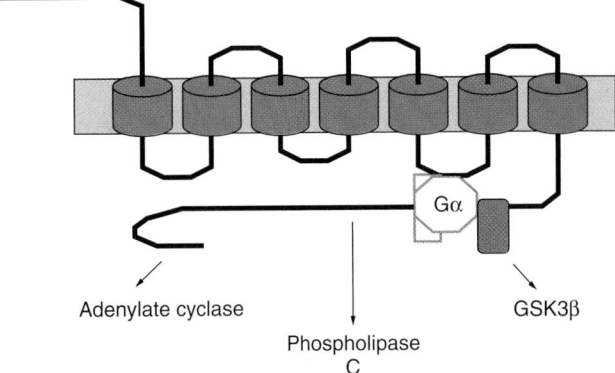

FIGURE 13-12 Prostaglandin receptors are seven-transmembrane G protein–coupled receptors.

and function by dietary salt intake has also been reported.[177] These studies also suggested an important role for luminal TP receptors in the distal tubule in indirect enhancement of glomerular vasoconstriction via effects on the macula densa and tubuloglomerular feedback.[178] However, other studies reveal no significant difference in tubuloglomerular feedback between wild-type and TP receptor knockout mice.[43]

	Renal expression	Knockout phenotype	References
DP	Minimal?	No reduced allergic **asthma**	T. Matsuoka, et al., 2000
IP	+ + Afferent arteriole	± Reduced **inflammation, pain,** increased thrombosis	T. Murata, et al., 1997
TP	+ Glomerulus, tubules?	No prolonged bleeding time, platelet defect	D. Thomas, et al., 1998
FP	+ + + Distal tubules	No failure of **partuition**	Y. Sugimoto, et al., 1997
EP1	+ + + + MCD	No decreased, pain sensation	K. Watanabe, et al., 1997
EP2	+ + interstital, stromal	Impaired **ovulation**, salt sensitive **hypertension (?)**	Kennedy, et al., 1999; Tilley, et al., 1999; Hizaki, et al., 1999; Guan, 2002
EP3	+ + + + TAL, MCD	± Impaired **febrile** response, mild **diluting** defect	Ushikubi, et al., 1998; Reming, et al., 1998
EP4	+ + + Glomerulus, + distal tubules	± Perinatal death from persistent **patent ductus arteriosus**	Nguyen, et al., 1997; Segi, et al., 1998

FIGURE 13-13 Published phenotypes of prostanoid receptor knockout mice.

A major phenotype of TP receptor disruption in mice and humans appears to be reduced platelet aggregation and prolonged bleeding time.[172] Thromboxane may also modulate the glomerular fibrinolytic system by increasing the production of an inhibitor of plasminogen activator (PAI-1) in mesangial cells.[179] Although a specific renal phenotype in the TP receptor knockout mouse has not yet been reported, important pathogenic roles for TXA₂ and glomerular TP receptors in mediating renal dysfunction in glomerulonephritis, diabetes mellitus, and sepsis seem likely.

In an angiotensin II–dependent mouse model of hypertension, deletion of the TP receptor gene ameliorated hypertension and reduced cardiac hypertrophy, but had no effect on proteinuria.[180] Although blockade of NO synthase in an NG-nitro-L-arginine methyl ester model of hypertension in which deletion of the TP receptor also ameliorated hypertension and did not decrease GFR, it led to an increase in worsening of histopathologic features and significant renal hypertrophy. This suggests that the TP receptor may play a renal protective role in some settings.[181]

IP Receptors

The cDNA for the prostacyclin (IP) receptor encodes a transmembrane protein of approximately 41 kDa. The IP receptor is selectively activated by the analog cicaprost.[182] Iloprost and carbaprostacyclin potently activate the IP receptor but also activate the EP1 receptor. Most evidence suggests that the PGI₂ receptor signals via stimulation of cAMP generation; however, at 1000-fold higher concentrations the cloned mouse PGI₂ receptor also signaled via PIP₂.[183] It remains unclear whether PIP₂ hydrolysis plays any significant role in the physiologic action of PGI₂.

IP receptor mRNA is highly expressed in mouse thymus, heart, and spleen[183] and in human kidney, liver, and lung.[184] In situ hybridization shows IP receptor mRNA predominantly in neurons of the dorsal root ganglia and vascular tissue, including aorta, pulmonary artery, and renal interlobular and glomerular afferent arterioles.[185] The expression of IP receptor mRNA in the dorsal root ganglia is consistent with a role for prostacyclin in pain sensation. Mice with IP receptor gene disruption exhibit a predisposition to arterial thrombosis, diminished pain perception, and inflammatory responses.[133]

PGI₂ has been demonstrated to play an important vasodilator role in the kidney,[186] including in the glomerular microvasculature,[187] as well as in regulation of renin release.[188,189] The capacity of PGI₂ and PGE₂ to stimulate cAMP generation in the glomerular microvasculature is distinct and additive,[190] which demonstrates that the effects of these two prostanoids are mediated via separate receptors. IP receptor knockout mice also exhibit salt-sensitive hypertension.[191] Prostacyclin is a potent stimulus of renal renin release, and studies using IP⁻/⁻ mice confirm an important role for the IP receptor in the development of renin-dependent hypertension of renal artery stenosis.[64]

Renal epithelial effects of PGI₂ in the thick ascending limb have also been suggested,[192] and IP receptors have been reported in the collecting duct,[193] but the potential expression and role of prostacyclin in these segments are less well established. Of interest, in situ hybridization also demonstrated significant expression of prostacyclin synthase in medullary collecting ducts,[194] consistent with a role for this metabolite in this region of the kidney. In summary, although IP receptors appear to play an important role in the regulation of renin release and as a vasodilator in the kidney, their role in regulating renal epithelial function remains to be firmly identified.

DP Receptors

The prostaglandin DP1 receptor has been cloned, and like the IP, EP2, and EP4 receptors, the DP receptor predominantly signals by increasing cAMP generation. The human DP receptor binds PGD₂ with a high-affinity binding of

$K_d = 300$ pmol/L and a lower-affinity binding at another site of $K_d = 13.4$ nmol/L.[195] DP-selective PGD_2 analogs include the agonist BW 245C.[196] DP receptor mRNA is highly expressed in leptomeninges, retina, and ileum but was not detected in the kidney.[197] Northern blot analysis of the human DP receptor demonstrated mRNA expression in the small intestine and retina,[198] whereas in the mouse DP receptor mRNA was detected in the ileum and lung.[195] PGD_2 has also been shown to affect the sleep-wake cycle,[199] pain sensation,[136] and body temperature.[200] Peripherally, PGD_2 has been shown to mediate vasodilation as well as possibly inhibiting platelet aggregation. Consistent with this latter finding, the DP receptor knockout mice displayed reduced inflammation in the ovalbumin model of allergic asthma.[201] Although the kidney appears capable of synthesizing PGD_2, its role in the kidney remains poorly defined. Intrarenal infusion of PGD_2 resulted in a dose-dependent increase in renal artery flow, urine output, creatinine clearance, and sodium and potassium excretion.[202]

More recently, another G protein–coupled receptor capable of binding and being activated by PGD_2 was cloned as an orphan chemoattractant receptor from eosinophils and T cells (type 2 helper T cell subset) and designated the CRTH2 receptor.[203] This receptor, now designated as the DP2 receptor, bears no significant sequence homology with the family of prostanoid receptors discussed earlier and couples to increased cell calcium rather than increased cAMP. The use of DP-selective agonists should help clarify whether the renal effects of PGD_2 are mediated by DP1 receptors or DP2 receptors. The recognition of this molecularly unrelated receptor allows for the possible existence of a distinct and new family of prostanoid-activated membrane receptors.

FP Receptors

The cDNA encoding the FP receptor was cloned from a human kidney cDNA library and encodes a protein of 359 amino acid residues. The bovine and murine FP receptors, cloned from corpora lutea, similarly encode proteins of 362 and 366 amino acid residues, respectively. Transfection of HEK293 (human embryonic kidney) cells with the human FP receptor cDNA conferred preferential hydrogen 3–labeled $PGF_{2\alpha}$ (^3H-$PGF_{2\alpha}$) binding with a K_d of 4.3 ± 1.0 nmo/L.[164,204] Selective activation of the FP receptor may be achieved using fluprostenol or latanoprost.[164] The binding of ^3H-$PGF_{2\alpha}$ was displaced by a panel of ligands with the following rank order potency: $PGF_{2\alpha}$ = fluprostenol > PGD_2 > PGE_2 > U 46619 > iloprost.[182] When expressed in oocytes, $PGF_{2\alpha}$ or fluprostenol induced a Ca^{2+}-dependent Cl^- current. Increased cell calcium has also been observed in fibroblasts expressing an endogenous FP receptor.[205] Some studies suggest that FP receptors may also activate protein kinase C–dependent and rho-mediated/protein kinase C–independent signaling pathways.[206] An alternatively spliced isoform with a shorter carboxy-terminal tail has been identified that appears to signal in a manner similar to that of the originally described FP receptor.[207] More recent studies suggest that these two isoforms may exhibit differential desensitization and may also activate a glycogen synthase kinase/β-catenin–coupled signaling pathway.[208]

Tissue distribution of FP receptor mRNA shows highest expression in ovarian corpus luteum followed by kidney, with lower expression in lung, stomach, and heart.[209] Expression of the FP receptor in corpora lutea is critical for normal birth, and homozygous disruption of the murine FP receptor gene results in failure of parturition in females, apparently due to failure of the normal preterm decline in progesterone levels.[210] $PGF_{2\alpha}$ is a potent constrictor of smooth muscle in the uterus, bronchi, and blood vessels; however, an endothelial FP receptor may also play a dilator role.[211] The FP receptor is also highly expressed in skin, where it may play an important role in carcinogenesis.[212] A clinically important role of the FP receptor in the eye in increasing uveoscleral outflow and reducing ocular pressure has been demonstrated. The FP-selective agonist latanoprost has been used clinically as an effective treatment for glaucoma.[213]

The role of FP receptors in regulating renal function is only partially defined. FP receptor expression has been mapped to the cortical collecting duct in mouse and rabbit kidney.[214] FP receptor activation in the collecting duct inhibits vasopressin-stimulated water absorption via a pertussis toxin–sensitive mechanism (which is presumably dependent on the inhibitory G protein G_i). Although $PGF_{2\alpha}$ increases cell Ca^{2+} in cortical collecting duct, the FP-selective agonists latanoprost and fluprostenol did not increase calcium level.[215] Since $PGF_{2\alpha}$ can also bind to EP1 and EP3 receptors,[182,216,217] these data suggest that the calcium increase activated by $PGF_{2\alpha}$ in the collecting duct may be mediated via an EP receptor. $PGF_{2\alpha}$ also increases Ca^{2+} in cultured glomerular mesangial cells and podocytes,[218,219] which suggests that an FP receptor may modulate glomerular contraction. In contrast to these findings, demonstration of glomerular FP receptors at the molecular level has not been forthcoming. Other vascular effects of $PGF_{2\alpha}$ have been described, including selective modulation of renal production of $PGF_{2\alpha}$ by sodium or potassium loading and AT_2 receptor activation.[144]

Recent studies have uncovered a role of the FP receptor in regulating renin expression. Interestingly, FP agonists increased renin mRNA expression in the juxtaglomerular apparatus in a dose-dependent manner, but unlike IP receptor agonists, they did not increase intracellular cAMP. Deletion of the FP receptor resulted in decreased renin levels and decreased systemic blood pressure. These data suggest that FP receptor blockade may be a novel means for the treatment of hypertension.[220]

EP Receptors

Four EP receptor subtypes have been identified.[221] Although these four receptors uniformly bind PGE_2 with a higher affinity than other endogenous prostanoids, the amino acid homology of each is more closely related to other prostanoid receptors that signal through similar mechanisms.[163] Thus the relaxant/cAMP–coupled EP2 receptor is more closely related to other relaxant prostanoid receptors such as the IP and DP receptors, whereas the constrictor/Ca^{2+}–coupled EP1 receptor is more closely related to the other Ca^{2+}-coupled prostanoid receptors such as the TP and FP receptors.[222] These receptors may also be selectively activated or antagonized by different analogs. EP receptor subtypes also exhibit differential expression along the nephron, which suggests distinct functional consequences of activating each EP receptor subtype in the kidney.[223]

EP1 Receptors

The human EP1 receptor cDNA encodes a 402–amino acid polypeptide that signals via inositol 1,4,5-trisphosphate (IP_3) generation and increased cell Ca^{2+} with IP_3 generation. Studies of EP1 receptors may use one of several relatively selective antagonists, including ONO-871, SC-19220, and SC-53122. EP1 receptor mRNA predominates in the kidney but also occurs to a lesser extent in the gastric muscularis mucosae and at even lower levels in the adrenals.[224] Renal EP1 mRNA expression determined by in situ hybridization is expressed primarily in the collecting duct and increases from the cortex to the papillae.[224] Activation of the EP1 receptor increases intracellular calcium and inhibits Na^+ and water reabsorption absorption in the collecting duct,[224] which suggests that renal EP1 receptor activation might contribute to the natriuretic and diuretic effects of PGE_2.

Hemodynamic, microvascular effects of EP1 receptors have also been supported. The EP1 receptor was originally described as a smooth muscle constrictor.[225] One report suggests that the EP1 receptor may also be present in cultured glomerular mesangial cells,[226] where it could play a role as a vasoconstrictor and a stimulus for mesangial cell proliferation. Although a constrictor PGE_2 effect has been reported in the afferent arteriole of rat,[227] apparently produced by EP1 receptor activation,[228] there does not appear to be very high expression of the EP1 receptor mRNA in preglomerular vasculature or other arterial resistance vessels in either mice or rabbits.[229] Other reports show that EP1 receptor knockout mice exhibit hypotension and hyperreninemia, which supports a role for this receptor in maintaining blood pressure.[230]

EP2 Receptors

Two cAMP-stimulating EP receptors, designated EP2 and EP4, have been identified. The EP2 receptor can be pharmacologically distinguished from the EP4 receptor by its sensitivity to butaprost.[231] In the literature prior to 1995 the cloned EP4 receptor was designated the EP2 receptor, but then a butaprost-sensitive EP receptor was cloned[232]; the original receptor was reclassified as the EP4 receptor and the newer butaprost sensitive protein designated the EP2 receptor.[233] A pharmacologically defined EP2 receptor has now also been cloned for the mouse, rat, rabbit, dog, and cow.[234] The human EP2 receptor cDNA encodes a 358–amino acid polypeptide, which signals through increased cAMP. The EP2 receptor may also be distinguished from the EP4 receptor, the other major relaxant EP receptor, by its relative insensitivity to the EP4 agonist PGE_1-OH and insensitivity to the weak EP4 antagonist AH23848,[231] as well as the high-affinity EP4 antagonists ONO-AE3-208 and L-161,982.[235]

The precise distribution of EP2 receptor mRNA has been partially characterized. This characterization reveals a major mRNA species of approximately 3.1 kb that is most abundant in the uterus, lung, and spleen and exhibits only low levels of expression in the kidney.[234] EP2 mRNA is expressed at much lower levels than EP4 mRNA in most tissues.[236] There is scant evidence to suggest segmental distribution of the EP2 receptor along the nephron.[234] Interestingly, it is expressed in cultured renal interstitial cells, which supports the possibility that the EP2 receptor is predominantly expressed in this portion of the nephron.[234] Studies in knockout mice demonstrate

a critical role for the EP2 receptor role in ovulation and fertilization.[237] In addition these studies suggest a potential role for the EP2 receptor in salt-sensitive hypertension.[237] This latter finding supports an important role for the EP2 receptor in protecting systemic blood pressure, perhaps via its vasodilator effect or effects on renal salt excretion. Evidence for the latter role has been revealed in studies demonstrating that a high-salt diet increases PGE_2 production, and infusion of EP-selective agonists identified the EP2 receptor as mediating PGE_2-evoked natriuresis. Moreover, deletion of the EP2 receptor ablated the natriuretic effect of PGE_2.[238]

EP3 Receptors

The EP3 receptor generally acts as a constrictor of smooth muscle.[239] Nuclease protection and Northern blot analysis demonstrate relatively high levels of EP3 receptor expression in several tissues, including kidney, uterus, adrenal, and stomach, with riboprobes hybridizing to major mRNA species at approximately 2.4 and approximately 7.0 kb.[240] This receptor is unique in that multiple (more than eight) alternatively spliced variants exist, differing only in their carboxy-terminal cytoplasmic tails.[241-243] The EP3 splice variants bind PGE_2 and the EP3 agonists MB28767 and sulprostone with similar affinity, and although they exhibit common inhibition of cAMP generation via a pertussis toxin–sensitive G_i-coupled mechanism, the tails may recruit different signaling pathways, including Ca^{2+}-dependent signaling[163,231] and the small G protein rho.[244] Differences in agonist-independent activity have been observed for several of the splice variants, which suggests that they may play a role in constitutive regulation of cellular events.[245] The physiologic roles of these different carboxy-terminal splice variants and sites of expression within the kidney remain uncertain.

In situ hybridization demonstrates that EP3 receptor mRNA is abundant in the thick ascending limb and collecting duct.[246] This distribution has been confirmed by reverse transcriptase polymerase chain reaction testing of microdissected rat and mouse collecting ducts and corresponds to the major binding sites for radioactive PGE_2 in the kidney.[247] An important role for a G_i-coupled PGE receptor in regulating water and salt transport along the nephron has been recognized for many years. PGE_2 directly inhibits salt and water absorption in both microperfused thick ascending limbs and collecting ducts. PGE_2 directly inhibits Cl^- absorption in the mouse or rabbit medullary thick ascending limb from either the luminal or basolateral surfaces.[248] PGE_2 also inhibits hormone-stimulated cAMP generation in the thick ascending limb. Good and George demonstrated that PGE_2 modulates ion transport in the rat thick ascending limb by a pertussis toxin–sensitive mechanism.[248] Interestingly, these effects also appear to involve protein kinase C activation,[249] which possibly reflects activation of a novel EP3 receptor signaling pathway that may correspond to alternative signaling pathways as described earlier.[244] Taken together, these data support a role for the EP3 receptor in regulating transport in both the collecting duct and thick ascending limb.

Blockade of endogenous PGE_2 synthesis by NSAIDs enhances urinary concentration. It is likely that PGE_2-mediated antagonism of vasopressin-stimulated salt absorption in the thick ascending limb and water absorption in the collecting duct contributes to its diuretic effect. In the in vitro microperfused collecting duct, PGE_2 inhibits both vasopressin-stimulated osmotic water absorption and vaso-pressin-stimulated cAMP generation.[215] Furthermore PGE$_2$ inhibition of water absorption and cAMP generation are both blocked by pertussis toxin, which suggests effects mediated by G$_i$.[215] When administered in the absence of vasopressin, PGE$_2$ actually stimulates water absorption in the collecting duct from either the luminal or the basolateral side.[250] These stimulatory effects of PGE$_2$ on transport in the collecting duct appear to be related to activation of the EP4 receptor.[250] Despite the presence of this absorption-enhancing EP receptor, in vivo studies suggest that, in the presence of vasopressin, the predominant effects of endogenous PGE$_2$ on water transport are diuretic. Based on the preceding functional considerations, one would expect EP3$^{-/-}$ mice to exhibit inappropriately enhanced urinary concentration. Surprisingly, EP3$^{-/-}$ mice exhibited a comparable urinary concentration after administration of desmopressin (DDAVP), with similar 24-hour water intake and similar maximal and minimal urinary osmolality.[59] The only clear difference was that in mice allowed free access to water, indomethacin increased urinary osmolality in normal mice but not in the knockout animals. These findings raise the possibility that some of the renal actions of PGE$_2$ normally mediated by the EP3 receptor have been coopted by other receptors (such as the EP1 or FP receptor) in the EP3 knockout mouse. This proposition remains to be formally tested.

Study of the importance of EP3 receptor activation in animal physiology has been significantly advanced by the availability of mice with targeted disruption of the associated gene.[18] Mice with targeted deletion of the EP3 receptor exhibit an impaired febrile response, which suggests that EP3 receptor antagonists could be effective antipyretic agents.[251] Other studies suggest that the EP3 receptor plays an important vasopressor role in the peripheral circulation of mice.[229] Studies in knockout mice also support a potential role for the EP3 receptor as an important systemic vasopressor.[229,252] In the intrarenal circulation, PGE$_2$ has variable effects, acting as a vasoconstrictor in the larger proximal portion of the intralobular arteries and changing to a vasodilator effect in the smaller distal intralobular arteries and afferent arterioles.[253]

EP4 Receptor

Like the EP2 receptor, the EP4 receptor signals through increased cAMP.[254] The human EP4 receptor cDNA encodes a 488–amino acid polypeptide with a predicted molecular mass of approximately 53 kDa.[255] Note that care must be taken in reviewing the literature prior to 1995, when, as noted earlier, this receptor was generally referred to as the *EP2 receptor*.[233] In addition to the human EP4 receptor, EP4 receptors for the mouse, rat, rabbit, and dog have been cloned. EP4 receptors can be pharmacologically distinguished from EP1 and EP3 receptors by their insensitivity to sulprostone and from EP2 receptors by the latter's insensitivity to butaprost and relatively selective activation by PGE$_1$-OH.[164] EP4-selective agonists (ONO-AE1-329, ONO-4819) and antagonists (ONO-AE3-208, L-161,982) have been generated[231]; however, to date, their use has not been widely reported.

EP4 receptor mRNA is highly expressed relative to EP2 receptor mRNA and widely distributed, with a major species of approximately 3.8 kb detected by Northern blot analysis in the thymus, ileum, lung, spleen, adrenal, and kidney.[236,256] Dominant vasodilator effects of EP4 receptor activation have

been described in venous and arterial beds.[196,239] A critical role for the EP4 receptor in regulating the perinatal closure of the pulmonary ductus arteriosus has also been suggested by studies of mice with targeted disruption of the EP4 receptor gene.[154,257] On a 129-strain background, EP4$^{-/-}$ mice had nearly 100% perinatal mortality due to persistent patent ductus arteriosus.[257] Interestingly, when bred on a mixed genetic background, only 80% of EP4$^{-/-}$ mice died, whereas approximately 21% underwent closure of the ductus and survived.[154] Preliminary studies in these survivors support an important role for the EP4 receptor as a systemic vasodepressor[258]; however, their heterogeneous genetic background complicates the interpretation of these results, since survival may select for modifier genes that not only allow ductus closure but also alter other hemodynamic responses.

Other roles for the EP4 receptor in controlling blood pressure have been suggested, including the ability to stimulate aldosterone release from zona glomerulosa cells.[259] In the kidney, EP4 receptor mRNA expression is primarily in the glomerulus, where its precise function is uncharacterized,[256,260] but it might contribute to regulation of the renal microcirculation as well as renin release.[261] Studies in mice with genetic deletion of selective prostanoid receptors indicated that in EP4$^{-/-}$ mice, as well as in IP$^{-/-}$ mice to a lesser extent, renin production failed to increase in response to loop diuretic administration, which indicates that macula densa–derived PGE$_2$ increased renin primarily through EP4 activation.[262] This corresponds to the results of studies suggesting that EP4 receptors are expressed in cultured podocytes and juxtaglomerular apparatus cells.[218,261] PGE$_2$ may mediate increased podocyte COX-2 expression through EP4–mediated increased cAMP, which activates p38 through a protein kinase A–independent process.[263] Finally, the EP4 receptor in the renal pelvis may participate in the regulation of salt excretion by altering afferent renal nerve output.[264]

Regulation of Renal Function by EP Receptors

PGE$_2$ exerts myriad effects in the kidney, presumably mediated by EP receptors. PGE$_2$ not only dilates the glomerular microcirculation and vasa rectae, supplying the renal medulla,[265] but also modulates salt and water transport in the distal tubule (see Figure 13-5).[266] The maintenance of normal renal function during physiologic stress is particularly dependent on endogenous prostaglandin synthesis. In this setting, the vasoconstrictor effects of angiotensin II, catecholamines, and vasopressin are more effectively buffered by prostaglandins in the kidney than in other vascular beds, which preserves normal renal blood flow, GFR, and salt excretion. Administration of cyclooxygenase-inhibiting NSAIDs in the setting of volume depletion interferes with these dilator effects and may result in a catastrophic decline in GFR that leads to overt renal failure.[267]

Other evidence points to vasoconstrictor and prohypertensive effects of endogenous PGE$_2$. PGE$_2$ stimulates renin release from the juxtaglomerular apparatus,[268] which leads to a subsequent increase in the level of the vasoconstrictor angiotensin II. In conscious dogs, long-term intrarenal PGE$_2$ infusion increases renal renin secretion, which results in hypertension.[269] Treatment of salt-depleted rats with indomethacin not only decreases plasma renin activity, but also reduces blood pressure, which suggests that prostaglandins support blood pressure during salt depletion via their capacity to increase renin secretion.[270] Direct vasoconstrictor effects of PGE_2 on the vasculature have also been observed.[229] It is conceivable that these latter effects might predominate in circumstances in which the kidney is exposed to excessively high perfusion pressures. Thus, depending on the setting, the primary effect of PGE_2 may be either to increase or to decrease vascular tone, effects that appear to be mediated by distinct EP receptors.

RENAL CORTICAL HEMODYNAMICS

The expression of the EP4 receptor in the glomerulus suggests that it may play an important role in the regulation of renal hemodynamics. Prostaglandins regulate the renal cortical microcirculation, and as alluded to earlier, both glomerular constrictor and dilator effects of prostaglandins have been observed.[229,271] In the setting of volume depletion, endogenous PGE_2 helps maintain GFR by dilating the afferent arteriole.[271] Some data suggest roles for EP and IP receptors coupled to increased cAMP generation in mediating vasodilator effects in the preglomerular circulation.[42,261,272] PGE_2 exerts a dilator effect on the afferent arteriole but not on the efferent arteriole, consistent with the presence of an EP2 or EP4 receptor in the preglomerular microcirculation.

RENIN RELEASE

Other data suggest that the EP4 receptor may also stimulate renin release. Soon after the introduction of NSAIDs it was recognized that endogenous prostaglandins play an important role in stimulating renin release.[42] Treatment of salt-depleted rats with indomethacin not only decreases plasma renin activity, but also causes blood pressure to fall, which suggests that prostaglandins support blood pressure during salt depletion via their capacity to increase renin secretion. Prostanoids also play a central role in the pathogenesis of renovascular hypertension, and administration of NSAIDs lowers blood pressure in both animals and humans with renal artery stenosis.[273] PGE_2 induces renin release in isolated preglomerular juxtaglomerular apparatus cells.[268] Like the effect of β-adrenergic agents, this effect appears to be through a cAMP-coupled response, which supports a role for an EP4 or EP2 receptor.[268] EP4 receptor mRNA has been detected in microdissected juxtaglomerular apparatus cells,[274] which supports the possibility that renal EP4 receptor activation contributes to enhanced renin release. Finally, regulation of plasma renin activity and intrarenal renin mRNA does not appear to be different in wild-type and EP2 knockout mice,[275] a finding that argues against a major role for the EP2 receptor in regulating renin release. Conversely, one report suggests that EP3 receptor mRNA is localized to the macula densa, which suggests that this cAMP-inhibiting receptor may also contribute to the control of renin release.[260]

RENAL MICROCIRCULATION

The EP2 receptor also appears to play an important role in regulating afferent arteriolar tone.[271] In the setting of systemic hypertension, the normal response of the kidney is to increase salt excretion, which mitigates the increase in blood pressure. This so-called pressure natriuresis plays a key role in the ability of the kidney to protect against hypertension.[276] Increased blood pressure is accompanied by increased renal perfusion pressure and enhanced urinary PGE_2 excretion.[277] Inhibition of prostaglandin synthesis markedly blunts (although it does not eliminate) pressure natriuresis.[278] The mechanism by which PGE_2 contributes to pressure natriuresis may involve changes

in resistance of the renal medullary microcirculation.[279] PGE_2 directly dilates the descending vasa recta, and increased medullary blood flow may contribute to the increased interstitial pressure observed as renal perfusion pressure increases, which leads to enhanced salt excretion.[265] The identity of the dilator PGE_2 receptor controlling the contractile properties of the descending vasa recta remains uncertain, but EP2 or EP4 receptors seem likely candidates.[196] Studies demonstrating salt-sensitive hypertension in mice with targeted disruption of the EP2 receptor[237] suggest that the EP2 receptor facilitates the ability of the kidney to increase sodium excretion and thereby protect systemic blood pressure from a high-salt diet. Given its defined role in vascular smooth muscle,[237] these effects of EP2 receptor disruption seem more likely to relate to its effects on renal vascular tone. In particular, loss of a vasodilator effect in the renal medulla might modify pressure natriuresis and could contribute to hypertension in EP2 knockout mice. Nonetheless, a role for either the EP2 or the EP4 receptor in regulating renal medullary blood flow remains to be established. In conclusion, direct vasomotor effects of EP4 receptors as well as effects on renin release may play critical roles in regulating systemic blood pressure and renal hemodynamics.

Effects of COX-1 and COX-2 Metabolites on Salt and Water Transport

COX-1 and COX-2 metabolites of arachidonate have important direct epithelial effects on salt and water transport along the nephron.[280] Thus, functional effects can be observed that are thought to be independent of any hemodynamic changes produced by these compounds. Because biologically active AA metabolites are rapidly metabolized, they act predominantly in an autocrine or paracrine fashion, and thus their locus of action will be quite close to their point of generation. Therefore, one can expect that direct epithelial effects of these compounds will result when they are produced by the tubule cells themselves or the neighboring interstitial cells, and the tubules possess an appropriate receptor for the ligand.

Proximal Tubule

Neither the proximal convoluted tubule nor the proximal straight tubule appears to produce amounts of biologically active cyclooxygenase metabolites of AA. As is discussed in a subsequent section, the dominant arachidonate metabolites produced by proximal convoluted and straight tubules are metabolites of the cytochrome P450 pathway.[281]

Early whole-animal studies suggested that PGE_2 might have an action in the proximal tubule because of its effects on urinary phosphate excretion. PGE_2 blocked the phosphaturic action of calcitonin infusion in thyroparathyroidectomized rats. Nevertheless, studies utilizing in vitro perfused proximal tubules failed to show an effect of PGE_2 on NaCl or phosphate transport in the proximal convoluted tubule. More recent studies suggest that PGE_2 may play a key role in the phosphaturic action of fibroblast growth factor 23,[282] because phosphaturia in Hyp mice with X-linked hyperphosphaturia is associated with markedly increased urine PGE_2 excretion, and phosphaturia was normalized by indomethacin administration.[283] Nevertheless, there are very few data on the actions of other cyclooxygenase metabolites in proximal tubules and scant molecular evidence for expression of classic G protein–coupled prostaglandin receptors in this segment of the nephron.

Loop of Henle

The nephron segments making up the loop of Henle also display limited metabolism of exogenous AA through the cyclooxygenase pathway, although given the realization that COX-2 is expressed in this segment, it is of note that PGE_2 was uniformly greater in the cortical segment than in the medullary thick ascending limb. The thick ascending limb has been shown to exhibit PGE_2 receptors in high density.[284] Studies have also demonstrated high expression levels of mRNA for the EP3 receptor in medullary thick ascending limb of both rabbit and rat[217] (see earlier section on the EP3 receptor). Subsequent to the demonstration that PGE_2 inhibits NaCl absorption in the medullary thick ascending limb of the rabbit perfused in vitro, it was shown that PGE_2 blocks antidiuretic hormone– but not cAMP-stimulated NaCl absorption in the medullary thick ascending limb of the mouse. It is likely that the mechanism involves activation of G_i and inhibition of adenyl cyclase by PGE_2, possibly via the EP3 receptors expressed in this segment.

Collecting Duct System

In vitro perfusion studies of rabbit cortical collecting tubule demonstrated that PGE_2 directly inhibits sodium transport in the collecting duct when applied to the basolateral surface of this nephron segment. It is now apparent that PGE_2 utilizes multiple signal transduction pathways in the cortical collecting duct, including those that modulate intracellular cAMP levels and Ca^{2+}. PGE_2 can stimulate or suppress cAMP accumulation. The latter may also involve stimulation of phosphodiesterase. Although modulation of cAMP levels appears to play an important role in PGE_2 effects on water transport in the cortical collecting duct (see following section), it is less clear that PGE_2 affects sodium transport via modulation of cAMP levels.[215] PGE_2 has been shown to increase cell calcium possibly coupled with protein kinase C activation in perfused cortical collecting ducts in vitro.[285] This effect may be mediated by the EP1 receptor subtype coupled to phosphatidylinositol hydrolysis.[224]

Water Transport

Vasopressin-regulated water transport in the collecting duct is markedly influenced by cyclooxygenase products, especially prostaglandins. When cyclooxygenase inhibitors are administered to humans, rats, or dog, the antidiuretic action of arginine vasopressin (AVP) is markedly augmented. Because vasopressin also stimulates endogenous PGE_2 production by the collecting duct, these results suggest that PGE_2 participates in a negative feedback loop, whereby endogenous PGE_2 production dampens the action of AVP.[286] In agreement with this model, the early classical studies of Grantham and Orloff directly demonstrated that PGE_1 blunted the water permeability response of the cortical collecting duct to vasopressin. In

these early studies, the action of PGE_1 appeared to be at a pre-cAMP step. Interestingly, when administered by itself, PGE_1 modestly augmented basal water permeability. These earlier studies have been confirmed with respect to PGE_2. PGE_2 also stimulates basal hydraulic conductivity and suppresses the hydraulic conductivity response to AVP in rabbit cortical collecting duct.[287,288] Inhibition of both AVP-stimulated cAMP generation and water permeability appears to be mediated by the EP1 and EP3 receptors, whereas the increase in basal water permeability may be mediated by the EP4 receptor.[250] These data are consistent with functional redundancy between EP1 and EP3 with respect to their effects on vasopressin-stimulated water absorption in the collecting duct.

Metabolism of Prostaglandins

15-Keto Dehydrogenase

The half-life of prostaglandins is 3 to 5 minutes and that of TXA_2 is approximately 30 seconds. Elimination of PGE_2, $PGF_{2\alpha}$, and PGI_2 proceeds through enzymatic and nonenzymatic pathways, whereas that of TXA_2 is nonenzymatic. The end products of all of these degradative reactions generally have minimal biologic activity, although this is not uniformly the case (see later). The principal enzyme involved in the transformation of PGE_2, PGI_2, and $PGF_{2\alpha}$ is 15-hydroxy-prostaglandin dehydrogenase (15-PGDH), which converts the 15 alcohol group to a ketone.[289]

15-PGDH is an enzyme dependent on $NAD^+/NADP^+$ (oxidized nicotinamide adenine dinucleotide/oxidized nicotinamide adenine dinucleotide phosphate) that is 30 to 49 times more active in the kidney of the young rat (3 weeks of age) than in the adult. Its K_m is 8.4 μmol/L for PGE_2 and 22.6 μmol/L for $PGF_{2\alpha}$.[289] It is mainly localized in cortical and juxtamedullary zones,[290] with little activity detected in papillary slices. At baseline, it is present in the proximal tubule, thick ascending limb, and collecting duct. However, it was found in the macula densa in COX-2 knockout mice and with consumption of a high-salt diet, and in cultured macula densa cells cyclooxygenase inhibition increased expression.[291] Disruption of the 15-PGDH gene in mice results in persistent patent ductus arteriosus, thought to be a result of failure of circulating PGE_2 levels to fall in the immediately peripartum period.[292] Thus administration of cyclooxygenase-inhibiting NSAIDs rescues the knockout mice by decreasing prostaglandins and allowing the animals to survive.

Subsequent catalysis of 15-hydroxy products by a Δ13-reductase leads to the formation of 13,14-dihydro compounds. PGI_2 and TXA_2 undergo rapid degradation to 6-keto-$PGF_{1\alpha}$ and TXB_2, respectively.[289] These stable metabolites are usually measured and their rates of formation taken as representative of those of the parent molecules.

ω/ω-1–Hydroxylation of Prostaglandins

Both PGA_2 and PGE_2 have been shown to undergo hydroxylation of the terminal or subterminal carbons by a cytochrome P450–dependent mechanism.[293] This reaction may be mediated by a CYP4A family member or CYP4F enzyme. Both CYP4A and CYP4F members have been mapped along the nephron.[294,295] Some of these derivatives have been shown to exhibit biologic activity.

Cyclopentenone Prostaglandins

The cyclopentenone prostaglandins include PGA_2, a PGE_2 derivative, and PGJ_2, a derivative of PGD_2. Although it remains uncertain whether these compounds are actually produced in vivo, this possibility has received increasing attention, because some cyclopentenone prostanoids have been shown to be activating ligands for nuclear transcription factors, including peroxisome proliferator–activated receptors δ and γ (PPARδ and PPARγ).[296-298] The realization that the antidiabetic thiazolidinedione drugs act through PPARγ to exert their antihyperglycemic and insulin-sensitizing effects[299] has generated intense interest in the possibility that the cyclopentenone prostaglandins might serve as the endogenous ligands for these receptors. An alternative biologic activity of these compounds has been recognized in their capacity to covalently modify thiol groups, forming adducts with cysteine of several intracellular proteins, including thioredoxin 1, vimentin, actin, and tubulin.[300] Studies investigating the biologic activity of cyclopentenone prostanoids abound, and the reader is referred to several excellent sources in the literature.[301-303] Although evidence exists supporting the presence of these compounds in vivo,[304] it remains uncertain whether they can be formed enzymatically or are an unstable spontaneous dehydration product of the E and D ring prostaglandins.[305]

Nonenzymatic Metabolism of Arachidonic Acid

It has long been recognized that oxidant injury can result in peroxidation of lipids. In 1990, Morrow and colleagues reported that a series of prostaglandin-like compounds can be produced by free radical–catalyzed peroxidation of AA that is independent of cyclooxygenase activity.[306] These compounds, which are termed *isoprostanes*, are increasingly used as a sensitive marker of oxidant injury in vitro and in vivo.[307] In addition, at least two of these compounds, 8-iso-$PGF_{2\alpha}$ (15-F_2-isoprostane) and 8-iso-PGE_2 (15-E_2-isoprostane) are potent vasoconstrictors when administered exogenously.[308] The compound 8-iso-$PGF_{2\alpha}$ has been shown to constrict the renal microvasculature and decrease GFR, an effect that is prevented by thromboxane receptor antagonism.[309] However, the role of endogenous isoprostanes as mediators of biologic responses remains unclear.

Prostaglandin Transport and Urinary Excretion

It is notable that most of the prostaglandin synthetic enzymes have been localized to the intracellular compartment, yet extracellular prostaglandins are potent autocoids and paracrine factors. Thus, prostanoids must be transported extracellularly to achieve efficient metabolism and termination of their signaling. Similarly, enzymes that metabolize PGE_2 to inactive compounds are also intracellular, requiring uptake of the prostaglandin for its metabolic inactivation. The molecular bases of these extrusion and uptake processes are only now being defined.

As fatty acids, prostaglandins may be classified as an organic anion at physiologic pH. Early microperfusion studies documented that basolateral PGE_2 could be taken up into proximal tubules cells and actively secreted into the lumen. Furthermore, this process could be inhibited by a variety of inhibitors of organic anion transport, including *p*-aminohippurate, probenecid, and indomethacin. Studies of basolateral renal membrane vesicles also supported the notion that this transport process was via an electroneutral anion exchanger. These studies are of note, since renal prostaglandins enter the urine in the loop of Henle, and late proximal tubule secretion could provide an important entry mechanism.[1]

A molecule that mediates PGE_2 uptake in exchange for lactate has now been cloned and christened *PGT* for "prostaglandin transporter."[310] PGT is a member of the SLC21/SLCO organic anion transporting family, and its cDNA encodes a transmembrane protein of 100 amino acids that exhibits broad tissue distribution (heart, placenta, brain, lung, liver, skeletal muscle, pancreas, kidney, spleen, prostate, ovary, small intestine, and colon).[311-313] Immunocytochemical studies of PGT expression in rat kidneys suggest expression primarily in glomerular endothelial and mesangial cells, arteriolar endothelial and muscularis cells, principal cells of the collecting duct, medullary interstitial cells, medullary vasa rectae endothelia, and papillary surface epithelium.[314] PGT appears to mediate PGE_2 uptake rather than release,[315] allowing target cells to metabolize this molecule and terminate signaling.[316] PGT expression is decreased with low salt and increased with high salt in the collecting duct; this may allow regulation of prostaglandin excretion by uptake of more prostaglandins excreted from the luminal surface, the site of the prostaglandin transporter, which would thereby permit more accumulation at the basolateral surface.[317]

Other members of the organic cation-anion-zwitterion transporter family SLC22 have also been shown to transport prostaglandins[310] and have been suggested to mediate prostaglandin excretion into the urine. Specifically, organic anion transporters 1 and 3 (OAT1 and OAT3) are localized on the basolateral proximal tubule membrane, where they likely participate in urinary excretion of PGE_2.[318,319] Conversely, members of the multidrug resistance–associated protein (MRP) family have been shown to transport prostaglandins in an adenosine triphosphate (ATP)–dependent fashion.[320,321] MRP2 (also designated *ATP-binding cassette, subfamily C, member 2* [ABCC2]) is expressed in kidney proximal tubule brush borders and may contribute to the transport (and urinary excretion) of glutathione-conjugated prostaglandins.[322,323] This transporter has more limited tissue expression, restricted to the kidney, liver, and small intestine, and could contribute not only to renal *p*-aminohippurate excretion but to prostaglandin excretion as well.[324]

Involvement of Cyclooxygenase Metabolites in Renal Pathophysiology

Experimental and Human Glomerular Injury

Glomerular Inflammatory Injury

Cyclooxygenase metabolites have been implicated in functional and structural alterations in glomerular and tubulointerstitial inflammatory diseases.[325] Essential fatty acid deficiency totally prevents the structural and functional consequences of administration of nephrotoxic serum to rats, an experimental model of anti–glomerular basement membrane (anti-GBM) glomerulonephritis.[326] Changes in arteriolar tone during the course of this inflammatory lesion are mediated principally by locally released cyclooxygenase and lipoxygenase metabolites of AA.[326]

TXA$_2$ release appears to play an essential role in mediating the increased renovascular resistance observed during the early phase of this disease.[1] Subsequently, increasing rates of PGE$_2$ generation may account for progressive dilation of renal arterioles and increases in renal blood flow at later stages of the disease. Consistent with this hypothesis, TXA$_2$ antagonism ameliorated the falls in renal blood flow and GFR 2 hours after administration of nephrotoxic serum, but not 24 hours after administration. During the later, heterologous phase of nephrotoxic serum–induced injury, cyclooxygenase metabolites mediate both the renal vasodilation and the reduction in K$_f$ that characterize this phase.[326] The net functional result of cyclooxygenase inhibition during this phase of experimental glomerulonephritis, therefore, depends on whether renal perfusion or the preservation of K$_f$ is more important to the maintenance of GFR. Evidence also indicates that cyclooxygenase metabolites are mediators of pathologic lesions and the accompanying proteinuria in this model.[1] COX-2 expression in the kidney increases in experimental anti-GBM glomerulonephritis[327,328] and after systemic administration of lipopolysaccharide.[329]

Fish oil diets (enriched in eicosapentaenoic acid), with an accompanying reduction in the generation of cyclooxygenase products, have been demonstrated to have a beneficial effect on the course of genetic murine lupus (in MRL/lpr mice). In subsequent studies, enhanced renal TXA$_2$ and PGE$_2$ generation was demonstrated in this model, as well as in New Zealand black (NZB) mice, another genetic model of lupus.[1] In addition, studies in humans demonstrated an inverse relation between TXA$_2$ biosynthesis and GFR as well as improvement of renal function following short-term therapy with a thromboxane receptor antagonist in patients with lupus nephritis.[1] More recently, studies have indicated that in humans, as well as in NZB mice, COX-2 expression was upregulated in individuals with active lupus nephritis, with co-localization to infiltrating monocytes, which suggests that monocytes infiltrating the glomeruli contribute to the exaggerated local synthesis of TXA$_2$.[330,331] COX-2 inhibition selectively decreased thromboxane production, and long-term treatment of NZB mice with a COX-2 inhibitor and mycophenolate mofetil significantly prolonged survival.[331] Taken together, these data, as well as others from animal and human studies, support a major role for the intrarenal generation of TXA$_2$ in mediating renal vasoconstriction during inflammatory and lupus-associated glomerular injury. In contrast, an EP4-selective agonist was shown to reduce glomerular injury in a mouse model of anti-GBM disease.[332]

The demonstration of a functionally significant role for cyclooxygenase metabolites in experimental and human inflammatory glomerular injury has raised the question of the cellular sources of these eicosanoids in the glomerulus. In addition to infiltrating inflammatory cells, resident glomerular macrophages, glomerular mesangial cells, and glomerular epithelial cells represent likely sources for eicosanoid generation. In the anti-Thy1.1 (antibody to thymocyte differentiation antigen) model of mesangioproliferative glomerulonephritis, COX-1 staining was transiently increased in diseased glomeruli at day 6 and was localized mainly to proliferating mesangial cells. COX-2 expression in the macula densa region also transiently increased at day 6.[333,334] Glomerular COX-2 expression in this model has been controversial, with one group reporting increased podocyte COX-2 expression[328] and two other groups reporting minimal, if any, glomerular COX-2 expression.[333,334] However, it is of interest that selective COX-2 inhibitors have been reported to inhibit glomerular repair in the anti-Thy1.1 model.[334] In both anti-Thy1.1 and anti-GBM models of glomerulonephritis, the nonselective cyclooxygenase inhibitor indomethacin increased levels of monocyte chemoattractant protein-1 (MCP-1), which suggests that prostaglandins may repress recruitment of monocytes/macrophages in experimental glomerulonephritis.[335]

A variety of cytokines have been reported to stimulate PGE$_2$ synthesis and COX-2 expression in cultured mesangial cells. Furthermore, complement components, in particular C5b-9, which are known to be involved in the inflammatory models described earlier, have been implicated in the stimulation of PGE$_2$ synthesis in glomerular epithelial cells. Cultured glomerular epithelial cells express predominantly COX-1, but exposure to C5b-9 significantly increased COX-2 expression.[1]

Glomerular Noninflammatory Injury

Studies have suggested that prostanoids may also mediate altered renal function and glomerular damage following subtotal renal ablation, and glomerular prostaglandin production may be altered in such conditions. Glomeruli from remnant kidneys, as well as from animals fed a high-protein diet, have increased prostanoid production.[1] These studies suggested an increase in cyclooxygenase enzyme activity per se rather than, or in addition to, increased substrate availability, since increases in prostanoid production were noted when excess exogenous AA was added.

Following subtotal renal ablation, there are selective increases in renal cortical and glomerular COX-2 mRNA and immunoreactive protein expression, without significant alterations in COX-1 expression.[336] This increased COX-2 expression is most prominent in the macula densa and surrounding the cortical thick ascending limb of the loop of Henle. In addition, COX-2 immunoreactivity is also present in podocytes of remnant glomeruli, and increased prostaglandin production in isolated glomeruli from remnant kidneys is inhibited by a COX-2–selective inhibitor but was not decreased by a COX-1–selective inhibitor.[336] Of interest, in the fawn-hooded rat, which develops spontaneous glomerulosclerosis, increased cortical thick ascending limb and macula densa COX-2 and neuronal NO synthase expression as well as increased juxtaglomerular cell renin expression precede the development of sclerotic lesions.[337] Recent studies have indicated that selective overexpression of COX-2 in podocytes in mice increases sensitivity to development of glomerulosclerosis, an effect that is mediated by thromboxane receptor activation.[338-340]

When given 24 hours after subtotal renal ablation, the nonselective NSAID indomethacin normalized increases in renal blood flow and single-nephron GFR; similar decreases in hyperfiltration were noted when indomethacin was administered short term to rats 14 days after subtotal nephrectomy, although in this latter study, the increased glomerular capillary pressure was not altered because both afferent and efferent arteriolar resistances increased.[1] Previous studies have also suggested that nonselective cyclooxygenase inhibitors may acutely decrease hyperfiltration in diabetes and inhibit proteinuria and/or structural injury.[1] More recent studies have indicated that selective COX-2 inhibitors decrease the hyperfiltration seen in rats with experimental diabetes or increased dietary protein.[341,342] Of note, NSAIDs have also been reported to be effective in reducing proteinuria in patients with refractory nephrotic syndrome.[1] Similarly, selective COX-2 inhibition decreased proteinuria in patients with both diabetic and nondiabetic renal disease without alterations in blood pressure.[343]

The prostanoids involved have not yet been completely characterized, although it is presumed that vasodilatory prostanoids are involved in mediation of the altered renal hemodynamics. Defective autoregulation of renal blood flow due to decreased myogenic tone of the afferent arteriole is seen after either subtotal ablation or excessive dietary protein intake and is corrected by inhibition of cyclooxygenase activity. In these hyperfiltering states, tubuloglomerular feedback is reset at a higher distal tubular flow rate.[1] Such a resetting dictates that afferent arteriolar vasodilatation will be maintained in the face of increased distal solute delivery. It has previously been shown that the alterations in tubuloglomerular feedback sensitivity after reduction in renal mass are prevented by administration of the nonselective cyclooxygenase inhibitor indomethacin.[1] An important role has been suggested for neuronal NO synthase, which is localized to the macula densa, in the vasodilatory component of tubuloglomerular feedback.[344-346] Of interest, studies by Ishihara and colleagues have determined that this neuronal NO synthase–mediated vasodilation is inhibited by the selective COX-2 inhibitor NS-398, which suggests that COX-2–mediated prostanoids may be essential for arteriolar vasodilation.[45,66]

Administration of COX-2–selective inhibitors decreased proteinuria and inhibited development of glomerular sclerosis in rats with reduced functioning renal mass.[347,348] In addition, COX-2 inhibition decreased mRNA expression of TGF-β_1 and types III and IV collagen in the remnant kidney.[347] Similar protection was observed with administration of nitroflurbiprofen, a NO–releasing NSAID without gastrointestinal toxicity.[349] Prior studies have also demonstrated that thromboxane synthase inhibitors retarded progression of glomerulosclerosis, with decreased proteinuria and glomerulosclerosis in rats with remnant kidneys and in diabetic nephropathy, in association with increased renal prostacyclin production and lower systolic blood pressure.[332] Studies in models of type 1 and type 2 diabetes indicated that COX-2–selective inhibitors retarded the progression of diabetic nephropathy.[350,351] Schmitz and colleagues confirmed increases in TXB_2 excretion in the remnant kidney and correlated decreases in arachidonic and linoleic acid levels with increased thromboxane production, because the thromboxane synthase inhibitor U-63557A restored fatty acid levels and retarded progressive glomerular destruction.[352]

Enhanced glomerular synthesis and/or urinary excretion of both PGE_2 and TXA_2 have been demonstrated in passive Heymann's nephritis and doxorubicin (Adriamycin)–induced glomerulopathies in rats. Both COX-1 and COX-2 expression are increased in glomeruli with passive Heymann's nephritis.[353] Both thromboxane synthase inhibitors and selective COX-2 inhibitors also decreased proteinuria in passive Heymann's nephritis.[1]

In contrast to the putative deleterious effects of thromboxane, the prostacyclin analog cicaprost retarded renal damage

in uninephrectomized dogs fed a high-sodium and high-protein diet, an effect that was not mediated by amelioration of systemic hypertension.[354] Similarly, both EP2 and EP4 agonists decrease glomerular and tubulointerstitial fibrosis in a model of subtotal renal ablation.[343] Recent studies have also indicated that in models of polycystic kidney disease, there is increased COX-2 expression and increased PGE_2 and thromboxane in cyst fluid. Either COX-2 inhibition or EP2 receptor inhibition decreased cyst growth and interstitial fibrosis.[355,356]

Prostanoids have also been shown to alter extracellular matrix production by mesangial cells in culture. TXA_2 stimulates matrix production by both TGF-β–dependent and TGF-β–independent pathways.[357] PGE_2 has been reported to decrease steady-state mRNA levels of α_1I and α_1III procollagens, but not α_1IV procollagen and fibronectin mRNA, and to reduce secretion of all studied collagen types into the cell culture supernatants. Of interest, this effect did not appear to be mediated by cAMP.[358] PGE_2 has also been reported to increase production of matrix metalloproteinase 2 (MMP-2) and to mediate angiotensin II–induced increases in MMP-2.[359] Whether vasodilatory prostaglandins mediate decreased fibrillar collagen production and increased matrix-degrading activity in glomeruli in vivo has not yet been studied; however, there is compelling evidence that prostanoids may either mediate or modulate matrix production in nonrenal cells.[360] Cultured lung fibroblasts isolated from patients with idiopathic pulmonary fibrosis exhibit decreased ability to express COX-2 and to synthesize PGE_2.[361]

Acute Renal Failure

When cardiac output is compromised, as in extracellular fluid volume depletion or congestive heart failure, systemic blood pressure is preserved by the action of high circulating levels of systemic vasoconstrictors (norepinephrine, angiotensin II, AVP). Amelioration of their effects within the renal vasculature serves to blunt the development of otherwise concomitant marked depression of renal blood flow. Intrarenal generation of vasodilator products of AA, including PGE_2 and PGI_2, is a central part of this protective adaptation. Increased renal vascular resistance induced by exogenously administered angiotensin II or renal nerve stimulation (increased adrenergic tone) is exaggerated during concurrent inhibition of prostaglandin synthesis. Experiments in animals with volume depletion have demonstrated the existence of intrarenal AVP-prostaglandin interactions similar to those described earlier for angiotensin II.[1] Studies in patients with congestive heart failure have confirmed that enhanced prostaglandin synthesis is crucial in protecting kidneys from various vasoconstrictor influences in this condition.

Acute renal failure accompanying the short-term administration of endotoxin in rats is characterized by progressive reductions in renal blood flow and GFR in the absence of hypotension. Renal histologic features in such animals are normal, but cortical generation of cyclooxygenase metabolites is markedly elevated. A number of reports have provided evidence of a role for TXA_2-induced renal vasoconstriction in this model of renal dysfunction.[362] In addition, roles for prostaglandins and TXA_2 in modulating or mediating renal injury have been suggested in ischemia-reperfusion[363] and models of toxin-mediated acute tubular injury, including those induced by uranyl nitrate[364] amphotericin B,[365] aminoglycosides,[366] and glycerol.[367] In experimental acute renal failure, administration of vasodilator prostaglandins has been shown to ameliorate injury.[368] Similarly, administration of either nonselective or COX-2–selective NSAIDs exacerbates experimental ischemia-reperfusion injury.[369]

COX-2 expression decreases in the kidney in response to acute ischemic injury.[370] There is some controversy about the role of cyclooxygenase products in ischemia-reperfusion injury. Roles for prostaglandins and TXA_2 in modulating or mediating renal injury have been suggested in ischemia-reperfusion[363] and in models of toxin-mediated acute tubular injury, including those induced by uranyl nitrate,[364] amphotericin B,[365] aminoglycosides,[366] and glycerol.[367] Furthermore, fibrosis resulting from prolonged ischemic injury has been shown to be ameliorated by nonspecific cyclooxygenase inhibition.[371] In contrast, renal injury in response to ischemia-reperfusion is worsened by COX-2–selective inhibitors and in COX-2$^{-/-}$ mice,[369] and administration of vasodilator prostaglandins has been shown to ameliorate injury,[368] possibly through a PPARδ-dependent mechanism.[372]

Urinary Tract Obstruction

After induction of long-term (more than 24 hours) ureteral obstruction, renal prostaglandin and TXA_2 synthesis is markedly enhanced, particularly in response to stimuli such as endotoxin or bradykinin. Enhanced prostanoid synthesis likely arises from infiltrating mononuclear cells, proliferating fibroblast-like cells, interstitial macrophages, and interstitial medullary cells. Considerable evidence, derived from studies using specific enzyme inhibitors, suggests a causal relationship between increased renal generation of this eicosanoid and the intense vasoconstriction that characterizes the kidney with hydronephrosis or after obstruction (reviewed in Klahr and Morrissey[325]). In this sense, therefore, hydronephrotic injury can be regarded as a form of subacute inflammatory insult in which intrarenal eicosanoid generation from infiltrating leukocytes contributes to the pathophysiologic process. Finally, TXA_2 has been implicated in the resetting of the tubuloglomerular feedback mechanism observed in hydronephrotic kidneys.[373] More recent studies have also suggested that selective COX-2 inhibitors may prevent renal damage in response to unilateral ureteral obstruction.[374,375] Prostaglandins derived from medullary COX-2 are mediators of the early phase of diuresis seen after relief of ureteral obstruction, because COX-2 inhibition prevents the acute (24-hour) phase of postobstructive diuresis. However, more persistent, chronic postobstructive diuresis is not prostaglandin dependent but results from downregulation of Na$^+$-K$^+$-2Cl$^-$ cotransporter type 2 (NKCC2) and decreases aquaporin-2 phosphorylation and translocation to the collecting duct membrane.[376,377]

Allograft Rejection and Cyclosporine Nephrotoxicity

Allograft Rejection

Coffman and colleagues demonstrated that short-term administration of a TXA_2 synthesis inhibitor was associated with significant improvement in rat renal allograft function.[378] A number of other experimental and clinical studies have also demonstrated increased TXA_2 synthesis during allograft rejection,[379,380] which has led some to suggest that increased urinary TXA_2 excretion may be an early indicator of renal and cardiac allograft rejection.

Calcineurin Inhibitor Nephrotoxicity

Numerous investigators have demonstrated effects of cyclosporine A on renal prostaglandin and TXA_2 synthesis and have provided evidence of a major role for renal and leukocyte TXA_2 synthesis in mediating acute as well as chronic cyclosporine A nephrotoxicity in rats.[381] Fish oil–rich diets, TXA_2 antagonists, and administration of cyclosporine A in fish oil as a vehicle have all been shown to reduce renal TXA_2 synthesis and afford protection against nephrotoxicity. Moreover, cyclosporine A has been reported to decrease renal COX-2 expression.[382]

Hepatic Cirrhosis and Hepatorenal Syndrome

Patients with cirrhosis of the liver show an increased renal synthesis of vasodilating prostaglandins, as indicated by the high urinary excretion of prostaglandins and/or their metabolites. Urinary excretion of 2-3-dinor-6-keto-PGF$_{1\alpha}$, an index of systemic PGI$_2$ synthesis, is increased in patients with cirrhosis and hyperdynamic circulation, which thus raises the possibility that systemic synthesis of PGI$_2$ may contribute to the arterial vasodilatation seen in these patients. Inhibition of cyclooxygenase activity in these patients may cause a profound reduction in renal blood flow and GFR, a reduction in sodium excretion, and an impairment of free water clearance.[383] The sodium-retaining properties of NSAIDs are particularly exaggerated in patients with cirrhosis of the liver, which attests to the dependence of renal salt excretion on vasodilatory prostaglandins. In the kidneys of rats with cirrhosis, COX-2 expression increases, whereas COX-1 expression is unchanged; however, in these animals, selective inhibition of COX-1 leads to impaired renal hemodynamics and natriuresis, whereas COX-2 inhibition has no effect.[384,385]

Diminished renal prostaglandin synthesis has been implicated in the pathogenesis of the severe sodium retention seen in hepatorenal syndrome, as well as in the resistance to diuretic therapy.[386,387] There is reduced renal synthesis of vasodilating PGE$_2$ in the face of activation of endogenous vasoconstrictors and a maintained or increased renal production of TXA_2.[383,388] Therefore, an imbalance between vasoconstricting systems and the renal vasodilator PGE$_2$ has been proposed as a factor contributing to the renal failure observed in this condition. However, administration of exogenous prostanoids to patients with cirrhosis is not effective either in improving renal function or in preventing the deleterious effect of NSAIDs.[383]

Diabetes Mellitus

In the streptozotocin-induced model of diabetes in rats, COX-2 expression is increased in the cortical thick ascending limb and macula densa region.[341,350] COX-2 immunoreactivity has also been detected in the macula densa region in human diabetic nephropathy.[39] Studies suggest that the vasodilator prostanoids PGI_2 and PGE_2 play an important role in the hyperfiltration seen early in diabetes mellitus.[389] Previous studies indicated that short-term use of nonselective cyclooxygenase inhibitors decreases hyperfiltration in diabetes and inhibits proteinuria and/or structural injury,[390] and more recent studies have also indicated that short-term administration of a selective COX-2 inhibitor decreased hyperfiltration.[341] The increased COX-2 expression appears to be mediated at least in part by increased ROS production in diabetes, because the superoxide dismutase analog tempol blocks the increased expression.[391] At least in cultured mesangial cells, the ROS that mediate increased COX-2 expression in response to high glucose level are derived from the mitochondria.[392]

Long-term administration of a selective COX-2 inhibitor significantly decreased proteinuria and reduced extracellular matrix deposition, as indicated by decreases in immunoreactive fibronectin expression and in mesangial matrix expansion. In addition, COX-2 inhibition reduced expression of TGF-β, PAI-1, and vascular endothelial growth factor in the kidneys of diabetic hypertensive animals.[350] The vasoconstrictor TXA_2 may play a role in the development of albuminuria and basement membrane changes in diabetic nephropathy. In addition, administration of a selective PGE_2 EP1 receptor antagonist prevented development of experimental diabetic nephropathy.[393] In contrast to the proposed detrimental effects of these vasoconstrictive prostanoids, administration of a prostacyclin analog decreased hyperfiltration and reduced macrophage infiltration in early diabetic nephropathy by increasing endothelial NO synthase expression in afferent arterioles and glomerular capillaries.[394]

Pregnancy

Most, though not all, investigators do not report increases in vasodilator prostaglandin synthesis in pregnancy or suggest an essential role for prostanoids in the mediation of the increased GFR and renal plasma flow of normal pregnancy[395]; however, diminished synthesis of PGI_2 has been demonstrated in humans and in animal models of pregnancy-induced hypertension.[396] In the latter, inhibition of TXA_2 synthetase has been associated with resolution of the hypertension, which suggests a possible pathophysiologic role.[397] Low-dose (60 to 100 mg/day) aspirin therapy has been demonstrated to have a moderate beneficial effect in reducing TXA_2 generation while preserving PGI_2 synthesis in patients at high risk of pregnancy-induced hypertension and preeclampsia.[398,399]

Lithium Nephrotoxicity

Lithium chloride is a mainstay of the treatment of bipolar illness in psychiatry. However, lithium therapy is routinely complicated by polyuria and even frank nephrogenic diabetes insipidus. In vitro and in vivo studies demonstrated that lithium induced renal medullary interstitial cell COX-2 protein expression via inhibition of glycogen synthase kinase-3β. COX-2 inhibition prevented lithium-induced polyuria. COX-2 inhibition also resulted in upregulation of aquaporin-2 and NKCC2.[400,401]

Role of Reactive Oxygen Species as Mediators of COX-2 Actions

Like NADPH oxidase, NO synthase, and xanthine oxidase, COX-2 can also be a source of oxygen radicals.[402] COX-2 enzymatic activity is commonly accompanied by associated oxidative mechanisms (cooxidation) and free-radical production.[403] The catalytic activity of cyclooxygenase consists of a series of radical reactions that use molecular oxygen and generate intermediate ROS.[404] Elevated levels of COX-2 protein are associated with increased ROS production and apoptosis in cultured renal cortical cells[405] and human mesangial cells.[392] It has been suggested that COX-2–mediated lipid peroxidation, rather than prostaglandins, can induce DNA damage via adduct formation.[406] The COX-2–specific inhibitor NS-398 was able to reduce the oxidative activity and prevent oxidant stress.[407]

Not only may ROS be generated by cyclooxygenase per se, but prostanoids may also activate intracellular pathways that generate ROS. Locally generated ROS may damage cell membranes, which leads to lipid peroxidation and release of AA. Prostanoids released during inflammatory reactions cause rapid degenerative changes in some cultured cells, and their potential cytotoxic effect has been suggested to occur through the acceleration of intracellular oxidative stress.[408] Thromboxane[409] and PGE_2 acting through the EP1 receptor[410] have been reported to induce NADPH oxidase and ROS production. Of interest, PGE_2 acting through the EP4 receptor inhibits macrophage oxidase activity.[411,412] As mentioned previously, there is also evidence for crosstalk between COX-2 and ROS, so that ROS may induce COX-2 expression.[406] Interestingly, during aging there is ROS-mediated NF-κB expression, which increases COX-2 expression in the kidney.[413] Furthermore, this appears to induce a vicious cycle, since COX-2 then serves as a source of ROS. The amount of renal ROS resulting from cyclooxygenase activity increases with age, and up to 25% of total kidney ROS production in aged rat kidneys is inhibited by NSAID administration.

Lipoxygenase Pathway (Figure 13-14)

The lipoxygenase enzymes metabolize AA to form leukotrienes, HETEs, and lipoxins. These lipoxygenase metabolites are primarily produced by leukocytes, mast cells, and macrophages in response to inflammation and injury. There are three lipoxygenase enzymes, 5-, 12-, and 15-lipoxygenase (5-LOX, 12-LOX, and 15-LOX), so named for the carbon of AA at which they insert an oxygen. The lipoxygenases are products of separate genes and have distinct distributions and patterns of regulation. Glomeruli, mesangial cells, cortical tubules, and vessels also produce the 12-LOX product, 12(S)-HETE, and the 15-LOX product, 15-HETE. Recent studies have localized 15-LOX mRNA primarily to the distal nephron, and 12-LOX mRNA to the glomerulus. 5-LOX mRNA and 5-LOX–activating protein (FLAP) mRNA were expressed in the glomerulus and the vasa recta.[414] In polymorphonuclear leukocytes (PMNs), macrophages, and mast cells, 5-LOX mediates the formation of leukotrienes.[415] 5-LOX, which is regulated by FLAP, catalyzes the conversion of AA to 5-hydroperoxyeicosatetraenoic acid (5-HPETE) and then to leukotriene A_4 (LTA_4).[416] LTA_4 is then further metabolized

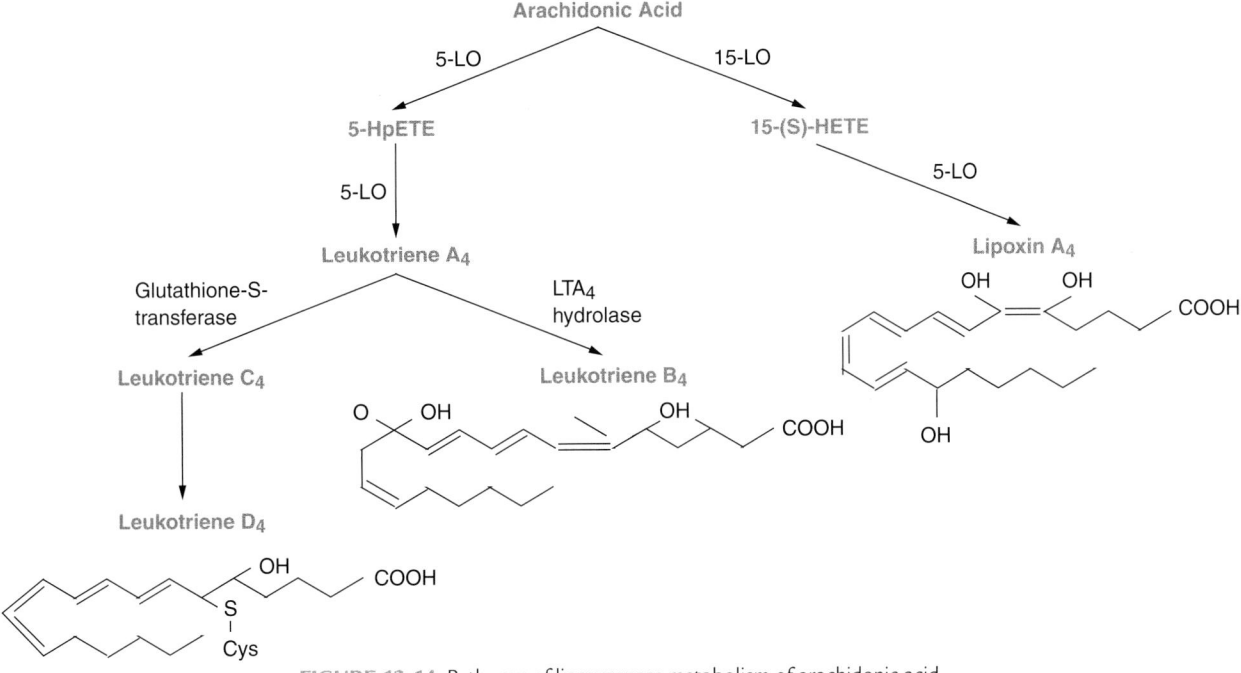

FIGURE 13-14 Pathways of lipoxygenase metabolism of arachidonic acid.

to either the peptidyl leukotrienes (LTC$_4$ and LTD$_4$) by glutathione S-transferase or to LTB$_4$ by LTA$_4$ hydrolase. Although glutathione S-transferase expression is limited to inflammatory cells, LTA$_4$ hydrolase is also expressed in glomerular mesangial cells and endothelial cells[417]; polymerase chain reaction analysis has actually demonstrated ubiquitous LTA$_4$ hydrolase mRNA expression throughout the rat nephron.[414] LTC$_4$ synthase mRNA could not be found in any nephron segment.[414]

Two cysteinyl leukotriene receptors have now been cloned and have been identified as members of the G protein–coupled superfamily of receptors. They have been localized to vascular smooth muscle and endothelium of the pulmonary vasculature.[418-420] In the kidney cysteinyl leukotriene receptor type 1 is expressed in the glomerulus, whereas cysteinyl receptor type 2 mRNA has not been detected in any nephron segment to date.[414]

The peptidyl leukotrienes are potent mediators of inflammation and vasoconstrictors of vascular, pulmonary, and gastrointestinal smooth muscle. In addition, they increase vascular permeability and promote mucus secretion.[421] Because of the central role that peptidyl leukotrienes play in the inflammatory triggering of asthma exacerbation, effective receptor antagonists have been developed and are now an important component of the treatment of asthma.[422]

In the kidney, LTD$_4$ administration has been shown to decrease renal blood flow and GFR, and peptidyl leukotrienes are thought to be mediators of decreased renal blood flow and GFR associated with acute glomerular inflammation. Micropuncture studies have revealed that the decreases in GFR are the result of both afferent and arteriolar vasoconstriction, with more pronounced efferent vasoconstriction and a decrease in K_f.[1] In addition both LTC$_4$ and LTD$_4$ increase proliferation of cultured mesangial cells.

The LTB$_4$ receptor is also a seven-transmembrane G protein–coupled receptor. On PMNs, receptor activation promotes chemotaxis, aggregation, and attachment to endothelium. In the kidney LTB$_4$ mRNA is localized to the glomerulus.[414] A second, low-affinity LTB$_4$ receptor is also expressed,[423] which may mediate calcium influx into PMNs and thereby lead to activation. LTB$_4$ receptor blockers lessen acute renal ischemic-reperfusion injury[424] and nephrotoxic nephritis in rats,[425] and PMN infiltration and structural and functional evidence of organ injury by ischemia-reperfusion are magnified in transgenic mice overexpressing the LTB$_4$ receptor.[426] In addition to activating cell surface receptors, LTB$_4$ has also been shown to be a ligand for the nuclear receptor PPARα.[427]

15-LOX leads to the formation of 15(S)-HETE. In addition, dual oxygenation in activated PMNs and macrophages by 5-LOX and 15-LOX leads to formation of the lipoxins. Lipoxin synthesis can also occur via transcellular metabolism of the leukocyte-generated intermediate, LTA$_4$, by 12-LOX in platelets or adjoining cells, including glomerular endothelial cells.[428,429]

15(S)-HETE is a potent vasoconstrictor in the renal microcirculation[430]; however, 15-LOX–derived metabolites antagonize the proinflammatory actions of leukotrienes, both by inhibiting PMN chemotaxis, aggregation, and adherence and by counteracting the vasoconstrictive effects of the peptidyl leukotrienes.[431,432] Administration of 15(S)-HETE reduced LTB$_4$ production by glomeruli isolated from rats with acute nephrotoxic serum–induced glomerulonephritis, and it has been proposed that 15-LOX may regulate 5-LOX activity in chronic glomerular inflammation, since it is known that in experimental glomerulonephritis, lipoxin A$_4$ (LXA$_4$) administration increased renal blood flow and GFR, in large measure by inducing afferent arteriolar vasodilation, an effect mediated in part by release of vasodilator prostaglandins.[1] LXA$_4$ also antagonized the effects of LTD$_4$ to decrease GFR, although not renal blood flow, even though administration of LXA$_4$ and LXB$_4$ directly into the renal artery induced vasoconstriction. In glomerular micropuncture studies administration of LXA$_4$ led to moderate decreases in K_f.[431] Lipoxins signal through a specific

G protein–coupled receptor denoted *ALXR*. This receptor is related at the nucleotide sequence level to both chemokine and chemotactic peptide receptors, such as *N*-formyl peptide receptor.[433] It is also noteworthy that in isolated perfused canine renal arteries and veins, LTC_4 and LTD_4 were found to be vasodilators, an effect that was partially dependent on an intact endothelium and was mediated by NO production.[434]

A potential interaction between cyclooxygenase- and lipoxygenase-mediated pathways has been reported. Although aspirin inhibits prostaglandin formation by both COX-1 and COX-2, aspirin-induced acetylation converts COX-2 to a selective generator of 15(*R*)-HETE. This product can then be released, taken up in a transcellular route by PMNs, and converted to 15-epi-lipoxins, which have biologic actions similar to those of the lipoxins.[435]

Similar to 15-HETE, 12(*S*)-HETE also potently vasoconstricts glomerular and renal vasculature.[428] 12(*S*)-HETE increases protein kinase C levels and depolarizes cultured vascular smooth muscle cells. Afferent arteriolar vasoconstriction and increases in smooth muscle calcium in response to 12(*S*)-HETE were partially inhibited by voltage-gated L-type calcium channel inhibitors.[436] 12(*S*)-HETE has also been proposed to be an angiogenic factor, since in cultured endothelial cells, 12-LOX inhibition reduces cell proliferation and 12-LOX overexpression stimulates cell migration and endothelial tube formation.[437] 12/15-LOX inhibitors and elective elimination of the leukocyte 12-LOX enzyme also ameliorate the development of diabetic nephropathy in mice.[438] There is also interaction between 12/15-LOX pathways and TGF-β–mediated pathways in the diabetic kidney.[439] 12(*S*)-HETE has also been proposed to be a mediator of renal vasoconstriction by angiotensin II, with inhibition of the 12-LOX pathway attenuating angiotensin II–mediated afferent arteriolar vasoconstriction and decreased renal blood flow.[440] Lipoxygenase inhibition also blunted renal arcuate artery vasoconstriction by norepinephrine and KCl.[441] However, 12-LOX products have also been implicated as inhibitors of renal renin release.[442,443]

Although the major influence of lipoxygenase products in the kidney derives from their release from infiltrating leukocytes or resident cells of macrophage/monocyte origin, there is evidence to suggest that intrinsic renal cells are capable of generating leukotrienes and lipoxins either directly or through transcellular metabolism of intermediates.[444] Human and rat glomeruli can generate 12- and 15-HETE, although the cells of origin are unclear. LTB_4 can be detected in supernatants of normal rat glomeruli, and its synthesis could be markedly diminished by maneuvers that depleted glomeruli of resident macrophages, such as irradiation or fatty acid deficiency. In addition, 5-, 12-, and 15-HETEs were detected in pig glomeruli and their structural identity confirmed by mass spectrometry.[1] 12-LOX products are increased in mesangial cells exposed to hyperglycemia and in diabetic nephropathy.[445] There also appears to be crosstalk between 12/15-LOX and COX-2. Both are increased in diabetes and with high glucose levels, and in cultured cells, 12(*S*)-HETE increases COX-2 whereas PGE_2 increases 12/15-LOX. Knockdown of 12/15-LOX expression with short hairpin RNA decreases COX-2 expression, whereas 12/15-LOX overexpression increases COX-2 expression.[446]

Glomeruli subjected to immune injury release LTB_4,[447] and LTB_4 generation was suppressed by resident macrophage depletion. Synthesis of peptidyl leukotrienes by inflamed

glomeruli has also been demonstrated,[448] but leukocytes could not be excluded as its primary source. LXA_4 is generated by immune-injured glomeruli.[449] Rat mesangial cells generate LXA_4 when provided with LTA_4 as substrate, which provides a potential intraglomerular source of lipoxins during inflammatory reactions. In nonglomerular tissue, 12-HETE production has been reported by rat cortical tubules and epithelial cells and 12- and 15-HETE by rabbit medulla.[1]

Biologic Activities of Lipoxygenase Products in the Kidney

In early experiments, systemic administration of LTC_4 in the rat and administration of LTC_4 and LTD_4 in the isolated perfused kidney revealed potent renal vasoconstrictor actions of these eicosanoids. Subsequently, micropuncture measurements revealed that LTD_4 exerts preferential constrictor effects on postglomerular arteriolar resistance and depresses K_f and GFR. The latter is likely due to receptor-mediated contraction of glomerular mesangial cells, which has been demonstrated for LTC_4 and LTD_4 in vitro (see earlier). These actions of LTD_4 in the kidney are consistent with its known smooth muscle contractile properties. LTB_4, a potent chemotactic and leukocyte-activating agent, is devoid of constrictor action in the normal rat kidney. LXA_4 dilates afferent arterioles when infused into the renal artery without affecting efferent arteriolar tone. This results in elevations in intraglomerular pressure and plasma flow rate, which augments GFR.[1]

Involvement of Lipoxygenase Products in Renal Pathophysiology

Increased generation rates of LTC_4 and LTD_4 have been documented in glomeruli from rats with immune complex nephritis and mice with spontaneously developing lupus nephritis.[415,449] Moreover, results from numerous physiologic studies using specific LTD_4 receptor antagonists have provided strong evidence for the release of these eicosanoids during glomerular inflammation. In four animal models of glomerular immune injury (anti-GBM nephritis, anti-Thy1.1 antibody–mediated mesangiolysis, passive Heymann's nephritis, and murine lupus nephritis) acute antagonism of LTD_4 by receptor-binding competition or inhibition of LTD_4 synthesis led to highly significant increases in GFR in nephritic animals.[450] The principal mechanism underlying the improvement in GFR was reversal of the depressed values of the glomerular ultrafiltration coefficient (K_f), which is characteristically compromised in immune-injured glomeruli. In other studies in rats with passive Heymann's nephritis, Katoh and colleagues provided evidence that endogenous LTD_4 not only mediates reductions in K_f and GFR, but that LTD_4-evoked increases in intraglomerular pressure underlie, to a large extent, the accompanying proteinuria.[450] Cysteinyl leukotrienes have been implicated in cyclosporine nephrotoxicity.[451] Of interest, 5-LOX deficiency accelerates renal allograft rejection.[452]

LTB_4 synthesis, measured in the supernates of isolated glomeruli, is markedly enhanced early in the course of several forms of glomerular immune injury.[453] Cellular sources of LTB_4 in injured glomeruli include PMNs and macrophages. All studies concur as to the *transient* nature of LTB_4 release. LTB_4

production decreases 24 hours after onset of the inflammation, which coincides with macrophage infiltration, a major source of 15-LOX activity.[454] 15-HPETE incubation decreased lipopolysaccharide-induced tumor necrosis factor expression in a human monocytic cell line,[455] and hemagglutinating virus of Japan (HVJ) liposome–mediated glomerular transfection of 15-LOX in rats decreased markers of injury (blood urea nitrogen level, proteinuria) and accelerated functional (GFR, renal blood flow) recovery in experimental glomerulonephritis.[456] In addition, MK-591, a FLAP antagonist, restored size selectivity and decreased glomerular permeability in acute GN.[457]

The suppression of LTB$_4$ synthesis beyond the first 24 hours of injury is rather surprising, because both PMNs and macrophages are capable of effecting the total synthesis of LTB$_4$ (they contain the two necessary enzymes that convert AA to LTB$_4$, namely, 5-LOX and LTA$_4$ hydrolase). It has therefore been suggested, based on in vitro evidence, that the major route for LTB$_4$ synthesis in inflamed glomeruli is through transcellular metabolism of leukocyte-generated LTA$_4$ to LTB$_4$ by the LTA$_4$ hydrolase present in glomerular mesangial, endothelial, and epithelial cells. Since the transformation of LTA$_4$ to LTB$_4$ is rate limiting, regulation of the LTB$_4$ synthetic rate might relate to regulation of LTA$_4$ hydrolase gene expression or catalytic activity in these parenchymal cells, rather than to the number of infiltrating leukocytes. In any case, leukocytes represent an indispensable source for LTA$_4$, the initial 5-LOX product and the precursor for LTB$_4$, because endogenous glomerular cells do not express the 5-LOX gene.[458] Thus, it was demonstrated that the PMN cell-specific activator N-formyl-methionine-leucine-phenylalanine stimulated LTB$_4$ production in isolated perfused kidneys harvested from nephrotoxic serum–treated rats to a significantly greater degree than in those from control animals treated with nonimmune rabbit serum.[459] The renal production of LTB$_4$ correlated directly with renal myeloperoxidase activity, which suggests interdependence of LTB$_4$ generation and PMN infiltration.

The acute and long-term significance of LTB$_4$ generation in conditioning the extent of glomerular structural and functional deterioration has been highlighted in studies in which LTB$_4$ was exogenously administered or in which its endogenous synthesis was inhibited. Intrarenal administration of LTB$_4$ to rats with mild nephrotoxic serum–induced injury was associated with an increase in PMN infiltration, a reduction in renal plasma flow rate, and marked exacerbation of the fall in GFR, the latter correlating strongly with the number of infiltrating PMNs per glomerulus; inhibition of 5-LOX, on the other hand, led to preservation of GFR and abrogation of proteinuria.[459] Similarly, both 5-LOX knockout mice and wild-type mice treated with the 5-LOX inhibitor zileuton had reduced renal injury in response to ischemia-reperfusion.[460] Thus, although LTB$_4$ is devoid of vasoconstrictor actions in the normal kidney, increased intrarenal generation of LTB$_4$ during early glomerular injury amplifies leukocyte-dependent reductions in glomerular perfusion and filtration rates and inflammatory injury, likely due to enhancement of PMN recruitment and/or activation.

Cytochrome P450 Pathway (Figure 13-15)

Following their elucidation and characterization as endogenous metabolites of AA, numerous studies have investigated the possibility that cytochrome P450 (CYP450) AA metabolites subserve physiologic and/or pathophysiologic roles in the kidney. In whole-animal physiology, CYP450 AA metabolites have been implicated in mediating the release of peptide hormones, regulation of vascular tone, and regulation of volume homeostasis. On the cellular level, CYP450 AA metabolites

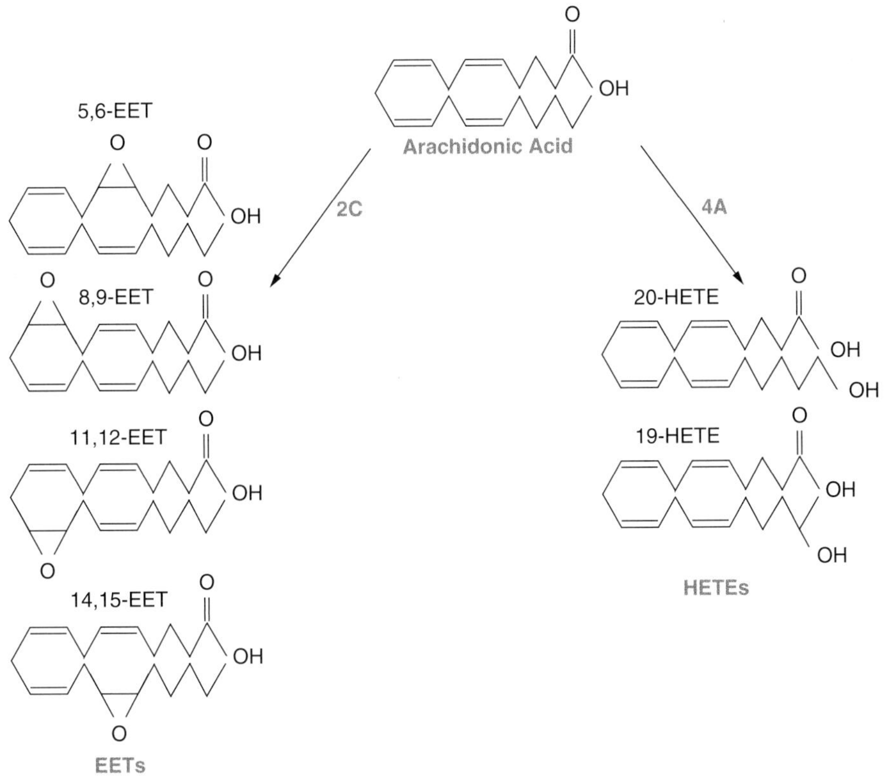

FIGURE 13-15 Pathways of cytochrome P450 (CYP450) metabolism of arachidonic acid.

have been proposed to regulate ion channels and transporters and to act as mitogens.

CYP450 monooxygenases are mixed-function oxidases that utilize molecular oxygen and NADPH as cofactors[461,462] and add an oxygen molecule to AA in a regionally specific and stereospecific geometry. CYP450 monooxygenase pathways metabolize AA to generate HETEs and EETs, the latter of which can be hydrolyzed to dihydroxyeicosatrienoic acids (DHETs).[461,463,464] The kidney displays one of the highest levels of CYP450 activity of any organ and produces CYP450 AA metabolites in significant amounts.[436,461,465] HETEs are formed primarily via CYP450 hydroxylase enzymes, and EETs and DHETs are formed primarily via CYP450 epoxygenase enzymes.[465] The CYP4A gene family is the major pathway for synthesis of hydroxylase metabolites, especially 20-HETE and 19-HETE,[281,465] whereas the production of epoxygenase metabolites is primarily via the 2C gene family.[436,461] A member of the 2J family that is an active epoxygenase is also expressed in the kidney.[466] CYP450 enzymes have been localized to both vasculature and tubules.[281] The 4A family of hydroxylases is expressed in the preglomerular renal arteriole, glomerulus, proximal tubule, the thick ascending limb of the loop of Henle, and macula densa.[467]

The 2C and 2J families of epoxygenases are expressed at highest levels in the proximal tubule and collecting duct.[466,468] When isolated nephron segments expressing CYP450 protein have been incubated with AA, production of CYP450 AA metabolites can be detected. 20-HETE and EETs are both produced in the afferent arteriole,[469] glomerulus,[470] and proximal tubule.[471] 20-HETE is the predominant CYP450 AA metabolite produced by the thick ascending limb of the loop of Henle and in the pericytes surrounding vasa recta capillaries,[472,473] whereas EETs are the predominant CYP450 AA metabolites produced by the collecting duct.[474]

Renal production of both epoxygenase and hydroxylase metabolites has been shown to be regulated by hormones and growth factors, including angiotensin II, endothelin, bradykinin, parathyroid hormone, and EGF.[281,436,462] Alterations in dietary salt intake also modulate CYP450 expression and activity.[475] Alterations in the production of CYP450 metabolites have been reported with uninephrectomy and in diabetes mellitus and hypertension.[281,463] Recent studies have shown that glycerol-containing epoxygenase metabolites are produced endogenously and serve as high-affinity ligands for cannabinoid receptors, which implicates these compounds as "endocannabinoids."[476]

Vasculature

20-Hydroxyeicosatetraenoic Acid

In rat and dog renal arteries and afferent arterioles, 20-HETE is a potent vasoconstrictor,[477] whereas it is a vasodilator in rabbit renal arterioles. The vasoconstriction is associated with membrane depolarization and a sustained rise in intracellular calcium level. 20-HETE is produced in the smooth muscle cells, and its afferent arteriolar vasoconstrictive effects are mediated by closure of calcium-activated potassium (K_{Ca}) channels through a tyrosine kinase– and extracellular signal–regulated kinase (ERK)–dependent mechanism (Figure 13-16).

An interaction between CYP450 AA metabolites and NO has also been demonstrated. NO can inhibit the formation of 20-HETE in renal vascular smooth muscle cells; a significant portion of NO's vasodilator effects in the preglomerular vasculature appear to be mediated by the inhibition of tonic 20-HETE vasoconstriction, and inhibition of 20-HETE formation attenuates the pressor response and fall in renal blood flow seen with NO synthase inhibition.[478,479]

Epoxides

Unlike CYP450 hydroxylase metabolites, epoxygenase metabolites of AA increase renal blood flow and GFR.[281,436,462] 11,12-EET and 14,15-EET vasodilate the preglomerular

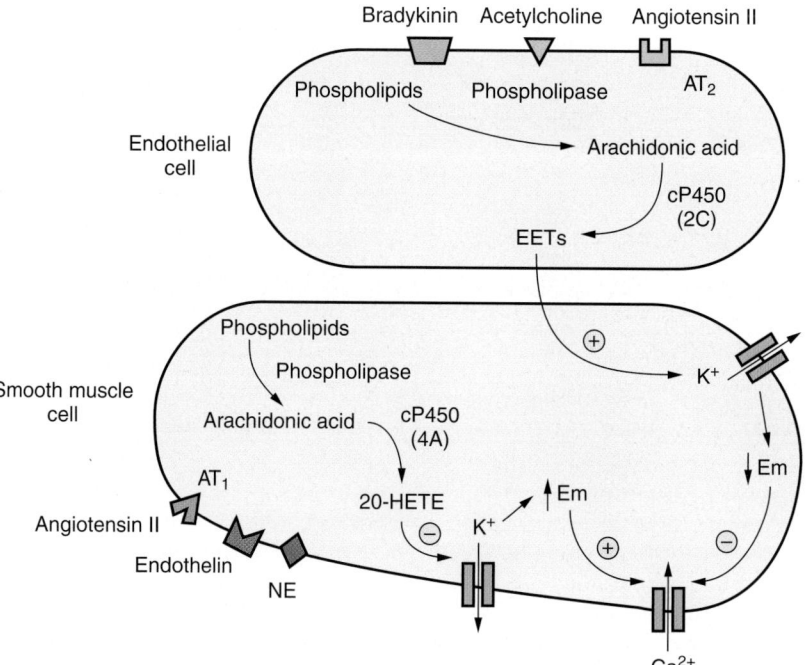

FIGURE 13-16 Proposed interactions of cytochrome P450 (CYP450) arachidonic acid metabolites derived from vascular endothelial cells and smooth muscle cells in the regulation of vascular tone.

arterioles independently of cyclooxygenase activity, whereas 5,6-EET and 8,9-EET cause cyclooxygenase-dependent vasodilation or vasoconstriction.[477] It is possible that these cyclooxygenase-dependent effects are mediated by cyclooxygenase conversion of 5,6-EET and 8,9-EET to prostaglandin- or thromboxane-like compounds.[480] EETs are produced primarily in the endothelial cells and exert their vasoactive effects on the adjacent smooth muscle cells. In this regard, it has been suggested that EETs, and specifically 11,12-EET, may serve as an endothelium-derived hyperpolarizing factor in the renal microcirculation.[436,481] EET-induced vasodilation is mediated by activation of K_{Ca} channels through cAMP-dependent stimulation of protein kinase C.

CYP450 metabolites may serve as either second messengers or modulators of the actions of hormonal and paracrine agents. Vasopressin increases renal production of CYP450 metabolites,[482] and increases in intracellular calcium and proliferation in cultured renal mesangial cells are augmented by EET administration.[482] CYP450 metabolites also may serve to modulate the renal hemodynamic responses of endothelin-1, with 20-HETE as a possible mediator of the vasoconstrictive effects and EETs counteracting the vasoconstriction.[483,484] Formation of 20-HETE does not affect the ability of endothelin-1 to increase free intracellular calcium transients in renal vascular smooth muscle but appears to enhance the sustained elevations that represent calcium influx through voltage-sensitive channels.

CYP450 metabolites have also been implicated in mediation of renal vascular responses to angiotensin II. In the presence of AT_1 receptor blockers, angiotensin II produces an endothelium-dependent vasodilation in rabbit afferent arterioles that is reliant on production of CYP450 epoxygenase metabolites by AT_2 receptor activation.[485] With intact AT_1 receptors, angiotensin II increases 20-HETE release from isolated preglomerular microvessels through an endothelium-independent mechanism.[486] The vasoconstrictive effects of angiotensin II are in part the result of 20-HETE–mediated inhibition of K_{Ca}, which enhances sustained increases in intracellular calcium concentration by calcium influx through voltage-sensitive channels. Inhibition of 20-HETE production reduces the vasoconstrictor response to angiotensin II by more than 50% in rat renal interlobular arteries from which the endothelium has been removed.[486]

Autoregulation

CYP450 metabolites of AA have been shown to be mediators of renal blood flow autoregulatory mechanisms. When prostaglandin production was blocked in canine arcuate arteries, AA administration enhanced myogenic responsiveness, and renal blood flow autoregulation was blocked by CYP450 inhibitors.[281,436] Similarly, in a rat juxtamedullary preparation, selective blockade of 20-HETE formation significantly decreased afferent arteriolar vasoconstrictor responses to elevations in perfusion pressure, and inhibition of epoxygenase activity enhanced vasoconstriction.[487] This suggests that 20-HETE is involved in afferent arteriolar autoregulatory adjustment, whereas release of vasodilatory epoxygenase metabolites in response to increases in renal perfusion pressure acts to attenuate the vasoconstriction. in vivo studies have also implicated 20-HETE as a mediator of the autoregulatory response to increased perfusion pressure.[488] Bradykinin-induced efferent

arteriolar vasodilation has been shown to be mediated in part by direct release of EETs from this vascular segment. In addition, bradykinin-induced release of 20-HETE from the glomerulus can modulate the EET-mediated vasodilation.[489]

Tubuloglomerular Feedback

CYP450 metabolites may also be involved in the tubuloglomerular feedback response.[281] As noted, 20-HETE is produced by both the afferent arteriole and macula densa, and studies have suggested the possibility that 20-HETE may serve as either a vasoconstrictive mediator of tubuloglomerular feedback released by the macula densa or a second messenger in the afferent arteriole in response to mediators released by the macula densa, such as adenosine or ATP.[490] 20-HETE may also mediate regulation of intrarenal distribution of blood flow.[491,492] In addition, there is recent evidence for connecting tubule–glomerular feedback in which increased sodium reabsorption in the connecting segment, which abuts the afferent arteriole, leads to increased AA release, which in turn increases production of EETs and vasodilatory prostaglandins. These then diffuse to the adjacent afferent arteriole and dilate it.[493]

Tubules

20-HETE and EETs both inhibit tubular sodium reabsorption.[281,462] Renal cortical interstitial infusion of the nonselective CYP450 inhibitor 17-octadecynoic acid (17-ODYA) increases papillary blood flow, renal interstitial hydrostatic pressure, and sodium excretion without affecting total renal blood flow or GFR. High dietary salt intake in rats increases expression of the renal epoxygenase CYP2C23 and production and urinary excretion of EETs, while decreasing 20-HETE production in renal cortex.[461,475] 14,15-EET has also been shown to inhibit renin secretion[494]; however, clotrimazole, which is a relatively selective epoxygenase inhibitor, induced hypertension in rats fed a high salt diet, suggesting a role in regulation of blood pressure.[475]

Proximal Tubule

The proximal tubule contains the highest concentration of CYP450 enzymes in the mammalian kidney and expresses minimal cyclooxygenase and lipoxygenase activity.[461] The 4A CYP450 family of hydroxylases that produce 19- and 20-HETE is highly expressed in mammalian proximal tubule.[294] CYP450 enzymes of both the 2C and 2J families that catalyze the formation of EETs are also expressed in the proximal tubule.[461] Both EETs and 20-HETE have been shown to be produced in the proximal tubule and have been proposed to be modulators of sodium reabsorption in the proximal tubule.

Studies in isolated perfused proximal tubule indicate that 20-HETE inhibits sodium transport whereas 19-HETE stimulates sodium transport, which suggests that 19-HETE may serve as a competitive antagonist of 20-HETE.[471,495] Administration of EETs inhibits amiloride-sensitive sodium transport in primary cultures of proximal tubule cells[496] and in LLC-PK$_1$ cells, a nontransformed, immortalized cell line from pig kidney with proximal tubule characteristics.[497,498]

20-HETE has been proposed to be a mediator of hormonal inhibition of proximal tubule reabsorption by PTH, dopamine, angiotensin II, and EGF. Although the mechanisms of 20-HETE's inhibition have not yet been completely elucidated, there is evidence that it can inhibit Na^+-K^+-ATPase activity by phosphorylation of the Na^+-K^+-ATPase α-subunit through a protein kinase C–dependent pathway.[499,500]

EETs may also serve as second messengers in the proximal tubule for EGF[501] and angiotensin II.[502] In the proximal tubule, angiotensin II has been noted to exert a biphasic response on net sodium uptake via AT_1 receptors, with low (10^{-10} to 10^{-11}) concentrations stimulating and high (10^{-7}) concentrations inhibiting net uptake.[502] Such high concentrations are not normally seen in plasma but may exist in the proximal tubule lumen as a result of the local production of angiotensin II by the proximal tubule.[503] The mechanisms by which CYPP450 AA metabolites modulate proximal tubule reabsorption have not been completely elucidated and may involve both luminal (Na^+/H^+ exchanger 3) and basolateral (Na^+-K^+ATPase) transporters.[496,499] CYP450 AA metabolites may modulate the proximal tubule component of the pressure-natriuretic response.[504]

Thick Ascending Limb of the Loop of Henle

20-HETE also serves as a second messenger for regulation of transport in the thick ascending limb. It is produced in this nephron segment[467] and can inhibit net Na^+-K^+-Cl^- cotransport by directly inhibiting the transporter and by blocking the 70-picosiemens apical K^+ channel.[472,505] In addition, 20-HETE has been implicated as a mediator of the inhibitory effects of angiotensin II[506] and bradykinin[507] on transport in the thick ascending limb of the loop of Henle.

Collecting Duct

In the collecting duct, EETs and/or their diol metabolites serve as inhibitors of the hydroosmotic effects of vasopressin, as well as inhibitors of sodium transport in this segment.[474,508] The latter effects were specific for 5,6-EET and may be secondary to formation of 5,6-epoxy-PGE_1.[508,509] Patch clamp studies have indicated that epithelial sodium channel activity in the cortical collecting duct is inhibited by 11,12-EET.[510,511]

Role in Mitogenesis

In rat mesangial cells, endogenous noncyclooxygenase metabolites of AA modulate the proliferative responses to phorbol esters, vasopressin, and EGF, and agonist-induced expression of the immediate early response genes c-fos and Egr-1 is inhibited by ketoconazole or nordihydroguaiaretic acid (NDGA), but not by specific lipoxygenase inhibitors.[512] EET-mediated increases in rat mesangial cell proliferation was the first direct evidence that CYP450 AA metabolites are cellular mitogens.[513] In cultured rabbit proximal tubule cells, CYP450 inhibitors blunted EGF-stimulated proliferation in proximal tubule cells.[501] In LLC-PKcl$_4$ cells (an established renal proximal tubule epithelial cell line derived from pig kidney) EETs were found to be potent mitogens, cytoprotective agents, and second messengers for EGF signaling. 14,15-EET-mediated signaling and mitogenesis are dependent on EGFR

transactivation, which is mediated by metalloproteinase-dependent release of heparin-binding EGF.[514] Not only the EETs but also 20-HETE has been shown to increase thymidine incorporation in primary cultures of rat proximal tubule and LLC-PK_1 cells[515] and vascular smooth muscle cells.[516]

Role in Hypertension

There is increasing evidence that the renal production of CYP450 AA metabolites is altered in a variety of models of hypertension and that blockade of the formation of compounds can alter blood pressure in several of these models. CYP450 AA metabolites may have both prohypertensive and antihypertensive properties. At the level of the renal tubule, both 20-HETE and EETs inhibit sodium transport. However, in the vasculature, 20-HETE promotes vasoconstriction and hypertension, whereas EETs are endothelium-derived vasodilators that have antihypertensive properties. Rats fed a high-salt diet show increased expression of the CYP450 epoxygenase 2C23[517] and develop hypertension if treated with a relatively selective epoxygenase inhibitor. Since EETs have antihypertensive properties, efforts are underway to develop selective inhibitors of soluble epoxide hydrolase, which converts active EETs to their inactive metabolites, DHETs, and thereby to increase EET levels. Studies in rats indicated that one such soluble epoxide hydrolase inhibitor, 1-cyclohexyl-3-dodecylurea, lowered blood pressure and reduced glomerular and tubulointerstitial injury in an angiotensin II–mediated model of hypertension in rats.[518]

In deoxycorticosterone acetate–salt hypertension, administration of a CYP450 inhibitor prevented the development of hypertension.[484,519] Angiotensin II stimulates the formation of 20-HETE in the renal circulation,[520] and inhibition of 20-HETE synthesis attenuated angiotensin II–mediated renal vasoconstriction[486,521] and reduced angiotensin II–mediated hypertension.[519]

The CYP4A2 gene is regulated by salt and is overexpressed in spontaneously hypertensive rats,[522] and production of both 20-HETE and diHETEs (dihydroxyeicosatetraenoic acids) is increased and production of EETs is reduced.[294,523] CYP450 inhibitors or antisense oligonucleotides directed against CYP4A1 and CYP4A2 lowered blood pressure in spontaneously hypertensive rats.[479,524] Conversely, studies in humans have indicated that a variant of the human CYP4A11 with reduced 20-HETE synthase activity is associated with hypertension.[525]

In Dahl salt-sensitive (Dahl S) rats, pressure natriuresis in response to salt loading is shifted so that the kidney requires a higher perfusion pressure to excrete the same amount of sodium as normotensive salt-resistant (Dahl R) rats.[281,461,462] This is due at least in part to increased reabsorption in the thick ascending limb of the loop of Henle. The production of 20-HETE and the expression of CYP4A protein are reduced in the outer medulla and thick ascending limb of Dahl S rats relative to Dahl R rats, which is consistent with the observed effect of 20-HETE to inhibit thick ascending limb transport. In addition, Dahl S rats do not show increased EET production in response to salt loading.

Studies have indicated that angiotensin II acts on AT_2 receptors on renal vascular endothelial cells to release EETs that may then counteract AT_1-induced renal vasoconstriction and may influence pressure natriuresis.[477,526,527] AT$_2$ receptor knockout mice develop hypertension,[528] which is associated with blunted pressure natriuresis, reduced renal blood flow and GFR, and defects in kidney 20-HETE production.[528]

There has been recent interest in the role of soluble epoxide hydrolase, which is the major enzyme mediating the metabolism of EETs to the inactive diHETEs, in the regulation of blood pressure. Angiotensin II induces soluble epoxide hydrolase in vasculature, which may contribute to the hypertensive effects by increasing EET metabolism.[529] Progressively more selective soluble epoxide hydrolase inhibitors are being developed and have been shown to be effective in reducing blood pressure in a number of experimental models of hypertension.[530]

Acknowledgments

The writing of this chapter was supported by grants from the Veterans Administration and the National Institute of Diabetes and Digestive and Kidney Diseases to Raymond Harris (DK62794 and DK79341) and Richard Breyer (DK37097 and DK46205).

References

1. Harris RC, Breyer MD. Arachidonic acid metabolites and the kidney. In: Brenner BM, ed. *Brenner and Rector's the kidney.* 7th ed. Philadelphia: Saunders; 2004:727-776.
2. Murakami M, Kudo I. Phospholipase A2. *J Biochem (Tokyo).* 2002;131:285-292.
3. Boulven I, Palmier B, Robin P, et al. Platelet-derived growth factor stimulates phospholipase C-γ 1, extracellular signal-regulated kinase, and arachidonic acid release in rat myometrial cells: contribution to cyclic 3′,5′-adenosine monophosphate production and effect on cell proliferation. *Biol Reprod.* 2001;65:496-506.
4. Fujishima H, Sanchez Mejia RO, Bingham 3rd CO, et al. Cytosolic phospholipase A$_2$ is essential for both the immediate and the delayed phases of eicosanoid generation in mouse bone marrow-derived mast cells. *Proc Natl Acad Sci U S A.* 1999;96:4803-4807.
5. Balsinde J, Winstead MV, Dennis EA. Phospholipase A$_2$ regulation of arachidonic acid mobilization. *FEBS Lett.* 2002;531:2-6.
6. Murakami M, Yoshihara K, Shimbara S, et al. Cellular arachidonate-releasing function and inflammation-associated expression of group IIF secretory phospholipase A$_2$. *J Biol Chem.* 2002;277:19145-19155.
7. Smith WL, Langenbach R. Why there are two cyclooxygenase isozymes. *J Clin Invest.* 2001;107:1491-1495.
8. Fitzpatrick FA, Soberman R. Regulated formation of eicosanoids. *J Clin Invest.* 2001;107:1347-1351.
9. FitzGerald GA, Patrono C. The coxibs, selective inhibitors of cyclooxygenase-2. *N Engl J Med.* 2001;345:433-442.
10. Bonazzi A, Mastyugin V, Mieyal PA, et al. Regulation of cyclooxygenase-2 by hypoxia and peroxisome proliferators in the corneal epithelium. *J Biol Chem.* 2000;275:2837-2844.
11. Hayama M, Inoue R, Akiba S, et al. ERK and p38 MAP kinase are involved in arachidonic acid release induced by H$_2$O$_2$ and PDGF in mesangial cells. *Am J Physiol Renal Physiol.* 2002;282:F485-F491.
12. Basavappa S, Pedersen SF, Jorgensen NK, et al. Swelling-induced arachidonic acid release via the 85-kDa cPLA2 in human neuroblastoma cells. *J Neurophysiol.* 1998;79:1441-1449.
13. Deleted in page proofs.
14. Hansen RA, Ogilvie GK, Davenport DJ, et al. Duration of effects of dietary fish oil supplementation on serum eicosapentaenoic acid and docosahexaenoic acid concentrations in dogs. *Am J Vet Res.* 1998;59:864-868.
15. Grande JP, Donadio Jr JV. Dietary fish oil supplementation in IgA nephropathy: a therapy in search of a mechanism?. *Nutrition.* 1998;14:240-242.
16. Kujubu DA, Fletcher BS, Varnum BC, et al. TIS10, a phorbol ester tumor promoter-inducible mRNA from Swiss 3T3 cells, encodes a novel prostaglandin synthase/cyclooxygenase homologue. *J Biol Chem.* 1991;266:12866-12872.
17. O'Banion M, Winn V, Young D. cDNA cloning and functional activity of a glucocorticoid-regulated inflammatory cyclooxygenase. *Proc Nat Acad Sci U S A.* 1992;89:4888-4892.
18. Jang BC, Munoz-Najar U, Paik JH, et al. Leptomycin B, an inhibitor of the nuclear export receptor CRM1, inhibits COX-2 expression. *J Biol Chem.* 2003;278:2773-2776.
19. Dixon DA, Tolley ND, King PH, et al. Altered expression of the mRNA stability factor HuR promotes cyclooxygenase-2 expression in colon cancer cells. *J Clin Invest.* 2001;108:1657-1665.
20. Inoue H, Taba Y, Miwa Y, et al. Transcriptional and posttranscriptional regulation of cyclooxygenase-2 expression by fluid shear stress in vascular endothelial cells. *Arterioscler Thromb Vasc Biol.* 2002;22:1415-1420.
21. Hla T, Bishop-Bailey D, Liu CH, et al. Cyclooxygenase-1 and -2 isoenzymes. *Int J Biochem Cell Biol.* 1999;31:551-557.
22. Mestre JR, Mackrell PJ, Rivadeneira DE, et al. Redundancy in the signaling pathways and promoter elements regulating cyclooxygenase-2 gene expression in endotoxin-treated macrophage/monocytic cells. *J Biol Chem.* 2001;276:3977-3982.
23. Tanabe T, Tohnai N. Cyclooxygenase isozymes and their gene structures and expression. *Prostaglandins Other Lipid Mediat.* 2002;68-69:95-114.
24. Inoue H, Tanabe T. Transcriptional role of the nuclear factor kappa B site in the induction by lipopolysaccharide and suppression by dexamethasone of cyclooxygenase-2 in U937 cells. *Biochem Biophys Res Commun.* 1998;244:143-148.
25. Dixon DA, Kaplan CD, McIntyre TM, et al. Post-transcriptional control of cyclooxygenase-2 gene expression. The role of the 3′-untranslated region. *J Biol Chem.* 2000;275:11750-11757.
26. Vezza R, Mezzasoma AM, Venditti G, et al. Prostaglandin endoperoxides and thromboxane A$_2$ activate the same receptor isoforms in human platelets. *Thromb Haemost.* 2002;87:114-121.
27. Garavito MR, Malkowski MG, et al. The structures of prostaglandin endoperoxide H synthases-1 and -2. *Prostaglandins Other Lipid Mediat.* 2002;68-69:129-152.
28. Kalgutkar AS, Crews BC, Rowlinson SW, et al. Aspirin-like molecules that covalently inactivate cyclooxygenase-2. *Science.* 1998;280:1268-1270.
29. Yu Y, Fan J, Chen X-S, et al. Genetic model of selective COX2 inhibition reveals novel heterodimer signaling. *Nat Med.* 2006;12:699-704.
30. Crofford LJ. Specific cyclooxygenase-2 inhibitors: what have we learned since they came into widespread clinical use? *Curr Opin Rheumatol.* 2002;14:225-230.
31. Li S, Ballou LR, Morham SG, et al. Cyclooxygenase-2 mediates the febrile response of mice to interleukin-1β. *Brain Res.* 2001;910:163-173.
32. Turini ME, DuBois RN. Cyclooxygenase-2: a therapeutic target. *Annu Rev Med.* 2002;53:35-57.
33. Pasinetti GM. From epidemiology to therapeutic trials with anti-inflammatory drugs in Alzheimer's disease: the role of NSAIDs and cyclooxygenase in beta-amyloidosis and clinical dementia. *J Alzheimers Dis.* 2002;4:435-445.
34. Harris RC, McKanna JA, Akai Y, et al. Cyclooxygenase-2 is associated with the macula densa of rat kidney and increases with salt restriction. *J Clin Invest.* 1994;94:2504-2510.
35. Guan Y, Chang M, Cho W, et al. Cloning, expression, and regulation of rabbit cyclooxygenase-2 in renal medullary interstitial cells. *Am J Physiol.* 1997;273:F18-F26.
36. Yang T, Schnermann JB, Briggs JP. Regulation of cyclooxygenase-2 expression in renal medulla by tonicity in vivo and in vitro. *Am J Physiol.* 1999;277:F1-F9.
37. Nantel F, Meadows E, Denis D, et al. Immunolocalization of cyclooxygenase-2 in the macula densa of human elderly. *FEBS Lett.* 1999;457:475-477.
38. Adegboyega PA, Ololade O. Immunohistochemical expression of cyclooxygenase-2 in normal kidneys. *Appl Immunohistochem Mol Morphol.* 2004;12:71-74.
39. Khan KN, Stanfield KM, Harris RK, et al. Expression of cyclooxygenase-2 in the macula densa of human kidney in hypertension, congestive heart failure, and diabetic nephropathy. *Ren Fail.* 2001;23:321-330.
40. Komhoff M, Jeck ND, Seyberth HW, et al. Cyclooxygenase-2 expression is associated with the renal macula densa of patients with Bartter-like syndrome. *Kidney Int.* 2000;58:2420-2424.
41. Harris RC, Breyer MD. Physiological regulation of cyclooxygenase-2 in the kidney. *Am J Physiol Renal Physiol.* 2001;281:F1-F11.
42. Schnermann J. Juxtaglomerular cell complex in the regulation of renal salt excretion. *Am J Physiol.* 1998;274:R263-279.
43. Schnermann J, Traynor T, Pohl H, et al. Vasoconstrictor responses in thromboxane receptor knockout mice: tubuloglomerular feedback and ureteral obstruction. *Acta Physiol Scand.* 2000;168:201-207.
44. Qi Z, Hao CM, Langenbach RI, et al. Opposite effects of cyclooxygenase-1 and -2 activity on the pressor response to angiotensin II. *J Clin Invest.* 2002;110:61-69.

45. Ichihara A, Imig JD, Inscho EW, et al. Cyclooxygenase-2 participates in tubular flow-dependent afferent arteriolar tone: interaction with neuronal NOS. *Am J Physiol*. 1998;275:F605-F612.
46. Perazella MA, Tray K. Selective cyclooxygenase-2 inhibitors: a pattern of nephrotoxicity similar to traditional nonsteroidal anti-inflammatory drugs. *Am J Med*. 2001;111:64-67.
47. Peti-Peterdi J, Komlosi P, Fuson AL, et al. Luminal NaCl delivery regulates basolateral PGE_2 release from macula densa cells. *J Clin Invest*. 2003;112:76-82.
48. Cheng HF, Wang JL, Zhang MZ, et al. Role of p38 in the regulation of renal cortical cyclooxygenase-2 expression by extracellular chloride. *J Clin Invest*. 2000;106:681-688.
49. Yang T, Park JM, Arend L, et al. Low chloride stimulation of prostaglandin E_2 release and cyclooxygenase-2 expression in a mouse macula densa cell line. *J Biol Chem*. 2000;275:37922-37929.
50. Zhang MZ, Yao B, McKanna JA, et al. Cross talk between the intrarenal dopaminergic and cyclooxygenase-2 systems. *Am J Physiol Renal Physiol*. 2005;288:F840-F845.
51. Hanner F, Chambrey R, Bourgeois S, et al. Increased renal renin content in mice lacking the Na^+/H^+ exchanger NHE2. *Am J Physiol Renal Physiol*. 2008;294:F937-F944.
52. Cheng HF, Wang JL, Zhang MZ, et al. Angiotensin II attenuates renal cortical cyclooxygenase-2 expression. *J Clin Invest*. 1999;103:953-961.
53. Harding P, Sigmon DH, Alfie ME, et al. Cyclooxygenase-2 mediates increased renal renin content induced by low-sodium diet. *Hypertension*. 1997;29:297-302.
54. Stichtenoth DO, Marhauer V, Tsikas D, et al. Effects of specific COX-2-inhibition on renin release and renal and systemic prostanoid synthesis in healthy volunteers. *Kidney Int*. 2005;68:2197-2207.
55. Traynor TR, Smart A, Briggs JP, et al. Inhibition of macula densa–stimulated renin secretion by pharmacological blockade of cyclooxygenase-2. *Am J Physiol*. 1999;277:F706-F710.
56. Cheng HF, Wang JL, Zhang MZ, et al. Genetic deletion of COX-2 prevents increased renin expression in response to ACE inhibition. *Am J Physiol Renal Physiol*. 2001;280:F449-F456.
57. Yang T, Endo Y, Huang YG, et al. Renin expression in COX-2-knockout mice on normal or low-salt diets. *Am J Physiol Renal Physiol*. 2000;279:F819-F825.
58. Cheng HF, Wang SW, Zhang MZ, et al. Prostaglandins that increase renin production in response to ACE inhibition are not derived from cyclooxygenase-1. *Am J Physiol Regul Integr Comp Physiol*. 2002;283:R638-R646.
59. Athirakul K, Kim HS, Audoly LP, et al. Deficiency of COX-1 causes natriuresis and enhanced sensitivity to ACE inhibition. *Kidney Int*. 2001;60:2324-2329.
60. Matzdorf C, Kurtz A, Hocherl K. COX-2 activity determines the level of renin expression but is dispensable for acute upregulation of renin expression in rat kidneys. *Am J Physiol Renal Physiol*. 2007;292:F1782-F1790.
61. Kim SM, Chen L, Mizel D, et al. Low plasma renin and reduced renin secretory responses to acute stimuli in conscious COX-2–deficient mice. *Am J Physiol Renal Physiol*. 2007;292:F415-F422.
62. Nguyen G. Increased cyclooxygenase-2, hyperfiltration, glomerulosclerosis, and diabetic nephropathy: put the blame on the (pro)renin receptor? *Kidney Int*. 2006;70:618-620.
63. Wang JL, Cheng HF, Harris RC. Cyclooxygenase-2 inhibition decreases renin content and lowers blood pressure in a model of renovascular hypertension. *Hypertension*. 1999;34:96-101.
64. Fujino T, Nakagawa N, Yuhki K, et al. Decreased susceptibility to renovascular hypertension in mice lacking the prostaglandin I_2 receptor IP. *J Clin Invest*. 2004;114:805-812.
65. El-Achkar TM, Plotkin Z, Marcic B, et al. Sepsis induces an increase in thick ascending limb Cox-2 that is TLR4 dependent. *Am J Physiol Renal Physiol*. 2007;293:F1187-F1196.
66. Ichihara A, Imig JD, Navar LG. Cyclooxygenase-2 modulates afferent arteriolar responses to increases in pressure. *Hypertension*. 1999;34:843-847.
67. Araujo M, Welch WJ. Cyclooxygenase 2 inhibition suppresses tubuloglomerular feedback: roles of thromboxane receptors and nitric oxide. *Am J Physiol Renal Physiol*. 2009;296:F790-F794.
68. He W, Miao FJ, Lin DC, et al. Citric acid cycle intermediates as ligands for orphan G-protein–coupled receptors. *Nature*. 2004;429:188-193.
69. Toma I, Kang JJ, Sipos A, et al. Succinate receptor GPR91 provides a direct link between high glucose levels and renin release in murine and rabbit kidney. *J Clin Invest*. 2008;118:2526-2534.
70. Vargas SL, Toma I, Kang JJ, et al. Activation of the succinate receptor GPR91 in macula densa cells causes renin release. *J Am Soc Nephrol*. 2009;20:1002-1011.
71. Hao CM, Yull F, Blackwell T, et al. Dehydration activates an NF-κB-driven, COX2-dependent survival mechanism in renal medullary interstitial cells. *J Clin Invest*. 2000;106:973-982.
72. Khan KN, Stanfield KM, Trajkovic D, et al. Expression of cyclooxygenase-2 in canine renal cell carcinoma. *Vet Pathol*. 2001;38:116-119.
73. Bishop-Bailey D, Calatayud S, Warner TD, et al. Prostaglandins and the regulation of tumor growth. *J Environ Pathol Toxicol Oncol*. 2002;21:93-101.
74. Toyota M, Shen L, Ohe-Toyota M, et al. Aberrant methylation of the cyclooxygenase 2 CpG island in colorectal tumors. *Cancer Res*. 2000;60:4044-4048.
75. Ichitani Y, Holmberg K, Maunsbach AB, et al. Cyclooxygenase-1 and cyclooxygenase-2 expression in rat kidney and adrenal gland after stimulation with systemic lipopolysaccharide: in situ hybridization and immunocytochemical studies. *Cell Tissue Res*. 2001;303:235-252.
76. Yang T, Huang Y, Heasley LE, et al. MAPK mediation of hypertonicity-stimulated cyclooxygenase-2 expression in renal medullary collecting duct cells. *J Biol Chem*. 2000;275:23281-23286.
77. Yang T, Zhang A, Pasumarthy A, et al. Nitric oxide stimulates COX-2 expression in cultured collecting duct cells through MAP kinases and superoxide but not cGMP. *Am J Physiol Renal Physiol*. 2006;291:F891-F895.
78. Kuper C, Bartels H, Fraek ML, et al. Ectodomain shedding of pro-TGF-α is required for COX-2 induction and cell survival in renal medullary cells exposed to osmotic stress. *Am J Physiol Cell Physiol*. 2007;293:C1971-C1982.
79. Yang T, Zhang A, Honeggar M, et al. Hypertonic induction of COX-2 in collecting duct cells by reactive oxygen species of mitochondrial origin. *J Biol Chem*. 2005;280:34966-34973.
80. Jaimes EA, Zhou MS, Pearse DD, et al. Upregulation of cortical COX-2 in salt-sensitive hypertension: role of angiotensin II and reactive oxygen species. *Am J Physiol Renal Physiol*. 2008;294:F385-F392.
81. Rocca B, Secchiero P, Ciabattoni G, et al. Cyclooxygenase-2 expression is induced during human megakaryopoiesis and characterizes newly formed platelets. *Proc Natl Acad Sci U S A*. 2002;99:7634-7639.
82. Taniura S, Kamitani H, Watanabe T, et al. Transcriptional regulation of cyclooxygenase-1 by histone deacetylase inhibitors in normal human astrocyte cells. *J Biol Chem*. 2002;277:16823-16830.
83. Brater DC. Effects of nonsteroidal anti-inflammatory drugs on renal function: focus on cyclooxygenase–2–selective inhibition. *Am J Med*. 1999;107:65S-70S:discussion 70S-71S.
84. Catella-Lawson F, McAdam B, Morrison BW, et al. Effects of specific inhibition of cyclooxygenase-2 on sodium balance, hemodynamics, and vasoactive eicosanoids. *J Pharmacol Exp Ther*. 1999;289:735-741.
85. Whelton A, Fort JG, Puma JA, et al. Cyclooxygenase-2–specific inhibitors and cardiorenal function: a randomized, controlled trial of celecoxib and rofecoxib in older hypertensive osteoarthritis patients. *Am J Ther*. 2001;8:85-95.
86. Swan SK, Rudy DW, Lasseter KC, et al. Effect of cyclooxygenase-2 inhibition on renal function in elderly persons receiving a low-salt diet. A randomized, controlled trial. *Ann Intern Med*. 2000;133:1-9.
87. Rossat J, Maillard M, Nussberger J, et al. Renal effects of selective cyclooxygenase-2 inhibition in normotensive salt-depleted subjects. *Clin Pharmacol Ther*. 1999;66:76-84.
88. Stokes JB. Effect of prostaglandin E_2 on chloride transport across the rabbit thick ascending limb of Henle. *J Clin Invest* 1979;64:495-502.
89. Whelton A, Schulman G, Wallemark C, et al. Effects of celecoxib and naproxen on renal function in the elderly. *Arch Intern Med*. 2000;160:1465-1470.
90. Muscara MN, Vergnolle N, Lovren F, et al. Selective cyclo-oxygenase-2 inhibition with celecoxib elevates blood pressure and promotes leukocyte adherence. *Br J Pharmacol*. 2000;129:1423-1430.
91. Atta MG, Whelton A. Acute renal papillary necrosis induced by ibuprofen. *Am J Ther*. 1997;4:55-60.
92. DeBroe M, Elseviers M. Analgesic nephropathy. *N Engl J Med*. 1998;338:446-452.
93. Segasothy M, Samad S, Zulfigar A, et al. Chronic renal disease and papillary necrosis associated with the long-term use of nonstroidal anti-inflammatory drugs as the sole or predominant analgesic. *Am J Kidney Dis*. 1994;24:17-24.
94. Black HE. Renal toxicity of non-steroidal anti-inflammatory drugs. *Toxicol Pathol*. 1986;14:83-90.
95. Hao CM, Redha R, Morrow J, et al. Peroxisome proliferator–activated receptor delta activation promotes cell survival following hypertonic stress. *J Biol Chem*. 2002;277:21341-21345.
96. Akhund L, Quinet RJ, Ishaq S. Celecoxib-related renal papillary necrosis. *Arch Intern Med*. 2003;163:114-115.
97. Ahmad SR, Kortepeter C, Brinker A, et al. Renal failure associated with the use of celecoxib and rofecoxib. *Drug Saf*. 2002;25:537-544.
98. Kleinknecht D. Interstitial nephritis, the nephrotic syndrome, and chronic renal failure secondary to nonsteroidal anti-inflammatory drugs. *Semin Nephrol*. 1995;15:228-235.
99. Henao J, Hisamuddin I, Nzerue CM, et al. Celecoxib-induced acute interstitial nephritis. *Am J Kidney Dis*. 2002;39:1313-1317.

100. Alper Jr AB, Meleg-Smith S, Krane NK. Nephrotic syndrome and interstitial nephritis associated with celecoxib. *Am J Kidney Dis.* 2002;40:1086-1090.

101. Tietjen DP. Recurrence and specificity of nephrotic syndrome due to tolmetin. *Am J Med.* 1989;87:354-355.

102. Radford Jr MG, Holley KE, Grande JP, et al. Reversible membranous nephropathy associated with the use of nonsteroidal anti-inflammatory drugs. *JAMA.* 1996;276:466-469.

103. Peruzzi L, Gianoglio B, Porcellini MG, et al. Neonatal end-stage renal failure associated with maternal ingestion of cyclo-oxygenase-type-2 selective inhibitor nimesulide as tocolytic. *Lancet.* 1999;354:1615:[letter, comment].

104. Komhoff M, Wang JL, Cheng HF, et al. Cyclooxygenase-2–selective inhibitors impair glomerulogenesis and renal cortical development. *Kidney Int.* 2000;57:414-422.

105. Dinchuk JE, Car BD, Focht RJ, et al. Renal abnormalities and an altered inflammatory response in mice lacking cyclooxygenase II. *Nature.* 1995;378:406-409.

106. Morham SG, Langenbach R, Loftin CD, et al. Prostaglandin synthase 2 gene disruption causes severe renal pathology in the mouse. *Cell.* 1995;83:473-482.

107. Langenbach R, Morham SG, Tiano HF, et al. Prostaglandin synthase 1 gene disruption in mice reduces arachidonic acid–induced inflammation and indomethacin-induced gastric ulceration. *Cell.* 1995;83:483-492.

108. Zhang MZ, Wang JL, Cheng HF, et al. Cyclooxygenase-2 in rat nephron development. *Am J Physiol.* 1997;273:F994-F1002.

109. Avner ED, Sweeney Jr WE, Piesco NP, et al. Growth factor requirements of organogenesis in serum-free metanephric organ culture. *In Vitro Cell Dev Biol.* 1985;21:297-304.

110. Sugimoto Y, Narumiya S, Ichikawa A. Distribution and function of prostanoid receptors: studies from knockout mice. *Prog Lipid Res.* 2000;39:289-314.

111. Bagai S, Rubio E, Cheng JF, et al. Fibroblast growth factor-10 is a mitogen for urothelial cells. *J Biol Chem.* 2002;277:23828-23837.

112. Gimbrone Jr MA, Topper JN, Nagel T, et al. Endothelial dysfunction, hemodynamic forces, and atherogenesis. *Ann N Y Acad Sci.* 2000;902:230-239:discussion 239-240.

113. McAdam BF, Catella-Lawson F, Mardini IA, et al. Systemic biosynthesis of prostacyclin by cyclooxygenase (COX)-2: the human pharmacology of a selective inhibitor of COX-2. *Proc Natl Acad Sci U S A.* 1999;96:272-277.

114. Fitzgerald GA. Coxibs and cardiovascular disease. *N Engl J Med.* 2004;351:1709-1711.

115. Bea F, Blessing E, Bennett BJ, et al. Chronic inhibition of cyclooxygenase-2 does not alter plaque composition in a mouse model of advanced unstable atherosclerosis. *Cardiovasc Res.* 2003;60:198-204.

116. Pratico D, Tillmann C, Zhang ZB, et al. Acceleration of atherogenesis by COX-1–dependent prostanoid formation in low density lipoprotein receptor knockout mice. *Proc Natl Acad Sci U S A.* 2001;98:3358-3363.

117. Burleigh ME, Babaev VR, Oates JA, et al. Cyclooxygenase-2 promotes early atherosclerotic lesion formation in LDL receptor-deficient mice. *Circulation.* 2002;105:1816-1823.

118. Belton OA, Duffy A, Toomey S, et al. Cyclooxygenase isoforms and platelet vessel wall interactions in the apolipoprotein E knockout mouse model of atherosclerosis. *Circulation.* 2003;108:3017-3023.

119. Burleigh ME, Babaev VR, Yancey PG, et al. Cyclooxygenase-2 promotes early atherosclerotic lesion formation in ApoE-deficient and C57BL/6 mice. *J Mol Cell Cardiol.* 2005;39:443-452.

120. Egan KM, Wang M, Fries S, et al. Cyclooxygenases, thromboxane, and atherosclerosis: plaque destabilization by cyclooxygenase-2 inhibition combined with thromboxane receptor antagonism. *Circulation.* 2005;111:334-342.

121. Hansson GK. Inflammation, atherosclerosis, and coronary artery disease. *N Engl J Med.* 2005;352:1685-1695.

122. Sato T, Sawada S, Tsuda Y, et al. The mechanism of thrombin-induced prostacyclin synthesis in human endothelial cells with reference to the gene transcription of prostacyclin-related enzymes and Ca^{2+} kinetics. *J Pharmacol Toxicol Methods.* 1999;41:173-182.

123. Okahara K, Sun B, Kambayashi J. Upregulation of prostacyclin synthesis–related gene expression by shear stress in vascular endothelial cells. *Arterioscler Thromb Vasc Biol.* 1998;18:1922-1926.

124. Guan Z, Buckman SY, Miller BW, et al. Interleukin-1β–induced cyclooxygenase-2 expression requires activation of both c-Jun NH_2-terminal kinase and p38 MAPK signal pathways in rat renal mesangial cells. *J Biol Chem.* 1998;273:28670-28676.

125. Soler M, Camacho M, Sola R, et al. Mesangial cells release untransformed prostaglandin H_2 as a major prostanoid. *Kidney Int.* 2001;59:1283-1289.

126. Guan Y, Zhang Y, Schneider A, et al. Urogenital distribution of a mouse membrane-associated prostaglandin E_2 synthase. *Am J Physiol Renal Physiol.* 2001;281:F1173-F1177.

127. Hao CM, Komhoff M, Guan Y, et al. Selective targeting of cyclooxygenase-2 reveals its role in renal medullary interstitial cell survival. *Am J Physiol.* 1999;277:F352-F359.

128. Chevalier D, Lo-Guidice JM, Sergent E, et al. Identification of genetic variants in the human thromboxane synthase gene (CYP5A1). *Mutat Res.* 2001;432:61-67.

129. Nusing R, Fehr PM, Gudat F, et al. The localization of thromboxane synthase in normal and pathological human kidney tissue using a monoclonal antibody Tu 300. *Virchows Arch.* 1994;424:69-74.

130. Wilcox CS, Welch WJ. Thromboxane synthase and TP receptor mRNA in rat kidney and brain: effects of salt intake and ANG II. *Am J Physiol Renal Physiol.* 2003;284:F525-F531.

131. Quest DW, Wilson TW. Effects of ridogrel, a thromboxane synthase inhibitor and receptor antagonist, on blood pressure in the spontaneously hypertensive rat. *Jpn J Pharmacol.* 1998;78:479-486.

132. Yokoyama C, Yabuki T, Shimonishi M, et al. Prostacyclin-deficient mice develop ischemic renal disorders, including nephrosclerosis and renal infarction. *Circulation.* 2002;106:2397-2403.

133. Murata T, Ushikubi F, Matsuoka T, et al. Altered pain perception and inflammatory response in mice lacking prostacyclin receptor. *Nature.* 1997;388:678-682.

134. Urade Y, Eguchi N. Lipocalin-type and hematopoietic prostaglandin D synthases as a novel example of functional convergence. *Prostaglandins Other Lipid Mediat.* 2002;68-69:375-382.

135. Urade Y, Hayaishi O. Prostaglandin D synthase: structure and function. *Vitam Horm.* 2000;58:89-120.

136. Eguchi N, Minami T, Shirafuji N, et al. Lack of tactile pain (allodynia) in lipocalin-type prostaglandin D synthase–deficient mice. *Proc Natl Acad Sci U S A.* 1999;96:726-730.

137. Vitzthum H, Abt I, Einhellig S, et al. Gene expression of prostanoid forming enzymes along the rat nephron. *Kidney Int.* 2002;62:1570-1581.

138. Ogawa M, Hirawa N, Tsuchida T, et al. Urinary excretions of lipocalin-type prostaglandin D_2 synthase predict the development of proteinuria and renal injury in OLETF rats. *Nephrol Dial Transplant.* 2006;21:924-934.

139. Ragolia L, Palaia T, Hall CE, et al. Accelerated glucose intolerance, nephropathy, and atherosclerosis in prostaglandin D_2 synthase knock-out mice. *J Biol Chem.* 2005;280:29946-29955.

140. Watanabe K. Prostaglandin F synthase. *Prostaglandins Other Lipid Mediat.* 2002;68-69:401-407.

141. Roberts 2nd LJ, Seibert K, Liston TE, et al. PGD_2 is transformed by human coronary arteries to 9α,11β-PGF_2, which contracts human coronary artery rings. *Adv Prostaglandin Thromboxane Leukot Res.* 1987;17A:427-429.

142. Sharif NA, Xu SX, Williams GW, et al. Pharmacology of [³H] prostaglandin E_1/[³H]prostaglandin E_2 and [³H]prostaglandin $F_{2α}$ binding to EP3 and FP prostaglandin receptor binding sites in bovine corpus luteum: characterization and correlation with functional data. *J Pharmacol Exp Ther.* 1998;286:1094-1102.

143. Wallner EI, Wada J, Tramonti G, et al. Relevance of aldo-keto reductase family members to the pathobiology of diabetic nephropathy and renal development. *Ren Fail.* 2001;23:311-320.

144. Siragy HM, Inagami T, Ichiki T, et al. Sustained hypersensitivity to angiotensin II and its mechanism in mice lacking the subtype-2 (AT_2) angiotensin receptor. *Proc Natl Acad Sci U S A.* 1999;96:6506-6510.

145. Siragy HM, Senbonmatsu T, Ichiki T, et al. Increased renal vasodilator prostanoids prevent hypertension in mice lacking the angiotensin subtype-2 receptor. *J Clin Invest.* 1999;104:181-188.

146. Siragy HM, Carey RM. The subtype 2 angiotensin receptor regulates renal prostaglandin F2 alpha formation in conscious rats. *Am J Physiol.* 1997;273:R1103-R1107.

147. Tanikawa N, Ohmiya Y, Ohkubo H, et al. Identification and characterization of a novel type of membrane-associated prostaglandin E synthase. *Biochem Biophys Res Commun.* 2002;291:884-889.

148. Jakobsson PJ, Thoren S, Morgenstern R, et al. Identification of human prostaglandin E synthase: a microsomal, glutathione-dependent, inducible enzyme, constituting a potential novel drug target. *Proc Natl Acad Sci U S A.* 1999;96:7220-7225.

149. Trebino CE, Stock JL, Gibbons CP, et al. Impaired inflammatory and pain responses in mice lacking an inducible prostaglandin E synthase. *Proc Natl Acad Sci U S A.* 2003;100:9044-9049.

150. Engblom D, Saha S, Engstrom L, et al. Microsomal prostaglandin E synthase-1 is the central switch during immune-induced pyresis. *Nat Neurosci.* 2003;6:1137-1138.

151. Ouellet M, Falgueyret JP, Hien Ear P, et al. Purification and characterization of recombinant microsomal prostaglandin E synthase-1. *Protein Expr Purif.* 2002;26:489-495.

152. Uematsu S, Matsumoto M, Takeda K, et al. Lipopolysaccharide-dependent prostaglandin E_2 production is regulated by the glutathione-dependent prostaglandin E_2 synthase gene induced by the Toll-like receptor 4/MyD88/NF-IL6 pathway. *J Immunol.* 2002;168:5811-5816.

153. Dinchuk JE, Car BD, Focht RJ, et al. Renal abnormalities and an altered inflammatory response in mice lacking cyclooxygenase II. *Nature.* 1995;378:406-409.

154. Nguyen M, Camenisch T, Snouwaert JN, et al. The prostaglandin receptor EP4 triggers remodelling of the cardiovascular system at birth. *Nature.* 1997;390:78-81.

155. Tanioka T, Nakatani Y, Semmyo N, et al. Molecular identification of cytosolic prostaglandin E_2 synthase that is functionally coupled with cyclooxygenase-1 in immediate prostaglandin E_2 biosynthesis. *J Biol Chem.* 2000;275:32775-32782.

156. Zhang Y, Schneider A, Rao R, et al. Genomic structure and genitourinary expression of mouse cytosolic prostaglandin E_2 synthase gene. *Biochim Biophys Acta.* 2003;1634:15-23.

157. Murakami M, Nakatani Y, Tanioka T, et al. Prostaglandin E synthase. *Prostaglandins Other Lipid Mediat.* 2002;68-69:383-399.

158. Hirata M, Hayashi Y, Ushikubi F, et al. Cloning and expression of cDNA for a human thromboxane A_2 receptor. *Nature.* 1991;349:617-620.

159. Raychowdhury MK, Yukawa M, Collins LJ, et al. Alternative splicing produces a divergent cytoplasmic tail in the human endothelial thromboxane A_2 receptor. *J Biol Chem.* 1994;269:19256-19261:[published erratum appears in *J Biol Chem* 270(12):7011, 1995].

160. Pierce KL, Regan JW. Prostanoid receptor heterogeneity through alternative mRNA splicing. *Life Sci.* 1998;62:1479-1483.

161. Wilson RJ, Rhodes SA, Wood RL, et al. Functional pharmacology of human prostanoid EP2 and EP4 receptors. *Eur J Pharmacol.* 2004;501:49-58.

162. Morinelli TA, Oatis Jr JE, Okwu AK, et al. Characterization of an ^{125}I-labeled thromboxane A_2/prostaglandin H_2 receptor agonist. *J Pharmacol Exp Ther.* 1989;251:557-562.

163. Narumiya S, Sugimoto Y, Ushikubi F. Prostanoid receptors: structures, properties, and functions. *Physiol Rev.* 1999;79:1193-1226.

164. Abramovitz M, Adam M, Boie Y, et al. The utilization of recombinant prostanoid receptors to determine the affinities and selectivities of prostaglandins and related analogs. *Biochim Biophys Acta.* 2000;1483:285-293.

165. Audoly LP, Rocca B, Fabre JE, et al. Cardiovascular responses to the isoprostanes iPF$_{2\alpha}$-III and iPE$_2$-III are mediated via the thromboxane A_2 receptor in vivo. *Circulation.* 2000;101:2833-2840.

166. Welch WJ. Effects of isoprostane on tubuloglomerular feedback: roles of TP receptors, NOS, and salt intake. *Am J Physiol Renal Physiol.* 2005;288:F757-F762.

167. Morrow JD. Quantification of isoprostanes as indices of oxidant stress and the risk of atherosclerosis in humans. *Arterioscler Thromb Vasc Biol.* 2005;25:279-286.

168. Abe T, Takeuchi K, Takahashi N, et al. Rat kidney thromboxane A_2 receptor: molecular cloning signal transduction and intrarenal expression localization. *J Clin Invest.* 1995;96:657-664.

169. Namba T, Sugimoto Y, Hirata M, et al. Mouse thromboxane A_2 receptor: cDNA cloning, expression and Northern blot analysis. *Biochem Biophys Res. Commun.* 1992;184:1197-1203.

170. Hirata T, Kakizuka A, Ushikubi F, et al. Arg60 to Leu mutation of the human thromboxane A_2 receptor in a dominantly inherited bleeding disorder. *J Clin Invest.* 1994;94:1662-1667.

171. Mannon RB, Coffman TM, Mannon PJ. Distribution of binding sites for thromboxane A_2 in the mouse kidney. *Am J Physiol.* 1996;271:F1131-F1138.

172. Thomas DW, Mannon RB, Mannon PJ, et al. Coagulation defects and altered hemodynamic responses in mice lacking receptors for thromboxane A_2. *J Clin Invest.* 1998;102:1994-2001.

173. Spurney RF, Onorato JJ, Albers FJ, et al. Thromboxane binding and signal transduction in rat glomerular mesangial cells. *Am J Physiol.* 1993;264:F292-F299.

174. Nasjletti A, Arthur C. Corcoran Memorial Lecture. The role of eicosanoids in angiotensin-dependent hypertension. *Hypertension.* 1998;31:194-200.

175. Kawada N, Dennehy K, Solis G, et al. TP receptors regulate renal hemodynamics during angiotensin II slow pressor response. *Am J Physiol Renal Physiol.* 2004;287:F753-F759.

176. Boffa J-J, Just A, Coffman TM, et al. Thromboxane receptor mediates renal vasoconstriction and contributes to acute renal failure in endotoxemic mice. *J Am Soc Nephrol.* 2004;15:2358-2365.

177. Welch WJ, Peng B, Takeuchi K, et al. Salt loading enhances rat renal TxA$_2$/PGH$_2$ receptor expression and TGF response to U-46,619. *Am J Physiol.* 1997;273:F976-F983.

178. Welch WJ, Wilcox CS. Potentiation of tubuloglomerular feedback in the rat by thromboxane mimetic. Role of macula densa. *J Clin Invest.* 1992;89:1857-1865.

179. Coffman TM, Spurney RF, Mannon RB, et al. Thromboxane A_2 modulates the fibrinolytic system in glomerular mesangial cells. *Am J Physiol.* 1998;275:F262-F269.

180. Francois H, Athirakul K, Mao L, et al. Role for thromboxane receptors in angiotensin-II–induced hypertension. *Hypertension.* 2004;43:364-369.

181. Francois H, Makhanova N, Ruiz P, et al. A role for the thromboxane receptor in L-NAME hypertension. *Am J Physiol Renal Physiol.* 2008;295:F1096-F1102.

182. Kiriyama M, Ushikubi F, Kobayashi T, et al. Ligand binding specificities of the eight types and subtypes of the mouse prostanoid receptors expressed in Chinese hamster ovary cells. *Br J Pharmacol.* 1997;122:217-224.

183. Namba T, Oida H, Sugimoto Y, et al. cDNA cloning of a mouse prostacyclin receptor: multiple signaling pathways and expression in thymic medulla. *J Biol Chem.* 1994;269:9986-9992.

184. Boie Y, Rushmore TH, Darmon-Goodwin A, et al. Cloning and expression of a cDNA for the human prostanoid IP receptor. *J Biol Chem.* 1994;269:12173-12178.

185. Oida H, Namba T, Sugimoto Y, et al. In situ hybridization studies on prostacyclin receptor mRNA expression in various mouse organs. *Br J Pharmacol.* 1995;116:2828-2837.

186. Nasrallah R, Hebert RL. Prostacyclin signaling in the kidney: implications for health and disease. *Am J Physiol Renal Physiol.* 2005;289:F235-F246.

187. Edwards A, Silldforff EP, Pallone TL. The renal medullary microcirculation. *Front Biosci.* 2000;5:E36-E52.

188. Bugge JF, Stokke ES, Vikse A, et al. Stimulation of renin release by PGE$_2$ and PGI$_2$ infusion in the dog: enhancing effect of ureteral occlusion or administration of ethacrynic acid. *Acta Physiol Scand.* 1990;138:193-201.

189. Ito S, Carretero OA, Abe K, et al. Effect of prostanoids on renin release from rabbit afferent arterioles with and without macula densa. *Kidney Int.* 1989;35:1138-1144.

190. Chaudhari A, Gupta S, Kirschenbaum M. Biochemical evidence for PGI$_2$ and PGE$_2$ receptors in the rabbit renal preglomerular microvasculature. *Biochim Biophys Acta.* 1990;1053:156-161.

191. Francois H, Athirakul K, Howell D, et al. Prostacyclin protects against elevated blood pressure and cardiac fibrosis. *Cell Metab.* 2005;2:201-207.

192. Hébert R, Regnier L, Peterson L. Rabbit cortical collecting ducts express a novel prostacyclin receptor. *Am J Physiol.* 1995;268:F145-F154.

193. Komhoff M, Lesener B, Nakao K, et al. Localization of the prostacyclin receptor in human kidney. *Kidney Int.* 1998;54:1899-1908.

194. Tone Y, Inoue H, Hara S, et al. The regional distribution and cellular localization of mRNA encoding rat prostacyclin synthase. *Eur J Cell Biol.* 1997;72:268-277.

195. Hirata M, Kakizuka A, Aizawa M, et al. Molecular characterization of a mouse prostaglandin D receptor and functional expression of the cloned gene. *Proc Natl Acad Sci U S A.* 1994;91:11192-11196.

196. Coleman RA, Grix SP, Head SA, et al. A novel inhibitory prostanoid receptor in piglet saphenous vein. *Prostaglandins.* 1994;47:151-168.

197. Oida H, Hirata M, Sugimoto Y, et al. Expression of messenger RNA for the prostaglandin D receptor in the leptomeninges of the mouse brain. *FEBS Lett.* 1997;417:53-56.

198. Boie Y, Sawyer N, Slipetz DM, et al. Molecular cloning and characterization of the human prostanoid DP receptor. *J Biol Chem.* 1995;270:18910-18916.

199. Urade Y, Hayaishi O. Prostaglandin D2 and sleep regulation. *Biochim Biophys Acta.* 1999;1436:606-615.

200. Sri Kantha S, Matsumura H, Kubo E, et al. Effects of prostaglandin D$_2$, lipoxins and leukotrienes on sleep and brain temperature of rats. *Prostaglandins Leukot Essent Fatty Acids.* 1994;51:87-93.

201. Matsuoka T, Hirata M, Tanaka H, et al. Prostaglandin D$_2$ as a mediator of allergic asthma. *Science.* 2000;287:2013-2017.

202. Rao PS, Cavanagh D, Dietz JR, et al. Dose-dependent effects of prostaglandin D$_2$ on hemodynamics, renal function, and blood gas analyses. *Am J Obstet Gynecol.* 1987;156:843-851.

203. Hirai H, Tanaka K, Takano S, et al. Cutting edge: agonistic effect of indomethacin on a prostaglandin D$_2$ receptor, CRTH2. *J Immunol.* 2002;168:981-985.

204. Abramovitz M, Boie Y, Nguyen T, et al. Cloning and expression of a cDNA for the human prostanoid FP receptor. *J Biol Chem.* 1994;269:2632-2636.

205. Woodward DF, Fairbairn CE, Lawrence RA. Identification of the FP-receptor as a discrete entity by radioligand binding in biosystems that exhibit different functional rank orders of potency in response to prostanoids. *Adv Exp Med Biol.* 1997;400A:223-227.

206. Pierce KL, Bailey TJ, Hoyer PB, et al. Cloning of a carboxyl-terminal isoform of the prostanoid FP receptor. *J Biol Chem.* 1997;272:883-887.

207. Pierce KL, Fujino H, Srinivasan D, et al. Activation of FP prostanoid receptor isoforms leads to Rho-mediated changes in cell morphology and in the cell cytoskeleton. *J Biol Chem.* 1999;274:35944-35949.

208. Fujino H, Srinivasan D, Regan JW. Cellular conditioning and activation of beta-catenin signaling by the FPB prostanoid receptor. *J Biol Chem.* 2002;277:48786-48795.

209. Sugimoto Y, Yamasaki A, Segi E, et al. Failure of parturition in mice lacking the prostaglandin F receptor. *Science.* 1997;277:681-683.

210. Hasumoto K, Sugimoto Y, Gotoh M, et al. Characterization of the mouse prostaglandin F receptor gene: a transgenic mouse study of a regulatory region that controls its expression in the stomach and kidney but not in the ovary. *Genes Cells.* 1997;2:571-580.
211. Chen J, Champa-Rodriguez ML, Woodward DF. Identification of a prostanoid FP receptor population producing endothelium-dependent vasorelaxation in the rabbit jugular vein. *Br J Pharmacol.* 1995;116:3035-3041.
212. Muller K, Krieg P, Marks F, et al. Expression of $PGF_{2\alpha}$ receptor mRNA in normal, hyperplastic and neoplastic skin. *Carcinogenesis.* 2000;21:1063-1066.
213. Linden C, Alm A. Prostaglandin analogues in the treatment of glaucoma. *Drugs Aging.* 1999;14:387-398.
214. Hebert RL, Carmosino M, Saito O, et al. Characterization of a rabbit PGF2α (FP) receptor exhibiting Gi-restricted signaling and that inhibits water absorption in renal collecting duct. *J Biol Chem.* 2005.
215. Hebert RL, Jacobson HR, Fredin D, et al. Evidence that separate PGE_2 receptors modulate water and sodium transport in rabbit cortical collecting duct. *Am J Physiol.* 1993;265:F643-F650.
216. Funk C, Furchi L, FitzGerald G, et al. Cloning and expression of a cDNA for the human prostaglandin E receptor EP_1 subtype. *J Biol Chem.* 1993;268:26767-26772.
217. Breyer MD, Jacobson HR, Davis LS, et al. In situ hybridization and localization of mRNA for the rabbit prostaglandin EP3 receptor. *Kidney Int.* 1993;44:1372-1378.
218. Bek M, Nusing R, Kowark P, et al. Characterization of prostanoid receptors in podocytes. *J Am Soc Nephrol.* 1999;10:2084-2093.
219. Breshnahan BA, Kelefiotis D, Stratidakis I, et al. $PGF_{2\alpha}$-induced signaling events in glomerular mesangial cells. *Proc Soc Exp Biol Med.* 1996;212:165-173.
220. Yu Y, Lucitt MB, Stubbe J, et al. Prostaglandin $F_{2\alpha}$ elevates blood pressure and promotes atherosclerosis. *Proc Natl Acad Sci U S A.* 2009;106:7985-7990.
221. Hata AN, Breyer RM. Pharmacology and signaling of prostaglandin receptors: multiple roles in inflammation and immune modulation. *Pharmacol Ther.* 2004;103:147-166.
222. Toh H, Ichikawa A, Narumiya S. Molecular evolution of receptors for eicosanoids. *FEBS Lett.* 1995;361:17-21.
223. Breyer MD, Breyer RM. G protein–coupled prostanoid receptors and the kidney. *Annu Rev Physiol.* 2001;63:579-605.
224. Guan Y, Zhang Y, Breyer RM, et al. Prostaglandin E_2 inhibits renal collecting duct Na^+ absorption by activating the EP1 receptor. *J Clin Invest.* 1998;102:194-201.
225. Coleman RA, Kennedy I, Humphrey PPA, et al. Prostanoids and their receptors. In: Emmet JC, ed. *Comprehensive medicinal chemistry.* Oxford, UK: Pergamon Press; 1990:643-714.
226. Ishibashi R, Tanaka I, Kotani M, et al. Roles of prostaglandin E receptors in mesangial cells under high-glucose conditions. *Kidney Int.* 1999;56:589-600.
227. Inscho E, Carmines P, Navar L. Prostaglandin influences on afferent arteriolar responses to vasoconstrictor agonists. *Am J Physiol.* 1990;259:F157-F163.
228. Purdy KE, Arendshorst WJ. EP_1 and EP_4 receptors mediate prostaglandin E_2 actions in the microcirculation of rat kidney. *Am J Physiol Renal Physiol.* 2000;279:F755-F764.
229. Zhang Y, Guan Y, Scheider A, et al. Characterization of murine vasopressor and vasodepressor prostaglandin E_2 receptors. *Hypertension.* 2000;35:1129-1134.
230. Stock JL, Shinjo K, Burkhardt J, et al. The prostaglandin E_2 EP1 receptor mediates pain perception and regulates blood pressure. *J Clin Invest.* 2001;107:325-331.
231. Tsuboi K, Sugimoto Y, Ichikawa A. Prostanoid receptor subtypes. *Prostaglandins Other Lipid Mediat.* 2002;68-69:535-556.
232. Regan JW, Bailey TJ, Pepperl DJ, et al. Cloning of a novel human prostaglandin receptor with characteristics of the pharmacologically defined EP2 subtype. *Mol Pharmacol.* 1994;46:213-220.
233. Nishigaki N, Negishi M, Honda A, et al. Identification of prostaglandin E receptor "EP2" cloned from mastocytoma cells as EP4 subtype. *FEBS Lett.* 1995;364:339-341.
234. Guan Y, Stillman BA, Zhang Y, et al. Cloning and expression of the rabbit prostaglandin EP2 receptor. *BMC Pharmacol.* 2002;2:14.
235. Kabashima K, Saji T, Murata T, et al. The prostaglandin receptor EP4 suppresses colitis, mucosal damage and CD4 cell activation in the gut. *J Clin Invest.* 2002;109:883-893.
236. Katsuyama M, Ikegami R, Karahashi H, et al. Characterization of the LPS-stimulated expression of EP2 and EP4 prostaglandin E receptors in mouse macrophage-like cell line, J774.1. *Biochem Biophys Res Commun.* 1998;251:727-731.
237. Kennedy CR, Zhang Y, Brandon S, et al. Salt-sensitive hypertension and reduced fertility in mice lacking the prostaglandin EP2 receptor. *Nat Med.* 1999;5:271-220.
238. Chen J, Zhao M, He W, et al. Increased dietary NaCl induces renal medullary PGE2 production and natriuresis via the EP2 receptor. *Am J Physiol Renal Physiol.* 2008;295:F818-F825.
239. Coleman RA, Smith WL, Narumiya S. VIII. International union of pharmacology classification of prostanoid receptors: properties, distribution, and structure of the receptors and their subtypes. *Pharmacol Rev.* 1994;46:205-229.
240. Boie Y, Stocco R, Sawyer N, et al. Molecular cloning and characterization of the four rat prostaglandin E_2 prostanoid receptor subtypes. *Eur J Pharmacol.* 1997;340:227-241.
241. Breyer RM, Emeson RB, Tarng JL, et al. Alternative splicing generates multiple isoforms of a rabbit prostaglandin E_2 receptor. *J Biol Chem.* 1994;269:6163-6169.
242. Kotani M, Tanaka I, Ogawa Y, et al. Molecular cloning and expression of multiple isoforms of human prostaglandin E receptor EP3 subtype generated by alternative messenger RNA splicing: multiple second messenger systems and tissue-specific distributions. *Mol Pharmacol.* 1995;48:869-879.
243. Irie A, Sugimoto Y, Namba T, et al. Third isoform of the prostaglandin-E-receptor EP3 subtype with different C-terminal tail coupling to both stimulation and inhibition of adenylate cyclase. *Eur J Biochem.* 1993;217:313-318.
244. Aoki J, Katoh H, Yasui H, et al. Signal transduction pathway regulating prostaglandin EP3 receptor–induced neurite retraction: requirement for two different tyrosine kinases. *Biochem J.* 1999;340:365-369.
245. Hasegawa H, Negishi M, Ichikawa A. Two isoforms of the prostaglandin E receptor EP3 subtype different in agonist-independent constitutive activity. *J Biol Chem.* 1996;271:1857-1860.
246. Breyer MD, Davis L, Jacobson HR, et al. Differential localization of prostaglandin E receptor subtypes in human kidney. *Am J Physiol.* 1996;270:F912-F918.
247. Taniguchi S, Watanabe T, Nakao A, et al. Detection and quantitation of EP3 prostaglandin E_2 receptor mRNA along mouse nephron segments by RT-PCR. *Am J Physiol.* 1994;266:C1453-C1458.
248. Good DW, George T. Regulation of HCO_3-absorption by prostaglandin E_2 and G-proteins in rat medullary thick ascending limb. *Am J Physiol.* 1996;270:F711-F717.
249. Good D. PGE_2 reverses AVP inhibition of HCO_3-absorption in rat MTAL by activation of protein kinase C. *Am J Physiol.* 1996;270:F978-F985.
250. Sakairi Y, Jacobson HR, Noland TD, et al. Luminal prostaglandin E receptors regulate salt and water transport in rabbit cortical collecting duct. *Am J Physiol.* 1995;269:F257-F265.
251. Ushikubi F, Segi E, Sugimoto Y, et al. Impaired febrile response in mice lacking the prostaglandin E receptor subtype EP3. *Nature.* 1998;395:281-284.
252. Audoly LP, Ruan X, Wagner VA, et al. Role of EP2 and EP3 PGE2 receptors in control of murine renal hemodynamics. *Am J Physiol Heart Circ Physiol.* 2001;280:H327-H333.
253. van Rodijnen WF, Korstjens IJ, Legerstee N, et al. Direct vasoconstrictor effect of prostaglandin E2 on renal interlobular arteries: role of the EP3 receptor. *Am J Physiol Renal Physiol.* 2007;292:F1094-F1101.
254. Castleberry TA, Lu B, Smock SL, et al. Molecular cloning and functional characterization of the canine prostaglandin E_2 receptor EP4 subtype. *Prostaglandins.* 2001;65:167-187.
255. Bastien L, Sawyer N, Grygorczyk R, et al. Cloning, functional expression, and characterization of the human prostaglandin E_2 receptor EP_2 subtype. *J Biol Chem.* 1994;269:11873-11877.
256. Breyer RM, Davis LS, Nian C, et al. Cloning and expression of the rabbit prostaglandin EP4 receptor. *Am J Physiol.* 1996;270:F485-F493.
257. Segi E, Sugimoto Y, Yamasaki A, et al. Patent ductus arteriosus and neonatal death in prostaglandin receptor EP4-deficient mice. *Biochem Biophys Res Commun.* 1998;246:7-12.
258. Audoly LP, Tilley SL, Goulet J, et al. Identification of specific EP receptors responsible for the hemodynamic effects of PGE2. *Am J Physiol.* 1999;277:H924-H930.
259. Csukas S, Hanke C, Rewolinski D, et al. Prostaglandin E_2-induced aldosterone release is mediated by an EP2 receptor. *Hypertension.* 1998;31:575-581.
260. Sugimoto Y, Namba T, Shigemoto R, et al. Distinct cellular localization of mRNAs for three subtypes of prostaglandin E receptor in kidney. *Am J Physiol.* 1994;266:F823-F828.
261. Jensen BL, Stubbe J, Hansen PB, et al. Localization of prostaglandin E_2 EP2 and EP4 receptors in the rat kidney. *Am J Physiol Renal Physiol.* 2001;280:F1001-F1009.
262. Nusing RM, Treude A, Weissenberger C, et al. Dominant role of prostaglandin E_2 EP4 receptor in furosemide-induced salt-losing tubulopathy: a model for hyperprostaglandin E syndrome/antenatal Bartter syndrome. *J Am Soc Nephrol.* 2005;16:2354-2362.
263. Faour WH, Gomi K, Kennedy CR. PGE2 induces COX-2 expression in podocytes via the EP_4 receptor through a PKA-independent mechanism. *Cell Signal.* 2008;20:2156-2164.
264. Kopp UC, Cicha MZ, Nakamura K, et al. Activation of EP4 receptors contributes to prostaglandin E_2-mediated stimulation of renal sensory nerves. *Am J Physiol Renal Physiol.* 2004;287:F1269-F1282.

265. Silldorf E, Yang S, Pallone T. Prostaglandin E_2 abrogates endothelin-induced vasoconstriction in renal outer medullary descending vasa recta of the rat. *J Clin Invest.* 1995;95:2734-2740.

266. Breyer M, Breyer R, Fowler B, et al. EP1 receptor antagonists block PGE_2 dependent inhibition of Na^+ absorption in the cortical collecting duct. *J Am Soc Nephrol.* 1996;7:1645.

267. Schlondorff D. Renal complications of nonsteroidal anti-inflammatory drugs. *Kidney Int.* 1993;44:643-653.

268. Jensen B, Schmid C, Kurtz A. Prostaglandins stimulate renin secretion and renin mRNA in mouse renal juxtaglomerular cells. *Am J Physiol.* 1996;271:F659-F669.

269. Hockel G, Cowley A. Prostaglandin E_2-induced hypertension in conscious dogs. *Am J Physiol.* 1979;237:H449-H454.

270. Francisco L, Osborn J, Dibona G. Prostaglandins in renin release during sodium deprivation. *Am J Physiol.* 1982;243:F537-F542.

271. Imig JD, Breyer MD, Breyer RM. Contribution of prostaglandin EP_2 receptors to renal microvascular reactivity in mice. *Am J Physiol Renal Physiol.* 2002;283:F415-F422.

272. Schnermann J. Cyclooxygenase-2 and macula densa control of renin secretion. *Nephrol Dial Transplant.* 2001;16:1735-1738.

273. Imanishi M, Tsuji T, Nakamura S, et al. Prostaglandin i_2/e_2 ratios in unilateral renovascular hypertension of different severities. *Hypertension.* 2001;38:23-29.

274. Jensen BL, Mann B, Skott O, et al. Differential regulation of renal prostaglandin receptor mRNAs by dietary salt intake in the rat. *Kidney Int.* 1999;56:528-537.

275. Tilley SL, Audoly LP, Hicks EH, et al. Reproductive failure and reduced blood pressure in mice lacking the EP2 prostaglandin E_2 receptor. *J Clin Invest.* 1999;103:1539-1545.

276. Guyton A. Blood pressure control-special role of the kidneys and body fluids. *Science.* 1991;252:1813-1816.

277. Carmines P, Bell P, Roman R, et al. Prostaglandins in the sodium excretory response to altered renal arterial pressure in dogs. *Am J Phyisol.* 1985;248:F8-F14.

278. Roman R, Lianos E. Influence of prostaglandins on papillary blood flow and pressure-natriuretic response. *Hypertension.* 1990;15:29-35.

279. Pallone TL, Silldorff EP. Pericyte regulation of renal medullary blood flow. *Exp Nephrol.* 2001;9:165-170.

280. Breyer MD, Breyer RM. Prostaglandin E receptors and the kidney. *Am J Physiol Renal Physiol.* 2000;279:F12-F23.

281. Roman RJ. P-450 metabolites of arachidonic acid in the control of cardiovascular function. *Physiol Rev.* 2002;82:131-185.

282. Syal A, Schiavi S, Chakravarty S, et al. Fibroblast growth factor-23 increases mouse PGE_2 production in vivo and in vitro. *Am J Physiol Renal Physiol.* 2006;290:F450-F455.

283. Baum M, Loleh S, Saini N, et al. Correction of proximal tubule phosphate transport defect in Hyp mice in vivo and in vitro with indomethacin. *Proc Natl Acad Sci U S A.* 2003;100:11098-11103.

284. Eriksson LO, Larsson B, Andersson KE. Biochemical characterization and autoradiographic localization of $[^3H]PGE_2$ binding sites in rat kidney. *Acta Physiol Scand.* 1990;139:405-415.

285. Hebert RL, Jacobson HR, Breyer MD. Prostaglandin E_2 inhibits sodium transport in rabbit cortical collecting duct by increasing intracellular calcium. *J Clin Invest.* 1991;87:1992-1998.

286. Breyer MD, Jacobson HR, Hebert RL. Cellular mechanisms of prostaglandin E_2 and vasopressin interactions in the collecting duct. *Kidney Int.* 1990;38:618-624.

287. Nadler SP, Hebert SC, Brenner BM. PGE_2, forskolin, and cholera toxin interactions in rabbit cortical collecting tubule. *Am J Physiol.* 1986;250:F127-F135.

288. Hebert RL, Jacobson HR, Breyer MD. PGE_2 inhibits AVP-induced water flow in cortical collecting ducts by protein kinase C activation. *Am J Physiol.* 1990;259:F318-F325.

289. Tai HH, Ensor CM, Tong M, et al. Prostaglandin catabolizing enzymes. *Prostaglandins Other Lipid Mediat.* 2002;68-69:483-493.

290. Sakuma S, Fujimoto Y, Hikita E, et al. Effects of metal ions on 15-hydroxy prostaglandin dehydrogenase activity in rabbit kidney cortex. *Prostaglandins.* 1990;40:507-514.

291. Yao B, Xu J, Harris RC, et al. Renal localization and regulation of 15-hydroxyprostaglandin dehydrogenase. *Am J Physiol Renal Physiol.* 2008;294:F433-F439.

292. Coggins KG, Latour A, Nguyen MS, et al. Metabolism of PGE_2 by prostaglandin dehydrogenase is essential for remodeling the ductus arteriosus. *Nat Med.* 2002;8:91-92.

293. Oliw E. Oxygenation of polyunsaturated fatty acids by cytochrome P450 monooxygenases. *Prog Lipid Res.* 1994;33:329-354.

294. Schwartzman ML, da Silva JL, Lin F, et al. Cytochrome P450 4A expression and arachidonic acid omega-hydroxylation in the kidney of the spontaneously hypertensive rat. *Nephron.* 1996;73:652-663.

295. Stec DE, Flasch A, Roman RJ, et al. Distribution of cytochrome P-450 4A and 4F isoforms along the nephron in mice. *Am J Physiol Renal Physiol.* 2003;284:F95-F102.

296. Yu K, Bayona WK, Kallen CB, et al. Differential activation of peroxisome proliferator activated receptors by eicosanoids. *J Biol Chem.* 1995;270:23975-23983.

297. Forman B, Tontonoz P, Chen J, et al. 15-Deoxy-$\Delta^{12,14}$-prostaglandin J_2 is a ligand for the adipocyte determination factor PPAR-γ. *Cell.* 1995;83:803-812.

298. Kliewer S, Lenhard J, Wilson T, et al. A prostaglandin J_2 metabolite binds peroxisome proliferator-activated receptor gamma and promotes adipocyte differentiation. *Cell.* 1995;83:813-819.

299. Witzenbichler B, Asahara T, Murohara T, et al. Vascular endothelial growth factor-C (VEGF-C/VEGF-2) promotes angiogenesis in the setting of tissue ischemia. *Am J Pathol.* 1998;153:381-394.

300. Stamatakis K, Sanchez-Gomez FJ, Perez-Sala D. Identification of novel protein targets for modification by 15-deoxy-$\Delta^{12,14}$-prostaglandin J_2 in mesangial cells reveals multiple interactions with the cytoskeleton. *J Am Soc Nephrol.* 2006;17:89-98.

301. Straus DS, Glass CK. Cyclopentenone prostaglandins: new insights on biological activities and cellular targets. *Med Res Rev.* 2001;21:185-210.

302. Negishi M, Katoh H. Cyclopentenone prostaglandin receptors. *Prostaglandins Other Lipid Mediat.* 2002;68-69:611-617.

303. Rossl A, Kapahl P, Natoli G, et al. Anti-inflammatory cyclopentenone prostaglandins are direct inhibitors of IκB kinase. *Nature.* 2000;403:103-108.

304. Shibata T, Kondo M, Osawa T, et al. 15-Deoxy-$\Delta^{12,14}$-prostaglandin J_2. A prostaglandin D_2 metabolite generated during inflammatory processes. *J Biol Chem.* 2002;277:10459-10466.

305. Fam SS, Murphey LJ, Terry ES, et al. Formation of highly reactive A-ring and J-ring isoprostane-like compounds (A4/J4-neuroprostanes) in vivo from docosahexaenoic acid. *J Biol Chem.* 2002;277:36076-36084.

306. Morrow JD, Harris TM, Roberts 2nd LJ. Noncyclooxygenase oxidative formation of a series of novel prostaglandins: analytical ramifications for measurement of eicosanoids. *Anal Biochem.* 1990;184:1-10.

307. Roberts 2nd LJ, Morrow JD. Products of the isoprostane pathway: unique bioactive compounds and markers of lipid peroxidation. *Cell Mol Life Sci.* 2002;59:808-820.

308. Morrow JD, Roberts LJ. The isoprostanes: unique bioactive products of lipid peroxidation. *Prog Lipid Res.* 1997;36:1-21.

309. Takahashi K, Nammour T, Fukunaga M, et al. Glomerular actions of a free radical–generated novel prostaglandin, 8-epi-prostaglandin $F_{2\alpha}$, in the rat. Evidence for interaction with thromboxane A_2 receptors. *J Clin Invest.* 1992;90:136-141.

310. Schuster VL. Prostaglandin transport. *Prostaglandins Other Lipid Mediat.* 2002;68-69:633-647.

311. Chan BS, Satriano JA, Pucci M, et al. Mechanism of prostaglandin E_2 transport across the plasma membrane of HeLa cells and *Xenopus* oocytes expressing the prostaglandin transporter "PGT." *J Biol Chem.* 1998;273:6689-6697.

312. Lu R, Kanai N, Bao Y, et al. Cloning, in vitro expression, and tissue distribution of a human prostaglandin transporter cDNA(hPGT). *J Clin Invest.* 1996;98:1142-1149.

313. Kanai N, Lu R, Satriano JA, et al. Identification and characterization of a prostaglandin transporter. *Science.* 1995;268:866-869.

314. Bao Y, Pucci ML, Chan BS, et al. Prostaglandin transporter PGT is expressed in cell types that synthesize and release prostanoids. *Am J Physiol Renal Physiol.* 2002;282:F1103-F1110.

315. Chi Y, Khersonsky SM, Chang Y-T, et al. Identification of a new class of prostaglandin transporter inhibitors and characterization of their biological effects on prostaglandin E_2 transport. *J Pharmacol Exp Ther.* 2006;316:1346-1350.

316. Nomura T, Chang HY, Lu R, et al. Prostaglandin signaling in the renal collecting duct: release, reuptake, and oxidation in the same cell. *J Biol Chem.* 2005;280:28424-28429.

317. Chi Y, Pucci ML, Schuster VL. Dietary salt induces transcription of the prostaglandin transporter gene in renal collecting ducts. *Am J Physiol Renal Physiol.* 2008;295:F765-F771.

318. Kimura H, Takeda M, Narikawa S, et al. Human organic anion transporters and human organic cation transporters mediate renal transport of prostaglandins. *J Pharmacol Exp Ther.* 2002;301:293-298.

319. Sauvant C, Holzinger H, Gekle M. Prostaglandin E_2 inhibits its own renal transport by downregulation of organic anion transporters rOAT1 and rOAT3. *J Am Soc Nephrol.* 2006;17:46-53.

320. Touhey S, O'Connor R, Plunkett S, et al. Structure-activity relationship of indomethacin analogues for MRP-1, COX-1 and COX-2 inhibition: identification of novel chemotherapeutic drug resistance modulators. *Eur J Cancer.* 2002;38:1661-1670.

321. Homem de Bittencourt Jr PI, Curi R. Antiproliferative prostaglandins and the MRP/GS-X pump role in cancer immunosuppression and insight into new strategies in cancer gene therapy. *Biochem Pharmacol.* 2001;62:811-819.

322. Jedlitschky G, Keppler D. Transport of leukotriene C4 and structurally related conjugates. *Vitam Horm.* 2002;64:153-184.

323. Nies AT, Konig J, Cui Y, et al. Structural requirements for the apical sorting of human multidrug resistance protein 2 (ABCC2). *Eur J Biochem.* 2002;269:1866-1876.

324. Van Aubel RA, Peters JG, Masereeuw R, et al. Multidrug resistance protein mrp2 mediates ATP-dependent transport of classic renal organic anion p-aminohippurate. *Am J Physiol Renal Physiol.* 2000;279:F713-F717.

325. Klahr S, Morrissey JJ. The role of growth factors, cytokines, and vasoactive compounds in obstructive nephropathy. *Semin Nephrol.* 1998;18:622-632.

326. Takahashi K, Kato T, Schreiner GF, et al. Essential fatty acid deficiency normalizes function and histology in rat nephrotoxic nephritis. *Kidney Int.* 1992;41:1245-1253.

327. Chanmugam P, Feng L, Liou S, et al. Radicicol, a protein tyrosine kinase inhibitor, suppresses the expression of mitogen-inducible cyclooxygenase in macrophages stimulated with lipopolysaccharide and in experimental glomerulonephritis. *J Biol Chem.* 1995;270:5418-5426.

328. Hirose S, Yamamoto T, Feng L, et al. Expression and localization of cyclooxygenase isoforms and cytosolic phospholipase A_2 in anti-Thy-1 glomerulonephritis. *J Am Soc Nephrol.* 1998;9:408-416.

329. Yang T, Sun D, Huang YG, et al. Differential regulation of COX-2 expression in the kidney by lipopolysaccharide: role of CD14. *Am J Physiol.* 1999;277:F10-F16.

330. Tomasoni S, Noris M, Zappella S, et al. Upregulation of renal and systemic cyclooxygenase-2 in patients with active lupus nephritis. *J Am Soc Nephrol.* 1998;9:1202-1212.

331. Zoja C, Benigni A, Noris M, et al. Mycophenolate mofetil combined with a cyclooxygenase-2 inhibitor ameliorates murine lupus nephritis. *Kidney Int.* 2001;60:653-663.

332. Nagamatsu T, Imai H, Yokoi M, et al. Protective effect of prostaglandin EP4-receptor agonist on anti-glomerular basement membrane antibody-associated nephritis. *J Pharmacol Sci.* 2006;102:182-188.

333. Hartner A, Pahl A, Brune K, et al. Upregulation of cyclooxygenase-1 and the PGE_2 receptor EP2 in rat and human mesangioproliferative glomerulonephritis. *Inflamm Res.* 2000;49:345-354.

334. Kitahara M, Eitner F, Ostendorf T, et al. Selective cyclooxygenase-2 inhibition impairs glomerular capillary healing in experimental glomerulonephritis. *J Am Soc Nephrol.* 2002;13:1261-1270.

335. Schneider A, Harendza S, Zahner G, et al. Cyclooxygenase metabolites mediate glomerular monocyte chemoattractant protein-1 formation and monocyte recruitment in experimental glomerulonephritis. *Kidney Int.* 1999;55:430-441:[see comments].

336. Wang J-L, Cheng H-F, Zhang M-Z, et al. Selective increase of cyclooxygenase-2 expression in a model of renal ablation. *Am J Physiol.* 1998;275:F613-F622.

337. Weichert W, Paliege A, Provoost AP, et al. Upregulation of juxtaglomerular NOS1 and COX-2 precedes glomerulosclerosis in fawn-hooded hypertensive rats. *Am J Physiol Renal Physiol.* 2001;280:F706-F714.

338. Cheng H, Fan X, Guan Y, et al. Distinct roles for basal and induced COX-2 in podocyte injury. *J Am Soc Nephrol.* 2009;20:1953-1562.

339. Jo YI, Cheng H, Wang S, et al. Puromycin induces reversible proteinuric injury in transgenic mice expressing cyclooxygenase-2 in podocytes. *Nephron Exp Nephrol.* 2007;107:e87-e94.

340. Cheng H, Wang S, Jo YI, et al. Overexpression of cyclooxygenase-2 predisposes to podocyte injury. *J Am Soc Nephrol.* 2007;18:551-559.

341. Komers R, Lindsley JN, Oyama TT, et al. Immunohistochemical and functional correlations of renal cyclooxygenase-2 in experimental diabetes. *J Clin Invest.* 2001;107:889-898.

342. Bing Y, Xu J, Qi Z, et al. The role of renal cortical cyclooxygenase-2 (COX-2) expression in hyperfiltration in rats with high protein intake. *Am J Physiol Renal Physiol.* 2006;291:F368-F374.

343. Vogt L, de Zeeuw D, Woittiez AJ, et al. Selective cyclooxygenase-2 (COX-2) inhibition reduces proteinuria in renal patients. *Nephrol Dial Transplant.* 2009;24:1182-1189.

344. Wilcox CS, Welch WJ, Murad F, et al. Nitric oxide synthase in macula densa regulates glomerular capillary pressure. *Pro Natl Acad Sci U S A.* 1992;89:11993-11997.

345. Welch WJ, Wilcox CS, Thomson SC. Nitric oxide and tubuloglomerular feedback. *Semin Nephrol.* 1999;19:251-262.

346. Thorup C, Erik A, Persson G. Macula densa derived nitric oxide in regulation of glomerular capillary pressure. *Kidney Int.* 1996;49:430-436.

347. Wang JL, Cheng HF, Shappell S, et al. A selective cyclooxygenase-2 inhibitor decreases proteinuria and retards progressive renal injury in rats. *Kidney Int.* 2000;57:2334-2342.

348. Goncalves AR, Fujihara CK, Mattar AL, et al. Renal expression of COX-2, ANG II, and AT1 receptor in remnant kidney: strong renoprotection by therapy with losartan and a nonsteroidal anti-inflammatory. *Am J Physiol Renal Physiol.* 2004;286:F945-F954.

349. Fujihara CK, Malheiros DM, Donato JL, et al. Nitroflurbiprofen, a new nonsteroidal anti-inflammatory, ameliorates structural injury in the remnant kidney. *Am J Physiol.* 1998;274:F573-F579.

350. Cheng HF, Wang CJ, Moeckel GW, et al. Cyclooxygenase-2 inhibitor blocks expression of mediators of renal injury in a model of diabetes and hypertension. *Kidney Int.* 2002;62:929-939.

351. Dey A, Maric C, Kaesemeyer WH, et al. Rofecoxib decreases renal injury in obese Zucker rats. *Clin Sci (Lond).* 2004;107:561-570.

352. Schmitz PG, Krupa SM, Lane PH, et al. Acquired essential fatty acid depletion in the remnant kidney: amelioration with U-63557A. *Kidney Int.* 1994;46:1184-1191.

353. Takano T, Cybulsky AV. Complement C5b-9-mediated arachidonic acid metabolism in glomerular epithelial cells: role of cyclooxygenase-1 and -2. *Am J Pathol.* 2000;156:2091-2101.

354. Villa E, Martinez J, Ruilope L, et al. Cicaprost, a prostacyclin analog, protects renal function in uninephrectomized dogs in the absence of changes in blood pressure. *Am J Hypertension.* 1992;6:253-257.

355. Sankaran D, Bankovic-Calic N, Ogborn MR, et al. Selective COX-2 inhibition markedly slows disease progression and attenuates altered prostanoid production in Han:SPRD-cy rats with inherited kidney disease. *Am J Physiol Renal Physiol.* 2007;293:F821-F830.

356. Elberg G, Elberg D, Lewis TV, et al. EP2 receptor mediates PGE_2-induced cystogenesis of human renal epithelial cells. *Am J Physiol Renal Physiol.* 2007;293:F1622-F1632.

357. Studer R, Negrete H, Craven P, et al. Protein kinase C signals thromboxane induced increases in fibronectin synthesis and TGF-β bioactivity in mesangial cells. *Kidney Int.* 1995;48:422-430.

358. Zahner G, Disser M, Thaiss F, et al. The effect of prostaglandin E_2 on mRNA expression and secretion of collagens I, III, and IV and fibronectin in cultured rat mesangial cells. *J Am Soc Nephrol.* 1994;4:1778-1785.

359. Singhal P, Sagar S, Garg P, et al. Vasoactive agents modulate matrix metalloproteinase-2-activity by mesangial cells. *Am J Med Sci.* 1995;310:235-241.

360. Varga J, Diaz-Perez A, Rosenbloom J, et al. PGE_2 causes a coordinate decrease in the steady state levels of fibronectin and types I and III procollagen mRNAs in normal human dermal fibroblasts. *Biochem Biophys Res Comm.* 1987;147:1282-1288.

361. Wilborn J, Crofford LJ, Burdick MD, et al. Cultured lung fibroblasts isolated from patients with idiopathic pulmonary fibrosis have a diminished capacity to synthesize prostaglandin E_2 and to express cyclooxygenase-2. *J Clin Invest.* 1995;95:1861-1868.

362. Wise WC, Cook JA, Tempel GE, et al. The rat in sepsis and endotoxic shock. *Prog Clin Biol Res.* 1989;299:243-252.

363. Ruschitzka F, Shaw S, Noll G, et al. Endothelial vasoconstrictor prostanoids, vascular reactivity, and acute renal failure. *Kidney Int Suppl.* 1998;67:S199-S201.

364. Chaudhari A, Kirschenbaum MA. Altered glomerular eicosanoid biosynthesis in uranyl nitrate-induced acute renal failure. *Biochim Biophys Acta.* 1984;792:135-140.

365. Hardie WD, Ebert J, Frazer M, et al. The effect of thromboxane A_2 receptor antagonism on amphotericin B–induced renal vasoconstriction in the rat. *Prostaglandins.* 1993;45:47-56.

366. Higa EM, Schor N, Boim MA, et al. Role of the prostaglandin and kallikrein-kinin systems in aminoglycoside-induced acute renal failure. *Braz J Med Biol Res.* 1985;18:355-365.

367. Papanicolaou N, Hatziantoniou C, Bariety J. Selective inhibition of thromboxane synthesis partially protected while inhibition of angiotensin II formation did not protect rats against acute renal failure induced with glycerol. *Prostaglandins Leukot Med.* 1986;21:29-35.

368. Vargas AV, Krishnamurthi V, Masih R, et al. Prostaglandin E_1 attenuation of ischemic renal reperfusion injury in the rat. *J Am Coll Surg.* 1995;180:713-717.

369. Patel NS, Cuzzocrea S, Collino M, et al. The role of cycloxygenase-2 in the rodent kidney following ischaemia/reperfusion injury in vivo. *Eur J Pharmacol.* 2007;562:148-154.

370. Villanueva S, Cespedes C, Gonzalez AA, et al. Effect of ischemic acute renal damage on the expression of COX-2 and oxidative stress-related elements in rat kidney. *Am J Physiol Renal Physiol.* 2007;292:F1364-F1371.

371. Feitoza CQ, Goncalves GM, Semedo P, et al. Inhibition of COX 1 and 2 prior to renal ischemia/reperfusion injury decreases the development of fibrosis. *Mol Med.* 2008;14:724-730.

372. Hsu YH, Chen CH, Hou CC, et al. Prostacyclin protects renal tubular cells from gentamicin-induced apoptosis via a PPARα-dependent pathway. *Kidney Int.* 2008;73:578-587.

373. Morsing P, Stenberg A, Persson AE. Effect of thromboxane inhibition on tubuloglomerular feedback in hydronephrotic kidneys. *Kidney Int.* 1989;36:447-452.

374. Miyajima A, Ito K, Asano T, et al. Does cyclooxygenase-2 inhibitor prevent renal tissue damage in unilateral ureteral obstruction? *J Urol.* 2001;166:1124-1129.

375. Ozturk H, Ozdemir E, Otcu S, et al. Renal effects on a solitary kidney of specific inhibition of cyclooxygenase-2 after 24 h of complete ureteric obstruction in rats. *Urol Res.* 2002;30:223-226.

376. Norregaard R, Jensen BL, Topcu SO, et al. COX-2 activity transiently contributes to increased water and NaCl excretion in the polyuric phase after release of ureteral obstruction. *Am J Physiol Renal Physiol.* 2007;292:F1322-F1333.

377. Norregaard R, Jensen BL, Topcu SO, et al. Cyclooxygenase type 2 is increased in obstructed rat and human ureter and contributes to pelvic pressure increase after obstruction. *Kidney Int.* 2006;70:872-881.

378. Coffman TM, Yarger WE, Klotman PE. Functional role of thromboxane production by acutely rejecting renal allografts in rats. *J Clin Invest.* 1985;75:1242-1248.

379. Tonshoff B, Busch C, Schweer H, et al. In vivo prostanoid formation during acute renal allograft rejection. *Nephrol Dial Transplant.* 1993;8:631-636.

380. Coffman TM, Yohay D, Carr DR, et al. Effect of dietary fish oil supplementation on eicosanoid production by rat renal allografts. *Transplantation.* 1988;45:470-474.

381. Coffman TM, Carr DR, Yarger WE, et al. Evidence that renal prostaglandin and thromboxane production is stimulated in chronic cyclosporine nephrotoxicity. *Transplantation.* 1987;43:282-285.

382. Hocherl K, Dreher F, Vitzthum H, et al. Cyclosporine A suppresses cyclooxygenase-2 expression in the rat kidney. *J Am Soc Nephrol.* 2002;13:2427-2436.

383. Laffi G, La Villa G, Pinzani M, et al. Arachidonic acid derivatives and renal function in liver cirrhosis. *Semin Nephrol.* 1997;17:530-548.

384. Lopez-Parra M, Claria J, Planaguma A, et al. Cyclooxygenase-1 derived prostaglandins are involved in the maintenance of renal function in rats with cirrhosis and ascites. *Br J Pharmacol.* 2002;135:891-900.

385. Bosch-Marce M, Claria J, Titos E, et al. Selective inhibition of cyclooxygenase 2 spares renal function and prostaglandin synthesis in cirrhotic rats with ascites. *Gastroenterology.* 1999;116:1167-1175.

386. Medina JF, Prieto J, Guarner F, et al. Effect of spironolactone on renal prostaglandin excretion in patients with liver cirrhosis and ascites. *J Hepatol.* 1986;3:206-211.

387. Epstein M, Lifschitz M. Renal eicosanoids as determinants of renal function in liver disease. *Hepatology.* 1987;7:1359-1367.

388. Moore K, Ward PS, Taylor GW, et al. Systemic and renal production of thromboxane A2 and prostacyclin in decompensated liver disease and hepatorenal syndrome. *Gastroenterology.* 1991;100:1069-1077.

389. DeRubertis FR, Craven PA. Eicosanoids in the pathogenesis of the functional and structural alterations of the kidney in diabetes. *Am J Kidney Dis.* 1993;22:727-735.

390. Hommel E, Mathiesen E, Arnold-Larsen S, et al. Effects of indomethacin on kidney function in type 1 (insulin-dependent) diabetic patients with nephropathy. *Diabetologia.* 1987;30:78-81.

391. Li J, Chen YJ, Quilley J. Effect of Tempol on renal cyclooxygenase expression and activity in experimental diabetes in the rat. *J Pharmacol Exp Ther.* 2005;314:818-824.

392. Kiritoshi S, Nishikawa T, Sonoda K, et al. Reactive oxygen species from mitochondria induce cyclooxygenase-2 gene expression in human mesangial cells: potential role in diabetic nephropathy. *Diabetes.* 2003;52:2570-2577.

393. Makino H, Tanaka I, Mukoyama M, et al. Prevention of diabetic nephropathy in rats by prostaglandin E receptor EP1-selective antagonist. *J Am Soc Nephrol.* 2002;13:1757-1765.

394. Yamashita T, Shikata K, Matsuda M, et al. Beraprost sodium, prostacyclin analogue, attenuates glomerular hyperfiltration and glomerular macrophage infiltration by modulating ecNOS expression in diabetic rats. *Diabetes Res Clin Pract.* 2002;57:149-161.

395. Baylis C. Cyclooxygenase products do not contribute to the gestational renal vasodilation in the nitric oxide synthase inhibited pregnant rat. *Hypertens Pregnancy.* 2002;21:109-114.

396. Khalil RA, Granger JP. Vascular mechanisms of increased arterial pressure in preeclampsia: lessons from animal models. *Am J Physiol Regul Integr Comp Physiol.* 2002;283:R29-R45.

397. Keith Jr JC, Thatcher CD, Schaub RG. Beneficial effects of U-63,557A, a thromboxane synthetase inhibitor, in an ovine model of pregnancy-induced hypertension. *Am J Obstet Gynecol.* 1987;157:199-203.

398. Klockenbusch W, Rath W. [Prevention of pre-eclampsia by low-dose acetylsalicylic acid—a critical appraisal]. *Z Geburtshilfe Neonatol.* 2002;206:125-130.

399. Heyborne KD. Preeclampsia prevention: lessons from the low-dose aspirin therapy trials. *Am J Obstet Gynecol.* 2000;183:523-528.

400. Rao R, Zhang MZ, Zhao M, et al. Lithium treatment inhibits renal GSK-3 activity and promotes cyclooxygenase 2–dependent polyuria. *Am J Physiol Renal Physiol.* 2005;288:F642-F649.

401. Kim GH, Choi NW, Jung JY, et al. Treating lithium-induced nephrogenic diabetes insipidus with a COX-2 inhibitor improves polyuria via upregulation of AQP2 and NKCC2. *Am J Physiol Renal Physiol.* 2008;294:F702-F709.

402. Virdis A, Colucci R, Fornai M, et al. Cyclooxygenase-2 inhibition improves vascular endothelial dysfunction in a rat model of endotoxic shock: role of inducible nitric-oxide synthase and oxidative stress. *J Pharmacol Exp Ther.* 2005;312:945-953.

403. Xu Z, Choudhary S, Voznesensky O, et al. Overexpression of COX-2 in human osteosarcoma cells decreases proliferation and increases apoptosis. *Cancer Res.* 2006;66:6657-6664.

404. Marnett LJ, Rowlinson SW, Goodwin DC, et al. Arachidonic acid oxygenation by COX-1 and COX-2. Mechanisms of catalysis and inhibition. *J Biol Chem.* 1999;274:22903-22906.

405. Rockwell P, Martinez J, Papa L, et al. Redox regulates COX-2 upregulation and cell death in the neuronal response to cadmium. *Cell Signal.* 2004;16:343-353.

406. Lee SH, Williams MV, Dubois RN, et al. Cyclooxygenase-2–mediated DNA damage. *J Biol Chem.* 2005;280:28337-28346.

407. Mouithys-Mickalad A, Deby-Dupont G, Dogne JM, et al. Effects of COX-2 inhibitors on ROS produced by *Chlamydia pneumoniae*–primed human promonocytic cells (THP-1). *Biochem Biophys Res Commun.* 2004;325:1122-1130.

408. Prasad KN, Hovland AR, La Rosa FG, et al. Prostaglandins as putative neurotoxins in Alzheimer's disease. *Proc Soc Exp Biol Med.* 1998;219:120-125.

409. Wilcox CS. Oxidative stress and nitric oxide deficiency in the kidney: a critical link to hypertension? *Am J Physiol Regul Integr Comp Physiol.* 2005;289:R913-R935.

410. Jaimes EA, Tian RX, Pearse D, et al. Up-regulation of glomerular COX-2 by angiotensin II: role of reactive oxygen species. *Kidney Int.* 2005;68:2143-2153.

411. Serezani CH, Chung J, Ballinger MN, et al. Prostaglandin E2 suppresses bacterial killing in alveolar macrophages by inhibiting NADPH oxidase. *Am J Respir Cell Mol Biol.* 2007;37:562-570.

412. Jia Z, Guo X, Zhang H, et al. Microsomal prostaglandin synthase-1–derived prostaglandin E2 protects against angiotensin II-induced hypertension via inhibition of oxidative stress. *Hypertension.* 2008;52:952-959.

413. Kim HJ, Kim KW, Yu BP, et al. The effect of age on cyclooxygenase-2 gene expression: NF-κB activation and IκBα degradation. *Free Radic Biol Med.* 2000;28:683-692.

414. Reinhold SW, Vitzthum H, Filbeck T, et al. Gene expression of 5-, 12-, and 15-lipoxygenases and leukotriene receptors along the rat nephron. *Am J Physiol Renal Physiol.* 2006;290:F864-F872.

415. Clarkson MR, McGinty A, Godson C, et al. Leukotrienes and lipoxins: lipoxygenase-derived modulators of leukocyte recruitment and vascular tone in glomerulonephritis. *Nephrol Dial Transplant.* 1998;13:3043-3051.

416. Dixon RA, Diehl RE, Opas E, et al. Requirement of a 5-lipoxygenase–activating protein for leukotriene synthesis. *Nature.* 1990;343:282-284.

417. Albrightson CR, Short B, Dytko G, et al. Selective inhibition of 5-lipoxygenase attenuates glomerulonephritis in the rat. *Kidney Int.* 1994;45:1301-1310.

418. Lynch KR, O'Neill GP, Liu Q, et al. Characterization of the human cysteinyl leukotriene CysLT1 receptor. *Nature.* 1999;399:789-793.

419. Sarau HM, Ames RS, Chambers J, et al. Identification, molecular cloning, expression, and characterization of a cysteinyl leukotriene receptor. *Mol Pharmacol.* 1999;56:657-663.

420. Hui Y, Funk CD. Cysteinyl leukotriene receptors. *Biochem Pharmacol.* 2002;64:1549-1557.

421. Bigby TD. The yin and the yang of 5-lipoxygenase pathway activation. *Mol Pharmacol.* 2002;62:200-202.

422. Hallstrand TS, Henderson Jr WR. Leukotriene modifiers. *Med Clin North Am.* 2002;86:1009-1033:vi.

423. Yokomizo T, Kato K, Terawaki K, et al. A second leukotriene B4 receptor, BLT2. A new therapeutic target in inflammation and immunological disorders. *J Exp Med.* 2000;192:421-432.

424. Noiri E, Yokomizo T, Nakao A, et al. An in vivo approach showing the chemotactic activity of leukotriene B4 in acute renal ischemic-reperfusion injury. *Proc Natl Acad Sci U S A.* 2000;97:823-828.

425. Suzuki S, Kuroda T, Kazama JI, et al. The leukotriene B4 receptor antagonist ONO-4057 inhibits nephrotoxic serum nephritis in WKY rats. *J Am Soc Nephrol.* 1999;10:264-270.

426. Chiang N, Gronert K, Clish CB, et al. Leukotriene B4 receptor transgenic mice reveal novel protective roles for lipoxins and aspirin-triggered lipoxins in reperfusion. *J Clin Invest.* 1999;104:309-316.

427. Devchand P, Keller H, Peters J, et al. The PPARα-leukotriene B4 pathway to inflammation control. *Nature.* 1996;384:39-43.

428. Badr KF. Glomerulonephritis: roles for lipoxygenase pathways in pathophysiology and therapy. *Curr Opin Nephrol Hypertens.* 1997;6:111-118.

429. Papayianni A, Serhan CN, Brady HR. Lipoxin A4 and B4 inhibit leukotriene-stimulated interactions of human neutrophils and endothelial cells. *J Immunol.* 1996;156:2264-2272.

430. Nassar GM, Badr KF. Role of leukotrienes and lipoxygenases in glomerular injury. *Miner Electrolyte Metab.* 1995;21:262-270.

431. Katoh T, Takahashi K, DeBoer DK, et al. Renal hemodynamic actions of lipoxins in rats: a comparative physiological study. *Am J Physiol.* 1992;263:F436-F442.

432. Brady HR, Lamas S, Papayianni A, et al. Lipoxygenase product formation and cell adhesion during neutrophil-glomerular endothelial cell interaction. *Am J Physiol.* 1995;268:F1-F12.

433. Chiang N, Fierro IM, Gronert K, et al. Activation of lipoxin A$_4$ receptors by aspirin-triggered lipoxins and select peptides evokes ligand-specific responses in inflammation. *J Exp Med.* 2000;191:1197-1208.

434. Pawloski JR, Chapnick BM. Leukotrienes C4 and D4 are potent endothelium-dependent relaxing agents in canine splanchnic venous capacitance vessels. *Circ Res.* 1993;73:395-404.

435. Claria J, Lee MH, Serhan CN. Aspirin-triggered lipoxins (15-epi-LX) are generated by the human lung adenocarcinoma cell line (A549)-neutrophil interactions and are potent inhibitors of cell proliferation. *Mol Med.* 1996;2:583-596.

436. Imig JD. Eicosanoid regulation of the renal vasculature. *Am J Physiol Renal Physiol.* 2000;279:F965-F981.

437. Nie D, Tang K, Diglio C, et al. Eicosanoid regulation of angiogenesis: role of endothelial arachidonate 12-lipoxygenase. *Blood.* 2000;95:2304-2311.

438. Ma J, Natarajan R, LaPage J, et al. 12/15-Lipoxygenase inhibitors in diabetic nephropathy in the rat. *Prostaglandins Leukot Essent Fatty Acids.* 2005;72:13-20.

439. Kim YS, Xu ZG, Reddy MA, et al. Novel interactions between TGF-β1 actions and the 12/15-lipoxygenase pathway in mesangial cells. *J Am Soc Nephrol.* 2005;16:352-362.

440. Imig JD, Deichmann PC. Afferent arteriolar responses to ANG II involve activation of PLA2 and modulation by lipoxygenase and P-450 pathways. *Am J Physiol.* 1997;273:F274-F282.

441. Wu XC, Richards NT, Michael J, et al. Relative roles of nitric oxide and cyclo-oxygenase and lipoxygenase products of arachidonic acid in the contractile responses of rat renal arcuate arteries. *Br J Pharmacol.* 1994;112:369-376.

442. Stern N, Nozawa K, Kisch E, et al. Tonic inhibition of renin secretion by the 12 lipoxygenase pathway: augmentation by high salt intake. *Endocrinology.* 1996;137:1878-1884.

443. Antonipillai I, Nadler J, Vu EJ, et al. A 12-lipoxygenase product, 12-hydroxyeicosatetraenoic acid, is increased in diabetics with incipient and early renal disease. *J Clin Endocrinol Metab.* 1996;81:1940-1945.

444. Brady HR, Papayianni A, Serhan CN. Transcellular pathways and cell adhesion as potential contributors to leukotriene and lipoxin biosynthesis in acute glomerulonephritis. *Adv Exp Med Biol.* 1997;400B:631-640.

445. Kang SW, Adler SG, Nast CC, et al. 12-Lipoxygenase is increased in glucose-stimulated mesangial cells and in experimental diabetic nephropathy. *Kidney Int.* 2001;59:1354-1362.

446. Xu ZG, Li SL, Lanting L, et al. Relationship between 12/15-lipoxygenase and COX-2 in mesangial cells: potential role in diabetic nephropathy. *Kidney Int.* 2006;69:512-519.

447. Rahman MA, Nakazawa M, Emancipator SN, et al. Increased leukotriene B4 synthesis in immune injured rat glomeruli. *J Clin Invest.* 1988;81:1945-1952.

448. Badr KF. Five-lipoxygenase products in glomerular immune injury. *J Am Soc Nephrol.* 1992;3:907-915.

449. Papayianni A, Serhan CN, Phillips ML, et al. Transcellular biosynthesis of lipoxin A4 during adhesion of platelets and neutrophils in experimental immune complex glomerulonephritis. *Kidney Int.* 1995;47:1295-1302.

450. Katoh T, Lianos EA, Fukunaga M, et al. Leukotriene D4 is a mediator of proteinuria and glomerular hemodynamic abnormalities in passive Heymann nephritis. *J Clin Invest.* 1993;91:1507-1515.

451. Butterly DW, Spurney RF, Ruiz P, et al. A role for leukotrienes in cyclosporine nephrotoxicity. *Kidney Int.* 2000;57:2586-2593.

452. Goulet JL, Griffiths RC, Ruiz P, et al. Deficiency of 5-lipoxygenase accelerates renal allograft rejection in mice. *J Immunol.* 2001;167:6631-6636.

453. Fauler J, Wiemeyer A, Marx KH, et al. LTB4 in nephrotoxic serum nephritis in rats. *Kidney Int.* 1989;36:46-50.

454. Lianos EA. Synthesis of hydroxyeicosatetraenoic acids and leukotrienes in rat nephrotoxic serum glomerulonephritis. Role of anti–glomerular basement membrane antibody dose, complement, and neutrophiles. *J Clin Invest.* 1988;82:427-435.

455. Ferrante JV, Huang ZH, Nandoskar M, et al. Altered responses of human macrophages to lipopolysaccharide by hydroperoxy eicosatetraenoic acid, hydroxy eicosatetraenoic acid, and arachidonic acid. Inhibition of tumor necrosis factor production. *J Clin Invest.* 1997;99:1445-1452.

456. Munger KA, Montero A, Fukunaga M, et al. Transfection of rat kidney with human 15-lipoxygenase suppresses inflammation and preserves function in experimental glomerulonephritis. *Proc Natl Acad Sci U S A.* 1999;96:13375-13380.

457. Guasch A, Zayas CF, Badr KF. MK-591 acutely restores glomerular size selectivity and reduces proteinuria in human glomerulonephritis. *Kidney Int.* 1999;56:261-267.

458. Makita N, Funk CD, Imai E, et al. Molecular cloning and functional expression of rat leukotriene A4 hydrolase using the polymerase chain reaction. *FEBS Lett.* 1992;299:273-277.

459. Yared A, Albrightson-Winslow C, Griswold D, et al. Functional significance of leukotriene B4 in normal and glomerulonephritic kidneys. *J Am Soc Nephrol.* 1991;2:45-56.

460. Patel NS, Cuzzocrea S, Chatterjee PK, et al. Reduction of renal ischemia-reperfusion injury in 5-lipoxygenase knockout mice and by the 5-lipoxygenase inhibitor zileuton. *Mol Pharmacol.* 2004;66:220-227.

461. Capdevila JH, Harris RC, Falck JR. Microsomal cytochrome P450 and eicosanoid metabolism. *Cell Mol Life Sci.* 2002;59:780-789.

462. Capdevila JH, Falck JR, Harris RC. Cytochrome P450 and arachidonic acid bioactivation: molecular and functional properties of the arachidonate monooxygenase. *J Lipid Res.* 2000;41:163-181.

463. Capdevila JH, Falck JR. Biochemical and molecular characteristics of the cytochrome P450 arachidonic acid monooxygenase. *Prostaglandins Other Lipid Mediat.* 2000;62:271-292.

464. Roman RJ. P-450 metabolites of arachidonic acid in the control of cardiovascular function. *Physiol Rev.* 2002;82:131-185.

465. McGiff JC, Quilley J. 20-HETE and the kidney: resolution of old problems and new beginnings. *Am J Physiol.* 1999;277:R607-R623.

466. Ma J, Qu W, Scarborough PE, et al. Molecular cloning, enzymatic characterization, developmental expression, and cellular localization of a mouse cytochrome P450 highly expressed in kidney. *J Biol Chem.* 1999;274:17777-17788.

467. Ito O, Alonso-Galicia M, Hopp KA, et al. Localization of cytochrome p-450 4A isoforms along the rat nephron. *Am J Physiol.* 1998;274:F395-F404.

468. Yokose T, Doy M, Taniguchi T, et al. Immunohistochemical study of cytochrome P450 2C and 3A in human non-neoplastic and neoplastic tissues. *Virchows Arch.* 1999;434:401-411.

469. Imig JD, Zou AP, Stec DE, et al. Formation and actions of 20-hydroxyeicosatetraenoic acid in rat renal arterioles. *Am J Physiol.* 1996;270:R217-R227.

470. Ito O, Roman RJ. Regulation of P-450 4A activity in the glomerulus of the rat. *Am J Physiol.* 1999;276:R1749-R1757.

471. Quigley R, Baum M, Reddy KM, et al. Effects of 20-HETE and 19(S)-HETE on rabbit proximal straight tubule volume transport. *Am J Physiol Renal Physiol.* 2000;278:F949-F953.

472. Escalante B, Erlij D, Falck JR, et al. Effect of cytochrome P450 arachidonate metabolites on ion transport in rabbit kidney loop of Henle. *Science.* 1991;251:799-802.

473. Ito O, Roman RJ. Role of 20-HETE in elevating chloride transport in the thick ascending limb of Dahl SS/Jr rats. *Hypertension.* 1999;33:419-423.

474. Hirt DL, Capdevila J, Falck JR, et al. Cytochrome P450 metabolites of arachidonic acid are potent inhibitors of vasopressin action on rabbit cortical collecting duct. *J Clin Invest.* 1989;84:1805-1812.

475. Makita K, Falck J, Capdevila J. Cytochrome P450, the arachidonic acid cascade, and hypertension: new vistas for an old enzyme system. *FASEB J.* 1996;10:1456-1463.

476. Chen JK, Chen J, Imig JD, et al. Identification of novel endogenous cytochrome p450 arachidonate metabolites with high affinity for cannabinoid receptors. *J Biol Chem.* 2008;283:24514-24524.

477. Imig JD, Navar LG, Roman RJ, et al. Actions of epoxygenase metabolites on the preglomerular vasculature. *J Am Soc Nephrol.* 1996;7:2364-2370.

478. Alonso-Galicia M, Sun CW, Falck JR, et al. Contribution of 20-HETE to the vasodilator actions of nitric oxide in renal arteries. *Am J Physiol.* 1998;275:F370-F378.

479. Sun CW, Alonso-Galicia M, Taheri MR, et al. Nitric oxide-20-hydroxyeicosatetraenoic acid interaction in the regulation of K$^+$ channel activity and vascular tone in renal arterioles. *Circ Res.* 1998;83:1069-1079.

480. Katoh T, Takahashi K, Capdevila J, et al. Glomerular stereospecific synthesis and hemodynamic actions of 8,9-epoxyeicosatrienoic acid in rat kidney. *Am J Physiol.* 1991;261:F578-F586.

481. Campbell WB, Gauthier KM. What is new in endothelium-derived hyperpolarizing factors? *Curr Opin Nephrol Hypertens.* 2002;11:177-183.

482. Vazquez B, Rios A, Escalante B. Arachidonic acid metabolism modulates vasopressin-induced renal vasoconstriction. *Life Sciences.* 1995;56:1455-1466.

483. Imig JD. Epoxygenase metabolites. Epithelial and vascular actions. *Mol Biotechnol.* 2000;16:233-251.

484. Oyekan AO, McAward K, Conetta J, et al. Endothelin-1 and CYP450 arachidonate metabolites interact to promote tissue injury in DOCA-salt hypertension. *Am J Physiol.* 1999;276:R766-R775.

485. Arima S, Endo Y, Yaoita H, et al. Possible role of P-450 metabolite of arachidonic acid in vasodilator mechanism of angiotensin II type 2 receptor in the isolated microperfused rabbit afferent arteriole. *J Clin Invest.* 1997;100:2816-2823.

486. Alonso-Galicia M, Maier KG, Greene AS, et al. Role of 20-hydroxyeicosatetraenoic acid in the renal and vasoconstrictor actions of angiotensin II. *Am J Physiol Regul Integr Comp Physiol.* 2002;283:R60-R68.

487. Imig JD, Falck JR, Inscho EW. Contribution of cytochrome P450 epoxygenase and hydroxylase pathways to afferent arteriolar autoregulatory responsiveness. *Br J Pharmacol.* 1999;127:1399-1405.

488. Zou AP, Fleming JT, Falck JR, et al. 20-HETE is an endogenous inhibitor of the large-conductance Ca^{2+}-activated K$^+$ channel in renal arterioles. *Am J Physiol.* 1996;270:R228-R237.

489. Wang H, Garvin JL, Falck JR, et al. Glomerular cytochrome P-450 and cyclooxygenase metabolites regulate efferent arteriole resistance. *Hypertension.* 2005;46:1175-1179.
490. Schnermann J. Adenosine mediates tubuloglomerular feedback. *Am J Physiol Regul Integr Comp Physiol.* 2002;283:R276-R277:discussion R278-R279.
491. Zou AP, Imig JD, Kaldunski M, et al. Inhibition of renal vascular 20-HETE production impairs autoregulation of renal blood flow. *Am J Physiol.* 1994;266:F275-F282.
492. Hercule HC, Oyekan AO. Cytochrome P450 ω/ω-1 hydroxylase–derived eicosanoids contribute to endothelin_A and endothelin_B receptor-mediated vasoconstriction to endothelin-1 in the rat preglomerular arteriole. *J Pharmacol Exp Ther.* 2000;292:1153-1160.
493. Ren Y, D'Ambrosio MA, Garvin JL, et al. Possible mediators of connecting tubule glomerular feedback. *Hypertension.* 2009;53:319-323.
494. Henrich WL, Falck JR, Campbell WB. Inhibition of renin release by 14,15-epoxyeicosatrienoic acid in renal. *Am J Physiol.* 1990;258:E269-E274.
495. Alonso-Galicia M, Falck JR, Reddy KM, et al. 20-HETE agonists and antagonists in the renal circulation. *Am J Physiol.* 1999;277:F790-F796.
496. Romero MF, Madhun ZT, Hopfer U, et al. An epoxygenase metabolite of arachidonic acid 5,6 epoxy-eicosatrienoic acid mediates angiotensin-induced natriuresis in proximal tubular epithelium. *Adv Prostaglandin Thromboxane Leukot Res.* 1991;21:205-208.
497. Escalante BA, Staudinger R, Schwartzman M, et al. Amiloride-sensitive ion transport inhibition by epoxyeicosatrienoic acids in renal epithelial cells. *Adv Prostaglandin Thromboxane Leukot Res.* 1995;23:207-209.
498. Staudinger R, Escalante B, Schwartzman ML, et al. Effects of epoxyeicosatrienoic acids on 86Rb uptake in renal epithelial cells. *J Cell Physiol.* 1994;160:69-74.
499. Nowicki S, Chen SL, Aizman O, et al. 20-Hydroxyeicosa-tetraenoic acid (20 HETE) activates protein kinase C. Role in regulation of rat renal Na+, K+-ATPase. *J Clin Invest.* 1997;99:1224-1230.
500. Carroll M, Balazy M, Margiotta P, et al. Cytochrome p-450 dependent HETEs: profile of biological activity and stimulation by vasoactive peptides. *Am J Physiol.* 1996;271:R863-R869.
501. Burns K, Capdevila J, Wei S, et al. Role of cytochrome P-450 epoxygenase metabolites in EGF signaling in renal proximal tubules. *Am J Physiol.* 1995;269:C831-C840.
502. Houillier P, Chambrey R, Achard JM, et al. Signaling pathways in the biphasic effect of angiotensin II on apical Na/H antiport activity in proximal tubule. *Kidney Int.* 1996;50:1496-1505.
503. Navar LG, Lewis L, Hymel A, et al. Tubular fluid concentrations and kidney contents of angiotensins I and II in anesthetized rats. *J Am Soc Nephrol.* 1994;5:1153-1158.
504. Zhang YB, Magyar CE, Holstein-Rathlou NH, et al. The cytochrome P-450 inhibitor cobalt chloride prevents inhibition of renal Na, K-ATPase and redistribution of apical NHE-3 during acute hypertension. *J Am Soc Nephrol.* 1998;9:531-537.
505. Wang W, Lu M, Balazy M, et al. Phospholipase A_2 is involved in mediating the effect of extracellular Ca^{2+} on apical K+ channels in rat TAL. *Am J Physiol.* 1997;273:F421-F429.
506. Good DW, George T, Wang DH. Angiotensin II inhibits HCO_3 absorption via a cytochrome P-450–dependent pathway in MTAL. *Am J Physiol.* 1999;276:F726-F736.
507. Grider JS, Falcone JC, Kilpatrick EL, et al. P450 arachidonate metabolites mediate bradykinin-dependent inhibition of NaCl transport in the rat thick ascending limb. *Can J Physiol Pharmacol.* 1997;75:91-96.
508. Sakairi Y, Jacobson HR, Noland TD, et al. 5,6-EET inhibits ion transport in collecting duct by stimulating endogenous prostaglandin synthesis. *Am J Physiol.* 1995;268:F931-F939.
509. Nusing RM, Schweer H, Fleming I, et al. Epoxyeicosatrienoic acids affect electrolyte transport in renal tubular epithelial cells: dependence on cyclooxygenase and cell polarity. *Am J Physiol Renal Physiol.* 2007;293:F288-F298.
510. Wei Y, Lin DH, Kemp R, et al. Arachidonic acid inhibits epithelial Na channel via cytochrome P450 (CYP) epoxygenase-dependent metabolic pathways. *J Gen Physiol.* 2004;124:719-727.
511. Nakagawa K, Holla VR, Wei Y, et al. Salt-sensitive hypertension is associated with dysfunctional Cyp4a10 gene and kidney epithelial sodium channel. *J Clin Invest.* 2006;116:1696-1702.
512. Sellmayer A, Uedelhoven WM, Weber PC, et al. Endogenous non-cyclooxygenase metabolites of arachidonic acid modulate growth and mRNA levels of immediate-early response genes in rat mesangial cells. *J Biol Chem.* 1991;266:3800-3807.
513. Harris RC, Homma T, Jacobson HR, et al. Epoxyeicosatrienoic acids activate Na+/H+ exchange and are mitogenic in cultured rat glomerular mesangial cells. *J Cell Physiol.* 1990;144:429-437.
514. Chen JK, Capdevila J, Harris RC. Heparin-binding EGF-like growth factor mediates the biological effects of P450 arachidonate epoxygenase metabolites in epithelial cells. *Proc Natl Acad Sci U S A.* 2002;99:6029-6034.
515. Lin F, Rios A, Falck JR, et al. 20-Hydroxyeicosatetraenoic acid is formed in response to EGF and is a mitogen in rat proximal tubule. *Am J Physiol.* 1995;269:F806-F816.
516. Uddin MR, Muthalif MM, Karzoun NA, et al. Cytochrome P-450 metabolites mediate norepinephrine-induced mitogenic signaling. *Hypertension.* 1998;31:242-247.
517. Holla VR, Makita K, Zaphiropoulos PG, et al. The kidney cytochrome P-450 2C23 arachidonic acid epoxygenase is upregulated during dietary salt loading. *J Clin Invest.* 1999;104:751-760.
518. Imig JD. Epoxide hydrolase and epoxygenase metabolites as therapeutic targets for renal diseases. *Am J Physiol Renal Physiol.* 2005;289:F496-F503.
519. Muthalif MM, Benter IF, Khandekar Z, et al. Contribution of Ras GTPase/MAP kinase and cytochrome P450 metabolites to deoxycorticosterone-salt–induced hypertension. *Hypertension.* 2000;35:457-463.
520. Croft KD, McGiff JC, Sanchez-Mendoza A, et al. Angiotensin II releases 20-HETE from rat renal microvessels. *Am J Physiol Renal Physiol.* 2000;279:F544-F551.
521. Joly E, Seqqat R, Flamion B, et al. Increased renal vascular reactivity to ANG II after unilateral nephrectomy in the rat involves 20-HETE. *Am J Physiol Regul Integr Comp Physiol.* 2006;291:R977-R986.
522. Iwai N, Inagami T. Identification of a candidate gene responsible for the high blood pressure of spontaneously hypertensive rats. *J Hypertension.* 1992;10:1155-1157.
523. Stec DE, Trolliet MR, Krieger JE, et al. Renal cytochrome P4504A activity and salt sensitivity in spontaneously hypertensive rats. *Hypertension.* 1996;27:1329-1336.
524. Wang MH, Zhang F, Marji J, et al. CYP4A1 antisense oligonucleotide reduces mesenteric vascular reactivity and blood pressure in SHR. *Am J Physiol Regul Integr Comp Physiol.* 2001;280:R255-R261.
525. Gainer JV, Bellamine A, Dawson EP, et al. Functional variant of CYP4A11 20-hydroxyeicosatetraenoic acid synthase is associated with essential hypertension. *Circulation.* 2005;111:63-69.
526. Imig JD, Zou AP, Ortiz de Montellano PR, et al. Cytochrome P-450 inhibitors alter afferent arteriolar responses to elevations in pressure. *Am J Physiol.* 1994;266:H1879-H1885.
527. Muller C, Endlich K, Helwig JJ. AT2 antagonist–sensitive potentiation of angiotensin II-induced constriction by NO blockade and its dependence on endothelium and P450 eicosanoids in rat renal vasculature. *Br J Pharmacol.* 1998;124:946-952.
528. Gross V, Schunck WH, Honeck H, et al. Inhibition of pressure natriuresis in mice lacking the AT2 receptor. *Kidney Int.* 2000;57:191-202.
529. Ai D, Fu Y, Guo D, et al. Angiotensin II up-regulates soluble epoxide hydrolase in vascular endothelium in vitro and in vivo. *Proc Natl Acad Sci U S A.* 2007;104:9018-9023.
530. Chiamvimonvat N, Ho CM, Tsai HJ, et al. The soluble epoxide hydrolase as a pharmacological target for hypertension. *J Cardiovasc Pharmacol.* 2007;50:225-237.

Disorders of Body Fluid Volume and Composition

Disorders of Sodium Balance

Itzchak N. Slotki and Karl L. Skorecki

Sodium (Na+) and water balance and their distribution among the various body compartments are essential for the maintenance of fluid homeostasis, particularly intravascular volume. Disturbances of either or both of these components have serious medical consequences, are relatively frequent, and are among the most common conditions encountered in hospital clinical practice. In fact, abnormalities of Na+ and water balance are responsible for, or associated with, a wide spectrum of medical and surgical admissions or complications. The principal disorders of Na+ balance are manifested clinically as either hypovolemia or hypervolemia, whereas disruption in water balance can be diagnosed only in the laboratory as either hyponatremia or hypernatremia. Although disorders of Na+ and water balance are often interrelated, the latter are considered in a separate chapter. In this chapter the physiologic and pathophysiologic features of Na+ balance are discussed. Because Na+ is restricted predominantly to the extracellular compartment, this chapter also addresses perturbations of extracellular fluid (ECF) volume homeostasis.

Physiology

Approximately 60% of adult body mass is composed of solute-containing fluids that can be divided into extracellular and intracellular compartments. Because water flows freely across cell membranes in accordance with the prevailing osmotic forces on either side of the membrane, the solute/water ratios in the intracellular fluid (ICF) and ECF are almost equal. However, the solute compositions of the ICF and ECF are quite different, as shown in Figure 14-1. The principal ECF cation is sodium; minor cations are potassium (K+), calcium, and magnesium. In contrast, potassium is the major ICF cation. The accompanying anions in the ECF are chloride, bicarbonate, and plasma proteins (mainly albumin), whereas electroneutrality of the ICF is maintained by phosphate and the negative charges on organic molecules. The difference in cationic composition of the two compartments is maintained by a pump-leak mechanism consisting of sodium-potassium adenosine triphosphatase (Na+-K+-ATPase), which operates in concert with sodium and potassium conductance pathways in the cell membrane.

The free movement of water across the membrane ensures that the ECF and ICF osmolalities are the same. However, the intracellular volume is greater because the amount of potassium salts inside the cell is larger than that of sodium salts outside the cell. The movement of water is determined by the "effective osmolality," or tonicity, of each compartment, so that if tonicity of the ECF rises—for example, as a result of excess Na+—water will move from the ICF to ECF to restore tonicity. On the other hand, addition of solute-free water leads to a proportionate decrease in both osmolality and tonicity of all body fluid compartments (see Chapter 15 for

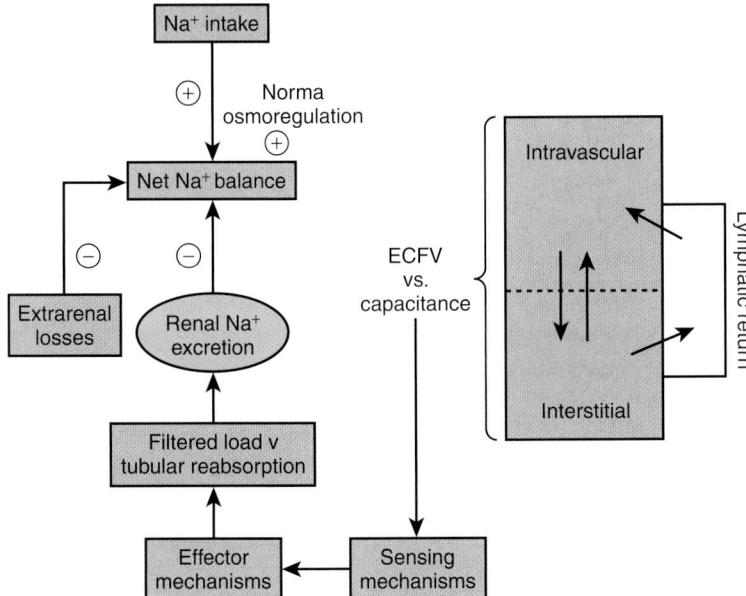

FIGURE 14-1 Overall scheme for body sodium balance and partitioning of extracellular fluid volume (ECFV). In the setting of normal osmoregulation, extracellular Na^+ content is the primary determinant of ECFV. Overall Na^+ homeostasis depends on the balance between losses (extrarenal and renal) and intake. Renal Na^+ excretion is determined by the balance between filtered load and tubule reabsorption. This latter balance is modulated under the influence of effector mechanisms, which, in turn, are responsive to sensing mechanisms that monitor the relation between ECFV and capacitance. In rats, a high-salt diet leads to interstitial hypertonic Na^+ accumulation in skin, resulting in increased density and hyperplasia of the lymphatic capillary network.

detailed discussion). The restriction of Na^+ to the ECF compartment by the pump-leak mechanism, in combination with maintenance of the osmotic equilibrium between ECF and ICF, ensures that ECF volume is determined mainly by total body Na^+ content.

The same mechanisms also govern the partitioning of fluid between the two compartments and are crucial for preservation of near constancy of ECF and ICF volume in the presence of variations in dietary intake and extrarenal losses of Na^+ and water. In order to maintain constancy of the ECF and ICF and thereby safeguard hemodynamic stability, cell volume, and solute composition, even minute changes in these parameters can be detected by a number of sensing mechanisms. These sensory signals lead to activation of neural and hormonal factors, which, in turn, cause appropriate adjustments in urinary Na^+ and water excretion and, hence, restoration of fluid balance. Constancy of ECF volume ensures a high degree of circulatory stability, whereas constancy of ICF volume protects against significant brain cell swelling or shrinkage.

Sodium Balance

Na^+ balance is the difference between intake (diet or supplementary fluids) and output (renal, gastrointestinal, perspiratory, and respiratory). In healthy humans in steady state, dietary intake is closely matched by urinary output of Na^+. Thus, a person consuming a chronically low-Na^+ diet (20 mmol/day, or approximately 1.2 g/day) excretes, in the steady state, a similar quantity of Na^+ in the urine (minus extrarenal losses). Conversely, on a high-Na^+ diet (200 mmol/day, or 12 g/day), approximately 200 mmol of Na^+ is excreted in the urine. Any perturbation of this balance leads to activation of the sensory and effector mechanisms outlined in the following discussions. In practice, any deviation in ECF volume in relation to its capacitance is sensed and translated, under the influence of neural and hormonal factors, into the appropriate

change in Na^+ excretion, principally through the kidneys but also, to a much lesser degree, through stool and sweat.

For normal functioning of the afferent sensing and efferent effector mechanisms that regulate ECF volume, the integrity of the intravascular and extravascular subcompartments of the ECF[1] is crucial (see Figure 14-1). Although the composition and concentration of small, noncolloid electrolyte solutes in these two subcompartments are approximately equal (slight differences are due to the Gibbs-Donnan effect), the concentration of colloid osmotic particles (mainly albumin and globulin) is higher in the intravascular compartment. The balance between transcapillary hydraulic and colloid osmotic (oncotic) gradients (Starling forces) favors the net transudation of fluid from the intravascular to interstitial compartment. However, this is countered by movement of lymphatic fluid from the interstitial to the intravascular compartment via the thoracic duct. The net effect is to restore and maintain the intravascular subcompartment at 25% of the total ECF volume (corresponding to 3.5 L of plasma); the remaining 75% is contained in the interstitial space (equivalent to 10.5 L in a 70-kg man). The constancy of ECF volume and the appropriate partitioning of the fluid between intravascular and interstitial subcompartments are crucial for maintaining hemodynamic stability. In particular, intravascular volume in relation to overall vascular capacitance is a major determinant of left ventricular filling volume and, hence, cardiac output and mean arterial pressure.

Effective Arterial Blood Volume

In order to understand the mechanisms regulating ECF volume, it is important to appreciate that what is sensed is the effective arterial blood volume (EABV). This can be defined as the part of the ECF in the arterial blood system that effectively perfuses the tissues. More specifically, in physiologic terms, what is sensed is the pressure induced by the EABV that perfuses the arterial baroceptors in the carotid sinus and glomerular afferent arterioles. Any change in perfusion pressure (or stretch) at these sites evokes appropriate compensatory responses. EABV is often, although not always, correlated with actual ECF volume and is proportional to total body Na^+. This means that the regulation of Na^+ balance and the maintenance of EABV are closely related functions. Na^+ loading generally leads to EABV expansion, whereas loss leads to depletion. However, in several situations, EABV and actual blood volume are not well correlated (see Table 14-5 later in the chapter). For example, in congestive heart failure (CHF), a primary decrease in cardiac output leads to lowered pressure in the perfusion of the baroceptors; that is, reduced EABV is sensed. This leads to renal Na^+ retention and ECF volume expansion. The net result is a state of increased plasma and total ECF volume, in association with reduced EABV.

The increase in plasma volume is partially appropriate in that intraventricular filling pressure rises and, by increasing myocardial stretching, leads to improved ventricular contractility, thereby raising cardiac output and restoring systemic blood pressure and baroceptor perfusion. However, this response is also maladaptive in that the elevated intraarterial pressure promotes fluid movement out of the intravascular space and into the tissues, which leads to both peripheral and pulmonary edema. In CHF, EABV is dependent on cardiac output; in other disease settings, however, these two parameters may be dissociated. Dissociation occurs in the presence of an arteriovenous fistula, when cardiac output rises in proportion to the blood flow through the fistula. However, the flow through the fistula shunts blood away from the capillaries perfusing the tissues, and therefore the EABV does not rise in conjunction with the rise in cardiac output. Similarly, a fall in systemic vascular resistance—which, together with cardiac output, is a determinant of blood pressure—leads to reductions in blood pressure and EABV.

Another situation in which cardiac output and EABV change in opposite directions is advanced cirrhosis with ascites. ECF volume expands because of the ascites, and plasma volume is increased as a result of fluid accumulation in the splanchnic venous circulation, in which the vessels are dilated but flow is sluggish. Although cardiac output may increase modestly as a result of arteriovenous shunting, marked peripheral vasodilation leads to a fall in systemic vascular resistance, with reductions in EABV and blood pressure. In the presence of reduced EABV, renal perfusion is impaired; under the influence of hormones, such as renin, norepinephrine, and antidiuretic hormone (or arginine vasopressin [AVP])—released in response to the perceived hypovolemia—further Na^+ and water retention ensue (see "Efferent Limb: Effector Mechanisms for Maintaining Effective Arterial Blood Volume" section).

To summarize, EABV is an unmeasured index of tissue perfusion that usually, but not always, reflects actual arterial blood volume. Therefore, EABV can be viewed as a functional parameter of organ perfusion. The diagnostic hallmark of reduced EABV is evidence of renal sodium retention, manifested as urinary sodium (U_{Na}) less than 15 to 20 mmol/L. This relationship holds true with the following exceptions: If renal Na^+ wasting occurs because of either diuretic therapy or intrinsic tubular disease or injury, then U_{Na} is relatively high, despite low EABV. Conversely, the presence of selective renal or glomerular ischemia (e.g., as a result of bilateral renal artery stenosis or acute glomerular injury) will be misinterpreted as

TABLE 14-1 Mechanisms for Sensing Regional Changes in Effective Arterial Blood Volume
Sensors of Cardiac Filling
Atrial
Neural pathways
Humoral pathways
Ventricular
Pulmonary
Sensors of Cardiac Output
Carotid and aortic baroceptors
Sensors of Organ Perfusion
Renal sensors
CNS sensors
GI tract sensors
Hepatic receptors
Guanylin peptides

CNS, Central nervous system; *GI*, gastrointestinal.

indicative of poor renal perfusion and is associated with renal Na^+ retention (low U_{Na}).

Regulation of Effective Arterial Blood Volume

Regulation of EABV can be divided into two stages: afferent sensing and efferent effector mechanisms. A number of mechanisms for sensing low EABV exist, all of them primed to stimulate renal Na^+ retention.

Afferent Limb: Sensing of Effective Arterial Blood Volume

Volume sensors are strategically situated at critical points in the circulation (Table 14-1). Each sensor reflects a specific characteristic of overall circulatory function so that atrial and ventricular sensors sense cardiac filling; arterial sensors respond to cardiac output; and renal, central nervous system (CNS), and gastrointestinal tract sensors monitor perfusion of the kidneys, brain, and gut, respectively. The common mechanism whereby volume is monitored is by physical alterations in the vessel wall such as stretch or tension. How exactly this occurs is still not fully elucidated, but the process of mechanosensing probably is dependent on both afferent sensory nerve endings in the vessel wall and activation of endothelial cells. Signal transduction mechanisms in endothelial cells include stretch-activated ion channels, cytoskeleton-associated protein kinases, integrin-cytoskeletal interactions, cytoskeletal-nuclear interactions, and generation of reactive oxygen species.[2,3] In addition, mechanical stretch and tension of blood vessel walls, as well as the frictional forces of the circulation or shear stress, can lead to alterations in gene expression that are mediated by specific recognition sites in the upstream promoter elements of responsive genes.[4,5] These signals induce efferent effector mechanisms that lead to modifications in renal Na^+ excretion, appropriate to the volume status.

SENSORS OF CARDIAC FILLING
Atrial Sensors. The pioneering experiments of Henry and associates[6] and Goetz and colleagues[7] in conscious dogs provided a clear demonstration that increased atrial wall tension leads to diuresis and natriuresis. The role of the atria in

volume regulation in humans has been elucidated in experiments involving head-out water immersion (HWI) and exposure to head-down tilt or nonhypotensive lower body negative pressure (LBNP). During HWI, the increased hydrostatic pressure of the water on the lower limbs leads to redistribution of the intravascular fluid from the peripheral to central circulation. The resulting increase in central blood volume causes a rise in cardiac output, which in turn produces a brisk increase in Na+ and water excretion, in an attempt to restore euvolemia.[8] In contrast, LBNP results in a redistribution of blood to the lower limbs, thereby reducing central venous and cardiac filling pressures without affecting arterial pressure, heart rate, or atrial diameter. The resulting retention of Na+ and water occurs without any change in renal plasma flow rate (RPF).[9]

Central hypervolemia may not be the only mechanism of HWI-induced Na+ and water diuresis. The external hydrostatic pressure of the water also reduces the hydrostatic pressure gradient across the capillary wall in the legs, leading to a net transfer of fluid from the interstitial to intravascular compartment. The resulting hemodilution causes a fall in the colloid osmotic pressure. The hemodilution effect may actually predominate, inasmuch as its abolition by placement of a tight inflated cuff (80 mm Hg) during HWI abrogates the natriuresis.[10,11] Regardless of which effect is dominant, a combination of hemodilution and central hypervolemia, through atrial stretch, induces neural and humoral changes that bring about the subsequent diuresis and natriuresis.

Neural Pathways. Two types of neural receptors in the atrium have been described: type A and type B. They are thought to be branching ends of small medullated fibers running in the vagus nerve. Only type B receptor activity is increased by atrial filling and stretch; type A receptors are not affected.[12] The signal is then thought to travel along cranial nerves IX and X to the hypothalamic and medullary centers, where a series of responses is initiated: inhibition of AVP release (left atrial signal)[13]; a selective decrease in renal but not lumbar sympathetic nerve discharge[14,15]; and decreased tone in peripheral precapillary and postcapillary resistance vessels. Conversely, reduction in central venous pressure and atrial volume, as illustrated by LBNP, stimulates renal nerve activity, as assessed by renal norepinephrine spillover and plasma norepinephrine concentration.[16,17]

The effects just described occur in response to acute atrial stretch, whereas chronic atrial stretch leads to adaptation and downregulation of the neural responses. This phenomenon has been described in rhesus monkeys exposed to 10-degree head-down tilt. In this model, natriuresis after saline infusion occurs at lower central venous and, hence, lower cardiac filling pressures.[17] Cardiac nerves appear to be essential only for restoration of Na+ balance in states of repletion, but not for the renal response to acute volume depletion.[18] For example, after human cardiac transplantation, a natural model of cardiac denervation, the expected suppression of the renin-angiotensin-aldosterone (RAAS) system in response to chronic volume expansion is not observed.[19]

Humoral Pathways. Cardiac denervation does not abolish the natriuresis and diuresis during atrial distension. This implies that additional factors other than cardiac nerves are involved in the response to volume repletion. The discovery of a factor in atrial extracts with strong natriuretic and vasodilatory activity led to the isolation and characterization of natriuretic peptides of cardiac origin.[20,21] The natriuretic peptide family comprises atrial natriuretic peptide (ANP), brain natriuretic peptide (BNP), C-type natriuretic peptide (CNP), *Dendroaspis* natriuretic peptide (DNP), and urodilatin. Although their structures are quite similar, each is encoded by different genes and has distinct, albeit overlapping, functions.[22-25] The actions of natriuretic peptides and their interaction with other hormone systems are discussed in detail later in the "Efferent Limb: Effector Mechanisms for Maintaining Effective Arterial Blood Volume" section, as well as in Chapter 12. This section is confined to a discussion of the afferent mechanisms of natriuretic peptide stimulation.

From studies in both animals and humans, it has become abundantly clear that any acute increment in atrial stretch or pressure causes a brisk release in ANP. Every 1–mm Hg rise in atrial pressure results in an approximate rise in ANP of 10 to 15 pmol/L. The process involves the cleavage of the prohormone, located in preformed stores in atrial granules, to the mature 28–amino acid C-terminus peptide in a sequence-specific manner by corin, a transmembrane serine protease.[26] Release of the hormone appears to occur in two steps: the first a Ca2+-sensitive K+ channel–dependent release of ANP from myocytes into the intercellular space, and then a Ca2+-independent translocation of the hormone into the atrial lumen.[27] The afferent mechanism for ANP release is activated by intravascular volume expansion, as well as by supine posture, HWI, saline administration, exercise, angiotensin II, tachycardia, and ventricular dysfunction.[28,29] Conversely, volume depletion induced by Na+ restriction, furosemide administration, or LNBP-mediated reduction in central venous pressure causes a fall in plasma ANP concentration.

In contrast to the effects of acute changes in atrial pressure on ANP release, the role of this peptide in the long-term regulation of plasma volume appears to be modest, at best. For example, although incremental oral salt-loading was associated with correspondingly higher baseline plasma ANP levels, only intravenous (not oral) salt loading led to increased ANP levels.[30] Moreover, in humans subjected to either intravenous or oral salt loading, no correlation could be found between changes in ANP levels and the degree of natriuresis.[31-33] The contrasting relationships among acute and chronic Na+ loading, plasma ANP levels, and natriuresis have been elegantly demonstrated in ANP gene–knockout mice. These mice display a reduced natriuretic response to acute ECF volume expansion in comparison with their wild-type counterparts. However, no differences in cumulative Na+ and water excretion were observed between the knockout and wild-type mice after a high- or low-Na+ diet for 1 week. The only difference between the two types of mice was a significant increase in mean arterial pressure. Further experiments utilizing disruptions of either the genes for ANP or its receptor, guanylate cyclase A (GC-A), showed the importance of this system in the maintenance of normal blood pressure and in modulating cardiac hypertrophy.[34]

In contrast to ANP, the other members of the natriuretic peptide family appear not to be involved in the physiologic regulation of Na+ excretion. Thus, results of gene-disruption studies involving BNP, CNP, or the guanylyl cyclase B (GC-B) receptor[35] indicated that these proteins exert local paracrine/autocrine cyclic guanosine monophosphate (cGMP)–mediated effects on cellular proliferation and differentiation in various tissues.[22,24,36] In summary, of the various natriuretic peptides, only ANP appears to have a direct role in sensing volume in the atria.

Ventricular and Pulmonary Sensors. Volume sensors have been found in the ventricles, coronary arteries, main pulmonary artery and bifurcation,[37] and juxtapulmonary capillaries in the interstitium of the lungs[38] but not in the intrapulmonary circulation.[39] These sensors have generally been considered as mediating reflex changes in heart rate and systemic vascular resistance, through modulation of the sympathetic nervous system (SNS) and of ANP. This also appears to be true for the coronary baroceptor reflex described in anesthetized dogs, by which changes in coronary artery pressure lead to alterations in lumbar and renal sympathetic discharge[40] and a coronary artery response much slower than that of the carotid and aortic barocéptors.[40] However, some evidence, also in dogs, suggests that ventricular and pulmonary sensors may also detect changes in blood volume through increased left ventricular pressure that causes a reflex inhibition of plasma renin activity.[41,42]

SENSORS OF CARDIAC OUTPUT

The receptors described so far are situated in low-pressure sites where they sense the fullness of the circulation and are probably more important for defending against excessive volume expansion and the consequent congestive manifestations of cardiac failure. The arterial (high-pressure) sensors, on the other hand, are geared more toward detecting low cardiac output or systemic vascular resistance, which manifest as underfilling of the vascular tree (i.e., EABV depletion) and as signaling the kidneys to retain Na^+. These high-pressure sensors are found in the aortic arch, in the carotid sinus, and in the renal vessels.

Carotid and Aortic Baroceptors. Histologic and molecular analysis of the carotid baroreceptor has revealed a large content of elastic tissue in the tunica media, which makes the vessel wall highly distensible in response to changes in intraluminal pressure, thereby facilitating transmission of the stimulus intensity to sensory nerve terminals. A change in the mean arterial pressure induces depolarization of these sensory endings, which results in action potentials. Afferent signals from the baroreceptors are integrated in the nucleus tractus solitarius of the medulla oblongata,[43] which leads to reflex changes in both systemic and renal sympathetic nerve activity (RSNA) and, to a lesser degree, release of AVP. A role for endocannabinoids has been postulated in baroceptor reflex modulation. In this regard, a significant increase in the endocannabinoid anandamide in the nucleus tractus solitarius was observed after an increase in blood pressure. Also, anandamide microinjections into the nucleus tractus solitarius induced prolonged baroreflex inhibition of RSNA. These results, along with other studies, support the hypothesis that endogenous anandamide can modulate the baroreflex through cannabinoid CB_1 receptor activation within the nucleus tractus solitarius.[44] An important additional function of the carotid baroreceptors is to maintain adequate cerebral perfusion. The aortic baroreceptor appears to behave in a way similar to that of the carotid baroreceptor.

SENSORS OF ORGAN PERFUSION

Renal Sensors. The kidney not only is the major effector target responding to signals that indicate the need for adjustments in Na^+ excretion but also has a central role in the afferent sensing of volume homeostasis, by virtue of the local sympathetic innervation. However, despite considerable knowledge concerning the mechanisms of renal sensing of EABV, the molecular identity and exact cellular location of the renal sensor or sensors remain elusive.[45] The integral relationship between both afferent and efferent renal sympathetic activities and the central arterial barocéptors was highlighted by Kopp and colleagues.[46] They showed that a high-Na^+ diet increases afferent RSNA, which then decreases efferent RSNA and leads to natriuresis. Using dorsal rhizotomy to induce afferent renal denervation in rats maintained on a high-Na^+ diet, they demonstrated increased mean arterial pressure that was dependent on impaired arterial baroreflex suppression of efferent RSNA activity. Animals fed a normal-Na^+ diet displayed no changes in arterial baroceptor function. Kopp and colleagues concluded that arterial baroreflex function contributes to increased efferent RSNA, which, in the absence of intact afferent RSNA, would eventually lead to Na^+ retention and hypertension. The role of RSNA in Na^+ regulation is further discussed in the "Mechanisms: Renal Nerves and Sympathetic Nervous System" section.

An additional level of renal sensing depends on the close anatomic proximity of the sensor and effector limbs to one another: Volume changes may be sensed through alterations in both glomerular hemodynamics and renal interstitial pressure. These alterations result simultaneously in adjustments in physical forces governing tubular Na^+ handling (further discussed in the "Efferent Limb: Effector Mechanisms for Maintaining Effective Arterial Blood Volume" section).

The kidneys, along with other organs, have the ability to maintain constant blood flow and constant glomerular filtration rate (GFR) at varying arterial pressures. This phenomenon, known as *autoregulation,* operates over a wide range of renal perfusion pressures (RPP). Autoregulation of renal blood flow (RBF) occurs through three mechanisms: the myogenic response, tubuloglomerular feedback, and a third mechanism. In the myogenic response, changes in RPP are sensed by smooth muscle elements that serve as baroreceptors in the afferent glomerular arteriole and dynamically respond by adjusting transmural pressure and tension across the arteriolar wall.[47]

The second mechanism, tubuloglomerular feedback, is operated by the juxtaglomerular apparatus, which comprises the afferent arteriole and, to a lesser extent, the cells of the macula densa in the early distal tubule.[47-49] The juxtaglomerular apparatus is also important because of its involvement in the synthesis and release of renin.[48] The physiologic release of renin from the cells of the juxtaglomerular apparatus is controlled by three pathways, all of which are driven by EABV status. First, renin release is inversely related to RPP and directly related to intrarenal tissue pressure. When RPP falls below the autoregulatory range, renin release is further enhanced. Second, renin secretion is influenced by solute delivery to the macula densa. Increased NaCl delivery past the macula densa leads to inhibition of renin release, whereas a decrease has the opposite effect. Sensing at the macula densa is mediated by NaCl entry through the Na^+-K^+-$2Cl^-$ cotransporter (NKCC2),[50,51] which leads to alterations in intracellular Ca^{2+}, together with production of prostaglandin E_2 (PGE_2),[52,53] adenosine,[54] and, subsequently, renin release. Third, changes in renal nerve activity influence renin release. Renal nerve stimulation increases renin release through direct activation of β-adrenergic receptors on juxtaglomerular cells. This effect is independent of major changes in renal hemodynamics.[55,56] Sympathetic stimulation also affects intrarenal baroreceptor input, the composition of the fluid delivered to the macula densa, and the renal actions of angiotensin II, so that renal nerves may serve primarily to potentiate other regulatory signals.[55-57]

The nature of the third mechanism of RBF autoregulation is still unclear, but Seeliger and associates,[58] using a normotensive angiotensin II clamp in anesthetized rats, were able to abolish the resetting of autoregulation during incremental shaped RPP changes. Under control conditions, the initial tubuloglomerular feedback response was dilatory after total occlusions but constrictive after partial occlusions. The initial third mechanism response was a mirror image of tubuloglomerular feedback: it was constrictive after total occlusions but dilatory after partial occlusions. The angiotensin clamp suppressed the tubuloglomerular feedback and turned the initial third mechanism response after total occlusions into dilation. Seeliger and associates concluded that (1) pressure-dependent renin-angiotensin system (RAS) stimulation was a major factor behind hypotensive resetting of autoregulation; (2) tubuloglomerular feedback sensitivity depended strongly on pressure-dependent changes in RAS activity; (3) the third mechanism was modulated, but not mediated, by the RAS; and (4) the third mechanism acted as a counterbalance to tubuloglomerular feedback.[58] They proposed that their findings might be related to the connecting tubule glomerular feedback.[59-61] Tubuloglomerular feedback is discussed further in the "Integration of Changes in Glomerular Filtration Rate and Tubular Reabsorption" section.

Central Nervous System Sensors. Certain areas in the CNS appear to act as sensors to detect alterations in body salt balance. This was suggested originally by results of experiments in rats, in which intracerebral injection of hypertonic saline led to reduced renal nerve activity and natriuresis.[62,63] Subsequently, DiBona[64] showed that administration of angiotensin II into the cerebral ventricles and changes in dietary Na+ modulate baroreflex regulation of RSNA. Similarly, stimulation of neurons located in the paraventricular nucleus and in a region extending to the anteroventral third ventricle led to ANP release, inducing angiotensin II blockade and inhibition of salt and water intake. Conversely, disruption of these neurons, as well as of the median eminence or neural lobe, led to decreased ANP release and impaired response to volume expansion.[65] Overall, despite the substantial evidence for CNS sensing of ECF volume status, the exact nature, mode of operation, and relative importance of this aspect of sensing remains unclear.

Gastrointestinal Tract Sensors. Under normal physiologic conditions, Na+ and water reach the ECF by absorption in the gastrointestinal tract. Therefore, it is not surprising that sensing and regulatory mechanisms of ECF volume have been found in the GI tract itself. The evidence for this phenomenon comes from experiments that showed more rapid natriuresis after an oral salt load than after a similar intravenous load. Moreover, infusions of hypertonic saline into the portal vein led to greater natriuresis than similar infusions into the femoral vein. These findings were consistent with the presence of Na+-sensing mechanisms in the splanchnic or portal circulation, or both.[66] In fact, these mechanisms appear to be located primarily in the portal system and are probably important in the pathogenesis of the hepatorenal syndrome, discussed later.

Hepatoportal Receptors. The two main neural reflexes, referred to as the *hepatorenal* and *hepatointestinal* reflexes, originate from receptors in the hepatoportal region. They transduce portal plasma Na+ concentration into hepatic afferent nerve activity; before a measurable increase in systemic Na+ concentration occurs, the hepatointestinal reflex attenuates intestinal Na+ absorption via the vagus nerve, and the hepatorenal reflex augments Na+ excretion.[67-69] These reflexes have been observed both in rats and in rabbits, as well as in humans, and have been shown to be impaired in the chronic bile duct ligation model of cirrhosis and portal hypertension.[70] In addition, the hepatic artery shows significant autoregulatory capacity, dilating when perfusion pressure falls and constricting when pressure rises, thereby maintaining hepatic arterial blood flow over a wide range of perfusion pressures. Moreover, there is extensive crosstalk between the portal and systemic circulations. For example, when portal blood flow decreases, the hepatic artery dilates, which is indicative of the presence of a sensor in the hepatic artery, which responds to changes in the contribution of the portal vein to total hepatic blood flow (see review by Oliver and Verna[71]). Clues to the mechanism of hepatic autoregulation come from models of reduced portal venous blood flow and acute hepatic injury, in which reduced Na+ excretion was abolished by administration of an adenosine A1 receptor antagonist; thus, these receptors probably have a role in the hepatorenal reflex.[72,73]

The observation that intraportal infusion of bumetanide or furosemide suppresses the response of hepatic afferent nerve activity to intraportal hypertonic saline suggests that the NKCC2 may be involved in sensing portal Na+ concentration.[74] In addition to hepatoportal Na+-sensing chemoreceptors, the liver also contains mechanoreceptors (baroreceptors). Increased intrahepatic hydrostatic pressure has been shown to be associated with enhanced RSNA and renal Na+ retention in various experimental models.[75,76] For example, when increased intrahepatic pressure was induced by thoracic caval constriction in dogs, raising venous pressure led to positive Na+ balance that was inhibited by liver denervation.[75] A clinical model for increased intrahepatic pressure is the Budd-Chiari syndrome,[77] and it is in situations such as this that hepatic volume-sensing mechanisms probably play a role in renal Na+ retention (see "Specific Treatments Based on the Pathophysiology of Sodium Retention in Cirrhosis" section).

Intestinal Natriuretic Hormones: Guanylin Peptides. As described previously, the natriuretic response of the kidneys to a Na+ load is more rapid when the load is delivered orally than when the same load is administered intravenously.[55] The different responses are observed without accompanying differences in plasma aldosterone.[78] This observation led to the idea that the gut produced a substance that signaled the kidneys to excrete excess Na+. The discovery of the guanylin family of cGMP-regulating peptides, or "intestinal natriuretic hormones," has shed light on this phenomenon.[79,80] Of the four currently known guanylin peptides, guanylin and uroguanylin are the ones best studied. They are small (15 to 16 amino acids), heat-stable peptides with intramolecular disulfide bridges that share similarity with the bacterial heat-stable enterotoxins that cause traveler's diarrhea and are found in mammals, birds, and fish.[79]

Both guanylin and uroguanylin are synthesized as prepropeptides, primarily in the intestine. The former, produced mainly by the ileum through proximal colon, circulates as proguanylin; the latter, which is expressed principally in the jejunum, circulates in its active form (see Sindic and Schlatter[80] and references therein). A physiologically important difference between guanylin and uroguanylin lies in their sensitivity to proteases. Because of a tyrosine residue at the ninth amino acid, guanylin is sensitive to protease digestion in the kidneys, which leads to its inactivation, whereas uroguanylin can be locally activated by the same proteases.[79] After an oral salt load, guanylin and uroguanylin released in the intestine lead to increased intestinal secretion of Cl^-, HCO_3^-, and water and to inhibition of Na^+ absorption.

In the kidneys, Na^+, K^+, and water excretion is increased, without any change in RBF or GFR and independently of RAAS, AVP, or ANPs.[79] The signaling pathway of guanylin peptides in the intestine involves binding to and activation of the receptor guanylyl cyclase C (GC-C), one of the eight guanylyl cyclases.[80] GC-C is a transmembrane protein, 1050 to 1053 amino acids in length, that is present in the intestinal brush border. Propagation of the signal occurs through the second messenger cGMP, which inhibits Na^+/H^+ exchange and activates protein kinase G II and protein kinase A, which in turn activate the cystic fibrosis transmembrane conductance regulator (CFTR), leading to Cl^- secretion; CFTR then activates the Cl^-/HCO_3^- exchanger, which leads to HCO_3^- secretion.

The best evidence for a link between the gut and the kidneys comes from mice lacking the uroguanylin gene, which display an impaired natriuretic response to oral salt loading but not to intravenous NaCl infusion.[81] However, because plasma prouroguanylin levels do not rise but urinary uroguanylin levels do increase after a high-salt meal, locally released peptide by the kidneys could still play a role in uroguanylin-associated natriuresis.[82,83] In the kidneys, both GC-C–dependent and –independent signaling pathways for guanylin peptides exist, inasmuch as knockout of GC-C in mice does not affect the high-salt diet–induced increase in uroguanylin.[79] From experiments on cell lines and isolated tubules, it appears that uroguanylin acts on the proximal tubule and principal cells of the cortical collecting duct.

In proximal cell lines, guanylin peptides increase cGMP and decrease cyclic adenosine monophosphate (cAMP), which leads to inhibition of Na^+/H^+ exchange and Na^+-K^+-ATPase; such events are consistent with decreased Na^+ reabsorption in this segment (see Sindic and Schlatter[79] and references therein). Crosstalk between guanylin peptides and ANPs may also occur in the proximal tubule.[84] In the principal cell, uroguanylin activation of a G protein–coupled receptor results in phospholipase A_2–dependent inhibition of the renal outer medullary potassium (ROMK) channel, which leads to depolarization and a reduced driving force for Na^+ reabsorption.[79] There is also evidence that guanylin may cause cell shrinkage in the inner medullary collecting duct (IMCD), which is suggestive of water secretion from this segment and a role in water diuresis.[79] Together, these data are highly suggestive of a role at least for uroguanylin, as a natriuretic hormone, in adjusting U_{Na} excretion to balance the levels of NaCl absorbed via the gastrointestinal tract.[79,80] The importance of this system in the control of renal Na^+ excretion in humans awaits further clarification.

A final point is that although multiple receptors are clearly involved in regulation of EABV, their functions appear to be considerably redundant. For example, cardiac or renal denervation in nonhuman primates and chronic aldosterone administration do not significantly affect the maintenance of Na^+ balance.[85,86]

Efferent Limb: Effector Mechanisms for Maintaining Effective Arterial Blood Volume

The maintenance of Na^+ homeostasis is achieved by adjustment of renal Na^+ excretion according to the body's needs. Like the mechanisms sensing changes in EABV, the pathways that enable the required adjustments in renal Na^+ excretion are multiple. The adjustments are made by integrated changes in both GFR and tubular reabsorption, so that changes in one component lead to appropriate changes in the other in order to maintain Na^+ homeostasis. In addition, tubular reabsorption is regulated by local peritubular and luminal factors, as well as by neural and humoral mechanisms (Table 14-2).

Integration of Changes in Glomerular Filtration Rate and Tubular Reabsorption

In humans, normal GFR leads to the delivery of approximately 24,000 mmol of Na^+ per day for downstream processing by the tubules. More than 99% of the filtrate is reabsorbed; only a tiny amount escapes into the final urine. Therefore, it is clear that even minute changes in the relationship between filtered load and fraction of Na^+ absorbed can exert a profound cumulative influence on net Na^+ balance. However, even marked perturbations in GFR are not necessarily associated with drastic alterations in U_{Na} excretion; thus, overall Na^+ balance is usually preserved. Such preservation results from appropriate adjustments in two important protective mechanisms: tubuloglomerular feedback, in which changes in tubular fluid Na^+ inversely affect GFR, and glomerulotubular balance, whereby changes in tubular flow rate, resulting from changes in GFR, directly affect tubular reabsorption.[48,49,87]

TABLE 14-2 Major Renal Effector Mechanisms for Regulating Effective Arterial Blood Volume

Glomerular Filtration Rate and Tubular Reabsorption

Tubuloglomerular feedback
Glomerulotubular balance
    Peritubular capillary Starling forces
    Luminal composition
    Physical factors beyond proximal tubule
    Medullary hemodynamics (pressure natriuresis)

Neural Mechanisms

Sympathetic nervous system
Renal nerves

Humoral Mechanisms

Renin-angiotensin-aldosterone system
Vasopressin
Prostaglandins
Natriuretic peptides
Endothelium-derived factors
    Endothelins
    Nitric oxide
Others (see text)

TUBULOGLOMERULAR FEEDBACK

A remarkable feature of nephron architecture is that, after emerging from Bowman's capsule and descending deep into the medulla, each tubule returns to its parent glomerulus. Guyton and associates[88] envisioned a functional relationship between the tubule and glomerulus; this idea led to a wealth of experimental evidence supporting the existence of tubuloglomerular feedback (reviewed by Schnermann and Briggs[89]). Tubuloglomerular feedback operates by changes in tubular fluid Na^+ at the macula densa (the point of contact between the specialized tubular cells of the cortical thick ascending limb of Henle adjacent to the extraglomerular mesangium), which elicit adjustments in glomerular arteriolar resistance. The system is constructed as a negative feedback loop in which an increase in NaCl concentration leads to increases in afferent arteriolar resistance and a consequent fall in GFR. This, in turn, leads to an increase in proximal reabsorption and a reduction in distal delivery of solute. In that manner, NaCl delivery to the distal nephron is maintained within narrow limits.[89]

The complexities of tubuloglomerular feedback have been unraveled slowly, initially by elaborate micropuncture studies that clearly established the tubular-glomerular link and, subsequently, by imaging and electrophysiologic techniques in isolated perfused tubule/glomerulus preparations. With these techniques, investigators elucidated the detailed mechanisms of changes in epithelial function in response to luminal NaCl composition. However, the signaling mechanisms linking changes in tubular composition with altered glomerular arteriolar tone only much later became evident through experiments in gene-manipulated mice.[89] The primary detection mechanism of tubuloglomerular feedback appears to be uptake of salt by means of the NKCC2, located in the apical membrane of macula densa cells. The evidence comes from tubuloglomerular feedback inhibition by inhibitors of the cotransporter, furosemide and bumetanide (reviewed by Castrop[90]), and by deletions in mice of the A or B isoform of NKCC2, both of which are expressed in macula densa cells.[50,89] In fact, complete inactivation of the NKCC2 gene leads to the severe salt-losing phenotype of antenatal Bartter's syndrome.[91] Similarly, inhibition or deletion of the ROMK channel in mice abolishes tubuloglomerular feedback (see Schnermann and Briggs[89]).

The next step in the juxtaglomerular cascade is less clear. One possibility is direct coupling of NKCC2-dependent NaCl uptake to the mediation step. Results of studies in the isolated perfused rabbit juxtaglomerular apparatus have indicated depolarization, alkalinization, and various ionic compositional changes occur after increased NaCl uptake; thus, one or more of these changes could trigger the signal.[92] A second possibility is that signal propagation is the consequence of transcellular NaCl transport and Na^+-K^+-ATPase–dependent basolateral extrusion. Early studies of this mechanism, in which pharmacologic inhibition with ouabain was used, yielded inconsistent evidence; however, this was probably a result of ouabain resistance of the α_1-subunit, the main isoform in the kidneys. Only the much less abundant α_2-subunit is sensitive to cardiac glycosides, whereas there is no specific inhibitor of the α_1-subunit. This stumbling block appears to have been overcome by the use of double-knockout mice, in which the α_1-subunit was made sensitive and the α_2-subunit resistant to ouabain. Results of these studies have clearly

indicated an important role for Na^+-K^+-ATPase in supporting tubuloglomerular feedback and that adenosine triphosphate (ATP) consumption is required for tubuloglomerular feedback (see Schnermann and Briggs[89]).

There is strong evidence that ATP release and degradation, rather than use, may be the link in the chain connecting NaCl changes in the macula densa with alteration of glomerular arteriolar tone. According to the current working model, after NaCl uptake and transcellular transport, ATP is released from macula densa cells and undergoes stepwise hydrolysis and dephosphorylation by ecto-ATPases and nucleotidases, to adenosine diphosphate, adenosine monophosphate, and then adenosine, which, in a paracrine manner, causes A_1 adenosine receptor–dependent afferent arteriolar constriction. Although the evidence for ATP breakdown is as yet incomplete, that for the effects of adenosine as a mediator of tubuloglomerular feedback is very strong. For example, isolated perfused mouse afferent arterioles exposed to adenosine display vigorous vasoconstriction, an effect not seen in A_1 adenosine receptor–deficient mice.[93,94] This effect is mediated by G_i-dependent activation of phospholipase C, release of Ca^{2+} from intracellular stores, and subsequent entry of Ca^{2+} through L-type Ca^{2+} channels.[93,95] Of particular interest is the fact that vasodilatory A_2 adenosine receptor is more abundant than the A_1 adenosine receptor in the renal vasculature, and continuous exogenous application of adenosine to mouse kidneys is indeed vasodilatory.[96] However, the generation of adenosine in the confines of the juxtaglomerular interstitium and its exclusive delivery to the afferent arteriole, where A_1 adenosine receptor expression predominates, ensures the appropriate response for tubuloglomerular feedback.

Other factors appear to be involved in tubuloglomerular feedback, both co-constrictors and modulators. Angiotensin II has been shown to act as an important cofactor in the vasoconstrictive action of adenosine. In this regard, deletions of the angiotensin II receptor or angiotensin converting enzyme (ACE) in mice abolished tubuloglomerular feedback. The effect may result from nonresponsiveness to adenosine in the absence of an intact RAS (reviewed by Schnermann and Briggs[89]). The high levels of neuronal nitric oxide synthase (nNOS, or NOS1) expression in macula densa cells are indicative of a role for nitric oxide in tubuloglomerular feedback.[97] Nitric oxide is thought to counterbalance angiotensin II–induced efferent arteriolar vasoconstriction and to modulate renin secretion by the juxtaglomerular apparatus.[98,99] Consistent with this idea is the finding that chronic absence of functional nNOS in macula densa cells is associated with enhanced vasoconstriction in the subnormal flow range, probably as a result of proportional increases in preglomerular and postglomerular tone. In addition, increased delivery of fluid to the macula densa induces nitric oxide release from these cells (see Patzak and Persson[98] and references therein).

Inhibition of the nitric oxide system by nonselective blockers of nitric oxide synthase (NOS) results in an exaggerated tubuloglomerular feedback response that leads to even further renal vasoconstriction, Na^+ and water retention, and arterial hypertension.[99] Also, tubuloglomerular feedback responses are absent in mice with concurrent deficiencies in nNOS and A_1 adenosine receptor, which implies that nNOS deficiency does not overcome deficient A_1 adenosine receptor signaling. Moreover, nitric oxide modulation of tubuloglomerular feedback can be mediated by ecto 5′-nucleotidase, the enzyme responsible for adenine formation.[100] Together, these data suggest that A_1 adenosine receptor signaling is primary and that nNOS plays a modulatory role in tubuloglomerular feedback.[89]

Afferent arteriolar A_1 adenosine receptor may not be the sole mediator of tubuloglomerular feedback. Activation by adenosine of A_2 adenosine receptor has been shown to dilate mouse cortical efferent receptors. The effect appeared to be mediated by the low-affinity A_{2b} adenosine receptor.[96] It is remarkable that this highly specific effect occurred despite the presence of A_1 adenosine receptor in the efferent arteriole. Apparently, therefore, the relative abundance of the various adenosine receptor subtypes in afferent and efferent arterioles ultimately allows fine-tuning of tubuloglomerular feedback by concerted changes in glomerular vascular tone.[101] Connexin 40, which plays a predominant role in the formation of gap junctions in the vasculature, also participates in the autoregulation of RBF and, therefore in tubuloglomerular feedback. Connexin-40–knockout mice displayed impaired steady-state autoregulation to a sudden-step increase in RPP. A marked reduction in tubuloglomerular feedback in connexin 40–knockout mice was thought to be responsible. The authors of this work showed that connexin 40 mediated RBF autoregulation occurred by transducing tubuloglomerular feedback–mediated signals to the afferent arteriole, independently of nitric oxide.[102]

A final point in the complexity of tubuloglomerular feedback is that there is evidence for three sites in addition to the macula densa that are in contact with the efferent arteriole: the terminal cortical thick ascending limb of Henle, the early distal tubule, and the connecting tubule. In particular, perimacular cells and oscillatory cells of the early distal tubule may be involved in the intracellular Ca^{2+} signaling required for adenosine-induced afferent vasoconstriction. On the other hand, the effect of the connecting tubule on the afferent arteriolar tone appears to be modulatory in that elevations in luminal NaCl, and cellular Na^+ entry via the epithelial sodium channel (ENaC), lead to afferent arteriolar dilation through the release of prostaglandins and epoxyeicosatrienoic acids.[59,103]

GLOMERULOTUBULAR BALANCE

Several factors are involved in the phenomenon of glomerulotubular balance, which describes the ability of proximal tubular reabsorption to adapt proportionally to the changes in filtered load.

Peritubular Capillary Starling Forces. Researchers have studied the natriuretic response to ECF volume expansion by examining the effects of acute infusions of saline or albumin in experimental animals and in humans. Therefore, their relevance to chronic regulation of ECF sodium balance is questionable. Nevertheless, the findings from these studies led to the notion that alterations in hydraulic and oncotic pressures (Starling forces) in the peritubular capillary play an important role in the regulation of Na^+ and water transport, especially in the proximal nephron. The peritubular capillary network is anatomically connected in series with the glomerular capillary bed of cortical glomeruli through the efferent arteriole; thus, changes in the physical determinants of GFR critically influence Starling forces in the peritubular capillaries.

Of importance is that about 10% of glomeruli, mainly those at the corticomedullary junction, are connected in series to the vasa recta of the medulla. In the proximal tubule—whose peritubular capillaries receive 90% of blood flow from glomeruli—the relation of hydraulic and oncotic driving forces to the transcapillary fluid flux is given by the Starling relationship

$$\text{Rate}_{abs} = K_r[(\pi_c - \pi_i) - (P_c - P_i)]$$

in which Rate_{abs} is the absolute rate of reabsorption of proximal tubule absorbate by the peritubular capillary; K_r is the capillary reabsorption coefficient (the product of capillary hydraulic conductivity and absorptive surface area); π_c and P_c are the local capillary colloid osmotic (oncotic) and hydraulic pressures, respectively; and π_i and P_i are the corresponding interstitial pressures. Whereas π_i and P_c oppose fluid absorption, π_c and P_i tend to favor uptake of reabsorbate. By simultaneously determining these driving forces, investigators can analyze the net pressure favoring fluid absorption or filtration. As a consequence of the anatomic relationship of the postglomerular efferent arteriole to the peritubular capillary, the hydraulic pressure is significantly lower in the peritubular capillary than in the glomerular capillary. The function of the efferent arteriole as a resistance vessel contributes to a decrease in hydraulic pressure between the glomerulus and the peritubular capillary.

Also, because the peritubular capillary receives blood from the glomerulus, the plasma oncotic pressure is high at the outset as a result of prior filtration of protein-free fluid. It follows that the greater the GFR is in relation to plasma flow rate, the greater the protein concentration in the efferent arteriolar plasma is and the lower the hydraulic pressure in the proximal peritubule capillary is; as a consequence, proximal fluid reabsorption is enhanced (Figure 14-2). Therefore, in contradistinction to the glomerular and peripheral capillary, the peritubular capillary is characterized by high values of $\pi_c - \pi_i$ that greatly exceed $P_c - P_i$, which results in net reabsorption of fluid.

The ratio of GFR to RBF defines the filtration fraction. The relationship of proximal reabsorption to filtration fraction may contribute to Na^+-retaining and edema-forming states, such as heart failure (see Figure 14-2). A series of in vivo micropuncture and microperfusion studies[104-107] yielded compelling experimental evidence for the relationship between proximal peritubular Starling forces and proximal fluid reabsorption. As a result of these studies, as well as studies in which the isolated perfused tubule model was used,[108] the role of peritubular forces in the setting of increased ECF volume can be summarized as follows:

1. Acute saline expansion results in dilution of plasma proteins and reduction in efferent arteriolar oncotic pressure. Single-nephron glomerular filtration rate (SNGFR) and peritubular P_c may be increased as well, but the decrease in peritubular π_c by itself results in a decreased net peritubular capillary reabsorptive force and decreased Rate_{abs}. Glomerulotubular balance is disrupted because Rate_{abs} falls despite the tendency for SNGFR to rise, and this development allows the excess Na^+ to be excreted and plasma volume to be restored.

2. Iso-oncotic plasma infusions tend to raise SNGFR and peritubular P_c but lead to relative constancy of efferent arteriolar oncotic pressure. Rate_{abs} may therefore decrease slightly, resulting in less disruption of glomerulotubular balance and natriuresis of lesser magnitude than that observed with saline expansion.

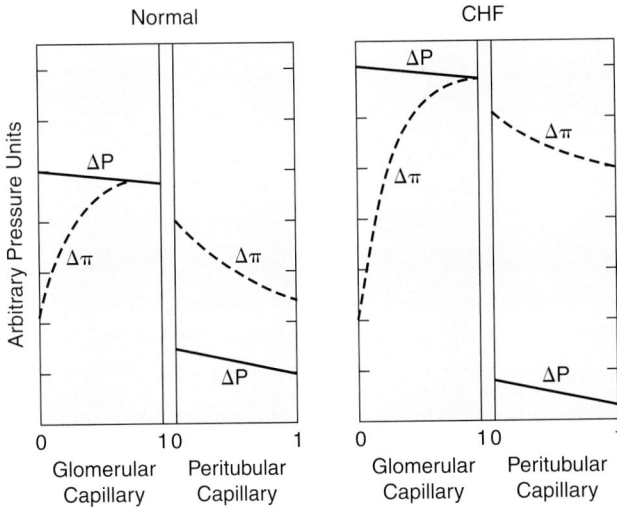

Normal   CHF

DIMENSIONLESS DISTANCES ALONG CAPILLARY SEGMENTS

FIGURE 14-2 The glomerular and peritubular microcirculations. **Left,** Approximate transcapillary pressure profiles for the glomerular and peritubular capillaries in normal humans. Vessel lengths are given in normalized, nondimensional terms, with 0 being the most proximal portion of the capillary bed and 1 the most distal portion. Thus, for the glomerulus, 0 corresponds to the afferent arteriolar end of the capillary bed, and 1 corresponds to the efferent arteriolar end. The transcapillary hydraulic pressure difference (ΔP) is relatively constant with distance along the glomerular capillary, and the net driving force for ultrafiltration ($\Delta P - \Delta \pi$) diminishes primarily as a consequence of the increase in the opposing colloid osmotic pressure difference ($\Delta \pi$), the latter resulting from the formation of an essentially protein-free ultrafiltrate. As a result of the drop in pressure along the efferent arteriole, the net driving pressure in the peritubular capillaries ($\Delta P - \Delta \pi$, in which $\Delta \pi$ is the change in transcapillary oncotic pressure) becomes negative, favoring reabsorption. **Right,** Hemodynamic alterations in the renal microcirculation in congestive heart failure (HF). The fall in renal plasma flow rate (RPF) in heart failure is associated with a compensatory increase in ΔP for the glomerular capillary, which is conducive to a greater-than-normal rise in the plasma protein concentration and, hence, in $\Delta \pi$ along the glomerular capillary. This increase in $\Delta \pi$ by the distal end of the glomerular capillary also translates to an increase in $\Delta \pi$ in the peritubular capillaries, resulting in increased net driving pressure for enhanced proximal tubule fluid absorption, believed to take place in heart failure. The increased peritubular capillary absorptive force in heart failure also probably results from the decline in ΔP, a presumed consequence of the rise in renal vascular resistance. (From Humes HD, Gottlieb M, Brenner BM: *The kidney in congestive heart failure: contemporary issues in nephrology,* vol 1, New York, 1978, Churchill Livingstone, pp 51-72.)

3. Hyperoncotic expansion usually increases both SNGFR (because of volume expansion) and efferent arteriolar oncotic pressure; as a result, Rate$_{abs}$ is enhanced. Glomerulotubular balance therefore tends to be better preserved than with iso-oncotic plasma or saline expansion.
4. Changes in π_i can directly alter proximal tubular reabsorption, independently of the peritubular capillary bed.

The alterations in proximal peritubular Starling forces that modulate fluid and electrolyte movements across the peritubular basement membrane into the surrounding capillary bed appear to be accompanied by corresponding changes in the structure of the peritubular interstitial compartment. Ultrastructural data from rats suggest that the peritubular capillary wall is in tight apposition to the tubule basement membrane for about 60% of the tubule basolateral surface. However, irregularly shaped wide portions of peritubular interstitium also exist over about 40% of the tubule basolateral surface;

thus, a major portion of reabsorbed fluid has to cross a true interstitial space before entering the peritubular capillaries. Alterations in the physical properties of the interstitial compartment could conceivably modulate either passive or active components of net fluid transport in the proximal tubule. Starling forces in the peritubular capillary are thought to regulate the rate of volume entry from the peritubular interstitium into the capillary. Any change in this rate of flux could lead to changes in interstitial pressure that secondarily modify proximal tubule solute transport. This formulation could explain why experimental maneuvers known to raise P_i (e.g., infusion of renal vasodilators, renal venous constriction, renal lymph ligation) were associated with a natriuretic response, whereas the opposite effect was obtained with renal decapsulation, which lowers P_i (see also the "Medullary Hemodynamics and Interstitial Pressure in the Control of Na$^+$ Excretion: Pressure Natriuresis" section).

Because of the relatively high permeability of the proximal tubule, changes in interstitial Starling forces are likely to be transduced mainly through alterations in passive bidirectional paracellular flux through the tight junctions.[109] The claudin family of adhesion molecules has clearly proved that the tight junction is a dynamic, multifunctional complex that may be amenable to physiologic regulation by cellular second messengers or in pathologic states.[110-112] Among the 24 known mammalian claudin family members, at least three—claudin-2, claudin-10, and claudin-11—are located in the proximal nephron of the mouse, and others are located at more distal nephron sites.[111,113] Claudin-2 is selectively expressed in the proximal nephron.[114] However, the exact role of the claudin family members in the influence of Starling forces on fluid reabsorption remains to be elucidated.

Luminal Composition. In addition to peritubular capillary and interstitial Starling forces, luminal factors may also play a role in the regulation of proximal tubule transport. For example, Romano and colleagues[115] showed that glomerulotubular balance could be fully expressed even when the native peritubular environment was kept constant while the rate of perfusion of proximal tubular segments with native tubular fluid was changed. Moreover, studies in isolated perfused rabbit proximal tubules indicated that the presence of a transtubular anion gradient, normally present in the late portion of the proximal nephron, was necessary for the flow dependence to occur.[116] A potential mechanism for modulation of proximal Na$^+$ reabsorption in response to changes in filtered load depends on the close coupling of Na$^+$ transport with the cotransport of glucose, amino acids, and other organic solutes. The increased delivery of organic solutes that accompanies increases in GFR, together with the preferential reabsorption of Na$^+$ with bicarbonate in the early proximal tubule, would lead to increased delivery of both Cl$^-$ and organic solutes to the late proximal tubule. The resulting transtubular anion gradient would then facilitate the "passive" reabsorption of both the organic solutes and NaCl in this segment, but, overall, net reabsorption would be reduced.

In summary, regardless of the exact mechanism, ECF volume expansion impairs the integrity of glomerulotubular balance, thus allowing increased delivery of salt and fluid to more distal parts of the nephron. The major factors acting on the proximal nephron during a decrease in ECF and effective arterial circulating volume are outlined schematically in Figure 14-3.

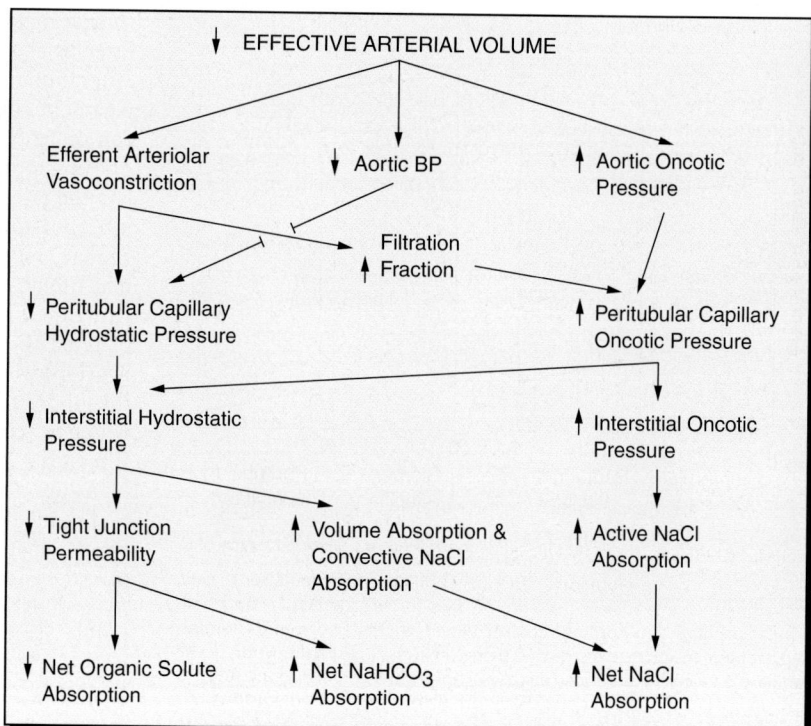

FIGURE 14-3 Effects of hemodynamic changes on proximal tubule solute transport. (From Seldin DW, Preisig PA, Alpern RJ: Regulation of proximal reabsorption by effective arterial blood volume, *Semin Nephrol* 11:212-219, 1991.)

Physical Factors Beyond the Proximal Tubule. Because the final urinary excretion of Na^+, in response to volume expansion or depletion, can be dissociated from the amount delivered out of the superficial proximal nephron, more distal or deeper segments of the nephron contribute to the modulation of Na^+ and water excretion. Several sites along the nephron, such as the loop of Henle, distal nephron, and cortical and papillary collecting ducts, were found (by micropuncture and microcatheterization techniques) to increase or decrease the rate of Na^+ reabsorption in response to enhanced delivery from early segments of the nephron. However, direct evidence that these transport processes are mediated by changes in Starling forces per se is lacking. Jamison and associates[117] provided a detailed review of these experiments.

In summary, the intrarenal control of Na^+ excretion can be generalized as follows: If ECF volume is held relatively constant, an increase in GFR leads to little or no increase in salt excretion because of a close coupling between the GFR and the intrarenal physical forces acting at the peritubular capillary to control $Rate_{abs}$. In addition, changes in the filtered load of small organic solutes, and perhaps other as-yet-uncharacterized glomerulus-borne substances in tubule fluid, may influence $Rate_{abs}$. To the extent that changes, if any, in the load of Na^+ delivered to more distal segments also occur, parallel changes in distal reabsorptive rates also occur, to ensure a high degree of glomerulotubular balance for the kidneys as a whole. Conversely, ECF volume expansion leads to large increases in Na^+ excretion even in the presence of reduced GFR. Changes in Na^+ reabsorption in the proximal tubule alone cannot account for this natriuresis of volume expansion, and a number of mechanisms for suppressing renal Na^+ reabsorption at more distal sites have been invoked.

Medullary Hemodynamics and Interstitial Pressure in the Control of Sodium Excretion: Pressure Natriuresis. The idea that changes in renal medullary hemodynamics may be involved in the natriuresis evoked by volume expansion was

initially proposed in the 1960s by Earley and Friedler.[118,119] According to their theory, ECF volume expansion results in an increase in RPP that is transmitted as an increase in medullary plasma flow and leads to a subsequent loss of medullary hypertonicity, elimination of the medullary osmotic gradient ("medullary washout"), and, thereby, decreased water reabsorption in the thin descending loop of Henle. The decrease in water reabsorption in the thin descending limb lowers the Na^+ concentration in the fluid entering the ascending loop of Henle, thus decreasing the transepithelial driving force for salt transport in this nephron segment. At the same time, a similar mechanism was proposed to explain the natriuresis after elevations in systemic blood pressure, a phenomenon termed *pressure natriuresis.*

The concept that alterations in the solute composition of the renal medulla and papilla play a key role in regulation of Na^+ transport gained significant support in the 1970s and 1980s, when results of micropuncture studies suggested that volume expansion, renal vasodilation, and increased RPP produced a greater inhibition of salt reabsorption in the loops of Henle within juxtamedullary nephrons than in those within superficial nephrons. Measurement of medullary plasma flow with laser Doppler flowmetry and videomicroscopy in experimental animals provided strong evidence for the redistribution of intrarenal blood flow toward the medulla after volume expansion and renal vasodilation. These studies were of particular interest with regard to the role of medullary hemodynamics in the control of Na^+ excretion, especially in the context of pressure natriuresis.[120-124]

The importance of pressure natriuresis in the long-term control of arterial blood pressure and ECF volume regulation was first recognized by Hall and associates.[123,124] According to this view, the kidneys alter Na^+ excretion in response to changes in arterial blood pressure. For instance, an increase in RPP results in a concomitant increase in Na^+ excretion, thereby decreasing circulating blood volume and restoring arterial pressure. The coupling between arterial pressure and Na⁺ excretion was found to occur in the setting of preserved cortical autoregulation (i.e., in the absence of changes in total RBF, GFR, or filtered load of Na⁺). This led to the suggestion that the pressure natriuresis mechanism was triggered by changes in medullary circulation.[118,121,125-127] Laser Doppler flowmetry and servo-null measurements of capillary pressure in volume-expanded rats revealed that papillary blood flow was directly related to RPP over a wide range of pressures studied.

As mentioned earlier, increase in medullary plasma flow might lead to medullary "washout" with a consequent reduction in the driving force for Na⁺ reabsorption in the ascending loop of Henle, particularly in the deep nephrons. In addition, the increase in medullary perfusion may be associated with a rise in P_i. In fact, increasing P_i by ECF volume expansion, by infusion of renal vasodilatory agents, by long-term mineralocorticoid escape, or by hilar lymph ligation resulted in a significant increase in Na⁺ excretion.[128,129] Moreover, prevention of the increase in P_i by removal of the renal capsule significantly attenuated, but did not completely block, the natriuretic response to elevations in RPP. Thus, as depicted in Figure 14-4, elevation in RPP is associated with an increase in medullary plasma flow and increased vasa recta capillary pressure, which results in an increase in medullary P_i. This increase of P_i is thought to be transmitted to the renal cortex in the encapsulated kidneys and to provide a signal that inhibits Na⁺ reabsorption along the nephron. In that regard, the renal medulla may be viewed as a sensor that can detect changes in RPP and initiate the pressure natriuresis mechanism.

In order to explain how changes in systemic blood pressure are transmitted to the medulla in the presence of efficient RBF and GFR autoregulation, it has been suggested that shunt pathways connect preglomerular vessels of juxtamedullary

nephrons directly to the postglomerular capillaries of the vasa recta.[118] Alternatively, autoregulation of RBF might lead to increased shear stress in the preglomerular vasculature, triggering the release of nitric oxide and perhaps cytochrome P450 products of arachidonic acid metabolism (see later discussion), thereby driving the cascade of events that inhibit Na⁺ reabsorption.[130,131] The mechanisms by which changes in P_i and U_{Na} excretion decrease tubular Na⁺ reabsorption, as well as the nephron sites responding to the alterations in P_i, have not been fully clarified.[128] As pointed out earlier, it was postulated that elevations in P_i may increase passive backleak or the paracellular pathway hydraulic conductivity, with a resultant increase in back flux of Na⁺ through the paracellular pathways.[129] However, the absolute changes in P_i, in the range of 3 to 8 mm Hg in response to increments of about 50 to 90 mm Hg in RPP, are probably not sufficient to account for the decrease in tubular Na⁺ reabsorption even in the proximal tubule, the nephron segment with the highest transepithelial hydraulic conductivity.[120] Nevertheless, considerable evidence from micropuncture studies indicates that pressure natriuresis is associated with significant changes in proximal fluid reabsorption particularly in deep nephrons, with enhanced delivery to the loop of Henle, alterations in the pars recta and thin descending limb.[129]

Pressure-induced changes in tubular reabsorption may also occur in more distal parts of the nephron, such as the ascending loop of Henle, distal nephron, and collecting duct.[132] Therefore, elevations in RPP can affect tubular Na⁺ reabsorption by both proximal and distal mechanisms. The finding that small changes in P_i are associated with significant alterations in tubular Na⁺ reabsorption led to the hypothesis that the changes in P_i may be amplified by various hemodynamic, hormonal, and paracrine factors.[115,118,121,125,129] Specifically, the phenomenon of pressure natriuresis is demonstrable particularly in states of volume expansion and renal vasodilation and is significantly attenuated in states of volume depletion.[129] Among a variety of hormonal and paracrine systems that have been documented to play a role in modulating pressure natriuresis, changes in the activity of the RAAS and local production of prostaglandins within the kidneys have received considerable attention.[129] Removal of the influence of angiotensin II, by either ACE inhibitors or angiotensin II type 1 (AT₁) receptor antagonists, potentiates the pressure natriuretic response, and inhibitors of cyclooxygenase attenuate it.[129,133] Of importance, however, is that pharmacologic blockade of these systems only attenuates but does not completely eliminate the pressure natriuresis response, which indicates that they act as modulators and not as mediators of the phenomenon.

The importance of endothelium-derived factors in the regulation of renal circulatory and excretory function has been recognized. Evidence suggests that endothelium-derived nitric oxide and P-450 eicosanoids play a role in the mechanism of pressure natriuresis.[120,125,130,131,134-136] Nitric oxide, generated in large amounts in the renal medulla, appears to play a critical role in the regulation of medullary blood flow and Na⁺ excretion.[126,127] Several studies showed that inhibition of intrarenal nitric oxide production can reduce Na⁺ excretion and markedly suppress the pressure natriuretic response, whereas administration of a nitric oxide precursor improves transmission of perfusion pressure into the renal interstitium and normalizes the defect in pressure natriuresis

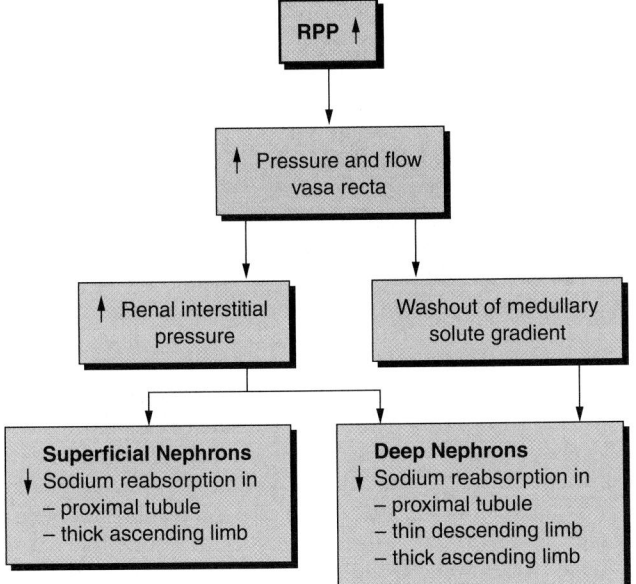

FIGURE 14-4 Role of the renal medulla in modulating tubular reabsorption of sodium in response to changes in renal perfusion pressure (RPP). (Adapted from Cowley AW Jr: Role of the renal medulla in volume and arterial pressure regulation, *Am J Physiol* 273:R1-R15, 1997.)

response in Dahl salt-sensitive rats.[120,132,137,138] Likewise, a positive correlation between urinary excretion of nitrites and nitrates (metabolites of nitric oxide) and changes in renal arterial pressure or U_{Na} excretion were observed both in dogs[139] and in rats.[134] Hydrogen peroxide (H_2O_2) has also been invoked in the mediation of RPP-induced changes in outer medullary blood flow and natriuresis. The response appears to be localized to the medullary thick ascending limb of Henle, in contrast to the nitric oxide effect, which occurs in the vasa recta.[134] Other factors involved in the regulation of medullary blood flow include superoxide and heme oxygenase, both of which are released in the renal medulla in response to increased RPP.[135,140]

The cytochrome P450 eicosanoids, particularly 20-hydroxyeicosatetraenoic acid (20-HETE), are additional endothelium-derived factors that may participate in the mechanism of pressure natriuresis.[130,131,141] These agents play an important role in the regulation of renal Na^+ transport and of renal and systemic hemodynamics.[142] These observations support the hypothesis that alterations in the production of renal nitric oxide, reactive oxygen species, and eicosanoids may be involved in mediation of the pressure-induced natriuretic response.

It is tempting to speculate that acute elevations in RPP in the autoregulatory range result in increased blood flow velocity and shear stress, leading to increased endothelial release of nitric oxide and reactive oxygen species. Enhanced renal production of these molecules may increase U_{Na} excretion either by acting directly on tubular Na^+ reabsorption or through its vasodilatory effect on renal vasculature. ATP is another paracrine factor that is involved in pressure natriuresis. ATP is an important regulator of renal salt and water homeostasis. ATP release appears to be mediated by connexin 30, inasmuch as release in response to increased tubular flow or hypotonicity was abolished in connexin 30–deficient mice. Moreover, increased arterial pressure, induced by ligation of the distal aorta, led to diuresis and natriuresis in normal mice, but the response was attenuated in connexin 30–knockout mice. These data imply that mechanosensitive connexin 30 hemichannels play an integral role in pressure natriuresis by releasing ATP into the tubular fluid, thereby inhibiting salt and water reabsorption.[143] Finally, Magyar and colleagues[144] reported that, in response to an increase in RPP, the apical Na^+/H^+ exchanger in the proximal tubules may be redistributed out of the brush border into intracellular compartments. Concomitantly, basolateral Na^+-K^+-ATPase activity decreased significantly. The mechanisms of these cellular events have not been fully elucidated, but they may be related directly to changes in P_i or to changes in the intrarenal paracrine agents described previously.

A major assumption of the pressure natriuresis theory is that changes in systemic and RPP mediate the natriuretic response by the kidneys. As pointed out in comprehensive reviews, acute regulatory changes in renal salt excretion may occur without measurable elevation in arterial blood pressure.[33,145-147] Of interest is that in many of these studies, the natriuresis was accompanied by a decrease in the activity of the RAAS without changes in plasma ANP levels.[33,58,145-147] Thus, whereas increases in arterial blood pressure can drive renal Na^+ excretion, other "pressure-independent" control mechanisms must also operate to mediate the "volume natriuresis."[33]

NEURAL MECHANISMS: RENAL NERVES AND SYMPATHETIC NERVOUS SYSTEM

Extensive autonomic innervation of the kidneys makes an important contribution to the physiologic regulation of all aspects of renal function.[55,148] Sympathetic nerves, predominantly adrenergic, have been observed at all segments of the renal vasculature and tubule.[149] Adrenergic nerve endings reach vascular smooth muscle cells and mesangial cells, cells of the juxtaglomerular apparatus, and all segments of the tubule: proximal, loop of Henle, and distal. Only the basolateral membrane separates the nerve endings from the tubular cells. Initial studies determined that the greatest innervation was found in the renal vasculature, mostly at the level of the afferent arterioles, followed by the efferent arterioles and outer medullary descending vasa recta.[150] However, high-density tubular innervation was found in the ascending limb of the loop of Henle, and the lowest density was observed in the collecting duct, inner medullary vascular elements, and papilla.[57,151] The magnitude of the tubular response to renal nerve activation may thus be proportional to the differential density of innervation. In accordance with these anatomic observations, stimulation of the renal nerve results in vasoconstriction of afferent and efferent arterioles[148,151] that is mediated by the activation of postjunctional α_1-adrenoreceptors.[152]

The presence of high-affinity adrenergic receptors in the nephron is also indicative of a significant role of the renal nerves in tubular function. The α_1-adrenergic receptors and most of the α_2-adrenergic receptors are localized in the basolateral membranes of the proximal tubule.[153] In the rat, β-adrenoreceptors have been found in the cortical thick ascending limb of Henle and are subtyped as β_1-adrenoceptors.[154] The predominant neurotransmitters in renal sympathetic nerves are noradrenaline and, to a lesser extent, dopamine and acetylcholine.[151] There is abundant evidence that changes in the activity of the renal sympathetic nerve play an important role in controlling body fluid homeostasis and blood pressure.[55,148,149] Renal sympathetic nerve activity can influence renal function and Na^+ excretion through several mechanisms: (1) changes in renal and glomerular hemodynamics, (2) effect on renin release from juxtaglomerular cells with increased formation of angiotensin II, and (3) direct effect on renal tubular fluid and electrolyte reabsorption.[55] Graded direct electrical stimulation of renal nerves produces frequency-dependent changes in RBF and GFR, reabsorption of renal tubular Na^+ and water, and secretion of renin.[55,149] The lowest frequency (0.5 to 1.0 Hz) stimulates renin secretion, and frequencies of 1.0 to 2.5 Hz increase renal tubule Na^+ and water reabsorption. Increasing the frequency of stimulation to 2.5 Hz and higher results in decreases in RBF and GFR.[55,148]

The decrease in SNGFR in response to enhanced renal nerve activity has been attributed to a combination of increases in both afferent and efferent glomerular resistance, the change in glomerular capillary hydrostatic pressure (ΔP)—in this case, a decrease—and a decrease in the glomerular ultrafiltration coefficient (K_f).[148,149] In Munich-Wistar rats, micropuncture experiments before and after renal nerve stimulation at different frequencies revealed that the effector loci for vasomotor control by renal nerves were in the afferent and efferent arteriole. In addition, although urine flow and Na^+ excretion declined with renal nerve stimulation, there was no change in absolute proximal fluid reabsorption rate, which suggests that reabsorption is increased in the more distal segments of the nephron.

Results of studies of the response of the kidneys to reflex activation of renal nerves also indicate that the SNS has a role in regulating renal hemodynamic function and Na^+ excretion. In rats receiving diets with different Na^+ levels, DiBona and Kopp[148] measured renal nerve activity in response to isotonic saline volume expansion and furosemide-induced volume contraction. A low-Na^+ diet resulted in a reduction in right atrial pressure and an increase in renal nerve activity. The magnitude of the increase in renal nerve activity was approximately 20% for each 1–mm Hg fall in atrial pressure. The high-Na^+ diet resulted in quantitatively similar changes in the opposite direction: that is, an increase in right atrial pressure and a reduction in renal nerve activity. Other studies in conscious animals in which researchers used maneuvers such as HWI and left atrial balloon inflation (reviewed by DiBona[55]) yielded evidence of the importance of reflex regulation of renal nerve activity.

Collectively, these studies demonstrated the reciprocal relationship between ECF volume and renal nerve activity, which is consistent with the role of central cardiopulmonary mechanoreceptors governing renal nerve activity. Moreover, the contribution of efferent renal nerve activity is of greater significance during conditions of dietary Na^+ restriction, when the need for renal Na^+ conservation is maximal. When this linkage between the renal SNS and the excretory renal function is defective, abnormalities in the regulation of ECF volume and blood pressure may develop.[151,155] Several studies in which the response of denervated kidneys to various physiologic maneuvers was examined also yielded evidence that renal nerves played a role in regulating renal hemodynamic function and Na^+ excretion.

Early studies showed that acute denervation of the kidneys is associated with increased urine flow and Na^+ excretion.[148] Micropuncture techniques showed that in euvolemic animals, elimination of renal innervation does not alter any of the determinants of SNGFR, which indicates that renal nerves contribute little to the vasomotor tone of normal animals under baseline physiologic conditions. However, absolute proximal reabsorption was significantly reduced, in the absence of changes in peritubular capillary oncotic pressure, hydraulic pressure, and renal interstitial pressure.[148] The decrease in tubular electrolyte and water reabsorption after renal denervation was also observed in the loop of Henle and segments of the distal nephron.[148]

In another micropuncture study in control rats and in rats with experimentally induced heart failure or acute volume depletion, measurements obtained before and after denervation demonstrated that denervation resulted in diuresis and natriuresis in normal rats but failed to alter any of the parameters of renal cortical microcirculation (reviewed by DiBona and Kopp[148]). In rats with heart failure, in contrast, denervation caused both an amelioration of renal vasoconstriction by decreasing afferent and efferent arteriolar resistance and, again, natriuresis. This study indicates that in situations in which efferent neural tone is heightened above baseline level, renal nerve activity may profoundly influence renal circulatory dynamics. However, although the basal level of renal nerve activity in normal rats or conscious animals is apparently insufficient to influence renal hemodynamics, it is sufficient to exert a tonic stimulation on renal tubular epithelial Na^+ reabsorption and renin release.[148] Classical studies, in which guanethidine was given to achieve autonomic blockade or in

patients with idiopathic autonomic insufficiency, revealed that intact adrenergic innervation is required for the normal renal adaptive response to dietary Na^+ restriction.[156]

More direct examination of efferent RSNA in humans has been made possible by the measurement of renal norepinephrine spillover to elucidate the kinetics of norepinephrine release. Friberg and associates[157] determined that in normal subjects, a low-Na^+ diet resulted in a fall in U_{Na} excretion and an increase in norepinephrine spillover, with no change in cardiac norepinephrine uptake; these findings support the concept of a true increase of efferent renal nerve activity secondary to Na^+ restriction. Similarly, low-dose infusion of norepinephrine to normal salt-replete volunteers resulted in a physiologic plasma increment of this neurotransmitter in association with antinatriuresis.[158] This reduction in Na^+ excretion occurred without any change in GFR but was associated with a significant decline in Li^+ clearance, an indication of enhanced proximal tubule reabsorption.

The cellular mechanisms mediating the tubular actions of norepinephrine appear to include stimulation of Na^+-K^+-ATPase activity and Na^+/H^+ exchange in proximal tubular epithelial cells.[148] It is assumed that α_1-adrenoreceptor stimulation, mediated by phospholipase C, causes an increase in intracellular Ca^{2+} that activates the Ca^{2+} calmodulin–dependent calcineurin phosphatase. Calcineurin converts Na^+-K^+-ATPase from its inactive phosphorylated form to its active dephosphorylated form.[159] The stimulatory effect of renal nerves on Na^+/H^+ exchange is mediated through stimulation of the α_2-adrenoreceptor.[148]

In addition to the direct action of Na^+ on epithelial cell transport and renal hemodynamics, interactions of renal nerve input with other effector mechanisms may contribute to the regulation of renal handling of Na^+. Efferent sympathetic nerve activity influences the rate of renin secretion in the kidneys by a variety of mechanisms, either directly or by interacting with the macula densa and vascular baroreceptor mechanisms for renin secretion.[148] The increase in renin secretion is mediated primarily by direct stimulation of β_1-adrenergic receptors located on juxtaglomerular granular cells.[148] Sympathetic activation of renin release is augmented during RPP reduction.[148] Results of studies in the isolated perfused rat kidney suggest that intrarenal generation of angiotensin II has an important prejunctional action on renal sympathetic nerve terminals to facilitate norepinephrine release during renal nerve stimulation.[148] However, the physiologic significance of this facilitatory interaction on tubular Na^+ reabsorption remains controversial. Thus, administration of an ACE inhibitor or an angiotensin receptor blocker (ARB) attenuated the antinatriuretic response to electrical renal nerve stimulation in anesthetized rats.[148] In contrast, when nonhypotensive hemorrhage was used to produce reflex increase in RSNA in conscious dogs, the associated antinatriuresis was unaffected by ACE inhibition or angiotensin II receptor blockade.[160]

Sympathetic activity is also a stimulus for the production and release of renal prostaglandins, coupled in series to the adrenergic-mediated renal vasoconstriction.[148] Evidence indicates that renal vasodilatory prostaglandins attenuate the renal hemodynamic vasoconstrictive response to activation of the renal adrenergic system in vivo and on isolated renal arterioles.[148] In Munich-Wistar rats, results of micropuncture experiments indicated that the primary factor responsible for the reduction in the glomerular K_f during renal nerve

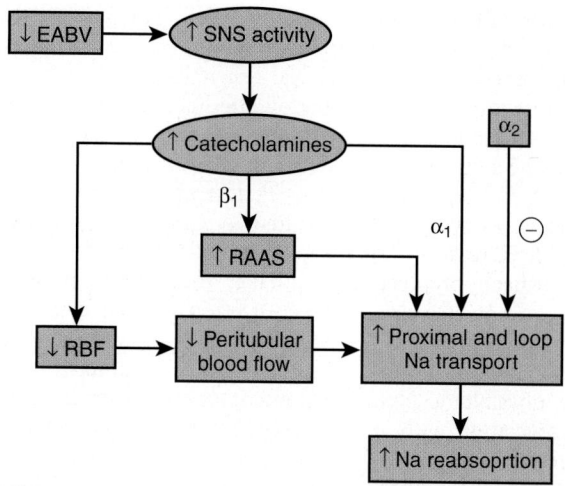

FIGURE 14-5 Sympathetic nervous system (SNS)-mediated effects of decreased effective arterial blood volume (EABV) on the kidneys. α_1, α_2, and β_1 refer to α_1-, α_2-, and β_1-adrenergic receptors, respectively. –, inhibitory effect; RAAS, renin-angiotensin-aldosterone system; RBF, renal blood flow.

stimulation may be angiotensin II rather than norepinephrine and that endogenously produced prostaglandins neutralize the vasoconstrictive effects of renal nerve stimulation at an intraglomerular locus rather than at the arteriolar level.

Another interaction examined is that between the renal SNS and AVP. Studies in conscious animals showed that AVP exerted a dose-related effect on the arterial baroreflex: Low doses of AVP might have sensitized the central baroreflex neurons to afferent input, whereas higher doses caused direct excitations of these neurons, which resulted in a reduction in sympathetic outflow.[148] In addition, AVP suppresses renal sympathetic outflow, and this response depends on the number of afferent inputs from baroreceptors.[161] Conversely, renal nerve stimulation resulted in elevations of plasma AVP levels and arterial pressure in conscious, baroreceptor-intact Wistar rats.[162] Many studies demonstrated, in both normal and pathologic situations, that increased RNSA can antagonize the natriuretic/diuretic response to ANP and that removal of the influence of sympathetic activity enhances the natriuretic action of the peptide (see DiBona and Kopp[148] and references therein). Conversely, renal denervation in Wistar rats increased ANP receptors and cGMP generation in glomeruli, which resulted in an increase in K_f after ANP infusion.[163]

In summary, renal sympathetic nerves can regulate U_{Na} and water excretion by changing renal vascular resistance, by influencing renin release from the juxtaglomerular granular cells, and through a direct effect on tubular epithelial cells (Figure 14-5). These effects may be modulated through interactions with various other hormonal systems, including ANP, prostaglandins, and AVP.

HUMORAL MECHANISMS

Renin-Angiotensin-Aldosterone System. The RAAS plays a central role in the regulation of ECF volume, Na^+ homeostasis, and cardiac function.[164] The system is activated in situations that compromise hemodynamic stability, such as blood loss, reduced EABV, low Na^+ intake, hypotension, and increase in sympathetic nerve activity. The RAAS comprises a coordinated hormonal cascade whose synthesis is initiated by the release of renin from the juxtaglomerular apparatus in

response to reduced renal perfusion or decrease in arterial pressure.[165] Messenger RNA for renin exists in juxtaglomerular cells and in renal tubule cells.[166] Renin acts on its circulating substrate, angiotensinogen, which is produced and secreted mainly by the liver but also by the kidneys.[164] Angiotensin converting enzyme 1 (ACE1), which cleaves angiotensin I to angiotensin II, exists in large amounts in the microvasculature of the lungs but also on endothelial cells of other vasculature beds and cell membrane of the brush border of the proximal nephron, heart, and brain.[164] Angiotensin II is the principal effector of the RAAS, although other smaller metabolic products of angiotensin II also have biologic activities.[167,168] Nonrenin (cathepsin G, plasminogen-activating factor, tonin) and non-ACE pathways (chymase, cathepsin G) also exist in these tissues and may contribute to tissue angiotensin II synthesis.[164]

In addition to its important function as a circulating hormone, angiotensin II produced locally acts as a paracrine agent in an organ-specific mode (reviewed by Paul et al[169]). In that regard, the properties of angiotensin II as a growth-promoting agent in the cardiovascular system and the kidneys have been increasingly appreciated.[164,169] For instance, local generation of angiotensin II in the kidneys results in higher intrarenal levels of this peptide in proximal tubular fluid, interstitial fluid, and renal medulla than in the circulation. The epithelial cells of the proximal nephron may be an important source for the in situ generation of angiotensin II, because these cells show abundant expression of the messenger RNA for angiotensinogen.[170] Furthermore, angiotensin II is apparently secreted from tubular epithelial cells into the lumen of the proximal nephron.[171] This may account for the fact that concentrations of angiotensin II are approximately 1000 times higher in the proximal tubular fluid than in the plasma.[171,172] Moreover, the mechanisms regulating intrarenal levels of angiotensin II may be dissociated from those controlling the systemic concentrations of the peptide.[170]

The biologic actions of angiotensin II are mediated through activation of at least two receptor subtypes, AT_1 and AT_2, encoded by different genes residing on different chromosomes.[173,174] Both receptors are G protein–coupled, seven-transmembrane polypeptides containing approximately 360 amino acids.[164,174] In the adult organism, the AT_1 receptor mediates most of the biologic activities of angiotensin II, whereas the AT_2 receptor appears to have a vasodilatory and antiproliferative effect.[167,175] AT_1 is expressed in the vascular poles of glomeruli, juxtaglomerular apparatus, and mesangial cells, whereas the quantitatively lower expression of AT_2 is confined to renal arteries and tubular structures.[173] Besides their functional distinction, the two receptor types employ different downstream pathways. Stimulation of the AT_1 receptor activates phospholipases A_2, C, and D, which results in increased cytosolic Ca^{2+} and inositol triphosphate and inhibition of adenylate cyclase. In contrast, activation of the AT_2 receptor results in increases in nitric oxide and bradykinin levels, which lead to elevation in cGMP concentrations and to vasodilation.[176]

Besides being an important source of several components of the RAAS, the kidney acts as a major target organ for the principal hormonal mediators of this cascade, angiotensin II and aldosterone. In the past, it was believed that the major contribution of angiotensin II to Na^+ homeostasis was the result of its action as a circulating vasoconstrictor hormone and through stimulation of aldosterone release from the adrenal cortex with subsequent tubular action of aldosterone. However, it is now abundantly clear that angiotensin II, through AT_1 receptors, exerts multiple direct intrarenal influences, including renal vasoconstriction, stimulation of tubular epithelial Na^+ reabsorption, augmentation of tubuloglomerular feedback sensitivity, modulation of pressure natriuresis, and stimulation of mitogenic pathways.[164] Moreover, exogenous infusion of angiotensin II that results in relatively low circulating levels of angiotensin II (picomolar range) is highly effective in modulating renal hemodynamic and tubular function, in comparison with the 10- to 100-fold higher concentrations required for its extrarenal effects. Thus, the kidneys appear to be uniquely sensitive to the actions of angiotensin II.

Furthermore, the synergistic interactions that exist between the renal vascular and tubular actions of angiotensin II significantly amplify the influence of angiotensin II on Na^+ excretion.[170] Among the direct renal actions of angiotensin II, its effect on renal hemodynamics appears to be of critical importance. Angiotensin II elicits a dose-dependent decrease in RBF but slightly augments GFR, as a result of its preferential vasoconstrictive effect on the efferent arteriole, and therefore increases filtration fraction. In turn, the increased filtration fraction may further modulate peritubular Starling forces, possibly by decreasing hydraulic pressure and increasing colloid osmotic pressure in the interstitium. These peritubular changes eventually lead to enhanced reabsorption of proximal Na^+ and fluid. Of importance, however, is that changes in preglomerular resistance have also been described during angiotensin II infusion or blockade.[177] These may be secondary either to changes in systemic arterial pressure (myogenic reflex) or to increased sensitivity of tubuloglomerular feedback, because angiotensin II does not alter preglomerular resistance when RPP is clamped or adjustments in tubuloglomerular feedback are prevented.[177]

In addition, angiotensin II may affect GFR by reducing K_f, thereby altering the filtered load of Na^+.[178] This effect is believed to reflect the action of the hormone on mesangial cell contractility and increasing permeability to macromolecules.[177] Finally, angiotensin II may also influence Na^+ excretion through its action on the medullary circulation. Because angiotensin II receptors are highly abundant in the renal medulla, this peptide may contribute significantly to the regulation of medullary blood flow.[177,179] In fact, use of fiberoptic probes revealed that angiotensin II usually reduces cortical blood flow and medullary blood flow and decreases Na^+ and water excretion.[177,179] As pointed out earlier, changes in medullary blood flow may affect medullary tonicity, which determines the magnitude of passive salt reabsorption in the loop of Henle, and may also modulate pressure natriuresis through alterations in renal interstitial pressure.[180]

The other well-characterized renal effect of angiotensin II is a direct action on proximal tubular epithelial transport. Infusions of angiotensin II to achieve systemic concentrations of 10^{-12} to 10^{-11} mol markedly stimulated Na^+ and water transport, independently of changes in renal or systemic hemodynamics.[164,181] Angiotensin II exerts a dose-dependent biphasic effect on proximal Na^+ reabsorption. Peritubular capillary infusion with solutions containing low concentrations of angiotensin II (10^{-12} to 10^{-10} mol) stimulated, whereas perfusion at higher concentrations of angiotensin II (>10^{-7} mol) inhibited proximal Na^+ reabsorption rate. Addition of either the AT_1 receptor antagonist losartan or the ACE inhibitor enalaprilat directly into the luminal fluid of the proximal nephron resulted in a significant decrease in proximal fluid reabsorption, which is indicative of tonic regulation of proximal tubule transport by endogenous angiotensin II.[182]

The specific mechanisms by which angiotensin II influences proximal tubule transport include increases in reabsorption of Na^+ and HCO_3^- by stimulation of the apical Na^+-H^+ antiporter, Na^+/H^+ exchanger isoform 3 (NHE3), basolateral Na^+-$3HCO_3^-$ symporter, and Na^+-K^+-ATPase.[183,184] Thus, angiotensin II can affect NaCl absorption by two mechanisms: (1) Activation of NHE3 can directly increase NaCl absorption. (2) Conditions that increase the rate of $NaHCO_3$ absorption can stimulate passive NaCl absorption by increasing the concentration gradient for passive Cl^- diffusion.[185] Na^+ reabsorption is further promoted by the action of angiotensin II on NHE3 and Na^+-K^+-ATPase in the medullary thick ascending limb of Henle.[164]

In both the early and late portions of the distal tubule, as well as the connecting tubule, angiotensin II regulates Na^+ and HCO_3^- reabsorption by stimulating NHE3 and the amiloride-sensitive Na^+ channel.[186-188] Two additional mechanisms may amplify the antinatriuretic effects of angiotensin II that are mediated by the direct actions of the peptide on renal hemodynamics and tubular transport. The first concerns the increased sensitivity of the tubuloglomerular feedback mechanism in the presence of angiotensin II, and the second concerns the effect of angiotensin II on pressure natriuresis. The decrease in distal delivery produced by the action of angiotensin II on renal hemodynamics and proximal fluid reabsorption could elicit afferent arteriolar vasodilation by means of the tubuloglomerular feedback mechanism, which, in turn, could antagonize the angiotensin II–mediated increase in proximal reabsorption. This effect, however, is minimized because angiotensin II increases the responsiveness of the tubuloglomerular feedback mechanism, thus maintaining GFR at a lower delivery rate to the macula densa.[61] The second mechanism by which the antinatriuretic effects of angiotensin II may be amplified is blunting of the pressure natriuresis mechanism so that higher pressures are needed to induce a given amount of Na^+ excretion.[130,164] This "shift to the right" in the pressure natriuresis curve may be viewed as an important Na^+-conserving mechanism in situations of elevated arterial pressure.

The use of ACE inhibitors and highly specific ARBs provided additional insight into the mechanisms of action of angiotensin II in the kidneys, and the findings suggested that most of the known intrarenal actions of angiotensin II, particularly regulation of renal hemodynamics and proximal tubule reabsorption of Na^+ and HCO_3^-, are mediated by the AT_1 receptor.[173] However, functional studies showed that some of the actions of angiotensin II at the renal level are mediated by AT_2 receptors.[173] The AT_2 receptor subtype plays a counterregulatory protective role against the AT_1 receptor–mediated antinatriuretic and pressor actions of angiotensin II. The accepted concept that angiotensin I was converted solely to angiotensin II was revised through the demonstration that angiotensin I is also a substrate for the formation of angiotensin-(1-7).[168] Moreover, a recently discovered homolog of ACE, angiotensin converting enzyme 2 (ACE2), is responsible for the formation of angiotensin-(1-7) from angiotensin II and for the conversion of angiotensin I to angiotensin-(1-9), which may be converted to angiotensin-(1-7) by ACE.[167,168]

Angiotensin-(1-7), through its G protein–coupled receptor, Mas, may play an important role as a regulator of cardiovascular and renal function by opposing the effects of angiotensin II; it does this through vasodilation, diuresis, and an antihypertrophic action (see Santos et al[167] and references therein). Thus, the RAAS can currently be envisioned as a dual-function system in which the vasoconstrictor/proliferative or vasodilator/antiproliferative actions are driven primarily by the ACE/ACE2 balance. According to this model, an increased ACE/ACE2 activity ratio leads to increased generation of angiotensin II and increased catabolism of angiotensin-(1-7), which is conducive to vasoconstriction; conversely, a decreased ACE/ACE2 ratio reduces angiotensin II and increases angiotensin-(1-7) levels, facilitating vasodilation. The additional effect of angiotensin-(1-7)/Mas to directly antagonize the actions of angiotensin II adds a further level of counterregulation.[167]

The final component of the RAAS, aldosterone, also plays an important physiologic role in the maintenance of ECF and Na^+ homeostasis.[189] The primary sites of aldosterone action are the principal cells of the cortical collecting tubule and convoluted distal tubule, in which the hormone promotes the reabsorption of Na^+ and the secretion of K^+ and protons.[189] Aldosterone may also enhance electrogenic Na^+ transport, but not K^+ secretion, in the IMCD.[190] Aldosterone exerts its effects on ionic transport by increasing the number of open Na^+ and K^+ channels in the luminal membrane and the activity of Na^+-K^+-ATPase in the basolateral membrane.[191] The effect of aldosterone on Na^+ permeability appears to be the primary event because blockade of the ENaC with amiloride prevents the initial increase in Na^+ permeability and Na^+-K^+-ATPase activity.[191] This effect on Na^+ permeability is mediated by changes in intracellular Ca^{2+} levels, intracellular pH, and methylation of channel proteins, thus increasing mean open probability of ENaC.[192] However, the long-term effect of aldosterone on Na^+-K^+-ATPase activity involves de novo protein synthesis, which is regulated at the transcriptional level by serum and glucocorticoid-induced kinase-1.[192]

It has become clear that aldosterone specifically regulates the α-subunit of ENaC and that changes in expression of a variety of genes are important intermediates in this process. Using microarray analysis in a mouse IMCD line, Gumz and associates[193] examined the acute transcriptional effects of aldosterone. They found that the most prominent transcript was period homolog 1 (Per1), an important component of the circadian clock. Gumz and associates[194] also showed that disruption of the Per1 gene leads to attenuated expression of messenger RNA encoded by the α-subunit of ENaC and increased U_{Na} excretion. They also noted that messenger RNA encoded by the α-subunit of ENaC was expressed in an apparent circadian pattern that was dramatically altered in mice lacking functional Per1 genes. These results imply that the circadian clock has a previously unknown role in the control of Na^+ balance. Perhaps of more importance is that they provide molecular insight into how the circadian cycle directly affects Na^+ homeostasis.

The Na^+-retaining effect of aldosterone in the collecting tubule induces an increase in the transepithelial potential difference, which is conducive to K^+ excretion. In terms of overall body fluid homeostasis, the actions of aldosterone in the defense of ECF result from the net loss of an osmotically active particle confined primarily to the intracellular compartment (K^+) and its replacement with a corresponding particle confined primarily to the ECF (Na^+). The effect of a given circulating level of aldosterone on overall Na^+ excretion depends on the volume of filtrate reaching the collecting duct and the composition of luminal and intracellular fluids. As noted earlier, this delivery of filtrate is in turn determined by other effector mechanisms (angiotensin II, sympathetic nerve activity, and peritubular physical forces) acting at more proximal nephron sites.

It is not surprising that Na^+ balance can be regulated over a wide range of intake, even in subjects without adrenal glands and despite fixed low or high supplemental doses of mineralocorticoids. Under these circumstances, other effector mechanisms predominate in controlling urinary Na^+ excretion, although often in a setting of altered ECF volume or K^+ concentration. In this regard, how renal Na^+ reabsorption and K^+ excretion are coordinately regulated by aldosterone has long been a puzzle. In states of EABV depletion, aldosterone release stimulated by angiotensin II induces maximal Na^+ reabsorption without significantly affecting plasma K^+ levels. Conversely, hyperkalemia-induced aldosterone secretion stimulates maximum K^+ excretion without major effects on renal Na^+ handling.

Elegant studies on the intracellular signaling pathways involved in renal Na^+ and K^+ transport have shed light on this puzzle. The key elements in this transport regulation are the Ste20/SPS1-related proline/alanine-rich kinase (SPAK), the with-no-lysine kinases (WNKs) and their effectors, the thiazide-sensitive NaCl cotransporter, and the K^+ secretory channel ROMK. According to the proposed model, when EABV is reduced or dietary salt intake is low, angiotensin II, mediated by the AT_1 receptor, leads to phosphorylation of WNK4, which stimulates phosphorylation of SPAK. In turn, SPAK phosphorylates the NaCl cotransporter, inducing Na^+ transport and conservation. Simultaneous phosphorylation of the full-length isoform of WNK1, WNK1-L, causes endocytosis of the ROMK channel, thereby enabling K^+ conservation, despite high aldosterone levels. In contrast, in the presence of hyperkalemia or low dietary salt, angiotensin II levels are low so that WNK4 cannot be activated, SPAK and NaCl cotransporter are not phosphorylated, and NaCl cotransporter trafficking to the apical membrane is inhibited. At the same time, K^+-induced kidney-specific WNK1 leads to suppression of WNK1-L, which allows ROMK trafficking to the apical membrane and maximal K^+ secretion. For further details, the reader is referred to an excellent recent review.[195]

In terms of blood pressure maintenance, systemic vasoconstriction—another major extrarenal action of angiotensin II—may be considered the appropriate response to perceived ECF volume contraction. As mentioned previously, higher concentrations of angiotensin II are needed to elicit this response than those that govern the renal antinatriuretic actions of angiotensin II, a situation analogous to the discrepancy between antidiuretic and pressor actions of vasopressin. Transition from an antinatriuretic to a natriuretic action of angiotensin II at high infusion rates can be attributed almost entirely to a concomitant rise in blood pressure.[196] There is now clear evidence that, besides the adrenal glomerulosa, aldosterone may also be produced by the heart and vasculature. It exerts powerful effects on blood vessels,[197] independently of actions that can be attributed to the blood pressure rise through regulation of salt and water balance. As observed with angiotensin II, aldosterone also possesses significant mitogenic and fibrogenic properties. It directly increases the expression and production of transforming growth factor-β and thus is involved in the development of glomerulosclerosis, hypertension, and cardiac injury/hypertrophy.[164,189,197]

In summary, angiotensin II, the principal effector of the RAAS, regulates extracellular volume and renal Na^+ excretion through intrarenal and extrarenal mechanisms. The intrarenal hemodynamic and tubular actions of the peptide and its main extrarenal actions (systemic vasoconstriction and aldosterone release) act in concert to adjust U_{Na} excretion under a variety of circumstances associated with alterations in ECF volume. Many of these mechanisms are synergistic and tend to amplify the overall influence of the RAAS. However, additional counterregulatory mechanisms, induced directly or indirectly by angiotensin II, provide a buffer against the unopposed actions of the primary components of the RAAS.

Vasopressin. AVP is a nonapeptide (nine–amino acid) hormone, synthesized in the brain, that is secreted from the posterior pituitary gland into the circulation in response to an increase in plasma osmolality (through osmoreceptor stimulation) or a decrease in EABV and blood pressure (through baroreceptor stimulation).[198] Thus, AVP plays a major role in the regulation of water balance and the support of blood pressure and EABV. AVP exerts its biologic actions through at least three different G protein–coupled receptors. Two of these receptors, V_{1A} and V_2, are abundantly expressed in the cardiovascular system and the kidneys; V_{1B} receptors are expressed on the surfaces of corticotrophic cells of the anterior pituitary gland, in the pancreas, and in the adrenal medulla. V_{1A} and V_2 receptors mediate the two main biologic actions of the hormone: vasoconstriction and increased water reabsorption by the kidneys, respectively. (V_2 receptor–mediated effects on hemostasis are discussed in Chapter 56). The V_{1A} and V_{1B} receptors operate through the phosphoinositide signaling pathway, causing release of intracellular Ca^{2+}. Found in vascular smooth muscle cells, hepatocytes, and platelets, the V_{1A} receptor mediates vasoconstriction, glycogenolysis, and platelet aggregation, respectively. The V_2 receptor, found mainly in the renal collecting duct epithelial cells, is linked to the adenylate cyclase pathway, and cAMP is used as its second messenger.

Under physiologic conditions, AVP functions primarily to regulate water content in the body by adjusting water reabsorption in the collecting duct according to plasma tonicity. A change in plasma tonicity by as little as 1% causes a parallel change in AVP release. This change, in turn, alters the water permeability of the collecting duct. The antidiuretic action of AVP results from complex effects of this hormone on principal cells of the collecting duct. First, AVP provokes the insertion of aquaporin-2 (AQP2)[199] water channels into the luminal membrane (short-term response) and increases synthesis of AQP2 messenger RNA and protein[200]; both responses increase water permeability along the collecting duct. This is considered in detail in Chapter 9. In brief, activation of V_2 receptors localized to the basolateral membrane of the principal cells increases cytosolic cAMP, which stimulates the activity of protein kinase A. The latter triggers a series of phosphorylation events that promotes the translocation of AQP2 from intracellular stores to the apical membrane,[201] which allows the reabsorption of water from the lumen to the cells. Then the water exits the cell to the hypertonic interstitium via aquaporin-3 and aquaporin-4, localized at the basolateral membrane.[202]

The second complex effect of AVP on the collecting duct is to increase the permeability of the IMCD to urea, through activation of the urea transporter UT-A1, which enables the accumulation of urea in the interstitium; there, it contributes, along with Na^+, to the hypertonicity of the medullary interstitium, which is a prerequisite for maximum urine concentration and water reabsorption.[203] AVP exerts several effects on Na^+ handling at different segments of the nephron, in which it increases Na^+ reabsorption through activation of ENaC, mainly in the cortical and outer medullary collecting duct.[204]

In addition, AVP may influence renal hemodynamics and reduce RBF, especially to the inner medulla.[205] The latter effect is mediated by the V_{1A} receptor and may be modulated by the local release of nitric oxide and prostaglandins. At higher concentrations,[206] AVP may also decrease total RBF and GFR, as part of the generalized vasoconstriction induced by the peptide.[200,207]

The role of the V_{1A} receptor in the kidneys has been further elaborated. In V_{1A} receptor–deficient ($V_{1A}R^{-/-}$) mice, plasma volume and blood pressure were decreased.[207] Also, urine volume of $V_{1A}R^{-/-}$ mice was greater than that of wild-type mice, particularly after a water load; however, GFR, U_{Na} excretion, AVP-dependent cAMP generation, levels of V_2 receptor, and AQP2 expression in the kidneys were lower, which indicates that the diminishment of GFR and the V_2 receptor–AQP2 system led to impaired urinary concentration in $V_{1A}R^{-/-}$ mice. This result is interesting because classic models implicate the V_2 receptors in water handling by the nephron. Moreover, plasma renin and angiotensin II levels were decreased, as was renin expression in granule cells. In addition, the expression of renin stimulators such as nNOS and cyclooxygenase-2 (COX-2) in macula densa cells, where $V_{1A}R$ is specifically expressed, was decreased in $V_{1A}R^{-/-}$ mice. Aoyagi and colleagues[207] concluded that AVP regulates body fluid homeostasis and GFR through the $V_{1A}R$ in macula densa cells by activating the RAAS and subsequently the V_2 receptor–AQP2 system.

A third receptor for AVP, V_3,[208] is found predominantly in the anterior pituitary gland and is involved in the regulation of adrenocorticotropic hormone (ACTH) release. In addition to its renal effects, AVP also regulates extrarenal vascular tone through the V_{1A} receptor. Stimulation of this receptor by AVP results in a potent arteriolar vasoconstriction in various vascular beds with a significant increase in systemic vascular resistance.[209] However, physiologic increases in AVP do not usually cause a significant increase in blood pressure, because AVP also potentiates the sinoaortic baroreflexes that subsequently reduce heart rate and cardiac output.[209] Nevertheless, at supraphysiologic concentrations of AVP, such as those that occur when EABV is severely compromised (e.g., in shock or heart failure), AVP plays an important role in supporting arterial pressure and maintaining adequate perfusion to vital organs such as the brain and myocardium. AVP also has a direct, V_1 receptor–mediated, inotropic effect in the isolated heart.[210] In vivo, however, AVP has been reported to decrease myocardial function[211]; this effect is attributed to either cardioinhibitory reflexes or coronary vasoconstriction induced by the peptide. Of more importance is that AVP has been shown to stimulate cardiomyocyte hypertrophy and protein synthesis in neonatal rat cardiomyocytes and in intact myocardium through a V_1-dependent mechanism.[212] These effects are very similar to those obtained with exposure of cardiomyocytes to angiotensin II or catecholamines, although not necessarily through the same cellular mechanisms. By this growth-promoting property, AVP may contribute to the induction of cardiac hypertrophy and remodeling.[213]

Controversy exists regarding the effect of AVP on natriuresis; some authors have found a natriuretic response with infusions, and others have found Na^+ retention.[214,215] These variations may result from differences between species or from acute changes in volume status.[216] Regardless of the effects of AVP on Na^+ excretion, in terms of overall volume homeostasis, the predominant influence of the hormone is indirectly through water accumulation or vasoconstriction. In fact, the vasoconstrictive V_1 receptor effect of AVP overrides the osmotically driven effect (see Chapter 15) in the presence of an ECF volume deficit of 20% or more. Nevertheless, in this regard, potential hypertensive effects of AVP are buffered by a concomitant increase in baroreflex-mediated sympathoinhibition or by an increase in PGE_2, which results in a blunting of vasoconstriction, and by a direct vasodepressor action of V_2 receptor activation.[217]

Prostaglandins. Prostaglandins, or cyclooxygenase-derived prostanoids, possess complex and diverse regulatory functions in the kidneys, including hemodynamics, renin secretion, growth response, tubular transport processes, and immune response in both health and disease (Table 14-3).[218,219] Currently, two known principal isoforms of cyclooxygenase (COX-1 and COX-2) catalyze the synthesis of prostaglandin H_2 (PGH_2) from arachidonic acid, released from membrane phospholipids. PGH_2 is then metabolized to the five major prostanoids—PGE_2; prostaglandins I_2, D_2, and $F_2\alpha$ (PGI_2, PGD_2, and $PGF_{2\alpha}$); and thromboxane A_2 (TXA_2)—through specific synthases[219] (see also Chapter 11). An additional splice variant of the COX-1 gene, COX-3, has been identified, but its function in humans is yet to be fully elucidated.[220]

Prostanoids are rapidly degraded so that their effect is localized strictly to their site of synthesis, which accounts for the predominance of their autocrine and paracrine mode of action. Each prostanoid has a specific cell surface G protein–coupled receptor, distinct for a given location, that determines the specific function of the prostaglandin in the given cell type.[219] COX-1 is constitutively expressed and serves in a housekeeping role in many cell types; it is expressed abundantly and is highly immunoreactive in the kidneys, especially in the collecting duct but also in medullary interstitial, mesangial, and arteriolar endothelial cells of most species.[219] In contrast, the expression of COX-2 is inducible and cell-type specific, and its renal expression is prominent in medullary interstitial cells, cortical cells of the thick ascending limb of Henle, and cells of the macula densa, in which expression is regulated in response to varying amounts of salt intake (see Hao and Breyer[219] and references therein). Furthermore, the profile of sensitivity to pharmacologic inhibitors differs between the two isoforms.[221] The principal prostanoid in the kidneys is PGE_2; others present are PGI_2, PGF_2, and TXA_2.[219] PGI_2 and PGE_2 are the main products in the cortex of normal kidneys, and PGE_2 predominates in the medulla.[219] Metabolism of arachidonic acid by other pathways (lipoxygenase, epoxygenase) leads to products that are involved in crosstalk with cyclooxygenase (see Nasrallah et al[218]). The major sites for prostaglandin production (and hence for local actions) are the renal arteries and arterioles and glomeruli in the cortex and interstitial cells in the medulla, with additional contributions from epithelial cells of the cortical and medullary collecting tubules.[222,223]

The two major roles for prostaglandins in volume homeostasis are (1) their effect on RBF and GFR and (2) their effect on tubular handling of salt and water, on the other. Table 14-3 lists target structures, mode of action, and major biologic effects of the active renal prostanoids. PGI_2 and PGE_2 have predominantly vasodilating and natriuretic activities; they also modulate the action of AVP and tend to stimulate renin secretion. TXA_2 has been shown to cause vasoconstriction, although the importance of the physiologic effects of TXA_2 on the kidneys is still controversial. The end results of the stimulation of renal prostaglandin secretion in the kidneys are vasodilation, increased renal perfusion, natriuresis, and facilitation of water excretion.

The role of prostaglandins as vasodilators in the glomerular microcirculation is now well established. The cellular targets for vasoactive hormones in the glomerular microcirculation are vascular smooth muscle cells of the afferent and efferent arterioles and mesangial cells within the glomeruli. Action at these sites governs renal vascular resistance, glomerular function, and downstream microcirculatory function in peritubular capillaries and vasa recta. In vivo studies showed that intrarenal infusions of PGE_2 and PGI_2 cause vasodilation and increased RBF.[222] In agreement with these findings, in vitro experiments with isolated renal microvessels showed that both PGE_2 and prostaglandin E_1 (PGE_1) attenuate angiotensin II–induced afferent arteriolar vasoconstriction, and PGI_2 antagonizes angiotensin II–induced efferent arteriolar vasoconstriction.[224] Similarly, PGE_2 has been shown to counteract

TABLE 14-3 Major Renal Biologic Effects of Prostaglandins and Thromboxane

AGENT	TARGET STRUCTURE	MODE OF ACTION	DIRECT CONSEQUENCES
PGE_2, PGI_2	Intrarenal arterioles	Vasodilation	Increased renal perfusion (more pronounced in inner cortical and medullary regions)
PGI_2	Glomeruli	Vasodilation	Increased filtration rate
PGE_2, PGI_2	Efferent arterioles	Vasodilation	Increased Na^+ excretion through increased postglomerular perfusion
PGE_2, PGI_2, $PGF_{2\alpha}$	Distal tubules	Decreased transport	Increased Na^+ excretion, decreased maximum medullary hypertonicity
PGE_2, PGI_2, $PGF_{2\alpha}$	Distal tubules	Inhibition of cAMP synthesis	Interference with AVP action
PGE_2, PGI_2	Juxtaglomerular apparatus	cAMP stimulation (?)	Increased renin release
TXA_2	Intrarenal arterioles	Vasoconstriction	Decreased renal perfusion

AVP, Arginine vasopressin; *cAMP,* cyclic adenosine monophosphate; *PGE_2,* prostaglandin E_2; *PGF_{2\alpha},* prostaglandin $F_{2\alpha}$; *PGI_2,* prostaglandin I_2; *TXA_2,* thromboxane A_2.

angiotensin II–induced contraction of isolated glomeruli and glomerular mesangial cells in culture, and conversely, cyclooxygenase inhibition augments these contractile responses. An inhibitory counterregulatory role of prostaglandins with regard to renal nerve stimulation has also been demonstrated from micropuncture studies.[148] Furthermore, in volume-contracted states, COX-2 expression and PGE_2 release in the macula densa and cortical thick ascending limb of Henle dramatically increase in response to decreased luminal Cl^- delivery. In addition to its direct vasodilator effect on afferent arterioles, PGE_2 leads to increased renin release from the macula densa (see Hao and Breyer[219]). The resulting rise in angiotensin II and consequent efferent arteriolar constriction also ensure maintenance of GFR.

In the clinical situation, in volume-replete states, the renal vasoconstrictive influences of angiotensin II and norepinephrine are mitigated by their simultaneous stimulation of vasodilatory renal prostaglandins so that RBF and GFR are maintained.[225] However, in the setting of heightened vasoconstrictor input from the RAAS, SNS, and AVP, as occurs during states of EABV depletion, the vasorelaxant action of PGE_2 and PGI_2 is overwhelmed, with the concomitant risk for the development of acute kidney injury.[219] Similarly, when this prostaglandin-mediated counterregulatory mechanism is suppressed by nonselective or COX-2–selective inhibitors, the unopposed actions of angiotensin II and norepinephrine can also lead to a rapid deterioration in renal function.[226] Moreover, COX-2–derived prostanoids also promote natriuresis and stimulate renin secretion.[219] Therefore, during states of volume depletion, low Na^+ intake, or the use of loop diuretics, COX-2 inhibitors (such as celecoxib or rofecoxib), as well as the nonselective cyclooxygenase inhibitors diclofenac and naproxen, can cause Na^+ and K^+ retention, edema formation, heart failure, and hypertension.[223]

Whereas the role of prostaglandins in modulating glomerular vasoreactivity in states of varying salt balance is firmly established, the effects of prostaglandins on salt excretion per se are still being unraveled. Certainly, the aforementioned vascular effects of prostaglandins can be expected to have secondary effects on tubular function through the various physical factors described previously in this chapter. One particular consequence of prostaglandin-induced renal vasodilation may be medullary interstitial solute washout. Such a change in medullary interstitial composition could potentially account for the observed increase in U_{Na} excretion with intrarenal infusion of PGE_2.[222] The natriuretic response to PGE_2 may also be attenuated by preventing an increase in renal interstitial hydraulic pressure, even in the presence of a persistent increase in RBF.[227] In addition, in rats, the natriuresis usually accompanying direct expansion of renal interstitial volume can be significantly attenuated by inhibition of prostaglandin synthesis.[227] These findings are consistent with the proposal that changes in prostaglandins have a significant effect on renal Na^+ excretion.

Results of a number of micropuncture and microcatheterization studies in vivo suggested that prostaglandins affected U_{Na} excretion independently of hemodynamic changes.[222] Subsequently, direct effects of PGE_2 on epithelial transport processes were demonstrated and were found to vary considerably in different nephron segments. In the medullary thick ascending limb of Henle and collecting tubule, PGE_2 caused a decrease in the reabsorption of water, Na^+, and Cl^- that was correlated with reduced Na^+-K^+-ATPase activity. In contrast, in the distal convoluted tubule, PGE_2 caused increased Na^+-K^+-ATPase activity.[228] The net effect of locally produced prostaglandins on tubular Na^+ handling is probably inhibitory because complete blockade of prostaglandin synthesis by indomethacin in rats receiving a normal or salt-loaded diet increased fractional Na^+ reabsorption and enhanced the activity of the renal medullary Na^+-K^+-ATPase.[229] In addition, PGE_2 inhibits AVP-stimulated NaCl reabsorption in the medullary thick ascending limb of Henle and AVP-stimulated water reabsorption in the collecting duct.[224,224,230] Both these effects tend to antagonize the overall hydroosmotic response to AVP. However, because no such effect is seen in the cortical thick ascending limb of Henle, which is capable of augmenting NaCl reabsorption in response to an increased delivered load, and because the effects of prostaglandins on solute transport in the collecting tubule remain controversial, no conclusions can be reached from these studies with regard to the contribution of direct epithelial effects of prostaglandins to overall Na^+ excretion.[224]

In whole animal and clinical balance studies, researchers have examined the effect of prostaglandin infusion or prostaglandin synthesis inhibition on urinary Na^+ excretion, or they have attempted to correlate changes in urinary prostaglandin excretion with changes in salt balance; these studies have also yielded conflicting and inconclusive results. Nevertheless, as elaborated earlier, prostaglandins have an important role in states of Na^+ imbalance (real or perceived Na^+ depletion) wherein they are involved to preserve GFR by countervailing renal vasoconstrictive influences.

The influence of changes in Na^+ intake on renal COX-1 and COX-2 expression has been studied extensively. The expression of COX-2 in the macula densa and thick ascending limb of Henle is increased by a low-salt diet, inhibition of RAAS, and renal hypoperfusion. In contrast, a high-salt diet has been reported to decrease COX-2 expression in the renal cortex.[218,219] None of these changes on Na^+ intake affected the expression of COX-1 in the cortex. In the medulla, whereas a low-salt diet downregulated both COX-1 and COX-2, a high-salt diet enhanced the expression of these cyclooxygenase isoforms.[218,219] In vitro studies showed that high osmolarity of the medium of cultured IMCD cells induces the expression of COX-2.[223] Infusion of nimesulide (a selective COX-2 inhibitor) into anesthetized dogs on normal Na^+ diet reduced U_{Na} excretion and urine flow rate, despite the lack of effect on renal hemodynamics or systemic blood pressure.[223]

Collectively, the differential regulation of COX-2 in the renal cortex and medulla can be integrated into a physiologically relevant model, in which upregulation of COX-2 in the cortical thick ascending limb of Henle and macula densa is induced in volume-contracted or vasoconstrictory states. In the cortical thick ascending limb of Henle, the effect is by direct inhibition of Na^+ excretion, whereas in the macula densa, COX-2 stimulates renin release, which leads to angiotensin II–mediated Na^+ retention. In contrast, medullary COX-2 is induced by a high-salt diet, which leads to net Na^+ excretion.[219]

Finally, in addition to the hemodynamically mediated and potential direct epithelial effects of prostaglandins, these agents may mediate the physiologic responses to other hormonal agents. The intermediacy of prostaglandins in renin release responses has already been cited. As another example, some, but not all, of the known physiologic effects of bradykinin and other products of the kallikrein-kinin system are mediated through bradykinin-stimulated prostaglandin production (e.g., inhibition of AVP-stimulated osmotic water permeability in the cortical collecting tubule).[224] In addition, the renal and systemic actions of angiotensin II appear to be differentially regulated by prostaglandin production that is catalyzed by COX-1 and COX-2. For instance, COX-2 deficiency in mice, induced by COX-2 inhibitors or knockout, dramatically augmented the systemic pressor effect of angiotensin II, whereas COX-1 deficiency abolished this pressor effect. Similarly, angiotensin II infusion reduced medullary blood flow in COX-2–deficient animals, but not in COX-1–deficient animals, which suggests that COX-2–dependent vasodilators are synthesized in the renal medulla. Moreover, the diuretic and natriuretic effects of angiotensin II were absent in COX-2–deficient animals, but they remained in COX-1–deficient animals. Thus, COX-1 and COX-2 exert opposite effects on systemic blood pressure and renal function.[231]

Natriuretic Peptides. The physiologic and pathophysiologic roles of the natriuretic peptide family in the regulation of Na^+ and water balance have become better understood since the discovery of ANP by de Bold and colleagues.[20] ANP is an endogenous 28–amino acid peptide secreted mainly by the right atrium. Besides ANP, two other natriuretic peptides have renal effects: BNP and CNP.[22] Although encoded by different genes, these peptides are highly similar in chemical structure, gene regulation, and degradation pathways, constituting a hormonal system that exerts various biologic actions on the renal, cardiac, and blood vessel tissues.[232] ANP plays an important role in blood pressure and volume homeostasis through its ability to induce natriuretic/diuretic and vasodilatory responses.[233,234] BNP has an amino acid sequence similar to that of ANP, with an extended NH_2-terminus. In humans, BNP is produced from pro–brain natriuretic peptide (proBNP), which contains 108 amino acids and, in accordance with a proteolytic process, releases a mature 32–amino acid molecule and N-terminal fragment into the circulation. Although BNP was originally cloned from the brain, it is now considered a circulating hormone produced mainly in the cardiac ventricles.[235] CNP, which is produced mostly by endothelial cells, shares the ring structure common to all natriuretic peptide members; however, it lacks the C-terminal tail.

The biologic effects of the natriuretic peptides are mediated by binding the peptide to specific membrane receptors localized to numerous tissues, including vasculature, renal arteries, glomerular mesangial and epithelial cells, collecting ducts, adrenal zona glomerulosa, and the CNS.[22] At least three different subtypes of natriuretic peptide receptors have been identified: NP-A, NP-B, and NP-C.[232] NP-A and NP-B, single-transmembrane proteins with molecular weights of approximately 120 to 140 kDa, mediate most of the biologic effects of natriuretic peptides. Both are coupled to guanylate cyclase in their intracellular portions.[232] After binding to their receptors, all three natriuretic peptide isoforms markedly increase cGMP in target tissues and in plasma. Therefore, analogs of cGMP or inhibitors of degradation of this second messenger mimic the vasorelaxant and renal effects of natriuretic peptides. The third class of natriuretic peptide–binding receptors, NP-C (molecular weight of 60 to 70 kDa), is believed to serve as a clearance receptor because it is not coupled to any known second-messenger system.[236] ANP-C

is the most abundant type of natriuretic peptide receptor in many key target organs of these peptides.[236]

Additional routes for the removal of natriuretic peptides includes enzymatic degradation by neutral endopeptidase (NEP) 24.11, a metalloproteinase located mainly in the lungs and the kidneys.[236]

Atrial Natriuretic Peptide. Both in vivo and in vitro studies, in humans as well as in experimental animals, established the role of ANP in the regulation of ECF volume and the control of blood pressure by acting on all organs and tissues involved in the homeostasis of Na^+ and blood pressure (Table 14-4).[233] Therefore, it is not surprising that ANP and NH_2-terminal ANP levels are increased in (1) conditions associated with enhanced atrial pressure, (2) systolic or diastolic cardiac dysfunction, (3) cardiac hypertrophy/remodeling, and (4) severe myocardial infarction.[22] In the kidneys, ANP exerts hemodynamic/glomerular effects that increase Na^+ and water delivery to the tubule, in combination with inhibitory effects on tubular Na^+ and water reabsorption, which lead to remarkable diuresis and natriuresis.[233]

In addition to its powerful diuretic and natriuretic activities, ANP also relaxes vascular smooth muscle and leads to vasodilation, by antagonizing the concomitant vasoconstrictive influences of angiotensin II, endothelin, AVP, and α_1-adrenergic input.[233] This vasodilation reduces preload, which results in a fall in cardiac output.[233] In addition, ANP reduces cardiac output by shifting fluid from the intravascular to the extravascular compartment, an effect mediated by increased capillary hydraulic conductivity for water.[237] Studies in endothelial-restricted GC-A–knockout mice have yielded evidence that ANP, through GC-A, enhances microvascular endothelial macromolecule permeability in vivo. Because such mice exhibit chronic hypervolemic hypertension, the authors hypothesized that modulation of transcapillary protein and

TABLE 14-4 Physiologic Actions of the Natriuretic Peptides

TARGET ORGAN	BIOLOGIC EFFECTS

Kidneys	Increased GFR
	  Afferent arteriolar vasodilation
	  Efferent arteriolar vasoconstriction
	Natriuresis
	  Inhibition of Na^+/H^+ exchanger (proximal tubule)
	  Inhibition of Na^+-Cl^- cotransporter (distal tubule)
	  Inhibition of Na^+ channels (collecting duct)
	Diuresis
	  Inhibition of AVP-induced aquaporin-2 incorporation into collecting duct apical membrane

Cardiac	Reduction in preload, leading to reduced cardiac output Inhibition of cardiac remodeling
Hemodynamic	Vasorelaxation Elevating capillary hydraulic conductivity Decreased cardiac preload and afterload
Endocrine	Suppression of RAAS Suppression of sympathetic outflow Suppression of AVP Suppression of endothelin
Mitogenesis	Inhibition of mitogenesis in vascular smooth muscle cells Inhibition of growth factor–mediated hypertrophy of cardiac fibroblasts

AVP, Arginine vasopressin; *GFR*, glomerular filtration rate; *RAAS*, renin-angiotensin-aldosterone system.

fluid transport might represent one of the most important hypovolemic actions of ANP.[238]

ANP has also been shown to exert antiproliferative, growth-regulatory properties in cultured glomerular mesangial cells, vascular smooth muscle cells, and endothelial cells.[233] Within the kidneys, ANP causes afferent vasodilation, efferent vasoconstriction, and mesangial relaxation, which lead to increases in glomerular capillary pressure, GFR, and filtration fraction (see Houben et al[235]). In combination with increased medullary blood flow, these hemodynamic effects enhance diuresis and natriuresis. However, the overall natriuretic effect of ANP infusion does not require these changes in glomerular function (except in response to larger doses of the peptide). At the tubular level, ANP inhibits the stimulatory effect of angiotensin II on the luminal Na^+/H^+ exchanger of the proximal tubule (see Houben et al[235] and references therein). Likewise, ANP, acting through cGMP, inhibits the thiazide-sensitive NaCl cotransporter in the distal tubule and ENaC in the collecting duct, along with inhibition of AVP-induced AQP2 incorporation into the apical membrane of these segments of the nephron (see Houben et al[235] and references therein; see Table 14-4).

Brain Natriuretic Peptide. The physiologic function of BNP, in contrast to that of ANP, remains unclear. Findings since 2005 suggest that BNP is produced by activated satellite cells in ischemic skeletal muscle or by cardiomyocytes in response to pressure load, thereby regulating the regeneration of neighboring endothelia through GC-A. Kuhn and associates[239] proposed that the BNP-mediated paracrine communication may be critically involved in coordinating muscle regeneration or hypertrophy and angiogenesis. However, administration of BNP to human subjects induces natriuretic, endocrine, and hemodynamic responses similar to those induced by ANP (see Houben et al[235] and references therein).

BNP is produced and secreted mainly by the ventricles, but also, in small amounts, by the atrium (see Houben et al[235] and references therein). Increased volume or pressure overload states such as CHF and hypertension enhance the secretion of BNP from the ventricles. Despite the comparable elevation in plasma levels of ANP and BNP in patients with CHF and other chronic volume-expanded conditions, acute intravenous saline loading or infusion of pressor doses of angiotensin II yields different patterns of ANP and BNP secretion.[240,241] Whereas plasma levels of ANP increase rapidly, the changes in plasma BNP of atrial origin are negligible, as expected in view of the minimal atrial content of BNP, in contrast to the abundance of ANP.[235] Moreover, plasma levels of BNP rise with age, from 26 ± 2 pg/mL in subjects aged 55 to 64 years to 31 ± 2 pg/mL in patients aged 65 to 74 years and to 64 ± 6 pg/mL in patients aged 75 years or older.[242]

Studies in animals and humans have demonstrated the natriuretic effects of pharmacologic doses of BNP. When administered to normal volunteers and hypertensive subjects at low doses, BNP induces a significant increase in U_{Na} excretion and, to a lesser extent, in urinary flow. Significant natriuresis and diuresis were observed after the infusion of either ANP or BNP to normal subjects. The combination of ANP and BNP did not produce a synergistic renal effect, which suggests that these peptides share similar mechanisms of action (see Houben et al[235] and references therein). Moreover, like ANP, BNP exerts a hypotensive effect in both animals and humans. For instance, transgenic mice that overexpress the

BNP gene exhibit significant and lifelong hypotension to the same extent as do transgenic mice that overexpress the ANP gene (see Hall[243] and references therein). Therefore, it is clear that BNP induces its biologic actions through mechanisms similar to those of ANP.[235]

This notion is supported by several findings: (1) Both ANP and BNP act through the same receptors, and both induce similar renal, cardiovascular, and endocrine actions in association with an increase in cGMP production (see Table 14-4); and (2) BNP suppresses ACTH-induced aldosterone generation both in cell culture and when BNP is infused in vivo. The latter action may be attributed to BNP inhibition of renin secretion, at least in dogs, although apparently not in humans (see Hall[243] and references therein). Like the hemodynamic effects of ANP, those of BNP vary according to the dose and species. When injected as a bolus at high doses, BNP caused a profound fall in systolic blood pressure in humans; however, when infused at low doses, this peptide failed to change blood pressure or heart rate (see Houben et al[235] and references therein). The effects of BNP have been used in the clinical setting both in the diagnosis and treatment of the volume overload state of CHF. This aspect is discussed in the "Specific Treatments Based on the Pathophysiology of Congestive Heart Failure" section.

C-Type Natriuretic Peptide. Although CNP is considered a neurotransmitter in the CNS, considerable amounts of this natriuretic peptide are produced by endothelial cells, where it plays a role in the local regulation of vascular tone.[236] Smaller amounts of CNP are produced in the kidneys, heart ventricles, and intestines.[236] In addition, CNP, which could be of endothelial or cardiac origin, has been found in human plasma. The physiologic stimuli for CNP production have not been identified, although enhanced expression of CNP messenger RNA has been reported after volume overload.[236] Intravenous infusion of CNP decreases blood pressure, cardiac output, urinary volume, and Na^+ excretion. Furthermore, the hypotensive effects of CNP are less pronounced compared to those of ANP and BNP, but CNP strongly stimulates cGMP production and inhibits vascular smooth muscle cells proliferation.[236]

Although all three natriuretic peptide forms inhibit the RAAS, CNP failed to induce significant changes in cardiac output, blood pressure, and plasma volume in sheep.[236] This finding supports the widely accepted concept that ANP and BNP are the major circulating natriuretic peptides, whereas CNP is a local regulator of vascular structure and tone. Although all forms of natriuretic peptides exist in the brain, the role and significance of their CNS expression in the regulation of salt and water balance are not understood. Together, the various biologic actions of natriuretic peptides lead to reduction of EABV, an expected response to perceived overfilling of the central intrathoracic circulation. Furthermore, all natriuretic peptides counteract the adverse effects of RAAS, which suggests that the two systems are acting in opposite directions in the regulation of body fluid and cardiovascular homeostasis.

Endothelium-Derived Factors. The endothelium is a major source of active substances that regulate vascular tone in healthy states and disease.[244] The best known representatives are endothelin, nitric oxide, and PGI_2. These vasoconstricting and vasodilating factors regulate the perfusion pressure of multiple organ systems that are strongly involved in water and Na^+ balance, such as the kidneys, heart, and vasculature.

This section summarizes some of the concepts regarding actions of endothelin and nitric oxide that are relevant to volume homeostasis.

Endothelin. The endothelin system consists of three vasoactive peptides: endothelin 1 (ET-1), endothelin 2 (ET-2), and endothelin 3 (ET-3). These peptides are synthesized and released mainly by endothelial cells and act in a paracrine and autocrine manner.[245-248] ET-1, the major representative of the endothelin family, is still the most potent vasoconstrictor known[249] (however, see also the "Urotensin" section). All endothelins are synthesized by proteolytic cleavage from specific prepro-endothelins that are further cleaved to form 37– to 39–amino acid precursors, called *big endothelin*. Big endothelin is then converted into the biologically active, 21–amino acid peptide by a highly specific endothelin converting enzyme (ECE), a phosphoramidon-sensitive membrane-bound metalloprotease. To date, two isoforms of ECE have been identified: ECE-1 and ECE-2.[250] ECE-2 is localized mainly to vascular smooth muscle cells and is probably an intracellular enzyme. In ECE-1–knockout mice, tissue levels of ET-1 are reduced by about one third, which suggests that ECE-independent pathways are involved in the synthesis of this peptide (see Barton and Yanagisawa[250] and references therein). In this regard, both chymase[251] and carboxypeptidase A[252] have been shown to be involved in mature endothelin production.

The endothelins bind to two distinct receptors, designated endothelin types A and B (ET-A and ET-B).[246-248] The ET-A receptor shows a higher affinity for ET-1 than for ET-2 or ET-3. The ET-B receptor shows equal affinity for each of the three endothelins. ET-A receptors are found mainly on vascular smooth muscle cells, on which their activation leads to vasoconstriction through an increase in cytosolic Ca^{2+}. ET-B receptors are also found on vascular smooth muscle cells, on which they can mediate vasoconstriction, but they are found predominantly on vascular endothelium, in which their activation results in vasodilation through prostacyclin and nitric oxide.[248] Endothelin is detectable in the plasma of human subjects and many experimental animals and therefore may also act as a circulating vasoactive hormone.[249]

Selective ET-A receptor antagonism is associated with vasodilation and a reduction in blood pressure, whereas selective ET-B antagonism is accompanied by vasoconstriction and a rise in blood pressure.[248] These data suggest complementary roles for the endothelin receptor subtypes in the maintenance of vascular tone. In addition to its vasoconstrictive action, endothelin has a variety of effects on the kidneys.[246-248,253] The kidney (mainly the inner medulla) is both a source and an important target organ of endothelin. ET-1 is synthesized by the endothelial cells of the renal vessels, whereas ET-1 and ET-3 are produced by various cell types of the nephron. ET-2 and ET-3 are produced at a rate of one to two orders of magnitude lower than ET-1, which appears to be the principal subtype involved in renal functional regulation.[246]

In relation to volume homeostasis, three major aspects of renal function are affected by ET-1 in a paracrine or autocrine manner: (1) renal and intrarenal blood flow, (2) glomerular hemodynamics, and (3) renal tubular transport of salt and water. Both ET-A and ET-B receptors are present in the glomerulus, renal vessels, and tubular epithelial cells, but most ET-B receptors are found in the medulla.[254] The renal vasculature, in comparison with other vascular beds, appears to be most sensitive to the vasoconstrictor action of ET-1. Infusion of ET-1 into the renal artery of anesthetized rabbits decreases RBF, GFR, natriuresis, and urine volume.[255] Micropuncture studies demonstrated that ET-1 increases afferent and efferent arteriolar resistance (afferent more than efferent), which results in a reduction in glomerular plasma flow rate. In addition, K_f is reduced because of mesangial cell contraction, resulting in a diminished SNGFR.

The profound reduction of RBF and concomitant lesser reduction in GFR should result in a rise in filtration fraction, but the effect of ET-1 on the filtration fraction appears to be variable: Some groups, using low doses in a canine model, reported a rise,[256] and others reported no significant effect.[257] Infusion of ET-1 for 8 days into conscious dogs increased plasma levels of endothelin by twofold to threefold and resulted in increased renal vascular resistance and decreased GFR and RBF.[206] Interestingly, the effect of endothelin on regional intrarenal blood flow is not homogeneous. Using laser Doppler flowmetry, Gurbanov and colleagues[258] found that administration of ET-1 in control rats produced a sustained cortical vasoconstriction and a transient medullary vasodilatory response. These results are in line with the medullary predominance of ET-B receptors, and the high density of ET-A–binding sites in the cortex.[246]

The effect of endothelin on Na^+ and water excretion varies and depends on the dose and source of endothelin. Systemic infusion of endothelin in high doses results in profound antinatriuresis and antidiuresis, apparently secondary to the decrease in GFR and RBF. However, in low doses or when produced locally in tubular epithelial cells, endothelin has been claimed to decrease the reabsorption of salt and water, which suggests that ET-1 target sites are present on renal tubules.[259] Also, administration of the endothelin precursor, big endothelin, has been shown to cause natriuresis, which supports the notion of a direct inhibitory autocrine action of endothelin on tubular salt reabsorption.

The natriuretic and diuretic actions of big ET-1 can be significantly reduced by ET-B–specific blockade.[260] Similar results were reported when the same ET-B antagonist was given chronically by osmotic minipump (reviewed by Pollock and Pollock[245]). Furthermore, ET-B–knockout rats have salt-sensitive hypertension that is reversed by luminal ENaC blockade with amiloride, which suggests that, in vivo, ET-B in the collecting duct tonically inhibits ENaC activity, the final regulator of Na^+ balance.[261] Similarly, mice with collecting duct–specific knockout of the ET-1 gene have impaired Na^+ excretion in response to Na^+ load and develop hypertension with high salt intake.[246] These mice also have heightened sensitivity to AVP and reduced ability to excrete an acute water load. These findings are in line with in vitro observations that ET-B mediates the inhibitory effects of ET-1 on Na^+ and water transport in the collecting duct and thick ascending limb of Henle.[246]

Thus, if vascular and mesangial endothelin exerts a greater physiologic effect than does tubule-derived endothelin, then RBF is diminished and net fluid retention occurs, whereas if the tubule-derived endothelin effect predominates, salt and water excretion is increased. The ability of ET-1 to reversibly inhibit AVP-stimulated water permeability was first shown in the isolated perfused IMCD[262] Moreover, ET-1 reduces AVP-stimulated cAMP accumulation and water permeability in the IMCD.[246] In addition, ET-1 mitigates the hydroosmotic effect of AVP in the cortical collecting duct and the outer medullary collecting duct. Furthermore, studies in rabbit cortical collecting duct have demonstrated that ET-1 may inhibit the luminal amiloride-sensitive ENaC by a Ca^{2+}-dependent effect. Moreover, collecting duct–specific ET-1–knockout mice were shown to have an impaired ability to excrete both Na^+ and water loads in comparison with their wild-type counterparts. Taking into account the facts that the medulla contains ET-B receptors and the highest endothelin concentrations in the body, and that endothelins also inhibit Na^+-K^+-ATPase in IMCD,[246] these effects may contribute to the diuretic and natriuretic actions of locally produced ET-1. This may also explain the natriuretic effect of ET-1 reported by some investigators, despite the reduction in RBF and GFR.[263]

Endothelin production in the kidneys is regulated differently than that in the vasculature. Whereas vascular (and mesangial) endothelin generation is controlled by thrombin, angiotensin II, and transforming growth factor–β, tubular endothelin production seems to depend on entirely different mechanisms, of which medullary tonicity may be particularly important. Volume expansion in humans increased urinary endothelin excretion, which was suggestive of an inhibitory action of renal endothelin on water reabsorption, particularly in the collecting duct.[254] Also, a high-salt diet, by raising medullary tonicity, stimulates ET-1 release, which in turn leads to increased endothelial NOS (eNOS, or NOS3) expression and natriuresis.[264] (The NOS-dependent ET-1 effects are discussed further in the following "Nitric Oxide" section). Therefore, both salt and water balance appear to regulate renal endothelin production and collecting duct fluid reabsorption by altering medullary tonicity. The signaling mechanisms for these phenomena, as well other renal actions of ET-1, continue be a subject of intensive research, and the interested reader is referred to a review that summarizes the current state of knowledge.[254]

Nitric Oxide. Nitric oxide is a diffusible gaseous molecule produced from its precursor L-arginine by the enzyme NOS, which exists in three distinct isoforms: nNOS, inducible NOS (iNOS, or NOS2), and eNOS.[245] NOS is expressed in endothelial cells of the renal vasculature (mainly eNOS), tubular epithelial and mesangial cells, and macula densa (mainly nNOS). There is controversy regarding the renal expression of iNOS in normal kidneys, but upregulation of this isoform is clearly seen in pathologic conditions such as ischemia-reperfusion injury (reviewed by Mount and Power[265]).

The availability of selective NOS inhibitors and NOS–knockout mice has improved the ability to investigate the individual role of the NOS isoforms in the regulation of renal function.[99] However, the role of a specific nitric oxide isoform in a given cell type is not yet fully understood. Therefore, this discussion refers to the renal effects of nitric oxide regardless of its enzymatic isoform source, unless the source has been determined.

The action of nitric oxide is mediated by activation of a soluble guanylyl cyclase, thereby increasing intracellular levels of its second messenger, cGMP.[266] In the kidneys, the physiologic roles of nitric oxide include the regulation of glomerular hemodynamics, attenuation of tubuloglomerular feedback, mediation of pressure natriuresis, maintenance of medullary perfusion, inhibition of tubular Na^+ reabsorption, and modulation of RSNA.[245] Renal NOS activity is regulated by several humoral factors, such as angiotensin II (see "Tubuloglomerular Feedback" section) and salt intake.[98]

The role of nitric oxide in the regulation of renal hemodynamics and excretory function is best illustrated by the fact that inhibition of intrarenal nitric oxide production results in increased blood pressure and impaired renal function.[267] Infusion of the NOS inhibitor, N_G monomethyl-L-arginine (L-NMMA), into one kidney in anesthetized dogs resulted in a dose-dependent decrease in urinary cGMP levels, decreases in RBF and GFR, Na^+ and water retention, and a decline in fractional Na^+ excretion in the ipsilateral kidney, in comparison with the contralateral kidney.[267] In addition, acute nitric oxide blockade amplified the renal vasoconstrictive action of angiotensin II in isolated micoperfused rabbit afferent arterioles and in conscious rats, which suggests that nitric oxide and angiotensin II interact in the control of renal vasculature (see Lai et al,[94] Patzak and Persson,[98] and Mount and Power[265] and references therein). This notion is supported by the findings that L-NMMA–induced vasoconstriction led to decreased RBF and K_f and was prevented by RAAS blockade; thus, some of the major effects of nitric oxide are to counterbalance the vasoconstrictive action of angiotensin II.

Nitric oxide has also been shown to exert a vasodilatory action on afferent arterioles and to mediate the renal vasorelaxant actions of acetylcholine and bradykinin (reviewed by Mount and Power[265]). The counterbalancing effect of nitric oxide on angiotensin II–induced efferent arteriolar vasoconstriction and its role in regulating tubuloglomerular feedback and in modulating renin secretion by the juxtaglomerular apparatus are discussed in the "Tubuloglomerular Feedback" section.[98,99]

The involvement of nitric oxide in the regulation of Na^+ balance is well characterized. In conscious dogs on a normal Na^+ diet, nitric oxide inhibition induced a significant decrease in natriuresis and diuresis without a change in arterial pressure. In dogs receiving a high-Na^+ diet and treatment with the nitric oxide inhibitor, L-nitroarginine methyl ester (L-NAME), both arterial pressure and cumulative Na^+ balance were higher than in dogs receiving a comparable diet but no treatment with nitric oxide inhibitors.[268] Exposure of rats to high-salt intake (1% NaCl drinking water) for 2 weeks induced increased serum concentration and urinary excretion of the nitric oxide metabolites, $NO_2 + NO_3$. Urinary $NO_2 + NO_3$ and Na^+ excretion were significantly correlated. The increase in urinary nitric oxide metabolites is attributed to the enhanced expression of all three NOS isoforms in the renal medulla by high-salt intake.[99] These findings suggest that nitric oxide may have a role in promoting diuresis and natriuresis in both normal and increased salt intake/volume-expanded states.[245]

As just mentioned, L-NAME infused directly into the renal medullary interstitium of anesthetized rats reduced papillary blood flow, in association with decreased Na^+ and water excretion, which indicates that nitric oxide exerts a vasodilatory effect on the renal medullary circulation and promotes Na^+ excretion.[126] Consistent with these data are the findings of high levels of eNOS in the renal medulla and the inhibitory effect of nitric oxide on Na^+-K^+-ATPase in the collecting duct.[269] Additional evidence of the involvement of the nitric oxide system in Na^+ homeostasis is derived from studies in which researchers examined the mechanism of salt-sensitive hypertension. According to these studies, activity of NOS, mainly nNOS, is significantly lower in salt-sensitive rats than in salt-resistant rats maintained on a high-salt diet.[270,271] In another study, the impaired activity of NOS in salt-sensitive rats was evidenced by decreased $NO_2 + NO_3$ excretion[272] Intravenous L-arginine increased nitric oxide production and prevented the development of salt-induced hypertension in Dahl salt-sensitive rats.[272] These findings suggest that nNOS plays an important role in Na^+ handling and that decreases in nNOS activity may in part be involved in the mechanism of salt-sensitive hypertension.

The involvement of nitric oxide in the abnormal Na^+ handling in hypertension could result from an inadequate direct effect on tubular Na^+ reabsorption in proximal and distal segments. However, attenuated inhibitory actions of nitric oxide on renin secretion and tubuloglomerular feedback may also contribute to salt retention and subsequent hypertension. In this context, investigators concluded that nitric oxide originating from the macula densa blunted the tubuloglomerular feedback–mediated vasoconstriction during high-salt intake in salt-resistant rats, whereas in salt-sensitive rats, this response was lost.[273] As already mentioned, there is strong evidence that both the medullary and other effects of nitric oxide occur in response to local endothelin production.[245] For example, the inhibition of NOS by L-NAME or the highly selective ET-B antagonist A-192621 abolished the diuretic and natriuretic effects of big ET-1 in the kidneys of anesthetized rats.[260] In addition, ET-1 acutely activated eNOS in the isolated medullary thick ascending limb of Henle and nNOS in isolated IMCD cells, via ET-B activation. Studies in ET-B receptor–deficient rats have shown that this activation of nNOS and eNOS is accompanied by an increase in nNOS protein but no change in messenger RNA expression (see Pollock and Pollock[245] and references therein). These data suggest that nNOS and eNOS activation occur by post-transcriptional pathways.

Activation of eNOS in the IMCD is also associated with inhibition of Na^+ reabsorption in the medullary thick ascending limb of Henle through phosphatidylinositol 3-kinase (PI3K)–stimulated Akt activity, leading to eNOS phosphorylation at Ser1177.[274] Thus, ET-1 has a paracrine effect on eNOS expression in the IMCD. However, the functional corollary of nNOS activation in the IMCD remains to be determined. A further action of nitric oxide is the inhibition of AVP-enhanced Na^+ reabsorption and hydroosmotic water permeability of the cortical collecting duct.[275] The signaling mechanisms involved in the nitric oxide effects on AVP have not been studied in detail. The role of nitric oxide in pressure natriuresis and RSNA is discussed in the relevant sections.

Kinins. The kallikrein-kinin system is a complex cascade responsible for the generation and release of vasoactive kinins. The active peptides bradykinin and kallidin are formed from precursors (kininogens) that are cleaved by tissue and circulatory kinin-forming enzymes.[276] Kinins are produced by many cell types and can be detected in urine, saliva, sweat, interstitial fluid, and, in rare cases, venous blood. The levels of bradykinin in the circulation are almost undetectable because of rapid metabolism by kininases, particularly kininase II/ACE1. The renal kallikrein-kinin system can produce local concentrations of bradykinin much higher than those present in blood. In the kidneys, bradykinin is metabolized by NEP.[277]

Kinins play an important role in hemodynamic and excretory processes through their G protein–coupled receptors,

BK-B_1 and BK-B_2. The BK-B_2 receptors mediate most of the actions of kinins[277] and are located mainly in the kidneys, although they are also detectable in the heart, lungs, brain, uterus, and testes. Activation of BK-B_2 receptors results in vasodilation, probably through a nitric oxide– or arachidonic acid metabolite–dependent mechanism.[276,278] Bradykinin is known for its multiple effects on the cardiovascular system, particularly vasodilation and plasma extravasation.[276]

Besides the vasculature, the kidney is an important target organ of kinins, in which they induce diuresis and natriuresis through activation of BK-B_2 receptors. These effects are attributed to an increase in RBF and to inhibition of Na^+ and water reabsorption in the distal nephron.[279,280] The latter effect is secondary to the observed action of kinins in reducing vascular resistance. Unlike many vasodilators, bradykinin increases RBF without significantly affecting GFR or Na^+ reabsorption at the proximal tubule level, but this increase is accompanied by a marked decrease in the water and salt reabsorption in the distal nephron, thus contributing to increased urine volume and Na^+ excretion.

Studies with transgenic animals have enriched the understanding of the physiologic role of the kinins and the interaction between the kallikrein-kinin system and the RAAS.[279] For instance, in the kidneys, angiotensin II acting through the AT_2 receptor stimulates a vasodilator cascade of bradykinin, nitric oxide, and cGMP during conditions of increased angiotensin II, such as Na^+ depletion.[267] In the absence of the AT_2 receptor, pressor and antinatriuretic hypersensitivity to angiotensin II is associated with bradykinin and nitric oxide deficiency.[267] Furthermore, involvement of the renal kinins in pressure natriuresis has been documented.[128] Bradykinin also mediates the biologic actions of angiotensin-(1-7), as shown in rats transgenic for the kallikrein gene, which display significantly augmented angiotensin-(1-7) mediated diuresis and natriuresis.[279] Because ACE is involved in the degradation of kinins, ACE inhibitors not only attenuate the formation of angiotensin II but also may lead to the accumulation of kinins. The latter are believed to be responsible in part for the beneficial effects of ACE inhibitors in patients with CHF, but also for their troublesome side effect of cough.[281] On the basis of the results of these studies, as well as those in which BKB_2 specific antagonists were used, the kallikrein-kinin system is believed to play a pivotal role in the regulation of fluid and electrolyte balance, mainly by acting as a counterregulatory modulator of vasoconstrictor and Na^+-retaining mechanisms.

Adrenomedullin. Human adrenomedullin is a 52–amino acid peptide that was discovered in 1993 by Kitamura and associates[282] in extracts of human pheochromocytoma cells. Adrenomedullin is approximately 30% homologous in structure with calcitonin gene–related peptide and amylin.[282,283] Adrenomedullin is produced from a 185–amino acid prepro-hormone that also contains a unique 20–amino acid sequence in the NH_2-terminus, termed *proadrenomedulin NH_2-terminal 20 peptide.* This sequence exists in vivo and has biologic activity similar to that of adrenomedullin.

Adrenomedullin messenger RNA is expressed in several tissues, including those of the atria, ventricles, vascular tissue, lungs, kidneys, pancreas, smooth muscle cells, small intestine, and brain. The synthesis and secretion of adrenomedullin are stimulated by chemical factors and physical stress. Among these stimulants are cytokines, corticosteroids, thyroid hormones, angiotensin II, norepinephrine, endothelin, bradykinin, and shear stress.[284] Adrenomedullin immunoreactivity has been localized in high concentrations in pheochromocytoma cells, the adrenal medulla, the atria, the pituitary gland, and, at lower levels, in cardiac ventricles, vascular smooth muscle cells, endothelial cells, glomeruli, distal and medullary collecting tubules, and the digestive, respiratory, reproductive, and endocrine systems.[284,285]

Adrenomedullin acts through a 395–amino acid membrane receptor that structurally resembles a G protein–coupled receptor and contains seven transmembrane domains. Adrenomedullin receptors constitute the calcitonin receptor–like receptor and a family of receptor-activity–modifying proteins.[286] Activation of these receptors increases intracellular cAMP, which probably serves as a second messenger for the peptide.[283,287] The most impressive biologic effect of adrenomedullin is long-lasting and dose-dependent vasodilation of the vascular system, including coronary arteries.[283,287,288] Injection of adrenomedullin into anesthetized rats, cats, or conscious sheep induced a potent and long-lasting hypotensive response associated with reduction in vascular resistance in the kidneys, brain, lungs, hind limbs, and mesentery.[284] The hypotensive action of adrenomedullin is accompanied by increases in heart rate and cardiac output caused by positive inotropic effects.[284] The vasodilating effect of adrenomedullin can be blocked by inhibiting NOS, which suggests that nitric oxide partly mediates the decrease in systemic vascular resistance.[283]

Besides its hypotensive action, adrenomedullin increases RBF through preglomerular and postglomerular arteriolar vasodilation.[287,289] The adrenomedullin-induced hyperperfusion is associated with dose-dependent diuresis and natriuresis.[284,287] These effects result from a decrease in tubular Na^+ reabsorption despite the adrenomedullin-induced hyperfiltration[289] and may be mediated partially by the locally released nitric oxide[290,291] and prostaglandins.[292] In addition, NEP inhibition potentiates exogenous adrenomedullin-induced natriuresis without affecting GFR.[293] Like natriuretic peptides, adrenomedullin suppresses aldosterone secretion in response to angiotensin II and high potassium levels.[283] Furthermore, in cultured vascular smooth muscle cells, adrenomedullin inhibits endothelin production induced by various stimuli.[284] Adrenomedullin acts in the CNS to inhibit both water and salt intake.[294] In the hypothalamus, adrenomedullin inhibits the secretion of AVP, an effect that may also contribute to its diuretic and natriuretic actions.[294]

Together, these findings show that adrenomedullin is a vasoactive peptide that may be involved in the physiologic control of renal, adrenal, vascular, and cardiac function. Furthermore, the existence of adrenomedullin-like immunoreactivity in the glomerulus and in the collecting tubule, in association with detectable amounts of adrenomedullin messenger RNA in the kidneys, suggests that adrenomedullin plays a renal paracrine role.[295]

In 2008, a new member of the adrenomedullin family, adrenomedullin-2 or intermedin, was identified. Adrenomedullin-2 is about 30% homologous with adrenomedullin. Because its renal and cardiovascular effects are similar to those of adrenomedullin-1, they are not discussed further here. The interested reader is referred to a comprehensive review.[296]

Urotensin. Urotensin II is a highly conserved peptide which binds to the human orphan G protein–coupled receptor GPR14, now named the urotensin II receptor. The parent peptide, prepro–urotensin II, is widely expressed in human tissues, including those of the CNS and peripheral nervous system, the GI tract, the vascular system, and the kidneys.[297] In the kidneys, immunoreactive staining for urotensin II was detected in the epithelial cells of the tubules, mostly in the distal tubule, with moderate staining in endothelial cells of the renal capillaries.[298] The C-terminus of the prohormone is cleaved to produce urotensin II, an 11–amino acid residue peptide. The human form of urotensin II includes a cyclic hexapeptide sequence that is fundamental for the action of this compound. The metabolic pathway leading to the production of urotensin II still remains incompletely characterized. Substantial urotensin II arteriovenous gradients (36% to 44%) have been demonstrated in the heart, liver, and kidneys, which is indicative of local urotensin II production.[299]

In vivo in humans, systemic infusion of urotensin II range led to local vasoconstriction in the forearm, no effect, or cutaneous vasodilation (reviewed by Richards and Charles[300]). These dissimilarities are probably attributable to many factors, including species variation, site and modality of injection, dose, vascular bed, and functional conditions of the experimental model.[300] Because urotensin II has been described as the most potent vasoconstrictor (see "Endothelin" section), it is reasonable to postulate that the vasoconstrictive action is direct, whereas the vasodilatory response may be mediated by other factors such as cyclooxygenase products and nitric oxide.

The involvement of the urotensin II system in the regulation of renal function in mammals has not been thoroughly investigated, and the data reported to date are as contradictory as those for vascular tone. In normal rats, intravenous boluses in the 1-nmol range caused minor reductions in GFR and no effect on Na^+ excretion.[301] However, in another study in which the same model was used, continuous infusion of urotensin II at doses in the 1-nmol/kg range elicited clear increases in GFR and nitric oxide–dependent diuresis and natriuresis.[302] In contrast, bolus injections in the 1-nmol range produced a dose-dependent decrease in GFR associated with reduced urine flow and Na^+ excretion.[303] Studies in rats with an aortocaval fistula (a model of chronic volume overload) showed that urotensin II boluses in the 1-nmol range exerted favorable, nitric oxide–dependent, renal hemodynamic effects.[301] Thus, the effect of urotensin II on renal function seems dependent on the modality of administration (bolus vs. continuous infusion) and on the experimental condition being investigated (normal rats vs. those with heart failure).

The variability in renal and vascular responses to urotensin II administration may also depend on the fact that the action of this peptide is regulated at the receptor level. The binding density of urotensin II is correlated with vasoconstrictor response in rats, and small changes in receptor density may result in pathophysiologic effects. Under normal conditions, most urotensin II receptors are already occupied by urotensin II. Changes in unoccupied receptor reserve—perhaps in response to alterations in urotensin II levels generated in experimental models or observed in disease states—might explain, at least in part, the observed variability in studies of renal and vascular function.[304]

Selective urotensin II receptor antagonists have been developed, the most potent of which is currently urantide. In normal rats, continuous administration of this compound increases GFR, as well as urine flow and Na^+ excretion.[303] On the basis of experimental results indicating that urotensin

II increases epithelial Na^+ transport in fish, it appears likely that urotensin II exerts a direct tubular effect, inasmuch as its receptor is expressed in the distal tubule.[303] Overall, urotensin II seems to have a tonic influence on renal function. To date, no data in humans are available.

Digitalis-Like Factors. In the early 1960s, Hugh de Wardener hypothesized the existence of endogenous digitalis-like factors, and an endogenous ouabain-like compound in human and other mammalian plasma was initially reported in the late 1970s.[304a,304b] Since 2000, interest in such factors—also known as endogenous cardiotonic steroids—has expanded considerably. In particular, two specific cardiotonic steroids in humans have been characterized extensively: endogenous cardenolide (or ouabain) and bufadienolide (marinobufagenin). An alternative mechanism by which cardiotonic steroids can signal through the Na^+-K^+-ATPase has also been described.[305] The main site of synthesis of these compounds is the adrenal cortex,[10] and the main consequences of Na^+ pump inhibition are attenuation of renal Na^+ transport and increased cytosolic Ca^{2+} in vascular smooth muscle cells, which lead to increased vascular resistance.[306] The latter mechanism has been implicated in the pathogenesis of hypertension. More recent work has also implicated these hormones in the regulation of cell growth, differentiation, apoptosis, and fibrosis; in the modulation of immunity and of carbohydrate metabolism; and in the control of various central nervous functions, including behavior.[305,307]

Neuropeptide Y. Neuropeptide Y, a 36-residue peptide, is a sympathetic cotransmitter stored and released together with noradrenaline by adrenergic nerve terminals of the SNS. Structurally, neuropeptide Y is highly homologous to two other members of the pancreatic polypeptide family, peptide YY and pancreatic polypeptide. These two closely related peptides are produced and released by the intestinal endocrine and pancreatic islet cells, respectively, and act as hormones.[308,309] Although neuropeptide Y was originally isolated from the brain and is highly expressed in the CNS, the peptide exhibits a wide spectrum of biologic activities in the cardiovascular system, GI tract, and kidneys[310-312] through multiple $G_{i/o}$ protein–coupled receptors: Y1, Y2, Y4, and Y5.[313]

In numerous studies, both in vivo and in vitro techniques demonstrated the capacity of the neuropeptide Y to reduce RBF and increase renal vascular resistance in various species, including rats, rabbits, pigs, and humans.[310] Despite the potent vasoconstrictor effect of the peptide on renal vasculature, this effect does not appear to be associated with any significant change in GFR. In view of the potent renal vasoconstrictor action of neuropeptide Y, a decrease in electrolyte and water excretion could be expected after its administration. However, the available data suggest that neuropeptide Y may exert either a natriuretic[314] or an antinatriuretic[315] action, depending on the experimental conditions and the species studied. In the absence of any new data since the publication of the previous edition of this book, the role of neuropeptide Y in the physiologic regulation of renal hemodynamics and electrolyte excretion remains enigmatic.

Apelin. Apelin is the endogenous ligand of the angiotensin-like receptor 1, a G protein–coupled receptor found to be involved in various physiologic events, such as water homeostasis, regulation of cardiovascular tone, and cardiac contractility (see Principe et al[316] and references therein). Apelin and its receptor are widely expressed in the CNS and in peripheral tissues, especially in endothelial cells. Apelin is also expressed in endothelial and vascular smooth muscle cells of glomerular arterioles and, to a lesser extent, in other parts of the nephron.[317]

Angiotensin-like receptor 1 activation leads to inhibition of cAMP production and activation of the Na^+/H^+ exchanger type 1. Through the former pathway, apelin enhances vascular dilation after the induction of eNOS, whereas the burst of Na^+/H^+ exchanger type 1 activity in cardiomyocytes leads to a dose-dependent increase in myocardial contractility (see Principe et al[316] and references therein). With regard to the renal effects of apelin, direct injection into the hypothalamus of lactating rats inhibited AVP release and reduced circulating AVP. Conversely, water deprivation led to increased systemic AVP and decreased apelin levels (see Principe et al[316] and references therein). These findings suggest that AVP and apelin have a reciprocal relationship in controlling water diuresis.

Apelin appears to also counter-regulate several effects of angiotensin II. For example, intravenous injection of apelin caused a nitric oxide–dependent fall in arterial pressure. Moreover, apelin receptor–knockout mice displayed an enhanced vasopressor response to systemic angiotensin II.[318] In addition, apelin modulated the abnormal aortic vascular tone in response to angiotensin II through eNOS phosphorylation in diabetic mice; this finding provided further evidence of a role for apelin in vascular function.[319] Intravenous injection of apelin also induced a significant diuresis and caused vasorelaxation of angiotensin II–preconstricted efferent and afferent arterioles. Activation of endothelial apelin receptors caused release of nitric oxide, which inhibited the angiotensin II–induced rise in intracellular Ca^{2+} levels. Furthermore, apelin had a direct receptor-mediated vasoconstrictive effect on vascular smooth muscle.[318] These results show that apelin has complex effects on the preglomerular and postglomerular microvasculature regulating renal hemodynamics. A direct role in tubular function remains to be determined but is suggested by collecting duct expression in close proximity to the vasopressin V_2 receptor.[317]

EXTRARENAL MECHANISMS OF VOLUME REGULATION: INTERSTITIAL HYPERTONIC SODIUM ACCUMULATION IN THE SKIN

The traditional two-compartment model of volume regulation, according to which the intravascular and interstitial spaces are in equilibrium, has been challenged. Results of initial studies indicated that Na^+ can be bound to and stored on proteoglycans in interstitial sites, where it becomes osmotically inactive; accordingly, a novel mechanism of volume regulation has been elucidated.[320-327] In rats fed a high-salt diet, this uniquely bound Na^+ was found to induce a state of subcutaneous interstitial hypertonicity and systemic hypertension.[322] Machnik and colleagues[320] offered compelling experimental evidence that this hypertonicity is sensed by macrophages, which then produce vascular endothelial growth factor C (VEGF-C), an angiogenic protein. In turn, VEGF-C stimulates increased numbers and density of lymphatic capillaries. Using cultured macrophage cell lines, subjected to osmotic stress, Go and associates[328] demonstrated activation of a transcription factor, tonicity-responsive enhancer–binding protein (TonEBP). This factor is known to activate osmoprotective genes in other hypertonic environments, such as the renal medulla.[328] Moreover, analysis of the VEGF-C promoter revealed two TonEBP binding sites and, in subsequent experiments, parallel upregulation of TonEBP and VEGF-C was observed. The effect of TonEBP on VEGF-C was shown to be specific, inasmuch as small interfering RNA for TonEBP, but not nonspecific small interfering RNA, inhibited the VEGF-C upregulation. Furthermore, macrophage depletion or inhibition of VEGF-C signaling led to exacerbation of high-salt diet–induced hypertension, clearly demonstrating the importance of this pathway in blood pressure regulation.[320] Finally, in humans with relatively resistant hypertension, elevated levels of VEGF-C were found,[320] which is consistent with a potential role of this growth factor in the redistribution of excess volume to the intravascular space and exacerbation of hypertension.[329]

Sodium Balance Disorders

Hypovolemia

Definition

Hypovolemia is the condition in which the volume of the ECF compartment is reduced in relation to its capacitance. As already discussed, the reduction may be absolute or relative. In states of absolute hypovolemia, the Na^+ balance is truly negative, reflecting past or ongoing losses. Hypovolemia is described as *relative* when there is no Na^+ deficit but the capacitance of the ECF compartment is increased. In this situation of reduced EABV, the ECF intravascular and extravascular (interstitial) compartments may vary in the same or opposite directions. ICF volume, reflected by measurements of plasma Na^+ or osmolality, may or may not be concomitantly disturbed; thus, hypovolemia may be classified as normonatremic, hyponatremic, or hypernatremic (see also Chapter 15, "Disorders of Water Balance").

Etiology

The causes of hypovolemia are summarized in Table 14-5. Both absolute and relative hypovolemia, in turn, can have either extrarenal or renal causes. *Absolute hypovolemia* results either from massive blood loss or from fluid loss from the skin, the gastrointestinal or respiratory system, or the kidneys. *Relative hypovolemia* results from states of vasodilation, generalized edema, or third-space loss. In both absolute and relative hypovolemia, the perceived reduction in intravascular volume prompts the compensatory hemodynamic changes and renal responses described in the "Physiology" section; the familiar clinical manifestations include tachycardia, hypotension, and renal retention of Na^+ and water.

Pathophysiology

ABSOLUTE HYPOVOLEMIA

Extrarenal. Massive bleeding, either gastrointestinal or a result of trauma, is the most frequent cause of absolute hypovolemia. The reduction in ECF volume is isotonic inasmuch as there is a proportionate loss of erythrocytes and plasma. The consequent fall in systemic blood pressure leads to compensatory tachycardia and vasoconstriction, and the ensuing altered transcapillary Starling hydraulic forces enable a shift of fluid from the interstitial to intravascular compartment.

TABLE 14-5 Causes of Absolute and Relative Hypovolemia

Absolute

Extrarenal

Bleeding
Gastrointestinal fluid loss
Skin fluid loss
Respiratory fluid loss
Extracorporeal ultrafiltration

Renal

Diuretics
Na^+ wasting tubulopathies
  Genetic
  Acquired tubulointerstitial disease
Obstructive uropathy/postobstructive diuresis
Hormone deficiency
  Hypoaldosteronism
  Adrenal insufficiency

Relative

Extrarenal

Edematous states
  Heart failure
  Cirrhosis
Generalized vasodilation
  Drugs
  Sepsis
  Pregnancy
Third-space loss

Renal

Severe nephrotic syndrome

In addition, the neural and hormonal responses to hypovolemia, described in the "Physiology" section, result in renal Na^+ and water retention, with the aim of restoring intravascular volume and hemodynamic stability.

Similar compensatory mechanisms become activated after fluid losses from the skin, the gastrointestinal system, and the respiratory system. Because of the large surface area of the skin, large amounts of fluid can be lost from this tissue. This can result from burns or excessive perspiration. Severe burns allow the loss of large volumes of plasma and interstitial fluid and can lead rapidly to profound hypovolemia. In the absence of medical intervention, hemoconcentration and hypoalbuminemia supervene. As after massive bleeding, the fluid loss is isotonic, and so plasma Na^+ concentration and osmolality remain normal. In contrast, excessive sweating, induced by exertion in hot environments, leads to hypotonic fluid loss as a result of the relatively low Na^+ concentration in this fluid (20 to 50 mmol/L). The resulting hypovolemia may, therefore, be accompanied by hypernatremia and hyperosmolality, and the type of fluid replacement must be tailored accordingly (see also Chapter 15).

Besides oral intake, the gastrointestinal tract is characterized by the entry of approximately 7 L of isotonic fluid, the overwhelming majority of which is reabsorbed in the large intestine. Hence, in normal conditions, fecal fluid loss is minimal. However, in the presence of pathologic conditions, such as vomiting, diarrhea, colostomy, and ileostomy secretions, especially those caused by infection, considerable or even massive fluid loss may occur. The ionic composition, osmolality, and pH of secretions vary according to the part of the gastrointestinal tract; therefore, the resulting hypovolemia is associated with a large spectrum of electrolyte and acid-base abnormalities (see appropriate chapters for further discussion).

In contrast to the massive losses that can occur from the skin and gastrointestinal system, fluid loss from the respiratory tract—as occurs in febrile states and patients who receive mechanical ventilation with inadequate humidification—is usually modest, and hypovolemia ensues only in the presence of accompanying causes. Finally, a special situation in which hypovolemia can occur is after excessive ultrafiltration in dialysis patients (see Chapter 64)

Renal. As described earlier, when the GFR and plasma Na^+ concentration are normal, approximately 24,000 mmol of Na^+ is filtered per day. Even when GFR is markedly impaired, the amount of filtered Na^+ far exceeds the dietary intake. In order to maintain Na^+ balance, all but 1% of the filtered load is reabsorbed. However, if the integrity of one or more of the tubular reabsorptive mechanisms is impaired, serious Na^+ deficit and absolute volume depletion can occur. The causes of absolute renal Na^+ losses include pharmacologic agents, renal structural disorders, endocrine disorders, and systemic disorders (see Table 14-5). All the diuretics widely used to treat hypervolemic states may induce hypovolemia if administered in excess or inappropriately. In particular, the powerful loop diuretics furosemide, bumetanide, torsemide, and ethacrynic acid are often given in combination with diuretics acting on other tubular segments (thiazides, aldosterone antagonists, distal ENaC blockers, and carbonic anhydrase inhibitors). Patients receiving these combinations need to be carefully monitored and fluid balance scrupulously adjusted in order to prevent hypovolemia. Patients commonly at risk are those with CHF or underlying hypertension who develop intercurrent infections.

Na^+ reabsorption may also be disrupted in inherited and acquired tubular disorders. Inherited disorders of both the proximal tubules (e.g., Fanconi's syndrome) and the distal tubules (e.g., Bartter's and Gitelman's syndromes) may lead to salt-wasting states in association with other electrolyte or acid-base disturbances. Acquired disorders of Na^+ reabsorption may be acute, as in nonoliguric acute kidney injury, the time immediately after renal transplantation, the polyuric recovery phase of acute kidney injury, and postobstructive diuresis (see relevant chapters for further details), or they may be chronic as a result of tubulointerstitial diseases with a propensity for salt wasting. In fact, chronic kidney disease of any cause is associated with heightened vulnerability to Na^+ losses because the ability to match tubular reabsorption with the sum of filtered load minus dietary intake is impaired.

In patients with hypertension, the frequent administration of diuretics for treatment further increases the risk of volume depletion. Osmotic diuretics, endogenous or exogenous, may also reduce tubular Na^+ reabsorption. Endogenous agents include urea—the principle molecule involved in the polyuric recovery phase of acute kidney injury and postobstructive diuresis—and glucose in hyperglycemia. In patients with raised intracranial pressure, exogenous agents, such as mannitol or glycerol, may be used to induce translocation of fluid from the ICF compartment to the ECF compartment and decrease brain swelling. The resulting polyuria may be associated with electrolyte and acid-base disturbances, the nature of which depends on the complex interplay between fluid intake and intercompartmental fluid shifts.

In addition to intrinsic tubular disorders, endocrine and other systemic disturbances may lead to impaired Na^+ reabsorption. The principal endocrine causes are mineralocorticoid deficiency and resistance states. A controversial cause is the systemic disturbance known as cerebral salt wasting. In this condition, salt wasting is thought to occur in response to an as-yet-unidentified factor released in the setting of acute head injury or intracranial hemorrhage.[330,331] The condition is usually diagnosed because of concomitant hyponatremia, and some experts doubt its independent existence, regarding cerebral salt wasting as essentially indistinguishable from the syndrome of inappropriate AVP.[332]

An underappreciated but not uncommon clinical setting for renal Na^+ loss is after the administration of large volumes of intravenous saline to patients over several days after surgery or after trauma. In this situation, tubular reabsorption of Na^+ is downregulated. If intravenous fluids are stopped before full reabsorptive capacity is restored, volume depletion may ensue. The phenomenon can be minimized by graded reduction in the infusion rate, which allows Na^+ reabsorptive pathways to be restored gradually.

In the context of volume depletion, mention should be made of diabetes insipidus. However, because this results from a deficiency of or tubular resistance to AVP, water loss is the main consequence, and the impact on ECF volume is only minor. AVP-related disorders are considered in Chapter 15.

RELATIVE HYPOVOLEMIA

Extrarenal. As outlined previously, the principal causes of relative hypovolemia are edematous states, vasodilation, and third-space loss (see Table 14-5). Vasodilation may be physiologic, as in normal pregnancy, or induced by drugs (hypotensive agents, such as hydralazine or minoxidil, that cause arteriolar vasodilation), or it may occur in sepsis during the phases of peripheral vasodilation and consequent low systemic vascular resistance.[333]

Edematous states in which the EABV and, hence, tissue perfusion are reduced include heart failure, decompensated cirrhosis with ascites, and nephrotic syndrome. In severe heart failure, low cardiac output and resulting low systemic blood pressure lead to a fall in RPP. As in absolute hypovolemia, the kidneys respond by retaining Na^+. Because the increased venous return cannot raise the cardiac output, a vicious cycle is created in which edema is further exacerbated and the persistently reduced cardiac output leads to further Na^+ retention. In decompensated cirrhosis, splanchnic venous pooling leads to decreased venous return, a consequent fall in cardiac output, and compensatory renal Na^+ retention. The pathophysiologic features of edematous states are discussed in more detail in the "Hypervolemia" section. Third-space loss occurs when fluid is sequestered into compartments not normally perfused with fluids, as in states of gastrointestinal obstruction, after trauma, in burns, in pancreatitis, in peritonitis, or in malignant ascites. The end result is that even though total body Na^+ is markedly increased, the EABV is severely reduced.

Renal. Approximately 10% of patients with the nephrotic syndrome—especially children with minimal change disease, but also any patient with serum albumin levels lower than 2 g/dL—manifest the clinical signs of hypovolemia. The low plasma oncotic pressure is conducive to movement of fluid from the ECF compartment to the interstitial space, thereby leading to reduced EABV.[334,335]

Clinical Manifestations

The clinical manifestations of hypovolemia depend on the magnitude and rate of volume loss, solute composition of the net fluid loss (i.e., the difference between input and output), and vascular and renal responses. The clinical features can be considered as being related to the underlying pathophysiologic process, the hemodynamic consequences, and the electrolyte and acid-base disturbances that attend the renal response to hypovolemia. A detailed history often reveals the cause of volume depletion (bleeding, vomiting, diarrhea, polyuria, diaphoresis, medications).

The symptoms and physical signs of hypovolemia appear only when intravascular volume is decreased by 5% to 15% and are often related to tissue hypoperfusion. Symptoms include generalized weakness, muscle cramps, and postural lightheadedness. Thirst is prominent if concomitant hypertonicity is present (hypertonic hypovolemia). Physical signs are related to the hemodynamic consequences of hypovolemia and include tachycardia; hypotension, which may be postural, absolute, or relative to the usual blood pressure; and low central venous pressure or jugular venous pressure. Elevation of jugular venous pressure, however, does not rule out hypovolemia, because of the possible confounding effects of underlying heart failure or lung disease. When volume depletion exceeds 10% to 20%, circulatory collapse is liable to occur, with severe supine hypotension, peripheral cyanosis, cold extremities, and impaired consciousness, extending even to coma. This is especially possible if fluid loss is rapid or occurs against a background of comorbid conditions. When the source of volume loss is extrarenal, oliguria also occurs. The traditional signs—reduced skin turgor, sunken eyes, and dry mucous membranes—are inconstant findings, and their absence is not considered useful for ruling out hypovolemia.

Diagnosis

The diagnosis of hypovolemia is based essentially on the clinical findings. Nevertheless, when the clinical findings are equivocal, various laboratory parameters may be helpful for confirming the diagnosis or for elucidating other changes that may be associated with volume depletion.

LABORATORY FINDINGS

Hemoglobin may decrease if significant bleeding has occurred or is ongoing, but this change, which is caused by hemodilution that results from translocation of fluid from the interstitial to intravascular compartment, may take up to 24 hours. Therefore, stable hemoglobin does not rule out significant bleeding. Moreover, the adaptive response of hemodilution may moderate the severity of hemodynamic compromise and the resulting physical signs. In hypovolemic situations that do not arise from bleeding, hemoconcentration is often seen, although this too is not universal, inasmuch as underlying chronic diseases that cause anemia may mask the differential loss of plasma.

Hemoconcentration may also be manifested as a rise in *plasma albumin* concentration, if albumin-free fluid is lost from the skin, gastrointestinal tract, or kidneys. On the other hand, when albumin is lost, either in parallel with other extracellular fluids (as in proteinuria, hepatic disease, protein-losing enteropathy, or catabolic states) or in protein-rich fluid

(third-space sequestration, burns), significant hypoalbuminemia is observed.

Plasma Na^+ concentration may be low, normal, or high, depending on the solute composition of the fluid lost and the replacement solution administered by either the patient or the treating physician. For example, the hypovolemic stimulus for AVP release may lead to preferential water retention and hyponatremia, especially if hypotonic replacement fluid is used. In contrast, the fluid content of diarrhea may be hypotonic or hypertonic, resulting, respectively, in hypernatremia or hyponatremia. Plasma Na^+ concentration reflects tonicity of plasma and provides no direct information about volume status, which is a clinical diagnosis.

Plasma K^+ and *acid-base* parameters can also change in hypovolemic conditions. After vomiting and also some forms of diarrhea, loss of K^+ and Cl^- may lead to hypokalemic alkalosis. More often, the principal anion lost in diarrhea is bicarbonate, which leads to hyperchloremic (non–anion gap) acidosis. When diuretics or Bartter's and Gitelman's syndromes (the inherited tubulopathies; Chapter 44) are the cause of hypovolemia, hypokalemic alkalosis is again typically seen. On the other hand, U_{Na} loss that occurs in adrenal insufficiency or is caused by aldosterone hyporesponsiveness is accompanied by a tendency for hyperkalemia and metabolic acidosis. Finally, when hypovolemia is sufficiently severe to impair tissue perfusion, high anion gap acidosis caused by lactic acid accumulation may be observed.

Blood urea and *creatinine* levels frequently rise in hypovolemic states, and this elevation reflects impaired renal perfusion. If tubular integrity is preserved, then the rise in urea level is typically disproportionate to that of creatinine (see Chapter 30). This results mainly because AVP enhances reabsorption of urea in the medullary collecting duct and as an effect of increased filtration fraction on proximal tubule handling of urea (reviewed by Blantz[336]). In the presence of severe hypovolemia, acute kidney injury may ensue, leading to loss of the differential rise in urea level. Proportional rises in urea and creatinine are also observed when hypovolemia occurs against a background of underlying renal functional impairment, as in chronic kidney disease stages 3 to 5 (Chapter 51).

Urine biochemical parameters can be extremely useful in establishing the diagnosis of hypovolemia caused by extrarenal fluid losses if there is no intrinsic renal injury and the patient is oliguric. The expected renal response of Na^+ and water conservation, by enhanced renal tubular reabsorption, results in oliguria, urine specific gravity exceeding 1.020, Na^+ concentration higher than 10 mmol/L, and osmolality higher than 400 mOsm/kg. When Na^+ concentration is 20 to 40 mmol/L, the finding of a fractional excretion of Na^+ (Na^+ clearance × 100/creatinine clearance) of less than 1% in the presence of a reduced GFR may be helpful. In a patient who previously received diuretic therapy, especially with loop diuretics, these indices may merely reflect the U_{Na} losses. In that case, fractional excretion of urea from less than 30% to 35% may help in the diagnosis of hypovolemia, although the specificity of this test is rather low.[337-339]

When hypovolemia occurs in the presence of arterial vasodilation, as observed in sepsis, some, but not all, of the clinical manifestations of hypovolemia are observed. Thus, tachycardia and hypotension are usually present, but the extremities are warm, which suggests that perfusion is maintained. This finding is misleading because vital organs, particularly the brain and kidneys, are underperfused as a result of the hypotension. The presence of lactic acidosis helps establish the correct diagnosis. Reduction in the EABV, as manifested by relative hypotension, may be observed in generalized edematous states, even though there is an overall excess of Na^+ and water; however, this excess is maldistributed between the extracellular and interstitial spaces.

Treatment

Absolute Hypovolemia

General Principles. The goals of treatment of hypovolemia are to restore normal hemodynamic status and tissue perfusion. These goals are achieved by reversal of the clinical symptoms and signs, described previously. Treatment can be divided into three stages: (1) initial replacement of the immediate fluid deficit; (2) maintenance of the restored ECF volume in the presence of ongoing losses; and (3) treatment of the underlying cause whenever possible. The main strategies to be addressed by the clinician are the route, volume, rate of administration, and composition of the replacement and maintenance fluids. These are liable to change according to the patient's response.

In general, when hypovolemia is associated with significant hemodynamic disturbance, intravenous rehydration is required. (The use of oral electrolyte solutions in the management of infant diarrhea is discussed in Chapters 73 through 77.) The volume of fluid and rate of administration should be determined on the basis of the urgency of the threat to circulatory integrity, adequacy of the clinical response, and underlying cardiac function. Elderly patients are especially vulnerable to aggressive fluid challenge, and careful monitoring is required, particularly to prevent acute left ventricular failure and pulmonary edema that result from overzealous correction.

Sometimes the clinical signs do not point unequivocally to the diagnosis of hypovolemia, even though the history is strongly suggestive. Because invasive monitoring of central venous and pulmonary venous pressures has not been shown to improve outcomes in this situation,[340,341] a "diagnostic fluid challenge" can be performed. If the patient improves clinically, blood pressure and urine output increase, and no overt signs of heart failure appear over the succeeding 6 to 12 hours, then the diagnosis is substantiated and fluid therapy can be cautiously continued. Conversely, if overt signs of fluid overload appear, the fluid challenge can be stopped and diuretic therapy reinstituted.

The initial calculations for replacing the fluid deficit are based on hemodynamic status. It is notoriously difficult to calculate volume deficits; therefore, good clinical judgment is necessary for successful management. Patients with life-threatening circulatory collapse and hypovolemic shock require rapid intravenous replacement through the cannula with the widest bore possible. This replacement should continue until blood pressure is corrected and tissue perfusion is restored. In the second stage of fluid replacement, the rate of administration should be reduced to maintain blood pressure and tissue perfusion. In elderly patients and those with underlying cardiac dysfunction, the risk of overrapid correction and precipitating pulmonary edema is heightened; therefore, slower treatment is preferable, to allow gradual filling of the ECF volume rather than causing pulmonary edema and

the threat of mechanical ventilation that are associated with adverse outcomes.[342]

Composition of Replacement Fluids. The composition of replacement fluid is less critical than the rate of infusion. The two main categories of replacement solution are crystalloid and colloid solutions. *Crystalloid solutions* are based largely on either NaCl of varying tonicity or dextrose. Isotonic (0.9%) saline, containing 154 mmol of Na^+ per liter, is the mainstay of volume replacement therapy inasmuch as it is confined to the ECF compartment in the absence of deviations in Na^+ concentration. One liter of isotonic saline increases plasma volume by approximately 300 mL; the rest is distributed to the interstitial compartment. In contrast, 1 L of 5% dextrose in water (D_5W), which is also isosmotic (277 mOsm/L), is eventually distributed throughout all the body fluid compartments, so that only 10% to 15% (100 to 150 mL) remains in the ECF. Therefore, D_5W should not be used for volume replacement.

Administration of 1 L of 0.45% saline (77 mmol of Na^+ per liter) in D_5W is equivalent to giving 500 mL of isotonic saline and the same volume of solute-free water. The distribution of the solute-free compartment throughout all the fluid compartments would result in plasma dilution and reduction in the plasma Na^+. Therefore, this solution should be reserved for the management of hypernatremic hypovolemia. Even in that situation, it must be remembered that volume replacement is less efficient than with isotonic saline and, early on during the treatment course, may cause plasma tonicity to fall too rapidly.

When hypovolemia is accompanied by severe metabolic acidosis (pH <7.10, plasma HCO_3^- <10 mmol/L), bicarbonate supplementation may be indicated. (For detailed discussion of the indications for bicarbonate administration, see Chapter 16). Because this anion is manufactured as 8.4% sodium bicarbonate (1000 mmol/L) for use in cardiac resuscitation, appropriate dilution is required for the treatment of acidosis associated with hypovolemia. Nephrologists are frequently called upon for consultation in these situations, and they should be ready to provide detailed protocols for the preparation of isotonic $NaHCO_3$. Two convenient methods are suggested: Either 75 mL (75 mmol) of 8.4% $NaHCO_3$ can be added to 1 L of 0.45% saline or 150 mL of concentrated bicarbonate can be added to 1 L of D_5W. Although the latter is hypertonic in the short term, it is unlikely to be harmful.

In the presence of accompanying hypokalemia, especially if metabolic alkalosis is also present, volume replacement solutions must be supplemented with K^+. Commercially available 1-L solutions of isotonic saline supplemented with 10 or 20 mmol of KCl make this option safe and convenient. (For details, see Chapters 16 and 17). On the other hand, other commercially available crystalloid solutions containing lactate (converted by the liver to bicarbonate) and low concentrations of KCl offer no advantage and less flexibility than isotonic saline.

Colloid solutions include plasma itself, albumin, or high-molecular-weight carbohydrate molecules, such as hydroxyethyl starch and dextrans, at concentrations that exert colloid osmotic pressures equal to or greater than that of plasma. Because the transcapillary barrier is impermeable to these large molecules, in theory they expand the intravascular compartment more rapidly and efficiently than do crystalloid solutions. Colloid solutions may be useful in the management of burns and severe trauma, when plasma protein losses are substantial and rapid plasma expansion with relatively small volumes is efficacious. However, when capillary permeability is increased, as in states of multiorgan failure or the systemic inflammatory response syndrome, colloid administration is ineffective. Moreover, randomized controlled studies in which crystalloid solutions were compared with colloid solutions have shown no survival benefit with colloid solutions,[343] except in certain very specialized clinical situations, such as cirrhosis with spontaneous bacterial peritonitis.[344] Therefore, the much cheaper and more readily available isotonic saline should remain the mainstay of therapy.

Relative Hypovolemia

Treatment of relative hypovolemia is more difficult than that of absolute hypovolemia because there is no real fluid deficit. If the relative hypovolemia is caused by peripheral vasodilation, as in a septic patient, it may be necessary to cautiously administer a crystalloid solution, such as isotonic saline, to maintain ECF volume until the systemic vascular resistance and venous capacitance return to normal. The excess volume administered can then be excreted by the kidneys. When vasodilation is more severe, vasoconstrictor agents may be needed to maintain systemic blood pressure. In the edematous states of severe CHF, advanced cirrhosis with portal hypertension, and severe nephrotic syndrome, when EABV is low but there is an overall excess of Na$^+$ and water, treatment may be extremely problematic. Administration of crystalloid solution will, in all likelihood, lead to worsening interstitial edema without significantly affecting the EABV. In these situations, prognosis is determined by whether the underlying condition can be reversed.

Hypervolemia

Definition

Hypervolemia is the condition in which the volume of the ECF compartment is expanded in relation to its capacitance. In most people, increments in Na$^+$ intake are matched by corresponding changes in Na$^+$ excretion as a result of the actions of the compensatory mechanisms detailed in the "Physiology" section. In these cases, no clinically detectable changes are observed. However, in the approximately 20% of the population who are "salt sensitive," the upward shift in ECF volume induced by high salt intake leads to a persistent rise in systemic arterial pressure, albeit without other overt signs of fluid retention (see Chapter 46 for a detailed discussion). In the following sections, the discussion is confined to the strict definition of hypervolemia in which Na$^+$ retention is ongoing and inappropriate for the prevailing ECF volume, with the appearance of clinical signs of volume overload.

Etiology

The causes of hypervolemia can be conveniently divided into two major categories: primary renal Na$^+$ retention and secondary retention resulting from compensatory mechanisms activated as a result of disease in other major organs (Table 14-6). *Primary renal Na$^+$ retention* can be further subclassified as caused by either intrinsic kidney disease or primary mineralocorticoid excess. Of the primary renal diseases causing Na$^+$ retention, oliguric renal failure limits the ability to excrete Na$^+$ and water, and affected patients are at risk for rapidly developing ECF volume overload (see Chapter 30).

TABLE 14-6 Causes of Renal Sodium Retention

Primary

Oliguric acute kidney injury
Chronic kidney disease
Glomerular disease
Severe bilateral renal artery stenosis
Salt-retaining tubulopathies (genetic)
Mineralocorticoid excess

Secondary

Heart failure
Cirrhosis
Idiopathic edema

In contrast, in chronic kidney disease, renal tubular adaptation to salt intake is usually efficient until late stage 4 and stage 5. However, in some primary glomerular diseases, especially in the presence of nephrotic range proteinuria, significant Na$^+$ retention may occur even when GFR is close to normal (see the following "Pathophysiology" section and Chapter 31). Primary mineralocorticoid excess or enhanced activity, in their early phases, lead to transient Na$^+$ retention. However, because of the phenomenon of "mineralocorticoid escape," the dominant clinical expression of these diseases is hypertension. Mineralocorticoid excess as a cause of secondary hypertension is discussed in Chapter 46.

Secondary renal Na$^+$ retention occurs in both low- and high-output cardiac failure, as well as in systolic and diastolic dysfunction. Hepatic cirrhosis with portal hypertension and nephrotic syndrome are also accompanied by renal Na$^+$ retention. In this chapter, only CHF and cirrhosis are considered. Nephrotic syndrome is discussed in detail in Chapter 31.

Pathophysiology

The cause of primary renal Na$^+$ retention is clearly disruption of normal renal function. In contrast, secondary renal Na$^+$ retention occurs either because of reduced EABV in the presence of total ECF volume expansion or in response to factors, as yet only partially defined, that are secreted by either the heart or liver that signal the kidneys to retain Na$^+$. In all conditions associated with secondary Na$^+$ retention, the renal effector mechanisms that normally operate to conserve Na$^+$ and protect against a Na$^+$ deficit are exaggerated, and their actions continue despite subtle or overt expansion of ECF volume. The pathophysiologic process of hypervolemia comprises local mechanisms of edema formation and systemic factors stimulating renal Na$^+$ retention; systemic factors can be further subclassified as abnormalities of the afferent sensing limb or of the efferent effector limb.

Local Mechanisms of Edema Formation

Peripheral interstitial fluid accumulation, which is common to all conditions that cause ECF volume expansion, results from disruption of the normal balance of transcapillary Starling forces. Transcapillary fluid and solute transport can be viewed as consisting of two types of flow: convective and diffusive. Bulk water movement occurs via convective transport induced by hydraulic and osmotic pressure gradients.[345] Capillary hydraulic pressure is under the influence of a number of factors, including systemic arterial and venous blood pressures, local blood flow, and the resistances imposed by the precapillary and postcapillary sphincters.

Systemic arterial blood pressure, in turn, is determined by cardiac output, intravascular volume, and systemic vascular resistance; systemic venous pressure is determined by right atrial pressure, intravascular volume, and venous capacitance. Na^+ balance is a key determinant of these latter hemodynamic parameters. Also, massive accumulation of fluid in the peripheral interstitial compartment (anasarca) can itself diminish venous compliance and, hence, alter overall cardiovascular performance.[346]

The balance of Starling forces prevailing at the arteriolar end of the capillary ($\Delta P > \Delta\pi$, in which $\Delta\pi$ is the change in transcapillary oncotic pressure) is favorable for the net filtration of fluid into the interstitium. Net outward movement of fluid along the length of the capillary is associated with an axial decrease in P_c and an increase in the π_c. Nevertheless, the local ΔP continues to exceed the opposing $\Delta\pi$ throughout the length of the capillary bed in several tissues; thus, filtration occurs along its entire length.[347] In such capillary beds, a substantial volume of filtered fluid must, therefore, return to the circulation via lymphatic vessels. In view of the importance of lymphatic drainage, the lymphatic vessels must be able to expand and proliferate, and the lymphatic flow must be able to increase in response to increased interstitial fluid formation; these mechanisms help minimize edema formation.

Several other mechanisms for minimizing edema formation have been identified. First, precapillary vasoconstriction tends to lower P_c and to diminish the filtering surface area in a given capillary bed. In fact, in the absence of appropriate regulation of microcirculatory myogenic reflex, excessive precapillary vasodilation appears to account for interstitial edema in the lower extremities that is associated with some Ca^{2+} entry blocker vasodilators.[348] Second, increased net filtration itself is associated with dissipation of P_c, dilution of interstitial fluid protein concentration, and a corresponding rise in intracapillary plasma protein concentration. The resulting change in the profile of Starling forces in association with increased filtration therefore tends to mitigate further interstitial fluid accumulation.[1,349] Finally, P_i is normally subatmospheric; however, even small increases in interstitial fluid volume tend to augment P_i, again opposing further transudation of fluid into the interstitial space.[350] The appearance of generalized edema therefore implies that one or more disturbances in microcirculatory hemodynamics is present in association with expansion of the ECF volume: increased venous pressure transmitted to the capillary, unfavorable adjustments in precapillary and postcapillary resistances, or inadequacy of lymphatic flow for draining the interstitial compartment and replenishing the intravascular compartment.

Insofar as the continued net accumulation of interstitial fluid without renal Na^+ retention might result in prohibitive intravascular volume contraction and cessation of interstitial fluid formation, generalized edema therefore is indicative of substantial renal Na^+ retention. In fact, the volume of accumulated interstitial fluid required for clinical detection of generalized edema (>2 to 3 L) necessitates that all states of generalized edema are associated with expansion of ECF volume and, hence, body exchangeable Na^+ content. In summary, all states of generalized edema reflect past or ongoing renal Na^+ retention.

RENAL SODIUM RETENTION
Reduced Effective Arterial Blood Volume. Renal Na^+ (and water retention) in edematous disorders occurs despite an increase in total blood and ECF volumes. In stark contrast,

healthy individuals with the same degree of Na^+ retention readily increase Na^+ and water excretion. Moreover, intrinsic renal function, in the absence of underlying renal disease, is normal in edematous states. This fact is dramatically illustrated by the observation that, after heart transplantation in patients with CHF[351] or liver transplantation in patients with hepatic cirrhosis,[352] Na^+ excretion is restored to normal. Similarly, when kidneys from patients with end-stage liver disease are transplanted into patients with normal liver function, Na^+ retention no longer occurs.

The paradox of Na^+ retention in the presence of expanded total and ECF volume is explained by the concept of EABV, described earlier. In brief, because 85% of blood circulates in the venous compartment and only 15% in the arterial compartment, expansion of the venous compartment leads to overall ECF volume excess that could occur concurrently with arterial underfilling. Arterial underfilling could result from either low cardiac output or peripheral arterial vasodilation, or a combination of the two. In turn, low cardiac output could result from true ECF volume depletion (see earlier discussion), cardiac failure, or decreased π_c with or without increased capillary permeability. All these stimuli would cause activation of ventricular and arterial sensors. Similarly, conditions such as high-output cardiac failure, sepsis, cirrhosis, and, in fact, normal pregnancy lead to peripheral arterial vasodilation and activation of arterial baroceptors. Activation of these afferent mechanisms would then induce the neurohumoral mechanisms that result in renal Na^+ and water retention (Figure 14-6).[353,354]

Although the mechanisms leading to Na^+ retention in CHF and cirrhosis are quite similar, specific differences between the two conditions have been observed, and these findings are discussed separately in the following sections.

Renal Sodium Retention in Heart Failure
Abnormalities of Sensing Mechanisms in Congestive Heart Failure. There is strong evidence that both the cardiopulmonary and baroceptor reflexes are blunted in CHF, so that they cannot exert an adequate tonic inhibitory effect on sympathetic outflow.[355,356] The resulting activated SNS triggers renal Na^+ retention by the mechanisms already described. With regard to cardiopulmonary receptor reflexes, several researchers, using a variety of models of CHF, have shown marked attenuation of atrial receptor firing in CHF in response to volume expansion.[357,358] In addition, loss of nerve ending arborization has been observed directly. Similarly, researchers using maneuvers that selectively alter central cardiac filling pressures (head-up tilt, LBNP) showed that patients with CHF, in contrast to normal subjects, usually do not demonstrate significant alterations in limb blood flow, circulating catecholamines, AVP, or renin activity in response to postural stimuli.[359,360] This diminished reflex responsiveness may be most impaired in patients with the greatest ventricular dysfunction.

Arterial baroceptor reflex impairment in CHF has been observed both in humans and in experimental models of CHF. High baseline values of muscle sympathetic activity were found in patients with CHF who failed to respond to activation and deactivation of arterial baroceptors by infusion of phenylephrine and Na^+ nitroprusside, respectively.[361] Function of carotid and aortic baroceptors was also depressed in experimental models of cardiac failure.[355,356] These changes were associated with upward resetting of receptor threshold and a reduced range of pressures over which the receptors functioned.

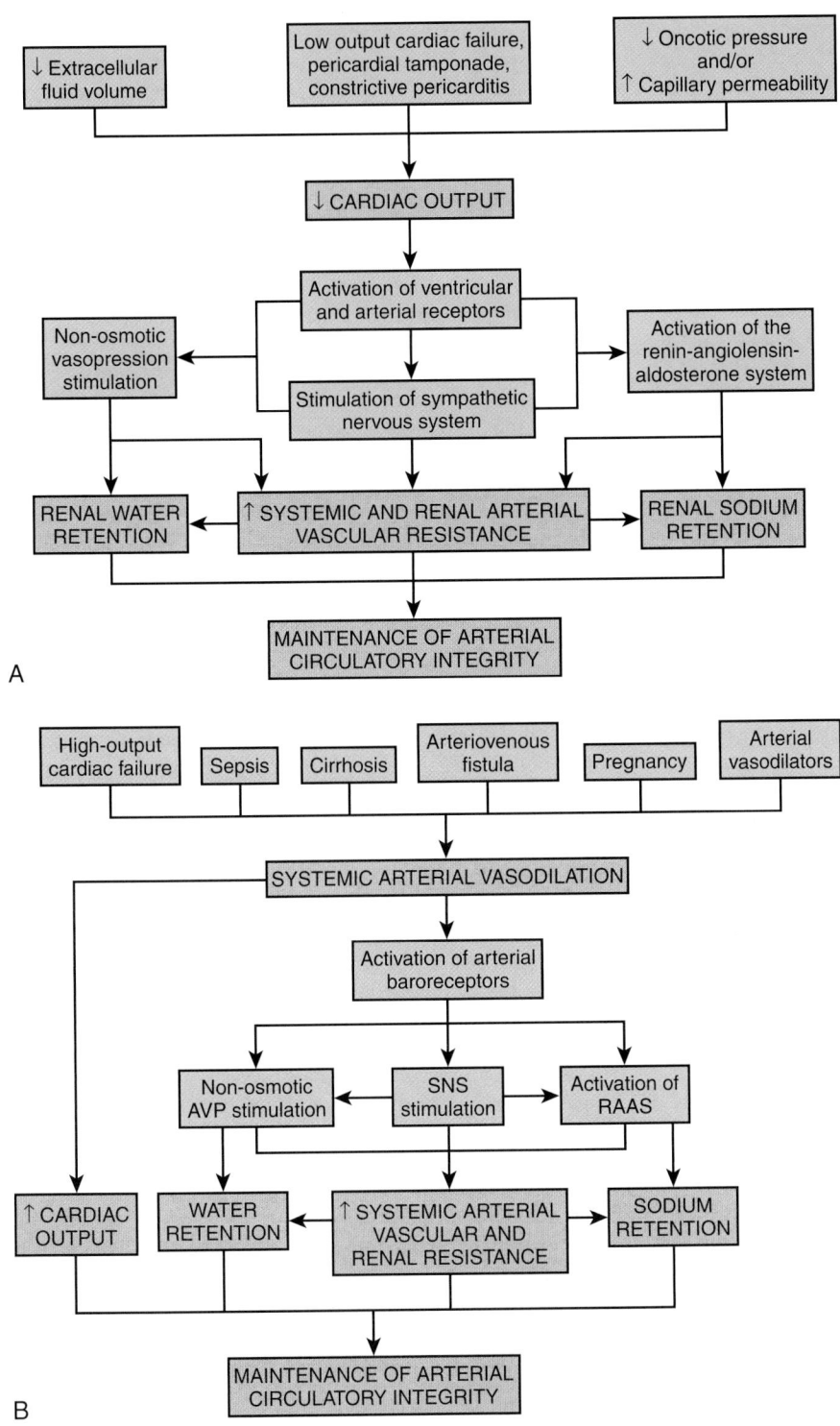

FIGURE 14-6 Sensing mechanisms that initiate and maintain renal sodium and water retention in various clinical conditions in which arterial underfilling, with resultant neurohumoral activation and renal sodium and water retention, is caused by a decrease in cardiac output (**A**) and by systemic arterial vasodilation (**B**). In addition to activating the neurohumoral axis, adrenergic stimulation causes renal vasoconstriction and enhances sodium and fluid transport by the proximal tubule epithelium. (From Schrier RW: Decreased effective blood volume in edematous disorders: what does this mean? *J Am Soc Nephrol* 18:2028-2031, 2007.)

Multiple abnormalities have been described in cardiopulmonary and arterial baroreceptor control of RSNA in CHF. Thus, rats with coronary ligation displayed an increased basal level of efferent RSNA that failed to decrease normally during volume expansion (see DiBona[55] and DiBona and Kopp[148] and references therein). Similarly, in sinoaortic denervated dogs with pacing-induced CHF, the cardiopulmonary baroreflex control of efferent RSNA became markedly attenuated in response to cardiopulmonary receptor stimulation by volume expansion. Left atrial baroreceptor stimulation produced by inflation of small balloons at the junction of the left atrial-pulmonary vein produced the same effect (see Zucker et al[362] and references therein). The abnormal regulation of efferent RSNA was caused by impaired function of both aortic and cardiopulmonary baroreflexes; the defect in cardiopulmonary baroreceptors was functionally more important.[55,148]

Several mechanisms have been implicated in the pathogenesis of the abnormal cardiopulmonary and arterial baroreflexes in CHF. Zucker and colleagues[362] suggested that loss of compliance in the dilated hearts, as well as gross changes in the structure of the receptors themselves, were the mechanisms underlying the depressed atrial receptor discharge in dogs with aortocaval fistula (see Zucker et al and references therein). In dogs with pacing-induced CHF, the decrease in carotid sinus baroreceptor sensitivity was related to augmented Na^+-K^+-ATPase activity in the baroreceptor membranes (see Zucker et al[362] and references therein). Increased activity of angiotensin II through the AT_1 receptor has also been invoked to explain depressed baroreflex sensitivity in CHF. Specifically, intracerebral or systemic administration of AT_1 receptor antagonists to rats or rabbits with CHF significantly improved arterial baroreflex control of RSNA or heart rate, respectively (see Zucker et al[362] and references therein). Moreover, angiotensin II injected into the vertebral artery of normal rabbits significantly attenuated arterial baroreflex function. This effect of angiotensin II could be blocked by the central α_1-adrenoreceptor prazosin.[363] In addition, ACE inhibition augmented arterial and cardiopulmonary baroreflex control of sympathetic nerve activity in patients with CHF.[364]

Newer data indicate that angiotensin II in the paraventricular nucleus potentiates—and AT_1 receptor antisense messenger RNA normalizes—enhanced the cardiac sympathetic afferent reflex in rats with chronic heart failure.[65,365] AT_1 receptors in the nucleus tractus solitarii are thought to mediate the interaction between the baroreflex and the cardiac sympathetic afferent reflex.[366] AT_2 receptor in the rostral ventrolateral medulla exhibited an inhibitory effect on sympathetic outflow, which was mediated at least partially by an arachidonic acid metabolic pathway. These data implied that a downregulation in the AT_2 receptor was a contributory factor in the sympathetic neural excitation in CHF.[367]

Together, these data provide evidence of the role of high endogenous levels of angiotensin II, acting through the AT_1 receptor in concert with downregulation of the AT_2 receptor, in the impaired baroreflex sensitivity observed in CHF, both in the afferent limb of the reflex arch and at more central sites. The central effect may be mediated through a central α_1-adrenoreceptor. The blunted cardiopulmonary and arterial baroreceptor sensitivity in CHF may also lead to an increase in AVP release and renin secretion. However, data on this link are scarce.

Another hypothesis, for which there is scant support, is that the secretory capacity of ANP in response to atrial stretch in CHF is reduced because of limited reserve of the hormone as a result of a tonically increased stimulus for release of the hormone. First, circulating levels of ANP are not depressed but instead elevated in CHF in proportion to the severity of cardiac dysfunction (reviewed by Krupicka et al[368]). Second, the ventricles become a major source of ANP secretion in CHF[369-371]; expression is normally limited to the atria. Third, the Na^+ retention of CHF is not reversed when plasma ANP levels are further increased by exogenous administration of the peptide.[372-374] Thus, the main abnormality of ANP in CHF is the development of "resistance" rather than impaired secretion of the peptide.

The disturbances in the sensing mechanisms that initiate and maintain renal Na^+ retention in CHF are summarized in Figure 14-6. As indicated, a decrease in cardiac output or a diversion of systemic blood flow[49] diminishes the blood flow to the critical sites of the arterial circuit with pressure- and flow-sensing capabilities. The responses to diminished blood flow culminate in renal Na^+ retention, mediated by the

effector mechanisms to be described. An increase in systemic venous pressure promotes the transudation of fluid from the intravascular to the interstitial compartment by increasing the peripheral transcapillary ΔP. These processes augment the perceived loss of volume and flow in the arterial circuit. In addition, distortion of the pressure-volume relationships as a result of chronic dilation in the cardiac atria attenuates the normal natriuretic response to central venous congestion. This attenuation is manifested predominantly as diminished neural suppressive response to atrial stretch, which results in increased sympathetic nerve activity and augmented release of renin and AVP.

Abnormalities of Effector Mechanisms in Heart Failure. CHF is also characterized by a series of adaptive changes in the efferent limb of the volume-control system, many of which are similar to those that govern renal function in states of true Na^+ depletion. These include adjustments in glomerular hemodynamics and tubular transport, which, in turn, are brought about by alterations in neural, humoral, and paracrine systems. However, in contrast to true volume depletion, CHF is also associated with activation of vasodilatory natriuretic agents, which tend to oppose the effects of the vasoconstrictor/antinatriuretic systems. The final effect on urinary Na^+ excretion is determined by the balance between these antagonistic effector systems, which, in turn, may shift during the evolution of heart failure toward a dominance of Na^+-retaining systems. The abnormal regulation of the efferent limb of the volume-control system reflects not only the exaggerated activity of the antinatriuretic systems but also the failure of vasodilatory/natriuretic systems that are activated in the course of the deterioration in cardiac function.

Alterations in Glomerular Hemodynamics. CHF in patients and experimental models is characterized by an increase in renal vascular resistance and a reduction in GFR, but also an even more marked reduction of RPF, so that the filtration fraction is increased.[375,376] In rats with CHF induced by coronary ligation or aortocaval fistula, SNGFR was lower than in control rats, but glomerular plasma flow was disproportionately reduced in such a way that single-nephron filtration fraction was markedly elevated. K_f was diminished, and both afferent and efferent arteriolar resistances were elevated, accounting for the diminished single-nephron glomerular plasma flow.[377,378] The rise in single-nephron filtration fraction was caused by a disproportionate increase in efferent arteriolar resistance.

In Figure 14-7, a comparison of the glomerular capillary hemodynamic profile in the normal state versus the CHF state is illustrated on the left graph of each panel. First, ΔP declines along the length of the glomerular capillary in both the normal and CHF states, but much more so in CHF, because of the increased efferent arteriolar resistance. Second, $\Delta\pi$ increases over the length of the glomerular capillary in both states as fluid is filtered into Bowman's space, but again to a greater extent in CHF because of the increased filtration fraction. As outlined the "Renin-Aldosterone System" section of this chapter, this preferential increase in efferent arteriolar resistance is mediated principally by angiotensin II and is critical for the preservation of GFR in the presence of reduced RPF.[379-381] Because of the intense efferent arteriolar vasoconstriction, further compensation is not possible if RPP falls as a result of systemic hypotension, causing in a sharp decline in GFR. A dramatic clinical correlate of this phenomenon is the marked decline in GFR seen in patients with CHF whose angiotensin II drive

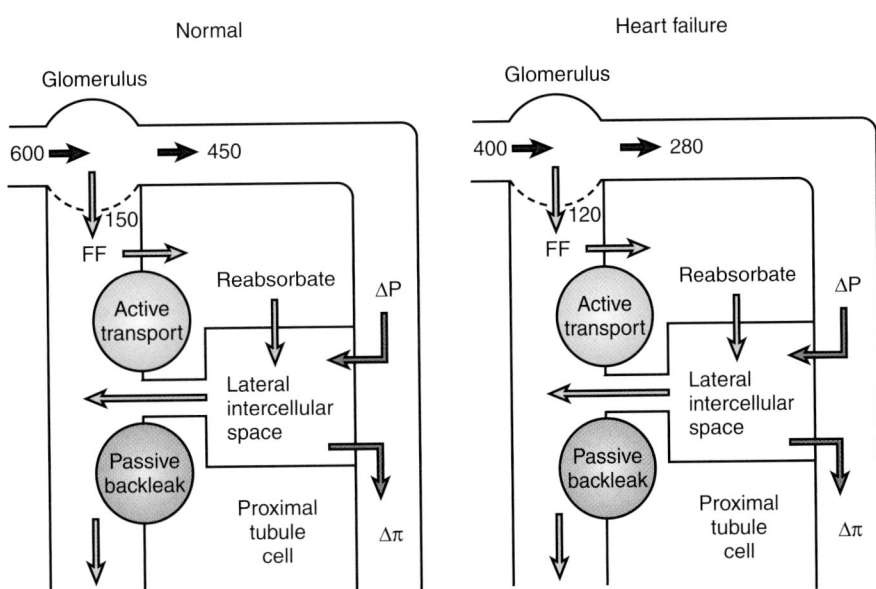

FIGURE 14-7 Peritubular control of proximal tubule fluid reabsorption. Fluid reabsorption in the normal state (**left**) and in patients with heart failure (**right**) is shown. Increased postglomerular arteriolar resistance in heart failure is depicted as narrowing. Numbers and *red block arrows* depict blood flow in preglomerular and postglomerular capillaries. ΔP and $\Delta \pi$ are the transcapillary hydraulic and oncotic pressure differences across the peritubular capillary, respectively; *yellow block arrows* indicate transtubular transport; *pink block arrows* represent the effect of peritubular capillary Starling forces on uptake of proximal reabsorbate; the thickness and font size of block arrows depict relative magnitude of effect. The increase in filtration fraction in heart failure causes $\Delta \pi$ to rise. The increase in renal vascular resistance in heart failure is believed to reduce ΔP. Both the increase in $\Delta \pi$ and the fall in ΔP enhance peritubular capillary uptake of proximal reabsorbate and thus increase absolute Na^+ reabsorption by the proximal tubule. (Adapted from Humes HD, Gottlieb M, Brenner BM: *The kidney in congestive heart failure: contemporary issues in nephrology*, vol 1, New York, 1978, Churchill Livingstone, pp 51-72.)

is removed by ACE inhibitors. In this situation, blood pressure may fall below the level necessary to maintain renal perfusion,[382] particularly in patients with preexisting renal failure, massive diuretic treatment, and limited cardiac reserve.[379]

Enhanced Tubular Reabsorption of Sodium. Enhanced tubular reabsorption of Na^+ in CHF is both secondary to the altered glomerular function described above and a direct result of neurohumeral mechanisms. A direct consequence of the glomerular hemodynamic alterations, and of augmented single-nephron filtration fraction, is an increase in the fractional reabsorption of filtered Na^+ at the level of the proximal tubule, as shown in several classical experimental and clinical studies.[377,383,384] In Figure 14-2, the peritubular capillary hemodynamic profile of the normal state is compared with that of CHF in each panel. In CHF, in comparison with the normal state, the average value of $\Delta \pi$ along the peritubular capillary is increased and that of ΔP is decreased. These values are favorable for fluid movement into the capillary and may also help reduce backleak of fluid into the tubule via paracellular pathways, promoting overall net reabsorption.

The peritubular control of proximal fluid reabsorption in normal and CHF states is illustrated schematically in Figure 14-7. A critical mediator of the enhanced tubular reabsorption of Na^+ is angiotensin II, which acts by modulating physical factors through its effect on efferent resistance, as well as by augmenting proximal epithelial transport directly, thereby amplifying the overall increase in proximal Na^+ reabsorption. This is clearly illustrated by experiments with ACE inhibitors, in which the increased single-nephron filtration fraction observed in heart failure was improved, which led to normalization of proximal peritubular capillary Starling forces and Na^+ reabsorption.[377]

Distal nephron sites also participate in the enhanced tubule Na^+ reabsorption in experimental models of CHF. In dogs and in rats with arteriovenous fistulas[385,386] and in dogs with

pericardial constriction[387] or chronic partial thoracic vena caval obstruction,[388] micropuncture studies demonstrated enhanced distal nephron Na^+ reabsorption. Levy[389] showed that the inability of dogs with chronic vena caval obstruction to excrete a Na^+ load is a consequence of enhanced reabsorption of Na^+ at the loop of Henle. Because renal vasodilation and elevation of RPP by saline loading prevented the enhanced reabsorption by the loop of Henle, altered renal hemodynamics appear to determine this response, much as in the proximal tubule.[390]

Neurohumoral Mediators. The primary neurohumoral mediators of Na^+ and water retention in CHF include the RAAS, SNS, AVP, and endothelins, which are vasoconstrictor/antinatriuretic (and antidiuretic) systems. In addition, several vasodilator/natriuretic substances, such as nitric oxide, prostaglandins, and adrenomedullin, are also activated. Upregulation of urotensin II and neuropeptide Y also appears to have a vasodilator/natriuretic effect, in contrast to the physiologic tonic effects of these peptides. In the final analysis, salt and water homeostasis is determined by the fine balance between these opposing systems, and the development of positive Na^+ balance and edema formation in CHF represents a turning point at which the balance is in favor of the vasoconstrictor/antinatriuretic forces (Figure 14-8). The dominant activity of Na^+-retaining systems in CHF is clinically important because impaired renal function is a strong predictor of mortality[391] and reversal of the neurohumoral impairment is associated with improved outcomes.[392]

Vasoconstrictor/Antinatriuretic (Antidiuretic) Systems

RENIN-ANGIOTENSIN-ALDOSTERONE SYSTEM

The activity of the RAAS is enhanced in most patients with CHF in correlation with the severity of cardiac dysfunction[393]; therefore, the activity of this system provides

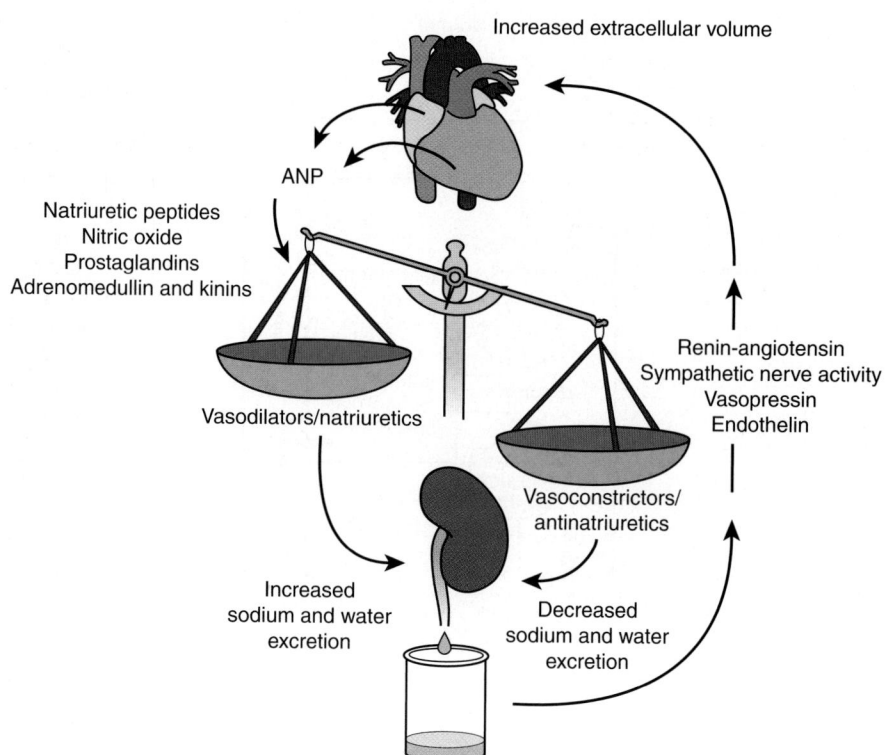

FIGURE 14-8 Efferent limb of extracellular fluid (ECF) volume control in heart failure. Volume homeostasis in heart failure is determined by the balance between natriuretic and antinatriuretic forces. In decompensated heart failure, enhanced activities of the Na⁺-retaining systems overwhelm the effects of the vasodilatory/natriuretic systems, which leads to a net reduction in Na⁺ excretion and an increase in ECF volume. (Adapted from Winaver J, Hoffman A, Abassi Z, et al: Does the heart's hormone, ANP, help in congestive heart failure? *News Physiol Sci* 10:247-253, 1995.)

a prognostic index for CHF patients. It is now abundantly clear that, despite providing initial benefits in hemodynamic support, continued activation of RAAS contributes to the progression and worsening of the primary cardiac component of the CHF syndrome as well, through maladaptive myocardial remodeling.[394,395] RAAS activation induces direct systemic vasoconstriction and activates other neurohormonal systems such as AVP, which contribute to maintaining adequate intravascular volume.[396] However, numerous studies in patients and in experimental models of CHF have established the deleterious role of the RAAS in the progression of cardiovascular and renal dysfunction in CHF (see Bekheirnia and Schrier[41] and Schrier[353,354] and references therein).

The kidneys in particular are highly sensitive to the action of vasoconstrictor agents, especially angiotensin II, and a decrease in RPF is one of the most common pathophysiologic alterations in clinical and experimental CHF. Micropuncture techniques demonstrated that rats with chronic stable CHF display depressed glomerular plasma flow rates and depressed SNGFR, as well as elevations in efferent arteriolar resistance and in filtration fraction. Direct renal administration of an ACE inhibitor did not affect renal function in sham-operated control rats, but it did normalize it in rats with experimental CHF. Using the aortocaval fistula model of CHF, Winaver and associates[397] showed that only some animals developed Na⁺ retention, whereas the rest maintained Na⁺ balance. The former subgroup was characterized by a marked increase in plasma renin activity and plasma aldosterone levels. In contrast, plasma renin activity and aldosterone levels in compensated animals were not different from those in sham-operated controls. Treatment with the ACE inhibitor enalapril resulted in a dramatic natriuretic response in rats with Na⁺ retention. Similarly, most patients with CHF maintain normal Na⁺ balance when placed on a low-salt diet, but about 50% develop

positive Na⁺ balance when fed a normal-salt diet.[398] A common feature of both animals and patients with Na⁺ retention was the activation of the RAAS. In dogs with experimental high-output CHF, the initial period of Na⁺ retention was associated with a profound activation of the RAAS, and the return to normal Na⁺ balance was accompanied by a progressive fall in plasma renin activity.[397]

In summary, these findings clearly demonstrate that activation of the RAAS contributes to the pathogenesis of Na⁺ and water retention in CHF. The deleterious effects of the RAAS on renal function are not surprising in view of the previously mentioned actions of angiotensin II and aldosterone on renal hemodynamics and excretory function. Activation of angiotensin II in response to the decreased pumping capacity of the failing myocardium promotes systemic vasoconstriction in association with the preferential vasoconstriction of efferent and afferent arterioles and mesangial cells.[164,394] In addition, angiotensin II both exerts a negative influence on renal cortical circulation in rats with CHF and increases tubular Na⁺ reabsorption directly and indirectly by augmenting aldosterone release.[394] In combination, these hemodynamic and tubular actions lead to avid Na⁺ and water retention, thus promoting circulatory congestion and edema formation.

Not all studies revealed a consistent relationship between RAAS and positive Na⁺ balance. For instance, in dogs with pulmonary artery or thoracic inferior vena caval constriction, the RAAS was activated to a striking degree during the early phase of constriction and was necessary for the support of systemic blood pressure. Administration of the ACE inhibitor captopril resulted in systemic hypotension. Over subsequent days, Na⁺ retention and ECF volume expansion were pronounced, and ACE inhibition was no longer accompanied by significant hypotension. However, animals with severe impairment of cardiac output remained sensitive to the hypotensive effects of ACE inhibition. Similarly, among patients with CHF, plasma renin activity and levels of vasoconstrictor hormones were most elevated in patients with acute, severe, and poorly compensated CHF. Levels declined when CHF became stable in the chronic stage.[399]

The foregoing experimental and clinical data thus indicate that the influence of the RAAS in maintaining circulatory homeostasis may depend on the stage of CHF, being most pronounced in acute and decompensated CHF and least pronounced in chronic stable CHF. However, even though the circulating RAAS is not activated in chronic stable CHF, alterations in renal function can still be corrected by ACE inhibition.[400] These and other supporting data are consistent with the activation of local RAAS in various tissues, including the heart, vasculature, kidneys, and brain, in the absence of alterations in the circulating hormone.[399] Moreover, results of several studies suggested that activation of the local RAAS in these tissues may play a crucial role in the pathogenesis of CHF.[399,401]

In addition to the mechanical stress exerted on the myocardium due to angiotensin II–mediated increased afterload, pressure overload activates the production of local angiotensin II, as a result of upregulation of angiotensinogen and tissue ACE.[394] Local angiotensin II acts through AT_1 in a paracrine/autocrine manner, leading to cardiac hypertrophy (because of its growth properties), remodeling and fibrosis (mediated by transforming growth factor-β), and reduced coronary flow, hallmarks of severe CHF.[402,403] In support of these observations are the improved cardiac function, prolonged survival, prevention of end-organ damage, and prevention or regression of cardiac hypertrophy in humans and animals with CHF treated with ACE inhibitors and ARBs.[165,394] In addition, ACE inhibitors and ARBs may improve endothelial dysfunction, vascular remodeling, and potentiation of the vasodilatory effects of the kinins.[164,404-406]

Like angiotensin II, aldosterone also acts directly on the myocardium, inducing structural remodeling of the interstitial collagen matrix (reviewed by Cowley and Skelton[10]). Moreover, cardiac aldosterone production is increased in patients with CHF, especially when caused by systolic dysfunction. Convincing evidence for the local production of aldosterone was provided by the finding that CYP11B2 messenger RNA (aldosterone synthase) is expressed in cultured neonatal rat cardiac myocytes. The adverse contribution of aldosterone to the functional and structural alterations of the failing heart was elegantly proved by the use of eplerenone, a specific aldosterone antagonist, which prevented progressive left ventricular systolic and diastolic dysfunction in association with reduced interstitial fibrosis, cardiomyocyte hypertrophy, and left ventricular chamber sphericity in dogs with CHF. Similarly, eplerenone attenuated the development of ventricular remodeling and reactive (but not reparative) fibrosis after myocardial infarction in rats.[407,408] These findings are in agreement with the results of clinical trials (see "Specific Treatments Based on the Pathophysiology of Congestive Heart Failure" section).[409,410]

As noted previously, in addition to its renal and cardiovascular hemodynamic effects, the RAAS is involved directly in the exaggerated Na+ reabsorption by the tubule in CHF. Angiotensin II has a dose-dependent direct effect on the proximal tubular epithelium that is favorable for active Na+ reabsorption.[411-413] The predominant effect of the RAAS on distal nephron function is mediated by the action of aldosterone, which acts on cortical and medullary portions of the collecting duct to enhance Na+ reabsorption, as outlined previously. Numerous researchers reported elevations in plasma aldosterone concentration, in urinary aldosterone secretion, or in natriuretic effects of aldosterone antagonists in animal models and human subjects with CHF, despite further activation of other antinatriuretic systems; these findings provide evidence of the pivotal role of this hormone in the mediation of Na+ retention in CHF.[393]

As with angiotensin II, the relative importance of mineralocorticoid action in the Na+ retention of CHF varies with stage and severity of disease. Further evidence for the involvement of the RAAS in the development of positive Na+ balance comes from studies showing that the renal and hemodynamic response to ANP is impaired in CHF and that administration of either angiotensin receptor blockade or ACE inhibition restores the blunted response to ANP (for further details, see the "Natriuretic Peptides" section).[397] Although patients with CHF have low plasma osmolarity, they display increased thirst, probably because of the high concentrations of angiotensin II, which stimulates thirst center cells in the hypothalamus.[393] This behavior may contribute to the positive water balance and hyponatremia in these patients (see also the "Arginine Vasopressin" section).

SYMPATHETIC NERVOUS SYSTEM

Patients with CHF experience progressive activation of the SNS with progressive decline of cardiac function.[414,415] Plasma norepinephrine levels are frequently elevated in CHF, and a strong consensus exists as to the adverse influence of sympathetic overactivity on the progression and outcome of patients with CHF.[414,416] Thus, sympathetic neural activity is significantly correlated with intracardiac pressures, cardiac hypertrophy, and left ventricular ejection fraction (LVEF).[415] Direct intraneural recordings in patients with CHF also showed increased neural traffic, which correlated with the increased plasma norepinephrine levels (reviewed by Kaye and Esler[416]). Activation of the SNS not only precedes the appearance of congestive symptoms but also is preferentially directed toward the heart and kidneys. Clinical investigations revealed that patients with mild CHF have higher plasma norepinephrine in the coronary sinus than in the renal veins.[417] At the early stages of CHF, increased activity of the SNS ameliorates the hemodynamic abnormalities—including hyperfusion, diminished plasma volume, and impaired cardiac function—by producing vasoconstriction and avid Na+ reabsorption.[402,415] However, chronic exposure to this system induces several long-term adverse myocardial effects, including induction of apoptosis and hypertrophy, with an overall reduction in cardiac function, which reduces contractility. Some of these effects may be mediated, in turn, by activation of the RAAS.[393,402]

Measurements made with catecholamine spillover techniques revealed that the basal sympathetic outflow to the kidneys is significantly increased in patients with CHF.[416] The activation of the SNS and increased efferent RSNA may be involved in the alterations in renal function in CHF. For example, exaggerated RSNA contributes to the increased renal vasoconstriction, avid Na+ and water retention, renin secretion, and attenuation of the renal actions of ANP.[418] Experimental studies demonstrated that in rats with experimental CHF caused by coronary artery ligation, renal denervation resulted in an increase in RPF and SNGFR and a decrease in afferent and efferent arteriolar resistance.[419] Similarly, in dogs with low cardiac output induced by vena caval constriction, administration of a ganglionic blocker resulted in a marked increase in Na^+ excretion.[416] In rats with CHF induced by coronary ligation, the decrease in RSNA in response to an acute saline load was less than that of control rats.[148] Bilateral renal denervation restored the natriuretic response to volume expansion; this finding implicates increased RSNA in the Na^+ avidity characteristic of CHF.[416]

Studies in dogs with high-output CHF induced by aortocaval fistula demonstrated that total postprandial urinary Na^+ excretion was approximately twofold higher in dogs with renal denervation than in control dogs with intact nerves.[420,421] In line with these observations, clinical investigation showed that administration of the α-adrenoreceptor blocker dibenamine to patients with CHF caused an increase in fractional Na^+ excretion, without a change in RPF or GFR. Treatment with ibopamine, an oral dopamine analog, resulted in vasodilation and positive inotropic and diuretic effects in patients with CHF.[421] Moreover, for a given degree of cardiac dysfunction, the concentration of norepinephrine is significantly higher in patients with concomitant abnormal renal function than in patients with preserved renal function.[422,423] These findings suggest that the association between renal function and prognosis in patients with CHF is linked by neurohormonal activation, including that in the CNS.

An additional mechanism by which RSNA may affect renal hemodynamics and Na^+ excretion in CHF is through its antagonistic interaction with ANP. On the one hand, ANP has sympathoinhibitory effects[424-427]; on the other, the SNS-induced salt and water retention in CHF may play a role in reducing renal responsiveness to ANP. For example, the blunted diuretic/natriuretic response to ANP in rats with CHF could be restored by prior renal denervation[420] or by administration of clonidine,[428] a centrally acting $α_2$-adrenoreceptor agonist, which decreases RSNA in CHF. These experimental and clinical data indicate that the SNS may play a role in the regulation of Na^+ excretion and glomerular hemodynamics in CHF, either by a direct renal action or by attenuating the action of ANP. However, studies in conscious dogs failed to show an ameliorative effect of renal denervation on renal hemodynamics and Na^+ excretion in CHF.[429] The discrepancies in these results probably arose because of species differences, the presence or absence of anesthesia, and the method of inducing CHF. It is also possible that high circulating catecholamines could interfere with the effects of renal denervation.

In summary, the perturbation of SNS activity in the efferent limb of volume homeostasis in CHF is a result of a complex interplay between the SNS itself and other neurohormonal mechanisms that act on the glomeruli and the renal tubules.

Vasopressin

Since the early 1980s, numerous studies have demonstrated that plasma levels of AVP are elevated in patients with CHF, mostly in those with advanced CHF with hyponatremia, but also in asymptomatic patients with left ventricular dysfunction (see Finley et al[430] and references therein). The high plasma levels of AVP are not suppressed after administration of an oral water load, despite the induction of marked hypo-osmolality.[431]

The mechanisms underlying the enhanced secretion of AVP in CHF are related to nonosmotic factors such as attenuated compliance of the left atrium, hypotension, and activation of the RAAS.[353,393] Impairment of the baroreflex control mechanism for AVP release was shown not to be involved.[432] Data on angiotensin II–stimulated release of AVP are conflicting. Early evidence of this mechanism[433] was later refuted.[434] Treatment with either an ACE inhibitor (captopril) or an α-blocker (prazosin) resulted in suppression of AVP and improved water excretion in response to water loading in patients with CHF, with only a small decline in blood pressure.[435] Therefore, improved cardiac function in response to afterload reduction (e.g., pulse pressure, stroke volume) was probably responsible for removal of the nonosmotic stimulus to AVP release.

The high circulating levels of AVP in CHF adversely affect both the kidneys and the cardiovascular system. In fact, raised levels of the C-terminal portion of the AVP prohormone (copeptin) at the time of diagnosis of acute decompensated heart failure are highly predictive of 1-year mortality.[436] The prognostic power of raised copeptin in CHF is similar to that of BNP levels (see the later "Brain Natriuretic Peptide" section). The most recognized renal effect of AVP in CHF is the development of hyponatremia, which usually occurs in advanced stages of the disease and may occur at AVP concentrations much lower than those required to produce vasoconstriction.[437] Hyponatremia most probably results from impaired solute-free water excretion in the presence of sustained release of AVP, irrespective of plasma osmolality. In accordance with this notion, studies in animal models of CHF demonstrated increased collecting duct expression of AQP2.[438,439] In addition, administration of specific V_2 receptor antagonists has been consistently associated with improvement in plasma Na^+ levels in both animals and patients with hyponatremia.[430,440] The improvement is associated with correction of the impaired urinary dilution in response to acute water load,[441] increased plasma osmolarity, and downregulation of renal AQP2 expression.[439] Treatment of CHF with selective V_2 receptor antagonists is discussed further in the "Specific Treatments Based on the Pathophysiology of Congestive Heart Failure" section.

Apart from hyponatremia, CHF is characterized by other alterations in renal function, including a decrease in RBF, especially to the cortex, a decrease in GFR, and Na^+ retention. The potential role of enhanced levels of AVP in these renal manifestations remains largely unknown.

The adverse effects of AVP on cardiac function (see Finley et al[430] and references therein) occur through its V_{1A} receptor on systemic vascular resistance (increased cardiac afterload), as well as by V_2-receptor–mediated water retention, which leads to systemic and pulmonary congestion (increased preload). In addition, AVP, through its V_{1A} receptor, acts directly on cardiomyocytes, causing a rise in intracellular Ca^{2+} and activation of mitogen-activated kinases and protein kinase C. These signaling mechanisms appear to mediate the observed cardiac remodeling, dilation, and hypertrophy. The remodeling might be further exacerbated by the aforementioned abnormalities in preload and afterload.

In summary, the data suggest (1) that AVP is involved in the pathogenesis of water retention and hyponatremia that characterize CHF and (2) that AVP receptor antagonists result in remarkable diuresis in both experimental and clinical CHF.

ENDOTHELIN

There is considerable evidence that ET-1 is involved in the development and progression of CHF. Furthermore, this peptide is probably involved in the reduced renal function that characterizes CHF, by inducing renal remodeling, interstitial fibrosis, glomerulosclerosis, hypoperfusion/hypofiltration, and positive salt and water balance.[442] The pathophysiologic role of ET-1 in CHF is supported by two major lines of evidence: (1) The endothelin system is activated in CHF, and (2) ET-1 receptor antagonists modify this pathophysiologic process.[443,444] The first line of evidence is based on the demonstration that plasma ET-1 and big ET-1 concentrations in both clinical CHF and experimental models of CHF are elevated and are correlated with hemodynamic severity and symptoms (see Ertl and Bauersachs[443] and references therein). Also, a negative correlation between plasma ET-1 concentration and LVEF has been reported (see Ertl and Bauersachs[443] and references therein). In another study, the degree of pulmonary hypertension was the strongest predictor of plasma ET-1 level in patients with CHF.[445] Moreover, plasma levels of big endothelin and ET-1 were independent markers of mortality and morbidity in the Valsartan Heart Failure Trial.[446] These prognostic reports are in line with the observation that plasma ET-1 is elevated only in patients with moderate and severe CHF, but not in patients with asymptomatic CHF.[447]

The increase in plasma levels of ET-1 may be caused by enhanced synthesis of the peptide in the lungs, heart, and circulation by several stimuli such as angiotensin II and thrombin, or it may be caused by decreased clearance by the pulmonary system.[443] In parallel to ET-1 levels, ET-A receptors are upregulated, whereas ET-B receptors are downregulated in the failing human heart.[448] The pathophysiologic significance of ET-1 activation in CHF remains speculative. In normal animals, increasing plasma ET-1 levels to concentrations found in CHF is associated with significant reduction in RBF and increased vascular resistance,[206] which is exactly what occurs in CHF.[449]

A cause-and-effect relationship between these hemodynamic abnormalities and ET-1 in CHF was demonstrated with the development of selective and highly specific endothelin receptor antagonists.[443] In this regard, acute administration of the mixed ET-A/ET-B receptor antagonists, bosentan and tezosentan, significantly improved renal cortical perfusion, reversed the profoundly increased renal vascular resistance and increased RBF and Na+ excretion in rats with severe decompensated CHF.[450,451] In addition, chronic blockade of ET-A by selective or dual ET-A/ET-B receptor antagonists attenuated the magnitude of Na+ retention and prevented the decline in GFR in experimental CHF[443,452] These effects are in line with observations that infusion of ET-1 in normal rats produced a sustained cortical vasoconstrictor and a transient medullary vasodilatory response.[258,431] In contrast, rats with decompensated CHF displayed severely blunted cortical vasoconstriction but significantly prolonged and preserved medullary vasodilation.[269] The significance of these attenuated renovascular effects of ET-1 and big endothelin in CHF experimental animals is uncertain, but the effect could result from activation of vasodilatory systems such as prostaglandins and nitric oxide. In fact, the medullary tissue of rats with decompensated CHF contains higher eNOS immunoreactive levels was comparable with that in sham-treated controls.[269] These findings indicate that endothelin may be involved in the altered renal hemodynamics and the pathogenesis of cortical vasoconstriction in CHF.

Vasodilatory/Natriuretic Systems

NATRIURETIC PEPTIDES

In decompensated heart failure, renal Na+ and water retention occurs despite expansion of the ECF volume and when the natriuretic peptide system is activated. Results of many clinical and experimental studies have implicated both ANP and BNP in the pathophysiologic process of the deranged cardiorenal axis in CHF.

Atrial Natriuretic Peptide. Plasma levels of ANP and NH2-terminal ANP are frequently elevated in patients with CHF and are correlated positively with the severity of cardiac failure, as well as with the elevated atrial pressure and other parameters of left ventricular dysfunction.[372,436,453-455] In this context, the concentration of circulating ANP was proposed as a diagnostic tool in the determination of cardiac dysfunction and as a prognostic marker in the prediction of survival of patients with CHF.[28] Although this proposal was clearly demonstrated, ANP has since been superseded by BNP as a diagnostic and prognostic tool (see later "Brain Natriuretic Peptide" section).

The high levels of plasma ANP are attributed to increased production rather than to decreased clearance. Although volume-induced atrial stretch is the main source for the elevated circulating ANP levels in CHF, enhanced synthesis and release of the hormone by the ventricular tissue in response to angiotensin II and endothelin also contribute to this phenomenon.[456,457] Despite the high levels of this potent natriuretic and diuretic agent, patients and experimental animals with CHF retain salt and water because renal responsiveness to natriuretic peptides is attenuated.[372,458,459] However, infusion of ANP to patients with CHF does lead to hemodynamic improvement and inhibition of activated neurohumoral systems. These data are in line with findings in both patients and animals that ANP is a weak counterregulatory hormone, insufficient to overcome the substantial vasoconstriction mediated by the SNS, RAAS, and AVP.[460,461] However, despite the blunted renal response to ANP in CHF, elimination of ANP production by atrial appendectomy in dogs with CHF aggravated the activation of these vasoconstrictive hormones and resulted in marked Na+ and water retention.[462] These data suggest that ANP plays a critical role as a suppressor of Na+-retaining systems and as an important adaptive or compensatory mechanism aimed at reducing pulmonary vascular resistance and hypervolemia.

Actually, the maintenance of Na+ balance in the initial compensated phase of CHF has been attributed in part to the elevated levels of ANP and BNP.[234] This notion is supported by the findings that inhibition of natriuretic peptide receptors in experimental CHF induces Na+ retention.[463] In addition, natriuretic peptides inhibit the angiotensin II–induced systemic vasoconstriction,[464] proximal tubule Na+ reabsorption,[465] and the secretion of aldosterone[464] and endothelin.[466] Furthermore, in an experimental model of CHF, inhibition of the natriuretic peptides by specific antibodies to their receptors caused further impairment in renal function, as indicated by increased renal vascular resistance and decreased GFR, RBF, urine flow, Na+ excretion, and activation of the RAAS.[466,467]

In view of the remarkable activation of the natriuretic peptide system and the ability of natriuretic peptides to counter the effects of the vasoconstrictor/antinatriuretic neurohormonal systems, why, then, do salt and water retention occur in overt CHF? Several mechanisms have been suggested to explain this apparent discrepancy:

1. Appearance of abnormal circulating peptides such as β-ANP and inadequate secretory reserves in comparison with the degree of CHF. However, the fact that circulating levels of native biologically active natriuretic peptides are clearly elevated in CHF indicates that these putative factors cannot account for the exaggerated salt and water retention.

2. Decreased availability of natriuretic peptides by upregulation of NEP and clearance receptors.[467] So far, no convincing evidence suggests that upregulation of clearance receptors exists in the renal tissue of CHF animals or patients, although increased abundance of clearance receptors for natriuretic peptides in platelets of patients with advanced CHF has been reported.[468] In contrast, several studies have demonstrated enhanced expression and activity of NEP in experimental CHF.[469,470] Moreover, numerous reports have shown that NEP inhibitors improve the vascular and renal response to natriuretic peptides in CHF (see the "Specific Treatments Based on the Pathophysiology of Congestive Heart Failure" section).

3. Activation of vasoconstrictor/antinatriuretic factors and development of renal hyporesponsiveness to ANP. Renal resistance to ANP may be present even in the early presymptomatic stage of the disease, but it progresses proportionately as CHF worsens.[471] In advanced CHF, when RPF is markedly impaired, the ability of natriuretic peptides to antagonize the renal effects of angiotensin II may be limited.[472] This point was clearly demonstrated in an animal model of CHF, in which chronic blockade by enalapril of the profoundly activated RAAS partially, but significantly, improved the natriuretic response to endogenous and exogenous ANP.[473] The favorable effects of ACE inhibition were especially evident in decompensated heart failure. These findings are in line with the fact that activation of RAAS in CHF largely contributes to Na+ and water retention by antagonizing the renal actions of ANP. The mechanisms underlying the attenuated renal effects of ANP in CHF are not completely understood, but they are known to include angiotensin II–induced afferent and efferent vasoconstriction, mesangial cell contraction, activation of cGMP phosphodiesterases that attenuate the accumulation of the second messenger of natriuretic peptides in target organs, and stimulation of Na+,H+-exchanger and Na+ channels in the proximal tubule and collecting duct.[473]

Activation of the SNS also can overwhelm the renal effects of ANP. As described earlier, overactivity of the SNS leads to vasoconstriction of the peripheral circulation and of the afferent and efferent arterioles, which causees reduction of RPF and GFR. These actions, together with the direct stimulatory effects of SNS on Na+ reabsorption in the proximal tubule and loop of Henle, contribute to the attenuated renal responsiveness to ANP in CHF. Moreover, the SNS-induced renal hypoperfusion/hypofiltration stimulates renin secretion, thus aggravating the positive Na+ and water balance. In rat models of CHF, the diuretic and natriuretic response to ANP was increased after sympathetic inhibition by low-dose clonidine[428] or bilateral renal denervation.[474] The beneficial effects of renal denervation could be attributed to upregulation of natriuretic peptide receptors and cGMP production, as was demonstrated in normal rats.[163]

In summary, the development of renal hyporesponsiveness to natriuretic peptides is paralleled closely by overreactivity of both the RAAS and SNS and represents a critical point in the development of positive salt balance and edema formation in advanced CHF.

Brain Natriuretic Peptide. As noted previously, BNP is structurally similar to ANP but is produced mainly by the ventricles in response to stretch and pressure overload (reviewed by Richards[232]). As with ANP, plasma levels of BNP and N-terminal (NT)–proBNP are elevated in patients with CHF in proportion to the severity of myocardial systolic and diastolic dysfunction and New York Heart Association classification.[233,368] Plasma levels of BNP are elevated only in severe CHF, whereas circulating concentrations of ANP are high in both mild and severe cases.[475,476] The extreme elevation of plasma BNP in severe CHF probably stems from the increased synthesis of BNP, predominantly by the hypertrophied ventricular tissue, although the contribution of the atria is significant.[477]

Although echocardiography remains the "gold standard" for the evaluation of left ventricular dysfunction, numerous studies have shown that plasma levels of BNP and NT-proBNP are reliable markers and, in fact, superior to ANP and NT-proANP for the diagnosis and prognosis of CHF.[23,232,368,436,478-480] The diagnostic capability of NT-proBNP is impressive, with high sensitivity, specificity, and negative predictive value, in patients with an ejection fraction of less than 35%. Similar high predictive values are found in patients with concomitant left ventricular hypertrophy, either in the absence of or after myocardial infarction (reviewed by several authors[232,368,436,481]). Moreover, the added presence of renal dysfunction appears to enhance these predictive values.[482] In addition, elevated plasma BNP (or NT-proBNP) and LVEF lower than 40% are complementary independent predictors of death, CHF, and new myocardial infarction at 3 years after an initial myocardial infarction. Risk stratification with the combination of LVEF lower than 40% and high levels of NT-proBNP is substantially better than that provided by either alone.[483] The plasma level of BNP is also a powerful marker for prognosis and risk stratification in the setting of CHF,[368,481] with graded increases in mortality throughout each quartile of BNP levels both in the Valsartan in Heart Failure Trial[446] and the Carvedilol Prospective Randomized, Cumulative Survival (COPERNICUS) NT-proBNP study (reviewed by Krupicka et al[368]).

As many as 40% to 50% of patients with CHF have normal systolic function. In these patients, even those who have no symptoms, elevated BNP levels are correlated with diastolic abnormalities on Doppler studies. Conversely, a reduction in BNP levels with treatment are associated with a reduction in left ventricular filling pressures, a lower readmission rate, and a better prognosis; thus, monitoring of BNP levels may provide valuable information regarding treatment efficacy and expected patient outcomes.[484,485]

Another diagnostic role for BNP is in the clear distinction of dyspnea caused by CHF from that caused by noncardiac entities.[486-491] This point was dramatically illustrated by the N-terminal Pro-BNP Investigation of Dyspnea in the Emergency Department (PRIDE) study, in which the median NT-proBNP level among 209 patients who had acute CHF was 4054 pg/mL, in contrast to 131 pg/mL among 390 patients (65%) who did not have acute CHF. At cutpoints of more than 450 pg/mL for patients younger than 50 years and more than 900 pg/mL for patients at least 50 years of age, NT-proBNP levels were highly sensitive and specific for the diagnosis of acute CHF. An NT-proBNP level lower than 300 pg/mL was optimal for ruling out acute CHF, with a negative predictive value of 99%. Increased level of NT-proBNP was the strongest independent predictor of a final diagnosis of acute CHF. NT-proBNP testing alone was superior to clinical judgment alone for diagnosing acute CHF; NT-proBNP plus clinical judgment was superior to NT-proBNP or clinical judgment alone.[488] Thus, the predictive accuracy of circulating BNP for distinguishing dyspnea caused by CHF from dyspnea with noncardiac causes equals and even exceeds the accuracy of classic examinations such as radiography and physical examination. Moreover, NT-proBNP levels perform better than both the National Health and Nutrition Examination score and Framingham clinical parameters (the most established criteria in use for the diagnosis of CHF).

In addition, the median time to discharge and cost of treatment were significantly lower in patients assessed by BNP levels than in those assessed in a conventional manner.[492,493] Circulating BNP and NT-proBNP levels have also been used as a guide in determining the therapeutic efficacy of drugs typically prescribed for CHF patients, including ACE inhibitors, ARBs, diuretics, digitalis, and β-blockers.[494-497] For example, in the Carvedilol Or Metoprolol European Trial, patients monitored for up to 5 years who achieved an NT-proBNP lower than 400 pg/mL after treatment with either β-blocker had a more favorable prognosis than did nonresponders.[498] Similarly, both BNP (intact or NT-proBNP) and ANP levels accurately reflected the improvement in ejection fraction of CHF patients treated with conventional therapy including ACE inhibitors. Addition of an ARB to the regimen led to further reductions in peptide levels and ejection fraction.[499,500] Conversely, the first cardiovascular event after 6 months of therapy was less frequent in CHF patients whose plasma BNP levels decreased in response to medical treatment.[496]

Together, these findings suggest that a simple and rapid determination of plasma levels of BNP or NT-proBNP in patients with CHF can be used to assess cardiac dysfunction, serve as a diagnostic and prognostic marker, and assist in titrating relevant therapy. However, it should be emphasized that plasma levels of both ANP and BNP are affected by several factors, including age, salt intake, gender, obesity, hemodynamic status, and renal function, and there is considerable overlap among different diagnostic groups (reviewed by Krupicka et al[368]). Therefore, a combination of conventional parameters such as clinical and echocardiographic measures assessed together with plasma levels of BNP yield better clinical guidelines in patients with CHF than each tool alone.[501]

C-Type Natriuretic Peptide. As mentioned earlier ("Physiology" section), CNP is synthesized mainly by endothelial cells, but small amounts are also produced by cardiac tissue.[502] In contrast to other natriuretic peptides, CNP is predominantly a vasodilator and has little effect on or may even reduce urinary flow and Na^+ excretion.[503,504] However, the production of CNP by the endothelium in proximity to its receptors in vascular smooth muscle cells suggests that this peptide may play a role in the control of vascular tone and growth.[505]

Like those of ANP and BNP, plasma CNP levels were found to be increased in CHF, although early studies showed no difference in plasma CNP levels between healthy individuals and patients with CHF.[505,506] CNP levels were directly correlated with New York Heart Association classification; with levels of BNP, ET-1, and adrenomedullin; and with pulmonary capillary wedge pressure, ejection fraction, and left ventricular end-diastolic diameter.[506-509] Higher levels of CNP have been found in the coronary sinuses than in the adjacent aorta, which is indicative of CNP release from the myocardium.[509,510] The demonstration of a CNP-induced inhibitory effect on cultured cardiac myocyte hypertrophy suggests that overexpression of CNP in the myocardium during CHF may be involved in counteracting cardiac remodeling.[502] In contrast to the diminished physiologic responses to ANP and BNP in animals with CHF in comparison with control animals, CNP elicited twice as much guanylyl cyclase activity as did ANP, which was shown to result from dramatic reductions in natriuretic peptide receptor A (NPR-A) activity without any change in natriuretic peptide receptor B (NPR-B) activity.[511] These novel findings imply a significant role for NPR-B–mediated natriuretic peptide activity in the failing heart and may explain the modest effects of nesiritide (BNP) treatment in CHF, inasmuch as the latter is NPR-A selective.[511]

Higher CNP levels in the renal vein than in the adjacent aorta have been reported in normal humans, but this difference was blunted in patients with CHF.[512] The physiologic significance of these data currently remains unexplained. Overall, the evidence available points to a possible peripheral vascular compensatory response to CHF by overexpression of CNP. Alternately, CNP may be involved in mitigating the cardiac remodeling so characteristic of CHF. Elaboration of the exact role of CNP in CHF is crucial for the design of potentially effective natriuretic peptide analogs for the management of CHF.

NITRIC OXIDE

After the discovery that nitric oxide is the prototypic endothelium-derived relaxing factor, this signaling molecule was implicated in the increased vascular resistance and impaired endothelium-dependent vascular responses characteristic of CHF.[513-518] Thus, the response to acetylcholine, an endothelium-dependent vasodilator that acts by releasing nitric oxide, was found to be markedly attenuated in CHF, both in human patients[519] and in experimental animals,[520] as well as in isolated resistance arteries from patients with CHF.[521] The mechanisms mediating the impaired activity of the nitric oxide system in CHF remain enigmatic. Possibilities include a reduction in shear stress associated with the decreased cardiac output,[522] downregulation of NOS,[523] decreased availability of the nitric oxide precursor L-arginine,[518] increased levels of the endogenous NOS inhibitor asymmetric dimethyl arginine (ADMA)[524] and overriding activity of counterregulatory vasoconstrictor systems such as the RAAS.[518,520]

In view of the role of nitric oxide in regulating RBF, altered activity of the nitric oxide system may be involved in the pathogenesis of the renal hypoperfusion in CHF. In line with this idea, rats with CHF induced by aortocaval fistula had attenuated nitric oxide–mediated renal vasodilation, which was reversed by pretreatment with an AT_1 receptor antagonist. This suggests that angiotensin II may be involved in mediating the impaired nitric oxide–dependent renal vasodilation.[520] The resulting imbalance between nitric oxide and excessive activation of the RAAS and endothelin systems could explain some of the beneficial effects of ACE inhibitors, ARBs, and aldosterone antagonists.[517]

The fact that patients with CHF have higher plasma levels of $NO_2 + NO_3$ and exhibit augmented responsiveness to NOS inhibitors suggests that the nitric oxide system in CHF is an ineffective counterregulatory mechanism in the presence of overwhelming vasoconstrictor forces.[518,525] Support for this concept came from a model of experimental CHF in rats, which overexpress eNOS in the renal medulla and, to a lesser extent, in the renal cortex.[269] It was speculated that this eNOS might play a role in the preservation of intact medullary perfusion and could attenuate the severe cortical vasoconstriction. Another explanation for the impaired renal hemodynamics in CHF is the accumulation of ADMA. In this context, plasma ADMA concentrations in patients with normotensive CHF were significantly higher than in controls, and in multiple regression analysis, ADMA levels were independently predictive of reduced effective RBF.[524]

An additional issue is that the myocardium contains all three NOS isoforms, and the locally generated nitric oxide is believed to play a modulatory role on cardiac function.[393,526] Thus, alterations in the cardiac nitric oxide system in CHF might contribute to the pathogenesis of cardiac dysfunction and, thereby, indirectly, to the impaired renal function.[527] Alteration in expression of cardiac NOS isoforms in CHF is complex, and the functional consequences of these changes depend on a balance among various factors, including disruption of the unique subcellular localization of each isoform and nitroso-redox imbalance.[528] Detailed discussion of this topic is beyond the scope of this review; the interested reader is referred to the cardiology literature (e.g., Espiner et al[28] and Bauersachs and Widder[513]).

In summary, endothelium-dependent vasodilation is attenuated in various vascular beds in CHF. This attenuation may occur in the presence of increased nitric oxide production, which suggests that the vascular nitric oxide may be another example of a failed vasodilator system in CHF.

Prostaglandins

Although the contribution of prostaglandins to renal function in euvolemic states is minimal, they play an important role in maintaining renal function in the setting of impaired RBF, as occurs in CHF. Renal hypoperfusion, either directly or by activation of the RAAS, stimulates the release of prostaglandins that exert a vasodilatory effect, predominantly at the level of the afferent arteriole, and promote Na^+ excretion by inhibiting Na^+ transport in the thick ascending limb of Henle and the medullary collecting duct.[529,530] Evidence of the compensatory role of prostaglandins in both experimental and clinical CHF comes from two sources. First, plasma levels of PGE_2, PGE_2 metabolites, and 6-keto-PGF_1 were higher in CHF patients than in normal subjects.[531] Moreover, studies in experimental and human CHF demonstrated a direct linear relationship between plasma renin activity and angiotensin II concentrations and levels of circulating and urinary PGE_2 and PGI_2 metabolites.[532] This correlation probably reflects both angiotensin II–induced stimulation of prostaglandin synthesis and prostaglandin-mediated increased renin release.

A similar counterregulatory role of prostaglandins with regard to the other vasoconstrictors (catecholamines and AVP) may also be inferred. An inverse correlation between plasma Na^+ concentrations and plasma levels of PGE_2 metabolites has also been demonstrated. The second approach that established the protective role of renal and vascular prostaglandins in CHF was derived from studies of nonsteroidal antiinflammatory drugs (NSAIDs), which inhibit the synthesis of prostaglandins. In various experimental models of CHF, inhibition of prostaglandin synthesis by indomethacin was associated with an elevation in urinary excretion of PGE_2, a significant increase in body weight, a profound increase in renal vascular resistance. and a resultant decrease in RBF, related mainly to afferent arteriolar constriction.[531,533] Serum creatinine and urea levels rose, and urine flow rate declined significantly.[533] In accordance with these observations, patients with CHF and hyponatremia, in whom extreme activation of the SNS and the RAAS occurred, were most susceptible to the adverse glomerular hemodynamic consequences of indomethacin treatment.[531] Such patients developed significant decreases in RBF and GFR accompanied by reduced urinary Na^+ excretion.[534] These effects were prevented by intravenous infusion of PGE_2. Moreover, pretreatment with indomethacin before captopril administration attenuated the captopril-induced increase in RBF. These results suggest that prostaglandins have a significant role in the regulation of renal function in patients with CHF and that captopril-induced improvement in renal hemodynamics is mediated in part by increased prostaglandin synthesis.

Renal prostaglandins may also play an important role in mediating the natriuretic effects of ANP. For example, in dogs with experimental CHF,[535] indomethacin reduced ANP-induced Na^+ excretion and creatinine clearance by 75% and 35%, respectively. Collectively, the results of both human and animal studies indicate that CHF is a "prostaglandin-dependent" state, in which elevated angiotensin II level and enhanced RSNA stimulate renal synthesis of PGE_2 and PGI_2, which would counteract the vasoconstrictor effects of these stimuli to maintain GFR and RBF. Therefore, administration of NSAIDs to patients or animals with CHF would leave these vasoconstrictor systems unopposed, leading to hypoperfusion, hypofiltration, and subsequent Na^+ and water retention.[530]

Clinical data amply bear out the close relationship between the consumption of NSAIDs, both nonselective cyclooxygenase inhibitors and selective COX-2 inhibitors, and a significant worsening of chronic CHF, especially in elderly patients taking diuretics.[536-540] The deleterious effects of selective COX-2 inhibitors on cardiac and renal functions are consistent with the relative abundance of COX-2 in renal tissue and, to a lesser extent, in the myocardium in patients with CHF.[541,542] Moreover, the significant increase in the risk of myocardial infarction and death with the COX-2 inhibitor rofecoxib raised serious safety problems in the use of these drugs and led to the withdrawal of rofecoxib from the market and a "black box" warning from the U.S. Food and Drug Administration about celecoxib.[543,544] The adverse cardiovascular effects are thought to be related to an imbalance between platelet COX-1–derived prothrombotic TXA_2 and endothelial COX-2–derived antithrombotic PGI_2, although maladaptive renal effects cannot be ruled out.[545] This would explain why not only selective COX-2 inhibitors but also nonselective cyclooxygenase inhibitors increase cardiovascular morbidity and mortality.[545] However, epidemiologic studies carried out since the withdrawal of rofecoxib indicate a decrease in the relative risk for hospitalization in CHF patients receiving NSAIDs, which suggests that physicians are prescribing these drugs more judiciously than in the past.[546] In addition, there is some evidence that celecoxib is safer than either rofecoxib or nonselective cyclooxygenase inhibitors in elderly patients with CHF.[537-540] The adverse effects of celecoxib may also be dose dependent.[547]

In summary, patients with preexisting CHF are dependent on adequate local prostaglandin levels in order to maintain RPF, GFR, and Na$^+$ excretion. Consequently, they are at high risk of volume overload, edema, and deterioration of cardiac function after the use of either COX-2 or nonselective cyclooxygenase inhibitors.

ADRENOMEDULLIN

Evidence suggests that adrenomedullin plays a role in the pathophysiology of CHF. In comparison with healthy subjects, patients with CHF have plasma levels of the mature form of adrenomedullin, as well as of the glycine-extended form, that are elevated up to fivefold and in proportion to the severity of cardiac and hemodynamic impairment.[284,548] High levels of midregional pro-adrenomedullin are also strong predictors of mortality in CHF.[549] In accordance with the correlation between plasma adrenomedullin levels and the severity of CHF, plasma adrenomedullin levels are also correlated with pulmonary arterial pressure, pulmonary capillary wedge pressure, norepinephrine level, ANP level, BNP level, and plasma renin activity in these patients. Plasma levels of the peptide fell with effective anti-CHF treatment, such as carvedilol.[288]

The origin of the increased amount of circulating adrenomedullin appears to be the failing myocardium itself, including both the ventricles and, to a lesser extent, the atria.[288] Similar findings have been reported for adrenomedullin-2.[550] Not only cardiac but also renal adrenomedullin level was significantly increased, in some but not all experimental models of CHF, in comparison with normal animals.[551,552] Although the significance of this renal upregulation of adrenomedullin in CHF is unclear, there is accumulating evidence that adrenomedullin has favorable effects on salt and water balance, as well as on hemodynamic abnormalities characterizing CHF. Both experimental and clinical studies showed that infusion of adrenomedullin produced beneficial renal effects in CHF-related volume overload. For example, in sheep with CHF caused by rapid pacing, brief administration (90 minutes) of adrenomedullin produced a threefold increase in Na$^+$ excretion with maintenance of urine output and a rise in creatinine clearance, in comparison with baseline levels in normal sheep.[288] Prolonged (for 4 days) administration of adrenomedullin in sheep with CHF produced a significant and sustained increase in cardiac output in association with enhanced urine volume.[288]

In contrast to the results in experimental CHF, acute administration of adrenomedullin to patients with CHF increased forearm blood flow but to a lesser extent than in normal subjects, which suggests that the vascular effects of adrenomedullin are significantly attenuated in CHF (see Rademaker et al[288]). In addition, adrenomedullin had no significant effect on urine volume and Na$^+$ excretion in patients with CHF, but it did reduce plasma aldosterone levels.[288] Also, adrenomedullin infusion led to increased stroke index,

dilation of resistance arteries, and urinary Na$^+$ excretion.[288] The improvement in cardiac function after adrenomedullin infusion is not surprising in view of its beneficial effects on preload and afterload and cardiac contractility.[284] Collectively, the vasodilatory and natriuretic activities of adrenomedullin, and its origin from the failing heart, suggest that adrenomedullin acts as a compensatory agent to balance the elevation in systemic vascular resistance and volume expansion in this disease state.

Because the favorable effects of adrenomedullin alone are rather modest, recent attempts at combination therapy with other vasodilatory/natriuretic substances have been made. In this regard, adrenomedullin in combination with other therapies such as BNP, ACE inhibitors, and NEP inhibitors resulted in hemodynamic and renal benefits greater than those achieved by each agent administered separately.[288] A small pilot trial of combined long-term human ANP and adrenomedullin in patients with acute decompensated heart failure demonstrated significant reductions in mean arterial pressure, pulmonary arterial pressure, systemic vascular resistance, and pulmonary vascular resistance without changing heart rate; cardiac output was also increased in comparison with baseline. In addition, the combination of adrenomedullin and human ANP reduced amounts of aldosterone, BNP, and free-radical metabolites, as well as increasing urine volume and Na$^+$ excretion over baseline values.[553]

These promising results should pave the way for larger controlled trials of adrenomedullin in combination with other vasodilator/natriuretic agents. However, in view of the known phenomenon of compensatory rises in vasoconstrictor/antinatriuretic mechanisms such as the RAAS, SNS, and endothelin, caution is needed with the use of adrenomedullin with ANP after natriuretic peptide therapy for CHF.

UROTENSIN

A role for urotensin II and its receptor, GPR14, in the pathogenesis of CHF has been suggested on the basis of the following findings: First, some but not all studies revealed that plasma levels of urotensin II are elevated in patients with CHF, in correlation with levels of other markers, such as NT-proBNP and ET-1.[554-556] Second, strong expression of urotensin II was demonstrated in the myocardium of patients with end-stage CHF, in correlation with the impairment of cardiac function.[557] This suggests that upregulation of the urotensin II/GPR14 system could play a part in the cardiac dysfunction associated with CHF. The upregulated urotensin II/GPR14 system in CHF may also have a role in the regulation of renal function in CHF. In rat models of CHF, urotensin II was shown to act primarily as a renal vasodilator, apparently by a nitric oxide–dependent mechanism.[301,302] Moreover, human urotensin II increased GFR in rats with CHF but did not alter urinary Na$^+$ excretion in either control or CHF rats. However, in contrast to the negligible renal vasodilatory effect in control rats, the peptide produced a prominent and prolonged decrease in renal vascular resistance in association with a significant increase in RPF and GFR in CHF rats. Thus, under conditions of increased baseline renal vascular tone found in CHF, human urotensin II has the capacity to act as a potent vasodilator in the kidneys. The clinical application of these data remains to be elucidated and is likely to be complicated, because this peptide might also be the most powerful known vasoconstrictor (see the "Physiology" section).

NEUROPEPTIDE Y

In contrast to the enigma surrounding its function in normal physiology, there is abundant evidence that neuropeptide Y has a significant role in the pathophysiologic process of CHF. Because neuropeptide Y co-localizes and is released with the adrenergic neurotransmitters, it is not surprising that the activated peripheral SNS, with high circulating norepinephrine levels in CHF, is also accompanied by excessive co-release of neuropeptide Y.[558] In fact, numerous studies demonstrated elevated plasma levels of neuropeptide Y of patients with CHF, regardless of the cause of the disease.[559,560] This increase is correlated with the severity the disease, which suggests that neuropeptide Y might serve as an independent prognostic factor for severity and outcome of CHF.[561]

Although circulating levels of neuropeptide Y are elevated in patients with CHF, local concentrations of neuropeptide Y, like those of norepinephrine, in the myocardium appear to be lower than normal.[562] Using an aortocaval fistula model of CHF in rats, Callanan and colleagues[313] demonstrated that the lower levels of myocardial neuropeptide Y are associated with decreased Y1 and increased Y2 receptor expression. Moreover, cardiac Y1 receptor expression decreased in proportion to the severity of cardiac hypertrophy and decompensation. Because Y1 receptor activation is associated with cardiomyocyte hypertrophy[563-566] and Y2 receptor activation with angiogenesis,[566] the data in this model suggest that neuropeptide Y may simultaneously attenuate the maladaptive cardiac remodeling observed in CHF and stimulate angiogenesis in the ischemic heart.[566] Similar patterns of receptor expression change were observed in the kidneys that were proportional to the degree of renal failure and Na^+ retention.[313] In contrast, administration of neuropeptide Y was shown in experimental models of CHF to exert diuretic and natriuretic properties,[567] probably by increasing the release of ANP and inhibiting the RAAS (Table 14-7),[568] thereby facilitating water and electrolyte clearance and reducing congestion. Therefore, in CHF, the higher circulating levels, together with the reduced tissue levels of neuropeptide Y, could be a counterregulatory mechanism to modulate the vasoconstrictive and Na^+ retaining, as well as the cardiac remodeling, effects of the RAAS and the SNS.

In addition, the downregulation of Y1 receptors, by reducing vascular constriction, could contribute to reductions in vascular resistance, in both the coronary and renal circulations. However, once the stage of decompensated heart failure is reached, the likelihood is that RAAS and SNS effects dominate, thereby overwhelming any favorable effects of neuropeptide Y. The precise role of neuropeptide Y in the pathogenesis of CHF progression, cardiac remodeling, and renal Na^+ and water retention, via Y1, Y2 and, possibly also, Y5 receptors, requires further clarification.

PHARMACOLOGIC AGENTS: PEROXISOME PROLIFERATOR-ACTIVATED RECEPTOR Γ AGONISTS AND CONGESTIVE HEART FAILURE

Peroxisome proliferator-activated receptors (PPARs) are nutrient-sensing nuclear transcription factors, of which PPARγ is of special interest in the context of Na^+ and water retention because of its ligands, the thiazolidinediones. Thiazolidinediones, by virtue of their ability to increase insulin sensitivity, are clinically used for the management of type 2 diabetes mellitus. In addition, thiazolidinediones decrease amounts of circulating free fatty acids and triglycerides, lower blood pressure, reduce levels of inflammatory markers, and reduce atherosclerosis in insulin-resistant patients and animal models. Moreover, they have been shown to be beneficial for cardiac remodeling in models of myocardial ischemia.[569] However, one of the troubling side effects of thiazolidinediones is fluid retention; therefore, CHF is one of the major contraindications to the clinical use of thiazolidinediones.

The site of PPARγ-induced fluid retention appears to involve the collecting duct, inasmuch as mice with collecting duct knockout of PPARγ were able to excrete salt loads more easily than were wild-type controls. Because PPARγ knockout also blocked the effect of thiazolidinediones on messenger RNA expression of the γ-subunit of the ENaC, the Na^+-retaining effect of thiazolidinediones appear to result from PPARγ stimulation of ENaC-mediated renal salt reabsorption.[570,571] In clinical terms, the Na^+-retaining effect of thiazolidinediones translates into increased incidence of heart failure in patients receiving these drugs, in comparison with controls.[572] Because of the Na^+- and fluid-retaining effects, as well as other concerns related to increased cardiovascular events,[572] the exact role of thiazolidinediones in the management of diabetes is currently undetermined.

In summary, the alterations in the efferent limb of volume regulation in CHF include enhanced activities of vasoconstrictor/Na^+-retaining systems and activation of counterregulatory vasodilatory/natriuretic systems. The magnitude of Na^+ excretion by the kidneys and, therefore, the disturbance in volume homeostasis in CHF are largely determined by the balance between these antagonistic systems. In the early stages of CHF, the balancing effect of the vasodilatory/natriuretic systems is of importance in the maintenance of circulatory and renal function. However, with the progression of CHF, this balance shifts toward dysfunction of the vasodilatory/natriuretic systems and marked activation of the vasoconstrictor/antinatriuretic systems. These disturbances are translated at the renal circulatory and tubular level to alterations that result in avid retention of salt and water, thereby leading to edema formation.

TABLE 14-7 Renal Effects of RAAS Inhibition in Heart Failure

Factors Favoring Improvement in Renal Function

Maintenance of Na^+ balance
   Reduction in diuretic dosage
   Increase in Na^+ intake
   Mean arterial pressure >80 mm Hg
Minimal neurohumoral activation
Intact counterregulatory mechanisms

Factors Favoring Deterioration in Renal Function

Evidence of Na^+ depletion or poor renal perfusion
   Large doses of diuretics
   Increased urea/creatinine ratio
   Mean arterial pressure <80 mm Hg
Evidence of maximal neurohumoral activation
   AVP-induced hyponatremia
Interruption of counterregulatory mechanisms
   Coadministration of prostaglandin inhibitors
   Adrenergic dysfunction (e.g., as in diabetes mellitus)

AVP, Arginine vasopressin; *RAAS*, renin-angiotensin-aldosterone system.

Renal Sodium Retention in Cirrhosis with Portal Hypertension

Abnormalities in renal Na$^+$ and water excretion commonly occur with cirrhosis, in humans as well as in experimental animal models.[573,574] Avid Na$^+$ and water retention may lead eventually to ascites, a common complication of cirrhosis and a major cause of morbidity and mortality, with the occurrence of spontaneous bacterial peritonitis, variceal bleeding, and development of the hepatorenal syndrome.[344,574] As in CHF, the pathogenesis of renal Na$^+$ and water retention in cirrhosis is related not to an intrinsic abnormality of the kidneys but to extrarenal mechanisms that regulate renal Na$^+$ and water handling.

ABNORMALITIES OF VOLUME-SENSING MECHANISMS IN CIRRHOSIS

Several formulations have been forwarded to explain the mechanisms of Na$^+$ and water retention in cirrhosis, of which the two major ones are the "overflow" and "underfilling" hypotheses. According to the "overflow" hypothesis, an extrarenal signal, possibly from the abnormal liver, induces primary renal Na$^+$ and water retention and plasma volume expansion, even before the appearance of clinical signs such as ascites. Conversely, the classic "underfilling" theory posits that ascites formation causes hypovolemia, which further initiates secondary renal Na$^+$ and water retention.

In 1988, Schrier and associates[575] proposed the "peripheral arterial vasodilation" hypothesis as the basis for relative hypovolemia.[576] The concept of peripheral arterial vasodilation was promoted in the 1990s as a unifying hypothesis to explain the mechanism of renal Na$^+$ and water retention in such diverse states of edema formation as cirrhosis and pregnancy.[41,353,354] At the same time, the importance of nitric oxide in the induction of peripheral arterial vasodilation and the hemodynamic abnormalities that mediate salt and water retention in cirrhosis became increasingly evident.[577,578] The contribution of nitric oxide, as well as other vasodilatory mechanisms, to the generation of the "hyperdynamic" circulation in cirrhosis was further demonstrated by numerous other investigators (see Iwakiri and Groszmann[579]). In the following sections, these competing theories of the disturbance in volume sensing in cirrhosis are briefly presented and followed by a description of the efferent limb of the volume-control system.

Overflow Hypothesis. On the basis of findings in patients with cirrhosis, Lieberman and colleagues[580] postulated non–volume-dependent renal Na$^+$ retention as the primary disturbance in Na$^+$ homeostasis in cirrhosis. In turn, this type of renal Na$^+$ retention leads to total plasma volume expansion, and the resulting increased hydrostatic pressure in the portosplanchnic bed promotes "overflow" ascites. Strong support for the overflow theory came from extensive and carefully designed studies in dogs with experimental cirrhosis (see Levy[581] and references therein). Results of these studies indicated that renal Na$^+$ retention and volume expansion could precede ascites formation by 10 days. The Na$^+$ retention occurred independently of measurable changes in cardiac output, mean arterial pressure, splanchnic blood volume, hepatic arterial blood flow, GFR, RPF, aldosterone level, and increased RSNA.[582] Also, elimination of ascites with the peritoneojugular LeVeen shunt did not prevent Na$^+$ retention during liberal salt intake. In additional studies in dogs with cirrhosis induced

by common bile duct ligation, Na$^+$ retention and ascites formation occurred only in dogs with partially or fully occluded portocaval fistulas, but not in animals with patent portocaval anastomosis and normal intrahepatic pressure. These results suggested that intrahepatic hypertension secondary to hepatic venous outflow obstruction was the primary stimulus for renal salt retention.[581]

In addition to the well-characterized increase in intrahepatic vascular resistance and sinusoidal pressure in cirrhosis, portal venous blood flow is decreased, and hepatic arterial blood flow is either increased or normal. Moreover, the lower the portal venous flow, the higher the hepatic arterial flow (Figure 14-9A). Of note, a similar response in portal venous and hepatic arterial flow is observed during hemorrhage-induced hypotension (reviewed by Oliver and Verna[71]). Therefore, it is abundantly clear that the liver is integrally involved in volume sensing. However, the exact anatomic interactions among hepatic arterioles, presinusoidal portal vein branches, and hepatic sinusoids in both the normal liver and cirrhotic liver remain to be elucidated.

Afferent Sensing of Intrahepatic Hypertension. The pathway by which intrahepatic hypertension could stimulate renal Na$^+$ retention, without the intermediary of underfilling, would probably involve the hepatic volume-sensing mechanisms mentioned earlier. These sensing mechanisms would respond specifically to elevated hepatic venous pressure with increased hepatic afferent nerve activity. The relays for these impulses consist of two autonomic nerve plexuses: one surrounding the hepatic artery and the other surrounding the portal vein.[583] These neural networks connect hepatic venous congestion to enhanced renal and cardiopulmonary sympathetic activity.

Occlusion of the inferior vena cava at the diaphragm was associated with rises in hepatic, portal, and renal venous pressures and resulted in markedly increased hepatic afferent nerve traffic and renal and cardiopulmonary sympathetic efferent nerve activity. Section of the anterior hepatic nerves eliminated the reflex increase in renal efferent nerve activity.[583] Similarly, denervation of the liver in dogs with vena caval constriction increased urinary Na$^+$ excretion.[75] More recently, intrahepatic administration of an adenosine receptor antagonist, 8-phenyltheophylline, to cirrhotic rats produced an effect similar to that of hepatic denervation.[584] Subsequently, the adenosine effect was shown to be mediated by the A$_1$ receptor, inasmuch as a selective antagonist of the A$_1$ receptor, but not of the A$_2$ receptor, inhibited Na$^+$ retention. Of importance is that the adenosine-dependent effects were abolished by hepatic denervation.[72]

Apart from the adenosine-mediated hepatorenal reflex, other, currently undefined humoral pathways could provide an anatomic or physiologic basis for the primary effects of alterations in intrahepatic hemodynamics on renal function. Only a rapid rise in sinusoidal pressure triggers the hepatorenal reflex and ascites formation (e.g., as in Budd-Chiari syndrome). However, chronically increased sinusoidal pressure, to levels even higher than those induced acutely, is usually not associated with ascites formation.[585] Despite the wealth of information on hepatic volume sensing, the molecular identity of the sensor, the cellular location of the sensor, and what is sensed remain elusive. Therefore, much work remains to completely unravel the role of overflow in the pathogenesis of Na$^+$ retention in cirrhosis.

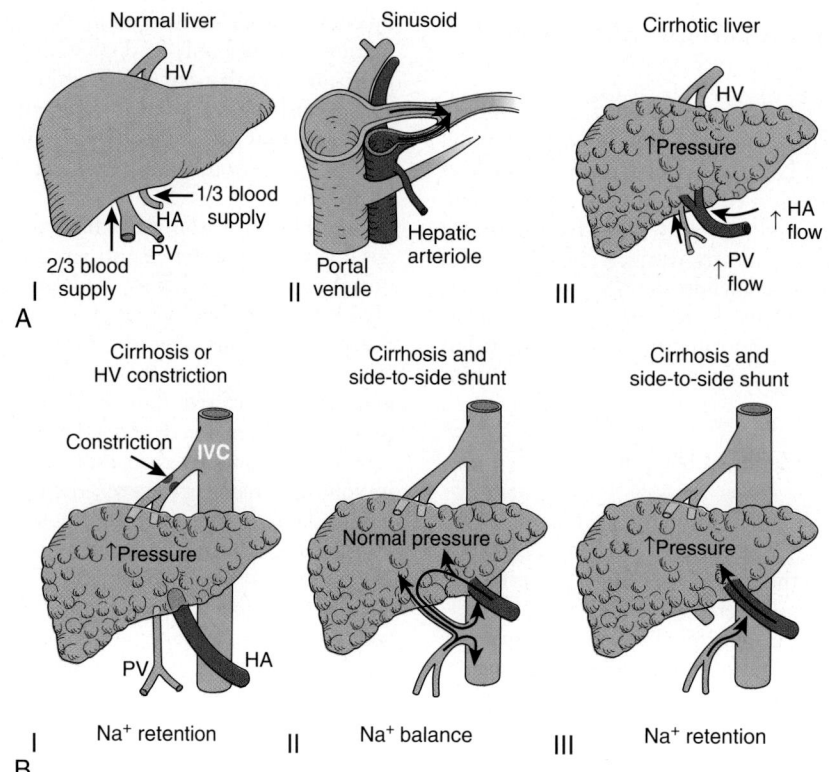

FIGURE 14-9 Characteristics of hepatic blood flow. **A,** Hepatic circulation. **i,** The normal liver receives two thirds of its blood flow from the portal vein (PV) and the remaining third from the hepatic artery (HA). **ii,** Both the portal venules and hepatic arterioles drain into hepatic sinusoids, but the exact arrangement that allows forward flow of the mixed venous and arterial bloods remains unclear. **iii,** Cirrhosis increases intrahepatic vascular resistance and sinusoidal pressure. In addition, PV flow is markedly decreased, and HA flow is either unchanged or increased. **B,** Hepatic vascular hemodynamics and sodium balance. **i,** Cirrhosis or restriction of HV flow increases intrahepatic vascular resistance and sinusoidal pressure, markedly decreasing PV flow and increasing HA flow. Changes in the physical forces or in the composition of the hepatic blood trigger Na⁺ retention and edema formation. **ii,** Insertion of a side-to-side portocaval shunt decreases sinusoidal pressure and maintains mixing of PV and HA blood, irrigating the liver. Under these conditions and despite cirrhosis, there is no Na⁺ retention. **iii,** Insertion of an end-to-side portocaval shunt only partially decreases the elevated sinusoidal pressure and prevents mixing of PV and HA blood supplies, inasmuch as the PV blood is diverted to the inferior vena cava. Under these conditions and, despite normalization of PV pressure, Na⁺ retention continues unabated. (Adapted from Oliver JA, Verna EC: Afferent mechanisms of sodium retention in cirrhosis and hepatorenal syndrome, *Kidney Int* 77:669-680, 2010.)

Underfilling Hypothesis. In contrast to the "overflow" concept, classic "underfilling" theory holds that during the development of cirrhosis, transudation of fluid and its accumulation in the peritoneal cavity as ascites result in true intravascular hypovolemia. The reduced EABV, in turn, is sensed by the various components of the afferent volume-control system described earlier. Subsequent activation of the efferent limb of the volume-control system, including the RAAS, SNS, and the nonosmotic release of AVP, results in enhanced renal Na⁺ and water retention, failure to escape from the Na⁺-retaining effect of aldosterone, and impaired excretion of solute-free water. The ultimate consequence of this mechanism is the development of positive Na⁺ balance and exacerbation of ascites formation.[578]

Several mechanisms have been invoked to account for the development of the hypovolemia. One such mechanism arose as a consequence of the disruption in normal Starling relationships that govern fluid movement in the hepatic sinusoids. These, unlike capillaries elsewhere in the body, are highly permeable for plasma proteins. As a result, partitioning of ECF between the intravascular (intrasinusoidal) and interstitial (space of Disse and lymphatic) compartments of the liver is determined predominantly by the ΔP along the length of the hepatic sinusoids. Obstruction of hepatic venous outflow promotes enhanced efflux of a protein-rich filtrate into the space of Disse and results in augmented hepatic lymph formation. Such augmented hepatic lymph flow, the main mechanism of ascites formation, has been observed in human subjects with cirrhosis and in experimental models of liver disease.[586,587]

Vastly increased hepatic lymph formation is accompanied by increased flow through the thoracic duct.[588] When the rate of enhanced hepatic lymph formation exceeds the capacity for return to the intravascular compartment via the thoracic duct, hepatic lymph accumulates as ascites, and the intravascular compartment is further compromised. As liver disease progresses, a fibrotic process surrounds the Kupffer cells lining the sinusoids, rendering the sinusoids less permeable for serum proteins. Under such circumstances, termed *capillarization of sinusoids*, a decrease in oncotic pressure also promotes transudation of ECF within the hepatic lymph space, much as it does in other vascular beds.[586]

Additional consequences of intrahepatic hypertension have also been postulated to contribute to perceived volume contraction. Among these, transmission of elevated intrasinusoidal pressures to the portal vein leads to expansion of the splanchnic venous system, collateral vein formation, and portosystemic shunting. This results in increased vascular capacitance and diversion of blood flow from the arterial circuit.[589] Vasodilation seems to occur not only in the splanchnic circulation but also in the systemic circulation and has been attributed to refractoriness to the pressor effects of vasoconstrictor hormones, such as angiotensin II and catecholamines, although the mechanism remains unknown.[590] Along with diminished hepatic reticuloendothelial cell function, portosystemic shunting allows various products of intestinal metabolism and absorption to bypass the liver and escape hepatic elimination. Among these products, endotoxins are thought to contribute to perturbations in renal function in cirrhosis, possibly secondary to the hemodynamic consequences of endotoxemia or through direct renal effects.[591]

Levels of conjugated bilirubin and bile acids may become elevated as a result of intrahepatic cholestasis or extrahepatic biliary obstruction. In experimental studies of bile duct ligation, it is difficult to distinguish the effects on renal function of jaundice itself from the effects of cirrhosis that ensue after the bile duct ligation. However, bile acids actually decrease proximal tubular reabsorption of Na^+, a direct renal action that would tend to promote natriuresis.[592] Nevertheless, the diuretic-like effect of bile salts may also contribute to the underfilling state in cirrhotic patients.[592,593]

Hypoalbuminemia could also contribute to the development of hypovolemia, by diminishing colloid osmotic forces in the systemic capillaries and hepatic sinusoids.[594] Hypoalbuminemia was believed to occur as a result of both decreased synthesis of albumin by the liver and dilution caused by ECF volume expansion. The development of hypoalbuminemia is a relatively late event in the course of chronic liver disease. Likewise, a relative impairment of cardiac function could contribute to diminished arterial blood pressure in some cirrhotic patients.[593,595] In these patients, tense ascites might reduce venous return (preload) to the heart.

Other factors that may also adversely affect cardiac performance include diminished β-adrenergic receptor signal transduction, cardiomyocyte cellular plasma membrane dysfunction, and increased activity or levels of cardiodepressant substances, such as cytokines, endocannabinoids, and nitric oxide. Although the cardiac dysfunction, termed *cirrhotic cardiomyopathy*, usually is clinically mild or silent, overt heart failure can be precipitated by stresses such as liver transplantation or transjugular intrahepatic portosystemic shunt (TIPS) insertion.[595] Finally, volume depletion in cirrhotic patients may be aggravated by vomiting, occult variceal bleeding, and excessive use of diuretics. Therefore, patients with cirrhosis tolerate hemorrhage or fluid loss very poorly, and they are prone to suffer cardiovascular collapse in the setting of hemodynamic disturbances.

Table 14-8 summarizes the various etiologic factors contributing to underfilling of the circulation in patients with advanced liver disease. Two major arguments have been provided in support of the underfilling theory. First, the progression of cirrhosis is characterized by increased neurohumoral activity with stimulation of the RAAS, increased sympathetic activity, and elevated plasma AVP levels. These classic markers of hypovolemia cannot be explained by the overflow hypothesis. Second, a salutary improvement in volume homeostasis was observed after volume replenishment in cirrhotic patients. For example, volume expansion could suppress the RAAS, increase the GFR, and cause natriuresis and negative salt balance in such patients. In fact, several maneuvers of volume

TABLE 14-8 Factors Causing Underfilling of the Circulation in Cirrhosis
Peripheral vasodilation and blunted vasoconstrictor response to reflex, chemical, and hormonal influences
Arteriovenous shunts, particularly in portal circulation
Increased vascular capacity of portal and systemic circulation
Hypoalbuminemia
Impaired left ventricular function, cirrhotic cardiomyopathy
Diminished venous return secondary to advanced tense ascites
Occult gastrointestinal bleeding from ulcers, gastritis, or varices
Volume losses resulting from vomiting and excessive use of diuretics

expansion, such as reinfusion of ascitic fluid, placement of LeVeen shunt, and HWI, were found to cause a brisk diuretic/natriuretic response in patients with cirrhosis. Conversely, the main argument against the underfilling theory was that measured plasma volume in most patients with compensated cirrhosis was increased, and this increase frequently antedated ascites formation.[596] In addition, although volume repletion by diverse measures, as described previously, could result in a dramatic improvement and natriuresis, such an improvement was, at best, temporary and occurred only in 30% to 50% of affected patients. Some of the variability could be a result of inadequate volume replenishment. Nevertheless, it appears that underfilling cannot be the entire explanation for the renal Na^+ and water retention that characterizes cirrhotic patients. However, underfilling appears to contribute to Na^+ retention in cirrhosis at specific stages of the disease.

Peripheral Arterial Vasodilation. Irrespective of the initial trigger, the hallmark of fluid retention in cirrhosis is peripheral arterial vasodilation, in association with renal vasoconstriction. Initially, vasodilation occurs in the splanchnic vascular bed and later in the systemic and pulmonary circulations, leading to "relative arterial underfilling."[575,579] This "relative" underfilling unloads the arterial high-pressure baroreceptors and other volume receptors, which, in turn, stimulate a compensatory neurohumoral response. This response includes activation of the RAAS and the SNS, as well as the nonosmotic release of AVP.[354,575] Thus, increased hepatic resistance to portal flow causes the gradual development of portal hypertension, collateral vein formation, and shunting of blood to the systemic circulation.

As portal hypertension develops, local production of vasodilators—mainly nitric oxide but also carbon monoxide, glucagon, prostacyclin, adrenomedullin, and endogenous opiates—increases, leading to splanchnic vasodilation.[574,577] In the early stages of cirrhosis, arterial pressure is maintained through increases in plasma volume and cardiac output, in the form of a "hyperdynamic" circulation. However, as the disease progresses, vasodilation in the splanchnic and, presumably, other vascular beds is so pronounced that EABV decreases markedly, leading to sustained neurohumoral activation, renal (as well as brachial, femoral, and cerebral) vasoconstriction, and further Na^+ and fluid retention.[574,575] This hypothesis could, therefore, potentially explain the increased cardiac output and the enhanced neurohumoral changes over the entire spectrum of cirrhosis.[596]

Thus, decreases in systemic vascular resistance associated with low arterial blood pressure and high cardiac output are clinical manifestations of the hyperdynamic circulation that are commonly seen in patients with cirrhosis. In fact, the combination of warm extremities, cutaneous vascular spiders, wide pulse pressure, and capillary pulsations in the nail bed has been known in cirrhotic patients since the early 1950s.[578,579] Pulmonary vasodilation, associated with the hepatopulmonary syndrome, one of the most severe complications of chronic liver disease, may also be considered an example of the hyperdynamic circulation caused by increased production of nitric oxide (and possibly also carbon monoxide in the lungs.[579,597]

The hepatorenal syndrome may also develop when the heart is not able to compensate any longer for the progressive decrease in systemic vascular resistance.[598] Thus, the hyperdynamic syndrome of chronic liver disease should be considered as a "progressive vasodilatory syndrome" that finally leads to multiorgan involvement.[579] As pointed out earlier, increased production of nitric oxide in the splanchnic vasculature plays a cardinal role in initiating this process.

Nitric Oxide. Considerable evidence indicates that aberrations in the endothelial vasodilator nitric oxide system are involved in the pathogenesis of the hyperdynamic circulation and Na$^+$ and water retention in cirrhosis, as well as in hepatic encephalopathy, hepatopulmonary syndrome, and cirrhotic cardiomyopathy.[579,599,600] Nitric oxide is produced in excess by the vasculature of different animal models of portal hypertension, as well as in cirrhotic patients (see Wiest and Groszmann[599] and references therein). In animal models, the increased production of nitric oxide can be detected at the onset of Na$^+$ retention and before the appearance of ascites,[601] and nitric oxide has been implicated in the impaired vascular responsiveness to vasoconstrictors. Moreover, removal of the vascular endothelial layer has been demonstrated to abolish the difference in vascular reactivity between cirrhotic and control vessels (see Iwakiri and Groszmann[579]).

Inhibition of NOS has beneficial effects both in experimental models of cirrhosis and in humans with the disease. Thus, low dose L-NAME treatment for 7 days[602] reversed the high nitric oxide production to control levels and corrected the hyperdynamic circulation in cirrhotic rats with ascites. The normalization of nitric oxide production was accompanied by a marked increase in urinary Na$^+$ and water excretion, a concomitant decrease of ascites, and decreases in plasma renin activity and in the concentrations of aldosterone and vasopressin.[603] In patients with cirrhosis, the vascular hyporesponsiveness of the forearm circulation to norepinephrine could be reversed by the NOS inhibitor L-NMMA.[604] Inhibition of nitric oxide production also corrected the hypotension and hyperdynamic circulation, led to improved renal function and Na$^+$ excretion, and led to a decrease in plasma norepinephrine levels, in these patients.[605]

The main enzymatic source of the increased systemic vascular nitric oxide generation in cirrhosis has been demonstrated to be eNOS in the arterial and splanchnic circulations.[577] The upregulation of eNOS appears to be, at least in part, caused by increased shear stress as a result of portal venous hypertension with increased flow in the splanchnic circulation.[577,579,599] However, in rats with portal vein ligation, eNOS upregulation and increased nitric oxide release in the superior mesenteric arteries were found to precede the development of the hyperdynamic splanchnic circulation (see Wiest and Groszmann[599] and references therein). In marked contrast to the increased nitric oxide generation in the splanchnic and systemic circulation, there is evidence for impaired nitric oxide production and endothelial dysfunction in the intrahepatic microcirculation in cirrhotic rats (see Wiest

and Groszmann[599] and references therein). The mechanism of this paradoxical behavior of the intrahepatic vascular bed is unknown. However, it has been speculated that this intrahepatic endothelial dysfunction and nitric oxide deficiency may play a significant role in the pathogenesis of the increased hepatic vascular resistance, as well as in the increased intrahepatic thrombosis and collagen synthesis in cirrhosis (reviewed by Wiest and Groszmann[599]). In fact, it is currently believed that the increase in intrahepatic vascular resistance does not result merely from mechanical distortion of the vasculature by fibrosis; rather, a dynamic process, contraction of myofibroblasts and stellate cells, is believed to determine the degree of intrahepatic vascular resistance.[586,599]

The decrease in nitric oxide production that results from endothelial dysfunction may shift the balance in favor of vasocostrictors (e.g., endothelin, leukotrienes, TXA$_2$, angiotensin II), thus causing an increase in intrahepatic vascular resistance.[599] In accordance with this idea, upregulation of either eNOS or nNOS expression in livers of rats with experimental cirrhosis was associated with a decrease in portal hypertension.[606,607] It has been clearly shown that eNOS protein is increased in animal models of portal hypertension and that this increase is already detectable in cirrhotic rats without ascites.[599] However, mice with targeted deletion of eNOS alone, or with combined deletions of eNOS and iNOS, may develop a hyperdynamic circulation in association with portal hypertension[608] This suggests that other vasodilatory agents may be activated in these mice. In fact, some evidence indicates that PGI$_2$,[609] endothelium-derived hyperpolarizing factor,[610] carbon monoxide,[611] adrenomedullin,[612] and other vasodilators may participate in the pathogenesis of the hyperdynamic circulation in experimental cirrhosis (see Iwakiri and Groszmann[579]).

Evidence that other isoforms of NOS may be involved in the generation of the hyperdynamic circulation and fluid retention in experimental cirrhosis is inconclusive.[613] Increased expression of nNOS has been thought to partially compensate for the endothelial isoform deficiency in the eNOS–knockout mouse.[614] In contrast, the role of iNOS remains controversial; some researchers have shown increased iNOS in arteries of animals with experimental biliary cirrhosis[615] but not in other forms of experimental cirrhosis.[577,616] Although nonspecific inhibition of NOS may correct the hyperdynamic circulation, preferential iNOS inhibition was shown to be generally ineffective (see Iwakiri and Groszmann[579]). Overall, the available data point to a predominant role for eNOS.

In experimental cirrhosis, several cellular mechanisms have been implicated in the upregulation of splanchnic eNOS activity and in the downregulation of intrahepatic eNOS activity. Elevation in shear stress as a result of the hyperdynamic circulation and portal hypertension has already been mentioned and is consistent with this well-documented mechanism for upregulating eNOS gene transcription in general. However, additional factors related to the hepatic dysfunction could further stimulate this upregulation. For example, eNOS activity is posttranscriptionally regulated by tetrahydrobiopterin[617] and by direct phosphorylation of eNOS protein.[618] For example, in rats with experimental cirrhosis, circulating endotoxins may increase the enzymatic production of tetrahydrobiopterin, thereby enhancing eNOS activity in the mesenteric vascular bed.[619]

Conversely, potential contributors to intrahepatic eNOS downregulation include interactions with other proteins such as caveolin, calmodulin, heat shock protein 90 (see Wiest and Groszmann[599] and Langer and Shah[600] and references therein) and eNOS trafficking inducer.[620] In addition, disorders of guanylyl cyclase activity have been described.[620] Increased levels of ADMA have been reported, and these levels correlate with the severity of portal hypertension during hepatic inflammation. Moreover, higher ADMA levels have been found in patients with decompensated cirrhosis than in those with compensated disease.[620] The raised ADMA levels have been linked to reduced activity of dimethylarginine dimethylhydrolases (DDAHs) that normally metabolize ADMA to citrulline. In this regard, targeted disruption of the DDAH-1 gene in mice or chemical inhibition of DDAH-1 in a model of endotoxin shock was associated with increased plasma and tissue levels of ADMA and decreased nitric oxide–dependent vasodilation.[621] Similarly, patients with alcoholic cirrhosis and superimposed inflammatory alcoholic hepatitis had higher plasma and tissue levels of ADMA, higher portal venous pressures, and decreased DDAH expression.[622] The therapeutic potential for increasing DDAH activity has been shown in an animal model of traumatic vascular injury. Transgenic overexpression of DDAH in this model led to reduced plasma ADMA levels, enhanced endothelial cell regeneration, and reduced neointima formation.[623] These data raise the possibility of translating the favorable effects of DDAH into the management of decompensated portal hypertension.[620] In the final analysis, the relative importance of the various mechanisms involved in the reduced intrahepatic and increased splanchnic and systemic NOS activity in cirrhosis remains to be determined.

Endocannabinoids. Endogenous cannabinoids are lipid-signaling molecules mimicking the activity of Δ9-tetrahydrocannabinol, the main psychotropic constituent of marijuana. They influence neuroprotection, pain and motor function, energy balance and food intake, cardiovascular function, immune and inflammatory responses, and cell proliferation. N-arachidonoylethanolamide, or anandamide, and 2-arachidonoylglycerol are the two most widely studied endocannabinoids that bind the two specific receptors CB_1 and CB_2. CB_1 is expressed mainly in the brain, whereas the CB_2 receptor is found mostly in cells of the immune system; both receptors are also expressed in many peripheral tissues under physiologic and pathologic conditions. Anandamide is also able to interact with the vanilloid receptor.[624] Although both hepatocytes and nonparenchymal liver cells are capable of producing endocannabinoids, the physiologic expression of CB_1 and CB_2 receptors in the adult liver is very low or even absent.

A compelling series of experimental and clinical studies has shown that the hepatic expression of CB_1 and CB_2 receptors and endocannabinoid production are greatly upregulated in chronic and acute liver damage (see Caraceni et al[625] and references therein). Of relevance to this discussion is that endocannabinoids have been implicated in portal hypertension and the hyperdynamic circulatory syndrome. In this regard, anandamide caused a dose-dependent increase in intrahepatic vascular resistance in the isolated perfused rat liver. This effect was magnified in cirrhotic livers and appeared to be mediated by enhanced production of cyclooxygenase-derived vasoconstrictive eicosanoids. In addition, chronic antagonism of

the CB_1 receptor reversed the upregulation of several vasoconstrictive eicosanoids in rat bile duct ligation–induced cirrhosis. With regard to the splanchnic vasodilation observed in cirrhosis, administration of the CB_1 receptor antagonist rimonabant to cirrhotic rats reversed arterial hypotension and increased vascular resistance; with a concomitant decrease in mesenteric arterial blood flow and portal venous pressure. The reduction in splanchnic blood flow was enhanced by the vanilloid receptor capsazepine. These findings indicate that the transient receptor potential vanilloid type 1 protein and the CB_1 receptor have a dual role in the splanchnic vasodilation characteristic of cirrhosis (see Caraceni et al[625] and references therein).

A role for endotoxin in the endocannabinoid effects was suggested by the demonstration that infusion of monocytes isolated from cirrhotic rats but not from control rats induced marked hypotension in normal animals (see Caraceni et al[625] and references therein). Also, the amount of anandamide was significantly higher in monocytes isolated from patients or rats with cirrhosis than in those from healthy subjects or animals. Because endotoxin represents a major stimulus for endocannabinoid generation in monocytes and platelets, it has been hypothesized that these cells are stimulated to produce large amounts of endocannabinoids by the elevated circulating endotoxin levels frequently found in patients with advanced cirrhosis. This production could then trigger splanchnic and peripheral vasodilation and arterial hypotension, together with intrahepatic vasoconstriction, through activation of the CB_1 receptors located in the vascular wall and in the perivascular nerves (see Caraceni et al[625] and references therein). The role for endocannabinoid antagonism in the treatment of human hepatorenal syndrome remains to be explored.

In summary, afferent sensing of volume in cirrhosis is characterized by increased intrahepatic vascular resistance and sinusoidal pressure, decreased portal venous blood flow, and increased hepatic arterial flow. Either because of changes in intrahepatic physical forces or in composition of the "mixed" intrahepatic blood, abnormal Na^+ retention is initiated, and edema develops (see Figure 14-9A). Cirrhosis alone is not sufficient to induce edema, inasmuch as a side-to-side portocaval shunt prevents (if inserted before induction of cirrhosis) or corrects (if inserted after induction of cirrhosis) renal Na^+ retention. This outcome could result from decreases in sinusoidal pressure or maintenance of the mixing of portal venous and hepatic arterial blood perfusing the liver. In contrast, end-to-side portocaval shunting only partially decreases elevated sinusoidal pressure and prevents mixing of portal venous and arterial hepatic blood supplies, inasmuch as the portal venous blood is diverted to the inferior vena cava. Under these conditions, and despite normalization of portal venous pressure, Na^+ retention continues unabated (see Figure 14-9B).

Available data are most consistent with the view that the putative EABV volume sensor in the hepatic circulation is pathologically activated in cirrhosis, failing to respond to the expanded ECF volume. Therefore, as the disease advances, edema worsens (see review by Oliver and Verna[71]).

ABNORMALITIES OF EFFECTOR MECHANISMS IN CIRRHOSIS
The efferent limb of volume regulation in cirrhosis is similar to that in CHF, consisting of adjustments in glomerular hemodynamics and tubule transport that are mediated by vasoconstrictor/antinatriuretic forces (RAAS, SNS, AVP, and

endothelin) and counterbalanced by vasodilator/natriuretic systems (natriuretic peptides and prostaglandins). Therefore, as in CHF, tilting the balance in favor of Na^+ retaining forces leads to renal Na^+ and water retention.[344,573,574]

Vasoconstrictors/Antinatriuretics

Renin-Angiotensin-Aldosterone System. As in other states of secondary Na^+ retention, the RAAS plays a central role in mediating renal Na^+ retention in cirrhosis, as demonstrated both in patients and animal models. Elevated plasma renin activity and aldosterone levels were noted in parallel with the progressive severity of cirrhosis and the increase in Na^+ retention. Activation of the RAAS is more prominent in patients with ascites than in pre-ascitic patients, which suggests that activation of the RAAS occurs at a relatively advanced stage of the disease. Results of studies in animal models of cirrhosis, in general, support this notion.[626] Nevertheless, positive Na^+ balance may already be evident in the pre-ascitic phase of the disease,[627] although plasma renin activity and aldosterone levels either remain within the normal range or may even be depressed.

As mentioned earlier, these observations were long believed to be evidence of the role of the overflow theory in the mechanism of ascites formation. However, Bernardi and associates[628] found elevated aldosterone levels that were inversely correlated with renal Na^+ excretion in pre-ascitic cirrhotic patients, particularly in the upright position. This finding suggested that posture-induced activation of the RAAS could already exist in the pre-ascitic phase. In accordance with this notion, renal Na^+ retention induced by LBNP was associated with a prominent increase in renal renin and angiotensin II excretion.[629] Moreover, treatment with the ARB losartan, at a dosage that did not affect systemic and renal hemodynamics or glomerular filtration, was associated with a significant natriuretic response.[630] The losartan-induced natriuresis in the presence of normal plasma renin activity was attributed to inhibition of the local intrarenal RAAS.[628,630] In fact, it has been demonstrated in rats with chronic bile duct ligation that activation of the intrarenal RAAS may precede activation of the circulating system.[631] In addition, losartan has been shown to cause a decrease in portal venous pressure in cirrhotic patients with portal hypertension.[632] The postural-induced activation of the RAAS, as well as the beneficial effects of low-dose losartan treatment, in patients with pre-ascitic cirrhosis may be explained by compartmentalization of the expanded blood volume within the splanchnic venous bed during standing and translocation toward the central and arterial circulatory beds during recumbence.[628]

In contrast, in Na^+-retaining cirrhotic patients with ascites, angiotensin II inhibition has deleterious effects. For example, administration of captopril, even in low doses, to such patients resulted in a decrease in both GFR and urinary Na^+ excretion.[633] At this stage of the disease, activation of the RAAS serves to support arterial pressure and maintain adequate circulation. Therefore, blockade of the RAAS by ACE inhibition or angiotensin receptor blockade may lead to a profound decrease in RPP. This scenario might be important in the pathogenesis of the hepatorenal syndrome, which is regularly preceded by a state of Na^+ retention and may be precipitated by a hypovolemic insult. Abnormalities of the renal circulation characteristic of this syndrome include marked diminution of RPF with renal cortical ischemia and increased renal vascular resistance, abnormalities consistent with the known actions of angiotensin II on the renal microcirculation. In this regard, several groups correlated activation of the RAAS with worsening hepatic hemodynamics and decreased rates of survival in patients with cirrhosis (reviewed by Wadei et al[573]). For this reason, ACE inhibitors and ARBs should be avoided in patients with cirrhosis and ascites.

Sympathetic Nervous System. Activation of the SNS is a common feature in patients with cirrhosis and ascites.[634] Circulating norepinephrine levels, as well as urinary excretion of catecholamines and their metabolites, are elevated in patients with cirrhosis and usually are correlated with the severity of the disease. Moreover, high levels of plasma norepinephrine in patients with decompensated cirrhosis are predictive of increased rate of mortality.[634] The source of the increase in norepinephrine levels is enhanced SNS activity, rather than reduced disposal, with nerve terminal spillover from the liver, heart, kidneys, muscle, and cutaneous innervation.[634,635] Elevated plasma norepinephrine levels were shown to be correlated closely with Na^+ and water retention in cirrhotic patients.[636] In addition, increased efferent renal sympathetic tone,[637] perhaps as a result of defective arterial and cardiopulmonary baroreflex control, was observed by direct recordings in experimental cirrhosis.[638] This scenario could explain why volume expansion fails to suppress the enhanced RSNA in cirrhosis.

Concomitantly with the increase in norepinephrine release, cardiovascular responsiveness to reflex autonomic stimulation may be impaired in patients with cirrhosis.[639] This impairment includes impeded vasoconstrictor responses to a variety of stimuli, such as mental arithmetic, LBNP, and the Valsalva maneuver. Such interference in the peripheral and central autonomic nervous system in cirrhosis could be explained partially by increased occupancy of endogenous catecholamine receptors, by downregulation of adrenergic receptors, or by a defect at the level of postreceptor signaling.[634] It is also possible that the excessive nitric oxide–dependent vasodilation found in cirrhosis could account for the vascular hyporesponsiveness. This assumption is supported by the finding that the hyporesponsiveness to pressor agents is not limited to norepinephrine but may also be observed in response to angiotensin II in patients and experimental animals.[590,640]

Metabolic derangements due to hepatic dysfunction, such as hypoglycemia and hyperinsulinemia, could also elicit sympathetic overactivity in cirrhosis.[634] Although hyperinsulinemia in cirrhotic models has been shown to stimulate Na^+ retention,[641] overt hypoglycemia is seldom observed in patients with compensated cirrhosis. Hypoxia may stimulate the SNS in patients with cirrhosis, as indicated by a negative correlation between circulating norepinephrine levels and arterial oxygen tension. Moreover, inhalation of oxygen significantly reduced circulating levels of norepinephrine, which suggests that a causal relationship exists between hypoxia and increased SNS activity in these patients.[634]

The increase in renal sympathetic tone and plasma norepinephrine levels could contribute to the antinatriuresis of cirrhosis by decreasing total RBF, or its intrarenal distribution, or by acting directly at the tubular epithelial level to enhance Na^+ reabsorption. In fact, patients with compensated cirrhosis may have decreased RBF even in the early stages, and as the disease progresses, RBF tends to decline further, concomitantly with the increase in sympathetic activity.[634] In this regard, activation of the SNS in cirrhotic patients was shown to be associated with a rightward and downward shift of the RBF/RPP autoregulatory curve in such a way that RBF became critically dependent on RPP. Moreover, this phenomenon was found to contribute to the development of the hepatorenal syndrome. Furthermore, insertion of a TIPS to reduce portal venous pressure in patients with hepatorenal syndrome leads to a fall in plasma norepinephrine levels and to an upward shift in the RBF/RPP curve.[642]

The centrality of SNS overactivity in cirrhosis was illustrated by the finding that in patients with cirrhosis and increased SNS activity, addition of clonidine to diuretic treatment induced an earlier diuretic response, with fewer diuretic requirements and complications.[643] In parallel with the increase in sympathetic activity, patients with progressive cirrhosis also showed an increase in the activities of the RAAS and AVP.[353,596] The marked neurohumoral activation that occurs at relatively advanced stages of cirrhosis probably represents a shift toward decompensation, characterized by a severe decrease in EABV and, perhaps, true volume depletion. A correlation also exists between plasma norepinephrine and AVP levels; thus, the increased activity of the SNS may stimulate the release of AVP.[596,636] In addition, a direct relationship exists between plasma norepinephrine and activity of the RAAS.

Together, the evidence suggests that the three pressor systems might be activated by the same mechanisms and operate in concert to counteract the low arterial blood pressure and decrease in EABV.[596,634]

Arginine Vasopressin. Patients and experimental animals with advanced hepatic cirrhosis frequently exhibit impaired renal water excretion as a result of nonosmotic release of AVP and, consequently, develop water retention with hyponatremia.[353,354,575,596] For example, cirrhotic patients who were unable to normally excrete a water load had high immunoreactive levels of AVP in comparison with cirrhotic patients who exhibited a normal response.[644] Affected patients also had higher plasma renin and aldosterone levels and lower urinary Na^+ excretion, which suggests that the inability to suppress vasopressin was secondary to a decrease in EABV.[644] In rats with experimental cirrhosis, plasma levels of AVP were elevated in association with overexpression of hypothalamic AVP messenger RNA, together with a diminished pituitary AVP content.[645] In addition, the expression of AQP2, the AVP-regulated water channel in the collecting duct, was significantly increased in rats with carbon tetrachloride (CCl_4)–induced cirrhosis. This finding was explained by increased AVP secretion, inasmuch as an AVP receptor antagonist significantly diminished AQP2 expression. It is, therefore, possible that upregulation of AQP2 plays an important role in water retention associated with hepatic cirrhosis, as well as in other pathologic states.[199]

As noted earlier in this chapter, AVP supports arterial blood pressure through its action on the V_1 receptors found on vascular smooth muscle cells, whereas the V_2 receptor is responsible for water transport in the collecting duct.[209] The availability of selective blockers of these receptors provided clear evidence for the dual roles of AVP in pathogenesis of cirrhosis.[208,646,647] Thus, the administration of a V_2 receptor antagonist to cirrhotic patients, as well as to rats with experimental cirrhosis, increased urine volume, decreased urine osmolality, and corrected hyponatremia.[430,647-650] Clinical applications of V_2 receptor antagonists are discussed in the

"Specific Treatments Based on the Pathophysiology of Congestive Heart Failure" section.

The V_1 receptor is important for the maintenance of arterial pressure and circulatory integrity, as shown in a rat model of cirrhosis and ascites.[651] After the actions of angiotensin II were blocked with saralasin, a selective V_1 receptor antagonist produced a pronounced fall in arterial blood pressure. These data serve to illustrate the effectiveness of selective V_2 receptor antagonists in the management of fluid retention in cirrhosis.

AVP also increases the synthesis of the vasodilatory PGE_2 and PGI_2 in several vascular beds, including the kidneys. This increase, in turn, may offset the vasoconstrictor action, as well as the hydroosmotic effect of AVP. In fact, urinary PGE_2 was found to be markedly increased in cirrhotic patients with positive free water clearance, despite an impaired ability to directly suppress AVP.[652,653] These data suggest that urinary diluting capacity is enhanced after a water load by increased synthesis of PGE_2 in the collecting duct.[652,653]

Endothelin. Plasma levels of immunoreactive endothelin are markedly elevated in patients with cirrhosis who have ascites and in the hepatorenal syndrome (see Angus[654] and references therein). However, the role of endothelin in the pathogenesis of the hemodynamic disturbances, fluid retention, and Na^+ retention in cirrhosis is still under debate. Although endothelins function as autocrine or paracrine agents by interacting with specific receptors at or near the site of synthesis, a fraction may spill over into the general circulation, in which it can have systemic effects. In fact, a number of studies have shown that there is a net hepatosplanchnic release of endothelins in cirrhosis that is correlated positively with portal venous pressure and cardiac output and inversely with central blood volume.[654,655] Increased local intrahepatic production of endothelin is also believed to contribute to the development of portal hypertension, probably through contraction of the stellate cells and a concomitant decrease in sinusoidal blood flow.[655]

In an attempt to provide further insight into the pathogenic significance of ET-1 in cirrhosis, Martinet and associates[656] measured ET-1 and its precursor, big ET-1, in the systemic circulation and in the splanchnic and renal venous beds of patients with cirrhosis and refractory ascites before and after TIPS insertion. They found that the blood levels of both peptides were higher in the vena cava, hepatic vein, portal vein, and renal vein of cirrhotic patients than in those of normal controls. One to 2 months after TIPS insertion, creatinine clearance and urinary Na^+ excretion increased, whereas ET-1 and big ET-1 levels were significantly reduced in portal and renal veins. The authors suggested that the hemodynamic changes occurring in patients with cirrhosis and refractory ascites could be related to local production of ET-1 by the splanchnic and renal vascular beds.

However, alteration in the status of other hormones (e.g., renin, aldosterone) after TIPS insertion might also contribute to these hemodynamic changes. An opposite effect—namely, an increase in plasma ET-1—was reported in response to acute temporary occlusion of TIPS by angioplasty balloon inflation, with a transient increase in portal venous pressure.[657] Interestingly, this was associated with a marked reduction of RPF and increased generation of ET-1 by the kidneys. Because the kidneys are uniquely sensitive to the vasoconstrictor effect of ET-1, ET-1 may play an important role in the pathogenesis of the hepatorenal syndrome.[655] This possibility is supported by the findings that the high plasma ET-1 levels in patients with the hepatorenal syndrome decreased within 1 week after successful orthotopic liver transplantation and that this decrease was accompanied by an improvement in renal function.[658]

The importance of the intrarenal endothelin system was demonstrated in a rat model of acute liver failure induced by galactosamine, in which renal failure also developed, despite normal renal histologic findings.[659] This situation reasonably mimics the hepatorenal syndrome in humans. Plasma concentrations of ET-1 were increased twofold after the onset of liver and renal failure, and the ET-A receptor was upregulated significantly in the renal cortex. Administration of bosentan, a nonselective endothelin receptor antagonist, prevented the development of renal failure when given before or 24 hours after the onset of liver injury.[659] Although it is possible that activation of the intrarenal endothelin system may play a role in the pathogenesis of the hepatorenal syndrome,[660] there is, so far, scant clinical evidence to support this view.

Apelin.   As mentioned earlier, apelin is the endogenous ligand of the angiotensin-like receptor 1, found to be involved in Na+ and water homeostasis and in regulation of cardiovascular tone and cardiac contractility, through a reciprocal relationship with angiotensin II and AVP (see Principe et al[316] and references therein). Because of these properties, apelin is potentially involved in the pathogenesis of advanced liver disease. Evidence for this hypothesis includes raised plasma apelin levels in patients and experimental animals with cirrhosis. In addition, an apelin receptor antagonist led to a reduction in the raised cardiac index, reversal of the increased total peripheral resistance, and improvement in Na+ and water excretion in rats with experimental cirrhosis.[316] These data raise the possibility for a therapeutic role of apelin antagonism in the management of severe hepatorenal syndrome. However, in view of the complex effects of apelin on glomerular hemodynamics, apelin antagonists should be used cautiously.

Vasodilators/Natriuretics
Natriuretic Peptides
Atrial Natriuretic Peptide.   Plasma levels of ANP are elevated in patients with cirrhosis, despite the reduction in effective circulating volume in late stages of the disease.[661,662] In the pre-ascitic stage of cirrhosis, the increase in plasma ANP may be important for the maintenance of Na+ homeostasis, but with progression of the disease, patients develop resistance to the natriuretic action of the peptide.[661,662] The high levels of ANP reflect mostly increased cardiac release rather than impaired clearance of the peptide.[663] The stimulus for increased cardiac ANP synthesis and release in cirrhosis has not been fully clarified. Overfilling of the circulation in early cirrhosis, secondary to intrahepatic hypertension–related renal Na+ retention, could trigger the increased plasma ANP concentrations at these early stages. In fact, increased left atrial size, in association with increased intravascular volume and plasma ANP concentration, has been reported in both ascitic and nonascitic alcoholic cirrhotic patients.[664]

Pre-ascitic patients also had significantly elevated circulating blood volumes with higher left and right pulmonary volumes, despite having normal blood pressure and normal renin, aldosterone, and norepinephrine levels.[665] High Na+ intake over a 5-week period in pre-ascitic patients resulted in weight gain and positive Na+ balance for 3 weeks, followed by a return to normal Na+ balance thereafter. Interestingly, the RAAS and SNS were suppressed, whereas ANP levels were elevated. Thus, despite continued high Na+ intake, pre-ascitic patients reach a new steady state of Na+ balance, thereby preventing fluid retention and the development of ascites. These findings also suggest that ANP plays an important role in preventing the transition from the pre-ascitic stage to ascites in these patients.[666] The factors responsible for maintaining relatively high levels of ANP during the later stages of cirrhosis, in association with arterial underfilling, also have not been determined. However, ANP levels do not increase further as patients proceed from early compensated to late decompensated stages of cirrhosis.

As pointed out earlier, with progression of the disease, many patients with cirrhosis and ascites lose the ability to respond normally to exogenous administration of ANP or to the high endogenous levels of the peptide.[661,662] The potential basis for this apparent resistance to ANP was extensively investigated by Skorecki and colleagues.[667] For example, in a series of patients with cirrhosis, they showed that HWI led to an increase in ANP and plasma and urinary cGMP, the second messenger for ANP in all subjects. However, not all subjects responded with a natriuresis. No difference in the cGMP response was observed between those who developed natriuresis (responders) and those who did not (nonresponders). In addition, nonresponders also tended to have more severe and advanced disease.[668,669] These findings suggest that the interference with the natriuretic action of ANP occurs at a stage of cellular signaling beyond cGMP production and that ANP receptors in the collecting duct are not defective.

A number of experimental interventions were shown to ameliorate ANP resistance in cirrhosis. These interventions included infusion of endopeptidase inhibitors, bradykinin, kininase II inhibitors, and mannitol; renal sympathetic denervation; peritoneovenous shunting; and orthotopic liver transplantation.[670-675] The results of these and other studies suggested that antinatriuretic factors, especially the SNS and RAAS, counterbalance and overcome the natriuretic effect of ANP in later stages of cirrhosis.[669] As discussed previously, excessive activation of the SNS in cirrhosis, characterized by increased circulating norepinephrine and efferent RNSA, may lead to a decrease in RPF and excessive proximal reabsorption of Na+. In fact, renal denervation was found to reverse the blunted diuretic and natriuretic responses to ANP in cirrhotic rats.[675]

With regard to the RAAS, overactivation of the system and failure to suppress the RAAS with HWI or ANP infusion was clearly associated with resistance to the natriuretic effects of ANP.[667] Furthermore, infusion of angiotensin II mimicked the nonresponder state by causing patients in the early stages of cirrhosis who still responded to ANP to become unresponsive[676] (Figure 14-10). This effect of angiotensin II infusion was reversible and occurred at both proximal (decreased distal delivery of Na+) and distal nephron sites to abrogate ANP-induced natriuresis. The importance of distal Na+ delivery was further confirmed in other studies, which showed that the administration of mannitol to increase distal delivery (as measured by lithium clearance) resulted in an improved natriuretic response to ANP in responders but not in nonresponders.[672,677]

All the available evidence indicates that ANP resistance is best explained by an effect of decreased delivery of Na+ to ANP-responsive distal nephron sites (glomerulotubular imbalance caused by abnormal systemic hemodynamics and

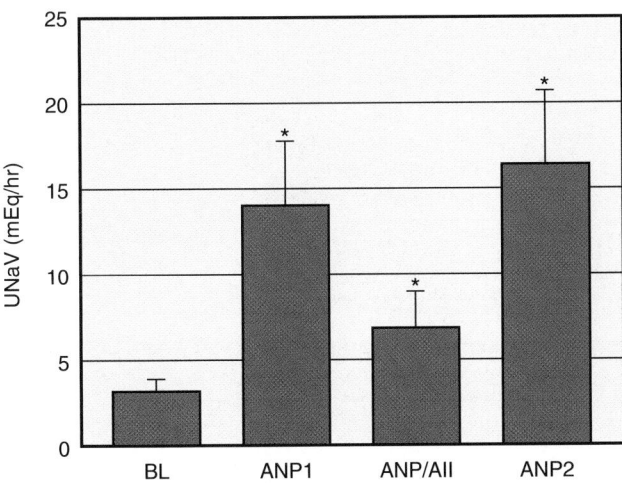

FIGURE 14-10 Effect of antiotensin II (AII) infusion in atrial natriuretic peptide (ANP)–induced natriuresis. Sodium excretion during the four experimental protocols is depicted. Response was defined by natriuresis greater than 0.83 mmol/hr (20 mmol/day). Note that urinary sodium excretion dropped to almost baseline levels with combined ANP/angiotensin II infusion and returned to ANP levels when angiotensin II was discontinued. *$P < 0.05$ from previous phase of experiment. ANP/AII, infusion of ANP and angiotensin II combined; ANP1, ANP infusion alone; ANP2, ANP alone; BL, baseline. (Adapted from Tobe SW, Blendis LM, Morali GA, et al: Angiotensin II modulates ANP induced natriuresis in cirrhosis with ascites, *Am J Kidney Dis* 21:472-479, 1993.)

activation of the RAAS) combined with an effective antinatriuretic factor's overcoming the natriuretic action of ANP at its site of action in the medullary collecting tubule.[669] The latter effect could result from decreased delivery or may be an effect of permissive cofactors such as prostaglandins and kinins. An overall formulation for the role of ANP in cirrhosis and the interrelationship of the peptide with antinatriuretic influences are summarized at the end of this section and in Figure 14-11.
Brain Natriuretic Peptide and C-Type Natriuretic Peptide. BNP levels have also been found to be elevated in patients with cirrhosis and ascites and, like that of ANP, its natriuretic effect is also blunted in cirrhotic patients with Na+ retention and ascites.[678-680] Plasma BNP levels may be correlated with cardiac dysfunction[680,681] and with severity of disease and may be of prognostic value in the progression of cirrhosis.[679,680,682] Plasma CNP levels in cirrhotic pre-ascitic patients, although not elevated in comparison to healthy controls, were found to be directly correlated with 24-hour natriuresis and urine volume[683] and inversely correlated with arterial compliance but not with systemic vascular resistance.[684] These data suggested that compensatory downregulation of CNP occurs in cirrhosis when vasodilation persists and that regulation of large and small arteries by CNP may differ.

In contrast to the pre-ascitic stage, patients with more advanced disease and impaired renal function had lower plasma and higher urinary CNP levels than did those with intact renal function. Moreover, urinary CNP was correlated inversely with urinary Na+ excretion. In patients with refractory ascites or hepatorenal syndrome treated with terlipressin infusion or TIPS (see "Specific Treatments Based on the Pathophysiology of Sodium Retention in Cirrhosis" section), urinary CNP declined and urinary Na+ excretion increased 1 week later.[685] Thus, CNP may have a significant role in renal Na+ handling in cirrhosis.

Finally, *Dendroapsis* natriuretic peptide levels were found to be increased in cirrhotic patients with ascites, but not in those without, and levels were correlated with disease severity.[686] The significance of these findings remains unknown.
Prostaglandins. As noted previously, prostaglandins make important contributions to the modulation of the hydro-osmotic effect of AVP and to the protection of RPF and GFR when activity of endogenous vasoconstrictor systems is increased. These properties of prostaglandins appear to be critical in patients with decompensated cirrhosis who have ascites but not renal failure. Such patients excrete greater amounts of vasodilatory prostaglandins than do healthy subjects, which suggests that renal production of prostaglandins is increased.[225,687] Likewise, in experimental models of cirrhosis, there is evidence for increased synthesis and activity of renal and vascular prostaglandins.[687,688] Conversely, it is not surprising that administration of agents that inhibit prostaglandin synthesis results in a clinically important deterioration of renal function in these patients. In fact, administration of nonselective cyclooxygenase inhibitors, such as the NSAIDs indomethacin and ibuprofen, resulted in a significant decrement in GFR and RPF in patients with cirrhosis and ascites, in contrast to healthy subjects. The decrement in renal hemodynamics varied directly with the degree of Na+ retention and neurohumoral activation, so that patients with high plasma renin and norepinephrine levels were particularly sensitive to these adverse effects.[687,689] However, the deleterious effects of NSAIDs on renal function were also observed in cirrhotic patients without ascites.[225,690-692]

As in other situations associated with decreased EABV, the COX-2 isoform was strongly upregulated in kidneys from rats with experimental cirrhosis with ascites. Nevertheless, the negative effects of prostaglandin inhibition on renal function appear to be solely COX-1 dependent, because studies in both in human and experimental cirrhosis with ascites showed that administration of selective COX-2 antagonists spared renal function, whereas nonselective cyclooxygenase inhibition led to a fall in GFR.[687,691,693] In these studies, in both patients and experimental animals, administration of the selective COX-2 inhibitor was carried out on a short-term basis. Additional long-term studies are required in order to establish the safety of these drugs in patients with advanced cirrhosis.

In contrast to nonazotemic patients with cirrhosis and ascites, it has been suggested that patients with hepatorenal syndrome have reduced renal synthesis of vasodilatory prostaglandins.[694] This situation would exacerbate renal vasoconstriction and Na+ and fluid retention and may be an important factor in the pathogenesis of hepatorenal syndrome.[687] However, an attempt to improve renal function in these patients by treatment with intravenous infusion of PGE₂ or its oral analog, misoprostol, was unsuccessful.[695]

An Integrated View of the Pathogenesis of Sodium Retention in Cirrhosis

Two general explanations for Na+ retention that complicates cirrhosis have been offered. According to the overflow mechanism of ascites formation in cirrhosis, a volume-independent stimulus is responsible for renal Na+ retention. Possible mediators include adrenergic reflexes activated by hepatic sinusoidal hypertension and increased systemic concentrations of an unidentified antinatriuretic factor as a result of impaired liver

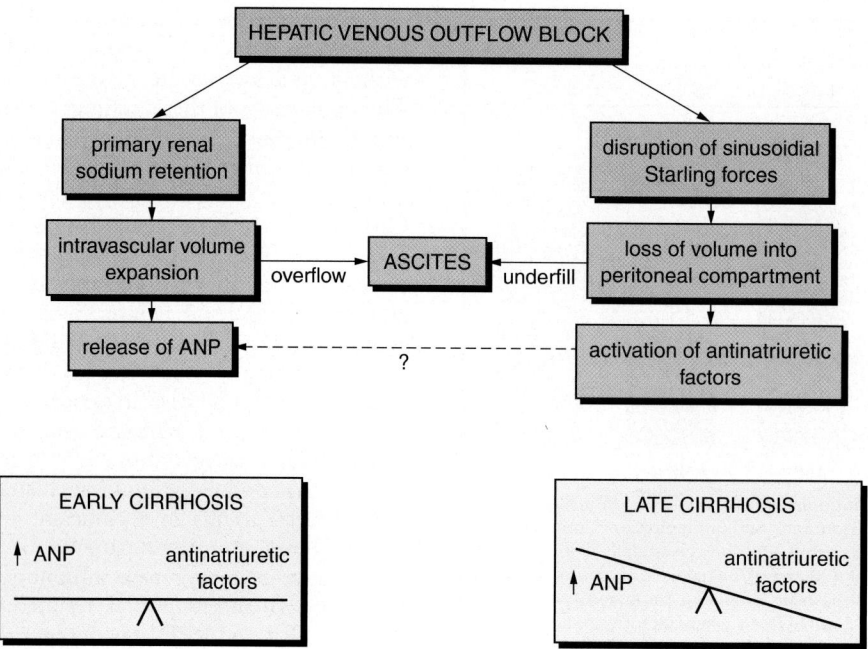

FIGURE 14-11 Working formulation for the role of atrial natriuretic peptide (ANP) in the renal sodium retention of cirrhosis. The primary hepatic abnormality for renal Na$^+$ retention is blockade of hepatic venous outflow. In early disease, this signals renal Na$^+$ retention with consequent intravascular volume expansion and a compensatory rise in plasma ANP. The rise in ANP is sufficient to counterbalance the primary antinatriuretic influences, but the expanded intravascular volume provides the potential for overflow ascites. With progression of disease, intrasinusoidal Starling forces are disrupted, volume is lost from the vascular compartment into the peritoneal compartment. This underfilling of the circulation may attenuate further increases in ANP levels and promote the activation of antinatriuretic factors. Whether the antinatriuretic factors activated by underfilling are the same as or different from those promoting primary renal Na$^+$ retention in early disease remains to be determined. At this later stage of disease, increased levels of ANP may not be sufficient to counterbalance antinatriuretic forces. (From Warner LC, Leung WM, Campbell P, et al: The role of resistance to atrial natriuretic peptide in the pathogenesis of sodium retention in hepatic cirrhosis, in Brenner BM, Laragh JH [editors]: *Advances in atrial peptide research,* vol 3 of *American Society of Hypertension series,* New York, 1989, Raven Press, pp 185-204.)

metabolism. According to the underfilling theory, in contrast, EABV depletion is responsible for renal Na$^+$ retention. The peripheral arterial vasodilation hypothesis is that reduced systemic vascular resistance lowers blood pressure and activates arterial baroreceptors, initiating Na$^+$ retention. The retained fluid extravasates from the hypertensive splanchnic circulation, preventing arterial repletion, and Na$^+$ retention and ascites formation continue.

It is quite obvious that neither the underfilling nor the overflow theory can account exclusively for all the observed derangements in volume regulation in cirrhosis. Rather, elements of the two concepts may occur simultaneously or sequentially in cirrhotic patients (see Figure 14-11). Thus, there is sufficient evidence that, early in cirrhosis, intrahepatic hypertension caused by hepatic venous outflow obstruction signals primary renal Na$^+$ retention, with consequent intravascular volume expansion. Whether underfilling of the arterial circuit is also a consequence of vasodilation at this stage remains to be determined. Because of expansion of the intrathoracic venous compartment at this stage, plasma ANP levels rise. This rise is sufficient to counterbalance the renal Na$^+$ retaining forces, but at the expense of an expanded intravascular volume, with the potential for overflow ascites. The propensity for the accumulation of volume in the peritoneal compartment and the splanchnic bed results from altered intrahepatic hemodynamics. With progression of disease, intrasinusoidal Starling forces are disrupted, and volume is lost from the vascular compartment into the peritoneal compartment. These events, coupled with other factors such as portosystemic shunting,

hypoalbuminemia, and vascular refractoriness to pressor hormones, lead to underfilling of the arterial circuit, without measurably affecting the venous compartment.

This arterial underfilling may attenuate further increases in ANP levels and promote the activation of antinatriuretic factors. Whether these antinatriuretic factors activated by underfilling are the same as, or different from, those that promote primary renal Na$^+$ retention in early disease remains to be determined. At this later stage of disease, elevated levels of ANP may not be sufficient to counterbalance antinatriuretic influences. In early cirrhosis, salt retention is isotonic, and so normonatremia is maintained. However, with advancing cirrhosis, defective water excretion supervenes, resulting in hyponatremia, which reflects combined ECF and ICF space expansion. The impaired water excretion and hyponatremia in cirrhotic patients with ascites is a marker of the severity of the hemodynamic abnormalities that initiate Na$^+$ retention and eventuate in the hepatorenal syndrome. The pathogenesis is related primarily to nonosmotic stimuli for release of vasopressin acting together with additional factors such as impaired distal Na$^+$ delivery.

Clinical Manifestations of Hypervolemia

Apart from the clinical manifestations of the underlying disease, the symptoms and signs of hypervolemia per se also depend on the amount and relative distribution of the fluid between the intravascular (arterial and venous) and interstitial space. Arterial volume overload is manifested as hypertension, whereas venous overload is manifested as raised jugular venous pressure. Interstitial fluid accumulation appears as peripheral edema, effusions in the pleural or peritoneal cavity (ascites) or in the alveolar space (pulmonary edema), or combinations of these manifestations. If cardiac and hepatic functions are normal and transcapillary Starling forces are intact, the excess volume is distributed proportionately throughout the ECF compartments. In this situation, the earliest sign of hypervolemia is hypertension, followed by peripheral edema and raised jugular venous pressure. Peripheral edema appears only when the interstitial volume overload exceeds 3 L and, because plasma volume itself is approximately 3 L, the presence of edema indicates substantial hypervolemia with prior or ongoing renal Na^+ retention.

When cardiac systolic function is impaired, as a result of myocardial, valvular, or pericardial disease, pulmonary and systemic venous hypertension predominate, and systemic blood pressure may be low as a result of disproportionate fluid accumulation in the venous rather than the arterial circulation. Disruption in transcapillary Starling forces, as found in both advanced cardiac and hepatic disease, may lead to fluid transudation into the pleural and peritoneal spaces, manifested as pleural effusions and ascites, respectively.

As already mentioned, the constellation of advanced liver cirrhosis or fulminant hepatic failure, ascites and oliguric renal failure in the absence of significant renal histopathologic disease is the hepatorenal syndrome. Two subtypes have been defined: type 1 is characterized by a rapid decline in renal function (doubling of serum creatinine level to >2.5 mg/dL or 50% reduction in creatinine clearance to <20 mL/min) over a 2-week period. Typically, an acute precipitating factor can be identified. Type 2 develops spontaneously and progressively over months (serum creatinine level >1.5 mg/dL or creatinine clearance <40 mL/min). Hepatorenal syndrome is discussed in detail in Chapter 30

Diagnosis

The diagnosis of hypervolemia is usually evident from the clinical history and physical examination. Any combination of peripheral edema, raised jugular venous pressure, pulmonary crepitations, and pleural effusions is likely to be diagnostic for hypervolemia. In the presence of these findings, the systemic blood pressure is crucial for distinguishing primary renal Na^+ retention from secondary Na^+ retention caused by reduced EABV. For example, in advanced primary renal failure, the blood pressure is high, whereas in severe congestive heart failure or advanced hepatic cirrhosis, blood pressure is likely to be relatively low. In more enigmatic cases, in which dyspnea is the sole complaint and clinical findings are minimal, measurement of plasma BNP or proBNP may help to distinguish between cardiac and pulmonary causes of the dyspnea.[478]

Simple laboratory tests may aid in confirming the clinical diagnosis. Elevated cardiac troponin level is consistent with, although not diagnostic of, myocardial damage.[696,697] Transaminase levels may be raised in hepatic disease, and hypoalbuminemia would be consistent with either hepatic cirrhosis or nephrotic-range proteinuria caused by glomerular disease. The latter, of course, would be confirmed by appropriate urine testing.

When blood pressure is low, evidence of prerenal azotemia (increased ratio of blood urea nitrogen to creatinine) may

be found, and in advanced cardiac or hepatic failure (the so-called cardiorenal and hepatorenal syndromes), intrinsic renal failure—proportionate increases in blood urea nitrogen and creatinine—may occur (see Chapter 30 for detailed discussion). In the urine, low EABV in the presence of hypervolemia is confirmed by low Na^+ concentration or low fractional excretion of Na^+, indicative of secondary renal Na^+ retention.

Treatment

Therapy for volume overload can be divided broadly into management of the volume overload itself and prevention or minimization of its occurrence and the associated morbidity and mortality. Clearly, recognition and treatment of the underlying disease causing hypervolemia is the critical first step. Thus, when EABV is significantly reduced, as in cardiac and hepatic failure, as well as in severe nephrotic syndrome, hemodynamic parameters should be optimized. Otherwise, therapy to induce negative Na^+ balance is associated with enhanced risk for worsening hemodynamic compromise.

Once the EABV is adjusted, three basic strategies can be used to induce negative Na^+ balance: dietary Na^+ restriction, diuretics, and extracorporeal ultrafiltration. The degree of hypervolemia and the clinical urgency for Na^+ removal determine which modality should be used. Therefore, in a patient with life-threatening pulmonary edema, immediate intravenous loop diuretics are indicated; if high doses of these drugs do not induce significant diuresis, then extracorporeal ultrafiltration may be life-saving. At the other extreme, a hypertensive patient with mild volume overload and preserved renal function may require only dietary salt restriction and a thiazide diuretic.

Once the acute stage of hypervolemia has been controlled, therapy must be directed toward the prevention or minimization of further acute episodes and improvement in overall prognosis. In addition to maintenance diuretic treatment, several strategies, based on the pathophysiologic process of Na^+ retention, are available clinically or are under experimental development.

SODIUM RESTRICTION

Effective management of hypervolemia of any cause must include Na^+ restriction. Without this intervention, the success of diuretic therapy is limited because the relative hypovolemia induced by diuretics leads to compensatory Na^+ retention and the potential creation of a vicious cycle consisting of increased diuretic dosage, further reduction in EABV, and yet greater renal Na^+ retention. A reasonable goal is to restrict Na^+ intake to 50 to 80 mmol (approximately 3 to 5 g of salt) per day. Because of the generally poor palatability of salt-restricted diets, salt substitutes may be used; however, because these preparations usually contain high concentrations of potassium, they must be used with caution by patients with renal impairment or those taking potassium-retaining drugs such as ACE inhibitors, ARBs, or aldosterone antagonists.

In hospitalized patients, extra attention must be paid to amounts and types of intravenous fluids administered. A frequent phenomenon encountered by nephrologists called for consultation in internal medicine departments is the scenario in which a patient is receiving intravenous saline together with high-dose diuretics. The usual rationale offered for this combination is that the saline will expand the intravascular volume and the diuretic will mobilize the excess interstitial volume. This logic has no sound physiologic or therapeutic basis, inasmuch as both modalities operate principally on the intravascular space. Furthermore, water restriction is also inappropriate except in the presence of accompanying hyponatremia (plasma Na^+ <135 mmol/L). In stark contrast to these recommendations, one research group has shown that intravenously infusing small volumes of hypertonic saline during diuretic dosing and liberalizing dietary salt intake while continuing to limit water consumption resulted in improved fluid removal in patients with CHF. Furthermore, less deterioration in renal function, shorter hospitalizations, reduced readmission rates, and even reductions in mortality were observed.[698,699] These novel findings stimulated the design of another clinical trial (Concentrated Saline Infusions and Increased Dietary Sodium with Diuretics for Heart Failure with Kidney Dysfunction; ClinicalTrials.gov Identifier: NCT00575484) in which the effects of this highly unconventional combination for the treatment of heart failure were examined in patients with renal dysfunction. This study was terminated in July 2010 and the results are eagerly anticipated.

Diuretics

Diuretics are classified according to their sites of action along the nephron and are discussed in detail in Chapter 50. They are described briefly here in relation to the treatment of hypervolemia.

Proximal Tubule Diuretics. The prototype of a proximal tubular diuretic is acetazolamide, a carbonic anhydrase inhibitor that inhibits proximal reabsorption of sodium bicarbonate. Prolonged use may cause hyperchloremic metabolic acidosis. This drug is more typically used in the management of chronic glaucoma rather than for reducing volume overload. Another proximally acting diuretic is metolazone, which, as a member of the thiazide class of diuretics, also inhibits the NaCl cotransporter in the distal tubule. The proximal action of metolazone may be associated with phosphate loss greater than that seen with traditional thiazides.[700] In general, metolazone is used as an adjunct to loop diuretics in resistant heart failure.[701] Mannitol also inhibits proximal tubular reabsorption,[702] but it is used mainly to reduce increased intracranial pressure.

Loop Diuretics. This group comprises the most powerful diuretics and includes furosemide, bumetanide, torsemide, and ethacrynic acid. Their mode of action is to inhibit transport via the $NKCC_2$ in the apical membrane of the thick ascending limb of the loop of Henle,[703] which is responsible for the reabsorption of about 25% of filtered Na^+ (see Chapter 5). They are used for the treatment of both severe hypervolemia and hypertension, especially in stages 4 and 5 of chronic kidney disease. Because of their powerful action, loop diuretics may lead to hypokalemia, intravascular volume depletion, and worsening prerenal azotemia, especially in elderly patients and in patients with reduced EABV.

Distal Tubule Diuretics. Diuretics that operate in this segment operate by blockade of the apical NaCl cotransporter. The group consists of hydrochlorothiazide, chlorthalidone, and metolazone (see earlier "Proximal Tubule Diuretics" section). They are typically used as first-line treatment of hypertension and also, particularly metolazone, as adjuncts to loop diuretics in resistant heart failure. Thiazides are also useful for reducing hypercalciuria in recurrent nephrolithiasis,[704] in

contrast to loop diuretics that are hypercalciuric.[705] Inhibition of Na^+ reabsorption by diuretics that work in the proximal tubule (except for carbonic anhydrase inhibitors), loop of Henle, and distal tubule leads to increased solute delivery to the collecting duct. Consequently, rates of potassium and proton secretion are accelerated, which may lead to hypokalemia and metabolic alkalosis.[703]

Collecting Duct Diuretics. Collecting duct (K^+-sparing) diuretics operate either by competing with aldosterone for occupation of the mineralocorticoid receptor[409] or by direct inhibition of the ENaC (amiloride and triamterene). As their alternative name implies, important side effects of this group are hyperkalemia and metabolic acidosis, which result from concomitant suppression of K^+ and proton secretion. Therefore, they are widely used in combination with both thiazide and loop diuretics to minimize hypokalemia. The aldosterone antagonists are especially useful in the management of disorders characterized by secondary hyperaldosteronism, such as cirrhosis with ascites. Moreover, aldosterone antagonists have been shown to have cardioprotective and renoprotective effects, through nonepithelial mineralocorticoid receptor blockade (see "Pathophysiology" and "Specific Treatments Based on the Pathophysiology of Congestive Heart Failure" sections in this chapter; also see Chapter 61).

Other Diuretic Agents. Natiuretic peptides are discussed in the "Specific Treatments Based on the Pathophysiology of Congestive Heart Failure" section. Patients with cirrhosis and ascites, who typically have little Na^+ in their urine, may have a natriuretic response to HWI as a result of effective volume depletion (see earlier "Underfilling Hypothesis" section), despite elevated plasma volume and cardiac output.[667] This modality has not been used outside the research setting.

Diuretic Resistance. As already mentioned, when Na^+ retention is severe and resistant to conventional doses of loop diuretics, combinations of diuretics acting at different nephron sites may produce effective natriuresis. Another method for overcoming diuretic resistance is the administration of a bolus dose of loop diuretic to yield a high plasma level, followed by high-dose continuous infusion. Alternately, high doses given intermittently may be successful in reversing diuretic resistance.

Whichever method is used to treat diuretic resistant hypervolemia, it is important to monitor carefully plasma Na^+, K^+, Mg^{2+}, Ca^{2+}, phosphate, blood urea nitrogen, and creatinine levels and correct any deviations appropriately. Other less common side effects of diuretics include cutaneous allergic reactions, acute interstitial nephritis (see Chapter 35), pancreatitis and rarely, blood dyscrasias.[706]

Extracorporeal Ultrafiltration

On occasion, extreme resistance to diuretics occurs, often accompanied by renal functional impairment. In such cases, removal of volume excess may be achieved by ultrafiltration through the use of hemofiltration, hemodialysis, or peritoneal dialysis (see Chapters 64 to 66). Chronic ambulatory peritoneal dialysis may yield symptomatic relief from pulmonary edema and anasarca in patients with resistant congestive cardiac failure, who are not candidates for surgical intervention.[707] The effect of these therapies on prognosis remains unproven.[708,709]

Specific Treatments Based on the Pathophysiology of Congestive Heart Failure

Because the clinical situation of a patient with CHF at any given time depends on the delicate balance between vasoconstrictor/antinatriuretic and vasodilator/natriuretic factors, any treatment that can tip the balance in favor of the latter should be efficacious. Thus, either increasing the activity of the natriuretic peptides or reducing the influence of the antinatriuretic mechanisms by pharmacologic means may achieve a shift in the balance in favor of Na$^+$ excretion in CHF. In the interplay between the RAAS and ANP in CHF, the approaches used in experimental studies and in clinical practice included reducing the activity of the RAAS by means of ACE inhibitors or ARBs, increasing the activity of ANP or its second messenger, cGMP, or combinations of approaches.

Inhibition of Renin-Angiotensin-Aldosterone System

The maladaptive actions of locally produced or circulatory angiotensin II have been examined in numerous studies, which have shown unequivocally that ACE inhibition and angiotensin receptor blockade improve renal function, cardiac performance, and life expectancy of patients with CHF.[710-712] In the few studies in which renal functional deterioration was observed, the blockade of angiotensin II–induced preferential efferent arteriolar constriction probably led to a sharp fall in glomerular capillary pressure and, hence, in GFR.[382] Because patients with CHF cannot overcome the Na$^+$-retaining action of aldosterone and continue to retain Na$^+$ in response to aldosterone, blockade of the latter by spironolactone induces substantial natriuresis in these patients.[393]

Overall, the effect of angiotensin II receptor blockade or ACE inhibition on renal function in CHF depends on a multiplicity of interacting factors. On the one hand, RBF may improve as a result of lower efferent arteriolar resistance. Systemic vasodilation may be associated with a rise in cardiac output. Under such circumstances, reversal of hemodynamically mediated effects of angiotensin II on Na$^+$ reabsorption would promote natriuresis. Moreover, inhibition of the RAAS could theoretically facilitate the action of natriuretic peptides to improve GFR and enhance Na$^+$ excretion. On the other hand, the aim of angiotensin II–induced elevation of the single-nephron filtration fraction is to preserve GFR in the presence of diminished RPF. In patients with precarious renal hemodynamics, a fall in systemic arterial pressure below the autoregulatory range combined with removal of the angiotensin II effect on glomerular hemodynamics may cause severe deterioration of renal function. The net result depends on the integrated sum of these physiologic effects, which, in turn, depends on the severity and stage of heart disease (see Table 14-5).

In addition, the other active component of the RAAS, aldosterone, plays a pivotal role in the pathogenesis of CHF by promoting Na$^+$ retention and contributing to vascular and cardiac remodeling by inducing perivascular and interstitial fibrosis.[713] In accordance with this notion, two clinical trials have shown that the addition of small doses of aldosterone inhibitors to standard therapy substantially reduces the mortality rate and the degree of morbidity in CHF patients. The Randomized Aldactone Evaluation Study (RALES) showed that therapy with spironolactone reduced overall mortality among patients with advanced CHF by 30% in comparison with placebo.[410] In addition, the study of eplerenone in patients with heart failure caused by systolic dysfunction, Eplerenone Post-AMI Heart Failure Efficacy and Survival Study (EPHESUS), showed that addition of eplerenone to optimal medical therapy reduced morbidity and mortality among patients with acute myocardial infarction complicated by left ventricular dysfunction and CHF.[409] Aldosterone inhibitors are now routinely used in the management of CHF. Caution is, of course required in the presence of renal dysfunction, because of the significant risk of hperkalemia.[714]

β-Blockade

Insofar as β-blockade is now standard of care in the management of CHF, this review would not be complete without mention of this class of drugs. However, because their effect in CHF is not directly related to Na$^+$ and water, this important therapy is not elaborated further in this chapter. The reader is referred to recent cardiology texts (e.g., Dickstein et al[712]).

Nitric Oxide Donor and Reactive Oxygen Species/Peroxynitrite Scavengers

Because nitric oxide signaling is disrupted in CHF, achieving nitric oxide balance by either nitric oxide donors or selective NOS inhibitors has emerged as an important therapeutic concept in addressing and correcting the pathophysiologic process of CHF.[528] In this regard, the beneficial effects of combined isosorbide dinitrate (nitric oxide donor)/hydralazine (reactive oxygen species and peroxynitrite scavenger) therapy, particularly in African-American patients, are noteworthy.[715,716] However, the question still remains as to the efficacy of this combination in other ethnic groups.[715]

Endothelin Antagonists

Initial clinical studies showed that acute endothelin antagonism by bosentan decreased vascular resistance and increased cardiac index and cardiac output in patients with CHF, which suggested that ET-1 played a role in the pathogenesis of CHF by increasing systemic vascular resistance.[717] However, in contrast to early studies, more recent comprehensive clinical trials demonstrated, at best, no benefits or, at worst, increased hepatic transaminase levels and mortality rate in patients with CHF that was treated with ET-A receptor antagonists (see Ertl and Bauersachs[443] and references therein). These disappointing results may be explained by the observation that ET-A receptor antagonism in experimental CHF further activates the RAAS in association with sustained Na$^+$ retention.[718] In summary, the increased local cardiac-pulmonary-renal production of ET-1 in CHF, together with the marked vasoconstrictor and mitogenic properties of the molecule, suggests that ET-1 contributes directly and indirectly to the enhanced Na$^+$ retention and edema formation by aggravating renal and cardiac functions, respectively.[444,719] However, the fact that ET-1 receptor antagonists were ineffective in clinical trials and that they led to secondary activation of the RAAS in animals indicates that these drugs are unlikely to be of significant benefit in the management of CHF.

Natriuretic Peptides

As noted previously, circulating levels of natriuretic peptides are elevated in CHF in proportion to the severity of the disease. However, the renal actions of these peptides are attenuated and even blunted in severe CHF. Nevertheless, several studies demonstrated that elimination of natriuretic peptide action through the use of blockers of NPR-A or surgical removal of the atrium disrupts renal function and cardiac performance in experimental CHF.[462,466] Therefore, increasing circulating levels of natriuretic peptides by the administration of exogenous synthetic peptides was tested in both clinical and experimental CHF and appeared to be beneficial under certain circumstances. For example, intravenous administration of ANP to patients with acute CHF improved their clinical status.[720] Similarly, injection of BNP reduced pulmonary arterial pressure, pulmonary capillary wedge pressure, right atrial pressure, systemic vascular resistance, and systemic blood pressure, in association with increased cardiac output and diuresis.[721,722] The hemodynamic and natriuretic effects of exogenous BNP administration were significantly greater than those obtained after similar doses of ANP in patients with CHF.

Suppressed plasma levels of norepinephrine and aldosterone have also been observed. In view of its beneficial effects, BNP (nesiritide) was approved for the treatment of acute decompensated CHF in the United States in 2001. However, more recent controlled studies have shown that, overall, the natriuretic effects of nesiritide are minimal in comparison with placebo. Moreover, up to one third of patients do not exhibit increased Na^+ excretion after BNP infusion, a phenomenon also observed with ANP.[723] A further limitation of nesiritide treatment is dose-related hypotension,[722] which would be enhanced if nesiritide were given with other vasodilators, such as ACE inhibitors.[494] Also, nesiritide leads to worsening renal function in more than 20% of patients, which could increase the risk of death, as occurs in other situations complicated by renal impairment.[723] Therefore, the role of BNP in the management of CHF is currently unclear, and further investigation is required.[724,725]

Neutral Endopeptidase Inhibitors and Vasopeptidase Inhibitors

Correcting the imbalance between the RAAS and the natriuretic peptide systems could also be achieved by inhibiting the enzymatic degradation of ANP by NEP or blocking CNP. Several specific and differently structured NEP inhibitors were developed and tested in experimental models and clinical trials. Most studies revealed enhanced plasma ANP and BNP levels in association with vasodilation, natriuresis, diuresis, and, subsequently, reduced cardiac preload and afterload.[726] Because NEP degrades other peptides (e.g., kinins), the latter may also be involved in the beneficial effects of NEP inhibitors. Candoxatril, the first NEP inhibitor released for clinical trials, produced favorable hemodynamic and neurohormonal effects in patients with CHF.[727,728] In addition, acute NEP inhibition in mild CHF resulted in marked increases in RPF and Na^+ excretion, which exceeded the increase observed either in control animals or in severe CHF; thus, NEP inhibition has a potential therapeutic role in enhancing renal function in mild CHF.[729]

In later studies of CHF, apparently the more marked activation of the RAAS served to attenuate the beneficial renal and hemodynamic actions of NEP inhibitors; thus, mechanisms other than exaggerated NEP activity were thought to be involved in the renal resistance to natriuretic peptides. Moreover, NEP inhibitors did not reduce afterload. On the basis of the foregoing findings, investigators predicted that a combination of RAAS and NEP inhibitors would be more effective than each treatment alone. This was indeed confirmed in dogs with pacing-induced CHF, in which NEP inhibition prevented the ACE inhibitor–induced decrease in GFR.[730] These findings led to the development of dual NEP and ACE inhibitors, known as vasopeptidase inhibitors.[727,731,732]

Of the various vasopeptidase inhibitors, omapatrilat has been the most studied. In fact, results in both experimental and clinical CHF suggested beneficial hemodynamic and renal effects mediated by the synergistic ACE and NEP inhibition offered by this drug.[733-737] This was thought to be a potential advantage because renal function frequently deteriorates during the progression of chronic CHF, and renal impairment is one of the most powerful prognostic indicators in patients with CHF.[391] However, as the results of definitive clinical trials emerged, it became evident that neither vasopeptidase inhibitors nor NEP inhibitors as add-on therapy to ACE inhibitors were more effective than ACE inhibitors alone in the treatment of CHF (reviewed by Iyengar and Abraham[738]). Furthermore, the combination was associated with more side effects, especially angioedema. Possible reasons for their failure include disproportionate increase in RAAS and endothelin activity over time, the development of tolerance to NEP inhibitors with chronic treatment, and downregulation of natriuretic peptide receptors in response to degradation of NEP inhibitors. A potential explanation for the angioedema that appears with the combination is an excessive accumulation of bradykinin that results from both ACE and NEP inhibition.[738]

Despite the failure of omapatrilat to live up to its initial promise, the evaluation of vasopeptidase inhibitors has greatly increased the understanding of the neurohumoral mechanisms involved in the pathogenesis of CHF.

Vasopressin Receptor Antagonists

The development of AVP receptor antagonists, known collectively as *vaptans*, has dramatically increased the understanding of the contribution of AVP to the alterations in renal and cardiac function.[739] and opened the way for their therapeutic use in CHF. Vaptans are small, orally active, nonpeptide molecules that lack agonist effects and display high affinity for and specificity to their corresponding receptors.[740] Highly selective and potent antagonists for the V_{1A}, V_2, and V_{1B} receptor subtypes and mixed V_{1A}/V_2 receptor antagonists are now available.[208] Vaptans have been clearly shown to produce hemodynamic improvement with transient decrease in systemic vascular resistance, increased cardiac output, and improved water diuresis in both experimental models of CHF and clinical trials (see Finley et al[430] and Farmakis et al[440] and references therein).

Several clinical trials have amply demonstrated the efficacy of AVP receptor antagonists in reversing hyponatremia, hemodynamic disturbances, and renal dysfunction in both compensated and decompensated CHF.[430,440] In CHF with hyponatremia, three randomized controlled trials involving tolvaptan[741-743] and one involving conivaptan[744] demonstrated normalization and maintenance of plasma Na[+] levels, decreases in body weight and edema, and increases in urine output, after treatment for up to 60 days. There was subjective improvement in dyspnea in some but not all patients. In contrast to the detrimental effects of aggressive therapy with loop diuretics on renal function, no significant changes in blood urea nitrogen and creatinine were reported after vaptan therapy (reviewed by Finley et al[430]). The positive effects were observed regardless of whether LVEF was less or greater than 40%. In one trial, tolvaptan, but not fluid restriction, corrected hyponatremia.[742] However, in the sole trial in which all-cause mortality was the primary endpoint, no significant effects of tolvaptan given for 60 days were seen after 9 months of follow-up.[743] In general, the patients participating in these trials had decompensated CHF.

Another trial (Treatment of Hyponatremia Based on Lixivaptan in NYHA Class III/IV Cardiac Patient Evaluation [BALANCE]) in which lixivaptan is used for decompensated CHF was completed in June 2010; results were not yet available at the time of this book going to press.[745] In four trials, researchers have examined the role of vaptans in stable class II or III CHF; tolvaptan was used in three trials (one published as an abstract only)[746,747] and conivaptan in one (published as an abstract only). As in decompensated CHF, decrease in body weight, increase in urine output, and a rise in plasma Na[+] (within the normal range) were observed. However, there was no improvement in functional capacity, exercise tolerance, or overall quality of life.[430]

In contrast to furosemide, tolvaptan did not reduce RBF.[430] Moreover, in the Multicenter Evaluation of Tolvaptan Effect on Remodelling (METEOR) trial, no beneficial or adverse effects of tolvaptan on cardiac remodeling or LVEF were observed after 1 year of treatment in patients receiving optimal evidence-based background therapies for CHF (ACE inhibitors, ARBs, and β-blockers).[747] These results are reassuring because tolvaptan is highly selective for the V_2 receptor, which raises the theoretical possibility that unopposed V_1 receptor–mediated effects under the influence of raised AVP levels may result from tolvaptan treatment.

With regard to hemodynamic effects of vaptans, two studies have been published on patients with advanced CHF and systolic dysfunction who received a single intravenous dose of either conivaptan or placebo.[748,749] The active drug modestly reduced pulmonary capillary wedge pressure and significantly reduced right atrial pressure in comparison with placebo, without affecting cardiac index, pulmonary arterial pressure, systemic or pulmonary vascular resistance, systemic arterial pressure, or heart rate. Urine output rose and osmolarity fell significantly.

In view of the impressive diuretic effect of vaptans, there is considerable interest in the potential loop diuretic–sparing effect mentioned previously. This idea was evaluated in one preliminary study.[430] In patients with chronic CHF who had signs of congestion, background diuretic therapy was withdrawn, salt restriction was instituted, and the patients were then randomly assigned to receive a 7-day regimen of tolvaptan, 30 mg/day; furosemide, 80 mg/day; or a combination of the two. Tolvaptan, but not furosemide, led to a significant decline in body weight, with no effect on plasma K[+]. This favorable effect of tolvaptan may result from its 24-hour action, in contrast to furosemide, the effect of which lasts only approximately 6 hours, thus allowing 18 hours of compensatory salt and water retention. Further studies are needed to explore the potential for vaptans as loop diuretic–sparing agents.

Adverse effects of vaptans appear to be relatively few and, on the whole, minor. Thirst and dry mouth are not unexpected; hypokalemia occurs in fewer than 10% of recipients, which is favorably comparable with loop diuretics. In the largest study to date, Efficacy of Vasopressin Antagonism in Heart Failure Outcome Study with Tolvaptan (EVEREST), involving more than 4000 patients, there was a small but significant increase in reported strokes; however, there was also a small but significant reduction in myocardial infarction rate (see Finley et al[430]).

In summary, AVP receptor antagonists appear to be promising in the treatment of advanced heart failure. Many unanswered questions remain regarding the exact role of AVP receptor antagonists in the management of CHF. These include the potential for long-term efficacy, the use in volume overload in the setting of preserved ejection fraction with a nondilated ventricle, the role in possible loop diuretic dose sparing, the duration of treatment, and dosing over the shorter and longer term.[430] Finally, and perhaps most important, is the question of whether AVP receptor antagonists improve longer term prognosis and reduce the high rate of mortality among patients with CHF who are already receiving optimal doses of ACE inhibitors, ARBs, and β-blockers.

Specific Treatments Based on the Pathophysiology of Sodium Retention in Cirrhosis

The prognosis of type 1 hepatorenal syndrome is dismal; the mortality rate is as high as 80% in the first 2 weeks, and only 10% of patients survive longer than 3 months.[573,587] Therefore, specific aggressive therapy in these patients is usually indicated in preparation for liver transplantation.[344,573,574] Patients with type 2 hepatorenal syndrome have a better prognosis; the median length of survival is approximately 6 months.[750] Aggressive management may be considered for such patients, regardless of transplantation candidacy. There are four major therapeutic interventions for hepatorenal syndrome: pharmacologic therapy, TIPS insertion, renal replacement therapies (RRTs), and liver transplantation.

Pharmacologic Treatment

The goals of pharmacologic therapy are to reverse the functional renal failure and prolong survival until suitable candidates can undergo liver transplantation. On the basis of the pathophysiologic features of renal vasoconstriction against a background of systemic and, specifically, splanchnic arterial vasodilation, specific treatments consist broadly of renal vaso-dilators and systemic vasoconstrictors. The former group includes direct renal vasodilators (dopamine, fenoldopam, and prostaglandins) and antagonists of endogenous renal vasocon-strictors (ACE inhibitors, ARBs, aldosterone antagonists, and endothelin antagonists). Systemic vasoconstrictors comprise vasopressin analogs (ornipressin, terlipressin), the somatosta-tin analog octreotide, and the α-adrenergic agonists.[751] In addition, the nonosmotically stimulated rise in plasma AVP levels and resulting impaired water excretion and hyponatre-mia can be potentially reversed by V_2 receptor antagonists.

Renal Vasodilators and Renal Vasoconstrictor Antagonists

Although these agents are theoretically attractive for the man-agement of Na+ retention in cirrhosis, none of the studies of renal vasodilators showed improvement in renal perfusion or GFR (see Wadei et al[573] and references therein). Low-dose dopamine infused for up to 24 hours improved cortical blood flow and the angiographic appearance of renal cortical vascu-lature without improvement in GFR or urine flow. Responses were the same both in refractory ascites and in hepatorenal syndrome. Dopamine in combination with vasoconstrictors proved more successful, but this could be attributed to vaso-constrictor therapy alone. Similarly, neither the oral PGE_1 analog misoprostol nor intravenous prostaglandin infusion induced significant changes in GFR or Na+ excretion. The ET-A antagonist BQ-123 produced dose-dependent renal improvement in one study on three patients, but subsequent studies showed a paradoxical vasodilating effect of endothe-lin in patients with cirrhosis (see Wadei et al[573] and refer-ences therein). Therefore, the role of endothelin blockers in hepatorenal syndrome remains controversial. With regard to RAAS blockade, a single study revealed that 1-week treat-ment with the ARB losartan led to increased Na+ excretion and an improvement in renal function in cirrhotic patients with and without ascites (see Wadei et al[573] and references therein). Further confirmatory studies are awaited.

In general, because of adverse effects and lack of benefit, the use of renal vasodilators in hepatorenal syndrome has largely been abandoned.

Systemic Vasoconstrictors

Systemic vasoconstrictors are the most promising pharmaco-logic agents in the management of hepatorenal syndrome, by virtue of their predominant action on the vasodilated splanch-nic circulation without affecting the renal circulation. Three groups of vasoconstrictors have been studied: vasopressin V_1 receptor analogs (ornipressin and terlipressin), the somatosta-tin analog (octreotide), and the α-adrenergic agonists.[751]

VASOPRESSIN V_1 RECEPTOR ANALOGS
These agents cause marked vasoconstriction through their action on the V_1 receptors present in the smooth muscle of the arterial wall. They are used extensively for the management of acute variceal bleeding in patients with cirrhosis and portal hypertension. Ornipressin infusion in combination with vol-ume expansion or low-dose dopamine was associated with a remarkable improvement in renal function and an increase in RPF, GFR, and Na+ excretion in almost half of the treated

patients (see Wadei et al[573] and references therein). Unfor-tunately, ornipressin had to be abandoned because of signifi-cant ischemic adverse effects that occurred in almost 30% of treated patients.[750]

Terlipressin, on the other hand, has favorable effects simi-lar to those of ornipressin without the accompanying adverse ischemic reactions. The administration of terlipressin and albumin in type 1 hepatorenal syndrome was associated with significant improvement in GFR, increase in arterial pres-sure, near-normalization of neurohumoral levels, and reduc-tion of serum creatinine level in 42% to 77% of cases.[573,574] The length of survival was also improved over that of historic cases, but it remained dismal: the median length was only 25 to 40 days. In nonresponders, who tended to have more severe cirrhosis (Child-Pugh score >13), length of survival was notably reduced.[752] The rates of response to terlipressin in type 2 hepatorenal syndrome were better than those in type 1, with 100% survival at 3 months.[753,754] Despite hepatorenal syndrome relapses in 50% of cases, reintroduction of therapy produced a further response.

From the results of two randomized controlled trials, it is now clear that both terlipressin alone and the combination of terlipressin and albumin are superior to albumin alone in improving renal function and reversing hepatorenal syndrome type 1.[755,756] However, these relatively small studies were unable to show a survival benefit for terlipressin. Attempts to prevent relapse of type 2 hepatorenal syndrome with mido-drine after terlipressin-induced improvement were also unsuc-cessful.[757] The optimum duration of terlipressin therapy is not clear. In all studies, terlipressin was given until serum creati-nine levels decreased to less than 1.5 mg/dL or for a maximum of 15 days. Whether extending the therapy beyond 15 days will add any benefit is not known. Moreover, the apparent sur-vival advantage of terlipressin, seen in the cohort studies, was poor; 80% of patients who did not receive a transplant died of their liver disease within 3 months of therapy. Therefore, terlipressin and albumin infusion may be appropriate only for patients awaiting liver transplantation.

The importance of V_1 receptor analogs is underscored by the observation that pretransplantation normalization of renal function in patients with hepatorenal syndrome by this ther-apy confers similar posttransplantation outcomes on patients with normal renal function who received transplants.[758] Despite the favorable effects of terlipressin, a major drawback is its unavailability in many countries, including the United States and Canada. In these countries, vasopressin itself may be a reasonable alternative.[759]

SOMATOSTATIN ANALOGS AND α-ADRENERGIC AGONISTS
Octreotide, an inhibitor of glucagon and other vasodilator peptide release, is currently the only available somatostatin analog. In small cohort studies, octreotide with albumin infu-sion or midodrine alone had no effect on renal function in hepatorenal syndrome.[576,760] However, both agents in combi-nation with albumin infusion led to a significant improvement in renal function and survival in both types 1 and 2 hepa-torenal syndrome, in comparison to historical controls.[761] A literature review concluded that the exact role of combined octreotide/midodrine therapy in hepatorenal syndrome man-agement remains to be determined.[762]

Whether vasopressin analogs or combined therapy with octreotide and midodrine are more efficacious in reversing hepatorenal syndrome remains an open question. Patients treated with vasopressin had a significantly higher recovery rate from type 1 hepatorenal syndrome, had improved length of survival, and were more likely to receive a liver transplant.[759] Finally, the administration of intravenous norepinephrine in association with albumin and furosemide resulted in reversal of hepatorenal syndrome in 10 (83%) of 12 patients with type 1 hepatorenal syndrome, and ischemic episodes were observed in only two.[763] It is interesting that in two of the responders to norepinephrine, terlipressin therapy had previously failed. Regression of renal failure was associated with improvement in patient survival, and four of the responders did not require liver transplantation 6 to 18 months after recovery of renal function. Although norepinephrine use seems to be counterintuitive because of already elevated levels in patients with hepatorenal syndrome, a recently published pilot randomized controlled trial showed that norepinephrine was a safe and effective as terlipressin.[763a]

Vasopressin V_2 Receptor Antagonists

As already mentioned hyponatremia is often seen in advanced cirrhosis with ascites and hepatorenal syndrome and is a marker of poor prognosis.[764] Therefore, attaining a water diuresis and reversing hyponateremia through the use of V_2 receptor antagonists are potentially important therapeutic goals. To date, the few cohort studies performed in animals and patients with cirrhosis have yielded promising results (reviewed by several authors[765-767]). Moreover, in the only randomized controlled trial so far reported, the V_2 receptor antagonist satavaptan given for 15 days improved the control of ascites and increased serum Na^+ in patients with cirrhosis, ascites, and hyponatremia who were already receiving spironolactone (100 mg/day). The only notable adverse effect, thirst, was significantly more common in the satavaptan than in the placebo group.[646] Further studies of vaptans in cirrhosis with ascites and hyponatremia are under way, and the results are eagerly awaited.

Transjugular Intrahepatic Portosystemic Shunt

The efficacy of TIPS in the reduction of portal venous pressure in patients with cirrhosis and refractory ascites with either type 1 or type 2 hepatorenal syndrome has been demonstrated in several small cohort studies.[768,769] Significant improvement in renal hemodynamics, GFR, and vasoconstrictive neurohumoral factors were observed in most patients[770,771] (reviewed by Wadei et al[573]). The rates of survival at 3, 6, 12, and 18 months were 81%, 71%, 48%, and 35%, respectively, a marked improvement in comparison with historical controls.[771] Of importance was that among patients who had type 1 hepatorenal syndrome and were treated with TIPS, the rate of 10-week survival was 53%, a significant improvement over that in historical cases and better than that reported after terlipressin and albumin infusion.[753] A novel finding was the ability to discontinue dialysis in four of seven dialysis-dependent patients after TIPS insertion. Moreover, liver transplantation was performed in two patients 7 months and 2 years, respectively, after TIPS insertion, when the medical condition that precluded transplantation had resolved.[771]

The mechanism by which TIPS exerts its favorable effects appears to be the result of reduction in sinusoidal hypertension, possible suppression of the putative hepatorenal reflex discussed earlier, improvement of the EABV by shunting portal venous blood into the systemic circulation, or amelioration of cardiac dysfunction.[769] Despite the encouraging beneficial effects of TIPS on reversal of hepatorenal syndrome and improvement in patient survival, some unanswered questions remain. First, the clinical, biochemical and neurohumoral parameters, although improved, are not normalized after TIPS insertion; thus, other factors in the pathogenetic pathway of hepatorenal syndrome may remain active. Second, the maximum renal recovery is delayed for up to 2 to 4 weeks after TIPS insertion, and renal Na^+ excretory capacity is still subnormal. The cause of this delay and the inability to normalize salt excretion are not clear, although one possibility is related to the proportionately greater action of TIPS to reduce presinusoidal pressure, as opposed to postsinusoidal and intrasinusoidal pressure. Third, patients with advanced cirrhosis are at risk for worsening liver failure, hepatic encephalopathy, or both and are not candidates for TIPS insertion. Fourth, TIPS has the potential for worsening the existing hyperdynamic circulation or precipitating acute heart failure in at risk patients; therefore, careful attention to cardiac status is mandatory (see Wadei et al[573] and references therein). Finally, TIPS is associated with a high incidence of portosystemic encephalopathy when used for the treatment of refractory ascites. Of interest is that this complication is far less frequent when TIPS is used for treating variceal hemorrhage.[768]

Notwithstanding these unsolved dilemmas, there is clearly a group of patients with hepatorenal syndrome for whom TIPS might prolong survival enough either to enable liver transplantation or, if they are not candidates, to remain dialysis independent. The possibility of combination or sequential therapies has also been examined in preliminary studies. For example, treatment with octreotide, midodrine, and albumin infusion, followed by TIPS insertion, in selected patients with preserved liver function was associated with persistent improvements in serum creatinine levels, RPF, GFR, natriuresis, plasma renin activity, and aldosterone levels.[751] Another group of 11 patients with type 2 hepatorenal syndrome showed similar improvement after sequential terlipressin and TIPS insertion. Whether combination therapy can preclude the need for liver transplantation or significantly improve survival remains to be investigated.

Renal Replacement Therapy

Conventional hemodialysis and continuous RRT have been extensively assessed in patients with hepatorenal syndrome (reviewed by Wadei et al[573]). The benefits, if any, in terms of prolonging survival, are dubious, and the rate of morbidity resulting from these therapies is high (see Wadei et al[573] and references therein). In oliguric patients awaiting liver transplantation who do not respond to vasoconstrictors or TIPS and who develop diuretic-resistant volume overload, hyperkalemia, or intractable metabolic acidosis, RRT may be a reasonable option as a bridge to transplantation. In view of the dismal prognosis of hepatorenal syndrome, especially type 1, decisions on RRT in patients who are not transplantation candidates should be carefully deliberated on an individual basis.

In contrast to conventional RRT, molecular adsorbent recirculating system (MARS) offers the potential advantage of removing albumin-bound water-soluble vasoactive agents, toxins, and proinflammatory cytokines. Relevant molecules include bile acids, tumor necrosis factor-α, interleukin-6, and nitric oxide that are known to be implicated in the pathogenesis of advanced cirrhosis.[574] The uniqueness of MARS lies in its ability to enable partial recovery of hepatic function, and results of preliminary studies are consistent with this idea.[772] In one study, MARS treatment led to a decrease in renal vascular resistance and improvement in splenic resistance index, a parameter related to portal resistance. The authors hypothesized that the hemodynamic effects were probably mediated by clearance of vasoactive substances.[773] Other researchers have shown that MARS leads to significantly reduced bilirubin levels, reduced grade of encephalopathy, decreased serum creatinine levels, and increased serum Na levels.[774] Finally, one study demonstrated a survival benefit; the mortality rate was reduced from 100% in the control group to 62.5% in the MARS-treated patients. At 30 days, 75% of the MARS group had survived.[774] However, all these studies were conducted with no more than 12 or 13 patients; thus, MARS, like the pharmacologic therapies described previously, should probably be considered currently as only a bridge to transplantation.

Liver Transplantation

Liver transplantation is the best option for treating hepatorenal syndrome because it offers a cure for both the liver disease and the renal dysfunction. The outcomes are somewhat worse in transplant recipients with hepatorenal syndrome than in those without the syndrome (3-year survival rates of 60% vs. 70% to 80%) and may be improved by the bridging therapies described previously (see Angeli and Merkel[574] and references therein). More data are needed to confirm the initial favorable reports.

With respect to renal function after transplantation in patients with hepatorenal syndrome, GFR decreases in the first month as a result of the stress of surgery, infections, immunosuppressive therapy, and other factors. Dialysis in the first month is required in 35% of patients with hepatorenal syndrome, as opposed to only 5% of patients without hepatorenal syndrome. Despite the prompt correction of hemodynamic and neurohumoral parameters, GFR recovers incompletely to 30-40 mL/min at 1 to 2 months, and renal functional impairment often persists over the long term. Overall, the rate of posttransplantation reversal of hepatorenal syndrome has been estimated to be no greater than 58%. Predictors of renal recovery included younger recipient and donor, nonalcoholic liver disease, and low posttransplantation bilirubin level.[775]

Perhaps surprisingly, duration of dialysis pre-transplantation did not influence renal recovery after transplantation. In this regard, the question of combined liver-kidney transplantation becomes critical. Data from the United Network for Organ Sharing showed better rates of 5-year survival of 62.2% after liver-kidney transplantation than after liver transplantation alone among patients with pretransplantation serum creatinine levels higher than 2.2 mg/dL. In contrast, single center results were similar, regardless of pretransplantation renal function.[776] The introduction of MELD (model of end-stage liver disease) scores for allocation of livers has increased the number of transplantations in patients with impaired renal function, but more liver-kidney transplantation are also performed.[777] More data are needed to enable a rational decision about who should receive liver-kidney transplants, as opposed to liver transplants alone.

For a general review of all aspects of liver transplantation, the reader is referred to several excellent recent reviews.[777-779]

References

1. Aukland K, Nicolaysen G. Interstitial fluid volume: local regulatory mechanisms. *Physiol Rev.* 1981;61:556-643.
2. Ali MH, Schumacker PT. Endothelial responses to mechanical stress: where is the mechanosensor? *Crit Care Med.* 2002;30:S198-S206.
3. Ali MH, Mungai PT, Schumacker PT. Stretch-induced phosphorylation of focal adhesion kinase in endothelial cells: role of mitochondrial oxidants. *Am J Physiol Lung Cell Mol Physiol.* 2006;291:L38-L45.
4. Gaucher C, Devaux C, Boura C, et al. in vitro impact of physiological shear stress on endothelial cells gene expression profile. *Clin Hemorheol Microcirc.* 2007;37:99-107.
5. Li YS, Haga JH, Chien S. Molecular basis of the effects of shear stress on vascular endothelial cells. *J Biomech.* 2005;38:1949-1971.
6. Henry JP, Gauer OH, Reeves JL. Evidence of the atrial location of receptors influencing urine flow. *Circ Res.* 1956;4:85-90.
7. Goetz KL, Hermreck AS, Slick GL, et al. Atrial receptors and renal function in conscious dogs. *Am J Physiol.* 1970;219:1417-1423.
8. Epstein M. Renal effects of head-out water immersion in humans: a 15-year update. *Physiol Rev.* 1992;72:563-621.
9. Miller JA, Floras JS, Skorecki KL, et al. Renal and humoral responses to sustained cardiopulmonary baroreceptor deactivation in humans. *Am J Physiol.* 1991;260:R642-R648.
10. Cowley Jr AW, Skelton MM. Dominance of colloid osmotic pressure in renal excretion after isotonic volume expansion. *Am J Physiol.* 1991;261:H1214-H1225.
11. Johansen LB, Pump B, Warberg J, et al. Preventing hemodilution abolishes natriuresis of water immersion in humans. *Am J Physiol.* 1998;275:R879-R888.
12. Kappagoda CT, Linden RJ, Sivananthan N. The nature of the atrial receptors responsible for a reflex increase in heart rate in the dog. *J Physiol.* 1979;291:393-412.
13. Quail AW, Woods RL, Korner PI. Cardiac and arterial baroreceptor influences in release of vasopressin and renin during hemorrhage. *Am J Physiol.* 1987;252:H1120-H1126.
14. DiBona GF, Sawin LL. Renal nerve activity in conscious rats during volume expansion and depletion. *Am J Physiol.* 1985;248:F15-F23.
15. Myers BD, Peterson C, Molina C, et al. Role of cardiac atria in the human renal response to changing plasma volume. *Am J Physiol.* 1988;254:F562-F573.
16. Wurzner G, Chiolero A, Maillard M, et al. Renal and neurohormonal responses to increasing levels of lower body negative pressure in men. *Kidney Int.* 2001;60:1469-1476.
17. Tidgren B, Hjemdahl P, Theodorsson E, et al. Renal responses to lower body negative pressure in humans. *Am J Physiol.* 1990;259:F573-F579.
18. Kaczmarczyk G, Schmidt E. Sodium homeostasis in conscious dogs after chronic cardiac denervation. *Am J Physiol.* 1990;258:F805-F811.
19. Braith RW, Mills Jr RM, Wilcox CS, et al. Breakdown of blood pressure and body fluid homeostasis in heart transplant recipients. *J Am Coll Cardiol.* 1996;27:375-383.
20. de Bold AJ, Borenstein HB, Veress AT, et al. A rapid and potent natriuretic response to intravenous injection of atrial myocardial extract in rats. *Life Sci.* 1981;28:89-94.
21. de Bold AJ, de Bold ML. Determinants of natriuretic peptide production by the heart: basic and clinical implications. *J Investig Med.* 2005;53:371-377.
22. Rubattu S, Sciarretta S, Valenti V, et al. Natriuretic peptides: an update on bioactivity, potential therapeutic use, and implication in cardiovascular diseases. *Am J Hypertens.* 2008;21:733-741.
23. Potter LR, Yoder AR, Flora DR, et al. Natriuretic peptides: their structures, receptors, physiologic functions and therapeutic applications. *Handb Exp Pharmacol.* 2009(191):341-366.
24. Piechota M, Banach M, Jacon A, et al. Natriuretic peptides in cardiovascular diseases. *Cell Mol Biol Lett.* 2008;13:155-181.
25. Woodard GE, Rosado JA. Natriuretic peptides in vascular physiology and pathology. *Int Rev Cell Mol Biol.* 2008;268:59-93.
26. Wu Q, Xu-Cai YO, Chen S, et al. Corin: new insights into the natriuretic peptide system. *Kidney Int.* 2009;75:142-146.

27. Cho KW, Kim SH, Seul KH, et al. Effect of extracellular calcium depletion on the two-step ANP secretion in perfused rabbit atria. *Regul Pept.* 1994;52:129-137.
28. Espiner EA, Richards AM, Yandle TG, et al. Natriuretic hormones. *Endocrinol Metab Clin North Am.* 1995;24:481-509.
29. Levin ER, Gardner DG, Samson WK. Natriuretic peptides. *N Engl J Med.* 1998;339:321-328.
30. Singer DR, Markandu ND, Buckley MG, et al. Contrasting endocrine responses to acute oral compared with intravenous sodium loading in normal humans. *Am J Physiol.* 1998;274:F111-F119.
31. Andersen LJ, Norsk P, Johansen LB, et al. Osmoregulatory control of renal sodium excretion after sodium loading in humans. *Am J Physiol.* 1998;275:R1833-R1842.
32. Andersen LJ, Andersen JL, Pump B, et al. Natriuresis induced by mild hypernatremia in humans. *Am J Physiol Regul Integr Comp Physiol.* 2002;282:R1754-R1761.
33. Bie P, Wamberg S, Kjolby M. Volume natriuresis vs. pressure natriuresis. *Acta Physiol Scand.* 2004;181:495-503.
34. John SW, Veress AT, Honrath U, et al. Blood pressure and fluid-electrolyte balance in mice with reduced or absent ANP. *Am J Physiol.* 1996;271:R109-R114.
35. Montoliu C, Kosenko E, Del Olmo JA, et al. Correlation of nitric oxide and atrial natriuretic peptide changes with altered cGMP homeostasis in liver cirrhosis. *Liver Int.* 2005;25:787-795.
36. Kuhn M. Cardiac and intestinal natriuretic peptides: insights from genetically modified mice. *Peptides.* 2005;26:1078-1085.
37. Doe CP, Self DA, Drinkhill MJ, et al. Reflex vascular responses in the anesthetized dog to large rapid changes in carotid sinus pressure. *Am J Physiol.* 1998;275:H1169-H1177.
38. Paintal AS. Vagal sensory receptors and their reflex effects. *Physiol Rev.* 1973;53:159-227.
39. McMahon NC, Drinkhill MJ, Hainsworth R. Absence of early resetting of coronary baroreceptors in anaesthetized dogs. *J Physiol.* 1998;513(pt 2):543-549.
40. Tavi P, Laine M, Weckstrom M, et al. Cardiac mechanotransduction: from sensing to disease and treatment. *Trends Pharmacol Sci.* 2001;22:254-260.
41. Bekheirnia MR, Schrier RW. Pathophysiology of water and sodium retention: edematous states with normal kidney function. *Curr Opin Pharmacol.* 2006;6:202-207.
42. Kockskämper J, von Lewinski D, Khafaga M, et al. The slow force response to stretch in atrial and ventricular myocardium from human heart: functional relevance and subcellular mechanisms. *Prog Biophys Mol Biol.* 2008;97:250-267.
43. Andresen MC, Doyle MW, Jin YH, et al. Cellular mechanisms of baroreceptor integration at the nucleus tractus solitarius. *Ann N Y Acad Sci.* 2001;940:132-141.
44. Brozoski DT, Dean C, Hopp FA, et al. Uptake blockade of endocannabinoids in the NTS modulates baroreflex-evoked sympathoinhibition. *Brain Res.* 2005;1059:197-202.
45. Gomez RA, Sequeira Lopez ML. Who and where is the renal baroreceptor? The connexin hypothesis. *Kidney Int.* 2009;75:460-462.
46. Kopp UC, Jones SY, DiBona GF. Afferent renal denervation impairs baroreflex control of efferent renal sympathetic nerve activity. *Am J Physiol Regul Integr Comp Physiol.* 2008;295:R1882-R1890.
47. Navar LG. Integrating multiple paracrine regulators of renal microvascular dynamics. *Am J Physiol.* 1998;274:F433-F444.
48. Schnermann J. Juxtaglomerular cell complex in the regulation of renal salt excretion. *Am J Physiol.* 1998;274:R263-R279.
49. Schnermann J, Homer W. Smith Award lecture. The juxtaglomerular apparatus: from anatomical peculiarity to physiological relevance. *J Am Soc Nephrol.* 2003;14:1681-1694.
50. Oppermann M, Mizel D, Huang G, et al. Macula densa control of renin secretion and preglomerular resistance in mice with selective deletion of the B isoform of the Na, K,2Cl co-transporter. *J Am Soc Nephrol.* 2006;17:2143-2152.
51. Castrop H, Lorenz JN, Hansen PB, et al. Contribution of the basolateral isoform of the Na-K-2Cl$^-$ cotransporter (NKCC1/BSC2) to renin secretion. *Am J Physiol Renal Physiol.* 2005;289:F1185-F1192.
52. Persson AE, Ollerstam A, Liu R, et al. Mechanisms for macula densa cell release of renin. *Acta Physiol Scand.* 2004;181:471-474.
53. Komlosi P, Fintha A, Bell PD. Current mechanisms of macula densa cell signalling. *Acta Physiol Scand.* 2004;181:463-469.
54. Oppermann M, Friedman DJ, Faulhaber-Walter R, et al. Tubuloglomerular feedback and renin secretion in NTPDase1/CD39–deficient mice. *Am J Physiol Renal Physiol.* 2008;294:F965-F970.
55. DiBona GF. Physiology in perspective: The Wisdom of the Body. Neural control of the kidney. *Am J Physiol Regul Integr Comp Physiol.* 2005;289:R633-R641.
56. DiBona GF. Nervous kidney. Interaction between renal sympathetic nerves and the renin-angiotensin system in the control of renal function. *Hypertension.* 2000;36:1083-1088.
57. DiBona GF. Neural control of the kidney: functionally specific renal sympathetic nerve fibers. *Am J Physiol Regul Integr Comp Physiol.* 2000;279:R1517-R1524.
58. Seeliger E, Wronski T, Ladwig M, et al. The renin-angiotensin system and the third mechanism of renal blood flow autoregulation. *Am J Physiol Renal Physiol.* 2009;296:F1334-F1345.
59. Ren Y, Garvin JL, Liu R, et al. Crosstalk between the connecting tubule and the afferent arteriole regulates renal microcirculation. *Kidney Int.* 2007;71:1116-1121.
60. Capasso G. A new cross-talk pathway between the renal tubule and its own glomerulus. *Kidney Int.* 2007;71:1087-1089.
61. Komlosi P, Bell PD, Zhang ZR. Tubuloglomerular feedback mechanisms in nephron segments beyond the macula densa. *Curr Opin Nephrol Hypertens.* 2009;18:57-62.
62. Bolanos L, Colina I, Purroy A. Intracerebroventricular infusion of hypertonic NaCl increases urinary cGMP in healthy and cirrhotic rats. *Arch Physiol Biochem.* 1999;107:323-333.
63. Hansell P, Isaksson B, Sjoquist M. Renal dopamine and noradrenaline excretion during CNS-induced natriuresis in spontaneously hypertensive rats: influence of dietary sodium. *Acta Physiol Scand.* 2000;168:257-266.
64. DiBona GF. Central angiotensin modulation of baroreflex control of renal sympathetic nerve activity in the rat: influence of dietary sodium. *Acta Physiol Scand.* 2003;177:285-289.
65. Zhu GQ, Gao L, Patel KP, et al. ANG II in the paraventricular nucleus potentiates the cardiac sympathetic afferent reflex in rats with heart failure. *J Appl Physiol.* 2004;97:1746-1754.
66. Carey RM. Evidence for a splanchnic sodium input monitor regulating renal sodium excretion in man. Lack of dependence upon aldosterone. *Circ Res.* 1978;43:19-23.
67. Morita H, Matsuda T, Tanaka K, et al. Role of hepatic receptors in controlling body fluid homeostasis. *Jpn J Physiol.* 1995;45:355-368.
68. Morita H, Matsuda T, Furuya F, et al. Hepatorenal reflex plays an important role in natriuresis after high-NaCl food intake in conscious dogs. *Circ Res.* 1993;72:552-559.
69. Morita H, Ohyama H, Hagiike M, et al. Effects of portal infusion of hypertonic solution on jejunal electrolyte transport in anesthetized dogs. *Am J Physiol.* 1990;259:R1289-R1294.
70. Matsuda T, Morita H, Hosomi H, et al. Response of renal nerve activity to high NaCl food intake in dogs with chronic bile duct ligation. *Hepatology.* 1996;23:303-309.
71. Oliver JA, Verna EC. Afferent mechanisms of sodium retention in cirrhosis and hepatorenal syndrome. *Kidney Int.* 2010;77:669-680.
72. Ming Z, Lautt WW. Intrahepatic adenosine-mediated activation of hepatorenal reflex is via A$_1$ receptors in rats. *Can J Physiol Pharmacol.* 2006;84:1177-1184.
73. Ming Z, Fan YJ, Yang X, et al. Contribution of hepatic adenosine A$_1$ receptors to renal dysfunction associated with acute liver injury in rats. *Hepatology.* 2006;44:813-822.
74. Morita H, Fujiki N, Hagiike M, et al. Functional evidence for involvement of bumetanide-sensitive Na$^+$K$^+$2Cl$^-$ cotransport in the hepatoportal Na$^+$ receptor of the Sprague-Dawley rat. *Neurosci Lett.* 1999;264:65-68.
75. Levy M, Wexler MJ. Sodium excretion in dogs with low-grade caval constriction: role of hepatic nerves. *Am J Physiol.* 1987;253:F672-F678.
76. Koyama S, Kanai K, Aibiki M, et al. Reflex increase in renal nerve activity during acutely altered portal venous pressure. *J Auton Nerv Syst.* 1988;23:55-62.
77. Blendis L. Budd-Chiari syndrome: a clinical model of the hepatorenal reflex? *Gastroenterology.* 2006;131:671-672.
78. Thomas L, Kumar R. Control of renal solute excretion by enteric signals and mediators. *J Am Soc Nephrol.* 2008;19:207-212.
79. Sindic A, Schlatter E. Renal electrolyte effects of guanylin and uroguanylin. *Curr Opin Nephrol Hypertens.* 2007;16:10-15.
80. Sindic A, Schlatter E. Cellular effects of guanylin and uroguanylin. *J Am Soc Nephrol.* 2006;17:607-616.
81. Lorenz JN, Nieman M, Sabo J, et al. Uroguanylin knockout mice have increased blood pressure and impaired natriuretic response to enteral NaCl load. *J Clin Invest.* 2003;112:1244-1254.
82. Kinoshita H, Fujimoto S, Nakazato M, et al. Urine and plasma levels of uroguanylin and its molecular forms in renal diseases. *Kidney Int.* 1997;52:1028-1034.
83. Fukae H, Kinoshita H, Fujimoto S, et al. Changes in urinary levels and renal expression of uroguanylin on low or high salt diets in rats. *Nephron.* 2002;92:373-378.
84. Santos-Neto MS, Carvalho AF, Monteiro HS, et al. Interaction of atrial natriuretic peptide, urodilatin, guanylin and uroguanylin in the isolated perfused rat kidney. *Regul Pept.* 2006;136:14-22.
85. Peterson TV, Jones CE. Renal responses of the cardiac-denervated nonhuman primate to blood volume expansion. *Circ Res.* 1983;53:24-32.
86. Peterson TV, Chase NL, Gray DK. Renal effects of volume expansion in the renal-denervated nonhuman primate. *Am J Physiol.* 1984;247:H960-H966.

87. Thomson SC, Blantz RC. Glomerulotubular balance, tubuloglomerular feedback, and salt homeostasis. *J Am Soc Nephrol.* 2008;19:2272-2275.

88. Guyton AC, Langston JB, Navar G. Theory for renal autoregulation by feedback at the juxtaglomerular apparatus. *Circ Res.* 1964;15(suppl):97.

89. Schnermann J, Briggs JP. Tubuloglomerular feedback: mechanistic insights from gene-manipulated mice. *Kidney Int.* 2008;74:418-426.

90. Castrop H. Mediators of tubuloglomerular feedback regulation of glomerular filtration: ATP and adenosine. *Acta Physiol (Oxf).* 2007;189:3-14.

91. Takahashi N, Chernavvsky DR, Gomez RA, et al. Uncompensated polyuria in a mouse model of Bartter's syndrome. *Proc Natl Acad Sci U S A.* 2000;97:5434-5439.

92. Bell PD, Lapointe JY, Peti-Peterdi J. Macula densa cell signaling. *Annu Rev Physiol.* 2003;65:481-500.

93. Hansen PB, Castrop H, Briggs J, et al. Adenosine induces vasoconstriction through G_i-dependent activation of phospholipase C in isolated perfused afferent arterioles of mice. *J Am Soc Nephrol.* 2003;14:2457-2465.

94. Lai EY, Patzak A, Steege A, et al. Contribution of adenosine receptors in the control of arteriolar tone and adenosine–angiotensin II interaction. *Kidney Int.* 2006;70:690-698.

95. Hansen PB, Friis UG, Uhrenholt TR, et al. Intracellular signalling pathways in the vasoconstrictor response of mouse afferent arterioles to adenosine. *Acta Physiol (Oxf).* 2007;191:89-97.

96. Al-Mashhadi RH, Skott O, Vanhoutte PM, et al. Activation of A(2) adenosine receptors dilates cortical efferent arterioles in mouse. *Kidney Int.* 2009;75:793-799.

97. Blantz RC, Deng A, Lortie M, et al. The complex role of nitric oxide in the regulation of glomerular ultrafiltration. *Kidney Int.* 2002;61:782-785.

98. Patzak A, Persson AE. Angiotensin II–nitric oxide interaction in the kidney. *Curr Opin Nephrol Hypertens.* 2007;16:46-51.

99. Herrera M, Garvin JL. Recent advances in the regulation of nitric oxide in the kidney. *Hypertension.* 2005;45:1062-1067.

100. Satriano J, Wead L, Cardus A, et al. Regulation of ecto-5′-nucleotidase by NaCl and nitric oxide: potential roles in tubuloglomerular feedback and adaptation. *Am J Physiol Renal Physiol.* 2006;291:F1078-F1082.

101. Bell TD, Welch WJ. Regulation of renal arteriolar tone by adenosine: novel role for type 2 receptors. *Kidney Int.* 2009;75:769-771.

102. Just A, Kurtz L, de Wit C, et al. Connexin 40 mediates the tubuloglomerular feedback contribution to renal blood flow autoregulation. *J Am Soc Nephrol.* 2009;20:1577-1585.

103. Ren Y, D'Ambrosio MA, Garvin JL, et al. Possible mediators of connecting tubule glomerular feedback. *Hypertension.* 2009;53:319-323.

104. Brenner BM, Troy JL. Postglomerular vascular protein concentration: evidence for a causal role in governing fluid reabsorption and glomerulotubular balance by the renal proximal tubule. *J Clin Invest.* 1971;50:336-349.

105. Ichikawa I, Brenner BM. Importance of efferent arteriolar vascular tone in regulation of proximal tubule fluid reabsorption and glomerulotubular balance in the rat. *J Clin Invest.* 1980;65:1192-1201.

106. Ichikawa I, Brenner BM. Mechanism of inhibition of proximal tubule fluid reabsorption after exposure of the rat kidney to the physical effects of expansion of extracellular fluid volume. *J Clin Invest.* 1979;64:1466-1474.

107. Skorecki KL, Brenner BM. Body fluid homeostasis in congestive heart failure and cirrhosis with ascites. *Am J Med.* 1982;72:323-338.

108. Imai M, Kokko JP. Effect of peritubular protein concentration on reabsorption of sodium and water in isolated perfused proximal tubules. *J Clin Invest.* 1972;51:314-325.

109. Garcia NH, Ramsey CR, Knox FG. Understanding the role of paracellular transport in the proximal tubule. *News Physiol Sci.* 1998;13:38-43.

110. Angelow S, Ahlstrom R, Yu AS. Biology of claudins. *Am J Physiol Renal Physiol.* 2008;295:F867-F876.

111. Angelow S, Yu AS. Claudins and paracellular transport: an update. *Curr Opin Nephrol Hypertens.* 2007;16:459-464.

112. Balkovetz DF. Tight junction claudins and the kidney in sickness and in health. *Biochim Biophys Acta.* 2009;1788:858-863.

113. Kiuchi-Saishin Y, Gotoh S, Furuse M, et al. Differential expression patterns of claudins, tight junction membrane proteins, in mouse nephron segments. *J Am Soc Nephrol.* 2002;13:875-886.

114. Enck AH, Berger UV, Yu AS. Claudin-2 is selectively expressed in proximal nephron in mouse kidney. *Am J Physiol Renal Physiol.* 2001;281:F966-F974.

115. Romano G, Favret G, Damato R, et al. Proximal reabsorption with changing tubular fluid inflow in rat nephrons. *Exp Physiol.* 1998;83:35-48.

116. Andreoli TE. An overview of salt absorption by the nephron. *J Nephrol.* 1999;12(suppl 2):S3-S15.

117. Jamison RL, Sonnenberg H, Stein JH. Questions and replies: role of the collecting tubule in fluid, sodium, and potassium balance. *Am J Physiol.* 1979;237:F247-F261.

118. Earley LE, Friedler RM. Changes in renal blood flow and possibly the intrarenal distribution of blood during the natriuresis accompanying saline loading in the dog. *J Clin Invest.* 1965;44:929-941.

119. Early LE, Friedler RM. Observations on the mechanism of decreased tubular reabsorption of sodium and water during saline loading. *J Clin Invest.* 1964;43:1928-1937.

120. Cowley Jr AW. Role of the renal medulla in volume and arterial pressure regulation. *Am J Physiol.* 1997;273:R1-R15.

121. Navar LG, Majid DS. Interactions between arterial pressure and sodium excretion. *Curr Opin Nephrol Hypertens.* 1996;5:64-71.

122. Roman RJ, Zou AP. Influence of the renal medullary circulation on the control of sodium excretion. *Am J Physiol.* 1993;265:R963-R973.

123. Hall JE. The kidney, hypertension, and obesity. *Hypertension.* 2003;41:625-633.

124. Hall JE, Guyton AC, Brands MW. Pressure-volume regulation in hypertension. *Kidney Int Suppl.* 1996;55:S35-S41.

125. Cowley Jr AW, Mattson DL, Lu S, et al. The renal medulla and hypertension. *Hypertension.* 1995;25:663-673.

126. Cowley Jr AW, Mori T, Mattson D, et al. Role of renal NO production in the regulation of medullary blood flow. *Am J Physiol Regul Integr Comp Physiol.* 2003;284:R1355-R1369.

127. Mattson DL. Importance of the renal medullary circulation in the control of sodium excretion and blood pressure. *Am J Physiol Regul Integr Comp Physiol.* 2003;284:R13-R27.

128. Granger JP, Alexander BT, Llinas M. Mechanisms of pressure natriuresis. *Curr Hypertens Rep.* 2002;4:152-159.

129. Granger JP. Pressure natriuresis. Role of renal interstitial hydrostatic pressure. *Hypertension.* 1992;19:I9-I17.

130. Evans RG, Majid DS, Eppel GA. Mechanisms mediating pressure natriuresis: what we know and what we need to find out. *Clin Exp Pharmacol Physiol.* 2005;32:400-409.

131. Dos Santos EA, Dahly-Vernon AJ, Hoagland KM, et al. Inhibition of the formation of EETs and 20-HETE with 1-aminobenzotriazole attenuates pressure natriuresis. *Am J Physiol Regul Integr Comp Physiol.* 2004;287:R58-R68.

132. Majid DS, Navar LG. Blockade of distal nephron sodium transport attenuates pressure natriuresis in dogs. *Hypertension.* 1994;23:1040-1045.

133. Kline RL, Liu F. Modification of pressure natriuresis by long-term losartan in spontaneously hypertensive rats. *Hypertension.* 1994;24:467-473.

134. Jin C, Hu C, Polichnowski A, et al. Effects of renal perfusion pressure on renal medullary hydrogen peroxide and nitric oxide production. *Hypertension.* 2009;53:1048-1053.

135. Cowley Jr AW. Renal medullary oxidative stress, pressure-natriuresis, and hypertension. *Hypertension.* 2008;52:777-786.

136. Kompanowska-Jezierska E, Wolff H, Kuczeriszka M, et al. Renal nerves and nNOS: roles in natriuresis of acute isovolumetric sodium loading in conscious rats. *Am J Physiol Regul Integr Comp Physiol.* 2008;294:R1130-R1139.

137. Salom MG, Lahera V, Miranda-Guardiola F, et al. Blockade of pressure natriuresis induced by inhibition of renal synthesis of nitric oxide in dogs. *Am J Physiol.* 1992;262:F718-F722.

138. Patel AR, Granger JP, Kirchner KA. L-arginine improves transmission of perfusion pressure to the renal interstitium in Dahl salt-sensitive rats. *Am J Physiol.* 1994;266:R1730-R1735.

139. Majid DS, Godfrey M, Grisham MB, et al. Relation between pressure natriuresis and urinary excretion of nitrate/nitrite in anesthetized dogs. *Hypertension.* 1995;25:860-865.

140. Li N, Yi F, Dos Santos EA, et al. Role of renal medullary heme oxygenase in the regulation of pressure natriuresis and arterial blood pressure. *Hypertension.* 2007;49:148-154.

141. Williams JM, Sarkis A, Lopez B, et al. Elevations in renal interstitial hydrostatic pressure and 20-hydroxyeicosatetraenoic acid contribute to pressure natriuresis. *Hypertension.* 2007;49:687-694.

142. Sarkis A, Lopez B, Roman RJ. Role of 20-hydroxyeicosatetraenoic acid and epoxyeicosatrienoic acids in hypertension. *Curr Opin Nephrol Hypertens.* 2004;13:205-214.

143. Sipos A, Vargas SL, Toma I, et al. Connexin 30 deficiency impairs renal tubular ATP release and pressure natriuresis. *J Am Soc Nephrol.* 2009;20:1724-1732.

144. Magyar CE, Zhang Y, Holstein-Rathlou NH, et al. Proximal tubule Na transporter responses are the same during acute and chronic hypertension. *Am J Physiol Renal Physiol.* 2000;279:F358-F369.

145. Reinhardt HW, Seeliger E. Toward an integrative concept of control of total body sodium. *News Physiol Sci.* 2000;15:319-325.

146. Rasmussen MS, Simonsen JA, Sandgaard NC, et al. Mechanisms of acute natriuresis in normal humans on low sodium diet. *J Physiol.* 2003;546:591-603.

147. Sandgaard NC, Andersen JL, Bie P. Hormonal regulation of renal sodium and water excretion during normotensive sodium loading in conscious dogs. *Am J Physiol Regul Integr Comp Physiol.* 2000;278:R11-R18.

148. DiBona GF, Kopp UC. Neural control of renal function. *Physiol Rev.* 1997;77:75-197.

149. Denton KM, Luff SE, Shweta A, et al. Differential neural control of glomerular ultrafiltration. *Clin Exp Pharmacol Physiol*. 2004;31:380-386.
150. Barajas L, Powers K. Monoaminergic innervation of the rat kidney: a quantitative study. *Am J Physiol*. 1990;259:F503-F511.
151. Eppel GA, Malpas SC, Denton KM, et al. Neural control of renal medullary perfusion. *Clin Exp Pharmacol Physiol*. 2004;31:387-396.
152. Jeffries WB, Pettinger WA. Adrenergic signal transduction in the kidney. *Miner Electrolyte Metab*. 1989;15:5-15.
153. Matsushima Y, Akabane S, Ito K. Characterization of alpha 1– and alpha 2–adrenoceptors directly associated with basolateral membranes from rat kidney proximal tubules. *Biochem Pharmacol*. 1986;35:2593-2600.
154. Summers RJ, Stephenson JA, Kuhar MJ. Localization of beta adrenoceptor subtypes in rat kidney by light microscopic autoradiography. *J Pharmacol Exp Ther*. 1985;232:561-569.
155. DiBona GF. Sympathetic nervous system and the kidney in hypertension. *Curr Opin Nephrol Hypertens*. 2002;11:197-200.
156. Gill JR, Bartter FC. Adrenergic nervous system in sodium metabolism. II. Effects of guanethidine on the renal response to sodium deprivation in normal man. *N Engl J Med*. 1966;275:1466-1471.
157. Friberg P, Meredith I, Jennings G, et al. Evidence for increased renal norepinephrine overflow during sodium restriction in humans. *Hypertension*. 1990;16:121-130.
158. McMurray JJ, Seidelin PH, Balfour DJ, et al. Physiological increases in circulating noradrenaline are antinatriuretic in man. *J Hypertens*. 1988;6:757-761.
159. Aperia A, Ibarra F, Svensson LB, et al. Calcineurin mediates α-adrenergic stimulation of Na+, K+-ATPase activity in renal tubule cells. *Proc Natl Acad Sci U S A*. 1992;89:7394-7397.
160. Nelson LD, Osborn JL. Role of intrarenal ANG II in reflex neural stimulation of plasma renin activity and renal sodium reabsorption. *Am J Physiol*. 1993;265:R392-R398.
161. Nishida Y, Bishop VS. Vasopressin-induced suppression of renal sympathetic outflow depends on the number of baroafferent inputs in rabbits. *Am J Physiol*. 1992;263:R1187-R1194.
162. Simon JK, Kasting NW, Ciriello J. Afferent renal nerve effects on plasma vasopressin and oxytocin in conscious rats. *Am J Physiol*. 1989;256:R1240-R1244.
163. Awazu M, Kon V, Harris RC, et al. Renal sympathetic nerves modulate glomerular ANP receptors and filtration. *Am J Physiol*. 1991;261:F29-F35.
164. Brewster UC, Perazella MA. The renin-angiotensin-aldosterone system and the kidney: effects on kidney disease. *Am J Med*. 2004;116:263-272.
165. Schmieder RE. Mechanisms for the clinical benefits of angiotensin II receptor blockers. *Am J Hypertens*. 2005;18:720-730.
166. Inagami T, Mizuno K, Kawamura M, et al. Localization of components of the renin-angiotensin system within the kidney and sustained release of angiotensins from isolated and perfused kidney. *Tohoku J Exp Med*. 1992;166:17-26.
167. Santos RA, Ferreira AJ, Simoes E, et al. Recent advances in the angiotensin-converting enzyme 2–angiotensin(1-7)–Mas axis. *Exp Physiol*. 2008;93:519-527.
168. Schindler C, Bramlage P, Kirch W, et al. Role of the vasodilator peptide angiotensin-(1-7) in cardiovascular drug therapy. *Vasc Health Risk Manag*. 2007;3:125-137.
169. Paul M, Poyan MA, Kreutz R. Physiology of local renin-angiotensin systems. *Physiol Rev*. 2006;86:747-803.
170. Kobori H, Nangaku M, Navar LG, et al. The intrarenal renin-angiotensin system: from physiology to the pathobiology of hypertension and kidney disease. *Pharmacol Rev*. 2007;59:251-287.
171. Braam B, Mitchell KD, Fox J, et al. Proximal tubular secretion of angiotensin II in rats. *Am J Physiol*. 1993;264:F891-F898.
172. Seikaly MG, Arant Jr BS, Seney Jr FD. Endogenous angiotensin concentrations in specific intrarenal fluid compartments of the rat. *J Clin Invest*. 1990;86:1352-1357.
173. Fogo AB. Angiotensin receptors: beyond number one. *Curr Opin Nephrol Hypertens*. 2004;13:275-277.
174. Thomas WG, Mendelsohn FA. Angiotensin receptors: form and function and distribution. *Int J Biochem Cell Biol*. 2003;35:774-779.
175. Katovich MJ, Grobe JL, Raizada MK. Angiotensin-(1-7) as an antihypertensive, antifibrotic target. *Curr Hypertens Rep*. 2008;10:227-232.
176. Arima S, Ito S. New insights into actions of the renin-angiotensin system in the kidney: concentrating on the Ang II receptors and the newly described Ang-(1-7) and its receptor. *Semin Nephrol*. 2001;21:535-543.
177. Navar LG, Inscho EW, Majid SA, et al. Paracrine regulation of the renal microcirculation. *Physiol Rev*. 1996;76:425-536.
178. Pagtalunan ME, Rasch R, Rennke HG, et al. Morphometric analysis of effects of angiotensin II on glomerular structure in rats. *Am J Physiol*. 1995;268:F82-F88.
179. Duke LM, Widdop RE, Kett MM, et al. AT(2) receptors mediate tonic renal medullary vasoconstriction in renovascular hypertension. *Br J Pharmacol*. 2005;144:486-492.
180. Zhao D, Navar LG. Acute angiotensin II infusions elicit pressure natriuresis in mice and reduce distal fractional sodium reabsorption. *Hypertension*. 2008;52:137-142.
181. Cogan MG. Angiotensin II: a powerful controller of sodium transport in the early proximal tubule. *Hypertension*. 1990;15:451-458.
182. Quan A, Baum M. Endogenous angiotensin II modulates rat proximal tubule transport with acute changes in extracellular volume. *Am J Physiol*. 1998;275:F74-F78.
183. Xu L, Dixit MP, Nullmeyer KD, et al. Regulation of Na+/H+ exchanger-NHE3 by angiotensin-II in OKP cells. *Biochim Biophys Acta*. 2006;1758:519-526.
184. Zhou Y, Boron WF. Role of endogenously secreted angiotensin II in the CO2-induced stimulation of HCO3 reabsorption by renal proximal tubules. *Am J Physiol Renal Physiol*. 2008;294:F245-F252.
185. Seldin DW, Preisig PA, Alpern RJ. Regulation of proximal reabsorption by effective arterial blood volume. *Semin Nephrol*. 1991;11:212-219.
186. Wang T, Giebisch G. Effects of angiotensin II on electrolyte transport in the early and late distal tubule in rat kidney. *Am J Physiol*. 1996;271:F143-F149.
187. Levine DZ, Iacovitti M, Buckman S, et al. Role of angiotensin II in dietary modulation of rat late distal tubule bicarbonate flux in vivo. *J Clin Invest*. 1996;97:120-125.
188. Loffing J, Korbmacher C. Regulated sodium transport in the renal connecting tubule (CNT) via the epithelial sodium channel (ENaC). *Pflugers Arch*. 2009;458:111-135.
189. Goodfriend TL. Aldosterone—a hormone of cardiovascular adaptation and maladaptation. *J Clin Hypertens (Greenwich)*. 2006;8:133-139.
190. Rad AK, Balment RJ, Ashton N. Rapid natriuretic action of aldosterone in the rat. *J Appl Physiol*. 2005;98:423-428.
191. Williams GH. Aldosterone biosynthesis, regulation, and classical mechanism of action. *Heart Fail Rev*. 2005;10:7-13.
192. Rossier BC. Hormonal regulation of the epithelial sodium channel ENaC: N or P(o)? *J Gen Physiol*. 2002;120:67-70.
193. Gumz ML, Popp MP, Wingo CS, et al. Early transcriptional effects of aldosterone in a mouse inner medullary collecting duct cell line. *Am J Physiol Renal Physiol*. 2003;285:F664-F673.
194. Gumz ML, Stow LR, Lynch IJ, et al. The circadian clock protein Period 1 regulates expression of the renal epithelial sodium channel in mice. *J Clin Invest*. 2009;119:2423-2434.
195. Welling PA, Chang YP, Delpire E, et al. Multigene kinase network, kidney transport, and salt in essential hypertension. *Kidney Int*. 2010;77:1063-1069.
196. Hall JE, Brands MW, Henegar JR. Angiotensin II and long-term arterial pressure regulation: the overriding dominance of the kidney. *J Am Soc Nephrol*. 1999;10(suppl 12):S258-S265.
197. Schiffrin EL. Effects of aldosterone on the vasculature. *Hypertension*. 2006;47:312-318.
198. Robertson GL. Physiology of ADH secretion. *Kidney Int Suppl*. 1987;21:S20-S26.
199. Fujita N, Ishikawa SE, Sasaki S, et al. Role of water channel AQP-CD in water retention in SIADH and cirrhotic rats. *Am J Physiol*. 1995;269:F926-F931.
200. Bankir L. Antidiuretic action of vasopressin: quantitative aspects and interaction between V1a and V2 receptor–mediated effects. *Cardiovasc Res*. 2001;51:372-390.
201. Brown D, Hasler U, Nunes P, et al. Phosphorylation events and the modulation of aquaporin 2 cell surface expression. *Curr Opin Nephrol Hypertens*. 2008;17:491-498.
202. Nielsen S, Kwon TH, Frokiaer J, et al. Regulation and dysregulation of aquaporins in water balance disorders. *J Intern Med*. 2007;261:53-64.
203. Yang B, Bankir L. Urea and urine concentrating ability: new insights from studies in mice. *Am J Physiol Renal Physiol*. 2005;288:F881-F896.
204. Bankir L, Fernandes S, Bardoux P, et al. Vasopressin-V2 receptor stimulation reduces sodium excretion in healthy humans. *J Am Soc Nephrol*. 2005;16:1920-1928.
205. Cowley Jr AW. Control of the renal medullary circulation by vasopressin V1 and V2 receptors in the rat. *Exp Physiol*. 2000;85(Spec No):223S-231S.
206. Wilkins Jr FC, Alberola A, Mizelle HL, et al. Systemic hemodynamics and renal function during long-term pathophysiological increases in circulating endothelin. *Am J Physiol*. 1995;268:R375-R381.
207. Aoyagi T, Izumi Y, Hiroyama M, et al. Vasopressin regulates the renin-angiotensin-aldosterone system via V1a receptors in macula densa cells. *Am J Physiol Renal Physiol*. 2008;295:F100-F107.
208. Serradeil-Le GC, Wagnon J, Valette G, et al. Nonpeptide vasopressin receptor antagonists: development of selective and orally active V1a, V2 and V1b receptor ligands. *Prog Brain Res*. 2002;139:197-210.
209. Maybauer MO, Maybauer DM, Enkhbaatar P, et al. Physiology of the vasopressin receptors. *Best Pract Res Clin Anaesthesiol*. 2008;22:253-263.
210. Huot SJ, Hansson JH, Dey H, et al. Utility of captopril renal scans for detecting renal artery stenosis. *Arch Intern Med*. 2002;162:1981-1984.

211. Cheng CP, Igarashi Y, Klopfenstein HS, et al. Effect of vasopressin on left ventricular performance. *Am J Physiol.* 1993;264:H53-H60.

212. Hiroyama M, Wang S, Aoyagi T, et al. Vasopressin promotes cardiomyocyte hypertrophy via the vasopressin V_{1A} receptor in neonatal mice. *Eur J Pharmacol.* 2007;559:89-97.

213. Bishara B, Shiekh H, Karram T, et al. Effects of novel vasopressin receptor antagonists on renal function and cardiac hypertrophy in rats with experimental congestive heart failure. *J Pharmacol Exp Ther.* 2008;326:414-422.

214. Andersen SE, Engstrom T, Bie P. Effects on renal sodium and potassium excretion of vasopressin and oxytocin in conscious dogs. *Acta Physiol Scand.* 1992;145:267-274.

215. Inaba M, Katayama S, Itabashi A, et al. Effects of arginine vasopressin on blood pressure and renal prostaglandin E_2 in rabbits. *Endocrinol Jpn.* 1991;38:505-509.

216. Walter SJ, Tennakoon V, McClune JA, et al. Role of volume status in vasopressin-induced natriuresis: studies in Brattleboro rats. *J Endocrinol.* 1996;151:49-54.

217. Holmes CL, Landry DW, Granton JT. Science review: vasopressin and the cardiovascular system part 1—receptor physiology. *Crit Care.* 2003;7:427-434.

218. Nasrallah R, Clark J, Hebert RL. Prostaglandins in the kidney: developments since Y2K. *Clin Sci (Lond).* 2007;113:297-311.

219. Hao CM, Breyer MD. Physiological regulation of prostaglandins in the kidney. *Annu Rev Physiol.* 2008;70:357-377.

220. Kis B, Snipes JA, Busija DW. Acetaminophen and the cyclooxygenase-3 puzzle: sorting out facts, fictions, and uncertainties. *J Pharmacol Exp Ther.* 2005;315:1-7.

221. Flier S, Buhre W. Selective COX-2 inhibitors: new insights into mechanisms of side effects? *Crit Care Med.* 2008;36:2694-2695.

222. Simmons DL, Botting RM, Hla T. Cyclooxygenase isozymes: the biology of prostaglandin synthesis and inhibition. *Pharmacol Rev.* 2004;56:387-437.

223. Kramer BK, Kammerl MC, Komhoff M. Renal cyclooxygenase-2 (COX-2). Physiological, pathophysiological, and clinical implications. *Kidney Blood Press Res.* 2004;27:43-62.

224. Bonilla-Felix M. Development of water transport in the collecting duct. *Am J Physiol Renal Physiol.* 2004;287:F1093-F1101.

225. Laffi G, La Villa G, Pinzani M, et al. Arachidonic acid derivatives and renal function in liver cirrhosis. *Semin Nephrol.* 1997;17:530-548.

226. Perazella MA, Eras J. Are selective COX-2 inhibitors nephrotoxic? *Am J Kidney Dis.* 2000;35:937-940.

227. Haas JA, Hammond TG, Granger JP, et al. Mechanism of natriuresis during intrarenal infusion of prostaglandins. *Am J Physiol.* 1984;247:F475-F479.

228. Bonvalet JP, Pradelles P, Farman N. Segmental synthesis and actions of prostaglandins along the nephron. *Am J Physiol.* 1987;253:F377-F387.

229. Rubinger D, Wald H, Scherzer P, et al. Renal sodium handling and stimulation of medullary Na-K-ATPase during blockade of prostaglandin synthesis. *Prostaglandins.* 1990;39:179-194.

230. Breyer MD, Hao C, Qi Z. Cyclooxygenase-2 selective inhibitors and the kidney. *Curr Opin Crit Care.* 2001;7:393-400.

231. Qi Z, Hao CM, Langenbach RI, et al. Opposite effects of cyclooxygenase-1 and -2 activity on the pressor response to angiotensin II. *J Clin Invest.* 2002;110:61-69.

232. Richards AM. Natriuretic peptides: update on peptide release, bioactivity, and clinical use. *Hypertension.* 2007;50:25-30.

233. Silver MA. The natriuretic peptide system: kidney and cardiovascular effects. *Curr Opin Nephrol Hypertens.* 2006;15:14-21.

234. Abassi Z, Karram T, Ellaham S, et al. Implications of the natriuretic peptide system in the pathogenesis of heart failure: diagnostic and therapeutic importance. *Pharmacol Ther.* 2004;102:223-241.

235. Houben AJ, van der Zander K, de Leeuw PW. Vascular and renal actions of brain natriuretic peptide in man: physiology and pharmacology. *Fundam Clin Pharmacol.* 2005;19:411-419.

236. Scotland RS, Ahluwalia A, Hobbs AJ. C-type natriuretic peptide in vascular physiology and disease. *Pharmacol Ther.* 2005;105:85-93.

237. Curry FR. Atrial natriuretic peptide: an essential physiological regulator of transvascular fluid, protein transport, and plasma volume. *J Clin Invest.* 2005;115:1458-1461.

238. Schreier B, Borner S, Volker K, et al. The heart communicates with the endothelium through the guanylyl cyclase-A receptor: acute handling of intravascular volume in response to volume expansion. *Endocrinology.* 2008;149:4193-4199.

239. Kuhn M, Volker K, Schwarz K, et al. The natriuretic peptide/guanylyl cyclase—a system functions as a stress-responsive regulator of angiogenesis in mice. *J Clin Invest.* 2009;119:2019-2030.

240. Sagnella GA. Measurement and significance of circulating natriuretic peptides in cardiovascular disease. *Clin Sci (Lond).* 1998;95:519-529.

241. Davidson NC, Struthers AD. Brain natriuretic peptide. *J Hypertens.* 1994;12:329-336.

242. Cowie MR, Jourdain P, Maisel A, et al. Clinical applications of B-type natriuretic peptide (BNP) testing. *Eur Heart J.* 2003;24:1710-1718.

243. Hall C. Essential biochemistry and physiology of (NT-pro)BNP. *Eur J Heart Fail.* 2004;6:257-260.

244. Mensah GA. Healthy endothelium: the scientific basis for cardiovascular health promotion and chronic disease prevention. *Vascul Pharmacol.* 2007;46:310-314.

245. Pollock JS, Pollock DM. Endothelin and NOS1/nitric oxide signaling and regulation of sodium homeostasis. *Curr Opin Nephrol Hypertens.* 2008;17:70-75.

246. Kohan DE. The renal medullary endothelin system in control of sodium and water excretion and systemic blood pressure. *Curr Opin Nephrol Hypertens.* 2006;15:34-40.

247. Ohkita M, Takaoka M, Matsumura Y. Drug discovery for overcoming chronic kidney disease (CKD): the endothelin ET B receptor/nitric oxide system functions as a protective factor in CKD. *J Pharmacol Sci.* 2009;109:7-13.

248. Dhaun N, Goddard J, Webb DJ. The endothelin system and its antagonism in chronic kidney disease. *J Am Soc Nephrol.* 2006;17:943-955.

249. Levin ER. Endothelins. *N Engl J Med.* 1995;333:356-363.

250. Barton M, Yanagisawa M. Endothelin: 20 years from discovery to therapy. *Can J Physiol Pharmacol.* 2008;86:485-498.

251. Wypij DM, Nichols JS, Novak PJ, et al. Role of mast cell chymase in the extracellular processing of big-endothelin-1 to endothelin-1 in the perfused rat lung. *Biochem Pharmacol.* 1992;43:845-853.

252. Seyrantepe V, Hinek A, Peng J, et al. Enzymatic activity of lysosomal carboxypeptidase (cathepsin) A is required for proper elastic fiber formation and inactivation of endothelin-1. *Circulation.* 2008;117:1973-1981.

253. Sorokin A, Kohan DE. Physiology and pathology of endothelin-1 in renal mesangium. *Am J Physiol Renal Physiol.* 2003;285:F579-F589.

254. Kohan DE. Biology of endothelin receptors in the collecting duct. *Kidney Int.* 2009;76:481-486.

255. Katoh T, Chang H, Uchida S, et al. Direct effects of endothelin in the rat kidney. *Am J Physiol.* 1990;258:F397-F402.

256. Tsuchiya K, Naruse M, Sanaka T, et al. Renal and hemodynamic effects of endothelin in anesthetized dogs. *Am J Hypertens.* 1990;3:792-795.

257. Stacy DL, Scott JW, Granger JP. Control of renal function during intrarenal infusion of endothelin. *Am J Physiol.* 1990;258:F1232-F1236.

258. Gurbanov K, Rubinstein I, Hoffman A, et al. Differential regulation of renal regional blood flow by endothelin-1. *Am J Physiol.* 1996;271:F1166-F1172.

259. Kon V, Yoshioka T, Fogo A, et al. Glomerular actions of endothelin in vivo. *J Clin Invest.* 1989;83:1762-1767.

260. Hoffman A, Haramati A, Dalal I, et al. Diuretic-natriuretic actions and pressor effects of big-endothelin (1-39) in phosphoramidon-treated rats. *Proc Soc Exp Biol Med.* 1994;205:168-173.

261. Gariepy CE, Ohuchi T, Williams SC, et al. Salt-sensitive hypertension in endothelin-B receptor–deficient rats. *J Clin Invest.* 2000;105:925-933.

262. Oishi R, Nonoguchi H, Tomita K, et al. Endothelin-1 inhibits AVP-stimulated osmotic water permeability in rat inner medullary collecting duct. *Am J Physiol.* 1991;261:F951-F956.

263. Abassi ZA, Ellahham S, Winaver J, et al. The intrarenal endothelin system and hypertension. *News Physiol Sci.* 2001;16:152-156.

264. Herrera M, Garvin JL. A high-salt diet stimulates thick ascending limb eNOS expression by raising medullary osmolality and increasing release of endothelin-1. *Am J Physiol Renal Physiol.* 2005;288:F58-F64.

265. Mount PF, Power DA. Nitric oxide in the kidney: functions and regulation of synthesis. *Acta Physiol (Oxf).* 2006;187:433-446.

266. Bryan NS, Bian K, Murad F. Discovery of the nitric oxide signaling pathway and targets for drug development. *Front Biosci.* 2009;14:1-18.

267. Carey RM, Jin X, Wang Z, et al. Nitric oxide: a physiological mediator of the type 2 (AT_2) angiotensin receptor. *Acta Physiol Scand.* 2000;168:65-71.

268. Salazar FJ, Alberola A, Pinilla JM, et al. Salt-induced increase in arterial pressure during nitric oxide synthesis inhibition. *Hypertension.* 1993;22:49-55.

269. Abassi Z, Gurbanov K, Rubinstein I, et al. Regulation of intrarenal blood flow in experimental heart failure: role of endothelin and nitric oxide. *Am J Physiol.* 1998;274:F766-F774.

270. Tolins JP, Shultz PJ. Endogenous nitric oxide synthesis determines sensitivity to the pressor effect of salt. *Kidney Int.* 1994;46:230-236.

271. Ikeda Y, Saito K, Kim JI, et al. Nitric oxide synthase isoform activities in kidney of Dahl salt-sensitive rats. *Hypertension.* 1995;26:1030-1034.

272. Hu L, Manning Jr RD. Role of nitric oxide in regulation of long-term pressure-natriuresis relationship in Dahl rats. *Am J Physiol.* 1995;268:H2375-H2383.

273. Wilcox CS, Welch WJ. TGF and nitric oxide: effects of salt intake and salt-sensitive hypertension. *Kidney Int Suppl.* 1996;55:S9-S13.

274. Herrera M, Hong NJ, Ortiz PA, et al. Endothelin-1 inhibits thick ascending limb transport via Akt-stimulated nitric oxide production. *J Biol Chem.* 2009;284:1454-1460.

275. Garcia NH, Pomposiello SI, Garvin JL. Nitric oxide inhibits ADH-stimulated osmotic water permeability in cortical collecting ducts. *Am J Physiol*. 1996;270:F206-F210.

276. Madeddu P, Emanueli C, El-Dahr S. Mechanisms of disease: the tissue kallikrein-kinin system in hypertension and vascular remodeling. *Nat Clin Pract Nephrol*. 2007;3:208-221.

277. Kakoki M, Smithies O. The kallikrein-kinin system in health and in diseases of the kidney. *Kidney Int*. 2009;75:1019-1030.

278. Cachofeiro V, Nasjletti A. Increased vascular responsiveness to bradykinin in kidneys of spontaneously hypertensive rats. Effect of *N* omega-nitro-L-arginine. *Hypertension*. 1991;18:683-688.

279. Souza Dos Santos RA, Passaglio KT, Pesquero JB, et al. Interactions between angiotensin-(1-7), kinins, and angiotensin II in kidney and blood vessels. *Hypertension*. 2001;38:660-664.

280. Sivritas SH, Ploth DW, Fitzgibbon WR. Blockade of renal medullary bradykinin B2 receptors increases tubular sodium reabsorption in rats fed a normal-salt diet. *Am J Physiol Renal Physiol*. 2008;295:F811-F817.

281. Liu YH, Yang XP, Sharov VG, et al. Effects of angiotensin-converting enzyme inhibitors and angiotensin II type 1 receptor antagonists in rats with heart failure. Role of kinins and angiotensin II type 2 receptors. *J Clin Invest*. 1997;99:1926-1935.

282. Kitamura K, Sakata J, Kangawa K, et al. Cloning and characterization of cDNA encoding a precursor for human adrenomedullin. *Biochem Biophys Res Commun*. 1993;194:720-725.

283. Kitamura K, Eto T. Adrenomedullin—physiological regulator of the cardiovascular system or biochemical curiosity? *Curr Opin Nephrol Hypertens*. 1997;6:80-87.

284. Kitamura K, Kangawa K, Eto T. Adrenomedullin and PAMP: discovery, structures, and cardiovascular functions. *Microsc Res Tech*. 2002;57:3-13.

285. Hanna FW, Buchanan KD. Adrenomedullin: a novel cardiovascular regulatory peptide. *QJM*. 1996;89:881-884.

286. Mukoyama M, Sugawara A, Nagae T, et al. Role of adrenomedullin and its receptor system in renal pathophysiology. *Peptides*. 2001;22:1925-1931.

287. Schell DA, Vari RC, Samson WK. Adrenomedullin: a newly discovered hormone controlling fluid and electrolyte homeostasis. *Trends Endocrinol Metab*. 1996;7:7-13.

288. Rademaker MT, Cameron VA, Charles CJ, et al. Adrenomedullin and heart failure. *Regul Pept*. 2003;112:51-60.

289. Hirata Y, Hayakawa H, Suzuki Y, et al. Mechanisms of adrenomedullin-induced vasodilation in the rat kidney. *Hypertension*. 1995;25:790-795.

290. Majid DS, Kadowitz PJ, Coy DH, et al. Renal responses to intra-arterial administration of adrenomedullin in dogs. *Am J Physiol*. 1996;270:F200-F205.

291. Miura K, Ebara T, Okumura M, et al. Attenuation of adrenomedullin-induced renal vasodilatation by NG-nitro L-arginine but not glibenclamide. *Br J Pharmacol*. 1995;115:917-924.

292. Jougasaki M, Aarhus LL, Heublein DM, et al. Role of prostaglandins and renal nerves in the renal actions of adrenomedullin. *Am J Physiol*. 1997;272:F260-F266.

293. Lisy O, Jougasaki M, Schirger JA, et al. Neutral endopeptidase inhibition potentiates the natriuretic actions of adrenomedullin. *Am J Physiol*. 1998;275:F410-F414.

294. Taylor MM, Samson WK. Adrenomedullin and the integrative physiology of fluid and electrolyte balance. *Microsc Res Tech*. 2002;57:105-109.

295. Nishikimi T. Adrenomedullin in the kidney—renal physiological and pathophysiological roles. *Curr Med Chem*. 2007;14:1689-1699.

296. Bell D, McDermott BJ. Intermedin (adrenomedullin-2): a novel counter-regulatory peptide in the cardiovascular and renal systems. *Br J Pharmacol*. 2008;153(suppl 1):S247-S262.

297. Ashton N. Renal and vascular actions of urotensin II. *Kidney Int*. 2006;70:624-629.

298. Shenouda A, Douglas SA, Ohlstein EH, et al. Localization of urotensin-II immunoreactivity in normal human kidneys and renal carcinoma. *J Histochem Cytochem*. 2002;50:885-889.

299. Charles CJ, Rademaker MT, Richards AM, et al. Urotensin II: evidence for cardiac, hepatic and renal production. *Peptides*. 2005;26:2211-2214.

300. Richards AM, Charles C. Urotensin II in the cardiovascular system. *Peptides*. 2004;25:1795-1802.

301. Ovcharenko E, Abassi Z, Rubinstein I, et al. Renal effects of human urotensin-II in rats with experimental congestive heart failure. *Nephrol Dial Transplant*. 2006;21:1205-1211.

302. Zhang AY, Chen YF, Zhang DX, et al. Urotensin II is a nitric oxide–dependent vasodilator and natriuretic peptide in the rat kidney. *Am J Physiol Renal Physiol*. 2003;285:F792-F798.

303. Song W, Abdel-Razik AE, Lu W, et al. Urotensin II and renal function in the rat. *Kidney Int*. 2006;69:1360-1368.

304. Douglas SA, Dhanak D, Johns DG. From "gills to pills": urotensin-II as a regulator of mammalian cardiorenal function. *Trends Pharmacol Sci*. 2004;25:76-85

304a.Clarkson EM, Raw SM, de Wardener HE. Two natriuretic substances in extracts of urine from normal man when salt-depleted and salt-loaded. *Kindney Int*. 1976;10:381-394

304b.Clarkson EM, Raw SM, De Wardener HE. Further observations on a low-molecular-weight natriuretic substance in the urine of normal man. *Kidney Int*. 1979;16:710-721.

305. Bagrov AY, Shapiro JI, Fedorova OV. Endogenous cardiotonic steroids: physiology, pharmacology, and novel therapeutic targets. *Pharmacol Rev*. 2009;61:9-38.

306. Blaustein MP. Endogenous ouabain: role in the pathogenesis of hypertension. *Kidney Int*. 1996;49:1748-1753.

307. Bagrov AY, Shapiro JI. Endogenous digitalis: pathophysiologic roles and therapeutic applications. *Nat Clin Pract Nephrol*. 2008;4:378-392.

308. Hazelwood RL. The pancreatic polypeptide (PP-fold) family: gastrointestinal, vascular, and feeding behavioral implications. *Proc Soc Exp Biol Med*. 1993;202:44-63.

309. Larhammar D. Evolution of neuropeptide Y, peptide YY and pancreatic polypeptide. *Regul Pept*. 1996;62:1-11.

310. Winaver J, Abassi Z. Role of neuropeptide Y in the regulation of kidney function. *EXS*. 2006;(95):123-132.

311. Persson PB, Gimpl G, Lang RE. Importance of neuropeptide Y in the regulation of kidney function. *Ann N Y Acad Sci*. 1990;611:156-165.

312. Bischoff A, Michel MC. Renal effects of neuropeptide Y. *Pflugers Arch*. 1998;435:443-453.

313. Callanan EY, Lee EW, Tilan JU, et al. Renal and cardiac neuropeptide Y and NPY receptors in a rat model of congestive heart failure. *Am J Physiol Renal Physiol*. 2007;293:F1811-F1817.

314. Smyth DD, Wilson JR, Seidlitz E, et al. Effects of central and peripheral neuropeptide Y on sodium and water excretion in the rat. *Physiol Behav*. 1989;46:9-11.

315. Echtenkamp SF, Dandridge PF. Renal actions of neuropeptide Y in the primate. *Am J Physiol*. 1989;256:F524-F531.

316. Principe A, Melgar-Lesmes P, Fernandez-Varo G, et al. The hepatic apelin system: a new therapeutic target for liver disease. *Hepatology*. 2008;48:1193-1201.

317. Hus-Citharel A, Bouby N, Frugiere A, et al. Effect of apelin on glomerular hemodynamic function in the rat kidney. *Kidney Int*. 2008;74:486-494.

318. Ishida J, Hashimoto T, Hashimoto Y, et al. Regulatory roles for APJ, a seven-transmembrane receptor related to angiotensin-type 1 receptor in blood pressure in vivo. *J Biol Chem*. 2004;279:26274-26279.

319. Zhong JC, Yu XY, Huang Y, et al. Apelin modulates aortic vascular tone via endothelial nitric oxide synthase phosphorylation pathway in diabetic mice. *Cardiovasc Res*. 2007;74:388-395.

320. Machnik A, Neuhofer W, Jantsch J, et al. Macrophages regulate salt-dependent volume and blood pressure by a vascular endothelial growth factor-C–dependent buffering mechanism. *Nat Med*. 2009;15:545-552.

321. Schafflhuber M, Volpi N, Dahlmann A, et al. Mobilization of osmotically inactive Na$^+$ by growth and by dietary salt restriction in rats. *Am J Physiol Renal Physiol*. 2007;292:F1490-F1500.

322. Titze J, Lang R, Ilies C, et al. Osmotically inactive skin Na$^+$ storage in rats. *Am J Physiol Renal Physiol*. 2003;285:F1108-F1117.

323. Titze J, Ritz E. Salt and its effect on blood pressure and target organ damage: new pieces in an old puzzle. *J Nephrol*. 2009;22:177-189.

324. Titze J. Water-free Na$^+$ retention: interaction with hypertension and tissue hydration. *Blood Purif*. 2008;26:95-99.

325. Titze J, Luft FC, Bauer K, et al. Extrarenal Na$^+$ balance, volume, and blood pressure homeostasis in intact and ovariectomized deoxycorticosterone-acetate salt rats. *Hypertension*. 2006;47:1101-1107.

326. Titze J, Shakibaei M, Schafflhuber M, et al. Glycosaminoglycan polymerization may enable osmotically inactive Na$^+$ storage in the skin. *Am J Physiol Heart Circ Physiol*. 2004;287:H203-H208.

327. Ziomber A, Machnik A, Dahlmann A, et al. Sodium-, potassium-, chloride-, and bicarbonate-related effects on blood pressure and electrolyte homeostasis in deoxycorticosterone acetate-treated rats. *Am J Physiol Renal Physiol*. 2008;295:F1752-F1763.

328. Go WY, Liu X, Roti MA, et al. NFAT5/TonEBP mutant mice define osmotic stress as a critical feature of the lymphoid microenvironment. *Proc Natl Acad Sci U S A*. 2004;101:10673-10678.

329. Marvar PJ, Gordon FJ, Harrison DG. Blood pressure control: salt gets under your skin. *Nat Med*. 2009;15:487-488.

330. Rivkees SA. Differentiating appropriate antidiuretic hormone secretion, inappropriate antidiuretic hormone secretion and cerebral salt wasting: the common, uncommon, and misnamed. *Curr Opin Pediatr*. 2008;20:448-452.

331. Sherlock M, O'Sullivan E, Agha A, et al. Incidence and pathophysiology of severe hyponatraemia in neurosurgical patients. *Postgrad Med J*. 2009;85:171-175.

332. Sterns RH, Silver SM. Cerebral salt wasting versus SIADH: what difference? *J Am Soc Nephrol*. 2008;19:194-196.

333. Hotchkiss RS, Karl IE. The pathophysiology and treatment of sepsis. *N Engl J Med*. 2003;348:138-150.

334. Koomans HA. Pathophysiology of oedema in idiopathic nephrotic syndrome. *Nephrol Dial Transplant*. 2003;18(suppl 6):vi30-vi32.

335. Rodriguez-Iturbe B, Herrera-Acosta J, Johnson RJ. Interstitial inflammation, sodium retention, and the pathogenesis of nephrotic edema: a unifying hypothesis. *Kidney Int*. 2002;62:1379-1384.

336. Blantz RC. Pathophysiology of pre-renal azotemia. *Kidney Int*. 1998;53:512-523.

337. Carvounis CP, Nisar S, Guro-Razuman S. Significance of the fractional excretion of urea in the differential diagnosis of acute renal failure. *Kidney Int*. 2002;62:2223-2229.

338. Diskin CJ, Stokes TJ, Dansby LM, et al. The evolution of the fractional excretion of urea as a diagnostic tool in oliguric states. *Am J Kidney Dis*. 2008;51:869-870.

339. Pepin MN, Bouchard J, Legault L, et al. Diagnostic performance of fractional excretion of urea and fractional excretion of sodium in the evaluations of patients with acute kidney injury with or without diuretic treatment. *Am J Kidney Dis*. 2007;50:566-573.

340. Andrews FJ, Nolan JP. Critical care in the emergency department: monitoring the critically ill patient. *Emerg Med J*. 2006;23:561-564.

341. Pinsky MR. Hemodynamic monitoring over the past 10 years. *Crit Care*. 2006;10:117.

342. Cotter G, Metra M, Milo-Cotter O, et al. Fluid overload in acute heart failure—re-distribution and other mechanisms beyond fluid accumulation. *Eur J Heart Fail*. 2008;10:165-169.

343. Hartog C, Reinhart K. CONTRA: hydroxyethyl starch solutions are unsafe in critically ill patients. *Intensive Care Med*. 2009;35:1337-1342.

344. Kashani A, Landaverde C, Medici V, et al. Fluid retention in cirrhosis: pathophysiology and management. *QJM*. 2008;101:71-85.

345. Crone C, Christensen O. Transcapillary transport of small solutes and water. *Int Rev Physiol*. 1979;18:149-213.

346. Magrini F, Niarchos AP. Hemodynamic effects of massive peripheral edema. *Am Heart J*. 1983;105:90-97.

347. Intaglietta M, Zweifach BW. Microcirculatory basis of fluid exchange. *Adv Biol Med Phys*. 1974;15:111-159.

348. Messerli FH. Calcium antagonists in hypertension: from hemodynamics to outcomes. *Am J Hypertens*. 2002;15:94S-97S.

349. Fauchald P. Colloid osmotic pressures, plasma volume and interstitial fluid volume in patients with heart failure. *Scand J Clin Lab Invest*. 1985;45:701-706.

350. Guyton AC, Taylor AE, Brace RA. A synthesis of interstitial fluid regulation and lymph formation. *Fed Proc*. 1976;35:1881-1885.

351. Singer DR, Markandu ND, Buckley MG, et al. Blood pressure and endocrine responses to changes in dietary sodium intake in cardiac transplant recipients. Implications for the control of sodium balance. *Circulation*. 1994;89:1153-1159.

352. Iwatsuki S, Popovtzer MM, Corman JL, et al. Recovery from "hepatorenal syndrome" after orthotopic liver transplantation. *N Engl J Med*. 1973;289:1155-1159.

353. Schrier RW. Water and sodium retention in edematous disorders: role of vasopressin and aldosterone. *Am J Med*. 2006;119:S47-S53.

354. Schrier RW. Decreased effective blood volume in edematous disorders: what does this mean? *J Am Soc Nephrol*. 2007;18:2028-2031.

355. Zucker IH, Wang W, Brandle M, et al. Neural regulation of sympathetic nerve activity in heart failure. *Prog Cardiovasc Dis*. 1995;37:397-414.

356. Thames MD, Kinugawa T, Smith ML, et al. Abnormalities of baroreflex control in heart failure. *J Am Coll Cardiol*. 1993;22:56A-60A.

357. Greenberg TT, Richmond WH, Stocking RA, et al. Impaired atrial receptor responses in dogs with heart failure due to tricuspid insufficiency and pulmonary artery stenosis. *Circ Res*. 1973;32:424-433.

358. Zucker IH, Earle AM, Gilmore JP. The mechanism of adaptation of left atrial stretch receptors in dogs with chronic congestive heart failure. *J Clin Invest*. 1977;60:323-331.

359. Goldsmith SR, Francis GS, Levine TB, et al. Regional blood flow response to orthostasis in patients with congestive heart failure. *J Am Coll Cardiol*. 1983;1:1391-1395.

360. Creager MA, Faxon DP, Rockwell SM, et al. The contribution of the renin-angiotensin system to limb vasoregulation in patients with heart failure: observations during orthostasis and alpha-adrenergic blockade. *Clin Sci (Lond)*. 1985;68:659-667.

361. Ferguson DW, Berg WJ, Roach PJ, et al. Effects of heart failure on baroreflex control of sympathetic neural activity. *Am J Cardiol*. 1992;69:523-531.

362. Zucker IH, Schultz HD, Li YF, et al. The origin of sympathetic outflow in heart failure: the roles of angiotensin II and nitric oxide. *Prog Biophys Mol Biol*. 2004;84:217-232.

363. Nishida Y, Ryan KL, Bishop VS. Angiotensin II modulates arterial baroreflex function via a central alpha 1–adrenoceptor mechanism in rabbits. *Am J Physiol*. 1995;269:R1009-R1016.

364. Dibner-Dunlap ME, Smith ML, Kinugawa T, et al. Enalaprilat augments arterial and cardiopulmonary baroreflex control of sympathetic nerve activity in patients with heart failure. *J Am Coll Cardiol*. 1996;27:358-364.

365. Zhu GQ, Gao L, Li Y, et al. AT$_1$ receptor mRNA antisense normalizes enhanced cardiac sympathetic afferent reflex in rats with chronic heart failure. *Am J Physiol Heart Circ Physiol*. 2004;287:H1828-H1835.

366. Wang WZ, Gao L, Pan YX, et al. AT$_1$ receptors in the nucleus tractus solitarii mediate the interaction between the baroreflex and the cardiac sympathetic afferent reflex in anesthetized rats. *Am J Physiol Regul Integr Comp Physiol*. 2007;292:R1137-R1145.

367. Gao L, Wang WZ, Wang W, et al. Imbalance of angiotensin type 1 receptor and angiotensin II type 2 receptor in the rostral ventrolateral medulla: potential mechanism for sympathetic overactivity in heart failure. *Hypertension*. 2008;52:708-714.

368. Krupicka J, Janota T, Kasalova Z, et al. Natriuretic peptides—physiology, pathophysiology and clinical use in heart failure. *Physiol Res*. 2009;58:171-177.

369. Edwards BS, Ackermann DM, Lee ME, et al. Identification of atrial natriuretic factor within ventricular tissue in hamsters and humans with congestive heart failure. *J Clin Invest*. 1988;81:82-86.

370. Saito Y, Nakao K, Arai H, et al. Augmented expression of atrial natriuretic polypeptide gene in ventricle of human failing heart. *J Clin Invest*. 1989;83:298-305.

371. Thibault G, Nemer M, Drouin J, et al. Ventricles as a major site of atrial natriuretic factor synthesis and release in cardiomyopathic hamsters with heart failure. *Circ Res*. 1989;65:71-82.

372. Cody RJ, Atlas SA, Laragh JH, et al. Atrial natriuretic factor in normal subjects and heart failure patients. Plasma levels and renal, hormonal, and hemodynamic responses to peptide infusion. *J Clin Invest*. 1986;78:1362-1374.

373. Scriven TA, Burnett Jr JC. Effects of synthetic atrial natriuretic peptide on renal function and renin release in acute experimental heart failure. *Circulation*. 1985;72:892-897.

374. Winaver J, Hoffman A, Burnett Jr JC, et al. Hormonal determinants of sodium excretion in rats with experimental high-output heart failure. *Am J Physiol*. 1988;254:R776-R784.

375. De Santo NG, Cirillo M, Perna A, et al. The kidney in heart failure. *Semin Nephrol*. 2005;25:404-407.

376. Bellomo R, Ronco C. The kidney in heart failure. *Kidney Int Suppl*. 1998;66:S58-S61.

377. Ichikawa I, Kon V, Pfeffer MA, et al. Role of angiotensin II in the altered renal function of heart failure. *Kidney Int Suppl*. 1987;20:S213-S215.

378. Nishikimi T, Frohlich ED. Glomerular hemodynamics in aortocaval fistula rats: role of renin-angiotensin system. *Am J Physiol*. 1993;264:R681-R686.

379. Suki WN. Renal hemodynamic consequences of angiotensin-converting enzyme inhibition in congestive heart failure. *Arch Intern Med*. 1989;149:669-673.

380. Packer M. Adaptive and maladaptive actions of angiotensin II in patients with severe congestive heart failure. *Am J Kidney Dis*. 1987;10:66-73.

381. Badr KF, Ichikawa I. Prerenal failure: a deleterious shift from renal compensation to decompensation. *N Engl J Med*. 1988;319:623-629.

382. Packer M, Lee WH, Medina N, et al. Functional renal insufficiency during long-term therapy with captopril and enalapril in severe chronic heart failure. *Ann Intern Med*. 1987;106:346-354.

383. Bennett WM, Bagby Jr GC, Antonovic JN, et al. Influence of volume expansion on proximal tubular sodium reabsorption in congestive heart failure. *Am Heart J*. 1973;85:55-64.

384. Johnston CI, Davis JO, Robb CA, et al. Plasma renin in chronic experimental heart failure and during renal sodium "escape" from mineralocorticoids. *Circ Res*. 1968;22:113-125.

385. Schneider EG, Dresser TP, Lynch RE, et al. Sodium reabsorption by proximal tubule of dogs with experimental heart failure. *Am J Physiol*. 1971;220:952-957.

386. Stumpe KO, Solle H, Klein H, et al. Mechanism of sodium and water retention in rats with experimental heart failure. *Kidney Int*. 1973;4:309-317.

387. Mandin H, Davidman M. Renal function in dogs with acute cardiac tamponade. *Am J Physiol*. 1978;234:F117-F122.

388. Auld RB, Alexander EA, Levinsky NG. Proximal tubular function in dogs with thoracic caval constriction. *J Clin Invest*. 1971;50:2150-2158.

389. Levy M. Effects of acute volume expansion and altered hemodynamics on renal tubular function in chronic caval dogs. *J Clin Invest*. 1972;51:922-938.

390. Friedler RM, Belleau LJ, Martino JA, et al. Hemodynamically induced natriuresis in the presence of sodium retention resulting from constriction of the thoracic inferior vena cava. *J Lab Clin Med*. 1967;69:565-583.

391. Damman K, Navis G, Voors AA, et al. Worsening renal function and prognosis in heart failure: systematic review and meta-analysis. *J Card Fail*. 2007;13:599-608.

392. Rea ME, Dunlap ME. Renal hemodynamics in heart failure: implications for treatment. *Curr Opin Nephrol Hypertens.* 2008;17:87-92.
393. Schrier RW, Abraham WT. Hormones and hemodynamics in heart failure. *N Engl J Med.* 1999;341:577-585.
394. Pagliaro P, Penna C. Rethinking the renin-angiotensin system and its role in cardiovascular regulation. *Cardiovasc Drugs Ther.* 2005;19:77-87.
395. Packer M. The neurohormonal hypothesis: a theory to explain the mechanism of disease progression in heart failure. *J Am Coll Cardiol.* 1992;20:248-254.
396. Chatterjee K. Neurohormonal activation in congestive heart failure and the role of vasopressin. *Am J Cardiol.* 2005;95:8B-13B.
397. Winaver J, Hoffman A, Abassi Z, et al. Does the heart's hormone, ANP, help in congestive heart failure?. *News Physiol Sci.* 1995;10:247-253.
398. Selektor Y, Weber KT. The salt-avid state of congestive heart failure revisited. *Am J Med Sci.* 2008;335:209-218.
399. Hirsch AT, Pinto YM, Schunkert H, et al. Potential role of the tissue renin-angiotensin system in the pathophysiology of congestive heart failure. *Am J Cardiol.* 1990;66:22D-30D.
400. Butler J, Forman DE, Abraham WT, et al. Relationship between heart failure treatment and development of worsening renal function among hospitalized patients. *Am Heart J.* 2004;147:331-338.
401. Weber KT, Swamynathan SK, Guntaka RV, et al. Angiotensin II and extracellular matrix homeostasis. *Int J Biochem Cell Biol.* 1999;31:395-403.
402. Kjaer A, Hesse B. Heart failure and neuroendocrine activation: diagnostic, prognostic and therapeutic perspectives. *Clin Physiol.* 2001;21:661-672.
403. Rosenkranz S. TGF-beta1 and angiotensin networking in cardiac remodeling. *Cardiovasc Res.* 2004;63:423-432.
404. Schafer A, Fraccarollo D, Tas P, et al. Endothelial dysfunction in congestive heart failure: ACE inhibition vs. angiotensin II antagonism. *Eur J Heart Fail.* 2004;6:151-159.
405. Cohn JN. ACE inhibition and vascular remodeling of resistance vessels: vascular compliance and cardiovascular implications. *Heart Dis.* 2000;2:S2-S6.
406. Tschope C, Schultheiss HP, Walther T. Multiple interactions between the renin-angiotensin and the kallikrein-kinin systems: role of ACE inhibition and AT$_1$ receptor blockade. *J Cardiovasc Pharmacol.* 2002;39:478-487.
407. Rudolph AE, Rocha R, McMahon EG. Aldosterone target organ protection by eplerenone. *Mol Cell Endocrinol.* 2004;217:229-238.
408. Delyani JA, Robinson EL, Rudolph AE. Effect of a selective aldosterone receptor antagonist in myocardial infarction. *Am J Physiol Heart Circ Physiol.* 2001;281:H647-H654.
409. Pitt B, Williams G, Remme W, et al. The EPHESUS trial: eplerenone in patients with heart failure due to systolic dysfunction complicating acute myocardial infarction. Eplerenone Post-AMI Heart Failure Efficacy and Survival Study. *Cardiovasc Drugs Ther.* 2001;15:79-87.
410. Pitt B, Zannad F, Remme WJ, et al. The effect of spironolactone on morbidity and mortality in patients with severe heart failure. Randomized Aldactone Evaluation Study Investigators. *N Engl J Med.* 1999;341:709-717.
411. Navar LG, Nishiyama A. Why are angiotensin concentrations so high in the kidney? *Curr Opin Nephrol Hypertens.* 2004;13:107-115.
412. Saccomani G, Mitchell KD, Navar LG. Angiotensin II stimulation of Na$^+$-H$^+$ exchange in proximal tubule cells. *Am J Physiol Renal Physiol.* 1990;258:F1188-F1195.
413. Geibel J, Giebisch G, Boron WF. Angiotensin II stimulates both Na$^+$-H$^+$ exchange and Na$^+$/HCO$_3^-$ cotransport in the rabbit proximal tubule. *Proc Natl Acad Sci U S A.* 1990;87:7917-7920.
414. Grassi G, Seravalle G, Quarti-Trevano F, et al. Sympathetic activation in congestive heart failure: evidence, consequences and therapeutic implications. *Curr Vasc Pharmacol.* 2009;7:137-145.
415. Davila DF, Nunez TJ, Odreman R, et al. Mechanisms of neurohormonal activation in chronic congestive heart failure: pathophysiology and therapeutic implications. *Int J Cardiol.* 2005;101:343-346.
416. Kaye D, Esler M. Sympathetic neuronal regulation of the heart in aging and heart failure. *Cardiovasc Res.* 2005;66:256-264.
417. Esler M, Lambert G, Brunner-La Rocca HP, et al. Sympathetic nerve activity and neurotransmitter release in humans: translation from pathophysiology into clinical practice. *Acta Physiol Scand.* 2003;177:275-284.
418. Bryan PM, Xu X, Dickey DM, et al. Renal hyporesponsiveness to atrial natriuretic peptide in congestive heart failure results from reduced atrial natriuretic peptide receptor concentrations. *Am J Physiol Renal Physiol.* 2007;292:F1636-F1644.
419. Kon V. Neural control of renal circulation. *Miner Electrolyte Metab.* 1989;15:33-43.
420. Villarreal D, Freeman RH, Johnson RA, et al. Effects of renal denervation on postprandial sodium excretion in experimental heart failure. *Am J Physiol.* 1994;266:R1599-R1604.
421. Lieverse AG, van Veldhuisen DJ, Smit AJ, et al. Renal and systemic hemodynamic effects of ibopamine in patients with mild to moderate congestive heart failure. *J Cardiovasc Pharmacol.* 1995;25:361-367.
422. Hillege HL, Girbes AR, de Kam PJ, et al. Renal function, neurohormonal activation, and survival in patients with chronic heart failure. *Circulation.* 2000;102:203-210.
423. Marenzi G, Lauri G, Guazzi M, et al. Cardiac and renal dysfunction in chronic heart failure: relation to neurohumoral activation and prognosis. *Am J Med Sci.* 2001;321:359-366.
424. Yusof AP, Yusoff NH, Suhaimi FW, et al. Role of supraspinal vasopressin neurones in the effects of atrial natriuretic peptide on sympathetic nerve activity. *Auton Neurosci.* 2009;148:50-54.
425. O'Tierney PF, Tse MY, Pang SC. Elevated renal norepinephrine in proANP gene–disrupted mice is associated with increased tyrosine hydroxylase expression in sympathetic ganglia. *Regul Pept.* 2007;143:90-96.
426. Kasama S, Toyama T, Kumakura H, et al. Effects of intravenous atrial natriuretic peptide on cardiac sympathetic nerve activity in patients with decompensated congestive heart failure. *J Nucl Med.* 2004;45:1108-1113.
427. Azevedo ER, Newton GE, Parker AB, et al. Sympathetic responses to atrial natriuretic peptide in patients with congestive heart failure. *J Cardiovasc Pharmacol.* 2000;35:129-135.
428. Feng QP, Hedner T, Hedner J, et al. Blunted renal response to atrial natriuretic peptide in congestive heart failure rats is reversed by the alpha 2–adrenergic agonist clonidine. *J Cardiovasc Pharmacol.* 1990;16:776-782.
429. Lohmeier TE, Reinhart GA, Mizelle HL, et al. Influence of the renal nerves on sodium excretion during progressive reductions in cardiac output. *Am J Physiol.* 1995;269:R678-R690.
430. Finley JJ, Konstam MA, Udelson JE. Arginine vasopressin antagonists for the treatment of heart failure and hyponatremia. *Circulation.* 2008;118:410-421.
431. Pruszczynski W, Vahanian A, Ardaillou R, et al. Role of antidiuretic hormone in impaired water excretion of patients with congestive heart failure. *J Clin Endocrinol Metab.* 1984;58:599-605.
432. Manthey J, Dietz R, Opherk D, et al. Baroreceptor-mediated release of vasopressin in patients with chronic congestive heart failure and defective sympathetic responsiveness. *Am J Cardiol.* 1992;70:224-228.
433. Bonjour JP, Malvin RL. Stimulation of ADH release by the renin-angiotensin system. *Am J Physiol.* 1970;218:1555-1559.
434. Henrich WL, Walker BR, Handelman WA, et al. Effects of angiotensin II on plasma antidiuretic hormone and renal water excretion. *Kidney Int.* 1986;30:503-508.
435. Bichet DG, Kortas C, Mettauer B, et al. Modulation of plasma and platelet vasopressin by cardiac function in patients with heart failure. *Kidney Int.* 1986;29:1188-1196.
436. Gegenhuber A, Struck J, Dieplinger B, et al. Comparative evaluation of B-type natriuretic peptide, mid-regional pro–A-type natriuretic peptide, mid-regional pro-adrenomedullin, and copeptin to predict 1-year mortality in patients with acute destabilized heart failure. *J Card Fail.* 2007;13:42-49.
437. Martin PY, Schrier RW. Sodium and water retention in heart failure: pathogenesis and treatment. *Kidney Int Suppl.* 1997;59:S57-S61.
438. Ishikawa SE, Schrier RW. Pathophysiological roles of arginine vasopressin and aquaporin-2 in impaired water excretion. *Clin Endocrinol (Oxf).* 2003;58:1-17.
439. Xu DL, Martin PY, Ohara M, et al. Upregulation of aquaporin-2 water channel expression in chronic heart failure rat. *J Clin Invest.* 1997;99:1500-1505.
440. Farmakis D, Filippatos G, Kremastinos DT, et al. Vasopressin and vasopressin antagonists in heart failure and hyponatremia. *Curr Heart Fail Rep.* 2008;5:91-96.
441. Verbalis JG. Vasopressin V$_2$ receptor antagonists. *J Mol Endocrinol.* 2002;29:1-9.
442. Meier-Kriesche H, Cibrik DM, Ojo AO, et al. Interaction between donor and recipient age in determining the risk of chronic renal allograft failure. *J Am Geriatr Soc.* 2002;50:14-17.
443. Ertl G, Bauersachs J. Endothelin receptor antagonists in heart failure: current status and future directions. *Drugs.* 2004;64:1029-1040.
444. Boerrigter G, Burnett JC. Endothelin in neurohormonal activation in heart failure. *Coron Artery Dis.* 2003;14:495-500.
445. Cody RJ, Haas GJ, Binkley PF, et al. Plasma endothelin correlates with the extent of pulmonary hypertension in patients with chronic congestive heart failure. *Circulation.* 1992;85:504-509.
446. Masson S, Latini R, Anand IS, et al. The prognostic value of big endothelin-1 in more than 2,300 patients with heart failure enrolled in the Valsartan Heart Failure Trial (Val-HeFT). *J Card Fail.* 2006;12:375-380.
447. Wei CM, Lerman A, Rodeheffer RJ, et al. Endothelin in human congestive heart failure. *Circulation.* 1994;89:1580-1586.
448. Zolk O, Quattek J, Sitzler G, et al. Expression of endothelin-1, endothelin-converting enzyme, and endothelin receptors in chronic heart failure. *Circulation.* 1999;99:2118-2123.
449. Lerman A, Kubo SH, Tschumperlin LK, et al. Plasma endothelin concentrations in humans with end-stage heart failure and after heart transplantation. *J Am Coll Cardiol.* 1992;20:849-853.

450. Gurbanov K, Rubinstein I, Hoffman A, et al. Bosentan improves renal regional blood flow in rats with experimental congestive heart failure. *Eur J Pharmacol.* 1996;310:193-196.
451. Qiu C, Ding SS, Hess P, et al. Endothelin mediates the altered renal hemodynamics associated with experimental congestive heart failure. *J Cardiovasc Pharmacol.* 2001;38:317-324.
452. Ding SS, Qiu C, Hess P, et al. Chronic endothelin receptor blockade prevents renal vasoconstriction and sodium retention in rats with chronic heart failure. *Cardiovasc Res.* 2002;53:963-970.
453. Burnett Jr JC, Kao PC, Hu DC, et al. Atrial natriuretic peptide elevation in congestive heart failure in the human. *Science.* 1986;231:1145-1147.
454. Raine AE, Erne P, Burgisser E, et al. Atrial natriuretic peptide and atrial pressure in patients with congestive heart failure. *N Engl J Med.* 1986;315:533-537.
455. Randa Abdel KM, Grace BD. Badawi NE: Plasma levels of adrenomedullin and atrial natriuretic peptide in patients with congestive heart failure of various etiologies. *Ital J Biochem.* 2007;56:18-27.
456. Hensen J, Abraham WT, Lesnefsky EJ, et al. Atrial natriuretic peptide kinetic studies in patients with cardiac dysfunction. *Kidney Int.* 1992;41:1333-1339.
457. Poulos JE, Gower Jr WR, Sullebarger JT, et al. Congestive heart failure: increased cardiac and extracardiac atrial natriuretic peptide gene expression. *Cardiovasc Res.* 1996;32:909-919.
458. Moe GW, Forster C, de Bold AJ, et al. Pharmacokinetics, hemodynamic, renal, and neurohormonal effects of atrial natriuretic factor in experimental heart failure. *Clin Invest Med.* 1990;13:111-118.
459. Eiskjaer H, Bagger JP, Danielsen H, et al. Attenuated renal excretory response to atrial natriuretic peptide in congestive heart failure in man. *Int J Cardiol.* 1991;33:61-74.
460. Hirsch AT, Creager MA, Dzau VJ. Relation of atrial natriuretic factor to vasoconstrictor hormones and regional blood flow in congestive heart failure. *Am J Cardiol.* 1989;63:211-216.
461. Kanamori T, Wada A, Tsutamoto T, et al. Possible regulation of renin release by ANP in dogs with heart failure. *Am J Physiol.* 1995;268:H2281-H2287.
462. Lohmeier TE, Mizelle HL, Reinhart GA, et al. Atrial natriuretic peptide and sodium homeostasis in compensated heart failure. *Am J Physiol.* 1996;271:R1353-R1363.
463. Stevens TL, Burnett Jr JC, Kinoshita M, et al. A functional role for endogenous atrial natriuretic peptide in a canine model of early left ventricular dysfunction. *J Clin Invest.* 1995;95:1101-1108.
464. Laragh JH. Atrial natriuretic hormone, the renin-aldosterone axis, and blood pressure–electrolyte homeostasis. *N Engl J Med.* 1985;313:1330-1340.
465. Harris PJ, Thomas D, Morgan TO. Atrial natriuretic peptide inhibits angiotensin-stimulated proximal tubular sodium and water reabsorption. *Nature.* 1987;326:697-698.
466. Wada A, Tsutamoto T, Matsuda Y, et al. Cardiorenal and neurohumoral effects of endogenous atrial natriuretic peptide in dogs with severe congestive heart failure using a specific antagonist for guanylate cyclase–coupled receptors. *Circulation.* 1994;89:2232-2240.
467. Charloux A, Piquard F, Doutreleau S, et al. Mechanisms of renal hyporesponsiveness to ANP in heart failure. *Eur J Clin Invest.* 2003;33:769-778.
468. Andreassi MG, Del RS, Palmieri C, et al. Up-regulation of "clearance" receptors in patients with chronic heart failure: a possible explanation for the resistance to biological effects of cardiac natriuretic hormones. *Eur J Heart Fail.* 2001;3:407-414.
469. Wegner M, Hirth-Dietrich C, Stasch JP. Role of neutral endopeptidase 24.11 in AV fistular rat model of heart failure. *Cardiovasc Res.* 1996;31:891-898.
470. Knecht M, Pagel I, Langenickel T, et al. Increased expression of renal neutral endopeptidase in severe heart failure. *Life Sci.* 2002;71:2701-2712.
471. Clerico A, Iervasi G, Del Chicca MG, et al. Circulating levels of cardiac natriuretic peptides (ANP and BNP) measured by highly sensitive and specific immunoradiometric assays in normal subjects and in patients with different degrees of heart failure. *J Endocrinol Invest.* 1998;21:170-179.
472. Sosa RE, Volpe M, Marion DN, et al. Relationship between renal hemodynamic and natriuretic effects of atrial natriuretic factor. *Am J Physiol.* 1986;250:F520-F524.
473. Abassi Z, Haramati A, Hoffman A, et al. Effect of converting-enzyme inhibition on renal response to ANF in rats with experimental heart failure. *Am J Physiol.* 1990;259:R84-R89.
474. Pettersson A, Hedner J, Hedner T. Relationship between renal sympathetic activity and diuretic effects of atrial natriuretic peptide (ANP) in the rat. *Acta Physiol Scand.* 1989;135:323-333.
475. Wei CM, Heublein DM, Perrella MA, et al. Natriuretic peptide system in human heart failure. *Circulation.* 1993;88:1004-1009.
476. Rademaker MT, Charles CJ, Espiner EA, et al. Natriuretic peptide responses to acute and chronic ventricular pacing in sheep. *Am J Physiol.* 1996;270:H594-H602.
477. Luchner A, Stevens TL, Borgeson DD, et al. Differential atrial and ventricular expression of myocardial BNP during evolution of heart failure. *Am J Physiol.* 1998;274:H1684-H1689.
478. Chang AM, Maisel AS, Hollander JE. Diagnosis of heart failure. *Heart Fail Clin.* 2009;5:25-35:vi.
479. de Sa DD, Chen HH. The role of natriuretic peptides in heart failure. *Curr Cardiol Rep.* 2008;10:182-189.
480. Clerico A, Fontana M, Zyw L, et al. Comparison of the diagnostic accuracy of brain natriuretic peptide (BNP) and the N-terminal part of the propeptide of BNP immunoassays in chronic and acute heart failure: a systematic review. *Clin Chem.* 2007;53:813-822.
481. Masson S, Latini R. Amino-terminal pro–B-type natriuretic peptides and prognosis in chronic heart failure. *Am J Cardiol.* 2008;101:56-60.
482. Luchner A, Hengstenberg C, Lowel H, et al. Effect of compensated renal dysfunction on approved heart failure markers: direct comparison of brain natriuretic peptide (BNP) and N-terminal pro-BNP. *Hypertension.* 2005;46:118-123.
483. Richards AM, Nicholls MG, Espiner EA, et al. B-type natriuretic peptides and ejection fraction for prognosis after myocardial infarction. *Circulation.* 2003;107:2786-2792.
484. Abhayaratna WP, Marwick TH, Becker NG, et al. Population-based detection of systolic and diastolic dysfunction with amino-terminal pro–B-type natriuretic peptide. *Am Heart J.* 2006;152:941-948.
485. Scardovi AB, Coletta C, Aspromonte N, et al. Brain natriuretic peptide plasma level is a reliable indicator of advanced diastolic dysfunction in patients with chronic heart failure. *Eur J Echocardiogr.* 2007;8:30-36.
486. Arques S, Roux E, Sbragia P, et al. Usefulness of bedside tissue Doppler echocardiography and B-type natriuretic peptide (BNP) in differentiating congestive heart failure from noncardiac cause of acute dyspnea in elderly patients with a normal left ventricular ejection fraction and permanent, nonvalvular atrial fibrillation: insights from a prospective, monocenter study. *Echocardiography.* 2007;24:499-507.
487. Belovicova M, Kinova S, Hrusovsky S. Brain natriuretic peptide (BNP) in differential diagnosis of dyspnea. *Bratisl Lek Listy.* 2005;106:203-206.
488. Januzzi Jr JL, Camargo CA, Anwaruddin S, et al. The N-terminal Pro-BNP Investigation of Dyspnea in the Emergency Department (PRIDE) study. *Am J Cardiol.* 2005;95:948-954.
489. Murray H, Cload B, Collier CP, et al. Potential impact of N-terminal pro-BNP testing on the emergency department evaluation of acute dyspnea. *CJEM.* 2006;8:251-258.
490. Sanz MP, Borque L, Rus A, et al. Comparison of BNP and NT-proBNP assays in the approach to the emergency diagnosis of acute dyspnea. *J Clin Lab Anal.* 2006;20:227-232.
491. Worster A, Balion CM, Hill SA, et al. Diagnostic accuracy of BNP and NT-proBNP in patients presenting to acute care settings with dyspnea: a systematic review. *Clin Biochem.* 2008;41:250-259.
492. Mueller C, Laule-Kilian K, Schindler C, et al. Cost-effectiveness of B-type natriuretic peptide testing in patients with acute dyspnea. *Arch Intern Med.* 2006;166:1081-1087.
493. Mueller C, Scholer A, Laule-Kilian K, et al. Use of B-type natriuretic peptide in the evaluation and management of acute dyspnea. *N Engl J Med.* 2004;350:647-654.
494. Bhatia V, Nayyar P, Dhindsa S. Brain natriuretic peptide in diagnosis and treatment of heart failure. *J Postgrad Med.* 2003;49:182-185.
495. Richards AM, Lainchbury JG, Nicholls MG, et al. BNP in hormone-guided treatment of heart failure. *Trends Endocrinol Metab.* 2002;13:151-155.
496. Troughton RW, Frampton CM, Yandle TG, et al. Treatment of heart failure guided by plasma aminoterminal brain natriuretic peptide (N-BNP) concentrations. *Lancet.* 2000;355:1126-1130.
497. Mueller C, Buser P. B-type natriuretic peptide (BNP): can it improve our management of patients with congestive heart failure? *Swiss Med Wkly.* 2002;132:618-622.
498. Olsson LG, Swedberg K, Cleland JG, et al. Prognostic importance of plasma NT-pro BNP in chronic heart failure in patients treated with a beta-blocker: results from the Carvedilol Or Metoprolol European Trial (COMET) trial. *Eur J Heart Fail.* 2007;9:795-801.
499. White M, Lepage S, Lavoie J, et al. Effects of combined candesartan and ACE inhibitors on BNP, markers of inflammation and oxidative stress, and glucose regulation in patients with symptomatic heart failure. *J Card Fail.* 2007;13:86-94.
500. Falcao LM, Pinto F, Ravara L, et al. BNP and ANP as diagnostic and predictive markers in heart failure with left ventricular systolic dysfunction. *J Renin Angiotensin Aldosterone Syst.* 2004;5:121-129.
501. Packer M. Should B-type natriuretic peptide be measured routinely to guide the diagnosis and management of chronic heart failure? *Circulation.* 2003;108:2950-2953.
502. Tokudome T, Horio T, Soeki T, et al. Inhibitory effect of C-type natriuretic peptide (CNP) on cultured cardiac myocyte hypertrophy: interference between CNP and endothelin-1 signaling pathways. *Endocrinology.* 2004;145:2131-2140.

503. Clavell AL, Stingo AJ, Wei CM, et al. C-type natriuretic peptide: a selective cardiovascular peptide. *Am J Physiol.* 1993;264:R290-R295.

504. Stingo AJ, Clavell AL, Aarhus LL, et al. Cardiovascular and renal actions of C-type natriuretic peptide. *Am J Physiol.* 1992;262:H308-H312.

505. Del RS, Passino C, Emdin M, et al. C-type natriuretic peptide and heart failure. *Pharmacol Res.* 2006;54:326-333.

506. Wright SP, Prickett TC, Doughty RN, et al. Amino-terminal pro-C-type natriuretic peptide in heart failure. *Hypertension.* 2004;43:94-100.

507. Del RS, Maltinti M, Cabiati M, et al. C-type natriuretic peptide and its relation to non-invasive indices of left ventricular function in patients with chronic heart failure. *Peptides.* 2008;29:79-82.

508. Del RS, Passino C, Maltinti M, et al. C-type natriuretic peptide plasma levels increase in patients with chronic heart failure as a function of clinical severity. *Eur J Heart Fail.* 2005;7:1145-1148.

509. Kalra PR, Clague JR, Bolger AP, et al. Myocardial production of C-type natriuretic peptide in chronic heart failure. *Circulation.* 2003;107:571-573.

510. Del RS, Maltinti M, Piacenti M, et al. Cardiac production of C-type natriuretic peptide in heart failure. *J Cardiovasc Med (Hagerstown).* 2006;7:397-399.

511. Dickey DM, Flora DR, Bryan PM, et al. Differential regulation of membrane guanylyl cyclases in congestive heart failure: natriuretic peptide receptor (NPR)–B, not NPR-A, is the predominant natriuretic peptide receptor in the failing heart. *Endocrinology.* 2007;148:3518-3522.

512. Kalra PR, Clague JR, Coats AJ, et al. C type natriuretic peptide production by the human kidney is blunted in chronic heart failure. *Clin Sci (Lond).* 2009.

513. Bauersachs J, Widder JD. Endothelial dysfunction in heart failure. *Pharmacol Rep.* 2008;60:119-126.

514. Lapu-Bula R, Ofili E. From hypertension to heart failure: role of nitric oxide–mediated endothelial dysfunction and emerging insights from myocardial contrast echocardiography. *Am J Cardiol.* 2007;99:7D-14D.

515. Ferdinand KC. African American Heart Failure trial: role of endothelial dysfunction and heart failure in African Americans. *Am J Cardiol.* 2007;99:3D-6D.

516. Tousoulis D, Charakida M, Stefanadis C. Inflammation and endothelial dysfunction as therapeutic targets in patients with heart failure. *Int J Cardiol.* 2005;100:347-353.

517. Bauersachs J, Schafer A. Endothelial dysfunction in heart failure: mechanisms and therapeutic approaches. *Curr Vasc Pharmacol.* 2004;2: 115-124.

518. Mendes Ribeiro AC, Brunini TM, Ellory JC, et al. Abnormalities in L-arginine transport and nitric oxide biosynthesis in chronic renal and heart failure. *Cardiovasc Res.* 2001;49:697-712.

519. Rabelo ER, Ruschel K, Moreno Jr H, et al. Venous endothelial function in heart failure: comparison with healthy controls and effect of clinical compensation. *Eur J Heart Fail.* 2008;10:758-764.

520. Abassi ZA, Gurbanov K, Mulroney SE, et al. Impaired nitric oxide–mediated renal vasodilation in rats with experimental heart failure: role of angiotensin II. *Circulation.* 1997;96:3655-3664.

521. Angus JA, Ferrier CP, Sudhir K, et al. Impaired contraction and relaxation in skin resistance arteries from patients with congestive heart failure. *Cardiovasc Res.* 1993;27:204-210.

522. Vanhoutte PM. Endothelium-dependent responses in congestive heart failure. *J Mol Cell Cardiol.* 1996;28:2233-2240.

523. Gaballa MA, Goldman S. Overexpression of endothelium nitric oxide synthase reverses the diminished vasorelaxation in the hindlimb vasculature in ischemic heart failure in vivo. *J Mol Cell Cardiol.* 1999;31:1243-1262.

524. Kielstein JT, Bode-Boger SM, Klein G, et al. Endogenous nitric oxide synthase inhibitors and renal perfusion in patients with heart failure. *Eur J Clin Invest.* 2003;33:370-375.

525. Habib F, Dutka D, Crossman D, et al. Enhanced basal nitric oxide production in heart failure: another failed counter-regulatory vasodilator mechanism? *Lancet.* 1994;344:371-373.

526. Schulz R, Rassaf T, Massion PB, et al. Recent advances in the understanding of the role of nitric oxide in cardiovascular homeostasis. *Pharmacol Ther.* 2005;108:225-256.

527. Cooke JP, Dzau VJ. Derangements of the nitric oxide synthase pathway, L-arginine, and cardiovascular diseases. *Circulation.* 1997;96:379-382.

528. Saraiva RM, Hare JM. Nitric oxide signaling in the cardiovascular system: implications for heart failure. *Curr Opin Cardiol.* 2006;21:221-228.

529. Winkelmayer WC, Waikar SS, Mogun H, et al. Nonselective and cyclooxygenase-2–selective NSAIDs and acute kidney injury. *Am J Med.* 2008;121:1092-1098.

530. Eras J, Perazella MA. NSAIDs and the kidney revisited: are selective cyclooxygenase-2 inhibitors safe? *Am J Med Sci.* 2001;321:181-190.

531. Dzau VJ, Packer M, Lilly LS, et al. Prostaglandins in severe congestive heart failure. Relation to activation of the renin-angiotensin system and hyponatremia. *N Engl J Med.* 1984;310:347-352.

532. Castellani S, Paladini B, Paniccia R, et al. Increased renal formation of thromboxane A$_2$ and prostaglandin F$_{2\alpha}$ in heart failure. *Am Heart J.* 1997;133:94-100.

533. Riegger GA, Elsner D, Hildenbrand J, et al. Prostaglandins, renin and atrial natriuretic peptide in the control of the circulation and renal function in heart failure in the dog. *Prog Clin Biol Res.* 1989;301:455-458.

534. Townend JN, Doran J, Lote CJ, et al. Peripheral haemodynamic effects of inhibition of prostaglandin synthesis in congestive heart failure and interactions with captopril. *Br Heart J.* 1995;73:434-441.

535. Villarreal D, Freeman RH, Habibullah AA, et al. Indomethacin attenuates the renal actions of atrial natriuretic factor in dogs with chronic heart failure. *Am J Med Sci.* 1997;314:67-72.

536. Gislason GH, Rasmussen JN, Abildstrom SZ, et al. Increased mortality and cardiovascular morbidity associated with use of nonsteroidal anti-inflammatory drugs in chronic heart failure. *Arch Intern Med.* 2009;169: 141-149.

537. Hudson M, Rahme E, Richard H, et al. Risk of congestive heart failure with nonsteroidal antiinflammatory drugs and selective cyclooxygenase 2 inhibitors: a class effect? *Arthritis Rheum.* 2007;57:516-523.

538. Hudson M, Richard H, Pilote L. Differences in outcomes of patients with congestive heart failure prescribed celecoxib, rofecoxib, or non-steroidal anti-inflammatory drugs: population based study. *BMJ.* 2005;330:1370.

539. Bernatsky S, Hudson M, Suissa S. Anti-rheumatic drug use and risk of hospitalization for congestive heart failure in rheumatoid arthritis. *Rheumatology (Oxford).* 2005;44:677-680.

540. Mamdani M, Juurlink DN, Lee DS, et al. Cyclo-oxygenase–2 inhibitors versus non-selective non-steroidal anti-inflammatory drugs and congestive heart failure outcomes in elderly patients: a population-based cohort study. *Lancet.* 2004;363:1751-1756.

541. Harris RC. COX-2 and the kidney. *J Cardiovasc Pharmacol.* 2006;47 (suppl 1):S37-S42.

542. Abassi Z, Brodsky S, Gealekman O, et al. Intrarenal expression and distribution of cyclooxygenase isoforms in rats with experimental heart failure. *Am J Physiol Renal Physiol.* 2001;280:F43-F53.

543. Solomon SD, McMurray JJ, Pfeffer MA, et al. Cardiovascular risk associated with celecoxib in a clinical trial for colorectal adenoma prevention. *N Engl J Med.* 2005;352:1071-1080.

544. Waxman HA. The lessons of Vioxx—drug safety and sales. *N Engl J Med.* 2005;352:2576-2578.

545. Vardeny O, Solomon SD. Cyclooxygenase-2 inhibitors, nonsteroidal anti-inflammatory drugs, and cardiovascular risk. *Cardiol Clin.* 2008;26:589-601.

546. McGettigan P, Han P, Jones L, et al. Selective COX-2 inhibitors, NSAIDs and congestive heart failure: differences between new and recurrent cases. *Br J Clin Pharmacol.* 2008;65:927-934.

547. Solomon SD, Wittes J, Finn PV, et al. Cardiovascular risk of celecoxib in 6 randomized placebo-controlled trials: the cross trial safety analysis. *Circulation.* 2008;117:2104-2113.

548. Nishikimi T, Matsuoka H. Cardiac adrenomedullin: its role in cardiac hypertrophy and heart failure. *Curr Med Chem Cardiovasc Hematol Agents.* 2005;3:231-242.

549. Adlbrecht C, Hulsmann M, Strunk G, et al. Prognostic value of plasma midregional pro-adrenomedullin and C-terminal-pro-endothelin-1 in chronic heart failure outpatients. *Eur J Heart Fail.* 2009;11:361-366.

550. Hirose T, Totsune K, Mori N, et al. Increased expression of adrenomedullin 2/intermedin in rat hearts with congestive heart failure. *Eur J Heart Fail.* 2008;10:840-849.

551. Jougasaki M, Heublein DM, Sandberg SM, et al. Attenuated natriuretic response to adrenomedullin in experimental heart failure. *J Card Fail.* 2001;7:75-83.

552. Totsune K, Takahashi K, Mackenzie HS, et al. Increased gene expression of adrenomedullin and adrenomedullin-receptor complexes, receptor-activity modifying protein (RAMP)2 and calcitonin-receptor–like receptor (CRLR) in the hearts of rats with congestive heart failure. *Clin Sci (Lond).* 2000;99:541-546.

553. Nishikimi T, Karasawa T, Inaba C, et al. Effects of long-term intravenous administration of adrenomedullin (AM) plus hANP therapy in acute decompensated heart failure. *Circ J.* 2009;73:892-898.

554. Ng LL, Loke I, O'Brien RJ, et al. Plasma urotensin in human systolic heart failure. *Circulation.* 2002;106:2877-2880.

555. Richards AM, Nicholls MG, Lainchbury JG, et al. Plasma urotensin II in heart failure. *Lancet.* 2002;360:545-546.

556. Russell FD, Meyers D, Galbraith AJ, et al. Elevated plasma levels of human urotensin-II immunoreactivity in congestive heart failure. *Am J Physiol Heart Circ Physiol.* 2003;285:H1576-H1581.

557. Douglas SA, Tayara L, Ohlstein EH, et al. Congestive heart failure and expression of myocardial urotensin II. *Lancet.* 2002;359:1990-1997.

558. Feuerstein GZ, Zukowska Z. NPY family of peptides, receptors and processing enzymes. In: Zukowska Z, Feuerstein GZ, eds. *NPY family of peptides in neurobiology, cardiovascular and metabolic disorders: from genes to therapeutics.* Boston: EXS Birkhäuser; 2005:7-33.

559. Madsen BK, Husum D, Videbaek R, et al. Plasma immunoreactive neuropeptide Y in congestive heart failure at rest and during exercise. *Scand J Clin Lab Invest.* 1993;53:569-576.

560. Ullman B, Jensen-Urstad M, Hulting J, et al. Neuropeptide Y, noradrenaline and invasive haemodynamic data in mild to moderate chronic congestive heart failure. *Clin Physiol*. 1993;13:409-418.

561. Ullman B, Hulting J, Lundberg JM. Prognostic value of plasma neuropeptide-Y in coronary care unit patients with and without acute myocardial infarction. *Eur Heart J*. 1994;15:454-461.

562. Anderson FL, Port JD, Reid BB, et al. Myocardial catecholamine and neuropeptide Y depletion in failing ventricles of patients with idiopathic dilated cardiomyopathy. Correlation with beta-adrenergic receptor downregulation. *Circulation*. 1992;85:46-53.

563. Pons J, Lee EW, Li L, et al. Neuropeptide Y: multiple receptors and multiple roles in cardiovascular diseases. *Curr Opin Investig Drugs*. 2004;5:957-962.

564. Li L, Lee EW, Ji H, et al. Neuropeptide Y–induced acceleration of postangioplasty occlusion of rat carotid artery. *Arterioscler Thromb Vasc Biol*. 2003;23:1204-1210.

565. Millar BC, Schluter KD, Zhou XJ, et al. Neuropeptide Y stimulates hypertrophy of adult ventricular cardiomyocytes. *Am J Physiol*. 1994;266:C1271-C1277.

566. Lee EW, Michalkiewicz M, Kitlinska J, et al. Neuropeptide Y induces ischemic angiogenesis and restores function of ischemic skeletal muscles. *J Clin Invest*. 2003;111:1853-1862.

567. Allen JM, Raine AE, Ledingham JG, et al. Neuropeptide Y: a novel renal peptide with vasoconstrictor and natriuretic activity. *Clin Sci (Lond)*. 1985;68:373-377.

568. Waeber B, Burnier M, Nussberger J, et al. Role of atrial natriuretic peptides and neuropeptide Y in blood pressure regulation. *Horm Res*. 1990;34:161-165.

569. Duan SZ, Ivashchenko CY, Usher MG, et al. PPAR-gamma in the cardiovascular system. *PPAR Res*. 2008;2008:745-804.

570. Guan Y, Hao C, Cha DR, et al. Thiazolidinediones expand body fluid volume through PPARgamma stimulation of ENaC-mediated renal salt absorption. *Nat Med*. 2005;11:861-866.

571. Zhang H, Zhang A, Kohan DE, et al. Collecting duct–specific deletion of peroxisome proliferator–activated receptor gamma blocks thiazolidinedione-induced fluid retention. *Proc Natl Acad Sci U S A*. 2005;102:9406-9411.

572. Home PD, Pocock SJ, Beck-Nielsen H, et al. Rosiglitazone Evaluated for Cardiovascular Outcomes in Oral Agent Combination Therapy for Type 2 Diabetes (RECORD): a multicentre, randomised, open-label trial. *Lancet*. 2009;373:2125-2135.

573. Wadei HM, Mai ML, Ahsan N, et al. Hepatorenal syndrome: pathophysiology and management. *Clin J Am Soc Nephrol*. 2006;1:1066-1079.

574. Angeli P, Merkel C. Pathogenesis and management of hepatorenal syndrome in patients with cirrhosis. *J Hepatol*. 2008;48(suppl 1):S93-S103.

575. Schrier RW, Arroyo V, Bernardi M, et al. Peripheral arterial vasodilation hypothesis: a proposal for the initiation of renal sodium and water retention in cirrhosis. *Hepatology*. 1988;8:1151-1157.

576. Angeli P, Volpin R, Piovan D, et al. Acute effects of the oral administration of midodrine, an alpha-adrenergic agonist, on renal hemodynamics and renal function in cirrhotic patients with ascites. *Hepatology*. 1998;28:937-943.

577. Martin PY, Gines P, Schrier RW. Nitric oxide as a mediator of hemodynamic abnormalities and sodium and water retention in cirrhosis. *N Engl J Med*. 1998;339:533-541.

578. Martin PY, Schrier RW. Pathogenesis of water and sodium retention in cirrhosis. *Kidney Int Suppl*. 1997;59:S43-S49.

579. Iwakiri Y, Groszmann RJ. The hyperdynamic circulation of chronic liver diseases: from the patient to the molecule. *Hepatology*. 2006;43:S121-S131.

580. Lieberman FL, Denison EK, Reynolds TB. The relationship of plasma volume, portal hypertension, ascites and renal sodium retention in cirrhosis: the overflow theory of ascites formation. *Ann N Y Acad Sci*. 1970;170:202-212.

581. Levy M. Pathogenesis of sodium retention in early cirrhosis of the liver: evidence for vascular overfilling. *Semin Liver Dis*. 1994;14:4-13.

582. Levy M. Sodium retention in dogs with cirrhosis and ascites: efferent mechanisms. *Am J Physiol*. 1977;233:F586-F592.

583. Kostreva DR, Castaner A, Kampine JP. Reflex effects of hepatic baroreceptors on renal and cardiac sympathetic nerve activity. *Am J Physiol*. 1980;238:R390-R394.

584. Ming Z, Smyth DD, Lautt WW. Decreases in portal flow trigger a hepatorenal reflex to inhibit renal sodium and water excretion in rats: role of adenosine. *Hepatology*. 2002;35:167-175.

585. Jimenez-Saenz M, Soria IC, Bernardez JR, et al. Renal sodium retention in portal hypertension and hepatorenal reflex: from practice to science. *Hepatology*. 2003;37:1494-1495.

586. Cardenas A, Arroyo V. Mechanisms of water and sodium retention in cirrhosis and the pathogenesis of ascites. *Best Pract Res Clin Endocrinol Metab*. 2003;17:607-622.

587. Arroyo V, Fernandez J, Gines P. Pathogenesis and treatment of hepatorenal syndrome. *Semin Liver Dis*. 2008;28:81-95.

588. Parasher VK, Meroni E, Malesci A, et al. Observation of thoracic duct morphology in portal hypertension by endoscopic ultrasound. *Gastrointest Endosc*. 1998;48:588-592.

589. Sikuler E, Kravetz D, Groszmann RJ. Evolution of portal hypertension and mechanisms involved in its maintenance in a rat model. *Am J Physiol*. 1985;248:G618-G625.

590. Bomzon A, Rosenberg M, Gali D, et al. Systemic hypotension and decreased pressor response in dogs with chronic bile duct ligation. *Hepatology*. 1986;6:595-600.

591. Levy M, Wexler MJ. Subacute endotoxemia in dogs with experimental cirrhosis and ascites: effects on kidney function. *Can J Physiol Pharmacol*. 1984;62:673-677.

592. Better OS, Guckian V, Giebisch G, et al. The effect of sodium taurocholate on proximal tubular reabsorption in the rat kidney. *Clin Sci (Lond)*. 1987;72:139-141.

593. Green J, Better OS. Systemic hypotension and renal failure in obstructive jaundice—mechanistic and therapeutic aspects. *J Am Soc Nephrol*. 1995;5:1853-1871.

594. Castell DO. Ascites in cirrhosis. Relative importance of portal hypertension and hypoalbuminemia. *Am J Dig Dis*. 1967;12:916-922.

595. Alqahtani SA, Fouad TR, Lee SS. Cirrhotic cardiomyopathy. *Semin Liver Dis*. 2008;28:59-69.

596. Schrier RW, Ecder T. Gibbs memorial lecture. Unifying hypothesis of body fluid volume regulation: implications for cardiac failure and cirrhosis. *Mt Sinai J Med*. 2001;68:350-361.

597. Rodriguez-Roisin R, Krowka MJ. Hepatopulmonary syndrome—a liver-induced lung vascular disorder. *N Engl J Med*. 2008;358:2378-2387.

598. Ruiz-del-Arbol L, Monescillo A, Arocena C, et al. Circulatory function and hepatorenal syndrome in cirrhosis. *Hepatology*. 2005;42:439-447.

599. Wiest R, Groszmann RJ. The paradox of nitric oxide in cirrhosis and portal hypertension: too much, not enough. *Hepatology*. 2002;35:478-491.

600. Langer DA, Shah VH. Nitric oxide and portal hypertension: interface of vasoreactivity and angiogenesis. *J Hepatol*. 2006;44:209-216.

601. Niederberger M, Gines P, Tsai P, et al. Increased aortic cyclic guanosine monophosphate concentration in experimental cirrhosis in rats: evidence for a role of nitric oxide in the pathogenesis of arterial vasodilation in cirrhosis. *Hepatology*. 1995;21:1625-1631.

602. Niederberger M, Martin PY, Gines P, et al. Normalization of nitric oxide production corrects arterial vasodilation and hyperdynamic circulation in cirrhotic rats. *Gastroenterology*. 1995;109:1624-1630.

603. Martin PY, Ohara M, Gines P, et al. Nitric oxide synthase (NOS) inhibition for one week improves renal sodium and water excretion in cirrhotic rats with ascites. *J Clin Invest*. 1998;101:235-242.

604. Campillo B, Chabrier PE, Pelle G, et al. Inhibition of nitric oxide synthesis in the forearm arterial bed of patients with advanced cirrhosis. *Hepatology*. 1995;22:1423-1429.

605. La Villa G, Barletta G, Pantaleo P, et al. Hemodynamic, renal, and endocrine effects of acute inhibition of nitric oxide synthase in compensated cirrhosis. *Hepatology*. 2001;34:19-27.

606. Yu Q, Shao R, Qian HS, et al. Gene transfer of the neuronal NO synthase isoform to cirrhotic rat liver ameliorates portal hypertension. *J Clin Invest*. 2000;105:741-748.

607. Van de Casteele M, Omasta A, Janssens S, et al. In vivo gene transfer of endothelial nitric oxide synthase decreases portal pressure in anaesthetised carbon tetrachloride cirrhotic rats. *Gut*. 2002;51:440-445.

608. Iwakiri Y, Cadelina G, Sessa WC, et al. Mice with targeted deletion of eNOS develop hyperdynamic circulation associated with portal hypertension. *Am J Physiol Gastrointest Liver Physiol*. 2002;283:G1074-G1081.

609. Sitzmann JV, Campbell K, Wu Y, et al. Prostacyclin production in acute, chronic, and long-term experimental portal hypertension. *Surgery*. 1994;115:290-294.

610. Barriere E, Tazi KA, Rona JP, et al. Evidence for an endothelium-derived hyperpolarizing factor in the superior mesenteric artery from rats with cirrhosis. *Hepatology*. 2000;32:935-941.

611. Chen YC, Gines P, Yang J, et al. Increased vascular heme oxygenase-1 expression contributes to arterial vasodilation in experimental cirrhosis in rats. *Hepatology*. 2004;39:1075-1087.

612. Kojima H, Sakurai S, Uemura M, et al. Adrenomedullin contributes to vascular hyporeactivity in cirrhotic rats with ascites via a release of nitric oxide. *Scand J Gastroenterol*. 2004;39:686-693.

613. Xu L, Carter EP, Ohara M, et al. Neuronal nitric oxide synthase and systemic vasodilation in rats with cirrhosis. *Am J Physiol Renal Physiol*. 2000;279:F1110-F1115.

614. Biecker E, Neef M, Sagesser H, et al. Nitric oxide synthase 1 is partly compensating for nitric oxide synthase 3 deficiency in nitric oxide synthase 3 knock-out mice and is elevated in murine and human cirrhosis. *Liver Int*. 2004;24:345-353.

615. Moreau R, Barriere E, Tazi KA, et al. Terlipressin inhibits in vivo aortic iNOS expression induced by lipopolysaccharide in rats with biliary cirrhosis. *Hepatology.* 2002;36:1070-1078.

616. Cahill PA, Redmond EM, Hodges R, et al. Increased endothelial nitric oxide synthase activity in the hyperemic vessels of portal hypertensive rats. *J Hepatol.* 1996;25:370-378.

617. Sessa WC. eNOS at a glance. *J Cell Sci.* 2004;117:2427-2429.

618. Iwakiri Y, Tsai MH, McCabe TJ, et al. Phosphorylation of eNOS initiates excessive NO production in early phases of portal hypertension. *Am J Physiol Heart Circ Physiol.* 2002;282:H2084-H2090.

619. Wiest R, Cadelina G, Milstien S, et al. Bacterial translocation up-regulates GTP–cyclohydrolase I in mesenteric vasculature of cirrhotic rats. *Hepatology.* 2003;38:1508-1515.

620. Mookerjee RP, Vairappan B, Jalan R. The puzzle of endothelial nitric oxide synthase dysfunction in portal hypertension: the missing piece? *Hepatology.* 2007;46:943-946.

621. Leiper J, Nandi M, Torondel B, et al. Disruption of methylarginine metabolism impairs vascular homeostasis. *Nat Med.* 2007;13:198-203.

622. Mookerjee RP, Malaki M, Davies NA, et al. Increasing dimethylarginine levels are associated with adverse clinical outcome in severe alcoholic hepatitis. *Hepatology.* 2007;45:62-71.

623. Konishi H, Sydow K, Cooke JP. Dimethylarginine dimethylaminohydrolase promotes endothelial repair after vascular injury. *J Am Coll Cardiol.* 2007;49:1099-1105.

624. Pacher P, Batkai S, Kunos G. The endocannabinoid system as an emerging target of pharmacotherapy. *Pharmacol Rev.* 2006;58:389-462.

625. Caraceni P, Domenicali M, Giannone F, et al. The role of the endocannabinoid system in liver diseases. *Best Pract Res Clin Endocrinol Metab.* 2009;23:65-77.

626. Lopez C, Jimenez W, Arroyo V, et al. Temporal relationship between the decrease in arterial pressure and sodium retention in conscious spontaneously hypertensive rats with carbon tetrachloride–induced cirrhosis. *Hepatology.* 1991;13:585-589.

627. Bernardi M, Trevisani F, Gasbarrini A, et al. Hepatorenal disorders: role of the renin-angiotensin-aldosterone system. *Semin Liver Dis.* 1994;14:23-34.

628. Bernardi M, Li BS, Arienti V, et al. Systemic and regional hemodynamics in pre-ascitic cirrhosis: effects of posture. *J Hepatol.* 2003;39:502-508.

629. Wong F, Sniderman K, Blendis L. The renal sympathetic and renin-angiotensin response to lower body negative pressure in well-compensated cirrhosis. *Gastroenterology.* 1998;115:397-405.

630. Wong F, Liu P, Blendis L. The mechanism of improved sodium homeostasis of low-dose losartan in preascitic cirrhosis. *Hepatology.* 2002;35:1449-1458.

631. Ubeda M, Matzilevich MM, Atucha NM, et al. Renin and angiotensinogen mRNA expression in the kidneys of rats subjected to long-term bile duct ligation. *Hepatology.* 1994;19:1431-1436.

632. Schneider AW, Kalk JF, Klein CP. Effect of losartan, an angiotensin II receptor antagonist, on portal pressure in cirrhosis. *Hepatology.* 1999;29:334-339.

633. Gentilini P, Romanelli RG, La Villa G, et al. Effects of low-dose captopril on renal hemodynamics and function in patients with cirrhosis of the liver. *Gastroenterology.* 1993;104:588-594.

634. Henriksen JH, Moller S, Ring-Larsen H, et al. The sympathetic nervous system in liver disease. *J Hepatol.* 1998;29:328-341.

635. Floras JS, Legault L, Morali GA, et al. Increased sympathetic outflow in cirrhosis and ascites: direct evidence from intraneural recordings. *Ann Intern Med.* 1991;114:373-380.

636. Bichet DG, Van Putten VJ, Schrier RW. Potential role of increased sympathetic activity in impaired sodium and water excretion in cirrhosis. *N Engl J Med.* 1982;307:1552-1557.

637. DiBona GF, Sawin LL, Jones SY. Characteristics of renal sympathetic nerve activity in sodium-retaining disorders. *Am J Physiol.* 1996;271:R295-R302.

638. Rodriguez-Martinez M, Sawin LL, DiBona GF. Arterial and cardiopulmonary baroreflex control of renal nerve activity in cirrhosis. *Am J Physiol.* 1995;268:R117-R129.

639. Laffi G, Lagi A, Cipriani M, et al. Impaired cardiovascular autonomic response to passive tilting in cirrhosis with ascites. *Hepatology.* 1996;24:1063-1067.

640. Ryan J, Sudhir K, Jennings G, et al. Impaired reactivity of the peripheral vasculature to pressor agents in alcoholic cirrhosis. *Gastroenterology.* 1993;105:1167-1172.

641. Wong F, Logan A, Blendis L. Hyperinsulinemia in preascitic cirrhosis: effects on systemic and renal hemodynamics, sodium homeostasis, forearm blood flow, and sympathetic nervous activity. *Hepatology.* 1996;23:414-422.

642. Stadlbauer V, Wright GA, Banaji M, et al. Relationship between activation of the sympathetic nervous system and renal blood flow autoregulation in cirrhosis. *Gastroenterology.* 2008;134:111-119.

643. Lenaerts A, Codden T, Meunier JC, et al. Effects of clonidine on diuretic response in ascitic patients with cirrhosis and activation of sympathetic nervous system. *Hepatology.* 2006;44:844-849.

644. Bichet D, Szatalowicz V, Chaimovitz C, et al. Role of vasopressin in abnormal water excretion in cirrhotic patients. *Ann Intern Med.* 1982;96:413-417.

645. Kim JK, Summer SN, Howard RL, et al. Vasopressin gene expression in rats with experimental cirrhosis. *Hepatology.* 1993;17:143-147.

646. Gines P, Wong F, Watson H, et al. Effects of satavaptan, a selective vasopressin V(2) receptor antagonist, on ascites and serum sodium in cirrhosis with hyponatremia: a randomized trial. *Hepatology.* 2008;48:204-213.

647. Ferguson JW, Therapondos G, Newby DE, et al. Therapeutic role of vasopressin receptor antagonism in patients with liver cirrhosis. *Clin Sci (Lond).* 2003;105:1-8.

648. Bray BA, Sutcliffe IC, Harrington DJ. Expression of the MtsA lipoprotein of *Streptococcus agalactiae* A909 is regulated by manganese and iron. *Antonie Van Leeuwenhoek.* 2009;95:101-109.

649. Jimenez W, Gal CS, Ros J, et al. Long-term aquaretic efficacy of a selective nonpeptide V(2)-vasopressin receptor antagonist, SR121463, in cirrhotic rats. *J Pharmacol Exp Ther.* 2000;295:83-90.

650. Tsuboi Y, Ishikawa S, Fujisawa G, et al. Therapeutic efficacy of the non-peptide AVP antagonist OPC-31260 in cirrhotic rats. *Kidney Int.* 1994;46:237-244.

651. Claria J, Jimenez W, Arroyo V, et al. Effect of V_1-vasopressin receptor blockade on arterial pressure in conscious rats with cirrhosis and ascites. *Gastroenterology.* 1991;100:494-501.

652. Arroyo V, Claria J, Salo J, et al. Antidiuretic hormone and the pathogenesis of water retention in cirrhosis with ascites. *Semin Liver Dis.* 1994;14:44-58.

653. Perez-Ayuso RM, Arroyo V, Camps J, et al. Evidence that renal prostaglandins are involved in renal water metabolism in cirrhosis. *Kidney Int.* 1984;26:72-80.

654. Angus PW. Role of endothelin in systemic and portal resistance in cirrhosis. *Gut.* 2006;55:1230-1232.

655. Moore K. Endothelin and vascular function in liver disease. *Gut.* 2004;53:159-161.

656. Martinet JP, Legault L, Cernacek P, et al. Changes in plasma endothelin-1 and big endothelin-1 induced by transjugular intrahepatic portosystemic shunts in patients with cirrhosis and refractory ascites. *J Hepatol.* 1996;25:700-706.

657. Kapoor D, Redhead DN, Hayes PC, et al. Systemic and regional changes in plasma endothelin following transient increase in portal pressure. *Liver Transpl.* 2003;9:32-39.

658. Vaughan RB, Angus PW, Chin-Dusting JP. Evidence for altered vascular responses to exogenous endothelin-1 in patients with advanced cirrhosis with restoration of the normal vasoconstrictor response following successful liver transplantation. *Gut.* 2003;52:1505-1510.

659. Anand R, Harry D, Holt S, et al. Endothelin is an important determinant of renal function in a rat model of acute liver and renal failure. *Gut.* 2002;50:111-117.

660. Moller S, Bendtsen F, Henriksen JH. Pathophysiological basis of pharmacotherapy in the hepatorenal syndrome. *Scand J Gastroenterol.* 2005;40:491-500.

661. Wong F, Blendis L. Pathophysiology of sodium retention and ascites formation in cirrhosis: role of atrial natriuretic factor. *Semin Liver Dis.* 1994;14:59-70.

662. Levy M. Atrial natriuretic peptide: renal effects in cirrhosis of the liver. *Semin Nephrol.* 1997;17:520-529.

663. Poulos JE, Gower WR, Fontanet HL, et al. Cirrhosis with ascites: increased atrial natriuretic peptide messenger RNA expression in rat ventricle. *Gastroenterology.* 1995;108:1496-1503.

664. Rector Jr WG, Adair O, Hossack KF, et al. Atrial volume in cirrhosis: relationship to blood volume and plasma concentration of atrial natriuretic factor. *Gastroenterology.* 1990;99:766-770.

665. Wong F, Liu P, Tobe S, et al. Central blood volume in cirrhosis: measurement with radionuclide angiography. *Hepatology.* 1994;19:312-321.

666. Wong F, Liu P, Blendis L. Sodium homeostasis with chronic sodium loading in preascitic cirrhosis. *Gut.* 2001;49:847-851.

667. Skorecki KL, Leung WM, Campbell P, et al. Role of atrial natriuretic peptide in the natriuretic response to central volume expansion induced by head-out water immersion in sodium-retaining cirrhotic subjects. *Am J Med.* 1988;85:375-382.

668. Legault L, Warner LC, Leung WM, et al. Assessment of atrial natriuretic peptide resistance in cirrhosis with head-out water immersion and atrial natriuretic peptide infusion. *Can J Physiol Pharmacol.* 1993;71:157-164.

669. Warner L, Skorecki K, Blendis LM, et al. Atrial natriuretic factor and liver disease. *Hepatology.* 1993;17:500-513.

670. MacGilchrist A, Craig KJ, Hayes PC, et al. Effect of the serine protease inhibitor, aprotinin, on systemic haemodynamics and renal function in patients with hepatic cirrhosis and ascites. *Clin Sci (Lond).* 1994;87:329-335.

671. Legault L, Cernacek P, Levy M. Attempts to alter the heterogeneous response to ANP in sodium-retaining caval dogs. *Can J Physiol Pharmacol.* 1992;70:897-904.

672. Morali GA, Tobe SW, Skorecki KL, et al. Refractory ascites: modulation of atrial natriuretic factor unresponsiveness by mannitol. *Hepatology.* 1992;16:42-48.

673. Tobe SW, Morali GA, Greig PD, et al. Peritoneovenous shunting restores atrial natriuretic factor responsiveness in refractory hepatic ascites. *Gastroenterology.* 1993;105:202-207.

674. Piccinni P, Rossaro L, Graziotto A, et al. Human natriuretic factor in cirrhotic patients undergoing orthotopic liver transplantation. *Transpl Int.* 1995;8:51-54.

675. Koepke JP, Jones S, DiBona GF. Renal nerves mediate blunted natriuresis to atrial natriuretic peptide in cirrhotic rats. *Am J Physiol.* 1987;252:R1019-R1023.

676. Tobe SW, Blendis LM, Morali GA, et al. Angiotensin II modulates atrial natriuretic factor-induced natriuresis in cirrhosis with ascites. *Am J Kidney Dis.* 1993;21:472-479.

677. Abraham WT, Lauwaars ME, Kim JK, et al. Reversal of atrial natriuretic peptide resistance by increasing distal tubular sodium delivery in patients with decompensated cirrhosis. *Hepatology.* 1995;22:737-743.

678. La Villa G, Riccardi D, Lazzeri C, et al. Blunted natriuretic response to low-dose brain natriuretic peptide infusion in nonazotemic cirrhotic patients with ascites and avid sodium retention. *Hepatology.* 1995;22:1745-1750.

679. Radvan M, Svoboda P, Radvanova J, et al. Brain natriuretic peptide in decompensation of liver cirrhosis in non-cardiac patients. *Hepatogastroenterology.* 2009;56:181-185.

680. Henriksen JH, Gotze JP, Fuglsang S, et al. Increased circulating pro–brain natriuretic peptide (proBNP) and brain natriuretic peptide (BNP) in patients with cirrhosis: relation to cardiovascular dysfunction and severity of disease. *Gut.* 2003;52:1511-1517.

681. Bernal V, Pascual I, Esquivias P, et al. Cardiac hemodynamic profiles and pro–B-type natriuretic peptide in cirrhotic patients undergoing liver transplantation. *Transplant Proc.* 2009;41:985-986.

682. Yildiz R, Yildirim B, Karincaoglu M, et al. Brain natriuretic peptide and severity of disease in non-alcoholic cirrhotic patients. *J Gastroenterol Hepatol.* 2005;20:1115-1120.

683. Zambruni A, Trevisani F, Gulberg V, et al. Daily profile of circulating C-type natriuretic peptide in pre-ascitic cirrhosis and in normal subjects: relationship with renal function. *Scand J Gastroenterol.* 2007;42:642-647.

684. Henriksen JH, Gulberg V, Gerbes AL, et al. Increased arterial compliance in cirrhosis is related to decreased arterial C-type natriuretic peptide, but not to atrial natriuretic peptide. *Scand J Gastroenterol.* 2003;38:559-564.

685. Gulberg V, Moller S, Henriksen JH, et al. Increased renal production of C-type natriuretic peptide (CNP) in patients with cirrhosis and functional renal failure. *Gut.* 2000;47:852-857.

686. Fabrega E, Crespo J, Rivero M, et al. *Dendroaspis* natriuretic peptide in hepatic cirrhosis. *Am J Gastroenterol.* 2001;96:2724-2729.

687. Claria J, Arroyo V. Prostaglandins and other cyclooxygenase-dependent arachidonic acid metabolites and the kidney in liver disease. *Prostaglandins Other Lipid Mediat.* 2003;72:19-33.

688. Niederberger M, Gines P, Martin PY, et al. Increased renal and vascular cytosolic phospholipase A_2 activity in rats with cirrhosis and ascites. *Hepatology.* 1998;27:42-47.

689. Epstein M. Renal prostaglandins and the control of renal function in liver disease. *Am J Med.* 1986;80:46-55.

690. Lopez-Parra M, Claria J, Planaguma A, et al. Cyclooxygenase-1 derived prostaglandins are involved in the maintenance of renal function in rats with cirrhosis and ascites. *Br J Pharmacol.* 2002;135:891-900.

691. Claria J, Kent JD, Lopez-Parra M, et al. Effects of celecoxib and naproxen on renal function in nonazotemic patients with cirrhosis and ascites. *Hepatology.* 2005;41:579-587.

692. Wong F, Massie D, Hsu P, et al. Indomethacin-induced renal dysfunction in patients with well-compensated cirrhosis. *Gastroenterology.* 1993;104:869-876.

693. Bosch-Marce M, Claria J, Titos E, et al. Selective inhibition of cyclooxygenase 2 spares renal function and prostaglandin synthesis in cirrhotic rats with ascites. *Gastroenterology.* 1999;116:1167-1175.

694. Govindarajan S, Nast CC, Smith WL, et al. Immunohistochemical distribution of renal prostaglandin endoperoxide synthase and prostacyclin synthase: diminished endoperoxide synthase in the hepatorenal syndrome. *Hepatology.* 1987;7:654-659.

695. Gines A, Salmeron JM, Gines P, et al. Oral misoprostol or intravenous prostaglandin E_2 do not improve renal function in patients with cirrhosis and ascites with hyponatremia or renal failure. *J Hepatol.* 1993;17:220-226.

696. Jaffe AS. The clinical impact of the universal diagnosis of myocardial infarction. *Clin Chem Lab Med.* 2008;46:1485-1488.

697. Tate JR. Troponin revisited 2008: assay performance. *Clin Chem Lab Med.* 2008;46:1489-1500.

698. Licata G, Di PP, Parrinello G, et al. Effects of high-dose furosemide and small-volume hypertonic saline solution infusion in comparison with a high dose of furosemide as bolus in refractory congestive heart failure: long-term effects. *Am Heart J.* 2003;145:459-466.

699. Paterna S, Parrinello G, Amato P, et al. Tolerability and efficacy of high-dose furosemide and small-volume hypertonic saline solution in refractory congestive heart failure. *Adv Ther.* 1999;16:219-228.

700. Winaver J, Teredesai P, Anast C, et al. Investigations into the mechanism of the phosphaturia induced by chlorothiazide. *J Pharmacol Exp Ther.* 1981;218:46-54.

701. Rosenberg J, Gustafsson F, Galatius S, et al. Combination therapy with metolazone and loop diuretics in outpatients with refractory heart failure: an observational study and review of the literature. *Cardiovasc Drugs Ther.* 2005;19:301-306.

702. Chiandussi L, Bartoli E, Arras S. Reabsorption of sodium in the proximal renal tubule in cirrhosis of the liver. *Gut.* 1978;19:497-503.

703. Greenberg A. Diuretic complications. *Am J Med Sci.* 2000;319:10-24.

704. Escribano J, Balaguer A, Pagone F, et al. Pharmacological interventions for preventing complications in idiopathic hypercalciuria. *Cochrane Database Syst Rev.* 2009(1):CD004754.

705. Lee CT, Chen HC, Lai LW, et al. Effects of furosemide on renal calcium handling. *Am J Physiol Renal Physiol.* 2007;293:F1231-F1237.

706. Prichard BN, Owens CW, Woolf AS. Adverse reactions to diuretics. *Eur Heart J.* 1992;13(suppl G):96-103.

707. Tormey V, Conlon PJ, Farrell J, et al. Long-term successful management of refractory congestive cardiac failure by intermittent ambulatory peritoneal ultrafiltration. *QJM.* 1996;89:681-683.

708. Liang KV, Greene EL, Williams AW, et al. Exploratory study of relationship between hospitalized heart failure patients and chronic renal replacement therapy. *Nephrol Dial Transplant.* 2009;24:2518-2523.

709. London GM, Pannier B. Renal replacement therapy for heart failure patients: in whom, when and which therapy to use? *Nephrol Dial Transplant.* 2009;24:2314-2315.

710. Hunt SA, Abraham WT, Chin MH, et al. 2009 Focused update incorporated into the ACC/AHA 2005 Guidelines for the Diagnosis and Management of Heart Failure in Adults: a report of the American College of Cardiology Foundation/American Heart Association Task Force on Practice Guidelines: developed in collaboration with the International Society for Heart and Lung Transplantation. *Circulation.* 2009;119:e391-e479.

711. Garg R, Yusuf S. Overview of randomized trials of angiotensin-converting enzyme inhibitors on mortality and morbidity in patients with heart failure. Collaborative Group on ACE Inhibitor Trials. *JAMA.* 1995;273:1450-1456.

712. Dickstein K, Cohen-Solal A, Filippatos G, et al. ESC guidelines for the diagnosis and treatment of acute and chronic heart failure 2008: the Task Force for the Diagnosis and Treatment of Acute and Chronic Heart Failure 2008 of the European Society of Cardiology. Developed in collaboration with the Heart Failure Association of the ESC (HFA) and endorsed by the European Society of Intensive Care Medicine (ESICM). *Eur Heart J.* 2008;29:2388-2442.

713. Gaddam KK, Pimenta E, Husain S, et al. Aldosterone and cardiovascular disease. *Curr Probl Cardiol.* 2009;34:51-84.

714. Desai A. Hyperkalemia associated with inhibitors of the renin-angiotensin-aldosterone system: balancing risk and benefit. *Circulation.* 2008;118:1609-1611.

715. Flack JM. Editorial commentary on fixed combination isosorbide dinitrate/hydralazine for nitric-oxide–enhancing therapy in heart failure. *Expert Opin Pharmacother.* 2007;8:275-277.

716. Franciosa JA. Fixed combination isosorbide dinitrate-hydralazine for nitric-oxide–enhancing therapy in heart failure. *Expert Opin Pharmacother.* 2006;7:2521-2531.

717. Kiowski W, Sutsch G, Hunziker P, et al. Evidence for endothelin-1–mediated vasoconstriction in severe chronic heart failure. *Lancet.* 1995;346:732-736.

718. Schirger JA, Chen HH, Jougasaki M, et al. Endothelin A receptor antagonism in experimental congestive heart failure results in augmentation of the renin-angiotensin system and sustained sodium retention. *Circulation.* 2004;109:249-254.

719. Kedzierski RM, Yanagisawa M. Endothelin system: the double-edged sword in health and disease. *Annu Rev Pharmacol Toxicol.* 2001;41:851-876.

720. Korinek J, Boerrigter G, Mohammed SF, et al. Insights into natriuretic peptides in heart failure: an update. *Curr Heart Fail Rep.* 2008;5:97-104.

721. Colucci WS, Elkayam U, Horton DP, et al. Intravenous nesiritide, a natriuretic peptide, in the treatment of decompensated congestive heart failure. Nesiritide Study Group. *N Engl J Med.* 2000;343:246-253.

722. Colucci WS. Nesiritide for the treatment of decompensated heart failure. *J Card Fail.* 2001;7:92-100.

723. Vesely DL. Which of the cardiac natriuretic peptides is most effective for the treatment of congestive heart failure, renal failure and cancer? *Clin Exp Pharmacol Physiol.* 2006;33:169-176.

724. Ezekowitz JA, Hernandez AF, Starling RC, et al. Standardizing care for acute decompensated heart failure in a large megatrial: the approach for the Acute Studies of Clinical Effectiveness of Nesiritide in Subjects with Decompensated Heart Failure (ASCEND-HF). *Am Heart J.* 2009;157:219-228.

725. Mohammed SF, Korinek J, Chen HH, et al. Nesiritide in acute decompensated heart failure: current status and future perspectives. *Rev Cardiovasc Med.* 2008;9:151-158.

726. Margulies KB, Burnett Jr JC. Neutral endopeptidase 24.11: a modulator of natriuretic peptides. *Semin Nephrol.* 1993;13:71-77.

727. McClean DR, Ikram H, Garlick AH, et al. The clinical, cardiac, renal, arterial and neurohormonal effects of omapatrilat, a vasopeptidase inhibitor, in patients with chronic heart failure. *J Am Coll Cardiol.* 2000;36:479-486.

728. McClean DR, Ikram H, Mehta S, et al. Vasopeptidase inhibition with omapatrilat in chronic heart failure: acute and long-term hemodynamic and neurohumoral effects. *J Am Coll Cardiol.* 2002;39:2034-2041.

729. Chen HH, Schirger JA, Chau WL, et al. Renal response to acute neutral endopeptidase inhibition in mild and severe experimental heart failure. *Circulation.* 1999;100:2443-2448.

730. Margulies KB, Perrella MA, McKinley LJ, et al. Angiotensin inhibition potentiates the renal responses to neutral endopeptidase inhibition in dogs with congestive heart failure. *J Clin Invest.* 1991;88:1636-1642.

731. Dawson A, Struthers AD. Vasopeptidase inhibitors in heart failure. *J Renin Angiotensin Aldosterone Syst.* 2002;3:156-159.

732. Rouleau JL, Pfeffer MA, Stewart DJ, et al. Comparison of vasopeptidase inhibitor, omapatrilat, and lisinopril on exercise tolerance and morbidity in patients with heart failure: IMPRESS randomised trial. *Lancet.* 2000;356:615-620.

733. Abassi ZA, Yahia A, Zeid S, et al. Cardiac and renal effects of omapatrilat, a vasopeptidase inhibitor, in rats with experimental congestive heart failure. *Am J Physiol Heart Circ Physiol.* 2005;288:H722-H728.

734. Burnett JC. Vasopeptidase inhibition. *Curr Opin Nephrol Hypertens.* 2000;9:465-468.

735. Molinaro G, Rouleau JL, Adam A. Vasopeptidase inhibitors: a new class of dual zinc metallopeptidase inhibitors for cardiorenal therapeutics. *Curr Opin Pharmacol.* 2002;2:131-141.

736. Sagnella GA. Vasopeptidase inhibitors. *J Renin Angiotensin Aldosterone Syst.* 2002;3:90-95.

737. Weber MA. Vasopeptidase inhibitors. *Lancet.* 2001;358:1525-1532.

738. Iyengar S, Abraham WT. Neutral endopeptidase inhibitors and endothelin antagonists. *Cardiol Clin.* 2008;26:41-48:vi.

739. Goldsmith SR, Gheorghiade M. Vasopressin antagonism in heart failure. *J Am Coll Cardiol.* 2005;46:1785-1791.

740. Thibonnier M, Coles P, Thibonnier A, et al. Molecular pharmacology and modeling of vasopressin receptors. *Prog Brain Res.* 2002;139:179-196.

741. Gheorghiade M, Gattis WA, O'Connor CM, et al. Effects of tolvaptan, a vasopressin antagonist, in patients hospitalized with worsening heart failure: a randomized controlled trial. *JAMA.* 2004;291:1963-1971.

742. Gheorghiade M, Gottlieb SS, Udelson JE, et al. Vasopressin V(2) receptor blockade with tolvaptan versus fluid restriction in the treatment of hyponatremia. *Am J Cardiol.* 2006;97:1064-1067.

743. Konstam MA, Gheorghiade M, Burnett Jr JC, et al. Effects of oral tolvaptan in patients hospitalized for worsening heart failure: the EVEREST Outcome Trial. *JAMA.* 2007;297:1319-1331.

744. Goldsmith SR, Elkayam U, Haught WH, et al. Efficacy and safety of the vasopressin V_{1A}/V_2-receptor antagonist conivaptan in acute decompensated heart failure: a dose-ranging pilot study. *J Card Fail.* 2008;14:641-647.

745. Ku E, Nobakht N, Campese VM. Lixivaptan: a novel vasopressin receptor antagonist. *Expert Opin Investig Drugs.* 2009;18:657-662.

746. Costello-Boerrigter LC, Smith WB, Boerrigter G, et al. Vasopressin-2–receptor antagonism augments water excretion without changes in renal hemodynamics or sodium and potassium excretion in human heart failure. *Am J Physiol Renal Physiol.* 2006;290:F273-F278.

747. Udelson JE, McGrew FA, Flores E, et al. Multicenter, randomized, double-blind, placebo-controlled study on the effect of oral tolvaptan on left ventricular dilation and function in patients with heart failure and systolic dysfunction. *J Am Coll Cardiol.* 2007;49:2151-2159.

748. Udelson JE, Smith WB, Hendrix GH, et al. Acute hemodynamic effects of conivaptan, a dual V(1A) and V(2) vasopressin receptor antagonist, in patients with advanced heart failure. *Circulation.* 2001;104:2417-2423.

749. Udelson JE, Orlandi C, Ouyang J, et al. Acute hemodynamic effects of tolvaptan, a vasopressin V_2 receptor blocker, in patients with symptomatic heart failure and systolic dysfunction: an international, multicenter, randomized, placebo-controlled trial. *J Am Coll Cardiol.* 2008;52:1540-1545.

750. Gines P, Guevara M, Arroyo V, et al. Hepatorenal syndrome. *Lancet.* 2003;362:1819-1827.

751. Wong F, Pantea L, Sniderman K. Midodrine, octreotide, albumin, and TIPS in selected patients with cirrhosis and type 1 hepatorenal syndrome. *Hepatology.* 2004;40:55-64.

752. Colle I, Durand F, Pessione F, et al. Clinical course, predictive factors and prognosis in patients with cirrhosis and type 1 hepatorenal syndrome treated with terlipressin: a retrospective analysis. *J Gastroenterol Hepatol.* 2002;17:882-888.

753. Ortega R, Gines P, Uriz J, et al. Terlipressin therapy with and without albumin for patients with hepatorenal syndrome: results of a prospective, nonrandomized study. *Hepatology.* 2002;36:941-948.

754. Alessandria C, Venon WD, Marzano A, et al. Renal failure in cirrhotic patients: role of terlipressin in clinical approach to hepatorenal syndrome type 2. *Eur J Gastroenterol Hepatol.* 2002;14:1363-1368.

755. Martin-Llahi M, Pepin MN, Guevara M, et al. Terlipressin and albumin vs albumin in patients with cirrhosis and hepatorenal syndrome: a randomized study. *Gastroenterology.* 2008;134:1352-1359.

756. Sanyal AJ, Boyer T, Garcia-Tsao G, et al. A randomized, prospective, double-blind, placebo-controlled trial of terlipressin for type 1 hepatorenal syndrome. *Gastroenterology.* 2008;134:1360-1368.

757. Alessandria C, Debernardi-Venon W, Carello M, et al. Midodrine in the prevention of hepatorenal syndrome type 2 recurrence: a case-control study. *Dig Liver Dis.* 2009;41:298-302.

758. Restuccia T, Ortega R, Guevara M, et al. Effects of treatment of hepatorenal syndrome before transplantation on posttransplantation outcome. A case-control study. *J Hepatol.* 2004;40:140-146.

759. Kiser TH, Fish DN, Obritsch MD, et al. Vasopressin, not octreotide, may be beneficial in the treatment of hepatorenal syndrome: a retrospective study. *Nephrol Dial Transplant.* 2005;20:1813-1820.

760. Pomier-Layrargues G, Paquin SC, Hassoun Z, et al. Octreotide in hepatorenal syndrome: a randomized, double-blind, placebo-controlled, crossover study. *Hepatology.* 2003;38:238-243.

761. Angeli P, Volpin R, Gerunda G, et al. Reversal of type 1 hepatorenal syndrome with the administration of midodrine and octreotide. *Hepatology.* 1999;29:1690-1697.

762. Karwa R, Woodis CB. Midodrine and octreotide in treatment of cirrhosis-related hemodynamic complications. *Ann Pharmacother.* 2009;43:692-699.

763. Duvoux C, Zanditenas D, Hezode C, et al. Effects of noradrenalin and albumin in patients with type I hepatorenal syndrome: a pilot study. *Hepatology.* 2002;36:374-380

763a. Alessandria C, Ottobrelli A, Debernardi-Venon W, et al. Noradrenalin vs terlipressin in patients with hepatorenal syndrome: a prospective, randomized, unblinded, pilot study. *J Hepatol.* 2007;47:499-505.

764. Guevara M, Baccaro ME, Torre A, et al. Hyponatremia is a risk factor of hepatic encephalopathy in patients with cirrhosis: a prospective study with time-dependent analysis. *Am J Gastroenterol.* 2009;104:1382-1389.

765. Moreau R. Hyponatremia in cirrhosis. Pathophysiology, prevalence, prognostic value, treatment. *Acta Gastroenterol Belg.* 2008;71:379-385.

766. Gines P, Guevara M. Hyponatremia in cirrhosis: pathogenesis, clinical significance, and management. *Hepatology.* 2008;48:1002-1010.

767. Gines P, Cardenas A. The management of ascites and hyponatremia in cirrhosis. *Semin Liver Dis.* 2008;28:43-58.

768. Colombato L. The role of transjugular intrahepatic portosystemic shunt (TIPS) in the management of portal hypertension. *J Clin Gastroenterol.* 2007;41(suppl 3):S344-S351.

769. Garcia-Tsao G. The transjugular intrahepatic portosystemic shunt for the management of cirrhotic refractory ascites. *Nat Clin Pract Gastroenterol Hepatol.* 2006;3:380-389.

770. Guevara M, Gines P, Bandi JC, et al. Transjugular intrahepatic portosystemic shunt in hepatorenal syndrome: effects on renal function and vasoactive systems. *Hepatology.* 1998;28:416-422.

771. Brensing KA, Textor J, Perz J, et al. Long term outcome after transjugular intrahepatic portosystemic stent-shunt in non-transplant cirrhotics with hepatorenal syndrome: a phase II study. *Gut.* 2000;47:288-295.

772. Choi JY, Bae SH, Yoon SK, et al. Preconditioning by extracorporeal liver support (MARS) of patients with cirrhosis and severe liver failure evaluated for living donor liver transplantation—a pilot study. *Liver Int.* 2005;25:740-745.

773. Donati G, Piscaglia F, Coli L, et al. Acute systemic, splanchnic and renal haemodynamic changes induced by molecular adsorbent recirculating system (MARS) treatment in patients with end-stage cirrhosis. *Aliment Pharmacol Ther.* 2007;26:717-726.

774. Mitzner SR, Stange J, Klammt S, et al. Improvement of hepatorenal syndrome with extracorporeal albumin dialysis MARS: results of a prospective, randomized, controlled clinical trial. *Liver Transpl.* 2000;6:277-286.

775. Marik PE, Wood K, Starzl TE. The course of type 1 hepato-renal syndrome post liver transplantation. *Nephrol Dial Transplant.* 2006;21:478-482.

776. Jeyarajah DR, Gonwa TA, McBride M, et al. Hepatorenal syndrome: combined liver kidney transplants versus isolated liver transplant. *Transplantation.* 1997;64:1760-1765.

777. Bloom RD, Bleicher M. Simultaneous liver-kidney transplantation in the MELD era. *Adv Chronic Kidney Dis.* 2009;16:268-277.

778. Gallegos-Orozco JF, Vargas HE. Liver transplantation: from Child to MELD. *Med Clin North Am.* 2009;93:931-950:ix.

779. Adam R, Hoti E. Liver transplantation: the current situation. *Semin Liver Dis.* 2009;29:3-18.

Disorders of Water Balance

Joseph G. Verbalis

Disorders of body fluids are among the most commonly encountered problems in clinical medicine. This is in large part because many different disease states can potentially disrupt the finely balanced mechanisms that control the intake and output of water and solute. Since body water is the primary determinant of the osmolality of the extracellular fluid, disorders of water metabolism can be broadly divided into hyperosmolar disorders, in which there is a deficiency of body water relative to body solute, and hypo-osmolar disorders, in which there is an excess of body water relative to body solute. Because sodium is the main contributor to plasma osmolality, these disorders are typically characterized by hypernatremia and hyponatremia, respectively. Before discussing specific aspects of these disorders, this chapter first briefly reviews the regulatory mechanisms underlying water metabolism that, in concert with sodium metabolism, maintain body fluid homeostasis.

Body Fluids: Compartmentalization, Composition, and Turnover

Water comprises approximately 55% to 65% of body weight, varying with age, sex, and amount of body fat, and therefore is the largest single constituent of the body. Total body water

(TBW) is distributed between the intracellular fluid (ICF) and the extracellular fluid (ECF) compartments. Estimates of the relative sizes of these two pools differ significantly depending on the tracer used to measure the ECF volume, but most studies in animals and humans have indicated that 55% to 65% of TBW resides in the ICF and 35% to 45% is in the ECF. Approximately 75% of the ECF compartment is interstitial fluid and only 25% is intravascular fluid (i.e., blood volume).[1,2] Figure 15-1 summarizes the estimated body fluid spaces of an average-weight adult.

The solute composition of the ICF and ECF differs considerably, because most cell membranes possess multiple transport systems that actively accumulate or expel specific solutes. Thus, membrane-bound Na^+–K^+–adenosine triphosphatase (Na^+-K^+-ATPase) maintains Na^+ in a primarily extracellular location and K^+ in a primarily intracellular location.[3] Similar transporters effectively result in confining Cl^- largely to the ECF and Mg^{2+}, organic acids, and phosphates to the ICF. Glucose, which requires an insulin-activated transport system to enter most cells, is present in significant amounts only in the ECF, because it is rapidly converted intracellularly to glycogen or metabolites. HCO_3^- is present in both compartments, but is approximately three times more concentrated in the ECF. Urea is unique among the major naturally occurring and to express the result relative to a standard solution of known concentration using units of either osmolality (milliosmoles of solute per kilogram of water, mOsm/kg H_2O), or osmolarity (milliosmoles of solute per liter of water, mOsm/L H_2O). Plasma osmolality (P_{osm}) can be measured directly as described earlier or calculated by summing the concentrations of the major solutes present in the plasma:

$$P_{osm} (mOsm / kg\ H_2O) = [2 \times plasma\ [Na^+]\ (mEq / L)] + [glucose\ (mg / dL) / 18] + [blood\ urea\ nitrogen\ (mg / dL) / 2.8]$$

The two methods produce comparable results under most conditions (the value obtained using the preceding formula is generally within 1% to 2% of that obtained by direct osmometry), as will simply doubling the plasma $[Na^+]$, since sodium and its accompanying anions are the predominant solutes present in plasma. However, the total osmolality of plasma is not always equivalent to the *effective* osmolality, often referred to as the *tonicity* of the plasma, because the latter is a function of the relative solute permeability properties of the membranes separating the ICF and ECF compartments.

Solutes to which cell membranes are impermeable (e.g., Na^+, mannitol) are restricted to the ECF compartment and are effective solutes, because they create osmotic pressure gradients across cell membranes leading to osmotic movement of water from the ICF to the ECF compartment. Solutes to which cell membranes are permeable (e.g., urea, ethanol, methanol) are ineffective solutes, because they do not create osmotic pressure gradients across cell membranes and therefore are not associated with such water shifts.[9] Glucose is a unique solute, since at normal physiologic plasma concentrations it is taken up by cells via active transport mechanisms and therefore acts as an ineffective solute, but under conditions of impaired cellular uptake (e.g., insulin deficiency) it becomes an effective extracellular solute.[10]

The importance of this distinction between total and effective osmolality is that only the effective solutes in plasma are determinants of whether clinically significant hyperosmolality or hypo-osmolality is present. An example of this is uremia: a patient with a blood urea nitrogen concentration that has increased by 56 mg/dL will have a corresponding 20 mOsm/kg H_2O elevation in plasma osmolality, but the effective osmolality will remain normal, since the increased urea is proportionally distributed across both the ECF and ICF. In contrast, a patient whose plasma $[Na^+]$ has increased by 10 mEq/L will also have a 20 mOsm/kg H_2O elevation of plasma osmolality, since the increased cation must be balanced by an equivalent increase in plasma anions, but in this case the effective osmolality will also be elevated by 20 mOsm/kg H_2O because the Na^+ and accompanying anions will largely remain restricted to the ECF due to the relative impermeability of cell membranes to Na^+ and other ions. Thus, elevations of solutes such as urea, unlike elevations of sodium, do not cause cellular dehydration and consequently do not activate mechanisms that defend body fluid homeostasis by increasing body water stores.

Both body water and solutes are in a state of continuous exchange with the environment. The magnitude of the turnover varies considerably depending on physical, social, and environmental factors, but in healthy adults it averages 5% to 10% of the total body content each day. For the most part, daily intake of water and electrolytes is not determined by physiologic requirements but is more a function of dietary

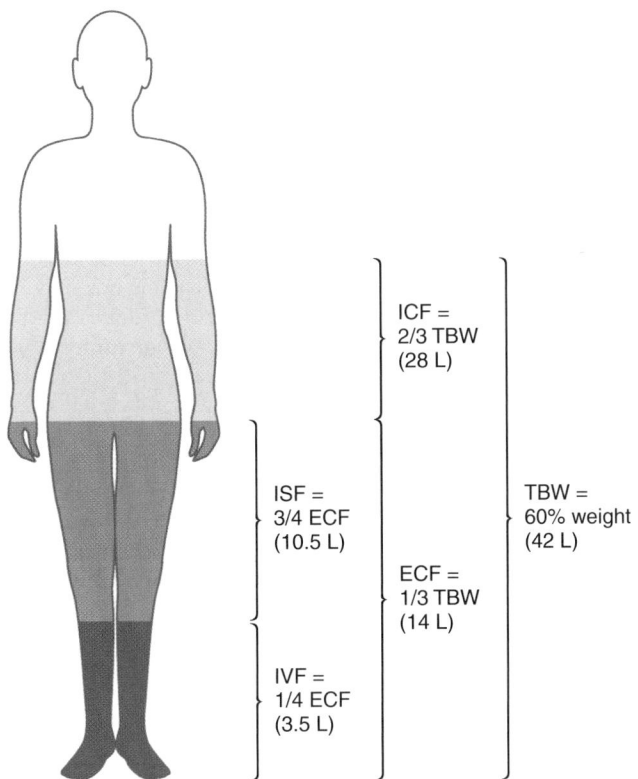

FIGURE 15-1 Schematic representation of body fluid compartments in humans. The *shaded areas* depict the approximate size of each compartment as a function of body weight. The *numbers* indicate the relative sizes of the various fluid compartments and the approximate absolute volumes of the compartments (in liters) in a 70-kg adult. ECF, Extracellular fluid; ICF, intracellular fluid; ISF, interstitial fluid; IVF, intravascular fluid; TBW, total body water. (From Verbalis JG: Body water and osmolality, in Wilkinson B, Jamison R [editors]: *Textbook of nephrology*, London, 1997, Chapman & Hall, pp 89-94.)

solutes in that it diffuses freely across most cell membranes[4]; therefore, it is present in similar concentrations in virtually all body fluids, except in the renal medulla, where it is concentrated by urea transporters (see Chapter 10).

Despite their very different solute compositions, the ICF and ECF have equivalent osmotic pressures.[5] This is a function of the total concentration of all solutes in a fluid compartment, because most biologic membranes are semipermeable (i.e., freely permeable to water but not to aqueous solutes). Thus, water will flow across membranes into a compartment with a higher solute concentration until a steady state is reached in which the osmotic pressures have equalized on both sides of the cell membrane.[6] An important consequence of this thermodynamic law is that the volume of distribution of body Na^+ and K^+ is actually the TBW rather than just the ECF or ICF volume, respectively.[7] For example, any increase in ECF sodium concentration (Na^+) will cause water to shift from the ICF to the ECF until the ICF and ECF osmotic pressures are equal, which thus effectively distributes the Na^+ across both extracellular and intracellular water.

Osmolality is defined as the concentration of all of the solutes in a given weight of fluid. The total solute concentration of a fluid can be determined and expressed in several different ways. The most common method is to measure its freezing point or vapor pressure, since these are colligative properties of the number of free solute particles in a volume of fluid,[8] preferences and cultural influences. Healthy adults have an average daily fluid ingestion of approximately 2 to 3 L, but with considerable individual variation. Approximately one third of this is derived from food or the metabolism of fat, and the rest is from discretionary ingestion of fluids. Similarly, of the 1000 mOsm of solute ingested or generated by the metabolism of nutrients each day, nearly 40% is intrinsic to food, another 35% is added to food as a preservative or flavoring, and the rest is mostly urea.

In contrast to basal intakes, which are largely unregulated, the urinary excretion of both water and solute is highly regulated to preserve body fluid homeostasis. Thus, under normal circumstances almost all ingested Na+, Cl−, and K+, as well as both ingested and metabolically generated urea, are excreted in the urine under the control of specific regulatory mechanisms. Other ingested solutes (e.g., divalent minerals) are excreted primarily by the gastrointestinal tract. Urinary excretion of water is also tightly regulated by the secretory and renal effects of arginine vasopressin, which is discussed in greater detail in Chapters 10 and 11 and in the following section on water metabolism.

Water Metabolism

Water metabolism is responsible for the balance between the intake and excretion of water. Each side of this balance equation can be considered to consist of a *regulated* and an *unregulated* component, the magnitudes of which can vary quite markedly under different physiologic and pathophysiologic conditions.

The unregulated component of water intake consists of the intrinsic water content of ingested foods and of beverages consumed primarily for reasons of palatability or desired secondary effects (e.g., caffeinated beverages) or for social or habitual reasons (e.g., alcoholic beverages), whereas the regulated component of water intake consists of fluids consumed in response to a perceived sensation of thirst. Studies of middle-aged subjects have found mean fluid intakes of 2.1 L/24 hr, and analysis of the fluids consumed indicates that the vast majority of the fluid ingestion is associated with meal consumption or is determined by influences such as taste or psychosocial factors rather than true thirst.[11]

The unregulated component of water excretion occurs via insensible water losses from a variety of sources (cutaneous losses from sweating, evaporative losses in exhaled air, gastrointestinal losses) as well as the obligate amount of water that the kidneys must excrete to eliminate solutes generated by body metabolism, whereas the regulated component of water excretion is comprised of the renal excretion of free water in excess of the obligate amount necessary to excrete metabolic solutes. Unlike solutes, a relatively large proportion of body water is excreted by evaporation from skin and lungs. This amount varies markedly depending on several factors, including dress, humidity, temperature, and exercise.[12]

Under the sedentary and temperature-controlled indoor conditions typical of modern urban life, daily insensible water loss in healthy adults is minimal at approximately 8 to 10 mL/kg body water (0.5 to 0.7 L in a 70-kg adult man or woman). However, insensible losses can increase to twice this level (i.e., 20 mL/kg body water) simply under conditions of increased activity and temperature, and if environmental temperature or activity is even greater, such as in arid environments, the rate of insensible water loss can even approximate the maximal rate of free water excretion by the kidney.[12] Thus, in quantitative terms, insensible loss and the factors that influence it can be just as important to body fluid homeostasis as regulated urine output.

Another major determinant of unregulated water loss is the rate of urine solute excretion, which cannot be reduced below a minimal obligatory level required to excrete the solute load. The volume of urine required depends not only on the solute load but also on the degree of antidiuresis. At a typical basal level of urinary concentration (urine osmolality = 600 mOsm/kg H_2O) and a typical solute load of 900 to 1200 mOsm/day, a 70-kg adult would require a total urine volume of 1.5 to 2.0 L (21 to 29 mL/kg body water) to excrete the solute load. However, under conditions of maximal antidiuresis (urine osmolality = 1200 mOsm/kg H_2O) the same solute load would require a minimal obligatory urine output of only 0.75 to 1.0 L/day. Conversely, a decrease in urine concentration to minimal levels (urine osmolality = 60 mOsm/kg H_2O) would require a proportionately larger urine volume of 15 to 20 L/day for excretion of the same solute load.

The previous discussion emphasizes that both water intake and water excretion have very substantial unregulated components, and these can vary tremendously as a result of factors that are unrelated to maintenance of body fluid homeostasis. In effect, the regulated components of water metabolism are those that act to maintain body fluid homeostasis by compensating for whatever perturbations result from unregulated water losses or gains. Within this framework, the major mechanisms responsible for regulating water metabolism are the pituitary secretion and renal effects of vasopressin, and thirst, each of which is discussed in greater detail in the following sections.

Vasopressin Synthesis and Secretion

The primary determinant of free water excretion in animals and humans is the regulation of urinary water excretion by circulating levels of *arginine vasopressin* (AVP) in plasma. The renal effects of AVP are covered extensively in Chapters 10 and 11. This chapter focuses on the regulation of AVP synthesis and secretion.

Structure and Synthesis

Before AVP was biochemically characterized, early studies used the general term *antidiuretic hormone* (ADH) to describe this substance. Now that AVP is known to be the only naturally occurring antidiuretic substance, it is more appropriate to refer to it by its correct hormonal designation. AVP is a nine–amino acid peptide that is synthesized in the hypothalamus. It is composed of a six–amino acid ringlike structure formed by a disulfide bridge, with a three–amino acid tail at the end of which the terminal carboxyl group is amidated. Substitution of lysine for arginine in position 8 yields lysine vasopressin, the antidiuretic hormone found in pigs and other members of the suborder Suina. Substitution of isoleucine for phenylalanine at position 3 and of leucine for arginine at position 8 yields oxytocin, a hormone found in all mammals as well as many submammalian species.[13] Oxytocin has weak antidiuretic activity,[14] but is a potent constrictor of smooth muscle in mammary glands and uterus.

As implied by their names, arginine and lysine vasopressin also cause constriction of blood vessels, which was the property that led to their original discovery in the late nineteenth century.[15] This pressor effect occurs only at concentrations many times those required to produce antidiuresis and is probably of little physiologic or pathologic importance in humans except under conditions of severe hypotension and hypovolemia, where it acts to supplement the vasoconstrictive actions of angiotensin II and the sympathetic nervous system.[16] The multiple actions of AVP are mediated by different G protein–coupled receptors,[17] designated V_{1a}, V_{1b}, and V_2 (see Chapter 11).

AVP and oxytocin are produced by the *neurohypophysis*, often referred to as the *posterior pituitary gland* because the neural lobe is located centrally and posterior to the adenohypophysis, or anterior pituitary gland, in the sella turcica. However, it is important to understand that the posterior pituitary gland consists only of the distal axons of the magnocellular

neurons that comprise the neurohypophysis. The cell bodies of these axons are found in specialized (magnocellular) neural cells located in two discrete areas of the hypothalamus, the paired supraoptic nucleus (SON) and paraventricular nucleus (PVN) (Figure 15-2). In adults the posterior pituitary is connected to the brain by a short stalk through the diaphragma sellae.

The neurohypophysis is supplied with blood by branches of the superior and inferior hypophysial arteries, which arise from the posterior communicating and intracavernous portion of the internal carotid artery. In the posterior pituitary, the arterioles break up into localized capillary networks that drain directly into the jugular vein via the sellar, cavernous, and lateral venous sinuses. Many of the neurosecretory neurons that terminate higher in the infundibulum and median eminence originate in parvicellular neurons in the PVN and are functionally distinct from the magnocellular neurons that terminate in the posterior pituitary, since they primarily enhance secretion of adrenocorticotropic hormone (ACTH) from the anterior pituitary. AVP-containing neurons also project from

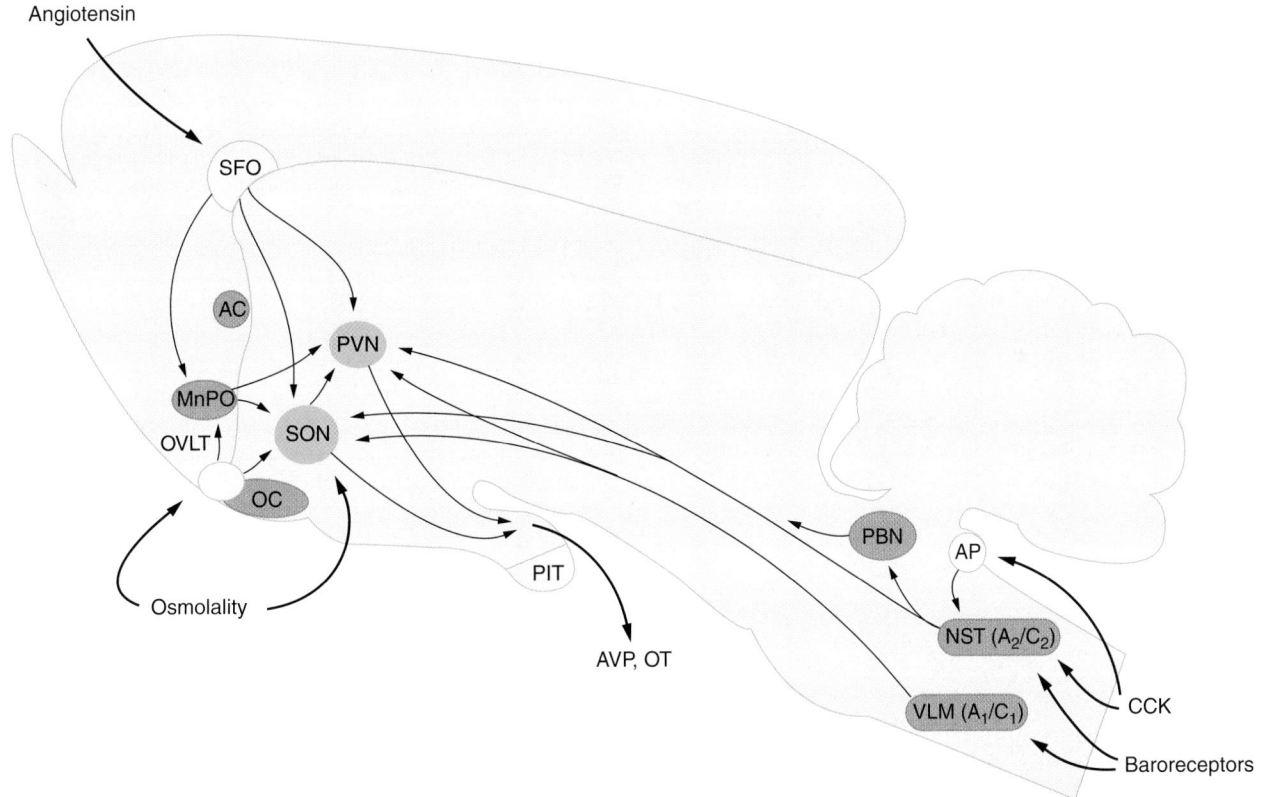

FIGURE 15-2 Summary of the main anterior hypothalamic pathways that mediate secretion of arginine vasopressin (AVP) and oxytocin (OT). The vascular organ of the lamina terminalis (OVLT) is especially sensitive to hyperosmolality. Hyperosmolality also activates other neurons in the anterior hypothalamus, such as those in the subfornical organ (SFO) and median preoptic nucleus (MnPO), as well as magnocellular neurons, which are intrinsically osmosensitive. Circulating angiotensin II (Ang II) activates neurons of the SFO, an essential site of Ang II action, as well as cells throughout the lamina terminalis and MnPO. In response to hyperosmolality or Ang II, projections from the SFO and OVLT to the MnPO activate excitatory and inhibitory interneurons that project to the supraoptic nucleus (SON) and paraventricular nucleus (PVN) to modulate direct inputs to these areas from the circumventricular organs. Cholecystokinin (CCK) acts primarily on gastric vagal afferents that terminate in the nucleus of the solitary tract (NST), but at higher doses, it can also act at the area postrema (AP). Although neurons are apparently activated in the ventrolateral medulla (VLM) and NST, most neurohypophyseal secretion appears to be stimulated by monosynaptic projections from A_2/C_2 cells, and possibly also noncatecholaminergic somatostatin/inhibin B cells, of the NST. Baroreceptor-mediated stimuli, such as hypovolemia and hypotension, are more complex. The major projection to magnocellular AVP neurons appears to arise from A_1 cells of the VLM that are activated by excitatory interneurons from the NST. Other areas, such as the parabrachial nucleus (PBN), may contribute multisynaptic projections. Cranial nerves IX and X, which terminate in the NST, also contribute input to magnocellular AVP neurons. It is unclear whether baroreceptor-mediated secretion of OT results from projections from VLM neurons or from NST neurons. AC, Anterior commissure; OC, optic chiasm; PIT, anterior pituitary. (From Stricker EM, Verbalis JG: Water intake and body fluids, in Squire LR, Bloom FE, McConnell SK, et al [editors]: *Fundamental neuroscience*, San Diego, 2003, Academic Press, pp 1011-1029.)

parvicellular neurons of the PVN to other areas of the brain, including the limbic system, the nucleus tractus solitarius (NTS), and the lateral gray matter of the spinal cord. The full extent of the functions of these extrahypophysial projections are still under study.

The genes that encode the AVP and oxytocin precursors are located in close proximity on chromosome 20, but are expressed at the messenger RNA (mRNA) level in mutually exclusive populations of neurohypophyseal neurons.[18] The AVP gene consists of approximately 2000 base pairs and contains three exons separated by two intervening sequences (Figure 15-3). Each exon encodes one of the three functional domains of the preprohormone, although small parts of the nonconserved sequences of *neurophysin* are located in the first and third exons that code for AVP and the C-terminal glycoprotein, called *copeptin*, respectively. The 5'-flanking region of the gene, which is upstream of the start site of transcription and regulates expression of the gene, shows extensive sequence homology across several species but is markedly different from that of the otherwise closely related gene for oxytocin.

The promoter region of the AVP gene in the rat contains several putative regulatory elements, including a glucocorticoid response element, a cyclic adenosine monophosphate (cAMP) response element, and four activating protein-2 (AP-2) binding sites.[19] Experimental data have suggested that the DNA sequences between the AVP and oxytocin genes, the intergenic region, may contain critical sites for cell-specific expression of these two hormones.[20]

The gene for AVP is also expressed in a number of other neurons, including but not limited to the parvicellular neurons of the PVN and SON. AVP and oxytocin genes are also expressed in several peripheral tissues, including the adrenal medulla, ovary, testis, thymus, and certain sensory ganglia.[21] However, the AVP mRNA in these tissues appears to be shorter (620 bases) than its hypothalamic counterpart (720 bases), apparently because of tissue-specific differences in the length of the poly(adenylic acid) tails. More importantly, the levels of AVP in peripheral tissues are generally two to three orders of magnitude lower than those in the neurohypophysis, which suggests that AVP in these tissues likely has paracrine

rather than endocrine functions. This is consistent with the observation that destruction of the neurohypophysis essentially eliminates AVP from the plasma despite the presence of these multiple peripheral sites of AVP synthesis.

Secretion of AVP and its associated neurophysin and copeptin peptide fragments occurs by a calcium-dependent exocytotic process similar to that described for other neurosecretory systems. Secretion is triggered by propagation of an electrical impulse along the axon that causes depolarization of the cell membrane, an influx of Ca^{2+}, fusion of secretory granules with the cell membrane, and extrusion of their contents. This view of the process is supported by the observation that AVP, neurophysin, and the glycoprotein copeptin are released simultaneously in response to many stimuli.[22] However, at the physiologic pH of plasma there is no binding of either AVP or oxytocin to their respective neurophysins, so after secretion each peptide circulates independently in the bloodstream.[23]

Stimuli for secretion of AVP or oxytocin also stimulate transcription and increase the mRNA content of both prohormones in the magnocellular neurons. This has been well documented in rats, in which dehydration, which stimulates secretion of AVP, accelerates transcription and increases the levels of AVP (and oxytocin) mRNA,[24,25] and hypo-osmolality, which inhibits secretion of AVP, produces a decrease in the content of AVP mRNA.[26] These and other data indicate that the major control of AVP synthesis most likely resides at the level of transcription.[27] Antidiuresis occurs via interaction of the circulating hormone with AVP V_2 receptors in the kidney, which results in increased water permeability of the collecting duct through the insertion of the aquaporin-2 (AQP2) water channel into the apical membranes of collecting tubule principal cells (see Chapter 10).

The importance of AVP for maintaining water balance is underscored by the fact that the normal pituitary stores of this hormone are very large, providing more than a week's supply of hormone for maximal antidiuresis under conditions of sustained dehydration.[27] Knowledge of the different conditions that stimulate pituitary AVP release in humans is therefore essential for an understanding of water metabolism.

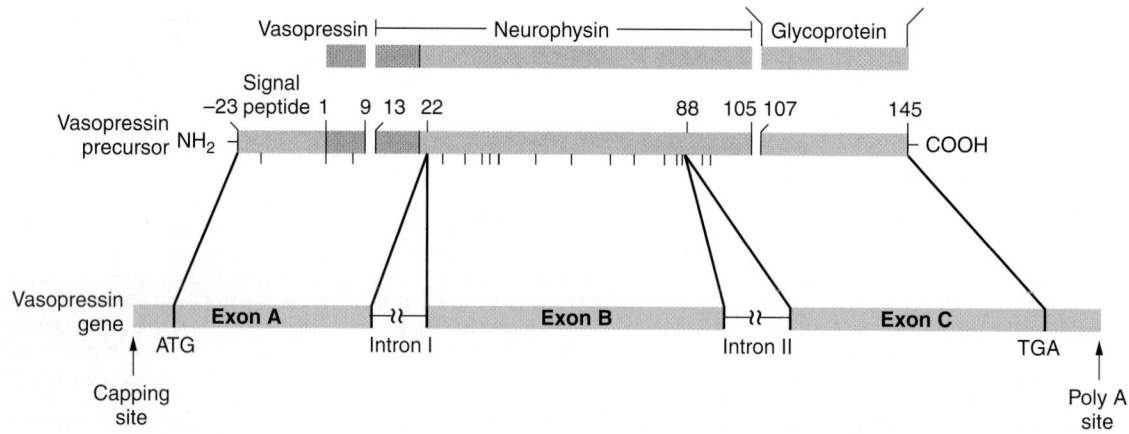

FIGURE 15-3 Arginine vasopressin (AVP) gene and its protein products. The three exons encode a 145–amino acid prohormone with an amino-terminal signal peptide. The prohormone is packaged into neurosecretory granules of magnocellular neurons. During axonal transport of the granules from the hypothalamus to the posterior pituitary, enzymatic cleavage of the prohormone generates the final products: AVP, neurophysin, and a COOH-terminal glycoprotein. When afferent stimulation depolarizes the AVP-containing neurons, the three products are released into capillaries of the posterior pituitary. (Adapted from Richter D, Schmale H: The structure of the precursor to arginine vasopressin, a model preprohormone, *Prog Brain Res* 60:227-233, 1983.)

Osmotic Regulation

AVP secretion is influenced by many different stimuli, but since the pioneering studies of antidiuretic hormone secretion by Verney, it has been clear that the most important under physiologic conditions is the osmotic pressure of plasma. With further refinement of radioimmunoassays for AVP, the unique sensitivity of this hormone to small changes in osmolality, as well as the corresponding sensitivity of the kidney to small changes in plasma AVP levels, have become apparent.

Although the magnocellular neurons themselves have been found to have intrinsic osmoreceptive properties,[28] research over the last several decades has clearly shown that the most sensitive osmoreceptive cells that are able to sense small changes in plasma osmolality and transduce these changes into AVP secretion are located in the anterior hypothalamus, likely in or near the circumventricular organ called the *organum vasculosum laminae terminalis* (OVLT)[29] (see Figure 15-2). Perhaps the strongest evidence for location of the primary osmoreceptors in this area of the brain are the multiple studies that have demonstrated that destruction of this area disrupts osmotically stimulated AVP secretion and thirst without affecting the neurohypophysis or its response to nonosmotic stimuli.[30,31]

Although some debate still exists with regard to the exact pattern of osmotically stimulated AVP secretion, most studies to date have supported the concept of a discrete osmotic threshold for AVP secretion above which a linear relationship between plasma osmolality and AVP levels occurs (Figure 15-4).[32] At plasma osmolalities below a threshold level, AVP secretion is suppressed to low or undetectable levels; above this point, AVP secretion increases linearly in direct proportion to plasma osmolality. The slope of the regression line relating AVP secretion to plasma osmolality can vary significantly across individual human subjects, in part because of genetic factors,[33] but also in relation to other factors. In general, each 1 mOsm/kg H_2O increase in plasma osmolality

causes an increase in plasma AVP level ranging from 0.4 to 1.0 pg/mL.

The renal response to circulating AVP is similarly linear, with urinary concentration that is directly proportional to AVP levels between 0.5 and 4 to 5 pg/mL, after which urinary osmolality is maximal and cannot increase further even with additional increases in AVP level (Figure 15-5). Thus, changes of as little as 1% in plasma osmolality are sufficient to cause significant increases in plasma AVP levels with proportional increases in urine concentration, and maximal antidiuresis is achieved after increases in plasma osmolality of only 5 to 10 mOsm/kg H_2O (i.e., 2% to 4%) above the threshold for AVP secretion.

Even this analysis, however, underestimates the sensitivity of this system in regulating free water excretion. Urinary osmolality is directly proportional to plasma AVP levels as a consequence of the fall in urine flow induced by the AVP, but urine volume is inversely related to urine osmolality (see Figure 15-5). An increase in plasma AVP concentration from 0.5 to 2 pg/mL has a much greater relative effect in decreasing urine flow than does a subsequent increase in AVP concentration from 2 to 5 pg/mL, which thus magnifies the physiologic effects of small changes in lowering plasma AVP levels. Furthermore, the rapid response of AVP secretion to changes in plasma osmolality coupled with the short half-life of AVP in human plasma (10 to 20 minutes) allows the kidneys to

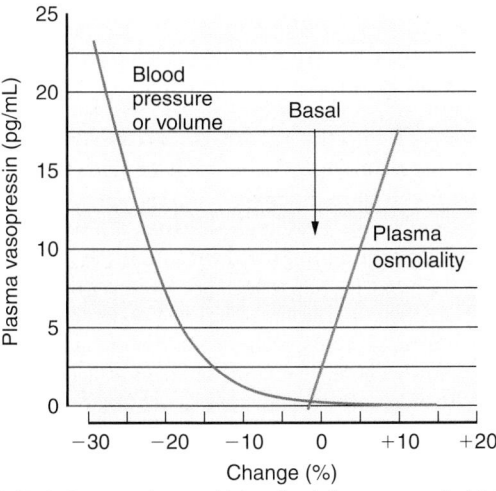

FIGURE 15-4 Comparative sensitivity of arginine vasopressin (AVP) secretion in response to increases in plasma osmolality and decreases in blood volume or blood pressure in human subjects. The *arrow* indicates the low plasma AVP concentrations found at basal plasma osmolality. Note that AVP secretion is much more sensitive to small changes in blood osmolality than to changes in volume or pressure. (Adapted from Robertson GL: Posterior pituitary, in Felig P, Baxter J, Frohman LA [editors]: *Endocrinology and metabolism,* New York, 1986, McGraw Hill, pp 338-386.)

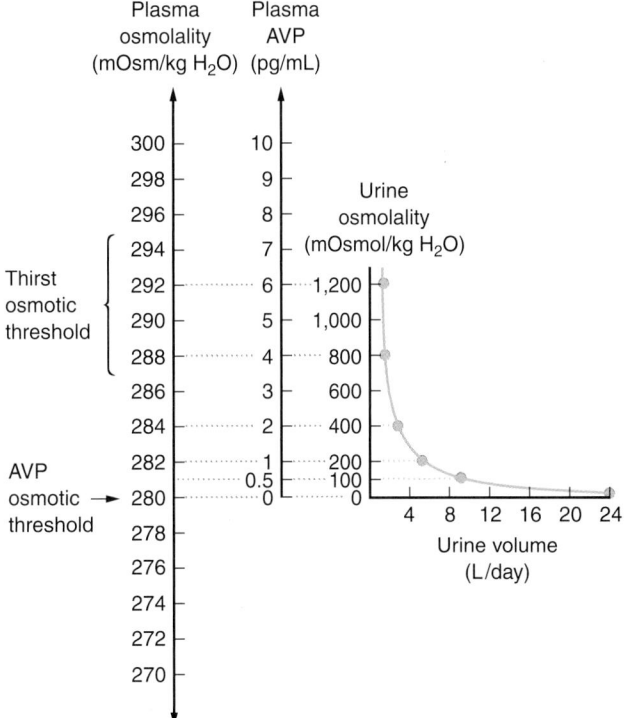

FIGURE 15-5 Relationship of plasma osmolality, plasma arginine vasopressin (AVP) concentrations, urine osmolality, and urine volume in humans. Note that the osmotic threshold for AVP secretion defines the point at which urine concentration begins to increase, but the osmotic threshold for thirst is significantly higher and approximates the point at which maximal urine concentration has already been achieved. Note also that, because of the inverse relationship between urine osmolality and urine volume, changes in plasma AVP concentrations have much larger effects on urine volume at low plasma AVP concentrations than at high plasma AVP concentrations. (Adapted from Robinson AG: Disorders of antidiuretic hormone secretion, *J Clin Endocrinol Metab* 14:55-88, 1985.)

respond to changes in plasma osmolality on a minute-to-minute basis. The net result is a finely tuned osmoregulatory system that adjusts the rate of free water excretion accurately to the ambient plasma osmolality primarily via changes in pituitary AVP secretion.

The set point of the osmoregulatory system also varies from person to person. In healthy adults, the osmotic threshold for AVP secretion ranges from 275 to 290 mOsm/kg H_2O (averaging approximately 280 to 285 mOsm/kg H_2O). As with sensitivity, individual differences in the set point of the osmoregulatory system are relatively constant over time and appear to be genetically determined.[33] However, multiple factors in addition to genetic influences can alter the sensitivity and/or the set point of the osmoregulatory system for AVP secretion.[33]

Foremost among these factors are acute changes in blood pressure, effective arterial blood volume, or both, which are discussed in the following section. Aging has been found to increase the sensitivity of the osmoregulatory system in multiple studies.[34,35] Metabolic factors such as serum Ca^{2+} and various drugs can alter the slope of the plasma AVP-osmolality relationship as well.[36] Lesser degrees of shifting of the osmosensitivity and set point for AVP secretion have been noted with alterations in gonadal hormones. Some studies have found increased osmosensitivity in women, particularly during the luteal phase of the menstrual cycle,[37] and in estrogen-treated men,[38] but these effects were relatively minor, and others have found no significant sex differences.[33] The set point of the osmoregulatory system is reduced more dramatically and reproducibly during pregnancy.[39] Some evidence has suggested the possible involvement of the placental hormone relaxin,[40] rather than gonadal steroids or human chorionic gonadotropin hormone, in pregnancy-associated resetting of the osmostat for AVP secretion.

That multiple factors can influence the set point and sensitivity of osmotically regulated AVP secretion is not surprising in view of the fact that AVP secretion reflects a balance of bimodal inputs—i.e., inhibitory as well as stimulatory[41]—from multiple different afferent inputs to the neurohypophysis (Figure 15-6).[42]

Understanding the osmoregulatory mechanism also requires addressing the observation that AVP secretion is not equally sensitive to all plasma solutes. Sodium and its anions, which normally contribute more than 95% of the osmotic pressure of plasma, are the most potent solutes in terms of their capacity to stimulate AVP secretion and thirst, although certain sugars such as mannitol and sucrose are equally effective when infused intravenously.[9] In contrast, increases in plasma osmolality caused by noneffective solutes such as urea or glucose cause little or no increase in plasma AVP levels in humans or animals.[9,43] These differences in response to various plasma solutes are independent of any recognized nonosmotic influence, which indicates that they are a property of the osmoregulatory mechanism itself.

According to current concepts, the osmoreceptor neuron is stimulated by osmotically induced changes in its water content. In such a case, the stimulatory potency of any given solute would be an inverse function of the rate at which it moves from the plasma to the inside of the osmoreceptor neuron. Solutes that penetrate slowly, or not at all, create an osmotic gradient that causes an efflux of water from the osmoreceptor, and the resultant shrinkage of the osmoreceptor neuron

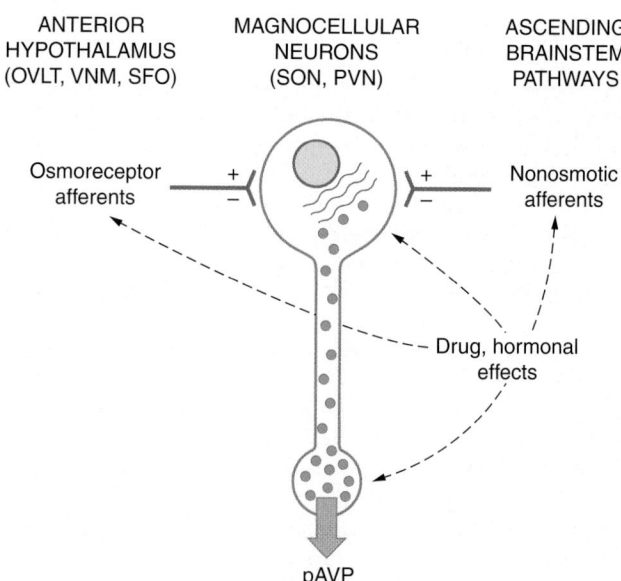

FIGURE 15-6 Schematic model of the regulatory control of the neurohypophysis. The secretory activity of individual magnocellular neurons is determined by an integration of the activities of both excitatory and inhibitory osmotic and nonosmotic afferent inputs. Superimposed on this are the effects of hormones and drugs, which can act at multiple levels to modulate the output of the system. (Adapted from Verbalis JG: Osmotic inhibition of neurohypophyseal secretion, *Ann N Y Acad Sci* 689:227-233, 1983.)

activates a stretch-inactivated noncationic channel that initiates depolarization and firing of the neuron.[44] Conversely, solutes that penetrate the cell readily create no gradient, and thus have no effect on the water content and cell volume of the osmoreceptors. This mechanism agrees well with the observed relationship between the effect of certain solutes like Na^+, mannitol, and glucose on AVP secretion and the rate at which they penetrate the blood-brain barrier.[29]

Many neurotransmitters have been implicated in mediating the actions of the osmoreceptors on the neurohypophysis. The SON is richly innervated by multiple pathways, including those utilizing acetylcholine, catecholamines, glutamate, γ-aminobutyric acid (GABA), histamine, opioids, angiotensin II, and dopamine (see review in Sladek and Kapoor[45]). Studies have supported a potential role for all of these, and others, in the regulation of AVP secretion, as has the detection of local secretion of AVP into the hypothalamus from dendrites of the AVP-secreting neurons.[46] Although it remains unclear which of these are involved in the normal physiologic control of AVP secretion, in view of the likelihood that the osmoregulatory system is bimodal and integrated with multiple different afferent pathways (see Figure 15-6), it seems likely that magnocellular AVP neurons are influenced by a very complex mixture of neurotransmitter systems, rather than by only a few.

Exactly how cells sense volume changes is a critical question for all of the mechanisms activated to achieve osmoregulation. Some of the most exciting new data have come from studies of brain osmoreceptors.[29] The cellular osmosensing mechanism utilized by the OVLT cells is an intrinsic depolarizing receptor potential, which these cells generate via a molecular transduction complex. Recent results suggest that this likely includes members of the *transient receptor potential vanilloid* (TRPV) family of cation channel proteins. These channels are generally activated by cell membrane stretch to produce a nonselective conductance of cations, with a preference for Ca^{2+}.

Multiple studies have characterized various members of the TRPV family as cellular mechanoreceptors in different tissues.[47] Both in vitro and in vivo studies of the TRPV family of cation channel proteins have provided evidence supporting roles for TRPV1, TRPV2, and TRPV4 proteins in the transduction of osmotic stimuli in mammals that are important for sensing cell volume.[48] Newer studies even indicate that genetic heterogeneity at or near the genomic locations of these mechanoreceptors contributes to interindividual differences in the propensity for disorders of water homeostasis, especially hyponatremia. Although the details of exactly how and where various members of the TRPV family of cation channel proteins participate in osmoregulation in different species remains to be ascertained by additional studies, a strong case can already be made for their involvement in the transduction of osmotic stimuli in the neural cells in the OVLT and surrounding hypothalamus that regulate osmotic homeostasis, and they appear to have been highly conserved throughout evolution.[48]

Nonosmotic Regulation

HEMODYNAMIC STIMULI

Not surprisingly, hypovolemia also is a potent stimulus for AVP secretion in humans,[32,49] because an appropriate response to volume depletion should include renal water conservation. In humans as well as multiple animal species, lowering blood pressure suddenly by any of several methods increases plasma AVP levels by an amount that is proportional to the degree of hypotension achieved.[32,50] This stimulus-response relationship follows an exponential pattern, such that small reductions in blood pressure, on the order of 5% to 10%, usually have little effect on plasma AVP, whereas blood pressure decreases of 20% to 30% result in hormone levels many times those required to produce maximal antidiuresis (see Figure 15-4).

The AVP response to acute reductions in blood volume appears to be quantitatively and qualitatively similar to the response to blood pressure. In rats, plasma AVP increases as an exponential function of the degree of hypovolemia. Thus, little increase in plasma AVP can be detected until blood volume falls by 5% to 8%; beyond that point, plasma AVP increases at an exponential rate in relation to the degree of hypovolemia and usually reaches levels 20 to 30 times normal when blood volume is reduced by 20% to 40%.[51,52] The volume-AVP relationship has not been as thoroughly characterized in other species, but it appears to follow a similar pattern humans.[53] Conversely, acute increases in blood volume or pressure suppress AVP secretion. This response has been characterized less well than that of hypotension or hypovolemia, but it seems to have a similar quantitative relationship (i.e., relatively large changes, on the order of 10% to 15%, are required to alter hormone secretion appreciably).[54]

The minimal to absent effect of small changes in blood volume and pressure on AVP secretion contrasts sharply with the extraordinary sensitivity of the osmoregulatory system (see Figure 15-4). Recognition of this difference is essential for understanding the relative contribution of each system to the control of AVP secretion under physiologic and pathologic conditions. Because day-to-day variations in TBW rarely exceed 2% to 3%, their effect on AVP secretion must be mediated largely, if not exclusively, by the osmoregulatory system. Nonetheless, modest changes in blood volume

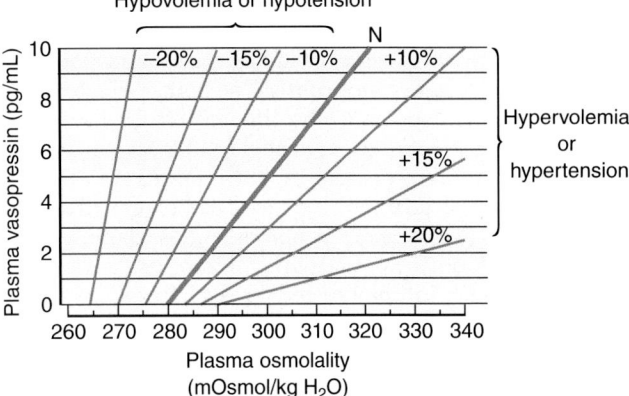

FIGURE 15-7 Relation between the osmolality of plasma and the concentration of arginine vasopressin (AVP) in plasma as modulated by blood volume and pressure. The line labeled *N* shows plasma AVP concentration across a range of plasma osmolality in an adult with normal intravascular volume (euvolemic) and normal blood pressure (normotensive). The lines to the left of *N* show the relationship between plasma AVP concentration and plasma osmolality in adults whose low intravascular volume (hypovolemia) or blood pressure (hypotension) is 10%, 15%, and 20% below normal. The lines to the right of *N* indicate volumes and blood pressures 10%, 15%, and 20% above normal. Note that hemodynamic influences do not disrupt the osmoregulation of AVP but rather raise or lower the set point of AVP secretion, and possibly the sensitivity as well, in proportion to the magnitude of the change in blood volume or pressure. (Adapted from Robertson GL, Athar S, Shelton RL: Osmotic control of vasopressin function, in Andreoli TE, Grantham JJ, Rector FC Jr [editors]: *Disturbances in body fluid osmolality*, Bethesda, Md, 1977, American Physiological Society, p 125.)

and pressure do, in fact, influence AVP secretion indirectly, even though they are weak stimuli by themselves. This occurs through shifting of the sensitivity of AVP secretion to osmotic stimuli, so that a given increase in osmolality causes a greater secretion of AVP during hypovolemic conditions than during euvolemic states (Figure 15-7).[55,56]

In the presence of a negative hemodynamic stimulus, plasma AVP continues to respond appropriately to small changes in plasma osmolality and can still be fully suppressed if the osmolality falls below the new (lower) set point. The retention of the threshold function is a vital aspect of the interaction, because it ensures that the capacity to regulate the osmolality of body fluids is not lost, even in the presence of significant hypovolemia or hypotension. Consequently, it is reasonable to conclude that the major effect of moderate degrees of hypovolemia on both AVP secretion and thirst is to modulate the gain of the osmoregulatory responses, with direct effects on thirst and AVP secretion occurring only during more severe degrees of hypovolemia (e.g., more than 10% to 20% reductions in blood pressure or volume).

These hemodynamic influences on AVP secretion are mediated at least in part by neural pathways that originate in stretch-sensitive receptors, generally called *baroreceptors*, in the cardiac atria, aorta, and carotid sinus (see Figure 15-2; reviewed in detail in Chapter 14). Afferent nerve fibers from these receptors ascend in the vagus and glossopharyngeal nerves to the nuclei of the NTS in the brainstem.[57] A variety of postsynaptic pathways from the NTS then project, both directly and indirectly via the ventrolateral medulla and the lateral parabrachial nucleus, to the PVN and SON in the hypothalamus.[58]

Early studies suggested that the input from these pathways was predominantly inhibitory under basal conditions, because interrupting them acutely resulted in large increases in plasma AVP levels as well as in arterial blood pressure.[59] However, as with most neural systems, including the neurohypophysis, innervation is complex and consists of both excitatory and inhibitory inputs. Consequently, different effects have been observed under different experimental conditions.

The baroreceptor mechanism also appears to mediate a large number of pharmacologic and pathologic effects on AVP secretion (Table 15-1). Among them are diuretics, isoproterenol, nicotine, prostaglandins, nitroprusside, trimethaphan, histamine, morphine, and bradykinin, all of which stimulate AVP at least in part by lowering blood volume or pressure,[49] and norepinephrine, which suppresses AVP by raising blood pressure.[60] In addition, upright posture, sodium depletion, congestive heart failure, cirrhosis, and nephrotic syndrome likely stimulate AVP secretion by reducing effective arterial blood volume.[61,62] Symptomatic orthostatic hypotension, vasovagal reactions, and other forms of syncope more markedly stimulate AVP secretion via greater and more acute decreases in blood pressure, with the exception of orthostatic hypotension associated with loss of afferent baroregulatory function.[63] Almost every hormone, drug, or condition that affects blood volume or pressure also affects AVP secretion, but in most cases the degree of change of blood pressure or volume is modest and results in a shift of the set point and/or sensitivity of the osmoregulatory response rather than marked stimulation of AVP secretion (see Figure 15-7).

DRINKING

Peripheral neural sensors other than baroreceptors also can affect AVP secretion. In humans as well as dogs, drinking lowers plasma AVP before there is any appreciable decrease in plasma osmolality or serum [Na+]. This is clearly a response to the act of drinking itself, because it occurs independently of the composition of the fluid ingested.[64,65] It may be influenced by the temperature of the fluid, however, since the degree of suppression appears to be greater in response to colder fluids.[66] The pathways responsible for this effect have not been delineated, but likely include sensory afferents originating in the oropharynx and transmitted centrally via the glossopharyngeal nerve.

NAUSEA

Among other nonosmotic stimuli to AVP secretion in humans, nausea is the most prominent. The sensation of nausea, with or without vomiting, is by far the most potent stimulus to AVP secretion known in humans. Although 20% increases in osmolality typically elevate plasma AVP levels to the range of 5 to 20 pg/mL and 20% decreases in blood pressure to 10 to 100 pg/mL, nausea has been described to cause AVP elevations in excess of 200 to 400 pg/mL.[67]

The pathway mediating this effect has been mapped to the chemoreceptor zone in the area postrema of the brainstem in animal studies (see Figure 15-2). It can be activated by a variety of drugs and conditions, including apomorphine, morphine, nicotine, alcohol, and motion sickness. Its effect on AVP is instantaneous and extremely potent (Figure 15-8), even when the nausea is transient and not accompanied by vomiting or changes in blood pressure. Pretreatment with fluphenazine, haloperidol, or promethazine in doses sufficient to prevent nausea completely abolishes the AVP response. The inhibitory effect of these dopamine antagonists is specific for

TABLE 15-1 Drugs and Hormones That Affect Vasopressin Secretion

STIMULATORY	INHIBITORY
Acetylcholine	Norepinephrine
Nicotine	Fluphenazine
Apomorphine	Haloperidol
Morphine (high doses)	Promethazine
Epinephrine	Oxilorphan
Isoproterenol	Butorphanol
Histamine	Opioid agonists
Bradykinin	Morphine (low doses)
Prostaglandin	Ethanol
β-Endorphin	Carbamazepine
Cyclophosphamide (intravenous)	Glucocorticoids
Vincristine	Clonidine
Insulin	Muscimol
2-Deoxyglucose	Phencyclidine
Angiotensin II	Phenytoin
Lithium	
Corticotropin-releasing factor	
Naloxone	
Cholecystokinin	

emetic stimuli, because they do not alter the AVP response to osmotic and hemodynamic stimuli. Water loading blunts, but does not abolish, the effect of nausea on AVP release, which suggests that osmotic and emetic influences interact in a manner similar to that for osmotic and hemodynamic pathways. Species differences also affect the response to emetic stimuli. Whereas dogs and cats appear to be even more sensitive than humans to emetic stimulation of AVP release, rodents have little or no AVP response to emetic stimuli but release large amounts of oxytocin instead.[68]

The emetic response probably mediates many pharmacologic and pathologic effects on AVP secretion. In addition to the effects of the drugs and conditions already noted, it may be responsible, at least in part, for the increase in AVP secretion that has been observed with vasovagal reactions, diabetic ketoacidosis, acute hypoxia, and motion sickness. Because nausea and vomiting are frequent side effects of many other drugs and diseases, many additional situations likely occur as well.

The reason for this profound stimulation is not known (although it has been speculated that the AVP response assists evacuation of stomach contents via contraction of gastric smooth muscle, AVP is not necessary for vomiting to occur); however, it is responsible for the intense vasoconstriction that produces the pallor often associated with this state.

HYPOGLYCEMIA

Acute hypoglycemia is a less potent but reasonably consistent stimulus for AVP secretion.[69,70] The receptor and pathway that mediate this effect are unknown; however, they appear separate from those of other recognized stimuli, because hypoglycemia stimulates AVP secretion even in patients who have selectively lost the capacity to respond to hypernatremia,

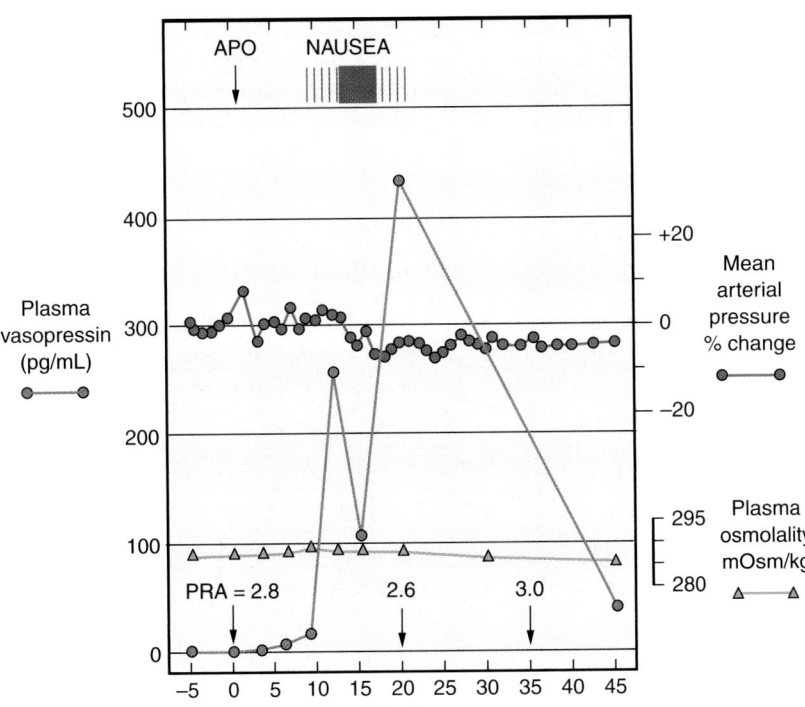

FIGURE 15-8 Effect of nausea on arginine vasopressin (AVP) secretion. Apomorphine (APO) was injected at the point indicated by the *vertical arrow*. Note that the rise in plasma AVP coincided with the occurrence of nausea and was not associated with detectable changes in plasma osmolality or blood pressure. *PRA,* Plasma renin activity. (Adapted from Robertson GL: The regulation of vasopressin function in health and disease, *Recent Prog Horm Res* 33:333-385, 1977.)

hypotension, or nausea.[70] The factor that actually triggers the release of AVP is likely intracellular deficiency of glucose or adenosine triphosphate, because 2-deoxyglucose is also an effective stimulus.[71] Generally, more than a 20% decrease in glucose level is required to significantly increase plasma AVP levels. The rate of fall in glucose is probably the critical stimulus, because the rise in plasma AVP is not sustained with persistent hypoglycemia.[69] Glucopenic stimuli are unlikely to be important in the physiology or pathology of AVP secretion, however, since there are probably few drugs or conditions that lower plasma glucose rapidly enough to stimulate release of the hormone. Importantly, this effect is also transient.

Renin-Angiotensin System

The renin-angiotensin system has also been intimately implicated in the control of AVP secretion.[72] Animal studies have indicated dual sites of action. Blood-borne angiotensin II stimulates AVP secretion by acting in the brain at the circumventricular subfornical organ (SFO),[73] a small structure located in the dorsal portion of the third cerebral ventricle (see Figure 15-2). Because circumventricular organs lack a blood-brain barrier, the densely expressed angiotensin II AT_1 receptors of the SFO can detect very small increases in blood levels of angiotensin II.[74] Neural pathways from the SFO to the hypothalamic SON and PVN mediate AVP secretion and also appear to use angiotensin II as a neurotransmitter.[75] This accounts for the observation that the most sensitive site for angiotensin-mediated AVP secretion and thirst is intracerebroventricular injection into the cerebrospinal fluid. Further evidence in support of angiotensin II as a neurotransmitter is that intraventricular administration of angiotensin receptor antagonists inhibits the AVP response to osmotic and hemodynamic stimuli.[76]

The level of plasma angiotensin II required to stimulate AVP release is quite high, which leads some to argue that this stimulus is active only under pharmacologic conditions.

This is consistent with observations that even pressor doses of angiotensin II increase plasma AVP only about twofold to fourfold[72] and may account for the failure of some investigators to demonstrate stimulation of thirst by exogenous angiotensin administration. However, the latter procedure may underestimate the physiologic effects of angiotensin, since the increased blood pressure caused by exogenously administered angiotensin II appears to blunt the induced thirst via activation of inhibitory baroreceptive pathways.[77]

Stress

Nonspecific stress caused by factors such as pain, emotion, or physical exercise has long been thought to cause AVP secretion, but it has never been determined whether this effect is mediated by a specific pathway or is secondary to the hypotension or nausea that often accompanies stress-induced vasovagal reactions. In rats[78] and humans,[79] a variety of noxious stimuli capable of activating the pituitary-adrenal axis and sympathetic nervous system do not stimulate AVP secretion unless they also lower blood pressure or alter blood volume. The marked rise in plasma AVP elicited by manipulation of the abdominal viscera in anesthetized dogs has been attributed to nociceptive influences,[80] but mediation by emetic pathways cannot be excluded in this setting. Endotoxin-induced fever stimulates AVP secretion in rats, and data support possible mediation of this effect by circulating cytokines such as interleukin-1 and interleukin-6.[81] Clarification of the possible role of nociceptive and thermal influences on AVP secretion is particularly important in view of the frequency with which painful or febrile illnesses are associated with osmotically inappropriate secretion of the hormone.

Hypoxia and Hypercapnia

Acute hypoxia and hypercapnia also stimulate AVP secretion.[82,83] In conscious humans, however, the stimulatory effect of moderate hypoxia (arterial oxygen pressure [Pao_2]

of >35 mm Hg) is inconsistent and seems to occur mainly in subjects who develop nausea or hypotension. In conscious dogs, more severe hypoxia (Pao_2 of <35 mm Hg) consistently increases AVP secretion without reducing arterial pressure.[84] Studies of anesthetized dogs suggest that the AVP response to acute hypoxia depends on the level of hypoxemia achieved. At a Pao_2 of 35 mm Hg or lower, plasma AVP increases markedly, even though there is no change or even an increase in arterial pressure, but less severe hypoxia (Pao_2 of >40 mm Hg) has no effect on AVP levels.[85] These results indicate that there is likely a hypoxemic threshold for AVP secretion and suggest that severe hypoxemia alone may also stimulate AVP secretion in humans. If so, it may be responsible, at least in part, for the osmotically inappropriate AVP elevations noted in some patients with acute respiratory failure.[86]

In conscious or anesthetized dogs, acute hypercapnia, independent of hypoxia or hypotension, also increases AVP secretion.[84,85] It has not been determined whether this response also exhibits threshold characteristics or otherwise depends on the degree of hypercapnia, nor is it known whether hypercapnia has similar effects on AVP secretion in humans or other animals. The mechanisms by which hypoxia and hypercapnia release AVP remain undefined, but they likely involve peripheral chemoreceptors and/or baroreceptors, because cervical vagotomy abolishes the response to hypoxemia in dogs.[87]

DRUGS

As is discussed more extensively in the sections on clinical disorders, a variety of drugs also stimulate AVP secretion, including nicotine (see Table 15-1). Drugs and hormones can potentially impact AVP secretion at many different sites, as depicted in Figure 15-6. As already discussed, many excitatory stimulants such as isoproterenol, nicotine, high doses of morphine, and cholecystokinin act, at least in part, by lowering blood pressure and/or producing nausea. Others, like substance P, prostaglandin, endorphin, and other opioids, have not been studied sufficiently to define their mechanism of action, but they may also work by one or both of the same mechanisms.

Inhibitory stimuli similarly have multiple modes of action. Vasopressor drugs like norepinephrine inhibit AVP secretion indirectly by raising arterial pressure. In low doses, a variety of opioids of all subtypes, including morphine, metenkephalin, and κ-agonists inhibit AVP secretion in rats and humans.[88] Endogenous opioid peptides interact with the magnocellular neurosecretory system at several levels to inhibit basal as well as stimulated secretion of AVP and oxytocin. Opioid inhibition of AVP secretion has been found to occur in isolated posterior pituitary tissue, and the action of morphine as well as several opioid agonists such as butorphanol and oxilorphan likely occurs via activation of κ-opioid receptors located on nerve terminals of the posterior pituitary.[89] The well-known inhibitory effect of ethanol on AVP secretion may be mediated at least in part by endogenous opiates, since it is due to an elevation in the osmotic threshold for AVP release[90] and can be blocked in part by treatment with naloxone.[91] Carbamazepine inhibits AVP secretion by diminishing the sensitivity of the osmoregulatory system; this effect occurs independently of changes in blood volume, blood pressure, or blood glucose level.[92] Other drugs that inhibit AVP secretion include clonidine, which appears to act via both central and peripheral adrenoreceptors,[93] muscimol,[94] which acts as a GABA

antagonist, and phencyclidine,[95] which probably acts by raising blood pressure. Despite the importance of these stimuli in pathologic conditions, however, none of them is a significant determinant of physiologic regulation of AVP secretion in humans.

Distribution and Clearance

Plasma AVP concentration is determined by the difference between the rates of secretion from the posterior pituitary gland and removal of the hormone from the vascular compartment via metabolism and urinary clearance. In healthy adults, intravenously injected AVP distributes rapidly into a space equivalent in size to the ECF compartment. This initial, or mixing, phase has a half-time of 4 to 8 minutes and is virtually complete in 10 to 15 minutes. The rapid mixing phase is followed by a second, slower decline that corresponds to the metabolic clearance of AVP. Most studies of this phase have yielded mean values of 10 to 20 minutes using both steady-state and non–steady-state techniques[32]; this is consistent with the observed rates of change in urine osmolality after water loading and injection of AVP, which also support a short half-life.[96] In pregnant women, the metabolic clearance rate of AVP increases nearly fourfold,[97] which becomes significant in the pathophysiology of gestational diabetes insipidus (see later discussion). Smaller animals such as rats clear AVP much more rapidly than humans because their cardiac output is higher relative to their body weight and surface area.[96]

Although many tissues have the capacity to inactivate AVP, metabolism in vivo appears to occur largely in the liver and kidney.[96] The enzymatic processes by which the liver and kidney inactivate AVP involve an initial reduction of the disulfide bridge followed by aminopeptidase cleavage of the bond between amino acid residues 1 and 2. The extent of further degradation and the peptide products that escape into plasma and urine are currently unknown.

Some AVP is excreted intact in the urine, but there is disagreement about the amounts and the factors that affect it. For example, in healthy, normally hydrated adults, the urinary clearance of AVP ranges from 0.1 to 0.6 mL/kg/min under basal conditions and has never been found to exceed 2 mL/kg/min, even in the presence of solute diuresis.[32] The mechanisms involved in the excretion of AVP have not been defined with certainty, but the hormone is probably filtered at the glomerulus and variably reabsorbed at sites along the nephron. The latter process may be linked to the reabsorption of Na^+ or other solutes in the proximal nephron, because the urinary clearance of AVP has been found to vary by as much as 20-fold in direct relation to the solute clearance.[32] Consequently, measurements of urinary AVP excretion in humans do not provide a consistently reliable index of changes in plasma AVP and should be interpreted cautiously when glomerular filtration or solute clearance are inconstant or abnormal.

Thirst

Thirst is the body's defense mechanism to increase water consumption in response to perceived deficits of body fluids. It can be most easily defined as a consciously perceived desire for water. True thirst must be distinguished from other determinants of fluid intake such as taste, dietary preferences, and social customs, as discussed previously. Thirst can be stimulated in animals and humans either by intracellular dehydration caused by increases in the effective osmolality of the ECF or by intravascular hypovolemia caused by losses of ECF.[98,99] As would be expected, these are many of the same variables that provoke AVP secretion. Of these, hypertonicity is clearly the most potent. As with AVP secretion, substantial evidence to date has supported mediation of osmotic thirst by osmoreceptors located in the anterior hypothalamus of the brain,[30,31] whereas hypovolemic thirst appears to be stimulated both by activation of low- and/or high-pressure baroreceptors[100] and by circulating angiotensin II.[101]

Osmotic Thirst

In healthy adults, an increase in effective plasma osmolality of only 2% to 3% above basal levels produces a strong desire to drink.[102] This response is not dependent on changes in ECF or plasma volume, since it occurs similarly regardless of whether plasma osmolality is raised by infusion of hypertonic solutions or by water deprivation. The absolute level of plasma osmolality at which a person develops a conscious urge to seek and drink water is called the *osmotic thirst threshold*. This threshold varies appreciably among individuals, probably due to genetic factors,[33] but in healthy adults it averages approximately 295 mOsm/kg H_2O. Of physiologic significance is the fact that this level is above the osmotic threshold for AVP release and approximates the plasma osmolality at which maximal concentration of the urine is normally achieved (see Figure 15-5).

The brain pathways that mediate osmotic thirst have not been well defined, but it is clear that initiation of drinking requires osmoreceptors located in the anteroventral hypothalamus in the same area that the osmoreceptors that control osmotic AVP secretion are located.[30,31] Whether the osmoreceptors for AVP and thirst are the same cells or simply are located in the same general area remains unknown.[29] However, the properties of the osmoreceptors are very similar. Ineffective plasma solutes such as urea and glucose, which have little or no effect on AVP secretion, are equally ineffective in stimulating thirst, whereas effective solutes such as NaCl and mannitol are.[9,103]

The sensitivities of the thirst and AVP osmoreceptors cannot be compared precisely, but they are probably also similar. Thus, in healthy adults, the intensity of thirst increases rapidly in direct proportion to serum [Na^+] or plasma osmolality and generally becomes intolerable at levels only 3% to 5% above the threshold level.[104] Water consumption also appears to be proportional to the intensity of thirst in both humans and animals, and under conditions of maximal osmotic stimulation can reach rates as high as 20 to 25 L/day. The dilution of body fluids by ingested water complements the retention of water that occurs during AVP-induced antidiuresis, and both responses occur concurrently when drinking water is available.

As with AVP secretion, the osmoregulation of thirst appears to be bimodal, because a modest decline in plasma osmolality induces a sense of satiation and reduces the basal rate of spontaneous fluid intake.[104,105] This effect is sufficient to prevent hypotonic overhydration even when antidiuresis is fixed at maximal levels for prolonged periods, which suggests that osmotically inappropriate secretion of AVP (syndrome of inappropriate antidiuretic hormone secretion, or SIADH)

should not result in the development of hyponatremia unless the satiety mechanism is impaired or fluid intake is inappropriately high for some other reason, such as the unregulated components of fluid intake discussed earlier.[105] Also as with AVP secretion, thirst can be influenced by oropharyngeal or upper gastrointestinal receptors that respond to the act of drinking itself.[65] In humans, however, the rapid relief provided by this mechanism lasts only a matter of minutes, and thirst quickly recurs until enough of the water is absorbed to lower plasma osmolality to normal. Therefore, although local oropharyngeal sensations may have a significant short-term influence on thirst, it is the hypothalamic osmoreceptors that ultimately determine the volume of water intake in response to dehydration.

Hypovolemic Thirst

In contrast to the threshold for osmotic thirst, the threshold for producing hypovolemic, or extracellular, thirst is significantly higher in both animals and humans. Studies in several species have shown that sustained decreases in plasma volume or blood pressure of at least 4% to 8%, and in some species 10% to 15%, are necessary to consistently stimulate drinking.[106,107] In humans, the degree of hypovolemia or hypotension required to produce thirst has not been precisely defined, but it has been difficult to demonstrate any effects of mild to moderate hypovolemia on stimulation of thirst independently of osmotic changes occurring with dehydration. This blunted sensitivity to changes in ECF volume or blood pressure in humans probably represents an adaptation that occurred as a result of the erect posture of primates, which predisposes them to wider fluctuations in blood and atrial filling pressures as a result of orthostatic pooling of blood in the lower body. Stimulation of thirst (and AVP secretion) by such transient postural changes in blood pressure might lead to overdrinking and inappropriate antidiuresis in situations in which the ECF volume was actually normal but only transiently maldistributed.

Consistent with a blunted response to baroreceptor activation, studies have also shown that systemic infusion of angiotensin II to pharmacologic levels is a much less potent stimulus to thirst in humans[108] than in animals, in which it is one of the most potent dipsogens known. Nonetheless, this response is not completely absent in humans, as demonstrated by rare cases of polydipsia in patients with pathologic causes of hyperreninemia.[109]

The pathways by which hypovolemia or hypotension produces thirst have not been well defined, but probably involve the same brainstem baroreceptive pathways that mediate hemodynamic effects on AVP secretion,[100] as well as a contribution from circulating levels of angiotensin II in some species.[110]

Integration of Vasopressin Secretion and Thirst

A synthesis of what is presently known about the regulation of AVP secretion and thirst in humans leads to a relatively simple but elegant system to maintain water balance. Under normal physiologic conditions, the sensitivity of the osmoregulatory system for AVP secretion accounts for maintenance of plasma osmolality within narrow limits by adjustment of renal water excretion in response to small changes in osmolality. Stimulated thirst does not represent a major regulatory mechanism under these conditions, and unregulated fluid ingestion supplies water in excess of true "need"; this excess is then excreted in keeping with osmoregulated pituitary AVP secretion. However, when unregulated water intake cannot adequately supply body needs in the presence of plasma AVP levels sufficient to produce maximal antidiuresis, then plasma osmolality rises to levels that stimulate thirst (see Figure 15-5), and water intake increases proportional to the elevation of osmolality above this thirst threshold.

In such a system, thirst essentially represents a backup mechanism called into play when pituitary and renal mechanisms prove insufficient to maintain plasma osmolality within a few percent of basal levels. This arrangement has the advantage of freeing humans from frequent episodes of thirst that would require a diversion of activities toward behavior oriented to seeking water when water deficiency is sufficiently mild to be compensated for by renal water conservation, but would stimulate water ingestion once water deficiency reaches potentially harmful levels. Stimulation of AVP secretion at plasma osmolalities below the threshold for subjective thirst acts to maintain an excess of body water sufficient to eliminate the need to drink whenever slight elevations in plasma osmolality occur.

This system of differential effective thresholds for thirst and AVP secretion nicely fits with the results of many studies that have demonstrated excess unregulated, or "need-free," drinking in both humans and animals. Only when this mechanism becomes inadequate to maintain body fluid homeostasis does thirst-induced regulated fluid intake become the predominant defense mechanism for the prevention of severe dehydration.

Disorders of Insufficient Vasopressin or Vasopressin Effect

Disorders of insufficient AVP or AVP effect are associated with inadequate urine concentration and increased urine output (*polyuria*). If thirst mechanisms are intact, this is accompanied by compensatory increases in fluid intake (*polydipsia*) as a result of stimulation of thirst to preserve body fluid homeostasis. The net result is polyuria and polydipsia with preservation of normal plasma osmolality and serum electrolyte concentrations. If thirst is impaired, however, or if fluid intake is insufficient for any reason to compensate for the increased urine excretion, then hyperosmolality and hypernatremia can result, with the consequent complications associated with these disorders.

The quintessential disorder of insufficient AVP is *diabetes insipidus* (DI), which is a clinical syndrome characterized by excretion of abnormally large volumes of urine (i.e., diabetes) that is dilute (i.e., hypotonic) and devoid of taste from dissolved solutes (e.g., insipid), in contrast to the hypertonic sweet-tasting urine characteristic of diabetes mellitus (*mellitus* means "honey" in Latin). Several different pathophysiologic mechanisms can cause hypotonic polyuria (Table 15-2). *Central* (also called *hypothalamic, neurogenic,* or *neurohypophyseal*) *diabetes insipidus* (CDI) is due to inadequate secretion, and usually deficient synthesis, of AVP in the hypothalamic neurohypophyseal system. Lack of AVP-stimulated activation of the V_2 subtype of AVP receptors in the kidney collecting tubules (see Chapters 10 and 11) causes excretion of large

TABLE 15-2 Causes of Hypotonic Polyuria

Central (Neurogenic) Diabetes Insipidus
Congenital disorders (congenital malformations, autosomal dominant AVP–neurophysin gene mutations)
Drug or toxin exposure (ethanol, diphenylhydantoin, snake venom)
Granulomatous diseases (histiocytosis, sarcoidosis)
Neoplastic disorders (craniopharyngioma, germinoma, lymphoma, leukemia, meningioma, pituitary tumor; metastases)
Infections (meningitis, tuberculosis, encephalitis)
Inflammatory/autoimmune disorders (lymphocytic infundibuloneurohypophysitis)
Trauma (neurosurgery, deceleration injury)
Vascular disorders (cerebral hemorrhage or infarction, brain death)
Idiopathic

Osmoreceptor Dysfunction
Granulomatous diseases (histiocytosis, sarcoidosis)
Neoplastic disorders (craniopharyngioma, pinealoma, meningioma, metastases)
Vascular disorders (anterior communicating artery aneurysm or ligation, intrahypothalamic hemorrhage)
Other disorders (hydrocephalus, ventricular/suprasellar cyst, trauma, degenerative diseases)
Idiopathic

Increased AVP Metabolism
Pregnancy

Nephrogenic Diabetes Insipidus
Congenital disorder (X-linked recessive AVP V_2 receptor gene mutations, autosomal recessive or dominant aquaporin-2 water channel gene mutations)
Drug exposure (demeclocycline, lithium, cisplatin, methoxyflurane)
Hypercalcemia
Hypokalemia
Infiltrating lesions (sarcoidosis, amyloidosis)
Vascular disorders (sickle cell anemia)
Mechanical disorders (polycystic kidney disease, bilateral ureteral obstruction)
Solute diuresis (glucose, mannitol, sodium, radiocontrast dyes)
Idiopathic

Primary Polydipsia
Psychogenic (schizophrenia, obsessive-compulsive behaviors)
Dipsogenic (downward resetting of thirst threshold, idiopathic or similar lesions as with central diabetes insipidus)

AVP, Arginine vasopressin.

volumes of dilute urine. In most cases thirst mechanisms are intact, which leads to compensatory polydipsia. However, in a variant of CDI called *osmoreceptor dysfunction,* thirst is also impaired, which leads to hypodipsia. *Diabetes insipidus of pregnancy* is a transient disorder due to an accelerated metabolism of AVP as a result of increased activity of the enzyme oxytocinase/vasopressinase in the serum of pregnant females, which again leads to polyuria and polydipsia; accelerated metabolism of AVP during pregnancy may also cause a patient with subclinical DI from other causes to shift from a relatively asymptomatic state to a symptomatic state as a result of the more rapid AVP degradation. *Nephrogenic diabetes insipidus* (NDI) is due to inappropriate renal responses to AVP. This produces excretion of dilute urine despite normal pituitary AVP secretion and secondary polydipsia, as in CDI. The final cause of hypotonic polyuria, *primary polydipsia,* differs significantly from the other causes because it is not deficient AVP secretion or impaired renal responses to AVP, but rather excessive ingestion of fluids. This can result from either an abnormality in the thirst mechanism, in which case it is sometimes called *dipsogenic diabetes insipidus,* or to psychiatric disorders, in which case it is generally referred to as *psychogenic polydipsia.*

Central Diabetes Insipidus

Etiology

Central diabetes insipidus (CDI) is caused by inadequate secretion of AVP from the posterior pituitary in response to osmotic stimulation. In most cases this is due to destruction of the neurohypophysis by a variety of acquired or congenital anatomic lesions that destroy or damage the neurohypophysis by pressure or infiltration (see Table 15-2). The severity of the resulting hypotonic diuresis depends on the degree of destruction of the neurohypophysis, which can lead to either complete or partial deficiency of AVP secretion. Despite the wide variety of lesions that can potentially cause CDI, it is much more common for CDI *not* to occur in the presence of such lesions than for the syndrome to be produced. This apparent inconsistency can be understood by considering several common principles of neurohypophyseal physiology and pathophysiology that are relevant in all of these cases.

The first is that the synthesis of AVP occurs in the hypothalamus (see Figure 15-2); the posterior pituitary simply represents the site of storage and secretion of the neurosecretory granules that contain AVP. Consequently, lesions contained within the sella turcica that destroy only the posterior pituitary generally do not cause CDI, because the cell bodies of the magnocellular neurons that synthesize AVP remain intact and the site of release of AVP shifts more superiorly, typically into the blood vessels of the median eminence at the base of the brain. Perhaps the best examples of this phenomenon are large pituitary macroadenomas that completely destroy the anterior and posterior pituitary. DI is a distinctly unusual presentation for such pituitary adenomas, because destruction of the posterior pituitary by such slowly enlarging intrasellar lesions merely destroys the nerve terminals, but not the cell bodies, of the AVP neurons. As this occurs, the site of release of AVP shifts more superiorly to the pituitary stalk and median eminence. Sometimes this can be detected on noncontrast magnetic resonance imaging (MRI) as a shift of the pituitary "bright spot" more superiorly to the level of the infundibulum or median eminence,[111] but often this process is too diffuse to be detected in this manner. The occurrence of DI from a pituitary adenoma is so uncommon, even with macroadenomas that obliterate sellar contents sufficiently completely to cause panhypopituitarism, that its presence should lead to consideration of alternative diagnoses, such as craniopharyngioma, which often causes damage to the median eminence by virtue of adherence of the capsule to the base of the hypothalamus; more rapidly enlarging sellar or suprasellar masses that do not allow sufficient time for the site of AVP release to be shifted more superiorly (e.g., metastatic lesions); or granulomatous disease with more diffuse hypothalamic involvement (e.g., sarcoidosis, histiocytosis). With very large pituitary adenomas that produce ACTH deficiency, it is actually more likely that patients will show hypo-osmolality from an SIADH-like picture as a result of the impaired free water excretion that accompanies hypocortisolism, as is discussed later.

A second general principle is that the capacity of the neurohypophysis to synthesize AVP is greatly in excess of the body's daily needs for maintenance of water homeostasis. Carefully controlled studies of surgical section of the pituitary stalk in dogs have clearly demonstrated that destruction of 80% to 90% of the magnocellular neurons in the hypothalamus is required to produce polyuria and polydipsia in this species.[112]

Thus, even lesions that do cause destruction of the AVP magnocellular neuron cell bodies must cause a large degree of destruction to produce DI. The most illustrative example of this is surgical section of the pituitary stalk in humans. Necropsy studies of these patients have revealed atrophy of the posterior pituitary and loss of the magnocellular neurons in the hypothalamus.[113] This loss of magnocellular cells presumably results from retrograde degeneration of neurons whose axons were cut during surgery. As is generally true for all neurons, the likelihood of retrograde neuronal degeneration depends on the proximity of the axotomy, in this case section of the pituitary stalk, to the cell body of the neuron. This was shown clearly in studies of human subjects in which section of the pituitary stalk at the level of the diaphragma sellae (i.e., a low stalk section) produced transient but not permanent DI, and section at the level of the infundibulum (i.e., a high stalk section) was required to cause permanent DI in most cases.[114]

In recent years, several genetic causes of AVP deficiency have also been characterized. Prior to the application of techniques for amplification of genomic DNA, the only experimental model for studying the mechanism of hereditary hypothalamic DI was the Brattleboro rat, a strain that was found serendipitously to have CDI.[115] In this animal, the disease demonstrates a classic pattern of autosomal recessive inheritance in which DI is expressed only in the homozygotes. The hereditary basis of the disease has been found to be a single base deletion producing a translational frameshift beginning in the third portion of the neurophysin coding sequence. Because the gene lacks a stop codon, there is a modified neurophysin, no glycopeptide, and a long polylysine tail.[116] Although the mutant prohormone accumulates in the endoplasmic reticulum, sufficient AVP is produced by the normal allele that the heterozygotes are asymptomatic.

In contrast, in humans almost all families with genetic CDI that have been described to date demonstrate an autosomal dominant mode of inheritance.[117-119] In this case, DI is exhibited despite the expression of one normal allele, which is sufficient to prevent the disease in the heterozygous Brattleboro rats. Numerous studies have been directed at understanding this apparent anomaly. Two potentially important clues as to the etiology of the DI in familial genetic CDI are that (1) severe to partial deficiencies of AVP and overt signs of DI do not develop in these patients until several months to several years after birth and then gradually progress over the ensuing decades,[117,120] which suggests adequate initial function of the normal allele with later decompensation; and (2) a limited number of autopsy studies suggest that some of these cases are associated with gliosis and a marked loss of magnocellular AVP neurons in the hypothalamus,[121] although other studies have shown normal neurons with decreased expression of AVP or no hypothalamic abnormality. In most of these cases, the hyperintense signal normally emitted by the neurohypophysis in T1-weighted magnetic resonance images (see later discussion) is also absent, although some exceptions have been reported.[122] Another interesting, but as yet unexplained, observation is that some adults in these families have been described in whom DI was clinically apparent during childhood but went into remission in adulthood, without evidence that the remissions could be attributed to renal or adrenal insufficiency, or to increased AVP synthesis.[123]

The autosomal dominant form of familial CDI is caused by diverse mutations in the gene that codes for the

AVP-neurophysin precursor (Figure 15-9). All of the mutations identified to date have been in the coding region of the gene and affect only one allele. They are located in all three exons and are predicted to alter or delete amino acid residues in the signal peptide, AVP, and neurophysin moieties of the precursor. Only the C-terminal glycopeptide, or copeptin moiety, has not been found to be affected. Most are missense mutations, but nonsense mutations (premature stop codons) and deletions also occur. One characteristic shared by all the mutations is that they are predicted to alter or delete one or more amino acids known, or reasonably presumed, to be crucial for processing, folding, and oligomerization of the precursor protein in the endoplasmic reticulum.[117,119]

Because of the related functional effects of the mutations, the common clinical characteristics of the disease, the dominant-negative mode of transmission, and the autopsy and hormonal evidence of postnatal neurohypophysial degeneration, it has been postulated that all of the mutations act by causing production of an abnormal precursor protein that accumulates and eventually kills the neurons because it cannot be correctly processed, folded, and transported out of the endoplasmic reticulum. Therefore the production of AVP from the normal genomic allele is also affected.

Expression studies of mutant DNA from several human mutations in cultured neuroblastoma cells support this misfolding-neurotoxicity hypothesis by demonstrating abnormal trafficking and accumulation of mutant prohormone in the endoplasmic reticulum with low or absent expression in the Golgi apparatus, which suggests difficulty with packaging into neurosecretory granules.[124] However, cell death may not be necessary to decrease available AVP. Normally proteins retained in the endoplasmic reticulum are selectively degraded, but if excess mutant is produced and the selective normal degradative process is overwhelmed, an alternate nonselective degradative system (autophagy) is activated. As more and more mutant precursor builds up in the endoplasmic reticulum, normal wild-type protein is trapped with the mutant protein and degraded by the activated nonspecific degradative system. In such a case, the amount of AVP that matures and

is packaged would be markedly reduced.[125,126] This explanation is consistent with those cases in which little pathology is found in the magnocellular neurons and also with cases of DI in which some small amount of AVP can still be detected.

Idiopathic forms of AVP deficiency represent a large pathogenic category in both adults and children. One study in children revealed that over half (54%) of all cases of CDI were classified as idiopathic.[127] These patients do not have historical or clinical evidence of any injury or disease that can be linked to their DI, and MRI of the pituitary-hypothalamic area generally reveals no abnormality other than absence of the posterior pituitary bright spot and sometimes varying degrees of thickening of the pituitary stalk.

Several lines of evidence have suggested that many of these patients may have had an autoimmune destruction of the neurohypophysis that accounts for their DI. First, the entity of *lymphocytic infundibuloneurohypophysitis* has been documented to be present in a subset of patients with idiopathic DI.[128] Lymphocytic infiltration of the anterior pituitary, or lymphocytic hypophysitis, has been recognized as a cause of anterior pituitary deficiency for many years, but it was not until an autopsy called attention to a similar finding in the posterior pituitary of a patient with DI that this pathology was recognized to occur in the neurohypophysis as well.[129] Since that initial report a number of similar cases have been described, including cases in the postpartum period, which is characteristic of lymphocytic hypophysitis.[130]

With the advent of MRI, lymphocytic infundibuloneurohypophysitis has been diagnosed based on the appearance of a thickened stalk and/or enlargement of the posterior pituitary mimicking a pituitary tumor. In these cases the characteristic bright spot on MRI T1-weighted images is lost. The enlargement of the stalk can so mimic a neoplastic process that some of these patients underwent surgery based on suspicion of a pituitary tumor, but lymphocytic infiltration of the pituitary stalk was found. Since then, a number of patients who were suspected of having infundibuloneurohypophysitis and who had no other obvious cause of DI have been followed and have shown regression of the thickened pituitary stalk over

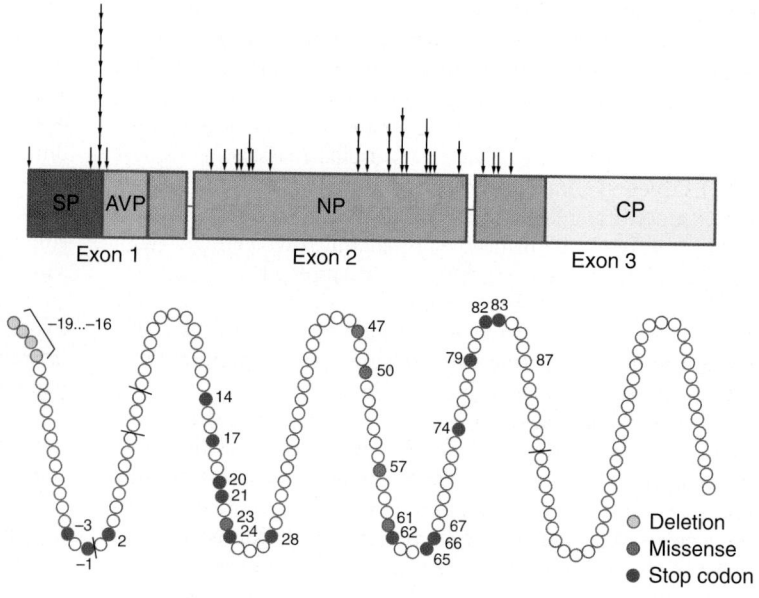

FIGURE 15-9 Location and type of mutations in the gene that codes for the arginine vasopressin (AVP)–neurophysin precursor in kindreds with the autosomal dominant form of familial central diabetes insipidus (CDI). *Each arrow* indicates the location of the mutation in a different kindred. The various portions of the precursor protein are designated by the following abbreviations: *AVP*, vasopressin; *CP*, copeptin; *NP*, neurophysin; and *SP*, signal peptide. Deletion and missense mutations are those expected to remove or replace one or more amino acid residues in the precursor. Mutations designated as stop codons are expected to cause premature termination of the precursor. Note that none of the mutations causes a frameshift or affects the part of the gene that encodes the copeptin moiety, that all of the stop codons are in the distal part of the neurophysin moiety, and that only one of the mutations affects the AVP moiety. All these findings are consistent with the concept that the mutant precursor is produced but cannot be folded properly because of interference with either (1) the binding of AVP to neurophysin, (2) the formation of intrachain disulfide bonds, or (3) the extreme flexibility or rigidity normally required at crucial places in the protein. (Adapted from Rittig S, Robertson GL, Siggaard C, et al: Identification of 13 new mutations in the vasopressin-neurophysin gene in 17 kindreds with familial autosomal dominant neurohypophyseal DI, *Am J Hum Genet* 58:107-117, 1996; and from Hansen LK, Rittig S, Robertson GL: Genetic basis of familial neurohypophyseal diabetes insipidus, *Trends Endocrinol Metab* 8:363-372, 1997.)

time.[127,128] Several cases have been reported of the coexistence of CDI and adenohypophysitis, and these presumably represent cases of combined lymphocytic infundibuloneurohypophysitis and hypophysitis.[131,132]

A second line of evidence supporting an autoimmune etiology in many cases of idiopathic DI is the finding of AVP antibodies in the sera of as many as one third of patients with idiopathic DI and two thirds of those with Langerhans cell histiocytosis X, but not in patients with DI caused by tumors.[133] More recently, 878 patients with autoimmune endocrine diseases but without hypothalamic DI were screened, and 9 patients were found to have AVP antibodies. Upon further testing, 4 of these patients were found to have partial DI and 5 had normal posterior pituitary function. After a 4-year follow-up, 3 of the subjects who had shown normal posterior pituitary function also had developed partial DI, and 1 had progressed to complete DI. Interestingly, 2 of the patients who had partial DI at entry were treated with desmopressin and after 1 year tested negative for AVP antibodies and had recovered normal posterior pituitary function.[134]

Pathophysiology

The normal inverse relationship between urine volume and urine osmolality (see Figure 15-5) means that initial decreases in maximal AVP secretion will not cause an increase in urine volume sufficient to be detected clinically by polyuria. In general, basal AVP secretion must fall to less than 10% to 20% of normal before basal urine osmolality decreases to less than 300 mOsm/kg H_2O and urine flow increases to symptomatic levels (i.e., >50 mL/kg body water per day). This resulting loss of body water produces a slight rise in plasma osmolality that stimulates thirst and induces a compensatory polydipsia. The resultant increase in water intake restores balance with urine output and stabilizes the osmolality of body fluids at a new, slightly higher but still normal level. As the AVP deficit increases, this new steady state level of plasma osmolality approximates the osmotic threshold for thirst (see Figure 15-5).

It is important to recognize that the deficiency of AVP need not be complete for polyuria and polydipsia to occur; it is only necessary that the maximal plasma AVP concentration achievable at or below the osmotic threshold for thirst be inadequate to concentrate the urine.[135] The degree of neurohypophysial destruction at which such failure occurs varies considerably from person to person, largely because of individual differences in the set point and sensitivity of the osmoregulatory system.[33] In general, functional tests of AVP levels in patients with DI of variable severity, duration, and cause indicate that AVP secretory capacity must be reduced by at least 75% to 80% for significant polyuria to occur; this agrees with the findings of neuroanatomic studies of cell loss in the supraoptic nuclei of dogs with experimental pituitary stalk section[112] and studies of patients who have undergone pituitary surgery.[113]

Because renal mechanisms for sodium conservation are unimpaired with impaired or absent AVP secretion, there is no accompanying sodium deficiency. Although untreated DI can lead to both hyperosmolality and volume depletion, until the water losses become severe, volume depletion is minimized by osmotic shifts of water from the ICF compartment to the more osmotically concentrated ECF compartment. This

phenomenon is not as evident following increases in ECF [Na+], since such osmotic shifts result in a slower increase in the serum [Na+] than would otherwise occur. However, when nonsodium solutes such as mannitol are infused, this effect is more obvious due to the progressive dilutional decrease in serum [Na+] caused by translocation of intracellular water to the ECF compartment. Because patients with DI do not have impaired urine Na+ conservation, the ECF volume is generally not markedly decreased, and regulatory mechanisms for maintenance of osmotic homeostasis are primarily activated: stimulation of thirst and AVP secretion (to whatever degree the neurohypophysis is still able to secrete AVP). In cases in which AVP secretion is totally absent (complete DI), patients are dependent entirely on water intake for maintenance of water balance. However, when some residual capacity to secrete AVP remains (partial DI), plasma osmolality can eventually reach levels that allow moderate degrees of urinary concentration (Figure 15-10).

The development of DI following surgical or traumatic injury to the neurohypophysis represents a unique situation and can follow any of several different well-defined patterns. In some patients, polyuria develops 1 to 4 days after injury and resolves spontaneously. Less often, the DI is permanent and continues indefinitely (see previous discussion on the relation between the level of pituitary stalk section and the development of permanent DI). Most interestingly, a *triphasic response* can occur as a result of pituitary stalk transection.[114] The initial DI (first phase) is due to axon shock and lack of function of the damaged neurons. This phase lasts from several hours to several days and then is followed by an antidiuretic phase (second phase) that is due to the uncontrolled release of AVP from the disconnected and degenerating posterior pituitary, or from the remaining severed neurons.[136] Overly aggressive administration of fluids during this second phase does not suppress the AVP secretion and can lead to hyponatremia.

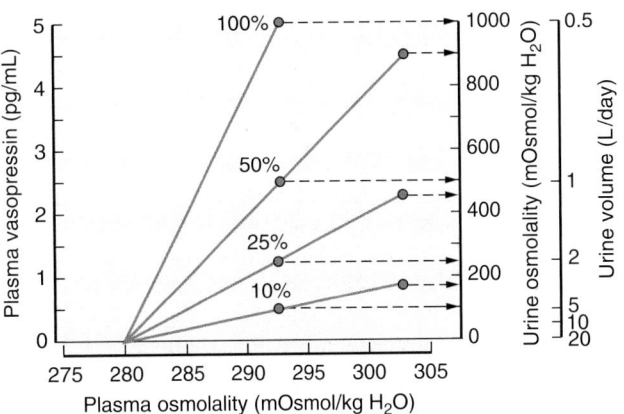

FIGURE 15-10 Relation between plasma arginine vasopressin (AVP) levels, urine osmolality, and plasma osmolality in subjects with normal posterior pituitary function (100%) compared with patients with graded reductions in AVP-secreting neurons (to 50%, 25%, and 10% of normal). Note that the patient with a 50% secretory capacity can achieve only half the plasma AVP level and half the urine osmolality of normal subjects at a plasma osmolality of 293 mOsm/kg H_2O, but with increasing plasma osmolality, this patient can nonetheless eventually stimulate sufficient AVP secretion to reach a near maximal urine osmolality. In contrast, patients with more severe degrees of AVP-secreting neuron deficits are unable to reach maximal urine osmolalities at any level of plasma osmolality. (Adapted from Robertson GL: Posterior pituitary, in Felig P, Baxter J, Frohman LA [editors]: *Endocrinology and metabolism*, New York, 1986, McGraw Hill, pp 338-386.)

The antidiuresis can last from 2 to 14 days, after which DI recurs following depletion of the AVP from the degenerating posterior pituitary gland (third phase).[137]

Transient hyponatremia without preceding or subsequent DI has been reported following transsphenoidal surgery for pituitary microadenomas[138] and generally occurs 5 to 10 days postoperatively. The incidence may be as high as 30% when such patients are carefully followed, although in the majority of cases the condition is mild and self-limited.[139,140] This phenomenon is due to inappropriate AVP secretion via the same mechanism as in the triphasic response, except that in these cases only the second phase occurs (*isolated second phase*) because the initial neural lobe/pituitary stalk damage is not sufficient to impair AVP secretion enough to produce clinical manifestations of DI.[141]

Once a deficiency of AVP secretion has been present for more than a few days or weeks, it rarely improves even if the underlying cause of the neurohypophysial destruction is eliminated. The major exception to this is in patients with postoperative DI, in whom spontaneous resolution is the rule. Although recovery from DI that persists more than several weeks postoperatively is less common, well-documented cases of long-term recovery have nonetheless been reported.[137] The reason for amelioration and resolution is apparent from pathologic and histologic examination of neurohypophyseal tissue following pituitary stalk section.[142,143] Neurohypophyseal neurons that have intact perikarya are able to regenerate axons and form new nerve terminal endings capable of releasing AVP into nearby capillaries. In animals this may be accompanied by a bulbous growth at the end of the severed stalk that represents a new, albeit small, neural lobe. In humans the regeneration process appears to proceed more slowly, and formation of a new neural lobe has not been noted. Nonetheless, histologic examination of a severed human stalk from a patient 18 months after hypophysectomy has demonstrated reorganization of neurohypophyseal fibers with neurosecretory granules in close proximity to nearby blood vessels, which closely resembles the histologic characteristics of a normal posterior pituitary.[143]

Recognition of the fact that almost all patients with CDI retain a limited capacity to secrete AVP allows an understanding of some otherwise perplexing features of the disorder. For example, in many patients, restricting water intake long enough to raise plasma osmolality by only 1% to 2% induces sufficient AVP secretion to concentrate the urine (Figures 15-10 and 15-11). As the plasma osmolality increases further, some patients with partial DI can even secrete enough AVP to achieve near maximal urine osmolalities (Figure 15-12). This should not cause confusion about the diagnosis of DI, however, because in such patients the urine osmolality will still be inappropriately low at plasma osmolalities within the normal range, and they will respond to exogenous AVP administration with further increases in urine osmolality. These responses to dehydration illustrate the relative nature of the AVP deficiency in most cases and underscore the importance of the thirst mechanism in restricting the use of residual secretory capacity under basal conditions of ad libitum water intake.

CDI is also associated with changes in the renal response to AVP. The most obvious change is a reduction in maximal concentrating capacity, which has been attributed to washout of the medullary concentration gradient caused by the chronic polyuria. The severity of this defect is proportional to the

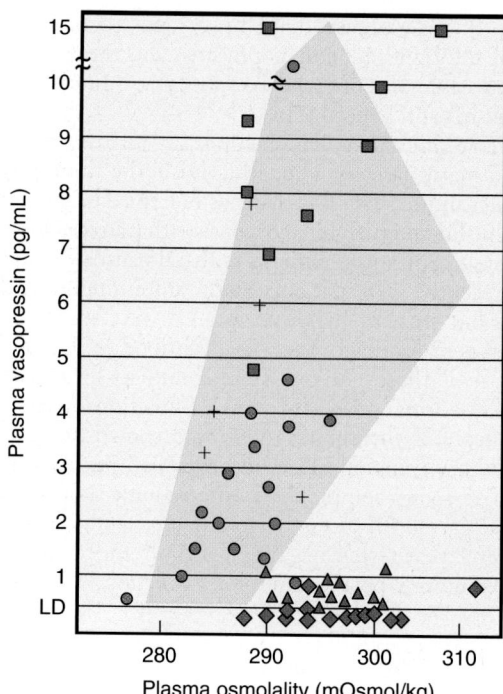

FIGURE 15-11 Relation between plasma arginine vasopressin (AVP) and concurrent plasma osmolality in patients with polyuria of diverse causes. All measurements were made at the end of a standard dehydration test. The *shaded area* represents the range of normal. In patients with severe (♦) or partial (▲) central diabetes insipidus (DI), plasma AVP was almost always subnormal relative to plasma osmolality. In contrast, the values from patients with dipsogenic (●) or nephrogenic (■) DI were consistently within or above the normal range. (From Robertson GL: Diagnosis of diabetes insipidus, in Czernichow AP, Robinson A [editors]: *Diabetes insipidus in man,* Basel, Switzerland, 1985, Karger, p 176.)

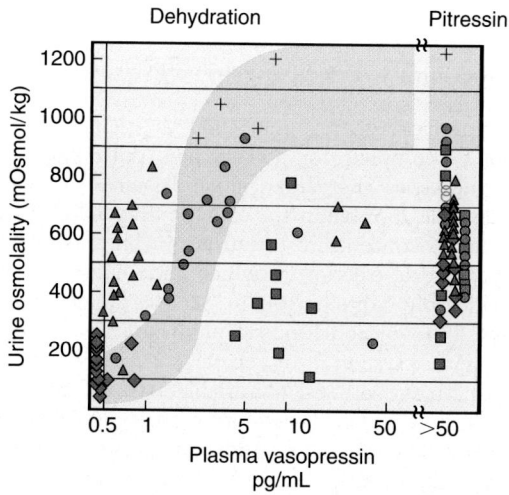

FIGURE 15-12 Relation between urine osmolality and concurrent plasma arginine vasopressin (AVP) in patients with polyuria of diverse causes. All measurements were made at the end of a standard dehydration test. The *shaded area* represents the range of normal. In patients with severe (♦) or partial (▲) central diabetes insipidus (DI), urine osmolality is normal or supranormal relative to plasma AVP when the latter is submaximal. In patients with nephrogenic DI (■), urine osmolality is always subnormal relative to plasma AVP. In patients with dipsogenic DI (●), the relation is normal at submaximal levels of plasma AVP but is usually subnormal when plasma AVP is high. (From Robertson GL: Diagnosis of diabetes insipidus, in Czernichow AP, Robinson A [editors]: *Diabetes insipidus in man,* Basel, Switzerland, 1985, Karger, p 176.)

magnitude of the polyuria and is independent of its cause.[135] Because of this, the level of urinary concentration achieved at maximally effective levels of plasma AVP is reduced in all types of DI. In patients with CDI this concentrating abnormality is offset to some extent by an apparent increase in renal sensitivity to low levels of plasma AVP (see Figure 15-12). The cause of this supersensitivity is unknown, but it may reflect upward regulation of AVP V_2 receptor expression or function secondary to a long-term deficiency of the hormone.[144]

Osmoreceptor Dysfunction

Etiology

An extensive literature in animals indicates that the primary osmoreceptors controlling AVP secretion and thirst are located in the anterior hypothalamus; lesions of this region, called the *anteroventral third ventricle (AV3V) area,* cause hyperosmolality in animals through a combination of impaired thirst and osmotically stimulated AVP secretion.[30,31] Initial reports in humans described this syndrome as *essential hypernatremia,*[145] and subsequent studies used the term *adipsic hypernatremia* in recognition of the profound thirst deficits found in most of the patients.[146] Based on the known pathophysiology, all of these syndromes can be grouped together as disorders of *osmoreceptor dysfunction.*[147]

Although the pathologies responsible for this condition can be quite varied, all of the cases reported to date have been due to various degrees of osmoreceptor destruction associated with a variety of different brain lesions, as summarized in Table 15-2. Many of these are the same types of lesions that can cause CDI, but in contrast to those in CDI, these lesions usually occur more rostrally in the hypothalamus, consistent with the anterior hypothalamic location of the primary osmoreceptor cells (see Figure 15-2). One lesion that is unique to this disorder is an anterior communicating cerebral artery aneurysm. Because the small arterioles that feed the anterior wall of the third ventricle originate from the anterior communicating cerebral artery, an aneurysm in this region[148]—or, more often, surgical repair of such an aneurysm, which typically involves ligation of the anterior communicating artery[149]—produces infarction of the part of the hypothalamus containing the osmoreceptor cells.

Pathophysiology

The cardinal defect in patients with this disorder is lack of the osmoreceptors that regulate thirst. With rare exceptions the osmoregulation of AVP is also impaired, although the hormonal response to nonosmotic stimuli remains intact (Figure 15-13).[150,151] Four major patterns of osmoreceptor dysfunction have been described as characterized by defects in thirst and/or AVP secretory responses: (1) upward resetting of the osmostat for both thirst and AVP secretion (normal AVP and thirst responses but at an abnormally high plasma osmolality), (2) partial osmoreceptor destruction (blunted AVP and thirst responses at all plasma osmolalities), (3) total osmoreceptor destruction (absent AVP secretion and thirst regardless of plasma osmolality), and (4) selective dysfunction of thirst osmoregulation with intact AVP secretion.[147] Regardless of the actual pattern, the hallmark of this disorder is an abnormal thirst response in addition to variable defects in AVP secretion.

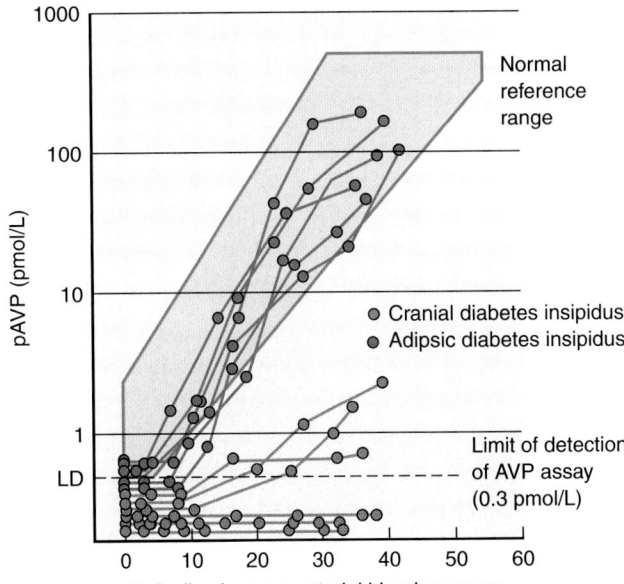

FIGURE 15-13 Plasma arginine vasopressin (AVP) responses to arterial hypotension produced by infusion of trimethaphan in patients with central diabetes insipidus ("cranial diabetes insipidus") and osmoreceptor dysfunction ("adipsic diabetes insipidus"). Normal responses in healthy volunteers are shown by the *shaded area.* Note that despite absent or markedly blunted AVP responses to hyperosmolality, patients with osmoreceptor dysfunction respond normally to baroreceptor stimulation induced by hypotension. (From Baylis PH, Thompson CJ: Diabetes insipidus and hyperosmolar syndromes, in Becker KL [editor]: *Principles and practice of endocrinology and metabolism,* Philadelphia, 1995, JB Lippincott, p 257.)

Because of this, such patients fail to drink sufficiently as their plasma osmolality increases, and as a result the new set point for plasma osmolality rises far above the normal thirst threshold. Unlike patients with CDI, whose polydipsia maintains their plasma osmolality within normal ranges, patients with osmoreceptor dysfunction typically have osmolalities in the range of 300 to 340 mOsm/kg H_2O. This again underscores the critical role played by normal thirst mechanisms in maintaining body fluid homeostasis; intact renal function alone is insufficient to maintain plasma osmolality within normal limits in such cases.

The rate of development and the severity of hyperosmolality and hypertonic dehydration in patients with osmoreceptor dysfunction are influenced by a number of factors. First is the ability to maintain some degree of osmotically stimulated thirst and AVP secretion, which will determine the new set point for plasma osmolality. Second are environmental influences that affect the rate of water output. When physical activity is minimal and ambient temperature is not elevated, the overall rates of renal and insensible water loss are low, and the patient's diet may be sufficient to maintain a relatively normal balance for long periods of time. Anything that increases perspiration, respiration, or urine output greatly accelerates the rate of water loss and thereby uncovers the patient's inability to mount an appropriate compensatory increase in water intake.[12] Under these conditions, severe and even fatal hypernatremia can develop relatively quickly. When the dehydration is only moderate (plasma osmolality of 300 to 330 mOsm/kg H_2O), the patient is usually asymptomatic and signs of volume depletion are minimal, but if the dehydration becomes severe the patient can exhibit symptoms and signs of hypovolemia, including weakness, postural dizziness, paralysis, confusion, coma, azotemia, hypokalemia, hyperglycemia, and secondary hyperaldosteronism (see later section on clinical manifestations). In severe cases, there may also be rhabdomyolysis with marked serum elevations in muscle enzymes and occasionally acute renal failure.

A third factor also influences the degree of hyperosmolality and dehydration present in these patients, however. For all cases of osmoreceptor dysfunction it is important to remember that afferent pathways from the brainstem to the hypothalamus remain intact; therefore, these patients usually have normal AVP and renal concentrating responses to baroreceptor-mediated stimuli such as hypovolemia and hypotension (see Figure 15-13)[151] and to other nonosmotic stimuli such as nausea (see Figure 15-8).[146,150] This has the effect of preventing severe dehydration, since as hypovolemia develops it will stimulate AVP secretion via baroreceptive pathways through the brainstem (see Figure 15-2). Although protective, this effect often causes confusion, since at some times these patients appear to have DI, yet at other times they can concentrate their urine quite normally. Nonetheless, the presence of refractory hyperosmolality with absent or inappropriate thirst should alert clinicians to the presence of osmoreceptor dysfunction regardless of apparent normal urine concentration at some times.

In a few patients with osmoreceptor dysfunction, forced hydration has been found to lead to hyponatremia in association with inappropriate urine concentration.[145,146] This paradoxical defect resembles that seen in SIADH and has been postulated to be due to two different pathogenic mechanisms. One is continuous or fixed secretion of AVP because of loss of the capacity for osmotic inhibition and stimulation of hormone secretion. These observations, as well as electrophysiologic data,[41] strongly suggest that the osmoregulatory system is bimodal (i.e., it is composed of inhibitory as well as stimulatory input to the neurohypophysis, see Figure 15-6). The other cause of the diluting defect appears to be hypersensitivity to the antidiuretic effects of AVP, because in some patients, urine osmolality may remain high even when the hormone is undetectable.[146]

Hypodipsia is also a common occurrence in elderly persons in the absence of any overt hypothalamic lesion.[152] In such cases, it is not clear whether the defect is in the hypothalamic osmoreceptors, in their projections to the cortex, or in some other regulatory mechanism. However, in most cases the osmoreceptor is probably not involved, because both basal and stimulated plasma AVP levels have been found to be normal, or even high, in relation to plasma osmolality in aged humans, except in only a few studies that showed decreased plasma levels of AVP relative to plasma osmolality.[153]

Gestational Diabetes Insipidus

Etiology

A relative deficiency of plasma AVP can also result from an increase in the rate of AVP metabolism.[97,154] This condition has been observed only in pregnancy, and therefore it is generally referred to as *gestational diabetes insipidus*. It is due to the action of a circulating enzyme called *cysteine aminopeptidase* (*oxytocinase* or *vasopressinase*) that is normally produced by the placenta to degrade circulating oxytocin and prevent premature

uterine contractions.[155] Because of the close structural similarity between AVP and oxytocin, this enzyme degrades both peptides. In some patients with gestational DI plasma levels of oxytocinase/vasopressinase are markedly elevated above those found normally in pregnancy.[154,156] In others, however, oxytocinase/vasopressinase levels are relatively normal but the effect of the increase in AVP metabolism may be exacerbated by an underlying subclinical deficiency of AVP secretion.[157] Some of these patients have been noted to have accompanying preeclampsia, acute fatty liver, and coagulopathies, but causal relations between the DI and these abnormalities have not been identified. The relationship of this disorder to the transient nephrogenic DI of pregnancy[158] is not clear.

Pathophysiology

The pathophysiology of gestational DI is similar to that of CDI. The only exception is that the polyuria is usually not corrected by administration of AVP, since this is rapidly degraded just as is endogenous AVP; however, it can be controlled by treatment with desmopressin, the AVP V_2 receptor agonist that is more resistant to degradation by oxytocinase/vasopressinase.[155] It should be remembered that patients with partial CDI in whom only low levels of AVP can be maintained, or patients with compensated NDI in whom the lack of response of the kidney to AVP may be not be absolute, can be relatively asymptomatic with regard to polyuria, but with accelerated destruction of AVP during pregnancy the underlying DI may become manifest. Consequently, patients who have gestational DI should not be assumed simply to have excess oxytocinase/vasopressinase; rather, these patients should be evaluated for other possible underlying pathologic conditions (see Table 15-2).[157]

Nephrogenic Diabetes Insipidus

Etiology

Resistance to the antidiuretic action of AVP is usually due to some defect within the kidney and is commonly referred to as *nephrogenic diabetes insipidus* (NDI). The condition was first recognized in 1945 in several patients with the familial, sex-linked form of the disorder. Subsequently, additional kindreds with the X-linked form of familial NDI were identified. Clinical studies of NDI indicate that symptomatic polyuria is present from birth, plasma AVP levels are normal or elevated, resistance to the antidiuretic effect of AVP can be partial or virtually complete, and the disease affects mostly males and is usually, although not always,[159] mild or absent in carrier females.

More than 90% of cases of congenital NDI are caused by mutations of the AVP V_2 receptor (see the review in Morello and Bichet[160] and Chapter 44). Most mutations occur in the part of the receptor that is highly conserved among species and/or is conserved among similar receptors, for example, homologies with AVP V_{1a} or oxytocin receptors. The effect of some of these mutations on receptor synthesis, processing, trafficking, and function has been studied using in vitro expression.[161,162] These studies show that the various mutations cause several different defects in cellular processing and function of the receptor, which can be classified into four general categories based on differences in transport to the cell surface and AVP binding and/or stimulation of adenylyl cyclase: (1) the mutant receptor is not inserted into the membrane, (2) the mutant receptor is inserted into the membrane but does not bind or respond to AVP, (3) the mutant receptor is inserted into the membrane and binds AVP but does not activate adenylyl cyclase, and (4) the mutant protein is inserted into the membrane and binds AVP but responds subnormally in terms of adenylyl cyclase activation.

Several studies have shown a relation between the clinical phenotype and the genotype and/or cellular phenotype.[161,163] Approximately 10% of the V_2 receptor defects causing congenital NDI are thought to arise de novo. This high incidence of de novo cases coupled with the large number of mutations that have been identified hinders the clinical use of genetic identification, because it is necessary to sequence the entire open reading frame of the receptor gene rather than short sequences of DNA; nonetheless, use of automated gene-sequencing techniques in selected families has been shown to successfully identify mutations in both patients with clinical disease and asymptomatic carriers.[164] Although most female carriers of the X-linked V_2 receptor defects have no clinical disease, some females have been reported with symptomatic NDI.[159] Carriers can have a decreased maximum urine osmolality in response to plasma AVP levels, but are generally asymptomatic because of the absence of overt polyuria. Occasionally a girl manifests severe NDI due to a V_2 receptor mutation, which is likely due to skewed inactivation of the normal X chromosome.[165]

Congenital NDI can also result from mutations of the autosomal gene that codes for AQP2, the protein which forms the water channels in renal medullary collecting tubules. When the proband is a girl, it is likely that the defect is a mutation of the AQP2 gene on chromosome 12, region q12-q13.[166] More than 20 different mutations of the AQP2 gene have been described (see the review by Knoers and Deen[167] and Chapter 44). The patients may be heterozygous for two different recessive mutations[168] or homozygous for the same abnormality from both parents.[169] Because most of these mutations are recessive, the patients usually do not present with a family history of DI unless consanguinity is present. Functional expression studies of these mutations show that

all of them result in varying degrees of reduced water transport, because the mutant aquaporins either are not expressed in normal amounts, are retained in various cellular organelles, or simply do not function effectively as water channels.

Regardless of the type of mutation, the phenotype of NDI from AQP2 mutations is identical to that produced by V_2 receptor mutations. Some of the defects in cellular routing and water transport can be reversed by treatment with chemicals that act like *chaperones*,[170] which suggests that misfolding of the mutant AQP2 may be responsible for misrouting. Similar salutary effects of chaperones have been found to reverse defects in cell surface expression and function of selected mutations of the AVP V_2 receptor.[171]

NDI can also be caused by a variety of drugs, diseases, and metabolic disturbances, among them lithium, hypokalemia, and hypercalcemia (see Table 15-2). Some of these disorders (e.g., polycystic kidney disease) act to distort the normal architecture of the kidney and interfere with the normal urine concentration process. However, experimental studies in animal models have suggested that many have in common a downregulation of AQP2 expression in the renal collecting tubules (Figure 15-14; see also Chapters 10 and 11).[172,173] The polyuria associated with potassium deficiency develops in parallel with decreased expression of kidney AQP2, and repletion of potassium reestablishes the normal urinary concentrating mechanism and normalizes renal expression of AQP2.[174] Similarly, hypercalcemia has also been found to be associated with downregulation of AQP2.[175] Consumption of a low-protein diet diminishes the ability to concentrate the urine primarily by decreased delivery of urea to the inner medulla, thus decreasing medullary concentration gradient, but rats on a low-protein diet also appear to downregulate AQP2, which could be an additional component of the decreased ability to concentrate the urine.[176] Bilateral urinary tract obstruction causes inability to produce a maximum concentration the urine, and rat models have demonstrated a downregulation of AQP2, which persists for several days after release of the obstruction.[177] However, it is not yet clear which of these effects on AQP2 expression are primary or secondary, and what cellular mechanisms are responsible for the downregulation of AQP2 expression.

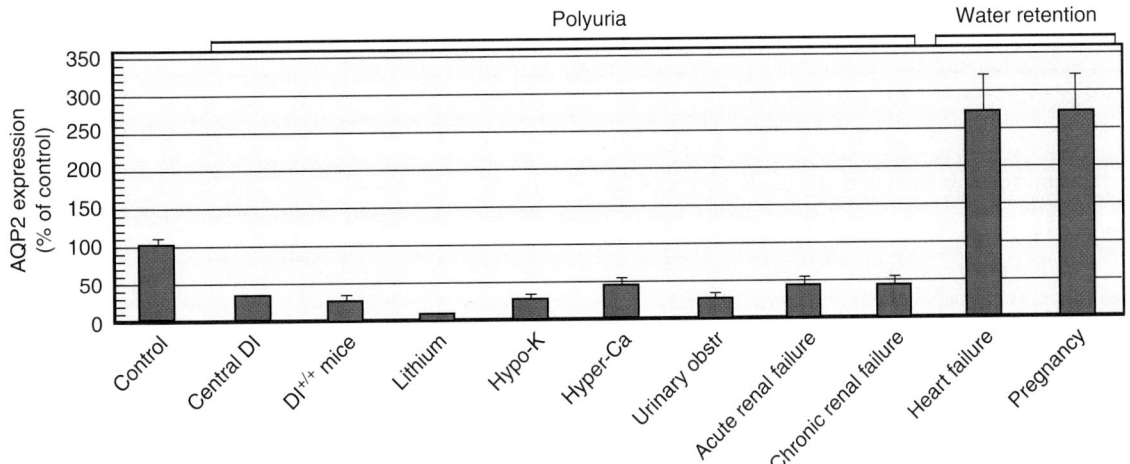

FIGURE 15-14 Kidney expression of the water channel aquaporin-2 in various animal models of polyuria and water retention. Note that kidney aquaporin-2 expression is uniformly downregulated relative to levels in controls in all animal models of polyuria, but upregulated in animal models of inappropriate antidiuresis. *DI*[+/+], Genetic diabetes insipidus; *Hyper-Ca*, hypercalcemia; *Hypo-K*, hypokalemia; Urinary obstr, ureteral obstruction. (From Nielsen S, Kwon TH, Christensen BM, et al: Physiology and pathophysiology of renal aquaporins, *J Am Soc Nephrol* 10:647-663, 1999.)

Administration of lithium to treat psychiatric disorders is the most common cause of drug-induced NDI and illustrates the multiple mechanisms likely involved in producing this disorder. As many as 10% to 20% of patients taking lithium long term develop some degree of NDI.[178] Lithium is known to interfere with the production of cAMP[179] and produces a dramatic (95%) reduction in kidney AQP2 levels in animals.[180] The defect of aquaporins is slow to correct both in experimental animals and in humans, and in some cases it can be permanent[181] in association with glomerular or tubulointerstitial nephropathy.[182] Several other drugs that are known to induce renal concentrating defects have also been associated with abnormalities of AQP2 synthesis.[183]

Pathophysiology

As in CDI, renal insensitivity to the antidiuretic effect of AVP in NDI also results in the excretion of an increased volume of dilute urine, a decrease in body water, and a rise in plasma osmolality, which by stimulating thirst induces a compensatory increase in water intake. As a consequence, the osmolality of body fluid stabilizes at a slightly higher level that approximates the osmotic threshold for thirst. As in patients with CDI, the magnitude of polyuria and polydipsia varies greatly depending on a number of factors, including the degree of renal insensitivity to AVP, individual differences in the set points and sensitivity of thirst and AVP secretion, as well as total solute load. It is important to note that the renal insensitivity to AVP need not be complete for polyuria to occur; the defect need only be great enough to prevent concentration of the urine at plasma AVP levels achievable under ordinary conditions of ad libitum water intake (i.e., at plasma osmolalities near the osmotic threshold for thirst). Calculations similar to those used for states of AVP deficiency indicate that this requirement is not met until the renal sensitivity to AVP is reduced by more than 10-fold. Because renal insensitivity to the hormone is often incomplete, especially in cases of acquired rather than congenital NDI, many patients with NDI are able to concentrate their urine to varying degrees when they are deprived of water or given large doses of desmopressin.

New knowledge about the renal concentration mechanism from studies of AQP2 expression in experimental animals (see Chapters 10 and 11) has suggested that a form of NDI is likely associated with all types of DI, as well as with primary polydipsia. Brattleboro rats have been found to have low levels of kidney AQP2 expression compared with Long-Evans control rats; AQP2 levels are corrected by treatment with AVP or desmopressin, but this process takes 3 to 5 days, during which time urine concentration remains subnormal despite pharmacologic concentrations of AVP.[184] Similarly, physiologic suppression of AVP by long-term overadministration of water produces a downregulation of AQP2 in the renal collecting duct.[184] Clinically, it is well known that patients with both CDI and primary polydipsia often fail to achieve maximally concentrated urine when they are given desmopressin during a water deprivation test to differentiate among the various causes of DI. This effect has long been attributed to a washout of the medullary concentration gradient as a result of the high urine flow rates in polyuric patients, but based on the results of animal studies it seems certain that at least part of the decreased response to AVP is due to a downregulation of kidney AQP2 expression. This also explains why it takes time,

typically several days, to restore normal urinary concentration after patients with primary polydipsia and CDI are treated with water restriction or antidiuretic therapy.[185]

Primary Polydipsia

Etiology

Excessive fluid intake also causes hypotonic polyuria and is, by definition, polydipsia. Consequently, this disorder must be differentiated from DI due to various other causes. Furthermore, it is apparent that despite normal pituitary and kidney function, patients with this disorder nonetheless share many characteristics of both CDI (i.e., AVP secretion is suppressed as a result of the decreased plasma osmolality) and NDI (i.e., kidney AQP2 expression is decreased as a result of the suppressed plasma AVP levels). Many different names have been used to describe patients with excessive fluid intake, but *primary polydipsia* remains the best descriptor, because it does not presume any particular etiology for the increased fluid intake.

Primary polydipsia is often due to a severe mental illness such as schizophrenia, mania, or an obsessive-compulsive disorder,[186] in which case it is called *psychogenic polydipsia*. These patients usually deny true thirst and attribute their polydipsia to bizarre motives such as a need to cleanse their body of poisons. Studies of patients in psychiatric hospitals have shown that as many as 42% of patients have some form of polydipsia, and in most reported cases there is no obvious explanation for the polydipsia.[187]

Primary polydipsia can also be caused by an abnormality in the osmoregulatory control of thirst, in which case it has been termed *dipsogenic diabetes insipidus*.[188] These patients have no overt psychiatric illness and invariably attribute their polydipsia to a nearly constant thirst. Dipsogenic DI is usually idiopathic, but it can also be secondary to organic structural lesions in the hypothalamus identical to those in any of the disorders described as causes of CDI, such as sarcoidosis of the hypothalamus, tuberculous meningitis, multiple sclerosis, or trauma. Consequently, all polydipsic patients should be evaluated by performing MRI of the brain before concluding that excessive water intake is due to an idiopathic or psychiatric cause.

Primary polydipsia can also be produced by drugs that cause a dry mouth or by any peripheral disorder causing pathologic elevations of renin and/or angiotensin.[109] Finally, primary polydipsia is sometimes caused by physicians, nurses, lay practitioners, or health writers who recommend a high fluid intake for valid causes (e.g., recurrent nephrolithiasis) or for unsubstantiated reasons of health.[189] These patients lack overt signs of mental illness, but also deny thirst and usually attribute their polydipsia to habits acquired from years of adherence to their drinking regimen.

Pathophysiology

The pathophysiology of primary polydipsia is essentially the reverse of that in CDI: the excessive intake of water expands and slightly dilutes body fluids, suppresses AVP secretion, and dilutes the urine. The resultant increase in the rate of water excretion balances the increase in intake, and the osmolality of body water stabilizes at a new, slightly lower level that approximates the osmotic threshold for AVP secretion. The magnitude of the polyuria and polydipsia vary considerably, depending on the nature or intensity of the stimulus to drink. In patients with abnormal thirst, the polydipsia and polyuria are relatively constant from day to day. However, in patients with psychogenic polydipsia, water intake and urine output tend to fluctuate widely, and at times can be quite large. Occasionally fluid intake rises to such extraordinary levels that the excretory capacity of the kidneys is exceeded and dilutional hyponatremia develops.[190]

There is little question that excessive water intake alone can sometimes be sufficient to override renal excretory capacity and produce severe hyponatremia. Although the water excretion rate of normal adult kidneys can generally exceed 20 L/day, maximum hourly rates are rarely more than 1000 mL/hour. Because many psychiatric patients drink predominantly during the day or during intense drinking binges,[191] they can transiently achieve symptomatic levels of hyponatremia with total daily volumes of water intake under 20 L if the water is ingested sufficiently rapidly. This likely accounts for many of the cases in which such patients have maximally dilute urine, which includes as many as 50% of patients in some studies, and show a quick correction via a free water diuresis.[192]

The prevalence of this disorder as derived from hospital admissions for acute symptomatic hyponatremia may have been underestimated, because studies of polydipsic psychiatric patients have shown a marked diurnal variation in serum [Na+] (from 141 mEq/L at 7 AM to 130 mEq/L at 4 PM), which suggests that many such patients drink excessively during the daytime but then correct themselves via a water diuresis at night.[193] Because of this and other considerations, this disorder has been defined as the *psychosis–intermittent hyponatremia–polydipsia (PIP) syndrome.*[191] However, many other cases of hyponatremia with psychogenic polydipsia have been found to meet the criteria for a diagnosis of SIADH, which suggests the presence of nonosmotically stimulated AVP secretion.

As might be expected in the face of much higher than normal water intakes, virtually any impairment of urinary dilution and water excretion can exacerbate the development of a positive water balance and thereby produce hypo-osmolality. Acute psychosis itself can also cause AVP secretion,[194] which often appears to take the form of a reset osmostat.[186] It is therefore apparent that no single mechanism can completely explain the occurrence of hyponatremia in polydipsic psychiatric patients; however, the combination of higher than normal water intakes plus modest elevations of plasma AVP levels due to a variety of potential sources appears to account for a significant portion of such cases.

Clinical Manifestations of Diabetes Insipidus

The characteristic clinical symptoms of DI are the polyuria and polydipsia that result from the underlying impairment of urinary concentrating mechanisms, which have already been covered in the previous sections discussing the pathophysiology of specific types of DI. Interestingly, patients with DI typically describe a craving for cold water, which appears to quench their thirst better.[66] Patients with CDI also typically describe a precipitous onset of their polyuria and polydipsia, which simply reflects the fact that urinary concentration can be maintained fairly well until the number of AVP-producing neurons in the hypothalamus decreases to 10% to 15% of normal, after which plasma AVP levels decrease to the range at which urine output increases dramatically.

Patients with DI, however, particularly those with osmoreceptor dysfunction syndromes, can also show varying degrees of hyperosmolality and dehydration depending on their overall hydration status. It is therefore important to be aware of the clinical manifestations of hyperosmolality as well. These can be divided into the signs and symptoms produced by dehydration, which are largely cardiovascular, and those caused by the hyperosmolality itself, which are predominantly neurologic and reflect brain dehydration as a result of osmotic water shifts out of the central nervous system (CNS). Cardiovascular manifestations of hypertonic dehydration include hypotension, azotemia, acute tubular necrosis secondary to renal hypoperfusion or rhabdomyolysis, and shock.[195,196] Neurologic manifestations range from nonspecific symptoms such as irritability and cognitive dysfunction to more severe manifestations of *hypertonic encephalopathy* such as disorientation, decreased level of consciousness, obtundation, chorea, seizures, coma, focal neurologic deficits, subarachnoid hemorrhage, and cerebral infarction.[195,197]

The severity of symptoms can be roughly correlated with the degree of hyperosmolality, but individual variability is marked, and for any single patient the level of serum [Na+] at which symptoms will appear cannot be accurately predicted. As with hypo-osmolar syndromes, the length of time over which hyperosmolality develops can markedly affect the clinical symptomatology. Rapid development of severe hyperosmolality is frequently associated with marked neurologic symptoms, whereas gradual development over several days or weeks generally causes milder symptoms.[195,198] In this case, the brain counteracts osmotic shrinkage by increasing intracellular content of solutes. These include electrolytes such as potassium and a variety of *organic osmolytes*, which previously had been called *idiogenic osmoles*. For the most part these are the same organic osmolytes that are lost from the brain during adaptation to hypo-osmolality.[199] The net effect of this process is to protect the brain against excessive shrinkage during sustained hyperosmolality. However, once the brain has adapted by increasing its solute content, rapid correction of the hyperosmolality can produce brain edema, because it takes a certain time (24 to 48 hours in animal studies) to dissipate the accumulated solutes, and until this process has been completed the brain will accumulate excess water as plasma osmolality is normalized.[200] This effect is most often seen in dehydrated pediatric patients, who can develop seizures with rapid rehydration[201]; it has been described only rarely in adults, including the most severely hyperosmolar patients with nonketotic hyperglycemic hyperosmolar coma.

Differential Diagnosis of Polyuria

Before complex diagnostic testing is initiated to differentiate among the various forms of DI and primary polydipsia, the presence of true hypotonic polyuria should be established by 24-hour measurement of urine for volume and osmolality. Generally accepted standards are that 24-hour urine volume should exceed 50 mL/kg body water with an osmolality of less than 300 mOsm/kg H_2O.[202] Simultaneously, there should be a determination of whether the polyuria is due to an osmotic agent such as glucose or to intrinsic renal disease. Routine laboratory studies and the clinical setting will usually distinguish these disorders; diabetes mellitus and other forms of solute diuresis usually can be excluded by the history, a routine urinalysis for glucose, or measurement of the solute excretion rate (urine osmolality × urine volume in liters of <15 mOsm/kg body water per day).

There is universal agreement that the diagnosis of DI requires stimulating AVP secretion osmotically and then measuring the adequacy of the secretion using either direct measurement of plasma AVP levels or indirect assessment by urine osmolality. In a patient who is already hyperosmolar with submaximally concentrated urine (i.e., urine osmolality of <800 mOsm/kg H_2O), the diagnosis is straightforward and simple: primary polydipsia is ruled out by the presence of hyperosmolality,[202] which confirms a diagnosis of DI. CDI can then be distinguished from NDI by evaluating the response to administered AVP (5 U subcutaneously) or, preferably, the AVP V_2 receptor agonist *desmopressin* (1 to 2 μg subcutaneously or intravenously). A significant increase in urine osmolality within 1 to 2 hours after injection indicates insufficient endogenous AVP secretion and therefore CDI, whereas an absent response indicates renal resistance to AVP effects and therefore NDI.

Although testing is conceptually simple, interpretational difficulties can arise because the water diuresis produced by AVP deficiency in CDI results in a washout of the renal medullary concentrating gradient as well as downregulation of kidney AQP2 water channels, as discussed previously, so that initial increases in urine osmolality in response to administered AVP or desmopressin are not as great as would be expected. Generally, increases in urine osmolality of more than 50% reliably indicate CDI and responses of less than 10% indicate NDI, but responses between 10% and 50% are indeterminate.[135] For this reason, plasma AVP levels should be measured to aid in making the distinction: hyperosmolar patients with NDI will have clearly elevated plasma AVP levels, whereas those with CDI will have absent (complete) or blunted (partial) AVP responses relative to the plasma osmolality (Figure 15-15). Since it will not be known beforehand which patients will have diagnostic versus indeterminate responses to AVP or desmopressin, a blood specimen for determination of plasma AVP level should be drawn prior to AVP or desmopressin administration in patients presenting with hyperosmolality and inadequately concentrated urine without a solute diuresis.

Because patients with DI have intact thirst mechanisms, most often they do not present with hyperosmolality, but rather with a normal plasma osmolality and serum [Na+] and symptoms of polyuria and polydipsia. In these cases it is most appropriate to perform a *fluid deprivation test*. The relative merits of the indirect fluid deprivation test (also know as the *Miller-Moses test*[203]) versus direct measurement of plasma AVP levels after a period of fluid deprivation[135] have been debated in the literature for the last several decades, with substantial pros and cons cited for each of these tests. On the one hand, the standard indirect test has a long track record of successfully indicating the appropriate diagnosis in the large majority of cases, generally yields interpretable results by the end of the test, and does not require sensitive assays for the notoriously difficult measurement of plasma AVP levels.[204,205] However, maximum urine concentrating capacity is well known to be variably reduced in all forms of DI as well as in primary polydipsia,[135] and as a result the absolute levels of urine osmolality achieved during fluid deprivation and after AVP administration are reduced to overlapping degrees in patients with partial CDI, partial NDI, and primary polydipsia (see Figure 15-15). Measurements of basal plasma osmolality or serum [Na+] are of little use, because they also overlap considerably in patients with these disorders.[202] And although association with certain diseases, surgical procedures, or family history often helps to differentiate among these disorders, sometimes the clinical setting may not be helpful because certain diseases such as sarcoidosis, tuberculous meningitis, and other hypothalamic pathologies can cause more than one type of DI (see Table 15-2).

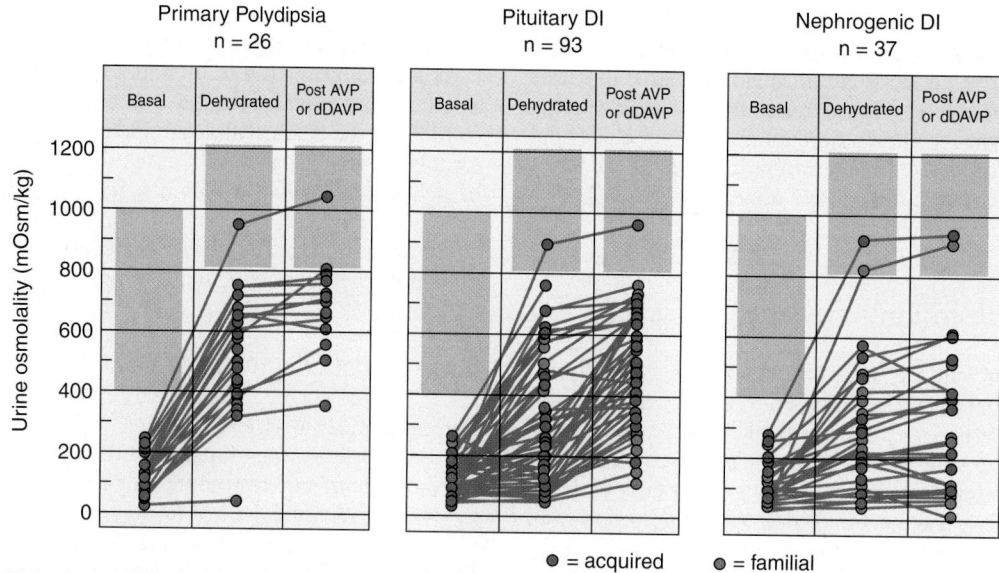

FIGURE 15-15 Effects of fluid deprivation and subsequent administration of vasopressin (AVP [Pitressin]) on urine osmolality in 156 patients with polyuria of diverse causes. The *shaded areas* indicate the range of values in healthy adults. Note that, although AVP responses tended to be greater in patients with central (neurogenic) diabetes insipidus (DI), the overlap between the three groups was significant.

As a consequence, a simpler approach that has been proposed is to measure plasma or urine AVP before and during exposure to a suitable osmotic stimulus such as fluid restriction or hypertonic NaCl infusion and plot the results as a function of the concurrent plasma osmolality or plasma [Na⁺] concentration (see Figures 15-11 and 15-12).[206,207] Using a highly sensitive and validated research assay for plasma AVP determinations, this approach has been shown to yield a definite diagnosis in most cases, provided the final level of plasma osmolality or sodium achieved is above the normal range (>295 mOsm/kg H₂O or 145 mmol/L, respectively). The diagnostic effectiveness of this approach derives from the fact that the magnitude of the AVP response to osmotic stimulation is not appreciably diminished by longer-term overhydration[186] or dehydration. Hence, the relationship of plasma AVP to plasma osmolality is usually within or above normal limits in NDI and primary polydipsia. In most cases, these two disorders can then be distinguished by measuring urine osmolality before and after the dehydration test and relating these values to the concurrent plasma AVP concentrations (see Figure 15-12). However, because maximal concentrating capacity can be severely blunted in patients with primary polydipsia, it is often better to analyze the relationship under basal, nondehydrated conditions when plasma AVP is not elevated. Because of the solute diuresis that often ensues following infusion of hypertonic NaCl, measurements of urine osmolality or AVP excretion are unreliable indicators of changes in hormone secretion and are of little or no diagnostic value when this procedure is used to increase osmolality to more than 295 mOsm/kg H₂O.

Given the proven usefulness of both the indirect and the direct approaches, a combined fluid deprivation test that synthesizes the crucial aspects of both tests can easily be performed (Table 15-3) and in many cases allows interpretation of both the plasma AVP levels and the response to an AVP challenge. The recent development of a commercial assay for the C-terminal glycoprotein of the AVP prohormone, *copeptin* (see Figure 15-3), offers the possibility of using a more stable and easier to measure marker of AVP secretion in response to induced dehydration and hypertonicity.[208] However, the clinical use of copeptin levels as a surrogate marker of AVP secretion during fluid deprivation tests will require standardization of normal and abnormal responses relative to plasma AVP levels.

When the fluid deprivation test with plasma AVP determinations is used, more than 95% of all cases of polyuria and polydipsia can be diagnosed accurately. A useful approach in the remaining indeterminate cases is to conduct a closely monitored trial of standard therapeutic doses of desmopressin. If this treatment abolishes thirst and polydipsia as well as polyuria for 48 to 72 hours without producing water intoxication, the patient most likely has uncomplicated CDI. On the other hand, if the treatment abolishes the polyuria but has no or a lesser effect on thirst or polydipsia and results in the development of hyponatremia, it is more likely that the patient has some form of primary polydipsia. If desmopressin has no effect over this time interval, even when given by injection, it is virtually certain that the patient has some form of NDI.

As might be expected, most patients with DI also exhibit a subnormal increase in AVP secretion in response to nonosmotic stimuli such as hypotension, nausea, and hypoglycemia.[206] For diagnostic purposes, however, these nonosmotic

tests of neurohypophyseal function do not provide any advantage over dehydration or hypertonic NaCl infusion, because orthostatic, emetic, and glucopenic stimuli are difficult to control or quantitate and generally cause a markedly variable AVP response. A more fundamental disadvantage of all nonosmotic stimuli is the possibility of a false-positive or false-negative results, since there are patients who exhibit little or no rise in AVP after hypotension or emesis yet lack polyuria and have a normal response to osmotic stimuli. Conversely, patients with osmoreceptor dysfunction exhibit little or no AVP response to hypertonic NaCl but have a normal increase in response to induced hypotension (see Figure 15-13).[151]

MRI has also proved to be useful in diagnosing DI. In normal subjects, the posterior pituitary produces a characteristic bright signal in the posterior part of the sella turcica on T1-weighted images, usually best seen in sagittal views.[209] This was originally thought to represent fatty tissue, but more recent evidence indicates that the bright spot is actually due to the stored hormone in neurosecretory granules.[210] An experimental study performed in rabbits subjected to dehydration for varying periods of time showed a linear correlation between pituitary AVP content and the signal intensity of the posterior pituitary on MRI images.[211] As might be expected from the fact that destruction of more than 85% to 90% of the neurohypophysis is necessary to produce clinical symptoms of

---

TABLE 15-3 Fluid Deprivation Test for the Diagnosis of Diabetes Insipidus (DI)

Procedure

1. Initiation of the deprivation period depends on the severity of the DI; in routine cases, the patient should take nothing by mouth after dinner the day before the test, whereas in cases of more severe polyuria and polydipsia, this may be too long a period without fluids, and the water deprivation should be begun early on the morning of the test (e.g., 6 AM).
2. Obtain plasma and urine osmolality measurements, serum electrolyte levels, and a plasma arginine vasopressin (AVP) level at the start of the test.
3. Measure urine volume and osmolality hourly or with each voided urine.
4. Stop the test when body weight decreases by ≥3%, the patient develops orthostatic blood pressure changes, the urine osmolality reaches a plateau (i.e., <10% change over two or three consecutive measurements), or the serum Na⁺ is >145 mmol/L.
5. Obtain plasma and urine osmolality measurements, serum electrolyte levels, and a plasma AVP level at the end of the test, when the plasma osmolality is elevated, preferably >300 mOsm/kg H₂O.
6. If the serum Na⁺ is <146 mmol/L or the plasma osmolality is <300 mOsm/kg H₂O when the test is stopped, then consider a short infusion of hypertonic saline (3% NaCl at a rate of 0.1 mL/kg/min for 1-2 hr) to reach these endpoints.
7. If hypertonic saline infusion is not required to achieve hyperosmolality, administer AVP (5 U) or desmopressin (DDAVP) (1 μg) subcutaneously and continue measuring urine osmolality and volume for an additional 2 hr.

Interpretation

1. An unequivocal urine concentration after AVP/DDAVP (>50% increase) indicates central DI and an unequivocal absence of urine concentration (<10%) strongly suggests nephrogenic DI (NDI) or primary polydipsia (PP).
2. In cases in which NDI must be differentiated from PP, as well as in cases in which the increase in urine osmolality after AVP/DDAVP administration is more equivocal (e.g., 10% to 50%), diagnosis is best made by examining the relation between plasma AVP levels and plasma osmolality obtained at the end of the dehydration period and/or hypertonic saline infusion and the relation between plasma AVP levels and urine osmolality under basal conditions (see Figures 15-11 and 15-12).

DI, this signal has been found almost always to be absent in patients with CDI in multiple studies.[212]

As with any diagnostic test, however, clinical usefulness depends on the sensitivity and specificity of the test. Although earlier studies using small numbers of subjects demonstrated the presence of the bright spot in all normal subjects, subsequent larger studies reported an age-related absence of a pituitary bright spot in up to 20% of normal subjects.[213] Conversely, some studies have reported the presence of a bright spot in patients with clinical evidence of DI.[214] This may be because some patients with partial CDI have not yet progressed to the point of depletion of all neurohypophyseal reserves of AVP, or a persistent bright spot in patients with DI might be due to pituitary content of oxytocin rather than AVP. In support of the latter explanation, it is known that oxytocinergic neurons are more resistant to destruction by trauma than are vasopressinergic neurons in both rats[215] and humans.[22] The presence of a posterior pituitary bright spot has been variably reported in other polyuric disorders. In primary polydipsia the bright spot usually is seen,[212] which is consistent with studies in animals in which even prolonged lack of secretion of AVP caused by hyponatremia did not cause a decreased AVP content in the posterior pituitary.[26] In NDI the bright spot has been reported to be absent in some patients but present in others.[122] Consequently, specificity is lacking to use MRI routinely as a diagnostic screening test for DI. Nonetheless, its sensitivity is sufficient to support an approximately 95% probability that a patient with a bright spot on MRI does not have CDI. Thus, MRI is more useful for ruling out than for ruling in a diagnosis of CDI.

Additional useful information can be gained through MRI via assessment of the pituitary stalk. Enlargement of the stalk beyond 2 to 3 mm is generally considered to be pathologic[216] and can be due to multiple disease processes.[217] Consequently, when the MRI scan reveals thickening of the stalk, especially with absence of the posterior pituitary bright spot, a diligent search should be made for systemic diseases, including measurement of cerebrospinal fluid and plasma β-human chorionic gonadotropin and α-fetoprotein for evaluation of suprasellar germinoma; chest imaging and measurement of cerebrospinal fluid and plasma angiotensin converting enzyme (ACE) levels for evaluation of sarcoidosis; and bone and skin surveys for identification of histiocytosis. When the diagnosis is still in doubt, the MRI evaluation should be repeated every 3 to 6 months. Continued enlargement, especially in children over the first three years of follow-up, suggests a germinoma and mandates biopsy, whereas a decrease in the size of the stalk over time is more indicative of an inflammatory process such as lymphocytic infundibuloneurohypophysitis.[218]

Treatment of Diabetes Insipidus

The general goals of treatment of all forms of DI are (1) a correction of any preexisting water deficits, and (2) a reduction in the ongoing excessive urinary water losses. The specific therapy required (Table 15-4) varies according to both the type of DI present and the clinical situation. Awake, ambulatory patients with normal thirst have relatively little body water deficit, but benefit greatly from alleviation of the polyuria and polydipsia that disrupt their normal daily activities. In contrast, comatose patients with acute DI after head trauma are

TABLE 15-4 Therapies for the Treatment of Diabetes Insipidus
Water
Antidiuretic agents
Arginine vasopressin (Pitressin)
Desmopressin (1-deamino-8-D-arginine vasopressin [DDAVP])
Antidiuresis-enhancing agents
Chlorpropamide
Prostaglandin synthetase inhibitors (indomethacin, ibuprofen, tolmetin)
Natriuretic agents
Thiazide diuretics
Amiloride

unable to drink in response to thirst, and in these patients, progressive hyperosmolality can be life-threatening.

The TBW deficit in a hyperosmolar patient can be estimated using the following formula:

$$\text{Total body water deficit} = 0.6 \times \text{Premorbid weight} \times (1 - 140 / [Na^+])$$

where $[Na^+]$ is the serum sodium concentration in milliequivalents per liter and weight is in kilograms. This formula depends on threeep up with ongoing losses until a definitive response to treatment has occurred.assumptions: (1) TBW is approximately 60% of the premorbid body weight, (2) no body solute was lost as the hyperosmolality developed, and (3) the premorbid serum $[Na^+]$ was 140 mEq/L.

To reduce the risk of CNS damage from protracted exposure to severe hyperosmolality, in most cases the plasma osmolality should be rapidly lowered in the first 24 hours to the range of 320 to 330 mOsm/kg H_2O, or by approximately 50%. Plasma osmolality may be estimated most easily as twice the serum $[Na^+]$ if there is no hyperglycemia, and measured osmolality may be substituted if azotemia is not present. As discussed earlier, the brain increases intracellular osmolality by increasing the content of a variety organic osmolytes as a protection against excessive shrinkage during hyperosmolality.[199] Because these osmolytes cannot be immediately dissipated, further correction to a normal plasma osmolality should be spread over the next 24 to 72 hours to avoid producing cerebral edema during treatment.[200] This is especially important in children,[219] and several studies have indicated that limiting correction of hypernatremia to a maximal rate of no more than 0.5 mmol/L/hr prevents the occurrence of symptomatic cerebral edema with seizures.[201,220] In addition, the possibility of associated thyroid or adrenal insufficiency should be kept in mind, because patients with CDI caused by hypothalamic masses can have associated deficiencies of anterior pituitary function.

The previous formula does not take into account ongoing water losses and is, at best, a rough estimate. Frequent serum and urine electrolyte determinations should be made, and the rate of administration of oral water, or intravenous 5% dextrose in water, should be adjusted accordingly. Note, for example, that the estimated deficit of a 70-kg patient whose serum $[Na^+]$ is 160 mEq/L is 5.25 L of water. In such an individual, administration of water at a rate greater than 200 mL/hr would be required simply to correct the established deficit over 24 hours. Additional fluid would be needed to keep up with ongoing losses until a definitive response to treatment has occurred.

Agents for Treatment

The therapeutic agents available for the treatment of DI are shown in Table 15-4. Water should be considered a therapeutic agent, since when it is ingested or infused in sufficient quantity there is no abnormality of body fluid volume or composition. As noted previously, in most patients with DI thirst remains intact, and patients will drink sufficient fluid to maintain a relatively normal fluid balance. Patients with known DI should therefore be treated to decrease the patient's polyuria and polydipsia to acceptable levels that allow the patient to maintain a normal lifestyle. Because the major goal of therapy is improvement in symptoms, the therapeutic regimen prescribed should be individually tailored to each patient to accommodate the patient's needs. The safety of the prescribed agent and the use of a regimen that avoids potential detrimental effects of overtreatment are primary considerations because of the relatively benign course of DI in most cases and the potential adverse consequences of hyponatremia. Available treatments are summarized in the following sections, and their use is discussed separately for different types of DI.

ARGININE VASOPRESSIN

Pitressin is a commercially available synthetic form of naturally occurring human AVP. The aqueous solution contains 20 U/mL. Because of the drug's relatively short half-life (2- to 4-hour duration of antidiuretic effect) and propensity to cause acute increases in blood pressure when given as a bolus intravenously, this route of administration should generally be avoided. This agent is mainly used for acute situations such as postoperative DI. However, repeated dosing is required unless a continuous infusion is used, and the frequency of dosing or the infusion rate must be titrated to achieve the desired reduction in urine output (see later discussion of postoperative DI).

DESMOPRESSIN

Desmopressin (deamino-8-D-arginine vasopressin; trade name, DDAVP) is an agonist of the AVP V_2 receptor that was developed for therapeutic use because it has a significantly longer half-life than AVP (8- to 20-hour duration of antidiuretic effect) and is devoid of the latter's pressor activity because it does not activate AVP V1a receptors on vascular smooth muscle.[221] As a result of these advantages, it is the drug of choice for both short- and long-term administration in patients with CDI.[222] Several different preparations are available. The intranasal form is provided either as an aqueous solution containing 100 µg/mL packaged in a bottle with a calibrated rhinal tube, which requires specific training to use properly, or as a nasal spray packaged in a pump device that delivers a metered dose of 10 µg in 0.1 mL. An oral preparation is also available in doses of 0.1 or 0.2 mg.

Neither the intranasal nor oral preparation should be used in an acute emergency setting, in which it is essential that the patient achieve a therapeutic dose of the drug; in this case, the parenteral form should always be used. This is supplied as a solution containing 4 µg/mL and may be given by the intravenous, intramuscular, or subcutaneous route. The parenteral form is approximately 5 to 10 times more potent than the intranasal preparation, and the recommended dosage is 1 to 2 µg every 8 to 12 hours. For both the intranasal and parenteral preparations, increasing the dose generally has the effect of prolonging the duration of antidiuresis for several hours rather than increasing its magnitude; consequently, altering the dose can be useful to reduce the required frequency of administration.

CHLORPROPAMIDE

Chlorpropamide (Diabinese), a sulfonylurea primarily used as an oral hypoglycemic agent, also potentiates the hydro-osmotic effect of AVP in the kidney. Chlorpropamide has been reported to reduce polyuria by 25% to 75% in patients with CDI. This effect appears to be independent of the severity of the disease and is associated with a proportional rise in urine osmolality, correction of dehydration, and elimination of the polydipsia similar to that caused by small doses of AVP or desmopressin.[202] The major site of action of chlorpropamide appears to be the renal tubule, where it potentiates the hydro-osmotic action of circulating AVP, but there is also evidence of a pituitary effect to increase release of AVP as well. The latter effect may account for the observation that chlorpropamide can produce significant antidiuresis even in patients with severe CDI and presumed near-total AVP deficiency.[202] The usual dose is 250 to 500 mg/day, with a response noted in 1 to 2 days and a maximum antidiuresis in 4 days.

It should be remembered that this is an off-label use of chlorpropamide. The drug should not be used in pregnant women or in children, it should never be used in an acute emergency setting in which achievement of rapid antidiuresis is necessary, and it should be avoided in patients with concurrent hypopituitarism because of the increased risk of hypoglycemia. Other sulfonylureas share chlorpropamide's effect but generally are less potent. In particular, the newer-generation oral hypoglycemic agents such as glipizide and glyburide are virtually devoid of any AVP-potentiating effects.

PROSTAGLANDIN SYNTHASE INHIBITORS

Prostaglandins have complex effects both in the CNS and in the kidney, most of which are incompletely understood at this time due to the variety of different prostaglandins and their multiplicity of cellular effects. In the brain, intracerebroventricular infusion of E prostaglandins stimulates AVP secretion,[223] and administration of prostaglandin synthase inhibitors attenuates osmotically stimulated AVP secretion.[224] However, in the kidney prostaglandin E_2 (PGE_2) has been reported to inhibit AVP-stimulated generation of cAMP in the cortical collecting tubule by interacting with inhibitory G protein (G_i).[225] Thus, the effect of prostaglandin synthase inhibitors in sensitizing AVP effects in the kidney likely results from enhanced cAMP generation upon AVP binding to the V_2 receptor. The predominantly renal effects of these agents are demonstrated by the fact that clinically these agents successfully reduce urine volume and free water clearance even in patients with NDI of different etiologies.[226]

NATRIURETIC AGENTS

Thiazide diuretics have a paradoxical antidiuretic effect in patients with CDI.[227] However, because better antidiuretic agents are available for treatment of CDI, their main therapeutic use is in NDI. Hydrochlorothiazide at dosages of 50 to 100 mg/day usually reduces urine output by approximately 50%, and efficacy can be further enhanced by restricting sodium intake. Unlike desmopressin or the other antidiuresis-enhancing drugs, these agents are equally effective in most forms of NDI (see later).

Treatment of Different Types of Diabetes Insipidus

CENTRAL DIABETES INSIPIDUS

Patients with CDI should generally be treated with intranasal or oral desmopressin. Unless the hypothalamic thirst center is also affected by the primary lesion causing superimposed osmoreceptor dysfunction, these patients will develop thirst when the plasma osmolality increases by only 2% to 3%.[202] Severe hyperosmolality is therefore not a risk in patients who are alert, ambulatory, and able to drink in response to perceived thirst. In these cases polyuria and polydipsia are inconvenient and disruptive, but not life-threatening. However, hypo-osmolality is largely asymptomatic and may be progressive if water intake continues during a period of continuous antidiuresis. Therefore, treatment must be designed to minimize polyuria and polydipsia but without an undue risk of hyponatremia from overtreatment. Treatment should be individualized to determine optimal dosage and dosing interval. Although tablets offer greater convenience and are generally preferred by patients, it is useful to start with the nasal spray initially because of its greater consistency of absorption and physiologic effect, and then switch to the oral tablets only after the patient is comfortable with use of the intranasal preparation to produce antidiuresis. After the patient has tried both preparations, the patient can then choose which he or she prefers for long-term usage.

Because of variability in response among patients, it is desirable to determine the duration of action of individual doses in each patient.[228] A satisfactory schedule can generally be determined using modest doses, and the maximum dosage needed is rarely above 0.2 μg orally or 10 μg intranasally (one nasal spray) given two or occasionally three times daily.[229] These dosages generally produce plasma desmopressin levels many times those required to yield maximum antidiuresis but obviate the need for more frequent treatment. Once-daily dosing suffices in rare patients. In a few patients, the effect of intranasal or oral desmopressin is erratic, probably as a result of variable interference with absorption from the gastrointestinal tract or nasal mucosa. This variability can be reduced and the duration of action prolonged by administering the drug on an empty stomach[230] or after thorough cleansing of the nostrils. Resistance caused by antibody production has not been reported to date.

Hyponatremia is a rare complication of desmopressin therapy and only occurs if the patient is continually antidiuretic while maintaining a fluid intake sufficient to become volume expanded and natriuretic. Absence of thirst in this circumstance is protective; but also, most patients with CDI who receive standard therapy are not continuously maximally antidiuretic. There are reports of hyponatremia in patients with normal AVP function, and presumably normal thirst, when they are given desmopressin to treat hemophilia or von Willebrand's disease[231] as well as in children treated with desmopressin for primary enuresis.[232] In these cases the hyponatremia can develop rapidly and is often first noted by the onset of convulsions and coma.[233] Severe hyponatremia in patients with DI being treated with desmopressin can be avoided by monitoring serum electrolyte levels frequently during initiation of therapy. Patients who show a tendency to develop low serum [Na+] who do not respond to recommended decreases in fluid intake should then be instructed to delay a scheduled dose of desmopressin once or twice a week

so that polyuria recurs, which allows any excess retained fluid to be excreted.[205]

Acute postsurgical DI occurs relatively frequently following surgery that involves the suprasellar hypothalamic area, but several confounding factors must be considered. These patients often receive stress doses of glucocorticoids, and the resulting hyperglycemia with glucosuria may confuse a diagnosis of DI. Thus, the blood glucose level must first be brought under control to eliminate an osmotic diuresis as the cause of the polyuria. In addition, excess fluids administered intravenously may be retained perioperatively, but then excreted normally postoperatively. If this large output is matched with continued intravenous input, an incorrect diagnosis of DI may be made based on the resulting polyuria. Therefore, if the serum [Na+] is not elevated concomitantly with the polyuria, the rate of parenterally administered fluid should be slowed with careful monitoring of serum [Na+] and urine output to establish the diagnosis.

Once a diagnosis of DI is confirmed, the only acceptable pharmacologic therapy is an antidiuretic agent. However, because many neurosurgeons fear water overload and brain edema after this type of surgery, the patient is sometimes treated only with intravenous fluid replacement for a considerable time before the institution of antidiuretic hormone therapy (see the discussion of the potential benefits of this approach later). If the patient is awake and able to respond to thirst, one can treat with an antidiuretic hormone and allow the patient's thirst to be the guide for water replacement. However, if the patient is unable to respond to thirst, because of either a decreased level of consciousness or hypothalamic damage to the thirst center, fluid balance must be maintained by intravenously administered fluid. The urine osmolality and serum [Na+] must be checked every several hours during the initial therapy, and then at least daily until the DI is stabilized or resolves. Caution must also be exercised regarding the volume of water replacement, because excess water administered during continued administration of AVP or desmopressin can create a syndrome of inappropriate antidiuresis and potentially severe hyponatremia. Studies in experimental animals have indicated that desmopressin-induced hyponatremia markedly impairs survival of AVP neurons after pituitary stalk compression,[215] which suggests that overhydration with subsequent decreased stimulation of the neurohypophysis may also increase the likelihood of permanent DI.

Postoperatively, desmopressin may be given parenterally in a dose of 1 to 2 μg subcutaneously, intramuscularly, or intravenously. The intravenous route is preferable, because it obviates any concern about absorption, is not associated with significant pressor activity, and is associated with the same total duration of action as the other parenteral routes. A prompt reduction in urine output should occur, and the duration of antidiuretic effect is generally 6 to 12 hours. Usually the patient is hypernatremic with relatively dilute urine when therapy is started. The urine osmolality and urine volume should be followed to be certain the dose was effective, and the serum [Na+] should be checked at frequent intervals to ensure that some improvement of hypernatremia occurs.

It is generally advisable to allow some return of the polyuria before administration of subsequent doses of desmopressin, because postoperative DI is often transient, and return of endogenous AVP secretion will become apparent by a lack of return of the polyuria. Also, in some cases, transient post-operative DI is part of a triphasic pattern that has been well described after pituitary stalk transection (see previous discussion). Because of this possibility, allowing a return of polyuria before redosing with desmopressin will permit earlier detection of a potential second phase of inappropriate antidiuresis and decrease the likelihood of producing symptomatic hyponatremia by continuing antidiuretic therapy and intravenous fluid administration when it is not required.

Some clinicians have recommended using a continuous intravenous infusion of a dilute solution of AVP to control DI postoperatively. Algorithms for continuous AVP infusion to treat postoperative and posttraumatic DI in pediatric patients have begun at infusion rates of 0.25 to 1.0 mU/kg/hr and titrated the rate using urine specific gravity (goal of 1.010 to 1.020) and urine volume (goal of 2 to 3 mL/kg/hr) as a guide to the adequacy of the antidiuresis.[234] Although pressor effects have not been reported at these infusion rates and the antidiuretic effects are quickly reversible in 2 to 3 hours, it should be remembered that use of continuous infusions instead of intermittent dosing will not allow one to assess when the patent has recovered from transient DI or entered the second phase of a triphasic response. If DI persists, the patient should eventually be switched to maintenance therapy with intranasal or oral preparations of desmopressin for the treatment of chronic DI.

Acute traumatic DI can occur after injuries to the head, usually in a motor vehicle accident. DI is more common with deceleration injuries that result in a shearing action on the pituitary stalk and/or cause hemorrhagic ischemia of the hypothalamus and/or posterior pituitary.[137] As with postsurgical DI, posttraumatic DI is usually recognized by hypotonic polyuria in the face of increased plasma osmolality. The clinical management is similar to that of postsurgical DI as outlined earlier, except that the possibility of anterior pituitary insufficiency must also be considered in such cases, and the patient should be given stress doses of glucocorticoids (e.g., hydrocortisone, 100 mg intravenously every 8 hours) until anterior pituitary function can be definitively evaluated.

OSMORECEPTOR DYSFUNCTION

In the short term, patients with hypernatremia due to osmoreceptor dysfunction should be treated the same as any other hyperosmolar patient by replacing the underlying free water deficit as described at the beginning of the "Treatment" section. The long-term management of osmoreceptor dysfunction syndromes requires a thorough search for a potentially treatable cause (see Table 15-2) in conjunction with the use of measures to prevent recurrence of dehydration. Because the hypodipsia cannot be cured and rarely, if ever, improves spontaneously, the mainstay of management is education of the patient and the patient's family about the importance of continuously regulating the patient's fluid intake in accordance with the hydration status. This is never accomplished easily in such patients, but can be done most efficaciously by establishing a daily schedule of water intake based on changes in body weight and regardless of the patient's thirst. In effect, a "prescription" for daily fluid intake must be written for these patients, because they will not drink spontaneously. In addition, if the patient has polyuria, desmopressin should also be given as for any patient with DI. The success of this regimen should be monitored periodically by measuring serum [Na+] (weekly at first, then monthly depending on the stability of the patient's condition). In addition, the target weight (at which hydration status and serum [Na+] concentration are normal) may need to be recalculated periodically to allow for growth in children or changes in body fat in adults.

GESTATIONAL DIABETES INSIPIDUS

The polyuria of gestational DI is usually not corrected by administration of AVP itself, since the AVP is rapidly degraded by high circulating levels of oxytocinase/vasopressinase just as is endogenous AVP. The treatment of choice is desmopressin, because this synthetic AVP V_2 receptor agonist is not destroyed by the oxytocinase/vasopressinase in the plasma of pregnant women[235] and to date appears to be safe for both the mother and the child.[236,237] Desmopressin has only 2% to 25% the oxytocic activity of AVP[222] and can be used with minimal stimulation of the oxytocin receptors in the uterus. Dosages should be customized to individual patients, since higher doses and more frequent dosing intervals are sometimes required because of the increased degradation of the peptide. However, physicians should remember that the naturally occurring volume expansion and resetting of the osmostat that occur in pregnancy maintain the serum [Na+] at a lower level during pregnancy.[39]

During delivery these patients can maintain adequate oral intake and administration of desmopressin can continue, but physicians should be cautious about overadministration of fluid parenterally during delivery, because these patients are not able to excrete the fluid and are susceptible to the development of water intoxication and hyponatremia. After delivery, oxytocinase/vasopressinase decreases in plasma within several days, and depending on the cause of the DI patients may experience disappearance of the disorder or become asymptomatic with regard to fluid intake and urine volume.[238]

NEPHROGENIC DIABETES INSIPIDUS

By definition, patients with NDI are resistant to the effects of AVP. Some patients with NDI can be treated by eliminating the drug (e.g., lithium) or disease (e.g., hypercalcemia) responsible for the disorder. For many others, however, including those with the genetic forms, the only practical form of treatment at present is to restrict sodium intake and administer a thiazide diuretic, either alone[227] or in combination with prostaglandin synthetase inhibitors[239] or amiloride.[240,241] The natriuretic effect of the thiazide class of diuretics is conferred by their ability to block sodium absorption in the renal cortical diluting site. When combined with dietary sodium restriction, the drugs cause modest hypovolemia. This stimulates isotonic proximal tubular solute reabsorption and diminishes solute delivery to the more distal diluting site, where experimental studies have indicated that thiazides also act to enhance water reabsorption in the inner medullary collecting duct independently of AVP.[242] Together, these effects markedly diminish renal diluting ability and free water clearance independently of any action of AVP. Thus, agents of this class are the mainstay of therapy for NDI. Monitoring for hypokalemia is recommended, and potassium supplementation is occasionally required. Any drug of the thiazide class may be used with equal potential for benefit, and clinicians should employ the one with which they are most familiar from use in treating other conditions.

Care must be exercised when treating patients taking lithium with diuretics, since the induced contraction of plasma volume may increase lithium concentrations and worsen potential toxic effects of the therapy. In the acute setting, diuretics are of no use in treating NDI, and only free water administration can reverse hyperosmolality. Indomethacin, tolmetin, and ibuprofen have been used in this setting,[239,243,244] although the last may be less effective than the others. The combination of thiazides and a nonsteroidal antiinflammatory agent will not increase urinary osmolality above that of plasma, but the lessening of polyuria is nonetheless beneficial to patients. In many cases the combination of thiazides with the potassium-sparing diuretic amiloride is preferred to lessen the potential side effects associated with long-term use of nonsteroidal antiinflammatory agents.[240,241] Amiloride also has the advantage of decreasing lithium entrance into cells in the distal tubule, and because of this may be preferable action in the treatment of lithium-induced NDI.[245,246]

Although desmopressin is generally not effective in the treatment of NDI, a few patients may have receptor mutations that allow partial responses to AVP or desmopressin,[247] with increases in urine osmolality following much higher dosages of these agents than are typically used to treat CDI (e.g., 6 to 10 μg intravenously), and it is generally worth a trial of desmopressin at these doses to ascertain whether this is a potentially useful therapy in selected patients in whom the responsiveness of other affected family members is not already known. Potential therapies involving administration of chaperones to bypass defects in cellular routing of misfolded aquaporin[170] and AVP V_2 receptor[171] proteins are an exciting future possibility.[160]

PRIMARY POLYDIPSIA

At present, there is no completely satisfactory treatment for primary polydipsia. Fluid restriction would seem to be the obvious treatment of choice. However, patients with a reset thirst threshold will be resistant to fluid restriction because of the resulting thirst from stimulation of brain thirst centers at higher plasma osmolalities.[248] In some cases, the use of alternative methods to ameliorate the sensation of thirst (e.g., wetting the mouth with ice chips or using sour candies to increase salivary flow) can help to reduce fluid intake. Fluid intake in patients with psychogenic causes of polydipsia is driven by psychiatric factors that have responded variably to behavioral modification and pharmacologic therapy. Several recent reports have suggested potential efficacy of the antipsychotic drug clozapine as an agent to reduce polydipsia and prevent recurrent hyponatremia in at least a subset of these patients.[249] Administration of any antidiuretic hormone or thiazides to decrease polyuria is hazardous because they invariably produce water intoxication.[202] Therefore, if the diagnosis of DI is uncertain, any trial of antidiuretic therapy should be conducted with close monitoring, preferably in the hospital with frequent evaluation of fluid balance and serum electrolyte levels. If a patient with primary polydipsia is troubled by nocturia, it may be reduced or eliminated by administering a small dose of desmopressin at bedtime. Since thirst and fluid intake are reduced during sleep, this treatment is less likely to cause water intoxication provided the dose is titrated to allow resumption of a water diuresis as soon as the patient awakens the next morning. This approach cannot be recommended for patients with psychogenic polydipsia, however, because of the unpredictability of their fluid intake.

Disorders of Excess Vasopressin or Vasopressin Effect

The disorders of the renal concentrating mechanism that have been described in the previous section can lead to water depletion, sometimes in association with hyperosmolality and hypernatremia. In contrast, disorders of the renal diluting mechanism most frequently present as hyponatremia and hypo-osmolality. Hyponatremia is among the most common electrolyte disorders encountered in clinical medicine, with an incidence of 0.97% and a prevalence of 2.48% in hospitalized adult patients when a serum [Na$^+$] of less than 130 mEq/L is the diagnostic criterion,[250] and a prevalence as high as 15% to 30% when a serum [Na$^+$] of less than 135 mEq/L is used.[251] The prevalence may be somewhat lower in the hospitalized pediatric population (between 0.34% and 1.38%),[252] but the incidence is higher than originally recognized in the geriatric population.[251,253]

Relation between Hypo-Osmolality and Hyponatremia

Because plasma osmolality is most often measured to assist in the evaluation of hyponatremic disorders, it is useful to bear in mind the basic relationship of plasma osmolality to plasma or serum [Na$^+$]. As reviewed in the introduction to this chapter, Na$^+$ and its associated anions account for nearly all of the osmotic activity of plasma. Therefore, changes in plasma [Na$^+$] are usually associated with comparable changes in plasma osmolality. The osmolality calculated from the concentrations of Na$^+$, urea, and glucose is usually in close agreement with that obtained from a measurement of osmolality.[254] When the measured osmolality exceeds the calculated osmolality by more than 10 mOsm/kg H_2O, an osmolar gap is present.[254] This occurs in two circumstances: (1) with a decrease in the water content of the serum, and (2) with addition of a solute other than urea or glucose to the serum. A decrease in the water content of serum is usually due to its displacement by excessive amounts of protein or lipids, which can occur in severe hyperlipidemia or hyperglobulinemia. Normally, 92% to 94% of plasma volume is water, and the remaining 6% to 8% is lipids and protein.

Because of its ionic nature, Na$^+$ dissolves only in the water phase of plasma. Thus, when a greater than normal proportion of plasma is accounted for by solids, the concentration of Na$^+$ in plasma water remains normal, but the concentration in the total volume, as measured by flame photometry, is artifactually low. Such a discrepancy can be avoided if the Na$^+$ concentration is measured with an ion-selective electrode, which that is now widely available.[255] However, the sample needs to remain undiluted (direct potentiometry) for accurate measurement of the serum [Na$^+$]. Although the flame photometer measures the concentration of Na$^+$ in the total plasma volume, the ion-selective electrode measures it only in the plasma water. Normally, this difference is only 3 mmol/L, but in the settings under discussion, the difference can be much greater. Because the large lipid and protein molecules contribute only minimally to the total osmolality, the measurement of osmolality by freezing point depression remains normal in these patients.

Hyponatremia associated with normal osmolality has been termed *factitious hyponatremia* or *pseudohyponatremia*. The most common causes of pseudohyponatremia are primary or secondary hyperlipidemic disorders. The serum need not appear lipemic, because increments in cholesterol alone can cause the same discrepancy.[255] Plasma protein elevations above 10 g/dL, as seen in multiple myeloma or macroglobulinemia, can also cause pseudohyponatremia. More recently the administration of intravenous immune globulin has been reported to be associated with hyponatremia without hypoosmolality in several patients.[256]

The second setting in which an osmolar gap occurs is the presence in plasma of an exogenous low-molecular-weight substance such as ethanol, methanol, ethylene glycol, or mannitol.[257] Undialyzed patients with chronic renal failure, as well as critically ill patients,[258] also have an increment in the osmolar gap of unknown cause. Whereas all of these exogenous substances, as well as glucose and urea, elevate measured osmolality, the effect they have on the plasma [Na$^+$] and intracellular hydration depends on the solute in question. As previously discussed, substances such as glucose, in the presence of relative insulin deficiency, do not penetrate cells readily and remain in the ECF. As a consequence, they draw water from the ICF compartment, which causes cell shrinkage, and this translocation of water commensurately decreases the extracellular [Na^{++}]. In this setting, therefore, the plasma [Na$^+$] can be low while plasma osmolality is normal or high. It is generally estimated that for every 100 mg/dL rise in plasma glucose level, the osmotic shift of water causes plasma [Na$^+$] to fall by 1.6 mEq/L. However, a more recent assessment suggests that this may represent an underestimate of the decrease caused by hyperglycemia and recommends a 2.4-mEq/L correction factor.[259]

Similar "translocational" hyponatremia occurs with mannitol or maltose or with the absorption of glycine during transurethral prostate resection and gynecologic and orthopedic procedures. A potential toxicity of glycine in this setting also requires consideration.[260] The introduction of new bipolar retroscopes that allow NaCl to be used as the irrigant should result in the disappearance of this clinical entity.

When the plasma solute is readily permeable (e.g., urea, ethylene glycol, methanol, ethanol), it enters cells and so does not establish an osmotic gradient for water movement. There is no cellular dehydration despite the hyperosmolar state, and the plasma [Na$^+$] remains unchanged. The relationship between plasma osmolality, plasma tonicity, and serum [Na$^+$] in the presence of various substances is summarized in Table 15-5.

Variables that Influence Water Excretion

In considering clinical disorders that result from excessive or inappropriate secretion of AVP, it is helpful to remember the many other variables that also influence water excretion (Figure 15-16). These factors fall into three broad categories.

Fluid Delivery from the Proximal Tubule

In spite of the fact that proximal fluid reabsorption is isosmotic and therefore does not contribute directly to urine dilution, the volume of tubule fluid that is delivered to the distal nephron determines in large measure the volume of dilute urine that can be excreted. Thus, if glomerular filtration is decreased or proximal tubule reabsorption is greatly enhanced, the resulting diminution in the amount of fluid delivered to the distal

TABLE 15-5 Relationship between Serum Tonicity and Sodium Concentration in the Presence of Other Conditions or Substances

CONDITION OR SUBSTANCE	PLASMA OSMOLALITY	PLASMA TONICITY	SERUM [NA$^+$]
Hyperglycemia	↑	↑	↓
Mannitol, maltose, glycine	↑	↑	↓
Azotemia (high blood urea concentration)	↑	↔	↔
Ingestion of ethanol, methanol, ethylene glycol	↑	↔	↔
Elevated serum lipid or protein	↔	↔	↓

↑, Increased; ↓, decreased; ↔, unchanged.

tubule itself limits the rate of renal water excretion even if other components of the diluting mechanism are intact.

Dilution of Tubular Fluid

The excretion of urine that is hypotonic to plasma requires that some segment of the nephron reabsorb solute in excess of water. The water impermeability of the entire ascending limb of the loop of Henle, as well as the capacity of its thick segment to reabsorb NaCl, actively endows this segment of the nephron with the characteristics required by the diluting process. Thus, the transport of NaCl by the Na$^+$-K$^+$-2Cl$^-$ cotransporter converts the hypertonic tubule fluid that is delivered from the descending limb of the loop of Henle to a distinctly hypotonic fluid (approximately 100 mOsm/kg H$_2$O). Interference with reabsorption of Na$^+$ and Cl$^-$ in the ascending limb therefore will impair urine dilution.

Water Impermeability of the Collecting Duct

The excretion of urine that is more dilute than the fluid that is delivered to the distal convoluted tubule requires continued solute reabsorption and minimal water reabsorption in the terminal segments of the nephron. Because the water permeability of the collecting duct epithelium is primarily dependent on the presence or absence of AVP, this hormone plays a pivotal role in determining the fate of the fluid delivered to the collecting duct and thus the concentration or dilution of the final urine (see Chapter 10). In the absence of AVP, the collecting duct remains essentially impermeable to water, even though some water is still reabsorbed. The continued reabsorption of solute then results in the excretion of a maximally dilute urine (approximately 50 mOsm/kg H$_2$O). Because the medullary interstitium is always hypertonic, the absence of circulating AVP, which renders the collecting duct impermeable to water, is critical to the normal diluting process. This diluting mechanism allows the intake and subsequent excretion of large volumes of water without major alterations in the tonicity of body water.[261] Rarely, this limit can be exceeded, which causes water intoxication. Much more commonly, however, hyponatremia occurs at lower rates of water intake, owing either to an intrarenal defect in urine dilution or to persistent

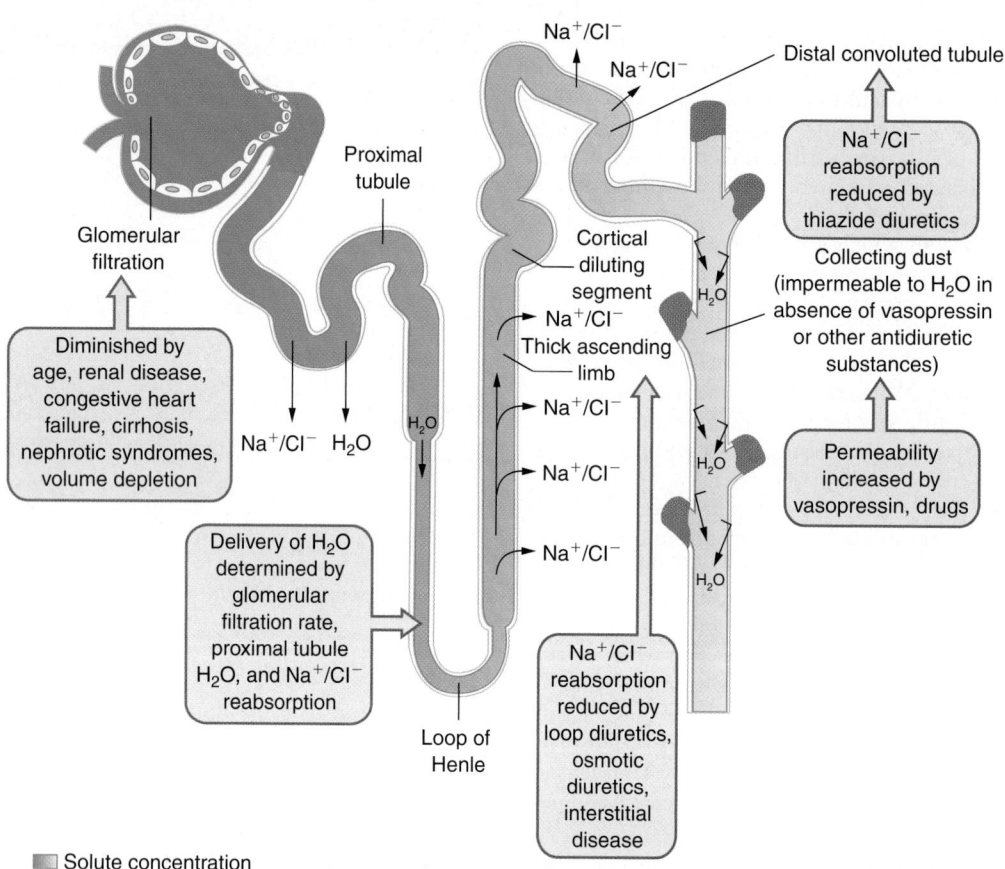

MECHANISMS OF URINE DILUTION

FIGURE 15-16 Urinary dilution mechanisms. Normal determinants of urinary dilution and disorders causing hyponatremia. (From Cogan M: Normal water homeostasis, in Cogan M [editor]: *Fluid and electrolytes,* Norwalk, Conn, 1991, Appleton & Lange, pp 98-106.)

secretion of AVP in the circulation. Because hypo-osmolality normally suppresses AVP secretion,[262] the hypo-osmolar state frequently reflects the persistent secretion of AVP in response to hemodynamic or other nonosmolar stimuli.[262]

Pathogenesis and Causes of Hyponatremia

The plasma or serum [Na+] is determined by the body's total content of sodium, potassium, and water:

$$\text{Serum }[Na^+] = \frac{\text{Total body exchangeable }Na^+ + \text{Total body exchangeable }K^+}{\text{Total body water}}$$

This formula has been simplified from the observations made by Edelman in the 1950s. This simplification introduces some errors in the prediction of changes in serum [Na+] based on the previous formula and has been the subject of some reinterpretation by Nguyen and Kurtz.[263] Although their revision of the formula is more accurate, as pointed out by Sterns,[264] there are so many inaccuracies in the measurement of sodium, potassium, and water losses as well as intake that there is no substitute for frequent measurements of serum [Na+] in rapidly changing clinical settings. As the previous relationship depicts, hyponatremia can occur through an increase in TBW, a decrease in body solutes (either Na+ or K+), or any

combination of these. In most cases, more than one of these mechanisms is operant. Therefore, a classification system to separate the various causes of hyponatremia should be based on factors other than the level of serum [Na+] itself.

In approaching the patient with hyponatremia, the physician's first task is to ensure that hyponatremia in fact reflects a hypo-osmotic state and does not result from one of the causes of pseudohyponatremia or translocational hyponatremia, discussed earlier. Thereafter, since a low serum [Na+] can be associated with decreased, normal, or high total body sodium,[265,266] the most useful means of classifying the cause of the hyponatremia is through assessment of ECF volume, namely, (1) hyponatremia with ECF volume depletion, (2) hyponatremia with excess ECF volume, and (3) hyponatremia with normal ECF volume.

Hyponatremia with Extracellular Fluid Volume Depletion

Patients with hyponatremia who have ECF volume depletion have sustained a deficit in total body Na+ that exceeds the deficit in TBW. The decrease in ECF volume is manifested by physical findings such as flat neck veins, decreased skin turgor, dry mucous membranes, orthostatic hypotension, and tachycardia. If sufficiently severe, volume depletion is a potent stimulus to AVP secretion. When the osmoreceptors and

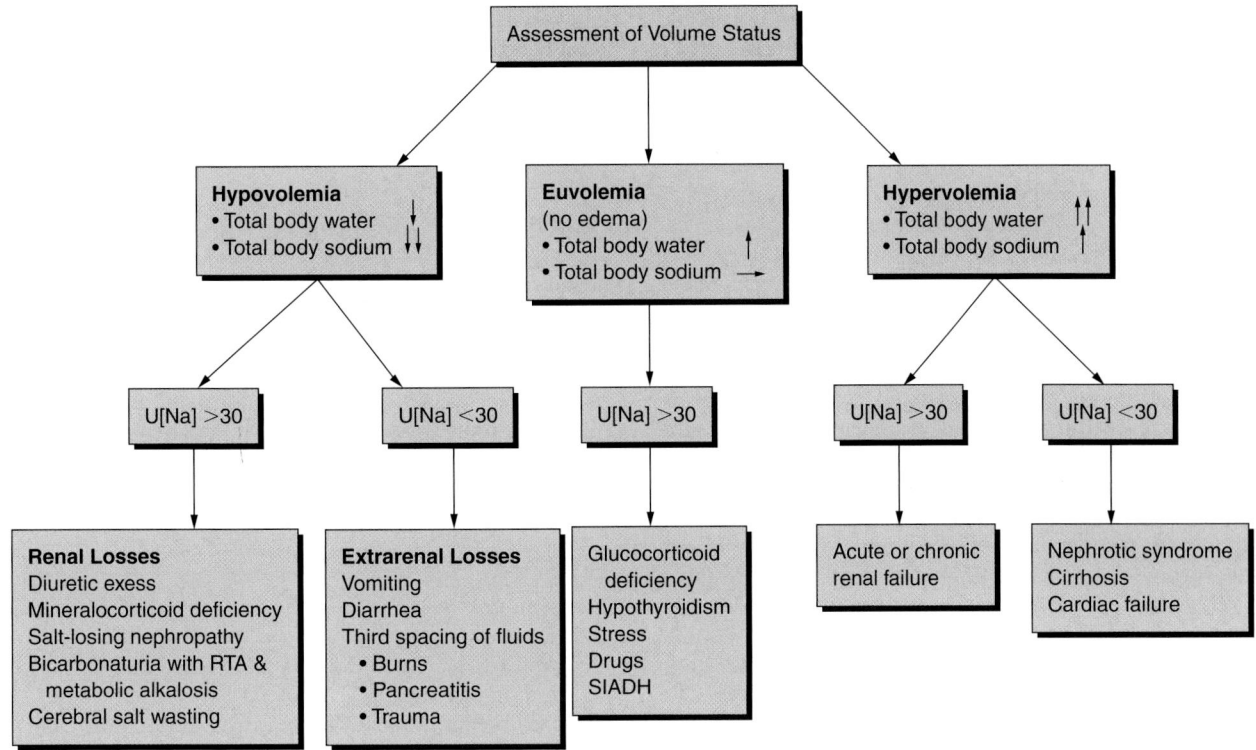

FIGURE 15-17 Diagnostic approach to the hyponatremic patient. (Modified from Halterman R, Berl T: Therapy of dysnatremic disorders, in Brady H, Wilcox C [editors]: *Therapy in nephrology and hypertension*, Philadelphia, 1999, Saunders, p 256.)

volume receptors receive opposing stimuli, the former remain fully active but the set point of the system is lowered. Thus, in the presence of hypovolemia, AVP is secreted and water is retained despite hypo-osmolality. Whereas the hyponatremia in this setting clearly involves a depletion of body solutes, the concomitant AVP-mediated retention of water is critical to the pathologic process producing hyponatremia.

As depicted in the flow chart in Figure 15-17, measurement of the urinary Na^+ concentration is helpful in assessing whether the fluid losses are renal or extrarenal in origin. A urinary Na^{++} concentration of less than 30 mEq/L reflects a normal renal response to volume depletion and points to an extrarenal source of fluid loss. This is most commonly seen in patients with gastrointestinal disease with vomiting or diarrhea. Other causes include loss of fluid into the third space, such as the abdominal cavity in pancreatitis or the bowel lumen in ileus. Burns and muscle trauma can also be associated with large fluid and electrolyte losses. Because many of these pathologic states are associated with thirst, an increase in either orally ingested or parenterally infused free water leads to hyponatremia.

A urinary Na^{++} concentration of more than 30 mEq/L in patients with hypovolemic hyponatremia points to the kidney as the source of the fluid losses. Diuretic-induced hyponatremia, a commonly observed clinical entity, accounts for a significant proportion of symptomatic hyponatremia in hospitalized patients. It occurs almost exclusively with thiazide rather than loop diuretics, most likely because the former have no effect on urine concentrating ability but the latter do. The hyponatremia is usually evident within 14 days in most patients, but can occur up to 2 years later in some.[267] Underweight women appear to be particularly prone to this complication,[268] and advanced age has been found to be a risk factor

in some,[267,269] but not all,[268] studies. A careful study on diluting ability in the elderly revealed that thiazide diuretics exaggerate the already slower recovery from hyponatremia induced by water ingestion in this population.[270]

Diuretics can cause hyponatremia by a variety of mechanisms[271]: (1) volume depletion, which results in impaired water excretion due to both enhanced AVP release and decreased fluid delivery to the diluting segment; (2) a direct effect of diuretics on the diluting segment; and (3) K^+ depletion, which causes a decrease in the water permeability of the collecting duct as well as an increase in water intake. K^+ depletion leads to hyponatremia independently of the Na^+ depletion that frequently accompanies diuretic use.[272] The concomitant administration of potassium-sparing diuretics does not prevent the development of hyponatremia. Although the diagnosis of diuretic-induced hyponatremia is frequently obvious, surreptitious diuretic abuse is being increasingly recognized and should be considered in patients in whom other electrolyte abnormalities and high urinary Cl^- excretion suggest this possibility.

Salt-losing nephropathy occurs in some patients with advanced renal insufficiency. In the majority of these patients, the Na^+-wasting tendency is not one that manifests itself at normal rates of sodium intake; however, some patients with interstitial nephropathy, medullary cystic disease, polycystic kidney disease, or partial urinary obstruction with sufficient Na^+ wasting exhibit hypovolemic hyponatremia.[273] Patients with proximal renal tubular acidosis exhibit renal sodium and potassium wasting despite modest renal insufficiency because bicarbonaturia obligates these cation losses.

It has long been recognized that adrenal insufficiency is associated with impaired renal water excretion and hyponatremia. This diagnosis should be considered in the volume-contracted hyponatremic patient whose urinary Na$^+$ concentration is not low, particularly when the serum [K$^+$], urea, and creatinine levels are elevated. Separate mechanisms for mineralocorticoid and glucocorticoid deficiency have been defined.[274] Observations in glucocorticoid-replete adrenalectomized experimental animals provide evidence to support a role of mineralocorticoid deficiency in abnormal water excretion, because both AVP release and intrarenal factors appear to be causal mechanisms. Conscious adrenalectomized dogs given physiologic doses of glucocorticoids developed hyponatremia. Either saline or physiologic doses of mineralocorticoids corrected the defect in association with both ECF volume repletion and improvement in renal hemodynamics. Immunoassayable AVP levels were elevated in a similarly treated group of mineralocorticoid-deficient dogs despite hypo-osmolality.[275] The decreased ECF volume thus provides the nonosmotic stimulus for AVP release.

More direct evidence for the role of AVP was provided in studies employing an AVP receptor antagonist. When glucocorticoid-replete, adrenally insufficient rats were given an AVP antagonist, the minimal urine osmolality was significantly lowered.[276] Urine dilution was not corrected, unlike in the mineralocorticoid-replete rats, which supports a role for an AVP-independent mechanism. These findings are in agreement with those from studies of adrenalectomized homozygous Brattleboro rats, which also have a defect in water excretion that can be partially corrected by administration of mineralocorticoids or by normalization of volume. In summary, therefore, the defect in water excretion associated with mineralocorticoid deficiency is mediated by AVP and by AVP-independent intrarenal factors, both of which are activated by decrements of ECF volume, rather than by deficiency of the hormone per se.

The presence in the urine of an osmotically active nonreabsorbable or poorly reabsorbable solute causes renal excretion of Na$^+$ and culminates in volume depletion. Glycosuria secondary to uncontrolled diabetes mellitus, mannitol infusion, or urea diuresis after relief of obstruction is a common setting for this disorder. In patients with diabetes, the Na$^+$ wasting caused by the glycosuria can be aggravated by ketonuria, because hydroxybutyrate and acetoacetate also cause urinary electrolyte losses. In fact, ketonuria can contribute to the renal Na$^+$ wasting and hyponatremia seen in starvation and alcoholic ketoacidosis.

Na$^+$ and water excretion are also increased when a nonreabsorbable anion appears in the urine. This is observed principally with the metabolic alkalosis and bicarbonaturia that accompany severe vomiting or nasogastric suction. In these patients, the excretion of HCO$_3^-$ requires the excretion of cations, including Na$^+$ and K$^+$, for the maintenance of electroneutrality. Whereas the renal losses in these clinical settings may be hypotonic, the volume contraction–stimulated thirst and water intake can result in the development of hyponatremia.

Cerebral salt wasting is a rare syndrome described primarily in patients with subarachnoid hemorrhage, but also in those with other types of CNS lesions. It leads to renal salt wasting and volume contraction.[277] Although hyponatremia is increasingly reported in these patients, true cerebral salt wasting is probably less common than reported.[278] In fact, one critical review found no conclusive evidence for volume contraction or renal salt wasting in any of the patients.[279]

The mechanism of this natriuresis is unknown, but an increased release of brain natriuretic peptides has been suggested.[280]

Hyponatremia with Excess Extracellular Fluid Volume

In advanced stages, the edematous states listed in Figure 15-17 are associated with a decrease in plasma [Na$^+$]. Patients generally have an increase in total body Na$^+$ content, but the rise in TBW exceeds that of Na$^+$. With the exception of renal failure, these states are characterized by avid Na$^+$ retention (urinary Na^{++} concentration of <10 mEq/L). This avid retention may be obscured by the concomitant use of diuretics, which are frequently prescribed in treating these patients. These agents can further contribute to the abnormal water excretion seen in these states.

Congestive Heart Failure

The common association between congestive heart failure and Na$^+$ and water retention is well established. A mechanism mediated by decreased delivery of tubule fluid to the distal nephron or increased release of AVP has been proposed. In an experimental model of low cardiac output, both AVP and diminished delivery to the diluting segment were found to be important in mediating the abnormality in water excretion. It thus appears that the decrement in "effective" arterial blood volume and the decrease in arterial filling are sensed by aortic and carotid sinus baroreceptors that stimulate AVP secretion.[281] This stimulation must supersede the inhibition of AVP release that accompanies acute distention of the left atrium. In fact, there is evidence that chronic distention of the atria blunts the sensitivity of this baroreceptor, so high-pressure baroreceptors can act in an uninhibited manner to stimulate AVP release. The importance of AVP in hyponatremia in experimental models of heart failure is underscored by the correction of the water excretory defect by an AVP antagonist in rats with inferior vena cava constriction.[282]

High plasma AVP levels have been demonstrated in patients with congestive heart failure, in both the presence and the absence of diuretics.[283] Likewise, the hypothalamic mRNA for the AVP preprohormone is elevated in rats with chronic heart failure.[284] Although the human studies do not exclude a role for intrarenal factors in the pathogenesis of the abnormal water retention, they complement the experimental observations that demonstrate a critical role for AVP in the pathologic process. It is most likely that nonosmotic pathways, whose activation is suggested by the increase in sympathetic activity seen in congestive heart failure,[285] are the mediators of AVP secretion in edema-forming states. These neurohumoral factors further contribute to the hyponatremia by decreasing the glomerular filtration rate (GFR) and enhancing tubular Na$^+$ reabsorption, thereby decreasing fluid delivery to the distal diluting segments of the nephron. The degree of neurohumoral activation correlates with the clinical severity of left ventricular dysfunction.[286] Hyponatremia is a powerful prognostic factor in these patients.[287]

The role of the AVP-regulated water channel (AQP2) has been examined in heart failure as well. Two groups have described an upregulation of this water channel in rats with heart failure.[288,289] In one study,[289] the nonpeptide V$_2$ receptor antagonist OPC31260 reversed the upregulation, which suggests that a receptor-mediated function, most likely enhanced cAMP generation, is responsible for the process. Consistent with these observations, a selective V_2 antagonist decreases AQP2 excretion[290] and increases urine flow in patients with heart failure.

Hepatic Failure

Patients with advanced cirrhosis and ascites frequently present with hyponatremia as a consequence of their inability to excrete a water load.[291] The classic view suggests that a decrement in effective arterial blood volume leads to avid Na^+ and water retention in an attempt to restore volume toward normal.[292] In this regard, a number of the pathologic derangements in cirrhosis, including splanchnic venous pooling, diminished plasma oncotic pressure secondary to hypoalbuminemia, and the decrease in peripheral resistance, could all contribute to a decrease in effective arterial blood volume.[293] This classic theory was challenged by observations that suggested primary renal Na^+ retention, the *overflow hypothesis*.[294] A proposal that unifies these views has been put forth: Na^+ retention occurs early in the process, but is a consequence of the severe vasodilation-mediated arterial underfilling.[295]

As with cardiac failure, the relative role of intrarenal versus extrarenal factors in impaired water excretion has been a matter of some controversy. The observation that expansion of intravascular volume with saline, mannitol, ascites fluid, water immersion, or peritoneovenous shunting improves water excretion in cirrhosis could be interpreted as implicating an intrarenal mechanism in the impaired water excretion, because these maneuvers increase GFR and improve distal delivery. Such maneuvers could also suppress baroreceptor-mediated AVP release and cause an osmotic diuresis, which would also improve water excretion.[292]

Experimental models of deranged liver function, including acute portal hypertension by vein constriction, bile duct ligation, and chronic cirrhosis produced by administration of carbon tetrachloride, have demonstrated a predominant role for AVP secretion in the pathogenesis of the disorder. In the latter model, an increment in hypothalamic AVP mRNA has also been demonstrated.[296] A study employing an AVP antagonist also points to a central role for AVP in the process.[297] As is the case in heart failure, increased expression of AQP2 has been reported in cirrhotic rats,[298] but dysregulation of AQP1 and AQP3 is also present in carbon tetrachloride–induced cirrhosis.[299] In contrast, in the common bile duct model of cirrhosis, no increase in AQP2 was observed.[300]

Although patients with cirrhosis who have no edema or ascites excrete a water load normally, those with ascites usually do not. Several studies have demonstrated elevated AVP levels in such patients.[291] Patients who had a defect in water excretion had higher levels of AVP, plasma renin activity, plasma aldosterone, and norepinephrine,[301] as well as lower rates of PGE_2 production. Likewise, their serum albumin level was lower, as was their urinary excretion of Na^+, all of which suggest a decrease in effective arterial blood volume. As is the case in heart failure, sympathetic tone is high in cirrhosis.[302] In fact, the plasma concentration of norepinephrine, a good index of baroreceptor activity in humans, appears to correlate well with the levels of AVP

and the excretion of water. These studies, therefore, offer strong support for the view that effective arterial blood volume is contracted, rather than expanded, in decompensated cirrhosis.[295]

This view is further strengthened by observations of subjects during head-out water immersion. This maneuver, which translocates fluid to the central blood volume, caused a decrease in AVP levels and improved water excretion,[303] but in this study, it was surprising that peripheral resistance decreased further. When head-out water immersion was combined with norepinephrine administration in an effort to increase systemic pressure and peripheral resistance, water excretion was completely normalized.[304]

Such observations underscore the critical role of peripheral vasodilation in the pathologic process. The observation that inhibition of nitric oxide corrects the arterial hyporesponsiveness to vasodilators[305] and the abnormal water excretion in cirrhotic rats provides strong evidence of a role for nitric oxide in the vasodilation.[306,307]

Nephrotic Syndrome

The incidence of hyponatremia in nephrotic syndrome is lower than that in either congestive heart failure or cirrhosis, most likely as a consequence of the higher blood pressure, higher GFR, and more modest impairment in Na^+ and water excretion in nephrotic syndrome than in the latter disorders.[308] Because lipids are frequently elevated, a direct measurement of plasma osmolality should always be obtained. Diminished excretion of free water was first noted in children with nephrotic syndrome, and since then, other investigators[309] have noted elevated plasma levels of AVP in these patients.

In view of the alterations in Starling's forces that accompany hypoalbuminemia and allow transudation of salt and water across capillary membranes to the interstitial space, patients with nephrotic syndrome have been believed to have intravascular volume contraction. The finding of increased levels of neurohumoral markers of reduced effective arterial blood volume also support this underfilling theory.[310] The possibility that this nonosmotic pathway stimulates AVP release was suggested by studies in which head-out water immersion and blood volume expansion[309] increased water excretion in nephrotic subjects. However, these pathogenic events may not be applicable to all patients with the disorder. Some patients with the nephrotic syndrome in fact have increased plasma volumes with suppressed plasma renin activity and aldosterone levels.[311] The cause of these discrepancies is not immediately evident, but this overfill view has been subject to some criticism.[312] It is most likely that the underfilling mechanism is operative in patients with normal GFR and with the histologic lesion of minimal change disease, and that hypervolemia may be more prevalent in patients with underlying glomerular pathology and decreased renal function. In such patients, an intrarenal mechanism probably causes Na^+ retention, as has been described in an experimental model of nephrotic syndrome.[313]

Also, in contrast to the increase in AQP2 found in the previously described Na^+- and water-retaining states, in two animal models of nephrotic syndrome induced with either puromycin aminonucleoside[314] or doxorubicin,[315] the expression of AQP2 was decreased. The animals were not hyponatremic and most likely had expanded ECF volumes to explain the discrepancy.

Renal Failure

Hyponatremia with edema can occur with either acute or chronic renal failure. It is clear that in the setting of either experimental or human renal disease, the ability to excrete free water is maintained better than the ability to reabsorb water. Nonetheless, the patient's GFR still determines the maximal rate of free water formation. Thus, whenever minimal urine osmolality is reduced to 150 to 250 mOsm/kg H_2O and fractional water excretion approaches 20% to 30% of the filtered load, the uremic patient with a GFR of 2 mL/min can excrete only 300 mL/day. Intake of more fluid than this culminates in hyponatremia. Thus, a decrement in GFR with an increase in thirst underlies the hyponatremia of patients with renal insufficiency in most cases.[316]

Hyponatremia with Normal Extracellular Fluid Volume

Figure 15-17 lists the clinical entities that must be considered in patients with hyponatremia whose volume is neither contracted nor expanded and who are, at least by clinical assessment, euvolemic. These entities are considered individually in the following sections.

Glucocorticoid Deficiency

Considerable evidence exists of an important role for glucocorticoids in the abnormal water excretion of adrenal insufficiency.[317] The water-excretory defect of anterior pituitary insufficiency, and particularly ACTH deficiency, is associated with elevated AVP levels[318,319] and is corrected by physiologic doses of glucocorticoids. Likewise, adrenalectomized dogs receiving replacement of mineralocorticoids still have abnormal water excretion.

The relative importance of intrarenal factors and AVP in defective water excretion has been a matter of considerable controversy. Studies employing a sensitive radioimmunoassay for plasma AVP and the Brattleboro rat with hypothalamic DI have provided evidence that both factors are involved. Support for a role of AVP has been obtained in studies of conscious adrenalectomized, mineralocorticoid-replaced dogs[320] and rats[321] and in research using an inhibitor of the hydro-osmotic effect of AVP.[276] Because plasma AVP was elevated despite a fall in plasma osmolality, the hormone's release was likely nonosmotically mediated. Although ECF volume was normal in these studies, a decrease in systemic pressure and cardiac function[320,321] could well have provided the hemodynamic stimulus for AVP release.

In addition, there may be a direct effect of glucocorticoids that inhibits AVP secretion. In this regard, AVP gene expression is increased in glucocorticoid-deficient rats.[322] The presence of a glucocorticoid-responsive element on the AVP gene promoter may be responsible for the inhibition of AVP gene transcription by glucocorticoids.[323] Also, glucocorticoid receptors are present in magnocellular neurons and their expression is increased during hypo-osmolality.[324]

A role for AVP-independent intrarenal factors was defined in studies involving the antidiuretic-deficient, adrenalectomized

Brattleboro rat[321] and the use of AVP receptor antagonists.[276] It appears that prolonged glucocorticoid deficiency (14 to 17 days) is accompanied by decreases in renal hemodynamics that impair water excretion. A direct effect of glucocorticoid deficiency that enhances water permeability of the collecting duct has been proposed, but this hypothesis is not supported by studies of anuran membranes, which suggest that glucocorticoids enhance rather than inhibit water movement. Anura is an order of animals in the class Amphibia that includes frogs and toads. Also, in vitro perfusion studies of the collecting duct of adrenalectomized rabbits show an impaired rather than enhanced AVP response,[325] a defect that may be related to enhanced cAMP metabolism.[326] In fact, AQP2 and AQP3 abundance appears not to be sensitive to glucocorticoids.[327]

In summary, the defect in glucocorticoid deficiency is primarily AVP dependent, but an AVP-independent mechanism becomes evident with more prolonged hormone deficiency. It appears likely that alterations in systemic hemodynamics account for the nonosmotic release of AVP, but a direct effect of glucocorticoid hormone on AVP release has not been entirely excluded. The AVP-independent renal mechanism probably involves alterations in renal hemodynamics and not a direct increase in collecting duct permeability. It should be remembered that secondary hypoadrenalism, as occurs in hypopituitarism and after long-term immunosuppressive steroid therapy, can also be associated with hyponatremia.[328,329]

Hypothyroidism

Patients and experimental animals with hypothyroidism often have impaired water excretion and sometimes develop hyponatremia.[317,330] The dilution defect is reversed by treatment with thyroid hormones. Both decreased delivery of filtrate to the diluting segment and persistent secretion of AVP, alone or combination, have been proposed as mechanisms responsible for the defect.

Hypothyroidism has been shown to be associated with decreases in GFR and renal plasma flow.[330] In the AVP-free Brattleboro rat, the decrement in maximal free water excretion can be entirely accounted for by the decrease in GFR. The osmotic threshold for AVP release appears not to be altered in hypothyroidism.[331] The normal suppression of AVP release with water loading and the normal response to hypertonic saline,[332] coupled with the failure to observe upregulation of hypothalamic AVP gene expression in hypothyroid rats,[333] are evidence for an AVP-independent mechanism. There is also, however, evidence for a role of AVP in impairing water excretion in hypothyroidism. In both experimental animals[334] and humans with advanced hypothyroidism,[330] elevated AVP levels were found in the basal state and after a water load.

Although increased sensitivity to AVP in hypothyroidism has been proposed, experimental evidence suggests the contrary, because urine osmolality is relatively low for the circulating levels of the hormone,[334] and AVP-stimulated cyclase is impaired in the renal medulla of hypothyroid rats,[335] which possibly leads to decreased AQP2 expression.[336] However, the predominant defect is one of water of excretion with increased AQP2 expression and reversal with a V_2 receptor antagonist.[337] It appears, therefore, that diminished distal fluid delivery and persistent AVP release mediate the impaired water excretion in this disorder, but the relative contributions of these two factors remain undefined and may depend on the severity of the endocrine disorder.

Psychosis—Primary Polydipsia

It has long been recognized that patients with psychiatric disease demonstrate generous water intake. Although such polydipsia is normally not associated with hyponatremia, these patients have been found to be at increased risk of developing hyponatremia when they are acutely psychotic.[338] Most such patients have schizophrenia, but some have psychotic depression. The frequency of hyponatremia in this population of patients is unknown, but in a survey conducted at one large psychiatric hospital, 20 polydipsic patients with a plasma [Na$^+$] of less than 124 mEq/L were reported,[339] and another survey found hyponatremia in 8 of 239 patients.[340]

Elucidation of the mechanism of the impaired water excretion has been confounded by the effects of antipsychotic drug treatment (see later). The relative contributions of the pharmacologic agent and the psychosis are difficult to define, because thiazides and carbamazepine are frequently implicated.[341] Nonetheless, there are several reports of psychotic patients who experienced water intoxication when free of medication.[342]

The mechanism responsible for the hyponatremia in psychosis appears to be multifactorial.[184] In a comprehensive study of water metabolism in eight psychotic hyponatremic patients and seven psychotic normonatremic control subjects, no unifying defect emerged. The investigators found a small defect in osmoregulation in the hyponatremic patients that caused AVP to be secreted at plasma osmolalities somewhat lower than those of the control group, but they did not observe a true resetting of the osmostat. Also, the hyponatremic patients had a mild urine dilution defect even in the absence of AVP. When AVP was present, the renal response was somewhat enhanced, which suggests increased renal sensitivity to the hormone. Psychotic exacerbations appear to be associated with increased AVP levels in schizophrenic patients with hyponatremia.[343] Finally, thirst perception is also increased, because excessive water intake that exceeds excretory capacity is responsible for most episodes of hyponatremia in these patients. However, concurrent nausea caused increased AVP levels in some of the subjects.[344] Although each of these derangements by itself would remain clinically unimportant, it is possible that during exacerbation of the psychosis the defects are more pronounced, and that, in combination, they can culminate in hyponatremia.[345]

Hyponatremia also occurs in beer drinkers (so-called beer potomania). Although this has been ascribed to an increase in fluid intake in the setting of very low solute intake,[346] one report suggests that such patients may also have sustained significant solute losses.[347]

Postoperative Hyponatremia

The incidence of hospital-acquired hyponatremia is high, both in adults[205] and in children,[348] and it is particularly prevalent in the postoperative stage[349,350] (incidence of approximately 4%). The majority of affected patients appear clinically euvolemic and have measurable levels of AVP in their circulation.[349,351] Although this hyponatremia occurs primarily as a consequence of administration of hypotonic fluids,[352] a decrease in serum [Na$^+$] can occur in this high-AVP state,

even when isotonic fluids are given.[353] Hyponatremia has also been reported following cardiac catheterization in patients receiving hypotonic fluids.[354] Although the presence of hyponatremia is a marker for poor outcomes, this is likely a consequence not of the hyponatremia per se but of the severe underlying diseases associated with it. As discussed in more detail later, there is a subgroup of postoperative hyponatremic patients, almost always premenstrual women, who develop catastrophic neurologic events, frequently accompanied by seizures and hypoxia.[355,356]

Endurance Exercise

There is increasing recognition that strenuous endurance exercise, such as military training[357] and marathons and long-distance triathlons,[358] can cause hyponatremia that is frequently symptomatic. A review of 57 patients with exercise-induced hyponatremia found a mean serum [Na$^+$] of 121 mEq/L.[359] A prospective study of 488 runners in the Boston Marathon revealed that 13% of the runners had a serum [Na$^+$]$^+$ of less than 130 mEq/L. A multivariate analysis revealed that weight gain related to excessive fluid intake was the strongest single predictor of the hyponatremia. Longer racing times and very low body mass indices were also predictors.[360] Composition of the consumed fluids and use of nonsteroidal antiinflammatory agents were not predictive. Symptomatic hyponatremia is even more frequent in ultraendurance events.[361]

Pharmacologically Induced Hyponatremia

Table 15-6 lists drugs associated with water retention. Some of the more clinically important ones are discussed here. An increasing number of patients who receive the AVP V$_2$ agonist desmopressin for indications such as von Willebrand disease[362] and nocturnal enuresis[363,364] are developing severe hyponatremia.

TABLE 15-6 Drugs Associated with Hyponatremia

Antidiuretic hormone analogs
Desmopressin
Oxytocin

Drugs that Enhance Arginine Vasopressin (AVP) Secretion
Chlorpropamide
Clofibrate
Carbamazepine, oxcarbazepine
Vincristine
Nicotine
Narcotics (μ-opioid receptor agonists)
Antipsychotics, antidepressants
Ifosfamide
Selective serotonin reuptake inhibitors
Ecstasy (amphetamine related)

Drugs That Potentiate Renal Action of AVP
Chlorpropamide
Cyclophosphamide
Nonsteroidal antiinflammatory drugs
Acetaminophen

Drugs That Cause Hyponatremia by Unknown Mechanisms
Haloperidol
Fluphenazine
Amitriptyline
Thioridazine

Data from Berl T, Schrier RW: Disorders of water metabolism, in Schrier RW (editor): *Renal and electrolyte disorders*, ed 6, Philadelphia, 2003, Lippincott Williams & Wilkins.

CHLORPROPAMIDE

The incidence of at least mild hyponatremia in patients taking chlorpropamide may be as high as 7%, but severe hyponatremia (<130 mEq/L) occurs in 2% of patients so treated.[365] As noted earlier, the drug exerts its action primarily by potentiating the renal action of AVP.[366] Studies of toad urinary bladder have demonstrated that, although chlorpropamide alone has no effect, it enhances both AVP- and theophylline-stimulated water flow but decreases cAMP-mediated flow. The enhanced response may be due to upregulation of the hormone's receptor.[367] On the other hand, studies of chlorpropamide-treated animals suggest that the drug enhances solute reabsorption in the medullary ascending limb (thereby increasing interstitial tonicity and the osmotic drive for water reabsorption) rather than a cAMP-mediated alteration in collecting duct water permeability.[368]

CARBAMAZEPINE AND OXCARBAZEPINE

The anticonvulsant drug carbamazepine is well known to possess antidiuretic properties. The incidence of hyponatremia in carbamazepine-treated patients was believed to be as high as 21%, but a survey of patients with mental retardation reported a lower incidence of 5%.[369] Cases continue to be reported.[370] The antiepileptic oxcarbazepine, of the same class as carbamazepine, has also been reported to cause hyponatremia.[371] Evidence exists for both a mechanism mediated by AVP secretion[90] and for renal enhancement of the hormone's action[372] to explain carbamazepine's antidiuretic effect. Paradoxically, the drug also appears to decrease the sensitivity of the AVP response to osmotic stimulation.[373]

PSYCHOTROPIC DRUGS

An increasing number of psychotropic drugs have been associated with hyponatremia, and they are frequently held to explain the water intoxication in psychotic patients. Among the agents implicated are the phenothiazines,[374] the butyrophenone haloperidol,[375] and the tricyclic antidepressants.[376] An increasing number of cases of amphetamine (Ecstasy)–related hyponatremia have been described.[377,378] Likewise, the widely used antidepressants fluoxetine,[379] sertraline,[380] and paroxetine[381] have been associated with hyponatremia. In a study of the latter drug involving 75 patients, 12% were found to develop hyponatremia (serum [Na+] of <135 mmol/L). The elderly appear to be particularly susceptible,[382,383] with an incidence as high as 22% to 28%.[384,385] The tendency for these drugs to cause hyponatremia is further compounded by their anticholinergic effects. By drying the mucous membranes, they can stimulate water intake. The role of the drugs in impaired water excretion has not, in most cases, been dissociated from the role of the underlying disorder for which the drug is given. Furthermore, evaluation of the effect of the drugs on AVP secretion has frequently revealed a failure to increase the levels of the hormone, particularly if mean arterial pressure remained unaltered. Therefore, although a clinical association between antipsychotic drugs and hyponatremia is frequently encountered, the pharmacologic agents themselves may not be the principal factors responsible for the water retention.[184]

ANTINEOPLASTIC DRUGS

Several drugs used in cancer therapy cause antidiuresis. The effect of vincristine may be mediated by the drug's neurotoxic effect on the hypothalamic microtubule system, which then alters normal osmoreceptor control of AVP release.[386] A retrospective survey suggests that this may be more common in Asian patients given the drug.[387] The mechanism of the diluting defect that results from cyclophosphamide administration is not fully understood. It may act, at least in part, to enhance action, because the drug does not increase hormone levels.[388] It is known that the antidiuresis has its onset 4 to 12 hours after injection of the drug, lasts as long as 12 hours, and seems to be temporally related to excretion of a metabolite. The importance of anticipating potentially severe hyponatremia in cyclophosphamide-treated patients who are vigorously hydrated to avert urologic complications cannot be overstated. The synthetic analog of cyclophosphamide, ifosfamide, has also been associated with hyponatremia and AVP secretion.[389]

NARCOTICS

Since the 1940s, it has been known that the administration of opioid agonists, such as morphine, reduces urine flow by causing the release of an antidiuretic substance. The possibility that endogenous opioids could serve as potential neurotransmitters has been suggested by the discovery of enkephalins in nerve fibers projecting from the hypothalamus to the neurohypophysis. The reported effects vary, however, and range from stimulation to no change and even to inhibition of AVP secretion. The reasons for these diverse observations may be that the opiates and their receptors are widely distributed in the brain, which implies that the site of action of the opiate can differ markedly depending on the route of administration. Likewise, there are multiple opiate peptides and receptor types. It has now been determined that agonists of μ-receptors have antidiuretic properties, whereas agonists of δ-receptors have the opposite effect.

MISCELLANEOUS

Several case reports suggest an association between the use of ACE inhibitors and hyponatremia.[390-392] Of interest is that all three reported patients were women in their sixties. The use of ACE inhibition was also a concomitant risk factor for the development of hyponatremia in a survey of veterans who received chlorpropamide.[365] Given the widespread use of these agents, however, the true incidence of hyponatremia must be vanishingly low. An association with angiotensin receptor blockers has not been reported to date. Four patients have been reported to develop hyponatremia during amiodarone loading.[393]

Syndrome of Inappropriate Antidiuretic Hormone Secretion

The syndrome of inappropriate antidiuretic hormone secretion (SIADH) is the most common cause of hyponatremia in hospitalized patients.[250] As first described by Schwartz and associates[394] in two patients with bronchogenic carcinoma and later further characterized by Bartter and Schwartz,[395] patients with this syndrome have serum hypo-osmolality when excreting urine that is less than maximally dilute (>100 mOsm/kg H2O). Thus, a diagnostic criterion for this syndrome is the presence of inappropriate urinary concentration.

The development of hyponatremia with a dilute urine (<100 mOsm/kg H2O) should raise suspicion of a primary polydipsic disorder. Although large volumes of fluid must be ingested to overwhelm normal water-excretory ability, if there are concomitant decreases in solute intake, this volume need not be excessively high.[396] In SIADH, the urinary Na+ is dependent on intake, because Na+ balance is well maintained. Because of this, urinary Na+ concentration is usually high, but it may be low in patients with the syndrome who are consuming a low-sodium diet.

The presence of Na+ in the urine is helpful in excluding extrarenal causes of hypovolemic hyponatremia, but low urinary Na+ concentration does not exclude SIADH. Before the diagnosis of SIADH is made, other causes of a decreased diluting capacity, such as renal, pituitary, adrenal, thyroid, cardiac, or hepatic disease, must be excluded. In addition, nonosmotic stimuli for AVP release, particularly hemodynamic derangements (e.g., due to hypotension, nausea, or drugs), need to be ruled out. Another clue to the presence of SIADH is the finding of hypouricemia. In one study, 16 of 17 patients had levels below 4 mg/dL, whereas in 13 patients with hyponatremia due to other causes the level was higher than 5 mg/dL. Hypouricemia appears to occur as a consequence of increased urate clearance.[397] Measurement of an elevated level of AVP can confirm the clinical diagnosis, but is not necessary. It should be noted, however, that the majority of patients with SIADH have AVP levels in the "normal" range (≤10 pg/mL); however, the presence of any measurable AVP is abnormal in the hypo-osmolar state. Because the presence of hyponatremia is itself evidence of abnormal dilution, a formal urine-diluting test need not be performed. The water loading test is helpful in determining whether an abnormality remains in a patient whose serum [Na+] has been corrected by water restriction.

Because Brattleboro rats receiving AVP,[398] as well as an animal model of SIADH, display upregulation of AQP2 expression, the excretion of AQP2 has been investigated as a marker for the persistent secretion of AVP. Excretion of the water channel remains elevated in patients with SIADH; however, this is not specific to this entity, because a similar pattern was observed in patients with hyponatremia due to hypopituitarism.[399]

PATHOPHYSIOLOGY

In 1953, Leaf and associates[400] described the effects of long-term AVP administration on Na+ and water balance. They noted that high-volume water intake was required for the development of hyponatremia. Concomitant with the water retention, an increment in urinary Na+ excretion was noted. The relative contributions of the water retention and Na+ loss to the development of hyponatremia were subsequently investigated. Acute water loading causes transient natriuresis, but when water intake is increased more slowly, no significant negative Na+ loss can be documented. Such studies clearly demonstrate that the hyponatremia is, in large measure, a consequence of water retention. However, it must be noted that the net increase in water balance fails to account entirely for the decrement in serum [Na+].[400]

In a carefully studied model of SIADH in rats, the retained water was found to be distributed in the intracellular space and to be in equilibrium with the tonicity of ECF.[401] The natriuresis and kaliuresis that occur early in the development of this model contribute to a decrement of body solutes and account, in part, for the observed hyponatremia.[402] Studies involving analysis of whole-body water and electrolyte content demonstrate that the relative contributions of water retention and solute losses vary with the duration of induced hyponatremia; the former is central to the process, but with more prolonged

hyponatremia, Na+ depletion becomes predominant.[403] In this regard, it has even been suggested that the natriuresis and volume contraction are an important component of the syndrome that maintains the secretion of AVP,[404] with atrial natriuretic peptide as a mediator of the Na+ loss.[405] Therefore, although natriuresis frequently accompanies the syndrome, the secretion of AVP is essential.

Finally, patients with the syndrome must also have a defect in thirst regulation whereby the osmotic inhibition of water intake is not operant. The mechanism of this failure to suppress thirst is not fully understood. After the initial retention of water, loss of Na+, and development of hyponatremia, continued administration of AVP is accompanied by the reestablishment of Na+ balance and a decline in the hydro-osmotic effect of the hormone. The integrity of renal regulation of Na+ balance is manifested by the ability to conserve Na+ during Na+ restriction and by the normal excretion of an Na+ load. Thus, the mechanisms that regulate Na+ excretion are intact. Loss of the hydro-osmotic effect of AVP, albeit to varying degrees, is evident in many studies,[400,402] because urine flow increased and urine osmolality decreased despite continued administration of the hormone (Figure 15-18). This effect has been termed *vasopressin escape*.[406] Several studies have demonstrated that hypotonic ECF volume expansion rather than chronic administration of AVP per se is needed for escape to occur, because the escape phenomenon is seen only when positive water balance is achieved.[406]

The cellular mechanisms responsible for vasopressin escape have been the subject of some investigation. Studies of toad urinary bladder revealed downregulation of AVP receptors[407] as well as decreased AVP binding in the inner medulla.[408] Post-cAMP mechanisms are probably also operant. In this regard, a decrease in the expression of AQP2 has been reported in the process of escape from desmopressin-induced antidiuresis, without a concomitant change in basolateral AQP3 and AQP4 expression.[409,410] The decrement in AQP2 was associated with decreased V2 responsiveness.[409] The distal tubule also has an increase in sodium transporters, including the α- and γ-subunits of the epithelial sodium channel and the thiazide-sensitive Na+-Cl− cotransporter.[411] In addition, it appears that chronic hyponatremia causes a decrement in hypothalamic AVP mRNA production, a process that could ameliorate the syndrome in the clinical setting.[27]

CLINICAL SETTINGS

It is now apparent that the previously described pathophysiologic sequence occurs in a variety of clinical settings characterized by persistent AVP secretion. Since the original report of Schwartz and colleagues,[394] SIADH has been described in an increasing number of clinical settings (Table 15-7). These fall into three general categories[412]: (1) malignancies, (2) pulmonary disease, and (3) CNS disorders. In addition, an increasing number of patients with acquired immunodeficiency syndrome have been reported to have hyponatremia. The frequency may be as high as 35% of hospitalized patients with the disease, and in as many as two thirds, SIADH may be the underlying cause of the hyponatremia.[413] As was noted previously, hyponatremia caused by excessive water repletion can occur after moderate and severe exercise.[358,359,414,415] Finally, it is increasingly recognized that an idiopathic form is common in the elderly.[416-419] As many as 25% of elderly patients admitted to a rehabilitation center had a serum [Na+]

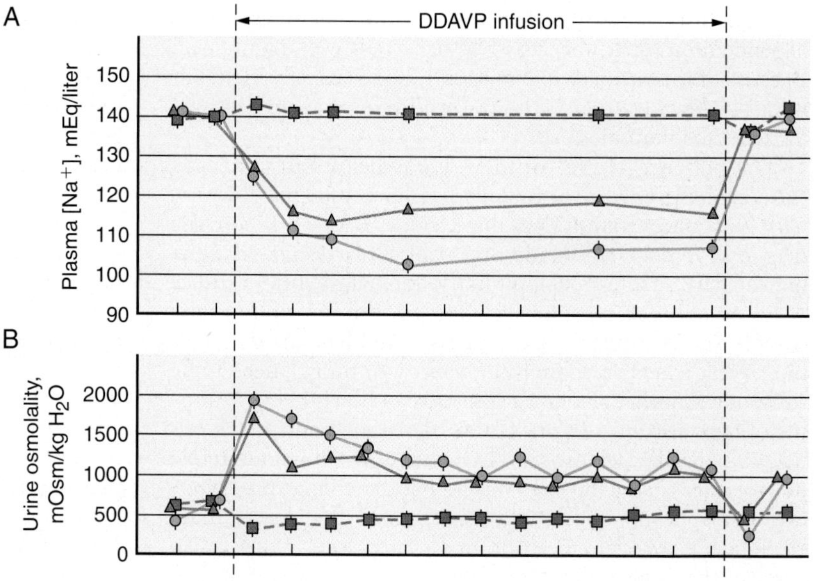

FIGURE 15-18 Effects of desmopressin (DDAVP) and water administration in two groups of normal rats (*circles* and *triangles*). Note that urine osmolality decreases and plasma Na stabilizes. Data for sham-treated control animals are indicated by *squares*. (From Verbalis JG, Drutarosky M: Adaptation to chronic hypo-osmolality in rats, *Kidney Int* 34:351-360, 1988.)

TABLE 15-7 Disorders Associated with the Syndrome of Inappropriate Antidiuretic Hormone Secretion			
CARCINOMAS	**PULMONARY DISORDERS**	**CENTRAL NERVOUS SYSTEM DISORDERS**	**OTHER**
Bronchogenic carcinoma	Viral pneumonia	Encephalitis (viral or bacterial)	Acquired immunodeficiency syndrome
Carcinoma of the duodenum	Bacterial pneumonia	Meningitis (viral, bacterial, tuberculous, fungal)	Prolonged exercise
Carcinoma of the pancreas	Pulmonary abscess	Head trauma	Idiopathic (in elderly)
Carcinoma of the ureter	Tuberculosis	Brain abscess	
Thymoma	Aspergillosis	Guillain-Barré syndrome	
Carcinoma of the stomach	Positive pressure breathing	Acute intermittent porphyria	
Lymphoma	Asthma	Subarachnoid hemorrhage or subdural hematoma	
Ewing's sarcoma	Pneumothorax	Cerebellar and cerebral atrophy	
Carcinoma of the bladder	Mesothelioma	Cavernous sinus thrombosis	
Prostatic carcinoma	Cystic fibrosis	Neonatal hypoxia	
Oropharyngeal tumor		Shy-Drager syndrome	
		Rocky Mountain spotted fever	
		Delirium tremens	
		Cerebrovascular accident (cerebral thrombosis or hemorrhage)	
		Acute psychosis	
		Peripheral neuropathy	
		Multiple sclerosis	

Data from Berl T, Schrier RW: Disorders of water metabolism, in Schrier RW (editor): *Renal and electrolyte disorders,* ed 6, Philadelphia, 2003, Lippincott Williams & Wilkins.

of less than 135 mEq/L.[417] In a significant proportion of these patients, no underlying cause was discovered. The incidence of the disorder in the elderly may be related to an increase in AQP2 production and excretion in this age group.[420]

A substance with antidiuretic properties has been extracted from some of the tumors or metastases of patients with malignancy-associated SIADH. However, AVP is not present in the tumors of all patients with the syndrome. A number of the tumors have also been found to produce the carrier hormone of AVP, neurophysin, which suggests that repression of normal genetic information has occurred.

Of the tumors that cause SIADH secretion, bronchogenic carcinoma, and particularly small cell lung cancer, is the most common, with a reported incidence of 11%.[421] It appears that patients with bronchogenic carcinoma have higher plasma AVP levels in relation to plasma osmolality, even if they do not manifest full-blown SIADH, although the levels of the hormone are higher in patients with the syndrome. The possibility that the hormone could serve as a marker of bronchogenic carcinoma has been suggested, and in fact, SIADH has been reported occasionally to precede the diagnosis of the tumor by several months.[422] In view of the potential to treat patients with this tumor, it is important that patients with unexplained SIADH be fully investigated and evaluated for the presence of this malignancy. Head and neck malignancies are the second most common tumors associated with SIADH, which occurs in approximately 3% of such patients. The mechanism whereby AVP is produced in other pulmonary disorders is not known, but the associated abnormalities in blood gas concentrations could act as mediators of the effect. Antidiuretic activity has also been assayed in tuberculous lung tissue. The syndrome can also occur in the setting of miliary rather than only lung-limited tuberculosis.[423]

In CNS disorders, AVP is most likely released from the neurohypophysis. Studies of monkeys have shown that elevations of intracranial pressure cause AVP secretion, and this may be the mechanism that mediates the syndrome in at least some CNS disorders. The magnocellular vasopressin-secreting cells in the hypothalamus are subject to numerous excitatory inputs, and therefore it is conceivable that a large variety of neurologic disorders can stimulate the secretion of AVP.

Finally, hyponatremia was described in two infants with undetectable AVP levels who were found to have a gain-of-function mutation at the X-linked vasopressin receptor in which a missense mutation in codon 137 resulted in a change from arginine to cysteine or leucine. The authors termed this *nephrogenic syndrome of inappropriate antidiuresis.*[424]

Zerbe and colleagues have studied osmoregulation of AVP secretion in a large group of patients with SIADH.[425] In the great majority, the plasma AVP concentration was inadequately suppressed relative to the hypotonicity present. In most patients, the plasma AVP concentration ranged between 1 and 10 pg/mL, the same range as in normally hydrated healthy adults. Inappropriate secretion, therefore, can often be demonstrated only by measuring AVP under hypotonic conditions. Even with this approach, however, abnormalities in plasma AVP were not apparent in almost 10% of the patients with clinical evidence of SIADH.

To better define the nature of the osmoregulatory defect in these patients, plasma AVP was measured during infusion of hypertonic saline. When this method of analysis was applied to 25 patients with SIADH, four different types of osmoregulatory defects were identified. As shown in Figure 15-19, in the type A osmoregulatory defect, infusion of hypertonic saline was associated with large and erratic fluctuations in plasma AVP, which bore no relationship to the rise in plasma osmolality. This pattern was found in 6 of 25 patients studied, who had acute respiratory failure, bronchogenic carcinoma, pulmonary tuberculosis, schizophrenia, or rheumatoid arthritis. This pattern indicates that the secretion of AVP either had been totally divorced from osmoreceptor control or was responding to some periodic nonosmotic stimulus.

A completely different type of osmoregulatory defect is exemplified by the type B response (see Figure 15-19). The infusion of hypertonic saline resulted in prompt and progressive rises in plasma osmolality. Regression analysis showed that the precision and sensitivity of this response were essentially the same as those in healthy subjects, except that the intercept or threshold value at 253 mOsm/kg was well below the normal range. This pattern, which reflects the resetting of the osmoreceptor, was found in 9 of the 25 patients who had a diagnosis of bronchogenic carcinoma, cerebrovascular disease, tuberculous meningitis, acute respiratory disease, or carcinoma

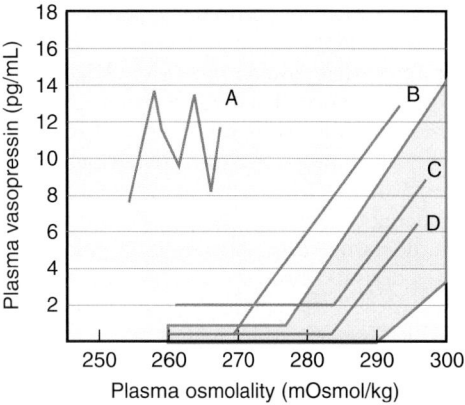

FIGURE 15-19 Plasma vasopressin level as a function of plasma osmolality during the infusion of hypertonic saline in four groups of patients with clinical syndrome of inappropriate antidiuretic hormone secretion (SIADH). The *shaded area* indicates the range of normal values. See text for descriptions of each group. (From Zerbe R, Stropes L, Robertson G: Vasopressin function in the syndrome of inappropriate antidiuresis, *Annu Rev Med* 31:315-327, 1980.)

of the pharynx. Another patient has been reported with hyponatremia and acute idiopathic polyneuritis who reacted in an identical manner to the hypertonic saline infusion and was determined to have resetting of the osmoreceptor. Because their threshold function is retained when they receive a water load, this patient and the others with reset osmostats are able to dilute their urine maximally and sustain a urine flow sufficient to prevent a further increase in body water. Thus, an abnormality in AVP regulation can exist in spite of the ability to maximally dilute the urine and excrete a water load.

In the type C response (see Figure 15-19), plasma AVP was elevated initially but did not change during the infusion of hypertonic saline until plasma osmolality reached the normal range. At that point, plasma AVP began to rise appropriately, which indicates a normally functioning osmoreceptor mechanism. This response was found in 8 of the 25 patients with a diagnosis of CNS disease, bronchogenic carcinoma, carcinoma of the pharynx, pulmonary tuberculosis, or schizophrenia. Its pathogenesis is unknown, but the authors speculate that it may be due to a constant, nonsuppressible leak of AVP despite otherwise normal osmoregulatory function. Unlike the type B response (resetting of the osmostat), the type C response results in impaired urine dilution and water excretion at all levels of plasma osmolality.

In the type D response (see Figure 15-19), the osmoregulation of AVP appears to be completely normal despite a marked inability to excrete a water load. The plasma AVP is appropriately suppressed under hypotonic conditions and does not rise until plasma osmolality reaches the normal threshold level. When this procedure is reversed by water loading, plasma osmolality and plasma AVP again fall normally, but urine dilution does not occur, and the water load is not excreted. This defect was present in 2 of 25 patients with the diagnosis of bronchogenic carcinoma, which indicates that, in these patients, the antidiuretic defect is caused by some abnormality other than SIADH. It could be due either to increased renal tubule sensitivity to AVP or to the existence of an antidiuretic substance other than AVP. Alternatively, it is possible that the presently available assays are not sufficiently sensitive to detect significant levels of AVP. Perhaps some of these subjects have the nephrogenic syndrome of antidiuresis described previously.[424]

It is of interest that patients with bronchogenic carcinoma, which has generally been believed to be associated with ectopic production of AVP, manifested every category of osmoregulatory defect, including resetting of the osmostat. It has been suggested that many of these tumors probably cause SIADH not by producing the hormone ectopically but rather by interfering with the normal osmoregulation of AVP secretion from the neurohypophysis through direct invasion of the vagus nerve, metastatic implants in the hypothalamus, or some other more generalized neuropathic changes.

Hyponatremia Symptoms, Morbidity, and Mortality

Symptoms of hyponatremia correlate both with the degree of decrease in the serum [Na+] and with the chronicity of the hyponatremia. Most clinical manifestations of hyponatremia begin at a serum [Na+] of less than 130 mEq/L. Although gastrointestinal complaints often occur early, the majority of the manifestations are neurologic, including lethargy, confusion, disorientation, obtundation, and seizures, designated as *hyponatremic encephalopathy*.[426] Many of the symptoms of hyponatremic encephalopathy are caused by cerebral edema, which may be mediated, at least in part, by AQP4.[427] In its most severe form, the cerebral edema can lead to tentorial herniation; in such cases, death can occur as a result of brainstem compression with respiratory arrest. The cerebral edema can also cause neurogenic pulmonary edema and hypoxemia,[428] which in turn can increase the severity of brain swelling.[429] In a retrospective study of 168 hyponatremic patients, most of them acute, there was a strong (13-fold) association between the development of hypoxemia and the risk of mortality.[430] The most severe life-threatening clinical features of hyponatremic encephalopathy are generally seen in cases of acute hyponatremia, defined as hyponatremia of less than 48 hours' duration. These symptoms can occur abruptly, sometimes with little warning.[426] A number of acutely hyponatremic patients have been reported also to develop rhabdomyolysis.[414]

The development of neurologic symptoms also depends on age, gender, and the magnitude and acuteness of the process. Elderly persons and young children with hyponatremia are most likely to develop symptoms. It has also become apparent that neurologic complications occur more frequently in menstruating women. In a case-control study, Ayus and colleagues noted that despite an approximately equal incidence of postoperative hyponatremia in males and females, 97% of those with permanent brain damage were women and 75% of them were menstruant.[356] The view that menstruating women and the elderly are more frequently affected is not universally accepted, however, because others have not found increased postoperative hyponatremia in this population,[431] and the aforementioned retrospective study did not reveal a gender or age association with mortality.[430]

The degree of clinical impairment is related not to the absolute measured level of lowered serum [Na+], but to both the rate and the extent of the fall in ECF osmolality. In a survey of hospitalized patients with hyponatremia (serum [Na+] of <128 mEq/L), 46% had CNS symptoms and 54% were asymptomatic.[432] It is notable, however, that the authors thought that the hyponatremia was the cause of the symptoms in only 31% of the symptomatic patients. In this subgroup of symptomatic patients, the mortality was no different from that of asymptomatic patients (9% to 10%). In contrast, the mortality of patients whose CNS symptoms were not caused by hyponatremia was high (64%), which suggests that the mortality of these patients is more often due to the associated disease than to the electrolyte disorder itself. This is in agreement with the report of Anderson,[250] who noted a 60-fold increase in mortality in hyponatremic patients over that in normonatremic control subjects. In the hyponatremic patients, death frequently occurred after the plasma [Na+] had returned toward normal and was generally felt to be due to progression of severe underlying disease. This suggests that the hyponatremia is an indicator of severe disease and poor prognosis. In fact, a number of recent studies further point out that even mild hyponatremia is an independent predictor of higher mortality in patients with a wide variety of disorders. These include patients with acute ST elevation myocardial infarctions, heart failure, and liver disease.[433]

The mortality of patients with acute symptomatic hyponatremia has been reported to be as high as 55% and as low as 5%.[434,435] The former figure reflects the small number of symptomatic hyponatremic patients encountered in a consultative setting, whereas the latter estimate is from a broad-based literature survey. Equally controversial is the mortality rate associated with hyponatremia in children. One series found no in-hospital deaths attributable to hyponatremia, but others described an 8.4% mortality rate in children after surgery and estimated that more than 600 children die as a result of hyponatremia in the United States yearly.[252] The mortality associated with chronic hyponatremia has been reported to be between 14% and 27%.[436,437]

The observed CNS symptoms are most likely related to the cellular swelling and cerebral edema that result from acute lowering of ECF osmolality, which leads to movement of water into cells. In fact, such cerebral edema occasionally causes herniation, as has been noted in postmortem examination of both humans and experimental animals. The increase in brain water, however, is much less marked than would be predicted from the decrease in tonicity were the brain to operate as a passive osmometer. The volume-regulatory responses that protect against cerebral edema, and that probably occur throughout the body, have been extensively studied and reviewed.[438] Studies of rats demonstrate a prompt loss of both electrolyte and organic osmolytes after the onset of hyponatremia.[439] Some of the osmolyte losses occur very quickly, within 24 hours,[440] but the loss of water becomes more marked in subsequent days (Figure 15-20).

The rate at which the brain restores the lost electrolytes and osmolytes when hyponatremia is corrected is also of pathophysiologic importance. Na+ and Cl− recover quickly and even overshoot normal brain levels.[441] However, the reaccumulation of osmolytes is considerably delayed (see Figure 15-20). This process likely accounts for the more remarked cerebral dehydration that accompanies the correction in previously adapted animals.[442] It has been observed that urea may prevent the myelinosis associated with this pathology. This may be due to the more rapid reaccumulation of organic osmolytes, and particularly myoinositol, in the azotemic state.[443]

In contrast to acute hyponatremia, chronic hyponatremia is much less symptomatic, and the reason for the profound

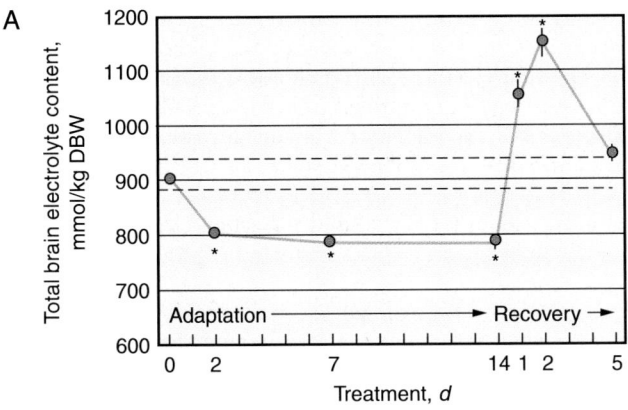

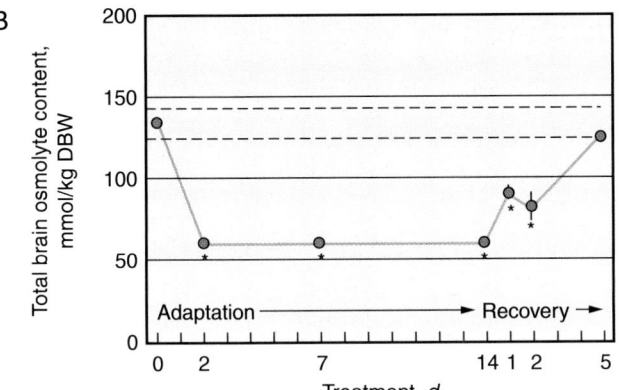

FIGURE 15-20 Comparison of changes in brain electrolyte (**A**) and organic osmolyte (**B**) contents during adaptation to hyponatremia and after rapid correction of hyponatremia in rats. Both electrolytes and organic osmolytes are lost quickly after the induction of hyponatremia beginning on day 0. Brain content of both solutes remains depressed during maintenance of hyponatremia from days 2 through 14. After rapid correction of the hyponatremia on day 14, electrolytes reaccumulate rapidly and overshoot normal brain levels on the first 2 days after correction before returning to normal levels by the fifth day after correction. In contrast, brain organic osmolytes recover much more slowly and do not return to normal brain levels until the fifth day after correction. The *dashed lines* indicate ± the standard error of the mean values of normonatremic rats on day 0. *Statistically significant difference compared with brain contents of normonatremic rats at the $P < 0.01$ level. DBW, Dry brain weight. (Data from Verbalis JG, Gullans SR: Hyponatremia causes large sustained reductions in brain content of multiple organic osmolytes in rats, *Brain Res* 567:274-282, 1991; and from Verbalis JG, Gullans SR: Rapid correction of hyponatremia produces differential effects on brain osmolyte and electrolyte reaccumulation in rats, *Brain Res* 606:19-27, 1993.)

differences between the symptoms of acute and chronic hyponatremia is now well understood to be the process of *brain volume regulation* described earlier.[444] Despite this powerful adaptation process, chronic hyponatremia is frequently associated with neurologic symptoms, albeit milder and more subtle than those in acute hyponatremia.

One report found a fairly high incidence of symptoms in 223 patients with chronic hyponatremia caused by thiazide administration: 49% experienced malaise or lethargy, 47% had dizzy spells, 35% had vomiting, 17% showed confusion or obtundation, 17% experienced falls, 6% had headaches, and 0.9% had seizures.[445] Although dizziness can potentially be attributed to diuretic-induced hypovolemia, symptoms such as confusion, obtundation, and seizures are more consistent with hyponatremic symptomatology. Because thiazide-induced hyponatremia can be readily corrected by stopping

the thiazide and/or administering sodium, this situation is an ideal one in which to assess improvement in hyponatremia symptoms with normalization of the serum [Na+]. In the aforementioned study, all of the enumerated symptoms improved with correction of the hyponatremia. This is one of the best examples demonstrating reversal of the symptoms associated with chronic hyponatremia by correction of the hyponatremia, because the patients in this study did not, in general, have severe underlying comorbid conditions that might complicate interpretation of their symptoms, as is often the case in patients with SIADH.

Even in patients judged to be "asymptomatic" by virtue of normal neurologic examination findings, accumulating evidence suggests that there may be previously unrecognized adverse effects as a result of chronic hyponatremia. In one study, 16 patients with hyponatremia secondary to SIADH in the range of 124 to 130 mmol/L demonstrated a significant gait instability that normalized after correction of the hyponatremia to normal ranges.[446] The functional significance of the gait instability was illustrated in a study of 122 Belgian patients with a variety of levels of hyponatremia, which was judged to be asymptomatic in all patients at the time of their visits to an emergency department (ED). These patients were compared with 244 age-, sex-, and disease-matched controls who also came to the emergency department during the same time period. Researchers found that 21% of the hyponatremic patients came to the ED because of a recent fall, compared with only 5% of the controls; this difference was highly significant and remained so after multivariable adjustment.[446] Consequently, this study clearly documented an increased incidence of falls in so-called asymptomatic hyponatremic patients.

The clinical significance of the gait instability and fall data were further evaluated in a study that compared 553 patients with fractures to an equal number of age- and sex-matched controls. Hyponatremia was found in 13% of the patients who had fractures compared with only 4% of the control patients.[447] Similar findings were reported in 364 elderly patients with large-bone fractures in New York[448] and in 1408 female patients with early chronic renal failure in Ireland.[449]

More recently published studies have shown that hyponatremia is associated with increased bone loss in experimental animals and a significantly increased odds ratio for osteoporosis of the femoral neck (odd ratio = 2.87; $P < 0.003$) in humans older than age 50 in the Third National Health and Nutrition Examination Survey (NHANES III) database.[450] Thus, the major clinical significance of chronic hyponatremia may lie in the increased morbidity and mortality associated with falls and fractures in the elderly population.

Treatment of Hyponatremia

Correction of hyponatremia is associated with markedly improved neurologic outcomes in patients with severely symptomatic hyponatremia. According to a retrospective review, in patients who had severe neurologic symptoms and a serum [Na+] of less than 125 mEq/L, prompt therapy with isotonic or hypertonic saline resulted in a correction in the range of 20 mEq/L over several days and neurologic recovery in almost all cases. In contrast, in patients who were treated with fluid restriction alone, there was very little correction over the study period (<5 mEq/L over 72 hours), and the neurologic outcomes were much worse, with most of these patients either dying or entering a persistently vegetative state.[451] Consequently, based on this and many similar retrospective analyses, prompt therapy to rapidly increase the serum [Na+] represents the standard of care for treatment of patients with severe life-threatening symptoms of hyponatremia.

As discussed earlier, chronic hyponatremia is much less symptomatic as a result of the process of brain volume regulation. Because of this adaptation process, chronic hyponatremia is arguably a condition that clinicians feel they may not need to be as concerned about, and this view has been reinforced by the common use of the descriptor *asymptomatic* to describe the hyponatremia in many such patients. As discussed previously, however, it is clear that many such patients very often do have neurologic symptoms, even if they are milder and more subtle, including headaches, nausea, mood disturbances, depression, difficulty concentrating, slowed reaction times, unstable gait, increased falls, confusion, and disorientation.[446] Consequently, all patients with hyponatremia who manifest any neurologic symptoms that could possibly be related to the hyponatremia should be considered as potential candidates for treatment of the hyponatremia, regardless of the chronicity of the hyponatremia or the serum [Na+] value.

Currently Available Therapies for Treatment of Hyponatremia

Conventional management strategies for hyponatremia range from saline infusion and fluid restriction to pharmacologic measures to adjust fluid balance. Consideration of treatment options should always include an evaluation of the benefits as well as the potential toxicities of any therapy, and therapies must be individualized for each patient.[452] It should always be remembered that sometimes simply stopping treatment with an agent that is associated with hyponatremia is sufficient to reverse a low serum [Na+].

Isotonic Saline

The treatment of choice for depletional hyponatremia (i.e., hypovolemic hyponatremia) is isotonic saline ([Na+] = 154 mmol/L) to restore ECF volume and ensure adequate organ perfusion. This initial therapy is appropriate for patients who either have clinical signs of hypovolemia or in whom a spot urine Na+ concentration is less than 30 mEq/L. However, this therapy is ineffective for dilutional hyponatremias such as SIADH,[394] and continued inappropriate administration of isotonic saline to a euvolemic patient may worsen the hyponatremia[454] and/or cause fluid overload. Although isotonic saline may improve the serum [Na+] in some patients with hypervolemic hyponatremia, their volume status generally worsens with this therapy, so unless the hyponatremia is profound isotonic saline should be avoided.

Hypertonic Saline

Acute hyponatremia presenting with severe neurologic symptoms is life-threatening and should be treated promptly with hypertonic solutions, typically 3% NaCl ([Na+] = 513 mmol/L), because this is the most reliable method to raise the serum [Na+] quickly. A continuous infusion of hypertonic

NaCl is generally used in inpatient settings. Various formulas have been suggested for calculating the initial rate of infusion of hypertonic solutions,[455] but until now there has been no consensus regarding optimal infusion rates of 3% NaCl. One of the simplest methods to estimate an initial 3% NaCl infusion rate utilizes the following relationship[452]:

$$\text{Patient's weight (kg)} \times \text{Desired correction rate (mEq/L/hr)}$$
$$= \text{Infusion rate of 3\% NaCl (mL/hr)}$$

Depending on individual hospital policies, the administration of hypertonic solutions may require that special procedures be followed (e.g., placement in the intensive care unit, sign-off by a consultant, etc.), of which each clinician must be aware to optimize patient care. An alternative option for more emergent situations is administration of a 100-mL bolus of 3% NaCl, repeated once if there is no clinical improvement in 30 minutes, an intervention which has been recommended by a consensus conference organized to develop guidelines for the prevention and treatment of exercise-induced hyponatremia, an acute and potentially lethal condition.[456] Injecting this amount of hypertonic saline intravenously raises the serum [Na+] by an average of 2 to 4 mEq/L, which is well below the recommended maximal daily rate of change of 10 to 12 mEq/24 hr or 18 mEq/48 hr.[457] Because the brain can only accommodate an average increase of approximately 8% in brain volume before herniation occurs, quickly increasing the serum [Na+] by as little as 2 to 4 mEq/L in acute hyponatremia can effectively reduce brain swelling and intracranial pressure.[458]

Many physicians are hesitant to use hypertonic saline in patients with chronic hyponatremia, because it can cause an overly rapid correction of serum sodium levels that can lead to osmotic demyelination syndrome.[459] Nonetheless, this remains the treatment of choice for patients with severe neurologic symptoms, even when the time course of the hyponatremia is nonacute or unknown. The administration of hypertonic saline is generally not recommended for most patients with edema-forming disorders because it acts as a volume expander and may exacerbate volume overload; consequently, as with isotonic NaCl, unless the hyponatremia is profound hypertonic saline should be avoided.

Fluid Restriction

For patients with chronic hyponatremia, fluid restriction has been the most popular and most widely accepted treatment. When SIADH is present, fluids should generally be limited to 500 to 1000 mL/24 hr. Because fluid restriction increases the serum [Na+] largely by underreplacing the fluid excreted by the kidneys, some have advocated an initial restriction to 500 mL less than the 24-hour urine output.[460] When fluid restriction is instituted, it is important for the nursing staff and the patient to understand that this includes *all* fluids that are consumed, not just water. Generally the water content of ingested food is not included in the restriction because it is balanced by insensible water losses (perspiration, exhaled air, feces, etc.), but caution should be exercised with foods that have high fluid concentrations (such as fruits and soups).

Restricting fluid intake can be effective when properly applied and managed in selected patients, but serum [Na+] is increased only slowly (1 to 2 mEq/L/day) even with severe restriction.[394] In addition, this therapy is often poorly tolerated because of an associated increase in thirst, which leads to poor adherence to a long-term restriction regimen. It is economically advantageous, however, and some patients do respond well to this option.

Fluid restriction should not be used in hypovolemic patients and is particularly difficult to maintain in patients with very elevated urine osmolalities secondary to high AVP levels. In general, if the sum of urine Na^+ and K^+ concentrations exceeds the serum $[Na^+]$, patients will not respond to fluid restriction in most cases, since electrolyte-free water clearance will be difficult to achieve.[461-463] In addition, fluid restriction is not practical for some patients, particularly patients in intensive care settings, who often require administration of significant volumes of fluids as part of their therapies.

Demeclocycline

Demeclocycline, a tetracycline antibiotic, inhibits adenylyl cyclase activation after AVP binds to its V_2 receptor in the kidney and thus targets the underlying pathophysiology of SIADH. This therapy is typically used when patients find severe fluid restriction unacceptable and the underlying disorder cannot be corrected. Demeclocycline is not approved by the U.S. Food and Drug Administration (FDA) for the treatment of hyponatremia, however, and can cause nephrotoxicity in patients with heart failure and cirrhosis, although this is usually reversible if caught quickly enough.[464]

Mineralocorticoids

Administration of mineralocorticoids, such as fludrocortisone, has been shown to be useful in a small number of elderly patients.[465] However, the initial studies of SIADH did not show it to be of benefit in patients with SIADH, and it carries the risk of fluid overload and hypertension. Consequently, it is rarely used to treat hyponatremia in the United States.

Urea

Administration of urea has been used successfully to treat hyponatremia because it induces osmotic diuresis and augments free water excretion. Effective dosages of urea for the treatment of hyponatremia are 30 to 90 g daily in divided doses.[466] Unfortunately, its use is limited because there is no United States Pharmacopeia formulation of urea, and it is not approved by the FDA for the treatment of hyponatremia. For this reason, urea has not been used extensively in the United States, and data to support its long-term use are limited. Furthermore, urea is associated with poor palatability, which leads to patient adherence problems. However, patients with feeding tubes may be excellent candidates for urea therapy since palatability is not a concern in this case, and the use of fluid restriction may be difficult in some patients with high obligate intake of fluids as part of their nutritional and medication therapy. Although mild increases in blood urea concentration can be seen with urea therapy, it rarely reaches clinically significant levels.

Furosemide and NaCl

The use of furosemide (40 mg/day) coupled with a high salt intake (200 mEq/day), which represents an extension of the treatment of acute symptomatic hyponatremia to the long-term management of euvolemic hyponatremia, has also been reported to be successful in selected cases.[467] However, the long-term efficacy and safety of this approach is unknown.

Arginine Vasopressin Receptor Antagonists

Clinicians have used all of the aforementioned conventional therapies for hyponatremia over the past decades. However, conventional therapies for hyponatremia, although effective in specific circumstances, are suboptimal for many different reasons, including variable efficacy, slow responses, intolerable side effects, and serious toxicities. But perhaps the most striking deficiency of most conventional therapies is that, with the exception of demeclocycline, these therapies do not directly target the underlying cause of almost all dilutional hyponatremias, namely, inappropriately elevated plasma AVP levels. A new class of pharmacologic agents, AVP receptor (AVPR) antagonists, that directly block AVP-mediated receptor activation have recently been approved by the FDA for the treatment of euvolemic and hypervolemic hyponatremia.[468]

Conivaptan and tolvaptan are competitive receptor antagonists of the AVP V_2 (antidiuretic) receptor and have been approved by the FDA for the treatment of euvolemic and hypervolemic hyponatremia. These agents, also known as *vaptans*, compete with AVP/ADH for binding at its site of action in the kidney, thereby blocking the antidiuresis caused by elevated AVP levels and directly attacking the underlying pathophysiology of dilutional hyponatremia. AVPR antagonists produce electrolyte free water excretion (called *aquaresis*) without affecting renal sodium and potassium excretion.[469] The overall result is a reduction in body water without natriuresis, which leads to an increase in the serum $[Na^+]$. One of the major benefits of this class of drugs is that serum $[Na^+]$ is significantly increased by an average of 4 to 8 mEq/L within 24 to 48 hours,[470,471] which is considerably faster than the effects of fluid restriction, which can take many days. Also, patient adherence has not been shown to be problem for vaptan therapy, whereas it is a major problem with attempted long-term use of fluid restriction.

Conivaptan is FDA approved for treatment of euvolemic and hypervolemic hyponatremia in hospitalized patients. It is available only as an intravenous preparation and is given as a 20-mg loading dose over 30 minutes, followed by a continuous infusion of 20 or 40 mg/day.[472] Generally, the 20-mg/day continuous infusion is used for the first 24 hours to gauge the initial response. If the correction of serum $[Na^+]$ is felt to be inadequate (e.g., <5 mEq/L), then the infusion rate can be increased to 40 mg/day. Therapy is limited to a maximum duration of 4 days because of drug interaction with other agents metabolized by hepatic cytochrome P450 isoenzyme 3A4.

Importantly, for conivaptan and all other vaptans, it is critical that the serum $[Na^+]$ concentration be measured frequently during the active phase of correction of the hyponatremia (a minimum of every 6 to 8 hours for conivaptan, but more frequently in patients with risk factors for the development of osmotic demyelination, such as severely low serum $[Na^+]$, malnutrition, alcoholism, or hypokalemia).[452] If the correction approaches 12 mEq/L in the first 24 hours, the infusion should be stopped and the patient monitored on fluid restriction. If the correction exceeds 12 mEq/L, consideration should be given to administering sufficient water, either orally or as intravenous 5% dextrose in water, to bring the overall correction below 12 mEq/L. The maximum correction limit should be reduced to 8 mEq/L over the first 24 hours in patients with risk factors for the development of osmotic demyelination, as mentioned previously. The most common adverse effects are injection-site reactions, which are generally mild and usually do not lead to treatment discontinuation; headache; thirst; and hypokalemia.[470]

Tolvaptan, an oral AVPR antagonist, is FDA approved for the treatment of dilutional hyponatremias. In contrast to conivaptan, it can be used for both short- and long-term treatment of hyponatremia because it is administered orally.[471] As with conivaptan, treatment with tolvaptan must be initiated in the hospital so that the rate of correction can be monitored carefully. Patients with a serum [Na+] of less than 125 mEq/L are eligible for therapy with tolvaptan as primary treatment; if the serum [Na+] is 125 mEq/L or more, tolvaptan therapy is indicated only if the patient has symptoms that could be attributable to the hyponatremia and the patient is resistant to attempts at fluid restriction.[473] The starting dose of tolvaptan is 15 mg on the first day, and the dose can be titrated to 30 mg and 60 mg at 24-hour intervals if the serum [Na+] remains below 135 mEq/L or the increase in serum [Na+] has been 5 mEq/L or less in the previous 24 hours.

As with conivaptan, it is essential that the serum [Na+] value be measured frequently during the active phase of correction of the hyponatremia (a minimum of every 6 to 8 hours, but more frequently in patients with risk factors for the development of osmotic demyelination). Limits for safe correction of hyponatremia and methods to compensate for overly rapid corrections are the same as described previously for conivaptan. One additional factor that helps to avoid overly rapid correction with tolvaptan is the recommendation that fluid restriction not be used during the active phase of correction, which allows the patient's thirst to compensate for an overly vigorous aquaresis. Common side effects include dry mouth, thirst, increased urinary frequency, dizziness, nausea, and orthostatic hypotension, which were relatively similar in placebo and tolvaptan groups in clinical trials.[471,473]

Because induction of increased renal fluid excretion via either diuresis or aquaresis can cause or worsen hypotension in patients with hypovolemic hyponatremia, vaptans are contraindicated in this patient population.[452] However, clinically significant hypotension was not observed in the clinical trials of either conivaptan or tolvaptan in euvolemic and hypervolemic hyponatremic patients. Although vaptans are not contraindicated in patients with decreased renal function, these agents generally will not be effective if the serum creatinine level is more than 2.5 mg/dL.

Hyponatremia Treatment Guidelines

Although various authors have published recommendations on the treatment of hyponatremia,[452,455,474-476] no standardized treatment algorithms have yet been widely accepted. The field is in need of evidence-based strategies. A synthesis of existing expert recommendations for treatment of hyponatremia is presented in Figure 15-21. This algorithm is based primarily on the symptomatology of hyponatremic patients, rather than the serum [Na+] or the chronicity of the hyponatremia, the latter of which is often difficult to ascertain. A careful neurologic history taking and assessment should always be done to identify potential causes for the patient's symptoms other than hyponatremia, although it will not always be possible to exclude an additive contribution from the hyponatremia to an underlying neurologic condition. In this model, patients are divided into three groups based on their presenting symptoms.

Level 1 symptoms include seizures, coma, respiratory arrest, obtundation, and vomiting, and usually imply a more acute onset or worsening of hyponatremia requiring immediate

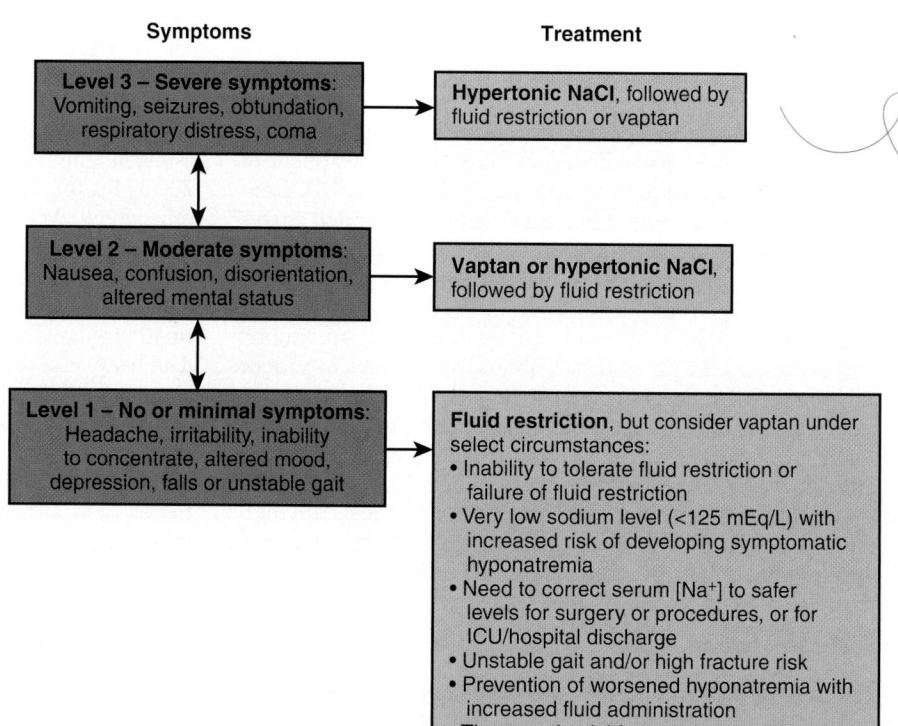

FIGURE 15-21 Algorithm for treatment of patients with hyponatremia based on presenting symptoms. The arrows between the symptom levels emphasize that patients often move between symptom levels as hyponatremia progresses or resolves.

active treatment. Therapies that will quickly raise serum sodium levels are required to reduce cerebral edema and decrease the risk of potentially fatal herniation.

Level 2 symptoms, which are more moderate, include nausea, confusion, disorientation, and altered mental status. These symptoms may be either chronic or acute, but the patient's condition allows time to elaborate a more deliberate approach to treatment.

Level 3 symptoms range from minimal symptoms such as a headache, irritability, inability to concentrate, altered mood, and depression to a virtual absence of discernible symptoms, and indicate that the patient may have chronic or slowly evolving hyponatremia. These symptoms call for a cautious approach, especially when patients have underlying comorbid conditions.

Patients with severe symptoms (level 1) should be treated with hypertonic saline as first-line therapy, followed by fluid restriction with or without AVPR antagonist therapy. Patients with moderate symptoms can benefit from a regimen of vaptan therapy or limited hypertonic saline administration, followed by fluid restriction or long-term vaptan therapy. Although moderate neurologic symptoms can indicate that a patient is in an early stage of acute hyponatremia, they more often indicate a chronically hyponatremic state with sufficient brain volume adaptation to prevent marked symptoms from cerebral edema. Regardless, close monitoring of these patients in a hospital setting is warranted until the symptoms improve or stabilize. Patients with no or minimal symptoms should be managed initially with fluid restriction, although treatment with vaptans may be appropriate for a wide range of specific clinical conditions, foremost of which is a failure of the serum [Na⁺] to improve despite reasonable attempts at fluid restriction (see Figure 15-21).

A special case is that in which spontaneous correction of hyponatremia occurs at an undesirably rapid rate as a result of the onset of water diuresis. This can occur following cessation of desmopressin therapy in a patient who has become hyponatremic, replacement of glucocorticoids in a patient with adrenal insufficiency, replacement of solutes in a patient with diuretic-induced hyponatremia, or spontaneous resolution of transient SIADH. Brain damage from osmotic demyelination syndrome can clearly ensue in this setting if the preceding period of hyponatremia has been of sufficient duration (usually ≥48 hours) to allow brain volume regulation to occur. If the previously discussed correction parameters have been exceeded and the correction is proceeding more rapidly than planned (usually because of abrupt excretion of hypotonic urine), the pathologic events leading to demyelination can be reversed by readministration of hypotonic fluids and desmopressin. The efficacy of this approach is suggested by both animal studies[477] and case reports in humans,[475,478] even when patients are overtly symptomatic.[479]

Although the aforementioned classification is based on presenting symptoms at the time of initial evaluation, it should be remembered that in some cases patients initially exhibit more moderate symptoms because they are in the early stages of hyponatremia. In addition, some patients with minimal symptoms are prone to develop more symptomatic hyponatremia during periods of increased fluid ingestion. In support of this observation, in approximately 70% of 31 patients who came to a university hospital with symptomatic hyponatremia and a mean serum [Na⁺] of 119 mmol/L, preexisting "asymptomatic" hyponatremia was the most common

risk factor identified.[480] Consequently, treatment of hyponatremia should also be considered to prevent progression from lower to higher levels of symptomatic hyponatremia, particularly in patients with a history of repeated presentations with symptomatic hyponatremia.

Monitoring of Serum [Na⁺] in Hyponatremic Patients

The frequency of serum [Na⁺] monitoring depends on both the severity of the hyponatremia and the therapy chosen. In all hyponatremic patients neurologic symptoms should be carefully assessed very early in the diagnostic evaluation to establish the symptomatic severity of the hyponatremia and to determine whether the patient requires more urgent therapy. In all patients undergoing active treatment with hypertonic saline for level 1 or 2 symptomatic hyponatremia, serum [Na⁺] and ECF volume status should be monitored frequently (every 2 to 4 hours) to ensure that the serum [Na⁺] does not exceeded the recommended levels during the active phase of correction[452]; overly rapid correction of serum sodium can cause damage to the myelin sheath of nerve cells, resulting in central pontine or basal ganglia myelinolysis, also known as *osmotic demyelination syndrome.*[459]

In patients treated with vaptans for level 2 or 3 symptoms, serum [Na⁺] should be monitored every 6 to 8 hours during the active phase of correction, which is generally the first 24 to 48 hours of therapy. Active treatment with hypertonic saline or vaptans should be stopped when the patient's symptoms are no longer present, a safe serum [Na⁺] (usually >120 mEq/L) has been achieved, or the rate of correction has reached 12 mEq/L within 24 hours or 18 mEq/L within 48 hours.[452,457] Importantly, osmotic demyelination syndrome has not yet been reported either in clinical trials of vaptans or with therapeutic use of any vaptan to date.

In patients with a stable level of serum [Na⁺] treated with fluid restriction or therapies other than hypertonic saline, measurement of serum [Na⁺] daily is generally sufficient, since levels will not change that quickly in the absence of active therapy or large changes in fluid intake or administration.

Long-Term Treatment of Chronic Hyponatremia

Some patients benefit from continued treatment of hyponatremia after discharge from the hospital. In many cases, such treatment consists of continued fluid restriction. However, as discussed previously, long-term adherence to this therapy regimen is poor due to the increased thirst that occurs with more severe degrees of fluid restriction. Thus, for selected patients whose hyponatremia has responded to tolvaptan in the hospital, consideration should be given to continuing the treatment on an outpatient basis after discharge. In patients with established chronic hyponatremia, tolvaptan has been shown to be effective in maintaining a normal [Na⁺] for as long as 4 years with continued daily therapy.[481]

Many patients who experience hyponatremia in the hospital, however, have a transient form of SIADH and do not need long-term therapy. In the conivaptan open-label study, approximately 70% of patients treated as inpatients for 4 days had normal serum [Na⁺] concentrations 7 and 30 days after

Etiology of SIADH	Likely duration of SIADH*	Relative risk of chronic SIADH
Tumors producing vasopressin ectopically (small-cell lung carcinoma, head and neck carcinoma)	Indefinite	**High**
Drug-induced, with continuation of offending agent (carbamazepine, SSRI)	Duration of drug therapy	
Brain tumors	Indefinite	
Idiopathic (senile)	Indefinite	
Subarachnoid hemorrhage	1–4 weeks	
Stroke	1–2 weeks	
Inflammatory brain lesions	Dependent on response to therapy	**Medium**
Respiratory failure (chronic obstructive lung disease)	Dependent on response to therapy	
HIV infection	Dependent on response to therapy	
Traumatic brain injury	2–7 days to indefinite	
Drug-induced, with cessation of offending agent	Duration of drug therapy	
Pneumonia	2–5 days	
Nausea, pain, prolonged exercise	Variable depending on cause	
Post-operative hyponatraemia	2–3 days postoperatively	**Low**
*Time frames are based on clinical experience.		

FIGURE 15-22 Estimated probability of need for long-term treatment of syndrome of inappropriate antidiuretic hormone secretion (SIADH) depending on underlying cause.

cessation of the vaptan therapy in the absence of long-term therapy for hyponatremia. Determination of which patients with hyponatremia during hospitalization are candidates for long-term therapy should be based on the cause of the SIADH. Figure 15-22 shows estimates of the relative probability that inpatients with SIADH due to different causes will have persistent hyponatremia that may benefit from long-term treatment with tolvaptan after discharge from the hospital. Nonetheless, for any individual patient this simply represents an estimate of the likelihood that long-term therapy will be required. In all cases, consideration should be given to a trial of stopping the drug at 2 to 4 weeks after discharge to see if hyponatremia is still present.

A reasonable period of tolvaptan cessation to evaluate for the presence of continued SIADH is 7 days, since this period was sufficient to demonstrate a recurrence of hyponatremia in the tolvaptan clinical trials.[471,481] Serum [Na$^+$] should be monitored every 2 or 3 days following cessation of tolvaptan so that the drug can be resumed as quickly as possible in those patients with recurrent hyponatremia, because the longer the patient is hyponatremic, the greater the risk of subsequent osmotic demyelination with overly rapid correction of the low serum [Na$^+$].

Future of Hyponatremia Treatment

Guidelines for the appropriate treatment of hyponatremia, and particularly the role of vaptan therapy, are still evolving and will undoubtedly change substantially over the next several years. Of special interest will be studies to assess whether more effective treatment of hyponatremia can decrease the incidence of falls and fractures in elderly patients, can reduce utilization of health care resources by both inpatients and outpatients with hyponatremia, and can lower the markedly increased morbidity and mortality of patients with hyponatremia across multiple disease states. The potential use of vaptans in the treatment of heart failure has already been studied. A large trial, Efficacy of Vasopressin Antagonism in Heart Failure Outcome Study with Tolvaptan (EVEREST), demonstrated short-term improvement in dyspnea, but no long-term survival benefit.[482] However, this trial was not powered to evaluate the outcomes of hyponatremic patients with heart failure. Consequently, the potential therapeutic role of these antagonists in the treatment of water-retaining disorders must await further studies specifically designed to assess the outcomes of hyponatremic patients treated with vaptans, as well as clinical experience that better delineates efficacies as well as potential toxicities of all treatments for hyponatremia. Nonetheless, it is abundantly clear that the vaptans have ushered in a new era in the evaluation and treatment of hyponatremic disorders.

References

1. Edelman IS, Leibman J. Anatomy of body water and electrolytes. *Am J Med.* 1959;27:256-277.
2. Fanestil DD. Compartmentation of body water. In: Narins RG, ed. *Clinical disorders of fluid and electrolyte metabolism.* New York: McGraw-Hill; 1994: pp 3-20.

3. Thomas RC. Electrogenic sodium pump in nerve and muscle cells. *Physiol Rev.* 1972;52:563.

4. Wolf AV, McDowell ME. Apparent and osmotic volumes of distribution of sodium, chloride, sulfate and urea. *Am J Physiol.* 1954;176:207.

5. Maffly RH, Leaf A. The potential of water in mammalian tissues. *J Gen Physiol.* 1959;42:1257.

6. Leaf A, Chatillon JY, Tuttle EPJ. The mechanism of the osmotic adjustment of body cells as determined in vivo by the volume of distribution of a large water load. *J Clin Invest.* 1954;33:1261.

7. Rose BD. New approach to disturbances in the plasma sodium concentration. *Am J Med.* 1986;81:1033-1040.

8. Hendry EB. Osmolarity of human serum and of chemical solutions of biologic importance. *Clin Chem.* 1961;7:156.

9. Zerbe RL, Robertson GL. Osmoregulation of thirst and vasopressin secretion in human subjects: effect of various solutes. *Am J Physiol.* 1983;244:E607-E614.

10. Vokes TP, Aycinena PR, Robertson GL. Effect of insulin on osmoregulation of vasopressin. *Am J Physiol.* 1987;252:E538-E548.

11. de Castro J. A microregulatory analysis of spontaneous fluid intake in humans: evidence that the amount of liquid ingested and its timing is mainly governed by feeding. *Physiol Behav.* 1988;3:705-714.

12. Adolph EF. *Physiology of man in the desert.* New York: Hafner Publishing; 1969.

13. Du Vigneaud V. Hormones of the posterior pituitary gland: Oxytocin and vasopressin. In: DuVigneaud V, Bing RJ, Oncley JL, eds. *The Harvey Lectures, 1954-55.* New York: Academic Press; 1956:p 1.

14. Edwards BR, LaRochelle Jr FT. Antidiuretic effect of endogenous oxytocin in dehydrated Brattleboro homozygous rats. *Am J Physiol.* 1984;247(3 pt 2):F453-F465.

15. Oliver G, Schaefer EA. On the physiological actions of extracts of the pituitary body and certain other glandular organs. *J Physiol (Lond).* 1895;18:277-279.

16. Cowley Jr AW. Vasopressin and blood pressure regulation. *Clin Physiol Biochem.* 1988;6(3-4):150-162.

17. Thibonnier M, Conarty DM, Preston JA, et al. Molecular pharmacology of human vasopressin receptors. *Adv Exp Med Biol.* 1998;449:251-276.

18. Mohr E, Bahnsen U, Kiessling C, et al. Expression of the vasopressin and oxytocin genes in rats occurs in mutually exclusive sets of hypothalamic neurons. *FEBS Lett.* 1988;242(1):144-148.

19. Mohr E, Richter D. Sequence analysis of the promoter region of the rat vasopressin gene. *FEBS Lett.* 1990;260(2):305-308.

20. Gainer H, Yamashita M, Fields RL, et al. The magnocellular neuronal phenotype: cell-specific gene expression in the hypothalamo-neurohypophysial system. *Prog Brain Res.* 2002;139:1-14.

21. Richter D. Molecular events in expression of vasopressin and oxytocin and their cognate receptors. *Am J Physiol.* 1988;255(2 pt 2):F207-F219.

22. Robinson AG, Haluszczak C, Wilkins JA, et al. Physiologic control of two neurophysins in humans. *J Clin Endocrinol Metab.* 1977;44(2):330-339.

23. Nowycky MC, Seward EP, Chernevskaya NI. Excitation-secretion coupling in mammalian neurohypophysial nerve terminals. *Cell Mol Neurobiol.* 1998;18(1):65-80.

24. Herman JP, Schafer MK, Watson SJ, et al. In situ hybridization analysis of arginine vasopressin gene transcription using intron-specific probes.

25. Majzoub JA, Rich A, van Boom J, et al. Vasopressin and oxytocin mRNA regulation in the rat assessed by hybridization with synthetic oligonucleotides. *J Biol Chem.* 1983;258(23):14061-14064.

26. Robinson AG, Roberts MM, Evron WA, et al. Hyponatremia in rats induces downregulation of vasopressin synthesis. *J Clin Invest.* 1990;86:1023-1029.

27. Fitzsimmons MD, Roberts MM, Robinson AG. Control of posterior pituitary vasopressin content: implications for the regulation of the vasopressin gene. *Endocrinology.* 1994;134(4):1874-1878.

28. Leng G, Mason WT, Dyer RG. The supraoptic nucleus as an osmoreceptor. *Neuroendocrinology.* 1982;34(1):75-82.

29. Verbalis JG. How does the brain sense osmolality? *J Am Soc Nephrol.* 2007;18(12):3056-3059.

30. Buggy J, Jonhson AK. Preoptic-hypothalamic periventricular lesions: thirst deficits and hypernatremia. *Am J Physiol.* 1977;233(1):R44-R52.

31. Thrasher TN, Keil LC, Ramsay DJ. Lesions of the organum vasculosum of the lamina terminalis (OVLT) attenuate osmotically-induced drinking and vasopressin secretion in the dog. *Endocrinology.* 1982;110(5):1837-1839.

32. Robertson GL. The regulation of vasopressin function in health and disease. *Rec Prog Horm Res.* 1976;33:333-385.

33. Zerbe RL, Miller JZ, Robertson GL. The reproducibility and heritability of individual differences in osmoregulatory function in normal human subjects. *J Lab Clin Med.* 1991;117:51-59.

34. Helderman JH, Vestal RE, Rowe JW, et al. The response of arginine vasopressin to intravenous ethanol and hypertonic saline in man: the impact of aging. *J Gerontol.* 1978;33:39-47.

35. Ledingham JGG, Crowe MJ, Forsling ML. Effects of aging on vasopressin secretion, water excretion, and thirst in man. *Kidney Int.* 1987;32(Suppl):S90-S92.

36. Baylis PH. Osmoregulation and control of vasopressin secretion in healthy humans. *Am J Physiol.* 1987;253(5 pt 2):R671-R678.

37. Vokes TJ, Weiss NM, Schreiber J, et al. Osmoregulation of thirst and vasopressin during normal menstrual cycle. *Am J Physiol.* 1988;254:R641-R647.

38. Vallotton MB, Merkelbach U, Gaillard RC. Studies of the factors modulating antidiuretic hormone excretion in man in response to the osmolar stimulus: effects of oestrogen and angiotensin II. *Acta Endocrinol (Copenh).* 1983;104(3):295-302.

39. Davison JM, Gilmore EA, et al. Altered osmotic thresholds for vasopressin secretion and thirst in human pregnancy. *Am J Physiol.* 1984;246:F105-F109.

40. Weisinger RS, Burns P, Eddie LW, et al. Relaxin alters the plasma osmolality-arginine vasopressin relationship in the rat. *J Endocrinol.* 1993;137(3):505-510.

41. Leng G, Brown CH, Bull PM, et al. Responses of magnocellular neurons to osmotic stimulation involves coactivation of excitatory and inhibitory input: an experimental and theoretical analysis. *J Neurosci.* 2001;21(17):6967-6977.

42. Verbalis JG. Osmotic inhibition of neurohypophysial secretion. *Ann N Y Acad Sci.* 1993;689:146-160.

43. Thrasher TN. Osmoreceptor mediation of thirst and vasopressin secretion in the dog. *Fed Proc.* 1982;41(9):2528-2532.

44. Bourque CW, Voisin DL, Chakfe Y. Stretch-inactivated cation channels: cellular targets for modulation of osmosensitivity in supraoptic neurons. *Prog Brain Res.* 2002;139:85-94.

45. Sladek CD, Kapoor JR. Neurotransmitter/neuropeptide interactions in the regulation of neurohypophyseal hormone release. *Exp Neurol.* 2001;171(2):200-209.

46. Ludwig M, Sabatier N, Dayanithi G, et al. The active role of dendrites in the regulation of magnocellular neurosecretory cell behavior. *Prog Brain Res.* 2002;139:247-256.

47. Liedtke W, Kim C. Functionality of the TRPV subfamily of TRP ion channels: add mechano-TRP and osmo-TRP to the lexicon!. *Cell Mol Life Sci.* 2005;62(24):2985-3001.

48. Liedtke W. Role of TRPV ion channels in sensory transduction of osmotic stimuli in mammals. *Exp Physiol.* 2007;92(3):507-512.

49. Schrier RW, Berl T, Anderson RJ. Osmotic and nonosmotic control of vasopressin release. *Am J Physiol.* 1979;236:F321-F332.

50. Raff H, Merrill D, Skelton M, et al. Control of ACTH and vasopressin in neurohypophysectomized conscious dogs. *Am J Physiol.* 1985;249(2 pt 2):R281-R284.

51. Dunn FL, Brennan TJ, Nelson AE, et al. The role of blood osmolality and volume in regulating vasopressin secretion in the rat. *J Clin Invest.* 1973;52:3212-3219.

52. Stricker EM, Verbalis JG. Interaction of osmotic and volume stimuli in regulation of neurohypophyseal secretion in rats. *Am J Physiol.* 1986;250:R267-R275.

53. Goldsmith SR, Francis GS, Cowley AW, et al. Response of vasopressin and norepinephrine to lower body negative pressure in humans. *Am J Physiol.* 1982;243(6):H970-H973.

54. Goldsmith SR, Cowley Jr AW, Francis GS, et al. Effect of increased intracardiac and arterial pressure on plasma vasopressin in humans. *Am J Physiol.* 1984;246(5 pt 2):H647-H651.

55. Robertson GL, Athar S. The interaction of blood osmolality and blood volume in regulating plasma vasopressin in man. *J Clin Endocrinol Metab.* 1976;42:613-620.

56. Quillen Jr EW, Cowley Jr AW. Influence of volume changes on osmolality-vasopressin relationships in conscious dogs. *Am J Physiol.* 1983;244(1):H73-H79.

57. Andresen MC, Doyle MW, Jin YH, et al. Cellular mechanisms of baroreceptor integration at the nucleus tractus solitarius. *Ann N Y Acad Sci.* 2001;940:132-141.

58. Renaud LP. CNS pathways mediating cardiovascular regulation of vasopressin. *Clin Exp Pharmacol Physiol.* 1996;23(2):157-160.

59. Blessing WW, Sved AF, Reis DJ. Destruction of noradrenergic neurons in rabbit brainstem elevates plasma vasopressin, causing hypertension. *Science.* 1982;217(4560):661-663.

60. Berl T, Cadnapaphornchai P, Harbottle JA, et al. Mechanism of suppression of vasopressin during alpha-adrenergic stimulation with norepinephrine. *J Clin Invest.* 1974;53(1):219-227.

61. Schrier RW. Pathogenesis of sodium and water retention in high-output and low-output cardiac failure, nephrotic syndrome, cirrhosis, and pregnancy (1). *N Engl J Med.* 1988;319:1065-1072.

62. Schrier RW. Pathogenesis of sodium and water retention in high-output and low-output cardiac failure, nephrotic syndrome, cirrhosis, and pregnancy (2). *N Engl J Med.* 1988;319:1127-1134.

63. Zerbe RL, Henry DP, Robertson GL. Vasopressin response to orthostatic hypotension. Etiologic and clinical implications. *Am J Med.* 1983;74(2):265-271.

64. Seckl JR, Williams TD, Lightman SL. Oral hypertonic saline causes transient fall of vasopressin in humans. *Am J Physiol.* 1986;251(2 pt 2):R214-R217.

65. Thompson CJ, Burd JM, Baylis PH. Acute suppression of plasma vasopressin and thirst after drinking in hypernatremic humans. *Am J Physiol.* 1987;252(6 pt 2):R1138-R1142.
66. Salata RA, Verbalis JG, Robinson AG. Cold water stimulation of oropharyngeal receptors in man inhibits release of vasopressin. *J Clin Endocrinol Metab.* 1987;65:561-567.
67. Rowe JW, Shelton RL, Helderman JH, et al. Influence of the emetic reflex on vasopressin release in man. *Kidney Int.* 1979;16:729-735.
68. Verbalis JG, McHale CM, Gardiner TW, et al. Oxytocin and vasopressin secretion in response to stimuli producing learned taste aversions in rats. *Behav Neurosci.* 1986;100:466-475.
69. Baylis PH, Robertson GL. Rat vasopressin response to insulin-induced hypoglycemia. *Endocrinology.* 1980;107:1975-1979.
70. Baylis PH, Zerbe RL, Robertson GL. Arginine vasopressin response to insulin-induced hypoglycemia in man. *J Clin Endocrinol Metab.* 1981;53:935-940.
71. Thompson DA, Campbell RG, Lilavivat U, et al. Increased thirst and plasma arginine vasopressin levels during 2-deoxy-D-glucose-induced glucoprivation in humans. *J Clin Invest.* 1981;67:1083-1093.
72. Keil LC, Summy-Long J, Severs WB. Release of vasopressin by angiotensin II. *Endocrinology.* 1975;96(4):1063-1065.
73. Ferguson AV, Renaud LP. Systemic angiotensin acts at subfornical organ to facilitate activity of neurohypophysial neurons. *Am J Physiol.* 1986;251(4 pt 2):R712-R717.
74. McKinley MJ, McAllen RM, Pennington GL, et al. Physiological actions of angiotensin II mediated by AT1 and AT2 receptors in the brain. *Clin Exp Pharmacol Physiol Suppl.* 1996;3:S99-S104.
75. McKinley MJ, Allen AM, Mathai ML, et al. Brain angiotensin and body fluid homeostasis. *Jpn J Physiol.* 2001;51(3):281-289.
76. Yamaguchi K, Sakaguchi T, Kamoi K. Central role of angiotensin in the hyperosmolality- and hypovolaemia-induced vasopressin release in conscious rats. *Acta Endocrinol (Copenh).* 1982;101(4):524-530.
77. Stocker SD, Stricker EM, Sved AF. Acute hypertension inhibits thirst stimulated by ANG II, hyperosmolality, or hypovolemia in rats. *Am J Physiol Regul Integr Comp Physiol.* 2001;280(1):R214-R224.
78. Keil LC, Severs WB. Reduction in plasma vasopressin levels of dehydrated rats following acute stress. *Endocrinology.* 1977;100(1):30-38.
79. Edelson JT, Robertson GL. The effect of the cold pressor test on vasopressin secretion in man. *Psychoneuroendocrinology.* 1986;11:307-316.
80. Ukai M, Moran Jr WH, Zimmermann B. The role of visceral afferent pathways on vasopressin secretion and urinary excretory patterns during surgical stress. *Ann Surg.* 1968;168(1):16-28.
81. Chikanza IC, Petrou P, Chrousos G. Perturbations of arginine vasopressin secretion during inflammatory stress. Pathophysiologic implications. *Ann N Y Acad Sci.* 2000;917:825-834.
82. Baylis PH, Stockley RA, Heath DA. Effect of acute hypoxaemia on plasma arginine vasopressin in conscious man. *Clin Sci Mol Med.* 1977;53(4):401-404.
83. Claybaugh JR, Hansen JE, Wozniak DB. Response of antidiuretic hormone to acute exposure to mild and severe hypoxia in man. *J Endocrinol.* 1978;77(2):157-160.
84. Rose Jr CE, Anderson RJ, Carey RM. Antidiuresis and vasopressin release with hypoxemia and hypercapnia in conscious dogs. *Am J Physiol.* 1984;247(1 pt 2):R127-R134.
85. Raff H, Shinsako J, Keil LC, et al. Vasopressin, ACTH, and corticosteroids during hypercapnia and graded hypoxia in dogs. *Am J Physiol.* 1983;244(5):E453-E458.
86. Farber MO, Weinberger MH, Robertson GL, et al. Hormonal abnormalities affecting sodium and water balance in acute respiratory failure due to chronic obstructive lung disease. *Chest.* 1984;85:49-54.
87. Anderson RJ, Pluss RG, Berns AS, et al. Mechanism of effect of hypoxia on renal water excretion. *J Clin Invest.* 1978;62(4):769-777.
88. Miller M. Role of endogenous opioids in neurohypophysial function of man. *J Clin Endocrinol Metab.* 1980;50(6):1016-1020.
89. Oiso Y, Iwasaki Y, Kondo K, et al. Effect of the opioid kappa-receptor agonist U50488H on the secretion of arginine vasopressin. Study on the mechanism of U50488H-induced diuresis. *Neuroendocrinology.* 1988;48(6):658-662.
90. Eisenhofer G, Johnson RH. Effect of ethanol ingestion on plasma vasopressin and water balance in humans. *Am J Physiol.* 1982;242(5):R522-R527.
91. Oiso Y, Robertson GL. Effect of ethanol on vasopressin secretion and the role of endogenous opioids. In: Schrier R, ed. *Water balance and antidiuretic hormone.* New York: Raven Press; 1985:p 265.
92. Stephens WP, Coe JY, Baylis PH. Plasma arginine vasopressin concentrations and antidiuretic action of carbamazepine. *Br Med J.* 1978;1(6125):1445-1447.
93. Reid IA, Ahn JN, Trinh T, et al. Mechanism of suppression of vasopressin and adrenocorticotropic hormone secretion by clonidine in anesthetized dogs. *J Pharmacol Exp Ther.* 1984;229(1):1-8.
94. Iovino M, De Caro G, Massi M, et al. Muscimol inhibits ADH release induced by hypertonic sodium chloride in rats. *Pharmacol Biochem Behav.* 1983;19(2):335-338.
95. Zerbe RL, Bayorh MA, Quirion R, et al. The role of vasopressin suppression in phencyclidine-induced diuresis. *Pharmacology.* 1983;26(2):73-78.
96. Lausen HD. Metabolism of the neurohypophyseal hormones. In: Greep RO, Astwood EB, Knobil E, et al. eds. *Handbook of physiology.* Washington, DC: American Physiological Society; 1974:pp 287-393.
97. Davison JM, Sheills EA, Barron WM, et al. Changes in the metabolic clearance of vasopressin and in plasma vasopressinase throughout human pregnancy. *J Clin Invest.* 1989;83(4):1313-1318.
98. Andersson B. Thirst—and brain control of water balance. *Am Sci.* 1971;59(4):408-415.
99. Fitzsimons JT. Thirst. *Physiol Rev.* 1972;52(2):468-561.
100. Quillen EW, Reid IA, Keil LC. Carotid and arterial baroreceptor influences on plasma vasopressin and drinking. In: Cowley AWJ, Liard JF, Ausiello DA, eds. *Vasopressin: cellular and integrative functions.* New York: Raven Press; 1988:pp 405-411.
101. Stricker EM, Verbalis JG. Water intake and body fluids. In: Zigmond MJ, Bloom FE, Landis SC, et al. eds. *Fundamental neuroscience.* 1st ed. San Diego: Academic Press; 1999:1111-1126.
102. Phillips PA, Rolls BJ, Ledingham JG, et al. Osmotic thirst and vasopressin release in humans: a double-blind crossover study. *Am J Physiol.* 1985;248(6 pt 2):R645-R650.
103. Szczepanska-Sadowska E, Kozlowski S. Equipotency of hypertonic solutions of mannitol and sodium chloride in eliciting thirst in the dog. *Pflugers Arch.* 1975;358(3):259-264.
104. Robertson GL. Disorders of thirst in man. In: Ramsay DJ, Booth DA, eds. *Thirst: physiological and psychological aspects.* London: Springer-Verlag; 1991:p 453.
105. Verbalis JG. Inhibitory controls of drinking. In: Ramsay DJ, Booth DA, eds. *Thirst: physiological and psychological aspects.* London: Springer-Verlag; 1991:pp 313-334.
106. Fitzsimons JT. Drinking by rats depleted of body fluid without increases in osmotic pressure. *J Physiol (Lond).* 1961;159:297-309.
107. Thrasher TN, Keil LC, Ramsay DJ. Hemodynamic, hormonal, and drinking responses to reduced venous return in the dog. *Am J Physiol.* 1982;243(3):R354-R362.
108. Phillips PA, Rolls BJ, Ledingham JG, et al. Angiotensin II-induced thirst and vasopressin release in man. *Clin Sci (Lond).* 1985;68(6):669-674.
109. Rogers PW, Kurtzman NA. Renal failure, uncontrollable thirst, and hyperreninemia. Cessation of thirst with bilateral nephrectomy. *JAMA.* 1973;225(10):1236-1238.
110. Stricker EM, Sved AF. Thirst. *Nutrition.* 2000;16(10):821-826.
111. Root AW, Martinez CR, Muroff LR. Subhypothalamic high-intensity signals identified by magnetic resonance imaging in children with idiopathic anterior hypopituitarism. Evidence suggestive of an "ectopic" posterior pituitary gland. *Am J Dis Child.* 1989;143(3):366-367.
112. Heinbecker P, White HL. Hypothalamico-hypophyseal system and its relation to water balance in the dog. *Am J Physiol.* 1941;133:582-593.
113. Maccubbin DA, Van Buren JM. A quantitative evaluation of hypothalamic degeneration and its relation to diabetes insipidus following interruption of the human hypophyseal stalk. *Brain.* 1963;86:443.
114. Lippsett MB, MacLean IP, West CD, et al. An analysis of the polyuria induced by hypophysectomy in man. *J Clin Endocrinol Metab.* 1956;16:183-195.
115. Valtin H, North WG, Edwards BR, et al. Animal models of diabetes insipidus. In: Czernichow P, Robinson AG, eds. *Diabetes insipidus in man.* Basel, Switzerland: Karger; 1985:pp 105-126.
116. Schmale H, Richter D. Single base deletion in the vasopressin gene is the cause of diabetes insipidus in Brattleboro rats. *Nature.* 1984;308(5961):705-709.
117. Hansen LK, Rittig S, Robertson GL. Genetic basis of familial neurohypophyseal diabetes insipidus. *Trends Endocrinol Metab.* 1997;8:363.
118. Repaske DR, Phillips III JA, Kirby LT, et al. Molecular analysis of autosomal dominant neurohypophyseal diabetes insipidus. *J Clin Endocrinol Metab.* 1990;70(3):752-757.
119. Rittig S, Robertson GL, Siggaard C, et al. Identification of 13 new mutations in the vasopressin-neurophysin II gene in 17 kindreds with familial autosomal dominant neurohypophyseal diabetes insipidus. *Am J Hum Genet.* 1996;58(1):107-117.
120. Repaske DR, Medlej R, Gultekin EK, et al. Heterogeneity in clinical manifestation of autosomal dominant neurohypophyseal diabetes insipidus caused by a mutation encoding ala-1→val in the signal peptide of the arginine vasopressin/neurophysin II/copeptin precursor. *J Clin Endocrinol Metab.* 1997;82(1):51-56.
121. Bergeron C, Kovacs K, Ezrin C, et al. Hereditary diabetes insipidus: an immunohistochemical study of the hypothalamus and pituitary gland. *Acta Neuropathol.* 1991;81(3):345-348.
122. Maghnie M, Villa A, Arico M, et al. Correlation between magnetic resonance imaging of posterior pituitary and neurohypophyseal function in children with diabetes insipidus. *J Clin Endocrinol Metab.* 1992;74(4):795-800.
123. Kaplowitz PB, D'Ercole AJ, Robertson GL. Radioimmunoassay of vasopressin in familial central diabetes insipidus. *J Pediatr.* 1982;100:76-81.

124. Siggaard C, Rittig S, Corydon TJ, et al. Clinical and molecular evidence of abnormal processing and trafficking of the vasopressin preprohormone in a large kindred with familial neurohypophyseal diabetes insipidus due to a signal peptide mutation. *J Clin Endocrinol Metab.* 1999;84:2933-2941.

125. Si-Hoe SL, de Bree FM, Nijenhuis M, et al. Endoplasmic reticulum derangement in hypothalamic neurons of rats expressing a familial neurohypophyseal diabetes insipidus mutant vasopressin transgene. *FASEB J.* 2000;14(12):1680-1684.

126. Davies J, Murphy D. Autophagy in hypothalamic neurones of rats expressing a familial neurohypophysial diabetes insipidus transgene. *J Neuroendocrinol.* 2002;14(8):629-637.

127. Maghnie M, Cosi G, Genovese E, et al. Central diabetes insipidus in children and young adults. *N Engl J Med.* 2000;343(14):998-1007.

128. Imura H, Nakao K, Shimatsu A, et al. Lymphocytic infundibuloneurohypophysitis as a cause of central diabetes insipidus. *N Engl J Med.* 1993;329(10):683-689.

129. Kojima H, Nojima T, Nagashima K, et al. Diabetes insipidus caused by lymphocytic infundibuloneurohypophysis. *Arch Pathol Lab Med.* 1989;113(12):1399-1401.

130. Van Havenbergh T, Robberecht W, Wilms G, et al. Lymphocytic infundibulohypophysitis presenting in the postpartum period: case report. *Surg Neurol.* 1996;46(3):280-284.

131. Nishioka H, Ito H, Sano T, et al. Two cases of lymphocytic hypophysitis presenting with diabetes insipidus: a variant of lymphocytic infundibulo-neurohypophysitis. *Surg Neurol.* 1996;46(3):285-290.

132. Thodou E, Asa SL, Kontogeorgos G, et al. Clinical case seminar: lymphocytic hypophysitis: clinicopathological findings. *J Clin Endocrinol Metab.* 1995;80(8):2302-2311.

133. Scherbaum WA, Bottazzo GF, Czernichow P. Role of autoimmunity in central diabetes insipidus. In: Czernichow P, Robinson AG, eds. *Diabetes insipidus in man.* Basel, Switzerland: Karger; 1985:pp 232-239.

134. De Bellis A, Colao A, Di Salle F, et al. A longitudinal study of vasopressin cell antibodies, posterior pituitary function, and magnetic resonance imaging evaluations in subclinical autoimmune central diabetes insipidus. *J Clin Endocrinol Metab.* 1999;84(9):3047-3051.

135. Zerbe RL, Robertson GL. A comparison of plasma vasopressin measurements with a standard indirect test in the differential diagnosis of polyuria. *N Engl J Med.* 1981;305:1539-1546.

136. Hollinshead WH. The interphase of diabetes insipidus. *Mayo Clin Proc.* 1964;39:92-100.

137. Verbalis JG, Robinson AG, Moses AM. Postoperative and post-traumatic diabetes insipidus. In: Czernichow P, Robinson AG, eds. *Diabetes insipidus in man.* Basel, Switzerland: Karger; 1984:pp 247-265.

138. Cusick JF, Hagen TC, Findling JW. Inappropriate secretion of antidiuretic hormone after transsphenoidal surgery for pituitary tumors. *N Engl J Med.* 1984;311:36-38.

139. Olson BR, Rubino D, Gumowski J, et al. Isolated hyponatremia after transsphenoidal pituitary surgery. *J Clin Endocrinol Metab.* 1995;80(1):85-91.

140. Olson BR, Gumowski J, Rubino D, et al. Pathophysiology of hyponatremia after transsphenoidal pituitary surgery. *J Neurosurg.* 1997;87(4):499-507.

141. Ultmann MC, Hoffman GE, Nelson PB, et al. Transient hyponatremia after damage to the neurohypophyseal tracts. *Neuroendocrinology.* 1992;56(6):803-811.

142. Daniel PM, Prichard MM. Regeneration of hypothalamic nerve fibres after hypophysectomy in the goat. *Acta Endocrinol (Copenh).* 1970;64(4):696-704.

143. Daniel PM, Prichard MM. The human hypothalamus and pituitary stalk after hypophysectomy or pituitary stalk section. *Brain.* 1972;95(4):813-824.

144. Block LH, Furrer J, Locher RA, et al. Changes in tissue sensitivity to vasopressin in hereditary hypothalamic diabetes insipidus. *Klin Wochenschr.* 1981;59(15):831-836.

145. DeRubertis FR, Michelis MF, Davis BB. "Essential" hypernatremia. Report of three cases and review of the literature. *Arch Intern Med.* 1974;134(5):889-895.

146. Halter JB, Goldberg AP, Robertson GL, et al. Selective osmoreceptor dysfunction in the syndrome of chronic hypernatremia. *J Clin Endocrinol Metab.* 1977;44:609-616.

147. Baylis PH, Thompson CJ. Osmoregulation of vasopressin secretion and thirst in health and disease. *Clin Endocrinol (Oxf).* 1988;29(5):549-576.

148. Takaku A, Shindo K, Tanaka S, et al. Fluid and electrolyte disturbances in patients with intracranial aneurysms. *Surg Neurol.* 1979;11(5):349-356.

149. McIver B, Connacher A, Whittle I, et al. Adipsic hypothalamic diabetes insipidus after clipping of anterior communicating artery aneurysm. *Br Med J.* 1991;303(6815):1465-1467.

150. DeRubertis FR, Michelis MF, Beck N, et al. "Essential" hypernatremia due to ineffective osmotic and intact volume regulation of vasopressin secretion. *J Clin Invest.* 1971;50(1):97-111.

151. Smith D, McKenna K, Moore K, et al. Baroregulation of vasopressin release in adipsic diabetes insipidus. *J Clin Endocrinol Metab.* 2002;87(10):4564-4568.

152. Phillips PA, Bretherton M, Johnston CI, et al. Reduced osmotic thirst in healthy elderly men. *Am J Physiol.* 1991;261(1 pt 2):R166-R171.

153. Hodak SP, Verbalis JG. Abnormalities of water homeostasis in aging. *Endocrinol Metab Clin North Am.* 2005;34(4):1031-1046:xi.

154. Durr JA, Hoggard JG, Hunt JM, et al. Diabetes insipidus in pregnancy associated with abnormally high circulating vasopressinase activity. *N Engl J Med.* 1987;316(17):1070-1074.

155. Durr JA. Diabetes insipidus in pregnancy. *Am J Kidney Dis.* 1987;9(4):276-283.

156. Gordge MP, Williams DJ, Huggett NJ, et al. Loss of biological activity of arginine vasopressin during its degradation by vasopressinase from pregnancy serum. *Clin Endocrinol (Oxf).* 1995;42(1):51-58.

157. Baylis PH, Thompson C, Burd J, et al. Recurrent pregnancy-induced polyuria and thirst due to hypothalamic diabetes insipidus: an investigation into possible mechanisms responsible for polyuria. *Clin Endocrinol (Oxf).* 1986;24(4):459-466.

158. Barron WM, Cohen LH, Ulland LA, et al. Transient vasopressin-resistant diabetes insipidus of pregnancy. *N Engl J Med.* 1984;310(7):442-444.

159. van Lieburg AF, Verdijk MA, Schoute F, et al. Clinical phenotype of nephrogenic diabetes insipidus in females heterozygous for a vasopressin type 2 receptor mutation. *Hum Genet.* 1995;96(1):70-78.

160. Morello JP, Bichet DG. Nephrogenic diabetes insipidus. *Annu Rev Physiol.* 2001;63:607-630.

161. Sadeghi H, Robertson GL, Bichet DG, et al. Biochemical basis of partial nephrogenic diabetes insipidus phenotypes. *Mol Endocrinol.* 1997;11(12):1806-1813.

162. Wildin RS, Cogdell DE, Valadez V. AVPR2 variants and V2 vasopressin receptor function in nephrogenic diabetes insipidus. *Kidney Int.* 1998;54(6):1909-1922.

163. Pasel K, Schulz A, Timmermann K, et al. Functional characterization of the molecular defects causing nephrogenic diabetes insipidus in eight families. *J Clin Endocrinol Metab.* 2000;85(4):1703-1710.

164. Wildin RS, Cogdell DE. Clinical utility of direct mutation testing for congenital nephrogenic diabetes insipidus in families. *Pediatrics.* 1999;103(3):632-639.

165. Chan Seem CP, Dossetor JF, Penney MD. Nephrogenic diabetes insipidus due to a new mutation of the arginine vasopressin V2 receptor gene in a girl presenting with non-accidental injury. *Ann Clin Biochem.* 1999;36(pt 6):779-782.

166. Deen PM, Knoers NV. Vasopressin type-2 receptor and aquaporin-2 water channel mutants in nephrogenic diabetes insipidus. *Am J Med Sci.* 1998;316(5):300-309.

167. Knoers NV, Deen PM. Molecular and cellular defects in nephrogenic diabetes insipidus. *Pediatr Nephrol.* 2001;16(12):1146-1152.

168. Canfield MC, Tamarappoo BK, Moses AM, et al. Identification and characterization of aquaporin-2 water channel mutations causing nephrogenic diabetes insipidus with partial vasopressin response. *Hum Mol Genet.* 1997;6(11):1865-1871.

169. van Os CH, Deen PM. Aquaporin-2 water channel mutations causing nephrogenic diabetes insipidus. *Proc Assoc Am Physicians.* 1998;110(5):395-400.

170. Tamarappoo BK, Verkman AS. Defective aquaporin-2 trafficking in nephrogenic diabetes insipidus and correction by chemical chaperones. *J Clin Invest.* 1998;101(10):2257-2267.

171. Morello JP, Salahpour A, Laperriere A, et al. Pharmacological chaperones rescue cell-surface expression and function of misfolded V2 vasopressin receptor mutants. *J Clin Invest.* 2000;105(7):887-895.

172. Knepper MA, Verbalis JG, Nielsen S. Role of aquaporins in water balance disorders. *Curr Opin Nephrol Hypertens.* 1997;6(4):367-371.

173. Nielsen S, Kwon TH, Christensen BM, et al. Physiology and pathophysiology of renal aquaporins. *J Am Soc Nephrol.* 1999;10(3):647-663.

174. Marples D, Frokiaer J, Dorup J, et al. Hypokalemia-induced downregulation of aquaporin-2 water channel expression in rat kidney medulla and cortex. *J Clin Invest.* 1996;97(8):1960-1968.

175. Earm JH, Christensen BM, Frokiaer J, et al. Decreased aquaporin-2 expression and apical plasma membrane delivery in kidney collecting ducts of polyuric hypercalcemic rats. *J Am Soc Nephrol.* 1998;9(12):2181-2193.

176. Sands JM, Naruse M, Jacobs JD, et al. Changes in aquaporin-2 protein contribute to the urine concentrating defect in rats fed a low-protein diet. *J Clin Invest.* 1996;97(12):2807-2814.

177. Frokiaer J, Christensen BM, Marples D, et al. Downregulation of aquaporin-2 parallels changes in renal water excretion in unilateral ureteral obstruction. *Am J Physiol.* 1997;273(2 pt 2):F213-F223.

178. Bendz H, Aurell M. Drug-induced diabetes insipidus: incidence, prevention and management. *Drug Saf.* 1999;21(6):449-456.

179. Christensen S, Kusano E, Yusufi AN, et al. Pathogenesis of nephrogenic diabetes insipidus due to chronic administration of lithium in rats. *J Clin Invest.* 1985;75(6):1869-1879.

180. Marples D, Christensen S, Christensen EI, et al. Lithium-induced downregulation of aquaporin-2 water channel expression in rat kidney medulla. *J Clin Invest.* 1995;95(4):1838-1845.

181. Bendz H, Sjodin I, Aurell M. Renal function on and off lithium in patients treated with lithium for 15 years or more. A controlled, prospective lithium-withdrawal study. *Nephrol Dial Transplant.* 1996;11(3):457-460.

182. Markowitz GS, Radhakrishnan J, Kambham N, et al. Lithium nephrotoxicity: a progressive combined glomerular and tubulointerstitial nephropathy. *J Am Soc Nephrol.* 2000;11(8):1439-1448.

183. Fernandez-Llama P, Andrews P, Ecelbarger CA, et al. Concentrating defect in experimental nephrotic syndrome: altered expression of aquaporins and thick ascending limb Na$^+$ transporters. *Kidney Int.* 1998;54(1):170-179.

184. Terris J, Ecelbarger CA, Nielsen S, et al. Long-term regulation of four renal aquaporins in rats. *Am J Physiol.* 1996;271(2 pt 2):F414-F422.

185. Harrington AR, Valtin H. Impaired urinary concentration after vasopressin and its gradual correction in hypothalamic diabetes insipidus. *J Clin Invest.* 1968;47:502.

186. Goldman MB, Luchins DJ, Robertson GL. Mechanisms of altered water metabolism in psychotic patients with polydipsia and hyponatremia. *N Engl J Med.* 1988;318(7):397-403.

187. de Leon J, Verghese C, Tracy JI, et al. Polydipsia and water intoxication in psychiatric patients: a review of the epidemiological literature. *Bio Psych.* 1994;35:408-419.

188. Robertson GL. Differential diagnosis of polyuria. *Annu Rev Med.* 1988;39:425-442.

189. Valtin H. "Drink at least eight glasses of water a day." Really? Is there scientific evidence for "8 × 8"? *Am J Physiol Regul Integr Comp Physiol.* 2002;283(5):R993-R1004.

190. Goldman MB, Robertson GL, Luchins DJ, et al. The influence of polydipsia on water excretion in hyponatremic, polydipsic, schizophrenic patients. *J Clin Endocrinol Metab.* 1996;81(4):1465-1470.

191. Vieweg WV, Carey RM, Godleski LS, et al. The syndrome of psychosis, intermittent hyponatremia, and polydipsia: evidence for diurnal volume expansion. *Psych Med.* 1990;8:135-144.

192. Cheng JC, Zikos D, Skopicki HA, et al. Long-term neurologic outcome in psychogenic water drinkers with severe symptomatic hyponatremia: the effect of rapid correction. *Am J Med.* 1990;88:561-566.

193. Vieweg WV, Robertson GL, Godleski LS, et al. Diurnal variation in water homeostasis among schizophrenic patients subject to water intoxication. *Schizophrenia Res.* 1988;1:351-357.

194. Goldman MB, Robertson GL, Luchins DJ, et al. Psychotic exacerbations and enhanced vasopressin secretion in schizophrenic patients with hyponatremia and polydipsia. *Arch Gen Psychiatry.* 1997;54(5):443-449.

195. Adrogue HJ, Madias NE. Hypernatremia. *N Engl J Med.* 2000;342(20):1493-1499.

196. Palevsky PM, Bhagrath R, Greenberg A. Hypernatremia in hospitalized patients. *Ann Intern Med.* 1996;124(2):197-203.

197. Riggs JE. Neurologic manifestations of fluid and electrolyte disturbances. *Neurol Clin.* 1989;7(3):509-523.

198. Palevsky PM. Hypernatremia. *Semin Nephrol.* 1998;18(1):20-30.

199. Gullans SR, Verbalis JG. Control of brain volume during hyperosmolar and hypo-osmolar conditions. *Annu Rev Med.* 1993;44:289-301.

200. Ayus JC, Armstrong DL, Arieff AI. Effects of hypernatraemia in the central nervous system and its therapy in rats and rabbits. *J Physiol.* 1996;492(pt 1):243-255.

201. Kahn A, Brachet E, Blum D. Controlled fall in natremia and risk of seizures in hypertonic dehydration. *Intensive Care Med.* 1979;5(1):27-31.

202. Robertson GL. Diabetes insipidus. *Endocrinol Metab Clin North Am.* 1995;24(3):549-572.

203. Miller M, Dalakos T, Moses AM, et al. Recognition of partial defects in antidiuretic hormone secretion. *Ann Intern Med.* 1970;73(5):721-729.

204. Moses AM. Clinical and laboratory observations in the adult with diabetes insipidus and related syndromes. In: Czernichow P, Robinson AG, eds. *Diabetes insipidus in man.* Basel, Switzerland: Karger; 1985:pp 156-175.

205. Robinson AG. Disorders of antidiuretic hormone secretion. *Clin Endocrinol Metab.* 1985;14:55-88.

206. Baylis PH, Gaskill MB, Robertson GL. Vasopressin secretion in primary polydipsia and cranial diabetes insipidus. *QJM.* 1981;50:345-358.

207. Milles JJ, Spruce B, Baylis PH. A comparison of diagnostic methods to differentiate diabetes insipidus from primary polyuria: a review of 21 patients. *Acta Endocrinol (Copenh).* 1983;104(4):410-416.

208. Morgenthaler NG, Struck J, Jochberger S, et al. Copeptin: clinical use of a new biomarker. *Trends Endocrinol Metab.* 2008;19(2):43-49.

209. Fujisawa I, Asato R, Nishimura K, et al. Anterior and posterior lobes of the pituitary gland: assessment by 1.5 T MR imaging. *J Comput Assist Tomogr.* 1987;11(2):214-220.

210. Arslan A, Karaarslan E, Dincer A. High intensity signal of the posterior pituitary. A study with horizontal direction of frequency-encoding and fat suppression MR techniques. *Acta Radiol.* 1999;40(2):142-145.

211. Kurokawa H, Fujisawa I, Nakano Y, et al. Posterior lobe of the pituitary gland: correlation between signal intensity on T1-weighted MR images and vasopressin concentration. *Radiology.* 1998;207(1):79-83.

212. Moses AM, Clayton B, Hochhauser L. Use of T1-weighted MR imaging to differentiate between primary polydipsia and central diabetes insipidus. *AJNR Am J Neuroradiol.* 1992;13:1273-1277:[Comment in *AJNR Am J Neuroradiol* 14(6):1443-1445, 1993; *AJNR Am J Neuroradiol* 13(5):1279-1291, 1992].

213. Brooks BS, el Gammal T, Allison JD, et al. Frequency and variation of the posterior pituitary bright signal on MR images. *AJNR Am J Neuroradiol.* 1989;10(5):943-948.

214. Maghnie M, Genovese E, Bernasconi S, et al. Persistent high MR signal of the posterior pituitary gland in central diabetes insipidus. *AJNR Am J Neuroradiol.* 1997;18(9):1749-1752.

215. Dohanics J, Hoffman GE, Verbalis JG. Chronic hyponatremia reduces survival of magnocellular vasopressin and oxytocin neurons following axonal injury. *J Neurosci.* 1996;16:2372-2380.

216. Bonneville JF, Cattin F, Dietemann JL. *The pituitary stalk. Computed tomography of the pituitary gland.* New York: Springer-Verlag; 1986: pp 106-114.

217. Leger J, Velasquez A, Garel C, et al. Thickened pituitary stalk on magnetic resonance imaging in children with central diabetes insipidus. *J Clin Endocrinol Metab.* 1999;84(6):1954-1960.

218. Czernichow P, Garel C, Leger J. Thickened pituitary stalk on magnetic resonance imaging in children with central diabetes insipidus. *Horm Res.* 2000;53(suppl 3):61-64.

219. Bruck E, Abal G, Aceto Jr T. Pathogenesis and pathophysiology of hypertonic dehydration with diarrhea. A clinical study of 59 infants with observations of respiratory and renal water metabolism. *Am J Dis Child.* 1968;115(2):122-144.

220. Blum D, Brasseur D, Kahn A, et al. Safe oral rehydration of hypertonic dehydration. *J Pediatr Gastroenterol Nutr.* 1986;5(2):232-235.

221. Fjellestad-Paulsen A, Hoglund P, Lundin S, et al. Pharmacokinetics of 1-deamino-8-D-arginine vasopressin after various routes of administration in healthy volunteers. *Clin Endocrinol (Oxf).* 1993;38(2):177-182.

222. Robinson AG. DDAVP in the treatment of central diabetes insipidus. *N Engl J Med.* 1976;294(10):507-511.

223. Sklar AH, Schrier RW. Central nervous system mediators of vasopressin release. *Physiol Rev.* 1983;63(4):1243-1280.

224. Hoffman PK, Share L, Crofton JT, et al. The effect of intracerebroventricular indomethacin on osmotically stimulated vasopressin release. *Neuroendocrinology.* 1982;34(2):132-139.

225. Nadler SP, Hebert SC, Brenner BM. PGE$_2$, forskolin, and cholera toxin interactions in rabbit cortical collecting tubule. *Am J Physiol.* 1986;250:F127-F135.

226. Allen HM, Jackson RL, Winchester MD, et al. Indomethacin in the treatment of lithium-induced nephrogenic diabetes insipidus. *Arch Intern Med.* 1989;149(5):1123-1126.

227. Magaldi AJ. New insights into the paradoxical effect of thiazides in diabetes insipidus therapy. *Nephrol Dial Transplant.* 2000;15(12):1903-1905.

228. Richardson DW, Robinson AG. Desmopressin. *Ann Intern Med.* 1985;103(2):228-239.

229. Lam KS, Wat MS, Choi KL, et al. Pharmacokinetics, pharmacodynamics, long-term efficacy and safety of oral 1-deamino-8-D-arginine vasopressin in adult patients with central diabetes insipidus. *Br J Clin Pharmacol.* 1996;42(3):379-385.

230. Rittig S, Jensen AR, Jensen KT, et al. Effect of food intake on the pharmacokinetics and antidiuretic activity of oral desmopressin (DDAVP) in hydrated normal subjects. *Clin Endocrinol (Oxf).* 1998;48(2):235-241.

231. Dunn AL, Powers JR, Ribeiro MJ, et al. Adverse events during use of intranasal desmopressin acetate for haemophilia A and von Willebrand disease: a case report and review of 40 patients. *Haemophilia.* 2000;6(1):11-14.

232. Robson WL, Norgaard JP, Leung AK. Hyponatremia in patients with nocturnal enuresis treated with DDAVP. *Eur J Pediatr.* 1996;155(11):959-962.

233. Schwab M, Wenzel D, Ruder H. Hyponatraemia and cerebral convulsion due to short term DDAVP therapy for control of enuresis nocturna. *Eur J Pediatr.* 1996;155(1):46-48.

234. Lugo N, Silver P, Nimkoff L, et al. Diagnosis and management algorithm of acute onset of central diabetes insipidus in critically ill children. *J Pediatr Endocrinol Metab.* 1997;10(6):633-639.

235. Davison JM, Sheills EA, Philips PR, et al. Metabolic clearance of vasopressin and an analogue resistant to vasopressinase in human pregnancy. *Am J Physiol.* 1993;264(2 pt 2):F348-F353.

236. Kallen BA, Carlsson SS, Bengtsson BK. Diabetes insipidus and use of desmopressin (Minirin) during pregnancy. *Eur J Endocrinol.* 1995;132(2):144-146.

237. Ray JG. DDAVP use during pregnancy: an analysis of its safety for mother and child. *Obstet Gynecol Surv.* 1998;53(7):450-455.

238. Iwasaki Y, Oiso Y, Kondo K, et al. Aggravation of subclinical diabetes insipidus during pregnancy. *N Engl J Med.* 1991;324(8):522-526.

239. Libber S, Harrison H, Spector D. Treatment of nephrogenic diabetes insipidus with prostaglandin synthesis inhibitors. *J Pediatr.* 1986;108(2):305-311.

240. Kirchlechner V, Koller DY, Seidl R, et al. Treatment of nephrogenic diabetes insipidus with hydrochlorothiazide and amiloride. *Arch Dis Child.* 1999;80(6):548-552.

241. Uyeki TM, Barry FL, Rosenthal SM, et al. Successful treatment with hydrochlorothiazide and amiloride in an infant with congenital nephrogenic diabetes insipidus. *Pediatr Nephrol.* 1993;7(5):554-556.

242. Cesar KR, Magaldi AJ. Thiazide induces water absorption in the inner medullary collecting duct of normal and Brattleboro rats. *Am J Physiol.* 1999;277(5 pt 2):F756-F760.

243. Usberti M, Dechaux M, Guillot M, et al. Renal prostaglandin E$_2$ in nephrogenic diabetes insipidus: effects of inhibition of prostaglandin synthesis by indomethacin. *J Pediatr.* 1980;97(3):476-478.

244. Chevalier RL, Rogol AD. Tolmetin sodium in the management of nephrogenic diabetes insipidus. *J Pediatr.* 1982;101(5):787-789.

245. Batlle DC, von Riotte AB, Gaviria M, et al. Amelioration of polyuria by amiloride in patients receiving long-term lithium therapy. *N Engl J Med.* 1985;312(7):408-414.

246. Singer I, Oster JR, Fishman LM. The management of diabetes insipidus in adults. *Arch Intern Med.* 1997;157(12):1293-1301.

247. Postina R, Ufer E, Pfeiffer R, et al. Misfolded vasopressin V2 receptors caused by extracellular point mutations entail congenital nephrogenic diabetes insipidus. *Mol Cell Endocrinol.* 2000;164(1-2):31-39.

248. Robertson GL. Abnormalities of thirst regulation. *Kidney Int.* 1984;25:460-469.

249. Canuso CM, Goldman MB. Clozapine restores water balance in schizophrenic patients with polydipsia-hyponatremia syndrome. *J Neuropsychiatry Clin Neurosci.* 1999;11(1):86-90.

250. Anderson RJ. Hospital-associated hyponatremia. *Kidney Int.* 1986;29:1237.

251. Hawkins RC. Age and gender as risk factors for hyponatremia and hypernatremia. *Clin Chim Acta.* 2003;337:169-172.

252. Wattad A, Chiang ML, Hill LL. Hyponatremia in hospitalized children. *Clin Pediatr (Phila).* 1992;31:153.

253. Saito T. Hyponatremia in elderly patients. *Intern Med.* 2001;40:851.

254. Kumar S, Berl T. Sodium. *Lancet.* 1998;352:220-228.

255. Turchin A, Seifter JL, Seely EW. Clinical problem-solving. Mind the gap. *N Engl J Med.* 2003;349:1465-1469.

256. Steinberger BA, Ford SM, Coleman TA. Intravenous immunoglobulin therapy results in post-infusional hyperproteinemia, increased serum viscosity, and pseudohyponatremia. *Am J Hematol.* 2003;73:97-100.

257. Perez-Perez AJ, Pazos B, Sobrado J, et al. Acute renal failure following massive mannitol infusion. *Am J Nephrol.* 2002;22:573-575.

258. Guglielminotti J, Pernet P, Maury E, et al. Osmolar gap hyponatremia in critically ill patients: evidence for the sick cell syndrome? *Crit Care Med.* 2002;30:1051-1055.

259. Hillier TA, Abbott RD, Barrett EJ. Hyponatremia: evaluating the correction factor for hyperglycemia. *Am J Med.* 1999;106:399-403.

260. Ayus JC, Arieff AI. Glycine induced hypo-osmolar hyponatremia. *Arch Intern Med.* 1997;557:223.

261. Berl T, Schrier RW. Disorders of water metabolism. In: Schrier RW, ed. *Renal and electrolyte disorders.* 6th ed. Philadelphia: Lippincott Williams & Wilkins; 2003.

262. Robertson GL. Physiopathology of ADH secretion. In: Tolis G, Labrie F, Martin JB, et al. eds. *Clinical neuroendocrinology: a pathophysiological approach.* New York: Raven Press; 1979:p 247.

263. Nguyen MK, Kurtz I. New insights into the pathophysiology of the dysnatremias: a quantitative analysis. *Am J Physiol Renal Physiol.* 2004;287:F172-F180.

264. Sterns R. Sodium and water balance disorders. *Nephrol Self Assess Program.* 2006;5:35-50.

265. Parikh C, Kumar S, Berl T. Disorders of water metabolism. In: Feehally J, Floege J, Johnson RR, eds. *Comprehensive clinical nephrology.* 3rd ed. St. Louis: Mosby; 2006.

266. Androgue HJ, Madias NE. Hyponatremia. *N Engl J Med.* 2000;342:1581-1589.

267. Chow KM, Kwan BC, Szeto CC. Clinical studies of thiazide-induced hyponatremia. *J Natl Med Assoc.* 2004;96:1305-1308.

268. Sonnenblick M, Friedlander Y, Rosin AJ. Diuretic induced severe hyponatremia. Review and analysis of 129 reported patients. *Chest.* 1993;103:601.

269. Sharabi Y, Illan R, Kamari Y, et al. Diuretic induced hyponatraemia in elderly hypertensive women. *J Hum Hypertens.* 2002;16:631-635.

270. Clark B, Shannon R, Rosa R, et al. Increased susceptibility to thiazide induced hyponatremia in the elderly. *J Am Soc Nephrol.* 1994;5:1106.

271. Berl T. Water metabolism in potassium depletion. *Miner Electrolyte Metab.* 1980;4:209.

272. Fichman MP, Vorherr H, Kleeman CR, et al. Diuretic induced hyponatremia. *Ann Intern Med.* 1971;75:853.

273. Danovitch GM, Bourgoignie J, Bricker NS. Reversibility of the salt losing tendency of chronic renal failure. *N Engl J Med.* 1977;296:14.

274. Schrier RW, Linas SL. Mechanisms of the defect in water excretion in adrenal insufficiency. *Miner Electrolyte Metab.* 1980;4:1.

275. Boykin J, McCool A, Robertson G, et al. Mechanisms of impaired water excretion in mineralocorticoid deficient dogs. *Miner Electrolyte Metab.* 1979;2:310.

276. Schrier RW. Body water homeostasis: clinical disorders of urinary dilution and concentration. *J Am Soc Nephrol.* 2006;17:1820-1832.

277. Palmer BF. Hyponatremia in patients with central nervous system disease: SIADH versus CSW. *Trends Endocrinol Metab.* 2003;14:182-187.

278. Bohn S, Carlotti P, Cusimono M, et al: Cerebral salt wasting: truth, fallacies theories and challenges. *Crit Care Med.* 30:2575-2002.

279. Oh MS, Carroll HJ. Cerebral salt-wasting syndromes. *Crit Care Clin.* 2001;17:125-138.

280. McGirt MJ, Blessing R, Nimjee SM, et al. Correlation of serum brain natriuretic peptide with hyponatremia and delayed ischemic neurological deficits after subarachnoid hemorrhage. *Neurosurgery.* 2004;54:1369-1373:discussion, 1373-1364.

281. Schrier RW, Gurevich AK, Cadnapaphornchai MA. Pathogenesis and management of sodium and water retention in cardiac failure and cirrhosis. *Semin Nephrol.* 2002;2:157-172.

282. Ishikawa S, Saito S, Okada K, et al. Effect of vasopressin antagonist on water excretion in vena cava constriction. *Kidney Int.* 1986;30:49.

283. Szatalowicz VL, Arnold PE, Chaimovitz C, et al. Radioimmunoassay of plasma arginine vasopressin in hyponatremic patients with congestive heart failure. *N Engl J Med.* 1981;305:263.

284. Kim JK, Michel JB, Soubrier F, et al. Arginine vasopressin gene expression in chronic cardiac failure in rats. *Kidney Int.* 1990;38:818.

285. Ferguson DW, Berg WJ, Sanders JS. Clinical and hemodynamic correlates of sympathetic nerve activity in normal humans and patients with heart failure. Evidence from direct microneurographic recordings. *J Am Coll Cardiol.* 1990;16:1125.

286. Benedict C, Johnston D, Weiner D, et al. Relation of neurohumoral activation to clinical variables and degrees of ventricular dysfunction. *J Am Coll Cardiol.* 1994;23:1410.

287. Lee W, Packer M. Prognostic importance of serum sodium concentration and its modification by converting enzyme inhibitors. *Circulation.* 1986;73:257.

288. Nielsen S, Torris D, Andersen C. Congestive heart failure in rats is associated with increased expression and targeting of aquaporin 2 water channel in collecting duct. *Proc Natl Acad Sci U S A.* 1997;94:5450.

289. Xu DL, Martin P-Y, Ohara M, et al. Upregulation of aquaporin 2 water channel expression in chronic heart failure rat. *J Clin Invest.* 1997;99:1500.

290. Martin PY, Abraham WT, Lieming X, et al. Selective V2-receptor vasopressin antagonism decreases urinary aquaporin-2 excretion in patients with chronic heart failure. *J Am Soc Nephrol.* 1999;10:2165-2170.

291. Gines P, Berl T, Bernardi M, et al. Hyponatremia in cirrhosis: from pathogenesis to treatment. *Hepatology.* 1998;28:851-864.

292. Schrier RW. Mechanisms of disturbed renal water excretion in cirrhosis. *Gastroenterology.* 1983;84:870.

293. Arroyo V, Jimenez W. Complications of cirrhosis: renal and circulatory dysfunction, light shadows in an important clinical problem. *J Hepatol.* 2000;32(suppl 1):157.

294. Unikowsky B, Wexler JJ, Levy M. Dogs with experimental cirrhosis of the liver but without intrahepatic hypertension do not retain sodium or form ascites. *J Clin Invest.* 1983;72:1594.

295. Rahman SN, Abraham W, Schrier RW. Peripheral arterial vasodilation in cirrhosis. *Gastroenterol Int.* 1992;5:192.

296. Kim J, Summer S, Howard R, et al. Vasopressin gene expression in rats with experimental cirrhosis. *Hepatology.* 1993;17:143.

297. Claria J, Jimenez W, Arroyo V, et al. Blockade of the hydrosmotic effect of vasopressin normalizes water excretion in cirrhotic rats. *Gastroenterology.* 1989;97:1294.

298. Fujita N, Ishikawa S, Sasaki S. Role of water channel AQP-CD in water retention in SIADH and cirrhotic rats. *Am J Physiol.* 1994;269:F926.

299. Fernandez-Llama P, Jimenez W, et al. Dysregulation of renal aquaporins and Na-Cl cotransporter in CCl4-induced cirrhosis. *Kidney Int.* 2000;58:216-228.

300. Fernandez-Llama P, Turner R, Dibona G, et al. Renal expression of aquaporins in liver cirrhosis induced by chronic common bile duct ligation in rats. *J Am Soc Nephrol.* 1999;10:1950-1957.

301. Bichet D, Van Putten VJ, Schrier RW. Potential role of increased sympathetic activity in impaired sodium and water excretion in cirrhosis. *N Engl J Med.* 1982;307:1552.

302. Floras J, Legaut L, Morali GA. Increased sympathetic outflow in cirrhosis and ascites. Direct evidence from intraneural recordings. *Ann Intern Med.* 1991;114:373.

303. Bichet DG, Groves BM, Schrier RW. Mechanism of improvement of water and sodium excretion by enhancement of central hemodynamics in decompensated cirrhosis. *Kidney Int.* 1983;24:788.

304. Shapiro M, Nichols K, Groves B, et al. Interrelationship between cardiac output and vascular resistance as determinants of effective arterial blood volume in cirrhotic patients. *Kidney Int*. 1985;28:201.

305. Weigert A, Martin P, Niederberger M. Endothelium dependent vascular hyporesponsiveness without detection of nitric oxide synthase induction in aorta of cirrhotic rats. *Hepatology*. 1856;22:1997.

306. Martin P-Y, Ohara M, Gines P. Nitric oxide synthase (NOS) inhibition for one week improves sodium and water excretion in cirrhotic rats with ascites. *J Clin Invest*. 1998;201:235.

307. Martin P-Y, Gines P, Schrier RW. Nitric oxide as a mediator of hemodynamic abnormalities and sodium and water retention in cirrhosis. *N Engl J Med*. 1998;339:533.

308. Abraham W, Cadnapopornchai M, Schrier RW. Cardiac failure, liver disease and nephrotic syndrome. In: Schrier RW, Gottschalk CW, eds. *Diseases of the kidney*. 7th ed. Philadelphia: Lippincott Williams & Wilkins; 2001:p 2465.

309. Usberti M, Federico S, Mecariello S, et al. Role of plasma vasopressin in the impairment of water excretion in nephrotic syndrome. *Kidney Int*. 1984;25:422.

310. Kimagi H, Onayma K, Isehi K. Role of renin-angiotensin-aldosterone in minimal change nephrotic syndrome. *Clin Nephrol*. 1985;25:229.

311. Meltzer JI, Keim HJ, Laragh JH, et al. Nephrotic syndrome: vasoconstriction and hypervolemic types indicated by renin-sodium profiling. *Ann Intern Med*. 1979;91:688.

312. Schrier RW, Fasset RG. A critique of the overfill hypothesis of sodium and water retention in the nephrotic syndrome. *Kidney Int*. 1998;53:1111.

313. Ichikawa I, Rennke HG, Hoyer JR, et al. Role of intrarenal mechanisms in the impaired salt excretion in experimental nephrotic syndrome. *J Clin Invest*. 1983;71:91.

314. Apostol E, Ecelbarger CA, Terris J, et al. Reduced renal medullary water channel expression in puromycin aminonucleoside–induced nephrotic syndrome. *J Am Soc Nephrol*. 1997;8:15-24.

315. Fernandez-Llama P, Andrews P, Ecelbarger CA, et al. Concentrating defect in experimental nephrotic syndrome: altered expression of aquaporins and thick ascending limb Na$^+$ transporters. *Kidney Int*. 1998;54:170-179.

316. Gross P, Raascher W. Vasopressin and hyponatremia in renal insufficiency. *Contrib Nephrol*. 1986;50:54.

317. Weiss NM, Robertson GL. Water metabolism in endocrine disorders. *Semin Nephrol*. 1987;4:303.

318. Ishikawa S, Fujisawa G, Tsuboi Y, et al. Role of antidiuretic hormone in hyponatremia in patients with isolated adrenocorticotropic hormone deficiency. *Endocrinol Jpn*. 1991;38:325.

319. Oelkers W. Hyponatremia and inappropriate secretion of vasopressin in patients with hypopituitarism. *N Engl J Med*. 1989;321:492.

320. Boykin J, de Torrente A, Erickson A, et al. Role of plasma vasopressin in impaired water excretion of glucocorticoid deficiency. *J Clin Invest*. 1978;62:738.

321. Linas SL, Berl T, Robertson GL, et al. Role of vasopressin in the impaired water excretion of glucocorticoid deficiency. *Kidney Int*. 1980;18:58.

322. Pyo HI, Summer SN, Kim JK. Vasopressin gene expression in glucocorticoid hormone deficient rats. *Ann N Y Acad Sci*. 1993;689:659.

323. Kim JK, Summer SN, Wood WM, et al. Role of glucocorticoid hormones in arginine vasopressin gene regulation. *Biochem Biophys Res Commun*. 2001;289:1252-1256.

324. Berghorn KA, Knapp LT, Hoffman GE, et al. Induction of glucocorticoid receptor expression in hypothalamus neurons during chronic hypo-osmolality. *Endocrinology*. 1995;136:804.

325. Schwartz MJ, Kokko JP. Urinary concentrating defect of adrenal insufficiency. Permissive role of adrenal steroids on the hydroosmotic response across the rabbit collecting tubule. *J Clin Invest*. 1980;66:234.

326. Jackson BA, Braun-Werness J, Kusano E, et al. Concentrating defect in adrenalectomized rat. *J Clin Invest*. 1983;72:997.

327. Kwon TH, Nielson J, Masilamani S, et al. Regulation of collection duct AQP3 expression response to mineralocorticoid. *Am J Physiol Renal Physiol*. 2002;283:F1403-F1421.

328. Olchovsky D, Ezra D, Vered I, et al. Symptomatic hyponatremia as a presenting sign of hypothalamic-pituitary disease: a syndrome of inappropriate secretion of antidiuretic hormone (SIADH)–like glucocorticosteroid responsive condition. *J Endocrinol Invest*. 2005;28:151-156.

329. Diederich S, Franzen NF, Bahr V, et al. Severe hyponatremia due to hypopituitarism with adrenal insufficiency: report on 28 cases. *Eur J Endocrinol*. 2003;148:609-617.

330. Hanna F, Scanlon M. Hyponatremia, hypothyroidism and role of arginine vasopressin. *Lancet*. 1997;350:755.

331. Hochberg Z, Benderly A. Normal osmotic threshold for vasopressin release in the hyponatremia of hypothyroidism. *Horm Res*. 1983;18:128.

332. Iwasaki Y, Oiso Y, Yamauchi K. Osmoregulation of plasma vasopressin in myxedema. *J Clin Endocrinol Metab*. 1990;70:534.

333. Howard R, Summer S, Rossi N. Short term hypothyroidism and vasopressin gene expression in the rat. *Am J Kidney Dis*. 1992;19:573.

334. Seif SM, Robinson AG, Zenser TV, et al. Neurohypophyseal peptides in hypothyroid rats: plasma levels and kidney response. *Metabolism*. 1979;28:137.

335. Harckom TM, Kim JK, Palumbo PJ, et al. Medullary effect of thyroid function on enzymes of the vasopressin-sensitive adenosine 3′,5′-monophosphate system in renal medulla. *Endocrinology*. 1978;102:1475.

336. Cadnapaphornchai MA, Kim YW, Gurevich AK, et al. Urinary concentrating defect in hypothyroid rats: role of sodium, potassium, 2-chloride co-transporter, and aquaporins. *J Am Soc Nephrol*. 2003;14:566-574.

337. Chen YC, Cadnapaphornchai MA, Yang J, et al. Nonosmotic release of vasopressin and renal aquaporins in impaired urinary dilution in hypothyroidism. *Am J Physiol Renal Physiol*. 2005;289:F672-F678.

338. Riggs AT, Dysken MW, Kim SW, et al. A review of disorders of water homeostasis in psychiatric patients. *Psychosomatics*. 1991;32:133.

339. Hariprasad MK, Eisinger RP, Nadler IM, et al. Hyponatremia in psychogenic polydipsia. *Arch Intern Med*. 1980;140:1639-1642.

340. Jose CJ, Perez Crult J. Incidence and morbidity of self-induced water intoxication in state mental hospital patients. *Am J Psychiatry*. 1979;136:221.

341. Shah PJ, Greenberg WM. Water intoxication precipitated by thiazide diuretics in polydipsic psychiatric patients. *Am J Psychiatry*. 1991;148:1424-1425.

342. Brows RP, Koesis JM, Cohen SK. Delusional depression and inappropriate antidiuretic hormone secretion. *Biol Psychiatry*. 1983;18:1059.

343. Goldman MB, Robertson GL, Luchins DJ, et al. Psychotic exacerbations and enhanced vasopressin secretion in schizophrenic patients with hyponatremia and polydipsia. *Arch Gen Psychiatry*. 1997;54:443-449.

344. Kawai N, Atsuomi B, Toshihito S, et al. Roles of arginine vasopressin and atrial natriuretic peptide in polydipsia-hyponatremia of schizophrenic patients. *Psychiatry Res*. 2001;101:37-45.

345. Berl T. Psychosis and water balance. *N Engl J Med*. 1988;318:441.

346. Fenves AZ, Thomas S, Knochel JP. Beer potomania: two cases and review of the literature. *Clin Nephrol*. 1996;45:61-64.

347. Musch W, Xhaet O, Decaux G. Solute loss plays a major role in polydipsia-related hyponatraemia of both water drinkers and beer drinkers. *QJM*. 2003;96:421-426.

348. Hoorn EJ, Geary D, Robb M, et al. Acute hyponatremia related to intravenous fluid administration in hospitalized children: an observational study. *Pediatrics*. 2004;113:1279-1284.

349. Chung H-M, Kluge R, Schrier RW, et al. Post-operative hyponatremia. *Arch Intern Med*. 1986;146:333.

350. Tambe AA, Hill R, Livesley PJ. Post-operative hyponatraemia in orthopaedic injury. *Injury*. 2003;34:253-255.

351. Anderson RJ, Chung H-M, Kluge R, et al. Hyponatremia: a prospective analysis of its epidemiology and the pathogenetic role of vasopressin. *Ann Intern Med*. 1985;102:164.

352. Shafiee MA, Charest AF, Cheema-Dhadli S, et al. Defining conditions that lead to the retention of water: the importance of the arterial sodium concentration. *Kidney Int*. 2005;67:613-621.

353. Steele A, Growishankar A, Abramson S, et al. Postoperative hyponatremia despite near isotonic saline infusion. A phenomenon of desalination. *Ann Intern Med*. 1997;126:20.

354. Aronson D, Dragu RE, Nakhoul F, et al. Hyponatremia as a complication of cardiac catheterization: a prospective study. *Am J Kidney Dis*. 2002;40:940-946.

355. Arieff AI. Permanent neurological disability from hyponatremia in healthy women undergoing elective surgery. *N Engl J Med*. 1986;314:1529.

356. Ayus JC, Wheeler J, Arieff AI. Postoperative hyponatremic encephalopathy in menstruant women. *Ann Intern Med*. 1992;117:891.

357. O'Brien KK, Montain SJ, Corr WP, et al. Hypernatremia associated with hyponatremia in US Army trainees. *Mil Med*. 2001;166:405-410.

358. Davis DP, Videen JS, Marino A, et al. Exercise associated hyponatremia in marathon runners: a two year experience. *J Emerg Med*. 2001;21:47-57.

359. Montain SJ, Sawka MN, Wenger CB. Hyponatremia associated with exercise: risk factors and pathogenesis. *Exerc Sports Sci Rev*. 2001;29:113-117.

360. Almond CS, Shin AY, Fortescue EB, et al. Hyponatremia among runners in the Boston Marathon. *N Engl J Med*. 2005;352:1550-1556.

361. Noakes TD, Sharwood K, Collins M, et al. The dipsomania of great distance: water intoxication in an Ironman triathlete. *Br J Sports Med*. 2004;38:E16.

362. Bertholini DM, Butler CS. Severe hyponatraemia secondary to desmopressin therapy in von Willebrand's disease. *Anaesth Intensive Care*. 2000;28:199-201.

363. Schwab M, Wenzel D, Ruder H. Hyponatraemia and cerebral convulsion due to short term DDAVP therapy for control of enuresis nocturna. *Eur J Pediatr*. 1996;155:46-48.

364. Shindel A, Tobin G, Klutke C. Hyponatremia associated with desmopressin for the treatment of nocturnal polyuria. *Urology*. 2002;60:344.

365. Hirokawa CA, Gray DR. Chlorpropamide-induced hyponatremia in the veteran population. *Ann Pharmacother*. 1992;26:1243.

366. Mendoza SA, Brown Jr CF. Effect of chlorpropamide on osmotic water flow across toad bladder and the response to vasopressin, theophylline and cyclic AMP. *J Clin Endocrinol Metab.* 1974;38:883-889.

367. Durr JA, Hensen J, Ehnis T, et al. Chlorpropamide upregulates antidiuretic hormone receptors and unmasks constitutive receptor signaling. *Am J Physiol Renal Physiol.* 2000;278:F799-F808.

368. Kusano B, Brain-Werness JL, Vich DJ, et al. Chlorpropamide action on renal concentrating mechanism in rats with hypothalamic diabetes insipidus. *J Clin Invest.* 1983;72:1298.

369. Kastner T, Friedman DL, Pond WS. Carbamazepine-induced hyponatremia in patients with mental retardation. *Am J Ment Retard.* 1992;96:536.

370. Cooney JA. Carbamazepine and SIADH. *Am J Psychiatry.* 1990;147:1101.

371. Steinhoff BJ, Stoll KD, Stodieck SR, et al. Hyponatremic coma under oxcarbazepine therapy. *Epilepsy Res.* 1995;11:67.

372. Meinders HE, Cejka V, Robertson GL. Antidiuretic action of carbamazepine. *Clin Sci Mol Med.* 1974;47:289.

373. Gold PW, Robertson GL, Ballenger J, et al. Carbamazepine diminishes the sensitivity of the plasma arginine vasopressin response to osmotic stimulation. *J Clin Endocrinol Metab.* 1983;57:952.

374. Kosten TR, Camp W. Inappropriate secretion of antidiuretic hormone in a patient receiving piperazine phenothiazines. *Psychosomatics.* 1980;21:351.

375. Peck V, Shenkman L. Haloperidol-induced syndrome of inappropriate secretion of antidiuretic hormone. *Clin Pharmacol Ther.* 1979;26:442.

376. Beckstrom D, Reding R, Cerletti J. Syndrome of inappropriate antidiuretic hormone secretion associated with amitriptyline administration. *JAMA.* 1979;241:133.

377. Cherney DZ, Davids MR, Halperin ML. Acute hyponatremia and "ecstasy": insights from a quantitative and integrated analysis. *QJM.* 2002;95:475-483.

378. Budisavljevic MN, Stewart L, Sahn SA, et al. Hyponatremia associated with 3,4-methylenedioxymethamphetamine ("Ecstasy") abuse. *Am J Med Sci.* 2003;326:89-93.

379. Vishwanath BM, Vavalgund A, Cusando W, et al. Fluoxetine as a cause of SIADH. *Am J Psychiatry.* 1991;148:542.

380. Kessler J, Samuels S. Sertraline and hyponatremia. *N Engl J Med.* 1996;335:524:[letter].

381. Fabian TJ, Amico JA, Kroboth PD, et al. Paroxetine-induced hyponatremia in the elderly due to the syndrome of inappropriate secretion of antidiuretic hormone (SIADH). *J Geriatr Psychiatry Neurol.* 2003;16:160-164.

382. Spigset O, Hedermalm K. Hyponatremia in relation to treatment with antidepressants. *Pharmacotherapy.* 1997;17:348.

383. Kirby D, Harrigan S, Ames D. Hyponatremia in elderly psychiatric patients treated with selective serotonin reuptake inhibitors and venlafaxine: a retrospective controlled study in an inpatient unit. *Int J Geriatr Psychiatry.* 2002;17:231-237.

384. Strachan J, Shepherd J. Hyponatraemia associated with the use of selective serotonin reuptake inhibitors. *Aust N Z J Psychiatry.* 1998;32:295-298.

385. Bouman WP, Pinner G, Johnson H. Incidence of selective serotonin reuptake inhibitor (SSRI) induced hyponatraemia due to the syndrome of inappropriate antidiuretic hormone (SIADH) secretion in the elderly. *Int J Geriatr Psychiatry.* 1998;13:12-15.

386. Robertson GL, Bhoopalam N, Zelkowitz LJ. Vincristine neurotoxicity and abnormal secretion of antidiuretic hormone. *Arch Intern Med.* 1973;132:717.

387. Hammond IW, Ferguson JA, Kwong K, et al. Hyponatremia and syndrome of inappropriate anti-diuretic hormone reported with the use of vincristine: an over-representation of Asians? *Pharmacoepidemiol Drug Saf.* 2002;11:229-234.

388. Bode U, Seif SM, Levine AS. Studies on the antidiuretic effect of cyclophosphamide, vasopressin release and sodium excretion. *Med Pediatr Oncol.* 1980;8:295.

389. Culine S, Ghosn M, Droz J. Inappropriate antidiuretic hormone secretion induced by ifosfamide. *Eur J Cancer.* 1990;26:922.

390. Subramanian D, Ayus JC. Case report: severe symptomatic hyponatremia associated with lisinopril therapy. *Am J Med Sci.* 1992;303:177.

391. Castrillon JL, Mediavilla A, Mendez MA, et al. Syndrome of inappropriate antidiuretic hormone secretion (SIADH) and enalapril. *J Intern Med.* 1993;233:89.

392. Gonzalex-Martinez H, Gaspard JJ, Espino DV. Hyponatremia due to enalapril in an elderly patient. A case report. *Arch Fam Med.* 1993;2:791.

393. Aslam MK, Gnaim C, Kutnick J, et al. Syndrome of inappropriate antidiuretic hormone secretion induced by amiodarone therapy. *Pacing Clin Electrophysiol.* 2004;27:831-832.

394. Schwartz WB, Bennett W, Curelop S, et al. A syndrome of renal sodium loss and hyponatremia probably resulting from inappropriate secretion of antidiuretic hormone. *Am J Med.* 1957;23:529.

395. Bartter FE, Schwartz WB. The syndrome of inappropriate secretion of antidiuretic hormone. *Am J Med.* 1967;42:790.

396. Thaler S, Teitelbaum I, Berl T. "Beer potomania" in beer drinkers. Effect of low dietary solute intake. *Am J Kidney Dis.* 1998;31:1028.

397. Passamonte PM. Hypouricemia, inappropriate secretion of antidiuretic hormone, and small cell carcinoma of the lung. *Arch Intern Med.* 1984;144:1569.

398. DiGiovanni SR, Nielsen S, Christensen E, et al. Regulation of collection duct water channel expression by vasopressin in Brattleboro rat. *Proc Natl Acad Sci U S A.* 1994;91:8984.

399. Saito T, Ishikawa S, Ando F, et al. Exaggerated urinary excretion of aquaporin 2 in the pathological state of impaired water excretion dependent upon arginine vasopressin. *J Clin Endocrinol Metab.* 1998;83:4043.

400. Leaf A, Bartter FC, Santos RF, et al. Evidence in man that urine electrolyte loss induced by Pitressin is a function of water retention. *J Clin Invest.* 1953;32:868.

401. Verbalis J. An experimental model of syndrome of inappropriate antidiuretic hormone secretion in the rat. *Am J Physiol.* 1984;247:E540.

402. Verbalis JG, Drutarosky M. Adaptation to chronic hypo-osmolality in rats. *Kidney Int.* 1988;34:351.

403. Verbalis JG. Pathogenesis of hyponatremia in an experimental model of inappropriate antidiuresis. *Am J Physiol.* 1994;267:R1617.

404. Nelson PB, Seif SM, Maroon JC, et al. Hyponatremia in intracranial disease: perhaps not the syndrome of inappropriate secretion of antidiuretic hormone. *J Neurosurg.* 1991;55:938.

405. Diringer MN, Lim JS, Kirsch JR, et al. Suprasellar and intraventricular blood predicts elevated plasma atrial natriuretic factor in subarachnoid hemorrhage. *Stroke.* 1991;22:577.

406. Anderson RJ. Arginine vasopressin escape. In vivo and in vitro studies. In: Cowley AW, Liard JK, Ausiello DA, eds. *Vasopressin: cellular and integrative function.* New York: Raven Press; 1988:p 215.

407. Eggena P, Ma CL. Downregulation of vasopressin receptors in toad bladder. *Am J Physiol.* 1986;250:C453.

408. Tian Y, Sandberg K, Murase T, et al. Vasopressin receptor binding is downregulated during renal escape from vasopressin antidiuresis. *Endocrinology.* 2000;141:307.

409. Ecelbarger C, Chou C, Lee A, et al. Escape from vasopressin-induced antidiuresis: role of vasopressin resistance of the collecting duct. *Am J Physiol.* 1998;274:F1161.

410. Ecelbarger C, Nielsen S, Olson BR, et al. Role of renal aquaporins in escape from vasopressin antidiuresis in rat. *J Clin Invest.* 1997;99:1852.

411. Ecelbarger C, Verbalis J, Knepper M. Increased abundance of distal sodium transporters in rat kidney during vasopressin escape. *J Am Soc Nephrol.* 2001;12:207.

412. Berl T, Schrier RW. Disorders of water metabolism. In: Schrier RW, ed. *Renal and electrolyte disorders.* 6th ed. Philadelphia: Lippincott William & Wilkins; 2003:p 1.

413. Tang WW, Kaptein EM, Feinstein EI, et al. Hyponatremia in hospitalized patients with the acquired immunodeficiency syndrome and the AIDS related complex. *Am J Med.* 1993;94:169.

414. Putterman C, Levy L, Rubinger D. Transient exercise induced water intoxication and rhabdomyolysis. *Am J Kidney Dis.* 1993;21:206.

415. Irving RA, Noakes TD, Buck R, et al. Evaluation of renal function and fluid homeostasis during recovery from exercise induced hyponatremia. *J Appl Physiol.* 1991;70:342.

416. Miller M, Hecker MS, Friedlander DA, et al. Apparent idiopathic hyponatremia in an ambulatory geriatric population. *J Am Geriatr Soc.* 1996;44:404-408.

417. Anpalahan M. Chronic idiopathic hyponatremia in older people due to the syndrome of inappropriate antidiuretic hormone secretion (SIADH) possibly related to aging. *J Am Geriatr Soc.* 2001;49:788-792.

418. Hirshberg B, Ben-Yehuda A. The syndrome of inappropriate antidiuretic hormone secretion in the elderly. *Am J Med.* 1997;103:270-273.

419. Arinzon Z, Feldman J, Jarchowsky J, et al. A comparative study of the syndrome of inappropriate antidiuretic hormone secretion in community-dwelling patients and nursing home residents. *Aging Clin Exp Res.* 2003;15:6-11.

420. Ishikawa SE, Saito T, Fukagawa A, et al. Close association of urinary excretion of aquaporin-2 with appropriate and inappropriate arginine vasopressin-dependent antidiuresis in hyponatremia in elderly subjects. *J Clin Endocrinol Metab.* 2001;86:1665-1671.

421. List AF, Hainsworth JD, Davis BW, et al. The syndrome of inappropriate secretion of antidiuretic hormone (SIADH) in small cell lung cancer. *J Clin Oncol.* 1986;4:1191.

422. Coyle S, Penney MD, Masters PW, et al. Early diagnosis of ectopic arginine vasopressin secretion. *Clin Chem.* 1993;39:152.

423. Hussain SF, Irfan M, Abbasi M, et al. Clinical characteristics of 110 miliary tuberculosis patients from a low HIV prevalence country. *Int J Tuberc Lung Dis.* 2004;8:493-499.

424. Feldman BJ, Rosenthal SM, Vargas GA, et al. Nephrogenic syndrome of inappropriate antidiuresis. *N Engl J Med.* 2005;352:1884-1890.

425. Zerbe R, Stropes L, Robertson G. Vasopressin function in the syndrome of inappropriate antidiuresis. *Annu Rev Med.* 1980;31:315.

426. Fraser CL, Arieff AI. Epidemiology, pathophysiology, and management of hyponatremic encephalopathy. *Am J Med.* 1997;102:67-77.

427. Manley GT, Fujimura M, Ma T, et al. Aquaporin-4 deletion in mice reduces brain edema after acute water intoxication and ischemic stroke. *Nat Med.* 2000;6(2):159-163.

428. Ayus JC, Varon J, Arieff AI. Hyponatremia, cerebral edema, and noncardiogenic pulmonary edema in marathon runners. *Ann Intern Med.* 2000;132(9):711-714.

429. Ayus JC, Arieff AI. Pulmonary complications of hyponatremic encephalopathy. noncardiogenic pulmonary edema and hypercapnic respiratory failure. *Chest.* 1995;107(2):517-521:[comment in *Chest* 107(2):300-301, 1995].

430. Nzerue CM, Baffoe-Bonnie H, You W, et al. Predictors of outcome in hospitalized patients with severe hyponatremia. *J Natl Med Assoc.* 2003;95(5):335-343.

431. Wijdicks EF, Larson TS. Absence of postoperative hyponatremia syndrome in young, healthy females. *Ann Neurol.* 1994;35:626-628.

432. Baran D, Hutchinson TA. The outcome of hyponatremia in a general hospital population. *Clin Nephrol.* 1984;22:72-76.

433. Upadhyay A, Jaber BL, Madias NE. Incidence and prevalence of hyponatremia. *Am J Med.* 2006;119(7 suppl 1):S30-S35.

434. Sterns RH. Severe symptomatic hyponatremia: treatment and outcome. A study of 64 cases. *Ann Int Med.* 1987;107:656-664.

435. Berl T. Treating hyponatremia: what is all the controversy about? *Ann Intern Med.* 1990;113:417-419:[review; comment in *Ann Intern Med* 114(3):248-249, 1991].

436. Sterns RH. The treatment of hyponatremia: first, do no harm. *Am J Med.* 1990;88:557-560.

437. Tierney WM, Martin DK, Greenlee MC, et al. The prognosis of hyponatremia at hospital admission. *J Gen Intern Med.* 1986;1:380-385.

438. Pasantes-Morales H, Franco R, Ordaz B, et al. Mechanisms counteracting swelling in brain cells during hyponatremia. *Arch Med Res.* 2002;33(3):237-244.

439. Lien YH, Shapiro JI, Chan L. Study of brain electrolytes and organic osmolytes during correction of chronic hyponatremia. Implications for the pathogenesis of central pontine myelinolysis. *J Clin Invest.* 1991;88:303-309.

440. Verbalis JG, Gullans SR. Hyponatremia causes large sustained reductions in brain content of multiple organic osmolytes in rats. *Brain Res.* 1991;567:274-282.

441. Verbalis JG, Gullans SR. Rapid correction of hyponatremia produces differential effects on brain osmolyte and electrolyte reaccumulation in rats. *Brain Res.* 1993;606:19-27.

442. Berl T. Treating hyponatremia: damned if we do and damned if we don't. *Kidney Int.* 1990;37:1006-1018.

443. Soupart A, Silver S, Schroeeder B, et al. Rapid (24-hour) reaccumulation of brain organic osmolytes (particularly myo-inositol) in azotemic rats after correction of chronic hyponatremia. *J Am Soc Nephrol.* 2002;13(6):1433-1441.

444. Gullans SR, Verbalis JG. Control of brain volume during hyperosmolar and hypo-osmolar conditions. *Annu Rev Med.* 1993;44:289-301.

445. Chow KM, Kwan BC, Szeto CC. Clinical studies of thiazide-induced hyponatremia. *J Natl Med Assoc.* 2004;96(10):1305-1308.

446. Renneboog B, Musch W, Vandemergel X, et al. Mild chronic hyponatremia is associated with falls, unsteadiness, and attention deficits. *Am J Med.* 2006;119(1):71.

447. Gankam KF, Andres C, Sattar L, et al. Mild hyponatremia and risk of fracture in the ambulatory elderly. *QJM.* 2008;101(7):583-588.

448. Sandhu HS, Gilles E, DeVita MV, et al. Hyponatremia associated with large-bone fracture in elderly patients. *Int Urol Nephrol.* 2009;41(3):733-737.

449. Kinsella S, Moran S, Sullivan MO, et al. Hyponatremia independent of osteoporosis is associated with fracture occurrence. *Clin J Am Soc Nephrol.* 2010;5(2):275-280.

450. Verbalis JG, Barsony J, Sugimura Y, et al. Hyponatremia-induced osteoporosis. *J Bone Miner Res.* 2010;25(3):554-563.

451. Ayus JC. Diuretic-induced hyponatremia. *Arch Intern Med.* 1986;146(7):1295-1296:[editorial].

452. Verbalis JG, Goldsmith SR, Greenberg A, et al. Hyponatremia treatment guidelines 2007: expert panel recommendations. *Am J Med.* 2007;120 (11 suppl 1):S1-S21.

453. Deleted in page proofs.

454. Steele A, Gowrishankar M, Abrahamson S, et al. Postoperative hyponatremia despite near-isotonic saline infusion: a phenomenon of desalination. *Ann Intern Med.* 1997;126(1):20-25:[comment in *Ann Intern Med* 126(12):1005-1006, 1997].

455. Adrogue HJ, Madias NE. Hyponatremia. *N Engl J Med.* 2000;342(21):1581-1589.

456. Hew-Butler T, Ayus JC, Kipps C, et al. Statement of the Second International Exercise-Associated Hyponatremia Consensus Development Conference, New Zealand, 2007. *Clin J Sport Med.* 2008;18(2):111-121.

457. Sterns RH, Cappuccio JD, Silver SM, et al. Neurologic sequelae after treatment of severe hyponatremia: a multicenter perspective. *J Am Soc Nephrol.* 1994;4:1522-1530.

458. Battison C, Andrews PJ, Graham C, et al. Randomized, controlled trial on the effect of a 20% mannitol solution and a 7.5% saline/6% dextran solution on increased intracranial pressure after brain injury. *Crit Care Med.* 2005;33(1):196-202.

459. Sterns RH, Riggs JE, Schochet Jr SS. Osmotic demyelination syndrome following correction of hyponatremia. *N Engl J Med.* 1986;314:1535-1542.

460. Robertson GL. Regulation of arginine vasopressin in the syndrome of inappropriate antidiuresis. *Am J Med.* 2006;119(7 suppl 1):S36-S42.

461. Furst H, Hallows KR, Post J, et al. The urine/plasma electrolyte ratio: a predictive guide to water restriction. *Am J Med Sci.* 2000;319(4):240-244.

462. Decaux G. The syndrome of inappropriate secretion of antidiuretic hormone (SIADH). *Semin Nephrol.* 2009;29(3):239-256.

463. Berl T. Impact of solute intake on urine flow and water excretion. *J Am Soc Nephrol.* 2008;19(6):1076-1078.

464. Singer I, Rotenberg D. Demeclocycline-induced nephrogenic diabetes insipidus. In-vivo and in-vitro studies. *Ann Intern Med.* 1973;79(5):679-683.

465. Ishikawa S, Fujita N, Fujisawa G, et al. Involvement of arginine vasopressin and renal sodium handling in pathogenesis of hyponatremia in elderly patients. *Endocr J.* 1996;43(1):101-108.

466. Decaux G, Genette F. Urea for long-term treatment of syndrome of inappropriate secretion of antidiuretic hormone. *Br Med J Clin Res.* 1981;283:1081-1083.

467. Decaux G, Waterlot Y, Genette F, et al. Treatment of the syndrome of inappropriate secretion of antidiuretic hormone with furosemide. *N Engl J Med.* 1981;304:329-330.

468. Greenberg A, Verbalis JG. Vasopressin receptor antagonists. *Kidney Int.* 2006;69(12):2124-2130.

469. Ohnishi A, Orita Y, Okahara R, et al. Potent aquaretic agent. A novel nonpeptide selective vasopressin 2 antagonist (OPC-31260) in men. *J Clin Invest.* 1993;92(6):2653-2659.

470. Zeltser D, Rosansky S, van Rensburg H, et al. Assessment of the efficacy and safety of intravenous conivaptan in euvolemic and hypervolemic hyponatremia. *Am J Nephrol.* 2007;27(5):447-457.

471. Schrier RW, Gross P, Gheorghiade M, et al. Tolvaptan, a selective oral vasopressin V2-receptor antagonist, for hyponatremia. *N Engl J Med.* 2006;355(20):2099-2112.

472. *Vaprisol (conivaptan hydrochloride injection) prescribing information.* Deerfield, Ill: Astellas Pharma US; 2006.

473. *Samsca (tolvaptan) prescribing information.* Tokyo: Otsuka Pharmaceutical Co; 2009.

474. Ellison DH, Berl T. Clinical practice. The syndrome of inappropriate antidiuresis. *N Engl J Med.* 2007;356(20):2064-2072.

475. Sterns RH, Nigwekar SU, Hix JK. The treatment of hyponatremia. *Semin Nephrol.* 2009;29(3):282-299.

476. Verbalis JG. Hyponatremia and hypo-osmolar disorders. In: Greenberg A, Cheung AK, Coffman TM, eds. *Primer on kidney diseases.* 5th ed. Philadelphia: Saunders; 2009:pp 52-59.

477. Soupart A, Penninckx R, Crenier L, et al. Prevention of brain demyelination in rats after excessive correction of chronic hyponatremia by serum sodium lowering. *Kidney Int.* 1994;45:193-200.

478. Goldszmidt MA, Iliescu EA. DDAVP to prevent rapid correction in hyponatremia. *Clin Nephrol.* 2000;53(3):226-229.

479. Oya S, Tsutsumi K, Ueki K, et al. Reinduction of hyponatremia to treat central pontine myelinolysis. *Neurology.* 2001;57(10):1931-1932.

480. Bissram M, Scott FD, Liu L, et al. Risk factors for symptomatic hyponatraemia: the role of pre-existing asymptomatic hyponatraemia. *Intern Med J.* 2007;37(3):149-155.

481. Berl T, Quittnat-Pelletier F, Verbalis JG, et al. Oral tolvaptan is safe and effective in chronic hyponatremia. *J Am Soc Nephrol.* 2010;21(4):705-712.

482. Konstam MA, Gheorghiade M, Burnett Jr JC, et al. Effects of oral tolvaptan in patients hospitalized for worsening heart failure: the EVEREST Outcome Trial. *JAMA.* 2007;297(12):1319-1331.

Disorders of Acid-Base Balance

Thomas D. DuBose Jr.

The appropriate diagnosis and management of acid-base disorders requires accurate interpretation of the specific acid-base disorder. Appropriate interpretation requires simultaneous measurement of plasma electrolyte levels and arterial blood gas (ABG) concentrations, as well as an appreciation by the clinician of the physiologic adaptations and compensatory responses that occur with specific acid-base disturbances. In most circumstances, these compensatory responses can be predicted through an analysis of the prevailing disorder in a stepwise manner. The maintenance of systemic pH requires the integration of a number of physiologic mechanisms, including cellular and extracellular buffering and the compensatory actions of the kidneys and lungs.

This chapter reviews acid-base homeostasis as a consequence of acid-base chemistry and physiology but places major emphasis on the pathophysiologic basis, diagnosis, and management of clinical acid-base disorders. The diagnosis of acid-base disorders is reviewed in detail, with emphasis on a simple stepwise approach founded on appreciation of the anion gap and the limits of physiologic compensation, especially in critically ill patients, in whom complex acid-base disturbances occur regularly.

Acid-Base Homeostasis

Acid-base homeostasis operates to maintain systemic arterial pH within a narrow range. Although clinical laboratories consider the normal range to be between 7.35 and 7.45 pH units, pH in vivo in an individual is maintained within a much narrower range. This degree of tight regulation is accomplished through (1) chemical buffering in the extracellular fluid (ECF) and the intracellular fluid (ICF), and (2) regulatory responses that are under the control of the respiratory and renal systems. Those chemical buffers, respiration, and renal processes efficiently dispose of the physiologic daily load of carbonic acid (as volatile CO_2) and nonvolatile acids, mainly derived from dietary protein intake, and defend against the occasional addition of pathologic quantities of acid and alkali. Therefore, chemical buffers within the extracellular and intracellular compartments serve to blunt changes in pH that would occur with retention of either acids or bases. In addition, the control of CO_2 tension (P_{CO_2}) by the central nervous system and respiratory system and the control of the plasma HCO_3^- by the kidneys constitute the regulatory processes that act in concert to stabilize the arterial pH.

The major buffer system in the body comprises a base (H^+ acceptor), which is predominantly HCO_3^-, and an acid (H^+ donor), which is predominantly carbonic acid (H_2CO_3):

$$H^+ + HCO_3^- \Leftrightarrow H_2CO_3 \quad (1)$$

Extracellular H^+ concentration ($[H^+]_e$) throughout the body is constant in the steady state. The HCO_3^-/H_2CO_3 ratio is proportional to the ratio of all the other extracellular buffers such as PO_4^{3-} and plasma proteins:

$$[H^+]_e \propto \frac{HCO_3^-}{H_2CO_3} \propto \frac{B^-}{HB} \quad (2)$$

The intracellular H^+ concentration ($[H^+]_i$), or pH_i, is also relatively stable. Both cellular ion exchange mechanisms and intracellular buffers (hemoglobin, tissue proteins, organophosphate complexes, and bone apatite) participate in the blunting of changes in both $[H^+]_i$ and $[H^+]_e$. Extracellular and intracellular buffers provide the *first line of defense* against the addition of acid or base to the body (see "Mechanisms of pH Buffering" section later).

The second line of defense is the respiratory system. Pulmonary participation in acid-base homeostasis relies on the excretion of CO_2 by the lungs. The reaction is catalyzed by the enzyme carbonic anhydrase:

$$H^+ + HCO_3^- \leftrightarrow H_2CO_3 \xleftrightarrow[\text{anhydrase}]{\text{Carbonic}} H_2O + CO_2 \quad (3)$$

Large amounts of CO_2 (10 to 12 mol/day) accumulate as metabolic end products of tissue metabolism. This CO_2 load is transported in the blood to the lungs as hemoglobin-generated HCO_3^- and hemoglobin-bound carbamino groups.[1]

$$\text{Metabolism} \rightarrow CO_2 \xleftrightarrow[\text{transport}]{\text{Blood}} \text{Lungs} \quad (4)$$

Conventionally, H^+ concentration is expressed in two different ways, either directly as $[H^+]$ or indirectly as pH. The relationship between these two factors can be written in mathematically equivalent forms:

$$pH = -\log_{10}[H^+] \quad (5)$$

$$[H^+] (Eq/L) = 10^{-pH} \quad (6)$$

When $[H^+]$ is expressed (for numeric convenience) in nanomoles per liter (nmol/L) or nanomolars (nM), then

$$[H^+] = 10^{9-pH} \quad (7)$$

Buffer Systems

Acid-base chemistry deals with molecular interactions that involve the transfer of H^+. A large variety of molecules, both inorganic and organic, contain hydrogen atoms that can dissociate to yield H^+. The relationship between an undissociated acid (HA) and its conjugate, disassociated base (A^-) may be represented as follows:

$$HA \Leftrightarrow H^+ + A^- \quad (8)$$

In addition to the many inorganic and organic acid-base substances encountered in biologic systems, many protein molecules (e.g., hemoglobin) contain acidic groups that may dissociate, yielding a corresponding conjugate base.

Mechanisms of pH Buffering

Buffer systems are critical to the physiology and pathophysiology of acid-base homeostasis and, in their broadest definition, are systems that attenuate the pH change in a solution or tissue by reversibly combining with or releasing H^+. Thus, the pH change of a solution during the addition of acid or base equivalents is smaller in the presence of a buffer system than it would have been if no buffer systems were present. The acid or base load can be *extrinsic*, such as during systemic acid or base infusion, or *intrinsic*, resulting from net generation of new acid or base equivalents that are added to the extracellular or intracellular space.

Chemical Equilibria of Physicochemical Buffer Systems

As an example of a physicochemical buffer pair, consider a neutral weak acid (HA) and its conjugate weak base (A^-). Examples of such buffer pairs are acetic acid and acetate and the carboxyl groups on proteins. Another example of a physicochemical buffer pair is a neutral weak base (B) and its conjugate weak acid (BH^+):

$$BH^+ \Leftrightarrow B + H^+ \quad (9)$$

Examples of such buffer pairs are NH_3 and NH_4^+ and the imidazole group in proteins. A rigorous analysis of the kinetics of reversible reactions in solution yields the law of mass action, which states that, at equilibrium (i.e., when the velocities of the forward and backward reactions are equal), the ratio of the concentration products of opposing reactions is a constant.

$$K_a' = \frac{[H^+][A^-]}{HA} \quad (10)$$

$$K_b' = \frac{[H^+][B^-]}{BH} \quad (11)$$

K_a' and K_b' are the equilibrium or dissociation constants for equations 10 and 11, respectively.

Taking logarithms of both sides of equations 10 and 11 and defining $pK_a' = -\log_{10}(K_a')$ and $pK_b' = -\log_{10}(K_b')$ yields

$$pH = pK_a' + \log_{10}\frac{[A^-]}{[HA]} \quad (12)$$

$$pH = pK_b' + \log_{10}\frac{[B^-]}{[BH]} \quad (13)$$

The dissociation constants K_a' and K_b' provide an estimate of the strength of the acid and base, respectively. From equations 12 and 13, it can be seen that the buffer pairs are half dissociated at $pH = pK'$. In other words, pK' of a buffer pair is defined as the pH at which 50% of the buffer pair exists as the weak acid (HA) and 50% as the anion (A^-).

Chemical Equilibria for the Carbon Dioxide–Bicarbonate System

When CO_2 is dissolved in water, H_2CO_3 is formed according to the reaction

$$CO_2 + H_2O \Leftrightarrow H_2CO_3 \quad (14)$$

The rate of this reaction, in the absence of the enzyme carbonic anhydrase, is slow, with a half-time of about 8 seconds at 37°C. The major portion of CO_2 remains as dissolved CO_2; only about 1 part in 1000 forms H_2CO_3, a nonvolatile acid. Because H_2CO_3 is a weak acid, it dissociates to yield H^+ and HCO_3^-.

$$H_2CO_3 \Leftrightarrow H^+ + HCO_3^- \tag{15}$$

The concentration of dissolved CO_2 is given by Henry's law:

$$[CO_2]_{dis} = \alpha_{CO_2} P_{CO_2} \tag{16}$$

where α_{CO_2} is the physical solubility coefficient for CO_2, which has a value of 0.0301 mmol/L in most body fluids, including plasma. Because the concentration of H_2CO_3 is low and proportional to the concentration of dissolved CO_2, equations 14 and 15 can be combined and treated as a single reaction:

$$CO_2 + H_2O \Leftrightarrow H^+ + HCO_3^- \tag{17}$$

The equilibrium constant for this reaction is given by

$$K = \frac{[H^+][HCO_3^-]}{[CO_2][H_2O]} \tag{18}$$

Defining $K' = K[H_2O]$ as the apparent equilibrium constant and using equation 17,

$$K' = \frac{[H^+][HCO_3^-]}{\alpha_{CO_2} P_{CO_2}} \tag{19}$$

Taking logarithms of both sides of equation 19 and recognizing that $pK' = \log_{10}(K')$ allows the familiar Henderson-Hasselbalch equation to be derived:

$$pH = pK' + \log_{10} \frac{[HCO_3^-]}{(\alpha_{CO_2} P_{CO_2})} \tag{20}$$

When $pK' = 6.1$ is used in equation 20, the Henderson equation is derived, which may be used in clinical interpretation of acid-base data:

$$[H^+](nmol/L) = 24 \frac{P_{CO_2}(mm\,Hg)}{[HCO_3^-](mmol/L)} \tag{21}$$

Physiologic Advantage of an Open Buffer System

The quantitative behavior of an open system buffer pair differs considerably from that of a buffer pair confined to a closed system. In an open system, the buffer pair may be envisioned as occurring in two separate but communicating compartments (internal and external). The external compartment provides an effective infinite reservoir of the uncharged buffer pair component, to which the barrier between the internal and the external compartments (e.g., plasma cell membrane, vascular capillary endothelium) is freely permeable.

Physiologically, the most important open system buffer is the CO_2-HCO_3^- system. Adjustments in alveolar ventilation serve to maintain a constant arterial CO_2 pressure (P_{aCO_2}):

$$\begin{array}{ccc} \text{Acid (H}^+\text{)} & & \text{(expired gas)} \\ \downarrow & & \uparrow\uparrow \\ H^+ + HCO_3^- \rightarrow & H_2CO_3 \rightarrow & H_2O + CO_2 \end{array} \tag{22}$$

The CO_2-HCO_3^- buffer system has a pK' of 6.1 and a base/acid ($[HCO_3^-]/[H_2CO_3]$) ratio of 20:1 at pH 7.4. Because buffer efficiency is greatest in the pH range near pK'_a, it appears at first glance that the CO_2-HCO_3^- system would not function as an effective buffer in the physiologic pH range. The potency and efficacy of the CO_2-HCO_3^- buffer system are due largely to the augmentation of buffer capacity that accompanies operation in an open system. Because CO_2 is freely diffusible across biologic barriers and cell membranes, its concentration in biologic fluids can be modulated rapidly through participation of the respiratory system. When acid (H^+) is added to an HCO_3^--containing fluid, H^+ combines with HCO_3^- to generate H_2CO_3, which, in the presence of the enzyme carbonic anhydrase, is rapidly dehydrated to CO_2 (equation 22). The CO_2 produced can escape rapidly from the fluid and be excreted in the lung, which prevents accumulation of CO_2 concentrations in biologic fluids.

Regulation of Buffers

The plasma HCO_3^- concentration is protected by both metabolic and renal regulatory mechanisms. In addition, the pH of blood can be affected by respiratory adjustments in P_{aCO_2}. Primary changes in P_{aCO_2} may result in acidosis or alkalosis, depending on whether CO_2 is elevated above or depressed below the normal value: 40 mm Hg. Such disorders are termed *respiratory acidosis* and *respiratory alkalosis,* respectively. A primary change in the plasma HCO_3^- concentration owing to metabolic or renal factors results in commensurate changes in ventilation. The respiratory response to acidemia or alkalemia blunts the change in blood pH that would occur otherwise. Such respiratory alterations that adjust blood pH toward normal are referred to as *secondary* or *compensatory* alterations, because they occur in response to primary metabolic changes.

Humans are confronted, under most physiologic circumstances, with an acid challenge. "Acid production" in biologic systems is represented by the milliequivalents (mEq) of protons (H^+) added to body fluids. Conversely, proton removal is equivalent to equimolar addition of base, OH^- (generation of HCO_3^- from dissolved CO_2). Metabolism generates a daily load of relatively strong acids (lactate, citrate, acetate, and pyruvate), which must be removed by other metabolic reactions. The oxidation of these organic acids in the Krebs cycle, for example, generates CO_2, which must be excreted by the lungs. The oxidation of carbon-containing fuels produces as much as 16,000 to 20,000 mmol of CO_2 gas daily. Nevertheless, the complete combustion of carbon involves the intermediate generation and metabolism of 2000 to 3000 mmol of relatively strong organic acids, such as lactic acids, tricarboxylic acids, ketoacids, or other acids, depending on the type of fuel consumed. These organic acids do not accumulate in the body under most circumstances, with concentrations remaining in the low millimolar range. If production and consumption rates become mismatched, however, these organic acids can accumulate (e.g., lactic acid accumulation with strenuous exertion). Correspondingly, the HCO_3^- in the ECF will decline as the organic acid concentration increases. During recovery, the organic acids reenter metabolic pathways to CO_2 production, removal of H^+, and generation of HCO_3^-. Nevertheless, if the organic anions are excreted (e.g., ketonuria), these entities are no longer available for regeneration of HCO_3^-. The metabolism of some body constituents such as proteins, nucleic acids, and small fractions of lipids and certain carbohydrates generates specific organic acids that cannot be burned to CO_2 (e.g., uric, oxalic, glucuronic, hippuric acids). In addition, the inorganic acids H_2SO_4 and H_3PO_4, derived respectively from sulfur-containing amino acids and organophosphates, must be excreted by the kidneys or the gastrointestinal tract.

In summary, in the steady state, as a result of the buffering power of the HCO_3^-/H_2CO_3 buffer system and its preeminence over other body buffer systems, addition or removal of H^+ results in equimolar changes in the HCO_3^- concentration according to the relationship outlined in equation 3. Moreover, because this buffer system is open to air, the concentration of CO_2 remains essentially fixed. Therefore, the evidence for H^+ addition or removal can be found in reciprocal changes in the numerator of the Henderson-Hasselbalch equation (equation 20), or the $[HCO_3^-]$.

Integration of Regulatory Processes

Three physiologic processes militate against changes in the HCO_3^-/CO_2 ratio: (1) metabolic regulation, (2) respiratory regulation, and (3) renal regulation. Metabolic regulation is of minor importance in terms of overall physiologic regulation of acid-base balance. Nevertheless, regulatory enzymes, whose activity may be pH sensitive, may catalyze metabolic reactions that either generate or consume organic acids. Such a process constitutes a negative feedback regulatory system. The best example is phosphofructokinase, the pivotal enzyme in the glycolytic pathway. Phosphofructokinase is a kinase enzyme that phosphorylates fructose 6-phosphate in glycolysis. The activity of phosphofructokinase is inhibited by low pH and enhanced by high pH. Thus, an increase in pH_i accelerates glycolysis and generates pyruvate and lactate. It follows, therefore, that the generation of lactic acid in patients with lactic acidosis and the generation of ketoacids in patients with keto-acidosis are impeded by acidemia.

Because, under most circumstances, CO_2 excretion and CO_2 production are matched, the usual steady-state $Paco_2$ is maintained at 40 mm Hg. Underexcretion of CO_2 produces hypercapnia, and overexcretion produces hypocapnia. Production and excretion are again matched but at a new steady-state Pco_2. Therefore, the $Paco_2$ is regulated primarily by neurorespiratory factors and is not subject to regulation by the rate of metabolic CO_2 production. Hypercapnia is primarily the result of hypoventilation, not increased CO_2 production. Increases or decreases in Pco_2 represent derangements of control of neurorespiratory regulation or can result from compensatory changes in response to a primary alteration in the plasma HCO_3^- concentration.

Renal Regulation

Although temporary relief from changes in the pH of body fluids may be accomplished by chemical buffering or respiratory compensation, the ultimate defense against the addition of nonvolatile acid or of alkali resides in the kidneys. The addition of a strong acid (HA) to the ECF titrates plasma HCO_3^-:

$$HA + NaHCO_3 \Leftrightarrow NaA + H_2O + CO_2 \qquad (23)$$

The CO_2 is expired by the lungs, and body HCO_3^- buffer stores are diminished. This process occurs constantly as endogenous metabolic acids are generated. To maintain a normal plasma HCO_3^- in the face of constant accession of metabolic acids, the kidneys must (1) conserve the HCO_3^- present in glomerular filtrate, and (2) regenerate the HCO_3^- decomposed by reaction with metabolic acids (equation 23). The first process (HCO_3^- reclamation) is accomplished predominantly in the proximal tubule, with an additional contribution by the loop of Henle and a minor contribution by more distal nephron segments. Under most circumstances, the filtered load of HCO_3^- is absorbed almost completely, especially during an acid load. Nevertheless, when less acid is generated or when the plasma HCO_3^- concentration increases above the normal value of 25 mEq/L, HCO_3^- will be excreted efficiently into the urine. The second process, HCO_3^- regeneration, is represented by the renal output of acid or net acid excretion (Figure 16-1).

$$\text{Net acid excretion} = NH_4^+ + \text{Titratable acid} - HCO_3^- \qquad (24)$$

On balance, each milliequivalent of net acid excreted corresponds to 1 mEq of HCO_3^- returned to the ECF. This process of HCO_3^- regeneration is necessary to replace the HCO_3^- lost by the entry of fixed acids into the ECF or, less commonly, the HCO_3^- excreted in stool or urine. Because a typical North American diet generates fixed acids at 50 to 70 mEq/day, net acid excretion must be affected to maintain acid-base balance. Therefore, net acid excretion approximates 50 to 70 mEq/day. If acid production remained increased and unabated by net acid excretion, metabolic acidosis would ensue. Conversely, an increase in net acid excretion above the level of net acid production results in metabolic alkalosis. Daily acid-base balance can be estimated, therefore, by subtracting net acid excretion plus any base absorbed from the gut from the amount of acid produced daily. The daily production of acid is represented by the amount of H_2SO_4 and noncombustible organic acids generated. In other words, net acid production is represented by the milliequivalents of SO_4^{2-} and organic acid anions (A^-) excreted in the urine.

Systemic Response to Changes in Carbon Dioxide Tension

Acute Response: Generation of Respiratory Acidosis or Alkalosis

Intrinsic disturbances in the respiratory system can alter the relationship of CO_2 production and excretion and give rise to abnormal values of $Paco_2$. Some stimuli evoke a primary increase in ventilation, which lowers systemic $Paco_2$. These stimuli include hypoxemia, fever, anxiety, central nervous system disease, acute cardiopulmonary processes, septicemia, liver failure, pregnancy, and drugs (e.g., salicylates).[2] Conversely, $Paco_2$ increases if the respiratory system is depressed by suppression of the respiratory control center or of the respiratory apparatus itself (neuromuscular, parenchymal, and airway components).[3] In both kinds of acute respiratory disorders, CO_2 is added to or subtracted from the body until the $Paco_2$ assumes a new steady state so that pulmonary CO_2 excretion equals CO_2 production. The accumulation or loss of CO_2 causes changes in blood pH within minutes. The

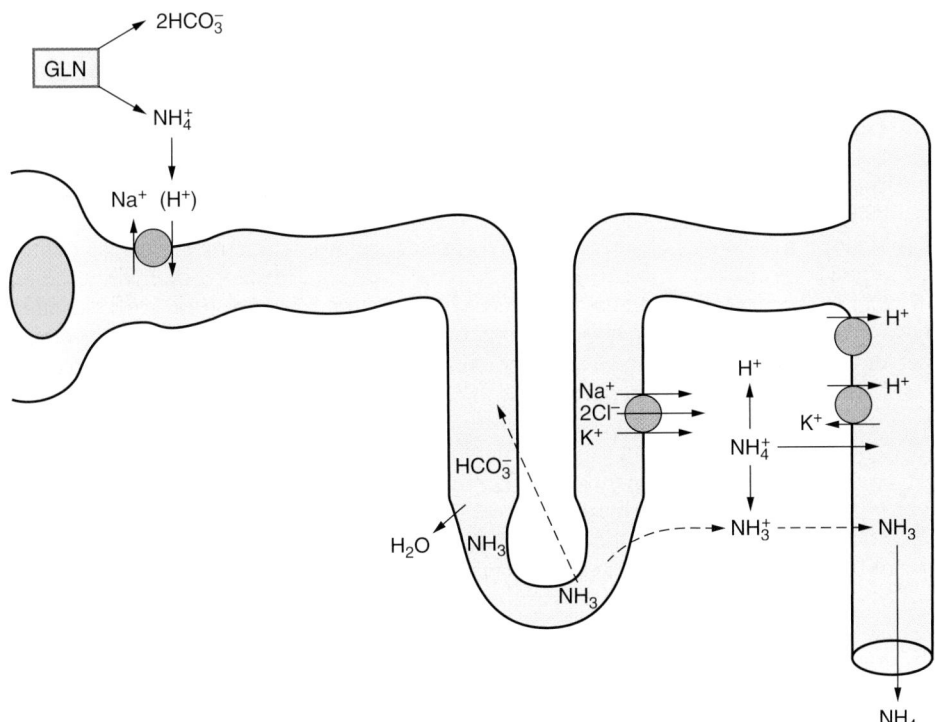

FIGURE 16-1 Synchrony of regulation of ammonium production (from glutamine [GLN] precursors, and excretion). Process allows generation of "new" HCO_3^- by the kidney. NH_4^+ excretion is regulated in response to changes in systemic acid-base and K^+ balance. Contributing segments include the proximal convoluted tubule, proximal straight tubule, thin descending limb, thick ascending limb, and medullary collecting duct. Upregulated by acidosis and hypokalemia. Inhibited by hyperkalemia.

plasma HCO_3^- decreases slightly as the $Paco_2$ is reduced in acute respiratory alkalosis and increases slightly in acute respiratory acidosis.[1-4] The small changes in HCO_3^- concentration are due to buffering by nonbicarbonate buffers.[1-4] The estimated change in blood HCO_3^- concentration is approximately equal to 0.1 mEq/L of $[HCO_3^-]$ for each millimeter of mercury increase in Pco_2 and 0.25 mEq/L for each millimeter of mercury decrease in Pco_2.[3] Acute alterations in Pco_2 in either direction within the physiologic range do not change the blood HCO_3^- concentration by more than a total of about 4 to 5 mEq/L from normal. Organic acid production, especially of lactic and citric acids, increases modestly during acute hypocapnia, decreasing the blood HCO_3^- concentration and blunting the respiratory response to metabolic alkalosis.[1-4]

Chronic Response

Although the blood pH is relatively poorly defended during acute changes in $Paco_2$, during chronic changes, the kidneys are recruited to excrete or retain HCO_3^- and return blood pH toward normal. The persistence of hypocapnia reduces renal bicarbonate absorption to achieve a further decrease in the plasma HCO_3^- concentration. Hypocapnia decreases renal HCO_3^- reabsorption[2] by inhibiting acidification in both the proximal[4] and the distal nephrons. The resulting decrease in plasma HCO_3^- concentration is equal to about 0.4 to 0.5 mEq/L for each millimeter of mercury decrease in Pco_2.[3] Thus, the arterial pH falls toward but not completely back to normal.

Several hours to days are required for full expression of the renal response to chronic hypocapnia,[3,4] which includes a reduction in the rate of H^+ secretion, an increase in urine pH, a decrease in NH_4^+ and titratable acid excretion, and a modest bicarbonaturia. An increase in blood Cl^- concentration occurs

simultaneously by means of several mechanisms: a shift of Cl^- out of red blood cells, ECF volume contraction, and enhanced Cl^- reabsorption. An overshoot in HCO_3^- generation and sustained reabsorption may occur on occasion, so that blood pH may become alkaline with severe chronic hypercapnia (values of ≤70 mm Hg).[3,4] One example of this phenomenon is the increment in renal HCO_3^- generation caused by nocturnal CO_2 retention in patients with obstructive sleep apnea. Both blood Pco_2 and HCO_3^- concentration increase during the night. Later in the morning, alkalotic blood gas values are often obtained, because $Paco_2$ has declined more rapidly than HCO_3^- concentration to values characteristic of wakefulness. In chronic hypercapnia, the blood HCO_3^- concentration increases about 0.25 to 0.50 mEq/L for each millimeter of mercury elevation in $Paco_2$.[3,4]

The increase in generation of HCO_3^- by the kidney during chronic hypercapnia takes several days for completion. The mechanism of HCO_3^- retention involves increased H^+ secretion by both proximal and distal nephron segments, regardless of sodium bicarbonate or sodium chloride intake, mineralocorticoid levels, or K^+ depletion.[1,3-5]

Chronic hypercapnia results in sustained increases in renal cortical Pco_2, and the increase in renal cortical Pco_2 that occurs with chronic hypercapnia stimulates acidification.[4,5] The increased Pco_2 enhances distal H^+ secretion so that increased NH_4^+ excretion occurs even with a low-salt diet or with hypoxemia. However, if hyperkalemia ensues or is present initially, the renal adaptation to chronic hypercapnia is blunted significantly. Hyperkalemia decreases NH_4^+ production and excretion even in the face of acidemia.[5,6] The effect of an elevated Pco_2 to augment tubule HCO_3^- reabsorption may also be mediated by hemodynamic changes, especially by systemic vasodilatation, so that a decreased effective ECF status is sensed by the kidney. Hypercapnia also decreases proximal sodium chloride reabsorption and causes chloruresis, which can further compromise ECF.[4,5] If the hemodynamic alterations induced by hypercapnia are corrected, the direct effect of acute hypercapnia to increase net renal HCO_3^- transport is abated. Thus, with time an adaptation occurs in the proximal nephron: HCO_3^- reabsorption is stimulated after several days of hypercapnia.[7]

In summary, although primary alterations in systemic $Paco_2$ cause relatively marked changes in blood pH, renal homeostatic mechanisms allow the blood pH to return toward normal over a sufficient period. The renal response to chronic hypercapnia is manifest primarily by an increase in net acid excretion and HCO_3^- absorption, which is accomplished by augmented H^+ secretion in both proximal and distal nephron segments.[8]

Systemic Response to Addition of Nonvolatile Acids

In addition to generating large quantities of CO_2, the metabolic processes of the body produce a smaller quantity of nonvolatile acids. The lungs readily excrete CO_2, and this process can respond rapidly to changes in production. In contrast, the kidneys must excrete nonvolatile acids through a much slower adaptive response. The time course of compensation for addition of acid or alkali to the body is displayed schematically in Figure 16-2. The hypothetical completion of each process is plotted as a function of time and progresses in the following sequence: (1) distribution and buffering in the ECF, (2) cellular buffering, (3) respiratory compensation, and (4) renal acid or base excretion.

Sources of Endogenous Acids

Pathologically, acid loads may be derived from endogenous acid production (e.g., generation of ketoacids and lactic acids) or loss of base (e.g., diarrhea) or from exogenous sources (e.g., ammonium chloride or toxin ingestion). Under normal physiologic circumstances, a daily input of acid derived from the diet and metabolism confronts the body. The net result of

these processes amounts to the entry of about 1.0 mEq of new H^+ per kilogram per day into the ECF.[1,4]

Sulfuric acid is formed when organic sulfur from methionine and cysteine residues of proteins are oxidized to SO_4^{2-}. The metabolism of sulfur-containing amino acids is the primary source of acid in the usual Western diet, accounting for approximately 50%. The quantity of sulfuric acid generated is equal to the SO_4^{2-} excreted in the urine.

Organic acids are derived from intermediary metabolites formed by partial combustion of dietary carbohydrates, fats, and proteins as well as from nucleic acids (uric acid). Organic acid generation contributes to net endogenous acid production when the conjugate bases are excreted in the urine as organic anions. If full oxidation of these acids can occur, however, H^+ is reclaimed and eliminated as CO_2 and water. The net amount of H^+ added to the body from this source can be estimated by the amount of organic anions excreted in the urine.

Phosphoric acid can be derived from hydrolysis of PO_4^{3-} esters in proteins and nucleic acids if it is not neutralized by mineral cations (e.g., Na^+, K^+, and Mg^{2+}). The contribution of dietary phosphates to acid production is dependent on the kind of protein ingested. Some proteins generate phosphoric acid, whereas others generate only neutral phosphate salts.[1,4] Hydrochloric acid is generated by metabolism of cationic amino acids (lysine, arginine, and some histidine residues) into neutral products. Other potential acid or base sources in the diet can be estimated from the amount of unidentified cations and anions ingested.

Potential sources of bases are also found in the diet (e.g., acetate, lactate, citrate) and can be absorbed to neutralize partially the H^+ loads from the three sources just mentioned. These potential base equivalents may be estimated by subtracting the unmeasured anions in the stool ($Na^+ + K^+ + Ca^{2+} + Mg^{2+} - Cl^- = 1.8$ P) from those measured in the diet. The net base absorbed by the gastrointestinal tract is derived from the anion gap (AG) of the diet minus that of the stool. Acid production is partially offset by HCO_3^- produced when organic anions combine with H^+ and are oxidized to CO_2 and H_2O or when dibasic phosphoesters combine with H^+ during hydrolysis. The gastrointestinal tract may modify the amount of these

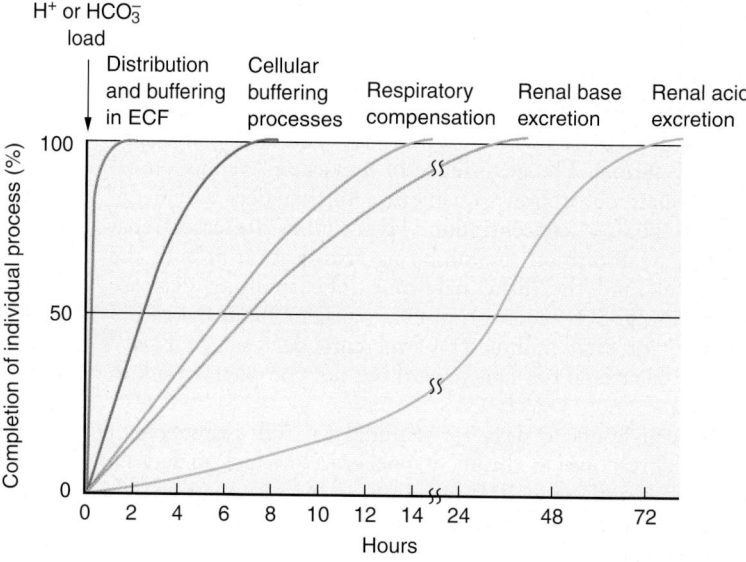

FIGURE 16-2 Time course of acid-base compensatory mechanisms in response to a metabolic acid or alkaline load. Component processes in completion of the distribution and extracellular buffering mechanisms, cellular buffering events, and respiratory and renal regulatory processes are presented as a function of time. *ECF,* Extracellular fluid.

potential bases reabsorbed under particular circumstances of acidosis or growth. It has been confirmed in patients ingesting an artificial diet that urinary $[NH_4^+ + $ titratable acid $(TA) - HCO_3^-]$ is equal to urinary $[SO_4^{2-} + $ organic $A^- + $ dietary phosphoester-derived $H^+]$.[1,4,9]

In summary, dietary foodstuffs contain many sources of acids and bases. These can be estimated by the urinary excretion of SO_4^{2-} and organic anions minus the unmeasured anions. The usual North American diet represents a daily source of acid generation for which the body must compensate constantly.

Hepatic and Renal Roles in Acid-Base Homeostasis

The generation of acid by protein catabolism is balanced by the generation of new HCO_3^- through renal NH_4^+ and titratable acid excretion. Hepatic catabolism of proteins, with the exception of sulfur- and PO_4^{3-}-containing amino acids, can be considered a neutral process. The products of these neutral reactions are HCO_3^- and NH_4^+. Most of the NH_4^+ produced by metabolism of amino acids reacts with HCO_3^- or forms urea and thus has no impact on acid-base balance. A portion of this NH_4^+ is diverted to glutamine synthesis, the amount of which is regulated by pH. Acidemia promotes and alkalemia inhibits glutamine synthesis. Glutamine enters the circulation and reaches the kidney, where it is deaminated to form glutamate. Renal glutamine deamination results in NH_4^+ production and initiates a metabolic process that generates new HCO_3^- through α-ketoglutarate. Glutamine deamination in the kidney is also highly regulated by systemic pH, so that acidemia augments and alkalemia inhibits NH_4^+ and HCO_3^- production. The ultimate control, however, resides in the renal excretion of NH_4^+, because the NH_4^+ must be excreted to escape entry into the hepatic urea synthetic pool. Hepatic urea synthesis would negate the new HCO_3^- realized from α-ketoglutarate in the kidney. Hepatic regulation of NH_4^+ metabolic pathways appears to facilitate glutamine production when NH_4^+ excretion is stimulated by acidemia or, conversely, blunts glutamine production when excretion is inhibited by alkalemia.[9]

Neurorespiratory Response to Acidemia

A critically important response to an acid load is the neurorespiratory control of ventilation. Although the precise mechanism for this response is debated,[1,3,4,9] the prevailing view is that a fall in systemic arterial pH is sensed by the chemoreceptors that stimulate ventilation and, therefore, reduce $Paco_2$. The fall in blood pH that would otherwise occur in uncompensated metabolic acidosis is therefore blunted. The pH is not restored to normal; however, $Paco_2$ declines by an average of 1.25 mm Hg for each 1.0 mEq/L drop in HCO_3^- concentration. The appropriate $Paco_2$ in steady-state metabolic acidosis can be estimated from the prevailing HCO_3^- concentration according to the following expression[10]:

$$Paco_2 = 1.5 [HCO_3^-] + 8 (\pm 2 \text{ mm Hg}) \qquad (25)$$

It is convenient to remember that the predicted (or compensatory) $Paco_2$ can be approximated by adding to the patient's $[HCO_3^-]$ the number 15 (valid in the pH range of 7.2 to 7.5). Because the $Paco_2$ cannot fall below about 10 to 12 mm Hg, the blood pH is less well defended by respiration after very large reductions in the plasma HCO_3^- concentration (Table 16-1).

Approximately 12 to 24 hours is required to achieve full respiratory compensation for metabolic acidosis (see Figure 16-2).

TABLE 16-1 Acid-Base Abnormalities and Appropriate Compensatory Responses for Simple Disorders					
PRIMARY ACID-BASE DISORDERS	**PRIMARY DEFECT**	**EFFECT ON pH**	**COMPENSATORY RESPONSE**	**EXPECTED RANGE OF COMPENSATION**	**LIMITS OF COMPENSATION**
Respiratory acidosis	Alveolar hypoventilation ($\uparrow Pco_2$)	$\downarrow$	$\uparrow$ Renal HCO_3^- reabsorption ($HCO_3^- \uparrow$)	Acute $\Delta[HCO_3^-] = +1$ mEq/L for each $\uparrow$ ΔPco_2 of 10 mm Hg	$[HCO_3^-] = 38$ mEq/L
				Chronic $\Delta[HCO_3^-] = +4$ mEq/L for each $\uparrow$ ΔPco_2 of 10 mm Hg	$[HCO_3^-] = 45$ mEq/L
Respiratory alkalosis	Alveolar hyperventilation ($\downarrow Pco_2$)	$\uparrow$	$\downarrow$ Renal HCO_3^- reabsorption ($HCO_3^- \downarrow$)	Acute $\Delta[HCO_3^-] = -2$ mEq/L for each $\downarrow$ ΔPco_2 of 10 mm Hg	$[HCO_3^-] = 18$ mEq/L
				Chronic $\Delta[HCO_3^-] = -5$ mEq/L for each $\downarrow$ ΔPco_2 of 10 mm Hg	$[HCO_3^-] = 15$ mEq/L
Metabolic acidosis	Loss of HCO_3^- or gain of H^+ ($\downarrow HCO_3^-$)	$\downarrow$	Alveolar hyperventilation to $\uparrow$ pulmonary CO_2 excretion ($\downarrow Pco_2$)	$Pco_2 = 1.5[HCO_3^-] + 8 \pm 2$ $Pco_2 = $ last 2 digits of pH $\times$ 100 $Pco_2 = 15 + [HCO_3^-]$	$Pco_2 = 15$ mm Hg
Metabolic alkalosis	Gain of HCO_3^- or loss of H^+ ($\uparrow HCO_3^-$)	$\uparrow$	Alveolar hypoventilation to $\downarrow$ pulmonary CO_2 excretion ($\uparrow Pco_2$)	$Pco_2 = +0.6$ mm Hg for $\Delta[HCO_3^-]$ of 1 mEq/L $Pco_2 = 15 + [HCO_3^-]$	$Pco_2 = 55$ mm Hg

Pco_2, Carbon dioxide pressure.
Adapted from Bidani A, Tauzon DM, Heming TA: Regulation of whole body acid-base balance, in DuBose TD, Hamm LL (editors): *Acid-base and electrolyte disorders: a companion to Brenner and Rector's the kidney,* Philadelphia, 2002, Saunders, pp 1-2.)

Renal Excretion

As already discussed, the kidneys eliminate the acid that is produced daily by metabolism and diet and have the capacity to increase urinary net acid excretion (and, hence, HCO_3^- generation) in response to endogenous or exogenous acid loads. Renal excretion of acid is usually matched to the net production of metabolic and dietary acids, about 55 to 70 mEq/day, so little disturbance in systemic pH or HCO_3^- concentration occurs.

As an acid load is incurred, the kidneys respond to restore balance by increasing NH_4^+ excretion (titratable acid excretion has limited capacity for regulation). With continued acid loading, renal net acid excretion increases over the course of 3 to 5 days (see Figure 16-2) but does not quite achieve the level of acid production. Progressive positive acid balance ensues, buffered presumably by bone carbonate.

Thus, the renal response to an acid load requires (1) reclamation of the filtered HCO_3^- by the proximal tubule, and (2) augmentation of NH_4^+ production and excretion by the distal nephron. In this way, the kidneys efficiently retain all filtered base and attempt to generate enough new base to restore the arterial pH toward normal.

In summary, acidosis enhances proximal HCO_3^- absorption, decreasing delivery of HCO_3^- out of the proximal tubule, and enhances distal acidification. Net acid excretion is increased by stimulation of NH_4^+ production and excretion.

Systemic Response to Gain of Alkali

Whereas the major goal of the body in defense of an acid challenge is to conserve body buffer stores and to generate new base, the response to an alkali load is to eliminate base as rapidly as possible. The response is dependent on the same three responses outlined for defense of an acid challenge, namely, cellular buffering and distribution within the ECF, respiratory compensation, and renal excretion.

Distribution and Cellular Buffering

Ninety-five percent of a base load in the form of HCO_3^- is distributed in the ECF within about 25 minutes[1,4,9,11] (see Figure 16-2). Simultaneously, the various processes of cellular buffering serve to dissipate this HCO_3^- load. Cellular buffering of the HCO_3^- load has a half-time of 3.3 hours. The apparent distribution volume for the administered HCO_3^- is inversely proportional to the preexisting plasma HCO_3^- concentration. A lesser fraction of base is buffered via cellular processes than occurs when a comparable amount of acid is administered (see Figure 16-2). Two thirds of the administered HCO_3^- is retained in the ECF; a third is buffered in cells, principally by Na^+/H^+ exchange, and a small amount is buffered by increased lactate production and Cl^-/HCO_3^- exchange.[1] Modest hypokalemia occurs as a result of K^+ shifts into cells and is approximately equal to 0.4 to 0.5 mEq/L of K^+ per 0.1 unit pH increase above 7.40.

In summary, the cellular defense against an alkaline load is somewhat less effective than the defense against an acid load. There is also poorer stabilization of intracellular pH in the alkaline than in the acid range.[1,11]

Respiratory Compensation

The pulmonary response to an acute increase in HCO_3^- concentration is biphasic. Neutralization of sodium bicarbonate by buffers (H^+ buffer$^-$) results in CO_2 liberation and an increase in Pco_2:

$$Na^+HCO_3^- + H^+buffer^- \Leftrightarrow Na^+buffer^- + H_2CO_3 \Leftrightarrow H_2O + CO_2 \quad (26)$$

The increased Pco_2 stimulates ventilation acutely to return Pco_2 toward normal. If the pulmonary system is compromised or the ventilation rate is controlled artificially, increased CO_2 production from infused sodium bicarbonate can lead to hazardous hypercapnia.[1,4,11]

About an hour after an abrupt increment in the HCO_3^- concentration, when the increased generation of CO_2 subsides, stimulation of respiration is transformed into suppression of respiration, and Pco_2 increases. This secondary hypercapnic response takes several hours and partially compensates for the elevated HCO_3^- concentration so that arterial pH is returned toward (although not completely to) normal (see Figure 16-2).

The hypercapnic response to metabolic alkalosis is difficult to reliably predict. Attempts to substantiate a role for K^+ deficiency in preventing hypoventilation have not been illuminating.[9,11,12] Moreover, studies of alkalotic patients taking diuretics demonstrate a predictable hypoventilatory response and cast doubt on a significant role of K^+ deficiency in blunting alkalosis-induced hypoventilation.[11] Most studies have found that an increase in Pco_2 regularly occurs in response to alkalosis. The hypoventilatory response can lead to borderline or even frank hypoxemia in patients with chronic lung disease.[11,12] In general, the increase in $Paco_2$ can be predicted to equal 0.75 mm Hg per 1.0 mEq/L increase in plasma HCO_3^-; or more simply, add the value of 15 to the measured plasma $[HCO_3^-]$[12] to predict the expected $Paco_2$ (see Table 16-1).

Renal Excretion

With Extracellular Volume Expansion

The addition of sodium bicarbonate to the body results in prompt cellular buffering and respiratory compensation. However, as with an acid load, the kidneys have the ultimate responsibility for the disposal of base and restoration of base stores to normal. The renal response is more rapid with HCO_3^- addition than with acid ingestion (see Figure 16-2). The speed and efficiency with which HCO_3^- can be excreted by the kidneys are such that it is difficult to render a patient with normal renal function more than mildly alkalotic on a long-term basis, even when as much as 24 mEq/kg/day of sodium bicarbonate is ingested for several weeks.[11,12]

The type B intercalated cell in the collecting tubule is capable of HCO_3^-/Cl^- exchange. However, the role of HCO_3^- secretion in chronic alkali loading has never been quantitated precisely in whole-organ clearance studies. Presumably HCO_3^- secretion by the type B intercalated cell militates against more severe alkalosis and participates in the HCO_3^- excretory response.

The proximal tubule is responsible principally for HCO_3^- excretion when the blood HCO_3^- concentration increases. Absolute proximal HCO_3^- reabsorption does not increase in proportion to HCO_3^- load in the rat kidney because of suppression of proximal acidification by alkalemia[5] so that HCO_3^- delivery to the distal nephron increases. The limited capacity of the distal nephron to secrete H^+ can be overwhelmed easily, and bicarbonaturia increases progressively. NH_4^+ and titratable acid excretion are mitigated in response to the increasing urine pH.[5,12] Acute graded HCO_3^- loads that concomitantly increase ECF also function in humans subjects to increase urinary HCO_3^- excretion progressively as plasma HCO_3^- concentration increases.[5]

In summary, an acute base load is excreted entirely, and the blood HCO_3^- concentration is returned to normal within 12 to 24 hours because of depression of fractional proximal HCO_3^- reabsorption. In addition to suppression of reabsorption of the filtered HCO_3^- load, direct HCO_3^- secretion in the cortical collecting tubule (CCT) has been proposed as another mechanism for mediating HCO_3^- disposal during metabolic alkalosis.[12]

The increased delivery of HCO_3^- out of the proximal tubule in response to an increased blood HCO_3^- concentration (and, hence, filtered HCO_3^- load) in the setting of ECF expansion facilitates HCO_3^- excretion and the return of blood pH toward normal. However, other factors may independently enhance distal H^+ secretion sufficiently to prevent HCO_3^- excretion and thus counterbalance the suppressed fractional proximal HCO_3^- reabsorptive capacity. Under these circumstances, the alkalosis is maintained. For example, in the setting of primary hyperaldosteronism, despite the expanded ECF, a stable mild alkalotic condition persists in most experimental models owing to augmented collecting duct H^+ secretion.[12] In such cases, concurrent hypokalemia facilitates the generation and maintenance of metabolic alkalosis by enhancing NH_4^+ production and excretion.[5,12] Moreover, chronic hypokalemia dramatically enhances the abundance and functionality of the H^+-K^+-adenosine triphosphatase (H^+-K^+-ATPase) in the medullary collecting tubule, thus increasing rather than decreasing bicarbonate absorption.[12-15] Enhanced nonreabsorbable anion delivery, as with drug anions such as penicillins, also increases net collecting tubule H^+ secretion by increasing the effective luminal negative potential difference or by suppressing HCO_3^- secretion in the cortical collecting duct (CCD).

With Extracellular Volume Contraction and Potassium Ion Deficiency

The renal response to an increase in plasma HCO_3^- concentration can be modified significantly in the presence of ECF contraction and K^+ depletion.[15,16] Because the volume of distribution of Cl^- is approximately equal to the ECF, the depletion of the ECF is roughly equivalent to the depletion of Cl^-. The critical role of effective ECF and K^+ stores in modifying net HCO_3^- reabsorption has been demonstrated in numerous experimental models.

Deficiency of both Cl^- and K^+ is common in metabolic alkalosis because of renal and/or gastrointestinal losses that occur concurrently with the generation of the alkalosis.[14,16] With Cl^- depletion alone, the normal bicarbonaturic response to an increase in plasma HCO_3^- is prevented and metabolic alkalosis can develop. K^+ depletion, even without mineralocorticoid administration, can cause metabolic alkalosis in rats and humans. When Cl^- and K^+ depletion coexist, severe metabolic alkalosis may develop in all species studied.

Two general mechanisms exist by which the bicarbonaturic response to hyperbicarbonatemia can be prevented by Cl^- and/or K^+ depletion: (1) As the plasma HCO_3^- concentration increases, there is a reciprocal fall in the glomerular filtration rate (GFR). If the fall in GFR were inversely proportional to the rise in the plasma HCO_3^- concentration, the filtered HCO_3^- load would not exceed the normal level. In this case, normal rates of proximal and distal HCO_3^- reabsorption would suffice to prevent bicarbonaturia. (2) Cl^- deficiency or K^+ deficiency increases overall renal HCO_3^- reabsorption in the setting of a normal GFR and high filtered HCO_3^- load. In this case, overall renal HCO_3^- reabsorption and, therefore, acidification would be increased. An increase in renal acidification might occur as a result of an increase in H^+ secretion by the proximal or the distal nephron or by both nephron segments.[12-14]

The possibility that Cl^- or K^+ depletion might decrease GFR or increase proximal HCO_3^- reabsorption has been evaluated in experimental animals. That extracellular and plasma volume depletion decreases GFR is well described. GFR can also be decreased by K^+ depletion in rats and dogs. The reduction in GFR by K^+ depletion is assumed to be the result of increased production of the vasoconstrictors angiotensin II and thromboxane B_2.[13,15] These results, taken together, provide support for the first mechanism: that metabolic alkalosis can be maintained by a depression in GFR.[12-16]

The combination of an elevated and stable plasma HCO_3^- concentration, negligible urinary HCO_3^- excretion, and normal or only slightly depressed GFR suggests that renal HCO_3^- reabsorption is enhanced. An increase in renal acidification appears to be a major mechanism by which metabolic alkalosis is maintained in models of the chronic disorder. Animals with experimental forms of chronic metabolic alkalosis display increased HCO_3^- reabsorption in both the proximal and the distal tubules. The increase in HCO_3^- absorption in the proximal tubule is due, at least in part, to an increase in the delivered load of HCO_3^-. The augmented HCO_3^- absorption in distal nephron segments appears to be due to a primary increase in H^+ secretion that is independent of the HCO_3^- load delivered. Chronic hypokalemia dramatically enhances the abundance and function of the colonic isoform of the H^+-K^+-ATPase in the medullary collecting tubule. Therefore, upregulation of the H^+-K^+-ATPase by hypokalemia may be a significant factor in the maintenance of chronic metabolic alkalosis.[13,17,18]

The maintenance of a high plasma HCO_3^- concentration by the kidney can be repaired by repletion of Cl^-.[19] The mechanism by which Cl^- repairs metabolic alkalosis could include normalization of the low GFR that was induced by ECF repletion. In addition, Cl^- repletion might result in a decrease in proximal HCO_3^- reabsorption, an increase in HCO_3^- secretion by the distal nephron, or other less well-defined mechanisms that favor enhanced Cl^- reabsorption in preference to HCO_3^- reabsorption.

Repletion of K^+ alone (without Cl^- repletion) only partially corrects metabolic alkalosis. Indeed, several experimental studies have shown that Cl^- repletion can repair the alkalosis despite persisting K^+ deficiency. Full correction of metabolic alkalosis by Cl^- but not K^+ supplementation does not necessarily prove that K^+ deficiency has no role in maintaining the alkalosis. In fact, in most studies of repair of hyperbicarbonatemia by Cl^- repletion alone (without K^+ repletion), normalization of blood pH occurred only after significant volume expansion occurred. There is complete agreement that, with simultaneous repair of K^+ and Cl^- deficiencies in metabolic alkalosis, correction of the alteration in renal HCO_3^- reabsorption ensues as a result of normalization of GFR, which allows increased HCO_3^- delivery from the proximal tubule and thus excretion of the excess HCO_3^-.

In summary, the physiologic response by the kidney to a base load associated with volume expansion is to excrete the base. Base is retained, however, if there is enhanced distal HCO_3^- reabsorption as a result of K^+ and/or Cl^- deficiency.

Stepwise Approach to the Diagnosis of Acid-Base Disorders

The four cardinal acid-base disorders reviewed thus far, and the predicted compensatory responses and their limits, are summarized in Table 16-1.

Suspicion that an acid-base disorder exists is usually based on clinical judgment or on the finding of an abnormal blood pH, $Paco_2$, or HCO_3^- concentration. In the era of transcutaneous pulse oximetry measurement of oxygen saturation it is important to remember that determination of blood pH, $Paco_2$, and HCO_3^- is vital in the management of critically ill patients. A normal hemoglobin oxygen saturation does not exclude serious perturbations in blood pH and $Paco_2$. Obviously, acid-base disorders require careful analysis of laboratory parameters along with the clinical processes occurring in the patient as revealed in the history and physical examination. The precise diagnosis is determined by proceeding in a step-wise fashion (Table 16-2).

TABLE 16-2 Systematic Method for Diagnosis of Simple and Mixed Acid-Base Disorders

1. Measure arterial blood gas and electrolyte concentrations simultaneously.

2. Compare the $[HCO_3^-]$ obtained on the electrolyte panel with the calculated value from the arterial blood gas analysis. Because the latter is obtained using the Henderson-Hasselbalch equation, agreement of the two values rules out laboratory error or error due to time discrepancy between the drawing of samples for blood gas analysis and for electrolyte levels.

3. Estimate the compensatory response for either carbon dioxide pressure (Pco_2) or HCO_3^- (see Table 16-1).

4. Calculate the anion gap (AG) (correct for low albumin level if necessary).

5. Appreciate the four major categories of high AG acidoses:
   Ketoacidosis
   Lactic acidosis
   Renal failure acidosis
   Toxin- or poison-induced acidosis

6. Appreciate the two major causes of non-AG acidoses:
   Gastrointestinal loss of HCO_3^-
   Renal loss of HCO_3^-
   Estimate the compensatory response for either Pco_2 or HCO_3^- (see Table 16-1)

7. Look for a mixed disorder.

   Compare the ΔAG and the ΔHCO_3^- (see text).

   Compare the $\Delta[Cl^-]$ and the ΔNa^+ (see text).

Step 1: Measure Arterial Blood Gas and Electrolyte Values Simultaneously

To avoid errors in diagnosis, ABG values should be measured simultaneously with the plasma electrolyte levels in all patients with component acid-base abnormalities. This is necessary because changes in plasma HCO_3^-, Na^+, K^+, and Cl^- do not allow precise diagnosis of specific acid-base disturbances. When drawing a specimen for ABG analysis, care should be taken to obtain the arterial blood sample without excessive heparin, and analysis should proceed expeditiously with the capped syringe stored on ice for transport.

Step 2: Verify Acid-Base Laboratory Values

A careful analysis of the blood gas indices (pH, $Paco_2$) should begin with a check to determine whether the concomitantly measured plasma HCO_3^- (total CO_2 concentration from the electrolyte panel results) is consistent with the ABG values. In the determination of ABG concentrations by the clinical laboratory, both pH and $Paco_2$ are measured, but the reported HCO_3^- concentration is calculated from the Henderson-Hasselbalch equation (equation 20) by the blood gas analyzer. The calculated value for HCO_3^- or (total CO_2) reported with the blood gas results should be compared with the measured HCO_3^- concentration (total CO_2) obtained on the electrolyte panel. The two values should agree within ±2 to 3 mEq/L. If these values do not agree, the clinician should suspect that the samples were not obtained simultaneously or that a laboratory error is present. The stepwise analysis of all available laboratory values to determine whether the patient has a *mixed* or *simple* acid-base disturbance is emphasized in the following sections.

On occasion, it may be necessary to compute the third value (pH, Pco_2, or HCO_3^-) when only two are available. From the Henderson equation, derived previously in this chapter (equation 21), several caveats of clinical significance are apparent. First, the normal H^+ concentration in blood is 40 nmol/L (conveniently remembered as the last two digits of the normal blood pH, 7.40), and the corresponding H^+ concentration at a pH of 7.00 is 100 nmol/L. Second, the H^+ concentration increases by about 10 nmol/L for each decrease in the blood pH of 0.10 unit (in the range of 7.20 to 7.50). An acidotic patient with a pH of 7.30 (a reduction of 0.10 pH unit, or an increase of 10 nmol/L H^+ concentration to 50 nmol/L) and a Pco_2 of 25 mm Hg would have a HCO_3^- concentration of 12 mEq/L:

$$[HCO_3^-] = 24 \times \frac{Paco_2}{[H^+]} = 24 \times \frac{25}{50} = 12 \text{ mEq}/L \qquad (27)$$

Although the Henderson equation and H^+ concentration have been suggested as the most physiologic way to portray acid-base equilibrium, the logarithmic transformation of the Henderson equation to the familiar Henderson-Hasselbalch equation is used more commonly (see equation 20). This equation is useful because acidity is measured in the clinical laboratory as pH rather than H^+ concentration.

Implicit in equations 20 and 21 is the concept that the final pH, or H^+ concentration, is determined by the ratio of HCO_3^- and $Paco_2$, not by the absolute value of either. Thus, a normal concentration of HCO_3^- does not necessarily mean that the pH is normal, nor does a normal $Paco_2$ denote a normal pH. Conversely, a normal pH does not imply that either HCO_3^- or $Paco_2$ is normal. Once again, a normal hemoglobin oxygen saturation value as determined by pulse oximetry does not exclude serious perturbations in blood pH and $Paco_2$.

Step 3: Define the Limits of Compensation to Distinguish Simple from Mixed Acid-Base Disorders

After verifying the blood acid-base values by either the Henderson equation (equation 21) or the Henderson-Hasselbalch equation (equation 20), one can define the precise acid-base disorder. If the HCO_3^- concentration is low and the Cl^- concentration is high, either chronic respiratory alkalosis or hyperchloremic metabolic acidosis is present. The ABG determination serves to differentiate the two conditions. Although both have a decreased $Paco_2$, the pH is high with a primary respiratory disorder and low in a metabolic disorder. Chronic respiratory acidosis and metabolic alkalosis are both associated with high HCO_3^- and low Cl^- concentration in plasma. Again, a pH measurement distinguishes the two conditions. In many clinical situations, however, a mixture of acid-base disorders may exist. Diagnosis of these disturbances requires additional information and a more complex analysis of data.

A convenient, but not always reliable, approach is an acid-base map, such as the one displayed in Figure 16-3, which defines the 95% confidence limits of simple acid-base sdisorders.[1,4,20] If the arterial acid-base values fall within one of the blue bands in Figure 16-3, one may assume that a simple acid-base disturbance is present, and a tentative diagnostic category can be assigned. Values that fall outside the blue areas imply, but do not prove, that a mixed disorder exists.

The two broad types of acid-base disorders are metabolic and respiratory. Metabolic acidosis and alkalosis are disorders characterized by primary disturbances in the concentration of HCO_3^- in plasma (numerator of equation 20), whereas respiratory disorders involve primarily alteration of $Paco_2$ (denominator of equation 20). The most commonly encountered clinical disturbances are simple acid-base disorders, that is, one of the four cardinal acid-base disturbances—metabolic acidosis, metabolic alkalosis, respiratory acidosis, or respiratory alkalosis—occurring in a pure or simple form. More complicated clinical situations, especially in severely ill patients, may give rise to *mixed acid-base disturbances.*[20] The possible combinations of mixed acid-base disturbances are outlined in Table 16-2.

To appreciate and recognize a mixed acid-base disturbance, it is important to understand the physiologic compensatory responses that occur in the simple acid-base disorders. Primary respiratory disturbances (denominator of equation 20) invoke secondary metabolic responses (numerator of equation 20), and primary metabolic disturbances evoke a predictable respiratory response (see Table 16-1). To illustrate, metabolic acidosis as a result of gain of endogenous acids (e.g., lactic acid or ketoacidosis) lowers the concentration of HCO_3^- in the ECF and thus extracellular pH. As a result of *acidemia,* the medullary chemoreceptors are stimulated and invoke an increase in ventilation. As a result of the hypocapnic response, the ratio of HCO_3^- to $Paco_2$ and the subsequent pH are returned toward, but not completely to, normal. The degree of compensation expected in a simple form of metabolic acidosis can be predicted from the relationship depicted in equation 26. Thus, a patient with metabolic acidosis and a plasma HCO_3^- concentration of 12 mEq/L would be expected to have a $Paco_2$ between 24 and 28 mm Hg. Values of $Paco_2$ below 24 or higher than 28 mm Hg define a *mixed metabolic-respiratory*

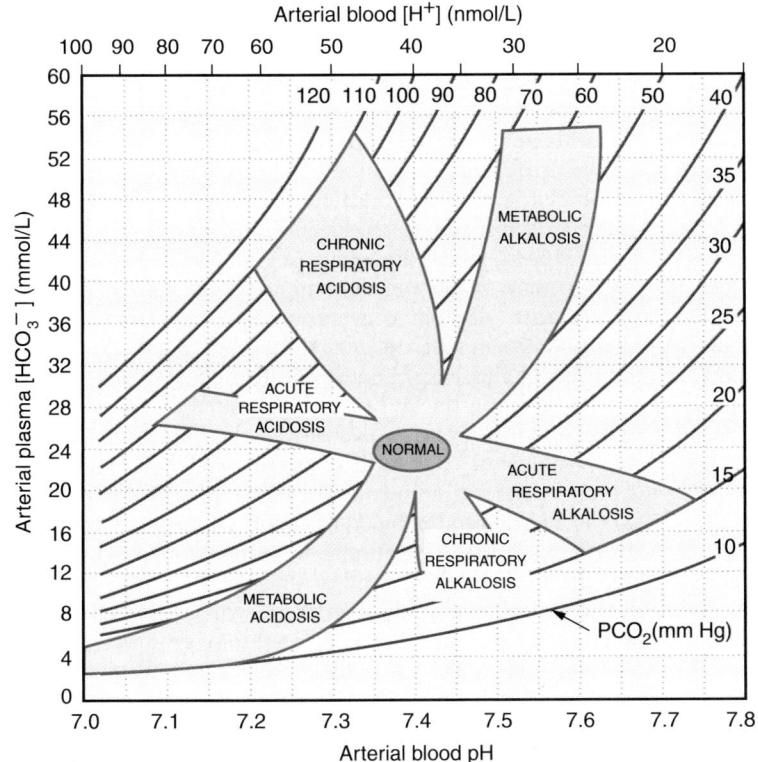

FIGURE 16-3 Acid-base nomogram (map). *Shaded areas* represent the 95% confidence limits of the normal respiratory and metabolic compensations for primary acid-base disturbances. Data falling *outside the shaded areas* denote a mixed disorder if a laboratory error is not present (see text).

disturbance (metabolic acidosis and respiratory alkalosis or metabolic acidosis and respiratory acidosis, respectively). Therefore, by definition, mixed acid-base disturbances exceed the physiologic limits of compensation.

Similar considerations are examined for each type of acid-base disturbance as these disorders are discussed in detail separately. It should be emphasized that compensation is a predictable physiologic consequence of the primary disturbance and does not represent a secondary acidosis or alkalosis (see Figure 16-3 and Table 16-1). As emphasized in the following sections, the recognition of mixed disturbances demands of the alert physician consideration of additional clinical disorders that may require immediate attention or additional therapy.

Clinical and Laboratory Parameters in Acid-Base Disorders

For correct diagnosis of a simple or mixed acid-base disorder, it is imperative that a careful history be obtained. Patients with pneumonia, sepsis, or cardiac failure frequently have a respiratory alkalosis, and patients with chronic obstructive pulmonary disease or a sedative drug overdose often display respiratory acidosis. The patient's drug history assumes importance because patients taking loop or thiazide diuretics may have metabolic alkalosis and patients receiving acetazolamide frequently have metabolic acidosis. Physical findings are often helpful as well. Tetany may occur with alkalemia, cyanosis with respiratory acidosis, and volume contraction with metabolic alkalosis. For example, the plasma HCO_3^- concentration rarely falls below 12 to 15 mEq/L as a result of compensation for respiratory alkalosis and rarely exceeds 45 mEq/L as a result of compensation for respiratory acidosis.[20]

The plasma K^+ value is often useful but should be considered only in conjunction with the HCO_3^- concentration and blood pH. It is generally appreciated that the serum K^+ value can be altered by primary acid-base disturbances as a result of shifts of K^+ either into the extracellular compartment or into the intracellular compartment. Metabolic acidosis leads to hyperkalemia. It has been reported that for each decrease in blood pH of 0.10 pH unit, the K^+ concentration should increase by 0.6 mEq/L. Thus, a patient with a pH of 7.20 would be expected to have a plasma K^+ value of 5.2 mEq/L. However, considerable variation in this relationship has been reported in several conditions, especially diabetic ketoacidosis (DKA) and lactic acidosis, which are often associated with K^+ depletion. The lack of correlation between the degree of acidemia and the plasma K^+ level is a result of several factors, including the nature and cellular permeability of the accompanying anion, the magnitude of the osmotic diuresis, the level of renal function, the presence or absence of preexisting changes in K^+ homeostasis, and the degree of catabolism. It is important to appreciate that the relationship between arterial blood pH and plasma K^+ is complex and therefore often variable. Nevertheless, the failure of a patient with severe acidosis to exhibit hyperkalemia or, conversely, the failure of a patient with severe metabolic alkalosis to exhibit hypokalemia suggests a significant derangement of body K^+ homeostasis. The combination of a low plasma K^+ and elevated HCO_3^- suggests metabolic alkalosis, whereas the combination of an elevated plasma K^+ and low HCO_3^- suggests metabolic acidosis.

It is helpful to compare the serum Cl^- concentration with the Na^+ concentration. The serum Na^+ concentration changes only as a result of changes in hydration or water homeostasis. The Cl^- concentration changes for two reasons: (1) changes in hydration and (2) changes in acid-base balance. Thus, changes in Cl^- not reflected by proportional changes in Na^+ suggest the presence of an acid-base disorder. For example, consider a patient with a history of vomiting, volume depletion, a Cl^- concentration of 85 mEq/L, and an Na^+ concentration of 130 mEq/L. In this case, both Na^+ and Cl^- are reduced, but the reduction in Cl^- is proportionally greater (15% versus 7%). A disproportionate decrease in Cl^- suggests metabolic alkalosis or respiratory acidosis, and a disproportionate increase in Cl^- suggests metabolic acidosis or respiratory alkalosis.

Step 4: Calculate the Anion Gap

All evaluations of acid-base disorders should include a simple calculation of the AG. The AG is calculated from the serum electrolytes and is defined as follows:

$$AG = Na^+ - (Cl^- + HCO_3^-) = 10 \pm 2 \, mEq/L \quad (28)$$

The AG represents the unmeasured anions normally present in plasma and unaccounted for by the serum electrolytes exclusive of K^+ that are measured on the electrolyte panel. The unmeasured anions normally present in serum include anionic proteins (principally albumin and, to lesser extent, α- and β-globulins), PO_4^{3-}, SO_4^{2-}, and organic anions. When acid anions, such as acetoacetate and lactate, are produced endogenously in excess and accumulate in ECF, the AG increases above the normal value. This is referred to as a *high anion gap* acidosis.[20,21] If it is assumed that the serum albumin level is within the normal range, for each milliequivalent per liter increase in the AG, there should be an equal decrease in the plasma HCO_3^- concentration. Serum protein at 1 g/dL has a negative charge equivalence of approximately 1.7 to 2.4 mEq/L.[22] The contribution of other unmeasured anions includes 2 mEq/L for PO_4^{3-}, 1 mEq/L for SO_4^{2-}, and 5 mEq/L for lactate and other organic anions.

An increase in the AG may be due to a decrease in unmeasured cations or an increase in unmeasured anions. Combined severe hypocalcemia and hypomagnesemia represent a decrease in the contribution of unmeasured cations (Table 16-3). In addition, the AG may increase secondary to an increase in anionic albumin, as a consequence of either an increased albumin concentration or alkalemia.[20,21] The increased AG in severe alkalemia can be explained in part by the effect of alkaline pH on the electrical charge of albumin.

A decrease in the AG can be generated by an increase in unmeasured cations or a decrease in the unmeasured anions (see Table 16-3). A decrease in the AG can result from (1) an increase in unmeasured cations (Ca^{2+}, Mg^{2+}, K^+), or (2) the addition to the blood of abnormal cations, such as Li^+ (Li^+ intoxication) or cationic immunoglobulins (immunoglobulin G as in plasma cell dyscrasias). Because albumin is the major unmeasured anion, the AG will also decrease if the quantity of albumin is low (e.g., nephrotic syndrome, protein malnutrition, capillary leak in intensive care unit patients).[22] In general, each decline in the serum albumin level by 1 g/dL from the normal value of 4.5 g/dL decreases the AG by 2.5 mEq/L. Therefore, when hypoalbuminemia exists, it is

TABLE 16-3 The Anion Gap	
ANION GAP = $Na^+ - (Cl^- + HCO_3^-)$ = 9 ± 3 mEq/L	
DECREASED ANION GAP	**INCREASED ANION GAP**
Increased Cations (Not Na^+)	**Increased Anions (Not Cl^- or HCO_3^-)**
↑ Ca^{2+}, Mg^{2+}	↑ Albumin
↑ Li^+	Alkalosis
↑ Immunoglobulin G	↑ Inorganic anions
Decreased Anions (Not Cl^- or HCO_3^-)	Phosphate
↓ Hypoalbuminemia*	Sulfate
Acidosis	↑ Organic anions
Laboratory Error	L-Lactate
Hyperviscosity	D-Lactate
Bromism	Ketones
	Uremic
	↑ Exogenously supplied anions
	Toxins
	Salicylate
	Paraldehyde
	Ethylene glycol
	Propylene glycol
	Methanol
	Toluene
	Pyroglutamic acid
	↑ Unidentified anions
	Other toxins
	Uremic
	Hyperosmolar, nonketotic states
	Myoglobinuric acute renal failure
	Decreased Cations (Not Na^+)
	↓ Ca^{2+}, Mg^{2+}

*For each decline in albumin by 1 g/dL from normal (4.5 g/dL), the anion gap decreases by 2.5 mEq/L.

possible to underestimate the AG and even miss an increased AG unless correction for the low albumin and its effect on the AG is taken into account. For example, in a patient with an albumin level of 1.5 g/dL and an uncorrected AG of 10 mEq/L, the corrected AG would be 17.5 mEq/L.

Laboratory errors can create a falsely low AG. Hyperviscosity and hyperlipidemia lead to an underestimation of the true Na^+ concentration, and bromide (Br^-) intoxication causes an overestimation of the true Cl^- concentration.[20]

In the presence of a normal serum albumin level, elevation of unmeasured anions is usually due to addition to the blood of non–Cl^--containing acids. Thus, in most clinical circumstances, a high AG indicates that a metabolic acidosis is present. The anions accompanying such acids include inorganic (PO_4^{3-}, SO_4^{2-}), organic (ketoacids, lactate, uremic organic anions), exogenous (salicylate or ingested toxins with organic acid production), or unidentified anions.[20] When

these non–Cl^--containing acids are added to the blood in excess of the rate of removal, HCO_3^- is titrated (consumed), and the accompanying anion is retained to balance the preexisting cationic (Na^+) charge:

$$H^+ anion^- + NaHCO_3 \Leftrightarrow H_2O + CO_2 + Na^+ anion^- \quad (29)$$

The preexisting Cl^- concentration is unchanged when the new acid anion is added to the blood. Therefore, the high AG acidoses exhibit normochloremia as well as a high gap. If the kidney does not excrete the anion, the magnitude of the decrement in HCO_3^- concentration will match the increment in the AG. If the retained anion can be metabolized to HCO_3^- directly or indirectly (e.g., ketones or lactate, after successful treatment), normal acid-base balance is restored as the AG returns toward the normal value. Alternatively, if the anion can be excreted, ECF contraction occurs, which leads to renal sodium chloride retention. Cl^- replaces the excreted anion, effectively bicarbonate is lost, and hyperchloremic acidosis emerges as the anion is excreted and the AG disappears.

In summary, after the titration of HCO_3^-, the ability of the kidney to excrete the anion of an administered acid determines the type of acidosis that develops. If the anion is filtered and is nonreabsorbable (e.g., SO_4^{2-}) ECF contraction, Cl^- retention, and hyperchloremic acidosis with a normal AG develop (non-AG acidosis). Conversely, if the anion is poorly filtered (e.g., uremic anions) or is produced endogenously, filtered, and reabsorbed (e.g., lactate and other organic anions), no change in Cl^- concentration occurs. The retained anion replaces the HCO_3^- lost when titrated by acid, which creates a high AG acidosis.

Step 5: Compare Delta Values

By definition, a high AG acidosis has two identifying features: a low HCO_3^- concentration and an elevated AG. This means, therefore, that the elevated AG will remain evident even if another disorder coincides to modify the HCO_3^- concentration independently. Simultaneous metabolic acidosis of the high AG variety plus either metabolic alkalosis or chronic respiratory acidosis is an example of such a situation. The HCO_3^- concentration may be normal or even high in such a setting. However, the AG is normal, and the Cl^- concentration is relatively depressed. Consider a patient with chronic obstructive pulmonary disease with compensated respiratory acidosis ($Paco_2$ of 65 mm Hg and HCO_3^- concentration of 40 mEq/L) in whom acute bronchopneumonia and respiratory decompensation develop. If this patient has an HCO_3^- concentration of 24 mEq/L, Na^+ of 145 mEq/L, K^+ of 4.8 mEq/L, and Cl^- of 96 mEq/L, it would be incorrect to assume that this "normal" HCO_3^- concentration represents improvement in acid-base status toward normal. Indeed, the arterial pH would probably be low (7.19), as a result of a more serious degree of hypercapnia than observed previously (e.g., if the Pco_2 increased from 65 to 80 mm Hg as a result of pneumonia). Even without blood gas measurements, prompt recognition that the AG was elevated to 25 mEq/L should suggest that a life-threatening lactic acidosis is superimposed on a preexisting chronic respiratory acidosis, which necessitates immediate therapy.

Similarly, a normal arterial HCO_3^- concentration, $Paco_2$, and pH do not ensure the absence of an acid-base disturbance. For example, an alcoholic patient who has been vomiting may develop a metabolic alkalosis with a pH of 7.55, HCO_3^- concentration of 40 mEq/L, Pco_2 of 48 mm Hg, Na^+ of 135 mEq/L, Cl^- of 80 mEq/L, and K^+ of 2.8 mEq/L. If such a patient were then to develop a superimposed alcoholic keto-acidosis (AKA) with a β-hydroxybutyrate concentration of 15 mmol/L, the arterial pH would fall to 7.40, HCO_3^- concentration to 25 mEq/L, and Pco_2 to 40 mm Hg. Although the blood gas values are normal, the AG (assuming no change in Na^+ or Cl^-) is elevated (25 mEq/L), which indicates the existence of a mixed metabolic acid-base disorder (mixed metabolic alkalosis and metabolic acidosis). The combination of metabolic acidosis and metabolic alkalosis is not uncommon and is most easily recognized when the AG is elevated but the HCO_3^- concentration and pH are near normal ($\Delta AG > \Delta HCO_3^-$).

Mixed Acid-Base Disorders

Mixed acid-base disorders—defined as independently coexisting disorders, not merely compensatory responses—are often seen in patients in critical care units and can lead to dangerous extremes of pH. A patient with DKA (metabolic acidosis) may develop an independent respiratory problem, leading to respiratory acidosis or alkalosis. Patients with underlying pulmonary disease may not respond to metabolic acidosis with an appropriate ventilatory response because of insufficient respiratory reserve. Such imposition of respiratory acidosis on metabolic acidosis can lead to severe acidemia and a poor outcome. When metabolic acidosis and metabolic alkalosis coexist in the same patient, the pH may be normal or near normal. When the pH is normal, an elevated AG denotes the presence of a metabolic acidosis. A discrepancy in the ΔAG (prevailing minus normal AG) and the ΔHCO_3^- (normal minus prevailing HCO_3^-) indicates the presence of a mixed high gap acidosis–metabolic alkalosis (see example later). A diabetic patient with ketoacidosis may have renal dysfunction resulting in simultaneous metabolic acidosis. Patients who have ingested an overdose of drug combinations such as sedatives and salicylates may have mixed disturbances as a result of the acid-base response to the individual drugs (metabolic acidosis mixed with respiratory acidosis or respiratory alkalosis, respectively).

Even more complex are triple acid-base disturbances. For example, patients with metabolic acidosis due to AKA may develop metabolic alkalosis due to vomiting and superimposed respiratory alkalosis due to the hyperventilation of hepatic dysfunction or alcohol withdrawal. Conversely, when hyperchloremic acidosis and metabolic alkalosis occur concomitantly, the increase in Cl^- is out of proportion to the change in HCO_3^- concentration ($\Delta Cl^- > \Delta HCO_3^-$).[20]

In summary, an AG exceeding that expected for a patient's albumin concentration and blood pH denotes the existence of either a simple high AG metabolic acidosis or a complex acid-base disorder in which an organic acidosis is superimposed on another acid-base disorder.

Step 6: Recognize Conditions Causing Acid-Base Abnormalities with High or Normal Anion Gap

Appreciation that the AG is elevated requires knowledge of the four causes of a high AG acidosis: (1) ketoacidosis, (2) lactic acidosis, (3) renal failure acidosis, and (4) toxin-induced metabolic acidosis (Table 16-4). Accordingly, if the

TABLE 16-4   Clinical Causes of High Anion Gap and Normal Anion Gap Acidosis
High Anion Gap Acidosis
Ketoacidosis
Diabetic ketoacidosis (acetoacetate)
Alcoholic ketoacidosis (hydroxybutyrate)
Starvation ketoacidosis
Lactic acidosis
L-Lactic acidosis (types A and B)
D-Lactic acidosis
Toxin-induced acidosis
Ethylene glycol
Methyl alcohol
Salicylate
Propylene glycol
Pyroglutamic acid
Normal Anion Gap Acidosis
Gastrointestinal loss of HCO_3^- (negative urine anion gap)
Diarrhea
External fistula
Renal loss of HCO_3^- or failure to excrete NH_4^+
Positive urine anion gap = low net acid excretion
Proximal renal tubular acidosis (RTA)
Classical distal renal tubular acidosis (low serum K^+)
Generalized distal renal tubular defect (high serum K^+)
Drugs that cause RTA
Carbonic anhydrase inhibitors (proximal RTA)
Amphotericin B ("gradient" classical distal RTA)
Miscellaneous
NH_4Cl ingestion
Sulfur ingestion
Dilutional acidosis

AG is normal in the face of metabolic acidosis, a hyperchloremic or non-AG acidosis exists. The specific causes of hyperchloremic acidosis that must be appreciated are outlined in a later section. Table 16-4 displays the directional changes in pH, Pco_2, and HCO_3^- for the four simple acid-base disorders. With this stepwise approach, in the next sections, the specific causes of the major types of acid-base disorders are reviewed in detail.

Respiratory Disorders

Respiratory Acidosis

Respiratory acidosis occurs as the result of severe pulmonary disease, respiratory muscle fatigue, or depression in ventilatory control. An increase in $Paco_2$ owing to reduced alveolar ventilation is the primary abnormality leading to acidemia. In acute respiratory acidosis, there is an immediate compensatory elevation in HCO_3^- (due to cellular buffering mechanisms), which increases 1 mEq/L for every 10 mm Hg increase in $Paco_2$. In chronic respiratory acidosis (>24 hours), renal adaption is achieved and the HCO_3^- increases by 4 mEq/L for every 10 mm Hg increase in $Paco_2$. The serum bicarbonate concentration usually does not increase above 38 mEq/L, however.

The clinical features of respiratory acidosis vary according to the severity, duration, underlying disease, and presence or absence of accompanying hypoxemia. A rapid increase in $Paco_2$ may result in anxiety, dyspnea, confusion,

TABLE 16-5 Respiratory Acid-Base Disorders

ALKALOSIS	ACIDOSIS

Central nervous system stimulation
  Pain
  Anxiety, psychosis
  Fever
  Cerebrovascular accident
  Meningitis, encephalitis
  Tumor
  Trauma
	Central nervous system depression
	Drugs (anesthetics, morphine, sedatives)
	Stroke
	Infection
	Airway
	  Obstruction
	  Asthma
	  Parenchyma

Hypoxemia or tissue hypoxia
  High-altitude acclimatization
  Pneumonia, pulmonary edema
  Aspiration
  Severe anemia
	Emphysema/chronic obstructive pulmonary disease
	Pneumoconiosis
	Bronchitis
	Adult respiratory distress syndrome
	Barotrauma

Drugs or hormones
  Pregnancy (progesterone)
  Salicylates
  Nikethamide
	Mechanical ventilation
	  Hypoventilation
	  Permissive hypercapnia
	Neuromuscular

Stimulation of chest receptors
  Hemothorax
  Flail chest
  Cardiac failure
  Pulmonary embolism
	Poliomyelitis
	Kyphoscoliosis
	Myasthenia
	Muscular dystrophies
	Multiple sclerosis

Miscellaneous
  Septicemia
  Hepatic failure
  Mechanical hyperventilation
  Heat exposure
  Recovery from metabolic acidosis
	Miscellaneous
	  Obesity
	  Hypoventilation

psychosis, and hallucinations and may progress to coma. Lesser degrees of dysfunction in chronic hypercapnia include sleep disturbances, loss of memory, daytime somnolence, and personality changes. Coordination may be impaired, and motor disturbances such as tremor, myoclonic jerks, and asterixis may develop. The sensitivity of the cerebral vasculature to the vasodilating effects of CO_2 can cause headaches and other signs that mimic increased intracranial pressure, such as papilledema, abnormal reflexes, and focal muscle weakness.

The causes of respiratory acidosis are displayed in Table 16-5 (*right column*). A reduction in ventilatory drive from depression of the respiratory center by a variety of drugs, injury, or disease can produce respiratory acidosis. Acutely, this may occur with general anesthetics, sedatives, narcotics, alcohol, and head trauma. Chronic causes of respiratory center depression include sedatives, alcohol, intracranial tumors, and the syndromes of sleep-disordered breathing, including the primary alveolar and obesity-hypoventilation syndromes. Neuromuscular disorders involving abnormalities or disease in the motor neurons, neuromuscular junction, and skeletal muscle can cause hypoventilation. Although a number of diseases should be considered in the differential diagnosis, drugs and electrolyte disorders should always be ruled out.

Mechanical ventilation, when not properly adjusted and supervised or when complicated by barotrauma or displacement of the endotracheal tube, may result in respiratory acidosis. This occurs if carbon dioxide production suddenly rises (because of fever, agitation, sepsis, or overfeeding) or if alveolar ventilation falls because of worsening pulmonary function. High levels of positive end-expiratory pressure in the presence of reduced cardiac output may cause hypercapnia as a result of large increases in alveolar dead space. Permissive hypercapnia has been utilized in the critical care setting with increasing frequency; lower tidal volumes are now used with the rationale of mitigating the barotrauma and volutrauma associated with high airways pressure and peak airway pressures in mechanically ventilated patients with respiratory distress syndrome.[23,24] Acute hypercapnia of any cause can lead to severe acidemia, neurologic dysfunction, and death. However, when CO_2 levels are allowed to increase gradually, the resulting acidosis is less severe, and the elevation in arterial Pco_2 is tolerated more readily. Although hypercapnia is not the goal of this approach, but secondary to the attempt to limit airway pressures, the arterial pH will decline, and the degree of acidemia may be evident. The magnitude of the acidemia associated with permissive hypercapnia may be augmented if superimposed on metabolic acidosis, such as lactic acidosis. This combination is not uncommon in the setting of the critical care unit. Bicarbonate therapy may be indicated with mixed metabolic acidosis–respiratory acidosis, but the goal of therapy with alkali is to not increase the bicarbonate and pH to normal. With low tidal volume ventilation, a reasonable therapeutic target for arterial pH is approximately 7.30.[23] Moreover, with hypercapnia in the range of 60 mm Hg, a larger amount of bicarbonate will be necessary to achieve this goal. Bicarbonate administration will further increase the Pco_2, especially in patients with fixed rates of ventilation, and will add to the magnitude of the hypercapnia. Use of a continuous bicarbonate infusion in this setting should be avoided if possible.

Disease and obstruction of the airways, when severe or long-standing, causes respiratory acidosis. Acute hypercapnia follows sudden occlusion of the upper airway or the more generalized bronchospasm that occurs with severe asthma, anaphylaxis, and inhalational burn or toxin injury. Chronic hypercapnia and respiratory acidosis occur in end-stage obstructive lung disease.[3]

Restrictive disorders involving both the chest wall and the lungs can cause acute and chronic hypercapnia. Rapidly progressing restrictive processes in the lung can lead to respiratory acidosis, because the high cost of breathing causes ventilatory muscle fatigue. Intrapulmonary and extrapulmonary restrictive defects present as chronic respiratory acidosis in their most advanced stages.

The diagnosis of respiratory acidosis requires, by definition, the measurement of arterial $Paco_2$ and pH. Detailed history and physical examination often provide important diagnostic clues to the nature and duration of the acidosis. When a diagnosis of respiratory acidosis is made, its cause should be investigated. Chest radiography is an initial step. Pulmonary function studies, including spirometry, diffusing capacity for carbon monoxide, lung volumes, and arterial $Paco_2$ and oxygen saturation usually provide adequate assessment of whether respiratory acidosis is secondary to lung disease. Workup for nonpulmonary causes should include a detailed drug history, measurement of hematocrit, and assessment of upper airway, chest wall, pleura, and neuromuscular function.[3]

The treatment of respiratory acidosis depends on its severity and rate of onset. Acute respiratory acidosis can be life-threatening, and measures to reverse the underlying cause should be undertaken simultaneously with restoration of adequate alveolar ventilation to relieve severe hypoxemia and acidemia. Temporarily, this may necessitate tracheal intubation and assisted mechanical ventilation. Oxygen level should be carefully titrated in patients with severe chronic obstructive pulmonary disease and chronic CO_2 retention who are breathing spontaneously. When oxygen is used injudiciously, these patients may experience progression of the respiratory acidosis when ventilation is driven by oxygen pressure (Pao_2) and not the normal parameters of $Paco_2$ and pH. Aggressive and rapid correction of hypercapnia should be avoided, because the falling $Paco_2$ may provoke the same complications noted with acute respiratory alkalosis (i.e., cardiac arrhythmias, reduced cerebral perfusion, and seizures). It is advisable to lower the $Paco_2$ gradually in chronic respiratory acidosis, with the aim of restoring the $Paco_2$ to baseline levels while at the same time providing sufficient chloride and potassium to enhance the renal excretion of bicarbonate.[3]

Chronic respiratory acidosis is frequently difficult to correct, but general measures aimed at maximizing lung function, including cessation of smoking; use of oxygen, bronchodilators, corticosteroids, and/or diuretics; and physiotherapy can help some patients and can forestall further deterioration. The use of respiratory stimulants may prove useful in selected cases, particularly if the patient appears to have hypercapnia out of proportion to his or her level of lung function.

Respiratory Alkalosis

Alveolar hyperventilation decreases $Paco_2$ and increases the $HCO_3^-/Paco_2$ ratio, thus increasing pH (alkalemia). Non-bicarbonate cellular buffers respond by consuming HCO_3^-. Hypocapnia develops whenever a sufficiently strong ventilatory stimulus causes CO_2 output in the lungs to exceed its metabolic production by tissues. Plasma pH and HCO_3^- concentration appear to vary proportionately with $Paco_2$ over a range from 40 to 15 mm Hg. The relationship between arterial hydrogen ion concentration and $Paco_2$ is about 0.7 nmol/L/mm Hg (or 0.01 pH unit/mm Hg) and that for plasma $[HCO_3^-]$ is 0.2 mEq/L/mm Hg, or the $[HCO_3^-]$ will decrease approximately 2 mEq/L for each 10 mm Hg.[2]

Beyond 2 to 6 hours, sustained hypocapnia is further compensated by a decrease in renal ammonium and titratable acid excretion and a reduction in filtered HCO_3^- reabsorption. The full expression of renal adaptation may take several days and depends on a normal volume status and renal function. The kidneys appear to respond directly to the lowered $Paco_2$ rather than to the alkalemia per se. A 1 mm Hg fall in $Paco_2$ causes a 0.4 to 0.5 mEq/L drop in HCO_3^- and a 0.3 nmol/L fall (or 0.003 unit rise in pH) in hydrogen ion concentration, or the $[HCO_3^-]$ will decrease 4 mEq/L for each 10 mm Hg decrease in $Paco_2$.[2]

The effects of respiratory alkalosis vary according to its duration and severity but, in general, are primarily those of the underlying disease. A rapid decline in $Paco_2$ may cause dizziness, mental confusion, and seizures, even in the absence of hypoxemia, as a consequence of reduced cerebral blood flow. The cardiovascular effects of acute hypocapnia in the awake human are generally minimal, but in the anesthetized or mechanically ventilated patient, cardiac output and blood pressure may fall because of the depressant effects of anesthesia and positive pressure ventilation on heart rate, systemic resistance, and venous return. Cardiac rhythm disturbances may occur in patients with coronary artery disease as a result of changes in oxygen unloading by blood from a left shift in the hemoglobin-oxygen dissociation curve (Bohr effect). Acute respiratory alkalosis causes minor intracellular shifts of sodium, potassium, and phosphate and reduces serum free calcium by increasing the protein-bound fraction. Hypocapnia-induced hypokalemia is usually minor.[2]

Respiratory alkalosis is among the most common acid-base disturbances encountered in critically ill patients (often as a component of a mixed disorder) and, when severe, portends a poor prognosis. Many cardiopulmonary disorders manifest respiratory alkalosis in their early to intermediate stages. Hyperventilation usually results in hypocapnia. The finding of normocapnia and hypoxemia may herald the onset of rapid respiratory failure and should prompt an assessment to determine whether the patient is becoming fatigued. Respiratory alkalosis is a common occurrence during mechanical ventilation.

The causes of respiratory alkalosis are summarized in Table 16-5 (*left column*). The hyperventilation syndrome may mimic a number of serious conditions and may be disabling. Paresthesias, circumoral numbness, chest wall tightness or pain, dizziness, inability to take an adequate breath, and, rarely, tetany may be themselves sufficiently stressful to perpetuate a vicious circle. ABG analysis demonstrates an acute or chronic respiratory alkalosis, often with hypocapnia in the range of 15 to 30 mm Hg and no hypoxemia. Central nervous system diseases or injury can produce several patterns of hyperventilation with sustained arterial $Paco_2$ levels of 20 to 30 mm Hg. Conditions such as hyperthyroidism, high caloric loads, and exercise raise the basal metabolic rate, but usually ventilation rises in proportion so that ABGs are unchanged and respiratory alkalosis does not develop. Salicylates, the most common cause of drug-induced respiratory alkalosis, stimulate the medullary chemoreceptor directly. The methylxanthine drugs theophylline and aminophylline stimulate ventilation and increase the ventilatory response to CO_2. High progesterone levels increase ventilation and decrease the arterial $Paco_2$ by as much as 5 to 10 mm Hg. Thus, chronic respiratory alkalosis is an expected feature of pregnancy. Respiratory alkalosis is a prominent feature in liver failure, and its severity correlates well with the degree of hepatic insufficiency and mortality. Respiratory alkalosis is common in patients with gram-negative septicemia, and it is often an early finding, before fever, hypoxemia, and hypotension develop. It is presumed that some bacterial product or toxin acts as a respiratory center stimulant, but the precise mechanism remains unknown.

The diagnosis of respiratory alkalosis requires measurement of arterial pH and $Paco_2$ (higher and lower than normal, respectively). The plasma K^+ concentration is often reduced, and the serum Cl^- concentration increased. In the acute phase, respiratory alkalosis is not associated with increased renal HCO_3^- excretion, but within hours, net acid excretion is reduced. In general, the HCO_3^- concentration falls by 2.0 mEq/L for each 10 mm Hg decrease in $Paco_2$.

Chronic hypocapnia reduces the serum bicarbonate concentration by 5.0 mEq/L for each 10 mm Hg decrease in $Paco_2$. It is unusual to observe a plasma bicarbonate concentration below 12 mEq/L as a result of a pure respiratory alkalosis. When a diagnosis of hyperventilation or respiratory alkalosis is made, its cause should be investigated. The diagnosis of hyperventilation syndrome is made by exclusion. In difficult cases, it may be important to rule out other conditions such as pulmonary embolism, coronary artery disease, and hyperthyroidism.

The treatment of respiratory alkalosis is primarily directed toward alleviation of the underlying disorder. Because respiratory alkalosis is rarely life-threatening, direct measures to correct it will be unsuccessful if the stimulus remains unchecked. If respiratory alkalosis complicates ventilator management, changes in dead space, tidal volume, and frequency can minimize the hypocapnia. Patients with hyperventilation syndrome may benefit from reassurance, rebreathing from a paper bag during symptomatic attacks, and attention to underlying psychologic stress. Antidepressants and sedatives are not recommended, although in a few patients, β-adrenergic blockers may help to ameliorate distressing peripheral manifestations of the hyperadrenergic state.

Metabolic Disorders

Metabolic Acidosis

Metabolic acidosis occurs as a result of a marked increase in endogenous production of acid (such as L-lactic acid and ketoacids), loss of HCO_3^- or potential HCO_3^- salts (diarrhea or renal tubular acidosis [RTA]), or progressive accumulation of endogenous acids.

The AG, which should be corrected for the prevailing albumin concentration (equation 28),[20,21] serves a useful role in the initial differentiation of the metabolic acidoses and should always be considered. Metabolic acidosis with a normal AG (hyperchloremic or non-AG acidosis) suggests that HCO_3^- has been effectively replaced by Cl^-. Thus, the AG does not change.

In contrast, metabolic acidosis with a high AG (see Table 16-3) indicates addition of an acid other than hydrochloric acid or its equivalent to the ECF. If the attendant non-Cl^- acid anion cannot be readily excreted and is retained after HCO_3^- titration, the anion replaces titrated HCO_3^- without disturbing the Cl^- concentration (equation 29). Hence, the acidosis is normochloremic and the AG increases. The relationship between the rate of addition to the blood of a non–Cl^--containing acid and the rate of excretion of the accompanying anion with secondary Cl^- retention determines whether the resultant metabolic acidosis is expressed as a high AG or hyperchloremic variety.[19,20]

Hyperchloremic (Normal Anion Gap) Metabolic Acidoses

The diverse clinical disorders that may result in a hyperchloremic metabolic acidosis are outlined in Table 16-6. Because a reduced plasma HCO_3^- and elevated Cl^- concentration may also occur in chronic respiratory alkalosis, it is important to confirm the acidemia by measuring arterial pH.

TABLE 16-6   Differential Diagnosis of Hyperchloremic Metabolic Acidosis

Gastrointestinal Bicarbonate Loss

Diarrhea
External pancreatic or small bowel drainage
Uterosigmoidostomy, jejunal loop
Drugs
  Calcium chloride (acidifying agent)
  Magnesium sulfate (diarrhea)
  Cholestyramine (bile acid diarrhea)

Renal Acidosis

Hypokalemia

Proximal RTA (type 2)
Distal (classical) RTA (type 1)
Drug-induced acidosis
  Acetazolamide and topiramate (proximal RTA)
  Amphotericin B (distal RTA)

Hyperkalemia

Generalized distal nephron dysfunction (type 4 RTA)
  Mineralocorticoid deficiency
  Mineralocorticoid resistance (PHA-1 autosomal dominant)
  Voltage defects (PHA-1, autosomal recessive)
  PHA-2
  ↓ Na^+ delivery to distal nephron
  Tubulointerstitial disease
Drug-induced acidosis
  Potassium-sparing diuretics (amiloride, triamterene, spironolactone)
  Trimethoprim
  Pentamidine
  Angiotensin converting enzyme inhibitors, angiotensin II receptor blockers
  Nonsteroidal antiinflammatory drugs
  Cyclosporine, tacrolimus

Normokalemia

Early renal insufficiency

Other

Acid loads (ammonium chloride, hyperalimentation)
Loss of potential bicarbonate: ketosis with ketone excretion
Dilution acidosis (rapid saline administration)
Hippurate
Cation exchange resins

PHA, Pseudohypoaldosteronism; *RTA*, renal tubular acidosis.

Hyperchloremic metabolic acidosis occurs most often as a result of loss of HCO_3^- from the gastrointestinal tract or as a result of a renal acidification defect. The majority of disorders in this category can be attributed to one of two major causes: (1) loss of bicarbonate from the gastrointestinal tract (diarrhea) or from the kidney (proximal RTA), or (2) inappropriately low renal acid excretion (classical distal RTA [cDRTA], type 4 RTA, or renal failure). Hypokalemia may accompany both gastrointestinal loss of HCO_3^- and proximal RTA and cDRTA. Therefore, the major challenge in distinguishing these causes is to be able to define whether the response of renal tubular function to the prevailing acidosis is appropriate (gastrointestinal origin) or inappropriate (renal origin).

Diarrhea results in the loss of large quantities of HCO_3^- decomposed by reaction with organic acids. Because diarrheal stools contain a higher concentration of HCO_3^- and decomposed HCO_3^- than plasma, volume depletion and metabolic acidosis develop. Hypokalemia exists because large quantities of K^+ are lost from stool and because volume depletion causes elaboration of renin and aldosterone, which enhances renal K^+ secretion by the nephron. Instead of an acid urine pH as might be anticipated with chronic diarrhea, a pH of 6.0 or more may be found. This occurs because chronic metabolic acidosis and hypokalemia increase renal NH_4^+ synthesis and excretion, which thus provides more urinary buffer that accommodates an increase in urine pH. Therefore, the urine pH, when 6.0 or higher, may erroneously suggest a nonrenal cause. Nevertheless, metabolic acidosis caused by gastrointestinal losses with a high urine pH can be differentiated from RTA. Because urinary NH_4^+ excretion is typically low in patients with RTA and high in patients with diarrhea,[5,6,25] the level of urinary NH_4^+ excretion (not usually measured by clinical laboratories) in metabolic acidosis can be assessed indirectly[6] by calculating the urine anion gap (UAG):

$$UAG = [Na^+ + K^+]_u - [Cl^-]_u \qquad (30)$$

where u denotes the urine concentration of these electrolytes. The rationale for using the UAG as a surrogate for ammonium excretion is that, in chronic metabolic acidosis, ammonium excretion should be elevated if renal tubular function is intact. Because ammonium is a cation, it should balance part of the negative charge of chloride in the previous expression assuming there is not a lot of HCO_3^- in the urine as in an alkaline urine. Therefore, the UAG should become progressively negative as the rate of ammonium excretion increases in response to acidosis or to acid loading.[6,19] NH_4^+ can be assumed to be present if the sum of the major cations ($Na^+ + K^+$) is less than the concentration of Cl^- in urine. A negative UAG (more than −20 mEq/L) provides evidence that sufficient NH_4^+ is present in the urine, as might occur with an extrarenal origin of the hyperchloremic acidosis. Conversely, urine estimated to contain little or no NH_4^+ has more $Na^+ + K^+$ than Cl^- (UAG is positive),[6,19,25] which indicates a renal mechanism for the hyperchloremic acidosis, such as in cDRTA (with hypokalemia) or hypoaldosteronism with hyperkalemia. Note that this qualitative test is useful only in the differential diagnosis of a hyperchloremic metabolic acidosis. If the patient has ketonuria or drug anions (penicillins or aspirin) in large quantity in the urine, the test is not reliable.

In this situation, the urinary ammonium (U_{NH4+}) may also be estimated from the measured urine osmolality (U_{osm}), urine [$Na^+ + K^+$], which will take into account the salts of β-hydroxybutyrate and other ketoacids, and urine urea and glucose (all expressed in mmol/L):

$$U_{NH_4^+} = 0.5 (U_{osm} - [2(Na^+ + K^+)_u + urea_u + glucose_u] \qquad (31)$$

Urinary ammonium concentrations of 75 mEq/L or more would be anticipated if renal tubular function is intact and the kidney is responding to the prevailing metabolic acidosis by increasing ammonium production and excretion. Conversely, values below 25 mEq/L denote inappropriately low urinary ammonium concentrations. In addition to the UAG, the fractional excretion of Na^+ may be helpful and would be expected to be low (<1% to 2%) in patients with HCO_3^- loss from the gastrointestinal tract but usually exceeds 2% to 3% in patients with RTA.[6,25]

Gastrointestinal HCO_3^- loss, as well as proximal RTA (type 2) and cDRTA (type 1), results in ECF contraction and stimulation of the renin-aldosterone system, which leads typically to hypokalemia. The serum K^+ concentration therefore serves to distinguish the previous disorders, which have a low K^+, from either generalized distal nephron dysfunction (e.g., type 4 RTA), in which the renin–aldosterone–distal nephron axis is abnormal and hyperkalemia exists, or the acidosis of progressive chronic kidney disease, in which normokalemia is common (see later).

In addition to gastrointestinal tract HCO_3^- loss, external loss of pancreatic and biliary secretions can cause a hyperchloremic acidosis. Cholestyramine, calcium chloride, and magnesium sulfate ingestion can also result in a hyperchloremic metabolic acidosis (see Table 16-6), especially in patients with renal insufficiency. Coexistent L-lactic acidosis is common in severe diarrheal illnesses but increases the AG.

Severe hyperchloremic metabolic acidosis with hypokalemia may occur in patients with ureteral diversion procedures. Because the ileum and the colon are both endowed with Cl^-/HCO_3^- exchangers, when the Cl^- from the urine enters the gut, or pouch, the HCO_3^- concentration increases as a result of the exchange process.[19] Moreover, K^+ secretion is stimulated, which, together with HCO_3^- loss, can result in a hyperchloremic hypokalemic metabolic acidosis. This defect is particularly common in patients with ureterosigmoidostomies and is more common with this type of diversion because of the prolonged transit time of urine caused by stasis in the colonic segment.

Dilutional acidosis, acidosis caused by exogenous acid loads and the posthypocapnic state, can usually be excluded by the history. When isotonic saline is infused rapidly, particularly in patients with temporary or permanent renal functional impairment, the serum HCO_3^- declines reciprocally in relation to Cl^-.[19] Addition of acid or acid equivalents to blood results in metabolic acidosis. Examples include infusion of arginine or lysine hydrochloride during parenteral hyperalimentation or ingestion of ammonium chloride. A similar situation may arise from endogenous addition of ketoacids during recovery from ketoacidosis when the sodium salts of ketones may be excreted by the kidneys and lost as potential HCO_3^-.[26]

This sequence may also occur in mild, chronic ketoacidosis if GFR is maintained with sodium replenishment and renal ketone excretion is high. This may be accentuated by a defect in tubule ketone reabsorption.[27] The plasma ketone concentration is maintained at low levels. Continued titration of HCO_3^- with Cl^- retention and excretion of potential base (ketones) may result in hyperchloremic acidosis. Metabolism of sulfur to sulfuric acid and excretion of SO_4^{2-} with Cl^- retention represents another example of a hyperchloremic acidosis resulting from increased acid loading and anion excretion.[26]

Loss of functioning renal parenchyma in progressive kidney disease is known to be associated with metabolic acidosis. Typically, the acidosis is hyperchloremic when the GFR is between 20 and 50 mL/min but may convert to the typical high AG acidosis of uremia with more advanced renal failure, that is, when the GFR is less than 20 mL/min.[28] It is generally assumed that such progression is observed more commonly in patients with tubulointerstitial forms of renal disease, but hyperchloremic metabolic acidosis can also occur with advanced glomerular disease. The principal defect in acidification of advanced renal failure is that ammoniagenesis is reduced in proportion to the loss of functional renal mass. In addition, medullary NH_4^+ accumulation and trapping in the outer medullary collecting tubule may be impaired.[28]

Because of adaptive increases in K⁺ secretion by the collecting duct and colon, the acidosis of chronic renal insufficiency is typically normokalemic.[28] Hyperchloremic metabolic acidosis accompanied by hyperkalemia is almost always associated with a generalized dysfunction of the distal nephron.[6,25] However, K⁺-sparing diuretics (amiloride, triamterene), as well as pentamidine, cyclosporine, tacrolimus, nonsteroidal antiinflammatory drugs (NSAIDs), angiotensin converting enzyme (ACE) inhibitors, angiotensin II receptor blockers (ARBs), β-blockers, and heparin may mimic or cause this disorder, resulting in hyperkalemia and a hyperchloremic acidosis.[6,25] Because hyperkalemia augments the development of acidosis by suppressing urinary net acid excretion, discontinuing these agents while reducing the serum K⁺ allows ammonium production and excretion to increase, which will help repair the acidosis.

Disorders of Impaired Renal Bicarbonate Reclamation: Proximal Renal Tubular Acidosis

Physiology

Because the first phase of acidification by the nephron involves reabsorption of the filtered HCO_3^- 80% of the filtered HCO_3^- is normally returned to the blood by the proximal convoluted tubule.[5] If the capacity of the proximal tubule is reduced,

less of the filtered HCO_3^- is reabsorbed in this segment and more is delivered to the more distal segments. This increased HCO_3^- delivery overwhelms the limited capacity for bicarbonate reabsorption by the distal nephron, and bicarbonaturia ensues, net acid excretion ceases, and metabolic acidosis follows. Enhanced Cl^- reabsorption, stimulated by ECF volume contraction, results in a hyperchloremic form of chronic metabolic acidosis. With progressive metabolic acidosis and decreased serum HCO_3^- levels, the filtered HCO_3^- load declines progressively. As the plasma HCO_3^- concentration decreases, the absolute amount of HCO_3^- entering the distal nephron eventually reaches the low level approximating the distal HCO_3^- delivery in normal individuals (at the normal threshold). At this point, the quantity of HCO_3^- entering the distal nephron can be reabsorbed completely (Figure 16-4), and the urine pH declines. A new steady state in which acid excretion equals acid production is then reached. As a consequence, the serum HCO_3^- concentration usually reaches a nadir of 15 to 18 mEq/L, so that systemic acidosis is not progressive. Therefore, in proximal RTA, in the steady state, the serum HCO_3^- is usually low and the urine pH acid (<5.5). With bicarbonate administration, the amount of bicarbonate in the urine increases the fractional excretion of bicarbonate (FE_{HCO3^-}) 10% to 15%, and the urine pH becomes alkaline.[25]

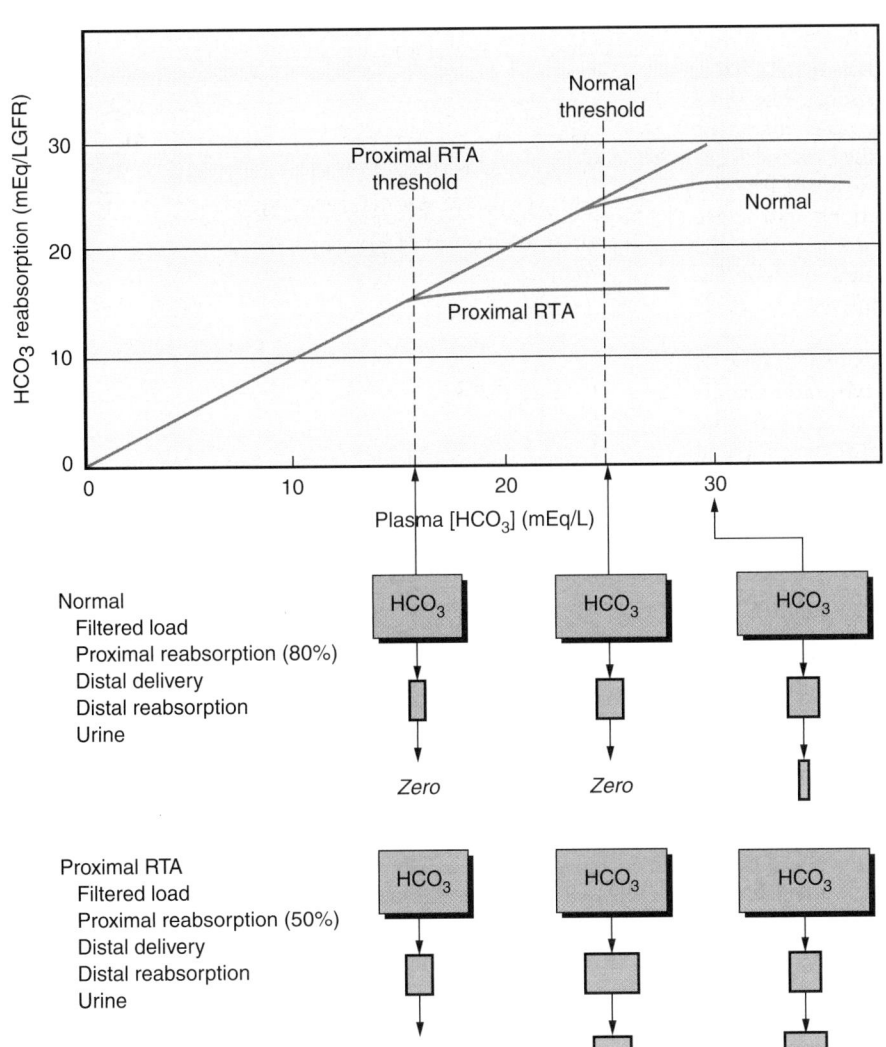

FIGURE 16-4 Schematic representation of the single-nephron correlates of whole-kidney HCO_3^- titration curves (*top*) in normal subjects and in patients with proximal renal tubular acidosis (proximal RTA). The impact of these relationships on bicarbonaturia is displayed below the graph. Bicarbonate will not appear in the urine when reabsorption is complete at the plasma HCO_3^- concentration threshold, and distal H⁺ secretory processes are capable of reabsorbing the HCO_3^- delivered out of the proximal nephron. The relationship shows that the fractional proximal HCO_3^- reabsorptive capacity is reduced in patients with proximal RTA (50% versus the normal 80%), so the new steady state is achieved at the expense of systemic metabolic acidosis. *GFR*, Glomerular filtration rate.

PATHOGENESIS

Proximal RTA can present in two ways: one in which acidification is the only defective function and one in which there is a more generalized proximal tubule dysfunction. A proximal tubule defect involving only acidification is rare. Such a disorder would be assumed to involve a selective defect in the Na^+-H^+ antiporter, H^+-ATPase, or the Na^+-HCO_3^--CO_3^{2-} symporter. Abnormalities of cell depolarization or abnormalities of the enzymes carbonic anhydrase II or IV could also cause a selective defect.[25]

In contradistinction to a selective defect, the majority of cases of proximal RTA fit into the category of generalized proximal tubule dysfunction with glycosuria, aminoaciduria, hypercitraturia, and phosphaturia, often referred to as *Fanconi's syndrome*. Numerous experimental studies in animal models demonstrate that the nephropathies induced by maleic acid and cystine involve disruption of active transcellular absorption of HCO_3^-, amino acids, and other solutes. Such a defect could be due to a generalized disorder of the Na^+-coupled apical membrane transporters, a selective disorder of the basolateral Na^+-K^+-ATPase, or a specific metabolic disorder that lowers intracellular adenosine triphosphate (ATP) concentration.

Development of Fanconi's syndrome by intracellular PO_4^{3-} depletion has also been proposed in hereditary fructose intolerance, in which ingestion of fructose leads to accumulation of fructose 1-phosphate in the proximal tubule. Because these patients lack the enzyme fructose 1-phosphate aldolase, fructose 1-phosphate cannot be further metabolized, and intracellular PO_4^{3-} is sequestered in this form. The renal lesion is confined to the proximal tubule because this is the only segment in the kidney that possesses the enzyme fructokinase. Administration of large parenteral loads of fructose to rats leads to high intracellular concentrations of fructose 1-phosphate and low concentrations of ATP and guanosine triphosphate (GTP), as well as of total adenine nucleotides. Prior PO_4^{3-} loading prevents reductions in intracellular ATP, PO_4^{3-}, and total adenine nucleotides.[25,29]

Numerous investigators have noted an association between vitamin D deficiency and a proximal RTA with aminoaciduria and hyperphosphaturia. In these studies, correction of the vitamin D deficiency has allowed correction of the proximal tubule dysfunction.[25] Similar results have been obtained in patients with vitamin D–dependent and vitamin D–resistant rickets treated with dihydrotachysterol.[25] The mechanisms involved in the proximal tubule dysfunction are not yet clear.

Another model for isolated proximal tubule acidosis is inherited carbonic anhydrase deficiency. Sly and associates[30] have reported an inherited syndrome with osteopetrosis, cerebral calcification, and RTA caused by an inherited deficiency of carbonic anhydrase II. These patients may have combined proximal and distal RTA but have no other evidence for proximal tubule dysfunction, and carbonic anhydrase IV is intact.[30] As already discussed, carbonic anhydrase II is present in the cytoplasm of renal cells, and thus an acidification defect occurring in association with its deficiency is not unexpected. A defect of carbonic anhydrase IV (the membrane-bound form) has not been reported.

CLINICAL SPECTRUM

In general, proximal RTA is more common in children. The two most common causes of acquired proximal RTA in adults are multiple myeloma, in which increased excretion of immunoglobulin light chains injures the proximal tubule epithelium, and chemotherapeutic drug injury of the proximal tubule (e.g., ifosfamide). The light chains that cause injury in multiple myeloma may have a biochemical characteristic in the variable domain that is resistant to degradation by proteases in lysosomes in proximal tubule cells. Accumulation of the variable domain fragments may be responsible for the impairment in tubular function. In contrast, idiopathic RTA and RTA due to ifosfamide toxicity, lead intoxication, and cystinosis are more common in children. Carbonic anhydrase inhibitors cause pure bicarbonate wasting but not Fanconi's syndrome.

A comprehensive list of the disorders associated with proximal RTA is presented in Table 16-7.[25] Some of the entities on this list are no longer seen and are of only historic interest. For example, application of sulfanilamide to the skin of patients with large-surface-area burns is no longer practiced in most centers, but sulfanilamide, a carbonic anhydrase inhibitor, is

TABLE 16-7 Disorders with Dysfunction of Renal Acidification—Defective HCO_3^- Reclamation: Proximal Renal Tubular Acidosis

Selective (Unassociated with Fanconi's Syndrome)

Primary
  Transient (infants)
  Idiopathic or genetic
Carbonic anhydrase deficiency, inhibition, or alteration
  Drugs
    Acetazolamide
    Sulfanilamide
    Mafenide acetate
  Carbonic anhydrase II deficiency with osteopetrosis

Generalized (Associated with Fanconi's Syndrome)

Primary (without associated systemic disease)
  Genetic
  Sporadic
Genetically transmitted systemic diseases
  Cystinosis
  Lowe's syndrome
  Wilson's syndrome
  Tyrosinemia
  Galactosemia
  Hereditary fructose intolerance (during fructose ingestion)
  Metachromatic leukodystrophy
  Pyruvate carboxylase deficiency
  Methylmalonic acidemia
Dysproteinemic states
  Multiple myeloma
  Monoclonal gammopathy
Secondary hyperparathyroidism with chronic hypocalcemia
  Vitamin D deficiency or resistance
  Vitamin D dependency
Drugs or toxins
  Ifosfamide
  Outdated tetracycline
  3-Methylchromone
  Streptozotocin
  Lead
  Mercury
  Amphotericin B (historic)
Tubulointerstitial diseases
  Sjögren's syndrome
  Medullary cystic disease
  Renal transplantation
Other renal and miscellaneous diseases
  Nephrotic syndrome
  Amyloidosis
  Paroxysmal nocturnal hemoglobinuria

absorbed from burned skin. Pharmaceutical manufacturing techniques have improved, and outdated tetracycline is no longer associated with proximal RTA. Some of the agents and disorders on this list—such as ifosfamide, Sjögren's syndrome, renal transplantation, and amyloidosis—also appear as causes of distal RTA (see Table 16-7).

DIAGNOSIS

The diagnosis of proximal RTA relies initially on the documentation of a chronic hyperchloremic metabolic acidosis. In the steady state these patients generally show chronic metabolic acidosis, an acid urine pH, and a low fractional excretion of HCO_3^-. With alkali therapy or slow infusion of sodium bicarbonate intravenously, when the plasma HCO_3^- increases above the threshold in these patients, bicarbonaturia ensues, and the urine becomes alkaline (Figure 16-5). When the plasma bicarbonate concentration is increased with an intravenous infusion of sodium bicarbonate at a rate of 0.5 to 1.0 mEq/kg/hr, the urine pH, even if initially acid, will increase once the reabsorptive threshold for bicarbonate has been exceeded. Thus, the urine pH may exceed 7.5 and FE_{HCO3}^- will increase to 15% to 20%. Therefore it is very difficult to increase serum HCO_3^- levels to the normal range.

The hyperchloremic metabolic acidosis of the steady state is usually seen in association with hypokalemia. If bicarbonate administration has been high in an attempt to repair the acidosis, the bicarbonaturia will drive kaliuresis and the hypokalemia may be severe.[25] Patients with proximal tubule dysfunction exhibit intact distal nephron function (generate steep urine pH gradients and titrate luminal buffers) when the serum HCO_3^- concentration and hence distal HCO_3^- delivery are sufficiently reduced. A low HCO_3^- threshold exists. Below this plasma HCO_3^- concentration, distal acidification can compensate for defective proximal acidification, although at the expense of systemic metabolic acidosis. When the plasma HCO_3^- concentration is raised to normal values, a large fraction of the filtered HCO_3^- is inappropriately excreted because the limited reabsorptive capacity of the distal nephron cannot compensate for the reduced proximal nephron reabsorption.

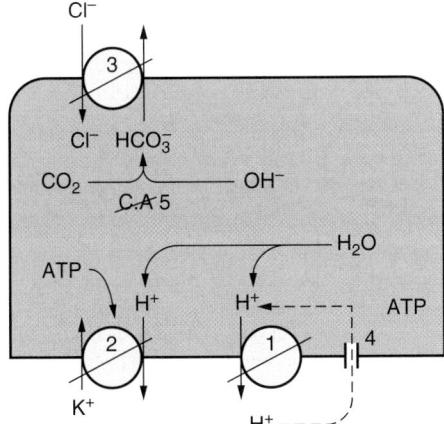

FIGURE 16-5 Type A intercalated cell of the collecting duct displaying five pathophysiologic defects that could result in classical distal renal tubular acidosis: (1) defective H+–adenosine triphosphatase (H+-ATPase), (2) defective H+-K+-ATPase, (3) defective HCO_3^-/Cl^- exchanger, (4) H+ leak pathway, and (5) defective intracellular carbonic anhydrase (type II). *ATP*, Adenosine triphosphate.

ASSOCIATED CLINICAL FEATURES

K+ excretion is typically high in patients with proximal RTA, especially during $NaHCO_3$ administration.[25] Kaliuresis is promoted by the increased delivery of a relatively impermeant anion, HCO_3^-, to the distal nephron in the setting of secondary hyperaldosteronism, which is due to mild volume depletion. Therefore, correction of acidosis in such patients leads to an exaggeration of the kaliuresis and K+ deficiency.

If the acidification defect is part of a generalized proximal tubule dysfunction (Fanconi's syndrome), such patients will have hypophosphatemia, hyperphosphaturia, hypouricemia, hyperuricosuria, glycosuria, aminoaciduria, hypercitraturia, hypercalciuria, and proteinuria.

Although Ca^{2+} excretion may be high in patients with proximal RTA, nephrocalcinosis and renal calculi are rare. This may be related to the high rate of citrate excretion in patients with proximal RTA compared with that of most patients with acidosis from other causes. Osteomalacia, rickets, abnormal gut Ca^{2+} and phosphorus absorption, and abnormal vitamin D metabolism in children are common, although not invariantly present. Adults tend to have osteopenia without pseudofractures.[25]

The proximal reabsorption of filtered low-molecular-weight proteins may also be abnormal in proximal RTA. Lysozymuria and increased urinary excretion of immunoglobulin light chains can occur.[25]

TREATMENT

The magnitude of the bicarbonaturia (>10% of the filtered load) at a normal HCO_3^- concentration requires that large amounts of HCO_3^- be administered. At least 10 to 30 mEq/kg/day of HCO_3^- or its metabolic equivalent (citrate) is required to maintain plasma HCO_3^- concentration at normal levels. Correcting the HCO_3^- to near normal values (22 to 24 mEq/L) is desirable in children to reestablish normal growth. Correction to this level is less desirable in adults. Large supplements of K+ are often necessary because of the kaliuresis induced by high distal HCO_3^- delivery when the plasma HCO_3^- concentration is normalized. Thiazides have proved useful in diminishing therapeutic requirements for HCO_3^- supplementation by causing ECF contraction to stimulate proximal absorption. However, K+ wasting continues to be a problem, often requiring the addition of a K+-sparing diuretic.[25] Vitamin D and PO_4^{3-} may be supplemented and in some patients even improve the acidification defect. Fructose should be restricted in patients with fructose intolerance.[29]

Disorders of Impaired Net Acid Excretion with Hypokalemia: Classical Distal Renal Tubule Acidosis

PATHOPHYSIOLOGY

The mechanisms involved in the pathogenesis of hypokalemic cDRTA have been more clearly elucidated by appreciation of the genetic and molecular bases of the inherited forms of this disease in the recent years. The observation that these patients tend to be hypokalemic (rather than hyperkalemic) demonstrates that generalized CCT dysfunction or aldosterone deficiency is not causative. Most studies suggest that the acquired or inherited forms of cDRTA are due to defects in the basolateral HCO_3^-/Cl^- exchanger, or subunits of the H+-ATPase. Other mechanisms are an abnormal leak pathway (e.g., amphotericin B induced)[6,19,25] or abnormalities of H^+-K^+-ATPase. Defects in these transport pathways and an increase in apical membrane permeability are displayed in Figure 16-5, which depicts acid-base transporters of a type A intercalated cell in the medullary collecting duct and the possible abnormalities causing cDRTA. Although the classical feature of this entity is an inability to acidify the urine maximally (to a pH of <5.5) in the face of systemic acidosis, attention to urine ammonium excretion rather than urine pH alone is necessary to diagnose this disorder.[6,25]

The pathogenesis of the acidification defect in most patients is evident by the response of the urine P_{CO_2} to sodium bicarbonate infusion. When normal subjects are given large infusions of sodium bicarbonate to produce a high HCO_3^- excretion, distal nephron H^+ secretion leads to the generation of a high P_{CO_2} in the renal medulla and final urine.[31] The magnitude of the urinary P_{CO_2} (often referred to as the *urine minus blood P_{CO_2}* or $U - B$ P_{CO_2}) can be used as an index of distal nephron H^+ secretory capacity.[32,33] The $U - B$ P_{CO_2} is generally subnormal in classical hypokalemic distal RTA, with the notable exception of amphotericin B–induced distal RTA, which remains the most common example of the "gradient" defect.[31,33,34]

Inherited Defects in the Bicarbonate/Chlorine Ion Exchanger. Three groups of investigators have independently demonstrated an association between mutations in the *AE1* gene, which encodes the basolateral HCO_3^-/Cl^- exchanger in the collecting duct, and the occurrence of autosomal dominant cDRTA (example 3 in Figure 16-5).[35-38] Surprisingly, however, when these point mutations were expressed in vitro, abnormalities in HCO_3^-/Cl^- exchange were not observed. It was hypothesized that misdirection of the HCO_3^-/Cl^- exchanger to the apical, rather than the basolateral, membrane might occur in this disorder, resulting in impaired net H^+ secretion.[36,37,39] For a more detailed discussion, see Alper.[40]

Hydrogen Ion–Secretory Defects (Inherited and Acquired). Alternatively, the rate of proton secretion could be affected by an abnormality in a specific transporter or mechanism involved in apical membrane proton extrusion. These include apical H^+-ATPase or H^+-K^+-ATPase (see Figure 16-5). Impairment of H^+-ATPase in cDRTA has been documented in both acquired and inherited disorders. Acquired defects of H^+-ATPase have been demonstrated in renal biopsy specimens of patients with Sjögren's syndrome with evidence of classical hypokalemic distal RTA.[25] These biopsy specimens revealed an absence of H^+-ATPase protein in the apical membrane of type A intercalated cells. Karet and colleagues[41] have described two different mutations in the *ATP6VIB1* gene encoding the B1 subunit of H^+-ATPase. One defect is associated with sensorineural deafness (*rdRTA1*) and the other with normal hearing (*rdRTA2*).[42] The former recessive disorder is manifest in the first year of life as a failure to thrive; bilateral sensorineural hearing deficits; hyperchloremic, hypokalemic metabolic acidosis; severe nephrolithiasis; nephrocalcinosis; and osteodystrophy. The H^+-ATPase is critical for maintaining pH in the cochlea and endolymph, and its loss in this disorder explains the hearing deficit as well as the renal tubule acidification defect. The latter defect is rare but is associated with normal hearing and has been localized to chromosome band 7q33-34. This group also identified the

gene *ATP6N1B*, which encodes an 840–amino acid novel kidney-specific isoform of ATP6N1A, the 116-kD noncatalytic accessory subunit of the proton pump. Through this work, they described a new kidney-specific proton pump accessory subunit that is highly expressed in proton-secreting cells in the distal nephron.[43,44] The genetic and molecular basis of distal RTA is outlined in Table 16-8.

Alternatively, abnormalities in H^+-K^+-ATPase could result in both hypokalemia and metabolic acidosis. A role for H^+-K^+-ATPase involvement in cDRTA was suggested by the observation that long-term administration of vanadate in rats decreased H^+-K^+-ATPase activity and was associated with metabolic acidosis, hypokalemia, and an inappropriately alkaline urine.[45] In addition, an unusually high incidence of hypokalemic distal RTA (endemic RTA) has been observed in northeastern Thailand. To date, no genetic linkages between H^+-K^+-ATPase genes and inherited forms of cDRTA have been documented. Nevertheless, such an abnormality has been suggested in an infant with severe metabolic acidosis and hypokalemia.[25]

Patients with impaired collecting duct H^+ secretion and cDRTA also exhibit uniformly low excretory rates of NH_4^+ when the degree of systemic acidosis is taken into account.[5,6,25] Low NH_4^+ excretion equates with inappropriately low renal regeneration of HCO_3^-, which indicates that the kidney is responsible for causing or perpetuating the chronic metabolic acidosis. Low NH_4^+ excretion in classical hypokalemic distal RTA occurs because of the failure to trap NH_4^+ in the medullary collecting duct as a result of higher than normal tubule fluid pH in this segment and loss of the disequilibrium pH (pH > 6.0).[46] The high urine pH indicates impaired H^+ secretion.

TABLE 16-8   Genetic and Molecular Bases of Distal Renal Tubular Acidoses

Classical Distal RTA

Inherited	
Autosomal dominant	Defect in *AE1* gene encodes for missense mutation in the HCO_3^-/Cl^- exchanger (band 3 protein)
	Transporter may be mistargeted to apical membrane
Autosomal recessive	Mutations in *ATP6V1B1*, encoding
With deafness	
With normal hearing	B-subunit of the apical H^+-ATPase in distal tubule (*rdRTA1*)
	Mutations in *ATP6N1B* (*rdRTA2*)
Carbonic anhydrase II	Defect in carbonic anhydrase II in red blood cells, bone kidney
Endemic (Northeastern Thailand)	Possible abnormality in H^+-K^+-ATPase
Acquired	Reduced expression of H^+-ATPase (Sjögren's syndrome)

Generalized Distal Nephron Dysfunction

Pseudohypoaldosteronism type 1	
Autosomal recessive	Loss-of-function mutation of ENaC; four known mutations of genes encoding three subunits of ENaC
Autosomal dominant	Heterozygous mutations of mineralocorticoid receptor gene
Pseudohypoaldosteronism type 2	WNK1 and WNK4 constitutively activate NCCT, protein kinase increasing NaCl absorption in cortical collecting tubule

ATPase, Adenosine triphosphatase; *ENaC,* epithelial sodium channel; *NCCT,* Na^+-Cl^- cotransporter in the connecting tubule; *WNK1, WNK4,* with no lysine (K) isoforms 1 and 4.

In summary, hypokalemic distal RTA is characterized by the inability to acidify the urine below pH 5.5. In some patients, this is attributable to an enhanced leakage pathway caused by an amphotericin B lesion; in rare patients, it occurs without exposure to the antibiotic.[47] However, in most patients, the defect cannot be attributed to such a leak. In these patients, a decreased rate of distal H^+ secretion is the likely mechanism. When the defect is a result of an abnormal H^+-ATPase, hypokalemia occurs secondarily as a result of volume depletion–induced hyperreninemic hyperaldosteronism and the acidosis that accompanies this disorder.

CLINICAL SPECTRUM AND ASSOCIATED FEATURES

The hallmark of classical hypokalemic distal RTA has been the inability to acidify the urine appropriately during spontaneous or chemically induced metabolic acidosis. The defect in acidification by the collecting duct impairs NH_4^+ and titratable acid excretion and results in positive acid balance, hyperchloremic metabolic acidosis, and volume depletion.[25,48-50] Moreover, medullary interstitial disease, which commonly occurs in conjunction with distal RTA, may impair NH_4^+ excretion by interrupting the medullary countercurrent system for NH_4^+.[6,25,48,49] Hypokalemia and hypercalciuria are typically present,[6] but proximal tubule reabsorptive function is preserved. The dissolution of bone, which may on occasion accompany distal RTA, appears to be the result of a chronic positive acid balance that causes Ca^{2+}, Mg^{2+}, and PO_4^{3-} wasting.[25] Because chronic metabolic acidosis also decreases renal production of citrate,[5,6,25] the resulting hypocitraturia in combination with hypercalciuria creates an environment favorable for urinary stone formation and nephrocalcinosis. Nephrocalcinosis appears to be a reliable marker for cDRTA, because nephrocalcinosis does not occur in proximal RTA or with generalized dysfunction of the nephron associated with hyperkalemia.[6,25] Nephrocalcinosis probably aggravates further the reduction in net acid excretion by impairing the transfer of ammonia from the loop of Henle into the collecting duct. Pyelonephritis is a common complication of distal RTA, especially in the presence of nephrocalcinosis, and eradication of the causative organism may be difficult.[25] Distal RTA occurs frequently in patients with Sjögren's syndrome.[51]

The clinical spectrum of cDRTA is outlined in detail in Table 16-9.[6,25,50]

TREATMENT

Correction of chronic metabolic acidosis can usually be achieved readily in patients with cDRTA by administration of alkali in an amount sufficient to neutralize the production of metabolic acids derived from the diet.[25] In adult patients with distal RTA, this amount may be equal to no more than 1 to 3 mEq/kg/day.[52] In growing children, endogenous acid production is usually between 2 and 3 mEq/kg/day but may, on occasion, exceed 5 mEq/kg/day. Larger amounts of bicarbonate must be administered to correct the acidosis and maintain normal growth.[6,25] The various forms of alkali replacement are outlined in Table 16-10.

In adult patients with distal RTA, correction of acidosis with alkali therapy reduces urinary K^+ excretion and prevents hypokalemia and Na^+ depletion.[25] Therefore, in most adult patients with distal RTA, K^+ supplementation is not necessary. Frank wasting of K^+ may occur in a minority of adult patients and in

TABLE 16-9 Disorders with Dysfunction of Renal Acidification—Selective Defect in Net Acid Excretion: Classical Distal Renal Tubular Acidosis

Primary

Familial

  Autosomal dominant

    AE1 gene

  Autosomal recessive

    With deafness (*rdRTA1* or *ATP6V1B1* gene)

    Without deafness (*rdRTA2* or *ATP6N1B*)

Sporadic

Endemic

Northeastern Thailand

Secondary to Systemic Disorders

Autoimmune Diseases

Hyperglobulinemic purpura	Fibrosing alveolitis
Cryoglobulinemia	Chronic active hepatitis
Sjögren's syndrome	Primary biliary cirrhosis
Thyroiditis	Polyarthritis nodosa
Human immunodeficiency syndrome nephropathy	

Hypercalciuria and Nephrocalcinosis

Primary hyperparathyroidism	Vitamin D intoxication
Hyperthyroidism	Idiopathic hypercalciuria
Medullary sponge kidney	Wilson's disease
Fabry's disease	Hereditary fructose intolerance
X-linked hypophosphatemia	

Drug- and Toxin-Induced Disease

Amphotericin B	Toluene
Cyclamate	Mercury
Hepatic cirrhosis	Vanadate
Ifosfamide	Lithium
	Classical analgesic nephropathy
Foscarnet	

Tubulointerstitial Diseases

Balkan nephropathy	Kidney transplantation
Chronic pyelonephritis	Leprosy
Obstructive uropathy	Jejunoileal bypass with hyperoxaluria
Vesicoureteral reflux	

Associated with Genetically Transmitted Diseases

Ehlers-Danlos syndrome	Hereditary elliptocytosis
Sickle cell anemia	Marfan's syndrome
Medullary cystic disease	Jejunal bypass with hyperoxaluria
Hereditary sensorineural deafness	Carnitine palmitoyltransferase deficiency
Osteopetrosis with carbonic anhydrase II deficiency	

TABLE 16-10 Forms of Alkali Replacement

Shohl's Solution	
Na⁺ citrate 500 mg	Each 1 mL contains 1 mEq sodium and is equivalent to 1 mEq of bicarbonate
Citric acid 334 mg/5 mL	
NaHCO₃ Tablets	3.9 mEq/tablet (325 mg)
	7.8 mEq/tablet (650 mg)
Baking Soda	60 mEq/teaspoon
K-Lyte	25-50 mEq/tablet
Potassium Citrate (PolyCitra, K-Shohl's)	
Na⁺ citrate 500 mg	Each 1 mL contains 1 mEq potassium and 1 mEq sodium and is equivalent to 2 mEq bicarbonate
K⁺ citrate 550 mg	
Citric acid 334 mg/5 mL	
Polycitra-K Crystals	
K⁺ citrate 3300 mg	Each packet contains 30 mEq potassium and is equivalent to 30 mEq bicarbonate
Citric acid 1002 mg/packet	
Urocit-K Tablets	
K⁺ citrate	5 or 10 mEq/tablet

some children in association with secondary hyperaldosteronism despite correction of the acidosis by alkali therapy, so that K⁺ supplementation is needed. If required, potassium can be administered as potassium bicarbonate (K-Lyte 25 or 50 mEq), potassium citrate (Urocit-K), or potassium citrate combination products (PolyCitra, K-Shohl's solution)[6,25] Maintenance of a normal serum bicarbonate concentration with alkali therapy also raises urinary citrate level, reduces urinary calcium level, lowers the frequency of nephrolithiasis, and tends to correct bone disease and restore normal growth in children.[52,53] Therefore, every attempt should be made to correct and maintain a near-normal serum [HCO₃⁻] in all patients with cDRTA.

Severe hypokalemia with flaccid paralysis, metabolic acidosis, and hypocalcemia may occur in some patients under extreme circumstances and require immediate therapy. Because the hypokalemia may result in respiratory depression, increasing systemic pH with alkali therapy may worsen the hypokalemia. Therefore, immediate intravenous potassium replacement should be achieved prior to alkali administration.

Disorders of Impaired Net Acid Excretion with Hyperkalemia: Generalized Distal Nephron Dysfunction (Type 4 Renal Tubular Acidosis)

The coexistence of hyperkalemia and hyperchloremic acidosis indicates a generalized dysfunction in the cortical and medullary collecting tubules. In the differential diagnosis, it is important to evaluate the functional status of the renin-aldosterone system and of ECF volume. The specific disorders causing hyperkalemic hyperchloremic metabolic acidosis are outlined in detail in Table 16-11.[6,25]

TABLE 16-11 Disorders with Dysfunction of Renal Acidification—Generalized Abnormality of Distal Nephron with Hyperkalemia

Mineralocorticoid Deficiency

Primary Mineralocorticoid Deficiency

Combined deficiency of aldosterone, desoxycorticosterone, and cortisol
  Addison's disease
  Bilateral adrenalectomy
  Bilateral adrenal destruction
  Hemorrhage or carcinoma
Congenital enzymatic defects
  21-hydroxylase deficiency
  3β-hydroxydehydrogenase deficiency
  Desmolase deficiency
Isolated (selective) aldosterone deficiency
  Chronic idiopathic hypoaldosteronism
  Heparin (low molecular weight or unfractionated) administration in critically ill patient
  Familial hypoaldosteronism
  Corticosterone methyl oxidase deficiency types 1 and 2
  Primary zona glomerulosa defect
  Transient hypoaldosteronism of infancy
  Persistent hypotension and/or hypoxemia in critically ill patient
Angiotensin II converting enzyme inhibition
  Endogenous
  Angiotensin converting enzyme inhibitors and angiotensin II receptor antagonists

Secondary Mineralocorticoid Deficiency

Hyporeninemic hypoaldosteronism
  Diabetic nephropathy
  Tubulointerstitial nephropathies
  Nephrosclerosis
  Nonsteroidal antiinflammatory agents
  Acquired immunodeficiency syndrome
  Immunoglobulin M monoclonal gammopathy

Mineralocorticoid Resistance

PHA-1—autosomal dominant (human mineralocorticoid receptor defect)

Renal Tubular Dysfunction (Voltage Defect)

PHA-1—autosomal recessive
PHA-2—autosomal dominant
Drugs that interfere with Na⁺ channel function in the CCT
  Amiloride
  Triamterene
  Trimethoprim
  Pentamidine
Drugs that interfere with Na⁺-K⁺-ATPase in the CCT
  Cyclosporine, tacrolimus
Drugs that inhibit aldosterone effect on the CCT
  Spironolactone
Disorders associated with tubulointerstitial nephritis and renal insufficiency
  Lupus nephritis
  Methicillin nephrotoxicity
  Obstructive nephropathy
  Kidney transplant rejection
  Sickle cell disease
  Williams' syndrome with uric acid nephrolithiasis

ATPase, Adenosine triphosphatase; *CCT,* cortical collecting tubule; *PHA-1, PHA-2,* pseudohypoaldosteronism types 1 and 2.

The regulation of potassium excretion is primarily the result of regulation of potassium secretion, which responds to hyperkalemia, aldosterone, sodium delivery, and nonreabsorbable anions in the CCD. Therefore, a clinical estimate of K⁺ transfer into that segment could be helpful to recognize hyperkalemia of renal origin. An abnormally low fractional excretion of potassium or transtubular potassium gradient

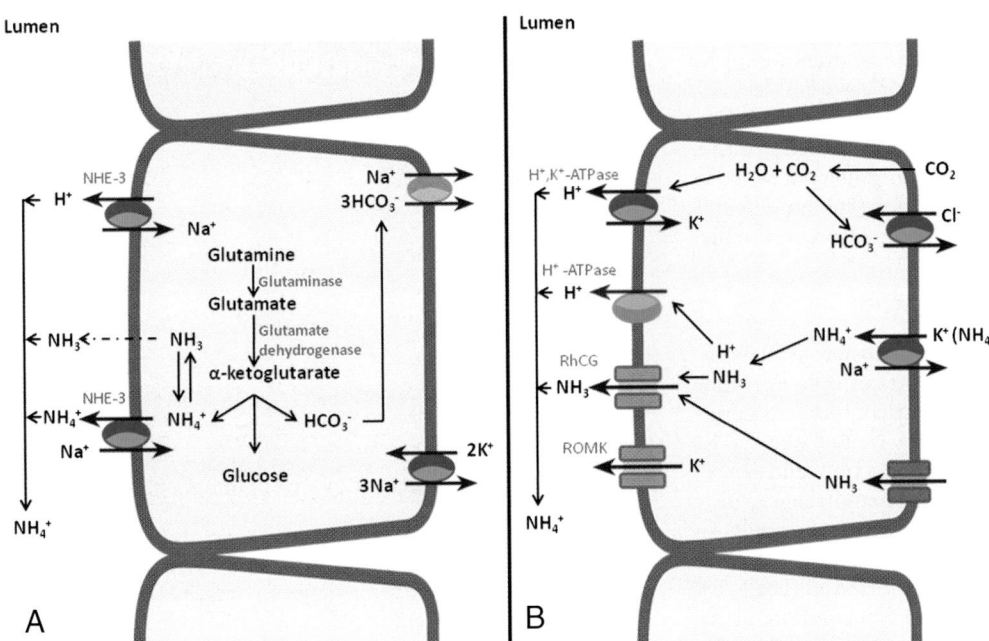

FIGURE 16-6 Cell models of ammonia synthesis and excretion pathways. **A,** Proximal convoluted tubule. Ammonia is derived from glutamine precursors to produce two NH_4^+ and two HCO_3^- molecules through an enzymatic pathway activated by acidemia and hypokalemia and inhibited by alkalemia and hyperkalemia. **B,** Type A intercalated cell in collecting tubule. Ammonium entry across basolateral membrane through substitution of K^+ for NH_4^+ in K^+ conductance and secreted across apical membrane via ROMK or RhCG (see the text). In both **A** and **B**, NH_3 diffusion coupled with H^+ secretion traps NH_4^+ in the tubule lumen.

(TTKG) in the face of hyperkalemia defines hyperkalemia of renal origin. When the TTKG is low (<8) in a hyperkalemic patient, it reveals that the collecting tubule is not responding appropriately to the prevailing hyperkalemia and that potassium secretion is impaired. In contrast, in hyperkalemia of nonrenal origin, the kidney should respond by increasing K^+ secretion, as evidenced by a sharp increase in the TTKG. The TTKG assumes that there is no significant net addition or absorption of K^+ between the CCD and the final urine, that CCD tubular fluid osmolality is approximately the same as plasma osmolality, that "osmoles" are not extracted between CCD and the final urine, and that plasma $[K^+]$ approximates peritubular fluid $[K^+]$. It is important to note that under certain clinical conditions, some or none of these assumptions may be entirely correct. With high urine flow rates, for example, the TTKG underestimates K^+ secretory capacity in the hyperkalemic patient.

Hyperkalemia should also be regarded as an important mediator of the renal response to acid-base balance. Potassium status can affect distal nephron acidification by both direct and indirect mechanisms. First, the level of potassium in systemic blood is an important determinant of aldosterone elaboration, which is also an important determinant of distal H^+ secretion. Chronic potassium deficiency was demonstrated in studies in the author's laboratory to stimulate ammonium production, whereas chronic hyperkalemia suppressed ammoniagenesis.[54,55] These changes in ammonium production may also affect medullary interstitial ammonium concentration and buffer availability.[55] Hyperkalemia has no effect on ammonium transport in the superficial proximal tubule but markedly impairs ammonium absorption in the thick ascending limb of the loop of Henle (TAL), reducing inner medullary concentrations of total ammonia and decreasing secretion of NH_3 into the inner medullary collecting duct. It is important to remember that the luminal membrane of the medullary thick ascending limb (mTAL) is very impermeable to both H_2O and NH_3. The mechanism for impaired absorption of NH_4^+ in the TAL is competition between K^+ and NH_4^+ for the K^+-secretory site on the $Na^+ - K^+ - 2Cl^-$

TABLE 16-12 Effects of Hyperkalemia on Ammonium Excretion
Decrease in NH_4^+ production
Decrease in NH_4^+ absorption in thick ascending limb of loop of Henle
Decrease in interstitial NH_4^+ concentration
Impaired countercurrent multiplication
Decrease in NH_3/NH_4^+ secretion into outer and inner medullary collecting ducts

transporter.[56,57] Hyperkalemia may also decrease entry of NH_4^+ into the medullary collecting duct through competition of NH_4^+ and K^+ for the K^+-secretory site on the basolateral membrane sodium pump (Figure 16-6).[57]

In summary, hyperkalemia may have a dramatic impact on ammonium production and excretion (Table 16-12). Chronic hyperkalemia decreases ammonium production in the proximal tubule and whole kidney, inhibits absorption of NH_4^+ in the mTAL, reduces medullary interstitial concentrations of NH_4^+ and NH_3, and decreases entry of NH_4^+ and NH_3 into the medullary collecting duct. This same series of events leads, in the final analysis, to a marked reduction in urinary ammonium excretion. The potential for development of a hyperchloremic metabolic acidosis is greatly augmented when a reduction in functional renal mass (GFR of <60 mL/min) coexists with hyperkalemia or when aldosterone deficiency or resistance is present.

CLINICAL DISORDERS
Generalized distal nephron dysfunction is manifest as a hyperchloremic, hyperkalemic metabolic acidosis in which urinary ammonium excretion is invariably depressed (positive UAG) and renal function is often compromised. Although hyperchloremic metabolic acidosis and hyperkalemia occur with regularity in advanced renal insufficiency, patients selected because of severe hyperkalemia (>5.5 mEq/L) with, for example, diabetic nephropathy and tubulointerstitial disease

have hyperkalemia that is disproportionate to the reduction in the GFR. The TTKG and/or the fractional excretion of K^+ (FE_{K^+}) is usually low in patients with this disorder. In such patients, a unique dysfunction of potassium and acid secretion by the collecting tubule coexists and can be attributed to either mineralocorticoid deficiency, resistance to mineralocorticoid, or a specific type of renal tubular dysfunction (voltage defects). The clinical spectrum of generalized abnormalities in the distal nephron is summarized in Table 16-11.

PRIMARY MINERALOCORTICOID DEFICIENCY

Although a number of factors modulate aldosterone elaboration, including angiotensin II, adrenocorticotropic hormone (ACTH), endothelin, dopamine, acetylcholine, epinephrine, plasma K^+, and Mg^{2+}, angiotensin II and plasma K^+ remain the principal modulators of production and secretion. Destruction of the adrenal cortex by hemorrhage, infection, invasion by tumors, or autoimmune processes results in Addison's disease. This causes combined glucocorticoid and mineralocorticoid deficiency and is recognized clinically by hypoglycemia, anorexia, weakness, hyperpigmentation, and a failure to respond to stress. These defects can occur in association with renal salt wasting and hyponatremia, hyperkalemia, and metabolic acidosis. The most common congenital adrenal defect in steroid biosynthesis is 21-hydroxylase deficiency, which is associated with salt wasting, hyperkalemia, and metabolic acidosis in a fraction of patients. Causes of Addison's disease include tuberculosis, autoimmune adrenal failure, fungal infections, adrenal hemorrhage, metastasis, lymphoma, acquired immunodeficiency syndrome (AIDS), amyloidosis, and drug toxicity (ketoconazole, fluconazole, phenytoin, rifampin, and barbiturates). These disorders are associated with low plasma aldosterone levels and high levels of plasma renin activity.[25] The metabolic acidosis of mineralocorticoid deficiency results from a decrease in hydrogen ion secretion in the collecting duct secondary to decreased H^+-ATPase pump number and function. The hyperkalemia of mineralocorticoid deficiency decreases ammonium production and excretion.

HYPORENINEMIC HYPOALDOSTERONISM

In contrast to patients with the primary adrenal disorder, patients in this group exhibit low plasma renin activity, are usually older (mean age 65 years), and frequently have mild to moderate renal insufficiency (70%) and acidosis (50%) in association with chronic hyperkalemia in the range of 5.5 to 6.5 mEq/L (Table 16-13).[25] Although the hyperkalemia may be asymptomatic, it is important to recognize that both the metabolic acidosis and the hyperkalemia are out of proportion to the level of reduction in GFR. The most frequently associated renal diseases are diabetic nephropathy and tubulointerstitial disease. Additional disorders associated with hyporeninemic hypoaldosteronism include obstructive uropathy, systemic lupus erythematosus, and human immunodeficiency virus (HIV) infection. For 80% to 85% of such patients, there is a reduction in plasma renin activity that does not respond to the usual physiologic maneuvers. Because approximately 30% of patients with hyporeninemic hypoaldosteronism are hypertensive, the finding of a low plasma renin activity in such patients suggests a volume-dependent form of hypertension with physiologic suppression of renin elaboration.

Impaired ammonium excretion is the combined result of hyperkalemia, impaired ammoniagenesis, a reduction

TABLE 16-13 Hyporeninemic Hypoaldosteronism: Typical Clinical Features
Mean age 65 yr
Asymptomatic hyperkalemia (75%)
Weakness (25%)
Arrhythmia (25%)
Hyperchloremic metabolic acidosis (>50%)
Renal insufficiency (70%)
Diabetes mellitus (50%)
Cardiac disorders
Arrhythmia (25%)
Hypertension (75%)
Congestive heart failure (50%)

in nephron mass, reduced proton secretion, and impaired transport of ammonium by nephron segments in the inner medulla.[6,25,58] Hyperchloremic metabolic acidosis occurs in approximately 50% of patients with hyporeninemic hypoaldosteronism. Drugs that may result in similar manifestations are reviewed later.

ISOLATED HYPOALDOSTERONISM IN CRITICALLY ILL PATIENTS

Isolated hypoaldosteronism, which may occur in critically ill patients, particularly in the setting of severe sepsis or cardiogenic shock, is manifest by markedly elevated ACTH and cortisol levels in concert with a decrease in aldosterone elaboration in response to angiotensin II. This may be secondary to selective inhibition of aldosterone synthase as a result of hypoxia or in response to cytokines such as tumor necrosis factor-α or interleukin-1 or, alternatively, as a result of high circulating levels of atrial natriuretic peptide (ANP).[6,25,59] ANP, a powerful suppressor of aldosterone secretion, may be elevated in congestive heart failure (CHF), with atrial arrhythmias, in subclinical cardiac disease, and in volume expansion. The tendency to manifest the features of hypoaldosteronism, including hyperkalemia and metabolic acidosis, is often potentiated by the administration of potassium-sparing diuretics, potassium loads in parenteral nutrition solutions, or heparin. The latter suppresses aldosterone synthesis in the critically ill patient (Table 16-14).

RESISTANCE TO MINERALOCORTICOID AND VOLTAGE DEFECTS

Autosomal dominant pseudohypoaldosteronism type 1 (PHA-1) is an example of a voltage defect in the collecting tubule and is due to aldosterone resistance. This disorder, which is clinically less severe than the autosomal recessive form discussed later, is associated with hyperkalemia (which can be attributed to impaired potassium secretion), renal salt wasting, elevated levels of renin and aldosterone, and hypotension. Physiologic mineralocorticoid replacement therapy does not correct the hyperkalemia. The autosomal dominant disorder has been shown to be the result of a mutation in the intracellular mineralocorticoid receptor in the collecting tubule.[60] Unlike in the autosomal recessive disorder, this defect is not expressed in organs other than the kidney and becomes less severe with advancing age. Because the decrease in mineralocorticoid reduces apical Na^+ absorption and the activity of the epithelial sodium channel (ENaC),

TABLE 16-14 Isolated Hypoaldosteronism in the Critically Ill Patient
Elevated adrenocorticotropic hormone and cortisol levels in association with a decrease in aldosterone elaboration
Inhibition of aldosterone synthase
Heparin
Hypoxia
Cytokines
Atrial natriuretic peptide
Manifestations of hypoaldosteronism
Hyperkalemia
Metabolic acidosis
Potentiated by K^+-sparing diuretics, K^+ loads, or heparin

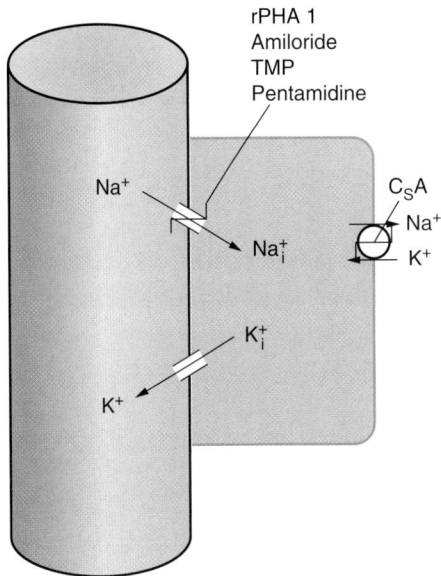

FIGURE 16-7 Examples of "voltage" defects in the cortical collecting tubule (CCT) causing abnormal Na^+ transport (and K^+ secretion) across the apical membrane of a principal cell: (1) the Na^+ channel (ENaC) is blocked or occupied by amiloride, trimethoprim (TMP), or pentamidine or is inoperative (autosomal recessive pseudohypoaldosteronism type 1 [rPHA-1]), and (2) basolateral Na^+-K^+–adenosine triphosphatase (Na^+-K^+-ATPase) activity is inhibited by calcineurin-cyclosporine (C_SA). As a consequence of impaired Na^+ uptake, transepithelial K^+ secretion is compromised, which leads to hyperkalemia. The pathogenesis of metabolic acidosis, when present, is the unfavorable voltage (which impairs H^+ secretion by the type A intercalated cell, not shown) or the inhibition of NH_4^+ production and transport and H^+-K^+-ATPase as a consequence of hyperkalemia.

transepithelial potential difference declines and K^+ secretion is impaired. Four hours after administration of fludrocortisone (0.1 mg orally) the TTKG will *not* increase, which reveals clearly that resistance to mineralocorticoid causes the hyperkalemia.

The prototype of a voltage defect is autosomal recessive PHA-1 (Figure 16-7). This disorder is the result of a loss-of-function mutation of the gene that encodes one of the α-, β-, or γ-subunits of the ENaC.[61-65] Children with this disorder have severe hyperkalemia and renal salt wasting because of impaired sodium absorption in principal cells of the CCT. In addition, the hyperchloremic metabolic acidosis may be severe and is associated with hypotension and marked elevations of plasma renin and aldosterone. These children also manifest vomiting, hyponatremia, failure to thrive, and respiratory distress. The latter is due to involvement of ENaC in the alveolus, which prevents Na^+ and water absorption in the lungs.[64,66] Patients with this disease respond to a high salt intake and correction of the hyperkalemia. Unlike the autosomal dominant form, autosomal recessive PHA-1 persists throughout life.

A number of additional adult patients have been reported with a rare form of autosomal dominant low-renin hypertension that is invariably associated with hyperkalemia, hyperchloremic metabolic acidosis, mild volume expansion, normal renal function, and low aldosterone levels. This syndrome has been designated *familial hyperkalemic hypertension* but is also known as *pseudohypoaldosteronism type 2* (PHA-2)[67] or *Gordon's syndrome.* Lifton's group[68,69] identified two genes causing PHA-2. Both genes encode members of the WNK (*with no lysine [K]*) family of serine-threonine kinases. WNK1 and WNK4 localize to the CCT. WNK4 negatively regulates surface expression of the Na^+-Cl^- cotransporter in the connecting tubule (NCCT).[69] Loss of regulation of NCCT by WNK4 results in a gain in NCCT function, which causes volume expansion, shunting of voltage, and therefore reduced K^+ secretion in the CCT.[69-71] PHA-2 may be distinguished from selective hypoaldosteronism by the presence of normal renal function and hypertension, the absence of diabetes mellitus and salt wasting, and a kaliuretic response to mineralocorticoids. The acidosis in these patients is mild and can be accounted for by the magnitude of hyperkalemia; the acidosis and renal potassium excretion are resistant to mineralocorticoid administration. Thiazide diuretics consistently correct the hyperkalemia and metabolic acidosis, as well as the hypertension, plasma aldosterone level, and plasma renin level.

SECONDARY RENAL DISEASES ASSOCIATED WITH ACQUIRED VOLTAGE DEFECTS

In addition to the inherited voltage defects discussed previously, there are a number of acquired renal disorders caused by drugs or tubulointerstitial diseases that are often associated with hyperkalemia (Table 16-15).[25] Examples of the former include amiloride and the structurally related compounds trimethoprim (TMP) and pentamidine. As discussed earlier, this explains the occurrence of hyperkalemic hyperchloremic acidosis in patients receiving higher doses of these agents. TMP and pentamidine occupy the Na^+ channel, as does amiloride, causing hyperkalemia, which contributes to the acidosis. Additional drugs not related to amiloride that are associated with hyperkalemia include cyclooxygenase-2 (COX-2) inhibitors, cyclosporine, tacrolimus, and NSAIDs.[72,73]

In these disorders, the frequency with which hyperkalemia is associated with metabolic acidosis and decreased net acid excretion as a result of impaired ammonium production or excretion cannot be presumed to be a result of the severity of impairment in renal function. Hyperkalemia that is out of proportion to the degree of renal insufficiency is typically observed in the nephropathies associated with sickle cell disease, HIV infection, systemic lupus erythematosus, obstructive uropathy, acute and chronic renal allograft rejection,

TABLE 16-15 Causes of Drug-induced Hyperkalemia
Impaired Renin-Aldosterone Elaboration or Function
Cyclooxygenase inhibitors (nonsteroidal antiinflammatory agents)
β-Adrenergic antagonists
Spironolactone
Angiotensin converting enzyme inhibitors and angiotensin receptor blockers
Heparin
Inhibition of Renal Potassium Secretion
Potassium-sparing diuretics (amiloride, triamterene)
Trimethoprim
Pentamidine
Cyclosporine
Digitalis overdose
Lithium
Altered Potassium Distribution
Insulin antagonists (somatostatin, diazoxide)
β-Adrenergic antagonists
α-Adrenergic agonists
Hypertonic solutions
Digitalis
Succinylcholine
Arginine hydrochloride, lysine hydrochloride

hypoaldosteronism, multiple myeloma, and amyloidosis.[25,74] Tubulointerstitial disease with hyperkalemia and hyperchloremic metabolic acidosis with or without salt wasting may be associated with analgesic abuse, sickle cell disease, obstructive uropathy, nephrolithiasis, nephrocalcinosis, and hyperuricemia.[25]

Hyperkalemic Distal Renal Tubular Acidosis

A generalized defect in CCD secretory function that results in hyperkalemic hyperchloremic metabolic acidosis has been designated as *hyperkalemic distal RTA* because of the coexistence of an inability to acidify the urine (urine pH of >5.5) during spontaneous acidosis or following an acid load and hyperkalemia. The hyperkalemia is the result of impaired renal K^+ secretion, and the TTKG or FE_K^+ is invariably lower than expected for hyperkalemia. Urine ammonium excretion is reduced, but aldosterone levels may be low, normal, or even increased.

Hyperkalemic distal RTA may be observed in a wide variety of renal diseases, including systemic lupus erythematosus, sickle cell disease, obstructive uropathy, and amyloidosis, as well as in transplantation. Drugs may be associated with a number of tubular defects that can be manifested as hyperkalemic distal RTA. Hyperkalemic distal RTA can be distinguished from selective hypoaldosteronism because plasma renin and aldosterone levels are usually high or normal. Typically in selective hypoaldosteronism, the urine pH is low and the defect in urinary acidification can be attributed to the decrease in ammonium excretion. In contrast with hypokalemic distal RTA or cDRTA, patients with hyperkalemic distal RTA do not show increased H^+ or K^+ excretion in response to nonreabsorbable anions (SO_4^{2-}) or furosemide.

Drug-Induced Renal Tubular Secretory Defects

Impaired Renin-Aldosterone Elaboration. Drugs may impair renin or aldosterone elaboration or cause mineralocorticoid resistance and produce effects that mimic the clinical manifestations of the acidification defect seen in the generalized form of distal RTA with hyperkalemia (see Table 16-15).

COX inhibitors (NSAIDs or COX-2 inhibitors) can generate hyperkalemia and metabolic acidosis as a result of inhibition of renin release.[73] β-Adrenergic antagonists cause hyperkalemia by altering potassium distribution and by interfering with the renin-aldosterone system. Heparin impairs aldosterone synthesis as a result of direct toxicity to the zona glomerulosa and inhibition of aldosterone synthase. ACE inhibitors and ARBs interrupt the renin-aldosterone system and result in hypoaldosteronism with hyperkalemia and acidosis, particularly in patients with advanced renal insufficiency or in patients with a tendency to develop hyporeninemic hypoaldosteronism (diabetic nephropathy). The combination of potassium-sparing diuretics and ACE inhibitors should be avoided in diabetic patients.

Inhibitors of Potassium Secretion in the Collecting Duct. Spironolactone acts as a competitive inhibitor of aldosterone and inhibits aldosterone biosynthesis. This drug may cause hyperkalemia and metabolic acidosis when administered to patients with significant renal insufficiency, patients with advanced liver disease, or patients with unrecognized renal hemodynamic compromise. Similarly, amiloride and triamterene may be associated with hyperkalemia, but through an entirely different mechanism. Both potassium-sparing diuretics occupy and thus block the apical Na^+-selective channel (ENaC) in the collecting duct principal cell (see Figure 16-7). Occupation of ENaC inhibits Na^+ absorption and reduces the negative transepithelial voltage, which alters the driving force for K^+ secretion.

Amiloride is the prototype for a growing number of agents, including TMP and pentamidine, that act similarly to cause hyperkalemia, particularly in patients with AIDS. TMP and pentamidine are related structurally to amiloride and triamterene. The protonated forms of both TMP and pentamidine have been demonstrated by Kleyman's group[75,76] to inhibit ENaC in A6 distal nephron cells. This effect in A6 cells has been verified in rat late distal tubules perfused in vivo.[77] Hyperkalemia has been observed in 20% to 50% of HIV-infected patients receiving high-dose trimethoprim-sulfamethoxazole (TMP-SMX) or TMP-dapsone for the treatment of opportunistic infections and as many as 100% of patients with AIDS-associated infections (due to *Pneumocystis jiroveci*) receiving pentamidine for longer than 6 days.[77] Because both TMP and pentamidine decrease the electrochemical driving force for both K^+ and H^+ secretion in the CCT, metabolic acidosis may accompany the hyperkalemia even in the absence of severe renal failure, adrenal insufficiency, tubulointerstitial disease, or hypoaldosteronism. Whereas it has been assumed that such a "voltage" defect could explain the decrease in H^+ secretion, it is likely that, in addition, hyperkalemia plays a significant role in the development of metabolic acidosis by direct inhibition of ammonium production and excretion (see Figure 16-6 and Table 16-12).

Cyclosporine A and tacrolimus may be associated with hyperkalemia in the transplant recipient as a result of inhibition of the basolateral Na^+-K^+-ATPase and the consequent decrease in intracellular $[K^+]$ and the transepithelial potential, which together reduce the driving force for K^+ secretion (see Figure 16-7).[73] It has been suggested that the specific mechanism of inhibition of the Na^+ pump is inhibition by these agents of calcineurin activity.[78] Either drug could also decrease the filtered load of K^+ through hemodynamic mechanisms such as vasoconstriction, which decrease GFR and alter the filtration fraction.

TABLE 16-16 Treatment of Generalized Dysfunction of the Nephron with Hyperkalemia
Alkali therapy (Shohl's solution or NaHCO₃)
Loop diuretic (furosemide, bumetanide)
Sodium polystyrene sulfonate (Kayexalate)
Low-potassium diet
Fludrocortisone (0.1-0.3 mg/day)
Avoid in hypertension, volume expansion, heart failure
Combine with loop diuretic
Avoid drugs associated with hyperkalemia
In pseudohypoaldosteronism type 1, add NaCl supplement

TREATMENT

In hyperkalemic hyperchloremic metabolic acidosis, documentation of the underlying disorder is necessary, and therapy should be based on a precise diagnosis if possible. Of particular importance is obtaining a thorough drug and dietary history. Contributing or precipitating factors should be considered, including low urine flow or decreased distal Na⁺ delivery, a rapid decline in GFR (especially in acute superimposed on chronic renal failure), hyperglycemia or hyperosmolality, and unsuspected sources of exogenous K⁺ intake.[25] The workup should include evaluation of the TTKG or the fractional excretion of potassium, an estimate of renal ammonium excretion (UAG, osmolar gap, and urine pH), and evaluation of plasma renin activity and aldosterone secretion. The latter may be assessed under stimulated conditions with dietary salt restriction and furosemide-induced volume depletion, and measurement of the response of potassium excretion to furosemide and fludrocortisone. An increase in the TTKG to a value of more than 6 measured 4 hours after a single oral dose of fludrocortisone (0.05 mg) suggests that mineralocorticoid deficiency, but not resistance, is causative.

The decision to treat is often based on the severity of the hyperkalemia. Reduction in the serum potassium level will often improve the metabolic acidosis by increasing ammonium excretion as potassium levels return to the normal range. Correction of hyperkalemia with sodium polystyrene can correct the metabolic acidosis as the serum potassium level declines.[6,25] Patients with combined glucocorticoid and mineralocorticoid deficiency should receive both adrenal steroids in replacement dosages. Additional measures may include use of laxatives, alkali therapy, or treatment with a loop diuretic to induce renal potassium and salt excretion (Table 16-16). Volume depletion should be avoided unless the patient is volume overexpanded or hypertensive. Supraphysiologic doses of mineralocorticoids are rarely necessary and, if administered, should be given cautiously in combination with a loop diuretic to avoid volume overexpansion or aggravation of hypertension and to increase potassium excretion.[25]

Infants with autosomal recessive or dominant PHA-1 should receive salt supplements in amounts sufficient to correct the volume depletion, hypotension, and other features of the syndrome and to allow normal growth. In contrast, patients with PHA-2 should receive thiazide diuretics along with dietary salt restriction.

Although it may be prudent to discontinue drugs that are identified as the most likely cause of the hyperkalemia, this may not always be feasible in patients with life-threatening disorders, for example, during TMP-SMX or pentamidine therapy in AIDS patients with *Pneumocystis jiroveci* pneumonia. Based on the previous analysis of the mechanism by which TMP and pentamidine cause hyperkalemia (voltage defect), it might also be reasoned that the delivery to the CCD of a poorly reabsorbed anion might improve the electrochemical driving force favoring K⁺ and H⁺ secretion. The combined use of acetazolamide along with sufficient sodium bicarbonate to deliver HCO₃⁻ to the CCT and thereby increase the negative transepithelial voltage could theoretically increase K⁺ and H⁺ secretion. Obviously with such an approach, aggravation of metabolic acidosis by excessive acetazolamide or insufficient NaHCO₃ administration must be avoided.

DISTINGUISHING THE TYPES OF RENAL TUBULAR ACIDOSIS

The contrasting findings and diagnostic features of the three types of RTA discussed in this chapter are summarized in Table 16-17.

Disorders of Impaired Net Acid Excretion and Impaired Bicarbonate Reclamation with Normokalemia: Acidosis of Progressive Renal Failure

A reduction in functional renal mass by disease has long been known to be associated with acidosis.[28] The metabolic acidosis is initially hyperchloremic (GFR in the range of 20 to 30 mL/min) but may convert to the normochloremic, high AG variety as renal insufficiency progresses and GFR falls below 15 mL/min.[28,79] The major defect in acidification is due to impaired net acid excretion. When the plasma HCO₃ concentration is in the normal range, urine pH is relatively high (≥6.0), and net acid excretion is low. Unlike patients with distal RTA, patients with primary renal disease have a normal ability to lower the urine pH during acidosis.[28] The distal H⁺ secretory capacity is qualitatively normal and can be increased by buffer availability in the form of PO₄³⁻ or by nonreabsorbable anions. Also in contrast to distal RTA, the U − B PcO₂ gradient is normal in patients with reduced GFR, which reflects intact distal H⁺ secretory capacity.

The principal defect in net acid excretion in patients with reduced GFR is thus not an inability to secrete H⁺ in the distal nephron, but rather an inability to produce or to excrete NH₄⁺. Consequently, the kidneys cannot quantitatively excrete all the metabolic acids produced daily, and metabolic acidosis supervenes.[28] Although the acidosis of chronic progressive kidney disease is rarely severe, the argument can be made that the progressive dissolution of bone[28] and the impaired hydroxylation of 25-hydroxycholecalciferol by acidosis[28,79] warrant treatment.

Moreover, chronic metabolic acidosis due to chronic progressive kidney disease has other deleterious effects, including insulin resistance, suppression of the growth hormone/insulin-like growth factor-1 cascade, increase in glucocorticoid levels, renal osteodystrophy, protein degradation, and muscle wasting. In general, it is accepted that alkali therapy helps to reverse these deleterious effects. An amount of alkali slightly in excess (1 to 2 mEq/kg/day) of dietary metabolic acid production usually restores acid-base equilibrium and prevents acid retention.[28] Fear of Na⁺ retention in chronic renal failure

TABLE 16-17 Contrasting Features and Diagnostic Studies in Renal Tubular Acidosis

FINDING	TYPE OF RENAL TUBULAR ACIDOSIS		
	PROXIMAL	CLASSICAL DISTAL	GENERALIZED DISTAL DYSFUNCTION
Plasma [K⁺]	Low	Low	High
Urine pH with acidosis	<5.5	>5.5	<5.5 or >5.5
Urine net charge	Positive	Positive	Positive
Fanconi's lesion	Present	Absent	Absent
Fractional bicarbonate excretion	10%-15%	2%-5%	5%-10%
U – B P_{CO_2}	Normal	Low*	Low
H⁺-ATPase defect		Low	
HCO₃⁻/Cl⁻ defect		High	
Amphotericin B		Normal	
Response to therapy	Least responsive	Responsive	Less responsive
Associated features	Fanconi's syndrome	Nephrocalcinosis/hyperglobulinemia	Renal insufficiency

*See specific defects below.
ATPase, Adenosine triphosphatase; *U – B P_{CO_2},* Urine minus blood CO_2 tension.

as a result of sodium bicarbonate administration appears ill founded. Unlike the case with sodium chloride therapy, patients with chronic renal disease retain administered sodium bicarbonate only as long as acidosis is present. Further sodium bicarbonate then exceeds the reabsorptive threshold and is excreted without causing an increase in weight or in blood pressure unless very large amounts are administered.

The clinical guidelines endorsed by the National Kidney Foundation Kidney Disease Outcomes Quality Initiative (KDOQI) recommend monitoring of total CO_2 in patients with chronic kidney disease with a goal of maintaining the [HCO₃⁻] above 22 mEq/L. Such therapy is based on the view that chronic metabolic acidosis has an adverse impact on muscle and bone metabolism.

Also of concern in chronic progressive kidney disease is the use of sevelamer hydrochloride, which has been shown in patients receiving long-term hemodialysis to result in significantly lower [HCO₃⁻] than do Ca^{2+}-containing phosphate binders.[80] Although it is associated with a lower intake of potential alkali, sevelamer may also provide an acid load.[81] Therefore, the clinician should be alert for changes in the [HCO₃⁻] when the patient is treated with sevelamer.

A number of potential mechanisms exist for the acidosis associated with sevelamer. This agent binds monovalent phosphate in exchange for chloride in the gastrointestinal tract. For each molecule of monovalent phosphate bound, one molecule of HCl is liberated. Upon entry of the polymer into the small intestine, exposure to bicarbonate secreted by the pancreas would result in the binding of bicarbonate by the polymer in exchange for chloride—much like the mechanism in chloride diarrhea. There may be other drug effects on bicarbonate in the colon as well.[82] As kidney disease progresses below a GFR of 15 mL/min, the non-AG acidosis typically evolves into the usual high AG acidosis of end-stage renal disease (see later).[80]

Sevelamer carbonate is a recent formulation of sevelamer in a buffered form which compares favorably to sevelamer hydrochloride in terms of serum phosphorus control but without causing a decline in serum [HCO₃⁻].

High Anion Gap Acidoses

The addition to the body of an acid load in which the attendant non-Cl⁻ anion is not excreted rapidly results in the development of a high AG acidosis. The normochloremic acidosis is maintained as long as the anion that was part of the original acid load remains in the blood. AG acidosis is caused by the accumulation of organic acids. This may occur if the anion does not undergo glomerular filtration (e.g., uremic acid anions), if the anion is filtered but is readily reabsorbed, or if, because of alteration in metabolic pathways (ketoacidosis, L-lactic acidosis), the anion cannot be utilized in the body. Theoretically, with a pure AG acidosis, the increment in the AG (ΔAG) above the normal value of 10 mEq/L should equal the decrease in bicarbonate concentration (ΔHCO₃⁻) below the normal value of 25 mEq/L. When this relationship is considered, circumstances in which the increment in the AG exceeds the decrement in bicarbonate (ΔAG > ΔHCO₃⁻) suggest the coexistence of a metabolic alkalosis. Such findings are not unusual when uremia or ketoacidosis leads to vomiting, for example.

Identification of the underlying cause of a high AG acidosis is facilitated by consideration of the clinical setting and associated laboratory values. The common causes are outlined in Table 16-18 and include (1) lactic acidosis (e.g., L-lactic acidosis and D-lactic acidosis), (2) ketoacidosis (e.g., diabetic, alcoholic, and starvation ketoacidoses), (3) toxin- or poison-induced acidosis (e.g., ethylene glycol, methyl alcohol, propylene glycol, or pyroglutamic acidosis), and (4) uremic acidosis.

Initial screening to differentiate the high AG acidoses should focus on (1) a history or other evidence of drug or toxin ingestion and ABG measurement to detect coexistent respiratory alkalosis (as with salicylates), (2) historical evidence of diabetes mellitus (DKA), (3) evidence of alcoholism or increased levels of β-hydroxybutyrate (AKA), (4) observation for clinical signs of uremia and determination of the blood urea and creatinine levels (uremic acidosis), (5) inspection of the urine for oxalate crystals (ethylene glycol), and, finally, (6) recognition of the numerous settings in which lactic acid

TABLE 16-18 Metabolic Acidosis with High Anion Gap

Conditions Associated with Type A Lactic Acidosis

Hypovolemic shock
Cholera
Septic shock
Cardiogenic shock
   Low-output heart failure
   High-output heart failure
Regional hypoperfusion
Severe hypoxia
   Severe asthma
   Carbon monoxide poisoning
   Severe anemia

Conditions Associated with Type B Lactic Acidosis

Liver disease
Diabetes mellitus
Catecholamine excess
   Endogenous
   Exogenous
Thiamine deficiency
Intracellular inorganic phosphate depletion
   Intravenous fructose
   Intravenous xylose
   Intravenous sorbitol
Alcohols and other ingested compounds metabolized by alcohol
   Dehydrogenase
   Ethanol
   Methanol
   Ethylene glycol
   Propylene glycol
Mitochondrial toxins
   Salicylates
   Cyanide
   2,4-dinitrophenol
   Nonnucleoside anti–reverse transcriptase drugs
Other drugs
Malignancy
Seizure
Inborn errors of metabolism

D-Lactic Acidosis

Short bowel syndrome
Ischemic bowel
Small-bowel obstruction

Ketoacidosis

Diabetic
Alcoholic
Starvation

Other Toxins

Salicylates
Paraldehyde
Pyroglutamic acid

Uremia (Late Renal Failure)

levels may be increased (hypotension, cardiac failure, ischemic bowel, intestinal obstruction and bacterial overgrowth, leukemia, cancer, and exposure to certain drugs).

Lactic Acidosis

PHYSIOLOGY

Lactic acid can exist in two forms: L-lactic acid and D-lactic acid. In mammals, only the levorotatory form is a product of metabolism. D-lactate can accumulate in humans as a by-product of metabolism by bacteria, which accumulate and overgrow in the gastrointestinal tract with jejunal bypass or

short bowel syndrome. Thus, D-lactic acidosis is a rare cause of high AG acidosis. Hospital chemical laboratories routinely measure L-lactic acid levels, not D-lactic acid levels. Thus, most of the remarks that follow apply to L-lactic acid metabolism and acidosis except as noted. L-lactic acidosis is one of the most common forms of a high AG acidosis.

Although lactate metabolism bears a close relationship to that of pyruvate,[83] lactic acid is in a metabolic cul-de-sac with pyruvate as its only outlet. In most cells, the major metabolic pathway for pyruvate is oxidation in the mitochondria to acetyl–coenzyme A by the enzyme pyruvate dehydrogenase within the mitochondria. The overall reaction is usually expressed as

$$\text{Pyruvate}^- + \text{NADH} \leftrightarrow \text{lactate}^- + \text{NAD} + \text{H}^+ \quad (32)$$

Normally, this cytosolic reaction catalyzed by the enzyme lactate dehydrogenase (LDH) is close to equilibrium, so that the law of mass action applies and the equation is rearranged as

$$[\text{Lactate}^-] = \text{Keq}[\text{pyruvate}^-][\text{H}^+]\frac{[\text{NADH}]}{[\text{NAD}^+]} \quad (33)$$

The lactate concentration is a function of the equilibrium constant (K_{eq}), the pyruvate concentration, the cytosolic pH, and the intracellular redox state represented by the concentration ratio of reduced to oxidized nicotinamide adenine dinucleotide or [NADH]/[NAD+].[83]

After rearranging the mass action equation, the ratio of lactate concentration to pyruvate concentration may be expressed as

$$\frac{[\text{Lactate}^-]}{[\text{pyruvate}^-]} = \text{Keq}[\text{H}^+]\frac{[\text{NADH}]}{[\text{NAD}^+]} \quad (34)$$

Because K_{eq} and intracellular H+ concentration are relatively constant, the normal lactate/pyruvate concentration ratio (1.0/0.1 mEq/L) is proportional to the NADH/NAD+ concentration ratio. Therefore the lactate/pyruvate ratio is regulated by the oxidation-reduction potential of the cell.

NADH/NAD+ is also involved in many other metabolic redox reactions.[83] Moreover, the steady-state concentrations of all these redox reactants are related to one another. Important in considerations of acid-base pathophysiology are the redox pairs β-hydroxybutyrate–acetoacetate and ethanol-acetaldehyde. The ratio of the reduced to the oxidized forms of these molecules is thus a function of the cellular redox potential:

$$\frac{[\text{NADH}]}{[\text{NAD}^+]} \propto \frac{[\text{Lactate}]}{[\text{Pyruvate}]} \propto \frac{[\beta\text{-hydroxybutyrate}]}{[\text{acetoacetate}]}$$
$$\propto \frac{[\text{ethanol}]}{[\text{acetaldehyde}]} \quad (35)$$

If the lactate concentration is high compared with that of pyruvate, NAD+ will be depleted, and the NADH/NAD+ ratio will increase. Likewise, all the other related redox ratios previously listed would be similarly affected; that is, both the β-hydroxybutyrate/acetoacetate and the ethanol/acetaldehyde ratios would increase. In clinical practice, these considerations are of practical importance. If lactate levels are increased as a result of lactic acidosis concurrently with ketone overproduction as a result of diabetic acidosis, the ketones exist primarily in the form of β-hydroxybutyrate. The results of tests for ketones that measure only acetoacetate (such as the nitroprusside reaction, e.g., Acetest tablets and reagent sticks), therefore may be misleadingly low or even negative despite high total ketone concentrations. Some hospital laboratories no longer use the nitroprusside reaction to estimate total ketones, and measurement of β-hydroxybutyrate and acetoacetate are the preferred tests. This assumes importance because high levels of alcohol plus ketones shift the redox ratio, so that the NADH/NAD$^+$ ratio is increased. Again, ketones would then be principally in the form of β-hydroxybutyrate. This situation is commonly found in AKA, in which the results of qualitative ketone tests that are more sensitive to acetoacetate are frequently only trace positive or negative, despite markedly increased β-hydroxybutyrate levels.

The L-lactate concentration can be increased in two ways relative to the pyruvate concentration. First, when pyruvate production is increased at a constant intracellular pH and redox stage, the lactate concentration increases at a constant lactate/pyruvate ratio of 10. In contrast, in states in which the production of lactate exceeds the ability to convert to pyruvate, so that the NADH/NAD$^+$ redox ratio is increased, an increased L-lactic acid concentration is observed, but with a lactate/pyruvate ratio greater than 10. This defines an *excess lactate* state. Therefore, the concentration of lactate must be viewed in terms of cellular determinants (e.g., the intracellular pH and redox state) as well as the total body production and removal rates. Normally, the rates of lactate entry and exit from the blood are in balance, so that net lactate accumulation is zero. This dynamic aspect of lactate metabolism is termed the *Cori cycle*:

$$2\text{Lactate}^+2\text{H}^+ \xleftarrow[\substack{\text{Muscle, brain, skin,}\\ \text{red blood cells, gut}}]{\text{Liver, kidney, heart}} \text{Glucose} \qquad (36)$$

As can be envisioned from this relationship, either net overproduction of lactic acid from glucose by some tissues or underutilization by others results in net addition of L-lactic acid to the blood and lactic acidosis. However, ischemia both accelerates lactate production and simultaneously decreases lactate utilization.

The production of lactic acid has been estimated to be about 15 to 20 mEq/kg/day in normal humans.[28] This enormous quantity contrasts with total ECF buffer base stores of about 10 to 15 mEq/kg, and with enhanced production lactic acid can accumulate. The rate of lactic acid production can be increased by ischemia, seizures, extreme exercise, leukemia, and alkalosis.[83] The increase in production occurs principally through enhanced phosphofructokinase activity.

Decreased lactate consumption may also lead to L-lactic acidosis. The principal organs for lactate removal during rest are the liver and kidneys. Both the liver and the kidneys and perhaps muscle have the capacity for increased lactate removal under the stress of increased lactate loads.[83] Hepatic utilization of lactate can be impeded by several factors: poor perfusion of the liver; defective active transport of lactate into cells; and inadequate metabolic conversion of lactate into pyruvate because of altered intracellular pH, redox state, or enzyme activity. Examples of states causing impaired hepatic lactate removal include primary diseases of the liver, enzymatic defects, tissue anoxia or ischemia, severe acidosis, and altered redox states, as occurs with alcohol intoxication, fructose

consumption by fructose-intolerant individuals, or administration of nucleoside (analog) reverse transcriptase inhibitors (NRTIs) such as zidovudine and stavudine in patients with HIV infection[83-85] or biguanides such as metformin.[83,86,87] Deaths have been reported due to refractory lactic acidosis secondary to thiamine deficiency in patients receiving parenteral nutrition formulations without thiamine.[88] Thiamine is a cofactor for pyruvate dehydrogenase that catalyzes the oxidative decarboxylation of pyruvate to acetyl–coenzyme A under aerobic conditions. Pyruvate cannot be metabolized in this manner in the presence of thiamine deficiency, so that excess pyruvate is converted to hydrogen ions and lactate.

The quantitative aspects of normal lactate production and consumption in the Cori cycle demonstrate how the development of lactic acidosis can be the most rapid and devastating form of metabolic acidosis.[83,89]

DIAGNOSIS

Because lactic acid has a pK$_a$ of 3.8, addition of lactic acid to the blood leads to a reduction in blood HCO$_3^-$ concentration and an equivalent elevation in lactate concentration, which is associated with an increase in the AG. Lactate concentrations are mildly increased in various nonpathologic states (e.g., exercise), but the magnitude of the elevation is generally small. In practical terms, a lactate concentration greater than 4 mmol/L (normal is 0.67 to 1.8 mmol/L) is generally accepted as evidence that the metabolic acidosis is ascribable to net lactic acid accumulation.

CLINICAL SPECTRUM

In the classical classification of the L-lactic acidoses (see Table 16-18), type A L-lactic acidosis is due to tissue hypoperfusion or acute hypoxia, whereas type B L-lactic acidosis is associated with common diseases, drugs and toxins, and hereditary and miscellaneous disorders.[83]

Tissue underperfusion and acute underoxygenation at the tissue level (tissue hypoxia) are the most common causes of type A lactic acidosis. Severe arterial hypoxemia even in the absence of decreased perfusion can generate L-lactic acidosis. Inadequate cardiac output, of either the low-output or the high-output variety, is the usual pathogenetic factor. The prognosis is related directly to the increment in plasma L-lactate and the severity of the acidemia.[83,87,89]

Numerous medical conditions (without tissue hypoxia) predispose to type B L-lactic acidosis (see Table 16-18). Hepatic failure reduces hepatic lactate metabolism, and leukemia increases lactate production. Severe anemia, especially as a result of iron deficiency or methemoglobulinemia, may cause lactic acidosis. Among the most common causes of L-lactic acidosis is bowel ischemia and infarction in patients in the medical intensive care unit. Malignant cells produce more lactate than normal cells even under aerobic conditions. This phenomenon is magnified if the tumor expands rapidly and outstrips the blood supply. Therefore, exceptionally large tumors may be associated with severe L-lactic acidosis. Seizures, extreme exertion, heat stroke, and tumor lysis syndrome may all cause L-lactic acidosis.

Several drugs and toxins predispose to L-lactic acidosis (see Table 16-18). Of these, metformin and other biguanides (such as phenformin) are the most widely reported to have this effect.[83,86,87] The occurrence of phenformin-induced lactic acidosis prompted the withdrawal of the drug from U.S. markets in 1977. Although much less frequent than phenformin-induced lactic acidosis, metformin-induced lactic acidosis has been reported in association with volume depletion and with contrast dye administration. Fructose causes intracellular ATP depletion and lactate accumulation.[83] Inborn errors of metabolism may also cause lactic acidosis, primarily by blocking gluconeogenesis or by inhibiting the oxidation of pyruvate.[83] Carbon monoxide poisoning produces lactic acidosis frequently by reduction of the oxygen-carrying capacity of hemoglobin. Cyanide binds cytochrome *a* and a_3 and blocks the flow of electrons to oxygen. In patients with HIV infection nucleoside analogs can induce toxic effects on mitochondria by inhibiting DNA polymerase-γ. Hyperlactatemia is common with NRTI therapy, especially stavudine and zidovudine, but the serum L-lactate level is usually only mildly elevated and compensated.[83-85,90] Nevertheless, with severe concurrent illness, pronounced lactic acidosis may occur in association with hepatic steatosis.[83,85] This combination carries a high mortality. Propylene glycol is used as a vehicle for intravenous medications and some cosmetics and is metabolized to lactic acid in the liver by alcohol dehydrogenase. The lactate is metabolized to pyruvic acid and shunted to the glycolytic pathway. Scattered case reports have described hyperosmolality with or without L-lactic acidosis when propylene glycol was used as a vehicle to deliver topical silver sulfadiazine cream, intravenous diazepam or lorazepam (in alcohol withdrawal), intravenous nitroglycerin, and etomidate.[91,92] A prospective study of nine patients receiving high-dose lorazepam infusions[91] showed elevated plasma propylene levels and an elevated osmolar gap. Six of nine patients had moderate degrees of metabolic acidosis.[91]

ASSOCIATED CLINICAL FEATURES

Hyperventilation, abdominal pain, and disturbances in consciousness are frequently present, as are signs of inadequate cardiopulmonary function in type A L-lactic acidosis. Leukocytosis, hyperphosphatemia, hyperuricemia, and hyperaminoacidemia (especially excess of alanine) are common, and hypoglycemia may occur.[83] Hyperkalemia may or may not accompany acute lactic acidosis.

TREATMENT OF L-LACTIC ACIDOSIS

General Supportive Care. The overall mortality of patients with L-lactic acidosis is 60% to 70% and approaches 100% in those with coexisting hypotension.[83] Therapy for this condition has not advanced substantively in the last 2 decades. The basic principle and only effective form of therapy for L-lactic acidosis is first to correct the underlying condition initiating the disruption in normal lactate metabolism. In type A L-lactic acidosis, cessation of acid production by improvement of tissue oxygenation, restoration of the circulating fluid volume, improvement or augmentation of cardiac function, resection of ischemic tissue, and amelioration of sepsis are necessary in many cases. Septic shock requires control of the underlying infection and volume resuscitation in hypovolemic shock. Hypothetically, interruption of the cytokine cascade may be advantageous but is not yet possible. High L-lactate levels portend a poor prognosis almost uniformly, and sodium bicarbonate administration is of little value. Use of vasoconstricting agents is problematic because they may potentiate the hypoperfused state. Dopamine is preferred to epinephrine if pressure support is required, but the vasodilator nitroprusside has been suggested because it may enhance cardiac output and hepatic and renal blood flow to augment lactate

removal.[83] Nevertheless, nitroprusside therapy may result in cyanide toxicity and has no proven efficacy in the treatment of this disorder.

Alkali Therapy. Alkali therapy is generally advocated for acute, severe acidemia (pH of <7.1) to improve inotropy and lactate utilization. However, in experimental models and clinical examples of lactic acidosis, it has been shown that $NaHCO_3$ therapy in large amounts can depress cardiac performance and exacerbate the acidemia. Paradoxically, bicarbonate therapy activates phosphofructokinase, which is regulated by intracellular pH, thereby increasing lactate production. The use of alkali in states of moderate L-lactic acidemia is therefore controversial, and it is generally agreed that attempts to normalize the pH or HCO_3^- concentration by intravenous $NaHCO_3$ therapy is both potentially deleterious and practically impossible. Thus, raising the plasma HCO_3^- to approximately 15 mEq/L and the pH to 7.2 to 7.25 is a reasonable goal to improve tissue pH. Constant infusion of hypertonic bicarbonate has many disadvantages and is discouraged. Fluid overload occurs rapidly with $NaHCO_3$ administration because of the massive amounts required in some cases. In addition, central venoconstriction and decreased cardiac output are common. The accumulation of lactic acid may be relentless and may necessitate administration of diuretics, ultrafiltration, or dialysis. Hemodialysis can simultaneously deliver HCO_3^-, remove lactate, remove excess ECF volume, and correct electrolyte abnormalities. The use of continuous renal replacement therapy as a means of lactate removal and simultaneous alkali addition is a promising adjunctive treatment in critically ill patients with L-lactic acidosis.

If the underlying cause of the L-lactic acidosis can be remedied, blood lactate will be reconverted to HCO_3^-. HCO_3^- derived from lactate conversion and any new HCO_3^- generated by renal mechanisms during acidosis and from exogenous alkali therapy are additive and may result in an overshoot alkalosis.

Other Agents. Dichloroacetate, an activator of pyruvate dehydrogenase, was suggested in an uncontrolled study to be a potentially useful therapeutic agent. In experimental L-lactic acidosis, dichloroacetate stimulated lactate consumption in muscle and hence decreased lactate production and improved survival. In nonacidotic diabetic patients, it successfully lowered lactate level as well as glucose, lipid, and amino acid levels. Despite encouraging results of its short-term clinical use in acute lactic acidosis, a prospective multicenter trial failed to substantiate any beneficial effect of dichloroacetate therapy.[93] Administration of methylene blue was once advocated as a means of reversing the altered redox state to enhance lactate metabolism. There is no evidence from controlled studies to support its use. THAM (0.3 mol/L tromethamine) and other preparations of this type are not effective.[83] Tribonat, a mixture of THAM, acetate, $NaHCO_3$, and phosphate, although apparently an effective clinical buffer, has produced no survival advantage in limited clinical trials.[94] Lactated Ringer's solution and lactate-containing peritoneal dialysis solutions should be avoided.

D-LACTIC ACIDOSIS

The manifestations of D-lactate acidosis are typically episodic encephalopathy and high AG acidosis in association with short bowel syndrome. Features include slurred speech, confusion, cognitive impairment, clumsiness, ataxia, hallucinations, and behavioral disturbances. D-Lactic acidosis has been described in patients with bowel obstruction, jejunal bypass, short bowel, or ischemic bowel disease. These disorders have in common ileus or stasis associated with overgrowth of flora in the gastrointestinal tract, which is exacerbated by a high-carbohydrate diet.[83] D-lactate acidosis therefore occurs when fermentation by colonic bacteria in the intestine causes D-lactate to accumulate so that it can be absorbed into the circulation. D-lactate is not measured by the typical clinical laboratory, which reports the L-isomer. The disorder should be suspected in patients with an unexplained AG acidosis and some of the typical features noted previously. While results of specific testing are awaited, the patient should be under orders to receive nothing by mouth. Serum D-lactate levels of greater than 3 mmol/L confirm the diagnosis. Treatment with a low-carbohydrate diet and antibiotics (neomycin, vancomycin, or metronidazole) is often effective.[95-98]

Ketoacidosis

DIABETIC KETOACIDOSIS

DKA is due to increased fatty acid metabolism and the accumulation of ketoacids (acetoacetate and β-hydroxybutyrate) as a result of insulin deficiency or resistance in association with elevated glucagon levels. DKA is usually seen in insulin-dependent diabetes mellitus in association with cessation of insulin therapy or an intercurrent illness, such as an infection, gastroenteritis, pancreatitis, or myocardial infarction, which increases insulin requirements temporarily and acutely. The accumulation of ketoacids accounts for the increment in the AG, which is accompanied, most often, by evidence of hyperglycemia (glucose level of >300 mg/dL). In comparison to patients with AKA, described later, patients with DKA have metabolic profiles characterized by a higher plasma glucose level and lower β-hydroxybutyrate/acetoacetate and lactate/pyruvate ratios.[27,98,99]

Treatment. Most, if not all, patients with DKA require correction of the volume depletion that almost invariably accompanies the osmotic diuresis in DKA. In general, it seems prudent to initiate therapy with intravenous isotonic saline at a rate of 1000 mL/hr, especially in the severely volume-depleted patient. When the pulse and blood pressure have stabilized and the corrected serum Na⁺ concentration is in the range 130 to 135 mEq/L, switch to 0.45% sodium chloride and slow the infusion rate. Lactated Ringer's solution should be avoided. If the blood glucose level falls below 300 mg/dL, 0.45% sodium chloride with 5% dextrose should be administered.[27,98]

Low-dose intravenous insulin therapy (0.1 U/kg/hr) smoothly corrects the biochemical abnormalities and minimizes hypoglycemia and hypokalemia.[27,98] Usually, in the first hour, a loading dose of the same amount is given initially as a bolus intravenously. Intramuscular insulin is not effective in patients with volume depletion, which often occurs in ketoacidosis.

Total body K⁺ depletion is usually present, although the K⁺ level on admission may be elevated or normal. A normal or reduced K⁺ value on admission indicates severe K⁺ depletion and should be approached with caution. Administration of fluid, insulin, and alkali may cause the K⁺ level to plummet. When urine output has been established, 20 mEq of potassium chloride should be administered in each liter of fluid as long as the K⁺ value is less than 4.0 mEq/L. Equal caution should be exercised in the presence of hyperkalemia, especially if the patient has renal insufficiency, because the usual therapy does not always correct hyperkalemia. Never administer potassium chloride empirically.

Young patients with a pure AG acidosis (ΔAG = ΔHCO$_3^-$) usually do not require exogenous alkali because the metabolic acidosis should be entirely reversible. Elderly patients, patients with severe high AG acidosis (pH of <7.15), or patients with a superimposed hyperchloremic component may receive small amounts of sodium bicarbonate by slow intravenous infusion (no more than 44 to 88 mEq in 60 minutes). Thirty minutes after this infusion is completed, ABG measurement should be repeated. Alkali administration can be repeated only if the pH remains at 7.20 or less, or if the patient exhibits a significant hyperchloremic component, but additional NaHCO$_3$ is rarely necessary. The AG should be followed closely during therapy because it is expected to decline as ketones are cleared from the plasma and projects an increase in plasma HCO$_3^-$ as the acidosis is repaired. Therefore, it is not necessary to monitor blood ketone levels continuously. Hypokalemia and other complications of alkali therapy dramatically increase when amounts of sodium bicarbonate exceeding 400 mEq are administered. However, the effect of alkali therapy on arterial blood pH needs to be reassessed regularly and the total administered kept at a minimum, if alkali therapy is necessary.[27,98,99]

Routine administration of PO$_4^{3-}$ (usually as potassium phosphate) is not advised because of the potential for hyperphosphatemia and hypocalcemia.[27,98] A significant proportion of patients with DKA have significant hyperphosphatemia before initiation of therapy. In the volume-depleted, malnourished patient, however, a normal or elevated PO$_4^{3-}$ concentration on admission may be followed by a rapid fall in plasma PO$_4^{3-}$ levels within 2 to 6 hours after initiation of therapy.

ALCOHOLIC KETOACIDOSIS

Some patients with chronic alcoholism, especially binge drinkers, who discontinue solid food intake while continuing alcohol consumption develop the alcoholic form of ketoacidosis when alcohol ingestion is curtailed abruptly.[27,98,99] Usually the onset of vomiting and abdominal pain with dehydration leads to cessation of alcohol consumption before the patient comes to the hospital.[27,99] The metabolic acidosis may be severe but is accompanied by only modestly deranged glucose levels, which are usually low but may be slightly elevated.[27,99] Typically, insulin levels are low and levels of triglyceride, cortisol, glucagon, and growth hormone are increased. The net result of this deranged metabolic state is ketosis. The acidosis is primarily due to elevated levels of ketones, which exist predominantly in the form of β-hydroxybutyrate because of the altered redox state induced by the metabolism of alcohol. Compared with patients with DKA, patients with AKA have lower plasma glucose concentrations and higher β-hydroxybutyrate/acetoacetate and lactate/pyruvate ratios.[27,99] This disorder is not rare and is underdiagnosed. The clinical presentation in AKA may be complex because a mixed disorder is often present caused by metabolic alkalosis (vomiting), respiratory alkalosis (alcoholic liver disease), lactic acidosis (hypoperfusion), and hyperchloremic acidosis (renal excretion of ketoacids). Finally, the osmolar gap is elevated if the blood alcohol level is elevated, but the differential diagnosis should always include ethylene glycol and/or methanol intoxication.

Treatment. Therapy includes intravenous glucose and saline administration, but insulin should be avoided. K^+, PO_4^{3-}, Mg^{2+}, and vitamin supplementation (especially thiamine) are frequently necessary. Glucose in isotonic saline, not saline alone, is the mainstay of therapy. Because of superimposed starvation, patients with AKA often develop hypophosphatemia within 12 to 18 hours of admission. Treatment with glucose-containing intravenous fluids increases the risk of severe hypophosphatemia. Levels should be checked on admission and at 4, 6, 12, and 18 hours. Profound hypophosphatemia may provoke aspiration, platelet dysfunction, hemolysis, and rhabdomyolysis. Therefore, phosphate replacement should be provided promptly when indicated. Hypokalemia and hypomagnesemia are also common and should not be overlooked.[27,99]

STARVATION KETOACIDOSIS
Ketoacidosis occurs within the first 24 to 48 hours of fasting, is accentuated by exercise and pregnancy, and is rapidly reversible by glucose or insulin administration. Starvation-induced hypoinsulinemia and accentuated hepatic ketone production have been implicated pathogenetically.[27,99] Fasting alone can increase ketoacid levels, although not usually above 10 mEq/L. High-protein weight-loss diets typically cause mild ketosis but not ketoacidosis. Patients typically respond to glucose and saline infusion.

Drug- and Toxin-Induced Acidosis

SALICYLATE
Intoxication with salicylates, although more common in children than in adults, may result in the development of a high AG metabolic acidosis, but the acid-base abnormality most commonly associated with salicylate intoxication in adults is respiratory alkalosis due to direct stimulation of the respiratory center by salicylates.[98] Adult patients with salicylate intoxication usually have pure respiratory alkalosis or mixed respiratory alkalosis–metabolic acidosis.[98] Metabolic acidosis occurs due to uncoupling of oxidative phosphorylation and enhances the transit of salicylates into the central nervous system. Only part of the increase in the AG is due to the increase in plasma salicylate concentration, because a toxic salicylate level of 100 mg/dL would account for an increase in the AG of only 7 mEq/L. High ketone concentrations have been reported to be present in as many as 40% of adult salicylate-intoxicated patients, sometimes as a result of salicylate-induced hypoglycemia.[100] L-Lactic acid production is also often increased, partly as a direct drug effect[98] and partly as a result of the decrease in Pco_2 induced by salicylate. Proteinuria and pulmonary edema may occur.

Treatment. General treatment should always consist of initial vigorous gastric lavage with isotonic saline followed by administration of activated charcoal via nasogastric tube. Treatment of the metabolic acidosis may be necessary, because acidosis can enhance the entry of salicylate into the central nervous system. Alkali should be given cautiously, and frank alkalemia should be avoided. Coexisting respiratory alkalosis can make this form of therapy hazardous. The renal excretion of salicylate is enhanced by an alkaline diuresis accomplished with intravenous administration of $NaHCO_3$. Caution is urged if the patient exhibits concomitant respiratory alkalosis with frank alkalemia, because $NaHCO_3$ may cause severe alkalosis and hypokalemia may result from alkalinization of the urine. To minimize the administration of $NaHCO_3$, acetazolamide may be administered to the alkalemic patient, but this can cause acidosis and impair salicylate elimination. Hemodialysis may be necessary in severe poisoning, especially if renal failure coexists; it is preferred in cases of severe intoxication (>700 mg/L) and is superior to hemofiltration, which does not correct the acid-base abnormality.[98,100]

TOXINS
The Osmolar Gap in Toxin-Induced Acidosis. Under most physiologic conditions, Na^+, urea, and glucose generate the osmotic pressure of blood. Serum osmolality is calculated according to the following expression:

$$\text{Osmolality} = 2[Na^+] + \frac{BUN}{2.8} + \frac{\text{glucose (mg/dL)}}{18} \quad (37)$$

The calculated and determined osmolalities should agree within 10 mOsm/kg. When the measured osmolality exceeds the calculated osmolality by more than 10 mOsm/kg, one of two circumstances prevails. First, the serum Na^+ may be spuriously low, as occurs with hyperlipidemia or hyperproteinemia (pseudohyponatremia). Second, osmolytes other than sodium salts, glucose, or urea may have accumulated in plasma. Examples are infused mannitol, radiocontrast media, or other solutes, including the alcohols, ethylene glycol, and acetone, which can increase the osmolality in plasma. For these examples, the difference between the osmolality calculated from equation 37 and the measured osmolality is proportional to the concentration of the unmeasured solute. Such differences in these clinical circumstances have been referred to as the *osmolar gap*. In the presence of an appropriate clinical history and index of suspicion, the osmolar gap becomes a very reliable and helpful screening tool in assessing for toxin-associated high AG acidosis.

Ethanol. Ethanol, after absorption from the gastrointestinal tract, is oxidized to acetaldehyde, acetyl–coenzyme A, and CO_2. A blood ethanol level over 500 mg/dL is associated with high mortality. Acetaldehyde levels do not increase appreciably unless the load is exceptionally high or the acetaldehyde dehydrogenase step is inhibited by compounds such as disulfiram, insecticides, or sulfonylurea hypoglycemia agents. In the presence of ethanol such agents result in severe toxicity. The association of ethanol with the development of AKA and lactic acidosis has been discussed in the previous section, but in general, ethanol intoxication does not cause a high AG acidosis.

Ethylene Glycol. Ingestion of ethylene glycol, used in antifreeze, leads to a high AG metabolic acidosis in addition to severe central nervous system, cardiopulmonary, and renal damage.[98,101,102] The high AG is attributable to ethylene glycol metabolites, especially oxalic acid, glycolic acid, and other incompletely identified organic acids.[102] L-Lactic acid production also increases as a result of a toxic depression in the reaction rates of the citric acid cycle and altered intracellular redox state.[102] Recognition of oxalate crystals in the urine facilitates diagnosis. Fluorescence of the urine by Wood's light (if the ingested ethylene glycol contains a fluorescent vehicle) has been suggested as a diagnostic indicator but is neither specific nor sensitive.[101,102] A disparity between the measured blood osmolality and that calculated (high osmolar gap) is often present.

Treatment includes prompt institution of osmotic diuresis, thiamine and pyridoxine supplementation, administration of 4-methylpyrazole (fomepizole),[103] or ethyl alcohol administration and dialysis.[98,101,103] Fomepizole is the drug of choice and should be given intravenously. Competitive inhibition of alcohol dehydrogenase with either fomepizole or ethyl alcohol is absolutely necessary in all patients to lessen toxicity, because ethanol and fomepizole compete for metabolic conversion of ethylene glycol and alter the cellular redox state. Fomepizole (initiated as a loading dose of 15 mg/kg, followed by 10 mg/kg every 12 hours), offers the advantages of a predictable decline in ethylene glycol levels without the adverse effect of excessive obtundation, as seen with ethyl alcohol infusion. When these measures have been accomplished, hemodialysis may be initiated to remove the ethylene glycol metabolites. The intravenous ethanol infusion should be increased during hemodialysis to allow maintenance of the blood alcohol level in the range of 100 to 150 mg/dL or more than 22 mmol/L. Ethanol can also be added to the dialysate bath. The indications for hemodialysis include (1) arterial pH of less than 7.3, (2) HCO_3^- concentration of more than 20 mEg/L, (3) osmolal gap of more than 10 mOsm/kg, and (4) oxalate crystalluria.[101]

Methanol. Ingestion of methanol (wood alcohol) causes metabolic acidosis in addition to severe optic nerve and central nervous system manifestations resulting from its metabolism to formic acid from formaldehyde.[98,101] Lactic acids and ketoacids as well as other unidentified organic acids may contribute to the acidosis. Because of the low molecular mass of methanol (32 Da), an osmolar gap is usually present. Therapy is generally similar to that for ethylene glycol intoxication, including general supportive measures, ethanol or fomepizole administration, and hemodialysis.[103]

Isopropyl Alcohol. Rubbing alcohol poisoning is usually the result of accidental oral ingestion or absorption through the skin. Although isopropyl alcohol is metabolized by the enzyme alcohol dehydrogenase, as are methanol and ethanol, isopropyl alcohol is *not metabolized to a strong acid* and *does not elevate the AG*. Isopropyl alcohol is metabolized to acetone, and the osmolar gap increases as the result of accumulation of both acetone and isopropyl alcohol. Despite a positive nitroprusside reaction from acetone, the AG, as well as the blood glucose level, are typically normal, not elevated, and the plasma HCO_3^- concentration is not depressed. Thus, isopropyl alcohol intoxication does not typically cause metabolic acidosis. Treatment is supportive, with attention to removal of unabsorbed alcohol from the gastrointestinal tract and administration of intravenous fluids. Hemodialysis is effective but not usually necessary. Although patients with significant isopropyl alcohol intoxication (blood levels of >100 mg/dL) may develop cardiovascular collapse and lactic acidosis, watchful waiting with a conservative approach (intravenous fluids, electrolyte replacement, and tracheal intubation) is often sufficient. Very severe intoxication (>400 mg/dL) is an indication for hemodialysis.[98]

Paraldehyde. Intoxication with paraldehyde is very rare and of historic interest. It is a result of the accumulation of acetic acid, the metabolic product of the drug from acetaldehyde, and other organic acids.

Pyroglutamic Acid. Pyroglutamic acid, or 5-oxoproline, is an intermediate in the γ-glutamyl cycle for the synthesis of glutathione. Acetaminophen ingestion can in rare cases deplete glutathione, which results in increased formation of γ-glutamyl cysteine, which is metabolized to pyroglutamic acid.[104] Accumulation of this intermediate, first appreciated in the rare patients with congenital glutathione synthetase deficiency, has been observed recently in an acquired variety. Those patients observed thus far have severe high AG acidosis and alterations in mental status.[104] Many were septic and were receiving full therapeutic dosages of acetaminophen. All had elevated blood levels of pyroglutamic acid, which increased in proportion to the increase in the AG. It is conceivable that the heterozygote state for glutathione synthetase deficiency could predispose to pyroglutamic acidosis, because only a minority of critically ill patients receiving acetaminophen develop this newly appreciated form of metabolic acidosis.[104]

PROPYLENE GLYCOL

Numerous intravenous preparations contain propylene glycol as the vehicle (lorazepam, diazepam, pentobarbital, phenytoin, nitroglycerin, and TMP-SMX). Propylene glycol may accumulate and cause a high AG, osmolar gap acidosis in patients receiving continuous infusion or high dosages of these agents, especially in the presence of chronic kidney disease, chronic liver disease, alcohol abuse, or pregnancy. The acidosis is the result of accumulation of L-lactic acid, D-lactic acid and L-acetaldehyde. Propylene glycol metabolism utilizes alcohol dehydrogenase. The acidosis typically abates with cessation of the offending agent.[105]

UREMIA

Advanced renal insufficiency eventually converts the hyperchloremic acidosis discussed earlier to a typical high AG acidosis.[28] Poor filtration plus continued reabsorption of poorly identified uremic organic anions contributes to the pathogenesis of this metabolic disturbance.

Classical uremic acidosis is characterized by a reduced rate of NH_4^+ production and excretion because of cumulative and significant loss of renal mass.[4,5,19,28] Usually, acidosis does not occur until a major portion of the total functional nephron population (>75%) has been destroyed, because of the ability of surviving nephrons to increase ammoniagenesis. Eventually, however, there is a decrease in total renal ammonia excretion as renal mass is reduced to a level at which the GFR is 20 mL/min or less. PO_4^{3-} balance is maintained as a result of both hyperparathyroidism, which decreases proximal PO_4^{3-} absorption, and an increase in plasma PO_4^{3-} as GFR declines. Protein restriction and the administration of phosphate binders reduce the availability of PO_4^{3-}.

Treatment of Acidosis of Chronic Renal Failure. The uremic acidosis of renal failure requires oral alkali replacement to maintain the HCO_3^- concentration above 20 mEq/L. This can be accomplished with relatively modest amounts of alkali (1.0 to 1.5 mEq/kg/day). Shohl's solution or sodium bicarbonate tablets (325- or 650-mg tablets) are equally effective. It is assumed that alkali replacement serves to prevent the harmful effects of prolonged positive H^+ balance, especially progressive catabolism of muscle and loss of bone. Because sodium citrate (Shohl's solution) has been shown to enhance the absorption of aluminum from the gastrointestinal tract, it should never be administered to patients receiving aluminum-containing antacids because of the risk of aluminum intoxication. When hyperkalemia is present, furosemide (60 to 80 mg/day) should be added. Occasionally a patient may require long-term oral sodium polystyrene sulfonate (Kayexalate) therapy (15 to 30 g/day). The pure powder preparation is better tolerated long term than the commercially available syrup preparation and avoids sorbitol (which may cause bowel necrosis).

Metabolic Alkalosis

Diagnosis of Simple and Mixed Forms of Metabolic Alkalosis

Metabolic alkalosis is a primary acid-base disturbance that is manifest in the most pure or simple form as alkalemia (elevated arterial pH) and an increase in $Paco_2$ as a result of compensatory alveolar hypoventilation. Metabolic alkalosis is one of the more common acid-base disturbances in hospitalized patients and occurs as both a simple and a mixed disorder.[11,106] A patient with a high plasma HCO_3^- concentration and a low plasma Cl^- concentration has either metabolic alkalosis or chronic respiratory acidosis. The arterial pH establishes the diagnosis, because it is increased in metabolic alkalosis and is typically decreased in respiratory acidosis. Modest increases in the $Paco_2$ are expected in metabolic alkalosis. A combination of the two disorders is not unusual, because many patients with chronic obstructive lung disease are treated with diuretics, which promote ECF contraction, hypokalemia, and metabolic alkalosis. Metabolic alkalosis is also frequently observed not as a pure or simple acid-base disturbance, but in association with other disorders such as respiratory acidosis, respiratory alkalosis, and metabolic acidosis (*mixed disorders*). *Mixed metabolic alkalosis–metabolic acidosis can be appreciated only if the accompanying metabolic acidosis is a high AG acidosis.* The mixed disorder can be appreciated by comparison of the increment in the AG above the normal value of 10 mEq/L (ΔAG = Patient's AG – 10) with the decrement in the $[HCO_3^-]$ below the normal value of 25 mEq/L (ΔHCO_3^- = 25 – Patient's HCO_3^-). A mixed metabolic alkalosis–high AG metabolic acidosis is recognized because the delta values are not similar. Often, there is no bicarbonate deficit, yet the AG is significantly elevated. Thus, in a patient with an AG of 20 but a near-normal bicarbonate concentration, mixed metabolic alkalosis–metabolic acidosis should be considered. Common examples include renal failure acidosis (uremic) with vomiting or DKA with vomiting.

Respiratory compensation for metabolic alkalosis is less predictable than that for metabolic acidosis. In general the anticipated Pco_2 can be estimated by adding 15 to the patient's serum $[HCO_3^-]$ in the range of HCO_3^- from 25 to 40 mEq/L. Further elevation in Pco_2 is limited by hypoxemia and, to some extent, hypokalemia, which accompanies metabolic alkalosis with regularity. Nevertheless, if a patient has a Pco_2 of only 40 mm Hg while the $[HCO_3^-]$ is frankly elevated (e.g., 35 mEq/L) and the pH is in the alkalemic range, then respiratory compensation is inadequate and a mixed metabolic alkalosis–respiratory alkalosis exists.

In assessing a patient with metabolic alkalosis, two questions must be considered: (1) What is the source of alkali gain (or acid loss) that *generated* the alkalosis? (2) What renal mechanisms are operating to prevent excretion of excess HCO_3^-, thereby *maintaining*, rather than correcting, the alkalosis? In the following discussion, the entities responsible for generating alkalosis are discussed individually and reference is made to the mechanisms necessary to sustain the increase in blood HCO_3^- concentration in each case. The general mechanisms responsible for the *maintenance of alkalosis* have been discussed in detail earlier in this chapter, and are a result of the combined effects of chloride, ECF volume, and potassium depletion (Figure 16-8).

Hypokalemia is an important participant in the maintenance phase of metabolic alkalosis and has selective effects on (1) H^+ secretion and (2) ammonium excretion. The former is a result, in part, of stimulation of the H^+-K^+-ATPase in type A intercalated cells of the collecting duct by hypokalemia. The latter is a direct result of enhanced ammoniagenesis and ammonium transport (proximal convoluted tubule, TAL, medullary collecting duct) in response to hypokalemia. Finally, hyperaldosteronism (primary or secondary) participates in sustaining the alkalosis by increasing activity of the H^+-K^+-ATPase in type A intercalated cells as well as the ENaC and the Na^+-K^+-ATPase in principal cells in the collecting duct. The net result of the latter process is to stimulate K^+ secretion through K^+-selective channels in this same cell, which thus maintains the alkalosis.[105]

Under normal circumstances, the kidneys display an impressive capacity to excrete HCO_3^-. For HCO_3^- to be added to the ECF, HCO_3^- must be administered exogenously or retained in some manner. Thus, *the development of metabolic alkalosis represents a failure of the kidneys to eliminate HCO_3^- at the normal capacity.* The kidneys retain, rather than excrete, the excess alkali and maintain the alkalosis if one of several mechanisms is operative (see Figure 16-8):

1. Cl^- deficiency (ECF contraction) exists concurrently with K^+ deficiency to decrease GFR and/or enhance proximal and distal HCO_3^- absorption. This combination of

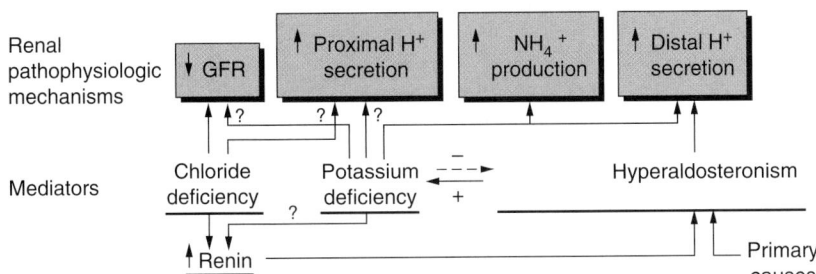

MAINTENANCE OF METABOLIC ALKALOSIS

FIGURE 16-8 Pathophysiologic basis and approach to treatment of the maintenance phase of chronic metabolic alkalosis. Paradoxical stimulation of bicarbonate absorption (H^+ secretion) and NH_4^+ production and excretion is the combined result of Cl^- deficiency, K^+ deficiency, and secondary hyperaldosteronism. *GFR,* Glomerular filtration rate.

disorders evokes secondary hyperreninemic hyperaldosteronism and stimulates H^+ secretion in the collecting duct and ammoniagenesis. Repair of the alkalosis may be accomplished by saline and K^+ administration.

2. Hypermineralocorticoidism and hypokalemia are induced by autonomous factors unresponsive to increased ECF. The stimulation of distal H^+ secretion is then sufficient to reabsorb the increased filtered HCO_3^- load and to overcome the decreased proximal HCO_3^- reabsorption caused by ECF expansion. Repair of the alkalosis in this case rests with removal of the excess autonomous mineralocorticoid; saline administration is ineffective.

The various causes of metabolic alkalosis are summarized in Table 16-19. In attempting to establish the cause of metabolic alkalosis, one must assess the status of the ECF, blood pressure, serum K^+ concentration, and renin-aldosterone system. For example, the presence of hypertension and hypokalemia in an alkalotic patient suggests that either the patient has some form of primary mineralocorticoid excess (see Table 16-19) or the patient is hypertensive and is taking diuretics. Low plasma renin activity and normal urinary Na^+ and Cl^- values in a patient not taking diuretics would also indicate a primary mineralocorticoid excess syndrome. The combination of hypokalemia and alkalosis in a normotensive, nonedematous patient can pose a difficult diagnostic problem. The possible causes to be considered include Bartter's or Gitelman's syndrome, Mg^{2+} deficiency, surreptitious vomiting, exogenous alkali, and diuretic ingestion. Urine electrolyte determinations and urine screening for diuretics are helpful diagnostic tools (Table 16-20). If the urine is alkaline, with high values for Na^+ and K^+ concentrations but low values for Cl^- concentration, the diagnosis is usually either active (continuous) vomiting (overt or surreptitious) or alkali ingestion. On the one hand, if the urine is relatively acid, with low concentrations of Na^+, K^+, and Cl^-, the most likely possibilities are prior (discontinuous) vomiting, a posthypercapnic state, or prior diuretic ingestion. If, on the other hand, the urinary Na^+, K^+, and Cl^- concentrations are not depressed, one must consider Mg^{2+} deficiency, Bartter's or Gitelman's syndrome, or current diuretic ingestion. In most patients, Gitelman's syndrome is characterized by a low urine Ca^{2+} concentration in addition to a low serum Mg^{2+} level. In contrast, the urine calcium level is elevated in Bartter's syndrome. The diagnostic approach to metabolic alkalosis is summarized in the flow diagram in Figure 16-9.

Exogenous Bicarbonate Loads

Long-term administration of alkali to individuals with normal renal function results in minimal, if any, alkalosis. In patients with chronic renal insufficiency, however, overt alkalosis can develop after alkali administration, presumably because the capacity to excrete HCO_3^- is exceeded or because coexistent hemodynamic disturbances have caused enhanced fractional HCO_3^- reabsorption.

BICARBONATE AND BICARBONATE-PRECURSOR ADMINISTRATION
The propensity of patients who have ECF contraction or renal disease plus alkali loads to develop alkalosis is exemplified by patients who receive oral or intravenous HCO_3^-, acetate loads in parenteral hyperalimentation solutions, sodium citrate loads (via regional anticoagulation, transfusions, or infant formula), or antacids plus cation exchange resins. The use of trisodium

citrate solution for regional anticoagulation has been reported to be a cause of metabolic alkalosis in patients receiving continuous renal replacement therapy.[107,108] Citrate metabolism consumes a hydrogen ion and thereby generates HCO_3^- in liver and skeletal muscle. Dilute (0.1 normal) HCl is often required for correction in this setting.[108] In the author's experience, the risk of alkalosis is reduced when anticoagulant citrate dextrose formula A is used, because less bicarbonate is generated than with hypertonic trisodium citrate administration.

TABLE 16-19   Causes of Metabolic Alkalosis

Exogenous HCO_3^- Loads

Acute alkali administration
Milk-alkali syndrome

Effective ECV Contraction, Normotension, K^+ Deficiency, and Secondary Hyperreninemic Hyperaldosteronism

Gastrointestinal origin
  Vomiting
  Gastric aspiration
  Congenital chloridorrhea
  Villous adenoma
    Combined administration of sodium polystyrene sulfonate (Kayexalate and aluminum hydroxide)
Renal origin
  Diuretics (especially thiazides and loop diuretics)
  Edematous states
  Posthypercapnic state
  Hypercalcemia-hypoparathyroidism
  Recovery from lactic acidosis or ketoacidosis
  Nonreabsorbable anions such as penicillin, carbenicillin
  Mg^{2+} deficiency
  K^+ depletion
  Bartter's syndrome (loss of function mutations in thick ascending limb of loop of Henle)
  Gitelman's syndrome (loss-of-function mutation in Na^+-Cl^- cotransporter)
  Carbohydrate refeeding after starvation

ECV Expansion, Hypertension, K^+ Deficiency, and Hypermineralocorticoidism

Associated with high renin level
  Renal artery stenosis
  Accelerated hypertension
  Renin-secreting tumor
  Estrogen therapy
Associated with low renin level
  Primary aldosteronism
    Adenoma
    Hyperplasia
    Carcinoma
    Glucocorticoid suppressible
  Adrenal enzymatic defects
    11β-hydroxylase deficiency
    17α-hydroxylase deficiency
  Cushing's syndrome or disease
    Ectopic corticotropin
    Adrenal carcinoma
    Adrenal adenoma
    Primary pituitary
  Other
    Licorice
    Carbenoxolone
    Chewer's tobacco
    Lydia Pinkham tablets

Gain-of-Function Mutation of ENaC with ECV Expansion, Hypertension, K^+ Deficiency, and Hyporeninemic Hypoaldosteronism

Liddle's syndrome

ECV, Extracellular fluid volume; *ENaC*, epithelial sodium channel.

MILK-ALKALI SYNDROME

Another cause of metabolic alkalosis is long-standing excessive ingestion of milk and antacids. The incidence of milk-alkali syndrome is now increasing because of the use of calcium supplementation (e.g., calcium carbonate) by women

for osteoporosis treatment or prevention. Older women with poor dietary intake ("tea and toasters") are especially prone. In Asia, betel nut chewing is a cause because the erosive nut is often wrapped in calcium hydroxide. Both hypercalcemia and vitamin D excess have been suggested to increase renal HCO_3^- reabsorption. Patients with these disorders are prone to develop nephrocalcinosis, renal insufficiency, and metabolic alkalosis.[105] Discontinuation of alkali ingestion or administration is usually sufficient to repair the alkalosis.

Normal Blood Pressure, Extracellular Volume Contraction, Potassium Depletion, and Hyperreninemic Hyperaldosteronism

GASTROINTESTINAL ORIGIN

Vomiting and Gastric Aspiration. Gastrointestinal loss of H^+ results in retention of HCO_3^- in the body fluids. Increased H^+ loss through gastric secretions can be caused by vomiting due to physical or psychiatric reasons, nasogastric tube aspiration, or a gastric fistula (see Table 16-19).[105]

The fluid and sodium chloride loss in vomitus or in nasogastric suction results in ECF contraction with an increase in plasma renin activity and aldosterone.[105] These factors decrease GFR and enhance the capacity of the renal tubule to reabsorb HCO_3^-.[11] During the active phase of vomiting, there is continued addition of HCO_3^- to plasma in exchange for Cl^-. The plasma HCO_3^- concentration increases to a level that exceeds the reabsorptive capacity of the proximal tubule. The excess

TABLE 16-20 Diagnosis of Metabolic Alkalosis	
SALINE-RESPONSIVE ALKALOSIS	**SALINE-UNRESPONSIVE ALKALOSIS**
LOW URINARY [Cl⁻] (<10 mEq/L)	*HIGH OR NORMAL URINARY [Cl⁻] (>15-20 mEq/L)*
Normotensive	Hypertensive
Vomiting	Primary aldosteronism
Nasogastric aspiration	Cushing's syndrome
Diuretic use (distant)	Renal artery stenosis
Posthypercapnia	Renal failure plus alkali therapy
Villous adenoma	Normotensive
Bicarbonate treatment of organic acidosis	Mg^{2+} deficiency
K^+ deficiency	Severe K^+ deficiency
Hypertensive	Bartter's syndrome
Liddle's syndrome	Gitelman's syndrome
	Diuretic use (recent)

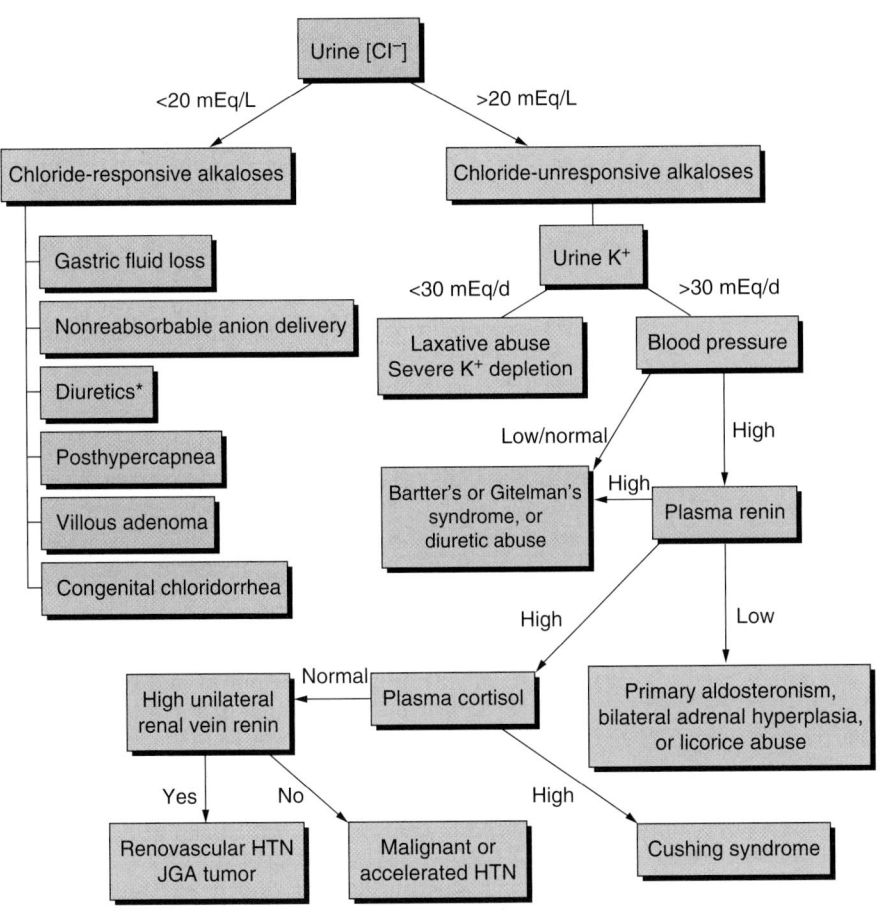

FIGURE 16-9 Diagnostic algorithm for metabolic alkalosis, based on the spot urine Cl^- and K^+ concentrations. *HTN,* Hypertension; *JGA,* juxtaglomerular apparatus.

* After diuretic therapy

sodium bicarbonate enters the distal tubule, where, under the influence of the increased level of aldosterone, K^+ and H^+ secretion is stimulated. Because of ECF contraction and hypochloremia, the kidney avidly conserves Cl^-. Consequently, in this disequilibrium state generated by active vomiting, the urine contains large quantities of Na^+, K^+, and HCO_3^- but has a low concentration of Cl^-. On cessation of vomiting, the plasma HCO_3^- concentration falls to the HCO_3^- threshold, which is markedly elevated by the continued effects of ECF contraction, hypokalemia, and hyperaldosteronism. The alkalosis is maintained at a slightly lower level than during the phase of active vomiting, and the urine is now relatively acidic with low concentrations of Na^+, HCO_3^-, and Cl^-.

Correction of the ECF contraction with sodium chloride may be sufficient to reverse these events, with restoration of normal blood pH even without repair of K^+ deficits.[11] Good clinical practice, however, dictates K^+ repletion as well.[105]

CONGENITAL CHLORIDORRHEA

Congenital chloridorrhea is a rare autosomal recessive disorder associated with severe diarrhea, fecal acid loss, and HCO_3^- retention. The pathogenesis is loss of the normal ileal HCO_3^-/Cl^- anion exchange mechanism so that Cl^- cannot be reabsorbed. The parallel Na^+/H^+ ion exchanger remains functional, which allows Na^+ to be reabsorbed and H^+ to be secreted. Subsequently, net H^+ and Cl^- exit in the stool, which causes Na^+ and HCO_3^- retention in the ECF.[11,105] Alkalosis results and is sustained by concomitant ECF contraction with hyperaldosteronism and K^+ deficiency. Therapy consists of oral supplements of sodium and potassium chloride. The use of proton pump inhibitors has been advanced as a means of reducing chloride secretion by the parietal cells and thus reducing the diarrhea.[109]

VILLOUS ADENOMA

Metabolic alkalosis has been described in cases of villous adenoma and is ascribed to high adenoma-derived K^+ secretory rates. K^+ and volume depletion likely cause the alkalosis, because colonic secretion is alkaline.

Renal Origin

DIURETICS

Drugs that induce chloruresis without bicarbonaturia, such as thiazides and loop diuretics (furosemide, bumetanide, and torsemide), acutely diminish the ECF space without altering the total body HCO_3^- content. The HCO_3^- concentration in the blood and ECF increases. The Pco_2 does not increase commensurately, and a "contraction" alkalosis results.[105] The degree of alkalosis is usually small, however, because of cellular and non-HCO_3^- ECF buffering processes.[11,105]

Administration of diuretics long term tends to generate an alkalosis by increasing distal salt delivery, so that both K^+ and H^+ secretion are stimulated. Diuretics, by blocking Cl^- reabsorption in the distal tubule or by increasing H^+ pump activity, may also stimulate distal H^+ secretion and increase net acid excretion. Maintenance of alkalosis is ensured by the persistence of ECF contraction, secondary hyperaldosteronism, K^+ deficiency, enhanced ammonium production, stimulation of H^+-K^+-ATPase, and the direct effect of the diuretic as long as diuretic administration continues. Repair of the alkalosis is achieved by providing Cl^- to normalize the ECF deficit.

EDEMATOUS STATES

In diseases associated with edema formation (CHF, nephrotic syndrome, cirrhosis), effective arterial blood volume is diminished, although total ECF is increased. Common to these diseases is diminished renal plasma flow and GFR with limited distal Na^+ delivery. Net acid excretion is usually normal, and alkalosis does not develop, even with an enhanced proximal HCO_3^- reabsorptive capacity. However, the distal H^+ secretory mechanism is primed by hyperaldosteronism to excrete excessive net acid if GFR can be increased to enhance distal Na^+ delivery or if K^+ deficiency or diuretic administration supervenes.

POSTHYPERCAPNIA

Prolonged CO_2 retention with chronic respiratory acidosis enhances renal HCO_3^- absorption and the generation of new HCO_3^- (increased net acid excretion). If the Pco_2 is returned to normal, metabolic alkalosis, caused by the persistently elevated HCO_3^- concentration, emerges. Alkalosis develops immediately if the elevated Pco_2 is abruptly returned toward normal by a change in mechanically controlled ventilation. There is a brisk bicarbonaturic response proportional to the change in Pco_2. The accompanying cation is predominantly K^+, especially if dietary potassium is not limited. Secondary hyperaldosteronism in states of chronic hypercapnia may be responsible for this pattern of response. Associated ECF contraction does not allow complete repair of the alkalosis by normalization of the Pco_2 alone. Alkalosis persists until Cl^- supplementation is provided. Enhanced proximal acidification as a result of conditioning induced by the previous hypercapnic state may also contribute to the maintenance of the posthypercapnic alkalosis.[5]

BARTTER'S SYNDROME

Both classical Bartter's syndrome and antenatal Bartter's syndrome are inherited as autosomal recessive disorders and involve impaired TAL salt absorption, which results in salt wasting, volume depletion, and activation of the renin-angiotensin system.[110] These manifestations are the result of loss-of-function mutations of one of the genes that encode three transporters involved in vectorial NaCl absorption in the TAL. The most prevalent disorder is the inheritance from both parents of mutations of the gene *NKCC2* that encodes the bumetanide-sensitive Na^+-$2Cl^-$-K^+ cotransporter on the apical membrane. Other mutations have also been described in rare families. For example, a mutation has been discovered in the gene *KCNJ1* that encodes the ATP-sensitive apical K^+ conductance channel (ROMK) that operates in parallel with the Na^+-$2Cl^-$-K^+ transporter to recycle K^+. Both defects can be associated with classical Bartter's syndrome. A third mutation of the *CLCNKb* gene encoding the voltage-gated basolateral chloride channel (ClC-Kb) is associated only with classical Bartter's syndrome and is milder and rarely associated with nephrocalcinosis. All three defects have the same net effect, loss of Cl^- transport in the TAL.[111]

Antenatal Bartter's syndrome has been observed in consanguineous families in association with sensorineural deafness, a syndrome linked to chromosome band 1p31. The responsible gene, *BSND*, encodes a subunit, barttin, that co-localizes with the ClC-Kb channel in the TAL and K-secreting epithelial cells in the inner ear. Barttin appears to be necessary for the function of the voltage-gated chloride channel. Expression of

ClC-Kb is lost when coexpressed with mutant barttins. Thus, mutations in *BSND* represent a fourth category of patients with Bartter's syndrome.[110] Such defects would predictably lead to ECF contraction, hyperreninemic hyperaldosteronism, and increased delivery of Na^+ to the distal nephron and, thus, alkalosis and renal K^+ wasting and hypokalemia. Secondary overproduction of prostaglandins, juxtaglomerular apparatus hypertrophy, and vascular pressor unresponsiveness would then ensue. Most patients have hypercalciuria and normal serum magnesium levels, which distinguishes this disorder from Gitelman's syndrome.

Bartter's syndrome is inherited as an autosomal recessive defect, and most patients studied with mutations in these genes have been homozygotes or compound heterozygotes for different mutations in one of these genes. A few patients with the clinical syndrome have no discernible mutation in any of these four genes. Plausible explanations include unrecognized mutations in other genes, a dominant-negative effect of a heterozygous mutation, or other mechanisms.

Recently, two groups of investigators have reported features of Bartter's syndrome in patients with autosomal dominant hypocalcemia and activating mutations in the calcium-sensing receptor (CaSR). Activation of the CaSR on the basolateral cell surface of the TAL inhibits the function of ROMK. Thus, mutations in CaSR may represent a fifth gene associated with Bartter's syndrome.[90]

Many of the features of Bartter's syndrome (e.g., elevated prostaglandin E_2 and kallikrein levels) that historically were considered potentially causative are now realized to be secondary to the genetic defects in TAL solute transport. Distinction from surreptitious vomiting, diuretic administration, and laxative abuse is necessary to make the diagnosis of Bartter's syndrome. The finding of a low urinary Cl^- concentration is helpful in identifying the vomiting patient. The urinary Cl^- concentration in Bartter's syndrome would be expected to be normal or increased, rather than depressed.

The treatment of Bartter's syndrome is generally focused on repair of the hypokalemia by inhibition of the renin-angiotensin-aldosterone or prostaglandin-kinin system. K^+ supplementation, Mg^{2+} repletion, and administration of propranolol, spironolactone, amiloride, prostaglandin inhibitors, or ACE inhibitors have been used with limited success.

GITELMAN'S SYNDROME

Patients with Gitelman's syndrome have a phenotype resembling that of Bartter's syndrome in that an autosomal recessive chloride-resistant metabolic alkalosis is associated with hypokalemia, a normal to low blood pressure, volume depletion with secondary hyperreninemic hyperaldosteronism, and juxtaglomerular hyperplasia.[111,112] However, hypocalciuria and symptomatic hypomagnesemia are consistently useful in distinguishing Gitelman's syndrome from Bartter's syndrome on clinical grounds.[112] These unique features mimic the effect of long-term thiazide diuretic administration. A number of missense mutations in the gene *SLC12A3*, which encodes the thiazide-sensitive sodium-chloride cotransporter in the distal convoluted tubule, have been described and account for the clinical features, including the classical finding of hypocalciuria.[113] It is not clear, however, why these patients have pronounced hypomagnesemia.

Gitelman's syndrome becomes symptomatic later in life and is associated with milder salt wasting than that occurring with Bartter's syndrome. A large study of adults with proven Gitelman's syndrome and *NCCT* mutations showed that salt craving, nocturia, cramps, and fatigue were more common than in sex- and age-matched controls.[113] Women experienced exacerbation of symptoms during menses, and many had complicated pregnancies. Salt craving seems to be a near universal feature and aggravates renal K^+ wasting.

Treatment of Gitelman's syndrome, as of Bartter's syndrome, consists of potassium supplementation (KCl 40 mEq, three or four times daily, or more), but also magnesium supplementation in most patients. Amiloride (5 to 10 mg twice daily) is more effective than spironolactone. ACE inhibitors have been suggested as helpful in selected patients but may cause symptomatic hypotension. Discouraging *excessive* dietary salt intake requires dietary counseling and may be a challenging component of management.

AFTER TREATMENT OF LACTIC ACIDOSIS OR KETOACIDOSIS

When an underlying stimulus for the generation of lactic acid or ketoacid is removed rapidly, as occurs with repair of circulatory insufficiency or with insulin administration, the lactate or ketones can be metabolized to yield an equivalent amount of HCO_3^-. Thus, the initial process of HCO_3^- titration that induced the metabolic acidosis is effectively reversed. In the oxidative metabolism of ketones or lactate, HCO_3^- is not directly produced; rather, H^+ is consumed by metabolism of the organic anions, with the liberation of an equivalent amount of HCO_3^-. This process regenerates HCO_3^- if the organic acids can be metabolized to HCO_3^- before their renal excretion. Other sources of new HCO_3^- are additive with the original amount of HCO_3^- regenerated by organic anion metabolism to create a surfeit of HCO_3^-. Such sources include (1) new HCO_3^- added to the blood by the kidneys as a result of enhanced net acid excretion during the preexisting acidotic period, and (2) alkali therapy during the treatment phase of the acidosis. The coexistence of acidosis-induced ECF contraction and K^+ deficiency acts to sustain the alkalosis.[11,105]

NONREABSORBABLE ANIONS AND MAGNESIUM ION DEFICIENCY

Administration of large amounts of nonreabsorbable anions, such as penicillin or carbenicillin, can enhance distal acidification and K^+ excretion by increasing the luminal potential difference attained or possibly by allowing Na^+ delivery to the CCT without Cl^-, which favors H^+ secretion without Cl^--dependent HCO_3^- secretion.[105] Mg^{2+} deficiency also results in hypokalemic alkalosis by enhancing distal acidification through stimulation of renin and hence aldosterone secretion.

POTASSIUM ION DEPLETION

Pure K^+ depletion causes metabolic alkalosis, although generally of only modest severity. One reason that the alkalosis is usually mild is that K^+ depletion also causes positive sodium chloride balance with or without mineralocorticoid administration. The salt retention, in turn, antagonizes the degree of alkalemia. When access to salt as well as to K^+ is restricted, more severe alkalosis develops. Activation of the renal H^+-K^+-ATPase in the collecting duct by chronic hypokalemia likely plays a role in maintenance of the alkalosis. The alkalosis is maintained in part by reduction in GFR without a change in tubule HCO_3^- transport. The pathophysiologic basis of the alkalosis has not been well defined in humans, but the alkalosis associated with severe K^+ depletion is resistant to salt administration. Repair of the K^+ deficiency is necessary to correct the alkalosis.

Extracellular Volume Expansion, Hypertension, and Hypermineralocorticoidism (see Table 16-17)

As previously discussed, mineralocorticoid administration increases net acid excretion and tends to create metabolic alkalosis. The degree of alkalosis is augmented by the simultaneous increase in K^+ excretion, which leads to K^+ deficiency and hypokalemia. Salt intake for sufficient distal Na^+ delivery is also a prerequisite for the development of both the hypokalemia and the alkalosis. Hypertension develops partly as a result of ECF expansion from salt retention. The alkalosis is not progressive and is generally mild. Volume expansion tends to antagonize the decrease in GFR and/or increase in tubule acidification induced by hypermineralocorticoidism and K^+ deficiency. Increased mineralocorticoid hormone levels may be the result of autonomous primary adrenal overproduction of mineralocorticoid or of secondary aldosterone release by primary renal overproduction of renin. In both cases, the normal feedback by ECF on net mineralocorticoid production is disrupted and volume retention results in hypertension.

HIGH RENIN LEVELS

States accompanied by inappropriately high renin levels may be associated with hyperaldosteronism and alkalosis. Renin levels are elevated because of primary elaboration of renin or, secondarily, by diminished effective circulating blood volume. Total ECF may not be diminished. Examples of high-renin hypertension include renovascular, accelerated, and malignant hypertension. Estrogens increase renin substrate and hence angiotensin II formation. Primary tumor overproduction of renin is another rare cause of hyperreninemic hyperaldosterone–induced metabolic alkalosis.[105]

LOW RENIN LEVELS

In some disorders, primary adrenal overproduction of mineralocorticoid suppresses renin elaboration. Hypertension occurs as the result of mineralocorticoid excess with volume overexpansion.

Primary Aldosteronism. Tumor involvement (adenoma or, rarely, carcinoma) or hyperplasia of the adrenal gland is associated with aldosterone overproduction. Mineralocorticoid administration or excess production (primary aldosteronism of Cushing's syndrome and adrenal cortical enzyme defects) increases net acid excretion and may result in metabolic alkalosis, which may be worsened by associated K^+ deficiency. ECF volume expansion from salt retention causes hypertension and antagonizes the reduction in GFR and/or increases tubule acidification induced by aldosterone and by K^+ deficiency. The kaliuresis persists and causes continued K^+ depletion with polydipsia, inability to concentrate the urine, and polyuria. Increased aldosterone levels may be the result of autonomous primary adrenal overproduction or of secondary aldosterone release due to renal overproduction of renin. In both situations, the normal feedback of ECF volume on net aldosterone production is disrupted, and hypertension from volume retention can result. The glucocorticoid-remediable form has an autosomal dominant inheritance pattern.

Glucocorticoid-Remediable Hyperaldosteronism. Glucocorticoid-remediable hyperaldosteronism is an autosomal dominant form of hypertension, the features of which resemble those of primary aldosteronism (hypokalemic metabolic alkalosis and volume-dependent hypertension). In this disorder, however, glucocorticoid administration corrects the hypertension as well as the excessive excretion of 18-hydroxysteroid in the urine. Dluhy and associates have demonstrated that this disorder results from unequal crossing over between two genes located in close proximity on chromosome 8.[114] This region contains the glucocorticoid-responsive promoter region of the gene encoding 11β-hydroxylase (*CYP11B1*) where it is joined to the structural portion of the *CYP11B2* gene encoding aldosterone synthase.[114] The chimeric gene produces excess amounts of aldosterone synthase, unresponsive to serum potassium or renin levels, but it is suppressed by glucocorticoid administration. Although a rare cause of primary aldosteronism, the syndrome is important to distinguish because treatment differs and it can be associated with severe hypertension, stroke, and accelerated hypertension during pregnancy.

Cushing's Disease or Syndrome. Abnormally high glucocorticoid production caused by adrenal adenoma or carcinoma or ectopic corticotropin production causes metabolic alkalosis. The alkalosis may be ascribed to coexisting mineralocorticoid (deoxycorticosterone and corticosterone) hypersecretion. Glucocorticoids also have the ability to enhance net acid secretion and NH_4^+ production by occupancy of mineralocorticoid receptors.

Liddle's Syndrome. Liddle's syndrome is associated with severe hypertension presenting in childhood, accompanied by hypokalemic metabolic alkalosis. These features resemble those of primary hyperaldosteronism, but the renin and aldosterone levels are suppressed (pseudohyperaldosteronism).[114] The defect is constitutive activation of the ENaC at the apical membrane of principal cells in the CCD. Liddle originally described patients with low renin and low aldosterone levels that did not respond to spironolactone. The defect in Liddle's syndrome is inherited as an autosomal dominant form of monogenic hypertension. This disorder has been attributed to an inherited abnormality in the gene that encodes the β- or the γ-subunit of renal ENaC. Either mutation results in deletion of the cytoplasmic tails of the β- or γ-subunit. The C termini contain PY amino acid motifs that are highly conserved, and essentially all mutations in Liddle's syndrome patients involve disruption or deletion of this motif. These PY motifs are important in regulating the number of sodium channels in the luminal membrane by binding to the WW domains of the Nedd4 (neural developmentally downregulated isoform 4)–like family of ubiquitin-protein ligases.[115] Disruption of the PY motif dramatically increases the surface localization of ENaC complex, because these channels are not internalized or degraded (Nedd4 pathway), but remain activated on the cell surface.[115] Persistent Na^+ absorption eventuates in volume expansion, hypertension, hypokalemia, and metabolic alkalosis.[114]

Miscellaneous Conditions. Ingestion of licorice, carbenoxolone, chewer's tobacco, or nasal spray can cause a typical pattern of hypermineralocorticoidism. These substances inhibit 11β-hydroxysteroid dehydrogenase (which normally metabolizes cortisol to an inactive metabolite), so that cortisol is allowed to occupy type I renal mineralocorticoid receptors, mimicking aldosterone. Genetic apparent mineralocorticoid excess resembles excessive ingestion of licorice: volume expansion, low renin level, low aldosterone level, and a salt-sensitive form of hypertension, which may include metabolic alkalosis and hypokalemia. The hypertension responds to thiazides and spironolactone but without abnormal steroid products in the urine. Licorice and carbenoxolone contain glycyrrhetinic acid, which inhibits 11β-hydroxysteroid dehydrogenase. This enzyme is responsible for converting cortisol to cortisone, an essential step in protecting the mineralocorticoid receptor from cortisol, and protects normal individuals from exhibiting apparent mineralocorticoid excess. Without the renal-specific form of this enzyme, monogenic hypertension develops.

Symptoms

Symptoms of metabolic alkalosis include changes in central and peripheral nervous system function similar to those in hypocalcemia: mental confusion, obtundation, and a predisposition to seizures, as well as paresthesias, muscular cramping, and even tetany. Aggravation of arrhythmias and hypoxemia in chronic obstructive pulmonary disease is also a problem. Related electrolyte abnormalities, including hypokalemia and hypophosphatemia, are common, and patients may show symptoms of these deficiencies.

Treatment

The maintenance of metabolic alkalosis represents a failure of the kidney to excrete bicarbonate efficiently because of chloride or potassium deficiency or continuous mineralocorticoid elaboration or both. Treatment is primarily directed at correcting the underlying stimulus for HCO_3^- generation and at restoring the ability of the kidney to excrete the excess bicarbonate. Assistance is gained in the diagnosis and treatment of metabolic alkalosis by paying attention to the urinary chloride concentration, the arterial blood pressure, and the volume status of the patient (particularly the presence or absence of orthostasis) (see Figure 16-9). Particularly helpful in the history is the presence or absence of vomiting, diuretic use, or alkali therapy. A high urine chloride level and hypertension suggest that mineralocorticoid excess is present. If primary aldosteronism is present, correction of the underlying cause (adenoma, bilateral hyperplasia, Cushing's syndrome) will reverse the alkalosis. Patients with bilateral adrenal hyperplasia may respond to spironolactone. Normotensive patients with a high urine chloride concentration may have Bartter's or Gitelman's syndrome if diuretic use or vomiting can be excluded. A low urine chloride level and relative hypotension suggests a chloride-responsive metabolic alkalosis such as vomiting or nasogastric suction. [H^+] loss by the stomach or kidneys can be mitigated by the use of proton pump inhibitors or the discontinuation of diuretics. The second aspect of treatment is to remove the factors that sustain HCO_3^- reabsorption, such as ECF volume contraction or K^+ deficiency. Although K^+ deficits should be corrected, NaCl therapy is usually sufficient to reverse the alkalosis if ECF volume contraction is present, as indicated by a low urine [Cl^-].

Patients with CHF or unexplained volume overexpansion represent special challenges in the critical care setting. Patients with a low urine chloride concentration, usually indicative of a "chloride-responsive" form of metabolic alkalosis, may not tolerate normal saline infusion. Renal HCO_3^- loss can be accelerated by administration of acetazolamide

(250 to 500 mg intravenously), a carbonic anhydrase inhibitor, if associated conditions that preclude infusion of saline (e.g., elevated pulmonary capillary wedge pressure, or evidence of CHF) are present.[105] Acetazolamide is usually very effective in patients with adequate renal function, but can exacerbate urinary K^+ losses. Dilute hydrochloric acid (0.1 normal HCl) is also effective but must be infused slowly centrally because it may cause hemolysis and is difficult to titrate. If it is used, the goal should be not to restore the pH to normal, but to reduce the pH to approximately 7.50. Patients receiving continuous renal replacement therapy in the intensive care unit typically develop metabolic alkalosis when high-bicarbonate dialysate is used or when citrate regional anticoagulation is employed. Therapy should include reduction of alkali loads via dialysis by reducing the bicarbonate concentration in the dialysate or, if citrate is being used, by infusion of 0.1 normal HCl postfiltration.

References

1. Bidani A, Tauzon DM, Heming TA. Regulation of whole body acid-base balance. In: DuBose TD, Hamm LL, eds. *Acid-base and electrolyte disorders: a companion to Brenner and Rector's the kidney*. Philadelphia: Saunders; 2002: 1-21.
2. Madias NE, Adrogue HJ. Respiratory alkalosis. In: DuBose TD, Hamm LL, eds. *Acid-base and electrolyte disorders: a companion to Brenner and Rector's the kidney*. Philadelphia: Saunders; 2002:147-164.
3. Toews GB. Respiratory acidosis. In: DuBose TD, Hamm LL, eds. *Acid-base and electrolyte disorders: a companion to Brenner and Rector's the kidney*. Philadelphia: Saunders; 2002:129-146.
4. Bidani A, DuBose Jr TD. Acid-base regulation: cellular and whole body. In: Arieff AI, DeFronzo RA, eds. *Fluid, electrolyte, and acid base disorders*. 2nd ed. New York: Churchill Livingstone; 1995:69.
5. Alpern RJ, Hamm LL. Urinary acidification. In: DuBose TD, Hamm LL, eds. *Acid-base and electrolyte disorders: a companion to Brenner and Rector's the kidney*. Philadelphia: Saunders; 2002:23-40.
6. DuBose TD, McDonald GA. Renal tubular acidosis. In: DuBose TD, Hamm LL, eds. *Acid-base and electrolyte disorders: a companion to Brenner and Rector's the kidney*. Philadelphia: Saunders; 2002:189-206.
7. Krapf R. Mechanisms of adaptation to chronic respiratory acidosis in the proximal tubule. *J Clin Invest*. 1989;83:890-896.
8. Schwartz GJ, Al-Awqati Q. Carbon dioxide causes exocytosis of vesicles containing H^+ pumps in isolated perfused proximal and collecting tubules. *J Clin Invest*. 1985;75:1638-1644.
9. Gennari FJ, Maddox DA. Renal regulation of acid-base homeostasis. integrated response. In: Seldin DW, Giebisch G, eds. *The kidney: physiology and pathophysiology*. 3rd ed. Philadelphia: Lippincott Williams & Wilkins; 2000:2015-2054.
10. Albert MS, Dell RB, Winters RW. Quantitative displacement of acid-base equilibrium in metabolic acidosis. *Ann Intern Med*. 1967;66:312.
11. Galla JH. Metabolic alkalosis. In: DuBose TD, Hamm LL, eds. *Acid-base and electrolyte disorders: a companion to Brenner and Rector's the kidney*. Philadelphia: Saunders; 2002:109-128.
12. DuBose TD. Metabolic alkalosis. In: Greenberg A, ed. *Primer on kidney diseases*. Philadelphia: Saunders; 2005:90-96.
13. DuBose Jr TD, Codina J, Burges A, et al. Regulation of H^+, K^+-ATPase expression in kidney. *Am J Physiol*. 1995;269:F500.
14. Wesson DE. Na/H exchange and H-K-ATPase increase distal tubule acidification in chronic alkalosis. *Kidney Int*. 1998;53:945-951.
15. Wesson DE, Dolson GM. Endothelin-1 increases rat distal tubule acidification in vivo. *Am J Physiol*. 1997;273:F586-F594.
16. Wesson DE. Combined K^+ and Cl^- repletion corrects augmented H^+ secretion by distal tubules in chronic alkalosis. *Am J Physiol*. 1994;266: F592-F603.
17. Guntupalli J, Onuigbo M, Wall SM, et al. Adaptation to low K^+ media increases H^+, K^+-ATPase but not H^+, K^+-ATPase-mediated pH_i recovery in $OMCD_1$ cells. *Am J Physiol*. 1997;273:C558-C571.
18. Wall SM, Mehta P, DuBose Jr TD. Dietary K^+ restriction upregulates total and Sch-28080–sensitive bicarbonate absorption in rat tIMCD. *Am J Physiol*. 1998;275:F543-F549.
19. Krapf R, Alpern RJ, Seldin DW. Clinical syndromes of metabolic acidosis. In: Seldin DW, Giebisch G, eds. *The kidney*. Philadelphia: Lippincott Williams & Wilkins; 2000:2055-2072.

20. Emmett M. Diagnosis of simple and mixed disorders. In: DuBose TD, Hamm LL, eds. *Acid–base and electrolyte disorders: a companion to Brenner and Rector's the kidney.* Philadelphia: Saunders; 2002:41-54.
21. Oh MS, Carroll HJ. The anion gap. *N Engl J Med.* 1977;297:814.
22. Feldman M, Soni N, Dickson B. Influence of hypoalbuminemia or hyperalbuminemia on the serum anion gap. *J Lab Clin Med.* 2005;146:317-320.
23. Acute Respiratory Distress Syndrome Network. Ventilation with lower tidal volumes as compared with traditional tidal volumes for acute lung injury and the acute respiratory distress syndrome. *N Engl J Med.* 2000;342:1301.
24. Slutsky AS, Tremblay LN. Multiple system organ failure. Is mechanical ventilation a contributing factor? *Am J Respir Crit Care Med.* 1998;157:1721-1725.
25. DuBose TD, Alpern RJ. Renal tubular acidosis. In: Scriver CR, Beaudet AL, Sly WS, et al. eds. *The metabolic and molecular bases of inherited disease.* 8th ed. New York: McGraw-Hill; 2001:4983-5021.
26. Wong KM, Chak WL, Cheung CY, et al. Hypokalemic metabolic acidosis attributed to cough mixture abuse. *Am J Kidney Dis.* 2001;38:390.
27. Halperin M, Kamel KS, Cherny DZI. Ketoacidosis. In: DuBose TD, Hamm LL, eds. *Acid–base and electrolyte disorders: a companion to Brenner and Rector's the kidney.* Philadelphia: Saunders; 2002:67-82.
28. Gauthier P, Simon EE, Lemann J. Acidosis of chronic renal failure. In: DuBose TD, Hamm LL, eds. *Acid–base and electrolyte disorders: a companion to Brenner and Rector's the kidney.* Philadelphia: Saunders; 2002:207-216.
29. Morris Jr RC, Nigon K, Reed EB. Evidence that the severity of depletion of inorganic phosphate determines the severity of the disturbance of adenine nucleotide metabolism in the liver and renal cortex of the fructose-loaded rat. *J Clin Invest.* 1978;61:209.
30. Sly WS, Whyte MP, Sundaram V, et al. Carbonic anhydrase II deficiency in 12 families with the autosomal recessive syndrome of osteopetrosis with renal tubular acidosis and cerebral calcification. *N Engl J Med.* 1985;313:139.
31. Morris RC. Jr: Renal tubular acidosis. Mechanisms, classification and implications. *N Engl J Med.* 1969;281:1405.
32. DuBose TD. Jr: Hydrogen ion secretion by the collecting duct as a determinant of the urine to blood Pco$_2$ gradient in alkaline urine. *J Clin Invest.* 1982;69:145.
33. DuBose Jr TD, Caflisch CR. Validation of the difference in urine and blood CO$_2$ tension during bicarbonate loading as an index of distal nephron acidification in experimental models of distal renal tubular acidosis. *J Clin Invest.* 1985;75:1116.
34. Batlle DC. Segmental characterization of defects in collecting tubule acidification. *Kidney Int.* 1986;30:546-554.
35. Bruce LJ, Cope DL, Jones GK, et al. Familial distal renal tubular acidosis is associated with mutations in red cell anion exchanger (Band 3, *AE1*) gene. *J Clin Invest.* 1997;100:1693.
36. Alper SL. Genetic diseases of acid-base transporters. *Annu Rev Physiol.* 2002;64:899.
37. Karet FE, Gainza FJ, Gyory AZ, et al. Mutations in the chloride-bicarbonate exchanger gene AE1 cause autosomal dominant but not autosomal recessive distal renal tubular acidosis. *Proc Natl Acad Sci U S A.* 1998;95:6337.
38. Jarolim P, Shayakul C, Prabakaran D, et al. Autosomal dominant distal renal tubular acidosis is associated in three families with heterozygosity for the R589H mutation in the AE1 (band 3) Cl–/HCO$_3$– exchanger. *J Biol Chem.* 1998;273:6380.
39. DuBose TD. Autosomal dominant distal renal tubular acidosis and the *AE1* gene. *Am J Kidney Dis.* 1999;33:1191-1197.
40. Alper SL. Molecular physiology of SLC4 anion exchangers. *Exp Physiol.* 2006;91:153-161.
41. Karet FE, Finberg KE, Nelson RD, et al. Mutations in the gene encoding B1 subunit of H$^+$-ATPase cause renal tubular acidosis with sensorineural deafness. *Nat Genet.* 1999;21:84.
42. Karet FE, Finberg KE, Nayir A, et al. Localization of a gene for autosomal recessive distal renal tubular acidosis with normal hearing (rdRTA2) to 7q33-34. *Am J Hum Genet.* 1999;65:1656.
43. Smith AN, Finberg KE, Wagner CA, et al. Molecular cloning and characterization of Atp6n1b. *J Biol Chem.* 2001;276:42382.
44. Smith AN, Skaug J, Choate KA, et al. Mutations in Atp6n1b, encoding a new kidney vacuolar proton pump 116-kD subunit, cause recessive distal renal tubular acidosis with preserved hearing. *Nat Genet.* 2000;26:71.
45. Kaitwatcharachai C, Vasuvattakul S, Yenchitsomanus P, et al. Distal renal tubular acidosis and high urine carbon dioxide tension in a patient with Southeast Asian ovalocytosis. *Am J Kidney Dis.* 1999;33:1147-1152.
46. DuBose Jr TD, Lucci MS, Hogg RJ, et al. Comparison of acidification parameters in superficial and deep nephrons of the rat. *Am J Physiol.* 1983;244:F497.
47. Bonilla-Felix M. Primary distal renal tubular acidosis as a result of a gradient defect. *Am J Kidney Dis.* 1996;27:428.
48. DuBose Jr TD, Good DW. Role of the thick ascending limb and inner medullary collecting duct in the regulation of urinary acidification. *Semin Nephrol.* 1991;11:120.
49. DuBose Jr TD, Good DW, Hamm LL, et al. Ammonium transport in the kidney: new physiologic concepts and their clinical implications. *J Am Soc Nephrol.* 1991;1:1193.
50. Laing CM, Toye AM, Capasso G, et al. Renal tubular acidosis: developments in our understanding of the molecular basis. *Int J Biochem Cell Biol.* 2005;37:1151-1161.
51. Pessler F, Emery H, Dai L, et al. The spectrum of renal tubular acidosis in paediatric Sjögren syndrome. *Rheumatology.* 2006;45:85-91.
52. Morris Jr RC, Sebastian A. Alkali therapy in renal tubular acidosis: who needs it? *J Am Soc Nephrol.* 2002;13:2186-2188.
53. Wrong O, Henderson JE, Kaye M. Distal renal tubular acidosis: alkali heals osteomalacia and increases net production of 1,25-dihydroxyvitamin D. *Nephron Physiol.* 2005;101:72-76.
54. DuBose Jr TD, Good DW. Effects of chronic chloride depletion metabolic alkalosis on proximal tubule transport and renal production of ammonium. *Am J Physiol.* 1995;269:F508.
55. DuBose Jr TD, Good DW. Chronic hyperkalemia impairs ammonium transport and accumulation in the inner medulla of the rat. *J Clin Invest.* 1992;90:1443.
56. Good DW. Ammonium transport by the thick ascending limb of Henle's loop. *Annu Rev Physiol.* 1994;56:623.
57. Watts BA, Good DW. Effects of ammonium on intracellular pH in rat medullary thick ascending limb: mechanisms of apical membrane NH$_4^+$ transport. *J Gen Physiol.* 1994;103:917.
58. DuBose Jr TD, Caflisch CR. Effect of selective aldosterone deficiency on acidification in nephron segments of the rat inner medulla. *J Clin Invest.* 1988;82:1624.
59. Antonipillai I, Wang Y, Horton R. Tumor necrosis factor and interleukin-1 may regulate renin secretion. *Endocrinology.* 1990;126:273.
60. Geller DS, Rodriguez-Soriano J, Valla Boado A, et al. Mutations in the mineralocorticoid receptor gene cause autosomal dominant pseudohypoaldosteronism type 1. *Nat Genet.* 1998;19:279.
61. Chang SS, Grunder S, Hanukoglu A, et al. Mutations in subunits of the epithelial sodium channel cause salt wasting with hyperkalemic acidosis, pseudohypoaldosteronism type 1. *Nat Genet.* 1996;12:248.
62. Grunder S, Firsou D, Chang SS, et al. A mutation causing pseudohypoaldosteronism type 1 identifies a conserved glycine that is involved in the gating of the epithelial sodium channel. *EMBO J.* 1997;16:899.
63. Viemann M, Peter M, Lopez-Siguero JP, et al. Evidence for genetic heterogeneity of pseudohypoaldosteronism type 1: identification of a novel mutation in the human mineralocorticoid receptor in one sporadic case and no mutations in two autosomal dominant kindreds. *J Clin Endocrinol Metab.* 2001;86:2056.
64. Adachi M, Tachibana K, Asakura Y, et al. Compound heterozygous mutations in the gamma subunit gene of ENaC (1627delG and 1570-1G→A) in one sporadic Japanese patient with a systemic form of pseudohypoaldosteronism type 1. *J Clin Endocrinol Metab.* 2001;86:9.
65. Thomas CP, Zhou J, Liu KZ, et al. Systemic pseudohypoaldosteronism from deletion of the promoter region of the human beta epithelial Na$^+$ channel subunit. *Am J Respir Cell Mol Biol.* 2002;27:314-319.
66. Barker PM, Nguyen MS, Gatzy JT, et al. Role of gamma ENaC subunit in lung liquid clearance and electrolyte balance in newborn mice: insights into perinatal adaptation and pseudohypoaldosteronism. *J Clin Invest.* 1998;102:1634.
67. Achard JM, Disse-Nicodem S, Fiquet-Kempf B, et al. Phenotypic and genetic heterogeneity of familial hyperkalaemic hypertension (Gordon syndrome). *Clin Exp Pharmacol Physiol.* 2001;28:1048.
68. Wilson FH, Disse-Nicodeme S, Choate KA, et al. Human hypertension caused by mutations in WNK kinases. *Science.* 2001;293:1107-1112.
69. Wilson FH, Kahle KT, Sabath E, et al. Molecular pathogenesis of inherited hypertension with hyperkalemia: the Na-Cl cotransporter is inhibited by wild-type but not mutant WNK4. *Proc Natl Acad Sci U S A.* 2003;100:680-684.
70. Kahle KT, Macgregor GG, Wilson FH, et al. Paracellular Cl$^-$ permeability is regulated by WNK4 kinase: insight into normal physiology and hypertension. *Proc Natl Acad Sci U S A.* 2004;101:14877-14882.
71. Kahle KT, Wilson FH, Leng Q, et al. WNK4 regulates the balance between renal NaCl reabsorption and K$^+$ secretion. *Nat Genet.* 2003;35:372-376.
72. Braden GL, O'Shea MH, Mulhern JG, et al. Acute renal failure and hyperkalaemia associated with cyclooxygenase-2 inhibitors. *Nephrol Dial Transplant.* 2004;19:1149-1153.
73. Caliskan Y, Kalayoglu-Besisik S, Sargin D, et al. Cyclosporine-associated hyperkalemia: report of four allogeneic blood stem-cell transplant cases. *Transplantation.* 2003;75:1069-1072.
74. Caramelo C, Bello E, Ruiz E, et al. Hyperkalemia in patients infected with the human immunodeficiency virus: involvement of a systemic mechanism. *Kidney Int.* 1999;56:198-205.

75. Schlanger LE, Kleyman TR, Ling BN. K$^+$-Sparing diuretic actions of trimethoprim: inhibition of Na$^+$ channels in A6 distal nephron cells. *Kidney Int.* 1994;45:1070-1076.
76. Kleyman TR, Roberts C, Ling BN. A mechanism for pentamidine-induced hyperkalemia: inhibition of distal nephron sodium transport. *Ann Intern Med.* 1995;122:103-106.
77. Valázquez H, Perazella MN, Wright FS, et al. Renal mechanisms of trimethoprim-induced hyperkalemia. *Ann Intern Med.* 1993;119:296-301.
78. Sands JM, McMahon SJ, Tumlin JA. Evidence that the inhibition of Na$^+$/K$^+$-ATPase activity by FK506 involves calcineurin. *Kidney Int.* 1994;46:647-652.
79. Kraut JA, Kurtz I. Metabolic acidosis of CKD: diagnosis, clinical characteristics, and treatment. *Am J Kidney Dis.* 2005;45:978-993.
80. Qunibi WY, Hootkins RE, McDowell LL, et al. Treatment of hyperphosphatemia in hemodialysis patients: the Calcium Acetate Renagel Evaluation (CARE Study). *Kidney Int.* 2004;65:1914-1926.
81. Sonikan MA, Pani IT, Iliopoulos AN, et al. Metabolic acidosis aggravation and hyperkalemia in hemodialysis patients treated by sevelamer hydrochloride. *Ren Fail.* 2005;27:143-147.
82. Wrong O, Harland C. Sevelamer-induced acidosis. *Kidney Int.* 2005;67:776-777.
83. Laski ME, Wesson DE. Lactic acidosis. In: DuBose TD, Hamm LL, eds. *Acid-base and electrolyte disorders: a companion to Brenner and Rector's the kidney.* Philadelphia: Saunders; 2002:68-83.
84. John M, Mallal S. Hyperlactatemia syndromes in people with HIV infection. *Curr Opin Infect Dis.* 2002;15:23.
85. Cote HC, Brumme ZL, Craig KJ, et al. Changes in mitochondrial DNA as a marker of nucleoside toxicity in HIV-infected patients. *N Engl J Med.* 2002;346:811.
86. Lalau JD, Race JM. Lactic acidosis in metformin therapy. *Drugs.* 1999;1:55.
87. Calabrese AT, Coley KC, DaPos SV, et al. Evaluation of prescribing practices: risk of lactic acidosis with metformin therapy. *Arch Intern Med.* 2002;162:434-437.
88. Romanski SA, McMahon MM. Metabolic acidosis and thiamine deficiency. *Mayo Clin Proc.* 1999;74:259-263.
89. Luft FC. Lactic acidosis update for critical care clinicians. *J Am Soc Nephrol.* 2001;12:S15.
90. Gerard Y, Maulin L, Yazdanpanah T, et al. Symptomatic hyperlactataemia: an emerging complication of antiretroviral therapy. *AIDS.* 2000;14:2723-2730.
91. Wilson KC, Reardon C, Farber HW. Propylene glycol toxicity in a patient receiving intravenous diazepam. *N Engl J Med.* 2000;343:815.
92. Arroliga AC, Shehab N, McCarthy K, et al. Relationship of continuous infusion lorazepam to serum propylene glycol concentration in critically ill adults. *Crit Care Med.* 2004;32:1709-1714.
93. Stacpoole PW, Wright EC, Baumgartner TG, et al. A controlled clinical trial of dichloroacetate for treatment of lactic acidosis in adults. The Dichloroacetate-Lactic Acidosis Study Group. *N Engl J Med.* 1992;327:1564.
94. Bjerneroth G. Alkaline buffers for correction of metabolic acidosis during cardiopulmonary resuscitation with focus on Tribonat—a review. *Resuscitation.* 1998;37:161-171.
95. Uchida H, Yamamoto H, Kisaki Y, et al. D-Lactic acidosis in short-bowel syndrome managed with antibiotics and probiotics. *J Pediatr Surg.* 2004;39:634-636.
96. Jorens PG, Demey HE, Schepens PJ, et al. Unusual d-lactic acid acidosis from propylene glycol metabolism in overdose. *J Toxicol Clin Toxicol.* 2004;42:163-169.
97. Lalive PH, Hadengue A, Mensi N, et al. [Recurrent encephalopathy after small bowel resection. Implication of d-lactate]. *Rev Neurol (Paris).* 2001;157:679.
98. Whitney GM, Szerlip HM. Acid-base disorders in the critical care setting. In: DuBose TD, Hamm LL, eds. *Acid-base and electrolyte disorders: a companion to Brenner and Rector's the kidney.* Philadelphia: Saunders; 2002:165-187.
99. Umpierrez GE, DiGirolamo M, Tuvlin JA, et al. Differences in metabolic and hormonal milieu in diabetic- and alcohol-induced ketoacidosis. *J Crit Care.* 2000;15:52.
100. Proudfoot AT, Krenzelok EP, Brent J, et al. Does urine alkalinization increase salicylate elimination? If so, why? *Toxicol Rev.* 2003;22:129-136.
101. Brent J. Fomepizole for ethylene glycol and methanol poisoning. *N Engl J Med.* 2009;360:2216-2223.
102. Fraser AD. Clinical toxicologic implications of ethylene glycol and glycolic acid poisoning. *Ther Drug Monit.* 2002;24:232-238.
103. Velez LI, Shepherd G, Lee YC, et al. Ethylene glycol ingestion treated only with fomepizole. *J Med Toxicol.* 2007;3:125-138.
104. Mizock BA, Belyaev S, Mecher C. Unexplained metabolic acidosis in critically ill patients: the role of pyroglutamic acid. *Intensive Care Med.* 2004;30:502-505.
105. DuBose TD. Metabolic alkalosis. In: Greenberg A, ed. *Primer on kidney diseases.* Philadelphia: Saunders; 2005:90-96.
106. Zar T, Yusufzai I, Sullivan A, et al. Acute kidney injury, hyperosmolality, and metabolic acidosis associated with lorazepam. *Nat Clin Pract Nephrol.* 2007;3:515-520.
107. Gupta M, Wadhwa NK, Bukovsky R. Regional citrate anticoagulation for continuous venovenous hemodiafiltration using calcium-containing dialysate. *Am J Kidney Dis.* 2004;43:67-73.
108. Meier-Kriesche H, Gitomer J, Finkel K, et al. Increased total to ionized calcium ratio during continuous venovenous hemodialysis with regional citrate anticoagulation. *Crit Care Med.* 2001;29:748-752.
109. Aichbichler BW, Zerr CH, Santa Ana CA, et al. Proton-pump inhibition of gastric chloride secretion in congenital chloridorrhea. *N Engl J Med.* 1997;336:106.
110. Simon DB, Karet FE, Rodriguez-Soriano J, et al. Genetic heterogeneity of Bartter's syndrome revealed by mutations in the K$^+$ channel, ROMK. *Nat Genet.* 1996;14:152-156.
111. Herbert SC, Gullans SR. The molecular basis of inherited hypokalemic alkalosis: Bartter's and Gitelman's syndromes. *Am J Physiol Renal Physiol.* 1996;271:F957-F959.
112. Shaer AJ. Inherited primary renal tubular hypokalemic alkalosis: a review of Gitelman and Bartter syndromes. *Am J Med Sci.* 2001;322:316-332.
113. Monkawa T, Kurihara I, Kobayashi K, et al. Novel mutations in thiazide-sensitive Na-Cl cotransporter gene of patients with Gitelman's syndrome. *J Am Soc Nephrol.* 2000;11:65.
114. Dluhy RG, Anderson B, Harlin B. Glucocorticoid-remediable aldosteronism is associated with hypertension in early childhood. *J Pediatr.* 2001;138:715.
115. Kamynina E, Staub O. Concerted action of ENaC, Nedd4-2, and Sgkl in transepithelial Na$^+$ transport. *Am J Physiol Renal Physiol.* 2002;283:F377.

Disorders of Potassium Balance

David B. Mount and Kambiz Zandi-Nejad

The diagnosis and management of potassium disorders are central skills in clinical nephrology, relevant not only to consultative nephrology but also to dialysis and renal transplantation. An understanding of the underlying physiology is critical to the diagnostic and management approach to hyperkalemia and hypokalemia. This chapter reviews those aspects of the physiology of potassium homeostasis judged to be relevant to the understanding of potassium disorders; a more detailed review of renal potassium transport is provided in Chapter 5.

Knowledge of the pathophysiology of potassium disorders continue to evolve. The expanding list of drugs with a potential to affect plasma potassium concentration (K^+) has both complicated clinical management and provided new insight. The evolving molecular understanding of rare disorders affecting plasma K^+ has also uncovered novel pathways of regulation.[1-4] Although none of these disorders constitutes a "public health menace"[5] they are experiments of nature that have provided new windows on critical aspects of potassium homeostasis. Finally, the increasing availability of knockout and transgenic mice with precisely defined genetic modifications has provided the unprecedented opportunity to extend the relevant molecular physiology to whole-animal studies. These advances can be incorporated into an increasingly mechanistic, molecular understanding of potassium disorders.

Normal Potassium Balance

The dietary intake of potassium ranges from less than 35 to more than 110 mmol/day in U.S. men and women. Despite this widespread variation in intake, homeostatic mechanisms serve to precisely maintain plasma K^+ between 3.5 and 5.0 mmol/L. In a healthy individual at steady state, the entire daily intake of potassium is excreted, approximately 90% in the urine and 10% in the stool.

More than 98% of total body potassium is intracellular, chiefly in muscle (Figure 17-1). Buffering of extracellular K^+ by this large intracellular pool plays a crucial role in the regulation of plasma K^+.[6] Thus within 60 minutes of an intravenous load of 0.5 mmol/kg of K^+-Cl^- only 41% appears in the urine, yet plasma K^+ rises by no more than 0.6 mmol/L[7]; adding the equivalent 35 mmol exclusively to the extracellular space of a 70-kg human would be expected to raise plasma K^+ by approximately 2.5 mmol/L.[8] Changes in cellular distribution also serve to defend plasma K^+ during K^+ depletion. For example, military recruits have been shown to maintain a normal plasma K^+ after 11 days of basic training, despite a profound K^+ deficit generated by renal and extrarenal loss.[9] The rapid exchange of intracellular K^+ with extracellular K^+ plays a crucial role in maintaining plasma K^+ within such a

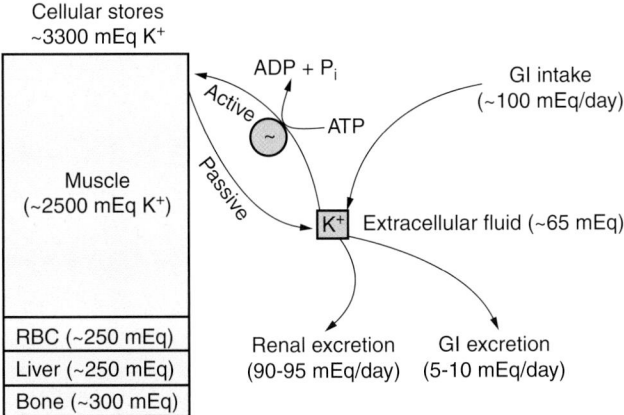

FIGURE 17-1 Body K+ distribution and cellular K+ flux. (From Wingo CS, Weiner ID: Disorders of potassium balance, in Brenner BM [editor]: *Brenner and Rector's the kidney,* ed 6, Philadelphia, 2000, Saunders, pp 998-1035.)

narrow range; this is accomplished by overlapping and synergistic[10] regulation of a number of renal and extrarenal transport pathways.

Potassium Transport Mechanisms

The intracellular accumulation of K+ against its electrochemical gradient is an energy-consuming process, mediated by the ubiquitous Na+–K+–adenosine triphosphatase (Na+-K+-ATPase) enzyme. Na+-K+-ATPase functions as an electrogenic pump, since the stoichiometry of transport is three intracellular Na+ ions to two extracellular K+ ions. The enzyme complex is made up of a tissue-specific combination of multiple α-, β-, and γ-subunits, which are further subject to tissue-specific patterns of regulation.[11] The Na+-K+-ATPase proteins share significant homology with the corresponding subunits of the H+-K+-ATPase enzymes (see "Potassium Transport in the Distal Nephron" section).

Cardiac glycosides—that is, digoxin and ouabain—bind to the α-subunits of Na+-K+-ATPase at an exposed extracellular hairpin loop that also contains the major binding sites for extracellular K+.[12] The binding of digoxin and K+ to the Na+-K+-ATPase complex is thus mutually antagonistic. This explains, in part, the potentiation of digoxin toxicity by hypokalemia.[13] Although the four α-subunits have equivalent affinity for ouabain, they differ significantly in intrinsic K+-ouabain antagonism.[14] Ouabain binding to isozymes containing the ubiquitous α1-subunit is relatively insensitive to K+ concentrations within the physiologic range, so that this isozyme is protected from digoxin under conditions in which cardiac α2- and α3-subunits, the probable therapeutic targets,[15] are inhibited.[14] Genetic reduction in cardiac α1 content has a negative ionotropic effect,[15] so that the relative resistance of this subunit to digoxin at physiologic plasma K+ concentrations has an additional cardioprotective effect.

Notably, the digoxin-ouabain binding site of α-subunits is highly conserved, which suggests a potential role in the physiologic response to endogenous ouabain- and digoxin-like compounds. Novel knock-in mice have been generated that express α2-subunits with engineered resistance to ouabain. These mice are strikingly resistant to ouabain-induced hypertension and to adrenocorticotropic hormone (ACTH)–dependent hypertension,[16] the latter of which is known to involve an increase in circulating ouabain-like glycosides. These provocative data lend new credence to the controversial role of such ouabain-like molecules in hypertension and cardiovascular disease. Furthermore, modulation of the K+-dependent binding of circulating ouabain-like compounds to Na+-K+-ATPase may underlie at least some of cardiovascular complications of hypokalemia[17] (see "Consequences of Hypokalemia" section).

Skeletal muscle contains as much as 75% of body potassium (see Figure 17-1) and exerts considerable influence on extracellular K+ concentration. Exercise is thus a well-described cause of transient hyperkalemia. Interstitial K+ in human muscle can reach levels as high as 10 mmol/L after fatiguing exercise.[18] Not surprisingly, therefore, changes in skeletal muscle Na+-K+-ATPase activity and abundance are major determinants of the capacity for extrarenal K+ homeostasis. Hypokalemia induces a marked decrease in muscle K+ content and Na+-K+-ATPase activity,[19] an "altruistic"[6] mechanism to regulate plasma K+ concentration. This is primarily due to dramatic decreases in the protein abundance of the α2-subunit of Na+-K+-ATPase.[20] In contrast, hyperkalemia due to potassium loading is associated with adaptive *increases* in muscle K+ content and Na+-K+-ATPase activity.[21]

These interactions are reflected in the relationship between physical activity and the ability to regulate extracellular K+ during exercise.[22] For example, exercise training is associated with increases in muscle Na+-K+-ATPase concentration and activity, with reduced interstitial K+ in trained muscles[23] and an enhanced recovery of plasma K+ after defined amounts of exercise.[22] Potassium can also accumulate in cells by coupling to the gradient for Na+ entry, entering via the electroneutral Na+-K+-2Cl− cotransporters NKCC1 and NKCC2. The NKCC2 protein is found only at the apical membrane of thick ascending limb (TAL) and macula densa cells (Figure 17-2 and Figure 17-10), where it functions in transepithelial salt transport and tubular regulation of renin release,[24] respectively. In contrast, NKCC1 is widely expressed in multiple tissues,[24] including muscle.[25] The cotransport of K+-Cl− by the four K+-Cl− cotransporters (KCC1 to KCC4) can also function in the transfer of K+ across membranes. Although the KCCs typically function as efflux pathways, they can mediate influx when extracellular K+ increases.[24]

The efflux of K+ out of cells is largely accomplished by K+ channels, which comprise the largest family of ion channels in the human genome. There are three major subclasses of mammalian K+ channels: the six–transmembrane domain (TMD) family, which encompasses both the voltage-sensitive and Ca2+-activated K+ channels; the two-pore, four-TMD family; and the two-TMD family of inwardly rectifying K+ (Kir) channels.[26]

There is tremendous genomic variety in human K+ channels, with 26 separate genes encoding principal subunits of the voltage-gated Kv channels and 16 genes encoding the principal Kir subunits. Further complexity is generated by the presence of multiple accessory subunits and alternative patterns of messenger RNA splicing. Not surprisingly, an increasing number and variety of K+ channels have been implicated in the control of K+ homeostasis and the membrane potential of excitable cells such as muscle and heart cells, and understanding of their important roles in the pathophysiology of potassium disorders continues to evolve.[27,28]

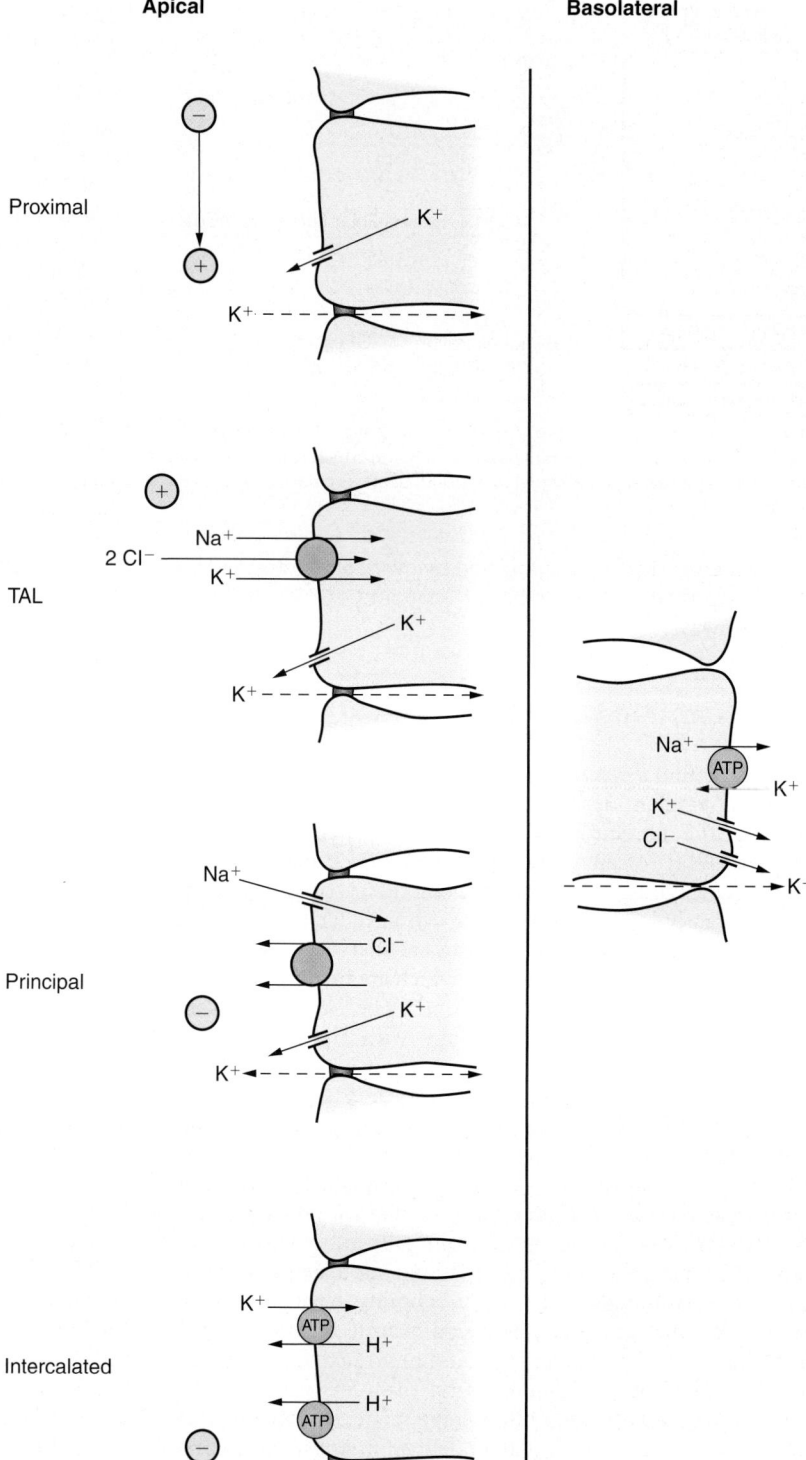

FIGURE 17-2 Schematic cell models of potassium transport along the nephron. Cell types are as specified. Note the differences in luminal potential difference along the nephron. TAL, Thick ascending limb. (From Giebisch G: Renal potassium transport: mechanisms and regulation, *Am J Physiol* 274:F817-F833, 1998.)

Factors Affecting Internal Distribution of Potassium

A number of hormones and physiologic conditions have acute effects on the distribution of K^+ between the intracellular and extracellular space (Table 17-1). Some of these factors are of particular clinical relevance and are therefore reviewed in detail.

Insulin

The hypokalemic effect of insulin has been known since the early twentieth century.[29] The impact of insulin on plasma K^+ and plasma glucose concentrations is separable at multiple levels, which suggests independent mechanisms.[19,30] Notably, the hypokalemic effect of insulin is not kidney dependent.[31] Insulin and K^+ appear to form a feedback loop of sorts, in that

TABLE 17-1 Factors Affecting Distribution of Potassium between Intracellular and Extracellular Compartments

ACUTE	
FACTOR	**EFFECT ON POTASSIUM**
Insulin	Enhanced cell uptake
β-Catecholamines	Enhanced cell uptake
α-Catecholamines	Impaired cell uptake
Acidosis	Impaired cell uptake
Alkalosis	Enhanced cell uptake
External potassium balance	Loose correlation
Cell damage	Impaired cell uptake
Hyperosmolality	Enhanced cell efflux
CHRONIC	
FACTOR	**EFFECT ON ATP PUMP DENSITY**
Thyroid	Enhanced
Adrenal steroids	Enhanced
Exercise(training)	Enhanced
Growth	Enhanced
Diabetes	Impaired
Potassium deficiency	Impaired
Chrome renal failure	Impaired

ATP, Adenosine triphosphate.

From Giebisch G: Renal potassium transport: mechanisms and regulation, *Am J Physiol* 274:F817-F833, 1998.

TABLE 17-2 Sustained Effects of β- and α-Adrenergic Agonists and Antagonists on Serum Potassium Concentration

CATECHOLAMINE SPECIFICITY	SUSTAINED EFFECT ON SERUM K^+
β_1- + β_2-Agonist (epinephrine, isoproterenol)	Decreased
Pure β_1-agonist (ITP)	None
Pure β_2-agonist (salbutamol, soterenol, terbutaline)	Decreased
β_1- + β_2-Antagonist (propranolol, sotalol)	Increased; blocks the effect of β-agonists
β_1-Antagonist (practolol, metoprolol, atenolol)	None; does not block effect of β-agonists
β_2-Antagonist (butoxamine, H 35/25)	Blocks hypokalemic effect of β-agonists
α-Agonist (phenylephrine)	Increased
α-Antagonist (phenoxybenzamine)	None; blocks effect of α-agonists

Results refer to the late (after 5 min) sustained effect.

ITP, Isopropylamino-3-(2-thiazoloxy)-2-propanol.

From Giebisch G: Renal potassium transport: mechanisms and regulation, *Am J Physiol* 274:F817-F833, 1998.

increases in plasma K^+ have a marked stimulatory effect on insulin levels.[19,32] Insulin-stimulated K^+ uptake, measured in rats using a K^+ clamp technique, is rapidly reduced by 2 days of K^+ depletion, prior to a modest drop in plasma K^+ concentration[33]; however, *no* change in plasma K^+ concentration was seen in rats subjected to a lesser K^+ restriction for 14 days.[10] Insulin-mediated K^+ uptake is thus modulated by the factors that serve to preserve plasma K^+ in the setting of K^+ deprivation (see also "Potassium Intake" section).

Inhibition of basal insulin secretion in normal subjects by somatostatin infusion increases plasma K^+ concentration by up to 0.5 mmol/L in the absence of a change in urinary excretion, which emphasizes the crucial role of circulating insulin in the regulation of plasma K^+.[34] Clinically, inhibition of insulin secretion by the somatostatin agonist octreotide can cause significant hyperkalemia in both anephric patients[35] and patients with normal renal function.[36]

Insulin stimulates the uptake of K^+ by several tissues, most prominently liver, skeletal muscle, cardiac muscle, and fat.[19,37] It does so by activating several K^+ transport pathways, with particularly well-documented effects on Na^+-K^+-ATPase.[38] Insulin activates Na^+/H^+ exchange and/or Na^+-K^+-$2Cl^-$ cotransport in several tissues. Although the ensuing increase in intracellular Na^+ was postulated to have a secondary activating effect on Na^+-K^+-ATPase,[26] it is clear that this is not the primary mechanism in most cell types.[39] Insulin induces translocation of the Na^+-K^+-ATPase α_2-subunit to the plasma membrane of skeletal muscle cells, with a lesser effect on the α_1-subunit.[40] This translocation is dependent on the activity of phosphoinositide-3-kinase (PI3K),[40] which itself also binds

to a proline-rich motif in the N terminus of the α-subunit.[41] The activation of PI3K by insulin thus induces phosphatase enzymes to dephosphorylate a specific serine residue adjacent to the PI3K binding domain. Trafficking of Na^+-K^+-ATPase to the cell surface also appears to require the phosphorylation of an adjacent tyrosine residue, perhaps catalyzed by the tyrosine kinase activity of the insulin receptor itself.[42] Finally, serum- and glucocorticoid-regulated kinase 1 (SGK1) plays a critical role in insulin-stimulated K^+ uptake, presumably via the known stimulatory effects of this kinase on Na^+-K^+-ATPase activity and/or Na^+-K^+-$2Cl^-$ cotransport.[43] The hypokalemic effect of insulin plus glucose is blunted in SGK1 knockout mice, with a marked reduction in hepatic insulin-stimulated K^+ uptake.[43]

Sympathetic Nervous System

The sympathetic nervous system plays a prominent role in regulating the balance between extracellular and intracellular K^+. Again, as is the case for insulin, the effect of catecholamines on plasma K^+ has been known for some time[44]; however, a complicating issue is the differential effect of stimulating α- and β-adrenergic receptors (Table 17-2). Uptake of K^+ by liver and muscle, with resultant hypokalemia, is stimulated via β_2-receptors.[26] The hypokalemic effect of catecholamines appears to be largely independent of changes in circulating insulin[26] and has been reported in nephrectomized animals.[45]

The cellular mechanisms whereby catecholamines induce K^+ uptake in muscle include an activation of Na^+-K^+-ATPase,[46] likely via increases in cyclic adenosine monophosphate (cAMP).[47] However, β-adrenergic receptors in skeletal muscle also activate the inwardly directed Na^+-K^+-$2Cl^-$ cotransporter NKCC1, which may account for as much as one third of the uptake response to catecholamines.[19,25] In contrast to β-adrenergic stimulation, α-adrenergic agonists impair the ability to buffer increases in K^+ induced by intravenous loading or by exercise[48]; the cellular mechanisms through which this occurs are not known. It is thought that β-adrenergic stimulation increases K[+] uptake during exercise to avoid hyperkalemia, whereas α-adrenergic mechanisms help blunt the ensuing postexercise nadir.[48] The clinical consequences of the sympathetic control of extrarenal K[+] homeostasis are reviewed elsewhere in this chapter.

Acid-Base Status

The association between changes in pH and plasma K[+] was observed some time ago.[49] It has long been held that acute disturbances in acid-base equilibrium result in changes in plasma K[+], so that alkalemia shifts K[+] into cells whereas acidemia is associated with K[+] release.[50,51] It is thought that this effective K[+]/H[+] exchange serves to help maintain extracellular pH. Rather limited data exist for the durable concept that a change of 0.1 unit in plasma pH results in 0.6 mmol/L change in plasma K[+] in the opposite direction.[52]

Despite the complexities of changes in K[+] homeostasis associated with various acid-base disorders, a few general observations can be made. The induction of metabolic acidosis by the infusion of mineral acids (NH_4^+-Cl^- or H^+-Cl^-) consistently increases plasma K[+],[50-54] whereas organic acidosis generally fails to increase plasma K[+].[51,53,55,56] Notably, a more recent report failed to detect an increase in plasma K[+] in normal human subjects with acute acidosis secondary to duodenal NH_4^+-Cl^- infusion, in which a modest acidosis was accompanied by an increase in circulating insulin.[57] However, as noted by Adrogué and Madias,[58] the concomitant infusion of 350 mL of 5% dextrose in water in these fasting subjects may have served to increase circulating insulin, which thus blunted the potential hyperkalemic response to NH_4^+-Cl^-.

Clinically, use of the oral phosphate binder sevelamer hydrochloride in patients with end-stage renal disease (ESRD) is associated with acidosis, due to effective gastrointestinal absorption of H^+-Cl^-. In hemodialysis patients this acidosis has been associated with an increase in plasma K[+], which is ameliorated by an increase in dialysis bicarbonate concentration.[59] Of note, hyperkalemia is not an expected complication of administration of sevelamer carbonate, which has recently supplanted sevelamer hydrochloride as a phosphate binder.

Metabolic alkalosis induced by sodium bicarbonate infusion usually results in a modest reduction in plasma K[+].[50-52,54,60] Respiratory alkalosis reduces plasma K[+] by a magnitude comparable to that of metabolic alkalosis.[50-52,61] Finally, acute respiratory acidosis increases plasma K[+]; the absolute increase is smaller than that induced by metabolic acidosis secondary to inorganic acids.[50-52] Again, however, some studies have failed to show a change in plasma K[+] following acute respiratory acidosis.[51,62]

Renal Potassium Excretion

Potassium Transport in the Distal Nephron

The proximal tubule and loop of Henle mediate the bulk of potassium reabsorption, so that a considerable fraction of filtered potassium is reabsorbed prior to entry into the superficial distal tubules.[63] Renal potassium excretion is primarily determined by regulated secretion in the distal nephron, specifically

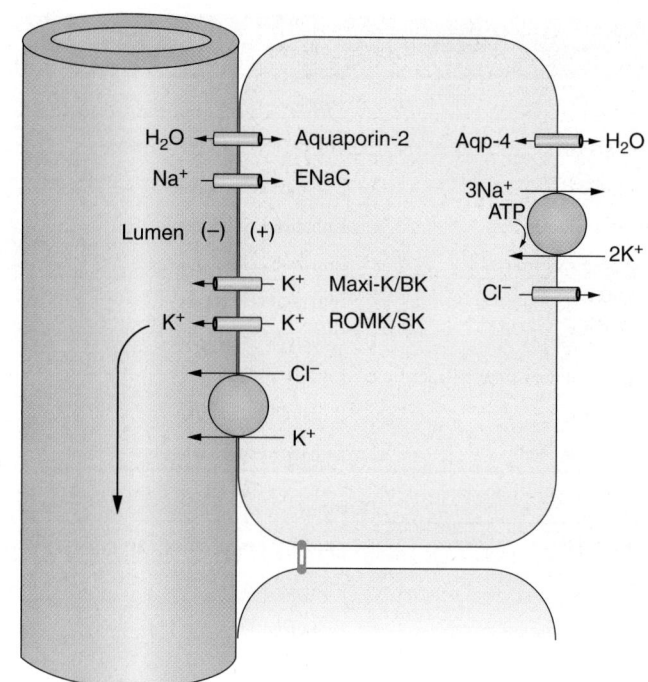

FIGURE 17-3 K[+]-secretory pathways in principal cells of the connecting segment (CNT) and cortical collecting duct (CCD). The absorption of Na[+] via the amiloride-sensitive epithelial sodium channel (ENaC) generates a lumen-negative potential difference, which drives K[+] excretion through the apical secretory K[+] channel ROMK. Flow-dependent K[+] secretion is mediated by an apical voltage-gated, calcium-sensitive Maxi-K/BK channel. Chloride-dependent electroneutral K[+] secretion is likely mediated by a K[+]-Cl[-] cotransporter.

within the connecting segment (CNT) and cortical collecting duct (CCD). The principal cells of the CNT and CCD play a dominant role in K[+] secretion; the relevant transport pathways are shown in Figures 17-2 and 17-3. Apical Na[+] entry via the amiloride-sensitive epithelial Na[+] channel (ENaC)[64] results in the generation of a lumen-negative potential difference in the CNT and CCD, which drives passive K[+] exit through apical K[+] channels.

A critical, clinically relevant consequence of this relationship is that K[+] secretion is dependent on delivery of adequate luminal Na[+] to the CNT and CCD.[65,66] K[+] secretion by the CCD essentially ceases as luminal Na[+] drops below 8 mmol/L.[67] Selective increases in thiazide-sensitive Na[+]-Cl[-] cotransport in the distal convoluted tubule (DCT), as seen in familial hyperkalemia with hypertension (FHHt; see "Hereditary Tubular Defects and Potassium Excretion" section), reduce Na[+] delivery to principal cells in the downstream CNT and CCD, which leads to hyperkalemia.[68] Dietary Na[+] intake also influences K[+] excretion; excretion is enhanced by excess Na[+] intake and reduced by Na[+] restriction (Figure 17-4).[65,66]

Basolateral exchange of Na[+] and K[+] is mediated by Na[+]-K[+]-ATPase, which provides the driving force for both Na[+] entry and K[+] exit at the apical membrane (see Figures 17-2 and 17-3). Under basal conditions of high Na[+]-Cl[-] and low K[+] intake, the bulk of aldosterone-stimulated Na[+] and K[+] transport occurs in the CNT, prior to the entry of tubular fluid into the CCD.[69] The density of both Na[+] and K[+] channels is thus considerably greater in the CNT than in the CCD,[70,71] and the capacity of the CNT for Na[+] reabsorption may be as much as 10 times greater than that of the CCD.[71]

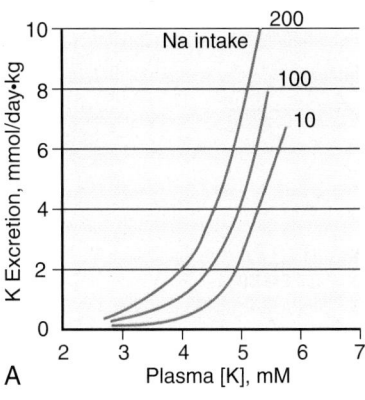
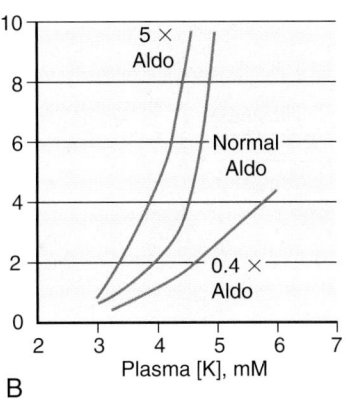

FIGURE 17-4 **A,** Relationship between steady-state serum K⁺ concentration and urinary K⁺ excretion in the dog, as a function of dietary Na⁺ intake (millimoles per day). Animals were adrenalectomized and given replacement aldosterone; dietary K⁺ and Na⁺ content were varied as specified. **B,** Relationship between steady-state serum K⁺ concentration and urinary K⁺ excretion as a function of circulating aldosterone level. Animals were adrenalectomized and variably given replacement aldosterone; dietary K⁺ content was varied. (**A** from Young DB, Jackson TE, Tipayamontri U, et al: Effects of sodium intake on steady-state potassium excretion, *Am J Physiol* 246:F772-F778, 1984; **B** from Young DB: Quantitative analysis of aldosterone's role in potassium regulation, *Am J Physiol* 255:F811-F822, 1988.)

The recruitment of ENaC subunits in response to dietary Na⁺ restriction begins in the CNT, with progressive recruitment of subunits to the apical membrane of the CCD at lower levels of dietary Na⁺.[72] The activity of secretory K⁺ channels in the CNT is also influenced by changes in dietary K⁺.[73] Again, this is consistent with progressive axial recruitment of transport capacity for the absorption of Na⁺ and secretion of K⁺ along the distal nephron.

Electrophysiologic characterization has documented the presence of several subpopulations of apical K⁺ channels in the CCD and CNT, most prominently a small-conductance (SK) 30-picosiemens channel[70,74] and a large-conductance Ca²⁺-activated 150-picosiemens (BK) channel[70,75] (see Figure 17-3). The SK channel is thought to mediate K⁺ secretion under baseline conditions, hence its designation as the "secretory" K⁺ channel. SK channel activity is mediated by the ROMK (renal outer medullary K⁺ channel) protein, encoded by the *Kcnj1* gene; targeted deletion of this gene in mice results in complete loss of SK activity within the CCD.[75]

Increased distal flow has a significant stimulatory effect on K⁺ secretion. This is due, in part, both to enhanced delivery and absorption of Na⁺ and to increased removal of secreted K⁺.[65,66] The apical Ca²⁺-activated BK channel plays a critical role in flow-dependent K⁺ secretion by the CNT and CCD.[74] BK channels have a heteromeric structure, with α-subunits that form the ion channel pore and modulatory β-subunits.[74] The β₁-subunits of BK channels are restricted to principal cells within the CNT,[74,76] whereas β₄-subunits are detectable at the apical membranes of TAL, DCT, and intercalated cells.[76] Flow-dependent K⁺ secretion is reduced in mice with targeted deletion of the α₁- and β₁-subunits,[74,77,78] consistent with a dominant role for BK channels. In addition to apical K⁺ channels, considerable evidence implicates apical K⁺-Cl⁻ cotransport in distal K⁺ secretion.[65,79,80] Pharmacologic studies of perfused tubules are consistent with K⁺-Cl⁻ cotransport mediated by the KCC proteins.[79]

A recent provocative study underlines the importance of ENaC-independent K⁺ excretion, be it mediated by apical K⁺-Cl⁻ cotransport and/or by other mechanisms.[81] Rats were infused with amiloride via osmotic minipumps, which generated urinary concentrations considered sufficient to inhibit more than 98% of ENaC activity. Whereas amiloride almost abolished K⁺ excretion in rats with a normal K⁺ intake, short- and long-term high-K⁺ diets led to an increasing fraction of K⁺ excretion that was independent of ENaC activity (approximately 50% after 7 to 9 days on a high-K⁺ diet).[81]

In addition to secretion, the distal nephron is capable of considerable reabsorption of K⁺, particularly during restriction of dietary K⁺.[19,63,82,83] This reabsorption is accomplished primarily by intercalated cells in the outer medullary collecting duct (OMCD), via the activity of apical H⁺-K⁺-ATPase pumps (see Figure 17-2). The molecular physiology of H⁺-K⁺-ATPase–mediated K⁺ reabsorption is reviewed in Chapter 5.

Control of Potassium Secretion

Aldosterone

Aldosterone is well established as an important regulatory factor in K⁺ excretion, and increases in plasma K⁺ concentration are an important stimulus for aldosterone secretion (see also "Regulation of Renal Renin and Adrenal Aldosterone" section). However, an increasingly dominant theme is that aldosterone plays a permissive and synergistic role in K⁺ homeostasis.[84-86] This is reflected clinically in the frequent absence of hyperkalemia or hypokalemia in disorders associated with a deficiency or an overabundance of circulating aldosterone, respectively (see "Hyperaldosteronism" and "Hypoaldosteronism" sections). Regardless, it is clear that aldosterone and downstream effectors of this hormone have clinically relevant effects on plasma K⁺ levels and that the ability to excrete K⁺ is modulated by systemic aldosterone levels (see Figure 17-4).

Aldosterone has no effect on the density of apical SK channels in the CCD or CNT; rather, the hormone induces a marked increase in the density of apical Na⁺ channels,[87] thus increasing the driving force for apical K⁺ excretion. The apical amiloride-sensitive ENaC is comprised of three subunits, α, β, and γ, that assemble together to synergistically traffic to the cell membrane and mediate Na⁺ transport.[64]

Aldosterone activates ENaC channel complexes by multiple mechanisms. First, it induces transcription of the ENaC α-subunit,[88,89] which increases its availability for coassembly with the more abundant β- and γ-subunits.[90] Second, aldosterone and dietary Na⁺-Cl⁻ restriction stimulate a significant redistribution of ENaC subunits in the CNT and early CCD, from a largely cytoplasmic location during dietary Na⁺-Cl⁻ excess to a purely apical distribution after aldosterone or Na⁺-Cl⁻ restriction.[72,91,92] Third, aldosterone induces the expression of serine-threonine kinase SGK1.[93] Coexpression of SGK1 with ENaC subunits results in increased expression at the plasma membrane.[91]

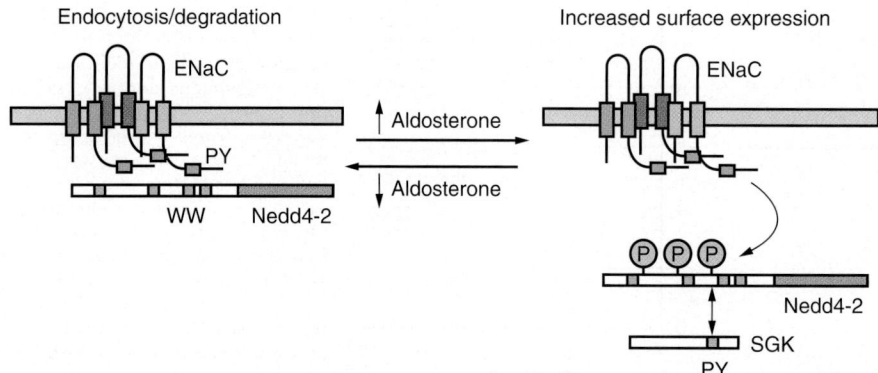

FIGURE 17-5 Coordinated regulation of the epithelial sodium channel (ENaC) by the aldosterone-induced kinase SGK (serum- and glucocorticoid-regulated kinase) and the ubiquitin ligase Nedd4-2 (neural developmentally downregulated isoform 4-2). Nedd4-2 binds via its WW domains to ENaC subunits via their PPXY domains (denoted *PY* here), ubiquitinating the channel subunits and targeting them for removal from the cell membrane and destruction in the proteosome. Aldosterone induces SGK, which phosphorylates and inactivates Nedd4-2, and thus surface expression of ENaC channels is increased. Mutations that cause Liddle's syndrome affect the interaction between ENaC and Nedd4-2. (From Snyder PM, Olson DR, Thomas BC: Serum and glucocorticoid-regulated kinase modulates Nedd4-2–mediated inhibition of the epithelial Na+ channel, *J Biol Chem* 277:5-8, 2002.)

SGK1 modulates membrane expression of ENaC by interfering with regulated endocytosis of its channel subunits. Specifically, the kinase interferes with interactions between ENaC subunits and the ubiquitin ligase Nedd4-2 (neural developmentally downregulated isoform 4-2).[90] The so-called PPxY domains in the C termini of all three ENaC subunits bind to WW domains of Nedd4-2.[94] These PPxY domains are deleted, truncated, or mutated in patients with Liddle's syndrome[95] (see "Liddle's Syndrome" section), leading to a gain-of-function in channel activity.[96] Nedd4-2 ubiquitinates ENaC subunits, thus inducing removal of channel subunits from the cell membrane followed by degradation in lysosomes and the proteosome.[90] A PPxY domain in SGK1 also binds to Nedd4-2, which is a phosphorylation substrate for the kinase. Phosphorylation of Nedd4-2 by SGK1 abrogates the inhibitory effect of this ubiquitin ligase on ENaC subunits[97] (Figure 17-5).

The importance of SGK1 in K^+ and Na^+ homeostasis is illustrated by the phenotype of SGK1 knockout mice.[98,99] On a normal diet, homozygous SGK1$^{-/-}$ mice exhibit normal blood pressure and a normal plasma K^+ concentration, with only a mild elevation of circulating aldosterone. However, dietary Na^+-Cl^- restriction in these mice results in relative Na^+ wasting and hypotension, marked weight loss, and a drop in glomerular filtration rate (GFR), despite considerable increases in circulating aldosterone.[99] In addition, dietary K^+ loading over 6 days leads to a 1.5 mmol/L increase in plasma K^+, also accompanied by a considerable increase in circulating aldosterone (approximately fivefold greater than that in wild-type littermate controls).[98] This hyperkalemia occurs despite evident increases in apical ROMK expression, compared with normokalemic littermate controls. The amiloride-sensitive, lumen-negative potential difference generated by ENaC is reduced in these SGK1 knockout mice,[98] which results in a decreased driving force for distal K^+ secretion and the observed susceptibility to hyperkalemia.

Another mechanism whereby aldosterone activates ENaC involves proteolytic cleavage of the channel proteins by serine proteases. A "channel-activating protease" that increases channel activity of ENaC was initially identified in *Xenopus laevis* A6 cells.[100] The mammalian ortholog, denoted *CAP1* (channel-activating protease 1) or prostasin, is an aldosterone-induced protein in principal cells.[101] Urinary excretion of CAP1 is increased in hyperaldosteronism, with a reduction after adrenalectomy.[101] CAP1 is membrane associated, via a glycosylphosphatidylinositol linkage.[100] Mammalian principal cells also express two transmembrane proteases, denoted CAP2 and CAP3, with homology to CAP1.[102] These and other proteases (furin, plasmin, etc.) activate ENaC by excising extracellular inhibitory domains from the α- and γ-subunits, which increases the open probability of channels at the plasma membrane.[102,103] Because SGK1 increases channel expression at the cell surface,[91] one would expect synergistic activation by coexpressed CAP1 through CAP3 and SGK, and this is indeed the case.[102]

Therefore, aldosterone activates ENaC by at least four separate synergistic mechanisms: induction of the ENaC α-subunit, induction of SGK1, repression of Nedd4-2, and induction of channel-activating proteases. Clinically, the inhibition of channel-activating proteases by the protease inhibitor nafamostat, a newer anticoagulant, causes hyperkalemia due to inhibition of ENaC activity.[104,105]

Potassium Intake

Changes in K^+ intake strongly modulate K^+ channel activity in the CNT and CCD (secretory capacity), in addition to H^+-K^+-ATPase activity in the OMCD (reabsorptive capacity). Increased dietary K^+ rapidly increases the activity of SK channels in the CCD and CNT,[73,106] along with a modest increase in Na^+ channel (ENaC) activity[87]; this is associated with an increase in apical expression of the ROMK channel protein.[107] The increase in ENaC and SK channel density in the CCD occurs within hours of assuming a high-K^+ diet, with a minimal associated increase in circulating aldosterone.[106]

BK channels in the CNT and CCD are also activated by dietary K^+ loading. Trafficking of BK subunits is thus affected by dietary K^+, with largely intracellular distribution of α-subunits in K^+-restricted rats and prominent apical expression in K^+-loaded rats.[108] Again, aldosterone does not contribute to the regulation of BK channel activity or expression in response to high-K^+ diet.[109]

A complex, synergistic mix of signaling pathways regulates K^+ channel activity in response to changes in dietary K^+ (see also Chapter 5). In particular, the WNK (*with no lysine [K]*) kinases play a critical role in modulating distal

K[+] secretion. *WNK1* and *WNK4* were initially identified as the causative genes for FHHt (see also "Hereditary Tubular Defects and Potassium Excretion" section). ROMK expression at the membrane of *Xenopus* oocytes is reduced by coexpression of WNK4. FHHt-associated mutations increase this effect, which suggests a direction inhibition of SK channels in FHHt.[4]

Transcription of the WNK1 gene generates several different isoforms. The predominant intrarenal WNK1 isoform is generated by a distal nephron transcriptional site that bypasses the N-terminal exons which encode the kinase domain, yielding a kinase-deficient "short" isoform[110] (WNK1-S). Full-length WNK1 (WNK1-L) inhibits ROMK by inducing endocytosis of the channel protein; the shorter, kinase-deficient WNK1-S isoform inhibits this effect of WNK1-L.[111,112] The ratio of WNK1-S to WNK1-L transcripts is reduced by K[+] restriction (greater endocytosis of ROMK)[112,113] and increased by K[+] loading (reduced endocytosis of ROMK),[111,113] which suggests that this ratio between WNK1-S and WNK1-L functions as a molecular "switch" to regulate distal K[+] secretion. The membrane trafficking of ROMK is also modulated by tyrosine phosphorylation of the channel protein, such that tyrosine phosphorylation stimulates endocytosis and tyrosine dephosphorylation induces exocytosis.[114,115] Intrarenal activity of the cytoplasmic tyrosine kinases c-src and c-yes is inversely related to dietary K[+] intake, with a decrease under high-K[+] conditions and a marked increase after several days of K[+] restriction.[116,117]

Several studies have implicated the intrarenal generation of superoxide anions in the activation of cytoplasmic tyrosine kinases by K[+] depletion.[118-120] Potential candidates for the upstream hormonal signals include angiotensin II and growth factors such as insulin-like growth factor-1.[118] In particular, angiotensin II inhibits ROMK activity in K[+]-restricted rats, but not in rats consuming a normal-K[+] diet.[121] This inhibition by angiotensin II involves downstream activation of superoxide production and c-src activity, so that the induction of angiotensin II by a low-K[+] diet appears to play a major role in reducing distal tubular K[+] secretion.[122]

Integrated Regulation of Distal Sodium Absorption and Potassium Secretion

Under certain physiologic conditions associated with marked induction of aldosterone, such as dietary sodium restriction, Na[+] balance can be maintained without significant effects on K[+] excretion. Yet by activating ENaC and generating a more lumen-negative potential difference, increases in aldosterone should lead to an obligatory kaliuresis. How is this physiologic consequence avoided? The mechanisms that underlie this "aldosterone paradox," the independent regulation of Na[+] and K[+] handling by the aldosterone-sensitive distal nephron, have recently begun to emerge. The major factors that allow for integrated but independent control of Na[+] and K[+] transport appear to include electroneutral thiazide-sensitive Na[+]-Cl[-] transport within the CCD,[123-125] ENaC-independent K[+] excretion within the distal nephron,[81] and the differential regulation of various signaling pathways by aldosterone, angiotensin II, and dietary K[+] intake[1,126] (see also Chapter 5).

Electroneutral Na[+]-Cl[-] transport in the CCD and ENaC-independent K[+] secretion may play important roles in disconnecting Na[+] and K[+] transport within the distal nephron.

Electroneutral, thiazide-sensitive, and amiloride-resistant Na[+]-Cl[-] transport within the CCD[123-125] are mediated by the combined activity of the Na[+]-dependent SLC4A8 (solute carrier family 4, subfamily A, isoform 8) Cl[-]/HCO_3[-] exchanger and the SLC26A4 Cl[-]/HCO_3[-] exchanger[125] (see also Chapter 5). This transport mechanism is apparently responsible for as much 50% of Na[+]-Cl[-] transport in mineralocorticoid-stimulated rat CCD,[123,124] which allows for ENaC-independent, electroneutral Na[+] absorption that will not directly affect K[+] secretion. The converse effect emerges after dietary K[+] loading, which increases the fraction of ENaC-independent, amiloride-resistant K[+] excretion to approximately 50%.[81]

Recent reports have indicated a key role in K[+] homeostasis for NCC, the thiazide-sensitive Na[+]-Cl[-] cotransporter in the DCT. Selective increases in DCT and NCC activity, as seen in FHHt, reduce Na[+] delivery to principal cells in the downstream CNT and CCD, leading to hyperkalemia.[68] Angiotensin II also activates NCC via WNK-dependent activation of the kinase SPAK (STE20/SPS1-related proline/alanine-rich kinase) and phosphorylation of the transporter protein,[127,128] which reduce delivery of Na[+] to the CNT and limit K[+] secretion.

In contrast, angiotensin II inhibits ROMK activity via several mechanisms, including downstream activation of c-src tyrosine kinases (see earlier).[120-122] Whereas K[+] restriction induces renin and circulating angiotensin II (see "Consequences of Hypokalemia" section), increases in dietary K[+] are suppressive.[122,129] A high-K[+] diet also inactivates NCC,[130] due the associated decrease in angiotensin II, in addition to the increase in the ratio of WNK1-S to WNK1-L isoforms that occurs with increased K[+] intake.[111-113] WNK1-S antagonizes the effect of WNK1-L on NCC, which leads to inhibition of NCC in conditions with a relative excess of WNK1-S.[1]

Finally, within principal cells, increases in aldosterone induce the SGK1 kinase, which phosphorylates WNK4 and attenuates the effect of WNK4 on ROMK,[131] while activating EnaC.[90,91,93] When dietary K[+] intake is reduced, however, c-src tyrosine kinase activity increases under the influence of increased angiotensin II, which causes direction inhibition of ROMK activity via tyrosine phosphorylation of the channel.[114,132,133] The increase in c-src tyrosine kinase activity also abrogates the inhibitory effect of SGK1 on WNK4.[126] Again, angiotensin II appears to mediate part of its inhibitory effect on ROMK through activation of c-src,[122] so that c-src serves as an important component of the "switch" that regulates K[+] secretion in response to changes in dietary K[+].

To summarize this important physiology, the differential effects of K[+] intake on angiotensin II versus aldosterone appear to be critical in resolving the aldosterone paradox; so too are the differential effects of K[+] intake on NCC-dependent Na[+]-Cl[-] transport in the DCT and on secretory K[+] channels within the downstream CNT and CCD (Figure 17-6). Under conditions of low Na[+] intake but moderate K[+] intake, angiotensin II and aldosterone are both strongly induced, which leads to enhanced Na[+]-Cl[-] transport via NCC, increased ENaC activity, and decreased secretory K[+] channel activity. Although ENaC is activated, the relative inhibition of ROMK by the increased angiotensin II prevents excessive kaliuresis. Angiotensin II–dependent activation of c-src kinases has direct inhibitory effects on ROMK trafficking and also abrogates the inhibitory effect of SGK1 on WNK4,[126] which leads to unopposed inhibition of ROMK by WNK4. In addition, the

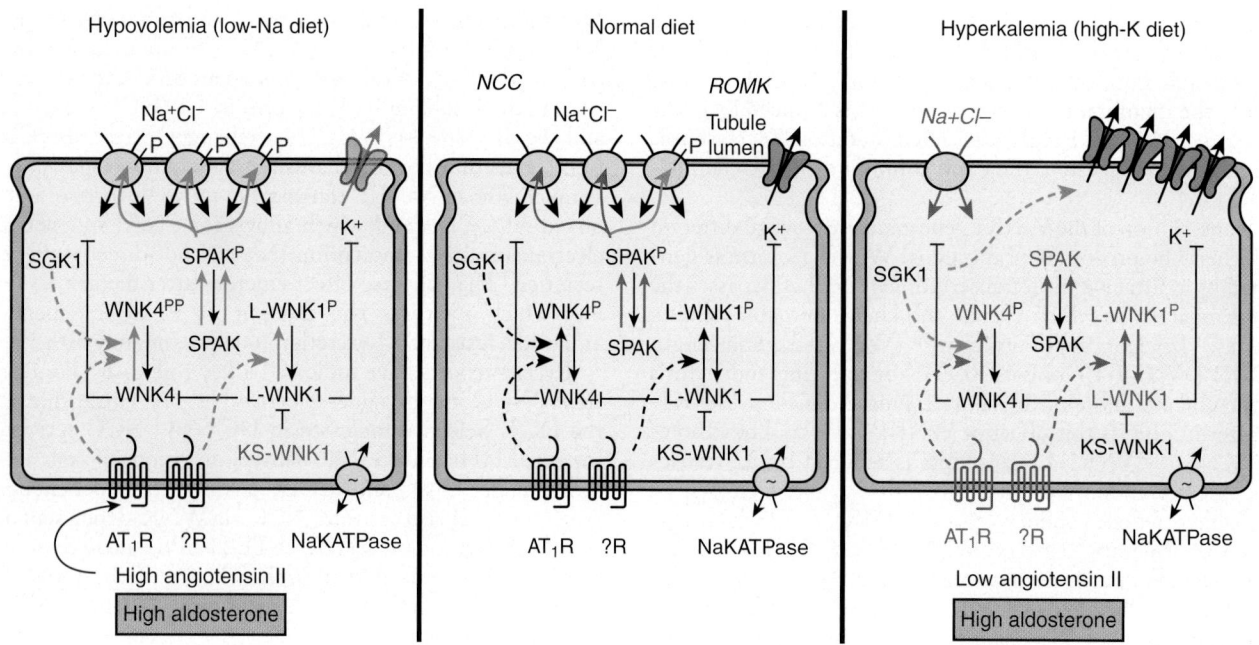

FIGURE 17-6 Integrated regulation of Na^+-Cl^- and K^+ transport in the distal convoluted tubule (DCT), connecting segment (CNT), and cortical collecting duct (CCD). The *green arrowheads* indicate activating pathways, and the *red blunt end* indicates an inhibitory pathway. **Left,** The pathway in the setting of a low-Na^+ diet, in which angiotensin II and SGK1 (serum- and glucocorticoid-regulated kinase 1) signaling leads to phosphorylation of WNK4 (*with no lysine* [*K*] 4). This stimulates phosphorylation of SPAK (STE20/SPS1-related proline/alanine-rich kinase), which in turn phosphorylates and activates thiazide-sensitive Na^+-Cl^- cotransport in the DCT via NCC (Na^+-Cl^- cotransporter). Stimulation of unknown receptors is hypothesized to cause phosphorylation of full-length WNK1 (L-WNK1), which can also stimulate SPAK phosphorylation. L-WNK1 has other functions: (1) it blocks the NCC-inhibitory form of WNK4, thus activating NCC, and (2) it inhibits secretion of K^+ via ROMK (renal outer medullary potassium) channels. **Right,** The pathway in the setting of high dietary K^+ intake, in which aldosterone is stimulated and angiotensin II is low. In the absence of sufficient angiotensin II, its type 1 receptor (AT_1R) cannot activate WNK4. This reduces SPAK activation and NCC phosphorylation. Dietary potassium loading also increases the level of a kidney-specific, kinase-deficient short isoform of WNK1 (KS-WNK1) to suppress the activity of L-WNK1. In consequence, the inhibitory effect of WNK4 on NCC dominates, blocking traffic of NCC to the apical membrane and thereby reducing NCC activity. KS-WNK1 also blocks the effect of L-WNK1 on ROMK endocytosis, which causes ROMK to increase at the apical membrane. The net effect is that K^+ secretion in the DCT and CNT/CCD is maximized, whereas NCC is suppressed. Aldosterone stimulation of the epithelial sodium channel (ENaC; not shown) offsets the decreased Na^+ reabsorption by NCC, which allows robust potassium secretion without changes in sodium balance. The roles of WNK3, SGK1, and c-src cytoplasmic tyrosine kinases are not shown in the interest of clarity; see text for further details. (From Welling PA, Chang YP, Delpire E: Multigene kinase network, kidney transport, and salt in essential hypertension, *Kidney Int* 77:1063-1069, 2010.)

aldosterone-dependent induction of electroneutral Na^+-Cl^- transport within the CCD[123-125] increases Na^+-Cl^- reabsorption but blunts the effect on the lumen-negative potential, thus limiting kaliuresis. When dietary K^+ increases, circulating aldosterone is moderately induced, but angiotensin II is suppressed. This leads to inhibition of NCC and increased downstream delivery of Na^+ to principal cells in the CNT and CCD, where ENaC activity is increased and ROMK and BK channels are significantly activated. ENaC-independent K^+ secretion is also strongly induced by increased dietary K^+ intake,[81] which contributes significantly to the ability to excrete K^+ in the urine.

Regulation of Renal Renin and Adrenal Aldosterone

Modulation of the renin-angiotensin-aldosterone system (RAAS) has profound clinical effects on K^+ homeostasis. Although multiple tissues are capable of renin secretion, renin of renal origin has a dominant physiologic impact. Renin secretion by juxtaglomerular cells within the afferent arteriole is initiated in response to a signal from the macula densa,[134] specifically a decrease in luminal chloride[135] transported through the Na^+-K^+-$2Cl^-$ cotransporter (NKCC2) at the apical membrane of macula densa cells.[24] In addition to

this macula densa signal, decreased renal perfusion pressure and renal sympathetic tone stimulate renal renin secretion.[19]

The various inhibitors of renin release include angiotensin II, endothelin-1,[136] adenosine,[137] atrial natriuretic peptide (ANP),[138] tumor necrosis factor-α,[139] and vitamin D.[140] Cyclic guanosine monophosphate–dependent protein kinase type II (cGKII) tonically inhibits renin secretion, in that renin secretion in response to several stimuli is exaggerated in homozygous *cGKII* knockout mice.[141] Activation of cGKII by ANP and/or nitric oxide has a marked inhibitory effect on the release of renin from juxtaglomerular cells.[138] Local factors that stimulate renin release from juxtaglomerular cells include prostaglandins,[142] adrenomedullin,[143] catecholamines (β1-receptors),[144] and succinate (GPR91 receptor).[145]

The relationship between renal renin release, the RAAS, and cyclooxygenase-2 (COX-2) is an interesting one.[142] COX-2 is heavily expressed in the macula densa,[142] with a significant recruitment of COX-2(+) cells seen with salt restriction or furosemide treatment.[19,142] Reduced intracellular chloride in macula densa cells appears to stimulate COX-2 expression via p38 mitogen-activated protein kinase,[146] whereas both aldosterone and angiotensin II reduce its expression.[142] Prostaglandins derived from COX-2 in the macula densa play a dominant role in the stimulation of renal renin release by salt restriction, furosemide, renal artery occlusion,

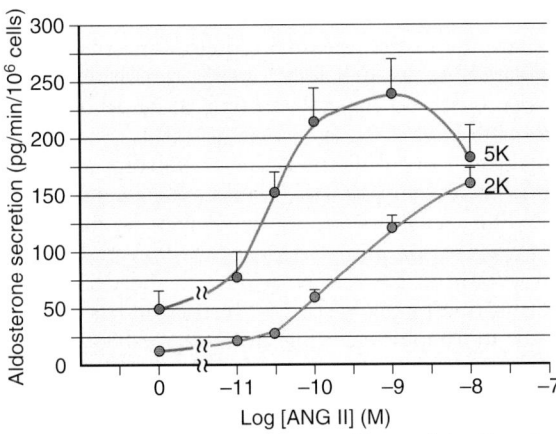

FIGURE 17-7 Synergistic effect of increased extracellular K⁺ and angiotensin II (ANG II) in inducing aldosterone release from bovine adrenal glomerulosa cells. Dose-response curves for ANG-II were measured at extracellular K⁺ concentrations of 2 mmol/L (*open circles*) and 5 mmol/L (*filled circles*). (From Chen XL, Bayliss DA, Fern RJ, et al: A role for T-type Ca²⁺ channels in the synergistic control of aldosterone production by ANG II and K⁺, *Am J Physiol* 276:F674-F683, 1999.)

or angiotensin converting enzyme (ACE) inhibition.[19,147] Specifically, COX-2–derived prostaglandins appear to play a role in tonic expression of renin in juxtaglomerular cells via modulation of intracellular cAMP and calcium, rather than functioning in the acute regulation of renin release.[142]

Renin released from the kidney ultimately stimulates aldosterone release from the adrenal via angiotensin II. Hyperkalemia per se is also an independent and synergistic stimulus (Figure 17-7) for aldosterone release from the adrenal gland.[19,148] Importantly, dietary K⁺ loading is less potent than dietary Na⁺-Cl⁻ restriction in increasing circulating aldosterone.[84] The resting membrane potential of adrenal glomerulosa cells is hyperpolarized, due to the activity of the "leak" K⁺ channels TASK-1 and TASK-3 (tandem of P domains in weak inward rectifier K⁺ channel [TWIK]–related acid-sensitive K⁺ channels). Combined deletion of genes encoding these channels leads to baseline depolarization of adrenal glomerulosa cells and an increase in plasma aldosterone that is resistant to dietary sodium loading.[149]

Angiotensin II and K⁺ both activate Ca²⁺ entry into glomerulosa cells via voltage-sensitive T-type Ca²⁺ channels,[19,150] primarily Cav 3.2.[151] Elevations in extracellular K⁺ thus depolarize glomerulosa cells and activate these Ca²⁺ channels, which are independently and synergistically activated by angiotensin II.[150] Calcium-dependent activation of calcium-calmodulin (CaM)–dependent protein kinase in turn activates the synthesis and release of aldosterone via induction of aldosterone synthase.[152] K⁺ and angiotensin II also enhance transcription of the Cav 3.2 Ca²⁺ channel by abrogating repression of this gene by neuron restrictive silencing factor; this ultimately amplifies the induction of aldosterone synthase.[151]

The adrenal release of aldosterone due to increased K⁺ is dependent on an intact *adrenal* renin-angiotensin system,[153] particularly during Na⁺ restriction. ACE inhibitors and angiotensin-receptor blockers (ARBs) thus markedly abrogate the effect of high K⁺ on salt-restricted adrenals.[154] Direct G protein–dependent activation of the TASK-1 and/or TASK-3 K⁺ channels by type 1A or 1B angiotensin II receptors (AT_{1A}, AT_{1B}) is thought to underlie the effect of angiotensin II on adrenal aldosterone release,[149] with abrogation of this effect

by ARBs or ACE inhibitors. Other clinically relevant activators of adrenal aldosterone release include prostaglandins[155] and catecholamines,[156] via increases in cAMP.[157,158]

Finally, ANP exerts a potent negative effect on aldosterone release induced by K⁺ and other stimuli,[159] at least in part by inhibiting early events in aldosterone synthesis.[160] ANP is therefore capable of inhibiting both renal renin release and adrenal aldosterone release, functions that may be central to the pathophysiology of hyporeninemic hypoaldosteronism.

Urinary Indices of Potassium Excretion

A bedside test to directly measure distal tubular K⁺ secretion in humans would be ideal; however, for obvious reasons this not technically feasible. A widely used surrogate is the transtubular K⁺ gradient (TTKG), which is defined as follows:

$$TTKG = \frac{[K^+]_{urine} \times Osmolality_{blood}}{[K^+]_{blood} \times Osmolality_{urine}}$$

The expected values of the TTKG are based largely on historical data and are less than 3 to 4 in the presence of hypokalemia and higher than 6 to 7 in the presence of hyperkalemia. The shifting opinions regarding the physiologically appropriate TTKG in hyperkalemia were recently reviewed.[161] Clearly water absorption in the CCD and medullary collecting duct is an important determinant of the absolute K⁺ concentration in the final urine; hence, the use of a ratio of urine/plasma osmolality. Indeed, water absorption may in large part determine the TTKG, so that it far exceeds the limiting K⁺ gradient.[162] The TTKG may be less useful in patients ingesting diets of changing K⁺ and mineralocorticoid content.[163] There is, however, a linear relationship between plasma aldosterone level and the TTKG, which suggests that it provides a rough approximation of the ability to respond to aldosterone with kaliuresis.[164] The response of the TTKG to mineralocorticoid administration, typically fludrocortisone, can thus be utilized in the diagnostic approach to hyperkalemia.[161] In hypokalemic patients, a TTKG of less than 2 to 3 separates patients with redistributive hypokalemia from those with hypokalemia due to renal potassium wasting, who will have TTKG values that are higher than 4.[165] The determination of urinary electrolyte levels for calculation of the TTKG provides the opportunity for the measurement of urinary Na⁺, the value of which determines whether significant prerenal stimuli are limiting distal Na⁺ delivery and thus K⁺ excretion (see also Figure 17-4). Measurement of urinary electrolyte levels also affords the opportunity to calculate the urinary anion gap, an indirect index of urinary NH_4^+ content and thus the ability to respond to acidemia.[166]

Consequences of Hyperkalemia and Hypokalemia

Consequences of Hypokalemia

Excitable Tissues: Muscle and Heart

Hypokalemia is a well-described risk factor for both ventricular and atrial arrhythmias.[26,167,168] For example, in patients undergoing cardiac surgery, a plasma K⁺ concentration of less than 3.5 mmol/L is a predictor of serious intraoperative arrhythmia, perioperative arrhythmia, and postoperative atrial fibrillation.[169] Moderate hypokalemia does not appear to increase the risk of serious arrhythmia during exercise stress testing, however.[170]

Electrocardiographic changes in hypokalemia include broad, flat T waves, ST depression, and QT prolongation. These are most marked when plasma K^+ concentration is less than 2.7 mmol/L.[171] Hypokalemia, often accompanied by hypomagnesemia, is an important cause of the long QT syndrome (LQTS) and torsades de pointes, either alone or in combination with drug toxicity[172] or with LQTS-associated mutations in cardiac K^+ and Na^+ channels.[173]

In a landmark study, Guo and colleagues recently demonstrated that hypokalemia accelerates the clathrin-dependent internalization and degradation of the *HERG* (human ether-à-go-go–related gene) K^+ channel protein.[28] *HERG* encodes pore-forming subunits of the cardiac rapidly activating delayed rectifier K^+ channel (I_{Kr}); I_{Kr} is largely responsible for potassium efflux during phases 2 and 3 of the cardiac action potential.[174] Loss-of-function mutations in *HERG* reduce I_{Kr} and cause type 2 LQTS.[28] Downregulation of *HERG* and I_{Kr} by hypokalemia provides an elegant explanation for the association with LQTS and torsades de pointes.

In muscle, hypokalemia causes hyperpolarization, thus impairing the capacity to depolarize and contract. Weakness and paralysis are therefore a not-infrequent consequence of hypokalemia of diverse etiologies.[175,176] On a historical note, the realization in 1946 that K^+ replacement reversed the hypokalemic diaphragmatic paralysis induced by treatment of diabetic ketoacidosis was a milestone in diabetes care.[177] Pathologically, muscle biopsy specimens in hypokalemic myopathy demonstrate phagocytosis of degenerating muscle fibers, fiber regeneration, and atrophy of type 2 fibers.[178] Most patients with significant myopathy have elevations in creatine kinase levels, and hypokalemia of diverse causes predisposes to rhabdomyolysis with acute renal failure.

Renal Consequences

Hypokalemia causes a host of structural and functional changes in the kidney, which are reviewed in detail elsewhere.[179] In humans, the renal pathology includes a relatively specific proximal tubular vacuolization,[179,180] interstitial nephritis,[181] and renal cysts.[182] Hypokalemic nephropathy can cause ESRD, mostly in patients with long-standing hypokalemia due to eating disorders and/or laxative abuse.[183] Acute renal failure with proximal tubular vacuolopathy has also been described.[184] In animal models, hypokalemia increases susceptibility to acute renal failure induced by ischemia, gentamicin, and amphotericin.[19] Potassium restriction in rats induces cortical angiotensin II and medullary endothelin-1 expression, with an ischemic pattern of renal injury.[185]

The prominent functional changes in renal physiology that are induced by hypokalemia include Na^+-Cl^- retention, polyuria,[180] phosphaturia,[26] hypocitraturia,[186] and increased ammoniagenesis.[179] Many of these clinical features are not broadly appreciated. K^+ depletion in rats causes proximal tubular hyperabsorption of Na^+-Cl^-, in association with an upregulation of angiotensin II,[185] the AT_1 receptor,[26] and the α_2-adrenergic receptor[26] in this nephron segment.

Na^+/H^+ exchanger isoform 3 (NHE3), the dominant apical Na^+ entry site in the proximal tubule, is massively (>700%) upregulated in K^+-deficient rats,[187] which is consistent with the observed hyperabsorption of both Na^+-Cl^- and bicarbonate.[179]

Polyuria in hypokalemia is due to polydipsia[188] and to a vasopressin-resistant defect in urinary concentrating ability.[179] This renal concentrating defect is multifactorial, with evidence for both a reduced hydroosmotic response to vasopressin in the collecting duct[179] and decreased Na^+-Cl^- absorption by the TAL.[26] K^+ restriction has been shown to result in a rapid, reversible decrease in the expression of aquaporin-2 in the collecting duct,[189] beginning in the CCD and extending to the medullary collecting duct within the first 24 hours.[190] In the TAL, the marked reductions seen during K^+ restriction in both the apical K^+ channel ROMK and the apical Na^+-K^+-$2Cl^-$ cotransporter NKCC2[187] reduce Na^+-Cl^- absorption and thus inhibit countercurrent multiplication and the driving force for water absorption by the collecting duct.

Cardiovascular Consequences

A large body of experimental and epidemiologic evidence implicates hypokalemia and/or reduced dietary K^+ in the genesis or worsening of hypertension, heart failure, and stroke.[191] K^+ depletion in young rats induces hypertension,[192] with a salt sensitivity that persists after K^+ levels are normalized; presumably this salt sensitivity is due to the significant tubulointerstitial injury induced by K^+ restriction.[185] Short-term K^+ restriction in healthy humans and patients with essential hypertension also induces Na^+-Cl^- retention and hypertension,[26] and abundant epidemiologic data link dietary K^+ deficiency and/or hypokalemia with hypertension.[168,191] Correction of hypokalemia is particularly important in hypertensive patients treated with diuretics; blood pressure in this setting is improved with the establishment of normokalemia,[193] and the cardiovascular benefits of diuretic agents are blunted by hypokalemia.[26,194] Hypokalemia reduces insulin secretion; this effect may be important in thiazide-associated diabetes.[195] Finally, K^+ depletion may play significant roles in the pathophysiology and progression of heart failure.[191]

Consequences of Hyperkalemia

Excitable Tissues: Muscle and Heart

Hyperkalemia constitutes a medical emergency, primarily due to its effect on the heart. Hyperkalemia depolarizes cardiac myocytes, reducing the membrane potential from −90 mV to approximately −80 mV. This brings the membrane potential closer to the threshold for generation of an action potential. Mild and/or rapid-onset hyperkalemia will initially increase cardiac excitability, since a lesser depolarizing stimulus is required to generate an action potential. Mild increases in extracellular K^+ also affect the repolarization phase of the cardiac action potential via increases in I_{Kr}, as discussed earlier (see "Consequences of Hypokalemia" section). I_{Kr} is highly sensitive to changes in extracellular K^+.[28] This effect on repolarization is thought to underlie the "early" signs of hyperkalemia,[196] including ST-T segment depression, peaked

TABLE 17-3 Approximate Relationship between Hyperkalemic Electrocardiographic (ECG) Changes and Serum Potassium Concentration

SERUM K+ CONCENTRATION	ECG ABNORMALITY
5.5-6.5 mmol/L	Tall peaked T waves with narrow base, best seen in precordial leads
6.5-8.0 mmol/L	Peaked T waves Prolonged PR interval Decreased amplitude of P waves Widening of QRS complex
>8.0 mmol/L	Absence of P waves Intraventricular blocks, fascicular blocks, bundle branch blocks, QRS axis shift Progressive widening of the QRS complex "Sine-wave" pattern (sinoventricular rhythm), ventricular fibrillation, asystole

From Mattu A, Brady WJ, Robinson DA: Electrocardiographic manifestations of hyperkalemia, *Am J Emerg Med* 18:721-729, 2000.

T waves, and QT interval shortening.[174] Persistent and increasing depolarization inactivates cardiac sodium channels, thus reducing the rate of phase 0 of the action potential (V_{max}). The decrease in V_{max} results in a reduction in myocardial conduction, with progressive prolongation of the P wave, PR interval, and QRS complex.[174] Severe hyperkalemia results in loss of the P wave and a progressive widening of the QRS complex; fusion with T waves causes a "sine-wave" sinoventricular rhythm. Cardiac arrhythmias associated with hyperkalemia include sinus bradycardia, sinus arrest, slow idioventricular rhythms, ventricular tachycardia, ventricular fibrillation, and asystole.[196,197]

The differential diagnosis and treatment of a wide-complex tachycardia in hyperkalemia can be particularly problematic; moreover, hyperkalemia potentiates the blocking effect of lidocaine on the cardiac Na+ channel, so that use of this agent may precipitate asystole or ventricular fibrillation in this setting.[198] Hyperkalemia can also cause a type 1 Brugada pattern in the electrocardiogram (ECG), with a pseudo–right bundle branch block and persistent "coved" ST segment elevation in at least two precordial leads. This "hyperkalemic Brugada sign" occurs in critically ill patients with significant hyperkalemia (plasma K+ > 7 mmol/L) and can be differentiated from genetic Brugada syndrome by an absence of P waves, marked QRS widening, and an abnormal QRS axis.[199]

The classical ECG manifestations in the progress of hyperkalemia are given in Table 17-3. These changes are notoriously insensitive, however, so that only 55% of patients with plasma K+ concentrations of more than 6.8 mmol/L in one case series manifested peaked T waves.[200] There is large interpatient variability in the absolute potassium level leading to ECG changes and cardiac toxicity of hyperkalemia. Relevant variables include the rapidity of the onset of hyperkalemia[201,202] and the presence or absence of concomitant hypocalcemia, acidemia, and/or hyponatremia.[203,204] Hemodialysis patients[204] and patients with chronic renal failure,[205] in particular, may not demonstrate ECG changes. Care should also be taken to adequately distinguish the symmetrically peaked "church steeple" T waves induced by hyperkalemia from T wave changes due to other causes.[206]

Hyperkalemia can also rarely present with ascending paralysis,[19] denoted *secondary hyperkalemic paralysis* to differentiate it from familial hyperkalemic periodic paralysis (HYPP). This presentation of hyperkalemia can mimic Guillain-Barré syndrome and may include diaphragmatic paralysis and respiratory failure.[207] Hyperkalemia from a diversity of causes can cause paralysis, as reviewed by Evers and colleagues.[208] The mechanism is not entirely clear; however, nerve conduction studies in one case suggested a neurogenic mechanism, rather than a direct effect on muscle excitability.[208]

In contrast to secondary hyperkalemic paralysis, HYPP is a primary myopathy. Patients with HYPP develop myopathic weakness during hyperkalemia induced by increased K+ intake or rest after heavy exercise.[209] The hyperkalemic trigger in HYPP serves to differentiate this syndrome from *hypokalemic* periodic paralysis (HOKP). A further distinguishing feature is the presence of myotonia in HYPP.[209] Depolarization of skeletal muscle by hyperkalemia unmasks an inactivation defect in a tetrodotoxin-sensitive Na+ channel in patients with HYPP, and autosomal dominant mutations in the *SCN4A* gene encoding this channel cause most forms of the disease.[210] Mild muscle depolarization (5 to 10 mV) in HYPP results in a persistent inward Na+ current through the mutant channel; the normal, allelic SCN4 channels quickly recover from inactivation and can then be reactivated, which results in myotonia. When muscle depolarization is more marked (i.e. 20 to 30 mV), all of the Na+ channels are inactivated, which renders the muscle inexcitable and causing weakness (Figure 17-8).

Related disorders due to mutations within the large SCN4A channel protein include HOKP type II,[211] paramyotonia congenita,[210] and K+-aggravated myopathy.[210] American quarter horses have a high incidence (4.4%) of HYPP due to a mutation in equine *SCN4A* traced to the sire Impressive (see Figure 17-8).[210]

Finally, loss-of-function mutations in the muscle-specific K+ channel subunit MinK-related peptide 2 (MiRP2) have also been shown to cause HYPP. MiRP2 and the associated voltage-sensitive K+ channel Kv 3.4 play a role in setting the resting membrane potential of skeletal muscle.[212]

Renal Consequences

Hyperkalemia has a significant effect on the ability to excrete an acid urine due to interference with the urinary excretion of ammonium (NH_4^+). Potassium loading in humans results in modest reduction in urinary NH_4^+ excretion and an impaired response to acid loading.[213] In rats, chronic potassium loading leads to hyperkalemia and a metabolic acidosis, due to a 40% reduction in urinary NH_4^+ excretion.[214] Proximal tubular ammonia generation falls, but without a significant effect on proximal tubular secretion of NH_4^+.[214]

The TAL absorbs NH_4^+ from the tubular lumen, followed by countercurrent multiplication and ultimately excretion from the medullary interstitium.[215] Hyperkalemia appears to inhibit renal acid excretion by competition of K+ with NH_4^+ for reabsorption by the TAL.[216] The NH_4^+ ion has the same ionic radius as K+ and can be transported in lieu of K+ by NKCC2,[217] the apical Na+-K+/NH_4^+-2Cl− cotransporter of the TAL. NH_4^+ exits the TAL via the basolateral Na+/H+ exchanger NHE4.[218] As is the case for other cations,

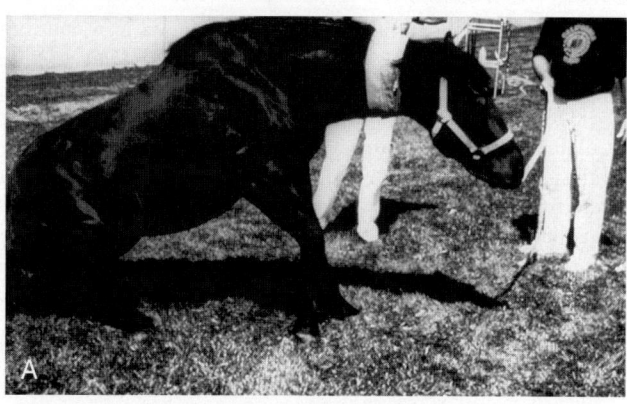

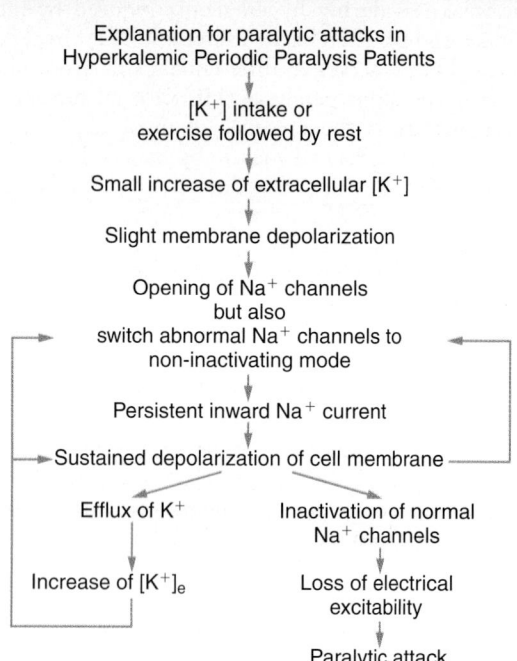

FIGURE 17-8 Hyperkalemic periodic paralysis (HYPP) due to mutations in the voltage-gated Na$^+$ channel of skeletal muscle. **A,** This disorder is particularly common in thoroughbred quarter horses. An affected horse is shown during a paralytic attack, triggered by rest after heavy exercise. **B,** Mechanistic explanation of muscle paralysis in HYPP. (**A** courtesy of Dr. Eric Hoffman; **B** from Lehmann-Horn F, Jurkat-Rott K: Voltage-gated ion channels and hereditary disease, *Physiol Rev* 79:1317-1372, 1999.)

countercurrent multiplication of NH$_4^+$ by the TAL greatly increases the concentration of NH$_4^+$/NH$_3$ available for secretion in the collecting duct. The NH$_4^+$ produced by the proximal tubule in response to acidosis is thus reabsorbed across the TAL, concentrated by countercurrent multiplication in the medullary interstitium, and secreted in the collecting duct. The capacity of the TAL to reabsorb NH$_4^+$ is increased during acidosis, due to an induction of NKCC2[217] and NHE4 expression.[218] Hyperkalemia induces acidosis in rats by reducing the NH$_4^+$ between the vasa recta (surrogate for interstitial fluid) and collecting duct,[216] due to interference with absorption of NH$_4^+$ by the TAL.

Clinically, patients with hyperkalemic acidosis due to hyporeninemic hypoaldosteronism demonstrate an increase in urinary NH$_4^+$ excretion in response to normalization of plasma K$^+$ levels with cation-exchange resins,[219,220] which indicates a significant role for hyperkalemia in generation of the acidosis.

Hypokalemia

Epidemiology

Hypokalemia is a relatively common finding in both outpatients and inpatients, perhaps the most common electrolyte abnormality encountered in clinical practice.[221] When defined as a plasma K$^+$ concentration of less than 3.6 mmol/L, it is found in up to 20% of hospitalized patients.[222] Hypokalemia is usually mild, with K$^+$ levels in the 3.0 to 3.5 mmol/L range, but in up to 25% it can be moderate to severe (<3.0 mmol/L).[222,223]

The most common causative factors in hospitalized patients with hypokalemia are gastrointestinal losses of potassium, diuretic therapy, and hypomagnesemia.[224] Hypokalemia is a particularly prominent problem in patients receiving thiazide diuretics for hypertension, with an incidence of up to 48% (average = 15% to 30%).[26,225] The thiazide-type diuretic metolazone is frequently used the management of heart failure refractory to loop diuretics alone and causes moderate (K$^+$ ≤ 3.0 mmol/L) or severe (K$^+$ ≤ 2.5 mmol/L) hypokalemia in approximately 40% and 10% of patients, respectively.[226] Hypokalemia is also a common finding in patients receiving peritoneal dialysis, with 10% to 20% requiring potassium supplementation.[227] Hypokalemia in itself can increase the in-hospital mortality rate up to 10-fold,[223] likely due to the profound effects on arrhythmogenesis, blood pressure, and cardiovascular morbidity.[191,228]

Spurious Hypokalemia

Delayed sample analysis is a well-recognized cause of spurious hypokalemia, due to increased cellular uptake; this may become clinically relevant if ambient temperature is increased.[26,229,230] Very rarely, patients with profound leukocytosis due to acute leukemia present with artifactual hypokalemia caused by time-dependent uptake of K$^+$ by the large white cell mass.[229] Such patients do not develop clinical or ECG complications of hypokalemia, and plasma K$^+$ level is normal if measured immediately after venipuncture.

Redistribution and Hypokalemia

Manipulation of the factors affecting internal distribution of K$^+$ (see "Factors Affecting Internal Distribution of Potassium" section) can cause hypokalemia due to redistribution of K$^+$ between the extracellular and intracellular compartments. Endogenous insulin is only rarely a cause of hypokalemia; however, administered insulin is a frequent cause of iatrogenic hypokalemia[222] and may be a factor in the "dead in bed syndrome" associated with aggressive glycemic control.[231] Insulin also may play a significant role in the hypokalemia associated with refeeding syndrome.[232]

Alterations in the activity of the endogenous sympathetic nervous system can cause hypokalemia in several settings, including alcohol withdrawal,[233] acute myocardial infarction,[191,234] and head injury.[235,236] Redistributive hypokalemia after severe head injury can be truly profound, with reported plasma K$^+$ concentrations of 1.2 mmol/L[235] and 1.9 mmol/L,[236] and marked rebound hyperkalemia after repletion.

Due to their ability to activate both Na^+-K^+-ATPase[46] and the Na^+-K^+-$2Cl^-$ cotransporter NKCC1,[19,25] β_2-agonists are powerful activators of cellular K^+ uptake. These agents are chiefly encountered in the treatment of asthma; however, tocolytics such as ritodrine can induce hypokalemia and arrhythmias during maternal labor.[237] The long-acting β_2-agonist clenbuterol, not approved for medical use in the United States, has caused hypokalemia in poisonings, including a recent outbreak of toxicity due to clenbuterol-adulterated heroin in the East Coast of the United States.[238] Occult sources of sympathomimetics, such as pseudoephedrine and ephedrine in cough syrup[176] or weight-loss agents,[239] can be an overlooked cause of hypokalemia. Finally, downstream activation of cAMP by xanthines such as theophylline[19,240] and dietary caffeine[241] may induce hypokalemia and may be synergistic in this respect with β_2-agonists.[242]

Whereas β_2-agonists activate K^+ uptake via Na^+-K^+-ATPase, one would expect that inhibition of passive K^+ efflux would also lead to hypokalemia; this is accomplished by barium, a potent inhibitor of K^+ channels. This rare cause of hypokalemia is usually associated with ingestion of the rodenticide barium carbonate, either unintentionally or during a suicide attempt.[243] Suicidal ingestion of barium-containing shaving powder[244] and hair remover[245] has also been reported. Barium salts are widely used in industry, and poisoning by various mechanisms has been described in industrial accidents.[19,246] Treatment of barium poisoning with K^+ serves both to increase plasma K^+ and to displace barium from affected K^+ channels[243]; hemodialysis is also an effective treatment.[247] Hypokalemia is also common with chloroquine toxicity or overdose,[248] although the mechanism is not entirely clear.

Hypokalemic Periodic Paralysis

The periodic paralyses have both genetic and acquired causes, and are further subdivided into hyperkalemic and hypokalemic forms.[19,209-211] The genetic and secondary forms of hyperkalemic paralysis were discussed earlier (see "Consequences of Hyperkalemia" section). Autosomal dominant mutations in the *CACNA1S* gene encoding the α_1-subunit of L-type calcium channels are the most common genetic cause of HOKP type I, whereas type II HOKP is due to mutations in the *SCN4A* gene encoding the skeletal Na^+ channel.[249]

In Andersen's syndrome, autosomal dominant mutations in the *KCNJ2* gene encoding the inwardly rectifying K^+ channel Kir 2.1 cause periodic paralysis, cardiac arrhythmias, and dysmorphic features.[250] Paralysis in Andersen's syndrome can be normokalemic, hypokalemic, or hyperkalemic; however, the symptomatic trigger is consistent within individual kindreds.[250]

The pathophysiology of HOKP is not entirely clear. Structurally, more than 90% of the HOKP-associated mutations result in loss of positively charged arginine residues in the S4 voltage-sensor domains of L-type calcium channels and the skeletal Na^+ channel.[211] This generates a so-called gating current, generated by a cation leak through an aberrant pore. This abnormal cation leak may directly lead to K^+-dependent paradoxical depolarization and hypokalemic weakness.[251] Alternatively, changes in insulin-sensitive transport events may cause the hypokalemic weakness.

Reversible attacks of paralysis with hypokalemia in HOKP are typically precipitated by rest after exercise and/or meals rich in carbohydrate.[211] Although the induction of endogenous insulin by carbohydrate meals is thought to reduce plasma K^+, thus triggering weakness, insulin can precipitate paralysis in HOKP in the absence of significant hypokalemia.[252] The generation of action potentials and muscle contraction are reduced in type I and II HOKP muscle fibers exposed to insulin in vitro.[249,253] This effect is seen at an extracellular K^+ concentration of 4.0 mmol/L and is potentiated as K^+ level decreases.[253]

Type I HOKP muscles show reduced activity of adenosine triphosphate (ATP)–sensitive, inwardly rectifying K^+ channels (K_{ATP}),[254] which likely contributes to hypokalemia due to the resultant unopposed activity of muscle Na^+-K^+-ATPase.[255] Insulin inhibits the remaining K_{ATP} activity in muscle fibers of both patients with type I HOKP[253] and hypokalemic rats[256]; this leads to a depolarizing shift toward the equilibrium potential for the Cl^- ion (approximately 50 mV). At this potential, voltage-dependent Na^+ channels are largely inactivated, which results in paralysis.

Paralysis is associated with multiple other causes of hypokalemia, both acquired and genetic.[175,176,257] Renal causes of hypokalemia with paralysis include Fanconi's syndrome,[258] Gitelman's syndrome,[257] and the various causes of hypokalemic distal renal tubular acidosis.[26,259] The activity and regulation of skeletal muscle K_{ATP} channels is aberrant in animal models of hypokalemia, which suggests a muscle physiology parallel to that in genetic HOKP (see earlier). However, the pathophysiology of thyrotoxic periodic paralysis (TPP), a particularly important cause of hypokalemic paralysis, is distinctly different from that of HOKP; for example, despite the clinical similarities between the two syndromes, thyroxine has no effect on HOKP.

TPP is classically seen in patients of Asian origin, but also occurs at higher frequencies in Hispanic patients.[260] This shared predisposition has recently been linked to genetic variation in Kir 2.6, a muscle-specific, thyroid hormone–responsive K^+ channel.[27] Patients typically have weakness of the extremities and limb girdles, with attacks occurring most frequently between 1 and 6 AM. As in HOKP, paralytic attacks in TPP may be precipitated by rest and/or by carbohydrate-rich meals. Clinical signs and symptoms of hyperthyroidism are not invariably present.[260,261] Hypokalemia is profound, ranging between 1.1 and 3.4 mol/L, and is frequently accompanied by hypophosphatemia and hypomagnesemia.[260] All three abnormalities presumably contribute to the associated weakness.

Diagnostically, a TTKG of less than 2 to 3 separates patients with TPP from those with hypokalemia due to renal potassium wasting, who have TTKG values that are above 4.[165] This distinction is of considerable therapeutic relevance: patients with large potassium deficits require aggressive repletion with K^+-Cl^-, which has a significant risk of rebound hyperkalemia in patients with TPP and related disorders.[262] The hypokalemia in TPP is most likely due to both direct and indirect activation of Na^+-K^+-ATPase, given the evidence for increased activity in erythrocytes and platelets in TPP patients.[26,263] Thyroid hormone clearly induces expression of multiple subunits of the Na^+-K^+-ATPase in skeletal muscle.[264] Increases in β-adrenergic response due to hyperthyroidism also play an important role, since high-dose propranolol

(3 mg/kg) rapidly reverses the hypokalemia, hypophosphatemia, and paralysis seen in acute attacks.[265,266] Of particular importance, no rebound hyperkalemia is associated with this treatment, whereas aggressive K^+ replacement in TPP is associated with an incidence of approximately 25%[262]; repletion-associated rebound hyperkalemia in TPP can be fatal.[267]

Nonrenal Potassium Loss

The loss of K^+ from skin is typically low, with the exception of extremes in physical exertion.[9] Direct gastric loss of K^+ due to vomiting or nasogastric suctioning is also typically minimal; however, the ensuing hypochloremic alkalosis results in persistent kaliuresis due to secondary hyperaldosteronism and bicarbonaturia.[268,269] Intestinal loss of K^+ due to diarrhea is a quantitatively important cause of hypokalemia, given the worldwide prevalence of diarrheal disease, and may be associated with acute complications such as myopathy and flaccid paralysis.[270] The presence of a non–anion gap metabolic acidosis with a negative urinary anion gap[166] (consistent with an intact ability to increase NH_4^+ excretion) should strongly suggest diarrhea as a cause of hypokalemia. Polyethylene glycol–based bowel preparation regimens for colonoscopy can also lead to hypokalemia in elderly patients.[271]

Noninfectious gastrointestinal processes such as celiac disease,[272] ileostomy,[273] and chronic laxative abuse can present with acute hypokalemic syndromes or with chronic complications such as ESRD.[19] Three recent reports have identified a novel association between colonic pseudo-obstruction (Ogilvie's syndrome) and hypokalemia due to secretory diarrhea with an abnormally high K^+ content.[274-276] In one patient with concomitant ESRD, immunohistochemical analysis revealed massive upregulation of the apical BK channel throughout the surface-crypt axes.[274] Colonic BK channels may play a significant role in intestinal K^+ secretion in a variety of pathologic conditions, including ESRD.[277] Several hypotheses have been put forward to explain the association between Ogilvie's syndrome and enhanced intestinal K^+ secretion, including active stimulation by catecholamines induced by colonic pseudo-obstruction.[276] BK channels appear to mediate adrenaline-induced colonic K^+ secretion.[278]

Renal Potassium Loss

Drugs

Diuretics are an especially important cause of hypokalemia, due to their ability to increase distal flow rate and distal delivery of Na^+. Thiazides generally cause more hypokalemia[19,193,225] than do loop diuretics, despite their lower natriuretic efficacy. One potential explanation is the differential effect of loop diuretics and thiazides on calcium excretion. Whereas thiazides and loss-of-function mutations in the Na^+-Cl^- cotransporter decrease Ca^{2+} excretion,[279] loop diuretics cause a significant calciuresis.[280] Increases in luminal Ca^{2+} in the distal nephron serve to reduce the lumen-negative driving force for K^+ excretion,[281] perhaps by direct inhibition of ENaC in principal cells. A mechanistic explanation is provided by the presence of the apical calcium-sensing receptor (CaSR) in the collecting duct.[282] Analogous to the evident decrease in the apical trafficking of aquaporin-2 induced by luminal

Ca^{2+}, tubular Ca^{2+} may stimulate endocytosis of ENaC via the CaSR and thus limit generation of the lumen-negative potential difference that is so critical for distal K^+ excretion. Regardless of the underlying mechanism, the increase in distal delivery of Ca^{2+} induced by loop diuretics may serve to blunt kaliuresis. Such a mechanism would not occur with thiazides, which reduce distal delivery of Ca^{2+}, with unopposed activity of ENaC and increased kaliuresis.

Another drug associated with hypokalemia due to kaliuresis is acetaminophen, which at toxic levels causes dose-dependent hypokalemia.[283,284] High doses of penicillin-related antibiotics are another important cause of hypokalemia, increasing obligatory K^+ excretion by acting as nonreabsorbable anions in the distal nephron. In addition to penicillin, implicated antibiotics include nafcillin, dicloxacillin, ticarcillin, oxacillin, and carbenecillin.[285] Increased distal delivery of other anions such as SO_4^{2-} and HCO_3^- also induces kaliuresis. The usual explanation is that K^+ excretion increases so as to balance the negative charge of these nonreabsorbable anions. However, increased delivery of such anions also increases the electrochemical gradient for K^+-Cl^- exit via apical K^+-Cl^- cotransport or parallel K^+/H^+ and Cl^-/HCO_3^- exchange[65,79,80] (see also "Potassium Transport in the Distal Nephron" section).

Drugs are also an important cause of Fanconi's syndrome,[286] which is often associated with significant hypokalemia (see "Renal Tubular Acidosis" section). Several tubular toxins result in both K^+ and magnesium wasting. These include gentamicin, which can cause tubular toxicity with hypokalemia that can masquerade as Bartter's syndrome.[287] Other drugs that can cause mixed magnesium and K^+ wasting include amphotericin, foscarnet (an antiviral drug),[288] and cisplatin[19,289] and ifosfamide (both chemotherapeutic agents).[290]

One intriguing cause of hypomagnesemia and hypokalemia is cetuximab, a humanized monoclonal antibody specific for the receptor for epidermal growth factor (EGF).[291] Paracrine EGF stimulates magnesium transport via the apical TRPM6 cation channel in the DCT, with magnesium wasting and hypomagnesemia seen in patients treated with cetuximab.[292] Aggressive replacement of magnesium is obligatory in the treatment of combined hypokalemia and hypomagnesemia, because successful K^+ replacement depends on treatment of the hypomagnesemia.

Hyperaldosteronism

Increases in circulating aldosterone (hyperaldosteronism) may be primary or secondary. Increased levels of circulating renin in secondary forms of hyperaldosteronism lead to increased levels of angiotensin II and thus aldosterone, and can be associated with hypokalemia. Causes include renal artery stenosis,[293] Page kidney (renal compression by a subcapsular mass or hematoma with hyperreninemia),[294] a paraneoplastic process,[295] and renin-secreting renal tumors.[296] The incidence of hypokalemia in renal artery stenosis is thought to be less than 20%.[293] An unusual presentation of renal artery stenosis and renal ischemia is hyponatremic hypertensive syndrome, in which the concurrent hypokalemia may be profound.[297]

Primary hyperaldosteronism (PA) may be genetic or acquired. Hypertension and hypokalemia, generally attributed to increases in circulating 11-deoxycorticosterone,[298] are seen in patients with congenital adrenal hyperplasia due to defects in either steroid 11β-hydroxylase[298] or steroid

17α-hydroxylase.[299] Deficient 11β-hydroxylase results in virilization and other signs of androgen excess,[298] whereas reduced sex steroids in 17α-hydroxylase deficiency result in hypogonadism.[299]

The two major forms of isolated PA are denoted *familial hyperaldosteronism type I* (FH-I, also known as *glucocorticoid-remediable hyperaldosteronism* or GRA)[300] and *familial hyperaldosteronism type II* (FH-II), in which aldosterone production is not repressible by exogenous glucocorticoids. Patients with FH-II are clinically indistinguishable from those with sporadic forms of PA due to bilateral adrenal hyperplasia; a gene has been localized to chromosome region 7p22 by linkage analysis, but has yet to be characterized.[301] A kindred with a third form of familial hyperaldosteronism (FH-III) has also been recently described, with hyporeninemia, hyperaldosteronism resistant to dexamethasone, and very high levels of 18-oxocortisol and 18-hydroxycortisol.[302]

Patients with FH-I/GRA are generally hypertensive, with the disease typically manifesting at an early age; the severity of hypertension is variable, however, and some affected individuals are normotensive.[300] Aldosterone levels are modestly elevated and regulated solely by ACTH. The diagnosis can be biochemically confirmed by a dexamethasone suppression test, and a suppression of aldosterone level to less than 4 ng/dL is consistent with the diagnosis.[303] Patients also have high levels of abnormal "hybrid" 18-hydroxylated steroids, generated by transformation of steroids typically formed in the zona fasciculata by aldosterone synthase, an enzyme that is normally expressed in the zona glomerulosa.[304,305]

FH-I has been shown to be caused by a chimeric gene duplication between the homologous 11β-hydroxylase (*CYP11B1*) and aldosterone synthase (*CYP11B2*) genes, in which the ACTH-responsive 11β-hydroxylase promoter is fused to the coding region of aldosterone synthase. This chimeric gene is thus under the control of ACTH and is expressed in a glucocorticoid-repressible fashion.[304] Ectopic expression of the hybrid *CYP11B1-CYP11B2* gene in the zona fasciculata has been reported in a single case in which adrenal tissue became available for molecular analysis.[306] Direct genetic testing for the hybrid *CYP11B1-CYP11B2* has largely supplanted biochemical screening for FH-I; genetic testing for FH-I should be pursued in patients with PA and a family history of PA and/or of strokes at a young age, and in young patients with PA (<20 years of age).[307]

Although the first patients reported with FH-I were hypokalemic, the majority are in fact normokalemic,[305,308] albeit perhaps with a propensity to develop hypokalemia while taking thiazide diuretics.[305] Patients with FH-I are able to appropriately increase K[+] excretion in response to K[+] loading or fludrocortisone administration, but fail to increase plasma aldosterone level in response to hyperkalemia.[309] This may reflect the ectopic expression of the chimeric aldosterone synthase in the adrenal fasciculata, which likely lack the appropriate constellation of ion channels to respond to increases in extracellular K[+] with an increase in aldosterone secretion.

Acquired causes of PA include aldosterone-producing adenomas (APAs, 35% of cases), primary or unilateral adrenal hyperplasia (PAH, 2% of cases), idiopathic hyperaldosteronism (IHA) due to bilateral adrenal hyperplasia (60% of cases), and adrenal carcinoma (<1% of cases).[310] A rare case involving paraneoplastic overexpression of aldosterone synthase in lymphoma has also been described.[311]

Increasing use of the plasma aldosterone concentration (PAC)/plasma renin activity (PRA) ratio in hypertension clinics has led to reports of a much higher incidence of PA than previously appreciated, with incidence rates in patients with hypertension ranging from 0% to 72%[312]; however, the prevalence was 3.2% in a large, multicenter study of patients with mild to moderate hypertension without hypokalemia.[313]

Regardless, the PAC/PRA ratio is a screening tool, and results must be confirmed by aldosterone suppression testing in which PAC or aldosterone secretion is measured after loading with salt or intravenous saline.[307,310] After hypertension and hypokalemia are controlled, oral salt loading over 3 days is followed by measurement of 24-hour urine aldosterone, sodium, and creatinine excretion. The 24-hour sodium excretion should exceed 200 mmol/day for adequate suppression, and a urinary aldosterone level of more than 33 nmol/day is consistent with PA.

Alternatively, in the saline infusion test, recumbent patients are infused with 2 L of isotonic saline over 4 hours, and PAC is then measured. In patients without PA, the measured PAC after saline infusion should decrease to less than 139 pmol/L. The measured PAC in patients with PA usually does not suppress to less than 277 pmol/L. Indeterminate values between 139 and 277 pmol/L can been seen in patients with IHA.[310]

Because surgery can be curative in APA, adequate differentiation of APA from IHA is critical. this requires both adrenal imaging and adrenal venous sampling (Figure 17-9). Contemporary reports and recommendations have thus emphasized the continued importance of adrenal vein sampling in subtype differentiation.[307]

Laparoscopic adrenalectomy is increasingly the preferred surgical management in APA or PAH.[307,310] Mineralocorticoid receptor antagonists are indicated for medical treatment of PA, with carefully monitored use of glucocorticoid to suppress ACTH in some patients with FH-I/GRA.[307,310]

The true incidence of hypokalemia in patients with acquired forms of PA remains difficult to evaluate, due to a variety of factors. First, historically, patients have only been screened for hyperaldosteronism when hypokalemia is present; hence, even recent case series from clinics with such a referral pattern may suffer from a selection bias; other recent series have concentrated on hypertensive patients, which is also a selection bias. Second, the incidence of hypokalemia is higher in adrenal adenomas than in IHA, likely due to higher average levels of aldosterone.[314] Third, since increased kaliuresis in hyperaldosteronism can be induced by dietary Na[+]-Cl[-] loading or diuretic use, dietary factors and/or medications may play a role in the incidence of hypokalemia at presentation.

Regardless, it is clear that hypokalemia is not a universal feature of PA. This is perhaps not unexpected, because aldosterone does not appear to affect the hypokalemic response of H[+]-K[+]-ATPase,[315] the major reabsorptive pathway for K[+] in the distal nephron (see also Chapter 5). A related issue is whether PA is underdiagnosed when hypokalemia is used as a criterion for further investigation. The utility of the PAC/PRA ratio in screening for hyperaldosteronism is an active issue in hypertension research.[312,313]

Finally, hypokalemia may also occur with systemic increases in glucocorticoids.[316,317] In bona fide Cushing's syndrome caused by increases in pituitary ACTH the incidence of hypokalemia is only 10%,[316] whereas it is 57%[317] to 100%[316] in patients with ectopic ACTH expression, despite a

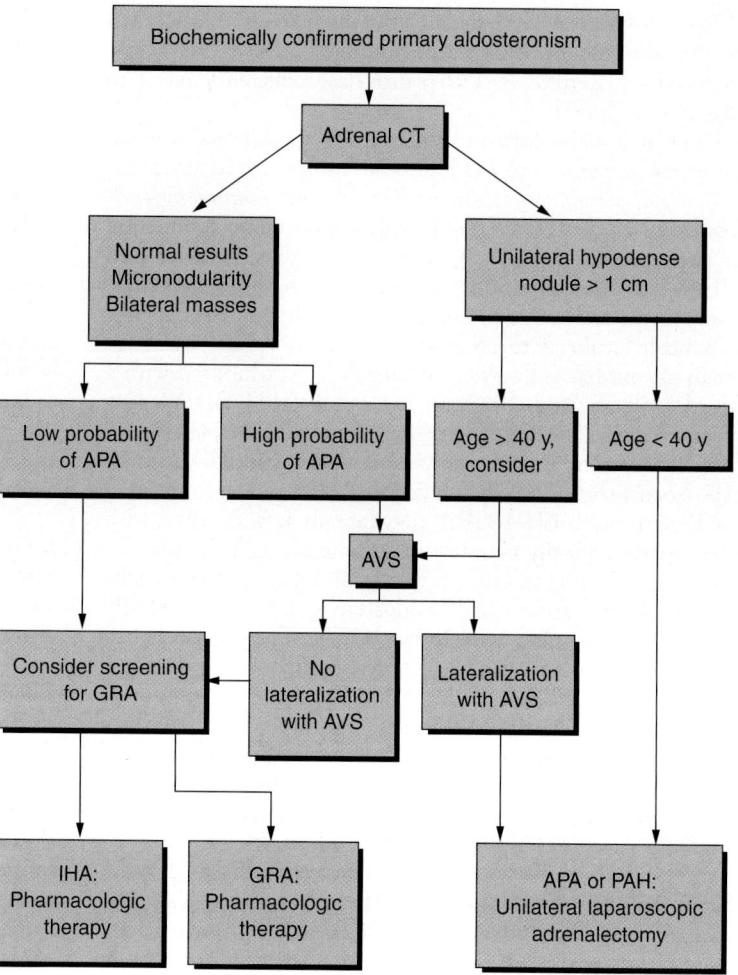

FIGURE 17-9 Diagnostic algorithm for patients with primary hyperaldosteronism. Hyperaldosteronism caused by adrenal adenoma (APA) must be distinguished from glucocorticoid-remediable hyperaldosteronism (GRA, or familial hyperaldosteronism type I [FH-I], primary or unilateral adrenal hyperplasia (PAH), and idiopathic hyperaldosteronism (IHA). This requires computed axial tomography (CT), adrenal venous sampling (AVS), and the relevant diagnostic biochemical and hormonal assays (see text). (From Young WF Jr: Adrenalectomy for primary aldosteronism, *Ann Intern Med* 138[2]:157-159, 2003.)

similar incidence of hypertension. Ectopic ACTH expression is associated primarily with neuroendocrine malignancies, most commonly bronchial carcinoid tumors, small cell lung cancer, and other neuroendocrine tumors.[318]

Indirect evidence suggests that the activity of renal 11β-hydroxysteroid dehydrogenase type 2 (11β-HSD2) is lower in patients with ectopic ACTH expression than in those with Cushing's syndrome,[319] which results in a syndrome of apparent mineralocorticoid excess (see next section). Whether this reflects a greater degree of saturation of the enzyme by circulating cortisol or direct inhibition of 11β-HSD2 by ACTH is not entirely clear, and there is evidence for both mechanisms[317]; however, indirect indices of 11β-HSD2 activity in patients with ectopic ACTH expression correlate with hypokalemia and other measures of mineralocorticoid activity.[320] Similar mechanisms likely underlie the severe hypokalemia reported in patients with familial glucocorticoid resistance, in which loss-of-function mutations in the glucocorticoid receptor result in marked hypercortisolism without cushingoid features, accompanied by very high ACTH levels.[321]

Syndromes of Apparent Mineralocorticoid Excess

The syndromes of apparent mineralocorticoid excess (AME) have a self-explanatory label. In the classical form of AME, recessive loss-of-function mutations in the 11β-HSD2 gene cause a defect in the peripheral conversion of cortisol to the inactive glucocorticoid cortisone. The resulting increase in the half-life of cortisol is associated with a marked decrease in synthesis, so that plasma levels of cortisol are normal and patients do not have cushingoid features.[322]

The 11β-HSD2 protein is expressed in epithelial cells that are targets for aldosterone. In the kidney, these include cells of the DCT, CNT, and CCD.[323] Since the mineralocorticoid receptor has equivalent affinity for aldosterone and cortisol, generation of cortisone by 11β-HSD2 serves to protect mineralocorticoid-responsive cells from illicit activation by cortisol.[324] In patients with AME, the unregulated mineralocorticoid effect of glucocorticoids results in hypertension, hypokalemia, and metabolic alkalosis, with suppressed PRA and aldosterone.[322] Biochemical diagnosis entails measuring the urinary free cortisol/urinary free cortisone ratio in a 24-hour urine collection.

Biochemical studies of mutant enzymes usually indicate a complete loss of function. Lesser enzymatic defects in patients with AME are associated with altered ratios of urinary cortisone/cortisol metabolites,[325] lesser impairment in the peripheral conversion of cortisol to cortisone,[326] and/or older age at presentation.[327]

Mice with a homozygous targeted deletion of the 11β-HSD2 gene exhibit hypertension, hypokalemia, and polyuria; the polyuria is likely secondary to the hypokalemia (see "Renal Consequences" section under "Consequences of Hypokalemia"), which reaches 2.4 mmol/mL in 11β-HSD2–null mice.[328] As expected, both PRA and plasma aldosterone in the 11β-HSD2–null mice are profoundly suppressed, with a decreased urinary Na+/K+ ratio that is increased by dexamethasone (given to suppress endogenous cortisol). These knockout mice have significant nephromegaly, due to a massive hypertrophy and hyperplasia of DCTs.

The relative effect of genotype on the morphology of cells in the DCT, CNT, and CCD was not determined by the appropriate phenotypic studies[329]; however, it is known that both the DCT and the CCD are target cells for aldosterone[330,331] and both cell types express 11β-HSD2. The induction of ENaC activity by unregulated glucocorticoid likely causes the Na+ retention and the marked increase in K+ excretion in 11β-HSD2–null mice. Results of distal tubular micropuncture studies in rats treated with a systemic inhibitor of 11β-HSD2 are consistent with such a mechanism.[332]

In addition, the cellular "gain of-function" in the DCT would be expected to be associated with hypercalciuria, given the phenotype of pseudohypoaldosteronism type 2 and Gitelman's syndrome (see "Hereditary Tubular Defects of Potassium Excretion" and "Gitelman's Syndrome" sections); indeed, patients with AME are reported to exhibit nephrocalcinosis.[322]

Pharmacologic inhibition of 11β-HSD2 is also associated with hypokalemia and AME. The most infamous offender is licorice, in its multiple guises (licorice root, tea, candies, herbal remedies, and so on). The early observations that licorice required small amounts of cortisol to exert its kaliuretic effect, in the addisonian absence of endogenous glucocorticoid,[333] presaged the observations that its active ingredients (glycyrrhetinic/glycyrrhizinic acid and carbenoxolone) inhibit 11β-HSD2 and related enzymes.[322] Licorice intake remains considerable in European countries, particularly Iceland, The Netherlands, and Scandinavia.[334] Pontefract cakes, eaten both as sweets and as a laxative, are a continued source of licorice in the United Kingdom,[334] and licorice is an ingredient in several popular sweeteners and preservatives in Malaysia.[335] Glycyrrhizinic acid is used in Japan to treat hepatitis and has been under evaluation elsewhere for the management of hepatitis C; AME has been reported with its use for this indication.[336] Glycyrrhizinic acid is also a component of Chinese herbal remedies, prescribed for disorders such as allergic rhinitis.[337] Pharmacologic inhibition of 11β-HSD2 has also been tested in patients with ESRD as a novel mechanism to control hyperkalemia (see "Treatment of Hyperkalemia" section).[338] Carbenoxolone in turn is used in some countries in the management of peptic ulcer disease.[322]

Finally, a mechanistically distinct form of AME has been reported caused by a gain-of-function mutation in the mineralocorticoid receptor.[339] A single kindred was described with autosomal dominant inheritance of severe hypertension and hypokalemia. The causative mutation involves a serine residue that is conserved in the mineralocorticoid receptor from multiple species, yet differs in other nuclear steroid receptors. This mutation results in constitutive activation of the mineralocorticoid receptor in the absence of ligand and induces significant affinity for progesterone.[339] The mineralocorticoid receptor is thus constitutively "on" in these patients, with a marked stimulation by progesterone. Of interest, pregnancies in the affected female members of the family have all been complicated by severe hypertension, due to marked increases in plasma progesterone induced by the gravid state.[339] Spironolactone can paradoxically activate this mutant receptor.

Liddle's Syndrome

Liddle's syndrome is associated with an autosomal dominant gain-in-function mutation in ENaC, the amiloride-sensitive Na+ channel of the CNT and CCD.[340] Patients manifest severe hypertension with hypokalemia, unresponsive to spironolactone yet sensitive to triamterene and amiloride. Liddle's syndrome could therefore also be classified as a syndrome of AME. Both hypertension and hypokalemia are variable aspects of the Liddle's phenotype. Consistent features include a blunted aldosterone response to ACTH and reduced urinary aldosterone excretion.[95,341] The differential diagnosis for Liddle's syndrome, as a cause of hereditary hypertension with hypokalemia and suppressed aldosterone levels, includes AME due to deficient 11β-HSD2; however, whereas patients with a Liddle's syndrome phenotype are resistant to blockade of the mineralocorticoid receptor with spironolactone and sensitive to amiloride, AME patients are sensitive to both drugs. Commercial genetic testing for both syndromes is available in the United States.

The overwhelming majority of mutations target the C terminus of either the β or γ ENaC subunit. ENaC channels containing Liddle's syndrome mutations are constitutively overexpressed at the cell membrane.[96,342] Unlike wild-type ENaC channels, they are not sensitive to inhibition by intracellular Na+,[343] an important regulator of endogenous channel activity in the CCD.[344] The mechanism whereby mutations in the C terminus of ENaC subunits lead to this channel phenotype were discussed earlier in this chapter (see Figure 17-5 and "Aldosterone" section).

In addition to effects on interaction with Nedd4-2–dependent retrieval from the plasma membrane, Liddle's-associated mutations increase proteolytic cleavage of ENaC at the cell membrane.[3] Aldosterone-induced channel-activating proteases activate ENaC channels at the plasma membrane. This important result provides a mechanistic explanation for the long-standing observation that Liddle's-associated mutations in ENaC appear to have a dual activating effect: on both the open probability of the channel (i.e., on channel activity) and on expression at the cell membrane.[96]

Given the overlapping and synergistic mechanisms that regulate ENaC activity, it stands to reason that mutations in ENaC that give rise to Liddle's syndrome might do so by a variety of means. Indeed, mutation of a residue within the extracellular domain of ENaC increases the open probability of the channel without changing surface expression; the patient with this mutation has a typical Liddle's syndrome phenotype.[345]

Extensive searches for more common mutations and polymorphisms in ENaC subunits that correlate with blood pressure in the general population have essentially been negative. However, there are a handful of genetic studies that correlate specific variants in ENaC subunits with biochemical evidence of greater in vivo activity of the channel, that is, suppression of PRA and aldosterone, and/or increased ratios of urinary K+ level to aldosterone or to PRA.[346,347]

Familial Hypokalemic Alkalosis

Bartter's and Gitelman's syndromes are the two major variants of familial hypokalemic alkalosis. Gitelman's syndrome is a much more common cause of hypokalemia than is Bartter's syndrome.[348] Although a clinical subdivision of these syndromes has been used in the past, a genetic classification is increasingly in use, due in part to phenotypic overlap.

Bartter's Syndrome

Patients with classical Bartter's syndrome typically have polyuria and polydipsia, and manifest a hypokalemic, hypochloremic alkalosis. They may have an increase in urinary calcium (Ca^{2+}) excretion, and 20% are hypomagnesemic.[349] Other features include marked elevation of plasma angiotensin II, plasma aldosterone, and plasma renin levels. Patients with antenatal Bartter's syndrome present earlier in life with a severe systemic disorder characterized by marked electrolyte wasting, polyhydramnios, and significant hypercalciuria with nephrocalcinosis. Prostaglandin synthesis and excretion are significantly increased and may account for many of the systemic symptoms.

Decreasing prostaglandin synthesis by cyclooxygenase inhibition can improve polyuria in patients with Bartter's syndrome by reducing the amplifying inhibition of urinary concentrating mechanisms by prostaglandins. Indomethacin also increases plasma K^+ concentration and decreases plasma renin activity, but does not correct the basic tubular defect. It does, however, appear to help increase the growth of Bartter's syndrome patients.[350] Of interest, COX-2 immunoreactivity is increased in the TAL and macula densa of patients with Bartter's syndrome,[351] and reports indicate a clinical benefit of COX-2 inhibitors.[352]

Early studies of Bartter's syndrome suggested that these patients had a defect in the function of the TAL.[353] Many of the clinical features are mimicked by the administration of loop diuretics, to which at least a subset of patients with antenatal Bartter's syndrome do not respond.[354] The apical Na^+-K^+-$2Cl^-$ cotransporter (NKCC2/SLC12A1) of the mammalian TAL[24] (Figure 17-10) was thus an early candidate gene. In 1996, disease-associated mutations were found in the human NKCC2 gene in four kindreds with antenatal Bartter's syndrome.[355] In the genetic classification of Bartter's syndrome, these patients are considered to have Bartter's syndrome type 1. Although the functional consequences of disease-associated NKCC2 mutations have not been comprehensively studied, the first[355] and subsequent reports[26] included patients with frameshift mutations and premature stop codons that predict the absence of a functional NKCC2 protein.

Bartter's syndrome is a genetically heterogeneous disease and shows allelic heterogeneity. Given the role of apical K^+ permeability in the TAL, encoded at least in part by ROMK,[75,356] this K^+ channel was another early candidate gene. K^+ recycling via the Na^+-K^+-$2Cl^-$ cotransporter and apical K^+ channels generates a lumen-positive potential difference in the TAL, which drives the paracellular transport of Na^+ and other cations[357] (see Figure 17-10). Multiple disease-associated mutations in ROMK have been reported in patients with Bartter's syndrome type 2, most of whom exhibit the antenatal phenotype.[350,358]

Finally, mutations in Bartter's syndrome type 3 have been reported in the chloride channel ClC-NKb,[359] which is expressed at the basolateral membrane of at least the TAL and DCT.[360] Patients with mutations in CLCNKB typically have the classical Bartter's phenotype, with a relative absence of nephrocalcinosis.

In a significant fraction of patients with Bartter's syndrome the NKCC2, ROMK, and CLCNKB genes are not involved.[359] For example, a subset of patients with associated sensorineural deafness exhibit linkage to chromosome band 1p31.[26] The gene for this syndrome, denoted BARTTIN, encodes a protein that is an obligatory subunit for the ClC-NKb chloride channel.[361] The occurrence of deafness in these patients suggests that barttin functions in the regulation or function of Cl^- channels in the inner ear. Notably, the CLCNKB gene is immediately adjacent to that for another epithelial Cl^- channel, denoted ClC-NKa. Digenic inactivation was described in two siblings with deafness and Bartter's syndrome,[362] which suggests that ClC-NKa plays an important role in barttin-dependent Cl^- transport in the inner ear.

Patients with autosomal dominant activating mutations in the CaSR have been described with hypocalcemia and hypokalemic alkalosis.[363,364] The CaSR is heavily expressed at the basolateral membrane of the TAL,[365] where it is thought to play an important inhibitory role in regulating the transcellular transport of both Na^+-Cl^- and Ca^{2+}. For example, activation of the basolateral CaSR in the TAL is known to reduce apical K^+ channel activity,[366] which would induce a Bartter's-like syndrome (see Figure 17-10). Genetic activation of the CaSR by these mutations was also expected to increase urinary Ca^{2+} excretion by inhibiting generation of the lumen-positive potential difference that drives paracellular Ca^{2+} transport in the TAL. In addition, the set point of the CaSR

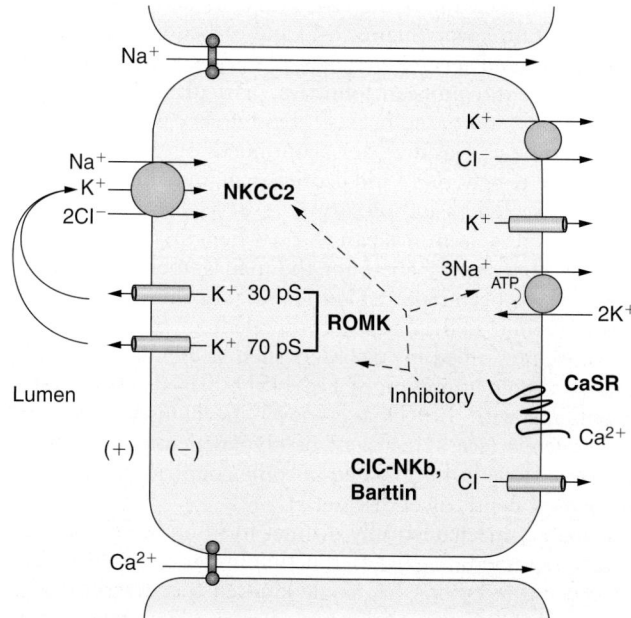

FIGURE 17-10 Bartter's syndrome and the thick ascending limb. Bartter's syndrome can result from loss-of-function mutations in the Na^+-K^+-$2Cl^-$ cotransporter NKCC2, the ROMK (renal outer medullary potassium) subunit of the K^+ channel, or the ClC-NKb and barttin subunits of the Cl^- channel (causing Bartter's syndrome types 1 to 4, respectively). Gain-of-function mutations in the calcium-sensing receptor CaSR can also cause a Bartter's syndrome phenotype (type 5). The CaSR has an inhibitory effect on salt transport by the thick ascending limb, targeting several transport pathways. ROMK encodes the low-conductance 30-picosiemens K^+ channel in the apical membrane and also appears to function as a critical subunit of the higher-conductance 70-picosiemens channel. The loss of K^+ channel activity in Bartter's syndrome type 2 leads to reduced apical K^+ recycling and reduced Na^+-K^+-$2Cl^-$ cotransport. Decrease in apical K^+ channels also leads to a decrease in the lumen-positive potential difference, which drives paracellular Na^+, Ca^{2+}, and Mg^{2+} transport.

response to Ca^{2+} in the parathyroid is shifted to the left, which inhibits parathyroid hormone (PTH) secretion by this gland. No doubt the positional cloning of other Bartter's syndrome genes will have a considerable impact on mechanistic understanding of the TAL.

Despite the reasonable correlation between the disease gene involved and the associated subtype of familial alkalosis, there is significant phenotypic overlap and phenotypic variability in hereditary hypokalemic alkalosis. For example, patients with mutations in *CLCNKB* most frequently exhibit classical Bartter's syndrome, but can present with a more severe antenatal phenotype, or even with a phenotype similar to that of Gitelman's syndrome.[26,367] With respect to Bartter's syndrome due to mutations in *NKCC2*, a number of patients have been described with variant presentations, including an absence of hypokalemia.[26] Two brothers were described with a late onset of mild Bartter's syndrome; these patients were found to be compound heterozygotes for a mutant form of *NKCC2* that exhibits partial function, with a loss-of-function mutation on the other *NKCC2* allele.[368]

Bartter's syndrome type 2 is particularly relevant to K^+ homeostasis, given that ROMK is the SK secretory channel of the CNT and CCD (see "Potassium Transport in the Distal Nephron" section). Patients with Bartter's syndrome type 2 typically have slightly higher plasma K^+ concentrations than those with the other genetic forms of Bartter's syndrome.[358,367] Patients with severe (9.0 mmol/L) transient neonatal hyperkalemia have also been described.[369] It is likely that this reflects a transient, developmental deficit in the other K^+ channels involved in distal K^+ secretion, including the apical maxi-K/BK channel responsible for flow-dependent K^+ secretion in the distal nephron.[74,370] Distal K^+ secretion in ROMK knockout mice is primarily mediated by maxi-K/BK channel activity,[371] so that developmental deficits in this channel would indeed lead to hyperkalemia in Bartter's syndrome type 2. The mammalian TAL has two major apical K^+ channels with different conductances, the 30-picosiemens channel corresponding to ROMK, and a 70-picosiemens channel.[372] Both are thought to play a role in transepithelial salt transport by the TAL. ROMK is evidently a subunit of the 70-picosiemens channel, given the absence of this conductance in TAL segments of ROMK knockout mice.[373] The identity of the other putative subunit of this 70-picosiemens channel is not yet known. One would assume that deficiencies in the associated gene would also be a cause of Bartter's syndrome.

Finally, Bartter's syndrome must be clinically differentiated from "pseudo–Bartter's syndrome." The common causes of the latter include laxative abuse, furosemide abuse, and bulimia (see "Clinical Approach to Hypokalemia" section). Other reported causes include gentamicin nephrotoxicity,[287] Sjögren's syndrome,[26] and cystic fibrosis.[26,374] Fixed loss of Na^+-Cl^- in sweat is likely the dominant predisposing factor for hypokalemic alkalosis in patients with cystic fibrosis. Patients with this presentation generally respond promptly to administration of intravenous fluids and electrolyte replacement. However, the cystic fibrosis transmembrane regulator (CFTR) protein coassociates with ROMK in the TAL and confers sensitivity to both ATP and glibenclamide to apical K^+ channels in this nephron segment.[375] Lu and colleagues have proposed that this interaction serves to modulate the response of ROMK to cAMP and vasopressin, so that in patients with CFTR deficiency K^+ excretion would not be appropriately reduced during water diuresis, which would predispose such patients to the development of hypokalemic alkalosis.[375]

Gitelman's Syndrome

A major advance in the understanding of hereditary alkaloses was the realization that a subset of patients exhibit marked hypocalciuria, rather than the hypercalciuria typically seen in Bartter's syndrome. Patients in this hypocalciuric subset are universally hypomagnesemic.[279] Such patients are now clinically classified as having Gitelman's syndrome. Although plasma renin activity may be increased, renal prostaglandin excretion is not elevated in these hypocalciuric patients,[376] another feature distinguishing Bartter's and Gitelman's syndromes.

Gitelman's syndrome is a milder disorder than Bartter's syndrome; however, patients do report significant morbidity, mostly related to muscular symptoms and fatigue.[377] The QT interval is frequently prolonged in Gitelman's syndrome, which suggests an increased risk of cardiac arrhythmia[378]; however, a more exhaustive cardiac evaluation of a large group of patients failed to detect significant abnormalities of cardiac structure or rhythm.[379] Nevertheless, presyncope and/or ventricular tachycardia has been observed in at least two patients with Gitelman's syndrome,[26,173] one with concomitant LQTS due to a mutation in the cardiac KCNQ1 K^+ channel.[173]

The hypocalciuria detected in Gitelman's syndrome is an expected consequence of inactivation of the thiazide-sensitive Na^+-Cl^- cotransporter NCC (SLC12A2), and loss-of-function mutations in the human gene have been reported.[380] Many of these mutations lead to a defect in cellular trafficking when introduced into the human NCC protein.[381]

Gitelman's syndrome is genetically homogeneous, except for the occasional patient with mutations in *CLCNKB* and an overlapping phenotype.[26,173,367] However, genetic analysis is not generally available, given the significant number of exons in SLC12A2 and the absence of "hot-spot" mutations in this disorder. One diagnostic alternative is to assess the physiologic response to thiazides; patients with Gitelman's syndrome have a blunted excretion of chloride after the administration of hydrochlorothiazide.[382]

The NCC protein has been localized to the apical membrane of epithelial cells in the DCT and CNT. A mouse strain with targeted deletion of the *Slc12a2* gene encoding NCC exhibits hypocalciuria and hypomagnesemia, with a mild alkalosis and marked increase in circulating aldosterone.[383] These knockout mice exhibit marked morphologic defects in the early DCT,[383] with both a reduction in absolute number of DCT cells and changes in ultrastructural appearance. That Gitelman's syndrome is a disorder of cellular development and/or cellular apoptosis should perhaps not be a surprise, given the observation that thiazide treatment promotes marked apoptosis of this nephron segment.[384] This cellular deficit leads to downregulation of the DCT magnesium channel TRPM6,[385] which results in the magnesium wasting and hypomagnesemia seen in Gitelman's syndrome.

The downstream CNT tubules are hypertrophied in NCC-deficient mice,[383] reminiscent of the hypertrophic DCT and CNT segments seen in furosemide-treated animals.[26] These CNT cells also exhibit an increased expression of ENaC at their apical membranes compared with littermate controls.[383] This is likely due to activation of SGK1-dependent trafficking of ENaC by the increase in circulating aldosterone (see "Aldosterone" section). Hypokalemia does not occur in NCC$^{-/-}$ mice on a standard rodent diet, but emerges on a K$^+$-restricted diet. The plasma K$^+$ concentration of these mice is approximately 1 mmol/L lower than that of K$^+$-restricted littermate controls.[386]

Several mechanisms account for the hypokalemia seen in Gitelman's syndrome and NCC$^{-/-}$ mice. The distal delivery of both Na$^+$ and fluid is decreased in NCC$^{-/-}$ mice, at least with consumption of a normal diet; however, the increased circulating aldosterone and CNT hypertrophy likely compensate, which leads to increased kaliuresis. As discussed earlier with regard to thiazides, decreased luminal Ca^{2+} in NCC deficiency may augment baseline ENaC activity,[281] further exacerbating the kaliuresis. Of particular interest, NCC-deficient mice develop considerable polydipsia and polyuria on a K$^+$-restricted diet.[386] This is reminiscent perhaps of the polydipsia that has been implicated in thiazide-associated hyponatremia.[387]

Hypocalciuria in Gitelman's syndrome is not accompanied by changes in plasma calcium, phosphate, vitamin D, or PTH levels,[388] which suggests a direct effect on renal calcium transport. The late DCT is morphologically intact in NCC-deficient mice, with preserved expression of epithelial calcium channel 1 (ECaC1, or TRPV5) and the basolateral Na$^+$/Ca^{2+} exchanger.[383] Furthermore, the hypocalciuric effect of thiazides persists in mice deficient in TRPV5,[385] which argues against the putative effects of this drug on distal Ca^{2+} absorption. Rather, several lines of evidence suggest that the hypocalciuria of Gitelman's syndrome and thiazide treatment is due to increased absorption of Na$^+$ by the proximal tubule,[383,385] with secondary increases in proximal Ca^{2+} absorption.

Regardless, reminiscent of the clinical effect of thiazides on bone, there are clear differences in bone density between affected and unaffected members of specific Gitelman kindreds. Thus homozygous patients have much higher bone densities than unaffected family members with wild-type genes, whereas heterozygotes have intermediate values of both bone density and calcium excretion.[388] An interesting association has repeatedly been described between chondrocalcinosis, the abnormal deposition of calcium pyrophosphate dihydrate in joint cartilage, and Gitelman's syndrome.[389] Patients have also been reported with ocular choroidal calcification.[390]

Finally, as in Bartter's syndrome, there are reports of patients with acquired tubular defects that mimic Gitelman's syndrome. These include patients with hypokalemic alkalosis, hypomagnesemia, and hypocalciuria after chemotherapy with cisplatin.[391] Patients have also been described with acquired Gitelman's syndrome due to Sjögren's syndrome and tubulointerstitial nephritis,[26,392] with a documented absence of coding sequence mutations in NCC.[392]

Renal Tubular Acidosis

Renal tubular acidosis (RTA) and related tubular defects can be associated with hypokalemia. Proximal RTA is characterized by a reduction in proximal bicarbonate absorption, with a reduced plasma bicarbonate concentration. Isolated proximal RTA is quite rare; genetic causes include loss of function due to mutations in the basolateral Na$^+$-HCO$_3^-$ transporter. More commonly, proximal RTA occurs in the context of multiple proximal tubular transport defects, encompassing Fanconi's syndrome.[286]

The cardinal features of Fanconi's syndrome are hyperaminoaciduria, glycosuria with a normal plasma glucose concentration, and phosphate wasting. Associated defects include proximal RTA, hypouricemia, hypercalciuria, hypokalemia, salt wasting, and increased excretion of low molecular weight proteins. Fanconi's syndrome is most commonly drug associated. Important contemporary causes include aristolochic acid, ifosfamide, and the acyclic nucleoside phosphonates (tenofovir, cidofovir, and adefovir).[286]

Prior to treatment with bicarbonate, patients with proximal RTA typically demonstrate mild hypokalemia, due primarily to baseline hyperaldosteronism[393]; however, patients have been described with profound hypokalemia on presentation, before treatment.[394] Regardless, treatment with oral sodium bicarbonate markedly increases distal tubular Na$^+$ and HCO$_3^-$ delivery, causing a marked increase in renal potassium wasting.[393] Patients often require mixed base replacement with oral citrate and bicarbonate, in addition to aggressive K$^+$-Cl$^-$ supplementation.

Hypokalemia is also associated with distal RTA, the so-called type 1 RTA. Hypokalemic distal RTA is most commonly due to a secretory defect, with reduced H$^+$-ATPase activity and decreased ability to acidify the urine. For example, hereditary defects in subunits of H$^+$-ATPase are associated with profound hypokalemia, in addition to acidosis and hypercalciuria.[395] The pathophysiology of the associated hypokalemia is multifactorial, due to the loss of electrogenic H$^+$ secretion (with enhanced K$^+$ secretion to maintain electroneutrality in the distal nephron), loss of H$^+$-K$^+$-ATPase activity, and increases in aldosterone.[396,397] Sjögren's syndrome is perhaps the most common cause of hypokalemic distal RTA in adults. The associated hypokalemia can be truly profound, often resulting in marked weakness and respiratory arrest.[397]

Magnesium Deficiency

Magnesium deficiency results in refractory hypokalemia, particularly if the plasma Mg^{2+} is less than 0.5 mmol/L[222]; in hypomagnesemic patients hypokalemia is thus resistant to K$^+$ replacement in the absence of Mg^{2+} repletion.[398,399] Magnesium deficiency is also a common concomitant of hypokalemia, in part because associated tubular disorders (e.g., aminoglycoside nephrotoxicity) may cause both kaliuresis and magnesium wasting. Plasma Mg^{2+} levels thus must be checked routinely in patients with hypokalemia.[221,400]

Several mechanisms appear to contribute to the effect of magnesium depletion on plasma K$^+$ concentration. Magnesium depletion has inhibitory effects on muscle Na$^+$-K$^+$-ATPase activity,[401] which results in significant efflux from muscle and a secondary kaliuresis. Distal K$^+$ secretion also appears to be enhanced due to a reduction in the normal physiologic inward rectification of ROMK secretory K$^+$ channels, with a subsequent increase in outward conductance.[402] ROMK and other Kir channels are inwardly rectifying, that is, K$^+$ flows inward more readily than outward. Even though outward conductance is usually less than inward conductance, K$^+$ efflux predominates in the CNT and CCD because the membrane potential is more positive than the equilibrium potential for K$^+$. Intracellular Mg^{2+} plays a key role in inward rectification, binding and blocking the pore of the channel from the cytoplasmic side.[402] The hypomagnesemia-associated reduction in cytoplasmic Mg^{2+} in principal cells reduces inward rectification of ROMK, which increases outward conductance and increases K$^+$ secretion. Finally, it has been suggested that the repletion of intracellular K$^+$ is impaired in hypomagnesemia, even in normokalemic patients.[400] Decreased intracellular Mg^{2+} enhances K$^+$ efflux from the cytoplasm of cardiac and perhaps skeletal myocytes, likely due to reduced intracellular blockade of inwardly rectifying K$^+$ channels (increased efflux) and inhibition of Na$^+$-K$^+$-ATPase (decreased influx). Plasma K$^+$ levels thus remain normal at the expense of intracellular K$^+$.[19,400,403] This phenomenon is particularly important in patients with cardiac disease who are taking both diuretics and digoxin. In such patients hypokalemia and arrhythmias will respond to correction of magnesium deficiency and potassium supplementation.[19,400]

Clinical Approach to Hypokalemia

The initial priority in the evaluation of hypokalemia is an assessment for signs and/or symptoms (muscle weakness, ECG changes, etc.) suggestive of an impending emergency that requires immediate treatment. The cause of hypokalemia is usually obvious from the history, physical examination, and/or results of basic laboratory tests. However, persistent hypokalemia despite appropriate initial intervention requires a more rigorous workup. In most cases, a systematic approach reveals the underlying cause (Figure 17-11).

The history should focus on medications (e.g., diuretics, laxatives, antibiotics, herbal medications), diet and dietary supplements (e.g., licorice), and associated symptoms (e.g., diarrhea). During the physical examination, particular attention should be paid to blood pressure, volume status, and signs suggestive of specific disorders associated with hypokalemia (hyperthyroidism, Cushing's syndrome, etc.).

Initial laboratory tests should include plasma electrolyte, urea, and creatinine levels; plasma osmolality; plasma Mg^{2+} and Ca^{2+} concentrations; a complete blood count; and urinary pH, osmolality, creatinine level, and electrolyte levels. Plasma and urine osmolality are required for calculation of the TTKG[161] (see "Urinary Indices of Potassium Excretion" section). A TTKG of less than 2 to 3 separates patients with redistributive hypokalemia from those with hypokalemia due to renal potassium wasting, who will have TTKG values that are above 4.[165] Further tests such as urinary Mg^{2+} and Ca^{2+} and plasma renin and aldosterone levels may be necessary in specific cases (see Figure 17-11). The timing and evolution of hypokalemia is also helpful in differentiating the cause, particularly in hospitalized patients; for example, hypokalemia due to transcellular shift usually occurs in a matter of hours.[404]

The most common causes of chronic, difficult-to-diagnose hypokalemia are Gitelman's syndrome, surreptitious vomiting, and diuretic abuse.[405] Alternatively, an associated acidosis suggests the diagnosis of hypokalemic distal or proximal RTA. Hypokalemia was found to occur in 5.5% of patients with eating disorders in an American study in the mid-1990s,[406] mostly in those with surreptitious vomiting (bulimia) or laxative abuse (the purging[269] subtype of anorexia nervosa). These patients may have a constellation of associated symptoms and signs, including dental erosion and depression.[407] Hypokalemic patients with bulimia will have an associated metabolic alkalosis, with an obligatory natriuresis accompanying the loss of bicarbonate; urinary Cl$^-$ concentration is typically less than 10 mmol/L, and this clue can often yield the diagnosis.[405,408] Urinary electrolyte levels, however, are generally unremarkable in unselected, mostly normokalemic patients with bulimia.[407]

Urinary excretion of Na$^+$, K$^+$, and Cl$^-$ is high in patients who abuse diuretics, albeit not to the levels seen in Gitelman's syndrome. Marked variability in urinary electrolyte levels is an important clue to diuretic abuse, which can be verified using urinary drug screens. Clinically, nephrocalcinosis is very common in furosemide abuse, due to the increase in urinary calcium excretion.[409]

Differentiation of Gitelman's syndrome from Bartter's syndrome requires a 24-hour urine collection to assess calcium excretion, because hypocalciuria is a distinguishing feature of the former.[279] Patients with Gitelman's syndrome are also invariably hypomagnesemic. Bartter's syndrome must be differentiated from pseudo–Bartter's syndrome due to gentamicin toxicity,[287,410] mutations in the cystic fibrosis gene (CFTR),[374,411] or Sjögren's syndrome with tubulointerstitial nephritis.[412] Acquired forms of Gitelman's syndrome have been reported after cisplatin therapy[391] and in patients with Sjögren's syndrome.[26,392]

Finally, although laxative abuse is perhaps a less common cause of chronic hypokalemia, an accompanying metabolic acidosis with a negative urinary anion gap should raise suspicion for this diagnosis.[166]

Treatment of Hypokalemia

The goals of therapy in hypokalemia are to prevent life-threatening conditions (diaphragmatic weakness, rhabdomyolysis, and cardiac arrhythmias), to replace any K$^+$ deficit, and to diagnose and correct the underlying cause. The urgency of therapy depends upon the severity of hypokalemia, associated conditions and settings (e.g., a patient with heart failure taking digoxin, or a patient with hepatic encephalopathy), and the rate of decline in plasma K$^+$ concentration. A rapid drop to less than 2.5 mmol/L poses a high risk of cardiac arrhythmias and calls for urgent replacement.[413]

Although replacement therapy is usually limited to patients with a true deficit, it should be considered in patients with hypokalemia due to redistribution (e.g., hypokalemic periodic paralysis) when serious complications such as muscle weakness, rhabdomyolysis, and cardiac arrhythmias are present or imminent.[414] The risk of arrhythmia from hypokalemia is highest in older patients, patients with evidence of organic heart disease, and patients taking digoxin or antiarrhythmic drugs.[221] In these high-risk patients, an increased incidence of arrhythmias may occur at even mild to modest degrees of hypokalemia.

It is also crucial to diagnose and eliminate the underlying cause, so as to tailor therapy to the pathophysiology involved. For example, the risk of overcorrection or rebound hyperkalemia in patients with hypokalemia caused by redistribution is particularly high, with the potential for fatal hyperkalemic arrhythmias.[222,235,267,414,415] When increased sympathetic tone or increased sympathetic response is thought to play a dominant role, the use of nonspecific β-adrenergic blockade with propranolol generally avoids this complication and should be considered. The relevant causes of hypokalemia include TPP,[265] theophylline overdose,[416] and acute head injury.[235]

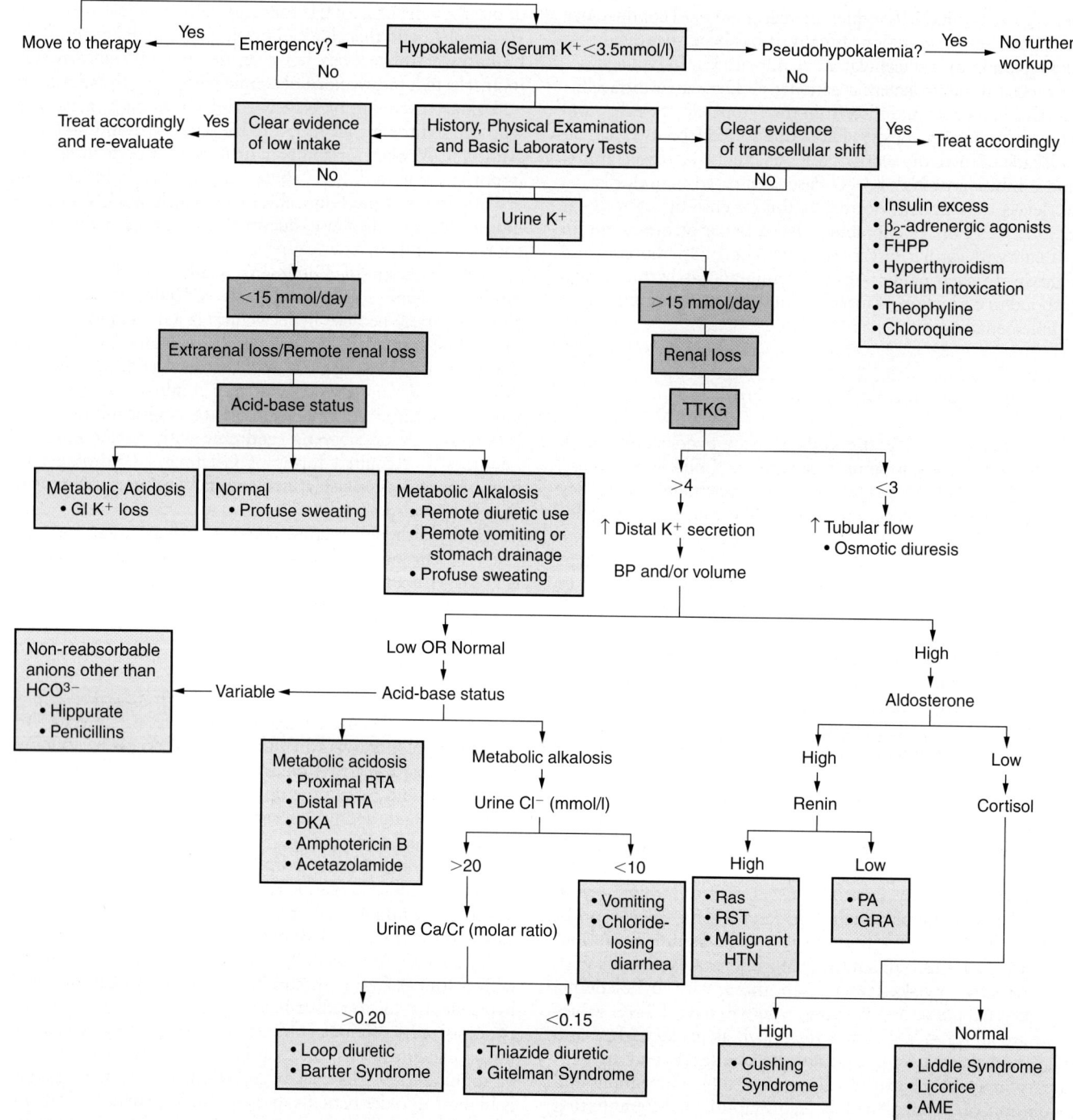

FIGURE 17-11 Clinical approach to hypokalemia. See text for details. AME, Apparent mineralocorticoid excess; BP, blood pressure; CCD, cortical collecting duct; DKA, diabetic ketoacidosis; FHPP, familial hypokalemic periodic paralysis; GI, gastrointestinal; GRA, glucocorticoid-remediable hyperaldosteronism; HTN, hypertension; PA, primary hyperaldosteronism; RAS, renal artery stenosis; RST, renin-secreting tumor; RTA, renal tubular acidosis; TTKG, transtubular potassium gradient.

K^+ replacement is the mainstay of therapy in hypokalemia. However, in hypomagnesemic patients hypokalemia can be refractory to K^+ replacement alone,[399] and concomitant Mg^{2+} deficiency should always be addressed with oral or parenteral repletion. To prevent hyperkalemia due to excessive supplementation, the deficit and the rate of correction should be estimated as accurately as possible. Renal function, medications, and comorbid conditions such as diabetes (with a risk of both insulinopenia and autonomic neuropathy) should also

be considered, to gauge the risk of overcorrection. Arbitrary adjustments in the dose of administered K^+-Cl^- replacement based on estimated GFR can potentially reduce the risk of hyperkalemia.[417] The goal is to raise the plasma K^+ to a safe range rapidly and then replace the remaining deficit at a slower rate over days to weeks.[221,222,414]

In the absence of abnormal K^+ redistribution, the total deficit correlates with plasma K^+ concentration,[222,414,418] so that plasma K^+ drops by approximately 0.27 mmol/L for every

100-mmol reduction in total body stores. Loss of 400 to 800 mmol of body K+ results in a reduction in plasma K+ concentration of approximately 2.0 mmol/L.[418] These values can be used to estimate replacement goals. However, such estimates are just an approximation of the amount of K+ replacement required to normalize plasma K+ concentration, with as much as a one in six risk of overreplacement.[224] Plasma K+ concentration should also be closely monitored during replacement, and K+ replacement withdrawn or adjusted if necessary.

Although the treatment of asymptomatic patients with borderline or low-normal plasma K+ concentration remains controversial, supplementation is recommended for patients with a plasma K+ concentration lower than 3 mmol/L. In high-risk patients (i.e., those with heart failure, cardiac arrhythmias, myocardial infarction, or ischemic heart disease, and those taking digoxin), plasma K+ concentration should be maintained at 4.0 mmol/L or higher[221] or even at 4.5 mmol/L or higher.[228] Patients with severe hepatic disease may not be able to tolerate mild to moderate hypokalemia due to the associated augmentation in ammoniagenesis, and thus plasma K+ should be maintained at approximately 4.0 mmol/L.[419,420] In asymptomatic patients with mild to moderate hypertension, an attempt should be made to maintain plasma K+ concentration above 4.0 mmol/L[221] and potassium supplementation should be considered when plasma K+ falls below 3.5 mmol/L.[221]

Notably, prospective studies have shown an inverse relationship between dietary potassium intake and both fatal and nonfatal stroke, independent of the associated antihypertensive effect.[221,421,422] Potassium is available in the form of potassium chloride, potassium phosphate, potassium bicarbonate or its precursors (potassium citrate, potassium acetate), and potassium gluconate.[221,222,414]

Potassium phosphate is indicated when phosphate deficit accompanies K+ depletion (e.g., in diabetic ketoacidosis).[414] Potassium bicarbonate (or its precursors) should be considered in patients with hypokalemia and metabolic acidosis.[221,414] Potassium chloride should otherwise be the default salt of choice for most patients, for several reasons. First, metabolic alkalosis typically accompanies chloride loss from the kidney (e.g., diuretics) or upper gastrointestinal tract (e.g., vomiting) and contributes significantly to renal K+ wasting.[222] In this setting, replacing chloride along with K+ is essential in treating the alkalosis and preventing further kaliuresis. Because dietary K+ is mainly in the form of potassium phosphate or potassium citrate, it usually does not suffice. Second, potassium bicarbonate may offset the benefits of K+ administration by aggravating concomitant alkalosis. Third, potassium chloride raises plasma K+ concentration at a faster rate than does potassium bicarbonate, a factor that is crucial in patients with marked hypokalemia and related symptoms. In all likelihood, this faster rise in plasma K+ occurs because Cl− is mainly an extracellular fluid anion that does not enter cells to the same extent as bicarbonate, which keeps the K+ in the extracellular fluid compartment.[423]

Parenteral (intravenous) K+ administration should be limited to patients unable to utilize the enteral route or patients experiencing associated signs and symptoms of hypokalemia. However, rapid correction of hypokalemia through oral supplementation is possible and may be faster than intravenous K+ supplementation, due to limitations in the rapidity with which intravenous K+ can be infused. For example, plasma K+ concentration can be increased by 1.0 to 1.4 mmol/L in 60 to 90 minutes after the oral intake of 75 mmol of K+[424]; the ingestion of approximately 125 to 165 mmol of K+ as a single oral dose can increase plasma K+ by approximately 2.5 to 3.5 mmol/L in 60 to 120 minutes.[425] The oral route is thus both effective and appropriate in patients with asymptomatic severe hypokalemia. If the patient is experiencing life-threatening signs and symptoms of hypokalemia, however, the maximum possible intravenous infusion of K+ should be administered acutely for symptom control, followed by rapid oral supplementation.

The usual intravenous dose is 20 to 40 mmol of K+-Cl− in a liter of vehicle solution.[414] The vehicle solution should be dextrose free to prevent a transient reduction in plasma K+ level of 0.2 to 1.4 mmol/L due to an enhanced endogenous insulin secretion induced by the dextrose.[426] Higher concentrations of K+-Cl− (up to 400 mmol/L, as 40 mmol in 100 mL of normal saline) have been used in life-threatening circumstances.[427,428] In these cases, the amount of K+ per intravenous bag should be limited (e.g., 20 mmol in 100 mL of saline solution) to prevent inadvertent infusion of a large dose.[428,429] These solutions are best given through a large central vein. Femoral veins are preferable, since infusion through upper body central lines can acutely increase the local concentration of K+ with deleterious effects on cardiac conduction.[428,429] As a general rule, and to avoid venous pain, irritation, and sclerosis, concentrations of more than 60 mmol/L should not be given through a peripheral vein.[414]

Although the recommended rate of administration is 10 to 20 mmol/hr, rates of 40 to 100 mmol/hr or even higher (for a short period) have been used in patients with life-threatening conditions.[427,429-431] However, a rapid increase in plasma K+ concentration associated with ECG changes may occur with higher rates of infusion (e.g., ≥80 mmol/hr).[432] Intravenous administration of K+ at a rate of more than 10 mmol/hr requires continuous ECG monitoring.[414] In patients infused at such high rates, close monitoring of the appropriate physiologic consequences of hypokalemia is essential; after these effects have abated, the rate of infusion should be decreased to the standard dosage of 10 to 20 mmol/hr.[429]

It is important to remember that, in patients with moderate to severe hypokalemia and Cl−-responsive metabolic alkalosis, volume expansion should be performed cautiously and with close follow-up of plasma K+ levels, since bicarbonaturia associated with volume expansion may aggravate renal K+ wasting and hypokalemia.[413] In patients with combined severe hypokalemia and hypophosphatemia (e.g., diabetic ketoacidosis), intravenous K+ phosphate can be used. However, this solution should be infused at a rate of less than 50 mmol over 8 hours to prevent the risk of hypocalcemia and metastatic calcification.[413] A combination of potassium phosphate and potassium chloride may be necessary to correct hypokalemia effectively in these patients.

The easiest and most straightforward method of oral K+ supplementation is to increase dietary intake of potassium-rich foods[222] (Table 17-4). One study compared the effectiveness of diet versus medication supplementation in cardiac surgery patients receiving diuretics in hospital and found no difference between the two groups with respect to maintenance of plasma K+ concentration. However, this study had limitations, including a small number of subjects, relatively short duration, and lack of information on acid-base status, which makes its results less than conclusive and not generalizable.[433]

TABLE 17-4   Foods with High Potassium Content

Highest content(>1000 mg [25 mmol]/100 g)

    Dried figs
    Molasses
    Seaweed

Very high content(>500 mg [12.5 mmol]/100 g)

    Dried fruits (dates, prunes)
    Nuts
    Avocados
    Bran Cereals
    Wheat germ
    Lima beans

High content(>250 mg [6.2 mmol]/100 g)

    Vegetables
      Spinach
      Tomatoes
      Broccoli
      Winter squash
      Beets
      Carrots
      Cauliflower
      Potatoes
    Fruits
      Bananas
      Cantaloupe
      Kiwis
      Oranges
      Mangos
    Meats
      Ground beef
      Steak
      Pork
      Veal
      Lamb

From Gennari FJ: Hypokalemia, *N Engl J Med* 339:451-458, 1998.

TABLE 17-5 Oral Preparations of Potassium Chloride	
SUPPLEMENT	**ATTRIBUTES**
Controlled-release microencapsulated tablets	Disintegrate better in stomach than encapsulated microparticles; less adherent and less cohesive
Encapsulated controlled-release microencapsulated particles	Fewer gastrointestinal tract erosions than with wax-matrix tablets
Potassium chloride elixir	Inexpensive, tastes bad, poor patient adherence; few gastrointestinal tract erosions; immediate effect
Potassium chloride (effervescent tablets) for solution	Convenient, but more expensive than elixir; immediate effect
Wax-matrix extended-release tablets	Easier to swallow; more gastrointestinal tract erosions than with microencapsulated formulas

From Cohn JN, Kowey PR, Whelton PK, et al: New guidelines for potassium replacement in clinical practice: a contemporary review by the National Council on Potassium in Clinical Practice, *Arch Intern Med* 160:2429-2436, 2000.

Regardless, dietary K^+ is mainly in the form of potassium phosphate or potassium citrate and is inadequate in the majority of patients who have concomitant K^+ and Cl^- deficiency. Most patients therefore need to combine a high-K^+ diet with a prescribed dose of K^+-Cl^-.[222] Salt substitutes are an inexpensive and potent source of K^+-Cl^-. Each gram contains 10 to 13 mmol of K^+[434]; however, patients, particularly those with an impaired ability to excrete potassium, need to be counseled regarding the appropriate amount and the potential for hyperkalemia.[435]

Potassium chloride is also available in either liquid or tablet form (Table 17-5).[221] In general, the available preparations are well absorbed.[222] Liquid forms are less expensive but are less well tolerated. Slow-release forms are more palatable and better tolerated; however, they have been associated with gastrointestinal ulceration and bleeding, which have been ascribed to local accumulation of high concentrations of K^+.[222,429] Notably, this risk is rather low, and lower still when the microencapsulated forms are used.[222] The chance of overdose and hyperkalemia is higher with slow-release formulations; unlike the immediate-release forms, these tablets are less irritating to the stomach and less likely to induce vomiting.[436]

The usual dose is 40 to 100 mmol of K^+ (as K^+-Cl^-) per day, divided into 2 or 3 doses, in patients taking diuretics[222] (K^+-Cl^- can be toxic in doses of more than 2 mmol/kg[436]). This dosage is effective in maintaining plasma K^+ concentration in up to 90% of patients. In the 10% of patients who remain hypokalemic, increasing the oral dose or adding a K^+-sparing diuretic is an appropriate choice.[222]

In addition to potassium supplementation, strategies to minimize K^+ losses should be considered. These measures may include minimizing the dose of non–K^+-sparing diuretics and restricting Na^+ intake more rigorously instead, and using a combination of non–K^+-sparing and K^+-sparing medications (e.g., ACE inhibitors, ARBs, K^+-sparing diuretics, β-blockers).[193,221] The use of a K^+-sparing diuretic is of particular importance in hypokalemia resulting from primary hyperaldosteronism and related disorders, such as Liddle's syndrome and AME; K^+ supplementation alone may be ineffective in these settings.[437-439] In patients with hypokalemia due to loss through upper gastrointestinal secretion (continuous nasogastric tube suction, continuous or self-induced vomiting), proton pump inhibitors are reportedly useful in helping to correct the metabolic alkalosis and reduce hypokalemia.[440] Care should be taken when discontinuing these agents.

Hyperkalemia

Epidemiology

Hyperkalemia is usually defined as a potassium level of 5.5 mmol/L or higher,[441,442] although in some studies levels of 5.0 to 5.4 mmol/L qualify for the diagnosis.[443] Hyperkalemia has been reported in 1.1% to 10% of all hospitalized patients,[200,441-444] with approximately 1.0% of patients (8% to 10% of hyperkalemic patients) having significant hyperkalemia (≥6.0 mmol/L).[441] Hyperkalemia has been associated with a higher mortality rate (14.3% to 41%)[26,441,442] and accounted for approximately 1 death per 1000 patients in one case series in the mid-1980s.[445] In most hospitalized patients, the pathophysiology of hyperkalemia is multifactorial, with reduced renal function, medications, older age (≥60 years), and hyperglycemia being the most common contributing factors.[200,441,442]

In patients with ESRD, the prevalence of hyperkalemia is 5% to 10%.[446-448] The prevalence increased from 2% to 42% as GFR decreased from 60 to 90 mL/min/1.73 m^2 to less than 20 mL/min/1.73 m^2 in one study.[449] The risk of hyperkalemia is higher in males with chronic kidney disease (CKD) and is tripled by treatment with ACE inhibitors or ARBs.[449] It has been argued that hyperkalemia accounts for or contributes to 1.9% to 5% of deaths among patients with ESRD.[200,448] Notably, however, the risk of death from hyperkalemia is reduced as CKD progresses, presumably due to as-yet-uncharacterized cardiac adaptation to chronic hyperkalemia.[450] Hyperkalemia is the reason for emergency hemodialysis in 24% of patients with ESRD who are receiving hemodialysis,[448] and renal failure is the most common cause of hyperkalemia diagnosed in the emergency room.[446]

The prevalence of marked hyperkalemia ($K^+ \geq 5.8$ mmol/L) is approximately 1% in a general medicine outpatient setting. Alarmingly, the management of outpatient hyperkalemia is often suboptimal, with approximately 25% of the patients lacking any follow-up, electrocardiography performed in only 36% of cases, and frequent delays in repeating plasma K^+ determinations.[451]

Pseudohyperkalemia

Factitious hyperkalemia, or pseudohyperkalemia, is an artifactual increase in plasma K^+ concentration due to the release of K^+ during or after venipuncture. There are several potential causes for pseudohyperkalemia.[452] First, forearm contraction,[453] fist clenching,[19] or tourniquet use[452] may increase K^+ efflux from local muscle and thus raise the measured plasma K^+ level. Second, thrombocytosis,[454] leukocytosis,[455] and/or erythrocytosis[456] may cause pseudohyperkalemia due to release of K^+ from these cellular elements. Third, acute anxiety during venipuncture may provoke respiratory alkalosis and hyperkalemia due to redistribution.[50-52,61] Fourth, sample contamination with potassium ethylenediaminetetraacetic acid (K^+-EDTA), used as a sample anticoagulant for some laboratory assays, can cause spurious hyperkalemia.[457]

There are several mechanisms for sample contamination with K^+-EDTA during blood draws or sample handling.[457] Gross contamination with K^+-EDTA usually results in spurious hypocalcemia and hypomagnesemia; lesser contamination is less obvious, which has led to the practice in some laboratories to perform EDTA assays on samples with a plasma K^+ level of more than 6 mmol/L when K^+-EDTA was used as an anticoagulant.

Fifth, mechanical and physical factors may induce pseudohyperkalemia after blood has been drawn. For example, pneumatic tube transport was shown to induce pseudohyperkalemia in a specimen from one patient with leukemia and massive leukocytosis.[458] Cooling of blood prior to the separation of cells from plasma or cooling of plasma is also a well-recognized cause of artifactual hyperkalemia.[459] The converse is the risk of increased uptake of K^+ by cells at high ambient temperatures, which leads to normal values in hyperkalemic patients and/or to spurious hypokalemia in patients who are normokalemic.[26,230] This issue is particularly important for samples drawn in the outpatient primary practice setting that are transported offsite and analyzed at a central facility.[26] This phenomenon leads to "seasonal pseudohyperkalemia and pseudohypokalemia"[26,460] with fluctuations in outpatient samples as a function of season and ambient temperature.

Finally, there are several hereditary subtypes of pseudohyperkalemia, caused by an increase in the passive K^+ permeability of erythrocytes. Abnormal red cell morphology, varying degrees of hemolysis, and/or perinatal edema can accompany hereditary pseudohyperkalemia, but in many kindreds there are no overt hematologic consequences. Plasma K^+ concentration increases in pseudohyperkalemia patient samples that have been left at room temperature, due to the abnormal K^+ permeability of erythrocytes.

Several subtypes have been defined, based on differences in the temperature-dependence curve of this red cell leak pathway.[26,461] The disorder is genetically heterogeneous, with a characterized gene on chromosome band 17q21 and uncharacterized loci on chromosome bands 16q23-ter and 2q35-36.[26] Of particular interest, eleven pedigrees of patients with autosomal dominant hemolysis, pseudohyperkalemia, and temperature-dependent loss of red cell K^+ were found to have heterozygous mutations in the *SLC4A1* gene on chromosome band 17q21, which encodes the band 3 anion exchanger, AE1.[461] The mutations that were detected all cluster within exon 17 of the gene,[461] between transmembrane domains 8 and 10 of the AE1 protein. These mutations reduce anion transport in both red cells and *Xenopus* oocytes injected with AE1, with the novel acquisition of a nonselective transport pathway for both Na^+ and K^+. Pseudohyperkalemia in these patients thus results from a genetic event that endows AE1 with the ability to transport K^+. That single point mutations can convert an anion exchanger to a nonselective cation channel serves to underline the narrow boundaries that separate exchangers and transporters from ion channels.[461]

More recently, mutations in the red cell Rh A glycoprotein (RhAG) have been linked to the monovalent cation leak associated with overhydrated hereditary stomatocytosis.[462] These mutations cause an exaggerated cation leak in the RhAG, which is thought to function as an NH_3 or NH_4^+ transporter RhAG.

Excess Intake of Potassium and Tissue Necrosis

Increased intake of even small amounts of K^+ may provoke severe hyperkalemia in patients with predisposing factors. For example, the oral administration of 32 mmol to a diabetic patient with hyporeninemic hypoaldosteronism resulted in an increase in plasma K^+ concentration from 4.9 mmol/L to a peak of 7.3 mmol/L within 3 hours.[463] Increased intake or changes in intake of dietary sources rich in K^+ (see Table 17-4) may also provoke hyperkalemia in susceptible patients. Very rarely, marked intake of K^+, for example in sports beverages,[464] may provoke severe hyperkalemia in individuals free of predisposing factors.

Other occult sources of K^+ must also be considered, including salt substitutes,[434] alternative medicines,[465] and alternative diets.[466] Geophagia with ingestion of K^+-rich clay[26] and cautopyreiophagia[467] (ingestion of burnt matchsticks) are two forms of pica that have been reported to cause hyperkalemia in dialysis patients. Sustained-release K^+-Cl^- tablets can cause hyperkalemia in suicidal overdoses.[436] Such pills are radiopaque and may thus be seen on radiographs; whole bowel irrigation should be used for gastrointestinal decontamination.[436]

Iatrogenic causes include simple overreplacement with K^+-Cl^-, as can occur commonly in hypokalemic patients,[224] or administration of a potassium-containing medication, such as

K^+-penicillin,[468] to a susceptible patient. Red cell transfusion is a well-described cause of hyperkalemia, with such a complication typically seen in children or in patients receiving massive transfusions. Risk factors for transfusion-related hyperkalemia include a higher rate and volume of transfusion, the use of central venous infusion and/or pressure pumping, the use of irradiated blood, and the use of older blood.[19,469] Whereas 7-day-old blood has a free K^+ concentration of approximately 23 mmol/L, the concentration rises to the 50-mmol/L range in 42-day-old blood.[470]

Hyperkalemia is a common occurrence in patients with severe trauma, with a period prevalence of 29% seen in massively traumatized patients at a U.S. military combat support hospital in Iraq.[471] Although red cell and/or blood product transfusion plays an important role, this and other studies indicate a complex pathophysiology for resuscitative hyperkalemia, with low cardiac output, acidosis, hypocalcemia, and other factors contributing to the risk of hyperkalemia in patients with severe trauma.[469,471]

Tissue necrosis is an important cause of hyperkalemia. Hyperkalemia due to rhabdomyolysis is particularly common, due the enormous store of K^+ in muscle (see Figure 17-1). In many cases, volume depletion, medications (statins, in particular), and metabolic predisposition contribute to the genesis of rhabdomyolysis. Hypokalemia is an important metabolic predisposing factor in rhabdomyolysis (see "Consequences of Hypokalemia" section); others include hypophosphatemia, hypernatremia and hyponatremia, and hyperglycemia. Those patients with hypokalemia-associated rhabdomyolysis in whom redistribution is the cause of hypokalemia are at particular risk of subsequent hyperkalemia as the rhabdomyolysis evolves and renal function worsens.[19,245] Finally, massive release of K^+ and other intracellular contents may occur as a result of acute tumor lysis.[463]

Redistribution and Hyperkalemia

Several different mechanisms can induce an efflux of intracellular K^+, resulting in hyperkalemia. The infusion of hypertonic mannitol or saline, but not hypertonic bicarbonate, generates an increase in plasma K^+ concentration.[472] Potential mechanisms include dilutional acidosis with subsequent shift in K^+, increased passive exit of K^+ due to an increase in intracellular K^+ activity from intracellular water loss, acute hemolysis, and a "solvent drag" effect as water exits cells.[473,474] Regardless of the cause, severe hyperkalemia, typically with an acute dilutional hyponatremia, is a well-described complication of mannitol administration for the treatment or prevention of cerebral edema.[474-476] Diabetic patients are prone to severe hyperkalemia in response to intravenous administration of hypertonic glucose in the absence of adequate coadministration of insulin, due to a similar osmotic effect.[477,478] Finally, a retrospective report documented considerable increases in plasma K^+ concentration after intravenous injection of contrast dye in five patients with CKD, four being maintained on dialysis and one with stage 4 CKD.[479] Again, the acute osmolar load was the likely cause of the acute hyperkalemia in these patients. The implications of this provocative study are not entirely clear; however, one would expect the development or worsening of hyperkalemia in dialysis patients exposed to large volumes of hyperosmolar contrast dye.

Two reports have appeared regarding the risk of hyperkalemia with the use of ε-aminocaproic acid (Amicar),[480,481] a cationic amino acid that is structurally similar to lysine and arginine. Cationic but not anionic amino acids induce efflux of K^+ from cells, although the transport pathways involved are unknown.[19]

Muscle plays a dominant role in extrarenal K^+ homeostasis, primarily via regulated uptake by Na^+-K^+-ATPase. Although exercise is a well-described cause of acute hyperkalemia, this effect is usually transient, and its clinical relevance is difficult to judge. In one study, ESRD patients maintained on dialysis did not have an exaggerated increase in plasma K^+ concentration with maximal exercise, perhaps due to greater insulin, catecholamine, and aldosterone responses to exercise and/or to their preexisting hyperkalemia.[482] The results and design of this and other studies of exercise-associated hyperkalemia in ESRD have been criticized by a more recent report, which linked abnormal extrarenal K^+ homeostasis to increased fatigue in ESRD.[483] In any event, exercise-associated hyperkalemia is not a major clinical cause of hyperkalemia.

Dialysis patients are susceptible to modest increases in plasma K^+ concentration after prolonged fasting, due to the relative insulinopenia in this setting.[484] This may be clinically relevant in preoperative ESRD patients, for whom intravenous glucose infusions with or without insulin are appropriate measures to prevent the development of hyperkalemia.[484] Insulin stimulates the uptake of K^+ by several tissues, primarily via stimulation of Na^+-K^+-ATPase activity.[26,38,40,43] Reduction in circulating insulin level is thus an important factor or cofactor in the generation of hyperkalemia in diabetic patients.

Patients with DKA typically present with plasma K^+ levels that are within normal limits or moderately elevated, but with profound whole-body potassium deficits. However, significant hyperkalemia (plasma K^+ > 6.0 to 6.5 mmol/L) is not uncommon in DKA,[485,486] due to a variety of potential factors: insulinopenia, renal dysfunction, and the hyperosmolar effect of severe hyperglycemia.[485-487]

Inhibition of insulin secretion by the somatostatin agonist octreotide can also cause significant hyperkalemia in both anephric patients[35] and patients with normal renal function.[36] Digoxin inhibits Na^+-K^+-ATPase and thus impairs the uptake of K^+ by skeletal muscle (see "Factors Affecting Internal Distribution of Potassium" section); thus digoxin overdose can result in hyperkalemia.

The skin and venom gland of the cane toad *Bufo marinus* contains high concentrations of bufadienolide, which is structurally similar to the cardioactive glycoside digoxin. The direct ingestion of such toads[488] or of toad extracts can result in fatal hyperkalemia. Certain herbal aphrodisiac pills, in particular, contain appreciable amounts of toad venom and have lead to several case reports of poisoning in the United States.[19,489] The toxin may be detected in the plasma of such patients using standard digoxin assays, since bufadienolide is immunologically similar to digoxin. Administration of digoxin-specific Fab fragment, indicated for the treatment of digoxin overdoses, may be effective and life-saving in bufadienolide toxicity.[19,489]

Finally, fluoride ions also inhibit Na^+-K^+-ATPase, so that fluoride poisoning is typically associated with hyperkalemia.[490]

Succinylcholine depolarizes muscle cells, which results in the efflux of K^+ through acetylcholine receptors (AChRs) and a rapid, but usually transient, hyperkalemia. The use of this agent is contraindicated in patients with thermal trauma, neuromuscular injury (upper or lower motor neuron), disuse atrophy, mucositis, or prolonged immobilization in an intensive care unit setting; the efflux of K$^+$ induced by succinylcholine is enhanced in these patients and can result in significant hyperkalemia.[491] These disorders share a 2- to 100-fold upregulation of AChRs at the plasma membrane of muscle cells, with loss of the normal clustering at the neuromuscular junction.[491] Depolarization of these upregulated AChRs by succinylcholine results in an exaggerated efflux of K$^+$ through the receptor-associated cation channels that are spread throughout the muscle cell membrane (Figure 17-12). Concomitant upregulation of the neuronal α$_7$-subunit of the AChR has also been observed in denervated muscle. The α$_7$-containing AChR is a homomeric, pentameric channel that depolarizes in response to both succinylcholine and choline, its metabolite.[491] Depolarization of α$_7$-AChRs in response to choline is not subject to desensitization, and this may explain in part the hyperkalemic effect that persists in some patients well after the paralytic effect of succinylcholine has subsided.[491] Consistent perhaps with this neuromuscular pathophysiology, patients with renal failure do not appear to have an increased risk of succinylcholine-associated hyperkalemia.[492]

A report of three patients suggested the possibility that drugs which share the ability to open K$_{ATP}$ channels may have an underappreciated propensity to cause hyperkalemia in critically ill patients. The implicated drugs included cyclosporine, isoflurane, and nicorandil.[493] These patients exhibited hyperkalemia that resisted the usual therapies (insulin/dextrose with or without hemofiltration), with a temporal hypokalemic response to the K$_{ATP}$ inhibitor glibenclamide (glyburide). The daring, off-label use of glibenclamide was presumably instigated by the senior author's observation that cyclosporine activates K$_{ATP}$ channels in vascular smooth muscle.[494] K$_{ATP}$ channels are widely distributed, including in skeletal muscle, so that activation of such channels is indeed a plausible cause of acute hyperkalemia. However, it still remains to be seen whether this is a common or important mechanism for acute hyperkalemia.

Finally, β-blockers cause hyperkalemia, in part by inhibiting cellular uptake but also through the hyporeninemic hypoaldosteronism induced by the effect of these drugs on both renal renin release and adrenal aldosterone release (see "Regulation of Renal Renin and Adrenal Aldosterone" section). Labetalol, a broadly reactive sympathetic blocker, is a particularly common cause of hyperkalemia in susceptible patients.[19,495] However, both nonspecific and cardiospecific β-blockers have been shown to reduce PRA, angiotensin II level, and aldosterone level,[496] so that β-blockade in general increases susceptibility to hyperkalemia.

Reduced Renal Excretion of Potassium

Hypoaldosteronism

Aldosterone promotes kaliuresis by activating apical amiloride-sensitive Na$^+$ currents in the CNT and CCD and thus increasing the lumen-negative driving force for K$^+$ excretion (see "Aldosterone" section). Aldosterone release from the adrenal glands may be reduced by hyporeninemic hypoaldosteronism and its multiple causes, by medications, or by isolated deficiency of ACTH. The isolated loss of pituitary secretion of ACTH leads to a deficit in circulating cortisol; variable defects in other pituitary hormones are likely secondary to this reduction in cortisol level.[497] Concomitant hyporeninemic hypoaldosteronism is frequent[26]; however, hyperkalemia is less common in secondary hypoaldosteronism than in Addison's disease.[497]

Primary hypoaldosteronism may be genetic or acquired.[498] The X-linked disorder adrenal hypoplasia congenita is caused by loss-of-function mutations in the transcriptional repressor DAX-1 (dosage-sensitive sex-reversal, adrenal hypoplasia congenita, critical region on the X chromosome, gene 1). Patients with adrenal hypoplasia congenita present with primary adrenal failure and hyperkalemia either shortly after birth or much later in childhood.[499] This bimodal presentation pattern does not appear to be influenced by *DAX1* genotype; rather, if patients survive the early neonatal period the diagnosis will then be missed until much later in life, when patients either show delayed puberty (see later) or experience an adrenal crisis. Steroidogenic factor 1 (SF-1), a functional partner for DAX-1, is also required for adrenal development in both mice and humans. Both genes are involved in gonadal development, with DAX-1 deficiency leading to hypogonadotropic hypogonadism[499] and SF-1 deficiency causing male-to-female sex reversal, in addition to adrenal insufficiency.

Reduced steroidogenesis causes two other important forms of primary hypoaldosteronism.[498] Congenital lipoid adrenal hyperplasia is a severe autosomal recessive syndrome characterized by impaired synthesis of mineralocorticoids, glucocorticoids, and gonadal steroids.[19] The disorder manifests in early infancy with adrenal crisis, including severe hyperkalemia.[500] Genotypically male 46,XY patients with congenital lipoid adrenal hyperplasia have female external genitalia due to the

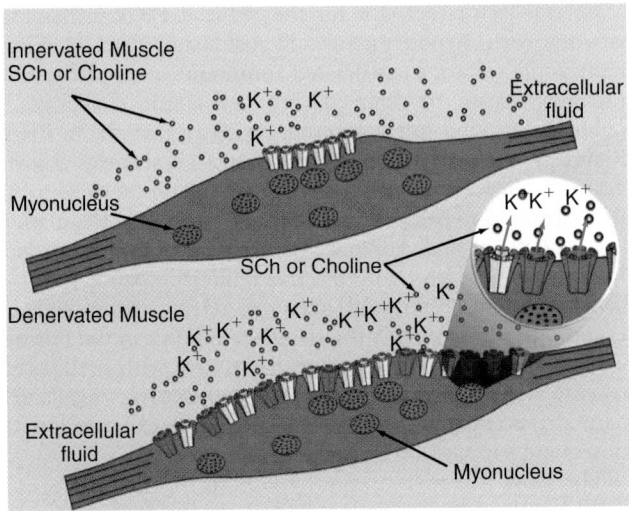

FIGURE 17-12 Increase in succinylcholine-induced efflux of potassium in denervated muscle. In innervated muscle, succinylcholine interacts with the entire plasma membrane, but depolarizes only the junctional (α$_1$, β$_1$, δ, and ε [*multicolored*]) acetylcholine receptors (AChRs). This leads to a modest transient hyperkalemia. With denervation, there is a considerable upregulation of muscle AChRs, with increased extrajunctional AChRs (α$_1$, β$_1$, δ, and γ [*multicolored*]) and acquisition of homomeric, neuronal-type α$_7$-AChRs. Depolarization of denervated muscle leads to an exaggerated K$^+$ efflux, due to the upregulation and redistribution of these AChRs. In addition, choline generated from the metabolism of succinylcholine maintains the depolarization mediated by α$_7$-AChRs, thus enhancing and prolonging the K$^+$ efflux after paralysis has subsided. (From Martyn JA, Richtsfeld M: Succinylcholine-induced hyperkalemia in acquired pathologic states: etiologic factors and molecular mechanisms, *Anesthesiology* 104:158-169, 2006.)

developmental absence of testosterone. Congenital lipoid adrenal hyperplasia is caused by loss-of-function mutations in steroidogenic acute regulatory protein, a small mitochondrial protein that helps shuttle cholesterol from the outer to the inner mitochondrial membrane and thus initiates steroidogenesis.[501] Some patients may alternatively have mutations in the side-chain cleavage P450 enzyme.[502]

The classical salt-wasting form of congenital adrenal hyperplasia due to 21-hydroxlase deficiency is associated with marked reductions in both cortisol and aldosterone levels, which leads to adrenal insufficiency.[503] 21-Hydroxylase is a cytochrome P450 enzyme encoded by the gene *CYP21B* that is involved in the bioconversion of progesterone to 11-deoxycorticosterone, a shared precursor for aldosterone and cortisol. Concomitant overproduction of androgenic steroids results in virilization in female patients with this form of congenital adrenal hyperplasia.

Isolated deficits in aldosterone synthesis with hyperreninemia are caused by loss-of-function mutations in aldosterone synthase, although genetic heterogeneity has been reported.[504] The disorder typically manifests in childhood with volume depletion and hyperkalemia.[505] Much as in pseudohypoaldosteronism due to loss-of-function mutations in the mineralocorticoid receptor (see later), patients tend to become asymptomatic in adulthood.

Acquired hyperreninemic hypoaldosteronism has been described in association with critical illness,[19] type 2 diabetes,[506] and amyloidosis due to familial Mediterranean fever,[507] as well as after metastasis of carcinoma to the adrenal gland.[19]

Finally, aldosterone synthesis is selectively reduced by heparin, with a 7% incidence of hyperkalemia associated with heparin therapy.[508] Both unfractionated[508] and low-molecular-weight[19,509] heparin can cause hyperkalemia. Hyperkalemia due to prophylactic subcutaneous administration of unfractionated heparin (5000 U twice daily) has also been reported.[510] Heparin reduces the adrenal aldosterone response to both angiotensin II and hyperkalemia, which results in hyperreninemic hypoaldosteronism. Histologic findings in experimental animals include a marked diminution in the size of the zona glomerulosa and an attenuated hyperplastic response to salt depletion.[508]

Most primary adrenal insufficiency is due to autoimmunity, either in Addison's disease or in the context of a polyglandular endocrinopathy.[498,511] Antiphospholipid syndrome may also cause bilateral adrenal hemorrhage and adrenal insufficiency.[512] Another renal syndrome in which there should be a high index of suspicion for adrenal insufficiency is renal amyloidosis.[513]

Finally, human immunodeficiency virus (HIV) infection has surpassed tuberculosis as the most important infectious cause of adrenal insufficiency. The most common cause of adrenalitis in HIV disease is cytomegalovirus; however, a long list of infectious, degenerative, and infiltrative processes may involve the adrenal glands in these patients.[514] Although the adrenal involvement in HIV disease is usually subclinical, adrenal insufficiency may be precipitated by stress, drugs such as ketoconazole that inhibit steroidogenesis, or the acute withdrawal of steroid agents such as megestrol. Megestrol is a progesterone derivative with antineoplastic properties used in the treatment of advanced carcinoma of the breast dind endometrium that can increase appetite at higher dosages.

Contemporary estimates of the risk of hyperkalemia in patients with Addison's disease are lacking; however, the incidence is likely 50% to 60%.[19] The absence of hyperkalemia in such a high percentage of hypoadrenal patients underscores the importance of aldosterone-independent modulation of K^+ excretion by the distal nephron. A high-K^+ diet and high peritubular K^+ concentration serve to increase apical Na^+ reabsorption and K^+ secretion in the CNT and CCD (see "Renal Potassium Excretion" section); in most patients with reductions in circulating aldosterone this homeostatic mechanism appears to be sufficient to regulate plasma K^+ concentration to within normal limits.

Hyporeninemic Hypoaldosteronism

Hyporeninemic hypoaldosteronism[515] is a very common predisposing factor in several large, overlapping subsets of hyperkalemic patients: diabetic patients,[516] the elderly,[19,159,517] and patients with renal insufficiency.[19] Hyporeninemic hypoaldosteronism has also been described in patients with systemic lupus erythematosus,[19,518] multiple myeloma,[26] and acute glomerulonephritis.[26] Classically, patients should show suppression of PRA and aldosterone level, which do not respond to typical maneuvers such as furosemide administration or sodium restriction.[515] Approximately 50% of patients have an associated acidosis, with reduced renal excretion of NH_4^+, a positive urinary anion gap, and a urine pH of less than 5.5.[166,220] Although the cause of this acidosis is clearly multifactorial,[519] strong clinical[219,220,520] and experimental[216] evidence suggests that hyperkalemia per se is the dominant factor, due to competitive inhibition of NH_4^+ transport in the TAL and reduced distal excretion of NH_4^+[521] (see also "Consequences of Hyperkalemia" section).

Several factors account for the reduced PRA in diabetic patients with hyporeninemic hypoaldosteronism.[516] First, many patients have an associated autonomic neuropathy, with impaired release of renin during orthostatic challenges.[19] Failure to respond to isoproterenol with an increase in PRA, despite an adequate cardiovascular response, suggests a postreceptor defect in the ability of the juxtaglomerular apparatus to respond to β-adrenergic stimuli[19] (see also "Regulation of Renal Renin and Adrenal Aldosterone" section). Second, the conversion of prorenin to active renin is impaired in some diabetic patients,[516] despite adequate release of prorenin in response to furosemide[19]; this suggests a defect in the normal processing of prorenin. Third, as is the case with perhaps all patients with hyporeninemic hypoaldosteronism (see later), many diabetic patients appear to be volume expanded, with subsequent suppression of PRA.

The most attractive current hypothesis for the suppression of PRA in hyporeninemic hypoaldosteronism is that primary volume expansion increases the level of circulating ANP, which then exerts a negative effect on both renal renin release and adrenal aldosterone release (see also "Regulation of Renal Renin and Adrenal Aldosterone" section). There is evidence that these patients are volume expanded, and many respond to either Na^+-Cl^- restriction or furosemide with an increase in PRA; that is, renin is physiologically rather than pathologically suppressed.[522-524] Patients with hyporeninemic hypoaldosteronism due to a diversity of underlying causes have elevated ANP levels,[19,26,159,523,525] which is also an indicator of their underlying volume expansion. Patients who respond to furosemide with an increase in PRA exhibit a concomitant decrease in ANP.[523] Furthermore, the infusion of exogenous ANP can suppress the adrenal aldosterone response to both hyperkalemia[159] and dietary Na^+-Cl^- depletion.[526]

Acquired Tubular Defects and Potassium Excretion

Unlike hyporeninemic hypoaldosteronism, hyperkalemic distal RTA is associated with a normal or increased aldosterone level and/or PRA. Urine pH in these patients is higher than 5.5, and they are unable to increase acid or K^+ excretion in response to furosemide, Na^+-SO_4^{2-}, or fludrocortisones.[527-529] Classical causes include systemic lupus erythematosus,[527] sickle cell anemia,[19,529] and amyloidosis.[19]

Hereditary Tubular Defects and Potassium Excretion

Hereditary tubular causes of hyperkalemia have overlapping clinical features with hypoaldosteronism; hence, the shared label *pseudohypoaldosteronism*. Pseudohypoaldosteronism type 1 (PHA-1) has both an autosomal recessive and an autosomal dominant form. The autosomal dominant form is due to loss-of-function mutations in the mineralocorticoid receptor.[530] These patients require aggressive salt supplementation during early childhood; however, as in the hypoaldosteronism due to mutations in aldosterone synthase, they typically become asymptomatic in adulthood.[340] Of interest, the lifelong increases in circulating levels of aldosterone, angiotensin II, and renin seen in this syndrome do not appear to have untoward cardiovascular consequences.[530]

The recessive form of PHA-1 is caused by various combinations of mutations in all three subunits of ENaC, resulting in impairment in its channel activity.[340] Patients with this syndrome show severe salt wasting, hypotension, and hyperkalemia in the neonatal period. In contrast to the autosomal dominant form of PHA-1, the syndrome does not improve in adulthood.[340] One unexpected result in the physiologic characterization of ENaC is that mice with a targeted deletion of the α-ENaC subunit were found to die within 40 hours of birth due to pulmonary edema.[26] Patients with recessive PHA-1 may have pulmonary symptoms, which can occasionally be very severe[531]; however, it appears that, unlike in ENaC-deficient mice, the modest residual activity associated with heteromeric PHA-1 channels is generally sufficient to mediate pulmonary Na^+ and fluid clearance in humans with loss-of-function mutations in ENaC.[532]

Pseudohypoaldosteronism type 2 (PHA-2; also known as *Gordon's syndrome* and, more recently, as *familial hyperkalemia with hypertension*, or FHHt) is in every respect the mirror image of Gitelman's syndrome. The clinical phenotype includes hypertension, hyperkalemia, hyperchloremic metabolic acidosis, suppressed PRA and aldosterone, hypercalciuria, and reduced bone density.[533] FHHt behaves like a gain of function in the thiazide-sensitive Na^+-Cl^- cotransporter NCC, and treatment with thiazides typically results in resolution of all clinical manifestations.[533] FHHt is an extreme form of hyporeninemic hypoaldosteronism due to volume expansion; aggressive salt restriction decreases ANP levels and increases PRA, with resolution of the hypertension, hyperkalemia, and metabolic acidosis.[525]

FHHt is an autosomal dominant syndrome, with as many as four genetic loci.[19] In a landmark paper, mutations in two related serine-threonine kinases were detected in various kindreds with FHHt.[534] The catalytic sites of these kinases lack specific catalytic lysines conserved in other kinases, hence the designation *WNK* (*with no lysine [K]*). Whereas FHHt mutations in WNK4 affect the C terminus of the coding sequence, large intronic deletions in the WNK1 gene result in increased expression. Both kinases are expressed within the distal nephron in both DCT and CCD cells. Whereas WNK1 localizes to the cytoplasm and basolateral membrane, WNK4 protein is found at the apical tight junctions.[534]

WNK-dependent phosphorylation and activation of the downstream SPAK and OSR1 (oxidative stress–responsive kinase 1) kinases leads to phosphorylation of a cluster of N-terminal threonines in NCC, which results in activation of Na^+-Cl^- cotransport[1] (see also Figure 17-6). However, coexpression of WNK4 with NCC reveals an additional *inhibitory* influence of the kinase on NCC, effects that are blocked by FHHt-associated point mutations in the kinase.[535] In particular, the inhibitory effects of WNK4 appear to dominate in mouse models with overexpression of wild-type WNK4 compared with those with FHHt mutant WNK4.[68] These competing, divergent mechanisms can be reconciled by the likelihood that the physiologic context determines whether WNK4 will have an activating or inhibitory effect on NCC.[1,535] For example, the *activation* of NCC by the AT_1 angiotensin II receptor appears to require the downstream activation of SPAK by WNK4.[127]

A key insight from study of the mechanisms of FHHt is that the activation of NCC in the DCT in this syndrome serves to reduce Na^+ delivery to principal cells in the downstream CNT and CCD, which leads to hyperkalemia.[68] This and other effects of the WNK pathways on distal K^+ secretion were discussed earlier in this chapter (see "Potassium Intake" section).

Medication-Related Hyperkalemia

Cyclooxygenase Inhibitors

Hyperkalemia is a well-recognized complication of the use of nonsteroidal antiinflammatory drugs (NSAIDs) that inhibit cyclooxygenases. NSAIDs cause hyperkalemia by a variety of mechanisms, as would be predicted from the relevant physiology. By decreasing GFR and increasing sodium retention they decrease distal delivery of Na^+ and reduce distal flow rate. Moreover, the flow-activated apical maxi-K/BK channel in the CNT and CCD is activated by prostaglandins[536]; hence, NSAIDs will reduce its activity and the flow-dependent component of K^+ excretion.[74,370] NSAIDs are also a classical cause of hyporeninemic hypoaldosteronism.[537,538] The administration of indomethacin to normal volunteers thus attenuates furosemide-induced increases in PRA.[147,539] Finally, NSAIDs would not cause hyperkalemia with such regularity if they did not also blunt the adrenal response to hyperkalemia, which is at least partially dependent on prostaglandins acting though prostaglandin EP2 receptors and cAMP.[158]

The physiology reviewed earlier in this chapter (see "Regulation of Renal Renin and Adrenal Aldosterone" section) suggests that COX-2 inhibitors would be equally likely to cause hyperkalemia. Indeed, COX-2 inhibitors can clearly cause sodium retention and a decrease in GFR,[540,541] which implies NSAID-like effects on renal pathophysiology.

COX-2–derived prostaglandins stimulate renal renin release[19] and COX-2 inhibitors reduce PRA in both dogs[26] and humans.[147] Salt restriction potentiates the hyperkalemia seen in dogs treated with COX-2 inhibitors,[26] so that hypovolemic patients may be particularly prone to hyperkalemia in this setting. The COX-2 inhibitor celecoxib and the nonselective NSAID ibuprofen have equivalent negative effects on K$^+$ excretion after a defined oral load.[542] Not surprisingly, clinical reports have begun to emerge of hyperkalemia and acute renal failure associated with the use of COX-2 inhibitors.[19,543,544] Where the data have been reported, circulating PRA and/or aldosterone levels have been reduced in hyperkalemia associated with COX-2 inhibitors.[26,544]

Cyclosporine and Tacrolimus

Both cyclosporine[545] and tacrolimus[546] cause hyperkalemia. The risk of sustained hyperkalemia may be higher in renal transplant patients treated with tacrolimus than in those treated with cyclosporine.[547] Cyclosporine is perhaps the most versatile of all drugs in the variety of mechanisms by which it causes hyperkalemia. It causes hyporeninemic hypoaldosteronism,[548] due in part to its inhibitory effect on COX-2 expression in the macula densa.[549] Cyclosporine inhibits apical SK secretory K$^+$ channels in the distal nephron,[550] in addition to basolateral Na$^+$-K$^+$-ATPase.[19] Finally, cyclosporine causes redistribution of K$^+$ and hyperkalemia, particularly when used in combination with β-blockers.[551] A provocative but preliminary report has linked acute hyperkalemia secondary to cyclosporine administration to indirect activation of K$_{ATP}$ channels (see also earlier)[493]; this is particularly intriguing given the reported response of cyclosporine-associated hyperkalemia to K$_{ATP}$ inhibition with glibenclamide infusion.

Inhibition of the Epithelial Sodium Channel

Inhibition of apical ENaC activity in the distal nephron by amiloride and other K$^+$-sparing diuretics predictably results in hyperkalemia. Amiloride is structurally similar to the antibiotics trimethoprim and pentamidine, which can also inhibit ENaC.[552-554] Trimethoprim thus inhibits Na$^+$ reabsorption and K$^+$ secretion in perfused CCDs.[555] Both trimethoprim-sulfamethoxazole (Bactrim) and pentamidine were reported to cause hyperkalemia during high-dose treatment of *Pneumocystis* pneumonia in HIV patients,[19,554] who are otherwise predisposed to hyperkalemia. However, this side effect is not restricted to high-dose intravenous therapy. In a study of hospitalized patients treated with standard doses of trimethoprim, significant hyperkalemia occurred in more than 50%, with severe hyperkalemia (>5.5 mmol/L) in 21%.[556] Risk factors for hyperkalemia due to normal-dose trimethoprim include renal insufficiency,[556] hyporeninemic hypoaldosteronism,[557] and concomitant use of ACE inhibitors and ARBs.[558]

Although trimethoprim and pentamidine directly inhibit ENaC, a novel indirect mechanism for ENaC inhibition associated hyperkalemia has been reported.[19,104] Aldosterone induces expression of the membrane-associated proteases CAP1 to CAP3 (see "Aldosterone" section). Nafamostat, a protease inhibitor widely used in Japan for pancreatitis and other indications, is known to cause hyperkalemia.[104] Indirect evidence suggests that the mechanism involves inhibition of amiloride-sensitive Na$^+$ channels in the CCD.[19] Treatment

of rats with nafamostat was also shown to reduce the urinary excretion of CAP1/prostasin, in contrast to the reported effect of aldosterone.[101] Thus inhibition of the protease activity of CAP1 by nafamostat appears to abrogate its activating effect on ENaC (Figure 17-13) and may reduce expression of the protein in the CCD.[105]

ACE Inhibitors and Mineralocorticoid and Angiotensin Antagonists

Hyperkalemia is a predictable and common effect of ACE inhibition, direct renin inhibition, and antagonism of the mineralocorticoid and angiotensin receptors[559] (Figure 17-14). The oral contraceptive agent Yasmin 28 and related products contain the progestin drospirenone, which inhibits the mineralocorticoid receptor[560] and can potentially cause hyperkalemia in susceptible patients.

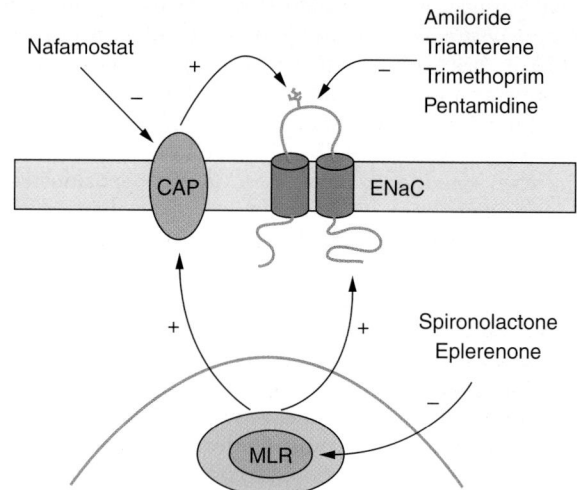

FIGURE 17-13 Pharmacologic inhibition of the epithelial sodium channel (ENaC). Whereas amiloride and related compounds directly inhibit the channel, the protease inhibitor nafamostat inhibits membrane-associated proteases such as CAP1 (channel-activating protease 1), thus indirectly inhibiting the channel. Spironolactone and related drugs inhibit the mineralocorticoid receptor, thus reducing transcription of the α-subunit of ENaC, the ENaC-activating kinase SGK (serum- and glucocorticoid-regulated kinase), and several other target genes (see text for details).

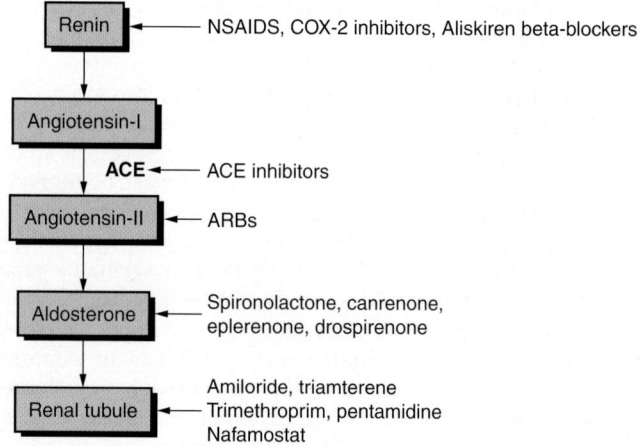

FIGURE 17-14 Medications that target the renin-angiotensin-aldosterone axis are common causes of hyperkalemia, as are drugs that inhibit epithelial sodium channels (ENaCs) in the renal tubule (collecting segment [CNT] or cortical collecting duct [CCD]).

As with many other causes of hyperkalemia, that induced by pharmacologic targeting of the RAAS axis depends on concomitant inhibition of adrenal aldosterone release by hyperkalemia. The adrenal release of aldosterone due to increased K^+ is clearly dependent on an intact adrenal renal-angiotensin system, so that this response is abrogated by systemic ACE inhibitors and ARBs[153] (see "Regulation of Renal Renin and Adrenal Aldosterone" section).

Dual treatment with lisinopril and spironolactone in patients with CKD is also associated with a reduction in extrarenal potassium disposition, given that reduced K^+ excretion alone does not explain the substantial increase in plasma K^+ after a defined oral potassium load.[561] ACE inhibitors and ARBs have the additional potential to cause acute renal failure and acute hyperkalemia in patients with an angiotensin-dependent GFR. Aliskiren has also been reported to cause acute renal failure with acute hyperkalemia, albeit in conjunction with spironolactone.[562]

RAAS inhibitors are an increasingly important cause of hyperkalemia, given the increasing indications for combining spironolactone or aliskiren with ACE inhibitors and/or ARBs in renal and cardiac disease,[563,564] in addition to the development of mineralocorticoid receptor antagonists with perhaps a greater potential for causing hyperkalemia.[565] Heart failure, diabetes, and CKD increase the risk of hyperkalemia from these agents.[559,566,567]

The prevalence of hyperkalemia associated with the combined use of mineralocorticoid receptor antagonists and ACE inhibitors and ARBs appears to be much higher in clinical practice (approximately 10%)[568] than that reported in large clinical trials,[559] in part due to the use of higher than recommended dosages.[19] Notably, Juurlink and colleagues[569] studied the correlation between the rate of prescription of spironolactone for Canadian patients with heart failure who were taking ACE inhibitors and the occurrence of hyperkalemia and associated morbidity before and after publication of the results of the Randomized Aldactone Evaluation Study (RALES).[570] Their provocative study found an abrupt increase in the rate of prescription of spironolactone after release of the RALES findings, with a temporal correlation with increases in the rate of hyperkalemia in patients admitted to hospital[569]; the association remained statistically significant for admissions in which hyperkalemia was the primary diagnosis.[571] However, a study in the United Kingdom found a similar increase in spironolactone use after the publication of RALES results, but without an increase in hyperkalemia or hyperkalemia-associated admissions to hospital.[572] It should also be emphasized that the development of hyperkalemia—or, for that matter, the presence of predisposing factors for hyperkalemia—does not appear to mitigate the mortality benefits of eplerenone in treatment of heart failure.[567]

Given the mounting evidence supporting the combined use of ACE inhibitors, ARBs, and/or mineralocorticoid receptor antagonists, it is prudent to systematically adhere to measures that will minimize the chance of associated hyperkalemia and therefore allow patients to benefit from the cardiovascular and renal effects of these agents. The patients at risk for the development of hyperkalemia in response to drugs that target the RAAS, singly or in combination therapy, are those in whom the ability of the kidneys to excrete the potassium load is markedly diminished due to one or a combination of the following: (1) decreased delivery of sodium to the CCD (as in congestive heart failure, volume depletion, etc.); (2) decreased circulating aldosterone level (hyporeninemic hypoaldosteronism, drugs such as heparin or ketoconazole, etc.); (3) inhibition of amiloride-sensitive Na^+ channels in the CNT and CCD, by coadministration of trimethoprim-sulfamethoxazole, pentamidine, or amiloride; (4) chronic tubulointerstitial disease, with associated dysfunction of the distal nephron; and (5) increased potassium intake (salt substitutes, high-potassium diet, etc.).

Overall, patients with diabetes, heart failure, and/or CKD are at particular risk for hyperkalemia from RAAS inhibition.[559,566,567] In these susceptible patients, the following approach is recommended to prevent or minimize the occurrence of hyperkalemia in response to medications that interfere with the RAAS[26,573]:

A. Estimate GFR using the Modification of Diet in Renal Disease (MDRD) equation, Cockcroft-Gault equation, and/or 24-hour creatinine clearance.

B. Inquire about diet and dietary supplements (e.g., salt substitutes, licorice) and prescribe a low-potassium diet.

C. Inquire about medications used, particularly those that can interfere with renal K^+ excretion (e.g., NSAIDS, COX-2 inhibitors, K^+-sparing diuretics) and, if appropriate, discontinue these agents.

D. Continue or initiate use of loop or thiazide-like diuretics depending upon the GFR.

E. Correct acidosis with sodium bicarbonate.

F. Initiate treatment with a low dose of only one of the following agents: ACE inhibitor, ARB, or mineralocorticoid receptor antagonist.

G. Check plasma K^+ concentration 3 to 5 days after initiation of the therapy and after each dosage increment, followed by another measurement 1 week later.

H. If the plasma K^+ concentration is above 5.6 mmol/L, ACE inhibitors, ARBs, and/or mineralocorticoid receptor blockers should be stopped and the patient should be treated for hyperkalemia.

I. If the plasma K^+ concentration is increased but is less than 5.6 mmol/L, reduce the drug dosage and reassess the possible contributing factors. If the patient is taking a combination of ACE inhibitors, ARBs, and/or mineralocorticoid receptor blockers, all but one should be stopped and potassium level rechecked.

J. A combination of a mineralocorticoid receptor blocker and either an ACE inhibitor or an ARB should not be prescribed to patients with stage 4 or 5 CKD (estimated GFR of <30 mL/min/1.73m².)

K. The dosage of spironolactone in combination with ACE inhibitors or ARBs should be no more than 25 mg/day.

Clinical Approach to Hyperkalemia

The first priority in the management of hyperkalemia is to assess the need for emergency treatment (e.g., presence of ECG changes, $K^+ \geq 6.5$ mmol/L). This should be followed by a comprehensive workup to determine the cause (Figure 17-15). The history and physical examination should focus on medications (e.g., ACE inhibitors, NSAIDs, trimethoprim-sulfamethoxazole), diet and dietary supplements (e.g., salt substitute), risk factors for kidney failure, reduction in urine output, blood pressure, and volume status.

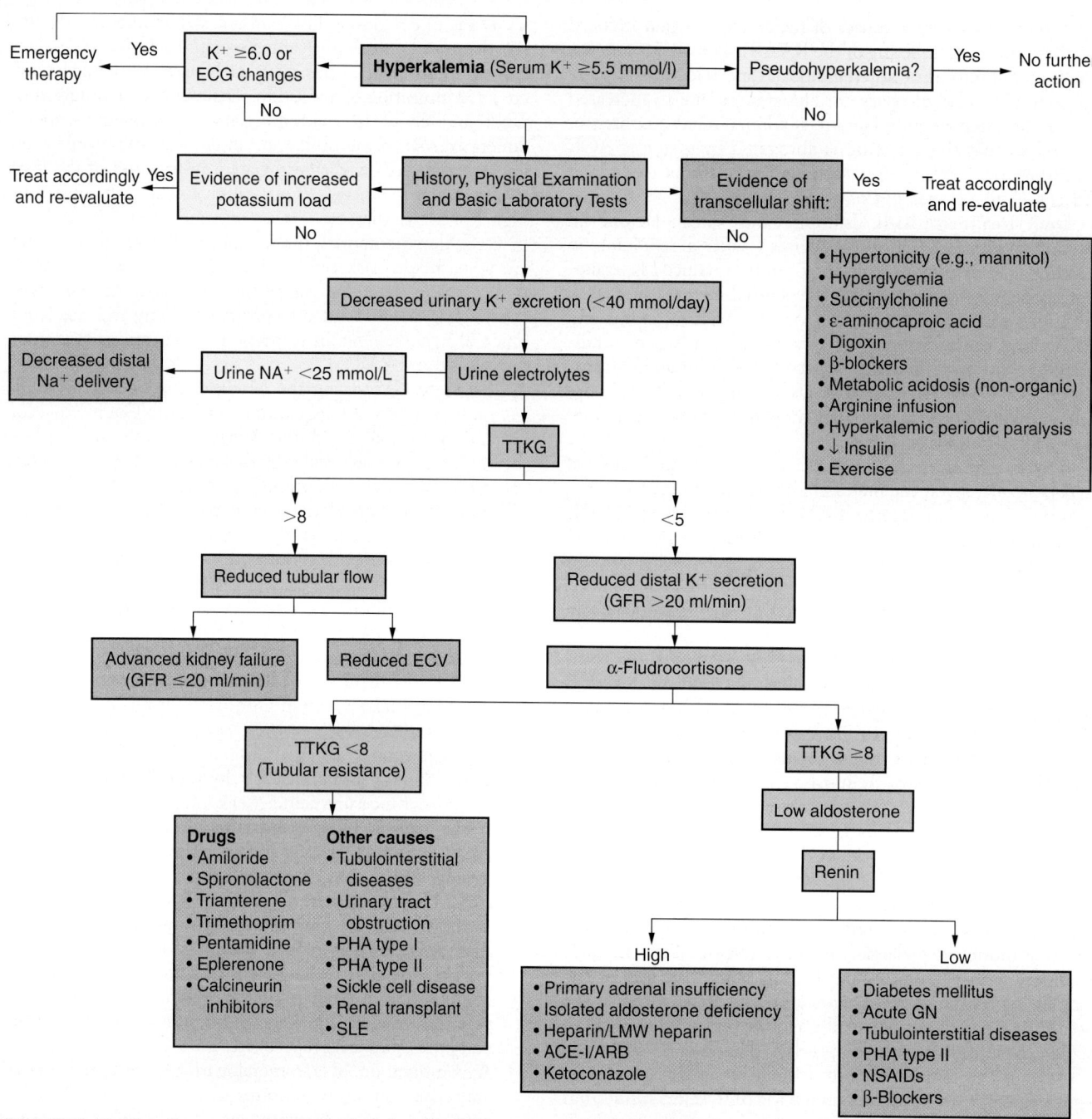

FIGURE 17-15 Clinical approach to hyperkalemia. See text for details. ACE-I, Angiotensin converting enzyme inhibitor; ARB, angiotensin receptor blocker; CCD, cortical collecting duct; ECG, electrocardiogram; ECV, effective circulatory volume; GFR, glomerular filtration rate; GN, glomerulonephritis; HIV, human immunodeficiency virus; LMW, low-molecular-weight; NSAIDs, nonsteroidal antiinflammatory drugs; PHA, pseudohypoaldosteronism; SLE, systemic lupus erythematosus; TTKG, transtubular potassium gradient.

Initial laboratory tests should include plasma levels of electrolytes, blood urea nitrogen, and creatinine; plasma osmolality; plasma Mg^{2+} and Ca^{2+} levels; a complete blood count; and urinary pH, osmolality, creatinine level, and electrolyte levels. Plasma and urine osmolality are required for calculation of the transtubular K^+ gradient (see "Urinary Indices of Potassium Excretion" section). Plasma renin activity, plasma aldosterone level, and the response of the TTKG to fludrocortisone may be necessary to determine the specific cause of an inappropriately low TTKG in hyperkalemia. Serial measurements of blood potassium concentration are key to

appreciating the kinetics of any changes and assessing the response to therapy.

Treatment of Hyperkalemia

Indications for the hospitalization of patients with hyperkalemia are poorly defined, in part because there is no universally accepted definition for mild, moderate, or severe hyperkalemia. The clinical sequelae of hyperkalemia, which are primarily cardiac and neuromuscular, depend on many other variables (e.g., plasma calcium level, acid-base status, and the rate of change in plasma K⁺ concentration[201-204]), in addition to the absolute value of the plasma K⁺ level.[444,574] These factors are likely to influence management decisions.

Plasma K⁺ ≥ 8.0 mmol/L, ECG changes other than peaked T waves, acute deterioration of renal function, and the existence of additional medical problems have been suggested as appropriate criteria for hospitalization.[444] However, hyperkalemia in patients with any ECG manifestation should be considered a true medical emergency and treated urgently.[197,443,575,576] Adequate management and serial monitoring of plasma K⁺ concentration generally requires hospital admission. Given the limitations of ECG changes as a predictor of cardiac toxicity (see "Consequences of Hyperkalemia" section), patients with severe hyperkalemia (K⁺ ≥ 6.5 to 7.0 mmol/L) in the absence of ECG changes should be managed aggressively.[174,197,443,576-578] Urgent management of hyperkalemia constitutes recording of a 12-lead ECG, admission to the hospital, continuous ECG monitoring, and immediate treatment.

The treatment of hyperkalemia is generally divided into three categories: (1) antagonism of the cardiac effects of hyperkalemia, (2) rapid reduction in K⁺ concentration by redistribution into cells, and (3) removal of K⁺ from the body. The necessary measures to treat the underlying conditions causing hyperkalemia should be undertaken to minimize the factors that are contributing to the hyperkalemia and to prevent future episodes.[197] Dietary restriction (usually 60 mEq/day) with emphasis on the K⁺ content of total parenteral nutrition solutions and enteral feeding products (typically 25 to 50 mmol/L) and adjustment of medications and intravenous fluids are necessary. Hidden sources of K⁺, such as intravenous antibiotics,[468] should not be overlooked.

Antagonism of Cardiac Effects

Intravenous calcium is the first-line drug in the emergency management of hyperkalemia, even in patients with normal calcium levels. The mutually antagonistic effects of Ca^{2+} and K⁺ on the myocardium and the protective role of Ca^{2+} in hyperkalemia have long been known.[579] Calcium raises the action potential threshold to a less negative value without changing the resting membrane potential; restoring the usual 15-mV difference between resting and threshold potentials reduces myocyte excitability.[174,580] Administration of calcium also alters the relationship between V_{max} and the resting membrane potential, maintaining a more normal V_{max} at less negative resting membrane potentials and thus restoring myocardial conduction.[174]

Calcium is available as calcium chloride or calcium gluconate (10-mL ampules of 10% solutions) for intravenous infusion. Each milliliter of 10% calcium gluconate and calcium chloride has 8.9 mg (0.22 mmol) and 27.2 mg (0.68 mmol) of elemental calcium, respectively.[581] Calcium gluconate[582] is less irritating to the veins and can be administered through a peripheral intravenous line; calcium chloride can cause tissue necrosis if it extravasates and must be administered through a central line.

A study of patients undergoing cardiac surgery with extracorporeal perfusion (with concomitant high gluconate infusion) suggested that the increase in the ionized calcium level is significantly lower with calcium gluconate.[583] This finding was attributed to a requirement for hepatic metabolism for the release of ionized calcium from calcium gluconate, so that less ionized calcium would be bioavailable in cases of liver failure or diminished hepatic perfusion.[583] However, further studies in vitro, in animals, in humans with normal hepatic function, and during the anhepatic stage of liver transplantation have shown equal and rapid dissociation of ionized calcium from equal doses of calcium chloride and calcium gluconate, which indicates that the release of ionized calcium from calcium gluconate is independent of hepatic metabolism.[26]

The recommended dose is 10 mL of 10% calcium gluconate (3 to 4 mL of calcium chloride), infused intravenously over 2 to 3 minutes and under continuous ECG monitoring. The effect of the infusion starts in 1 to 3 minutes and lasts 30 to 60 minutes.[448,578] The dose should be repeated if there is no change in ECG findings or if the ECG abnormalities recur after initial improvement.[448,578] Calcium should be used with extreme caution in patients taking digitalis, because hypercalcemia potentiates the toxic effects of digitalis on the myocardium.[582] In this case, 10 mL of 10% calcium gluconate should be added to 100 mL of 5% dextrose in water and infused over 20 to 30 minutes to avoid hypercalcemia and to allow for an even distribution of calcium in the extracellular compartment.[446,577,580] To prevent the precipitation of calcium carbonate, calcium should not be administered in solutions containing bicarbonate.

Redistribution of Potassium into Cells

Sodium bicarbonate, β₂-agonists, and insulin with glucose all are used in the treatment of hyperkalemia to induce a redistribution of K⁺. Of these treatments, insulin with glucose is the most constant and reliable, whereas bicarbonate is the most controversial. However, they are all temporary measures and should not be substituted for the definitive treatment of hyperkalemia, which is removal of K⁺ from the body.

Insulin and Glucose

Insulin has the ability to lower plasma K⁺ level by shifting K⁺ into cells, particularly into skeletal myocytes and hepatocytes (see "Factors Affecting Internal Distribution of Potassium" section). This effect is reliable, reproducible, concentration dependent,[448] and effective, even in patients with CKD and ESRD[584-586] and in those in the anhepatic stage of liver transplantation.[587] The effect of insulin on plasma K⁺ levels is independent of age, of adrenergic activity,[588] and of its hypoglycemic effect, which in fact may be impaired in patients with CKD and/or ESRD.[26]

Insulin can be administered with glucose as a constant infusion or as a bolus injection.[585,586] The recommended dose of insulin with glucose infusion is 10 U of regular insulin in 500 mL of 10% dextrose, given over 60 minutes (there is no further drop in plasma K⁺ concentration after 90 minutes of insulin infusion[580,588]). However, a bolus injection is easier to administer, particularly under emergency conditions.[197] The recommended dose is 10 U of regular insulin administered intravenously followed immediately by 50 mL of 50% dextrose (25 g of glucose).[575,585,589,590] The effect of insulin on K⁺ level begins in 10 to 20 minutes, peaks at 30 to 60 minutes, and lasts for 4 to 6 hours.[448,577,585,591] In almost all patients, the plasma K⁺ drops by 0.5 to 1.2 mmol/L after this treatment.[586,587,590,591] The dose can be repeated as necessary.

Despite glucose administration, hypoglycemia may occur in up to 75% of patients treated with the bolus regimen described earlier, typically 1 hour after the infusion.[585] The likelihood of hypoglycemia is greater when the dose of glucose given is less than 30 g.[446] To prevent this, infusion of 10% dextrose at 50 to 75 mL/hr and close monitoring of the blood glucose levels is recommended.[575,589] Administration of glucose without insulin is not recommended, because the endogenous insulin release may be variable.[484] Administration of glucose in the absence of insulin may in fact increase plasma K^+ concentration by increasing plasma osmolality.[477,478,589] In hyperglycemic patients with glucose levels of 200 to 250 mg/dL or more, insulin should be administered without glucose and with close monitoring of plasma glucose level.[580] Combined treatment with β_2-agonists, in addition to providing a synergistic effect with insulin in lowering plasma K^+, may reduce the level of hypoglycemia.[585] Of note, the combined regimen may increase the heart rate by 15.1 ± 6.0 beats/min.[585]

β_2-ADRENERGIC AGONISTS

β_2-Agonists are an important but underutilized group of agents for the acute management of hyperkalemia. They exert their effect by activating Na^+-K^+-ATPase and the NKCC1 Na^+-K^+-$2Cl^-$ cotransporter, shifting K^+ into hepatocytes and skeletal myocytes (see also "Factors Affecting Internal Distribution of Potassium" section).

Albuterol (Salbutamol), a selective β_2-agonist, is the most widely studied and used. It is available in oral, inhaled, and intravenous forms; both the intravenous and inhaled or nebulized forms are effective.[592] The recommended dose for intravenous administration, which is not available in the United States, is 0.5 mg of albuterol in 100 mL of 5% dextrose, given over 10 to 15 minutes.[580,592,593] Its K^+-lowering effect starts in few minutes, is maximal at about 30 to 40 minutes[592,593] and lasts for 2 to 6 hours.[446] It reduces plasma K^+ levels by approximately 0.9 to 1.4 mmol/L.[446] The recommended dose for inhaled albuterol is 10 to 20 mg of nebulized albuterol in 4 mL of normal saline, inhaled over 10 minutes[585] (nebulized levalbuterol is as effective as albuterol[594]). Its kaliopenic effect starts at about 30 minutes, reaches its peak at about 90 minutes,[585,592] and lasts for 2 to 6 hours.[446,592]

Inhaled albuterol reduces plasma K^+ levels by approximately 0.5 to 1.0 mmol/L[446]; albuterol administered by metered-dose inhaler with spacer reduces plasma K^+ level by approximately 0.4 mmol/L.[595] Albuterol (in inhaled or parenteral form) and insulin with glucose have additive effects in reducing plasma K^+ levels, and can decrease plasma K^+ concentration by approximately 1.2 to 1.5 mmol/L in total.[446,585,591] A subset of patients with ESRD (approximately 20% to 40%) are not responsive to the K^+-lowering effect of albuterol ($\Delta K^+ \le 0.4$ mmol/L); therefore, albuterol (or other β_2-agonists) should not be used as a single agent in the treatment of hyperkalemia.[448,484] In an attempt to reduce pharmacokinetic variability, one study tested the effects of weight-based dosing on plasma K^+ levels, using 7 µg/kg of subcutaneous terbutaline (a β_2-agonist) in a group of ESRD patients.[596] The results showed a significant decline in plasma K^+ levels in almost all patients (mean = 1.31 ± 0.5 mmol/L; range = 0.5 to 2.3 mmol/L) in 30 to 90 minutes; of note, heart rate increased by an average of 25.8 ± 10.5 beats/min (range = 6.5 to 48).[596]

Treatment with albuterol may result in an increase in plasma glucose level (approximately 2 to 3 mmol/L) and, as noted earlier, in heart rate. The increase in heart rate is more pronounced with the intravenous form (approximately 20 beats/min) than with the inhaled form (approximately 6 to 10 beats/min).[484,592] There is no significant increase in systolic or diastolic blood pressure with nebulized or intravenous administration of albuterol.[592] However, it is prudent to use these agents with caution in patients with ischemic heart disease.[446]

SODIUM BICARBONATE

Bicarbonate prevailed as a preferred treatment modality for hyperkalemia for decades. For example, in a survey of nephrology training program directors in 1989, it was ranked as the second-line treatment, after Ca^{2+}.[597] Its use to treat acute hyperkalemia was based mainly on the results of small, older, uncontrolled clinical studies with a very limited number of patients,[52,60,598] in which bicarbonate was typically administered as a long infusion over many hours (not by intravenous push, which later became the routine).[599] One of these studies, which is frequently quoted, concluded that the K^+-lowering effect of bicarbonate is independent of changes in pH.[60] However, confounding variables included the duration of infusion, the use of glucose-containing solutions, and infrequent monitoring of plasma K^+ level.[60,600]

The role of bicarbonate in the acute treatment of hyperkalemia has been challenged.[586,599,601] Blumberg and colleagues compared different K^+-lowering modalities (Figure 17-16) and showed that bicarbonate infusion (isotonic or hypertonic) for up to 60 minutes had no effect on plasma K^+ level in their cohort of ESRD patients on hemodialysis[586]; there is, however, an effect of isotonic bicarbonate at 4 to 6 hours.[599] These observations were later confirmed by others, who failed to show any acute K^+-lowering effects (within 60 to 120 minutes) for bicarbonate.[599-601]

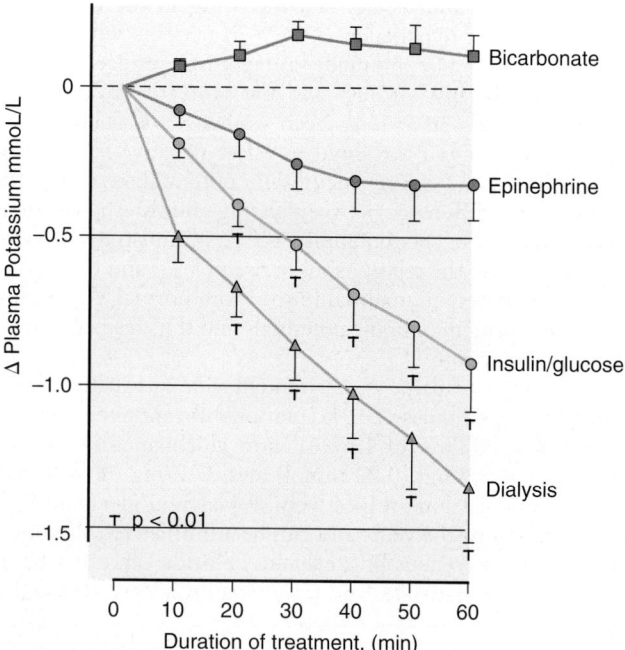

FIGURE 17-16 Changes in serum K^+ during intravenous infusion of bicarbonate, epinephrine, or insulin in glucose, and during hemodialysis. (From Blumberg A, Weidmann P, Shaw S, et al: Effect of various therapeutic approaches on plasma potassium and major regulating factors in terminal renal failure, *Am J Med* 85:507-512, 1988.)

A few studies have shown that metabolic acidosis may attenuate the physiologic responses to insulin and β_2-agonists.[448,601] The combined effect of bicarbonate and insulin with glucose has been studied with conflicting results.[601] In addition, bicarbonate and albuterol coadministration failed to show any additional benefit over albuterol alone.[601]

In summary, administration of bicarbonate, especially as a single agent, has no role in the contemporary treatment of acute hyperkalemia. Prolonged infusion of isotonic bicarbonate in ESRD patients does reduce plasma K^+ concentration at 5 to 6 hours by up to 0.7 mmol/L; approximately half of this effect is due to volume expansion.[599] Regardless of the mechanism, bicarbonate infusion may have a limited role in the *subacute* control of hyperkalemia, for example in the nondialytic management of patients with severe hyperkalemia.[602] The acute effect of bicarbonate infusion on plasma K^+ level in severely acidemic patients is not clear; however, it may be of some benefit in this setting.[197,575]

Of note, the infusion of sodium bicarbonate may reduce serum ionized calcium levels and cause volume overload, issues of relevance in patients with renal failure.[448,577] When bicarbonate administration is used to treat hyperkalemia, the authors recommend isotonic infusion of sodium bicarbonate; although hypertonic sodium bicarbonate does not increase plasma K^+ level,[472] it has been reported to cause hypernatremia.[586]

Removal of Potassium

DIURETICS

Diuretics have a relatively modest effect on urinary K^+ excretion in patients with CKD,[603] particularly in an acute setting.[578] However, these medications are useful in correcting hyperkalemia in patients with the syndrome of hyporeninemic hypoaldosteronism[604] or selective renal K^+ secretory problems (e.g., after transplantation or administration of trimethoprim).[605,606]

In patients with impaired renal function, use of the following agents is recommended: (1) oral diuretics with the highest bioavailability (e.g., torsemide) and the least renal metabolism, (e.g., torsemide, bumetanide) to minimize the chance of accumulation and toxicity; (2) intravenous agents (short-term treatment) with the least hepatic metabolism (e.g., furosemide rather than bumetanide); (3) combinations of loop and thiazide-like diuretics for better efficacy, although this may decrease GFR due to activation of tubuloglomerular feedback.[607] Use of the maximal effective "ceiling" dose is recommended.[603,607]

MINERALOCORTICOIDS

Limited data are available on the role of mineralocorticoids in the management of acute hyperkalemia.[26,608] However, these agents have been used to treat chronic hyperkalemia in patients with hypoaldosteronism with or without hyporeninism, in those with systemic lupus erythematosus,[609] in kidney transplant patients taking cyclosporine,[610] and in ESRD patients maintained on hemodialysis who have interdialytic hyperkalemia.[611,612]

The recommended dose is 0.1 to 0.3 mg/day of fludrocortisone, a synthetic glucocorticoid with potent mineralocorticoid activity and modest glucocorticoid activity (0.3 mg of fludrocortisone is equal to 1 mg of prednisone with regard to glucocorticoid activity).[26,610-612] In patients with ESRD maintained on hemodialysis, this regimen reduces plasma K^+ concentration by 0.5 to 0.7 mmol/L and has not been associated with significant changes in blood pressure or weight (as a surrogate for fluid retention).[611] However, more recent studies of a regimen of 0.1 mg/day of fludrocortisone in patients receiving long-term hemodialysis have shown statistically significant but clinically inconsequential effects on plasma K^+ concentration.[613,614] The long-term safety of fludrocortisone treatment in patients with ESRD has not been established, and given the minimal effect on plasma K^+ concentration the authors do not recommend its use for the management of interdialytic hyperkalemia.

Pharmacologic inhibition of 11β-HSD2 with glycyrrhetinic acid has also been tested as a novel mechanism to control hyperkalemia in patients with ESRD.[338] As in other aldosterone-sensitive epithelia, the 11β-HSD2 enzyme protects colonic epithelial cells from illicit activation of the mineralocorticoid receptor by cortisol. Hypothesizing that glycyrrhetinic acid would activate extrarenal potassium secretion by the colon and other tissues, Farese and colleagues tested the effect of the drug in a double-blind, placebo-controlled trial involving 10 ESRD patients.

Treatment with glycyrrhetinic acid significantly increased the plasma ratio of cortisol to cortisone, consistent with successful inhibition of 11β-HSD2. This effect was associated with a significant reduction in mean plasma K^+ concentration, with 70% of predialysis values in the normal range (3.5 to 4.7 mmol/L) in the glycyrrhetinic acid phase of the trial, versus 24% in the placebo phase.[338] Plasma renin activity and aldosterone levels also dropped, perhaps due to the lower median plasma K^+ level. Glycyrrhetinic acid is thus a promising agent for long-term management of plasma K^+ in ESRD patients; however, more extensive clinical testing is clearly required before widespread utilization.

CATION-EXCHANGE RESINS

Ion-exchange resins are cross-linked polymers containing acidic or basic structural units that can exchange either anions or cations on contact with a solution. They are capable of binding to a variety of monovalent and divalent cations. Cation-exchange resins are classified based on the cation (i.e., hydrogen, ammonium, sodium, potassium, or calcium) that is cycled during the synthesis of the resin to saturate sulfonic or carboxylic groups. In 1950 Elkinton and colleagues successfully used a carboxylic resin in ammonium cycle in three patients with hyperkalemia.[615] However, hydrogen- and ammonium-cycled resins were associated with metabolic acidosis[616] and mouth ulcers,[617] which made the sodium-cycled resins preferable.[618] Calcium-cycled resins may have other potential benefits, including a phosphate-lowering effect; however, this requires large, potentially toxic, doses of resin[619]; moreover, these resins have been associated with hypercalcemia.[620]

The dominant resin clinically available in the United States is sodium polystyrene sulfonate (SPS). SPS exchanges Na^+ for K^+ in the gastrointestinal tract, mainly in the colon,[575,617,621] and has been shown to increase the fecal excretion of K^+.[617] Occasional constipation, easily controlled with enema or cathartics, has been reported with oral administration of SPS in water.[617] To prevent constipation and to facilitate the passage of the resin through the gastrointestinal tract, Flinn and colleagues added sorbitol to the resin,[622] even though the occurrence of constipation and impaction had not been reported in an earlier study[618] of SPS use cited by these authors. It has since become routine to administer SPS with sorbitol, with approximately 5 million doses administered annually in the United States alone.[623] Notably, although *SPS* is used in this chapter to denote sodium polystyrene sulfonate, SPS is in fact also a brand name for sodium polystyrene sulfonate in sorbitol, which indicates the frequency with which these agents are administered together.[576]

The effect of ingested SPS on plasma K^+ concentration is slow; it may take from 4 to 24 hours to see a significant effect on plasma K^+ level.[577,578,617] The oral dose is usually 15 to 30 g, which can be repeated every 4 to 6 hours. Each gram of resin binds 0.5 to 1.2 mEq of K^+ in exchange for 2 to 3 mEq of Na^+.[578,617,624,625] The discrepancy is caused in part by the binding of small amounts of other cations.[617]

The hypokalemic effect may be due partly to the coadministered laxative. One study of healthy subjects compared the rate of fecal excretion of K^+ by different laxatives with or without SPS and found that the combination of phenolphthalein/ docusate with resin produced greater fecal excretion of K^+ (49 mmol in 12 hours) than did phenolphthalein/docusate alone (37 mmol in 12 hours) or other laxative-resin combinations.[624]

Earlier studies of SPS, mostly before the era of long-term hemodialysis, used multiple doses of the exchange resin orally or rectally as an enema and were associated with declines in plasma K^+ levels of 1 mmol/L and 0.8 mmol/L in 24 hours, respectively.[617] With the advent of routine hemodialysis, however, it has become common to order only a single dose of resin-cathartic in the management of acute hyperkalemia. One study has addressed the efficacy of this practice, evaluating the effect of four different single-dose resin-cathartic regimens on the plasma K^+ levels of six patients with CKD on maintenance hemodialysis. None of the regimens used reduced the plasma K^+ concentration below the initial baseline.[625] Notably, the subjects in this study were normokalemic. Regardless, if SPS is judged to be appropriate in the management of hyperkalemia (see later), repeated doses are usually required for an adequate effect.

SPS can be administered rectally as a retention enema in patients unable to take or tolerate the oral form. The recommended dose is 30 to 50 g of resin as an emulsion in 100 mL of an aqueous vehicle (e.g., 20% dextrose in water) every 6 hours. It should be administered warm (body temperature), after a cleansing enema with body-temperature tap water, through a rubber tube placed at about 20 cm from the rectum with the tip well into the sigmoid colon. The emulsion should be introduced by gravity, flushed with an additional 50 to 100 mL of non–sodium-containing fluid, retained for at least 30 to 60 minutes, and followed by a cleansing enema (250 to 1000 mL of body-temperature tap water).[626] SPS in sorbitol should not be used for enemas, given the risk of colonic necrosis.[578,627]

An increasing concern with oral SPS in sorbitol is intestinal necrosis caused by the administration of this preparation[623,627-630]; this is frequently a fatal complication.[623,627,629] Studies in experimental animals suggest that sorbitol is required for the intestinal injury[627]; however, SPS crystals can often be detected in human pathologic specimens, adherent to the injured mucosa.[629,630] A case of colonic necrosis following oral SPS alone, without sorbitol, has also been reported,[631] which directly implicates SPS in the intestinal injury. The risk of intestinal necrosis appears to be greatest when SPS is given with sorbitol within the first week after surgery. For example, out of 117 patients who received SPS with sorbitol within a week of surgery, two patients developed intestinal necrosis.[628] Notably, however, in a recent case series examining intestinal necrosis associated with SPS in sorbitol, only 2 out of 11 confirmed cases occurred in the postoperative setting.[629] Although most cases of intestinal necrosis have occurred in patients receiving SPS in 70% sorbitol it has also been reported in patients receiving SPS in 33% sorbitol.[623]

In response to these reports, the U.S. Food and Drug Administration (FDA) removed recommendations for concomitant or postdosing use of sorbitol from the labeling of SPS in 2005.[623] However, the FDA allowed continued marketing of the most frequently used premixed SPS in sorbitol suspension, given that it contained only 33% sorbitol. After this labeling change, more cases of intestinal necrosis were reported, including some associated with the use of SPS in 33% sorbitol, as noted earlier.[623] As a result, in September 2009 the FDA changed the safety labeling for SPS powder, stating that concomitant administration of sorbitol is not recommended.[623]

Given these serious concerns, clinicians must carefully consider whether emergency treatment with SPS is actually necessary for the management of hyperkalemia.[576,623,632] There are minimal data on the efficacy of SPS within the first 24 hours after administration for hyperkalemia[623]; at best, the effect occurs within 4 to 6 hours of administration.[577,578,617] This temporal limitation should be taken into consideration when deciding whether or not to administer SPS in acute hyperkalemia. In patients with intact renal function alternative measures such as hydration to increase distal tubular delivery of Na^+ and distal tubular flow rate, and/or administration of diuretics are often sufficient for potassium removal. In patients with advanced renal failure, the use of SPS is reasonable as a temporizing maneuver while awaiting hemodialysis; however, if hemodialysis is available within 1 to 4 hours the authors question the need for SPS, given the delayed hypokalemic response and the risk of potentially fatal intestinal necrosis. Furthermore, if the patient has existing vascular access for hemodialysis the risk of intestinal necrosis outweighs that of the dialysis procedure.

If SPS is administered, the preparation ideally should not contain sorbitol. SPS without sorbitol is typically available as a powder that must be reconstituted with water. If a laxative other than sorbitol is coadministered, it should not contain potassium or other cations such as magnesium or calcium, which can compete with potassium for binding to the resin. In patients with renal insufficiency, the laxative should not contain phosphorus. Reasonable laxatives for this purpose include lactulose and some preparations of polyethylene glycol 3350. However, data demonstrating the efficacy and safety of these laxatives when used with SPS are not available.[576] It should also be noted that administering SPS without sorbitol might not eliminate the risk of intestinal necrosis, given the role of the SPS resin itself in this complication.[629-631]

SPS without sorbitol is rarely available in the United States. Many pharmacies and hospitals stock only SPS premixed with sorbitol.[623] Although there are indications that SPS preparations with 33% sorbitol carry a lesser risk, cases of intestinal necrosis have also been described with this preparation. Clinicians must weigh the relative risk of using this preparation in the management of acute hyperkalemia.[623] In any case, SPS with sorbitol should not be used in patients at higher risk for intestinal necrosis, including postoperative patients, patients with a history of bowel obstruction, patients with slow intestinal transit, patients with ischemic bowel disease, and renal transplant recipients.

Finally, oral SPS with sorbitol can also injure the upper gastrointestinal tract, although the clinical significance of these findings is not known.[633] Other potential complications include reduction of plasma calcium level,[634] volume overload,[616] interference with lithium absorption,[635] and iatrogenic hypokalemia.[626]

DIALYSIS

All modes of acute renal replacement therapy are effective in removing K^+. Continuous hemodiafiltration is increasingly used in the management of critically ill and hemodynamically unstable patients.[636] Peritoneal dialysis, although not very effective in an acute setting, has been used effectively in cases of cardiac arrest complicating acute hyperkalemia.[637] Peritoneal dialysis is capable of removing significant amounts of K^+ (5 mmol/hr or 240 mmol in 48 hours) using 2-L exchanges, with each exchange taking almost an hour.[580] However, hemodialysis is the preferred mode when rapid correction of a hyperkalemic episode is desired.[638]

An average 3- to 5-hour hemodialysis session removes approximately 40 to 120 mmol of K^+.[26,638-645] Approximately 15% of the total K^+ removal results from ultrafiltration, with the remaining clearance from dialysis.[642,646] Of the total K^+ removed, about 40% is from extracellular space, and the remainder is from intracellular compartments.[640,642,643] In most patients, the greatest decline in plasma K^+ (1.2 to 1.5 mmol/L) and the largest amount of K^+ removal occur during the first hour; the plasma K^+ concentration usually reaches its nadir at about 3 hours. Despite a relatively constant plasma K^+ concentration thereafter, K^+ removal continues until the end of the hemodialysis session, although at significantly lower rate.[26,641,642]

The amount of K^+ removed depends primarily on the type and surface area of the dialyzer used, blood flow rate, dialysate flow rate, dialysis duration, and plasma/dialysate K^+ gradient. However, about 40% of the difference in removal cannot be explained by the aforementioned factors and may instead be related to the relative distribution of K^+ between intracellular and extracellular spaces.[640] Glucose-free dialysates are more efficient in removing K^+.[640,643] This effect may be caused by alterations in endogenous insulin levels, with concomitant intracellular shift of K^+; the insulin level is 50% lower when glucose-free dialysates are used.[640] Furthermore, these findings imply that K^+ removal may be greater if hemodialysis is performed with the patient in a fasting state.[646] Treatment with β_2-agonists also reduces the total K^+ removal by approximately 40%.[638]

The change in pH during dialysis has been thought to have no significant effect on K^+ removal.[638,646] A recent study evaluated this issue in detail, examining the effect of dialysate bicarbonate concentration on both plasma K^+ level and K^+ removal. Dialysates with bicarbonate concentrations of 39 mmol/L (high), 35 mmol/L (standard), and 27 mmol/L (low) were utilized. The use of a high concentration of bicarbonate was associated with a more rapid decline in plasma K^+ level; this difference was statistically significant for comparisons of both high-bicarbonate versus standard-bicarbonate dialysates

and high-bicarbonate versus low-bicarbonate dialysates at 60 and 240 minutes. However, the total amount of K^+ removed was higher with the low-bicarbonate dialysate (116.4 ± 21.6 mmol per dialysis) than with the standard-bicarbonate dialysate (73.2 ± 12.8 mmol per dialysis) and high-bicarbonate dialysate (80.9 ± 15.4 mmol per dialysis), although neither of these differences was statistically significant.[647] Therefore, although high-bicarbonate dialysis may *acutely* have a more rapid effect on plasma K^+ level, this advantage is potentially mitigated by a lower total removal of the ion over the course of a typical treatment session.

One of the major determinants of total K^+ removal is the K^+ gradient between the plasma and dialysate. Dialysates with a lower K^+ concentration are more effective at reducing plasma K^+ concentration.[641,645] Many nephrologists use the "rule of 7s" to set the dialysate K^+ concentration: the plasma K^+ concentration plus the dialysate K^+ concentration should equal approximately 7. If this rule were followed, however, then dialysate with a K^+ concentration of 0.0 or 1.0 mEq/L ("0K" or "1K" bath) would need to be used for patients with plasma K^+ concentrations exceeding 6 to 7 mmol/L. A rapid decline in plasma K^+ concentration due to the use of 0K or 1K dialysate can have deleterious effects due to several mechanisms. First, an acute decrease in plasma K^+ level can be associated with rebound hypertension (i.e., a significant increase in blood pressure 1 hour after dialysis),[639] which is attributed in part to the peripheral vasoconstriction that is a direct result of the change in plasma K^+ concentration.[639] Second, a low plasma K^+ concentration can alter the rate of tissue metabolism—the so-called Solandt effect[648]—and decrease tissue oxygen consumption, which promotes arteriolar constriction.[639] This vasoconstriction, in turn, may reduce the efficiency of dialysis,[26] although a randomized, prospective study did not confirm this finding.[641] Discrepencies among reported findings are likely due to differences in the glucose content of the dialysate utilized; differences in circulating insulin may have had additional, unrelated effects on muscle blood flow.[649] Finally, dialysates with a very low K^+ concentration may increase the risk of significant arrhythmia.[645,650]

Several studies have found an increased incidence of significant arrhythmia with hemodialysis, occurring during and immediately after treatment.[650-652] An incidence of up to 76% has been reported.[653] However, many investigators do not consider the hemodialysis procedure to be significantly arrhythmogenic.[654-656] Some have suggested that a relationship exists between decreases in plasma K^+ concentration, dialysate K^+ concentration, and the incidence of significant arrhythmias.[650] Despite the controversy, it seems prudent to recommend that dialysates with a very low K^+ concentration (0 or 1 mmol/L) be used cautiously, particularly in patients at high risk. This definition includes patients receiving digitalis; those with a history of arrhythmia, coronary artery disease, left ventricular hypertrophy, or high systolic blood pressure; and those of advanced age. Continuous cardiac monitoring for all patients undergoing dialysis with a 0- or 1-mmol/L K^+ bath is strongly recommended.[448]

Given the risk of inducing arrhythmias with very low-K^+ dialysates, an alternative approach has been proposed for the treatment of significant hyperkalemia.[448,657] In this regimen, dialysis is initiated with a 3- to 4-mEq/L K^+ bath, which will immediately lower the plasma K^+ concentration in a slower and perhaps safer manner.[650] The K^+ concentration of the dialysate may then be lowered in a stepwise fashion with each subsequent hour of dialysis. A more sophisticated approach uses potassium profiling to maintain a constant K^+ gradient during dialysis.[657-659] Potassium profiling results in more sustained, even removal of potassium[658] than dialysis using a fixed-K^+ bath (2.5 mEq/L), with less effect on ventricular ectopy.[657-659]

For the management of severe hyperkalemia (plasma $K^+ \geq$ 7.0 mEq/L) the authors favor the use of stepped reduction or potassium profiling of dialysate K^+ concentrations. We rarely encounter the need to use 1K or 0K dialysate baths, which we also avoid at the beginning of dialysis sessions for treatment of acute hyperkalemia. We recommend restricting the upfront use of these low-K^+ baths to patients with life-threatening hyperkalemic arrhythmias and/or life-threatening conduction abnormalities.

A rebound increase in plasma K^+ concentration can occur after hemodialysis. This phenomenon can be especially marked in cases of massive release from devitalized tissues (e.g., tumor lysis, rhabdomyolysis) and requires frequent monitoring of plasma K^+ and further hemodialysis. However, a rebound increase may also occur in ESRD patients during regular maintenance hemodialysis, despite technically adequate treatment,[642] particularly in those patients with a high predialysis K^+ concentration. Factors that attenuate K^+ removal and thus increase the risk and magnitude of postdialysis rebound include pretreatment with β_2-agonists,[638] pretreatment with insulin and glucose, food consumption early in the dialysis session,[646] a high predialysis plasma K^+ concentration,[642] and higher dialysate Na^+ concentrations.[644]

References

1. Welling PA, Chang YP, Delpire E, et al. Multigene kinase network, kidney transport, and salt in essential hypertension. *Kidney Int.* 2010;77:1063-1069.
2. Zhou R, Patel SV, Snyder PM. Nedd4-2 catalyzes ubiquitination and degradation of cell surface ENaC. *J Biol Chem.* 2007;282:20207-20212.
3. Knight KK, Olson DR, Zhou R, et al. Liddle's syndrome mutations increase Na^+ transport through dual effects on epithelial Na^+ channel surface expression and proteolytic cleavage. *Proc Natl Acad Sci U S A.* 2006;103:2805-2808.
4. Kahle KT, et al. WNK4 regulates the balance between renal NaCl reabsorption and K^+ secretion. *Nat Genet.* 2003;35:372-376.
5. Warnock DG, Bubien JK. Liddle's syndrome: a public health menace? *Am J Kidney Dis.* 1995;25:924-927.
6. McDonough AA, Thompson CB, Youn JH. Skeletal muscle regulates extracellular potassium. *Am J Physiol Renal Physiol.* 2002;282:F967-F974.
7. Williams ME, Rosa RM, Silva P, et al. Impairment of extrarenal potassium disposal by α-adrenergic stimulation. *N Engl J Med.* 1984;311:145-149.
8. Rosa RM, Epstein FH. Extrarenal potassium metabolism. In: Seldin DW, Giebisch G, eds. *The kidney: physiology and pathophysiology.* 3rd ed. vol 2. Philadelphia: Lippincott Williams & Wilkins; 2000:1552-1573.
9. Knochel JP, Dotin LN, Hamburger RJ. Pathophysiology of intense physical conditioning in a hot climate. I. Mechanisms of potassium depletion. *J Clin Invest.* 1972;51:242-255.
10. Chen P, et al. Modest dietary K^+ restriction provokes insulin resistance of cellular K^+ uptake and phosphorylation of renal outer medulla K^+ channel without fall in plasma K^+ concentration. *Am J Physiol Cell Physiol.* 2006;290:C1355-C1363.
11. Therien AG, Blostein R. Mechanisms of sodium pump regulation. *Am J Physiol Cell Physiol.* 2000;279:C541-C566.
12. Lingrel JB, Croyle ML, Woo AL, et al. Ligand binding sites of Na, K-ATPase. *Acta Physiol Scand Suppl.* 1998;643:69-77.
13. McDonough AA, Wang J, Farley RA. Significance of sodium pump isoforms in digitalis therapy. *J Mol Cell Cardiol.* 1995;27:1001-1009.
14. Crambert G, et al. Transport and pharmacological properties of nine different human Na, K-ATPase isozymes. *J Biol Chem.* 2000;275:1976-1986.
15. James PF, et al. Identification of a specific role for the Na, K-ATPase alpha 2 isoform as a regulator of calcium in the heart. *Mol Cell.* 1999;3:555-563.
16. Lorenz JN, et al. ACTH-induced hypertension is dependent on the ouabain-binding site of the α2-Na^+-K^+-ATPase subunit. *Am J Physiol Heart Circ Physiol.* 2008;295:H273-H280.
17. Akimova O, Tremblay J, Hamet P, et al. The Na^+/K^+-ATPase as $[K^+]_o$ sensor: role in cardiovascular disease pathogenesis and augmented production of endogenous cardiotonic steroids. *Pathophysiology.* 2006;13(4):209-216.
18. Juel C, Pilegaard H, Nielsen JJ, et al. Interstitial K(+) in human skeletal muscle during and after dynamic graded exercise determined by microdialysis. *Am J Physiol Regul Integr Comp Physiol.* 2000;278:R400-R406.
19. Mount DB, Zandi-Nejad K. Disorders of potassium balance. In: Brenner BM, ed. *Brenner and Rector's the kidney.* 7th ed. Philadelphia: Saunders; 2004:997-1040.
20. Clausen T. Clinical and therapeutic significance of the Na^+, K^+ pump*. *Clin Sci (Lond).* 1998;95:3-17.
21. Bundgaard H, Schmidt TA, Larsen JS, et al. K^+ supplementation increases muscle [Na^+-K^+-ATPase] and improves extrarenal K^+ homeostasis in rats. *J Appl Physiol.* 1997;82:1136-1144.
22. McKenna MJ. Effects of training on potassium homeostasis during exercise. *J Mol Cell Cardiol.* 1995;27:941-949.
23. Nielsen JJ, et al. Effects of high-intensity intermittent training on potassium kinetics and performance in human skeletal muscle. *J Physiol.* 2004;554:857-870.
24. Hebert SC, Mount DB, Gamba G. Molecular physiology of cation-coupled Cl^- cotransport: the SLC12 family. *Pflugers Arch.* 2004;447:580-593.
25. Gosmanov AR, Wong JA, Thomason DB. Duality of G protein–coupled mechanisms for β-adrenergic activation of NKCC activity in skeletal muscle. *Am J Physiol Cell Physiol.* 2002;283:C1025-C1032.
26. Mount DB, Zandi-Nejad K. Disorders of potassium balance. In: Brenner BM, ed. *Brenner and Rector's the kidney.* Philadelphia: Saunders; 2007:547-587.
27. Ryan DP, et al. Mutations in potassium channel Kir2.6 cause susceptibility to thyrotoxic hypokalemic periodic paralysis. *Cell.* 2010;140:88-98.
28. Guo J, et al. Extracellular K^+ concentration controls cell surface density of IKr in rabbit hearts and of the HERG channel in human cell lines. *J Clin Invest.* 2009;119:2745-2757.
29. Briggs AP, Koechig I, Doisy EA, et al. Some changes in the composition of blood due the injection of insulin. *J Biol Chem.* 1924;58:721-730.
30. Ferrannini E, et al. Independent stimulation of glucose metabolism and Na^+-K^+ exchange by insulin in the human forearm. *Am J Physiol.* 1988;255:E953-E958.
31. Rossetti L, Klein-Robbenhaar G, Giebisch G, et al. Effect of insulin on renal potassium metabolism. *Am J Physiol.* 1987;252:F60-F64.
32. Dluhy RG, Axelrod L, Williams GH. Serum immunoreactive insulin and growth hormone response to potassium infusion in normal man. *J Appl Physiol.* 1972;33:22-26.
33. Choi CS, Thompson CB, Leong PK, et al. Short-term K(+) deprivation provokes insulin resistance of cellular K(+) uptake revealed with the K(+) clamp. *Am J Physiol Renal Physiol.* 2001;280:F95-F102.
34. DeFronzo RA, et al. Influence of basal insulin and glucagon secretion on potassium and sodium metabolism. Studies with somatostatin in normal dogs and in normal and diabetic human beings. *J Clin Invest.* 1978;61:472-479.
35. Adabala M, Jhaveri KD, Gitman M. Severe hyperkalaemia resulting from octreotide use in a haemodialysis patient. *Nephrol Dial Transplant.* 2010;25:3439-3442.
36. Sargent AI, Overton CC, Kuwik RJ, et al. Octreotide-induced hyperkalemia. *Pharmacotherapy.* 1994;14:497-501.
37. DeFronzo RA, Felig P, Ferrannini E, et al. Effect of graded doses of insulin on splanchnic and peripheral potassium metabolism in man. *Am J Physiol.* 1980;238:E421-E427.
38. Clausen T, Everts ME. Regulation of the Na, K-pump in skeletal muscle. *Kidney Int.* 1989;35:1-13.
39. Li D, Sweeney G, Wang Q, et al. Participation of PI3K and atypical PKC in Na^+-K^+-pump stimulation by IGF-I in VSMC. *Am J Physiol.* 1999;276:H2109-H2116.
40. Al-Khalili L, Yu M, Chibalin AV. Na(+), K(+)-ATPase trafficking in skeletal muscle: insulin stimulates translocation of both alpha(1)- and alpha(2)-subunit isoforms. *FEBS Lett.* 2003;536:198-202.
41. Yudowski GA, et al. Phosphoinositide-3 kinase binds to a proline-rich motif in the Na^+, K^+-ATPase alpha subunit and regulates its trafficking. *Proc Natl Acad Sci U S A.* 2000;97:6556-6561.
42. Feraille E, et al. Insulin-induced stimulation of Na^+-K^+-ATPase activity in kidney proximal tubule cells depends on phosphorylation of the α-subunit at Tyr-10. *Mol Biol Cell.* 1999;10:2847-2859.
43. Boini KM, Graf D, Kuhl D, et al. SGK1 dependence of insulin induced hypokalemia. *Pflugers Arch.* 2009;457:955-961.
44. D'Silva JL. The action of adrenaline on serum potassium. *J Physiol.* 1934;82:393-398.
45. Olsson AM, Persson S, Schoder R. Effects of terbutaline and isoproterenol on hyperkalemia in nephrectomized rabbits. *Scand J Urol Nephrol.* 1978;12:35-38.

46. Ballanyi K, Grafe P. Changes in intracellular ion activities induced by adrenaline in human and rat skeletal muscle. *Pflugers Arch.* 1988;411:283-288.

47. Scheid CR, Fay FS. Beta-adrenergic stimulation of 42K influx in isolated smooth muscle cells. *Am J Physiol.* 1984;246:C415-C421.

48. Williams ME, et al. Catecholamine modulation of rapid potassium shifts during exercise. *N Engl J Med.* 1985;312:823-827.

49. Fenn WO, Cobb DM. The potassium equilibrium in muscle. *J Gen Physiol.* 1934;17:629-656.

50. Simmons DH, Avedon M. Acid-base alterations and plasma potassium concentration. *Am J Physiol.* 1959;197:319-326.

51. Adrogué HJ, Madias NE. Changes in plasma potassium concentration during acute acid-base disturbances. *Am J Med.* 1981;71:456-467.

52. Burnell JM, Villamill MF, Uyeno BT, et al. The effect in humans of extracellular PH change on the relationship between serum potassium concentration and intracellular potassium. *J Clin Invest.* 1956;35:935-939.

53. Oster JR, Perez G, Castro A, et al. Plasma potassium response to acute metabolic acidosis induced by mineral and nonmineral acids. *Miner Electrolyte Metab.* 1980;4:28-36.

54. Abrams WB, Lewis DW, Bellet S. The effect of acidosis and alkalosis on the plasma potassium concentration and the electrocardiogram of normal and potassium depleted dogs. *Am J Med Sci.* 1951;222:506-515.

55. Fulop M. Serum potassium in lactic acidosis and ketoacidosis. *N Engl J Med.* 1979;300:1087-1089.

56. Orringer CE, Eustace JC, Wunsch CD, et al. Natural history of lactic acidosis after grand-mal seizures. A model for the study of an anion-gap acidosis not associated with hyperkalemia. *N Engl J Med.* 1977;297:796-799.

57. Wiederseiner JM, Muser J, Lutz T, et al. Acute metabolic acidosis: characterization and diagnosis of the disorder and the plasma potassium response. *J Am Soc Nephrol.* 2004;15:1589-1596.

58. Adrogué HJ, Madias NE. PCO2 and [K+]p in metabolic acidosis: certainty for the first and uncertainty for the other. *J Am Soc Nephrol.* 2004;15:1667-1668.

59. Sonikian M, Metaxaki P, Vlassopoulos D, et al. Long-term management of sevelamer hydrochloride–induced metabolic acidosis aggravation and hyperkalemia in hemodialysis patients. *Ren Fail.* 2006;28:411-418.

60. Fraley DS, Adler S. Correction of hyperkalemia by bicarbonate despite constant blood pH. *Kidney Int.* 1977;12:354-360.

61. Krapf R, Caduff P, Wagdi P, et al. Plasma potassium response to acute respiratory alkalosis. *Kidney Int.* 1995;47:217-224.

62. Natalini G, et al. Acute respiratory acidosis does not increase plasma potassium in normokalaemic anaesthetized patients. A controlled randomized trial. *Eur J Anaesthesiol.* 2001;18:394-400.

63. Malnic G, Klose RM, Giebisch G. Micropuncture study of renal potassium excretion in the rat. *Am J Physiol.* 1964;206:674-686.

64. Canessa CM, et al. Amiloride-sensitive epithelial Na+ channel is made of three homologous subunits. *Nature.* 1994;367:463-467.

65. Giebisch G. Renal potassium transport: mechanisms and regulation. *Am J Physiol.* 1998;274:F817-F833.

66. Muto S. Potassium transport in the mammalian collecting duct. *Physiol Rev.* 2001;81:85-116.

67. Stokes JB. Potassium secretion by cortical collecting tubule: relation to sodium absorption, luminal sodium concentration, and transepithelial voltage. *Am J Physiol.* 1981;241:F395-F402.

68. Lalioti MD, et al. Wnk4 controls blood pressure and potassium homeostasis via regulation of mass and activity of the distal convoluted tubule. *Nat Genet.* 2006;38:1124-1132.

69. Meneton P, Loffing J, Warnock DG. Sodium and potassium handling by the aldosterone-sensitive distal nephron: the pivotal role of the distal and connecting tubule. *Am J Physiol Renal Physiol.* 2004;287:F593-F601.

70. Frindt G, Palmer LG. Apical potassium channels in the rat connecting tubule. *Am J Physiol Renal Physiol.* 2004;287:F1030-F1037.

71. Frindt G, Palmer LG. Na channels in the rat connecting tubule. *Am J Physiol Renal Physiol.* 2004;286:F669-F674.

72. Loffing J, et al. Differential subcellular localization of ENaC subunits in mouse kidney in response to high- and low-Na diets. *Am J Physiol Renal Physiol.* 2000;279:F252-F258.

73. Frindt G, Shah A, Edvinsson J, et al. Dietary K regulates ROMK channels in connecting tubule and cortical collecting duct of rat kidney. *Am J Physiol Renal Physiol.* 2009;296:F347-F354.

74. Pluznick JL, Sansom SC. BK channels in the kidney: role in K(+) secretion and localization of molecular components. *Am J Physiol Renal Physiol.* 2006;291:F517-F529.

75. Lu M, et al. Absence of small conductance K+ channel (SK) activity in apical membranes of thick ascending limb and cortical collecting duct in ROMK (Bartter's) knockout mice. *J Biol Chem.* 2002;277:37881-37887.

76. Grimm PR, Foutz RM, Brenner R, et al. Identification and localization of BK-β subunits in the distal nephron of the mouse kidney. *Am J Physiol Renal Physiol.* 2007;293:F350-F359.

77. Rieg T, et al. The role of the BK channel in potassium homeostasis and flow-induced renal potassium excretion. *Kidney Int.* 2007;75:566-573.

78. Grimm PR, Irsik DL, Settles DC, et al. Hypertension of Kcnmb1−/− is linked to deficient K secretion and aldosteronism. *Proc Natl Acad Sci U S A.* 2009;106:11800-11805.

79. Amorim JB, Bailey MA, Musa-Aziz R, et al. Role of luminal anion and pH in distal tubule potassium secretion. *Am J Physiol Renal Physiol.* 2003;284:F381-F388.

80. Mount DB, Gamba G. Renal K-Cl cotransporters. *Curr Opin Nephrol Hypertens.* 2001;10:685-692.

81. Frindt G, Palmer LG. K+ secretion in the rat kidney: Na+channel–dependent and –independent mechanisms. *Am J Physiol Renal Physiol.* 2009;297:F389-F396.

82. Wingo CS, Armitage FE. Rubidium absorption and proton secretion by rabbit outer medullary collecting duct via H-K-ATPase. *Am J Physiol.* 1992;263:F849-F857.

83. Okusa MD, Unwin RJ, Velazquez H, et al. Active potassium absorption by the renal distal tubule. *Am J Physiol.* 1992;262:F488-F493.

84. Palmer LG, Frindt G. Aldosterone and potassium secretion by the cortical collecting duct. *Kidney Int.* 2000;57:1324-1328.

85. Giebisch GH. A trail of research on potassium. *Kidney Int.* 2002;62:1498-1512.

86. Gennari FJ, Segal AS. Hyperkalemia: an adaptive response in chronic renal insufficiency. *Kidney Int.* 2002;62:1-9.

87. Palmer LG, Antonian L, Frindt G. Regulation of apical K and Na channels and Na/K pumps in rat cortical collecting tubule by dietary K. *J Gen Physiol.* 1994;104:693-710.

88. Mick VE, et al. The α-subunit of the epithelial sodium channel is an aldosterone-induced transcript in mammalian collecting ducts, and this transcriptional response is mediated via distinct cis-elements in the 5′-flanking region of the gene. *Mol Endocrinol.* 2001;15:575-588.

89. Reisenauer MR, et al. AF17 competes with AF9 for binding to Dot1a to up-regulate transcription of epithelial Na+ channel alpha. *J Biol Chem.* 2009;284:35659-35669.

90. Snyder PM. Minireview: regulation of epithelial Na+ channel trafficking. *Endocrinology.* 2005;146:5079-5085.

91. Loffing J, et al. Aldosterone induces rapid apical translocation of ENaC in early portion of renal collecting system: possible role of SGK. *Am J Physiol Renal Physiol.* 2001;280:F675-F682.

92. Nielsen J, et al. Sodium transporter abundance profiling in kidney: effect of spironolactone. *Am J Physiol Renal Physiol.* 2002;283:F923-F933.

93. Naray-Fejes-Toth A, Canessa C, Cleaveland ES, et al. sgk is an aldosterone-induced kinase in the renal collecting duct. Effects on epithelial Na+ channels. *J Biol Chem.* 1999;274:16973-16978.

94. Kamynina E, Tauxe C, Staub O. Distinct characteristics of two human Nedd4 proteins with respect to epithelial Na(+) channel regulation. *Am J Physiol Renal Physiol.* 2001;281:F469-F477.

95. Findling JW, Raff H, Hansson JH, et al. Liddle's syndrome: prospective genetic screening and suppressed aldosterone secretion in an extended kindred. *J Clin Endocrinol Metab.* 1997;82:1071-1074.

96. Firsov D, et al. Cell surface expression of the epithelial Na channel and a mutant causing Liddle syndrome: a quantitative approach. *Proc Natl Acad Sci U S A.* 1996;93:15370-15375.

97. Snyder PM, Olson DR, Thomas BC. Serum and glucocorticoid-regulated kinase modulates Nedd4-2-mediated inhibition of the epithelial Na+ channel. *J Biol Chem.* 2002;277:5-8.

98. Huang DY, et al. Impaired regulation of renal K+ elimination in the sgk1-knockout mouse. *J Am Soc Nephrol.* 2004;15:885-891.

99. Wulff P, et al. Impaired renal Na(+) retention in the sgk1-knockout mouse. *J Clin Invest.* 2002;110:1263-1268.

100. Vallet V, Chraibi A, Gaeggeler HP, et al. An epithelial serine protease activates the amiloride-sensitive sodium channel. *Nature.* 1997;389:607-610.

101. Narikiyo T, et al. Regulation of prostasin by aldosterone in the kidney. *J Clin Invest.* 2002;109:401-408.

102. Vuagniaux G, Vallet V, Jaeger NF, et al. Synergistic activation of ENaC by three membrane-bound channel-activating serine proteases (mCAP1, mCAP2, and mCAP3) and serum- and glucocorticoid-regulated kinase (Sgk1) in *Xenopus* oocytes. *J Gen Physiol.* 2002;120:191-201.

103. Kleyman TR, Carattino MD, Hughey RP. ENaC at the cutting edge: regulation of epithelial sodium channels by proteases. *J Biol Chem.* 2009;284:20447-20451.

104. Kitagawa H, Chang H, Fujita T. Hyperkalemia due to nafamostat mesylate. *N Engl J Med.* 1995;332:687.

105. Iwashita K, et al. Inhibition of prostasin secretion by serine protease inhibitors in the kidney. *J Am Soc Nephrol.* 2003;14:11-16.

106. Palmer LG, Frindt G. Regulation of apical K channels in rat cortical collecting tubule during changes in dietary K intake. *Am J Physiol.* 1999;277:F805-F812.

107. Lin DH, et al. Protein tyrosine kinase is expressed and regulates ROMK1 location in the cortical collecting duct. *Am J Physiol Renal Physiol.* 2004;286:F881-F892.

108. Najjar F, et al. Dietary K⁺ regulates apical membrane expression of maxi-K channels in rabbit cortical collecting duct. *Am J Physiol Renal Physiol.* 2005;289:F922-F932.

109. Estilo G, et al. Effect of aldosterone on BK channel expression in mammalian cortical collecting duct. *Am J Physiol Renal Physiol.* 2008;295:F780-F788.

110. Delaloy C, et al. Multiple promoters in the WNK1 gene: one controls expression of a kidney-specific kinase-defective isoform. *Mol Cell Biol.* 2003;23:9208-9221.

111. Wade JB, et al. WNK1 kinase isoform switch regulates renal potassium excretion. *Proc Natl Acad Sci U S A.* 2006;103:8558-8563.

112. Lazrak A, Liu Z, Huang CL. Antagonistic regulation of ROMK by long and kidney-specific WNK1 isoforms. *Proc Natl Acad Sci U S A.* 2006;103:1615-1620.

113. O'Reilly M, et al. Dietary electrolyte-driven responses in the renal WNK kinase pathway in vivo. *J Am Soc Nephrol.* 2006;17:2402-2413.

114. Lin DH, et al. K depletion increases protein tyrosine kinase-mediated phosphorylation of ROMK. *Am J Physiol Renal Physiol.* 2002;283:F671-F677.

115. Sterling H, et al. Inhibition of protein-tyrosine phosphatase stimulates the dynamin-dependent endocytosis of ROMK1. *J Biol Chem.* 2002;277:4317-4323.

116. Mount DB, Yu AS. Transport of inorganic solutes: sodium, potassium, calcium, magnesium, and phosphate. In: Brenner BM, ed. *Brenner and Rector's the kidney.* 8th ed. Philadelphia: Saunders; 2007:156-213.

117. Wei Y, Bloom P, Lin D, Gu R, et al. Effect of dietary K intake on apical small-conductance K channel in CCD: role of protein tyrosine kinase. *Am J Physiol Renal Physiol.* 2001;281:F206-F212.

118. Babilonia E, et al. Superoxide anions are involved in mediating the effect of low K intake on c-Src expression and renal K secretion in the cortical collecting duct. *J Biol Chem.* 2005;280:10790-10796.

119. Babilonia E, et al. Role of gp91phox-containing NADPH oxidase in mediating the effect of K restriction on ROMK channels and renal K excretion. *J Am Soc Nephrol.* 2007;18:2037-2045.

120. Wang ZJ, et al. Decrease in dietary K intake stimulates the generation of superoxide anions in the kidney and inhibits K secretory channels in the CCD. *Am J Physiol Renal Physiol.* 2010;298:F1515-F1522.

121. Wei Y, Zavilowitz B, Satlin LM, et al. Angiotensin II inhibits the ROMK-like small conductance K channel in renal cortical collecting duct during dietary potassium restriction. *J Biol Chem.* 2007;282:6455-6462.

122. Jin Y, Wang Y, Wang ZJ, et al. Inhibition of angiotensin type 1 receptor impairs renal ability of K conservation in response to K restriction. *Am J Physiol Renal Physiol.* 2009;296:F1179-F1184.

123. Tomita K, Pisano JJ, Burg MB, et al. Effects of vasopressin and bradykinin on anion transport by the rat cortical collecting duct. Evidence for an electroneutral sodium chloride transport pathway. *J Clin Invest.* 1986;77:136-141.

124. Terada Y, Knepper MA. Thiazide-sensitive NaCl absorption in rat cortical collecting duct. *Am J Physiol.* 1990;259:F519-F528.

125. Leviel F, et al. The Na⁺-dependent chloride-bicarbonate exchanger SLC4A8 mediates an electroneutral Na⁺ reabsorption process in the renal cortical collecting ducts of mice. *J Clin Invest.* 2010;120:1627-1635.

126. Yue P, et al. Src family protein tyrosine kinase (PTK) modulates the effect of SGK1 and WNK4 on ROMK channels. *Proc Natl Acad Sci U S A.* 2009;106:15061-15066.

127. San-Cristobal P, et al. Angiotensin II signaling increases activity of the renal Na-Cl cotransporter through a WNK4-SPAK-dependent pathway. *Proc Natl Acad Sci U S A.* 2009;106:4384-4389.

128. Sandberg MB, Riquier AD, Pihakaski-Maunsbach K, et al. ANG II provokes acute trafficking of distal tubule Na⁺-Cl⁻ cotransporter to apical membrane. *Am J Physiol Renal Physiol.* 2007;293:F662-F669.

129. Sealey JE, Clark I, Bull MB, et al. Potassium balance and the control of renin secretion. *J Clin Invest.* 1970;49:2119-2127.

130. Vallon V, Schroth J, Lang F, et al. Expression and phosphorylation of the Na⁺-Cl⁻ cotransporter NCC in vivo is regulated by dietary salt, potassium, and SGK1. *Am J Physiol Renal Physiol.* 2009;297:F704-F712.

131. Ring AM, et al. An SGK1 site in WNK4 regulates Na⁺ channel and K⁺ channel activity and has implications for aldosterone signaling and K⁺ homeostasis. *Proc Natl Acad Sci U S A.* 2007;104:4025-4029.

132. Sterling D, Brown NJ, Supuran CT, et al. The functional and physical relationship between the DRA bicarbonate transporter and carbonic anhydrase II. *Am J Physiol Cell Physiol.* 2002;283:C1522-C1529.

133. Lin DH, Sterling H, Wang WH. The protein tyrosine kinase-dependent pathway mediates the effect of K intake on renal K secretion. *Physiology (Bethesda).* 2005;20:140-146.

134. Skott O, Briggs JP. Direct demonstration of macula densa–mediated renin secretion. *Science.* 1987;237:1618-1620.

135. Lorenz JN, Weihprecht H, Schnermann J, et al. Renin release from isolated juxtaglomerular apparatus depends on macula densa chloride transport. *Am J Physiol.* 1991;260:F486-F493.

136. Wagner C, Jensen BL, Kramer BK, et al. Control of the renal renin system by local factors. *Kidney Int Suppl.* 1998;67:S78-S83.

137. Schweda F, Wagner C, Kramer BK, et al. Preserved macula densa–dependent renin secretion in A1 adenosine receptor knockout mice. *Am J Physiol Renal Physiol.* 2003;284:F770-F777.

138. Henrich WL, McAlister EA, Smith PB, et al. Direct inhibitory effect of atriopeptin III on renin release in primate kidney. *Life Sci.* 1987;41:259-264.

139. Todorov V, Muller M, Schweda F, et al. Tumor necrosis factor-α inhibits renin gene expression. *Am J Physiol Regul Integr Comp Physiol.* 2002;283:R1046-R1051.

140. Li YC, et al. 1,25-Dihydroxyvitamin D₃ is a negative endocrine regulator of the renin-angiotensin system. *J Clin Invest.* 2002;110:229-238.

141. Wagner C, Pfeifer A, Ruth P, et al. Role of cGMP-kinase II in the control of renin secretion and renin expression. *J Clin Invest.* 1998;102:1576-1582.

142. Peti-Peterdi J, Harris RC. Macula densa sensing and signaling mechanisms of renin release. *J Am Soc Nephrol.* 2010;21:1093-1096.

143. Jensen BL, Kramer BK, Kurtz A. Adrenomedullin stimulates renin release and renin mRNA in mouse juxtaglomerular granular cells. *Hypertension.* 1997;29:1148-1155.

144. Boivin V, et al. Immunofluorescent imaging of β₁- and β₂-adrenergic receptors in rat kidney. *Kidney Int.* 2001;59:515-531.

145. Vargas SL, Toma I, Kang JJ, et al. Activation of the succinate receptor GPR91 in macula densa cells causes renin release. *J Am Soc Nephrol.* 2009;20:1002-1011.

146. Cheng HF, Wang JL, Zhang MZ, et al. Role of p38 in the regulation of renal cortical cyclooxygenase-2 expression by extracellular chloride. *J Clin Invest.* 2000;106:681-688.

147. Stichtenoth DO, Marhauer V, Tsikas D, et al. Effects of specific COX-2-inhibition on renin release and renal and systemic prostanoid synthesis in healthy volunteers. *Kidney Int.* 2005;68:2197-2207.

148. Dluhy RG, Axelrod L, Underwood RH, et al. Studies of the control of plasma aldosterone concentration in normal man. II. Effect of dietary potassium and acute potassium infusion. *J Clin Invest.* 1972;51:1950-1957.

149. Davies LA, et al. TASK channel deletion in mice causes primary hyperaldosteronism. *Proc Natl Acad Sci U S A.* 2008;105:2203-2208.

150. Chen XL, Bayliss DA, Fern RJ, et al. A role for T-type Ca²⁺ channels in the synergistic control of aldosterone production by ANG II and K⁺. *Am J Physiol.* 1999;276:F674-F683.

151. Somekawa S, et al. Regulation of aldosterone and cortisol production by the transcriptional repressor neuron restrictive silencer factor. *Endocrinology.* 2009;150:3110-3117.

152. Condon JC, Pezzi V, Drummond BM, et al. Calmodulin-dependent kinase I regulates adrenal cell expression of aldosterone synthase. *Endocrinology.* 2002;143:3651-3657.

153. Hilbers U, et al. Local renin-angiotensin system is involved in K⁺-induced aldosterone secretion from human adrenocortical NCI-H295 cells. *Hypertension.* 1999;33:1025-1030.

154. Mazzocchi G, Malendowicz LK, Markowska A, et al. Role of adrenal renin-angiotensin system in the control of aldosterone secretion in sodium-restricted rats. *Am J Physiol Endocrinol Metab.* 2000;278:E1027-E1030.

155. Saruta T, Kaplan NM. Adrenocortical steroidogenesis: the effects of prostaglandins. *J Clin Invest.* 1972;51:2246-2251.

156. Gordon RD, Kuchel O, Liddle GW, et al. Role of the sympathetic nervous system in regulating renin and aldosterone production in man. *J Clin Invest.* 1967;46:599-605.

157. Gupta P, Franco-Saenz R, Mulrow PJ. Regulation of the adrenal renin angiotensin system in cultured bovine zona glomerulosa cells: effect of catecholamines. *Endocrinology.* 1992;130:2129-2134.

158. Csukas S, Hanke CJ, Rewolinski D, et al. Prostaglandin E₂–induced aldosterone release is mediated by an EP2 receptor. *Hypertension.* 1998;31:575-581.

159. Clark BA, Brown RS, Epstein FH. Effect of atrial natriuretic peptide on potassium-stimulated aldosterone secretion: potential relevance to hypoaldosteronism in man. *J Clin Endocrinol Metab.* 1992;75:399-403.

160. Cherradi N, et al. Atrial natriuretic peptide inhibits calcium-induced steroidogenic acute regulatory protein gene transcription in adrenal glomerulosa cells. *Mol Endocrinol.* 1998;12:962-972.

161. Choi MJ, Ziyadeh FN. The utility of the transtubular potassium gradient in the evaluation of hyperkalemia. *J Am Soc Nephrol.* 2008;19:424-426.

162. Weinstein AM. A mathematical model of rat cortical collecting duct: determinants of the transtubular potassium gradient. *Am J Physiol Renal Physiol.* 2001;280:F1072-F1092.

163. Chacko M, Fordtran JS, Emmett M. Effect of mineralocorticoid activity on transtubular potassium gradient, urinary [K]/[Na] ratio, and fractional excretion of potassium. *Am J Kidney Dis.* 1998;32:47-51.

164. Joo KW, et al. Transtubular potassium concentration gradient (TTKG) and urine ammonium in differential diagnosis of hypokalemia. *J Nephrol.* 2000;13:120-125.

165. Lin SH, et al. Laboratory tests to determine the cause of hypokalemia and paralysis. *Arch Intern Med.* 2004;164:1561-1566.

166. Batlle DC, Hizon M, Cohen E, et al. The use of the urinary anion gap in the diagnosis of hyperchloremic metabolic acidosis. *N Engl J Med.* 1988;318:594-599.
167. Cohen JD, Neaton JD, Prineas RJ, et al. Diuretics, serum potassium and ventricular arrhythmias in the Multiple Risk Factor Intervention Trial. *Am J Cardiol.* 1987;60:548-554.
168. He FJ, MacGregor GA. Fortnightly review: beneficial effects of potassium. *BMJ.* 2001;323:497-501.
169. Wahr JA, et al. Preoperative serum potassium levels and perioperative outcomes in cardiac surgery patients. Multicenter Study of Perioperative Ischemia Research Group. *JAMA.* 1999;281:2203-2210.
170. Modesto KM, et al. Safety of exercise stress testing in patients with abnormal concentrations of serum potassium. *Am J Cardiol.* 2006;97:1247-1249.
171. Slovis C, Jenkins R. ABC of clinical electrocardiography: conditions not primarily affecting the heart. *BMJ.* 2002;324:1320-1323.
172. Roden DM. A practical approach to torsade de pointes. *Clin Cardiol.* 1997;20:285-290.
173. Darbar D, Sile S, Fish FA, et al. Congenital long QT syndrome aggravated by salt-wasting nephropathy. *Heart Rhythm.* 2005;2:304-306.
174. Parham WA, Mehdirad AA, Biermann KM, et al. Hyperkalemia revisited. *Tex Heart Inst J.* 2006;33:40-47.
175. Tang NL, et al. Severe hypokalemic myopathy in Gitelman's syndrome. *Muscle Nerve.* 1999;22:545-547.
176. Wong KM, et al. Hypokalemic metabolic acidosis attributed to cough mixture abuse. *Am J Kidney Dis.* 2001;38:390-394.
177. Tattersall RB. A paper which changed clinical practice (slowly). Jacob Holler on potassium deficiency in diabetic acidosis (1946). *Diabet Med.* 1999;16:978-984.
178. Comi G, Testa D, Cornelio F, et al. Potassium depletion myopathy: a clinical and morphological study of six cases. *Muscle Nerve.* 1985;8:17-21.
179. Mujais SK, Katz AI. Potassium deficiency. In: Seldin DW, Giebisch G, eds. *The kidney: physiology and pathophysiology.* 3rd ed. vol 2. Philadelphia: Lippincott Williams & Wilkins; 2000:1615-1646.
180. Schwartz WB, Relman AS. Effects of electrolyte disorders on renal structure and function. *N Engl J Med.* 1967;276:383-389:contd.
181. Cremer W, Bock KD. Symptoms and course of chronic hypokalemic nephropathy in man. *Clin Nephrol.* 1977;7:112-119.
182. Torres VE, Young Jr WF, Offord KP, et al. Association of hypokalemia, aldosteronism, and renal cysts. *N Engl J Med.* 1990;322:345-351.
183. Yasuhara D, et al. "End-stage kidney" in longstanding bulimia nervosa. *Int J Eat Disord.* 2005;38:383-385.
184. Menahem SA, Perry GJ, Dowling J, et al. Hypokalaemia-induced acute renal failure. *Nephrol Dial Transplant.* 1999;14:2216-2218.
185. Suga SI, et al. Hypokalemia induces renal injury and alterations in vasoactive mediators that favor salt sensitivity. *Am J Physiol Renal Physiol.* 2001;281:F620-F629.
186. Levi M, McDonald LA, Preisig PA, et al. Chronic K depletion stimulates rat renal brush-border membrane Na-citrate cotransporter. *Am J Physiol.* 1991;261:F767–F673.
187. Elkjaer ML, et al. Altered expression of renal NHE3, TSC, BSC-1, and ENaC subunits in potassium-depleted rats. *Am J Physiol Renal Physiol.* 2002;283:F1376-F1388.
188. Berl T, Linas SL, Aisenbrey GA, et al. On the mechanism of polyuria in potassium depletion. The role of polydipsia. *J Clin Invest.* 1977;60:620-625.
189. Marples D, Frokiaer J, Dorup J, et al. Hypokalemia-induced downregulation of aquaporin-2 water channel expression in rat kidney medulla and cortex. *J Clin Invest.* 1996;97:1960-1968.
190. Amlal H, Krane CM, Chen Q, et al. Early polyuria and urinary concentrating defect in potassium deprivation. *Am J Physiol Renal Physiol.* 2000;279:F655-F663.
191. Coca SG, Perazella MA, Buller GK. The cardiovascular implications of hypokalemia. *Am J Kidney Dis.* 2005;45:233-247.
192. Ray PE, Suga S, Liu XH, et al. Chronic potassium depletion induces renal injury, salt sensitivity, and hypertension in young rats. *Kidney Int.* 2001;59:1850-1858.
193. Kaplan NM, Carnegie A, Raskin P, et al. Potassium supplementation in hypertensive patients with diuretic-induced hypokalemia. *N Engl J Med.* 1985;312:746-749.
194. Cohen HW, Madhavan S, Alderman MH. High and low serum potassium associated with cardiovascular events in diuretic-treated patients. *J Hypertens.* 2001;19:1315-1323.
195. Shafi T, Appel LJ, Miller 3rd ER, et al. Changes in serum potassium mediate thiazide-induced diabetes. *Hypertension.* 2008;52:1022-1029.
196. Mattu A, Brady WJ, Robinson DA. Electrocardiographic manifestations of hyperkalemia. *Am J Emerg Med.* 2000;18:721-729.
197. Greenberg A. Hyperkalemia: treatment options. *Semin Nephrol.* 1998;18:46-57.
198. McLean SA, Paul ID, Spector PS. Lidocaine-induced conduction disturbance in patients with systemic hyperkalemia. *Ann Emerg Med.* 2000;36:615-618.
199. Littmann L, Monroe MH, Taylor 3rd L, et al. The hyperkalemic Brugada sign. *J Electrocardiol.* 2007;40:53-59.
200. Acker CG, Johnson JP, Palevsky PM, et al. Hyperkalemia in hospitalized patients: causes, adequacy of treatment, and results of an attempt to improve physician compliance with published therapy guidelines. *Arch Intern Med.* 1998;158:917-924.
201. Surawicz B, Chlebus H, Mazzoleni A. Hemodynamic and electrocardiographic effects of hyperpotassemia. Differences in response to slow and rapid increases in concentration of plasma K. *Am Heart J.* 1967;73:647-664.
202. Paice B, Gray JM, McBride D, et al. Hyperkalaemia in patients in hospital. *Br Med J (Clin Res Ed).* 1983;286:1189-1192.
203. Montague BT, Ouellette JR, Buller GK. Retrospective review of the frequency of ECG changes in hyperkalemia. *Clin J Am Soc Nephrol.* 2008;3:324-330.
204. Aslam S, Friedman EA, Ifudu O. Electrocardiography is unreliable in detecting potentially lethal hyperkalaemia in haemodialysis patients. *Nephrol Dial Transplant.* 2002;17:1639-1642.
205. Szerlip HM, Weiss J, Singer I. Profound hyperkalemia without electrocardiographic manifestations. *Am J Kidney Dis.* 1986;7:461-465.
206. Somers MP, Brady WJ, Perron AD, et al. The prominent T wave: electrocardiographic differential diagnosis. *Am J Emerg Med.* 2002;20:243-251.
207. Freeman SJ, Fale AD. Muscular paralysis and ventilatory failure caused by hyperkalaemia. *Br J Anaesth.* 1993;70:226-267.
208. Evers S, Engelien A, Karsch V, et al. Secondary hyperkalaemic paralysis. *J Neurol Neurosurg Psychiatry.* 1998;64:249-252.
209. Miller TM, et al. Correlating phenotype and genotype in the periodic paralyses. *Neurology.* 2004;63:1647-1655.
210. Lehmann-Horn F, Jurkat-Rott K. Voltage-gated ion channels and hereditary disease. *Physiol Rev.* 1999;79:1317-1372.
211. Raja Rayan DL, Hanna MG. Skeletal muscle channelopathies: nondystrophic myotonias and periodic paralysis. *Curr Opin Neurol.* 2010;23:466-476.
212. Abbott GW, et al. MiRP2 forms potassium channels in skeletal muscle with Kv3.4 and is associated with periodic paralysis. *Cell.* 2001;104:217-231.
213. Tannen RL, Wedell E, Moore R. Renal adaptation to a high potassium intake. The role of hydrogen ion. *J Clin Invest.* 1973;52:2089-2101.
214. DuBose Jr TD, Good DW. Effects of chronic hyperkalemia on renal production and proximal tubule transport of ammonium in rats. *Am J Physiol.* 1991;260:F680-F687.
215. Good DW. Ammonium transport by the thick ascending limb of Henle's loop. *Annu Rev Physiol.* 1994;56:623-647.
216. DuBose Jr TD, Good DW. Chronic hyperkalemia impairs ammonium transport and accumulation in the inner medulla of the rat. *J Clin Invest.* 1992;90:1443-1449.
217. Attmane-Elakeb A, et al. Stimulation by in vivo and in vitro metabolic acidosis of expression of rBSC1, the Na-K(NH₄)-2Cl cotransporter of the rat medullary thick ascending limb. *J Biol Chem.* 1998;273:33681-33691.
218. Bourgeois S, et al. NHE4 is critical for the renal handling of ammonia in rodents. *J Clin Invest.* 2010;120:1895-1904.
219. Matsuda O, et al. Primary role of hyperkalemia in the acidosis of hyporeninemic hypoaldosteronism. *Nephron.* 1988;49:203-209.
220. Szylman P, Better OS, Chaimowitz C, et al. Role of hyperkalemia in the metabolic acidosis of isolated hypoaldosteronism. *N Engl J Med.* 1976;294:361-365.
221. Cohn JN, Kowey PR, Whelton PK, et al. New guidelines for potassium replacement in clinical practice: a contemporary review by the National Council on Potassium in Clinical Practice. *Arch Intern Med.* 2000;160:2429-2436.
222. Gennari FJ. Hypokalemia. *N Engl J Med.* 1998;339:451-458.
223. Paltiel O, Salakhov E, Ronen I, et al. Management of severe hypokalemia in hospitalized patients: a study of quality of care based on computerized databases. *Arch Intern Med.* 2001;161:1089-1095.
224. Crop MJ, Hoorn EJ, Lindemans J, et al. Hypokalaemia and subsequent hyperkalaemia in hospitalized patients. *Nephrol Dial Transplant.* 2007;22:3471-3477.
225. Schnaper HW, et al. Potassium restoration in hypertensive patients made hypokalemic by hydrochlorothiazide. *Arch Intern Med.* 1989;149:2677-2681.
226. Rosenberg J, Gustafsson F, Galatius S, et al. Combination therapy with metolazone and loop diuretics in outpatients with refractory heart failure: an observational study and review of the literature. *Cardiovasc Drugs Ther.* 2005;19:301-306.
227. Tziviskou E, et al. Prevalence and pathogenesis of hypokalemia in patients on chronic peritoneal dialysis: one center's experience and review of the literature. *Int Urol Nephrol.* 2003;35:429-434.
228. Macdonald JE, Struthers AD. What is the optimal serum potassium level in cardiovascular patients? *J Am Coll Cardiol.* 2004;43:155-161.
229. Masters PW, Lawson N, Marenah CB, et al. High ambient temperature: a spurious cause of hypokalaemia. *BMJ.* 1996;312:1652-1653.

230. Ulahannan TJ, McVittie J, Keenan J. Ambient temperatures and potassium concentrations. *Lancet.* 1998;352:1680-1681.

231. Heller SR, Robinson RT. Hypoglycaemia and associated hypokalaemia in diabetes: mechanisms, clinical implications and prevention. *Diabetes Obes Metab.* 2000;2:75-82.

232. Fuentebella J, Kerner JA. Refeeding syndrome. *Pediatr Clin North Am.* 2009;56:1201-1210.

233. Laso FJ, Gonzalez-Buitrago JM, Martin-Ruiz C, et al. Inter-relationship between serum potassium and plasma catecholamines and 3':5' cyclic monophosphate in alcohol withdrawal. *Drug Alcohol Depend.* 1990;26:183-188.

234. Madias JE, Shah B, Chintalapally G, et al. Admission serum potassium in patients with acute myocardial infarction: its correlates and value as a determinant of in-hospital outcome. *Chest.* 2000;118:904-913.

235. Schaefer M, Link J, Hannemann L, et al. Excessive hypokalemia and hyperkalemia following head injury. *Intensive Care Med.* 1995;21:235-237.

236. Tse HF, Yeung CK. From profound hypokalemia to fatal rhabdomyolysis after severe head injury. *Am J Med.* 2000;109:599-600.

237. Braden GL, von Oeyen PT, Germain MJ, et al. Ritodrine- and terbutaline-induced hypokalemia in preterm labor: mechanisms and consequences. *Kidney Int.* 1997;51:1867-1875.

238. Hoffman RS, Kirrane BM, Marcus SM. A descriptive study of an outbreak of clenbuterol-containing heroin. *Ann Emerg Med.* 2008;52:548-553.

239. de Wijkerslooth LR, Koch BC, Malingre MM, et al. Life-threatening hypokalaemia and lactate accumulation after autointoxication with Stacker 2, a "powerful slimming agent." *Br J Clin Pharmacol.* 2008;66:728-731.

240. Amitai Y, Lovejoy Jr FH. Hypokalemia in acute theophylline poisoning. *Am J Emerg Med.* 1988;6:214-218.

241. Rice JE, Faunt JD. Excessive cola consumption as a cause of hypokalaemic myopathy. *Intern Med J.* 2001;31:317-318.

242. Whyte KF, Reid C, Addis GJ, et al. Salbutamol induced hypokalaemia: the effect of theophylline alone and in combination with adrenaline. *Br J Clin Pharmacol.* 1988;25:571-578.

243. Ahlawat SK, Sachdev A. Hypokalaemic paralysis. *Postgrad Med J.* 1999;75:193-197.

244. Downs JC, Milling D, Nichols CA. Suicidal ingestion of barium-sulfide–containing shaving powder. *Am J Forensic Med Pathol.* 1995;16:56-61.

245. Sigue G, et al. From profound hypokalemia to life-threatening hyperkalemia: a case of barium sulfide poisoning. *Arch Intern Med.* 2000;160:548-551.

246. Jacobs IA, Taddeo J, Kelly K, et al. Poisoning as a result of barium styphnate explosion. *Am J Ind Med.* 2002;41:285-288.

247. Wells JA, Wood KE. Acute barium poisoning treated with hemodialysis. *Am J Emerg Med.* 2001;19:175-177.

248. Bradberry SM, Vale JA. Disturbances of potassium homeostasis in poisoning. *J Toxicol Clin Toxicol.* 1995;33:295-310.

249. Jurkat-Rott K, et al. Voltage-sensor sodium channel mutations cause hypokalemic periodic paralysis type 2 by enhanced inactivation and reduced current. *Proc Natl Acad Sci U S A.* 2000;97:9549-9554.

250. Plaster NM, et al. Mutations in Kir2.1 cause the developmental and episodic electrical phenotypes of Andersen's syndrome. *Cell.* 2001;105:511-519.

251. Jurkat-Rott K, et al. K+-dependent paradoxical membrane depolarization and Na+ overload, major and reversible contributors to weakness by ion channel leaks. *Proc Natl Acad Sci U S A.* 2009;106:4036-4041.

252. Ruff RL. Skeletal muscle sodium current is reduced in hypokalemic periodic paralysis. *Proc Natl Acad Sci U S A.* 2000;97:9832-9833.

253. Ruff RL. Insulin acts in hypokalemic periodic paralysis by reducing inward rectifier K+ current. *Neurology.* 1999;53:1556-1563.

254. Tricarico D, Servidei S, Tonali P, et al. Impairment of skeletal muscle adenosine triphosphate–sensitive K+ channels in patients with hypokalemic periodic paralysis. *J Clin Invest.* 1999;103:675-682.

255. Renaud JM. Modulation of force development by Na+, K+, Na+ K+ pump and KATP channel during muscular activity. *Can J Appl Physiol.* 2002;27:296-315.

256. Tricarico D, Capriulo R, Conte Camerino D. Insulin modulation of ATP-sensitive K+ channel of rat skeletal muscle is impaired in the hypokalaemic state. *Pflugers Arch.* 1999;437:235-240.

257. Cheng NL, Kao MC, Hsu YD, et al. Novel thiazide-sensitive Na-Cl cotransporter mutation in a Chinese patient with Gitelman's syndrome presenting as hypokalaemic paralysis. *Nephrol Dial Transplant.* 2003;18:1005-1008.

258. Yang SS, Chu P, Lin YF, et al. Aristolochic acid–induced Fanconi's syndrome and nephropathy presenting as hypokalemic paralysis. *Am J Kidney Dis.* 2002;39:E14.

259. Feldman M, et al. Molecular investigation and long-term clinical progress in Greek Cypriot families with recessive distal renal tubular acidosis and sensorineural deafness due to mutations in the ATP6V1B1 gene. *Clin Genet.* 2006;69:135-144.

260. Manoukian MA, Foote JA, Crapo LM. Clinical and metabolic features of thyrotoxic periodic paralysis in 24 episodes. *Arch Intern Med.* 1999;159:601-606.

261. Goh SH. Thyrotoxic periodic paralysis: reports of seven patients presenting with weakness in an Asian emergency department. *Emerg Med J.* 2002;19:78-79.

262. Ko GT, et al. Thyrotoxic periodic paralysis in a Chinese population. *QJM.* 1996;89:463-468.

263. Chan A, Shinde R, Chow CC, et al. In vivo and in vitro sodium pump activity in subjects with thyrotoxic periodic paralysis. *BMJ.* 1991;303:1096-1099.

264. Azuma KK, Hensley CB, Tang MJ, et al. Thyroid hormone specifically regulates skeletal muscle Na(+)-K(+)-ATPase alpha 2- and beta 2-isoforms. *Am J Physiol.* 1993;265:C680-C687.

265. Lin SH, Lin YF. Propranolol rapidly reverses paralysis, hypokalemia, and hypophosphatemia in thyrotoxic periodic paralysis. *Am J Kidney Dis.* 2001;37:620-623.

266. Birkhahn RH, Gaeta TJ, Melniker L. Thyrotoxic periodic paralysis and intravenous propranolol in the emergency setting. *J Emerg Med.* 2000;18:199-202.

267. Ahmed I, Chilimuri SS. Fatal dysrhythmia following potassium replacement for hypokalemic periodic paralysis. *West J Emerg Med.* 2010;11:57-59.

268. Kassirer JP, Schwartz WB. The response of normal man to selective depletion of hydrochloric acid. Factors in the genesis of persistent gastric alkalosis. *Am J Med.* 1966;40:10-18.

269. Coghill NF, McAllen PM, Edwards F. Electrolyte losses associated with the taking of purges investigated with aid of sodium and potassium radioisotopes. *BMJ.* 1959;1:14-19.

270. Orman RA, Lewis Jr JB. Flaccid quadriparesis associated with *Yersinia enterocolitis*-induced hypokalemia. *Arch Intern Med.* 1989;149:1193-1194.

271. Ho JM, Juurlink DN, Cavalcanti RB. Hypokalemia following polyethylene glycol–based bowel preparation for colonoscopy in older hospitalized patients with significant comorbidities. *Ann Pharmacother.* 2010;44:466-470.

272. Wolf I, Mouallem M, Farfel Z. Adult celiac disease presented with celiac crisis: severe diarrhea, hypokalemia, and acidosis. *J Clin Gastroenterol.* 2000;30:324-326.

273. Diekmann F, et al. Hypokalemic nephropathy after pelvic pouch procedure and protective loop ileostomy. *Z Gastroenterol.* 2001;39:579-582.

274. Simon M, et al. Over-expression of colonic K+ channels associated with severe potassium secretory diarrhoea after haemorrhagic shock. *Nephrol Dial Transplant.* 2008;23:3350-3352.

275. Blondon H, Bechade D, Desrame J, et al. Secretory diarrhoea with high faecal potassium concentrations: a new mechanism of diarrhoea associated with colonic pseudo-obstruction? Report of five patients. *Gastroenterol Clin Biol.* 2008;32:401-404.

276. van Dinter Jr TG, et al. Stimulated active potassium secretion in a patient with colonic pseudo-obstruction: a new mechanism of secretory diarrhea. *Gastroenterology.* 2005;129:1268-1273.

277. Sandle GI, Hunter M. Apical potassium (BK) channels and enhanced potassium secretion in human colon. *QJM.* 2010;103:85-89.

278. Sorensen MV, et al. Adrenaline-induced colonic K+ secretion is mediated by KCa1.1 (BK) channels. *J Physiol.* 2010;588:1763-77.

279. Bettinelli A, et al. Use of calcium excretion values to distinguish two forms of primary renal tubular hypokalemic alkalosis: Bartter and Gitelman syndromes. *J Pediatr.* 1992;120:38-43:[see comments].

280. Suki WN, et al. Acute treatment of hypercalcemia with furosemide. *N Engl J Med.* 1970;283:836-840.

281. Okusa MD, Velazquez H, Ellison DH, et al. Luminal calcium regulates potassium transport by the renal distal tubule. *Am J Physiol.* 1990;258:F423-F428.

282. Sands JM, et al. Apical extracellular calcium/polyvalent cation–sensing receptor regulates vasopressin-elicited water permeability in rat kidney inner medullary collecting duct. *J Clin Invest.* 1997;99:1399-1405.

283. Pakravan N, Bateman DN, Goddard J. Effect of acute paracetamol overdose on changes in serum and urine electrolytes. *Br J Clin Pharmacol.* 2007;64:824-832.

284. Waring WS, Stephen AF, Malkowska AM, et al. Acute acetaminophen overdose is associated with dose-dependent hypokalaemia: a prospective study of 331 patients. *Basic Clin Pharmacol Toxicol.* 2008;102:325-328.

285. Johnson DW, Kay TD, Hawley CM. Severe hypokalaemia secondary to dicloxacillin. *Intern Med J.* 2002;32:357-358.

286. Izzedine H, Launay-Vacher V, Isnard-Bagnis C, et al. Drug-induced Fanconi's syndrome. *Am J Kidney Dis.* 2003;41:292-309.

287. Landau D, Kher KK. Gentamicin-induced Bartter-like syndrome. *Pediatr Nephrol.* 1997;11:737-740.

288. Malin A, Miller RF. Foscarnet-induced hypokalaemia. *J Infect.* 1992;25:329-330.

289. Milionis HJ, Bourantas CL, Siamopoulos KC, et al. Acid-base and electrolyte abnormalities in patients with acute leukemia. *Am J Hematol.* 1999;62:201-207.

290. Husband DJ, Watkin SW. Fatal hypokalaemia associated with ifosfamide/mesna chemotherapy. *Lancet.* 1988;1:1116.

291. Cao Y, Liu L, Liao C, et al. Meta-analysis of incidence and risk of hypokalemia with cetuximab-based therapy for advanced cancer. *Cancer Chemother Pharmacol.* 2010;66:37-42.

292. Groenestege WM, et al. Impaired basolateral sorting of pro-EGF causes isolated recessive renal hypomagnesemia. *J Clin Invest.* 2007;117:2260-2267.

293. Bunchman TE, Sinaiko AR. Renovascular hypertension presenting with hypokalemic metabolic alkalosis. *Pediatr Nephrol.* 1990;4:169-170.

294. Pintar TJ, Zimmerman S. Hyperreninemic hypertension secondary to a subcapsular perinephric hematoma in a patient with polyarteritis nodosa. *Am J Kidney Dis.* 1998;32:503-507.

295. Ringrose TR, Phillips PA, Lindop GB. Renin-secreting adenocarcinoma of the colon. *Ann Intern Med.* 1999;131:794-795.

296. Corvol P, Pinet F, Plouin PF, et al. Renin-secreting tumors. *Endocrinol Metab Clin North Am.* 1994;23:255-270.

297. Nicholls MG. Unilateral renal ischemia causing the hyponatremic hypertensive syndrome in children—more common than we think? *Pediatr Nephrol.* 2006;21:887-890.

298. White PC. Steroid 11β-hydroxylase deficiency and related disorders. *Endocrinol Metab Clin North Am.* 2001;30:61-79:vi.

299. Goldsmith O, Solomon DH, Horton R. Hypogonadism and mineralocorticoid excess. The 17-hydroxylase deficiency syndrome. *N Engl J Med.* 1967;277:673-677.

300. Dluhy RG, Lifton RP. Glucocorticoid-remediable aldosteronism. *J Clin Endocrinol Metab.* 1999;84:4341-4344.

301. Sukor N, et al. Further evidence for linkage of familial hyperaldosteronism type II at chromosome 7p22 in Italian as well as Australian and South American families. *J Hypertens.* 2008;26:1577-1582.

302. Geller DS, et al. A novel form of human mendelian hypertension featuring nonglucocorticoid-remediable aldosteronism. *J Clin Endocrinol Metab.* 2008;93:3117-3123.

303. Litchfield WR, New MI, Coolidge C, et al. Evaluation of the dexamethasone suppression test for the diagnosis of glucocorticoid-remediable aldosteronism. *J Clin Endocrinol Metab.* 1997;82:3570-3573.

304. Lifton RP, et al. A chimaeric 11β-hydroxylase/aldosterone synthase gene causes glucocorticoid-remediable aldosteronism and human hypertension. *Nature.* 1992;355:262-265.

305. Rich GM, et al. Glucocorticoid-remediable aldosteronism in a large kindred: clinical spectrum and diagnosis using a characteristic biochemical phenotype. *Ann Intern Med.* 1992;116:813-820.

306. Pascoe L, et al. Glucocorticoid-suppressible hyperaldosteronism and adrenal tumors occurring in a single French pedigree. *J Clin Invest.* 1995;96:2236-2246.

307. Funder JW, et al. Case detection, diagnosis, and treatment of patients with primary aldosteronism: an endocrine society clinical practice guideline. *J Clin Endocrinol Metab.* 2008;93:3266-3281.

308. Jamieson A, et al. Clinical, biochemical and genetic features of five extended kindred's with glucocorticoid-suppressible hyperaldosteronism. *Endocr Res.* 1995;21:463-469.

309. Litchfield WR, et al. Impaired potassium-stimulated aldosterone production: a possible explanation for normokalemic glucocorticoid-remediable aldosteronism. *J Clin Endocrinol Metab.* 1997;82:1507-1510.

310. Young WF. Primary aldosteronism: renaissance of a syndrome. *Clin Endocrinol (Oxf).* 2007;66:607-618.

311. Mulatero P, Rabbia F, Veglio F. Paraneoplastic hyperaldosteronism associated with non-Hodgkin's lymphoma. *N Engl J Med.* 2001;344:1558-1559.

312. Montori VM, Young Jr WF. Use of plasma aldosterone concentration–to–plasma renin activity ratio as a screening test for primary aldosteronism. A systematic review of the literature. *Endocrinol Metab Clin North Am.* 2002;31:619-632:xi.

313. Williams JS, et al. Prevalence of primary hyperaldosteronism in mild to moderate hypertension without hypokalaemia. *J Hum Hypertens.* 2006;20:129-136.

314. Blumenfeld JD, et al. Diagnosis and treatment of primary hyperaldosteronism. *Ann Intern Med.* 1994;121:877-885.

315. Eiam-Ong S, Kurtzman NA, Sabatini S. Regulation of collecting tubule adenosine triphosphatases by aldosterone and potassium. *J Clin Invest.* 1993;91:2385-2392.

316. Howlett TA, et al. Diagnosis and management of ACTH-dependent Cushing's syndrome: comparison of the features in ectopic and pituitary ACTH production. *Clin Endocrinol (Oxf).* 1986;24:699-713.

317. Torpy DJ, Mullen N, Ilias I, et al. Association of hypertension and hypokalemia with Cushing's syndrome caused by ectopic ACTH secretion: a series of 58 cases. *Ann N Y Acad Sci.* 2002;970:134-144.

318. Isidori AM, et al. The ectopic adrenocorticotropin syndrome: clinical features, diagnosis, management, and long-term follow-up. *J Clin Endocrinol Metab.* 2006;91:371-377.

319. Stewart PM, Walker BR, Holder G, et al. 11β-Hydroxysteroid dehydrogenase activity in Cushing's syndrome: explaining the mineralocorticoid excess state of the ectopic adrenocorticotropin syndrome. *J Clin Endocrinol Metab.* 1995;80:3617-3620.

320. Koren W, et al. Enhanced Na+/H+ exchange in Cushing's syndrome reflects functional hypermineralocorticoidism. *J Hypertens.* 1998;16:1187-1191.

321. Mendonca BB, et al. Female pseudohermaphroditism caused by a novel homozygous missense mutation of the GR gene. *J Clin Endocrinol Metab.* 2002;87:1805-1809.

322. White PC, Mune T, Agarwal AK. 11β-Hydroxysteroid dehydrogenase and the syndrome of apparent mineralocorticoid excess. *Endocr Rev.* 1997;18:135-156.

323. Bostanjoglo M, et al. 11β-hydroxysteroid dehydrogenase, mineralocorticoid receptor, and thiazide-sensitive Na-Cl cotransporter expression by distal tubules. *J Am Soc Nephrol.* 1998;9:1347-1358:[published erratum in *J Am Soc Nephrol* 9(11):2179, 1998].

324. Funder JW, Pearce PT, Smith R, et al. Mineralocorticoid action: target tissue specificity is enzyme, not receptor, mediated. *Science.* 1988;242:583-585.

325. Li A, et al. Molecular basis for hypertension in the "type II variant" of apparent mineralocorticoid excess. *Am J Hum Genet.* 1998;63:370-379.

326. Wilson RC, et al. A genetic defect resulting in mild low-renin hypertension. *Proc Natl Acad Sci U S A.* 1998;95:10200-10205.

327. Nunez BS, et al. Mutants of 11β-hydroxysteroid dehydrogenase (11-HSD2) with partial activity: improved correlations between genotype and biochemical phenotype in apparent mineralocorticoid excess. *Hypertension.* 1999;34:638-642.

328. Kotelevtsev Y, et al. Hypertension in mice lacking 11β-hydroxysteroid dehydrogenase type 2. *J Clin Invest.* 1999;103:683-689.

329. Loffing J, et al. Distribution of transcellular calcium and sodium transport pathways along mouse distal nephron. *Am J Physiol Renal Physiol.* 2001;281:F1021-F1027.

330. Kim GH, et al. The thiazide-sensitive Na-Cl cotransporter is an aldosterone-induced protein. *Proc Natl Acad Sci U S A.* 1998;95:14552-14557.

331. Masilamani S, Kim GH, Mitchell C, et al. Aldosterone-mediated regulation of ENaC alpha, beta, and gamma subunit proteins in rat kidney. *J Clin Invest.* 1999;104:R19-R23.

332. Biller KJ, Unwin RJ, Shirley DG. Distal tubular electrolyte transport during inhibition of renal 11β-hydroxysteroid dehydrogenase. *Am J Physiol Renal Physiol.* 2001;280:F172-F179.

333. Borst JGG, Ten Holt SP, de Vries LA, et al. Synergistic action of liquorice and cortisone in Addison's and Simmond's disease. *Lancet.* 1953;1:657-663.

334. Woywodt A, Herrmann A, Haller H, et al. Severe hypokalaemia: is one reason enough? *Nephrol Dial Transplant.* 2004;19:2914-2917.

335. Hamidon BB, Jeyabalan V. Exogenously-induced apparent hypermineralocorticoidism associated with ingestion of "asam boi." *Singapore Med J.* 2006;47:156-158.

336. van Rossum TG, de Jong FH, Hop WC, et al. 'Pseudo-aldosteronism' induced by intravenous glycyrrhizin treatment of chronic hepatitis C patients. *J Gastroenterol Hepatol.* 2001;16:789-795.

337. Iida R, Otsuka Y, Matsumoto K, et al. Pseudoaldosteronism due to the concurrent use of two herbal medicines containing glycyrrhizin: interaction of glycyrrhizin with angiotensin-converting enzyme inhibitor. *Clin Exp Nephrol.* 2006;10:131-135.

338. Farese S, et al. Glycyrrhetinic acid food supplementation lowers serum potassium concentration in chronic hemodialysis patients. *Kidney Int.* 2009;76:877-884.

339. Geller DS, et al. Activating mineralocorticoid receptor mutation in hypertension exacerbated by pregnancy. *Science.* 2000;289:119-123.

340. Lifton RP, Gharavi AG, Geller DS. Molecular mechanisms of human hypertension. *Cell.* 2001;104:545-556.

341. Botero-Velez M, Curtis JJ, Warnock DG. Brief report: Liddle's syndrome revisited—a disorder of sodium reabsorption in the distal tubule. *N Engl J Med.* 1994;330:178-181.

342. Pradervand S, et al. Dysfunction of the epithelial sodium channel expressed in the kidney of a mouse model for Liddle syndrome. *J Am Soc Nephrol.* 2003;14:2219-2228.

343. Kellenberger S, Gautschi I, Rossier BC, et al. Mutations causing Liddle syndrome reduce sodium-dependent downregulation of the epithelial sodium channel in the *Xenopus* oocyte expression system. *J Clin Invest.* 1998;101:2741-2750.

344. Frindt G, Silver RB, Windhager EE, et al. Feedback regulation of Na channels in rat CCT. II. Effects of inhibition of Na entry. *Am J Physiol.* 1993;264:F565-F574.

345. Hiltunen TP, et al. Liddle's syndrome associated with a point mutation in the extracellular domain of the epithelial sodium channel gamma subunit. *J Hypertens.* 2002;20:2383-2390.

346. Hannila-Handelberg T, et al. Common variants of the beta and gamma subunits of the epithelial sodium channel and their relation to plasma renin and aldosterone levels in essential hypertension. *BMC Med Genet.* 2005;6:4.

347. Ambrosius WT, et al. Genetic variants in the epithelial sodium channel in relation to aldosterone and potassium excretion and risk for hypertension. *Hypertension.* 1999;34:631-637.

348. Gladziwa U, et al. Chronic hypokalaemia of adults: Gitelman's syndrome is frequent but classical Bartter's syndrome is rare. *Nephrol Dial Transplant.* 1995;10:1607-1613.

349. Guay-Woodford LM. Bartter syndrome: unraveling the pathophysiologic enigma. *Am J Med.* 1998;105:151-161.

350. Brochard K, et al. Phenotype-genotype correlation in antenatal and neonatal variants of Bartter syndrome. *Nephrol Dial Transplant.* 2009;24:1455-1464.

351. Komhoff M, et al. Cyclooxygenase-2 expression is associated with the renal macula densa of patients with Bartter-like syndrome. *Kidney Int.* 2000;58:2420-2424.

352. Reinalter SC, et al. Role of cyclooxygenase-2 in hyperprostaglandin E syndrome/antenatal Bartter syndrome. *Kidney Int.* 2002;62:253-260.

353. Gill Jr JR, Bartter FC. Evidence for a prostaglandin-independent defect in chloride reabsorption in the loop of Henle as a proximal cause of Bartter's syndrome. *Am J Med.* 1978;65:766-772.

354. Kockerling A, Reinalter SC, Seyberth HW. Impaired response to furosemide in hyperprostaglandin E syndrome: evidence for a tubular defect in the loop of Henle. *J Pediatr.* 1996;129:519-528.

355. Simon DB, et al. Bartter's syndrome, hypokalaemic alkalosis with hypercalciuria, is caused by mutations in the Na-K-2Cl cotransporter NKCC2. *Nat Genet.* 1996;13:183-188.

356. Xu JZ, et al. Localization of the ROMK protein on apical membranes of rat kidney nephron segments. *Am J Physiol.* 1997:F739-F748.

357. Sun A, Grossman EB, Lombardi M, et al. Vasopressin alters the mechanism of apical Cl⁻ entry from Na⁺:Cl⁻ to Na⁺:K⁺:2Cl⁻ cotransport in mouse medullary thick ascending limb. *J Membr Biol.* 1991;120:83-94.

358. Simon DB, et al. Genetic heterogeneity of Bartter's syndrome revealed by mutations in the K⁺ channel, ROMK. *Nat Genet.* 1996;14:152-156.

359. Simon DB, et al. Mutations in the chloride channel gene,CLCNKB, cause Bartter's syndrome type III. *Nat Genet.* 1997;17:171-178.

360. Vandewalle A, et al. Localization and induction by dehydration of ClC-K chloride channels in the rat kidney. *Am J Physiol.* 1997;272:F678-F688.

361. Estevez R, et al. Barttin is a Cl⁻ channel β-subunit crucial for renal Cl⁻ reabsorption and inner ear K⁺ secretion. *Nature.* 2001;414:558-561.

362. Schlingmann KP, et al. Salt wasting and deafness resulting from mutations in two chloride channels. *N Engl J Med.* 2004;350:1314-1319.

363. Watanabe S, et al. Association between activating mutations of calcium-sensing receptor and Bartter's syndrome. *Lancet.* 2002;360:692-694.

364. Vargas-Poussou R, et al. Functional characterization of a calcium-sensing receptor mutation in severe autosomal dominant hypocalcemia with a Bartter-like syndrome. *J Am Soc Nephrol.* 2002;13:2259-2266.

365. Riccardi D, et al. Localization of the extracellular Ca²⁺/polyvalent cation–sensing protein in rat kidney. *Am J Physiol.* 1998;274:F611-F622.

366. Wang WH, Lu M, Hebert SC. Cytochrome P-450 metabolites mediate extracellular Ca²⁺-induced inhibition of apical K⁺ channels in the TAL. *Am J Physiol.* 1996;271:C103-C111.

367. Peters M, et al. Clinical presentation of genetically defined patients with hypokalemic salt-losing tubulopathies. *Am J Med.* 2002;112:183-190.

368. Pressler CA, et al. Late-onset manifestation of antenatal Bartter syndrome as a result of residual function of the mutated renal Na⁺-K⁺-2Cl⁻ Co-transporter. *J Am Soc Nephrol.* 2006;17:2136-2142.

369. Finer G, et al. Transient neonatal hyperkalemia in the antenatal (ROMK defective) Bartter syndrome. *J Pediatr.* 2003;142:318-323.

370. Woda CB, Bragin A, Kleyman TR, et al. Flow-dependent K⁺ secretion in the cortical collecting duct is mediated by a maxi-K channel. *Am J Physiol Renal Physiol.* 2001;280:F786-F793.

371. Bailey MA, et al. Maxi-K channels contribute to urinary potassium excretion in the ROMK-deficient mouse model of type II Bartter's syndrome and in adaptation to a high-K diet. *Kidney Int.* 2006;70:51-59.

372. Lu M, Wang W. Two types of K⁺ channels are present in the apical membrane of the thick ascending limb of the mouse kidney. *Kidney Blood Press Res.* 2000;23:75-82.

373. Lu M, et al. ROMK is required for expression of the 70-pS K channel in the thick ascending limb. *Am J Physiol Renal Physiol.* 2004;286:F490-F495.

374. Dave S, Honney S, Raymond J, et al. An unusual presentation of cystic fibrosis in an adult. *Am J Kidney Dis.* 2005;45:e41-e44.

375. Lu M, et al. CFTR is required for PKA-regulated ATP sensitivity of Kir1.1 potassium channels in mouse kidney. *J Clin Invest.* 2006;116:797-807.

376. Luthy C, et al. Normal prostaglandinuria E₂ in Gitelman's syndrome, the hypocalciuric variant of Bartter's syndrome. *Am J Kidney Dis.* 1995;25:824-828.

377. Cruz DN, Shaer AJ, Bia MJ, et al. Gitelman's syndrome revisited: an evaluation of symptoms and health-related quality of life. *Kidney Int.* 2001;59:710-717.

378. Bettinelli A, et al. Electrocardiogram with prolonged QT interval in Gitelman disease. *Kidney Int.* 2002;62:580-584.

379. Foglia PE, et al. Cardiac work up in primary renal hypokalaemia-hypomagnesaemia (Gitelman syndrome). *Nephrol Dial Transplant.* 2004;19:1398-1402.

380. Simon DB, et al. Gitelman's variant of Bartter's syndrome, inherited hypokalaemic alkalosis, is caused by mutations in the thiazide-sensitive Na-Cl cotransporter. *Nat Genet.* 1996;12:24-30.

381. De Jong JC, et al. Functional expression of mutations in the human NaCl cotransporter: evidence for impaired routing mechanisms in Gitelman's syndrome. *J Am Soc Nephrol.* 2002;13:1442-1448.

382. Colussi G, et al. A thiazide test for the diagnosis of renal tubular hypokalaemic disorders. *Clin J Am Soc Nephrol.* 2007;2:454-460.

383. Loffing J, et al. Altered renal distal tubule structure and renal Na⁺ and Ca²⁺ handling in a mouse model for Gitelman's syndrome. *J Am Soc Nephrol.* 2004;15:2276-2288.

384. Loffing J, et al. Thiazide treatment of rats provokes apoptosis in distal tubule cells. *Kidney Int.* 1996;50:1180-1190.

385. Nijenhuis T, et al. Enhanced passive Ca²⁺ reabsorption and reduced Mg²⁺ channel abundance explains thiazide-induced hypocalciuria and hypomagnesemia. *J Clin Invest.* 2005;115:1651-1658.

386. Morris RG, Hoorn EJ, Knepper MA. Hypokalemia in a mouse model of Gitelman's syndrome. *Am J Physiol Renal Physiol.* 2006;290:F1416-F1420.

387. Friedman E, Shadel M, Halkin H, et al. Thiazide-induced hyponatremia. Reproducibility by single dose rechallenge and an analysis of pathogenesis. *Ann Intern Med.* 1989;110:24-30.

388. Cruz D, Simon D, Lifton RP. Inactivating mutations in the Na-Cl cotransporter is associated with high bone density. *J Am Soc Nephrol.* 1999;10:597A.

389. Cobeta-Garcia JC, Gascon A, Iglesias E, et al. Chondrocalcinosis and Gitelman's syndrome. A new association? *Ann Rheum Dis.* 1998;57:748-749.

390. Vezzoli G, Soldati L, Jansen A, et al. Choroidal calcifications in patients with Gitelman's syndrome. *Am J Kidney Dis.* 2000;36:855-858.

391. Panichpisal K, Angulo-Pernett F, Selhi S, et al. Gitelman-like syndrome after cisplatin therapy: a case report and literature review. *BMC Nephrol.* 2006;7:10.

392. Chen YC, et al. Primary Sjögren's syndrome associated with Gitelman's syndrome presenting with muscular paralysis. *Am J Kidney Dis.* 2003;42:586-590.

393. Sebastian A, McSherry E, Morris Jr RC. On the mechanism of renal potassium wasting in renal tubular acidosis associated with the Fanconi syndrome (type 2 RTA). *J Clin Invest.* 1971;50:231-243.

394. Tsai CS, Chen YC, Chen HH, et al. An unusual cause of hypokalemic paralysis: aristolochic acid nephropathy with Fanconi syndrome. *Am J Med Sci.* 2005;330:153-155.

395. Karet FE, et al. Mutations in the gene encoding B1 subunit of H⁺-ATPase cause renal tubular acidosis with sensorineural deafness. *Nat Genet.* 1999;21:84-90.

396. Sebastian A, McSherry E, Morris Jr RC. Renal potassium wasting in renal tubular acidosis (RTA): its occurrence in types 1 and 2 RTA despite sustained correction of systemic acidosis. *J Clin Invest.* 1971;50:667-678.

397. Comer DM, Droogan AG, Young IS, et al. Hypokalaemic paralysis precipitated by distal renal tubular acidosis secondary to Sjögren's syndrome. *Ann Clin Biochem.* 2008;45:221-225.

398. Rodriguez M, Solanki DL, Whang R. Refractory potassium repletion due to cisplatin-induced magnesium depletion. *Arch Intern Med.* 1989;149:2592-2594.

399. Whang R, et al. Magnesium depletion as a cause of refractory potassium repletion. *Arch Intern Med.* 1985;145:1686-1689.

400. Whang R, Whang DD, Ryan MP. Refractory potassium repletion. A consequence of magnesium deficiency. *Arch Intern Med.* 1992;152:40-45.

401. Dorup I, Clausen T. Correlation between magnesium and potassium contents in muscle: role of Na⁺-K⁺ pump. *Am J Physiol.* 1993;264:C457-C463.

402. Huang CL, Kuo E. Mechanism of hypokalemia in magnesium deficiency. *J Am Soc Nephrol.* 2007;18:2649-2652.

403. Vandenberg CA. Inward rectification of a potassium channel in cardiac ventricular cells depends on internal magnesium ions. *Proc Natl Acad Sci U S A.* 1987;84:2560-2564.

404. Groeneveld JH, Sijpkens YW, Lin SH, et al. An approach to the patient with severe hypokalaemia: the potassium quiz. *QJM.* 2005;98:305-316.

405. Reimann D, Gross P. Chronic, diagnosis-resistant hypokalaemia. *Nephrol Dial Transplant.* 1999;14:2957-2961.

406. Greenfeld D, Mickley D, Quinlan DM, et al. Hypokalemia in outpatients with eating disorders. *Am J Psychiatry.* 1995;152:60-63.

407. Crow SJ, Rosenberg ME, Mitchell JE, et al. Urine electrolytes as markers of bulimia nervosa. *Int J Eat Disord.* 2001;30:279-287.

408. Woywodt A, Herrmann A, Eisenberger U, et al. The tell-tale urinary chloride. *Nephrol Dial Transplant.* 2001;16:1066-1068.

409. Kim YG, et al. Medullary nephrocalcinosis associated with long-term furosemide abuse in adults. *Nephrol Dial Transplant.* 2001;16:2303-2309.

410. Holmes AM, Hesling CM, Wilson TM. Drug-induced secondary hyperaldosteronism in patients with pulmonary tuberculosis. *Q J Med.* 1970;39:299-315.

411. Bates CM, Baum M, Quigley R. Cystic fibrosis presenting with hypokalemia and metabolic alkalosis in a previously healthy adolescent. *J Am Soc Nephrol.* 1997;8:352-355.

412. Casatta L, Ferraccioli GF, Bartoli E. Hypokalaemic alkalosis, acquired Gitelman's and Bartter's syndrome in chronic sialoadenitis. *Br J Rheumatol.* 1997;36:1125-1128.

413. Kone BC. Hypokalemia. In: DuBose Jr TD, Hamm LL, eds. *Acid-base and electrolyte disorders: a companion to Brenner and Rector's the kidney.* Philadelphia: Saunders; 2002:381-394.

414. Kim GH, Han JS. Therapeutic approach to hypokalemia. *Nephron.* 2002;92(suppl 1):28-32.

415. Zydlewski AW, Hasbargen JA. Hypothermia-induced hypokalemia. *Mil Med.* 1998;163:719-721.

416. Kearney TE, Manoguerra AS, Curtis GP, et al. Theophylline toxicity and the β-adrenergic system. *Ann Intern Med.* 1985;102:766-769.

417. Chapman SA, Kaufenberg AJ, Anderson P, et al. Safety and effectiveness of a modification of diet in renal disease equation-based potassium replacement protocol. *Ann Pharmacother.* 2009;43:436-443.

418. Sterns RH, Cox M, Feig PU, et al. Internal potassium balance and the control of the plasma potassium concentration. *Medicine (Baltimore).* 1981;60:339-354.

419. Gabduzda GJ, Hall 3rd PW. Relation of potassium depletion to renal ammonium metabolism and hepatic coma. *Medicine (Baltimore).* 1966;45:481-490.

420. Jaeger P, Karlmark B, Giebisch G. Ammonium transport in rat cortical tubule: relationship to potassium metabolism. *Am J Physiol.* 1983;245:F593-F600.

421. Khaw KT, Barrett-Connor E. Dietary potassium and stroke-associated mortality. A 12-year prospective population study. *N Engl J Med.* 1987;316:235-240.

422. Ascherio A, et al. Intake of potassium, magnesium, calcium, and fiber and risk of stroke among US men. *Circulation.* 1998;98:1198-1204.

423. Villamil MF, Deland EC, Henney RP, et al. Anion effects on cation movements during correction of potassium depletion. *Am J Physiol.* 1975;229:161-166.

424. Nicolis GL, Kahn T, Sanchez A, et al. Glucose-induced hyperkalemia in diabetic subjects. *Arch Intern Med.* 1981;141:49-53.

425. Keith NM, Osterberg AE, Burchell HB. Some effects of potassium salts in man. *Ann Intern Med.* 1942;16:879.

426. Kunin AS, Surawicz B, Sims EAH. Decrease in serum potassium concentrations and appearance of cardiac arrhythmias during infusion of potassium with glucose in potassium-depleted patients. *N Engl J Med.* 1962;266:228-233.

427. Hamill RJ, Robinson LM, Wexler HR, et al. Efficacy and safety of potassium infusion therapy in hypokalemic critically ill patients. *Crit Care Med.* 1991;19:694-699.

428. Kruse JA, Carlson RW. Rapid correction of hypokalemia using concentrated intravenous potassium chloride infusions. *Arch Intern Med.* 1990;150:613-617.

429. Rose BD, Post TW. Hypokalemia. In: Rose BD, Post TW, eds. *Clinical physiology of acid-base and electrolyte disorders.* vol 1. New York: McGraw-Hill; 2001:836-887.

430. Pullen H, Doig A, Lambie AT. Intensive intravenous potassium replacement therapy. *Lancet.* 1967;2:809-811.

431. Abramson E, Arky R. Diabetic acidosis with initial hypokalemia. Therapeutic implications. *JAMA.* 1966;196:401-403.

432. Seftel HC, Kew MC. Early and intensive potassium replacement in diabetic acidosis. *Diabetes.* 1966;15:694-696.

433. Norris W, Kunzelman KS, Bussell S, et al. Potassium supplementation, diet vs pills: a randomized trial in postoperative cardiac surgery patients. *Chest.* 2004;125:404-409.

434. Sopko JA, Freeman RM. Salt substitutes as a source of potassium. *JAMA.* 1977;238:608-610.

435. Doorenbos CJ, Vermeij CG. Danger of salt substitutes that contain potassium in patients with renal failure. *BMJ.* 2003;326:35-36.

436. Su M, et al. Sustained-release potassium chloride overdose. *J Toxicol Clin Toxicol.* 2001;39:641-648.

437. Ganguly A, Weinberger MH. Triamterene-thiazide combination: alternative therapy for primary aldosteronism. *Clin Pharmacol Ther.* 1981;30:246-250.

438. Brown JJ, et al. Comparison of surgery and prolonged spironolactone therapy in patients with hypertension, aldosterone excess, and low plasma renin. *Br Med J.* 1972;2:729–334.

439. Griffing GT, et al. Amiloride in primary hyperaldosteronism. *Clin Pharmacol Ther.* 1982;31:56-61.

440. Eiro M, Katoh T, Watanabe T. Use of a proton-pump inhibitor for metabolic disturbances associated with anorexia nervosa. *N Engl J Med.* 2002;346:140.

441. Stevens MS, Dunlay RW. Hyperkalemia in hospitalized patients. *Int Urol Nephrol.* 2000;32:177-180.

442. Moore ML, Bailey RR. Hyperkalaemia in patients in hospital. *N Z Med J.* 1989;102:557-558.

443. Rastegar A, Soleimani M, Rastergar A. Hypokalaemia and hyperkalaemia. *Postgrad Med J.* 2001;77:759-764.

444. Charytan D, Goldfarb DS. Indications for hospitalization of patients with hyperkalemia. *Arch Intern Med.* 2000;160:1605-1611.

445. Ponce SP, Jennings AE, Madias NE, et al. Drug-induced hyperkalemia. *Medicine (Baltimore).* 1985;64:357-370.

446. Ahee P, Crowe AV. The management of hyperkalaemia in the emergency department. *J Accid Emerg Med.* 2000;17:188-191.

447. Allon M, Dunlay R, Copkney C. Nebulized albuterol for acute hyperkalemia in patients on hemodialysis. *Ann Intern Med.* 1989;110:426-429.

448. Ahmed J, Weisberg LS. Hyperkalemia in dialysis patients. *Semin Dial.* 2001;14:348-356.

449. Moranne O, et al. Timing of onset of CKD-related metabolic complications. *J Am Soc Nephrol.* 2009;20:164-171.

450. Einhorn LM, et al. The frequency of hyperkalemia and its significance in chronic kidney disease. *Arch Intern Med.* 2009;169:1156-1162.

451. Moore CR, Lin JJ, O'Connor N, et al. Follow-up of markedly elevated serum potassium results in the ambulatory setting: implications for patient safety. *Am J Med Qual.* 2006;21:115-124.

452. Wiederkehr MR, Moe OW. Factitious hyperkalemia. *Am J Kidney Dis.* 2000;36:1049-1053.

453. Skiner S. A cause of erroneous potassium levels. *Lancet.* 1961;277:478-480.

454. Graber M, Subramani K, Corish D, et al. Thrombocytosis elevates serum potassium. *Am J Kidney Dis.* 1988;12:116-120.

455. Bellevue R, Dosik H, Spergel G, et al. Pseudohyperkalemia and extreme leukocytosis. *J Lab Clin Med.* 1975;85:660-664.

456. Sevastos N, et al. Pseudohyperkalemia in patients with increased cellular components of blood. *Am J Med Sci.* 2006;331:17-21.

457. Cornes MP, Ford C, Gama R. Spurious hyperkalaemia due to EDTA contamination: common and not always easy to identify. *Ann Clin Biochem.* 2008;45:601-603.

458. Kellerman PS, Thornbery JM. Pseudohyperkalemia due to pneumatic tube transport in a leukemic patient. *Am J Kidney Dis.* 2005;46:746-748.

459. Oliver Jr TK, Young GA, Bates GD, et al. Factitial hyperkalemia due to icing before analysis. *Pediatrics.* 1966;38:900-902.

460. Sodi R, Davison AS, Holmes E, et al. The phenomenon of seasonal pseudohypokalemia: effects of ambient temperature, plasma glucose and role for sodium-potassium-exchanging-ATPase. *Clin Biochem.* 2009;42:813-818.

461. Bruce LJ, et al. Monovalent cation leaks in human red cells caused by single amino-acid substitutions in the transport domain of the band 3 chloride-bicarbonate exchanger, AE1. *Nat Genet.* 2005;37:1258-1263.

462. Bruce LJ, et al. The monovalent cation leak in overhydrated stomatocytic red blood cells results from amino acid substitutions in the Rh-associated glycoprotein. *Blood.* 2009;113:1350-1357.

463. Arrambide K, Toto RD. Tumor lysis syndrome. *Semin Nephrol.* 1993;13:273-280.

464. Parisi A, et al. Complex ventricular arrhythmia induced by overuse of potassium supplementation in a young male football player. Case report. *J Sports Med Phys Fitness.* 2002;42:214-216.

465. Mueller BA, Scott MK, Sowinski KM, et al. Noni juice (*Morinda citrifolia*): hidden potential for hyperkalemia? *Am J Kidney Dis.* 2000;35:310-312.

466. Nagasaki A, Takamine W, Takasu N. Severe hyperkalemia associated with "alternative" nutritional cancer therapy. *Clin Nutr.* 2005;24:864-865.

467. Abu-Hamdan DK, Sondheimer JH, Mahajan SK. Cautopyreiophagia. Cause of life-threatening hyperkalemia in a patient undergoing hemodialysis. *Am J Med.* 1985;79:517-519.

468. Thiele A, Rehman HU. Hyperkalemia caused by penicillin. *Am J Med.* 2008;121:e1-e2.

469. Smith HM, Farrow SJ, Ackerman JD, et al. Cardiac arrests associated with hyperkalemia during red blood cell transfusion: a case series. *Anesth Analg.* 2008;106:1062-1069.

470. Baz EM, Kanazi GE, Mahfouz RA, et al. An unusual case of hyperkalaemia-induced cardiac arrest in a paediatric patient during transfusion of a "fresh" 6-day-old blood unit. *Transfus Med.* 2002;12:383-386.

471. Perkins RM, Aboudara MC, Abbott KC, et al. Resuscitative hyperkalemia in noncrush trauma: a prospective, observational study. *Clin J Am Soc Nephrol.* 2007;2:313-319.

472. Moreno M, Murphy C, Goldsmith C. Increase in serum potassium resulting from the administration of hypertonic mannitol and other solutions. *J Lab Clin Med.* 1969;73:291-298.

473. Makoff DL, da Silva JA, Rosenbaum BJ, et al. Hypertonic expansion: acid-base and electrolyte changes. *Am J Physiol.* 1970;218:1201-1207.

474. Flynn BC. Hyperkalemic cardiac arrest with hypertonic mannitol infusion: the strong ion difference revisited. *Anesth Analg.* 2007;104:225-226.

475. Hirota K, et al. Two cases of hyperkalemia after administration of hypertonic mannitol during craniotomy. *J Anesth.* 2005;19:75-77.

476. Hassan ZU, Kruer JJ, Fuhrman TM. Electrolyte changes during craniotomy caused by administration of hypertonic mannitol. *J Clin Anesth.* 2007;19:307-309.

477. Goldfarb S, Strunk B, Singer I, et al. Paradoxical glucose-induced hyperkalemia. Combined aldosterone-insulin deficiency. *Am J Med.* 1975;59:744-750.

478. Magnus Nzerue C, Jackson E. Intractable life-threatening hyperkalaemia in a diabetic patient. *Nephrol Dial Transplant.* 2000;15:113-114.

479. Sirken G, Raja R, Garces J, et al. Contrast-induced translocational hyponatremia and hyperkalemia in advanced kidney disease. *Am J Kidney Dis.* 2004;43:e31-e35.

480. Perazella MA, Biswas P. Acute hyperkalemia associated with intravenous ε-aminocaproic acid therapy. *Am J Kidney Dis.* 1999;33:782-785.

481. Nzerue CM, Falana B. Refractory hyperkalaemia associated with use of ε-aminocaproic acid during coronary bypass in a dialysis patient. *Nephrol Dial Transplant.* 2002;17:1150-1151.

482. Clark BA, Shannon C, Brown RS, et al. Extrarenal potassium homeostasis with maximal exercise in end-stage renal disease. *J Am Soc Nephrol.* 1996;7:1223-1227.

483. Sangkabutra T, et al. Impaired K^+ regulation contributes to exercise limitation in end-stage renal failure. *Kidney Int.* 2003;63:283-290.

484. Allon M. Hyperkalemia in end-stage renal disease: mechanisms and management. *J Am Soc Nephrol.* 1995;6:1134-1142.

485. Fulop M. Hyperkalemia in diabetic ketoacidosis. *Am J Med Sci.* 1990;299:164-169.

486. Van Gaal LF, De Leeuw IH, Bekaert JL. Diabetic ketoacidosis–induced hyperkalemia. Prevalence and possible origin. *Intensive Care Med.* 1986;12:416-418.

487. Milionis HJ, Dimos G, Elisaf MS. Severe hyperkalaemia in association with diabetic ketoacidosis in a patient presenting with severe generalized muscle weakness. *Nephrol Dial Transplant.* 2003;18:198-200.

488. Chi HT, Hung DZ, Hu WH, et al. Prognostic implications of hyperkalemia in toad toxin intoxication. *Hum Exp Toxicol.* 1998;17:343-346.

489. Gowda RM, Cohen RA, Khan IA. Toad venom poisoning: resemblance to digoxin toxicity and therapeutic implications. *Heart.* 2003;89:e14.

490. Baltazar RF, Mower MM, Reider R, et al. Acute fluoride poisoning leading to fatal hyperkalemia. *Chest.* 1980;78:660-663.

491. Martyn JA, Richtsfeld M. Succinylcholine-induced hyperkalemia in acquired pathologic states: etiologic factors and molecular mechanisms. *Anesthesiology.* 2006;104:158-169.

492. Thapa S, Brull SJ. Succinylcholine-induced hyperkalemia in patients with renal failure: an old question revisited. *Anesth Analg.* 2000;91:237-241.

493. Singer M, Coluzzi F, O'Brien A, et al. Reversal of life-threatening, drug-related potassium-channel syndrome by glibenclamide. *Lancet.* 2005;365:1873-1875.

494. Wilson AJ, Jabr RI, Clapp LH. Calcium modulation of vascular smooth muscle ATP-sensitive K(+) channels: role of protein phosphatase-2B. *Circ Res.* 2000;87:1019-1025.

495. McCauley J, et al. Labetalol-induced hyperkalemia in renal transplant recipients. *Am J Nephrol.* 2002;22:347-351.

496. Blumenfeld JD, et al. β-Adrenergic receptor blockade as a therapeutic approach for suppressing the renin-angiotensin-aldosterone system in normotensive and hypertensive subjects. *Am J Hypertens.* 1999;12:451-459.

497. Yamamoto T, Fukuyama J, Hasegawa K, et al. Isolated corticotropin deficiency in adults. Report of 10 cases and review of literature. *Arch Intern Med.* 1992;152:1705-1712.

498. Fujieda K, Tajima T. Molecular basis of adrenal insufficiency. *Pediatr Res.* 2005;57:62R-69R.

499. Achermann JC, Meeks JJ, Jameson JL. Phenotypic spectrum of mutations in DAX-1 and SF-1. *Mol Cell Endocrinol.* 2001;185:17-25.

500. Fujieda K, et al. Spontaneous puberty in 46, XX subjects with congenital lipoid adrenal hyperplasia. Ovarian steroidogenesis is spared to some extent despite inactivating mutations in the steroidogenic acute regulatory protein (StAR) gene. *J Clin Invest.* 1997;99:1265-1271.

501. Bose HS, Sugawara T, Strauss 3rd JF, et al. The pathophysiology and genetics of congenital lipoid adrenal hyperplasia. International Congenital Lipoid Adrenal Hyperplasia Consortium. *N Engl J Med.* 1996;335:1870-1878.

502. Hiort O, et al. Homozygous disruption of P450 side-chain cleavage (CYP11A1) is associated with prematurity, complete 46, XY sex reversal, and severe adrenal failure. *J Clin Endocrinol Metab.* 2005;90:538-541.

503. Speiser PW. Congenital adrenal hyperplasia owing to 21-hydroxylase deficiency. *Endocrinol Metab Clin North Am.* 2001;30:31-59:vi.

504. Kayes-Wandover KM, et al. Congenital hyperreninemic hypoaldosteronism unlinked to the aldosterone synthase (CYP11B2) gene. *J Clin Endocrinol Metab.* 2001;86:5379-5382.

505. Kayes-Wandover KM, Schindler RE, Taylor HC, et al. Type 1 aldosterone synthase deficiency presenting in a middle-aged man. *J Clin Endocrinol Metab.* 2001;86:1008-1012.

506. Morimoto S, et al. Selective hypoaldosteronism with hyperreninemia in a diabetic patient. *J Clin Endocrinol Metab.* 1979;49:742-747.

507. Agmon D, Green J, Platau E, et al. Isolated adrenal mineralocorticoid deficiency due to amyloidosis associated with familial Mediterranean fever. *Am J Med Sci.* 1984;288:40-43.

508. Oster JR, Singer I, Fishman LM. Heparin-induced aldosterone suppression and hyperkalemia. *Am J Med.* 1995;98:575-586.

509. Koren-Michowitz M, et al. Early onset of hyperkalemia in patients treated with low molecular weight heparin: a prospective study. *Pharmacoepidemiol Drug Saf.* 2004;13:299-302.

510. Liu AA, Bui T, Nguyen HV, et al. Subcutaneous unfractionated heparin-induced hyperkalaemia in an elderly patient. *Australas J Ageing.* 2009;28:97.

511. Oelkers W. Adrenal insufficiency. *N Engl J Med.* 1996;335:1206-1212.

512. Espinosa G, et al. Adrenal involvement in the antiphospholipid syndrome: clinical and immunologic characteristics of 86 patients. *Medicine (Baltimore).* 2003;82:106-118.

513. Danby P, Harris KP, Williams B, et al. Adrenal dysfunction in patients with renal amyloid. *Q J Med.* 1990;76:915-922.

514. Mayo J, Collazos J, Martinez E, et al. Adrenal function in the human immunodeficiency virus–infected patient. *Arch Intern Med.* 2002;162:1095-1098.

515. Schambelan M, Stockigt JR, Biglieri EG. Isolated hypoaldosteronism in adults. A renin-deficiency syndrome. *N Engl J Med.* 1972;287:573-578.

516. Lush DJ, King JA, Fray JC. Pathophysiology of low renin syndromes: sites of renal renin secretory impairment and prorenin overexpression. *Kidney Int.* 1993;43:983-999.

517. Michelis MF. Hyperkalemia in the elderly. *Am J Kidney Dis.* 1990;16:296-299.

518. Lee FO, et al. Mechanisms of hyperkalemia in systemic lupus erythematosus. *Arch Intern Med.* 1988;148:397-401.

519. DuBose Jr TD, Caflisch CR. Effect of selective aldosterone deficiency on acidification in nephron segments of the rat inner medulla. *J Clin Invest.* 1988;82:1624-1632.

520. Sebastian A, Schambelan M, Lindenfeld S, et al. Amelioration of metabolic acidosis with fludrocortisone therapy in hyporeninemic hypoaldosteronism. *N Engl J Med.* 1977;297:576-583.

521. DuBose TD. Hyperkalemic hyperchloremic metabolic acidosis: pathophysiologic insights. *Kidney Int.* 1997;51:591-602.

522. Sebastian A, Schambelan M. Amelioration of type 4 renal tubular acidosis in chronic renal failure with furosemide. *Kidney Int.* 1977;12:534.

523. Chan R, et al. Renin-aldosterone system can respond to furosemide in patients with hyperkalemic hyporeninism. *J Lab Clin Med.* 1998;132:229-235.

524. Oh MS, et al. A mechanism for hyporeninemic hypoaldosteronism in chronic renal disease. *Metabolism.* 1974;23:1157-1166.

525. Klemm SA, Gordon RD, Tunny TJ, et al. Biochemical correction in the syndrome of hypertension and hyperkalaemia by severe dietary salt restriction suggests renin-aldosterone suppression critical in pathophysiology. *Clin Exp Pharmacol Physiol.* 1990;17:191-195.

526. Tuchelt H, et al. Role of atrial natriuretic factor in changes in the responsiveness of aldosterone to angiotensin II secondary to sodium loading and depletion in man. *Clin Sci (Lond).* 1990;79:57-65.

527. DeFronzo RA, et al. Impaired renal tubular potassium secretion in systemic lupus erythematosus. *Ann Intern Med.* 1977;86:268-271.

528. DeFronzo RA, Taufield PA, Black H, et al. Impaired renal tubular potassium secretion in sickle cell disease. *Ann Intern Med.* 1979;90:310-316.

529. Batlle D, Itsarayoungyuen K, Arruda JA, et al. Hyperkalemic hyperchloremic metabolic acidosis in sickle cell hemoglobinopathies. *Am J Med.* 1982;72:188-192.

530. Geller DS, et al. Autosomal dominant pseudohypoaldosteronism type 1: mechanisms, evidence for neonatal lethality, and phenotypic expression in adults. *J Am Soc Nephrol.* 2006;17:1429-1436.

531. Akcay A, Yavuz T, Semiz S, et al. Pseudohypoaldosteronism type 1 and respiratory distress syndrome. *J Pediatr Endocrinol Metab.* 2002;15:1557-1561.

532. Bonny O, et al. Functional expression of a pseudohypoaldosteronism type I mutated epithelial Na^+ channel lacking the pore-forming region of its alpha subunit. *J Clin Invest.* 1999;104:967-974.

533. Mayan H, et al. Pseudohypoaldosteronism type II: marked sensitivity to thiazides, hypercalciuria, normomagnesemia, and low bone mineral density. *J Clin Endocrinol Metab.* 2002;87:3248-3254.

534. Wilson FH, et al. Human hypertension caused by mutations in WNK kinases. *Science.* 2001;293:1107-1112.

535. Ko B, Hoover RS. Molecular physiology of the thiazide-sensitive sodium-chloride cotransporter. *Curr Opin Nephrol Hypertens.* 2009;18:421-427.

536. Ling BN, Webster CL, Eaton DC. Eicosanoids modulate apical Ca^{2+}-dependent K^+ channels in cultured rabbit principal cells. *Am J Physiol.* 1992;263:F116-F126.

537. Mactier RA, Khanna R. Hyperkalemia induced by indomethacin and naproxen and reversed by fludrocortisone. *South Med J.* 1988;81:799-801.

538. Tan SY, Shapiro R, Franco R, et al. Indomethacin-induced prostaglandin inhibition with hyperkalemia. A reversible cause of hyporeninemic hypoaldosteronism. *Ann Intern Med.* 1979;90:783-785.

539. Tan SY, Mulrow PJ. Inhibition of the renin-aldosterone response to furosemide by indomethacin. *J Clin Endocrinol Metab*. 1977;45:174-176.
540. Harris Jr RC. Cyclooxygenase-2 inhibition and renal physiology. *Am J Cardiol*. 2002;89:10D-17D.
541. Swan SK, et al. Effect of cyclooxygenase-2 inhibition on renal function in elderly persons receiving a low-salt diet. A randomized, controlled trial. *Ann Intern Med*. 2000;133:1-9.
542. Preston RA, Afshartous D, Alonso AB. Effects of selective vs. nonselective cyclooxygenase inhibition on dynamic renal potassium excretion: a randomized trial. *Clin Pharmacol Ther*. 2008;84:208-211.
543. Braden GL, O'Shea MH, Mulhern JG, et al. Acute renal failure and hyperkalaemia associated with cyclooxygenase-2 inhibitors. *Nephrol Dial Transplant*. 2004;19:1149-1153.
544. Lam Q, Schneider HG. Hyperkalaemia with cyclooxygenase-2 inhibition and hypoaldosteronism. *Intern Med J*. 2005;35:572-573.
545. Perazella MA. Drug-induced hyperkalemia: old culprits and new offenders. *Am J Med*. 2000;109:307-314.
546. Oishi M, et al. A case of hyperkalemic distal renal tubular acidosis secondary to tacrolimus in living donor liver transplantation. *Transplant Proc*. 2000;32:2225-2226.
547. Higgins R, et al. Hyponatraemia and hyperkalaemia are more frequent in renal transplant recipients treated with tacrolimus than with cyclosporin. Further evidence for differences between cyclosporin and tacrolimus nephrotoxicities. *Nephrol Dial Transplant*. 2004;19:444-450.
548. Bantle JP, Nath KA, Sutherland DE, et al. Effects of cyclosporine on the renin-angiotensin-aldosterone system and potassium excretion in renal transplant recipients. *Arch Intern Med*. 1985;145:505-508.
549. Hocherl K, Dreher F, Vitzthum H, et al. Cyclosporine A suppresses cyclooxygenase-2 expression in the rat kidney. *J Am Soc Nephrol*. 2002;13:2427-2436.
550. Ling BN, Eaton DC. Cyclosporin A inhibits apical secretory K⁺ channels in rabbit cortical collecting tubule principal cells. *Kidney Int*. 1993;44:974-984.
551. Pei Y, Richardson R, Greenwood C, et al. Extrarenal effect of cyclosporine A on potassium homeostasis in renal transplant recipients. *Am J Kidney Dis*. 1993;22:314-319.
552. Choi MJ, et al. Brief report: trimethoprim-induced hyperkalemia in a patient with AIDS. *N Engl J Med*. 1993;328:703-706.
553. Kleyman TR, Roberts C, Ling BN. A mechanism for pentamidine-induced hyperkalemia: inhibition of distal nephron sodium transport. *Ann Intern Med*. 1995;122:103-106.
554. Velazquez H, Perazella MA, Wright FS, et al. Renal mechanism of trimethoprim-induced hyperkalemia. *Ann Intern Med*. 1993;119:296-301.
555. Muto S, Tsuruoka S, Miyata Y, et al. Effect of trimethoprim-sulfamethoxazole on Na⁺ and K⁺ transport properties in the rabbit cortical collecting duct perfused in vitro. *Nephron Physiol*. 2006;102:51-60.
556. Alappan R, Perazella MA, Buller GK. Hyperkalemia in hospitalized patients treated with trimethoprim-sulfamethoxazole. *Ann Intern Med*. 1996;124:316-320.
557. Elisaf M, Terrovitou C, Tomos P, et al. Severe hyperkalaemia after cotrimoxazole administration in a patient with hyporeninaemic hypoaldosteronism. *Nephrol Dial Transplant*. 1997;12:1254-1255.
558. Antoniou T, et al. Trimethoprim-sulfamethoxazole–induced hyperkalemia in patients receiving inhibitors of the renin-angiotensin system: a population-based study. *Arch Intern Med*. 2010;170:1045-1049.
559. Weir MR, Rolfe M. Potassium homeostasis and renin-angiotensin-aldosterone system inhibitors. *Clin J Am Soc Nephrol*. 2010;5:531-548.
560. Genazzani AR, Mannella P, Simoncini T. Drospirenone and its antialdosterone properties. *Climacteric*. 2007;10(suppl 1):11-18.
561. Preston RA, et al. Mechanisms of impaired potassium handling with dual renin-angiotensin-aldosterone blockade in chronic kidney disease. *Hypertension*. 2009;53:754-760.
562. Venzin RM, Cohen CD, Maggiorini M, et al. Aliskiren-associated acute renal failure with hyperkalemia. *Clin Nephrol*. 2009;71:326-328.
563. Mehdi UF, Adams-Huet B, Raskin P, et al. Addition of angiotensin receptor blockade or mineralocorticoid antagonism to maximal angiotensin-converting enzyme inhibition in diabetic nephropathy. *J Am Soc Nephrol*. 2009;20:2641-2650.
564. Cohen DL, Townsend RR. Is there added value to adding ARB to ACE inhibitors in the management of CKD? *J Am Soc Nephrol*. 2009;20:1666-1668.
565. Pitt B, et al. Eplerenone, a selective aldosterone blocker, in patients with left ventricular dysfunction after myocardial infarction. *N Engl J Med*. 2003;348:1309-1321.
566. Johnson ES, et al. Predicting the risk of hyperkalemia in patients with chronic kidney disease starting lisinopril. *Pharmacoepidemiol Drug Saf*. 2010;19:266-272.
567. Pitt B, Bakris G, Ruilope LM, et al. Serum potassium and clinical outcomes in the Eplerenone Post-Acute Myocardial Infarction Heart Failure Efficacy and Survival Study (EPHESUS). *Circulation*. 2008;118:1643-1650.
568. Gross P, Pistrosch F. Hyperkalaemia: again. *Nephrol Dial Transplant*. 2004;19:2163-2166.
569. Juurlink DN, et al. Rates of hyperkalemia after publication of the Randomized Aldactone Evaluation Study. *N Engl J Med*. 2004;351:543-551.
570. Pitt B, et al. The effect of spironolactone on morbidity and mortality in patients with severe heart failure. Randomized Aldactone Evaluation Study Investigators. *N Engl J Med*. 1999;341:709-717.
571. Goldfarb DS. Hyperkalemia after the publication of RALES. *N Engl J Med*. 2004;351:2448-2450:[author reply, 2448-2450].
572. Wei L, Struthers AD, Fahey T, et al. Spironolactone use and renal toxicity: population based longitudinal analysis. *BMJ*. 2010;340:c1768.
573. Palmer BF. Managing hyperkalemia caused by inhibitors of the renin-angiotensin-aldosterone system. *N Engl J Med*. 2004;351:585-592.
574. Levinsky NG. Management of emergencies. VI. *Hyperkalemia. N Engl J Med*. 1966;274:1076-1077.
575. Allon M. Treatment and prevention of hyperkalemia in end-stage renal disease. *Kidney Int*. 1993;43:1197-1209.
576. Mount DB. Treatment and prevention of hyperkalemia. In: Basow DS, ed. *UpToDate*. Waltham, MA; 2010, UpToDate.
577. Kim HJ, Han SW. Therapeutic approach to hyperkalemia. *Nephron*. 2002;92(suppl 1):33-40.
578. Evans KJ, Greenberg A. Hyperkalemia: a review. *J Intensive Care Med*. 2005;20:272-290.
579. Winkler AW, Hoff HE, Smith PK. Factors affecting the toxicity of potassium. *Am J Physiol*. 1939;127:430-436.
580. Pergola PE, DeFronzo R. Clinical disorders of hyperkalemia. In: Seldin DW, Giebisch G, eds. *The kidney: physiology and pathophysiology*. 3rd ed. vol 2. Philadelphia: Lippincott Williams & Wilkins; 2000:1647-1700.
581. Davey M, Caldicott D. Calcium salts in management of hyperkalaemia. *Emerg Med J*. 2002;19:92-93.
582. Bower JO, Mengle HAK. The additive effects of calcium and digitalis. *JAMA*. 1936;106:1151-1153.
583. White RD, Goldsmith RS, Rodriguez R, et al. Plasma ionic calcium levels following injection of chloride, gluconate, and glucepate salts of calcium. *J Thorac Cardiovasc Surg*. 1976;71:609-613.
584. Alvestrand A, Wahren J, Smith D, et al. Insulin-mediated potassium uptake is normal in uremic and healthy subjects. *Am J Physiol*. 1984;246:E174-E180.
585. Allon M, Copkney C. Albuterol and insulin for treatment of hyperkalemia in hemodialysis patients. *Kidney Int*. 1990;38:869-872.
586. Blumberg A, Weidmann P, Shaw S, et al. Effect of various therapeutic approaches on plasma potassium and major regulating factors in terminal renal failure. *Am J Med*. 1988;85:507-512.
587. De Wolf A, Frenette L, Kang Y, et al. Insulin decreases the serum potassium concentration during the anhepatic stage of liver transplantation. *Anesthesiology*. 1993;78:677-682.
588. Minaker KL, Rowe JW. Potassium homeostasis during hyperinsulinemia: effect of insulin level, beta-blockade, and age. *Am J Physiol*. 1982;242:E373-E377.
589. Perazella MA. Approach to hyperkalemic end-stage renal disease patients in the emergency department. *Conn Med*. 1999;63:131-136.
590. Emmett M. Non-dialytic treatment of acute hyperkalemia in the dialysis patient. *Semin Dial*. 2000;13:279-280.
591. Lens XM, Montoliu J, Cases A, et al. Treatment of hyperkalaemia in renal failure: salbutamol v. insulin. *Nephrol Dial Transplant*. 1989;4:228-232.
592. Liou HH, et al. Hypokalemic effects of intravenous infusion or nebulization of salbutamol in patients with chronic renal failure: comparative study. *Am J Kidney Dis*. 1994;23:266-271.
593. Montoliu J, Lens XM, Revert L. Potassium-lowering effect of albuterol for hyperkalemia in renal failure. *Arch Intern Med*. 1987;147:713-717.
594. Ostovar H, Jones J, Brown M. Best evidence topic report. Nebulised levalbuterol or albuterol for lowering serum potassium. *Emerg Med J*. 2005;22:366-367.
595. Mandelberg A, et al. Salbutamol metered-dose inhaler with spacer for hyperkalemia: how fast? How safe? *Chest*. 1999;115:617-622.
596. Sowinski KM, Cronin D, Mueller BA, et al. Subcutaneous terbutaline use in CKD to reduce potassium concentrations. *Am J Kidney Dis*. 2005;45:1040-1045.
597. Iqbal Z, Friedman EA. Preferred therapy of hyperkalemia in renal insufficiency: survey of nephrology training-program directors. *N Engl J Med*. 1989;320:60-61.
598. Schwarz KC, Cohen BD, Lubash GD, et al. Severe acidosis and hyperpotassemia treated with sodium bicarbonate infusion. *Circulation*. 1959;19:215-220.
599. Blumberg A, Weidmann P, Ferrari P. Effect of prolonged bicarbonate administration on plasma potassium in terminal renal failure. *Kidney Int*. 1992;41:369-374.
600. Gutierrez R, Schlessinger F, Oster JR, et al. Effect of hypertonic versus isotonic sodium bicarbonate on plasma potassium concentration in patients with end-stage renal disease. *Miner Electrolyte Metab*. 1991;17:297-302.

601. Allon M, Shanklin N. Effect of bicarbonate administration on plasma potassium in dialysis patients: interactions with insulin and albuterol. *Am J Kidney Dis.* 1996;28:508-514.
602. Carvalhana V, Burry L, Lapinsky SE. Management of severe hyperkalemia without hemodialysis: case report and literature review. *J Crit Care.* 2006;21:316-321.
603. Suki WN. Use of diuretics in chronic renal failure. *Kidney Int Suppl.* 1997;59:S33-S35.
604. Sebastian A, Schambelan M, Sutton JM. Amelioration of hyperchloremic acidosis with furosemide therapy in patients with chronic renal insufficiency and type 4 renal tubular acidosis. *Am J Nephrol.* 1984;4:287-300.
605. DeFronzo RA, et al. Investigations into the mechanisms of hyperkalemia following renal transplantation. *Kidney Int.* 1977;11:357-365.
606. Reiser IW, Chou SY, Brown MI, et al. Reversal of trimethoprim-induced antikaliuresis. *Kidney Int.* 1996;50:2063-2069.
607. Wilcox CS. New insights into diuretic use in patients with chronic renal disease. *J Am Soc Nephrol.* 2002;13:798-805.
608. Sherman DS, Kass CL, Fish DN. Fludrocortisone for the treatment of heparin-induced hyperkalemia. *Ann Pharmacother.* 2000;34:606-610.
609. Dreyling KW, Wanner C, Schollmeyer P. Control of hyperkalemia with fludrocortisone in a patient with systemic lupus erythematosus. *Clin Nephrol.* 1990;33:179-183.
610. Petersen KC, Silberman H, Berne TV. Hyperkalaemia after cyclosporin therapy. *Lancet.* 1984;1:1470.
611. Furuya R, Kumagai H, Sakao T, et al. Potassium-lowering effect of mineralocorticoid therapy in patients undergoing hemodialysis. *Nephron.* 2002;92:576-581.
612. Imbriano LJ, Durham JH, Maesaka JK. Treating interdialytic hyperkalemia with fludrocortisone. *Semin Dial.* 2003;16:5-7.
613. Kaisar MO, et al. A randomized controlled trial of fludrocortisone for the treatment of hyperkalemia in hemodialysis patients. *Am J Kidney Dis.* 2006;47:809-814.
614. Kim DM, Chung JH, Yoon SH, et al. Effect of fludrocortisone acetate on reducing serum potassium levels in patients with end-stage renal disease undergoing haemodialysis. *Nephrol Dial Transplant.* 2007;22:3273-3276.
615. Elkinton JR, Clark JK, Squires RD, et al. Treatment of potassium retention in uremia with cation exchange resin: preliminary report. *Am J Med Sci.* 1950;220:547-552.
616. Berlyne GM, Janabi K, Shaw AB. Dangers of resonium A in the treatment of hyperkalemia in renal failure. *Lancet.* 1966;1:167-169.
617. Scherr L, Ogden DA, Mead AW, et al. Management of hyperkalemia with cation-exchange resin. *N Engl J Med.* 1961;264:115-119.
618. Evans BM, Jones NC, Milne MD, et al. Ion-exchange resins in the treatment of anuria. *Lancet.* 1953;265:791-795.
619. Monzu B, Caramelo C, Traba ML, et al. Effect of potassium-chelating resins on phosphorus absorption. *Nephron.* 1994;68:148.
620. Papadimitriou M, Gingell JC, Chisholm GD. Hypercalcaemia from calcium ion-exchange resin in patients on regular haemodialysis. *Lancet.* 1968;2:948-950.
621. Agarwal R, Afzalpurkar R, Fordtran JS. Pathophysiology of potassium absorption and secretion by the human intestine. *Gastroenterology.* 1994;107:548-571.
622. Flinn RB, Merrill JP, Welzant WR. Treatment of the oliguric patient with a new sodium-exchange resin and sorbitol. *N Engl J Med.* 1961;264:111-115.
623. Sterns RH, Rojas M, Bernstein P, et al. Ion-exchange resins for the treatment of hyperkalemia: are they safe and effective? *J Am Soc Nephrol.* 2010;21:733-735.
624. Emmett M, et al. Effect of three laxatives and a cation exchange resin on fecal sodium and potassium excretion. *Gastroenterology.* 1995;108:752-760.
625. Gruy-Kapral C, et al. Effect of single dose resin-cathartic therapy on serum potassium concentration in patients with end-stage renal disease. *J Am Soc Nephrol.* 1998;9:1924-1930.
626. Gales MA, Gales BJ, Dyer ME, et al. Rectally administered sodium polystyrene sulfonate. *Am J Health Syst Pharm.* 1995;52:2813-2815.
627. Lillemoe KD, et al. Intestinal necrosis due to sodium polystyrene (Kayexalate) in sorbitol enemas: clinical and experimental support for the hypothesis. *Surgery.* 1987;101:267-272.
628. Gerstman BB, Kirkman R, Platt R. Intestinal necrosis associated with postoperative orally administered sodium polystyrene sulfonate in sorbitol. *Am J Kidney Dis.* 1992;20:159-161.
629. McGowan CE, Saha S, Chu G, et al. Intestinal necrosis due to sodium polystyrene sulfonate (Kayexalate) in sorbitol. *South Med J.* 2009;102:493-497.
630. Rashid A, Hamilton SR. Necrosis of the gastrointestinal tract in uremic patients as a result of sodium polystyrene sulfonate (Kayexalate) in sorbitol: an underrecognized condition. *Am J Surg Pathol.* 1997;21:60-69.
631. Cheng ES, Stringer KM, Pegg SP. Colonic necrosis and perforation following oral sodium polystyrene sulfonate (Resonium A/Kayexalate) in a burn patient. *Burns.* 2002;28:189-190.
632. Kamel KS, Wei C. Controversial issues in the treatment of hyperkalaemia. *Nephrol Dial Transplant.* 2003;18:2215-2218.
633. Abraham SC, Bhagavan BS, Lee LA, et al. Upper gastrointestinal tract injury in patients receiving Kayexalate (sodium polystyrene sulfonate) in sorbitol: clinical, endoscopic, and histopathologic findings. *Am J Surg Pathol.* 2001;25:637-644.
634. Ng YY, et al. Reduction of serum calcium by sodium sulfonated polystyrene resin. *J Formos Med Assoc.* 1990;89:399-402.
635. Linakis JG, et al. Sodium polystyrene sulfonate treatment for lithium toxicity: effects on serum potassium concentrations. *Acad Emerg Med.* 1996;3:333-337.
636. Amaya F, Fukui M, Tsuruta H, et al. Simulation of potassium extraction by continuous haemodiafiltration. *Anaesth Intensive Care.* 2002;30:198-201.
637. Jackson MA, Lodwick R, Hutchinson SG. Hyperkalaemic cardiac arrest successfully treated with peritoneal dialysis. *BMJ.* 1996;312:1289-1290.
638. Allon M, Shanklin N. Effect of albuterol treatment on subsequent dialytic potassium removal. *Am J Kidney Dis.* 1995;26:607-613.
639. Dolson GM, Ellis KJ, Bernardo MV, et al. Acute decreases in serum potassium augment blood pressure. *Am J Kidney Dis.* 1995;26:321-326.
640. Sherman RA, Hwang ER, Bernholc AS, et al. Variability in potassium removal by hemodialysis. *Am J Nephrol.* 1986;6:284-288.
641. Zehnder C, Gutzwiller JP, Huber R, et al. Low-potassium and glucose-free dialysis maintains urea but enhances potassium removal. *Nephrol Dial Transplant.* 2001;16:78-84.
642. Blumberg A, Roser HW, Zehnder C, et al. Plasma potassium in patients with terminal renal failure during and after haemodialysis; relationship with dialytic potassium removal and total body potassium. *Nephrol Dial Transplant.* 1997;12:1629-1634.
643. Ward RA, Wathen RL, Williams TE, et al. Hemodialysate composition and intradialytic metabolic, acid-base and potassium changes. *Kidney Int.* 1987;32:129-135.
644. De Nicola L, et al. Effect of dialysate sodium concentration on interdialytic increase of potassium. *J Am Soc Nephrol.* 2000;11:2337-2343.
645. Hou S, McElroy PA, Nootens J, et al. Safety and efficacy of low-potassium dialysate. *Am J Kidney Dis.* 1989;13:137-143.
646. Allon M. Medical and dialytic management of hyperkalemia in hemodialysis patients. *Int J Artif Organs.* 1996;19:697-699.
647. Heguilen RM, et al. The faster potassium-lowering effect of high dialysate bicarbonate concentrations in chronic haemodialysis patients. *Nephrol Dial Transplant.* 2005;20:591-597.
648. Solandt DY. The effect of potassium on the excitability and resting metabolism of frog's muscle. *J Physiol (Lond).* 1936;86:162-170.
649. Baron AD. Hemodynamic actions of insulin. *Am J Physiol.* 1994;267:E187-E202.
650. Morrison G, Michelson EL, Brown S, et al. Mechanism and prevention of cardiac arrhythmias in chronic hemodialysis patients. *Kidney Int.* 1980;17:811-819.
651. Kimura K, Tabei K, Asano Y, et al. Cardiac arrhythmias in hemodialysis patients. A study of incidence and contributory factors. *Nephron.* 1989;53:201-207.
652. Ramirez G, Brueggemeyer CD, Newton JL. Cardiac arrhythmias on hemodialysis in chronic renal failure patients. *Nephron.* 1984;36:212-218.
653. Rombola G, Colussi G, De Ferrari ME, et al. Cardiac arrhythmias and electrolyte changes during haemodialysis. *Nephrol Dial Transplant.* 1992;7:318-322.
654. Weber H, et al. Chronic hemodialysis: high risk patients for arrhythmias? *Nephron.* 1984;37:180-185.
655. Wizemann V, Kramer W, Funke T, et al. Dialysis-induced cardiac arrhythmias: fact or fiction? Importance of preexisting cardiac disease in the induction of arrhythmias during renal replacement therapy. *Nephron.* 1985;39:356-360.
656. Kyriakidis M, et al. Cardiac arrhythmias in chronic renal failure? Holter monitoring during dialysis and everyday activity at home. *Nephron.* 1984;38:26-29.
657. Redaelli B, et al. Effect of a new model of hemodialysis potassium removal on the control of ventricular arrhythmias. *Kidney Int.* 1996;50:609-617.
658. Santoro A, et al. Patients with complex arrhythmias during and after haemodialysis suffer from different regimens of potassium removal. *Nephrol Dial Transplant.* 2008;23:1415-1421.
659. Munoz RI, et al. Effect of acetate-free biofiltration with a potassium-profiled dialysate on the control of cardiac arrhythmias in patients at risk: a pilot study. *Hemodial Int.* 2008;12:108-113.

Disorders of Calcium, Magnesium, and Phosphate Balance

Miroslaw J. Smogorzewski, Robert K. Rude, and Alan S.L. Yu

Disorders of Calcium Homeostasis

The extracellular fluid (ECF) calcium concentration in the human body is tightly regulated by a complex process. Three organs, including the skeleton, kidney, and intestine, are involved in this process through their direct or indirect interaction with parathyroid hormone (PTH), parathyroid hormone–related protein (PTHrP), vitamin D,* and calcitonin. Phosphatonins such as fibroblast growth factor 23 (FGF-23), although they participate in phosphate and vitamin D homeostasis, do not modify extracellular calcium concentration.

This homeostatic system is modulated by dietary and environmental factors (including vitamins, hormones, medications, and mobility). Disorders of extracellular calcium homeostasis may be regarded as perturbations of this homeostatic system, either at the level of the genes controlling this system (as in, for example, familial hypocalciuric hypercalcemia, pseudohypoparathyroidism, or vitamin D–dependent rickets) or perturbations of this system induced by nongenetic means (as in lithium toxicity or postsurgical hypoparathyroidism).

Calcium fluxes between the ECF and one of the organs (skeleton, kidney, and intestine) or their combination as well as abnormal binding of the calcium to serum protein can cause hypercalcemia. PTH protects against hypocalcemia directly, by augmenting calcium mobilization from bone, by increasing renal tubular reabsorption of calcium, and by enhancing intestinal absorption of calcium, and indirectly, by its effect on vitamin D

metabolism. States with excess PTH may cause hypercalcemia, whereas PTH deficiency is associated with hypocalcemia. Similarly, PTHrP promotes bone resorption, enhances renal reabsorption of calcium, and decreases renal tubular reabsorption of phosphate. Excess of this hormone is responsible for the hypercalcemia of malignancy. Vitamin D and its metabolites increase intestinal absorption of calcium and cause bone resorption; therefore excess vitamin D induces hypercalcemia. Calcitonin inhibits bone resorption, but its physiologic role in protecting against hypercalcemia in humans is not proven.

Whole-Body Calcium Homeostasis

An adult human body contains approximately 1000 g to 1300 g of calcium with 99.3% in bone and teeth as hydroxyapatite crystal, 0.6% in soft tissues, and 0.1% in ECF, including 0.03% in plasma.[1] Maintenance of normal calcium balance and serum calcium levels depends on integrated regulation of calcium absorption and secretion by the intestinal tract, the excretion of calcium by the kidney, as well as calcium release from and calcium deposition into bone. In young adults calcium balance is neutral. Approximately 1000 mg of calcium is ingested per day, 200 mg is absorbed by the gut, mainly duodenum, and 800 mg is excreted. Out of 10 g of calcium filtrate produced by the kidney per day, only approximately 200 mg is excreted with the urine. At the same time 0.5 g of calcium is released from bone and same amount is deposited with new bone formation.

PTH, by stimulating bone resorption and kidney distal tubular calcium reabsorption as well as activation of renal hydroxylation of 25-hydroxyvitamin D (25[OH]D) to 1,25-dihydroxyvitamin D (1,25[OH]$_2$D), increases serum calcium levels. Depression in serum levels of calcium directly

---

*Vitamin D can be either vitamin D$_3$ (generated in the skin or acquired from food or animals or as a supplement) or vitamin D$_2$ (acquired from food or plants or as a supplement). Medications such as calcitriol are 1,25(OH)$_2$D$_3$ only. In this chapter we refer to all forms as vitamin D (or its metabolites) and omit the subscript.

stimulates, through the calcium-sensing receptor (CaSR) in the parathyroid gland, the secretion of preformed PTH from the parathyroid gland. This can occur within seconds. Subsequently PTH biosynthesis by the parathyroid gland increases over 24 to 48 hours, and it is followed by parathyroid gland hypertrophy and hyperplasia. Vitamin D metabolites and serum phosphorus levels also regulates PTH levels in blood.

The values for serum total calcium concentration in adults vary among clinical laboratories depending on the methods of measurement; the normal range is between 8.6 and 10.3 mg/dL (2.15 and 2.57 mmol/L).[2,3] Variations occur in serum calcium levels depending on age and gender, with a general trend toward lower serum calcium concentrations with aging.[4]

Calcium in blood exists in three distinct fractions: protein-bound calcium (40%), free (ionized) Ca^{2+} (48%), and calcium complexed to various anions such as phosphate, lactate, citrate, and bicarbonate (12%).[5] The latter two forms, complexed calcium and free calcium ions, together comprise the ultrafiltrable fraction of plasma calcium. Once again, 10 g is filtered every 24 hours. Plasma albumins are responsible for 90% and globulins for 10% of protein-bound calcium.

Free calcium is the physiologically active component of extracellular calcium with regard to cardiac myocyte contractility, neuromuscular activity, bone mineralization, and other calcium-dependent processes. Free Ca^{2+}, or ionized Ca^{2+}, is measured in most hospitals using ion-selective electrodes, and values in adults range between 4.65 and 5.28 mg/dL (1.16 and 1.32 mmol/L).[3,4]

Total calcium reflects the levels of free calcium if plasma levels of protein, pH, and anions are normal. The relationship between calcium ion and the concentration of protein in the serum is represented by a simple mass action expression:

$$([Ionized\ Ca^{2+}] \times [Protein])/[Calcium\ proteinate] = Kd$$

where *Protein* is the concentration of serum proteins, primarily albumin. Because Kd is constant, the numerator and denominator must change proportionately in any physiologic or pathologic state. A change in the concentration of total serum calcium will occur after a change in the concentration of serum proteins or alterations in their binding properties and after a primary change in the concentration of calcium ion. A fall in serum albumin reduces the protein and the calcium proteinate proportionately, which results in a fall in total serum calcium level, with the free calcium ion concentration remaining normal. If plasma levels of albumin are low, an adjustment (commonly but erroneously referred to as a "correction") of the measured serum levels of calcium should be made. For the routine clinical interpretation of serum calcium concentration needed for appropriate care of patients a simple formula for adjustment of total serum calcium concentration for changes in plasma albumin concentration is used by clinicians.

In conventional units:

$$Adjusted\ total\ calcium\ (mg/dL) = Total\ calcium\ (mg/dL) \\ + 0.8\ (4 - Albumin\ [g/dL])$$

In units of the International System of Units (SI):

$$Adjusted\ total\ calcium\ (mmol/L) = \\ Total\ calcium\ (mmol/L) + 0.02\ [40 - Albumin\ (g/L)]$$

This formula was endorsed in 1977 by an editorial in the *British Medical Journal*,[6] and the correction factor of 0.02 (in SI units) was chosen arbitrarily for simplicity from the range (0.018 to 0.025) available in the literature at that time. Other formulas have been developed, particularly for patients with chronic kidney disease (CKD), that have slightly better discriminatory ability (though not statistically significantly so) to make the diagnosis of hypocalcemia or hypercalcemia established by measurement of free calcium level.[7,8]

Also, a fall in pH of 0.1 unit will cause an approximately 0.1 mEq/L rise in the concentration of ionized Ca^{2+}, since hydrogen ions displace calcium from albumin, whereas alkalosis decreases free calcium by enhancing the binding of calcium to albumin.[4] There is no correction for this effect of pH in the previous formula, which also limits its accuracy.

Calcium binding to globulin is small (1.0 g of globulin binds 0.2 to 0.3 mg of calcium), and it is unusual to see a change in the total concentration of serum calcium as a result of alterations in the levels of globulin in the blood. However, in instances in which the globulin concentration in serum is extremely high (greater than 8.0 g/dL), such as in multiple myeloma, mild to moderate hypercalcemia may be seen because of an elevation of the globulin-bound calcium. In addition, immunoglobulin G myeloma proteins may have increased calcium-binding properties, and an elevation in the total level of serum calcium could occur with even a moderate increase in serum levels of globulins. In these circumstances, the ionized Ca^{2+} level in serum is normal, and therefore this kind of hypercalcemia would not require treatment.

Unfortunately, calcium status will be incorrectly predicted by the simple adjustment formula in 20% to 30% of individuals,[9] and the agreement between corrected and free calcium levels is only modest.[10] Thus, free calcium should be assessed, particularly in critically ill patients with acid-base disturbances, in patients exposed to a large amount of citrated blood, and in those with severe blood protein disorders.

Hypercalcemia

Hypercalcemia is relatively common and frequently overlooked, with an annual incidence in the population estimated to be 0.1% to 0.2% and a prevalence of 0.17% to 2.92% in the hospital population and 1.07% to 3.9% in the normal population.[11] Hypercalcemia results from an alteration in the net fluxes of calcium to and from four compartment: the bone, the gut, the kidney, and serum binding proteins (Table 18-1). Most commonly, hypercalcemia is caused by net calcium movement from the skeleton into the ECF through increased osteoclastic bone resorption, as in hyperparathyroidism or excess PTHrP production in malignancy. Excess circulating $1,25(OH)_2D$ from various causes also may contribute to excess bone resorption. Increased intestinal calcium absorption may lead to the development of hypercalcemia, as in vitamin D overdose or milk-alkali syndrome.

In general, the kidney does not contribute to hypercalcemia; rather, it defends against the development of hypercalcemia. Typically, hypercalciuria precedes hypercalcemia. Extracellular calcium itself in fact appears to have a calciuric effect on the renal tubule by its direct action on the CaSR of the thick ascending limb (TAL). Thus, in most hypercalcemic states, renal calcium handling is subject to competing influences: excess PTH or PTHrP acts on the PTH-PTHrP receptor to promote renal calcium reabsorption; excess calcium acts on the calcium receptor to promote calcium excretion.[12]

TABLE 18-1 Causes of Hypercalcemia

Malignancy
  Humoral hypercalcemia of malignancy (HHM) with secretion of
    parathyroid hormone (PTH)–related protein by the tumor
  Local osteolytic hypercalcemia (LOH)
  Tumor (lymphoma, germinoma) generation of 1,25-dihydroxyvitamin D_3
  Ectopic PTH secretion from tumor
Primary hyperparathyroidism
  Adenoma, hyperplasia, carcinoma
  Multiple endocrine neoplasia types 1 and 2a
Familial hypocalciuric hypercalcemia
Neonatal severe hyperparathyroidism
Other endocrine disorders
  Hyperthyroidism
  Acromegaly
  Pheochromocytoma
  Acute adrenal insufficiency
Granulomatous disorders
  Sarcoidosis
  Tuberculosis
  Berylliosis
  Disseminated coccidioidomycosis or candidiasis
  Histoplasmosis
  Leprosy
  Granulomatous lipoid pneumonia
  Silicone-induced granuloma
  Eosinophilic granuloma
  Farmer's lung
Vitamin overdosages
  Vitamin D
  Vitamin A
Immobilization
Renal failure
  Diuretic phase of acute renal failure, especially that due to
    rhabdomyolysis
  Chronic renal failure
  After renal transplantation
Medications
  Therapies and supplements causing milk-alkali syndrome
  Thiazide diuretics
  Lithium
  Foscarnvet
  Growth hormone
  Theophylline and aminophylline
  Estrogen and selective estrogen receptor modulators
  Vasoactive intestinal polypeptide
  Hyperalimentation regimens
Idiopathic hypercalcemia of infancy
Increased serum protein level
  Hemoconcentration
  Hyperglobulinemia due to multiple myeloma

TABLE 18-2 Clinical Features of Hypercalcemia

General

Malaise, tiredness, weakness

Neuropsychiatric

Impaired concentration, loss of memory, headache, drowsiness, lethargy, disorientation, confusion, irritability, depression, paranoia, hallucinations, ataxia, speech defects, visual disturbances, deafness (due to calcification of the eardrum), pruritus, mental retardation (infants), stupor, coma

Neuromuscular

Muscle weakness, hyporeflexia or absent reflexes, hypotonia, myalgia, arthralgia, bone pain, joint effusion, chondrocalcinosis, dwarfism (infants)

Gastrointestinal

Loss of appetite, dry mouth, thirst, polydipsia, nausea, vomiting, constipation, abdominal pain, weight loss, acute pancreatitis (calcifying), peptic ulcer, acute gastric dilation

Renal

Polyuria, nocturia, nephrocalcinosis, nephrolithiasis, interstitial nephritis, acute and chronic renal failure

Cardiovascular

Arrhythmia, bradycardia, first-degree heart block, short QT interval, bundle branch block, cardiac arrest (rare), hypertension, vascular calcification

Metastatic Calcification

Band keratopathy, red eye syndrome, conjunctival calcification, nephrocalcinosis, vascular calcification, pruritus

and rate of increase than the underlying cause. Hypercalcemia may be classified based on total serum calcium concentration[13] as follow:
Mild: Ca concentration = 10.4 to 11.9 mg/dL
Moderate: Ca concentration = 12.0 to 13.9 mg/dL
Severe (hypercalcemic crisis): Ca concentration = 14.0 to 16.0 mg/dL
Signs and symptoms and complications of hypercalcemia are summarized in Table 18-2.

In as many as 10% of patients with elevated levels of serum calcium the hypercalcemia is detected by a routine blood chemistry screening test, and such patients are considered to have "asymptomatic hypercalcemia." But even very mild hypercalcemia may be of clinical significance inasmuch as some studies have suggested an increased cardiovascular risk from quite mild, but prolonged, calcium elevations.[14] In symptomatic patients, the spectrum of the clinical presentation is varied and can be nonspecific. Mild hypercalcemia may present with malaise, weakness, minor joint pain, and other vague symptoms. In patients with severe hypercalcemia, the psychoneurotic pattern may be minimal, and the major symptoms are more likely to be nausea, abdominal pain, vomiting, constipation, polyuria, and mental disturbances ranging from headache and lethargy to coma. Recent loss of memory can be prominent and can be a presenting symptom.

Hypercalciuria induced by hypercalcemia causes nephrogenic diabetes insipidus with polyuria and polydipsia leading to ECF volume depletion, decrease glomerular filtration rate (GFR), and further increase in serum calcium level. Nephrolithiasis and nephrocalcinosis are common complications of hypercalcemia and are seen in 15% to 20% of cases of PHPT.

In rare cases, the kidney can actively contribute to the development of hypercalcemia. Unlike in primary hyperparathyroidism (PHPT) and humoral hypercalcemia of malignancy, in which increases in renal calcium excretion are observed, renal calcium excretion is not elevated in familial hypocalciuric hypercalcemia because of a defective renal response to calcium itself. The hypercalcemia associated with thiazide use is also mediated by the kidney: in both thiazide use and its genetic counterpart, Gitelman's syndrome, renal calcium excretion is decreased.

Clinical Manifestations

Hypercalcemia adversely affects the function of nearly all organ systems, but in particular the kidney, central nervous system, and cardiovascular system. The clinical manifestations of hypercalcemia relate more to the degree of hypercalcemia

Laboratory Findings

Laboratory findings in patients with hypercalcemia include abnormalities related to the underlying disease causing the hypercalcemia, and these are beyond the scope of this chapter. Alterations in the electrocardiogram (ECG) and electroencephalogram (EEG) occur in hypercalcemic patients independent of the cause of the hypercalcemia. The ECG shows a shortened ST segment and therefore a reduced QT interval as a result of an increased rate of cardiac repolarization. In patients with severe hypercalcemia exceeding 16 mg/dL, there is a widening of the T waves, resulting in an increase in the QT interval. Bradycardia and first-degree heart block may be evident on the ECGs of patients with acute and severe hypercalcemia. The EEG displays slowing and other nonspecific changes.

Diagnosis

A careful history taking and physical examination, and results of routine laboratory tests will, in most patients, lead to the correct diagnosis of hypercalcemia. A flow diagram for the evaluation of hypercalcemia is shown in Figure 18-1. PHPT and malignancy-associated hypercalcemia together are responsible for 90% of cases of hypercalcemia, with malignancy being the most common cause in hospitalized patients and PHPT being

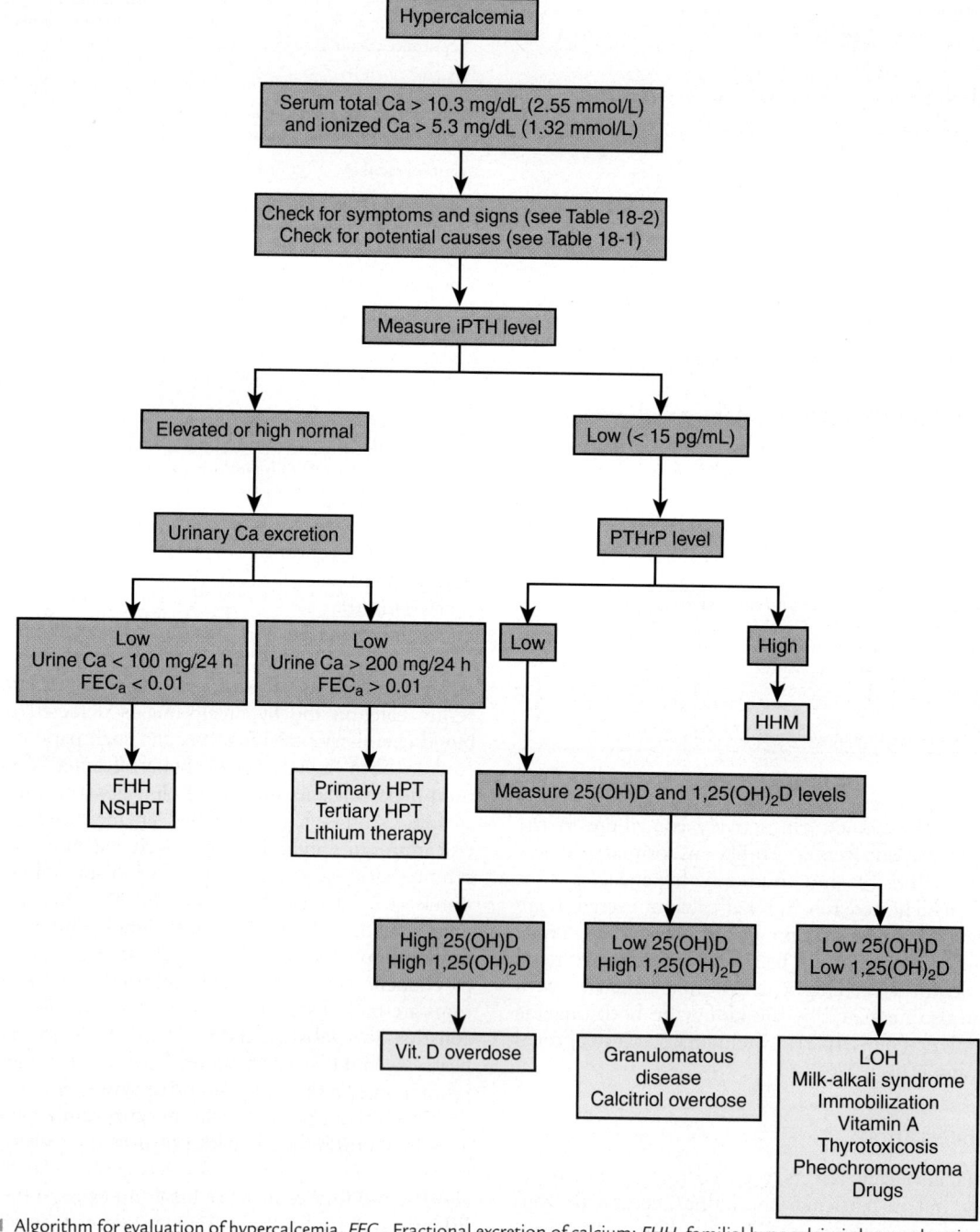

FIGURE 18-1 Algorithm for evaluation of hypercalcemia. *FEC_a,* Fractional excretion of calcium; *FHH,* familial hypocalciuric hypercalcemia; *HHM,* humoral hypercalcemia of malignancy; *HPT,* hyperparathyroidism; *LOH,* localized osteolytic hypercalcemia; *NSHPT,* neonatal severe hyperparathyroidism.

the most common in the outpatient clinic population.[13,15-17] It is generally easy to differentiate these two entities. Hypercalcemia is only rarely an early finding in occult malignancy. Assessment of PTH levels is essential in the diagnosis of hypercalcemia. Levels of "intact" and biologically active PTH hormone are measured by immunoradiometric or immunochemiluminometric assays. These assays also detect large carboxy-terminal fragments of PTH such as PTH (7-84) and may overestimate the amount of bioactive hormone in serum. There is no cross reactivity between PTH and PTHrP assays. In PHPT, levels of PTH are either frankly elevated or in the upper range of normal (Figure 18-2). Particularly in young individuals with PHPT, the PTH levels are more likely to be in the middle to upper normal range.

In patients with hypercalcemia and elevated PTH levels the differential diagnosis includes hyperparathyroidism due to thiazide diuretics or lithium, familial hypocalciuric hypercalcemia, and the tertiary hyperparathyroidism associated with renal failure and kidney transplantation. Patients with familial hypocalciuric hypercalcemia have a positive family history, onset of hypercalcemia at a young age, very low urinary calcium excretion, and specific genetic abnormalities.

In malignancy-associated hypercalcemia and hypercalcemia due to most other causes, PTH levels are low. Diagnosis of humoral hypercalcemia of malignancy frequently can be made on clinical grounds. In addition, PTHrP can now be assayed by commercial clinical laboratories either to support a diagnosis of humoral hypercalcemia of malignancy or to aid in diagnosis when the cause of hypercalcemia is obscure.

Approximately 10% of cases of hypercalcemia are due to causes other than PHPT and malignancy. Of particular importance in the evaluation of a hypercalcemic patient are the family history (because of familial syndromes characterized by hypercalcemia, including multiple endocrine neoplasia types 1 and 2, and familial hypocalciuric hypercalcemia), the medication history (because of the several medication-induced forms of hypercalcemia), and the presence of other disease (such as granulomatous or malignant disease). Plasma $1,25(OH)_2D$ level should be measured when granulomatous disorders or $1,25(OH)_2D$ lymphoma syndrome is considered. High $25(OH)D$ levels may suggest vitamin D intoxication as a cause of hypercalcemia.

Causes

PRIMARY HYPERPARATHYROIDISM

PHPT is caused by excessive and incompletely regulated secretion of PTH and consequent hypercalcemia and hypophosphatemia (see Table 18-1). It is the underlying cause of approximately 50% of cases of hypercalcemia in the general population. The estimated prevalence of PHPT is on the order of 1%, but may be as high as 2% in postmenopausal women.[18,19] The annual incidence is approximately 0.03% to 0.04%.[19-21]

A single enlarged parathyroid gland (adenoma) is the cause of PHPT in 80% to 85% of cases. These adenomas are benign, clonal neoplasms of parathyroid chief cells that lose their normal sensitivity to calcium. In about 15% to 20% of patients with PHPT all four parathyroid glands are hyperplastic. This occurs in sporadic PHPT or in conjunction with multiple endocrine neoplasia type 1 (MEN1) or type 2 (MEN2).[16] In diffuse hyperplasia, the "set point" for calcium is not changed in any given parathyroid cell, but the increased number of cells causes excess PTH production and hypercalcemia. Parathyroid carcinoma is seen in no more than 0.5% to 1% of patients with PHPT.[22]

PHPT occurs at all ages but is most common in older individuals, and peak incidence is in the sixth decade of life. After age 50, women are about three times more frequently affected than men. Sporadic PHPT is the most common. External neck irradiation during childhood is recognized as a risk factor for PHPT.

The genetic alterations underlying parathyroid adenomas are being partially elucidated.[23] Rearrangements and overexpression of the *PRAD1* (parathyroid adenomatosis 1)/cyclin D1 oncogene have been observed in about one fifth of parathyroid adenomas.[24,25] The *MEN1* tumor suppressor gene, *MENIN*, is inactivated in about 15% of adenomas.[26,27] Other chromosomal regions may also harbor parathyroid tumor suppressor genes.

PHPT typically presents in one of three ways. In 60% to 80%, there are minimal or no symptoms, and mild hypercalcemia is discovered during routine laboratory testing. Another 20% to 25% of patients have a chronic course manifested by mild or intermittent hypercalcemia, recurrent renal stones,

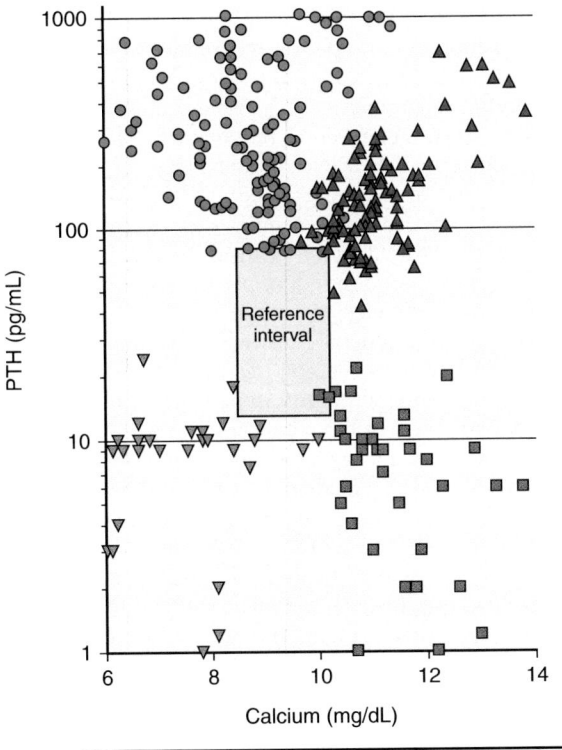

FIGURE 18-2 Relationship between total serum calcium and intact parathyroid hormone (PTH) concentrations. Values for patients with known primary hyperparathyroidism, secondary hyperparathyroidism, humoral hypercalcemia of malignancy or other PTH-independent cause of hypercalcemia, and hypoparathyroidism (Hypo) are plotted. The *rectangle* represents the normal reference range for the assays. (From O'Neill S, Gordon C, Guo R, et al: Multivariate analysis of clinical, demographic, and laboratory data for classification of patients with disorders of calcium homeostasis, *Am J Clin Pathol* 135[1]: 100-107, 2011.)

and complications of nephrolithiasis; in these patients the parathyroid tumor is small (less than 1.0 g) and slowly growing. Finally, 5% to 10% have severe and symptomatic hypercalcemia and overt osteitis fibrosa cystica; in these patients the parathyroid tumor is usually large (greater than 5.0 g). Patients with parathyroid carcinoma typically have severe hypercalcemia, with "classical" renal and bone involvement.[22]

The diagnosis of PHPT is now usually suggested by the incidental finding of hypercalcemia rather than by any of the sequelae of PTH excess such as skeletal and renal complications or symptomatic hypercalcemia.[15] Hypercalcemia may be quite mild and intermittent. Hypercalciuria was noted in 40% of patients with PHPT; nephrolithiasis in 19%; and classical bone disease, osteitis fibrosa cystica, in only 2% in studies performed between 1984 and 2000 in the United States.[14] But even in individuals with mild PHPT there is also progressive bone loss, as measured by bone mineral densitometry over 15 years of observation.[28]

The diagnosis of PHPT is established by laboratory testing showing hypercalcemia, inappropriately normal or elevated blood levels of PTH, hypercalciuria, hypophosphatemia, phosphaturia, and increased urinary excretion of cyclic adenosine monophosphate (cAMP). Hyperchloremic acidosis may be present, and the ratio of serum chloride to serum phosphorus is elevated. The serum levels of alkaline phosphatase and of uric acid also may be elevated. The serum concentration of magnesium is usually normal but may be low or high.

Some controversy surrounds the potential relationship between PHPT and increased mortality.[15] A number of studies have shown that PHPT may be associated with hypertension,[28,29] dyslipidemia,[30] diabetes,[31] increased thickness of the carotid artery,[32] and increased mortality,[33-35] primarily from cardiovascular disease.[37,38] The morbidity from PHPT can also be substantial, especially in symptomatic patients with severe hypercalcemia and with late diagnosis. The classic bone lesion in PHPT, osteitis fibrosa cystica, is now rarely seen. Diffuse osteopenia is more common.[39] Even in asymptomatic patients, increased rates of bone turnover are always present.[40]

Standard therapy for PHPT remains surgery.[15,29] It is generally agreed that parathyroidectomy is indicated in all patients with biochemically confirmed PHPT who have specific symptoms or signs of their disease, such as a history of life-threatening hypercalcemia, renal insufficiency, or kidney stones.

In 2008, the Third International Workshop on Hyperparathyroidism updated 2002 National Institutes of Health guidelines for the management of asymptomatic hyperparathyroidism.[29] Surgery is advised for asymptomatic disease in patients with a serum calcium level of more than 1 mg/dL above normal, reduced bone mass (T-score of less than −2.5 at any site), GFR of less than 60 mL/min, or age younger than 50 years. Hypercalciuria (>400 mg calcium per 24 hours) is no longer regarded as an indication for parathyroid surgery, since hypercalciuria in PHPT was not established as a risk factor for stone formation.

Patients older than 50 years with no obvious symptoms should receive close follow-up, including measurement of bone density every 1 or 2 years and determination of serum creatinine and calcium levels annually. All monitored patients should receive vitamin D supplementation to achieve a 25(OH)D level above 20 ng/dL, and calcium intake should be maintained at levels comparable to those of individuals without PHPT.

Preoperative localization of the parathyroid glands has generally been considered unnecessary in patients with uncomplicated disease who are undergoing surgery for the first time. Sestamibi scan is the most popular and sensitive technique to localize PTH glands, with accuracy rates up to 90%, followed by ultrasonography of the neck.[30] If a single adenoma is visualized, minimally invasive parathyroidectomy may be an option and is associated with a cure rate of 95% to 98%. This procedure requires the surgeon to visualize only one gland as long as resection results in a substantial intraoperative decline in PTH. Otherwise, all four parathyroid glands should be surgically identified. Although excision of a single enlarged gland is curative, the finding of more than one enlarged gland raises the possibility of diffuse parathyroid hyperplasia and MEN. When all glands are enlarged, subtotal parathyroidectomy of 3½ glands or total removal of 4 glands with autotransplantation of a portion of one gland is performed.[15]

Recurrence of hyperparathyroidism is rare after identification and removal of one enlarged gland.[31] If the initial exploration fails and hypercalcemia persists or recurs, more extensive preoperative parathyroid localization should be performed.[15,30] Complications are greater after reexploration of the neck than after the initial operation.

Although parathyroidectomy remains the definitive treatment for PHPT, patients who refuse surgery, have contraindications for surgery, or do not meet current operative guidelines can be treated pharmacologically. Four classes of medications can be useful: calcimimetic drugs, bisphosphonates, estrogens, and selective estrogen receptor modulators.[42] There are insufficient long-term data to recommend any of these medications as alternatives to surgery. The CaSR agonist cinacalcet is approved in some European countries for treatment of PHPT but not in the United States. Cinacalcet therapy in patients with PHPT was found to reduce plasma PTH levels, normalize serum calcium concentration in the short and long term, and preserve bone mineral density.[32-35] Bisphosphonates and hormone replacement therapy decreased bone turnover and increased bone mineral density in patients with PHPT without change in serum calcium concentration.[32]

Parathyroid carcinoma probably accounts for fewer than 1% of cases PHPT.[22] The diagnosis of parathyroid carcinoma may be difficult to make in the absence of metastases, because the histologic appearance of the tumor may be similar to that of atypical adenomas.[36] In general, parathyroid carcinomas are typically large (3 cm), irregular, hard tumors with a low degree of aggressive growth, and survival is common if the entire gland can be removed.[22,37] Cinacalcet is approved for patients with inoperable parathyroid cancer to control hypercalcemia.

MALIGNANCY

Hypercalcemia occurs in approximately 10% to 25% of patients with some cancer, especially during the last 4 to 6 weeks of life. It can be classified into four categories: humoral hypercalcemia of malignancy (HHM); local osteolytic hypercalcemia (LOH); $1,25(OH)_2D$-induced hypercalcemia; and ectopic secretion of authentic PTH.[38,39]

HHM from increased secretion of PTHrP by a malignant tumor accounts for approximately 80% of cases. Numerous types of malignancies are associated with HHM and secretion of PTHrP, including squamous cell cancer (e.g., of the head and neck, esophagus, cervix, or lung) and renal cell, breast, and ovarian carcinomas. Lymphomas associated with human T-lymphotropic virus type 1 infection may cause PTHrP-mediated HHM, and other non-Hodgkin's lymphomas may be associated with PTHrP-mediated hypercalcemia as well.[40,41]

PTHrP is a large protein encoded by a gene on chromosome 12. It is similar to PTH only at the N terminus, where the initial eight amino acids are identical.[41] PTHrP is widely expressed in a variety of tissues, including keratinocytes, mammary gland, placenta, cartilage, nervous system, vascular smooth muscle, and various endocrine sites.[42] Injection of PTHrP produces hypercalcemia in rats[43] and essentially reproduces the entire clinical syndrome of HHM, but other circulating factors such as cytokines may also be important. Normal circulating levels of PTHrP are negligible; it is probably unimportant in normal calcium homeostasis. However, mice with a targeted disruption in the PTHrP gene show a lethal defect in bone development,[44] which demonstrates its importance in normal development.

Circulating PTHrP interacts with the PTH-PTHrP receptor in bone and renal tubules. It activates bone resorption and suppresses osteoblastic bone formation, thus causing flux of calcium (up to 700 to 1000 mg/day) from bone into the ECF. The reason for this uncoupling of bone formation from bone resorption remains unclear.[41] PTHrP mimics the anticalciuric effect of PTH and thus exacerbates hypercalcemia. Other effects of PTHrP include phosphaturia and hypophosphatemia, and increased cAMP excretion by the kidney. HHM is associated with reduction in $1,25(OH)_2D$ levels (in contrast to PHPT), which may limit intestinal calcium absorption. Consistent with the physiologic role of PTHrP patients are hypercalcemic and hypophosphatemic and demonstrate increased osteoclastic bone resorption, increased urinary cAMP, and hypercalciuria.

LOH accounts for 20% of cases malignancy-associated hypercalcemia. LOH-producing tumors include breast and prostate cancers, and hematologic neoplasms (multiple myeloma, lymphoma/leukemia). LOH is caused by locally produced osteoclast–activating cytokines, including PTHrP and interleukins 1, 6, and 8. PTHrP increases RANK (receptor activator of nuclear factor κB) expression on osteoblasts and RANK-mediated osteoclast bone resorption. The resorbing bone releases transforming growth factor-β, which in turn stimulate PTHrP expression on tumor cells.[45,46] The bone metastases can be classified as osteolytic, osteoblastic, or mixed. Osteolytic lesions are caused by osteoclast activation by malignant cells and appear as areas of increased radiolucency on radiographs. LOH leads to predictable pathophysiologic events that include hypercalcemia, suppression of circulating PTH and $1,25(OH)_2D$, hyperphosphatemia, and hypercalciuria. Bone metastases may produce severe pain and pathologic fractures.

Hypercalcemia in breast cancer is associated with the presence of both extensive osteolytic metastases and HHM.[46,47] Extensive osteolytic bone destruction is seen in multiple myeloma.[45] Although bone lesions develop in all patients with myeloma, hypercalcemia occurs only in 15% to 20% of patients who are in later stages of disease and have impaired kidney function. The degree of hypercalcemia and bone destruction are not well correlated.[48] Treatment with bisphosphonates appears to protect against the development of skeletal complications (including hypercalcemia) in patients with myeloma and lytic bone lesions.[49]

Hypercalcemia due to $1,25(OH)_2D$ production by malignant lymphomas has been reported.[50,51] All types of lymphoma can cause this syndrome. The malignant cells or adjacent cells overexpress the enzyme 1α-hydroxylase, which converts $25(OH)D$ to $1,25(OH)_2D$. Hypercalcemia is mainly secondary to increased intestinal calcium, although decreased renal clearance and bone resorption may also develop. Ectopic production of authentic PTH by a nonparathyroid tumor may occur, but it is very rare.[52]

FAMILIAL PRIMARY HYPERPARATHYROIDISM SYNDROMES
Familial PHPT syndromes are defined by a combination of hypercalcemia and elevated or nonsuppressed serum PTH levels.

FAMILIAL HYPOCALCIURIC HYPERCALCEMIA AND NEONATAL SEVERE HYPERPARATHYROIDISM
Familial hypocalciuric (benign) hypercalcemia (FHH) is a rare disease (estimated prevalence of 1 per 78,000) with autosomal dominant inheritance, high penetrance for hypercalcemia, and relative hypocalciuria.[53-55] FHH was first described in 1966 by Jackson and Boonstra[56] and in 1972 by Foley and colleagues.[57] The hypercalcemia is typically mild to moderate (10.5 mg/dL to 12 mg/dL), and affected patients do not exhibit the typical complications associated with elevated serum calcium concentrations. Both total and ionized calcium concentrations are elevated, but the PTH level is generally "inappropriately normal," although mild elevations in approximately 15% to 20% of cases have been reported. Urinary calcium excretion is not elevated, as would be expected in hypercalcemia due to other causes. The fractional excretion of calcium is usually less than 1%.[54] Serum magnesium concentration is commonly mildly elevated and serum phosphate concentration is decreased. Bone mineral density is normal, as are vitamin D levels.

The finding of a right-shifted set point for Ca^{2+}-regulated PTH release in FHH pointed toward the role of CaSR in FHH.[58] Indeed, in most families with FHH, the disease is caused by autosomal dominant loss-of-function mutations in the *CASR* gene located on chromosome arm 3q, which encodes for CaSR. CaSR is a G protein–coupled membrane receptor widely expressed in mammalian tissues, particularly the parathyroid gland and the kidney. In the kidney, CaSR is expressed throughout the nephron, but most strongly in the TAL. The fact that relative hypocalciuria persists in FHH patients even after parathyroidectomy confirms the role of CaSR in regulating renal calcium handling.[59]

More than 257 mutations have been described for *CASR*, most of which are inactivating, missense, and found throughout the large predicted structure of the CaSR protein.[58,60,61] Expression studies of mutant CaSRs have shown great variability in their effect on calcium responsiveness. In some cases, CaSR mutations only slightly shift the set point for calcium; other mutations appear to render the receptor largely inactive.[62-64] In about 15% of patients with typical features of FHH, CaSR mutations have not been found. In some of these cases, CaSR mutations may be in noncoding sequences; in others, different gene defects may be responsible.

CaSR mutation analysis has an occasional role in the diagnosis of FHH in cases in which results of biochemical tests remain inconclusive and the distinction of FHH from mild PHPT is unclear. It is critical to make an accurate diagnosis, because the hypercalcemia in FHH does not respond to subtotal parathyroidectomy.

Hypercalcemia in FHH has a generally benign course and is resistant to medications, except for some cases successfully treated with the calcimimetic agent cinacalcet.[65] The potential benefit of calcimimetic agents in FHH is supported by in vitro studies using human CaSR mutants which show that the calcimimetic agent R-568 enhances the potency of extracellular Ca^{2+} toward the mutants.[66]

Patients who inherit two copies of CaSR alleles bearing inactivating mutations develop neonatal severe hyperparathyroidism. Neonatal severe hyperparathyroidism is an extremely rare disorder, is most commonly autosomal recessive, is often reported in the offspring of consanguineous FHH parents, and is characterized by severe hyperparathyroid hyperplasia, elevation of PTH levels, severe hyperparathyroid bone disease, and elevated extracellular calcium levels.[53,58,67,68] In a few affected infants, only one defective allele has been found, but it is unclear whether the finding of only one defective allele is due to the presence of an undetected defect in the other CaSR allele. Treatment is total parathyroidectomy, followed by vitamin D and calcium supplementation. This disease is usually lethal without surgical intervention.

MULTIPLE ENDOCRINE NEOPLASIAS

MEN1 is a rare autosomal dominant disorder with an estimated prevalence of 2 to 3 per 100,000, characterized by endocrine tumors in at least two of three main tissues: the parathyroid gland, the pituitary, and enteropancreatic tissue. It is the most common form of familial PHPT.[69] PHPT is present in 87% to 97% of patients, whereas pancreatic and pituitary tumors are more likely to be absent.[15,70] The responsible gene, *MENIN*,[71] encodes a nuclear protein whose function is not well understood, but which probably acts as a tumor suppressor.[72] MEN2A is a syndrome of heritable predisposition to medullary thyroid carcinoma, pheochromocytoma, and PHPT. Mutations in the RET (rearranged during transfection) proto-oncogene, which encodes a tyrosine kinase receptor, are responsible for MEN2A.[73] The biochemical diagnosis and indications for surgery in patients with PHPT associated with MEN1 or MEN2A are similar to those in patients with sporadic PHPT.[70]

HYPERPARATHYROIDISM–JAW TUMOR

Hyperparathyroidism–jaw tumor (HPT-JT) syndrome is a rare autosomal dominant disorder characterized by severe hypercalcemia, parathyroid adenoma, and fibro-osseous tumors of the mandible or maxilla.[74] Renal manifestations include cysts, hamartomas, and Wilms' tumors. Mutations in the *HRPT2* tumor suppressor gene are responsible for HPT-JT.[75]

NONPARATHYROID ENDOCRINOPATHIES

Hypercalcemia may occur in patients with other endocrine diseases. Mild hypercalcemia is present in up to 20% of the patients with hyperthyroidism, but severe hypercalcemia is uncommon.[76,77] Thyroid hormones (thyroxine and triiodothyronine) increase bone resorption and lead to hypercalcemia and/or hypercalciuria when bone resorption exceeds bone formation significantly.[78] Because of a possible increased association between hyperthyroidism and parathyroid adenoma, the latter must be ruled out in patients with thyrotoxicosis and hypercalcemia. Furthermore, the hypercalcemia in a patient

with thyrotoxicosis can be attributed to this disease only if it resolves after the patient achieves an euthyroid state.

Pheochromocytoma may be associated with hypercalcemia[79]; most commonly, it is due to coincident PHPT and MEN2A. In some patients hypercalcemia disappears after removal of the adrenal tumor, and some of these tumors produce PTHrP.[80] Acute adrenal insufficiency is a rare cause of hypercalcemia.[81] Because these patients may be dehydrated and have hemoconcentration, a rise in serum albumin concentration and increased binding of calcium to serum albumin secondary to hyponatremia may contribute to the increase in serum calcium level. In addition, isolated adrenocorticotropic hormone deficiency can result in hypercalcemia.[82] Growth hormone administration[83] and acromegaly[84] have both been associated with hypercalcemia. Acromegaly is often accompanied by mild hypercalcemia (15% to 20% of cases), which results from enhanced intestinal calcium absorption and augmented bone resorption.[85,86] In acromegalic patients with hypercalcemia, the serum levels of PTH are normal but may be inappropriately high for the levels of serum calcium.

VITAMIN D–MEDIATED HYPERCALCEMIA

Vitamin D is naturally generated in skin under exposure to ultraviolet B light or is acquired from the diet and medical supplements. Excess of vitamin D or its metabolites can cause hypercalcemia and hypercalciuria. The mechanism of hypercalcemia is a combination of increased intestinal calcium absorption and bone resorption induced by vitamin D, and decreased calcium renal clearance resulting from dehydration. Toxic effects occur from amounts of vitamin D that lead to an increase in plasma total 25(OH)D well in excess of 80 ng/mL, which exceeds the binding capacity of vitamin D–binding protein (DBP) for 25(OH)D. The resulting increase in "free" circulating $25(OH)D_3$ may activate the vitamin D nuclear receptor. Vitamin D metabolites may also displace $1,25(OH)_2D$ from DBP, increasing $1,25(OH)_2D$ free levels and thus increasing signal transduction.[87]

Hypercalcemia has been reported in cases of accidental overdose of vitamin D from fortified cow's milk[88,89] and from over-the-counter supplements.[90] Serum 25(OH)D levels were elevated, $1,25(OH)_2D$ levels were normal, and PTH levels were either depressed or normal in these cases. However, vitamin D well in excess of the tolerable upper intake of 2000 IU/day is required for this form of hypercalcemia to develop.[91] The diagnosis is made by the history and detection of elevated 25(OH)D levels. Vitamin D analogs, including $1,25(OH)_2D$ used in the treatment of hyperparathyroidism and metabolic bone disease in CKD patients, can also cause hypercalcemia.[92]

MEDICATIONS

Hypercalcemia and hyperparathyroidism are a long-recognized and well-described consequence of lithium therapy.[93-96] The prevalence of lithium-associated hypercalcemia in those taking the drug is estimated to be 4% to 6%.[94,95] Lithium probably interferes with signal transduction elicited by CaSR, which increases the set point for extracellular calcium to inhibit PTH secretion.[95-97] This leads to parathyroid hyperplasia or adenoma.[98] The spectrum of lithium-induced calcium disorders is wide and includes cases with overt hyperparathyroidism, mild or severe hypercalcemia, and elevated or normal

PTH levels. Hypocalciuria is common, although hypercalciuria was reported in a few case series. Hypercalcemia can be reversible after a few weeks of discontinuance of lithium in most patients receiving lithium treatment for a short period (fewer than 5 years). The CaSR agonist cinacalcet has also been used with good results in those patients for whom cessation of lithium therapy was not an option.[99] Symptomatic patients with hyperparathyroidism should be treated with parathyroidectomy.[95,96]

Vitamin A intake in dosages exceeding the recommended daily allowance of 5000 U/day over prolonged periods of time, especially in the elderly and in patients with impaired kidney function, may cause hypercalcemia with increased alkaline phosphatase levels, presumably from increased osteoclast-mediated bone resorption.[100-102] The hypercalcemia is accompanied by high retinol plasma levels, and discontinuation of vitamin A causes normalization of plasma calcium concentration. Vitamin A analogs, used in the management of dermatologic and hematologic malignant disease, have also been reported to cause hypercalcemia.[103,104]

Estrogens and the selective estrogen receptor modifier tamoxifen used in the management of breast cancer may cause hypercalcemia early in treatment in the presence of bone metastasis.[105] Hypercalcemia was noted in approximately 0.4% to 1.9% of patients treated with thiazide diuretics, with an annual incidence rate of 7.7 per 100,000 in the population of Olmsted County, Minnesota.[106,107] A reduction in urinary calcium excretion, volume contraction, and metabolic alkalosis are the major reasons for thiazide-induced hypercalcemia. In addition, thiazides may increase intestinal calcium absorption and unmask PHPT.[107-109] Hypercalcemia is usually mild, asymptomatic, and nonprogressive. Individuals with unsuppressed PTH levels despite hypercalcemia or with severe and continued hypercalcemia may have PHPT. Many other agents occasionally cause hypercalcemia, including theophylline, foscarnet, growth hormone, parenteral nutrition, manganese in toxic doses, and 8-chloro-cAMP.

Milk-Alkali Syndrome

Milk-alkali syndrome was originally described in patients with duodenal ulcers receiving therapy with sodium bicarbonate and large amounts of milk. These patients had hypercalcemia, hyperphosphatemia, hypocalciuria, and renal insufficiency, together with kidney and other soft tissue calcifications.[110] During the last 20 years, calcium supplements in the form of calcium carbonate for the prevention and treatment of osteoporosis have become the main cause of this syndrome.[111,112] In some studies, milk-alkali syndrome is the third most common cause of hypercalcemia in hospitalized patients without end-stage renal disease.[113]

The pathogenesis of milk-alkali syndrome can be divided into two phases: generation of hypercalcemia by intake of calcium (usually more than 4 g of elemental calcium), and the maintenance phase. Hypercalcemia activates the renal CaSR, which causes natriuresis and water diuresis with volume depletion and a decrease in GFR. Increased tubular reabsorption of calcium as a result of metabolic alkalosis and volume depletion contribute to maintenance of hypercalcemia.[112] The diagnosis is made largely by the history and may not be obvious because of atypical dietary sources of calcium and alkali. Hypercalcemia can be corrected, but renal damage may be permanent.

Immobilization

Immobilization, especially in high bone turnover states (youth, hyperparathyroidism, breast cancer with bone involvement, Paget's disease), suppresses osteoblastic bone formation and increases osteoclastic bone resorption, which leads to uncoupling of these two processes with subsequent release of calcium from the bone and thus to hypercalcemia.[114,115] Typically, from 10 days to a few weeks are required for the development of immobilization hypercalcemia. Administration of bisphosphonates may help decrease the hypercalcemia and osteopenia in this setting.[116] Mobilization remains the ultimate cure for this condition.

Granulomatous Disease

A variety of granulomatous diseases are associated with hypercalcemia. The most common is sarcoidosis (prevalence of hypercalcemia and hypercalciuria of 10% and 20%, respectively), but tuberculosis, berylliosis, histoplasmosis, coccidioidomycosis, pneumocystosis, leprosy, histiocytosis X, eosinophilic granulomatosis, and inflammatory bowel disease may present with hypercalcemia.[82,117-119] Hypercalcemia is more common in chronic and disseminated granulomatous diseases. Sun exposure, or even small doses of vitamin D supplementation, may precipitate or worsen this syndrome.

The hypercalcemia, which has been best studied in sarcoidosis, is caused by inappropriate extrarenal production of $1,25(OH)_2D$ by activated macrophages with increased 1α-hydroxylase activity.[120,121] Elevated levels of circulating $1,25(OH)_2D$ have been described in most granulomatous diseases during hypercalcemia, except in coccidioidomycosis. The $1,25(OH)_2D$ in turn leads to intestinal hyperabsorption of calcium, hypercalciuria, and hypercalcemia. Osteopontin, highly expressed by histiocytes in granulomas, may contribute to hypercalcemia via osteoclast activation and bone resorption. Bone mineral content tends to be reduced in these patients. Hypercalciuria may precede hypercalcemia and may be an early indicator of this complication.

Standard treatment consists of administration of glucocorticoids, which decreases the abnormal $1,25(OH)_2D$ production.[122] Chloroquine and ketoconazole, which also decrease $1,25(OH)_2D$ production by competitive inhibition of cytochrome P450–dependent 1α-hydroxylase, have been shown to be efficacious as well.[123,124]

Liver Disease

Hypercalcemia has been reported in patients with end-stage liver disease with hyperbilirubinemia who are awaiting liver transplantation, in the absence of hyperparathyroidism or hypervitaminosis D.[125]

Acute and Chronic Renal Failure

Hypercalcemia may be observed in patients with renal failure and in renal transplant recipients. These conditions are discussed in detail in Chapter 54.

Treatment

The therapy for hypercalcemia must be tailored to the degree of hypercalcemia, the clinical condition, and the underlying cause (Table 18-3).[13] Theoretically, a decrease in the serum levels of calcium can be achieved by enhancing its urinary excretion, augmenting net movement of calcium into bone,

TABLE 18-3 Pharmacologic Therapy for Hypercalcemia

INTERVENTION	DOSAGE	ADVERSE EFFECT
Hydration or Calciuresis		
Intravenous saline	200-500 mL/hr, depending on the cardiovascular and renal status of the patient	Congestive heart failure
Furosemide	20-40 mg intravenously, *after rehydration has been achieved*	Dehydration, hypokalemia, hypomagnesemia
First-Line Medications		
Intravenous bisphosphonates*		
Pamidronate	60-90 mg intravenously over a 2-hr period in a solution of 50-200 mL of saline or 5% dextrose in water[†]	Renal failure, transient flulike syndrome with aches, chills, and fever
Zoledronate	4 mg intravenously over a 15-min period in a solution of 50 mL of saline or 5% dextrose in water	Renal failure, transient flulike syndrome with aches, chills, and fever
Second-Line Medications		
Glucocorticoids[‡]	For example, prednisone, 60 mg orally daily for 10 days	Potential interference with chemotherapy; hypokalemia, hyperglycemia, hypertension, Cushing's syndrome, immunosuppression
Mithramycin	Single dose of 25 μg/kg of body weight over a 4- to 6-hr period in saline	Thrombocytopenia, platelet aggregation defect, anemia, leukopenia, hepatitis, renal failure[§]
Calcitonin	4-8 IU/kg subcutaneously or intramuscularly every 12 hr	Flushing, nausea, escape phenomenon
Gallium nitrate	100-200 mg/m² of body surface area intravenously given continuously over a 24-hr period for 5 days	Renal failure

*Pamidronate and zoledronate are approved by the Food and Drug Administration (FDA) for treatement of hypercalcemia. Ibandronate is approved by the FDA for postmenopausal osteoporosis. Clodronate is approved in Canada for hypercalcemia of malignancy. Ibandronate and clodronate are also available in continental Europe, the United Kingdom, and elsewhere. Bisphosphonates should be used with caution, if at all, when the serum creatinine level is >2.5-3.0 mg/dL (>221.0-265.2 μmol/L).
[†]Pamidronate is generally used at a dose of 90 mg, but the 60-mg dose may be used to treat patients of small stature or those with renal impairment or mild hypercalcemia.
[‡]These drugs have a slow onset of action compared with the bisphosphonates; approximately 4 to 10 days are required for a response.
[§]These effects have been reported in association with higher-dose regimens used to treat testicular cancer (50 μg/kg of body weight per day over a period of 5 days) and in patients receiving multiple doses of 25 μg/kg; they are not expected to occur with a single dose of 25 μg/kg unless preexisting liver, kidney, or hematologic disease is present. Many of the recommendations in this table are based on historical precedent and common practice rather than on results of randomized clinical trials. There are data from randomized trials comparing bisphosphonates to the other agents listed and to one another.
Modified from Stewart AF: Clinical practice. Hypercalcemia associated with cancer, *N Engl J Med* 352(4):373-379, 2005.

inhibiting bone resorption, reducing intestinal absorption of calcium, and/or removing calcium from the ECF by other means. Patients with mild hypercalcemia (<12 mg/dL) do not require immediate treatment. They should stop any medications implicated in causing hypercalcemia, avoid volume depletion and physical inactivity, and maintain adequate hydration. Moderate hypercalcemia (12 to 14 mg/dL), especially if acute and symptomatic, requires more aggressive therapy. Patients with severe hypercalcemia (>14 mg/dL), even without symptoms, should be treated intensively.

VOLUME REPLETION AND LOOP DIURETICS
Correction of the ECF volume is the first and the most important step in the treatment of severe hypercalcemia from any causes. It can be achieved with infusion of normal isotonic saline at 200 to 500 mL/hr, adjusted to obtain a urine output of 150 to 200 mL/hr and accompanied by appropriate hemodynamic monitoring.[13,126,127] Volume repletion can lower calcium concentration by approximately 1 to 3 mg/dL by increasing GFR and decreasing sodium and calcium reabsorption in proximal and distal tubules.

Once volume expansion is achieved, loop diuretics can be given concurrently with saline to increase the calciuresis by blocking the Na^+-K^+-$2Cl^-$ cotransporter in the TAL.[126] Most commonly furosemide is used at a dosage of 40 to 80 mg every 6 hours, and this treatment together with saline therapy may decrease serum calcium concentration by 2 to 4 mg/dL. Urinary losses of fluid, potassium, and magnesium should be evaluated at intervals of 2 to 4 hours and quantitatively replaced to prevent ECF volume contraction, hypokalemia, and hypomagnesemia. Usually, 20 to 40 mEq of KCl and 15 to 30 mg of magnesium ion per liter of saline infusate are adequate to replenish the urinary losses of these electrolytes.

Care must be taken to monitor the patient's volume status closely during the administration of large amounts of saline and diuretic, particularly in hospitalized patients with cardiac or pulmonary disease. It must be admitted that the use of loop diuretics for the treatment of hypercalcemia is not supported by any randomized controlled studies and lately has been criticized for this reason.[127] However, in the authors' opinion loop diuretics still remain an important tool in the management of hypercalcemia, especially in patients at risk of volume overload.

INHIBITION OF BONE RESORPTION
The increase in bone resorption, as the most common pathologic process leading to hypercalcemia, must be addressed concurrently with volume expansion and hydration. Bisphosphonates are currently the agents of choice in the treatment of mild to severe hypercalcemia, especially that associated with cancer. They are pyrophosphate analogs with a high affinity for hydroxyapatite and inhibit osteoclast function in areas of high bone turnover.[13]

In the United States, the Food and Drug Administration has approved two bisphosphonates for treatment of hypercalcemia: zoledronate (4 mg intravenously over at least 15 minutes) and pamidronate (60 to 90 mg intravenously over 2 to 24 hours). The clinical response takes 48 to 96 hours and is sustained for up to 3 weeks. Doses can be repeated no sooner than every 7 days. Both agents are effective in lowering calcium level. Zoledronate was slightly more efficacious than pamidronate in a randomized clinical trial.[128] In Europe other bisphosphonates such as clodronate and ibandronate are also approved.

Fever is observed in about one fifth of patients taking bisphosphonates; rare side effects include acute renal failure, collapsing glomerulopathy, and osteonecrosis of the jaw. The dosage of bisphosphonates should be adjusted in patients with preexisting kidney disease.[129] The renal component of hypercalcemia, which includes increased distal tubular calcium reabsorption driven by PTH-PTHrP, does not respond to bisphosphonates.

Calcitonin is also an effective inhibitor of osteoclast bone resorption. It has a rapid onset of action (within 12 hours), its effect is transient, and it has minimal toxicity.[130] Calcitonin is usually given at a dosage of 4 to 8 U/kg subcutaneously, every 6 to 12 hours. Its role is mainly to provide initial treatment of severe hypercalcemia while waiting for the more sustained effect of bisphosphonates to begin.

Gallium nitrate inhibits bone resorption by increasing the solubility of hydroxyapatite crystals. The usual dosage is 200 mg/m^2 intravenously over 24 hours with adequate hydration for 5 consecutive days, and the hypocalcemic effect is not generally observed until the end of this period. Gallium nitrate is effective, but can be nephrotoxic.[131,132]

Plicamycin (mithramycin) (25 µg/kg intravenously every 5 to 7 days) may be used in patients with severe renal failure. Other therapies for hypercalcemia, such as chelation with ethylenediaminetetraacetic acid (EDTA) and intravenous phosphate, have adverse side effect profiles and are no longer recommended. Glucocorticoids are useful therapy for hypercalcemia from a specific subset of causes. They are most effective in hematologic malignancies (multiple myeloma, Hodgkin's disease) and disorders of vitamin D metabolism (granulomatous disease, vitamin D toxicity).[117,122]

In severely hypercalcemic patients who are comatose, have ECG changes, have severe renal failure, or cannot receive aggressive hydration, hemodialysis with a low- or no-calcium dialysate is an effective treatment.[133] Continuous renal replacement therapy can also be used to treat severe hypercalcemia.[134] The effect of dialysis is transitory, and it must be followed by other measures.

As discussed in earlier sections, cinacalcet, an allosteric activator of CaSR, is approved for use in patients with inoperable parathyroid cancer to control hypercalcemia. The off-label use of cinacalcet has been reported for treatment of patients with PHPT who have mild disease, for whom parathyroid surgery has failed, or who have contraindications to surgery.[161] Other hypercalcemic disorders such as familial hypocalciuric hypercalcemia and lithium-induced hyperparathyroidism have been also treated with cinacalcet.

Hypocalcemia

Hypocalcemia is usually defined as a total serum calcium concentration, corrected for protein, of less than 8.4 mg/dL and/or an ionized Ca^{2+} concentration of less 1.16 mmol/L, although these values may vary slightly depending on the laboratory. Estimation of the ionized Ca^{2+} concentration based on the total serum calcium concentration corrected for albumin is encumbered with error, as discussed earlier. Thus ionized Ca^{2+} concentration should be measured directly before any major workup for the causes of hypocalcemia is undertaken.

TABLE 18-4 Clinical Features of Hypocalcemia
Neuromuscular Irritability
General fatigability and muscle weakness
Paresthesias, numbness
Circumoral and peripheral extremity tingling
Muscle twitching and cramping
Tetany, carpopedal spasms
Chvostek's sign, Trousseau's sign
Laryngeal and bronchial spasms
Altered Central Nervous System Function
Emotional disturbances: irritability, depression
Altered mental status, coma
Seizures: tonic-clonic
Papilledema, pseudotumor cerebri
Cerebral calcifications
Cardiovascular Features
Lengthening of the QTc interval
Dysrhythmias
Hypotension
Congestive heart failure
Dermatologic and Ocular Features
Dry skin, coarse hair, brittle nails
Cataracts

Hypocalcemia is highly prevalent in hospitalized patients (10% to 18%) and particularly common in the intensive care unit (ICU) (70% to 80%).[135,136]

Clinical Manifestations

Acute hypocalcemia can result in severe clinical symptoms that need rapid correction, whereas chronic hypocalcemia may be a laboratory finding in asymptomatic patients. The clinical features of hypocalcemia are summarized in Table 18-4. Their presentation reflects both the absolute calcium concentration and the rapidity of its fall. The threshold for overt symptoms depends also on serum pH, and the severity of any concurrent hypomagnesemia, hyponatremia, or hypokalemia.

The classical symptoms of hypocalcemia are neuromuscular excitability in the form of numbness, circumoral tingling, the reported sensation of "pins and needles" in the feet and hands, muscle cramps, carpopedal spasm, laryngeal stridor, or frank tetany. Tapping over the facial nerve anterior to the ear can induce facial muscle spasm (Chvostek's sign). However, Chvostek's sign may occur in 10% of normal people and was absent in 29% of patients with mild hypocalcemia. Trousseau's sign of *main d' accoucheur*, elicited by inflation of a sphygmomanometer cuff placed on the upper arm to 10 mm Hg above systolic blood pressure for 3 minutes, has greater than 90% sensitivity and specificity.[137]

Patients with hypocalcemia may experience emotional disturbances, irritability, impairment of memory, confusion, delusion, hallucination, paranoia, and depression. Epileptic, often Jacksonian, seizures may occur but are usually not associated with aura, loss of consciousness, and incontinence. Patients with chronic hypocalcemia, including those with idiopathic and postsurgical hypoparathyroidism and those with pseudohypoparathyroidism, may have papilledema, elevated cerebrospinal fluid pressure, and neurologic signs simulating a cerebral tumor. Bilateral cataracts affecting the anterior and posterior subcapsular areas of the cortical portions of the lens may develop after 1 year of hypocalcemia. The cataracts do not resolve after correction of the hypocalcemia.

In patients with idiopathic hypoparathyroidism, the skin may be dry and scaly, eczema and psoriasis may worsen, and moniliasis can occur. The eyelashes and eyebrows may be scanty, and axillary and pubic hair may be absent. Because some forms of this disease have an autoimmune etiology, manifestations of other autoimmune diseases such as adrenal, thyroid, and gonadal insufficiency; diabetes mellitus; pernicious anemia; vitiligo; and alopecia areata may be present and should be sought.

Long-lasting hypocalcemia in children and adults can cause congestive heart failure due to cardiomyopathy, which is reversible with correction of the calcium disorder.[138-140] Prolongation of the QTc on the ECG is a well-known effect of hypocalcemia on heart conduction. Hypoparathyroidism in children often causes tooth abnormalities such as defective enamel and root formation, dental hypoplasia, or failure of adult teeth to erupt. Severe skeletal mineralization may occur in the fetus of untreated pregnant women with hypoparathyroidism and hypocalcemia.

Laboratory Findings

The alterations in the levels of serum PTH and serum and urinary electrolytes in various hypocalcemic states depend on the mechanisms responsible for the hypocalcemia (see Figure 18-2), and knowledge of these changes aids in the differential diagnosis of these disorders. X-ray examination of the skull or computed axial tomographic scanning of the brain may reveal intracranial calcifications, especially of the basal ganglia.[141] These have been noted in up to 20% of hypocalcemic patients with idiopathic hypoparathyroidism but are less common in postsurgical hypoparathyroidism unless the disease is long-standing. Such calcifications are also encountered in patients with pseudohypoparathyroidism. Bone disease may be observed, but the specific findings differ for the various causes of hypocalcemia (see later).

Diagnosis

The most common causes of hypocalcemia in the nonacute setting are hypoparathyroidism, hypomagnesemia, renal failure, and vitamin D deficiencies (Table 18-5). These entities should be considered early in the diagnosis of hypocalcemic individuals. It is conceptually and clinically useful to subclassify hypocalcemic individuals into those with elevated PTH levels and those with either subnormal or inappropriately normal PTH concentrations, as in primary hypoparathyroidism. A thorough medical history and physical examination are diagnostically important, because hypocalcemia can be caused by postsurgical, pharmacologic, inherited, developmental, and nutritional problems, in addition to being part of complex syndromes.

Causes

The causes of hypocalcemia are summarized in Table 18-5. They can be broadly classified into three categories: PTH related (hypoparathyroidism and pseudohypoparathyroidism), vitamin D related (low production and vitamin D resistance), and miscellaneous.

TABLE 18-5 Causes of Hypocalcemia

Inherited and genetic syndromes with hypoparathyroidism
  PTH gene mutations/isolated congenital hypoparathyroidism
  Autosomal dominant hypoparathyroidism with activating mutation of the CaSR (MIM 146200)
  DiGeorge syndrome (MIM 188400)
  Other forms of familial hypoparathyroidism
Inherited and genetic syndromes with resistance to PTH action
  Pseudohypoparathyroidism, types 1a, 1b, and 2
  Hypomagnesemic syndromes
Acquired hypoparathyroidism/inadequate PTH production
  Damage or destruction of the parathyroid glands
    Postsurgical
    Autoimmune: isolated or with multiple endocrine dysfunction
      Acquired antibodies against CaSR
      Polyglandular failure syndrome type 1 (MIM 240300 and 607358)
    Irradiation
    Metastatic and infiltrative diseases
    Deposition of heavy metals: iron overload, copper overload
  Reversible impairment of PTH secretion
    Severe hypomagnesemia
    Hypermagnesemia
Inadequate vitamin D production
  Vitamin d deficiency: nutritional, lack of sunlight exposure
  Malabsorption
  End-stage liver disease and cirrhosis
  Chronic kidney disease
Vitamin D resistance
  Pseudo–vitamin D deficiency rickets (vitamin D–dependent rickets type 1)
  Vitamin D–resistant rickets (vitamin D–dependent rickets type 2)
Miscellaneous causes
  Hyperphosphatemia
  Phosphate retention caused by acute or chronic renal failure
  Excess phosphate absorption caused by enemas, oral supplements
  Massive phosphate release caused by tumor lysis or crush injury
Drugs
  Foscarnet
  Bisphosphonates (especially in patients with vitamin D deficiency)
Rapid transfusion of large volumes of citrate-containing blood
Acute critical illness (multiple contributing causes)
Hungry bone syndrome/recalcification tetany
  After thyroidectomy for Graves' disease
  After parathyroidectomy
Osteoblastic metastases
Acute pancreatitis
Rhabdomyolysis
Substances interfering with the laboratory assay for total Ca^{2+}
  Gadolinium salts in contrast agents given during magnetic resonance imaging or magnetic resonance angiography

CaSR, Calcium-sensing receptor; *MIM*, Mendelian Inheritance in Man; *PTH*, parathyroid hormone.

PARATHYROID HORMONE–RELATED DISORDERS: HYPOPARATHYROIDISM AND PSEUDOHYPOPARATHYROIDISM

The PTH-related disorders presents with hypocalcemia and hyperphosphatemia due to failure of the parathyroid gland to secrete adequate amounts of biologically active PTH or resistance to PTH action at the tissue level. Both entities can be either inherited or acquired. The levels of PTH are low or absent in hypoparathyroidism due to lack of PTH production, but elevated in pseudohypoparathyroidism due to secondary or adaptive increase in PTH secretion. The fractional calcium excretion is elevated in hypoparathyroidism and low in pseudohypoparathyroidism. Skeletal response in both categories of disorders is appropriate to the levels of circulating PTH, with low bone turnover in hypoparathyroidism and excessive bone remodeling in pseudohypoparathyroidism.[142,143]

			TABLE 18-6 Genetic Syndromes Associated with Hypoparathyroidism			
SYNDROME	OTHER CLINICAL FEATURES	PROCESS AFFECTED	MODE OF INHERITANCE	GENE MUTATED	SYNDROME MIM NO.	REFERENCE
Familial isolated hypoparathyroidism	None	Parathyroid gland development	AR	GCM2	146200	412
			X-linked	SOX3?	307700	413
		PTH gene mutation affecting its synthesis	AR	Prepro-PTH splice site		414
			AD	Prepro-PTH signal peptide		415
Autosomal dominant hypoparathyroidism	Hypocalcemia, hypomagnesemia, hypercalciuria	Calcium sensing	AD	CaSR	146200 601298	145
DiGeorge's/CATCH 22 syndrome	Cardiac anomalies, abnormal facies, thymic aplasia, cleft palate	Defective third and fourth branchial pouch development	Sporadic or AD	Chromosome band 22q11 deletions (including TBX1)	188400	416
HDR	Hypoparathyroid, deafness, renal anomalies	Parathyroid development	AD	GATA3 transcription factor	146255	417
Kenny-Caffey/ Sanjad-Sakati	Microcephaly, mental retardation, growth failure ± osteosclerosis		AR	TBCE (chaperone for tubulin folding)	241410 244460	418
Polyglandular failure syndrome type 1/autoimmune polyendocrinopathy– candidiasis– ectodermal dystrophy (APECED)	Chronic mucocutaneous candidiasis, Addison's disease	Immune tolerance	AR	AIRE (autoimmune transcriptional regulator)	240300	419

AD, Autosomal dominant; *AR*, autosomal recessive; *CaSR*, calcium-sensing receptor; *MIM*, Mendelian Inheritance in Man; *PTH*, parathyroid hormone.

Hypoparathyroidism is a rare disorder. One study in Japan found the prevalence to be 7.2 per million people.[144]

Genetic Causes of Hypoparathyroidism. At least four different mutations affecting either the PTH gene or genes involved in parathyroid development have been identified as a cause of familial isolated hypoparathyroidism (Table 18-6). All of these conditions present during the neonatal period with severe hypocalcemia without any other organ involvement and respond well to therapy with vitamin D analogs. Heterozygous gain-of-function mutations in the CaSR gene can activate CaSR or cause CaSR to be hyperresponsive to extracellular calcium.[145] The phenotype seen is essentially the opposite of FHH and has been termed *autosomal dominant hypoparathyroidism*. Patients have mild hypocalcemia, hypomagnesemia, and hypercalciuria, with low or inappropriately normal PTH levels. The set point for PTH secretion is shifted to the left.

Treatment with calcium supplements and vitamin D is warranted only for patients with severe symptomatic hypocalcemia. The goal should be to increase calcium level to render the patient asymptomatic, not necessarily to achieve a normal calcium level. Renal calcium excretion requires monitoring, because these patients may develop frank hypercalciuria and nephrocalcinosis.[146,147] Thiazide diuretics or injectable PTH can be used to decrease calciuria at any given level of serum calcium concentration.[148]

A number of rare congenital syndromes with multiple developmental abnormalities can also be associated with familial hypoparathyroidism, including DiGeorge syndrome, HDR syndrome (*h*ypoparathyroidism, sensorineural *d*eafness, and *r*enal anomalies), polyglandular failure syndrome

type 1 (presented most frequently APECED [(*a*utoimmune *p*olyendocrinopathy–*c*andidiasis–*e*ctodermal *d*ystrophy]), and mitochondrial disorders (see Table 18-6).

Genetic Syndromes with Resistance to Parathyroid Hormone Action. Individuals with pseudohypoparathyroidism are hypocalcemic and hyperphosphatemic but have elevated PTH levels. This condition, reported in 1942 by Albright, was the first described example of a hormone-resistance disease.[149] The patients exhibited a pattern of features of Albright's hereditary osteodystrophy that included short stature, round face, mental retardation, brachydactyly, and the lack of a phosphaturic response to parathyroid extract.

Pseudohypoparathyroidism is now recognized as a heterogeneous group of related disorders.[150,151] It may be inherited or sporadic. Pseudohypoparathyroidism is subdivided into two types depending on the renal tubular response to infused exogenous PTH. Pseudohypoparathyroidism type 1 (PHP-1) refers to complete resistance to the effects of PTH, as demonstrated by the absence of an increase serum calcium, urinary cAMP, and phosphate levels in response to PTH infusion in these patients.[152,153] The category of PHP-1 is subdivided into PHP-1a, with Albright's hereditary osteodystrophy, and PHP-1b, without Albright's hereditary osteodystrophy. The presence of Albright's hereditary osteodystrophy without hypocalcemia and endocrine dysfunction is called *pseudo-pseudohypoparathyroidism*.

PHP-1a and pseudo-pseudohypoparathyroidism result from loss-of-function mutations of the GNAS1 gene, which encodes the stimulatory G protein α-subunit (Gα$_s$) that couples the type 1 PTH receptor to the adenyl cyclase pathway.[154] Patients with GNAS1 gene mutation also have resistance to thyroid-stimulating hormone, gonadotropins, glucagons, calcitonin, and gonadotropin-releasing hormone because the same $G\alpha_s$ pathway is used by these hormones.

Promoter-specific and parent-of-origin allelic patterns of genomic imprinting of GNAS1 have been established and provide the probable explanation for the complex phenotypic expression of the dominantly inherited genetic defect. Maternal transmission of the mutation causes PHP-1a; paternal transmission leads to pseudo-pseudohypoparathyroidism.[155] PHP-1b appears to be due to mutations that affect the regulatory elements of GNAS1 mainly in the proximal tubules.[156,157] Patients with PHP-1c exhibit the features of PHP-1, but without defective $G\alpha_s$ activity.

PHP-2 is a heterogeneous group of disorders characterized by a reduced phosphaturic response to PTH but a normal increase in urinary cAMP.[158] The cause is unclear but may involve a defect in the intracellular response to cAMP or some other component of the PTH signaling pathway. PHP-2 does not appear to follow a clear familial pattern.

Hypomagnesemic Syndromes. Impaired PTH secretion and inadequate PTH response to hypocalcemia are typically observed in hypomagnesemic patients. This is corrected by magnesium replacement. Congenital defects leading to hypomagnesemia and hypocalcemia are discussed in the section of this chapter on magnesium disorders and in Chapters 44 and 74.

Acquired Hypoparathyroidism and Inadequate Parathyroid Hormone Production

Postsurgical Causes. The most common cause of acquired hypoparathyroidism in adults is surgical removal of or damage to the parathyroid glands. Transient hypocalcemia after thyroid surgery was observed in 2% to 23% of cases, whereas permanent hypocalcemia occurred in approximately 1% to 3% (0% to 5%).[159-161] Hypocalcemia was more likely to occur after total thyroidectomy for cancer, Graves' disease, radical neck dissection for other cancers, and repeated operations for parathyroid adenoma removal. Hypoparathyroidism may result from inadvertent removal of the parathyroids, damage from bleeding, or devascularization. Removal of a single hyperfunctioning parathyroid adenoma can result in transient hypocalcemia because of hypercalcemia-induced suppression of PTH secretion from the normal glands. Surgical experience and use of appropriate surgical technique may reduce the frequency of hypothyroidism.[161]

The "hungry bone" or recalcification syndrome represents an important cause of prolonged hypocalcemia after parathyroidectomy or thyroidectomy for any form of hyperparathyroidism or hyperthyroidism, respectively.[162] Postoperative withdrawal of PTH decreases osteoclastic bone resorption without affecting osteoblastic activity and leads to increased bone uptake of calcium, phosphate, and magnesium. Risk factors for the development of hungry bone syndrome include large parathyroid adenomas, age older than 60 years, and high preoperative levels of serum PTH, calcium, and alkaline phosphatase. There are reports that bisphosphonate therapy for Paget's disease and cinacalcet use for secondary hyperparathyroidism can also cause hungry bone syndrome.[163,164]

Nonsurgical Causes. Acquired hypoparathyroidism from nonsurgical causes is rare, except in autoimmune disorders and magnesium deficiency. Although metal overload diseases (hemochromatosis, Wilson's disease),[165,166] granulomatous diseases, miliary tuberculosis, amyloidosis, and neoplastic infiltrate are often mentioned as causes of hypoparathyroidism,

these entities are quite rare. Alcohol consumption has been reported to cause transient hypocalcemia.[167]

Magnesium Disorders. Both magnesium excess and magnesium deficiency can produce generally mild hypocalcemia and reversible hypoparathyroidism. Acute infusion of magnesium or hypermagnesemia inhibits PTH secretion.[168] Mg^{2+} is an extracellular CaSR agonist, although less potent than calcium. Hypermagnesemia when severe enough, as observed in patients with chronic renal failure or those receiving the short-term high doses of intravenous magnesium sulfate used in obstetrics, can activate the CaSR and inhibit PTH secretion.[169]

Hypomagnesemic patients typically have low or inappropriately normal PTH levels for the degree of hypocalcemia observed.[170] Moderate hypomagnesemia (serum magnesium levels of 0.8 to 1.0 mg/dL) primarily causes PTH resistance at the level of the target organ,[171] whereas severe hypomagnesemia also decreases PTH secretion.[172] The effect of chronic severe hypomagnesemia comes not from an extracellular effect on CaSR, but from intracellular magnesium depletion, which leads to G α-subunit activation, enhanced CaSR signalling, and hence blunted PTH secretion.[172] The appropriate therapy is magnesium replacement; in the absence of adequate magnesium replacement, the hypocalcemia is resistant to PTH or vitamin D therapy.

Autoimmune Disease. Autoimmune hypoparathyroidism can present either as an isolated finding or as a part of the APECED syndrome (also called *polyendocrinopathy type 1* and *autoimmune polyglandular syndrome type 1*). APECED can be sporadic or familial (see Table 18-6).[215] Autoantibodies against parathyroid tissue have been reported in a significant percentage of cases of hypoparathyroidism, but the causative role of these antibodies is unclear. The CaSR has been identified as a possible autoantigen in some cases of autoimmune hypoparathyroidism (either isolated or polyglandular).[217]

VITAMIN D–RELATED DISORDERS

Low Vitamin D Production. Both inherited and acquired disorders of vitamin D and its metabolites can be associated with hypocalcemia.[173] Vitamin D is a fat-soluble vitamin that is either produced in the skin under ultraviolet B radiation from 7-dehydrocholesterol or absorbed in the gastrointestinal tract from external sources. Vitamin D is present naturally in a few foods, is artificially added to others, and is available as a food supplement or drug.[174] Despite routine dietary supplementation in milk and other foods, vitamin D deficiency is common in a number of populations,[173,174] such as breast-feeding infants, older adults, people with dark skin and limited sun exposure, people with fat malabsorption,[175] and people who have undergone gastric bypass surgery.[176]

A study of hospitalized patients found a high prevalence of vitamin D deficiency, even in younger patients without risk factors who were consuming the recommended daily allowance of vitamin D_3.[177] Fat malabsorption syndromes, common in liver diseases, sprue, Whipple's disease, and Crohn's disease, may result in malabsorption of vitamin D.[178,179] Liver diseases may impair the hydroxylation of vitamin D to 25(OH)D (calcidiol), and drugs such as phenytoin and barbiturates stimulate the conversion of 25(OH)D to inactive metabolites.[180] Treatment of hepatic osteodystrophy with vitamin D and calcium is not fully effective.[181] Deficiency of 1α-hydroxylase, as observed in advanced CKD, leads to deficiency of $1,25(OH)_2D$

(calcitriol), the most important biologic form for maintaining calcium and phosphorus homeostasis. Vitamin D deficiency with hypocalcemia is commonly seen in patients with renal insufficiency (see Chapter 54). Patients with nephrotic syndrome may in addition have decreased 25(OH)D levels as a result of urinary loss, which leads to hypocalcemia, and secondary hyperparathyroidism.[182]

The level of 25(OH)D in the serum is the best indicator of vitamin D status. Levels of 1,25(OH)$_2$D do not decrease until vitamin D deficiency is severe. Prolonged vitamin D deficiency causes rickets (a disorder of mineralization of growing bone) in children and osteomalacia (a disorder of mineralization of formed bone) in adults. The combination of calcium deficiency and vitamin D deficiency accelerates skeletal abnormalities and hypocalcemia.

The diagnosis of vitamin D deficiency is confirmed by measurement of serum 25(OH)D levels. Hypocalcemia is usually observed only when vitamin D deficiency is severe (25[OH]D levels of <10 ng/mL) and when skeletal stores of calcium are depleted; otherwise the compensatory rise of PTH would be able to mobilize calcium from the bone.[173,174,183,184] The 24-hour urinary calcium excretion is low to very low. Hypophosphatemia, increased alkaline phosphatase levels, and normal levels of FGF-23 are typically seen with vitamin D deficiency.[173]

Vitamin D Resistance. The observation that some forms of rickets cannot be cured by regular doses of vitamin D led to the discovery of rare inherited abnormalities in vitamin D metabolism or the vitamin D receptor. Vitamin D–dependent rickets type 1 (VDDR-1) (MIM 26700) is characterized by autosomal recessive, childhood-onset rickets, hypocalcemia, secondary hyperparathyroidism, and aminoaciduria. The biochemical abnormality is defective 1α-hydroxylation of 25(OH)D, caused by mutations in the gene for the 25(OH)D–1α-hydroxylase.[185] Therapy with calcitriol or 1α-hydroxyvitamin D$_3$ (alphacalcidol) restores serum 1,25(OH)$_2$D levels and must be continued for life.

VDDR-2 (also called *hereditary vitamin D–resistant rickets*) is an autosomal recessive disorder (MIM 277440). Affected patients have extreme elevations in 1,25(OH)$_2$D levels, in addition to alopecia and the abnormalities seen in VDDR-1.[186] Biochemically, the disorder results from end-organ resistance to 1,25(OH)$_2$D. A number of different mutations have been found in the vitamin D receptor gene of affected individuals.[187] High-dose calcium intake and calcium infusion may be the only way to treat hypocalcemia and rickets in these children.

MISCELLANEOUS CAUSES

Medications. Medications are a relatively common cause of hypocalcemia, particularly in hospitalized patients.[188] Some of the gadolinium-based contrast agents (gadodiamide and gadoversetamide) used in magnetic resonance imaging studies cause pseudohypocalcemia by interfering with colorimetric assays for calcium. The calcium reading can be as low as 6 mg/dL but with no symptoms or signs of hypocalcemia.[188,189] Drug-induced hypomagnesemia (cisplatinum, aminoglycoside, amphotericin B, diuretics) and hypermagnesemia (magnesium sulfate infusion, magnesium-containing antacids) can cause hypocalcemia. Inhibitors of bone resorption (bisphosphonates, calcimimetics, mithramycin, and calcitonin) may depress serum calcium to subnormal levels.[188] Proton pump inhibitors and histamine 2 antagonists may reduce calcium

absorption and/or inhibit bone resorption and provoke hypocalcemia.[190] Citrate administration during transfusion of citrated blood or plasmapheresis may cause hypocalcemia. Transfusions of citrated blood rarely cause significant hypocalcemia, but it may occur in the course of massive transfusion.[191] Similarly, significant hypocalcemia occurs after plasmapheresis.[192] Foscarnet (trisodium phosphoformate) can cause hypocalcemia through the chelation of extracellular calcium ions, so that normal total calcium measurements may not reflect ionized hypocalcemia.[193] As stated previously, anticonvulsants, particularly phenytoin and phenobarbital, appear to interfere with vitamin D metabolism. Fluoride overdose is an exceedingly rare cause of hypocalcemia. Oral sodium phosphate–induced hyperphosphatemia may cause hypocalcemia, particularly in patients with renal failure.[188,194] Other drugs associated with hypocalcemia include antiinfectious agents (pentamidine, ketoconazole) and chemotherapeutic agents (asparaginase, cisplatin, doxorubicin).

Critical Illness. In patients with complicated, critical illnesses, total calcium measurements may be poor indicators of the ionized Ca^{2+} concentration because a large number of factors that may interfere with or alter calcium-protein binding may be present (albumin infusion, citrate administration, administration of intravenous fluids, acid-base disturbances, dialysis therapy). Thus, it is particularly important to measure ionized Ca^{2+} in this setting. Hypocalcemia is frequently noted in both gram-negative sepsis and toxic shock syndrome.[136,195] This entity is multifactorial; the primary cause is unclear, but a direct effect of interleukin-1 on parathyroid function may be partly responsible.[196]

Other Causes. Hypocalcemia is common in acute pancreatitis and is a poor prognostic indicator.[197] It is probably due to calcium chelation by free fatty acids generated by the action of pancreatic lipase. Massive tumor lysis, particularly from rapidly growing hematologic malignancies, may cause hyperphosphatemia, hyperuricemia, and hypocalcemia.[198] The early phase of rhabdomyolysis may include severe hyperphosphatemia and associated hypocalcemia; in contrast, hypercalcemia is common in the recovery phase. In hemodialysis patients, hypocalcemia is common and may result at least in part from reduced renal phosphate clearance and consequent hyperphosphatemia and reduced 1,25(OH)$_2$D production (see Chapter 54).

Treatment

The optimal management of hypocalcemia has not been examined in clinical trials, but accepted practices exist. The treatment depends on the speed of onset and the severity of clinical and laboratory features. Oral calcium supplementation may be sufficient treatment for mild hypocalcemia. Patients with acute, severe (Ca concentration of <7.0 to 7.5 mg/dL, ionized Ca^{2+} concentration of <0.8 mmol/L), symptomatic hypocalcemia, such as after parathyroidectomy, and with evidence of neuromuscular effects or tetany should be treated promptly with intravenous calcium. The preferred calcium salt is calcium gluconate (10 mL of 10% calcium gluconate contains 93 mg of elemental calcium). Initially, 1 to 2 g (93 to 186 mg of elemental calcium) of intravenous calcium gluconate in 50 mL of 5% dextrose is given over a period of 10 to 20 minutes, followed by slow infusion at a rate of 0.3 to 1.0 mg of elemental calcium per kilogram per hour.[171] The dose can be adjusted to maintain the serum calcium concentration at the lower end of normal values. The infusion solution should not contain phosphates or bicarbonates. Intravenous infusion may be needed until the patient's condition is stabilized and oral calcium and calcitriol therapy start working. Correction of hypomagnesemia and hyperphosphatemia should also be undertaken when present. Dialysis may be appropriate if hyperphosphatemia is also present.

Treatment of chronic hypocalcemia depends on the underlying cause. For instance, underlying hypomagnesemia or vitamin D deficiency should be corrected. The principal therapy for primary parathyroid dysfunction or PTH resistance is dietary calcium supplementation and vitamin D therapy. Oral calcium supplementation, beginning with 500 to 1000 mg of elemental calcium daily and increasing up to a maximum of 2000 mg daily, is a good strategy. Correction of serum calcium concentration to the low-normal range is generally advised; correction to normal levels may lead to frank hypercalciuria. Several preparations of vitamin D are available for the treatment of hypocalcemia. The role of vitamin D therapy in chronic kidney diseases is discussed separately.

Disorders of Magnesium Homeostasis

Hypomagnesemia and Magnesium Deficiency

The terms *hypomagnesemia* and *magnesium deficiency* tend to be used interchangeably. However, there is a complex relationship between total body Mg stores, serum Mg concentrations, and the Mg level in different intracellular compartments. Because ECF Mg accounts for only 1% of total body Mg, it is hardly surprising that serum Mg concentrations have been found to correlate poorly with overall Mg status. Indeed, in patients with Mg deficiency, serum Mg concentrations may be normal or may seriously underestimate the severity of the Mg deficit.[199] Approximately 50% to 60% of Mg is in the skeleton, of which two thirds is within the hydration shell and one third on the crystal surface,[200] and this may serve as a reservoir for maintaining extracellular and intracellular Mg. Except for 1% in the ECF, the rest is intracellular, and significant amounts of Mg are found in the nucleus, the mitochondria, the endoplasmic/sarcoplasmic reticulum, and the cytoplasm. The majority of Mg is bound to adenosine triphosphate (ATP). No satisfactory clinical test to assay body Mg stores is available.[201]

The Mg tolerance test is generally thought to be the best test of overall Mg status.[201] It is based on the observation that Mg-deficient patients tend to retain a greater proportion of a parenterally administered Mg load and excrete less in the urine than normal individuals do.[202] Clinical studies indicate that the results of an Mg tolerance test correlate well with Mg status as assessed by skeletal muscle Mg content and exchangeable Mg pools. However, test results are invalid in patients who have impaired renal function or a renal Mg-wasting syndrome and in patients who are taking diuretics or other medications that induce renal Mg wasting. For this reason and also because of the time and effort required to perform the Mg^{2+} tolerance test, it is used primarily as a research tool.

The serum Mg concentration, although an insensitive measure of Mg deficit, remains the only practical test of Mg status in widespread use. Surveys of serum Mg levels in hospitalized patients indicate a high incidence of hypomagnesemia (presumably an underestimate of the true incidence of Mg deficiency), ranging from 11% in inpatients in general wards[203] to 60% in patients admitted to ICUs.[204,205] Furthermore, among ICU patients, those with hypomagnesemia had increased mortality compared with normomagnesemic patients.[204] The functionally important value is believed to be the ionized Mg^{2+} concentration, which is less than total serum Mg due to protein binding. Measurements with ion-selective electrodes have found ionized Mg^{2+} concentrations that are approximately 70% of the total serum Mg, a proportion that is fairly constant among the general population.[201] In critically ill patients, however, there is a poor correlation between total and ionized serum Mg levels.[205]

Causes

Mg deficiency may be caused by decreased intake or intestinal absorption; by increased losses via the gastrointestinal tract, kidneys, or skin; and, rarely, by sequestration in the bone compartment (Figure 18-3). When the cause cannot be determined simply from the history and physical examination, it is often helpful to distinguish between renal Mg^{2+} wasting and extrarenal causes of Mg deficiency by assessing urinary Mg excretion. In the setting of Mg deficiency, a urine Mg excretion rate greater than 24 mg/day is abnormal and usually suggestive of renal Mg wasting.[206] If a 24-hour urine collection is unavailable, the fractional excretion of Mg (FE_{Mg}) can be calculated from a random urine specimen as follows:

$$FE_{Mg} = \frac{\text{Urine Mg concentration} \times \text{Plasma creatinine concentration}}{0.7 \times \text{Plasma total Mg concentration} \times \text{Urine creatinine concentration}}$$

Note that a correction factor of 0.7 is applied to the plasma total Mg concentration to estimate the free Mg^{2+}. In general, an FE_{Mg} of more than 2% in an individual with normal GFR is indicative of inappropriate urinary Mg loss.[207] If renal Mg wasting has been excluded, the losses must be extrarenal in origin, and the underlying cause can usually be identified from the case history.

EXTRARENAL CAUSES

Nutritional Deficiency. Human Mg deprivation studies have demonstrated that induction of severe Mg deficiency by dietary means in normal individuals is surprisingly difficult, because nearly all foods contain significant amounts of Mg and renal adaptation to conserve Mg is very efficient. The 1994 U.S. Department of Agriculture Continuing Survey of Food Intakes by Individuals (CSFII) indicated that the mean daily intake was 323 mg in males and 228 mg in females. These values fall below the current recommended daily allowance of approximately 420 mg for males and 320 mg for females.[208] It has been suggested that 75% of individuals in the United States have dietary Mg intake that is below the recommended level. Therefore, Mg deficiency of nutritional origin can be observed, particularly in two clinical settings: alcoholism and parenteral feeding.

In individuals with chronic alcoholism, the intake of ethanol substitutes for the intake of important nutrients.[209]

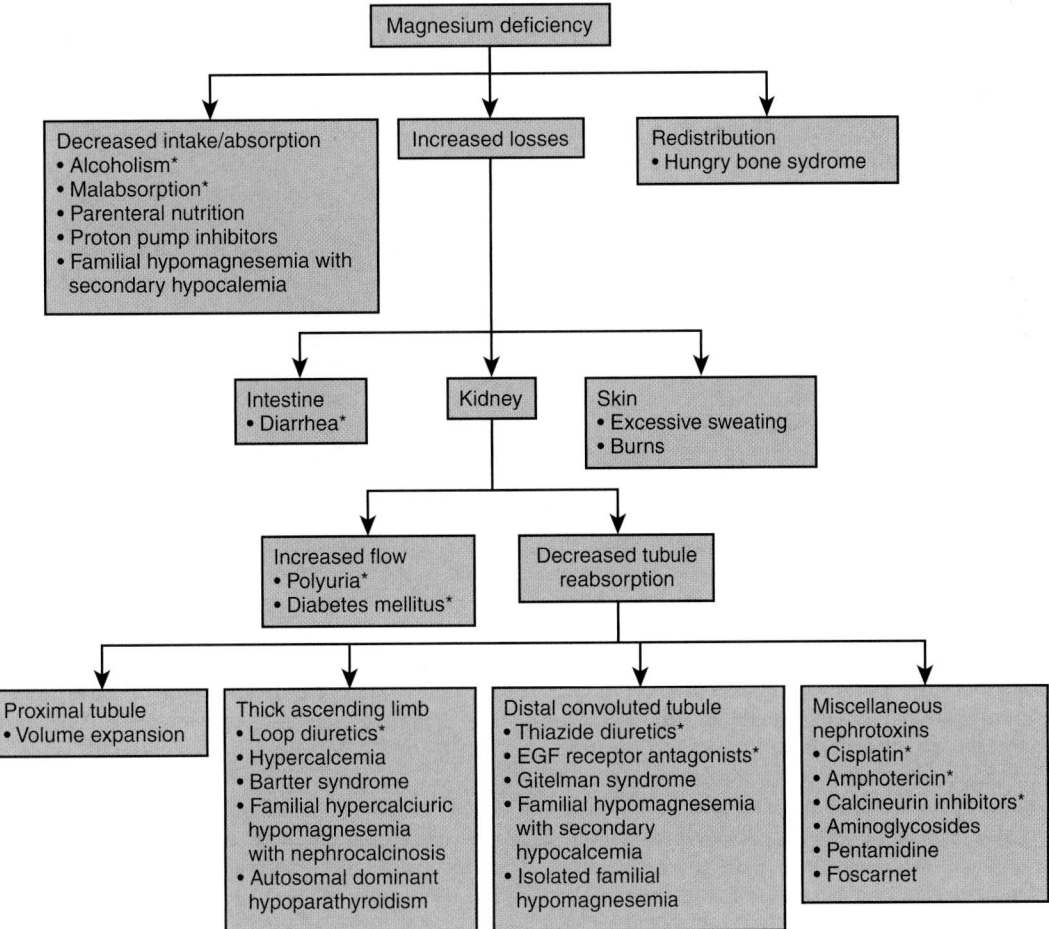

FIGURE 18-3 Etiology of magnesium deficiency. *Common causes.

Approximately 20% to 25% of alcoholic patients are frankly hypomagnesemic, and most can be shown to be Mg deficient using the Mg tolerance test.[202] Of note, some evidence suggests that alcohol also may impair renal Mg conservation.[210]

Patients receiving parenteral nutrition may develop hypomagnesemia.[211] In general, these patients are sicker than the average inpatient and are more likely to have other conditions associated with an Mg deficit and ongoing Mg losses. Hypomagnesemia may also occur as a part of the refeeding syndrome.[212] In this condition, overzealous parenteral feeding of severely malnourished patients causes hyperinsulinemia, as well as rapid cellular uptake of glucose and water, together with phosphorus, potassium, and Mg.

Intestinal Malabsorption. Generalized malabsorption syndromes caused by conditions such as celiac disease, Whipple's disease, and inflammatory bowel disease are frequently associated with intestinal Mg wasting and Mg deficiency.[213] In fat malabsorption with concomitant steatorrhea, free fatty acids in the intestinal lumen may combine with Mg to form nonabsorbable soaps, a process known as *saponification*, which contributes to impaired Mg absorption. Indeed, the severity of hypomagnesemia in patients with malabsorption syndrome correlates with the fecal fat excretion rate, and in rare patients, reduction of dietary fat intake alone, which reduces steatorrhea, can correct the hypomagnesemia. Previous intestinal resection, particularly of the distal part of the small intestine,

is also an important cause of Mg malabsorption[214] and a confounding factor in many studies of patients with Crohn's disease. Mg deficiency was a common complication of bariatric surgery by jejunoileal bypass,[215] but fortunately does not occur with gastric bypass.[216]

Recently, proton pump inhibitors have been reported to cause hypomagnesemia in some patients.[217] The evidence suggests that it is due to intestinal Mg malabsorption. A rare mutation of the TRPM6 (transient receptor potential cation channel, subfamily M, member 6) Mg transport channel can also lead to intestinal Mg^{2+} malabsorption along with renal Mg wasting, causing hypomagnesemia with secondary hypocalcemia.[218]

Diarrhea and Gastrointestinal Fistula. The Mg concentration of diarrheal fluid is high and ranges from 1 to 16 mg/dL,[214] so Mg deficiency may occur in patients with chronic diarrhea of any cause, even in the absence of concomitant malabsorption,[199] and in patients who abuse laxatives. By contrast, secretions from the upper gastrointestinal tract are low in Mg content, and significant Mg deficiency is therefore rarely observed in patients with an intestinal, biliary, or pancreatic fistula; ileostomy; or prolonged gastric drainage (except as a consequence of malnutrition).[214]

Cutaneous Losses. Hypomagnesemia may be observed after prolonged intense exertion. For example, serum Mg concentrations fall 20% on average after a marathon run.[219] About a quarter of the decrement in serum Mg can be accounted for by losses in sweat, which can contain up to 0.5 mg/dL of Mg, with the remainder most likely due to transient redistribution into the intracellular space. Mg supplementation may be indicated for those participating in a number of sports, especially if the athlete is consuming a diet with a suboptimal Mg level.[220] Hypomagnesemia occurs in 40% of patients with severe burn injuries during the early period of recovery. The major cause is loss of Mg in the cutaneous exudate, which can exceed 1 g/day.[221]

Redistribution to Bone Compartment. Hypomagnesemia may occasionally accompany the profound hypocalcemia of hungry bone syndrome observed in some patients with hyperparathyroidism and severe bone disease immediately after parathyroidectomy.[222] In such cases, a high bone turnover state exists, and sudden removal of excess PTH is believed to result in virtual cessation of bone resorption, with a continued high rate of bone formation and consequent sequestration of both Ca and Mg in bone mineral.

Diabetes Mellitus. Hypomagnesemia is common in patients with diabetes mellitus and has been reported to occur in 13.5% to 47.7% of nonhospitalized patients with type 2 diabetes.[223] The cause is thought to be multifactorial, with contributing factors that include decreased oral intake of Mg-rich foods, poor intestinal absorption due to diabetic autonomic neuropathy, and increased renal excretion. The latter could in turn be caused by glomerular hyperfiltration, osmotic diuresis, or decreased TAL and distal tubule Mg reabsorption due to functional insulin deficiency.[224,225] In addition, some studies have suggested that Mg deficiency might itself impair glucose tolerance, which would partly explain the association. A recent study suggested that genetic variants in the Mg transport channels TRPM6 and TRPM7 may increase the risk of type 2 diabetes mellitus in women consuming a diet containing less than 250 mg/day of Mg.[226]

RENAL MAGNESIUM WASTING

The diagnosis of renal Mg wasting is made by demonstrating an inappropriately high rate of renal Mg excretion in the face of hypomagnesemia, as described earlier. The causes are summarized in Figure 18-3.

Polyuria. Not surprisingly, increased urine output from any cause is often accompanied by increased renal losses of Mg. Renal Mg wasting occurs with osmotic diuresis, as in the severe hyperglycemic state of diabetic ketoacidosis.[227,228] Hypermagnesuria also occurs during the polyuric phase of recovery from acute renal failure in a native kidney, during recovery from ischemic injury in a transplanted kidney, and in postobstructive diuresis. In such cases, it is likely that residual tubule reabsorptive defects persisting from the primary renal injury play as important a role as polyuria itself in inducing renal Mg wasting.[229]

Extracellular Fluid Volume Expansion. In the proximal tubule, Mg reabsorption is passive and is driven by the reabsorption of sodium and water in this segment. Extracellular volume expansion, which decreases proximal sodium and water reabsorption, also increases urinary Mg excretion. Thus, long-term therapy with Mg-free parenteral fluids, either crystalloid or hyperalimentary,[230] can cause renal Mg wasting, as can hyperaldosteronism.[231]

Diuretics. Loop diuretics inhibit the apical membrane NaK2Cl cotransporter of the TAL and abolish the transepithelial potential difference, thereby inhibiting paracellular

Mg reabsorption. Hypomagnesemia is thus a frequent finding in patients receiving long-term loop diuretic therapy.[232] Long-term treatment with thiazide diuretics, which inhibit the NaCl cotransporter (NCC), also cause renal Mg wasting. Thiazide diuretics or knockout of NCC in mice causes downregulation of expression of TRPM6, the apical Mg entry channel in the distal convoluted tubule (DCT), which may explain the mechanism of the magnesuria.[233]

Epidermal Growth Factor Receptor Blockers. Hypomagnesemia is common in patients receiving cetuximab[234] and panitumumab,[235] monoclonal antibodies that block the epidermal growth factor (EGF) receptor, which are used in the treatment of metastatic colorectal cancer. The incidence of hypomagnesemia increases with the length of therapy, reaching almost 50% in patients treated for longer than 6 months.[236] The median time to onset of hypomagnesemia after beginning treatment is 99 days, and it generally reverses 1 to 3 months after discontinuance of therapy.[237] FE_{Mg} is inappropriately elevated, which suggests a defect in renal Mg reabsorption.[238]

Recent studies suggest that the EGF receptor is located basolaterally in the DCT.[238] Autocrine or paracrine activation of the receptor stimulates redistribution of TRPM6 to the apical membrane via a Rac1 (Ras-related C3 botulinum toxin substrate 1)–dependent signalling pathway[239] and presumably increases transepithelial Mg reabsorption. Thus EGF receptor blockade likely causes renal Mg wasting by antagonizing this pathway.

Hypercalcemia. Elevated serum ionized Ca^{2+} levels, for example in patients with malignant bone metastases, directly induce renal Mg wasting and hypomagnesemia,[240] probably by stimulating the basolateral calcium-sensing receptor in the TAL of the loop of Henle. In hyperparathyroidism, the situation is more complicated, because the hypercalcemia-induced tendency to Mg wasting is counteracted by the action of PTH in stimulating Mg reabsorption; therefore, renal Mg handling is usually normal and Mg deficiency is rare.[241]

Tubule Nephrotoxins. Cisplatin, a widely used chemotherapeutic agent for solid tumors, frequently causes renal Mg wasting. Hypomagnesemia is almost universal at a monthly dose of 50 mg/m^2.[242] The occurrence of Mg wasting does not appear to correlate with the incidence of cisplatin-induced acute renal failure.[243] Renal magnesuria continues after cessation of the drug for a mean of 4 to 5 months, but it can persist for years.[243] Although the nephrotoxic effects of cisplatin are manifested histologically as acute tubular necrosis confined to the S3 segment of proximal tubule, the magnesuria does not correlate temporally with the clinical development of acute renal failure secondary to acute tubular necrosis. Furthermore, patients who become hypomagnesemic are also subject to the development of hypocalciuria, which suggests that the reabsorption defect may actually be in the DCT. More recent data, however, suggest that the principal effect of cisplatin may be impairment of intestinal Mg absorption.[244] Carboplatin, an analog of cisplatin, is considerably less nephrotoxic and rarely causes either acute renal failure or hypomagnesemia.[245]

Amphotericin B is a well-recognized tubule nephrotoxin that can cause renal K wasting, distal renal tubular acidosis, and acute renal failure, with tubule necrosis and Ca deposition noted in the DCT and TAL on renal biopsy specimens.[246] Amphotericin B causes renal Mg wasting and hypomagnesemia that is related to the cumulative dose administered, but these effects may be observed after as little as a 200-mg total dose.[247] Interestingly, the amphotericin B–induced magnesuria is accompanied by the reciprocal development of hypocalciuria; thus, as with cisplatin, the serum Ca concentration is usually preserved, which again suggests that the functional tubule defect resides in the DCT.

Aminoglycosides cause a syndrome of renal Mg and K wasting with hypomagnesemia, hypokalemia, hypocalcemia, and tetany. Hypomagnesemia may occur despite levels in the appropriate therapeutic range.[248] In most patients reported to develop hypomagnesemia onset was delayed, occurring after at least 2 weeks of therapy, and these patients received total doses in excess of 8 g, which suggests that it is the cumulative dose of aminoglycoside that is the key predictor of toxicity. In addition, no correlation has been found between the occurrence of aminoglycoside-induced acute tubular necrosis and hypomagnesemia. Mg wasting persists after cessation of the aminoglycoside, often for several months. All aminoglycosides in clinical use have been implicated, including gentamicin, tobramycin, and amikacin, as well as neomycin when administered topically for extensive burn injuries. Symptomatic aminoglycoside-induced renal Mg wasting is now relatively uncommon because of heightened general awareness of the toxicity of these drugs. However, asymptomatic hypomagnesemia can be observed in a third of individuals treated with a single course of an aminoglycoside at standard dosages (3 to 5 mg/kg/day for a mean of 10 days). In these cases, the hypomagnesemia occurs on average 3 to 4 days after the start of therapy and readily reverses after cessation of therapy.[249]

Intravenous administration of pentamidine causes hypomagnesemia as a result of renal Mg wasting in most patients, typically in association with hypocalcemia.[250] The average onset of symptomatic hypomagnesemia is after 9 days of therapy, and the defect persists for at least 1 to 2 months after discontinuation of pentamidine.

Hypomagnesemia is also observed in two thirds of acquired immunodeficiency syndrome (AIDS) patients with cytomegalovirus retinitis treated intravenously with the pyrophosphate analog foscarnet.[251] As with aminoglycosides and pentamidine, foscarnet-induced hypomagnesemia is often associated with significant hypocalcemia.

The calcineurin inhibitors cyclosporine and tacrolimus cause renal Mg wasting and hypomagnesemia in patients after organ transplantation.[252] The mechanism is thought to be downregulation of the distal tubule Mg channel TRPM6.[253]

Tubulointerstitial Nephropathies. Renal Mg wasting has occasionally been reported in patients with acute or chronic tubulointerstitial nephritis not caused by nephrotoxic drugs; for example, in chronic pyelonephritis and acute renal allograft rejection. Other manifestations of tubule dysfunction, such as salt wasting, hypokalemia, renal tubular acidosis, and Fanconi's syndrome, also may be present and provide clues to the diagnosis.[229]

Inherited Renal Magnesium-Wasting Disorders

Primary Magnesium-Wasting Disorders. Primary Mg-wasting disorders are rare. These can be broadly classified into distinct clinical syndromes depending on whether the hypomagnesemia is isolated, occurs together with hypocalcemia, or is associated with hypercalciuria and nephrocalcinosis.[254] The pathogenesis and clinical features of these syndromes, which generally present in childhood, are discussed in detail in Chapter 74.

Bartter's and Gitelman's Syndromes (see also Chapter 44). Bartter's syndrome is an autosomal recessive disorder characterized by sodium wasting, hypokalemic metabolic alkalosis, and hypercalciuria, and it usually occurs in infancy or early childhood.[255] All patients with Bartter's syndrome are by definition hypercalciuric; in addition, a third have hypomagnesemia with inappropriate magnesuria, consistent with loss of the TAL transepithelial potential difference that drives paracellular divalent cation reabsorption. Thus, the physiology of Bartter's syndrome is essentially identical to that of long-term loop diuretic therapy.

Gitelman's syndrome is a variant of Bartter's syndrome that is distinguished primarily by hypocalciuria.[256] Patients with Gitelman's syndrome are identified later in life, usually after the age of 6 years, and have milder symptoms. The genetic defect in these families is caused by inactivating mutations in the DCT electroneutral thiazide-sensitive NaCl cotransporter NCC, and therefore resembles the effects of long-term thiazide diuretic therapy. Renal Mg wasting and hypomagnesemia are universally found in patients with Gitelman's syndrome.

Calcium-Sensing Disorders. In FHH, the hypercalcemia is due to inactivating mutations in CaSR (discussed earlier). As a consequence of the inactivated CaSR, the normal magnesuric response to hypercalcemia is impaired,[257] and thus patients with this disorder are paradoxically mildly hypermagnesemic. Activating mutations in CaSR cause the opposite syndrome, autosomal dominant hypoparathyroidism. As might be expected, most such patients are mildly hypomagnesemic, presumably because of TAL Mg wasting.[146]

Clinical Manifestations

Hypomagnesemia may cause symptoms and signs of disordered cardiac, neuromuscular, and central nervous system function. It is also associated with an imbalance of other electrolytes such as K and Ca. Many of the cardiac and neurologic manifestations attributed to Mg deficiency may be explained by the hypokalemia and hypocalcemia that frequently coexist in the same patient. Patients who have mild hypomagnesemia or who are Mg deficient with normal serum Mg levels may be completely asymptomatic.[258] Thus, the clinical importance of mild to moderate Mg depletion remains controversial, although it has been associated with a number of disorders such as hypertension and osteoporosis (see later).

CARDIOVASCULAR SYSTEM

Mg has protean and complex effects on myocardial ion fluxes, among which its effect on the sodium pump (Na-K-ATPase) is probably the most important. Because Mg is an obligate cofactor in all reactions that require ATP, it is essential for the activity of Na-K-ATPase.[259] During Mg deficiency, Na-K-ATPase function is impaired. The intracellular K concentration falls, which may potentially result in a relatively depolarized resting membrane potential; thus the excitation threshold for activation of an action potential is more easily attainable, and this predisposes to ectopic excitation and tachyarrhythmias.[260] Furthermore, the magnitude of the outward K gradient is decreased, which reduces the driving force for the K efflux needed to terminate the cardiac action potential, and as a result, repolarization is delayed.

ECG changes may be observed with isolated hypomagnesemia and usually reflect abnormal cardiac repolarization, including bifid T waves and other nonspecific abnormalities in T-wave morphology, U waves, prolongation of the QT or QU interval, and, rarely, electrical alternation of the T or U wave.[261] Numerous anecdotal reports indicate that hypomagnesemia alone can predispose to cardiac tachyarrhythmias, particularly of ventricular origin, including torsades de pointes, monomorphic ventricular tachycardia, and ventricular fibrillation, which may be resistant to standard therapy and respond only to Mg replenishment.[261] Many of the patients described in these reports also had a prolonged QT interval, an abnormality that is known to predispose to torsades de pointes and may also increase the period of vulnerability to R-on-T phenomena. In the setting of exaggerated cardiac excitability, hypomagnesemia may be the trigger for other types of ventricular tachyarrhythmias.[261] In addition, hypomagnesemia facilitates the development of digoxin cardiotoxicity.[262] Because both cardiac glycosides and Mg depletion inhibit Na-K-ATPase, their additive effects on intracellular K depletion may account for their enhanced toxicity in combination.

The existence of occasional patients with clear hypomagnesemia–induced arrhythmias is undisputed. The issue of whether mild hypomagnesemia and Mg depletion carry the same risk as severe hypomagnesemia does, and the relative importance of Mg deficiency versus coexistent hypokalemia or intrinsic cardiac disease in the pathogenesis of the arrhythmia, remain highly controversial.[263] Data on Mg deficiency and arrhythmia in individuals without overt heart disease is provocative. In one small prospective study, low dietary Mg level appeared to increase the risk for supraventricular and ventricular ectopy despite the absence of frank hypomagnesemia, hypokalemia, and hypocalcemia.[264] In the Framingham Offspring Study, lower levels of serum Mg were associated with higher prevalence of ventricular premature complexes.[265]

The role of Mg deficiency and the clinical utility of adjunctive Mg therapy has been studied extensively in acute myocardial infarction (AMI), which is the leading cause of death in the United States. Mg deficiency may be a risk factor, because it has been shown to play a role in systemic and coronary vascular tone, as well as in cardiac dysrhythmias as mentioned earlier, and it also inhibits steps in the coagulation process and platelet aggregation.

Although several small controlled trials suggested that adjunctive Mg therapy reduced mortality from AMI by 50%, three major trials define our understanding regarding Mg therapy in AMI.[268] The Second Leicester Intravenous Magnesium Intervention Trial (LIMIT-2) was the first study involving large numbers of participants.[266] Mg treatment was associated with an approximately 25% lower mortality rate. In the Fourth International Study of Infarct, unlike the LIMIT-2 study, however, the mortality rate in the Mg-treated group was not significantly different from that in the control group.[267] The most recently reported study, the Magnesium in Coronaries (MAGIC) Trial, was designed to investigate the effects of early intervention in higher-risk patients.[268] Over a 3-year period, 6213 participants were studied. The mortality of the Mg-treated group at 30 days was not significantly different from that of the placebo group. The overall evidence from clinical trials does not support the routine use of adjunctive Mg therapy in patients with AMI at this time.

A number of studies have demonstrated an inverse relationship between dietary Mg intake and blood pressure.[269,270]

Hypomagnesemia and/or reduction of intracellular Mg have also been inversely correlated with blood pressure. This may be especially important in individuals with diabetes mellitus. Patients with essential hypertension were found to have reduced free Mg concentrations in red blood cells. The Mg levels were inversely related to both systolic and diastolic blood pressure. Intervention studies examining Mg therapy in hypertension have led to conflicting results. Several have shown a positive blood pressure–lowering effect of supplements, whereas others have not. Other dietary factors may also play a role. In the Dietary Approaches to Stop Hypertension (DASH) study, consumption of a diet rich in fruits and vegetables, which increased Mg intake from 176 to 423 mg/day (along with increasing potassium), significantly lowered blood pressure.[271]

The mechanism by which Mg deficit may affect blood pressure is not clear, but Mg does regulates vascular tone and reactivity and attenuates agonist-induced vasoconstriction. Mg depletion may involve decreased production of prostacyclin, increased production of thromboxane A_2, and enhanced vasoconstrictive effect of angiotensin II and norepinephrine.

NEUROMUSCULAR SYSTEM

Symptoms and signs of neuromuscular irritability, including tremor, muscle twitching, Trousseau's and Chvostek's signs, and frank tetany, may develop in patients with isolated hypomagnesemia.[272] Hypomagnesemia is also frequently manifested as seizures, which may be generalized and tonic-clonic in nature or multifocal motor seizures, and they are sometimes triggered by loud noises.[272] Interestingly, noise-induced seizures and sudden death also occur in mice made hypomagnesemic by dietary Mg deprivation.

The effects of Mg deficiency on brain neuronal excitability are thought to be mediated by N-methyl-D-aspartate (NMDA)–type glutamate receptors.[273] Glutamate is the principal excitatory neurotransmitter in the brain; it acts as an agonist at NMDA receptors and opens a cation conductance channel that depolarizes the postsynaptic membrane. Extracellular Mg normally blocks NMDA receptors, so hypomagnesemia may release the inhibition of glutamate-activated depolarization of the postsynaptic membrane and thereby trigger epileptiform electrical activity.[274] As discussed later, hypocalcemia is often observed in Mg deficiency and may also contribute to the neuromuscular hyperexcitability.

Vertical nystagmus is a rare but diagnostically useful neurologic sign of severe hypomagnesemia.[275] In the absence of a structural lesion of the cerebellar or vestibular pathways, the only recognized metabolic causes are Wernicke's encephalopathy and severe Mg deficiency.[275]

SKELETAL SYSTEM

Dietary Mg depletion in animals has been shown to lead to a decrease in skeletal growth and increased skeletal fragility.[276] A decrease in osteoblastic bone formation and an increase in osteoclastic bone resorption are implicated as the cause of decreased bone mass. In humans, epidemiologic studies suggest a correlation between bone mass and dietary Mg intake.[277] Few studies have been conducted assessing Mg status in patients with osteoporosis. Low serum and red blood cell Mg concentrations as well as high retention of parenterally administered Mg have suggested a deficit. Low skeletal Mg content has been observed in some, but not all, studies.

Investigations of the effect of supplementation on bone mass have generally demonstrated an increase in bone mineral density, although study design limits useful information. Larger long-term placebo-controlled double-blind investigations are required.

There are several potential mechanisms that may account for a decrease in bone mass in Mg deficiency. Mg is mitogenic for bone cell growth, which may directly result in a decrease in bone formation. It also affects crystal formation; a lack results in a larger, more perfect crystal, which may affect bone strength. Mg deficiency may result in a fall in both serum PTH and $1,25(OH)_2D$ levels as discussed earlier. Since both hormones are trophic for bone, impaired secretion or skeletal resistance may result in osteoporosis. Low serum $1,25(OH)_2D$ may also result in decreased intestinal Ca absorption. Increased release of inflammatory cytokines in bone has been observed in rodents and may result in activation of osteoclasts and increased bone resorption.[276,278]

ELECTROLYTE HOMEOSTASIS

Patients with hypomagnesemia are frequently also hypokalemic. Many of the conditions associated with hypomagnesemia that have been outlined earlier can cause simultaneous Mg and K loss. However, hypomagnesemia by itself can induce hypokalemia in both humans and experimental animals, and in such patients the hypokalemia is often refractory to K administration until the Mg deficit is corrected.[279] The cause of the hypokalemia appears to be increased secretion in the distal nephron.[280] The mechanism has been attributed to cytosolic Mg depletion, which would release intracellular block of the apical secretory K channel, ROMK.[281]

Hypocalcemia is present in approximately half of patients with hypomagnesemia.[258] The major cause is impairment of PTH secretion by Mg deficiency, which is reversed within 24 hours by Mg replenishment.[171] In addition, hypomagnesemic patients also have low circulating $1,25(OH)_2D$ levels and end-organ resistance to both PTH and vitamin D.[171]

OTHER DISORDERS

Mg depletion has also been associated with several other disorders such as insulin resistance and metabolic syndrome in type 2 diabetes mellitus.[270,282] Mg deficiency has been associated with migraine headache, and Mg therapy has been reported to be effective in the treatment of migraine.[283] Because Mg deficiency results in smooth muscle spasm, it has also been implicated in asthma, and Mg therapy has been effective in treating asthma in some studies.[284,285] Finally, a high dietary Mg intake has been associated with reduced risk of colon cancer.[286,287]

Treatment

Mg deficiency may sometimes be prevented. Individuals whose dietary intake has been reduced or who are being maintained by parenteral nutrition should receive Mg supplementation. The recommended daily allowance of Mg in adults is 420 mg (35 mEq) for men and 320 mg (27 mEq) for women.[288] Thus, in the absence of dietary Mg intake, an appropriate supplement would be one 140-mg tablet of Mg oxide four to five times daily or the equivalent dose of an alternative oral Mg-containing salt. Because the oral bioavailability of Mg is approximately 33% in patients with normal intestinal

function, the equivalent parenteral maintenance requirement of Mg would be 10 mEq daily.

Once symptomatic Mg deficiency develops, patients should clearly receive Mg replacement therapy. However, the importance of treating asymptomatic Mg deficiency remains controversial. Given the clinical manifestations outlined earlier, it seems prudent to provide Mg replacement therapy to all Mg-deficient patients who have a significant underlying cardiac or seizure disorder, patients with concurrent severe hypocalcemia or hypokalemia, and patients with isolated asymptomatic hypomagnesemia if it is severe (<1.4 mg/dL).

INTRAVENOUS REPLACEMENT

In the inpatient setting, the intravenous route of administration of Mg is favored because it is highly effective, inexpensive, and usually well tolerated. The standard preparation is $MgSO_4 \cdot 7H_2O$. The initial rate of replacement depends on the urgency of the clinical situation. In a patient who is actively experiencing seizures or who has a cardiac arrhythmia, 8 to 16 mEq (1 to 2 g) may be administered intravenously over a 2- to 4-minute period; otherwise, a slower rate of replacement is safer. Because the added extracellular Mg equilibrates slowly with the intracellular compartment and because renal excretion of extracellular Mg exhibits a threshold effect, approximately 50% of parenterally administered Mg is excreted into urine.[289] A slower rate and prolonged course of replacement would be expected to decrease these urinary losses and therefore to be much more efficient and effective at replenishing body Mg stores.

The magnitude of the Mg deficit is difficult to gauge clinically and cannot be readily deduced from the serum Mg concentration. In general, though, the average deficit can be assumed to be 1 to 2 mEq/kg of body weight.[289] A simple regimen for nonemergency Mg replenishment is to administer 64 mEq (8 g) of $MgSO_4$ over the first 24 hours and then 32 mEq (4 g) daily for the next 2 to 6 days. It is important to remember that serum Mg levels rise early, whereas intracellular stores take longer to replenish, so Mg administration should continue for at least 1 to 2 days after the serum Mg level normalizes. In patients with renal Mg wasting, additional Mg may be needed to replace ongoing losses. In patients with reduced GFR, the rate of replenishment should be reduced by 25% to 50%,[289] the patient should be carefully monitored for signs of hypermagnesemia, and the serum Mg level should be checked frequently.

The main adverse effects of Mg replacement are due to hypermagnesemia resulting from Mg administration at an excessive rate or in an excessive amount. These effects include facial flushing, loss of deep tendon reflexes, hypotension, and atrioventricular block. Monitoring of tendon reflexes is a useful bedside test to detect Mg overdose. In addition, intravenous administration of large amounts of $MgSO_4$ results in an acute decrease in the serum ionized Ca^{2+} level[290] related to increased urinary Ca excretion and complexing of Ca by sulfate. Thus, in an asymptomatic patient who is already hypocalcemic, administration of $MgSO_4$ may further lower the ionized Ca^{2+} level and thereby precipitate tetany.[291]

Administration of Mg with sulfate as the anion may have an additional theoretical disadvantage. Because sulfate cannot be reabsorbed in the distal tubule, it favors the development of a negative luminal electrical potential, which increases K secretion. In Mg-depleted rats with hypokalemia, administration of Mg in the form of a nonsulfate salt was associated with correction of the hypokalemia, whereas administration of $MgSO_4$ resulted in persistent hypokalemia and kaliuresis.[292]

ORAL REPLACEMENT

Oral Mg administration is used either initially for correction of mild cases of hypomagnesemia or for continued replacement of ongoing losses in the outpatient setting after an initial course of intravenous replacement therapy. A number of oral Mg salts are available, but little is known about their relative oral bioavailability or efficacy, and all of them cause diarrhea in high dosages. The upper safe limit set by the Food Nutrition Board is 300 mg/day of elemental Mg.[208] This limit is based on the occurrence of diarrhea

Mg hydroxide and Mg oxide are alkalinizing salts with the potential to cause systemic alkalosis, whereas the sulfate and gluconate salts may potentially exacerbate K^+ wasting, as discussed earlier. The appropriate dosage of each salt can be estimated, if ongoing losses are known, by determining its content of elemental Mg and assuming a bioavailability of approximately 33% for patients with normal intestinal function. In patients with intestinal Mg malabsorption, this dosage may need to be increased twofold to fourfold.

POTASSIUM-SPARING DIURETICS

In patients with inappropriate renal Mg wasting, potassium-sparing diuretics that block the distal tubule epithelial Na channel, such as amiloride and triamterene, may reduce renal Mg losses.[293] These drugs may be particularly useful in patients whose hypomagnesemia is refractory to oral replacement or who require such high dosages of oral Mg that diarrhea develops. In rats, amiloride and triamterene can be demonstrated to reduce renal Mg clearance at baseline and after induction of Mg diuresis by furosemide, but the mechanism is unknown. One possibility is that these drugs, by reducing luminal Na uptake and inhibiting the development of a negative luminal transepithelial potential difference, may favor passive reabsorption of Mg in the late distal tubule or collecting duct.[294]

Hypermagnesemia

Causes

In states of body Mg excess, the kidney has a very large capacity for Mg excretion. Once the apparent renal threshold is exceeded, most of the excess filtered Mg is excreted unchanged into the final urine; the serum Mg concentration is then determined by the GFR. Thus, hypermagnesemia generally occurs in two clinical settings: compromised renal function and excessive Mg intake.

RENAL INSUFFICIENCY

In chronic renal failure, the remaining nephrons adapt to the decreased filtered load of Mg by markedly increasing their fractional excretion of Mg.[295] As a consequence, serum Mg levels are usually well maintained until the creatinine clearance falls below about 20 mL/min.[295] Even in advanced renal insufficiency, significant hypermagnesemia is rare unless the patient has received exogenous Mg in the form of antacids, cathartics, or enemas. Increasing age is an important risk factor for hypermagnesemia in individuals with apparently normal renal function; it presumably reflects the decline in GFR that normally accompanies old age.[296]

EXCESSIVE MAGNESIUM INTAKE

Hypermagnesemia can occur in individuals with a normal GFR when the rate of Mg intake exceeds the renal excretory capacity. It has been reported with excessive oral ingestion of Mg-containing antacids[297] and cathartics[298] and with the use of rectal $MgSO_4$ enemas,[299] and is common with large parenteral doses of Mg, such as those given for preeclampsia. Toxicity from enterally administered Mg salts is particularly common in patients with inflammatory disease, obstruction,[297] or perforation of the gastrointestinal tract, presumably because Mg absorption is enhanced.

MISCELLANEOUS CAUSES

Modest elevations in serum Mg concentration (less than 4 mEq/L) have occasionally been described in patients receiving lithium therapy, as well as in patients who have just undergone surgery and in those with bone metastases, milk-alkali syndrome, FHH,[257] hypothyroidism, pituitary dwarfism, and Addison's disease. In most patients cases, the mechanism is unknown.

Clinical Manifestations

Mg toxicity is a serious and potentially fatal condition. Progressive hypermagnesemia is usually associated with a predictable sequence of symptoms and signs.[300] Initial manifestations, observed once the serum Mg level exceeds 4 to 6 mg/dL, are hypotension, nausea, vomiting, facial flushing, urinary retention, and ileus. If untreated, Mg toxicity may progress to flaccid skeletal muscular paralysis and hyporeflexia, bradycardia and bradyarrhythmias, respiratory depression, coma, and cardiac arrest. An abnormally low (or even negative) serum anion gap may be a clue to hypermagnesemia,[296] but it is not consistently observed, and its occurrence probably depends on the nature of the anion that accompanies the excess body Mg.

CARDIOVASCULAR SYSTEM

Hypotension is one of the earliest manifestations of hypermagnesemia,[301] is often accompanied by cutaneous flushing, and is thought to be due to vasodilatation of vascular smooth muscle and inhibition of norepinephrine release by sympathetic postganglionic nerves. ECG changes are common but nonspecific.[301] Sinus or junctional bradycardia may develop, as well as varying degrees of sinoatrial, atrioventricular, and His bundle conduction block. Cardiac arrest as a result of asystole is often the terminal event.

NERVOUS SYSTEM

High levels of extracellular Mg inhibit acetylcholine release from the neuromuscular end plate,[302] which leads to the development of flaccid skeletal muscle paralysis and hyporeflexia when serum Mg level exceeds 8 to 12 mg/dL. Respiratory depression is a serious complication of advanced Mg toxicity.[301] Smooth muscle paralysis also occurs and is manifested as urinary retention, intestinal ileus, and pupillary dilatation. Signs of central nervous system depression, including lethargy, drowsiness, and eventually coma, are well described in severe hypermagnesemia, but they may also be entirely absent.

Treatment

Mild cases of Mg toxicity in individuals with good renal function may require no treatment other than cessation of Mg supplements, because renal Mg clearance is usually quite rapid. The normal half-life of serum Mg is approximately 28 hours. In the event of serious toxicity, particularly cardiac toxicity, temporary antagonism of the effect of Mg may be achieved by the administration of intravenous calcium (1 g of calcium chloride infused into a central vein over a period of 2 to 5 minutes or calcium gluconate infused through a peripheral vein, repeated after 5 minutes if necessary).[300] Renal excretion of Mg can be enhanced by saline diuresis and by the administration of furosemide, which inhibits tubule reabsorption of Mg in the medullary TAL.

In patients with renal failure, the only way to clear the excess Mg may be by dialysis. The typical dialysate for hemodialysis contains 0.6 to 1.2 mg/dL of Mg, but Mg-free dialysate can also be used and is generally well tolerated except for producing muscle cramps.[303] Hemodialysis is extremely effective in removing excess Mg and can achieve clearances of up to 100 mL/min.[303] As a rough rule of thumb, the expected change in serum Mg after a 3- to 4-hour dialysis session with a high-efficiency membrane is approximately a third to a half the difference between the dialysate Mg^{2+} concentration and predialysis serum ultrafilterable Mg (estimated at 70% of total serum Mg).[303] Note that when hemodialysis is performed using a bath with the same total concentration of Mg as in serum, net transfer of Mg into the patient occurs, because the ultrafilterable (and therefore free) Mg concentration in serum is less than the total concentration, and thus the gradient of free Mg^{2+} is directed from dialysate to blood.

Disorders of Phosphate Homeostasis

Body phosphate metabolism is regulated through plasma inorganic phosphorus (Pi) concentration. Of the total body phosphorus content (500 to 800 g), 85% is in the skeleton, 14% in soft tissues, and the rest is distributed between other tissues and the ECF. The ECF pool of phosphorus is about 600 mg. Two thirds of the phosphorus in blood exists as organic phosphates (mainly phospholipids) and one third as Pi. Pi in the blood, for practical purposes, occurs in the form of two orthophosphates: $H_2PO_4^-$ and HPO_4^{2-}. At a plasma pH of 7.4 there are four divalent HPO_4^{2-} ions for every one monovalent $H_2PO_4^-$ ion, so that the composite valence is 1.8 (i.e., 1 mmol Pi is equal to 1.8 mEq). Thus Pi in plasma circulates as phosphates, but is measured in the laboratory as phosphorus (normal value = 2.5 to 4.5 mg/dL).

There are great variations in Pi plasma levels with age, ranging up to 7.4 mg/dL in infants and up to 5.8 mg/dL in children aged 1 to 2 years.[4,304] Between 85% and 90% of plasma phosphorus is filterable by the kidneys (50% ionized Pi and 40% complexed Pi with cations) and the rest is bound to the protein.

The average daily phosphorus intake varies from 800 to 1500 mg, mostly as Pi. Approximately 60% of this is absorbed by the intestine through a sodium-dependent active transport mechanism stimulated by 1,25(OH)$_2$D and through passive diffusion of Pi. In addition, 150 to 200 mg of phosphorus is secreted daily by the colon. PTH and a low-Pi diet increase absorption, whereas a high-Pi diet decreases absorption, all through 1,25(OH)$_2$D. Low Pi stimulates 1α-hydroxylase activity in the kidney and increases 1,25(OH)$_2$D generation. Bone turnover of Pi is about 200 mg daily.[1]

As discussed in detail in Chapter 7, the kidney is the major organ regulating phosphate homeostasis. The net renal excretion of Pi under steady-state conditions is the same as the Pi absorbed by the gastrointestinal tract. Up to 80% of renal reabsorption of phosphate occurs in the proximal tubule by means of the NaPi cotransporter family of proteins—type IIa (NaPi-IIa) and type IIc (NaPi-IIc)—in the luminal brush border membrane.[305] The rest of the urinary phosphate is either reabsorbed in the distal tubules or excreted in the urine. PTH increases Pi excretion by decreasing the abundance of NaPi-IIa and NaPi-IIc in the brush border membrane. A low serum phosphate concentration stimulates renal NaPi cotransporters and hence phosphate reabsorption.[305] FGF-23, similar to PTH, acts to reduce phosphate reabsorption in the proximal tubules but, contrary to PTH, FGF-23 decreases the circulating level of 1,25(OH)$_2$D.

The urinary phosphate excretion can be measured from a 24-hour urine collection. It can be assessed by determining fractional excretion of filtered phosphate (FE$_{Pi}$) or by calculating the ratio of the renal tubular maximal reabsorption rate of phosphate (TmP) to the GFR[306]:

$$TmP/GFR_{Cr} (mg/dL) = Serum\ Pi - [(Urine\ Pi \times Serum\ creatinine)/Urine\ creatinine]$$

where GFR_{Cr} is the GFR as estimated by creatinine clearance. The latter method is the preferred one, since the TmP/GFR ratio is independent of kidney function. The normal range for TmP/GFR is 2.6 to 4.4 mg/dL; lower values indicate a lowered renal phosphate threshold, and hence excessive urinary phosphate loss.

Hyperphosphatemia

Hyperphosphatemia is generally defined as a serum phosphate level above 5 mg/dL. For children, the upper range of normal is 6 mg/dL. In infants, phosphorus levels as high as 7.4 mg/dL are considered normal.[304] The serum phosphorus level usually exhibits diurnal variation. Typically, phosphorus levels are lowest in the late morning and peak in the first morning hours.[307] The clinical causes of hyperphosphatemia[308] can be broadly classified into three groups: reduced phosphate excretion, excess intake of phosphorus, and redistribution of cellular phosphorus (Table 18-7).

Causes

DECREASED RENAL PHOSPHATE EXCRETION

Chronic Kidney Disease. Decreased renal function is by far the most common cause of hyperphosphatemia. In CKD stages 2 and 3, increased fractional excretion of PO$_4$, due to compensatory increased secretion of PTH and FGF-23, is able to compensate for decreased GFR. With further falls in GFR (CKD stage 4 or 5), Pi excretion can no longer be maintained, which leads to hyperphosphatemia. Hyperphosphatemia is observed in acute kidney injury as well as CKD. Hyperphosphatemia caused by decreased

TABLE 18-7 Causes of Hyperphosphatemia

Decreased Renal Excretion of Phosphorus

Chronic kidney disease stages 3-5
Acute renal failure/acute kidney injury
Hypoparathyroidism, pseudohypoparathyroidism
Acromegaly
Tumoral calcinosis
    Fibroblast growth factor 23 (FGF-23)–inactivating gene mutation
    GALNT3 mutation with aberrant FGF-23 glycosylation
    KLOTHO inactivating mutation with FGF-23 resistance
Bisphosphonates

Exogenous Phosphorus Administration

Ingestion of phosphate, phosphate-containing enemas
Intravenous phosphate delivery

Redistribution of Phosphorus

Respiratory acidosis/metabolic acidosis
Tumor lysis syndrome
Rhabdomyolysis
Hemolytic anemia
Catabolic state

Pseudohyperphosphatemia

Hyperglobulinemia, hyperlipidemia, hemolysis, hyperbilirubinemia

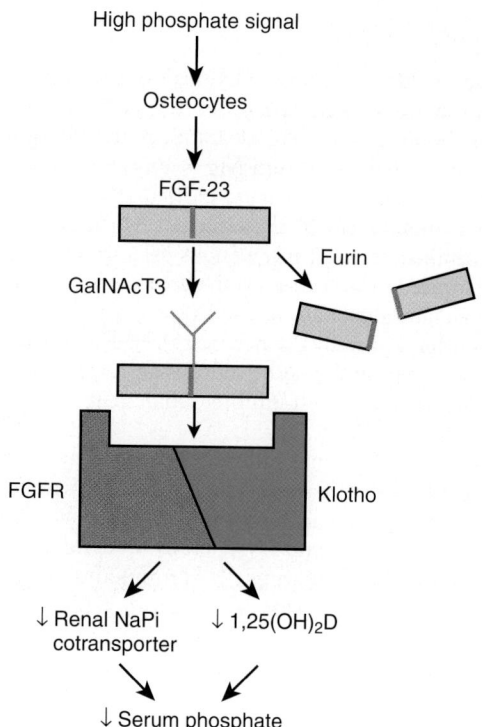

FIGURE 18-4 Current model of the physiology and pathophysiology of fibroblast growth factor 23 (FGF-23). FGF-23 (*yellow*) is normally released by osteocytes in response to a high-phosphate signal. It contains a cleavage site (*blue*) for degradation by furin and other subtilisin-like proteases. The glycosylation of FGF-23 (*red*) by N-acetyl-D-galactosamine transferase (GalNAcT3) protects it from cleavage. Intact (uncleaved) FGF-23 is able to bind to its receptor, a heteromer of FGF receptor (FGFR) and Klotho. In target cells such as the renal proximal tubule, it causes downregulation of NaPi cotransporters and of 1,25-dihydroxyvitamin D_3 (1,25[OH]$_2D_3$), thereby lowering serum phosphate level back to its normal set point. Hypophosphatemia may occur when the amount of intact FGF-23 is pathologically increased. This can be due to ectopic synthesis of FGF-23 by mesenchymal tumors (tumor-induced osteomalacia), mutation of the furin-cleavage site (autosomal dominant hypophosphatemic rickets [ADHR]), or upregulation of FGF-23 by *PHEX* (phosphate-regulating gene with homology to endopeptidases on the X chromosome) as occurs in X-linked hypophosphatemic rickets. Unlike other causes of hypophosphatemia, these disorders are all associated with suppressed levels of 1,25(OH)$_2$D. Familial tumoral calcinosis, which is associated with hyperphosphatemia, is caused by a decrease in the amount or function of intact FGF-23. This can be caused by mutations in FGF-23 that lead to reduced secretion or loss-of-function mutations in either GalNAcT3 or Klotho.

renal function is not discussed in detail here because it is reviewed extensively in Chapter 54 in the context of renal osteodystrophies.

Hypoparathyroidism and Pseudohypoparathyroidism. Either deficient secretion of PTH (hypoparathyroidism) or renal resistance to PTH (pseudohypoparathyroidism) decreases renal excretion of phosphate, leading to hyperphosphatemia and hypercalcemia. These entities are discussed earlier in this chapter. In primary hypoparathyroidism, circulating phosphorus generally reaches a higher than normal steady-state level (6 to 7 mg/dL), with a low serum calcium level.

Acromegaly. Some patients with acromegaly demonstrate hyperphosphatemia. Parathyroid function is usually normal or slightly increased in acromegaly.[84] The hyperphosphatemia observed appears to result from increased proximal tubule phosphate reabsorption. Growth hormone and insulin-like growth factor-1 directly stimulate proximal tubule phosphorus reabsorption and increase the tubular maximum excretory capacity for phosphorus.[309]

Familial Tumoral Calcinosis. Familial tumoral calcinosis (FTC; MIM 211900) is a rare autosomal recessive disorder noted for progressive deposition of calcium phosphate crystals in periarticular and soft tissues. The hyperphosphatemic form of this disease results from increased proximal tubular reabsorption of phosphorus due to loss-of-function mutations in a number of separate human genes, namely, the uridine diphosphate–N-acetyl-α-D-galactosamine (*GALNT3*) gene,[310] which encodes a glycosyltransferase; the FGF-23 gene[311,312]; and *KLOTHO*, which encodes a cofactor necessary for FGF-23 binding to its receptor.[313] FGF-23 normally inhibits proximal tubule reabsorption of phosphorus and causes renal phosphate wasting. The unifying pathogenic mechanism in FTC is abrogation of the effect of FGF-23. This is because the missense mutations in the FGF-23 gene inhibit its secretion, mutations in *GALNT3* cause aberrant FGF-23 glycosylation,[314] and mutations in *KLOTHO* lead to FGF-23 resistance (Figure 18-4).

FTC has been described mainly in families from Africa and the Mediterranean area. The FGF-23–null mouse model shows characteristics similar to those of FTC.[315] Thus, in many ways FTC is the phenotypic opposite of X-linked and autosomal dominant hypophosphatemic rickets (see later discussion). Together, a normal serum calcium concentration and elevated serum phosphorus concentration lead to an elevated calcium phosphate product and soft, painless, slow-growing tissue calcium phosphate deposition. Biochemically, in addition to a high Pi level, there is an increased 1,25(OH)$_2$D level[316] with normal serum calcium and alkaline phosphatase concentrations. Urinary phosphate reabsorption is supranormal.

Reduction of the phosphorus intake in the diet, use of phosphate binders such as aluminium hydroxide or sevelamer, as well as administration of acetazolamide have been reported to be effective treatment.[317] Occasionally surgical intervention is needed.

Bisphosphonates. Bisphosphonates can cause hyperphosphatemia. Mechanisms include phosphate redistribution and decreased urinary phosphate excretion.[318,319] This is not because of PTH since the levels of PTH in blood and urinary excretion of cAMP in response to exogenous PTH are normal in patients receiving bisphosphonates.

INCREASED PHOSPHORUS INTAKE

Severe hyperphosphatemia has been recognized for at least half a century as a complication of sodium phosphate administration either orally as a cathartic agent or in enemas (e.g., Fleet).[308] Acute renal failure, hypocalcemia, severe electrolyte disturbances, and death have been described as a part of the clinical picture. Despite that, sodium phosphate has been used since 1990 as the most effective and, in initial assessment, safe agent for bowel cleansing before colonoscopy. Initially an oral solution (Phospho-soda, two doses every 12 hours, 5.8 g of Pi each) was used, but currently oral tablets containing a similar amount of Pi are more popular.[320,321] In healthy volunteers these regimens cause a rise of the serum Pi to as high as 8.9 mg/dL (mean = 6.7 mg/dL), 3.1 to 3.5 mg/dL above baseline levels, during 24 hours of observation.[322]

Over the last 10 years, numerous case reports and case series have described an association between the use of oral sodium phosphate for bowel cleansing and *phosphate nephropathy*. Typically, patients who recently (days to weeks prior) had colonoscopy present with nonspecific symptoms and with deterioration of kidney function. Kidney biopsy specimens shows acute and chronic tubular injury with calcium phosphate deposits (tubular calcifications).[320,323] Most patients do not recover kidney function fully, and some progress to CKD stage 5.

Overall, such adverse renal effects are uncommon in patients treated with sodium phosphate, but for those few who develop them the consequences are serious. The risk factors for developing phosphate nephropathy are advanced age, female gender, impaired kidney function, volume contraction, ulceration of bowel mucosa, bowel obstruction or ileus, hypertension, and use of angiotensin converting enzyme inhibitors or angiotensin receptor blockers, or nonsteroidal antiinflammatory drugs.[320,324] Alternative methods of bowel preparation should be considered for patients with these risk factors.

Hyperphosphatemia has also been observed in the ICU setting when excessive amount of phosphate are given intravenously for hyperalimentation, particularly in patients with renal failure.

REDISTRIBUTION OF PHOSPHORUS

Respiratory Acidosis and Metabolic Acidosis. Respiratory acidosis can lead to hyperphosphatemia, renal resistance to the effect of PTH, and hypocalcemia.[325] The effect is more pronounced when respiratory acidosis is acute than when it is chronic. Respiratory acidosis does not appear to significantly alter the renal handling of phosphorus. Rather, efflux of phosphate from cells into the extracellular space is probably responsible for the hyperphosphatemia of respiratory acidosis.[326]

Lactic acidosis and to a lesser extent diabetic ketoacidosis also cause hyperphosphatemia.[327,328] Metabolic acidosis in general reduces glycolysis and Pi utilization. In lactic acidosis this effect is intensified by tissue hypoxia and intracellular Pi release. Patients with uncontrolled diabetes mellitus are intracellularly phosphate depleted despite hyperphosphatemia, an

abnormality that becomes unmasked once insulin therapy is initiated.

Tumor Lysis Syndrome and Rhabdomyolysis. Because phosphate is predominantly stored intracellularly, clinical conditions associated with increased catabolism and tissue destruction, such as rhabdomyolysis, fulminant hepatitis, hemolytic anemia, malignant hyperthermia, severe hyperthermia, and tumor lysis syndrome, can result in hyperphosphatemia. The severity of the hyperphosphatemia may be exacerbated by the development of acute kidney injury.

Tumor lysis syndrome is a constellation of metabolic abnormalities including hyperuricemia, hyperkalemia, and hyperphosphatemia that is caused by rapid and massive breakdown of tumor cells.[329,330] Clinical consequences may include acute kidney injury, pulmonary edema, cardiac arrhythmia, and seizures. The syndrome typically occurs from 3 days before to 7 days after initiation of chemotherapy. Hyperphosphatemia was seen in essentially all patients with Burkitt's lymphoma after treatment if they had any preexisting kidney disease and in approximately 30% of patients with normal renal function. It is also seen in patients with other forms of lymphoma, in those with lymphoblastic and myelogenous leukemias, and in patients with solid cancer with a high tumor burden. Malignant lymphoid cells may contain up to four times more intracellular phosphorus than mature lymphoid cells. The lactate dehydrogenase level before the initiation of therapy correlates with the development of hyperphosphatemia and azotemia.[331] Phosphate nephropathy with tubular calcifications has been reported in tumor lysis syndrome patients with extremely high serum Pi levels.[329]

To prevent tumor lysis syndrome, intensive volume expansion is generally recommended before chemotherapy to induce high urine output (120 to 150 mL/hr) and phosphate and uric acid excretion.[332] The usefulness of urine alkalinization (pH > 7.0) with bicarbonate infusion and/or acetazolamide is unclear, and this practice is controversial. Alkalinization may increase uric acid solubility in the tubules, but its use requires caution because, in the presence of a high calcium phosphate product, alkalinization increases the risk of nephrocalcinosis. Phosphate binders are also commonly prescribed. Early on in tumor lysis syndrome, daily or even twice-daily hemodialysis may be necessary to control severe hyperphosphatemia and acute renal failure. Continuous renal replacement therapy is the preferred treatment for tumor lysis and acute kidney injury in hemodynamically compromised patients.

PSEUDOHYPERPHOSPHATEMIA

Laboratory readings incorrectly indicating hyperphosphatemia in patient samples may occur in certain settings as a result of interference with the analysis. This problem is most common in cases of paraproteinemia (as in multiple myeloma or Waldenström's macroglobulinemia).[333] Liposomal amphotericin B,[334] hemolysis, and hyperlipidemia in the blood specimen can also lead to spuriously elevated measurements of phosphorus. Hyperbilirubinemia causes interference with Pi laboratory tests.

Clinical Manifestations and Treatment

Most of the major clinical manifestations of hyperphosphatemia stem from hypocalcemia, discussed earlier in this chapter. Chronic hyperphosphatemia of CKD and its metabolic consequences are discussed in Chapter 54. Treatment of chronic hyperphosphatemia is generally accomplished through dietary phosphate restriction, use of oral phosphate binders, and renal replacement therapy. Acute hyperphosphatemia in association with hypocalcemia requires rapid attention. Discontinuation of supplemental phosphates and initiation of hydration are indicated for patients with acute exogenous Pi overload. Severe hyperphosphatemia in patients with reduced renal function or acute kidney injury, particularly in those with tumor lysis syndrome, may require hemodialysis or a continuous form of renal replacement therapy. Volume expansion may increase urinary phosphate excretion, as can administration of acetazolamide. In diabetic ketoacidosis, treatment with insulin and correction of metabolic acidosis reverses the hyperphosphatemia.

Hypophosphatemia

Hypophosphatemia is a decrease in the concentration of Pi in plasma, and phosphate depletion is a decrease in the total body content of phosphorus. Hypophosphatemia can occur in the presence of a low, normal, or high total body content of phosphorus. Similarly, phosphate depletion may exist with low, normal, or high Pi levels in plasma. The incidence of hypophosphatemia is between 0.2% and 2.2% in the hospitalized population, but may be 2.5% to 30% in individuals with chronic alcoholism, 28% to 34% in patients in the ICU, and as high as 65% to 80% in patients with sepsis.[335,336] There is an association between hypophosphatemia and mortality among hospitalized patients[337] and between hypophosphatemia and all-cause mortality in the dialysis population.[338]

Clinical Manifestations

Moderate hypophosphatemia (plasma Pi between 2.5 and 1.0 mg/dL) usually occurs without significant phosphate depletion and without specific signs or symptoms. In severe hypophosphatemia (plasma Pi below 1.0 mg/dL), phosphates depletion is usually present, and it can have significant clinical consequences, including disturbances in multiple cellular functions and organ systems.

The clinical manifestations of hypophosphatemia and phosphate depletion generally result from a decrease in intracellular ATP levels. In addition, erythrocytes show a decrease in 2,3-diphosphoglycerate levels, which increases hemoglobin-oxygen affinity and alters oxygen transport efficiency.[339] Hypophosphatemia causes a rise in intracellular cytosolic calcium in cells such as leukocytes, pancreatic islet cells, and synaptosomes isolated from phosphate-depleted animals. These elevated cytosolic calcium levels were associated with decreased ATP and impaired cell response to stimuli.[340]

Hematologic consequences include a predisposition to hemolysis, thought to result from increased red cell rigidity.[341,342] Hemolysis is not typically seen in the absence of other exacerbating features. Phagocytosis and chemotaxis of polymorphonuclear cells is diminished, since impaired ATP production diminishes the phagocytic capability.[343]

Severe hypophosphatemia may result in proximal myopathy, weakness, and bone pain[335,344] and can be complicated by rhabdomyolysis.[345] Because cell breakdown may lead to

the release of intracellular phosphate, normophosphatemia or hyperphosphatemia in this setting may mask the existence of true phosphate depletion. Overt heart failure and respiratory failure as a result of decreased muscle performance may be observed.[346,347] Correction of Pi leads to improvement of myocardial function.[348,349] Neurologic manifestations of severe hypophosphatemia include paresthesias, tremor, and encephalopathy; these also improve with phosphate replacement.[335] Chronic phosphate depletion alters bone metabolism, which results in increased bone resorption, rickets, and osteomalacia.

Hypophosphatemia leads to proximal and distal tubular defects resulting in water diuresis, glucosuria, bicarbonaturia, hypercalciuria, and hypermagnesuria.[350] The hypercalciuria is not solely the result of altered renal calcium handling but also reflects increased calcium release from bone and increased intestinal calcium absorption.[351]

Metabolic consequences of hypophosphatemia include insulin resistance, diminished gluconeogenesis, hypoparathyroidism, and metabolic acidosis with reduced H^+ excretion and ammonia generation. Hypophosphatemia is also a potent stimulator of 1α-hydroxylation of 25(OH)D to $1,25(OH)_2D$.

Diagnosis

The probable cause of hypophosphatemia may be immediately apparent from the clinical findings (e.g., in a malnourished patient with alcoholism or anorexia). Shifts of phosphorus from the extracellular to the intracellular space generally occur in the acute setting (respiratory alkalosis, treatment of diabetic ketoacidosis). In hospitalized patients, hypophosphatemia caused by shifts of phosphorus into the intracellular compartment are much more common than hypophosphatemia caused by renal losses.[352] In situations in which the underlying diagnosis is not immediately apparent, it can be clinically useful to determine the rate of urine phosphorus excretion. High urine phosphorus levels in the face of hypophosphatemia suggest hyperparathyroidism, a renal tubule defect, or a form of rickets.

Causes

Hypophosphatemia may be due to increased renal phosphate excretion, decreased intestinal absorption, shift of phosphate from extracellular to intracellular fluid, or a combination of multiple mechanisms (Table 18-8).

INCREASED RENAL PHOSPHATE EXCRETION

Hypophosphatemia caused by increased urinary phosphate excretion is generally the result of either excess PTH, increased production or activity of FGF-23 in normal or dysplastic bone, or a disorder of renal phosphate handling in the proximal tubule.

Hyperparathyroidism. Both primary and secondary hyperparathyroidism may lead to hyperphosphaturia and hypophosphatemia. Primary hyperparathyroidism was discussed earlier in this chapter. The degree of hypophosphatemia observed is usually moderate in severity; increased urinary phosphate excretion is balanced by mobilization of Pi from the bone and enhanced intestinal absorption of Pi. The secondary hyperparathyroidism observed in patients with CKD is typically

TABLE 18-8 Causes of Hypophosphatemia

Increased urinary phosphate excretion
  Primary and secondary hyperparathyroidism
  Increased production or activity of fibroblast growth factor 23 (FGF-23)
    Inherited disorders
      X-linked hypophosphatemia (*PHEX* mutations)
      Autosomal dominant hypophosphatemic rickets (FGF-23 mutations)
      Autosomal recessive hypophosphatemic rickets (*DMP1* and *ENPP1* mutations)
    Acquired disorder
      Tumor-induced osteomalacia
  Disorders of proximal tubule inorganic phosphate reabsorption
    Hereditary hypophosphatemic rickets with hypercalciuria (*SLC34A3* mutations)
    Autosomal recessive renal phosphate wasting (*SLC34A1* mutations)
  Fanconi's syndrome
  Post–renal transplantation status
  Medications: Acetazolamide, calcitonin, glucocorticoids, diuretics, bicarbonate, acetaminophen, iron (intravenous), antineoplastics, antiretrovirals, aminoglycosides, anticonvulsants
  Acute tubular necrosis recovery, after urinary obstruction
  Miscellaneous: hepatectomy, colorectal surgery, volume expansion, osmotic diuresis
Decreased intestinal absorption of phosphate
  Malnutrition with low phosphate intake, anorexia, starvation
  Malabsorption of phosphate: chronic diarrhea, gastrointestinal tract diseases
  Intake of phosphate-binding agents
  Vitamin D deficiency or vitamin D resistance
    Nutritional deficiency: low dietary intake, low sun exposure
    Malabsorption
    Chronic kidney disease
    Chronic liver disease
    Vitamin D synthetic and vitamin D receptor defects
Altered phosphorus distribution/intracellular shift
  Acute respiratory alkalosis
  Refeeding of malnourished patients, alcoholic patients
  Hungry bone syndrome (after parathyroidectomy)
Hypophosphatemia resulting from multiple mechanisms
  Alcoholism
  Diabetic ketoacidosis, insulin therapy
  Miscellaneous
    Tumor consumption of phosphate: leukemia blast crisis, lymphoma
    Sepsis
    Heat stroke and hyperthermia

associated with hyperphosphatemia because of a decreased ability of the kidney to excrete phosphorus. However, some patients with secondary hyperparathyroidism, decreased intestinal calcium absorption, and vitamin D deficiency may have hypophosphatemia.

Increased Production or Activity of Phosphatonins. There are several rare syndromes of renal phosphate wasting with rickets or osteomalacia, but without vitamin D deficiency and without hypocalcemia, that are due to increased production or activity of FGF-23 or other phosphatonins.[353]

X-Linked Hypophosphatemia. X-linked hypophosphatemia (XLH; MIM 307800) is a rare X-linked dominant disorder characterized by hypophosphatemia, rickets and osteomalacia, growth retardation, decreased intestinal calcium and phosphate absorption, and decreased renal phosphate reabsorption.

Serum 1,25(OH)$_2$D levels are inappropriately normal or low, and calcium and PTH levels are normal. The prevalence of the disease is 1 per 20,000, penetrance is high, and

both females and males are affected.[354] The gene responsible, phosphate-regulating gene with homology to endopeptidases on the X chromosome (*PHEX*) was identified by positional cloning.[355] Its function is still unclear.[353] *PHEX* is predominantly expressed in bone.[356] It is involved in some way in the negative regulation of FGF-23,[357] so *PHEX* mutations lead to increased serum phosphatonin activity and increased urine phosphate excretion. Abnormal synthesis of 1,25(OH)$_2$D in XLH can be explained by increased activity of FGF-23, which leads to downregulation of 1α-hydroxylase.[358] Treatment of XLH patients with oral phosphate and calcitriol improves their growth rate. Treatment does not reduce renal phosphate excretion, but the major goal of therapy is to allow normal growth and reduce bone pain.[359]

Autosomal Dominant Hypophosphatemic Rickets. Autosomal dominant hypophosphatemic rickets (ADHR; MIM 193100) is an extremely rare disorder of phosphate wasting. The phenotype is similar to that of XLH. Some individuals are initially seen in childhood with lower-extremity deformities, as well as rickets and phosphate wasting. Others have bone pain, weakness, and phosphate wasting as adolescents or adults. In some individuals with early-onset disease, the phosphate wasting resolves after puberty.

The ADHR locus was mapped to chromosome band 12p13.3 and identified as the gene encoding FGF-23.[360] Missense mutations in FGF-23 appear to interfere with its proteolytic cleavage by furin or other subtilisin-like proprotein convertases,[357,361,362] causing prolonged or enhanced FGF-23 action on the kidney and phosphate wasting. Treatment is with phosphate replacement and calcitriol, similar to that for patients with XLH.

Tumor-Induced Osteomalacia. Tumor-induced osteomalacia (TIO), or oncogenic osteomalacia, is an acquired paraneoplastic syndrome of renal phosphate wasting. Most commonly this syndrome presents in adults in their sixth decade and has a protracted course. Hypophosphatemia with normal serum calcium and PTH levels, renal Pi wasting, low calcitriol levels, and decreased bone mineralization are the hallmarks of TIO.[363] It is caused by mesenchymal tumors that express and secrete FGF-23.[364] Other phosphatonin factors have been identified, including matrix extracellular phosphoglycoprotein (MEPE), frizzled-related protein 4 (FRP-4), and FGF-7.[365]

The definitive treatment of TIO is complete resection. However, the mesenchymal tumors are often small and difficult to localize. Therefore, medical management with phosphate supplementation and calcitriol is frequently necessary to improve bone healing. Cinacalcet has also been used with good response to induce hypoparathyroidism and to decrease phosphate wasting.[366]

Disorders of Proximal Tubule Phosphate Reabsorption
Hereditary Hypophosphatemic Rickets with Hypercalciuria. Hereditary hypophosphatemic rickets with hypercalciuria (HHRH; MIM 241530) is a rare autosomal recessive syndrome characterized by rickets, short stature, renal phosphate wasting, and hypercalciuria. HHRH is caused by mutations in *SLC34A3*, the gene encoding the NaPi-IIc cotransporter.[367] Patients have an appropriate elevation in 1,25(OH)$_2$D levels, which results in hypercalciuria. Patients are treated with phosphorus supplementation. A similar autosomal recessive disorder has been described in

two patients with loss-of-function mutations in the *SLC34A1* (*NPT2*) gene, which encodes the NaPi-IIa cotransporter. However, unlike patients with HHRH, these patients also had Fanconi's syndrome (see next section).[368]

Fanconi's Syndrome. Fanconi's syndrome is a disorder characterized by defects in the proximal tubular reabsorption of glucose, phosphate, calcium, amino acids, bicarbonate, uric acid, and other organic compounds.[369] The syndrome can be either genetic or acquired. Inherited causes of Fanconi's syndrome include cystinosis, tyrosinemia, and Wilson's disease. Acquired causes include monoclonal gammopathies, amyloidosis, collagen vascular diseases, kidney transplant rejection, and exposure to many drugs or toxins such as heavy metals, antineoplastic agents, antiretroviral agents, aminoglycosides, and anticonvulsants.[370,371] Severe hypophosphatemia in Fanconi's syndrome can lead to rickets or osteomalacia.

Renal Transplantation. Hypophosphatemia is observed in up to 90% of patients after kidney transplantation.[372,373] It is typically mild to moderate, and mostly occurs during the first weeks after surgery, but it may last up to 12 months and occasionally persists for many years.[372] These patients have phosphaturia and a decreased TmP/GFR ratio with well-preserved GFR. The causes of posttransplant hypophosphatemia include persistent (tertiary) hyperparathyroidism,[372] excess of FGF-23 in posttransplant period,[374] 25(OH)D and 1,25(OH)$_2$D deficiency, and immunosuppressive medications.[375]

Pretransplant levels of PTH and FGF-23 predict the severity of hypophosphatemia, and the hormones may act synergistically to increase phosphaturia.[376] It seems likely that in some patients the leading factor for phosphate wasting is PTH, whereas in others it is FGF-23. Cinacalcet has been found to correct urinary phosphate wasting and normalize Pi concentration in kidney transplant recipients by decreasing PTH without affecting high levels of FGF-23.[377] The major consequence of posttransplant hypophosphatemia is progressive bone loss and osteomalacia. Management of posttransplant hypophosphatemia concentrates on replacement of phosphate, correction of vitamin D deficiency, and treatment of hyperparathyroidism.

Drug-Induced Hypophosphatemia. There is an extensive and growing list of medications that can cause hypophosphatemia and phosphate urinary losses as part of Fanconi's syndrome, as discussed earlier, or by affecting only NaPi transporters in the kidney. Diuretics, including acetazolamide, loop diuretics, and some thiazides with carbonic anhydrase activity, such as metozalone, can increase phosphaturia. The volume contraction that accompanies the use of diuretics usually stimulates proximal tubular NaPi reabsorption and prevents the development of severe hypophosphatemia. Conversely, volume expansion with saline can cause phosphaturia and hypophosphatemia.[378] Corticosteroids both decrease intestinal phosphorus absorption and increase renal phosphorus excretion and thus may cause mild to moderate hypophosphatemia.[379] Hypophosphatemia has been reported in patients treated for malignancies with many of the novel tyrosine kinase inhibitors, including imatinib (50%)[380] and sorafenib (13%).[381] The mechanism is thought to be inhibition of Ca and Pi resorption from bone, together with secondary hyperparathyroidism leading to phosphaturia.[382] Parenteral iron administration has been associated with hypophosphatemia, phosphate wasting,

and inhibition of 1α-hydroxylation of vitamin D,[383] which were found to be mediated by an increase in FGF-23.[384] Hypophosphatemia has also been reported in acetaminophen toxicity, but the mechanism is not clear. Finally, the administration of large doses of estrogens in patients with metastatic prostate carcinoma can also produce hypophosphatemia.[385]

Miscellaneous Causes. Significant urinary losses of phosphate may lead to hypophosphatemia during recovery from acute tubular necrosis and during recovery from obstructive uropathy. Postoperative hypophosphatemia has been reported after liver resection, colorectal surgery, aortic bypass, and cardiothoracic surgery.[386-388] Posthepatectomy hypophosphatemia appears to be due to a transient increase in the renal fractional excretion of phosphate, rather than to increased metabolic demand by the regenerative liver.[389]

DECREASED INTESTINAL ABSORPTION

Malnutrition. Malnutrition and low phosphate intake are not a common cause of hypophosphatemia. Increased renal reabsorption of phosphorus can compensate for all but the most severe decreases in oral phosphate intake. However, if phosphate deprivation is prolonged and severe (<100 mg/day) or if it coexists with diarrhea, the continued colonic secretion of phosphate can lead to hypophosphatemia. Hypophosphatemia seen in children with protein malnutrition and kwashiorkor was found to be associated with increased mortality.[390]

Malabsorption. More common is hypophosphatemia resulting from malabsorption. Most phosphorus absorption occurs in the duodenum and jejunum, and intestinal disorders affecting the small intestine may lead to hypophosphatemia.[391] Phosphate-binding cations such as aluminium, calcium, magnesium, and iron form complexes with phosphorus in gastrointestinal tract, which results in decreased phosphate absorption. Hypophosphatemia can develop quickly, even in patients given a relatively moderate but sustained dosage. When combined with poor nutritional intake or extensive dialysis, this may result in overshoot hypophosphatemia. Prolonged use of phosphate-binding antacids can lead to clinically significant osteomalacia.[392]

Vitamin D–Mediated Disorders. Vitamin D is critical for normal control of phosphorus. Deficiency of vitamin D leads to decreased intestinal absorption of phosphorus. In addition, vitamin D deficiency leads to hypocalcemia, hyperparathyroidism, and a consequent PTH-mediated increase in renal phosphorus excretion. The vitamin D deficiency and vitamin D resistance syndromes characterized by hypophosphatemia, hypocalcemia, and bone disease were discussed earlier in this chapter in the section on hypocalcemia.

REDISTRIBUTION OF PHOSPHATE

Redistribution of phosphate from the extracellular space into cells is a common cause of hypophosphatemia in hospitalized patients. This shift of phosphate occurs due to various mechanisms, including elevated levels of insulin, glucose, and catecholamines; respiratory alkalosis; increased cell production (leukemia blast crisis, lymphoma); and rapid bone mineralization (hungry bone syndrome).

Respiratory Alkalosis. The fall in carbon dioxide during acute respiratory alkalosis causes carbon dioxide diffusion from the intracellular space, increases intracellular pH, and stimulates glycolysis. The consequent increase in formation of phosphorylated carbohydrates leads to a fall in extracellular phosphorus levels.[393] When the alkalosis is prolonged and severe, phosphorus levels can drop below 1 mg/dL.[394] Mild hypophosphatemia may occur in patients with asthma during the increased ventilation after treatment of an acute asthma episode[395] and in patients with panic disorders with intermittent hypocapnia. Hypophosphatemia is common in mechanically ventilated patients, particularly if they are also receiving glucose infusions. The urinary phosphate excretion can drop to undetectable levels, which indicates maximal urinary Pi reabsorption. This drop in phosphaturia contrasts with the high urine phosphate excretion and hypophosphatemia that may be observed with metabolic alkalosis from sodium bicarbonate administration.

Refeeding Syndrome. In chronically malnourished individuals, rapid refeeding can result in significant hypophosphatemia. The incidence of refeeding-related hypophosphatemia is quite high in hospitalized patients receiving parenteral nutrition, as high as one in three in one series.[396,397] Risk factors for refeeding syndrome include eating disorders, chronic alcoholism, kwashiorkor, cancer, and diabetes mellitus.[396] Refeeding after even very short periods of starvation can lead to hypophosphatemia.[397] The mechanism is related to insulin-induced increases in cellular phosphate uptake and utilization. The maintenance of serum Pi in the normal range is essential in the management of refeeding syndrome. Adequate phosphate in the parenteral nutrition formulation (20 to 30 mmol of Pi per liter) generally prevents this complication. Even higher amounts may be required in patients with diabetes or chronic alcoholism.

Hypophosphatemia Resulting from Multiple Mechanisms

Alcoholism. Hypophosphatemia and phosphate depletion are particularly common and often a severe problem in alcoholic patients with poor intake, vitamin D deficiency, and heavy use of phosphate-bindinsg antacids.[398] Alcohol-induced proximal tubule dysfunction also contributes to phosphate depletion.[210] Alcoholic patients frequently develop acute respiratory alkalosis due to alcohol withdrawal, sepsis, or cirrhosis. Phosphorus deficiency is often not manifested as hypophosphatemia at the initial evaluation for medical care. Typically, refeeding or administration of intravenous glucose (or both) in this patient population stimulates shifts of phosphorus into cells and thereby uncovers severe hypophosphatemia. Hypophosphatemic alcoholics are at high risk for development of rhabdomyolysis.[345]

Diabetic Ketoacidosis. In uncontrolled diabetes, phosphates are released from cells. These appear in the urine because concomitant glycosuria, ketonuria, acidosis, and osmotic diuresis all increase urinary phosphate excretion.[399] Although serum phosphate levels may be normal, total phosphate stores are usually low. The metabolic syndrome is also associated with hypophosphatemia.[400] During treatment of diabetic ketoacidosis, the development of hypophosphatemia is extremely common.[401] Administration of insulin stimulates the cellular uptake of phosphorus, and thus the serum phosphate level can fall dramatically with treatment.[328] However, routine administration of phosphate in this setting before the development of hypophosphatemia is discouraged, because it may lead to significant hypocalcemia.[402] Phosphate depletion can itself be a cause of insulin resistance, and decreases in insulin

requirements have been observed after phosphate replacement therapy.[400,403]

Miscellaneous Conditions. Moderate, and at times severe, hypophosphatemia may be observed in acute leukemia, in the leukemic phases of lymphomas,[404] and during hematopoietic reconstitution after stem cells transplantation.[405] Rapid cell growth with consequent phosphorus utilization is very likely responsible for the drop in extracellular phosphorus. Hypophosphatemia was observed in toxic shock syndrome[406] and in sepsis,[407] but the complicated clinical picture in septic patients makes it difficult to attribute the hypophosphatemia to a unique mechanism. Rapid volume expansion diminishes proximal tubule sodium phosphate reabsorption and may lead to transient hypophosphatemia.[378] Hypophosphatemia is seen in patients with heat stroke, as well as those with hyperthermia, mainly due to increased renal phosphorus excretion.

Treatment

The first step in the management of hypophosphatemia is to establish the cause of the low Pi concentration, followed by determination of whether Pi replacement is needed. There is little evidence that mild hypophosphatemia (2.0 to 2.5 mg/dL) has significant clinical consequences in humans or that aggressive Pi replacement is needed in such cases. This is particularly true when Pi shift is the major cause of the hypophosphatemia. Patients with symptomatic hypophosphatemia and phosphate depletion do require replacement therapy. Severe hypophosphatemia, with a plasma Pi concentration of less than 1 mg/dL, even in the absence of phosphate depletion, requires intravenous phosphate therapy.

Since the serum level of phosphorus may not be a good reflection of total body stores, it is essentially impossible to predict the amount of phosphorus necessary to correct phosphorus deficiency and hypophosphatemia.[408] In chronically malnourished patients (e.g., anorectic and alcoholic patients), significant phosphorus replenishment will be necessary, whereas in patients who are hypophosphatemic from other causes (antacid ingestion, acetazolamide use), correction of the underlying problem may be sufficient.

Phosphate can be administered either orally or parenterally. In mild or moderate hypophosphatemia, oral replenishment with low-fat milk (containing 0.9 mg Pi per milliliter) is well tolerated and effective. Alternatively, oral sodium or potassium phosphate tablets containing 250 mg (8 mmol) of phosphorus can be ordered. A typical patient with moderate or severe hypophosphatemia will probably need 1000 to 2000 mg (32 to 64 mmol) of phosphorus per day for body stores to be replenished within 7 to 10 days. Side effects include diarrhea, hyperkalemia, and volume overload.

Intravenous phosphorus replacement is generally reserved for individuals with severe (<1 mg/dL) hypophosphatemia. Various regimens are used in clinical practice, all based on uncontrolled observational studies. Some are more conservative in the amount of phosphate delivered to avoid side effects, which may include renal failure, hypocalcemic tetany, and hyperphosphatemia. One standard regimen is to administer 2.5 mg/kg of body mass of elemental phosphorus (0.08 mmol/kg of phosphate) over a 6-hour period for severe asymptomatic hypophosphatemia and 5 mg/kg of body mass of elemental phosphorus (0.16 mmol/kg of phosphate) over a 6-hour period for severe symptomatic hypophosphatemia.[409] A more intensive regimen is 10 mg/kg of body mass (0.32 mmol/kg of phosphate) administered over 12 hours.[410] Even with this regimen, however, only 58% of treated patients achieved serum Pi levels above 2 mg/dL. A graded dosing scheme for intravenous phosphate replacement (0.16 mmol/kg over 4 to 6 hours, 0.32 mmol/kg over 4 to 6 hours, and 0.64 mmol/kg over 6 to 8 hours for serum Pi concentrations of 2.1 to 2.5 mg/dL, 1.5 to 2.0 mg/dL, and <1.5 mg/dL, respectively) was used effectively to treat ICU patients without renal dysfunction and hypercalcemia.[411] Other intensive phosphate-replacement regimens have been reported and have been found to be effective and safe in the ICU for treatment of selected patients with severe hypophosphatemia.[337]

References

1. Nordin BE. Nutritional considerations. In: Nordin BE, ed. *Calcium, phosphate, and magnesium metabolism.* Edinburgh: Churchill Livingstone; 1976:1-112.
2. Elin RJ. Laboratory reference intervals and values. In: Goldman L, Ausiello D, eds. *Cecil medicine.* Philadelphia: Saunders; 2008:2983-2996.
3. Enders DB, Rude RK. Disorders of the bone. In: Burtis CA, Ashwood ER, Burns MD, eds. *Tietz fundamentals of clinical chemistry.* Philadelphia: Saunders; 2008:711-734.
4. Portale AA. Blood calcium, phosphorus, and magnesium. In: Favus MJ, ed. *Primer on the metabolic bone diseases and disorders of mineral metabolism.* Philadelphia: Lippincott Williams & Wilkins; 1999:115-118.
5. Moore EW. Ionized calcium in normal serum, ultrafiltrates, and whole blood determined by ion-exchange electrodes. *J Clin Invest.* 1970;49(2):318-334.
6. Correcting the calcium. *Br Med J.* 1977;1(6061):598.
7. Clase CM, Norman GL, Beecroft ML, et al. Albumin-corrected calcium and ionized calcium in stable haemodialysis patients. *Nephrol Dial Transplant.* 2000;15(11):1841-1846.
8. Jain A, Bhayana S, Vlasschaert M, et al. A formula to predict corrected calcium in haemodialysis patients. *Nephrol Dial Transplant.* 2008;23(9):2884-2888.
9. Ladenson JH, Lewis JW, Boyd JC. Failure of total calcium corrected for protein, albumin, and pH to correctly assess free calcium status. *J Clin Endocrinol Metab.* 1978;46(6):986-993.
10. Gauci C, Moranne O, Fouqueray B, et al. Pitfalls of measuring total blood calcium in patients with CKD. *J Am Soc Nephrol.* 2008;19(8):1592-1598.
11. Frolich A. Prevalence of hypercalcaemia in normal and in hospital populations. *Dan Med Bull.* 1998;45(4):436-439.
12. Motoyama HI, Friedman PA. Calcium-sensing receptor regulation of PTH-dependent calcium absorption by mouse cortical ascending limbs. *Am J Physiol Renal Physiol.* 2002;283(3):F399-F406.
13. Stewart AF. Clinical practice. Hypercalcemia associated with cancer. *N Engl J Med.* 2005;352(4):373-379.
14. Lind L, Skarfors E, Berglund L, et al. Serum calcium: a new, independent, prospective risk factor for myocardial infarction in middle-aged men followed for 18 years. *J Clin Epidemiol.* 1997;50(8):967-973.
15. Kinder BK, Stewart AF. Hypercalcemia. *Curr Probl Surg.* 2002;39(4):349-448.
16. Bilezikian JP, Silverberg SJ. Clinical spectrum of primary hyperparathyroidism. *Rev Endocr Metab Disord.* 2000;1(4):237-245.
17. Silverberg SJ, Lewiecki EM, Mosekilde L, et al. Presentation of asymptomatic primary hyperparathyroidism: proceedings of the third international workshop. *J Clin Endocrinol Metab.* 2009;94(2):351-365.
18. Lundgren E, Rastad J, Thrufjell E, et al. Population-based screening for primary hyperparathyroidism with serum calcium and parathyroid hormone values in menopausal women. *Surgery.* 1997;121(3):287-294.
19. Melton 3rd LJ. The epidemiology of primary hyperparathyroidism in North America. *J Bone Miner Res.* 2002;17(suppl 2):N12-N17.
20. Wermers RA, Khosla S, Atkinson EJ, et al. The rise and fall of primary hyperparathyroidism: a population-based study in Rochester, Minnesota, 1965-1992. *Ann Intern Med.* 1997;126(6):433-440.
21. Wermers RA, Khosla S, Atkinson EJ, et al. Incidence of primary hyperparathyroidism in Rochester, Minnesota, 1993-2001: an update on the changing epidemiology of the disease. *J Bone Miner Res.* 2006;21(1):171-177.
22. Marcocci C, Cetani F, Rubin MR, et al. Parathyroid carcinoma. *J Bone Miner Res.* 2008;23(12):1869-1880.
23. DeLellis RA, Mazzaglia P, Mangray S. Primary hyperparathyroidism: a current perspective. *Arch Pathol Lab Med.* 2008;132(8):1251-1262.
24. Hsi ED, Zukerberg LR, Yang WI, et al. Cyclin D1/PRAD1 expression in parathyroid adenomas: an immunohistochemical study. *J Clin Endocrinol Metab.* 1996;81(5):1736-1739.
25. Hemmer S, Wasenius VM, Haglund C, et al. Deletion of 11q23 and cyclin D1 overexpression are frequent aberrations in parathyroid adenomas. *Am J Pathol.* 2001;158(4):1355-1362.
26. Heppner C, Kester MB, Agarwal SK, et al. Somatic mutation of the MEN1 gene in parathyroid tumours. *Nat Genet.* 1997;16(4):375-378.
27. Farnebo F, Teh BT, Kytola S, et al. Alterations of the MEN1 gene in sporadic parathyroid tumors. *J Clin Endocrinol Metab.* 1998;83(8):2627-2630.
28. Rubin MR, Bilezikian JP, McMahon DJ, et al. The natural history of primary hyperparathyroidism with or without parathyroid surgery after 15 years. *J Clin Endocrinol Metab.* 2008;93(9):3462-3470.
29. Bilezikian JP, Khan AA, Potts Jr JT. Guidelines for the management of asymptomatic primary hyperparathyroidism: summary statement from the third international workshop. *J Clin Endocrinol Metab.* 2009;94(2):335-339.
30. Udelsman R, Pasieka JL, Sturgeon C, et al. Surgery for asymptomatic primary hyperparathyroidism: proceedings of the third international workshop. *J Clin Endocrinol Metab.* 2009;94(2):366-372.
31. Rudberg C, Akerstrom G, Palmer M, et al. Late results of operation for primary hyperparathyroidism in 441 patients. *Surgery.* 1986;99(6):643-651.
32. Khan A, Grey A, Shoback D. Medical management of asymptomatic primary hyperparathyroidism: proceedings of the third international workshop. *J Clin Endocrinol Metab.* 2009;94(2):373-381.
33. Silverberg SJ, Bone 3rd HG, Marriott TB, et al. Short-term inhibition of parathyroid hormone secretion by a calcium-receptor agonist in patients with primary hyperparathyroidism. *N Engl J Med.* 1997;337(21):1506-1510.
34. Peacock M, Bilezikian JP, Klassen PS, et al. Cinacalcet hydrochloride maintains long-term normocalcemia in patients with primary hyperparathyroidism. *J Clin Endocrinol Metab.* 2005;90(1):135-141.
35. Peacock M, Bolognese MA, Borofsky M, et al. Cinacalcet treatment of primary hyperparathyroidism: biochemical and bone densitometric outcomes in a five-year study. *J Clin Endocrinol Metab.* 2009;94(12):4860-4867.
36. Anderson BJ, Samaan NA, Vassilopoulou-Sellin R, et al. Parathyroid carcinoma: features and difficulties in diagnosis and management. *Surgery.* 1983;94(6):906-915.
37. Hoelting T, Weber T, Werner J, et al. Surgical treatment of parathyroid carcinoma (Review). *Oncol Rep.* 2001;8(4):931-934.
38. Stewart AF, Broadus AE. Malignancy-associated hypercalcemia. In: DeGroot LJ, Jameson JL, eds. *Endocrinology.* Philadelphia: Saunders; 2006.
39. Horwitz MJ, Hodak SP, Stewart AF. Non-parathyroid hypercalcemia. In: Rosen CJ, Compston JE, Lian JB, eds. *Primer on the metabolic bone diseases and disorders of mineral metabolism.* Hoboken, NJ: Wiley; 2008:307-312.
40. Kremer R, Shustik C, Tabak T, et al. Parathyroid-hormone-related peptide in hematologic malignancies. *Am J Med.* 1996;100(4):406-411.
41. Mundy GR, Edwards JR. PTH-related peptide (PTHrP) in hypercalcemia. *J Am Soc Nephrol.* 2008;19(4):672-675.
42. Wysolmerski JJ. Parathyroid hormone-related protein. In: Rosen CJ, Compston JE, Lian JB, eds. *Primer on the metabolic bone diseases and disorders of mineral metabolism.* Hoboken, NJ: Wiley; 2008:127-133.
43. Stewart AF, Mangin M, Wu T, et al. Synthetic human parathyroid hormone-like protein stimulates bone resorption and causes hypercalcemia in rats. *J Clin Invest.* 1988;81(2):596-600.
44. Karaplis AC, Luz A, Glowacki J, et al. Lethal skeletal dysplasia from targeted disruption of the parathyroid hormone-related peptide gene. *Genes Dev.* 1994;8(3):277-289.
45. Edwards CM, Zhuang J, Mundy GR. The pathogenesis of the bone disease of multiple myeloma. *Bone.* 2008;42(6):1007-1013.
46. Kakonen SM, Mundy GR. Mechanisms of osteolytic bone metastases in breast carcinoma. *Cancer.* 2003;97(3 suppl):834-839.
47. Grill V, Ho P, Body JJ, et al. Parathyroid hormone-related protein: elevated levels in both humoral hypercalcemia of malignancy and hypercalcemia complicating metastatic breast cancer. *J Clin Endocrinol Metab.* 1991;73(6):1309-1315.
48. Durie BG, Salmon SE, Mundy GR. Relation of osteoclast activating factor production to extent of bone disease in multiple myeloma. *Br J Haematol.* 1981;47(1):21-30.
49. Kyle RA, Yee GC, Somerfield MR, et al. American Society of Clinical Oncology 2007 clinical practice guideline update on the role of bisphosphonates in multiple myeloma. *J Clin Oncol.* 2007;25(17):2464-2472.
50. Breslau NA, McGuire JL, Zerwekh JE, et al. Hypercalcemia associated with increased serum calcitriol levels in three patients with lymphoma. *Ann Intern Med.* 1984;100(1):1-6.

51. Seymour JF, Gagel RF, Hagemeister FB, et al. Calcitriol production in hypercalcemic and normocalcemic patients with non-Hodgkin lymphoma. *Ann Intern Med.* 1994;121(9):633-640.

52. Nussbaum SR, Gaz RD, Arnold A. Hypercalcemia and ectopic secretion of parathyroid hormone by an ovarian carcinoma with rearrangement of the gene for parathyroid hormone. *N Engl J Med.* 1990;323(19):1324-1328.

53. Heath DA. Familial hypocalciuric hypercalcemia. *Rev Endocr Metab Disord.* 2000;1(4):291-296.

54. Marx SJ, Attie MF, Levine MA, et al. The hypocalciuric or benign variant of familial hypercalcemia: clinical and biochemical features in fifteen kindreds. *Medicine (Baltimore).* 1981;60(6):397-412.

55. Hinnie J, Bell E, McKillop E, et al. The prevalence of familial hypocalciuric hypercalcemia. *Calcif Tissue Int.* 2001;68(4):216-218.

56. Jackson CE, Boonstra CE. Hereditary hypercalcemia and parathyroid hyperplasia without definite hyperparathyroidism. *J Lab Clin Med.* 1966;68:883.

57. Foley Jr TP, Harrison HC, Arnaud CD, et al. Familial benign hypercalcemia. *J Pediatr.* 1972;81(6):1060-1067.

58. Egbuna OI, Brown EM. Hypercalcaemic and hypocalcaemic conditions due to calcium-sensing receptor mutations. *Best Pract Res Clin Rheumatol.* 2008;22(1):129-148.

59. Attie MF, Gill Jr JR, Stock JL, et al. Urinary calcium excretion in familial hypocalciuric hypercalcemia. Persistence of relative hypocalciuria after induction of hypoparathyroidism. *J Clin Invest.* 1983;72(2):667-676.

60. Pollak MR, Seidman CE, Brown EM. Three inherited disorders of calcium sensing. *Medicine (Baltimore).* 1996;75(3):115-123.

61. Hendy GN, D'Souza-Li L, Yang B, et al. Mutations of the calcium-sensing receptor (CASR) in familial hypocalciuric hypercalcemia, neonatal severe hyperparathyroidism, and autosomal dominant hypocalcemia. *Hum Mutat.* 2000;16(4):281-296.

62. Bai M, Quinn S, Trivedi S, et al. Expression and characterization of inactivating and activating mutations in the human Ca^{2+}-sensing receptor. *J Biol Chem.* 1996;271(32):19537-19545.

63. Bai M, Pearce SH, Kifor O, et al. In vivo and in vitro characterization of neonatal hyperparathyroidism resulting from a de novo, heterozygous mutation in the Ca^{2+}-sensing receptor gene: normal maternal calcium homeostasis as a cause of secondary hyperparathyroidism in familial benign hypocalciuric hypercalcemia. *J Clin Invest.* 1997;99(1):88-96.

64. Bai M, Janicic N, Trivedi S, et al. Markedly reduced activity of mutant calcium-sensing receptor with an inserted Alu element from a kindred with familial hypocalciuric hypercalcemia and neonatal severe hyperparathyroidism. *J Clin Invest.* 1997;99(8):1917-1925.

65. Timmers HJ, Karperien M, Hamdy NA, et al. Normalization of serum calcium by cinacalcet in a patient with hypercalcaemia due to a de novo inactivating mutation of the calcium-sensing receptor. *J Intern Med.* 2006;260(2):177-182.

66. Lu JY, Yang Y, Gnacadja G, et al. Effect of the calcimimetic R-568 [3-(2-chlorophenyl)-N-((1R)-1-(3-methoxyphenyl)ethyl)-1-propanamine] on correcting inactivating mutations in the human calcium-sensing receptor. *J Pharmacol Exp Ther.* 2009;331(3):775-786.

67. Pollak MR, Brown EM, Chou YH, et al. Mutations in the human Ca^{2+}-sensing receptor gene cause familial hypocalciuric hypercalcemia and neonatal severe hyperparathyroidism. *Cell.* 1993;75(7):1297-1303.

68. Pollak MR, Chou YH, Marx SJ, et al. Familial hypocalciuric hypercalcemia and neonatal severe hyperparathyroidism. Effects of mutant gene dosage on phenotype. *J Clin Invest.* 1994;93(3):1108-1112.

69. Guo SS, Sawicki MP. Molecular and genetic mechanisms of tumorigenesis in multiple endocrine neoplasia type-1. *Mol Endocrinol.* 2001;15(10):1653-1664.

70. Brandi ML, Gagel RF, Angeli A, et al. Guidelines for diagnosis and therapy of MEN type 1 and type 2. *J Clin Endocrinol Metab.* 2001;86(12):5658-5671.

71. Lemmens I, Van de Ven WJ, Kas K, et al. Identification of the multiple endocrine neoplasia type 1 (MEN1) gene. The European Consortium on MEN1. *Hum Mol Genet.* 1997;6(7):1177-1183.

72. Marx SJ, Agarwal SK, Kester MB, et al. Germline and somatic mutation of the gene for multiple endocrine neoplasia type 1 (MEN1). *J Intern Med.* 1998;243(6):447-453.

73. Donis-Keller H, Dou S, Chi D, et al. Mutations in the RET proto-oncogene are associated with MEN 2A and FMTC. *Hum Mol Genet.* 1993;2(7):851-856.

74. Jackson CE, Norum RA, Boyd SB, et al. Hereditary hyperparathyroidism and multiple ossifying jaw fibromas: a clinically and genetically distinct syndrome. *Surgery.* 1990;108(6):1006-1012:discussion, 1012-1013.

75. Carpten JD, Robbins CM, Villablanca A, et al. HRPT2, encoding parafibromin, is mutated in hyperparathyroidism–jaw tumor syndrome. *Nat Genet.* 2002;32(4):676-680.

76. Burman KD, Monchik JM, Earll JM, et al. Ionized and total serum calcium and parathyroid hormone in hyperthyroidism. *Ann Intern Med.* 1976;84(5):668-671.

77. Chow KM, Szeto CC. An unusual cause of hypercalcemia. *South Med J.* 2004;97(6):588-589.

78. Mundy GR, Shapiro JL, Bandelin JG, et al. Direct stimulation of bone resorption by thyroid hormones. *J Clin Invest.* 1976;58(3):529-534.

79. Stewart AF, Hoecker JL, Mallette LE, et al. Hypercalcemia in pheochromocytoma. Evidence for a novel mechanism. *Ann Intern Med.* 1985;102(6):776-779.

80. Mune T, Katakami H, Kato Y, et al. Production and secretion of parathyroid hormone–related protein in pheochromocytoma: participation of an α-adrenergic mechanism. *J Clin Endocrinol Metab.* 1993;76(3):757-762.

81. Diamond T, Thornley S. Addisonian crisis and hypercalcaemia. *Aust N Z J Med.* 1994;24(3):316.

82. Jacobs TP, Bilezikian JP. Clinical review: rare causes of hypercalcemia. *J Clin Endocrinol Metab.* 2005;90(11):6316-6322.

83. Knox JB, Demling RH, Wilmore DW, et al. Hypercalcemia associated with the use of human growth hormone in an adult surgical intensive care unit. *Arch Surg.* 1995;130(4):442-445.

84. Aloia J, Powell D, Mendizibal E, et al. Parathyroid function in acromegaly. *Horm Res.* 1975;6(3):145-149.

85. Nadarajah A, Hartog M, Redfern B, et al. Calcium metabolism in acromegaly. *Br Med J.* 1968;4(5634):797-801.

86. Ezzat S, Melmed S, Endres D, et al. Biochemical assessment of bone formation and resorption in acromegaly. *J Clin Endocrinol Metab.* 1993;76(6):1452-1457.

87. Jones G. Pharmacokinetics of vitamin D toxicity. *Am J Clin Nutr.* 2008;88(2):582S-586S.

88. Jacobus CH, Holick MF, Shao Q, et al. Hypervitaminosis D associated with drinking milk. *N Engl J Med.* 1992;326(18):1173-1177.

89. Blank S, Scanlon KS, Sinks TH, et al. An outbreak of hypervitaminosis D associated with the overfortification of milk from a home-delivery dairy. *Am J Public Health.* 1995;85(5):656-659.

90. Koutkia P, Chen TC, Holick MF. Vitamin D intoxication associated with an over-the-counter supplement. *N Engl J Med.* 2001;345(1):66-67.

91. Hathcock JN, Shao A, Vieth R, et al. Risk assessment for vitamin D. *Am J Clin Nutr.* 2007;85(1):6-18.

92. Bell NH, Stern PH. Hypercalcemia and increases in serum hormone value during prolonged administration of 1α,25-dihydroxyvitamin D. *N Engl J Med.* 1978;298(22):1241-1243.

93. Garfinkel PE, Ezrin C, Stancer HC. Hypothyroidism and hyperparathyroidism associated with lithium. *Lancet.* 1973;2(7824):331-332.

94. Bendz H, Sjodin I, Toss G, et al. Hyperparathyroidism and long-term lithium therapy—a cross-sectional study and the effect of lithium withdrawal. *J Intern Med.* 1996;240(6):357-365.

95. Szalat A, Mazeh H, Freund HR. Lithium-associated hyperparathyroidism: report of four cases and review of the literature. *Eur J Endocrinol.* 2009;160(2):317-323.

96. Khairallah W, Fawaz A, Brown EM, et al. Hypercalcemia and diabetes insipidus in a patient previously treated with lithium. *Nat Clin Pract Nephrol.* 2007;3(7):397-404.

97. Brown EM. Lithium induces abnormal calcium-regulated PTH release in dispersed bovine parathyroid cells. *J Clin Endocrinol Metab.* 1981;52(5):1046-1048.

98. Mallette LE, Khouri K, Zengotita H, et al. Lithium treatment increases intact and midregion parathyroid hormone and parathyroid volume. *J Clin Endocrinol Metab.* 1989;68(3):654-660.

99. Sloand JA, Shelly MA. Normalization of lithium-induced hypercalcemia and hyperparathyroidism with cinacalcet hydrochloride. *Am J Kidney Dis.* 2006;48(5):832-837.

100. Penniston KL, Tanumihardjo SA. The acute and chronic toxic effects of vitamin A. *Am J Clin Nutr.* 2006;83(2):191-201.

101. Ragavan VV, Smith JE, Bilezikian JP. Vitamin A toxicity and hypercalcemia. *Am J Med Sci.* 1982;283(3):161-164.

102. Bhalla K, Ennis DM, Ennis ED. Hypercalcemia caused by iatrogenic hypervitaminosis A. *J Am Diet Assoc.* 2005;105(1):119-121.

103. Valentic JP, Elias AN, Weinstein GD. Hypercalcemia associated with oral isotretinoin in the treatment of severe acne. *JAMA.* 1983;250(14):1899-1900.

104. Marabelle A, Sapin V, Rousseau R, et al. Hypercalcemia and 13-cis-retinoic acid in post-consolidation therapy of neuroblastoma. *Pediatr Blood Cancer.* 2009;52(2):280-283.

105. Mulvenna PM, Wright AJ, Podd TJ. Life-threatening tamoxifen-induced hypercalcaemia. *Clin Oncol (R Coll Radiol).* 1999;11(3):193-195.

106. Christensson T, Hellstrom K, Wengle B. Hypercalcemia and primary hyperparathyroidism. Prevalence in patients receiving thiazides as detected in a health screen. *Arch Intern Med.* 1977;137(9):1138-1142.

107. Wermers RA, Kearns AE, Jenkins GD, et al. Incidence and clinical spectrum of thiazide-associated hypercalcemia. *Am J Med.* 2007;120(10):911 e9-15.

108. Popovtzer MM, Subryan VL, Alfrey AC, et al. The acute effect of chlorothiazide on serum-ionized calcium. Evidence for a parathyroid hormone–dependent mechanism. *J Clin Invest.* 1975;55(6):1295-1302.

109. Bazzini C, Vezzoli V, Sironi C, et al. Thiazide-sensitive NaCl-cotransporter in the intestine: possible role of hydrochlorothiazide in the intestinal Ca^{2+} uptake. *J Biol Chem.* 2005;280(20):19902-19910.

110. Burnett CH, Commons RR, Albright F, et al. Hypercalcemia without hypercalcuria or hypophosphatemia, calcinosis and renal insufficiency; a syndrome following prolonged intake of milk and alkali. *N Engl J Med.* 1949;240(20):787-794.

111. Felsenfeld AJ, Levine BS. Milk alkali syndrome and the dynamics of calcium homeostasis. *Clin J Am Soc Nephrol.* 2006;1(4):641-654.

112. Beall DP, Henslee HB, Webb HR, et al. Milk-alkali syndrome: a historical review and description of the modern version of the syndrome. *Am J Med Sci.* 2006;331(5):233-242.

113. Picolos MK, Lavis VR, Orlander PR. Milk-alkali syndrome is a major cause of hypercalcaemia among non–end-stage renal disease (non-ESRD) inpatients. *Clin Endocrinol (Oxf).* 2005;63(5):566-576.

114. Stewart AF, Adler M, Byers CM, et al. Calcium homeostasis in immobilization: an example of resorptive hypercalciuria. *N Engl J Med.* 1982;306(19):1136-1140.

115. Minaire P, Neunier P, Edouard C, et al. Quantitative histological data on disuse osteoporosis: comparison with biological data. *Calcif Tissue Res.* 1974;17(1):57-73.

116. Sato Y, Asoh T, Kaji M, et al. Beneficial effect of intermittent cyclical etidronate therapy in hemiplegic patients following an acute stroke. *J Bone Miner Res.* 2000;15(12):2487-2494.

117. Sharma OP. Vitamin D, calcium, and sarcoidosis. *Chest.* 1996;109(2):535-539.

118. Caldwell JW, Arsura EL, Kilgore WB, et al. Hypercalcemia in patients with disseminated coccidioidomycosis. *Am J Med Sci.* 2004;327(1):15-18.

119. Lionakis MS, Samonis G, Kontoyiannis DP. Endocrine and metabolic manifestations of invasive fungal infections and systemic antifungal treatment. *Mayo Clin Proc.* 2008;83(9):1046-1060.

120. Barbour GL, Coburn JW, Slatopolsky E, et al. Hypercalcemia in an anephric patient with sarcoidosis: evidence for extrarenal generation of 1,25-dihydroxyvitamin D. *N Engl J Med.* 1981;305(8):440-443.

121. Mason RS, Frankel T, Chan YL, et al. Vitamin D conversion by sarcoid lymph node homogenate. *Ann Intern Med.* 1984;100(1):59-61.

122. Sandler LM, Winearls CG, Fraher LJ, et al. Studies of the hypercalcaemia of sarcoidosis: effect of steroids and exogenous vitamin D_3 on the circulating concentrations of 1,25-dihydroxy vitamin D_3. *Q J Med.* 1984;53(210):165-180.

123. Adams JS, Sharma OP, Diz MM, et al. Ketoconazole decreases the serum 1,25-dihydroxyvitamin D and calcium concentration in sarcoidosis-associated hypercalcemia. *J Clin Endocrinol Metab.* 1990;70(4):1090-1095.

124. O'Leary TJ, Jones G, Yip A, et al. The effects of chloroquine on serum 1,25-dihydroxyvitamin D and calcium metabolism in sarcoidosis. *N Engl J Med.* 1986;315(12):727-730.

125. Gerhardt A, Greenberg A, Reilly Jr JJ, et al. Hypercalcemia. A complication of advanced chronic liver disease. *Arch Intern Med.* 1987;147(2):274-277.

126. Suki WN, Yium JJ, Von Minden M, et al. Acute treatment of hypercalcemia with furosemide. *N Engl J Med.* 1970;283(16):836-840.

127. LeGrand SB, Leskuski D. Zama, I: Narrative review: furosemide for hypercalcemia: an unproven yet common practice. *Ann Intern Med.* 2008;149(4):259-263.

128. Major P, Lortholary A, Hon J, et al. Zoledronic acid is superior to pamidronate in the treatment of hypercalcemia of malignancy: a pooled analysis of two randomized, controlled clinical trials. *J Clin Oncol.* 2001;19(2):558-567.

129. Perazella MA, Markowitz GS. Bisphosphonate nephrotoxicity. *Kidney Int.* 2008;74(11):1385-1393.

130. Deftos LJ, First BP. Calcitonin as a drug. *Ann Intern Med.* 1981;95(2):192-197.

131. Warrell Jr RP, Israel R, Frisone M, et al. Gallium nitrate for acute treatment of cancer-related hypercalcemia. A randomized, double-blind comparison to calcitonin. *Ann Intern Med.* 1988;108(5):669-674.

132. Cvitkovic F, Armand JP, Tubiana-Hulin M, et al. Randomized, double-blind, phase II trial of gallium nitrate compared with pamidronate for acute control of cancer-related hypercalcemia. *Cancer J.* 2006;12(1):47-53.

133. Camus C, Charasse C, Jouannic-Montier I, et al. Calcium free hemodialysis: experience in the treatment of 33 patients with severe hypercalcemia. *Intensive Care Med.* 1996;22(2):116-121.

134. Kindgen-Milles D, Kram R, Kleinekofort W, et al. Treatment of severe hypercalcemia using continuous renal replacement therapy with regional citrate anticoagulation. *ASAIO J.* 2008;54(4):442-444.

135. Desai TK, Carlson RW, Geheb MA. Prevalence and clinical implications of hypocalcemia in acutely ill patients in a medical intensive care setting. *Am J Med.* 1988;84(2):209-214.

136. Zivin JR, Gooley T, Zager RA, et al. Hypocalcemia: a pervasive metabolic abnormality in the critically ill. *Am J Kidney Dis.* 2001;37(4):689-698.

137. Urbano FL. Signs of hypocalcemia: Chvostek's and Trousseau's signs. *Hosp Physician.* 2000;36:43-45.

138. Connor TB, Rosen BL, Blaustein MP, et al. Hypocalcemia precipitating congestive heart failure. *N Engl J Med.* 1982;307(14):869-872.

139. Kazmi AS, Wall BM. Reversible congestive heart failure related to profound hypocalcemia secondary to hypoparathyroidism. *Am J Med Sci.* 2007;333(4):226-229.

140. Maiya S, Sullivan I, Allgrove J, et al. Hypocalcaemia and vitamin D deficiency: an important, but preventable, cause of life-threatening infant heart failure. *Heart.* 2008;94(5):581-584.

141. Illum F, Dupont E. Prevalences of CT-detected calcification in the basal ganglia in idiopathic hypoparathyroidism and pseudohypoparathyroidism. *Neuroradiology.* 1985;27(1):32-37.

142. Nakamura Y, Matsumoto T, Tamakoshi A, et al. Prevalence of idiopathic hypoparathyroidism and pseudohypoparathyroidism in Japan. *J Epidemiol.* 2000;10(1):29-33.

143. Shoback D. Clinical practice. *Hypoparathyroidism. N Engl J Med.* 2008;359(4):391-403.

144. Shaw N. A practical approach to hypocalcemia in children. In: Allgrove J, Shaw NJ, eds. *Calcium and bone disorders in children and adolescents.* Basel, Switzerland: Karger; 2009:73-92.

145. Pollak MR, Brown EM, Estep HL, et al. Autosomal dominant hypocalcaemia caused by a Ca^{2+}-sensing receptor gene mutation. *Nat Genet.* 1994;8(3):303-307.

146. Pearce SH, Williamson C, Kifor O, et al. A familial syndrome of hypocalcemia with hypercalciuria due to mutations in the calcium-sensing receptor. *N Engl J Med.* 1996;335(15):1115-1122.

147. Lienhardt A, Bai M, Lagarde JP, et al. Activating mutations of the calcium-sensing receptor: management of hypocalcemia. *J Clin Endocrinol Metab.* 2001;86(11):5313-5323.

148. Winer KK, Yanovski JA, Sarani B, et al. A randomized, cross-over trial of once-daily versus twice-daily parathyroid hormone 1-34 in treatment of hypoparathyroidism. *J Clin Endocrinol Metab.* 1998;83(10):3480-3486.

149. Albright F, Burnett CH, Smith PH, et al. Pseudohypoparathyroidism—an example of "Seabright-Bantam syndrome": report of three cases. *Endocrinology.* 1942;30:922-932.

150. Rubin MR, Levine MA. Hypoparathyroidism and pseudohypoparathyroidism. In: Rosen CJ, Compston JE, Lian JB, eds. *Primer on the metabolic bone diseases and disorders of mineral metabolism.* Hoboken, NJ: Wiley; 2008:354-361.

151. Ringel MD, Schwindinger WF, Levine MA. Clinical implications of genetic defects in G proteins. The molecular basis of McCune-Albright syndrome and Albright hereditary osteodystrophy. *Medicine (Baltimore).* 1996;75(4):171-184.

152. Chase LR, Melson GL, Aurbach GD. Pseudohypoparathyroidism: defective excretion of 3',5'-AMP in response to parathyroid hormone. *J Clin Invest.* 1969;48(10):1832-1844.

153. Levine MA, Germain-Lee E. Jan de Beur, S: Genetic basis for resistance to parathyroid hormone. *Horm Res.* 2003;60(suppl 3):87-95.

154. Farfel Z, Brickman AS, Kaslow HR, et al. Defect of receptor-cyclase coupling protein in pseudohypoparathyroidism. *N Engl J Med.* 1980;303(5):237-242.

155. Nakamoto JM, Sandstrom AT, Brickman AS, et al. Pseudo-hypoparathyroidism type Ia from maternal but not paternal transmission of a $G_s\alpha$ gene mutation. *Am J Med Genet.* 1998;77(4):261-267.

156. Bastepe M, Frohlich LF, Hendy GN, et al. Autosomal dominant pseudohypoparathyroidism type Ib is associated with a heterozygous microdeletion that likely disrupts a putative imprinting control element of GNAS. *J Clin Invest.* 2003;112(8):1255-1263.

157. Bastepe M, Frohlich LF, Linglart A, et al. Deletion of the NESP55 differentially methylated region causes loss of maternal GNAS imprints and pseudohypoparathyroidism type Ib. *Nat Genet.* 2005;37(1):25-27.

158. Drezner M, Neelon FA. Lebovitz, HE: Pseudohypoparathyroidism type II: a possible defect in the reception of the cyclic AMP signal. *N Engl J Med.* 1973;289(20):1056-1060.

159. Demeester-Mirkine N, Hooghe L, Van Geertruyden J, et al. Hypocalcemia after thyroidectomy. *Arch Surg.* 1992;127(7):854-858.

160. Yamashita H, Noguchi S, Tahara K, et al. Postoperative tetany in patients with Graves' disease: a risk factor analysis. *Clin Endocrinol (Oxf).* 1997;47(1):71-77.

161. Page C, Strunski V. Parathyroid risk in total thyroidectomy for bilateral, benign, multinodular goitre: report of 351 surgical cases. *J Laryngol Otol.* 2007;121(3):237-241.

162. Brasier AR, Nussbaum SR. Hungry bone syndrome: clinical and biochemical predictors of its occurrence after parathyroid surgery. *Am J Med.* 1988;84(4):654-660.

163. Whitson HE, Lobaugh B, Lyles KW. Severe hypocalcemia following bisphosphonate treatment in a patient with Paget's disease of bone. *Bone.* 2006;39(4):954-958.

164. Lazar ES, Stankus N. Cinacalcet-induced hungry bone syndrome. *Semin Dial.* 2007;20(1):83-85.
165. Angelopoulos NG, Goula A, Rombopoulos G, et al. Hypoparathyroidism in transfusion-dependent patients with β-thalassemia. *J Bone Miner Metab.* 2006;24(2):138-145.
166. Carpenter TO, Carnes Jr DL, Anast. CS: Hypoparathyroidism in Wilson's disease. *N Engl J Med.* 1983;309(15):873-877.
167. Laitinen K, Lamberg-Allardt C, Tunninen R, et al. Transient hypoparathyroidism during acute alcohol intoxication. *N Engl J Med.* 1991;324(11):721-727.
168. Cholst IN, Steinberg SF, Tropper PJ, et al. The influence of hypermagnesemia on serum calcium and parathyroid hormone levels in human subjects. *N Engl J Med.* 1984;310(19):1221-1225.
169. Brown EM, Vassilev PM, Hebert SC. Calcium ions as extracellular messengers. *Cell.* 1995;83(5):679-682.
170. Elisaf M, Milionis H. Siamopoulos, KC: Hypomagnesemic hypokalemia and hypocalcemia: clinical and laboratory characteristics. *Miner Electrolyte Metab.* 1997;23(2):105-112.
171. Rude RK, Oldham SB, Singer FR. Functional hypoparathyroidism and parathyroid hormone end-organ resistance in human magnesium deficiency. *Clin Endocrinol (Oxf).* 1976;5(3):209-224.
172. Quitterer U, Hoffmann M, Freichel M, et al. Paradoxical block of parathormone secretion is mediated by increased activity of G alpha subunits. *J Biol Chem.* 2001;276(9):6763-6769.
173. Holick MF. Resurrection of vitamin D deficiency and rickets. *J Clin Invest.* 2006;116(8):2062-2072.
174. *Dietary supplement fact sheet: vitamin D.* Bethesda, Md: National Institutes of Health, Office of Dietary Supplements; 2009.
175. Honasoge M, Rao DS. Metabolic bone disease in gastrointestinal, hepatobiliary, and pancreatic disorders and total parenteral nutrition. *Curr Opin Rheumatol.* 1995;7(3):249-254.
176. Morgan DB, Paterson CR, Woods CG, et al. Search for osteomalacia in 1228 patients after gastrectomy and other operations on the stomach. *Lancet.* 1965;2(7422):1085-1088.
177. Thomas MK, Lloyd-Jones DM, Thadhani RI, et al. Hypovitaminosis D in medical inpatients. *N Engl J Med.* 1998;338(12):777-783.
178. Hajjar ET, Vincenti F, Salti IS. Gluten-induced enteropathy. Osteomalacia as its principal manifestation. *Arch Intern Med.* 1974;134(3):565-566.
179. Parfitt AM, Miller MJ, Frame B, et al. Metabolic bone disease after intestinal bypass for treatment of obesity. *Ann Intern Med.* 1978;89(2):193-199.
180. Hahn TJ. Drug-induced disorders of vitamin D and mineral metabolism. *Clin Endocrinol Metab.* 1980;9(1):107-127.
181. Crippin JS, Jorgensen RA, Dickson ER, et al. Hepatic osteodystrophy in primary biliary cirrhosis: effects of medical treatment. *Am J Gastroenterol.* 1994;89(1):47-50.
182. Barragry JM, France MW, Carter ND, et al. Vitamin-D metabolism in nephrotic syndrome. *Lancet.* 1977;2(8039):629-632.
183. Singh J, Moghal N, Pearce SH, et al. The investigation of hypocalcaemia and rickets. *Arch Dis Child.* 2003;88(5):403-407.
184. Preece MA, Tomlinson S, Ribot CA, et al. *Studies of vitamin D deficiency in man.* Q J Med. 1975;44(176):575-589.
185. Kitanaka S, Takeyama K, Murayama A, et al. Inactivating mutations in the 25-hydroxyvitamin D₃ 1α-hydroxylase gene in patients with pseudovitamin D–deficiency rickets. *N Engl J Med.* 1998;338(10):653-661.
186. Brooks MH, Bell NH, Love L, et al. Vitamin-D–dependent rickets type II. Resistance of target organs to 1,25-dihydroxyvitamin D. *N Engl J Med.* 1978;298(18):996-999.
187. Haussler MR, Haussler CA, Jurutka PW, et al. The vitamin D hormone and its nuclear receptor: molecular actions and disease states. *J Endocrinol.* 1997;154(suppl):S57-S73.
188. Liamis G, Milionis HJ. Elisaf, M: A review of drug-induced hypocalcemia. *J Bone Miner Metab.* 2009;27(6):635-642.
189. Prince MR, Erel HE, Lent RW, et al. Gadodiamide administration causes spurious hypocalcemia. *Radiology.* 2003;227(3):639-646.
190. Subbiah V, Tayek JA. Tetany secondary to the use of a proton-pump inhibitor. *Ann Intern Med.* 2002;137(3):219.
191. Rudolph R, Boyd CR. Massive transfusion: complications and their management. *South Med J.* 1990;83(9):1065-1070.
192. Silberstein LE, Naryshkin S, Haddad JJ, et al. Calcium homeostasis during therapeutic plasma exchange. *Transfusion.* 1986;26(2):151-155.
193. Jacobson MA, Gambertoglio JG, Aweeka FT, et al. Foscarnet-induced hypocalcemia and effects of foscarnet on calcium metabolism. *J Clin Endocrinol Metab.* 1991;72(5):1130-1135.
194. Heher EC, Thier SO, Rennke H, et al. Adverse renal and metabolic effects associated with oral sodium phosphate bowel preparation. *Clin J Am Soc Nephrol.* 2008;3(5):1494-1503.
195. Sperber SJ, Blevins DD, Francis JB. Hypercalcitoninemia, hypocalcemia, and toxic shock syndrome. *Rev Infect Dis.* 1990;12(5):736-739.
196. Boyce BF, Yates AJ, Mundy GR. Bolus injections of recombinant human interleukin-1 cause transient hypocalcemia in normal mice. *Endocrinology.* 1989;125(5):2780-2783.
197. Ranson JH, Rifkind KM, Roses DF, et al. Prognostic signs and the role of operative management in acute pancreatitis. *Surg Gynecol Obstet.* 1974;139(1):69-81.
198. Zusman J, Brown DM, Nesbit ME. Hyperphosphatemia, hyperphosphaturia and hypocalcemia in acute lymphoblastic leukemia. *N Engl J Med.* 1973;289(25):1335-1340.
199. Lim P, Jacob E. Tissue magnesium level in chronic diarrhea. *J Lab Clin Med.* 1972;80(3):313-321.
200. Wallach S. Availability of body magnesium during magnesium deficiency. *Magnesium.* 1988;7(5-6):262-270.
201. Arnaud MJ. Update on the assessment of magnesium status. *Br J Nutr.* 2008;99(suppl 3):S24-S36.
202. Ryzen E, Elbaum N, Singer FR, et al. Parenteral magnesium tolerance testing in the evaluation of magnesium deficiency. *Magnesium.* 1985;4:137-147.
203. Wong ET, Rude RK, Singer FR, et al. A high prevalence of hypomagnesemia and hypermagnesemia in hospitalized patients. *Am J Clin Pathol.* 1983;79(3):348-352.
204. Tong GM, Rude RK. Magnesium deficiency in critical illness. *J Intensive Care Med.* 2005;20(1):3-17.
205. Escuela MP, Guerra M, Anon JM, et al. Total and ionized serum magnesium in critically ill patients. *Intensive Care Med.* 2005;31(1):151-156.
206. Sutton RA, Domrongkitchaiporn S. Abnormal renal magnesium handling. *Miner Electrolyte Metab.* 1993;19(4-5):232-240.
207. Elisaf M, Panteli K, Theodorou J, et al. Fractional excretion of magnesium in normal subjects and in patients with hypomagnesemia. *Magnes Res.* 1997;10(4):315-320.
208. Standing Committee on the Scientific Evaluation of Dietary Reference Intakes of the Food and Nutrition Board of the Institute of Medicine. *Dietary reference intakes for calcium, phosphorus, magnesium, vitamin D and fluoride.* Washington, DC: National Academies Press; 1997.
209. Romani AM. Magnesium homeostasis and alcohol consumption. *Magnes Res.* 2008;21(4):197-204.
210. De Marchi S, Cecchin E, Basile A, et al. Renal tubular dysfunction in chronic alcohol abuse—effects of abstinence. *N Engl J Med.* 1993;329(26):1927-1934.
211. Ziegler TR. Parenteral nutrition in the critically ill patient. *N Engl J Med.* 2009;361(11):1088-1097.
212. Birmingham CL, Puddicombe D. Hlynsky, J: Hypomagnesemia during refeeding in anorexia nervosa. *Eat Weight Disord.* 2004;9(3):236-237.
213. Booth CC, Babouris N, Hanna S, et al. Incidence of hypomagnesaemia in intestinal malabsorption. *Br Med J.* 1963;2:141-144.
214. Thorén L. Magnesium deficiency in gastrointestinal fluid loss. *Acta Chir Scand Suppl.* 1963;306:1-65.
215. Hocking MP, Davis GL, Franzini DA, et al. Long-term consequences after jejunoileal bypass for morbid obesity. *Dig Dis Sci.* 1998;43(11):2493-2499.
216. Johansson HE, Zethelius B, Ohrvall M, et al. Serum magnesium status after gastric bypass surgery in obesity. *Obes Surg.* 2008;19(9):1250-1255.
217. Cundy T, Dissanayake A. Severe hypomagnesaemia in long-term users of proton-pump inhibitors. *Clin Endocrinol (Oxf).* 2008;69(2):338-341.
218. Schlingmann KP, Weber S, Peters M, et al. Hypomagnesemia with secondary hypocalcemia is caused by mutations in TRPM6, a new member of the TRPM gene family. *Nat Genet.* 2002;31(2):166-170.
219. Cohen L, Zimmerman AL. Changes in serum electrolyte levels during marathon running. *S Afr Med J.* 1978;53:449-453.
220. Nielsen FH, Lukaski HC. Update on the relationship between magnesium and exercise. *Magnes Res.* 2006;19(3):180-189.
221. Berger MM, Rothen C, Cavadini C, et al. Exudative mineral losses after serious burns: a clue to the alterations of magnesium and phosphate metabolism. *Am J Clin Nutr.* 1997;65(5):1473-1481.
222. Farese S. [The hungry bone syndrome—an update]. *Ther Umsch.* 2007;64(5):277-280.
223. Pham PC, Pham PM, Pham SV, et al. Hypomagnesemia in patients with type 2 diabetes. *Clin J Am Soc Nephrol.* 2007;2(2):366-373.
224. Dai LJ, Ritchie G, Bapty BW, et al. Insulin stimulates Mg²⁺ uptake in mouse distal convoluted tubule cells. *Am J Physiol.* 1999;277(6 pt 2):F907-F913.
225. Mandon B, Siga E, Chabardes D, et al. Insulin stimulates Na⁺, Cl⁻, Ca²⁺, and Mg²⁺ transports in TAL of mouse nephron: cross-potentiation with AVP. *Am J Physiol.* 1993;265(3 pt 2):F361-F369.
226. Song Y, Hsu YH, Niu T, et al. Common genetic variants of the ion channel transient receptor potential membrane melastatin 6 and 7 (TRPM6 and TRPM7), magnesium intake, and risk of type 2 diabetes in women. *BMC Med Genet.* 2009;10:4.
227. Nabarro JDN, Spencer AG, Stowers JM. Metabolic studies in severe diabetic ketosis. *Q J Mod.* 1952;82:225-243.
228. Martin HE, Smith K, Wilson ML. The fluid and electrolyte therapy of severe diabetic acidosis and ketosis: a study of twenty-nine episodes (twenty-six patients). *Am J Med.* 1958;24:376-389.

229. Rude RK. Magnesium disorders. In: Kokko JP, Tannen RL, eds. *Fluids and Electrolytes*. Philadelphia: Saunders; 1996:421-445.

230. Dickerson RN, Brown RO. Hypomagnesemia in hospitalized patients receiving nutritional support. *Heart Lung*. 1985;14(6):561-569.

231. Mader IJ, Iseri LT. Spontaneous hypopotassemia, hypomagnesemia, alkalosis and tetany due to hypersecretion of corticosterone-like mineralocorticoid. *Am J Med*. 1955;19:976-988.

232. Dyckner T, Wester PO. Renal excretion of electrolytes in patients on long-term diuretic therapy for arterial hypertension and/or congestive heart failure. *Acta Med Scand*. 1985;218(5):443-448.

233. Nijenhuis T, Vallon V, van der Kemp AW, et al. Enhanced passive Ca^{2+} reabsorption and reduced Mg^{2+} channel abundance explains thiazide-induced hypocalciuria and hypomagnesemia. *J Clin Invest*. 2005;115(6):1651-1658.

234. Schrag D, Chung KY, Flombaum C, et al. Cetuximab therapy and symptomatic hypomagnesemia. *J Natl Cancer Inst*. 2005;97(16):1221-1224.

235. Van Cutsem E, Peeters M, Siena S, et al. Open-label phase III trial of panitumumab plus best supportive care compared with best supportive care alone in patients with chemotherapy-refractory metastatic colorectal cancer. *J Clin Oncol*. 2007;25(13):1658-1664.

236. Fakih MG, Wilding G. Lombardo, J: Cetuximab-induced hypomagnesemia in patients with colorectal cancer. *Clin Colorectal Cancer*. 2006;6(2):152-156.

237. Tejpar S, Piessevaux H, Claes K, et al. Magnesium wasting associated with epidermal-growth-factor receptor–targeting antibodies in colorectal cancer: a prospective study. *Lancet Oncol*. 2007;8(5):387-394.

238. Groenestege WM, Thebault S, van der Wijst J, et al. Impaired basolateral sorting of pro-EGF causes isolated recessive renal hypomagnesemia. *J Clin Invest*. 2007;117(8):2260-2267.

239. Thebault S, Alexander RT, Tiel Groenestege WM, et al. EGF increases TRPM6 activity and surface expression. *J Am Soc Nephrol*. 2009;20(1):78-85.

240. Quamme GA. Effect of hypercalcemia on renal tubular handling of calcium and magnesium. *Can J Physiol Pharmacol*. 1982;60:1275-1280.

241. Johansson G, Danielson BG. Ljunghall, S: Magnesium homeostasis in mild-to-moderate primary hyperparathyroidism. *Acta Chir Scand*. 1980;146(2):85-91.

242. Buckley JE, Clark VL, Meyer TJ, et al. Hypomagnesemia after cisplatin combination chemotherapy. *Arch Intern Med*. 1984;144(12):2347-2348.

243. Brock PR, Koliouskas DE, Barratt TM, et al. Partial reversibility of cisplatin nephrotoxicity in children. *J Pediatr*. 1991;118(4 pt 1):531-534.

244. Lajer H, Kristensen M, Hansen HH, et al. Magnesium and potassium homeostasis during cisplatin treatment. *Cancer Chemother Pharmacol*. 2005;55(3):231-236.

245. Ettinger L, Gaynon P, Krailo M, et al. A phase II study of carboplatin in children with recurrent or progressive solid tumors. *A report from the Children's Cancer Group Cancer*. 1994;73(4):1297-1301.

246. Goldman RD, Koren G. Amphotericin B nephrotoxicity in children. *J Pediatr Hematol Oncol*. 2004;26(7):421-426.

247. Barton CH, Pahl M, Vaziri ND, et al. Renal magnesium wasting associated with amphotericin B therapy. *Am J Med*. 1984;77(3):471-474.

248. Wilkinson R, Lucas GL, Heath DA, et al. Hypomagnesaemic tetany associated with prolonged treatment with aminoglycosides. *Br Med J*. 1986;292(6523):818-819.

249. Zaloga GP, Chernow B, Pock A, et al. Hypomagnesemia is a common complication of aminoglycoside therapy. *Surg Gynecol Obstet*. 1984;158:561-565.

250. Mani S. [letter]. Pentamidine-induced renal magnesium wasting. *AIDS*. 1992;6(6):594-595.

251. Palestine AG, Polis MA, De Smet MD, et al. A randomized, controlled trial of foscarnet in the treatment of cytomegalovirus retinitis in patients with AIDS. *Ann Intern Med*. 1991;115(9):665-673.

252. Navaneethan SD, Sankarasubbaiyan S, Gross MD, et al. Tacrolimus-associated hypomagnesemia in renal transplant recipients. *Transplant Proc*. 2006;38(5):1320-1322.

253. Nijenhuis T, Hoenderop JG, Bindels RJ. Downregulation of Ca2+ and Mg2+ transport proteins in the kidney explains tacrolimus (FK506)–induced hypercalciuria and hypomagnesemia. *J Am Soc Nephrol*. 2004;15(3):549-557.

254. Naderi AS, Reilly RF. Jr. Hereditary etiologies of hypomagnesemia. *Nat Clin Pract Nephrol*. 2008;4(2):80-89.

255. Simon DB, Karet FE, Hamdan JM, et al. Bartter's syndrome, hypokalaemic alkalosis with hypercalciuria, is caused by mutations in the Na-K-2Cl cotransporter NKCC2. *Nat Genet*. 1996;13(2):183-188.

256. Simon DB, Lifton RP. The molecular basis of inherited hypokalemic alkalosis: Bartter's and Gitelman's syndromes. *Am J Physiol*. 1996;271(5 pt 2):F961-F966.

257. Kristiansen JH, Brochner Mortensen J, Pedersen KO. Familial hypocalciuric hypercalcaemia I: Renal handling of calcium, magnesium and phosphate. *Clin Endocrinol (Oxf)*. 1985;22(1):103-116.

258. Kingston ME, Al-Siba'i MB, Skooge WC. Clinical manifestations of hypomagnesemia. *Crit Care Med*. 1986;14(11):950-954.

259. Cowan JA. Structural and catalytic chemistry of magnesium-dependent enzymes. *Biometals*. 2002;15(3):225-235.

260. Whang R, Morosi HJ, Rodgers D, et al. The influence of sustained magnesium deficiency on muscle potassium repletion. *J Lab Clin Med*. 1967;70(6):895-902.

261. Agus ZS. Hypomagnesemia. *J Am Soc Nephrol*. 1999;10(7):1616-1622.

262. Seller RH, Cangiano J, Kim KE, et al. Digitalis toxicity and hypomagnesemia. *Am Heart J*. 1970;79(1):57-68.

263. Zehender M, Meinertz T, Faber T, et al. Antiarrhythmic effects of increasing the daily intake of magnesium and potassium in patients with frequent ventricular arrhythmias. Magnesium in Cardiac Arrhythmias (MAGICA) Investigators. *J Am Coll Cardiol*. 1997;29(5):1028-1034.

264. Klevay L, Milne D. Low dietary magnesium increases supraventricular ectopy. *Am J Clin Nutr*. 2002;75(3):550-554.

265. Tsuji H, Venditti Jr FJ, Evans JC, et al. The associations of levels of serum potassium and magnesium with ventricular premature complexes (the Framingham Heart Study). *Am J Cardiol*. 1994;74(3):232-235.

266. Woods KL, Fletcher S. Long-term outcome after intravenous magnesium sulphate in suspected acute myocardial infarction: the second Leicester Intravenous Magnesium Intervention Trial (LIMIT-2). *Lancet*. 1996;343(8901):816-819.

267. Fourth International Study of Infarct Survival Collaborative Group. ISIS-4: a randomised factorial trial assessing early oral captopril, oral mononitrate, and intravenous magnesium sulphate in 58,050 patients with suspected acute myocardial infarction. *Lancet*. 1995;345(8951):669-685.

268. Early administration of intravenous magnesium to high-risk patients with acute myocardial infarction in the Magnesium in Coronaries (MAGIC) Trial: a randomised controlled trial. *Lancet*. 2002;360(9341):1189-1196.

269. Sontia B, Touyz RM. Role of magnesium in hypertension. *Arch Biochem Biophys*. 2007;458(1):33-39.

270. Touyz RM. Role of magnesium in the pathogenesis of hypertension. *Mol Aspects Med*. 2003;24(1-3):107-136.

271. Appel LJ, Moore TJ, Obarzanek E, et al. A clinical trial of the effects of dietary patterns on blood pressure. DASH Collaborative Research Group. *N Engl J Med*. 1997;336(16):1117-1124.

272. Vallee BL, Wacker WEC, Ulmer DD. The magnesium-deficiency tetany syndrome in man. *New Engl J Med*. 1960;262:155-161.

273. McIntosh TK. Novel pharmacologic therapies in the treatment of experimental traumatic brain injury: a review. *J Neurotrauma*. 1993;10(3):215-261.

274. Mody I, Lambert JD, Heinemann U. Low extracellular magnesium induces epileptiform activity and spreading depression in rat hippocampal slices. *J Neurophysiol*. 1987;57(3):869-888.

275. Saul RF, Selhorst JB. Downbeat nystagmus with magnesium depletion. *Arch Neurol*. 1981;38(10):650-652.

276. Rude RK, Gruber HE. Magnesium deficiency and osteoporosis: animal and human observations. *J Nutr Biochem*. 2004;15(12):710-716.

277. Tong G, Rude RK. The role of dietary magnesium deficiency in osteoporosis. In: New SA, Bonjour JP, eds. *The Royal Society of Chemistry*. Cambridge, UK: Nutritional aspects of bone health; 2003:339-350.

278. Rude RK, Gruber HE, Norton HJ, et al. Reduction of dietary magnesium by only 50% in the rat disrupts bone and mineral metabolism. *Osteoporos Int*. 2006;17(7):1022-1032.

279. Whang R, Whang DD, Ryan MP. Refractory potassium repletion. A consequence of magnesium deficiency. *Arch Intern Med*. 1992;152(1):40-45.

280. Carney SL, Wong NL, Dirks JH. Effect of magnesium deficiency and excess on renal tubular potassium transport in the rat. *Clin Sci (Lond)*. 1981;60(5):549-554.

281. Huang CL, Kuo E. Mechanism of hypokalemia in magnesium deficiency. *J Am Soc Nephrol*. 2007;18(10):2649-2652.

282. Ford ES, Li C, McGuire LC, et al. Intake of dietary magnesium and the prevalence of the metabolic syndrome among U.S. adults. *Obesity (Silver Spring)*. 2007;15(5):1139-1146.

283. Sun-Edelstein C, Mauskop A. Role of magnesium in the pathogenesis and treatment of migraine. *Expert Rev Neurother*. 2009;9(3):369-379.

284. Cheuk DK, Chau TC, Lee SL. A meta-analysis on intravenous magnesium sulphate for treating acute asthma. *Arch Dis Child*. 2005;90(1):74-77.

285. Mohammed S, Goodacre S. Intravenous and nebulised magnesium sulphate for acute asthma: systematic review and meta-analysis. *Emerg Med J*. 2007;24(12):823-830.

286. Dai Q, Shrubsole MJ, Ness RM, et al. The relation of magnesium and calcium intakes and a genetic polymorphism in the magnesium transporter to colorectal neoplasia risk. *Am J Clin Nutr*. 2007;86(3):743-751.

287. Folsom AR, Hong CP. Magnesium intake and reduced risk of colon cancer in a prospective study of women. *Am J Epidemiol*. 2006;163(3):232-235.

288. Standing Committee on the Scientific Evaluation of Dietary Reference Intakes. Food and Nutrition Board, Institute of Medicine: Dietary reference intakes: calcium, phosphorus, magnesium, vitamin D and fluoride. Washington, DC: National Academies Press; 1999.

289. Oster JR, Epstein M. Management of magnesium depletion. *Am J Nephrol*. 1988;8(5):349-354.

290. Eisenbud E, LoBue CC. Hypocalcemia after therapeutic use of magnesium sulfate. *Arch Intern Med.* 1976;136(6):688-691.
291. Navarro J, Oster JR, Gkonos PJ, et al. Tetany induced on separate occasions by administration of potassium and magnesium in a patient with hungry-bone syndrome. *Miner Electrolyte Metab.* 1991;17(5):340-344.
292. Farkas RA, McAllister CT, Blachley JD. Effect of magnesium salt anions on potassium balance in normal and magnesium-depleted rats. *J Lab Clin Med.* 1987;110(4):412-417.
293. Bundy JT, Connito D, Mahoney MD, et al. *Treatment of idiopathic renal magnesium wasting with amiloride. Am J Nephrol.* 1995;15:75-77.
294. Dai LJ, Raymond L, Friedman PA, et al. Mechanisms of amiloride stimulation of Mg^{2+} uptake in immortalized mouse distal convoluted tubule cells. *Am J Physiol.* 1997;272(2 pt 2):F249-F256.
295. Coburn JW, Popovtzer MM, Massry SG, et al. The physicochemical state and renal handling of divalent ions in chronic renal failure. *Arch Intern Med.* 1969;124(3):302-311.
296. Clark BA, Brown RS. Unsuspected morbid hypermagnesemia in elderly patients. *Am J Nephrol.* 1992;12(5):336-343.
297. McLaughlin SA, McKinney PE. Antacid-induced hypermagnesemia in a patient with normal renal function and bowel obstruction. *Ann Pharmacother.* 1998;32(3):312-315.
298. Onishi S, Yoshino S. Cathartic-induced fatal hypermagnesemia in the elderly. *Intern Med.* 2006;45(4):207-210.
299. Tofil NM, Benner KW, Winkler MK. Fatal hypermagnesemia caused by an Epsom salt enema: a case illustration. *South Med J.* 2005;98(2):253-256.
300. Mordes JP, Wacker WE. *Excess magnesium.* 1977;29(4):273-300.
301. Touyz RM. Magnesium in clinical medicine. *Front Biosci.* 2004;9:1278-1293.
302. del Castillo J, Engbaek L. The nature of the neuromuscular block produced by magnesium. *J Physiol.* 1954;124:370-384.
303. Kelber J, Slatopolsky E, Delmez JA. Acute effects of different concentrations of dialysate magnesium during high-efficiency dialysis. *Am J Kid Dis.* 1994;24(3):453-460.
304. Burritt MF, Slockbower JM, Forsman RW, et al. Pediatric reference intervals for 19 biologic variables in healthy children. *Mayo Clin Proc.* 1990;65(3):329-336.
305. Murer H, Hernando N, Forster I, et al. Proximal tubular phosphate reabsorption: molecular mechanisms. *Physiol Rev.* 2000;80(4):1373-1409.
306. Barth JH, Jones RG, Payne RB. Calculation of renal tubular reabsorption of phosphate: the algorithm performs better than the nomogram. *Ann Clin Biochem.* 2000;37(pt 1):79-81.
307. Markowitz M, Rotkin L, Rosen JF. Circadian rhythms of blood minerals in humans. *Science.* 1981;213(4508):672-674.
308. Thatte L, Oster JR, Singer I, et al. Review of the literature: severe hyperphosphatemia. *Am J Med Sci.* 1995;310(4):167-174.
309. Quigley R, Baum M. Effects of growth hormone and insulin-like growth factor I on rabbit proximal convoluted tubule transport. *J Clin Invest.* 1991;88(2):368-374.
310. Topaz O, Shurman DL, Bergman R, et al. Mutations in GALNT3, encoding a protein involved in O-linked glycosylation, cause familial tumoral calcinosis. *Nat Genet.* 2004;36(6):579-581.
311. Araya K, Fukumoto S, Backenroth R, et al. A novel mutation in fibroblast growth factor 23 gene as a cause of tumoral calcinosis. *J Clin Endocrinol Metab.* 2005;90(10):5523-5527.
312. Chefetz I, Heller R, Galli-Tsinopoulou A, et al. A novel homozygous missense mutation in FGF23 causes familial tumoral calcinosis associated with disseminated visceral calcification. *Hum Genet.* 2005;118(2):261-266.
313. Ichikawa S, Imel EA, Kreiter ML, et al. A homozygous missense mutation in human KLOTHO causes severe tumoral calcinosis. *J Clin Invest.* 2007;117(9):2684-2691.
314. Kato K, Jeanneau C, Tarp MA, et al. Polypeptide GalNAc-transferase T3 and familial tumoral calcinosis. Secretion of fibroblast growth factor 23 requires O-glycosylation. *J Biol Chem.* 2006;281(27):18370-18377.
315. Shimada T, Kakitani M, Yamazaki Y, et al. Targeted ablation of Fgf23 demonstrates an essential physiological role of FGF23 in phosphate and vitamin D metabolism. *J Clin Invest.* 2004;113(4):561-568.
316. Mitnick PD, Goldfarb S, Slatopolsky E, et al. Calcium and phosphate metabolism in tumoral calcinosis. *Ann Intern Med.* 1980;92(4):482-487.
317. Yamaguchi T, Sugimoto T, Imai Y, et al. Successful treatment of hyperphosphatemic tumoral calcinosis with long-term acetazolamide. *Bone.* 1995;16(4 suppl):247S-250S.
318. Walton RJ, Russell RG, Smith R. Changes in the renal and extrarenal handling of phosphate induced by disodium etidronate (EHDP) in man. *Clin Sci Mol Med.* 1975;49(1):45-56.
319. McCloskey EV, Yates AJ, Gray RE, et al. Diphosphonates and phosphate homoeostasis in man. *Clin Sci (Lond).* 1988;74(6):607-612.
320. Markowitz GS, Perazella MA. Acute phosphate nephropathy. *Kidney Int.* 2009;76(10):1027-1034.
321. Mackey AC, Green L, Amand KS, et al. Sodium phosphate tablets and acute phosphate nephropathy. *Am J Gastroenterol.* 2009;104(8):1903-1906.
322. Caswell M, Thompson WO, Kanapka JA, et al. The time course and effect on serum electrolytes of oral sodium phosphates solution in healthy male and female volunteers. *Can J Clin Pharmacol.* 2007;14(3):e260-e274.
323. Desmeules S, Bergeron MJ. Isenring, P: Acute phosphate nephropathy and renal failure. *N Engl J Med.* 2003;349(10):1006-1007.
324. Brunelli SM, Lewis JD, Gupta M, et al. Risk of kidney injury following oral phosphosoda bowel preparations. *J Am Soc Nephrol.* 2007;18(12):3199-3205.
325. Krapf R, Jaeger P, Hulter HN. Chronic respiratory alkalosis induces renal PTH-resistance, hyperphosphatemia and hypocalcemia in humans. *Kidney Int.* 1992;42(3):727-734.
326. Thompson CH, Kemp GJ, Radda GK. Changes in high-energy phosphates in rat skeletal muscle during acute respiratory acidosis. *Acta Physiol Scand.* 1992;146(1):15-19.
327. O'Connor LR, Klein KL, Bethune JE. Hyperphosphatemia in lactic acidosis. *N Engl J Med.* 1977;297(13):707-709.
328. Kebler R, McDonald FD, Cadnapaphornchai P. Dynamic changes in serum phosphorus levels in diabetic ketoacidosis. *Am J Med.* 1985;79(5):571-576.
329. Cairo MS, Bishop M. Tumour lysis syndrome: new therapeutic strategies and classification. *Br J Haematol.* 2004;127(1):3-11.
330. Abu-Alfa AK, Younes A. Tumor lysis syndrome and acute kidney injury: evaluation, prevention, and management. *Am J Kidney Dis.* 2010;55(5 suppl. 3):S1-S13:quiz S14-S19.
331. Tsokos GC, Balow JE, Spiegel RJ, et al. Renal and metabolic complications of undifferentiated and lymphoblastic lymphomas. *Medicine (Baltimore).* 1981;60(3):218-229.
332. Coiffier B, Altman A, Pui CH, et al. Guidelines for the management of pediatric and adult tumor lysis syndrome: an evidence-based review. *J Clin Oncol.* 2008;26(16):2767-2778.
333. Larner AJ. Pseudohyperphosphatemia. *Clin Biochem.* 1995;28(4):391-393.
334. Lane JW, Rehak NN, Hortin GL, et al. Pseudohyperphosphatemia associated with high-dose liposomal amphotericin B therapy. *Clin Chim Acta.* 2008;387(1-2):145-149.
335. Gaasbeek A, Meinders AE. Hypophosphatemia: an update on its etiology and treatment. *Am J Med.* 2005;118(10):1094-1101.
336. Knochel JP. The pathophysiology and clinical characteristics of severe hypophosphatemia. *Arch Intern Med.* 1977;137(2):203-220.
337. Brunelli SM, Goldfarb S. Hypophosphatemia: clinical consequences and management. *J Am Soc Nephrol.* 2007;18(7):1999-2003.
338. Block GA, Klassen PS, Lazarus JM, et al. Mineral metabolism, mortality, and morbidity in maintenance hemodialysis. *J Am Soc Nephrol.* 2004;15(8):2208-2218.
339. Lichtman MA, Miller DR, Cohen J, et al. Reduced red cell glycolysis, 2,3-diphosphoglycerate and adenosine triphosphate concentration, and increased hemoglobin-oxygen affinity caused by hypophosphatemia. *Ann Intern Med.* 1971;74(4):562-568.
340. Massry SG, Fadda GZ, Perna AF, et al. Mechanism of organ dysfunction in phosphate depletion: a critical role for a rise in cytosolic calcium. *Miner Electrolyte Metab.* 1992;18(2-5):133-140.
341. Jacob HS, Amsden T. Acute hemolytic anemia with rigid red cells in hypophosphatemia. *N Engl J Med.* 1971;285(26):1446-1450.
342. Melvin JD, Watts RG. Severe hypophosphatemia: a rare cause of intravascular hemolysis. *Am J Hematol.* 2002;69(3):223-224.
343. Craddock PR, Yawata Y, VanSanten L, et al. Acquired phagocyte dysfunction. A complication of the hypophosphataemia of parenteral hyperalimentation. *N Engl J Med.* 1974;290(25):1403-1407.
344. Schubert L, DeLuca HF. Hypophosphatemia is responsible for skeletal muscle weakness of vitamin D deficiency. *Arch Biochem Biophys.* 2010;500(2):157-161.
345. Knochel JP. Hypophosphatemia and rhabdomyolysis. *Am J Med.* 1992;92(5):455-457.
346. Newman JH, Neff TA, Ziporin P. Acute respiratory failure associated with hypophosphatemia. *N Engl J Med.* 1977;296(19):1101-1103.
347. Fuller TJ, Nichols WW, Brenner BJ, et al. Reversible depression in myocardial performance in dogs with experimental phosphorus deficiency. *J Clin Invest.* 1978;62(6):1194-1200.
348. O'Connor LR, Wheeler WS, Bethune JE. Effect of hypophosphatemia on myocardial performance in man. *N Engl J Med.* 1977;297(17):901-903.
349. Zazzo JF, Troche G, Ruel P, et al. High incidence of hypophosphatemia in surgical intensive care patients: efficacy of phosphorus therapy on myocardial function. *Intensive Care Med.* 1995;21(10):826-831.
350. Goldfarb S, Westby GR, Goldberg M, et al. Renal tubular effects of chronic phosphate depletion. *J Clin Invest.* 1977;59(5):770-779.
351. Coburn JW, Massry SG. Changes in serum and urinary calcium during phosphate depletion: studies on mechanisms. *J Clin Invest.* 1970;49(6):1073-1087.
352. Juan D, Elrazak MA. Hypophosphatemia in hospitalized patients. *JAMA.* 1979;242(2):163-164.
353. Bastepe M, Juppner H. Inherited hypophosphatemic disorders in children and the evolving mechanisms of phosphate regulation. *Rev Endocr Metab Disord.* 2008;9(2):171-180.

354. Dixon PH, Christie PT, Wooding C, et al. Mutational analysis of PHEX gene in X-linked hypophosphatemia. *J Clin Endocrinol Metab.* 1998;83(10):3615-3623.

355. A gene (PEX) with homologies to endopeptidases is mutated in patients with X-linked hypophosphatemic rickets. The HYP Consortium. *Nat Genet.* 1995;11(2):130-136.

356. Meyer MH, Meyer Jr RA. MRNA expression of Phex in mice and rats: the effect of low phosphate diet. *Endocrine.* 2000;13(1):81-87.

357. Liu S, Guo R, Simpson LG, et al. Regulation of fibroblastic growth factor 23 expression but not degradation by PHEX. *J Biol Chem.* 2003;278(39):37419-37426.

358. Shimada T, Hasegawa H, Yamazaki Y, et al. FGF-23 is a potent regulator of vitamin D metabolism and phosphate homeostasis. *J Bone Miner Res.* 2004;19(3):429-435.

359. Sullivan W, Carpenter T, Glorieux F, et al. A prospective trial of phosphate and 1,25-dihydroxyvitamin D_3 therapy in symptomatic adults with X-linked hypophosphatemic rickets. *J Clin Endocrinol Metab.* 1992;75(3):879-885.

360. Autosomal dominant hypophosphataemic rickets is associated with mutations in FGF23. *Nat Genet.* 2000;26(3):345-348.

361. White KE, Carn G, Lorenz-Depiereux B, et al. Autosomal-dominant hypophosphatemic rickets (ADHR) mutations stabilize FGF-23. *Kidney Int.* 2001;60(6):2079-2086.

362. Benet-Pages A, Lorenz-Depiereux B, Zischka H, et al. FGF23 is processed by proprotein convertases but not by PHEX. *Bone.* 2004;35(2):455-462.

363. Jan de Beur SM. Tumor-induced osteomalacia. *JAMA.* 2005;294(10):1260-1267.

364. Shimada T, Mizutani S, Muto T, et al. Cloning and characterization of FGF23 as a causative factor of tumor-induced osteomalacia. *Proc Natl Acad Sci U S A.* 2001;98(11):6500-6205.

365. Schiavi SC, Moe OW. Phosphatonins: a new class of phosphate-regulating proteins. *Curr Opin Nephrol Hypertens.* 2002;11(4):423-430.

366. Geller JL, Khosravi A, Kelly MH, et al. Cinacalcet in the management of tumor-induced osteomalacia. *J Bone Miner Res.* 2007;22(6):931-937.

367. Bergwitz C, Roslin NM, Tieder M, et al. SLC34A3 mutations in patients with hereditary hypophosphatemic rickets with hypercalciuria predict a key role for the sodium-phosphate cotransporter NaPi-IIc in maintaining phosphate homeostasis. *Am J Hum Genet.* 2006;78(2):179-192.

368. Prie D, Huart V, Bakouh N, et al. Nephrolithiasis and osteoporosis associated with hypophosphatemia caused by mutations in the type 2a sodium-phosphate cotransporter. *N Engl J Med.* 2002;347(13):983-991.

369. Roth KS, Foreman JW, Segal S. : The Fanconi syndrome and mechanisms of tubular transport dysfunction. *Kidney Int.* 1981;20(6):705-716.

370. Izzedine H, Launay-Vacher V, Isnard-Bagnis C, et al. Drug-induced Fanconi's syndrome. *Am J Kidney Dis.* 2003;41(2):292-309.

371. Woodward CL, Hall AM, Williams IG, et al. Tenofovir-associated renal and bone toxicity. *HIV Med.* 2009;10(8):482-487.

372. Evenepoel P, Claes K, Kuypers D, et al. Natural history of parathyroid function and calcium metabolism after kidney transplantation: a single-centre study. *Nephrol Dial Transplant.* 2004;19(5):1281-1287.

373. Sakhaee K. Post-renal transplantation hypophosphatemia. *Pediatr Nephrol.* 2010;25(2):213-220.

374. Green J, Debby H, Lederer E, et al. Evidence for a PTH-independent humoral mechanism in post-transplant hypophosphatemia and phosphaturia. *Kidney Int.* 2001;60(3):1182-1196.

375. Sato T, Fukagawa M, Uchida K, et al. 1,25-dihydroxyvitamin D synthesis after renal transplantation: the role of fibroblast growth factor 23 and cyclosporine. *Clin Transplant.* 2009;23(3):368-374.

376. Evenepoel P, Meijers BK, de Jonge H, et al. Recovery of hyperphosphatoninism and renal phosphorus wasting one year after successful renal transplantation. *Clin J Am Soc Nephrol.* 2008;3(6):1829-1836.

377. Serra AL, Wuhrmann C, Wuthrich RP. Phosphatemic effect of cinacalcet in kidney transplant recipients with persistent hyperparathyroidism. *Am J Kidney Dis.* 2008;52(6):1151-1157.

378. Suki WN, Martinez-Maldonado M, Rouse D, et al. Effect of expansion of extracellular fluid volume on renal phosphate handling. *J Clin Invest.* 1969;48(10):1888-1894.

379. Turner ST, Kiebzak GM, Dousa TP. Mechanism of glucocorticoid effect on renal transport of phosphate. *Am J Physiol.* 1982;243(5):C227-C236.

380. Owen S, Hatfield A, Letvak L. Imatinib and altered bone and mineral metabolism. *N Engl J Med.* 2006;355(6):627:author reply 628-629.

381. Escudier B, Eisen T, Stadler WM, et al. Sorafenib in advanced clear-cell renal-cell carcinoma. *N Engl J Med.* 2007;356(2):125-134.

382. Berman E, Nicolaides M, Maki RG, et al. Altered bone and mineral metabolism in patients receiving imatinib mesylate. *N Engl J Med.* 2006;354(19):2006-2013.

383. Sato K, Shiraki M. Saccharated ferric oxide-induced osteomalacia in Japan: iron-induced osteopathy due to nephropathy. *Endocr J.* 1998;45(4):431-439.

384. Schouten BJ, Hunt PJ, Livesey JH, et al. FGF23 elevation and hypophosphatemia after intravenous iron polymaltose: a prospective study. *J Clin Endocrinol Metab.* 2009;94(7):2332-2337.

385. Citrin DL, Wallemark CB, Nadler R, et al. Estramustine affects bone mineral metabolism in metastatic prostate cancer. *Cancer.* 1986;58(10):2208-2213.

386. George R, Shiu MH. Hypophosphatemia after major hepatic resection. *Surgery.* 1992;111(3):281-286.

387. Cohen J, Kogan A, Sahar G, et al. Hypophosphatemia following open heart surgery: incidence and consequences. *Eur J Cardiothorac Surg.* 2004;26(2):306-310.

388. Salem RR, Tray K. Hepatic resection-related hypophosphatemia is of renal origin as manifested by isolated hyperphosphaturia. *Ann Surg.* 2005;241(2):343-348.

389. Nafidi O, Lapointe RW, Lepage R, et al. Mechanisms of renal phosphate loss in liver resection–associated hypophosphatemia. *Ann Surg.* 2009;249(5):824-827.

390. Manary MJ, Hart CA, Whyte MP. Severe hypophosphatemia in children with kwashiorkor is associated with increased mortality. *J Pediatr.* 1998;133(6):789-791.

391. Gannage MH, Abikaram G, Nasr F, et al. Osteomalacia secondary to celiac disease, primary hyperparathyroidism, and Graves' disease. *Am J Med Sci.* 1998;315(2):136-139.

392. Chines A, Pacifici R. Antacid and sucralfate-induced hypophosphatemic osteomalacia: a case report and review of the literature. *Calcif Tissue Int.* 1990;47(5):291-295.

393. Brautbar N, Leibovici H, Massry SG. On the mechanism of hypophosphatemia during acute hyperventilation: evidence for increased muscle glycolysis. *Miner Electrolyte Metab.* 1983;9(1):45-50.

394. Mostellar ME, Tuttle Jr EP. Effects of alkalosis on plasma concentration and urinary excretion of inorganic phosphate in man. *J Clin Invest.* 1964;43:138-149.

395. Laaban JP, Waked M, Laromiguiere M, et al. Hypophosphatemia complicating management of acute severe asthma. *Ann Intern Med.* 1990;112(1):68-69.

396. Boateng AA, Sriram K, Meguid MM, et al. Refeeding syndrome: treatment considerations based on collective analysis of literature case reports. *Nutrition.* 2010;26(2):156-167.

397. Marik PE, Bedigian MK. Refeeding hypophosphatemia in critically ill patients in an intensive care unit. A prospective study. *Arch Surg.* 1996;131(10):1043-1047.

398. Knochel JP. Hypophosphatemia in the alcoholic. *Arch Intern Med.* 1980;140(5):613-615.

399. Seldin DW, Tarail R. The metabolism of glucose and electrolytes in diabetic acidosis. *J Clin Invest.* 1950;29(5):552-565.

400. Haglin L. Hypophosphataemia: cause of the disturbed metabolism in the metabolic syndrome. *Med Hypotheses.* 2001;56(6):657-663.

401. Atchley DW, Loeb RF, Richards DW, et al. On diabetic acidosis: a detailed study of electrolyte balances following the withdrawal and reestablishment of insulin therapy. *J Clin Invest.* 1933;12(2):297-326.

402. Fisher JN, Kitabchi AE. A randomized study of phosphate therapy in the treatment of diabetic ketoacidosis. *J Clin Endocrinol Metab.* 1983;57(1):177-180.

403. Ravenscroft AJ, Valentine JM, Knappett PA. Severe hypophosphataemia and insulin resistance in diabetic ketoacidosis. *Anaesthesia.* 1999;54(2):198.

404. Zamkoff KW, Kirshner JJ. Marked hypophosphatemia associated with acute myelomonocytic leukemia. Indirect evidence of phosphorus uptake by leukemic cells. *Arch Intern Med.* 1980;140(11):1523-1524.

405. Steiner M, Steiner B, Wilhelm S, et al. Severe hypophosphatemia during hematopoietic reconstitution after allogeneic peripheral blood stem cell transplantation. *Bone Marrow Transplant.* 2000;25(9):1015-1016.

406. Chesney PJ, Davis JP, Purdy WK, et al. Clinical manifestations of toxic shock syndrome. *JAMA.* 1981;246(7):741-748.

407. Barak V, Schwartz A, Kalickman I, et al. Prevalence of hypophosphatemia in sepsis and infection: the role of cytokines. *Am J Med.* 1998;104(1):40-47.

408. Levenson SM, Adams MA, Rosen H, et al. Studies in phosphorus metabolism in man. III. The distribution, exchange and excretion of phosphorus in man using radioactive phosphorus (P32) as a tracer. *J Clin Invest.* 1953;32(6):497-509.

409. Lentz RD, Brown DM, Kjellstrand CM. Treatment of severe hypophosphatemia. *Ann Intern Med.* 1978;89(6):941-944.

410. Vannatta JB, Andress DL, Whang R, et al. High-dose intravenous phosphorus therapy for severe complicated hypophosphatemia. *South Med J.* 1983;76(11):1424-1426.

411. Clark CL, Sacks GS, Dickerson RN, et al. Treatment of hypophosphatemia in patients receiving specialized nutrition support using a graduated dosing scheme: results from a prospective clinical trial. *Crit Care Med.* 1995;23(9):1504-1511.

412. Ding C, Buckingham B, Levine MA. Familial isolated hypoparathyroidism caused by a mutation in the gene for the transcription factor GCMB. *J Clin Invest.* 2001;108(8):1215-1220.

413. Bowl MR, Nesbit MA, Harding B, et al. An interstitial deletion-insertion involving chromosomes 2p25.3 and Xq27.1, near SOX3, causes X-linked recessive hypoparathyroidism. *J Clin Invest.* 2005;115(10):2822-2831.

414. Parkinson DB, Thakker RV. A donor splice site mutation in the parathyroid hormone gene is associated with autosomal recessive hypoparathyroidism. *Nat Genet.* 1992;1(2):149-152.

415. Arnold A, Horst SA, Gardella TJ, et al. Mutation of the signal peptide-encoding region of the preproparathyroid hormone gene in familial isolated hypoparathyroidism. *J Clin Invest.* 1990;86(4):1084-1087.

416. Yagi H, Furutani Y, Hamada H, et al. Role of TBX1 in human del22q11.2 syndrome. *Lancet.* 2003;362(9393):1366-1373.

417. Van Esch H, Groenen P, Nesbit MA, et al. GATA3 haplo-insufficiency causes human HDR syndrome. *Nature.* 2000;406(6794):419-422.

418. Parvari R, Hershkovitz E, Grossman N, et al. Mutation of TBCE causes hypoparathyroidism-retardation-dysmorphism and autosomal recessive Kenny-Caffey syndrome. *Nat Genet.* 2002;32(3):448-452.

419. Neufeld M, Maclaren NK, Blizzard RM. Two types of autoimmune Addison's disease associated with different polyglandular autoimmune (PGA) syndromes. *Medicine (Baltimore).* 1981;60(5):355-362.

Epidemiology and Risk Factors in Kidney Disease

Chapter 19

Epidemiology of Kidney Disease

Chi-yuan Hsu

Epidemiology is defined as "the study of the incidence and distribution of diseases" by the *Oxford English Dictionary.* This chapter focuses on the epidemiology of end-stage renal disease (ESRD), chronic kidney disease (CKD), and acute kidney injury (AKI), the three most important clinical problems in nephrology, measured either by number of patients affected or by rates of associated morbidity and mortality. Some initial definitions are useful. The incidence rate of a disease is typically defined as number of new cases per person-year from longitudinal studies in which patients were enrolled without disease at baseline. The prevalence rate of a disease is typically defined as number of persons with disease per population at any one time in cross-sectional studies. Disease prevalence thus is dependent not only on disease incidence but also on how long the condition persists. Both incidence rates and prevalence rates are typically normalized to some underlying population (e.g., the total U.S. population). Hence, if the underlying population size increases, as the U.S. population has, absolute incidence (and prevalence) *count* can increase over time, even if the incidence (or prevalence) *rate* were unchanged.

This chapter also touches upon risk factors for kidney disease, which are discussed in greater detail in Chapters 20 ("Demographics of Kidney Disease") and 21 ("Risk Factors and Kidney Disease").

Epidemiology of End-Stage Renal Disease

In the study of kidney disease epidemiology, the traditional focus has been on ESRD. ESRD is the most serious and dramatic manifestation of kidney disease and naturally was the focus of much clinical attention in the early decades of nephrology in the 1950s and 1960s. During this time, with pioneering work in renal transplantation and dialysis, nephrology became recognized as a separate discipline. Several decades' worth of very strong data exist with regard to the epidemiology of ESRD, in large part because of the existence of ESRD registries such as the Michigan Kidney Registry[1] and the United States Renal Data System (USRDS). The USRDS provides powerful epidemiology data because it has nationally comprehensive patient-level data and tracks outcomes after the diagnosis of ESRD. Examples of registries in other countries include the Australia and New Zealand Dialysis and Transplant Registry, the Canadian Organ Replacement Register, and the United Kingdom Renal Registry.

Definition of End-Stage Renal Disease

The generally accepted definition of ESRD is an operational one: the receipt of maintenance dialysis (peritoneal dialysis or hemodialysis) or kidney transplantation. In other words, it is not defined by a certain glomerular filtration rate (GFR) or some other objective threshold. This point is important in interpreting trends in incidence (and prevalence) of ESRD because these trends may be substantially affected by practice patterns independent of underlying distribution of disease in the population. For example, it has been documented that in the United States, mean serum creatinine level at the start of maintenance renal replacement therapy decreased from 8.5 mg/dL in 1996 to 6.4 mg/dL in 2007 (Figure 19-1). Similarly, according to the Australia and New Zealand Dialysis and Transplant Registry, serum creatinine concentration at the start of ESRD treatment decreased from 1000 µmol/L (11.3 mg/dL) in 1992 to 750 µmol/L (8.5 mg/dL) in 2001.[2] These trends are probably attributable to earlier initiation of dialysis, driven by the belief that "healthy initiation" of dialysis—at a higher GFR before onset of gross uremic symptoms—is beneficial.[3] This may also reflect the fact that patients with multiple comorbid conditions who are malnourished (and hence have reduced production of creatinine) are being entered more liberally into dialysis programs. Although

the wisdom of this practice has been questioned by some,[4,5] this change in practice pattern has undoubtedly contributed to the rise in the number of new cases of "ESRD." This practice would also have other implications for secular trends in the epidemiology of ESRD. For example, the rate of mortality in the first year after onset of dialysis reflects outcome among some persons who would not have been initiated on dialysis in prior calendar years.

Incidence of End-Stage Renal Disease

According to the 2009 annual report by the USRDS, the annual incidence of ESRD in the United States was 354 per 1 million person-years (adjusted for age, gender, and race).[39,39a] This is actually a slight drop from the prior year. This secular trend is quite different from that observed in the 1980s and 1990s, in which the incidence of ESRD increased at a rapid rate (Figure 19-2). In fact, the incidence of ESRD has reached a plateau since 2001 (see Figure 19-2).

This encouraging trend may be attributed to more successes in retarding the progression of CKD as a result of more aggressive control of blood pressure with drugs such as those that block the renin-angiotensin system. Improved glycemic control among patients with diabetes mellitus may have also helped. The effect of such treatment is illustrated by a Finnish study in which outcome among young patients with type 1 diabetes was tracked over several decades.[6] In that study, those in whom type 1 diabetes was diagnosed between 1980 and 1999 had less than half the risk of developing ESRD of those in whom type 1 diabetes was diagnosed between 1965 and 1969. This favorable trend in disease incidence *rates* may not be apparent when data are presented as incidence *count*, in as much as the absolute number of new ESRD patients will continue to increase because of the enlarging size of the U.S. population, even if incidence *rate* were held constant.[7]

The incidence of ESRD varies considerably across patient subgroups. In the United States, the incidence of ESRD among African-Americans is strikingly higher (by 3.7-fold) than the incidence among white persons. Incidence rates are also higher among those of Asian descent and Hispanic ethnicity (Figure 19-3). The incidence of ESRD has been increasing most rapidly among people aged 75 and older and is now highest in this age group

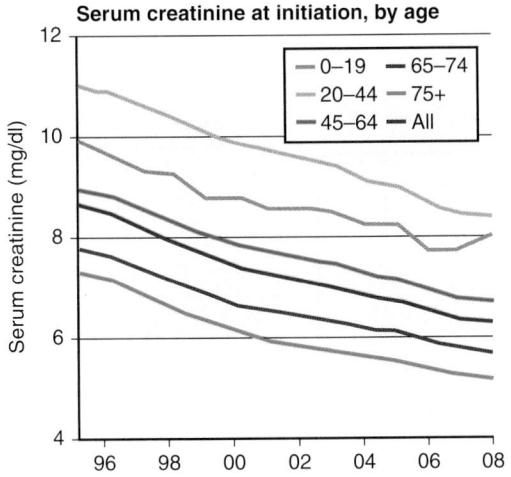

FIGURE 19-1 Mean serum creatinine (mg/dL) at the start of dialysis in the United States as reported to the U.S. Renal Data System. The drop in serum creatinine is almost certainly due to changes in secular changes in practice pattern and more liberal initiation of dialysis. (From U.S. Renal Data System: *USRDS 2009 annual data report: atlas of chronic kidney disease and end-stage renal disease in the United States,* Bethesda, MD, 2009, National Institutes of Health and National Institute of Diabetes and Digestive and Kidney Diseases, p 246.)

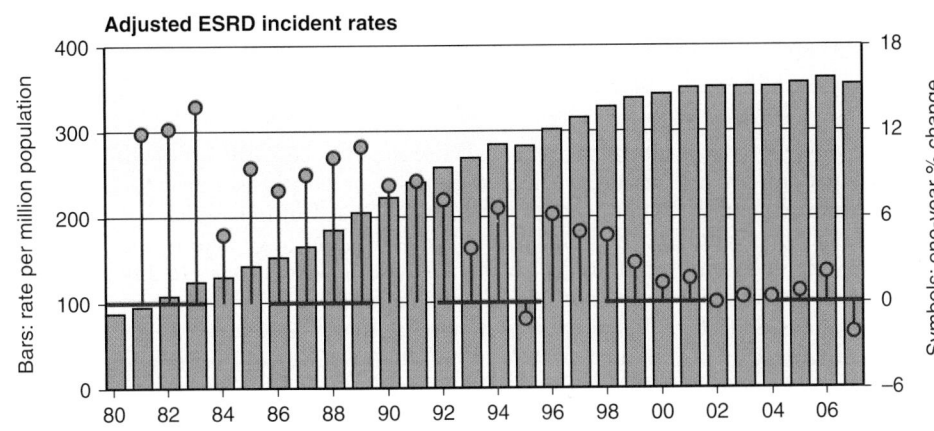

FIGURE 19-2 Trend over time in the United States in adjusted rates of incident ESRD. This rate (adjusted for age, gender, and race) had been relatively stable from 2000 to 2007. (From U.S. Renal Data System: *USRDS 2009 annual data report: atlas of chronic kidney disease and end-stage renal disease in the United States,* Bethesda, MD, 2009, National Institutes of Health and National Institute of Diabetes and Digestive and Kidney Diseases, p 206.)

ADJUSTED ESRD INCIDENT RATES, BY AGE AND RACE/ETHNICITY

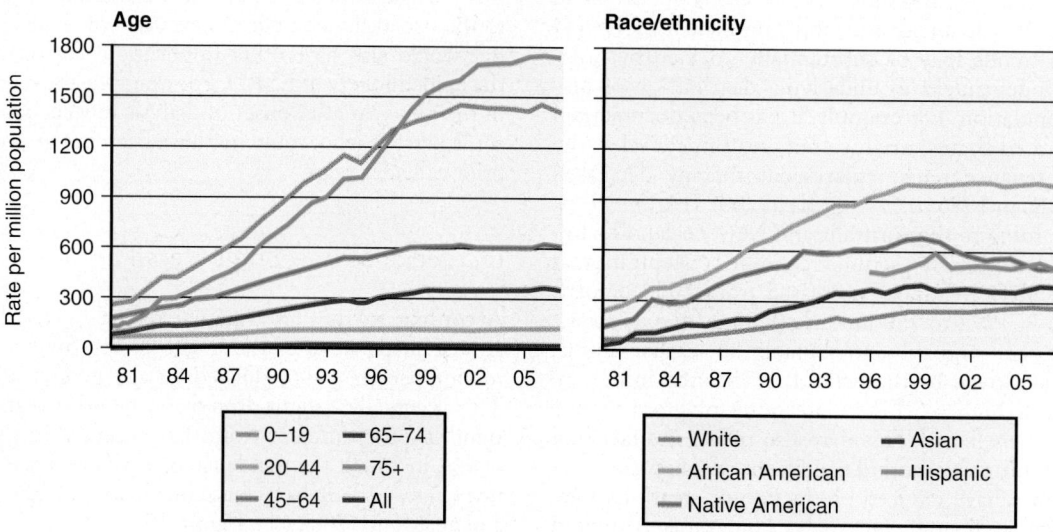

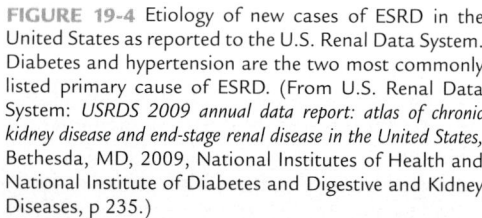

FIGURE 19-3 Differences in incidence of ESRD in the United States by age and race/ethnicity. In recent years, those older than 75 years have been observed to have the highest incidence of treated ESRD (1735 per million population in 2007). The adjusted ESRD incidence rates were 998 per million population for African Americans, 396 per million population for Asians/Pacific Islanders, and 273 per million population for Whites in 2007. (From U.S. Renal Data System: *USRDS 2009 annual data report: atlas of chronic kidney disease and end-stage renal disease in the United States,* Bethesda, MD, 2009, National Institutes of Health and National Institute of Diabetes and Digestive and Kidney Diseases, p 206.)

FIGURE 19-4 Etiology of new cases of ESRD in the United States as reported to the U.S. Renal Data System. Diabetes and hypertension are the two most commonly listed primary cause of ESRD. (From U.S. Renal Data System: *USRDS 2009 annual data report: atlas of chronic kidney disease and end-stage renal disease in the United States,* Bethesda, MD, 2009, National Institutes of Health and National Institute of Diabetes and Digestive and Kidney Diseases, p 235.)

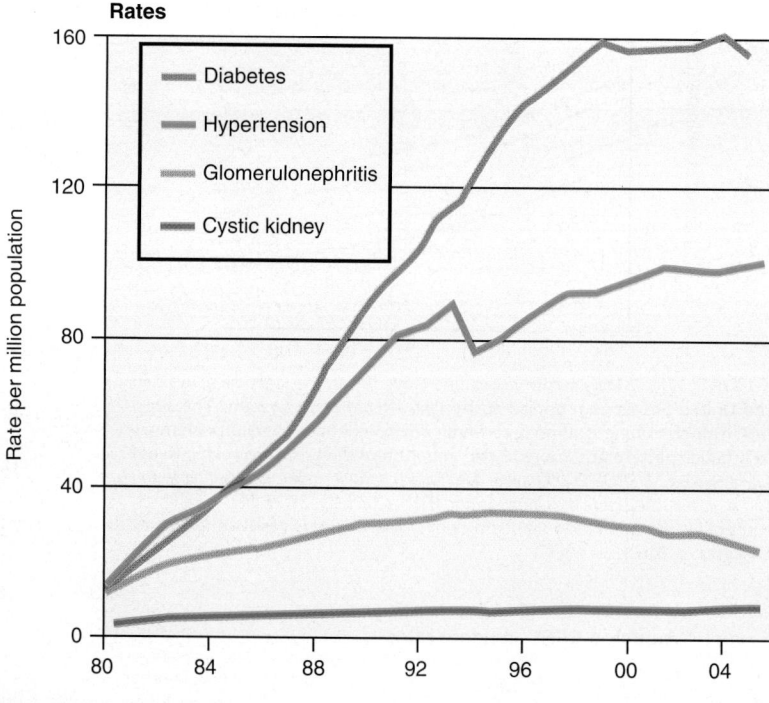

(see Figure 19-3). As alluded to previously, some of this rise may be attributed to the fact that elderly patients with more comorbid conditions are being entered more liberally into dialysis (and transplantation) programs. (See relevant sections in Chapters 20 and 21.) The most common listed cause of ESRD is diabetes (155 per 1 million population, or 45% of all cases of ESRD), followed by hypertension (99 per 1 million population, or 28% of all cases) (Figure 19-4). However, these are "primary diagnoses" for ESRD assigned by the treating physician at the start of dialysis when the original cause of disease may be difficult to discern. For example, numerous cases of ESRD ascribed to hypertension were preceded by clinical features highly suggestive of other renal parenchymal diseases (e.g., nephrotic range proteinuria).[8,9] Genetic studies have demonstrated that genetic variations accounted for much of the higher incidence of "hypertensive nephrosclerosis" observed among African-Americans.[10-12,12a,12b] These novel advances will undoubtedly force a rethinking of how physicians currently assign causes for ESRD.

Furthermore, the convention of ascribing only one primary cause to any case of ESRD may be inherently limited. For example, prospective studies have shown that patients with diabetes mellitus appear to be at several-fold higher risk for ESRD ascribed to nondiabetic causes.[13] At the same time, this convention cannot reflect the contribution of multiple disease processes to the final ESRD outcome (e.g., nonrecovery of renal function after acute tubular necrosis in a patient with underlying diabetic nephropathy). These considerations aside, it is clear that the rising number of patients who are overweight or obese and the rising number of patients with type 2 diabetes are of major concern for future increases in incidence of ESRD.[14-16] It remains unknown whether and to what extend this effect will be blunted by improved medical therapy among patients with these risk factors.[17]

Prevalence of End-Stage Renal Disease

According to the 2009 annual report by the USRDS, the annual prevalence of ESRD in the United States was 1665 per 1 million population (adjusted for age, gender, and race).[39,39a] As alluded to previously, the prevalence of disease depends not only on the number of new cases but also on the rate of survival of existing patients. Improved rates of survival both of patients on dialysis and of transplant recipients therefore increase the prevalence of disease (and "burden of ESRD"), but they actually reflect improvement in care. Indeed, the adjusted rates of mortality among patients on dialysis and among transplant recipients have improved (Figure 19-5). Another reflection of the difference between incidence and prevalence is the fact that although only 2% of incident ESRD patients are treated by kidney transplantation as the initial

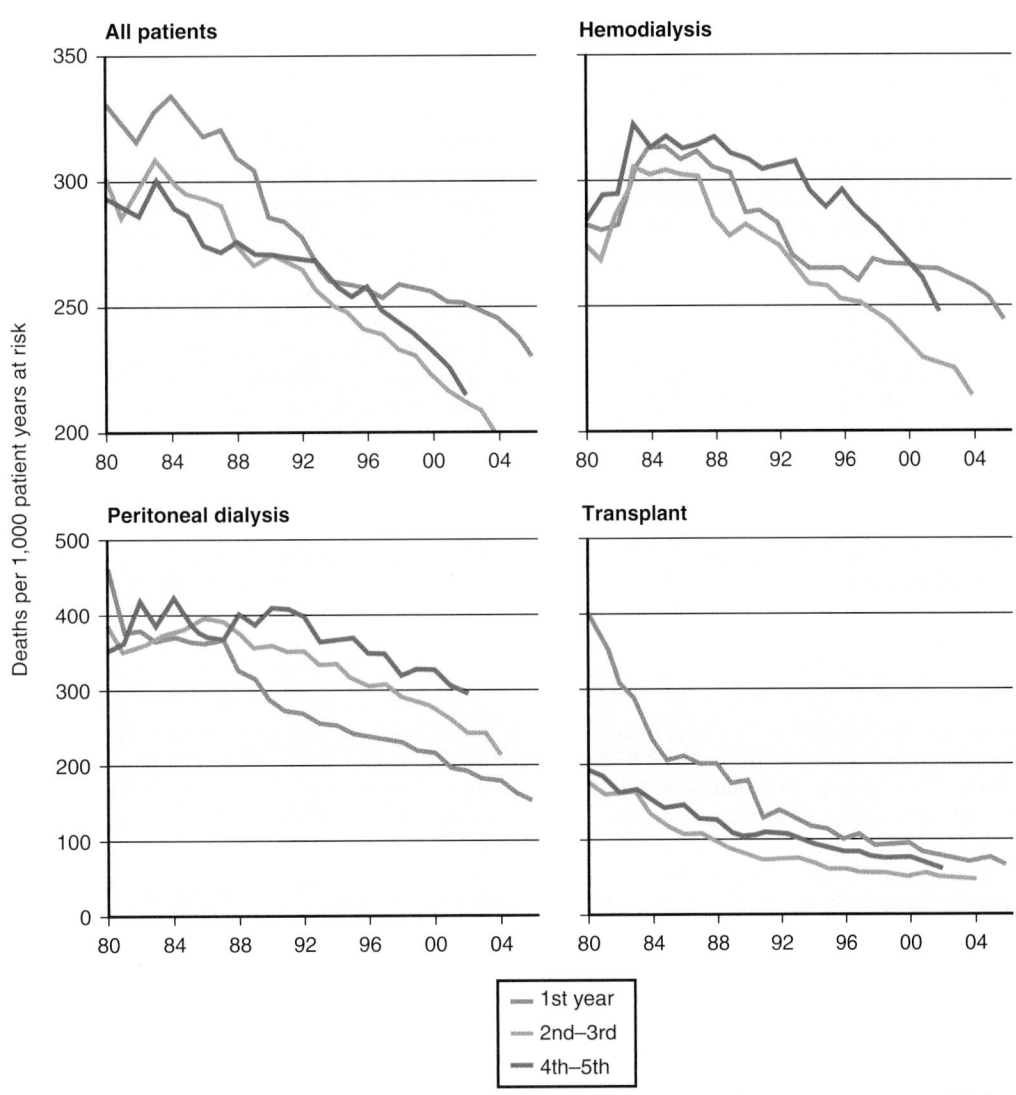

FIGURE 19-5 Risk of death in ESRD patients over time by different modalities of renal replacement therapy. From 1980 to 2006, the first-year mortality rate among incident dialysis and first transplant patients fell 30.5%: from 331.2 to 230.2 per 1000 patient years. After remaining quite stable in the late 1990s and early 2000s, mortality rates for hemodialysis patients have also fallen. (From U.S. Renal Data System: *USRDS 2009 annual data report: atlas of chronic kidney disease and end-stage renal disease in the United States,* Bethesda, MD, 2009, National Institutes of Health and National Institute of Diabetes and Digestive and Kidney Diseases, p 199.)

modality, 30% of prevalent ESRD patients are maintained with kidney transplants. This is because not only do numerous dialysis patients subsequently undergo kidney transplantation but also patients with kidney transplants survive longer. Similarly, the black-white disparity in ESRD is even more pronounced when prevalence ESRD is used as the metric instead of incidence ESRD because, on average, black patients survive longer with ESRD than do their white counterparts.

Rates of mortality among patients with ESRD, especially those on dialysis, remain alarmingly high: in excess of 20% per year. This high mortality rate is paralleled by high rates of hospitalization and health care utilization. Many epidemiology studies have sought to account for this. The burden of coexisting medical conditions already present at the start of dialysis appears to be a key problem. This is consistent with the observation that interventions to manipulate dialysis-related parameters—such as dose of dialysis per treatment,[18,19] use of more recombinant erythropoietin,[20] and newer phosphate binders[21]—have not succeeded in reducing mortality rates. A notable observation is that numerous risk factors for mortality in the general population, such as high blood pressure, high cholesterol level, and high body mass index, are paradoxically associated with lower risk of mortality among patients on maintenance dialysis.[22] Whether this is a result of confounding by factors such as underlying systolic cardiac dysfunction, malnutrition, or inflammation is an active area of investigation.[23] It is disappointing that numerous interventions to treat conventional Framingham risk factors *after* onset of ESRD, such as lipid lowering,[24,25] have been unsuccessful, and even the benefits of lowering blood pressure remain uncertain.[26,27]

Kidney Transplantation

Although no randomized controlled clinical trials have been performed, the best observational data indicate that, all else being equal, receipt of a kidney transplant confers reduced risk of mortality,[28] in addition to improved quality of life.[29] Currently, the rate of 1-year survival with a functioning allograft is 90% among recipients of deceased-donor transplants and 96% among recipients of living-donor transplants. In 2007, the number of kidney transplantations performed in the United States exceeded 17,513. Donations from deceased donors has increased, perhaps as a result of public education efforts and use of organs that would previously have been discarded (e.g., donation after cardiac death or expanded-criteria donor). After rising for nearly a decade, rates of living donor donations began declining during the 2000s (Figure 19-6). Shortage of transplant organs, however, remains a major problem and has resulted in longer waiting times. The pressure to increase the number of organs has led to numerous contentious discussions regarding proposed schemes to pay donors and the use of kidneys from living donors who have medical conditions such as hypertension which previously were considered contraindications to donation.

International Comparisons

Incidence and prevalence rates of ESRD vary considerably across different regions and countries. Taiwan (whose data include only patients on dialysis), Mexico (specifically

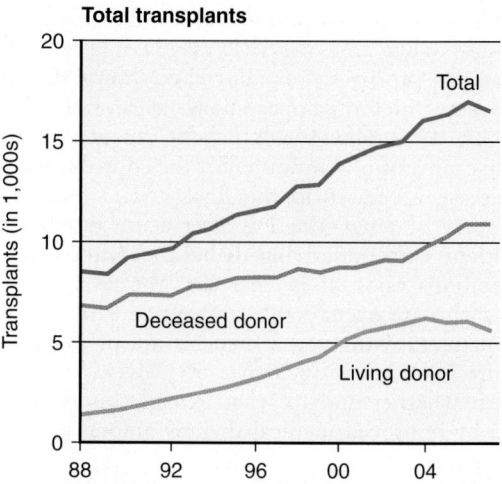

Total transplants

FIGURE 19-6 Number of transplants in the United States (limited to ESRD patients ages 20 and older). Shown are total number and breakdown by donor type. (From U.S. Renal Data System: *USRDS 2009 annual data report: atlas of chronic kidney disease and end-stage renal disease in the United States,* Bethesda, MD, 2009, National Institutes of Health and National Institute of Diabetes and Digestive and Kidney Diseases, p 283.)

Jalisco), and the United States report the highest rates of incident ESRD at 415, 372, and 361 per 1 million population, respectively (Figure 19-7). Interpreting rates of incidence of ESRD across countries, however, is complicated by lack of uniform data collection methods. Furthermore, because only treated ESRD cases are counted, differences in access to renal replacement therapy as a result of economics, public policy, or local practice patterns will greatly influence the statistics of incidence and prevalence rates.[30,31]

Despite these limitations, it is clear that the practice of renal replacement therapy varies considerably across the world. For example, in Hong Kong, the great majority of patients on dialysis are treated with peritoneal dialysis (reported to be 80% of prevalent patients vs. 36% in New Zealand, 26% in Iceland, and 7% in the United States). Home hemodialysis use also varies greatly (reported to be 16% in New Zealand, 10% in Australia, and 1% in the United States.) In terms of transplantation rates, the reported rates range widely: 58 per 1 million person-years in the United States; 38 per 1 million person-years in Israel and 23 per 1 million person-years in Argentina; and 3 per 1 million person-years in Romania. Finally, the economic model of delivery of dialysis also varies. In the United States, the majority of patients (nearly 60%) currently undergo dialysis at facilities owned by large dialysis companies. In other countries (such as Germany), the system is much more decentralized. Beyond registry data, international observational studies, such the Dialysis Outcomes and Practice Patterns Study (DOPPS), have documented noticeable practice variations. For example, in the late 1990s, arteriovenous fistula was used as the dialysis access by 80% of European but by only 24% of U.S. prevalent patients. The fistula was used as the access in 66% of European patients beginning hemodialysis, in comparison with 15% of such patients in the United States.[32] This and other differences may explain the much higher rate of mortality among U.S. patients than among patients elsewhere in the world.[33] (See also Section XIII, "Global Considerations in Kidney Disease.")

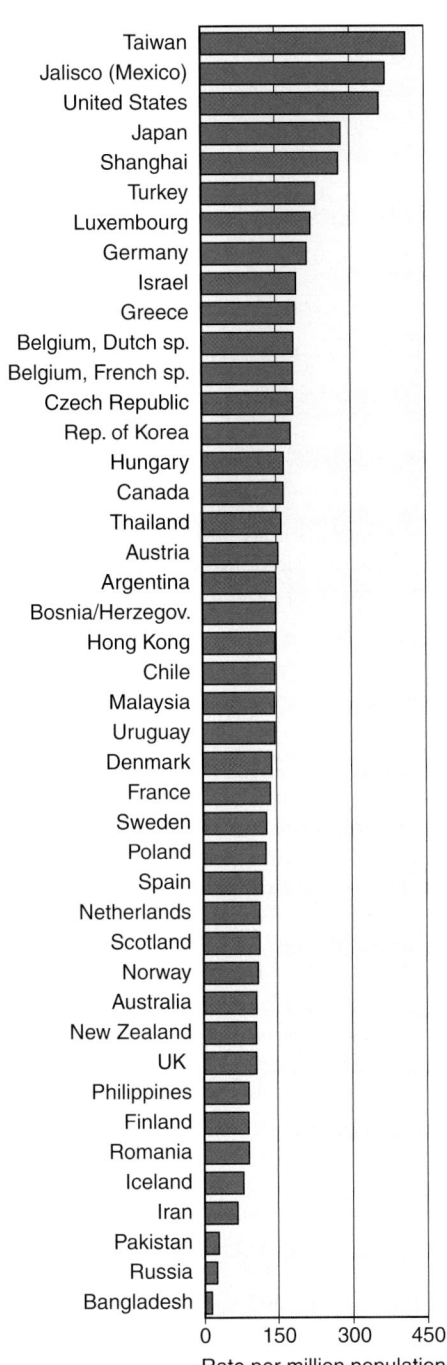

FIGURE 19-7 Reported incidence of ESRD in different countries in 2007. Incident rates of reported ESRD in 2007 were greatest in Taiwan (dialysis only), at 415 per million population, followed by Jalisco (Mexico), the United States, Japan (dialysis only), and Turkey, at 372, 361, 285, and 229, respectively. Rates of less than 100 per million were reported by Bangladesh, Iceland, Romania, Finland, and the Philippines. (From U.S. Renal Data System: *USRDS 2009 annual data report: atlas of chronic kidney disease and end-stage renal disease in the United States*, Bethesda, MD, 2009, National Institutes of Health and National Institute of Diabetes and Digestive and Kidney Diseases, p 348.)

Epidemiology of Chronic Kidney Disease

Since 2000, research into CKD has burgeoned. This field was codified in large part after the publication in 2002 of the National Kidney Foundation's Kidney Disease Outcomes Quality Initiative (KDOQI) definition and classification of CKD (Table 19-1).[34,35] Before this, no consensus definition of CKD had existed,[36] which made defining disease incidence and prevalence difficult. The National Kidney Foundation's CKD definition and classification have been very influential, widely disseminated, and widely adopted. Since the publication of the National Kidney Foundation CKD guidelines, the most common method used to estimate renal function is the simplified four-variable Modification of Diet in Renal Disease (MDRD) equation[37,38]:

$$GFR \ (mL/min/1.73 \ m^2) = 186 \times$$
$$[\text{serum creatinine level}]^{-1.154} \times [\text{age}]^{-0.203} \times$$
$$[0.742 \text{ if patient is female}] \times [1.212 \text{ if patient is black}]$$

This equation was derived from data from 1628 patients enrolled in the baseline period of the MDRD study, in whom GFR was measured directly with the use of urinary clearance of injected iodine-125–iothalamate. (See Chapter 25, "Laboratory Assessment of Kidney Disease: Glomerular Filtration Rate, Urinalysis, and Proteinuria.")

Prevalence of Chronic Kidney Disease

Most of the population study of CKD has focused on the prevalence of CKD. Probably the best data source for determining the prevalence of CKD in the population of an entire country has been the National Health and Nutrition Examination Surveys (NHANES) in the United States. Sponsored by the Centers for Disease Control and Prevention (CDC), NHANES is a series of surveys encompassing interviews with and physical examinations on a nationally representative sample of participants. The second series of NHANES (NHANES II) was conducted from 1976 to 1980; the third series (NHANES III) was conducted from 1988 to 1994; and the latest series was launched in 1999 as a continuous survey. According to data from NHANES from 1999 to 2004, the prevalence rate of CKD stages 1 to 4 among people aged 20 or older was 131,000 per 1 million persons (13.1%) (Figure 19-8). This translated into an absolute number of 26.3 million individuals and is therefore two orders of magnitude larger than the absolute number of patients with incident ESRD (104,962) or the absolute number of patients with prevalent ESRD (467,723; all 2004 data).[39,39a] This also represents an increase in the prevalence of CKD stages 1 to 4 from 100,000 per 1 million persons (10.0%), based on the NHANES III (1988 to 1994) survey.[40]

Two important caveats must be kept in mind in interpreting these data. First, the prevalence estimates vary greatly with the choice of equation to estimate renal function.[41] The MDRD equation is known to underestimate GFR among patients with more preserved renal function.[42,43] Newer equations have been devised to try to overcome this limitation. When one such equation—the CKD-EPI equation—was applied to the NHANES data for 1999 to 2004, the prevalence of stages 1 to 4 CKD dropped from 131,000 per 1 million to 115,000 per 1 million persons (or an absolute difference of 3 million, a margin of error much larger than the number of patients with ESRD).[44] This reduction is attributable primarily to a lower estimated prevalence of stage 3 disease (63,000 per 1 million vs. 78,000 per 1 million), which is what would be expected in view of the known bias in the MDRD equation.

TABLE 19-1 Classification and Staging of Chronic Kidney Disease by the National Kidney Foundation*		
STAGE	DESCRIPTION	GFR (ML/MIN/1.73 M²)
1	Kidney damage with normal or ↑ GFR	≥90
2	Kidney damage with mild ↓ GFR	60-89
3	Moderate ↓ GFR	30-59
4	Severe ↓ GFR	15-29
5	Kidney failure	<15 or dialysis

*This widely adopted classification required evidence of kidney damage (such as increased proteinuria) above a GFR level of 60 ml/min/1.73m² for the diagnosis of CKD but not below this threshold.

Chronic kidney disease is defined as either kidney damage or GFR <60 mL/min/1.73 m² for ≥ 3 months. Kidney damage is defined as pathologic abnormalities or markers of damage, including abnormalities in blood or urine tests or imaging studies.

GFR, Glomerular flow rate.

From National Kidney Foundation: K/DOQI clinical practice guidelines for chronic kidney disease: evaluation, classification, and stratification, *Am J Kidney Dis* 2002; 39(2, Suppl 2):S1-S266.

Second, interpreting temporal trends in CKD prevalence is complicated by problems with differences in calibration of creatinine measurement.[45,46] Until the mid to late 2000s, the same blood sample measured in different laboratories could yield serum creatinine concentration values that differed, commonly by 0.2 or 0.3 mg/dL.[47] In the past 2 decades of NHANES surveys, serum creatinine has been measured in several different laboratories in which different methods were used, which thus introduced systematic biases. A conservative trend analysis in which this bias was taken into account eliminated much, if not all, of the apparent increase in prevalence of CKD from the period 1988 to 1994 to the period 1999 to 2004.[40] (In fact, the exact method by which serum creatinine is calibrated also has substantial effects on the measurement of prevalence of disease.[40,48]) Further evidence that estimates of prevalence of CKD in NHANES over time were confounded by problems in creatinine calibration came from an analysis in which cystatin C was used as the measure of renal function. This cystatin C–based analysis showed that, in fact, the prevalence of CKD did not change from the period 1988 to 1994 to the period 1999 to 2004.[49]

Incidence of Chronic Kidney Disease

Less is known about incidence of CKD because few truly representative longitudinal cohorts are available for tracking and quantifying the development of new cases of CKD. According to one report based on the Atherosclerosis Risk in Communities (ARIC) study,[50] the incidence rate was 10,350 per 1 million person-years when incident CKD was defined as the MDRD equation's estimated GFR of less than 60 mL/min/1.73 m². This reported incidence is similar to that based on another analysis of data from both ARIC and the Cardiovascular Health Study: 13,000 per 1 million person-years.[51] In both ARIC and the Cardiovascular Health Study, researchers attempted to correct for creatinine calibration drift over time, which is important because these drifts are comparable in magnitude with creatinine changes caused by progression of CKD over several years. Estimates of disease incidence in other studies have been similar, and the reported incidence CKD was higher if new-onset albuminuria was also counted as a new case of CKD.[52] A common limitation of these studies is that only one observed low GFR is used to define new cases of CKD. (The KDOQI definition requires two low GFR readings, at least 3 months apart.) This is also a problem with the prevalence data. Because some patients may only have a transient drop in GFR, prevalence and incidence estimates would be lower if case definition required documentation of chronically low GFR levels.

Outcome by Stage of Chronic Kidney Disease

Although there is great interest in knowing outcome (such as incidence of dialysis vs. death) by level of CKD stage, it is clear that within the same stage of CKD, different subgroups of patients have rather different outcomes. In one study of patients enrolled in a health maintenance organization in the United States, over the 5-year observation period, rates of renal replacement therapy were 1.3% and 19.9%, for those with stages 3 and 4 CKD, and the corresponding rates of death were 24.3% and 45.7%.[53] This study and other studies of patients with CKD who received usual medical care[54] showed that in general, risk of death is much higher than risk of ESRD. This must also be true for the population as a whole, in view of the small number of incident ESRD cases in comparison with the much larger number of prevalent CKD cases (a difference of about two orders of magnitude). However, this ratio of death versus ESRD varies greatly with age. In one large study, male U.S. veterans with CKD stages 3 to 5 were monitored for a mean of 3.2 years; among patients of all ages, rates of both death and ESRD were inversely related to estimated GFR at baseline. However, among those with comparable levels of estimated GFR, older patients had higher rates of death and lower rates of ESRD than did younger patients. As a consequence, the level of estimated GFR below which the risk of ESRD exceeded the risk of death varied by age, ranging from 45 mL/min/1.73 m² for 18- to 44-year-old patients to 15 mL/min/1.73 m² for 65- to 84-year-old patients. Among those aged 85 years or older, the risk of death always exceeded the risk of ESRD (Figure 19-9).[55] Furthermore, among patients enrolled in randomized clinical trials of interventions to retard renal disease progression—such as the MDRD study,[56] the Reduction of Endpoints in NIDDM [non–insulin-dependent diabetes mellitus] with the Angiotensin II Antagonist Losartan (RENAAL),[57] and the Irbesartan in Diabetic Nephropathy Trial (IDNT)[58]—risk of ESRD was higher than risk of death. This is because trial enrollees are not representative of the general population with CKD.

PREVALENCE OF CHRONIC KIDNEY DISEASE (CKD) STAGES BY AGE GROUP IN NHAMES 1988–1994 AND 1999–2004

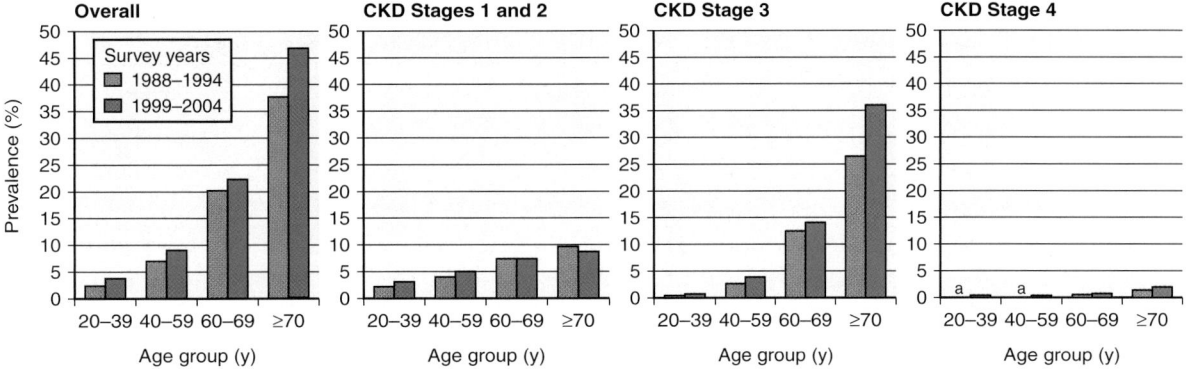

NHANES indicates National Health and Nutrition Examination Surveys.
^aThere were no cases in 1988–1994.

FIGURE 19-8 Prevalence of CKD stages by age group in NHANES surveys from 1988 to 1994 and 1999 to 2004. This analysis, based on serum creatinine measurements, estimated that overall the prevalence rate of CKD increased from 10.0% (95% CI, 9.1-10.9) to 13.1% (95% CI, 12.0-14.1). (From Coresh J, Selvin E, Stevens LA, et al: Prevalence of chronic kidney disease in the United States, *JAMA* 2007;298[17]:2038-2047.)

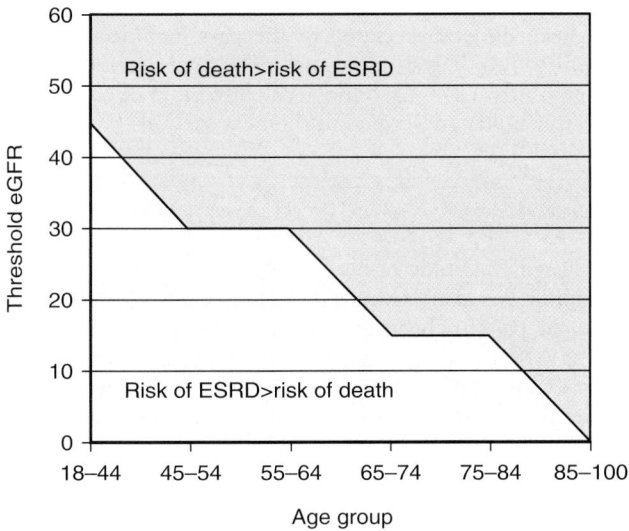

Baseline eGFR threshold below which risk for ESRD exceeded risk for death for each age group.

FIGURE 19-9 Relative risk of death vs. ESRD by age and estimated GFR threshold among U.S. male veterans. Among patients who were younger than 45 years, the incidence of treated ESRD was greater than that of death at all estimated GFR (eGFR) levels <45 ml/min per 1.73m². Conversely, among those aged 65 to 84, only at eGFR levels <15 ml/min per 1.73m² did risk for ESRD exceed risk for death. Among those ages 85 to 100, the risk for death exceeded risk for ESRD even at eGFR levels <15 ml/min per 1.73m². (From O'Hare AM, Choi AI, Berthenthal D, et al: Age affects outcomes in chronic kidney disease, *J Am Soc Nephrol* 2007;18[10]:2758-2765.)

Controversies Regarding Classification of Chronic Kidney Disease

Vocal criticism of the National Kidney Foundation's CKD classification system has been increasing.[59-63] The concerns focus mainly on a few issues. One is the contention that estimated GFR lower than 60 mL/min/1.73 m² alone (without other signs of renal parenchymal damage)—identified in a large number of elderly patients—does not truly represent CKD but merely reflects "normal" aging. This problem is compounded by the known bias in the MDRD equation, which is known to underestimate renal function, particularly

among patients with lower serum creatinine levels. More research regarding the implications of decreased GFR among elderly persons will be helpful in informing this debate. Thus, it is possible that in the future, there will be alternative definitions of CKD that will naturally lead to revisions in incidence and prevalence data. Changing the definition of CKD would have substantial implications. For example, screening for CKD has garnered much interest. The definition of "chronic kidney disease" affects estimates of disease prevalence and the natural history of "cases" detected through screening. These two factors will critically determine the value of any screening efforts[64,65] in which the benefits of early detection and intervention must be balanced against the risk of harm to patients whose cases were false-positive ones.[66] (Data from screening programs such as National Kidney Foundation's Kidney Early Evaluation Program [KEEP] are less reliable as guides to prevalence of disease because targeted screening and self-selection means that the observed rates of disease are unlikely to be representative of the general population.)

International Comparisons

The NHANES studies from the United States discussed previously are the most reliable and sophisticated analyses with regard to the prevalence of CKD in the general population. Direct international comparison is problematic because of lack of uniformity in calibration of serum creatinine or lack of representative community-based samples—two critical elements needed to obtain reliable estimates of disease prevalence in the population. As summarized in this chapter in the prior edition of *Brenner and Rector's The Kidney*,[67] the prevalence of GFRs of 60 mL/min/1.73 m² or lower has been reported to vary from less than 2% (20,000 per 1 million persons) to more than 40% (400,000 per 1 million persons) in different studies from different countries. One study of data from the population-based Health Survey of Nord-Trondelag County (HUNT II) in Norway[68] did show that the prevalence of CKD in the United States was similar to that in Norway (Table 19-2). In this study, investigators analyzed data explicitly by using the same methods used in NHANES, and creatinine measurements were calibrated.

TABLE 19-2 Estimated Prevalence of Chronic Kidney Disease, Stages 1 to 4 (Expressed as Percentage of Population) in Norway versus the United States

STAGE	NORWAY: 1995 to 1997* WHITE (*N* = 65,181)	UNITED STATES: 1988 to 1994* WHITE (*N* = 6635)	BLACK (*N* = 4163)	OVERALL (*N* = 15,625)
1	2.7 (0.3)	2.8 (0.3)	5.8 (0.3)	3.3 (0.3)
2	3.2 (0.4)	3.2 (0.3)	2.5 (0.3)	3.0 (0.3)
3	4.2 (0.1)	4.8 (0.3)	3.1 (0.2)	4.3 (0.3)
4	0.16 (0.01)	0.21 (0.03)	0.25 (0.08)	0.20 (0.03)
Total	10.2 (0.5)	11.0 (0.6)	11.6 (0.5)	11.0 (0.5)

*Expressed as a percentage of the population, with standard errors in parentheses.
  Total CKD prevalence in Norway was 10.2%, which closely approximates reported U.S. CKD prevalence. Thus lower progression to ESRD rather than a smaller pool of individuals at risk appears to explain the much lower incidence of ESRD in Norway compared with the United States.
  From Hallan SI, Coresh J, Astor BC, et al: International comparison of the relationship of chronic kidney disease prevalence and ESRD risk, *J Am Soc Nephrol* 2006;17(8):2275-2284.

Epidemiologic Relationship between Chronic Kidney Disease and End-Stage Renal Disease

The HUNT II study is also interesting because it highlighted another notable epidemiologic feature. Although the prevalence of CKD in Norway is similar to that in the United States, the incidence of ESRD in Norway is much lower than that in the United States (see Figure 19-7).[68] Similar dissociations between epidemiologic features of CKD and ESRD have been noted in the United States. For example, an analysis in which investigators juxtaposed CKD prevalence with ESRD incidence, using data from NHANES and the U.S. Renal Data System, revealed that although the incidence of ESRD in the United States is much higher among black persons than among white persons, the prevalence of CKD does not appear to be higher among black persons.[69] The lack of higher prevalence of stages 3 and 4 CKD among black persons in comparison with white persons has also been observed in other population-based studies.[70,71] Presumably the much higher incidence rate of ESRD among black persons is ascribable to more rapid progression from CKD to ESRD.[69]

There is also epidemiologic dissociation between CKD and ESRD over time. The rise in the incidence of ESRD in the 1980s and 1990s in the United States was not paralleled by a proportionate rise in the prevalence of underlying CKD. Rather, risk of ESRD per case of CKD had increased. Among every 1000 adults aged 20 to 74 with CKD stage 3 or 4 in 1978, 9 new cases of ESRD developed in 1983, but among every 1000 adults with CKD stage 3 or 4 in 1991, 16 new cases of ESRD developed in 1996 (relative risk = 1.7, 95% confidence interval = 1.1 to 2.7).[72] In an analysis of data of individual patients who underwent screening health examinations from 1964 to 1985 in Northern California, the crude incidence of ESRD increased from 140 per 1 million person-years among individuals examined in 1964 to 340 per 1 million person-years among those examined in 1985 (Figure 19-10).[73] This increase represents an 8% per-calendar-year higher risk for progressing to needing treatment for ESRD, and this risk was not explained by increases over time in the prevalence of CKD or risk factors for renal failure such as age, gender, race, diabetes, blood pressure, body mass index, proteinuria, serum creatinine level, or other comorbid conditions. These epidemiologic and individual patient-level data strongly

suggest that prevalence of CKD or prevalence of conventional risk factors for kidney disease (such as diabetes mellitus) is not the only determinant of future incidence of ESRD. Other potentially important factors that may have been underappreciated in the past include more liberal entry into dialysis programs (described previously) or a higher incidence of AKI and accelerated loss of renal function after injury (described in the next section).

Epidemiology of Acute Kidney Injury

The systematic study of acute renal failure (or AKI) in the population is a relatively new development. One limiting factor in the past has been the lack of consensus on the definition of AKI (or acute renal failure). Because different acute increases in serum creatinine level were used in different studies to define cases, it is difficult to compare disease incidence across different clinical settings, patient populations, and calendar years because it is not known how much of the observed variation results from differences in definition, as opposed to differences in true underlying disease frequency. This may be less of a problem when the outcome is AKI that necessitates dialysis. In these cases, however, an additional layer of complexity is that the criteria for initiating acute dialysis may vary by place and time. Some investigators have tried to define the incidence of acute renal failure by using International Classification of Diseases, Ninth Revision, Clinical Modification (ICD-9-CM) codes, such as 584.X (acute renal failure). These diagnostic codes, however, have been shown to be specific but quite insensitive.[74] Probably only the most severe cases were captured, and so these studies may give some idea about the lower bound of disease estimates. In addition, there may be "code creep," by which milder degrees of AKI are more likely to be diagnosed as awareness of this condition increases.[74] Temporal changes in incidence of AKI defined by diagnostic codes must therefore be interpreted with caution.

The proposed consensus definitions of acute renal failure or AKI have greatly improved the situation. In 2004, the Acute Dialysis Quality Initiative (ADQI) Group proposed the RIFLE (Risk, Injury, Failure, Loss and End-stage renal disease) classification schema for acute renal failure (Figure 19-11).[75] Three years later, the Acute Kidney Injury Network (AKIN) put forth its own system, which included replacing the

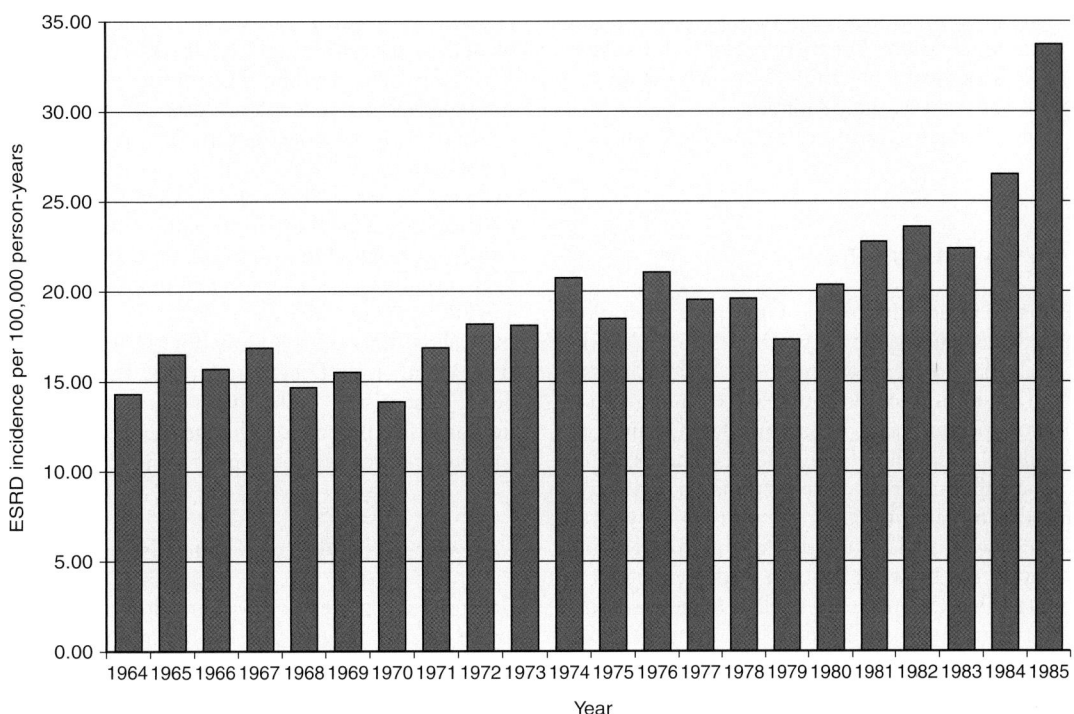

FIGURE 19-10 Crude incidence (per 100,000 person-years) of new cases of treated ESRD through 2000 by year of cohort entry (year of baseline examination). This progressive increase in rate does not appear to be accounted for by baseline differences renal function or risk factors for ESRD. In other words, an individual with a certain set of clinical characteristics from the 1980s was more likely to go on to receive treatment for ESRD compared with an individual with identical risk factors from the 1960s. (From Hsu CY, Go AS, McCulloch CE, et al: Exploring secular trends in the likelihood of receiving treatment for end-stage renal disease, *Clin J Am Soc Nephrol* 2007;2[1]:81-88.)

term *acute renal failure* with *acute kidney injury* and defining "abrupt" changes in renal function as those occurring within 48 hours. The AKIN staging system for AKI according to abrupt increases in serum creatinine levels is as follows[76]:

- Stage 1: increase of 0.3 mg/dL or more, or increase of 150% to 200% (1.5-fold to 2.0-fold) from baseline
- Stage 2: increase of more than 200% to 300% (more than 2.0- to 3.0-fold) from baseline
- Stage 3: increase of more than 300% (more than 3.0-fold) from baseline, or serum creatinine level of 4.0 mg/dL or higher with an acute rise of at least 0.5 mg/dL

Both the RIFLE and AKIN systems also allow changes in urine output to be included in the definitions of stages of AKI. However, reliable information on urine output is often not available in large epidemiologic data sets, and so this has rarely been used to define incidence of AKI in the population setting.

A second limitation in the past has been the fact that most studies were based on hospitalized patients or on the subgroup of hospitalized patients in the intensive care unit (ICU).[77-81] The denominator in these studies is often hospitalization or ICU admission, which are suboptimal criteria because rates of hospitalization (or ICU admission) per population are not defined and because they vary in different countries and across time. For example, one much-cited study of patients from Tufts–New England Medical Center in Boston from 1978 to 1979 revealed that the incidence of acute renal failure was 4.9% per hospitalization.[77] Applying the identical criteria to patients admitted to Rush Presbyterian–St. Luke's Medical Center in Chicago in 1996, the same investigative team found that the incidence of AKI was 7.2% per hospitalization.[78] However, it not possible to determine how much of this change is accounted for by variation in threshold for hospital

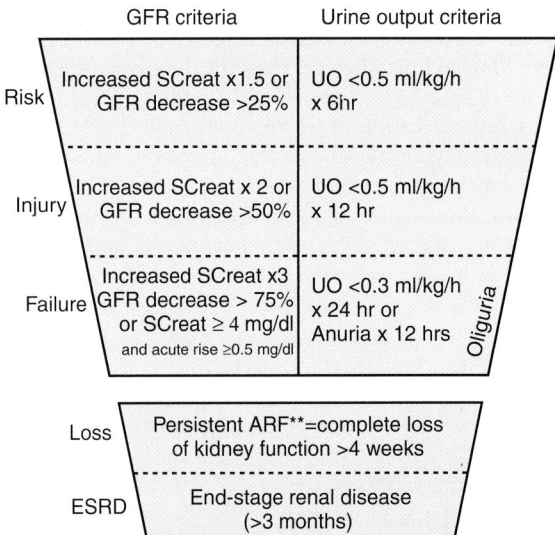

FIGURE 19-11 The RIFLE (Risk, Injury, Failure, Loss and End-stage renal disease) classification system for acute renal failure/acute kidney injury. The classification system includes separate criteria for creatinine and urine output (UO). A patient can fulfill the criteria through changes in serum creatinine (SCreat), changes in UO, or both. The criteria that lead to the worst possible classification should be used. Note that the F component of RIFLE (failure of kidney function) is present even if the increase in SCreat is under threefold as long as the new SCreat is greater than 4.0 mg/dL (350 μmol/L) in the setting of an acute increase of at least 0.5 mg/dL (44 μmol/L). Persistent ARF (loss) is defined as need for renal replacement therapy (RRT) for more than 4 weeks, whereas ESRD is defined by need for dialysis for longer than 3 months. (From Bellomo R, Ronco C, Kellum JA, et al: Acute renal failure—definition, outcome measures, animal models, fluid therapy and information technology needs: the Second International Consensus Conference of the Acute Dialysis Quality Initiative [ADQI] Group, *Crit Care* 2004;8[4]:R204-R212.)

admission in comparison with true underlying changes in the incidence of acute renal failure. For these reasons, the following discussions focuses mostly on studies in which the underlying population was used as the denominator and in which well-defined acute changes in serum creatinine level was used to define AKI.

Incidence of Acute Kidney Injury

A population-based study from the Grampian region of Scotland revealed that during the first 6 months of 2003, the incidence of AKI, diagnosed according to the RIFLE classification, was 2147 per 1 million person-years[82] (among which 336 per 1 million person-years were considered acute-on-chronic renal failure). Overall, 8.5% of the cases necessitated dialysis (183 per 1 million person-years). Sepsis was a precipitating factor in 47% of patients.

Several studies have provided incidence data on AKI that necessitated dialysis. An 11-week Scottish study conducted in 2000 demonstrated that the incidence of dialysis-necessitating AKI was 203 per 1 million person-years.[83] Another Scottish study from the Dumfries and Galloway area (from 1994 to 2000) produced a similar estimate of dialysis-necessitating AKI, at 176 patients per 1 million person-years.[84] These estimates are much higher than those reported in prior studies. For example, a 9-month study conducted in 1991 to 1992 in Madrid, Spain, reported that the community incidence of dialysis-necessitating AKI was only 75 per 1 million person-years.[85] The strong temporal trend in increase in incidence of dialysis-necessitating AKI was confirmed in an analysis of a nationally representative database of hospitalizations in the United States. This showed that the incidence of dialysis-necessitating AKI rose from 40 per 1 million person-years in 1988 to 270 per 1 million person-years in 2002.[86] Of interest was that despite an increase in the degree of comorbidity, in-hospital mortality rates had declined.

Finally, the community-based estimate of incidence of dialysis-necessitating AKI was reported out of a large integrated health care delivery system in Northern California (Kaiser Permanente). Between 1996 and 2003, the incidence of dialysis-necessitating AKI increased from 195 to 295 per 1 million person-years. This study provided evidence that the increase in this incidence was not simply a result of secular changes in practice pattern (i.e., initiating dialysis earlier in the course of AKI[87,88]), in as much as there was a parallel increase in the incidence of AKI that did not necessitate dialysis that was defined by documented abrupt changes in serum creatinine levels (Figure 19-12). Overall, AKI was more common among men and among elderly persons, although those aged 80 years or older were less likely to receive acute dialysis treatment. The exact reasons for the increasing incidence of AKI are unclear. They may include the increase in the incidence of sepsis,[80,89] a dominant risk factor for AKI.[90] In addition, invasive procedures that are nephrotoxic, such as cardiac catheterization, have been used more.[91-93]

Prevalence of Acute Kidney Injury

Because of the relatively short duration of AKI, defining prevalence of disease is probably not a meaningful parameter, and no reliable data on the population prevalence of AKI are available.

Linking Acute, Chronic, and End-Stage Renal Disease

A number of studies have demonstrated linkages between the epidemiologic features of acute, chronic, and end-stage renal disease. First, although CKD is well known to be a strong (probably the strongest) risk factor for AKI, this relationship was not quantified rigorously until 2008. It turned out that even patients with only stage "3a" CKD (estimated GFR = 45 to 59 mL/min/1.73 m²) are at nearly twice the risk of AKI as persons with estimated GFR ≥ 60 mL/min/1.73 m². Moreover, at every GFR level, patients with diabetes had higher risk than did patients without diabetes (Figure 19-13).[94] Second, data have shown that episodes of AKI accelerate

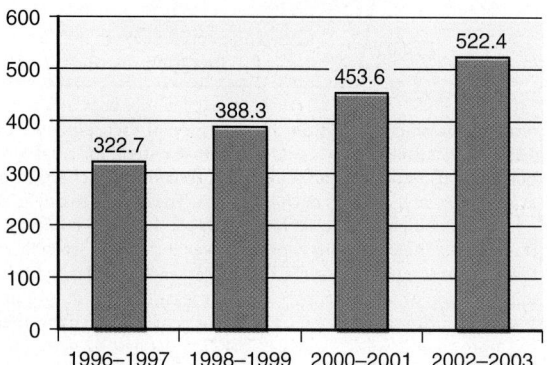

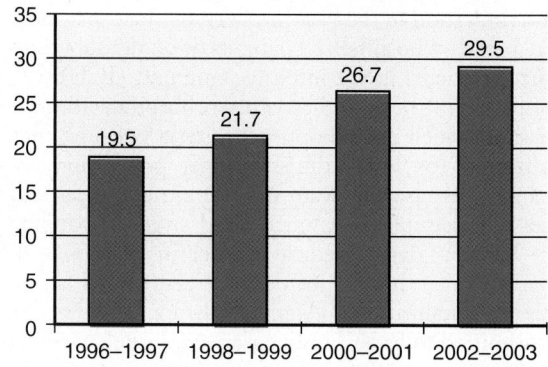

FIGURE 19-12 Secular trends in incidence of AKI. In this community-based study, incidences of both non–dialysis-requiring* and dialysis-requiring AKI have increased over time in parallel from 1996 to 2003. The former increased from 322.7 to 522.4 per 100,000 person-years; the latter from 19.5 to 29.5 per 100,000 person-years. *, Non–dialysis-requiring AKI defined using documented acute changes in serum creatinine and criteria defined in reference 77. (From Hsu CY, McCulloch CE, Fan D, et al: Community-based incidence of acute renal failure, *Kidney Int* 2007;72[2]:208-212.)

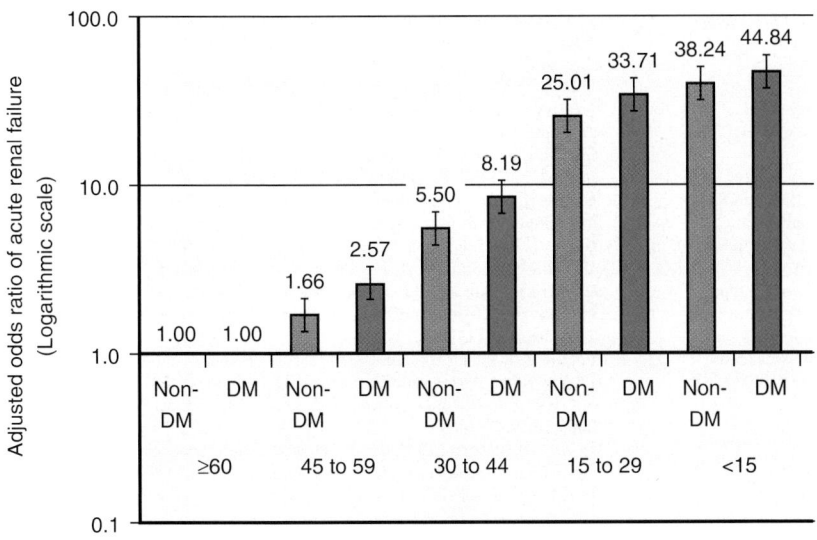

FIGURE 19-13 Baseline severity of CKD and risk of dialysis requiring AKI. Among both patients with and without diabetes, there was a strong association between level of preadmission eGFR and risk of AKI, which was evident at an eGFR as high as 60 ml/min/1.73m². (From Hsu CY, Ordonez JD, Chertow GM, et al: The risk of acute renal failure in patients with chronic kidney disease. *Kidney Int* 2008;74[1]:101-107.)

Multivariable association of baseline estimated GFR and dialysis-requiring ARF stratified by the presence or absence of diabetes mellitus (DM). Each model adjusted for age, sex, race/ethnicity, diagnosed hypertension, and documented proteinuria.

development or progression of CKD.[95] For example, one study demonstrated that among patients who suffered dialysis-necessitating AKI who had baseline stage "3b" CKD (preadmission estimated GFR = 15 to 44 mL/min/1.73 m²) or worse, approximately half of the survivors developed ESRD because they did not recover sufficient renal function to discontinue dialysis.[96] For those with baseline preadmission GFR of 45 mL/min/1.73 m² or higher, dialysis-necessitating AKI was independently associated with a 28-fold increase in the risk of developing stage 4 or 5 CKD in the subsequent months to years.[97] Also emerging is evidence that even AKI that does not necessitate dialysis does accelerate decrease in GFR and increases the risk of subsequent ESRD.[98-100] Renal parenchymal injury sustained during episodes of AKI may lead to permanent tubulointerstitial fibrosis and a reduction in the number of functioning nephrons.[101,102] Thus, the substantial increase in the incidence of AKI may explain some increase in the incidence of end-stage disease that is out of proportion to the increase in prevalence of CKD outlined previously. According to one estimate, 25% of the observed increased in ESRD incidence though the 1990s in the United States may be attributed to changes in incidence and outcome of patients with AKI.[103]

Conclusion

Much progress has been made since 2000 with regard to defining the epidemiologic features of kidney disease. Although the field had traditionally been dominated by research on ESRD, the study of the incidence and distribution of CKD is a rapidly maturing area. Ongoing investigations into the population epidemiologic features of AKI will fill important gaps in current knowledge.

References

1. Completeness and reliability of USRDS data: comparisons with the Michigan Kidney Registry. *Am J Kidney Dis.* 1992;20(5, Suppl 2):84-88.
2. Stewart JH, McCredie MR, Williams SM, et al. Interpreting incidence trends for treated end-stage renal disease: implications for evaluating disease control in Australia. *Nephrology (Carlton).* 2004;9(4):238-246.
3. Hakim RM, Lazarus JM. Initiation of dialysis. *J Am Soc Nephrol.* 1995;6(5):1319-1328.
4. Murtagh FE, Marsh JE, Donohoe P, et al. Dialysis or not? A comparative survival study of patients over 75 years with chronic kidney disease stage 5. *Nephrol Dial Transplant.* 2007;22(7):1955-1962.
5. Rosansky SJ, Clark WF, Eggers P, et al. Initiation of dialysis at higher GFRs: is the apparent rising tide of early dialysis harmful or helpful? *Kidney Int.* 2009;76(3):257-261.
6. Finne P, Reunanen A, Stenman S, et al. Incidence of end-stage renal disease in patients with type 1 diabetes. *JAMA.* 2005;294(14):1782-1787.
7. Gilbertson DT, Liu J, Xue JL, et al. Projecting the number of patients with end-stage renal disease in the United States to the year 2015. *J Am Soc Nephrol.* 2005;16(12):3736-3741.
8. Schlessinger SD, Tankersley MR, Curtis JJ. Clinical documentation of end-stage renal disease due to hypertension. *Am J Kidney Dis.* 1994;23:655-660.
9. Hsu CY. Does non-malignant hypertension cause renal insufficiency? Evidence-based perspective. *Curr Opin Nephrol Hypertens.* 2002;11(3):267-272.
10. Kao WH, Klag MJ, Meoni LA, et al. MYH9 is associated with nondiabetic end-stage renal disease in African Americans. *Nat Genet.* 2008;40(10):1185-1192.
11. Kopp JB, Smith MW, Nelson GW, et al. MYH9 is a major-effect risk gene for focal segmental glomerulosclerosis. *Nat Genet.* 2008;40(10):1175-1184.
12. Freedman BI, Sedor JR. Hypertension-associated kidney disease: perhaps no more. *J Am Soc Nephrol.* 2008;19(11):2047-2051.
12a. Genovese G, Friedman D, Ross MD, et al. Association of rypanolytic ApoL1 variants with kidney disease in African-Americans. *Science.* 2010;329(5993):841-845. Published online july 15, 2010.

12b. Tzur S, Rosset S, Shemer R, et al. Missense mutations in the APOL1 gene are highly associated with end stage kidney disease risk previously attributed to the MYH9 gene. *And Hum Genet.* 2010;128(3):345-350. Published online july 16, 2010.

13. Brancati FL, Whelton PK, Randall BL, et al. Risk of end-stage renal disease in diabetes mellitus: a prospective cohort study of men screened for MRFIT. *JAMA.* 1997;278(23):2069-2074.

14. Perneger TV, Brancati FL, Whelton PK, et al. End-stage renal disease attributable to diabetes mellitus. *Ann Intern Med.* 1994;121(12):912-918.

15. Humphrey LL, Ballard DJ, Frohnert PP, et al. Chronic renal failure in non–insulin-dependent diabetes mellitus. A population-based study in Rochester, Minnesota. *Ann Intern Med.* 1989;111(10):788-796.

16. Pavkov ME, Bennett PH, Knowler WC, et al. Effect of youth-onset type 2 diabetes mellitus on incidence of end-stage renal disease and mortality in young and middle-aged Pima Indians. *JAMA.* 2006;296(4):421-426.

17. Flegal KM, Graubard BI, Williamson DF, et al. Excess deaths associated with underweight, overweight, and obesity. *JAMA.* 2005;293(15):1861-1867.

18. Eknoyan G, Beck GJ, Cheung AK, et al. Effect of dialysis dose and membrane flux in maintenance hemodialysis. *N Engl J Med.* 2002;347(25):2010-2019.

19. Paniagua R, Amato D, Vonesh E, et al. Effects of increased peritoneal clearances on mortality rates in peritoneal dialysis: ADEMEX, a prospective, randomized, controlled trial. *J Am Soc Nephrol.* 2002;13(5):1307-1320.

20. Besarab A, Bolton WK, Browne JK, et al. The effects of normal as compared with low hematocrit values in patients with cardiac disease who are receiving hemodialysis and epoetin. *N Engl J Med.* 1998;339(9):584-590.

21. Suki WN, Zabaneh R, Cangiano JL, et al. Effects of sevelamer and calcium-based phosphate binders on mortality in hemodialysis patients. *Kidney Int.* 2007;72(9):1130-1137.

22. Kalantar-Zadeh K, Block G, Humphreys MH, et al. Reverse epidemiology of cardiovascular risk factors in maintenance dialysis patients. *Kidney Int.* 2003;63(3):793-808.

23. Liu Y, Coresh J, Eustace JA, et al. Association between cholesterol level and mortality in dialysis patients: role of inflammation and malnutrition. *JAMA.* 2004;291(4):451-459.

24. Wanner C, Krane V, Marz W, et al. Atorvastatin in patients with type 2 diabetes mellitus undergoing hemodialysis. *N Engl J Med.* 2005;353(3):238-248.

25. Fellstrom BC, Jardine AG, Schmieder RE, et al. Rosuvastatin and cardiovascular events in patients undergoing hemodialysis. *N Engl J Med.* 2009;360(14):1395-1407.

26. Heerspink HJ, Ninomiya T, Zoungas S, et al. Effect of lowering blood pressure on cardiovascular events and mortality in patients on dialysis: a systematic review and meta-analysis of randomised controlled trials. *Lancet.* 2009;373(9668):1009-1015.

27. Tomson CRV. Blood pressure and outcome in patients on dialysis. *Lancet.* 2009;373(9668):981-982.

28. Wolfe RA, Ashby VB, Milford EL, et al. Comparison of mortality in all patients on dialysis, patients on dialysis awaiting transplantation, and recipients of a first cadaveric transplant. *N Engl J Med.* 1999;341(23):1725-1730.

29. Evans RW, Manninen DL, Garrison Jr LP, et al. The quality of life of patients with end-stage renal disease. *N Engl J Med.* 1985;312(9):553-559.

30. Yang WC, Hwang SJ. Incidence, prevalence and mortality trends of dialysis end-stage renal disease in Taiwan from 1990 to 2001: the impact of national health insurance. *Nephrol Dial Transplant.* 2008;23(12):3977-3982.

31. Calderon-Margalit R, Gordon ES, Hoshen M, et al. Dialysis in Israel, 1989–2005—time trends and international comparisons. *Nephrol Dial Transplant.* 2008;23(2):659-664.

32. Pisoni RL, Young EW, Dykstra DM, et al. Vascular access use in Europe and the United States: results from the DOPPS. *Kidney Int.* 2002;61(1):305-316.

33. Foley RN, Hakim RM. Why is the mortality of dialysis patients in the United States much higher than the rest of the world? *J Am Soc Nephrol.* 2009;20(7):1432-1435.

34. National Kidney Foundation. K/DOQI clinical practice guidelines for chronic kidney disease: evaluation, classification, and stratification. *Am J Kidney Dis.* 2002;39(2, Suppl 2):S1-S266.

35. Levey AS, Coresh J, Balk E, et al. National Kidney Foundation practice guidelines for chronic kidney disease: evaluation, classification, and stratification. *Ann Intern Med.* 2003;139(2):137-147.

36. Hsu CY, Chertow GM. Chronic renal confusion: insufficiency, failure, dysfunction, or disease. *Am J Kidney Dis.* 2000;36(2):415-418.

37. Levey AS, Bosch JP, Lewis JB, et al. A more accurate method to estimate glomerular filtration rate from serum creatinine: a new prediction equation. *Ann Intern Med.* 1999;130(6):461-470.

38. Levey AS, Greene T, Kusek JW, et al. A simplified equation to predict glomerular filtration rate from serum creatinine [abstract]. *J Am Soc Nephrol.* 2000;11:155A.

39. U.S. Renal Data System: *2009 Annual data report. Section A: incidence of reported ESRD.* Available at: http://www.usrds.org/2009/ref/A_Ref_09.pdf. Accessed December 17, 2010.

39a. U.S. Renal Data System: *2009 Annual data report. Section B: prevalence of reported ESRD.* Available at: http://www.usrds.org/2009/ref/B_Ref_09.pdf. Accessed December 17, 2010.

40. Coresh J, Selvin E, Stevens LA, et al. Prevalence of chronic kidney disease in the United States. *JAMA.* 2007;298(17):2038-2047.

41. Snyder JJ, Foley RN, Collins AJ. Prevalence of CKD in the United States: a sensitivity analysis using the National Health and Nutrition Examination Survey (NHANES) 1999–2004. *Am J Kidney Dis.* 2009;53(2):218-228.

42. Ibrahim H, Mondress M, Tello A, et al. An alternative formula to the Cockcroft-Gault and the Modification of Diet in Renal Diseases formulas in predicting GFR in individuals with type 1 diabetes. *J Am Soc Nephrol.* 2005;16(4):1051-1060.

43. Poggio ED, Wang X, Greene T, et al. Performance of the Modification of Diet in Renal Disease and Cockcroft-Gault equations in the estimation of GFR in health and in chronic kidney disease. *J Am Soc Nephrol.* 2005;16(2):459-466.

44. Levey AS, Stevens LA, Schmid CH, et al. A new equation to estimate glomerular filtration rate. *Ann Intern Med.* 2009;150(9):604-612.

45. Hsu CY, Chertow GM, Curhan GC. Methodological issues in studying the epidemiology of mild to moderate chronic renal insufficiency. *Kidney Int.* 2002;61:1567-1576.

46. Coresh J, Astor BC, McQuillan G, et al. Calibration and random variation of the serum creatinine assay as critical elements of using equations to estimate glomerular filtration rate. *Am J Kidney Dis.* 2002;39:920-929.

47. Murthy K, Stevens LA, Stark PC, et al. Variation in the serum creatinine assay calibration: a practical application to glomerular filtration rate estimation. *Kidney Int.* 2005;68(4):1884-1887.

48. Coresh J, Astor BC, Greene T, et al. Prevalence of chronic kidney disease and decreased kidney function in the adult US population: Third National Health and Nutrition Examination Survey. *Am J Kidney Dis.* 2003;41(1):1-12.

49. Foley RN, Wang C, Snyder JJ, et al. Cystatin C levels in U.S. adults, 1988–1994 versus 1999–2002: NHANES. *Clin J Am Soc Nephrol.* 2009;4(5):965-972.

50. Bash LD, Coresh J, Kottgen A, et al. Defining incident chronic kidney disease in the research setting: the ARIC Study. *Am J Epidemiol.* 2009;170(4):414-424.

51. Kshirsagar AV, Bang H, Bomback AS, et al. A simple algorithm to predict incident kidney disease. *Arch Intern Med.* 2008;168(22):2466-2473.

52. Lucove J, Vupputuri S, Heiss G, et al. Metabolic syndrome and the development of CKD in American Indians: the Strong Heart Study. *Am J Kidney Dis.* 2008;51(1):21-28.

53. Keith DS, Nichols GA, Gullion CM, et al. Longitudinal follow-up and outcomes among a population with chronic kidney disease in a large managed care organization. *Arch Intern Med.* 2004;164(6):659-663.

54. Go AS, Chertow GM, Fan D, et al. Chronic kidney disease and the risks of death, cardiovascular events, and hospitalization. *N Engl J Med.* 2004;351(13):1296-1305.

55. O'Hare AM, Choi AI, Bertenthal D, et al. Age affects outcomes in chronic kidney disease. *J Am Soc Nephrol.* 2007;18(10):2758-2765.

56. Menon V, Wang X, Sarnak MJ, et al. Long-term outcomes in nondiabetic chronic kidney disease. *Kidney Int.* 2008;73(11):1310-1315.

57. Brenner BM, Cooper ME, de Zeeuw D, et al. Effects of losartan on renal and cardiovascular outcomes in patients with type 2 diabetes and nephropathy. *N Engl J Med.* 2001;345(12):861-869.

58. Lewis EJ, Hunsicker LG, Clarke WR, et al. Renoprotective effect of the angiotensin-receptor antagonist irbesartan in patients with nephropathy due to type 2 diabetes. *N Engl J Med.* 2001;345(12):851-860.

59. Winearls CG, Glassock RJ. Dissecting and refining the staging of chronic kidney disease. *Kidney Int.* 2009;75(10):1009-1014.

60. Glassock RJ, Winearls C. CKD in the elderly. *Am J Kidney Dis.* 2008;52(4):803:(author reply, Am J Kidney Dis 2008;52(4):803-804).

61. Bauer C, Melamed ML, Hostetter TH. Staging of chronic kidney disease: time for a course correction. *J Am Soc Nephrol.* 2008;19(5):844-846.

62. Poggio ED, Rule AD. A critical evaluation of chronic kidney disease—should isolated reduced estimated glomerular filtration rate be considered a "disease"? *Nephrol Dial Transplant.* 2009;24(3):698-700.

63. Ikizler TA. CKD classification: time to move beyond KDOQI. *J Am Soc Nephrol.* 2009;20(5):929-930.

64. Richards N, Harris K, Whitfield M, et al. Primary care–based disease management of chronic kidney disease (CKD), based on estimated glomerular filtration rate (eGFR) reporting, improves patient outcomes. *Nephrol Dial Transplant.* 2008;23(2):549-555.

65. Richards N, Harris K, Whitfield M, et al. The impact of population-based identification of chronic kidney disease using estimated glomerular filtration rate (eGFR) reporting. *Nephrol Dial Transplant.* 2008;23(2):556-561.

66. den Hartog JR, Reese PP, Cizman B, et al. The costs and benefits of automatic estimated glomerular filtration rate reporting. *Clin J Am Soc Nephrol.* 2009;4(2):419-427.

67. Coresh J, Eustace JA. Epidemiology of kidney disease. In: Brenner BM, ed. *Brenner and Rector's The Kidney*. Philadelphia: W.B. Saunders; 2008: pp 615-632.

68. Hallan SI, Coresh J, Astor BC, et al. International comparison of the relationship of chronic kidney disease prevalence and ESRD risk. *J Am Soc Nephrol*. 2006;17(8):2275-2284.

69. Hsu CY, Lin F, Vittinghoff E, et al. Racial differences in the progression from chronic renal insufficiency to end-stage renal disease in the United States. *J Am Soc Nephrol*. 2003;14(11):2902-2907.

70. McClellan W, Warnock DG, McClure L, et al. Racial differences in the prevalence of chronic kidney disease among participants in the Reasons for Geographic and Racial Differences in Stroke (REGARDS) cohort study. *J Am Soc Nephrol*. 2006;17(6):1710-1715.

71. Kramer H, Palmas W, Kestenbaum B, et al. Chronic kidney disease prevalence estimates among racial/ethnic groups: The Multi-Ethnic Study of Atherosclerosis. *Clin J Am Soc Nephrol*. 2008;3(5):1391-1397.

72. Hsu CY, Vittinghoff E, Lin F, et al. The incidence of end-stage renal disease is increasing faster than the prevalence of chronic renal insufficiency. *Ann Intern Med*. 2004;141(2):95-101.

73. Hsu CY, Go AS, McCulloch CE, et al. Exploring secular trends in the likelihood of receiving treatment for end-stage renal disease. *Clin J Am Soc Nephrol*. 2007;2(1):81-88.

74. Waikar SS, Wald R, Chertow GM, et al. Validity of International Classification of Diseases, Ninth Revision, Clinical Modification codes for acute renal failure. *J Am Soc Nephrol*. 2006;17(6):1688-1694.

75. Bellomo R, Ronco C, Kellum JA, et al. Acute renal failure—definition, outcome measures, animal models, fluid therapy and information technology needs: the Second International Consensus Conference of the Acute Dialysis Quality Initiative (ADQI) Group. *Crit Care*. 2004;8(4):R204-R212.

76. Levin A, Warnock DG, Mehta RL, et al. Improving outcomes from acute kidney injury: report of an initiative. *Am J Kidney Dis*. 2007;50(1):1-4.

77. Hou SH, Bushinsky DA, Wish JB, et al. Hospital-acquired renal insufficiency: a prospective study. *Am J Med*. 1983;74(2):243-248.

78. Nash K, Hafeez A, Hou S. Hospital-acquired renal insufficiency. *Am J Kidney Dis*. 2002;39(5):930-936.

79. Uchino S, Kellum JA, Bellomo R, et al. Acute renal failure in critically ill patients: a multinational, multicenter study. *JAMA*. 2005;294(7):813-818.

80. Xue JL, Daniels F, Star RA, et al. Incidence and mortality of acute renal failure in Medicare beneficiaries, 1992 to 2001. *J Am Soc Nephrol*. 2006;17(4):1135-1142.

81. Obialo CI, Okonofua EC, Tayade AS, et al. Epidemiology of de novo acute renal failure in hospitalized African Americans: comparing community-acquired vs hospital-acquired disease. *Arch Intern Med*. 2000;160(9):1309-1313.

82. Ali T, Khan I, Simpson W, et al. Incidence and outcomes in acute kidney injury: a comprehensive population-based study. *J Am Soc Nephrol*. 2007;18(4):1292-1298.

83. Metcalfe W, Simpson M, Khan IH, et al. Acute renal failure requiring renal replacement therapy: incidence and outcome. *Q J Med*. 2002;95(9):579-583.

84. Robertson S, Newbigging K, Isles CG, et al. High incidence of renal failure requiring short-term dialysis: a prospective observational study. *Q J Med*. 2002;95(9):585-590.

85. Liano F, Pascual J. Epidemiology of acute renal failure: a prospective, multicenter, community-based study. *Kidney Int*. 1996;50(3):811-818.

86. Waikar SS, Curhan GC, Wald R, et al. Declining mortality in patients with acute renal failure, 1988 to 2002. *J Am Soc Nephrol*. 2006;17(4):1143-1150.

87. Liu KD, Himmelfarb J, Paganini E, et al. Timing of initiation of dialysis in critically ill patients with acute kidney injury. *Clin J Am Soc Nephrol*. 2006;1(5):915-919.

88. Liu KD, Matthay MA, Chertow GM. Evolving practices in critical care and potential implications for management of acute kidney injury. *Clin J Am Soc Nephrol*. 2006;1(4):869-873.

89. Martin GS, Mannino DM, Eaton S, et al. The epidemiology of sepsis in the United States from 1979 through 2000. *N Engl J Med*. 2003;348(16):1546-1554.

90. Himmelfarb J, Ikizler TA. Acute kidney injury: changing lexicography, definitions, and epidemiology. *Kidney Int*. 2007;71(10):971-976.

91. Lucas FL, DeLorenzo MA, Siewers AE, et al. Temporal trends in the utilization of diagnostic testing and treatments for cardiovascular disease in the United States, 1993–2001. *Circulation*. 2006;113(3):374-379.

92. Alter DA, Stukel TA, Newman A. Proliferation of cardiac technology in Canada: a challenge to the sustainability of Medicare. *Circulation*. 2006;113(3):380-387.

93. Marenzi G, Assanelli E, Campodonico J, et al. Contrast volume during primary percutaneous coronary intervention and subsequent contrast-induced nephropathy and mortality. *Ann Intern Med*. 2009;150(3):170-177.

94. Hsu CY, Ordonez JD, Chertow GM, et al. The risk of acute renal failure in patients with chronic kidney disease. *Kidney Int*. 2008;74(1):101-107.

95. Wald R, Quinn RR, Luo J, et al. Chronic dialysis and death among survivors of acute kidney injury requiring dialysis. *JAMA*. 2009;302(11):1179-1185.

96. Hsu CY, Chertow GM, McCulloch CE, et al. Nonrecovery of kidney function and death after acute on chronic renal failure. *Clin J Am Soc Nephrol*. 2009;4:891-898.

97. Lo LJ, Go AS, Chertow GM, et al. Dialysis-requiring acute renal failure increases the risk of progressive chronic kidney disease. *Kidney Int*. 2009;76(8):893-899.

98. Newsome BB, Warnock DG, McClellan WM, et al. Long-term risk of mortality and end-stage renal disease among the elderly after small increases in serum creatinine level during hospitalization for acute myocardial infarction. *Arch Intern Med*. 2008;168(6):609-616.

99. Ishani A, Xue JL, Himmelfarb J, et al. Acute kidney injury increases risk of ESRD among elderly. *J Am Soc Nephrol*. 2009;20(1):223-228.

100. Amdur RL, Chawla LS, Amodeo S, et al. Outcomes following diagnosis of acute renal failure in U.S. veterans: focus on acute tubular necrosis. *Kidney Int*. 2009;76(10):1089-1097.

101. Pagtalunan ME, Olson JL, Tilney NL, et al. Late consequences of acute ischemic injury to a solitary kidney. *J Am Soc Nephrol*. 1999;10(2):366-373.

102. Lewers DT, Mathew TH, Maher JF, et al. Long-term follow-up of renal function and histology after acute tubular necrosis. *Ann Intern Med*. 1970;73(4):523-529.

103. Hsu CY. Linking the population epidemiology of acute renal failure, chronic kidney disease and end-stage renal disease. *Curr Opin Nephrol Hypertens*. 2007;16(3):221-226.

Demographics of Kidney Disease

Amanda Hyre Anderson, Jeffrey S. Berns, Melissa B. Bleicher, and Harold I. Feldman

Patterns in the prevalence, incidence, and progression of chronic kidney disease vary by certain demographic characteristics, including gender, race or ethnicity, and socioeconomic status. This chapter summarizes what is known of these patterns, describes consistent findings across sociodemographic groups, speculates on the genesis of variations across demographic groups, and highlights questions that still remain pertaining to kidney outcomes in these populations.

Gender and Chronic Kidney Disease

Differences between men and women in the incidence and prevalence of various kidney diseases and the rate of kidney disease progression may be influenced by gender differences in glomerular mass, responses to hormones, cytokines, apoptosis, vasoactive and other soluble circulating factors, as well as differences in the responses to aging and reductions in nephron mass. Women have been reported to have approximately 10% to 15% fewer glomeruli than men on average, but this is thought to be a function primarily of birth weight and body surface area (BSA) rather than gender.[1-4] Glomerular volume tends to be similar in men and women.[1,3] Glomerular filtration rate (GFR) is also similar in men and women when corrected for BSA and muscle mass,[5-9] although some have reported a somewhat lower BSA-adjusted GFR in women.[10] Thus, although some subtle differences in renal mass and structure have been reported in men compared with women, these are probably of little or no clinical significance and are more likely related to factors other than gender. Studies of experimental animal models and human studies have described gender differences and sex hormone influences in the synthesis and plasma levels of, and biologic responses to, a variety of circulating factors involved in the regulation of normal renal function. These same factors may also be involved in responses to renal injury and susceptibility to kidney disease. Some of these are angiotensinogen, angiotensin II, prorenin, renin, angiotensin converting enzyme, and angiotensin receptor. Gender differences have also been reported in synthesis of and responsiveness to nitric oxide and prostaglandin, lipid oxidation and oxidative stress, mesangial cell collagen synthesis and degradation, responses to transforming growth factor-β and tumor necrosis factor-α, and apoptotic and profibrotic signaling pathways.[11-13] High adiponectin levels have also been reported to predict chronic kidney disease (CKD) progression in men, but not in women.[14] Estradiol has been identified as having various effects on mesangial cells.[15-20] Neither androgens nor estrogens directly influence GFR or renal blood flow in humans.[21,22] The extent to which any of these factors is specifically and causally related to gender differences in kidney function or kidney disease incidence and progression is still uncertain.

Gender Differences in Glomerular Disease Incidence and Prevalence

Research assessments of glomerular disease incidence and prevalence in adults are made difficult by uncertainty about the population base from which these figures are derived, variations in study participants' ages, and varying indications for kidney biopsy. The overall incidence of primary glomerular diseases among residents of Olmstead County, Minnesota, which has a primarily white population, has been estimated based on renal biopsy records to be 7.9 per 100,000 person-years in men and 5.4 per 100,000 person-years in women.[23] A study in France reported a prevalence of primary glomerular disease of 8.2 per 1000 among men and 5.1 per 1000 among women during a 27-year period ending in 2002.[24] Men tend to predominate in many series of adult patients with focal segmental glomerulosclerosis (FSGS) and immunoglobulin A (IgA) nephropathy, with a more variable gender mix for adults with minimal change disease and membranous nephropathy.[25-31] The incidence rates for end-stage renal disease (ESRD) in the United States are approximately 60% higher among men than among women.[32] Although men have higher incidence rates of CKD and ESRD, the estimated prevalence of moderate (i.e., stage 3 or 4) CKD is higher among women (8.0% in women versus 5.4% in men).[8]

Gender Differences in Progression of Primary Glomerular Disease

Prognosis—namely, the rate of progression of the underlying renal disease—is generally considered to be worse in men than in women with membranous nephropathy, IgA nephropathy, FSGS, and lupus nephritis.[25,26,33-39] However, studies using multivariate analysis to evaluate the effect of gender on renal disease progression have produced discrepant findings.[33,34,40-44] Although none has found female gender to be associated with more rapid renal disease progression, the often-cited association of male gender with more rapid disease progression has been inconsistent. Much of this literature was analyzed in a recent meta-analysis by Neugarten and colleagues.[33] This meta-analysis considered 8 studies with over 2000 patients with nondiabetic "chronic renal disease" for which no specific etiology was identified and concluded that kidney disease progression was statistically significantly associated with male gender (Figure 20-1).[34,40-42,45-48] Of five studies excluded from this analysis because of incomplete reporting of effect size,[43,49-52] two concluded that kidney disease progression was more rapid in men, whereas three found no gender difference. Although this meta-analysis did not assess women's menopausal status, other studies have reported that the more favorable rate of progression in women is limited to those in the premenopausal period.[34,47] An association between male gender and progression of IgA nephropathy was demonstrated in the meta-analysis by Neugarten and colleagues,[33] which encompassed 25 studies and over 3000

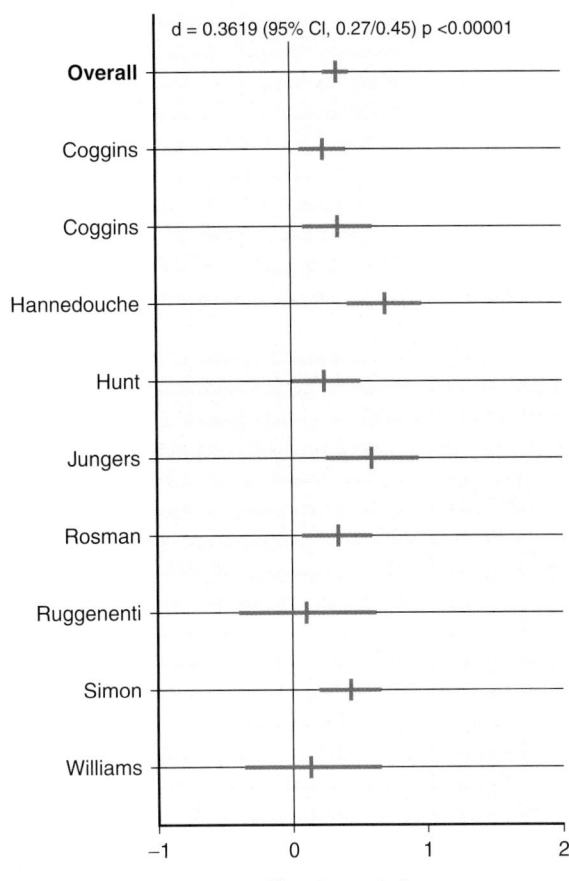

FIGURE 20-1 Effect size and 95% confidence interval (CI) for individual studies of the effect of gender on the progression of chronic renal disease of mixed etiology. The overall mean effect size and 95% CI are shown on top. A positive value indicates that male gender is associated with an adverse renal outcome. (From Neugarten J, Acharya A, Silbiger SR: Effect of gender on the progression of nondiabetic renal disease: a meta-analysis, *J Am Soc Nephrol* 11:319-329, 2000.)

patients (Figure 20-2).[47,53-74] Twenty-one of these 25 studies found more rapid progression in men. In all but a few of the studies in this meta-analysis, however, the association was not statistically significant. In addition, several studies suggested that men had better outcomes. Twelve of 13 studies excluded from this meta-analysis because of the inability to calculate effect size found no gender differences.[75-86] Combined, these data suggest that any association between gender and IgA nephropathy progression is likely to be weak. In 21 studies involving nearly 1900 patients with membranous nephropathy considered in the Neugarten and others meta-analysis,[47,87-106] male gender was significantly associated with disease progression (Figure 20-3). However, five studies that were excluded (due to inability to calculate effect sizes) reported no gender association with progression.[107-111] Other older pooled analyses have also reported an association of male gender with poorer renal outcome for membranous nephropathy.[112,113] Several other more recent meta-analyses have also considered gender influences on progression of renal disease with a variety of underlying causes. Jafar and colleagues performed a patient-level meta-analysis using pooled data from patients with nondiabetic kidney disease from 11 prospective randomized controlled trials on the use of angiotensin converting enzyme inhibitors to slow disease progression.[114]

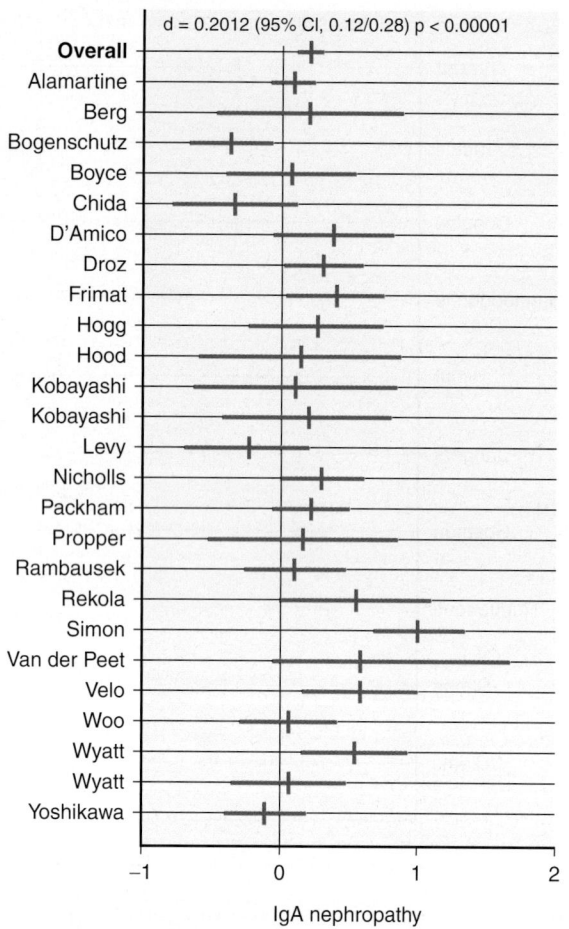

FIGURE 20-2 Effect size and 95% confidence interval (CI) for individual studies of the effect of gender on the progression of immunoglobulin A (IgA) nephropathy. The overall mean effect size and 95% CI are shown on top. A positive value indicates that male gender is associated with an adverse renal outcome. (From Neugarten J, Acharya A, Silbiger SR: Effect of gender on the progression of nondiabetic renal disease: a meta-analysis, *J Am Soc Nephrol* 11:319-329, 2000.)

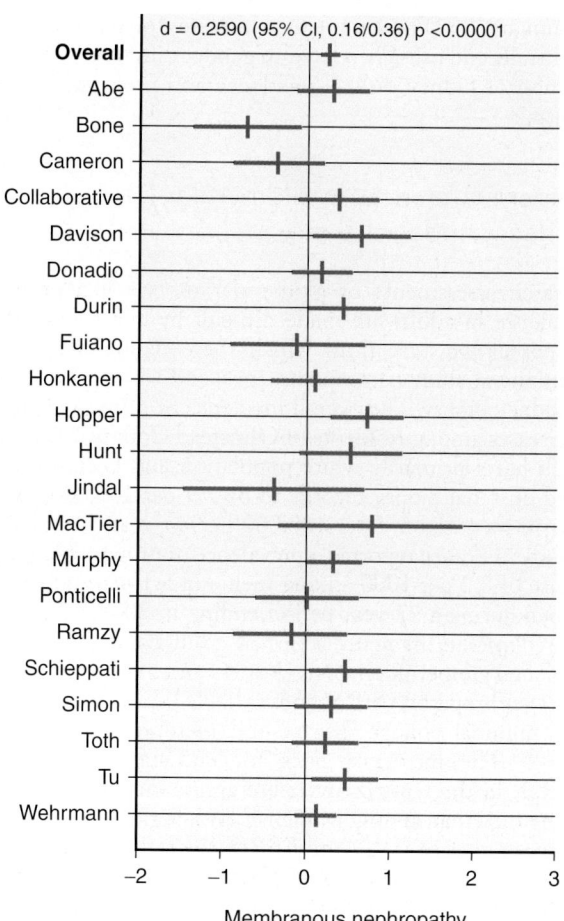

FIGURE 20-3 Effect size and 95% confidence interval (CI) for individual studies of the effect of gender on the progression of membranous nephropathy. The overall mean effect size and 95% CI are shown on top. A positive value indicates that male gender is associated with an adverse renal outcome. (From Neugarten J, Acharya A, Silbiger SR: Effect of gender on the progression of nondiabetic renal disease: a meta-analysis, *J Am Soc Nephrol* 11:319-329, 2000.)

Using doubling of serum creatinine level or onset of ESRD as a composite primary endpoint, these authors concluded that the risk of renal disease progression was no different in men and women in an unadjusted analysis, but that the risk was actually higher in women than in men after adjustment for baseline variables, including urine protein excretion and treatment assignment (relative risk [RR] = 1.30 to 1.36 depending on the model). The authors noted that most of the women in these trials were of postmenopausal age, which limits applicability of the results to younger premenopausal women. Several additional studies considering gender influences on renal disease progression have been published recently. Two large population-based studies reported a more favorable prognosis for women than for men with CKD in Norway and Sweden.[35,36] The Modification of Diet in Renal Disease (MDRD) study, which enrolled patients with autosomal dominant polycystic kidney disease (ADPKD), glomerulonephritis, or other nondiabetic kidney diseases, reported the rate of kidney disease progression to be slower in women than in men, particularly among younger premenopausal women.[47] This difference was markedly diminished and no longer statistically significant after adjustment for level of proteinuria and blood pressure. A more recent report of the MDRD study participants'

long-term outcomes also found similar kidney failure event rates for men and women.[115] Cattran and colleagues analyzed outcomes for over 1300 patients enrolled in the Toronto Glomerulonephritis Registry who had membranous nephropathy, FSGS, or IgA nephropathy.[39] After adjustment for blood pressure and proteinuria, no difference was found between men and women in disease progression and renal survival rates, except among those with proteinuria levels of more than 7 g/day. In this latter group, men had more rapid loss of GFR than women. Disease progression has been found to be similar for men and women with IgA nephropathy in most other studies as well.[53,54,74,80,82,83,86,116]

Gender Differences in Lupus Nephritis Progression

Recent studies of gender influences on lupus nephritis outcomes in adults have reported discrepant findings,[117-122] but are limited by small numbers of patients, variable outcome measures, and varying assessment of other covariates such as histopathologic disease class, proteinuria, blood pressure, and immunosuppressive treatment.

Gender Differences in Progression of Autosomal Dominant Polycystic Kidney Disease

In the meta-analysis by Neugarten and colleagues mentioned earlier,[33] in 12 studies enrolling over 3000 patients with ADPKD,[123-134] there was an apparent small protective effect of male gender on disease progression (Figure 20-4). However, this conclusion was largely the result of inclusion of a single Italian study that reported a highly statistically significant favorable association between male gender and disease progression.[133] Exclusion of this study resulted in the finding of a statistically significant association between male gender and more rapid progression, an effect seen in 10 of 12 studies (although all 4 excluded studies found no gender association with disease progression).[135-138] More recent studies published since this meta-analysis have also come to varying conclusions regarding the effects of gender on the progression of ADPKD.[139-142] Of two recent reports of magnetic resonance imaging of kidney and cyst growth, only one found male gender to be associated with more rapid growth.[143,144] The association between ADPKD genotype and progression of renal disease appears to be modified by gender. Gender does not appear to significantly influence renal outcomes in the more common variant of ADPKD caused by mutation in the polycystin 1 gene.[142,145,146] In contrast, women with ADPKD caused by mutations in the polycystin 2 gene tend to have more favorable renal outcomes than men.[146,147] The biologic basis for this difference is not presently known.

Gender Differences in Diabetic Nephropathy Progression

Influences of gender and sex hormones in diabetes and diabetic nephropathy have been reviewed recently.[148] There are relatively few data on the association of gender with rate of progression of diabetic nephropathy, and the studies that have been performed report inconsistent findings.[149-160] Girls with type 1 diabetes are more likely to develop microalbuminuria during puberty than are boys, and there tends to be a more rapid loss of GFR following puberty in women than in men.[150,156,159] In adults with childhood-onset type 1 diabetes, several studies have suggested that males have a greater likelihood of developing albuminuria, and among those with diabetic nephropathy, the rate of decline in GFR is faster.[149,152,160-165] One study found that, compared with men, women with type 1 diabetes were more likely to develop diabetic nephropathy while maintaining good metabolic control, a gender effect that was attenuated in the setting of poor metabolic control.[165] Other studies have not found an independent adverse influence of male gender on rate of progression of diabetic renal disease.[149,150,156,157,159,166] There are remarkably few data regarding gender influences on progression of diabetic nephropathy in patients with type 2 diabetes. The percentage of men and women with diabetic nephropathy starting dialysis is similar, although recent data from the United States Renal Data System (USRDS) indicate that the incidence of ESRD is slightly higher among white men with type 2 diabetes than among white women.[32] Studies also suggest a greater incidence and prevalence of microalbuminuria and macroalbuminuria in white men than in white women, with the opposite gender predilection among blacks.[148,167-170]

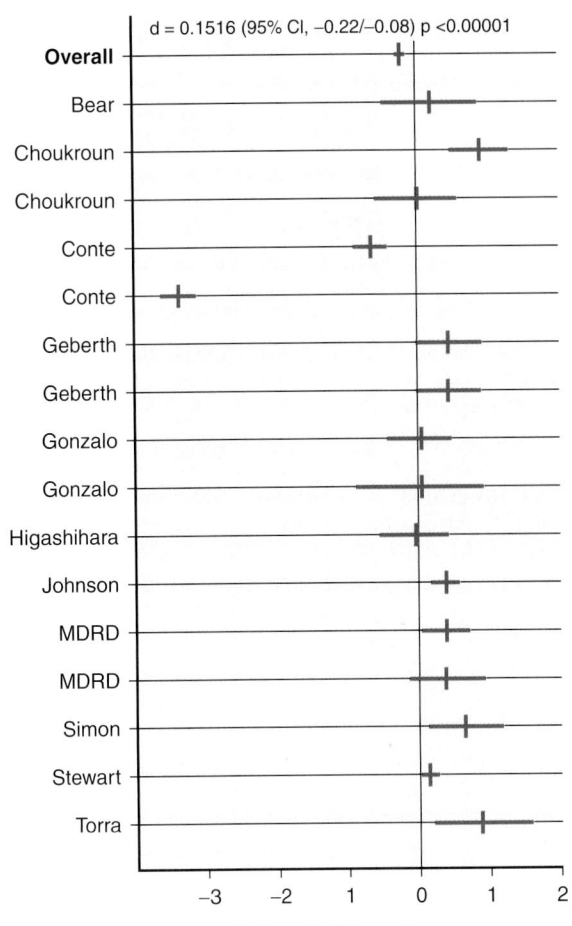

FIGURE 20-4 Effect size and 95% confidence interval (CI) for individual studies of the effect of gender on the progression of autosomal dominant polycystic kidney disease. The overall mean effect size and 95% CI are shown on top. A negative value indicates that female gender is associated with an adverse renal outcome. (From Neugarten J, Acharya A, Silbiger SR: Effect of gender on the progression of nondiabetic renal disease: a meta-analysis, *J Am Soc Nephrol* 11:319-329, 2000.)

Progression of diabetic nephropathy tends to be more rapid among women, however, although some studies have reported similar rates of disease progression and risk for development of renal endpoints including ESRD across gender.[148,167-176]

Oral Contraceptive or Hormone Replacement Therapy and Kidney Disease

Few studies have examined the influence of oral contraceptives and hormone replacement therapy (HRT) on kidney function in women with and without recognized kidney disease. Oral contraceptive use has been associated with a higher prevalence of microalbuminuria in women with diabetic nephropathy in some studies[177,178] but not others.[179] One study found a greater risk associated with higher estrogen strength and longer-term use (>5 years).[178] Oral contraceptive use has also been associated with a higher risk of microalbuminuria and decline of GFR in premenopausal women without CKD.[180] In a small, short-term prospective study, administration of a combination of estradiol and norgestrel for 3.5 months to 16 postmenopausal women with diabetes mellitus and hypertension was associated with a statistically significant reduction in mean level of proteinuria from 452 to 370 mg/day and an increase in creatinine clearance from 100.8 to 106.2 mL/min.[181] In a community-based case-control study, postmenopausal HRT was associated with a twofold higher odds ratio (OR) for microalbuminuria after adjustment for several clinical variables.[178] The odds ratio for microalbuminuria was similar in women receiving HRT with and without progestins. The association between HRT use and microalbuminuria was limited to women using HRT for longer than 5 years. In contrast, in another study postmenopausal HRT was associated with a lower mean urine albumin/creatinine ratio and a lower prevalence of microalbuminuria at a baseline examination and after 5 years of follow-up.[182]

More recently, Ahmed and colleagues studied nearly 6000 postmenopausal women for over 2 years to examine the effect of HRT on estimated GFR using the abbreviated MDRD equation.[183] After adjustment for age, diabetes, other comorbidities, and baseline estimated GFR (eGFR), HRT use was found to be associated with more rapid decline in eGFR and a 19% greater risk for eGFR to fall by 4 mL/min/1.73 m² per year or more. The higher rate of eGFR decline and risk of rapid GFR loss were limited to users of estrogen-only HRT; use of combined or progestin-only HRT was not associated with decline in eGFR. There was also a linear relationship between cumulative dose of estrogen and decline in mean eGFR. The risk associated with estrogen-containing HRT was limited to women using oral treatment; use of transvaginal estrogen was not associated with a statistically significant decline in eGFR. Thus, while women are considered to be at less risk for development and progression of many types of kidney disease, the influences of menopausal status and hormonal replacement have not been thoroughly investigated. The findings of Ahmed and colleagues[183] need to be further explored with consideration of factors not evaluated in that study, such as blood pressure, level of proteinuria, and obesity, before concluding with any certainty that oral estrogen-based HRT accelerates progression of CKD.

Summary

Patterns in the incidence of kidney disease across gender are generally consistent, with higher rates occurring in men than in women. Similarly, men are reported to have greater rates of progression of nondiabetic CKD for some specific types of kidney disease, especially compared with premenopausal women. More investigation into rates of progression of IgA nephropathy, lupus nephritis, and ADPKD across gender and into overall progression rates in postmenopausal women is warranted. Additional study of the effects of HRT in women on the incidence and progression of kidney disease is also needed.

Race, Ethnicity, and Chronic Kidney Disease

Defining Race and Ethnicity

The use of racial classifications in medicine and epidemiology is the subject of much debate, owing mainly to the many ways this information can be captured and interpreted. Nonetheless, classification by race-ethnicity in biomedical research facilitates several important activities, including the characterization of health statistics, the determination of the risk of adverse health outcomes, and the examination of delivery of health care services across subpopulations. Also, these classifications can be used as a proxy for unmeasured biologic and social factors.[184] The utility of describing race-ethnicity and relating it to outcomes of interest lies in the ability to capture information on differences in genetics and biology, behavior, exposure to environmental factors, and social and physical environments. However, the imperfect nature of the relationship between race and these attributes highlights the importance of supplementing race and ethnicity data, when possible, with data on individual-level factors that are often meant to be represented by race. To reflect most accurately factors related to social, cultural, and physical environments and exposures, individual race and ethnicity are often self-designated. This approach to classification was first adopted by the U.S. Census Bureau in 1960, followed by the opportunity to self-designate Hispanic ethnicity in 1970, and, finally, the ability to designate more than one racial category in 2000.[185,186] The increasing percentage of the American population that can trace its roots to multiracial or multiethnic sources has motivated researchers and demographers to collect and analyze self-designated racial-ethnic data in ways that reflect this racial and ethnic admixture. However, limited knowledge of ancestry as well as the large and increasing frequency of migration creates additional challenges to valid racial classification. Despite these limitations, when race is used as an explanatory factor to represent genetic and biologic determinants of disease, self-designated race may be informative as long as there is enough additional information on important socioeconomic, behavioral, and physical environment factors. Finally, it has been suggested that ethnic groups that share a unique history, language, customs, ancestry, geography, and/or religion, or specific genetic markers should replace traditional racial classifications in biomedical research.[187-189] These approaches may limit the usefulness of race as an explanatory factor in research and may not be suitable for all types of investigations.

Race-Ethnicity and the Incidence of Chronic Kidney Disease

An emphasis on defining and investigating CKD before patients become dependent on dialysis has only emerged in recent years. National guidelines were first established in 2002 to define and stage prevalent CKD.[190] To date, no such guidance has been provided to define and capture information on the incidence of CKD nationally or in the research setting. To address the lack of national data on the burden, awareness, risk factors, and health consequences of CKD, the National Chronic Kidney Disease Surveillance System is now under development after a pilot and feasibility phase as part of the Chronic Kidney Disease Initiative of the Centers for Disease Control and Prevention.[191] This system will use passive surveillance strategies incorporating a broad network of data sources and aims to disseminate information through fact sheets, reports, and a website. In research, large longitudinal studies are necessary to provide reliable estimates of the incidence of disease. However, no standards or guidelines exist to instruct researchers on how to combine longitudinal data on clinical outcomes with laboratory criteria to define incident CKD. Published definitions include data on serum creatinine, International Classification of Diseases (ICD) codes, and/ or death records, but do so in varied ways.[192-198] Variations in the definition of incident CKD can modify the relationship between race and CKD occurrence. For example, in the Atherosclerosis Risk in Communities (ARIC) study, incident CKD among participants aged 45 to 64 years at baseline occurred at a higher rate in blacks than in whites when the definition of CKD was based on a rise in serum creatinine level (8.0 versus 3.2 per 1000 person-years, respectively) and ICD codes (2.0 versus 1.0 per 1000 person-years), but at a lower rate when CKD was defined as a low eGFR (8.9 versus 10.8 per 1000 person-years).[199] A composite definition requiring both a low eGFR and at least a 25% drop in eGFR resulted in similar incidence rates for blacks and whites (6.9 versus 6.6 per 1000 person-years, respectively). Despite the lack of consistency in defining incident CKD, several estimates of CKD incidence rates for different racial and ethnic groups have been reported. According to the 2009 Annual Data Report from the USRDS, in the general Medicare population (mean age = 75.5 years) the incidence of CKD, based on diagnostic codes, was 5.6% among African Americans compared with 3.8% among whites in 2007.[200] A 1999 publication that included data for ARIC participants reported a CKD incidence of 28.4 per 1000 person-years among black participants with diabetes compared with 9.6 per 1000 person-years among whites with diabetes, and an age-, sex-, and baseline serum creatinine level–adjusted odds ratio of 3.2 (95% confidence interval [CI] = 1.9 to 5.3) for early kidney function decline among blacks compared with whites.[198] After further adjustment for potentially modifiable risk factors related to socioeconomic status and health behaviors, including education, household income, health insurance, fasting glucose level, mean systolic blood pressure, smoking history, and physical activity level, the odds ratio decreased to 1.4 (95% CI = 0.7 to 2.7), an 82% reduction in excess risk.[198] Although this and other studies have attributed a substantial proportion of the excess risk for kidney disease among black Americans to these nonracial factors, a difference in risk across race still remains in adjusted analyses.

Race-Ethnicity and the Prevalence of Chronic Kidney Disease

Estimates of CKD prevalence are reported much more frequently than estimates of incidence because they can be obtained with a single assessment of renal function. These estimates are associated with certain limitations as discussed in Chapter 19. Racial disparities in CKD were examined by collecting data at entry into the Reasons for Geographic and Racial Differences in Stroke (REGARDS) study, a population-based cohort study of adults older than 45 years. An eGFR of less than 60 mL/min/1.73 m^2 (i.e., stage 3 to 5 CKD) was found in 43.3% overall and was more prevalent among whites than among blacks (49.9 versus 33.7%, respectively; Table 20-1).[201] Although blacks were less likely than whites to have an eGFR between 30 and 60 mL/min/1.73 m^2; however, the reverse was true for an eGFR of less than 30 mL/min/1.73 m^2. When data from the National Health and Nutrition Examination Survey (NHANES) from 1988 to 1994 and 1999 to 2004 and the MDRD GFR estimating equation were used, the prevalence of CKD was found to increase from 10.5% to 13.8% among non-Hispanic whites, from 10.2% to 11.7% among non-Hispanic blacks, and from 6.3% to 8.0% among Mexican Americans over this time period.[202] The 1999 to 2004 estimates of the prevalence of stage 1 to 4 CKD among non-Hispanic whites and blacks in the United States were no longer significantly different when made using a more recently published GFR estimating equation known as the *Chronic Kidney Disease Epidemiology Collaboration (CKD-EPI) equation,*[8] results that emphasize the impact of the tool used to assess kidney function. A racial difference persisted in the prevalence of stage 3 and 4 CKD, however; estimates for blacks and whites shifted from 9.6% and 5.2%, respectively, using the MDRD GFR estimating equation to 7.8% and 5.4%, respectively, using the CKD-EPI equation. Even after multivariable adjustment, another analysis of NHANES data for 1988 to 1994 revealed a higher likelihood of albuminuria in African Americans and Mexican Americans with and without diabetes than in U.S. whites with and without diabetes (OR = 1.8 to 2.8).[203] Finally, in a study of adult Navajo Indians, 3% to 6% of nondiabetic individuals and 10% to 11% of diabetic individuals had an

eGFR (mL/min/1.73 m^2)	N (%)		OR (95% CI)	AOR[†] (95% CI)
	BLACK (N = 8139)	**WHITE (N = 11,620)**		
>60	5394 (66.3)	5817 (50.1)	Reference	Reference
50-59	1541 (18.9)	3611 (31.1)	0.46 (0.43-0.49)	0.42 (0.40-0.46)
40-49	693 (8.5)	1506 (13.0)	0.50 (0.45-0.55)	0.37 (0.33-0.41)
30-39	287 (3.5)	521 (4.5)	0.59 (0.51-0.67)	0.38 (0.32-0.45)
20-29	116 (1.4)	131 (1.1)	0.95 (0.74-1.22)	0.48 (0.36-0.64)
10-19	60 (0.7)	25 (0.2)	2.56 (1.62-4.13)	1.73 (1.02-2.94)
<10	48 (0.6)	9 (0.08)	5.75 (2.82-11.7)	4.19 (1.90-9.24)

TABLE 20-1   Racial Differences in Renal Function by Level of MDRD eGFR and Odds of a Low GFR in Black Compared with White Individuals*

*A total of 2029 participants were excluded from analyses because of missing values for MDRD components.

†Controlled for age, gender, hypertension, diabetes, previous stroke or myocardial infarction, region, and smoking status.

aOR, Adjusted odds ratio; *CI*, confidence interval; *eGFR*, estimated glomerular filtration rate; *GFR*, glomerular filtration rate; *MDRD*, Modification of Diet in Renal Disease (equation); *OR*, odds ratio.

From McClellan W, Warnock DG, McClure L, et al: Racial differences in the prevalence of chronic kidney disease among participants in the Reasons for Geographic and Racial Differences in Stroke (REGARDS) cohort study, *J Am Soc Nephrol* 17:1710-1715, 2006.

elevated serum creatinine level consistent with a creatinine clearance of 65 mL/min or less for men and 53 mL/min or less for women.[204] Individuals of Hispanic ethnicity are often aggregated into one group despite the fact that a wide variety of national origins and races are represented by this classification. Rodriguez and colleagues examined data from the Hispanic Health and Nutrition Examination Survey (HHANES) on differences in serum creatinine level and estimated creatinine clearances across Hispanic subgroups, including Mexican Americans, mainland Puerto Ricans, and Cuban Americans. Cuban Americans had the highest mean serum creatinine levels, and both Puerto Ricans (OR = 1.7; 95% CI = 1.2 to 2.6) and Cuban Americans (OR = 4.6; 95% CI = 2.5 to 8.3) were more likely than Mexican Americans to have estimated creatinine clearances of less than 60 mL/min/1.73 m². [205] These observations further highlight the heterogeneity of physiology within currently used racial and ethnic categorizations.

Race-Ethnicity and the Progression of Chronic Kidney Disease

Rates of progression of CKD to ESRD are higher among African American, Hispanic, and American Indian adults compared with white U.S. adults, as described in Chapter 19.[32,206,207] For example, among individuals with CKD, Hispanics had a significantly increased risk of ESRD (hazard ratio [HR] = 1.33; 95% CI = 1.2 to 1.5) compared with non-Hispanic whites in a recent large study of Kaiser Permanente of Northern California health plan enrollees.[208] Among African Americans, the rate of decline of GFR was greater (by 1.4 to 1.5 mL/min/year) and the risk of developing ESRD was twofold higher (RR = 2.0; 95% CI = 1.1 to 3.6) compared with whites.[209,210] This finding was reinforced recently by a longitudinal study of Medicare recipients aged 65 years and older who were followed for up to 10 years.[211] After adjustment for age and gender, black patients with diabetes were found to be 2.4 to 2.7 times more likely to develop ESRD than whites, and other racial-ethnic groups were 1.6 to 1.7 times more likely than whites to develop ESRD. Similar elevations in risk were noted among black and other racial-ethnic minorities with hypertension. Finally, among patients with neither diabetes nor hypertension, black patients were still 3.5 times more likely than

whites, and those with a designated race of "other" two times more likely than whites, to develop ESRD. The persistence of these racial disparities unexplainable by diabetes and hypertension underscores the existence of other responsible factors. The mechanisms accounting for this increased risk are still being elucidated, but it is apparent that a proportion is attributable to factors captured by self-designated race-ethnicity.

Potential Mechanisms of Racial-Ethnic Disparities

Racial disparities in kidney disease may partially be explained by a higher prevalence and lower levels of control of hypertension among African American adults (Figure 20-5).[212-217] Hypertension appears to occur earlier and with more severity in African Americans, which leads to greater end-organ damage.[216] Additional potential causes of kidney disease disparities between whites and blacks may be differences in the prevalence and control of diabetes,[213,218] the prevalence and severity of obesity,[219,220] cytokine production,[221,222] renal hemodynamics,[223,224] and electrolyte regulation[225]; differences in genetic factors; and differences in socioeconomic status, access to health care, behavioral factors, and physical environments. One such explanation was provided in a recent publication in which Hung and colleagues reported a higher risk of CKD progression among participants in the African American Study of Kidney Disease and Hypertension who had certain C-reactive protein polymorphisms.[226] Similar disparities exist between Hispanic adults and whites that may be partially explained by a higher prevalence, earlier onset, and increased severity of diabetes[227-230]; lower rates of awareness, treatment, and control of hypertension[215]; and a higher prevalence of obesity[231,232] in this ethnic minority population, among other biologic, social, behavioral, and communication factors. Several studies have also identified factors related to access to health care as being strongly predictive of the development of ESRD.[198,233] One recent ecologic study comparing areas in California defined by zip codes reported a higher incidence of ESRD caused by diabetes in areas with a higher proportion of hospitalizations of patients with no insurance or with Medicaid, and a lower incidence in areas with more hospitalizations of those with managed

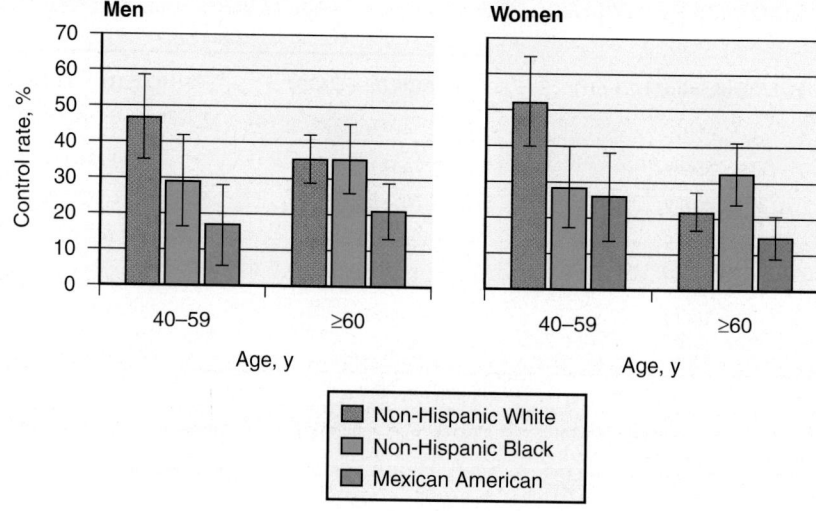

FIGURE 20-5 Overall hypertension control rates in 1999 and 2000 by age and race-ethnicity in men and women. Error bars indicate 95% confidence intervals. Data are weighted to the U.S. population. For comparisons between racial-ethnic groups (with non-Hispanic whites as the referent), *P* values are as follows: for Mexican Americans—men aged 40 to 59 years, *P* < 0.001; men aged 60 years and older, *P* = 0.003; women aged 40 to 59 years, *P* = 0.002; women aged 60 years and older, *P* = 0.04; for non-Hispanic blacks—men aged 40 to 59 years, *P* = 0.02; men aged 60 years and older, *P* = 0.51; women aged 40 to 59 years, *P* = 0.003; women aged 60 years and older, *P* = 0.98. (From Hajjar I, Kotchen TA: Trends in prevalence, awareness, treatment, and control of hypertension in the United States, 1988-2000, *JAMA* 290:199-206, 2003.)

care insurance plans.[234] Surprisingly, the unadjusted incidence rates were lower in zip codes with known shortages of health professionals than in zip codes with ample health professional populations (adjusted rates were not presented). In addition, incidence of ESRD was higher in areas with more hospitalizations for hyperglycemic complications, which suggests a role for ineffective or poor access to treatment in the development of ESRD caused by diabetes. Similarly, a recent report cited more abnormal laboratory values at the onset of ESRD treatment among those without medical insurance.[235] The persistence of variations in risk of CKD progression by race after adjustment for many of these factors has motivated investigation of previously unexplained genetic variation using new investigative tools. Recently, two independent groups performed genome-wide analyses for ESRD risk loci in incident African American ESRD patients. Both used admixture linkage dysequilibrium analysis, which is based on the premise that when two genetically diverse populations mix, the admixed population receives chromosomal regions from either ancestry that can be identified by genotyping markers with different allelic frequencies in the ancestral populations. The groups screened the genome of African Americans with ESRD to identify ESRD susceptibility loci, regions of the genome in which individuals with ESRD manifest more or less African ancestry than their nondiseased counterparts. The Family Investigation of Nephropathy and Diabetes Research Group identified an association between excess African ancestry and nondiabetic ESRD on chromosome band 22q12, but no association with diabetic ESRD.[236] In contrast, the presence of an allele of European origin at this locus was found to be protective, with individuals with this allele showing a relative risk of 0.5 compared with individuals carrying an allele of African origin. In this study, the majority of excess ESRD risk of African ancestry was correlated with a number of common single-nucleotide polymorphisms (SNPs) in or near the gene encoding nonmuscle myosin heavy-chain type II isoform A *(MYH9)*. Several investigators have found this region that encodes the *MYH9* and apolipoprotein L1 *(ApoL1)* genes to be associated with both biopsy-proven idiopathic FSGS and human immunodeficiency virus-1 (HIV-1)–associated FSGS in African Americans.[237,238] Recent publications by Genovese and others have since demonstrated that FSGS and nondiabetic ESRD in African Americans are even more strongly associated with two independent sequence variants encoded in the *ApoL1* gene on chromosome 22 compared to the *MYH9* gene (FSGS OR = 10.5, 95% CI = 6.0 to 18.4; hypertension-attributed ESRD OR = 7.3, 95% CI = 5.6 to 9.5).[238,238a,238b,238c] Additional genetic determinants of apparent racial differences in the progression of CKD, including the apolipoprotein E gene *(APOE)* e2 allele,[239] have been reported recently in the United States, and polymorphisms of paraoxonase-1 and multiple others have been identified as potential susceptibility loci in Japanese adults.[240,241]

Summary

There is little variation in reports of the patterns of incidence, prevalence, and progression of kidney disease across race and ethnicity. In general, despite a lower prevalence of CKD among African Americans and Hispanics than among whites, the incidence of CKD is higher in African Americans, and rates of progression are faster in African Americans, Hispanics, and American Indians than in non-Hispanic whites.

Socioeconomic Factors and Chronic Kidney Disease

Socioeconomic Exposures

Earlier in this chapter, racial disparities in the incidence and progression of CKD were discussed. Racial differences in kidney disease risk are partially mediated by factors related to socioeconomic status and social deprivation. This portion of the excess risk is potentially modifiable and therefore of particular interest for targeting prevention strategies. Socioeconomic status has been described as a distal risk factor for kidney disease that acts through several proximal factors, including poverty or low income, lack of nutrition, low educational level, exposure to heavy metals, substance abuse, and limited access to health care.[233] These factors can be investigated at both the individual and neighborhood level at any given point in time. As a result, several recent analyses have examined both individual- and area-level socioeconomic status.[196,242] A framework for considering the numerous social and cultural determinants of disparities in CKD is provided in Figure 20-6. In addition, as in many disease processes that develop over protracted periods of time, both past and present exposures are responsible for increases in risk. For this reason, life course (i.e., the cumulative effect of social environments over the course of a lifetime) and parental socioeconomic factors have also been investigated as contributors to the incidence and progression of kidney disease.[243] Full evaluation of these individual- and area-level factors in biomedical research is a key to unlocking the explanation for the observed racial and ethnic disparities in kidney disease.

Socioeconomic Factors and the Incidence of Chronic Kidney Disease

Very few studies have examined risk factors for the incidence of CKD, and fewer yet have investigated socioeconomic factors. Krop and colleagues observed that blacks with diabetes mellitus were three times more likely than whites with diabetes mellitus to develop CKD in unadjusted analyses.[198] Subsequent adjustment for additional covariates revealed that 6% of the excess risk for development of CKD in black adults compared with white adults with diabetes was explained by income and educational level. Suboptimal health behaviors and poor control of glucose level and blood pressure accounted for a substantial proportion of the remaining risk. Given the strong relationship among socioeconomic status, health behaviors, and glycemic and hypertensive control,[213,244,245] the overall effect of socioeconomic factors on the incidence of CKD is understated in the aforementioned figure of 6% excess risk. A similar constellation of risk factors has been described in conjunction with renal involvement in systemic lupus erythematosus (SLE). Higher incidences of lupus nephritis have been noted among minority populations. One recent publication including data for participants with recently diagnosed SLE in the Lupus in Minorities: Nature vs Nurture (LUMINA) Study reported the development of lupus nephritis among

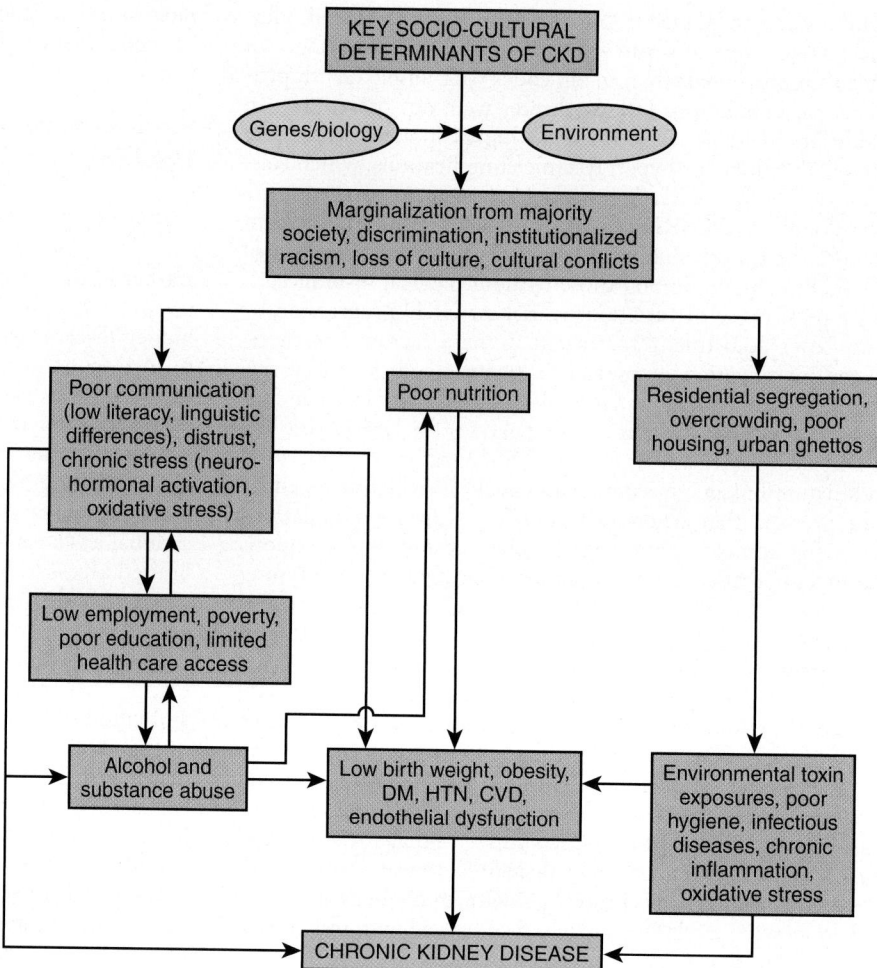

FIGURE 20-6 Framework for integrating key sociocultural determinants of chronic kidney disease (CKD). (From Norris K, Nissenson AR: Race, gender, and socioeconomic disparities in CKD in the United States, *J Am Soc Nephrol* 19:1261-1270, 2008; adapted from Norris KC, Agodoa LY: Unraveling the racial disparities associated with kidney disease, *Kidney Int* 68:914-924, 2005.)

44.6% of Texas Hispanics, 11.3% of Puerto Rican Hispanics, 45.8% of African Americans, and 18.3% of whites.[246] Upon further analysis, a composite socioeconomic status factor incorporating information on education, insurance, and poverty status was found to account for 14.5% of the variance due to ethnicity after adjustment, and socioeconomic status and genetic admixture together accounted for an additional 12.2% of the variance. Of note, an additional 36.8% of the variance in this model could be attributed to genetic admixture, which underscores the greater importance of genetic factors compared with socioeconomic factors in explaining the racial disparities in renal involvement in SLE. A population-based case-control study in Sweden provides additional evidence of the risk of incident CKD associated with low socioeconomic status. Odds ratios of incident CKD for families of solely unskilled workers were 2.1 (95% CI = 1.1 to 4.0) and 1.6 (95% CI = 1.0 to 2.6) for women and men, respectively, compared with families with at least one professional worker.[247] In addition, Swedish adults with 9 years or less of education were 30% more likely (OR = 1.3; 95% CI = 1.0 to 1.7) to develop CKD than adults with a college education. Finally, in parts of the United Kingdom, an approximately 50% increase in the incidence of CKD was reported among those in the highest quintile of social deprivation (i.e., living in an electoral ward with a high proportion of households without a car, unemployed, overcrowding, and housing not occupied by the owner) compared with the lowest quintile.[248]

Socioeconomic Factors and the Prevalence of Chronic Kidney Disease

The relationship between the prevalence of CKD and measures of socioeconomic status and social deprivation has been better characterized than the relationship between the incidence of CKD and these measures. Using data from the ARIC study, Shoham and colleagues found that being a member of the working class for some or all of one's life was associated with increased odds of CKD among both whites and blacks (OR = 1.4, 95% CI = 0.9 to 2.0; and OR = 1.9, CI = 1.3 to 2.9, respectively).[249] Martins and others cite a significant association (OR = 1.2; 95% CI = 1.1 to 1.3) between living at less than 200% of the federal poverty level and microalbuminuria using data from the Third National Health and Nutrition Examination Survey (NHANES III) after multivariable adjustment.[250] Another analysis of data from NHANES III confirmed these findings and revealed a higher prevalence of CKD among non-Hispanic whites and blacks with fewer than 12 years of education and with an income equivalence level (i.e., total household income divided by the square root of the number of people dependent on that income) of less than $12,000 compared with non-Hispanic whites only with an income equivalence level of $28,000 or more.[251] An even stronger relationship was observed between unemployment and CKD prevalence, but only among non-Hispanic blacks and Mexican Americans. Interestingly, these same associations could not be

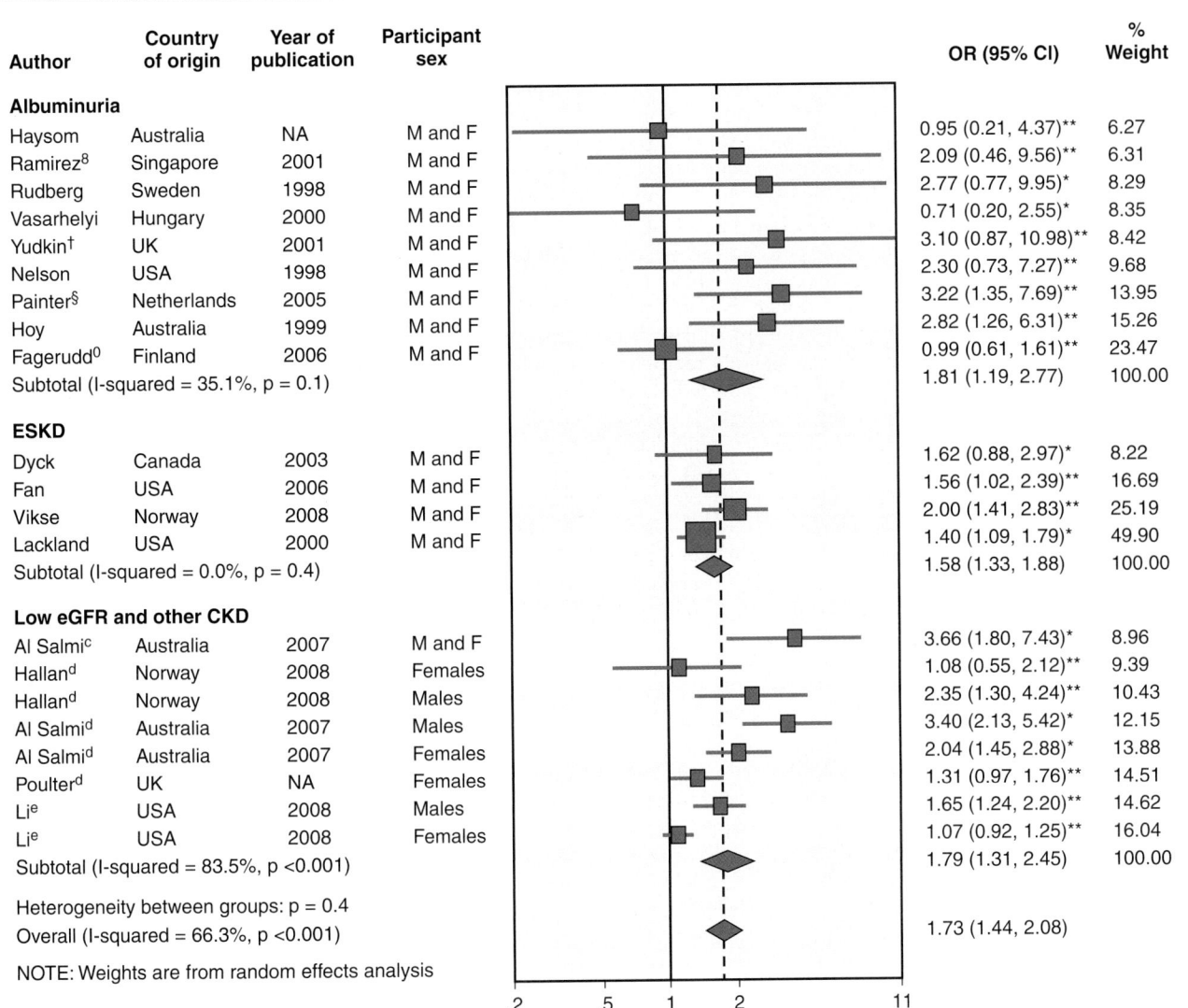

Author	Country of origin	Year of publication	Participant sex	OR (95% CI)	% Weight
Albuminuria					
Haysom	Australia	NA	M and F	0.95 (0.21, 4.37)**	6.27
Ramirez[ß]	Singapore	2001	M and F	2.09 (0.46, 9.56)**	6.31
Rudberg	Sweden	1998	M and F	2.77 (0.77, 9.95)*	8.29
Vasarhelyi	Hungary	2000	M and F	0.71 (0.20, 2.55)*	8.35
Yudkin[†]	UK	2001	M and F	3.10 (0.87, 10.98)**	8.42
Nelson	USA	1998	M and F	2.30 (0.73, 7.27)**	9.68
Painter[§]	Netherlands	2005	M and F	3.22 (1.35, 7.69)**	13.95
Hoy	Australia	1999	M and F	2.82 (1.26, 6.31)**	15.26
Fagerudd[0]	Finland	2006	M and F	0.99 (0.61, 1.61)**	23.47
Subtotal (I-squared = 35.1%, p = 0.1)				1.81 (1.19, 2.77)	100.00
ESKD					
Dyck	Canada	2003	M and F	1.62 (0.88, 2.97)*	8.22
Fan	USA	2006	M and F	1.56 (1.02, 2.39)**	16.69
Vikse	Norway	2008	M and F	2.00 (1.41, 2.83)**	25.19
Lackland	USA	2000	M and F	1.40 (1.09, 1.79)*	49.90
Subtotal (I-squared = 0.0%, p = 0.4)				1.58 (1.33, 1.88)	100.00
Low eGFR and other CKD					
Al Salmi[c]	Australia	2007	M and F	3.66 (1.80, 7.43)*	8.96
Hallan[d]	Norway	2008	Females	1.08 (0.55, 2.12)**	9.39
Hallan[d]	Norway	2008	Males	2.35 (1.30, 4.24)**	10.43
Al Salmi[d]	Australia	2007	Males	3.40 (2.13, 5.42)*	12.15
Al Salmi[d]	Australia	2007	Females	2.04 (1.45, 2.88)*	13.88
Poulter[d]	UK	NA	Females	1.31 (0.97, 1.76)**	14.51
Li[e]	USA	2008	Males	1.65 (1.24, 2.20)**	14.62
Li[e]	USA	2008	Females	1.07 (0.92, 1.25)**	16.04
Subtotal (I-squared = 83.5%, p <0.001)				1.79 (1.31, 2.45)	100.00
Heterogeneity between groups: p = 0.4					
Overall (I-squared = 66.3%, p <0.001)				1.73 (1.44, 2.08)	

NOTE: Weights are from random effects analysis

FIGURE 20-7 Odds ratios (ORs) and 95% confidence intervals (CIs) for risk of chronic kidney disease (CKD) associated with low versus normal birth weight. The statistical size of the study was defined in terms of the inverse of the variance of the regression coefficient, indicated by *blue squares*. *Dashed vertical line* is the inverse variance-weighted regression through the overall point estimate. *Individual study estimates not adjusted for confounders or estimates adjusted or controlled for age and/or sex only. **Estimates adjusted for additional factors. Outcome is [a]proteinuria; [b]diabetic nephropathy (albuminuria or end-stage renal disease); [c]CKD stages 2 to 5: estimated glomerular filtration rate (eGFR) of 60 to 90 mL/min/1.73 m² with proteinuria ± hematuria or eGFR of less than 60 mL/min/1.73 m² or patient on dialysis therapy; [d]eGFR less than 10th percentile for gender; and [e]albuminuria or eGFR less than 60 mL/min/1.73 m². Exposure measured as §exposure to famine midgestation (vs. not exposed) and †ponderal index in the lower 3rd percentile (versus highest 3rd). F, Female; M, male; NA, not applicable (unpublished analysis). (From White SL, Perkovic V, Cass A, et al: Is low birth weight an antecedent of CKD in later life? A systematic review of observational studies, *Am J Kidney Dis* 54:248-261, 2009.)

detected using data from similar surveys of adults in Australia and Thailand.[251] Some effects of socioeconomic status on CKD are mediated by more proximal factors such as nutritional status, health behaviors, and environmental exposures. Nutritional deprivation or physiologic insults in utero cause intrauterine growth restriction (IUGR). Building on the developmental origins of health and disease hypothesis put forward by Barker,[252] Brenner and Chertow hypothesized that IUGR causes a decrease in nephron number that leads to a susceptibility toward hypertension and reduced kidney function later in life.[253] A systematic review and meta-analysis of 32 observational studies evaluated the relationship between birth weight and CKD, assessed at age older than 12 months.[254] Combined weighted estimates of effect provided an odds ratio for CKD associated with low birth weight of 1.7 (95% CI = 1.4 to 2.1; Figure 20-7). These results were consistent across multiple

definitions of CKD, including albuminuria, ESRD, and low eGFR. Finally, numerous environmental exposures that impact kidney health occur disproportionately among certain populations, including those of low socioeconomic status. Exposure to cadmium and lead, even at low levels, is associated with a significantly increased prevalence of kidney disease.[255-263] Data on the renal effects of drinking water or residential environmental exposure to uranium are scarce, and very few studies have found a significant association between this type of exposure to uranium and renal outcomes, including kidney stones, chronic nephritis, and microalbuminuria.[264-266] Overcrowding in residences poses more risk for streptococcal infections, which may lead to poststreptococcal glomerulonephritis. Reductions in renal functional reserve, chronic renal disease, and development of ESRD have been reported in patients who have recovered from poststreptococcal glomerulonephritis.[267-269]

Socioeconomic Factors and the Progression of Chronic Kidney Disease

The association between race-ethnicity and the progression of CKD has been discussed earlier in this chapter. As noted previously, socioeconomic factors highly correlated with race-ethnicity account for a proportion of this excess risk. In particular, Tarver-Carr and others reported a 2.7-fold increased risk of ESRD among African Americans compared with whites.[209] Twelve percent of the excess risk of developing ESRD among African Americans was explained by sociodemographic factors, including education, poverty status, and marital status. A large longitudinal study involving over 170,000 members of Kaiser Permanente of Northern California reported a significant risk of developing ESRD among members who never attended college (HR = 1.6; 95% CI = 1.2 to 2.0) or completed some college (HR = 1.5; 95% CI = 1.1 to 1.9) compared with college graduates after multivariable adjustment.[270]

Recent studies have integrated neighborhood-level socioeconomic factors in the examination of the progression of CKD. One such study using data on the incidence of ESRD in Georgia, North Carolina, and South Carolina defined neighborhood poverty using the percentage of the census tract population living below the poverty level.[271] Unadjusted incidence rate ratios of ESRD increased from 1.5 to 4.5 in a dose-response manner for census tracts with 5.0% to 9.9%, 10.0% to 14.9%, 15.0% to 19.9%, 20.0% to 24.9%, and 25% or more of the population living below the poverty level, compared with tracts with fewer than 5% living below the poverty level. This marker of neighborhood poverty was significantly associated with a higher incidence of ESRD among both blacks and whites. However, there was a stronger relationship between incidence of ESRD and census tract poverty among blacks than among whites. Finally, Merkin and colleagues analyzed data from both the ARIC study and Cardiovascular Health Study separately to assess the relationship between individual- and neighborhood-level socioeconomic status and progressive CKD. In the ARIC study, age- and center-adjusted incidence rates of progressive CKD increased with declining area-level socioeconomic scores for African American women and white men, but not for African American men and white women.[196] Living in areas in the lowest quartile of area-level socioeconomic status was significantly associated with a 60% greater risk of progressive CKD (HR = 1.6; 95% CI = 1.0 to 2.5) only among white men after adjustment for multiple variables, including individual-level socioeconomic status. Among participants in the Cardiovascular Health Study, age- and center-adjusted incidence rates of progressive CKD were inversely related to area-level socioeconomic scores as well as to individual levels of income and education.[242] After adjustment for multiple variables, including individual-level socioeconomic status, living in areas in the lowest quartile of area-level socioeconomic status was found to be associated with a hazard ratio for progressive CKD of 1.5 (95% CI = 1.0 to 2.0) compared with living in areas in the highest quartile. The association with individual-level socioeconomic status no longer remained significant after adjustment in this elderly population.

Summary

Socioeconomic factors, especially income, education, and environmental factors, appear to explain a large proportion of the excess incidence and progression of CKD among African American and other racial-ethnic groups compared with whites. Additional studies are needed to clarify the influence of access to health care and early-life socioeconomic status on kidney health.

Conclusion

Although there are several studies and data sets reporting the incidence of CKD in the United States, more consistency in the definition of incident CKD is needed to facilitate the assessment of differences and disparities across sociodemographic groups. In addition, there is no single way to capture information on the progression of CKD, and this poses a challenge to researchers and clinicians trying to systematically review and interpret findings across studies. Examination of the pattern of kidney disease across gender has not yielded a consistent relationship. Although the prevalence of CKD appears to be higher among women, men are reported to have a higher incidence of glomerular disease and greater progression of nondiabetic CKD, especially compared with premenopausal women. Results are less consistent across gender, however, regarding progression of IgA nephropathy and progression overall in postmenopausal women. More studies are needed to elucidate any gender differences in the progression of lupus nephritis. Similarly, the reported relationships between gender and ADPKD progression, and gender and the development of microalbuminuria and macroalbuminuria and progression of diabetic nephropathy are not consistent and may be modified by age and race. Reported patterns of kidney disease across racial-ethnic groups have been more consistent than those reported across gender. A lower prevalence of CKD has been observed among African American and Hispanics than among whites. As eGFR levels decline, however, African Americans seem to have a higher prevalence of CKD and albuminuria than non-Hispanic whites, which is consistent with the long-observed pattern of higher rates of ESRD among African Americans. The incidence of CKD is higher in African Americans, and rates of progression are faster in African Americans, Hispanics, and American Indians than in non-Hispanic whites. A substantial proportion of the excess incidence and progression of CKD among African American and other racial-ethnic groups compared with whites is associated with socioeconomic determinants. Evidence of the impact of income, education, and environmental factors on kidney outcomes is consistent; however, the association between access to care and these same outcomes is less clearly documented. There is some suggestion of interactions between socioeconomic status and race for kidney outcomes, but this matter needs further study.

References

1. Hughson M, Farris III AB, Douglas-Denton R, et al. Glomerular number and size in autopsy kidneys: the relationship to birth weight. *Kidney Int.* 2003;63:2113-2122.
2. Hughson MD, Douglas-Denton R, Bertram JF, et al. Hypertension, glomerular number, and birth weight in African Americans and white subjects in the southeastern United States. *Kidney Int.* 2006;69: 671-678.
3. Neugarten J, Kasiske B, Silbiger SR, et al. Effects of sex on renal structure. *Nephron.* 2002;90:139-144.
4. Nyengaard JR, Bendtsen TF. Glomerular number and size in relation to age, kidney weight, and body surface in normal man. *Anat Rec.* 1992;232: 194-201.

5. Slack TK, Wilson DM. Normal renal function: CIN and CPAH in healthy donors before and after nephrectomy. *Mayo Clin Proc.* 1976;51:296-300.
6. Daugirdas JT, Meyer K, Greene T, et al. Scaling of measured glomerular filtration rate in kidney donor candidates by anthropometric estimates of body surface area, body water, metabolic rate, or liver size. *Clin J Am Soc Nephrol.* 2009;4:1575-1583.
7. Macdonald JH, Marcora SM, Kumwenda MJ, et al. The relationship between estimated glomerular filtration rate, demographic and anthropometric variables is mediated by muscle mass in non-diabetic patients with chronic kidney disease. *Nephrol Dial Transplant.* 2006;21:3488-3494.
8. Levey AS, Stevens LA, Schmid CH, et al. A new equation to estimate glomerular filtration rate. *Ann Intern Med.* 2009;150:604-612.
9. Levey AS, Bosch JP, Lewis JB, et al. A more accurate method to estimate glomerular filtration rate from serum creatinine: a new prediction equation. :Modification of Diet in Renal Disease Study Group. *Ann Intern Med.* 1999;130:461-470.
10. Poggio ED, Rule AD, Tanchanco R, et al. Demographic and clinical characteristics associated with glomerular filtration rates in living kidney donors. *Kidney Int.* 2009;75:1079-1087.
11. Verzola D, Villaggio B, Procopio V, et al. Androgen-mediated apoptosis of kidney tubule cells: role of c-Jun amino terminal kinase. *Biochem Biophys Res Commun.* 2009;387:531-536.
12. Verzola D, Gandolfo MT, Salvatore F, et al. Testosterone promotes apoptotic damage in human renal tubular cells. *Kidney Int.* 2004;65:1252-1261.
13. Metcalfe PD, Leslie JA, Campbell MT, et al. Testosterone exacerbates obstructive renal injury by stimulating TNF-alpha production and increasing proapoptotic and profibrotic signaling. *Am J Physiol Endocrinol Metab.* 2008;294:E435-E443.
14. Kollerits B, Fliser D, Heid IM, et al. Gender-specific association of adiponectin as a predictor of progression of chronic kidney disease: the Mild to Moderate Kidney Disease Study. *Kidney Int.* 2007;71:1279-1286.
15. Lei J, Silbiger S, Ziyadeh FN, et al. Serum-stimulated alpha 1 type IV collagen gene transcription is mediated by TGF-beta and inhibited by estradiol. *Am J Physiol.* 1998;274:F252-F258.
16. Kwan G, Neugarten J, Sherman M, et al. Effects of sex hormones on mesangial cell proliferation and collagen synthesis. *Kidney Int.* 1996;50:1173-1179.
17. Neugarten J, Silbiger SR. Effects of sex hormones on mesangial cells. *Am J Kidney Dis.* 1995;26:147-151.
18. Neugarten J, Ghossein C, Silbiger S. Estradiol inhibits mesangial cell-mediated oxidation of low-density lipoprotein. *J Lab Clin Med.* 1995;126:385-391.
19. Silbiger S, Lei J, Neugarten J. Estradiol suppresses type I collagen synthesis in mesangial cells via activation of activator protein-1. *Kidney Int.* 1999;55:1268-1276.
20. Silbiger S, Lei J, Ziyadeh FN, et al. Estradiol reverses TGF-beta1-stimulated type IV collagen gene transcription in murine mesangial cells. *Am J Physiol.* 1998;274:F1113-F1118.
21. Klopp C, Young NF, Taylor HC. The effects of testosterone and of testosterone propionate on renal functions in man. *J Clin Invest.* 1945;24:189-191.
22. Dignam WS, Voskian J, Ssali NS. Effects of estrogens on renal hemodynamics and excretion of electrolytes in human subjects. *J Clin Endocrinol Metab.* 1956;16:1032-1042.
23. Swaminathan S, Leung N, Lager DJ, et al. Changing incidence of glomerular disease in Olmsted County, Minnesota: a 30-year renal biopsy study. *Clin J Am Soc Nephrol.* 2006;1:483-487.
24. Simon P, Ramee MP, Boulahrouz R, et al. Epidemiologic data of primary glomerular diseases in western France. *Kidney Int.* 2004;66:905-908.
25. Silbiger SR, Neugarten J. The impact of gender on the progression of chronic renal disease. *Am J Kidney Dis.* 1995;25:515-533.
26. D'Amico G. Influence of clinical and histological features on actuarial renal survival in adult patients with idiopathic IgA nephropathy, membranous nephropathy, and membranoproliferative glomerulonephritis: survey of the recent literature. *Am J Kidney Dis.* 1992;20:315-323.
27. Korbet SM, Genchi RM, Borok RZ, et al. The racial prevalence of glomerular lesions in nephrotic adults. *Am J Kidney Dis.* 1996;27:647-651.
28. Hanko JB, Mullan RN, O'Rourke DM, et al. The changing pattern of adult primary glomerular disease. *Nephrol Dial Transplant.* 2009;24:3050-3054.
29. Wyatt RJ, Julian BA, Baehler RW, et al. Epidemiology of IgA nephropathy in central and eastern Kentucky for the period 1975 through 1994. :Central Kentucky Region of the Southeastern United States IgA Nephropathy DATABANK Project. *J Am Soc Nephrol.* 1998;9:853-858.
30. Braden GL, Mulhern JG, O'Shea MH, et al. Changing incidence of glomerular diseases in adults. *Am J Kidney Dis.* 2000;35:878-883.
31. Briganti EM, Dowling J, Finlay M, et al. The incidence of biopsy-proven glomerulonephritis in Australia. *Nephrol Dial Transplant.* 2001;16:1364-1367.
32. US Renal Data System. *USRDS 2009 annual data report: atlas of end stage renal disease in the United States.* Bethesda, Md: National Institutes of Health, National Institute of Diabetes and Digestive and Kidney Diseases; 2009.
33. Neugarten J, Acharya A, Silbiger SR. Effect of gender on the progression of nondiabetic renal disease: a meta-analysis. *J Am Soc Nephrol.* 2000;11:319-329.
34. Coggins CH, Breyer LJ, Caggiula AW, et al. Differences between women and men with chronic renal disease. *Nephrol Dial Transplant.* 1998;13:1430-1437.
35. Evans M, Fryzek JP, Elinder CG, et al. The natural history of chronic renal failure: results from an unselected, population-based, inception cohort in Sweden. *Am J Kidney Dis.* 2005;46:863-870.
36. Eriksen BO, Ingebretsen OC. The progression of chronic kidney disease: a 10-year population-based study of the effects of gender and age. *Kidney Int.* 2006;69:375-382.
37. Molina JF, Drenkard C, Molina J, et al. Systemic lupus erythematosus in males: a study of 107 Latin American patients. *Medicine (Baltimore).* 1996;75:124-130.
38. Moranne O, Watier L, Rossert J, et al. Primary glomerulonephritis: an update on renal survival and determinants of progression. *QJM.* 2008;101:215-224.
39. Cattran DC, Reich HN, Beanlands HJ, et al. The impact of sex in primary glomerulonephritis. *Nephrol Dial Transplant.* 2008;23:2247-2253.
40. Hannedouche T, Chauveau P, Kalou F, et al. Factors affecting progression in advanced chronic renal failure. *Clin Nephrol.* 1993;39:312-320.
41. Jungers P, Hannedouche T, Itakura Y, et al. Progression rate to end-stage renal failure in non-diabetic kidney diseases: a multivariate analysis of determinant factors. *Nephrol Dial Transplant.* 1995;10:1353-1360.
42. Hunt LP, Short CD, Mallick NP. Prognostic indicators in patients presenting with the nephrotic syndrome. *Kidney Int.* 1988;34:382-388.
43. Gerstoft J, Balslov JT, Brahm M, et al. Prognosis in glomerulonephritis. II. Regression analyses of prognostic factors affecting the course of renal function and the mortality in 395 patients. Calculation of a prognostic model. Report from a Copenhagen study group of renal diseases. *Acta Med Scand.* 1986;219:179-187.
44. D'Amico G, Gentile MG, Fellin G, et al. Effect of dietary protein restriction on the progression of renal failure: a prospective randomized trial. *Nephrol Dial Transplant.* 1994;9:1590-1594.
45. Rosman JB, Langer K, Brandl M, et al. Protein-restricted diets in chronic renal failure: a four year follow-up shows limited indications. *Kidney Int.* 1989;27(Suppl):S96-S102.
46. Ruggenenti P, Gaspari F, Perna A, et al. Cross sectional longitudinal study of spot morning urine protein:creatinine ratio, 24 hour urine protein excretion rate, glomerular filtration rate, and end stage renal failure in chronic renal disease in patients without diabetes. *BMJ.* 1998;316:504-509.
47. Simon P, Ramee MP, Autuly V, et al. Epidemiology of primary glomerular diseases in a French region. Variations according to period and age. *Kidney Int.* 1994;46:1192-1198.
48. Williams PS, Fass G, Bone JM. Renal pathology and proteinuria determine progression in untreated mild/moderate chronic renal failure. *Q J Med.* 1988;67:343-354.
49. Hannedouche T, Albouze G, Chauveau P, et al. Effects of blood pressure and antihypertensive treatment on progression of advanced chronic renal failure. *Am J Kidney Dis.* 1993;21:131-137.
50. Locatelli F, Marcelli D, Comelli M, et al. Proteinuria and blood pressure as causal components of progression to end-stage renal failure. Northern Italian Cooperative Study Group. *Nephrol Dial Transplant.* 1996;11:461-467.
51. Mallick NP, Short CD, Hunt LP. How far since Ellis? The Manchester Study of glomerular disease. *Nephron.* 1987;46:113-124.
52. Hannedouche T, Chauveau P, Fehrat A, et al. Effect of moderate protein restriction on the rate of progression of chronic renal failure. *Kidney Int.* 1989;27(Suppl):S91-S95.
53. Alamartine E, Sabatier JC, Guerin C, et al. Prognostic factors in mesangial IgA glomerulonephritis: an extensive study with univariate and multivariate analyses. *Am J Kidney Dis.* 1991;18:12-19.
54. Bogenschutz O, Bohle A, Batz C, et al. IgA nephritis: on the importance of morphological and clinical parameters in the long-term prognosis of 239 patients. *Am J Nephrol.* 1990;10:137-147.
55. Chida Y, Tomura S, Takeuchi J. Renal survival rate of IgA nephropathy. *Nephron.* 1985;40:189-194.
56. Droz D, Kramar A, Nawar T, et al. Primary IgA nephropathy: prognostic factors. *Contrib Nephrol.* 1984;40:202-207.
57. Frimat L, Briancon S, Hestin D, et al. IgA nephropathy: prognostic classification of end-stage renal failure. L'Association des Néphrologues de l'Est. *Nephrol Dial Transplant.* 1997;12:2569-2575.
58. Packham DK, Yan HD, Hewitson TD, et al. The significance of focal and segmental hyalinosis and sclerosis (FSHS) and nephrotic range proteinuria in IgA nephropathy. *Clin Nephrol.* 1996;46:225-229.

59. Rekola S, Bergstrand A, Bucht H. Deterioration of GFR in IgA nephropathy as measured by 51Cr-EDTA clearance. *Kidney Int.* 1991;40:1050-1054.
60. Hood SA, Velosa JA, Holley KE, et al. IgA-IgG nephropathy: predictive indices of progressive disease. *Clin Nephrol.* 1981;16:55-62.
61. Nicholls KM, Fairley KF, Dowling JP, et al. The clinical course of mesangial IgA associated nephropathy in adults. *Q J Med.* 1984;53:227-250.
62. Propper DJ, Power DA, Simpson JG, et al. The incidence, mode of presentation, and prognosis of IgA nephropathy in northeast Scotland. *Semin Nephrol.* 1987;7:363-366.
63. Velo M, Lozano L, Egido J, et al. Natural history of IgA nephropathy in patients followed-up for more than ten years in Spain. *Semin Nephrol.* 1987;7:346-350.
64. van der PJ, Arisz L, Brentjens JR, et al. The clinical course of IgA nephropathy in adults. *Clin Nephrol.* 1977;8:335-340.
65. Boyce NW, Holdsworth SR, Thomson NM, et al. Clinicopathological associations in mesangial IgA nephropathy. *Am J Nephrol.* 1986;6:246-252.
66. Woo KT, Chiang GS, Lau YK, et al. IgA nephritis in Singapore: clinical, prognostic indices, and treatment. *Semin Nephrol.* 1987;7:379-381.
67. Rambausek M, Rauterberg EW, et al. Evolution of IgA glomerulonephritis: relation to morphology, immunogenetics, and BP. *Semin Nephrol.* 1987;7:370-373.
68. Kobayashi Y, Fujii K, Hiki Y, et al. Steroid therapy in IgA nephropathy: a retrospective study in heavy proteinuric cases. *Nephron.* 1988;48:12-17.
69. Kobayashi Y, Hiki Y, Fujii K, et al. Moderately proteinuric IgA nephropathy: prognostic prediction of individual clinical courses and steroid therapy in progressive cases. *Nephron.* 1989;53:250-256.
70. Berg UB, Widstam-Attorps UC. Follow-up of renal function and urinary protein excretion in childhood IgA nephropathy. *Pediatr Nephrol.* 1993;7:123-129.
71. Wyatt RJ, Kritchevsky SB, Woodford SY, et al. IgA nephropathy: long-term prognosis for pediatric patients. *J Pediatr.* 1995;127:913-919.
72. Levy M, Gonzalez-Burchard G, Broyer M, et al. Berger's disease in children. Natural history and outcome. *Medicine (Baltimore).* 1985;64:157-180.
73. Yoshikawa N, Ito H, Nakamura H. Prognostic indicators in childhood IgA nephropathy. *Nephron.* 1992;60:60-67.
74. D'Amico G, Minetti L, Ponticelli C, et al. Prognostic indicators in idiopathic IgA mesangial nephropathy. *Q J Med.* 1986;59:363-378.
75. Syre G. IGA mesangial glomerulonephritis; significance and pathogenesis of segmental-focal glomerular lesions. *Virchows Arch A Pathol Anat Histopathol.* 1983;402:11-24.
76. Nieuwhof C, Kruytzer M, Frederiks P, et al. Chronicity index and mesangial IgG deposition are risk factors for hypertension and renal failure in early IgA nephropathy. *Am J Kidney Dis.* 1998;31:962-970.
77. Hoy WE, Hughson MD, Smith SM, et al. Mesangial proliferative glomerulonephritis in southwestern American Indians. *Am J Kidney Dis.* 1993;21:486-496.
78. Magil AB, Ballon HS. IgA nephropathy. Evaluation of prognostic factors in patients with moderate disease. *Nephron.* 1987;47:246-252.
79. Cattran DC, Greenwood C, Ritchie S. Long-term benefits of angiotensin-converting enzyme inhibitor therapy in patients with severe immunoglobulin A nephropathy: a comparison to patients receiving treatment with other antihypertensive agents and to patients receiving no therapy. *Am J Kidney Dis.* 1994;23:247-254.
80. Koyama A, Igarashi M, Kobayashi M. Natural history and risk factors for immunoglobulin A nephropathy in Japan. Research Group on Progressive Renal Diseases. *Am J Kidney Dis.* 1997;29:526-532.
81. Ibels LS, Gyory AZ. IgA nephropathy: analysis of the natural history, important factors in the progression of renal disease, and a review of the literature. *Medicine (Baltimore).* 1994;73:79-102.
82. Johnston PA, Brown JS, Braumholtz DA, et al. Clinico-pathological correlations and long-term follow-up of 253 United Kingdom patients with IgA nephropathy. A report from the MRC Glomerulonephritis Registry. *Q J Med.* 1992;84:619-627.
83. Katafuchi R, Oh Y, Hori K, et al. An important role of glomerular segmental lesions on progression of IgA nephropathy: a multivariate analysis. *Clin Nephrol.* 1994;41:191-198.
84. Lee HS, Koh HI, Lee HB, et al. IgA nephropathy in Korea: a morphological and clinical study. *Clin Nephrol.* 1987;27:131-140.
85. Mustonen J, Pasternack A, Helin H, et al. Clinicopathologic correlations in a series of 143 patients with IgA glomerulonephritis. *Am J Nephrol.* 1985;5:150-157.
86. Radford Jr MG, Donadio Jr JV, Bergstralh EJ, et al. Predicting renal outcome in IgA nephropathy. *J Am Soc Nephrol.* 1997;8:199-207.
87. Murphy BF, Fairley KF, Kincaid-Smith PS. Idiopathic membranous glomerulonephritis: long-term follow-up in 139 cases. *Clin Nephrol.* 1988;30:175-181.
88. Abe S, Amagasaki Y, Konishi K, et al. Idiopathic membranous glomerulonephritis: aspects of geographical differences. *J Clin Pathol.* 1986;39:1193-1198.
89. Cameron JS, Healy MJ, Adu D. The Medical Research Council trial of short-term high-dose alternate day prednisolone in idiopathic membranous nephropathy with nephrotic syndrome in adults. The MRC Glomerulonephritis Working Party. *Q J Med.* 1990;74:133-156.
90. A controlled study of short-term prednisone treatment in adults with membranous nephropathy. Collaborative Study of the Adult Idiopathic Nephrotic Syndrome. *N Engl J Med.* 1979;301:1301-1306.
91. Davison AM, Cameron JS, Kerr DN, et al. The natural history of renal function in untreated idiopathic membranous glomerulonephritis in adults. *Clin Nephrol.* 1984;22:61-67.
92. Fuiano G, Stanziale P, Balletta M, et al. Effectiveness of steroid therapy in different stages of membranous nephropathy. *Nephrol Dial Transplant.* 1989;4:1022-1029.
93. Honkanen E, Tornroth T, Gronhagen-Riska C, et al. Long-term survival in idiopathic membranous glomerulonephritis: can the course be clinically predicted? *Clin Nephrol.* 1994;41:127-134.
94. Hopper Jr J, Trew PA, Biava CG. Membranous nephropathy: its relative benignity in women. *Nephron.* 1981;29:18-24.
95. Jindal K, West M, Bear R, et al. Long-term benefits of therapy with cyclophosphamide and prednisone in patients with membranous glomerulonephritis and impaired renal function. *Am J Kidney Dis.* 1992;19:61-67.
96. MacTier R, Boulton Jones JM, Payton CD, et al. The natural history of membranous nephropathy in the West of Scotland. *Q J Med.* 1986;60:793-802.
97. Ponticelli C, Zucchelli P, Imbasciati E, et al. Controlled trial of methylprednisolone and chlorambucil in idiopathic membranous nephropathy. *N Engl J Med.* 1984;310:946-950.
98. Ramzy MH, Cameron JS, Turner DR, et al. The long-term outcome of idiopathic membranous nephropathy. *Clin Nephrol.* 1981;16:13-19.
99. Schieppati A, Mosconi L, Perna A, et al. Prognosis of untreated patients with idiopathic membranous nephropathy. *N Engl J Med.* 1993;329:85-89.
100. Toth T, Takebayashi S. Factors contributing to the outcome in 100 adult patients with idiopathic membranous glomerulonephritis. *Int Urol Nephrol.* 1994;26:93-106.
101. Tu WH, Petitti DB, Biava CG, et al. Membranous nephropathy: predictors of terminal renal failure. *Nephron.* 1984;36:118-124.
102. Wehrmann M, Bohle A, Bogenschutz O, et al. Long-term prognosis of chronic idiopathic membranous glomerulonephritis. An analysis of 334 cases with particular regard to tubulo-interstitial changes. *Clin Nephrol.* 1989;31:67-76.
103. Durin S, Barbanel C, Landais P, et al. [Long term course of idiopathic extramembranous glomerulonephritis. Study of predictive factors of terminal renal insufficiency in 82 untreated patients]. *Nephrologie.* 1990;11:67-71.
104. Donadio Jr JV, Torres VE, Velosa JA, et al. Idiopathic membranous nephropathy: the natural history of untreated patients. *Kidney Int.* 1988;33:708-715.
105. Bone JM, Rustom R, Williams PS. "Progressive" versus "indolent" idiopathic membranous glomerulonephritis. *QJM.* 1997;90:699-706.
106. Hunt LP. Statistical aspects of survival in membranous nephropathy. *Nephrol Dial Transplant.* 1992;1(suppl 7):53-59.
107. Cattran DC, Pei Y, Greenwood CM, et al. Validation of a predictive model of idiopathic membranous nephropathy: its clinical and research implications. *Kidney Int.* 1997;51:901-907.
108. Kibriya MG, Tishkov I, Nikolov D. Immunosuppressive therapy with cyclophosphamide and prednisolone in severe idiopathic membranous nephropathy. *Nephrol Dial Transplant.* 1994;9:138-143.
109. Pei Y, Cattran D, Greenwood C. Predicting chronic renal insufficiency in idiopathic membranous glomerulonephritis. *Kidney Int.* 1992;42:960-966.
110. Ponticelli C, Zucchelli P, Passerini P, et al. A randomized trial of methylprednisolone and chlorambucil in idiopathic membranous nephropathy. *N Engl J Med.* 1989;320:8-13.
111. Zucchelli P, Ponticelli C, Cagnoli L, et al. Long-term outcome of idiopathic membranous nephropathy with nephrotic syndrome. *Nephrol Dial Transplant.* 1987;2:73-78.
112. Hogan SL, Muller KE, Jennette JC, et al. A review of therapeutic studies of idiopathic membranous glomerulopathy. *Am J Kidney Dis.* 1995;25:862-875.
113. Reichert LJ, Koene RA, Wetzels JF. Prognostic factors in idiopathic membranous nephropathy. *Am J Kidney Dis.* 1998;31:1-11.
114. Jafar TH, Schmid CH, Stark PC, et al. The rate of progression of renal disease may not be slower in women compared with men: a patient-level meta-analysis. *Nephrol Dial Transplant.* 2003;18:2047-2053.
115. Menon V, Wang X, Sarnak MJ, et al. Long-term outcomes in nondiabetic chronic kidney disease. *Kidney Int.* 2008;73:1310-1315.
116. Haas M. Histologic subclassification of IgA nephropathy: a clinicopathologic study of 244 cases. *Am J Kidney Dis.* 1997;29:829-842.
117. Barr RG, Seliger S, Appel GB, et al. Prognosis in proliferative lupus nephritis: the role of socio-economic status and race/ethnicity. *Nephrol Dial Transplant.* 2003;18:2039-2046.

118. Abraham MA, Korula A, Jayakrishnan K, et al. Prognostic factors in diffuse proliferative lupus nephritis. *J Assoc Physicians India.* 1999;47:862-865.

119. Ward MM, Studenski S. Clinical prognostic factors in lupus nephritis. The importance of hypertension and smoking. *Arch Intern Med.* 1992;152:2082-2088.

120. Ward MM. Changes in the incidence of endstage renal disease due to lupus nephritis in the United States, 1996-2004. *J Rheumatol.* 2009;36:63-67.

121. Soni SS, Gowrishankar S, Adikey GK, et al. Sex-based differences in lupus nephritis: a study of 235 Indian patients. *J Nephrol.* 2008;21:570-575.

122. Vachvanichsanong P, Dissaneewate P, McNeil E. Diffuse proliferative glomerulonephritis does not determine the worst outcome in childhood-onset lupus nephritis: a 23-year experience in a single centre. *Nephrol Dial Transplant.* 2009;24:2729-2734.

123. Bear JC, Parfrey PS, Morgan JM, et al. Autosomal dominant polycystic kidney disease: new information for genetic counselling. *Am J Med Genet.* 1992;43:548-553.

124. Choukroun G, Itakura Y, Albouze G, et al. Factors influencing progression of renal failure in autosomal dominant polycystic kidney disease. *J Am Soc Nephrol.* 1995;6:1634-1642.

125. Johnson AM, Gabow PA. Identification of patients with autosomal dominant polycystic kidney disease at highest risk for end-stage renal disease. *J Am Soc Nephrol.* 1997;8:1560-1567.

126. Klahr S, Breyer JA, Beck GJ, et al. Dietary protein restriction, blood pressure control, and the progression of polycystic kidney disease. Modification of Diet in Renal Disease Study Group. *J Am Soc Nephrol.* 1995;5:2037-2047.

127. Stewart JH. End-stage renal failure appears earlier in men than in women with polycystic kidney disease. *Am J Kidney Dis.* 1994;24:181-183.

128. Higashihara E, Aso Y, Shimazaki J, et al. Clinical aspects of polycystic kidney disease. *J Urol.* 1992;147:329-332.

129. Torra R, Badenas C, Darnell A, et al. Linkage, clinical features, and prognosis of autosomal dominant polycystic kidney disease types 1 and 2. *J Am Soc Nephrol.* 1996;7:2142-2151.

130. Geberth S, Ritz E, Zeier M, et al. Anticipation of age at renal death in autosomal dominant polycystic kidney disease (ADPKD)? *Nephrol Dial Transplant.* 1995;10:1603-1606.

131. Gonzalo A, Gallego A, Rivera M, et al. Influence of hypertension on early renal insufficiency in autosomal dominant polycystic kidney disease. *Nephron.* 1996;72:225-230.

132. Gonzalo A, Gallego A, Tato A, et al. Age at renal replacement therapy in autosomal dominant polycystic kidney disease. *Nephron.* 1996;74:620.

133. Conte F, Serbelloni P, Milani S, et al. Clinical data of a cooperative Italian study of ADPKD. Italian ADPKd Cooperative Study Group. Autosomal Dominant Polycystic Kidney Disease. *Contrib Nephrol.* 1995;115:72-87.

134. Simon P. Prognosis of autosomal dominant polycystic kidney disease. *Nephron.* 1995;71:247-248.

135. Churchill DN, Bear JC, Morgan J, et al. Prognosis of adult onset polycystic kidney disease re-evaluated. *Kidney Int.* 1984;26:190-193.

136. Davies F, Coles GA, Harper PS, et al. Polycystic kidney disease re-evaluated: a population-based study. *Q J Med.* 1991;79:477-485.

137. Yium J, Gabow P, Johnson A, et al. Autosomal dominant polycystic kidney disease in blacks: clinical course and effects of sickle-cell hemoglobin. *J Am Soc Nephrol.* 1994;4:1670-1674.

138. Iglesias CG, Torres VE, Offord KP, et al. Epidemiology of adult polycystic kidney disease, Olmsted County, Minnesota: 1935-1980. *Am J Kidney Dis.* 1983;2:630-639.

139. Fick-Brosnahan GM, Belz MM, McFann KK, et al. Relationship between renal volume growth and renal function in autosomal dominant polycystic kidney disease: a longitudinal study. *Am J Kidney Dis.* 2002;39:1127-1134.

140. Ishikawa I, Maeda K, Nakai S, et al. Gender difference in the mean age at the induction of hemodialysis in patients with autosomal dominant polycystic kidney disease. *Am J Kidney Dis.* 2000;35:1072-1075.

141. Dicks E, Ravani P, Langman D, et al. Incident renal events and risk factors in autosomal dominant polycystic kidney disease: a population and family-based cohort followed for 22 years. *Clin J Am Soc Nephrol.* 2006;1:710-717.

142. Paterson AD, Magistroni R, He N, et al. Progressive loss of renal function is an age-dependent heritable trait in type 1 autosomal dominant polycystic kidney disease. *J Am Soc Nephrol.* 2005;16:755-762.

143. Harris PC, Bae KT, Rossetti S, et al. Cyst number but not the rate of cystic growth is associated with the mutated gene in autosomal dominant polycystic kidney disease. *J Am Soc Nephrol.* 2006;17:3013-3019.

144. Torres VE, King BF, Chapman AB, et al. Magnetic resonance measurements of renal blood flow and disease progression in autosomal dominant polycystic kidney disease. *Clin J Am Soc Nephrol.* 2007;2:112-120.

145. Rossetti S, Burton S, Strmecki L, et al. The position of the polycystic kidney disease 1 (PKD1) gene mutation correlates with the severity of renal disease. *J Am Soc Nephrol.* 2002;13:1230-1237.

146. Hateboer N, Dijk MA, Bogdanova N, et al. Comparison of phenotypes of polycystic kidney disease types 1 and 2. European PKD1-PKD2 Study Group. *Lancet.* 1999;353:103-107.

147. Magistroni R, He N, Wang K, et al. Genotype-renal function correlation in type 2 autosomal dominant polycystic kidney disease. *J Am Soc Nephrol.* 2003;14:1164-1174.

148. Maric C. Sex, diabetes and the kidney. *Am J Physiol Renal Physiol.* 2009;296:F680-F688.

149. Breyer JA, Bain RP, Evans JK, et al. Predictors of the progression of renal insufficiency in patients with insulin-dependent diabetes and overt diabetic nephropathy. The Collaborative Study Group. *Kidney Int.* 1996;50:1651-1658.

150. Holl RW, Grabert M, Thon A, et al. Urinary excretion of albumin in adolescents with type 1 diabetes: persistent versus intermittent microalbuminuria and relationship to duration of diabetes, sex, and metabolic control. *Diabetes Care.* 1999;22:1555-1560.

151. Hovind P, Tarnow L, Parving HH. Remission and regression of diabetic nephropathy. *Curr Hypertens Rep.* 2004;6:377-382.

152. Jacobsen P, Rossing K, Tarnow L, et al. Progression of diabetic nephropathy in normotensive type 1 diabetic patients. *Kidney Int.* 1999;71(Suppl):S101-S105.

153. Jones CA, Krolewski AS, Rogus J, et al. Epidemic of end-stage renal disease in people with diabetes in the United States population: do we know the cause? *Kidney Int.* 2005;67:1684-1691.

154. Laron-Kenet T, Shamis I, Weitzman S, et al. Mortality of patients with childhood onset (0-17 years) type I diabetes in Israel: a population-based study. *Diabetologia.* 2001;44(suppl 3):B81-B86.

155. Monti MC, Lonsdale JT, Montomoli C, et al. Familial risk factors for microvascular complications and differential male-female risk in a large cohort of American families with type 1 diabetes. *J Clin Endocrinol Metab.* 2007;92:4650-4655.

156. Orchard TJ, Dorman JS, Maser RE, et al. Prevalence of complications in IDDM by sex and duration. Pittsburgh Epidemiology of Diabetes Complications Study II. *Diabetes.* 1990;39:1116-1124.

157. Rossing P, Hougaard P, Parving HH. Risk factors for development of incipient and overt diabetic nephropathy in type 1 diabetic patients: a 10-year prospective observational study. *Diabetes Care.* 2002;25:859-864.

158. Ruggenenti P, Gambara V, Perna A, et al. The nephropathy of non-insulin-dependent diabetes: predictors of outcome relative to diverse patterns of renal injury. *J Am Soc Nephrol.* 1998;9:2336-2343.

159. Schultz CJ, Konopelska-Bahu T, Dalton RN, et al. Microalbuminuria prevalence varies with age, sex, and puberty in children with type 1 diabetes followed from diagnosis in a longitudinal study. Oxford Regional Prospective Study Group. *Diabetes Care.* 1999;22:495-502.

160. Sibley SD, Thomas W, de Boer I, et al. Gender and elevated albumin excretion in the Diabetes Control and Complications Trial/Epidemiology of Diabetes Interventions and Complications (DCCT/EDIC) cohort: role of central obesity. *Am J Kidney Dis.* 2006;47:223-232.

161. Hovind P, Tarnow L, Oestergaard PB, et al. Elevated vascular endothelial growth factor in type 1 diabetic patients with diabetic nephropathy. *Kidney Int.* 2000;75(Suppl):S56-S61.

162. Tolonen N, Forsblom C, Thorn L, et al. Lipid abnormalities predict progression of renal disease in patients with type 1 diabetes. *Diabetologia.* 2009;52:2522-2530.

163. Mangili R, Deferrari G, Di MU, et al. Arterial hypertension and microalbuminuria in IDDM: the Italian Microalbuminuria Study. *Diabetologia.* 1994;37:1015-1024.

164. Raile K, Galler A, Hofer S, et al. Diabetic nephropathy in 27,805 children, adolescents, and adults with type 1 diabetes: effect of diabetes duration, A1C, hypertension, dyslipidemia, diabetes onset, and sex. *Diabetes Care.* 2007;30:2523-2528.

165. Zhang L, Krzentowski G, Albert A, et al. Factors predictive of nephropathy in DCCT type 1 diabetic patients with good or poor metabolic control. *Diabet Med.* 2003;20:580-585.

166. Cotter J, Oliveira P, Cunha P, et al. Risk factors for development of microalbuminuria in diabetic and nondiabetic normoalbuminuric hypertensives with high or very high cardiovascular risk—a twelve-month follow-up study. *Nephron Clin Pract.* 2009;113:c8-15.

167. Gall MA, Hougaard P, Borch-Johnsen K, et al. Risk factors for development of incipient and overt diabetic nephropathy in patients with non–insulin dependent diabetes mellitus: prospective, observational study. *BMJ.* 1997;314:783-788.

168. Parving HH, Gall MA, Skott P, et al. Prevalence and causes of albuminuria in non–insulin-dependent diabetic patients. *Kidney Int.* 1992;41:758-762.

169. Ravid M, Brosh D, Ravid-Safran D, et al. Main risk factors for nephropathy in type 2 diabetes mellitus are plasma cholesterol levels, mean blood pressure, and hyperglycemia. *Arch Intern Med.* 1998;158:998-1004.

170. Savage S, Nagel NJ, Estacio RO, et al. Clinical factors associated with urinary albumin excretion in type II diabetes. *Am J Kidney Dis.* 1995;25:836-844.

171. Joshy G, Dunn P, Fisher M, et al. Ethnic differences in the natural progression of nephropathy among diabetes patients in New Zealand: hospital admission rate for renal complications, and incidence of end-stage renal disease and renal death. *Diabetologia*. 2009;52:1474-1478.
172. Xu J, Lee ET, Devereux RB, et al. A longitudinal study of risk factors for incident albuminuria in diabetic American Indians: the Strong Heart Study. *Am J Kidney Dis*. 2008;51:415-424.
173. Keane WF, Brenner BM, de Zeeuw D, et al. The risk of developing end-stage renal disease in patients with type 2 diabetes and nephropathy: the RENAAL study. *Kidney Int*. 2003;63:1499-1507.
174. Crook ED, Patel SR. Diabetic nephropathy in African-American patients. *Curr Diab Rep*. 2004;4:455-461.
175. Looker HC, Krakoff J, Funahashi T, et al. Adiponectin concentrations are influenced by renal function and diabetes duration in Pima Indians with type 2 diabetes. *J Clin Endocrinol Metab*. 2004;89:4010-4017.
176. Young BA, Maynard C, Boyko EJ. Racial differences in diabetic nephropathy, cardiovascular disease, and mortality in a national population of veterans. *Diabetes Care*. 2003;26:2392-2399.
177. Ahmed SB, Hovind P, Parving HH, et al. Oral contraceptives, angiotensin-dependent renal vasoconstriction, and risk of diabetic nephropathy. *Diabetes Care*. 2005;28:1988-1994.
178. Monster TB, Janssen WM, De Jong PE, et al. Oral contraceptive use and hormone replacement therapy are associated with microalbuminuria. *Arch Intern Med*. 2001;161:2000-2005.
179. Garg SK, Chase HP, Marshall G, et al. Oral contraceptives and renal and retinal complications in young women with insulin-dependent diabetes mellitus. *JAMA*. 1994;271:1099-1102.
180. Atthobari J, Gansevoort RT, Visser ST, et al. The impact of hormonal contraceptives on blood pressure, urinary albumin excretion and glomerular filtration rate. *Br J Clin Pharmacol*. 2007;63:224-231.
181. Szekacs B, Vajo Z, Varbiro S, et al. Postmenopausal hormone replacement improves proteinuria and impaired creatinine clearance in type 2 diabetes mellitus and hypertension. *BJOG*. 2000;107:1017-1021.
182. Agarwal M, Selvan V, Freedman BI, et al. The relationship between albuminuria and hormone therapy in postmenopausal women. *Am J Kidney Dis*. 2005;45:1019-1025.
183. Ahmed SB, Culleton BF, Tonelli M, et al. Oral estrogen therapy in postmenopausal women is associated with loss of kidney function. *Kidney Int*. 2008;74:370-376.
184. Mays VM, Ponce NA, Washington DL, et al. Classification of race and ethnicity: implications for public health. *Annu Rev Public Health*. 2003;24:83-110.
185. US Census Bureau, Population Division: *Racial and ethnic classifications used in Census 2000 and beyond*. Suitland, MD: US Census Bureau, Population Division; 2009.
186. Winker MA. Measuring race and ethnicity: why and how? *JAMA*. 2004;292:1612-1614.
187. Institute of Medicine. *The unequal burden of cancer: an assessment of NIH research and programs for ethnic minorities and the medically underserved*. Washington, DC: National Academy Press; 1999.
188. Freeman HP. The meaning of race in science—considerations for cancer research: concerns of special populations in the National Cancer Program. *Cancer*. 1998;82:219-225.
189. Gilbert W. A vision of the grail. In: Kevles DJ, Hood L, eds. *The code of codes: scientific and social issues in the Human Genome Project*. Cambridge, Mass: Harvard University Press; 1992:83.
190. National Kidney Foundation. KDOQI clinical practice guidelines for chronic kidney disease: evaluation, classification, and stratification. *Am J Kidney Dis*. 2002;39:S1-S266.
191. Saran R, Hedgeman E, Plantinga L, et al. Establishing a National Chronic Kidney Disease Surveillance System for the United States. *Clin J Am Soc Nephrol*. 2010;5:152-161.
192. Hsu CC, Kao WH, Coresh J, et al. Apolipoprotein E and progression of chronic kidney disease. *JAMA*. 2005;293:2892-2899.
193. Foster MC, Hwang SJ, Larson MG, et al. Overweight, obesity, and the development of stage 3 CKD: the Framingham Heart Study. *Am J Kidney Dis*. 2008;52:39-48.
194. Young JH, Klag MJ, Muntner P, et al. Blood pressure and decline in kidney function: findings from the Systolic Hypertension in the Elderly Program (SHEP). *J Am Soc Nephrol*. 2002;13:2776-2782.
195. Shoham DA, Vupputuri S, ez Roux AV, et al. Kidney disease in life-course socioeconomic context: the Atherosclerosis Risk in Communities (ARIC) study. *Am J Kidney Dis*. 2007;49:217-226.
196. Merkin SS, Coresh J, Roux AV, et al. Area socioeconomic status and progressive CKD: the Atherosclerosis Risk in Communities (ARIC) study. *Am J Kidney Dis*. 2005;46:203-213.
197. Hsu CC, Bray MS, Kao WH, et al. Genetic variation of the renin-angiotensin system and chronic kidney disease progression in black individuals in the atherosclerosis risk in communities study. *J Am Soc Nephrol*. 2006;17:504-512.
198. Krop JS, Coresh J, Chambless LE, et al. A community-based study of explanatory factors for the excess risk for early renal function decline in blacks vs whites with diabetes: the Atherosclerosis Risk in Communities study. *Arch Intern Med*. 1999;159:1777-1783.
199. Bash LD, Coresh J, Kottgen A, et al. Defining incident chronic kidney disease in the research setting: the ARIC study. *Am J Epidemiol*. 2009;170:414-424.
200. US Renal Data System. *USRDS 2009 annual data report: atlas of chronic kidney disease in the United States*. Bethesda, Md: National Institutes of Health, National Institute of Diabetes and Digestive and Kidney Diseases; 2009.
201. McClellan W, Warnock DG, McClure L, et al. Racial differences in the prevalence of chronic kidney disease among participants in the Reasons for Geographic and Racial Differences in Stroke (REGARDS) cohort study. *J Am Soc Nephrol*. 2006;17:1710-1715.
202. Coresh J, Selvin E, Stevens LA, et al. Prevalence of chronic kidney disease in the United States. *JAMA*. 2007;298:2038-2047.
203. Bryson CL, Ross HJ, Boyko EJ, et al. Racial and ethnic variations in albuminuria in the US Third National Health and Nutrition Examination Survey (NHANES III) population: associations with diabetes and level of CKD. *Am J Kidney Dis*. 2006;48:720-726.
204. Hoy W, Jim S, Warrington W, et al. Urinary findings and renal function in adult Navajo Indians and associations with type 2 diabetes. *Am J Kidney Dis*. 1996;28:339-349.
205. Rodriguez RA, Hernandez GT, O'Hare AM, et al. Creatinine levels among Mexican Americans, Puerto Ricans, and Cuban Americans in the Hispanic Health and Nutrition Examination Survey. *Kidney Int*. 2004;66:2368-2373.
206. Pugh JA, Stern MP, Haffner SM, et al. Excess incidence of treatment of end-stage renal disease in Mexican Americans. *Am J Epidemiol*. 1988;127:135-144.
207. Chiapella AP, Feldman HI. Renal failure among male Hispanics in the United States. *Am J Public Health*. 1995;85:1001-1004.
208. Peralta CA, Shlipak MG, Fan D, et al. Risks for end-stage renal disease, cardiovascular events, and death in Hispanic versus non-Hispanic white adults with chronic kidney disease. *J Am Soc Nephrol*. 2006;17:2892-2899.
209. Tarver-Carr ME, Powe NR, Eberhardt MS, et al. Excess risk of chronic kidney disease among African-American versus white subjects in the United States: a population-based study of potential explanatory factors. *J Am Soc Nephrol*. 2002;13:2363-2370.
210. Hunsicker LG, Adler S, Caggiula A, et al. Predictors of the progression of renal disease in the Modification of Diet in Renal Disease Study. *Kidney Int*. 1997;51:1908-1919.
211. Xue JL, Eggers PW, Agodoa LY, et al. Longitudinal study of racial and ethnic differences in developing end-stage renal disease among aged medicare beneficiaries. *J Am Soc Nephrol*. 2007;18:1299-1306.
212. Duru OK, Li S, Jurkovitz C, et al. Race and sex differences in hypertension control in CKD: results from the Kidney Early Evaluation Program (KEEP). *Am J Kidney Dis*. 2008;51:192-198.
213. McWilliams JM, Meara E, Zaslavsky AM, et al. Differences in control of cardiovascular disease and diabetes by race, ethnicity, and education: U.S. trends from 1999 to 2006 and effects of medicare coverage. *Ann Intern Med*. 2009;150:505-515.
214. Kalaitzidis R, Li S, Wang C, et al. Hypertension in early-stage kidney disease: an update from the Kidney Early Evaluation Program (KEEP). *Am J Kidney Dis*. 2009;53:S22-S31.
215. Hajjar I, Kotchen TA. Trends in prevalence, awareness, treatment, and control of hypertension in the United States, 1988-2000. *JAMA*. 2003;290:199-206.
216. Chobanian AV, Bakris GL, Black HR, et al. Seventh Report of the Joint National Committee on Prevention, Detection, Evaluation, and Treatment of High Blood Pressure. *Hypertension*. 2003;42:1206-1252.
217. Cutler JA, Sorlie PD, Wolz M, et al. Trends in hypertension prevalence, awareness, treatment, and control rates in United States adults between 1988-1994 and 1999-2004. *Hypertension*. 2008;52:818-827.
218. Ong KL, Cheung BM, Wong LY, et al. Prevalence, treatment, and control of diagnosed diabetes in the U.S. National Health and Nutrition Examination Survey 1999-2004. *Ann Epidemiol*. 2008;18:222-229.
219. Flegal KM, Carroll MD, Ogden CL, et al. Prevalence and trends in obesity among US adults, 1999-2000. *JAMA*. 2002;288:1723-1727.
220. Ogden CL, Carroll MD, Curtin LR, et al. Prevalence of overweight and obesity in the United States, 1999-2004. *JAMA*. 2006;295:1549-1555.
221. Iglesias-De La Cruz MC, Ruiz-Torres P, Alcami J, et al. Hydrogen peroxide increases extracellular matrix mRNA through TGF-beta in human mesangial cells. *Kidney Int*. 2001;59:87-95.
222. Suthanthiran M, Gerber LM, Schwartz JE, et al. Circulating transforming growth factor-beta1 levels and the risk for kidney disease in African Americans. *Kidney Int*. 2009;76:72-80.
223. Levy SB, Talner LB, Coel MN, et al. Renal vasculature in essential hypertension: racial differences. *Ann Intern Med*. 1978;88:12-16.

224. Lilley JJ, Hsu L, Stone RA. Racial disparity of plasma volume in hypertensive man. *Ann Intern Med.* 1976;84:707-708:(letter).
225. Aviv A, Gardner J. Racial differences in ion regulation and their possible links to hypertension in blacks. *Hypertension.* 1989;14:584-589.
226. Hung AM, Crawford DC, Griffin MR, et al. CRP polymorphisms and progression of chronic kidney disease in African Americans. *Clin J Am Soc Nephrol.* 2010;5:24-33.
227. Romero LJ, Lindeman RD, Liang HC, et al. Prevalence of self-reported illnesses in elderly Hispanic and non-Hispanic whites in New Mexico. *Ethn Dis.* 2001;11:263-272.
228. Raymond CA. Diabetes in Mexican-Americans: pressing problem in a growing population. *JAMA.* 1988;259:1772.
229. Baxter J, Hamman RF, Lopez TK, et al. Excess incidence of known non–insulin-dependent diabetes mellitus (NIDDM) in Hispanics compared with non-Hispanic whites in the San Luis Valley, Colorado. *Ethn Dis.* 1993;3:11-21.
230. Marshall JA, Hamman RF, Baxter J, et al. Ethnic differences in risk factors associated with the prevalence of non–insulin-dependent diabetes mellitus. The San Luis Valley Diabetes Study. *Am J Epidemiol.* 1993;137:706-718.
231. Samet JM, Coultas DB, Howard CA, et al. Diabetes, gallbladder disease, obesity, and hypertension among Hispanics in New Mexico. *Am J Epidemiol.* 1988;128:1302-1311.
232. Nichaman MZ, Garcia G. Obesity in Hispanic Americans. *Diabetes Care.* 1991;14:691-694.
233. Perneger TV, Whelton PK, Klag MJ. Race and end-stage renal disease. Socioeconomic status and access to health care as mediating factors. *Arch Intern Med.* 1995;155:1201-1208.
234. Ward MM. Access to care and the incidence of end-stage renal disease due to diabetes. *Diabetes Care.* 2009;32:1032-1036.
235. Ward MM. Laboratory abnormalities at the onset of treatment of end-stage renal disease: are there racial or socioeconomic disparities in care? *Arch Intern Med.* 2007;167:1083-1091.
236. Kao WH, Klag MJ, Meoni LA, et al. MYH9 is associated with nondiabetic end-stage renal disease in African Americans. *Nat Genet.* 2008;40:1185-1192.
237. Kopp JB, Smith MW, Nelson GW, et al. MYH9 is a major-effect risk gene for focal segmental glomerulosclerosis. *Nat Genet.* 2008;40:1175-1184.
238. Genovese G, Tonna SJ, knob AU, et al. A risk allele for focal segmental glomerulosclerosis in African Americans is located within a region containing ApoL1 and MYH9. *kidney Int.* 2010;78:698-704.
238a. Genovese G, Friedman DJ, Ross MD, et al. Association of trypanolytic ApoL1 variants with kidney disease in African Americans. *Science.* 2010;329:841-845.
238b. Freedman BI, Kopp JB, Langefeld CD, et al. The apolipoprotein L1 (ApoL1) gene and nondiabetic in African Americans. *J Am Soc Nephrol.* 2010;21:1422-1426.
238c. Tzur S, Rosset S, Shemer R, et al. Missense mutations in the APOL1 gene are highly associated with end stage kidney disease risk previously attributed to the MYH9 gene. *Hum Genet.* 2010;128:345-350.
239. Chu AY, Parekh RS, Astor BC, et al. Association of APOE polymorphism with chronic kidney disease in a nationally representative sample: a Third National Health and Nutrition Examination Survey (NHANES III) genetic study. *BMC Med Genet.* 2009;10:108.
240. Ichikawa K, Konta T, Emi M, et al. Genetic polymorphisms of paraoxonase-1 are associated with chronic kidney disease in Japanese women. *Kidney Int.* 2009;76:183-189.
241. Yoshida T, Kato K, Yokoi K, et al. Association of candidate gene polymorphisms with chronic kidney disease in Japanese individuals with hypertension. *Hypertens Res.* 2009;32:411-418.
242. Merkin SS, Roux AV, Coresh J, et al. Individual and neighborhood socioeconomic status and progressive chronic kidney disease in an elderly population: the Cardiovascular Health Study. *Soc Sci Med.* 2007;65:809-821.
243. Shoham DA, Vupputuri S, Kshirsagar AV. Chronic kidney disease and life course socioeconomic status: a review. *Adv Chronic Kidney Dis.* 2005;12:56-63.
244. Johnson EO, Novak SP. Onset and persistence of daily smoking: the interplay of socioeconomic status, gender, and psychiatric disorders. *Drug Alcohol Depend.* 2009;104(suppl 1):S50-S57.
245. Clarke PJ, O'Malley PM, Johnston LD, et al. Differential trends in weight-related health behaviors among American young adults by gender, race/ethnicity, and socioeconomic status: 1984-2006. *Am J Public Health.* 2009;99:1893-1901.
246. Alarcon GS, Bastian HM, Beasley TM, et al. Systemic lupus erythematosus in a multi-ethnic cohort (LUMINA) XXXII: [corrected] contributions of admixture and socioeconomic status to renal involvement. *Lupus.* 2006;15:26-31.
247. Fored CM, Ejerblad E, Fryzek JP, et al. Socio-economic status and chronic renal failure: a population-based case-control study in Sweden. *Nephrol Dial Transplant.* 2003;18:82-88.
248. Drey N, Roderick P, Mullee M, et al. A population-based study of the incidence and outcomes of diagnosed chronic kidney disease. *Am J Kidney Dis.* 2003;42:677-684.
249. Shoham DA, Vupputuri S, Kaufman JS, et al. Kidney disease and the cumulative burden of life course socioeconomic conditions: the Atherosclerosis Risk in Communities (ARIC) study. *Soc Sci Med.* 2008;67:1311-1320.
250. Martins D, Tareen N, Zadshir A, et al. The association of poverty with the prevalence of albuminuria: data from the Third National Health and Nutrition Examination Survey (NHANES III). *Am J Kidney Dis.* 2006;47:965-971.
251. White SL, McGeechan K, Jones M, et al. Socioeconomic disadvantage and kidney disease in the United States, Australia, and Thailand. *Am J Public Health.* 2008;98:1306-1313.
252. Barker DJ, Bull AR, Osmond C, et al. Fetal and placental size and risk of hypertension in adult life. *BMJ.* 1990;301:259-262.
253. Brenner BM, Chertow GM. Congenital oligonephropathy and the etiology of adult hypertension and progressive renal injury. *Am J Kidney Dis.* 1994;23:171-175.
254. White SL, Perkovic V, Cass A, et al. Is low birth weight an antecedent of CKD in later life? A systematic review of observational studies. *Am J Kidney Dis.* 2009;54:248-261.
255. Navas-Acien A, Tellez-Plaza M, Guallar E, et al. Blood cadmium and lead and chronic kidney disease in U.S. adults: a joint analysis. *Am J Epidemiol.* 2009;170:1156-1164.
256. Wedeen RP, Maesaka JK, Weiner B, et al. Occupational lead nephropathy. *Am J Med.* 1975;59:630-641.
257. Muntner P, Menke A, DeSalvo KB, et al. Continued decline in blood lead levels among adults in the United States: the National Health and Nutrition Examination Surveys. *Arch Intern Med.* 2005;165:2155-2161.
258. Muntner P, He J, Vupputuri S, et al. Blood lead and chronic kidney disease in the general United States population: results from NHANES III. *Kidney Int.* 2003;63:1044-1050.
259. Akesson A, Lundh T, Vahter M, et al. Tubular and glomerular kidney effects in Swedish women with low environmental cadmium exposure. *Environ Health Perspect.* 2005;113:1627-1631.
260. Hotz P, Buchet JP, Bernard A, et al. Renal effects of low-level environmental cadmium exposure: 5-year follow-up of a subcohort from the Cadmibel study. *Lancet.* 1999;354:1508-1513.
261. Hellstrom L, Elinder CG, Dahlberg B, et al. Cadmium exposure and end-stage renal disease. *Am J Kidney Dis.* 2001;38:1001-1008.
262. Tsaih SW, Korrick S, Schwartz J, et al. Lead, diabetes, hypertension, and renal function: the normative aging study. *Environ Health Perspect.* 2004;112:1178-1182.
263. Roels HA, Lauwerys RR, Buchet JP, et al. Health significance of cadmium induced renal dysfunction: a five year follow-up. *Br J Ind Med.* 1989;46:755-764.
264. Pinney SM, Freyberg RW, Levine GE, et al. Health effects in community residents near a uranium plant at Fernald, Ohio, USA. *Int J Occup Med Environ Health.* 2003;16:139-153.
265. Zamora ML, Zielinski JM, Moodie GB, et al. Uranium in drinking water: renal effects of long-term ingestion by an aboriginal community. *Arch Environ Occup Health.* 2009;64:228-241.
266. Institute of Medicine. *Gulf War and health: updated literature review of depleted uranium.* Washington, DC: National Academies Press; 2008.
267. Cleper R, Davidovitz M, Halevi R, et al. Renal functional reserve after acute poststreptococcal glomerulonephritis. *Pediatr Nephrol.* 1997;11:473-476.
268. Pinto SW, Sesso R, Vasconcelos E, et al. Follow-up of patients with epidemic poststreptococcal glomerulonephritis. *Am J Kidney Dis.* 2001;38:249-255.
269. White AV, Hoy WE, McCredie DA. Childhood post-streptococcal glomerulonephritis as a risk factor for chronic renal disease in later life. *Med J Aust.* 2001;174:492-496.
270. Hsu CY, Iribarren C, McCulloch CE, et al. Risk factors for end-stage renal disease: 25-year follow-up. *Arch Intern Med.* 2009;169:342-350.
271. Volkova N, McClellan W, Klein M, et al. Neighborhood poverty and racial differences in ESRD incidence. *J Am Soc Nephrol.* 2008;19:356-364.

Risk Factors and Chronic Kidney Disease

Maarten W. Taal

The Need to Define Risk in Chronic Kidney Disease

In 2002, a simple definition for chronic kidney disease (CKD) was proposed[1] and subsequently adopted worldwide. In addition, the four-variable formula from the Modification of Diet in Renal Disease (MDRD) study facilitated automated estimation of glomerular filtration rate (GFR) from a measurement of serum creatinine concentration. As a result, awareness of CKD has increased. Population-based studies from around the world have revealed a prevalence of up to 16.8%,[2] substantially higher than anticipated. The large number of people now known to be affected by CKD has major implications for the provision of health care and, in particular, nephrology services. Nephrologists traditionally provided highly specialized services to a relatively small number of patients with specific and relatively rare kidney diseases or advanced CKD; today, they must consider how best to provide care for less advanced CKD in a substantial proportion of the general population.

Furthermore, early-stage CKD is largely asymptomatic, and detection therefore requires a process of screening. Studies indicate that screening whole populations is not cost effective,[3] and subgroups at high risk who would benefit from targeted screening therefore must be identified. Successful screening programs are likely to identify large numbers of patients with previously undiagnosed CKD, but in most countries, nephrology services are unable to provide long-term care to all patients with CKD and the associated costs would be prohibitive.

A solution to this problem is suggested by evidence of substantial heterogeneity among patients who meet the diagnostic criteria for CKD: the majority are at relatively low risk of ever progressing to end-stage kidney disease (ESKD). The Kidney Disease Outcomes Quality Initiative (K/DOQI) classification system for CKD is now widely accepted and has proved valuable, particularly in identifying the prevalence of different stages of CKD in epidemiologic studies.[4] However, this classification provides little information about the risk of future decline in renal function.[5] Investigators have identified a wide range of rates of decline in GFR among patients with CKD, and up to 15% may even show an increase in GFR over time.[6] There is thus a need to develop methods for risk stratification within CKD to identify the relatively small subgroup of patients who are at risk for progression to ESKD and who may benefit from specialist intervention to slow or halt CKD progression. Such risk stratification would be equally important for identifying individuals who are at low risk for progression and could thus be reassured and spared unnecessary referral to a nephrologist.

An important additional aspect of CKD is its association with a substantially increased risk of future cardiovascular events, which in most patients with mild CKD substantially exceeds the risk of ESKD.[7] Whereas CKD is associated with a high prevalence of many traditional risk factors for cardiovascular disease such as hypertension and dyslipidemia, risk prediction tools such as the Framingham risk score substantially underestimate cardiovascular risk in patients with CKD.[8] This underestimation is a result of the role of several nontraditional cardiovascular risk factors that are specific to CKD.

From this discussion, it is clear that there is a need to identify and understand factors that are associated with an increased risk of developing CKD and, once it is diagnosed, factors that are associated with increased risks of progression to ESKD and of cardiovascular events. This chapter reviews current knowledge of these risk factors, as well as the methods being applied to achieve risk prediction among patients with CKD. Risk factors for cardiovascular disease in patients with CKD, many of which overlap with risk factors for CKD progression, are discussed in Chapter 55.

Definition of a Risk Factor

A *risk factor* is a variable that has a causal association with a disease or disease process; the presence of the variable in an individual or a population is associated with an increased risk of the presence or future development of the disease. Thus, risk factors may be useful for identifying subjects at increased risk for a disease or for a particular outcome that results from a disease process. In the course of epidemiologic research, many variables may appear to be associated with a disease of interest, but these may be chance associations, noncausal associations, or causal associations (true risk factors). The Bradford Hill criteria are the minimum requirements for identifying a causal relationship between a putative risk factor (exposure) and a disease (outcome) (Table 21-1). In complex diseases (such as CKD) that result from the combined effects of multiple factors, many risk factors probably do not fulfill all the criteria. Nevertheless, the criteria do provide a useful framework for assessing the strength of a proposed causal relationship between risk factor and disease.

Epidemiologic Methods for Identifying Risk Factors

Studies to investigate associations between putative risk factors and a disease may be classified as observational or experimental. Observational studies include cross-sectional, case-control, and cohort studies, whereas the randomized controlled trial (RCT) is the main experimental study.

Cross-Sectional Studies

In this study type, associations between putative risk factors and a disease are investigated in a study population at a single time point. Cross-sectional studies therefore have the advantage of being relatively quick and simple to perform, but because they are limited to a single point in time, they are unable to fulfill the Bradford and Hill criterion for temporality. Thus, associations may be identified, but inference regarding causality cannot be made. Nevertheless, these studies are useful as an initial search for putative risk factors and hypothesis generation.

Case-Control Studies

As in cross-sectional studies, subjects are examined at a single point in time; in a case-control design, however, subjects with a particular disease ("cases") are identified according to specific criteria and are compared with control subjects who are similar to the case subjects with regard to age, gender, and other variables but do not have the disease. Data from cases and controls are then compared with regard to the prevalence of a particular exposure or putative risk factor. One weakness of case-control studies is that they often rely on recollection of past exposure to the putative risk factor. An additional challenge is to match cases and controls adequately with regard to variables other than the putative risk factor or factors.

Cohort Studies

Cohort studies are prospective studies in which a population of subjects with and without exposure (or variable exposure) to a putative risk factor are monitored for a certain length of time, and the rates of disease occurrence in the two groups are compared. Advantages are that the temporality criterion for causality may be fulfilled and the incidence of disease measured directly. One weakness of cohort studies is the potential

TABLE 21-1 Bradford Hill Criteria of Causality	
CRITERIA	**EXPLANATION**
Strength of association	The stronger the association is, the more likely the relationship is to be causal.
Consistency	A causal association is consistent when replicated in different populations and studies.
Specificity	A single putative cause produces a single effect.
Temporality	Exposure precedes outcome (i.e., risk factor predates disease).
Biologic gradient	Increasing exposure to risk factor increases risk of disease, and reduction in exposure reduces risk.
Plausibility	The observed association is consistent with biologic mechanisms of disease processes.
Coherence	The observed association is compatible with existing theory and knowledge within a given field.
Experimental evidence	The factor under investigation is amenable to modification by an appropriate experimental approach.
Analogy	An established cause-and-effect relationship exists for a similar exposure or disease.

Modified from Hill AB: The environment and disease: association or causation? *Proc R Soc Med* 58:295300, 1965.

for confounding. This may occur when a variable is associated with both the putative risk factor (exposure) and the disease (outcome). Thus, the presence of a confounder may alter (strengthen, weaken, or mask) the association between exposure and outcome. Multivariable regression analysis may be used to adjust or control for potential confounding, but it may not completely eliminate the effects of confounding, and incomplete adjustment may result in residual confounding.

Randomized Controlled Trials

In this study design, subjects in a population are randomly assigned to one of two or more conditions involving treatments or interventions. After a fixed period of follow-up, the randomized groups are compared with regard to the rate of a predefined outcome. To reduce the potential for bias, subjects or investigators, or both, are not made aware of the treatment condition. In a single-blind study, only subjects are unaware of what treatment they receive, whereas in a double-blind study, both subjects and investigators are unaware, usually through the use of a matching placebo. Randomization, if successful, produces close matching of the groups with regard to a wide range of known and unknown variables at the time of baseline measurements, which reduces the possibility of confounding. Furthermore, the RCT is the only study design capable of fulfilling the causality criterion for experimental evidence. Nevertheless, although the RCT constitutes the "gold standard" for investigating the effect of a therapeutic intervention, it is not as definitive for evaluating putative risk factors. This is because a particular intervention may modify more than one risk factor; therefore, a change in the outcome cannot be attributed to the change in a single risk factor. Perhaps the best example of this limitation in CKD is treatment with an angiotension converting enzyme (ACE) inhibitor that

modifies both blood pressure and proteinuria. It is not possible to attribute the subsequent slowing of GFR decline to either lowering of blood pressure or reduction of proteinuria alone.

Data from RCTs may also be used to perform subgroup or post hoc analyses. Subgroup analyses may be prespecified in the trial design (preferable) or be performed post hoc. Although subgroup and post hoc analyses may be useful for exploratory analyses and hypothesis generation, they are prone to several weaknesses. First, they may be underpowered and therefore prone to type 2 errors (incorrect failure to reject the null hypothesis); second, if too many hypotheses are tested, they may be prone to type 1 errors (incorrect rejection of a true null hypothesis).

Risk Factors and Mechanisms of Progression of Chronic Kidney Disease

It has long been appreciated that once GFR has decreased to below a critical level, CKD tends to progress relentlessly toward ESKD. This observation suggests that loss of a critical number of nephrons provokes a vicious cycle of further nephron loss. Detailed studies have elucidated a number of interrelated mechanisms that together contribute to CKD progression, including glomerular hemodynamic responses to nephron loss (raised glomerular capillary hydraulic pressure and single-nephron GFR), proteinuria, and proinflammatory responses. A generally good prognosis after unilateral nephrectomy[9] attests to the fact that a single pathogenic factor may be insufficient to initiate progressive CKD, but multiple factors may interact to overcome renal reserve and provoke progressive nephron loss.[10] In order to meet the Bradford Hill criteria of plausibility and coherence, a putative risk factor should therefore in some way affect known mechanisms of CKD progression (see Chapter 51 for further details). Figure 21-1

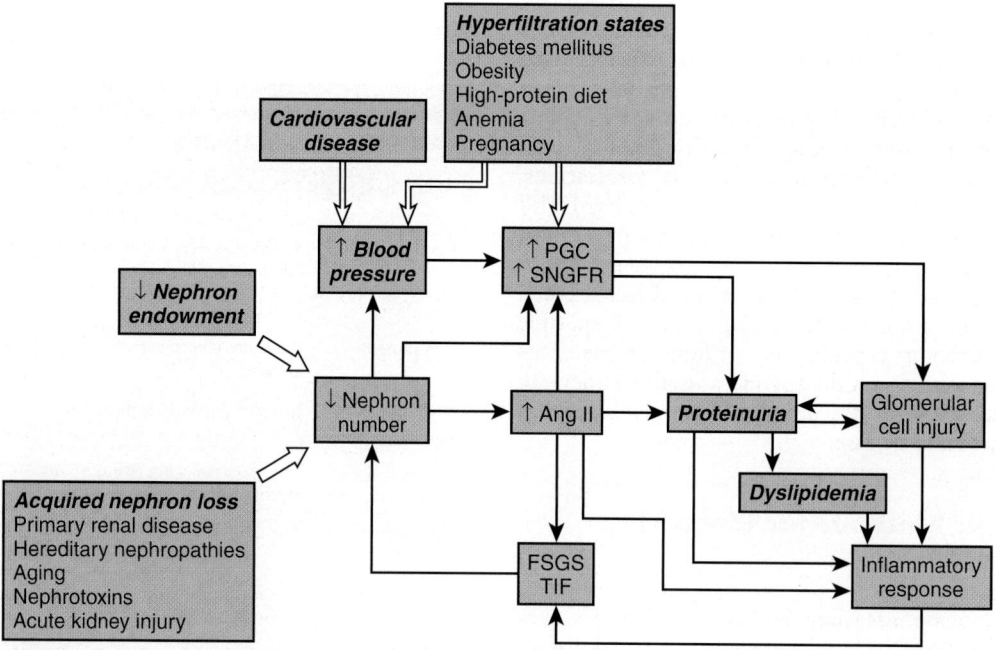

FIGURE 21-1 Schema showing the interaction of risk factors for progression of chronic kidney disease (CKD) with pathophysiologic mechanisms that contribute to a vicious cycle of progressive nephron loss. Ang II, angiotensin II; FSGS, focal and segmental glomerulosclerosis; PGC, glomerular capillary hydraulic pressure; SNGFR, single-nephron glomerular filtration rate; TIF, tubulointerstitial fibrosis. (Adapted from Taal MW, Brenner BM: Predicting initiation and progression of chronic kidney disease: developing renal risk scores, *Kidney Int* 70:1694-1705, 2006.)

shows how risk factors may interact with pathophysiologic mechanisms to initiate or accelerate CKD progression.

On the basis of the current understanding of the mechanisms underlying the pathogenesis of CKD and its progression, risk factors may be categorized as *susceptibility factors, initiation factors,* and *progression factors* (Table 21-2). However, distinguishing between these categories may be difficult in some cases because some factors—for example, diabetes mellitus—may act in all three ways, and in some studies it may be impossible to distinguish susceptibility factors from progression factors because participants were inadequate characterized at study entry.

Susceptibility Factors

Susceptibility risk factors are associated with an individual's increased risk for developing CKD after exposure to a factor that has potential to cause renal damage. An example is reduced nephron number after uninephrectomy, which is associated with an increased risk for developing diabetic nephropathy if the individual develops diabetes.[11] In studies of susceptibility factors, investigators should recruit subjects who are free of CKD at the time of baseline measurements, are exposed to an initiating factor, and are monitored over a prolonged period of time to allow ascertainment of outcomes. This could be achieved through a cohort study or subgroup analysis of an RCT.

Initiation Factors

Initiation factors directly cause or initiate kidney damage in a susceptible individual. Examples include exposure to nephrotoxic drugs, urinary tract obstruction, or primary glomerulopathies that may provoke CKD in some but not necessarily all exposed individuals. In studies of initiation factors, investigators should recruit subjects without CKD at entry or without known susceptibility factors, with variable exposure to a putative initiating factor. A cohort study design is best suited to investigating outcomes in subjects exposed and those not exposed to the factor of interest; an RCT design could be used to assess the potential nephrotoxicity of a new drug.

Progression Factors

Progression factors contribute to the progression of kidney damage once CKD has developed. An example is hypertension, which exacerbates raised intraglomerular hydraulic pressure and therefore accelerates glomerular damage. In studies of progression factors, investigators should recruit subjects with relatively early-stage CKD in a cohort study design. RCTs may also be used to study progression factors if the intervention being investigated modifies a putative progression factor. Outcomes may therefore be compared between the control subjects and the subjects in whom the risk factor was modified. Unfortunately, however, many interventions alter several risk factors, and it may therefore not be possible to attribute an improved outcome to changes in a single risk factor.

Demographic Variables

Age

The prevalence of CKD increases with age and is reported to be as high as 56% in people aged 75 years or older.[12] Longitudinal studies of subjects without kidney disease have demonstrated a decline in GFR with increasing age in some but not all subjects, which implies that nephron loss may be regarded as part of normal aging.[13] On the other hand, aging is associated with an increase in several other risk factors for CKD—including hypertension, obesity, and cardiovascular disease—that may contribute to the rise in prevalence of CKD. Several population-based studies have revealed a higher incidence of proteinuria and CKD,[14,15] as

TABLE 21-2 Risk Factors for Chronic Kidney Disease

RISK FACTOR	SUSCEPTIBILITY	INITIATION	PROGRESSION
Older age	+		
Gender	+		
Ethnicity	+		+
Family history of chronic kidney disease	+		
Metabolic syndrome	+		
Hemodynamic factors:			
Low nephron number	+		+
Diabetes mellitus	+	+	+
Hypertension	+		+
Obesity	+		+
High protein intake	+		+
Pregnancy		+	+
Primary renal disease		+	
Genetic renal disease		+	
Urologic disorders		+	
Acute kidney injury		+	+
Cardiovascular disease	+		+
Albuminuria			+
Hypoalbuminemia			+
Anemia	+		+
Dyslipidemia	+		+
Hyperuricemia	+		+
↑ ADMA level			+
Hyperphosphatemia			+
Smoking	+		+
Nephrotoxins		+	+

ADMA, Asymmetric dimethyl arginine.

well ESKD, with increasing age.[16] Similarly, the incidence of a decline in renal function over 5 years was higher among older patients with hypertension than among younger patients.[17]

Paradoxically, advanced age appears to be a negative predictor of ESKD among patients with CKD. The risk of progression to ESKD was decreased among older patients with stage 3 CKD (hazard ratio [HR] = 0.75; 95% confidence interval [CI] = 0.63 to 0.89 for each 10-year increase in age).[18] Nevertheless, older age was associated with a greater rate of decline in GFR.[18] This apparent contradiction is probably explained by the competing risks of death and ESKD in older patients, which is illustrated by the observation from one longitudinal study that for patients aged 65 years or older, the risk of ESKD exceeded the risk of death only when GFR was 15 mL/minute/1.73 m^2 or lower (Figure 21-2).[19]

On the other hand, another study revealed that among patients with stage 4 and 5 CKD, an age of 65 years or older was associated with slower decline in renal function than was an age younger than 45 years.[20] Thus, older age appears to act as a susceptibility factor for CKD but not necessarily a progression factor. Data from one community-based study of subjects 75 years of age or older indicate that CKD is associated with significant comorbidity in elderly patients; comorbid conditions include increased numbers of cardiovascular events, reduced physical and cognitive function, and a higher prevalence of potentially reversible factors such as anemia. Long-term follow-up of these subjects confirmed that, as in younger subjects, reduced GFR (particularly GFR < 45 mL/minute/1.73 m^2) was an independent risk factor for all-cause and cardiovascular mortality,[12] as well as for the need for hospitalization[21] in older people. These observations suggest that targeted screening for CKD in older subjects would be a cost-effective strategy; however, more studies are needed to investigate the extent to which the risks associated with CKD in elderly patients may be attenuated by intervention. For further discussion of CKD in elderly patients, see Chapters 20 and 23.

Gender

In experimental studies, male rodents were found to be more susceptible to age-related glomerulosclerosis than were females; this observation was independent of glomerular hemodynamics or hypertrophy and was attributable to a specific androgen effect.[22] Data regarding the effect of gender on the risk of CKD and progression in humans are, however, somewhat contradictory. Many reports indicate that male gender is associated with worse renal outcomes. Researchers have reported a higher incidence of proteinuria and CKD among men in the general population,[14] an increased risk of ESKD or death associated with CKD in men,[14,16,23] a higher risk of decline in renal function among male hypertensive patients,[17] a lower risk of ESKD among female patients with stage 3 CKD,[18] and a shorter time to the need for renal replacement therapy among male patients with stages 4 and 5 CKD.[20] Data from the United States Renal Data System show a substantially higher incidence of ESKD among men (413 per million population [pmp] in 2003) versus females (280 pmp).[24] Furthermore, a meta-analysis of 68 studies that included 11,345 patients with CKD revealed a higher rate of decline in renal function in men.[25]

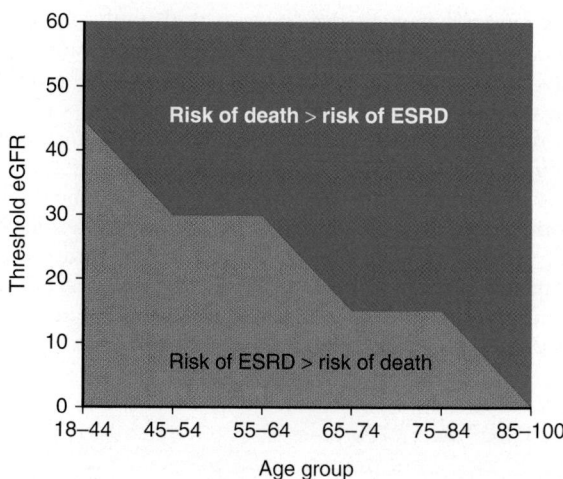

FIGURE 21-2 Baseline estimated glomerular filtration rate (eGFR) threshold below which the risk for end-stage kidney disease (ESKD) exceeded the risk for death in each age group among 209,622 U.S. veterans with stages 3 to 5 chronic kidney disease (CKD), monitored for a mean of 3.2 years. (From O'Hare AM, Choi AI, Bertenthal D, et al: Age affects outcomes in chronic kidney disease, *J Am Soc Nephrol* 18:2758-2765, 2007.)

In 11 randomized trials, the efficacy of ACE inhibitor in the treatment of CKD was evaluated. A meta-analysis of individual patient data from these trials did not reveal an increased risk of both doubling of serum creatinine levels and ESKD, or of ESKD alone, among men.[26] In fact, after adjustment for baseline variables, including blood pressure and urinary protein excretion, women evidenced a significantly higher risk for reaching these endpoints than did men.[26] One limitation of this and several of the other studies quoted is that menopausal status of the women was not documented. In the Chronic Renal Insufficiency in Birmingham (CRIB) study, female gender was identified as an independent risk factor for ESKD, but this finding may have resulted from reliance on serum creatinine level as a measure of GFR, because a given creatinine value represents a lower GFR in a woman than in a man.[27] For further discussion of the effect of gender on CKD, see Chapters 19, 20, and 51.

Ethnicity

African Americans are overrepresented in the population of dialysis recipients in the United States, which suggests that ethnicity is a strong risk factor for the progression of CKD to ESKD. Population-based studies have revealed a higher incidence of ESKD among African Americans that was attributable only in part to socioeconomic and other known risk factors.[4,16,28,29] Similarly, among diabetic adults, the risk of early decline in renal function (increase in serum creatinine level of ≥0.4 mg/dL) was approximately threefold higher (odds ratio [OR] = 3.15; 95% CI = 1.86 to 5.33) among black patients than among white patients, but 82% of this excess risk was attributable to socioeconomic and other known risk factors.[30]

The risk of renal function decline over 5 years among hypertensive patients was greater among African Americans,[17] and black race was independently associated with a greater rate of GFR decline in the Modification of Diet in Renal Disease (MDRD) study.[6] According to data from the

Reasons for Geographic and Racial Differences in Stroke (REGARDS) cohort study, an estimated GFR of 50 to 59 mL/minute/1.73 m² was less prevalent, but an estimated GFR of 10 to 19 mL/minute/1.73 m² was more prevalent, among African American subjects than among white subjects[31]; these findings suggest that African American ethnicity acts as a progression factor but not as a susceptibility factor. United States Renal Data System reports revealed a substantially higher incidence of ESKD among African Americans (3.6 times higher than among white persons), Hispanics (1.5 times higher than among non-Hispanic persons) and Native Americans (1.8 times higher than among white persons).[32] Similarly, in 2008, ESKD was more prevalent among minority groups: among African Americans, 5205 pmp; among Native Americans, 2700 pmp; among Hispanics, 2458 pmp; among Asians, 1992 pmp; and among white persons, 1248 pmp.[32] In other studies, CKD and ESKD have been reported to be more prevalent among ethnic groups such as Asians,[33] Hispanics,[34] Native Americans,[35] Mexican Americans,[36] and Australian Aboriginals.[37] The mechanisms underlying these associations remain to be elucidated, but possible explanations include genetic factors, increased prevalence of diabetes mellitus, lower nephron endowment, and increased susceptibility to salt-sensitive hypertension, as well as environmental, lifestyle, and socioeconomic differences. Ethnicity and CKD are discussed in further detail in Chapters 19, 20, and 51.

Hereditary Factors

Hereditary renal diseases resulting from a single gene defect—such as autosomal dominant polycystic kidney disease, Alport's disease, Fabry's disease, and congenital nephrotic syndrome—account for a relatively small but clinically important proportion of all cases of CKD. However, evidence is rapidly accumulating that genetic factors account for familial clustering of many other forms of CKD with multifactorial causes. Of 25,883 patients with incident ESKD, 22.8% reported a family history of ESKD,[38] and of the relatives of patients with ESKD, 49.3% were found by screening to have evidence of CKD.[39] In another case-control study of 689 patients with ESKD and 361 controls, having one first-degree relative with CKD increased the risk of ESKD by 1.3 (95% CI = 0.7 to 2.6), and having two such relatives increased the risk by 10.4 (95% CI = 2.7 to 40.2) after controlling for multiple known risk factors (including diabetes and hypertension).[40] Similarly, a case-control study of 103 white American patients with ESKD reported a 3.5-fold increase (95% CI = 1.5 to 8.4) in risk of ESKD with the presence of a first-, second-, or third-degree relative with ESKD.[41]

Investigators have identified specific gene polymorphisms that may explain the high prevalence of ESKD among African Americans. Some alleles of the gene for non–muscle myosin heavy chain 9 (*MYH9*) are associated with increased risk of ESKD and have been estimated to account for approximately 40% to 45% of cases of ESKD among African Americans.[42,43] Even stronger associations with CKD in African Americans have been reported with two independent sequence variants of the gene for apolipoprotein L-I, located in the chromosomal regions adjacent to *MYH9*. These gene variants confer resistance to trypanosomal infection and the associated sleeping sickness, which explains how selection probably resulted in a high prevalence of these variants in the population.[44]

Results of other studies suggest that genetic factors also increase susceptibility to early manifestations of CKD. In one study of 169 families in which one proband had type 2 diabetes, the diabetic siblings of the probands with microalbuminuria had a significantly higher risk of also having microalbuminuria after adjustment for confounding risk factors (OR = 3.94; 95% CI = 1.93 to 9.01) than did the diabetic siblings of probands without microalbuminuria.[45] Furthermore, the nondiabetic siblings of diabetic probands with microalbuminuria evidenced significantly higher urinary albumin excretion rates (but within the normal range) than did the nondiabetic siblings of normoalbuminuric diabetic probands.

Genomewide association studies have identified multiple novel loci that are significantly associated with elevated serum creatinine levels or with CKD,[46-48] which suggests that many new genetic risk factors for CKD are likely to be identified in the near future. From the previous discussion, it is clear that genetic factors may act as susceptibility factors in some persons, as initiating factors in patients with CKD caused by a single gene defect, or as progression factors in other affected patients. As a result of the rapid growth in knowledge of genetic aspects of CKD, genetic risk factors will become increasingly important in risk prediction for patients with CKD. For a more detailed discussion of genetic aspects of kidney disease, see Chapters 42, 43, and 44.

Hemodynamic Factors

Experimental studies have shown that glomerular hemodynamic responses (glomerular capillary hypertension and hyperfiltration) to nephron loss[49] and chronic hyperglycemia[50] are critical factors in establishing the vicious cycle of nephron loss that is characteristic of CKD. In addition, any factor that further increases glomerular hypertension, hyperfiltration, or both may be expected to exacerbate glomerular damage and accelerate the progression of CKD (see Figure 21-1).

Decreased Nephron Number

Nephron Endowment

Autopsy studies have revealed that the number of nephrons per kidney varies widely in humans: according to one series, from 210,332 to 2,702,079.[51] Multiple factors have been shown to influence nephron endowment; these include factors that affect the fetal-maternal environment, as well as genetic factors.[52] A substantial body of evidence exists to support the hypothesis that low nephron endowment predisposes individuals to CKD by provoking an increase in single-nephron GFR and, therefore, a reduction in renal reserve. It is not currently possible to ascertain nephron number in living human subjects, but autopsy studies have shown an association between reduced nephron number and both hypertension[53] and glomerulosclerosis.[54]

In human autopsy studies, low birth weight is directly associated with reduced nephron number,[55,56] and birth weight may therefore serve as a marker of nephron endowment. Low birth weight is also a risk factor for the development of hypertension and diabetes mellitus later in life, both of which further increase the risk of CKD.[57] One meta-analysis of 32 studies that included data from more than 2 million subjects revealed significant increases in the risk of albuminuria (OR = 1.81; 95% CI = 1.19 to 2.77) and that of ESKD (OR = 1.58; 95% CI = 1.33 to 1.88) in association with low birth weight.[58] Thus, low birth weight, acting as a marker of reduced nephron endowment, may be regarded as both a susceptibility risk factor and a progression risk factor for CKD. Factors affecting nephron endowment and the consequences of reduced nephron endowment are discussed in more detail in Chapter 22.

Acquired Nephron Deficit

In experimental models of acquired nephron deficit, severe nephron loss (as in 5/6 nephrectomy) alone can initiate a cycle of progressive injury in the remaining glomeruli that is mediated primarily through glomerular hypertension and hyperfiltration.[49] Of 14 humans subjected to similarly large reductions in nephron number after partial resection of a single kidney, 2 developed ESKD and 9 developed proteinuria, the extent of which was inversely correlated with the amount of renal tissue remaining.[59] Lesser degrees of acquired nephron loss, such as that occurring with removal of one of two previously normal kidneys (uninephrectomy), may not be sufficient to cause CKD in the majority of subjects[9,60,61] but may predispose affected individuals to other forms of CKD if they are subsequently exposed to other risk factors. This is perhaps best illustrated by the observation that uninephrectomy exacerbates renal injury in experimental diabetic nephropathy[62] and, in humans with diabetes, increases the risk of developing diabetic nephropathy.[11]

In most forms of human CKD, initial nephron loss caused by primary renal disease, multisystem disorders that involve the kidneys, or exposure to nephrotoxins is focal, but the hemodynamic adaptations in remaining glomeruli are thought to contribute to nephron loss by provoking further glomerulosclerosis (see Chapter 51). Results of several epidemiologic studies have supported this hypothesis by showing that patients with reduced GFR are at increased risk for a further decline in renal function. At least one study revealed an increased risk of developing CKD in association with an estimated GFR of less than 90 mL/minute/1.73 m² in participants without evidence of CKD at the time of baseline measurements (OR = 3.01; 95% CI = 1.98 to 4.58, in comparison with an estimated GFR of ≥120 mL/minute/1.73 m²).[15] Among patients known to have CKD, several longitudinal studies have reported an increased risk of ESKD with decreased GFR at the time of baseline measurements: 3047 patients with stage 3 CKD evidenced a hazard ratio of 2.5 (95% CI = 1.89 to 3.31) for ESKD with each 10 mL/minute/1.73 m² decrease in estimated GFR[18]; among 131 patients with CKD (mean estimated GFR 31 ± 15 mL/minute/1.73 m²), each 1 mL/minute/1.73 m² increase in estimated GFR was associated with a hazard ratio of 0.914 (95% CI = 0.864 to 0.968) for ESKD[63]; and among 920 patients with stages 4 and 5 CKD, an estimated GFR of 13.7 to 16.6 mL/minute/1.73 m² was associated with a relative risk for ESKD of 1.5 (95% CI = 1.21 to 1.91) in comparison with an estimated GFR of more than 18.5 mL/minute/1.73 m².[20]

In accordance with the findings of these individual studies, two large meta-analyses of cohort studies have identified baseline GFR as strong predictor of ESKD. Among 845,125 participants from the general population, estimated GFR was independently associated with an increased risk of developing ESKD when it fell below 75 mL/minute/1.73 m². For groups of patients with average estimated GFRs of 60, 45, and 15 mL/minute/1.73 m², the hazard ratios for developing ESKD were 4, 29, and 454, respectively, in comparison with a reference group with an estimated GFR of 95 mL/minute/1.73 m². Similar findings were reported in 173,892 other participants considered to be at increased risk for developing CKD (Figure 21-3).[64] Among 21,688 patients with CKD, lower estimated GFR was an independent risk factor for ESKD: A fall of 15 mL/minute/1.73 m² below a threshold of 45 mL/minute/1.73 m² was associated with a pooled hazard ratio of 6.24.[65] Furthermore, analysis of the risk for CKD progression among patients with type 2 diabetes mellitus and nephropathy identified elevated serum creatinine level as an independent predictor of progression to ESKD in the Reduction of Endpoints in NIDDM with the Angiotensin II Antagonist Losartan (RENAAL) study (HR = 3.59; 95% CI = 2.90 to 4.45),[66] and higher serum creatinine level was an independent risk factor for ESKD in a cohort study of 382 patients with stages 3, 4, and 5 CKD.[27]

On the other hand, detailed analysis of data from the MDRD study confirmed a wide range of rates of GFR decline among patients with CKD but demonstrated no association between the baseline GFR and the subsequent rate of decline.[6] Thus, in different contexts, acquired nephron deficit may be regarded as a susceptibility factor (e.g., after nephrectomy in a healthy kidney donor), an initiation factor (when severe nephron loss provokes glomerulosclerosis in remaining previously normal glomeruli), or a progression factor (when nephron loss accelerates preexisting damage in remaining glomeruli).

Acute Kidney Injury

Despite previous perceptions that patients who recover from acute kidney injury (AKI) regain normal renal function and have a good prognosis, several more recent cohort studies have revealed that recovery from AKI is associated with a substantially increased risk of CKD and death. Among 3769 adults who required dialysis for AKI and survived without dialysis for at least 30 days after hospital discharge, the incidence rate for chronic dialysis was 2.63 per 100 person years, in contrast to 0.91 per 100 person years in 13,598 matched controls (adjusted HR, 3.23; 95% CI = 2.70 to 3.86).[67] The relative risk was particularly high for those with no previous diagnosis of CKD (adjusted HR = 15.54; 95% CI = 9.65 to 25.03). There was no difference between the groups in rate of survival. In another study of similar design, outcomes were investigated in 343 patients with a pre-admission estimated GFR of more than 45 mL/minute/1.73 m² who required dialysis for AKI but survived for at least 30 days after hospital discharge without dialysis. After controlling for potential confounders, AKI that necessitated dialysis was associated with a 28-fold increase in the risk of developing stage 4 or 5 CKD (adjusted HR = 28.1; 95% CI = 21.1 to 37.6) and more than double the risk of death (adjusted HR = 2.3; 95% CI = 1.8 to 3.0), in comparison to 555,660 adult patients hospitalized during the same period but without AKI.[68]

Analysis of data from a cohort of 233,803 Medicare beneficiaries aged 67 years or older who were hospitalized in 2000 revealed substantially increased risk for developing ESKD

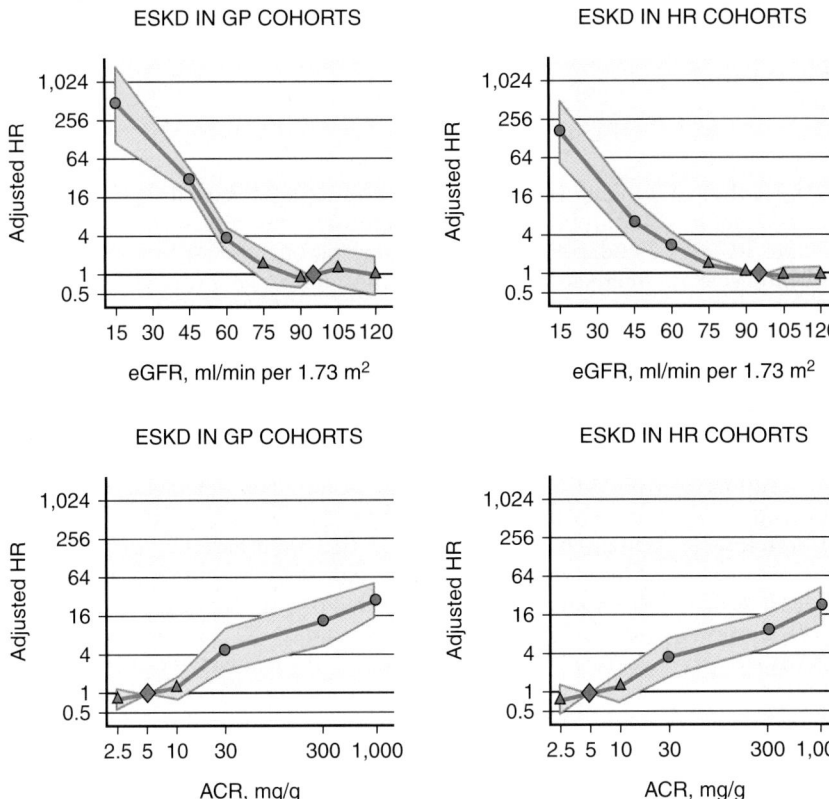

FIGURE 21-3 Pooled hazard ratios (95% confidence interval) for end-stage kidney disease (ESKD) according to spline estimated glomerular filtration rate (eGFR; *upper panels*) and ratio of urine albumin to creatinine (*lower panels*), adjusted for each other and for age, sex, and cardiovascular risk factors (continuous analyses). Reference categories are eGFR of 95 mL/minute/1.73 m², urine albumin/creatinine ratio of 5 mg/g, or negative or trace findings on dipstick testing. Results are shown for general population cohorts (*left panels*) and for those at high risk (*right panels*). *Dots* represent statistical significance; *triangles* represent nonsignificance; and *shaded areas* represent the 95% confidence interval. *ACR,* Urine albumin/creatinine ratio; *GP cohorts,* general population; *HR,* hazard ratio; *HR cohorts,* high-risk cohorts. (From Gansevoort RT, Matsushita K, van der Velde M, et al: Lower estimated GFR and higher albuminuria are associated with adverse kidney outcomes in both general and high-risk populations. A collaborative meta-analysis of general and high-risk population cohorts, *Kidney Int* 79:1341-1352, 2011.)

in patients who developed AKI on a background of CKD (HR = 41.2; 95% CI = 34.6 to 49.1) or without previous CKD (HR = 13.0; 95% CI = 10.6 to 16.0), in comparison with patients who did not develop AKI. The importance of AKI as a risk factor for CKD initiation was further illustrated by the observation that of the 4730 patients who had AKI without preexisting CKD, 72.1% developed CKD within 2 years of the AKI episode. Furthermore, 25.2% of those who developed ESKD had a history of AKI.[69] In a similar study, 113,272 patients hospitalized with a primary diagnosis of acute tubular necrosis, AKI, pneumonia, or myocardial infarction (control group) were studied. Overall, 11.4% progressed to stage 4 CKD during follow-up; that percentage included 20.0% of patients with acute tubular necrosis, 13.2% of those with AKI, 24.7% of those with preexisting CKD, and 3.3% of the control patients. After controlling for other variables, having a diagnosis of AKI, acute tubular necrosis, or CKD increased the risk of developing stage 4 CKD by 303%, 564%, and 550%, respectively, in comparison with controls. After controlling for covariates, AKI and CKD were associated with 12% and 20% increased risk of death, respectively, in comparison with controls.[70]

The multiplicative effect of AKI on CKD progression is further illustrated by a study of 39,805 patients with estimated GFRs of less than 45 mL/minute/1.73 m² before hospitalization. Those who survived an episode of dialysis-necessitating AKI had a very high risk of developing ESKD within 30 days of hospital discharge (i.e. nonrecovery from AKI) that was related to preadmission estimated GFR. The incidences of ESKD were 42% for estimated GFRs of 30 to 44 mL/minute/1.73 m² and as high as 63% for estimated GFRs of 15 to 29 mL/minute/1.73 m², whereas it was only 1.5% among those who did not have dialysis-necessitating AKI. Among patients who survived more than 30 days after hospital discharge without ESKD, the incidences of ESKD and death at 6 months were 12.7% and 19.7%, respectively, in comparison with 1.7% and 7.4% among the patients with CKD but no AKI. After adjustment for multiple risk factors, AKI was associated with a 30% increase in long-term risk for death or ESKD (adjusted HR = 1.30; 95% CI = 1.04 to 1.64).[71] Together, these data show that AKI should be regarded as an important risk factor for CKD initiation and progression. The mechanisms responsible for these observations require further elucidation, but those proposed include nephron loss, loss of peritubular capillaries, and interstitial fibrosis.[72] The incidence of AKI has increased over the past few decades and it is likely to become an increasingly important risk factor for CKD among older patients.

Blood Pressure

Hypertension is an almost universal consequence of reduced renal function, but it is also an important factor in the progression of CKD. In the hypothesis of CKD progression presented in Figure 21-1, it is clear that elevations in systemic blood pressure that are transmitted to the glomerulus contribute to glomerular hypertension and thus accelerate glomerular damage. Hypertension has been shown to be predictive of ESKD risk in several large population-based studies.[14,15,23,73] Furthermore, the magnitude of increased risk is closely associated with the level of blood pressure, according to several studies, so that even elevations in blood pressure below the threshold for the diagnosis of hypertension were associated with increased risk of ESKD.[14,23,74]

Among patients with CKD in the MDRD study, higher baseline measurements of mean arterial pressure were independently predictive of a greater rate of GFR decline.[6] These observations have prompted a call for blood pressure to be viewed as a continuous rather than a dichotomous risk factor for CKD, with less emphasis on traditional definitions of "hypertension" and "normotension."[75] Despite these close associations, the causality criterion for a risk factor requires evidence from an RCT. At least three large RCTs have been conducted to investigate the effect of "intensive" versus "standard" blood pressure lowering on CKD progression. Whereas the primary analysis of data from the MDRD study found no significant difference between the rate of decline in GFR between patients randomised to "intensive" (target MAP of <92 mm Hg, equivalent to <125/75mm Hg) versus "standard" blood pressure control (target MAP <107mm Hg, equivalent to 140/90 mm Hg), secondary analysis did show benefit associated with the low blood pressure target among patients with higher levels of proteinuria at baseline.[76]

Further secondary analysis showed that achieved lower blood pressure was also associated with a slower GFR decline, an effect that was more marked among patients with more severe proteinuria at the time of baseline measurements.[77] Moreover, long-term follow-up (mean 6.6 years) of patients from the MDRD study revealed a significant reduction in the risk of ESKD (adjusted HR = 0.68; 95% CI = 0.57 to 0.82) or in a combined endpoint of ESKD or death (adjusted HR = 0.77; 95% CI = 0.65 to 0.91) among patients randomly assigned to achieve "low" blood pressure targets, even though treatment and blood pressure data were not available beyond the 2.2 years of the original trial.[78]

In the African American Study of Kidney Disease and Hypertension (AASK), no significant difference in the rate of GFR decline was observed between subjects randomly assigned to achieve a mean arterial pressure of 92 mm Hg or lower and those assigned to achieve a pressure of 102 to 107 mm Hg. However, patients in AASK generally had mild proteinuria at the time of baseline measurements (mean urine protein level, 0.38 to 0.63 g/day).[79] Furthermore, prolonged follow-up of the AASK cohort after completion of the randomized trial revealed no significant differences in the primary outcome for the whole cohort; however, in subjects with a baseline urine protein/creatinine ratio higher than 0.22 who were initially randomly assigned to receive intensive blood pressure control, the risks of creatinine level doubling, ESKD, and death were significantly reduced.[80] Thus, the results of the MDRD study and AASK suggest a significant interaction between blood pressure and proteinuria as risk factors for CKD progression.

In a third study, patients with nondiabetic CKD who were taking ACE inhibitors were given a calcium channel blocker to further reduce blood pressure; this treatment failed to produce additional renoprotection, but the degree of additional blood pressure reduction was modest (4.1/2.8 mm Hg) and may have been insufficient to improve outcomes in patients already receiving optimal ACE inhibitor therapy.[81] Of interest is that blood pressure was not an independent predictor of ESKD among diabetic patients in the RENAAL study[66] or in predominantly nondiabetic subjects in the CRIB study.[27] This is probably because blood pressure was well controlled in all subjects (in the RENAAL study), which illustrates how risk

factors may vary in importance, depending on the population studied.

Obesity and Metabolic Syndrome

In experimental models, obesity is associated with hypertension, proteinuria, and progressive renal disease. Micropuncture studies have confirmed that obesity is another cause of glomerular hyperfiltration and glomerular hypertension, which can exacerbate the progression of CKD.[82,83] Furthermore, several other factors associated with obesity and the metabolic syndrome may contribute to renal damage; these factors include hormones and proinflammatory molecules produced by adipocytes,[84] increased mineralocorticoid levels or mineralocorticoid receptor activation by cortisol,[85] and reduced adiponectin levels.[86] In humans, severe obesity is associated with increased renal plasma flow, glomerular hyperfiltration, and albuminuria, abnormalities that are reversed by weight loss.[87] Obesity, as defined by a high body mass index (BMI), has been associated with increased risk of developing CKD in several large population-based studies.[15,88] Moreover, one study revealed a progressive increase in relative risk of developing ESKD in association with increasing BMI (relative risk = 3.57 and 95% CI = 3.05 to 4.18 for a BMI of 30.0 to 34.9 kg/m², in comparison with a BMI of 18.5 to 24.9 kg/m²) among 320,252 subjects confirmed to have no evidence of CKD at initial screening.[89]

There is evidence that obesity may directly cause a specific form of glomerulopathy characterized by proteinuria and histologic features of focal and segmental glomerulosclerosis,[90,91] but it is likely that it also acts as a risk factor in the development of several other forms of renal disease. Interest has focused on the role of the metabolic syndrome (insulin resistance)—defined by the presence of abdominal obesity, dyslipidemia, hypertension, and fasting hyperglycemia—in the development of CKD. An analysis of the Third National Health and Nutrition Examination Survey (NHANES) data revealed a significantly increased risk of CKD and microalbuminuria in patients with the metabolic syndrome, as well as a progressive increase in risk associated with the number of components of the metabolic syndrome present.[92] Furthermore, in a large longitudinal study of 10,096 patients without diabetes or CKD at the time of baseline measurements, metabolic syndrome was identified as an independent risk factor for the development of CKD over 9 years (adjusted OR = 1.43; 95% CI = 1.18 to 1.73). Again, there was a progressive increase in risk in association with the number of traits of the metabolic syndrome present (when one trait was present, OR = 1.13 and 95% CI = 0.89 to 1.45; in comparison, when five traits were present, OR = 2.45 and 95% CI = 1.32 to 4.54).[93]

In another study, a high hip/waist ratio, a marker of insulin resistance, was independently associated with impaired renal function, even in lean individuals (BMI < 25 kg/m²) among a population-based cohort of 7676 subjects.[94] The effect of obesity on the progression of established CKD is less well documented. Increased BMI has been identified as a risk factor for CKD progression among subjects with immunoglobulin A (IgA) nephropathy,[95] those who have undergone renal mass reduction surgery or have renal agenesis,[96] and those with renal transplants.[97] On the other hand, BMI was unrelated to the risk of ESKD among a cohort of patients with stage 4 and 5 CKD.[20]

It is widely recognized that weight loss is difficult to achieve in obese patients, but surgical intervention in the form of gastric banding or gastric bypass appears to offer the most effective long-term outcomes. Two large cohort studies showed significant survival benefit in subjects who underwent bariatric surgery[98,99]; unfortunately, renal endpoints were not reported in these studies. Beneficial renoprotective effects of weight loss were reported in a meta-analysis of observational studies. Weight loss was found to be associated with reduction in proteinuria, independently of blood pressure[100]; smaller studies have also revealed improvement or stabilization of renal function[101] or reduction in proteinuria[102] after bariatric surgery in subjects with CKD. The best method for assessing obesity in CKD remains to be determined. BMI is the most widely applied method but does not take account of body composition. One study demonstrated a high sensitivity but relatively low specificity of BMI for detecting obesity in subjects with CKD.[103]

High Dietary Protein Intake

Protein feeding provokes an increase in GFR in rodents[104] and in humans.[105] In accordance with the hypothesis that the glomerular hemodynamic changes associated with hyperfiltration accelerate glomerular injury, experimental studies have demonstrated that a high-protein diet accelerates renal disease progression, whereas dietary protein restriction[106,107] results in normalization of glomerular capillary hydraulic pressure, as well as normalization of single-nephron GFR and marked attenuation of glomerular damage.[49] Observational studies in humans have revealed an increased risk of microalbuminuria associated with higher dietary protein intake among subjects with diabetes and hypertension (OR = 3.3; 95% CI = 1.4 to 7.8) but not among healthy subjects or those with isolated diabetes or hypertension.[108] This finding illustrates, again, the interaction between risk factors for CKD. In another study, high intake of protein, particularly nondairy animal protein, was associated with a higher rate of GFR decline among women with an estimated GFR of 55 to 80 mL/minute/1.73 m^2 but not in those with an estimated GFR exceeding 80 mL/minute/1.73 m^2.[109]

Randomized trials for investigating the effects of high protein diet are lacking, but several researchers have sought to examine the potential renoprotective effects of dietary protein restriction. In the MDRD study, primary analysis revealed no significant difference in the mean rate of GFR decline in subjects randomly assigned to consume diets low or very low in protein,[76] but secondary analysis of outcomes, according to achieved dietary protein intake, showed that a reduction in protein intake of 0.2 g/kg/day was correlated with a 1.15 mL/minute/year reduction in the rate of GFR decline, equivalent to a 29% reduction in mean rate of GFR decline.[110] On the other hand, long-term follow-up of participants in study 2 of the MDRD trial revealed no renoprotective benefit among those consuming a diet very low in protein in the original study, but the risk of death in this group was higher (HR = 1.92; 95% CI = 1.15 to 3.20).[111] Nevertheless, three meta-analyses of smaller studies have all reported a significant renoprotective benefit associated with dietary protein restriction.[112-114] The role of dietary protein restriction in the management of CKD is discussed further in Chapters 51 and 60.

Pregnancy and Preeclampsia

Physiologic adaptations during pregnancy provoke glomerular hyperfiltration that usually does not cause renal damage. In the context of preexisting CKD, however, the glomerular hyperfiltration of pregnancy can exacerbate proteinuria and glomerular injury. Several studies have shown an increased risk of CKD progression during pregnancy, particularly when the pregestational serum creatinine level is 1.4 mg/dL or higher (≥124 μmol/L). In one study of 82 pregnancies in 67 women with primary renal disease and serum creatinine levels of 1.4 mg/dL or higher, blood pressure, serum creatinine level, and proteinuria increased during pregnancy. In 70 pregnancies with postpartum data available, persistent loss of maternal renal function at 6 months was reported in 22 women (31%), and by 12 months, 8 (36%) of these women had progressed to ESKD. Adverse obstetric outcomes were preterm delivery (in 59%) and low birth weight (in 37%), but the fetal survival rate was 93%.[115] In a more recent series of 49 women with stages 3 to 5 CKD before pregnancy, mean GFR declined during pregnancy (from 35 ± 12.2 to 30 ± 13.8 mL/minute/1.73 m^2), but the mean rate of GFR decline did not change post partum. Nevertheless, a pregestational GFR lower than 40 mL/minute/1.73 m^2, in combination with a protein level exceeding 1 g/day, was associated either with a more rapid postpartum GFR decline and a shorter time to ESKD or with halving of GFR and low birth weight.[116]

Although earlier reports had been suggestive of good outcomes, one more recent study revealed adverse effects associated even with early-stage CKD. In 91 pregnancies in which the mothers had predominantly stages 1 and 2 CKD, modest increases in hypertension, serum creatinine level, and proteinuria were observed. Adverse obstetric outcomes—including preterm delivery, lower birth weight, and need for admission to the neonatal intensive care unit—were more frequent than in pregnant controls at low risk, and this remained true even when only patients with stage 1 CKD were considered, although there were no perinatal deaths.[117] On the other hand, pregnancy was not associated with more rapid decline in GFR over 5 years in a cohort of 245 women of childbearing age who had IgA nephropathy and serum creatinine levels of 1.2 mg/dL or lower (in the majority).[118]

Complications of pregnancy, particularly preeclampsia, may also cause renal damage. In one large population-based study, renal outcomes were assessed in 570,433 women who had had at least one singleton pregnancy. Only 477 women developed ESKD at a mean of 17 ± 9 years after the first pregnancy (overall rate, 3.7 per 100,000 women per year), but preeclampsia was associated with a significant increase in the risk of ESKD; relative risk ranged from 4.7 (95% CI = 3.6 to 6.1) for preeclampsia in a single pregnancy to 15.5 (95% CI = 7.8 to 30.8) for preeclampsia in two or three pregnancies. The risk was further increased if the newborn had low birth weight or was preterm. Causes of ESKD were glomerulonephritis in 35%, hereditary or congenital disease in 21%, diabetic nephropathy in 14%, and interstitial nephritis in 12%.[119] Similarly, in women with diabetes before pregnancy, preeclampsia and preterm birth were associated with significantly increased risks of ESKD and death, which illustrates how different risk factors for CKD may interact to increase risk.[120]

Possible explanations for these observations include the presence of pathogenic factors common to CKD and preeclampsia, including obesity, hypertension, insulin resistance, and endothelial dysfunction; exacerbation by preeclampsia of preexisting subclinical CKD; and effects of preeclampsia on the kidney that increase the risk of CKD later in life.[121] The possibility that preeclampsia may provoke renal damage is suggested by several studies that demonstrated an increased incidence of microalbuminuria after preeclampsia. A meta-analysis of seven such studies revealed a 31% prevalence of microalbuminuria at a weighted mean of 7.1 years after preeclampsia, in comparison with a 7% prevalence among a control group with uncomplicated pregnancies.[122] More research is needed to identify which mechanisms are most relevant; however, even without further information, preeclampsia should be regarded as a risk factor for the development and progression of CKD.

Multisystem Disorders

Diabetes Mellitus

Diabetic nephropathy is rapidly becoming the most common cause of ESKD worldwide. In one population-based study of 23,534 subjects,[23] diabetes was associated with a substantially increased risk of ESKD or death related to CKD (relative HR = 7.5; 95% CI = 4.8 to 11.7). In another study of 1428 subjects with estimated creatinine clearance rate of more than 70 mL/minute at the time of baseline measurements,[123] diabetes was associated with an increased risk of moderate chronic renal impairment (estimated creatinine clearance rate, <50 mL/minute). Glycemic control is a key risk factor for the development of diabetic nephropathy, according to results of randomized trials that showed reduced risk of developing nephropathy in subjects with type 1 diabetes[124] and type 2 diabetes[125] who were randomly assigned to undergo tight glycemic control.

The pathogenesis of diabetic nephropathy is complex and involves multiple mechanisms, including glomerular hemodynamic factors,[50,126] advanced glycation end-product formation, generation of reactive oxygen species, and upregulation of profibrotic growth factors and cytokines.[127,128] (For further discussion of the pathogenesis of diabetic nephropathy, see Chapter 38.) In at least one study, diabetic nephropathy was associated with more rapid progression to ESKD than were other causes of CKD.[20] Thus, diabetes may be regarded as a susceptibility, initiation, and progression risk factor for CKD.

Primary Renal Disease

Whereas substantial variation in the rate of GFR decline has been observed between subjects with a common cause of CKD, there is also evidence that some forms of CKD may provoke more rapid progression than others. In the MDRD study, a diagnosis of autosomal dominant polycystic kidney disease was an independent predictor of a greater rate of GFR decline,[6] and in a cohort of patients with stages 4 and 5 CKD,

diabetic nephropathy was associated with shorter time to ESKD than were other diagnoses.[20]

Cardiovascular Disease

In multiple studies, investigators have reported that CKD is associated with a substantial increase in the risk of cardiovascular disease,[129] and it is therefore not surprising that cardiovascular disease is also associated with an increased risk of CKD. In a study of hospitalized Medicare beneficiaries, the prevalence of stage 3 or more severe CKD was 60.4% among those with heart failure and 51.7% among those with myocardial infarction. The presence of CKD in addition to heart disease was associated with significant increases in risk of progression to ESKD and risk of death.[130] These observations may be explained in part by the fact that cardiovascular disease and CKD share many risk factors, including obesity, metabolic syndrome, hypertension, diabetes mellitus, dyslipidemia, and smoking.

In addition, cardiovascular disease may exert effects on the kidneys that promote initiation and progression of CKD; these effects include decreased renal perfusion in heart failure and atherosclerosis of the renal arteries. For example, in patients undergoing elective coronary angiography, renal atherosclerosis was detected in 39% (≥70% stenosis in 7.3%).[131] Furthermore, arterial stiffness may result in greater transmission of elevated systemic blood pressure to glomerular capillaries and exacerbate glomerular hypertension. In one study, pulse wave velocity and augmentation index, markers of arterial stiffness, were identified as independent risk factors for progression to ESKD among subjects with stages 4 and 5 CKD[132]; and in another study, augmentation index was an independent determinant of rate of decline of creatinine clearance among subjects with stage 3 CKD.[133] On the other hand, neither pulse wave velocity nor augmentation index was a predictor of rate of GFR decline in a cohort of subjects with stages 2 to 4 CKD.[134] The interaction between cardiovascular and renal disease is further illustrated by the observation that among subjects with CKD, a diagnosis of cardiovascular disease is associated with an increased risk of progression to ESKD.[135,136] For further discussion of cardiovascular disease in patients with CKD, see Chapter 55.

Biomarkers

Urinary Protein Excretion

Abnormal excretion of protein in the urine indicates dysfunction of the glomerular filtration barrier and is therefore a marker of glomerulopathy, as well as an index of disease severity. Experimental evidence suggests that proteinuria may also contribute to progressive renal damage in CKD (see Chapter 52). Proteinuria is strongly associated with the risk of CKD progression, as well as with cardiovascular and all-cause mortality. In a mass screening of a general population of 107,192 participants by means of dipstick urinalysis, proteinuria was identified as the most powerful predictor of ESKD risk over 10 years (OR = 14.9; 95% CI = 10.9 to 20.2).[14] Similarly, among 12,866 middle-aged men enrolled in the Multiple Risk Factor Intervention Trial (MRFIT), proteinuria detected by dipstick test was associated with a significantly increased risk for developing ESKD over 25 years (for 1+ proteinuria, HR = 3.1 and 95% CI = 1.8 to 3.8; for ≥2+ proteinuria, HR = 15.7 and 95% CI = 10.3 to 23.9). Furthermore, detection of 2+ proteinuria or higher increased the hazard ratio for ESKD associated with an estimated GFR of less than 60 mL/minute/1.73 m^2 from 2.4 (95% CI = 1.5 to 3.8) without proteinuria to 41 (95% CI = 15.2 to 71.1) with proteinuria.[137]

Similar associations have been reported for measurements of urinary albumin in the general population. In the Nord-Trøndelag Health (HUNT 2) study, which included 65,589 adults, microalbuminuria and macroalbuminuria were independent predictors of ESKD after 10.3 years (HRs = 13.0 and 47.2, respectively), and the combination of reduced estimated GFR with albuminuria was substantially more predictive of ESKD.[138] In the Prevention of Renal and Vascular End-stage Disease (PREVEND) study, albuminuria was an independent predictor of a decline in estimated GFR to less than 60 mL/minute/1.73 m^2.[139,140] Among patients who had CKD with a wide variety of causes, proteinuria at the time of baseline measurements has consistently been predictive of renal outcomes.[63,141,142] In three large prospective studies that included patients with nondiabetic CKD (MDRD; Ramipril Efficacy In Nephropathy; and AASK), more severe proteinuria at the time of baseline measurements was strongly associated with a more rapid decline in GFR.[6,77,143,144] Similarly, among patients with diabetic nephropathy, baseline urinary albumin/creatinine ratio was a strong independent predictor of ESKD in the RENAAL study and in the Irbesartan in Diabetic Nephropathy Trial.[66,145]

The findings of these individual studies have been confirmed by two large meta-analyses. In an analysis that included nine general population cohorts (n = 845,125) and eight cohorts with increased risk of developing CKD (n = 173,892), urine albumin/creatinine ratios higher than 30 mg/g, higher than 300 mg/g and higher than 1000 mg/g were independently associated with progressive increases in the risk of ESKD, progressive CKD, and AKI (see Figure 21-3).[64] Among 21,688 patients known to have CKD from 13 studies, an eightfold increase in urine albumin/creatinine ratio or protein/creatinine ratio was associated with increased rates of all-cause mortality (pooled HR = 1.40) and risk of ESKD (pooled HR = 3.04).[65]

Secondary analyses of prospective RCTs have revealed that the extent of "residual proteinuria" that persists despite optimal treatment with an ACE inhibitor or angiotensin receptor blocker is also predictive of renal prognosis: In the Ramipril Efficacy In Nephropathy study, percentage reduction in proteinuria value over the first 3 months and the absolute level of proteinuria at 3 months were strong independent predictors of the subsequent rate of decline in GFR[146]; in the Irbesartan in Diabetic Nephropathy Trial, greater reduction in proteinuria value at 12 months was associated with a greater reduction in the risk of ESKD (HR = 0.44; 95% CI = 0.40 to 0.49 for each halving of baseline proteinuria value)[145]; and in AASK, change in proteinuria value from the times of baseline to 6-month measurements was predictive of subsequent progression of CKD.[144] Similarly, a meta-analysis of data from 1860 patients with nondiabetic CKD showed that during antihypertensive treatment, the current severity of proteinuria was a powerful predictor of the combined endpoint of doubling of baseline serum creatinine values or onset of ESKD (relative risk = 5.56; 95% CI = 3.87 to 7.98 for each 1.0-g/day increase in proteinuria value).[26] These data support the proposal that

proteinuria, like blood pressure, should be regarded as a continuous risk factor for CKD progression.[75]

Proteinuria thus appears to be a powerful predictor of renal risk in the general population, in patients with CKD before treatment, and in patients with CKD who are receiving treatment. Furthermore, analysis of data from the RENAAL study[34] revealed that the presence of albuminuria at the time of baseline measurements was the most important independent predictor of ESKD risk in all ethnic groups, including white, black, Asian, and Hispanic populations. Reduction in albuminuria at 6 months was also predictive of renoprotection in all ethnic groups.[34]

These important observations raise the question of how best to measure the magnitude of proteinuria. As discussed previously, all measurements of proteinuria are predictive of renal outcomes, including values obtained by dipstick urinalysis, urine albumin/creatinine ratio or protein/creatinine ratio, and the amount of urinary albumin or protein excretion over 24 hours. A secondary analysis of data from the RENAAL trial revealed that—in comparison with 24-hour urinary protein excretion, 24-hour urinary albumin excretion, or urinary albumin concentration—urine albumin/creatinine ratio measured on first morning void was a better predictor of time to doubling of serum creatinine level or of time to development of ESKD among patients with diabetes and CKD.[147] On the other hand, retrospective analysis of data from 5586 patients with CKD reported similar hazard ratios associated with urinary albumin/creatinine ratio and protein/creatinine ratio for the outcomes of all-cause mortality, start of renal replacement therapy, and doubling of serum creatinine concentration.[148] Further analysis of these data identified a cohort of patients with a normal urine albumin/creatinine ratio but an elevated urine protein/creatinine ratio in whom the risk of ESKD or death was intermediate between the groups in which both urine albumin/creatinine ratio and protein/creatinine ratio were abnormal or normal.[149]

Together these data imply that any measurement to establish the presence of proteinuria is better than no measurement. If the goal is to detect and monitor microalbuminuria, the urine albumin/creatinine ratio measured on the first morning void is best. For patients with CKD, urine albumin/creatinine ratio or protein/creatinine ratio may be measured, and there is some evidence that additional information may be obtained from both.[150]

Serum Albumin Concentration

Serum albumin concentration is widely regarded as a marker of nutritional status, but it may also be reduced as a result of proteinuria or inflammation. Several studies have identified lower serum albumin as a risk factor for CKD progression. In the MDRD study, a higher baseline concentration of serum albumin was associated with slower subsequent rate of GFR decline, but in a multivariable analysis, this association was displaced by a similar correlation with baseline concentration of serum transferrin, another marker of protein nutrition.[6] In three studies, researchers found associations between serum albumin and renal outcomes in patients with type 2 diabetes and CKD. Among 182 patients with a mean serum creatinine concentration of 1.5 mg/dL at the time of baseline measurement, hypoalbuminemia was an independent risk factor for ESKD.[151] In a long-term follow-up study of 343 patients, a lower baseline concentration of serum albumin was an independent predictor of CKD progression,[152] and in the RENAAL study, lower serum albumin was an independent predictor of ESKD.[66]

Similar observations have been reported in other forms of CKD. In a cohort of 2269 patients with IgA nephropathy, a lower concentration of serum total protein (composed largely of albumin) was an independent risk factor for ESKD,[153] and in a cohort of 3449 patients with CKD referred to a nephrology service, a lower concentration of serum albumin was an independent risk factor for ESKD.[154] In these studies, the predictive value of serum albumin concentration was independent of proteinuria, which indicates that it was not merely acting as a marker of albuminuria.

Anemia

Chronic anemia resulting from inherited hemoglobinopathy is associated with increased renal plasma flow, as well as with glomerular hyperfiltration and subsequent development of proteinuria, hypertension, and ESKD.[155,156] Anemia is a common complication of CKD of any cause, and several studies have shown that it is also an independent predictor of CKD progression. In the RENAAL study, baseline hemoglobin concentration was a significant independent predictor of ESKD among diabetic patients: Each 1-g/dL decrease in hemoglobin concentration was associated with a 11% increase in the risk of ESKD.[157] Baseline hemoglobin concentration was also one of four variables included in the renal risk score developed from the RENAAL data.[66] Similarly, a higher hemoglobin concentration was independently associated with lower risk of progression to ESKD (halving of GFR or need for dialysis) or death among 131 patients with all forms of CKD (HR = 0.778 and 95% CI = 0.639 to 0.948 for each 1-g/dL increase).[63] Furthermore, a time-averaged hemoglobin concentration of 12g/dL or lower was associated with a significantly increased risk of ESKD among 853 male veterans with stages 3 to 5 CKD (HR = 0.74 and 95% CI = 0.65-0.84 for each 1-g/dL increase in hemoglobin concentration).[158]

Two other cohort studies have identified lower hemoglobin concentration as an independent risk factor for more rapid decline in GFR among patients with stage 4 CKD[159] and for the development of ESKD among patients with stages 3 and 4 CKD.[160] In accordance with the hypothesis that anemia contributes directly to CKD progression, researchers in two small randomized studies reported renoprotective benefit associated with erythropoietin therapy. Among patients with serum creatinine concentrations of 2 to 4 mg/dL and hematocrit lower than 30%, erythropoietin treatment was associated with significantly improved renal survival.[161] In nondiabetic patients with serum creatinine concentrations of 2 to 6 mg/dL, early treatment (started when hemoglobin concentration < 11.6 g/dL) with erythropoietin alpha was associated with a 60% reduction in the risk of doubling serum creatinine concentration, ESKD, or death, in comparison with delayed treatment (started when hemoglobin concentration < 9.0 g/dL).[162]

On the other hand, two other studies in which left ventricular mass was the primary endpoint,[163,164] as well as the Trial to Reduce Cardiovascular Events with Aranesp Therapy (TREAT),[165] demonstrated no effect of high versus low hemoglobin target concentration on rate of decline in GFR.

Several investigators have, however, reported adverse outcomes associated with normalization of hemoglobin concentration in patients with CKD. In the Cardiovascular Risk Reduction by Early Anemia Treatment with Epoetin Beta (CREATE) randomized study, achievement of a higher hemoglobin target concentration (13 to 15 mg/dL) was associated with a shorter time to initiation of dialysis than was achievement of the lower target concentration (10.5 to 11.5 mg/dL).[166] In TREAT, a higher hemoglobin target concentration was associated with an increased risk of stroke,[165] and in the Correction of Hemoglobin and Outcomes in Renal Insufficiency (CHOIR) study, a higher hemoglobin target concentration was associated with increased incidence of the combined endpoint of all-cause mortality, myocardial infarction, or hospitalization for congestive cardiac failure.[167]

Dyslipidemia

Lipid abnormalities are common in patients with CKD. In several studies, dyslipidemia has been identified as both a susceptibility risk factor and a progression risk factor for CKD. In population-based studies, several lipid profile abnormalities have been associated with an increased risk of developing CKD; these abnormalities include elevated ratio of low-density lipoprotein (LDL) cholesterol to high-density lipoprotein (HDL) cholesterol[168]; higher triglyceride and lower HDL cholesterol levels[169]; lower HDL cholesterol levels[15]; and elevated total cholesterol, low HDL cholesterol, or elevated total cholesterol to HDL cholesterol levels.[170]

In several observational studies, dyslipidemia was reported to be a risk factor for CKD progression. In the MDRD study, lower HDL cholesterol levels were independently predictive of a more rapid decline in GFR[6]; in a smaller study of patients with CKD, elevated total cholesterol, LDL cholesterol, and apolipoprotein B levels were all associated with more rapid decline in GFR.[171] Among 223 patients with IgA nephropathy, hypertriglyceridemia was independently predictive of CKD progression.[172] Hypercholesterolemia was predictive of loss of renal function in patients with type 1 and type 2 diabetes,[173,174] and among nondiabetic patients, CKD advanced more rapidly in those with hypercholesterolemia and hypertriglyceridemia.[175]

RCTs of lipid-lowering treatment have produced mixed results with regard to renal outcomes. In data from a prospective randomized trial of pravastatin treatment in patients with previous myocardial infarction, subgroup analysis revealed that pravastatin slowed the rate of decline in patients with an estimated GFR lower than 40 mL/minute/1.73 m². an effect that was also more pronounced in patients with proteinuria.[176] Similarly, in the Heart Protection Study, patients with previous cardiovascular disease or diabetes who were randomly assigned to receive simvastatin treatment evidenced a smaller increase in serum creatinine concentration than did those who received placebo.[177] In a placebo-controlled open-label study of patients with CKD, proteinuria, and hypercholesterolemia, creatinine clearance was preserved with atorvastatin treatment, whereas it declined in patients receiving placebo.[178] On the other hand, lipid lowering with fibrates was not associated with renoprotection in two studies,[168,179] although one other study did show reduced incidence of microalbuminuria among patients with type 2 diabetes who received fenofibrate.[180]

One meta-analysis of 13 small controlled trials revealed that lipid-lowering therapy was associated with a significantly slower rate of GFR decline (0.156 mL/minute/month; 95% CI = 0.026 to 0.285 mL/minute/month; P = 0.008) among patients with CKD.[64] On the other hand, analysis of data from a relatively small subgroup with renal endpoints recorded in a meta-analysis of studies of statin therapy in patients with CKD showed that statin therapy was associated with a reduction in proteinuria but no improvement in creatinine clearance.[181] The Study of Heart and Renal Protection (SHARP) is the largest RCT conducted to investigate the cardiovascular and renoprotective effects of lipid lowering in CKD. Patients with CKD or who were receiving dialysis were randomly assigned to receive treatment with simvastatin and ezetimibe or placebo (n = 9438). Whereas the treatment recipients achieved a mean LDL cholesterol lowering of 43 mg/dL and a 17% reduction in major atherosclerotic events, no significant benefit was observed with regard to the incidence of the renal endpoints ESKD (risk ratio = 0.97; 95% CI = 0.89 to 1.05) and ESKD or doubling of creatinine level (risk ratio = 0.94; 95% CI = 0.86 to 1.01).[182] Patients in SHARP had relatively advanced CKD (mean estimated GFR of 27 ± 13 mL/minute/1.73 m²); therefore, it is possible that lipid lowering may be renoprotective in less advanced CKD. Mechanisms whereby dyslipidemia may contribute to CKD progression are discussed in Chapter 51.

Serum Uric Acid Concentration

Hyperuricemia is a common consequence of chronic renal failure and may also contribute to CKD progression. In several population-based studies, hyperuricemia was identified as an independent risk factor for subsequent increase in serum creatinine concentration,[183] decrease in estimated GFR (in blood donors),[184] and development of CKD (defined by estimated GFR of <60 mL/minute/1.73 m²).[185] In one such study, hyperuricemia was identified as an independent risk factor for ESKD among women, but not among men.[186] In patients with IgA nephropathy, hyperuricemia has emerged as a risk factor for CKD progression in two studies.[172,187] On the other hand, a prospective cohort study of 227 patients with nondiabetic CKD revealed that uric acid levels were predictive of progression in an unadjusted model, but this association disappeared when the analysis was adjusted for GFR and proteinuria.[188]

To date, only small, short-term randomized trials have been conducted to investigate the renoprotective potential of lowering serum uric acid levels. Among 54 patients with CKD, patients randomly assigned to receive treatment with allopurinol evidenced stable serum creatinine concentration over a 12-month period, whereas patients in a control group showed an increase. Of interest is that this benefit was not correlated with uric acid levels.[189] In a further study, 113 patients with CKD were randomly assigned to receive allopurinol or usual treatment. Allopurinol treatment was associated with a slower rate of GFR decline that was correlated inversely with change in uric acid concentration. Patients receiving allopurinol also evidenced a reduction in C-reactive protein, cardiovascular events, and hospitalizations.[190] Possible mechanisms whereby hyperuricemia may contribute to CKD progression are exacerbation of glomerular hypertension,[191,192] endothelial dysfunction,[193,194] and proinflammatory effects.[195]

Plasma Asymmetric Dimethyl Arginine Concentration

Asymmetric dimethyl arginine (ADMA) is formed by the breakdown of arginine-methylated proteins and acts as an endogenous inhibitor of nitric oxide synthase to reduce nitric oxide production. The increased ADMA concentrations observed with reduced GFR have been proposed as one mechanism for the endothelial dysfunction associated with CKD. Elevated ADMA concentrations are associated with cardiovascular disease and cardiovascular mortality in patients with CKD.[196] In animal models, administration of ADMA was associated with the development of hypertension; increased deposition of collagen I, collagen III, and fibronectin in glomeruli and in blood vessels; and rarefaction of peritubular capillaries.[197] Conversely, overexpression of dimethylarginine dimethylaminohydrolase (DDAH), the enzyme responsible for degradation of ADMA, was associated with reduced ADMA concentration and amelioration of renal injury in rats after 5/6 nephrectomy, which implies that ADMA may also promote CKD progression.[198]

In several relatively small studies, increased ADMA concentration was identified as a risk factor for CKD progression. Among 131 patients with CKD, a higher plasma ADMA concentration was an independent risk factor for ESKD or death (HR = 1.203 and 95% CI = 1.07 to 1.35 for each 0.1-μmol/L increase).[63] In 227 patients with mild to moderate nondiabetic CKD, higher ADMA concentrations were predictive of progression to the combined endpoint of creatinine concentration doubling or ESKD (HR = 1.47 and 95% CI = 1.12 to 1.93 for each 0.1-μmol/L increase).[199] Finally, retrospective analysis of data from 109 patients with IgA nephropathy revealed associations between ADMA concentration and both glomerular and tubulointerstitial injury. Furthermore, plasma ADMA concentration was an independent determinant of annual GFR reduction rate.[200]

Serum Phosphate Concentration

When rats were fed a high-phosphate diet after uninephrectomy, renal calcium and phosphate deposition and tubulointerstitial injury were observed within 5 weeks.[201] Furthermore, in both animals and humans with CKD, dietary phosphate restriction or treatment with oral phosphate binders is associated with reductions in proteinuria and glomerulosclerosis, as well as attenuation of CKD progression.[202-205] Together, these data suggest that phosphate loading or hyperphosphatemia exacerbates renal injury in CKD. In addition, higher levels of the phosphotonin fibroblast growth factor 23 have been identified as an independent predictor of CKD progression.[206,207] In three cohort studies of patients with CKD, higher serum phosphate concentration was identified as an independent risk factor for progression.[27,154,159]

Neutrophil Gelatinase–Associated Lipocalin

Neutrophil gelatinase–associated lipocalin (NGAL) is a small protein released by renal tubule cells in response to injury and has been proposed as an early marker of AKI (see Chapter 29). Studies have revealed that urine NGAL levels are elevated in proportion to the extent of renal damage in patients with various forms of CKD, including diabetic nephropathy and membranous glomerulonephritis.[208,209] Furthermore, in one study of 96 patients with CKD, serum and urine NGAL concentration were inversely correlated with GFR and were independently predictive of CKD progression.[210]

Nephrotoxins

Smoking

In population-based studies, cigarette smoking has been identified as an independent risk factor for various manifestations of CKD, including proteinuria,[211] elevated serum creatinine concentration,[212] decreased estimated GFR,[15,213] and development of ESKD or death in association with CKD (relative HR = 2.6; 95% CI = 1.8 to 3.7).[23] In the study by Haroun and associates,[23] smoking accounted for 31% of the attributable risk for the development of CKD. Smoking has also been shown to increase the risk of progression of CKD caused by diabetes,[214,215] hypertensive nephropathy,[216] glomerulonephritis,[217] lupus nephritis,[218] IgA nephropathy,[219] and autosomal dominant polycystic kidney disease.[219] Randomized trials of the effect of smoking cessation on CKD progression are lacking, but in one observational study, smoking cessation was associated with less progression to macroalbuminuria and a slower rate of GFR decline than was continued smoking among patients with diabetes.[220] Possible mechanisms whereby cigarette smoking may contribute to renal damage include sympathetic nervous system activation, glomerular capillary hypertension, endothelial cell injury, and direct tubulotoxocity.[221]

Alcohol and Recreational Drugs

The role of alcohol consumption as a potential risk factor for CKD remains unclear. One case-control study revealed a significant association between ESKD and consumption of more than two alcoholic drinks per day,[222] whereas another similar study demonstrated no association (with the exception of moonshine alcohol).[223] Some population-based studies have revealed that alcohol consumption is not related to CKD risk,[224,225] but one study demonstrated a significant association of heavy alcohol intake (more than four servings per day) with prevalent CKD, as well as with the risk of developing CKD among participants with normal GFR.[213] Furthermore, heavy alcohol intake substantially increased the risk of CKD progression associated with smoking: in participants who smoked and drank heavily, the risk of developing CKD was increased almost fivefold.[213]

The role of recreational drugs as a risk factor for CKD has not been widely investigated, but one case-control study demonstrated that the use of heroin, cocaine, or other psychedelic drugs was positively associated with the development of ESKD.[226] After reports of a specific renal lesion characterized by proteinuria and focal segmental glomerulosclerosis ("heroin nephropathy"), other investigators reported a wide range of renal lesions in patients with a history of heroin abuse. It is unclear whether the observed renal lesions resulted from direct effects of heroin or are attributable to impurities in the drug or associated blood-borne virus infections and endocarditis.

An association with renal amyloidosis, possibly due to chronic skin infections, has also been reported.[227] Of interest is that heroin abuse was not associated with an increased risk of mild CKD among 647 hypertensive patients, who did evidence an association between illicit drug abuse and CKD.[228]

Cocaine exerts several adverse effects that may induce renal injury, including rhabdomyolysis, vasoconstriction, activation of the renin-angiotensin system, oxidative stress, and increased collagen synthesis.[227] Furthermore, chronic administration of cocaine to rats resulted in multiple renal lesions, including glomerular atrophy and sclerosis, tubule cell necrosis, and areas of interstitial necrosis.[229] Among 647 patients attending a hypertension clinic, a history of any illicit drug use was independently associated with a relative risk of 2.3 (95% CI = 1.0 to 5.1) for mild CKD, whereas use of cocaine and psychedelic drugs was associated with relative risks of 3.0 (95% CI = 1.1 to 8.0) and 3.9 (95% CI = 1.1 to 14.4), respectively.[228]

Analgesics

Analgesic nephropathy is well described as a cause of CKD and ESKD that result from abuse of combination analgesics containing aspirin and phenacetin; this condition was prevalent in Australia and Switzerland until sale of these products was restricted[230] (see Chapter 83). Cohort studies of participants without CKD at the time of baseline measurements have, however, not reported strong associations between analgesic use and the development of CKD. Among 1697 women in the Nurses Health Study, consumption of more than 3000 g of acetaminophen was associated with an increased risk of GFR decline of more than 30 mL/minute/1.73 m² over 11 years (HR = 2.04; 95% CI = 1.28 to 3.24), but use of higher amounts of aspirin or nonsteroidal antiinflammatory drugs (NSAIDs) was not associated with increased risk.[231] Among 4494 male physicians, occasional to moderate use of aspirin, acetaminophen, and NSAIDs was not associated with GFR decline over 14 years.[232] Similarly, in the NHANES studies, habitual use of aspirin, acetaminophen, or ibuprofen was not significantly associated with prevalence of low GFR or albuminuria.[233]

On the other hand, analgesic use may exacerbate the progression of established CKD. In one large study of 19,163 patients with newly diagnosed CKD, use of aspirin, acetaminophen, or NSAIDs was associated with an increased risk of progression to ESKD in a dose-dependent manner. With regard to cyclooxygenase-2 inhibitors, use of rofecoxib—but not celecoxib—was associated with increased risk of ESKD.[234] The use of single-compound acetaminophen or aspirin, however, is reported not to accelerate progression among patients with stages 4 and 5 CKD.[235]

Lead

Overt lead toxicity results in the well-recognized entity of lead nephropathy, characterized by chronic interstitial nephritis and an association with gout. In addition, epidemiologic studies have demonstrated that mild elevations in blood lead levels are associated with moderate reductions in GFR, hypertension, or both in the general population.[236,237] Furthermore, in a prospective study, elevations in blood lead levels and body lead burden within the normal range were identified as important risk factors for CKD progression.[238] Similarly, body lead burden was a risk factor for progression among 108 patients with low-normal values of body lead burden and no history of lead exposure.[239] Moreover, subjects who were randomly assigned to receive chelation therapy exhibited a modest improvement in GFR over 24 months, in contrast to a small decline in those randomly assigned to control conditions (+6.6 ± 10.7 vs. −4.6 ± 4.3 mL/minute/1.73 m^2; $P < 0.001$).[239]

On the other hand, a case-control study of patients in Sweden with incident CKD, neither the CKD nor rate of GFR decline was associated with occupational exposure to lead.[240] In one NHANES study, serum cystatin C, concentration a multivariable equation, or a combined creatinine/cystatin C equation was used to estimate GFR; each equation identified greater reductions in GFR in association with doubling of blood lead levels than did creatinine-based estimates of GFR calculated with the MDRD or Chronic Kidney Disease Epidemiology Collaboration (CKD-EPI) equations.[241]

Cadmium

Chronic exposure to cadmium is also associated with a distinctive nephropathy characterized by proximal tubule damage and low molecular weight proteinuria.[242] Furthermore, low-level cadmium exposure resulting from environmental contamination was associated with tubular proteinuria,[243] and analysis of data from 14,778 participants in the NHANES studies revealed an independent increased risk of albuminuria, reduced GFR, or both between the highest and lowest quartiles of blood cadmium levels.[244] Comparison of the lowest and highest quartiles for blood cadmium and lead levels revealed an even greater increased risk of albuminuria, reduced GFR, or both.[244] In another NHANES study, blood and urine cadmium levels were positively correlated with urine albumin/creatinine ratio and negatively associated with GFR. Higher blood and urine cadmium levels were independently associated with albuminuria, and higher blood cadmium levels were associated with both albuminuria and reduced GFR.[242] Occupational exposure and low-level environmental exposure to cadmium were associated with an increased risk of ESKD in a population-based study in Sweden.[245]

Renal Risk Scores

The investigation of risk factors that predict the development and/or progression of CKD in diverse populations has led to the observation that a relatively small group of risk factors appears to be common to different forms of CKD. This observation supports the notion of a "common pathway" of mechanisms that underlie the progression of CKD. It has also led to the proposal that these common risk factors could be combined to develop a "renal risk score" to predict the development and future risk of progression of CKD in a manner analogous to the Framingham risk score for predicting cardiovascular risk in the general population.[246] Since 2006, considerable progress has been made in developing such risk scores. They may conveniently be divided into two groups: those that apply to the general population (i.e., persons without CKD at the time of baseline measurements) and those that predict the risk of progression in patients in whom CKD has already been

diagnosed. In addition, researchers in one study developed a risk score to predict the development of CKD after an episode of AKI (discussed below).[253]

Renal Risk Scores in the General Population

To date, six risk scores (summarized in Table 21-3) have been proposed to assess the risk of CKD in the general population and, in some cases, subsequent progression of the disease. In the first study, Bang and colleagues[247] used data from 8530 adults included in the NHANES studies to identify risk factors for prevalent CKD (defined as estimated GFR of <60 mL/minute/1.73 m^2). Bang and colleagues proposed a risk score that was based on nine variables: age, female sex, hypertension, anemia, diabetes, peripheral vascular disease, history of cardiovascular disease, congestive heart failure, and proteinuria. The area under the receiver operating characteristic (ROC) curve was high at 0.88, and a score of 4 or higher resulted in a sensitivity of 92% and specificity of 68%. The positive predictive value was low, at 18%, but the negative predictive value was 99%. External validation with data from the Atherosclerosis Risk in Communities (ARIC) study yielded an area under the ROC curve of 0.71.[247] ARIC was a cross-sectional study, and the risk score therefore does not predict the risk of future CKD; rather, it identifies individuals at increased risk of having current, undiagnosed CKD. As such, it would be useful for guiding efforts to screen populations for CKD, but it gives no information about the future risk of CKD progression. The applicability of the score to general populations is somewhat weakened by the inclusion of two variables that require prior laboratory testing: anemia and proteinuria. Furthermore, the presence of significant proteinuria is sufficient to diagnose CKD in the absence of any reduction in GFR

Another scoring system was developed to predict the risk of incident CKD through the use of combined data from 14,155 participants in the ARIC study and the Cardiovascular Health Study (CHS), aged 45 years or older, with baseline estimated GFR of more than 60 mL/minute/1.73 m^2. After identifying 10 predictors of incident CKD (defined as estimated GFR of <60 mL/minute/1.73 m^2 during follow-up of up to 9 years), Kshirsagar and colleagues[248] proposed a simplified model that was based on eight categorical variables: age, anemia, female sex, hypertension, diabetes mellitus, peripheral vascular disease, and history of congestive heart failure or cardiovascular disease. This formula yielded an area under the ROC curve of 0.69, and a score of 3 or higher resulted in 69% sensitivity and 58% specificity, but positive predictive value was low, at only 17%.[248]

In a similar study, O'Seaghdha and associates[249] used data from 2490 participants in the Framingham Heart Study to produce a risk score for incident CKD (defined as estimated GFR of <60 mL/minute/1.73 m^2). The final model included age, diabetes, hypertension, baseline estimated GFR, and albuminuria; the area under the ROC curve was 0.813. External validation was performed with data from the ARIC study (areas under the ROC curve = 0.79 and 0.75 in white and black patients, respectively).[249]

In one other study, Chien and colleagues[250] developed a risk score for incident CKD (defined as estimated GFR of <60 mL/minute/1.73 m^2) in 5168 Chinese participants. Age, BMI, diastolic blood pressure, type 2 diabetes, previous

TABLE 21-3   Renal Risk Scores for the General Population

DATA SOURCE	SCORED[247]	SCORED2[248]	CHINESE STUDY[250]	FRAMINGHAM[249]	QKIDNEY[251]	PREVEND[139]
Population	NHANES	CHS and ARIC	General population	Framingham Heart Study	QResearch	eGFR >45
Outcome	eGFR <60 (prevalent)	eGFR <60 (incident)	eGFR <60 (incident)	eGFR <60 (incident)	CKD ESKD	Rapid ↓ GFR
Factors	Age Female HT DM PVD CVD CCF Anemia Proteinuria	Age Female HT DM PVD CVD CCF Anemia	Age BMI Type 2 DM Stroke DBP Proteinuria Uric acid Hemoglobin A_{1C} Glucose level	Age HT DM eGFR Albuminuria	Age Ethnicity Deprivation Family history Smoking HT DM PVD CVD CCF RA SBP BMI Use of NSAIDs	Age HT SBP eGFR Albuminuria C-reactive protein
Area under ROC curve	0.88	0.69	0.77	0.81	0.88	0.84
Validation	ARIC	CHS and ARIC	General population	ARIC	THIN	Internal

ARIC, Atherosclerosis Risk in Communities; *BMI,* body mass index; *CCF,* congestive cardiac failure; *CHS,* Cardiovascular Health Study; *CKD,* chronic kidney disease; *CVD,* cardiovascular disease; *DBP,* diastolic blood pressure; *DM,* diabetes mellitus; eGFR, estimated glomerular filtration rate; *HT,* hypertension; *NHANES,* National Health and Nutrition Examination Survey; *NSAIDs,* nonsteroidal antiinflammatory drugs; *PREVEND,* Prevention of Renal and Vascular End-stage Disease; *PVD,* peripheral vascular disease; *RA,* rheumatoid arthritis; *ROC,* receiver operating characteristic; *SBP,* systolic blood pressure; *SCORED,* SCreening for Occult REnal Disease; *THIN,* The Health Improvement Network.

stroke, serum uric acid level, postprandial blood glucose level, hemoglobin A_{1C} concentration, and proteinuria with values exceeding 100 mg/dL were included in two risk scores (one using clinical variables only and a second with all variables) for which the area under the ROC curve was 0.77. The study was limited by relatively short follow-up (median, 2.2 years) and a low area under the ROC curve of 0.67 for external validation data.[250] These scores are useful in identifying individuals at higher risk of developing CKD for purposes of monitoring or intervention to reduce risk, but they do not distinguish the minority who are at risk of progressing to ESKD from the majority who are at low risk.

In an attempt to develop a risk score that would identify only individuals at high risk, another group evaluated data from patients (775,091 women and 799,658 men, aged 35 to 74 years, without a recorded diagnosis of CKD) in 368 primary care practices in the United Kingdom. Two outcomes were studied over a period of up to 7 years: moderate-severe CKD (defined as the need for kidney transplantation or dialysis; diagnosis of nephropathy; proteinuria; or estimated GFR of <45 mL/minute/1.73 m²) and ESKD (defined as the need for kidney transplantation or dialysis, or estimated GFR of <15 mL/minute/1.73 m²). Separate risk scores were developed for men and women. The variables in the final model for moderate-severe CKD included age, ethnicity, social deprivation, smoking, BMI, systolic blood pressure, diabetes, rheumatoid arthritis, cardiovascular disease, treated hypertension,

congestive cardiac failure, peripheral vascular disease, use of NSAIDs, and family history of kidney disease. For women, it also included systemic lupus erythematosus and history of kidney stones. The model for ESKD was similar but did not include NSAID use. Internal and external validation was performed, and the area under the ROC curve ranged from 0.818 to 0.878.[251] One important limitation of this study is that it was observational and is therefore likely to be subject to significant bias. Furthermore, in only 56% of participants was a serum creatinine concentration recorded at inclusion, and it is therefore probable that several had undiagnosed CKD. The composite outcome of "moderate to severe CKD" comprised several disparate variables and is therefore not clinically useful, but the ESKD outcome is relevant because it identifies only the minority at increased risk of severe progression. This study also illustrates the utility of a risk score that could be programmed into primary care computer systems to alert family practitioners to patients who are at risk of progression to ESKD.

Data from 6809 participants in the PREVEND study were used to develop a risk score with the primary outcome of progressive CKD over 6.4 years, defined as the 20% most rapid decline in GFR and estimated GFR of less than 60 mL/minute/1.73 m². The final risk score included baseline estimated GFR, age, albuminuria, systolic blood pressure, C-reactive protein concentration, and known hypertension. The area under the ROC curve was 0.84, and internal validation was

TABLE 21-4 Renal Risk Scores for Patients with Chronic Kidney Disease

DATA SOURCE	RENAAL STUDY[66]	AIPRD STUDY[252]	IGAN STUDY[153]	KAISER PERMANENTE COHORT[160]	CRIB STUDY[27]	SUNNYBROOK HOSPITAL COHORT[154]
Disease	Diabetic nephropathy	CKD	IgA nephropathy	CKD, stages 3 to 4	CKD, stages 3 to 5	CKD, stages 3 to 5
Variables		Age	Age Male	Age Male		Age Male
	Creatinine UACR	Creatinine UPE SBP	1/creatinine Proteinuria* SBP	Estimated GFR Not applicable Hypertension Diabetes mellitus	Female Creatinine UACR	eGFR UACR
	Serum albumin Hemoglobin		Serum total protein	Anemia		Serum albumin
					Serum phosphate	Calcium Serum phosphate Serum bicarbonate
			Histologic grade Hematuria			
Outcome	ESKD	ESKD or doubling of serum creatinine level	ESKD	RRT	ESKD	ESKD
Area under ROC curve		0.939	0.89		0.873	0.917
Validation	None	None	None	None	External	External

*Urine dipstick measurement.

AIPRD, ACE Inhibition in Progressive Renal Disease; *CRIB,* Chronic Renal Impairment in Birmingham; *ESKD,* end-stage kidney disease; e*GFR,* glomerular filtration rate; *IgAN,* IgA nephropathy; *RENAAL,* Reduction of Endpoints in NIDDM with the Angiotensin II Antagonist Losartan; *ROC,* receiver operating characteristic; *RRT,* renal replacement therapy; *SBP,* systolic blood pressure; *UACR,* urine albumin/creatinine ratio; *UPE,* urinary protein excretion (24-hour).

performed using a bootstrapping procedure.[139] Despite this, the risk score has relatively low sensitivity and positive predictive value. The proposed threshold score of 27 or higher identified 2.1% of the population as being at high risk but with only 15.7% sensitivity and a positive predictive value of 28.1%. The specificity and negative predictive value were high, at 98.4% and 96.7%, respectively. Thus, a low score is useful in identifying individuals at low risk, but a high score does not identify the majority of individuals at high risk. Selecting a lower threshold would improve sensitivity with some reduction in specificity and could be used to identify a group at intermediate risk for closer monitoring. Limitations of this study are that it was performed in a white population, and the data have not been validated externally. External validation in other populations is therefore required before this risk score can be considered for clinical use.

Risk Scores for Patients with Diagnosed Chronic Kidney Disease

At least six risk scores have been developed for patients with diagnosed CKD in a variety of study populations and are summarized in Table 21-4. In analysis of data from 1513 patients with diabetic nephropathy included in the RENAAL study,[66] urine albumin/creatinine ratio, serum albumin concentration, serum creatinine concentration, and hemoglobin concentration were identified as independent risk factors for ESKD. A risk score was derived from the coefficients of these variables in the Cox proportional hazards model, which successfully separated the participants into quartiles of ESKD risk (Figure 21-4), with a marked difference in risk between the first and last quartile (6.7 versus 257.2 per thousand patient years).[66]

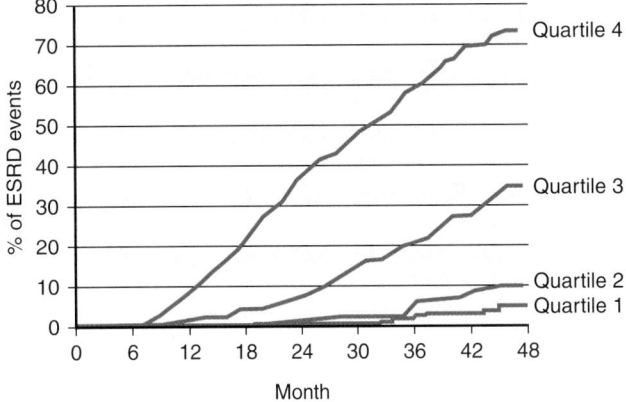

FIGURE 21-4 Kaplan-Meier curve for the end-stage kidney disease (ESKD) endpoint, stratified by quartile of risk score in 1513 patients with diabetic nephropathy from the Reduction of Endpoints in NIDDM with the Angiotensin II Antagonist Losartan (RENAAL) study. (From Keane WF, Zhang Z, Lyle PA, et al: Risk scores for predicting outcomes in patients with type 2 diabetes and nephropathy: the RENAAL Study, *Clin J Am Soc Nephrol* 1:761-767, 2006.)

Among 1860 patients with nondiabetic CKD from a combined database of 11 clinical trails, Cox proportional hazards analysis revealed age, serum creatinine concentration, proteinuria, and systolic blood pressure as independent risk factors for the combined endpoint of time to ESKD or doubling of creatinine concentration. Using methods similar to those used in the RENAAL study, Kent and colleagues[252] developed a risk model based on these variables to stratify patients into quartiles of risk. For control patients, the annual incidence of the combined endpoint was 0.4% in the lowest quartile, in contrast to 28.7% in the highest quartile; in those randomly assigned to receive ACE inhibitor treatment, the annual incidences were 0.2% and 19.7% in the lowest and highest quartiles, respectively.[252]

In analysis of data from 2269 patients with IgA nephropathy, Wakai and associates[153] identified systolic blood pressure, proteinuria (assessed with urine dipstick test), serum total protein concentration, 1/serum creatinine, and histologic grade at initial biopsy as predictors of time to ESKD. Age, gender, and severity of hematuria were added to these variables to develop a scoring system for estimating the 4- and 7-year cumulative incidences of ESKD. There was close agreement between estimated and observed risks (area under ROC curve = 0.939).[153]

In a retrospective study, data from 9782 patients with stages 3 and 4 CKD were analyzed with regard to a primary outcome of onset of renal replacement therapy (dialysis or transplantation). Six independent risk factors—age, male sex, estimated GFR, hypertension, diabetes, and anemia—were identified and incorporated into a risk score that stratified participants into quintiles of risk. The risk of progression to renal replacement therapy was 19% in the quintile at highest risk, in comparison with 0.2% in the quintile at lowest risk. Area under the ROC curve was 0.89, and observed risk differed from predicted by less than 1%.[160] One limitation of this study (apart from its retrospective design) was the lack of data regarding proteinuria. Among 382 patients with stages 3 to 5 CKD from the CRIB study, independent risk factors for progression to ESKD during a mean of 4.1 years of follow-up were female sex, serum creatinine concentration, serum phosphate concentration, and urine albumin/creatinine ratio. A risk score was derived from these variables (area under ROC curve = 0.873) and externally validated in a similar cohort of patients with stages 3 to 5 CKD (East Kent cohort); this score yielded an area under the ROC curve of 0.91, even though urine albumin/creatinine ratios were not available in the validation cohort.[27]

Last, a risk score for predicting ESKD was developed with data from a cohort of 3449 Canadian patients with stages 3 to 5 CKD (Sunnybrook Hospital cohort). The variables included age, male sex, estimated GFR, albuminuria, serum calcium level, serum phosphate concentration, serum bicarbonate concentration, and serum albumin concentration (area under ROC curve = 0.917). External validation was performed with data from a separate cohort of 4942 patients with stages 3 to 5 CKD (British Columbia CKD Registry), which yielded an area under the ROC curve of 0.841. There was close agreement between predicted and observed risk in the validation cohort (Figure 21-5).[154] The shared advantage of the latter two risk scores is that both have been externally validated. In addition, both include variables that are all available to a biochemistry laboratory; therefore, laboratories could report a risk score with each estimate of GFR.

Risk Scores for Predicting Chronic Kidney Disease after Acute Kidney Injury

The risk of CKD and progression to ESKD escalates after an episode of AKI. Researchers have therefore tried to develop a risk score to identify patients at highest risk. In one study population of 5351 predominantly male veterans with a primary admission diagnosis of AKI, three risk prediction models were

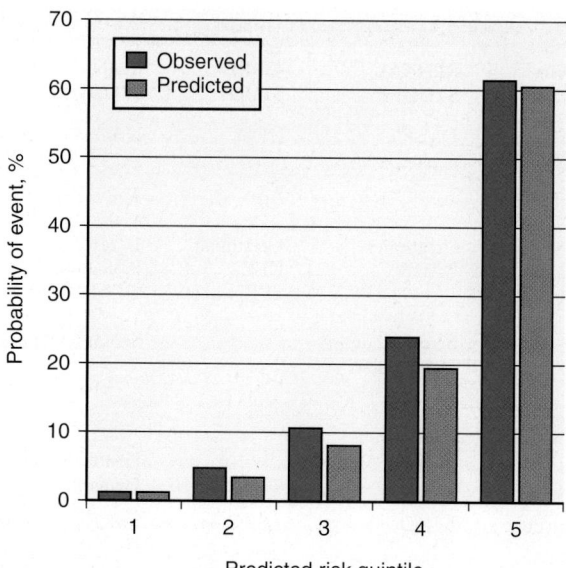

FIGURE 21-5 Renal risk score: predicted versus observed risk of developing end-stage kidney disease (ESKD) at 3 years in a validation cohort of patients with stages 3 to 5 chronic kidney disease (CKD). (From Tangri N, Stevens LA, Griffith J, et al: A predictive model for progression of chronic kidney disease to kidney failure, *JAMA* 305:1553-1559, 2011.)

developed to predict the risk of progression to CKD stage 4. Risk factors that entered the models included increased age, non–African American race, time at risk, low serum albumin concentration, diabetes, lower baseline estimated GFR, higher mean serum creatinine concentration during hospitalization, and severity of AKI, as assessed by the Risk, Injury, Failure, Loss and End-stage kidney disease (RIFLE) score or need for dialysis. Area under the ROC curve ranged from 0.77 to 0.82 for the three models. At the optimal cutpoint, sensitivity ranged from 0.71 to 0.77, and specificity ranged from 0.64 to 0.74. External validation was performed on a control population of 11,589 patients admitted for pneumonia or myocardial infarction and yielded good prediction accuracy (area under ROC curve ranged from 0.81 to 0.82). Sensitivity at the optimal cutpoint ranged from 0.66 to 0.71 and specificity from 0.61 to 0.70.[253]

Further validation in other populations that include a more representative proportion of women is required before these risk models can be applied. A validated risk score for patients recovering from AKI may prove very important for identifying patients at high risk so that closer follow-up and intervention can reduce the risk of progressive CKD. However, more trials are needed to evaluate the effect of renoprotective interventions in this setting.

Future Considerations

Considerable progress has been made since 2000 in identifying risk factors that help predict the progression of CKD in diverse cohorts from the general population and nephrology clinics. The variation between studies is probably attributable to differences in the populations and in the variables studied. Remarkably, a relatively small group of risk factors appears common to many studies, and much progress has been made in developing risk scores based on these variables to predict

CKD progression. Further evaluation of proposed risk scores is necessary to determine their applicability to unselected populations.

Separate risk scores will probably be required for patients without CKD to predict the future risk of developing CKD and for patients in whom CKD has already been diagnosed, although some variables included would clearly be common to both risk scores. It would be an advantage if a risk score applicable to the general population did not depend on laboratory variables, whereas for the population with CKD, a score based entirely on laboratory variables would facilitate automated reporting of a risk score.

Future studies will probably focus on the use of novel biomarkers and genetic factors as risk factors (see Chapter 29) and variables in risk scores, although measurement of such markers will probably be more expensive than that of the simple risk factors used to date. Further studies are also required to develop risk scores to predict cardiovascular risk in patients with CKD that take into account the close association between CKD and cardiovascular disease.

References

1. Kidney Disease Outcomes and Quality Initiative. K/DOQI clinical practice guidelines for chronic kidney disease: evaluation, classification, and stratification. *Am J Kidney Dis.* 2002;39:S1-S266.
2. Centers for Disease Control and Prevention. Prevalence of chronic kidney disease and associated risk factors—United States, 1999-2004. *MMWR Morb Mortal Wkly Rep.* 2007;56:161-165.
3. Boulware LE, Jaar BG, Tarver-Carr ME, et al. Screening for proteinuria in US adults: a cost-effectiveness analysis. *JAMA.* 2003;290:3101-3114.
4. Kiberd BA, Clase CM. Cumulative risk for developing end-stage renal disease in the US population. *J Am Soc Nephrol.* 2002;13:1635-1644.
5. Clase CM, Garg AX, Kiberd BA. Classifying kidney problems: can we avoid framing risks as diseases? *BMJ.* 2004;329:912-915.
6. Hunsicker LG, Adler S, Caggiula A, et al. Predictors of the progression of renal disease in the Modification of Diet in Renal Disease Study. *Kidney Int.* 1997;51:1908-1919.
7. Hallan SI, Dahl K, Oien CM, et al. Screening strategies for chronic kidney disease in the general population: follow-up of cross sectional health survey. *BMJ.* 2006;333:1047.
8. Weiner DE, Tighiouart H, Elsayed EF, et al. The Framingham predictive instrument in chronic kidney disease. *J Am Coll Cardiol.* 2007;50:217-224.
9. Ibrahim HN, Foley R, Tan L, et al. Long-term consequences of kidney donation. *N Engl J Med.* 2009;360:459-469.
10. Nenov VD, Taal MW, Sakharova OV, et al. Multi-hit nature of chronic renal disease. *Curr Opin Nephrol Hypertension.* 2000;9:85-97.
11. Jeon HG, Jeong IG, Lee JW, et al. Prognostic factors for chronic kidney disease after curative surgery in patients with small renal tumors. *Urology.* 2009;74:1064-1068.
12. Roderick PJ, Atkins RJ, Smeeth L, et al. CKD and mortality risk in older people: a community-based population study in the United Kingdom. *Am J Kidney Dis.* 2009;53:950-960.
13. Lindeman RD, Tobin J, Shock NW. Longitudinal studies on the rate of decline in renal function with age. *J Am Ger Soc.* 1985;33:278-285.
14. Iseki K, Iseki C, Ikemiya Y, et al. Risk of developing end-stage renal disease in a cohort of mass screening. *Kidney Int.* 1996;49:800-805.
15. Fox CS, Larson MG, Leip EP, et al. Predictors of new-onset kidney disease in a community-based population. *JAMA.* 2004;291:844-850.
16. Weller JM, Wu SC, Ferguson CW, et al. End-stage renal disease in Michigan. Incidence, underlying causes, prevalence, and modalities of treatment. *Am J Nephrol.* 1985;5:84-95.
17. Shulman NB, Ford CE, Hall WD, et al. Prognostic value of serum creatinine and effect of treatment of hypertension on renal function. Results from the Hypertension Detection and Follow-up Program. The Hypertension Detection and Follow-up Program Cooperative Group. *Hypertension.* 1989;13(5 suppl):I80-I93.
18. Eriksen BO, Ingebretsen OC. The progression of chronic kidney disease: a 10-year population-based study of the effects of gender and age. *Kidney Int.* 2006;69:375-382.
19. O'Hare AM, Choi AI, Bertenthal D, et al. Age affects outcomes in chronic kidney disease. *J Am Soc Nephrol.* 2007;18:2758-2765.
20. Evans M, Fryzek JP, Elinder CG, et al. The natural history of chronic renal failure: results from an unselected, population-based, inception cohort in Sweden. *Am J Kidney Dis.* 2005;46:863-870.
21. Nitsch D, Nonyane BA, Smeeth L, et al. CKD and Hospitalization in the elderly: a community-based cohort study in the United Kingdom. *Am J Kidney Dis.* 2011;57:664-672.
22. Baylis C. Age-dependent glomerular damage in the rat. Dissociation between glomerular injury and both glomerular hypertension and hypertrophy. Male gender as a primary risk factor. *J Clin Invest.* 1994;94:1823-1829.
23. Haroun MK, Jaar BG, Hoffman SC, et al. Risk factors for chronic kidney disease: a prospective study of 23,534 men and women in Washington County, Maryland. *J Am Soc Nephrol.* 2003;14:2934-2941.
24. United States Renal Data System. Incidence and prevalence, *USRDS Annual Data Report,* 2005:66-80. Available at: http://www.usrds.org/2005/pdf/02_incid_prev_05.pdf. Accessed June 24, 2011.
25. Neugarten J, Acharya A, Silbiger SR. Effect of gender on the progression of nondiabetic renal disease: a meta-analysis. *J Am Soc Nephrol.* 2000;11:319-329.
26. Jafar TH, Schmid CH, Stark PC, et al. The rate of progression of renal disease may not be slower in women compared with men: a patient-level meta-analysis. *Nephrol Dial Transplant.* 2003;18:2047-2053.
27. Landray MJ, Emberson JR, Blackwell L, et al. Prediction of ESRD and death among people with CKD: the Chronic Renal Impairment in Birmingham (CRIB) prospective cohort study. *Am J Kidney Dis.* 2010;56:1082-1094.
28. Klag MJ, Whelton PK, Randall BL, et al. End-stage renal disease in African-American and white men. 16-year MRFIT findings. *JAMA.* 1997;277:1293-1298.
29. Tarver-Carr ME, Powe NR, Eberhardt MS, et al. Excess risk of chronic kidney disease among African-American versus white subjects in the United States: a population-based study of potential explanatory factors. *J Am Soc Nephrol.* 2002;13:2363-2370.
30. Krop JS, Coresh J, Chambless LE, et al. A community-based study of explanatory factors for the excess risk for early renal function decline in blacks vs whites with diabetes: the Atherosclerosis Risk in Communities study. *Arch Intern Med.* 1999;159:1777-1783.
31. McClellan W, Warnock DG, McClure L, et al. Racial differences in the prevalence of chronic kidney disease among participants in the Reasons for Geographic and Racial Differences in Stroke (REGARDS) cohort study. *J Am Soc Nephrol.* 2006;17:1710-1715.
32. United States Renal Data System. *Annual data report: vol 2 atlas of ESRD,* 2010. Available at www.usrds.org/atlas.htm. Accessed June 24, 2011.
33. Roderick PJ, Raleigh VS, Hallam L, et al. The need and demand for renal replacement therapy in ethnic minorities in England. *J Epidemiol Comm Health.* 1996;50:334-339.
34. de Zeeuw D, Ramjit D, Zhang Z, et al. Renal risk and renoprotection among ethnic groups with type 2 diabetic nephropathy: a post hoc analysis of RENAAL. *Kidney Int.* 2006;69:1675-1682.
35. Hoy WE, Megill DM, Hughson MD. Epidemic renal disease of unknown etiology in the Zuni Indians. *Am J Kidney Dis.* 1987;9:485-496.
36. Pugh JA, Stern MP, Haffner SM, et al. Excess incidence of treatment of end-stage renal disease in Mexican Americans. *Am J Epidemiol.* 1988;127:135-144.
37. Spencer JL, Silva DT, Snelling P, et al. An epidemic of renal failure among Australian Aboriginals. *Med J Aust.* 1998;168:537-541.
38. Freedman BI, Volkova NV, Satko SG, et al. Population-based screening for family history of end-stage renal disease among incident dialysis patients. *Am J Nephrol.* 2005;25:529-535.
39. Jurkovitz C, Franch H, Shoham D, et al. Family members of patients treated for ESRD have high rates of undetected kidney disease. *Am J Kidney Dis.* 2002;40:1173-1178.
40. Lei HH, Perneger TV, Klag MJ, et al. Familial aggregation of renal disease in a population-based case-control study. *J Am Soc Nephrol.* 1998;9:1270-1276.
41. Spray BJ, Atassi NG, Tuttle AB, et al. Familial risk, age at onset, and cause of end-stage renal disease in white Americans. *J Am Soc Nephrol.* 1995;5:1806-1810.
42. Freedman BI, Hicks PJ, Bostrom MA, et al. Non–muscle myosin heavy chain 9 gene *MYH9* associations in African Americans with clinically diagnosed type 2 diabetes mellitus–associated ESRD. *Nephrol Dial Transplant.* 2009;24:3366-3371.
43. Freedman BI, Hicks PJ, Bostrom MA, et al. Polymorphisms in the non–muscle myosin heavy chain 9 gene (*MYH9*) are strongly associated with end-stage renal disease historically attributed to hypertension in African Americans. *Kidney Int.* 2009;75:736-745.
44. Li PK, Weening JJ, Dirks J, et al. Participants of ISNCWoPoPoRD: A report with consensus statements of the International Society of Nephrology 2004 Consensus Workshop on Prevention of Progression of Renal Disease, Hong Kong, June 29, 2004. *Kidney Int Suppl.* 2005;94:s2-s7:2005.

45. Faronato PP, Maioli M, Tonolo G, et al. Clustering of albumin excretion rate abnormalities in Caucasian patients with NIDDM. *Diabetologia.* 1997;40:816-823.

46. Boger CA, Chen MH, Tin A, et al. *CUBN* is a gene locus for albuminuria. *J Am Soc Nephrol.* 2011;22:555-570.

47. Chambers JC, Zhang W, Lord GM, et al. Genetic loci influencing kidney function and chronic kidney disease. *Nat Genet.* 2010;42:373-375.

48. Kottgen A, Pattaro C, Boger CA, et al. New loci associated with kidney function and chronic kidney disease. *Nat Genet.* 2010;42:376-384.

49. Hostetter TH, Olson JL, Rennke HG, et al. Hyperfiltration in remnant nephrons: a potentially adverse response to renal ablation. *J Am Soc Nephrol.* 2001;12:1315-1325.

50. Zatz R, Dunn BR, Meyer TW, et al. Prevention of diabetic glomerulopathy by pharmacological amelioration of glomerular capillary hypertension. *J Clin Invest.* 1986;77:1925-1930.

51. Hoy WE, Ingelfinger JR, Hallan S, et al. The early development of the kidney and the implications for future health. *J Develop Orig Health Dis.* 2010;1:216-233.

52. Puelles VG, Hoy WE, Hughson MD, et al. Glomerular number and size variability and risk for kidney disease. *Curr Opin Nephrol Hypertens.* 2011;20:7-15.

53. Keller G, Zimmer G, Mall G, et al. Nephron number in patients with primary hypertension. *N Engl J Med.* 2003;348:101-108.

54. McNamara BJ, Diouf B, Hughson MD, et al. Renal pathology, glomerular number and volume in a West African urban community. *Nephrol Dial Transplant.* 2008;23:2576-2585.

55. Manalich R, Reyes L, Herrera M, et al. Relationship between weight at birth and the number and size of renal glomeruli in humans: a histomorphometric study. *Kidney Int.* 2000;58:770-773.

56. Hughson M, Farris 3rd AB, Douglas-Denton R, et al. Glomerular number and size in autopsy kidneys: the relationship to birth weight. *Kidney Int.* 2003;63:2113-2122.

57. Godfrey KM, Barker DJ. Fetal programming and adult health. *Public Health Nutr.* 2001;4:611-624.

58. White SL, Perkovic V, Cass A, et al. Is low birth weight an antecedent of CKD in later life? A systematic review of observational studies. *Am J Kidney Dis.* 2009;54:248-261.

59. Novick AC, Gephardt G, Guz B, et al. Long-term follow-up after partial removal of a solitary kidney. *N Engl J Med.* 1991;325:1058-1062.

60. Kasiske BL, Ma JZ, Louis TA, et al. Long-term effects of reduced renal mass in humans. *Kidney Int.* 1995;48:814-819.

61. Lentine KL, Schnitzler MA, Xiao H, et al. Racial variation in medical outcomes among living kidney donors. *N Engl J Med.* 2010;363:724-732.

62. Steffes MW, Brown DM, Mauer SM. Diabetic glomerulopathy following unilateral nephrectomy in the rat. *Diabetes.* 1978;27:35-41.

63. Ravani P, Tripepi G, Malberti F, et al. Asymmetrical dimethylarginine predicts progression to dialysis and death in patients with chronic kidney disease: a competing risks modeling approach. *J Am Soc Nephrol.* 2005;16:2449-2455.

64. Gansevoort RT, Matsushita K, van der Velde M, et al. Lower estimated GFR and higher albuminuria are associated with adverse kidney outcomes in both general and high-risk populations. A collaborative meta-analysis of general and high-risk population cohorts. *Kidney Int.* 2011;79:1341-1352.

65. Astor BC, Matsushita K, Gansevoort RT, et al. Lower estimated glomerular filtration rate and higher albuminuria are associated with mortality and end-stage renal disease. A collaborative meta-analysis of kidney disease population cohorts. *Kidney Int.* 2011;79:1331-1340.

66. Keane WF, Zhang Z, Lyle PA, et al. Risk scores for predicting outcomes in patients with type 2 diabetes and nephropathy: The RENAAL study. *Clin J Am Soc Nephrol.* 2006;1:761-767.

67. Wald R, Quinn RR, Luo J, et al. Chronic dialysis and death among survivors of acute kidney injury requiring dialysis. *JAMA.* 2009;302:1179-1185.

68. Lo LJ, Go AS, Chertow GM, et al. Dialysis-requiring acute renal failure increases the risk of progressive chronic kidney disease. *Kidney Int.* 2009;76:893-899.

69. Ishani A, Xue JL, Himmelfarb J, et al. Acute kidney injury increases risk of ESRD among elderly. *J Am Soc Nephrol.* 2009;20:223-228.

70. Amdur RL, Chawla LS, Amodeo S, et al. Outcomes following diagnosis of acute renal failure in U.S. veterans: focus on acute tubular necrosis. *Kidney Int.* 2009;76:1089-1097.

71. Hsu CY, Chertow GM, McCulloch CE, et al. Nonrecovery of kidney function and death after acute on chronic renal failure. *Clin J Am Soc Nephrol.* 2009;4:891-898.

72. Basile DP, Donohoe D, Roethe K, et al. Renal ischemic injury results in permanent damage to peritubular capillaries and influences long-term function. *Am J Physiol Renal Physiol.* 2001;281:F887-F899.

73. Klag MJ, Whelton PK, Randall BL, et al. Blood pressure and end-stage renal disease in men. *New Engl J Med.* 1996;334:13-18.

74. Hsu CY, McCulloch CE, Darbinian J, et al. Elevated blood pressure and risk of end-stage renal disease in subjects without baseline kidney disease. *Arch Intern Med.* 2005;165:923-928.

75. Forman JP, Brenner BM. "Hypertension" and "microalbuminuria": the bell tolls for thee. *Kidney Int.* 2006;69:22-28.

76. Klahr S, Levey AS, Beck GJ, et al. The effects of dietary protein restriction and blood-pressure control on the progression of chronic renal disease. Modification of Diet in Renal Disease Study Group. *N Engl J Med.* 1994;330:877-884.

77. Peterson JC, Adler S, Burkart JM, et al. Blood pressure control, proteinuria, and the progression of renal disease. The Modification of Diet in Renal Disease Study. *Ann Intern Med.* 1995;123:754-762.

78. Sarnak MJ, Greene T, Wang X, et al. The effect of a lower target blood pressure on the progression of kidney disease: long-term follow-up of the modification of diet in renal disease study. *Ann Intern Med.* 2005;142:342-351.

79. Wright Jr JT, Bakris G, Greene T, et al. Effect of blood pressure lowering and antihypertensive drug class on progression of hypertensive kidney disease: results from the AASK trial. *JAMA.* 2002;288:2421-2431.

80. Appel LJ, Wright Jr JT, Greene T, et al. Intensive blood-pressure control in hypertensive chronic kidney disease. *N Engl J Med.* 2010;363:918-929.

81. Ruggenenti P, Perna A, Loriga G, et al. Blood-pressure control for renoprotection in patients with non-diabetic chronic renal disease (REIN-2): multicentre, randomised controlled trial. *Lancet.* 2005;365:939-946.

82. Schmitz PG, O'Donnell MP, Kasiske BL, et al. Renal injury in obese Zucker rats: glomerular hemodynamic alterations and effects of enalapril. *Am J Physiol.* 1992;263:F496-F502.

83. Park SK, Kang SK. Renal function and hemodynamic study in obese Zucker rats. *Korean J Intern Med.* 1995;10:48-53.

84. Wolf G. After all those fat years: renal consequences of obesity. *Nephrol Dial Transplant.* 2003;18:2471-2474.

85. Sowers JR, Whaley-Connell A, Epstein M. Narrative review: the emerging clinical implications of the role of aldosterone in the metabolic syndrome and resistant hypertension. *Ann Intern Med.* 2009;150:776-783.

86. Ix JH, Sharma K. Mechanisms linking obesity, chronic kidney disease, and fatty liver disease: the roles of fetuin-A, adiponectin, and AMPK. *J Am Soc Nephrol.* 2010;21:406-412.

87. Chagnac A, Weinstein T, Herman M, et al. The effects of weight loss on renal function in patients with severe obesity. *J Am Soc Nephrol.* 2003;14:1480-1486.

88. Gelber RP, Kurth T, Kausz AT, et al. Association between body mass index and CKD in apparently healthy men. *Am J Kidney Dis.* 2005;46:871-880.

89. Hsu CY, McCulloch CE, Iribarren C, et al. Body mass index and risk for end-stage renal disease. *Ann Intern Med.* 2006;144:21-28.

90. Kambham N, Markowitz GS, Valeri AM, et al. Obesity-related glomerulopathy: an emerging epidemic. *Kidney Int.* 2001;59:1498-1509.

91. Ritz E, Koleganova N, Piecha G. Is there an obesity-metabolic syndrome related glomerulopathy? *Curr Opin Nephrol Hypertens.* 2011;20:44-49.

92. Chen J, Muntner P, Hamm LL, et al. The metabolic syndrome and chronic kidney disease in U.S. adults. *Ann Intern Med.* 2004;140:167-174.

93. Kurella M, Lo JC, Chertow GM. Metabolic syndrome and the risk for chronic kidney disease among nondiabetic adults. *J Am Soc Nephrol.* 2005;16:2134-2140.

94. Pinto-Sietsma SJ, Navis G, Janssen WM, et al. A central body fat distribution is related to renal function impairment, even in lean subjects. *Am J Kidney Dis.* 2003;41:733-741.

95. Bonnet F, Deprele C, Sassolas A, et al. Excessive body weight as a new independent risk factor for clinical and pathological progression in primary IgA nephritis. *Am J Kidney Dis.* 2001;37:720-727.

96. Gonzalez E, Gutierrez E, Morales E, et al. Factors influencing the progression of renal damage in patients with unilateral renal agenesis and remnant kidney. *Kidney Int.* 2005;68:263-270.

97. Meier-Kriesche HU, Arndorfer JA, Kaplan B. The impact of body mass index on renal transplant outcomes: a significant independent risk factor for graft failure and patient death. *Transplantation.* 2002;73:70-74.

98. Adams TD, Gress RE, Smith SC, et al. Long-term mortality after gastric bypass surgery. *N Engl J Med.* 2007;357:753-761.

99. Sjostrom L, Narbro K, Sjostrom CD, et al. Effects of bariatric surgery on mortality in Swedish obese subjects. *N Engl J Med.* 2007;357:741-752.

100. Afshinnia F, Wilt TJ, Duval S, et al. Weight loss and proteinuria: systematic review of clinical trials and comparative cohorts. *Nephrol Dial Transplant.* 2010;25:1173-1183.

101. Alexander JW, Goodman HR, Hawver LR, et al. Improvement and stabilization of chronic kidney disease after gastric bypass. *Surg Obes Relat Dis.* 2009;5:237-241.

102. Agrawal V, Khan I, Rai B, et al. The effect of weight loss after bariatric surgery on albuminuria. *Clin Nephrol.* 2008;70:194-202.

103. Agarwal R, Bills JE, Light RP. Diagnosing obesity by body mass index in chronic kidney disease: an explanation for the "obesity paradox?" *Hypertension.* 2010;56:893-900.

104. Krishna GG, Newell G, Miller E, et al. Protein-induced glomerular hyperfiltration: role of hormonal factors. *Kidney Int.* 1988;33:578-583.

105. Bosch JP, Lew S, Glabman S, et al. Renal hemodynamic changes in humans. Response to protein loading in normal and diseased kidneys. *Am J Med.* 1986;81:809-815.

106. Zatz R, Meyer TW, Rennke HG, et al. Predominance of hemodynamic rather than metabolic factors in the pathogenesis of diabetic glomerulopathy. *Proc Natl Acad Sci U S A.* 1985;82:5963-5967.

107. Bertani T, Zoja C, Abbate M, et al. Age-related nephropathy and proteinuria in rats with intact kidneys exposed to diets with different protein content. *Lab Invest.* 1989;60:196-204.

108. Wrone EM, Carnethon MR, Palaniappan L, et al. Association of dietary protein intake and microalbuminuria in healthy adults: Third National Health and Nutrition Examination Survey. *Am J Kidney Dis.* 2003;41:580-587.

109. Knight EL, Stampfer MJ, Hankinson SE, et al. The impact of protein intake on renal function decline in women with normal renal function or mild renal insufficiency. *Ann Intern Med.* 2003;138:460-467.

110. Levey AS, Adler S, Caggiula AW, et al. Effects of dietary protein restriction on the progression of advanced renal disease in the Modification of Diet in Renal Disease study. *Am J Kidney Dis.* 1996;27:652-663.

111. Menon V, Kopple JD, Wang X, et al. Effect of a very low-protein diet on outcomes: long-term follow-up of the Modification of Diet in Renal Disease (MDRD) study. *Am J Kidney Dis.* 2009;53:208-217.

112. Fouque D, Wang P, Laville M, et al. Low protein diets delay end-stage renal disease in non-diabetic adults with chronic renal failure. *Nephrol Dial Transplant.* 2000;15:1986-1992.

113. Pedrini MT, Levey AS, Lau J, et al. The effect of dietary protein restriction on the progression of diabetic and nondiabetic renal diseases: a meta-analysis. *Ann Intern Med.* 1996;124:627-632.

114. Kasiske BL, Lakatua JD, Ma JZ, et al. A meta-analysis of the effects of dietary protein restriction on the rate of decline in renal function. *Am J Kidney Dis.* 1998;31:954-961.

115. Jones DC, Hayslett JP. Outcome of pregnancy in women with moderate or severe renal insufficiency. *N Engl J Med.* 1996;335:226-232.

116. Imbasciati E, Gregorini G, Cabiddu G, et al. Pregnancy in CKD stages 3 to 5: fetal and maternal outcomes. *Am J Kidney Dis.* 2007;49:753-762.

117. Piccoli GB, Attini R, Vasario E, et al. Pregnancy and chronic kidney disease: a challenge in all CKD stages. *Clin J Am Soc Nephrol.* 2010;5:844-855.

118. Limardo M, Imbasciati E, Ravani P, et al. Pregnancy and progression of IgA nephropathy: results of an Italian multicenter study. *Am J Kidney Dis.* 2010;56:506-512.

119. Vikse BE, Irgens LM, Leivestad T, et al. Preeclampsia and the risk of end-stage renal disease. *N Engl J Med.* 2008;359:800-809.

120. Sandvik MK, Iversen BM, Irgens LM, et al. Are adverse pregnancy outcomes risk factors for development of end-stage renal disease in women with diabetes? *Nephrol Dial Transplant.* 2010;25:3600-3607.

121. Cornelis T, Odutayo A, Keunen J, et al. The kidney in normal pregnancy and preeclampsia. *Semin Nephrol.* 2011;31:4-14.

122. McDonald SD, Han Z, Walsh MW, et al. Kidney disease after preeclampsia: a systematic review and meta-analysis. *Am J Kidney Dis.* 2010;55:1026-1039.

123. Hsu CY, Bates DW, Kuperman GJ, et al. Diabetes, hemoglobin A(1c), cholesterol, and the risk of moderate chronic renal insufficiency in an ambulatory population. *Am J Kidney Dis.* 2000;36:272-281.

124. The Diabetes Control and Complications Research Group. The effect of intensive treatment of diabetes on the development and progression of long-term complications in insulin-dependent diabetes mellitus. *N Engl J Med.* 1993;329:977-986.

125. UK Prospective Diabetes Study. Intensive blood-glucose control with sulphonylureas or insulin compared with conventional treatment and risk of complications in patients with type 2 diabetes (UKPDS 33). *Lancet.* 1998;352:837-853.

126. Amin R, Turner C, van Aken S, et al. The relationship between microalbuminuria and glomerular filtration rate in young type 1 diabetic subjects: the Oxford Regional Prospective Study. *Kidney Int.* 2005;68:1740-1749.

127. Sakharova OV, Taal MW, Brenner BM. Pathogenesis of diabetic nephropathy: focus on transforming growth factor-beta and connective tissue growth factor. *Curr Opin Nephrol Hypertension.* 2001;10:727-738.

128. Tesch GH, Lim AK. Recent insights into diabetic renal injury from the db/db mouse model of type 2 diabetic nephropathy. *Am J Physiol Renal Physiol.* 2010;300:F301-F310.

129. Matsushita K, van der Velde M, Astor BC, et al. Association of estimated glomerular filtration rate and albuminuria with all-cause and cardiovascular mortality in general population cohorts: a collaborative meta-analysis. *Lancet.* 2010;375:2073-2081.

130. McClellan WM, Langston RD, Presley R. Medicare patients with cardiovascular disease have a high prevalence of chronic kidney disease and a high rate of progression to end-stage renal disease. *J Am Soc Nephrol.* 2004;15:1912-1919.

131. Buller CE, Nogareda JG, Ramanathan K, et al. The profile of cardiac patients with renal artery stenosis. *J Am Coll Cardiol.* 2004;43:1606-1613.

132. Taal MW, Sigrist MK, Fakis A, et al. Markers of arterial stiffness are risk factors for progression to end-stage renal disease among patients with chronic kidney disease stages 4 and 5. *Nephron Clin Pract.* 2007;107:c177-c181.

133. Takenaka T, Mimura T, Kanno Y, et al. Qualification of arterial stiffness as a risk factor to the progression of chronic kidney diseases. *Am J Nephrol.* 2005;25:417-424.

134. Chue CD, Edwards NC, Davis LJ, et al. Serum phosphate but not pulse wave velocity predicts decline in renal function in patients with early chronic kidney disease. *Nephrol Dial Transplant.* Epub January 19, 2011.

135. Levin A, Djurdjev O, Barrett B, et al. Cardiovascular disease in patients with chronic kidney disease: getting to the heart of the matter. *Am J Kidney Dis.* 2001;38:1398-1407.

136. Chiu YL, Chien KL, Lin SL, et al. Outcomes of stage 3-5 chronic kidney disease before end-stage renal disease at a single center in Taiwan. *Nephron Clin Pract.* 2008;109:c109-c118.

137. Ishani A, Grandits GA, Grimm RH, et al. Association of single measurements of dipstick proteinuria, estimated glomerular filtration rate, and hematocrit with 25-year incidence of end-stage renal disease in the multiple risk factor intervention trial. *J Am Soc Nephrol.* 2006;17:1444-1452.

138. Hallan SI, Ritz E, Lydersen S, et al. Combining GFR and albuminuria to classify CKD improves prediction of ESRD. *J Am Soc Nephrol.* 2009;20:1069-1077.

139. Halbesma N, Jansen D, Heymans M, et al. Development and validation of a general population renal risk score. *Clin J Am Soc Nephrol.* 2011;6:1731-1738.

140. Verhave JC, Gansevoort RT, Hillege HL, et al. An elevated urinary albumin excretion predicts de novo development of renal function impairment in the general population. *Kidney Int Suppl.* 2004;92:S18-S21.

141. D'Amico G, Minetti L, Ponticelli C, et al. Prognostic indicators in idiopathic IgA mesangial nephropathy. *Q J Med.* 1986;59:363-378.

142. Vikse BE, Aasarod K, Bostad L, et al. Clinical prognostic factors in biopsy-proven benign nephrosclerosis. *Nephrol Dial Transplant.* 2003;18:517-523.

143. Randomised placebo-controlled trial of effect of ramipril on decline in glomerular filtration rate and risk of terminal renal failure in proteinuric, non-diabetic nephropathy. The GISEN Group (Gruppo Italiano di Studi Epidemiologici in Nefrologia). *Lancet.* 1997;349:1857-1863.

144. Lea J, Greene T, Hebert L, et al. The relationship between magnitude of proteinuria reduction and risk of end-stage renal disease: results of the African American Study of Kidney Disease and Hypertension. *Arch Intern Med.* 2005;165:947-953.

145. Atkins RC, Briganti EM, Lewis JB, et al. Proteinuria reduction and progression to renal failure in patients with type 2 diabetes mellitus and overt nephropathy. *Am J Kidney Dis.* 2005;45:281-287.

146. Ruggenenti P, Perna A, Remuzzi G. Retarding progression of chronic renal disease: the neglected issue of residual proteinuria. *Kidney Int.* 2003;63:2254-2261.

147. Lambers Heerspink HJ, Gansevoort RT, Brenner BM, et al. Comparison of different measures of urinary protein excretion for prediction of renal events. *J Am Soc Nephrol.* 2010;21:1355-1360.

148. Methven S, MacGregor MS, Traynor JP, et al. Comparison of urinary albumin and urinary total protein as predictors of patient outcomes in CKD. *Am J Kidney Dis.* 2011;57:21-28.

149. Methven S, Traynor JP, Hair MD, et al. Stratifying risk in chronic kidney disease: an observational study of UK guidelines for measuring total proteinuria and albuminuria. *QJM.* Epub March 7, 2011.

150. McIntyre NJ, Taal MW. How to measure proteinuria? *Curr Opin Nephrol Hypertens.* 2008;17:600-603.

151. Yokoyama H, Tomonaga O, Hirayama M, et al. Predictors of the progression of diabetic nephropathy and the beneficial effect of angiotensin-converting enzyme inhibitors in NIDDM patients. *Diabetologia.* 1997;40:405-411.

152. Leehey DJ, Kramer HJ, Daoud TM, et al. Progression of kidney disease in type 2 diabetes—beyond blood pressure control: an observational study. *BMC Nephrol.* 2005;6:8.

153. Wakai K, Kawamura T, Endoh M, et al. A scoring system to predict renal outcome in IgA nephropathy: from a nationwide prospective study. *Nephrol Dial Transplant.* 2006;21:2800-2808.

154. Tangri N, Stevens LA, Griffith J, et al. A predictive model for progression of chronic kidney disease to kidney failure. *JAMA.* 2011;305:1553-1559.

155. Ataga KI, Orringer EP. Renal abnormalities in sickle cell disease. *Am J Hematol.* 2000;63:205-211.

156. Scheinman JI. Sickle cell disease and the kidney. *Semin Nephrol.* 2003;23:66-76.
157. Mohanram A, Zhang Z, Shahinfar S, et al. Anemia and end-stage renal disease in patients with type 2 diabetes and nephropathy. *Kidney Int.* 2004;66:1131-1138.
158. Kovedsy CP, Trivedi BK, Kalantar-Zadeh K, et al. Association of anemia with outcomes in men with moderate and severe chronic kidney disease. *Kidney Int.* 2006;69:560-564.
159. Levin A, Djurdjev O, Beaulieu M, et al. Variability and risk factors for kidney disease progression and death following attainment of stage 4 CKD in a referred cohort. *Am J Kidney Dis.* 2008;52:661-671.
160. Johnson ES, Thorp ML, Platt RW, et al. Predicting the risk of dialysis and transplant among patients with CKD: a retrospective cohort study. *Am J Kidney Dis.* 2008;52:653-660.
161. Kuriyama S, Tomonari H, Yoshida H, et al. Reversal of anemia by erythropoietin therapy retards the progression of chronic renal failure, especially in nondiabetic patients. *Nephron.* 1997;77:176-185.
162. Gouva C, Nikolopoulos P, Ioannidis JP, et al. Treating anemia early in renal failure patients slows the decline of renal function: a randomized controlled trial. *Kidney Int.* 2004;66:753-760.
163. Levin A, Djurdjev O, Thompson C, et al. Canadian randomized trial of hemoglobin maintenance to prevent or delay left ventricular mass growth in patients with CKD. *Am J Kidney Dis.* 2005;46:799-811.
164. Roger SD, McMahon LP, Clarkson A, et al. Effects of early and late intervention with epoetin alpha on left ventricular mass among patients with chronic kidney disease (stage 3 or 4): results of a randomized clinical trial. *J Am Soc Nephrol.* 2004;15:148-156.
165. Pfeffer MA, Burdmann EA, Chen CY, et al. A trial of darbepoetin alfa in type 2 diabetes and chronic kidney disease. *N Engl J Med.* 2009;361:2019-2032.
166. Drueke TB, Locatelli F, Clyne N, et al. Normalization of hemoglobin level in patients with chronic kidney disease and anemia. *N Engl J Med.* 2006;355:2071-2084.
167. Singh AK, Szczech L, Tang KL, et al. Correction of anemia with epoetin alfa in chronic kidney disease. *N Engl J Med.* 2006;355:2085-2098.
168. Manttari M, Tiula E, Alikoski T, et al. Effects of hypertension and dyslipidemia on the decline in renal function. *Hypertension.* 1995;26:670-675.
169. Muntner P, Coresh J, Smith JC, et al. Plasma lipids and risk of developing renal dysfunction: the Atherosclerosis Risk in Communities study. *Kidney Int.* 2000;58:293-301.
170. Schaeffner ES, Kurth T, Curhan GC, et al. Cholesterol and the risk of renal dysfunction in apparently healthy men. *J Am Soc Nephrol.* 2003;14:2084-2091.
171. Samuelsson O, Mulec H, Knight-Gibson C, et al. Lipoprotein abnormalities are associated with increased rate of progression of human chronic renal insufficiency. *Nephrol Dial Transplant.* 1997;12:1908-1915.
172. Syrjanen J, Mustonen J, Pasternack A. Hypertriglyceridaemia and hyperuricaemia are risk factors for progression of IgA nephropathy. *Nephrol Dial Transplant.* 2000;15:34-42.
173. Krolewski AS, Warram JH, Christlieb AR. Hypercholesterolemia—a determinant of renal function loss and deaths in IDDM patients with nephropathy. *Kidney Int Suppl.* 1994;45:S125-S131.
174. Ravid M, Brosh D, Ravid-Safran D, et al. Main risk factors for nephropathy in type 2 diabetes mellitus are plasma cholesterol levels, mean blood pressure, and hyperglycemia. *Arch Intern Med.* 1998;158:998-1004.
175. Maschio G, Oldrizzi L, Rugiu C, et al. Serum lipids in patients with chronic renal failure on long-term, protein-restricted diets. *Am J Med.* 1989;87:51N-54N.
176. Tonelli M, Moye L, Sacks FM, et al. Effect of pravastatin on loss of renal function in people with moderate chronic renal insufficiency and cardiovascular disease. *J Am Soc Nephrol.* 2003;14:1605-1613.
177. Collins R, Armitage J, Parish S, et al. MRC/BHF Heart Protection Study of cholesterol-lowering with simvastatin in 5963 people with diabetes: a randomised placebo-controlled trial. *Lancet.* 2003;361:2005-2016.
178. Bianchi S, Bigazzi R, Caiazza A, et al. A controlled, prospective study of the effects of atorvastatin on proteinuria and progression of kidney disease. *Am J Kidney Dis.* 2003;41:565-570.
179. Tonelli M, Collins D, Robins S, et al. Effect of gemfibrozil on change in renal function in men with moderate chronic renal insufficiency and coronary disease. *Am J Kidney Dis.* 2004;44:832-839.
180. Ansquer JC, Foucher C, Rattier S, et al. Fenofibrate reduces progression to microalbuminuria over 3 years in a placebo-controlled study in type 2 diabetes: results from the Diabetes Atherosclerosis Intervention Study (DAIS). *Am J Kidney Dis.* 2005;45:485-493.
181. Navaneethan SD, Pansini F, Perkovic V, et al. HMG CoA reductase inhibitors (statins) for people with chronic kidney disease not requiring dialysis. *Cochrane Database Syst Rev.* (2):CD007784, 2009.
182. Baigent C, Landray MJ, Reith C, et al. The effects of lowering LDL cholesterol with simvastatin plus ezetimibe in patients with chronic kidney disease (Study of Heart and Renal Protection): a randomised placebo-controlled trial. *Lancet.* 2011;377:2181-2192.
183. Iseki K, Oshiro S, Tozawa M, et al. Significance of hyperuricemia on the early detection of renal failure in a cohort of screened subjects. *Hypertension Res Clin Exp.* 2001;24:691-697.
184. Bellomo G, Venanzi S, Verdura C, et al. Association of uric acid with change in kidney function in healthy normotensive individuals. *Am J Kidney Dis.* 2010;56:264-272.
185. Sonoda H, Takase H, Dohi Y, et al. Uric acid levels predict future development of chronic kidney disease. *Am J Nephrol.* 2011;33:352-357.
186. Iseki K, Ikemiya Y, Inoue T, et al. Significance of hyperuricemia as a risk factor for developing ESRD in a screened cohort. *Am J Kidney Dis.* 2004;44:642-650.
187. Ohno I, Hosoya T, Gomi H, et al. Serum uric acid and renal prognosis in patients with IgA nephropathy. *Nephron.* 2001;87:333-339.
188. Sturm G, Kollerits B, Neyer U, et al. Uric acid as a risk factor for progression of non-diabetic chronic kidney disease? The Mild to Moderate Kidney Disease (MMKD) study. *Exp Gerontol.* 2008;43:347-352.
189. Siu YP, Leung KT, Tong MK, et al. Use of allopurinol in slowing the progression of renal disease through its ability to lower serum uric acid level. *Am J Kidney Dis.* 2006;47:51-59.
190. Goicoechea M, de Vinuesa SG, Verdalles U, et al. Effect of allopurinol in chronic kidney disease progression and cardiovascular risk. *Clin J Am Soc Nephrol.* 2010;5:1388-1393.
191. Sanchez-Lozada LG, Tapia E, Santamaria J, et al. Mild hyperuricemia induces vasoconstriction and maintains glomerular hypertension in normal and remnant kidney rats. *Kidney Int.* 2005;67:237-247.
192. Sanchez-Lozada LG, Tapia E, Avila-Casado C, et al. Mild hyperuricemia induces glomerular hypertension in normal rats. *Am J Physiol Renal Physiol.* 2002;283:F1105-F1110.
193. Butler R, Morris AD, Belch JJ, et al. Allopurinol normalizes endothelial dysfunction in type 2 diabetics with mild hypertension. *Hypertension.* 2000;35:746-751.
194. Kanbay M, Yilmaz MI, Sonmez A, et al. Serum uric acid level and endothelial dysfunction in patients with nondiabetic chronic kidney disease. *Am J Nephrol.* 2011;33:298-304.
195. Sanchez-Lozada LG, Nakagawa T, Kang DH, et al. Hormonal and cytokine effects of uric acid. *Curr Opin Nephrol Hypertension.* 2006;15:30-33.
196. Young JM, Terrin N, Wang X, et al. Asymmetric dimethylarginine and mortality in stages 3 to 4 chronic kidney disease. *Clin J Am Soc Nephrol.* 2009;4:1115-1120.
197. Mihout F, Shweke N, Bige N, et al. Asymmetric dimethylarginine (ADMA) induces chronic kidney disease through a mechanism involving collagen and TGF-beta1 synthesis. *J Pathol.* 2011;223:37-45.
198. Matsumoto Y, Ueda S, Yamagishi S, et al. Dimethylarginine dimethylaminohydrolase prevents progression of renal dysfunction by inhibiting loss of peritubular capillaries and tubulointerstitial fibrosis in a rat model of chronic kidney disease. *J Am Soc Nephrol.* 2007;18:1525-1533.
199. Fliser D, Kronenberg F, Kielstein JT, et al. Asymmetric dimethylarginine and progression of chronic kidney disease: the Mild to Moderate Kidney Disease study. *J Am Soc Nephrol.* 2005;16:2456-2461.
200. Fujimi-Hayashida A, Ueda S, Yamagishi S, et al. Association of asymmetric dimethylarginine with severity of kidney injury and decline in kidney function in IgA nephropathy. *Am J Nephrol.* 2011;33:1-6.
201. Haut LL, Alfrey AC, Guggenheim S, et al. Renal toxicity of phosphate in rats. *Kidney Int.* 1980;17:722-731.
202. Barsotti G, Giannoni A, Morelli E, et al. The decline of renal function slowed by very low phosphorus intake in chronic renal patients following a low nitrogen diet. *Clin Nephrol.* 1984;21:54-59.
203. Delmez JA, Slatopolsky E. Hyperphosphatemia: its consequences and treatment in patients with chronic renal disease. *Am J Kidney Dis.* 1992;19:303-317.
204. Ritz E, Gross ML, Dikow R. Role of calcium-phosphorous disorders in the progression of renal failure. *Kidney Int Suppl.* 2005;99:S66-S70.
205. Shimamura T. Prevention of 11-deoxycorticosterone-salt–induced glomerular hypertrophy and glomerulosclerosis by dietary phosphate binder. *Am J Pathol.* 1990;136:549-556.
206. Fliser D, Kollerits B, Neyer U, et al. Fibroblast growth factor 23 (FGF23) predicts progression of chronic kidney disease: the Mild to Moderate Kidney Disease (MMKD) study. *J Am Soc Nephrol.* 2007;18:2600-2608.
207. Titan SM, Zatz R, Graciolli FG, et al. FGF-23 as a predictor of renal outcome in diabetic nephropathy. *Clin J Am Soc Nephrol.* 2010;6:241-247.
208. Bolignano D, Coppolino G, Lacquaniti A, et al. Pathological and prognostic value of urinary neutrophil gelatinase–associated lipocalin in macroproteinuric patients with worsening renal function. *Kidney Blood Press Res.* 2008;31:274-279.

209. Bolignano D, Lacquaniti A, Coppolino G, et al. Neutrophil gelatinase–associated lipocalin as an early biomarker of nephropathy in diabetic patients. *Kidney Blood Press Res.* 2009;32:91-98.
210. Bolignano D, Lacquaniti A, Coppolino G, et al. Neutrophil gelatinase–associated lipocalin (NGAL) and progression of chronic kidney disease. *Clin J Am Soc Nephrol.* 2009;4:337-344.
211. Halimi JM, Giraudeau B, Vol S, et al. Effects of current smoking and smoking discontinuation on renal function and proteinuria in the general population. *Kidney Int.* 2000;58:1285-1292.
212. Bleyer AJ, Shemanski LR, Burke GL, et al. Tobacco, hypertension, and vascular disease: risk factors for renal functional decline in an older population. *Kidney Int.* 2000;57:2072-2079.
213. Shankar A, Klein R, Klein BE. The association among smoking, heavy drinking, and chronic kidney disease. *Am J Epidemiol.* 2006;164:263-271.
214. Muhlhauser I, Overmann H, Bender R, et al. Predictors of mortality and end-stage diabetic complications in patients with Type 1 diabetes mellitus on intensified insulin therapy. *Diabet Med.* 2000;17:727-734.
215. Orth SR, Schroeder T, Ritz E, et al. Effects of smoking on renal function in patients with type 1 and type 2 diabetes mellitus. *Nephrol Dial Transplant.* 2005;20:2414-2419.
216. Regalado M, Yang S, Wesson DE. Cigarette smoking is associated with augmented progression of renal insufficiency in severe essential hypertension. *Am J Kidney Dis.* 2000;35:687-694.
217. Stengel B, Couchoud C, Cenee S, et al. Age, blood pressure and smoking effects on chronic renal failure in primary glomerular nephropathies. *Kidney Int.* 2000;57:2519-2526.
218. Ward MM, Studenski S. Clinical prognostic factors in lupus nephritis. The importance of hypertension and smoking. *Arch Intern Med.* 1992;152:2082-2088.
219. McLaughlin JK, Lipworth L, Chow WH, et al. Analgesic use and chronic renal failure: a critical review of the epidemiologic literature. *Kidney Int.* 1998;54:679-686.
220. Phisitkul K, Hegazy K, Chuahirun T, et al. Continued smoking exacerbates but cessation ameliorates progression of early type 2 diabetic nephropathy. *Am J Med Sci.* 2008;335:284-291.
221. Orth SR, Ritz E. The renal risks of smoking: an update. *Curr Opin Nephrol Hypertens.* 2002;11:483-488.
222. Perneger TV, Whelton PK, Puddey IB, et al. Risk of end-stage renal disease associated with alcohol consumption. *Am J Epidemiol.* 1999;150:1275-1281.
223. Vupputuri S, Sandler DP. Lifestyle risk factors and chronic kidney disease. *Ann Epidemiol.* 2003;13:712-720.
224. Knight EL, Stampfer MJ, Rimm EB, et al. Moderate alcohol intake and renal function decline in women: a prospective study. *Nephrol Dial Transplant.* 2003;18:1549-1554.
225. Stengel B, Tarver-Carr ME, Powe NR, et al. Lifestyle factors, obesity and the risk of chronic kidney disease. *Epidemiology.* 2003;14:479-487.
226. Perneger TV, Klag MJ, Whelton PK. Recreational drug use: a neglected risk factor for end-stage renal disease. *Am J Kidney Dis.* 2001;38:49-56.
227. Jaffe JA, Kimmel PL. Chronic nephropathies of cocaine and heroin abuse: a critical review. *Clin J Am Soc Nephrol.* 2006;1:655-667.
228. Vupputuri S, Batuman V, Muntner P, et al. The risk for mild kidney function decline associated with illicit drug use among hypertensive men. *Am J Kidney Dis.* 2004;43:629-635.
229. Barroso-Moguel R, Mendez-Armenta M, Villeda-Hernandez J. Experimental nephropathy by chronic administration of cocaine in rats. *Toxicology.* 1995;98:41-46.
230. Nanra RS. Analgesic nephropathy in the 1990s—an Australian perspective. *Kidney Int Suppl.* 1993;42:S86-S92.
231. Curhan GC, Knight EL, Rosner B, et al. Lifetime nonnarcotic analgesic use and decline in renal function in women. *Arch Intern Med.* 2004;164:1519-1524.
232. Kurth T, Glynn RJ, Walker AM, et al. Analgesic use and change in kidney function in apparently healthy men. *Am J Kidney Dis.* 2003;42:234-244.
233. Agodoa LY, Francis ME, Eggers PW. Association of analgesic use with prevalence of albuminuria and reduced GFR in US adults. *Am J Kidney Dis.* 2008;51:573-583.
234. Kuo HW, Tsai SS, Tiao MM, et al. Analgesic use and the risk for progression of chronic kidney disease. *Pharmacoepidemiol Drug Saf.* 2010;19:745-751.
235. Evans M, Fored CM, Bellocco R, et al. Acetaminophen, aspirin and progression of advanced chronic kidney disease. *Nephrol Dial Transplant.* 2009;24:1908-1918.
236. Muntner P, He J, Vupputuri S, et al. Blood lead and chronic kidney disease in the general United States population: results from NHANES III. *Kidney Int.* 2003;63:1044-1050.
237. Ekong EB, Jaar BG, Weaver VM. Lead-related nephrotoxicity: a review of the epidemiologic evidence. *Kidney Int.* 2006;70:2074-2084.
238. Yu CC, Lin JL, Lin-Tan DT. Environmental exposure to lead and progression of chronic renal diseases: a four-year prospective longitudinal study. *J Am Soc Nephrol.* 2004;15:1016-1022.
239. Lin JL, Lin-Tan DT, Li YJ, et al. Low-level environmental exposure to lead and progressive chronic kidney diseases. *Am J Med.* 2006;119:707.e1-707.e9.
240. Evans M, Fored CM, Nise G, et al. Occupational lead exposure and severe CKD: a population-based case-control and prospective observational cohort study in Sweden. *Am J Kidney Dis.* 2010;55:497-506.
241. Spector JT, Navas-Acien A, Fadrowski J, et al. Associations of blood lead with estimated glomerular filtration rate using MDRD, CKD-EPI and serum cystatin C–based equations. *Nephrol Dial Transplant.* Epub January 19, 2011.
242. Ferraro PM, Costanzi S, Naticchia A, et al. Low level exposure to cadmium increases the risk of chronic kidney disease: analysis of the NHANES 1999-2006. *BMC Public Health.* 2010;10:304.
243. Jarup L, Hellstrom L, Alfven T, et al. Low level exposure to cadmium and early kidney damage: the OSCAR study. *Occup Environ Med.* 2000;57:668-672.
244. Navas-Acien A, Tellez-Plaza M, Guallar E, et al. Blood cadmium and lead and chronic kidney disease in US adults: a joint analysis. *Am J Epidemiol.* 2009;170:1156-1164.
245. Hellstrom L, Elinder CG, Dahlberg B, et al. Cadmium exposure and end-stage renal disease. *Am J Kidney Dis.* 2001;38:1001-1008.
246. Taal MW, Brenner BM. Predicting initiation and progression of chronic kidney disease: developing renal risk scores. *Kidney Int.* 2006;70:1694-1705.
247. Bang H, Vupputuri S, Shoham DA, et al. SCreening for Occult REnal Disease (SCORED): a simple prediction model for chronic kidney disease. *Arch Intern Med.* 2007;167:374-381.
248. Kshirsagar AV, Bang H, Bomback AS, et al. A simple algorithm to predict incident kidney disease. *Arch Intern Med.* 2008;168:2466-2473.
249. O'Seaghdha CM, Lyass A, Massaro J, et al. Development of a risk score for chronic kidney disease in population-based studies. *ASN Renal Week F-P01920.* 2010:[Abstract]. Published online at http://www.asn-online.org/education_and_meetings/kidneyweek/archives/RW10Abstracts.pdf.
250. Chien KL, Lin HJ, Lee BC, et al. A prediction model for the risk of incident chronic kidney disease. *Am J Med.* 2010;123:836-846.e2.
251. Hippisley-Cox J, Coupland C. Predicting the risk of chronic kidney disease in men and women in England and Wales: prospective derivation and external validation of the QKidney scores. *BMC Fam Pract.* 2010;11:49.
252. Kent DM, Jafar TH, Hayward RA, et al. Progression risk, urinary protein excretion, and treatment effects of angiotensin-converting enzyme inhibitors in nondiabetic kidney disease. *J Am Soc Nephrol.* 2007;18:1959-1965.
253. Chawla LS, Amdur RL, Amodeo S, et al. The severity of acute kidney injury predicts progression to chronic kidney disease. *Kidney Int.* 2011;79:1361-1369.

Nephron Endowment

Valerie A. Luyckx and Barry M. Brenner

Genetic factors are important determinants of the development and function of major organ systems as well as of susceptibility to disease. Rare genetic and congenital abnormalities leading to abnormal kidney development are associated with the occurrence of subsequent renal dysfunction, often manifested very early in life.[1,2] Most renal disease in the general population, however, is not ascribable to genetic mutations. The most common causes of end-stage renal disease (ESRD) worldwide are the polygenic disorders of diabetes and hypertension. Hypertension and renal disease prevalence vary among populations of different ethnic backgrounds, with very high rates observed among Aboriginal Australians, Native Americans, and people of African descent.[3-5] Similarly, renal disease associated with hypertension and diabetes appears to run in families. It is well established that lifestyle factors pose significant risk for the development and persistence of hypertension and diabetes in the general population, with increasing obesity being the most concerning, especially in the developing world.[6] Searches for specific genetic polymorphisms or mutations, however, have not yielded "smoking genes" except in rare kindreds, but instead point to a likely complex interplay between polygenic predisposition and environmental factors in the development of diabetes, hypertension, and renal disease.[6-9] Furthermore, evidence highlighting the far-reaching effects of the intrauterine environment and early postnatal growth on organ development, organ function, and subsequent susceptibility to adult disease is becoming more and more compelling.[10] These data suggest that factors in fetal development may be the first in a succession of "hits" that ultimately manifest in overt disease expression. This chapter outlines the effects of fetal programming on renal development (nephrogenesis), nephron endowment, and the risks of hypertension and kidney disease in later life. Low birth weight also predicts later-life diabetes, and therefore renal function may be affected indirectly as well, through fetal programming effects on other organ systems that are beyond the scope of this discussion.[11]

Fetal Programming of Adult Disease

The process through which an environmental insult experienced early in life, particularly in utero, can predispose to adult disease is known as *fetal programming* or *developmental plasticity*. Fetal programming refers to the observation that an environmental stimulus experienced during a critical period of development in utero can induce long-term structural and functional effects in the developing organism.[12] Developmental plasticity is the process whereby different phenotypes may result on a background of a single genotype in response to different environmental stimuli experienced during intrauterine life.[13] These phenomena are intimately linked and have far-reaching implications, because their effects can be transferred and perpetuated across generations.[14] The association between adverse intrauterine events, for which low birth weight may be a surrogate marker, and subsequent cardiovascular disease has long been recognized.[12,13,15,16] Adults who had low weight at birth have higher cardiovascular morbidity and mortality than those who had normal birth weight.[17] Since then, a large body of evidence from different populations has not only confirmed these initial findings but also expanded them to include other conditions such as hypertension, impaired glucose tolerance, type 2 diabetes, obesity, and chronic kidney disease (CKD).[12,18-23] Of these, the relation between low birth weight and subsequent hypertension has been the most studied, as shown in Figure 22-1.[24-26] It is important to note that reported blood pressures tend to be higher in infants, children, and young adults of low birth weight than in those of normal birth weight, but do not reach overt hypertensive ranges until well

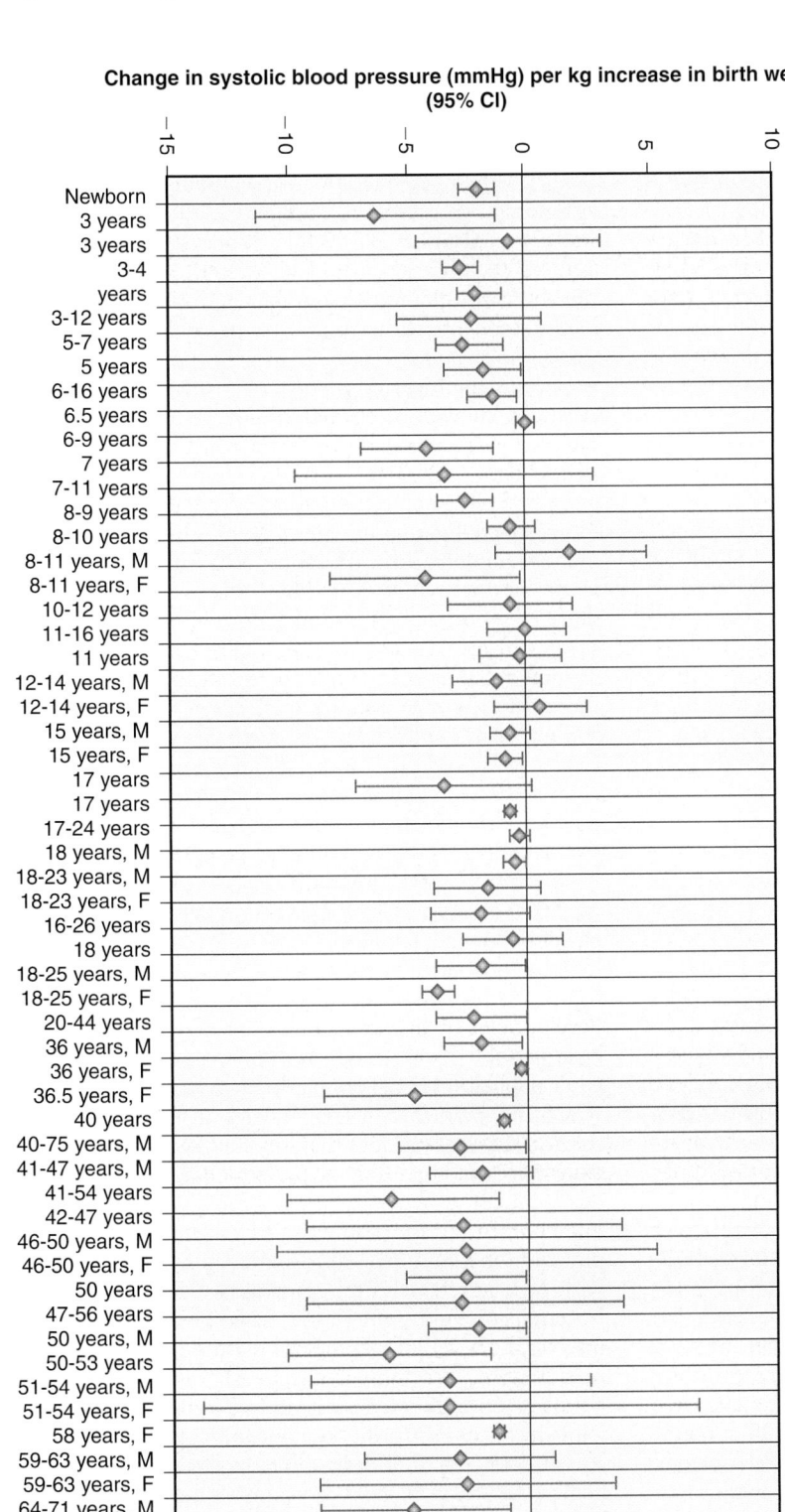

FIGURE 22-1 Studies reporting multiple regression analysis of change in systolic blood pressure (in millimeters of mercury) per kilogram increase in birth weight in children, adolescents, and adults. (For complete citations for individual studies, please refer to original source, Figure 1, p. 819.) (Adapted from Huxley RR, Shiell AW, Law CM: The role of size at birth and postnatal catch-up growth in determining systolic blood pressure: a systematic review of the literature, *J Hypertens* 18:815-831, 2000.)

into adulthood in most studies.[27-29] The majority of studies have been conducted in white populations. An association of higher blood pressure with lower birth weight in African American children has been reported in some studies, but not all, which suggests the presence of additional effects contributing to the greater severity of hypertension in those of African origin.[30-34] Consistently, however, in all populations, blood pressures are highest in those with low birth weight who "caught up" fastest in postnatal weight, which highlights the additional impact of early postnatal nutrition in developmental programming.[10,28,35] The differences in blood pressure between people who had low birth weight and those who had normal birth weight also become amplified with age, with the result that adults who had been of low birth weight often develop overt hypertension, which increases with age.[36] Recent evidence has shown a convincing association between low birth weight and risk of CKD in diverse populations.[21-23,37-39] Whether the increased risk for CKD is a direct consequence of altered renal development in utero or a cumulative process resulting from other effects of programming, such as diabetes and hypertension, superimposed upon renal abnormalities is not yet clear.

Nephron Number

The kidney is the organ central to the development of hypertension. The relationship among renal sodium handling, intravascular fluid volume homeostasis, and hypertension is well accepted.[40,41] In addition, all known monogenic mutations associated with hypertension involve proteins expressed in the kidney.[42,43] That factors intrinsic to the kidney itself affect blood pressure has been demonstrated clinically in renal transplantation cases, in which the blood pressure in the recipient after transplantation has been shown to be related to the blood pressure or hypertension risk factors of the donor; that is, hypertension "follows" the kidney.[44] In 1988 Brenner and colleagues[45] proposed that a congenital (programmed) reduction in nephron number may be a factor explaining why some individuals are susceptible to hypertension and renal injury, whereas others may seem relatively resistant under similar circumstances (e.g., sodium excess or diabetes mellitus). A reduction in nephron number and whole-kidney glomerular surface area would result in reduced sodium excretory capacity that enhances susceptibility to hypertension and reduces renal reserve, which limits compensation for renal injury. This hypothesis is attractive because an association between a reduced nephron number and low birth weight, a surrogate marker of an adverse intrauterine environment, for example, may explain some of the differences in hypertension and renal disease prevalence observed among populations of different ethnicity, among whom those who tend to have lower birth weights often have higher prevalences and more rapid progression of renal disease.[46-49]

An obstacle to investigation of the nephron number hypothesis has been the difficulty of accurately counting nephrons.[50] Review of early studies shows that humans were believed to have an average of approximately 1 million nephrons per kidney.[51] These studies, however, were performed using techniques such as acid maceration or traditional stereologic analysis, which are prone to bias because of required assumptions, extrapolations, and operator sensitivity.[50-52] More

recently, an "unbiased" fractionator-sampling/dissector-counting method has been developed that is believed to be more objective and reproducible.[50-52] It is important to recognize that all reported glomerular counting techniques have been applied to autopsy samples and that, to date, no validated technique permits determination of nephron number in vivo. Basgen and associates[53] attempted to develop an in vivo glomerular counting method and compared the fractionator technique with a combined renal biopsy and magnetic resonance imaging (MRI) method applied to excised canine kidneys. These authors found good agreement between the two methods in glomerular number on average, but within a given kidney, there was up to a 36% difference, which potentially makes the renal biopsy–MRI technique less useful in individual organs. When the fractionator technique was used, the average glomerular (nephron) number in 37 normal Danish adults was reported to be 617,000 per kidney (range of 331,000 to 1,424,000).[51] These authors also reported a positive correlation between glomerular number and kidney weight, which has subsequently been used as a surrogate marker for nephron number in vivo. Another study including 78 kidneys from subjects of multiple ethnic origins in the United States and Australia showed somewhat similar results, with a mean of 784,909 glomeruli per kidney, but with a very wide range of 210,332 to 1,825,380.[54] In both studies, numbers of viable glomeruli were reduced in kidneys from older subjects, owing to age-related glomerulosclerosis and obsolescence.[51,54] Glomerular number, therefore, appears to vary by up to eightfold in the normal population. This variability of mean nephron number reported in presumed normal subjects in different studies, from 617,000 to 1,429,200, should raise a note of caution about use of the fractionator technique.[51,55] Whether these differences reflect true differences in the populations studied or are reflections of small samples sizes will become clearer with time as more studies accumulate or as better techniques evolve. It is known that persons born with severe nephron deficits—for example, unilateral renal agenesis, bilateral renal hypoplasia, and oligomeganephronia—develop progressive proteinuria, glomerulosclerosis, and renal dysfunction with time.[2,56] Similarly, people born with nephron numbers at or below the median level may be more susceptible to superimposed postnatal factors that act as subsequent "hits"; thus, a significant proportion of the population may be at risk for the development of hypertension and renal disease.[57] This may be a plausible hypothesis, given that some 30% of the world's adult population is hypertensive.[6]

Consideration of experimental data in animals indicates that surgical removal of more than one kidney under different circumstances and in different species does not always lead to the development of hypertension and renal disease.[52] In humans, uninephrectomy is accompanied by compensatory hypertrophy and function of the remaining contralateral kidney, often with little adverse clinical consequence, although progressive hypertension and proteinuria have been reported.[58-60] Of interest, however, uninephrectomy on postnatal day 1 in rats or fetal uninephrectomy in sheep—that is, loss of nephrons at a time when nephrogenesis is not yet completed—does lead to adult hypertension prior to any evidence of renal injury.[61-63] These data support the hypothesis that intrauterine or congenital reduction in nephron number, because it takes place before nephrogenesis is completed, may be associated with different compensatory mechanisms or a reduced compensatory capacity than occurs in response to later nephron loss, and result in subsequent development or risk of hypertension. In support of this hypothesis, kidneys from rats that underwent uninephrectomy at 3 days of age showed a similar total glomerular number but a significantly reduced number of mature glomeruli compared with those who underwent nephrectomy at 120 days of age.[64] Furthermore, the mean glomerular volume in neonatally nephrectomized rats increased by 59% versus 20% in the rats nephrectomized as adults, which likely indicates a greater burden of compensatory hypertrophy and hyperfunction in response to neonatal nephrectomy.

Nephron Number and Glomerular Volume

Despite the large variation in nephron number seen in the normal population, it has been noted that glomerular volume consistently varies inversely with glomerular number as shown in Figure 22-2, although the correlation appears stronger among whites and Aboriginal Australians than in people of African origin.[55,65-67] This relationship suggests that larger glomeruli may reflect compensatory hyperfiltration and hypertrophy in subjects with fewer nephrons.[54,66] In fact, Hoy and colleagues[65] found that, although mean glomerular volume was increased in individuals with reduced nephron numbers, total glomerular tuft volume (a surrogate for total filtration surface area) was not different among groups with different nephron numbers (Table 22-1). This observation suggests that total filtration surface area may initially be maintained in the setting of a reduced nephron number but at the expense of glomerular hypertension and hypertrophy, which are maladaptive and predictors of poor outcomes.[68-70] Consistent with this possibility, glomerulomegaly is common in renal biopsy specimens from Aboriginal Australians, a population with high rates of low birth weight and renal disease, and has also been associated with faster rate of decline of glomerular filtration rate (GFR) in Pima Indians.[71-73] Furthermore, in a study of donor kidneys, maximal planar area of glomeruli was found to be higher in kidneys from African Americans than in those from whites and a predictor of poorer transplant function.[69] In populations at high risk of kidney failure, therefore, large glomeruli are a common finding at early stages of renal disease and may reflect programmed reductions in nephron number in these populations, in which access to prenatal and subsequent health care is often suboptimal.[74-76] An increase in glomerular volume is not always associated with a reduction in glomerular number, however.[67] Examination of adult kidneys obtained at autopsy demonstrated considerable variation in individual glomerular volume within kidneys, which was augmented in whites with lower nephron numbers, but was not significantly different in African Americans with low and with high nephron numbers.[67] Similarly, among Senegalese adults, although glomerular volume tended to be higher in those with lower nephron numbers, variability was high in all kidneys.[77,78] Nephron number, therefore, may not be the only factor predisposing to hypertension and renal disease in people of African origin, and other potentially programmable factors such as modulation of glomerular flow may augment the effect of nephron number in these populations.[67,77-79]

Evidence for Fetal Programming in the Kidney

Low birth weight is defined by the World Health Organization as a birth weight of less than 2500 g. Low birth weight can be the result of intrauterine growth restriction (IUGR;

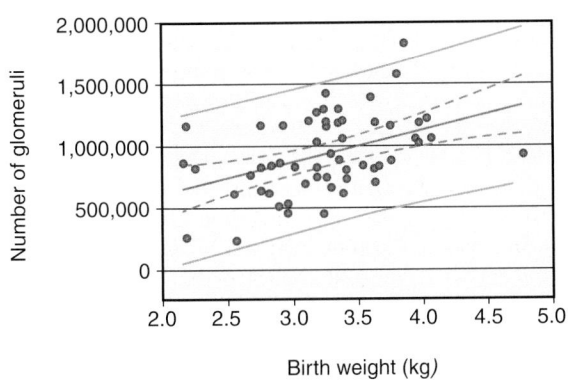
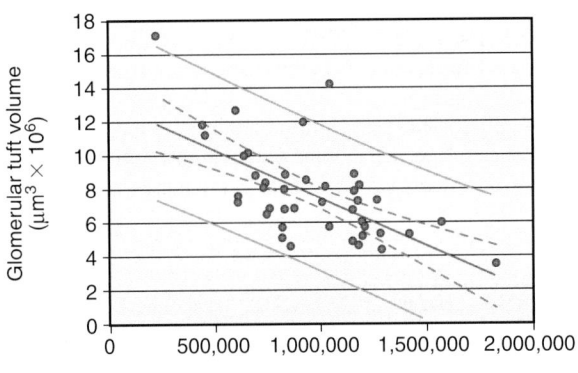

FIGURE 22-2 Birth weight, glomerular number, and glomerular volume in adults. (From Hughson M, Farris AB, Douglas-Denton R, et al: Glomerular number and size in autopsy kidneys: the relationship to birth weight, *Kidney Int* 63:2113-2122, 2003.)

TABLE 22-1 Glomerular Characteristics by Birth Weight in Humans				
MEAN BIRTH WEIGHT (RANGE)	N	MEAN NO. GLOMERULI (95% CI)*	MEAN GLOMERULAR TUFT VOLUME (µm² × 10⁶)	TOTAL GLOMERULAR TUFT VOLUME (cm²)
2.65 kg (1.81-3.12)	29	770,860 (658,757-882,963)	9.2	6.7
3.27 kg (3.18-3.38)	28	965,729 (885,714-1,075,744)	7.2	6.8
3.93 kg (3.41-4.94)	30	1,005,356 (900,094-1,110,599)	6.9	6.6

*Adjusted for age, gender, race, and body surface area.
 CI, Confidence interval.
From Hoy WE, Hughson MD, Bertram JF, et al: Nephron number, hypertension, renal disease, and renal failure, *J Am Soc Nephrol* 16:2557-2564, 2005.

birth weight of <10th percentile for gestational age) or premature birth. Low birth weight associated with IUGR generally reflects intrauterine stress during late gestation, whereas low birth weight associated with prematurity may be an appropriate weight for the duration of gestation. Low birth weight at full term (i.e., IUGR) has the strongest association with adult disease.[80] Low birth weight is more common among African Americans, Native Americans, and Aboriginal Australians than among whites, and the former are populations with disproportionately high rates of hypertension, CKD, type 2 diabetes, and cardiovascular disease.[3,47,81-83]

Multiple animal models have demonstrated the association of low birth weight (induced by gestational exposure to a low-protein diet, uterine ischemia, dexamethasone administration, vitamin A deprivation) with subsequent hypertension.[84-91] The link between adult hypertension and low birth weight in these animal models appears to be mediated, at least in part, by an associated congenital nephron deficit occurring with IUGR.[84,88,89] Vehaskari and colleagues[89] demonstrated an almost 30% reduction in glomerular number in offspring of pregnant rats fed a low-protein diet compared with offspring of those fed a normal-protein diet during pregnancy. As shown in Figure 22-3, the offspring of mothers fed a low-protein diet had systolic blood pressures that were 20 to 25 mm Hg higher by 8 weeks of age.[89] Similarly, Celsi and associates[84] found that prenatal administration of dexamethasone in rats was also associated with low birth weight and fewer glomeruli compared with controls. In these nephron-deficient rats, GFR was reduced, albuminuria was increased, and urinary sodium excretion was lower than in rats with a greater nephron complement.[84] Uteroplacental insufficiency, induced by maternal uterine artery ligation late in gestation, also resulted in low nephron number and was associated with profibrotic renal gene expression with age, although hypertension developed only in males.[92,93] Conversely, adequate postnatal nutrition, accomplished by cross-fostering growth-restricted pups onto normal lactating females at birth, restored nephron number and abrogated the development of subsequent hypertension in male rats.[93]

Taken together, these findings in animals lend credence to the hypothesis that a congenital deficit in nephron number, resulting in a decreased filtration surface area and thus a limitation in renal sodium excretion, is an independent factor determining susceptibility to essential hypertension and subsequent renal injury. Low nephron number alone, however, does not account for all observed programmed hypertension. Supplementation of a low-protein diet during gestation with glycine, urea, or alanine resulted in a normalization of nephron number in rat offspring, but blood pressure normalized only in those whose mothers were supplemented with glycine.[24] Likewise, augmentation of nephron number by postnatal hypernutrition resulted in a 20% increase in nephron number but also in obesity, hypertension, and glomerulosclerosis with age.[94] These findings therefore suggest that there may be other factors contributing to intrauterine and developmental programming of hypertension in addition to, or independent of, nephron number.

Programming of Nephron Number in Humans

As mentioned previously, nephron numbers vary widely in the normal human population (see Figure 22-2 and Table 22-1). More and more data are emerging that support a direct relationship between nephron number and birth weight and an inverse relationship between nephron number and glomerular volume.[66,95,96] After analysis of 56 kidneys, Hughson and colleagues[95] reported a linear relationship between glomerular number and birth weight and calculated a regression coefficient predicting an increase of 257,426 glomeruli per kilogram increase in birth weight. The applicability of the regression coefficient in populations in which the distribution of nephron number appears bimodal, however, may not be valid. It has also been calculated that in the normal population without renal disease, approximately 4500 glomeruli are lost per kidney per year after the age of 18.[65] Glomerular numbers tend to be lower in females than in males. A kidney starting with a lower nephron number therefore would conceivably reach a critical reduction of nephron mass, either with age or in response to a renal insult, earlier than a kidney with a greater nephron complement, which contributes to hypertension and/or renal dysfunction.

Kidney development in the human begins during the ninth week of gestation and continues until the thirty-fourth to thirty-sixth week.[65] Nephron number at birth is therefore largely dependent on the intrauterine environment and gestational age. It is generally believed that no new nephrons are formed in humans after birth. In an attempt to investigate whether glomerulogenesis does indeed continue postnatally in premature infants, Rodriguez and colleagues[97] studied kidneys at autopsy from 56 extremely premature infants and compared them with those from 10 full-term infants as controls. The radial glomerular counts were lower in premature than in full-term infants and correlated with gestational age. Furthermore, evidence of active glomerulogenesis, indicated by the presence of basophilic S-shaped bodies immediately under the renal capsule, was found in premature infants who died before 40 days but absent in those who died after 40 days of life. The authors concluded that nephrogenesis may continue for up to 40 days after birth in premature infants. Interestingly, these authors also stratified their cases by presence or absence of renal failure in the infants. Among infants surviving longer than 40 days, those with renal failure (serum creatinine level ≥2.0 mg/dL) had significantly fewer glomeruli than those

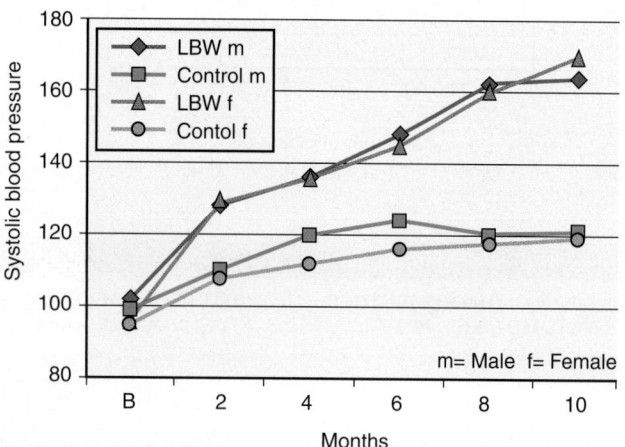

FIGURE 22-3 Fetal programming of hypertension in low-birth-weight rats. (Adapted from Vehaskari VM, Aviles DH, Manning J: Prenatal programming of adult hypertension in the rat, *Kidney Int* 59:238-245, 2001.)

without renal failure. This cross-sectional observation may suggest that renal failure inhibited glomerulogenesis or, conversely, that fewer glomeruli lowered the threshold for development of renal failure in these extremely ill infants. Those premature infants surviving longer than 40 days without renal failure exhibited glomerulomegaly, which may reflect, at least in the short term, a compensatory renoprotective response.

In studies whose results contrasted with these findings, Hinchliffe and associates[98,99] examined nephron number in premature or full-term stillbirths and in infants who died at 1 year of age and who either were born at an appropriate weight for gestational age or were small for gestational age. At both time points, growth-restricted infants had fewer nephrons than controls. In addition, the number of nephrons in growth-restricted infants dying at 1 year of age had not increased compared with the number in the growth-restricted stillbirths, which demonstrated a lack of postnatal compensation in nephron number (Figure 22-4*A*).

Manalich and colleagues[66] examined the kidneys of neonates dying within 2 weeks of birth in relation to their birth weights (see Figure 22-4*B*). A significant direct correlation was found between glomerular number and birth weight. In addition, there was also a strong inverse correlation between glomerular volume and glomerular number independent of sex and race.

These studies, therefore, support the hypothesis that an adverse intrauterine environment, manifested as low birth weight in infants, is associated with a congenital reduction in nephron number and an early compensatory increase in glomerular volume. Analysis of the relationship between renal mass and nephron number in infants younger than 3 months of age revealed a direct relationship (Figure 22-5).[100] Regression analysis predicted an increase of 23,459 nephrons per gram of kidney mass.[100] Renal mass is known to be proportional to nephron number, and renal volume is proportional to renal mass; therefore, renal volume has been analyzed as a surrogate for nephron endowment in infants in vivo.[51] Ultrasound evaluation of fetal renal function in utero revealed a reduction in hourly urine volume, higher prevalence of oligohydramnios, reduced renal perfusion, and reduced renal volume in growth-restricted fetuses.[101-103] These findings may represent reduced fetal perfusion in situations of uterine compromise and do not necessarily reflect altered renal development.

In a subsequent analysis, kidney size and growth postnatally were assessed by ultrasound in 178 children who were born prematurely or were small for gestational age and in 717 mature children with appropriate weight for gestational age at 0, 3, and 18 months; weight for gestational age was found to be positively associated with kidney volume at all three time

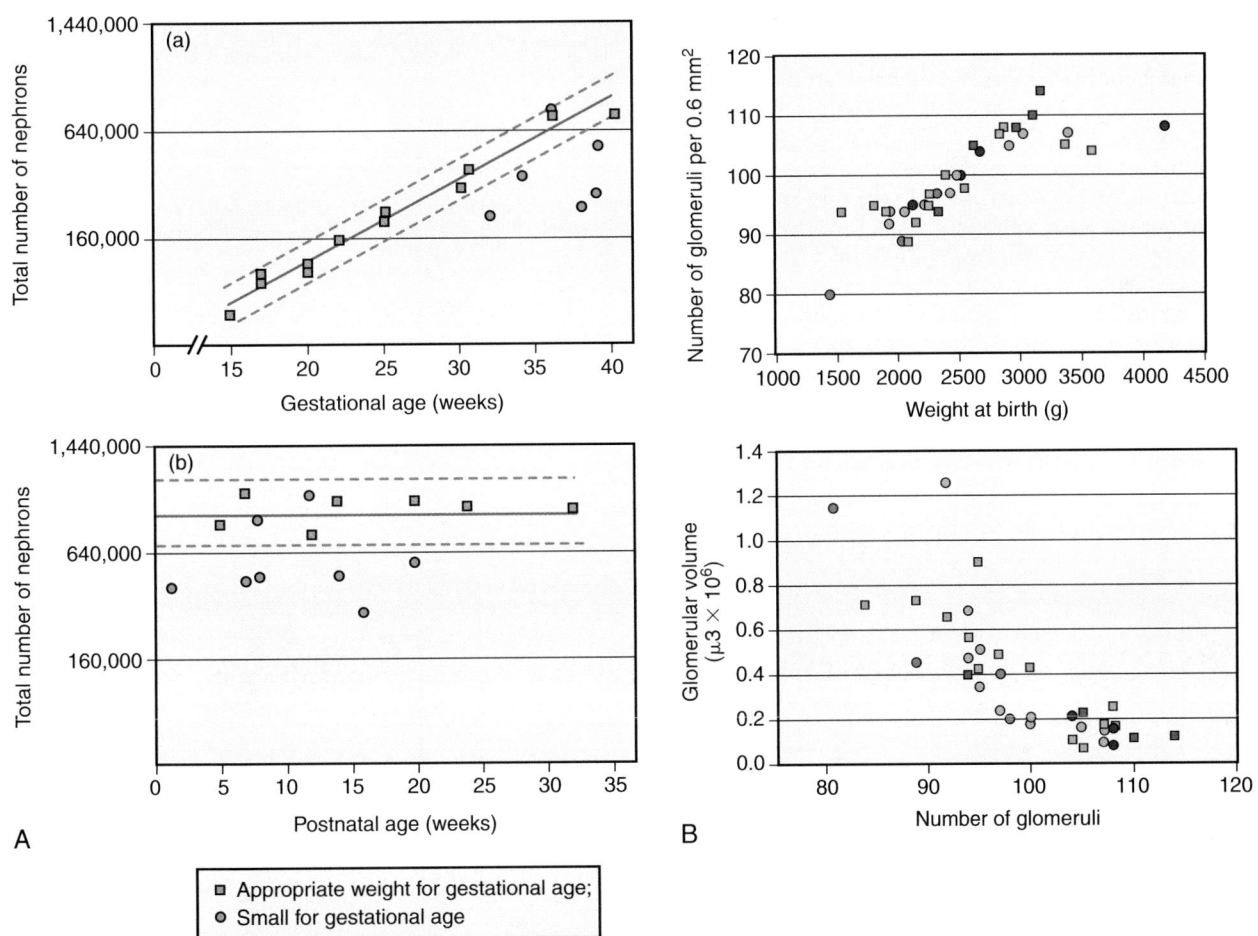

FIGURE 22-4 **A,** Effect of intrauterine growth restriction (IUGR) on nephron number in humans. *a,* Nephron number in relation to gestational age. *b,* Lack of postnatal catch-up in nephron number. **B,** Birth weight, glomerular volume, and glomerular number in neonates. (**A** from Hinchliffe SA, Lynch MR, Sargent PH, et al: The effect of intrauterine growth retardation on the development of renal nephrons, *Br J Obstet Gynaecol* 99:296-301, 1992; **B** from Manalich R, Reyes L, Herrera M, et al: Relationship between weight at birth and the number and size of renal glomeruli in humans: a histomorphometric study, *Kidney Int* 58:770-773, 2000.)

points.[104] Slight catch-up in kidney growth was observed in growth-retarded infants but not in premature infants. In Aboriginal Australian children, low birth weight was also found to be associated with lower renal volumes on ultrasonography.[105] Comparison of renal volume in children aged 9 to 12 years born prematurely, at either small or appropriate weight for gestational age, and in controls found that kidneys were smallest in those who had been preterm and small for gestational age, but when adjustment was made for body surface area, there were no significant differences between the groups.[106] A smaller kidney size, therefore, may be a surrogate marker for a reduced nephron endowment, but it must be borne in mind that the growth in kidney size on ultrasonography cannot distinguish between the components of normal growth with age and renal hypertrophy.

In a population of 140 adults aged 18 to 65 years who died of various causes, a significant correlation was also observed between birth weight and glomerular number.[96] Glomerular volume was again found to be inversely correlated with glomerular number. Mean glomerular numbers did not differ statistically between African American and white subjects, although the distribution among African Americans appeared bimodal, with a few outliers having very high nephron numbers and several subjects having nephron numbers below 500,000. No white subject had fewer than 500,000 nephrons. Significantly, however, none of the subjects in this study had been of low birth weight; therefore, no conclusion can be drawn as to whether an association with low birth weight and nephron number exists in either population group.[96] In addition, it may be argued that because low birth weight is more prevalent among African Americans, this cohort was more representative of the general white population than the general African American population, because it included only subjects of normal birth weight.[83]

In a European study comparing 26 individuals with non–insulin-dependent diabetes with 19 age-matched nondiabetic controls, no difference in glomerular number was found, but again, all subjects had birth weights above 3000 g, and therefore the impact of low birth weight on nephron number could not be assessed.[107] In support of a potential association between nephron number and hypertension, a study of whites aged 35 to 59 years who died in accidents found that in

10 subjects with a history of essential hypertension the number of glomeruli per kidney was significantly lower, and glomerular volume significantly higher, than in 10 normotensive matched controls (Figure 22-6).[55] Birth weights were not reported in this study, but the authors concluded that a reduced nephron number is associated with susceptibility to essential hypertension. Similarly, in a subset of 63 subjects for whom mean arterial pressures and birth weights were available, Hughson and colleagues[96] reported a significant correlation between birth weight and glomerular number, mean arterial pressure and glomerular number, and mean arterial pressure and birth weight in the white but not the African American subjects. Among African Americans having nephron numbers below the mean, however, twice as many were hypertensive as normotensive, which suggests a possible contribution of lower nephron number in this group as well.[96] No study has examined the relationship of low birth weight and nephron number in black subjects; therefore, it remains unknown whether a similar relationship between low birth weight and low nephron number exists in this population. Glomerular volumes were found to be higher in the hypertensive African American subjects than in hypertensive whites.[96] A similar finding was reported for donor kidney biopsy specimens, in which maximal planar area of glomeruli was found to be higher in African Americans than in whites.[70] In this study, glomerulomegaly emerged as an independent predictor of poor allograft function. The consistent finding of larger glomeruli in African Americans may suggest a greater

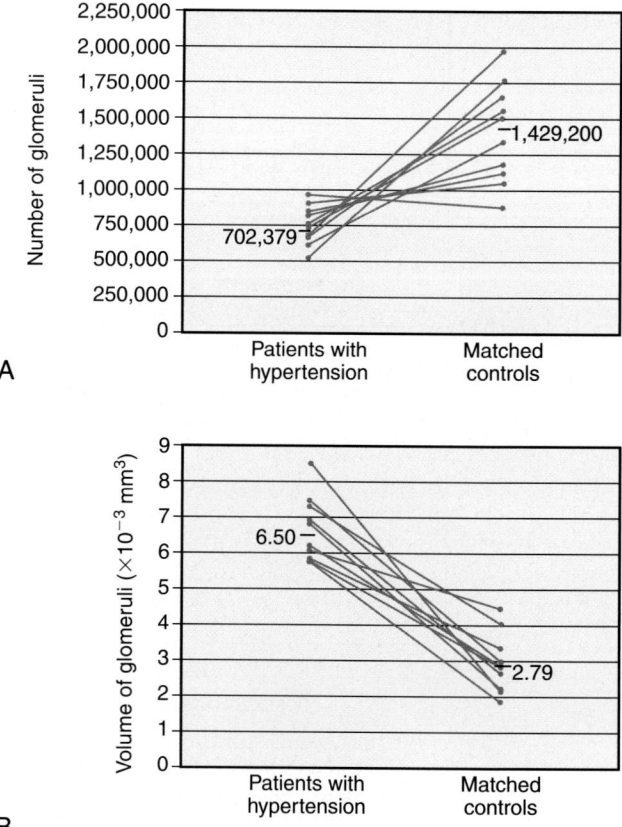

A

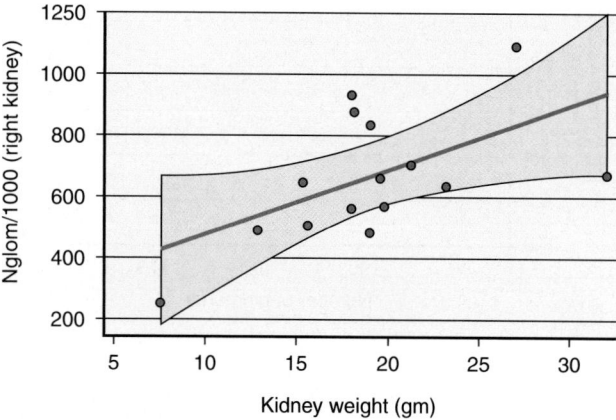

FIGURE 22-5 Relationship between nephron number and mass of the right kidney in white infants 3 months of age or younger who died within the first 3 months of life. (From Zhang Z, Quinlan J, Hoy W, et al: A common RET variant is associated with reduced newborn kidney size and function, *J Am Soc Nephrol* 19:2027-2034, 2008.)

B

FIGURE 22-6 Nephron number (**A**) and glomerular volume (**B**) in white subjects with primary hypertension compared with controls. (From Keller G, Zimmer G, Mall G, et al: Nephron number in patients with primary hypertension, *N Engl J Med* 348:101-108, 2003.)

prevalence of low nephron number in this population as a result of higher prevalence of low birth weight.

Programming of Renal Function and Disease

Experimental Evidence

Although nephron numbers have been shown to be reduced in infants of low birth weight, for adults there are no data on nephron number specifically in those who had been of low birth weight. The association between nephron number and birth weight does appear to be a consistent finding in infants, however, so the extrapolation that nephron numbers would also remain reduced in adults who had low birth weight seems reasonable.[95] As mentioned previously, the determination of nephron number in vivo is difficult and not yet reliable enough; therefore, the most frequently used in vivo surrogate marker available at present is birth weight. In some animal models, low nephron numbers have also been observed in the setting of normal birth weight; therefore, among humans, if birth weight is the only surrogate marker used, the impact of nephron number on any outcome is likely to be underestimated.[108] Other surrogates for an adverse intrauterine environment and low nephron numbers are outlined in Table 22-2.

TABLE 22-2 Clinical Surrogates for Low Nephron Number and Susceptibility to Hypertension and Renal Disease in Humans
Low birth weight[66,97,99]
Prematurity[97,99]
Short stature[141,239]
Low kidney mass[51,100]
Reduced kidney volume[104,105]
Glomerulomegaly[66,95,99]

Glomerulomegaly is also consistently observed in the setting of a low nephron number. Although this may be a compensatory mechanism to restore filtration surface area, it is conceivable that renal reserve in these kidneys is reduced.[65] If this is the case, these kidneys may be expected to be less able to compensate further in the setting of additional renal insults and to begin to manifest signs of renal dysfunction (i.e., proteinuria, elevations in serum creatinine level, and hypertension). In support of this hypothesis, in low-birth-weight rats, induction of glomerulonephritis by anti–Thy-1 antibody injection resulted in significant upregulation of inflammatory markers and development of sclerotic lesions by day 14 compared with normal-birth-weight controls.[109] Interestingly, however, blood pressure and urine protein excretion was no different between low- and normal-birth-weight rats, which suggests a programmed susceptibility to renal inflammation and fibrosis independent of these variables.

In a provocative study, diabetes was induced by streptozotocin injection in subgroups of rats of low birth weight (induced by maternal protein restriction) and normal birth weight.[110] Low-birth-weight rats, as expected, were found to have reduced nephron numbers and higher blood pressures than those of normal birth weight. Among those rendered diabetic, there was a greater proportional increase in renal size and glomerular hypertrophy in the low-birth-weight rats than in normal-birth-weight controls after 1 week (Figure 22-7).[110] This study demonstrates that the renal response to injury in the setting of a reduced nephron number may be exaggerated and could lead to accelerated loss of renal function. Subsequently, the same authors[111] reported outcomes in low-birth-weight versus normal-birth-weight diabetic rats at 40 weeks. Histologically, the podocyte density was reduced and the average area covered by each podocyte was greater in the low-birth-weight diabetic rats than in the normal-birth-weight controls. These findings correlated with urine albumin excretion rate, which was higher in low-birth-weight diabetic rats, although this effect did not reach statistical significance. In support of the role of altered podocyte physiology

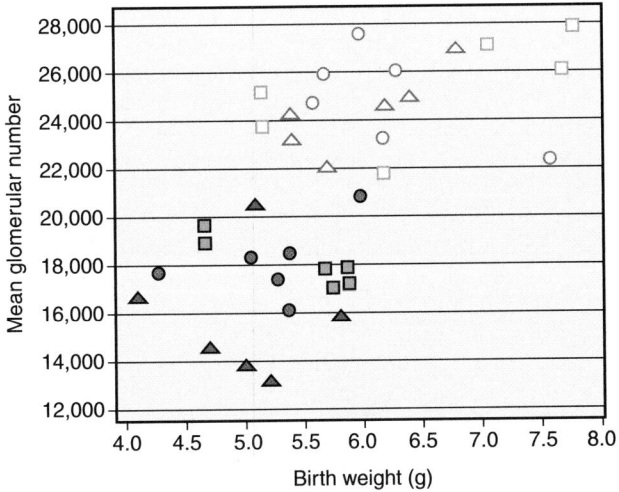

Solid symbols—Low protein diet offspring
Open symbols—Normal protein diet offspring

A

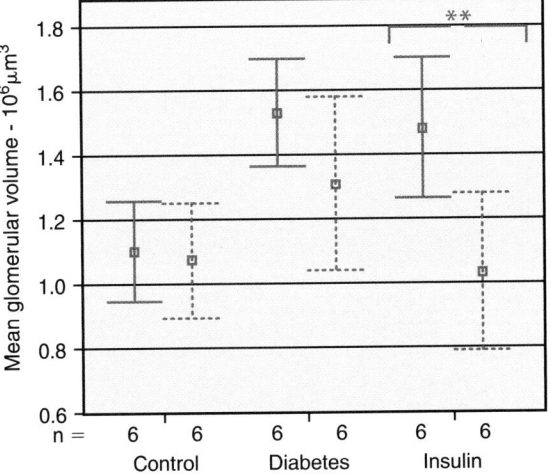

— Low protein diet offspring; - - Normal protein diet offspring

B

FIGURE 22-7 Influence of glomerular number on adaptation to diabetes in rats. (From Jones SE, Bilous RW, Flyvbjerg A, et al: Intra-uterine environment influences glomerular number and the acute renal adaptation to experimental diabetes, *Diabetologia* 44:721-728, 2001.)

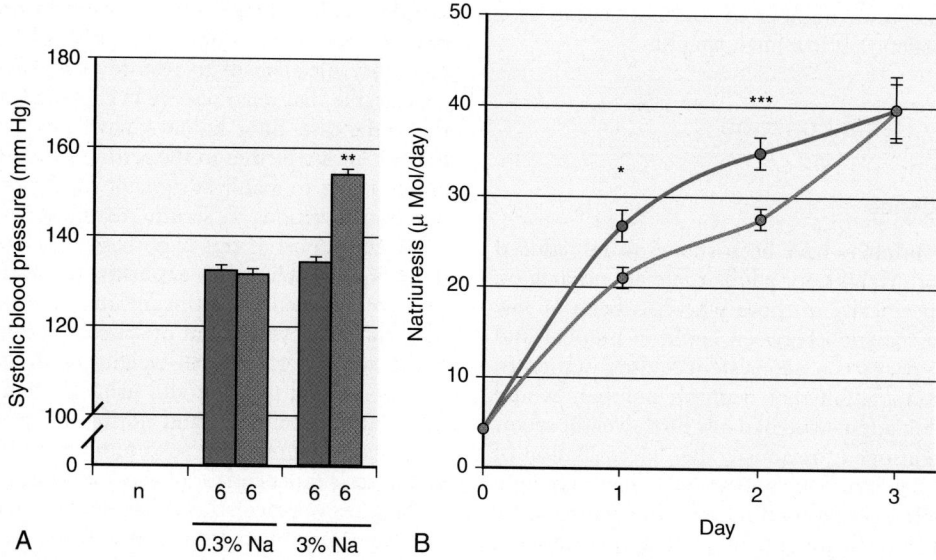

FIGURE 22-8 **A,** Effect of high-sodium diet on systolic blood pressure in 3-month-old rat offspring of control (*blue*) or diabetic (*red*) mothers on normal-salt (0.3%) or high-salt (3%) diet. **B,** Impairment of sodium excretion in offspring of diabetic mothers (*red line*) compared with controls (*blue line*) in the first 3 days after initiation of high-salt diet. (From Nehiri T, Duong Van Huyen J-P, Viltard M, et al: Exposure to maternal diabetes induces salt-sensitive hypertension and impairs renal function in adult rat offspring, *Diabetes* 57:2167-2175, 2008.)

in renal disease progression, similar findings were observed in the Munich-Wistar-Frömter rat,[112] a strain that has congenitally reduced nephron numbers and develops spontaneous renal disease (see later). Whether these podocyte changes are secondary to an increase in glomerular pressure in the setting of reduced nephron numbers or a primary programmed structural change leading to glomerular injury is not yet known.

As mentioned previously, hypertension has frequently been reported in low-birth-weight rats and sheep, but is not universally observed.[12,24,26,84,113] Some authors have reported the presence of salt-sensitive hypertension in rats in which low birth weight was induced by maternal uterine artery ligation, whereas others report no salt sensitivity in rats in which low birth weight was induced by maternal protein restriction, although age and timing of dietary intervention appear to play a role.[114-116] Elevations in blood pressure in response to a high-salt diet have been more consistently observed in aging than in young rats, which suggests an early adaptive mechanism that may decline with age or worsening salt sensitivity as nephron numbers decline with age.[117] In young rats, however, despite no change in blood pressure, an increase in plasma volume was observed, consistent with sodium retention.[118] Interestingly, early changes in sodium intake have been found to have a long-term impact on programming of hypertension in low-birth weight rats. Short-term feeding of a low-salt diet, from weaning to 6 weeks of age, abrogated hypertension at 10 and 51 weeks, whereas short-term high-salt feeding exacerbated hypertension, despite reinstitution of a normal-salt diet.[119,120] Similar salt sensitivity was observed in adult offspring of mothers with gestational diabetes (Figure 22-8).[121] The increase in salt sensitivity may result from a reduction in filtration surface area, but programmed changes in renal sodium transporters have also been reported, as discussed later.

In rats in which low birth weight was induced by maternal protein restriction, GFR was found to be reduced, concomitant with a reduction in nephron number.[90,122] Of interest, GFR was reduced by 10%, although nephron number was

reduced by 25%, which implies some degree of compensatory hyperfunction per nephron (Figure 22-9).[26] In contrast, in low-birth-weight rats exposed to prenatal dexamethasone and subsequently fed a high-protein diet, GFR was similar to that in normal-birth-weight controls.[123] Nephron numbers were reduced by 13% only in male low-birth-weight rats. This study may suggest that there is a threshold reduction in nephron number above which compensation is adequate or that the high-protein diet induced supranormal GFRs in both groups that masked subtle differences in baseline GFR.

Another study that measured GFR in rats with low birth weight, this time induced by maternal uterine artery ligation during gestation, also failed to demonstrate a difference in GFR in low-birth-weight rats, but they were significantly hypertensive compared with normal-birth-weight controls.[91] Conceivably, in this study, the higher intraglomerular pressure due to elevated blood pressure and reduced nephron mass in low-birth-weight rats may have led to a compensatory increase in single-nephron GFR (SNGFR) and thus normalization of whole-kidney GFR. In another study, low-birth-weight rats that had been subjected to gestational protein restriction had significantly higher blood pressures and urinary protein excretion at 20 weeks of age than controls, although again GFR was no different.[124]

Definitive understanding of the pathophysiologic impact of a reduction in nephron number is difficult to obtain from the existing literature, which includes studies with very varied experimental conditions. Overall, however, it is possible that, although whole-kidney GFR may not change, SNGFR is increased in the setting of a reduced nephron number. In support of this possibility, the Munich-Wistar-Frömter rat is known to develop spontaneous progressive glomerular injury. Interestingly, compared with the control Wistar rat strain, nephron numbers have been found to be significantly reduced, urine protein excretion and systolic blood pressure to be significantly higher, and, by micropuncture study, SNGFR to be significantly elevated.[112] A "naturally" occurring (i.e., not experimentally induced) congenital nephron deficit, therefore,

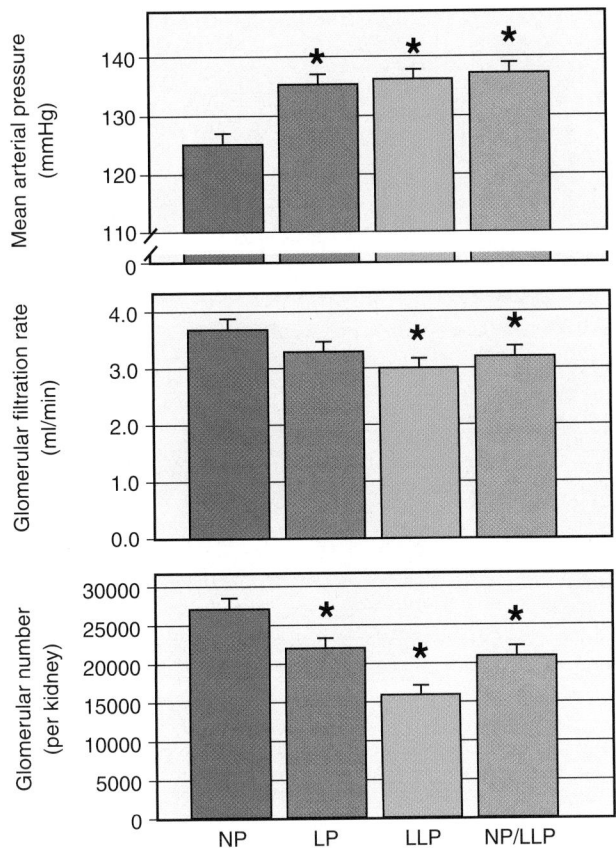

NP = 19% protein diet; LP = 8.5% protein diet; LLP = 5% protein diet; NP/LLP = 5% in last ¹/₂ of pregnancy.
*$P < 0.05$

FIGURE 22-9 Increased blood pressure, decreased glomerular filtration rate, and glomerular number in low-birth-weight adult male rats. (From Vehaskari VM, Woods LL: Prenatal programming of hypertension: lessons from experimental models, *J Am Soc Nephrol* 16:2545-2556, 2005.)

does appear to predispose to progressive renal functional decline.

Evidence in Humans

A recent case series of 6 patients, aged 15 to 52 years, who had been born prematurely at low birth weight described findings consistent with secondary focal and segmental glomerulosclerosis, associated with glomerulomegaly in all biopsy specimens (Figure 22-10).[39] The authors suggest a susceptibility to hyperfiltration and glomerulosclerosis associated with prematurity and low birth weight. One consequence of glomerular hyperfiltration is microalbuminuria. Studies from several countries have demonstrated an increased prevalence of microalbuminuria and proteinuria in adults who had been of low birth weight.[3,5,71,125-127] In long-term follow-up studies of children who had been extremely low-birth-weight premature infants, weighing less than 1000 g a birth, serum creatinine level was found to be higher and GFR reduced compared with those in age-matched normal-birth-weight children at ages 6 to12 years.[128] A similar study found a linear trend of increasing estimated GFR with birth weight in children when cystatin C, but not creatinine, was used for GFR estimation.[129] Studies applying creatinine-based formulas therefore may underestimate the impact of birth weight on

GFR. This study highlights the need to validate measures of renal function in low-birth weight individuals and potentially the need to use adapted formulas in this population.[130]

Another study compared blood pressures and renal function in females in their mid-twenties who had been preterm, small-for-gestational-age, or normal-weight full-term infants.[131] Blood pressures were significantly higher in those who had been preterm than in normal-birth-weight controls. There was no statistically significant difference in GFR or urinary albumin excretion between the groups, but GFR tended to be lower in the small-for-gestational-age group and albuminuria higher in the preterm and small-for-gestational-age groups. This study included fewer than 20 subjects in each group, which might suggest that, with larger numbers of subjects, statistical significance may have been reached. In a similar study, 422 19-year-old subjects who had been very premature were stratified according to whether they had been appropriate weight or small for gestational age at birth.[132] Birth weight was found to be negatively associated with serum creatinine level and albuminuria and positively associated with GFR. The authors concluded that IUGR is associated with poorer renal function in young adults.

The same authors examined renal functional reserve in 20-year-old subjects who had been premature and either small or appropriate for gestational age and in controls who were born at full term and had normal birth weight by measuring GFR and effective renal plasma flow (ERPF) before and after low-dose dopamine infusion or an oral amino acid load.[133] After renal stimulation, the relative increase in GFR tended to be lower in subjects who were small for gestational age compared with those who were appropriate weight for gestational age and with control subjects, and ERPF was lower in both groups of premature subjects, although statistical significance was not reached, probably because of small subject numbers. These results are potentially consistent with reduced renal reserve capacity in the kidneys of low-birth-weight and premature individuals. Consistent with this, an increase in salt sensitivity has also been described in children and adults who had low birth weight compared with those who had normal birth weight, independent of GFR, which demonstrates reduced renal adaptive capacity (Figure 22-11).[134,135]

Analysis of 724 subjects aged 48 to 53 who had been subjected to malnutrition in midgestation during the Dutch famine revealed an increased prevalence of microalbuminuria (12%) compared with those subjected to malnutrition during early gestation (9%) or late gestation (7%), or not exposed to famine (4% to 8%).[136] Interestingly, size at birth was not associated with the observed increase in microalbuminuria, which suggests that renal development may have been irreversibly affected in midgestation, although subsequent intrauterine whole-body growth was able to catch up with restoration of more normal nutrition. These data further emphasize the need for other surrogate markers of the intrauterine environment in addition to birth weight.

The importance of early extrauterine nutrition, in addition to intrauterine conditions, has been highlighted in a cohort of premature infants born either with very low birth weight (<1000 g) or before 30 weeks of gestation.[137] Cases were stratified based on whether the infants experienced IUGR and were small for gestational age; experienced extrauterine (i.e., postnatal) growth restriction; or were appropriate weight

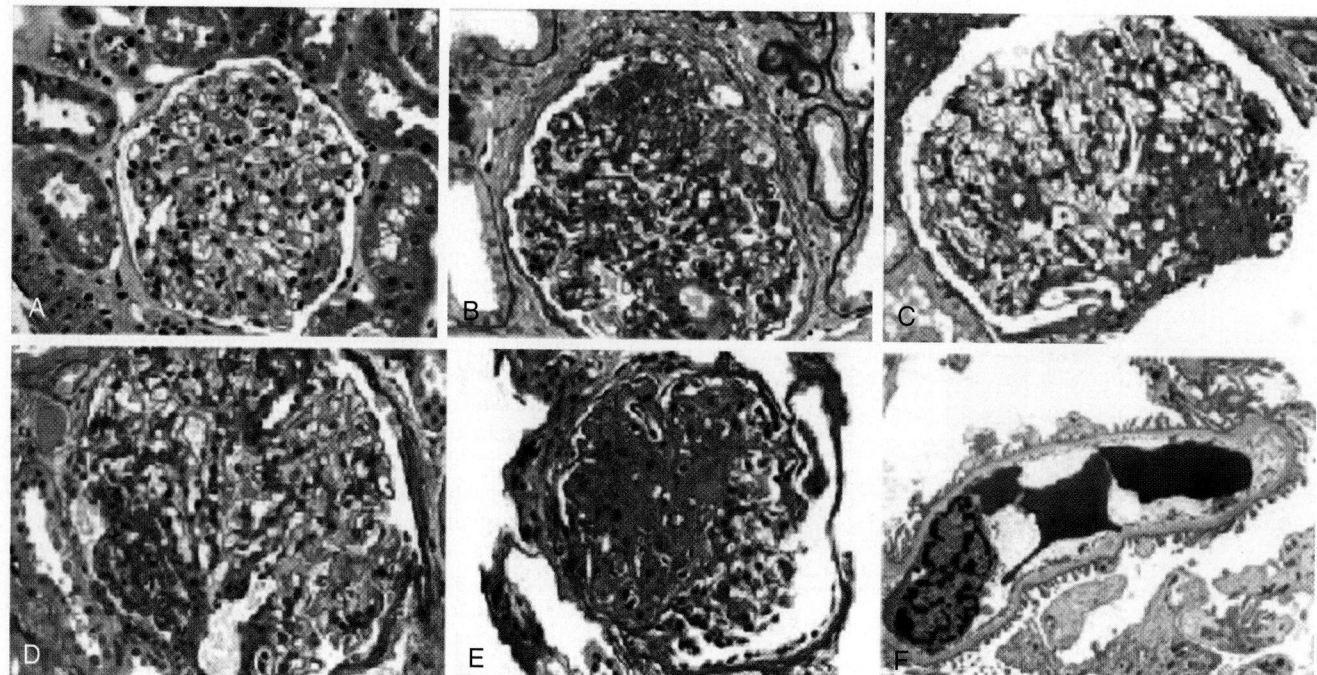

FIGURE 22-10 Renal biopsy findings. *a,* Normal-sized control glomerulus (hematoxylin and eosin stain, ×40). *b* through *e,* Representative glomeruli from four patients who had been premature and had very low birth weight, demonstrating glomerulomegaly and segmental occlusion of glomerular capillaries by matrix accumulation and hyalinosis (periodic acid–Schiff stain, ×40). *f,* Ultrastructural examination of glomerular capillary demonstrating foot process effacement (electron micrograph, ×5000). (From Hodgin JB, Rasoulpour M, Markowitz GS, et al: Very low birth weight is a risk factor for secondary focal segmental glomerulosclerosis, *Clin J Am Soc Nephrol* 4:71-76, 2009.)

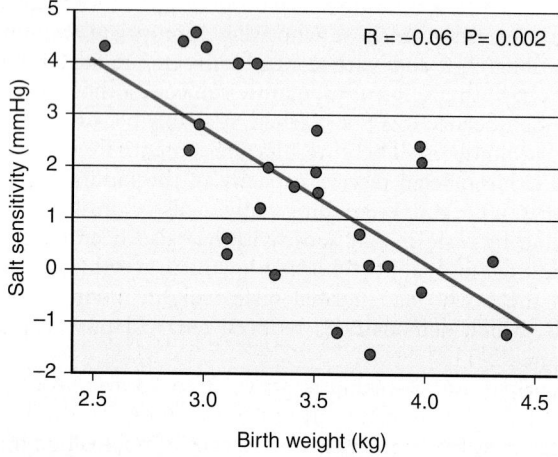

FIGURE 22-11 Correlation between birth weight and salt sensitivity in 27 normotensive adults. (From de Boer MP, Ijzerman RP, de Jongh RT, et al: Birth weight relates to salt sensitivity of blood pressure in healthy adults, *Hypertension* 51:928-932, 2008.)

for gestational age and grew normally. At 7.6 years of age, renal volumes were smaller than expected for height and iothalamate GFRs were significantly lower in both groups of children experiencing perinatal growth restriction. These data again emphasize the critical important of adequate protein intake during renal development.[137]

It is not easy to dissect the relative contributions of genetics and the fetal environment to the ultimate manifestation of disease. To address this question, Gielen and colleagues[138] studied 653 twins, comprising 265 twin pairs and 123 individuals whose twin did not participate in the study. Creatinine clearance was significantly lower in twins who had low birth weight than in those who had normal birth weight. Furthermore, intrapair birth weight differences were positively correlated with GFR in both monozygotic and dizygotic twin pairs; that is, the twin with the higher birth weight had a higher creatinine clearance. These authors concluded that fetoplacental factors have a greater impact than genetic factors on adult renal function. A genetic contribution, however, cannot be excluded. Common polymorphisms of genes involved in branching morphogenesis, *RET* (1476A allele) and *PAX* (AAA haplotypes), have been found to be associated with a 10% reduction in kidney volume and an increase in cord blood cystatin C in normal-birth-weight white newborns.[100,139] These polymorphisms were found in 25% and 18% of the cohort respectively, and therefore may be important contributors to the variability in nephron number in the white population independent of birth weight.

Early compelling evidence of the relationship between birth weight and renal function was published by Hoy and associates,[3,71,125,126] who studied the Aboriginal Australian population. These authors found that the odds ratio for overt albuminuria was 2.8 in those who had been of low birth weight, with a reference value of 1.0 for those of normal birth weight (Figure 22-12).[126] Furthermore, not only was albuminuria associated with low birth weight, but the degree of albuminuria predicted loss of renal function and was strongly correlated with both renal and nonrenal deaths.[71,72]

Similarly, among Pima Indians with type 2 diabetes, the prevalence of albuminuria was 63% in those who had had a birth weight of less than 2500 g, 41% in those of normal birth weight, and 64% in those of high birth weight (≥4500 g).[5] When the data analysis was controlled for maternal diabetes, however, the odds of albuminuria among those of high birth weight was not increased, which indicates a major role

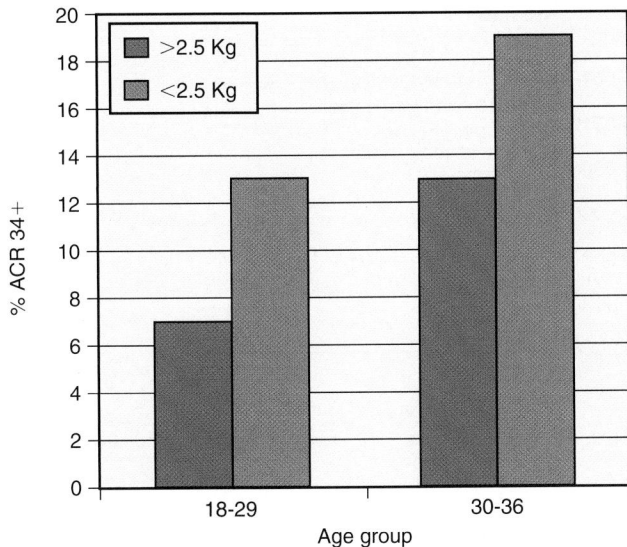

FIGURE 22-12 Birth weight and albumin/creatinine ratio in Tiwi adults. (From Hoy WE, Mathews JD, McCredie DA, et al: The multidimensional nature of renal disease: rates and associations of albuminuria in an Australian Aboriginal community, *Kidney Int* 54:1296-1304, 1998.)

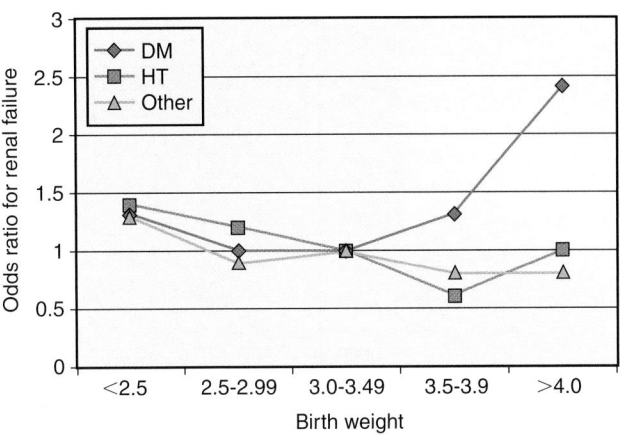

FIGURE 22-13 Birth weight and risk of end-stage renal disease. (From Lackland DT, Bendall HE, Osmond C, et al: Low birth weights contribute to high rates of early-onset chronic renal failure in the Southeastern United States, *Arch Intern Med* 160:1472-1476, 2000.)

for gestational exposure to diabetes in the programming of renal disease risk. This finding has been confirmed in other studies.[140]

Gestational hyperglycemia often results in high birth weight and, as is discussed later, is also associated with reduced nephron number in the offspring. A handful of studies have examined the relationship between birth weight and diabetic nephropathy and have found an increased susceptibility among subjects who had been of low birth weight.[5,141,142] Among women with type 1 diabetes mellitus, nephropathy was present in 75% of those with a birth weight below the 10th percentile (≤2700 g), compared with 35% of those with birth weights above the 90th percentile (≥4000 g).[141] This relationship was not present in men; however, men with diabetic nephropathy were significantly shorter than those without nephropathy, which possibly indicates some degree of growth restriction.[141]

A variety of generally small studies have reported a greater severity of renal disease and more rapid progression of diverse renal diseases, including immunoglobulin A nephropathy, membranous nephropathy, minimal change disease, nephrotic syndrome, and chronic pyelonephritis, in children and adults who had been of low birth weight.[142-148] Lackland and colleagues[47] were the first to examine the relationship of birth weight and ESRD, analyzing data for 1230 dialysis patients and 2460 age- and sex-matched normal controls in South Carolina. This population has a high prevalence of ESRD in young patients, with 70% attributable to hypertension or diabetes. In this cohort, the odds ratio for ESRD was 1.4 (95% confidence interval = 1.1 to 1.8) for those with birth weights under 2500 g compared with those of normal birth weight. This association was consistent for all causes of ESRD and was not affected by family history of ESRD.[47,149] Interestingly, the odds ratio for diabetic renal disease was 2.4 for those having birth weights higher than 4000 g, which may have reflected fetal diabetes exposure (Figure 22-13). Similarly, in a retrospective analysis of a cohort of over 2 million white children, the relative risk of developing ESRD was 1.7 in those

with birth weights at less than the 10th percentile (Figure 22-14).[22] Interestingly, a birth weight of 4.5 kg or more was associated with an increased risk of ESRD in females only. A recent meta-analysis of 31 studies encompassing over 2 million subjects (Figure 22-15) concluded that individuals who had low birth weight have a 70% increased risk of developing CKD, including albuminuria, reduced GFR, and ESRD, in later life.[23] As with the association of birth weight and blood pressures in humans and experimental animals, in some studies the birth weight effect was greater in males.[21-23]

Various hypotheses have been suggested for the programmed gender differences, but these are beyond the scope of this chapter and are reviewed elsewhere.[150] Importantly, the relationship between CKD and birth weight is U-shaped, with higher risk associated with both low and high birth weights; therefore, increased risk is not exclusive to low-birth-weight individuals.[5,21,47] Thus, epidemiologic data are accumulating in support of the impact of fetal programming on subsequent renal disease.

Importantly, the impact of programming may also have intergenerational implications. A mother who had been subjected to adverse intrauterine events as a fetus may have subtle changes in renal function and blood pressure that may impact the success of her own pregnancies. It has been shown that among mothers who experienced adverse perinatal outcomes, especially delivery of infants with birth weights of less than 1.5 kg or development of preeclampsia, the relative risk of requiring a kidney biopsy at a later time was 17.[151] Women who experience preeclampsia are also at increased risk of subsequent ESRD.[152] Conversely, mothers with estimated GFRs of less than 75 mL/min, or a GFR of less than 90 mL/min with hypertension had a significantly increased risk of preeclampsia, preterm birth, or delivery of infants small for gestational age.[153] It is plausible, therefore, that in turn these premature or low-birth-weight infants themselves will be at increased risk for hypertension and kidney disease, perpetuating a vicious circle.

The association between low birth weight and subsequent metabolic syndrome has been well described in many populations around the world.[13,17,154] Whether very early renal dysfunction, manifested as microalbuminuria, is a trigger or a consequence of the metabolic syndrome is a topic of significant interest. Recent evidence points to improved

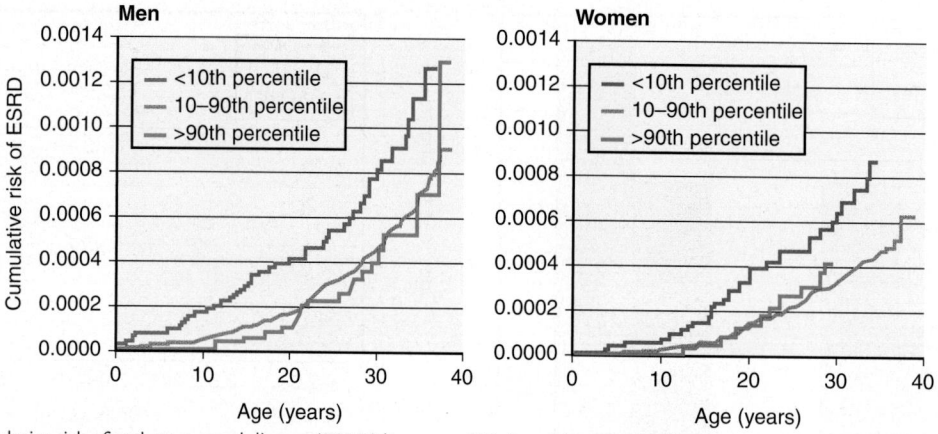

FIGURE 22-14 Cumulative risk of end-stage renal disease (ESRD) by age and birth weight. (From Vikse BE, Irgens LM, Leivestad T, et al: Low birth weight increases risk for end-stage renal disease, *J Am Soc Nephrol* 19:151-157, 2008.)

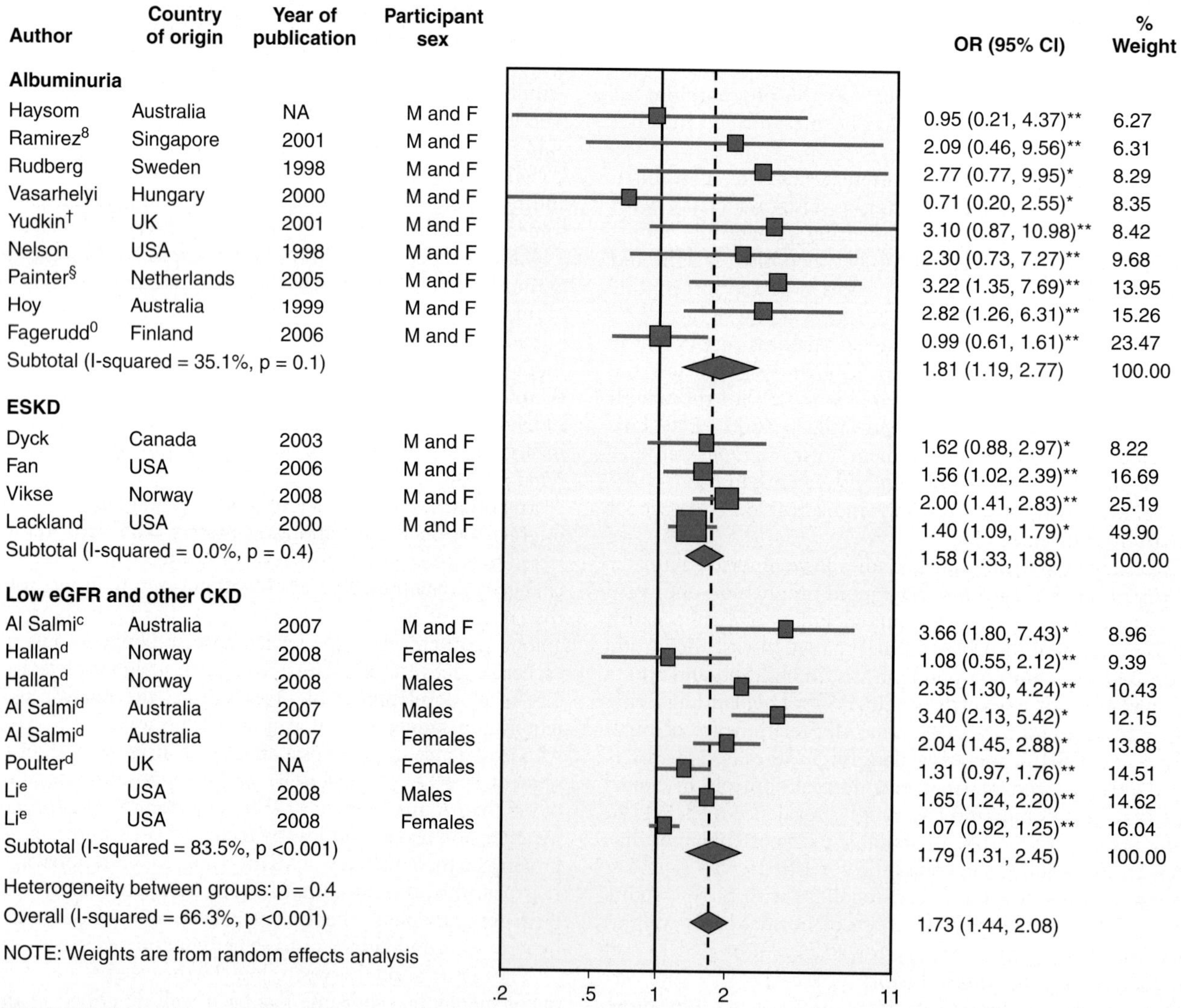

Author	Country of origin	Year of publication	Participant sex		OR (95% CI)	% Weight
Albuminuria						
Haysom	Australia	NA	M and F		0.95 (0.21, 4.37)**	6.27
Ramirez[8]	Singapore	2001	M and F		2.09 (0.46, 9.56)**	6.31
Rudberg	Sweden	1998	M and F		2.77 (0.77, 9.95)*	8.29
Vasarhelyi	Hungary	2000	M and F		0.71 (0.20, 2.55)*	8.35
Yudkin[†]	UK	2001	M and F		3.10 (0.87, 10.98)**	8.42
Nelson	USA	1998	M and F		2.30 (0.73, 7.27)**	9.68
Painter[§]	Netherlands	2005	M and F		3.22 (1.35, 7.69)**	13.95
Hoy	Australia	1999	M and F		2.82 (1.26, 6.31)**	15.26
Fagerudd[0]	Finland	2006	M and F		0.99 (0.61, 1.61)**	23.47
Subtotal (I-squared = 35.1%, p = 0.1)					1.81 (1.19, 2.77)	100.00
ESKD						
Dyck	Canada	2003	M and F		1.62 (0.88, 2.97)*	8.22
Fan	USA	2006	M and F		1.56 (1.02, 2.39)**	16.69
Vikse	Norway	2008	M and F		2.00 (1.41, 2.83)**	25.19
Lackland	USA	2000	M and F		1.40 (1.09, 1.79)*	49.90
Subtotal (I-squared = 0.0%, p = 0.4)					1.58 (1.33, 1.88)	100.00
Low eGFR and other CKD						
Al Salmi[c]	Australia	2007	M and F		3.66 (1.80, 7.43)*	8.96
Hallan[d]	Norway	2008	Females		1.08 (0.55, 2.12)**	9.39
Hallan[d]	Norway	2008	Males		2.35 (1.30, 4.24)**	10.43
Al Salmi[d]	Australia	2007	Males		3.40 (2.13, 5.42)*	12.15
Al Salmi[d]	Australia	2007	Females		2.04 (1.45, 2.88)*	13.88
Poulter[d]	UK	NA	Females		1.31 (0.97, 1.76)**	14.51
Li[e]	USA	2008	Males		1.65 (1.24, 2.20)**	14.62
Li[e]	USA	2008	Females		1.07 (0.92, 1.25)**	16.04
Subtotal (I-squared = 83.5%, p <0.001)					1.79 (1.31, 2.45)	100.00
Heterogeneity between groups: p = 0.4						
Overall (I-squared = 66.3%, p <0.001)					1.73 (1.44, 2.08)	

NOTE: Weights are from random effects analysis

.2   .5   1   2   11

FIGURE 22-15 Odds ratios and 95% confidence intervals for risk of chronic kidney disease associated with low versus normal birth weight. Outcome is [a]proteinuria; [b]diabetic nephropathy, albuminuria, or end stage renal disease; [c]chronic kidney disease stages 2 to 5; [d]estimated glomerular filtration rate (GFR) less than 10th percentile for sex; [e]albuminuria or estimated GFR less than 60 mL/min/1.73 m². (From White SL, Perkovic V, Cass A, et al: Is low birth weight an antecedent of CKD in later life? A systematic review of observational studies, *Am J Kidney Dis* 54:248-261, 2009.)

cardiovascular outcomes with reduction in microalbuminuria, which may support the former possibility, although experimental evidence also supports simultaneous programming of the endocrine pancreas and cardiovascular system during fetal development.[155]

Proposed Mechanisms of Fetal Programming of Nephron Number

Kidney development is a complex process involving tightly controlled expression of many genes and constant remodelling.[92,156] The molecular regulation of kidney development is exhaustively reviewed elsewhere.[92,157] Many experimental models, as outlined in Table 22-3, have been shown to result in a reduced nephron number. In many of the experimental models of programming, as mentioned previously, a reduced nephron number is associated often with low birth weight and often with subsequent hypertension and evidence of renal injury. Interestingly, in normal rat litters, those pups with naturally occurring low birth weight (i.e., birth weights below −2 standard deviations from the mean) have been found to have a 13% reduction in nephron number, which is also associated with glomerulomegaly and proteinuria.[158] Low birth weight in rodents, therefore, may be associated with a low nephron number even under nonexperimental conditions.

Low birth weight in humans is often associated with poor maternal nutrition, smoking, alcohol ingestion, infections, and low socioeconomic status, all factors that, in turn, may affect nephrogenesis.[65] In humans, kidney development begins at around 8 weeks of gestation and continues until 36 weeks. Approximately two thirds of the nephrons develop during the last trimester of gestation, which makes this the window during which the fetal kidney is most susceptible to adverse effects, but earlier insults can also have a major impact on subsequent nephrogenesis.[98,159]

In rodents, nephrogenesis continues for up to 10 days after birth, but in most animal studies, the major impact is noted when environmental stimuli are manipulated when nephrogenesis is most active, that is, mid to late gestation.[159] Three processes determine ultimate nephron number: branching of the ureteric bud, condensation of mesenchymal cells, and conversion of mesenchymal condensates into epithelium.[156] It has been estimated that a 2% decrease in ureteric bud branching efficiency would result in a 50% reduction in final nephron complement after 20 generations of branching.[160] The specific molecular mechanisms whereby nephron numbers may be affected and/or function altered, however, are not yet completely understood. Several potential mechanisms have been proposed and investigated thus far, as summarized in Table 22-4 and discussed later.

Maternal Nutrient Restriction

Experimental alterations in maternal dietary composition at different stages of gestation have been shown to program embryonic kidney gene expression early in the course of gestation, which later affects nephron number.[161] Fetal nutrient supply is also affected by alterations in placental blood flow.

Maternal *protein restriction* during pregnancy has been the most widely studied model, but because the manipulations

TABLE 22-3 Experimental Models of Reduced Nephron Number

EXPERIMENTAL MODEL	POSSIBLE MECHANISM OF NEPHRON NUMBER REDUCTION
Maternal low-protein diet	↑ Apoptosis in metanephros and postnatal kidney Altered gene expression in developing kidney Altered gene methylation ↓ Placental 11β-HSD2 expression
Maternal vitamin A restriction	↓ Branching of ureteric bud ? Maintenance of spatial orientation of vascular development ↓ c-ret expression
Maternal iron restriction	? Reduced oxygen delivery ? Altered glucocorticoid responsiveness ? Altered micronutrient availability
Gestational glucocorticoid exposure	↑ Fetal glucocorticoid exposure ? Enhanced tissue maturation ↑ Glucocorticoid receptor expression ↑ α_1 and β_1 adenosine triphosphatase expression ↓ Renal and adrenal 11β-HSD2 expression
Uterine artery ligation/embolization	↑ Proapoptotic gene expression in developing kidney: casepase-3, Bax, p53 ↓ Antiapoptotic gene expression: Pax-2, Bcl-2 Altered gene methylation Altered renin-angiotensin gene expression
Maternal diabetes/hyperglycemia	↓ IGF-2/mannose-6-phosphate receptor expression Altered IGF-2 activity or bioavailability Activation of nuclear factor kB
Gestational drug exposure Gentamicin β-lactams Cyclosporine Ethanol Cyclooxygenase-2 inhibitors	↓ Branching morphogenesis ↑ Mesenchymal apoptosis Arrest of nephron formation ? Reduced vitamin A levels Effect on prostaglandins

11β-HSD2, 11β-hydroxysteroid dehydrogenase type 2; *IGF-2*, insulin-like growth factor-2

occur at different times of gestation and for different periods during gestation, the results are not always easy to compare and interpret. Furthermore, not all low-protein diets have the same programming effects. It has been proposed that relative deficiencies of specific amino acids—methionine or glycine, for example—may have a greater impact on organ development than total protein restriction per se.[24,162] Interestingly, maternal protein restriction in rats results in intergenerational programming persisting into the F2 generation.[163] These effects have been proposed to be mediated largely by changes in DNA methylation, depending on amino acid availability, which results in epigenetic changes in gene expression.[12] In the rat model of uterine ischemia, restoration of good fetal nutrition postnatally, during ongoing nephrogenesis, has been shown to result in restoration of nephron number, a finding that further emphasizes the critical importance of maternal nutrition during renal development.[93]

Maternal *iron restriction* during pregnancy in rats has also been found to lead to a reduction in birth weight and nephron number and the development of subsequent hypertension in the offspring.[164] The authors of the study suggest that fetal anemia may result in reduced tissue oxygen delivery, altered

TABLE 22-4 Experimental and Human Associations with Reduced Nephron Numbers and Clinical Findings

MODEL	SUBJECT	GLOMERULAR NUMBER	BIRTH WEIGHT	BLOOD PRESSURE	RENAL FUNCTION
Maternal calorie restriction[168,171,202]	Rat	↓ 20-40%	↓	↑	↓ GFR Proteinuria
Uterine artery ligation[93,158,179]	Rat	↓ 20-30%	↓	↑	Impaired Proteinuria
Low-protein diet[89,124,169,240]	Rat	↓ 25% ↓ 17% ↓ 16%	↓/⇔	↑	↓ GFR Proteinuria ↓ Longevity
Iron deficiency[164]	Rat	↓ 22%	↓	↑	NA
Vitamin A deficiency[165]	Rat	↓ 20%	↔	NA	NA
Ethanol exposure[167]	Sheep	↓ 11%	↔	NA	NA
Glucocorticoid exposure[84,88,183,241]	Rat, sheep	↓ 20% ↓ 38%	↔ ↔	↑ ↑	Glomerulosclerosis ↑ Collagen deposition
Maternal diabetes[121,188]	Rat	↓ 10-35%	↔	↑	Salt sensitivity
Gentamicin exposure[194,196]	Rat	↓ 10-20%	↓	NA	NA
β-Lactam exposure[198]	Rat	↓ 5-10%	↔	NA	Tubular dilatation Interstitial inflammation
Cyclosporine exposure[200,242]	Rabbit	↓ 25-33%	↓/↔	↑	↓ GFR ↑ RVR Proteinuria
Dahl salt-sensitive rat[45]	Rat	↓ 15%	↔	↑ with Na intake	Accelerated FSGS
Munich-Wistar-Frömter rat[45,243]	Rat	↓ 40%		↑ with age	↑ SNGFR FSGS
Milan hypertensive rat[45]	Rat	↓ 17%		↑	NA
PVG/c[45]	Rat	↑ 122%		resistant	Resistant to FSGS
Os/+ mouse[244]	Mouse	↓ 50%		NA	Glomerular hypertrophy
PAX2 mutations[139,174,177]	Mouse, human	↓ 22%		NA	Renal coloboma syndrome in humans, small kidneys
GDNF heterozygosity[180,181]	Mouse	↓ 30%	↔	↑	Normal GFR Enlarged glomeruli
c-ret–null mutation[156]	Mouse	↓	NA	NA	Severe renal dysplasia
hIGFBP-1 overexpression[193]	Mouse	↓ 18-25%	↓	NA	Glomerulosclerosis
Bcl-2 deficiency[175]	Mouse	↓	NA	NA	↑ BUN and creatinine
BF-2–null mutation[156]	Mouse	↓ 75%	NA	NA	NA
BMP 7–null mutation[156,245,246]	Mouse	↓	NA	NA	Small kidneys
p53 transgenic mouse[178]	Mouse	↓ 50%	NA	NA	Glomerular hypertrophy Renal failure
Cyclooxygenase-2–null mutaton[247]	Mouse	NA	↔	↔	↓ GFR
Fibroblast growth factor receptor 2 deletion[248]	Mouse	↓	↔	↑	Glomerular and tubular injury
Fibroblast growth factor 7–null mutation[249]	Mouse	↓ 30%	NA	NA	Small kidneys
Pbx1-null mutation[250]	Mouse	↓	NA	NA	Embryonic lethal
Intrauterine growth retardation[66,99]	Human 0-1 yr	↓ 13-35%	↓	NA	NA
Hypertensive (relative to normotensive) whites[55,96]	Human 35-59 yr	↓ 19-50%	NA	↑	Glomerulosclerosis not ↑
Hypertensive (relative to normotensive) African Americans[96]	Human 35-59 yr	NS ↓	NA	↑	Glomerulosclerosis not ↑
Aboriginal Australians[52]	Human 0-85 yr	↓ 23%	↓	NA	
Senegalese Africans[77,78]	Human 5-70 yr	NA	NA	NA	↑ Variability of glomerular size with ↓ glomerular numbers

BUN, Blood urea nitrogen; *FSGS*, focal segmental glomerulosclerosis; *GFR*, glomerular filtration rate; *GDNF*, glial cell line–derived neurotrophic factor; *hIGFBP-1*, human insulin-like growth factor–binding protein-1; *NA*, not assessed; *NS*, nonsignificant; *RVR*, renal vascular resistance; *SNGFR*, single-nephron glomerular filtration rate; ↑, increased; ↓, decreased; ↔, no change.
Data from Brenner et al,[45] Kett and Bertram,[52] Clark and Bertram,[156] and Moritz et al.[246]

fetal kidney glucocorticoid sensitivity, or altered availability of other micronutrients that may affect nephrogenesis. These hypotheses remain to be proved.

Maternal *vitamin A restriction* has also been associated with a reduction in nephron number in the offspring.[87,165] Severe vitamin A deficiency during pregnancy is associated with congenital malformations and renal defects in the offspring. Vitamin A and all-*trans* retinoic acid have been shown to stimulate nephrogenesis through modulation of ureteric bud branching capacity in ureteric epithelial cell culture and in maintenance of spatial organization of blood vessel development in cultured renal cortical explants.[165] in vivo, a vitamin A–deficient diet sufficient to reduce circulating vitamin A levels by 50% in pregnant rats resulted in a 25% reduction in nephron number in the offspring.[165] Intriguingly, supplementation of vitamin A increased nephron numbers. Analysis of 21-day-old fetal rats (just before birth) revealed a direct correlation between plasma retinol concentration and nephron number, as shown in Figure 22-16.[165] The reduction in nephron number in the setting of vitamin A deficiency is likely mediated at least in part by modulation of genes regulating branching morphogenesis.[165] These genes are discussed in detail later. Supplemental retinoic acid was therefore studied as a means to stimulate nephrogenesis in postnatal preterm baboons, but no effect was observed.[166] It is interesting to note that smoking and alcohol intake are associated with reduced levels of circulating vitamin A, and both, during pregnancy, are associated with infant low birth weight.

In sheep, repeated *ethanol* exposure during the second half of pregnancy resulted in an 11% reduction in nephron number.[167] There has been a single abstract suggesting an impact of maternal alcohol ingestion on kidney development in children, but it is not known whether the effects are mediated by associated vitamin A deficiency or other mechanisms.[65] Subtle differences in vitamin A level during pregnancy, therefore, may be a significant factor contributing to the wide distribution of nephron number in the general population.[65]

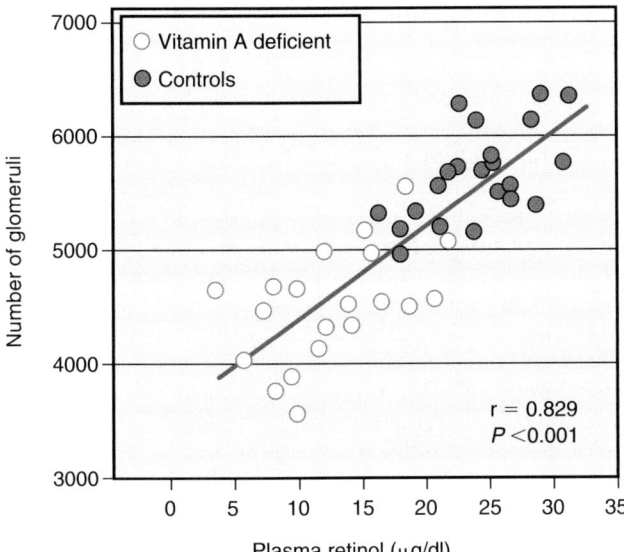

FIGURE 22-16 Nephron number and plasma retinol in term rat fetuses. (From Merlet-Benichou C: Influence of fetal environment on kidney development, *Int J Dev Biol* 43:453-456, 1999.)

Increased Apoptosis in the Kidney

Total calorie restriction and maternal dietary protein restriction in animals result in low birth weight of offspring and frequently associated hypertension and reduced nephron numbers.[12,89,168-172] Vehaskari and colleagues[89] reported a 29% reduction in nephron number in low-birth-weight rat offspring of mothers subjected to a 6% low-protein diet compared with offspring of mothers consuming a 20% normal-protein diet during pregnancy. Associated with this reduction, systolic blood pressures were 20 to 25 mm Hg higher at 8 weeks in pups in the low-protein-diet group than in those in the normal-protein-diet group (see Figure 22-3). These authors also found that, although the kidneys looked histologically normal at 8 weeks postnatally, there was evidence of increased apoptosis without an increase in proliferation in the low-protein-diet group.

Welham and colleagues[172] examined embryonic metanephroi to evaluate at which stage of development a low-protein diet affects nephrogenesis. At embryonic day 13, the metanephros has just formed, the ureteric bud has branched once, branch tips are surrounded by condensed mesenchyme that later transforms into tubule epithelium, and the ureteric stalk is surrounded by loose stromal mesenchyme.[161] By day 15, multiple branching cycles have occurred and primitive nephrons begin to be formed.[161] The authors therefore examined metanephroi at these two time points. At embryonic day 13, there was no difference in the number of cells in metanephroi from embryos whose mothers had received a normal-protein diet compared with those from embryos whose mothers had eaten a reduced-protein diet. At day 15, however, there were significantly fewer cells per metanephros in the low-protein group than in the normal-protein group. Furthermore, when the investigators examined apoptosis at these two time points, they observed a significant increase in the numbers of apoptotic cells in the low-protein group at day 13 but not at day 15. The authors concluded that the increase in early (day 13) apoptosis was most likely responsible for the reduced cell numbers later (day 15).

As mentioned previously, Vehaskari and colleagues[89] noted an increase in apoptosis at 8 weeks postnatally in offspring of rats fed a low-protein diet; therefore, there may be successive waves of apoptosis at different stages of nephrogenesis that may affect final nephron endowment. Welham and colleagues[172] described an increase in apoptosis in both the condensing and the loose mesenchyme of the metanephros but did not measure the relative amount of cell death in each compartment. They suggest two possible mechanisms whereby an increase in apoptosis observed in the offspring of low-protein-diet–fed dams at embryonic day 13 could lead to a reduction in nephron number: (1) directly through loss of actual nephron precursors (i.e., in the condensing mesenchyme), or (2) indirectly through loss of cells in the loose mesenchyme (i.e., the stromal compartment, which supports nephrogenesis but does not contribute actual cells to the final epithelial lineage).[172] These hypotheses are as yet unproved, but evidence for an impact of changes in the supporting metanephric stroma on nephron development and number is emerging. Mice deficient in the BF-2 transcription factor, expressed in metanephric stroma, have abnormal kidney development and reduced nephron numbers, associated with slower differentiation of condensed mesenchyme into tubule epithelium and decreased ureteric branching.[173] Nephron development therefore depends upon a close relationship between tubule epithelial precursors and surrounding tissue matrix. Both compartments are thus likely to be susceptible to programming effects.

Other studies have suggested that altered regulation of apoptosis in the developing kidney may be due to downregulation of antiapoptotic factors (e.g., Pax-2 or Bcl-2) and/or upregulation of proapoptotic factors in response to environmental or other stimuli (e.g., Bax, p53).[172,174-176] Humans with haploinsufficiency of PAX2 have renal coloboma syndrome, which includes renal hypoplasia and early renal failure as well as optic nerve colobomas.[139,174,177] PAX2 is an antiapoptotic transcriptional regulator that is highly expressed in the branching ureteric bud as well as in foci of induced nephrogenic mesenchyme during kidney development.[174] Heterozygous mice with Pax2 mutations were found to be very small at birth and to have significant reductions in nephron number. In addition, there was a significant increase in apoptotic cell death in the developing kidneys. Subsequent research demonstrated that loss of Pax2 antiapoptotic activity reduced ureteric bud branching and increased ureteric bud apoptosis.[177] Similarly, loss of the antiapoptotic factor Bcl-2 or gain of function of the proapoptotic factor p53 in Bcl-2 knockout mice and p53 transgenic mice is also associated with a significant reduction in nephron number, due to increased apoptosis in metanephric blastemas.[175,178]

Mutant mouse models, however, although providing evidence that an increase in apoptosis results in reduced nephron numbers, do not address the impact of environmental factors in renal programming. Pham and associates[179] examined gene expression in the kidneys of growth-retarded offspring of rats subjected to uterine artery ligation during gestation. These authors found a 25% reduction in glomerular number, associated with increased evidence of apoptosis and increased proapoptotic caspase-3 activity in the kidney at birth. Furthermore, they found evidence of increased messenger RNA (mRNA) expression of the proapoptotic genes Bax and p53 and decreased expression of the antiapoptotic gene Bcl-2. These authors also found evidence of hypomethylation of the p53 gene, which, in addition to a decrease in Bcl-2 expression, would lead to an increase in p53 activity. Alteration in gene methylation has also been proposed as a mechanism of low-protein diet–induced programming effects, as mentioned previously. The increase in apoptotic activity in the developing kidney subjected to various gestational insults therefore appears to be a consistent finding and to be mediated via modulation of gene expression in a number of different pathways.

Glial Cell Line–Derived Neurotrophic Factor and c-ret Receptor Function

Glial cell line–derived neurotrophic factor (GDNF), signalling through its receptor tyrosine kinase Ret, is known to be a key ligand-receptor interaction driving initiation of ureteric bud branching. The c-ret receptor is expressed on the tips of the ureteric bud branches, and knockout of this receptor in mice leads to severe renal dysplasia and reduction in nephron number.[156] Homozygous GDNF-null mutant mice have complete renal agenesis and die shortly after birth.[180] Heterozygous GDNF mice exhibit reduced branching morphogenesis and have approximately 30% fewer nephrons than wild-type

mice.[180,181] These mice also develop spontaneous hypertension and glomerulomegaly with time. Polymorphisms in GDNF are not associated with newborn renal size in humans, however.[182] As described previously, maternal dietary vitamin A level has a significant impact on nephrogenesis (see Figure 22-16). In cultured metanephroi, the expression of c-ret was found to be regulated by retinoic acid supplementation in a dose-dependent manner.[165] GDNF expression was not affected by vitamin A fluctuations. Modulation of c-ret expression is therefore likely to be a significant pathway through which vitamin A availability regulates nephrogenesis.

Fetal Exposure to Glucocorticoids

Under normal circumstances, the fetus is protected from exposure to excess maternal corticosteroids by the placental enzyme 11β-hydroxysteroid dehydrogenase type 2 (11β-HSD2), which metabolizes corticosterone to the inert 11-dehydrocorticosterone.[12] Prenatal administration of dexamethasone, a steroid not metabolized by 11β-HSD2, was found to lead to fetal growth restriction, a 20% to 60% reduction in nephron number, glomerulomegaly, and subsequent hypertension in rats and sheep.[84,88,123,183] Similar effects have been seen with lower levels of placental 11β-HSD2 in rats and humans with mutations in the 11β-HSD2 gene, in whom birth weights are low and hypertension develops prematurely.[184,185] Interestingly, a maternal low-protein diet during gestation has been shown to result in decreased placental expression of 11β-HSD2, which therefore likely increases the exposure of the fetus to maternal corticosteroids.[24,186] Treatment of pregnant rats fed a low-protein diet with an inhibitor of steroid synthesis abrogates the programming of hypertension in the offspring, which suggests a prominent role for fetal steroid exposure in the low-protein-diet model.[12,24] Excessive fetal steroid exposure may then drive inappropriate gene expression and affect growth and nephrogenesis, potentially through more rapid maturation of tissue structures.[24]

To investigate the molecular mechanisms through which glucocorticoid exposure may program hypertension, Bertram and associates[186] examined expression of steroid-responsive receptors in offspring of rats fed a low-protein diet during gestation. These authors found a greater than twofold increase in fetal and neonatal glucocorticoid receptor mRNA expression in offspring of mothers fed a low-protein diet compared with offspring of those fed a normal-protein diet. This difference increased to threefold as the offspring aged. In addition, the expression of the corticosteroid-responsive renal Na+/K+–adenosine triphosphatase (ATPase) α_1- and β_1-subunits was increased in these offspring. Expression of the mineralocorticoid receptors was no different in the two groups. Interestingly, levels of 11β-HSD2 in offspring kidney and adrenal gland were significantly reduced during fetal and postnatal life in those exposed to a low-protein diet in utero. These authors conclude that the observed changes would result in marked increases in glucocorticoid action in these tissues and is likely a significant mediator of programmed hypertension.[186] In another study, prenatal dexamethasone exposure was associated with increased proximal tubule transport, in part related to increased activity of tubular Na+/H+ exchanger isoform 3 (NHE3).[187] The mechanism of glucocorticoid-mediated reduction in nephron number has not yet been elucidated.

Fetal Exposure to Hyperglycemia and the Role of Insulin-like Growth Factors and Their Receptors

As discussed previously, in the South Carolina dialysis population and the Pima Indian population in Arizona, high birth weight is associated with an increased susceptibility to proteinuria and renal disease (see Figure 22-13).[5,47,140] High birth weight is a complication of gestational hyperglycemia and diabetes and may therefore also be a surrogate marker of abnormal intrauterine programming. To address the question of whether gestational diabetes affects nephrogenesis in the offspring, Amri and colleagues[188] studied offspring of rats rendered hyperglycemic during pregnancy either by inducing diabetes mellitus with streptozotocin or by infusing glucose from gestational days 12 to 16. Nephron numbers in offspring exposed to maternal hyperglycemia were reduced by 10% to 35%, and the degree of nephron number reduction correlated with the degree of maternal hyperglycemia (Figure 22-17). Furthermore, in vitro culture of metanephroi subjected to varying glucose concentrations demonstrated that tight glucose control is necessary for optimal metanephric growth and differentiation. In one study in mice, offspring of diabetic mothers had fewer nephrons, with evidence of increased apoptosis in tubules and podocytes.[189] The study authors suggested that the reduction in nephron number may be mediated by an increased renal angiotensinogen and renin mRNA expression and nuclear factor κB activation. With regard to function, study of adult rat offspring of diabetic mothers revealed glomerular hypertrophy, reduced GFR and renal plasma flow, hypertension, and decreased endothelium-mediated vasodilation, despite no reduction in nephron number.[190,191] These findings suggest that programming of hypertension in offspring of diabetic mothers may be multifactorial.

Offspring of diabetic pregnancies have a higher incidence of congenital malformations, resulting from defects in early organogenesis.[192] Furthermore, it is known that expression and bioavailability of the insulin-like growth factors (IGFs) are altered in diabetic pregnancies, and that IGFs and their binding proteins are important regulators of fetal development.[192] The impact of maternal diabetes on metanephros expression of IGFs and their receptors was studied in rats in which maternal diabetes was induced by streptozotocin and in gestational-age–matched normal controls.[192] In metanephroi from offspring subjected to maternal diabetes, there was no significant change in IGF-1 or IGF-2 or insulin receptor expression at any stage. Throughout nephrogenesis, however, there was a significantly increased expression of the IGF-2/mannose-6-phosphate receptor. The authors postulate that because this receptor tightly regulates the action of IGF-2, a reduction in its expression may lead to enhanced activity of IGF-2, a critical player in renal development. The same group of investigators has examined the impact of IGF-binding protein 1 on nephrogenesis in genetically modified mice.[193]

Overexpression of human IGF-binding protein 1 in adult mice results in glomerulosclerosis. Offspring of females overexpressing human IGF-binding protein 1 were found to be growth restricted and to have an 18% to 25% reduction in nephron number depending on whether human IGF binding protein-1 was overexpressed in the mother only, fetus only, or both. When metanephroi from these mice were cultured in the presence of IGF-1 or IGF-2, the authors found that IGF-2 increased nephron numbers by 25% to 40% in a concentration-dependent manner, whereas IGF-1 had no effect.[193] This study did not involve maternal diabetes or hyperglycemia, but the findings are consistent with a role for increased IGF-2 activity in nephrogenesis.

Fetal Drug Exposure

Several medications commonly used during pregnancy or in the early postnatal period have been studied for their effects on nephrogenesis. Administration of the aminoglycoside antibiotic *gentamicin* to pregnant rats results in a permanent nephron deficit in their offspring.[194] Subsequent experiments by the same authors demonstrated a significant reduction in nephron number in metanephric explants cultured in the presence of gentamicin.[195] In cultured metanephroi, within 8 hours of gentamicin administration, the drug was localized to the growing tips of ureteric buds and the surrounding blastema, and within 24 hours, the presence of gentamicin was associated with a significant reduction in the number of branching points.[196] These data suggest that the reduction in nephron number observed after administration of gentamicin during pregnancy is a result of a decrease in branching morphogenesis. Others, however, failed to find a reduction in nephron number in rat pups administered gentamicin intraperitoneally from birth to 14 days of age.[197] Although there is ongoing nephrogenesis after birth, these studies, taken together, may suggest a more proximal window of action for gentamicin in utero.

Another group of antibiotics that has been shown to result in impaired nephrogenesis is the β-*lactams*.[198] Administration of ampicillin to pregnant rats leads to an 11% average reduction in nephron number in the offspring, as well as evidence of focal cystic tubule dilatation and interstitial inflammation. The administration of ceftriaxone in vivo did not result in a nephron deficit, but histologically, there was evidence of renal interstitial inflammation. The penicillins were also found to inhibit nephrogenesis in cultured metanephroi in vitro in a

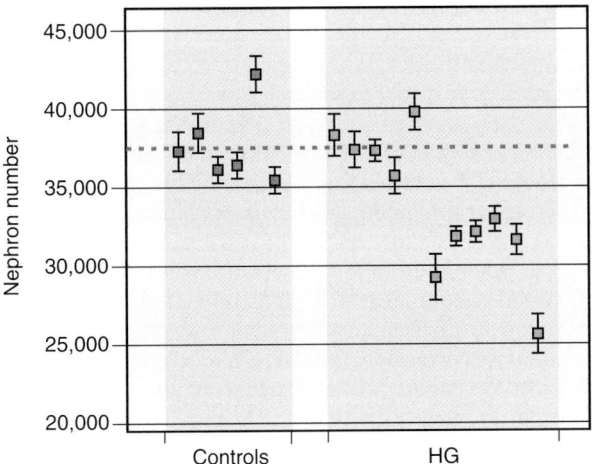

HG-hyperglycemia. Dotted line represents mean value in control group

FIGURE 22-17 Effects of maternal hyperglycemia on nephron number in rat offspring. (From Amri K, Freund N, Vilar J, et al: Adverse effects of hyperglycemia on kidney development in rats: in vivo and in vitro studies, *Diabetes* 48:2240-2245, 1999.)

dose-dependent fashion, an effect that was less evident with ceftriaxone. Importantly, nephrogenesis was affected even at therapeutic dosages of penicillins in the rat, which warrants further research on such frequently used antibiotics in human pregnancy. The mechanism whereby these antibiotics reduce nephron number is likely an increase in apoptosis observed in the induced mesenchyme in exposed developing kidneys.[87]

The immunosuppressive medication *cyclosporine* is a known nephrotoxin in humans, and this drug crosses the placenta.[151] Women treated with this medication may have successful pregnancies, but its effect on the fetal kidney is not well described, although infants of these women tend to have birth weights in the low range.[199] The effects of administration of this medication in varying dosages and at different stages of gestation were evaluated in pregnant rabbits, and results compared with those for rabbits receiving either vehicle or no drug.[199] Cyclosporine administration in the later period, but not the earlier period, of gestation resulted in smaller litters and growth-restricted pups. All pups exposed to cyclosporine in utero had a 25% to 33% reduction in nephron number compared with controls. The reduction in nephron number was accompanied by glomerulomegaly and was independent of birth weight. At 1 month of age, these kidneys also demonstrated foci of glomerulosclerosis. Subsequent functional evaluation of the kidneys of rabbits exposed to cyclosporine in utero demonstrated a reduction in GFR at 18 and 35 weeks of age and an increase in proteinuria at 11, 18, and 35 weeks of age.[200] Rabbits exposed to cyclosporine in utero developed spontaneous hypertension by 11 weeks of age, which worsened progressively with time.[200] It is important to recognize that, despite reduction in nephron number from birth, renal function did not deteriorate until later, an important factor to bear in mind when evaluating children exposed to cyclosporine in utero. Nephron formation was found to be arrested, potentially due to inhibition of conversion of metanephric mesenchyme to epithelium in the presence of cyclosporine.[87]

Nonsteroidal antiinflammatory drugs are sometimes used in premature children after birth. Their effect on nephrogenesis has been studied in rodents. Administration of a cyclooxygenase-2 inhibitor, but not a cyclooxygenase-1 inhibitor, postnatally in rats and mice resulted in reduced cortical volume, impairment of nephrogenesis, and reduced glomerular diameter.[201] Administration of indomethacin or ibuprofen postnatally did not affect nephron number in rats.[197] The impact of these medications on human nephrogenesis is not known.

Programmed Changes within the Kidney

The kidney is one of the major organs influencing blood pressure, and programming of hypertension does appear to be mediated at least in part by nephron endowment. That congenitally acquired nephron number is not the sole programmable factor responsible for subsequent hypertension has been shown in offspring of rats fed a low-protein diet in whom diets were supplemented with glycine, alanine, or urea.[24] As mentioned previously, nephron number was restored in all offspring, but hypertension was prevented only in the glycine supplementation group.

In humans, in the two studies that have examined nephron number in relation to presence or absence of essential hypertension in adults, a relationship between the two was found in whites but was weaker in African Americans.[55,96] These studies suggest that programming of hypertension may occur in the absence of an alteration in nephron number. The pressure-natriuresis curve is shifted to the right in most forms of hypertension, and prenatally programmed hypertension has been demonstrated by some investigators to be salt sensitive.[26,114,119,122,134,135] A reduction in filtration surface area associated with a reduction in nephron number is one plausible hypothesis to explain this observation, but other programmed effects have also been described that are likely to influence blood pressure and sodium homeostasis.

Renal Vascular Reactivity

An increase in baseline renal vascular resistance has been described by several authors using different models of fetal programming.[200,202,203] In addition, renal arterial responses to β-adrenergic stimulation and sensitivity to adenylyl cyclase were found to be increased in 21-day-old growth-restricted offspring of mothers subjected to uterine artery ligation during gestation.[204] The renal expression of β_2-adrenoreceptor mRNA was increased in the pups of rats subjected to reduced uteroplacental blood flow, but there was also evidence of adaptations to the signal transduction pathway contributing to the β-adrenergic hyperresponsiveness observed. Intriguingly, these findings were much more marked in the right than in the left kidney, an observation that remains unexplained but that is not without precedent: asymmetry of renal blood flow was found in 51% of a cohort of hypertensive individuals without renovascular disease.[204,205] Functionally, the growth-restricted rats in the aforementioned study had reduced glomerular numbers, exhibited hyperfiltration and hyperperfusion, and had significantly increased proteinuria compared with the controls. In children, low birth weight was associated with increased systolic blood pressure, elevated uric acid levels, and dilation mediated by reduced flow (Figure 22-18).[206] Uric acid level was inversely associated with flow-mediated dilation in the low-birth-weight group. It is not yet clear whether vascular function is programmed independently or whether subtle decreases in renal function may result in elevations in uric acid that affect vascular reactivity.

Renin-Angiotensin System

All of the components of the renin-angiotensin system are expressed in the developing kidney.[207] The importance of angiotensin II in nephrogenesis was demonstrated by the administration of the angiotensin II subtype 1 receptor (AT_1R) blocker losartan to normal rats during the first 12 days of life (while nephrogenesis is proceeding), which resulted in a reduction in final nephron number and subsequent development of hypertension.[208] Interestingly, administration of losartan or the angiotensin converting enzyme (ACE) inhibitor captopril to low-birth-weight rats from 2 to 4 weeks of age abrogated the development of adult hypertension in these animals.[12,93,209,210] These data suggest upregulation of the AT_1R postnatally, which could be a result of increased glucocorticoid exposure.[12] In support of this hypothesis, administration of angiotensin II or ACE inhibitor to adult rats subjected to a low-protein diet in utero resulted in an exaggerated

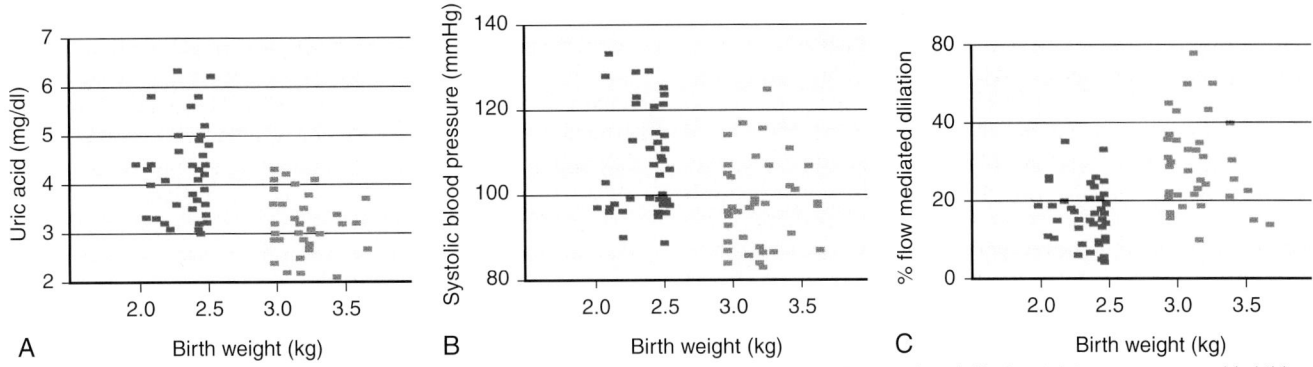

FIGURE 22-18 Correlations among birth weight, uric acid (**A**), systolic blood pressure (**B**) and flow-mediated dilation (**C**) in 8- to 13-year-old children. (From Franco MC, Christofalo DM, Sawaya AL, et al: Effects of low birth weight in 8- to 13-year old children: implications in endothelial function and uric acid levels, *Hypertension* 48:45-50, 2006.)

hypertensive or hypotensive response compared with control rats.[12,211-213]

Expression of angiotensinogen and renin mRNA was found to be decreased in neonatal kidneys of rats subjected to uterine ischemia, but increased in mouse offspring of diabetic mothers.[189,210] In neonates and young offspring of rats subjected to gestational protein restriction, renal renin, AT_1R, and angiotensin II mRNA and protein levels have all been found to be reduced compared with control rats, but the AT_1R expression increases above control levels as the rats reach the prehypertensive stage.[26,90,208,212-214] In contrast, AT_1R expression has been reported to be increased or unchanged in rats subjected to uterine ischemia and is further modulated by postnatal nutrition.[93,210]

Renal expression of the angiotensin II subtype 2 receptor (AT_2R) has been found to be downregulated in young rats and upregulated in neonatal sheep, an effect that may reflect different stages of renal maturation at birth in these species.[108,211] Angiotensin II can stimulate the expression of Pax-2 (an antiapoptotic factor) through AT_2R.[215] AT_2R expression therefore is likely to affect nephrogenesis and kidney development, but its role in programming is still unclear. Overall, programmed suppression of the intrarenal renin-angiotensin system during nephrogenesis is likely to contribute to the reduction in nephron number under adverse circumstances, and postnatal upregulation of the AT_1R, possibly mediated by an increase in glucocorticoid activity or sensitivity, may contribute to the subsequent development of hypertension. More detailed investigation is required, however, to dissect temporal changes in expression and differences among various programming models.

Altered Sodium Handling by the Kidney

As mentioned earlier, salt sensitivity has been reported in several animal models and humans in association with low birth weight and reduced nephron number. A potential contributor to a shift to the right of the pressure-natriuresis curve is an alteration of sodium transporter expression or activity in the kidney. Administration of dexamethasone to pregnant rats was associated with growth retardation in the offspring, lower nephron number, reduction in GFR, higher blood pressure, lower urinary sodium excretion rate, reduced fractional excretion of sodium, and higher tissue sodium content

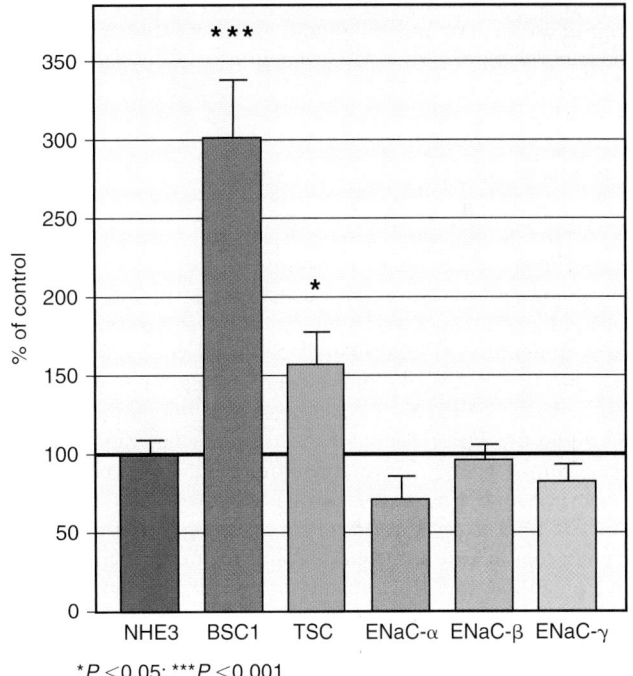

*P <0.05; ***P <0.001

FIGURE 22-19 Apical sodium transporter expression in 4-week-old offspring of mothers consuming a low-protein diet. BSC, Bumetanide-sensitive cotransporter; ENac, epithelial sodium channel; NHE3, Na$^+$/H$^+$ exchanger isoform 3; TSC, thiazide-sensitive contransporter. (From Vehaskari VM, Woods LL: Prenatal programming of hypertension: lessons from experimental models, *J Am Soc Nephrol* 16:2545-2556, 2005.)

in liver and skeletal muscle.[84] Similar findings were seen in growth-retarded piglets, in which low nephron number was associated with a reduced GFR but a normal fractional excretion of sodium.[216] A lower fractional excretion of sodium in the presence of reduced GFR is strong evidence of sodium retention by the kidney. Consistent with these whole-kidney observations, Manning and colleagues[217] found significant increases in expression of the sodium cotransporters Na-K-2Cl (bumetanide-sensitive cotransporter [BSC1], 302%) and Na-Cl (thiazide-sensitive cotransporter [TSC], 157%) in the offspring of rats fed a protein-restricted diet during gestation compared with controls (Figure 22-19).

Other authors reported an increase in glucocorticoid receptor expression and expression of the glucocorticoid responsive α_1- and β_1-subunits of Na$^+$/K$^+$-ATPase in offspring of pregnant rats fed a low-protein diet.[186] Prenatal dexamethasone administration was associated with increased expression of proximal tubular NHE3, as well as BSC1 and TSC, but no change was found in expression of components of the epithelial sodium channel (ENaC).[218] Intriguingly, renal denervation reduced systolic blood pressure together with sodium transporter expression in this model, which suggests an indirect regulation of these genes via sympathetic nerve activity in dexamethasone-exposed animals.[218] In rats subjected to maternal diabetes, however, expression of the β and γ ENaC subunits, but not the α ENaC subunit, as well as Na⁺/K⁺-ATPase were significantly increased compared with controls.[121] Expression of NHE3 and TSC were not changed, and BSC1 expression decreased in response to a high-salt diet in this study (Figure 22-20). Despite differences among models, these data, taken together, suggest that increased sodium avidity of the fetally programmed kidney, possibly in the setting of an increase in background glucocorticoid activity, is a likely contributor to the development of adult hypertension.

Impact of Nephron Endowment on Transplantation Outcomes

Assignment of donor kidneys is largely decided based on immunologic matching. In animal experiments of renal transplantation, however, an impact of transplanted nephron mass, independent of immunologic factors, on the subsequent development of chronic allograft nephropathy has been demonstrated.[219-222] Despite such evidence, assignment of kidneys on the basis of the physiologic capacity of the donor organ to meet the metabolic needs of the recipient has not generally been considered.[223] More and more data are accumulating, however, suggesting that transplanted renal mass has a significant impact on long-term posttransplantation outcomes. Demographic and anthropomorphic factors associated with late renal allograft loss include donor age, sex, and race, as well as recipient body surface area (BSA).[224-226] In general, kidneys from older, female, and African American donors fare worse and tend to have lower nephron numbers than those of younger, white, and male donors.[51,70,227,228] Indirectly, these observations suggest that the intrinsic nephron endowment of the transplanted kidney is likely to play a role in the development of chronic allograft nephropathy.

To investigate this question, several researchers have compared recipient and donor BSA as surrogates for metabolic demand and kidney size; others have used kidney weights or renal volumetric measurements by ultrasonography as surrogates for nephron mass. Mismatches between donor kidney size and recipient BSA have an impact on long-term allograft outcomes. A retrospective analysis of 32,083 patients who received a first cadaver kidney found that large recipients of kidneys from small donors had a 43% increased risk of late allograft failure compared with medium-sized recipients who received kidneys from medium-sized donors.[229] Outcomes were best in small recipients receiving kidneys from large donors. Other smaller, studies have not consistently found similar results.[229] One such study analyzed 378 paired recipients of cadaver kidneys from 189 donors, of which one recipient had a high and the other a low BSA.[230] These authors did not find a significant association between allograft loss and the ratio between donor and recipient BSA, but BSA ranges in the "larger" and "smaller" groups overlapped in this study, which limits the power to detect a true effect.[230]

Another study evaluated outcomes in patients receiving cadaveric kidneys from donors either younger or older than 60 years of age.[231] Kidneys from older donors have fewer viable nephrons and may be less able to recover from transplant-related injury.[51,232] Recipients were also subdivided into two groups according to mean body mass index (BMI) and mean BSA.[231] The authors found that, among patients receiving kidneys from donors older than age 60, graft survival at 5 years was significantly better in those with smaller BMI and BSA. This study demonstrates that an older kidney with fewer nephrons transplanted into a smaller recipient functions better than an older kidney in a larger recipient.

Kidney size may not always be directly proportional to BSA; therefore, determining the ratio of donor to recipient BSA may not be an ideal method of estimating mismatch between nephron mass and recipient. Kidney weight, however, is an acceptable surrogate for nephron mass.[51,233] Using this indicator, Kim and associates[234] analyzed the ratio of donor kidney weight to recipient body weight (DKW/RBW) in 259 live-donor transplants. These authors found that a DKW/RBW of greater than 4.5 g/kg was significantly associated with improved allograft function at 3 years compared with a ratio of less than 3.0 g/kg. A similar study that included 964 recipients of cadaveric kidneys, in whom proteinuria and

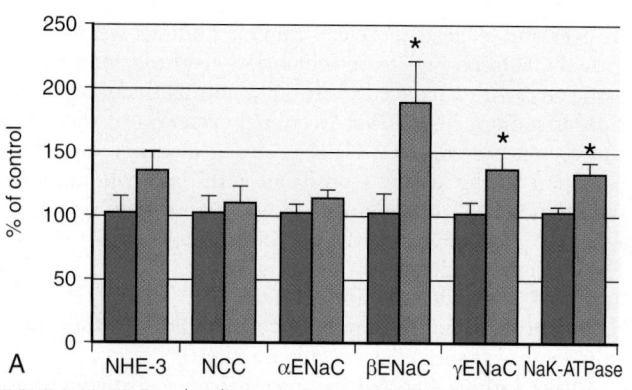
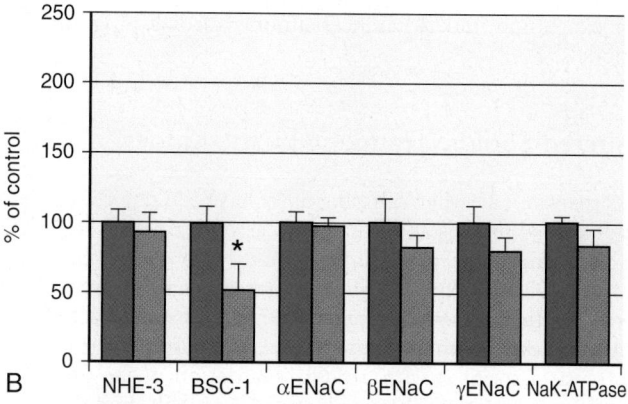

FIGURE 22-20 Renal sodium transporter abundance in the renal cortex (**A**) and medulla (**B**) of kidneys from 3-month-old controls (*blue*) or offspring of diabetic mothers (*red*). (From Nehiri T, Duong Van Huyen J-P, Viltard M, et al: Exposure to maternal diabetes induces salt-sensitive hypertension and impairs renal function in adult rat offspring, *Diabetes* 57:2167-2175, 2008.)

Cockcroft-Gault creatinine clearances were also determined, found that 10% of the recipients were "strongly" mismatched, with a DKW/RBW ratio of less than 2 g/kg.[228] The DKW/RBW ratio was lowest when male recipients received kidneys from female donors. The risk of having proteinuria higher than 0.5 g/kg was significantly greater, and proteinuria developed earlier, in those with DKW/RBW below 2 g/kg compared with those with higher ratios. In fact, proteinuria was present in 50% of those with a DKW/RBW of less than 2 g/kg, 33% of those with a DKW/RBW of 2 to 4 g/kg, and 23% of those with a DKW/RBW of 4 g/kg or higher. At 5-year follow-up, however, there was no difference in graft survival among the three DKW/RBW groups. The study authors concede that it is likely that longer follow-up is needed to determine the true impact of donor/recipient mismatch.[228]

Other investigators have used renal ultrasonography to measure cadaveric transplant kidney (Tx) cross-sectional area in relation to recipient body weight (W) to calculate a "nephron dose index," Tx/W.[235] These authors found that, during the first 5 years after transplantation, serum creatinine level was significantly lower in patients with a high Tx/W than in those with lower values, with a trend toward better graft survival. Therefore, the ratio between renal mass and the recipient's metabolic needs does appear to be a determinant of long-term allograft function. A small kidney transplanted into a large recipient may not have an adequate capacity to meet the metabolic needs of the recipient without imposing glomerular hyperfiltration, which ultimately leads to further nephron loss and eventual allograft failure.[25,232] Transplanted nephron mass not only may be a function of congenital endowment and attrition of nephrons with age but also may be affected by peritransplant renal injury (i.e., donor hypotension, prolonged cold and warm ischemia, administration of nephrotoxic immunosuppressive drugs). All of these factors, in addition to immunologic matching, need to be closely considered in selection of appropriate recipients in whom the allograft is likely to function for the longest time and therefore provide the best possible improvement in quality of life.

Conclusion

Evidence for the association between an adverse fetal environment and subsequent hypertension and kidney disease in later life is now quite compelling, and this association appears to be mediated, at least in part, by impaired nephrogenesis. Concomitant glomerular hypertrophy and altered expression of sodium transporters in the programmed kidney also contribute to the vicious circle of glomerular hypertension, glomerular injury, and sclerosis, which leads to worsening hypertension and ongoing renal injury (Figure 22-21). In addition, multiple other factors, such as increased oxidative stress, renal inflammation, accelerated senescence, and catch-up growth, are all likely contributors to ongoing nephron loss and eventual renal disease.[236-238] The number of nephrons in humans varies widely, which suggests that a significant proportion of the general population, especially in areas where high or low birth weights are prevalent, may be at increased risk of developing later-life hypertension and renal dysfunction. Measurement of nephron number in vivo remains an obstacle, with the best surrogate markers thus far being a low birth weight, a high birth weight, and, in the absence of other known renal diseases, reduced kidney volume on ultrasonography, especially in children, and glomerular enlargement on kidney biopsy specimens. A kidney with a reduced complement of nephrons has less renal reserve to adapt to dietary excesses or to compensate for renal injury. The molecular mechanisms through which fetal programming exerts its effects on nephrogenesis are varied and likely complementary and intertwined. Although in some animal studies nephron number and blood pressure can be "rescued" by good postnatal nutrition, the applicability of these findings to humans is somewhat doubtful at present. The fact that even seemingly minor influences, such as

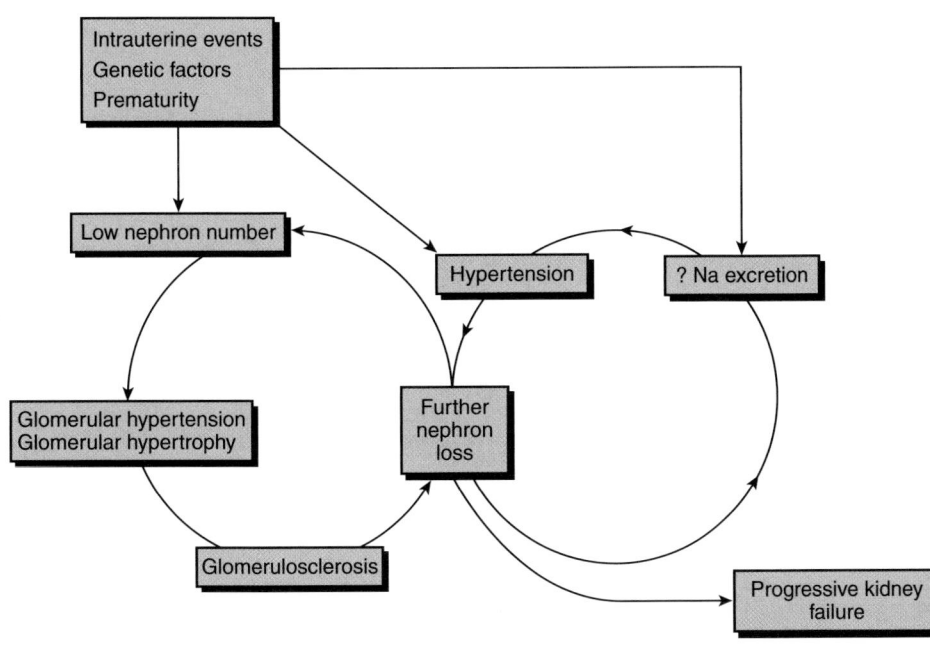

FIGURE 22-21 Proposed mechanism of fetal programming of hypertension and renal disease. (Adapted from Zandi-Nejad K, Luyckx VA, Brenner BM: Adult hypertension and kidney disease: the role of fetal programming, *Hypertension* 47: 502-508, 2006.)

composition of maternal diet during fetal life, can have major consequences on renal development in the offspring underscores the critical importance of optimizing perinatal care and early nutrition, which can have a major impact on population health in the future.

References

1. Kemper MJ, Muller-Wiefel DE. Renal function in congenital anomalies of the kidney and urinary tract. *Curr Opin Urol.* 2001;11:571-575.
2. Schreuder MF, Langemeijer ME, Bokenkamp A, et al. Hypertension and microalbuminuria in children with congenital solitary kidneys. *J Paediatr Child Health.* 2008;44:363-368.
3. Hoy WE, Rees M, Kile E, et al. Low birthweight and renal disease in Australian Aborigines. *Lancet.* 1998;352:1826-1827.
4. Lackland DT. Mechanisms and fetal origins of kidney disease. *J Am Soc Nephrol.* 2005;16:2531-2532.
5. Nelson RG, Morgenstern H, Bennett PH. Birth weight and renal disease in Pima Indians with type 2 diabetes mellitus. *Am J Epidemiol.* 1998;148: 650-656.
6. Kaplan NM, Opie LH. Controversies in hypertension. *Lancet.* 2006;367:168-176.
7. Bianchi G. Genetic variations of tubular sodium reabsorption leading to "primary" hypertension: from gene polymorphism to clinical symptoms. *Am J Physiol Regul Integr Comp Physiol.* 2005;289:R1536-R1549.
8. Hubner N, Yagil C, Yagil Y. Novel integrative approaches to the identification of candidate genes in hypertension. *Hypertension.* 2006;47:1-5.
9. Lifton RP, Gharavi AG, Geller DS. Molecular mechanisms of human hypertension. *Cell.* 2001;104:545-556.
10. Ben-Shlomo Y, McCarthy A, Hughes R, et al. Immediate postnatal growth is associated with blood pressure in young adulthood: the Barry Caerphilly Growth Study. *Hypertension.* 2008;52:638-644.
11. Hales CN, Barker DJ. Type 2 (non–insulin-dependent) diabetes mellitus: the thrifty phenotype hypothesis. *Diabetologia.* 1992;35:595-601.
12. McMillen IC, Robinson JS. Developmental origins of the metabolic syndrome: prediction, plasticity, and programming. *Physiol Rev.* 2005;85:571-633.
13. Barker DJ. Developmental origins of adult health and disease. *J Epidemiol Community Health.* 2004;58:114-115.
14. Drake AJ, Walker BR. The intergenerational effects of fetal programming: non-genomic mechanisms for the inheritance of low birth weight and cardiovascular risk. *J Endocrinol.* 2004;180:1-16.
15. Forsdahl A. Are poor living conditions in childhood and adolescence an important risk factor for arteriosclerotic heart disease? *Br J Prev Soc Med.* 1977;31:91-95.
16. Kermack WO, McKendrick AG, McKinlay PL. Death-rates in Great Britain and Sweden. Some general regularities and their significance. *Lancet.* 1934;i:698-703.
17. Barker DJ, Hales CN, Fall CH, et al. Type 2 (non–insulin-dependent) diabetes mellitus, hypertension and hyperlipidaemia (syndrome X): relation to reduced fetal growth. *Diabetologia.* 1993;36:62-67.
18. Bellinger L, Langley-Evans SC. Fetal programming of appetite by exposure to a maternal low protein diet in the rat. *Clin Sci (Lond).* 2005;109(4):13-20.
19. Gardner DS, Tingey K, Van Bon BW, et al. Programming of glucose-insulin metabolism in adult sheep after maternal undernutrition. *Am J Physiol Regul Integr Comp Physiol.* 2005;289(4):R947-954.
20. Wust S, Entringer S, Federenko IS, et al. Birth weight is associated with salivary cortisol responses to psychosocial stress in adult life. *Psychoneuroendocrinology.* 2005;30:591-598.
21. Li S, Chen SC, Shlipak M, et al. Low birth weight is associated with chronic kidney disease only in men. *Kidney Int.* 2008;73:637-642.
22. Vikse BE, Irgens LM, Leivestad T, et al. Low birth weight increases risk for end-stage renal disease. *J Am Soc Nephrol.* 2008;19:151-157.
23. White SL, Perkovic V, Cass A, et al. Is low birth weight an antecedent of CKD in later life? A systematic review of observational studies. *Am J Kidney Dis.* 2009;54:248-261.
24. Langley-Evans S, Langley-Evans A, Marchand M. Nutritional programming of blood pressure and renal morphology. *Arch Physiol Biochem.* 2003;111:8-16.
25. Luyckx VA, Brenner BM. Low birth weight, nephron number, and kidney disease. *Kidney Int Suppl.* 2005:S68-S77.
26. Vehaskari VM, Woods LL. Prenatal programming of hypertension: lessons from experimental models. *J Am Soc Nephrol.* 2005;16:2545-2556.
27. Barker DJ, Osmond C, Golding J, et al. Growth in utero, blood pressure in childhood and adult life, and mortality from cardiovascular disease. *Br Med J.* 1989;298:564-567.
28. Huxley RR, Shiell AW, Law CM. The role of size at birth and postnatal catch-up growth in determining systolic blood pressure: a systematic review of the literature. *J Hypertens.* 2000;18:815-831.
29. Launer LJ, Hofman A, Grobbee DE. Relation between birth weight and blood pressure: longitudinal study of infants and children. *Br Med J.* 1993;307:1451-1454.
30. Hemachandra AH, Klebanoff MA, Furth SL. Racial disparities in the association between birth weight in the term infant and blood pressure at age 7 years: results from the collaborative perinatal project. *J Am Soc Nephrol.* 2006;17:2576-2581.
31. Rostand SG, Cliver SP, Goldenberg RL. Racial disparities in the association of foetal growth retardation to childhood blood pressure. *Nephrol Dial Transplant.* 2005;20:1592-1597.
32. Vancheri F, Alletto M, Burgio A, et al. [Inverse relationship between fetal growth and arterial pressure in children and adults]. *G Ital Cardiol.* 1995;25:833-841.
33. Zhao M, Shu XO, Jin F, et al. Birthweight, childhood growth and hypertension in adulthood. *Int J Epidemiol.* 2002;31:1043-1051.
34. Cruickshank JK, Mzayek F, Liu L, et al. Origins of the "black/white" difference in blood pressure: roles of birth weight, postnatal growth, early blood pressure, and adolescent body size: the Bogalusa Heart Study. *Circulation.* 2005;111:1932-1937.
35. Hemachandra AH, Howards PP, Furth SL, et al. Birth weight, postnatal growth, and risk for high blood pressure at 7 years of age: results from the Collaborative Perinatal Project. *Pediatrics.* 2007;119:E1264-E1270.
36. Law CM, de Swiet M, Osmond C, et al. Initiation of hypertension in utero and its amplification throughout life. *Br Med J.* 1993;306:24-27.
37. Al Salmi I, Hoy WE, Kondalsamy-Chennakes S, et al. Birth weight and stages of CKD: a case-control study in an Australian population. *Am J Kidney Dis.* 2008;52:1070-1078.
38. Hallan S, Euser AM, Irgens LM, et al. Effect of intrauterine growth restriction on kidney function at young adult age: the Nord Trondelag Health (HUNT 2). *Study. Am J Kidney Dis.* 2008;51:10-20.
39. Hodgin JB, Rasoulpour M, Markowitz GS, et al. Very low birth weight is a risk factor for secondary focal segmental glomerulosclerosis. *Clin J Am Soc Nephrol.* 2009;4:71-76.
40. Guyton AC, Coleman TG, Young DB, et al. Salt balance and long-term blood pressure control. *Annu Rev Med.* 1980;31:15-27.
41. Guyton AC, Young DB, DeClue JW, et al. Fluid balance, renal function, and blood pressure. *Clin Nephrol.* 1975;4:122-126.
42. Lifton RP, Wilson FH, Choate KA, et al. Salt and blood pressure: new insight from human genetic studies. *Cold Spring Harb Symp Quant Biol.* 2002;67:445-450.
43. Xu J, Li G, Wang P, et al. Renalase is a novel, soluble monoamine oxidase that regulates cardiac function and blood pressure. *J Clin Invest.* 2005;115:1275-1280.
44. Guidi E, Menghetti D, Milani S, et al. Hypertension may be transplanted with the kidney in humans: a long-term historical prospective follow-up of recipients grafted with kidneys coming from donors with or without hypertension in their families. *J Am Soc Nephrol.* 1996;7:1131-1138.
45. Brenner BM, Garcia DL, Anderson S. Glomeruli and blood pressure. Less of one, more the other? *Am J Hypertens.* 1988;1:335-347.
46. Hsu CY, Lin F, Vittinghoff E, et al. Racial differences in the progression from chronic renal insufficiency to end-stage renal disease in the United States. *J Am Soc Nephrol.* 2003;14:2902-2907.
47. Lackland DT, Bendall HE, Osmond C, et al. Low birth weights contribute to high rates of early-onset chronic renal failure in the Southeastern United States. *Arch Intern Med.* 2000;160:1472-1476.
48. Lackland DT, Egan BM, Ferguson PL. Low birth weight as a risk factor for hypertension. *J Clin Hypertens (Greenwich).* 2003;5:133-136.
49. Lackland DT, Egan BM, Syddall HE, et al. Associations between birth weight and antihypertensive medication in black and white Medicaid recipients. *Hypertension.* 2002;39:179-183.
50. Bertram JF. Counting in the kidney. *Kidney Int.* 2001;59:792-796.
51. Nyengaard JR, Bendtsen TF. Glomerular number and size in relation to age, kidney weight, and body surface in normal man. *Anat Rec.* 1992;232: 194-201.
52. Kett MM, Bertram JF. Nephron endowment and blood pressure: what do we really know? *Curr Hypertens Rep.* 2004;6:133-139.
53. Basgen JM, Steffes MW, Stillman AE, et al. Estimating glomerular number in situ using magnetic resonance imaging and biopsy. *Kidney Int.* 1994;45:1668-1672.
54. Hoy WE, Douglas-Denton RN, Hughson MD, et al. A stereological study of glomerular number and volume: preliminary findings in a multiracial study of kidneys at autopsy. *Kidney Int Suppl.* 2003:S31-S37.
55. Keller G, Zimmer G, Mall G, et al. Nephron number in patients with primary hypertension. *N Engl J Med.* 2003;348:101-108.
56. Bhathena DB, Julian BA, McMorrow RG, et al. Focal sclerosis of hypertrophied glomeruli in solitary functioning kidneys of humans. *Am J Kidney Dis.* 1985;5:226-232.

57. Nenov VD, Taal MW, Sakharova OV, et al. Multi-hit nature of chronic renal disease. *Curr Opin Nephrol Hypertens.* 2000;9:85-97.
58. Flanigan WJ, Burns RO, Takacs FJ, et al. Serial studies of glomerular filtration rate and renal plasma flow in kidney transplant donors, identical twins, and allograft recipients. *Am J Surg.* 1968;116:788-794.
59. Kasiske BL, Ma JZ, Louis TA, et al. Long-term effects of reduced renal mass in humans. *Kidney Int.* 1995;48:814-819.
60. Ibrahim HN, Foley R, Tan L, et al. Long-term consequences of kidney donation. *N Engl J Med.* 2009;360:459-469.
61. Moritz KM, Wintour EM, Dodic M. Fetal uninephrectomy leads to postnatal hypertension and compromised renal function. *Hypertension.* 2002;39:1071-1076.
62. Woods LL, Weeks DA, Rasch R. Hypertension after neonatal uninephrectomy in rats precedes glomerular damage. *Hypertension.* 2001;38:337-342.
63. Singh RR, Denton KM, Bertram JF, et al. Development of cardiovascular disease due to renal insufficiency in male sheep following fetal unilateral nephrectomy. *J Hypertens.* 2009;27:386-396.
64. Nyengaard JR. Number and dimensions of rat glomerular capillaries in normal development and after nephrectomy. *Kidney Int.* 1993;43:1049-1057.
65. Hoy WE, Hughson MD, Bertram JF, et al. Nephron number, hypertension, renal disease, and renal failure. *J Am Soc Nephrol.* 2005;16:2557-2564.
66. Manalich R, Reyes L, Herrera M, et al. Relationship between weight at birth and the number and size of renal glomeruli in humans: a histomorphometric study. *Kidney Int.* 2000;58:770-773.
67. Zimanyi MA, Hoy WE, Douglas-Denton RN, et al. Nephron number and individual glomerular volumes in male Caucasian and African American subjects. *Nephrol Dial Transplant.* 2009;24:2428-2433.
68. Abdi R, Dong VM, Rubel JR, et al. Correlation between glomerular size and long-term renal function in patients with substantial loss of renal mass. *J Urol.* 2003;170:42-44.
69. Abdi R, Slakey D, Kittur D, et al. Baseline glomerular size as a predictor of function in human renal transplantation. *Transplantation.* 1998;66:329-333.
70. Abdi R, Slakey D, Kittur D, et al. Heterogeneity of glomerular size in normal donor kidneys: impact of race. *Am J Kidney Dis.* 1998;32:43-46.
71. Hoy WE, Wang Z, VanBuynder P, et al. The natural history of renal disease in Australian Aborigines. Part 1. Changes in albuminuria and glomerular filtration rate over time. *Kidney Int.* 2001;60:243-248.
72. Hoy WE, Wang Z, VanBuynder P, et al. The natural history of renal disease in Australian Aborigines. Part 2. Albuminuria predicts natural death and renal failure. *Kidney Int.* 2001;60:249-256.
73. Lemley KV. A basis for accelerated progression of diabetic nephropathy in Pima Indians. *Kidney Int Suppl.* 2003;83:S38-S42.
74. Lu MC, Halfon N. Racial and ethnic disparities in birth outcomes: a life-course perspective. *Matern Child Health J.* 2003;7:13-30.
75. Schmidt K, Pesce C, Liu Q, et al. Large glomerular size in Pima Indians: lack of change with diabetic nephropathy. *J Am Soc Nephrol.* 1992;3:229-235.
76. Young RJ, Hoy WE, Kincaid-Smith P, et al. Glomerular size and glomerulosclerosis in Australian Aborigines. *Am J Kidney Dis.* 2000;36:481-489.
77. McNamara BJ, Diouf B, Hughson MD, et al. Renal pathology, glomerular number and volume in a West African urban community. *Nephrol Dial Transplant.* 2008;23:2576-2585.
78. McNamara BJ, Diouf B, Hughson MD, et al. Associations between age, body size and nephron number with individual glomerular volumes in urban West African males. *Nephrol Dial Transplant.* 2009;24:1500-1506.
79. Hughson MD, Gobe GC, Hoy WE, et al. Associations of glomerular number and birth weight with clinicopathological features of African Americans and whites. *Am J Kidney Dis.* 2008;52:18-28.
80. Yiu V, Buka S, Zurakowski D, et al. Relationship between birthweight and blood pressure in childhood. *Am J Kidney Dis.* 1999;33:253-260.
81. Fang J, Madhavan S, Alderman MH. The influence of maternal hypertension on low birth weight: differences among ethnic populations. *Ethn Dis.* 1999;9:369-376.
82. Fuller KE. Low birth-weight infants: the continuing ethnic disparity and the interaction of biology and environment. *Ethn Dis.* 2000;10:432-445.
83. Lackland DT, Barker DJ. Birth weight: a predictive medicine consideration for the disparities in CKD. *Am J Kidney Dis.* 2009;54:191-193.
84. Celsi G, Kistner A, Aizman R, et al. Prenatal dexamethasone causes oligonephronia, sodium retention, and higher blood pressure in the offspring. *Pediatr Res.* 1998;44:317-322.
85. Gilbert T, Lelievre-Pegorier M, Merlet-Benichou C. Long-term effects of mild oligonephronia induced in utero by gentamicin in the rat. *Pediatr Res.* 1991;30:450-456.
86. Langley-Evans SC. Intrauterine programming of hypertension in the rat: nutrient interactions. *Comp Biochem Physiol A Physiol.* 1996;114:327-333.
87. Merlet-Benichou C. Influence of fetal environment on kidney development. *Int J Dev Biol.* 1999;43:453-456.
88. Ortiz LA, Quan A, Weinberg A, et al. Effect of prenatal dexamethasone on rat renal development. *Kidney Int.* 2001;59:1663-1669.
89. Vehaskari VM, Aviles DH, Manning J. Prenatal programming of adult hypertension in the rat. *Kidney Int.* 2001;59:238-245.
90. Woods LL, Ingelfinger JR, Nyengaard JR, et al. Maternal protein restriction suppresses the newborn renin-angiotensin system and programs adult hypertension in rats. *Pediatr Res.* 2001;49:460-467.
91. Alexander BT. Placental insufficiency leads to development of hypertension in growth-restricted offspring. *Hypertension.* 2003;41:457-462.
92. Moritz KM, Mazzuca MQ, Siebel AL, et al. Uteroplacental insufficiency causes a nephron deficit, modest renal insufficiency but no hypertension with ageing in female rats. *J Physiol.* 2009;587:2635-2646.
93. Wlodek ME, Mibus A, Tan A, et al. Normal lactational environment restores nephron endowment and prevents hypertension after placental restriction in the rat. *J Am Soc Nephrol.* 2007;18:1688-1696.
94. Boubred F, Buffat C, Feuerstein JM, et al. Effects of early postnatal hypernutrition on nephron number and long-term renal function and structure in rats. *Am J Physiol Renal Physiol.* 2007;293:F1944-F1949.
95. Hughson M, Farris AB, Douglas-Denton R, et al. Glomerular number and size in autopsy kidneys: The relationship to birth weight. *Kidney Int.* 2003;63:2113-2122.
96. Hughson MD, Douglas-Denton R, Bertram JF, et al. Hypertension, glomerular number, and birth weight in African Americans and white subjects in the southeastern United States. *Kidney Int.* 2006;69:671-678.
97. Rodriguez MM, Gomez AH, Abitbol CL, et al. Histomorphometric analysis of postnatal glomerulogenesis in extremely preterm infants. *Pediatr Dev Pathol.* 2004;7:17-25.
98. Hinchliffe SA, Howard CV, Lynch MR, et al. Renal developmental arrest in sudden infant death syndrome. *Pediatr Pathol.* 1993;13:333-343.
99. Hinchliffe SA, Lynch MR, Sargent PH, et al. The effect of intrauterine growth retardation on the development of renal nephrons. *Br J Obstet Gynaecol.* 1992;99:296-301.
100. Zhang Z, Quinlan J, Hoy W, et al. A common RET variant is associated with reduced newborn kidney size and function. *J Am Soc Nephrol.* 2008;19:2027-2034.
101. Deutinger J, Bartl W, Pfersmann C, et al. Fetal kidney volume and urine production in cases of fetal growth retardation. *J Perinat Med.* 1987;15:307-315.
102. Kurjak A, Kirkinen P, Latin V, et al. Ultrasonic assessment of fetal kidney function in normal and complicated pregnancies. *Am J Obstet Gynecol.* 1981;141:266-270.
103. Silver LE, Decamps PJ, Korst LM, et al. Intrauterine growth restriction is accompanied by decreased renal volume in the human fetus. *Am J Obstet Gynecol.* 2003;188:1320-1325.
104. Schmidt IM, Damgaard IN, Boisen KA, et al. Increased kidney growth in formula-fed versus breast-fed healthy infants. *Pediatr Nephrol.* 2004;19:1137-1144.
105. Spencer J, Wang Z, Hoy W. Low birth weight and reduced renal volume in Aboriginal children. *Am J Kidney Dis.* 2001;37:915-920.
106. Rakow A, Johansson S, Legnevall L, et al. Renal volume and function in school-age children born preterm or small for gestational age. *Pediatr Nephrol.* 2008;23:1309-1315.
107. Nyengaard JR, Bendtsen TF, Mogensen CE. Low birth weight—is it associated with few and small glomeruli in normal subjects and NIDDM patients? *Diabetologia.* 1996;39:1634-1637.
108. Gilbert JS, Lang AL, Grant AR, et al. Maternal nutrient restriction in sheep: hypertension and decreased nephron number in offspring at 9 months of age. *J Physiol.* 2005;565:137-147.
109. Plank C, Ostreicher I, Hartner A, et al. Intrauterine growth retardation aggravates the course of acute mesangioproliferative glomerulonephritis in the rat. *Kidney Int.* 2006;70:1974-1982.
110. Jones SE, Bilous RW, Flyvbjerg A, et al. Intra-uterine environment influences glomerular number and the acute renal adaptation to experimental diabetes. *Diabetologia.* 2001;44:721-728.
111. Jones SE, White KE, Flyvbjerg A, et al. The effect of intrauterine environment and low glomerular number on the histological changes in diabetic glomerulosclerosis. *Diabetologia.* 2006;49:191-199.
112. Macconi D, Bonomelli M, Benigni A, et al. Pathophysiologic implications of reduced podocyte number in a rat model of progressive glomerular injury. *Am J Pathol.* 2006;168:42-54.
113. Holemans K, Gerber R, Meurrens K, et al. Maternal food restriction in the second half of pregnancy affects vascular function but not blood pressure of rat female offspring. *Br J Nutr.* 1999;81:73-79.
114. Sanders MW, Fazzi GE, Janssen GM, et al. High sodium intake increases blood pressure and alters renal function in intrauterine growth-retarded rats. *Hypertension.* 2005;46:71-75.
115. Zimanyi MA, Bertram JF, Black MJ. Does a nephron deficit in rats predispose to salt-sensitive hypertension? *Kidney Blood Press Res.* 2004;27:239-247.

116. Gilbert JS. Sex, salt, and senescence: sorting out mechanisms of the developmental origins of hypertension. *Hypertension.* 2008;51:997-999.
117. Salazar F, Reverte V, Saez F, et al. Age- and sodium-sensitive hypertension and sex-dependent renal changes in rats with a reduced nephron number. *Hypertension.* 2008;51:1184-1189.
118. Magalhaes JC, da Silveira AB, Mota DL, et al. Renal function in juvenile rats subjected to prenatal malnutrition and chronic salt overload. *Exp Physiol.* 2006;91:611-619.
119. Manning J, Vehaskari VM. Postnatal modulation of prenatally programmed hypertension by dietary Na and ACE inhibition. *Am J Physiol Regul Integr Comp Physiol.* 2005;288:R80-R84.
120. Stewart T, Ascani J, Craver RD, et al. Role of postnatal dietary sodium in prenatally programmed hypertension. *Pediatr Nephrol.* 2009;24:1727-1733.
121. Nehiri T, Duong Van Huyen JP, Viltard M, et al. Exposure to maternal diabetes induces salt-sensitive hypertension and impairs renal function in adult rat offspring. *Diabetes.* 2008;57:2167-2175.
122. Woods LL, Weeks DA, Rasch R. Programming of adult blood pressure by maternal protein restriction: role of nephrogenesis. *Kidney Int.* 2004;65:1339-1348.
123. Martins JP, Monteiro JC, Paixao AD. Renal function in adult rats subjected to prenatal dexamethasone. *Clin Exp Pharmacol Physiol.* 2003;30:32-37.
124. Nwagwu MO, Cook A, Langley-Evans SC. Evidence of progressive deterioration of renal function in rats exposed to a maternal low-protein diet in utero. *Br J Nutr.* 2000;83:79-85.
125. Hoy WE, Mathews JD, McCredie DA, et al. The multidimensional nature of renal disease: rates and associations of albuminuria in an Australian Aboriginal community. *Kidney Int.* 1998;54:1296-1304.
126. Hoy WE, Rees M, Kile E, et al. A new dimension to the Barker hypothesis: low birthweight and susceptibility to renal disease. *Kidney Int.* 1999;56:1072-1077.
127. Yudkin JS, Martyn CN, Phillips DI, et al. Associations of microalbuminuria with intra-uterine growth retardation. *Nephron.* 2001;89:309-314.
128. Rodriguez-Soriano J, Aguirre M, Oliveros R, et al. Long-term renal follow-up of extremely low birth weight infants. *Pediatr Nephrol.* 2005;20:579-584.
129. Franco MC, Nishida SK, Sesso R. GFR estimated from cystatin C versus creatinine in children born small for gestational age. *Am J Kidney Dis.* 2008;51:925-932.
130. Ingelfinger JR. Weight for gestational age as a baseline predictor of kidney function in adulthood. *Am J Kidney Dis.* 2008;51:1-4.
131. Kistner A, Celsi G, Vanpee M, et al. Increased blood pressure but normal renal function in adult women born preterm. *Pediatr Nephrol.* 2000;15:215-220.
132. Keijzer-Veen MG, Schrevel M, Finken MJ, et al. Microalbuminuria and lower glomerular filtration rate at young adult age in subjects born very premature and after intrauterine growth retardation. *J Am Soc Nephrol.* 2005;16:2762-2768.
133. Keijzer-Veen MG, Kleinveld HA, Lequin MH, et al. Renal function and size at young adult age after intrauterine growth restriction and very premature birth. *Am J Kidney Dis.* 2007;50:542-551.
134. de Boer MP, Ijzerman RG, de Jongh RT, et al. Birth weight relates to salt sensitivity of blood pressure in healthy adults. *Hypertension.* 2008;51:928-932.
135. Simonetti GD, Raio L, Surbek D, et al. Salt sensitivity of children with low birth weight. *Hypertension.* 2008;52:625-630.
136. Painter RC, Roseboom TJ, van Montfrans GA, et al. Microalbuminuria in adults after prenatal exposure to the Dutch famine. *J Am Soc Nephrol.* 2005;16:189-194.
137. Bacchetta J, Harambat J, Dubourg L, et al. Both extrauterine and intrauterine growth restriction impair renal function in children born very preterm. *Kidney Int.* 2009;76:445-452.
138. Gielen M, Pinto-Sietsma SJ, Zeegers MP, et al. Birth weight and creatinine clearance in young adult twins: influence of genetic, prenatal, and maternal factors. *J Am Soc Nephrol.* 2005;16:2471-2476.
139. Quinlan J, Lemire M, Hudson T, et al. A common variant of the PAX2 gene is associated with reduced newborn kidney size. *J Am Soc Nephrol.* 2007;18:1915-1921.
140. Nelson RG, Morgenstern H, Bennett PH. Intrauterine diabetes exposure and the risk of renal disease in diabetic Pima Indians. *Diabetes.* 1998;47:1489-1493.
141. Rossing P, Tarnow L, Nielsen FS, et al. Short stature and diabetic nephropathy. *Br Med J.* 1995;310:296-297.
142. Sandeman D, Reza M, Phillips DI, et al. Why do some type 1 diabetic patients develop nephropathy? A possible role of birth weight. *Diabet Med.* 1992;9:A36.
143. Duncan RC, Bass PS, Garrett PJ, et al. Weight at birth and other factors influencing progression of idiopathic membranous nephropathy. *Nephrol Dial Transplant.* 1994:875.
144. Garrett P, Sandeman D, Reza M, et al. Weight at birth and renal disease in adulthood. *Nephrol Dial Transplant.* 1993;8:920.
145. Na YW, Yang HJ, Choi JH, et al. Effect of intrauterine growth retardation on the progression of nephrotic syndrome. *Am J Nephrol.* 2002;22:463-467.
146. Zidar N, Cavic MA, Kenda RB, et al. Effect of intrauterine growth retardation on the clinical course and prognosis of IgA glomerulonephritis in children. *Nephron.* 1998;79:28-32.
147. Zidar N, Cor A, Premru Srsen T, et al. Is there an association between glomerular density and birth weight in healthy humans? *Nephron.* 1998;80:97-98.
148. Teeninga N, Schreuder MF, Bokenkamp A, et al. Influence of low birth weight on minimal change nephrotic syndrome in children, including a meta-analysis. *Nephrol Dial Transplant.* 2008;23:1615-1620.
149. Fan ZJ, Lackland DT, Kenderes B, et al. Impact of birth weight on familial aggregation of end-stage renal disease. *Am J Nephrol.* 2003;23:117-120.
150. Grigore D, Ojeda NB, Alexander BT. Sex differences in the fetal programming of hypertension. *Gend Med.* 2008;5(Suppl A):S121-S132.
151. Vikse BE, Irgens LM, Bostad L, et al. Adverse perinatal outcome and later kidney biopsy in the mother. *J Am Soc Nephrol.* 2006;17:837-845.
152. Vikse BE, Irgens LM, Leivestad T, et al. Preeclampsia and the risk of end-stage renal disease. *N Engl J Med.* 2008;359:800-809.
153. Munkhaugen J, Lydersen S, Romundstad PR, et al. Kidney function and future risk for adverse pregnancy outcomes: a population-based study from HUNT II. Norway. *Nephrol Dial Transplant.* 2009;24(12):3744-3750.
154. Tian JY, Cheng Q, Song XM, et al. Birth weight and risk of type 2 diabetes, abdominal obesity and hypertension among Chinese adults. *Eur J Endocrinol.* 2006;155:601-607.
155. Ibsen H, Olsen MH, Wachtell K, et al. Reduction in albuminuria translates to reduction in cardiovascular events in hypertensive patients: losartan intervention for endpoint reduction in hypertension study. *Hypertension.* 2005;45:198-202.
156. Clark AT, Bertram JF. Molecular regulation of nephron endowment. *Am J Physiol.* 1999;276:F485-F497.
157. Hershkovitz D, Burbea Z, Skorecki K, et al. Fetal programming of adult kidney disease: cellular and molecular mechanisms. *Clin J Am Soc Nephrol.* 2007;2:334-342.
158. Schreuder MF, Nyengaard JR, Fodor M, et al. Glomerular number and function are influenced by spontaneous and induced low birth weight in rats. *J Am Soc Nephrol.* 2005;16:2913-2919.
159. Simeoni U, Zetterstrom R. Long-term circulatory and renal consequences of intrauterine growth restriction. *Acta Paediatr.* 2005;94:819-824.
160. Sakurai H, Nigam SK. in vitro branching tubulogenesis: implications for developmental and cystic disorders, nephron number, renal repair, and nephron engineering. *Kidney Int.* 1998;54:14-26.
161. Welham SJ, Riley PR, Wade A, et al. Maternal diet programs embryonic kidney gene expression. *Physiol Genomics.* 2005;22:48-56.
162. Langley-Evans SC. Nutritional programming of disease: unravelling the mechanism. *J Anat.* 2009;215:36-51.
163. Harrison M, Langley-Evans SC. Intergenerational programming of impaired nephrogenesis and hypertension in rats following maternal protein restriction during pregnancy. *Br J Nutr.* 2009;101:1020-1030.
164. Lisle SJ, Lewis RM, Petry CJ, et al. Effect of maternal iron restriction during pregnancy on renal morphology in the adult rat offspring. *Br J Nutr.* 2003;90:33-39.
165. Merlet-Benichou C, Vilar J, Lelievre-Pegorier M, et al. Role of retinoids in renal development: pathophysiological implication. *Curr Opin Nephrol Hypertens.* 1999;8:39-43.
166. Sutherland MR, Gubhaju L, Yoder BA, et al. The effects of postnatal retinoic acid administration on nephron endowment in the preterm baboon kidney. *Pediatr Res.* 2009;65:397-402.
167. Gray SP, Kenna K, Bertram JF, et al. Repeated ethanol exposure during late gestation decreases nephron endowment in fetal sheep. *Am J Physiol Regul Integr Comp Physiol.* 2008;295:R568-R574.
168. Almeida JR, Mandarim-de-Lacerda CA. Maternal gestational protein-calorie restriction decreases the number of glomeruli and causes glomerular hypertrophy in adult hypertensive rats. *Am J Obstet Gynecol.* 2005;192:945-951.
169. Langley-Evans A, Phillips GJ, Jackson AA. In utero exposure to maternal low protein diets induces hypertension in weanling rats, independently of maternal blood pressure changes. *Clin Nutr.* 1994;13:319-324.
170. Langley-Evans SC, Jackson AA. Rats with hypertension induced by in utero exposure to maternal low-protein diets fail to increase blood pressure in response to a high salt intake. *Ann Nutr Metab.* 1996;40:1-9.
171. Lucas SR, Costa Silva VL, Miraglia SM, et al. Functional and morphometric evaluation of offspring kidney after intrauterine undernutrition. *Pediatr Nephrol.* 1997;11:719-723.
172. Welham SJ, Wade A, Woolf AS. Protein restriction in pregnancy is associated with increased apoptosis of mesenchymal cells at the start of rat metanephrogenesis. *Kidney Int.* 2002;61:1231-1242.

173. Hatini V, Huh SO, Herzlinger D, et al. Essential role of stromal mesenchyme in kidney morphogenesis revealed by targeted disruption of Winged Helix transcription factor BF-2. *Genes Dev.* 1996;10:1467-1478.

174. Porteous S, Torban E, Cho NP, et al. Primary renal hypoplasia in humans and mice with PAX2 mutations: evidence of increased apoptosis in fetal kidneys of Pax2(1Neu)$^{+/-}$ mutant mice. *Hum Mol Genet.* 2000;9:1-11.

175. Sorenson CM, Rogers SA, Korsmeyer SJ, et al. Fulminant metanephric apoptosis and abnormal kidney development in bcl-2-deficient mice. *Am J Physiol.* 1995;268:F73-F81.

176. Torban E, Eccles MR, Favor J, et al. PAX2 suppresses apoptosis in renal collecting duct cells. *Am J Pathol.* 2000;157:833-842.

177. Dziarmaga A, Clark P, Stayner C, et al. Ureteric bud apoptosis and renal hypoplasia in transgenic PAX2-Bax fetal mice mimics the renal-coloboma syndrome. *J Am Soc Nephrol.* 2003;14:2767-2774.

178. Godley LA, Kopp JB, Eckhaus M, et al. Wild-type p53 transgenic mice exhibit altered differentiation of the ureteric bud and possess small kidneys. *Genes Dev.* 1996;10:836-850.

179. Pham TD, MacLennan NK, Chiu CT, et al. Uteroplacental insufficiency increases apoptosis and alters p53 gene methylation in the full-term IUGR rat kidney. *Am J Physiol Regul Integr Comp Physiol.* 2003;285:R962-R970.

180. Cullen-McEwen LA, Drago J, Bertram JF. Nephron endowment in glial cell line-derived neurotrophic factor (GDNF) heterozygous mice. *Kidney Int.* 2001;60:31-36.

181. Cullen-McEwen LA, Kett MM, Dowling J, et al. Nephron number, renal function, and arterial pressure in aged GDNF heterozygous mice. *Hypertension.* 2003;41:335-340.

182. Zhang Z, Quinlan J, Grote D, et al. Common variants of the glial cell–derived neurotrophic factor gene do not influence kidney size of the healthy newborn. *Pediatr Nephrol.* 2009;24:1151-1157.

183. Wintour EM, Moritz KM, Johnson K, et al. Reduced nephron number in adult sheep, hypertensive as a result of prenatal glucocorticoid treatment. *J Physiol.* 2003;549:929-935.

184. Dave-Sharma S, Wilson RC, Harbison MD, et al. Examination of genotype and phenotype relationships in 14 patients with apparent mineralocorticoid excess. *J Clin Endocrinol Metab.* 1998;83:2244-2254.

185. Seckl JR, Meaney MJ. Glucocorticoid programming. *Ann N Y Acad Sci.* 2004;1032:63-84.

186. Bertram C, Trowern AR, Copin N, et al. The maternal diet during pregnancy programs altered expression of the glucocorticoid receptor and type 2 11beta-hydroxysteroid dehydrogenase: potential molecular mechanisms underlying the programming of hypertension in utero. *Endocrinology.* 2001;142:2841-2853.

187. Dagan A, Gattineni J, Cook V, et al. Prenatal programming of rat proximal tubule Na$^+$/H$^+$ exchanger by dexamethasone. *Am J Physiol Regul Integr Comp Physiol.* 2007;292:R1230-R1235.

188. Amri K, Freund N, Vilar J, et al. Adverse effects of hyperglycemia on kidney development in rats: in vivo and in vitro studies. *Diabetes.* 1999;48:2240-2245.

189. Tran S, Chen YW, Chenier I, et al. Maternal diabetes modulates renal morphogenesis in offspring. *J Am Soc Nephrol.* 2008;19:943-952.

190. Rocha SO, Gomes GN, Forti AL, et al. Long-term effects of maternal diabetes on vascular reactivity and renal function in rat male offspring. *Pediatr Res.* 2005;58:1274-1279.

191. Magaton A, Gil FZ, Casarini DE, et al. Maternal diabetes mellitus—early consequences for the offspring. *Pediatr Nephrol.* 2007;22:37-43.

192. Amri K, Freund N, Van Huyen JP, et al. Altered nephrogenesis due to maternal diabetes is associated with increased expression of IGF-II/mannose-6-phosphate receptor in the fetal kidney. *Diabetes.* 2001;50:1069-1075.

193. Doublier S, Amri K, Seurin D, et al. Overexpression of human insulin-like growth factor binding protein-1 in the mouse leads to nephron deficit. *Pediatr Res.* 2001;49:660-666.

194. Gilbert T, Lelievre-Pegorier M, Merlet-Benichou C. Immediate and long-term renal effects of fetal exposure to gentamicin. *Pediatr Nephrol.* 1990;4:445-450.

195. Gilbert T, Gaonach S, Moreau E, et al. Defect of nephrogenesis induced by gentamicin in rat metanephric organ culture. *Lab Invest.* 1994;70:656-666.

196. Gilbert T, Cibert C, Moreau E, et al. Early defect in branching morphogenesis of the ureteric bud in induced nephron deficit. *Kidney Int.* 1996;50:783-795.

197. Kent AL, Douglas-Denton R, Shadbolt B, et al. Indomethacin, ibuprofen and gentamicin administered during late stages of glomerulogenesis do not reduce glomerular number at 14 days of age in the neonatal rat. *Pediatr Nephrol.* 2009;24:1143-1149.

198. Nathanson S, Moreau E, Merlet-Benichou C, et al. In utero and in vitro exposure to beta-lactams impair kidney development in the rat. *J Am Soc Nephrol.* 2000;11:874-884.

199. McKay DB, Josephson MA. Pregnancy in recipients of solid organs—effects on mother and child. *N Engl J Med.* 2006;354:1281-1293.

200. Tendron-Franzin A, Gouyon JB, Guignard JP, et al. Long-term effects of in utero exposure to cyclosporin A on renal function in the rabbit. *J Am Soc Nephrol.* 2004;15:2687-2693.

201. Komhoff M, Wang JL, Cheng HF, et al. Cyclooxygenase-2-selective inhibitors impair glomerulogenesis and renal cortical development. *Kidney Int.* 2000;57:414-422.

202. Franco Mdo C, Arruda RM, Fortes ZB, et al. Severe nutritional restriction in pregnant rats aggravates hypertension, altered vascular reactivity, and renal development in spontaneously hypertensive rats offspring. *J Cardiovasc Pharmacol.* 2002;39:369-377.

203. Paixao AD, Maciel CR, Teles MB, et al. Regional Brazilian diet-induced low birth weight is correlated with changes in renal hemodynamics and glomerular morphometry in adult age. *Biol Neonate.* 2001;80:239-246.

204. Sanders MW, Fazzi GE, Janssen GM, et al. Reduced uteroplacental blood flow alters renal arterial reactivity and glomerular properties in the rat offspring. *Hypertension.* 2004;43:1283-1289.

205. van Onna M, Houben AJ, Kroon AA, et al. Asymmetry of renal blood flow in patients with moderate to severe hypertension. *Hypertension.* 2003;41:108-113.

206. Franco MC, Christofalo DM, Sawaya AL, et al. Effects of low birth weight in 8- to 13-year-old children: implications in endothelial function and uric acid levels. *Hypertension.* 2006;48:45-50.

207. Guron G, Friberg P. An intact renin-angiotensin system is a prerequisite for normal renal development. *J Hypertens.* 2000;18:123-137.

208. Woods LL, Rasch R. Perinatal ANG II programs adult blood pressure, glomerular number, and renal function in rats. *Am J Physiol.* 1998;275:R1593-R1599.

209. Langley-Evans SC, Jackson AA. Captopril normalises systolic blood pressure in rats with hypertension induced by fetal exposure to maternal low protein diets. *Comp Biochem Physiol A Physiol.* 1995;110:223-228.

210. Grigore D, Ojeda NB, Robertson EB, et al. Placental insufficiency results in temporal alterations in the renin angiotensin system in male hypertensive growth restricted offspring. *Am J Physiol Regul Integr Comp Physiol.* 2007;293:R804-R811.

211. McMullen S, Gardner DS, Langley-Evans SC. Prenatal programming of angiotensin II type 2 receptor expression in the rat. *Br J Nutr.* 2004;91:133-140.

212. Sahajpal V, Ashton N. Increased glomerular angiotensin II binding in rats exposed to a maternal low protein diet in utero. *J Physiol.* 2005;563:193-201.

213. Vehaskari VM, Stewart T, Lafont D, et al. Kidney angiotensin and angiotensin receptor expression in prenatally programmed hypertension. *Am J Physiol Renal Physiol.* 2004;287:F262-F267.

214. Sahajpal V, Ashton N. Renal function and angiotensin AT1 receptor expression in young rats following intrauterine exposure to a maternal low-protein diet. *Clin Sci (Lond).* 2003;104:607-614.

215. Zhang SL, Moini B, Ingelfinger JR. Angiotensin II increases Pax-2 expression in fetal kidney cells via the AT2 receptor. *J Am Soc Nephrol.* 2004;15:1452-1465.

216. Bauer R, Walter B, Bauer K, et al. Intrauterine growth restriction reduces nephron number and renal excretory function in newborn piglets. *Acta Physiol Scand.* 2002;176:83-90.

217. Manning J, Beutler K, Knepper MA, et al. Upregulation of renal BSC1 and TSC in prenatally programmed hypertension. *Am J Physiol Renal Physiol.* 2002;283:F202-F206.

218. Dagan A, Kwon HM, Dwarakanath V, et al. Effect of renal denervation on prenatal programming of hypertension and renal tubular transporter abundance. *Am J Physiol Renal Physiol.* 2008;295:F29-F34.

219. Azuma H, Nadeau K, Mackenzie HS, et al. Nephron mass modulates the hemodynamic, cellular and molecular response of the rat renal allograft. *Transplantation.* 1997;63:519-528.

220. Heeman UW, Azuma H, Tullius SG, et al. The contribution of reduced functioning mass to chronic kidney allograft dysfunction in rats. *Transplantation.* 1994;58:1317-1321.

221. Mackenzie HS, Azuma H, Rennke HG, et al. Renal mass as a determinant of late allograft outcome: Insights from experimental studies in rats. *Kidney Int.* 1995;48:S38-S42.

222. Mackenzie HS, Azuma H, Troy JL, et al. Augmenting kidney mass at transplantation abrogates chronic renal allograft injury in rats. *Proc Assoc Am Phys.* 1996;108:127-133.

223. Brenner BM, Milford EL. Nephron underdosing: a programmed cause of chronic renal allograft failure. *Am J Kidney Dis.* 1993;21:66-72.

224. Chertow GM, Brenner BM, Mackenzie HS, et al. Non-immunologic predictors of chronic renal allograft failure: data from the United Network of Organ Sharing. *Kidney Int.* 1995;48:S48-S51.

225. Chertow GM, Brenner BM, Mori M, et al. Antigen-independent determinants of graft survival in living-related kidney transplantation. *Kidney Int.* 1997;52:S-84-S-86.

226. Chertow GM, Milford EL, Mackenzie HS, et al. Antigen-independent determinants of cadaveric kidney transplant failure. *JAMA.* 1996;276:1732-1736.

227. Fulladosa X, Moreso F, Narvaez JA, et al. Estimation of total glomerular number in stable renal transplants. *J Am Soc Nephrol*. 2003;14:2662-2668.
228. Giral M, Nguyen JM, Karam G, et al. Impact of graft mass on the clinical outcome of kidney transplants. *J Am Soc Nephrol*. 2005;16:261-268.
229. Kasiske BL, Snyder JJ, Gilbertson D. Inadequate donor size in cadaver kidney transplantation. *J Am Soc Nephrol*. 2002;13:2152-2159.
230. Gaston RS, Hudson SL, Julian BA, et al. Impact of donor/recipient size matching on outcomes in renal transplantation. *Transplantation*. 1996;61:383-388.
231. Nakatani T, Sugimura K, Kawashima H, et al. The influence of recipient body mass on the outcome of cadaver kidney transplants. *Clin Exp Nephrol*. 2002;6:158-162.
232. Vazquez MA, Jeyarajah DR, Kielar ML, et al. Long-term outcomes of renal transplantation: a result of the original endowment of the donor kidney and the inflammatory response to both alloantigens and injury. *Curr Opin Nephrol Hypertens*. 2000;9:643-648.
233. Taal MW, Tilney NL, Brenner BM, et al. Renal mass: an important determinant of late allograft outcome. *Transpl Rev*. 1998;12:74-84.
234. Kim YS, Kim MS, Han DS, et al. Evidence that the ratio of donor kidney weight to recipient body weight, donor age, and episodes of acute rejection correlate independently with live-donor graft function. *Transplantation*. 2002;72:280-283.
235. Nicholson ML, Windmill DC, Horsburgh T, et al. Influence of allograft size to recipient body-weight ratio on the long-term outcome of renal transplantation. *Br J Surg*. 2000;87:314-319.
236. Franco MC, Kawamoto EM, Gorjao R, et al. Biomarkers of oxidative stress and antioxidant status in children born small for gestational age: evidence of lipid peroxidation. *Pediatr Res*. 2007;62:204-208.
237. Jennings BJ, Ozanne SE, Dorling MW, et al. Early growth determines longevity in male rats and may be related to telomere shortening in the kidney. *FEBS Lett*. 1999;448:4-8.
238. Stewart T, Jung FF, Manning J, et al. Kidney immune cell infiltration and oxidative stress contribute to prenatally programmed hypertension. *Kidney Int*. 2005;68:2180-2188.
239. Hoy WE, Bertram JF, Denton RD, et al. Nephron number, glomerular volume, renal disease and hypertension. *Curr Opin Nephrol Hypertens*. 2008;17:258-265.
240. Hoppe CC, Evans RG, Bertram JF, et al. Effects of dietary protein restriction on nephron number in the mouse. *Am J Physiol Regul Integr Comp Physiol*. 2007;292:R1768-R1774.
241. Ortiz LA, Quan A, Zarzar F, et al. Prenatal dexamethasone programs hypertension and renal injury in the rat. *Hypertension*. 2003;41:328-334.
242. Tendron A, Decramer S, Justrabo E, et al. Cyclosporin A administration during pregnancy induces a permanent nephron deficit in young rabbits. *J Am Soc Nephrol*. 2003;14:3188-3196.
243. Fassi A, Sangalli F, Maffi R, et al. Progressive glomerular injury in the MWF rat is predicted by inborn nephron deficit. *J Am Soc Nephrol*. 1998;9:1399-1406.
244. Zalups RK. The Os/+ mouse: a genetic animal model of reduced renal mass. *Am J Physiol*. 1993;264:F53-F60.
245. Kazama I, Mahoney Z, Miner JH, et al. Podocyte-derived BMP7 is critical for nephron development. *J Am Soc Nephrol*. 2008;19:2181-2191.
246. Moritz KM, Wintour EM, Black MJ, et al. Factors influencing mammalian kidney development: implications for health in adult life. *Adv Anat Embryol Cell Biol*. 2008;196:1-78.
247. Norwood VF, Morham SG, Smithies O. Postnatal development and progression of renal dysplasia in cyclooxygenase-2 null mice. *Kidney Int*. 2000;58:2291-2300.
248. Poladia DP, Kish K, Kutay B, et al. Link between reduced nephron number and hypertension: studies in a mutant mouse model. *Pediatr Res*. 2006;59:489-493.
249. Qiao J, Uzzo R, Obara-Ishihara T, et al. FGF-7 modulates ureteric bud growth and nephron number in the developing kidney. *Development*. 1999;126:547-554.
250. Schnabel CA, Godin RE, Cleary ML. Pbx1 regulates nephrogenesis and ureteric branching in the developing kidney. *Dev Biol*. 2003;254:262-276.

Aging and Kidney Disease

Devasmita Choudhury, Moshe Levi, and Meryem Tuncel

The inevitable process of aging brings about changes in structure and function in the kidney that may translate to clinical outcomes associated with greater morbidity and mortality. Despite aging, the kidneys are remarkable in maintaining the internal milieu until renal reserve is challenged, adapting less well and recovering more slowly in the presence of intervening infections and toxin exposures, immunologic processes, and other organ failure. That older healthy kidney transplants are more prone to chronic allograft nephropathy compared with younger donor kidneys illustrates the impact of aging on the kidney and its function.[1-5] In addition, the presence of a decrease in renal function may increase hazards for all-cause and cardiovascular mortality in older adults.[6] The number of adults older than 65 years of age continues to climb and is estimated to reach more than 60 million by 2030,[7] and the number of elderly with chronic kidney disease (CKD)[8] and end-stage renal disease (ESRD) also continues to rise. Among hospitalized older adults, renal failure is estimated to exist in at least 30 percent of patients.[9] Therefore a basic understanding of how the kidney changes in structure, function, and response to acute and chronic physiologic and

pathophysiologic changes with aging becomes important to prevent unwanted outcomes.

Structural Changes

Gross and Microscopic Changes

The decrease in renal mass with age as noted by changes in size, weight, and volume from radiographic and postmortem studies appears to be age appropriate with a concurrent loss in body surface area.[10-13] Renal weight can change by as much as 15% to 20% from young adulthood (245 to 270 g) to the ninth decade (180 to 200 g).

Analysis of wedge biopsy specimens of allografts from aging deceased donors (>55 years) shows a greater prevalence of sclerotic glomeruli than in specimens from deceased donors younger than 40 years of age.[14] Glomerulosclerosis and tubulointerstitial fibrosis certainly contribute to the decrease in renal size. Senescence of the nephron and interstitium appear to be gradual and progressive, with intervening insults or comorbid conditions hastening this process. Sclerotic changes seen in the walls of the larger renal vessels can be made worse in the presence of hypertension. A higher degree of vascular sclerosis as noted by increased fibrointimal and medial sclerosis of sections of human cortical arteries is seen in 70-year-olds than in 6-year-olds.[15] In addition, more arteriolosclerosis of interlobular and arcuate arteries is found in older versus younger healthy donor kidneys. Cortical nephrons demonstrate ischemic changes by age 70. Glomeruli exhibit tuft lobulation, increased mesangial volume, capillary collapse, and obliteration. Hyaline deposits are noted in residual glomeruli with little cellular response[16,17] (Figure 23-1). Peritubular capillary density is decreased, which provides a reason for findings of low concentrations of proangiogenic vascular endothelial growth factors and increased expression of antiangiogenic factor thrombospondin in aging rats.[18] These changes with basement membrane thickening and wrinkling in both glomeruli and tubules force progressive reduction and simplification of vascular channels,[19,20] which results in the shunting of blood from afferent to efferent arterioles of the juxtamedullary glomeruli. Intact arteriolar vera rectae continue to provide adequate blood flow to the renal medulla.

With glomerular sclerosis, tubular atrophy follows, with tubules decreasing in size and number. Atrophied tubules creating distal diverticula may form the beginnings of early renal cysts frequently seen in older kidneys.[21] Furthermore, accumulation of debris and bacteria in these structures may be a reason for infection. Animal studies have also suggested that fibrosis of the tubulointerstitium may even precede development of focal glomerulosclerosis and tubular atrophy.[22,23] Morphometric evaluation of aging mice indicates more age-related tubulointerstitial fibrosis in males than in females.[24] Evidence for interstitial inflammation with fibroblast activation and accelerated apoptosis are found in aging rodents.[25]

Immunostaining for the adhesive proteins osteopontin and intracellular adhesion molecule-1 (ICAM-1) as well as collagen IV deposition are found in association with focal tubular proliferation, myofibroblast activation, and macrophage infiltration in aging rat kidneys. Altered endothelial nitric oxide synthase (eNOS) expression in the face of peritubular ischemia and injury may be the trigger for the inflammation leading to focal glomerulosclerosis and tubular atrophy.[25] Examination of renal tissues obtained at autopsy showed increased collagen I protein accumulation with age that correlated with the extent of interstitial fibrosis,[26,27] which perhaps suggests the importance of collagen I in age-associated interstitial fibrosis. Further probing of aged kidneys at the molecular level demonstrated increased levels of the cell cycle inhibitor p16INK4a with age, glomerulosclerosis, and tubulointerstitial fibrosis.[28] Other markers of replicative senescence, including critical telomere shortening, are found in the renal cortex with aging. Acting as mitotic clocks, telomere DNA repeats shorten with each cell replication; however, structural changes can also occur prematurely in response to stress, leading to early senescence.[29,30]

Mediators and Potential Modulators of Age-Associated Renal Fibrosis

Alterations in the activity of factors that mediate renal fibrosis (Figure 23-2), such as angiotensin II, transforming growth factor-β (TGF-β), nitric oxide (NO), advanced glycosylation end products (AGEs), oxidative stress, inflammation, and lipids, as well factors that prevent fibrosis, such as Klotho, vitamin D, the vitamin D receptor, and the farnesoid X receptor (FXR), are also evident in kidneys of aging animals and may be targets for modulating progression of sclerosis. Longitudinal studies in healthy elderly indicate that up to one third of individuals have little functional change in creatinine clearance, whereas two thirds show decline in function.[31] Thus it is possible that various factors hasten sclerosis in some more than others. The ability to modify these factors may result in preventing progressive age-related decline in renal function.

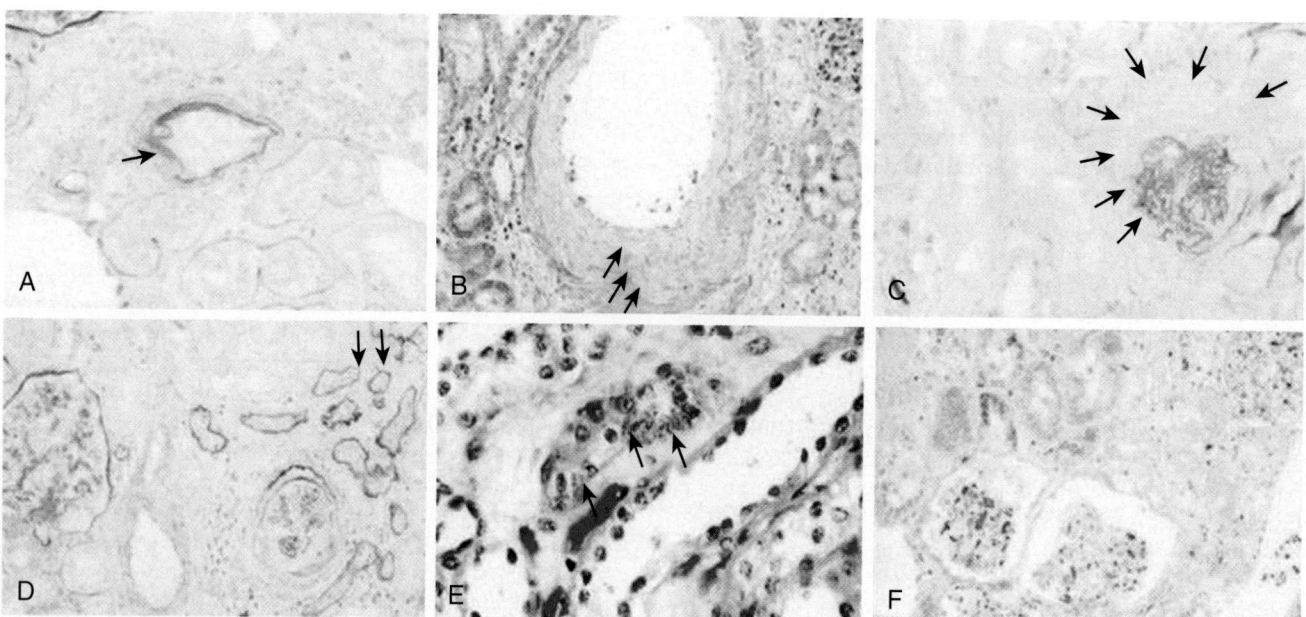

FIGURE 23-1 Histologic features of renal senescence. **A,** Arteriohyalinosis. **B,** Fibrous intimal thickening. **C,** Glomerulosclerosis. **D,** Tubular atrophy. **E,** Lipofuscin pigment. **F,** Interstitial fibrosis. (Courtesy of Dr. Marjan Afrouzian, Edmonton, Alberta, Canada.)

Angiotensin II

Diverse biologic effects of angiotensin II on the kidney, including proximal tubular transport of sodium and water,[32] glomerular and tubular growth,[33-35] decreased NO synthesis,[36] immunomodulation, growth factor induction, oxidative stress, inflammation, cell migration, apoptosis, and accumulation of extracellular matrix proteins. can affect glomerulosclerosis and tubulointerstitial fibrosis. Hemodynamic effects of angiotensin II in aging nephrons maintain filtration pressure through preferential efferent arteriolar vasoconstriction. These effects, however, are also implicated in inducing intraglomerular hypertension and subsequent glomerular damage.[37] When angiotensin converting enzyme inhibitors (ACEIs) are administered to aged rats, there is a decrease in intrarenal vascular resistance and intracapillary pressure, which reduces protein leak in aging rodents.[38] Chronic ACEI use decreases postprandial hyperfiltration, thus decreasing filtered load.[39] Glomerular capillary size selectivity or change in the distribution of negative charge within the glomerular barrier may also be affected by ACEIs.[38,40] ACEI-treated aged mice are noted to have a decrease in glomerular area, decrease in mesangial area, and overall total decrease in glomerulosclerosis compared with age-matched and sex-matched untreated mice.[40-44] It is interesting to note that although systemic changes in renin and ACEs may not be evident with aging, there is intrarenal downregulation of renin messenger RNA (mRNA) and ACE level with aging.[45] Nonhemodynamic growth effects of angiotensin II stimulate profibrotic cytokines. Angiotensin II induces synthesis and autocrine action of TGF-β to stimulate collagen IV transcription in the medullary collecting tubule.[46,47] Angiotensin II also promotes monocyte-macrophage influx, stimulates mRNA and protein expression of the chemokine RANTES in endothelial cells, and inhibits NO.[48] NO inhibition leads to transcription of the proinflammatory chemokine monocyte chemoattractant protein-1 (MCP-1). Tubulointerstitial fibrosis and α smooth muscle cell actin was significantly reduced in aged rats treated with the ACEI enalapril compared with either aged rats receiving the calcium channel blocker nifedipine or untreated aged rates, even though blood pressure control was similar.[49]

Another nonhemodynamic effect of angiotensin II in the aged kidney may be matrix accumulation by stimulation of plasminogen activator inhibitor-1 (PAI-1) from the endothelium.[50] Increased PAI-1 levels inhibit tissue plasminogen activator and urokinase plasminogen activator and lead to decreased proteolysis and fibrinolysis with increased matrix accumulation.[51] Angiotensin antagonist–treated rats had regression of age-related glomerular and vascular sclerosis with decrease in collagen content.[52] Use of angiotensin II antagonists also prevented age-associated decrease in mitochondrial energy production by lessening the age-related increases in mitochondrial oxidants.[53] The *Klotho* gene is primarily expressed in the kidney, and its protein product is associated with suppression of premature aging and arteriosclerosis. Angiotensin II appears to downregulate this gene expression. Mouse *Klotho* gene transfer via adenovirus vector into male Sprague-Dawley rats ameliorated angiotensin II–mediated renal morphologic damage. Also Klotho mRNA downregulation was reversed by administration of the angiotensin II receptor blocker (ARB) losartan but not by the use of other antipressor agents such as hydralazine.[54]

Several additional recent studies also demonstrate renal protective effects of ACEIs or ARBs in the aging kidney mediated by several complementary mechanisms, including prevention of age-related increases in oxidative stress and levels of AGEs, and prevention of age-related decreases in eNOS and Klotho.[55-61] In addition, a recent study demonstrated that disruption of the type 1 angiotensin II receptor ($AT_{1A}R$) promotes longevity in mice and prevents cardiovascular and renal pathology, and these effects are mediated in part by decreased oxidative stress and increase in the number of mitochondria and upregulation of the survival genes nicotinamide phosphoribosyltransferase (Nampt) and sirtuin 3 (Sirt3) in the kidney.[62] Given the diversity of the $AT_{1A}R$ signaling pathways in the kidney and in the cardiovascular system,[63] angiotensin II may indeed play a critical role in age-related decline in renal function, although conclusive data in humans are lacking.

Transforming Growth Factor-β

Renal fibrosis seen with aging may be the result of normal or pathologic tissue repair or both. The response to injury is wound healing and tissue repair. Persistent injury or insult may lead to tissue fibrosis. TGF-β, an active modulator of tissue repair, is associated with the structural changes of renal scarring as seen in the aging kidney. A number of factors can stimulate TGF-β, including increased angiotensin II activity, abnormal glucose metabolism, platelet-derived growth factors,

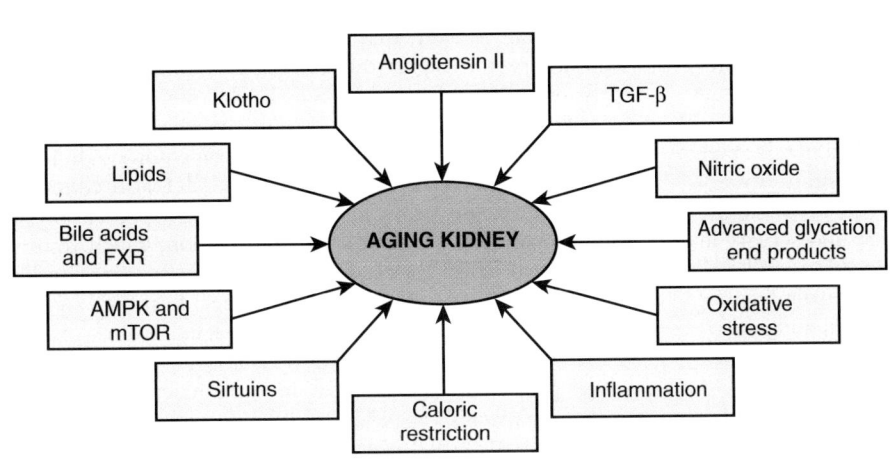

FIGURE 23-2 Factors that mediate and moderate age-related glomerulosclerosis and tubulointerstitial fibrosis.

hypoxic or oxidative stress, mesangial stretch, and increased levels of AGEs. TGF-β induces gene transcription and production of matrix proteins collagen III, IV, and I, fibronectin, tenascin, osteonectin, osteopontin, thrombospondin, and matrix glycosaminoglycans.[64] The net result is accumulation of extracellular matrix proteins with subsequent glomerulosclerosis and tubulointerstitial nephritis.[65-68] TGF-β mRNA is increased in the renal interstitium of aged rats.[23,69] Downregulation of TGF-β via angiotensin II antagonism results in decreased interstitial fibrosis.[69] Although increased expression of TGF-β may in part mediate age-related sclerosis, direct evidence is not available. Identification and use of antisense oligonucleotides inhibiting TGF-β expression or function such as decorin may provide better understanding of the role TGF-β plays in aging sclerosis and prevention. Recently identified functions of relaxin, a peptide hormone produced by the pregnant ovary and the prostate, include antifibrotic properties. Via direct actions on TGF-β–stimulated fibroblasts to decrease collagen I and III, treatment of relaxin-deficient 12-month-old male knockout mice with relaxin improved established interstitial fibrosis, glomerulosclerosis, and cortical thickening, with a decrease in collagen content.[70,71] Future studies may further clarify the clinical use of this peptide in age-related renal sclerosis.

Nitric Oxide

The role of NO goes beyond its effect on vascular reactivity. NO acts to decrease fibrosis by inhibiting the nuclear factor κ light-chain enhancer of activated B cells (NF-κB) family of transcription factors, which in the presence of reactive oxygen intermediates stimulates MCP-1 and promotes influx of monocytes-macrophages leading to inflammation and injury.[72,73] In the aging vasculature, however, levels of NO are decreased, as seen in urinary excretion of stable NO oxidation products (nitrites and nitrates) in aged rats.[74,75] Oxidant stress may also induce nicotinamide adenine dinucleotide phosphate-oxidase (NADPH oxidase)–mediated NO scavenging and NO depletion in aged kidneys.[76] In addition there is decreased expression of eNOS in peritubular capillaries of aged rats.[25] This can lead to chronic tubulointerstitial ischemia and fibrosis. Dietary supplementation with L-arginine in aging rats improves renal plasma flow (RPF) and glomerular filtration rate (GFR) and decreases proteinuria and glomerulosclerosis.[77] Supplementation with L-arginine also significantly decreases kidney collagen and N-ε-(carboxymethyl)lysine accumulation.[78] Suspected factors imposing on the age-related decrease in eNOS are increased angiotensin II activity, increased AGE levels, hypoxia, oxidative stress, increased dietary protein intake, and insulin resistance.[75,79-83] Angiotensin II antagonists and/or dietary protein restriction is associated with significant increases and normalization of urinary NO excretion.[75] The sexual dimorphism seen in the aging kidney is also attributed to lower eNOS levels and activity in male than in female rodents and humans.[84] In this regard glomerular arginine transport is decreased in older male rats but not in older female rats.[85] Alterations in estrogen and androgen activity can in part mediate these sex-dependent effects.

Recent studies indicate that Akt kinase–induced eNOS phosphorylation at serine 1177 plays a critical role in regulation of eNOS activity.[83] Aging is associated with decreased eNOS phosphorylation and activity in human umbilical vein endothelial cells.[86] Inhibition of oxidative stress by α-lipoic acid,[87] inhibition of ceramide levels,[88] and inhibition of arginase[89] reverses the age-related decreases in eNOS activity. Most recent studies in human subjects with vascular endothelial dysfunction[90] using endothelial cells obtained from the brachial artery and peripheral veins, however, suggest that increased endothelin-1 activity rather than decreased eNOS activity contributes to vascular endothelial dysfunction in aging.[91]

Advanced Glycosylation End Products

Cross-links of glycosylated proteins, lipids, and nucleic acids (AGEs) slowly accumulate and produce damage to the vascular and renal tissue with aging.[92,93] In the presence of hyperglycemia, these end products accumulate more rapidly and accelerate tissue damage.[94] These glycated proteins decrease vascular elasticity, induce endothelial cell permeability, and increase monocyte chemotactic activity via AGE-receptor ligand binding, which stimulates macrophage activation and secretion of cytokines and growth factors. AGE accumulation in the vascular endothelium and basement membrane results in defective NO vasodilation, possibly due to chemical inactivation of endothelium-derived relaxing factor.[95-98] Similar perturbations of the vascular endothelium are evident in diabetic patients and those with age-related vasculopathy. Both biochemical assays and histochemical studies have demonstrated increased levels of AGE and AGE receptor (RAGE) in aged kidneys of animals.[92] AGE deposition in the kidney is associated with increased mesangial matrix, increased basement thickening, increased vascular permeability, and induction of platelet-derived growth factor and TGF-β, resulting in glomerulosclerosis and tubulointerstitial fibrosis.[95] Several factors contribute to AGE and RAGE accumulation, including age-related decline in GFR and increased oxidative stress, which cause oxidative modifications of glycated proteins and accumulation of N-ε-(carboxymethyl)lysine. With age-related insulin resistance there is abnormal glucose metabolism and glycation of proteins. Recent studies also suggest that lifelong AGE-enriched food consumption and smoking can lead to increased AGE loads and increased AGE accumulation in tissues.[99,100]

Although mesangial cell response to AGE-RAGE interaction is increased in the kidney in the presence of hyperglycemia and oxidative stress, a newly identified mesangial cell receptor, AGER1, may act to counterregulate the proinflammatory mesangial cell response to increased AGEs. Supersaturation and possible receptor downregulation under increased AGE burden may prevent appropriate opposing regulatory control of this receptor.[101] Recent studies in human embryonic kidney cells indicate that AGER1 also counteracts cellular oxidant stress induced by AGEs via prevention of p66shc-dependent FKHRL1 phosphorylation, which results in inactivation of FKHRL1, and MnSOD suppression.[102] The importance of this pathway is further illustrated by the fact that p66shc knockout mice are protected against oxidative stress and oxidant-dependent renal injury.[103] AGER1 also provides protection against AGE-induced generation of reactive oxygen species via NADPH.[104] Interestingly, mice that are fed a low-AGE diet over the long term have lower RAGE and higher AGER1 levels (Figure 23-3) and develop less glomerulosclerosis and proteinuria (Figure 23-4).[105] Of clinical significance, AGER1 is suppressed in human subjects with CKD, and reduction of dietary AGEs results in restoration of AGER1.[106]

Studies of long-term aminoguanidine treatment in aged rats and rabbits show marked decreases in glomerulosclerosis and proteinuria,[107] as well as a decrease in age-related arterial stiffening and cardiac hypertrophy.[108] Furthermore, AGE-associated changes in vascular permeability as well as abnormal vasodilation to acetylcholine and nitroglycerin were reversed in aminoguanidine-treated animals.[109] In addition, mononuclear cell migration activity was prevented in these animals. Calorie restriction (CR) also seems to decrease the burden of AGE and other glycated proteins, including N-ε-(carboxymethyl)lysine and pentosidine, and to increase life span in rats restricted to 60% of the ad libitum dietary intake of control rats.[110,111] AGE content in the renal glomeruli and abdominal aorta of lean 30-month-old rats restricted to even 30% caloric intake was decreased compared with that of

control rats of similar age consuming an ad libitum diet.[112] Measures that decrease the burden of AGEs in the elderly may therefore be of high benefit in lessening age-related renal disease.

Oxidative Stress

Tissue injury in aging can occur from free radical production and/or antioxidant enzyme deficiency with subsequent lipid peroxidation and oxidative stress.[113-116] Increased urinary oxidized amino acid levels in aged rats indicate the presence of increased oxidized skeletal muscle proteins.[117] Aged kidneys show increased levels of reactive oxygen species and thiobarbiturate acid–reactive substances, which are associated with lipid oxidative damage.[118] In addition, other markers of oxidative stress and lipid peroxidation, such as isoprostanes, AGE, RAGE, and increased heme oxygenase, are also noted in aged rats.[119] Experimental studies evaluating oxidative stress on *Klotho* gene expression in mouse cells of the most

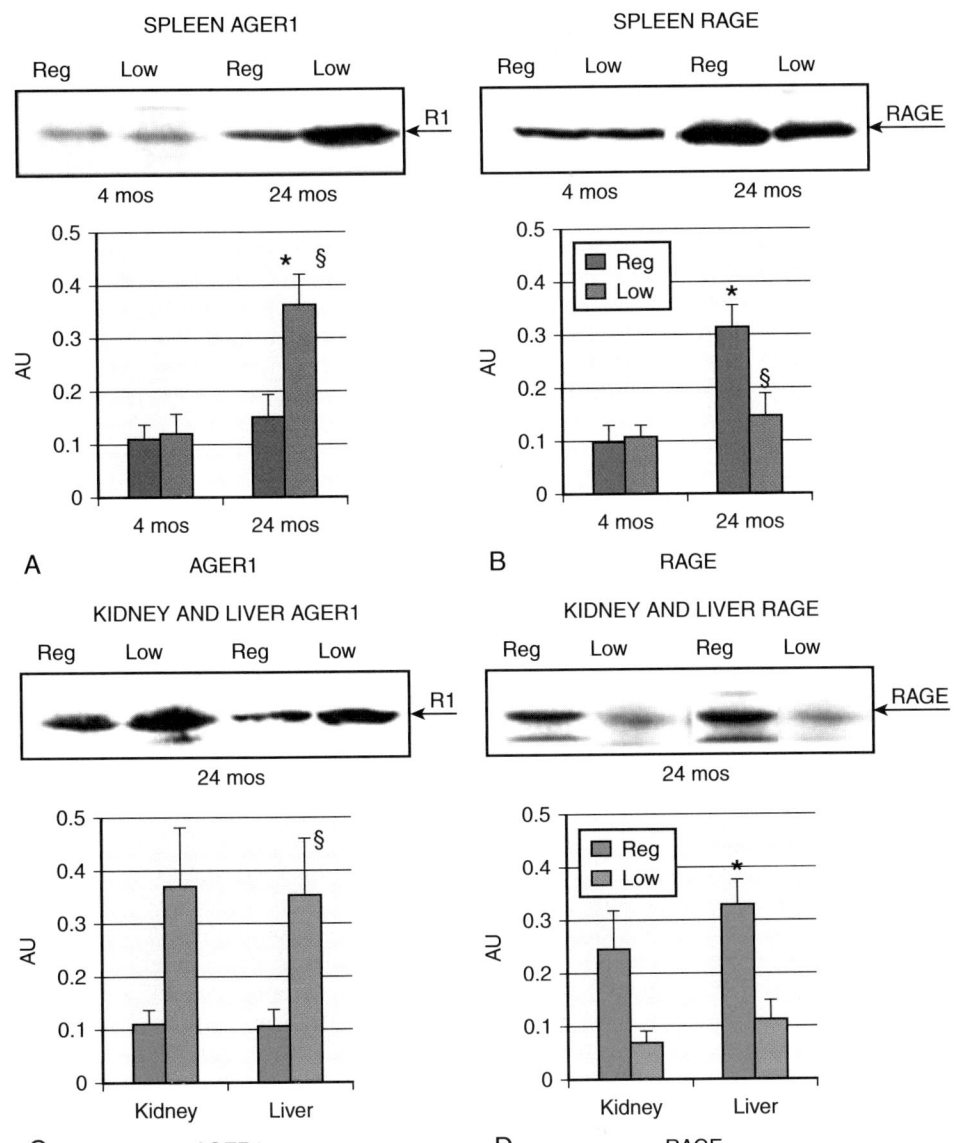

FIGURE 23-3 Effect of a low-glycotoxin diet on levels of the advanced glycosylation end product receptors AGER1 and RAGE. AGER1 (A) and RAGE (B) protein levels were assessed in spleen tissues from mice consuming either a diet with normal high AGE levels (Reg_AGE) or a low-AGE diet (Low_AGE) (n = 6 per group) at 4 and 24 months. AGER1 expression (C) in kidney and liver and RAGE expression (D) in kidney and liver of the same mouse groups were also assessed at 24 months by Western blotting and densitometric analysis. Data are shown as mean ± standard error for three independent experiments. *Statistically significant difference compared with 4-month Reg_AGE at the P < 0.01 level. §Statistically significant difference compared with 24-month Reg_AGE at the P < 0.01 level. (From Cai W, He JC, Zhu L, et al: Reduced oxidant stress and extended lifespan in mice exposed to a low glycotoxin diet: association with increased AGER1 expression, *Am J Pathol* 170[6]:1893-1902, 2007.)

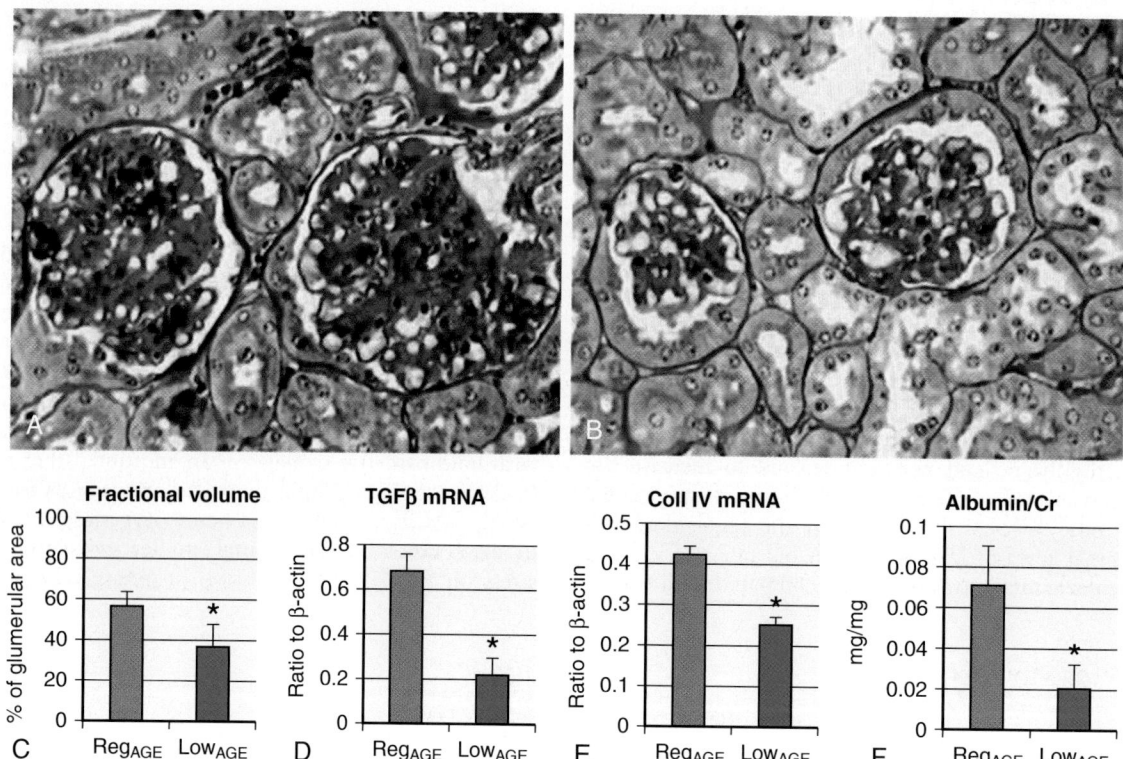

FIGURE 23-4 Effect of a low-glycotoxin diet on glomeruli and renal function in mice. Morphology of renal cortex (**A**) with consumption of a diet containing normal high levels of advanced glycosylation end products, or AGEs (Reg$_{AGE}$), and (**B**) after consumption of a low-AGE diet (Low$_{AGE}$) (n = 6 per group). (Periodic acid–Schiff stain, original magnification ×200.) **C,** Fractional mesangial volume (*P < 0.05) in Reg$_{AGE}$ versus Low$_{AGE}$ mice. **D,** Transforming growth factor-β (TGF-β) levels (*P < 0.05). **E,** Collagen type IV (Coll IV) messenger RNA (mRNA) levels (*P < 0.05). **F,** Albumin/creatinine ratio (*P < 0.05). Data are shown as mean ± standard error of triplicate values. (From Cai W, He JC, Zhu L, et al: Reduced oxidant stress and extended lifespan in mice exposed to a low glycotoxin diet: association with increased AGER1 expression, *Am J Pathol* 170[6]:1893-1902, 2007.)

distal part of the inner medullary collecting duct (IMCD3) show reduced *Klotho* expression,[120] which suggests another possible mechanism for renal aging. When an antioxidant vitamin E–enriched diet is fed to aged rats, markers of oxidative stress are lessened, with improvements noted in RPF and GFR, as well as decreased glomerulosclerosis.[119] Studies indicate that ACEI can increase antioxidant enzyme activity and block TGF-β induction by reactive oxygen species.[121,122] In addition, the antioxidant taurine also blocks reactive oxygen species in cultured mesangial cells.[123] A superoxide scavenger, tempol, restored the NO–mediated ability of ARBs to suppress oxygen consumption in renal cortical tissue.[76] These finding suggest the possibility that both angiotensin II antagonists and antioxidants may be potential therapeutic options in the future. Furthermore, CR is also noted to decrease age-related oxidative stress by suppressing activation of mitogen-activated protein kinase cellular signaling pathways, as well as to reduce mitochondrial lipid peroxidation and membrane damage with a concomitant decrease in apoptosis,[124,125] which suggests perhaps the need for dietary discrimination in the prevention of age-associated renal sclerosis. Recent evidence indicates an important role for mitochondria-generated reactive oxygen species in mediating age-related diseases.[126,127] In fact, in several genetic mouse models of longevity, including Ames and Snell dwarf mice, p66sch knockout mice, and mice heterozygous for insulin-like growth factor receptor, the increased life span has been correlated with increased resistance to oxidative stress.[128-132] A recent study investigating the effects of underexpression or overexpression of genes encoding

for antioxidant enzymes found that superoxide dismutase 1 (copper-zinc superoxide dismutase or SOD1) knockout mice had a decreased life span and increased oxidative stress. However, SOD1 transgenic mice did not have an increased life span.[133] This report did not mention the effects of superoxide dismutase deletion or overexpression in age-related renal disease and this is still an area of interest for intervention in age-related renal disease.

Calorie Restriction: Sirtuins, Adenosine Monophosphate–Activated Protein Kinase, Mammalian Target of Rapamycin, and Ribosomal Protein S6 Kinase 1

CR is usually defined as a 25% to 45% reduction in caloric intake compared with an ad libitum diet while the levels of all essential nutrients are maintained.[134] CR has been found to extend the life of many rat and mouse strains as well as yeast, worms, and fruit flies.[135-139] CR also decreases age-related diseases in rhesus monkeys, including insulin resistance, atherosclerosis, oxidative damage, and immune dysfunction.[140-147] A recent study has shown that in addition to reducing the incidence of diabetes, cancer, cardiovascular disease, and brain atrophy, CR also decreases mortality in rhesus monkeys.[148] Although the effect of CR on human longevity remains unknown, CR studies in humans show similar beneficial effects on health.[149,150] CR also decreases age-related proteinuria and glomerulosclerosis in rats and in mice.[151,152]

THE DIVERSE PHYSIOLOGICAL ROLES OF THE SIRTUINS

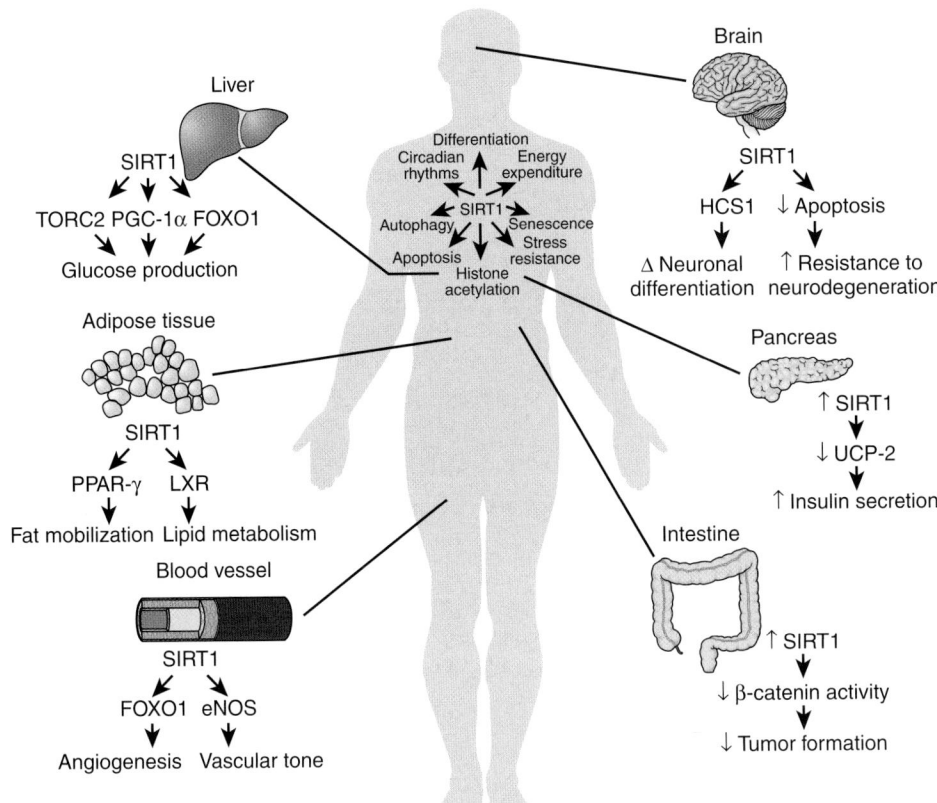

FIGURE 23-5 Examples of the organ-specific physiology of silent information regulator T1 (SIRT1), along with some of the direct and indirect targets of sirtuin regulation (see text for details). In addition, examples of some of the SIRT1-regulated intracellular parameters are presented, ranging from modulation of progenitor differentiation to alteration of the threshold for apoptosis. ↓, Decreasing; ↑, increasing; Δ, change in. (From Finkel T, Deng CX, Mostoslavsky R: Recent progress in the biology and physiology of sirtuins, *Nature* 460[7255]:587-591, 2009.)

Several potential mechanisms have been proposed for the beneficial effects of CR, including (1) reduced body fat content, (2) reduction of metabolic rate, (3) attenuation of oxidative stress, (4) attenuation of inflammation, (5) modulation of mitochondrial function, (6) increase in the activity of sirtuins, (7) increase in adenosine monophosphate–activated protein kinase (AMPK) signaling, and (8) decreases in mTOR (mammalian target of rapamycin) and S6K1 (ribosomal protein S6 kinase 1) signaling.[153-155] Sir2 (silent information regulator 2) was first identified in yeast and was found to mediate enzymatic histone deacetylase activity dependent on the oxidized form of nicotinamide adenine dinucleotide (NAD+). To date seven mammalian homologs have been identified, SIRT1 through SIRT7. These are present in different subcellular compartments, and sirtuin-mediated NAD+-dependent enzymatic histone deacetylation controls the activity of various proteins and genes that regulate cell survival, differentiation, metabolism, DNA repair, inflammation, and longevity.[156-158] Several studies have shown that SIRT1 activity is increased in most tissues, including the kidney, in response to CR.[159-164] In support of an important role for SIRT1 in mediating the effects of CR, studies have shown that SIRT1 knockout mice are resistant to the effects of a calorie-restricted diet.[165] In contrast, SIRT1 transgenic mice have a phenotype similar to that of mice on a calorie-restricted diet.[166-168] Mice treated with resveratrol, the synthetic activator of SIRT1, also display the transcriptional aspects of CR, including protection against age-related renal disease.[169-173] Most recently, CR has been shown to increase SIRT1-induced FOXO3 (forkhead box O3) deacetylation, which results in increases in Bnip3 (BCL2/adenovirus

E1B 19 kDa protein-interacting protein 3), mitochondrial autophagy, and prevention of age-dependent decrease in kidney function.[174] Sirtuins have diverse physiologic functions that extend beyond their important role in the aging process (Figure 23-5)[174]

Recent studies indicate a complex regulation of metabolic pathways in response to CR that integrates the effects of CR on insulin release, AMPK, SIRT1, and FOXO activation as well as inhibition of mTOR[175-177] (Figure 23-6). Interestingly these metabolic effects are similar to the effects of exercise and fasting, which also regulate AMPK, SIRT1, peroxisome proliferator–activated receptor γ coactivator 1α (PGC-1α), and FOXO activity (Figure 23-7). These findings are of great importance, because aging is associated with decreased SIRT1 activity due to a decline in systemic NAD+ synthesis,[178] and aging also is associated with reductions in AMPK activity and mitochondrial biogenesis.[179] Activation of SIRT1 and AMPK activity therefore holds great promise for the prevention of age-related metabolic defects and disease. Very interestingly, recent studies have revealed additional complexity of the metabolic regulation by showing that SIRT1 deacetylates and positively regulates the oxysterol-activated nuclear receptor LXR (liver X receptor),[180] which plays an important role in mediating reverse cholesterol efflux and inhibition of inflammation. SIRT1 also deacetylates the bile acid–activated nuclear receptor FXR,[181] which plays an important role in inhibiting sterol regulatory element–binding protein-1 (SREBP-1)–mediated fatty acid synthesis and also inflammation, oxidative stress, and fibrosis. In fact although the effects of LXR activation on renal disease remains to be determined, recent studies indicate

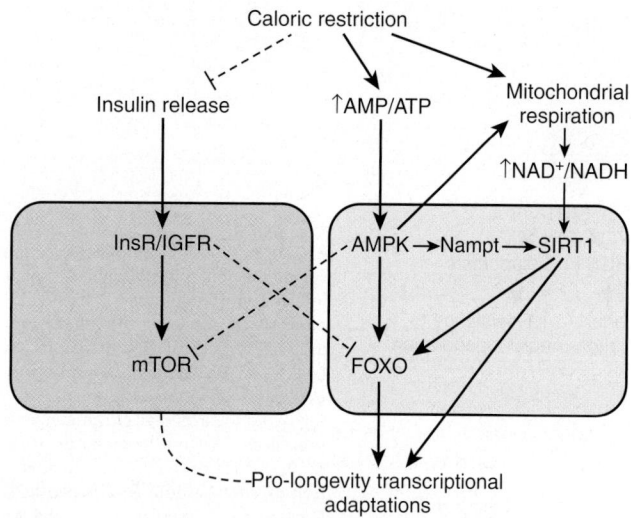

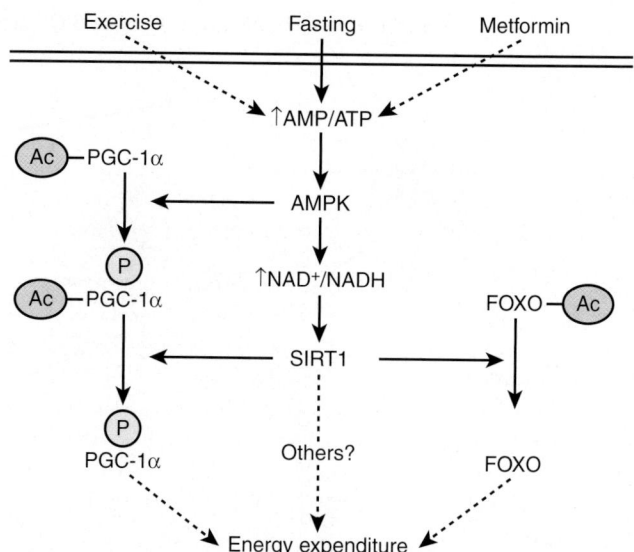

FIGURE 23-6 Integrative view of mammalian signaling pathways involved in regulating the effects of caloric restriction (CR). Despite evidence linking silent information regulator T1 (SIRT1) to the effects of CR in mammals, these effects might be due to SIRT1 acting in conjunction with other factors. For example, CR might be sensed not only by SIRT1 as a change in the ratio of oxidized to reduced nicotinamide adenine dinucleotide (NAD^+/NADH) but also by adenosine monophosphate–activated protein kinase (AMPK) as a change in the ratio of adenosine monophosphate (AMP) to adenosine triphosphate (ATP). AMPK can regulate mitochondrial respiration, which in turn can positively regulate SIRT1. Both AMPK and SIRT1 can impact the activity of forkhead box O1 (FOXO) transcription factors, which also have been extensively linked to the regulation of metabolism and longevity. In addition, CR promotes the downregulation of insulin-derived signals, which also interact with FOXO transcription factors. Hence, the metabolic and longevity responses to CR, rather than being defined by single elements, might be a consequence of the balance of these signaling networks. (From Canto C, Auwerx J: Caloric restriction, SIRT1 and longevity, *Trends Endocrinol Metab* 20[7]:325-331, 2009.)

FIGURE 23-7 Scheme illustrating the convergent actions of adenosine monophosphate–activated protein kinase (AMPK) and silent information regulator T1 (SIRT1) on peroxisome proliferator–activated receptor γ coactivator 1α (PGC-1α). Pharmacologic (metformin) and physiologic (fasting or exercise) activation of AMPK in muscle triggers an increase in the ratio of oxidized to reduced nicotinamide adenine dinucleotide (NAD^+/NADH), which activates SIRT1. AMPK also induces the phosphorylation of PGC-1α and primes it for subsequent deacetylation by SIRT1. The impact of AMPK and SIRT1 on the acetylation status of PGC-1α and other transcriptional regulators, such as the forkhead box O1 (FOXO) family of transcription factors, will then modulate mitochondrial function and lipid metabolism. (From Canto C, Gerhart-Hines Z, Feige JN, et al: AMPK regulates energy expenditure by modulating NAD^+ metabolism and SIRT1 activity, *Nature* 458[7241]:1056-1060, 2009.)

that activation of FXR using natural and synthetic bile acid analogs modulates renal lipid metabolism and prevents the development and progression of proteinuria and glomerulosclerosis in mouse models of type 2 diabetes mellitus and diet-induced obesity and insulin resistance.[182,183] Whether FXR agonists have similar effects in rodent or human aging kidney remains to be determined. Two recent studies also indicate potentially important roles for mTOR and S6K1 in regulating mammalian life span. Treatment of relatively old mice with rapamycin, an inhibitor of mTOR, extended life span in male and female mice.[184] Interestingly, the long-lived Ames dwarf mouse has reduced TOR signaling.[185,186] Mechanistic studies in yeast indicate that deletion or inhibition of TOR upregulates mitochondrial gene expression and prevent cellular accumulation of reactive oxygen species.[187] Similarly, deletion of S6K1, a component of the nutrient-responsive mTOR signaling pathway, results in increased life span and decreases in insulin resistance and age-related diverse pathologies.[188] Most intriguingly, deletion of S6K1-induced gene expression patterns similar to those seen with CR or activation of AMPK.

Lipid Metabolism

Animal studies indicate that the abnormal lipid metabolism in CKD and aging are mediated by altered expression of a number of transcriptional factors and nuclear hormone receptors. In animal models of CKD there is evidence for increased expression of SREBP-1 and SREBP-2 in the liver and in the adipose tissue. SREBP-1 and SREBP-2 are master regulators of fatty acid, triglyceride, and cholesterol synthesis and therefore mediate increased serum lipid levels as well as insulin resistance.[189-191] In addition there is decreased expression of peroxisome proliferator–activated receptor α (PPARα), which results in impaired fatty acid oxidation.[192] Similar changes also occur in the liver and kidneys of animals with the nephrotic syndrome[193-195] and in aging.[152,196,197] Recent studies indicate that expression and activity of FXR are decreased in the liver of aging mice.[198] FXR is a bile acid–activated nuclear hormone receptor that plays an important role in regulation of bile acid, fatty acid, cholesterol, and glucose metabolism in the liver and in the kidney.[182,199] Decreased FXR activity may mediate the increased expression and activity of SREBP-1 and decreased expression and activity of PPARα in aging. CR is known to prevent age-related alterations in metabolic function, and several studies have shown that CR prevents the age-related increased expression of SREBP-1 and decrease in PPARs.[134,200-202]

One important mediator of the metabolic effects of CR is the increased expression of the sirtuin SIRT1, an NAD-dependent deacetylase enzyme. There is now increasing evidence that sirtuin analogs replicate several of the beneficial effects of CR, including adipogenesis, insulin sensitivity and signaling, and lipid metabolism,[167,169,203,204] and SIRT1 transgenic mice show phenotypes resembling those caused by

CR.[166,195] Studies in animal models thus continue to be useful in understanding the complex changes in lipid metabolism in aging and CKD.

Although experimental data support a role for dyslipidemia in the progression of renal disease,[205,206] the data for humans come primarily from observational studies. High triglyceride and low HDL levels as seen in CKD predicted an increase in the risk of renal dysfunction when participants of the Atherosclerosis Risk in Communities study were followed for approximately 3 years.[207] Similarly, low HDL level and high LDL/HDL cholesterol ratio suggested greater risk for a rise in serum creatinine level or increase in the development of in stage 3 CKD (GFR of <60 mL/min) for individuals followed over time in the Physicians' Health Study and Framingham Offspring Study.[208-210] Samuelsson and colleagues observed a strong association between plasma triglyceride-rich apolipoprotein B–containing lipoproteins and rate of decline in GFR.[211] This association was also evident for participants with moderate to severe kidney disease in the Modification of Diet in Renal Disease (MDRD) study.[212] These data suggest, then, that lipid lowering may possibly benefit patients with CKD by slowing the rate of progression. In fact, subgroup post hoc analysis of the data from several prospective trials in which hyperlipidemia was treated with 3-hydroxy–3-methylglutaryl–coenzyme A reductase inhibitors (statins) suggest a slower decrease in renal function and reduced proteinuria, although this has not been observed for all statin trials. Combined data for 3402 participants with an estimated GFR (eGFR) of 30 to 59.9 mL/min from three randomized double-blinded trials with 18,569 participants comparing pravastatin 40 mg/day and placebo noted an absolute decrease in the eGFR, as calculated by the MDRD equation, of 0.22 mL/min/1.73 m^2 (95% confidence interval = 0.7 to 0.37).[213] Meta-analysis of other randomized trials suggests a 1.2 mL/min slower drop in GFR and less proteinuria in those subjects treated with statins.[214,215] The antiinflammatory effect of statins may be beneficial with regard to endothelial function and vessel stiffness; however, a beneficial effect of statin treatment in decreasing urine protein has not been uniformly seen.[216] In addition, patients randomly assigned to receive fluvastatin to prevent cardiac events were noted to have stable renal function. Although pooled data from 10,000 patients treated with rosuvastatin (5 to 40 mg) found a drop in renal function, study of long-term use has suggested either no change or an increase in GFR.[217] The effect of hyperlipidemia on renal disease progression remains yet to be clearly determined given that available data are primarily observational. Thus statin use in the elderly for renoprotection alone may be premature.

Bile Acid Metabolism and the Farnesoid X Receptor

Recent studies in a long-lived dwarf mutant mouse, the little mouse (Ghrhr$^{lit/lit}$), which fails to secret growth hormone (GH) and therefore has very low circulating levels of GH and insulin-like growth factor-1 (IGF-1), have identified a potential role for alterations in xenobiotic metabolism mediated by FXR in association with longevity in these mice.[218] A possible role for bile acids as endocrine regulators of aging has also been found in *Caenorhabditis elegans*, in which bile acid–like steroids influence life span via the DAF-12 nuclear receptor.[219] Although the age-related renal pathology in long-lived dwarf mutant mice has not been well studied, recent research involving diet-induced obesity in diabetic mice treated with FXR agonists indicates that FXR agonists decrease proteinuria and glomerulosclerosis by modulating renal lipid metabolism, oxidative stress, inflammation, and fibrosis.[182,183] Whether FXR can also modulate age-related renal disease remains to be determined.

Klotho

The Klotho gene has been identified as a novel gene that has multiple effects in regulating the aging process as well as mineral metabolism and endocrine functions.[220,221] Mice with defects in Klotho gene expression exhibit multiple aging-like phenotypes and die prematurely, whereas transgenic mice that overexpress the Klotho gene live longer than wild-type mice.[222,223] The mechanisms of the antiaging effects of Klotho are still being determined, but potential mechanisms include effects on antioxidative stress as well as modulation of insulin and IGF-1 signaling processes.[220,221] Although Klotho is very strongly expressed in the kidney and plays an important role in the regulation of fibroblast growth factor 23 signaling, phosphate transport activity, TRPV5 (transient receptor potential cation channel subfamily V member 5) activity, and ROMK1 (regulation of Kir 1.1 potassium channel) activity,[220,221] the exact role of Klotho in age-related renal disease remains to be determined. Recent studies, however, indicate that the renal actions of angiotensin II are mediated via modulation of renal Klotho expression.[54] In addition, the effects of the PPARγ agonists,[224] including their beneficial effects in age-related renal disease,[225] are mediated by regulation of intrarenal Klotho expression.

Functional Changes

Renal Plasma Flow

Measurement of changes in effective renal plasma flow (ERPF) using paraaminohippurate clearance indicate a 10% decline per decade as healthy adults age from 30 to 90 years, with a greater change noted in men than in women[226] (Figure 23-8). Medullary blood flow remains preserved, whereas cortical blood flow decreases in parallel with observed histologic changes. A small but definite decrease in the renal fraction of the cardiac output may be contributing, in addition to anatomic changes and changes in vascular responsiveness.[227,228] Administration of a potent vasodilator, including intraarterial acetylcholine or intravenous pyrogen or atrial natriuretic peptide (ANP), results in a blunted vasodilatory response in older compared with younger subjects.[229] Similarly amino acid plus low-dose dopamine infusion increases both RPF and GFR in healthy older subjects, but vasodilation is less than in younger subjects.[230,231] Higher levels of the endogenous nitric oxide synthase (NOS) inhibitor asymmetric dimethylarginine (ADMA) are noted with increasing age and are inversely associated with ERPF in healthy elderly and hypertensive elderly.[232] However, whether this results from tubular

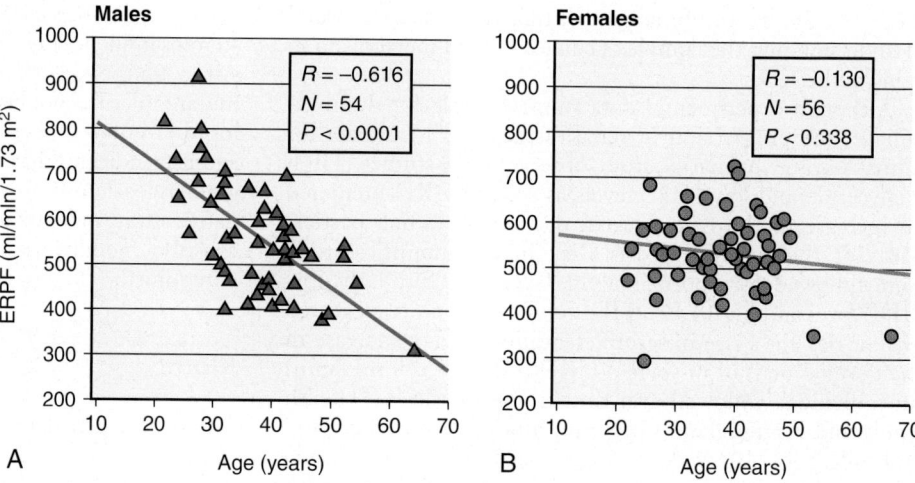

FIGURE 23-8 Relationship between age and relative effective renal plasma flow (ERPF, in milliliters per minute per 1.73 m² body surface area [BSA]) in males (**A**) and females (**B**). (From Berg UB: Differences in decline in GFR with age between males and females. Reference data on clearances of inulin and PAH in potential kidney donors, *Nephrol Dial Transplant* 21[9]:2577-2582, 2006.)

cell senescence and the inability to degrade ADMA remains unclear. Recent studies in 5/6 nephrectomized rats indicate that overexpression of the enzyme dimethyl aminohydrolase, responsible for the hydrolysis of ADMA to dimethylamine and citrulline, ameliorated sclerotic glomerular changes.[233] Thus cell senescence may be contributing to underlying vascular changes and response.

Altered intrarenal signaling from an imbalance between vasodilatory and vasoconstrictive mediators in the elderly can also affect renal vasculature and RPF. NO production from isolated conduit arteries decreases with age,[234-236] with low levels of NOS and L-arginine,[236,237] although gene expression for substrate synthesis is not affected.[238] Prostacyclin (prostaglandin I₂ [PGI₂]) is decreased in aging human vascular cells and older rat kidneys in comparison to vasoconstrictive thromboxanes.[239,240] Older subjects also excrete less vasodilatory natriuretic prostaglandins. However, forearm vasodilation after PGI₂ infusion, although lower in older healthy subjects than in younger comparison subjects, did not change with NOS inhibition in the older group, whereas young subjects had a blunted response.[241] While intraarterial angiotensin infusion results in a similar vasoconstrictive response in younger and older subjects, abrogation of angiotensin II–mediated vasoconstriction leads to an exaggerated or preserved vasodilation,[242,243] with increased RPF seen in rats.[244] Similar findings are noted with intravenous glycine infusion in older rats.[245] Competitive inhibition of NO results in significant vasoconstriction, increased renal vascular resistance, and decreased RPF in older compared with younger rats.[246] Thus, the renal vasculature appears to remain in a constant state of vasodilation to compensate for underlying sclerotic damage with aging. Renal function is then maintained despite a decrease in renal functional reserve.[247]

Although increases in preglomerular and efferent arteriolar resistances are noted in micropuncture studies in both young and old rats after angiotensin infusion, renal and glomerular plasma flow decrease in association with increased glomerular hydraulic pressure gradient and filtration fraction. Single-nephron GFR and GFR, however, are lower in older rats in association with a decreased glomerular capillary ultrafiltration coefficient (K_f). These parameters remain unchanged in younger rats. Angiotensin II–mediated glomerular mesangial

cell contraction and decreased K_f likely translate to decreased filtration surface.[248] Although larger nonsclerotic glomeruli in transplants from deceased aged donors had a larger filtration surface with higher K_f, overall allograft K_f was 45% lower with a marked decrease in the number of functioning glomeruli compared with organs from younger donors.[14] Thus the drop in K_f with age seen in healthy transplant donors is likely a function of both underlying structural changes that lower K_f and a decrease in the number of functioning glomeruli.[249] Relatively preserved medullary flow with decreased cortical flow in aging may allow for a higher filtration fraction in juxtamedullary nephrons than in cortical nephrons. Thus, despite a decrease in RPF, filtration fraction increases with age[247,249-251] (Figure 23-9).

Glomerular Filtration Rate

Measurements of inulin and iothalamate clearance in aging individuals confirm earlier findings based on urea and creatinine clearances, showing a progressive decline in GFR with aging, although the rate of change may vary based on measurement methodology[249] (Figure 23-10). Creatinine clearance in healthy elderly estimates a drop of 0.8 mL/min/1.73 m² per year, whereas iohexol clearance suggests a decrease of 1.0 mL/min/1.73 m² per year.[252,253] In addition, associated factors such as race, gender, genetic variation, and underlying risks of renal and vascular disease affect the rate of decline in a given individual. Some have suggested a greater decrease in GFR in healthy elderly men than in elderly women,[226] although others have noted that gender differences in the rate of decline in GFR are relatively small.[254] African Americans and Japanese elderly seem to have a greater rate of decline in GFR than whites.[12,255] Comorbid conditions of hypertension, glucose intolerance, diabetes, systemic or renal atherosclerosis, and lipid abnormalities can enhance loss of GFR in the elderly.[256-258] Elevated pulse pressure indicative of increased arterial stiffness in older individuals correlates inversely with GFR.[259] Older participants in the Cardiovascular Health Study with systemic microvascular disease as determined by retinal examination exhibited a greater decrease in GFR.[253] Despite a gradual decline in GFR, a parallel increase in serum creatinine level may not

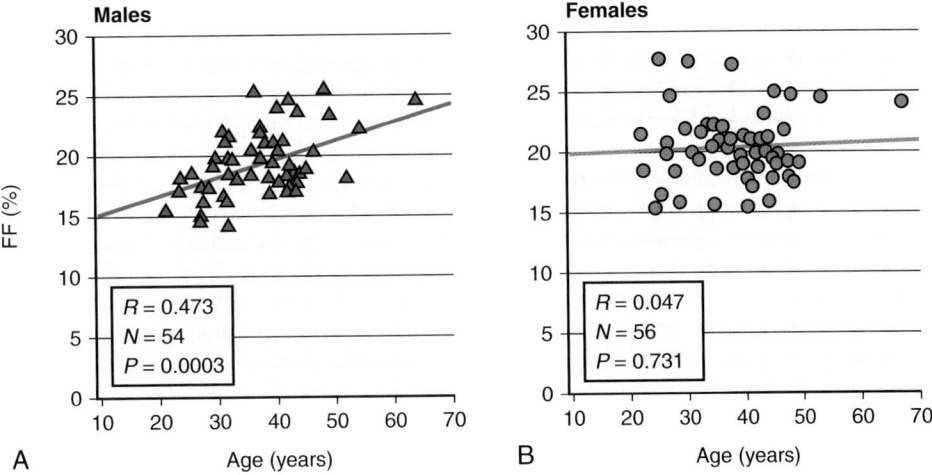

FIGURE 23-9 Relationship between age and filtration fraction (FF, in percent) in males (**A**) and females (**B**). (From Berg UB: Differences in decline in GFR with age between males and females. Reference data on clearances of inulin and PAH in potential kidney donors, *Nephrol Dial Transplant* 21[9]:2577-2582, 2006.)

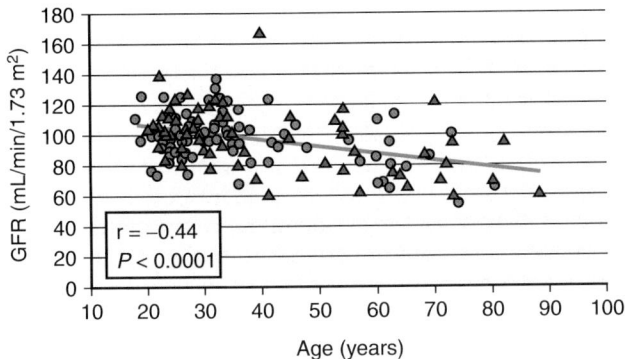

FIGURE 23-10 Glomerular filtration rate (GFR) plotted as a function of age in 164 healthy individuals. *Circles* are males; *triangles* are females. (From Hoang K, Tan JC, Derby G, et al: Determinants of glomerular hypofiltration in aging humans, *Kidney Int* 64[4]:1417-1424, 2003.)

be evident in the elderly because muscle mass decreases with age, which leads to overestimation of GFR. Measurement of steady-state 24-hour creatinine clearance, which depends on collected volume, diet, and appropriate collection times, is sometimes cumbersome for the elderly. Although technetium 99m–labeled diethylenetriamine-pentaacetic acid, iodine 125 iothalamate, or radiocontrast clearance with single-injection iohexol x-ray fluorescence analysis may be more accurate,[260] expense, radioactivity exposure, and test availability can be limiting factors in obtaining routine GFR measurements. Commonly used formulas to calculate GFR may either overestimate or underestimate actual GFR in older individuals, although the MDRD[261] and Chronic Kidney Disease Epidemiology Collaboration (CKD-EPI)[262] equations may provide a closer approximation than the standard Cockcroft-Gault equation.[262,263] Other clearance markers, including serum cystatin C, a cysteine proteinase with endogenous and constant production by nucleated cells that is freely filtered, catabolized, and reabsorbed but not secreted by renal tubules, are being more closely investigated for accuracy in predicting GFR in the elderly and may be comparable to the MDRD equation, although body mass index may affect the results and lead to discrepancies between the two estimations.[264-266]

Sodium Conservation

Tubular efficiency in reabsorbing filtered sodium diminishes with aging. With sodium restriction, subjects 60 years and older take 31 hours to decrease urine sodium versus 17.6 hours for those 30 years of age and younger.[267] Distal sodium conservation may be decreased,[268] because age-related interstitial scarring, lower nephron number, and increased medullary flow likely increase solute load per nephron as seen in those with chronic renal disease. Changes in hormonal levels and responses regulating sodium reabsorption with aging can also influence renal sodium conservation. Both plasma renin levels and aldosterone levels are lower in healthy elderly. Despite normal levels of renin substrate, there is a 30% to 50% decrease in basal renin activity. Maneuvers to increase renin activity, such as upright position, sodium restriction to 10 mEq/day, furosemide administration, and air jet stress, further amplify age-related difference in renin activity.[269] Even after hemorrhagic stress, plasma renin levels are lower in 15 month-old-rats than in 3-month-old rats, reflecting the age-related differences before the stress event.[45] Aged rats are found to have downregulation of renin mRNA abundance and decreased juxtamedullary single-nephron renin activity[270] as well as lower renal levels of ACE and type 1 angiotensin receptor mRNA.[45,271] In older rats the response to sodium deprivation with a fall in mean arterial pressure is blunted plasma renin activity with a delayed decrease in urinary sodium excretion. Measurement of plasma renin substrate in healthy aged adults suggests decreased conversion of inactive to active renin.[272]

Changes in plasma aldosterone in aging parallel changes in plasma renin activity, with a 30% to 50% decrease in older adults. Aldosterone and cortisol response to adrenocorticotropic hormone remains appropriate with aging, which negates the possibility of an intrinsic adrenal defect and suggests a greater likelihood of renin-angiotensin deficiency.[273] The sluggish tubular conservation of sodium in response to restricted dietary sodium can be reproduced with ACE inhibition and blocking of the renin-angiotensin-aldosterone system (RAAS).[274] Tubular sensitivity to aldosterone infusion appears preserved, with appropriate sodium reabsorption, a finding that supports an abnormal RAAS response as an important factor in delayed tubular sodium reabsorption in the elderly.

Sodium Excretion

Natriuretic response to sodium or volume loading is also blunted in the elderly.[275,276] Adults older than 40 years excrete a 2-L saline load much more slowly and excrete more during the night than gender-, size-, and race- matched younger adults[255,277] (Figure 23-11). Nocturia thus is more prevalent in older individuals. Older kidney donors with single kidneys exhibit a greater drop in natriuretic ability with saline loading than similar younger donors[274] (Figure 23-12).

A decreased response to ANP, important in the control of sodium excretion, is found with aging. Via specific cell surface receptors on renal vasculature and tubular epithelium, ANP induces hyperfiltration, inhibits luminal membrane sodium channels and reabsorption, and suppresses renin release. Although ANP is rapidly degraded, selective blockade of degradative enzymes or clearance receptors can prolong ANP serum half-life.[278] Older healthy adults have serum ANP levels that are three to five times higher than those in younger adults. ANP levels increase in response to increased salt load and head-out-of-water immersion in older subjects to a greater extent than in younger ones,[279-281] although decreased salt intake results in similar ANP levels in the old and young. Thus ANP secretion remains intact with aging. Higher basal levels result from decreased metabolic clearance.[282,283] Age-associated decrease in GFR likely does not contribute, given that patients with CKD and low GFR do not have high ANP levels.[284]

Levels of endopeptidases in the proximal tubular brush border that break down ANP are lower with aging. Blocking endopeptidases with an infusion of the endopeptidase inhibitor phosphoramidon in rats with reduced renal mass increases urinary cyclic guanosine monophosphate (cGMP), ANP second messenger, and urinary salt excretion.[285] Similar effects can also be seen in congestive heart failure patients when renal endopeptidase is inhibited by candoxatril: there is urinary excretion of ANP, cGMP, and sodium with no changes in renal hemodynamics,[286] which provides further support for a decrease in ANP response with age. Some have proposed that higher ANP levels are a homeostatic response to reduced ANP renal sensitivity with aging, because urinary sodium excretion reaches a plateau after a 2 ng/kg/min ANP infusion in older adults,[275,276] whereas younger subjects continue to have increased urinary sodium excretion with incremental increases in ANP.[275] Although cGMP and ANP levels are no different at baseline, low-dose ile-ANP increases cGMP but not urinary sodium excretion in older subjects,[282,287] which suggests that the problem occurs after cGMP. Furthermore, plasma renin and aldosterone levels during ANP infusion imply that the natriuretic properties of ANP are different than those caused by RAAS suppression. Age appears to influence each ANP action differently.[276,282]

Urinary Concentration

Older individuals are frequently unable to reach maximal urinary concentrating capacity.[252,288] The presence of an intact osmoreceptor and volume receptor sensitivity to arginine vasopressin (AVP) release as well as an intact collecting tubule response to AVP under maximum medullary tonicity is necessary for appropriate urinary concentration. With aging, a combination of processes may lead to impaired water excretion. Investigations suggest that both volume and osmotic stimulation of AVP remain intact with age, with osmoreceptor sensitivity for AVP actually enhanced in the elderly.[289,290] Older adults demonstrate increased basal circulating AVP levels after 24 hours of water deprivation.[291,292] A concentrating defect remains after AVP infusion, however, which suggests impaired intrarenal AVP response.[293] Medullary "washout" is suspected in light of increased solute and osmolar clearance

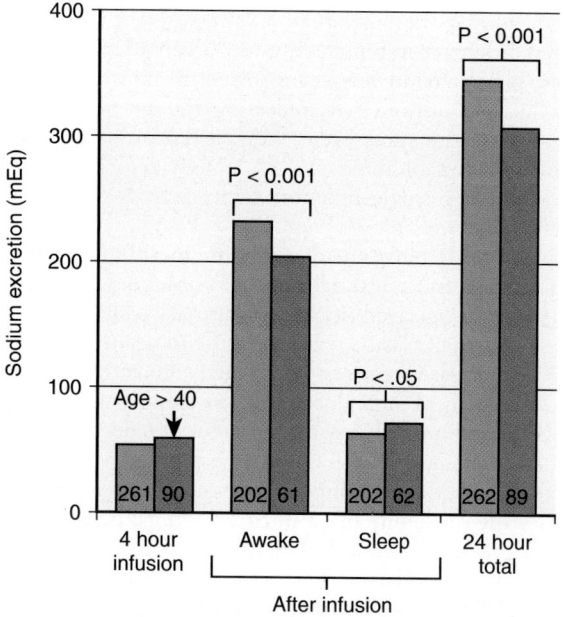

FIGURE 23-11 Comparison of urinary sodium excretion in younger (*yellow bars*) and older (*red bars*) subjects after administration of 2 L of intravenous normal saline. Numbers at the bottoms of bars are the number of subjects in each group. (From Luft FC, Grim CE, Fineberg N, et al: Effects of volume expansion and contraction in normotensive whites, blacks, and subjects of different ages, *Circulation* 59[4]:643-650, 1979.)

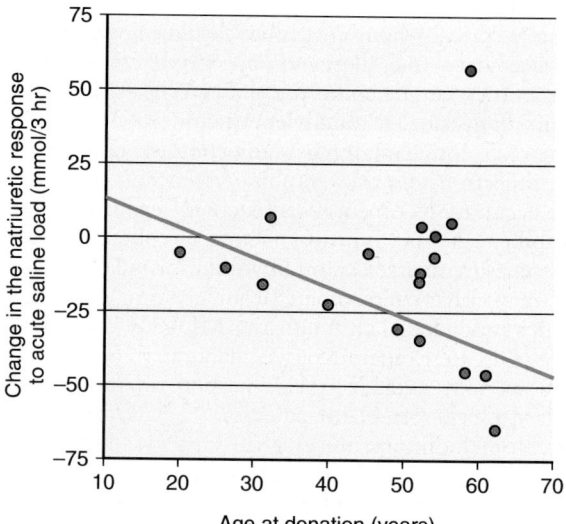

FIGURE 23-12 Influence of age at donation on change in natriuretic response to acute saline load in kidney donors after uninephrectomy. *Red circles* indicates normotensive; *blue circles* indicates de novo hypertensive. (From Mimran A, Ribstein J, Jover B: Aging and sodium homeostasis, *Kidney Int Suppl* 37:S107-S113, 1992.)

and decreased urine osmolality despite 12 hours of overnight water deprivation in healthy elderly.[252] Water diuresis results in decreased sodium chloride transport in the ascending loop of Henle.[294] Studies in aged rats, however, suggest AVP resistance in the collecting tubules. Solute-free water excretion remains normal after 40 hours of dehydration and exogenous AVP administration; however, solute-free water reabsorption is impaired. Young and aged rats maintain identical solute content in the inner medulla.[295] However, aged rats are noted to have decreased medullary abundance of Na-K-2CL cotransporter type 2 (NKCC2) and decreased cortical abundance of epithelial sodium channel β- and γ-subunits. Although restricted water intake increased the abundance of both NCCK2 and Na-Cl cotransporter in aging rats, the response remains significantly blunted.[296] Taken together, these findings imply that aging can impact both ascending limb solute transport and collecting tubule water transport.

In the collecting tubule, no change is noted in receptor number or affinity for AVP,[297] although higher AVP levels are needed to increase cyclic adenosine monophosphate (cAMP) because older animals have decreased cAMP levels.[298,299] Levels of postreceptor guanine nucleotide–binding protein (Gs protein) is also lower in older kidneys.[300] There is significantly less stimulation of adenylate cyclase in older rabbit cortical collecting tubules despite G protein stimulation with cholera toxin and forskolin stimulation of adenylate cyclase at the level of the catalytic unit and G protein interaction.[301] Thus abnormality of AVP response in aging may be at the level of interaction of the Gs catalytic subunit of adenylate cyclase. Further evaluation of collecting duct water channels suggested decreased expression of aquaporin-2 (AQP2)[288] and aquaporin-3 (AQP3) in older rats, although papillary cAMP content was no different than in young rats.[302] Increases in AQP2 mRNA appear to preserve AQP2 protein expression in the outer medulla where it is less downregulated with aging than the inner medullary collecting duct (IMCD), which suggests a posttranslational defect of AQP2 protein expression in older rats that can be compensated for by higher AQP2 mRNA levels in the outer medulla. With a significant 2-day water deprivation AQP2 and AQP3 expression increased markedly in both young and old rats, with age-related differences resolved in AQP2 regulation.[303] Vasopressin V2 receptor mRNA abundance is lower in aging rats, although equivalent plasma AVP levels are present in old and young rats.[288] Basolateral V2 receptors are similarly downregulated in dehydrated older and younger rats,[304] which perhaps explains the lower water permeability of the inner medullary collecting duct and decrease in urinary concentration seen in aging. Another possible cause of decreased urinary concentration in aging may be decreased expression of urea transporters UT-A1 and UT-B1 in the renal medulla with decreased papillary osmolality regardless of food restriction or an ad libitum feeding.[305] Papillary urea accumulation as well as urine osmolality and flow rates improved with upregulation of urea transporters when deamino-8-D-arginine vasopressin (DDAVP) was given.[306]

Urinary Dilution

Water diuresis in older individuals uncovers the inability to dilute urine maximally with increasing age.[307] Minimum urine osmolality reached by subjects older than 70 years is 92

mOsm/kg H_2O compared with 52 mOsm/kg H_2O in those younger than 40 years. Free water clearance after oral water loading of 20 mL/kg and overnight fluid fast is 6.0 ± 0.6 mL/min in the elderly compared with 10.1 ± 0.8 mL/min in the young. Maximum urinary dilution depends on several factors, including appropriate solute extraction, adequate AVP suppression, and distal delivery of the filtered load. Solute-free water clearance is decreased even when correction is made for the age-related decline in GFR.[307]

Acid-Base Balance

Homeostatic acid-base balance is well maintained in the elderly. It is only during acid loading that an impaired ability to excrete an acid load is evident. Although age-related loss of renal mass and GFR contribute, endogenous acid generation from acid diets can worsen a low-grade metabolic acidosis with age. Findings from a cross-sectional observational evaluation across different age groups showed lower net acid excretion capacity in healthy elderly in comparison with healthy younger adults.[308] Furthermore, net acid excretion was positively correlated with calcium and magnesium excretion in this same elderly group of patients.[309] Plasma bicarbonate and blood pH change as GFR changes with age[310] (Figure 23-13). Plasma chloride reciprocally increases, as seen in renal tubular acidosis or early renal disease.[311] Decreased ammonium excretion is noted with aging. Ammonium excretion increased

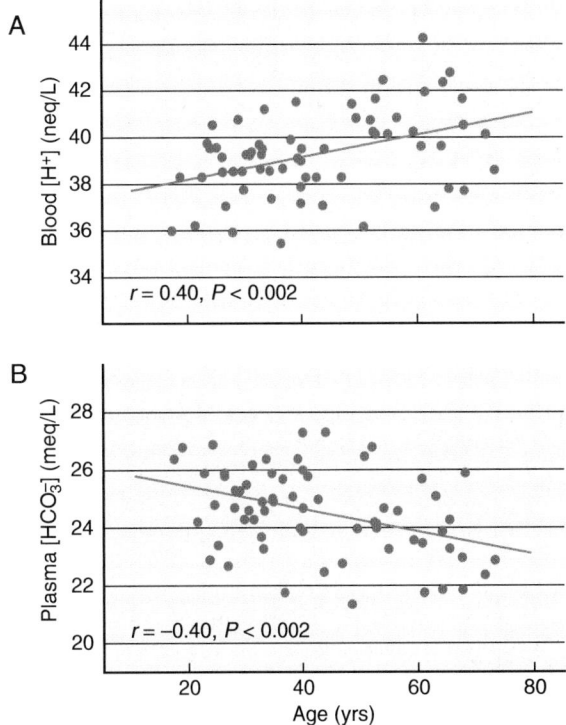

FIGURE 23-13 Relation between blood pH [(H+)b] and age (**A**) and between plasma bicarbonate concentration [(HCO3−)p] and age (**B**) in normal adult humans (*n* = 64). Each data point represents the mean steady-state value in a subject eating a constant diet. Regression equation: (H+)b = 0.045 × age + 37.2 (HCO3−)p = −0.038 × age + 26.0 (From Frassetto LA, Morris RC Jr, Sebastian A: Effect of age on blood acid-base composition in adult humans: role of age-related renal functional decline, *Am J Physiol* 271[6 pt 2]:F1114-F1122, 1996.)

similarly in both the young and old with glutamine intake.[312] However, ammonium loading resulted in lower ammonium excretion and inability to reach minimal urine pH even with correction for GFR in the older patients, which suggests the possibility of an intrinsic tubular defect.[313] In animal studies, sodium-hydrogen exchanger in the proximal tubule was noted to increase activity similarly in young and aged rats. Phosphate transport also decreased to the same extent in both groups.[314]

Although the degree of acidosis is subtle in the elderly, complications of chronic acidosis including bone demineralization and muscle wasting can be seen in the elderly. Higher protein intake can result in endogenous acid production. Muscle breakdown mediated by activation of the adenosine triphosphate–dependent ubiquitin and proteasome pathway is induced by acidosis.[315] Net acid excretion in healthy elderly correlates positively with changes in parathyroid hormone (PTH) and urinary calcium levels.[316] Acidemia regulates calcium and alkali mobilization from bone and inhibits renal calcium reabsorption. Higher protein intake in Western diets in conjunction with impaired acid excretion with age can negatively affect calcium balance and predispose to osteoporosis and increased incidence of muscle wasting and fractures even when bicarbonate levels are normal.[317] Bicarbonate supplementation corrected metabolic acidosis, improved serum albumin and prealbumin levels, and decreased whole-body protein degradation as evaluated by a decrease in normalized protein catabolic rate when given to elderly patients with chronic renal failure.[318] Although supplementation with potassium bicarbonate has improved nitrogen and calcium balance in postmenopausal women[319] and appears to have favorable effects on bone resorption and calcium excretion the older men and women,[320] the recommendation for bicarbonate supplementation in all elderly individuals to prevent complications of subtle acidosis needs further assessment.

Potassium Balance

Total body potassium decreases with age as muscle mass changes, and the decrease is more evident in women. Lower plasma renin and aldosterone levels reflect this change and lead to a relative hypoaldosteronism in the elderly. Potassium infusion results in a decreased aldosterone response in older individuals[321] (Figure 23-14), and less efficient potassium excretion is noted in aging rats on a high-potassium diet.[322] KCL infusion also leads to higher plasma potassium levels and inability to shift K into cells. Bilateral nephrectomy and high-K feedings in older rats were associated with a 38% decrease in the activity of the sodium-potassium exchange pump (Na$^+$/K$^+$–adenosine triphosphatase [ATPase]).[322] Insulin-mediated potassium uptake does not appear to be affected by age in humans, however.[323] Increase in potassium levels in the elderly during exercise suggests an impaired β-adrenergic–induced increase in the adenylate cyclase system resulting in decreased activity of the Na$^+$/K$^+$-ATPase pump in the skeletal muscle.[324] Older individuals are more prone to developing the syndrome of hyporeninemic hypoaldosteronism (type 4 renal tubular acidosis) given abnormalities in RAAS and renal acidification. Therefore medications that can further impair long-term potassium adaptation, including RAAS inhibitors (ACEIs, ARBs, heparin, calcineurin inhibitors, spironolactone, eplerenone), β-blockers, nonsteroidal antiinflammatory

drugs (NSAIDs), and sodium channel blockers (trimethoprim, pentamidine, amiloride, triamterene) may lead to significant hyperkalemia in the elderly, and their use should be carefully monitored.

Calcium Balance

Altered calcium homeostasis in the elderly may predispose older adults to both hyperparathyroidism and osteoporosis. Although renal tubular calcium absorption appears to remain relatively intact with aging, calcium metabolism is impaired. Proximal intestinal and distal tubular calcium absorption requires calcium entry from the apical membrane, calcium diffusion through the cytosol buffered by the calcium-binding proteins calbindin-D28K and calbindin-D9K, then basolateral calcium extrusion via basolateral membrane Na$^+$/Ca$^+$ exchanger and Ca^{2+}-ATPase in the kidneys and plasma membrane Ca^{2+}-ATPase in the intestine.[325] The luminal calcium channels TRPV5 of the distal and connecting tubule and TRPV6 in the duodenal brush border are highly selective for Ca^{2+} and constitutively active. The Klotho gene product, a β-glucuronidase Klotho hormone, can hydrolyze extracellular

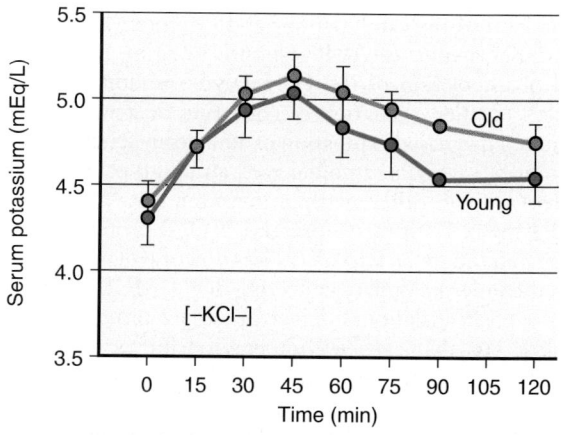

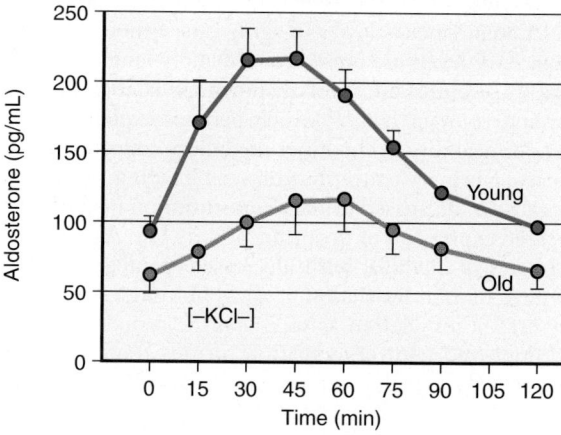

FIGURE 23-14 Serum potassium and aldosterone levels before, during, and after infusion of potassium chloride (0.05 mEq/kg body weight over 45 minutes) in six healthy young and six healthy elderly men. Changes in serum potassium levels were similar, but elderly subjects have a lower aldosterone responses ($P < 0.005$) by analysis of variance. (From Mulkerrin E, Epstein FH, Clark BA: Aldosterone responses to hyperkalemia in healthy elderly humans, *J Am Soc Nephrol* 6[5]:1459-1462, 1995.)

sugar moieties of TRPV5, thus entrapping this channel in the plasma membrane and increasing calcium translocation.[326] In addition, the α_1-subunit of Na$^+$/K$^+$-ATPase is also an α-Klotho–binding protein and is required for Na$^+$/K$^+$-ATPase recruitment to the cell surface in response to extracellular calcium.[327] Thus Na$^+$/K$^+$-ATPase–dependent secretion of PTH in response to low calcium levels may be decreased with Klotho deficiency. An age-related decrease in distal tubular epithelial calcium channel protein TRPV5 abundance is noted that corresponds to a decrease in TRPV5 mRNA and slight increases in 24-hour urine calcium excretion in older mice.[328] Klotho-deficient mice exhibit increased TRPV5 expression, decreased Na$^+$/Ca$^+$ exchanger, and calbindin-D28K, which suggests impaired distal and connecting tubule calcium reabsorption.[329] Changes in calcium metabolism can thus be also affected by decreases in Klotho protein with age.[330,331] However, both renal calcium excretion and reabsorption in response to decreased or increased calcium intake are reported to be appropriate, as are the filtered load of calcium and proximal tubular calcium reabsorption per nephron, in both old and young rats.[332,333] Intestinal calcium reabsorption, however, is decreased with aging, with associated decreased 1α-hydroxylase activity, decreased 1,25-dihydroxycholecalciferol (1,25[OH]$_2$D$_3$) and increased basal PTH levels. Levels of vitamin D–dependent calcium-binding proteins also decrease with age in association with the change in calcium absorption.[332,334] Although renal vitamin D production is lower with PTH stimulation, final concentrations of vitamin D are similar in both old and young. Urinary cAMP and fractional phosphorus also increase with PTH infusion as expected in both young and old, which suggests an intact renal response to PTH with aging.[335] PTH response to calcium infusion is altered with age, however. The calcium set point for PTH suppression is higher, as is the number of parathyroid cells. How the G protein–coupled calcium-sensing receptor plays a role in this changed set point is yet to be clarified.[336]

Phosphate Balance

Intrinsic renal tubular capacity for phosphate reabsorption decreases with age.[336,337] Older kidneys adapt less well to a phosphate-restricted diet.[338,339] In addition, intestinal absorption of phosphorus in the elderly is lower. Evaluation of maximal inorganic phosphate (Pi) transport capacity (TmPi) in older parathyroidectomized rats infused with graded levels of Pi suggests a significantly lower TmPi with age. There is an appropriate further decrease in TmPi with PTH infusion in these rats, although the magnitude of the response is less with age.[336]

Primary cultures of renal tubular cells from young and aged rats show an age-related impaired response in phosphate transport similar to that seen in vivo.[340] Maximum sodium-dependent phosphate transport velocity (Na/Pi cotransport) and the ability to adapt to low-phosphate culture media are decreased in cultured cells from older rats, accompanied by a decrease in type IIa Na/Pi cotransporter cortical mRNA levels and apical brush border membrane protein abundance.[339,341]

Increase in membrane cholesterol content may further act to decrease Na/Pi cotransport with aging.[342] Cholesterol enrichment in vitro of isolated brush border membranes of young adult rats reproduces the age-related impairment in

maximum velocity of Na/Pi cotransport activity.[342] Direct changes in opossum kidney cell cholesterol content seem to affect Na/Pi cotransport activity by changing expression of the apical membrane type II Na/Pi cotransport protein.[343] Thus changes in membrane cholesterol content with age may contribute to changes in phosphate transport.

The effect of age-related changes in 1,25(OH)$_2$D$_3$ metabolism on intestinal phosphate transport should be considered, given that vitamin D replacement improves renal and intestinal phosphate transport in vitamin D–deficient animals.[344-346] Interestingly, changes in phosphate transport resulting from vitamin D administration parallel significant changes in brush border membrane lipid composition and fluidity.[347] Thus, age-related effects of 1,25(OH)$_2$D$_3$ may possibly be mediated by lipid-modulating properties that improve renal and intestinal transport of phosphate (and calcium).

Osmolar Disorders

Hyponatremia

Hyponatremia can be a common finding in geriatric adults given the enhanced osmotic AVP release and impaired ability to dilute urine.[348,349] Many older ambulatory patients are also found to have an idiopathic form of the syndrome of inappropriate antidiuretic hormone.[350] This predisposition to hyponatremia can be further exacerbated by medications that can affect AVP action or release (Table 23-1). In addition, thiazide-type diuretics with distal tubular effects on solute reabsorption further impair urinary dilution in the elderly and can be implicated in nearly 20% to 30% of cases.[351] Aging-associated decreases in prostaglandin synthesis also inhibit water diuresis and increase susceptibility to hyponatremia with thiazide use.[351] Acute or significant hyponatremia can present subtly as apathy, disorientation, lethargy, muscle cramps, anorexia, or nausea and progress to more devastating symptoms of agitation, depressed deep tendon reflexes, pseudobulbar palsy, and seizures resulting from osmotic water shifts from the extracellular to intracellular space. Thus early recognition with prompt appropriate therapy is indicated to avoid severe neurologic sequela, including central pontine myelinolysis.

Hypernatremia

A concentrating defect in the presence of abnormal sodium conservation and a decreased thirst response with aging predisposes older individuals to dehydration and hypernatremia. Certainly inability to access free water because of altered level of consciousness or immobility in the elderly can lead to a marked rise in serum sodium and osmolality, with associated mortality reported as high as 46% to 70%, particularly with sodium levels higher than 160 mEq/L.[352] Medications like tranquilizers and sedatives that cloud sensorium and inhibit thirst or decrease AVP action in the renal tubules, such as lithium and demeclocycline, should be used with caution in older adults. In addition, osmotic diuretics, high-protein or glucose parenteral feedings, and bowel cathartics need to be used with carefully in older adults to avoid dehydration. The presence of systemic illness, infection, fever, or neurologic impairment

TABLE 23-1 Drugs and Mechanisms Leading to Impaired Water Metabolism in the Elderly				
CAUSE SALT AND WATER IMBALANCE	**INHIBIT AVP RELEASE**	**INHIBIT PERIPHERAL AVP ACTION**	**POTENTIATE AVP RELEASE**	**POTENTIATE PERIPHERAL AVP ACTION**
Indapamide	Fluphenazine	Lithium	Nicotine	Tolbutamide
Thiazides	Haloperidol	Colchicine	Vincristine	Chlorpropamide
	Promethazine	Vinblastine	Histamine	Nonsteroidal antiinflammatory agents
	Morphine (low dose)	Demeclocycline	Morphine (high dose)	Lamotrigine
	Alcohol	Glyburide	Epinephrine	
	Carbamazepine	Methoxyflurane	Cyclophosphamide	
	Norepinephrine	Acetohexamide	Angiotensin	
	Cisplatinum	Propoxyphene	Bradykinin	
	Clonidine	Loop diuretics		
	Glucocorticoids			

AVP, Arginine vasopressin.

may add to impaired AVP secretion and increase the underlying predisposition for hypernatremia. Symptomatic severe cellular dehydration can be associated with obtundation, stupor, coma, seizures, and death. Thus particular care and medication review are necessary in the older debilitated patient to avoid hypernatremia.

Renal Disease in the Aging Kidney

Acute Kidney Injury

Susceptibility to acute renal insult is notably greater with aging.[353,354] Older rats have a greater increase in renal vascular resistance, show a greater drop in glomerular filtration, and take longer to recover after renal artery occlusion than younger rats. Similarly, older euvolemic men consuming a constant-sodium diet show increased renal vascular resistance in the face of a blunted response to orthostatic change. Aged adults are unable to improve medullary oxygenation with water diuresis as are younger adults, which suggests a predisposition to hypoxic renal injury in older adults[355] (Figure 23-15). Older surgical patients undergoing cardiopulmonary bypass who had no clinical signs of acute renal failure excreted more kidney-specific proteins (N-acetyl-β-glucosaminidase, α_1-microglobulin, glutathione transferase-π, glutathione-α) and had a higher fractional excretion of sodium after surgery than before surgery, whereas younger patients did not show similar increases.[356]

Acute kidney injury (AKI) is reported to be 3.5 times more prevalent in patients older than 70 years, with increased morbidity and mortality found in older hospitalized patients.[357,358] An estimated 28% of adults older than 65 years are less likely to recover kidney function in the face of AKI.[359] Multifactorial and iatrogenic processes leading to AKI, whether prerenal, intrinsic, or postrenal, are poorly tolerated by aging individuals with decreased renal reserve and underlying comorbid conditions such as diabetes, hypertension, atherosclerosis, heart failure, or malignancies. Elderly individuals with generalized atherosclerosis are also more likely to have spontaneous and/or procedure-related cholesterol renal atheroemboli. In addition, acute vasculitis and rapidly progressive glomerulonephritis can

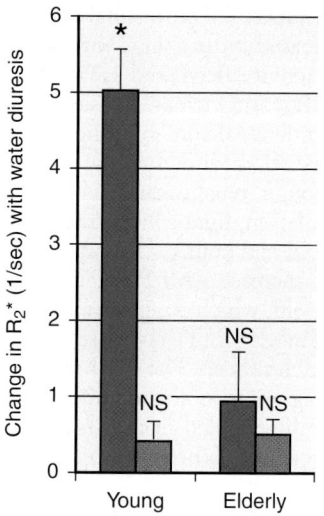

FIGURE 23-15 Comparison of changes in R_2^* (1/sec) in response to water load in nine young and nine elderly subjects. R_2^* reflects the apparent spin-spin relaxation of deoxygenated hemoglobin by magnetic resonance and is equal to the slope or equivalent to the concentration of deoxyhemoglobin or blood oxygen pressure (Po_2) or tissue Po_2. Because blood Po_2 is thought to be in rapid equilibrium with tissue Po_2, changes in blood oxygen level–dependent magnetic resonance imaging signal intensity or R_2^* should reflect changes in the Po_2 of the tissue. *Black bars* indicate medulla; *shaded bars* indicate cortex. Bar heights represent mean values with standard error indicated. NS, Not significant. *Statistically significant at the $P < 0.01$ level. (From Prasad PV, Epstein FH: Changes in renal medullary pO_2 during water diuresis as evaluated by blood oxygenation level–dependent magnetic resonance imaging: effects of aging and cyclooxygenase inhibition, *Kidney Int* 55[1]:294-298, 1999.)

be devastating in aging individuals who have with a nephritic picture.

Prerenal processes account for 50% of AKI in the elderly. Dehydration and volume depletion secondary to vomiting, diarrhea, bleeding, and excessive use of diuretics are frequent causes of prerenal AKI in the elderly. Impaired urinary concentration, sodium conservation, and thirst with aging can predispose to these processes. In addition, acute volume changes are less well tolerated by the aging kidney given the blunted autoregulation, decreased RPF, and decreased renal reserve of older kidneys. Renal hypoperfusion from decreased cardiac output, sepsis, and use of medications that interfere with renal autoregulatory mechanisms such as angiotensin antagonists (ACEIs, ARBs) and prostaglandin inhibitors (NSAIDs) can cause and exacerbate prerenal processes, leading to AKI in older adults. Use of NSAIDs by patients aged 65 years and older increases risk of AKI by 58%.[360] The usual indices differentiating prerenal from intrinsic causes such as urine sodium level, fractional sodium excretion, and urine osmolality need careful interpretation in the elderly, because tubular defects from aging may preclude a higher urine sodium excretion despite underlying hypoperfusion.[353] Prerenal AKI is usually reversible with careful volume management, discontinuation of exacerbating medications, and improvements in cardiac output. However, evolution of prerenal azotemia to acute tubular necrosis (ATN) is more common in older (23%) than in younger patients (15%).[361]

Intrinsic AKI results in acute structural insults that prolong recovery of renal clearance in the elderly. Among hospitalized older patients with intrinsic AKIs, ischemic and nephrotoxic tubular injury resulting in ATN is found in almost 50% of patients.[362] Decreased NO synthesis in aging vasculature associated with lower levels of the NO substrate L-arginine in the elderly[236,363] and higher ADMA levels[364,365] impairs vasodilation, predisposing the aged kidney to ischemia. This is supported by the findings that GFR, RPF, and RVR in older rats improved with L-arginine feeding prior to renal artery occlusion and that these effects were abolished with administration of the NO inhibitor L-NAME. Furthermore NO availability is improved, with an increase in eNOS mRNA and protein, when RhoA protein activation is partially inhibited, which decreases renal vasoconstriction and significantly attenuates ischemic lesions in older animals with ischemic acute renal failure, results that suggest the vulnerability of the aged kidney to AKI.

Biochemical and metabolic changes in the aging kidney may also play a role in making the older kidney prone to ischemic injury. These effects are noted in aged renal cortical slices exposed to anoxia, which are less able to uptake paraaminohippurate and tetraethylammonium than are renal cortical slices from younger rats.[354]

Approximately one third of AKI in the elderly results from surgical complications of hypotension before or after surgery, postsurgical fluid losses from gastrointestinal drainage, dysrhythmias, and myocardial infarction. In the hospital septic complications also account for one third of AKI cases in older individuals. Gram-negative endotoxemia inducing renal vasoconstriction increases the risk for ATN. Associated multiorgan failure and perioperative sepsis worsen catabolic demands, adding to the poor prognosis in the elderly.[237,366] Hemodynamic instability from sepsis coupled with the use of nephrotoxic antibiotics such as the aminoglycosides and amphotericin can prolong renal dysfunction.[367] Aminoglycoside nephrotoxicity is increased with age. Various cancer therapeutic agents are also associated with the development of ATN in the elderly.[368] Decreased clearance and tubular changes occurring in aging may enhance the toxic effects of antibiotics and chemotherapeutic agents. Therefore, antibiotic and chemotherapy dosing and monitoring need careful attention in the elderly, and best estimates of clearance should be employed. Radiocontrast infusions used for diagnostic and therapeutic imaging in the elderly can also result in acute and prolonged vasoconstriction and lead to ATN. Initial vasodilation with

the intraarterial or intravenous contrast injection shifts to significant vasoconstriction with delivery of the osmotic load to the macula densa, which triggers tubuloglomerular feedback with renin release and a drop in GFR that causes medullary hypoxia, impaired adaptive response, and cytotoxic tubular damage.[369] A rise in serum creatinine level is usually seen within 1 to 4 days after contrast administration. Attention to appropriate volume maintenance prior to contrast injection is crucial in preventing contrast-induced nephropathy in the elderly.[370,371] The benefit of isotonic bicarbonate infusion or use of the vasodilatory antioxidant N-acetylcysteine still needs to be clarified, although given the low risk these measures are used as prophylaxis by some.[372,373]

Intraarterial cannulation with any procedures in elderly patients who have generalized atherosclerosis poses a risk of atheroemboli to the kidney, although spontaneous cholesterol embolization may also occur in this high-risk population. Manipulation of the arterial vasculature for radiographic or surgical intervention, such as carotid, coronary, renal, or abdominal angiography, aortic surgery, or percutaneous transluminal angioplasty of coronary or renal arteries can result in both renal and systemic cholesterol plaque embolization to end arteries with resulting ischemia of the affected tissue. Atheroemboli are also associated with the use of anticoagulants and fibrinolytic agents.[374] Ensuing renal failure is frequently progressive and irreversible, and may or may not be associated with systemic symptoms such as purpura; livido reticularis of the abdomen, lumbosacrum, and lower extremities; distal digit necrosis; retinal occlusion with cholesterol plaques (Hollenhorst plaques); gastrointestinal bleeding; pancreatitis; myocardial infarction; and cerebral ischemia. Associated laboratory findings of hypocomplementemia and eosinophilia with atheroemboli, when present, can be clinically useful in diagnosis. Heightened awareness of the risks associated intraarterial procedures and anticoagulation in the elderly as well as supportive therapy remain primary elements of care for this disease process.

Tubulointerstitial inflammation and acute interstitial nephritis are particularly associated with the use of antibiotics such as penicillins, β-lactams, and sulfonamides but can be caused by various medications commonly used in older patients and may or may not present with typical features of pyuria, hematuria, fever, rash, and eosinophilia.[367] Infections with agents such as staphylococci, streptococci, *Legionella*, cytomegalovirus, and human immunodeficiency virus can also lead to tubulointerstitial inflammation and nephritis.[375] Inflammation activates the release of degradative enzymes from macrophages; these enzymes damage the basement membrane and delay regeneration and repair of tubules, which results in a fall in GFR.[375]

Interstitial nephritis caused by NSAIDs, ACEIs, and ARBs can present as nephrotic proteinuria either with or without pyuria. NSAIDs, particularly propionic acid derivatives, can lead to minimal change or membranous lesions, whereas the ACEI captopril has been associated with membranous lesions on renal biopsy specimens. Avoiding further exposure to the causative agent is the usual remedy, and there is little evidence supporting steroid use to minimize prolonged AKI.[376,377]

Acute urinary obstruction in the elderly can present simply as a rise in blood urea nitrogen and creatinine levels or with complaints of pain, bladder distension, dysuria, hesitancy, hematuria, dribbling, or incontinence. Numerous processes can contribute to acute obstruction in the elderly, although benign or malignant prostatic hypertrophy is common in men, and urethral strictures from chronic infection or inflammation are notable in women. Urogenital cancers, including pelvic tumors of the uterus and cervix in women as well as retroperitoneal fibrosis, metastatic tumors, and lymphomas, should be considered if elderly patients have acute obstruction. Bladder cancer is closely linked to increasing age.[378] Long-term use of combinations of analgesics such as aspirin, paracetamol, and pyrazolones, as well as use of the cyclooxygenase-2 inhibitor celecoxib have been associated with papillary sloughing and may lead to transient obstructive symptoms until tissue passage.[379,380]

Anticholinergic agents and inhibitors of the central nervous system can lead to bladder detrusor muscle overactivity or detrusor instability in the elderly, as can also occur in those with cerebrovascular accident or neurodegenerative disorders such as Parkinson's or Alzheimer's disease. Nerve injury or autonomic neuropathy associated with diabetes or chronic alcohol use causes detrusor underactivity with bladder outlet obstruction. Elderly patients can also have sphincter abnormalities leading to voiding difficulty and early obstruction. Postmenopausal women may have atrophy of supporting tissues due to low estrogen levels with prolapse of pelvic structures that leads to obstructive nephropathy. Because prolonged obstruction can result in irreversible renal loss, heightened sensitivity to presenting signs and symptoms is necessary, and the presence of such symptoms should prompt careful medication review and genitourinary evaluation with measurement of postvoid urine residual and noncontrast renal imaging by ultrasonography, computed tomography, or magnetic resonance imaging, with urologic intervention as indicated.

AKI also increases the risk of ESRD in the elderly. In a cohort of nearly 234,000 Medicare beneficiaries 67 years and older discharged from the hospital, the incidence of AKI was 3.1%, and 5.3 per 1000 developed ESRD.[381] Therefore early recognition of an increased susceptibility of elderly patients to AKI is crucial, with the aim of preventing AKI by avoiding nephrotoxic medications and interventions that increase risk. Early nephrology referral and management is prudent if these exposures cannot be avoided.

Although aging individuals have both greater risks for AKI and prolonged recovery from AKI, therapeutic intervention should not be based on age alone, because factors other than age can contribute to overall survival in the elderly.[366,382,383] Response to dialysis therapy for AKI in the elderly is frequently good, providing relief of uremic symptoms and complications such volume overload, bleeding, disorientation, catabolic state, and electrolyte disturbances.

Hypertension

Hypertension leading to kidney disease is a common problem in the elderly in most developed nations. National Health and Nutrition Examination Survey (NHANES) data from 1999 to 2004 indicate the presence of hypertension in 67% of U.S. adults aged 60 and older.[384] Overall there is a progressive increase in the incidence of coronary disease and stroke and cardiovascular mortality as blood pressure rises above 115/75 mm Hg, with some notable differences in risk based on age and underlying comorbid conditions. Between the ages of

40 and 69 years, a 20 mm Hg systolic blood pressure (SBP) change is associated with a twofold difference in the death rates from ischemic heart disease and other vascular causes, with an even greater difference noted in the stroke death rate.[385] As age increases, SBP and pulse pressure become better predictors of cardiovascular disease (CVD).[386] Elastic senescence, altered extracellular matrix cross-linking, and calcium deposition lead to fibrotic changes with medial elastocalcinosis and stiffness in the larger elastic aging vasculature, which decreases vascular capacitance and propagation of the pulse wave velocity, clinically evident as widened pulse pressure.[387] Impaired endothelial function and relaxation from low NO production with age is also noted to increase vascular stiffness.[388] With increased arterial stiffness in aging as diastolic blood pressure (DBP) decreases and pulse pressure increases, it becomes important to monitor a combination of blood pressure components, such as SBP + DBP or pulse pressure + mean arterial pressure, to gauge CVD risk.[389] Isolated systolic hypertension (ISH) with SBP over 160 mm Hg and DBP less than 90 mm Hg is evident in nearly 75% of hypertensive elderly.[390] Although hypertension independently increases the risk of ESRD, elevated systolic pressure appears to be associated with greater risk of ESRD.[391] ISH is a strong independent risk factor for a decline in kidney function in older individuals[392] (Figure 23-16).

Measurement of blood pressure in the elderly should follow standard guidelines in the American Heart Association recommendations,[393] although standing blood pressure should also be taken periodically in the elderly given the increased risk for postural hypotension. A thorough examination to assess underlying causes and end-organ involvement, including laboratory evaluation of renal function (serum creatinine level or eGFR), is important in those elderly diagnosed with hypertension.[394] Although treatment of elevated blood pressure in the elderly, including those over 80 years of age, is clearly beneficial,[395-397] the goal of SBP less than 140 mm Hg developed for the general population may need to be adjusted for those with ISH and for elderly patients 80 years and older. Blood pressure therapy that decreases DBP to 60 mm Hg or less in the elderly with ISH can impair tissue perfusion, increase cardiovascular risk, and reduce survival. Thus SBP goals should not be reached at the expense of excessive DBP reduction. The intention-to-treat Hypertension in the Very Elderly Trial (HYVET) supports a target blood pressure of 150/80 mm Hg in patients 80 years of age or older, noting a 21% reduction in all-cause mortality and a marked reduction in other cardiovascular morbidity, such as stroke and heart failure.[396]

Lifestyle modification with appropriate dietary salt restriction, exercise, and weight loss when necessary remains the primary treatment, with medications added as required and tailored to each patient. Various medications have been used and are tolerated in the elderly, including chlorthalidone, hydrochlorothiazide, ACEIs, ARBs, and calcium channel blockers.[398-401] These drugs should be initiated at lower dosages and titrated carefully, with awareness of the greater risk of postural and postprandial hypertension in the elderly given the exaggerated response in those with ISH.[402] In a random sample of individuals aged 75 years or older, SBP dropped by more than 50% when rising from a supine to a standing position. The total prevalence of orthostatic hypotension was 34% in this cohort,[403] which emphasizes the need to monitor

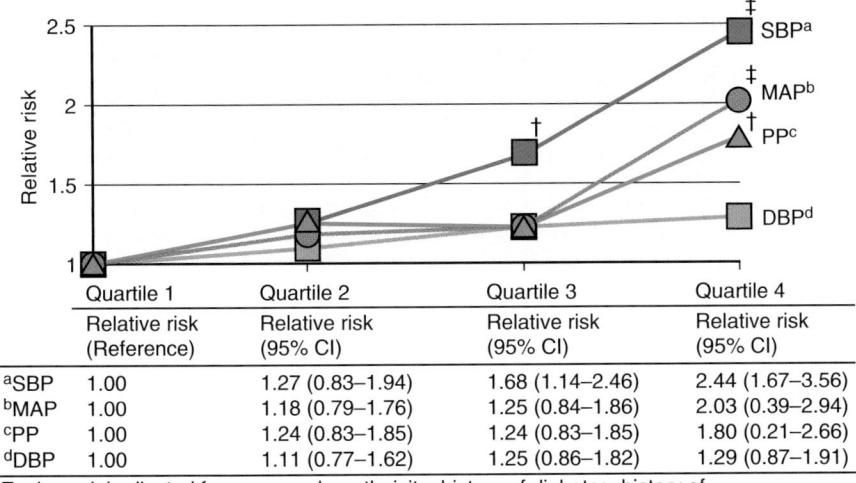

FIGURE 23-16 Adjusted relative risk of a decline in kidney function according to quartiles of blood pressure (BP) component in 2181 participants in the Systolic Hypertension in the Elderly Program (SHEP). (From Young JH, Klag MJ, Muntner P, et al: Blood pressure and decline in kidney function: findings from the Systolic Hypertension in the Elderly Program (SHEP), *J Am Soc Nephrol* 13[11]:2776-2782, 2002.)

	Quartile 1 Relative risk (Reference)	Quartile 2 Relative risk (95% CI)	Quartile 3 Relative risk (95% CI)	Quartile 4 Relative risk (95% CI)
[a]SBP	1.00	1.27 (0.83–1.94)	1.68 (1.14–2.46)	2.44 (1.67–3.56)
[b]MAP	1.00	1.18 (0.79–1.76)	1.25 (0.84–1.86)	2.03 (0.39–2.94)
[c]PP	1.00	1.24 (0.83–1.85)	1.24 (0.83–1.85)	1.80 (0.21–2.66)
[d]DBP	1.00	1.11 (0.77–1.62)	1.25 (0.86–1.82)	1.29 (0.87–1.91)

*Each model adjusted for age, gender, ethnicity, history of diabetes, history of cardiovascular disease, and current smoking.
†P value <0.01 for comparison with Quartile 1.
‡P value <0.001 for comparison with Quartile 1.

and initiate antihypertensive therapy carefully in the elderly. Furthermore, given that many elderly are taking a variety of medications, it is important to be wary of drug-drug interactions, which may either potentiate antihypertensive therapy, as do the α_1-blockers frequently used to treat benign prostatic hypertrophy, or inhibit antihypertensive therapy, as do the NSAIDs frequently used to manage antiinflammatory processes in the elderly.[404]

Renovascular Disease

Renovascular disease is an important cause of resistant hypertension and progressive renal insufficiency, often presenting in the elderly as part of a generalized atherosclerosis process rather than an isolated syndrome. Large numbers of patients with atherosclerotic renovascular disease (ARVD) are now reaching ESRD,[405] with the prevalence of renovascular disease estimated to be 6.8% in unselected community-dwelling African American and white men and women older than 65 years of age.[406] Angiographically determined stenosis of 75% or greater in the renal arteries is more likely to progress to occlusion.[407] Unexplained progressive azotemia, worsening or new-onset hypertension, and/or development of AKI with antihypertensive therapy should raise suspicion of renovascular disease in an elderly patient. These may be more evident when ACEIs and ARBs are used. Patients also may experience recurrent episodes of acute (flash) pulmonary edema or otherwise unexplained heart failure.[407,408] Patients with ARVD are at increased risk of death from CVD[409]; therefore, aggressive control of atherosclerotic risk factors is recommended. Screening and diagnostic tests should be performed for patients with moderate to high probability of ARVD[410] (see Chapter 47 for complete discussion). Treatment options for hemodynamically significant lesions, including medical therapy with antihypertensive drugs, revascularization with angioplasty with or without stenting, or surgery, should be individualized for each patient with consideration of the benefits and risks of each procedure. A recent randomized trial comparing endovascular revascularization plus medical therapy with medical therapy alone in older patients with ARVD found no clinical benefit for revascularization when the end points of renal function, blood pressure, time to renal and cardiovascular events, and mortality were assessed over 34 months of follow-up. Serious complications associated with revascularization occurred in 23 patients, including two deaths and three amputations of toes or limbs.[411] Revascularization also carries the risk of atheroemboli, although the reported incidence is low. There is no evidence that revascularization improves any outcomes in asymptomatic patients.[412]

Glomerular Disease

Renal biopsy findings in the elderly suggest that acute and chronic glomerular disease is common in this patient population[413-421] (Table 23-2). As in younger patients, AKI and/or nephrotic syndrome often are the reason for renal biopsy in the elderly.[419,420,422]

Nephritic presentations with acute or rapidly progressive renal failure can be devastating in the elderly. Several small case series suggest that pauci-immune glomerulonephritis (GN) is more evident in older adults over 60 years of age.[418,420,423,424] Of the pauci-immune biopsy specimens evaluated at a large referral center, 79% cases were noted in those older than 60 years of age.[425] Although fewer cases of anti–glomerular basement membrane GN and immune complex crescentic GN were noted in these reports, diagnostic workup for these processes must be included. Similarly, although the incidence of postinfectious or poststreptococcal diffuse proliferative GN has decreased in most developed nations, the disease is becoming more evident in the elderly in underdeveloped regions and in those elderly living under poor socioeconomic or debilitating conditions.[426,427] Therefore a careful history should be taken to identify possible exposure, and a history and/or examination findings suggesting the possibility of infection should prompt early diagnosis and supportive treatment in the elderly.

TABLE 23-2 Renal Pathology of the Elderly Presenting with Nephrotic Syndrome in Representative Studies

	STUDY					
	SHIN ET AL. (2001)[431]	PRAKASH ET AL. (2003)[427]	RIVERA ET AL. (2004)[421]	NAIR ET AL. (2004)[419]	NAIR ET AL. (2004)[419]	UEZONO ET AL. (2006)[420]
Number of patients	75	40	725	137	33	27
Age of study population (years)	≥60	≥60	≥65	66-79	≥80	≥65
Mean age ± standard deviation (years)	64.5 ± 4.4	64.2 ± 3.8	ND	71.5 ± 3.6	83.3 ± 2.8	72.88 ± 5.2
Primary glomerular disease	81.3%	60.0%	64.8%	45.5%	42.4%	63.0%
Minimal change disease	26.2%	5%	13.2%	12.1%	18.2%	18.5%
Focal/segmental glomerulosclerosis	ND	10.0%	9.7%	12.1%	15.2%	22.2%
Membranous nephropathy	44.3%	27.5%	28.0%	21.2%	6.1%	14.8%
Membranoproliferative glomerulonephritis	ND	7.5%	7.2%	0.0%	0.0%	0.0%
Mesangial proliferative glomerulonephritis*	ND	ND	5.9%	0.0%	3.0%	7.4%
Other	ND	10.0%	ND	ND	ND	ND
Secondary renal disease	18.7%	40.0%	35.2%	44.5%	57.6%	37.0%
Diabetic glomerulopathy	ND	22.5%	1.7%	15.2%	3.0%	11.1%
Nephrosclerosis	ND	0.0%	ND	24.2%	42.4%	7.4%
Primary amyloidosis	ND	15.0%	17.2%	9.1%	9.1%	7.4%
Lupus nephritis	ND	0.0%	1.4%	0.0%	0.0%	0.0%
Hepatitis B–associated glomerulopathy	42.9%	0.0%	ND	ND	0.0%	0.0%
Other	ND	2.5%	ND	6.1%	3.0%	3.7%

ND, No immunosuppressive therapy.
*Including immunoglobulin A nephropathy.
Modified from Uezono S, Hara S, Sato Y, et al: Renal biopsy in elderly patients: a clinicopathological analysis, *Ren Fail* 28(7):549-555, 2006.

Paraproteinemia, particularly multiple myeloma, can also present as AKI in the elderly with or without overt hypercalcemia.[428] Thus quantification of urine protein, immunoelectrophoresis, and immunofixation can be important early on, particularly if the cause of AKI remains unclear. A test result positive for monoclonal proteins should also be followed by further evaluation for the presence of amyloidosis or light-chain deposition disease. In addition, minimal change disease can present as AKI in the elderly with significant proteinuria and hypertension. Renal biopsy findings frequently suggest acute tubular injury in the presence of minimal change disease, although the cause remains speculative.[429,430]

Primary glomerular diseases appear to be more prevalent in the elderly than secondary diseases, although diabetic glomerulopathy may be underrepresented because biopsies often are not performed in cases of presumed diabetic renal disease.[422] Relative frequencies of various glomerular diseases are different in older than in younger patients. Membranous nephropathy is the most common histologic finding in numerous case series,[417,427,431] with 36% of 317 renal biopsy specimens of patients older than 60 years showing nephrotic syndrome. Minimal change disease (11%) and amyloidosis (10.7%) also were noted and were more frequent than other diagnoses in this large series.[417] In the very elderly (≥80 years), focal sclerosis from hypertension and hypertensive nephrosclerosis

seemed to be more prevalent, followed by immunoglobulin A and membranous nephropathy.[424] Nephrotic syndrome can coexist with or precede malignancy in up to 30% of the elderly. An immune response to tumor antigens is considered the possible pathologic cause. Solid tumors of the lung, breast, colon or rectum, kidney, and stomach have been commonly reported in association with membranous lesions in renal biopsy specimens, with resolution of the nephrosis after tumor treatment.[432] Minimal change lesions on renal biopsy specimens have also been noted in conjunction with Hodgkin's and non-Hodgkin's lymphoma in the elderly.[433,434] Given this association, a thorough history taking, physical examination, and basic screening to rule out a secondary malignant cause should be considered in elderly patients with new-onset nephrosis.

Use of steroids alone for the treatment of membranous lesions has little impact on the rate of renal functional decline in the elderly, although the incidence of CKD is noted to be greater in the elderly, likely due to decreased functional reserve. Although treatment with steroids and cytotoxic agents may lead to partial or complete remission, individual risk-benefit assessment is important given the high risk of infection in the elderly. Minimal change lesions in the elderly may respond to steroid use alone; however, the response to both steroids and cytotoxic agents is less than for younger patients. However, older patients with minimal change disease seem to experience relapse less frequently and have more stable remissions after cyclophosphamide treatment.[435]

Because systemic amyloidosis, either primary or secondary to paraproteinemia, can present as nephrosis in the elderly, serum and 24-hour urine collection for protein electrophoresis with immunofixation and quantitation of immunoglobulins is necessary in elderly patients who have unexplained proteinuria or nephrotic syndrome. Bone marrow should be examined to rule out myeloma. In experienced hands, Congo red staining of tissue obtained from abdominal fat pad biopsy may provide confirmation of amyloid; however, renal tissue obtained by biopsy may need to be evaluated for amyloid fibrils in many cases. In a small number of elderly patients generalized global sclerosis can also present with nephrotic proteinuria caused by undiagnosed processes that lead to renal scarring, with hypertension hastening this process. Based on limited data, recommendations for treatment of glomerular diseases are to select and tailor therapy for the elderly using the same criteria as for younger individuals. Treatment with medications requires cautious dosing and careful follow-up because drug metabolism and renal excretion are altered in the elderly, which increases the risk of drug toxicity.[436]

Chronic Kidney Disease

CKD increases in prevalence with age and heralds a poor outcome.[437-439] CKD is recognized as a global public health problem, and approximately 38% of U.S. adults aged 70 years and older have an eGFR of less than 60 mL/min/1.73 m².[440] CKD in the elderly is associated with a greater risk of kidney failure and CVD, including ischemic stroke and death.[439,441,442] A high risk for all-cause and CVD mortality has been described in community-dwelling elderly individuals with CKD, particularly in those with an eGFR of less than 45 mL/min/1.73 m² and in men.[6] Frailty is also more prevalent among older patients with CKD than among those with normal renal function,[443] and cognitive impairment increases in older CKD patients independent of other confounders,[444,445] although the full extent of the burden of CKD in the elderly is yet to be known.

Although the progression of longstanding medical disease such as diabetes, hypertension, chronic GN, and renovascular and obstructive nephropathy is known to contribute to worsening of CKD with age, the onset of AKI can hasten the CKD process. In addition, long-term use of combinations of analgesics, frequently seen in the elderly, may be associated with papillary necrosis and progression to CKD.[379,380] Similarly, decompensated medical illness can result from gradual CKD progression even though frank uremic symptoms are absent. Older individuals may experience episodes of volume overload and symptoms of heart failure, gastrointestinal bleeding, hypertension, or gradual confusion that indicate progression of renal loss. Interestingly, the most frequent cause of death in elderly patients with CKD is CVD rather than the progression of kidney disease to kidney failure.[442,446] Therefore cardiovascular risk management remains important in elderly patients with CKD. Estimates of renal function from serum creatinine levels alone may be inadequate in the elderly given the changes in muscle mass with age. Although the accuracy of available formulas for estimating GFR in the elderly continues to be investigated,[447-450] the MDRD and CKD-EPI equations may be useful.[262]

Renal Replacement Therapy

A significant number of elderly reaching ESRD require renal replacement therapy.[451,452] The number of octogenarians and nonagenarians starting dialysis has nearly doubled, rising from 7054 persons in 1996 to 13,577 persons in 2003.[453] In a retrospective analysis of patient survival among those older than 75 years who had stage 5 CKD, the 1- and 2-year survival rates were 84% and 76%, respectively, in the group receiving dialysis compared with 68% and 47%, respectively, in the group treated conservatively. The survival advantage was lost, however, in patients with multiple comorbid conditions, particularly in those with ischemic heart disease.[454]

In-center hemodialysis is the modality of choice for 96% of those older than 75 years.[455] Approximately 19% of the elderly undergo peritoneal dialysis.[455] Although no clear modality advantage exists in the elderly,[456-458] some studies suggest a higher mortality in elderly patients receiving peritoneal dialysis, particularly in those with diabetes.[459,460] For either modality, overall survival for the elderly is shorter than that for younger patients, as would be expected.[455,461] Thus, the choice between hemodialysis and peritoneal dialysis should remain individualized in the elderly, with consideration given to medical and psychosocial factors. Maintenance hemodialysis requires arteriovenous fistula (AVF) access, particularly in the elderly, because it is associated with a lower incidence of infectious complications.[462] Concern for fistula maturation is not unique to older patients, and thus age should not be a limiting factor in AVF creation given the equivalent procedural and fistula survival rates.[462] Similarly, peritoneal dialysis may be an option for elderly patients who experience hemodynamic instability during hemodialysis.[463,464] There is little difference between older and younger patients in the likelihood of technique failure, number of peritonitis episodes, and types of infections, and fewer peritoneal catheter replacements actually are required in older patients.[464,465]

Renal replacement in the elderly heralds important problems requiring careful medical management given the frequent presence of various comorbid conditions and the necessary and concurrent use of numerous medications that may have changed clearances in the face of ESRD and dialysis. Elderly dialysis patients may be more prone to hypoglycemia because of prolonged insulin clearance, poor intake, and decreased sympathetic response due to other medications. Therefore close monitoring of medications and careful attention to detect subtle changes in the elderly dialysis patient's clinical condition are essential.[466] Despite limited survival of some patients, many elderly patients have a high quality of life on dialysis, and they should not be denied treatment on the basis of chronologic age alone.[467-469] On the other hand, among 3702 nursing home residents in the United States for whom dialysis treatment was started between June 1998 and October 2000, the initiation of dialysis was associated with a substantial and sustained decline in functional status.[470] Dialysis should not be used only to prolong the dying process. Symptom relief and maintenance of independence should be considered the main goals of treatment.

Renal Transplantation

The categorization of people listed for kidney transplantation has shown a shift toward older candidates as the subset of older patients with ESRD increases[471] and kidney allocation remains skewed toward younger recipients. The 2007 Scientific Registry of Transplant Recipients reported that of all candidates listed for kidney transplantation, 59% were 50 years or older, and 14% were 65 years or older,[472] which suggests that age alone does not necessarily preclude candidacy for renal transplantation for those medically eligible. Although younger transplant patients experience a greater number of healthy life-years, older patients undergoing transplantation have a significant survival advantage over those remaining on dialysis.[473-475] The overall risk of death is 41% lower for older kidney transplant recipients than for wait-listed candidates, and the survival advantage is also seen for recipients of extended criteria donor (ECD) kidneys.[476]

Nontransplanted patients 60 years and older had an overall 2.54 times higher adjusted risk of death than that of transplanted patients of the same age, regardless of the type of graft; when data were stratified by donor graft type, risk of death was 3.78 times higher for patients receiving non–extended criteria deceased donor grafts and 2.31 times higher for those receiving ECD grafts.[477] Allograft type impacts recipient survival in recipients 65 years of age and older, with 2009 registry data suggesting better survival rates for living donor grafts compared to deceased non-ECD grafts and deceased ECD grafts (Table 23-3) at 3 months, 1 year, and 5 years. Allograft survival is similarly excellent after 3 months, 1 year, and 5 years for recipients 65 years and older, with living donor allografts faring best followed by deceased non-ECD grafts and deceased ECD grafts[472] (Table 23-4).

Increasing the kidney transplant donor pool for a growing number of wait-listed candidates forces consideration of graft procurement from older donors. Delayed graft function and some decrease in allograft survival, as well as in patient survival, can be associated with increasing donor age.[478,479] Graft survival at 3 and 5 years for living donor grafts from donors 55 years of age and older was noted to be 85% and 76%, respectively, compared with 89% and 82%, respectively, for grafts from living donors younger than 55 years, and 82% and 73%, respectively, for grafts from deceased donors younger than 55 years.[480] Although risk of acute rejection can be less in older recipients, the impact of acute rejection on overall long-term allograft function may be more significant.[481] Nevertheless, transplant graft loss in older recipients occurs primarily from patient death secondary to infection and CVD.[482-484] Thus a careful, thorough preoperative evaluation in the prospective elderly transplant patient is necessary.[485,486]

The use of immunosuppressive agents in the elderly can be challenging because of the increased incidence of associated comorbid conditions and altered pharmacokinetics in this age group.[481,482,487] Data from which to evaluate induction regimens and the optimal combination of medications for maintenance immunosuppression among the elderly remain limited at this time. In conclusion, in the absence of contraindications and in the presence of careful screening, transplantation may be offered to patients regardless of age, and expanded use of older living donors may help meet the demand for transplant organs.

Urinary Tract Infection

Urinary tract infection (UTI), whether symptomatic or asymptomatic, is relatively common and a frequent reason for hospital admission[488] in the elderly as various comorbid conditions, anatomic abnormalities, and weakened host defense mechanisms become evident. Mechanical and hormonal changes in the urinary tract with age often lead to urinary tract obstruction or urine stasis. Coexisting illnesses in the elderly, including cerebrovascular accidents, dementia, impaired mobility, and incontinence of bladder and bowel, often are associated with poor hygiene. Bladder dystonia, changes in the pelvic musculature, prostatic enlargement, and urethral stricture can contribute to obstructive uropathy. Decreased prostatic secretions in older men may predispose to infections of the lower urinary tract. Prostatic microcalculi can harbor bacteria and become a nidus for infection in men. Decreased vaginal estrogen levels in postmenopausal women may lead to increased vaginal pH by causing relative depletion of lactobacilli and increase the risk for bacterial colonization and infection in women.[489] Data are conflicting, however, on the role of systemic and topical estrogen therapy to decrease the incidence of UTI.

Classic signs and symptoms of UTI include urinary frequency, urinary urgency, dysuria, nocturia, and suprapubic discomfort as well as occasional hematuria with cystitis. Pyelonephritis usually presents with costovertebral angle tenderness, fever, and variable lower urinary tract symptoms.

TABLE 23-3 Adjusted Patient Survival Rates for Transplant Recipients 65 Years of Age and Older

	3 MONTHS	1 YEAR	5 YEARS
Recipients of living donor kidney transplants	99.2%	96.9%	79.2%
Recipients of deceased non–extended criteria donor kidneys	97.5%	93.3%	69.6%
Recipients of deceased extended criteria donor kidneys	95.5%	90.1%	61.3%

Data from The U.S. Organ Procurement and Transplantation Network and the Scientific Registry of Transplant Recipients 2009 annual report. Available at http://optn.transplant.hrsa.gov/ar2009/survival rates.htm. Accessed April 2011.

TABLE 23-4 Adjusted Allograft Survival Rates for Transplant Recipients 65 Years of Age and Older

	3 MONTHS	1 YEAR	5 YEARS
Living donor allograft	98%	95.4%	73.9%
Deceased non–extended criteria donor allograft	95.2%	89.4%	61.6%
Deceased extended criteria donor allograft	90.3%	83.2%	52.5%

Data from The U.S. Organ Procurement and Transplantation Network and the Scientific Registry of Transplant Recipients 2009 annual report. Available at http://optn.transplant.hrsa.gov/ar2009/survival rates.htm. Accessed April 2011.

However, a wide spectrum of nonspecific clinical symptoms is interpreted inappropriately as UTI in the elderly, which leads to a tendency to both overdiagnose and overtreat.[490] Even typical symptoms require cautious interpretation, because they are common in elderly people without infection.[491] A retrospective case series from one hospital suggests that in approximately 40% of cases, UTI is incorrectly diagnosed in hospitalized older people.[488] There has also been a tendency to manage all clinical deterioration in long-term care facility residents who have positive urine culture results as UTIs, which again contributes to excess antimicrobial use, heightens the problem of antimicrobial resistance, and exposes older patients to unnecessary antibiotic side effects.[492] On the other hand, cognitively impaired older patients may not recall or report symptoms and do not have classic genitourinary symptoms, which makes the diagnosis more problematic. A prospective cohort study of women and men in nursing homes addressed the question of clinical presentation of UTI in residents of long-term care facilities. Dysuria, change in the character of the urine, and altered mental status were the only clinical features significantly associated with bacteriuria plus pyuria. Of these features, dysuria most effectively discriminated between those with and those without bacteriuria plus pyuria.[493]

Atypical clinical manifestations can make diagnosis, prevention, and treatment of UTI in the older patient challenging (Table 23-5). The incidence of asymptomatic bacteriuria increases with increasing age. Bacteriuria without symptoms of infection implies isolation of a specified quantity of bacteria in a properly collected urine sample.[494] Although community-dwelling older women experience symptomatic UTI more often than older men, gender differences are less pronounced in older age groups than in younger age groups.[495] Estimated prevalence of asymptomatic bacteriuria in women older than 80 years living in the community is 20%, whereas 5% to 10% of similarly aged men are bacteriuric without symptoms. Nearly 25% to 50% of institutionalized elderly women and 15% to 40% of elderly institutionalized men, however, are found to have asymptomatic bacteriuria.[495] Because asymptomatic bacteriuria does not necessarily predict poor outcome or treatment impact on morbidity or mortality in the elderly,[494] routine screening for and treatment of asymptomatic bacteriuria, whether or not accompanied by pyuria, is not recommended for either community-dwelling or institutionalized elderly individuals.[491,494,496-498] Use of indwelling urinary catheters, although common in the elderly, raises concerns for bacterial colonization and biofilm formation on both external and internal catheter surfaces and is associated with a 5% per day infection rate. UTI most commonly presents as fever without localized genitourinary signs and symptoms in these patients and requires treatment. Asymptomatic catheter-acquired UTI does not require antimicrobials.

For elderly patients without an indwelling catheter, the minimum criterion for initiating antibiotic therapy according to consensus guidelines is acute dysuria alone or fever in the presence of at least one of the following: new or worsening urgency, frequency, suprapubic pain, gross hematuria, costovertebral angle tenderness, or urinary incontinence.[499] For treatment of symptomatic infection, selection of an antimicrobial should be delayed, wherever possible, until culture results are available. In patients with an indwelling catheter, the catheter should be removed and replaced with a new catheter before initiation of antimicrobial treatment for symptomatic infection.[500]

Escherichia coli remains the most common cause of symptomatic UTI in older men and women.[501] Nevertheless, a wide spectrum of organisms has been isolated from individuals with a long-term indwelling catheter, including yeast species.[500] A urine culture should be performed before initiation of antimicrobial therapy in older individuals with suspected UTI. In relatively healthy women living in the community, however, a short course of empiric antimicrobial therapy can be effective if the patient shows typical symptoms. A 3-day course of antibiotic therapy for uncomplicated symptomatic UTI in older women seems to offer efficacy similar to that of the more standard 7-day therapy, with significantly fewer adverse events.[502] Duration of therapy for men is usually 7 days for cystitis. Treatment is continued for 10 to 14 days for pyelonephritis for both men and women.

Chronic bacterial prostatitis is characterized by positive results on cultures of expressed prostatic fluid and is usually associated with recurrent UTIs. The initial treatment for

TABLE 23-5 Management of Urinary Tract Infection in the Elderly			
PRESENTATION	**CLINICAL SYMPTOMS**	**URINARY FINDINGS**	**TREATMENT**
Asymptomatic bacteriuria	None	± Pyuria	No treatment
Symptomatic bacteriuria	Dysuria, fever, new or worsened urgency, frequency, suprapubic pain, costovertebral angle tenderness, altered mental status, gross hematuria, urinary incontinence	Pyuria, bacteriuria	Antimicrobials, preferably after urine culture
In-dwelling catheter—symptomatic bacteriuria	Fever	Pyuria, bacteriuria	Insertion of new catheter, Antimicrobials after urine culture
In-dwelling catheter—asymptomatic bacteriuria	None	± Pyuria ± Bacteriuria	No antimicrobials
Recurrent symptomatic bacteriuria (two or more episodes within 6 mo)	Clinical symptoms of bacteriuria	Pyuria, bacteriuria	Genitourinary evaluation to rule out strictures and obstruction Consider at least 4 wk of appropriate antimicrobials for prostatitis Consider 6-12 mo low-dose antimicrobials for uncomplicated urinary tract infection in females

chronic bacterial prostatitis is the use of a prostate-penetrating antimicrobial agent (e.g., a fluoroquinolone or trimethoprim-sulfamethoxazole) that is effective against the pathogen identified by prostatic localization cultures. The usual course of therapy is 4 weeks.[503]

Long-term (6- to 12-month) low-dose prophylactic antimicrobial therapy can be used for prevention of recurrent uncomplicated UTI in older women in the community who are experiencing two or more UTI episodes in a 6-month period. A first-line regimen is nitrofurantoin 50 or 100 mg or trimethoprim-sulfamethoxazole one half a regular-strength tablet daily or every other day at bedtime.[495] The optimal duration of UTI therapy for residents of long-term care facilities is not known. In general, the diagnosis of UTI in frail elderly people should be made only after a careful clinical evaluation and thorough review of laboratory data.

Renal Cysts

Simple renal cysts occur commonly in aging kidneys.[504,505] One study reported prevalences of 11.5% in individuals aged 50 to 70 years and 22.1% in those aged 70 years and older,[506] whereas another found rates as high as 36.1% in the eighth decade of life, with a relative frequency of 2:1 in men compared with women.[507]

Simple cysts are benign and asymptomatic, and usually are an incidental finding in patients undergoing abdominal imaging for other causes. They may be solitary, or multiple and bilateral and generally have little clinical significance.[507] Rarely, however, they may be associated with pain, infection, rupture, hematuria, and hypertension.[508-510] Cysts that have smooth clear walls and are fluid-filled without internal echoes by ultrasonography usually require no further workup.[511-513] However, cysts that are filled with debris and/or internal echoes, are thick walled, or occur in association with a possible renal mass are considered complicated and need careful follow-up and investigation with further imaging,[512,514,515] cyst puncture, angiography, or surgical exploration as indicated.

Acknowledgements

The authors would like to thank the library and medical media staff at the Dallas VA Medical Center and Jolene Richardson for providing expert help in obtaining references and preparing figures.

References

1. Prommool S, Jhangri GS, Cockfield SM, et al. Time dependency of factors affecting renal allograft survival. *J Am Soc Nephrol.* 2000;11(3):565-573.
2. Terasaki PI, Gjertson DW, Cecka JM, et al. Significance of the donor age effect on kidney transplants. *Clin Transplant.* 1997;11(5 pt 1):366-372.
3. Kasiske BL, Snyder J. Matching older kidneys with older patients does not improve allograft survival. *J Am Soc Nephrol.* 2002;13(4):1067-1072.
4. Cecka JM. The UNOS renal transplant registry. *Clin Transpl.* 2001; 1-18. UCLA Immunogenetics, Los Angeles.
5. Asderakis A, Dyer P, Augustine T, et al. Effect of cold ischemic time and HLA matching in kidneys coming from "young" and "old" donors: do not leave for tomorrow what you can do tonight. *Transplantation.* 2001;72(4):674-678.
6. Roderick PJ, Atkins RJ, Smeeth L, et al. CKD and mortality risk in older people: a community-based population study in the United Kingdom. *Am J Kidney Dis.* 2009;53(6):950-960.
7. Knickman JR, Snell EK. The 2030 problem: caring for aging baby boomers. *Health Serv Res.* 2002;37(4):849-884.
8. Campbell KH, O'Hare AM. Kidney disease in the elderly: update on recent literature. *Curr Opin Nephrol Hypertens.* 2008;17(3):298-303.
9. Liangos O, Wald R, O'Bell JW, et al. Epidemiology and outcomes of acute renal failure in hospitalized patients: a national survey. *Clin J Am Soc Nephrol.* 2006;1(1):43-51.
10. Gourtsoyiannis N, Prassopoulos P, Cavouras D, et al. The thickness of the renal parenchyma decreases with age: a CT study of 360 patients. *AJR Am J Roentgenol.* 1990;155(3):541-544.
11. McLachlan M, Wasserman P. Changes in sizes and distensibility of the aging kidney. *Br J Radiol.* 1981;54(642):488-491.
12. Tauchi H, Tsuboi K, Okutomi J. Age changes in the human kidney of the different races. *Gerontologia.* 1971;17(2):87-97.
13. Kasiske BL, Umen AJ. The influence of age, sex, race, and body habitus on kidney weight in humans. *Arch Pathol Lab Med.* 1986;110(1):55-60.
14. Tan JC, Workeneh B, Busque S, et al. Glomerular function, structure, and number in renal allografts from older deceased donors. *J Am Soc Nephrol.* 2009;20(1):181-188.
15. Tracy RE, Berenson G, Wattigney W, et al. The evolution of benign arterionephrosclerosis from age 6 to 70 years. *Am J Pathol.* 1990;136(2):429-439.
16. Melk A, Halloran PF. Cell senescence and its implications for nephrology. *J Am Soc Nephrol.* Feb 2001;12(2):385-393.
17. Hill GS, Heudes D, Bariety J. Morphometric study of arterioles and glomeruli in the aging kidney suggests focal loss of autoregulation. *Kidney Int.* 2003;63(3):1027-1036.
18. Kang DH, Anderson S, Kim YG, et al. Impaired angiogenesis in the aging kidney: vascular endothelial growth factor and thrombospondin-1 in renal disease. *Am J Kidney Dis.* 2001;37(3):601-611.
19. Lindeman RD, Goldman R. Anatomic and physiologic age changes in the kidney. *Exp Gerontol.* 1986;21(4-5):379-406.
20. Takazakura E, Sawabu N, Handa A, et al. Intrarenal vascular changes with age and disease. *Kidney Int.* 1972;2(4):224-230.
21. Baert L, Steg A. Is the diverticulum of the distal and collecting tubules a preliminary stage of the simple cyst in the adult? *J Urol.* 1977;118(5):707-710.
22. Abrass CK, Adcox MJ, Raugi GJ. Aging-associated changes in renal extracellular matrix. *Am J Pathol.* 1995;146(3):742-752.
23. Ding G, Franki N, Kapasi AA, et al. Tubular cell senescence and expression of TGF-beta1 and p21(WAF1/CIP1) in tubulointerstitial fibrosis of aging rats. *Exp Mol Pathol.* 2001;70(1):43-53.
24. Yabuki A, Tanaka S, Matsumoto M, et al. Morphometric study of gender differences with regard to age-related changes in the C57BL/6 mouse kidney. *Exp Anim.* 2006;55(4):399-404.
25. Thomas SE, Anderson S, Gordon KL, et al. Tubulointerstitial disease in aging: evidence for underlying peritubular capillary damage, a potential role for renal ischemia. *J Am Soc Nephrol.* 1998;9(2):231-242.
26. Gagliano N, Arosio B, Santambrogio D, et al. Age-dependent expression of fibrosis-related genes and collagen deposition in rat kidney cortex. *J Gerontol A Biol Sci Med Sci.* 2000;55(8):B365-B372.
27. Eikmans M, Baelde HJ, de Heer E, et al. Effect of age and biopsy site on extracellular matrix mRNA and protein levels in human kidney biopsies. *Kidney Int.* 2001;60(3):974-981.
28. Melk A, Schmidt BM, Takeuchi O, et al. Expression of p16INK4a and other cell cycle regulator and senescence associated genes in aging human kidney. *Kidney Int.* 2004;65(2):510-520.
29. Melk A, Kittikowit W, Sandhu I, et al. Cell senescence in rat kidneys in vivo increases with growth and age despite lack of telomere shortening. *Kidney Int.* 2003;63(6):2134-2143.
30. Tsirpanlis G. Cellular senescence, cardiovascular risk, and CKD: a review of established and hypothetical interconnections. *Am J Kidney Dis.* 2008;51(1):131-144.
31. Lindeman RD, Tobin J, Shock NW. Longitudinal studies on the rate of decline in renal function with age. *J Am Geriatr Soc.* 1985;33(4):278-285.
32. Cogan MG. Angiotensin II: a powerful controller of sodium transport in the early proximal tubule. *Hypertension.* 1990;15(5):451-458.
33. Norman JT. The role of angiotensin II in renal growth. *Ren Physiol Biochem.* 1991;14(4-5):175-185.
34. Maric C, Aldred GP, Antoine AM, et al. Effects of angiotensin II on cultured rat renomedullary interstitial cells are mediated by AT1A receptors. *Am J Physiol.* 1996;271(5 pt 2):F1020-F1028.
35. Wolf G, Ziyadeh FN, Zahner G, et al. Angiotensin II is mitogenic for cultured rat glomerular endothelial cells. *Hypertension.* 1996;27(4):897-905.
36. Wolf G, Ziyadeh FN, Schroeder R, et al. Angiotensin II inhibits inducible nitric oxide synthase in tubular MCT cells by a posttranscriptional mechanism. *J Am Soc Nephrol.* 1997;8(4):551-557.

37. Anderson S, Brenner BM. Effects of aging on the renal glomerulus. *Am J Med.* 1986;80(3):435-442.
38. Heudes D, Michel O, Chevalier J, et al. Effect of chronic ANG I-converting enzyme inhibition on aging processes. I. Kidney structure and function. *Am J Physiol.* 1994;266(3 pt 2):R1038-R1051.
39. Corman B, Chami-Khazraji S, Schaeverbeke J, et al. Effect of feeding on glomerular filtration rate and proteinuria in conscious aging rats. *Am J Physiol.* 1988;255(2 pt 2):F250-F256.
40. Remuzzi A, Puntorieri S, Battaglia C, et al. Angiotensin converting enzyme inhibition ameliorates glomerular filtration of macromolecules and water and lessens glomerular injury in the rat. *J Clin Invest.* 1990;85(2):541-549.
41. Zoja C, Remuzzi A, Corna D, et al. Renal protective effect of angiotensin-converting enzyme inhibition in aging rats. *Am J Med.* 1992;92(4B):60S-63S.
42. Anderson S, Rennke HG, Zatz R. Glomerular adaptations with normal aging and with long-term converting enzyme inhibition in rats. *Am J Physiol.* 1994;267(1 pt 2):F35-F43.
43. Michel JB, Heudes D, Michel O, et al. Effect of chronic ANG I-converting enzyme inhibition on aging processes. II. Large arteries. *Am J Physiol.* 1994;267(1 pt 2):R124-R135.
44. Ferder L, Inserra F, Romano L, et al. Decreased glomerulosclerosis in aging by angiotensin-converting enzyme inhibitors. *J Am Soc Nephrol.* 1994;5(4):1147-1152.
45. Jung FF, Kennefick TM, Ingelfinger JR, et al. Down-regulation of the intrarenal renin-angiotensin system in the aging rat. *J Am Soc Nephrol.* 1995;5(8):1573-1580.
46. Wolf G, Killen PD, Neilson EG. Intracellular signaling of transcription and secretion of type IV collagen after angiotensin II-induced cellular hypertrophy in cultured proximal tubular cells. *Cell Regul.* 1991;2(3):219-227.
47. Wolf G, Zahner G, Schroeder R, et al. Transforming growth factor beta mediates the angiotensin-II-induced stimulation of collagen type IV synthesis in cultured murine proximal tubular cells. *Nephrol Dial Transplant.* 1996;11(2):263-269.
48. Wolf G, Ziyadeh FN, Thaiss F, et al. Angiotensin II stimulates expression of the chemokine RANTES in rat glomerular endothelial cells. Role of the angiotensin type 2 receptor. *J Clin Invest.* 1997;100(5):1047-1058.
49. Inserra F, Romano LA, de Cavanagh EM, et al. Renal interstitial sclerosis in aging: effects of enalapril and nifedipine. *J Am Soc Nephrol.* 1996;7(5):676-680.
50. Vaughan DE, Lazos SA, Tong K. Angiotensin II regulates the expression of plasminogen activator inhibitor-1 in cultured endothelial cells. A potential link between the renin-angiotensin system and thrombosis. *J Clin Invest.* 1995;95(3):995-1001.
51. Fogo AB. The role of angiotensin II and plasminogen activator inhibitor-1 in progressive glomerulosclerosis. *Am J Kidney Dis.* 2000;35(2):179-188.
52. Ma LJ, Nakamura S, Aldigier JC, et al. Regression of glomerulosclerosis with high-dose angiotensin inhibition is linked to decreased plasminogen activator inhibitor-1. *J Am Soc Nephrol.* 2005;16(4):966-976.
53. de Cavanagh EM, Piotrkowski B, Basso N, et al. Enalapril and losartan attenuate mitochondrial dysfunction in aged rats. *FASEB J.* 2003;17(9):1096-1098.
54. Mitani H, Ishizaka N, Aizawa T, et al. In vivo klotho gene transfer ameliorates angiotensin II–induced renal damage. *Hypertension.* 2002;39(4):838-843.
55. Basso N, Paglia N, Stella I, et al. Protective effect of the inhibition of the renin-angiotensin system on aging. *Regul Pept.* 2005;128(3):247-252.
56. Thomas MC, Tikellis C, Burns WM, et al. Interactions between renin angiotensin system and advanced glycation in the kidney. *J Am Soc Nephrol.* 2005;16(10):2976-2984.
57. Basso N, Paglia N, Cini R, et al. Effect of omapatrilat on the aging process of the normal rat. *Cell Mol Biol (Noisy-le-grand).* 2005;51(6):557-564.
58. Negri AL. The klotho gene: a gene predominantly expressed in the kidney is a fundamental regulator of aging and calcium/phosphorus metabolism. *J Nephrol.* 2005;18(6):654-658.
59. Monacelli F, Poggi A, Storace D, et al. Effects of valsartan therapy on protein glycoxidation. *Metabolism.* 2006;55(12):1619-1624.
60. Gilliam-Davis S, Payne VS, Kasper SO, et al. Long-term AT1 receptor blockade improves metabolic function and provides renoprotection in Fischer-344 rats. *Am J Physiol Heart Circ Physiol.* 2007;293(3):H1327-H1333.
61. Baumann M, Bartholome R, Peutz-Kootstra CJ, et al. Sustained tubulo-interstitial protection in SHRs by transient losartan treatment: an effect of decelerated aging? *Am J Hypertens.* 2008;21(2):177-182.
62. Benigni A, Corna D, Zoja C, et al. Disruption of the Ang II type 1 receptor promotes longevity in mice. *J Clin Invest.* 2009;119(3):524-530.
63. Mattson MP, Maudsley S. Live longer sans the AT1A receptor. *Cell Metab.* 2009;9(5):403-405.

64. Roberts AB, McCune BK, Sporn MB. TGF-beta: regulation of extracellular matrix. *Kidney Int.* 1992;41(3):557-559.
65. Wolf G. Link between angiotensin II and TGF-beta in the kidney. *Miner Electrolyte Metab.* 1998;24(2-3):174-180.
66. Noble NA, Border WA. Angiotensin II in renal fibrosis: should TGF-beta rather than blood pressure be the therapeutic target? *Semin Nephrol.* 1997;17(5):455-466.
67. Peters H, Noble NA, Border WA. Transforming growth factor-beta in human glomerular injury. *Curr Opin Nephrol Hypertens.* 1997;6(4):389-393.
68. Frishberg Y, Kelly CJ. TGF-beta and regulation of interstitial nephritis. *Miner Electrolyte Metab.* 1998;24(2-3):181-189.
69. Ruiz-Torres MP, Bosch RJ, O'Valle F, et al. Age-related increase in expression of TGF-beta1 in the rat kidney: relationship to morphologic changes. *J Am Soc Nephrol.* 1998;9(5):782-791.
70. Samuel CS, Zhao C, Bond CP, et al. Relaxin-1–deficient mice develop an age-related progression of renal fibrosis. *Kidney Int.* 2004;65(6):2054-2064.
71. Hewitson TD, Samuel CS. Relaxin: an endogenous renoprotective factor? *Ann N Y Acad Sci.* 2009;1160:289-293.
72. Wolf G. Molecular mechanisms of angiotensin II in the kidney: emerging role in the progression of renal disease: beyond haemodynamics. *Nephrol Dial Transplant.* 1998;13(5):1131-1142.
73. Satriano JA, Shuldiner M, Hora K, et al. Oxygen radicals as second messengers for expression of the monocyte chemoattractant protein, JE/MCP-1, and the monocyte colony-stimulating factor, CSF-1, in response to tumor necrosis factor-alpha and immunoglobulin G. Evidence for involvement of reduced nicotinamide adenine dinucleotide phosphate (NADPH)–dependent oxidase. *J Clin Invest.* 1993;92(3):1564-1571.
74. Hill C, Lateef AM, Engels K, et al. Basal and stimulated nitric oxide in control of kidney function in the aging rat. *Am J Physiol.* 1997;272(6 pt 2):R1747-R1753.
75. Sonaka I, Futami Y, Maki T. L-Arginine–nitric oxide pathway and chronic nephropathy in aged rats. *J Gerontol.* 1994;49(4):B157-B161.
76. Adler S, Huang H, Wolin MS, et al. Oxidant stress leads to impaired regulation of renal cortical oxygen consumption by nitric oxide in the aging kidney. *J Am Soc Nephrol.* 2004;15(1):52-60.
77. Reckelhoff JF, Kellum Jr JA, Racusen LC, et al. Long-term dietary supplementation with L-arginine prevents age-related reduction in renal function. *Am J Physiol.* 1997;272(6 pt 2):R1768-R1774.
78. Radner W, Hoger H, Lubec B, et al. L-Arginine reduces kidney collagen accumulation and N-epsilon-(carboxymethyl)lysine in the aging NMRI-mouse. *J Gerontol.* 1994;49(2):M44-M46.
79. Nakayama I, Kawahara Y, Tsuda T, et al. Angiotensin II inhibits cytokine-stimulated inducible nitric oxide synthase expression in vascular smooth muscle cells. *J Biol Chem.* 1994;269(15):11628-11633.
80. Arima S, Ito S, Omata K, et al. High glucose augments angiotensin II action by inhibiting NO synthesis in in vitro microperfused rabbit afferent arterioles. *Kidney Int.* 1995;48(3):683-689.
81. Hogan M, Cerami A, Bucala R. Advanced glycosylation endproducts block the antiproliferative effect of nitric oxide. Role in the vascular and renal complications of diabetes mellitus. *J Clin Invest.* 1992;90(3):1110-1115.
82. McQuillan LP, Leung GK, Marsden PA, et al. Hypoxia inhibits expression of eNOS via transcriptional and posttranscriptional mechanisms. *Am J Physiol.* 1994;267(5 pt 2):H1921-H1927.
83. Huang PL. eNOS, metabolic syndrome and cardiovascular disease. *Trends Endocrinol Metab.* 2009;20(6):295-302.
84. Baylis C. Sexual dimorphism in the aging kidney: differences in the nitric oxide system. *Nat Rev Nephrol.* 2009;5(7):384-396.
85. Schwartz IF, Chernichovski T, Krishtol N, et al. Sexual dimorphism in glomerular arginine transport affects nitric oxide generation in old male rats. *Am J Physiol Renal Physiol.* 2009;297(1):F80-F84.
86. Yoon HJ, Cho SW, Ahn BW, et al. Alterations in the activity and expression of endothelial NO synthase in aged human endothelial cells. *Mech Ageing Dev.* 2010;131(2):119-123.
87. Smith AR, Hagen TM. Vascular endothelial dysfunction in aging: loss of Akt-dependent endothelial nitric oxide synthase phosphorylation and partial restoration by (R)-alpha-lipoic acid. *Biochem Soc Trans.* 2003;31(pt 6):1447-1449.
88. Smith AR, Visioli F, Frei B, et al. Age-related changes in endothelial nitric oxide synthase phosphorylation and nitric oxide dependent vasodilation: evidence for a novel mechanism involving sphingomyelinase and ceramide-activated phosphatase 2A. *Aging Cell.* 2006;5(5):391-400.
89. Kim JH, Bugaj LJ, Oh YJ, et al. Arginase inhibition restores NOS coupling and reverses endothelial dysfunction and vascular stiffness in old rats. *J Appl Physiol.* 2009;107(4):1249-1257.
90. Donato AJ, Eskurza I, Silver AE, et al. Direct evidence of endothelial oxidative stress with aging in humans: relation to impaired endothelium-dependent dilation and upregulation of nuclear factor-kappaB. *Circ Res.* 2007;100(11):1659-1666.

91. Donato AJ, Gano LB, Eskurza I, et al. Vascular endothelial dysfunction with aging: endothelin-1 and endothelial nitric oxide synthase. *Am J Physiol Heart Circ Physiol.* 2009;297(1):H425-H432.
92. Verbeke P, Perichon M, Borot-Laloi C, et al. Accumulation of advanced glycation endproducts in the rat nephron: link with circulating AGEs during aging. *J Histochem Cytochem.* 1997;45(8):1059-1068.
93. Schleicher ED, Wagner E, Nerlich AG. Increased accumulation of the glycoxidation product N(epsilon)-(carboxymethyl)lysine in human tissues in diabetes and aging. *J Clin Invest.* 1997;99(3):457-468.
94. Raj DS, Choudhury D, Welbourne TC, et al. Advanced glycation end products: a nephrologist's perspective. *Am J Kidney Dis.* 2000;35(3):365-380.
95. Vlassara H. Advanced glycosylation in nephropathy of diabetes and aging. *Adv Nephrol Necker Hosp.* 1996;25:303-315.
96. McVeigh GE, Brennan GM, Johnston GD, et al. Impaired endothelium-dependent and independent vasodilation in patients with type 2 (non–insulin-dependent) diabetes mellitus. *Diabetologia.* 1992;35(8):771-776.
97. Gascho JA, Fanelli C, Zelis R. Aging reduces venous distensibility and the venodilatory response to nitroglycerin in normal subjects. *Am J Cardiol.* 1989;63(17):1267-1270.
98. Bucala R, Tracey KJ, Cerami A. Advanced glycosylation products quench nitric oxide and mediate defective endothelium-dependent vasodilatation in experimental diabetes. *J Clin Invest.* 1991;87(2):432-438.
99. He C, Sabol J, Mitsuhashi T, et al. Dietary glycotoxins: inhibition of reactive products by aminoguanidine facilitates renal clearance and reduces tissue sequestration. *Diabetes.* 1999;48(6):1308-1315.
100. Cerami C, Founds H, Nicholl I, et al. Tobacco smoke is a source of toxic reactive glycation products. *Proc Natl Acad Sci U S A.* 1997;94(25):13915-13920.
101. Lu C, He JC, Cai W, et al. Advanced glycation endproduct (AGE) receptor 1 is a negative regulator of the inflammatory response to AGE in mesangial cells. *Proc Natl Acad Sci U S A.* 2004;101(32):11767-11772.
102. Cai W, He JC, Zhu L, et al. AGE-receptor-1 counteracts cellular oxidant stress induced by AGEs via negative regulation of p66shc-dependent FKHRL1 phosphorylation. *Am J Physiol Cell Physiol.* 2008;294(1):C145-C152.
103. Menini S, Amadio L, Oddi G, et al. Deletion of p66Shc longevity gene protects against experimental diabetic glomerulopathy by preventing diabetes-induced oxidative stress. *Diabetes.* 2006;55(6):1642-1650.
104. Cai W, Torreggiani M, Zhu L, et al. AGER1 regulates endothelial cell NADPH oxidase-dependent oxidant stress via PKCδ: implications for vascular disease. *Am J Physiol Cell Physiol.* 2010;298(3):C624-34.
105. Cai W, He JC, Zhu L, et al. Reduced oxidant stress and extended lifespan in mice exposed to a low glycotoxin diet: association with increased AGER1 expression. *Am J Pathol.* 2007;170(6):1893-1902.
106. Vlassara H, Cai W, Goodman S, et al. Protection against loss of innate defenses in adulthood by low advanced glycation end products (AGE) intake: role of the antiinflammatory AGE receptor-1. *J Clin Endocrinol Metab.* 2009;94(11):4483-4491.
107. Li YM, Steffes M, Donnelly T, et al. Prevention of cardiovascular and renal pathology of aging by the advanced glycation inhibitor aminoguanidine. *Proc Natl Acad Sci U S A.* 1996;93(9):3902-3907.
108. Corman B, Duriez M, Poitevin P, et al. Aminoguanidine prevents age-related arterial stiffening and cardiac hypertrophy. *Proc Natl Acad Sci U S A.* 1998;95(3):1301-1306.
109. Vlassara H, Fuh H, Makita Z, et al. Exogenous advanced glycosylation end products induce complex vascular dysfunction in normal animals: a model for diabetic and aging complications. *Proc Natl Acad Sci U S A.* 1992;89(24):12043-12047.
110. Cefalu WT, Bell-Farrow AD, Wang ZQ, et al. Caloric restriction decreases age-dependent accumulation of the glycoxidation products, N epsilon-(carboxymethyl)lysine and pentosidine, in rat skin collagen. *J Gerontol A Biol Sci Med Sci.* 1995;50(6):B337-B341.
111. Novelli M, Masiello P, Bombara M, et al. Protein glycation in the aging male Sprague-Dawley rat: effects of antiaging diet restrictions. *J Gerontol A Biol Sci Med Sci.* 1998;53(2):B94-B101.
112. Teillet L, Verbeke P, Gouraud S, et al. Food restriction prevents advanced glycation end product accumulation and retards kidney aging in lean rats. *J Am Soc Nephrol.* 2000;11(8):1488-1497.
113. Xia E, Rao G, Van Remmen H, et al. Activities of antioxidant enzymes in various tissues of male Fischer 344 rats are altered by food restriction. *J Nutr.* 1995;125(2):195-201.
114. Oppenheim RW. Related mechanisms of action of growth factors and antioxidants in apoptosis: an overview. *Adv Neurol.* 1997;72:69-78.
115. Papa S, Skulachev VP. Reactive oxygen species, mitochondria, apoptosis and aging. *Mol Cell Biochem.* 1997;174(1-2):305-319.
116. Beckman KB, Ames BN. The free radical theory of aging matures. *Physiol Rev.* 1998;78(2):547-581.
117. Leeuwenburgh C, Hansen PA, Holloszy JO, et al. Oxidized amino acids in the urine of aging rats: potential markers for assessing oxidative stress in vivo. *Am J Physiol.* 1999;276(1 pt 2):R128-R135.
118. Ruiz-Torres P, Lucio J, Gonzalez-Rubio M, et al. Oxidant/antioxidant balance in isolated glomeruli and cultured mesangial cells. *Free Radic Biol Med.* 1997;22(1-2):49-56.
119. Reckelhoff JF, Kanji V, Racusen LC, et al. Vitamin E ameliorates enhanced renal lipid peroxidation and accumulation of F2-isoprostanes in aging kidneys. *Am J Physiol.* 1998;274(3 pt 2):R767-R774.
120. Mitobe M, Yoshida T, Sugiura H, et al. Oxidative stress decreases klotho expression in a mouse kidney cell line. *Nephron Exp Nephrol.* 2005;101(2):e67-e74.
121. Ushio-Fukai M, Zafari AM, Fukui T, et al. p22phox is a critical component of the superoxide-generating NADH/NADPH oxidase system and regulates angiotensin II-induced hypertrophy in vascular smooth muscle cells. *J Biol Chem.* 1996;271(38):23317-23321.
122. de Cavanagh EM, Inserra F, Ferder L, et al. Superoxide dismutase and glutathione peroxidase activities are increased by enalapril and captopril in mouse liver. *FEBS Lett.* 1995;361(1):22-24.
123. Cruz CI, Ruiz-Torres P, del Moral RG, et al. Age-related progressive renal fibrosis in rats and its prevention with ACE inhibitors and taurine. *Am J Physiol Renal Physiol.* 2000;278(1):F122-F129.
124. Kim HJ, Jung KJ, Yu BP, et al. Influence of aging and calorie restriction on MAPKs activity in rat kidney. *Exp Gerontol.* 2002;37(8-9):1041-1053.
125. Lee JH, Jung KJ, Kim JW, et al. Suppression of apoptosis by calorie restriction in aged kidney. *Exp Gerontol.* 2004;39(9):1361-1368.
126. Storz P. Reactive oxygen species–mediated mitochondria-to-nucleus signaling: a key to aging and radical-caused diseases. *Sci STKE.* 2006;2006(332):re3.
127. Miyazawa M, Ishii T, Yasuda K, et al. The role of mitochondrial superoxide anion (O2(-)) on physiological aging in C57BL/6J mice. *J Radiat Res (Tokyo).* 2009;50(1):73-83.
128. Liang H, Masoro EJ, Nelson JF, et al. Genetic mouse models of extended lifespan. *Exp Gerontol.* 2003;38(11-12):1353-1364.
129. Brown-Borg HM, Borg KE, Meliska CJ, et al. Dwarf mice and the ageing process. *Nature.* 1996;384(6604):33.
130. Murakami S, Salmon A, Miller RA. Multiplex stress resistance in cells from long-lived dwarf mice. *FASEB J.* 2003;17(11):1565-1566.
131. Migliaccio E, Giorgio M, Mele S, et al. The p66shc adaptor protein controls oxidative stress response and life span in mammals. *Nature.* 1999;402(6759):309-313.
132. Holzenberger M, Dupont J, Ducos B, et al. IGF-1 receptor regulates lifespan and resistance to oxidative stress in mice. *Nature.* 2003;421(6919):182-187.
133. Perez VI, Bokov A, Van Remmen H, et al. Is the oxidative stress theory of aging dead? *Biochim Biophys Acta.* 2009;1790(10):1005-1014.
134. Piper MD, Bartke A. Diet and aging. *Cell Metab.* 2008;8(2):99-104.
135. McCay CM, Crowell MF, Maynard LA. The effect of retarded growth upon the length of life span and upon the ultimate body size. 1935 *Nutrition.* 1989;5(3):155-171:discussion, 172.
136. Masoro EJ. Overview of caloric restriction and ageing. *Mech Ageing Dev.* 2005;126(9):913-922.
137. Lin SJ, Kaeberlein M, Andalis AA, et al. Calorie restriction extends *Saccharomyces cerevisiae* lifespan by increasing respiration. *Nature.* 2002;418(6895):344-348.
138. Henderson S. *Dissecting the process of aging using the nematode Caenorhabditis elegans.* ed 6. San Diego: Elsevier; 2006.
139. Partridge L, Piper MD, Mair W. Dietary restriction in. *Drosophila. Mech Ageing Dev.* 2005;126(9):938-950.
140. Roth GS, Ingram DK, Lane MA. Caloric restriction in primates and relevance to humans. *Ann N Y Acad Sci.* 2001;928:305-315.
141. Lane MA, Ingram DK, Roth GS. Calorie restriction in nonhuman primates: effects on diabetes and cardiovascular disease risk. *Toxicol Sci.* 1999;52(suppl 2):41-48.
142. Kemnitz JW, Roecker EB, Weindruch R, et al. Dietary restriction increases insulin sensitivity and lowers blood glucose in rhesus monkeys. *Am J Physiol.* 1994;266(4 pt 1):E540-E547.
143. Verdery RB, Ingram DK, Roth GS, et al. Caloric restriction increases HDL2 levels in rhesus monkeys (*Macaca mulatta*). *Am J Physiol.* 1997;273(4 pt 1):E714-E719.
144. Blanc S, Schoeller D, Kemnitz J, et al. Energy expenditure of rhesus monkeys subjected to 11 years of dietary restriction. *J Clin Endocrinol Metab.* 2003;88(1):16-23.
145. Lane MA, Baer DJ, Rumpler WV, et al. Calorie restriction lowers body temperature in rhesus monkeys, consistent with a postulated anti-aging mechanism in rodents. *Proc Natl Acad Sci U S A.* 1996;93(9):4159-4164.
146. Zainal TA, Oberley TD, Allison DB, et al. Caloric restriction of rhesus monkeys lowers oxidative damage in skeletal muscle. *FASEB J.* 2000;14(12):1825-1836.

147. Messaoudi I, Warner J, Fischer M, et al. Delay of T cell senescence by caloric restriction in aged long-lived nonhuman primates. *Proc Natl Acad Sci U S A.* 2006;103(51):19448-19453.
148. Colman RJ, Anderson RM, Johnson SC, et al. Caloric restriction delays disease onset and mortality in rhesus monkeys. *Science.* 2009;325(5937):201-204.
149. Fontana L, Meyer TE, Klein S, et al. Long-term calorie restriction is highly effective in reducing the risk for atherosclerosis in humans. *Proc Natl Acad Sci U S A.* 2004;101(17):6659-6663.
150. Holloszy JO, Fontana L. Caloric restriction in humans. *Exp Gerontol.* 2007;42(8):709-712.
151. Jiang T, Liebman SE, Lucia MS, et al. Calorie restriction modulates renal expression of sterol regulatory element binding proteins, lipid accumulation, and age-related renal disease. *J Am Soc Nephrol.* 2005;16(8):2385-2394.
152. Jiang T, Liebman SE, Lucia MS, et al. Role of altered renal lipid metabolism and the sterol regulatory element binding proteins in the pathogenesis of age-related renal disease. *Kidney Int.* 2005;68(6):2608-2620.
153. Russell SJ, Kahn CR. Endocrine regulation of ageing. *Nat Rev Mol Cell Biol.* 2007;8(9):681-691.
154. Mair W, Dillin A. Aging and survival: the genetics of life span extension by dietary restriction. *Annu Rev Biochem.* 2008;77:727-754.
155. Masoro EJ. Caloric restriction–induced life extension of rats and mice: a critique of proposed mechanisms. *Biochim Biophys Acta.* 2009;1790(10):1040-1048.
156. Westphal CH, Dipp MA, Guarente L. A therapeutic role for sirtuins in diseases of aging? *Trends Biochem Sci.* 2007;32(12):555-560.
157. Finkel T, Deng CX, Mostoslavsky R. Recent progress in the biology and physiology of sirtuins. *Nature.* 2009;460(7255):587-591.
158. Haigis MC, Sinclair DA. Mammalian sirtuins: biological insights and disease relevance. *Annu Rev Pathol.*5:253-295.
159. Imai S. SIRT1 and caloric restriction: an insight into possible trade-offs between robustness and frailty. *Curr Opin Clin Nutr Metab Care.* 2009;12(4):350-356.
160. Cohen HY, Miller C, Bitterman KJ, et al. Calorie restriction promotes mammalian cell survival by inducing the SIRT1 deacetylase. *Science.* 2004;305(5682):390-392.
161. Nisoli E, Tonello C, Cardile A, et al. Calorie restriction promotes mitochondrial biogenesis by inducing the expression of eNOS. *Science.* 2005;310(5746):314-317.
162. Chen D, Bruno J, Easlon E, et al. Tissue-specific regulation of SIRT1 by calorie restriction. *Genes Dev.* 2008;22(13):1753-1757.
163. Gerhart-Hines Z, Rodgers JT, Bare O, et al. Metabolic control of muscle mitochondrial function and fatty acid oxidation through SIRT1/PGC-1alpha. *EMBO J.* 2007;26(7):1913-1923.
164. Rodgers JT, Lerin C, Haas W, et al. Nutrient control of glucose homeostasis through a complex of PGC-1alpha and SIRT1. *Nature.* 2005;434(7029):113-118.
165. Boily G, Seifert EL, Bevilacqua L, et al. SirT1 regulates energy metabolism and response to caloric restriction in mice. *PLoS One.* 2008;3(3):e1759.
166. Bordone L, Cohen D, Robinson A, et al. SIRT1 transgenic mice show phenotypes resembling calorie restriction. *Aging Cell.* 2007;6(6):759-767.
167. Banks AS, Kon N, Knight C, et al. SirT1 gain of function increases energy efficiency and prevents diabetes in mice. *Cell Metab.* 2008;8(4):333-341.
168. Pfluger PT, Herranz D, Velasco-Miguel S, et al. Sirt1 protects against high-fat diet–induced metabolic damage. *Proc Natl Acad Sci U S A.* 2008;105(28):9793-9798.
169. Feige JN, Lagouge M, Canto C, et al. Specific SIRT1 activation mimics low energy levels and protects against diet-induced metabolic disorders by enhancing fat oxidation. *Cell Metab.* 2008;8(5):347-358.
170. Lagouge M, Argmann C, Gerhart-Hines Z, et al. Resveratrol improves mitochondrial function and protects against metabolic disease by activating SIRT1 and PGC-1alpha. *Cell.* 2006;127(6):1109-1122.
171. Baur JA, Pearson KJ, Price NL, et al. Resveratrol improves health and survival of mice on a high-calorie diet. *Nature.* 2006;444(7117):337-342.
172. Milne JC, Lambert PD, Schenk S, et al. Small molecule activators of SIRT1 as therapeutics for the treatment of type 2 diabetes. *Nature.* 2007;450(7170):712-716.
173. Pearson KJ, Baur JA, Lewis KN, et al. Resveratrol delays age-related deterioration and mimics transcriptional aspects of dietary restriction without extending life span. *Cell Metab.* 2008;2(2):157-168.
174. Kume S, Uzu T, Horiike K, et al. Calorie restriction enhances cell adaptation to hypoxia through Sirt1-dependent mitochondrial autophagy in mouse aged kidney. *J Clin Invest.* 2010;120(4):1043–1055.
175. Chaudhary N, Pfluger PT. Metabolic benefits from Sirt1 and Sirt1 activators. *Curr Opin Clin Nutr Metab Care.* 2009;12(4):431-437.
176. Canto C, Auwerx J. Caloric restriction, SIRT1 and longevity. *Trends Endocrinol Metab.* 2009;20(7):325-331.
177. Canto C, Gerhart-Hines Z, Feige JN, et al. AMPK regulates energy expenditure by modulating NAD⁺ metabolism and SIRT1 activity. *Nature.* 2009;458(7241):1056-1060.
178. Ramsey KM, Mills KF, Satoh A, et al. Age-associated loss of Sirt1-mediated enhancement of glucose-stimulated insulin secretion in beta cell-specific Sirt1-overexpressing (BESTO) mice. *Aging Cell.* 2008;7(1):78-88.
179. Reznick RM, Zong H, Li J, et al. Aging-associated reductions in AMP-activated protein kinase activity and mitochondrial biogenesis. *Cell Metab.* 2007;5(2):151-156.
180. Li X, Zhang S, Blander G, et al. SIRT1 deacetylates and positively regulates the nuclear receptor LXR. *Mol Cell.* 2007;28(1):91-106.
181. Kemper JK, Xiao Z, Ponugoti B, et al. FXR acetylation is normally dynamically regulated by p300 and SIRT1 but constitutively elevated in metabolic disease states. *Cell Metab.* 2009;10(5):392-404.
182. Jiang T, Wang XX, Scherzer P, et al. Farnesoid X receptor modulates renal lipid metabolism, fibrosis, and diabetic nephropathy. *Diabetes.* 2007;56(10):2485-2493.
183. Wang XX, Jiang T, Shen Y, et al. The farnesoid X receptor modulates renal lipid metabolism and diet-induced renal inflammation, fibrosis, and proteinuria. *Am J Physiol Renal Physiol.* 2009;297(6):F1587-F1596.
184. Harrison DE, Strong R, Sharp ZD, et al. Rapamycin fed late in life extends lifespan in genetically heterogeneous mice. *Nature.* 2009;460(7253):392-395.
185. Sharp ZD, Bartke A. Evidence for down-regulation of phosphoinositide 3-kinase/Akt/mammalian target of rapamycin (PI3K/Akt/mTOR)–dependent translation regulatory signaling pathways in Ames dwarf mice. *J Gerontol A Biol Sci Med Sci.* 2005;60(3):293-300.
186. Stanfel MN, Shamieh LS, Kaeberlein M, et al. The TOR pathway comes of age. *Biochim Biophys Acta.* 2009;1790(10):1067-1074.
187. Bonawitz ND, Chatenay-Lapointe M, Pan Y, et al. Reduced TOR signaling extends chronological life span via increased respiration and upregulation of mitochondrial gene expression. *Cell Metab.* 2007;5(4):265-277.
188. Selman C, Tullet JM, Wieser D, et al. Ribosomal protein S6 kinase 1 signaling regulates mammalian life span. *Science.* 2009;326(5949):140-144.
189. Korczynska J, Stelmanska E, Nogalska A, et al. Upregulation of lipogenic enzymes genes expression in white adipose tissue of rats with chronic renal failure is associated with higher level of sterol regulatory element binding protein-1. *Metabolism.* 2004;53(8):1060-1065.
190. Chmielewski M, Sucajtys-Szulc E, Kossowska E, et al. Increased gene expression of liver SREBP-2 in experimental chronic renal failure. *Atherosclerosis.* 2007;191(2):326-332.
191. Chmielewski M, Sucajtys E, Swierczynski J, et al. Contribution of increased HMG-CoA reductase gene expression to hypercholesterolemia in experimental chronic renal failure. *Mol Cell Biochem.* 2003;246(1-2):187-191.
192. Mori Y, Hirano T, Nagashima M, et al. Decreased peroxisome proliferator–activated receptor alpha gene expression is associated with dyslipidemia in a rat model of chronic renal failure. *Metabolism.* 2007;56(12):1714-1718.
193. Kim HJ, Vaziri ND. Sterol regulatory element-binding proteins, liver X receptor, ABCA1 transporter, CD36, scavenger receptors A1 and B1 in nephrotic kidney. *Am J Nephrol.* 2009;29(6):607-614.
194. Zhou Y, Zhang X, Chen L, et al. Expression profiling of hepatic genes associated with lipid metabolism in nephrotic rats. *Am J Physiol Renal Physiol.* 2008;295(3):F662-F671.
195. Kim CH, Kim HJ, Mitsuhashi M, et al. Hepatic tissue sterol regulatory element binding protein 2 and low-density lipoprotein receptor in nephrotic syndrome. *Metabolism.* 2007;56(10):1377-1382.
196. Nogalska A, Sucajtys-Szulc E, Swierczynski J. Leptin decreases lipogenic enzyme gene expression through modification of SREBP-1c gene expression in white adipose tissue of aging rats. *Metabolism.* 2005;54(8):1041-1047.
197. Pallottini V, Martini C, Cavallini G, et al. Modified HMG-CoA reductase and LDLr regulation is deeply involved in age-related hypercholesterolemia. *J Cell Biochem.* 2006;98(5):1044-1053.
198. Vila L, Roglans N, Alegret M, et al. Hypertriglyceridemia and hepatic steatosis in senescence-accelerated mouse associate to changes in lipid-related gene expression. *J Gerontol A Biol Sci Med Sci.* 2007;62(11):1219-1227.
199. Lefebvre P, Cariou B, Lien F, et al. Role of bile acids and bile acid receptors in metabolic regulation. *Physiol Rev.* 2009;89(1):147-191.
200. Martini C, Pallottini V, Cavallini G, et al. Caloric restrictions affect some factors involved in age-related hypercholesterolemia. *J Cell Biochem.* 2007;101(1):235-243.
201. Zhu M, Miura J, Lu LX, et al. Circulating adiponectin levels increase in rats on caloric restriction: the potential for insulin sensitization. *Exp Gerontol.* 2004;39(7):1049-1059.
202. Zhu M, de Cabo R, Lane MA, et al. Caloric restriction modulates early events in insulin signaling in liver and skeletal muscle of rat. *Ann N Y Acad Sci.* 2004;1019:448-452.

203. Brooks CL, Gu W. How does SIRT1 affect metabolism, senescence and cancer?. *Nat Rev Cancer.* 2009;9(2):123-128.
204. Lavu S, Boss O, Elliott PJ, et al. Sirtuins—novel therapeutic targets to treat age-associated diseases. *Nat Rev Drug Discov.* 2008;7(10):841-853.
205. Keane WF, Kasiske BL, O'Donnell MP. Lipids and progressive glomerulosclerosis. A model analogous to atherosclerosis. *Am J Nephrol.* 1988;8(4):261-271.
206. Joles JA, Kunter U, Janssen U, et al. Early mechanisms of renal injury in hypercholesterolemic or hypertriglyceridemic rats. *J Am Soc Nephrol.* 2000;11(4):669-683.
207. Muntner P, Coresh J, Smith JC, et al. Plasma lipids and risk of developing renal dysfunction: the Atherosclerosis Risk in Communities study. *Kidney Int.* 2000;58(1):293-301.
208. Schaeffner ES, Kurth T, Curhan GC, et al. Cholesterol and the risk of renal dysfunction in apparently healthy men. *J Am Soc Nephrol.* 2003;14(8):2084-2091.
209. Fox CS, Larson MG, Leip EP, et al. Predictors of new-onset kidney disease in a community-based population. *JAMA.* 2004;291(7):844-850.
210. Cases A, Coll E. Dyslipidemia and the progression of renal disease in chronic renal failure patients. *Kidney Int Suppl.* 2005;(99):S87-S93.
211. Samuelsson O, Mulec H, Knight-Gibson C, et al. Lipoprotein abnormalities are associated with increased rate of progression of human chronic renal insufficiency. *Nephrol Dial Transplant.* 1997;12(9):1908-1915.
212. Hunsicker LG, Adler S, Caggiula A, et al. Predictors of the progression of renal disease in the Modification of Diet in Renal Disease Study. *Kidney Int.* 1997;51(6):1908-1919.
213. Tonelli M, Isles C, Craven T, et al. Effect of pravastatin on rate of kidney function loss in people with or at risk for coronary disease. *Circulation.* 2005;112(2):171-178.
214. Sandhu S, Wiebe N, Fried LF, et al. Statins for improving renal outcomes: a meta-analysis. *J Am Soc Nephrol.* 2006;17(7):2006-2016.
215. Levi M. Do statins have a beneficial effect on the kidney? *Nat Clin Pract Nephrol.* 2006;2(12):666-667.
216. Asselbergs FW, Diercks GF, Hillege HL, et al. Effects of fosinopril and pravastatin on cardiovascular events in subjects with microalbuminuria. *Circulation.* 2004;110(18):2809-2816.
217. Vidt DG, Cressman MD, Harris S, et al. Rosuvastatin-induced arrest in progression of renal disease. *Cardiology.* 2004;102(1):52-60.
218. Amador-Noguez D, Dean A, Huang W, et al. Alterations in xenobiotic metabolism in the long-lived little mice. *Aging Cell.* 2007;6(4):453-470.
219. Gerisch B, Rottiers V, Li D, et al. A bile acid–like steroid modulates *Caenorhabditis elegans* lifespan through nuclear receptor signaling. *Proc Natl Acad Sci U S A.* 2007;104(12):5014-5019.
220. Kuro-o M. Klotho and aging. *Biochim Biophys Acta.* 2009;1790(10):1049-1058.
221. Kuro-o M. Klotho. *Pflugers Arch.* 459(2):333-343.
222. Kuro-o M, Matsumura Y, Aizawa H, et al. Mutation of the mouse klotho gene leads to a syndrome resembling ageing. *Nature.* 1997;390(6655):45-51.
223. Kurosu H, Yamamoto M, Clark JD, et al. Suppression of aging in mice by the hormone Klotho. *Science.* 2005;309(5742):1829-1833.
224. Zhang H, Li Y, Fan Y, et al. Klotho is a target gene of PPAR-gamma. *Kidney Int.* 2008;74(6):732-739.
225. Yang HC, Deleuze S, Zuo Y, et al. The PPARgamma agonist pioglitazone ameliorates aging-related progressive renal injury. *J Am Soc Nephrol.* 2009;20(11):2380-2388.
226. Berg UB. Differences in decline in GFR with age between males and females. Reference data on clearances of inulin and PAH in potential kidney donors. *Nephrol Dial Transplant.* 2006;21(9):2577-2582.
227. Kenney WL, Ho CW. Age alters regional distribution of blood flow during moderate-intensity exercise. *J Appl Physiol.* 1995;79(4):1112-1119.
228. Minson CT, Wladkowski SL, Cardell AF, et al. Age alters the cardiovascular response to direct passive heating. *J Appl Physiol.* 1998;84(4):1323-1332.
229. Mulkerrin EC, Brain A, Hampton D, et al. Reduced renal hemodynamic response to atrial natriuretic peptide in elderly volunteers. *Am J Kidney Dis.* 1993;22(4):538-544.
230. Clark B. Biology of renal aging in humans. *Adv Ren Replace Ther.* 2000;7(1):11-21.
231. Fuiano G, Sund S, Mazza G, et al. Renal hemodynamic response to maximal vasodilating stimulus in healthy older subjects. *Kidney Int.* 2001;59(3):1052-1058.
232. Kielstein JT, Bode-Boger SM, Frolich JC, et al. Asymmetric dimethylarginine, blood pressure, and renal perfusion in elderly subjects. *Circulation.* 2003;107(14):1891-1895.
233. Ueda S, Yamagishi S, Matsumoto Y, et al. Involvement of asymmetric dimethylarginine (ADMA) in glomerular capillary loss and sclerosis in a rat model of chronic kidney disease (CKD). *Life Sci.* 2009;84(23-24):853-856.
234. Kang CK, Park CA, Lee H, et al. Hypertension correlates with lenticulostriate arteries visualized by 7T magnetic resonance angiography. *Hypertension.* 2009;54(5):1050-1056.
235. Luscher TF, Bock HA. The endothelial L-arginine/nitric oxide pathway and the renal circulation. *Klin Wochenschr.* 1991;69(13):603-609.
236. Reckelhoff JF, Kellum JA, Blanchard EJ, et al. Changes in nitric oxide precursor, L-arginine, and metabolites, nitrate and nitrite, with aging. *Life Sci.* 1994;55(24):1895-1902.
237. Sarwar G, Botting HG, Collins M. A comparison of fasting serum amino acid profiles of young and elderly subjects. *J Am Coll Nutr.* 1991;10(6):668-674.
238. Mistry SK, Greenfeld Z, Morris Jr SM, et al. The "intestinal-renal" arginine biosynthetic axis in the aging rat. *Mech Ageing Dev.* 2002;123(8):1159-1165.
239. Tokunaga O, Yamada T, Fan JL, et al. Age-related decline in prostacyclin synthesis by human aortic endothelial cells. Qualitative and quantitative analysis. *Am J Pathol.* 1991;138(4):941-949.
240. Nakajima M, Hashimoto M, Wang F, et al. Aging decreases the production of PGI2 in rat aortic endothelial cells. *Exp Gerontol.* 1997;32(6):685-693.
241. Nicholson WT, Vaa B, Hesse C, et al. Aging is associated with reduced prostacyclin-mediated dilation in the human forearm. *Hypertension.* 2009;53(6):973-978.
242. Naeije R, Fiasse A, Carlier E, et al. Systemic and renal haemodynamic effects of angiotensin converting enzyme inhibition by zabicipril in young and in old normal men. *Eur J Clin Pharmacol.* 1993;44(1):35-39.
243. Hollenberg NK, Moore TJ. Age and the renal blood supply: renal vascular responses to angiotensin converting enzyme inhibition in healthy humans. *J Am Geriatr Soc.* 1994;42(8):805-808.
244. Baylis C. Renal responses to acute angiotensin II inhibition and administered angiotensin II in the aging, conscious, chronically catheterized rat. *Am J Kidney Dis.* 1993;22(6):842-850.
245. Baylis C, Fredericks M, Wilson C, et al. Renal vasodilatory response to intravenous glycine in the aging rat kidney. *Am J Kidney Dis.* 1990;15(3):244-251.
246. Tank JE, Vora JP, Houghton DC, et al. Altered renal vascular responses in the aging rat kidney. *Am J Physiol.* 1994;266(6 pt 2):F942-F948.
247. Esposito C, Plati A, Mazzullo T, et al. Renal function and functional reserve in healthy elderly individuals. *J Nephrol.* 2007;20(5):617-625.
248. Zhang XZ, Qiu C, Baylis C. Sensitivity of the segmental renal arterioles to angiotensin II in the aging rat. *Mech Ageing Dev.* 1997;97(2):183-192.
249. Hoang K, Tan JC, Derby G, et al. Determinants of glomerular hypofiltration in aging humans. *Kidney Int.* 2003;64(4):1417-1424.
250. DeSanto NG, Anastasio P, Coppola S, et al. Age-related changes in renal reserve and renal tubular function in healthy humans. *Child Nephrol Urol.* 1991;11(1):33-40.
251. Fliser D, Zeier M, Nowack R, et al. Renal functional reserve in healthy elderly subjects. *J Am Soc Nephrol.* 1993;3(7):1371-1377.
252. Rowe JW, Shock NW, DeFronzo RA. The influence of age on the renal response to water deprivation in man. *Nephron.* 1976;17(4):270-278.
253. Edwards MS, Wilson DB, Craven TE, et al. Associations between retinal microvascular abnormalities and declining renal function in the elderly population: the Cardiovascular Health Study. *Am J Kidney Dis.* 2005;46(2):214-224.
254. Rook M, van der Heide JJ, Navis G. Significant negative association with age and both GFR and ERPF in male and female living kidney donors. *Nephrol Dial Transplant.* 2007;22(1):283:author reply, 284.
255. Luft FC, Fineberg NS, Miller JZ, et al. The effects of age, race and heredity on glomerular filtration rate following volume expansion and contraction in normal man. *Am J Med Sci.* 1980;279(1):15-24.
256. Fliser D, Franek E, Joest M, et al. Renal function in the elderly: impact of hypertension and cardiac function. *Kidney Int.* 1997;51(4):1196-1204.
257. Tolbert EM, Weisstuch J, Feiner HD, et al. Onset of glomerular hypertension with aging precedes injury in the spontaneously hypertensive rat. *Am J Physiol Renal Physiol.* 2000;278(5):F839-F846.
258. Ribstein J, Du Cailar G, Mimran A. Glucose tolerance and age-associated decline in renal function of hypertensive patients. *J Hypertens.* 2001;19(12):2257-2264.
259. Verhave JC, Fesler P, du Cailar G, et al. Elevated pulse pressure is associated with low renal function in elderly patients with isolated systolic hypertension. *Hypertension.* 2005;45(4):586-591.
260. Baracskay D, Jarjoura D, Cugino A, et al. Geriatric renal function: estimating glomerular filtration in an ambulatory elderly population. *Clin Nephrol.* 1997;47(4):222-228.
261. Levey AS, Bosch JP, Lewis JB, et al. A more accurate method to estimate glomerular filtration rate from serum creatinine: a new prediction equation. Modification of Diet in Renal Disease Study Group. *Ann Intern Med.* 1999;130(6):461-470.
262. Levey AS, Stevens LA, Schmid CH, et al. A new equation to estimate glomerular filtration rate. *Ann Intern Med.* 2009;150(9):604-612.

263. Cockcroft DW, Gault MH. Prediction of creatinine clearance from serum creatinine. *Nephron.* 1976;16(1):31-41.
264. Dharnidharka VR, Kwon C, Stevens G. Serum cystatin C is superior to serum creatinine as a marker of kidney function: a meta-analysis. *Am J Kidney Dis.* 2002;40(2):221-226.
265. Fehrman-Ekholm I, Seeberger A, Bjork J, et al. Serum cystatin C: a useful marker of kidney function in very old people. *Scand J Clin Lab Invest.* 2009;69(5):606-611.
266. Vupputuri S, Fox CS, Coresh J, et al. Differential estimation of CKD using creatinine- versus cystatin C–based estimating equations by category of body mass index. *Am J Kidney Dis.* 2009;53(6):993-1001.
267. Epstein M, Hollenberg NK. Age as a determinant of renal sodium conservation in normal man. *J Lab Clin Med.* 1976;87(3):411-417.
268. Macias Nunez JF, Garcia Iglesias C, Bondia Roman A, et al. Renal handling of sodium in old people: a functional study. *Age Ageing.* 1978;7(3):178-181.
269. Bauer JH. Age-related changes in the renin-aldosterone system. Physiological effects and clinical implications. *Drugs Aging.* 1993;3(3):238-245.
270. Hayashi M, Saruta T, Nakamura R, et al. Effect of aging on single nephron renin content in rats. *Ren Physiol.* 1981;4(1):17-21.
271. Lu X, Li X, Li L, et al. Variation of intrarenal angiotensin II and angiotensin II receptors by acute renal ischemia in the aged rat. *Ren Fail.* 1996;18(1):19-29.
272. Tsunoda K, Abe K, Goto T, et al. Effect of age on the renin-angiotensin-aldosterone system in normal subjects: simultaneous measurement of active and inactive renin, renin substrate, and aldosterone in plasma. *J Clin Endocrinol Metab.* 1986;62(2):384-389.
273. Weidmann P, de Chatel R, Schiffmann A, et al. Interrelations between age and plasma renin, aldosterone and cortisol, urinary catecholamines, and the body sodium/volume state in normal man. *Klin Wochenschr.* 1977;55(15):725-733.
274. Mimran A, Ribstein J, Jover B. Aging and sodium homeostasis. *Kidney Int Suppl.* 1992;37:S107-S113.
275. Leosco D, Ferrara N, Landino P, et al. Effects of age on the role of atrial natriuretic factor in renal adaptation to physiologic variations of dietary salt intake. *J Am Soc Nephrol.* 1996;7(7):1045-1051.
276. Pollack JA, Skvorak JP, Nazian SJ, et al. Alterations in atrial natriuretic peptide (ANP) secretion and renal effects in aging. *J Gerontol A Biol Sci Med Sci.* 1997;52(4):B196-B202.
277. Luft FC, Grim CE, Fineberg N, et al. Effects of volume expansion and contraction in normotensive whites, blacks, and subjects of different ages. *Circulation.* 1979;59(4):643-650.
278. Brenner BM, Ballermann BJ, Gunning ME, et al. Diverse biological actions of atrial natriuretic peptide. *Physiol Rev.* 1990;70(3):665-699.
279. Ohashi M, Fujio N, Nawata H, et al. High plasma concentrations of human atrial natriuretic polypeptide in aged men. *J Clin Endocrinol Metab.* 1987;64(1):81-85.
280. Haller BG, Zust H, Shaw S, et al. Effects of posture and ageing on circulating atrial natriuretic peptide levels in man. *J Hypertens.* 1987;5(5):551-556.
281. Tajima F, Sagawa S, Iwamoto J, et al. Renal and endocrine responses in the elderly during head-out water immersion. *Am J Physiol.* 1988;254(6 pt 2):R977-R983.
282. Or K, Richards AM, Espiner EA, et al. Effect of low dose infusions of ile-atrial natriuretic peptide in healthy elderly males: evidence for a postreceptor defect. *J Clin Endocrinol Metab.* 1993;76(5):1271-1274.
283. Gillies AH, Crozier IG, Nicholls MG, et al. Effect of posture on clearance of atrial natriuretic peptide from plasma. *J Clin Endocrinol Metab.* 1987;65(6):1095-1097.
284. Rascher W, Tulassay T, Lang RE. Atrial natriuretic peptide in plasma of volume-overloaded children with chronic renal failure. *Lancet.* 1985;2(8450):303-305.
285. Lafferty HM, Gunning M, Silva P, et al. Enkephalinase inhibition increases plasma atrial natriuretic peptide levels, glomerular filtration rate, and urinary sodium excretion in rats with reduced renal mass. *Circ Res.* 1989;65(3):640-646.
286. Kimmelstiel CD, Perrone R, Kilcoyne L, et al. Effects of renal neutral endopeptidase inhibition on sodium excretion, renal hemodynamics and neurohormonal activation in patients with congestive heart failure. *Cardiology.* 1996;87(1):46-53.
287. Tan AC, Hoefnagels WH, Swinkels LM, et al. The effect of volume expansion on atrial natriuretic peptide and cyclic guanosine monophosphate levels in young and aged subjects. *J Am Geriatr Soc.* 1990;38(11):1215-1219.
288. Tian Y, Serino R, Verbalis JG. Downregulation of renal vasopressin V2 receptor and aquaporin-2 expression parallels age-associated defects in urine concentration. *Am J Physiol Renal Physiol.* 2004;287(4):F797-F805.
289. Helderman JH, Vestal RE, Rowe JW, et al. The response of arginine vasopressin to intravenous ethanol and hypertonic saline in man: the impact of aging. *J Gerontol.* 1978;33(1):39-47.
290. Ishikawa S, Fujita N, Fujisawa G, et al. Involvement of arginine vasopressin and renal sodium handling in pathogenesis of hyponatremia in elderly patients. *Endocr J.* 1996;43(1):101-108.
291. Phillips PA, Bretherton M, Risvanis J, et al. Effects of drinking on thirst and vasopressin in dehydrated elderly men. *Am J Physiol.* 1993;264(5 pt 2):R877-R881.
292. Faull CM, Holmes C, Baylis PH. Water balance in elderly people: is there a deficiency of vasopressin? *Age Ageing.* 1993;22(2):114-120.
293. Miller JH, Shock NW. Age differences in the renal tubular response to antidiuretic hormone. *J Gerontol.* 1953;8(4):446-450.
294. Macias Nunez JF, Garcia Iglesias C, Tabernero Romo JM, et al. Renal management of sodium under indomethacin and aldosterone in the elderly. *Age Ageing.* 1980;9(3):165-172.
295. Bengele HH, Mathias RS, Perkins JH, et al. Urinary concentrating defect in the aged rat. *Am J Physiol.* 1981;240(2):F147-F150.
296. Tian Y, Riazi S, Khan O, et al. Renal ENaC subunit, Na-K-2Cl and Na-Cl cotransporter abundances in aged, water-restricted F344 × Brown Norway rats. *Kidney Int.* 2006;69(2):304-312.
297. Davidson YS, Davies I, Goddard C. Renal vasopressin receptors in ageing C57BL/Icrfat mice. *J Endocrinol.* 1987;115(3):379-385.
298. Beck N, Yu BP. Effect of aging on urinary concentrating mechanism and vasopressin-dependent cAMP in rats. *Am J Physiol.* 1982;243(2):F121-F125.
299. Goddard C, Davidson YS, Moser BB, et al. Effect of ageing on cyclic AMP output by renal medullary cells in response to arginine vasopressin in vitro in C57BL/Icrfat mice. *J Endocrinol.* 1984;103(2):133-139.
300. Liang CT, Barnes J, Hanai H, et al. Decrease in Gs protein expression may impair adenylate cyclase activation in old kidneys. *Am J Physiol.* 1993;264(5 pt 2):F770-F773.
301. Wilson PD, Dillingham MA. Age-associated decrease in vasopressin-induced renal water transport: a role for adenylate cyclase and G protein malfunction. *Gerontology.* 1992;38(6):315-321.
302. Preisser L, Teillet L, Aliotti S, et al. Downregulation of aquaporin-2 and -3 in aging kidney is independent of V(2) vasopressin receptor. *Am J Physiol Renal Physiol.* 2000;279(1):F144-F152.
303. Combet S, Gouraud S, Gobin R, et al. Aquaporin-2 downregulation in kidney medulla of aging rats is posttranscriptional and is abolished by water deprivation. *Am J Physiol Renal Physiol.* 2008;294(6):F1408-F1414.
304. Terashima Y, Kondo K, Inagaki A, et al. Age-associated decrease in response of rat aquaporin-2 gene expression to dehydration. *Life Sci.* 1998;62(10):873-882.
305. Combet S, Teillet L, Geelen G, et al. Food restriction prevents age-related vasopressin-dependent recruitment of aquaporin-2. *Am J Physiol Renal Physiol.* 2001;281(6):F1123-F1131.
306. Combet S, Geffroy N, Berthonaud V, et al. Correction of age-related polyuria by dDAVP: molecular analysis of aquaporins and urea transporters. *Am J Physiol Renal Physiol.* 2003;284(1):F199-F208.
307. Crowe MJ, Forsling ML, Rolls BJ, et al. Altered water excretion in healthy elderly men. *Age Ageing.* 1987;16(5):285-293.
308. Berkemeyer S, Vormann J, Gunther AL, et al. Renal net acid excretion capacity is comparable in prepubescence, adolescence, and young adulthood but falls with aging. *J Am Geriatr Soc.* 2008;56(8):1442-1448.
309. Rylander R, Remer T, Berkemeyer S, et al. Acid-base status affects renal magnesium losses in healthy, elderly persons. *J Nutr.* 2006;136(9):2374-2377.
310. Frassetto LA, Morris Jr RC, Sebastian A. Effect of age on blood acid-base composition in adult humans: role of age-related renal functional decline. *Am J Physiol.* 1996;271(6 pt 2):F1114-F1122.
311. Frassetto L, Sebastian A. Age and systemic acid-base equilibrium: analysis of published data. *J Gerontol A Biol Sci Med Sci.* 1996;51(1):B91-B99.
312. Adler S, Lindeman RD, Yiengst MJ, et al. Effect of acute acid loading on urinary acid excretion by the aging human kidney. *J Lab Clin Med.* 1968;72(2):278-289.
313. Agarwal BN, Cabebe FG. Renal acidification in elderly subjects. *Nephron.* 1980;26(6):291-295.
314. Prasad R, Kinsella JL, Sacktor B. Renal adaptation to metabolic acidosis in senescent rats. *Am J Physiol.* 1988;255(6 pt 2):F1183-F1190.
315. Mitch WE, Medina R, Grieber S, et al. Metabolic acidosis stimulates muscle protein degradation by activating the adenosine triphosphate–dependent pathway involving ubiquitin and proteasomes. *J Clin Invest.* 1994;93(5):2127-2133.
316. Jajoo R, Song L, Rasmussen H, et al. Dietary acid-base balance, bone resorption, and calcium excretion. *J Am Coll Nutr.* 2006;25(3):224-230.
317. Alpern RJ, Sakhaee K. The clinical spectrum of chronic metabolic acidosis: homeostatic mechanisms produce significant morbidity. *Am J Kidney Dis.* 1997;29(2):291-302.

318. Verove C, Maisonneuve N, El Azouzi A, et al. Effect of the correction of metabolic acidosis on nutritional status in elderly patients with chronic renal failure. *J Ren Nutr.* 2002;12(4):224-228.

319. Sebastian A, Morris Jr RC. Improved mineral balance and skeletal metabolism in postmenopausal women treated with potassium bicarbonate. *N Engl J Med.* 1994;330:1776-1781.

320. Dawson-Hughes B, Harris SS, Palermo NJ, et al. Treatment with potassium bicarbonate lowers calcium excretion and bone resorption in older men and women. *J Clin Endocrinol Metab.* 2009;94(1):96-102.

321. Mulkerrin E, Epstein FH, Clark BA. Aldosterone responses to hyperkalemia in healthy elderly humans. *J Am Soc Nephrol.* 1995;6(5):1459-1462.

322. Bengele HH, Mathias R, Perkins JH, et al. Impaired renal and extrarenal potassium adaptation in old rats. *Kidney Int.* 1983;23(5):684-690.

323. Minaker KL, Rowe JW. Potassium homeostasis during hyperinsulinemia: effect of insulin level, beta-blockade, and age. *Am J Physiol.* 1982;242(6):E373-E377.

324. Ford GA, Blaschke TF, Wiswell R, et al. Effect of aging on changes in plasma potassium during exercise. *J Gerontol.* 1993;48(4):M140-M145.

325. Lewin E, Olgaard K. Klotho, an important new factor for the activity of Ca^{2+} channels, connecting calcium homeostasis, ageing and uraemia. *Nephrol Dial Transplant.* 2006;21(7):1770-1772.

326. Chang Q, Gyftogianni E, van de Graaf SF, et al. Molecular determinants in TRPV5 channel assembly. *J Biol Chem.* 2004;279(52):54304-54311.

327. Imura A, Tsuji Y, Murata M, et al. alpha-Klotho as a regulator of calcium homeostasis. *Science.* 2007;316(5831):1615-1618.

328. van Abel M, Huybers S, Hoenderop JG, et al. Age-dependent alterations in Ca^{2+} homeostasis: role of TRPV5 and TRPV6. *Am J Physiol Renal Physiol.* 2006;291(6):F1177-F1183.

329. Alexander RT, Woudenberg-Vrenken TE, Buurman J, et al. Klotho prevents renal calcium loss. *J Am Soc Nephrol.* 2009;20(11):2371-2379.

330. Kuro-o M. Klotho as a regulator of fibroblast growth factor signaling and phosphate/calcium metabolism. *Curr Opin Nephrol Hypertens.* 2006;15(4):437-441.

331. Xiao NM, Zhang YM, Zheng Q, et al. Klotho is a serum factor related to human aging. *Chin Med J (Engl).* 2004;117(5):742-747.

332. Armbrecht HJ, Zenser TV, Gross CJ, et al. Adaptation to dietary calcium and phosphorus restriction changes with age in the rat. *Am J Physiol.* 1980;239(5):E322-E327.

333. Corman B, Roinel N. Single-nephron filtration rate and proximal reabsorption in aging rats. *Am J Physiol.* 1991;260(1 pt 2):F75-F80.

334. Armbrecht HJ, Zenser TV, Bruns ME, et al. Effect of age on intestinal calcium absorption and adaptation to dietary calcium. *Am J Physiol.* 1979;236(6):E769-E774.

335. Halloran BP, Lonergan ET, Portale AA. Aging and renal responsiveness to parathyroid hormone in healthy men. *J Clin Endocrinol Metab.* 1996;81(6):2192-2197.

336. Mulroney SE, Woda C, Haramati A. Changes in renal phosphate reabsorption in the aged rat. *Proc Soc Exp Biol Med.* 1998;218(1):62-67.

337. Portale AA, Lonergan ET, Tanney DM, et al. Aging alters calcium regulation of serum concentration of parathyroid hormone in healthy men. *Am J Physiol.* 1997;272(1 pt 1):E139-E146.

338. Levi M, Jameson DM, van der Meer BW. Role of BBM lipid composition and fluidity in impaired renal Pi transport in aged rat. *Am J Physiol.* 1989;256(1 pt 2):F85-F94.

339. Kiebzak GM, Sacktor B. Effect of age on renal conservation of phosphate in the rat. *Am J Physiol.* 1986;251(3 pt 2):F399-F407.

340. Chen ML, King RS, Armbrecht HJ. Sodium-dependent phosphate transport in primary cultures of renal tubule cells from young and adult rats. *J Cell Physiol.* 1990;143(3):488-493.

341. Sorribas V, Lotscher M, Loffing J, et al. Cellular mechanisms of the age-related decrease in renal phosphate reabsorption. *Kidney Int.* 1996;50(3):855-863.

342. Levi M, Baird BM, Wilson PV. Cholesterol modulates rat renal brush border membrane phosphate transport. *J Clin Invest.* 1990;85(1):231-237.

343. Breusegem SY, Halaihel N, Inoue M, et al. Acute and chronic changes in cholesterol modulate Na-Pi cotransport activity in OK cells. *Am J Physiol Renal Physiol.* 2005;289(1):F154-F165.

344. Brandis M, Harmeyer J, Kaune R, et al. Phosphate transport in brush-border membranes from control and rachitic pig kidney and small intestine. *J Physiol.* 1987;384:479-490.

345. Kurnik BR, Hruska KA. Effects of 1,25-dihydroxycholecalciferol on phosphate transport in vitamin D–deprived rats. *Am J Physiol.* 1984;247(1 pt 2):F177-F184.

346. Liang CT, Barnes J, Cheng L, et al. Effects of 1,25-$(OH)_2D_3$ administered in vivo on phosphate uptake by isolated chick renal cells. *Am J Physiol.* 1982;242(5):C312-C318.

347. Brasitus TA, Dudeja PK, Eby B, et al. Correction by 1-25-dihydroxycholecalciferol of the abnormal fluidity and lipid composition of enterocyte brush border membranes in vitamin D–deprived rats. *J Biol Chem.* 1986;261(35):16404-16409.

348. Beck LH, Lavizzo-Mourey R. Geriatric hypernatremia [erratum in Ann Intern Med 108(1):161, 1988]. *Ann Intern Med.* 1987;107(5):768-769.

349. Upadhyay A, Jaber BL, Madias NE. Incidence and prevalence of hyponatremia. *Am J Med.* 2006;119(7 suppl 1):S30-S35.

350. Miller M, Hecker MS, Friedlander DA, et al. Apparent idiopathic hyponatremia in an ambulatory geriatric population. *J Am Geriatr Soc.* 1996;44(4):404-408.

351. Clark BA, Shannon RP, Rosa RM, et al. Increased susceptibility to thiazide-induced hyponatremia in the elderly. *J Am Soc Nephrol.* 1994;5(4):1106-1111.

352. Snyder NA, Feigal DW, Arieff AI. Hypernatremia in elderly patients. A heterogeneous, morbid, and iatrogenic entity. *Ann Intern Med.* 1987;107(3):309-319.

353. Beierschmitt WP, Keenan KP, Weiner M. Age-related increased susceptibility of male Fischer 344 rats to acetaminophen nephrotoxicity. *Life Sci.* 1986;39(24):2335-2342.

354. Miura K, Goldstein RS, Morgan DG, et al. Age-related differences in susceptibility to renal ischemia in rats. *Toxicol Appl Pharmacol.* 1987;87(2):284-296.

355. Prasad PV, Epstein FH. Changes in renal medullary pO_2 during water diuresis as evaluated by blood oxygenation level–dependent magnetic resonance imaging: effects of aging and cyclooxygenase inhibition. *Kidney Int.* 1999;55(1):294-298.

356. Boldt J, Brenner T, Lang J, et al. Kidney-specific proteins in elderly patients undergoing cardiac surgery with cardiopulmonary bypass. *Anesth Analg.* 2003;97(6):1582-1589.

357. Xue JL, Daniels F, Star RA, et al. Incidence and mortality of acute renal failure in Medicare beneficiaries, 1992 to 2001. *J Am Soc Nephrol.* 2006;17(4):1135-1142.

358. Pascual J, Orofino L, Liano F, et al. Incidence and prognosis of acute renal failure in older patients. *J Am Geriatr Soc.* 1990;38(1):25-30.

359. Schmitt R, Coca S, Kanbay M, et al. Recovery of kidney function after acute kidney injury in the elderly: a systematic review and meta-analysis. *Am J Kidney Dis.* 2008;52(2):262-271.

360. Griffin MR, Yared A, Ray WA. Nonsteroidal antiinflammatory drugs and acute renal failure in elderly persons. *Am J Epidemiol.* 2000;151(5):488-496.

361. Macias-Nunez JF, Lopez-Novoa JM, Martinez-Maldonado M. Acute renal failure in the aged. *Semin Nephrol.* 1996;16(4):330-338.

362. Pascual J, Liano F. Causes and prognosis of acute renal failure in the very old. Madrid Acute Renal Failure Study Group. *J Am Geriatr Soc.* 1998;46(6):721-725.

363. Cronin RE. Renal failure following radiologic procedures. *Am J Med Sci.* 1989;298(5):342-356.

364. Xiong Y, Yuan LW, Deng HW, et al. Elevated serum endogenous inhibitor of nitric oxide synthase and endothelial dysfunction in aged rats. *Clin Exp Pharmacol Physiol.* 2001;28(10):842-847.

365. Miyazaki H, Matsuoka H, Cooke JP, et al. Endogenous nitric oxide synthase inhibitor: a novel marker of atherosclerosis. *Circulation.* 1999;99(9):1141-1146.

366. Gentric A, Cledes J. Immediate and long-term prognosis in acute renal failure in the elderly. *Nephrol Dial Transplant.* 1991;6(2):86-90.

367. Choudhury D, Ahmed Z. Drug-associated renal dysfunction and injury. *Nat Clin Pract Nephrol.* 2006;2(2):80-91.

368. Sahni V, Choudhury D, Ahmed Z. Chemotherapy-associated renal dysfunction. *Nat Rev Nephrol.* 2009;5(8):450-462.

369. Efstratiadis G, Pateinakis P, Tambakoudis G, et al. Contrast media–induced nephropathy: case report and review of the literature focusing on pathogenesis. *Hippokratia.* 2008;12(2):87-93.

370. Bader BD, Berger ED, Heede MB, et al. What is the best hydration regimen to prevent contrast media–induced nephrotoxicity? *Clin Nephrol.* 2004;62(1):1-7.

371. Weisbord SD, Palevsky PM. Prevention of contrast-induced nephropathy with volume expansion. *Clin J Am Soc Nephrol.* 2008;3(1):273-280.

372. Merten GJ, Burgess WP, Gray LV, et al. Prevention of contrast-induced nephropathy with sodium bicarbonate: a randomized controlled trial. *JAMA.* 2004;291(19):2328-2334.

373. Tepel M, van der Giet M, Schwarzfeld C, et al. Prevention of radiographic-contrast-agent–induced reductions in renal function by acetylcysteine. *N Engl J Med.* 2000;343(3):180-184.

374. Gupta BK, Spinowitz BS, Charytan C, et al. Cholesterol crystal embolization–associated renal failure after therapy with recombinant tissue-type plasminogen activator. *Am J Kidney Dis.* 1993;21(6):659-662.

375. Michel DM, Kelly CJ. Acute interstitial nephritis. *J Am Soc Nephrol.* 1998;9(3):506-515.

376. Clarkson MR, Giblin L, O'Connell FP, et al. Acute interstitial nephritis: clinical features and response to corticosteroid therapy. *Nephrol Dial Transplant.* 2004;19(11):2778-2783.

377. Gonzalez E, Gutierrez E, Galeano C, et al. Early steroid treatment improves the recovery of renal function in patients with drug-induced acute interstitial nephritis. *Kidney Int.* 2008;73(8):940-946.

378. Shariat SF, Milowsky M, Droller MJ. Bladder cancer in the elderly. *Urol Oncol.* 2009;27(6):653-667.
379. De Broe ME, Elseviers MM. Over-the-counter analgesic use. *J Am Soc Nephrol.* 2009;20(10):2098-2103.
380. Akhund L, Quinet RJ, Ishaq S. Celecoxib-related renal papillary necrosis. *Arch Intern Med.* 2003;163(1):114-115.
381. Ishani A, Xue JL, Himmelfarb J, et al. Acute kidney injury increases risk of ESRD among elderly. *J Am Soc Nephrol.* 2009;20(1):223-228.
382. Druml W, Lax F, Grimm G, et al. Acute renal failure in the elderly 1975-1990. *Clin Nephrol.* 1994;41(6):342-349.
383. Pascual J, Liano F, Ortuno J. The elderly patient with acute renal failure. *J Am Soc Nephrol.* 1995;6(2):144-153.
384. Ostchega Y, Dillon CF, Hughes JP, et al. Trends in hypertension prevalence, awareness, treatment, and control in older U.S. adults: data from the National Health and Nutrition Examination Survey 1988 to 2004. *J Am Geriatr Soc.* 2007;55(7):1056-1065.
385. Lewington S, Clarke R, Qizilbash N, et al. Age-specific relevance of usual blood pressure to vascular mortality: a meta-analysis of individual data for one million adults in 61 prospective studies. *Lancet.* 2002;360(9349):1903-1913.
386. Franklin SS, Larson MG, Khan SA, et al. Does the relation of blood pressure to coronary heart disease risk change with aging? The Framingham Heart Study. *Circulation.* 2001;103(9):1245-1249.
387. Dao HH, Essalihi R, Bouvet C, et al. Evolution and modulation of age-related medial elastocalcinosis: impact on large artery stiffness and isolated systolic hypertension. *Cardiovasc Res.* 2005;66(2):307-317.
388. Taddei S, Virdis A, Mattei P, et al. Aging and endothelial function in normotensive subjects and patients with essential hypertension. *Circulation.* 1995;91(7):1981-1987.
389. Franklin SS, Lopez VA, Wong ND, et al. Single versus combined blood pressure components and risk for cardiovascular disease: the Framingham Heart Study. *Circulation.* 2009;119(2):243-250.
390. Franklin SS, Jacobs MJ, Wong ND, et al. Predominance of isolated systolic hypertension among middle-aged and elderly U.S. hypertensives: analysis based on National Health and Nutrition Examination Survey (NHANES) III. *Hypertension.* 2001;37(3):869-874.
391. Klag MJ, Whelton PK, Randall BL, et al. Blood pressure and end-stage renal disease in men. *N Engl J Med.* 1996;334(1):13-18.
392. Young JH, Klag MJ, Muntner P, et al. Blood pressure and decline in kidney function: findings from the Systolic Hypertension in the Elderly Program (SHEP). *J Am Soc Nephrol.* 2002;13(11):2776-2782.
393. Pickering TG, Hall JE, Appel LJ, et al. Recommendations for blood pressure measurement in humans and experimental animals. Part 1: Blood pressure measurement in humans: a statement for professionals from the Subcommittee of Professional and Public Education of the American Heart Association Council on High Blood Pressure Research. *Hypertension.* 2005;45(1):142-161.
394. Chobanian AV, Bakris GL, Black HR, et al. Seventh Report of the Joint National Committee on Prevention, Detection, Evaluation, and Treatment of High Blood Pressure. *Hypertension.* 2003;42(6):1206-1252.
395. Staessen JA, Gasowski J, Wang JG, et al. Risks of untreated and treated isolated systolic hypertension in the elderly: meta-analysis of outcome trials. *Lancet.* 2000;355(9207):865-872.
396. Beckett NS, Peters R, Fletcher AE, et al. Treatment of hypertension in patients 80 years of age or older. *N Engl J Med.* 2008;358(18):1887-1898.
397. Chobanian AV, Bakris GL, Black HR, et al. The Seventh Report of the Joint National Committee on Prevention, Detection, Evaluation, and Treatment of High Blood Pressure: the JNC 7 report. *JAMA.* 2003;289(19):2560-2572.
398. Prevention of stroke by antihypertensive drug treatment in older persons with isolated systolic hypertension. Final results of the Systolic Hypertension in the Elderly Program (SHEP). SHEP Cooperative Research Group. *JAMA.* 1991;265(24):3255-3264.
399. Staessen JA, Fagard R, Thijs L, et al. Randomised double-blind comparison of placebo and active treatment for older patients with isolated systolic hypertension. The Systolic Hypertension in Europe (Syst-Eur) Trial Investigators. *Lancet.* 1997;350(9080):757-764.
400. Jamerson K, Weber MA, Bakris GL, et al. Benazepril plus amlodipine or hydrochlorothiazide for hypertension in high-risk patients. *N Engl J Med.* 2008;359(23):2417-2428.
401. Major outcomes in high-risk hypertensive patients randomized to angiotensin-converting enzyme inhibitor or calcium channel blocker vs. diuretic: the Antihypertensive and Lipid-Lowering Treatment to Prevent Heart Attack Trial (ALLHAT). *JAMA.* 2002;288(23):2981-2997.
402. Applegate WB, Davis BR, Black HR, et al. Prevalence of postural hypotension at baseline in the Systolic Hypertension in the Elderly Program (SHEP) cohort. *J Am Geriatr Soc.* 1991;39(11):1057-1064.
403. Hiitola P, Enlund H, Kettunen R, et al. Postural changes in blood pressure and the prevalence of orthostatic hypotension among home-dwelling elderly aged 75 years or older. *J Hum Hypertens.* 2009;23(1):33-39.
404. Frishman WH. Effects of nonsteroidal anti-inflammatory drug therapy on blood pressure and peripheral edema. *Am J Cardiol.* 2002;89(6A):18D-25D.
405. Mailloux LU, Napolitano B, Bellucci AG, et al. Renal vascular disease causing end-stage renal disease, incidence, clinical correlates, and outcomes: a 20-year clinical experience. *Am J Kidney Dis.* 1994;24(4):622-629.
406. Hansen KJ, Edwards MS, Craven TE, et al. Prevalence of renovascular disease in the elderly: a population-based study. *J Vasc Surg.* 2002;36(3):443-451.
407. Jacobson HR. Ischemic renal disease: an overlooked clinical entity? *Kidney Int.* 1988;34(5):729-743.
408. Brammah A, Robertson S, Tait G, et al. Bilateral renovascular disease causing cardiorenal failure. *BMJ.* 2003;326(7387):489-491.
409. Chabova V, Schirger A, Stanson AW, et al. Outcomes of atherosclerotic renal artery stenosis managed without revascularization. *Mayo Clin Proc.* 2000;75(5):437-444.
410. Zucchelli PC. Hypertension and atherosclerotic renal artery stenosis: diagnostic approach. *J Am Soc Nephrol.* 2002;13(suppl 3):S184-S186.
411. Wheatley K, Ives N, Gray R, et al. Revascularization versus medical therapy for renal-artery stenosis. *N Engl J Med.* 2009;361(20):1953-1962.
412. Hirsch AT, Haskal ZJ, Hertzer NR, et al. ACC/AHA 2005 Practice Guidelines for the management of patients with peripheral arterial disease (lower extremity, renal, mesenteric, and abdominal aortic): a collaborative report from the American Association for Vascular Surgery/Society for Vascular Surgery, Society for Cardiovascular Angiography and Interventions, Society for Vascular Medicine and Biology, Society of Interventional Radiology, and the ACC/AHA Task Force on Practice Guidelines (Writing Committee to Develop Guidelines for the Management of Patients With Peripheral Arterial Disease): endorsed by the American Association of Cardiovascular and Pulmonary Rehabilitation; National Heart, Lung, and Blood Institute; Society for Vascular Nursing; TransAtlantic Inter-Society Consensus; and Vascular Disease Foundation. *Circulation.* 2006;113(11):e463-e654.
413. Moorthy AV, Zimmerman SW. Renal disease in the elderly: clinicopathologic analysis of renal disease in 115 elderly patients. *Clin Nephrol.* 1980;14(5):223-229.
414. Kingswood JC, Banks RA, Tribe CR, et al. Renal biopsy in the elderly: clinicopathological correlations in 143 patients. *Clin Nephrol.* 1984;22(4):183-187.
415. Davison AM, Johnston PA. Idiopathic glomerulonephritis in the elderly. *Contrib Nephrol.* 1993;105:38-48.
416. Simon P, Ramee MP, Autuly V, et al. Epidemiology of primary glomerular diseases in a French region. Variations according to period and age. *Kidney Int.* 1994;46(4):1192-1198.
417. Davison AM, Johnston PA. Glomerulonephritis in the elderly. *Nephrol Dial Transplant.* 1996;11(suppl 9):34-37.
418. Haas M, Spargo BH, Wit EJ, et al. Etiologies and outcome of acute renal insufficiency in older adults: a renal biopsy study of 259 cases. *Am J Kidney Dis.* 2000;35(3):433-447.
419. Nair R, Bell JM, Walker PD. Renal biopsy in patients aged 80 years and older. *Am J Kidney Dis.* 2004;44(4):618-626.
420. Uezono S, Hara S, Sato Y, et al. Renal biopsy in elderly patients: a clinicopathological analysis. *Ren Fail.* 2006;28(7):549-555.
421. Rivera F, Lopez-Gomez JM, Perez-Garcia R. Clinicopathologic correlations of renal pathology in Spain. *Kidney Int.* 2004;66(3):898-904.
422. Glassock RJ. Glomerular disease in the elderly population. *Geriatr Nephrol Urol.* 1998;8(3):149-154.
423. Bergesio F, Bertoni E, Bandini S, et al. Changing pattern of glomerulonephritis in the elderly: a change of prevalence or a different approach? *Contrib Nephrol.* 1993;105:75-80.
424. Moutzouris DA, Herlitz L, Appel GB, et al. Renal biopsy in the very elderly. *Clin J Am Soc Nephrol.* 2009;4(6):1073-1082.
425. Jennette JC. Rapidly progressive crescentic glomerulonephritis. *Kidney Int.* 2003;63(3):1164-1177.
426. Rodriguez-Iturbe B, Musser JM. The current state of poststreptococcal glomerulonephritis. *J Am Soc Nephrol.* 2008;19(10):1855-1864.
427. Prakash J, Singh AK, Saxena RK, et al. Glomerular diseases in the elderly in India. *Int Urol Nephrol.* 2003;35(2):283-288.
428. Haynes RJ, Read S, Collins GP, et al. Presentation and survival of patients with severe acute kidney injury and multiple myeloma: 20-year experience from a single centre. *Nephrol Dial Transplant.* 2009;25(2):419-426.
429. Waldman M, Crew RJ, Valeri A, et al. Adult minimal-change disease: clinical characteristics, treatment, and outcomes. *Clin J Am Soc Nephrol.* 2007;2(3):445-453.
430. Cameron MA, Peri U, Rogers TE, et al. Minimal change disease with acute renal failure: a case against the nephrosarca hypothesis. *Nephrol Dial Transplant.* 2004;19(10):2642-2646.
431. Shin JH, Pyo HJ, Kwon YJ, et al. Renal biopsy in elderly patients: clinicopathological correlation in 117 Korean patients. *Clin Nephrol.* 2001;56(1):19-26.

432. Maruenda J, Kallas H, Lowenthal DT. Nephrotic syndrome in the elderly. *Geriatr Nephrol Urol.* 1999;9(2):123-128.

433. Audard V, Larousserie F, Grimbert P, et al. Minimal change nephrotic syndrome and classical Hodgkin's lymphoma: report of 21 cases and review of the literature. *Kidney Int.* 2006;69(12):2251-2260.

434. Rault R, Holley JL, Banner BF, et al. Glomerulonephritis and non-Hodgkin's lymphoma: a report of two cases and review of the literature. *Am J Kidney Dis.* 1992;20(1):84-89.

435. Nolasco F, Cameron JS, Heywood EF, et al. Adult-onset minimal change nephrotic syndrome: a long-term follow-up. *Kidney Int.* 1986;29(6):1215-1223.

436. Bressler R, Bahl JJ. Principles of drug therapy for the elderly patient. *Mayo Clin Proc.* 2003;78(12):1564-1577.

437. Levey AS, Atkins R, Coresh J, et al. Chronic kidney disease as a global public health problem: approaches and initiatives—a position statement from Kidney Disease Improving Global Outcomes. *Kidney Int.* 2007;72(3):247-259.

438. Zhang QL, Rothenbacher D. Prevalence of chronic kidney disease in population-based studies: systematic review. *BMC Public Health.* 2008;8:117.

439. Stevens LA, Levey AS. Chronic kidney disease in the elderly—how to assess risk. *N Engl J Med.* 2005;352(20):2122-2124.

440. Coresh J, Selvin E, Stevens LA, et al. Prevalence of chronic kidney disease in the United States. *JAMA.* 2007;298(17):2038-2047.

441. Koren-Morag N, Goldbourt U, Tanne D. Renal dysfunction and risk of ischemic stroke or TIA in patients with cardiovascular disease. *Neurology.* 2006;67(2):224-228.

442. Yahalom G, Schwartz R, Schwammenthal Y, et al. Chronic kidney disease and clinical outcome in patients with acute stroke. *Stroke.* 2009;40(4):1296-1303.

443. Shlipak MG, Stehman-Breen C, Fried LF, et al. The presence of frailty in elderly persons with chronic renal insufficiency. *Am J Kidney Dis.* 2004;43(5):861-867.

444. Kurella M, Chertow GM, Fried LF, et al. Chronic kidney disease and cognitive impairment in the elderly: the Health, Aging, and Body Composition study. *J Am Soc Nephrol.* 2005;16(7):2127-2133.

445. Kurella Tamura M, Wadley V, Yaffe K, et al. Kidney function and cognitive impairment in U.S. adults: the Reasons for Geographic and Racial Differences in Stroke (REGARDS) study. *Am J Kidney Dis.* 2008;52(2):227-234.

446. O'Hare AM, Choi AI, Bertenthal D, et al. Age affects outcomes in chronic kidney disease. *J Am Soc Nephrol.* 2007;18(10):2758-2765.

447. Glassock RJ, Winearls C. Screening for CKD with eGFR: doubts and dangers. *Clin J Am Soc Nephrol.* 2008;3(5):1563-1568.

448. Winearls CG, Glassock RJ. Dissecting and refining the staging of chronic kidney disease. *Kidney Int.* 2009;75(10):1009-1014.

449. Poggio ED, Rule AD. A critical evaluation of chronic kidney disease—should isolated reduced estimated glomerular filtration rate be considered a "disease"? *Nephrol Dial Transplant.* 2009;24(3):698-700.

450. Glassock RJ, Winearls C. An epidemic of chronic kidney disease: fact or fiction? *Nephrol Dial Transplant.* 2008;23(4):1117-1121.

451. Jager KJ, van Dijk PC, Dekker FW, et al. The epidemic of aging in renal replacement therapy: an update on elderly patients and their outcomes. *Clin Nephrol.* 2003;60(5):352-360.

452. Stengel B, Billon S, Van Dijk PC, et al. Trends in the incidence of renal replacement therapy for end-stage renal disease in Europe, 1990-1999. *Nephrol Dial Transplant.* 2003;18(9):1824-1833.

453. Kurella M, Covinsky KE, Collins AJ, et al. Octogenarians and nonagenarians starting dialysis in the United States. *Ann Intern Med.* 2007;146(3):177-183.

454. Murtagh FE, Marsh JE, Donohoe P, et al. Dialysis or not? A comparative survival study of patients over 75 years with chronic kidney disease stage 5. *Nephrol Dial Transplant.* 2007;22(7):1955-1962.

455. Letourneau I, Ouimet D, Dumont M, et al. Renal replacement in end-stage renal disease patients over 75 years old. *Am J Nephrol.* 2003;23(2):71-77.

456. Balaskas EV, Yuan ZY, Gupta A, et al. Long-term continuous ambulatory peritoneal dialysis in diabetics. *Clin Nephrol.* 1994;42(1):54-62.

457. Lunde NM, Port FK, Wolfe RA, et al. Comparison of mortality risk by choice of CAPD versus hemodialysis among elderly patients. *Adv Perit Dial.* 1991;7:68-72.

458. Maiorca R, Vonesh EF, Cavalli P, et al. A multicenter, selection-adjusted comparison of patient and technique survivals on CAPD and hemodialysis. *Perit Dial Int.* 1991;11(2):118-127.

459. Bloembergen WE, Port FK, Mauger EA, et al. A comparison of mortality between patients treated with hemodialysis and peritoneal dialysis. *J Am Soc Nephrol.* 1995;6(2):177-183.

460. Winkelmayer WC, Glynn RJ, Mittleman MA, et al. Comparing mortality of elderly patients on hemodialysis versus peritoneal dialysis: a propensity score approach. *J Am Soc Nephrol.* 2002;13(9):2353-2362.

461. Yang X, Fang W, Kothari J, et al. Clinical outcomes of elderly patients undergoing chronic peritoneal dialysis: experiences from one center and a review of the literature. *Int Urol Nephrol.* 2007;39(4):1295-1302.

462. Lok CE, Oliver MJ, Su J, et al. Arteriovenous fistula outcomes in the era of the elderly dialysis population. *Kidney Int.* 2005;67(6):2462-2469.

463. Nissenson AR. Dialysis therapy in the elderly patient. *Kidney Int Suppl.* 1993;40:S51-S57.

464. Ismail N, Hakim RM, Oreopoulos DG, et al. Renal replacement therapies in the elderly. Part 1: Hemodialysis and chronic peritoneal dialysis. *Am J Kidney Dis.* 1993;22(6):759-782.

465. Wolcott DL, Nissenson AR. Quality of life in chronic dialysis patients: a critical comparison of continuous ambulatory peritoneal dialysis (CAPD) and hemodialysis. *Am J Kidney Dis.* 1988;11(5):402-412.

466. St. Peter WL, Clark JL, Levos OM. Drug therapy in haemodialysis patients. Special considerations in the elderly. *Drugs Aging.* 1998;12(6):441-459.

467. Tapson JS, Rodger RS, Mansy H, et al. Renal replacement therapy in patients aged over 60 years. *Postgrad Med J.* 1987;63(746):1071-1077.

468. Westlie L, Umen A, Nestrud S, et al. Mortality, morbidity, and life satisfaction in the very old dialysis patient. *Trans Am Soc Artif Intern Organs.* 1984;30:21-30.

469. Rebollo P, Ortega F, Baltar JM, et al. Is the loss of health-related quality of life during renal replacement therapy lower in elderly patients than in younger patients? *Nephrol Dial Transplant.* 2001;16(8):1675-1680.

470. Kurella Tamura M, Covinsky KE, Chertow GM, et al. Functional status of elderly adults before and after initiation of dialysis. *N Engl J Med.* 2009;361(16):1539-1547.

471. Ismail N, Hakim RM, Helderman JH. Renal replacement therapies in the elderly. Part II: Renal transplantation. *Am J Kidney Dis.* 1994;23(1):1-15.

472. U.S. Organ Procurement and Transplantation Network, Scientific Registry of Transplant Recipients: The 2007 annual report of the OPTN and SRTR: transplant data 1997-2006. Available at: http://www.ustransplant.org/annual_reports. Accessed August 2009.

473. Wolfe RA, Ashby VB, Milford EL, et al. Comparison of mortality in all patients on dialysis, patients on dialysis awaiting transplantation, and recipients of a first cadaveric transplant. *N Engl J Med.* 1999;341(23):1725-1730.

474. Johnson DW, Herzig K, Purdie D, et al. A comparison of the effects of dialysis and renal transplantation on the survival of older uremic patients. *Transplantation.* 2000;69(5):794-799.

475. Oniscu GC, Brown H, Forsythe JL. How great is the survival advantage of transplantation over dialysis in elderly patients? *Nephrol Dial Transplant.* 2004;19(4):945-951.

476. Rao PS, Merion RM, Ashby VB, et al. Renal transplantation in elderly patients older than 70 years of age: results from the Scientific Registry of Transplant Recipients. *Transplantation.* 2007;83(8):1069-1074.

477. Savoye E, Tamarelle D, Chalem Y, et al. Survival benefits of kidney transplantation with expanded criteria deceased donors in patients aged 60 years and over. *Transplantation.* 2007;84(12):1618-1624.

478. De La Vega LS, Torres A, Bohorquez HE, et al. Patient and graft outcomes from older living kidney donors are similar to those from younger donors despite lower GFR. *Kidney Int.* 2004;66(4):1654-1661.

479. Gill J, Bunnapradist S, Danovitch GM, et al. Outcomes of kidney transplantation from older living donors to older recipients. *Am J Kidney Dis.* 2008;52(3):541-552.

480. Gill JS, Gill J, Rose C, et al. The older living kidney donor: part of the solution to the organ shortage. *Transplantation.* 2006;82(12):1662-1666.

481. Danovitch GM, Gill J, Bunnapradist S. Immunosuppression of the elderly kidney transplant recipient. *Transplantation.* 2007;84(3):285-291.

482. Martins PN, Pratschke J, Pascher A, et al. Age and immune response in organ transplantation. *Transplantation.* 2005;79(2):127-132.

483. Nyberg G, Nilsson B, Hallste G, et al. Renal transplantation in elderly patients: survival and complications. *Transplant Proc.* 1993;25(1 pt 2):1062-1063.

484. Tesi RJ, Elkhammas EA, Davies EA, et al. Renal transplantation in older people. *Lancet.* 1994;343(8895):461-464.

485. Morris GE, Jamieson NV, Small J, et al. Cadaveric renal transplantation in elderly recipients: is it worthwhile? *Nephrol Dial Transplant.* 1991;6(11):887-892.

486. Kappes U, Schanz G, Gerhardt U, et al. Influence of age on the prognosis of renal transplant recipients. *Am J Nephrol.* 2001;21(4):259-263.

487. Meier-Kriesche HU, Ojo A, Hanson J, et al. Increased immunosuppressive vulnerability in elderly renal transplant recipients. *Transplantation.* 2000;69(5):885-889.

488. Woodford HJ, George J. Diagnosis and management of urinary tract infection in hospitalized older people. *J Am Geriatr Soc.* 2009;57(1):107-114.

489. Pabich WL, Fihn SD, Stamm WE, et al. Prevalence and determinants of vaginal flora alterations in postmenopausal women. *J Infect Dis.* 2003;188(7):1054-1058.

490. McMurdo ME, Gillespie ND. Urinary tract infection in old age: over-diagnosed and over-treated. *Age Ageing.* 2000;29(4):297-298.
491. Baldassarre JS, Kaye D. Special problems of urinary tract infection in the elderly. *Med Clin North Am.* 1991;75(2):375-390.
492. Nicolle LE. Urinary tract infection in geriatric and institutionalized patients. *Curr Opin Urol.* 2002;12(1):51-55.
493. Juthani-Mehta M, Quagliarello V, Perrelli E, et al. Clinical features to identify urinary tract infection in nursing home residents: a cohort study. *J Am Geriatr Soc.* 2009;57(6):963-970.
494. Nicolle LE, Bradley S, Colgan R, et al. Infectious Diseases Society of America guidelines for the diagnosis and treatment of asymptomatic bacteriuria in adults. *Clin Infect Dis.* 2005;40(5):643-654.
495. Nicolle LE. Urinary tract infections in the elderly. *Clin Geriatr Med.* 2009;25(3):423-436.
496. Abrutyn E, Mossey J, Berlin JA, et al. Does asymptomatic bacteriuria predict mortality and does antimicrobial treatment reduce mortality in elderly ambulatory women? *Ann Intern Med.* 1994;120(10): 827-833.
497. Abrutyn E, Berlin J, Mossey J, et al. Does treatment of asymptomatic bacteriuria in older ambulatory women reduce subsequent symptoms of urinary tract infection? *J Am Geriatr Soc.* 1996;44(3):293-295.
498. Nicolle LE, Mayhew WJ, Bryan L. Prospective randomized comparison of therapy and no therapy for asymptomatic bacteriuria in institutionalized elderly women. *Am J Med.* 1987;83(1):27-33.
499. Loeb M, Bentley DW, Bradley S, et al. Development of minimum criteria for the initiation of antibiotics in residents of long-term-care facilities: results of a consensus conference. *Infect Control Hosp Epidemiol.* 2001;22(2):120-124.
500. Nicolle LE. Catheter-related urinary tract infection. *Drugs Aging.* 2005;22(8):627-639.
501. Nicolle LE. Resistant pathogens in urinary tract infections. *J Am Geriatr Soc.* 2002;50(suppl 7):S230-S235.
502. Vogel T, Verreault R, Gourdeau M, et al. Optimal duration of antibiotic therapy for uncomplicated urinary tract infection in older women: a double-blind randomized controlled trial. *CMAJ.* 2004;170(4):469-473.
503. Schaeffer AJ. Clinical practice. Chronic prostatitis and the chronic pelvic pain syndrome. *N Engl J Med.* 2006;355(16):1690-1698.
504. Carrim ZI, Murchison JT. The prevalence of simple renal and hepatic cysts detected by spiral computed tomography. *Clin Radiol.* 2003;58(8):626-629.
505. Nahm AM, Ritz E. The simple renal cyst. *Nephrol Dial Transplant.* 2000;15(10):1702-1704.
506. Ravine D, Gibson RN, Donlan J, et al. An ultrasound renal cyst prevalence survey: specificity data for inherited renal cystic diseases. *Am J Kidney Dis.* 1993;22(6):803-807.
507. Terada N, Ichioka K, Matsuta Y, et al. The natural history of simple renal cysts. *J Urol.* 2002;167(1):21-23.
508. Papanicolaou N, Pfister RC, Yoder IC. Spontaneous and traumatic rupture of renal cysts: diagnosis and outcome. *Radiology.* 1986;160(1):99-103.
509. Chin HJ, Ro H, Lee HJ, et al. The clinical significances of simple renal cyst: is it related to hypertension or renal dysfunction? *Kidney Int.* 2006;70(8):1468-1473.
510. Babka JC, Cohen MS, Sode J. Solitary intrarenal cyst causing hypertension. *N Engl J Med.* 1974;291(7):343-344.
511. Clayman RV, Surya V, Miller RP, et al. Pursuit of the renal mass. Is ultrasound enough? *Am J Med.* 1984;77(2):218-223.
512. Bosniak MA. The current radiological approach to renal cysts. *Radiology.* 1986;158(1):1-10.
513. Israel GM, Bosniak MA. An update of the Bosniak renal cyst classification system. *Urology.* 2005;66(3):484-488.
514. Israel GM, Hindman N, Bosniak MA. Evaluation of cystic renal masses: comparison of CT and MR imaging by using the Bosniak classification system. *Radiology.* 2004;231(2):365-371.
515. Balci NC, Semelka RC, Patt RH, et al. Complex renal cysts: findings on MR imaging. *AJR Am J Roentgenol.* 1999;172(6):1495-1500.

Evaluation of the Patient with Kidney Disease

Approach to the Patient with Kidney Disease

Michael Emmett, Andrew Z. Fenves, and John C. Schwartz

Readers of this chapter are assumed already to be competent medical historians and to be very familiar with the essentials of the general physical examination. Furthermore, many of the topics that are briefly reviewed in this chapter are addressed in much greater detail in other parts of this textbook. Consequently, the focus here is on certain features of the history, physical examination, and laboratory testing that might be of specific utility to nephrologists and nephrology trainees. The chapter is divided into nine broad areas of kidney disorder and addresses those features of greatest importance to the early diagnostic and therapeutic phases of the patient's workup.

Hematuria

Hematuria is the excretion of abnormal amounts of red blood cells (RBCs) into the urine. Normal individuals excrete about 1 million RBCs per day in their urine. When translated to the sediment of a spun urine specimen, this equates to about 1 to 3 RBCs per high-power field (HPF). Therefore excretion of more than 3 RBCs per HPF is abnormal and may warrant further evaluation. Asymptomatic "microscopic hematuria" is very common; it may be detected in up to 13% of adults.[1] Although it is most often of no consequence, hematuria can be a sign of serious disease and should never be ignored. Gross hematuria occurs when enough blood is present in the urine to turn it red or brown. Although microscopic and gross hematuria are generally caused by the same conditions, there are marked differences in the relative frequencies with which various pathologic conditions manifest these two presentations. Therefore, the diagnostic approaches to these two conditions are different. Routine screening of healthy individuals for the presence of hematuria is not recommended by the U.S. Preventive Services Task Force.[2] However, asymptomatic microscopic hematuria may be detected when a urinalysis is performed during the evaluation of a patient for nonurinary complaints. Furthermore, despite official recommendations, urinalyses are nonetheless frequently ordered as a screening test. When such testing reveals hematuria, the person's age, gender, race, medical history, and physical findings should be considered in deciding whether to further evaluate this finding and, if so, in determining the most appropriate diagnostic studies and the sequence in which they should be performed. Asymptomatic microscopic hematuria should be confirmed in at least two of three midstream clean-catch voidings before the physician embarks on a potentially expensive workup, which can have significant adverse impact and complications. If microscopic hematuria spontaneously resolves, evaluation decisions are strongly influenced by the clinician's index of suspicion (see later). Microscopic hematuria associated with symptoms such as urinary frequency or pain is more worrisome and mandates further evaluation. Gross hematuria, especially if clots are passed, usually indicates a urologic source of bleeding. Even a single episode of gross hematuria mandates evaluation. The most common cause of gross hematuria in young women (<40 years of age) is urinary tract infection (UTI). Malignancy must be strongly considered and ruled out by appropriate studies in older patients.[3] Brown, "Coca-Cola"–colored, or smoky urine with RBCs present on microscopy is very suggestive of a glomerular source of bleeding.

History and Review of Systems

Three major factors influencing the workup are the patient's gender, race, and age. The common causes of hematuria in children and young adults are much different than those in older individuals. Hematuria in adults older than 40 years (some experts propose an age cutoff of older than 50 years) must be considered a sign of malignancy (of the bladder, upper urinary tract, or kidney) until proved otherwise. Although malignancy is much less frequent in young patients with hematuria, a Wilms' tumor should be considered. Bladder cancer is much more common in men and in whites. Hypercalciuria, and less commonly hyperuricosuria, cause hematuria frequently in children but less commonly in adults. Hematuria due to UTI is much more common in women, whereas older men may bleed from the prostate. In women, cyclic gross hematuria concurrent with the menses raises the strong possibility of genitourinary (GU) tract endometriosis. The combination of hematuria with fever, dysuria, or flank pain, or a prior history of these symptoms raises the likelihood of infection, stones, or malignancy. Colicky pain suggests ureteral obstruction from a stone, blood clot, or sloughed renal papilla. This is especially the case if the pain radiates to the testicle or labia. A family history of renal dysfunction or renal stones should be sought. When a patient with hematuria has family members with renal failure, polycystic kidney disease or Alport's disease should be considered. Familial hearing loss, especially in male relatives, also suggests Alport's disease. A very common cause of otherwise unexplained asymptomatic familial hematuria is thin basement membrane disease.[4] Sickle cell trait is a very common cause of hematuria in African Americans. Sickle cell anemia can also cause hematuria.[5]

Hematuria sometimes occurs after vigorous exercise or participation in contact or noncontact sports.[6] Mechanisms include direct recurrent trauma to the bladder or kidneys and pathologic renal hemodynamic effects. However, the fact that hematuria occurs after completing a long bicycle ride or running a marathon does not exclude the possibility of other potentially serious pathologic conditions, and generally a complete evaluation is necessary. Exercise-related hemoglobinuria, such as march hemoglobinuria, and postexercise myoglobinuria result in excretion of globin pigments

and positive results on dipstick testing without RBCs in the urine.

Travel history may be very important as, for example, when hematuria develops in patients who have traveled to areas where *Schistosoma haematobium* infection or tuberculosis is endemic. Although otherwise unexplained bleeding into the urine can occur in patients with hereditary or acquired coagulation disorders or in patients who take therapeutic anticoagulants, these conditions and drugs should not preclude consideration of other important underlying etiologies. Bleeding disorders and anticoagulants will cause any pathologic GU structures such as malignancies to bleed more readily. This is especially common in older patients.[7] A history of cigarette smoking (or second-hand smoke exposure) increases the risk of bladder cancer twofold to fourfold.[8] Occupational exposure to aniline dyes and aromatic amines and amides; treatment with some chemotherapeutic agents such as cyclophosphamide and mitotane; and radiation to the pelvis increase the risk for uroepithelial cancers. In the past, long-term use of analgesics did increase the risk of bladder cancer, but this was probably due to the presence of phenacetin, which has now been removed from these medications. Indeed, the use of aspirin and other nonsteroidal antiinflammatory drugs (NSAIDs) has been shown to reduce the likelihood of bladder cancer in some epidemiologic studies.[9]

A recent history of pharyngitis followed by hematuria raises the possibility of glomerulonephritis with synpharyngitic bleeding. Chronic glomerulonephritis, most commonly immunoglobulin A (IgA) nephropathy, is often exacerbated by an upper respiratory tract infection and may result in gross hematuria. This is distinct from poststreptococcal glomerulonephritis, which occurs 2 to 6 weeks following the infection.

With gross hematuria, it is useful to determine if the bleeding is more pronounced at the very beginning or at the termination of voiding. Although formal "three-glass" urine collections are rarely performed, a history of initiation hematuria suggests a urethral source, whereas termination hematuria is suggestive of bladder neck or prostatic urethra pathology. Blood clots in some the urine usually denote structural urologic pathology.

Physical Examination

Evaluation of blood pressure and volume status is especially important when glomerulonephritis is a consideration. If palpation of the abdomen reveals a mass, a renal tumor or hydronephrosis may exist. A palpable bladder after voiding indicates obstruction or retention. Atrial fibrillation raises the possibility of renal embolic infarction, especially if the patient has flank pain. Costovertebral angle tenderness is also suggestive of pyelonephritis, nephrolithiasis, or ureteropelvic junction obstruction. A bruit over the kidney suggests a vascular cause. Careful genital and rectal examination is necessary to diagnose prostatitis, prostate cancer, epididymitis, meatal stenosis, and other structural causes of hematuria.

Laboratory Tests

A diagnosis of gross hematuria is suggested by red or brown urine. Only about 1 mL of blood causes 1 L of urine to become red. However, many substances other than RBCs can produce red or brown urine. Many chemicals, medications, and food metabolites can produce a spectrum of urine colors. A chemical test for hemoglobin is very helpful in distinguishing among these possibilities. The most commonly used method of testing the urine for blood is the urine test strip or dipstick, which utilizes the peroxidase-like activity of hemoglobin to generate a color change. The test strip does not react with most nonhemoglobin pigments that can color the urine. In addition to detecting the hemoglobin within RBCs, however, the test reaction yields a positive result with free hemoglobin and myoglobin. Also, hypochlorite solutions, which are sometimes used to clean urine collection containers, can produce a false-positive test strip reaction for blood. Therefore, a positive test strip result must be followed by a microscopic examination of the urine to confirm the presence of RBCs. Some of the causes of red or brown urine are shown in Table 24-1.

It is crucial to separate hematuria caused by glomerular abnormalities from bleeding due to other pathologic kidney conditions (tumors or cysts) or pathologic processes distal to the glomerulus (interstitial disease, stones, or tumors, or other processes affecting the renal pelvis, ureters, bladder, urethra, prostate, or other lower GU system structures). When blood originates from glomeruli, the RBCs pass through the length of the renal tubules, where they are subjected to marked changes in osmolality, ionic strength, pH, and other forces. Compression of the RBCs together with urine proteins creates RBC casts (Figure 24-1), and identification of these casts on microscopic examination is excellent evidence of glomerular bleeding. Although quite specific, RBC casts often are not seen even with definite glomerular bleeding. A more common helpful finding in glomerular bleeding is the identification of dysmorphic RBCs of varying shape and sizes with blebs, budding, and especially the vesicle-shaped protrusions that characterize acanthocytes (i.e., "Mickey Mouse ears"; see Figure 24-1). For dysmorphic RBCs to be an excellent indicator of glomerular bleeding, most of the urine RBCs should be affected.[10] Acanthocytes are quite specific, however, and if they represent more than 5% of the RBCs, this is very a suggestive sign of glomerular bleeding. Another indication that bleeding is more likely of glomerular origin is coexistent significant proteinuria (>0.5 g/day or >0.5 g protein per gram of creatinine). The presence of pyuria with hematuria suggests inflammation or infection and warrants a urine culture. Table 24-2 highlights some of the features that can be used to differentiate glomerular and nonglomerular, or urologic, hematuria. Urine cytologic analysis is indicated when otherwise unexplained hematuria is documented. It has good specificity when results are positive and a sensitivity of about 80% for bladder cancer but a much lower sensitivity for upper tract malignancy.[11]

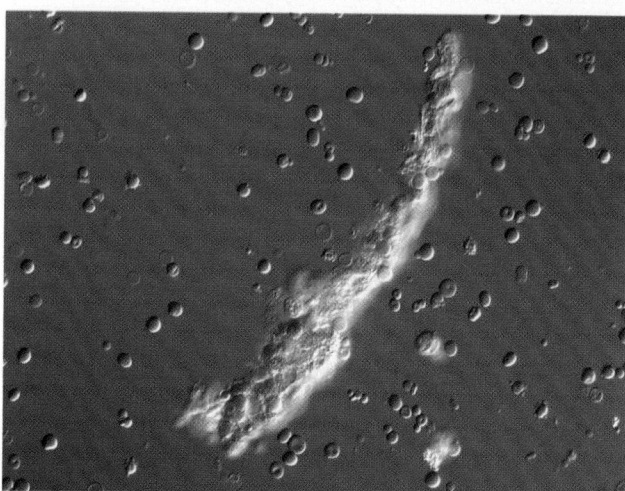

FIGURE 24-1 Red blood cell cast and acanthocytes consistent with glomerular bleeding (diffusion interference contrast optics). (Courtesy of Dr. Rajiv Agarwal, Nephrology Division, Indiana University School of Medicine.)

TABLE 24-1 Causes of Red or Brown Urine

ENDOGENOUS SUBSTANCES	FOODS	DRUGS
Red blood cells	Artificial food coloring	Adriamycin
Hemoglobin	Beets	Chloroquine
Myoglobin	Blackberries	Deferoxamine
Bilirubin	Blueberries	Levodopa
Porphyrins	Fava beans	Methyldopa
Melanin	Paprika	Metronidazole
	Rhubarb	Nitrofurantoin
		Phenazopyridine (Pyridium)
		Phenolphthalein
		Phenytoin
		Prochlorperazine
		Quinine
		Rifampin
		Sulfonamides

TABLE 24-2 Differentiation of Glomerular from Urologic Bleeding

	GLOMERULAR HEMATURIA	NONGLOMERULAR/ UROTHELIAL/ UROLOGIC HEMATURIA
Urine color	Dark red, brown, cola colored, smoky	Bright red
Clots	–	+
Proteinuria	+	–
Red blood cell morphology	Dysmorphic (especially acanthocytes)	Isomorphic
Hypertension	+	–
Edema	+	–
Urinary voiding symptoms	–	+
Back pain, flank pain	+	+
Renal function	Reduced	Normal
Family history	+	+
Trauma	–	+
Upper respiratory tract infection	+	–
Fever, rash	+	–

Imaging

When hematuria is not believed to be of glomerular origin, then computed tomography (CT) with and without intravenous (IV) contrast is currently the preferred initial imaging modality to evaluate microscopic and gross hematuria and has largely replaced intravenous pyelography (IVP). CT urography has excellent sensitivity for stones, identifies most kidney tumors, and reveals other non–GU tract abdominal pathologic processes. The major downside of a CT scan is the need for IV contrast and the significant radiation exposure. If CT cannot be done, then renal ultrasonography is the next best initial imaging test. If the explanation for hematuria is not evident on the initial study, the next diagnostic imaging test to perform is cystoscopy. Direct visualization of the bladder requires cystoscopy. Abnormal areas or lesions can be biopsied. Performing cystoscopy at the time of bleeding may localize the bleeding site. If no abnormality is noted and there is any suspicion of upper tract disease, retrograde pyelography may be performed. One diagnostic approach is illustrated in Figure 24-2. A major decision branch is based on the patient's age and other risk factors for bladder cancer. There is controversy about the specific age to be used for diagnostic stratification. Some experts believe it should be 40 years and others argue for 50 years. Figure 24-3 shows the frequency of renal, uroepithelial, and bladder cancers separated by gender and age in 1930 patients evaluated for hematuria.[3]

Nephritic Syndrome

Classic nephritic syndrome is characterized by glomerular hematuria and an active urine sediment, manifested by dysmorphic RBCs (especially acanthocytes) and RBC casts, and often white blood cells (WBCs) and WBC casts. In general, these are the result of an inflammatory process in the glomerulus. Usually, glomerular filtration rate (GFR) is reduced, and variable degrees of hypertension, oliguria, and edema occur. Proteinuria is common but often of relatively low magnitude. In many cases the degree of proteinuria is limited by the accompanying reduction in GFR. However,

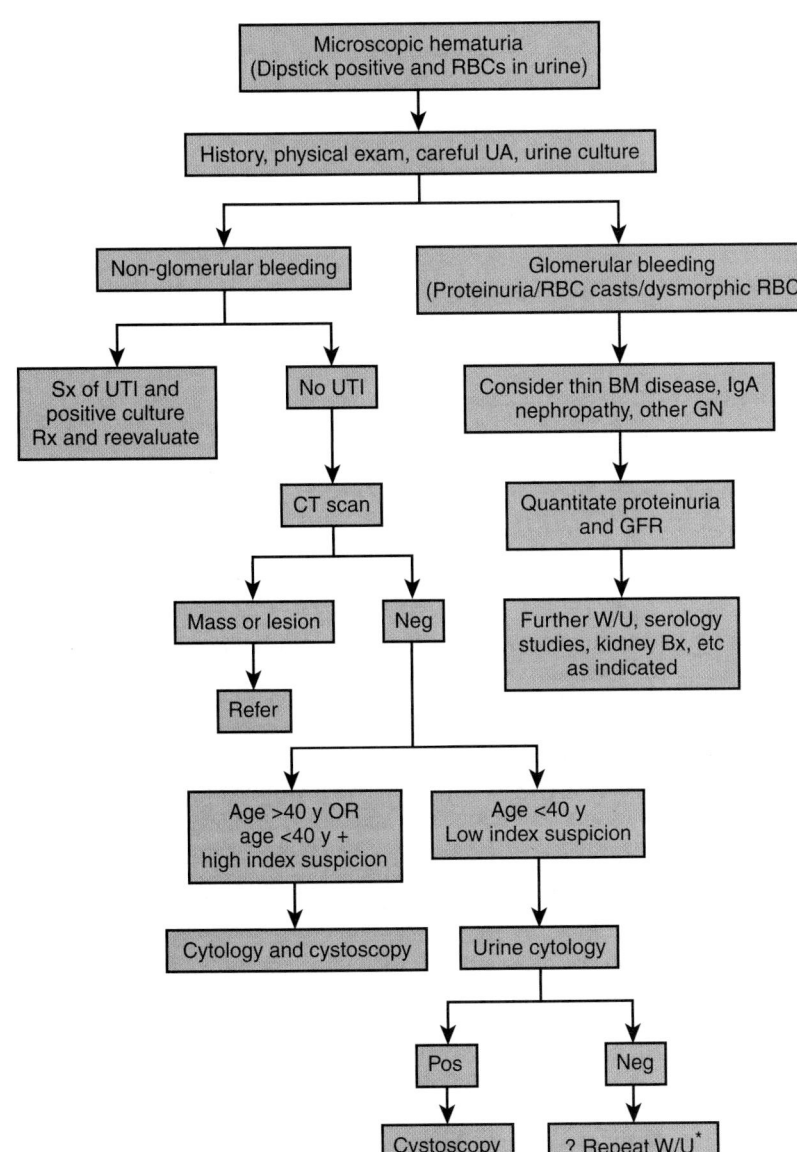

FIGURE 24-2 Diagnostic scheme for evaluation of microscopic hematuria. *Workup should be repeated if the patient develops new symptoms of gross hematuria.

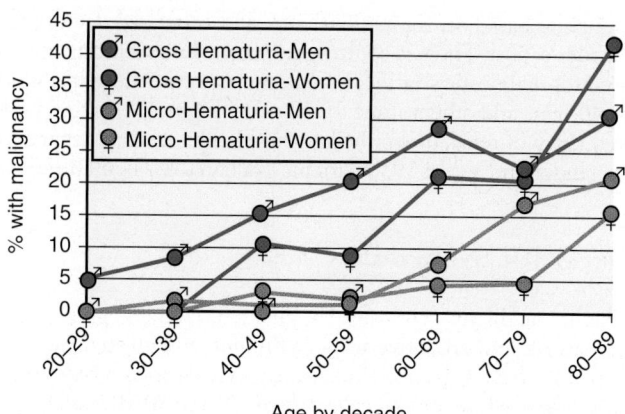

FIGURE 24-3 Prospective analysis of the risk of malignancy in 1930 patients undergoing workup for hematuria. (Adapted from Khadra MH, Pickard RS, Charlton M, et al: A prospective analysis of 1,930 patients with hematuria to evaluate current diagnostic practice, *J Urol* 163:524-527, 2000.)

high-grade proteinuria and even full-blown nephrotic syndrome can coexist with nephritic syndrome in some patients. The hematuria can be sporadic, intermittent, or persistent. It can be microscopic or gross. Isolated glomerular hematuria without inflammation (e.g., that which occurs with thin basement membrane disease) is generally not considered to be the result of a nephritic process. The character of the glomerular hematuria does not always predict the underlying cause of the disorder, nor does it predict the long-term renal outcome of the process.

Nephritic syndrome can occur as an isolated renal process or as a feature of a systemic disease or a hereditary disorder. Glomerular hematuria due to nephritic syndrome must be distinguished from bleeding caused by other kidney, interstitial, or lower GU tract pathology, including stones, benign or malignant mass lesions, and infections. The features that help differentiate these classes of hematuria have been discussed in the previous hematuria section and are listed in Table 24-2. When nephritic hematuria is identified, additional renal evaluation is required.

History and Review of Systems

The patient's history often helps to distinguish glomerular hematuria from urothelial or urologic hematuria. Glomerular hematuria, when visible, is often described as dark brown, tea or cola colored, or smoky as opposed to the overtly red color often seen with urologic pathology. Clots are almost never formed with glomerular hematuria. The patient may also note that the urine has become foamy as a result of the excretion of albumin, which has a soaplike action and reduces the surface tension of urine. Urinary voiding symptoms are distinctly uncommon. Back, flank, or abdominal pain does not distinguish glomerular hematuria from urothelial hematuria. There may be a history of an antecedent upper respiratory tract or skin infection in patients with poststreptococcal glomerulonephritis (postpharyngitic hematuria). In other patients with an underlying form of chronic glomerulonephritis, such as IgA glomerulonephritis, gross hematuria may occur simultaneously with, or immediately after, an episode of pharyngitis

(synpharyngitic hematuria). There may be a family history of glomerular disease. A history of hypertension, fluid retention, and/or edema formation suggests glomerular hematuria, particularly if renal function is reduced. Fever, skin rash, and joint symptoms raise the possibility of a systemic disease causing glomerular hematuria. Hearing loss and visual symptoms related to lens abnormalities can be seen with Alport's disease. Hemoptysis raises the possibility of vasculitis or anti–glomerular basement membrane (anti-GBM) disease.

Physical Examination

Hypertension is very frequent with glomerular hematuria. Most often this is due to renal salt retention and volume expansion. The salt retention is caused by enhanced reabsorption in the distal nephron, especially the cortical collecting tubule.[12] The renin-angiotensin-aldosterone system in most patients with nephritic syndrome is functioning normally.[13] Malignant hypertension with vital organ injury occurs in some patients. Careful eye-retinal examination may yield a specific diagnosis. High-frequency sensorineural hearing loss strongly suggests Alport's disease. Typical skin rashes and other abnormalities can be seen in systemic lupus erythematous, vasculitis, Fabry's disease, and Henoch-Schönlein purpura. Joint findings may suggest a rheumatologic–collagen vascular disease or vasculitis. Examination of the suprapubic area, the back, or the flanks is generally unrevealing.

Laboratory Tests

Urine Studies

The hallmark of nephritic syndrome is glomerular hematuria. Hematuria is most easily recognized by a positive result on a urine dipstick test for blood. See the preceding section on hematuria for further discussion. Proteinuria is a frequent accompaniment to hematuria in patients with nephritic syndrome but is usually absent in patients with urothelial hematuria. The proteinuria can range from low grade (<500 to 1000 mg/day) to overt nephrotic levels (>3000 mg/day). Protein excretion can be quantitated with 24-hour urine collection. Alternatively, a spot urine protein/creatinine ratio can be determined, which gives a reasonable estimate of the magnitude of proteinuria.[14]

Microscopic examination of the urine in the nephritic state reveals a variable number of free RBCs. Often a small pellet of RBCs can be noted at the bottom of a test tube of centrifuged urine. RBC casts are the definitive finding in the nephritic syndrome but very often cannot be seen. A more commonly identified characteristic of glomerular bleeding is dysmorphic urine RBCs with blebs, budding, and vesicle-shaped protrusions[10] (see Figure 24-1). Examination of the urine sediment with phase-contrast microscopy can be especially helpful. Kidney inflammation also generates pyuria and WBC casts. Hyaline casts can be seen, especially with marked proteinuria.

Blood Studies

Routine laboratory studies should include a complete blood count (CBC), electrolyte levels, blood urea nitrogen (BUN) concentration, creatinine concentration, and liver panel.

TABLE 24-3 Glomerular Filtration Rate (GFR)/Creatinine Clearance Estimating Formulas

Cockcroft-Gault Equation

(estimates creatinine clearance)

$$eGFR = \frac{(140 - age) \times wt\ (kg)}{Cr \times 72} \times .85 \ (if\ female)$$

Abbreviated MDRD Equation

(estimates body surface area–corrected GFR in mL/min/1.73 m^2)

$$eGFR = 186 \times Cr^{-1.154} \times Age^{-0.203} \times 1.21 \ (if\ black) \times .742 \ (if\ female)$$

Cr, Serum creatinine concentration (measured as mg/dL); *eGFR,* estimated glomerular filtration rate; *MDRD,* Modification of Diet in Renal Disease study.
   Data from National Kidney Foundation: K/DOQI clinical practice guidelines for chronic kidney disease: evaluation, classification, and stratification, *Am J Kidney Dis* 39(2 suppl 1):S1-S266, 2002.

TABLE 24-4 Complement Levels in Acute Nephritic Syndromes

Low Serum Complement Levels

Systemic Diseases (Low C3 and C4)

Systemic lupus erythematosus

Cryoglobulinemia (hepatitis C)

Bacterial endocarditis

Shunt nephritis

Renal Localized Diseases

Acute poststreptococcal glomerulonephritis (low C3; normal C4)

Membranoproliferative glomerulonephritis

   Type I (low C3 and C4)

   Type II (dense deposit disease) (low C3; normal C4)

Normal Serum Complement Levels

Systemic Diseases

Polyarteritis nodosa

Antineutrophil cytoplasmic antibody–positive granulomatosis vasculitis (Wegener's granulomatosis)

Hypersensitivity vasculitis

Henoch-Schönlein purpura

Goodpasture's syndrome

Renal Localized Diseases

Immunoglobulin A nephropathy

Rapidly progressive glomerulonephritis

Anti–glomerular basement membrane disease isolated to kidney

Pauci-immune glomerulonephritis (kidney localized)

Sedimentation rate and C-reactive protein level are often elevated regardless of the cause of nephritic syndrome. A determination of the GFR is required. Usually this is accomplished with a quantitative urine collection for measurement of creatinine clearance. Iothalamate clearance, if available, provides the most accurate measurement. Various formulas, such as the Cockcroft-Gault equation or one of the equations developed by the Modification of Diet in Renal Disease (MDRD) study, can estimate the GFR based on a single and presumably stable serum creatinine measurement (Table 24-3). However, all methods that rely on a single serum creatinine measurement will give erroneous results when renal function is rapidly changing and the serum creatinine concentration is not relatively stable.

Measurements of complement levels can be very helpful in patients with nephritic syndrome.[15] It is generally best to begin with a measure of total hemolytic complement (CH$_{50}$) and then proceed to measurement of C3 (a component of both the classic and alternative complement pathways) and C4 (a component of the classic pathway only). Table 24-4 separates the various forms of acute nephritic glomerulonephritis into those with normal and those with reduced complement levels. Low C3 with normal C4 levels suggest poststreptococcal glomerulonephritis or membranoproliferative glomerulonephritis, whereas low C3 and C4 levels are more consistent with postinfectious glomerulonephritis, systemic lupus erythematous, hepatitis C–associated membranoproliferative glomerulonephritis (type I), or mixed cryoglobulinemia.

Other serologic studies, mainly to measure various autoantibodies, are ordered when specific underlying systemic diseases are considered the possible cause. The antinuclear antibody (ANA) and anti-DNA, anti-Smith, and anti-Rho antibodies help confirm the diagnosis of systemic lupus erythematosus and other collagen vascular diseases. The perinuclear antineutrophil cytoplasmic antibody (P-ANCA) and cytoplasmic antineutrophil cytoplasmic antibody (C-ANCA) tests help to establish a diagnosis of vasculitis. Anti-GBM antibodies are seen in patients with Goodpasture's syndrome. A number of infectious diseases can produce an acute nephritic syndrome. It is also important to consider viral hepatitis, both B and C, as well as human immunodeficiency virus (HIV) infection and syphilis and, if plausible, to send blood specimens for diagnostic studies. Other infectious diseases that must always be considered are infectious endocarditis or another persistent bacterial infection such as an abscess or infected vascular

shunt. Blood cultures must be ordered for all patients with otherwise unexplained fever, heart murmurs, or leukocytosis.

The commonly ordered laboratory studies for patients with nephritic syndrome are shown in Table 24-5.

Imaging

Renal size is a very important parameter to define in patients with nephritic syndrome. This is most easily accomplished with renal ultrasonography. Although normal-sized kidneys do not definitively predict reversibility (even irreversible end-stage kidneys can be of normal size as a result of swelling or infiltration in patients with diabetes mellitus or amyloidosis), small kidneys do indicate that irreversible fibrosis and atrophy are probably present. The assessment of renal size is therefore especially important for determining renal prognosis and making decisions regarding renal biopsy. If the kidneys are small (<9 cm in a normal-sized adult) the likelihood of reversible disease decreases markedly, and the difficulty and risk of the biopsy procedure increase.

Renal Biopsy

Patients with glomerular hematuria who have normal blood pressure, normal renal function, and minimal proteinuria rarely require a renal biopsy unless the clinical presentation

TABLE 24-5 Blood Studies for Acute Nephritic Syndrome
Routine
Complete blood count
Electrolyte levels
Blood urea nitrogen and creatinine concentrations
Liver function studies
Complement levels (total hemolytic complement [CH_{50}], C3, C4)
As Clinical Findings Suggest
Anti-DNA antibody test
Antineutrophil cytoplasmic antibody (ANCA) titer
Anti–glomerular basement membrane antibody test
Antistreptolysin O titer or streptozyme test
Cryoglobulin titer
Hepatitis B and C antibody assay and viral load determination
Human immunodeficiency virus test
Blood cultures

TABLE 24-6 Causes of Secondary Nephrotic Syndrome
Systemic Diseases
Diabetes mellitus
Systemic lupus erythematosus
Amyloidosis
Carcinoma
Lymphoma and myeloma
Preeclampsia
Drugs
Gold
Antibiotics
Nonsteroidal antiinflammatory drugs
Penicillamine
Heroin
Infections
Human immunodeficiency virus infection
Hepatitis B and C
Malaria
Syphilis
Congenital/Inherited Disorders
Alport's syndrome
Congenital nephrotic syndrome
Nail-patella syndrome

suggests an underlying systemic illness causing secondary glomerular disease. Renal biopsy may be helpful when glomerular hematuria is associated with abnormal renal function and is especially so when it is important to establish the specific diagnosis to guide therapy.[16] When renal function is decreasing rapidly (rapidly progressive glomerulonephritis) and a nephritic picture exists, the biopsy may need to be obtained very rapidly.

Nephrotic Syndrome

Nephrotic syndrome has historically been considered to include five principal clinical findings:
1. High-grade, albumin-dominant proteinuria (generally >3 to 3.5 g/day or spot urine protein/creatinine ratio of >3 to 3.5 [grams of protein per gram of creatinine])
2. Hypoalbuminemia
3. Edema
4. Hyperlipidemia
5. Lipiduria

However, milder and earlier forms of many clinical disorders that can generate the full nephrotic syndrome may produce lower degrees of albuminuria in the range between 30 mg/day to 3500 mg/day with or without the other features. Also, the full spectrum of nephrotic syndrome may not develop in some patients despite high-grade albuminuria. The principal underlying abnormality responsible for all the other clinical features of nephrotic syndrome is increased permeability of the glomerular capillaries. Nephrotic syndrome may occur as an idiopathic and isolated condition, may be an inherited disorder, or may be a complication of an underlying systemic disease or allergic or immunologic disorder. It is always imperative to identify any underlying cause, when one exists (Table 24-6). This is accomplished by recognizing clues from the history and physical examination, reviewing a routine set of laboratory studies, and performing more specific tests suggested by the initial findings.

History and Review of Systems

The patient's history often helps elucidate the cause of nephrotic syndrome. The most common underlying systemic disease causing nephrotic syndrome is diabetes mellitus, and the syndrome can develop in those with all subtypes of this disorder. Although other glomerulopathies can also occur in patients with diabetes, atypical historical, physical, and laboratory findings usually cause the physician to consider another cause for nephrotic syndrome.[17] The history may also point to other relatively common disorders that generate nephrotic syndrome. These include systemic lupus erythematosus and the various forms of systemic amyloidosis—primary, secondary or reactive, and familial-hereditary. Infectious causes including viral hepatitis, HIV infection, *Mycoplasma* infection, and syphilis as well as parasitic causes such as malaria, schistosomiasis, filariasis, and toxoplasmosis must be considered. Many drugs can cause the syndrome, so it is extremely important to obtain a complete list of medications, including legally prescribed and over-the-counter medications, herbal or "natural" products, and illicit drugs. Drugs and drug classes that have been linked to nephrotic syndrome are the NSAIDs, penicillamine, several antibiotics, and, much more rarely, angiotensin converting enzyme inhibitors, tamoxifen, and lithium. A paraneoplastic nephrotic syndrome can be the presenting complaint with a variety of solid malignancies, lymphomas, and leukemias or can develop during treatment, sometimes as a treatment complication. Familial forms of nephrotic syndrome often present in infancy.[18] The nephrotic syndrome may rarely be a prominent feature in patients with

Alport's disease and nail-patella syndrome. Some patients can date the onset of major proteinuria, because they notice that their urine has become foamy. This phenomenon, which is most readily noticed by men, occurs because albumin has a soaplike effect that reduces the surface tension of urine. This can be a very useful sign in patients with recurring episodes of nephrotic syndrome.

Physical Examination

Edema is a major characteristic of nephrotic syndrome. The development of hypoalbuminemia reduces the oncotic pressure within the capillaries, and this favors the net translocation of fluid into the interstitial spaces. To the extent that this occurs, intravascular volume and blood pressure fall, and this triggers the sympathetic nervous system, activates the renin-angiotensin-aldosterone axis, elevates vasopressin levels, and modulates many other control systems that act together to promote net renal salt and water retention. This pathogenic sequence has been termed the *underfill mechanism* of salt and water retention in nephrotic syndrome. However, edema formation in many, perhaps most, nephrotic patients cannot be fully explained by underfill mechanisms. Although reduced intravascular oncotic pressures certainly exist in nephrotic patients, the net hydrostatic gradient for water movement across capillary beds is also influenced by the interstitial oncotic pressure, and this generally falls in parallel with reductions in plasma oncotic pressure. Consequently, the net hydrostatic pressure gradient from the intravascular compartment to the interstitial space may not significantly increase. Edema formation under these conditions may be the consequence of a primary form of renal salt and water retention. This pathogenic sequence for edema formation is called the *overfill mechanism*. Undoubtedly each of these mechanisms plays a role in various phases and forms of nephrotic syndrome. The mechanism that predominates is probably related to the specific renal lesion causing the nephrotic syndrome.[19,20] Also, these mechanisms may evolve from one form to the other. Regardless of which mechanism occurs initially, either will likely progress to a steady-state condition in which the initial effective arterial volume status is difficult or impossible to discern. Whether the initiating event is "underfill" of the effective arterial space leading to renal salt and water retention or "overfill" of this compartment causing excess salt and water to enter the interstitial spaces, the development of clinically apparent edema in an adult requires the net retention of about 8 to 10 pounds of fluid, which is equivalent to more than 4 L of normal saline.

Nephrotic edema is a form of pitting edema. When the thumb is pushed against a bony structure such as the tibia or sacrum, the resulting "pit" remains visible for a short period of time. Pitting edema is graded on a scale of 1 to 4 (from very slight to more apparent to deep pitting that persists for longer than 2 minutes).

Nephrotic edema is diffuse and to some degree probably affects virtually all tissues, but it is not equally distributed. The interstitial pressure in various locations has a major impact on edema formation. Thus the low ambient interstitial pressure often results in prominent periorbital edema. Gravitational force also causes nephrotic edema to accumulate in dependent body parts. Edema is generally worse in the lower legs and feet at the end of the day and becomes more prominent in the face after

nocturnal recumbency. Bedfast patients accumulate edema fluid in their back and sacral areas. The diurnal variation of edema formation becomes less prominent when the degree of edema worsens. Edema that is massive and generalized is termed *anasarca*. *Dropsy* is a historical term for generalized edema.

Nephrotic edema is usually symmetric (after adjustment for gravitational dependency), and unilateral edema should raise the possibility of edema due to local anatomic abnormalities such as venous thromboses, varicosities, or lymphatic obstruction. However, asymmetric nephrotic edema can be caused by upon an anatomic condition that generates greater local or asymmetrical edema. Severe edema can result in skin breakdown, blisters, weeping, and superinfection. Chronic (months to years) severe edema of any cause, including nephrotic syndrome, can produce fibrosis of the skin and subcutaneous tissues. The resulting "brawny" edema is usually pigmented, is very firm, and often will not pit.

Physical clues to other disorders that produce generalized edema should be sought during physical examination. The neck veins must be carefully evaluated to determine whether right-sided cardiac pressures are increased due to cardiac, pulmonary, or pericardial abnormalities. Elevated jugular venous pressures, pericardial knock, Kussmaul's sign (absence of inspiratory decline in jugular pressure), and prominent *x* and *y* descents suggest pericardial disease. Pulsus paradoxus (an exaggerated fall in systemic blood pressure of 10 mm Hg or more with inspiration) suggests pericardial or pulmonary disease. Although prominent ascites often indicates liver disease, whereas pulmonary congestion and pleural effusions suggest cardiac or pulmonary pathology, fluid may accumulate in these locations in patients with severe nephrotic syndrome in the absence of cardiac or liver abnormalities.

Many skin findings other than edema are associated with nephrotic syndrome itself and some suggest underlying primary diseases. Xanthelasma palpebrarum (periorbital-eyelid xanthomas) is associated with hypercholesterolemia about 50% of the time and may become very prominent in nephrotic patients. Eruptive xanthomas, usually associated with extreme hypertriglyceridemia, are much rarer but may also occur in patients with nephrotic syndrome. A number of relatively specific skin, nail, and scalp abnormalities are associated with various rheumatolgic conditions. These include a malar facial rash, scarring alopecia, mat telangiectasia, nail bed telangiectasia and nail fold capillary loops and vascular infarcts, and erythema nodosum. Sarcoidosis is also frequently associated with erythema nodosum and skin papules. Jaundice, angiomata, telangiectasia, and palmar erythema raise the likelihood of hepatic disorders. The vasculitides produce a number of skin manifestations, including leukocytoclastic rashes and skin infarctions.

Several nail findings occur in nephrotic patients. Transverse white lines, or leukonychia (sometimes called *Muehrcke's lines*) can develop during periods of marked hypoalbuminemia. Chronic hypoalbuminemia may cause more diffuse white nails (Terry's or half-and-half nails) or yellow nails.[21] None of these nail findings is specific, however, and they can also occur with other debilitating diseases, after chemotherapy, and so on. Nail-patella syndrome—characterized by dystrophic nails, hypoplastic patellae, and iliac horns—may present with nephrotic syndrome.

The eyes, in addition to being swollen, may be inflamed or show evidence of scleritis with systemic vasculitic disease. Of course the heart and liver must be carefully examined and the extremities must be carefully evaluated for evidence of arthritis and for deep vein thrombi, which occur with increased frequency in these patients.[22]

Laboratory Tests

Urine Studies

Proteinuria is readily detected using a semiquantitative urine dipstick test. The protein-detecting pad is impregnated with a protein-sensitive pH indicator dye and a strong pH buffer (which keeps the pad's pH constant independent of the actual urine pH). The pH indicator changes color when moistened with urine containing dissolved proteins (the phenomenon is called the *protein error* of pH indicators). Dipstick protein tests are most sensitive to albumin and react poorly to urine globulins and immunoglobulin light chains (Bence Jones protein). The dipstick results have the following approximate correlations with protein concentration:

Negative:<15mg/dL
Trace: 15-30 mg/dL
1+: 30-100 mg/dL
2+: 100-300 mg/dL
3+: 300-1000 mg/dL
4+: >1000 mg/dL

Extremely alkaline urine (i.e., infected urine) can overwhelm the acid buffer and thereby produce a false-positive dipstick protein test.

More recently albumin-specific urine dipstick tests have been marketed specifically to detect low-grade albuminuria (i.e., microalbuminuria). Some can simultaneously measure creatinine concentrations so that the albumin/creatinine ratio can be determined.

Albumin-specific dipstick tests are generally not used to diagnosis or follow patients with overt (macro) albuminuria or nephrotic syndrome. Sulfosalicylic acid precipitates most urine proteins, and the resulting turbidity is proportional to the protein concentration. The sulfosalicylic acid turbidity test detects albumin, globulins, and Bence Jones proteins. Although it was a very useful test, environmental safety concerns have eliminated it from most physician's offices.

If a high urine protein concentration is documented, a quantitative measurement of protein excretion will be required. This is usually achieved with a 24-hour urine collection. Alternatively, the protein/creatinine ratio (grams protein/gram creatinine) in a single morning specimen may be used.[14] If the creatinine excretion rate is assumed to be about 1 g/day, then the ratio of grams protein to 1 gram of creatinine will approximate the 24-hour protein excretion. Approximate corrections can be made depending on the patient's gender and body habitus. A timed quantitative urine collection has the advantage of permitting measurement of creatinine clearance, and this may be very useful.

The urine dipstick protein test, sulfosalicylic acid turbidity test, 24-hour protein excretion, and protein/creatinine ratio are all measures of total protein concentration or excretion. None of these will characterize the specific urine proteins (except that the urine dipstick tests are more sensitive to albumin, and the albumin sticks are specific to that class). Agarose gel protein electrophoresis of the urine defines the urine protein classes (i.e., albumin, α_1-globulin, α_2-globulin, β-globulin, γ-globulin), and monoclonal immunoglobulins and light chains can be identified. Electrophoresis results also allow stratification of nephrotic patients into those with selective proteinuria (mainly albumin) and those with nonselective proteinuria (both heavy albuminuria and globulinuria). This differentiation may have prognostic implications. Characterization of intact immunoglobulins, heavy chains, and light chains is also accomplished with either immunoelectrophoresis or immunofixation.

Hyaline casts are common in patients with nephrotic syndrome and represent precipitated Tamm-Horsfall protein together with abnormally filtered and excreted serum proteins.[23,24] Cellular casts are usually indicative of renal infection and/or interstitial inflammation (WBC casts) or glomerular inflammation, proliferation, and/or necrosis (when RBC casts are seen; see Figure 24-1). Such disorders may be idiopathic and isolated to the kidney, associated with systemic vasculitis, or related to another systemic inflammatory disease process such as systemic lupus erythematosus.

Lipiduria is a characteristic feature of nephrotic syndrome. The lipids in the urine sediment can be found in excreted tubule cells (oval fat bodies), within fatty casts, and/or as free-floating lipid globules. Some, but not all, of the urinary lipid is esterified cholesterol, and this component is birefringent and therefore is best seen with a polarizing microscope, which demonstrates their characteristic bright crosslike appearance[25] (Figure 24-4). Much of the urine fat originates from filtered high-density lipoprotein. The high-density lipoprotein is small enough to be filtered by "leaky" glomerular epithelial and is then partially reabsorbed by renal tubule epithelial cells, which subsequently degenerate and slough into the urine.[26]

Blood Studies

Initial studies should include a routine chemical profile (electrolytes, glucose, BUN, creatinine, total protein, albumin, calcium, phosphate, and liver enzymes), a lipid panel (total cholesterol, triglycerides, high-density lipoprotein cholesterol, and low-density lipoprotein cholesterol), and a CBC. The

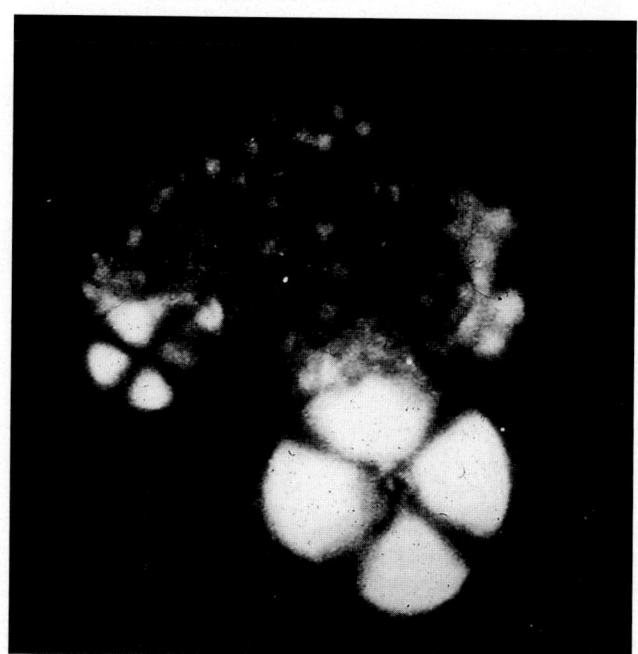

FIGURE 24-4 Lipiduria. Birefringent cholesterol crystals seen with polarizing light microscopy.

sodium concentration may be artifactually reduced (pseudo-hyponatremia) as a result of a displacement error caused by hyperlipidemia. This error occurs with flame photometry and with indirect potentiometry but not with direct potentiometry. The calcium concentration must also be corrected for the low albumin concentration, and measurement of ionized calcium concentration may be helpful. Additional testing is directed by the patient's clinical presentation and findings and the suspicions of the physician. Testing for syphilis and HIV and screening studies for viral hepatitis (hepatitis B and C) are generally performed. If a collagen vascular disease is suspected, then an ANA assay, anti–double-stranded DNA antibody assay, complement levels, and other more specific tests for autoimmune disorders are indicated. Although determination of sedimentation rate is sometimes helpful, it is usually elevated in all patients with nephrotic syndrome, regardless of cause.[27] If a paraproteinemia disorder (including primary amyloidosis) is suspected, a serum immunoelectrophoresis or immunofixation study should be performed (in addition to qualitative and quantitative urine protein studies). When clinical and historical features are suggestive, cryoglobulin and antistreptolysin O titers are obtained. Assessment of the GFR is mandatory and is usually accomplished with a timed urine collection for calculation of the creatinine clearance. Although estimation of GFR from the serum creatinine concentration using one of several equations, such as the MDRD equation, can be very helpful, collection of a timed urine specimen for measurement of protein and creatinine excretion is indicated in all nephrotic patients who are considered to be compliant and who can understand the instructions for accurate collection of such a specimen. When available, an iothalamate clearance may be very helpful; this remains the "gold standard" measure for GFR.

Imaging

A chest radiograph (CXR) is required to assess cardiac size and evaluate for pericardial disease, pleural effusions, and so on. A renal sonogram with Doppler study is required to determine the renal anatomy and status of the collection system and renal vasculature. Special attention is directed to the possibility of renal vein thrombosis. The finding of a single kidney, asymmetrical kidney size, or bilaterally small kidneys will direct subsequent evaluation. Patients should have routine age-indicated screening studies for malignancy such as mammography and colonoscopy. However, extensive studies to rule out occult malignancy are not indicated.

Renal Biopsy

Renal biopsy is not always indicated in patients with nephrotic syndrome. If the cause seems apparent, then treatment can be initiated without histologic confirmation. For example, biopsy is not usually required in a patient with long-standing diabetes mellitus who develops nephrotic syndrome after the expected time period. However, if atypical features exist, such as very active sediment with RBC casts, a very short time course, or absence of retinopathy and other end-organ involvement, then a biopsy may be required to rule out other causes of the syndrome. In young children with a classic clinical presentation,

the diagnosis of minimal change disease can be assumed and therapy initiated without histologic confirmation. This diagnosis is not as frequent in adults, and empiric therapy is less commonly initiated. Nonetheless, this course may be appropriate when contraindications to a biopsy exist or the patient is very reluctant to undergo an invasive procedure, and the clinical features are consistent with minimal change nephropathy. In the majority of adults with nephrotic syndrome, however, a biopsy is appropriate to define the disease, improve prognostication, and direct therapeutic intervention.

Obstructive Uropathy

Obstructive uropathy refers to structural or functional interference with normal urine flow anywhere from the renal pelvis to the urethra. The resultant increase in pressure within the urinary tract proximal to the obstruction leads to a number of structural and physiologic changes. The anatomic outcome of an obstructive process often includes dilatation of the calyces and renal pelvis, termed *hydronephrosis*, and, if the obstruction is distal to the ureteropelvic junction, *hydroureter*.

Obstructive uropathy is a common cause of acute or subacute renal failure. The early recognition of this clinical entity is essential both to improve prognosis and to identify the most appropriate therapy, which is quite different than that used to treat other forms of acute kidney injury. Untreated obstructive uropathy can result in a progressive and irreversible loss of renal function and eventually lead to end-stage renal disease. However, early recognition and treatment can allow a potentially full renal recovery. Obstructive uropathy is often described as acute (hours to a few days), subacute (several days to weeks), and chronic (months to years). The obstruction may be unilateral or bilateral, and either partial or complete. The clinician should establish the severity and chronicity of the condition so that appropriate therapy can be instituted. This is accomplished by means of careful history taking and physical examination, appropriate laboratory tests, and selected imaging studies depending on the clinical circumstances.

History and Review of Systems

Patients with acute obstructive uropathy may report abrupt onset of severe flank pain (if the obstruction is at the level of the ureter or above) or suprapubic pain and fullness (if there is lower-level obstruction). The pain is often colicky when the intraluminal process is due to nephrolithiasis or papillary necrosis. The pain may be accompanied by urinary frequency and urgency if there is partial urinary tract obstruction. Occasionally, nausea and even vomiting may occur when severe pain is present. A history of complete anuria should always alert the physician to the possibility of obstruction, especially in the appropriate clinical setting, for example, in an elderly man with a history of prostate cancer or prostatic hypertrophy. Gross hematuria may occur when obstructive uropathy is due to nephrolithiasis, papillary necrosis, or neoplasms of the urinary tract. Rarely, patients may report the passage of renal calculi or small pieces of tissue with the sudden cessation of pain after such an event. The history in patients with subacute or chronic obstruction is often negative or vague, but symptoms can include suprapubic fullness, frequency, polyuria, or nocturia. Patients may also complain of difficulty with initiating or stopping micturition if bladder outlet obstruction is present. Occasionally, urinary tract obstruction leads to an infection such as pyelonephritis, with accompanying high fever, flank pain, and dysuria.

Physical Examination

The physical examination can be very informative when bladder obstruction exists. The enlarged bladder may be detected with palpation and percussion. In rare cases a flank mass may be palpable from a hydronephrotic kidney. Prostatic enlargement and other prostatic pathology that may produce obstruction, such as malignancy or infection, can be detected via rectal examination. The physical examination is usually of limited value, however, for detecting obstruction of the ureters or pelvis of the kidney. Hypertension is occasionally caused by urinary tract obstruction. Several mechanisms have been proposed for this development. In acute, unilateral obstruction there can be activation of the renin-angiotensin system, with increased renin secretion by the obstructed kidney.[28,29] The plasma renin activity is typically normal with bilateral obstruction or with chronic unilateral obstruction. The hypertension that may occur in this setting has been attributed to renal failure with extracellular fluid (ECF) volume expansion.[30] In these instances, the diuresis that follows the correction of the obstruction often, but not always, eliminates the hypertension. Fever may be present if infection complicates obstruction.

Laboratory Tests

The initial laboratory evaluation may provide clues to the presence of obstructive uropathy. The urinalysis may reveal a few RBCs and WBCs. There may be evidence of impaired renal function in patients with complete or severe partial bilateral obstruction or in those with obstruction of a solitary kidney. The plasma creatinine concentration is usually normal in patients with unilateral obstruction due to the presence of the normal contralateral kidney. However, unilateral renal obstruction can very rarely lead to anuria and acute renal failure. This has been attributed to vascular or ureteral spasm.[31] Renal tubular acidosis with hyperkalemia is well described with obstructive uropathy.[32] Multiple defects in renin, aldosterone, and distal tubule function have been described. In some patients renin and aldosterone levels are reduced and the electrolyte abnormalities resolve in response to exogenous mineralocorticoids. In others, distal tubule injury diminishes sodium reabsorption and potassium secretion. The hyperchloremic acidosis is due to both hyperkalemia-induced suppression of ammoniagenesis and directly impaired proton secretion. Consequently, obstructive uropathy is a common cause of hyperkalemia and type 4 renal tubular acidosis.[32,33] Often, maximal urine concentrating capacity is also reduced.[33]

Acute obstruction causes an initial increase in renal blood flow, but this is soon followed by a reduction attributed to vasoconstriction.[33] This can sometimes increase the BUN/creatinine ratio similar to that seen in prerenal azotemia.

Imaging

Renal ultrasonography is the test of choice to diagnose obstructive uropathy. This modality avoids IV contrast exposure. It has an extremely high sensitivity (>95%) and very good specificity (75%) for the diagnosis of hydronephrosis.[34,35] In early obstruction (first 1 to 3 days), however, the collecting system can be relatively noncompliant, and therefore overt hydronephrosis may not occur. Furthermore, when extrinsic compression of the ureter exists, obstructive uropathy can develop without overt dilation of the ureter or the renal pelvis. This most often occurs in elderly men with malignancy involving the retroperitoneum or prostate or when retroperitoneal fibrosis exists.[36] Furthermore, hydronephrosis or hydroureter should not be equated with obstruction. Nonobstructive hydronephrosis can occur as a result of neuromuscular abnormalities of the bladder and/or ureters (megacystis-megaureter syndrome) and in other conditions such as vesicoureteral reflux and pregnancy.[37] Examination of the resistive index of the renal vasculature (vasoconstriction occurs with obstruction) and the response of the resistive index to a diuretic challenge can be a very helpful differentiator.[37] As Ellenbogen and colleagues stated, "It should be clear that the degree of hydronephrosis does not always correspond with the degree of obstruction."[35] When ultrasonographic results are inconclusive or the suspicion of obstruction is very high despite a nondiagnostic sonogram, CT scanning should be performed. The combination of renal ultrasonography and CT of the kidneys will establish the diagnosis of obstructive uropathy in the overwhelming majority of cases.[34,37] CT scans have generally replaced the IVP.

In some cases a retrograde study or percutaneous nephrostomy is necessary. Although much more invasive studies, they do not require IV contrast material, have a very high diagnostic yield, and also often treat the obstruction. Whenever a high degree of clinical suspicion of bladder obstruction exists, bladder catheterization, both a diagnostic and a therapeutic procedure, should be performed.

Hypertension

Systemic hypertension is one of the most common disorders seen in clinical practice. In the United States it affects about 20% of white adults, 40% of African American adults, and more than 80% of those older than 80 years of age. In addition, it is extremely common in patients with virtually any type of renal disease. The nephrologist must be an expert in the diagnosis and treatment of this disease and should have a rigorous and systematic approach for the diagnosis and treatment of hypertension. Over time the definition and classification of adult hypertension has been a moving target. The most recent diagnostic classification and therapeutic guidelines were published in the Seventh Report of the Joint National Committee on Prevention, Detection, Evaluation, and Treatment of High Blood Pressure.[38] Table 24-7 shows how this report classifies blood pressure, but these guidelines should always be viewed in the context of the individual patient's history and clinical circumstances. Also these blood pressure levels are for patients who are not acutely ill and are not taking antihypertensive medications. A patient with a consistently elevated blood pressure and no comorbid conditions is obviously treated quite differently than an individual with

TABLE 24-7 Classification of Blood Pressure in Adults		
HYPERTENSION CLASSIFICATION	SYSTOLIC PRESSURE (mm Hg)	DIASTOLIC PRESSURE (mm Hg)
Normal	<120	and <80
Prehypertension	120-139	or 80-89
Stage 1 hypertension	140-159	or 90-99
Stage 2 hypertension	≥160	or ≥100

TABLE 24-8 Causes of Secondary Hypertension
Renal parenchymal disease
Renovascular hypertension
Fibromuscular dysplasia
Atherosclerotic renal artery disease
Renal vasculitis
Renal infarction
Primary hyperaldosteronism
Renin-secreting tumor
Pheochromocytoma
Cushing's syndrome
Liddle's syndrome
Apparent mineralocorticoid excess
Geller's syndrome
Aortic coarctation
Thyroid disease
Drugs (e.g., corticosteroids, cocaine, amphetamines, oral contraceptives)
Sleep apnea

a similar degree of hypertension but with coexistent diabetes mellitus or other cardiovascular or renal disease. Chronic systemic hypertension is also associated with the development of cardiovascular disease, congestive heart failure, stroke, and chronic kidney disease (CKD). Appropriate treatment of the hypertension clearly reduces the risk of development of these complications, and it is therefore imperative to carefully evaluate and classify hypertensive patients so that appropriate therapy can be rendered.

History and Review of Systems

The evaluation of patients with hypertension should include an assessment of target organ function and/or damage, concomitant risk factors, and comorbid conditions, as well as a search to detect causes of secondary forms of hypertension, especially reversible conditions.[39] Obviously, a complete and detailed medical history is the first step in the evaluation. Particular attention should be paid to the presence of other cardiovascular risk factors such as age, African American ethnicity, underlying CKD, dyslipidemia, history of smoking, obesity, microalbuminuria, left ventricular hypertrophy, a family history of a myocardial infarction before age 50, and coincident arterial disease. The clinician should determine the duration and degree of hypertension and assess for any symptoms of severe hypertension such as blurry vision, visual loss, headaches, encephalopathy, or nausea. A thorough dietary history is also essential and should include an estimate of sodium, potassium, calcium, and fat intake. Other important factors to identify include tobacco use, alcohol consumption, all prescribed and over-the-counter medications taken, illicit drug use, the efficacy of previous antihypertensive drug therapy and any adverse effects, and the presence (or absence) of sexual dysfunction. It is remarkable that patients (and many physicians) remain unaware of the potential hypertensive effects of many over-the-counter medications, particularly the NSAID class of drugs. A family history of hypertension is also very important for the diagnosis of both familial monogenetic forms of hypertension and essential hypertension.

Nephrologists are very often asked to evaluate and treat hypertensive patients who are referred for a second opinion, particularly those with poor blood pressure control. In this population it is particularly important to identify any potential primary (and hopefully reversible) cause for secondary hypertension (Table 24-8). In this regard, symptoms characteristic of certain underlying causes of hypertension should be sought. Examples include paroxysmal hypertension, sweating, palpitations, and severe headache for pheochromocytomas; sweating, palpitations, and weight loss for thyrotoxicosis; and weight gain, edema, and polyuria for Cushing's syndrome.

A common form of secondary hypertension is that due to atherosclerotic renal artery stenosis. These patients may relate a history of recent worsening of their blood pressure control despite adherence to the antihypertensive medication regimen. They also very frequently have a history of generalized vascular disease. Primary hyperaldosteronism is now recognized as a very common condition, especially in patients with difficult to control or severe hypertension. Prevalence among hypertensive patients may be as high as 10%. Although spontaneous or drug-related hypokalemia suggests this diagnosis, it often presents with normal electrolytes.

Physical Examination

The physical examination begins with careful blood pressure measurement in the office setting. Patients should not smoke or ingest caffeine for at least 30 minutes prior to the examination. They should be comfortably seated in a chair with back support with the arm resting at heart level. An appropriately sized cuff must be used. Its width should be at least 40 percent of arm circumference and its length at least 80 percent of arm circumference.[40] Two or more readings should be taken 2 to 5 minutes apart and averaged. Blood pressure should also be measured in the supine and standing position if orthostatic hypotension is likely. When a coarctation is considered, blood pressure should be measured in each arm and also in the legs. Use of incorrect cuff size in obese individuals causes an overestimation of blood pressure. Although the use of mercury manometers is encouraged, these have largely been eliminated due to the environmental toxicity of mercury. A regularly calibrated aneroid or electronic device is acceptable. Overestimation of systolic blood pressure is common in elderly patients who have calcified and stiff arteries that cannot be compressed. This condition, called *pseudohypertension*, is suspected when the radial artery remains palpable after the cuff has been inflated above systolic blood pressure.

The next very important element of the physical examination is a thorough funduscopic evaluation. The presence and severity of hypertensive retinopathy provides an important clue to the duration and severity of the hypertension. Special note should be made of hemorrhage, arteriolar narrowing, papilledema, and/or cotton-wool spots.

The cardiovascular and pulmonary examination may reveal evidence of carotid and/or peripheral vascular disease, left ventricular hypertrophy (e.g., hyperdynamic precordium and the presence of a fourth heart sound), or congestive heart failure (e.g., jugular venous distention, peripheral edema, third heart sound, and/or rales). Coarctation of the aorta is suggested by differences in the intensity of the radial pulses or a radial-femoral arterial pulsation difference or temporal delay.

The abdominal and flank examination may reveal abdominal bruits suggesting renal artery stenosis. Neurologic examination in severely hypertensive patients may reveal findings consistent with encephalopathy. Abnormal findings on thyroid examination may suggest otherwise occult thyroid disease. The presence of hyperpigmentation and striae raises the possibility of Cushing's syndrome. Neurofibroma and café au lait spots suggest the possibility of neurofibromatosis (and either pheochromocytoma or renal vascular disease).

Laboratory Tests

The extent of laboratory evaluation depends on the clinical circumstances of the individual patient. The initial evaluation of a person with stage 1 hypertension includes measurement of serum electrolytes, BUN, creatinine, calcium, and glucose; a lipid profile; urinalysis; and CBC. If warranted by the clinical history and physical examination findings, additional testing such as thyroid studies, urine albumin/creatinine ratio, and quantitation of GFR with a timed urine collection for measurement of creatinine clearance or iothalamate clearance are measured. When a pheochromocytoma is suspected, 24-hour urine catecholamines and fractionated metanephrines, or fractionated plasma catecholamines or free metanephrines should be measured. A plasma aldosterone/plasma renin activity ratio is a reasonable screening test for the detection of primary hyperaldosteronism if this condition is clinically suspected. This test should be ordered for patients with unprovoked hypokalemia; those with severe diuretic-induced hypokalemia, unexpected metabolic alkalosis, or severe or resistant hypertension; or hypertensive patients with an incidentally discovered adrenal mass ("incidentaloma").

Imaging

A baseline CXR is appropriate for all hypertensive patients. Other imaging modalities are required when the history, physical examination, and laboratory results suggest that the hypertension may be secondary to anatomic abnormalities or when pathologic end-organ changes due to the hypertension must be determined. Renal sonography is an excellent non-invasive test for assessing renal size, identifying cysts, and detecting hydronephrosis. It is obviously indicated whenever enlarged kidneys or a mass can be palpated. When there is strong clinical suspicion of renovascular hypertension, several options are available to establish the diagnosis. They include spiral CT angiography, magnetic resonance angiography, and duplex Doppler ultrasonography. Which screening test is best is determined by the specific features of each patient and the skill of the imaging center that is used. Renal artery Doppler studies are very operator dependent, and results are often suboptimal in large patients. CT angiography of the renal arteries is an excellent diagnostic tool but carries the risk of contrast-related kidney injury in susceptible patients as well as considerable radiation exposure. Gadolinium-enhanced magnetic resonance angiography also yields excellent results, but is contraindicated in patients with reduced kidney function because of concerns about nephrogenic systemic fibrosis. Also it cannot be used when patients are claustrophobic or have metallic implants. Captopril renal perfusion scans are no longer recommended as a screening test because of their relatively low predictive value. It should be emphasized that one should proceed directly to catheter angiography if the clinical suspicion is very high, no matter what any screening tests show.

Other Studies

An electrocardiogram is necessary to screen for left ventricular hypertrophy and cardiac arrhythmias and to provide a baseline for future comparison.

Nephrolithiasis

Nephrolithiasis, or kidney stones, is an increasingly prevalent medical problem. Over 5% of the U.S. population is affected, and the lifetime risk of developing a stone is between 10% and 15%.[41] Patients who develop a first stone are very likely to have a second one (50% within 5 years and 80% within 20 years).[41] Therefore, every physician is likely to encounter patients with this problem.

History and Review of Systems

Kidney stones are strongly suspected when patients present with classic signs and symptoms such as gross hematuria associated with waves of flank and/or lower abdominal pain (colic), which may radiate into the genital region. However, symptoms are sometimes very vague. Either gross hematuria or microscopic hematuria is usually, but not always, present. The absence of hematuria does not exclude a diagnosis of nephrolithiasis.[42] Poorly localized abdominal pain, nausea, vomiting, and urinary frequency may occur. Often, patients are entirely asymptomatic, and the stones are noted incidentally when an imaging study is done for a different reason. When painful symptoms do develop, they generally indicate that an asymptomatic stone has passed from the renal pelvis into the ureter where it has caused obstruction, inflammation, and/or bleeding. These symptoms often first occur during the night or in the early morning, beginning abruptly with rapidly worsening pain. The paroxysms of pain probably reflect hyperperistalsis of the renal calyces, pelvis, and ureter. The site of pain and its referral pattern are clues to the stone's location. Upper ureteral obstruction usually produces flank pain and tenderness, and anterior abdominal radiation of pain. Lower ureteral obstruction produces lower abdominal pain, which frequently radiates into the testicle or labia. Very often stones lodge near the ureterovesical junction where they irritate the bladder, which produces urinary frequency, urinary urgency, suprapubic tenderness, and dysuria. If the stone enters the bladder and then obstructs its outlet, suprapubic pain and anuria may develop.

Potential kidney stone risk factors should be identified. The patient should be questioned about unusual dietary habits. Does the patient consume large amounts of oxalate-rich foods such as spinach, rhubarb, beets, or black tea? Is intake of animal protein, which reduces urine citrate excretion, excessive? High salt ingestion increases urine calcium excretion. Sardines, anchovies, and organ meat are rich sources of purines and thereby increase urine uric acid excretion. The medication history may reveal other important clues to stone pathogenesis. Some medications increase the risk of stones by reducing urine citrate excretion—carbonic anhydrase inhibitors such as acetazolamide and topiramate are important examples. Other medications that may directly precipitate as stones are the protease inhibitor indinavir, triamterene, and some sulfonamides.[43] Dietary supplements, vitamins, and minerals such as calcium salts and vitamin D can produce hypercalciuria.

A number of underlying medical conditions can generate kidney stones. These include most chronic disorders associated with hypercalciuria, such as hyperparathyroidism and sarcoidosis. Hypercalcemia-hypercalciuria of malignancy usually does not result in kidney stones because of its acute presentation and relatively short course. Any medical or surgical condition associated with significant steatorrhea (short gut disorders, cystic fibrosis, bile salt depletion from ileal disease, gastrointestinal bypass) may generate stones as a result of hyperoxaluria and reduced urine volume. Chronic diarrhea without steatorrhea causes chronic metabolic acidosis and persistent aciduria—a risk factor for uric acid stones. Strong epidemiologic associations with both calcium and uric acid kidney stones have been demonstrated for obesity, weight gain, diabetes mellitus, and metabolic syndrome.[44] The impact of occupations associated with reduced fluid intake and/or excessive sweating should be considered, because low urine volume is a major risk factor for stone formation. A history of recurrent kidney infections raises concern for infection (struvite) stones (see later). The age when the first kidney stone develops is also a clue to the etiologic diagnosis. Kidney stones associated with inherited disorders such as cystinuria and congenital hyperoxaluria often present in the young. Ethnicity has a major impact on risk. Over a 6-year period (1988 to 1994) in the United States, whites had the highest risk of kidney stones (5.9%), African Americans the lowest risk (1.7%), and Mexican Americans intermediate risk (2.6%).[41] The family history also may be helpful; first-degree relatives of patients with stones very often also have had stones.[45]

Physical Examination

The presence of fever is a sign of possible infection, which must be rapidly addressed. It is of critical importance to recognize an infection proximal to an obstructing stone. This is a medical-urologic emergency requiring urgent drainage of the renal pelvis (surgically or via interventional radiology) and appropriate antibiotic therapy. Fever and/or leukocytosis,

which do not usually occur with uncomplicated kidney stones, are red flags for this condition. The skin is generally pale and cool, and often clammy. The patient should be examined for costovertebral angle tenderness. Hypoactive bowel sounds and ileus may develop in these patients, but abdominal tenderness is unusual, and if rebound tenderness is present another cause should be sought. Bruits over the abdominal aorta and iliac vessels may be indicative of a leaking aortic abdominal aneurysm, which can mimic the symptoms of renal colic. In men, a rectal examination may reveal prostatitis, and in women, a pelvic examination may suggest ovarian pathology or an ectopic pregnancy.

Laboratory Tests

The routine initial laboratory battery includes a CBC. The WBC count may be slightly increased with an uncomplicated stone, but leukocytosis of more than 15,000 cells/mm^3 and a left shift suggests a complicating infection. The BUN and creatinine values are important markers of GFR, especially if renal mass is reduced, severe obstruction exists, or the patient is volume depleted. An electrolyte panel may provide clues that distal renal tubular acidosis exists (hyperchloremic acidosis and hypokalemia). The serum calcium, phosphate, and uric acid levels can indicate the existence of a hypercalcemic-hypercalciuric condition, renal phosphate wasting, or a hyperuricosuric condition. In women of childbearing age a pregnancy test must be performed.

Urine Studies

Hematuria with isomorphic RBCs is very common but not universal.[42] RBC casts should not be seen. Proteinuria should be absent or low grade. Although pyuria may occur without infection, it should always raise suspicion, and a urine culture should be performed. The urine pH may provide a helpful clue. A very high pH of freshly voided urine (i.e., >7.5) almost always indicates the existence of a UTI. Chronic UTIs may lead to the development of struvite stones, also called *triple phosphate*, *urease-related*, or *infection stones*. When the infecting bacteria produce the enzyme urease, the urea in urine is split into two molecules of NH_3 and one of CO_2. The CO_2 escapes from the urine, whereas each NH_3 molecule binds a proton and thereby elevates the urine pH above that under usual physiologic conditions. Abundant ammonium in an alkaline urine tends to precipitate with magnesium and phosphate to form struvite ($MgNH_4PO_4 \cdot 6H_2O$). Note that struvite is really a double phosphate crystal. The term *triple phosphate* derives from the fact that carbonate-apatite ($Ca_{10}[PO_4]_6 \cdot CO_3$) commonly coprecipitates with struvite, which results in a combination of three cations—calcium, magnesium, and ammonium—and the phosphate anion. Struvite stones often grow to large staghorn shapes. Urease-producing bacteria include *Ureaplasma urealyticum*, most *Proteus* species, and many *Staphylococcus*, *Klebsiella*, and *Pseudomonas* species. *Escherichia coli* does not generate urease.

A urine pH that is not appropriately acidic (<5.5) in a patient with hyperchloremic acidosis suggests distal renal tubular acidosis, a disorder often associated with calcium phosphate stones. Conversely, persistently acidic urine is associated with uric acid stones (because uric acid becomes increasingly insoluble as the pH falls below 6.5). When bacteriuria is identified, a urine sample must be sent for culture. If overt signs of infection exist, then hospital admission for additional evaluation is generally required.

Identification of crystals in the urine sediment can be helpful and sometimes diagnostic. Recognition of the "benzene ring" cysteine is virtually diagnostic of cystinuria. The "coffin lid" crystals of struvite are also very characteristic and indicate that an infection-related stone is likely. Although uric acid and calcium oxalate crystals are very common and relatively nonspecific, they may be helpful clues to etiology when kidney stones are recognized.[46] Twenty-four-hour urine collection for quantitation of nephrolithiasis-relevant chemicals can be very helpful. Several commercial laboratories offer stone risk profile or metabolic stone risk testing. These studies may identify abnormally high (e.g., calcium, oxalate, urate) and/or low (e.g., citrate) chemical concentrations and excretion rates. The saturation-supersaturation state of the urine for various stone-forming crystals is also routinely calculated. In general at least two samples should be collected for such studies because of significant day-to-day variation in excretion rates. Specimens should be sent for these studies whenever recurrent stones develop or when a first stone is documented in a patient with a higher than usual risk for recurrence (e.g., those with a family history of stones, patients with gastrointestinal disorders). Some suggest that 24-hour urine studies should be performed after the first kidney stone in all patients.

Imaging

The imaging procedure of choice is a noncontrast helical CT scan with relatively thin (3- to 5-mm) cuts. This modality has replaced IVP as the preferred imaging procedure. Although a plain radiograph of the abdomen (kidneys, ureters, bladder) is very inexpensive and may be diagnostic, it has generally also been replaced by the CT scan as the initial screening test.[47] The CT scan can detect radiopaque calculi as small as 1 mm in diameter. Calcium stones are opaque; cysteine and struvite stones are slightly radiopaque; and pure uric acid stones are radiolucent. Stones comprised of indinavir or triamterene are also radiolucent. The CT scan will also reveal renal anatomy, the presence of hydronephrosis, other abdominal and pelvic pathology, and other potential causes of the patient's symptoms. Although a renal-abdominal sonogram will demonstrate renal anatomy and reveal the presence of hydronephrosis and most stones in the renal pelvis, it will miss most ureteral stones. Therefore sonography is generally used to follow the progress of known stone disease but not as an initial study. However, sonography is indicated as the initial procedure in pregnant women and others for whom radiation exposure must be minimized. Magnetic resonance imaging (MRI) is generally not very good for the diagnosis of kidney stones.

Differential Diagnosis

Many conditions can mimic nephrolithiasis. Any form of renal bleeding associated with blood clots can cause ureteral obstruction and produce symptoms identical to those of a kidney stone. Other clinical mimics of kidney stones

are acute abdominal aneurysm, pyelonephritis, renal cancer, renal tuberculosis, papillary necrosis, renal infarction, and renal vein thrombosis. Papillary necrosis, which is more likely in patients with diabetes or sickle cell disease, can cause true renal colic when sloughed papillae obstruct the ureter. Ectopic pregnancy, appendicitis, and bowel obstruction must be considered. Finally, some patients complain of kidney stone symptoms because they are seeking analgesic drugs. Table 24-9 shows the differential diagnosis of urolithiasis-like pain.

Initial Treatment

Patients with renal colic can often be managed conservatively as outpatients with analgesics and fluids. However, admission and urgent urologic consultation is required if the patient is septic, has an infection proximal to an obstruction, has obstruction of a solitary kidney (including a renal transplant) or bilateral kidney obstruction, has high-grade obstruction with a large (> 7-mm) stone, has acute kidney failure, has urine extravasation, or has unrelenting pain despite analgesic use or pain responsive only to parenteral analgesics.

The most important determinant of the likelihood that a stone will pass is its size. Most kidney stones smaller than

TABLE 24-9 Differential Diagnosis of Urolithiasis-Like Pain

CATEGORY	DISORDERS
Renal	Pyelonephritis Blood clot Renal infarction Tumor (kidney or pelvis) Papillary necrosis
Ureteral	Tumor Blood clot Stricture
Bladder	Tumor Blood clot Urinary retention
Intraabdominal	Peritonitis Appendicitis Biliary disease Bowel obstruction Vascular disorder Aortic aneurysm Mesenteric insufficiency
Retroperitoneal	Lymphadenopathy Fibrosis Tumor
Gynecologic	Ectopic or tubal pregnancy Ovarian torsion/cyst rupture Pelvic inflammatory disease Cervical cancer Endometriosis Ovarian vein syndrome
Neuromuscular	Muscle pain Rib fracture Radiculitis
Infectious	Herpes zoster Pleuritis/pneumonia Fungal bezoar

4 mm in diameter will pass spontaneously. As stone size increases beyond a diameter of 4 mm, the chance of passing falls progressively until it becomes very unlikely at a diameter of 10 mm. Consequently, conservative outpatient therapy becomes less likely to be successful as the stone size increases beyond 4 to 5 mm.[48,49] Narcotics and/or NSAIDs are used for analgesia. If the patient is to be managed as an outpatient then NSAIDs are the preferred agents. If nausea and vomiting are prominent, a parenteral NSAID such as ketorolac can be used.[50] For severe pain IV morphine is generally given.[51] If the stone has a reasonable chance of passing without urologic intervention, then glucocorticosteroids, calcium channel blockers (usually nifedipine), and/or α_1-adrenergic antagonists (usually tamsulosin, which is used to treat benign prostatic hyperplasia) are often employed to relax ureteral muscles and thereby assist stone passage. Patients should always attempt to retrieve the passed stone for analysis. This can be accomplished by urinating through a filter or fine screen (an aquarium net is a good option). If none is available, the patient can urinate through a fine gauze pad or simply void into a glass jar so the calculus will be visible.

Acute Kidney Injury

Acute kidney injury (AKI) is a clinical syndrome broadly defined as an abrupt decline in renal function occurring over a period of hours to days resulting in the retention of nitrogenous and metabolic waste products and ECF volume. Very often, electrolyte and acid-base disorders also develop (hyperkalemia, hyponatremia, and metabolic acidosis). AKI develops as a result of a variety of pathophysiologic influences and may lead to varying degrees of damage to one or more anatomic divisions of the nephron with subsequent adverse functional consequences. Although the initial clinical manifestation of AKI may be oliguria, urine volume can remain normal or even increase, and patients can be completely asymptomatic. The diagnosis is often made when routine biochemical screening reveals a recent increase in serum creatinine and/or BUN concentrations.

There is no universally accepted operational definition of AKI, and more than 30 different criteria have been employed in various clinical studies.[52] Commonly used definitions include an absolute increase in serum creatinine concentration of 0.5 to 1.0 mg/dL, and relative increases of 25% to 100% over a period of 1 to several days. Although far from perfect, these approaches have proved to be useful in identifying patients with AKI in clinical practice. More recently a new classification and diagnostic system known by the acronym *RIFLE* (*R*isk, *I*njury, *F*ailure, *L*oss, *E*nd stage) has been introduced.[52] Table 24-10 shows this diagnostic and classification system.

The incidence of AKI depends greatly on the patient population studied and the criteria used to identify affected patients. The incidence of AKI in ambulatory patients is very low, but AKI develops in up to 7% of hospitalized patients and about 30% of those admitted to intensive care units.[53,54] United Kingdom population studies report that the annual incidence of AKI is between 486 and 620 per million.[54] Outcomes associated with AKI have changed little over the past 50 years. The in-hospital mortality rate of critically ill patients with AKI is higher than 50%. Older age, female gender, respiratory failure, liver failure, sepsis, and impaired consciousness all correlate with higher in-hospital mortality rates.

The causes of AKI can be broadly divided into three categories: prerenal azotemia (a disorder characterized by renal hypoperfusion in which renal parenchymal tissue integrity is preserved), intrinsic renal failure with parenchymal tissue injury, and postrenal failure (dysfunction due to acute obstruction of the urinary tract) (Table 24-11). Appropriate categorization of AKI requires the clinician to integrate the findings and results from a careful history, physical examination, and appropriate laboratory and imaging studies.

TABLE 24-11 Causes of Acute Kidney Injury

Prerenal

Gastrointestinal hemorrhage

Burns

Pancreatitis

Capillary leak

Diarrhea, vomiting, nasogastric suction, fistula fluid loss

Excessive sweating

Diuretics, nonsteroidal antiinflammatory drugs

Congestive heart failure

Cirrhosis

Intrinsic

Ischemia (e.g., postoperative acute tubular necrosis)

Nephrotoxins (e.g., radiocontrast agents, aminoglycosides)

Sepsis

Acute interstitial nephritis

Acute glomerulonephritis

Acute vascular syndrome (e.g., bilateral renal artery thromboembolism or dissection)

Atheroembolic disease

Postrenal

Bilateral upper tract obstruction (e.g., nephrolithiasis, papillary necrosis) or obstruction of solitary functioning kidney

Lower tract obstruction (e.g., prostatic hypertrophy, urethral stricture, bladder mass or stone, obstructed urinary catheter)

TABLE 24-10 RIFLE Criteria for Acute Kidney Injury (AKI)

CLASS	GFR	URINE OUTPUT
Risk	Creatinine increase ×1.5 or GFR fall of >25%	<0.5 mL/kg/hr >6 hr
Injury	Creatinine increase ×2 or GFR fall of >50%	<0.5 mL/kg/hr >12 hr
Failure	Creatinine increase ×3 or GFR fall of >75% *or* Creatinine ≥4 mg% (acute increase ≥0.5 mg%)	<0.3 mL/kg/hr >24 hr *or* Anuria >12 hr
Loss	Persistent AKI = complete loss of renal function >4 wk	
End stage	End-stage renal disease >3 mo	

GFR, Glomerular filtration rate.

History and Review of Systems

The initial goal of history taking is to establish whether the patient actually has AKI. In this regard, a careful review of clinical, pharmacy, nursing, and radiologic records is necessary. A relatively recent serum creatinine determination is invaluable but not always available. In some cases the clinician must make a presumptive diagnosis of AKI pending further data collection and investigation. A diagnosis of AKI can usually be more readily established when it occurs during a hospitalization because urine output is often recorded and laboratory values are measured frequently.

A history of anuria should raise the possibility of obstructive uropathy. The historical features that assist in the differentiation of AKI into the categories shown in Table 24-11 should be identified. One of the risk factors that most strongly predicts the development of AKI is the presence of CKD.[55] A history of salt and fluid losses such as occur with diarrhea, vomiting, or ECF loss into a third space as is seen with extensive burns, pancreatitis, or leaky capillaries suggests a prerenal etiology. NSAIDs, angiotensin converting enzyme inhibitors, and angiotensin receptor blockers, especially when combined with diuretics, can generate a renal hypoperfusion state and AKI. Therefore medication review is essential to identify such drugs and also any other potential nephrotoxic agents.

A history of heart failure or liver disease increases the likelihood that AKI is the result of reduced effective arterial volume. Often, the cause of AKI is multifactorial (e.g., a patient with a gastrointestinal hemorrhage may undergo a radiologic study with IV contrast). It is also critically important to identify any history of underlying CKD. Often, such patients develop superimposed AKI due to a variety of renal insults. A history of decreased urine output or anuria is important, but, as noted earlier, many patients have normal urine output despite AKI.

A history of voiding symptoms such as urinary frequency, hesitancy, or incontinence suggests the possibility of obstructive uropathy. Many patients with renal artery emboli and some with bilateral renal vein thrombosis may present with flank pain and a history of hematuria. It is also important to elicit any history of a recent interventional procedure, which raises the possibility of AKI as a result of IV or intraarterial contrast infusion or atheroembolic disease. A history of fever, skin rash, arthralgias, sinusitis, and/or hemoptysis raises the possibility of glomerulonephritis related to infection, collagen vascular disease, or vasculitis.

Physical Examination

An extremely important aspect of the physical examination in every patient with AKI is an assessment of ECF and effective arterial volume status. Overt hypotension is the strongest indicator of potential renal underperfusion. Less severe volume depletion is suggested by an orthostatic pulse increase of more than 30 beats/min (measured 1 minute after standing). Of note, orthostatic hypotension, defined as a drop in systolic blood pressure of more than 20 mm Hg after standing, is less helpful because it occurs in 10% of normal subjects.[56] Dry axillae and dry mucous membranes with a furrowed tongue are useful signs of volume depletion. However, poor skin turgor and slow capillary refill have not been shown to be helpful

signs in adults.[56] The neck veins are usually flat when volume contraction exists.

Renal perfusion is reduced as a result of heart failure or hepatic cirrhosis. Signs of the former condition include distended neck veins, pulmonary rales, an S_3 gallop, and pitting peripheral edema. Stigmata of chronic liver disease, including jaundice, hepatosplenomegaly, ascites, gynecomastia, nail clubbing, palmar erythema, vascular spiders, and testicular atrophy, should be sought. The presence of either true ECF volume depletion or reduced effective arterial volume raises the very strong possibility of a prerenal (and potentially readily reversible) cause of the AKI.

The physical examination may suggest a systemic disease associated with an intrinsic AKI, such as vasculitis, endocarditis, thrombotic thrombocytopenic purpura and hemolytic uremic syndrome, and so on. An important cause of AKI in the hospitalized or recently hospitalized patient is atheroembolic (cholesterol embolic) disease. This often overlooked condition generally occurs following an invasive procedure that requires intraarterial catheterization (e.g., cardiac catheterization, angiography) or cardiac or aortic surgeries. Skin findings include livedo reticularis, ulcers, purpura, petechiae, painful erythematous nodules, cyanosis, and gangrene. Retinal examination may reveal arterial atheroemboli (Hollenhorst plaques).

Flank tenderness or an enlarged palpable bladder indicates possible postrenal causes for AKI. A digital examination of the prostate should be performed in all men with AKI, and a bimanual pelvic examination to detect pelvic masses should be considered in women. If lower tract obstruction is a serious consideration in-and-out diagnostic postvoid bladder catheterization should be done. The normal postvoid residual urine volume is less than 50 mL. Any urine collected should be saved for potential additional studies.

Laboratory Tests

Initial testing in AKI must include urinalysis and an estimate of the GFR. ECF volume contraction causes marked urine concentration, which increases the urine specific gravity and may generate positive dipstick protein results. Microscopy often reveals hyaline casts, but there should be few cells and no cellular casts. Quantitative protein excretion is relatively low (<1 g/day). A "bland" finding on urinalysis is also consistent with an obstructive or postrenal cause for AKI, unless a complicating infection produces pyuria and bacteriuria, or hematuria results from stone disease. AKI due to intrinsic damage such as tubular necrosis will generate a "dirty" urinalysis with many epithelial cells and muddy brown granular and epithelial cell casts. The urine is generally isosthenuric (i.e., specific gravity is 1.010). Rhabdomyolysis causes myoglobinuria, and pigmented granular casts are seen. Acute glomerulonephritis produces proteinuria, hematuria, and RBC casts. Acute interstitial nephritis causes pyuria and white cell casts. If it is due to an allergic reaction, then urine eosinophils are often seen, but this is not a specific finding.[57]

Estimation of the GFR gives an approximate measure of the number of functioning nephrons. In the setting of AKI the GFR is, by definition, not in a steady state. This makes GFR estimates, especially those based on plasma creatinine, unreliable. However, a rising creatinine concentration indicates that the renal injury is stable or worsening, whereas a falling creatinine concentration is indicative of improvement. A daily rise in creatinine concentration of more than 1 mg/dL is usually associated with a GFR of less than 10 mL/min. A timed urine collection for determination of creatinine and/or urea clearance can be very helpful (but even here tubular secretion of creatinine can lead to overestimation of the GFR). When available, clearance values for radioisotopes such as iothalamate can be used as the most accurate measurement of GFR.

Routine studies of electrolytes, BUN, calcium, and phosphorus should be performed. Potentially life-threatening hyperkalemia and severe metabolic acidosis must be identified and treated. Table 24-12 lists a number of urine and plasma chemical measurements and calculations that help differentiate prerenal AKI from intrinsic renal injury. Although measurement of the urine sodium concentration can be helpful in distinguishing these disorders, the fractional excretion of sodium and/or urea is a better indicator. Important exceptions include AKI due to contrast nephropathy, rhabdomyolysis, acute myeloma kidney, and acute urate nephropathy in which the fractional excretion of sodium and urea are often very low despite the absence of an apparent prerenal cause.

Imaging

Imaging of the urinary tract by ultrasonography is an extremely helpful and important test in the setting of AKI. It will generally diagnose obstruction. However, it is not 100% sensitive nor specific; ultrasonography can produce negative results immediately following obstruction or in patients with ureteric encasement. Renal ultrasonography also provides an excellent measurement of kidney size. This helps to distinguish chronic renal failure (in which the kidneys are often small and echogenic) from AKI (in which renal size is expected to be normal). If contrast nephropathy is suspected, a plain radiograph of the abdomen (kidneys, ureters, bladder [KUB]) may reveal

a persistent nephrogram due to retained IV contrast material. Doppler ultrasonography can also be useful in the assessment of renal arterial and venous patency when vascular obstruction is suspected. Although CT, MRI, and angiography can be used when ultrasonography is insufficient, these modalities are limited because renal injury restricts the use of contrast agents.

Renal Biopsy

Renal biopsy is generally not necessary in the setting of AKI. However, renal biopsy can be useful when vasculitis, glomerulonephritis, or allergic interstitial nephritis is considered a possible cause of the AKI.[58]

Chronic Kidney Disease and Chronic Kidney Failure

CKD, regardless of the specific cause, is defined as an irreversible and usually progressive decline in nephron function and number generally quantitated as a reduction in GFR. As GFR falls from 90 mL/min to approximately 30 mL/min, retention in the plasma of substances that are handled primarily by glomerular filtration develops. The plasma concentrations of urea nitrogen and creatinine, two such substances that are routinely measured, increase. As the GFR falls from 30 to 15 mL/min, additional alterations in plasma composition develop, and additional pathophysiologic disturbances, including anemia, altered calcium and phosphate metabolism, and nutritional changes, occur. Although overt symptoms may be absent, careful evaluation generally reveals a wide spectrum of abnormalities in these patients. Then, as GFR falls below 10 mL/min, overt uremic signs and symptoms develop, and if the decline is irreversible, the patient will have reached end-stage kidney failure (ESKD). Uremic syndrome is the result of severely reduced excretory function with retention of metabolic products, fluid and acid-base derangements, hormonal abnormalities, and other consequences of the loss of renal function.

In 2002 the National Kidney Foundation proposed a new classification system for CKD based on the severity of GFR reduction and made recommendations for appropriate actions to be taken at each disease stage.[59] This system, known as the *Kidney Disease Outcomes Quality Initiative (KDOQI) Classification*, is shown in Table 24-13. Also shown in the table are the number of adults in the United States with each stage of chronic kidney disease (CKD). Most individuals with CKD have stage 1 or 2 disease. Patients with stage 3 CKD, numbering almost 8 million, comprise the most rapidly expanding group. In 2007 the incidence of ESKD in the United States was approximately 355,000 and the prevalence was 1665 per million population.[60,61] Mortality in patients with CKD is high, and in patients with stage 3 CKD the risk of death (usually from cardiovascular disease) is at least 10 times higher than the risk of progression to ESKD. Patients with ESKD have a mortality rate of about 50% after 3 years and 65% to 75% at 5 years. At least 60% of these deaths are also related to cardiovascular disease. CKD has manifestations and complications affecting virtually every organ system, including the central and peripheral nervous, neuropsychiatric, endocrine, hematologic, cardiovascular, gastrointestinal, peripheral

TABLE 24-12 Tests to Differentiate Prerenal from Intrinsic Kidney Damage

MEASURE	PRERENAL AKI	INTRINSIC KIDNEY DAMAGE (ATN, ETC.)
Urine Na (mEq/L)	<20	>40
Urine osmolality (mOsm/kg H_2O)	>500	<350
Serum BUN/creatinine (Cr) ratio	>20	10-15*
Fractional excretion of Na $\dfrac{[U_{Na} \times P_{Cr}]}{[P_{Na} \times U_{Cr}]} \times 100$	<1†	>2
Fractional excretion of urea $\dfrac{[U_{Urea} \times P_{Cr}]}{[P_{Urea} \times U_{Cr}]} \times 100$	<30†	>50

*A BUN/Cr ratio of <10 may occur with rhabdomyolysis because the Cr concentration increases sharply as a result of increased release from necrotic muscle. A low BUN/Cr ratio can also develop in malnourished individuals due to very low BUN.

†The fractional excretion of Na and fractional excretion of urea are often also very low with contrast nephropathy, rhabdomyolysis, acute myeloma kidney, and acute urate nephropathy.

AKI, Acute kidney injury; *ATN,* acute tubular necrosis; *BUN,* blood urea nitrogen; *P,* plasma; *U,* urinary.

TABLE 24-13 National Kidney Foundation Kidney Disease Outcomes Quality Initiative (KDOQI) Classification System, Disease Prevalence, and Action Plan

STAGE	DESCRIPTION	GFR (mL/min/1.73 m²)	PREVALENCE (IN MILLIONS)*	ACTION
	At increased risk	≥90 (with CKD risk factors)		Reduction of CKD risk factors
1	Kidney damage with normal or ↑ GFR	≥90	3.6	Treatment of comorbid conditions and reduction of CVD risks
2	Kidney damage with mild ↓ GFR	60-89	6.5	Estimation of progression rate
3	Moderate ↓ GFR	30-59	15.5	Evaluation and treatment of complications
4	Severe ↓ GFR	15-29	0.7	Preparation for kidney replacement therapy
5	Kidney failure (end-stage kidney disease)	<15 (or dialysis)	0.6	Kidney replacement (if uremic)

Chronic kidney disease is defined as kidney damage for ≥3 months defined by structural or functional abnormalities of the kidney, with or without decreased GFR. Damage may be documented as a pathologic abnormality or the presence of markers of kidney damage. These include abnormalities on blood or urine tests, abnormalities on kidney imaging tests, or a GFR of <60 mL/min/1.73 m².

CKD, Chronic kidney disease; *CVD*, cardiovascular disease; *GFR*, glomerular filtration rate.

Prevalence data from National Kidney Foundation,[59] United States Renal Data System,[60] and Coresh et al.[61] Data are for adults aged ≥20 years.

vascular, and skeletal systems. Consequently the diagnosis and treatment of CKD requires a broad, multifaceted approach.

The most common renal diseases that progress to ESKD (in order of both incidence and prevalence) are diabetic nephropathy, hypertensive nephrosclerosis, polycystic kidney disease, and chronic glomerulonephritis. The focus of the history, physical examination, and laboratory studies in these patients is establish the specific diagnosis, determine the severity of kidney dysfunction, identify any reversible component, identify and quantitate any comorbid conditions and complications, assess the risk for continued loss of kidney function, and assess the risk for cardiovascular disease.

History and Review of Symptoms

Patients are often referred to a nephrologist for evaluation of CKD when the BUN and creatinine concentrations are noted to be elevated on routine laboratory testing. The patient may have no knowledge of any kidney disorder or abnormal kidney function. Other patients may have had an extensive prior renal evaluation. In some the kidney disease is an isolated abnormality; in others an underlying disease known to be associated with kidney involvement such as systemic lupus erythematosus, hepatitis B or C, scleroderma, or vasculitis may exist. The duration of the kidney disease and the rate of progression must be established whenever possible. The patient might know of a specific diagnosis, the severity or stage of the kidney disease, and its pace. Any available laboratory data, biopsy reports, and imaging results should be obtained. Prior urologic interventions should be reviewed. Any previous discussions regarding treatment or renal replacement therapy should be discussed, and the patient's adherence to prior nephrologic recommendations should be determined.

A detailed family history of kidney disease can be extremely informative. Monogenic familial kidney diseases include polycystic kidney disease, Alport's disease, medullary cystic disease, certain forms of membranoproliferative glomerulonephritis, and Fabry's disease. Polygenic familial disorders include diabetes mellitus, hypertension, obesity, hyperlipidemia, and premature vascular disease. The patient's general health, ability to perform activities of daily living, energy level, appetite,

and any recent weight changes should be assessed. Mental acuity, memory, mood, and any change in sleep pattern must be evaluated. Sometimes family members can provide a more accurate assessment of these parameters than the patient.

Many symptoms do not become apparent until very late in the disease course. Patients with CKD may exhibit amazing adaptive ability. GU symptomatology should be identified. This includes voiding symptoms such as polyuria, nocturia, hesitancy, and frequency and any history of UTIs; back, flank, abdominal, or pelvic pain; renal calculi; or urologic manipulation. Any history of GU malignancy, including cancer of the bladder, prostate, kidney, or cervix, and any renal imaging procedures should be reviewed. Cardiovascular, peripheral vascular, and cerebrovascular disease history should be elicited. Coronary artery disease is the most important vascular complication in patients with CKD.[62] A history of myocardial infarction and/or congestive heart failure should be noted and left ventricular function assessed. A history of coronary artery interventions, significant arrhythmias, or insertion of a pacemaker or defibrillator should be identified. It is imperative that any history of resting or exertional chest pain and/or shortness of breath be recognized. Peripheral vascular disease is also very common in patients with CKD. A history of claudication, peripheral ulcers, revascularization, gangrenous extremities, or extremity amputation must be documented. Symptoms secondary to autonomic and sensorimotor neuropathy should be identified.

Nutritional status, appetite, and weight changes should be determined. The interpretation of weight change is complicated, however, because loss of body mass may be masked by fluid accumulation. Food may taste bad, and foul breath may develop. With overt uremia, anorexia, nausea, and vomiting develop. Occasionally diarrhea is present. In the diabetic patient with ESKD it may be difficult to distinguish between uremic symptoms and those of diabetic neuropathy and enteropathy. Musculoskeletal complaints occur frequently with CKD. Muscle cramps are often related to diuretic use. Muscle wasting and loss of muscle strength occur. Bone and joint pain may be due to osteodystrophy. Spontaneous fractures can occur.

All medications should be carefully reviewed and documented. The review should include current and prior medications, and over-the-counter and nonprescription medications. Medications should be reviewed for potential nephrotoxic effects and appropriate dosing. Calcineurin inhibitors (cyclosporine, tacrolimus), lithium, pamidronate, chemotherapy agents (cisplatin, mitomycin C), and various analgesics are several examples of drugs that can damage the kidneys. Recently, use of sodium phosphate bowel preparations before colonoscopy or surgical procedures has been found to cause irreversible renal disease.[63] Therefore, this has become an important line of questioning in patients with otherwise unexplained CKD.

Ophthalmic complications, largely related to diabetes and hypertension, are common in CKD. Lens abnormalities may occur in patients with Alport's disease. When diabetes exists, the date of onset, type of treatments, results of microalbuminuria studies, adequacy of control, hemoglobin A_{1C} levels, and so on, should be ascertained. In general, the onset of type 2 diabetes is difficult to determine, because it may be clinically silent for years. Hypertensive nephrosclerosis is the second leading cause of CKD resulting in ESKD, and hypertension is also a very common complication of virtually all forms of CKD. Differentiating primary hypertension that has caused CKD from a kidney disease complicated by hypertension is frequently very difficult. The duration of hypertension may also be difficult to establish. Hospitalization for an acute cardiovascular event may lead to recognition of hypertension. A history of high or low blood pressure extremes, as well as response to and adherence to antihypertensive medication regimens, should be documented. A history of gross or microscopic hematuria, proteinuria, or foamy urine suggests glomerulonephritis, the third most common cause of CKD progressing to ESKD. Back or flank pain may be presenting or prominent complaints. Fever, skin rash, inflammation of the eyes or sinuses, and joint pains raise the possibility of secondary forms of glomerulonephritis. Occasionally a family history of glomerulonephritis can be elicited.

Polycystic kidney disease is often diagnosed from the family history. Occasionally polycystic kidney disease is first recognized after an abdominal imaging procedure reveals the diagnosis. Shoulder, back, flank, and/or pelvic pain occur frequently. Abdominal fullness, bloating, and episodes of hematuria are often described. Sometimes the patient feels the enlarged kidneys. The multiple extrarenal manifestations of polycystic kidney disease include cerebral aneurysms, which are by far the most life-threatening extrarenal complication. Because they occur more commonly within families, a history of cerebral aneurysms, stroke, or sudden death at a young age among relatives should be sought. Colonic diverticula and abdominal wall or inguinal hernias are also common in these patients.

Physical Examination

Assessment of vital signs should include supine and upright pulse and blood pressure measurements. One primary focus of the physical examination in patients with CKD is the assessment of ECF and effective intraarterial volume status. This is not always straightforward. Physical findings that indicate volume depletion are also discussed in the section on acute kidney injury. Although overt hypotension is the strongest indicator of potential renal underperfusion, an orthostatic pulse increase of more than 30 beats/min (measured 1 minute after standing) is indicative of less severe volume depletion.[56] Orthostatic hypotension, defined as a drop in systolic blood pressure of more than 20 mm Hg after standing, is less

helpful because it is seen in 10% of normal subjects. Autonomic neuropathy also complicates the assessment of orthostatic hypotension. Dry axillae and dry mucous membranes with a furrowed tongue are useful signs of volume depletion. However, poor skin turgor and slow capillary refill have not been shown to be helpful signs in adults.[56] The neck veins are usually flat in the volume-contracted patient. If volume depletion is possible, a trial of ECF expansion with crystalloid solutions is indicated to determine if a reversible component of kidney dysfunction exists. At the other extreme, hypertension, peripheral edema, pleural effusions, and pulmonary rales may indicate volume overload and require treatment with diuretics or ultrafiltration. However, edema and effusions may also be the result of nephrotic syndrome. Heart failure and cirrhosis also generate total body salt and water expansion with effective intraarterial volume contraction.

Advanced CKD produces a sallow appearance. Generalized muscle wasting may be observed. Current body weight should be noted and compared with prior known weights.

Thorough evaluation of the cardiovascular system is mandatory. Retinal examination may reveal hypertensive or diabetic retinopathy. Carotid pulse should be evaluated and the presence of bruits identified. Cardiac examination may reveal left ventricular hypertrophy or decompensation. Flank or abdominal bruits may suggest renovascular disease.

Palpation of the abdomen may reveal an enlarged bladder or large kidneys. Costovertebral tenderness indicates possible inflammatory or infectious kidney disease.

Motor and/or sensory neuropathy can occur with CKD as well as diabetes. Muscle wasting is common. Neuromuscular irritability with tremor and myoclonic jerks can be seen when CKD is advanced or is complicated by hypocalcemia or hypomagnesemia.

Skin changes common in CKD include pallor related to anemia, hyperpigmentation, and scratch marks and excoriations produced as a result of pruritus. Uremic frost, representing residue from evaporated urea-rich sweat, occurs in severe untreated ESKD. Skin necrosis due to calcific arteriopathy and calciphylaxis is a dreaded complication.

Laboratory Tests

The urinalysis can provide important clues to the diagnosis. Hematuria with high-grade proteinuria suggests a glomerular process, either glomerulonephritis or diabetes, whereas low-grade proteinuria is consistent with nephrosclerosis, an interstitial disease, or polycystic disease. When the urine sediment reveals RBCs, their appearance as acanthocytes (see Figure 24-1) or RBC casts supports a glomerular origin.

The urine protein/creatinine ratio provides an estimate of protein excretion. With the assumption that urine creatinine excretion is about 1 g/day, this ratio, expressed as grams of protein per gram of creatinine, represent the daily protein excretion in grams per day. Adjustments can be made for very small or very large patients. Excretion of more than 3 g/day of protein (primarily albumin) is most consistent with a glomerular process. True quantitative measurement of protein and creatinine excretion may be very helpful in selected patients.

Blood studies should include a CBC, BUN and creatinine concentrations, electrolyte panel, calcium level, phosphate level, liver function studies, and a lipid panel. Sedimentation rate and C-reactive protein level provide information about the patient's inflammatory state. Based on the results of these tests and the patient's underlying conditions, the iron storage status, vitamin B_{12} and folate levels, and hemoglobin A_{1C} levels are often measured. Serologic testing to evaluate for the presence of systemic lupus erythematosus or other collagen vascular diseases, HIV infection, hepatitis B or C, and multiple myeloma is often done. Evaluation of complement levels may be helpful with certain types of glomerulonephritis.

An assessment of the GFR is an essential component of the evaluation of the patient with CKD. GFR can be estimated from the serum creatinine concentration using one of several standard formulas (see Table 24-3). These formulas produce inaccurate results for the very old, the very large, and patients with a relatively high GFR (normal serum creatinine concentration). In addition, the serum creatinine concentration must be relatively stable. A timed urine collection to measure creatinine clearance is the standard method for documenting renal function. A radioisotope clearance study (usually iothalmate) is the most accurate, gold standard method for determining GFR. Serum cystatin C level has recently been proposed as a better marker of renal function, but this test is not routinely done in most facilities. It may have some advantage relative to creatinine concentration, but this remains unproven.

Imaging

Renal ultrasonography should be done for all patients being evaluated for CKD. The sonogram provides a kidney size assessment, supplies information on cortical width and echogenicity, and demonstrates the presence or absence of scars and hydronephrosis as well as renal stones or masses. Renal Doppler ultrasound imaging is used to assess renovascular flow. If there is any suspicion of coexistent heart disease, an echocardiogram can be done to assess cardiac size, left ventricular function, regional wall motion abnormalities, pulmonary pressures, valvular function, and pericardial fluid.

Urinary Tract Infection

UTI is one of the most frequent infectious illnesses occurring in humans and is probably the most common bacterial infection.[64] It can occur in those of all ages, from the very young to the very old. It most often affects women in the reproductive age group. UTI presents in multiple ways, from asymptomatic bacteriuria, to bothersome local symptoms of pelvic pain and dysuria, to severe local symptoms of back or flank pain and fever, to severe overwhelming infection with septic shock and multiorgan failure.

It is useful to separate UTIs on an anatomic basis. Pyelonephritis represents an upper urinary tract infection of the kidney itself. Lower urinary tract infections may be separated into those of the bladder (cystitis), prostate, and urethra.

History and Review of Systems

The most common complaint of patients with an acute UTI is urinary frequency and dysuria. Other voiding symptoms such as difficulty voiding, polyuria, halting voiding symptoms, or frequent small voids also occur. Sometimes a change in the appearance of the urine is the presenting complaint. The patient may complain of grossly purulent, foul-smelling, and/or blood-tinged or frankly bloody urine. Passage of a stone or tissue debris may be reported. Patients with UTIs (other than asymptomatic bacteriuria) also often present with some localizing symptom. Back, flank, abdominal, and/or pelvic pain may be the presenting complaint. Fever, with or without chills, suggests a more serious illness.

A past history of similar symptoms associated with a documented UTI can often be elicited. The frequency of prior UTIs should be established. The patient's report of specific antibiotics used for treatment of previous UTIs is helpful. Some patients can describe prior infecting organisms as demonstrated on urine culture.

In addition to localizing symptoms of pain, with or without fever, some patients have constitutional symptoms of fatigue, malaise, and weight loss. Gastrointestinal symptoms of nausea and vomiting, constipation, or diarrhea may be present. With severe UTIs, symptoms of hypotension with orthostatic dizziness may be seen.

Asymptomatic bacteriuria can occur as the initial presentation. It must be distinguished from urinary contamination at the time of urine culture. It is often identified in patients with a history of UTIs and is sometimes noted when urine cultures are performed during follow-up of previously treated symptomatic UTIs. Most often it is detected in patients at high risk for UTIs in whom surveillance urine cultures are performed. High-risk groups include pregnant women; sexually active young women; elderly men and women, particularly in a nursing home setting; patients with indwelling urinary catheters or other drainage devices; patients with diabetes; and patients with spinal cord injury. However, current recommendations are that only pregnant women should be screened (and treated) for asymptomatic bacteriuria.[64] There is currently no evidence that the benefits of screening outweigh its potential negative impact in any other adult patient group.[65]

It is important to identify underlying risk factors for the development of the current UTI as well as previous episodes of UTI. Most young and middle-aged women have no apparent anatomic abnormality that might predispose them to UTIs. Recurrent UTIs in this group should prompt a discussion regarding the timing of the UTI with respect to sexual activity. The use of diaphragms and spermicides as well as delayed postcoital micturition has been associated with UTI. Vaginitis is an important risk factor for UTI in women, so a history of associated symptoms should be elicited. There is little evidence that tampon use or the method (direction of wiping) of cleansing after defecation have a significant impact on the risk of developing UTI. The frequency of UTI increases during pregnancy and is probably related to a combination of physiologic and anatomic changes, frequent glucosuria, and hormonal effects.

UTIs in men raise concern for an anatomic abnormality. The most common abnormalities that predispose men to UTI are prostatic enlargement and prostatitis. Sexual history regarding homosexual activity, and specifically anal intercourse, which increases UTI risk in men, is also important. Other anatomic abnormalities that predispose patients to UTI include bladder pathology (neurogenic bladder, especially in the setting of spinal cord injury; bladder cancer with disruption of the urothelium; bladder diverticula); enterovesical fistula; polycystic kidney disease; prostate cancer; urinary drainage devices and procedures (indwelling transurethral or suprapubic bladder catheters, percutaneous nephrostomy, ureteral stent, ileal conduit); renal calculi with or without urinary obstruction; vesicoureteral reflux; and urinary obstruction at any level.

Certain medical conditions also place patients at increased risk for developing UTIs and complications of these infections. These include pregnancy, diabetes, renal transplantation, and long-term immunosuppression.

Physical Examination

Physical examination findings in the setting of UTI are often nonspecific.[66] Fever may indicate a more serious or complicated UTI, as does hypotension and tachycardia. The patient with a severe systemic infection of urinary origin may have a toxic appearance and altered mentation. Careful attention should be given to the back, flank, abdomen, and pelvic areas to detect localized tenderness or palpable mass. The patient should be inspected for urinary drainage devices. In men a rectal examination for assessment of the prostate is important.

Laboratory Tests

The urinalysis results often confirm the presence of an active UTI.[67] Gross visual inspection of the urine may reveal turbidity or blood, and the urine often has a foul smell. On the urine dipstick test, the pH can be markedly alkaline (supraphysiologic level, i.e., >7.5) when the urine is infected with urea-splitting bacteria (see section on laboratory evaluation of nephrolithiasis). The dipstick result is often positive for occult blood. The nitrite test result is positive when the urine is infected with Enterobacteriaceae. These gram-negative bacilli have an enzyme that reduces urinary nitrate to nitrite. A false-negative nitrite test result can occur when the urine is very dilute (e.g., the patient is taking a diuretic) or the infecting bacteria do not produce the nitrate reductase enzyme (*Staphylococcus* or *Enterococcus* species or *Pseudomonas aeruginosa*). Urine granulocytes generally indicate inflammation, which may or may not be due to infection. They can be detected by a dipstick test for leukocyte esterase, an enzyme contained in the granules of neutrophils. More than 5 WBCs per HPF is needed for a positive test finding. In rare cases false-positive results are produced by strong oxidants in the urine collection container. High-grade proteinuria or glucosuria, some antibiotics, and high levels of ascorbic acid can produce false-negative results.

Simultaneous positive test results for nitrite and leukocyte esterase virtually guarantee the presence of a UTI. A finding of marked proteinuria raises the possibility of reflux nephropathy complicated by focal glomerulosclerosis, whereas moderate proteinuria (in the range of 1 to 1.5 g/day or less) can occur with chronic interstitial nephritis. The spun urine sediment shows neutrophils, often in clumps, and occasionally neutrophil casts. RBCs are also usually seen. Bacteria are generally easily observed when significant bacteriuria exists. A Gram-stained smear of either unspun urine or spun sediment can aid in identification of the bacteria and help target empiric therapy.

Urine culture will verify an active UTI. Good urine collection and culture techniques are necessary to avoid contamination. Midstream urine should be collected after careful washing of external genitalia followed by voiding into a sterile container. Bladder catheterization, suprapubic needle bladder aspiration, or sterile aspiration of urine from the tube of a closed catheter drainage system is sometimes required. Most true UTIs are caused by a single organism. Therefore demonstration of multiple organisms on urine culture strongly suggests contamination. A colony count of more than 10^5 organisms/mL (from voided specimens) correlates with active infection. However, colony counts of less than 10^5/mL may be significant in a symptomatic patient.

The vast majority (80% to 90%) of positive urine cultures in the outpatient setting grow *E. coli*. The presence of other gram-negative bacteria on urine culture suggests a complicated UTI possibly related to renal calculi or obstruction. *Proteus* infections occur in patients with staghorn calculi. Urine culture findings for hospitalized patients are much more diverse. UTIs caused by gram-positive cocci (usually *Enterococcus*) are uncommon, and those due to *Staphylococcus* species are extremely rare. *Staphylococcus aureus* UTI may suggest staphylococcal bacteremia, and UTI caused by coagulase-negative staphylococci can occur after instrumentation in elderly men. Mycobacterial and fungal UTIs are very rare. *Candida* infections may develop in immunocompromised patients or those with long-standing catheters. Anaerobic bacteria almost never cause UTIs.

An assessment of baseline renal function should be done. This is most commonly accomplished using a serum creatinine measurement and any one of several standard predictive formulas (see Table 24-3). If renal function is reduced, this may be an acute or chronic process. Acute renal failure occurs in patients with volume depletion and sepsis syndromes with hypotension. Infection with bilateral urinary obstruction or obstruction in a solitary functional kidney can present with AKI or kidney failure. Chronic renal dysfunction and failure can occur with vesicoureteral reflux, chronic pyelonephritis, or chronic urinary obstruction. In all patients with persistently reduced estimates of kidney function, formal measurements should be obtained using either a timed urine collection to assess creatinine clearance or an isotopic measurement of GFR.

A number of acid-base and potassium abnormalities may occur in patients with UTI. If UTI causes nausea and vomiting then metabolic alkalosis and hypokalemia ensue. Hyperkalemia can be caused by renal dysfunction or may be a component of type 4 renal tubular acidosis due to chronic renal interstitial disease or obstruction. Metabolic acidosis can be caused by lactic acidosis associated with sepsis or renal tubular acidosis.

Imaging

Kidney and GU tract imaging is usually done to diagnose vesicoureteral reflux, renal calculi, and other lesions that obstruct urine flow or otherwise cause stasis. In general, imaging studies are not required in adult women with an uncomplicated UTI that responds rapidly to antibiotic treatment. Imaging is generally recommended for all men with their first UTI. Imaging should also be done when patients have a complicated UTI, when bacteremia has developed, when the UTI has failed to respond to appropriate antibiotic therapy, and when urinary obstruction or stones are suspected. Women with unexplained recurrent UTIs and all patients with pyelonephritis serious enough to warrant hospitalization should undergo imaging. Also, if hematuria persists following resolution of a UTI, imaging is indicated.

Renal ultrasonography has now replaced IV urography as the standard renal imaging procedure in patients with UTI. Renal size, cortical width and echogenicity, obstruction, and stones can be readily determined with ultrasonography. Bladder and prostate anatomy can be assessed. CT with contrast infusion permits further assessment of renal and ureteral anatomy and pathology. Pyelonephritis in an obstructed kidney requires emergent intervention for drainage, and detection of a perinephric abscess usually also calls for surgical intervention.

Some patients require cystoscopy, retrograde pyelography, and/or voiding cystography to detect vesicoureteral reflux.

References

1. Mohr DN, Offord KP, Owen RA, Melton 3rd LJ. Asymptomatic microhematuria and urologic disease. A population-based study. *JAMA.* 1986;256:224-229.
2. U. S. Preventive Services Task Force. *Screening for bladder cancer in adults: recommendation statement.* June 2004. Available at http://www.uspreventiveservicestaskforce.org/3rduspstf/bladder/blacanrs.htm.Accessed March 12, 2011.
3. Khadra MH, Pickard RS, Charlton M, et al. A prospective analysis of 1,930 patients with hematuria to evaluate current diagnostic practice. *J Urol.* 2000;163:524-527.
4. Karl Tryggvason. Jaakko Patrakka: Thin basement membrane nephropathy. *J Am Soc Nephrol.* 2006;17:813-822.
5. Kiryluk K, Jadoon A, Gupta M, et al. Sickle cell trait and gross hematuria. *Kidney Int.* 2007;71:706-710.
6. Abarbanel J, Benet AE, Lask D, et al. Sports hematuria. *J Urol.* 1990;143:887-890.
7. Culclasure TF, Bray VJ, Hasbargen JA. The significance of hematuria in the anticoagulated patient. *Arch Intern Med.* 1994;154:649-652.
8. Brennan P, Bogillot O, Cordier S, et al. Cigarette smoking and bladder cancer in men: a pooled analysis of 11 case-control studies. *Int J Cancer.* 2000;86:289-294.
9. Fortuny J, Kogevinas M, Garcia-Closas M, et al. Use of analgesics and nonsteroidal anti-inflammatory drugs, genetic predisposition, and bladder cancer risk in Spain. *Cancer Epidemiol Biomarkers Prev.* 2006;15:1696-1702.
10. Pollock C, Liu PL, Gyory AZ, et al. Dysmorphism of urinary RBCs—value in diagnosis. *Kidney Int.* 1989;36:1045-1049.
11. Koss LG, Deitch D, Ramanathan R, et al. Diagnostic value of cytology of voided urine. *Acta Cytol.* 1985;29:810-816.
12. Juncos LI. Intrarenal mechanisms of salt and water retention in the nephritic syndrome. *Kidney Int.* 2002;61:1182-1195.
13. Rodríguez-Iturbe B, Baggio B, Colina-Chourio J, et al. Studies on the renin-aldosterone system in the acute nephritic syndrome. *Kidney Int.* 1981;19:445-453.
14. Ruggenenti P, Gaspari F, Perna A, et al. Cross sectional longitudinal study of spot morning urine protein:creatinine ratio, 24 hour urine protein excretion rate, glomerular filtration rate, and end stage renal failure in chronic renal disease in patients without diabetes. *BMJ.* 1998;316:504-509.
15. Brown KM, Sacks SH, Sheerin NS. Mechanisms of disease: the complement system in renal injury—new ways of looking at an old foe. *Nat Clin Pract Nephrol.* 2007;3:277-286.
16. Madaio MP, Harrington JT. Current concepts: the diagnosis of acute glomerulonephritis. *N Engl J Med.* 1983;309:1299-1302.
17. Olsen S. Identification of non-diabetic glomerular disease in renal biopsies from diabetics—a dilemma. *Nephrol Dial Transplant.* 1999;14:1846-1849.
18. Niaudet P. Genetic forms of nephrotic syndrome. *Pediatr Nephrol.* 2004;19:1313-1318.
19. Schrier RW, Fassett RG. A critique of the overfill hypothesis of sodium and water retention in the nephrotic syndrome. *Kidney Int.* 1998;53:1111-1117.
20. Koomans HA, Kortlandt W, Geers AB, et al. Lowered protein content of tissue fluid in patients with the nephrotic syndrome: observations during disease and recovery. *Nephron.* 1985;40:391-395.
21. Cockram CS, Richards P. Yellow nails and nephrotic syndrome. *Br J Dermatol.* 1979;101:707-709.
22. Llach F. Hypercoagulability, renal vein thrombosis, and other thrombotic complications of nephrotic syndrome. *Kidney Int.* 1985;28:429-439.
23. Venkataseshan VS, Faraggiana T, Grishman E, et al. Renal failure due to tubular obstruction by large protein casts in patients with massive proteinuria. *Clin Nephrol.* 1993;39:321-326.
24. Cohen AH. Morphology of renal tubular hyaline casts. *Lab Invest.* 1981;44:280-287.
25. Martin RS, Small DM. Physicochemical characterization of the urinary lipid from humans with nephrotic syndrome. *J Lab Clin Med.* 1984;103:798-810.
26. Blackburn V, Grignani S, Fogazzi GB. Lipiduria as seen by transmission electron microscopy. *Nephrol Dial Transplant.* 1998;13:2682-2684.
27. Liverman PC, Tucker FL, Bolton WK. Erythrocyte sedimentation rate in glomerular disease: association with urinary protein. *Am J Nephrol.* 1988;8:363-367.
28. Weidmann P, Beretta-Piccoli C, Hirsch D, et al. Curable hypertension with unilateral hydronephrosis. Studies on the role of circulating renin. *Ann Intern Med.* 1977;87:437-440.
29. Wanner C, Lüscher TF, Schollmeyer P, et al. Unilateral hydronephrosis and hypertension: cause or coincidence? *Nephron.* 1987;45:236-241.
30. Vaughn Jr ED, Bubler FR, Laragh JH. Normal renin secretion in hypertensive patients with primarily unilateral chronic hydronephrosis. *J Urol.* 1974;112:153.
31. Maletz R, Beman D, Peelle K, et al. Reflex anuria and uremia from unilateral ureteral obstruction. *Am J Kidney Dis.* 1993;22:870-873.
32. Batlle DC, Arruda JA, Kurtzman NA. Hyperkalemic distal renal tubular acidosis associated with obstructive uropathy. *N Engl J Med.* 1981;304:373-380.
33. Klahr S. Nephrology forum: pathophysiology of obstructive nephropathy. *Kidney Int.* 1983;23:414-426.
34. Webb JA. Ultrasonography and Doppler studies in the diagnosis of renal obstruction. *BJU Int.* 2000;86(suppl 1):25-32.
35. Ellenbogen PH, Scheible FW, Talner LB, et al. Sensitivity of gray-scale ultrasound in detecting urinary tract obstruction. *AJR Am J Roentgenol.* 1978;130:730-733.
36. Spital A, Valvo JR, Segal AJ. Nondilated obstructive uropathy. *Urology.* 1988;31:478-482.
37. Mostbeck GH, Zontsich T, Turetschek K. Ultrasound of the kidney: obstruction and medical diseases. *Eur Radiol.* 2001;11:1878-1889.
38. Chobanian AV, Bakris GL, Black HR, et al. National Heart, Lung, and Blood Institute Joint National Committee on Prevention, Detection, Evaluation, and Treatment of High Blood PressureNational High Blood Pressure Education Program Coordinating Committee, et al. The Seventh Report of the Joint National Committee on Prevention, Detection, Evaluation, and Treatment of High Blood Pressure: the JNC 7 report. *JAMA.* 2003;289:2560-2572.
39. Ram V, Fenves A. Hypertension. In: Rakel RE, ed. *Conn's current therapy 2000.* Philadelphia: Saunders; 1999:303-315.
40. Frolich ED, Grim C, Laberthe DR, et al. Recommendations for human blood pressure determination by sphygmomanometers; report of special task force appointed by the Steering Committee. *Circulation.* 1988;77:502A-514A.
41. Stamatelou KK, Francis ME, Jones CA, et al. Time trends in reported prevalence of kidney stones in the United States. *Kidney Int.* 2003;63:1951-1952.
42. Luchs JS, Katz DS, Lane MJ, et al. Utility of hematuria testing in patients with suspected renal colic: correlation with unenhanced helical CT results. *Urology.* 2002;59:839-842.
43. Daudon M, Jungers P. Drug-induced renal calculi: epidemiology, prevention and management. *Drugs.* 2004;64:245-275.
44. Taylor EN, Stampfer MJ, Curhan GC. Obesity, weight gain, and the risk of kidney stones. *JAMA.* 2005;293:455-462.
45. Ljunghall S, Danielson BG, Fellstrom B, et al. Family history of renal stones in recurrent stone patients. *Br J Urol.* 1985;57:370-374.
46. Daudon M, Jungers P. Clinical value of crystalluria and quantitative morphoconstitutional analysis of urinary calculi. *Nephron Physiol.* 2004;98:31-36.
47. Longo J, Akbar SA, Schaff T, et al. A prospective comparative study of noncontrast helical computed tomography and intravenous urogram for the assessment of renal colic. *Emerg Radiol.* 2001;8:285-292.
48. National Institutes of Health Consensus Development Conference on Prevention and Treatment of Kidney Stones, Bethesda, Maryland. *JAMA.* 1988;260:977-981.
49. Preminger GM, Tiselius HG, Assimos DG, et al. EAU/AUA Nephrolithiasis Guideline Panel: 2007 Guideline for the management of ureteral calculi. *J Urol.* 2007;178:2418-2434.
50. Larkin GL, Peacock 4th WF, Pearl SM, et al. Efficacy of ketorolac tromethamine versus meperidine in the ED treatment of acute renal colic. *Am J Emerg Med.* 1999;17:6-10.

51. Safdar B, Degutis LC, Landry K, et al. Intravenous morphine plus ketorolac is superior to either drug alone for treatment of acute renal colic. *Ann Emerg Med.* 2006;48:173-181.
52. Bellomo R, Ronco C, Kellum JA, et al. Acute Dialysis Quality Initiative workgroup: Acute renal failure—definition, outcome measures, animal models, fluid therapy and information technology needs: the Second International Consensus Conference of the Acute Dialysis Quality Initiative (ADQI) Group. *Crit. Care.* 2004;8:R204-R212.
53. Nash K, Hafeez A, Hon S. Hospital-acquired renal insufficiency. *Am J Kidney Dis.* 2002;39:930-936.
54. Khan IH, Catto GR, Edward N, et al. Acute renal failure: factors influencing nephrology referral and outcome. *QJM.* 1997;90:781-785.
55. Hsu CY, Ordoñez JD, Chertow GM, et al. The risk of acute renal failure in patients with chronic kidney disease. *Kidney Int.* 2008;74:101-107.
56. McGee S, Abernethy 3rd WB, Simel DL. The rational clinical examination. Is this patient hypovolemic? *JAMA.* 1999;281:1022-1029.
57. Nolan 3rd CR, Anger MS, Kelleher SP. Eosinophiluria—a new method of detection and definition of the clinical spectrum. *N Engl J Med.* 1986;315:1516-1519.
58. Solez K, Racusen LC. Role of the renal biopsy in acute renal failure. *Contrib Nephrol.* 2001;132:68-75.
59. National Kidney Foundation. K/DOQI clinical practice guidelines for chronic kidney disease: evaluation, classification, and stratification. *Am J Kidney Dis.* 2002;39(Suppl 1):S1-S266.
60. United States Renal Data System. *USRDS 2009 annual data report: atlas of chronic kidney disease and end-stage renal disease in the united states.* Bethesda, Md: National Institutes of Health, National Institute of Diabetes and Digestive and Kidney Diseases; 2009, Available at: http://www.usrds.org/adr.htm. Accessed March 17, 2011.
61. Coresh J, Selvin E, Stevens LA, et al. Prevalence of chronic kidney disease in the United States. *JAMA.* 2007;298:2038-2047.
62. Dikow R, Zeier M, Ritz E. Pathophysiology of cardiovascular disease and renal failure. *Cardiol Clin.* 2005;23:311-317.
63. Markowitz GS, Stokes MB, Radhakrishnan J, et al. Acute phosphate nephropathy following oral sodium phosphate bowel purgative: an under recognized cause of chronic renal failure. *J Am Soc Nephrol.* 2005;16: 3389-3396.
64. Foxman B. Epidemiology of urinary tract infections: incidence, morbidity, and economic costs. *Am J Med.* 2002;113(suppl 1A):5S-13S.
65. Lin K, Fajardo K. U.S. Preventive Services Task Force: Screening for asymptomatic bacteriuria in adults: evidence for the U.S. Preventive Services Task Force reaffirmation recommendation statement. *Ann Intern Med.* 2008;149:W20-W24.
66. Bent S, Nallamothu BK, Simel DL, et al. Does this woman have an acute uncomplicated urinary tract infection? *JAMA.* 2002;287:2701-2710.
67. Young JL, Soper DE. Urinalysis and urinary tract infection: update for clinicians. *Infect Dis Obstet Gynecol.* 2001;9:249-255.

Laboratory Assessment of Kidney Disease: Glomerular Filtration Rate, Urinalysis, and Proteinuria

Ajay K. Israni and Bertram L. Kasiske

Detection and Diagnosis of Kidney Disease

Because patients in early stages of chronic kidney disease (CKD) often exhibit few signs and symptoms, tests for screening and diagnosis are critical in nephrology. Directly or indirectly, these tests measure kidney structure and function. Ideally, they should detect abnormalities early enough to alert patients and physicians to the potential need for therapy that may prevent morbidity and mortality associated with kidney disease. In addition, testing can help establish a specific diagnosis that will suggest the correct therapy and the likelihood of response to treatment. Even in the absence of effective therapy, accurate diagnosis of kidney disease helps determine prognosis, which often serves a useful purpose in its own right.

Tests to determine kidney structure and function can also be important for measuring disease progression. Once disease has been detected and therapy begun, it is desirable to determine whether the therapy has been effective, so that ineffective therapy can be discontinued or altered. In any case, it is important to predict the clinical course of disease to better inform patients and to help determine when renal replacement therapy may be appropriate. Finally, data have now suggested that CKD is an important independent risk factor for cardiovascular disease. Individuals with mild to moderate reductions in kidney function are at increased risk for cardiovascular disease, and reduced kidney function is associated with a worse prognosis from cardiovascular disease.[1] Microalbuminuria, even in the absence of diabetes, has also been linked to cardiovascular disease.[2] Therefore, detection of kidney damage may help identify patients for cardiovascular disease risk factor management.

The tests that best detect abnormalities in kidney function are those that measure glomerular filtration rate (GFR). However, measurements of GFR may not be useful for screening purposes in many clinical settings. Patients with early kidney disease may have normal or even increased GFR. Because there is a large amount of physiologic variability among normal individuals, it is virtually impossible to define limits for normal GFR. Indeed, substantial differences in the amount of structural kidney damage can be demonstrated in patients with identical GFRs. Furthermore, measuring GFR is of little value in establishing a diagnosis once other abnormalities have been detected. Nevertheless, an accurate determination of GFR can provide useful prognostic information and can be particularly helpful in following the clinical course. Guidelines developed by the National Kidney Foundation's Kidney Disease Outcomes Quality Initiative (KDOQI) have defined stages of CKD largely on the basis of levels of GFR.[3]

Urinalysis is often the most useful test for detecting early kidney abnormalities. Measuring urine protein or examining the urine sediment can also help establish a diagnosis or determine whether a patient should undergo kidney biopsy. Examining the microscopic structure of kidney tissue is invaluable in detecting and diagnosing kidney disease. However, major limitations of kidney biopsy include the risk and inconvenience of the procedure as well as the potential for sampling errors. The selection of patients who should undergo biopsy can be aided by measurements in urine that help screen for kidney injury.

Renal Clearance—Glomerular Filtration Rate

Overview

GFR is traditionally measured as the renal clearance of a particular substance, or marker, from plasma. The clearance of an indicator substance is the amount removed from plasma, divided by the average plasma concentration over the time of measurement. Clearance is expressed in moles or weight of the indicator per volume per time. It can be thought of as the volume of plasma that can be completely cleared of the indicator in a unit of time.

Under the right conditions, measuring the amount of an indicator in both plasma and urine can allow the accurate calculation of GFR (Figure 25-1). Indeed, if we assume that there is no extrarenal elimination, tubular reabsorption, or tubular secretion of the marker, then GFR can be calculated as:

$$GFR = (U \times V)/(P \times T)$$

where U is the urine concentration, V is the urine volume, and P is the average plasma concentration of the marker over the time (T) of the urine collection.

Unfortunately, tubular secretion or tubular reabsorption of the indicator, or both, can cause renal clearance measurements to give estimates of the GFR that are falsely high or falsely low. Under the right conditions, plasma concentrations of an indicator substance can be completely dependent on renal clearance and can accurately reflect GFR. When the amount of an indicator added to the plasma from an exogenous or endogenous source is constant, and when there is no extrarenal elimination, tubular secretion, or tubular reabsorption, then the GFR is equal to the inverse plasma concentration of the indicator multiplied by a constant. That constant is the amount excreted by glomerular filtration, which, under steady-state conditions, must equal the amount added to the plasma (see Figure 25-1). In other words, under these conditions, $U \times V/T$ is equal to a constant (C) so that GFR = C/P, and changes in GFR must be inversely proportional to changes in P. This information can be used to define the characteristics of an ideal indicator for measuring GFR (Tables 25-1 and 25-2). Although such an indicator does not exist, its definition can serve as a useful benchmark for comparing the advantages and disadvantages of tests designed to measure GFR.

The ideal endogenous indicator would be produced at the same constant rate under all conditions, so that changes in the plasma levels are inversely proportional to changes in GFR multiplied by a constant. This constant would be uniquely determined for an individual patient by measuring the urine excretion rate of the marker (GFR equals the urine excretion

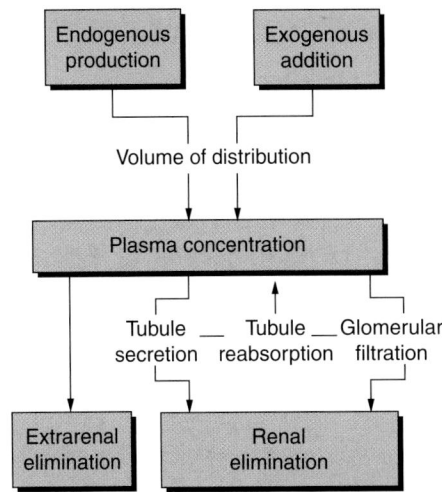

FIGURE 25-1 Factors influencing the relationship between an indicator used to measure renal function and true glomerular filtration rate (GFR). When tubular secretion and reabsorption of the indicator are nil and plasma concentration is constant, then GFR is equal to renal elimination divided by plasma concentration. Also, if the sum of endogenous production and exogenous addition minus extrarenal elimination is constant, then renal elimination is constant and the GFR is inversely proportional to plasma concentration.

rate divided by the plasma concentration). Thereafter, only a single plasma determination would be needed to accurately assess GFR in that patient, unless the renal function were changing so rapidly that a steady state was not achieved. An ideal exogenous indicator would have all of these same characteristics, but should also be safe, easy to administer, and inexpensive.

Whether endogenous or exogenous, an ideal indicator would distribute freely and instantaneously throughout the extracellular space. It would not bind to plasma proteins and would be freely filtered at the glomerulus. It would be subject to neither excretion nor reabsorption in the tubules or urinary collecting system. It would be completely resistant to degradation, and its elimination would be entirely dependent on glomerular filtration. It would be easy to measure in plasma and in urine, and nothing would interfere with the assay. Ideally, the interpatient and intrapatient coefficient of variation would be low.

Obviously, the ideal marker for measuring GFR has yet to be discovered. Nevertheless, a mythical gold standard obeys principles that should be considered in any discussion of methods used to measure GFR. Actual methods will violate these principles in different ways and with different tradeoffs in accuracy and practicality. In the end, these tradeoffs can be tailored to the clinical situation, with estimated prior probabilities taken into account, to achieve a maximum amount of information for a minimum cost. The question is not which test is best, but which test is best suited for the clinical situation at hand.

Plasma Urea

Urea was one of the first indicators used to measure GFR. Unfortunately, it has few of the attributes of an ideal marker, and plasma urea concentration has been shown to be a poor measure of GFR. Urea production is variable and is largely dependent on protein intake. Although one quarter of the

TABLE 25-1 Formulas for Estimating Glomerular Filtration Rate Using Serum Creatinine Level and Other Clinical Parameters

FORMULA	UNITS	REFERENCE
(100/Cr) − 12, *if male*	mL/min/1.73 m^2	Jelliffe[3] and Jelliffe[30]
(80/Cr) − 7, *if female*		
Wt × (29.3 − 0.203 × Age)/(Cr × 14.4), *if male*	mL/min	Kampmann et al.[32], Mawer et al.[34]
Wt × (25.3 − 0.175 × Age)/(Cr × 14.4), *if female*		
{98 − [16 × (Age − 20)/20]}/Cr, *multiply by* 0.90 *if female*	mL/min/1.73 m^2	Jelliffe[31]
[(140 − Age) × Wt]/(72 × Cr), *multiply by* 0.85 *if female*	mL/min	Cockcroft and Gault[28]
[(145 − Age)/Cr] − 3, *multiply by* 0.85 *if female*	mL/min/70 kg	Hull et al.[29]
[27 − (0.173 × Age)]/Cr, *if male*	mL/min	Bjornsson et al.[27]
[27 − (0.175 × Age)]/Cr, *if female*		
[7.58/(Cr × 0.0884)] − (0.103 × Age) + (0.096 × Wt) − 6.66, *if male*	(height^2)/3	Walser, Drew, and Guldan[35]
[6.05/(Cr × 0.0884)] − (0.080 × Age) + (0.080 × Wt) − 4.81, *if female*	(height^2)/3	
170 × Cr$^{-0.999}$ × Age$^{-0.176}$ × 0.762 (*if female*) × 1.180 (*if black*) × SUN$^{-0.170}$ × Alb$^{0.318}$	mL/min/1.73 m^2	Levey et al.[33] (MDRD study)
175 × Cr$^{-1.154}$ × Age$^{-0.203}$ × 0.742 (*if female*) × 1.212 (*if black*)	mL/min/1.73 m^2	*
141 × min(Cr/κ, 1)α × max(Cr/κ, 1)$^{-1.209}$ × 0.993^{Age} × 1.018 (*if female*) × 1.59 (*if black*), where κ is 0.7 for females and 0.9 for males, α is −0.329 for females and −0.411 for males, *min* indicates the minimum of Cr/κ or 1, and *max* indicates the maximum of Cr/κ or 1.	mL/min/1.73 m^2	Levey et al.[37] (CKD-EPI study)

*This revised MDRD equation uses the creatinine value obtained using the isotope dilution mass spectrometry–traceable creatinine assay.[234]

Alb, Serum albumin level (g/dL); *Cr,* serum creatinine level (mg/dL); *CKD-EPI,* Chronic Kidney Disease Epidemiology Collaboration; *GFR,* glomerular filtration rate; *MDRD,* Modification of Diet in Renal Disease; *SUN,* serum urea nitrogen level (mg/dL); *Wt,* body weight (kg).

TABLE 25-2 Characteristics of an Ideal Endogenous or Exogenous Marker for Measuring Glomerular Filtration Rate

Constant production
Safe
Convenient
Readily diffusible in extracellular space
No protein binding and freely filterable
No tubular reabsorption
No tubular secretion
No extrarenal elimination or degradation
Accurate and reproducible assay
No compounds interfere
Inexpensive
No influence on the glomerular filtration rate

urea produced is metabolized in the intestine, the ammonia produced is reconverted to urea. Thus, most of the urea is ultimately excreted by the kidneys. With a molecular weight of 60 Da, urea is freely filtered at the glomerulus. However, it can be readily reabsorbed, and the amount of tubular reabsorption is variable. Indeed, medullary collecting duct urea reabsorption is functionally linked to water reabsorption. In states of diuresis and low levels of antidiuretic hormone, the medullary collecting duct is relatively impermeable to urea. However, in states of decreased effective intravascular volume, low urine tubular flow, and increased antidiuretic hormone, urea reabsorption can be substantial.[4]

The concentration of urea, or blood urea nitrogen (BUN), in the plasma is affected by a number of factors other than alterations in GFR. As indicated previously, increased plasma urea levels accompany decreased urine flow in patients with intravascular volume depletion, as occurs after the administration of diuretics. Congestive heart failure also raises plasma urea level, probably by similar mechanisms. Increased plasma levels that are probably caused by increased production are seen with elevated dietary protein intake, gastrointestinal bleeding, and tetracycline use. On the other hand, reduced levels of plasma urea can be seen in patients with alcohol abuse and chronic liver disease.[4]

Urea Clearance

Because of tubular urea reabsorption, renal urea clearance usually underestimates GFR. Urea clearance can be as little as one half or less of the GFR as measured by other techniques. As with plasma urea, the state of hydration can markedly influence urea clearance. However, the degree of underestimation of glomerular filtration and the tendency for urea clearance to vary with the state of hydration are both less in patients with markedly reduced renal function. Moreover, because creatinine clearance overestimates GFR, some investigators have suggested that the mean of creatinine and urea clearance would be a reasonable estimate of GFR, at least in patients with low levels of renal function.[4] In a large enough sample of patients, errors from tubular reabsorption of urea may negate errors from tubular secretion of creatinine, so that mean urea and creatinine clearances may better approximate the true GFR. However, the factors that affect tubular creatinine secretion and urea reabsorption are different, and any tendency for "two wrongs to make a right" would likely be coincidental and infrequent in an individual patient.

Urea clearance determinations are made by measuring renal urea excretion. The accuracy of any clearance technique that relies on urine excretion measurements is compromised by problems associated with obtaining accurate urine collections. Twenty-four-hour collections are inconvenient and difficult for most patients to perform. Patients should be instructed to empty the bladder, note the time, and save all subsequent urine, including urine voided at exactly the same time 24 hours from the time of initiation. They should be warned to empty the bladder before defecation to avoid inadvertent loss of urine. The completeness of 24-hour urine collections can be examined by measuring creatinine excretion (see later). Shorter collection times enhance patient adherence but provide samples for only a portion of the day, during which GFR varies in a diurnal pattern. Incomplete bladder emptying can also reduce the accuracy of timed urine collections. Incomplete bladder emptying can be obviated by catheterization, but the discomfort, risk, and inconvenience often make it unacceptable.

Serum Creatinine

Creatinine is a metabolic product of creatine and phosphocreatine, both of which are found almost exclusively in muscle. Thus, creatinine production is proportional to muscle mass and varies little from day to day. However, production can change over longer periods of time if there is a change in muscle mass. Age- and gender-associated differences in creatinine production are also largely attributable to differences in muscle mass.[4]

Although diet ordinarily accounts for a relatively small proportion of overall creatinine excretion, it is another source of variability in serum creatinine levels. Creatine from ingested meat is converted to creatinine and can be the source of up to 30% of total creatinine excretion. Thus, variability in meat intake can also contribute to variability in serum creatinine levels. The conversion of creatine to creatinine can occur with cooking. Because creatinine is readily absorbed from the gastrointestinal tract, ingesting cooked meat can lead to a rapid increase in serum creatinine levels.[4]

Creatinine is small (molecular weight 113 Da), does not bind to plasma proteins, and is freely filtered by the renal glomerulus. However, it has long been appreciated that creatinine is also secreted by the renal tubule. Secretion is a saturable process that probably occurs via the organic cation pathway and is blocked by some commonly used medications, including cimetidine, trimethoprim, pyrimethamine, and dapsone.[4]

If tubular secretion of creatinine were constant, differences in serum creatinine concentration and renal clearance could still reflect differences in GFR. However, evidence suggests that measurements of the secretion of creatinine vary substantially in the same individuals over time, between individuals, and between laboratories. Particularly troublesome is the fact that the proportion of total renal creatinine excretion due to tubular secretion increases with decreasing renal function. This feature could have a dampening effect on serial measurements in individuals, because GFR could fall more rapidly than indicated by either serum creatinine level or creatinine clearance.

Although proportional tubular secretion of creatinine increases with decreasing GFR, total urine creatinine excretion actually declines owing to the fact that extrarenal creatinine degradation increases with declining renal function. Indeed, it has been shown that increased extrarenal creatinine degradation may be sufficient to account entirely for the decrease in urine creatinine excretion associated with declining GFR. The extrarenal degradation of creatinine has been attributed to its conversion to carbon dioxide and methylamine by bacteria in the intestine. Because of the increase in extrarenal creatinine degradation with declining kidney function, plasma creatinine concentration can be expected to underestimate declines in GFR.

A number of methods are used to measure creatinine such as alkaline picrate methods (Jaffé method), enzymatic methods, high-performance liquid chromatography (HPLC), isotope dilution mass spectrometry (IDMS), gas chromatography, and liquid chromatography.[5,6] The original Folin-Wu method used the Jaffé reaction, which has been employed with various modifications since that time.[4] The method of Hare involved the isolation of creatinine by absorption on Lloyd's reagent.[7] The direct alkaline picrate method of Bonsnes and Taussky[5] has been used. This method involves the complexing of creatinine with alkaline picrate and measurement using a colorimetric technique. The modified Jaffé reaction and enzymatic methods have also been adapted for use in autoanalyzers and thus are the most commonly used methods. Other methods may employ ortho-nitrobenzaldehyde (Sakaguchi reaction) and imidohydrolase.[6]

There is probably more variation in what laboratories report as the upper limit of normal for serum creatinine concentration than for any other standard chemistry value.[8] In the absence of procedures to remove noncreatinine chromogens, the upper limit of the normal measured by the Jaffé reaction may be as high as 1.6 to 1.9 mg/dL for adults (to covert milligrams per deciliter to millimolars per liter, multiply by 88.4). The upper limit of normal for serum creatinine measured by autoanalyzer or the imidohydrolase method is usually 1.2 to 1.4 mg/dL. Some laboratories report separate normal ranges for men and women and for adults and children.

Besides differences in methods, differences in equipment may also affect plasma creatinine concentrations. Miller and colleagues[9] evaluated over 5000 laboratories using 20 different instruments to measure creatinine by up to three different alkaline picrate methods and found that the mean serum creatinine concentration on a standardized sample ranged from 0.84 to 1.21 mg/dL. The bias, which describes the systematic deviation from the gold standard measure, was more strongly associated with the instrument manufacturer than with the use of a particular method such as the alkaline picrate method.

A number of normal plasma constituents can interfere with creatinine measurement. Glucose, fructose, pyruvate, acetoacetate, uric acid, ascorbic acid, and plasma proteins can all cause the Jaffé colorimetric assay to yield falsely high creatinine values.[4] The low levels of these substances generally do not interfere with the Jaffé assay of creatinine in urine. Normally, interfering chromogens increase the creatinine result by about 20%, but in some disease states, the interference can be much greater. In diabetic ketoacidosis, for example, spurious elevations in serum creatinine level can be significant.

Cephalosporin antibiotics can also interfere with the Jaffé reaction.[10-13] One study showed that, in marked renal insufficiency, serum creatinine rises and noncreatinine chromogens contribute proportionally less to the total reaction.[14] In individuals with normal kidney function, noncreatinine chromogens made up 14% (range = 4.5% to 22.3%) of the total, whereas in individuals with serum creatinine levels ranging from 5.6 to 29.4 mg/dL, noncreatinine chromogens contributed only 5% (range = 0% to 14.6%) to the total measured level.[14] This same study found no effect of the noncreatinine chromogens on the variability of plasma values.

Several modifications made to the classic Jaffé assay have been designed to remove interfering chromogens before analysis,[15] including deproteinization with specific adsorption of creatinine using fuller's earth and ion exchange resins, measurement of Jaffé-positive chromogens before and after the destruction of creatinine with bacteria, and dialysis separation. These methods have largely been replaced by less costly and more convenient autoanalyzer techniques. Autoanalyzer methods utilize the Jaffé reaction, but separate creatinine from noncreatinine chromogens by the rate of color development,[15] thus avoiding most of the interference seen with the standard Jaffé method.[16] However, very high serum bilirubin levels can cause falsely low creatinine levels.[17] Newer techniques measuring true serum creatinine give plasma levels that are slightly lower than those obtained using the Jaffé assay method.[15] The imidohydrolase method can be perturbed by extremely high glucose levels[6] and by the antifungal agent 5-flucytosine.[4]

KDOQI guidelines recommend that autoanalyzer manufacturers and clinical laboratories calibrate serum creatinine assays using an international standard.[3] The Creatinine Standardized Program, created by the National Kidney Disease Education Program of the U.S. National Institutes of Health, recommends using a creatinine measurement method that has its calibration traceable to the IDMS methods, and starting in 2008, most instrument manufacturers have agreed to this calibration.[18]

For research studies, the National Institute of Standards and Technology has a standard reference material to calibrate creatinine measurements for most commonly used methods to ensure commutability with native serum samples.[18] *Commutability* has been defined as the equivalence of the mathematical relationships between the results obtained by different measurement procedures for a reference material and for representative samples from healthy and diseased individuals. Commutability does not mean accuracy or trueness of results.

Serum creatinine concentration is probably the most widely used indirect measure of GFR, its popularity attributable to convenience and low cost. Unfortunately, serum creatinine is very insensitive to even substantial declines in GFR. The GFR as measured by more accurate techniques (described later) may be reduced by up to 50% before serum creatinine level becomes elevated.[4]

The correct interpretation of serum creatinine level in the clinical setting is problematic. Failure to consider variations in creatinine production due to differences in muscle mass frequently leads to misinterpretation of serum creatinine levels. This confusion may be compounded by the use of standard normal ranges for serum creatinine levels that appear on routine laboratory reports. For example, a serum creatinine value that falls within the "normal" range may indicate a normal GFR in a young, healthy individual. However, the same serum creatinine value in an elderly individual could indicate a twofold reduction in GFR owing to a comparable reduction in muscle mass.[4] Therefore, KDOQI guidelines recommend that clinical laboratories report serum creatinine with an estimated GFR using a serum creatinine–based formula[3] (see Table 25-1).

Muscle mass may also decline over a relatively short period of time. For example, significant declines in creatinine excretion were seen in patients undergoing kidney transplantation, especially those who had long-term declines in allograft function.[19] The decline in creatinine excretion was probably due to decreases in muscle mass from multiple causes, including the effects of corticosteroids. As a result of the reduction in muscle mass, changes in serum creatinine underestimated the amount of decline in kidney function.[4]

Failure to remember the potential effects of tubular secretion on serum creatinine, especially in patients with reduced kidney function, may lead the clinician to believe that renal function is better than it actually is. One study has suggested that tubular secretion of creatinine is significant in patients with nephritic syndrome and decreased serum albumin levels.[20]

Moreover, the potential for interference from plasma constituents and medications requires the clinician to know what assay is being used to measure serum creatinine. On the basis of whether the reported upper limit of normal for adults is high (1.4 to 1.9 mg/dL) or low (1.2 to 1.4 mg/dL), it may sometimes be possible to correctly surmise whether an unmodified alkaline picrate–Jaffé reaction (higher normal limits) or a newer method that removes interference with chromogens (lower normal limits) is being used. The clinician should also be aware of the precision of the assay. Precision is commonly measured by the coefficient of variation, which is the mean of replicate samples divided by the standard deviation.

Creatinine Clearance

Measuring creatinine clearance obviates some of the problems of using serum creatinine level as a marker of GFR, but creates others. Differences in steady-state creatinine production due to differences in muscle mass that affect serum creatinine concentration should not affect creatinine clearance. Extrarenal elimination of creatinine should have little influence on the ability of the creatinine clearance to estimate GFR. However, the reliability of creatinine clearance is greatly diminished by variability in tubular secretion of creatinine and by the inability of most patients to accurately collect timed urine samples.[20] Indeed, some investigators[21,22] have argued that the creatinine clearance rate is a less reliable measure of GFR than serum creatinine level and should be abandoned.

Tubular secretion of creatinine gives a creatinine clearance rate that overestimates the true GFR. The overestimation is reduced somewhat if serum and urine creatinine are both measured by the Jaffé method. As discussed, plasma constituents tend to falsely raise the serum creatinine level as measured by the Jaffé assay, whereas urine creatinine levels are largely unaffected. Thus, creatinine clearance determinations calculated from serum and urine creatinine levels measured with the Jaffé assay tend to be falsely low. In a given population of patients, this error will tend to cancel the error introduced by tubular creatinine secretion, and the creatinine clearance rate approximates GFR. However, the two errors are independent, and the occurrence of opposing errors of the same magnitude in the same patient is largely a result of chance.[4] Thus, variability in the precision of creatinine clearance rate as an estimate of true GFR is not reduced and may be increased by this fortuitous combination of errors. Indeed, the creatinine clearance rate determined in 30 patients using a total chromogen method was only 9% higher than inulin clearance, although the true creatinine clearance was 31% higher. However, the correlation coefficient for inulin clearance compared with the true creatinine clearance ($r = 0.96$) was much better than the correlation coefficient for inulin clearance compared with the total chromogen creatinine clearance ($r = 0.86$), which suggests that the latter technique was more accurate but less precise.[4]

Prolonged storage of the urine can introduce error in the creatinine clearance determination by perturbing urine creatinine levels. High temperature and low urine pH enhance the conversion of creatine to creatinine in urine.[23] Indeed, storing urine under adverse conditions for 24 hours was shown to cause a 20% increase in the amount of measured urine creatinine.[23] This problem can be obviated by refrigerating urine samples and by measuring the urine creatinine level without delay.

Tubular secretion of creatinine would cause little difficulty if it were constant, and a constant correction factor could be subtracted from creatinine clearance determinations to yield a more accurate estimate of GFR. Unfortunately, interpatient and intrapatient variability in tubular creatinine secretion makes such an approach impossible. The tendency for tubular secretion to rise proportionally with declining levels of kidney function, for example, decreases the usefulness of creatinine clearance determinations as accurate reflections of GFR in patients with kidney disease.[24]

As mentioned earlier in the discussion of urea clearance, all renal clearance techniques that rely on measuring a marker of GFR in the urine are subject to the vagaries of urine collection. Variability in the adequacy of timed urine samples can introduce substantial error in the clearance determination. Having patients perform urine collections under the direct supervision of trained personnel can enhance the accuracy of timed collections. However, decreasing the duration of urine collection may increase the contribution of errors due to incomplete bladder emptying, especially if urine volumes are not increased with water loading. In addition, short-interval urine collections negate the advantages of time-averaged GFR estimates made from 24-hour urine collection. The cost of the procedure can also be substantially higher if trained personnel are used to directly supervise urine collections in a clinic setting.

In principle, the renal clearance of creatinine is the urine creatinine excretion divided by the area under the plasma creatinine concentration time curve over the period of time in which the urine was sampled. In practice, creatinine clearance is usually measured by determining the urine creatinine excretion and sampling a single plasma creatinine value. It is then assumed that the plasma creatinine was constant over the time of the urine collection. Plasma creatinine remains relatively constant over 24 hours if food intake and activity are also constant. However, in a 24-hour period, there may be substantial variability in plasma creatinine levels, largely due to effects of diet.[4] Thus, under usual clinical conditions, the assumption that plasma creatinine levels are constant during the period of urine collection may not valid and may, in fact, be a source of error.

The day-to-day coefficient of variation for serum creatinine level is approximately 8%.[25] Because two creatinine determinations must be made to calculate a creatinine clearance, the coefficient of variation of the creatinine clearance should be higher than that of the serum creatinine level. Indeed, the coefficient of variation of creatinine clearance could be expected to be at least 11.3% (the square root of 2 times the square of 8%). This is, in fact, similar to the coefficient of variation for creatinine clearance reported in at least one investigation.[25] Other researchers[26] have reported a day-to-day coefficients of variation for creatinine clearance as high as 27% when the procedure is carried out in the routine clinical setting. Because tubular secretion of creatinine is a major limitation in the use of creatinine clearance method, several investigators tried to enhance the accuracy of creatinine clearance measurements by blocking tubular creatinine secretion with the histamine-2 receptor antagonist cimetidine. In many patients, however, tubular secretion of creatinine was not completely blocked, and the cimetidine-enhanced creatinine clearance value still overestimated GFR in these individuals. Therefore, the cimetidine-enhanced creatinine clearance technique will not replace other, more accurate methods for measuring GFR. Measurement of cimetidine-enhanced creatinine clearance could prove to be a cost-effective alternative in many clinical situations, however.

Serum Creatinine Formulas for Estimation of Kidney Function

The need to collect a urine sample remains a major drawback of the creatinine clearance technique, with or without cimetidine enhancement. Therefore, many attempts have been made to mathematically transform or correct serum creatinine level so that it may more accurately reflect GFR (see Table 25-1).[21,27-35] Under ideal conditions, GFR, as measured by a marker such as creatinine, should be equal to the inverse of the creatinine value multiplied by a constant rate of creatinine excretion. However, changes in creatinine production, extrarenal elimination, and tubular secretion of creatinine can all create errors in the use of inverse creatinine value to measure changes in GFR. Indeed, none of the shortcomings of using serum creatinine level as a marker of GFR is avoided by using inverse creatinine value.[4]

One of the problems with using creatinine or its inverse as a measure of GFR is that interpatient and intrapatient differences in creatinine production often occur. Variations in creatinine production due to age- and sex-related differences in muscle mass have been measured and have been incorporated in formulas to improve the ability of serum creatinine to estimate GFR.

A widely used formula is that of Cockcroft and Gault,[28] which reduces the variability of serum creatinine estimates of GFR measured in a population of men and women of different ages. However, the formula does not take into account differences in creatinine production between individuals of the same age and sex or even in the same individual over time. The formula systematically overestimates GFR in individuals who are obese or edematous. Moreover, it does not take into account extrarenal elimination, tubular handling, or inaccuracies in the laboratory measurement of creatinine that can contribute to error in the serum creatinine estimate of GFR.

Because of its relative simplicity and the ready availability of the required input data, the Cockcroft-Gault formula has maintained widespread support. In subjects screened for the African-American Study of Kidney Disease and Hypertension pilot study, outpatient 24-hour urine collections and timed creatinine clearance measurements offered no more precision than the Cockcroft-Gault formula and required substantially more time and effort.

The GFR has probably never been measured with more accuracy in a large population of patients than it was in the Modification of Diet in Renal Disease (MDRD) study. The investigators[36] used the isotopically measured GFR determinations from the MDRD study to derive a formula for estimating GFR using only readily measurable clinical variables. Significantly, they derived the formula based on data from a randomly selected subset of patients from the whole population, and then tested the formula in the remainder of the population. The formula, sometimes referred to as the *MDRD study equation* or the *Levey formula*, uses only serum chemistry values (creatinine, urea, and albumin) and patient characteristics (age, gender, and race). It was able to predict 90.3% of the variability in isotopically measured GFR in the validation sample (see Table 25-1).[33] A simplified version requiring only serum creatinine value, age, race, and gender was found to correlate similarly with measured GFR.

Levey and colleagues[33] cautioned against the immediate application of these formulas in patient subgroups not represented in the initial study, including individuals with normal kidney function, patients with type 1 diabetes, elderly persons, and kidney transplant recipients. It cannot be assumed that formulas to predict kidney function derived from data for one patient population will be valid when applied to another population. For example, few diabetic individuals were included in some of the original studies that examined formulas for predicting GFR. When these formulas were subsequently tested in diabetic patients, they were found to be inaccurate.

Several studies have indicated that the MDRD equation underestimates GFR for subjects with normal kidney function. Therefore, a recent study utilized GFR, measured as clearance of exogenous filtration markers obtained in 26 independent research projects, to develop a new creatinine equation to potentially replace the MDRD equation.[37] This new equation is referred to as the *Chronic Kidney Disease Epidemiology Collaboration* or *CKD-EPI equation*.[37] This new equation is substantially more accurate among subjects with higher GFRs[37] but needs to be validated for other groups.

Serum creatinine formulas for estimating the GFR may not be reliable in certain individuals. Individuals who follow a vegetarian diet, consume creatinine supplements, have unusual muscle mass, have an unusual weight (the morbidly obese, amputees), or are pregnant were not included in the study populations that were used to generate these formulas. Likewise, the formulas may not be accurate for individuals from different ethnic groups.[38]

Serum Cystatin C

Several low-molecular-weight (LMW) proteins have been evaluated as endogenous markers of GFR, with cystatin C commanding the most attention. The use of serum cystatin C concentration as a marker of GFR was first suggested in 1985, when Simonsen and colleagues[39-43] demonstrated a correlation between reciprocal cystatin C values and chromium 51–radiolabeled ethylenediaminetetraacetic acid (^{51}Cr-EDTA) clearance. Since then, numerous investigators[40,44-46] have shown that cystatin C may be a good marker of GFR.

Cystatin C is a 13-kDa basic protein of the cystatin superfamily of cysteine proteinase inhibitors. It is synthesized by all nucleated cells at a constant rate, which fulfills an important criterion for any endogenous marker of GFR. In most studies, production of cystatin C is not found to be altered by inflammatory processes, by muscle mass, or by gender.[4] One study did find higher levels of cystatin C in males, older patients, and those of greater height and weight. However, the study utilized 24-hour urine collections to determine creatinine clearance as the gold standard for kidney function.[47] Another study found that inflammation or immunosuppression therapy may affect cystatin C levels.

Concentrations of cystatin C are highest in the first days of life and rapidly decrease during the first 4 months, likely due to maturation of the glomerular filtration capacity. In children older than 1 year, cystatin C levels stabilize and approximate those of adults. An increase in levels after the fifth decade reflects the age-related decline in GFR and contrasts with stable serum creatinine values, which presumably are due to a decline in muscle mass with age.[48] Because of its low molecular weight and positive charge at physiologic pH, cystatin C freely passes the glomerular filter. It is not secreted, but proximal tubular cells reabsorb and catabolize the filtered cystatin C, which results in very low urinary concentrations.[49] Although calculation of GFR using urinary cystatin C is not possible, some investigators[50] have speculated that urinary cystatin C could serve as a marker for renal tubular dysfunction.

Cystatin C can be measured using any of a number of radioimmunoassays, fluorescent techniques, and enzymatic immunoassays.[42] Because these methods are slow and relatively imprecise, widespread clinical use is not feasible. Latex immunoassays employing latex particles conjugated with cystatin C–specific antibody demonstrate greater precision, produce more consistent reference intervals, and are far quicker.[42] Particle-enhanced turbidimetric immunoassay (PETIA)[44,45] and particle-enhanced nephelometric immunoassay (PENIA)[48] are the two available versions of latex immunoassay. On the basis of a 2002 meta-analysis, immunonephelometric methods appear to be superior to other assays when measuring cystatin C.[51]

Studies involving a number of patients have shown that serum cystatin C concentration may be more sensitive and specific than serum creatinine level for detecting early changes in isotopically determined GFR.[45,46,52] Receiver operating characteristic (ROC) analysis of the data from one of these studies demonstrated superior accuracy of cystatin C concentration over creatinine concentration in patients with reduced GFR.[44] In addition, small reductions in GFR appear to be detected more easily using cystatin C measurement than creatinine determination.[45,46]

Other studies have indicated that cystatin C determination has a greater ability to detect subclinical kidney dysfunction than creatinine measurement.[53] Coll and colleagues[53] demonstrated that cystatin C levels rose when GFR fell to 88 mL/min/1.73 m^2 and that creatinine levels did not rise until GFR dropped to 75 mL/min/1.73 m^2. However, ROC analysis showed no difference in the diagnostic accuracy of the two tests.[53] Likewise, several other studies have failed to show a significant difference between cystatin C and creatinine determinations, despite a trend toward greater accuracy with cystatin C.[43,54,55]

A meta-analysis[51] incorporating studies reported in 46 articles and 8 abstracts and using standard measures of GFR suggested superiority of reciprocal cystatin C value over reciprocal serum creatinine level as a marker of GFR.[51] Superior correlation coefficients and greater ROC plot area-under-the-curve values were calculated for cystatin C. The authors of this meta-analysis speculated that prior studies indicating a lack of superiority of cystatin C could reflect a type II error or differences caused by assay methods.

Cystatin C concentration has been examined in a diverse population. In children, cystatin C measurement appears to be at least as useful as serum creatinine determination in assessing GFR, although the number of children studied who were younger than 4 years is small. This age subgroup, for which serum creatinine levels have been unreliable, might arguably receive the most benefit from the measurement of cystatin C concentration to evaluate GFR. Cystatin C has been favorably evaluated in other similar subgroups, including patients with cirrhosis, spinal cord injury, and rheumatoid arthritis, as well as elderly patients.[56] In diabetic patients, results have been mixed.[57,58]

In kidney transplant recipients, cystatin C value has been found to be more sensitive than serum creatinine level in detecting decreases in GFR. However, some investigators have shown that cystatin C values underestimate GFR in this population.[59] In one study, levels of cystatin C were significantly higher in 54 pediatric kidney transplant recipients than in 56 control subjects with similar GFR values.[59] The reason for this result is not clear. However, corticosteroids have been implicated, given the finding of elevation of cystatin C level in asthmatic patients treated with corticosteroids[60] and the results of in vitro experiments demonstrating a dose-dependent rise in cystatin C production in HeLa cells treated with dexamethasone.[61] A case-control study of kidney transplant recipients showed a dose-dependent increase in cystatin C in individuals who were receiving corticosteroids compared with those who were not.[62] In contrast, corticosteroids did not raise levels of cystatin C in a group of children treated for nephritic syndrome.[63] Mixed conclusions of other studies evaluating cystatin C as a marker of GFR in transplant recipients[64] and the discrepancy in the effects of corticosteroids illustrate a need for further studies in this population.

The cost of the cystatin C assay, the difficulty in making the assay universally available, and the potentially high intra-individual variability in the determination of cystatin C levels are all issues that require attention if this particular marker is to be used in clinical practice.[65,66] Currently, there is no standard for serum cystatin C measurement.[67]

Inulin

Inulin was once considered the gold standard of exogenously administered markers of GFR. However, the scarcity and high cost of inulin all but eliminated its routine use. Inulin (molecular weight 5200 Da) is a polymer of fructose found in tubers such as the dahlia, the Jerusalem artichoke, and chicory. Inulin is inert and does not bind to plasma proteins. It distributes in extracellular fluid, is freely filtered at the glomerulus, and is neither reabsorbed nor secreted by renal tubules.

Inulin is readily measured in plasma and urine by one of several colorimetric assays. These assays are time consuming to perform but can be adapted for use on an autoanalyzer. Glucose is also detected by most inulin assays and must therefore be either removed beforehand or measured independently in the sample and subtracted. In any case, appropriate care must be taken in patients with high plasma or urine glucose levels, especially if the levels fluctuate during the GFR determination.[4]

The renal clearance method for using inulin to measure GFR was originally developed and championed by Homer Smith. Over the years, this technique has been used by many clinical investigators and has been modified only slightly. Generally, measurements are made under standardized conditions. Patients are typically studied in the morning, after an overnight fast. An oral water load of 10 to 15 mL/kg body weight is given before inulin is infused, and additional water is administered throughout the test to ensure a constant urine flow rate of at least 4 mL/min. When a good urine flow has been established, a loading dose of inulin is given, followed by a constant infusion to maintain plasma levels. Once a steady state has been achieved, several timed (generally 30-minute) urine collections are carried out. Ideally, a bladder catheter is used to ensure the accuracy of the timed urine collections. Serial plasma levels of inulin are also measured. Inulin clearance is calculated from the plasma level (time averaged), urine concentration, and urine flow rate.

Usually, an average of three to five separate determinations is made. Each of these measurements is subject to inaccuracies; indeed, the coefficient of variation between clearance periods is 10%,[36] and the coefficient of variation of inulin clearance measured on different days in the same individual is approximately 7.5%.[36] No doubt, some of the variability in inulin clearance determinations made in the same individual is due to error in measurement, and some is due to true fluctuation in GFR (see later). It has been estimated that a difference of 20 mL/1.73 m^2/min in the values of inulin clearances measured in the same individual on 2 separate days predicts a real difference in GFR at a statistical significance level of $P < 0.05$.[4] A difference of 27 mL/1.73 m^2/min between measurements predicts a real difference at the $P < 0.01$ level.[4]

The renal inulin clearance method has a number of drawbacks. Bladder catheterization is associated with some risk and is not readily accepted by many patients. Although inulin clearance measurements can be carried out using spontaneous voiding, incomplete bladder emptying can introduce additional variability. Unfortunately, no studies have compared inulin clearance results obtained using bladder catheterization with those obtained using spontaneous voiding. Problems with residual urine are most likely to occur in individuals with prostatism and in patients with neurogenic bladder dysfunction. High urine volumes probably help reduce the effect of incomplete bladder emptying, but water loading is itself uncomfortable for many patients. It has been noted that inulin clearance tends to decline during serial urine collections, in part as a result of the difficulty patients have in maintaining a high water intake throughout the procedure. Use of an intravenous cannula and a constant infusion is another source of discomfort and inconvenience. Thus, despite its accuracy, the renal inulin clearance technique is cumbersome and inconvenient.

To avoid problems related to urine collection, many investigators have turned to plasma clearance techniques. Plasma clearance can be measured with the use of either a constant infusion or a bolus injection.[68] If, during a constant infusion, both the distribution space and the plasma level of inulin are constant, the rate of infusion will be equal to the rate of elimination. The inulin clearance then becomes the rate of infusion divided by the plasma concentration. There is a high degree of correlation between results obtained using this technique and those obtained using the renal clearance method.[68] However, maintaining constant plasma concentrations is very difficult,[69,70] and the constant infusion technique is not always used. The bolus injection technique has been used with inulin,[71] and this technique is discussed in greater detail in the section on radionuclide and radiocontrast markers of GFR.

As previously noted, a number of problems limit the usefulness of inulin as a marker of GFR. Although most data suggest that inulin is freely filtered and is not handled by the renal tubules, this may not be true in all clinical situations. For example, it has been suggested that impaired filtration, back diffusion of inulin, or both can limit the usefulness of the inulin clearance method in kidney transplant recipients.[72] However, the decline in the use of inulin as a marker of GFR has been due largely to its scarcity and cost.

Radionuclide and Radiocontrast Markers of Glomerular Filtration Rate

Any of several radionuclide-labeled and unlabeled radiocontrast markers of GFR can be used in either renal or plasma clearance studies. Estimating GFR by plasma clearance of an indicator given by intravenous bolus injection is convenient and has been used more often than constant infusion or renal clearance techniques. The assumptions underlying the measurement of renal clearance using a single-injection technique are critical. Basically, renal clearance is measured as the plasma clearance, or the amount of indicator injected divided by the integrated area of the plasma concentration curve over time.[73] Because it is not possible to measure enough samples to accurately determine the area under the plasma concentration time curve, this area is estimated based on mathematical formulations that describe the decline in plasma levels over time.

Models used to estimate plasma clearance assume that the volume of distribution and renal excretion are constant over time and that there is no extrarenal excretion. A constant renal excretion has been demonstrated for at least two indicators, iodine 125m–radiolabeled iothalamate (^{125}I-iothalamate) and ^{51}Cr-EDTA.[74] However, GFR may be underestimated with the use of technetium 125m–radiolabeled diethylenetriaminepentaacetic acid (^{99m}Tc-DTPA), possibly due to plasma protein binding and decreasing renal clearance over time.[75,76] Other researchers[77] have shown that there is a small, constant overestimation of plasma clearance compared with renal clearance of ^{51}Cr-EDTA.

Although the indicator is eliminated directly from the arterial circulation, it is injected intravenously, and blood samples to measure the plasma clearance are drawn from the venous compartment. The assumption that there is instantaneous equilibration between the arterial and the venous circulation is incorrect.[4] Thus, any method used to calculate renal clearance must correct for inaccuracies due to delayed equilibration between the venous and the arterial compartments.

Because it is not possible to measure the entire plasma concentration time curve, a limited number of samples must be measured, and an appropriate curve fitted to these points must be used to measure the plasma clearance. Both one- and two-compartment models have been used to measure plasma clearance (Figure 25-2). In the two-compartment model, the first compartment can be thought of as corresponding to plasma and the second to extracellular fluid.[4] Two slopes and two intercepts are derived by plotting plasma values over time after injection.[78] One slope and intercept are derived from a straight line fit to the initial data when plotted on a logarithmic scale, and the other slope and intercept are derived from a line fit to the data of the terminal elimination phase.

Unfortunately, the two-compartment method, although more accurate than the one-compartment model, requires more frequent plasma sampling. Therefore, most investigators now use a one-compartment model, in which only values measured during the terminal elimination phase (generally commencing 90 to 120 minutes after injection) are sampled. In this model, the slope and intercept of a line plotted on a logarithmic scale are used to calculate clearance using the following formula:

$$Clearance = V_o[\ln(2)] / t_{1/2}$$

where V_o is the volume of distribution and $t_{1/2}$ is the half-time for decay in plasma levels. The value derived from this relationship is multiplied by a constant to correct for systematic errors attributable to overestimation of V_o and a higher concentration of marker in venous compared with arterial blood. The clearance calculated using this simple monoexponential model is surprisingly accurate.[4] Also surprising is the fact that as few as two samples yield results that seem to be as accurate as those based on multiple samples.[79]

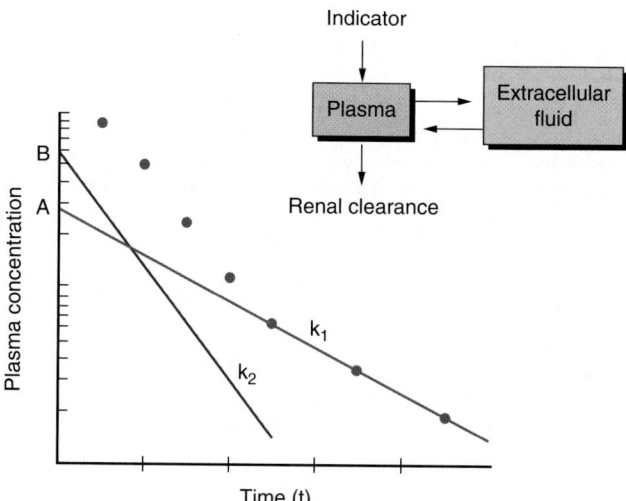

FIGURE 25-2 Plasma disappearance curve for the indicator of glomerular filtration rate (GFR) after bolus intravenous administration. *Dots* represent measured concentrations. The line with slope k_1 and intercept A is the least-squares best fit of the terminal elimination phase. The line with slope k_2 and intercept B represents the best fit of the difference between actual values and values calculated from the line fitted to the terminal elimination phase. GFR (one-compartment method) is calculated as Qk_1/A, where Q is the quantity of indicator administered. GFR (two-compartment method) is calculated as $Qk_1k_2/(Ak_2 + Bk_1)$.

Single-sample techniques have also been used to estimate plasma clearance.[80] One such method was based on the use of different sampling times dictated by the predicted GFR.[80] Tepe and colleagues[81] compared different sampling times using monoexponential models for GFR determinations in 139 subjects. They found that a single-sample method was accurate and that sampling between 60 and 240 minutes after injection was optimal. Other researchers have confirmed that single-sample techniques can give reasonably accurate estimates of GFR that are generally suitable for clinical practice.[82,83] Nevertheless, multiple sampling yields a GFR determination that is more accurate than that obtained by single-sample techniques and may therefore be more suitable for clinical investigations that must detect small differences in changes in GFR among patients.[84] There is some controversy over the applicability of standard adult formulas for calculating GFR in children using single-sample techniques,[85,86] and further study is required.

Whether single or multiple samples are used with a monoexponential model, it is probably important that the sampling time be adjusted to the level of kidney function.[73,84] To sample after only 2 hours may be too soon for patients with normal to moderately decreased kidney function[74]; a sampling time of 4 to 5 hours after injection is probably more appropriate for this group.[73] However, this interval may be too short for individuals with more marked declines in kidney function or for patients with ascites. In such patients, sampling times up to 24 hours may be appropriate.[73] The use of radiolabeling and very sensitive HPLC detection methods have reduced the amount of marker that needs to be administered, and this, in turn, has permitted subcutaneous administration.[87] It has been shown that reasonably predictable plasma concentrations can be achieved after subcutaneous injection of a radiolabeled marker such as ^{125}I-iothalamate. Thus, the renal clearance of such a marker can be measured after subcutaneous injection.

The measurement of plasma clearance need not require plasma sampling. A gamma camera positioned over the kidneys can be used to measure renal elimination of a radioactive indicator.[88,89] Quantitative renal imaging most commonly uses ^{99m}Tc-DTPA, radioiodinated iodohippuran (Hippuran), ^{123}I-ortho-iodohippurate, or ^{99m}Tc-mercaptoacetyltriglycine.[89,90] Estimation of GFR has now been combined with computed tomography using radiocontrast agents.[91] Magnetic resonance imaging (MRI) has also been proposed as a method for estimating GFR and renal blood flow.[92]

In general, GFR determination through quantitative renal imaging is not as precise as that arrived at through plasma sampling.[90,93] The advantage of quantitative renal imaging is that additional information pertaining to the anatomy of renal function can be obtained. Indeed, the "split function" or relative contribution of each kidney to total GFR can be calculated. This information can be important in the evaluation of some patients with renal vascular disease and can be crucial in certain circumstances (e.g., in deciding whether or not to carry out a unilateral nephrectomy). Although currently experimental, MRI techniques may someday provide quantitative information on regional cortical and medullary perfusion. Another potential application of techniques that measure isotopes externally which exploits the rapidity with which such measurements can be obtained is the monitoring of acute changes in kidney function. Indeed, miniaturized external monitoring devices have been used for real-time monitoring of kidney function using ^{99m}Tc-DTPA.[94]

It is assumed that, whatever indicator is used to measure plasma clearance, it is not extensively protein bound, is freely filtered, is neither secreted nor reabsorbed by the tubules, and is eliminated only by the kidneys. A number of radionuclide and radiocontrast markers have been developed to measure GFR. In general, they share most of the characteristics of inulin that make it a good indicator of GFR. The popularity of these radionuclide-labeled agents is attributable to their ready availability, ease of administration, relatively low cost, and accuracy of laboratory assay.

Probably the most extensively investigated radionuclide-bound indicator of GFR is ^{51}Cr-EDTA.[4] It is small (molecular weight 292 Da), appears to have little binding to plasma proteins, and is freely filtered by the glomerulus. Studies in humans have shown that the renal clearance of ^{51}Cr-EDTA is about 10% lower than that of inulin when both are measured simultaneously. Although the reason for these lower values is not known, they could be due to plasma protein binding, tubular reabsorption, or in vivo dissociation of the nuclide from EDTA.

Iothalamate sodium, a derivative of triiodobenzoic acid, is a high-osmolar ionic radiocontrast agent. It is small (molecular weight 614 Da) and appears to be only slightly bound to plasma proteins. Several studies in humans have found that simultaneously measured renal clearances of ^{125}I-iothalamate and inulin are similar,[4] but whether this finding resulted from similar renal handling of inulin and iothalamate or whether there was a fortuitous cancellation of errors due, for example, to plasma protein binding countering the effects of tubular secretion is unclear. The use of ^{125}I-iothalamate to measure kidney function is generally considered safe, although there are virtually no long-term follow-up data. The potential problem of thyroid uptake and concentration of the radionuclide can be avoided by administering a large dose of oral iodine (Lugol's solution) prior to the procedure. The half-life of ^{125}I is approximately 60 days.[4]

DTPA (molecular weight 393 Da) has frequently been chelated to radionuclides for use in renal imaging.[89] The one most commonly used to measure GFR is ^{99m}Tc-DTPA.[95,96] The radiolabeling of DTPA with ^{99m}Tc must be carried out immediately before use owing to the chelate's instability. The half-life of ^{99m}Tc is only 6 hours, so samples must be counted soon after the procedure.[89] Protein binding of ^{99m}Tc-DTPA may be a significant source of error in some patients.[75,76] A comparison of clearance measurements based on whole plasma and protein-free, ultrafiltered plasma found significant differences, especially in patients taking multiple medications.[93]

All radionuclide markers are radioactive. This fact has begun to erode their acceptance by patients and has caused them to be subjected to close monitoring by regulatory agencies. In the United States, the storage and disposal of all radioactive waste has come under growing scrutiny and regulation, and the use of isotopes now requires that a number of conditions be met. The actual amount of radiation delivered to patients is generally considered to be less than the amount received while undergoing most standard radiologic procedures.[4] However, the isotope is concentrated in the urine, so that exposure of the urinary collecting system may be greater.[89] To alleviate this potential problem, patients are advised to maintain a high fluid intake and urine volume after the procedure. There are no long-term follow-up studies to assess the risk of this exposure of the collecting system to radiation. In theory, the use of radioisotopes in children and pregnant women may carry an increased risk of potential problems.

In an effort to avoid the use of radiolabeled compounds, techniques have been developed to measure low levels of iodine in urine and plasma. These techniques permit the use of unlabeled radiocontrast agents, which are inherently rich in iodine, to measure GFR. Radiocontrast agents are of low molecular weight (600 to 1600 Da), are not protein bound, and are eliminated from plasma mainly by glomerular filtration. The HPLC assay has been used to measure renal clearance of iothalamate sodium (Conray), diatrizoate meglumine (Hypaque), and iohexol (Omnipaque). The sensitivity of the assay allows the use of as little as 1 mL of radiocontrast agent, which can be injected subcutaneously. The main disadvantage of HPLC is the expense, time, and labor needed to carry out the assay.

A rapid and convenient method has been developed to measure relatively low concentrations of iodine with the use of x-ray fluorescence, and the method has been applied to the measurement of the plasma clearance of iohexol.[97,98] The use of iohexol (molecular weight 821 Da) to measure GFR has grown in popularity, probably because of the low incidence of adverse effects, which is attributable to iohexol's low osmolality and nonionic properties. Plasma clearance determinations using iohexol appear to be comparable to those obtained with the use of other radionuclide-labeled markers and with inulin.[99,100] Up to 30 mL of iohexol may be required if samples are measured by x-ray fluorescence, but the amount administered is reduced in patients with decreased kidney function. As little as 5 mL may be needed if more sensitive techniques are used (e.g., HPLC). The technique appears to be safe, an observation that is not surprising because, even in very high-risk diabetic patients with markedly reduced kidney function, nephrotoxicity from radiocontrast agents occurred only at doses above those generally used to measure kidney function.[101] The incidence of extrarenal adverse reactions from higher doses of nonionic radiocontrast agents used in radiographic procedures is low.

All of the methods that use labeled or unlabeled radiocontrast agents share the risk of allergic reactions. Although this risk is low, none of these agents should be administered to patients who are allergic to iodine. Higher doses of iohexol can also be used when GFR is measured in conjunction with standard urography.[102] Extremely low levels of GFR can be measured, and the technique has been adapted to determine residual renal function in patients receiving maintenance hemodialysis.[103]

Normalization of Glomerular Filtration Rate

The measurement of GFR is usually better suited for monitoring disease progression than for detection or diagnosis, for two reasons. The first is the cost and inconvenience of the procedure. The second is the enormous physiologic variability of GFR in healthy individuals, which makes it difficult to define what a normal GFR should be for an individual patient.[4] An understanding of the factors that contribute to this normal variability is essential in interpreting the results of any test of GFR.

A number of investigators have attempted to normalize GFR in populations of humans who have no known kidney disease. For years, body surface area (BSA) has been used to normalize GFR.[4] Usually, GFR is indexed to BSA; that is, GFR is expressed per unit of BSA. However, at least one report suggested that a regression relationship is more accurate than indexing for normalization of GFR to BSA.[104] The rationale has been that the weight of the kidney and the basal metabolic rate are proportional to BSA in normal individuals of different ages and body sizes.[4] Generally, the DuBois formula for calculating BSA using power functions of height and weight has been used to estimate BSA.[4] This formula is less accurate at extremes of age. Obesity may also perturb the otherwise physiologic relationship between BSA and renal hemodynamic function.[105]

The argument has been made that extracellular fluid volume should be used to normalize GFR, because the purpose of the kidney is to maintain the composition of the extracellular fluid. A comparison of the use of extracellular volume and calculated BSA in normalizing GFR found that the two methods yielded very similar results.[106] Like extracellular fluid volume, blood volume is also closely correlated with calculated BSA in adult men and women.[4] In addition, both kidney and glomerular size correlate with BSA.[107] Thus, to the extent that GFR may be expected to correlate with kidney and glomerular size, the use of BSA to normalize GFR seems to be sound.

Blood volume, extracellular fluid volume, and basal metabolic rate can be more accurately predicted with the use of indices of lean body mass than with calculated BSA alone. Thus, measures of lean body mass could theoretically be better predictors of normal GFR, at least in adults. However, until this is clearly demonstrated to be the case, the more convenient calculated BSA will, no doubt, continue to be the standard for normalizing GFR.[4]

Although the variability of GFR measurements in normal individuals can be reduced by taking BSA differences into account, the residual variability is substantial. A number of factors may contribute to this variability. GFR normally declines with age, but does so to a variable extent.[4] It is well known that dietary protein intake can affect GFR. Similarly, salt intake, water consumption, posture, and normal diurnal variation can all affect GFR determinations in normal individuals. In women, the menstrual cycle can affect GFR and may be an additional source of physiologic variability.[4]

The concept of *renal functional reserve* was introduced in studies that demonstrated higher GFR after an oral protein load.[108] This development led to an unfortunate confusion between increased function due to structural changes after a reduction in kidney mass and acute increases in GFR of a functional nature (e.g., after an oral protein load).[108] In theory, the normal intraindividual physiologic variability in GFR could be reduced if the measurement were made after an acute maneuver that maximized kidney function. However, there are inadequate data to determine whether this is in fact the case. Moreover, such maneuvers substantially increase the complexity and expense of the measurement.

Applications

A number of factors should be considered in selecting a clinical test to measure GFR. Unfortunately, the necessary information on accuracy, precision, and expected prevalence of

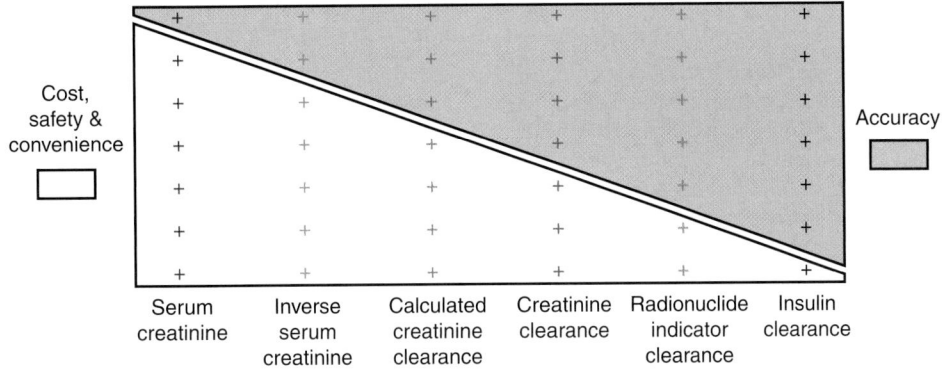

FIGURE 25-3 Conflict between practicality (cost, safety, and convenience) and accuracy of methods to estimate glomerular filtration rate (GFR). On one end of the spectrum, serum creatinine level is most practical but least accurate. On the other end of the spectrum, inulin clearance is most accurate but least practical.

abnormal results is usually not available for each test in each specific clinical situation. However, recognition of how these factors affect the utility of a test, along with crude estimations of these critical parameters, can provide guidance in test selection. Finally, the usefulness of a test to measure GFR is dictated not only by issues of accuracy and precision but also by cost, safety, and convenience. In general, the tests that are most accurate and precise are also those that are most costly and inconvenient (Figure 25-3). No single test of GFR is ideally suited for every clinical and research application. Rather, the goal should be to select the most accurate and precise test to answer the question being addressed in the safest, most cost-effective, and convenient manner possible in the population being studied.

In clinical practice, tests of GFR are most commonly used for (1) screening for the presence of kidney disease, (2) measuring disease progression to determine prognosis and effects of therapy, (3) confirming the need for treatment of end-stage renal disease with dialysis or transplantation, (4) estimating renal clearance of drugs to guide dosing, and (5) assessing GFR as a risk factor for cardiovascular disease.[4,109] For research purposes, tests of GFR are most commonly asked to distinguish differences in the rate of change between two or more experimental groups.

Although precise data do not exist, it is probable that none of the currently available tests of renal function is very well suited for detecting early or mild kidney disease in the general population. Nevertheless, there is a legitimate need for tests to identify patients with moderate or marked declines in kidney function in high-risk situations. The cost and inconvenience of creatinine clearance and radionuclide measurements of GFR ordinarily preclude their use for these screening purposes. Therefore, serum creatinine level has most often been used to screen for the presence of significant renal impairment. For example, serum creatinine level is commonly used to screen for impaired renal function to identify patients who are at increased risk of developing radiocontrast-induced acute renal failure. Serum creatinine has been shown to be useful in this situation. Clearly, the large number of patients who receive radiocontrast agents would preclude the use of other, more expensive and inconvenient tests for this purpose. Similarly, the high prevalence of essential hypertension in the Western world renders radionuclide determinations of GFR impractical as a first-line screening procedure to detect a renal cause of hypertension in low-risk individuals. Therefore,

most clinical laboratories report a calculated GFR using the MDRD equation along with the serum creatinine level. Such calculated GFR measurements serve as a screening tool in the general population.

In contrast to the situation for individuals who are unlikely to have kidney disease, the use of more expensive, but more accurate measures of GFR may be warranted in patients at high risk of kidney functional impairment. For example, the prevalence of kidney dysfunction in patients with systemic lupus erythematosus and low serum complement levels may be high enough to justify the use of a radionuclide determination of GFR to screen for kidney dysfunction that could suggest a need for therapy or additional diagnostic tests. Similarly, the high incidence of both acute and chronic kidney allograft rejection could make the use of relatively complex tests of kidney function cost effective in transplant patients.

Much effort has been devoted to defining methods for measuring progression of CKD. It has been noted that plots of inverse serum creatinine level over time can often be closely fitted (by least-squares method) to a straight line. The use of inverse creatinine value has generally been found to provide fits as good as or better than plots of logarithmically transformed serum creatinine values. Serial inverse creatinine values can be corrected for changes in creatinine excretion (measured less frequently than serum creatinine level) to reduce error attributable to changes in muscle mass over time.

Because changes in the rate of decline in inverse creatinine level may indicate an effect of therapeutic intervention, a method developed to determine whether there is a "break point" of two hinged regression lines has been applied to plots of inverse serum creatinine values.[4] Changes in kidney function estimated by plots of serial inverse serum creatinine levels can vary substantially from changes estimated by radionuclide-determined GFR.[110,111] Correlation between radionuclide measurements of GFR and changes in creatinine clearance are no better and may even be worse than that for inverse creatinine levels.[111,112] Because spontaneous changes in the slope of inverse creatinine values are frequent,[113] inverse serum creatinine plots are not reliable predictors of the time remaining to dialysis or transplantation or of changes in the rate of functional decline attributable to therapy.

Estimating renal clearance of drugs that are predominantly eliminated by glomerular filtration, in the absence of tubular secretion and reabsorption, is yet another potential application for tests of kidney function. In principle, the rate of drug elimination is often proportional to the GFR. However, because most drugs are either weak acids or weak bases, changes in urine pH can alter tubular handling and affect the relationship between GFR and renal elimination. Competition of drugs for the same secretory pathway can also perturb renal elimination. Nevertheless, impaired renal function is the most common way in which the kidney affects drug levels, and GFR can approximate renal excretion of many drugs. Cost, convenience, and timeliness make creatinine clearance and radionuclide determinations of GFR impractical for guiding drug dosing. Most investigators have used formulas for calculating GFR from age, sex, and serum creatinine values to dose drugs that are excreted primarily by the kidney. Although the accuracy of these calculated clearances has been studied by using other measures of kidney function as a gold standard, the ability of these formulas to predict pharmacokinetic profiles has not been determined for most therapeutic agents.

Many studies have attempted to examine changes in the rate of decline in GFR, determined by inverse creatinine plots or other techniques, to assess the effectiveness of therapeutic interventions. However, measuring changes in the rate of decline is problematic, as previously discussed. Moreover, it has also been shown that a substantial proportion of apparent amelioration in functional declines measured by inverse creatinine or radionuclide determinations of GFR can be attributed to regression toward the mean.[112] Therefore, comparing the rate of change in GFR between two or more experimental groups has become the most reliable method for studying interventions designed to delay or prevent progression of CKD.[114] Generally, cost and inconvenience are subordinated to the increased accuracy and precision of radionuclide measurements of GFR in a clinical trial, and these tests are routinely used in that setting. A study of 2250 patients participating in two large, randomized, controlled trials confirmed the reliability of serial determinations of the renal clearance of subcutaneously injected ^{125}I-iothalamate.[115]

A doubling of serum creatinine concentration has also been used as an endpoint in a number of clinical trials measuring progression of CKD. Using time to doubling of serum creatinine level as an endpoint avoids the difficult to prove assumption that the rate of decline in kidney function is uniformly linear in all patients. It also avoids problems with premature patient dropout. Although the low cost and convenience of using time to doubling of serum creatinine level makes this endpoint particularly attractive, it nevertheless has a number of important limitations.[116] First and foremost is the insensitivity of serum creatinine value to changes in GFR. False-positive results may also be problematic. It has been pointed out that an analysis based on changes in serum creatinine value would have given a positive result in the MDRD study, whereas no such benefit of intervention could be demonstrated when more accurate methods were used to measure changes in GFR.[116]

Furthermore, variation in serum creatinine assays and calibration method can have an important impact on the ability to accurately predict levels of kidney function. Coresh and colleagues[117] analyzed frozen sera from participants in both the MDRD study and the Third National Health and Nutrition Examination Survey (NHANES III) and showed substantial variation in calibration of serum creatinine values among laboratories and through time. These errors in calibration became more important with progressively higher GFR values. Therefore, both research and clinical laboratories should consider serum creatinine calibration traceable to IDMS methods.[18,118] Clearly, better techniques are still needed to measure the progression of CKD in clinical trials, techniques that can reduce the number of patients and duration of follow-up required to assess the effectiveness of therapies.

Urinalysis

Overview

There are three ways to obtain a urine specimen: spontaneous voiding, ureteral catheterization, and percutaneous bladder puncture. Although the safety and utility of suprapubic needle aspiration of the bladder has been demonstrated, its use is generally reserved to situations in which urine cannot easily be obtained by other means. It may be particularly useful in infants, for example.

Once a specimen is obtained, there are countless techniques for examining the urine and its contents. This section reviews only those analytic techniques that are readily available and in common use and focuses on three broad areas: (1) chemical content, (2) protein composition, and (3) formed elements. The discussion of chemical content is limited to tests readily available through the use of reagent strips, such as specific gravity, pH, bilirubin, urobilinogen, nitrite, leukocyte esterase, glucose, and ketoacetate. More specific chemical tests (e.g., tests to diagnose metabolic disorders) are not discussed. Similarly, the measurement and interpretation of urine electrolyte composition are excluded from this section. The discussion of protein composition focuses on proteins from both tubular and glomerular sources. Formed elements include commonly encountered blood cells and casts.[4]

As with all laboratory procedures and clinical tests, the usefulness of urinalysis techniques depends not only on accuracy and precision but also on prior probabilities of the occurrence of positive results. Studies have found that routine hospital admission or preoperative urinalysis that includes both reagent strip testing and microscopic examination rarely leads to better patient outcomes and is generally not cost effective.[119-121] As a result, most investigators have concluded that routine urinalysis should be abandoned in these settings. Whether a more limited approach to routine screening that relies on reagent strip testing without microscopy is more effective remains to be determined.[122,123]

The probability of a positive result on urinalysis is no doubt greater for patients who are already known to have proteinuria than for otherwise normal patients routinely admitted to a hospital. Therefore, the utility of examining the urine sediment may be quite different in patients with proteinuria and in routinely admitted patients. In one study, in patients who were believed to have kidney disease and therefore underwent biopsy, urine microscopy was highly predictive of abnormal kidney histologic findings.[124] Data such as these have led to the suggestion that examining the urine sediment is critical in assessing the implications of proteinuria.[125] Although accurate data on the sensitivity and specificity of urinalysis techniques for most clinical conditions are not available, an awareness of how individual tests are influenced by the underlying likelihood of disease can be helpful in determining the appropriate use of urinalysis and in assessing the implications of the results.

Chemical Characteristics

Color

The color of urine is determined by chemical content, concentration, and pH. Urine may be almost colorless if the output is high and the concentration is low. Cloudy urine is generally the result of phosphates (usually normal) or leukocytes and bacteria (usually abnormal). Black urine is seen in alkaptonuria.[4] Acute intermittent porphyria frequently causes dark urine. A number of exogenous chemicals and drugs can make urine green, but green urine may also be associated with *Pseudomonas* bacteriuria and urine bile pigments. The most common cause of red urine is hemoglobin. Red urine in the absence of red blood cells in the sediment usually indicates either free hemoglobin or myoglobin. Red urine with red sediment indicates hemoglobin. In contrast, red urine with clear sediment is most often the result of myoglobin but may also be seen in some porphyrias, with the use of the bladder analgesic phenazopyridine and a variety of other medications, with the ingestion of food dyes, and with the consumption of beets in some individuals. Finally, red-orange urine due to rifampin is one of the better-known drug effects. Among endogenous sources, bile pigments are the most common cause of orange urine.[4]

Specific Gravity

The measurement of urine specific gravity is usually included as part of the standard urinalysis. Specific gravity is a convenient and rapidly obtained indicator of urine osmolality. It can be measured accurately with a refractometer or a hygrometer or more crudely estimated with a dipstick.

The accuracy and usefulness of the reagent strip method has been debated. Measurement of specific gravity by dipstick depends on the ionic strength of the urine and the fact that there is generally a linear relationship between ionic strength and osmolality in urine. The strip contains a polyionic polymer with binding sites saturated with hydrogen ions. The release of hydrogen ions when they are competitively replaced with urinary cations causes a change in the pH-sensitive indicator dye. Specific gravity values measured by dipstick tend to be falsely high if the urine pH is less than 6 and falsely low if the pH is higher than 7. The effects of albumin, glucose, and urea on osmolality are not reflected by changes in the dipstick specific gravity. In newborns, specific gravity measurement with either a refractometer or a reagent strip is inaccurate.

The specific gravity of urine reflects the relative proportion of dissolved solutes to total volume and, as such, is a measure of urine concentration. The normal range for specific gravity is 1.003 to 1.030, but values decrease with age as the kidney's ability to concentrate urine decreases. Specific gravity can be used to crudely estimate how the concentration of other urine constituents may reflect total excretion of those constituents, because specific gravity correlates inversely with 24-hour urine volume. Indeed, self-monitoring of urine specific gravity may be useful for stone-forming patients, who benefit from maintaining a dilute urine. Specific gravity can be affected by protein, glucose, mannitol, dextrans, diuretics, radiographic contrast media, and some antibiotics. Most clinical decisions should be based only on more accurate determinations of urine osmolality.[4]

Urine pH

Urine pH is usually measured with a reagent test strip. Most commonly, the double indicators methyl red and bromthymol blue are used in the reagent strips to give a broad range of colors at different pH values. In conjunction with other specific urine and plasma measurements, urine pH is often invaluable in diagnosing systemic acid-base disorders. By itself, however, urine pH provides little useful diagnostic information. The normal range for urine pH is 4.5 to 7.8. A very alkaline urine (pH > 7.0) is suggestive of infection with a urea-splitting organism, such as *Proteus mirabilis*. Prolonged storage can lead to overgrowth of urea-splitting bacteria and a high urine pH. However, vegetarian diet, diuretic therapy, vomiting, gastric suction, and alkali therapy can also cause a high urine pH. Low urine pH (pH < 5.0) is seen most commonly in metabolic acidosis. A higher value may indicate the presence of one of the forms of renal tubular acidosis. Acidic urine is also associated with the ingestion of large amounts of meat.[4]

Bilirubin and Urobilinogen

Only conjugated bilirubin is passed into the urine. Thus, the result of a reagent test for bilirubin is typically positive in patients with obstructive jaundice or jaundice due to hepatocellular injury, whereas it is usually negative in patients with jaundice due to hemolysis. In patients with hemolysis, however, the urine urobilinogen result is often positive. Reagent test strips are very sensitive to bilirubin, detecting as little as 0.05 mg/dL. However, the presence of bilirubin in the urine is not very sensitive for detecting liver disease. False-positive test results for urine bilirubin can occur if the urine is contaminated with stool. Prolonged storage and exposure to light can lead to false-negative results.[4]

Leukocyte Esterase and Nitrites

Dipstick screening for urinary tract infection has been recommended for high-risk individuals, but the issue is controversial. The U.S. Preventive Services Task Force has recommended screening for asymptomatic bacteriuria in pregnant women at 12 to 16 weeks' gestation. The task force stated that there was insufficient evidence to recommend for or against the routine screening of elderly women, women with diabetes, or children who are asymptomatic.[126] However, the American College of Physicians and the Canadian Task Force on the Periodic Health Examination have recommended that urinalysis not be used to screen for bacteriuria in asymptomatic persons.[126]

In children, routine screening for bacteriuria has also been controversial. The American Academy of Pediatrics recommends screening in infancy, early childhood, late childhood, and adolescence.[127] However, on the basis of a cost-effectiveness analysis, Kaplan and colleagues[128] suggested that a single screening test at school entry would be more economically efficient.

Whether dipstick screening for bacteriuria is sufficient (without microscopic examination) has also been debated.[129] Craver and colleagues[130] found that dipstick testing (with microscopic confirmation of positive results) was sufficient and cost effective for children in an emergency department setting. In a study of 5486 urine samples, Bonnardeaux and colleagues[131] found that a negative dipstick result was probably sufficient to exclude microscopic abnormalities in the urine. Thus, it seems reasonable that a microscopic examination can be reserved for patients with an abnormal dipstick test result.

The esterase method relies on the fact that esterases are released from lysed urine granulocytes. These esterases liberate 3-hydroxy-5-phenylpyrrole after substrate hydrolysis. The pyrrole reacts with a diazonium salt, yielding a pink to purple color. The result is usually interpreted as negative, trace, small, moderate, or large. Allowing urine to stand indefinitely results in a greater lysis of leukocytes and a more intense reaction. False-positive results can occur with vaginal contamination. High levels of glucose, albumin, ascorbic acid, tetracycline, cephalexin, or cephalothin, or large amounts of oxalic acid may inhibit the reaction.[132]

Urinary bacteria convert nitrates to nitrites. In the reagent strip test, nitrite reacts with a p-arsanilic acid to form a diazonium compound; further reaction with 1,2,3,4-tetrahydrobenzo(h)quinolin-3-ol, results in a pink color endpoint.[133] Results are usually interpreted as positive or negative. High specific gravity and ascorbic acid may interfere with the test. False-negative results are common and may be due to low urine nitrates resulting from low diet intake. It may take up to 4 hours to convert nitrate to nitrite, so inadequate bladder retention time can also give false-negative results.[133] Prolonged storage of the sample can lead to degradation of nitrites, another source of false-negative results. Finally, several potential urinary pathogens such as *Streptococcus faecalis*, other gram-positive organisms, *Neisseria gonorrhea*, and *Mycobacterium tuberculosis* do not convert nitrate to nitrite.[133]

Studies have examined the sensitivity and specificity of reagent strip tests for urinary tract infection in different clinical settings and patient populations, including patients attending a general medicine clinic,[134] patients visiting an emergency department because of abdominal pain,[135] children with neurogenic bladders,[136] children attending a general medical outpatient clinic,[137] men being screened for sexually transmitted disease,[138] and women.[139] A meta-analysis of the results of 51 relevant studies compared the use of nitrite testing alone, leukocyte esterase testing alone, disjunctive pairing (either test result positive), and conjunctive pairing (both test results positive).[140] ROC curves were fitted to the data using logistic transformations and weighted linear regression. This analysis indicated that the disjunctive pairing of both tests is the most accurate approach to screening for infection. However, when the likelihood of infection is high (e.g., when signs and symptoms are present), negative results on both tests are still inadequate to exclude infection. These tests, in combination with other clinical information, may be more useful in situations in which the likelihood of infection is low.

Glucose

Reagent strip measurement of urine glucose level, once used to monitor diabetic therapy, has been almost completely replaced by more reliable methods that measure blood glucose level using finger stick. Urine glucose is less accurately quantitated than blood glucose and is dependent on urine volume. In addition, the appearance of glucose in the urine

always occurs later than blood glucose elevations. Thus, the value of the reagent strip glucose test is limited almost entirely to screening.

Most reagent strips use a glucose oxidase–peroxidase method, which generally detects levels of glucose as low as 50 mg/dL.[141] Because the renal threshold for glucose is generally 160 to 180 mg/dL, the presence of detectable urine glucose indicates a blood glucose level in excess of 210 mg/dL. Large quantities of ketones, ascorbate, and phenazopyridine hydrochloride (Pyridium) metabolites may interfere with the color reaction,[141] and urine peroxide contamination may cause false-positive results. Nevertheless, the appearance of glucose in the urine is a specific indicator of high serum glucose levels. Glucosuria due to a low renal threshold for glucose reabsorption is rare. As a screening test for diabetes, fasting urine glucose testing has a specificity of 98% but a sensitivity of only 17%.[142]

Ketones

Ketones (acetoacetate and acetone) are generally detected with the nitroprusside reaction.[143] Ascorbic acid and phenazopyridine can give false-positive reactions. β-Hydroxybutyrate (often 80% of total serum ketones in ketosis) is not normally detected by the nitroprusside reaction. Ketones may appear in the urine, but not in serum, with prolonged fasting or starvation. Ketones may also be measured in the urine in alcoholic or diabetic ketoacidosis.

Hemoglobin and Myoglobin

Reagent strips utilize the peroxidase-like activity of hemoglobin to catalyze the reaction of cumene hydroperoxide and 3,3′,5,5′-tetramethylbenzidine. Hematuria or contamination of the urine with menstrual blood produces a positive reaction. Oxidizing contaminants and povidone-iodine will cause false-positive reactions.[141] Myoglobin will also react positively.

Free hemoglobin is filtered at the renal glomerulus and thus will appear in the urine when the capacity for plasma protein binding with haptoglobin is exceeded. Some of the hemoglobin is catabolized by the proximal tubules. The principal cause of increased serum and urine free hemoglobin is hemolysis. Rhabdomyolysis gives rise to myoglobin. A positive dipstick test result for hemoglobin in the absence of red blood cells in the urine sediment may suggest either hemolysis or rhabdomyolysis. Often, the clinical history provides important differential diagnostic information. Hemolysis can usually be diagnosed by examining the peripheral blood smear and measuring levels of lactate dehydrogenase, haptoglobin, and serum free hemoglobin. Rhabdomyolysis is accompanied by increased levels of serum creatine phosphokinase. In the end, specific assays for hemoglobin and myoglobin can be used to measure urine levels.

Protein

Normal Physiology

Normally, large quantities of high-molecular-weight (HMW) plasma proteins traverse the glomerular capillaries, mesangium, or both without entering the urinary space. Both charge- and size-selective properties of the capillary wall prevent all but a tiny fraction of albumin, globulin, and other large plasma proteins from crossing. Smaller proteins (<20,000 Da) pass readily across the capillary wall. Because the plasma concentration of these proteins is much lower than that of albumin and globulins, however, the filtered load is small. Moreover, LMW proteins are normally reabsorbed by the proximal tubule. Thus, proteins such as α_2-microglobulin, apoproteins, enzymes, and peptide hormones are normally excreted in only very small amounts in the urine.[4] Most healthy individuals excrete between 30 and 130 mg/day of protein, and the upper limit of normal total urine protein excretion is generally given as 150 to 200 mg/day for adults.[144] The upper limit of normal albumin excretion is usually given as 30 mg/day.[144]

A very small amount of protein that normally appears in the urine is the result of normal tubular secretion. Tamm-Horsfall protein is an HMW glycoprotein (23×10^6 Da) that is formed on the epithelial surface of the thick ascending limb of the loop of Henle and early distal convoluted tubule.[4] Tamm-Horsfall protein, also known as *uromodulin*, binds and inactivates the cytokines interleukin-1 and tumor necrosis factor.[145,146] Immunoglobulin A (IgA) and urokinase are also secreted by the renal tubule and appear in the urine in small amounts.[4]

From a consideration of normal physiology, it is apparent that abnormal amounts of protein may appear in the urine as the result of three mechanisms. First, a disruption of the capillary wall barrier may lead to a large amount of HMW plasma proteins that overwhelm the limited capacity of tubular reabsorption and cause protein to appear in the urine. The resulting proteinuria can be classified as glomerular in origin. Second, tubular damage or dysfunction can inhibit the normal resorptive capacity of the proximal tubule, resulting in increased amounts of mostly LMW proteins in the urine. Such proteinuria can be classified as tubular proteinuria. Third, normal or abnormal plasma proteins produced in increased amounts can be filtered at the glomerulus and overwhelm the resorptive capacity of the proximal tubule. These filtered proteins can be especially numerous if their size is small or they are positively charged. Although increased urine protein excretion can also result from increased tubular production of protein, this is rarely the case.

Techniques to Measure Urine Protein

Protein can be measured in random samples, in timed or untimed overnight samples, or in 24-hour collections. Inaccurate urine collection is probably the greatest source of error in quantifying protein excretion in timed collections, particularly 24-hour collections. However, urine creatinine can be measured to judge the adequacy of the 24-hour collection. If creatinine excretion is similar to that in previous 24-hour samples, then the collection is likely to be reasonably accurate. If no other collections are available for comparison, then the adequacy of collection can be judged from the expected normal range of creatinine excretion. For hospitalized men aged 20 to 50 years, this range was found to be 18.5 to 25.0 mg/kg of body weight per day, and for women of the same age, 16.5 to 22.4 mg/kg/day (Figure 25-4). These values declined with age, so that for men aged 50 to 70 years, creatinine excretion was 15.7 to 20.2 mg/kg/day, and for women, 11.8 to 16.1 mg/kg/day (see Figure 25-4). Patients who are malnourished or who may have reduced

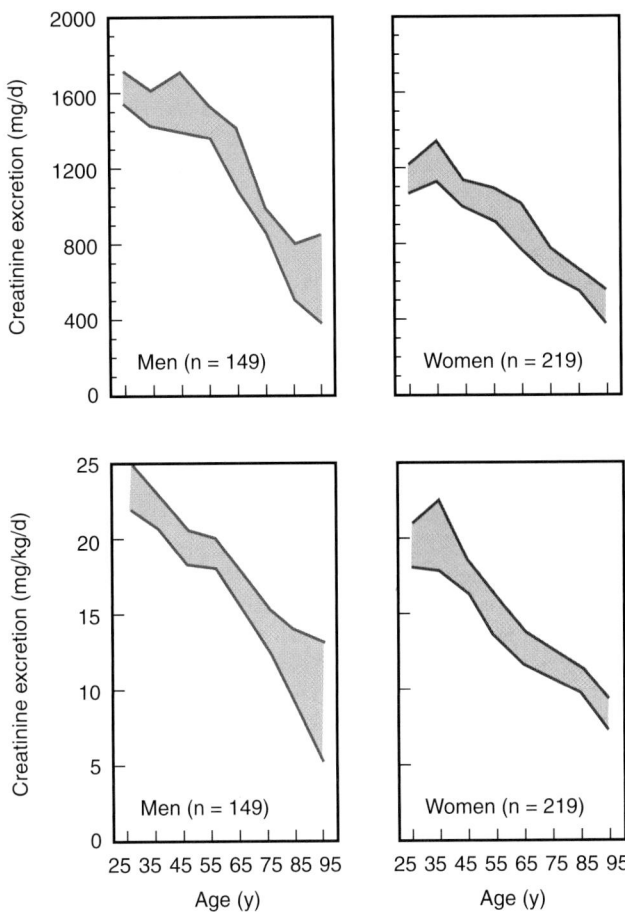

FIGURE 25-4 Age-related differences in urine creatinine excretion in healthy men (*left panels*) and healthy women (*right panels*). *Shaded areas* represent 95% confidence intervals calculated from the data of Kampmann and colleagues.[32] Values in the upper panels are in milligrams per day and values in the lower panels are in milligrams per kilogram of body weight per day.

muscle mass for other reasons can be expected to have lower than normal creatinine excretion rates.[4]

Tests to accurately quantitate total protein concentration in urine rely on precipitation. In the commonly used sulfosalicylic acid method, sulfosalicylic acid is added to a sample of urine, and the turbidity is measured with a photometer or nephelometer. Protein is quantified through comparison of the turbidity of the sample with that of a standard. This method lacks precision, and the coefficient of variation is as high as 20%. A number of proteins are detected with this method, including γ-globulin light chains and albumin. The method is more sensitive to albumin than to globulins. Trichloroacetic acid can be used in place of sulfosalicylic acid to increase the sensitivity to γ-globulin. False-positive reactions may occur from high levels of tolmetin sodium (Tolectin), tolbutamide, antibiotics, and radiocontrast agents.

Total protein can more accurately be quantified with the use of several monospecific antibodies to different types of urine protein, but this method is somewhat cumbersome and is seldom used in clinical laboratories.[4]

Total protein concentration in urine can be estimated using chemical-impregnated plastic strips. Most dipstick reagents contain a pH-sensitive colorimetric indicator that changes color when negatively charged proteins bind to it. Positively charged proteins, however, are less readily detected. Positively charged immunoglobulin light chains, for example, may escape urine dipstick detection even when present in large amounts in the urine. A very high urine pH (>7.0) can also give false-positive results, as can contamination of the urine with blood.

The dipstick technique is sensitive to very small urine protein concentrations (the lower limit of detection is 10 to 20 mg/dL). At these low levels, however, the major constituent of urine protein may be Tamm-Horsfall protein, and thus a positive test result may not reflect kidney injury. This is especially likely to occur when the urine volume is low and the concentration is high. When urine volume is high and the urine is maximally dilute, however, a relatively large amount of protein can go undetected. Indeed, total protein excretion approaching 1 g/day may not be detected if urine output is high. If, for example, urine volume is 10 L/day, then the concentration of 1 g of protein would be 10 mg/dL, or below the limit of detection of most reagent strip tests for total protein.[4]

The consistency of results when the same sample is assessed repeatedly or the precision of reagent strip tests in measuring urine total protein concentration is generally poor.[147] Variability in interpretation both by the same technologist and among technologists has been examined and has been found to be relatively high. For example, at low levels of urine protein concentration (e.g., 6 to 39 mg/dL), inconsistent results among different technologists were seen in 19% to 56% of the determinations. At higher concentrations (e.g., 196 to 328 mg/dL), inconsistencies were seen in 19% to 44% of the determinations.[4] Similar findings were reported in a later study that also found that inconsistencies depended somewhat on the experience of the operator and the type of reagent strip. Inconsistencies were found among experienced technologists in up to 33% of cases and among inexperienced technologists in up to 93% of cases.[147]

The sensitivity and specificity of reagent strip protein tests have also been assessed using more accurate quantitative determinations as gold standards. Interestingly, the sensitivity of these tests appears to be higher when assessing samples prepared by adding albumin and globulin to normal, protein-free urine than when assessing actual patient specimens.[147] This difference likely reflects the inability of reagent strips to react to many of the heterogeneous proteins found in human urine. When 20 to 25 mg/dL is used as the limit of detection in clinical specimens, the sensitivity of reagent strips has been found to be only 32% to 46%, and the specificity is 97% to 100%.[147] The effect of the sensitivity and specificity on the usefulness of these reagent strip tests also depends, of course, on the prevalence of proteinuria in the population being screened. In a population with a low prevalence of disease, the low sensitivity of the reagent strip tests suggests that the majority of cases of proteinuria would be missed.[4,147]

Urine albumin concentrations can be quantified by a number of assays, including the following:

1. Radioimmunoassay can be carried out using a double-antibody technique. Albumin in a urine sample competes with a known amount of radiolabeled albumin for fixed binding sites of antibodies. Free albumin can be separated from bound albumin by immunoabsorption of the (albumin-bound) antibody. Albumin concentration in the sample is inversely proportional to the radioactivity.[148]

2. The immunoturbidimetric technique depends on the turbidity of a solution when albumin in a sample of urine reacts with a specific antibody. The turbidity is measured using a spectrophotometer, and the absorbency is proportional to the albumin concentration.[149]

3. When albumin in the urine sample reacts with a specific antibody, it forms light-scattering antigen-antibody complexes that can be measured with a laser nephelometer. The amount of albumin is proportional to scatter in the signal.[150]

4. The competitive enzyme-linked immunosorbent assay (ELISA) has also been used to measure urine albumin.[151]

5. HPLC has also been used to measure urine albumin. This assay also measures the immuno-unreactive intact albumin that is not recognized by immunologic methods. However, the clinical significance of this immuno-unreactive intact albumin is not fully understood.[152]

Currently, there is no standardized procedure for measuring urine albumin and reporting results in standardized units. Although the correlation among results obtained using most of these quantitative assays is very good, a good correlation only indicates a strong linear relationship. For example, the correlation coefficients (r values) between radioimmunoassay and immunoturbidimetry and between radioimmunoassay and nephelometry were both 0.98.[153] Intraassay coefficients of variation for immunoturbidimetry and nephelometry were found to be 6.6% and 11.5% at low concentrations (10 to 60 mg/L) and 11.1% and 4.1% at high concentrations (90 to 120 mg/L), respectively.[153] Interassay coefficients of variation were 11.4% and 11.5% at low concentrations (10 to 60 mg/L) and 5.4% and 1.4% at high concentrations (90 to 120 mg/L), respectively, for these two techniques.[153] However, the study comparing these assays had few samples in the midrange of albumin concentration (16 to 90 mg/L), and here there were considerable differences in results between the radioimmunoassay and the nephelometry assay.[153] In another study, results obtained by radioimmunoassay, immunoturbidimetry, nephelometry, and HPLC varied by up to threefold.[154] Other studies have also found similar variations among different immunoassays.[155]

In contrast, the within-run coefficient of variation for an immunoturbidimetric method was found to be 3.5% at low albumin concentrations and 2.4% at high albumin concentrations.[156] The day-to-day coefficient of variation for the same assay was 5.1% at low and high albumin concentrations.[156] Therefore, ideally the same assay should be used when comparing the albuminuria results over time for a given patient. The choice of assay used to measure albuminuria is largely determined by issues of accuracy, cost, and convenience.

Reagent strip methods have recently been developed to screen qualitatively for urine albumin excretion. The Albustix (Bayer Diagnostik, Munich, Germany) reagent strip uses a protein error of indicators method that causes color changes in the presence of albumin.[157] Trace reactions indicate urine albumin concentrations between 50 and 200 mg/L. Thus, more positive reactions can be used to indicate albumin concentrations higher than those generally found in patients with microalbuminuria. In one study, the sensitivity and specificity of the Albustix were found to be only 81% and 55%, respectively.[157] Thus, there was almost a 50% chance of a false-negative result with the Albustix method.

Screening methods have been developed to detect low albumin excretion rates that are abnormal but that are below the level detectable by standard reagent strips (i.e., in the microalbuminuria range).[153,158-163] One of the most extensively investigated methods to screen for microalbuminuria is the immunometric dipstick Micral-Test (Boehringer Mannheim, Mannheim, Germany).[153,159] The strip is made up of a series of reagent pads through which the urine sample passes sequentially. Urine is first drawn into a wick fleece and then passes into a buffer fleece that adjusts the sample pH. Next, it passes into a third pad, in which albumin in the sample is bound by a soluble conjugate of antibodies linked to the enzyme β-galactosidase. Excess antibody is then adsorbed on immobilized albumin in the next pad, so that only albumin bound to antibody and enzyme reaches the color pad. There the β-galactosidase reacts with a chemical substrate to produce a red dye, the intensity of which is proportional to the concentration of bound albumin. The test strip must be read at precisely 5 minutes.[153,159]

Another qualitative test that has been examined in several investigations is the Micro-Bumintest (Ames Division, Miles Laboratories, Elkhart, Indiana). This test uses a reagent tablet containing the indicator dye bromphenol blue. The intensity of the bluish green color produced after a drop of urine is placed on the surface of the tablet is proportional to the concentration of albumin.[153] A latex agglutination method, Albusure (Cambridge Life Sciences, Cambridge, England), binds albumin in the urine sample to latex.[157] Agglutination occurs when the preparation is mixed with sheep antihuman antibody. When urine albumin concentrations are higher than 20 mg/L, agglutination is inhibited (antigen excess). Thus, agglutination indicates urine albumin concentration of less than 20 mg/L.

A number of studies have examined the sensitivity and specificity of screening methods designed to detect very low levels of albumin in urine.[153,158-163] Because these tests are only semiquantitative (i.e., nonparametric), a true coefficient of variation cannot be determined. Nevertheless, in one evaluation of the Micral-Test method, the estimated coefficient of variation for the same sample interpreted by different technicians was 12.4%.[161] Experience in reading the Micral-Test results was shown to be important.[160] Observer concordance for the Micro-Bumintest was found to be 95% in one study.[163] A new version of the Micral-Test, Micral-Test II, has been described[164]; it is designed to react faster, to be less dependent on timing, and to allow a better color comparison to reduce observer variance. Indeed, in one study, the interobserver concordance was 93% with the Micral-Test II.[164]

Several studies have examined the sensitivity and specificity of the newer reagent strips that measure very low concentrations of urine albumin. Most of these investigations studied patients with diabetes, and most examined the Micral-Test,[153,158-160,165] the Micro-Bumintest,[153,163] or both. In general, these albumin reagent strip tests are more sensitive than standard dipstick tests, but they also have a relatively high rate of false-positive results. Moreover, it should be remembered that, for the most part, these reagent strips were tested in populations of diabetic patients with a high prior probability of a positive result. The number of false-positive results would be expected to be much higher in populations in which the prevalence of albuminuria was lower. Because results of these strips may be in error owing to variation in urinary concentration, these tests should be used to approximate urinary protein only if the ability to directly measure protein is not available.[166,167]

All of the qualitative or semiquantitative urine protein and albumin screening tests discussed so far measure only total protein or albumin concentration. The sensitivity and specificity of these tests can be markedly influenced by fluid intake, the state of diuresis, and the resulting urine concentration. Indeed, in one study, albumin concentration had a low discriminant value for detection of increased albumin excretion in a 12-hour timed urine sample (Figure 25-5). In an effort to correct for problems arising out of variability in urine volume and concentration, many investigators have used the protein/creatinine or albumin/creatinine ratio in random or timed urine collections. There is a high degree of correlation between 24-hour urine protein excretion and protein/creatinine ratios in random, single-voided urine samples in patients with a variety of kidney diseases.[168] It has been suggested that a protein/creatinine ratio of more than 3.0 or 3.5 mg/mg or less than 0.2 mg/mg indicates protein excretion rates of more than 3.0 or 3.5 g/24 hours or less than 0.2 g/24 hours, respectively.[168] However, few studies have systematically examined the sensitivity and specificity or defined optimal levels of detection for protein/creatinine ratios in large numbers of patients in different clinical settings.

Much of the data on the usefulness of albumin/creatinine ratios have been derived from studies of patients with type 1 or type 2 diabetes.[169-172] In most of these investigations, the sensitivity and specificity of albumin/creatinine ratios were determined using albumin excretion rates from timed urine collections as the standard. Data from several studies were combined to examine the true- and false-positive rates for detection of albuminuria in overnight urine using albumin/creatinine ratios.[4] Independent of the albumin/creatinine

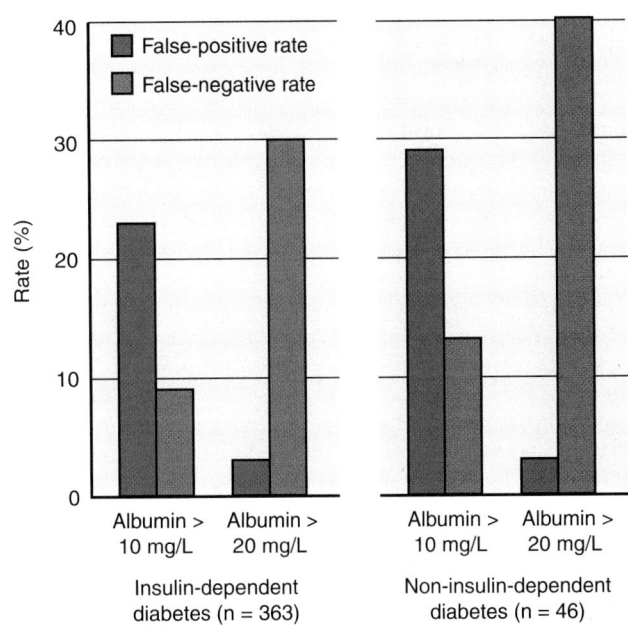

FIGURE 25-5 Comparison of false-positive and false-negative rates when urine albumin concentration was used to predict 12-hour (overnight) excretion of more than 15 µg/min in diabetic patients. At a concentration cutoff of more than 10 mg/L, the false-positive rate is high. At a concentration cutoff of more than 20 mg/L, the false-positive rate is reduced, but the false-negative rate is high. (Data from Kouri TT, Viikari JSA, Mattila KS, et al: Invalidity of simple concentration-based screening tests for early nephropathy due to urinary volumes of diabetic patients, *Diabetes Care* 14:591-593, 1991.)

ratio cutoff used, the sensitivities and specificities appeared to be reasonable.[4] Altogether, these data suggest that albumin/creatinine ratios may be useful as a screening test for kidney disease in populations in which the expected prevalence of disease is high (e.g., diabetic persons).

Less clear is their potential usefulness in other patient populations in which the prior likelihood of disease may be lower than in patients with diabetes.[173] A cross-sectional study by Ruggenenti and colleagues[174] found that morning protein/creatinine ratios in 177 nondiabetic outpatients with CKD were predictive of declining kidney function. In kidney transplant recipients, protein/creatinine ratios have been shown to correlate significantly with measurements of 24-hour urine protein and appear useful as both screening devices and longitudinal tests for following the level of proteinuria.[175] Use of the protein/creatinine ratio has also proved reliable in detecting significant proteinuria in pregnant women,[176,177] but the threshold for identifying significant proteinuria in pregnant women is controversial.[178-180]

There is a lack of data directly comparing the prognostic value of urinary albumin versus total protein excretion, and it is therefore not clear which test is most appropriate in different clinical settings. The KDOQI guidelines acknowledge the lack of data on the appropriate test for detecting proteinuric kidney disease. However, the guidelines recommend the albumin/creatinine ratio as a screening tool given that albuminuria has been associated with kidney disease in diabetes, hypertension, and glomerular disease.[3]

Although protein/creatinine and albumin/creatinine ratios may be more quantitative than a simple dipstick screening procedure, their use has a number of limitations. For example, determining the protein/creatinine or albumin/creatinine ratio from morning first-void samples may underestimate 24-hour protein excretion because of the reduction in proteinuria that normally occurs at night.[181] Storage time and temperature may also affect albumin levels in urine,[182] and specimens should be analyzed as soon as possible after collection. The fact that urine creatinine must be measured in addition to albumin introduces another source of error. Indeed, the combination of the errors of two measurements is greater than the error of either one alone (the combined coefficient of variation is the square root of the sum of the squares of the two individual coefficients of variation). Urine creatinine concentration is extremely variable, so that very different ratios can be obtained in individuals with similar protein excretion rates. Moreover, a number of variables that may interfere with creatinine determinations may affect the ratios.[183] Despite these limitations, the urine protein/creatinine or albumin/creatinine ratio may be useful, especially in individuals in whom 24-hour urine collection is difficult or impossible.

Given the day-to-day variability in albumin excretion and the potential limitations of the albumin/creatinine ratio, the American Diabetic Association recommends that a patient be deemed to have microalbuminuria only if at least two or three samples in a 3- to 6-month period show elevated levels.[167] Because creatinine levels vary based on muscle mass and ethnicity,[184] some have proposed using sex- and ethnicity-specific normal levels when assessing albumin/creatinine ratios; however, efforts are still under way to standardize these definitions.[184a]

A number of analytic tools have been developed to separate and identify individual urinary proteins.[185] These techniques include agarose gel electrophoresis, column gel chromatography, polyacrylamide gel electrophoresis, immunoelectrophoresis, and isoelectric focusing. Proteomic techniques employing mass spectrometry and peptide mass fingerprinting have expanded the number of identified urinary proteins. However, these latter techniques are generally designed to identify, but not accurately quantitate, urine proteins. Some have been used in clinical laboratories to determine the selectivity of urine protein or to identify monoclonal immunoglobulin heavy and light chains. Otherwise, they have been largely confined to research applications.

Applications of Urine Protein Measurement

SCREENING FOR KIDNEY DISEASE

Although urine protein measurement can be used to assist in the diagnosis of kidney disease and to assess progression and response to therapy (discussed later), it is most commonly used as a screening test. Because screening tests are generally applied to relatively large numbers of patients, convenience and cost are major considerations. To make screening more convenient, a number of methods have been developed to measure urine protein in a single-voided, or "spot," urine sample, so that timed urine collections can be avoided.

In 1982, Viberti and colleagues[186] reported that clinical (Albustix-positive) proteinuria subsequently developed in patients with insulin-dependent diabetes in whom albumin excretion rates of 30 to 140 μg/min were measured by radioimmunoassay in timed overnight urine collections. In contrast, patients with rates of less than 30 μg/min did not develop overt proteinuria.[186] These investigators[186] coined the term *microalbuminuria* to indicate increased urine albumin excretion rates in patients with normal urine total protein levels.

A more recent follow-up of the original cohort confirmed that the patients with microalbuminuria not only had a higher risk of developing overt proteinuria but also had a greater risk of dying from cardiovascular disease.[187] Similar findings have been reported by others in patients with insulin-dependent and non–insulin-dependent diabetes.[188-191] Some investigators have used 15 to 150 μg/min to define microalbuminuria,[191] whereas others have used 20 to 200 μg/min.[189,192] Microalbuminuria has also been defined as urine albumin excretion of 30 to 300 mg/day.[144] It has also been defined as a urine albumin/creatinine ratio of above 30 mg/g (or 0.03 mg/mg) in an untimed urine sample but may vary by race and gender. Others have defined microalbuminuria as 20 to 200 mg/g and 30 to 400 mg/g for males and females, respectively.[189]

Whatever definition is used, microalbuminuria appears to be an important risk factor for end-organ damage in patients with diabetes. Similarly, in patients with essential hypertension, increased urine albumin excretion (>30 mg/24 hours) is associated with increased cardiovascular mortality. Most studies showing a relationship between microalbuminuria and end-organ damage have used quantitative techniques to measure urine albumin excretion. Although few studies have examined whether other screening techniques predict outcome, there is no reason to believe that the results cannot be extrapolated to other screening tests, with differences in sensitivity and specificity taken into account. Indeed, albumin/creatinine ratios have been shown to predict the subsequent development of overt kidney disease. In a population of diabetic southwestern Native Americans, albumin/creatinine ratios of 0.03 to 0.30 mg/mg (microalbuminuria range) were a strong predictor of diabetic nephropathy.[193]

The recognition that microalbuminuria identifies diabetic patients at risk for subsequent renal and cardiovascular disease complications has given great impetus to efforts to develop effective screening tools. Borch-Johnsen and associates,[192] using published data, carried out a critical appraisal of screening for microalbuminuria in patients with diabetes. Making a number of assumptions, they performed a cost-benefit analysis of the impact of screening and antihypertensive treatment and concluded that screening and intervention programs are likely to lead to considerable reductions in cost and mortality.[192]

Even though assessment for microalbuminuria has been recommended as a routine test to screen for early diabetic nephropathy, it is important to realize that there are some patients with either type 1 or type 2 diabetes who have decreased GFR due to diabetic nephropathy in the absence of microalbuminuria.[194,195]

The use of dipstick tests for total protein excretion and microalbuminuria to screen for renal disease has not been rigorously examined in nondiabetic patient populations. Epidemiologic data suggest that even in nondiabetic individuals, proteinuria is a risk factor for cardiovascular disease,[2] perhaps because proteinuria is a sensitive indicator of kidney damage. However strong these correlations are statistically (low *P* value), the amount of unexplained variability (low *r* value) is great, which suggests that the sensitivity and specificity of proteinuria for detection of kidney injury in the general population could be too low to make urine protein testing a useful screening tool for an individual patient. Nevertheless, data to assess this are generally not available for individuals who are not diabetic.

A cost-effectiveness analysis compared a strategy of annual screening with no screening for proteinuria at age 50 years followed by treatment with an angiotensin converting enzyme inhibitor or an angiotensin II receptor blocker and found that annual screening was not cost effective unless selectively directed toward high-risk groups of patients older than 60 years and patients with hypertension.[196]

Regardless of whether or not measuring urine protein excretion in the general population is a cost-effective approach to the early detection of kidney disease, such screening may be useful when combined with other clinical parameters in estimating vascular disease risk. However, the prospective data needed to assess the utility of this application of urine protein excretion testing are also incomplete.

The appropriate manner in which to use various tests to screen for renal disease has not been extensively investigated. Because the number of false-positive results on dipstick tests for protein excretion is high, a positive test result should probably be followed by tests designed to more accurately quantitate urine protein excretion. In some clinical circumstances, however, the likelihood that a positive dipstick test result for urine protein excretion indicates CKD is so low that the screening test should be repeated at a later date before more costly quantitation procedures are undertaken. A positive dipstick test result for protein in a patient with a urinary tract infection, for example, can be dismissed if subsequent posttreatment tests give negative results. Fever can cause tubular and glomerular proteinuria that most often disappears when the fever resolves. Congestive heart failure and seizures can also cause transient proteinuria. Light or strenuous exercise is often associated with urine protein excretion that resolves spontaneously.[4]

It seems clear that, even in the absence of identifiable causes of transient proteinuria, some individuals have increases in urine protein excretion that are not associated with kidney disease.[197] This proteinuria can be classified in two categories: (1) intermittent and (2) persistent and postural. Several dipstick measurements of urine protein over time can be made to determine whether an individual patient fits in either of these two distinct patterns.

Intermittent proteinuria is less well characterized than postural proteinuria, but it appears to be relatively benign in otherwise healthy individuals. It has been shown, for example, that mortality after more than 40 years of follow-up among those who had intermittently positive urine protein screen results as college students was no different than that among individuals who did not have intermittently positive results. However, few histologic studies including sufficiently large numbers of patients have been carried out to precisely characterize intermittent proteinuria.[4]

Posture can cause an increase in urine protein excretion in otherwise healthy individuals.[197] This postural proteinuria should be distinguished from the increase in proteinuria seen in patients with kidney disease who assume an upright posture. Postural proteinuria usually does not exceed 1 g/24 hours. It is usually diagnosed by detecting protein excretion during the day that is absent at night while the patient is recumbent. Kidney histologic examination in patients with postural proteinuria generally yields normal or nonspecific findings.[198,199] Patients with postural proteinuria have been shown to have an excellent long-term prognosis.[200] Indeed, six patients diagnosed by Thomas Addis had no evidence of kidney disease after 42 to 50 years of follow-up.[201]

Even in individuals without postural proteinuria or renal disease, levels of urine protein excretion are lower at night than during the day.[202] Thus, the timing of urine collection is likely to influence the sensitivity and specificity of screening tests for urine protein excretion.

Diagnosis and Prognosis

Once proteinuria has been detected by screening, the clinician must not only confirm the results of screening but also precisely quantitate the amount of protein excretion in a timed urine collection. Quantifying urine protein excretion may help to distinguish glomerular from tubular proteinuria. If, for example, a patient's protein excretion is in the nephrotic range (e.g., >3 g/24 hours), a glomerular source is almost certain. Quantitation of urine protein excretion can also provide useful prognostic information and assist in monitoring the response to therapy.

After detection and quantification, determination of the composition of urine protein may provide diagnostic information. Higher amounts of albumin and HMW proteins suggest glomerular proteinuria, whereas isolated increases in LMW protein fractions are more suggestive of tubular proteinuria. It is unusual for tubular proteinuria to exceed 1 to 2 g/day, and only a small fraction of protein excretion due to tubular damage should be albumin. Tubular proteins are heterogeneous; however, α_2-microglobulin is often a major constituent.

β_2-Microglobulin is an LMW (11.8-kDa) protein that has been identified as the light chain of class I major histocompatibility antigens (e.g., human leukocyte antigens A, B, and C). β_2-Microglobulin is most commonly measured in urine using radioimmunoassay or ELISA. It is freely filtered at the glomerulus and is avidly taken up and catabolized by the proximal tubule. Not surprisingly, therefore, detectable urinary levels of β_2-microglobulin have been associated with many pathologic conditions involving the proximal tubule, including aminoglycoside-induced damage, Balkan endemic nephropathy, heavy metal nephropathies, radiocontrast nephropathy, and kidney transplant rejection. The sensitivity and specificity of this test of tubular injury have generally not been established in different clinical situations in which prior probabilities of various kidney disorders may strongly influence its usefulness.

Glomerular proteinuria can be further characterized as selective or nonselective. Patients with a clearance ratio of IgG (an HMW protein) to albumin that is less than 0.10 are said to have a selective glomerular proteinuria, whereas those with IgG/albumin clearance ratios of more than 0.50 have a nonselective pattern. In general, selective proteinuria is more often seen in patients with minimal change disease and predicts a good response to treatment with corticosteroids.[4] The sensitivity and specificity of determining the selectivity of glomerular proteinuria have not been systematically examined in large numbers of patients with different kidney diseases. Moreover, the cost of the protein separation procedures has limited their widespread clinical use.

Plasma cell dyscrasias may produce monoclonal proteins, immunoglobulin, free light chains, and a combination of these. Light chains are filtered at the glomerulus and may appear in the urine as Bence Jones protein. The detection of urine immunoglobulin light chains can be the first clue to a number of important clinical syndromes associated with plasma cell dyscrasias that involve the kidney.[4] Unfortunately, urine immunoglobulin light chains may not be detected by reagent strip tests for protein. However, plasma cell dyscrasias may also manifest as proteinuria or albuminuria when the glomerular deposition of light chains causes disruption of the normally impermeable capillary wall.[203] The diagnosis of a plasma cell dyscrasia can be suspected when a tall, narrow band on electrophoresis suggests the presence of a monoclonal γ-globulin or immunoglobulin light chain. However, monoclonal proteins are best detected using serum and urine immunoelectrophoresis.[4]

Once patients have been screened and a diagnosis of kidney disease has been established, measuring the amount of urine protein can provide additional prognostic information and can be used to monitor the response to therapy. The amount of urine protein excretion has consistently been shown to predict subsequent disease progression in different clinical settings: for example, protein excretion correlated with progression in patients presenting with the nephrotic syndrome[204] and in patients with mild renal insufficiency of various causes.[205] Similar findings have been reported in patients with IgA nephropathy, membranous nephropathy, and type I membranoproliferative glomerulonephritis.[206] The clinical course and effect of immunosuppressive therapy can also be monitored with sequential quantitation of urine protein excretion.[207]

Formed Elements

Urine Microscopy Methods

The examination of the urine by microscopy remains a useful qualitative and semiquantitative procedure. Efforts to more accurately quantitate formed elements in the urine have been made over the years. For example, Addis measured excretion rates of erythrocytes using timed urine collections. However, formed elements can quickly deteriorate in the urine, and timed collections are difficult for most patients to carry out with accuracy. Moreover, the excretion rate of many formed elements correlates with urine concentration, so that often little additional information is gained from the effort made to collect timed specimens.[4] For all of these reasons, the use of timed collections to obtain excretion rates of formed elements has not gained widespread acceptance. The number of formed elements can still be quantified using untimed specimens and a counting chamber.

A number of factors affect formed elements in the urine, and when possible, collection and handling conditions should be optimized to take account of these factors. Contamination with bacteria can be minimized through careful attention to collection technique. A midstream, clean-catch specimen should be collected when possible; the patient should be instructed to retract foreskin or labia. A high urine concentration and a low urine pH help to preserve formed elements.[4] Thus, a first-void morning specimen, which is most likely to be acidic and concentrated, should be used whenever possible. Strenuous exercise and bladder catheterization can cause hematuria, and urine specimens collected to detect hematuria should not be obtained under these conditions.

Urine should be examined as soon as possible after collection to avoid lysis of the formed elements and bacterial overgrowth. The specimen should not be refrigerated, because lowering the temperature causes the precipitation of phosphates and urates. It is helpful first to measure the urine specific gravity and pH, so as to judge the density of formed elements according to the concentration and acidity of the specimen. Specimens from concentrated and acidic urine may be expected to have a greater density of formed elements than dilute and alkaline specimens from the same patients. Urine should be centrifuged at approximately 2000 rpm for 5 to 10 minutes or 2500 to 3000 rpm for 3 to 5 minutes. The supernatant should be carefully poured off, the pellet resuspended by gentle agitation, and a drop placed on a slide under a coverslip.

Most commonly, urine is examined under an ordinary bright-field microscope. However, polarized light can be used to identify anisotropic crystals, and phase-contrast microscopy can enhance the contrast of cell membranes. The urine should first be examined under low power (100×) to best judge the number of formed elements. These elements can then be examined in detail under high power (400×). Generally, the urine is examined unstained, but occasionally stains can be helpful in distinguishing cell types.

Hematuria

Gross hematuria may first be detected by a change in urine color. Microscopic hematuria can be detected by dipstick methods, microscopic examination, or both. These latter methods may be applied as diagnostic tests in patients with known kidney disease or as screening tools in healthy or high-risk individuals. The sensitivity and specificity of screening tests for hematuria have not been thoroughly examined in many pertinent patient populations. Moreover, the cost/benefit ratio of screening is often unclear. Who and when to screen for microscopic hematuria are controversial.

The most cogent reason to screen for occult hematuria may be to facilitate the early and potentially life-saving detection of urologic malignancies. Results of a dipstick test in more than 10,000 adult men undergoing health screening were found to be positive in about 2.5%.[208] About one fourth of those who underwent further investigation had cystoscopic abnormalities, including bladder neoplasms in two men. However, more than one third of those found to have occult hematuria in this retrospective study did not undergo further investigation. In another study of over 2000 men, 4% were found to have occult hematuria, and one of these patients was found to have bladder carcinoma.[209] Higher detection rates have been reported by other investigators.[210]

The U.S. Preventive Services Task Force (http://www.prev entiveservices.ahrq.gov) no longer recommends screening for occult hematuria in the general population.[126] The value of screening for occult hematuria in other populations is questionable,[211] and the role of occult hematuria screening to detect parenchymal kidney disease is unclear.

Even when the urine is red, or when a dipstick screening test result is positive, the sediment should be examined to determine whether red cells are present. The presence of other pigments such as free hemoglobin and myoglobin can masquerade as hematuria. In addition, red blood cells can be detected in the urine sediment when screening test results are negative. An occasional red blood cell can be seen in normal individuals, but generally only one or two cells per high-power field.

The differential diagnosis of hematuria is broad, but for practical purposes hematuria can be categorized as originating in the upper or lower urinary tract. Hematuria that is accompanied by red blood cell casts, marked proteinuria, or both is most likely to be glomerular in origin. In the absence of these important findings, distinguishing glomerular from postglomerular bleeding can be difficult.

Red blood cells originating in glomeruli have been reported to have a distinctive dysmorphic appearance that is most readily appreciated using phase-contrast microscopy.[212-214] Automated blood cell analysis has also been used to determine the number of dysmorphic red cells in urine.[215,216] In vitro studies suggest that pH and osmolality changes found in the distal tubule can explain the higher number of dysmorphic red blood cells in patients with glomerular disease.[217]

The clinical utility of tests for distinguishing dysmorphic red cells in the urine has been examined in numerous studies.[215,218-221] Most investigators concluded that detecting dysmorphic red cells reliably identified patients with glomerular disease; however, one investigator-blinded, controlled trial found unacceptable interobserver variability.[220]

A number of investigators have attempted to develop automated methods to detect glomerular hematuria.[222-224] These techniques employ cell counters or more sophisticated flow cytometry methods. However, the use of automated cell size determination in testing the urine of individuals with low-grade hematuria may be particularly unreliable owing to interference from cell debris.[222]

A meta-analysis of 21 published studies using predetermined criteria for evaluation of dysmorphic urine red cells was carried out.[225] All studies originated in referral centers. The weighted average sensitivity and specificity of dysmorphic red cell test detection of glomerular disease were 0.88 (95% confidence interval [CI] = 0.86 to 0.91) and 0.95 (95% CI = 0.93 to 0.97), respectively. The sensitivity and specificity of abnormal red blood cell volumes (determined using

automated methods) for detection of glomerular disease were 1.00 (95% CI = 0.98 to 1.00) and 0.87 (95% CI = 0.80 to 0.91). The investigators in this meta-analysis concluded that the negative predictive value of these tests was probably not sufficient to rule out important urologic lesions, especially in a referral setting in which the prevalence of urologic disease may be relatively high.

The differential diagnosis of hematuria is shown in Table 25-3. Kidney vascular causes include arterial and venous thrombosis, arteriovenous malformations, arteriovenous fistula, and nutcracker syndrome (compression of the left renal vein between the aorta and the superior mesenteric artery).[226] Most patients receiving anticoagulant therapy who have hematuria can be found to have an underlying cause, especially if the hematuria is macroscopic. However, excessive anticoagulation or other coagulopathies can themselves be associated with hematuria. The source of hematuria in patients with sickle cell disease is

TABLE 25-3 Common Sources of Hematuria
Vascular
Coagulation abnormalities
Overanticoagulation
Arterial emboli or thrombosis
Arteriovenous malformation
Arteriovenous fistula
Nutcracker syndrome
Renal vein thrombosis
Loin-pain hematuria syndrome (vascular?)
Glomerular
Immunoglobulin A nephropathy
Thin basement membrane diseases (including Alport's syndrome)
Other causes of primary and secondary glomerulonephritis
Interstitial
Allergic interstitial nephritis
Analgesic nephropathy
Renal cystic diseases
Acute pyelonephritis
Tuberculosis
Renal allograft rejection
Uroepithelial
Malignancy
Vigorous exercise
Trauma
Papillary necrosis
Cystitis/urethritis/prostatitis (usually caused by infection)
Parasitic diseases (e.g., schistosomiasis)
Nephrolithiasis or bladder calculi
Multiple Sites or Source Unknown
Hypercalciuria
Hyperuricosuria
Sickle cell disease

often unclear, although occasionally sickle cells may actually be seen in the urine.[227,228]

Worldwide, the most common cause of glomerular hematuria is probably IgA nephropathy.[227] However, thin basement membrane diseases and other causes of glomerular nephritis are common as well. The differential diagnosis of glomerular hematuria is influenced by the geographic locale and the clinical setting. Thus, in Asia, IgA nephropathy is a very common cause of microscopic hematuria.[227] However, in another report, 25 of 30 otherwise healthy candidates for kidney donation who had asymptomatic microscopic hematuria were found to have hereditary nephritis.[229] Interstitial nephritis, whether allergic or infectious, is frequently associated with microscopic hematuria. Uroepithelial causes of hematuria include nephrolithiasis, acute and chronic infections, and malignancies. Malignancies are more common in patients who are male, are older, have macroscopic rather than microscopic hematuria, are white rather than black, or have a history of analgesic abuse or other toxic exposure. An approach to the patient with asymptomatic hematuria is presented in Chapter 24.

Leukocyturia

The number of white blood cells that can normally be found in the urine is controversial. A conservative approach is to consider more than one per high-power field to be abnormal. The differential diagnosis of leukocyturia is broad. White blood cells can enter the urine from anywhere along the excretory system. The presence of other formed elements (e.g., proteinuria and casts) suggests a glomerular source. In the absence of other formed elements, the clinician must look beyond the urine sediment for additional clues to find the origin of urine leukocytes. Unlike for red blood cells, there are no effective methods to identify the origin of white blood cells found in the urine.

Contamination is a common cause of leukocyturia that should always be considered in the absence of other suggestive clinical findings. Most often, leukocytes in the urine are polymorphonuclear. However, it should not be assumed that all urinary leukocytes are neutrophils. The presence of nonneutrophil white blood cells in the urine—for example, eosinophils—can sometimes be an important diagnostic clue. An association between eosinophiluria and drug-induced hypersensitivity reactions was first reported by Eisenstaedt in 1951. Since then, a number of investigators have reported on the association between eosinophiluria and kidney disease.[4]

Wright's stain can be used to detect urine eosinophils, but a urine pH less than 7 inhibits Wright's stain.[230] The use of Hansel's stain improves the sensitivity of urinary eosinophil detection over the standard Wright's stain.[231] In one retrospective investigation, the use of Hansel's stain rather than Wright's stain improved the sensitivity of using the presence of any urinary eosinophils for detection of acute interstitial nephritis from 25% to 63%[231]; the positive predictive value was improved from 25% to 50%.[231] However, not all patients in this study underwent renal biopsy to establish the diagnosis of interstitial nephritis, and the retrospective inclusion of only patients in whom urinary eosinophils were sought by clinicians makes interpretation of these data difficult.

The true sensitivity and specificity of urinary eosinophils for detecting different clinical kidney diseases are unclear. Indeed, the list of diseases that may be associated with eosinophiluria is long and continues to grow (Table 25-4). Moreover, the sensitivity and specificity of eosinophiluria for detecting kidney disease can be expected to vary with the threshold value used.[232]

Other Cells

It is difficult to identify the origin of cells that are neither leukocytes nor red blood cells without special stains. Most common are probably squamous epithelial cells. These are shed from the bladder or urethra and are rarely pathologic. Renal tubular cells may appear whenever there has been tubular damage. Transitional epithelial cells are rare but may be seen with collecting system infection or neoplasias.

Urine Fat

In the absence of contamination, urinary lipids are almost always pathologic. Lipids are not usually seen as an isolated finding; however, their presence is rarely diagnostic. Lipids usually appear as free fat droplets or oval fat bodies. They have a distinctive appearance and are most readily seen under polarized light as doubly refractile "Maltese crosses." The Maltese cross is indicative of cholesterol and cholesterol esters. Maltese crosses can also be seen with some crystals and with starch granules. Neutral fat can be identified with special lipid stains. Urinary lipids are most commonly associated with proteinuria and are particularly common in patients with nephrotic syndrome; they can also occur in the absence of heavy proteinuria. Urine fat can also be seen in bone marrow or fat embolization syndromes.[4]

TABLE 25-4 Diseases Associated with Eosinophiluria
Common
Acute allergic interstitial nephritis
Urinary tract infection (upper and lower tract)
Unusual
Acute tubular necrosis
Diabetic nephropathy
Focal segmental glomerulosclerosis
Polycystic kidney disease
Obstruction
Rapidly progressive glomerulonephritis
Postinfectious glomerulonephritis
Immunoglobulin A nephropathy
Acute cystitis
Acute prostatitis
Atheroembolic renal disease
Renal transplant rejection

From Silkensen JR, Kasiske BL: Laboratory assessment of renal disease: clearance, urinalysis, and renal biopsy, in Brenner BM (editor): *Brenner and Rector's the kidney*, ed 7, Philadelphia, 2004, Saunders, p 1131.

Casts

Casts are cylindrical bodies severalfold larger than leukocytes and red blood cells. They form in distal tubules and collecting ducts where Tamm-Horsfall glycoprotein precipitates and entraps cells present in the urinary space. Dehydration and the resulting increased tubular fluid concentration favor the formation of casts. An acid urine is also conducive to cast formation.

Detection of casts in the urine sediment often provides helpful diagnostic information. The differential diagnosis of cast formation is aided by first considering the type of cast found. A number of different types can be readily distinguished (Figure 25-6).[4] Hyaline or finely granular casts can be seen in normal individuals and provide little useful diagnostic information. Cellular casts are generally more helpful. Red blood cell casts, for example, are distinctive and most often indicate

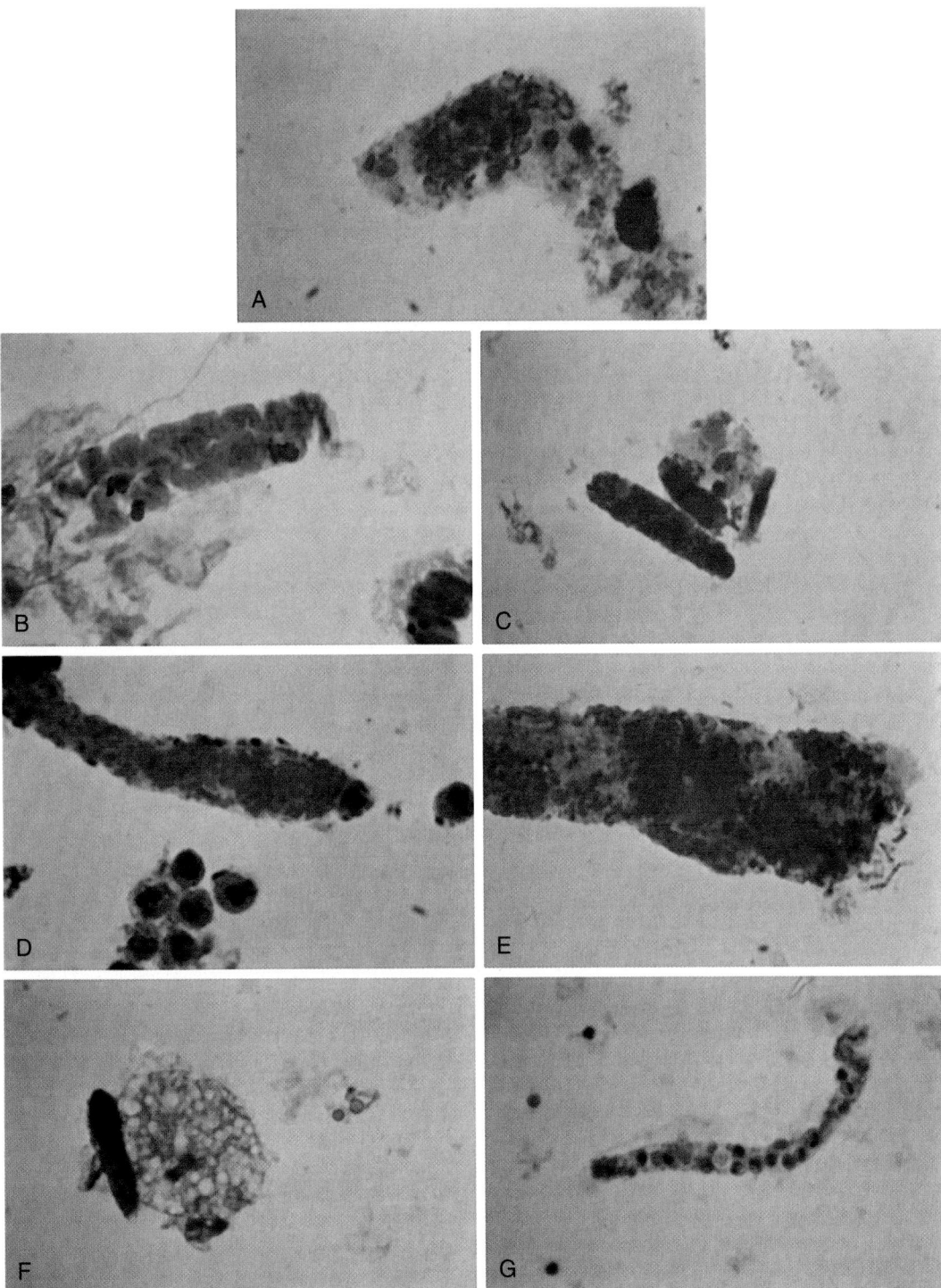

FIGURE 25-6 Abnormalities in urine sediment stained to enhance detail. **A,** Red blood cell cast. (×900.) **B,** Hyaline cast. (×900.) **C,** Hyaline and granular casts. (×400.) **D,** Coarse granular cast with adjacent white blood cells. (×750.) **E,** Fine and coarse granular cast. (×900.) **F,** Oval fat body with adjacent hyalin cast. (×400.) **G,** White blood cell cast. (×400.)

glomerular disease. White blood cell casts are most commonly associated with interstitial nephritis but can also be seen in glomerulonephritis. Casts made up of renal tubular epithelial cells are always indicative of tubular damage. Coarsely granular casts often result from the degeneration of different cellular casts. They also contain protein aggregates. Thus, the presence of granular casts is usually pathologic, but nonspecific. Waxy casts are also nonspecific. They are believed to result from the degeneration of cellular casts and thus can be seen in a variety of kidney diseases. Pigmented casts usually derive their distinctive color from bilirubin or hemoglobin, and they are found in hyperbilirubinemia and hemoglobinuria, respectively. Fatty casts contain lipid and oval fat bodies (see preceding section).

Crystals and Other Elements

A large variety of crystals can be seen in the urine sediment. Most result from urine concentration, acidification, and ex vivo cooling of the sample and have little pathologic significance. However, an experienced observer can gain useful information in patients with microhematuria, nephrolithiasis, or toxin ingestion by examining a freshly voided, warm specimen.[233] For example, a large number of calcium oxalate crystals may suggest ethylene glycol toxicity when seen in the right clinical setting. As another example, a large number of uric acid crystals in the setting of acute renal failure suggests tumor lysis syndrome.

Calcium oxalate crystals are uniform small double pyramids that often appear as crosses in a square. Calcium phosphate crystals, on the other hand, are usually narrow rectangular needles, often clumped in a flower-like configuration. Uric acid crystals form only in an acidic urine, which favors the conversion of relatively insoluble urate salts into insoluble uric acid. Calcium magnesium ammonium pyrophosphate (so-called triple phosphate) crystals form domed rectangles that take on the appearance of coffin lids. These magnesium ammonium phosphate (struvite) and calcium carbonate–apatite stones occur when ammonia production is increased and the urine pH is elevated, which thereby decreases the solubility of phosphate. This combination of events occurs when urease-producing organisms, such as *Proteus* or *Klebsiella*, are present in the urine.

Microorganisms

The most common cause of bacteria in the urine is contamination, particularly in specimens that have been improperly collected. The concomitant presence of leukocytes, however, suggests infection. Fungal elements may also be seen, especially in women. Like bacteria, fungi can be contaminants or pathogens. The most common protozoan seen in the urine is *Trichomonas vaginalis*. Urinary parasites are generally not seen in the urine sediment. In Africa and the Middle East, however, *Schistosoma haematobium* is common.

Conflicts and Support

Dr. Kasiske currently receives research support from the Merck/Schering Plough Joint Venture and Bristol-Myers Squibb. In the past 2 years, he received honoraria from AstraZeneca, Bristol-Myers Squibb, Fujisawa, Merck, Pfizer, and Wyeth.

Dr. Israni currently receives research support from Roche, Amgen, Genzyme, and Bristol-Myers Squibb.

This chapter was supported in part by a Robert Wood Johnson Physician Faculty Scholar grant to Dr. Israni (NIH ARRA grant SU19-AI070119).

References

1. Sarnak M, Levey AS, Schoolwerth AC, et al. Kidney disease as a risk factor for development of cardiovascular disease: a statement from the American Heart Association Councils on Kidney in Cardiovascular Disease, High Blood Pressure Research, Clinical Cardiology, and Epidemiology and Prevention. *Hypertension.* 2003;42:1050-1065.
2. Gerstein H, Mann JF, Yi Q, et al. Albuminuria and risk of cardiovascular events, death, and heart failure in diabetic and nondiabetic individuals. *JAMA.* 2001;286:421-426.
3. National Kidney Foundation Kidney. *K/DOQI clinical practice guidelines for chronic kidney disease: evaluation, classification and stratification.* 2002;39 (suppl 1):S1-S266.
4. Silkensen J, Kasiske BL. Laboratory assessment of renal disease: clearance, urinalysis, and renal biopsy. In: Brenner BM, ed. *Brenner and Rector's the kidney.* Philadelphia: Saunders; 2004:1107-1150.
5. Bonsnes R, Taussky HH. On the colorimetric determination of creatinine by Jaffé reaction. *J Biol Chem.* 1945;158:581-591.
6. Toffaletti J, Blosser N, Hall T, et al. An automated dry-slide enzymatic method evaluated for measurement of creatinine in serum. *Clin Chem.* 1983;29:684-687.
7. Hare R. Endogenous creatinine in serum and urine. *Proc Soc Exp Biol Med.* 1950;74:148-151.
8. Jacobs D, De Mott WR, Strobel SL, et al. Chemistry. In: Jacobs D, Kasten BL, De Mott WR, Wolfson WL, eds. *Laboratory test handbook.* Baltimore: Williams & Wilkins; 1990:171-172.
9. Miller W, Myers GL, Ashwood ER, et al. Creatinine measurement: state of the art in accuracy and interlaboratory harmonization. *Arch Pathol Lab Med.* 2005;129:297-304.
10. Durham S, Bignell AHC, Wise R. Interference of cefoxitin in the creatinine estimation and its clinical relevance. *J Clin Pathol.* 1979;32:1148-1151.
11. Saah A, Koch TR, Drusano GL. Cefoxitin falsely elevates creatinine levels. *JAMA.* 1982;247:205-206.
12. Swain R, Briggs SL. Positive interference with the Jaffé reaction by cephalosporin antibiotics. *Clin Chem.* 1977;23:1340-1342.
13. Young D. *Effects of drugs on clinical laboratory tests.* 3rd ed. Washington, DC: American Association of Clinical Chemistry Press; 1990, pp 3-128.
14. Doolan P, Alpen EL, Theil GB. A clinical appraisal of the plasma concentration and endogenous clearance of creatinine. *Am J Med.* 1962;32:65-79.
15. Fabiny D, Ertingshausen G. Automated reaction-rate method for determination of serum creatinine with the Centritichem. *Clin Chem.* 1971;17:696-700.
16. Gerard S, Khayam-Bashi H. Characterization of creatinine error in ketotic patients: a prospective comparison of alkaline picrate methods with an enzymatic method. *Am J Clin Pathol.* 1985;84:659-664.
17. Osberg I, Hammond KB. A solution to the problem of bilirubin interference with the kinetic Jaffé method for serum creatinine. *Clin Chem.* 1978;24:1196-1197.
18. Myers GL, Miller WG, Coresh J. Recommendations for improving serum creatinine measurement: a report from the laboratory working group of the National Kidney Disease Education Program. *Clin Chem.* 2006;52:5-18.
19. Kasiske B. Creatinine excretion after renal transplantation. *Transplantation.* 1989;48:424-428.
20. Coresh J, Toto RD, Kirk KA, et al. Creatinine clearance as a measure of GFR in screenees for the African-American Study of Kidney Disease and Hypertension pilot study. *Am J Kidney Dis.* 1998;32:32-42.
21. DeSanto N, Coppola S, Anastasio P, et al. Predicted creatinine clearance to assess glomerular filtration rate in chronic renal disease in humans. *Am J Nephrol.* 1991;11:181-185.
22. Payne R. Creatinine clearance: a redundant clinical investigation. *Ann Clin Biochem.* 1986;23:243-250.
23. Fuller N, Elia M. Factors influencing the production of creatinine: implications for the determination and interpretation of urinary creatinine and creatine in man. *Clin Chim Acta.* 1988;175:199-210.
24. Shemesh O, Golbetz H, Kriss JP, et al. Limitations of creatinine as a filtration marker in glomerulopathic patients. *Kidney Int.* 1985;28:830-838.
25. Rosano T, Brown HH. Analytical and biological variability of serum creatinine and creatinine clearance: implications for clinical interpretation. *Clin Chem.* 1982;28:2330-2331.

26. Bröchner-Mortensen J, Rödbro P. Selection of routine method for determination of glomerular filtration rate in adult patients. *Scand J Clin Lab Invest*. 1976;36:35-43.
27. Bjornsson T, Cocchetto DM, McGowan FX, et al. Nomogram for estimating creatinine clearance. *Clin Pharmacokinet*. 1983;8:365-369.
28. Cockcroft D, Gault MH. Prediction of creatinine clearance from serum creatinine. *Nephron*. 1976;16:31-41.
29. Hull J, Hak LJ, Koch GG, et al. Influence of range of renal function and liver disease on predictability of creatinine clearance. *Clin Pharmacol Ther*. 1981;29:516-521.
30. Jelliffe R, Jelliffe SM. Estimation of creatinine clearance from changing serum creatinine levels. *Lancet*. 1971;2:710.
31. Jelliffe R. Creatinine clearance: bedside estimate. *Ann Intern Med*. 1973;79:604-605.
32. Kampmann J, Siersbaek-Nielson K, Kristensen M, et al. Rapid evaluation of creatinine clearance. *Acta Med Scand*. 1974;196:517-520.
33. Levey A, Bosch JP, Lewis JB, et al. A more accurate method to estimate glomerular filtration rate from serum creatinine: a new prediction equation. Modification of Diet in Renal Disease Study Group. *Ann Intern Med*. 1999;130:461-470.
34. Mawer G, Knowles BR, Lucas SB, et al. Computer-assisted dosing of kanamycin for patients with renal insufficiency. *Lancet*. 1972;1:12-14.
35. Walser M, Drew HH, Guldan JL. Prediction of glomerular filtration rate from serum creatinine concentration in advanced chronic renal failure. *Kidney Int*. 1993;44:1145-1148.
36. Levey A. Use of glomerular filtration rate measurements to assess the progression of renal disease. *Semin Nephrol*. 1989;9:370-379.
37. Levey AS, Stevens LA, Schmid CH, et al. A new equation to estimate glomerular filtration rate. *Ann Intern Med*. 2009;150:604-612.
38. Li Z, Lew NL, Lazarus JM, et al. Comparing the urea reduction ratio and the urea product as outcome-based measures of hemodialysis dose. *Am J Kidney Dis*. 2000;35:598-605.
39. Simonsen O, Grubb A, Thysell H. The blood serum concentration of cystatin C (gamma-trace) as a measure of the glomerular filtration rate. *Scand J Clin Lab Invest*. 1985;45:97-101.
40. Grubb A. Diagnostic value of analysis of cystatin C and protein HC in biological fluids. *Clin Nephrol*. 1992;38(suppl 1):S20-S27.
41. Rule A, Bergstralh EJ, Slezak JM, et al. Glomerular filtration rate estimated by cystatin C among different clinical presentations. *Kidney Int*. 2006;69:399-405.
42. Laterza O, Price CP, Scott MG. Cystatin C: an improved estimator of glomerular filtration rate? *Clin Chem*. 2002;48:699-707.
43. Woitas R, Stoffel-Wagner B, Flommersfeld S, et al. Correlation of serum concentrations of cystatin C and creatinine to inulin clearance in liver cirrhosis. *Clin Chem*. 2000;46:712-715.
44. Kyhse-Andersen J, Schmidt C, Nordin G, et al. Serum cystatin C, determined by a rapid, automated particle-enhanced turbidimetric method, is a better marker than serum creatinine for glomerular filtration rate. *Clin Chem*. 1994;40:1921-1926.
45. Newman D, Thakkar H, Edwsards RG, et al. Serum cystatin C measured by automated immunoassay: a more sensitive marker of changes in GFR than serum creatinine. *Kidney Int*. 1995;47:312-318.
46. Tian S, Kusano E, Ohara T, et al. Cystatin C measurement and its practical use in patients with various renal diseases. *Clin Nephrol*. 1997;48:104-108.
47. Knight E, Verhave JC, Spiegelman D, et al. Factors influencing serum cystatin C levels other than renal function and the impact on renal function measurement. *Kidney Int*. 2004;65:1416-1421.
48. Finney H, Newman DJ, Price CP. Adult reference ranges for serum cystatin C, creatinine and predicted creatinine clearance. *Ann Clin Biochem*. 2000;37(pt 1):49-59.
49. Sawyer W, Canaday BR, Poe TE, et al. A multicenter evaluation of variables affecting the predictability of creatinine clearance. *Am J Clin Pathol*. 1982;78:832-838.
50. Uchida K, Gotoh A. Measurement of cystatin-C and creatinine in urine. *Clin Chim Acta*. 2002;323:121-128.
51. Dharnidharka V, Kwon C, Stevens G. Serum cystatin C is superior to serum creatinine as a marker of kidney function: a meta-analysis. *Am J Kidney Dis*. 2002;40:221-226.
52. Stevens LA, Coresh J, Schmid CH, et al. Estimating GFR using serum cystatin C alone and in combination with serum creatinine: a pooled analysis of 3,418 individuals with CKD. *Am J Kidney Dis*. 2009;51:395-406.
53. Coll E, Botey A, Alvarez L, et al. Serum cystatin C as a new marker for noninvasive estimation of glomerular filtration rate and as a marker for early renal impairment. *Am J Kidney Dis*. 2000;36:29-34.
54. Donadio C, Lucchesi A, Ardini M, et al. Cystatin C, beta 2-microglobulin, and retinol-binding protein as indicators of glomerular filtration rate: comparison with plasma creatinine. *J Pharm Biomed Anal*. 2001;24:835-842.
55. Stickle D, Cole B, Hock K, et al. Correlation of plasma concentrations of cystatin C and creatinine to inulin clearance in a pediatric population. *Clin Chem*. 1998;44:1334-1338.

56. Shlipak M, Sarnak MJ, Katz R, et al. Cystatin C and the risk of death and cardiovascular events among elderly persons. *N Engl J Med*. 2005;352:2049-2060.
57. Mussap M, Dalla VM, Fioretto P, et al. Cystatin C is a more sensitive marker than creatinine for the estimation of GFR in type 2 diabetic patients. *Kidney Int*. 2002;61:1453-1461.
58. Oddoze C, Morange S, Portugal H, et al. Cystatin C is not more sensitive than creatinine for detecting early renal impairment in patients with diabetes. *Am J Kidney Dis*. 2001;38:310-316.
59. Bokenkamp A, Domanetzki M, Zinck R, et al. Cystatin C serum concentrations underestimate glomerular filtration rate in renal transplant recipients. *Clin Chem*. 1999;45:1866-1868.
60. Cimerman N, Brguljan PM, Krasovec M, et al. Serum cystatin C, a potent inhibitor of cysteine proteinases, is elevated in asthmatic patients. *Clin Chim Acta*. 2000;300:83-95.
61. Bjarnadottir M, Grubb A, Olafsson I. Promoter-mediated, dexamethasone-induced increase in cystatin C production by HeLa cells. *Scand J Clin Lab Invest*. 1995;55:617-623.
62. Risch L, Blumberg A, Huber A. Rapid and accurate assessment of glomerular filtration rate in patients with renal transplants using serum cystatin C. *Nephrol Dial Transplant*. 1999;14:1991-1996.
63. Bokenkamp A, van Wijk JA, Lentze MJ, et al. Effect of corticosteroid therapy on serum cystatin C and beta2-microglobulin concentrations. *Clin Chem*. 2002;48:1123-1126.
64. Bokenkamp A, Ozden N, Dieterich C, et al. Cystatin C and creatinine after successful kidney transplantation in children. *Clin Nephrol*. 1999;52:371-376.
65. Deinum J, Derkx FH. Cystatin for estimation of glomerular filtration rate? *Lancet*. 2000;356:1624-1625.
66. Keevil B, Kilpatrick ES, Nichols SP, et al. Biological variation of cystatin C: implications for the assessment of glomerular filtration rate. *Clin Chem*. 1998;44:1535-1539.
67. Mussap M, Plebani M. Biochemistry and clinical role of human cystatin C. *Crit Rev Clin Lab Sci*. 2004;41:467-550.
68. Schnurr E, Lahme W, Küppers H. Measurement of renal clearance of inulin and PAH in the steady state without urine collection. *Clin Nephrol*. 1980;13(1):26-29.
69. van Acker B, Koomen GCM, Arisz L. Drawbacks of the constant-infusion technique for measurement of renal function. *Am J Physiol*. 1995;268(4 pt 2):F543-F552.
70. van Guldener C, Gans ROB, ter Wee PM. Constant infusion clearance is an inappropriate method for accurate assessment of an impaired glomerular filtration rate. *Nephrol Dial Transplant*. 1995;10:47-51.
71. Florijn K, Barendregt JNM, Lentjex EGWM, et al. Glomerular filtration rate measurement by "single-shot" injection of inulin. *Kidney Int*. 1994;46:252-259.
72. Rosenbaum R, Hruska KA, Anderson C, et al. Inulin: an inadequate marker of glomerular filtration rate in kidney donors and transplant recipients? *Kidney Int*. 1979;16:179-186.
73. Brochner-Mortensen J. Current status on assessment and measurement of glomerular filtration rate. *Clin Physiol*. 1985;5(1):1-17.
74. Pihl B. The single injection technique for determination of renal clearance. V. A comparison with the continuous infusion technique in the dog and in man. *Scand J Urol Nephrol*. 1974;8:147-154.
75. Carlsen J, Moller ML, Lund JO, et al. Comparison of four commercial Tc-99m(Sn)DTPA preparations used for the measurement of glomerular filtration rate: concise communication. *J Nucl Med*. 1980;21:126-129.
76. Russell C, Bischoff PG, Rowell KL, et al. Quality control of Tc-99m DTPA for measurement of glomerular filtration: concise communication. *J Nucl Med*. 1983;24:722-727.
77. Sambataro M, Thomaseth K, Pacini G, et al. Plasma clearance rate of ^{51}Cr-EDTA provides a precise and convenient technique for measurement of glomerular filtration rate in diabetic humans. *J Am Soc Nephrol*. 1996;7:118-127.
78. Bianchi C, Donadio C, Tramonti G. Noninvasive methods for the measurement of total renal function. *Nephron*. 1981;28:53-57.
79. Gaspari F, Mosconi L, Viganò G, et al. Measurement of GFR with a single intravenous injection of nonradioactive iothalamate. *Kidney Int*. 1992;41:1081-1084.
80. Tauxe W. Determination of glomerular filtration rate by single sample technique following injection of radioiodinated diatrizoate. *J Nucl Med*. 1986;27:45-50.
81. Tepe P, Tauxe WN, Bagchi A, et al. Comparison of measurement of glomerular filtration rate by single sample, plasma disappearance slope/intercept and other methods. *Eur J Nucl Med*. 1987;13:28-31.
82. Lundqvist S, Hietala SO, Groth S, et al. Evaluation of single sample clearance calculations of 902 patients. A comparison of multiple and single sample techniques. *Acta Radiol*. 1997;38:68-72.
83. Rydström M, Tengström B, Cederquist I, et al. Measurement of glomerular filtration rate by single-injection, single-sample techniques, using ^{51}Cr-EDTA or iohexol. *Scand J Urol Nephrol*. 1995;29:135-139.

84. Gaspari F, Guerini E, Perico N, et al. Glomerular filtration rate determined from a single plasma sample after intravenous iohexol injection: is it reliable? *J Am Soc Nephrol*. 1996;7:2689-2693.

85. Fleming J, Waller DG. Feasibility of estimating glomerular filtration rate on children using single-sample adult technique. *J Nucl Med*. 1997;38:1665-1667.

86. Ham H, Piepsz A. Feasibility of estimating glomerular filtration rate in children using single-sample adult technique. *J Nucl Med*. 1996;37:1805-1808.

87. Al-Uzri A, Holliday MA, Gambertoglio JG, et al. An accurate practical method for estimating GFR in clinical studies using a constant subcutaneous infusion. *Kidney Int*. 1992;41:1701-1706.

88. Blaufox M, Aurell M, Bubeck B, et al. Report of the Radionuclides in Nephrourology Committee on renal clearance. *J Nucl Med*. 1996;37:1883-1890.

89. Sanger J, Kramer EL. Radionuclide quantitation of renal function. *Urol Radiol*. 1992;14:69-78.

90. Oriuchi N, Inoue T, Hayashi I, et al. Evaluation of gamma camera–based measurement of individual kidney function using iodine-123 orthoiodohippurate. *Eur J Nucl Med*. 1996;23:371-375.

91. Blomley M, Dawson P. Review article: the quantification of renal function with enhanced computed tomography. *Br J Radiol*. 1996;69:989-995.

92. Niendorf E, Grist TM, Lee Jr FT, et al. Rapid in vivo measurement of single-kidney extraction fraction and glomerular filtration rate with MR imaging. *Radiology*. 1998;206:791-798.

93. Goates J, Morton KA, Whooten WW, et al. Comparison of methods for calculating glomerular filtration rate: technetium-99m-DTPA scintigraphic analysis, protein-free and whole-plasma clearance of technetium-99m-DTPA and iodine-125-iothalamate clearance. *J Nucl Med*. 1990;31:424-429.

94. Rabito C, Panico F, Rubin R, et al. Noninvasive, real-time monitoring of renal function during critical care. *J Am Soc Nephrol*. 1994;4:1421-1428.

95. Bianchi C, Bonadio M, Donadio C, et al. Measurement of glomerular filtration rate in man using DTPA-99mTc. *Nephron*. 1979;24:174-178.

96. Dubovsky E, Russell CD. Quantitation of renal function with glomerular and tubular agents. *Semin Nucl Med*. 1982;12:308-329.

97. O'Reilly P, Brooman PJC, Martin PJ, et al. Accuracy and reproducibility of a new contrast clearance method for the determination of glomerular filtration rate. *BMJ*. 1986;293:234-236.

98. O'Reilly P, Jones DA, Farah NB. Measurement of the plasma clearance of urographic contrast media for the determination of glomerular filtration rate. *J Urol*. 1988;139:9-11.

99. Gaspari F, Perico N, Matalone M, et al. Precision of plasma clearance of iohexol for estimation of GFR in patients with renal disease. *J Am Soc Nephrol*. 1998;9:310-313.

100. Lewis R, Kerr N, Van Buren C, et al. Comparative evaluation of urographic contrast media, inulin, and 99mTc-DTPA clearance methods for determination of glomerular filtration rate in clinical transplantation. *Transplantation*. 1989;48:790-796.

101. Manske C, Sprafka JM, Strony JT, et al. Contrast nephropathy in azotemic diabetic patients undergoing coronary angiography. *Am J Med*. 1990;89:615-620.

102. Lundqvist S, Hietala S-O, Berglund C, et al. Simultaneous urography and determination of glomerular filtration rate. A comparison of total plasma clearances of iohexol and 51Cr-EDTA in plegic patients. *Acta Radiol*. 1994;35:391-395.

103. Swan S, Halstenson CE, Kasiske BL, et al. Determination of residual renal function with iohexol clearance in hemodialysis patients. *Kidney Int*. 1996;49:232-235.

104. Turner S, Reilly SL. Fallacy of indexing renal and systemic hemodynamic measurements for body surface area. *Am J Physiol*. 1995;268(4 pt 2):R978-R988.

105. Schmieder R, Beil AH, Weihprecht H, et al. How should renal hemodynamic data be indexed in obesity? *J Am Soc Nephrol*. 1995;5:1709-1713.

106. White A, Strydom WJ. Normalisation of glomerular filtration rate measurements. *Eur J Nucl Med*. 1991;18:385-390.

107. Kasiske B, Umen AJ. The influence of age, sex, race, and body habitus on kidney weight in humans. *Arch Pathol Lab Med*. 1986;110:55-60.

108. Zuccalà A, Zucchelli P. Use and misuse of the renal functional reserve concept in clinical nephrology. *Nephrol Dial Transplant*. 1990;5:410-417.

109. Israni A, Snyder JJ, Skeans MA, et al. Predicting coronary heart disease after kidney transplantation: Patient Outcomes in Renal Transplantation (PORT) Study. *Am J Transpl*. 2010;10:338-353.

110. Viberti G, Bilous RW, Mackintosh D, et al. Monitoring glomerular function in diabetic nephropathy. *Am J Med*. 1983;74:256-264.

111. Walser M, Drew HH, LaFrance ND. Creatinine measurements often yielded false estimates of progression in chronic renal failure. *Kidney Int*. 1988;34:412-418.

112. Levey A, Gassman JJ, Hall PM, et al. Assessing the progression of renal disease in clinical studies: effects of duration of follow-up and regression to the mean. *J Am Soc Nephrol*. 1991;1:1087-1094.

113. Shah B, Levey AS. Spontaneous changes in the rate of decline in reciprocal serum creatinine: errors in predicting the progression of renal disease from extrapolation of the slope. *J Am Soc Nephrol*. 1992;2:1186-1191.

114. Walser M. Progression of chronic renal failure in man. *Kidney Int*. 1990;37:1195-1210.

115. Levey A, Greene T, Schluchter MD, et al. Glomerular filtration rate measurements in clinical trials. *J Am Soc Nephrol*. 1993;4:1159-1171.

116. Rossing P. Doubling of serum creatinine: is it sensitive and relevant? *Nephrol Dial Transplant*. 1998;13:244-246.

117. Coresh J, Astor BC, McQuillan G, et al. Calibration and random variation of the serum creatinine assay as critical elements of using equations to estimate glomerular filtration rate. *Am J Kidney Dis*. 2002;39:920-929.

118. Murthy K, Stevens LA, Stark PC, et al. Variation in the serum creatinine assay calibration: a practical application to glomerular filtration rate estimation. *Kidney Int*. 2005;68:1884-1887.

119. Akin B, Hubbell FA, Frye EB, et al. Efficacy of the routine admission urinalysis. *Am J Med*. 1987;82:719-722.

120. Kroenke K, Hanley JF, Copley JB, et al. The admission urinalysis: impact on patient care. *J Gen Intern Med*. 1986;1:238-242.

121. Mitchell N, Stapleton FB. Routine admission urinalysis examination in pediatric patients: a poor value. *Pediatrics*. 1990;86:345-349.

122. Khallid N, Haddad FH. Is routine urinalysis worthwhile? *Lancet*. 1988;1:747.

123. Schumann G, Greenberg NF. Usefulness of macroscopic urinalysis as a screening procedure. *Am J Clin Pathol*. 1979;71:452-456.

124. Györy A, Hadfield C, Lauer CS. Value of urine microscopy in predicting histological changes in the kidney: double blind comparison. *BMJ*. 1984;288:819-822.

125. Morrin P. Urinary sediment in the interpretation of proteinuria. *Ann Intern Med*. 1983;98:254-255.

126. U.S. Preventive Services Task Force. Screening for asymptomatic bacteriuria, hematuria and proteinuria. *Am Fam Physician*. 1990;42:389-395.

127. Recommendations for preventive pediatric health care. In: *Policy reference guide: a comprehensive guide to AAP policy statement*. Elk Grove Village, Ill: American Academy of Pediatrics; 1993.

128. Kaplan R, Springate JE, Feld LG. Screening dipstick urinalysis: a time to change. *Pediatrics*. 1997;100:919-921.

129. Arant BJ. Screening for urinary abnormalities: worth doing and worth doing well. *Lancet*. 1998;351:307-308.

130. Craver R, Abermanis JG. Dipstick only urinalysis screen for the pediatric emergency room. *Pediatr Nephrol*. 1997;11:331-333.

131. Bonnardeaux A, Somerville P, Kaye M. A study on the reliability of dipstick urinalysis. *Clin Nephrol*. 1994;41:167-172.

132. Jacobs D, De Mott WR, Willie GR. Urinalysis and clinical microscopy. In: Jacobs D, Kasten BL, De Mott WR, et al. eds. *Laboratory test handbook*. Baltimore: Williams & Wilkins; 1990:914-915.

133. Jacobs D, De Mott WR, Willie GR. Urinalysis and clinical microscopy. In: Jacobs D, Kasten BL, De Mott WR, et al. eds. *Laboratory test handbook*. Baltimore: Williams & Wilkins; 1990:919.

134. Ditchburn R, Ditchburn JS. A study of microscopical and chemical tests for the rapid diagnosis of urinary tract infections in general practice. *Br J Gen Pract*. 1990;40:406-408.

135. McGlone R, Lambert M, Clancy M, et al. Use of Ames SG10 Urine Dipstick for diagnosis of abdominal pain in the accident and emergency department. *Arch Emerg Med*. 1990;7:42-47.

136. Liptak G, Campbell J, Stewart R, et al. Screening for urinary tract infection in children with neurogenic bladders. *Am J Phys Med Rehabil*. 1993:122-126.

137. Lohr J, Portilla MG, Geuder TG, et al. Making a presumptive diagnosis of urinary tract infection by using a urinalysis performed in an on-site laboratory. *J Pediatr*. 1993;122:22-25.

138. McNagny S, Parker RM, Zenilman JM, et al. Urinary leukocyte esterase test: a screening method for the detection of asymptomatic chlamydial and gonococcal infections in men. *J Infect Dis*. 1992;165:573-576.

139. Blum R, Wright RA. Detection of pyuria and bacteriuria in symptomatic ambulatory women. *J Gen Intern Med*. 1992;7:140-144.

140. Hurlbut III T, Littenberg B. The diagnostic accuracy of rapid dipstick tests to predict urinary tract infection. *Am J Clin Pathol*. 1991;96:582-588.

141. Jacobs D, De Mott WR, Willie GR. Urinalysis and clinical microscopy. In: Jacobs D, Kasten BL, De Mott WR, et al. eds. *Laboratory test handbook*. Baltimore: Williams & Wilkins; 1990:906-909.

142. Singer D, Coley CM, Samet JH, et al. Tests of glycemia in diabetes mellitus: their use in establishing a diagnosis and in treatment. *Ann Intern Med*. 1990;110:125-137.

143. Jacobs D, De Mott WR, Willie GR. Urinalysis and clinical microscopy. In: Jacobs D, Kasten BL, De Mott WR, et al. eds. *Laboratory test handbook*. Baltimore: Williams & Wilkins; 1990:912.

144. Shihabi Z, Konen JC, O'Connor ML. Albuminuria vs urinary total protein for detecting chronic renal disorders. *Clin Chem.* 1991;37:621-624.

145. Hession C, Decker JM, Sherblom AP, et al. Uromodulin (Tamm-Horsfall glycoprotein): a renal ligand for lymphokines. *Science.* 1987;237:1479-1484.

146. Pennica D, Kohr WJ, Kuang W-J, et al. Identification of human uromodulin as the Tamm-Horsfall urinary glycoprotein. *Science.* 1987;236:83-88.

147. Allen J, Krauss EA, Deeter RG. Dipstick analysis of urinary protein. A comparison of Chemstrip-9 and Multistix-10SG. *Arch Pathol Lab Med.* 1991;115:34-37.

148. Rowe D, Dawnay A, Watts GF. Microalbuminuria in diabetes mellitus: review and recommendations for the measurement of albumin in urine. *Ann Clin Biochem.* 1990;27:297-312.

149. Harmoinen A, Vuorinen P, Jokela H. Turbidimetric measurement of microalbuminuria. *Clin Chim Acta.* 1987;166:85-89.

150. Stamp R. Measurement of albumin in urine by end-point immunonephelometry. *Ann Clin Biochem.* 1988;25:442-443.

151. Neuman R, Cohen MP. Improved competitive enzyme-linked immunoassay (ELISA) for albuminuria. *Clin Chim Acta.* 1989;179:229-238.

152. Comper W, Osicka TM, Jerums G. High prevalence of immuno-unreactive intact albumin in urine of diabetic patients. *Am J Kidney Dis.* 2003;41:336-342.

153. Tiu S, Lee SS, Cheng MW. Comparison of six commercial techniques in the measurement of microalbuminuria in diabetic patients. *Diabetes Care.* 1993;16:616-620.

154. Comper W, Jerums G, Osicka TM. Differences in urinary albumin detected by four immunoassays and high-performance liquid chromatography. *Clin Biochem.* 2004;37:105-111.

155. Giampietro O, Penno G, Clerico A, et al. Which method for quantifying "microalbuminuria" in diabetics? Comparison of several immunological methods (immunoturbidimetric assay, immunonephelometric assay, radioimmunoassay and two semiquantitative tests) for measurement of albumin in urine. *Acta Diabetol.* 1992;28:239-245.

156. Ballantyne F, Gibbons J, O'Reilly DS. Urine albumin should replace total protein for the assessment of glomerular proteinuria. *Ann Clin Biochem.* 1993;30(pt 1):101-103.

157. Sawicki P, Heinemann L, Berger M. Comparison of methods for determination of microalbuminuria in diabetic patients. *Diabet Med.* 1989;6:412-415.

158. Bangstad H, Try K, Dahl-Jørgensen K, et al. New semiquantitative dipstick test for microalbuminuria. *Diabetes Care.* 1991;14:1094-1097.

159. Marshall S, Schearing PA, Alberti KG. Micral-test strips evaluated for screening for albuminuria. *Clin Chem.* 1992;38:588-591.

160. Poulsen P, Hansen B, Amby T, et al. Evaluation of a dipstick test for microalbuminuria in three different clinical settings, including the correlation with urinary albumin excretion rate. *Diabetes Metab.* 1992;18:395-400.

161. Schaufelberger H, Caduff F, Engler H, et al. Evaluation eines Streifentests (Micral-TestR) zur semiquantitativen Erfassung der mikroalbinurie in der Praxis. *Schweiz Med Wochenschr.* 1992;122:576-581.

162. Schwab S, Dunn FL, Feinglos MN. Screening for microalbuminuria. *Diabetes Care.* 1992;15:1581-1584.

163. Tai J, Tze WJ. Evaluation of Micro-Bumintest reagent tablets for screening of microalbuminuria. *Diabetes Res Clin Pract.* 1990;9:137-142.

164. Mogensen C, Viberti GC, Peheim E, et al. Multicenter evaluation of the Micral-Test II test strip, an immunologic rapid test for the detection of microalbuminuria. *Diabetes Care.* 1997;20:1642-1646.

165. Minetti E, Cozzi MG, Granata S, et al. Accuracy of the urinary albumin titrator stick "Micral-Test" in kidney-disease patients. *Nephrol Dial Transplant.* 1997;12:78-80.

166. Gross J, de Azevedo MJ, Silveiro SP, et al. Diabetic nephropathy: diagnosis, prevention, and treatment. *Diabetes Care.* 2005;28:164-176.

167. Molitch M, Defronzo RA, Franz MJ, et al. Nephropathy in diabetes. *Diabetes Care.* 2004;27(suppl 1):S79-S83.

168. Schwab S, Christensen L, Dougherty K, et al. Quantitation of proteinuria by the use of protein-to-creatinine ratios in single urine samples. *Arch Intern Med.* 1987;147:934-943.

169. Cohen D, Close CF, Viberti GC. The variability of overnight urinary albumin excretion in insulin-dependent diabetic and normal subjects. *Diabet Med.* 1987;4:437-440.

170. Gatling W, Knight C, Hill RD. Screening for early diabetic nephropathy: which sample to detect microalbuminuria? *Diabet Med.* 1985;2:451-455.

171. Hutchison A, O'Reilly DS, MacCuish AC. Albumin excretion rate, albumin concentration, and albumin creatinine ratio compared for screening diabetics for slight albuminuria. *Clin Chem.* 1988;34:2019-2021.

172. Marshall S, Alberti KGMM. Screening for early diabetic nephropathy. *Ann Clin Biochem.* 1986;23:195-197.

173. Sessoms S, Mehta K, Kovarsky J. Quantitation of proteinuria in systemic lupus erythematosus by use of a random, spot urine collection. *Arthritis Rheum.* 1983;26:918-920.

174. Ruggenenti P, Gaspari F, Perna A, et al. Cross-sectional longitudinal study of spot morning urine protein:creatinine ratio, 24-hour urine protein excretion rate, glomerular filtration rate, and end-stage renal failure in chronic renal disease in patients without diabetes. *BMJ.* 1998;316:504-509.

175. Torng S, Rigatto C, Rush DN, et al. The urine protein to creatinine ratio (P/C) as a predictor of 24-hour urine protein excretion in renal transplant patients. *Transplantation.* 2001;72:1453-1456.

176. Ramos J, Martins-Costa SH, Mathias MM, et al. Urinary protein/creatinine ratio in hypertensive pregnant women. *Hypertens Pregnancy.* 1999;18:209-218.

177. Rodriguez-Thompson D, Lieberman ES. Use of a random urinary protein-to-creatinine ratio for the diagnosis of significant proteinuria during pregnancy. *Am J Obstet Gynecol.* 2001;185:808-811.

178. Al R, Baykal C, Karacay O, et al. Random urine protein-creatinine ratio to predict proteinuria in new-onset mild hypertension in late pregnancy. *Obstet Gynecol.* 2004;104:367-371.

179. Durnwald C, Mercer B. A prospective comparison of total protein/creatinine ratio versus 24-hour urine protein in women with suspected preeclampsia. *Am J Obstet Gynecol.* 2003;189:848-852.

180. Neithardt A, Dooley SL, Borensztajn J. Prediction of 24-hour protein excretion in pregnancy with a single voided urine protein-to-creatinine ratio. *Am J Obstet Gynecol.* 2002:883-886.

181. Zuppi C, Baroni S, Scribano D, et al. Choice of time for urine collection for detecting early kidney abnormalities in hypertensives. *Ann Clin Biochem.* 1995;32:373-378.

182. Hara F, Nakazato K, Shiba K, et al. Studies of diabetic nephropathy. I. Effects of storage time and temperature on microalbuminuria. *Biol Pharm Bull.* 1994;17:1241-1245.

183. Watts G, Pillay D. Effect of ketones and glucose on the estimation of urinary creatinine: implications for microalbuminuria screening. *Diabet Med.* 1990;7:263-265.

184. Mattix H, Hsu CY, Shaykevich S, et al. Use of the albumin/creatinine ratio to detect microalbuminuria: implications of sex and race. *J Am Soc Nephrol.* 2002;13:1034-1039.

184a. National Kidney Disease Education Program: Laboratory professionals: urine albumin standardization. Available at: http://www.nkdep.nih.gov/labprofessionals/urine_albumin_standardization.htm. Accessed January 27, 2010.

185. Weber M. Urinary protein analysis. *J Chromatogr.* 1988;429:315-344.

186. Viberti G, Jarrett RJ, Mahmud U, et al. Microalbuminuria as a predictor of clinical nephropathy in insulin-dependent diabetes mellitus. *Lancet.* 1982;1:1430-1431.

187. Messent J, Elliott TG, Hill RD, et al. Prognostic significance of microalbuminuria in insulin-dependent diabetes mellitus: a twenty-three year follow-up study. *Kidney Int.* 1992;41:836-839.

188. Jarrett R, Viberti CG, Argyropoulos A, et al. Microalbuminuria predicts mortality in non–insulin-dependent diabetes. *Diabet Med.* 1984;1:17-19.

189. Mattock M, Morrish NJ, Viberti G, et al. Prospective study of microalbuminuria as predictor of mortality in NIDDM. *Diabetes Care.* 1992;41:736-741.

190. Mogensen C. Microalbuminuria predicts clinical proteinuria and early mortality in maturity-onset diabetes. *N Engl J Med.* 1984;310:356-360.

191. Mogensen C, Christensen CK. Predicting diabetic nephropathy in insulin-dependent patients. *N Engl J Med.* 1984;311:89-93.

192. Borch-Johnsen K, Wenzel H, Viberti GC, et al. Is screening and intervention for microalbuminuria worthwhile in patients with insulin dependent diabetes? *Br Med J.* 1993;306:1722-1725.

193. Nelson R, Knowler WC, Pettitt DJ, et al. Assessment of risk of overt nephropathy in diabetic patients from albumin excretion in untimed urine specimens. *Arch Intern Med.* 1991;151:1761-1765.

194. Caramori M, Fioretto P, Mauer M. Low glomerular filtration rate in normoalbuminuric type 1 diabetic patients: an indicator of more advanced glomerular lesions. *Diabetes.* 2003;52:1036-1040.

195. MacIsaac R, Tsalamandris C, Panagiotopoulos S, et al. Nonalbuminuric renal insufficiency in type 2 diabetes. *Diabetes Care.* 2004;27:195-200.

196. Boulware L, Jaar BG, Tarver-Carr ME, et al. Screening for proteinuria in US adults: a cost-effectiveness analysis. *JAMA.* 2003;290:3101-3114.

197. Robinson R. Nephrology forum: isolated proteinuria in asymptomatic patients. *Kidney Int.* 1980;18:395-406.

198. Robinson R. Isolated proteinuria. *Contrib Nephrol.* 1981;24:53-62.

199. von Bonsdorff M, Koskenvuo K, Salmi HA, et al. Prevalence and causes of proteinuria in 20-year-old Finnish men. *Scand J Urol Nephrol.* 1981;15:285-290.

200. Springberg P, Garrett Jr LE, Thompson Jr AL, et al. Fixed and reproducible orthostatic proteinuria: results of a 20-year follow-up. *Ann Intern Med.* 1982;97:516-519.

201. Rytand D, Spreiter S. Prognosis in postural (orthostatic) proteinuria. *N Engl J Med.* 1981;305:618-621.

202. Houser M. Characterization of recumbent, ambulatory, and postexercise proteinuria in the adolescent. *Pediatr Res.* 1987;21:442-446.

203. Buxbaum J, Chuba JV, Hellman GC, et al. Monoclonal immunoglobulin deposition disease: light chain and light and heavy chain deposition diseases and their relation to light chain amyloidosis. *Ann Intern Med.* 1990;112:455-464.

204. Hunt L, Short CD, Mallick NP. Prognostic indicators in patients presenting with the nephrotic syndrome. *Kidney Int.* 1988;34:382-388.

205. Williams P, Fass G, Bone JM. Renal pathology and proteinuria determine progression in untreated mild/moderate chronic renal failure. *Q J Med.* 1988;67:343-354.

206. D'Amico G. Influence of clinical and histological features on actuarial renal survival in adult patients with idiopathic IgA nephropathy, membranous nephropathy, and membranoproliferative glomerulonephritis: survey of the recent literature. *Am J Kidney Dis.* 1992;20:315-323.

207. Brahm M, Brammer M, Balsløv JT, et al. Prognosis in glomerulonephritis. III. A longitudinal analysis of changes in serum creatinine and proteinuria during the course of disease: effect of immunosuppressive treatment. Report from Copenhagen Study Group of Renal Diseases. *J Intern Med.* 1992;231:339-347.

208. Ritchie C, Bevan EA, Collier SJ. Importance of occult haematuria found at screening. *BMJ.* 1986;292:681-683.

209. Thompson I. The evaluation of microscopic hematuria: a population-based study. *J Urol.* 1987;138:1189-1190.

210. Messing E, Vaillancourt A. Hematuria screening for bladder cancer. *J Occup Med.* 1990;32:838-845.

211. Lieu T, Grasmeder III HM, Kaplan BS. An approach to the evaluation and treatment of microscopic hematuria. *Pediatr Clin North Am.* 1991;38: 579-592.

212. Fairley K, Birch DF. Hematuria: a simple method for identifying glomerular bleeding. *Kidney Int.* 1982;21:105-108.

213. Fassett R, Horgan BA, Mathew TH. Detection of glomerular bleeding by phase contrast microscopy. *Lancet.* 1982;1:1432-1434.

214. Van Iseghem P, Hauglastaine D, Bollens W, et al. Urinary erythrocyte morphology in acute glomerulonephritis. *BMJ.* 1983;287:1183.

215. Goldwasser P, Antignani A, Mittman N, et al. Urinary red cell size: diagnostic value and determinants. *Am J Nephrol.* 1990,10:148-156.

216. Shichiri M, Nishio Y, Suenaga M, et al. Red-cell volume distribution curves in diagnosis of glomerular and non-glomerular haematuria. *Lancet.* 1988;1:908-911.

217. Schramek P, Moritsch A, Haschkowitz H, et al. in vitro generation of dysmorphic erythrocytes. *Kidney Int.* 1989;36:72-77.

218. Marcussen N, Schumann JL, Schumann GB, et al. Analysis of cytodiagnostic urinalysis findings in 77 patients with concurrent renal biopsies. *Am J Kidney Dis.* 1992;20:618-628.

219. Raman G, Pead L, Lee HA, et al. A blind controlled trial of phase-contrast microscopy by two observers for evaluating the source of hematuria. *Nephron.* 1986;44:304-308.

220. Sayer J, McCarthy MP, Schmidt JD. Identification and significance of dysmorphic versus isomorphic hematuria. *J Urol.* 1990;143:545-548.

221. Thal S, DeBellis CC, Iverson SA, et al. Comparison of dysmorphic erythrocytes with other urinary sediment parameters of renal bleeding. *Am J Clin Pathol.* 1986;86:784-787.

222. Apeland T. Flow cytometry of urinary erythrocytes for evaluating the source of haematuria. *Scand J Urol Nephrol.* 1995;29:33-37.

223. Hyodo T, Kumano K, Haga M, et al. Analysis of urinary red blood cells of healthy individuals by an automated urinary flow cytometer. *Nephron.* 1997;75:451-457.

224. Lettgen B, Hestermann C, Rascher W. Differentiation of glomerular and non-glomerular hematuria in children by measurement of mean corpuscular volume of urinary red cells using a semi-automated cell counter. *Acta Paediatr.* 1994;83:946-949.

225. Offringa M, Benbassat J. The value of urinary red cell shape in the diagnosis of glomerular and post-glomerular haematuria. A meta-analysis. *Postgrad Med J.* 1992;68:648-654.

226. Shaper K, Jackson JE, Williams G. The nutcracker syndrome: an uncommon cause of haematuria. *Br J Urol.* 1994;74:144-146.

227. Tanaka H, Kim S-T, Takasugi M, et al. Isolated hematuria in adults: IgA nephropathy is a predominant cause of hematuria compared with thin glomerular basement membrane nephropathy. *Am J Nephrol.* 1996;16: 412-416.

228. Fogazzi G, Leong SO, Cameron JS. Don't forget sickled cells in the urine when investigating a patient for haematuria. *Nephrol Dial Transplant.* 1996;11:723-725.

229. Sobh M, Moustafa FE, el-Din Saleh MA, et al. Study of asymptomatic microscopic hematuria in potential living related kidney donors. *Nephron.* 1993;65:190-195.

230. Jacobs D, De Mott WR, Willie GR. Urinalysis and clinical microscopy. In: Jacobs D, Kasten BL, De Mott WR, et al. eds. *Laboratory test handbook.* Baltimore: Williams & Wilkins; 1990:903-904.

231. Corwin H, Bray RA, Haber MH. The detection and interpretation of urinary eosinophils. *Arch Pathol Lab Med.* 1989;113:1256-1258.

232. Corwin H, Korbet SM, Schwartz MM. Clinical correlates of eosinophiluria. *Arch Intern Med.* 1985;145:1097-1099.

233. Jacobs D, De Mott WR, Willie GR. Urinalysis and clinical microscopy. In: Jacobs D, Kasten BL, De Mott WR, et al. eds. *Laboratory test handbook.* Baltimore: Williams & Wilkins; 1990:938.

234. National Kidney Disease Education Program: Laboratory professionals: pharmacists and authorized drug prescribers: creatinine standardization recommendations. Available at: http://www.nkdep.nih.gov/labprofessionals/ Pharmacists_and_Authorized_Drug_Prescribers.htm. Accessed January 27, 2010.

Interpretation of Electrolyte and Acid-Base Parameters in Blood and Urine

Kamel S. Kamel, Mogamat R. Davids, Shih-Hua Lin, and Mitchell L. Halperin

An analysis of laboratory data from samples of blood and urine is essential to make accurate diagnoses and to design optimal therapy for patients with disturbances of water, sodium (Na^+), potassium (K^+), and acid-base homeostasis.[1,2] The clinical approach and interpretation of these tests relies heavily on an understanding of concepts in renal physiology and on an integration of this information in a whole-body context. Hence each section in the chapter begins with a discussion of physiologic concepts that help to focus on the most important factors in the renal regulation of the homeostasis of the substances in question. This is followed by a discussion of the clinical tools, which employ the laboratory data to help determine the underlying pathophysiology of the disturbance. This information is then used to construct an approach to the evaluation of a patient with each of these disorders. At the end of each section, sample consults are presented succinctly to illustrate how this approach is used at the bedside.

Two principles must be emphasized. First, *there are no normal values for the urinary excretion of water and electrolytes*, because individuals in steady state excrete all ions that are consumed and not lost by nonrenal routes. The urine also contains the major nitrogenous metabolic waste, urea—the rate of excretion of which depends largely on protein intake in steady state. Second, *data should be interpreted by considering the prevailing stimulus and the "expected" renal response*. In this context, urine provided over short periods of time is more valuable than 24-hour urine collections, because the former more closely reflects the renal response to the stimulus present over a certain period of time.

Water and Sodium

This section illustrates how information about the composition and volume of the urine is used in the differential diagnosis and treatment of disorders causing polyuria and of those causing an abnormal intracellular fluid (ICF) volume and/or abnormal extracellular fluid (ECF) volume.

Polyuria

There are two definitions of polyuria:

Conventional definition: Polyuria is defined as a urine volume that is more than 2.5 L/day, but this is an arbitrary value based on a comparison to the usual 24-hour urine volume values observed in individuals who consume a typical Western diet.

Physiology-based definition: Polyuria is defined as a urine volume that is *higher than expected* in a specific setting (e.g., a patient with cirrhosis of the liver who consumes a diet containing little NaCl and protein; polyuria may be present if the urine volume is considerably less than 2.5 L/day).

Classification

There are two categories to consider: water diuresis and osmotic diuresis. Nevertheless, if one uses the physiology-based definition, polyuria is not possible by this definition if the P_{Na} is less than 136 mmol/L, because the urine flow rate cannot exceed its maximum value. Stated another way, there can only be the expected high urine flow rate in this setting.[3] A urine flow rate less than the expected value would be considered *oliguria*, even if the urine volume is greater than 2.5 L/day.

Water Diuresis

Concept 1

To move water across a membrane, there must be a channel that allows water to cross that membrane (an aquaporin) and a driving force for the movement of water (a difference in concentration of effective osmoles or a difference in hydrostatic pressure across that membrane).

Water Channels

There are two critically important aquaporin water channels in the luminal membranes of cells in the kidney, AQP1 and AQP2. AQP1 channels are nonregulated water channels that are present in tubules before the loop of Henle (what we call the *first functional nephron unit* involved in the control of water excretion).[3] AQP1 channels are also present in the descending thin limbs of the loop of Henle of juxtamedullary nephrons[4] (Figure 26-1). There are no AQP1 channels throughout the descending thin limbs of superficial nephrons (which constitute approximately 85% of the total[4]), in the medullary thick ascending limbs of the loop of Henle, or in the cortical distal nephron segments before the late distal convoluted tubule (what we call the *middle functional nephron unit* involved in the control of water excretion).[3]

Vasopressin is released when the concentration of Na^+ in plasma, or P_{Na}, is higher than 136 mmol/L. This hormone causes the insertion of AQP2 into the luminal membrane of principal cells in the late cortical distal nephron and the medullary collecting duct (MCD) (what we call the *third functional nephron unit* involved in the control of water excretion). AQP2 permits water to be reabsorbed when there is an osmotic driving force.[5] During a maximum water diuresis, AQP2 must be absent in the luminal membrane of principal cells in the final functional nephron unit. Notwithstanding, even in the absence of vasopressin, there is a small degree of water permeability in the inner medullary collecting duct (iMCD), called *basal* or *residual water permeability*.[6]

Driving Force

Water will be drawn from a compartment with a lower effective osmolality to one with a higher effective osmolality. The magnitude of the force is enormous (approximately 19.3 mm Hg when there is a difference of 1 mOsm/kg H_2O). Since the osmolality of fluid that reaches the late cortical distal nephron segments is close to 100 mOsm/L and since AQP2 are present in the luminal membranes of its cells when vasopressin acts, water is reabsorbed because the osmotic pressure difference is approximately 200 mOsm/L (interstitial osmolality equals the plasma osmolality, or P_{osm}, which is approximately 300 mOsm/L for easy math). Hence the osmotic driving force is almost 4000 mm Hg (19.3 mm Hg × 200 mOsm/L).

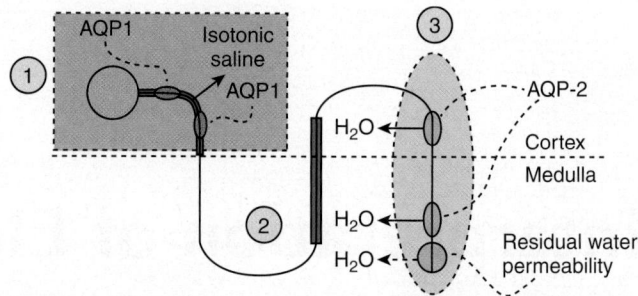

FIGURE 26-1 Functional units of the nephron based on the presence of aquaporin-1 (AQP1) or AQP2. The *stylized structure* represents a nephron; AQP1 is represented as an *oval with lighter shading* and AQP2 is represented as a *rectangle with darker shading*. The *thin line* represents the descending thin limbs of the loop of Henle (DtL). AQP1 is always present in luminal membranes in the initial functional nephron unit (shown within the *dashed rectangle*). Hence isotonic saline is reabsorbed in this unit and desalination does not occur. The second functional nephron unit of the majority of the nephrons lacks aquaporins AQP1 and AQP2 with one exception; the DtL of juxtamedullary nephrons always have AQP1, and reabsorption of Na^+ and Cl^- therefore occurs without water in all of the following nephron segments in this functional unit of the nephron, which includes the DtL of most of the nephrons in these superficial but not juxtamedullary nephrons, the medullary and cortical thick ascending limbs of the loop of Henle, and the early distal convoluted tubule (DCT). When there are no actions of vasopressin to insert AQP2 in the luminal membrane of the third functional unit of the nephron (i.e., the later DCT cortical and medullary collecting ducts) (inside the *dashed oval*), the luminal fluid is desalinated during a water diuresis. The inner medullary collecting duct (MCD) is always somewhat permeable to water (owing to residual or basal water permeability). Notwithstanding, reabsorption of water by this route is important only during water diuresis. Contraction of the renal pelvis augments reabsorption of water in the inner MCD, because it increases contact time and stirring.

Concept 2

The maximum volume of urine during water diuresis is equal to the volume of distal delivery of filtrate minus the volume of filtrate reabsorbed via residual water permeability in the IMCD:

Maximum urine flow rate during water diuresis =
Distal delivery of filtrate − Water reabsorbed via residual water permeability

The distal delivery of filtrate is equal to the glomerular filtration rate (GFR) minus the volume of filtrate reabsorbed in the initial functional nephron unit (i.e., largely the proximal convoluted tubule including its pars recta segment).

Distal delivery of filtrate = GFR − Water reabsorbed in the initial functional nephron unit

There is an enormous difference in osmotic pressure between the luminal and interstitial fluid compartments during water diuresis, which drives the reabsorption of water via residual water permeability in the iMCD.

Concept 3

There is a second component of the physiology of water diuresis, the "desalination" of luminal fluid in nephron segments that lack AQP1 and AQP2. This process occurs in the medullary thick ascending limb of the loop of Henle in the middle functional nephron unit and throughout the final functional nephron unit when vasopressin does not cause the insertion of AQP2.

Regulation of the reabsorption of Na^+ and Cl^- in the medullary thick ascending limb of the loop of Henle seems to be via dilution of the concentration of an inhibitor of this process in the medullary interstitial compartment (probably ionized calcium[7]) (Figure 26-2) by water reabsorption from the water-permeable nephron segments in the medulla (i.e., the MCD and the descending thin limbs of the loop of Henle of juxtamedullary nephrons). Thus, water reabsorption via residual water permeability during water diuresis may serve the function of diluting the concentration of this inhibitor to allow for this process of desalination to occur. Desalination of luminal fluid in the third functional unit is augmented by flow activation of the epithelial sodium channel (ENaC), which stimulates the reabsorption of Na^+ in this location.[8]

Concept 4

Since, in most clinical circumstances, there is no change in the number of osmoles in the ICF compartment, the volume of the ICF compartment is indirectly proportional to the P_{Na}.

When the P_{Na} rises, cell volume decreases. This is most important clinically for the brain, because part of its blood supply comes from blood vessels attached to the skull, and a hemorrhage into the brain owing to stretching and possibly rupture of these blood vessels may occur when the brain volume shrinks. When the P_{Na} falls, the volume of cells increases. This again is most important for brain cells, because the rigid skull ultimately increases intracranial pressure.

Tools

Urine Flow Rate

In individuals consuming a typical Western diet, the peak urine flow rate during a water diuresis is 10 to 15 mL/min (approximately 14 to 21 L/day). If the daily urine volume is considerably below 10 L, a reason should be sought for a low distal delivery of filtrate. Notwithstanding, the distal delivery of filtrate will fall ultimately as the effective circulating volume declines, and this high urine flow rate is not likely to be sustained.

The urine flow rate declines when desmopressin (dDAVP) is given to a patient with central diabetes insipidus. However, the urine flow rate in such a patient is still higher than that in a normal individual who consumes a typical Western diet if the osmole excretion rate is high (e.g., owing to infusions of large volumes of saline) and because the medullary interstitial osmolality is likely to be lower because of a prior washout during the water diuresis.[9]

Osmole Excretion Rate

The osmole excretion rate is equal to the product of the urine osmolality (U_{osm}) and the urine flow rate:

$$\text{Osmole excretion rate} = U_{osm} \times \text{Urine flow rate}$$

In individuals eating a typical Western diet, this excretion rate is 600 to 900 mOsm/day, with electrolytes and urea each accounting for close to half of the urine osmoles. In the absence of AQP2, a change in the rate of excretion of osmoles does *not* directly affect the urine volume; rather, there is a difference in the U_{osm}. Nevertheless, the rate of excretion of

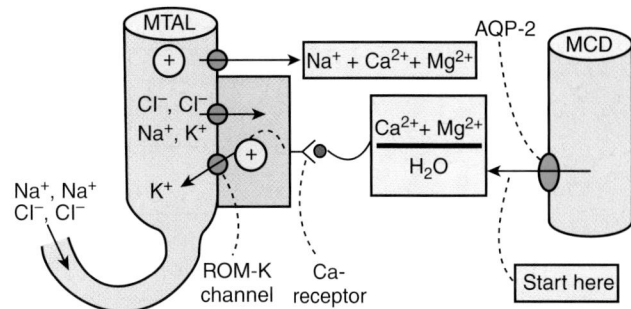

FIGURE 26-2 Regulation of the concentrating process in the renal medulla by the concentration of ionized calcium in the medullary interstitial compartment. To reabsorb Na^+ and Cl^- in the medullary thick ascending limb of the loop of Henle (mTAL), K^+ must enter its lumen via the rat outer medullary potassium (ROMK) channel to be a substrate for the Na^+-K^+-$2Cl^-$ cotransporter and to create the lumen-positive voltage that drives the passive reabsorption of Na^+, Mg^{2+}, and Ca^{2+} via the paracellular pathway. Once the activities of Mg^{2+} and Ca^{2+} rise sufficiently in the medullary interstitial compartment, a signal is generated to inhibit flux of K^+ through luminal ROMK and hence the further reabsorption of Na^+ + Cl^- in this nephron unit. When water is reabsorbed from the medullary collecting duct (MCD), the concentration of ionized Ca^{2+} in the medullary interstitial compartment falls. Thus more Na^+ and Cl^- (and also Ca^{2+} and Mg^{2+}) are reabsorbed until the sum of the activities of Ca^{2+} and Mg^{2+} rises sufficiently in the medullary interstitial compartment to complete this cycle of inhibitory control.

osmoles must be calculated in patients with a water diuresis, because it will affect the urine flow rate if dDAVP is administered and there is a renal response to its actions.

Urine Osmolality

The U_{osm} is equal to the number of excreted osmoles divided by the urine volume. Therefore during water diuresis, a change in the U_{osm} could reflect a change in the osmole excretion rate and/or in the volume of filtrate delivered to the late distal nephron (which largely determines the urine volume in this setting). For example, if the rate of excretion of osmoles is 800 mOsm/day, the U_{osm} will be 50 mOsm/L when the 24-hour urine volume is 16 L/day and 100 mOsm/L when the 24-hour urine volume is 8 L. A note of caution is needed: a rise in the U_{osm} following the administration of dDAVP may reflect a fall in the distal delivery of filtrate owing to a fall in blood pressure and the GFR rather than a renal response to the actions of dDAVP.[10]

Tonicity Balance

To decide what the basis is for a change in the P_{Na} and to define the proper therapy to return the volume and composition of the ECF and ICF compartments to their normal values, separate balances for water and Na^+ must be calculated.[11] To calculate tonicity balance, the input and output volumes and the quantity of Na^+ and K^+ infused and excreted over the period when the P_{Na} changed must be examined (Figure 26-3). In practical terms, tonicity balance can be determined only in a hospital setting where inputs and outputs are accurately recorded. With regard to the output, this can be restricted to the urine in an acute setting. In a febrile patient, balance calculations will not be as accurate because sweat losses are not measured. If the volume of the urine and the volume of the Na^+ plus K^+ in the fluid infused are known, the clinician can calculate the quantity of Na^+ plus K^+ in the urine and determine why the P_{Na} changed over that time.[11]

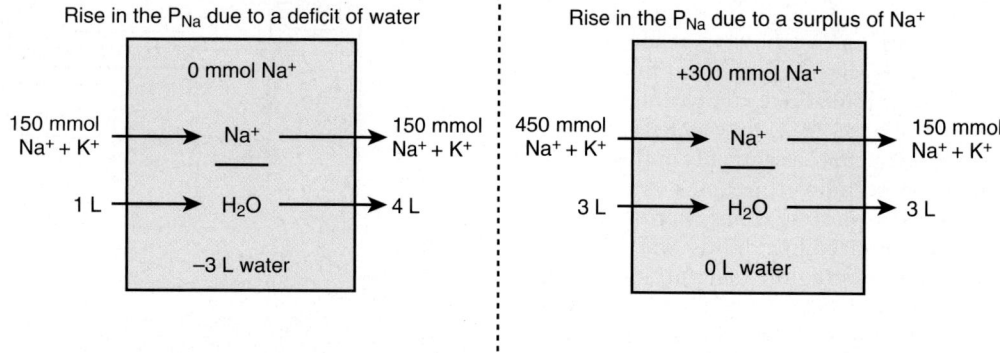

FIGURE 26-3 Tonicity balance to determine the basis for a rise in the plasma concentration of Na^+ (P_{Na}). To determine the tonicity balance, the input and output volumes and the quantity of Na^+ and K^+ infused and excreted in the urine are required. Two examples of an acute rise in the P_{Na} from 140 mmol/L to 150 mmol/L are shown. In the example in the left portion of the figure, there is a negative balance of 3 L of water. In contrast, in the example in the right portion of the figure, the rise in the P_{Na} is due to a positive balance of 300 mmol of Na^+. Note that if one were to calculate electrolyte-free water balance in each example, there would be a deficit of 3 L of electrolyte-free water in the example on the left and of 2 L of electrolyte-free water in the example on the right, because there is a net gain of 300 mmol of Na^+ without water.

CALCULATION OF ELECTROLYTE-FREE WATER BALANCE

To calculate electrolyte-free water balance, one must know the volume and concentrations of $Na^+ + K^+$ in the input and the urine. The first step is to decide how much water is needed to make all of the $Na^+ + K^+$ into an isotonic saline solution (e.g., 150 mmol in 1 L of water in molal terms if the P_{osm} is within the normal range). If the concentration of $Na^+ + K^+$ in a urine sample is lower than that in plasma, the remainder of the volume is called *electrolyte-free water*. Alternatively, had there been residual $Na^+ + K^+$, the excretion of the remaining electrolytes is given the very confusing name of *negative* electrolyte-free water. As shown in Table 26-1, an electrolyte-free water balance cannot distinguish between negative balances of water and positive balances for Na^+ as the cause of the rise in the P_{Na}. Accordingly, the authors do not use the calculation of electrolyte-free water balance, because although it correctly predicts the change in P_{Na}, it does not reveal its basis and hence it is not helpful in the design of therapy to return the volume and composition of the ECF and ICF compartments to their normal values.

Clinical Approach to the Patient with Water Diuresis

The steps to take to determine the diagnosis are outlined in Flow Chart 26-1.

STEP 1. APPLY THE CONCEPTS OF THE CONTROL OF THE URINE FLOW RATE

A large water diuresis is the expected physiologic response to a water intake that is large enough to cause the arterial P_{Na} to fall below 136 mmol/L. In this case, the diagnosis is primary polydipsia. Once the P_{Na} has returned to the normal range, the urine flow rate should decrease and the U_{osm} should rise appropriately, although it should be kept in mind that the prior water diuresis may have caused a lower medullary interstitial osmolality due to medullary washout. In contrast, diabetes insipidus is present when there is a water diuresis and the P_{Na} is higher than 140 mmol/L. This disorder could be because of a lesion in the hypothalamic–posterior pituitary axis that controls the production and/or release of vasopressin (central diabetes insipidus), a circulating vasopressinase, or a renal lesion that prevents vasopressin from

TABLE 26-1 Comparison of Tonicity Balance and Electrolyte-Free Water Balance in a Patient with Hypernatremia

	$NA^+ + K^+$ (mmol)	WATER (L)	ELECTROLYTE-FREE WATER (L)
Infusion of 3 L of isotonic saline			
Input	450	3	0
Output	150	3	2
Balance	**+300**	**0**	**–2**
Infusion of 4 L of isotonic saline			
Input	600	4	0
Output	150	3	2
Balance	**+450**	**+1**	**–2**
No intravenous fluid infusion			
Input	0	0	0
Output	150	3	2
Balance	**–150**	**–3**	**–2**

Three situations are illustrated in which the plasma Na^+ concentration rises from 140 to 150 mmol/L. The only difference is the volume of isotonic saline infused in each setting. In all three examples, there is a negative balance of 2 L of electrolyte-free water. Notwithstanding, the balances for Na^+ and for water are very different in these three examples. Accordingly, the goals for therapy to correct the hypernatremia and to return the volume and composition of the extracellular and intracellular fluid compartments to their normal values are different and become clear only after a tonicity balance is calculated.

causing the insertion of AQP2 in the luminal membrane of principal cells in the final functional unit of the nephron (see Figure 26-1).

Calculate the osmole excretion rate (see the equation in the "Osmole Excretion Rate" section earlier). The usual value is close to 0.5 mOsm/min in individuals consuming a typical Western diet. If the osmole excretion rate is appreciably higher, be careful, because an osmotic diuresis will ensue if the patient has a renal response to the administration of vasopressin or its dDAVP analog. This may lead to significant changes in the P_{Na} and hence brain cell volume depending on the concentrations of Na^+ and K^+ in the urine and the tonicity of administered fluids.

Examine the central water control system (Figure 26-4) for a lesion that has caused the defect in vasopressin biosynthesis or release. An important part of this workup is to determine

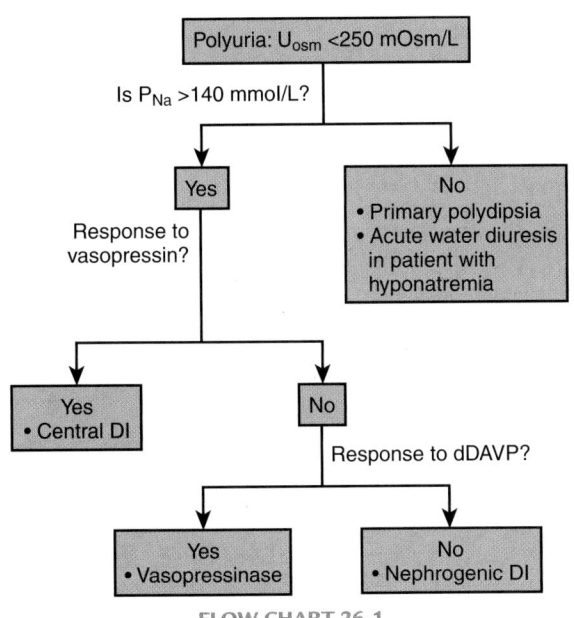

FLOW CHART 26-1

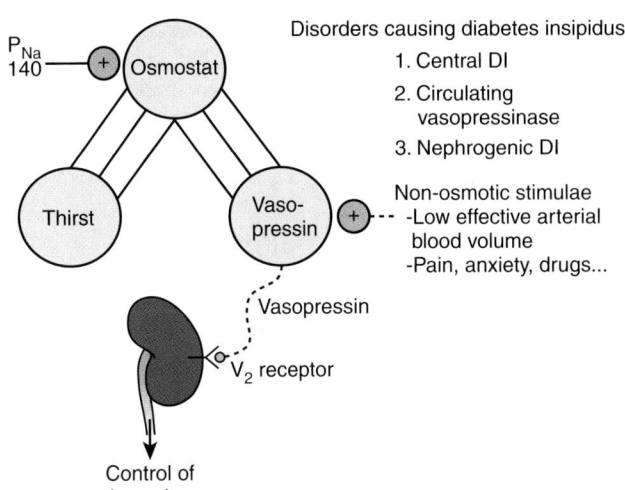

FIGURE 26-4 Water control system. The primary sensor is the osmostat (*top circle*), which detects a change in the plasma concentration of Na^+ (P_{Na}) via an effect on the volume of its cells. The osmostat is linked to the thirst center (*lower left circle*) and to the vasopressin release center (*lower right circle*). Nonosmotic stimuli (e.g., nausea, pain, anxiety) also influence the release of vasopressin. Vasopressin release is stimulated when there is a large decrease in the effective arterial blood volume; a lower P_{Na} is needed to suppress the release of vasopressin in this setting. When vasopressin acts, the urine flow rate is directly proportional to the number of effective osmoles that are excreted and indirectly proportional to the effective osmolality in the inner medullary interstitial compartment. The clinical disorders associated with a large excretion of electrolyte-free water (i.e., diabetes insipidus [DI]) and the sites of these lesions are listed on the right.

whether thirst is present; its absence suggests that the defect involves the hypothalamic osmostat.

STEP 2. EXAMINE THE RENAL RESPONSE TO VASOPRESSIN OR dDAVP

If the water diuresis is curtailed by the administration of dDAVP, the diagnosis is central diabetes insipidus or the release of an enzyme that hydrolyzes vasopressin in plasma (vasopressinase). If there is a reason to suspect the latter, examine the response to the administration of vasopressin after the actions of dDAVP have worn off and the patient is experiencing a water diuresis again. Although there was a response to dDAVP, the patient will not respond to administration of the usual dose of vasopressin.

STEP 3. ESTABLISH THE BASIS FOR NEPHROGENIC DIABETES INSIPIDUS

If dDAVP fails to cause the appropriate decrease in urine flow rate (depending on the rate of excretion of osmoles) and the appropriate rise in U_{osm} (depending on the value of medullary interstitial osmolality, which is usually lower from prior water diuresis), the diagnosis is an AQP2 deficiency type of nephrogenic diabetes insipidus. Hereditary nephrogenic diabetes insipidus could be caused by an X-linked recessive type 2 vasopressin receptor (V_2) mutation (more common) or an autosomal recessive or dominant AQP2 mutation. Among the acquired disorders, the most common cause of nephrogenic diabetes insipidus in an adult is the use of lithium to treat a bipolar affective disorder.

Consult 1: Does This Patient Have Polyuria?

A 22-year-old woman lives in a hot climate. She is concerned about her body image and runs several miles a day. To avoid "dehydration," she forces herself to drink large volumes of water. She is health conscious and consumes a low-salt, low-protein diet. She sought medical advice because she wakes up two or three times every night to urinate, passing large volumes in each voiding. On the past two visits, her laboratory results were very similar; her P_{Na} was 130 mmol/L, the 24-hour urine volume was 5 L/day, and the U_{osm} was 80 mOsm/kg H_2O.

Questions

Does this patient have polyuria?
What risks related to her P_{Na} value do you anticipate?

Discussion

DOES THIS PATIENT HAVE POLYURIA?

According to the conventional definition, polyuria is present in this patient. A water diuresis is present because the urine flow rate is 5 L/day and the U_{osm} is less than the P_{osm}. Because she has hyponatremia, polyuria is caused by primary polydipsia (see Flow Chart 26-1).

According to the physiology-based definition, the "expected" urine flow rate in a normal adult who lacks vasopressin actions (i.e., there is no stimulus for its release because the P_{Na} is 130 mmol/L) should be at least 10 mL/min or more than 14 L/day.[12] Hence a daily urine volume of 5 L in this setting is *low*; in fact, the patient has a diminished ability to excrete water. She has a low effective arterial blood volume because of ongoing losses of Na^+ and Cl^- in sweat and the low intake of salt (as can be deduced from her low osmole excretion rate, 80 mOsm/L × 5 L/day = 400 mOsm/day vs. the usual 600 to 900 mOsm/day). Because of a somewhat lower GFR and increased reabsorption of Na^+ in the initial functional unit of the nephron, she has a low distal delivery of filtrate.

The combination of this low distal delivery and the presence of residual water permeability in the iMCD leads to diminished ability to excrete water, even in the absence of detectable levels of vasopressin in plasma.[6] Hyponatremia will develop if her water intake exceeds her urine volume and the volume lost.[13]

WHAT RISKS RELATED TO HER P_{Na} VALUE DO YOU ANTICIPATE?

Since this is a chronic condition, she should be in balance, which means that her water intake equals her water loss. Her P_{Na} will fluctuate, however, because her intake of water and electrolytes is not likely to be constant throughout the day or from day to day. One route for water loss is her urine (5 L/day); she also has a large loss of water in sweat (volume is not known, perhaps 1 L/hr during vigorous exercise in a hot environment). Hence she has a daily intake and loss of many liters of water.

Herniation of the Brain. With such a large throughput of water, the patient could easily develop a large *positive* balance of water, which will cause acute hyponatremia and lead to brain cell swelling and a rise in intracranial pressure. There are three possible causes of this large positive balance of water: First, she may drink too much water on a given day (note that her water intake is not driven by thirst). Second, she may lose less water in sweat (e.g., she may not run every day). Third, water excretion may decrease suddenly owing to a nonosmotic stimulus for the release of vasopressin (e.g., pain, nausea, anxiety, intake of drugs such as Ecstasy [3,4-methylenedioxymethamphetamine][14]).

Osmotic Demyelination. The complication of osmotic demyelination may develop if the patient has a large *negative* balance of water and, consequently, too rapid a rise in her P_{Na}, especially if she is malnourished and/or K^+ depleted, because patients with a poor dietary intake are at greater risk of developing osmotic demyelination.[15] Because her urine flow rate is determined by the rate of delivery of filtrate to the distal nephron, this delivery may increase if she were to have a high salt intake (e.g., pizza with anchovies) or if she were given a large infusion of saline.

Consult 2: What Is "Partial" about Partial Central Diabetes Insipidus?

A healthy 32-year-old man recently experienced a basal skull fracture. His urine output has been consistently about 4 L/day since his head injury. His U_{osm} was approximately 200 mOsm/kg H_2O in multiple 24-hour urine collections. In blood samples drawn early in the morning, his P_{Na} was approximately 143 mmol/L, and vasopressin was not detectable. During the daytime, his U_{osm} was consistently approximately 90 mOsm/kg H_2O and his P_{Na} was 137 mmol/L. When he was given dDAVP, his urine flow rate decreased to 0.5 mL/min and the U_{osm} rose to 900 mOsm/kg H_2O. Two other facts, however, merit emphasis. First, he is always thirsty in the morning when he wakes up. Second, his sleep is not interrupted by a need to void. In fact his U_{osm} was approximately 425 mOsm/kg H_2O in several overnight urine samples. Moreover, his urine flow rate fell to 0.5 mL/min and his U_{osm} rose to 900 mOsm/kg H_2O after an infusion of hypertonic saline.

Questions

Is this a water diuresis?
What are the best options for therapy?

Discussion

IS THIS A WATER DIURESIS?

Since the patient's U_{osm} was 200 mOsm/kg H_2O and the urine volume was 4 L/day, this was a water diuresis with a usual osmole excretion rate for a person consuming a typical Western diet (800 mOsm/day) (see Flow Chart 26-1). The patient had an adequate renal response to dDAVP because his U_{osm} rose to 900 mOsm/kg H_2O. Hence he has central diabetes insipidus. Because his urine volume was 4 L/day and not 10 to 15 L/day, the diagnosis was *partial* central diabetes insipidus.

Interpretation

Central Diabetes Insipidus. Although the diagnosis of partial central diabetes insipidus was straightforward, there were two facts that have not yet been interpreted. First, because the patient was thirsty, his "osmostat" and thirst center as well as the majority of fibers connecting them appear to be functionally intact (Figure 26-5). Similarly, because his U_{osm} was higher than his P_{osm} (his overnight U_{osm} was 425 mOsm/kg H_2O) when his P_{Na} was 143 mmol/L, his vasopressin release center seemed to function, but only when there was a strong stimulus for the release of this hormone. Therefore a possibility for his lesion is destruction of some but not all of the fibers linking the osmostat to the vasopressin release center (see Figure 26-5).[16] The higher P_{Na} could also explain why polyuria was *not* present overnight (he stopped his oral water intake several hours before going to sleep). This clarifies the diagnosis of partial central diabetes insipidus, or at least the concept of what that diagnosis really implies.

Primary Polydipsia. Because the patient's P_{Na} was high enough early in the morning to stimulate the release of vasopressin (143 mmol/L), primary polydipsia is not present at

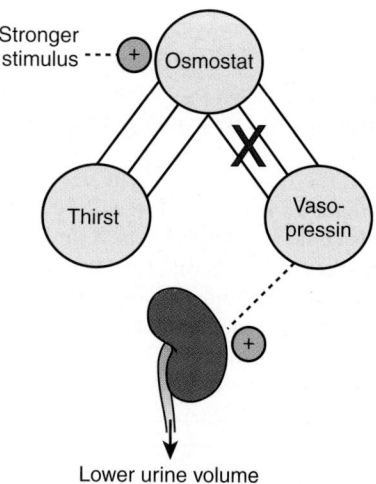

FIGURE 26-5 Lesion causing *partial* central diabetes insipidus in the patient described in Consult 2. The *upper circle* labeled "osmostat" is the sensor, the *lower left circle* is the thirst center, and the *lower right circle* is the vasopressin release center. The *X* symbol represents a hypothetical lesion due to a basal skull fracture that caused severing of some but not all of the fibers connecting the osmostat to the vasopressin release center.

this time. In contrast, during the daytime, his U_{osm} was consistently about 90 mOsm/kg H_2O and his P_{Na} was 137 mmol/L, which suggests that primary polydipsia is present while he is awake. It probably reflects a learned behavior to avoid the very uncomfortable feeling of thirst. This interpretation provides a rationale to understand the pathophysiology of and, importantly, the treatment options for his partial central diabetes insipidus.

WHAT ARE THE BEST OPTIONS FOR THERAPY?

The major point related to treatment options is that a higher P_{Na} can stimulate the release of vasopressin. There are two ways to raise the P_{Na}: induce a positive balance of Na^+ or induce a negative balance of water. The patient selected treatment with oral NaCl tablets to raise his P_{Na} and control his daytime polyuria because of their rapid and reproducible onset of action (Table 26-2). Moreover, this therapy avoids the risk of acute hyponatremia, which may occur if he were given dDAVP and he drank an excessive quantity of water. In contrast, to raise his P_{Na} overnight, the patient selected water deprivation to permit him to have undisturbed sleep, because he was able to tolerate the thirst that developed.

Consult 3: A Water Diuresis and an Osmotic Diuresis in the Same Patient

A craniopharyngioma was resected from a 16-year-old male (weight = 50 kg, total body water = 30 L). During neurosurgery, his urine flow rate rose to 10 mL/min (3 L in 300 min) and his P_{Na} rose from 140 to 150 mmol/L. During this period, he received of 3 L of isotonic saline. His U_{osm} was 120 mOsm/kg H_2O, and his urine Na^+ + K^+ concentration (U_{Na} + U_K) was 50 mmol/L. To confirm the diagnosis of central diabetes insipidus, he was given dDAVP, and his urine flow rate fell to 6 mL/min, his U_{osm} rose to 375 mOsm/kg H_2O, and the concentration of Na^+ plus K^+ in his urine rose to 175 mmol/L.

Questions

What is the *expected* renal response to dDAVP in this patient? Why did the patient's P_{Na} rise from 140 to 150 mmol/L during this large water diuresis?

TABLE 26-2 Options for Therapy for the Patient in Consult 2

OPTIONS	ADVANTAGES	DISADVANTAGES
1. Desmopressin (dDAVP)	Avoids thirst	Long duration of effect
	Rapid onset of effect	Acute hyponatremia if there is a large intake of water
		May downregulate V_2 receptors
2. Water restriction	Effect lasts until water intake	Thirst is present
	Conserves V_2 receptors	Slow onset of effect
3. Hypertonic NaCl	Rapid onset of effect	Thirst is present
	Conserves V_2 receptors	

Options 2 and 3 are designed to raise the plasma Na^+ concentration and thereby cause the release of endogenous vasopressin.
V_2, Vasopressin type 2 receptors.

Discussion

WHAT IS THE *EXPECTED* RENAL RESPONSE TO dDAVP IN THIS PATIENT?

The initial information available to assess the patient's response to dDAVP is his urine flow rate. When dDAVP acts, the urine flow rate is directly proportional to the osmole excretion rate and is inversely proportional to the medullary interstitial osmolality.

Osmole Excretion Rate. The osmole excretion rate before dDAVP was given is equal to the product of the U_{osm} (120 mOsm/kg H_2O) and urine flow rate (10 mL/min), or 1.2 mOsm/min; this is more than double the usual rate of 0.5 mOsm/min in individuals consuming a typical Western diet.

Urine Osmolality. It is important to recognize that because of a prior water diuresis, there will be a degree of washout of the patient's renal medulla. Hence the maximum U_{osm} in response to the administration of dDAVP will be significantly lower than that observed in normal subjects. In fact, the patient's U_{osm} was 375 mOsm/kg H_2O.

Nature of the Osmoles. Before the administration of dDAVP, five sixths of the osmoles in the urine were Na^+ plus K^+ salts: $2(U_{Na} + U_K) = 50$ mmol/L, U_{osm} 120 mOsm/kg H_2O). Because electrolytes are effective osmoles, whereas urea is not usually an effective osmole in the urine when vasopressin acts,[17,18] most of the osmoles in the patient's urine were effective osmoles, which will obligate the excretion of water after dDAVP acts. Based on all of these considerations, it is no surprise that the patient's urine flow rate was approximately 6 mL/min after administration of dDAVP. In fact, once the effect of the anesthetic agent, which diminished the tone of venous capacitance vessels, has disappeared, there may be an even higher effective osmole excretion rate—that is, a larger natriuresis driven by the higher central venous pressure.

WHY DID THE PATIENT'S P_{Na} RISE FROM 140 TO 150 mmol/L DURING THIS LARGE WATER DIURESIS?

Tonicity Balance. The patient received 3 L of water (as isotonic saline, but it is still 3 L of water in volume terms), and he excreted 3 L of urine (with a U_{Na} + U_K of 50 mmol/L, but it, too, is still water in volume terms). Accordingly, there is a zero balance of water.

Balance data for Na^+ plus K^+ reveal that the patient received 450 mmol (3 L × 150 mmol Na^+/L) and he excreted only 150 mmol (3 L × 50 mmol/ Na^+/L). Hence he has a positive balance of 300 mmol of Na^+ plus K^+. Dividing this surplus by the total body water (30 L) suggests that the rise in P_{Na} should be 10 mmol/L, a value equal to the actual rise in the P_{Na}. Therefore the basis for the rise in P_{Na} was a positive balance of Na^+ and not a deficit of water. The proper treatment to restore body tonicity and the volume and composition of the ECF and ICF compartments is to induce a negative balance of 300 mmol of Na^+ plus K^+.

Osmotic Diuresis

Concept 5

When AQP2 water channels are present in the luminal membrane of the late distal nephron, the U_{osm} should be equal to the medullary interstitial osmolality.

The volume of the urine during an osmotic diuresis is directly proportional to the rate of excretion of osmoles and indirectly proportional to the medullary interstitial osmolality.

Concept 6

Not all osmoles are equal in their ability to increase the urine volume.

The osmoles that cannot achieve equal concentrations in the lumen of the MCD and in the medullary interstitial compartment are called *effective osmoles;* they dictate what the urine flow rate will be when AQP2 channels are present in the luminal membranes of the principal cells in the MCD and thus are permeable to water.

Urea may be an *ineffective* urine osmole in some circumstances and an effective urine osmole in other circumstances. Because cells in the IMCD have urea transporters in their luminal membrane when vasopressin acts,[19] urea is usually an ineffective osmole (same concentration of urea on both sides of that membrane) and it does *not* cause water to be excreted.[17,18] The net result of excretion of some extra urea is a higher U_{osm} but not a higher effective U_{osm} or a higher urine flow rate.[18] Therefore, it is more correct to say that the urine flow rate is directly proportional to the number of nonurea or effective urine osmoles and inversely proportional to their concentration in the medullary interstitial compartment:

$$\text{Urine flow rate} = (\text{Effective urine osmoles}) / (\text{Effective } U_{osm})$$

In contrast, when the rate of excretion of urea rises by a large amount, urea might *not* be absorbed fast enough to achieve equal concentrations on both sides of a membrane. Hence, urea may become an effective osmole in the iMCD and obligate the excretion of water. The analysis is not always that simple, however, because urea is a partially effective urine osmole if the rate of excretion of electrolytes is low.[17,18]

Concept 7

The medullary interstitial osmolality falls during an osmotic diuresis because of medullary washout.

This washout occurs when a larger number of liters of water enter the medullary interstitial compartment from the MCD owing to the fact that more liters are delivered to the MCD. The expected medullary interstitial osmolality is approximately 600 mOsm/kg H_2O at somewhat high osmole excretion rates and reaches values closer to the P_{osm} at much higher osmole excretion rates.[20]

Tools

OSMOLE EXCRETION RATE

The osmole excretion rate should be much higher than 1000 mOsm/day (0.7 mOsm/min) in an adult during an osmotic diuresis (Flow Chart 26-2).

URINE OSMOLALITY

The U_{osm} should be higher than the P_{osm}. The absolute value for the U_{osm} depends on the osmole excretion rate and the urine flow rate.

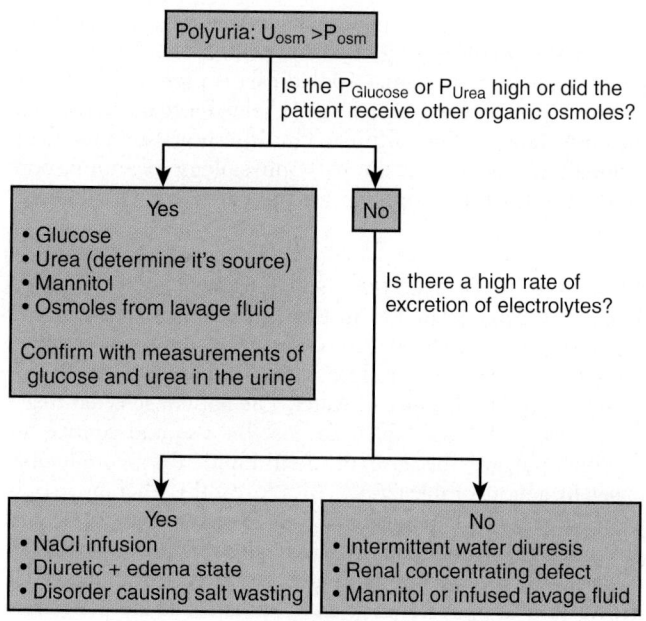

FLOW CHART 26-2

NATURE OF THE URINE OSMOLES

The nature of the urine osmoles should be determined by measuring the rate of excretion of the individual osmoles in the urine. As a quick test, however, which solute is likely to be responsible for the osmotic diuresis may be deduced by measuring the concentrations of the solutes in plasma (e.g., glucose and urea) and determining if mannitol or lavage fluid solutes were infused. Nevertheless, patients rarely are given a sufficiently large amount of mannitol for it to be the sole cause of a large and sustained osmotic diuresis. A saline-induced osmotic diuresis may occur if there was a large infusion of saline or in a patient who has cerebral or renal salt wasting. For a state of salt wasting to be diagnosed, there must be an appreciable excretion of Na^+ at a time when the effective circulating volume is *definitely* contracted.[21]

SOURCE OF THE URINE OSMOLES

In a patient with a glucose- or urea-induced osmotic diuresis, it is important to decide whether these osmoles were derived from an exogenous source or from catabolism of endogenous proteins.

Urea Appearance Rate. The rate of appearance of urea can be determined from the amount of urea that is retained in the body plus the amount excreted in the urine over a given period of time. The former can be calculated from the rise in the concentration of urea in plasma (P_{urea}) and the volume of distribution of urea (assumed to be equal to total body water; approximately 60% of body weight in the absence of obesity).

Source of Urea. Close to 16% of the weight of protein is nitrogen. Therefore if 100 g of protein were oxidized, 16 g of nitrogen would be formed. Since the molecular weight of nitrogen is 14, approximately 1140 mmol of nitrogen would be produced. Because urea contains two atoms of nitrogen, approximately 570 mmol of urea are produced from the oxidation of 100 g of protein. In terms of lean body mass, because water is its main constituent (80% of weight), each kilogram has 800 g of water and 180 g of protein.[22] Therefore, breakdown of 1 kg of lean mass will produce approximately

1000 mmol of urea. One can use this calculation to determine if the source of urea was exogenous or if the urea was produced by endogenous breakdown of protein.

Source of Glucose. If there is a large glucose-induced osmotic diuresis, the glucose will be from an exogenous source, such as the ingestion of fruit juice or sweetened soda pop.[23] The reason for this is that the production of glucose from endogenous sources is relatively small (i.e., to produce enough glucose from protein for 1 L of osmotic diuresis would require the catabolism of 90 g of protein, because 60% of the weight of protein can be converted to glucose; this is equivalent to the catabolism of 1 lb of lean body mass[22]).

Clinical Approach to the Patient with Osmotic Diuresis

The steps in the clinical approach to evaluation of the patient with osmotic diuresis are illustrated in Flow Chart 26-2.

STEP 1. CALCULATE THE OSMOLE EXCRETION RATE

If the U_{osm} is greater than the P_{osm} and the osmole excretion rate exceeds 1000 mOsm/day (0.7 mOsm/min), an osmotic diuresis is present. Make sure that the urine sample sent to the laboratory was not the last portion of urine collected over a long period.

STEP 2. DEFINE THE NATURE OF THE EXCRETED OSMOLES

One can make a reasonable assessment of a solute's likelihood to cause polyuria if its concentration in plasma is measured, the GFR is estimated, and the renal handling of that solute is known. One should also determine whether enough mannitol or lavage fluid was administered to cause the observed degree of polyuria. If Na^+ and Cl^- are excreted at very high rates and if they represent the majority of the urine osmoles, this could be the basis for the osmotic diuresis.

STEP 3. IDENTIFY THE SOURCE OF THE OSMOLES IN THE URINE

In a patient with a glucose- or urea-induced osmotic diuresis, it is important to decide whether these osmoles were derived from an endogenous source or from catabolism of exogenous proteins. When there is a glucose-induced osmotic diuresis, one must assess the plasma glucose concentration and the GFR to assess the magnitude of the possible osmotic diuresis. Be aware of "hidden" glucose in the lumen of the gastrointestinal (GI) tract, because this may soon be absorbed and contribute to the osmotic diuresis.[23]

In a patient with a saline-induced osmotic diuresis, one must determine why so much NaCl is being excreted. Some potential causes are prior excessive saline administration (a common situation in a hospital setting), administration of a loop diuretic in a patient with a significant degree of edema, and cerebral salt wasting or renal salt wasting.

Consult 4: An Unusually Large Osmotic Diuresis in a Diabetic Patient

A 50-kg, 14-year-old female adolescent has a long history of poorly controlled type 1 diabetes mellitus because she does not take insulin regularly. In the past 48 hours, she was thirsty and drank a large volume of fruit juice; her urine volume was very high. On physical examination, her effective arterial blood volume was not appreciably contracted. The urine flow rate was 10 mL/min over a 100-minute period. Other laboratory data include the following: pH = 7.33; plasma HCO_3^- concentration (P_{HCO_3}) = 24 mmol/L; plasma anion gap (P_{AG}) = 16 mEq/L; plasma K^+ concentration (P_K) = 4.8 mmol/L; plasma creatinine concentration (P_{Cr}) = 1.0 mg/dL (88 μmol/L; close to her usual values); blood urea nitrogen (BUN) concentration = 22 mg/dL (P_{urea} = 8 mmol/L); and hematocrit = 0.45. Of note, there was no decrease in her plasma glucose concentration (P_{Glu}) despite the excretion of a large amount of glucose in the urine.[24]

	ADMISSION		AFTER 100 min	
	PLASMA	URINE	PLASMA	URINE
Glucose in mg/dL (mmol/L)	1260 (70)	5400 (300)	1260 (70)	5400 (300)
Na^+ in mmol/L	125	50	123	50
Osmolality in mOsm/L	320	450	281	450

Questions

What is the basis of the polyuria?
What dangers do you anticipate for this patient?

Discussion

WHAT IS THE BASIS OF THE POLYURIA?

Osmole Excretion Rate. The product of the patient's U_{osm} (450 mOsm/L) and urine flow rate (10 mL/min) yields an osmole excretion rate of 4.5 mOsm/min, a value that is ninefold higher than the usual value in an adult (approximately 0.5 mOsm/min).

Urine Osmolality. The U_{osm} of 450 mOsm/kg H_2O indicates that this polyuria is due to an osmotic diuresis. In addition, this U_{osm} is lower than expected; this probably reflects the very high osmole excretion rate, which caused a larger fall in the patient's medullary interstitial osmolality due to a large volume of water reabsorption in the MCD.

Urine Flow Rate. The urine flow rate was extremely high for two reasons: the very high osmole excretion rate and the low osmolality in the patient's medullary interstitial compartment.

Nature of the Urine Osmoles. Because the patient's GFR was only modestly low and her P_{Glu} was extremely high (1260 mg/dL or 70 mmol/L), her filtered load of glucose will be markedly higher than the maximum tubular capacity for its reabsorption; hence, this is likely to be a glucose-induced osmotic diuresis (confirmed by the finding of a urine glucose concentration [U_{Glu}] of approximately 300 mmol/L).

Source of the Urine Osmoles. Special emphasis should be given to the fact that the patient's P_{Glu} did not decline despite such a high rate of excretion of glucose. In quantitative terms, the total content of glucose in her ECF compartment is 126 g [(1260 mg/dL × 10 to convert to milligrams per liter) × 10 L ECF volume ÷ 1000], and she excreted 54 g of glucose in the initial 100-min period [(5400 mg/dL × 10) × 1 L ÷ 1000]. Therefore, she excreted close to half of the content of glucose in her entire ECF compartment. To maintain this degree of hyperglycemia, she needed a large input of glucose in a short period of time. The only likely source of such a large amount of glucose is glucose that was retained in her stomach. As a reference, 1 L of apple juice contains approximately 135 g of glucose. For ingested glucose to cause an osmotic diuresis, this patient would need a rapid rate of exit of fluid from the stomach.[23] Although the usual effect of hyperglycemia is to slow gastric emptying, this did *not* occur in this patient.[24]

WHAT DANGERS DO YOU ANTICIPATE FOR THIS PATIENT?

Low Extracellular Fluid Volume. Since glucose is an effective osmole in the ECF compartment, it helped to maintain the patient's ECF volume and thereby her effective arterial blood volume. If she had discontinued her ingestion of glucose-containing beverages long before arriving in hospital, her ECF volume would now be obviously contracted, because she would have excreted urine with a large quantity of glucose.

Cerebral Edema. Brain cell swelling may occur if there is a significant fall in the patient's effective P_{osm}, which is defined as follows[25]:

$$Effective\ P_{osm} = 2\ (P_{Na}) + P_{Glu}\ (all\ values\ in\ mmol/L)$$

This could occur if glucose and water enter the body and the glucose is metabolized, leaving the water behind. This risk would be even greater if the patient had changed her intake to water rather than sugar-containing beverages.[23]

Defense of the Extracellular Fluid Volume

Concept 8

The volume of the ECF compartment is largely determined by its quantity of Na+.

The most reliable way to know how much Na+ is present in the ECF compartment is to measure the P_{Na} and to multiply this value by the ECF volume. This requires a *quantitative* assessment of the ECF volume, which can easily be obtained using the hematocrit[27] or the total plasma proteins if their values were normal to begin with.[28]

Concept 9

Na+ wasting can be diagnosed only if there is excretion of too much Na+ while the effective arterial blood volume is low.

To make a diagnosis of renal or cerebral salt wasting, one needs a *quantitative* estimate of the ECF volume as well as an assessment of the effective arterial blood volume.

Tools

QUANTITATIVE ASSESSMENT OF THE EXTRACELLULAR FLUID VOLUME

The physical examination findings; the concentrations of K+, HCO_3^-, creatinine, urea, and urate in plasma; and the fractional excretions of the latter two are useful at times to suggest that the effective arterial blood volume may be contracted. Nevertheless, none of these provide a quantitative estimate of the ECF volume. For the latter, one relies on the hematocrit (or a change in the hematocrit with therapy in a patient who has anemia or erythrocytosis) (Table 26-3).

TABLE 26-3 Use of the Hematocrit or the Concentration of Hemoglobin in Blood to Estimate the Extracellular Fluid (ECF) Volume

HEMATOCRIT	HEMOGLOBIN (g/L)	% CHANGE IN ECF VOLUME
0.40	140	0
0.50	170	−33
0.60	210	−60

The assumptions made when using this calculation are that the patient did not have anemia or erythrocytosis, the red blood cell (RBC) volume is 2 L, and the plasma volume is 3 L (blood volume is 5 L). The formula is as follows: Hematocrit = RBC volume/(RBC volume + Plasma volume). For clinical purposes, values between the ones listed can be deduced by iteration.

Sample Calculation. In a healthy adult, the usual hematocrit is 0.40; this represents a blood volume of 5 L (2 L of red blood cells [RBCs] and 3 L of plasma):

$$Hematocrit\ (0.40) = 2\ L\ RBCs / Blood\ volume$$
$$(2\ L\ RBC + 3\ L\ plasma)$$

When the hematocrit is 0.50, the analogous equation can be solved for *x*, the present blood volume:

$$Hematocrit\ (0.50) = 2\ L\ RBCs / x\ L\ blood\ volume$$

Because there are still 2 L of RBCs, the present blood volume is 4 L, and the plasma volume is therefore 2 L. Hence the plasma volume is reduced by 1 L from its normal 3 L value. When changes in Starling forces are ignored for simplicity, the ECF volume should have declined to approximately two thirds of its normal volume.

Basis for the Low Effective Arterial Blood Volume. Measuring urine electrolyte levels can be very helpful to gain insights into the basis for a contracted effective arterial blood volume (Table 26-4). As background, the expected response to a low effective circulating volume is to excrete as little Na+ and Cl− as possible. Because timed and complete urine collections to calculate absolute rates of excretion of Na+ and Cl− are seldom obtained, clinicians must interpret the U_{Na} and urine chloride concentration (U_{Cl}) in a spot urine sample. A low U_{Na} and/or a low U_{Cl} does not necessarily indicate a low rate of excretion of Na+ and/or Cl− if the urine flow rate is high. To avoid this type of error, the U_{Na} and U_{Cl} should be related to the concentration of creatinine in the urine (U_{Cr}).

Low Rate of Excretion of Na+ and Cl−. A pattern of low excretion of Na+ and Cl− may suggest a low intake of NaCl, or contraction of the effective arterial blood volume because of a loss of NaCl by a nonrenal route (e.g., by sweat or the intestinal tract), or a prior renal loss of Na+ and Cl− (e.g., remote use of diuretics).

High Rate of Excretion of Na+ but Little Excretion of Cl−. In a patient with a low effective arterial blood volume, an anion other than Cl− is being excreted with Na+. If the anion is HCO_3^- (the urine pH is alkaline), recent vomiting should be suspected. The anion could also be one that was ingested or administered (e.g., penicillin), in which case the urine pH is usually less than 6.

High Rate of Excretion of Cl− but Little Excretion of Na+. In a patient with a low effective arterial blood volume, a cation other than Na+ is being excreted with Cl−. Most often the

TABLE 26-4 Use of Urine Electrolyte Levels in the Differential Diagnosis of Hypokalemia in a Patient with a Contracted Effective Arterial Blood Volume

CONDITION	URINE Na$^+$	URINE Cl$^-$
Vomiting		
Recent	High	Low
Remote	Low	Low
Diuretic use		
Recent	High	High
Remote	Low	Low
Diarrhea or laxative abuse	Low	High
Renal tubular disorders (e.g., Bartter's or Gitelman's syndrome)	High	High

High, Urine concentration of >15 mmol/L; *low*, urine concentration of <15 mmol/L in the absence of a large urine flow rate.

cation is NH_4^+ and the setting is diarrhea or laxative abuse. Occasionally the cation can be K^+ if KCl was ingested.

Rates of Excretion of Na$^+$ and Cl$^-$ That Are Not Low. In a patient who has a low effective arterial blood volume, a high rate of excretion of both Na^+ and Cl^- suggests that the patient has a deficit of a stimulator of the reabsorption of Na^+ and Cl^- (e.g., aldosterone), that an inhibitor of the reabsorption of NaCl is present (e.g., a diuretic), or that the patient has an intrinsic renal lesion with effects that are similar to those of a diuretic (e.g., Bartter's syndrome or Gitelman's syndrome). The pattern of excretion of electrolytes throughout the day can also be very important. For example, if the U_{Na} and U_{Cl} in a spot urine sample are both very low, whereas at other times these excretion rates are high, this suggests that the patient is taking a diuretic.

FRACTIONAL EXCRETION OF SODIUM OR CHLORIDE
When a typical Western diet is consumed, the daily excretions of Na^+ and Cl^- are approximately 150 mmol. Because a normal GFR is approximately 180 L/day, the kidney filters approximately 27,000 mmol of Na^+ and 20,000 mmol of Cl^- per day (after adjusting the P_{Na} and P_{Cl} per plasma water). Rather than expressing this function in terms of fractional reabsorption (>99%), it is common to express it in terms of fractional excretion (fractional excretion of Na [FE_{Na}] is approximately 0.5%, and fractional excretion of Cl [FE_{Cl}] is approximately 0.75%). To make this calculation as simple as possible, the urine/plasma ratio for creatinine is used (all units in mmol/L):

$$FE_{Na} = 100 \times (U_{Na}/P_{Na})/(U_{Cr}/P_{Cr})$$
$$FE_{Cl} = 100 \times U_{Cl}/P_{Cl}/U_{Cr}/P_{Cr}$$

There are three practical points to bear in mind when using the FE_{Na} or FE_{Cl}. First, the excretions of Na^+ and Cl^- are directly related to the dietary intake of NaCl. Hence a low FE_{Na} or FE_{Cl} may represent either a low effective arterial blood volume or a low intake of NaCl or both. Second, FE_{Na} or FE_{Cl} may be high in a patient with a low effective ECF volume when there is an unusually large excretion of another anion (e.g., HCO_3^- in the case of Na^+) or another cation (e.g., NH_4^+ in the case of Cl^-). Third, the numeric values for the FE_{Na} and FE_{Cl} will be twice as high in a euvolemic patient with the same intake of NaCl if that individual has a GFR that is reduced by 50% of its original value. Hence the clinical significance of the FE_{Na} and FE_{Cl} numeric values must be

interpreted in light of the GFR at the time the measurements are made. Nevertheless, the use of these parameters may be of value in the differential diagnosis of prerenal azotemia versus acute tubular necrosis.[29] The advantage of using these parameters in this setting rather than U_{Na} and U_{Cl} is that using U_{Cr}/P_{Cr} adjusts these concentration terms for water reabsorption in the nephron.

DETERMINATION OF THE NEPHRON SITE WITH AN ABNORMAL REABSORPTION OF SODIUM
Failure to Reabsorb Other Substances. If a large amount of a compound or an ion that should have been reabsorbed in a given nephron segment is being excreted, one has presumptive evidence for a reabsorptive defect in that nephron segment. For example, if the defect is in the proximal convoluted tubule, one might find glucosuria in the absence of hyperglycemia.
Compensatory Effects in Downstream Nephron Segments. For example, when there is inhibition of the reabsorption of NaCl in upstream nephron segments, more Na^+ and Cl^- are delivered to the late cortical distal nephron, where the reabsorption of Na^+ may occur in conjunction with K^+ secretion.

Consult 5: Assessment of the Effective Extracellular Fluid Volume

A 25-year-old woman was assessed by her family physician because of progressive weakness. Although she admitted to being concerned about her body image, she denied vomiting or taking diuretics. Her blood pressure was 90/60 mm Hg, her pulse rate was 110 beats/min, and her jugular venous pressure was low. Acid-base measurements in arterial blood revealed a pH of 7.39, and a carbon dioxide partial pressure (Pco_2) of 39 mm Hg. In results from venous blood, her P_{HCO_3} was 24 mmol/L, P_{AG} was 17 mEq/L, P_K was 2.9 mmol/L, hematocrit was 0.50, and plasma albumin concentration (P_{Alb}) was 5.0 g/dL (50 g/L). The urine electrolyte levels before therapy were a U_{Na} of less than 5 mmol/L, a U_{Cl} of 42 mmol/L, and a U_K of 23 mmol/L.

Questions

How severe is the patient's ECF volume contraction?
What is the cause of the patient's low effective arterial blood volume?

Discussion

HOW SEVERE IS THE PATIENT'S ECF VOLUME CONTRACTION?
The elevated value for the hematocrit (0.50) provides quantitative information about the patient's ECF volume (see Table 26-3)[30]; her ECF volume is reduced by 33% if she did not have anemia before her ECF volume became low. If anemia were present, her ECF volume would be even more reduced.

WHAT IS THE CAUSE OF THE PATIENT'S LOW EFFECTIVE ARTERIAL BLOOD VOLUME?
The low U_{Na} implies that the effective arterial blood volume is low. Nevertheless, the high U_{Cl} (42 mmol/L) does not necessarily indicate an intrinsic renal abnormality. Rather, the fact that the patient's U_{Cl} exceeded the sum of her U_{Na} + U_K suggests that there is another cation in that urine, most likely NH_4^+.

Interpretation. Calculating the content of HCO_3^- in the patient's ECF volume reveals that she had a deficit of $NaHCO_3$ (see the section "Metabolic Acidosis" for more discussion). Loss of NaCl plus $NaHCO_3$ via the GI tract was suspected as the cause of contracted ECF volume. The patient later admitted to the frequent use of a laxative. Hence the hypokalemia and contracted effective arterial blood volume are easily accounted for. Hypokalemia stimulated ammoniagenesis, which raised the rate of excretion of the cation NH_4^+; this obligated the excretion of Cl^- despite the presence of a low effective arterial blood volume.

Assessment of the Intracellular Fluid Volume: An Emphasis on the Patient with Hyponatremia

Definition. *Hyponatremia is present when the P_{Na} is less than 135 mmol/L. This is almost always associated with an expanded ICF volume.*

From a clinical perspective, hyponatremia should be divided into three categories based on whether it is acute, chronic, or chronic with an acute component. This has important implications for the design of therapy.

1. When hyponatremia is acute (i.e., present for <48 hours): The major risk is an increase in intracranial pressure, which may lead to brain herniation. Urgent therapy with hypertonic saline is needed to draw water out of the cranium.
2. When hyponatremia is chronic (i.e., present for >48 hours) and there is no acute element: The major risk is the development of osmotic demyelination from too rapid a rise in the P_{Na}. If a water diuresis is likely to occur in a patient who is considered at a high risk for development of osmotic demyelination, consider giving dDAVP at the onset of therapy. Be aware that the administration of a large amount of K^+ may raise the P_{Na} after K^+ enters and Na^+ exits cells.
3. When an acute element of hyponatremia is present in a patient with chronic hyponatremia: The P_{Na} must be raised quickly to lower intracranial pressure, but this rise should not exceed the desired upper limit for the increase in P_{Na} over a 24-hour period to avoid causing osmotic demyelination.

Classification of Hyponatremia

Hyponatremia is not a specific disease; rather it is a diagnostic category with many different causes. The most important first step in the classification of hyponatremia is to determine whether there is an acute component of hyponatremia in the patient. Acute hyponatremia is an emergency, and steps must be taken immediately to lower a life-threatening rise in intracranial pressure and then additional measures must be taken to be certain that water does not return to its intracellular location inside the skull.

In patients with chronic hyponatremia, the major pathophysiology is an inability to excrete all the water that was ingested in the transition period while the P_{Na} was falling. In some patients, this limited capacity to excrete water is due to a low distal delivery of filtrate. To emphasize this point, this category is called the *syndrome of inappropriate antidiuresis* (SIAD). In others, the defect in water excretion is because of the presence of vasopressin, which leads to the insertion of AQP2 into the luminal membrane of the third functional unit of the nephron (see Figure 26-1). In contrast to the previous category, this category is called the *syndrome of inappropriate secretion of antidiuretic hormone* (SIADH). Since SIADH is a diagnosis of exclusion, it cannot be made if the patient has another condition that leads to a low distal delivery of filtrate.

There are two reasons for a low distal delivery of filtrate: enhanced proximal reabsorption of Na^+ and thereby water, and a very low GFR. Renal excretion of water will be even lower despite the absence of actions of vasopressin as a result of reabsorption of water in the iMCD via its residual water permeability.[31]

ENHANCED REABSORPTION OF FILTRATE IN THE PROXIMAL CONVOLUTED TUBULE

Enhanced reabsorption of filtrate in the proximal convoluted tubule can result from a deficit of Na^+ or a disorder that causes low cardiac output. Because there is an obligatory minimal loss of Na^+ in each liter of urine during a large water diuresis, a deficit of Na^+ can be created during the polyuria induced by a large intake of water in an individual who consumes little NaCl (e.g., patients with beer potomania). Therefore, both the intake of NaCl and the routes for its potential loss (i.e., via urine, the GI tract, and/or the skin) should be assessed. The magnitude of the deficit of NaCl rises progressively if the reasons for the negative balance of NaCl are not reversed. This will result in a progressive decline in the distal delivery of filtrate. Later in the course of the illness when the deficit of Na^+ and Cl^- is quite large, vasopressin may be released in response to hemodynamic stimuli.

Laboratory Tests in a Patient with Hyponatremia

The major diagnostic tests focus on the recognition of the presence of a low distal delivery of filtrate. A difficulty with the classification of SIAD is that many of these patients have a mild to modest degree of effective arterial blood volume contraction, but this cannot always be detected by the physical examination. The following laboratory tests may provide helpful clues in this context.

Tools to Detect a Low Effective Arterial Blood Volume

CONCENTRATIONS OF SODIUM AND CHLORIDE IN THE URINE
The U_{Na} and the U_{Cl} are very helpful to detect the presence of a low effective arterial blood volume, and they may also provide clues to its cause. This was presented in Table 26-4.

CONCENTRATIONS OF UREA AND URATE IN PLASMA
Patients with a low effective arterial blood volume tend to have a high P_{urea} and plasma urate concentration (P_{urate}), because reabsorption of urea and urate is increased in the proximal convoluted tubule. The converse is also true in patients with chronic hyponatremia owing to SIADH, because this subgroup has a somewhat larger degree of expansion of effective arterial blood volume. Because the reabsorption of urea is strongly influenced by the effective arterial blood volume whereas that of creatinine is not, the rise in P_{urea} is more pronounced than the rise in P_{Cr} in patients with low effective arterial blood volume. Therefore, the ratio of urea to creatinine in plasma is likely to be high in patients with hyponatremia as a result of a deficit of Na^+ that causes a low distal delivery of filtrate. This may not be the case, however, if protein intake is low.

Other Tests

A low P_K, a rise in P_{Cr}, and a high P_{HCO_3} may suggest that the effective arterial blood volume is low. One should be sure to consider the muscle mass of the patient when evaluating P_{Cr}.

Consult 6: Hyponatremia with Brown Spots

A 22-year-old woman has myasthenia gravis. In the past 6 months, she has noted a marked decline in her energy, and her weight has fallen from 110 lb to 103 lb (50 kg to 47 kg). She often feels faint when she stands up quickly. She reported no large recent intake of water. On physical examination, her blood pressure was 80/50 mm Hg, pulse rate was 126 beats/min, jugular venous column height was below the level of the sternal angle, and there was no peripheral edema. Brown pigmented spots were evident in her buccal mucosa. The electrocardiographic (ECG) findings were unremarkable. The biochemical data were as follows:

	PLASMA	URINE
Na^+	112 mmol/L	130 mmol/L
K^+	5.5 mmol/L	24 mmol/L
BUN (urea)	28 mg/dL (10 mmol/L)	130 mmol/L
Creatinine	1.7 mg/dL (150 μmol/L)	6.0 mmol/L
Osmolality	242 mOsm/kg H_2O	450 mOsm/kg H_2O

Questions

What is the most likely basis for the very low effective arterial blood volume?

Are emergency situations present on admission?

What dangers should be anticipated during therapy, and how can they be avoided?

Discussion

What Is the Most Likely Basis for the Very Low Effective Arterial Blood Volume?

In this case, the very contracted effective arterial blood volume (manifested by the low blood pressure and tachycardia), the low P_{Na}, the high P_K of 5.5 mmol/L, and the renal Na^+ wasting strongly suggest that the most likely diagnosis is adrenal insufficiency. This is likely due to autoimmune adrenalitis, because the patient has myasthenia gravis. The major basis for the renal wasting of Na^+ is a lack of aldosterone. The low effective arterial blood volume is also caused in part by a lesser degree of contraction of venous capacitance vessels because of the low glucocorticoid levels.

Are Emergency Situations Present on Admission?

There are two potential emergencies that dominate the initial management: a very contracted effective arterial blood volume and the lack of cortisol, because this patient likely has adrenal insufficiency. To deal with the former, the patient needs an infusion of a solution that is isotonic to the patient to reexpand her effective arterial blood volume without changing the P_{Na}. This saline solution should be infused quickly at the onset and then at a slower rate once the hemodynamic state improves.

The second potential emergency is not life threatening at this moment, and it can be dealt with by administering cortisol. There is one other possible emergency on admission—the presence of an acute element to the patient's hyponatremia. Such an acute element does not seem to be present because the patient reported no recent large water intake and she did not have significant symptoms that could be related to an acute component of hyponatremia.

What Dangers Should Be Anticipated during Therapy, and How Can They Be Avoided?

Reexpansion of the patient's effective arterial blood volume can lead to increased excretion of water due to an increased distal delivery of filtrate and suppression of the release of vasopressin. In addition, the administration of cortisol will improve her hemodynamic state and also inhibit the release of corticotropin-releasing factor and hence of vasopressin. The net result of this therapy is to cause a large excretion of water and thereby a dangerous and large rise in her P_{Na}. Because the patient has a small muscle mass (and hence a small total body water volume), a relatively smaller excretion of water can lead to a too-rapid rise in her P_{Na}. In addition, because of her poor nutritional state, which becomes even more evident if her weight loss is interpreted in conjunction with a large gain of water in her cells, one should set a much lower upper limit for the maximum allowable daily rise in her P_{Na}. Accordingly, dDAVP should be administered to prevent a water diuresis before beginning therapy.

Potassium

Hypokalemia and hyperkalemia are common electrolyte disorders in clinical practice that are associated with life-threatening cardiac arrhythmias. Data on the urine composition provide essential evidence to establish their underlying pathophysiology and to suggest options for therapy.

Concept 10

Three factors may regulate the movement of K^+ across cell membranes: the concentration difference for K^+, the electrical voltage across cell membranes, and the presence of open K^+ channels in cell membranes.

Close to 98% of K^+ in the body is in cells. A negative voltage is the force that retains K^+ in this location. This is due in part to the active transport of Na^+ out of cells by Na^+–K^+–adenosine triphosphatase (Na^+-K^+-ATPase), because this is an electrogenic pump that exports 3 Na^+ ions and imports only 2 K^+ ions.[32] More Na^+ will be exported by the Na^+-K^+-ATPase, and hence the voltage inside the cells will become more negative, if there is a higher concentration of intracellular Na^+ or if this ion pump has a higher activity because of the effect of β_2-adrenergics, thyroid hormone, and/or insulin (Figure 26-6).[33] For an increase in pump activity via an increase in intracellular Na^+ to result in an increase in negative voltage in the interior of cells, Na^+ entry must be electroneutral (e.g., via the Na^+/H^+ exchanger [NHE] in cell membranes). Insulin causes the insertion of more pump units into the cell membrane (major effect) and may also stimulate NHE (minor effect). It is important to recognize that NHE is almost always *inactive* in this location, but it can become active if there is a high concentration of insulin in plasma and/or a high concentration

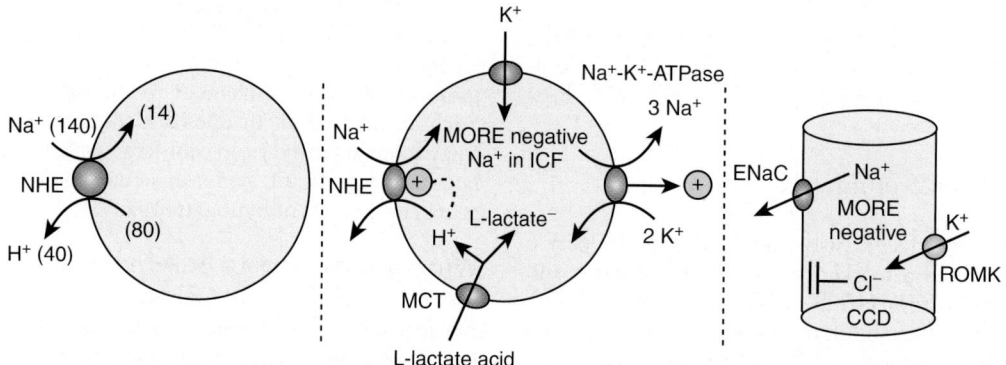

FIGURE 26-6 Physiology of the movement of K^+ across cell membranes. For details, see text. The *circles* in the center and left panels of the figure represent the cell membrane and the *cylinder* in the right panel represents the cortical collecting duct (CCD). To retain K^+ inside cells, the voltage inside the cell must be more negative. This occurs by increasing cation flux through the electrogenic Na^+-K^+ adenosine triphosphatase (Na^+-K^+-ATPase) in cell membranes, which can occur if there are more active units of this cation pump in the cell membrane and/or if there is a rise in the concentration of Na^+ in these cells, providing that the entry of Na^+ was electroneutral. As shown in the left panel, notice that Na^+/H^+ exchanger (NHE) in muscle cell membranes mediates an electroneutral entry of Na^+ into these cells, but it is inactive under basal conditions as evidenced by there being a much lower concentration of Na^+ in cells than in the extracellular fluid (ECF) and a higher concentration of H^+ in the intracellular fluid (ICF) compartment than in the ECF compartment. Insulin causes the insertion of more Na^+-K^+-ATPase pump units into the cell membrane (major effect), and it may also activate NHE. As shown in the central panel of the figure, uptake of acids on the monocarboxylic acid transporter (e.g., L-lactic acid), if it were to occur in the vicinity of NHE, this may cause a high submembrane concentration of H^+ and thereby activation of NHE. The subsequent exit of Na^+ via the Na^+-K^+-ATPase may cause an increase in the magnitude of the negative voltage inside cells. As shown in the right panel, K^+ secretion into the lumen of the CCD requires a negative luminal voltage and the presence of open K^+ channels in the luminal membrane of principal cells in the CCD.

of H^+ in the ICF compartment near NHE.[34] β_2-Adrenergics activate Na^+-K^+-ATPase via a cyclic adenosine monophosphate–dependant mechanism, which increases the affinity of the pump for Na^+, thus leading to electrogenic exit of preexisting intracellular Na^+.

Concept 11

There is no normal rate of K^+ excretion in the urine, because healthy individuals in steady state excrete all the K^+ they eat and absorb from the GI tract. This concept of steady state is particularly relevant in patients who have chronic hypokalemia or hyperkalemia.

The expected rate of K^+ excretion in a patient with hypokalemia is the rate observed in normal individuals who are deprived of K^+, whereas the expected rate of K^+ excretion in a patient with hyperkalemia is the rate observed in normal individuals who are given a very large load of KCl.

Concept 12

Long-term regulation of K^+ homeostasis is mediated primarily via the modulation of the rate of renal excretion of K^+.

Regulation of renal excretion of K^+ occurs primarily in the late cortical distal nephron, including the late distal convoluted tubule, the connecting segment, and the cortical collecting duct. The abbreviation *CCD* is used here to indicate all of these nephron segments. Secretion of K^+ in the CCD requires the generation of a lumen-negative voltage via the electrogenic reabsorption of Na^+ (more reabsorption of Na^+ than of its accompanying anions, which are usually Cl^- in a given time frame), and the presence of open K^+ channels in the luminal membranes of the principal cells. Once there is a high luminal concentration of K^+ in the CCD (K^+_{CCD}), the rate of excretion of K^+ will rise if there is an even further rise in the flow rate traversing the CCD.

Tools

Assessment of the Rate of Excretion of Potassium in the Urine

The appropriate renal response is to excrete as little K^+ as possible (i.e., <15 mmol/day) when there is a deficit of K^+,[35] and to excrete as much K^+ as possible (i.e., >200 mmol/day) when there is hyperkalemia due to a positive balance of K^+.[36] A 24-hour urine collection is not necessary to assess the rate of excretion of K^+. Because creatinine is excreted at a near-constant rate throughout the day,[37] the same information about the rate of excretion of K^+ acquired from a 24-hour urine collection can be obtained by determining the urinary concentration of K^+ divided by the concentration of creatinine in a spot urine sample (U_K/U_{Cr}). The use of U_K/U_{Cr} has advantages because the required data are available quickly and more relevant information is gathered because one knows the P_K, which influences the excretion of K^+ at that time. On the other hand, it has a limitation, because there is a diurnal variation in K^+ excretion[38]; nevertheless, this does not negate the advantages. The expected U_K/U_{Cr} ratio in a patient with hypokalemia is less than 15 mmol K^+ per gram of creatinine (or <1.5 mmol K^+ per mmol of creatinine), whereas this ratio should be above 200 mmol K^+ per gram of creatinine (>20 mmol K^+ per mmol of creatinine) in a patient with hyperkalemia.

Establishment of the Basis for the Abnormal Rate of Excretion of Potassium

In a patient with hypokalemia, a higher than expected rate of excretion of K^+ implies that the lumen voltage is abnormally more negative and that open luminal K^+ channels (likely ROMK) are present in the luminal membranes of the CCD.[39] The greater lumen-negative voltage is because of reabsorption of more Na^+ than Cl^- per unit time in the CCD. The converse is true in a patient with hyperkalemia, in whom the rate of excretion of K^+ is lower than expected.

TABLE 26-5 Use of Plasma Renin and Plasma Aldosterone Values to Assess the Basis of Hypokalemia or Hyperkalemia

	RENIN	ALDOSTERONE
Lesions That Cause Hypokalemia		
Adrenal Gland		
Primary hyperaldosteronism	Low	High
Glucocorticoid-remediable hyperaldosteronism	Low	High
Kidney		
Renal artery stenosis	High	High
Malignant hypertension	High	High
Renin-secreting tumor	High	High
Liddle's syndrome	Low	Low
Disorders involving 11β-hydroxysteroid dehydrogenase	Low	Low
Lesions That Cause Hyperkalemia		
Adrenal Gland		
Addison's disease	High	Low
Kidney		
Pseudohypoaldosteronism type 1	High	High
Hyporeninemic hypoaldosteronism	Low	Low

The clinical indices that help in the differential diagnosis of the pathophysiology of the abnormal rate of electrogenic reabsorption of Na^+ in the CCD are an assessment of the ECF volume and an assessment of the ability to conserve Na^+ and Cl^- in response to a contracted effective arterial blood volume. Measurement of the plasma activity of renin (P_{renin}) and the plasma level of aldosterone (P_{Aldo}) are also helpful in this setting (Table 26-5).[40]

Clinical Approach to the Patient with Hypokalemia

Step 1. Deal with Medical Emergencies That May Be Present on Presentation and Anticipate and Prevent Risks That May Arise During Therapy

Our first step in this clinical approach, as in all other sections, is to deal with emergencies and to anticipate dangers associated with each mode of therapy for the patient with hypokalemia (Flow Chart 26-3).

Step 2. Determine If the Major Basis for Hypokalemia Is an Acute Shift of Potassium into Cells

The most important initial step is to establish whether the duration of illness is short. The following characteristics should be present if the basis of hypokalemia is a shift of K^+ into cells. There should be a minimum rate of excretion of K^+. A significant degree of metabolic acidosis or metabolic alkalosis should not be present (Flow Chart 26-4).

The most important cause of an acute shift of K^+ into cells is an adrenergic surge that lasts for many hours or the presence of hyperthyroidism in an Asian or a Hispanic patient. Therefore, once it has been established that there is an acute shift of K^+ into cells, the next step is to determine if an adrenergic surge may have caused this shift (see Figure 26-6). In these settings, tachycardia, a wide pulse pressure, and systolic hypertension are often present. It is very important to recognize this group of patients, because the administration of nonselective β-blockers can lead to a very prompt recovery (i.e., within 2 hours) without the need for a large infusion of KCl, and hence

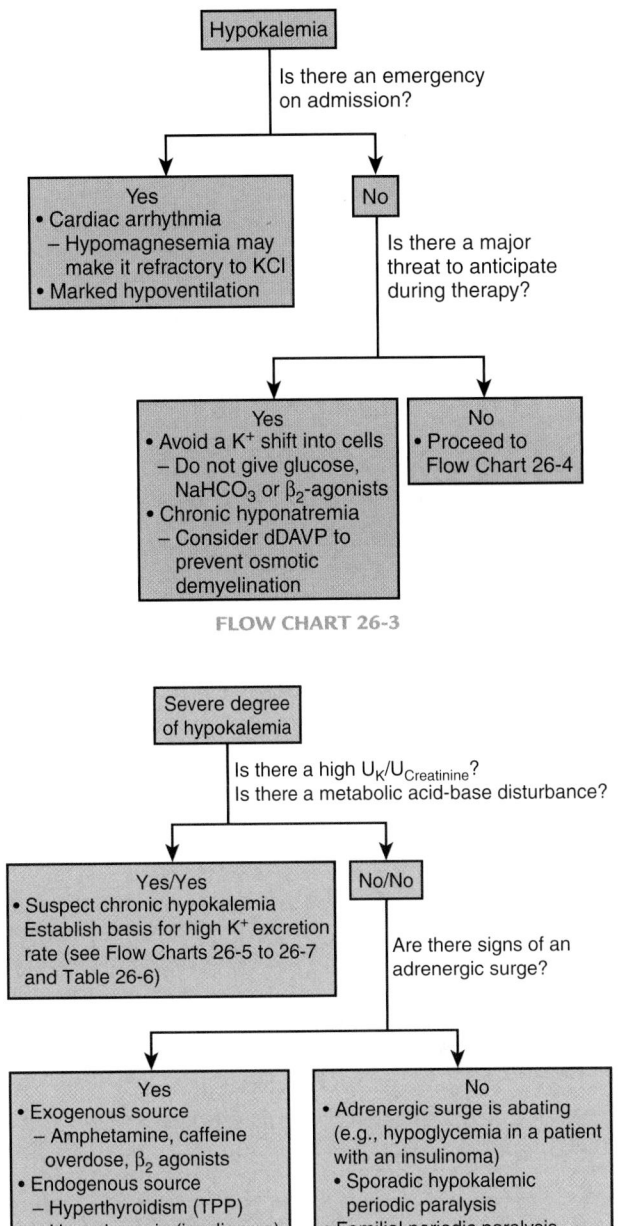

FLOW CHART 26-3

FLOW CHART 26-4

the development of rebound hyperkalemia when the stimulus for this shift of K^+ abates can be avoided.

Step 3. Determine the Acid-Base Status in Patients with Chronic Hypokalemia

If the patient has chronic hypokalemia, the first step is to examine the acid-base status in plasma (a list of causes of hypokalemia is provided in Table 26-6).

SUBGROUP WITH METABOLIC ACIDOSIS
The group of patients with hypokalemia and metabolic acidosis can be divided into two categories by examining the rate of excretion of NH_4^+ in the urine (Flow Chart 26-5). The rate of excretion of NH_4^+ can be estimated using the urine osmolal gap (see later).

TABLE 26-6 Causes of Hypokalemia

Shift of K^+ into Cells
Hormones (insulin and β_2-adrenergics are most important)
Alkalemia (not a major mechanism for hypokalemia)
Anabolic state (e.g., recovery from diabetic ketoacidosis)
Other (e.g., anesthesia, hypokalemic periodic paralysis)

Increased K^+ Loss Associated with Hyperchloremic Metabolic Acidosis
Gastrointestinal loss of $NaHCO_3$ (e.g., diarrhea, laxative abuse, fistula, ileus, ureteral diversion)
Overproduction of hippuric acid (e.g., toluene abuse)
Reduced reabsorption of $NaHCO_3$ in the proximal convoluted tubule (e.g., proximal renal tubular acidosis treated with large amounts of $NaHCO_3$, long-term use of acetazolamide)
Distal renal tubular acidosis
Low distal H^+ secretion subtype
High distal secretion of HCO_3^- (e.g., Southeast Asian ovalocytosis with second mutation involving the Cl^-/HCO_3^- anion exchanger)

Increased K^+ Loss Associated with Metabolic Alkalosis
Vomiting, nasogastric suction, some types of diarrhea
Diuretic use or abuse
Other disorders: can be classified based on blood pressure and/or plasma renin activity
    Conditions characterized by a low effective arterial blood volume, absence of hypertension, and high plasma renin activity (e.g., Bartter's syndrome, Gitelman's syndrome, ligand binding to calcium-sensing receptor (Ca-SR) in the thick ascending limb of the loop of Henle)
    Conditions characterized by a high effective arterial blood volume and hypertension (e.g., renal artery stenosis, malignant hypertension, primary hyperaldosteronism, glucocorticoid-remediable aldosteronism (GRA), Liddle's syndrome, apparent mineralocorticoid excess syndrome, Cushing's syndrome).

A decreased intake of K^+ is rarely a sole cause of chronic hypokalemia unless the intake of K^+ is very low and the duration of the low intake of K^+ is prolonged. Nevertheless, a low intake of K^+ can lead to a more severe degree of the hypokalemia if there is an ongoing K^+ loss.
Over a 24-hour period, both a normal individual and a patient with hyperkalemia reabsorb close to 70 mmol more Na^+ than Cl^- in CCD and secrete close to 70 mmol of K^+. Because of recycling of urea, 5 L of fluid exit the terminal CCD in both the normal subject and the patient with hyperkalemia.

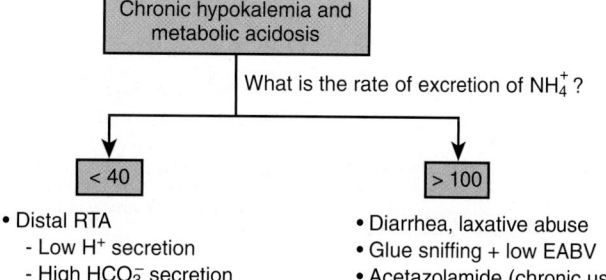

FLOW CHART 26-5

Chronic hypokalemia and metabolic acidosis

What is the rate of excretion of NH_4^+?

< 40
- Distal RTA
  - Low H^+ secretion
  - High HCO_3^- secretion
- Proximal RTA treated with large dose of $NaHCO_3$

> 100
- Diarrhea, laxative abuse
- Glue sniffing + low EABV
- Acetazolamide (chronic use)

SUBGROUP WITH METABOLIC ALKALOSIS

Patients with chronic hypokalemia and metabolic alkalosis can be divided into two major categories based on their rate of renal excretion of K^+ using the U_K/U_{Cr} ratio (Flow Chart 26-6). Those with a low value for this ratio (i.e., <30 mmol K^+ per gram of creatinine or <3 mmol per mmol of creatinine) will have conditions associated with a loss of K^+ by nonrenal routes, such as in sweat (e.g., in cystic fibrosis) or via the GI tract (e.g., in diarrhea fluid, in drainage fluids). On the other hand, in patients who have chronic hypokalemia, metabolic alkalosis, and a large renal excretion of K^+, the steps to take to determine the underlying pathophysiology are outlined in Flow Chart 26-7.

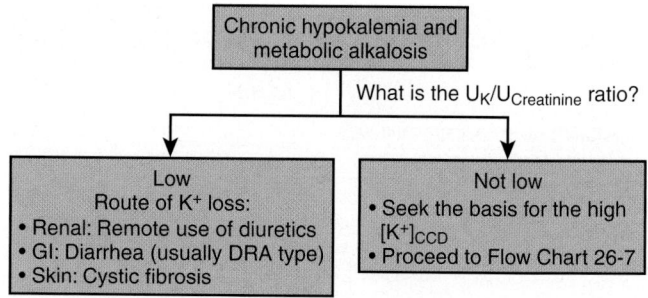

FLOW CHART 26-6

Chronic hypokalemia and metabolic alkalosis

What is the $U_K/U_{Creatinine}$ ratio?

Low
Route of K^+ loss:
- Renal: Remote use of diuretics
- GI: Diarrhea (usually DRA type)
- Skin: Cystic fibrosis

Not low
- Seek the basis for the high $[K^+]_{CCD}$
- Proceed to Flow Chart 26-7

In essence, one is attempting to categorize these patients on the basis of the pathophysiology of the high potassium concentration in the luminal fluid of CCD ($[K^+]_{CCD}$) into those with more reabsorption of Na^+ and those with less reabsorption of Cl^- in the CCD. The clinical indices that help in the differential diagnosis are an assessment of the effective arterial blood volume, the blood pressure, and the ability to conserve Na^+ and Cl^- in response to a contracted effective arterial blood volume.

More Reabsorption of Na^+ than of Cl^-. Patients with more reabsorption of Na^+ than of Cl^- are expected to have hypertension, an effective arterial blood volume that is not low, and the ability to conserve Na^+ and Cl^- in response to low effective arterial blood volume. This pathophysiology can be caused by two groups of disorders based on the P_{Aldo} value (Figure 26-7). One group consists of conditions with high P_{Aldo}, whereas the other includes the conditions in which the actions of aldosterone are mimicked and, as a result, the P_{Aldo} is low. A list of the conditions can be found in Table 26-6.

Less Reabsorption of Cl^- than of Na^+. Patients with less reabsorption of chloride than of sodium are expected to have a low effective arterial blood volume, the absence of hypertension, and the inability to conserve Na^+ and Cl^- in response to a low effective arterial blood volume. The most common causes are protracted vomiting and the use of diuretic agents.

Disorders that cause less reabsorption of Cl^- (than of Na^+) in the CCD can be divided into three groups. First are conditions characterized by the delivery of very little Cl^- to the CCD (e.g., delivery of Na^+ with HCO_3^-, as in recent vomiting, or with a drug anion like penicillin); second are disorders in which there is a decreased rate of reabsorption of Cl^- in the CCD (e.g., possibly because of the effect of HCO_3^- or an alkaline luminal pH[41]); third are disorders in which a combination of a high delivery of Na^+ and Cl^- to the CCD due to inhibition of their absorption in an upstream nephron segment together with a higher capacity for the reabsorption of Na^+ than Cl^- in the CCD (e.g., release of aldosterone in response to a low effective arterial blood volume). In patients with less reabsorption of Cl^- than of Na^+, the P_{renin} value should be high. The use of urine electrolyte levels in the differential diagnosis of hypokalemia in a patient with a contracted effective arterial blood volume is summarized in Table 26-4.

Consult 7: Hypokalemia and a Low Rate of Potassium Excretion

A 35-year-old obese Asian male developed extreme weakness progressing to paralysis over a period of 12 hours. It was preceded by his routine exercise after consumption of a

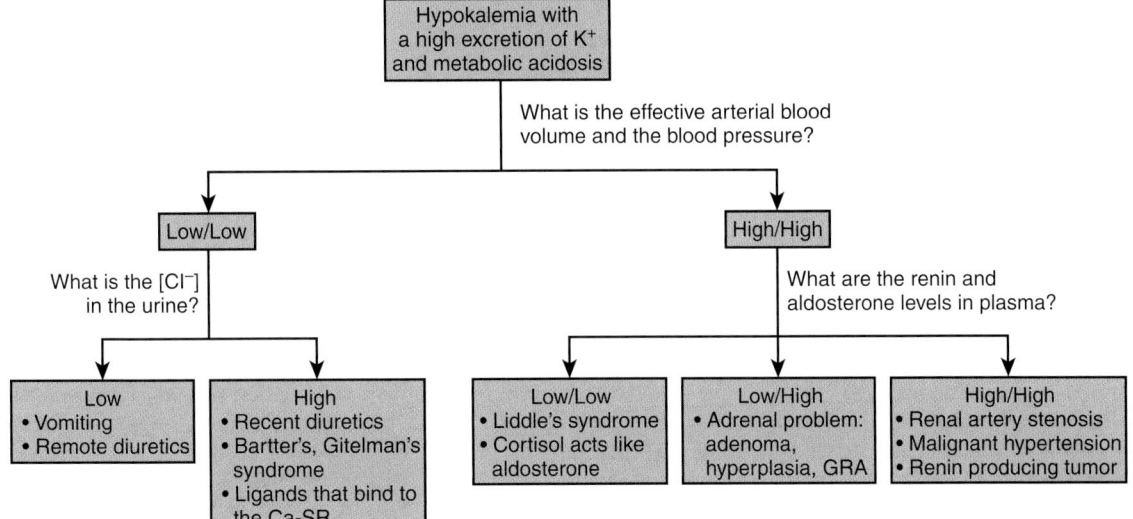

FLOW CHART 26-7

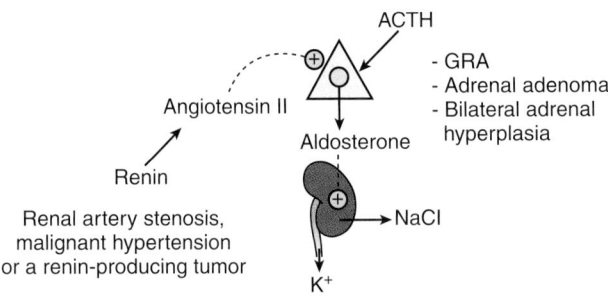

HIGH ALDOSTERONE CONCENTRATION

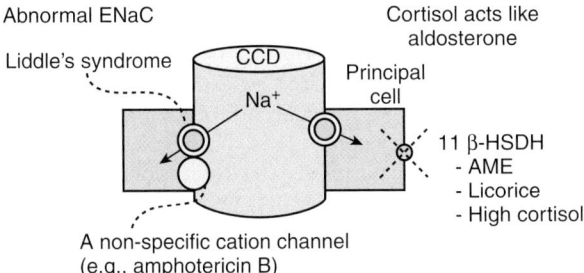

LOW ALDOSTERONE CONCENTRATION

FIGURE 26-7 Conditions causing hypokalemia with more reabsorption of Na⁺ than of Cl⁻. Conditions in which there is both hypokalemia and an abnormally high plasma aldosterone concentration (P_Aldo) are illustrated in the upper portion. In contrast, conditions with hypokalemia but low P_Aldo are illustrated in the lower portion. *ACTH,* Adrenocorticotropic hormone; *AME,* apparent mineralocorticoid excess syndrome; *ENaC,* epithelial sodium channel; *GRA,* glucocorticoid-remediable aldosteronism; *11β-HSDH,* 11β-hydroxysteroid dehydrogenase.

carbohydrate-rich meal. He has had three similar attacks of paralysis in the past 6 months, but there is no family history of hypokalemia, paralysis, or hyperthyroidism. He denied the use of laxatives or diuretics, but he did take amphetamines to induce weight loss. On physical examination, he was alert and oriented; blood pressure was 150/70 mm Hg, heart rate was 124 beats/min, and respiratory rate was 18 breaths/min. Symmetrical flaccid paralysis with areflexia was present in all four

limbs. There were no other abnormal findings on examination. The pH and Pco₂ in the following table were measured in arterial blood, whereas all other data are based on venous blood. The ECG showed prominent U waves. On subsequent evaluation, results of thyroid function tests were found to be normal.

	BLOOD	URINE		BLOOD
K⁺ (mmol/L)	1.8	10	pH	7.40
Creatinine (mg/dL)	0.6	100	PCO₂ (mm Hg)	40
Na⁺ (mmol/L)	140	100	HCO₃⁻ (mmol/L)	25
Cl⁻ (mmol/L)	103	92	Glucose (mg/dL)	84

Questions

Is there a medical emergency?
What is the basis of the hypokalemia?
What are the major options for therapy?

Discussion

IS THERE A MEDICAL EMERGENCY?

Because the ECG did not show significant changes due to hypokalemia and because respiratory muscle weakness was not present as evident from the arterial Pco₂, there are no emergencies that required immediate therapy (see Flow Chart 26-3).

WHAT IS THE BASIS OF THE HYPOKALEMIA?

The steps to follow are illustrated in Flow Chart 26-4.
Is the Major Basis of Hypokalemia an Acute Shift of K⁺ into Cells? Since the time course was short, the major basis for the patient's acute hypokalemia is a shift of K⁺ into cells. In support of this diagnosis, his U_K/U_Cr ratio was less than 15 mmol K⁺ per gram of creatinine (<1.5 mmol K⁺ per

mmol of creatinine).[42] There is a possible caveat, because a low rate of excretion of K^+ may represent the normal renal response to a prior renal K^+ loss or an extrarenal loss of K^+. The absence of an acid-base disorder, however, also suggests that the major basis for his hypokalemia is an acute shift of K^+ into cells.[42]

What Are the Reasons for K^+ to Shift into Cells? There are reasons to believe that K^+ may have shifted into cells (e.g., a large carbohydrate intake, because high insulin levels increase the number of Na^+-K^+-ATPase in cell membrane and may also activate NHE; and vigorous exercise, because β_2-adrenergic agonists activate Na^+-K^+-ATPase). On physical examination, there were findings supporting a high β-adrenergic state (e.g., tachycardia, systolic hypertension, and a wide pulse pressure). Other laboratory test results that were not available in this patient but are consistent with this diagnosis include the presence of hypophosphatemia along with a low ratio of urine phosphate concentration to urine calcium concentration.[43] There was no personal or family history of hypokalemic periodic paralysis or hyperthyroidism. Notwithstanding, the stimulus for the K^+ shift needs to be prolonged considering that his symptoms persisted for a long period of time. The absence of hypoglycemia makes it unlikely that there was a prolonged excessive release of insulin. Long-term β_2-adrenergic stimulation can be caused by the amphetamine used by this patient or by a large intake of caffeine, especially if the relevant cytochrome P450 isoenzyme for its metabolism is inhibited[44]; the latter was denied by the patient on careful questioning.

Interpretation. The cause of the hypokalemia seems to be an acute shift of K^+ into cells due to a large adrenergic surge produced by the use of amphetamines[44] (more detailed information about the causes of an acute shift of K^+ into cells can be found in Lin et al.[42]).

WHAT ARE THE MAJOR OPTIONS FOR THERAPY?

Because the diagnosis is an acute shift of K^+ into cells due to a large adrenergic surge related to amphetamine use, the patient was treated with a nonselective β-blocker and moderate K^+ supplementation[45]; the P_K returned to the normal range in 2 hours. Of great importance, large doses of K^+ should not be given because of the risk of life-threatening rebound hyperkalemia when the cause of the K^+ shift abates.

Consult 8: Hypokalemia and a High Rate of Potassium Excretion

A 76-year-old Asian man developed progressive muscle weakness over the previous 6 hours that became so severe that he was unable to move. He had no other neurologic symptoms. He reported no vomiting, diarrhea, or use of diuretics or laxatives. Hypokalemia (P_K of 3.3 mmol/L) and hypertension had been noted 1 year earlier, but had not been investigated further. There was no family history of hypertension or hypokalemia. His blood pressure was 160/96 mm Hg and his heart rate was 70 beats/min. The neurologic examination revealed symmetric flaccid paralysis with areflexia, but no other findings. The laboratory data before therapy are shown in the following table. Subsequent measurements revealed that his P_{renin} and P_{Aldo} were low and his plasma cortisol concentration was in the normal range.

	BLOOD	URINE		BLOOD	URINE
K^+ (mmol/L)	1.8	26	pH	7.55	—
Na^+ (mmol/L)	147	132	P_{CO_2} (mm Hg)	40	—
Cl^- (mmol/L)	90	138	HCO_3^- (mmol/L)	45	—
Creatinine (mg/dL)	0.8	60	Osmolality (mOsm/L)	302	482

The patient was treated initially with intravenous KCl; the weakness improved when his P_K reached 2.5 mmol/L. Treatment was continued with oral KCl supplementation. Two weeks later, his P_K and blood pressure had returned to normal levels, and his body weight had decreased from 78 to 74 kg.

Questions

Were there any emergencies on admission?
What is the cause of hypokalemia in this patient?

Discussion

WERE THERE ANY EMERGENCIES ON ADMISSION?

Always deal with emergencies first. The only potential emergency to deal with is the extreme weakness if it were to compromise ventilation. If KCl is to be administered via the intravenous route, do not give it with glucose because the release of insulin could cause the K in plasma to fall and induce a cardiac arrhythmia.

WHAT IS THE CAUSE OF HYPOKALEMIA IN THIS PATIENT?

Assess the Rate of Excretion of K^+. At presentation the patient had an acute symptom, extreme weakness of both upper and lower limbs. There was little to support the diagnosis of hypokalemic periodic paralysis because he had not had previous attacks of paralysis and there was no evidence of thyrotoxicosis. Most importantly, his U_K/U_{Cr} ratio was 5, a value that is fivefold higher than would be expected if the major basis for his hypokalemia were an acute shift of K^+ into cells. Moreover, he had metabolic alkalosis. Hence his hypokalemia was largely due to a disorder that caused excessive loss of K^+ into the urine.

Notwithstanding, his acute presentation with extreme weakness might be due to an acute shift of K^+ into cells in conjunction with a chronic disorder that caused excessive excretion of K^+. Since this patient had hypokalemia with metabolic alkalosis and a high U_K/U_{Cr} ratio, the approach to determining the pathophysiology of his hypokalemia follows the steps illustrated in Flow Chart 26-7.

On clinical assessment, the patient's ECF volume was not contracted and he had hypertension. Therefore the increased lumen-negative voltage in his CCD was likely due to a higher rate of reabsorption of Na^+ than of Cl^- in the CCD. Because both P_{Aldo} and P_{renin} were suppressed, the differential diagnosis was between disorders in which cortisol acts as a mineralocorticoid and those characterized by an open ENaC despite the undetectable levels of aldosterone. A chest radiograph did not reveal a lung mass, and cortisol levels were not elevated. Inherited disorders in which ENaC is constitutively active (e.g., Liddle's syndrome) seemed unlikely considering the patient's age. Although the patient denied consuming licorice or chewing tobacco, it turned out that he used an herbal sweetener to

TABLE 26-7 Causes of Hyperkalemia

High Intake of K$^+$
Only if combined with low excretion of K$^+$

Shift of K$^+$ Out of Cells
Cell necrosis; hemolysis in the blood drawn
Lack of insulin
Use of nonselective β-blockers (small effect if only factor)
Metabolic acidosis associated with anions that are largely restricted to the extracellular fluid compartment (e.g., HCl, citric acid)
Rare causes (e.g., hyperkalemic periodic paralysis)

Diminished K$^+$ Loss in the Urine
Advanced chronic renal insufficiency
Specific lesions that may lead to a low K$^+$ concentration in the CCD
Primary Decrease in the Flux of Na$^+$ through ENaC
Very low delivery of Na$^+$ to the CCD
Low levels of aldosterone (e.g., Addison's disease)
Blockade of the aldosterone receptor (e.g., spironolactone)
Low ENaC activity (type 1 pseudohypoaldosteronism)
Blockade of ENaC (e.g., amiloride, triamterene, trimethoprim)
Cl$^-$ and Na$^+$ Reabsorbed at Similar Rates in the CCD
Increased reabsorption of Na$^+$ and Cl$^-$ in the distal convoluted tubule (e.g., Gordon's syndrome)
Possible Cl$^-$ shunt in the CCD (e.g., some of the causes of hyporeninemic hypoaldosteronism, diabetic nephropathy, drugs such as cyclosporin)

CCD, Late cortical distal nephron, including the late distal convoluted tubule, the connecting segment, and the cortical collecting duct; *ENaC*, epithelial sodium channel.

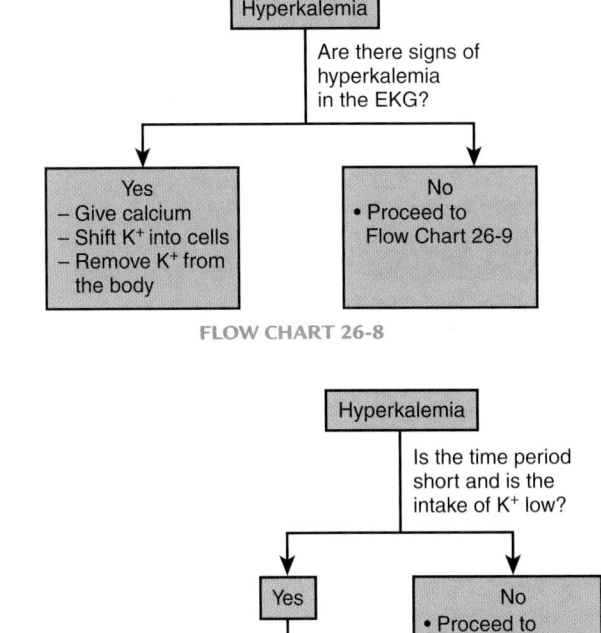

FLOW CHART 26-8

FLOW CHART 26-9

sweeten his tea which contained large amounts of glycyrrhizic acid (the active principle in licorice).[46] Discontinuing this intake led to a normal P_K and a natruresis and fall in his blood pressure.

Clinical Approach to the Patient with Hyperkalemia

A list of causes of hyperkalemia is provided in Table 26-7.

Step 1. Address Emergencies

It is imperative to recognize when hyperkalemia represents a medical emergency, because therapy must take precedence over diagnosis (Flow Chart 26-8). One must also anticipate the dangers associated with each mode of therapy and take steps to prevent them from occurring.

Step 2. Determine Whether the Cause of the Hyperkalemia is a Shift of Potassium Out of Cells in Vivo or in Vitro

Is the time period short and/or has the intake of K$^+$ been low? If the answer is yes, there are the following three options to consider.
1. The high P_K could be due to a shift of K$^+$ out of cells in the body or in the test tube in the laboratory; this is in vitro, which we call pseudohyperkalemia in Flow Chart 26-9. To see whether this has occurred, look for a reason for a less negative voltage in cells (Figure 26-8). The major causes include a lack of insulin, metabolic acidosis due to the addition of HCl or organic acids that are not the physiologic monocarboxylic acids (e.g., citric acid), and exhaustive exercise. A family history of acute hyperkalemia suggests that there may be a molecular basis for the disorder (e.g., hyperkalemic periodic paralysis).
2. There could be destruction of cells in the body. In this case, the diagnosis is usually obvious (e.g., crush injury).

3. Pseudohyperkalemia may be present (Flow Chart 26-9). In this setting, ECG changes will *not* be associated with hyperkalemia if this is its only cause. Conditions that can cause pseudohyperkalemia such as hemolysis, megakaryocytosis, fragile tumor cells, a K$^+$ channel disorder in red blood cells, and excessive fist clenching during blood sampling should be excluded. Pseudohyperkalemia can be present in cachectic patients, because the normal T tubule architecture in skeletal muscle may be disturbed. This permits more K$^+$ to be released into venous blood, even without excessive fist clenching during blood sampling.

Step 3. Assess the Rate of Renal Excretion of Potassium

In a patient with chronic hyperkalemia, pseudohyperkalemia should first be ruled out. To assess the renal response in a patient with hyperkalemia, one can use the expected rate of K$^+$ excretion in normal individuals who are given a K$^+$ load (Figure 26-9); these individuals can augment the rate of excretion of K$^+$ to more than 200 mmol/day. This is achieved with only a minor increase in the P_K. In contrast, patients with chronic hyperkalemia have a rate of excretion of K$^+$ that is equal to their current intake of K$^+$. Nevertheless, this can be achieved only while their P_K is elevated. It is common, but not necessary, to rely on a 24-hour urine collection to assess the rate of excretion of K$^+$. Because an exact value is

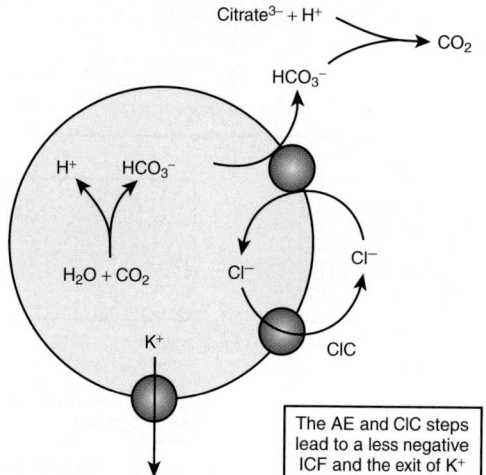

FIGURE 26-8 Role of the anion exchanger in the shift of K$^+$ out of cells. The H$^+$ from citric acid cannot enter cells via any of these transporters because it is not a substrate for the monocarboxylic acid cotransporter (citrate is a tricarboxylic anion). As shown in the right portion of the figure, when the anion exchanger (AE) is activated (AEs are normally *inactive* in cell membranes), the addition of citric acid will lower the plasma HCO$_3^-$ concentration (P$_{HCO_3}$), and this may cause more HCO$_3^-$ to be exported and more Cl$^-$ to enter cells during the period in which this anion exchanger is active. The rise in intracellular Cl$^-$ and the negative voltage inside the cell forces Cl$^-$ ions out of the cells down their electrochemical gradient via the specific Cl$^-$ ion channel (ClC). This exit of Cl$^-$ causes the intracellular fluid (ICF) voltage to become less negative, and as a result, K$^+$ may exit from cells if open K$^+$ channels are present in the cell membrane.

not needed, the ratio of the concentrations of K$^+$ and creatinine in spot urine samples (U$_K$/U$_{Cr}$) can be used even though there is a diurnal variation in K$^+$ excretion. Therefore, if fewer than 200 mmol K$^+$ per gram of creatinine or 20 mmol K$^+$ per mmol of creatinine are excreted in a patient with hyperkalemia, there is a renal defect in K$^+$ excretion.

Step 4. Determine the Basis for the Low U$_K$/U$_{Cr}$ Ratio

The most common explanation for a low U$_K$/U$_{Cr}$ ratio is a less negative voltage in the lumen of the CCD due to a lower rate of electrogenic reabsorption of Na$^+$ in the CCD. There are two major categories of conditions associated with low lumen-negative voltage: those with a diminished rate of reabsorption of Na$^+$ via ENaC, and those in which the reabsorption of Na$^+$ and Cl$^-$ occur at nearly equal rates (Flow Chart 26-10).

DIMINISHED REABSORPTION OF SODIUM VIA EPITHELIAL SODIUM CHANNELS IN THE CCD

The first subgroup of patients with diminished reabsorption of Na$^+$ via ENaC consists of those who have a marked decrease in the effective arterial blood volume. These patients may have a level of delivery of Na$^+$ to the CCD that is sufficiently low to limit the rate of secretion of K$^+$. The hallmark for this diagnosis is the excretion of urine with a very low concentration of Na$^+$.

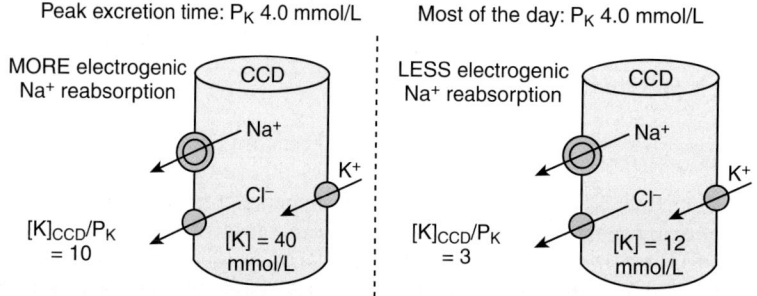

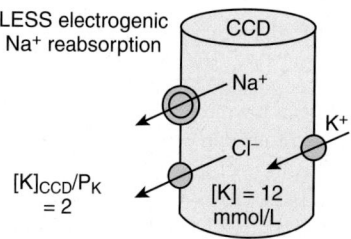

FIGURE 26-9 Excretion of K$^+$ in normal individuals and in patients with chronic hyperkalemia. The *barrel-shaped structures* represent the cortical collecting duct (CCD). The top portion of the figure describes normal subjects (plasma potassium concentration [P$_K$] = 4.0 mmol/L) and the bottom section describes patients with chronic hyperkalemia (P$_K$ = close to 6.0 mmol/L). Over a 24-hour period, both a normal individual and a patient with hyperkalemia reabsorb close to 70 mmol more Na$^+$ than Cl$^-$ in CCD and secrete close to 70 mmol of K$^+$. Because of recycling of urea, 5 L of fluid exit the terminal CCD in both the normal subject and the patient with hyperkalemia. The top left section illustrates the rate of excretion of K$^+$ when it is at its maximum rate (close to noon), whereas the top right section illustrates this secretory process when the rate of excretion of K$^+$ declines. If this peak excretion of K$^+$ were to be present for the time it takes for 1 L of fluid to exit terminal CCD, then 40 mmol of K$^+$ will be excreted. Even if the K CCD/PK declines to a value of 2 for the remainder of the day, K$^+$ balance will be maintained. In contrast, a patient with chronic hyperkalemia has a lower maximum ratio of the concentration of K$^+$ in the lumen of the CCD. As a result, the patient will need to maintain peak K$^+$ excretion rates for most of the day (that individual no longer has a diurnal variation in the excretion of K$^+$), and the price to pay is chronic hyperkalemia (lower portion of the figure). If the rate of flow in terminal CCD were to decrease to 4.5 L/day (less delivery of NaCl due to decreased effective circulating volume; less delivery of urea due to diminished urea recycling because of decreased protein intake), the plasma K$^+$ will need to rise to close to 7.5 mmol/L to maintain K$^+$ balance if K$^+$ intake remains the same.

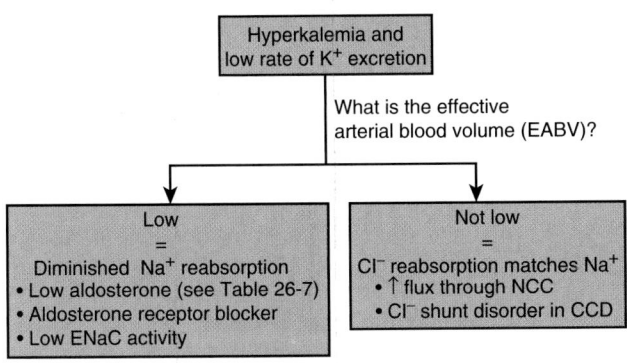

FLOW CHART 26-10

The second subgroup consists of patients who have lesions that diminish the number of open ENaC in the luminal membrane of principal cells in the CCD. Accordingly, the reabsorption of Na^+ cannot occur at a rate high enough to generate a large lumen-negative voltage in the CCD. In this case the reasons for the lower rate of reabsorption of Na^+ include low aldosterone action (e.g., adrenal insufficiency, the presence of blockers of the aldosterone receptor in principal cells), molecular defects that diminish the number of ENaC units in the luminal membrane of the CCD, and the presence of cationic compounds in the lumen of the CCD that block ENaC (e.g., the use of potassium-sparing diuretics such as amiloride or triamterene or of cationic antimicrobial agents such as trimethoprim). These patients have a low effective arterial blood volume and a higher than expected rate of excretion of Na^+ and Cl^-, as well as a high P_{renin}. Measurement of P_{Aldo} is helpful to determine the reason for this diminished Na^+ reabsorption via ENaC in the CCD.

REABSORPTION OF SODIUM AND CHLORIDE AT NEAR-EQUAL RATES IN THE CCD

One subgroup of patients with near-equal reabsorption of Na^+ and Cl^- seems to have an increased permeability for Cl^- in the CCD (a "Cl^- shunt disorder"). In another subgroup, the site of the lesion might be in the early distal convoluted tubule, where there is enhanced electroneutral reabsorption of Na^+ and Cl^- via the Na^+-Cl^- cotransporter. Accordingly, the delivery of Na^+ and Cl^- to the CCD is not sufficiently large to permit the rate of reabsorption of Na^+ to exceed the rate of reabsorption of Cl^- in the CCD by an appreciable amount. In addition, suppression of release of aldosterone by an expanded effective arterial blood volume leads to a diminished number of open ENaC units in the luminal membranes of principal cells. These patients are expected to have a rise in $[K^+]_{CCD}$ with administration of a thiazide diuretic. Patients with a Cl^- shunt disorder, on the other hand, are expected to have a rise in K^+ excretion with induction of bicarbonaturia (e.g., with administration of acetazolamide).

Consult 9: Hyperkalemia in a Patient Taking Trimethoprim

A 35-year-old cachectic man with human immunodeficiency virus (HIV) infection developed *Pneumocystis jiroveci* (formerly *Pneumocystis carinii*) pneumonia. On admission, he was febrile, but his ECF volume and all plasma electrolyte values were in the normal range. He was treated with cotrimoxazole (sulfamethoxazole and trimethoprim). Three days later, he was noted to have low blood pressure, his effective blood volume was low, and his P_K had risen to 6.8 mmol/L. His urine volume was 0.8 L/day and his U_{osm} was 350 mOsm/L. Laboratory values are shown in the table below. His ECG showed peaked, "tent shaped" T waves.

	BLOOD	URINE		BLOOD	URINE
K^+ (mmol/L)	6.8	14	pH	7.30	—
Na^+ (mmol/L)	130	60	Pco_2 (mm Hg)	30	—
Cl^- (mmol/L)	105	43	HCO_3^- (mmol/L)	15	—
Creatinine	0.9 mg/dL	0.8 g/L	BUN (mg/dL)	14	280

Questions

Why is hyperkalemia present?

Discussion

WHY IS HYPERKALEMIA PRESENT?

The steps to follow are provided in Flow Charts 26-8 to 26-10. Although an element of pseudohyperkalemia could be present in this cachectic patient, the presence of ECG changes indicates that he has true hyperkalemia.

Is the Time Period Short and/or Has the Intake of K^+ Been Low? Because the rise in P_K occurred over many days, one would be tempted to conclude that the major basis for the hyperkalemia was the low rate of excretion of K^+.

Because the patient consumed very little K^+, a shift of K^+ from cells rather than a large positive external balance for K^+ should be the major reason for the hyperkalemia.[40] The likely causes of this exit of K^+ from cells are cell necrosis, insulin deficiency, and/or metabolic acidosis (due to an acid that is not a substrate for the monocarboxylic acid cotransporter in cell membrane [e.g., HCl]).[47] Insulin deficiency could be due to the α-adrenergic effect of adrenaline released in response to the low ECF volume.[48] If the major basis of hyperkalemia is a shift of K^+ from cells, it would be an error to induce a large loss of K^+ when the total body K^+ surplus is small. It is important to realize that this patient could also have a defect in K^+ excretion.

What Is the Rate of Excretion of K^+? The rate of excretion of K^+ was extremely low in the face of hyperkalemia (U_K/U_{Cr} ratio was 17.5 mmol K^+ per gram of creatinine). The rate of excretion of K^+ is even lower than reflected by this ratio, considering his small muscle mass and hence a lower rate of excretion of creatinine.

What Is the Basis for the Low U_K/U_{Cr} Ratio? Because the patient had a low effective arterial blood volume and a U_{Na} and U_{Cl} that were inappropriately high in the presence of a contracted effective arterial blood volume, his low U_K/U_{Cr} ratio was due to diminished reabsorption of Na^+ in the CCD (see Flow Chart 26-10). The major groups of disorders that can cause diminished reabsorption of Na^+ in the CCD are listed in Table 26-8. Because the patient did not have a response to exogenous mineralocorticoids, the presumptive diagnosis was that his diminished Na^+ reabsorption in the CCD was due to inhibition of ENaC by the trimethoprim that was used to treat his *Pneumocystis jiroveci*.[49] Both his P_{renin} and P_{Aldo} (which became available later) were high, as expected in this setting (see Table 26-5).

Interpretation. Renal salt wasting due to blockade of ENaC by trimethoprim led to the development of a contracted ECF volume. As a result, there was a shift of K^+ out of cells, probably because of inhibition of insulin release by α-adrenergics.[48] Because of the low ECF volume (and the low intake of proteins), there was a low rate of flow in the CCD. This low flow rate, in addition to diminishing the rate of K^+ excretion, caused the trimethoprim concentration to be higher in the lumen of the CCD (same amount of trimethoprim in a smaller volume); hence trimethoprim became a more effective blocker of ENaC.

From a therapeutic point of view, the question arose as to whether trimethoprim treatment should be discontinued. Because the drug was needed to treat the patient's *Pneumocystis jiroveci*, a means to remove its renal ENaC-blocking effect was sought. The concentration of trimethoprim falls in the lumen of the CCD if flow in the CCD is enhanced by increasing the number of osmoles delivered to this nephron segment. To achieve this, one could increase the delivery of urea to the CCD by increasing the intake of protein or inhibit the reabsorption of Na^+ and Cl^- in the loop of Henle by administering a loop diuretic and infusing enough NaCl to reexpand the patient's ECF volume. Inducing bicarbonaturia could also be considered in order to lower the concentration of H^+ in the luminal fluid in the CCD and thereby reduce the level of the cationic form of the drug that blocks ENaC.[50]

TABLE 26-8 Causes of Metabolic Alkalosis

Causes Usually Associated with a Contracted Effective Arterial Blood Volume

Low Urine Chloride Concentration
Loss of gastric secretions (e.g., vomiting, nasogastric suction)
Remote use of diuretics
Delivery of Na^+ to the CCD with nonreabsorbable anions plus a reason for high avidity for reabsorption of Na^+ in the CCD
Posthypercapnic states
Loss of HCl via the lower gastrointestinal tract (e.g., congenital disorder with Cl^- loss in diarrhea, acquired forms of down-regulated Cl^-/HCO_3^- anion exchanger in adenoma/adenocarcinoma)

High Urine Chloride Concentration
Recent diuretic use
Endogenous diuretics (occupancy of the calcium-sensing receptor in the thick ascending limb of the loop of Henle; inborn errors affecting transporters of Na^+ and/or Cl^- in the nephron, such as Bartter's or Gitelman's syndrome)

Causes Associated with an Expanded Extracellular Volume and Possibly Hypertension

Disorders with enhanced ENaC activity causing hypokalemia
    Primary aldosteronism
    Primary hyperreninemic hyperaldosteronism (e.g., renal artery stenosis, malignant hypertension, renin-producing tumor)
Disorders with cortisol acting as a mineralocorticoid (e.g., apparent mineralocorticoid excess syndrome, licorice ingestion, adrenocorticotropic hormone–producing tumor)
Disorders with constitutively active ENaC in the CCD (e.g., Liddle's syndrome)
Large reduction in the glomerular filtration rate plus administration of NaHCO₃

CCD, Late cortical distal nephron, including the late distal convoluted tubule, the connecting segment, and the cortical collecting tubule; *ENaC,* epithelial sodium channel.

Metabolic Alkalosis

Metabolic alkalosis is an electrolyte disorder accompanied by changes in acid-base parameters in plasma, namely, an elevated concentration of HCO_3^- (P_{HCO_3}) and pH (see Table 26-8). Most patients with metabolic alkalosis have a deficit of NaCl, KCl, and/or HCl, each of which leads to a higher P_{HCO_3}. The following fundamental concepts are central to an understanding of why metabolic alkalosis develops. They also provide the basis for the clinical approach to this diagnostic category and the design of optimal therapy.

Concept 13

The concentration of HCO_3^- is the ratio of the content of HCO_3^- in the ECF compartment (numerator) to the ECF volume (denominator).

Hence, a rise in the concentration of HCO_3^- might be due to an increase in the numerator of this ratio (addition of HCO_3^-) and/or a decrease in the denominator (diminished ECF volume) (Figure 26-10). A quantitative estimate of the ECF volume is critical to determine the quantity of HCO_3^- in the ECF compartment and thereby to determine the basis of the metabolic alkalosis.

Concept 14

Electroneutrality must be present in every body compartment and in the urine.

Because electroneutrality must be present, terms such as *Cl^- depletion alkalosis* are misleading. Deficits must be defined as deficits in HCl, KCl, and/or NaCl.

Concept 15

Knowing the balances for Na^+, K^+, and Cl^- allows one to decide why the P_{HCO_3} has risen and what changes have occurred in the composition of the ECF and ICF compartments.

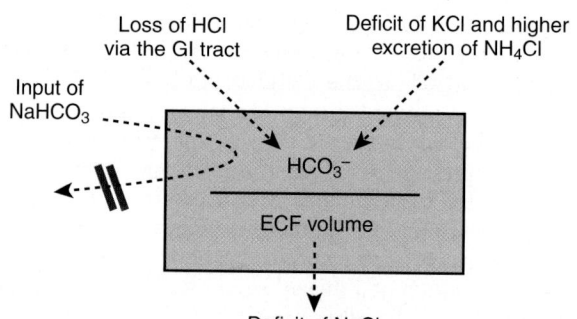

FIGURE 26-10 Basis of a high concentration of HCO_3^- in the extracellular fluid (ECF) compartment. The *rectangle* represents the ECF compartment. The concentration of HCO_3^- is the ratio of the content of HCO_3^- in the ECF compartment (numerator) to the ECF volume (denominator). The major causes of a rise in the content of HCO_3^- in the ECF compartment are a deficit of HCl and a deficit of KCl (upper portion of the figure). The major cause of a fall in the ECF volume is a deficit of NaCl. An intake of NaHCO₃ is not sufficient on its own to produce a sustained increase in the content of HCO_3^- in the ECF compartment, unless there is also a marked reduction in the glomerular filtration rate (GFR) or there is another lesion that leads to failure to remove the usual stimuli (see Concept 16) for the reabsorption of NaHCO₃ in the proximal convoluted tubule (*double bold lines* in the left portion of the figure indicate the reduced renal output of NaHCO₃).

Even though balance data are likely not to be available for most patients, a quantitative assessment of ECF volume can be obtained using the hematocrit and/or total protein concentration. Thus, it is possible to reach tentative conclusions about the contribution of individual deficits of the different Cl^--containing compounds to the development of metabolic alkalosis.

Concept 16

Critical to an understanding of the pathophysiology of metabolic alkalosis is the fact that there is no tubular maximum for HCO_3^- reabsorption in the kidney.

Angiotensin II and the usual pH in proximal convoluted tubule cells are the two major physiologic stimuli for $NaHCO_3$ reabsorption in this nephron segment. Both of these stimuli must be removed for $NaHCO_3$ to be excreted. Contrary to the widely held belief, there is no renal tubular maximum for the reabsorption of HCO_3^-. Rather HCO_3^- ions are retained unless their reabsorption is inhibited (a low angiotensin II level because of expansion of the effective arterial blood volume and/or an alkaline proximal convoluted tubule cell pH). Stated in a different way, ingesting $NaHCO_3$ will not cause metabolic alkalosis because it expands the effective arterial blood volume, lowers the angiotensin II level, and raises the ICF pH in cells of the proximal convoluted tubule. Nevertheless, $NaHCO_3$ can be retained when there is a significant decrease in its filtered load due to a fall in the GFR.[51]

$NaCl$ or HCl deficits, which can cause a higher P_{HCO_3}, can also lead to a secondary deficit of KCl and, thereby, to hypokalemia. A deficit of K^+ is associated with an acidified proximal convoluted tubule cell pH and can then both initiate and sustain a high P_{HCO_3} as a result of renal generation of new HCO_3^- (higher excretion of NH_4^+), reduced excretion of dietary HCO_3^- in the form of organic anions,[52] and enhanced reabsorption of HCO_3^- in the proximal convoluted tubule (Flow Chart 26-11).

Tools

Quantitative Estimate of the Extracellular Fluid Volume

It is critical to know the ECF volume to determine the content of HCO_3^- in the ECF compartment and thereby the reason for a rise in the P_{HCO_3}. One can often rely on the hematocrit for this purpose (see Table 26-3), but not in a patient who has anemia or erythrocytosis.

Balance Data for Sodium, Potassium, and Chloride

Balance data for Na^+, K^+, and Cl^- are essential to describe deficits in electroneutral terms, but they are not usually available in clinical settings. Nevertheless, they can be inferred if one knows the new ECF volume and the P_{Na}, P_{Cl}, and P_{HCO_3}. One cannot know the balances for K^+ from these calculations, but one can deduce their rough magnitude by comparing the differences in the content of Na^+ with that of Cl^- and HCO_3^- in the ECF compartment.[53]

Clinical Approach to the Patient with Metabolic Alkalosis

Our first step in this clinical approach, as in all other sections, is to deal initially with emergencies and to anticipate dangers associated with each mode of therapy. The next step is to examine a list of potential causes of hypokalemia.

A list of causes of metabolic alkalosis is provided in Table 26-8. Four aspects of the clinical picture in a patient with metabolic alkalosis merit careful attention: the medical history (e.g., vomiting, diuretic use), the presence of hypertension, the effective arterial blood volume status, and the P_K. The clinical approach to a patient with metabolic alkalosis is outlined in Flow Chart 26-12. The first step is to rule out the common causes of metabolic alkalosis—vomiting and the use of diuretics. Although this may be evident from the history, some patients may deny taking diuretics or inducing vomiting.

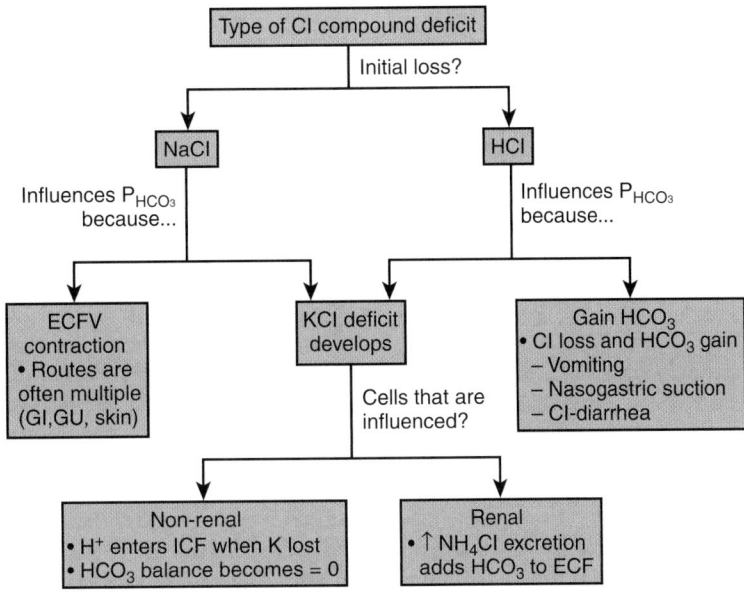

FLOW CHART 26-11

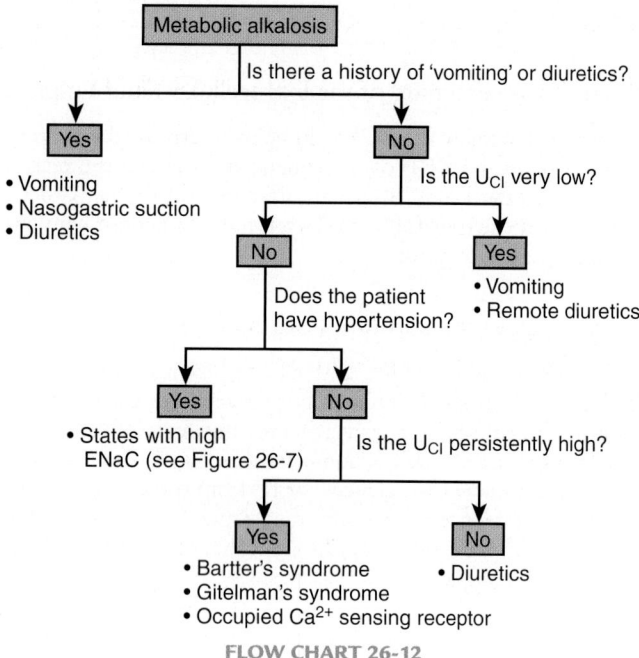

FLOW CHART 26-12

Examining urine electrolyte levels is particularly helpful if these diagnoses are suspected (see Table 26-4).

An excellent initial test is to determine the U_{Cl}. A very low U_{Cl} is expected when there is a deficit of HCl and/or NaCl, but a recent intake of diuretics causes the excretion of Na^+ and Cl^-. The U_{Na} is likely to be high if there is a recent episode of vomiting. If the U_{Cl} is not low, assessment of effective arterial blood volume and blood pressure helps separate patients with disorders of high ENaC activity (effective arterial blood volume is not low, hypertension is present) from those with Bartter's or Gitelman's syndrome (effective arterial blood volume is low, hypertension is absent). Serial measurements of U_{Cl} in spot urine samples are helpful to separate patients with Bartter's or Gitelman's syndrome (persistently high U_{Cl}) from those with diuretic abuse (intermittently high U_{Cl}).

Consult 10: Metabolic Alkalosis without Diuretic Use or Vomiting

After a forced 6-hour run in the desert in the heat of the day, the patient, an elite corps soldier, was the only one in his squad who collapsed. Although he perspired profusely during the run, he had free access to water and glucose-containing fluids. He did not vomit and reported no intake of medications. Physical examination revealed a markedly contracted ECF volume. Initial laboratory data were as follows:

P_{Na} (mmol/L)	140	pH	7.47
P_K (mmol/L)	2.7	P_{HCO_3} (mmol/L)	37
P_{Cl} (mmol/L)	90	Arterial Pco_2 (mm Hg)	47
Hematocrit	0.50		

Questions

What is the basis for the metabolic alkalosis?
What is the treatment for metabolic alkalosis in this patient?

Discussion

WHAT IS THE BASIS FOR THE METABOLIC ALKALOSIS?

Quantitative Estimate of the ECF Volume. This patient had an obvious degree of contraction of his ECF volume, but the physical examination cannot provide a quantitative dimension for this deficit. To distinguish between HCl, KCl, and NaCl deficits, a quantitative analysis of the degree of contraction of the ECF volume is needed—his hematocrit of 0.50 provides this information (see Table 26-3). With a hematocrit of 0.50, his ECF volume decreased by one third from its normal value of 15 L (because he weighed 80 kg) to approximately 10 L; accordingly, he lost 5 L of ECF in that period.

Balance Data for Na+, K+, and Cl⁻

Deficit of HCl. There was no history of vomiting, so an HCl deficit is a very unlikely cause of the metabolic alkalosis.

Deficit of KCl. The basis of hypokalemia could be a shift of K^+ into cells or a loss of KCl in the urine. To lower the P_K to 2.7 mmol/L due to a deficit of KCl, especially in this muscular elite soldier, the loss of KCl would have to be very large (at least several hundred mmol). Moreover, it is extremely unlikely that this would have happened over such a short period of time. Furthermore, even if there were a KCl deficit, it is difficult to attribute the rise in the P_{HCO_3} to the formation of new HCO_3^- due to the renal effects of hypokalemia (high excretion of NH_4^+) because the time course is too short.

Deficit of NaCl. The decrease in the patient's ECF volume was approximately 5 L. One can now calculate how much this degree of ECF volume contraction would raise his P_{HCO_3} by dividing the normal content of HCO_3^- in his ECF compartment (15 L × 25 mmol/L or 375 mmol) by his new ECF volume of 10 L, which yields 37.5 mmol/L. This value is remarkably close to the measured P_{HCO_3} of 37 mmol/L. Therefore, the major reason for his metabolic alkalosis is the NaCl deficit (a "contraction" form of metabolic alkalosis).

Balance for Na⁺. Multiplying the patient's P_{Na} (140 mmol/L) before the race by his normal ECF volume (15 L) yields an Na^+ content of approximately 2100 mmol in this compartment. After the race, his P_{Na} was 140 mmol/L and his ECF volume was 10 L; hence his ECF Na^+ content was now 1400 mmol. Accordingly, the deficit of Na^+ in his ECF compartment is approximately 700 mmol.

Balance for Cl⁻. Multiplying the patient's P_{Cl} before the race (103 mmol/L) by his normal ECF volume (15 L) yields a Cl^- content of approximately 1545 mmol in this compartment. After the race, his P_{Cl} was 90 mmol/L and his ECF volume was 10 L; hence his ECF Cl^- content was now 900 mmol. Accordingly, his deficit of Cl^- is approximately 645 mmol, a value that is similar to his deficit of Na^+.

Balance for K⁺. It is possible to have a loss of KCl in sweat in patients with cystic fibrosis with concentrations of K^+ as high as 20 to 30 mmol/L. Nevertheless, because there was little difference between the deficits of Na^+ and Cl^-, there is only a minor loss of K^+ and a total body deficit of K^+. Accordingly, the major mechanism for hypokalemia is likely to be a shift of K^+ into cells (due to β_2 adrenergic surge and possibly, but not likely, the alkalemia).

Interpretation. The deficits of Na^+ and Cl^- in the patient's ECF compartment are similar. The next step is to examine possible routes for a large loss of NaCl in such a short time period. Because neither diarrhea nor polyuria was present, the only route for a large NaCl loss is via sweat. For such a large loss of NaCl in sweat, the concentration of NaCl in sweat must be high (e.g., approximately 70 mmol/L for Na^+ and Cl^-); moreover, the patient would need to lose approximately 1 L of sweat per hour. The likely underlying lesion is cystic fibrosis; this diagnosis was confirmed later by molecular studies.[54]

WHAT IS THE TREATMENT FOR METABOLIC ALKALOSIS IN THIS PATIENT?
Because the basis for the metabolic alkalosis is largely a deficit of NaCl, the patient will need to receive NaCl as his major treatment. The goal is to replace the deficit that was calculated (approximately 700 mmol).

Metabolic Acidosis

Metabolic acidosis is a process that causes a fall in the P_{HCO_3} and a rise in the concentration of H^+ in plasma. Metabolic acidosis is a diagnostic category with many different causes (Table 26-9). The risks for the patient depend on the underlying disorder that caused the metabolic acidosis, the ill effects due to the H^+ load (binding of H^+ to intracellular proteins in vital organs such as the brain and heart), and possible dangers associated with the anions that accompanied the H^+ load (e.g., chelation of ionized calcium by citrate in a patient with metabolic acidosis due to ingestion of citric acid[55]) (Table 26-10).

The goal in this section is to provide a logical bedside approach to evaluation when the patient first seeks medical attention.[56] The initial decisions are to determine if an emergency is present and to anticipate and prevent threats that may develop during therapy. As in previous sections, the concepts that provide the underpinning for this approach are highlighted. After each is defined, the laboratory tests that are needed to better define the problem are outlined. Illustrative cases are provided to emphasize the concepts and the usefulness of these tools.

Concept 17

The P_{HCO_3} is the ratio of the content of HCO_3^- in the ECF compartment to the ECF volume:

$$[HCO_3^-]_{ECF} = \text{Concentration of } HCO_3^- \text{ in the ECF compartment / ECF volume}$$

It is important to distinguish between acidemia (lower plasma pH) and acidosis. The term *acidemia* simply indicates a high concentration of H^+ in plasma. Acidemia may not be present in a patient who has metabolic acidosis if there is a large decrease in the ECF volume,[28] which raises the concentration of HCO_3^- even when the HCO_3^- content in the ECF compartment is decreased (e.g., in patients with cholera[30] and certain patients with diabetic ketoacidosis[27]). To make a diagnosis of metabolic acidosis in this setting, a quantitative estimate of the ECF volume is needed to assess the *content* of HCO_3^- in this compartment.

Concept 18

H^+ ions must by removed by the bicarbonate buffer system (BBS) to avoid their binding to intracellular proteins.[57] The overwhelming majority of the BBS is located in the ECF and ICF of skeletal muscle.

TABLE 26-9 Causes of Metabolic Acidosis

Acid Gain

With Retention of Anions in Plasma
L-lactic acidosis
  Due predominantly to overproduction of L-lactic acid
    Hypoxic lactic acidosis
      Inadequate delivery of O_2, as in cardiogenic shock, shunting of blood past organs (e.g., sepsis), or excessive demand for oxygen (seizures)
      Miniseizures (e.g., isoniazid treatment causing vitamin B_6 deficiency)
      Metastatic tumors (especially large tumors with hypoxic areas plus liver involvement)
    Increased production of L-lactic acid in absence of hypoxia
    Overproduction of reduced nicotinamide adenine dinucleotide (NADH) and accumulation of pyruvate in the liver (e.g., metabolism of ethanol plus a deficiency of thiamin)
    Decreased pyruvate dehydrogenase activity (e.g., thiamin deficiency, inborn errors of metabolism)
    Compromised mitochondrial electron transport system (e.g., cyanide, riboflavin deficiency, inborn errors affecting the electron transport system)
    Excessive degree of uncoupling of oxidative phosphorylation (e.g., phenformin)
  Due predominantly to reduced removal of L-lactate
    Liver failure (e.g., severe acute viral hepatitis, shock liver, drugs)
  Due to a combination of reduced removal and overproduction of L-lactic acid
    Antiretroviral drugs (inhibition of mitochondrial electron transport plus hepatic steatosis)
    Metastatic tumors (especially large tumors with hypoxic areas plus liver involvement)
Ketoacidosis (diabetic ketoacidosis; alcoholic ketoacidosis; hypoglycemic ketoacidosis, including starvation; ketoacidosis due to a large supply of short-chain fatty acids, e.g., acetic acid from fermentation of poorly absorbed carbohydrate plus inhibition of acetyl–coenzyme A carboxylase)
Renal insufficiency (metabolism of dietary sulfur containing amino acids and decreased renal excretion of NH_4^+)
Metabolism of toxic alcohols (e.g., formic acid from metabolism of methanol, glycolic acid and oxalic acid from metabolism of ethylene glycol)
D-lactic acidosis (and increased concentration of other organic acids produced by gastrointestinal bacteria)
Pyroglutamic acidosis

With a High Rate of Excretion of Anions in Urine
Glue sniffing (hippuric acid overproduction)
Diabetic ketoacidosis with excessive ketonuria

$NaHCO_3$ Loss

Direct Loss of $NaHCO_3$
Via the gastrointestinal tract (e.g., diarrhea, ileus, fistula)
Via the urine (proximal renal tubular acidosis or low carbonic anhydrase II or IV activity)
Indirect Loss of $NaHCO_3$ (Low Urinary NH_4^+ Excretion)
Low glomerular filtration rate
Renal tubular acidosis
  Low availability of NH_3 (urine pH of ~5) leads to problem with proximal convoluted tubule ammoniagenesis: hyperkalemia, alkaline pH in proximal convoluted tubule cells
  Defect in net distal H^+ secretion (urine pH often ~7)

If buffering by the BBS is compromised in skeletal muscle, many more H^+ will be forced to bind to proteins in cells in vital organs (e.g., brain cells). If this occurs, these proteins will have a more positive charge, a change in their shape, and ultimately a diminution in their essential functions.[58]

Tools

The laboratory tools used in the diagnosis of the cause of metabolic acidosis are summarized in Table 26-11.

On Admission

Hemodynamic instability
  Marked decrease in myocardial contractility (e.g., cardiogenic shock)
  Very low intravascular volume (e.g., NaCl loss, hemorrhage)
Decreased peripheral vascular resistance (e.g., sepsis)
Cardiac arrhythmia
  Most frequently seen in patients with hyperkalemia or hypokalemia
Failure of ventilation (e.g., respiratory muscle weakness due to hypokalemia)
Presence of toxins (e.g., methanol, ethylene glycol)
Presence of reactive oxygen species (e.g., pyroglutamic acidosis)
Nutritional deficiency (especially of B vitamins)

During Treatment

Development of cerebral edema during treatment of diabetic ketoacidosis in children
  Overly rapid infusion of isotonic saline
  Failure to keep a constant effective plasma osmolality during therapy
Pulmonary edema (e.g., in patients with severe diarrhea if the extracellular fluid volume is expanded, but $NaHCO_3$ is not given)
Too rapid a rise in the plasma Na^+ concentration in patients with chronic hyponatremia
Development of a severe degree of acidemia in a patient with metabolic acidosis (see discussion in Consult 11)
Acute shift of K^+ into cells (e.g., administration of glucose to patients with hypokalemia, administration of insulin to patients with diabetic ketoacidosis and hypokalemia, administration of $NaHCO_3$ to patients with a low plasma potassium concentration)
Wernicke's encephalopathy due to failure to give thiamin (vitamin B_1) to patients with chronic alcoholism who have alcoholic ketoacidosis

QUANTITATIVE ASSESSMENT OF THE EXTRACELLULAR FLUID VOLUME

For quantitative assessment of the ECF, the hematocrit[27] (see Table 26-3) or the concentration of total proteins in plasma is used.[28] The assumptions are that the patient does not have a preexisting anemia or a low total plasma protein concentration.

TOOLS TO ASSESS THE REMOVAL OF HYDROGEN IONS BY THE BICARBONATE BUFFER SYSTEM

Arterial P_{CO_2}. For H^+ to be removed by the bicarbonate buffer system (BBS) in the ECF compartment, the arterial P_{CO_2} must be low as expected for the degree of acidemia. Although the arterial P_{CO_2} sets a *lower limit* on the possible value for the P_{CO_2} in cells, it is *not* a reliable indicator of the actual value of the intracellular P_{CO_2}.[57]

$$H^+ + HCO_3^- \rightarrow CO_2 + H_2O \quad (\text{"pulled" by a low capillary } CO_2 \text{ concentration})$$

Venous P_{CO_2}. To remove H^+ by the BBS in the ICF compartment, the P_{CO_2} must be low in cells. This latter P_{CO_2} is equal to the P_{CO_2} in capillaries draining individual organs. Because CO_2 is not added after the capillary, the *venous* P_{CO_2} reflects the capillary P_{CO_2} (Figure 26-11). There is one caveat, however: if an appreciable quantity of blood shunts from the arterial to the venous circulation, the venous P_{CO_2} will not reflect the P_{CO_2} in cells.

The venous P_{CO_2} may be considerably higher than the arterial P_{CO_2} when a larger quantity of CO_2 is produced and/or there is a very low rate of blood flow.[58] The P_{CO_2} measured in the brachial or femoral vein reflects the P_{CO_2} in skeletal muscle cells and interstitial space, the site where most of the buffering of H^+ by the BBS should occur.[58] If this venous P_{CO_2} is high, there is a failure of the BBS in muscle, which

QUESTION	PARAMETER ASSESSED	TOOLS TO USE
Is the content of HCO_3^- low in the extracellular fluid (ECF)?	ECF volume	Hematocrit or total plasma proteins
Have new acids accumulated?	Appearance of new anions in the body or the urine	Plasma anion gap
		Urine anion gap
Are toxic alcohols present?	Presence of alcohols as unmeasured osmoles	Plasma osmolal gap
Is the renal response to acidemia adequate?	Rate of excretion of NH_4^+	Osmolal gap in plasma
If NH_4^+ excretion is high, which anion was excreted?	Gastrointestinal loss of $NaHCO_3$	Urine $[Cl^-]$ is high
	Excretion of new anions of an added acid	Urine anion gap
What is the basis for a low rate of excretion of NH_4^+?	Low net distal H^+ secretion	Urine pH > 6.5
	Low NH_3 availability	Urine pH ~ 5.0
	If both of the above defects are present	Urine pH ~ 6.0
Is there a defect in H^+ secretion?	Distal H^+ secretion	P_{CO_2} in alkaline urine
	Proximal H^+ secretion	Fractional excretion of HCO_3, urine citrate concentration

indicates that more of the H^+ load was buffered in vital organs (e.g., the brain) (Figure 26-12). At the usual blood flow rate, the brachial venous P_{CO_2} is approximately 46 mm Hg when the arterial P_{CO_2} is 40 mm Hg, but much higher venous P_{CO_2} values were seen in patients with diabetic ketoacidosis because they have a very contracted ECF volume.[27] This tool can also be used during therapy; the high venous P_{CO_2} will fall appreciably when sufficient saline has been infused.

Clinical Approach: Initial Steps

Step 1. Identify threats for the patient, anticipate and prevent dangers that may arise during therapy (Flow Chart 26-13).
Step 2. Determine whether H^+ ions were buffered appropriately by the BBS.
Step 3. Determine whether the cause of the metabolic acidosis is added acids and/or a deficit of $NaHCO_3$.

Consult 11: Hyperglycemia without Obvious Appreciable Ketoacidosis

A 16-year-old 50-kg female adolescent has had several past admissions for diabetic ketoacidosis because she failed to take her insulin on a regular basis. Her present illness began

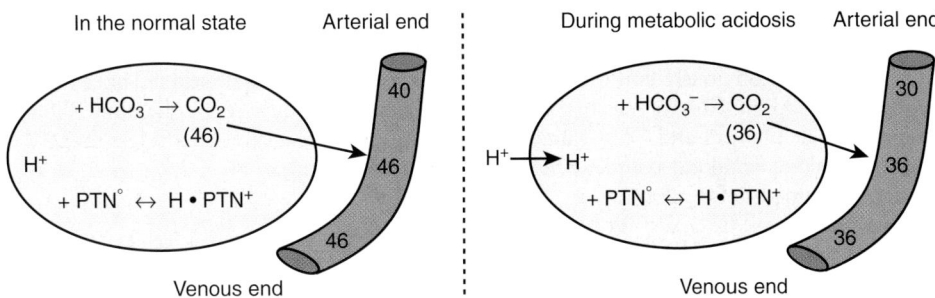

FIGURE 26-11 Effectiveness of the bicarbonate buffer system (BBS) in skeletal muscle. The *large oval* represents a skeletal muscle cell, and the *curved cylindrical structure* to its right represents its capillary. The normal state is shown on the left, and buffering of an H^+ load is shown on the right. Notice that a lower arterial Pco_2 favors the diffusion of CO_2 from cells into the capillary and that the venous Pco_2 is virtually equal to the Pco_2 in cells. Hence, new H^+ ions are forced to react with HCO_3^- in cells because the Pco_2 in cells has declined; of even greater importance, the concentration of H^+ in cells does not rise appreciably, and very few H^+ ions bind to proteins in cells.

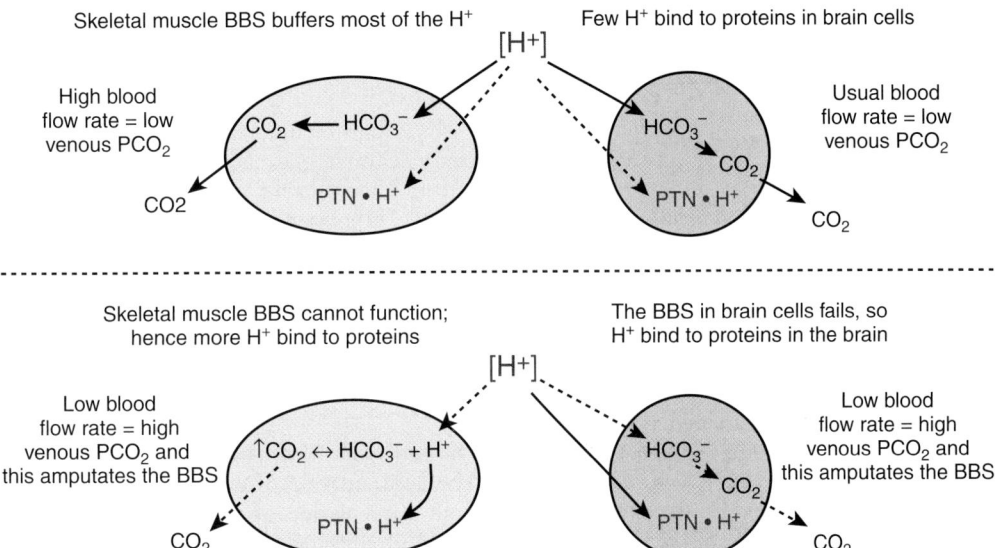

FIGURE 26-12 Buffering of H^+ in the brain in a patient with a contracted effective arterial blood volume. Buffering of H^+ in a patient with a normal effective arterial blood volume and thereby a low muscle venous Pco_2 is depicted in the top of the figure. The vast majority of H^+ removal occurs by the BBS in the interstitial space and in cells of skeletal muscles. Buffering of a H^+ load in a patient with a contracted effective arterial blood volume and thereby a high venous Pco_2 is depicted in the bottom of the figure. A high muscle venous Pco_2 prevents H^+ removal by the BBS in muscles. As a result, the circulating H^+ concentration rises (as illustrated by the larger font for $[H^+]$), which increases the H^+ burden for brain cells.

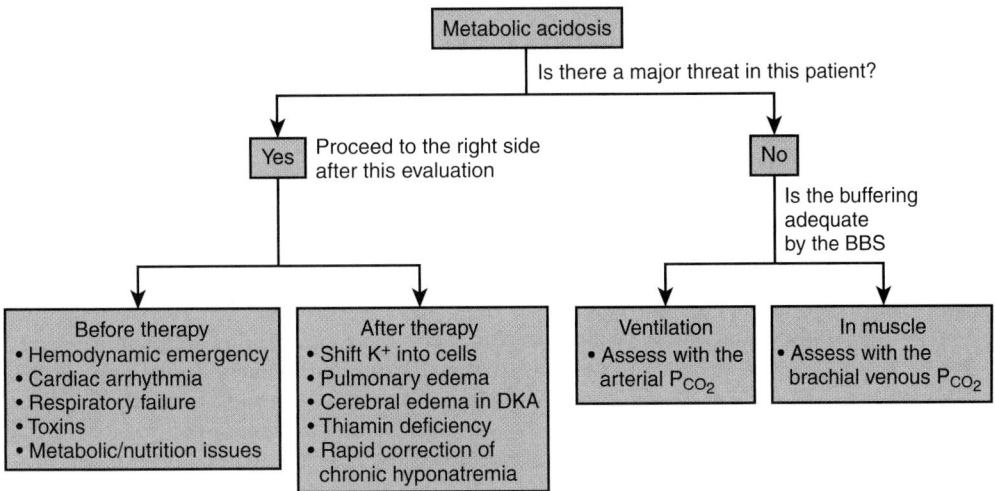

FLOW CHART 26-13

gradually. In response to thirst, she drank large volumes of predominantly fruit juice and she voided frequently. On examination, her ECF volume was obviously contracted, but she was not breathing deeply or rapidly. She was easily roused, but she was less alert than usual. The pH and Pco_2 values in the following table are from an *arterial* blood sample, whereas the remainder of the data, obtained before therapy, are from blood drawn from her brachial vein. The *venous* Pco_2 was 69 mm Hg. Although glucose appears twice, this was done to present units in plasma in SI units and in mg/dL, as the latter units may be more familiar to readers in some countries.

Glucose (mg/dL)	900	Glucose (mmol/L)	50
Na^+ (mmol/L)	120	K^+ (mmol/L)	5.5
Cl^- (mmol/L)	80	HCO_3^- (mmol/L)	21
pH	7.40	Pco_2 (mm Hg)	40
Albumin (g/dL)	5.1	Anion gap (mEq/L)	19
Creatinine (mg/dL)	2.0	Hematocrit	0.55

Questions

Does this patient have metabolic acidosis?
Is the H^+ buffering ability of the BBS in skeletal muscle cells diminished?

Discussion

DOES THIS PATIENT HAVE METABOLIC ACIDOSIS?

The patient's arterial pH, P_{HCO_3}, and Pco_2 were close to the normal range. However, the modestly elevated value for her P_{AG} suggests that added acids were present and that she may have metabolic acidosis. Because her ECF volume is contracted, the quantity of HCO_3^- in her ECF compartment must be calculated. When the hematocrit of 0.55 is used for this purpose, her plasma volume is calculated as close to 1.5 L instead of the normal value of 3 L; hence her ECF volume is reduced by approximately 50% (approximately 5 L instead of 10 L). This marked reduction in her ECF volume is due to the urinary loss of NaCl during the prolonged osmotic diuresis, which was driven by the large ingestion of sugar in fruit juice. This low ECF volume and near-normal P_{HCO_3} indicate that she has a significant deficit of $NaHCO_3$ in her ECF compartment (5 L × 21 mmol/L = 105 mmol HCO_3^-).

Upon reflection, the elevated value for her P_{AG} was due in large part to a high P_{Alb}, which represents the contracted ECF volume, and in part to the addition of new acids (confirmed later because the concentration of betahydroxybutyrate anions was somewhat elevated in plasma were not appreciably elevated). Thus the patient does have metabolic acidosis due to a deficit of $NaHCO_3$. This deficit of HCO_3^- represents an indirect loss of $NaHCO_3$ caused by the excretion of keto-acid anions along with Na^+ in the urine, because the rate of excretion of NH_4^+ is not high early in the course of diabetic ketoacidosis.

IS THE H^+ BUFFERING ABILITY OF THE BBS IN SKELETAL MUSCLE CELLS DIMINISHED?

Since the patient's brachial venous Pco_2 was 69 mm Hg, buffering of H^+ by the BBS in muscle was compromised. Hence there would be more H^+ binding to intracellular proteins in

vital organs (e.g., brain and heart). This is called a *tissue form* of respiratory acidosis.[30]

The venous Pco_2 should fall once tissue perfusion improves. As a clinical guide, enough saline should be given to lower venous Pco_2 to a value that is less than 10 mm Hg higher than the arterial Pco_2.

Metabolic Acidosis Due to Added Acids
Concept 19

When addition of acids is the cause of metabolic acidosis, one can detect the addition of H^+ by the appearance of new anions in plasma. These new anions may remain in the body or they may be excreted (e.g., in the urine or diarrhea fluid).

Concept 20

The new anions may be a cause of important dangers for the patient.

Examples include anions such as citrate that chelate ionized calcium in plasma[55] and anions that are excreted at a high rate and hence cause a very high rate of excretion of Na^+ and K^+ (e.g., hippurate anions in a patient with metabolic acidosis due to glue sniffing).

Tools

The laboratory tools used in the diagnosis of the cause of metabolic acidosis are summarized in Table 26-11.

DETECTION OF NEW ANIONS IN THE PLASMA

The accumulation of new anions in plasma can be detected from a calculation of the P_{AG}. When using this calculation, one must adjust the P_{AG} for the concentration of albumin, the major unmeasured anion in plasma. As a rough estimate, the baseline value for the P_{AG} rises (or falls) by 3 to 4 mEq/L for every 10 g/L or 1 g/dL rise (or fall) in the P_{Alb}.

Another approach to detecting new anions in plasma was recommended by Stewart.[59] It is called the *strong ion difference* approach. This method is rather complex and offers only a minor advantage over the P_{AG} in that it includes a correction for the net negative charge on plasma albumin. It suffers from the same limitations as the P_{AG} because it relies *only* on concentrations in plasma (rather than content in ECF volume) and does not include information from the venous Pco_2 to assess buffering of H^+ load by the BBS.

DETECTION OF NEW ANIONS IN THE URINE

New anions in the urine can be detected by calculating the urine anion gap:

$$\text{Urine anion gap} = (U_{Na} + U_K + U_{NH_4}) - U_{Cl}$$

The concentration of NH_4^+ in the urine (U_{NH_4}) is estimated from the urine osmolal gap (U_{OG}) (Figure 26-13) as discussed in the next section. The nature of these new anions may sometimes be deduced by comparing their filtered load with their excretion rate. For example, when there is a very large quantity of the new anion in the urine compared with the rise in the P_{AG}, one can suspect that this anion was secreted in the proximal convoluted tubule (e.g., hippurate anion from the metabolism of toluene[60]) or freely filtered and poorly reabsorbed by the proximal convoluted tubule (e.g., reabsorption of ketoacid anions may be inhibited by salicylate anions). On the other hand, a very low excretion of new anions suggests that they were avidly reabsorbed in the proximal convoluted tubule (e.g., L-lactate).

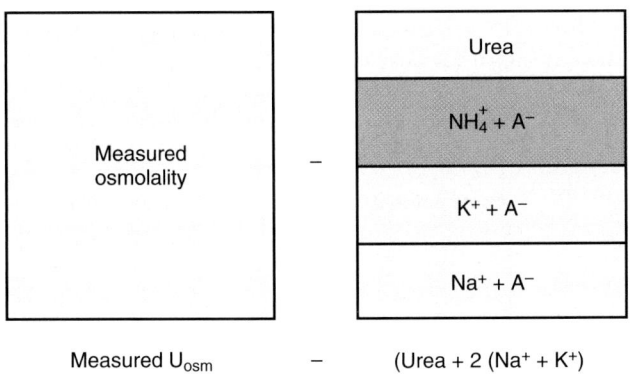

FIGURE 26-13 Indirect assessment of the concentration of NH_4^+ in the urine using the urine osmolal gap. The essence of the test is that a high concentration of NH_4^+ (shown in the *shaded region* in the right portion of the figure) is detected in the urine by its contribution to the urine osmolality (U_{osm}). In essence one measures the total osmolality of the urine and subtracts the osmolality attributed to the principal urine osmoles usually present, urea and Na^+ plus K^+ salts (i.e., double the concentrations of Na^+ and K^+). The concentration of NH_4^+ in the urine = $U_{OG}/2$.

DETECTION OF TOXIC ALCOHOLS

The presence of alcohols in plasma can be detected by finding a large increase in plasma osmolal gap (P_{OG}):

$$P_{OG} = \text{Measured } P_{osm} - ([\,2P_{Na}] + P_{Glu} + P_{urea})$$
$$\text{(all values in mmol/L)}$$

This occurs because alcohols are uncharged compounds that have a low molecular weight, and because large quantities are ingested.

Clinical Approach to the Patient with Metabolic Acidosis Due to Added Acids

The steps to follow in the diagnosis of the cause of metabolic acidosis caused by added acids are illustrated in Flow Chart 26-14. If metabolic acidosis develops over a short period of time, the likely causes are overproduction of L-lactic acid (e.g., shock) or ingested acids. The first situation is obvious hypoxic L-lactic acidosis (i.e., cases in which the supply of oxygen is too low to match the demand for ATP regeneration by aerobic fuel oxidation). The other setting in which H^+ input can be very fast is the ingestion of a large quantity of an acid (e.g., metabolic acidosis due to ingestion of citric acid).

Hyperchloremic Metabolic Acidosis

Concept 21

The expected renal response to chronic metabolic acidosis is a high rate of excretion of NH_4^+.

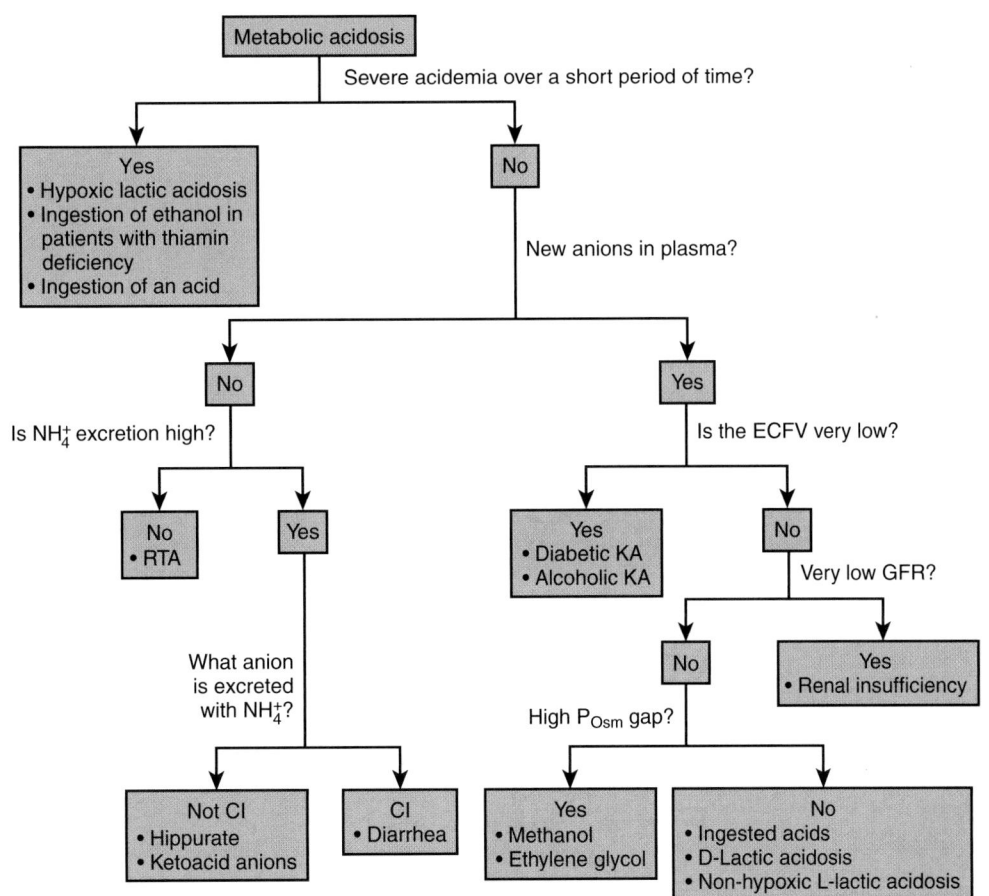

FLOW CHART 26-14

In this setting, the expected rate of excretion of NH_4^+ is more than 200 mmol/day.[61] The term *chronic* is stressed because there is a lag of a few days before very high rates of excretion of NH_4^+ can be achieved.

Concept 22

A low rate of excretion of NH_4^+ could be due a decreased medullary NH_3 or a decreased net H^+ secretion in the distal nephron.

A low rate of ammoniagenesis could be caused by an alkaline proximal convoluted tubule cell (e.g., hyperkalemia, or genetic and/or acquired disorders that cause a higher concentration of HCO_3^- in cells of the proximal convoluted tubule; these lesions diminish the exit of HCO_3^-) or decreased availability of adenosine diphosphate in these cells reflecting less work performed in proximal convoluted tubule cells because of a low filtered load of Na^+ due to a reduced GFR.[62] Another cause for a low rate of excretion of NH_4^+ is a low net secretion of H^+ in the distal nephron. This could be due to an H^+-ATPase defect (e.g., autoimmune and hypergammaglobulinemic disorders, including Sjögren's syndrome), backleak of H^+ (e.g., drugs such as amphotericin B), or disorders associated with the distal secretion of HCO_3^- (e.g., in certain patients with Southeast Asian ovalocytosis[63]).

Tools

ASSESSMENT OF THE RATE OF EXCRETION OF AMMONIUM IN THE URINE

Urine Osmolal Gap. Because the U_{OG} detects all NH_4^+ salts in the urine (Figure 26-13), it provides the best indirect estimate of U_{NH_4}, and hence the urine net charge (or urine anion gap) is no longer used for this purpose[64]:

$$U_{OG} = \text{Measured } U_{osm} - \text{Calculated } U_{osm}$$

$$\text{Calculated } U_{osm} = 2(U_{Na} + U_K) + U_{urea} + U_{Glu}$$
$$\text{(all values in mmol/L)}$$

$$\text{Concentration of } NH_4^+ \text{ in the urine} = U_{OG}/2$$

The premise of the test is that NH_4^+ is detected by its contribution to the U_{osm}.

The U_{NH_4}/U_{Cr} ratio in a spot urine sample is now used to assess the rate of excretion of NH_4^+. The rationale is that the rate of excretion of creatinine is relatively constant over the 24-hour period in complete timed urine collections.[37] In a patient with chronic metabolic acidosis the expected renal response is a U_{NH_4}/U_{Cr} ratio of more than 150 mmol of NH_4^+ per gram of creatinine (>15 mmol of NH_4^+ per mmol of creatinine).

DETERMINATION OF THE CAUSE OF THE LOW RATE OF AMMONIUM EXCRETION

Urine pH. The urine pH is *not* helpful in determining that the rate of excretion of NH_4^+ is low.[65] For example, at a urine pH of 6.0, the U_{NH_4} can be 20 mmol/L or 200 mmol/L (Figure 26-14). On the other hand, the basis for the low rate of excretion of NH_4^+ may be deduced from the urine pH. A urine pH that is approximately 5 suggests that the basis for a low rate of excretion of NH_4^+ is primarily a decreased availability of NH_3 in the medullary interstitial compartment. On the other hand, a urine pH that is above 6.5 suggests that

NH_4^+ excretion is low because there is a defect in H^+ secretion and/or that there was a high rate of excretion of HCO_3^- in the distal nephron.

Distal Hydrogen Ion Secretion. H^+ secretion in the distal nephron can be evaluated by measuring the Pco_2 in alkaline urine (U_{PCO_2}) during bicarbonate loading (Figure 26-15). A U_{PCO_2} that is approximately 70 mm Hg in a second-void alkaline urine indicates that H^+ secretion in the distal nephron is likely to be normal, whereas much lower U_{PCO_2} values suggest that distal H^+ secretion is impaired.[66] In patients with low net distal H^+ secretion, the U_{PCO_2} can be high if there is a lesion causing a backleak of H^+ from the lumen of the collecting ducts (e.g., use of amphotericin B[67]) or distal secretion of HCO_3^-, as in some patients with Southeast Asian ovalocytosis

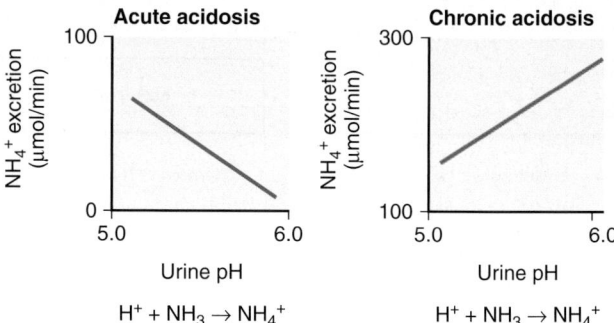

FIGURE 26-14 Failure of the urine pH to reveal the U_{NH_4}. As shown on the left, during acute metabolic acidosis, the NH_4^+ is only modestly higher, whereas the urine pH is low. This is because there is enhanced distal H^+ secretion, but a time lag exists before the rate of renal production of NH_4^+ is augmented. In contrast, during chronic metabolic acidosis as shown on the right, the rate of renal production of NH_4^+ is so high that the availability of NH_3 in the medullary interstitial compartment provides more NH_3 in the lumen of the medullary collecting duct than H^+ secretion in this nephron segment. Therefore, note the much higher NH_4^+ excretion rate at a urine pH of 6.

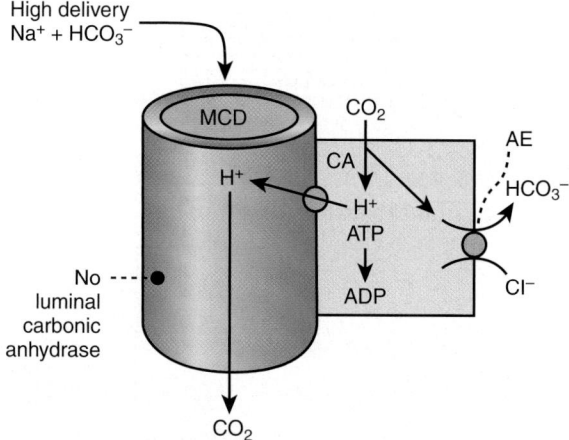

FIGURE 26-15 Use of the Pco_2 in alkaline urine to assess the distal secretion of H^+. The *cylinder* represents the medullary collecting duct (MCD), and the *rectangle* on its right side represents an α-intercalated cell, which contains a hydrogen-adenosine triphosphatase (H^+-ATPase) pump. The patient is given an oral load of $NaHCO_3$ to increase the filtered load of HCO_3^- and its delivery to the distal nephron. Because the luminal membranes of the MCD lack carbonic anhydrase, the carbonic acid formed is delivered to the lower urinary tract, where it decomposes to CO_2 and H_2O, and thereby causes the urine Pco_2 to be elevated (usually to approximately 70 mm Hg). An elevated Pco_2 in a second-void alkaline urine sample, indicates that there is no major defect in H^+ secretory capacity in this nephron segment.

who also have a second mutation in the Cl^-/HCO_3^- anion exchanger that leads to mistargeting of the exchanger to the luminal membrane of the α-intercalated cells.[58,63] A caveat with using this test is that the U_{PCO_2} is also influenced by the renal concentrating ability.[68]

Proximal Cell pH

Fractional Excretion of HCO_3^-. In patients with metabolic acidosis associated with a low capacity to reabsorb filtered HCO_3^- (e.g., disorders with defects in H^+ secretion in the proximal convoluted tubule, called *proximal renal tubular acidosis*), some would measure the fractional excretion of HCO_3^- after infusing $NaHCO_3$ to confirm this diagnosis. This is rarely needed in the authors' opinion. Often the results are far from clear (e.g., in a patient with an abnormal ECF volume or hypokalemia), and in addition, the test can impose a danger (e.g., in a patient with a low P_K). The condition will be detected clinically by failure to correct the metabolic acidosis despite administration of large amounts of $NaHCO_3$.

Rate of Citrate Excretion. The rate of excretion of citrate is a marker of pH in cells of the proximal convoluted tubule.[69] The daily rate of excretion of citrate in children and adults consuming their usual diets is approximately 400 mg (approximately 2 mmol citrate per gram [or per 10 mmol] of creatinine). Although the rate of excretion of citrate is very low during most forms of metabolic acidosis,[70] a notable exception is in disorders causing an alkaline proximal convoluted tubule cell pH.[71]

Clinical Approach to the Patient with Hyperchloremic Metabolic Acidosis

The steps in the clinical evaluation of patients with hyperchloremic metabolic acidosis based on the laboratory data detailed earlier are outlined in Flow Chart 26-15.

Consult 12: Determination of the Cause of Hyperchloremic Metabolic Acidosis

A 23-year-old woman has Southeast Asian ovalocytosis and was referred for assessment of hypokalemia. Findings of the physical examination were unremarkable. Results of laboratory tests on plasma and a spot urine sample are summarized in the following table. The U_{urea} was 220 mmol/L and the urine was glucose free.

	PLASMA	URINE		PLASMA	URINE
pH	7.35	6.8	Pco_2 (mm Hg)	30	—
HCO_3^- (mmol/L)	15	10	K^+ (mmol/L)	3.1	35
Na^+ (mmol/L)	140	75	Cl^- (mmol/L)	113	95
Anion gap (mEq/L)	12	15	Creatinine (mg/dL)	0.7	60
Osmolality (mOsm/L)	290	450	Citrate (mg/dL)	—	Low

Questions

What is the basis of the hyperchloremic metabolic acidosis?
What is the cause of the low rate of excretion of NH_4^+?

Discussion

WHAT IS THE BASIS OF THE HYPERCHLOREMIC METABOLIC ACIDOSIS?

The patient had a low U_{NH_4} because the measured U_{osm} (450 mOsm/kg H_2O) was very similar to the calculated U_{osm} of 440 mOsm/kg H_2O, that is, $2[U_{Na}$ (75 mmol/L) $+ U_K$

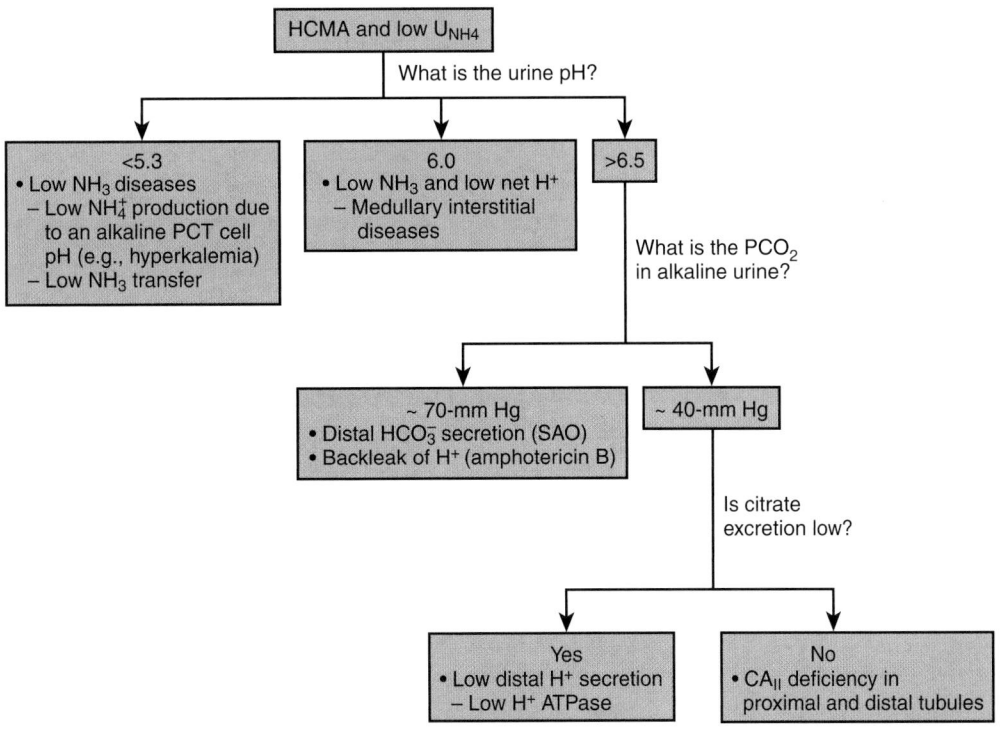

FLOW CHART 26-15

$(35 \text{ mmol/L})] + U_{urea}$ (220 mOsm/kg H_2O). Since the GFR was not very low, the diagnosis is a form of renal tubular acidosis.

WHAT IS THE CAUSE OF THE LOW RATE OF EXCRETION OF NH_4^+?

Urine pH. Because the urine pH is 6.8, the basis for the low rate of NH_4^+ excretion is a low *net* secretion of H^+ in the distal nephron (see Flow Chart 26-14).

Distal H^+ Secretion. After hypokalemia was corrected, the patient was given a load of $NaHCO_3$ to measure Pco_2 in alkaline urine. The Pco_2 in alkaline urine was 70 mm Hg (see Flow Chart 26-15). H^+ secretion by the proximal convoluted tubule seemed to be intact as the P_{HCO_3} remained in the normal range after she was given $NaHCO_3$. Because the U_{PCO_2} was unexpectedly high and a defect leading to a backleak of H^+ is unlikely, perhaps the patient's mutant Cl^-/HCO_3^- anion exchanger was targeted abnormally to the luminal membrane of α-intercalated cells. The U_{PCO_2} would be high due to distal secretion of HCO_3^- by alkaline intercalated cells.

Concluding Remarks

Given the tremendous advances in our understanding of the integrative physiology of the topics covered in this chapter and the many new insights gained from molecular and genetic advances, clinicians should now be able to pursue diagnoses right down to the enzyme or transporter that is defective. A physiology-based clinical approach is a crucial component to make more exact diagnoses and design more appropriate therapy for patients with disorders of water, Na^+, K^+, and/or acid-base homeostasis.

References

1. Kamel KS, Ethier JH, Richardson RMA, et al. Urine electrolytes and osmolality: when and how to use them. *Am J Nephrol.* 1990;10:89-102.
2. Halperin ML, Kamel KS. Use of the composition of the urine at the bedside: emphasis on physiological principles to provide insights into diagnostic and therapeutic issues. In: Seldin DW, Giebisch G, eds. *The kidney: physiology and pathophysiology.* ed 3. New York: Lippincott Williams & Wilkins; 2000.
3. Halperin ML, Kamel KS, Goldstein MB. *Fluid, electrolyte and acid-base physiology: a problem-based approach.* Philadelphia: Elsevier; 2010.
4. Zhai X, Fenton R, Andreasen A, et al. Aquaporin-1 is not expressed in descending thin limbs of short-loop nephrons. *J Am Soc Nephrol.* 2007;18:2937-2944.
5. Nielsen S, Frokiaer J, Marples D, et al. Aquaporins in the kidney: from molecules to medicine. *Physiol Rev.* 2002;82:205-244.
6. Halperin ML, Bichet DG, Oh MS. Integrative physiology of basal water permeability in the distal nephron: implications for the syndrome of inappropriate secretion of antidiuretic hormone. *Clin Nephrol.* 2001;56: 339-345.
7. Halperin ML, Kamel KS, Oh MS. Mechanisms to concentrate the urine: an opinion. *Curr Opin Nephrol Hypertens.* 2008;17:416-422.
8. Satlin LM, Carattino MD, Liu W, et al. Regulation of cation transport in the distal nephron by mechanical forces. *Am J Physiol Renal Physiol.* 2006;291:F923-F931.
9. Bohn D, Davids MR, Friedman O, et al. Acute and fatal hyponatraemia after resection of a craniopharyngioma: a preventable tragedy. *Quart J Med.* 2005;98:691-704.
10. Bichet DG, Mohammad R, Lonergan M, et al. Hemodynamic and coagulation responses to 1-desamino[8-D-arginine] vasopressin in patients with congenital nephrogenic diabetes insipidus. *N Engl J Med.* 1988;318:881-887.
11. Carlotti APCP, Bohn D, Mallie J-P, et al. Tonicity balance and not electrolyte-free water calculations more accurately guide therapy for acute changes in natremia. *Intensive Care Med.* 2001;27:921-924.
12. Shafiee MA, Charest AF, Cheema-Dhadli S, et al. Defining conditions that lead to the retention of water: the importance of the arterial sodium concentration. *Kidney Int.* 2005;67:613-621.
13. Oh MS, Carroll HJ, Roy A, et al. Chronic hyponatremia in the absence of ADH: possible role of decreased delivery of filtrate. *J Am Soc Nephrol.* 1997;8:108A.
14. Cherney DZI, Davids MR, Halperin ML. Acute hyponatraemia and MDMA ("Ecstasy"): insights from a quantitative and integrative analysis. *QJM.* 2002;95:475-483.
15. Laureno R, Karp BI. Pontine and extrapontine myelinolysis following rapid correction of hyponatremia. *Lancet.* 1988;1:1439-1441.
16. Kamel KS, Bichet DG, Halperin ML. Studies to clarify the pathophysiology of partial central diabetes insipidus. *Am J Nephrol.* 2001;37:1290-1293.
17. Gamble JL, McKhann CF, Butler AM, et al. An economy of water in renal function referable to urea. *Am J Physiol.* 1934;109:139-154.
18. Gowrishankar M, Lenga I, Cheung RY, et al. Minimum urine flow rate during water deprivation: importance of the permeability of urea in the inner medulla. *Kidney Int.* 1998;53:159-166.
19. Sands JM, Layton HE. The urine concentrating mechanism and urea transporters. In: Alpern RJ, Hebert SC, eds. *The kidney: physiology and pathophysiology.* ed 4. New York: Elsevier; 2008:1143-1178.
20. Deetjen P, Baeyer HV, Drexel H. Renal glucose transport. In: Seldin D, Giebisch G, eds. *The kidney: physiology and pathophysiology.* ed 2. New York: Raven Press; 1992:2873-2888.
21. Singh S, Bohn D, Cusimano M, et al. Cerebral salt wasting; truths, fallacies, theories and challenges. *Crit Care Med.* 2002;30:2575-2579.
22. Halperin ML, Rolleston FS. *Clinical detective stories: a problem-based approach to clinical cases in energy and acid-base metabolism.* ed 1. London: Portland Press; 1993.
23. Carlotti APCP, Guergerian A-M, Hyslop St Georgi, et al. Occult risk factor for the development of cerebral edema in children with diabetic ketoacidosis: possible role for stomach emptying. *Pediatr Diabetes.* 2009;10:26-37.
24. Davids MR, Edoute Y, Stock S, et al. Severe degree of hyperglycemia: novel insights revealed by the use of simple principles of integrative physiology. *QJM.* 2002;95:113-124.
25. Carlotti APCP, Bohn D, Halperin ML. Importance of timing of risk factors for cerebral oedema during therapy for diabetic ketoacidosis. *Arch Dis Child.* 2003;88:170-173.
26. Deleted in page proofs.
27. Napolova O, Urbach S, Davids MR, et al. How to assess the degree of extracellular fluid volume contraction in a patient with a severe degree of hyperglycemia. *Nephrol Dial Transplant.* 2003;18:2674-2677.
28. Watten RH, Morgan FM, Songkhla YN, et al. Water and electrolyte studies in cholera. *J Clin Invest.* 1959;38:1879-1889.
29. Mitch WE, Collier VU, Walser M. Creatinine metabolism in chronic renal failure. *Clin Sci.* 1980;58:327-335.
30. Zalunardo N, Lemaire M, Davids MR, et al. Acidosis in a patient with cholera: a need to redefine concepts. *QJM.* 2004;97:681-696.
31. Halperin ML, Oh MS, Kamel KS. Integrating effects of aquaporins, vasopressin, distal delivery of filtrate and residual water permeability on the magnitude of a water diuresis. *Nephron Physiol.* 2010;114(1):p11-p17.
32. Russell JM. Sodium-potassium-chloride cotransport. *Physiol Rev.* 2000;80:211-276.
33. Clausen T. Regulation of active Na^+-K^+ transport in skeletal muscle. *Physiol Rev.* 1986;66:542-580.
34. Solemani M, Burham C. Physiology and molecular aspects of the Na^+:HCO_3^- cotransporter in health and disease processes. *Kidney Int.* 2000;57:371-384.
35. Huth EJ, Squires RD, Elkinton JR. Experimental potassium depletion in normal human subjects. II. Renal and hormonal factors in the development of extracellular alkalosis during depletion. *J Clin Invest.* 1959;38:1149-1165.
36. Talbott JH, Schwab RS. Recent advances in the biochemistry and therapeutics of potassium salts. *N Engl J Med.* 1940;222:585-590.
37. Cockcroft DW, Gault MH. Prediction of creatinine clearance from serum creatinine. *Nephron.* 1976;16:31-41.
38. Steele A, deVeber H, Quaggin SE, et al. What is responsible for the diurnal variation in potassium excretion? *Am J Physiol.* 1994;36:R554-R560.
39. Cheema-Dhadli S, Lin S-H, Chong CK, et al. Requirements for a high rate of potassium excretion in rats consuming a low electrolyte diet. *J Physiol.* 2006;572(pt 2):493-501.
40. Halperin ML, Kamel KS. Potassium. *Lancet.* 1998;352:135-142.
41. Carlisle EJF, Donnelly SM, Ethier J, et al. Modulation of the secretion of potassium by accompanying anions in humans. *Kidney Int.* 1991;39:1206-1212.
42. Lin S-H, Lin Y-F, Halperin ML. Hypokalemia and paralysis: clues on admission to help in the differential diagnosis. *QJM.* 2001;94:133-139.
43. Lin S-H, Chu P, Cheng C-J, et al. Early diagnosis of thyrotoxic periodic paralysis: spot urine calcium to phosphate ratio. *Crit Care Med.* 2006 Dec;34(12):2984-2989.

44. Alazami M, Lin S-H, Chu C-J, et al. Unusual causes of hypokalaemia and paralysis. *QJM*. 2006;99:181-192.

45. Lin SH, Lin YF. Propranolol rapidly reverses paralysis, hypokalemia and hypophosphatemia in thyrotoxic periodic paralysis. *Am J Kidney Dis*. 2001;37:620-624.

46. Edwards CRW. Lessons from licorice. *N Engl J Med*. 1991;24:1242-1243.

47. Rosa RM, Williams ME, Epstein FH. Extrarenal potassium metabolism. In: Seldin DW, Giebisch G, eds. *The kidney: physiology and pathophysiology*. ed 2. New York: Raven Press; 1992:2165-2190.

48. Porte DJ. Sympathetic regulation of insulin secretion. *Arch Intern Med*. 1969;123:252-260.

49. Choi MJ, Fernandez PC, Patnaik A, et al. Trimethoprim induced hyperkalemia in a patient with AIDS. *N Engl J Med*. 1993;328:703-706.

50. Schreiber MS, Chen C-B, Lessan-Pezeshki M, et al. Antikaliuretic action of trimethoprim is minimized by raising urine pH. *Kidney Int*. 1996;49:82-87.

51. Rubin SI, Sonnenberg B, Zettle R, et al. Metabolic alkalosis mimicking the acute sequestration of HCl in rats: bucking the alkaline tide. *Clin Invest Med*. 1994;17:515-521.

52. Cheema-Dhadli S, Lin S-H, Halperin ML. Mechanisms used to dispose of a progressively increasing alkali load in the rat. *Am J Physiol*. 2002;282:F1049-F1055.

53. Shafiee MA, Napalova O, Charest AF, et al. When is sodium chloride the physiologically appropriate treatment for patients with metabolic alkalosis. *Indian J Nephrol*. 2003;13:45-54.

54. Smith HW, Dhatt G, Melia W, et al. Cystic fibrosis presenting as hyponatremic heat exhaustion. *BMJ*. 1995;310:579-580.

55. DeMars C, Hollister K, Tomassoni A, et al. Citric acidosis: a life-threatening cause of metabolic acidosis. *Ann Emerg Med*. 2001;38:588-591.

56. Kamel KS, Halperin ML. An improved approach to the patient with metabolic acidosis: a need for four amendments. *J Nephrol*. 2006;19(suppl 9):578-585.

57. Gowrishankar M, Kamel KS, Halperin ML. Buffering of a H+ load: A "brain-protein-centered" view. *J Am Soc Nephrol*. 2007;18:2278-2280.

58. Vasuvattakul S, Warner LC, Halperin ML. Quantitative role of the intracellular bicarbonate buffer system in response to an acute acid load. *Am J Physiol*. 1992;262:R305-R309.

59. Stewart PA. Modern quantitative acid-base chemistry. *Can J Physiol Pharmacol*. 1983;61:1444-1461.

60. Carlisle EJF, Donnelly SM, Vasuvattakul S, et al. Glue-sniffing and distal renal tubular acidosis: sticking to the facts. *J Am Soc Nephrol*. 1991;1:1019-1027.

61. Halperin ML. How much "new" bicarbonate is formed in the distal nephron in the process of net acid excretion? *Kidney Int*. 1989;35:1277-1281.

62. Halperin ML, Jungas RL, Pichette C, et al. A quantitative analysis of renal ammoniagenesis and energy balance: a theoretical approach. *Can J Physiol Pharmacol*. 1982;60:1431-1435.

63. Kaitwatcharachai C, Vasuvattakul S, Yenchitsomanus P, et al. Distal renal tubular acidosis in a patient with Southeast Asian ovalocytosis: possible interpretations of a high urine Pco$_2$. *Am J Kidney Dis*. 1999;33:1147-1152.

64. Dyck RF, Asthana S, Kalra J, et al. A modification of the urine osmolal gap: an improved method for estimating urine ammonium. *Am J Nephrol*. 1990;10:359-362.

65. Richardson RMA, Halperin ML. The urine pH: a potentially misleading diagnostic test in patients with hyperchloremic metabolic acidosis. *Am J Kidney Dis*. 1987;10:140-143.

66. Halperin ML, Goldstein MB, Haig A, et al. Studies on the pathogenesis of type I (distal) renal tubular acidosis as revealed by the urinary Pco$_2$ tensions. *J Clin Invest*. 1974;53:669-677.

67. Roscoe J, Goldstein M, Halperin M, et al. Effect of amphotericin B on urine acidification in rats: implications for the pathogenesis of distal renal tubular acidosis. *J Lab Clin Med*. 1977;89:463-470.

68. Berliner RW, DuBose TDJ. Carbon dioxide tension of alkaline urine. In: Seldin DW, Giebisch G, eds. *The kidney: physiology and pathophysiology*. ed 2. New York: Raven Press; 1992:2681-2694.

69. Simpson D. Citrate excretion: a window on renal metabolism. *Am J Physiol*. 1983;244:F223-F234.

70. Dedmond RE, Wrong O. The excretion of organic anion in renal tubular acidosis with particular reference to citrate. *Clin Sci*. 1962;22:19-32.

71. Halperin ML, Kamel KS, Ethier JH, et al. What is the underlying defect in patients with isolated, proximal renal tubular acidosis? *Am J Nephrol*. 1989;9:265-268.

Diagnostic Kidney Imaging

William D. Boswell, Jr., Hossein Jadvar, and Suzanne L. Palmer

Imaging has evolved since 1900, but the most changes have occurred since 1990, with marked improvements in technology. In the earliest forms of imaging, only anatomic information was available. Many different imaging examinations are now performed to evaluate the kidneys and the urinary tract; these methods provide not only anatomic but also functional and metabolic information. X-ray studies include plain radiography, intravenous urography (IVU), antegrade and retrograde pyelography, and computed tomography (CT). Most of these studies provide anatomic information, as does ultrasonography, which involves the use of high-frequency sound waves, not ionizing radiation. Magnetic resonance imaging (MRI) yields primarily anatomic information but has the potential for functional evaluation as well. Nuclear medicine studies contribute primarily functional information; positron emission tomography (PET) is a means of metabolic assessment. Each modality has something to offer in the evaluation of the kidneys, thanks to technical advances in all the areas. To properly evaluate the clinical situation in patients, it is important to understand the benefits, the limitations, and the diagnostic yields of each modality.

Imaging Techniques

Plain Radiograph of the Abdomen

Plain radiography of the abdomen has been used for years as the starting point or first step in the evaluation of the kidneys, as well as the rest of the abdomen. Radiography of the kidneys, ureters, and bladder (KUB) (Figure 27-1) is the first image of many studies of the abdomen, including IVU. The KUB examination alone yields little significant information. Renal size and contour may be estimated if the renal outlines can be seen, calcifications may be visualized, and other findings in the abdomen may be noted. If performed, it should be only the starting point in the evaluation of the kidneys. Intravenous iodinated contrast material is usually necessary for the opacification of the kidneys and urinary tract on radiographic examinations.

Intravenous Urography

IVU is still used by many physicians as the primary means of evaluating the kidneys and urinary tract.[1,2] IVU is also known as *intravenous pyelography*. The manner in which it is performed is best tailored to the clinical problem that is being studied. Scout or plain radiography of the abdomen (KUB) is performed before any contrast material is injected intravenously. This image provides a starting point for the investigation of the urinary tract, but it also serves as an overall assessment of the abdomen and pelvis in general. Subsequently, 25 to 40 g of iodine in the form of iodinated contrast material (generally 75 to 150 mL) is injected intravenously for the study. The method of choice is a bolus injection, which leads to peak iodine concentrations in the plasma. Infusion techniques for contrast medium injection have been used in the past, but the peak iodine concentration is lower,

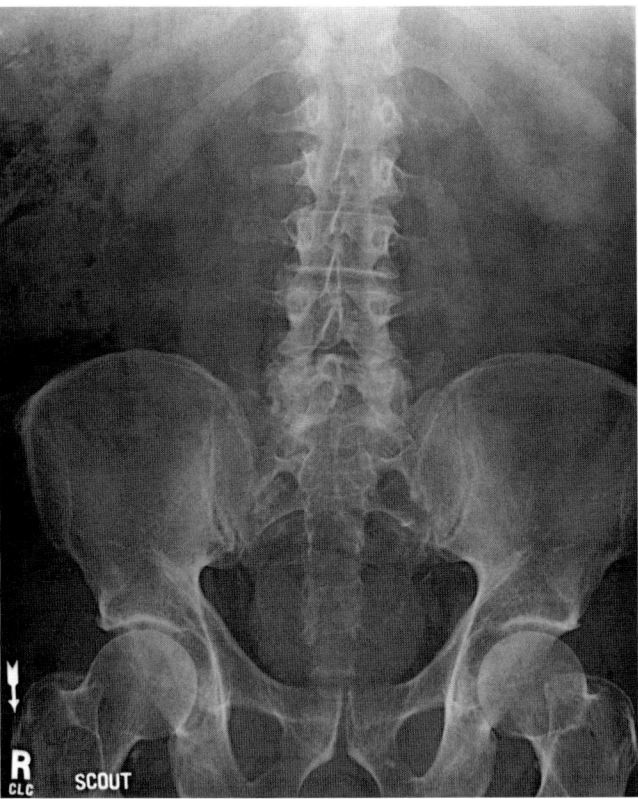

FIGURE 27-1 Plain radiograph of the abdomen: kidneys, ureters, and bladder (KUB). The kidneys lie posteriorly in the retroperitoneum in the upper abdomen. They are surrounded by fat. The ribs overlie the kidney, and bowel gas is visible in the right upper quadrant. The psoas muscles are also well viewed because retroperitoneal fat abuts them.

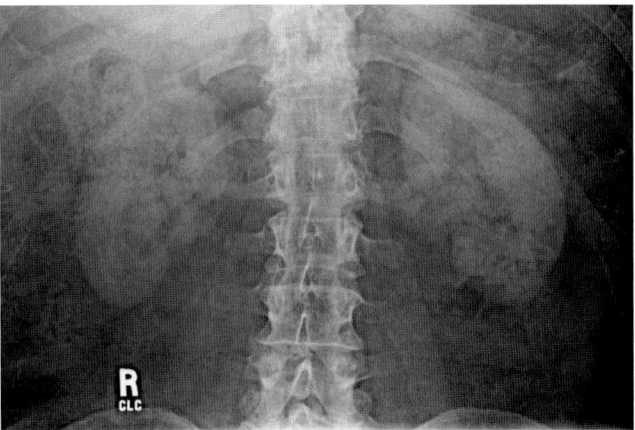

FIGURE 27-2 Intravenous urography: nephrogram. This image is obtained within 60 seconds after injection of contrast material. The kidneys are visible with smooth borders and the overlying bowel gas.

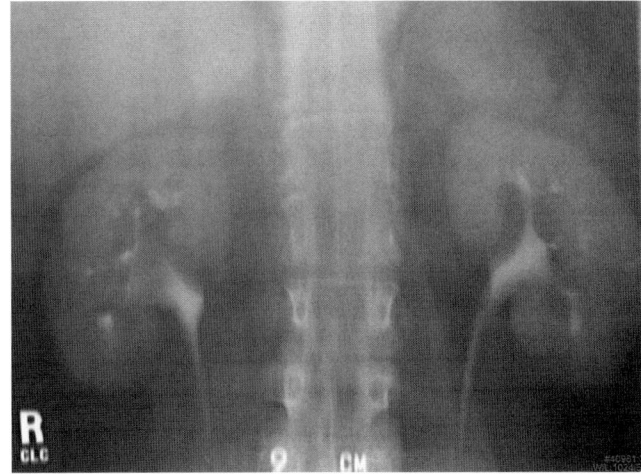

FIGURE 27-3 Intravenous urography: nephrotomogram. This image is obtained 5 to 7 minutes after the injection of contrast material. The overall outline of kidney is well depicted; the calyces, renal pelvis, and proximal ureter are opacified with the excreted contrast material.

and assessment findings overall are poorer. Timed sequential images of the kidneys and the remainder of the genitourinary system are then obtained.[3,4]

As the iodinated contrast medium is filtered by the glomerulus, the plasma iodine concentration determines the concentration of iodine in the glomerular filtrate. The higher the concentration of iodine injected, the greater the amount of iodine is within the kidneys, and thus the better the kidneys and subsequently the pelvicalyceal system are visualized.[5] The first image obtained in IVU is taken immediately after the injection of the contrast medium is completed (generally within 30 to 60 seconds). The nephrogram, or image of the kidneys, reflects the iodine concentration within the tubular system of the kidneys (Figure 27-2).[6] A higher plasma concentration of iodine leads to a higher iodine concentration in the glomerular filtrate. A higher iodine concentration in the tubular system results in a denser nephrogram, or better depiction of the kidneys. This nephrogram may be used to evaluate the size, shape, and contour of the kidneys. The overall appearance and density of the kidneys should be symmetric. The outlines of the kidneys are usually well depicted against the lower or darker appearance of perirenal fat. The presence of renal cortical scars and contour abnormalities caused by renal masses is usually well depicted. The kidneys are usually homogeneous in appearance throughout; a cyst or mass within a kidney causes an alteration in the overall density of the kidney.

By 3 to 5 minutes after the injection, the iodinated contrast material has reached the calyceal system. The excretion

of the contrast medium by the kidneys should always be symmetric, and the contrast material should appear in the calyces at similar times. The anatomic depiction of the calyces, infundibula, and pelvis is best displayed by 5 to 10 minutes after injection. Tomography may be performed, usually at 5 to 7 minutes, and it assists in the delineation of the renal contours, calyceal system, and renal pelvis (Figure 27-3). The calyces have a well-formed cup shape with sharp fornices and end in a thin, smooth infundibulum, which leads into the renal pelvis. The calyces may be compound or complex, whereby several end in one infundibulum. Abdominal compression may improve visualization of the renal elements early in the study; subsequent release allows for the drainage of the contrast material into the ureters and better visualization of the ureters. Imaging of the ureters is usually accomplished 10 to 15 minutes after injection. The drainage of the contrast material from the kidney and ureters allows for a global assessment of the urinary bladder (Figure 27-4). The total number of images needed for the complete study depends on the clinical question to be answered.[2-4]

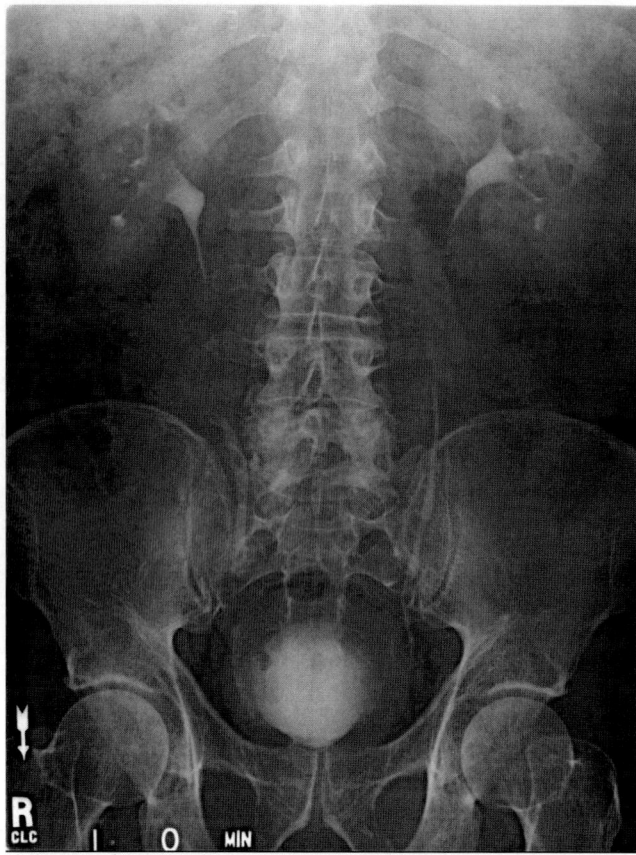

FIGURE 27-4 Intravenous urography: excretory phase. This image is obtained 10 minutes after the injection of the contrast material. The kidneys are well visualized; contrast material outlines the calyces, pelvis, ureters, and bladder.

Iodinated Contrast Media

Over the years, many different intravascular contrast media have been employed.[7] All these contrast agents contain iodine in the form of a triiodinated benzoic acid ring in solution. Contrast agents are characterized as either ionic or non-ionic and as either monomers or dimers. These agents are also known as *high osmolar contrast media* (HOCM), *low osmolar contrast media* (LOCM), or *isotonic contrast media* (IOCM), depending on their osmolality in relation to plasma. HOCM was used successfully from the 1960s through the 1990s for most intravascular applications, including IVU, CT, and angiographic applications. Since the introduction of LOCM in the mid-1980s and IOCM in the 1990s, there has been a gradual shift to these agents. Since the mid-2000s, virtually all studies involving intravascular injection of contrast material have been performed with LOCM or IOCM.

All the HOCM agents are ionic. They are categorized as diatrizoates, iothalamates, and metrizoates. These compounds are all water-soluble salt solutions, and all are hyperosmolar in relation to plasma. The osmolality of these compounds is generally five to eight times that of plasma (300 mOsm/L). The anion is the iodine-containing portion of the salt; the cation is generally either sodium or meglumine. Ionic media dissociate in water, whereas non-ionic media remain in solution. Within the bloodstream, these agents are not bound to any plasma proteins and are therefore filtered by the glomerulus directly. Virtually all of the contrast material injected is filtered by the glomerulus; in patients with normal renal function, there is no tubular reabsorption of excreted material.[7] In patients with renal failure, contrast media may be excreted via other routes, including the biliary system or gastrointestinal tract. All iodinated contrast agents are dialyzable.

Contrast material within the plasma has a half-life of 1 to 2 hours in patients with normal renal function. Virtually all contrast material is excreted by the kidneys within 24 hours. The volume of contrast material injected, the concentration of contrast material within the plasma, and the glomerular filtration rate (GFR) determine the amount of contrast material excreted into the collecting systems and, subsequently, the calyces, renal pelvis, and ureters. Thus, in patients with normal renal function, the concentration of iodine in the plasma ultimately determines the quality of the study findings. Other factors, most particularly the state of hydration, also come into play. Changes in the tubular reabsorption of water along the nephron affects the concentration of iodine within the tubule and thus the subsequent iodine concentration in the urine, which is visualized in the calyces and renal pelvis on the radiographic studies.

Most LOCM agents are non-ionic compounds, with the exception of Ioxaglate, which is an ionic dimer.[8] These compounds do not dissociate in solution. The LOCM are also hyperosmolar in relation to plasma but to a much lesser degree than HOCM. The osmolality of LOCM is generally two to three times that of plasma. These agents, like HOCM, are filtered by the glomerulus but have a higher concentration within the tubular system because less water is reabsorbed. The osmotic effect of LOCM is less than that of HOCM in the tubular system and at a higher overall concentration; therefore, within the urine, the quality of imaging studies is generally improved.[9] Iohexol, Iopamidol, and Ioversol make up the group of non-ionic LOCM agents.

IOCM agents are non-ionic dimers: Iodixanol and Iotrol. These agents are isotonic in relation to plasma. They, like HOCM and LOCM, are handled in the kidneys and filtered by the glomerulus with no tubular reabsorption or excretion. These agents are generally used not for renal imaging but almost exclusively for cardiac catheterizations. Cost is the major difference; IOCM are two to four times more expensive.

Reactions to the injection of any of the contrast agents may occur. These reactions are not "allergic" responses in the sense of an antigen-antibody reaction.[10] No antibodies to contrast media have ever been isolated. The reactions, however, have the appearance of allergic reactions. Although the majority of these reactions are mild or minor, severe reactions and deaths do occur. With ionic HOCM agents, the reaction rate in the general population is 5% to 6%.[11] Among patients with a history of allergy, the reaction rate is 10% to 12%, and among those who have had a previous reaction to intravenous administration of contrast material, the rate is 15% to 20%. The rates of reactions to LOCM and IOCM agents are much lower, in the range of 1% to 2%.[12,13] In children, the rate of adverse reaction to LOCM in very low (<0.5%).[14] Most reactions are mild, consisting of flushing, nausea, and vomiting, and treatment is not required. Mild dermal reactions, primarily urticaria, do occur and may or may not necessitate treatment. Moderate and severe reactions, which occur with considerably less frequency, include bronchospasm, laryngeal edema, seizures, arrhythmias, syncope shock, and cardiac arrest. All moderate and severe reactions necessitate treatment. The risk of death has decreased from 1 per 8000 to 1 per 12,000 with HOCM and from 1 per 75,000 to 1 per 100,000 with LOCM and IOCM.[12]

Because the reaction that occurs in patients after injection of contrast material is not antigen-antibody mediated, pretesting plays no role.[15] Neither the rate of injection nor the dose of contrast material has been clearly established as a determinant in the occurrence of contrast material–related reactions.[12,16] Premedication with antihistamines is used in some patients with a history of minor reactions. The use of glucocorticoids plus histamine-1 blockers and histamine-2 blockers is reserved for patients who need to be studied with iodinated contrast agents and have a history of prior contrast material–related reaction, usually moderate or severe in nature. Few if any controlled studies have yielded data with which to critically evaluate this pretreatment regimen.[17]

Contrast material–related nephropathy occurs with a significant frequency, especially among hospitalized patients. The administration of iodinated contrast agents is the third leading cause of hospital-acquired acute kidney injury (AKI)/acute renal failure (ARF), after surgery and hypotension.[18-20] Data from two studies, however, suggest that the risk of contrast material–related nephropathy is similar in patients who undergo a radiographic study but do not receive any iodinated contrast agent.[21,22]

The use of iso-osmolar contrast material does not appear to reduce the risk of contrast material–related nephropathy.[23] Contrast material–related nephropathy has been most frequently studied in patients with intraarterial injections of contrast media (i.e., cardiac catheterizations). The incidence among patients after intravenous administration of contrast material is believed to be much lower than among patients with intraarterially administered contrast material. Other studies have shown that the use of intravenous contrast agents in patients at high risk is not likely to produce a permanent decrease in renal function.[24] Patients at risk may be identified with estimated GFR.[25] The cause of contrast material–related nephropathy is unknown but believed to be multifactorial.[20] Contrast material–induced nephropathy is commonly defined as AKI occurring within 48 hours of the intravascular administration of iodinated contrast material, for which no other causes are readily apparent. The definition is actually quite variable within the literature, but the condition is most commonly associated with a rise in serum creatinine level of 0.5 mg/dL above a baseline value.[26,27]

Most cases of contrast material–related nephropathy manifest as an asymptomatic, transient decrease in renal function and are nonoliguric. The serum creatinine level usually peaks at 3 to 5 days and returns to baseline level within 10 to 14 days. Oliguric kidney injury occurs in a much smaller group of patients, with a peak creatinine elevation at 5 to 10 days and a return to baseline values by 14 to 21 days. In rare cases, oliguric kidney injury related to administration of contrast media may necessitate short- or long-term dialysis.

Risk factors for patients who may develop contrast material–induced AKI are well known.[28] These include preexisting renal impairment, diabetes with renal insufficiency, dehydration, advancing age, congestive heart failure, ongoing treatment with nephrotoxic drugs, peripheral vascular disease, multiple myeloma, cirrhosis and liver failure, prior load of contrast material within 48 to 72 hours, and use of diuretics, especially furosemide.[29,30] Contrast material–related

AKI/ARF rarely if ever occurs in individuals who are well hydrated and have normal renal function.[31,32] Although data are somewhat conflicting, contrast material–related nephropathy occurs with all types of contrast material.[26,33,34]

Contrast material–induced nephropathy is best prevented by recognition of the known risk factors.[35] Proper hydration is of paramount importance and must be begun 12 hours before the study with contrast material.[36,37] Various methods of pretreatment have been tried with variable success. These include mannitol, diuretics, calcium channel blockers, adenosine antagonists (theophylline), dopamine agonists, *N*-acetylcysteine, and sodium bicarbonate.[38-43] Morikawa and colleagues[44] suggested that atrial natriuretic peptide may of useful in preventing contrast material–related nephropathy in patients with chronic renal failure who were undergoing angiography with contrast media. Their work indicated that this peptide was more likely to be protective of glomerular function than renal tubular function. In our institution, patients with an estimated GFR of less than 60 mL/minute/1.73 m^2 are hydrated with 500 to 1000 mL of normal saline before the administration of contrast medium and continue to be hydrated after the examination with an additional 500 to 1000 mL of normal saline. *N*-acetylcysteine is added for patients with estimated GFR of less than 30 and for patients who will undergo major surgical procedures within 24 to 48 hours. All patients, regardless of estimated GFR, are encouraged to remain well hydrated both before and after contrast studies. Patients who are allowed nothing by mouth overnight are not allowed to become dehydrated before CT studies. Again, with appropriate hydration and normal renal function, contrast material–related nephropathy rarely occurs.

Ultrasonography

Ultrasonography is a leading diagnostic examination used in the investigation of the kidneys and urinary tract.[44a] It is noninvasive and requires little or no preparation of patients. It is the first-line examination in azotemic patients for assessing renal size and the presence or absence of hydronephrosis and obstruction. It is used to assess the vasculature of native and transplanted kidneys. Ultrasonography is also used to evaluate renal structure and to characterize renal masses. As a guide for renal biopsy, ultrasonography has helped to decrease morbidity and mortality.

Diagnostic ultrasonography is an outgrowth of sound navigation and ranging (sonar) technology, used first during World War II for the detection of objects under water. In medical ultrasonography, high-frequency sound waves are used to investigate diagnostic problems. In the abdomen and, more particularly, the kidneys, 2.5- to 4.0-mHz sound waves are generally employed.

The ultrasound unit consists of a transducer, which sends and receives the sound waves; a microprocessor or computer, which obtains and processes the returning signal; and an image display system or monitor, which displays the processed images. The piezoelectric transducer converts electrical energy into high-frequency sound waves that are transmitted through the patient's body. It converts the returning reflected sound waves back into electrical energy that can be processed by the computer. Sound travels as a waveform through the tissues being imaged. The speed of the sound wave depends on the

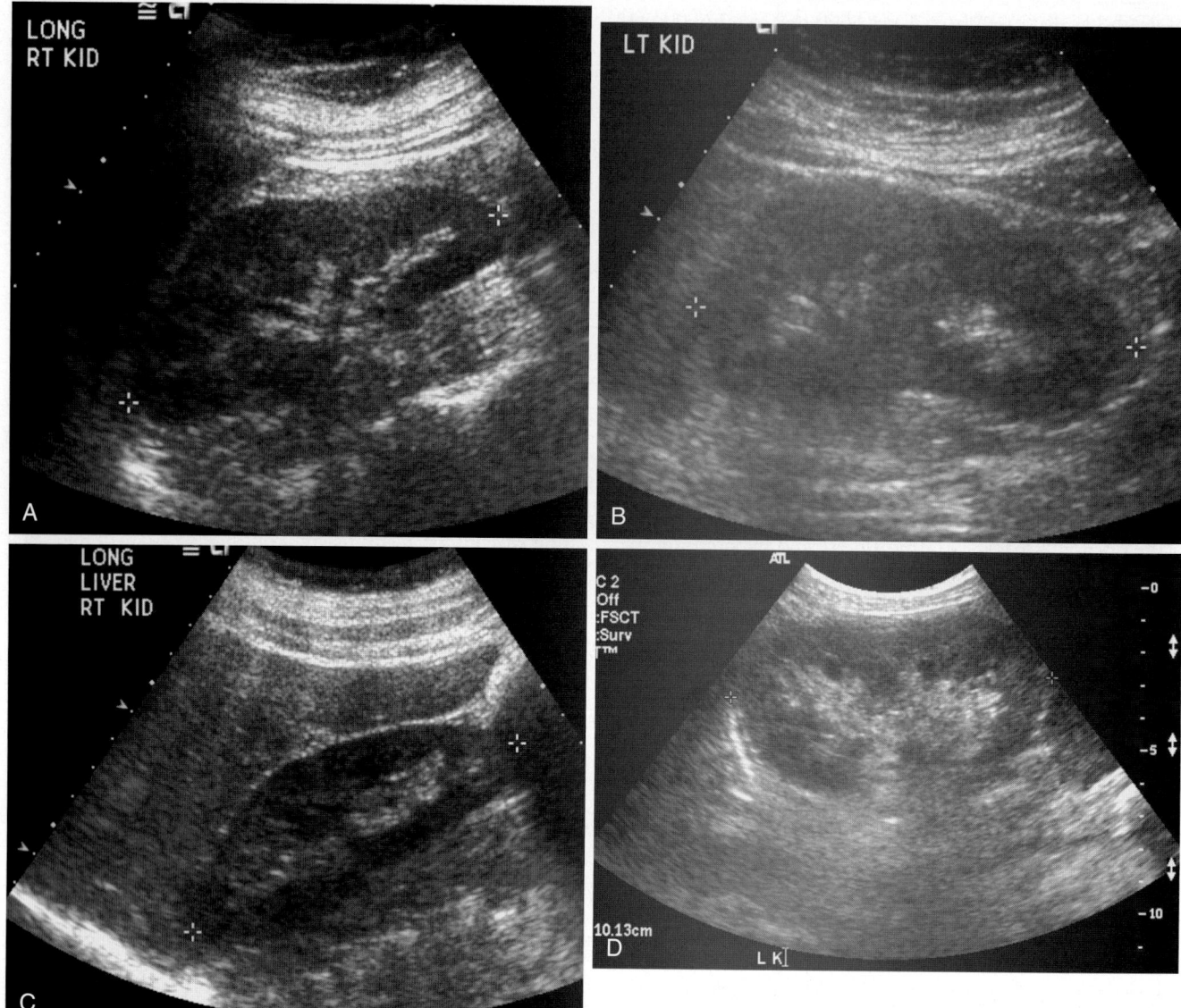

FIGURE 27-5 Renal ultrasonography: normal kidneys. Normal right kidneys (**A, C**) and normal left kidneys (**B, D**) are shown. The central echogenic structure represents the vascular elements, calyces, and renal sinus fat. The peripheral cortex is noted to be smooth and regular. Renal pyramids are depicted as hypoechoic structures between the central echo complex and the cortex in **D**.

tissue through which it is traveling. In air, sound travels at 331 m per second, and in the soft tissues of the body, it travels at approximately 1540 m per second.

Different tissues and the interface between these tissues have different acoustic impedance. As the sound wave travels through different tissues, part of the wave is reflected back to the transducer. The depth of the tissue interface is measured by the time the sound wave takes to return to the transducer. A gray-scale image is produced by the measured reflected sound, in which the intensity of the pixels (picture elements) are proportional to the intensities of the reflected sound (Figure 27-5). When the acoustic interfaces are quite large, strong echoes result. These are known as *specular reflectors* and are visible from the renal capsule and bladder wall. Nonspecular reflectors generate echoes of lower amplitude and are visible in the renal parenchyma. Strong reflection of sound by bone and air results in little or no information from the tissues beneath; this appearance is known as *shadowing*. Lack

of acoustic impedance as observed in fluid-filled structures, such as the urinary bladder and renal cysts, allows the sound waves to penetrate further, which results in a relative increase in intensity distal to the structures; this is known as *increased through-transmission*. Real-time ultrasonography, which provides sequential images at a rapid frame rate, allows the demonstration of motion of organs and pulsation of vessels.

Doppler ultrasonography, based on the Doppler frequency shift of the sound wave caused by moving objects, can be used to assess venous and arterial blood flow (Figure 27-6).[45,46] Assessment of the waveforms can be used in diagnosis. The peripheral arterial resistance can be measured within the kidneys as resistive index:

Resistive index = Peak systolic velocity − Lowest diastolic
velocity / Peak systolic velocity

(Figure 27-7). In general, a normal resistive index is 0.70 or less. Native and transplanted kidneys can be evaluated.

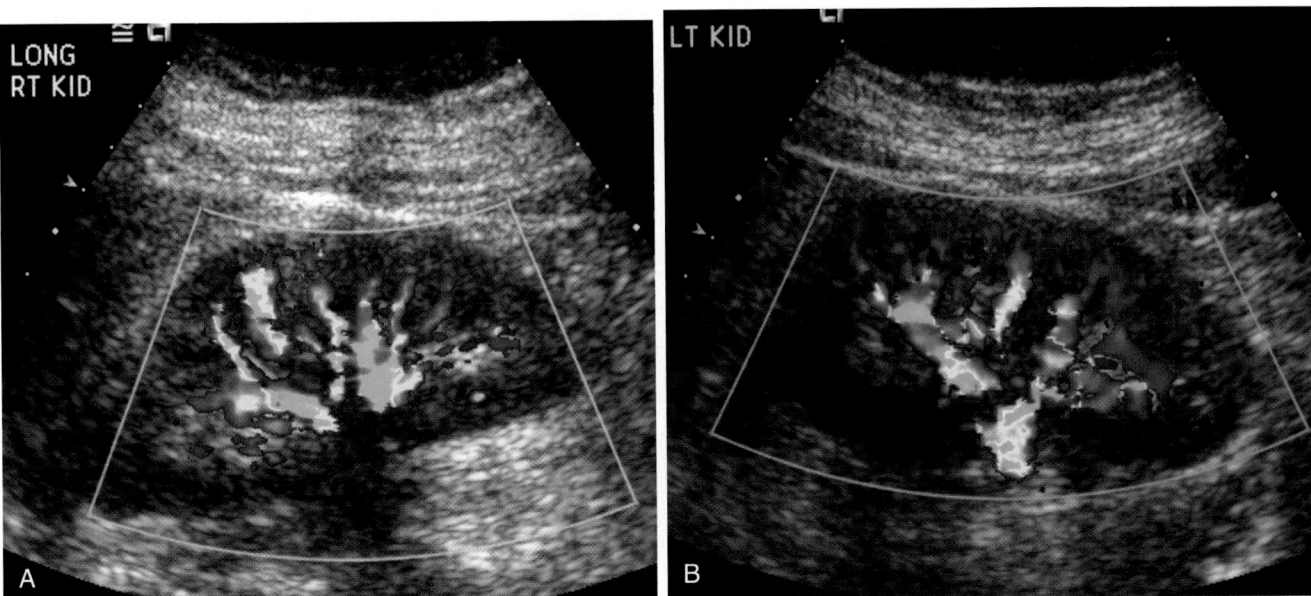

FIGURE 27-6 Color Doppler ultrasonography: normal kidneys. Normal right (**A**) and left (**B**) kidneys are visible. The red echogenic areas represent arterial flow (flow toward the transducer), and blue echogenic areas represent venous flow (flow away from the transducer).

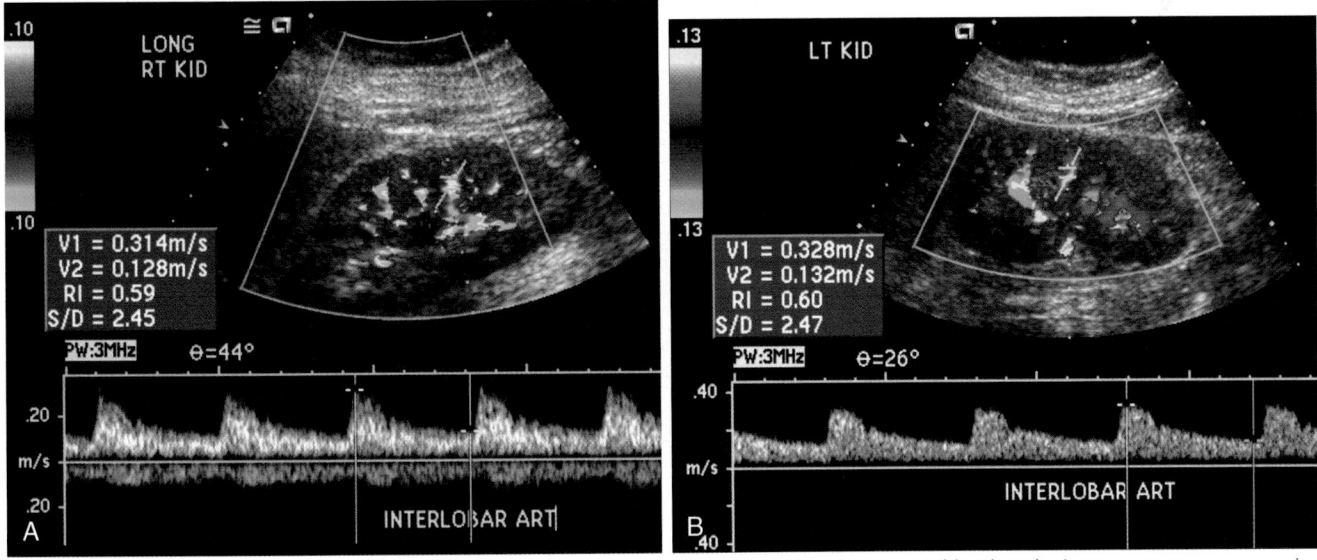

FIGURE 27-7 Power Doppler ultrasonography: normal kidneys. Normal right (**A**) and left (**B**) kidneys are visible. The color image represents a summation of all flow—arterial and venous—within the kidney.

Increased resistive index is a nonspecific indicator of disease and a sign of increased peripheral vascular resistance.[47] With color Doppler ultrasonography, the image is encoded with colors assigned to the pixels representing the direction, velocity, and volume of flow within vessels.[46] In power Doppler ultrasonography, the amplitude of the signal is used to produce a color map of the intrarenal vasculature and flow within the kidneys (Figure 27-8).[45]

Ultrasonography: Normal Anatomy

The kidneys are located within Gerota's fascia and are surrounded by perinephric fat in the retroperitoneum. Ultrasonographic images of the kidneys are generally obtained in the longitudinal, transverse, and parasagittal planes.[48] The appearance of the perinephric fat varies from slightly less echogenic to highly echogenic in comparison with the renal cortex. The renal capsule is visible as an echogenic line surrounding the kidney. The centrally located renal sinus and hilum, containing renal sinus fat, vessels, and the collecting system, are usually echogenic because of the presence of renal sinus fat (see Figure 27-5). The amount of renal sinus fat generally increases with age. Tubular structures corresponding to vessels and the collecting system may be visible in the renal hilum. Color Doppler ultrasonography may be used to differentiate the vessels from the collecting system.

Overall renal echogenicity of the liver on the right is generally compared with that of the spleen on the left (see Figure 27-5). The normal renal cortex is less echogenic than the liver and spleen. Underlying liver disease may alter this picture. The medullary pyramids are hypoechoic, and their triangular shape points to the renal hilum. The renal cortex lies peripherally,

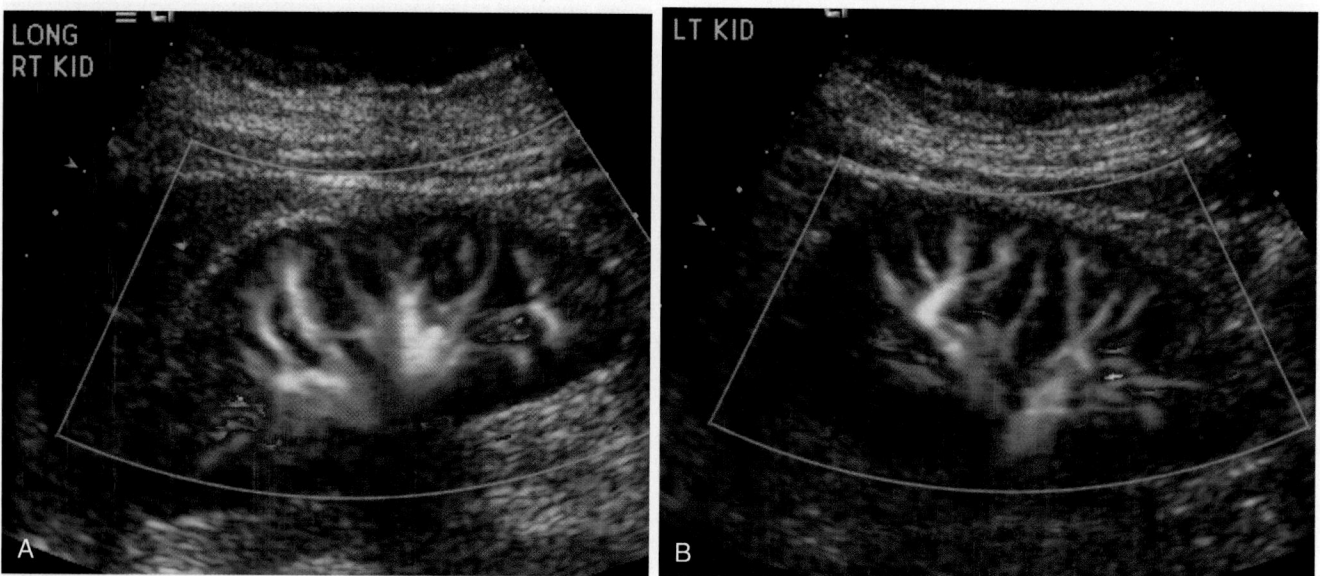

FIGURE 27-8 Power Doppler ultrasonography: normal kidneys. Normal right (**A**) and left (**B**) kidneys are visible. The waveforms within the interlobar arteries are visualized with the resistive indices calculated for each kidney.

and the separation from the medulla is usually demarcated by an echogenic focus attributable to the arcuate arteries along the corticomedullary junction. Columns of Bertin have the same echogenicity as the renal cortex and separate the renal pyramids. On occasion, a column of Bertin may appear large and simulates a mass, a "pseudotumor." Even when a column of Bertin is large or prominent, its echogenicity is similar to that of the cortex, and the vascular pattern observed on power Doppler images is also the same.

Renal size is easily measured ultrasonographically. The normal longitudinal dimension of the right kidney is 11 cm ± 1 cm, and that of the left kidney is 11.5 cm ± 1 cm. The contours of the kidneys are usually smooth; occasionally, some slight nodularity is present as a result of fetal lobulation. The renal arteries and veins may be visible extending from the renal hilum to the aorta and inferior vena cava (IVC). The veins lie anterior to the arteries. The renal arterial branching pattern within the kidneys may be visible on color Doppler ultrasonography (see Figure 27-6).[49] The resistive indices of the main, intralobar, and arcuate vessels may be calculated (see Figure 27-7). With power Doppler imaging, the intrarenal vasculature may be assessed; it demonstrates an overall increased pattern in the cortex in relation to the medulla, which corresponds to the normal arterial flow to the kidney (see Figure 27-8).[50,51] The renal calyces and collecting systems are not typically visible with ultrasonography unless fullness or distension caused by diuresis or obstruction is present. When visible, the collecting systems are branching anechoic structures in the renal sinus fat, connecting together to the renal pelvis. The urinary bladder is visible in the pelvis as a fluid-filled sonolucent structure. The entrance of the ureters into the bladder at the trigone may be visualized on color Doppler ultrasonography. Ureteral jets should be visible bilaterally.

When a kidney is not identified in its normal location in the retroperitoneum, the remainder of the abdomen and pelvis should be assessed. Ectopic kidneys may lie lower in the abdomen or within the pelvis and may also be located on the opposite side; the kidneys may even be fused (horseshoe kidneys). Horseshoe kidneys tend to lie lower in the

retroperitoneum, and their axes may be different from those of normal kidneys.

Increased echogenicity within the renal cortex may be suggestive of the presence of renal parenchymal disease.[51,52] The echogenicity of the renal cortex may be increased in patients with either acute or chronic kidney injury. This finding is nonspecific and is not correlated with the degree or severity of kidney injury. The finding is bilateral. The increased cortical echogenicity in patients with chronic kidney injury is generally related to interstitial fibrosis.[47] A patient with small, echogenic kidneys usually has end-stage kidney disease. Ultrasonography has been very useful in directing renal biopsy in patients with either acute or chronic kidney injury. Identification and localization of the kidneys greatly facilitate the procedure. The use of ultrasonography has decreased both the procedure time and rates of morbidity and mortality.

Computed Tomography

CT has become an essential tool for diagnosis in virtually all areas of the body. In the genitourinary tract, it has supplanted IVU, which had been the mainstay of diagnosis for years. Even in areas in which ultrasonography is employed, CT offers a complementary and sometimes superior means of imaging. CT is now the first examination to be performed in patients with renal colic, renal stone disease, renal trauma, renal infection and abscess, renal mass, hematuria, and urothelial abnormalities.

CT has been heralded as the greatest improvement in diagnostic radiology since Wilhelm Roentgen discovered x-rays in 1895. Sir Godfrey Hounsfield developed the first CT scanner in 1970.[53] The first clinical applications in 1971 were in the head. The first body CT scanner was installed in Georgetown University Medical Center in 1974. The field has grown rapidly since that time, with new technical innovations, image processing, and visualization methods. For his outstanding work in the field and for demonstrating the unique and remarkable clinical capabilities of CT, Hounsfield was awarded the Nobel Prize for Medicine in 1979.

CT is the computer reconstruction of a radiographically generated image that typically depicts a slice through the area being studied in the body. The x-ray tube produces a highly collimated fan-bean and is mounted opposite an array of electronic detectors. This system rotates in tandem around the patient. The detector system collects hundreds of thousands of samples representing the attenuation of the x-ray along the line formed from the x-ray source to the detector as the rotation occurs. These data are transferred to a computer, which reconstructs the image. The image may then be displayed on a computer monitor or transferred to radiographic film for reviewing.

The CT image is actually made up of numerous pixels (picture elements), each corresponding to a CT number representing the amount of x-rays absorbed by the patient at a particular point in the cross-sectional image. These pixels represent a two-dimensional display of a three-dimensional object. Each pixel element actually has a third dimension: the slice thickness or depth. Thus, the CT number is actually the average attenuation of x-rays of all the tissues within a specific volume element, a voxel, which is used to create the individual image or slice.

CT numbers are the x-ray attenuation of each voxel in relation to the x-ray attenuation of water (whose CT number is 0). Tissues that attenuate more x-rays than does water have positive CT numbers, and those with less x-ray attenuation than water have negative numbers. Bone may have a CT number higher than 1000, whereas air in the lungs has a CT number of approximately –1000. Different shades of gray on a scale of white to black are assigned to the CT numbers (highest number is depicted as white, lowest as black). The image of each slice is thus created on the monitor; the image may be manipulated to accentuate the regions being imaged. The image data is constant, but by varying the range of CT numbers, the appearance of the image may be changed; this ability is a key element of any digital image.

The initial CT scanners were relatively slow because the technology required a point-and-shoot process. One slice was obtained, the patient moved, and the next slice obtained. With this initial generation of body CT scanners, a scan of the abdomen took 4 minutes or more to complete. In 1990, helical/spiral technology was introduced in which the x-ray tube and detector system continuously rotated around the patient, and the patient moved continuously through the gantry. Scan time through the abdomen was reduced to 25 to 35 seconds. After helical/spiral CT, a two-detector system was introduced that produced two slices for every 360-degree rotation of the x-ray tube and detector system. This was the first scanner for multidetector CT (MDCT). By 1998, four-detector systems were introduced by all manufacturers. Today, 64-slice/detector systems are generally the standard; 128-, 256-, and 320-detector systems are also in use, primarily for advanced applications, such as computed tomographic angiography (CTA) for the coronary arteries. With MDCT, each 360-degree rotation results in the number of slices equal to the number of detectors (i.e., a 64-detector system produces 64 slices in one 360-degree rotation). These technologic advances have led to dramatic increase in the speed of scans (4 to 10 seconds), routine use of thin slices or collimation (1 to 2 mm thick), and marked improvement in spatial resolution (ability to display small objects clearly).[54]

As a result of the faster scanning times, enhancement by intravenous contrast material has improved and become more widely used.[55] For example, the kidneys can be scanned in the arterial, venous, nephrographic, and delay phases, which allows for a more complete assessment. With a 16- to 64-detector scan, a single acquisition of CT data takes from 3 to 7 seconds, and slice thickness is less than 1 mm. The images are normally displayed as transverse or axial images. As the slice thickness has been reduced to the point that the voxel has become a cube or near cube (isotropic voxel), sagittal, coronal, oblique, and off-axis images may be displayed with no loss of resolution. The data acquisition may also be displayed as a three-dimensional volumetric display with the regions of interest highlighted.[54] In scanning today, the patient holds his or her breath once, which helps eliminate virtually all motion artifacts and the misregistration artifacts observed with breathing. In imaging of the heart, electrocardiographic gated acquisition to the cardiac cycle produces an image in which the motion of the heart is frozen, which results in clear assessment of the coronary arteries, valves, and related anatomy. The kidneys are well suited for assessment with MDCT, inasmuch as sagittal, coronal, and three-dimensional displays add to the information content of the study.[55-59]

Computed tomographic urography (CTU), introduced in 1999 to 2000, is an outgrowth of the advances made with technology for MDCT and state-of-the-art workstations with their added computer processing and display capabilities.[54,60] CTU provides a complete examination of the kidneys and the remainder of genitourinary tract. CTU is used to assess the kidney as a whole (anatomic), the vascular tree (function and perfusion), and the excretory (urothelial) patterns. Noncontrast scans enable assessment of renal calculi, high-density cysts, and contour abnormalities.[61] Early phase scans (12 to 15 seconds) enable arterial assessment. Scanning at 25 to 30 seconds yields a combined arterial-venous phase image with clear corticomedullary differentiation. At 90 to 100 seconds, true nephrographic phase imaging of the kidneys is obtained.[55] Delayed imaging, typically at 3 to 7 minutes and up to 10 minutes, enables the evaluation of the urothelium (calyces, renal pelvis, ureters, and bladder) in the excretory phase.[62] Axial images, multiplanar reconstructions, maximum-intensity projection (MIP) images, and three-dimensional volumetric displays complement each other in CTU. Properly performed, CTU is superior to IVU.[63-66]

Computed Tomography Technique

Noncontrast images are obtained through the kidneys and the remainder of the genitourinary tract to the pelvic floor if stone disease is the primary problem. In the case of vascular problems and renal masses, arterial-venous phase imaging is usually required and accomplished by a rapid bolus injection of iodinated contrast medium, generally 4 to 5 mL/second and a volume of 100 to 120 mL, with scans in the arterial-venous phases 25 to 30 seconds after injection. When needed as in cases of suspected renal artery stenosis, true arterial phase imaging may begin 12 to 15 seconds after injection. Nephrographic imaging 90 to 100 seconds after injection is subsequently performed, with excretory imaging to follow. Slice thickness is generally 2 mm or less, which allows for workstation reconstruction as necessary. The radiation dose for this technique is approximately 1.5 times that of IVU, but the information content is exceedingly higher.

Computed Tomography Anatomy

The kidneys lie in the retroperitoneum, surrounded by Gerota's fascia in the perinephric space. Fat generally outlines the kidneys; the liver is anterior-superior on the right, the spleen superior on the left, and the spine, aorta, and IVC central between the kidneys (Figure 27-9). The abdominal contents lie anteriorly. This anatomy is easily viewed in all phases of scanning. With arterial and venous phase scans, the renal arteries are easily seen, generally posterior to the venous structures (Figure 27-10). The right renal artery is located behind the IVC (Figure 27-11). The left renal vein courses anterior to the aorta and then enters the IVC, and the right renal vein is generally viewed obliquely entering the IVC. The adrenal glands are found in a location superior to the upper poles of the kidneys. In venous phase imaging, it is easy to distinguish the renal cortex from the medulla. Cortical thickness and medullary appearance may be assessed easily (see Figure 27-10). The nephrographic phase should

demonstrate the symmetric enhancement for each of the kidneys (Figure 27-12).[55] At 7 to 10 minutes in the excretory phase, the calyces should be well depicted with sharp fornices, a cupped central section, and a narrow smooth infundibulum leading to the renal pelvis (Figure 27-13).[62] Coronal images in a slab MIP format display this to the best advantage. Three-dimensional volumetric reformations also may display the anatomic delay (Figure 27-14).[65] The excretory phase images also delineate the ureters from the renal pelvis to the bladder. A curved reformatted series of images or three-dimensional display is needed to display the ureters in their entirety. Proper tailoring of the examination to the diagnostic problem provides guidance for the correct imaging acquisition.[56,58,66]

Magnetic Resonance Imaging

Like CT, MRI is a computer-based, multiplanar imaging modality. Instead of ionizing radiation, however, electromagnetic radiation is used in MRI. MRI is an alternative to contrast material–enhanced CT, especially in patients with allergy to iodinated contrast material and in patients for whom reduction of radiation exposure is desired, such as pregnant women and children. MRI routinely allows detailed tissue characterization of the kidney and surrounding structures. The properties of physics underlying MRI are complex and are addressed only briefly.

Clinical MRI is based on the interaction of hydrogen ions (protons) and radiofrequency waves in the presence of a strong magnetic field.[67-69] The strong magnetic field, called the *external magnetic field*, is generated by a large-bore, high–field strength magnet. Most magnets in clinical use are superconducting magnets. The magnet strength is measured in teslas (T) and can range from 0.2 to 3 T for clinical imaging and up to 15 T for animal research. Renal imaging is performed best on high-field magnets (1.5 to 3 T) that allow for higher spatial resolution and faster imaging.

Images of the patient are obtained through a multistep process of energy transfer and signal transmission. When a patient is placed in the magnet, the mobile protons associated with fat and water molecules align longitudinal to the external magnetic field. No signal is obtained unless a

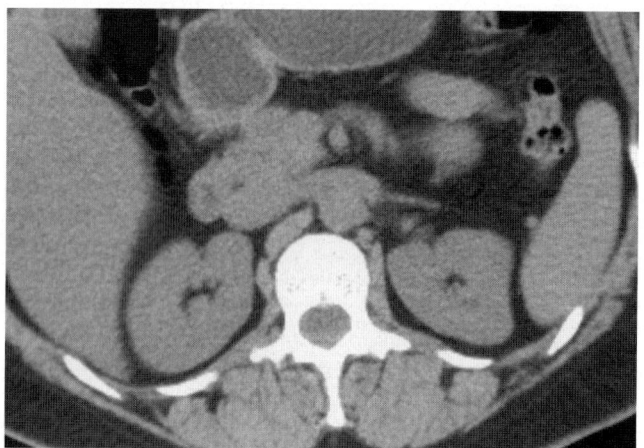

FIGURE 27-9 Noncontrast computed tomographic scan through the midportion of normal kidneys. The kidneys lie in the retroperitoneum with the lumbar spine and psoas muscles more centrally. The liver is anterolateral to the right kidney, and the spleen anterolateral to the left kidney.

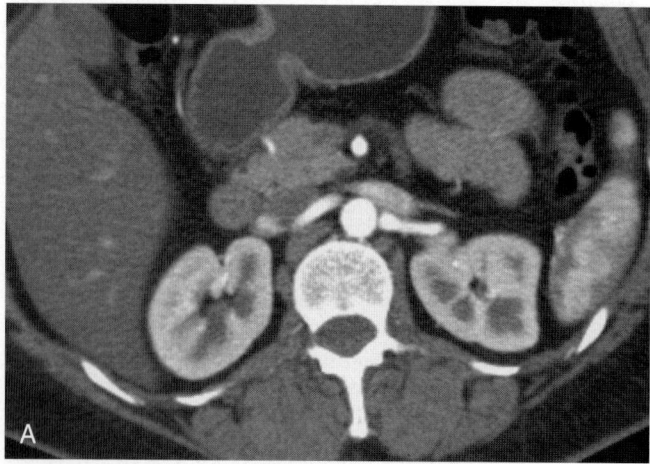
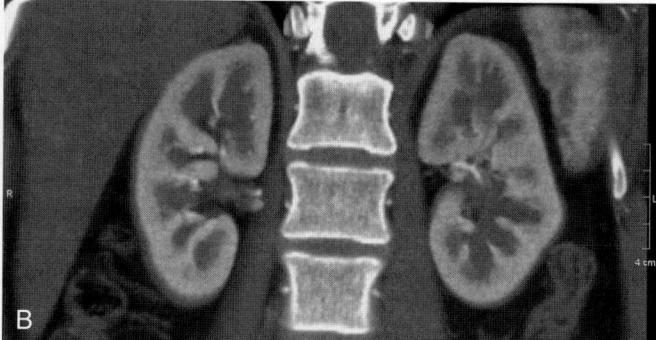

FIGURE 27-10 Computed tomographic scan: normal corticomedullary phase. Axial slice (**A**) and coronal image (**B**) demonstrate the dense enhancement of the cortex in relation to the medulla containing the renal pyramids.

resonant radiofrequency pulse is applied to the patient. The radiofrequency pulse causes the mobile protons within the patient to move from a lower, stable energy state to a higher, unstable energy state (*excitation*). When the radiofrequency pulse is removed, the protons return to the lower energy steady state while emitting frequency transmissions or signals (*relaxation*). In radiologic terms, an external radiofrequency pulse "excites" the protons, causing them to "flip" to a higher energy state. When the radiofrequency pulse is removed, the protons "relax" with emission of a "radio signal." The signals produced during proton relaxation are separated from one another with applied magnetic field gradients. The emitted signals are captured by a receiving coil and reconstructed into images through a complex computerized algorithm: the Fourier transform.[67-69]

Different tissues have different relaxation rates that lead to different levels of signal production or signal intensity.

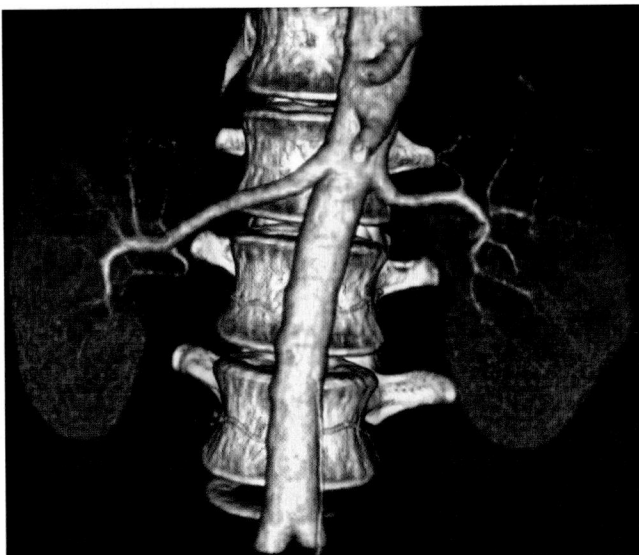

FIGURE 27-11 Renal computed tomographic angiogram: normal findings. The aorta and the exiting renal arteries on the right and left are visible. The kidneys are visible peripherally with the branching renal arteries.

The signal intensity of each tissue is determined by three characteristics:

1. *Proton density of the tissue.* The greater the number of mobile protons, the greater the signal produced by the tissue. For example: a volume of urine has more mobile protons than does the same volume of renal tissue; therefore, urine produces more signal than do the kidneys. Stones have far fewer mobile protons per unit volume and therefore produce little signal.
2. *T1 relaxation time.* The T1 time is how quickly a proton returns to the preexcitation energy state. The shortest T1 times (rapid relaxation) produce the strongest signal.
3. *T2 relaxation time.* The T2 time is how quickly the proton signal decays as a result of non-uniformity of the magnetic field. A non-uniform field accelerates signal decay and leads to signal loss.[67-69]

In MRI, multiple pulse sequences are obtained. A pulse sequence is a set of defined radiofrequency pulses and timing parameters used to obtain image data. These sequences include, but are not limited to, spin echo, gradient echo, inversion recovery, and steady-state precession. The data are obtained in volumes (voxels), reconstructed as two-dimensional pixels, and displayed in relation to variations in tissue signal intensity (tissue contrast). Tissue contrast, like signal intensity, is determined by proton density and relaxation times. T1 weighting is related to the rate of T1 relaxation and the time allowed for relaxation, also known as the *pulse repetition time* (TR). T2 weighting is related to the rate of T2 relaxation and the time at which the "radio signal" is sampled by the receiver coil, also known as the *time to echo* (TE). TR and TE are programmable parameters that can be altered to accentuate T1 and T2 weighting with contrast media.[67-69] For the general observer, T1-weighted sequences have short TR and TE and show simple fluid as black. T2-weighted sequences have long TR and TE and show simple fluid as white (Figure 27-15).

Many programmable parameters other than TR and TE are used to optimize imaging. These include, but are not limited to, choice of pulse sequence, coil types and gradients, slice orientation and thickness, field of view and matrix, gating to reduce motion, and use of intravenous contrast material.

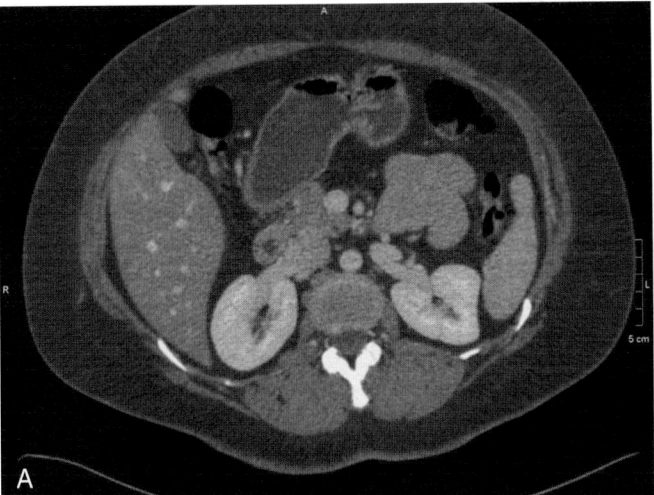
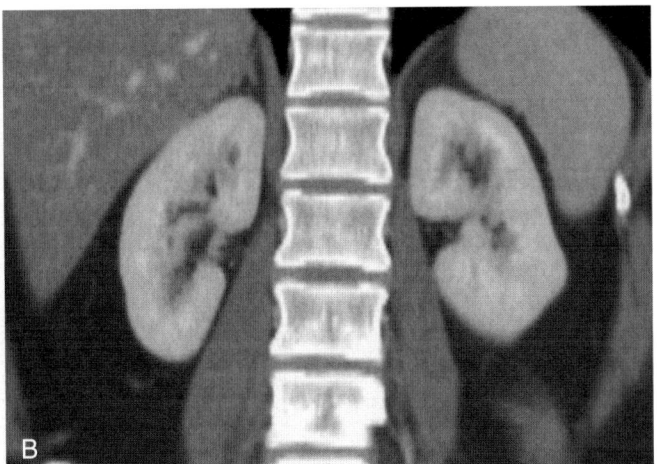

FIGURE 27-12 Computed tomographic scan: normal nephrographic phase. The axial image (**A**) and the coronal image (**B**) demonstrate the homogeneous appearance of the kidneys, with the cortex and medulla no longer differentially enhanced. These images are typically obtained 80 to 120 seconds after the injection of contrast material.

Although many pulse sequences are used in clinical MRI, ultrafast sequences are preferred for renal imaging. These fast sequences can be obtained in less than 30 seconds while the patients hold their breath. The benefits of rapid acquisition include improvement in image quality, as a result of reduction of motion artifact; reduction of total scan time; and the ability to perform dynamic imaging.[70]

MRI is not indicated for patients who have certain implanted medical devices, such as pacemakers, ferromagnetic aneurysm clips, and ferromagnetic stapedial implants. Not all implants or devices cause problems, but knowledge of the type of device is crucial for determining whether the patient can safely enter the magnet.[71]

Gadolinium Chelate Contrast Media and Nephrogenic Systemic Fibrosis

Intravenous contrast material is used routinely in renal imaging because it improves lesion detection and diagnostic accuracy. Gadolinium is a paramagnetic substance that shortens the T1 and T2 relaxation times, resulting in increased signal intensity on T1-weighted images and decreased signal intensity on T2-weighted sequences (Figure 27-16). The pharmacokinetics and enhancement patterns of intravenous gadolinium chelate (Gd-C) agents are similar to those of iodinated contrast agents used for radiograph examinations. Unlike iodinated contrast agents, the dose response to Gd-C is nonlinear; the signal intensity increases at low concentrations and then decreases at higher concentrations. Hence, the collecting systems, ureters, and bladder first brighten and then darken on T1-weighted sequences as the gadolinium concentration within the urine increases.

Gd-C agents are generally well tolerated; adverse reactions occur in approximately 0.07% to 2.4% of cases. Minor reactions include coldness, warmth, or pain at the injection site; nausea; vomiting; headache; paresthesias; dizziness; and itching. Rash, hives, or urticaria occurs in 0.004% to 0.07% of cases; and severe, life-threatening reactions occur in about 0.001% to 0.01%. Nephrotoxicity has not been reported with regard to the doses used for clinical MRI[72-75]; however, there

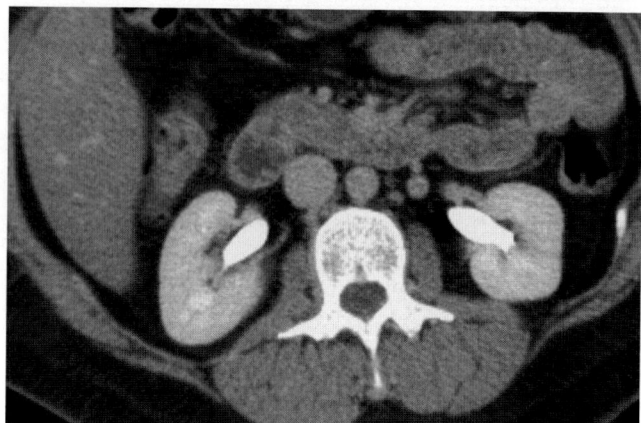

FIGURE 27-13 Computed tomographic scan: normal excretory phase. The calyces and renal pelvis are now easily noted because they are opacified by the excreted contrast material. This scan is obtained 5 to 10 minutes after the injection of contrast material.

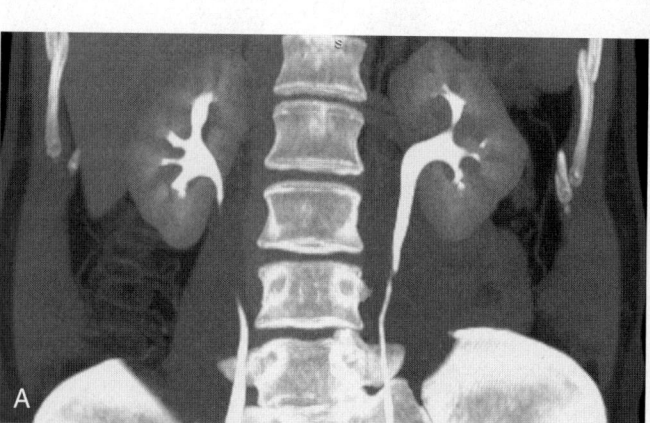
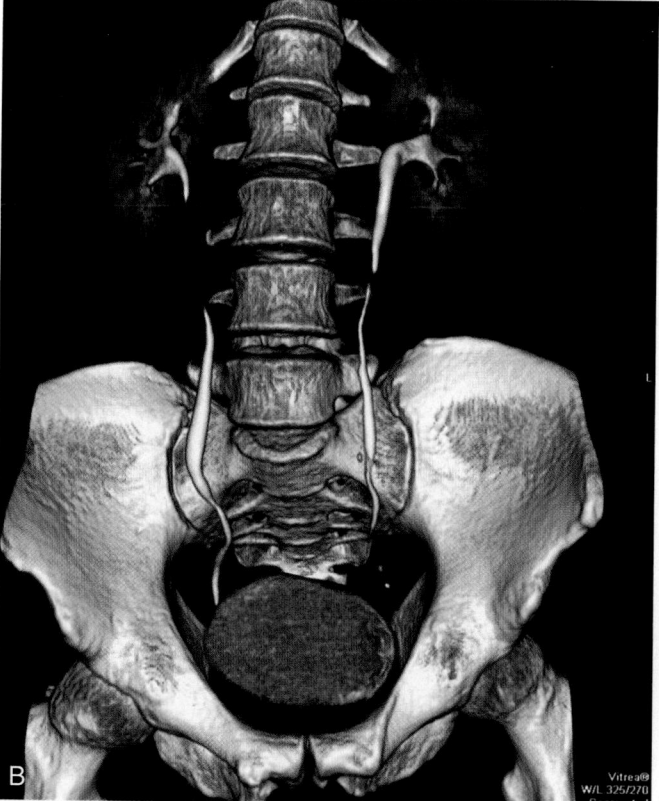

FIGURE 27-14 Computed tomographic urogram: normal findings. The maximum-intensity projection (MIP) image (**A**) and the volume-rendered image (**B**) demonstrate the calyces, renal pelvis, ureters, and bladder. The MIP image is a slab, 15 mm thick, in the coronal plane. The volume-rendered image was taken as the extraneous tissues adjacent to the kidneys were removed, and it highlights the genitourinary tract.

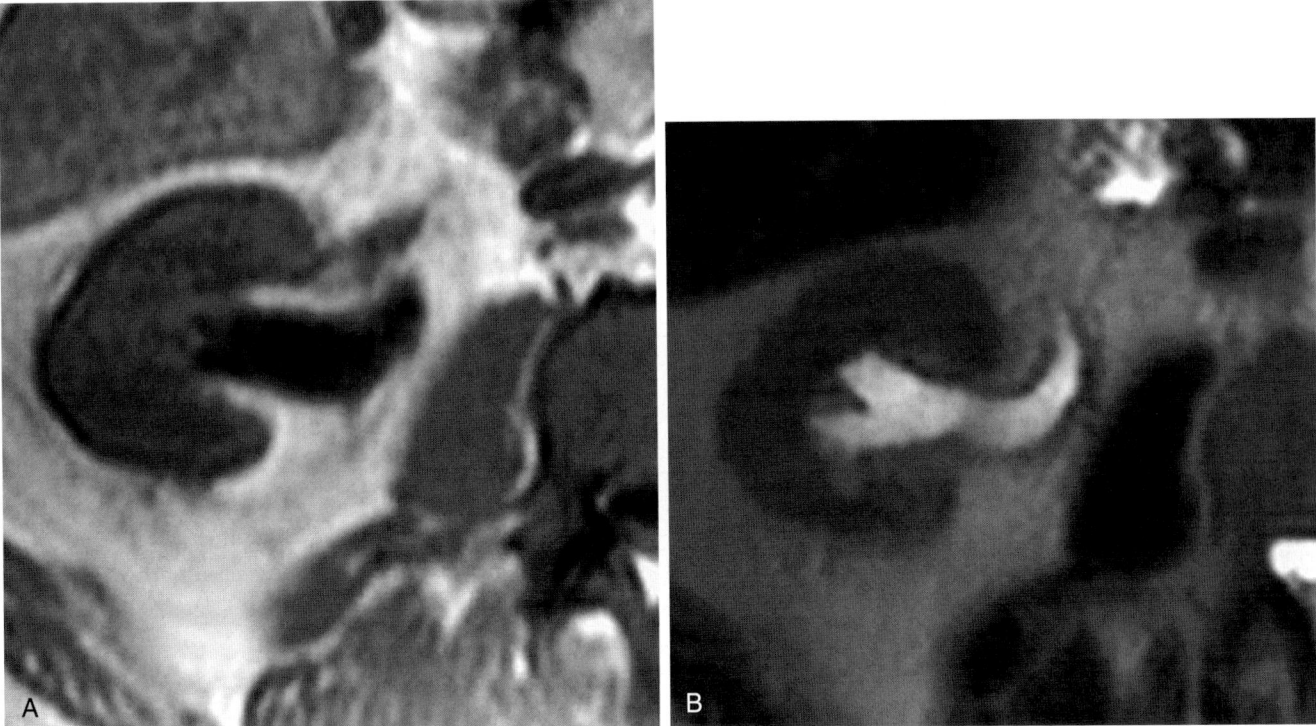

FIGURE 27-15 Normal signal characteristics of simple fluids on magnetic resonance imaging. Urine appears dark on T1-weighted sequences (**A**) and bright on T2-weighted sequences (**B**).

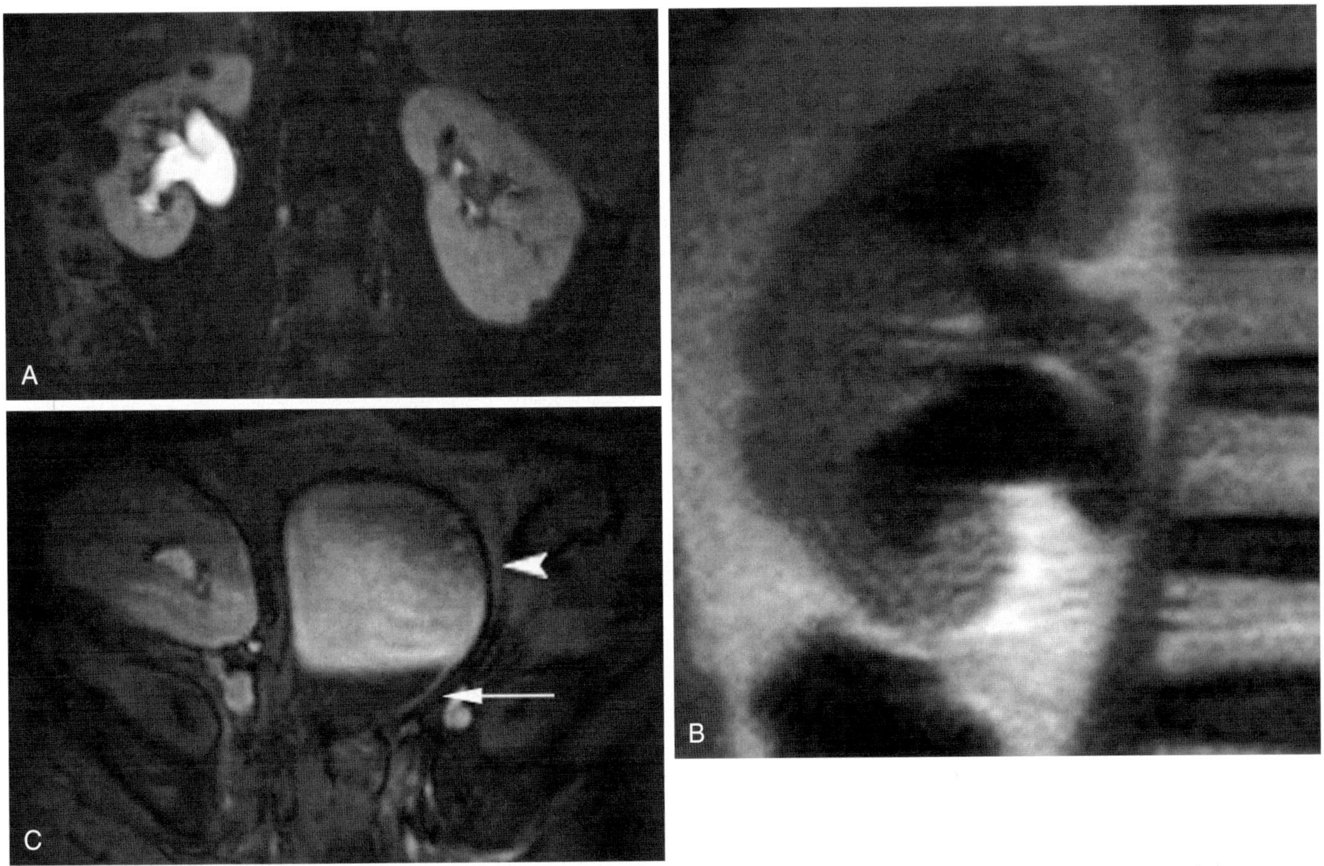

FIGURE 27-16 Paramagnetic effects of gadolinium on urine. **A,** Coronal T1-weighted image from a magnetic resonance urogram (MRU) demonstrates enhancement of the urine in the collection system. **B,** Coronal T2-weighted image from an MRU demonstrates low signal intensity of urine in the collecting system secondary to effects of gadolinium. **C,** Axial T1-weighted, delayed image after contrast medium enhancement demonstrates layering of contrast material. The denser, more concentrated gadolinium is dark (*arrow*). The less concentrated gadolinium is brighter and layers above (*arrowhead*).

have been some reports of nephrotoxicity with high doses of intravenous Gd-C in populations at high risk: those with moderate to severe kidney injury.[76,77] The relative risks associated with each Gd-C agent have not been elucidated clearly, and the agents cannot be differentiated on the basis of efficacy; therefore, most Gd-C agents approved by the U.S. Food and Drug Administration (FDA) are clinically interchangeable.[75] Gd-C may interfere with serum calcium and magnesium measurements, especially in patients with renal insufficiency.[78] As with iodinated contrast material, hemodialysis filters Gd-C effectively, and dialysis is therefore recommended after use of contrast material in patients already on hemodialysis.[79]

Although Gd-C agents were once considered the safest intravenous contrast agents to use in patients with renal disease, they are now thought to carry significant risk in patients with moderate to severe renal disease.[80-85] Gd-C agents have been associated with nephrogenic systemic fibrosis (NSF), a rare, multiorgan, fibrosing condition for which there is no known effective treatment.[86] Patients with NSF typically present with symmetric, dark red patches or papules on skin, swelling of extremities, and thickening of skin that sometimes is described as "woody" and like an "orange peel." The skin thickening can inhibit motion of joints, leading to contractures and immobility. Burning, itching, or severe pain in involved areas or "deep bone pain" in hips and ribs has been described, as has rapid, new-onset fluctuating hypertension. Other structures affected include the lungs, esophagus, skeletal muscles, and heart. These structures may become scarred, which leads to restriction of function; and although NSF is not by itself a cause of death, the resulting restriction of function may contribute to death.[87] Symptoms may develop over a period of days to months; however, in approximately 5% of patients, the course may be rapidly progressive.[87] Diagnosis is confirmed by full-thickness skin biopsy, which reveals thickened collagen bundles, mucin deposition, and proliferation of fibroblasts and elastic fibers without signs of inflammation. NSF tends to affect middle-aged patients without predilection for gender or ethnicity. Although no treatment is known to be consistently successful, improving renal function appears to slow or stop the progression of NSF.[87] To date, no cases of NSF have been documented in patients with normal renal function; NSF has been reported only in people with kidney disease.

NSF was first described in 1997, and the description was published in 2000.[88] It was not until January 2006 that a possible causal relationship between Gd-C and NSF was presented in the literature by Grobner.[80] As of June 2011, 335 cases of NSF have been reported to the International Center for Nephrogenic Fibrosing Dermopathy.[87] Currently, suspected risk factors for NSF include intravenous administration of a high dose of Gd-C, acute or chronic renal failure, venous thrombosis, coagulopathy, and vascular surgery.[89]

The potential for NSF to occur in association with all Gd-C agents is suspected but not proven. As more medical research data become available, recommendations for the usage of Gd-C in patients with moderate to severe renal disease will be modified.[85,89-91] The FDA and the American College of Radiology blue-ribbon panel[86] published recommendations for the use of all classes of Gd-C agents in high-risk patients. All patients should be questioned about a history of renal disease. For patients with renal disease (including neoplasm, transplanted kidney, and unilateral kidney); those older than 60 years; those with a history of hypertension; and those with a history of diabetes, an estimated GFR should be calculated within 6 weeks of an anticipated Gd-C study. For those with severe liver disease and liver transplants, or those who are hospitalized, an estimated GFR should be calculated nearly simultaneously with the anticipated Gd-C study. The recommendations are as follows:

- For patients with dialysis-dependent chronic renal failure: Contrast material–enhanced CT followed by dialysis should be considered instead of contrast material–enhanced MRI. If MRI is absolutely necessary, consider using techniques to reduce the dose of contrast material and perform the examination shortly before dialysis. Although Gd-C agents are effectively removed with hemodialysis, no published report has proved that early dialysis prevents the development of NSF.[89]
- For patients whose estimated GFR is lower than 30 mL/minute/1.73 m^2 (stage 4 or 5 chronic kidney disease [CKD]): Avoid Gd-C, if possible, by considering alternative studies. If MRI is absolutely necessary, use the lowest dose of Gd-C possible, and obtain informed consent regarding the risk of NSF (which is 3% to 5% in this patient population).
- For patients whose estimated GFR is 30 to 60 mL/minute/1.73 m^2 (stage 3 CKD): Follow standard dosing recommendations, because this patient population is considered to be at extremely low or no risk for developing NSF at FDA-recommended doses.
- For patients whose estimated GFR is 60 to 119 mL/minute/1.73 m^2 (stage 1 or 2 CKD): There is no evidence that patients in this group are at increased risk of developing NSF.
- For patients with ARF: All contrast material should be avoided. Gd-C should be administered only if absolutely necessary.

Suspected cases of NSF should be confirmed by skin biopsy and reported to the International Center for Nephrogenic Fibrosing Dermopathy to help further the understanding of NSF and its association with Gd-C. Further information on the different FDA-approved Gd-C agents, including their properties and how these properties may affect safety profiles, as well as a complete discussion on the relationship of NSF and Gd-C agents, were provided by Thomsen and colleagues[92] and by Kanal and associates.[86]

Magnetic Resonance Imaging Protocols

Diagnostic Magnetic Resonance Imaging: Routine Renal Examination

Routine MRI evaluation of the kidneys includes axial and coronal T1-weighted and T2-weighted sequences. Both can be obtained with and without fat suppression. Dynamic contrast material–enhanced T1-weighted sequences are also routinely obtained. In patients with normal renal function, the renal cortex and medullary pyramids are easily differentiated on sequences not enhanced by contrast material, because MRI provides excellent tissue differentiation. On T1-weighted sequences, the renal cortex has higher signal intensity than do the medullary pyramids. On T2-weighted sequences, the renal cortex has lower in signal intensity than do the medullary pyramids (Figure 27-17). With kidney injury, this corticomedullary differentiation disappears (Figure 27-18).[93,94] Urine, like

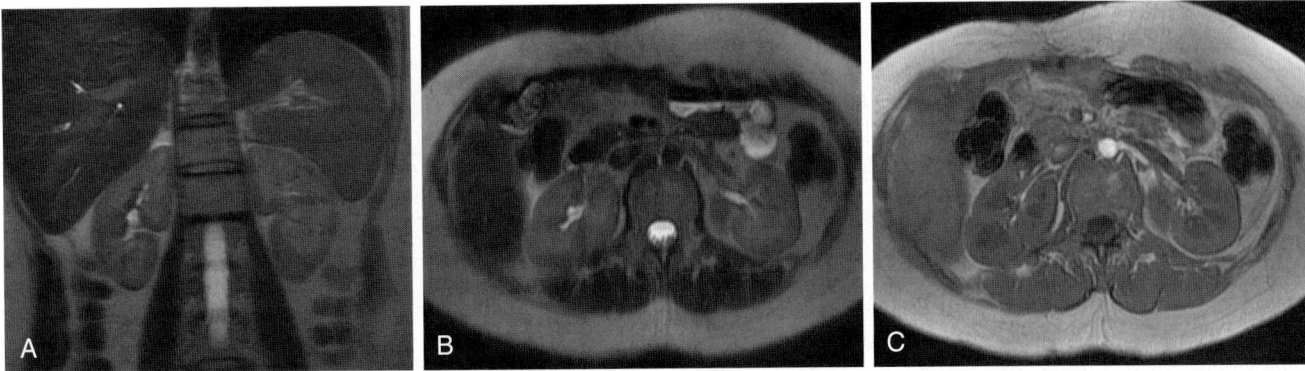

FIGURE 27-17 Normal appearance of corticomedullary differentiation on magnetic resonance imaging (MRI). Coronal (**A**) and axial (**B**) T2-weighted images demonstrate decreased signal intensity of the renal cortex in relation to the medullary pyramids. Axial T1-weighted image (**C**) demonstrates increased signal intensity of the renal cortex in relation to the medullary pyramids.

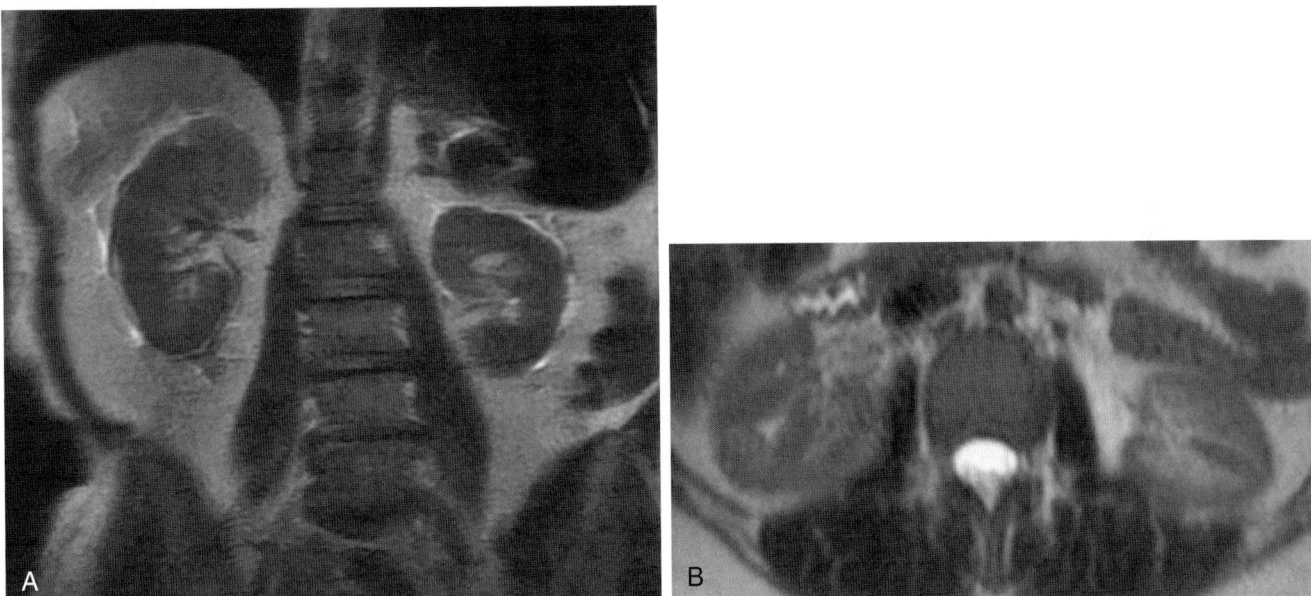

FIGURE 27-18 Coronal T2-weighted image demonstrates loss of corticomedullary differentiation in patient with elevated creatinine level. Also, the renal sizes are asymmetric.

water, normally appears black on T1-weighted sequences and white on T2-weighted sequences (see Figure 27-15).

Contrast material–enhanced MRI (CE-MRI) allows for dynamic evaluation of the kidneys and surrounding structures. Serial acquisitions are obtained after bolus injection of gadolinium (0.1 to 0.2 mmol per kilogram of body weight) at 2 mL/second.[95,96] The injection should be administered by means of an automatic, magnetic resonance–compatible power injector to ensure accuracy of the timed bolus, including volume and rate of injection.[96,97] The corticomedullary-arterial phase (approximately 20 seconds after injection) is best for evaluating the arterial structures and corticomedullary differentiation. In the nephrographic phase (70 to 90 seconds after injection), tumor detection is maximized, and the renal veins and surrounding structures are best demonstrated (Figure 27-19). Imaging can be performed in any plane, but the coronal plane is used most frequently for dynamic imaging because it allows imaging of the kidneys, ureters, vessels, and surrounding structures in the fewest number of images. The characteristics of parenchymal enhancement are similar to those observed on contrast material–enhanced CT.

Renal Vascular Evaluation: Magnetic Resonance Angiography/Venography

On routine imaging before use of contrast media, the vessels can be variable in signal intensity, ranging from white to black due to many factors including, but not limited to, flow-related parameters, location and orientation of the imaged vessel, and choice of pulse sequence. Pulse sequences not enhanced by contrast media can be used for angiography and venography, but until recently, their use has been limited in abdominal imaging. These sequences are sometimes called "bright-blood" sequences and include time-of-flight magnetic resonance angiography (MRA), which is based on flow-related enhancement, and phase-contrast MRA, which is based on velocity and direction of flow. Phase-contrast MRA can be used in conjunction with contrast material–enhanced MRA (CE-MRA) to detect turbulent flow and high velocities associated with stenoses.

Unlike the "bright blood" sequences, CE-MRA minimizes flow-related enhancement and motion. The success of CE-MRA depends on the T1-shortening properties of

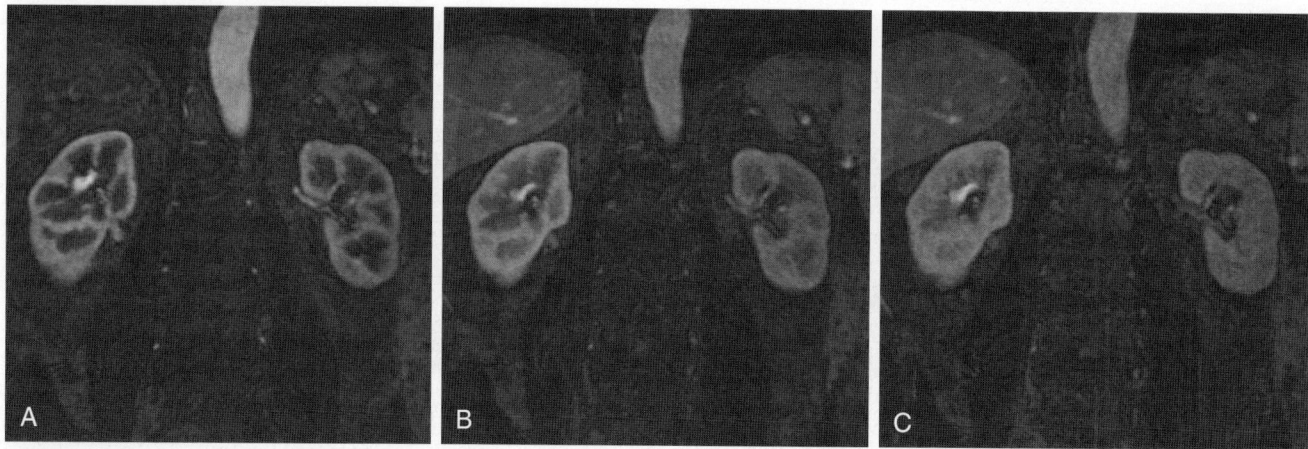

FIGURE 27-19 Magnetic resonance appearance of a normal kidney after bolus injection of gadolinium contrast material at 20 seconds (**A**), 50 seconds (**B**), and 80 seconds (**C**) after the start of the injection.

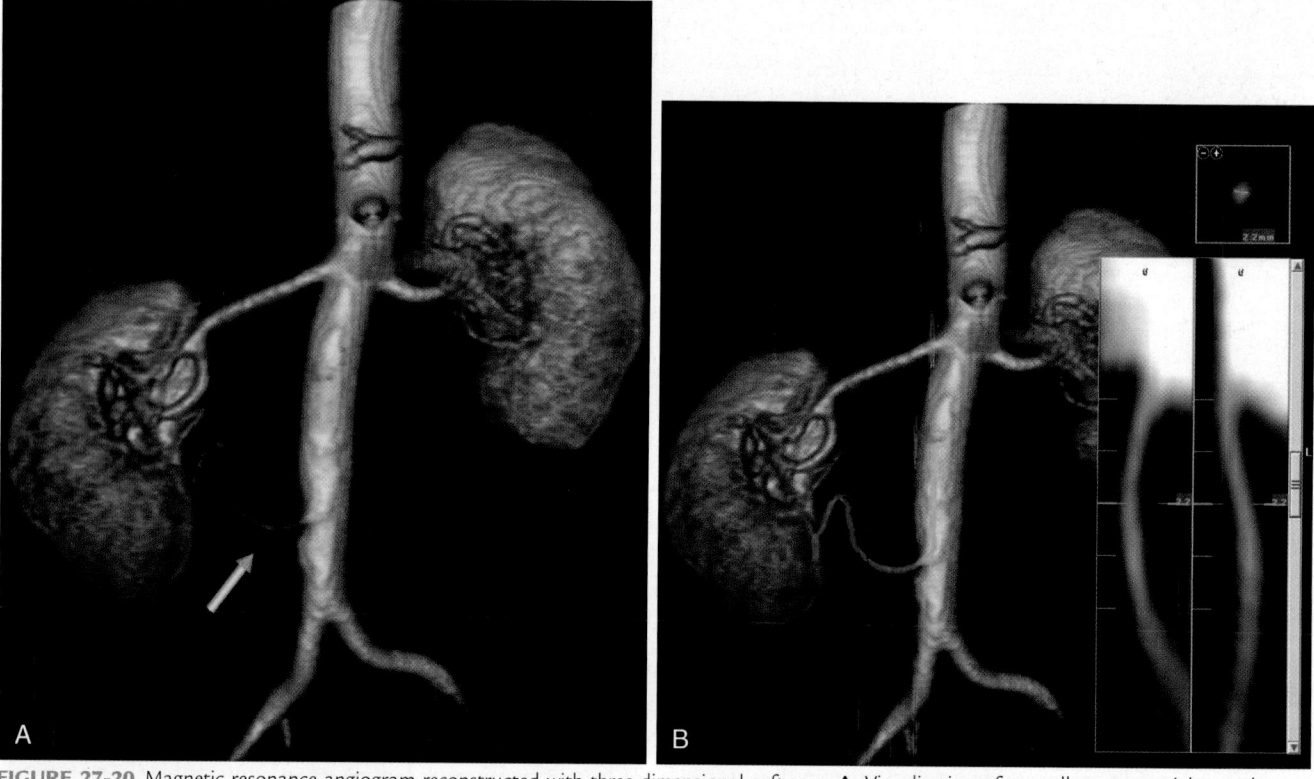

FIGURE 27-20 Magnetic resonance angiogram reconstructed with three-dimensional software. **A,** Visualization of a small accessory right renal artery (*arrow*) is excellent. **B,** The accessory artery is depicted in a way to make more accurate luminal measurements.

gadolinium, which allow for faster imaging, increased coverage, and improved resolution.[68,98] Accurate timing of the bolus injection is critical in CE-MRA. The time at which the bolus arrives at the renal arteries may be determined with a bolus injection of 1 mL of gadolinium, followed by a saline flush. A three-dimensional T1-weighted gradient-echo MRI pulse sequence is then obtained in the coronal plane during the injection of approximately 15 to 20 mL of gadolinium at 2 mL/second, timed to capture the arterial phase.[95,96] Sequential three-dimensional sequences are obtained to capture the venous phase (magnetic resonance venography). The data sets can be postprocessed into multiple formats, improving ease and accuracy of interpretation (Figure 27-20).[99-101]

Collecting System Evaluation: Magnetic Resonance Urography

Magnetic resonance urography (MRU) consists of protocols tailored to the evaluation of the renal collecting system and the disease found there. MRU can be performed with heavily T2-weighted sequences, where urine provides the intrinsic contrast, or with contrast material–enhanced T1-weighted sequences, which mimic conventional IVU and CTU. Heavily T2-weighted sequences are most useful in patients with dilated collecting systems, in whom all water-filled structures are bright (Figure 27-21), and in patients with impaired renal excretion, in whom urography with contrast media is most limited. Unfortunately, without adequate distension

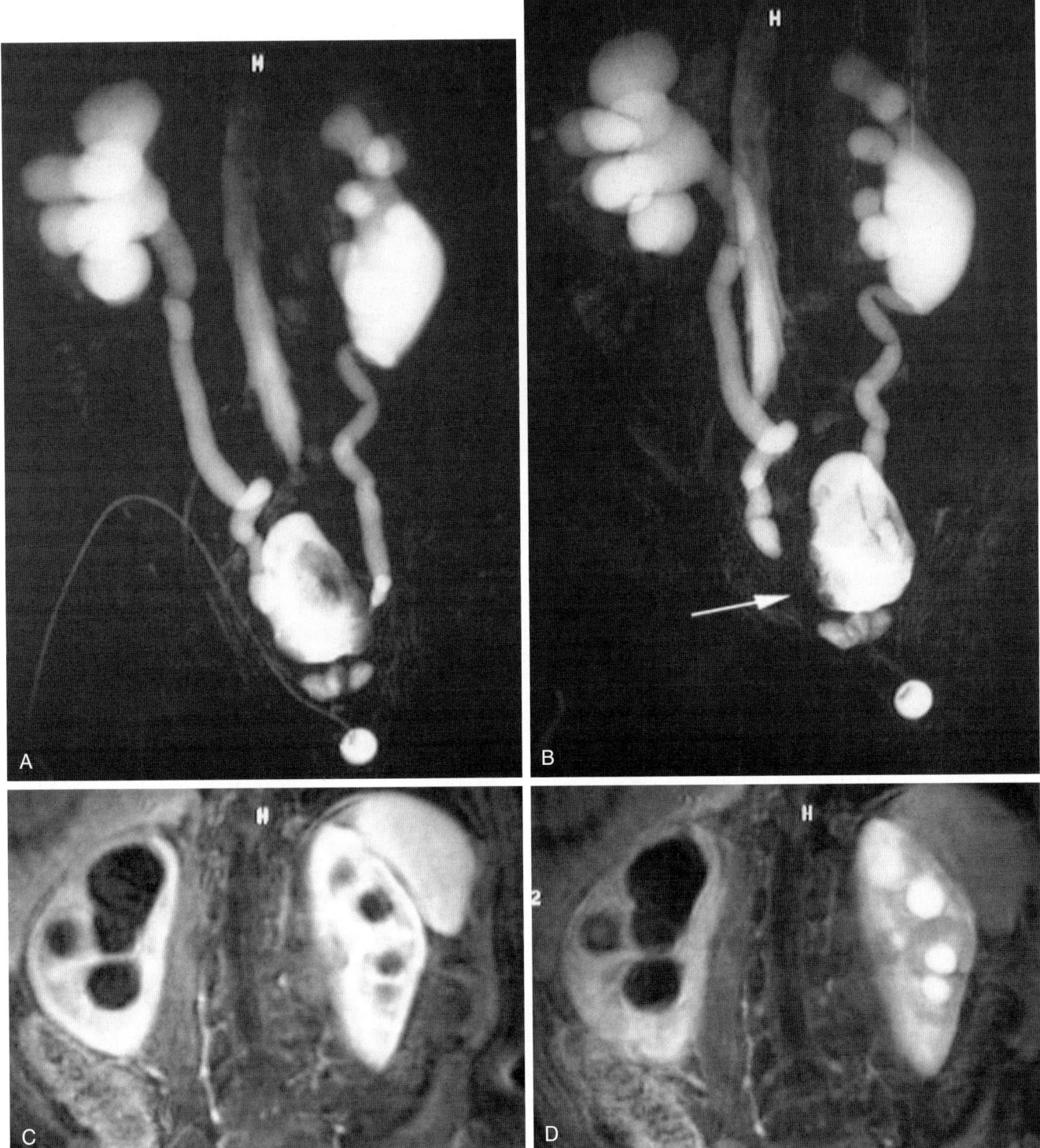

FIGURE 27-21 Bilateral hydronephrosis secondary to bladder tumor. **A** and **B,** Heavily T2-weighted magnetic resonance urograms (MRU) demonstrate bilateral hydronephrosis and hydroureter caused by bladder mass (*arrow*). **C,** Contrast medium–enhanced MRU in the nephrographic phase demonstrates asymmetric enhancement of the kidneys. **D,** MRU in the excretory phase demonstrates asymmetric excretion of gadolinium. There is no excretion on the right as demonstrated by unenhanced (dark) urine within the collecting system.

of the collecting system, T2-weighted evaluation is limited. Although it is a good morphologic examination, T2-weighted urography is ultimately limited by a lack of functional information. For example, T2-weighted urography cannot reliably differentiate between an obstructed system and an ectatic collecting system (Figure 27-22).[102] Contrast material–enhanced

T1-weighted urography in the excretory phase is superior to T2-weighted urography because both structure and function can be evaluated.[102-104]

T2-weighted sequences and contrast material–enhanced T1-weighted sequences are complementary and are frequently obtained together as part of a complete MRU examination.

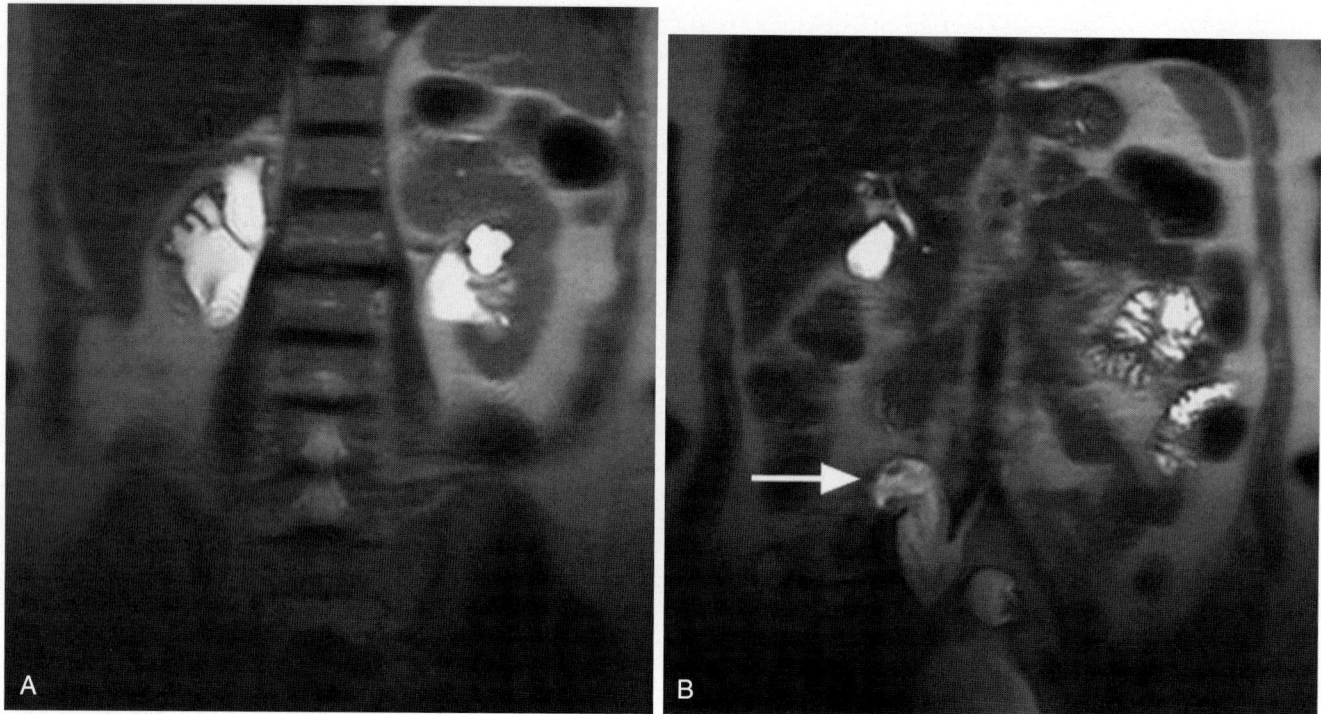

FIGURE 27-22 A and **B,** Coronal T2-weighted images demonstrate right renal atrophy and dilation of the right collecting system in a patient who had undergone bladder resection and iliocondiut reconstruction (*arrow*). On these static images, it is difficult to differentiate between an obstructed system and a nonobstructed system. The patient had pelvocaliectasis without obstruction, demonstrated on the contrast medium–enhanced portion of the examination.

In patients with nondilated systems, both techniques require hydration and furosemide for adequate distension of the renal collecting system.[102,105] Typical MRU starts with a coronal, heavily T2-weighted sequence in which simple fluid (urine, cerebrospinal fluid, ascites) is bright and all other tissues are dark (see Figure 27-21). This rapid breath-hold sequence takes less than 5 seconds to obtain and is presented as a urogram-like image. The T2-weighted sequence is used as an initial survey of fluid within the collecting system. Low-dose furosemide (0.1 mg per kilogram of body weight; maximum dose, 10 mg) is administered intravenously, 30 to 60 seconds before the intravenous administration of gadolinium (0.1 mmol/kg).[103,104] Furosemide is given to increase urine volume and dilute the gadolinium within the collecting system.[103,105] Coronal, three-dimensional, postcontrast T1-weighted sequences are obtained with the same technique as in renal MRA, in the corticomedullary-arterial phase, nephrographic phase, and excretory phase (see Figure 27-21).[104] Additional sequences may be obtained in any plane to better evaluate suspected disease.

By combining renal MRI and MRU, the clinician can obtain a comprehensive morphologic and functional evaluation of urinary tract. MRU helps accurately evaluate the upper urinary tract and is useful in the evaluation of anatomic anomalies, including duplications, ureteropelvic obstruction, anomalous crossing vessels, and ureteroceles[105,106] (Figure 27-23). Obstructive disease is well evaluated regardless of whether the cause is intrinsic or extrinsic to the collecting system.

Renal Functional Magnetic Resonance Imaging

Renal function can be evaluated with MRI. Techniques include contrast material–enhanced magnetic resonance renography, diffusion-weighted imaging (DWI), and blood

oxygen level–dependent (BOLD) MRI. Magnetic resonance renography is a contrast material–enhanced sequence in which dynamic images are obtained during the 7 to 10 minutes after administration of intravenous contrast material; tissue signal intensities are converted to tissue gadolinium concentrations, and these values are plotted against time. Current clinical applications include the evaluation of renal artery stenosis, both with and without the use of angiotensin converting enzyme (ACE) inhibitors, and the evaluation of early postoperative renal transplant dysfunction, to distinguish acute rejection from acute tubular necrosis. What prevents widespread clinical use, however, is the lack of consensus on optimal imaging technique and methods of data analysis.[107]

DWI is based on the brownian motion of water molecules in tissue and is a noncontrast MRI technique that is used for both structural and functional imaging. Initial experience with DWI has yielded reproducible information on renal function, with the possibility of determining the degree of dysfunction.[108] No large studies have been performed, and further research is required before the usefulness of DWI is confirmed. Animal research is being performed with the hope of using noninvasive DWI as a tool for monitoring early renal graft rejection after transplantation.[109]

BOLD MRI enables only indirect evaluation of renal oxygenation. Various researchers use this technique to explore renal artery stenosis, renal transplant dysfunction, and diabetic nephropathy. Sadowski and colleagues[110] demonstrated the feasibility of using BOLD MRI to evaluate the oxygen status of renal transplants and to detect the presence of acute rejection. They concluded that MRI may differentiate acute rejection from normal function and acute tubular necrosis, but further research is required.

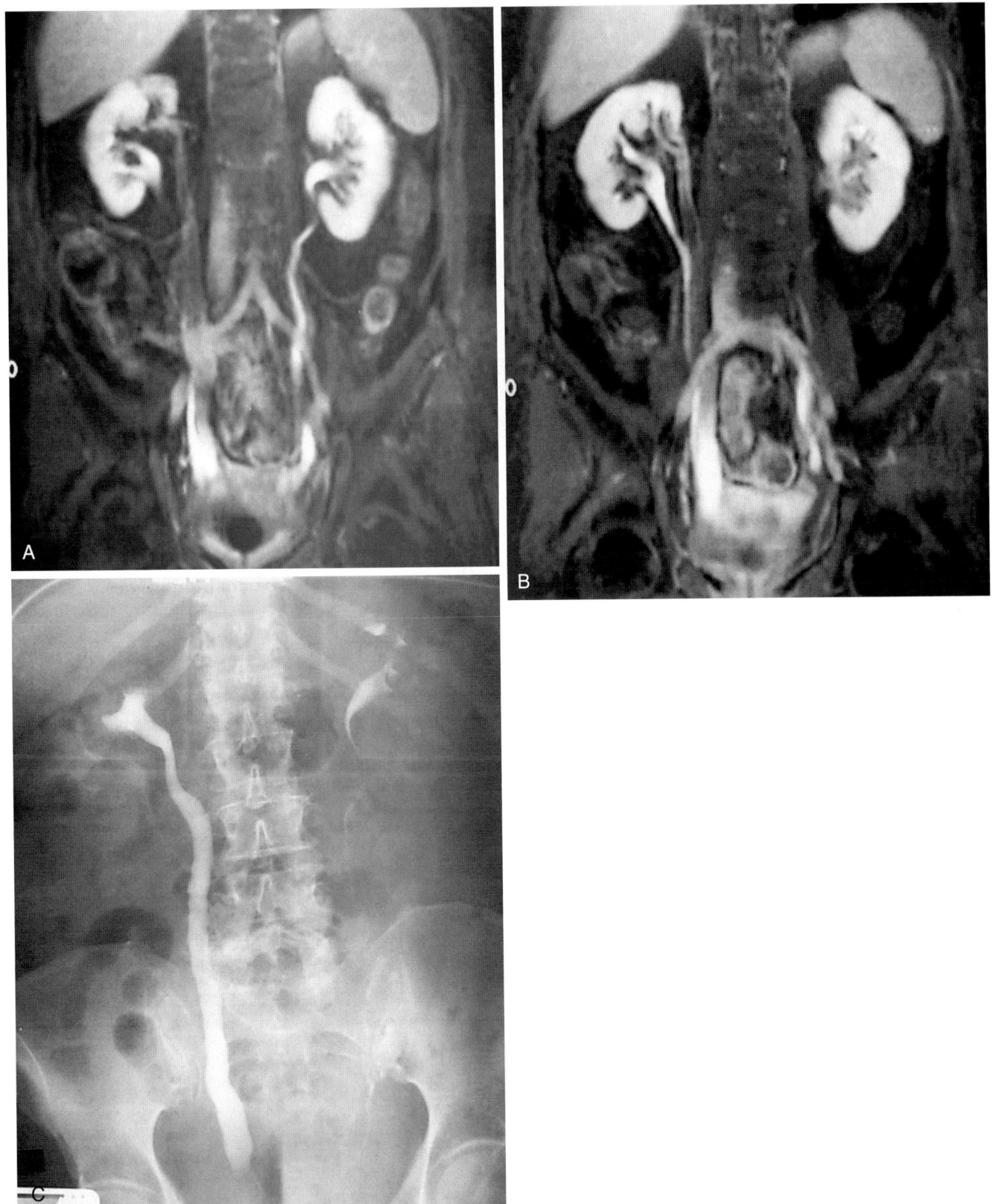

FIGURE 27-23 Duplicated collecting system. **A** and **B,** Contrast material–enhanced magnetic resonance urograms (MRUs) demonstrate a duplicated collecting system on the right with delayed excretion of the upper pole moiety. **C,** Obstruction of the upper pole moiety is confirmed on intravenous urogram.

Nuclear Medicine

Scintigraphy offers imaging-based diagnostic information on renal structure and function.[111] Many single-photon radiotracers have long been in routine clinical use in renal scintigraphy; they are tailored to provide physiologic information complementing the primarily anatomic and structural-based imaging modalities, such as ultrasonography, CT, and MRI. With the rapid expansion of PET and, more recently, hybrid structural-functional imaging systems such as PET-CT, additional unprecedented opportunities have developed for quantitative imaging evaluation of renal diseases in clinical medicine and in research.[112] Scintigraphy, including PET, makes a unique contribution to the imaging evaluation of renal structure and function. The common radiopharmaceuticals used in renal scintigraphy are described first.

Radiopharmaceuticals

Technetium 99m–Labeled Diethylenetriaminepentaacetic Acid (^{99m}Tc-DTPA)

Technetium 99m–labeled diethylenetriaminepentaacetic acid (^{99m}Tc-DTPA) is the common agent for assessing GFR. The ideal agent for measuring GFR would be cleared only by glomerular filtration and would not be secreted or reabsorbed. ^{99m}Tc-DTPA satisfies the first requirement but has variable degrees of protein binding, which deviates its kinetics from the ideal agent such as inulin. For a 20-mCi (740-MBq) dose, the radiation exposures of the kidneys and the urinary bladder are 1.8 and 2.3 rad, respectively.[113]

Iodine 131–Labeled Ortho-iodohippurate

The mechanisms underlying renal clearance of I 131–labeled ortho-iodohippurate (^{131}I-ortho-iodohippurate) are GFR (about 20%) and tubular secretion (about 80%). ^{131}I-ortho-iodohippurate is an acceptable alternative to *p*-aminohippuric acid (PAH) for determining renal plasma flow (RPF), although the amount cleared is 15% lower than that of PAH. PAH is not entirely cleared by the kidneys; about 10% of arterial PAH remains in the renal venous blood. Therefore, ^{131}I-ortho-iodohippurate helps measure *effective* RPF. The efficiency of tubular extraction of ^{131}I-ortho-iodohippurate is 90%, and there is no hepatobiliary excretion. Ortho-iodohippurate may also be labeled with iodine 123, which not only provides urinary kinetics equivalent to those provided by iodine 131 but also enables improved image quality because the administered dose is typically larger, in view of its more favorable profile of radiation exposure. For a 300-μCi (11.1 MBq) dose of ^{131}I-ortho-iodohippurate, the radiation exposures of the kidneys and the urinary bladder are 0.02 and 1.4 rad, respectively. A few drops of nonradioactive iodine (e.g., saturated solution of potassium iodide) administered orally help minimize the thyroid uptake of free iodine 131.[113]

Technetium 99m–Labeled Mercaptoacetyltriglycine

Technetium 99m–labeled mercaptoacetyltriglycine (^{99m}TC-MAG3) has properties similar to those of ^{131}I-ortho-iodohippurate but has significant advantages of better image quality and less radiation exposure. The tubular extraction fraction of ^{99m}Tc-MAG3 is lower than that of ^{131}I-ortho-iodohippurate, at about 60% to 70%. Also, hepatobiliary excretion is about 3%, which increases with renal insufficiency. Despite these features, however, ^{99}Tc-MAG3 is commonly used in scintigraphic evaluation of renal function. For a 10-mCi (370-MBq) dose, the radiation exposures of the kidneys and the urinary bladder are 0.15 and 4.4 rad, respectively.[113]

Technetium 99m–Labeled Dimercaptosuccinic Acid

Technetium 99m–labeled dimercaptosuccinic acid (^{99m}Tc-DMSA) localizes to renal cortex at high concentration and has a slow urinary excretion rate. About 50% of the injected dose accumulates in the renal cortex in 1 hour. The tracer is bound to the renal proximal tubular cells. In view of the high retention of ^{99m}Tc-DMSA in the renal cortex, it has become useful for imaging of the renal parenchyma. For a 6-mCi (222-MBq) dose, the radiation exposures of the kidneys and the urinary bladder are 3.78 and 0.42 rad, respectively.[113]

Fluorine 18 2-Fluoro-2-deoxy-D-glucose

Fluorine 18 2-fluoro-2-deoxy-D-glucose (FDG) is the most common positron-labeled radiotracer in PET. FDG is a modified form of glucose in which the hydroxyl group in the 2′ position is replaced by the fluorine 18 positron emitter. FDG accumulates in cells in proportion to glucose metabolism. Cell membrane glucose transporters facilitate the transport of glucose and FDG across the cell membrane. Both glucose and FDG are phosphorylated in the 6′ position by the hexokinase. The conversion of glucose-6-phosphate or FDG-6-phosphate back to glucose or FDG, respectively, is effected by the enzyme phosphatase. In most tissues, including cancer cells, there is little phosphatase activity. FDG-6-phosphate cannot undergo further conversions and is therefore trapped in the cell.

FDG is excreted in the urine. The typical FDG dose is 0.144 mCi/kg (minimum, 1 mCi; maximum, 20 mCi). The urinary bladder wall receives the highest radiation dose from FDG.[114,115] The radiation dose depends on the excretion rate, the varying size of the bladder, the bladder volume at the time of FDG administration, and an activity curve of estimated bladder time. For a typical 15-mCi dose of FDG and voiding at 1 hour after tracer injection, the average estimated radiation dose absorbed by the adult bladder wall is 3.3 rad (0.22 rad/mCi).[116] The doses absorbed by other organs are between 0.75 and 1.28 rad (0.050 to 0.085 rad/mCi); the average dose absorbed is 1.0 rad.[116] Renal failure may alter the FDG biodistribution, which may necessitate reduction of dose or image acquisition time after tracer administration, or both.[117] Specifically, in patients with suspected renal failure (blood serum creatinine level in excess of 1.1 mg/dL), the FDG accumulation in brain may decrease, whereas the blood pool activity is increased.[118]

Imaging in Clinical Nephrology

Normal Renal Function

GFR and effective RPF may be assessed by means of dynamic quantitative nuclear imaging techniques. The GFR quantifies the amount of filtrate formed per minute (normal: 125 mL/minute in adults). Only 20% of RPF is filtered through the semipermeable membrane of the glomerulus. The filtrate is protein free and almost completely reabsorbed in the tubules. Filtration is maintained over a range of arterial pressures with autoregulation. The ideal agent for the determination of GFR is inulin, which is only filtered but is neither secreted nor reabsorbed.[113,119]

In these studies, ^{99m}Tc-DTPA is often used to demonstrate renal perfusion and assess glomerular filtration, although 5% to 10% of injected ^{99m}Tc-DTPA is protein bound and 5% remains in the kidneys after 4 hours. A typical imaging protocol includes posterior 5-second flow images for 1 minute, followed by 1-minute-per-frame images for 20 minutes. The GFR may be obtained through the Gates method, in which images of renal uptake are obtained during the second and third minutes after ^{99m}Tc-DTPA administration. Regions of interest are drawn over the kidneys, and background activity correction is applied. A standard dose is counted by the gamma camera for normalization. Depth photon attenuation is corrected according to a formula relating body weight and height. A split GFR can be obtained for each kidney, which is not possible with the creatinine clearance method.[113,119]

The effective RPF (normal, 585 mL/minute in adults) can be obtained with ^{131}I-ortho-iodohippurate and ^{99m}Tc-MAG3 imaging.[120] However, ^{131}I-ortho-iodohippurate has been largely replaced by ^{99}Tc-MAG3 because MAG3 has better imaging characteristics and dosimetry (when radiolabeled with ^{99m}Tc). Currently, ^{99}Tc-MAG3 is the renal imaging agent of choice primarily because of the combined renal clearance of ^{99}Tc-MAG3 by both filtration and tubular extraction, which enables clinicians to obtain relatively high-quality images even in patients with impaired renal function. The imaging protocol includes posterior 1-second images for 60 seconds (flow study), followed by 1-minute images for 5 minutes and then 5-minute images for 30 minutes. The relative tubular function may be obtained by drawing renal regions of interest, corrected for background activity.[121,122] A renogram is constructed to depict the renal tracer uptake over time. The first portion of the renogram has a sharp upward slope occurring about 6 seconds after peak aortic activity (phase I); the upward slope represents perfusion. This is followed by extension to the peak value, which represents both renal perfusion and early renal clearance (phase II), which can be dependent on body position.[123] The next phase (phase III) is depicted by a downward slope, which represents excretion. Normal perfusion of the kidneys is symmetric (50% ± 5%). The peak of the renogram occurs at about 2 to 3 minutes (vs. 3 to 5 minutes with DTPA) in normal adults, and by 30 minutes, more than 70% of the tracer is cleared and present in the urinary bladder (Figure 27-24).[113,119,124]

Renal cortical structure can be imaged with ^{99m}Tc-DMSA; the appearance of these images is correlated strongly with differential GFR and differential renal blood flow. Imaging is started 90 to 120 minutes after administration of the tracer and can be obtained up to 4 hours later. Planar images are obtained in the anterior, posterior, left anterior oblique/right anterior oblique, and right posterior oblique/left posterior oblique projections. Single-photon computed tomography (SPECT) is also often performed. In a normal scan, renal cortical uptake is evenly distributed. Normal variations include dromedary hump (splenic impression on the left kidney), fetal lobulation, horseshoe kidney, crossed fused ectopy, and hypertrophied column of Bertin. The renal images also allow accurate assessment of the relative renal size, position, and axis.[113,119]

Kidney Injury: Acute and Chronic

AKI/ARF is characterized as prerenal, renal, or postrenal in origin. AKI/ARF is commonly encountered in the hospital setting. In affected patients, the prerenal and renal forms are

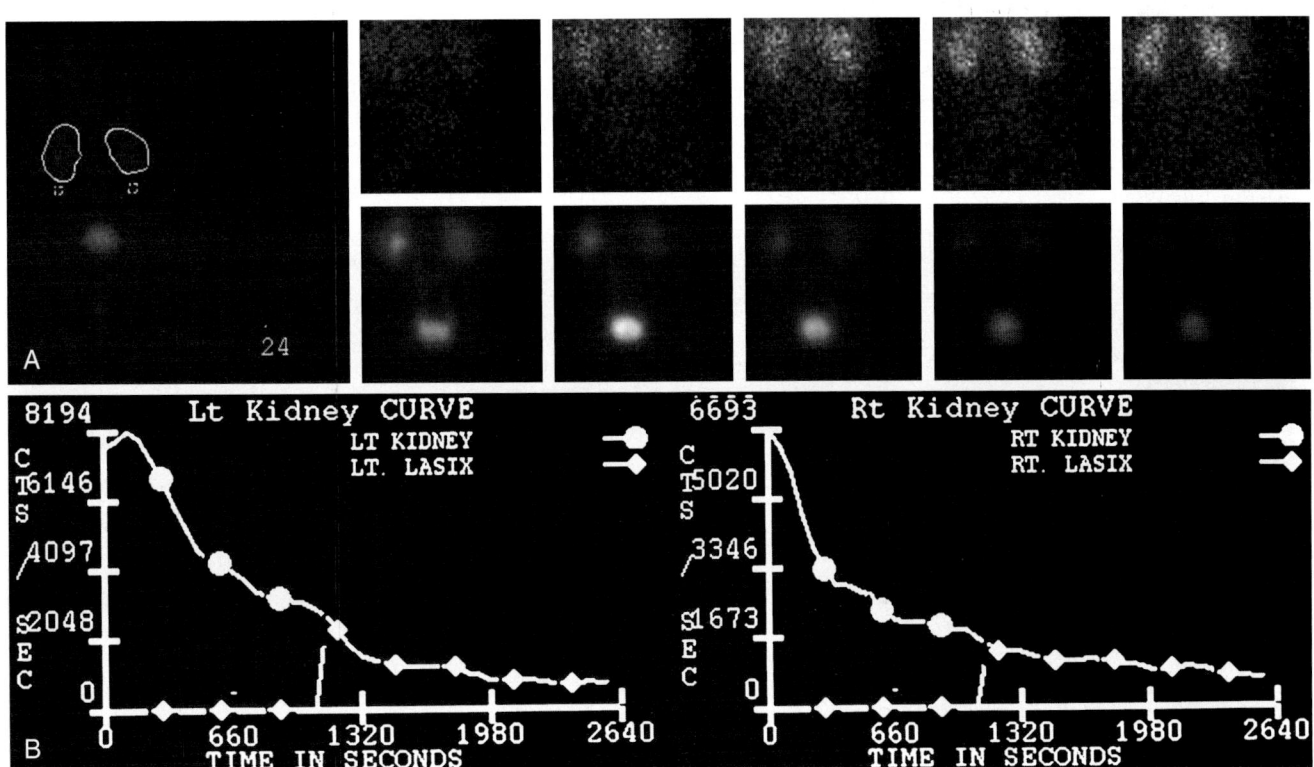

FIGURE 27-24 A and **B,** Normal-appearing renogram with technetium 99m-labeled mercaptoacetyltriglycine.

most frequently caused by hypotension, dehydration, nephrotoxic drugs, and hypoperfusion of the kidneys.[18] These prerenal and renal causes account for more than 90% of all cases. Although postrenal AKI/ARF is less common, it should be identified because it is often rapidly reversible. Postrenal AKI/ARF is most often caused by urinary tract obstruction or obstructive uropathy. Radiographic evaluation is performed to confirm or rule out postrenal AKI/ARF in the form of obstructed kidneys.

Plain radiographs offer little in the assessment of AKI/ARF; only renal size and the presence or absence of renal stones can be assessed. IVU plays no role in the assessment of AKI/ARF because iodinated contrast material is required for that study. Ultrasonography is the method of choice in evaluating patients with AKI/ARF. Renal size, echogenicity

of the kidneys, cortical thickness, and the presence or absence of hydronephrosis are generally imaged easily.[125] A thin rim of decreased echogenicity ("renal sweat") may surround the kidneys in patients with kidney injury.[126] For patients with AKI/ARF, ultrasonography is more than 95% accurate in detecting hydronephrosis (i.e., dilation of the collecting systems and renal pelvis).[127,128] A postrenal cause of AKI/ARF is diagnosed when both kidneys exhibit hydronephrosis.[129] The specific cause may not be elucidated with ultrasonography, and other methods, such as CT or MRI, must be used.

The principal ultrasonographic finding of hydronephrosis is the separation of the central renal sinus echo complex by a sonolucent fluid-filled renal pelvis, which is connected directly to the dilated calyces and infundibula in the more peripheral aspects of the kidney. Hydronephrosis is generally graded according to the extent of calyceal dilation and the degree of cortical thinning.[127,130,131] In mild (grade I) hydronephrosis, pelvicalyceal system is filled with fluid, which causes slight separation of the central renal sinus fat (Figure 27-25). The calyces are not distorted, and the thickness of the renal cortex appears normal. In moderate (grade II) hydronephrosis the pelvicalyceal system appears more distended with greater separation of the central echo complex. The contour of the calyces is rounded, but the cortical thickness is unaltered (Figure 27-26). With moderate-to-severe grade III hydronephrosis the calyces are more distended, and cortical thinning is recognized. In severe (grade IV) hydronephrosis, the calyceal system is markedly dilated (Figure 27-27). The calyces appear as large, ballooned, fluid-filled structures with a dilated renal pelvis of variable size. Cortical loss is evident, with the dilated calyces approaching or reaching the renal capsule. In general, the length and overall size of a hydronephrotic kidney is increased. Long-standing obstruction may, however, result in renal parenchymal atrophy, and the kidney may be somewhat small, with marked cortical thinning. The degree of hydronephrosis is not always correlated with the amount of obstruction.

Although hydronephrosis is usually easily diagnosed with ultrasonography, it must not be confused with renal cystic disease. In hydronephrosis, the dilated calyces have a visibly direct communication with the renal pelvis, which is also dilated.[48]

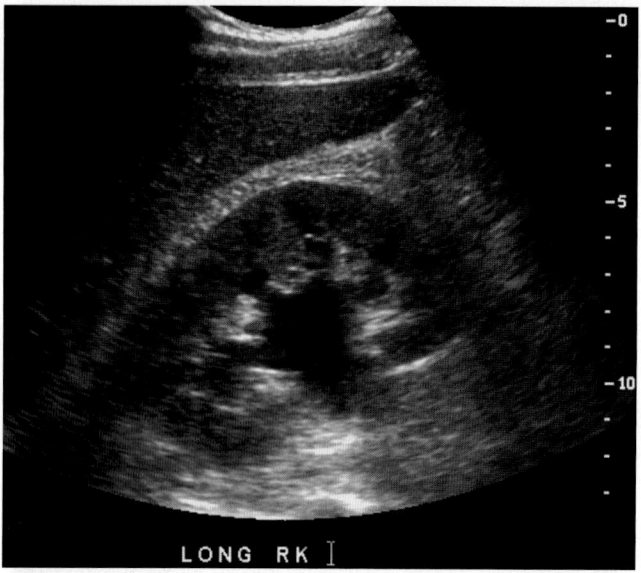

FIGURE 27-25 Mild (grade I) hydronephrosis: ultrasonography. The central echo complex is separated by the mildly distended calyces and renal pelvis. Notice the connection between the calyces and the renal pelvis. The thickness of the cortex is preserved, and the renal border remains smooth.

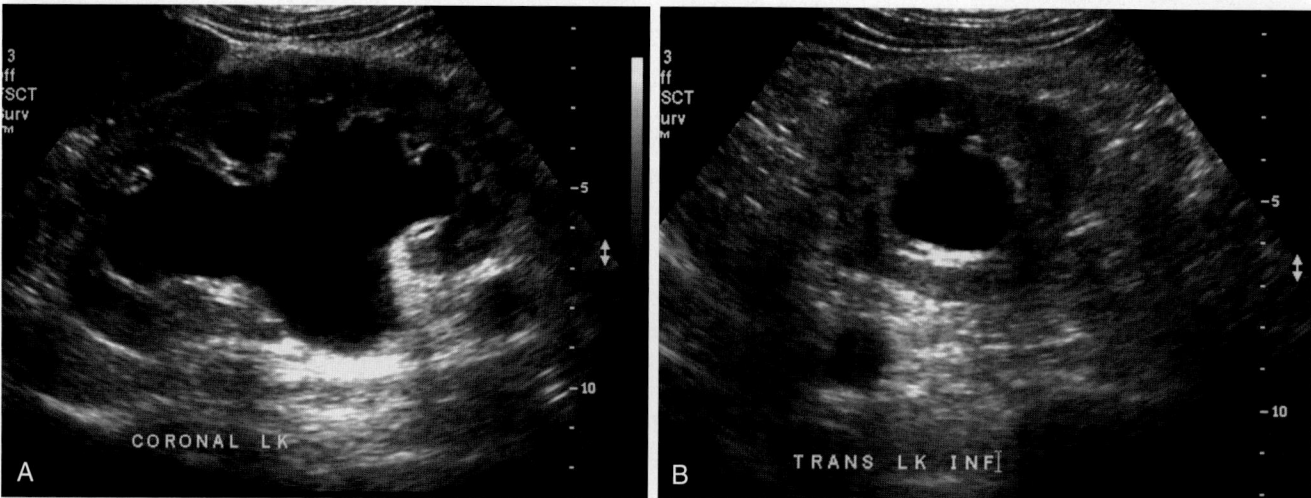

FIGURE 27-26 Moderate (grade II) hydronephrosis: ultrasonography, longitudinal image (**A**) and transverse image (**B**). The dilated calyces are rounded and filled with urine. The renal pelvis is dilated as well. Again, note the connection between the calyces and the renal pelvis. The cortex remains relatively normal in thickness, and the renal border is smooth.

In cystic disease, the round fluid-filled cysts have walls, and no direct communication is evident between each calyx and the renal pelvis. Cases of peripelvic cysts are frequently misdiagnosed as a dilated renal pelvis. Renal artery aneurysm may also be confused with a dilated renal pelvis, but it can be diagnosed correctly with added Doppler color-flow ultrasonography.

In nonobstructive hydronephrosis, the ultrasound image may be confusing.[132,133] Grade I hydronephrosis and possibly more severe grades may be observed in patients in whom no obstructive cause is found. Some authorities consider mild dilation of the pelvicalyceal system a normal variant. Nonobstructive causes of hydronephrosis include increased urine production and flow, such as that which occurs with diuresis from any cause and with pregnancy, acute and chronic infection, vesicoureteral reflux, papillary necrosis, congenital megacalyces, overdistended bladder, and postobstructive dilation.[134] In patients with repeated episodes of intermittent or partial obstruction, the calyces become quite distensible or compliant, which causes the appearance of hydronephrosis to vary, depending on the state of hydration and urine production. Patients with vesicoureteral reflux

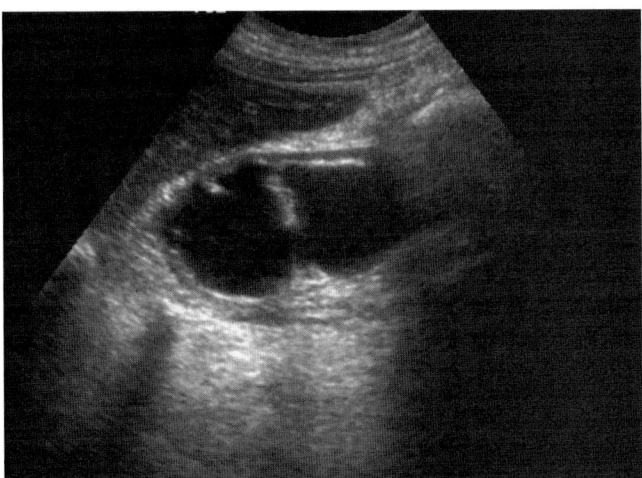

FIGURE 27-27 Severe (grade IV) hydronephrosis: ultrasonography. Longitudinal image of the right kidney demonstrates a large fluid-filled sac; with no normal elements of the kidney remain visible. The cortex is almost gone, but the outer border of the kidney remains smooth.

also demonstrate distensible pelvicalyceal systems. Duplex Doppler ultrasonography has been suggested as an additive means of differentiating obstructive from nonobstructive hydronephrosis.[135,136] The measurement of resistive indices has been investigated as a means of diagnosing acute renal obstruction, as well; the acutely obstructed kidney has an elevated resistive index, and the nonobstructed kidney has a normal resistive index of less than 0.70.[137,138] The results have been variable, and thus no consistent recommendation is available.[138,139]

Ultrasonography is also used in patients with CKD. Cortical echogenicity may be increased in both acute and chronic renal parenchymal disease (Figure 27-28).[140] The pattern should be bilateral. In chronic kidney injury, the degree of cortical echogenicity is correlated with the severity of the interstitial fibrosis, global sclerosis, focal tubular atrophy, and number of hyaline casts per glomerulus.[47] Similar correlation is observed with decreasing renal size. These findings, however, are nonspecific, and renal biopsy is required for diagnosis. The normal corticomedullary differentiation is lost with increasing cortical echogenicity.[52] Cortical echogenicity may also be increased in some patients with AKI/ARF, as in glomerulonephritis and lupus nephritis. Sequential studies over time may be used to assess the progression of disease by monitoring the renal size and cortical echogenicity.

The key to the diagnosis of renal parenchymal disease is renal core biopsy and resulting histopathologic study.[140] Ultrasonography facilitates the performance of renal biopsy by demonstrating the kidney and the proper location for biopsy. Ultrasonography may also be used to evaluate for complications associated with renal biopsy, such as perirenal hematoma and arteriovenous fistula.

In AKI/ARF and CKD, when ultrasound evaluation demonstrates bilateral hydronephrosis, it is usually followed by CT scanning. Noncontrast CT easily demonstrates the dilated pelvicalyceal systems in the kidney. The parenchymal thickness can be visualized in relation to the dilated collecting systems. The urine-filled calyces and pelvis are less dense than the surrounding parenchyma. The course of the dilated ureters may be followed distally to establish the site of obstruction. The cause is frequently visible, as in cases of pelvic tumors, distal ureteral stones, and retroperitoneal adenopathy or mass.

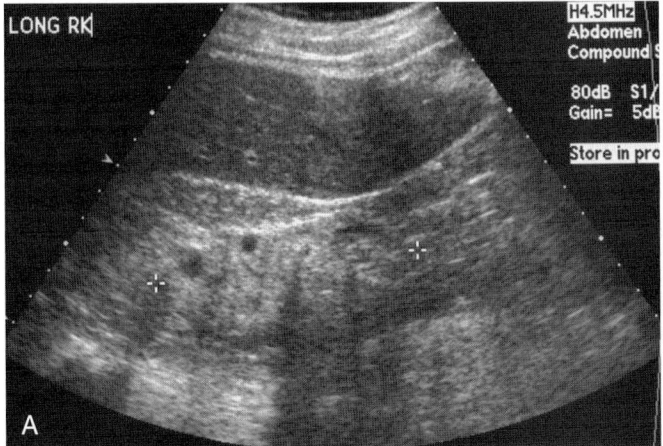
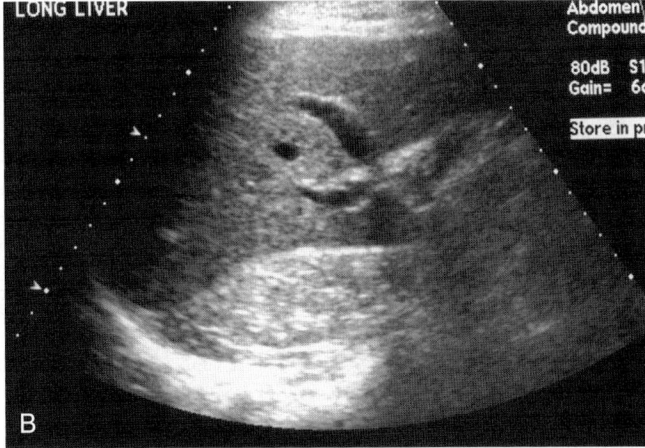

FIGURE 27-28 Chronic kidney injury: ultrasonography. End-stage kidney disease (ESKD) is noted (**A** and **B**); the kidneys are highly echogenic in relation to the adjacent liver. No normal renal structures are visible, but the kidneys remain smooth in overall contour. Note the two small hypoechoic renal cysts in the surface in **A**.

If obstruction is not the cause, other potential causes such as cirrhosis and ascites with accompanying hepatic failure may be evident. In end-stage kidney disease, CT usually demonstrates small, contracted kidneys, which may also show evidence of adulthood-acquired polycystic disease (Figure 27-29). In general, the overall size and thickness of the renal parenchyma appear to decrease with age.[141] In patients in whom chronic long-standing obstruction is the cause of kidney injury, CT generally demonstrates large, fluid-containing kidneys with little or no cortex remaining. Autosomal dominant polycystic kidney disease may also be observed on CT (Figure 27-30). The innumerable cysts are visible throughout the enlarged kidneys. Frequently, some of the cyst walls may contain thin rims of calcification. The density of the internal contents of the cysts may also vary as a result of hemorrhage or proteinaceous debris. For patients undergoing regular dialysis, iodinated contrast may be administered if necessary for CT scans, because the material is dialyzable.

Like CT, MRI is accurate in demonstrating renal structure, as well as prerenal and postrenal causes of kidney injury. MRI is sensitive for the detection of renal parenchymal disease, but the renal parenchymal causes of injury have nonspecific features, and biopsy is generally required (Figures 27-31 and 27-32).[142] Noncontrast MRI routinely allows for detailed tissue characterization of the kidney and surrounding structures. Gadolinium chelates should be avoided in patients with AKI/ARF and CKD stage 4 and 5; newer sequences, such as diffusion weighted and bright blood techniques, provide a way to increase the conspicuity of neoplastic and vascular causes of renal failure without the use of intravenous contrast agents (Figure 27-33).[89,143]

In kidney injury, glomerular and tubular dysfunctions are reflected by abnormal findings on renal scintigraphy and renography. Renal uptake of ^{99}Tc-MAG3 is prolonged, with tubular tracer stasis and little or no excretion. In patients with AKI, if ^{99}Tc-MAG3 has more renal activity than hepatic activity 1 to 3 minutes after injection, recovery is likely, whereas when renal uptake is less than the hepatic uptake, dialysis may be needed.[144] In chronic kidney injury, renal perfusion, cortical tracer extraction, and tracer excretion are diminished. However, this imaging pattern is nonspecific and must be interpreted in the clinical context.[113]

Unilateral Obstruction

Although ultrasonography is frequently the first imaging method used to detect the obstructed kidney, it usually cannot help clinicians establish the cause of the obstruction. Contrast studies, primarily IVU and CT, are the methods of choice for the patient with normal renal function. Antegrade or retrograde pyelography is used as secondary means of assessment. Of these three methods, CT is the most helpful in establishing the site and cause of unilateral obstruction.

IVU has been used for years in evaluating obstructed kidneys.[3] The scout image may give a hint as to the cause (e.g., mass in the pelvis). The obstructed kidney is usually larger than the normal contralateral kidney. The initial nephrogram and appearance of contrast material in the collecting system may be delayed. With time the nephrogram may be larger than that of the normal kidney.[3] Once the collecting system and renal pelvis are opacified with the excreted contrast material, they are dilated and distended. The ureter fills late in relation to the normal kidney. Delayed images may be required with prone or upright views to identify the site of obstruction. In IVU, the site of obstruction is visible, but, again, the cause may be only inferred; this is also true with the antegrade and retrograde pyelography.

Contrast material–enhanced CT and, more specifically, CTU are most useful in assessing the patient with unilateral obstruction.[59] The findings obtained with IVU are amplified with CTU. Small differences in the enhancement pattern of the kidney that are not notable on IVU may be viewed with CT (Figure 27-34). Differences in the excretion patterns by the kidneys are also more sensitively depicted on CT.[58,59] The urine-filled or contrast material–filled ureters point to the obstruction. In axial or coronal images, the course of the dilated ureters on the obstructed side may be followed to the cause. The multiple causes of unilateral obstruction—including both intraureteral and extraureteral causes—may

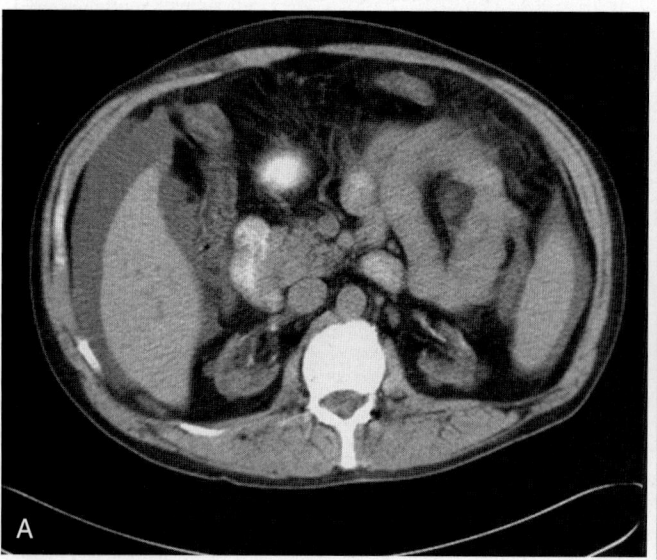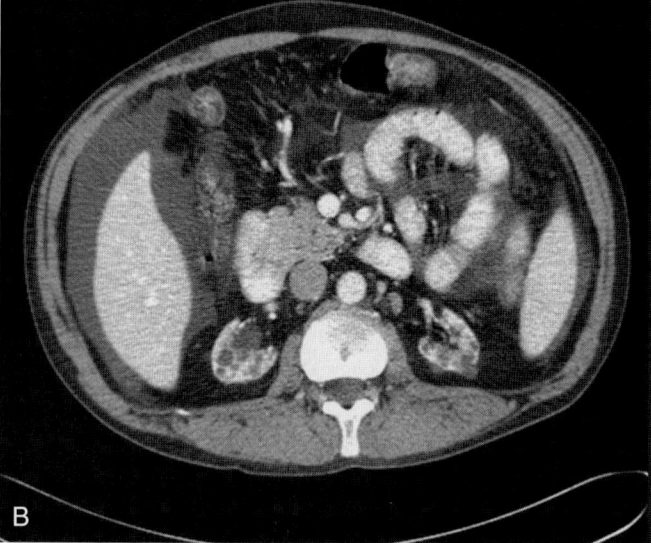

FIGURE 27-29 Adulthood-acquired polycystic kidney disease: computed tomographic scan, axial image without contrast material (**A**) and axial image after administration of contrast material (**B**). The kidneys are small bilaterally with multiple 1-cm cysts primarily in the cortex.

be visible on CT (Figure 27-35). MRI demonstrates similar findings and may be used when CT with contrast material is contraindicated.

Nuclear medicine assessment by means of diuretic renography may also be used to evaluate for obstructive uropathy. It is a noninvasive procedure and yields excellent results. In general, the patient should be well hydrated. In children and in adults with noncompliant bladder, catheterization of the bladder may be used to ensure drainage and reduce back pressure in the urinary system. Scintigraphy with ^{99m}Tc-MAG3 is

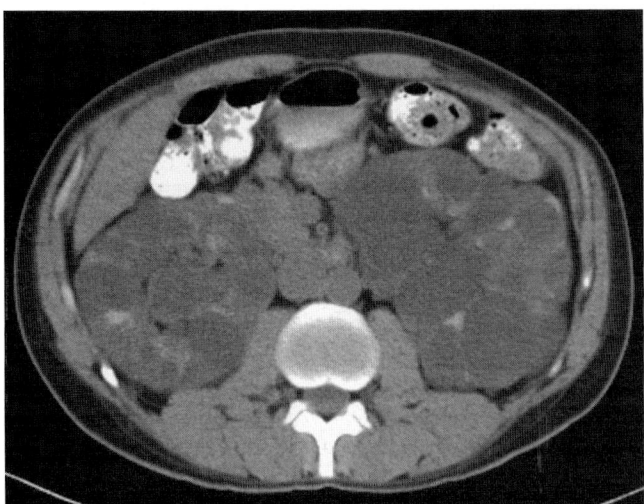

FIGURE 27-30 Autosomal dominant polycystic kidney disease: computed tomographic (CT) scan without contrast material. This CT image demonstrates the markedly enlarged kidney bilaterally with multiple low-density cysts throughout both kidneys. The little remaining renal parenchyma is noted by the sparse, higher density material squeezed by the cysts.

often employed. Furosemide (Lasix) is administered intravenously (1 mg/kg; higher dose in cases of renal insufficiency) when the renal pelvis and ureter are maximally distended.[145] It may be administered as early as 10 to 15 minutes, and as late as 30 to 40 minutes, after tracer administration. Regions of interest are drawn around each renal pelvis, with the background regions as crescent shapes lateral to each kidney. After furosemide administration, in cases of dilation without obstruction, the collecting system empties rapidly, with a subsequent steep decline in the renogram curve. Obstruction can be ruled out if the clearance half time of the renal pelvic emptying is less than 10 minutes. A curve that reaches a plateau or continues to rise after administration of furosemide is indicative of obstruction, with a clearance half time of more than 20 minutes (Figure 27-36). A slow downward slope after furosemide administration may be indicative of partial obstruction. An apparent poor response to furosemide may also occur in patients with severe pelvic dilation (reservoir effect). Other pitfalls include poor injection technique of either the diuretic or the radiotracer, impaired renal function, and dehydration, in which delayed tracer transit and excretion may not be overcome by the effect of a diuretic. Kidneys in neonates (<1 month of age) may be too immature to respond to furosemide, and neonates are thus not suitable candidates for diuretic renal scintigraphy.[113,146]

Various protocols in relation to the timing of furosemide administration have also been reported. In the F0 method, furosemide is injected simultaneously with ^{99}Tc-MAG3 administration. A 17-year clinical experience at one institution proved that this protocol is useful for patients of all ages and for all indications.[147] Taghavi and associates[148] compared diuresis renographic protocols with injection of furosemide 15 minutes before (F–15) and 20 minutes after (F+20)

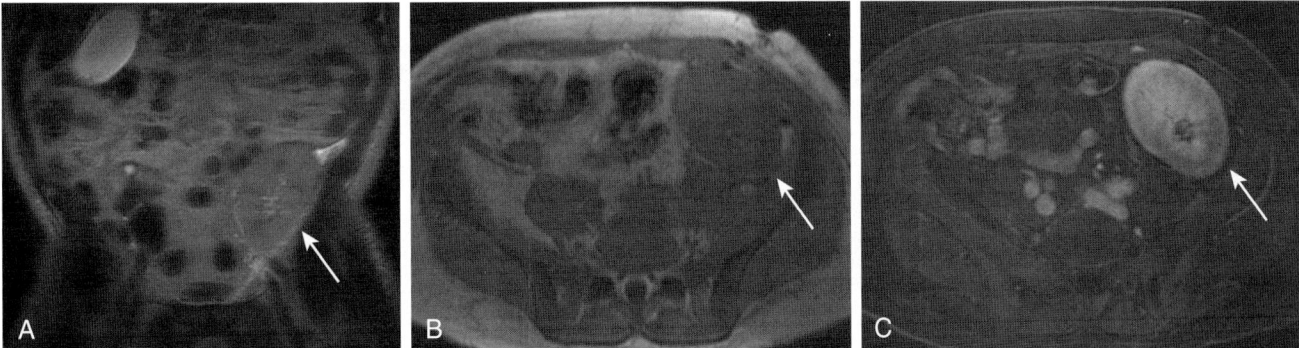

FIGURE 27-31 Renal transplant graft with acute tubular necrosis. Coronal T2-weighted image (**A**), axial T1-weighted image (**B**), and gadolinium-enhanced T1-weighted image (**C**) show reversal of the normal corticomedullary differentiation in a patient with biopsy-proven acute tubular necrosis.

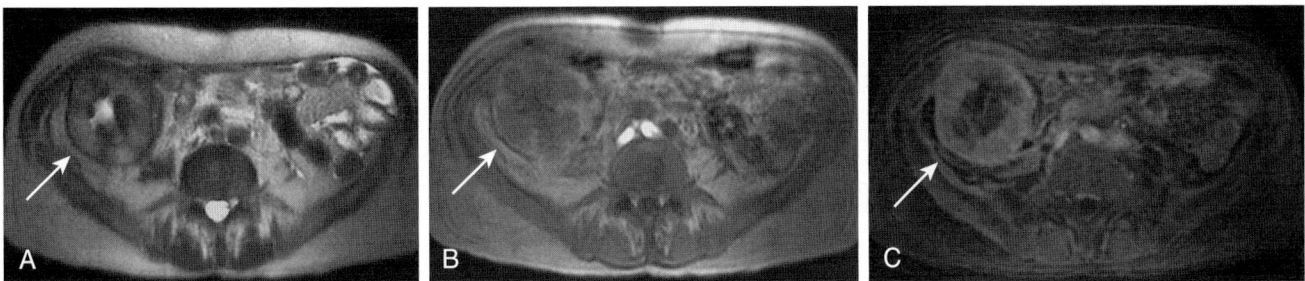

FIGURE 27-32 Renal transplant graft with chronic injury caused by immunoglobulin A (IgA) nephropathy. Axial T2-weighted image (**A**), axial T1-weighted image (**B**), and gadolinium-enhanced T1-weighted image (**C**) demonstrate accentuation of the corticomedullary differentiation.

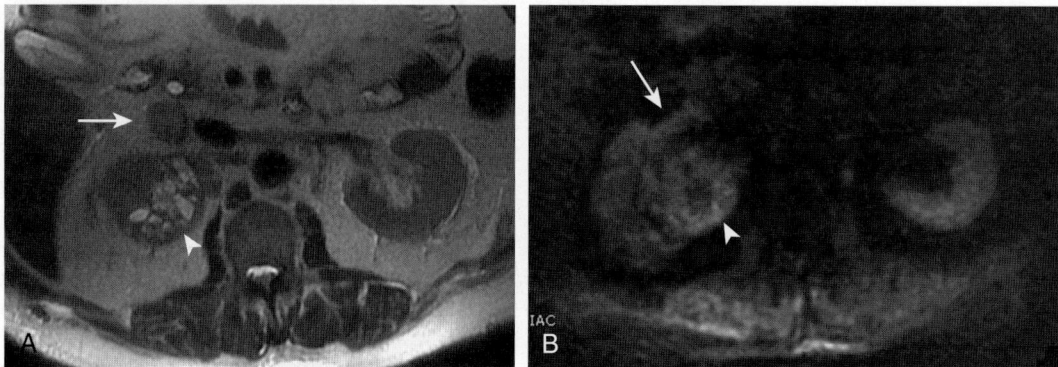

FIGURE 27-33 Diffusion-weighted imaging (DWI). **A,** Axial T2-weighted image demonstrates a heterogeneous renal mass with high signal intensity (*arrowhead*) and a structure of intermediate signal intensity adjacent to the inferior vena cava that is suspect for vascular invasion (*arrow*). **B,** Axial DWI demonstrates the renal mass (*arrowhead*) and increased signal intensity within the renal vein, which confirms renal vein invasion.

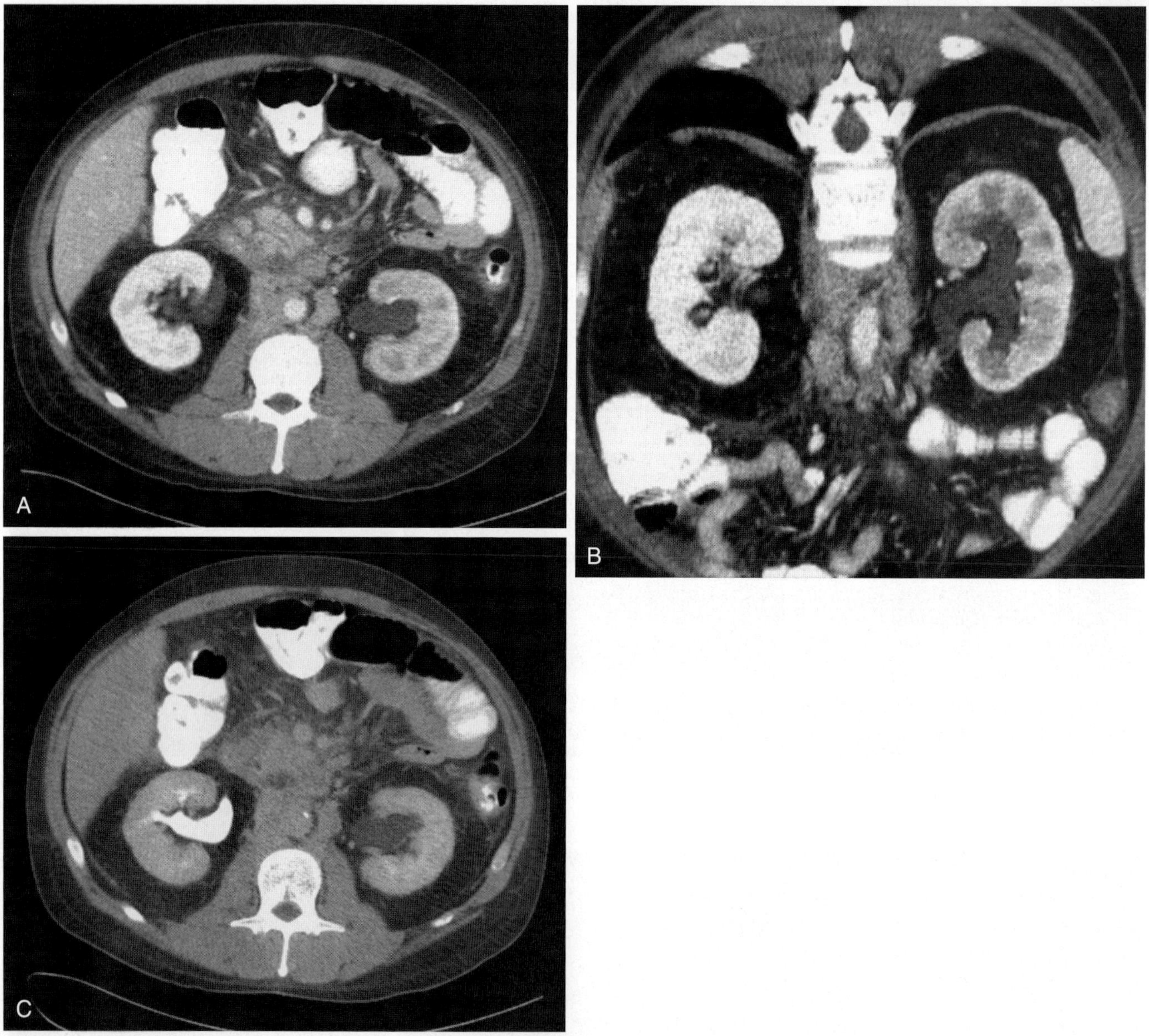

FIGURE 27-34 Unilateral hydronephrosis: contrast material–enhanced computed tomographic scan. Axial (**A**) and coronal (**B**) nephrographic phase images of an obstructed left kidney. The right kidney is in the nephrographic phase, whereas the left (obstructed) kidney is still in the corticomedullary phase; this is apparent with differential enhancement. In the excretory phase image (**C**), the right kidney has contrast material within the collecting system and the renal pelvis. The left kidney has no contrast material in the pelvocalyceal system and contains only nonopacified urine. The patient had lymphoma with retroperitoneal lymph nodes, which caused the obstruction more distally.

also calcify within the calyx. All these types of calcification may be visible on plain radiographs of the abdomen but are viewed to better advantage with noncontrast CT scans of the abdomen (Figure 27-37).

Cortical calcification is most often associated with cortical necrosis from any cause.[149] Dystrophic calcification develops in the damaged cortex after the episode of acute cortical necrosis. The calcifications tend to resemble tram tracks and to be circumferential. Other entities in which cortical calcification are found include hyperoxaluria, Alport's syndrome, and, in rare cases, chronic glomerulonephritis. The stippled calcifications of hyperoxaluria may be found in both the cortex and the medulla, as well as in other organs, such as the heart. In Alport's syndrome, only cortical calcifications are found.

Calcifications in the medulla are much more common than cortical calcifications.[149] The most common cause of medullary nephrocalcinosis is primary hyperparathyroidism. Intratubular deposition of calcium oxalate crystals occurs first; later deposits are in the interstitial renal parenchyma. The distribution appears to be within the renal pyramid. The radiologic picture may be either focal or diffuse and either unilateral or bilateral. Nephrolithiasis also occurs in patients with primary hyperparathyroidism. Nephrocalcinosis occurs in other diseases in which hypercalcemia or hypercalciuria occur, such as hyperthyroidism, sarcoidosis, hypervitaminosis D, immobilization, multiple myeloma, and metastatic neoplasms. These calcifications are nonspecific and punctate in appearance and are usually medullary in location.

In 70% to 75% of cases of renal tubular acidosis, there is evidence of nephrocalcinosis. The calcifications tend to be uniform and distributed throughout the renal pyramids bilaterally. With medullary sponge kidney and renal tubular ectasia, small calculi form in the distal collecting tubules, probably because of stasis. The appearance varies from involvement of only a single calyx to involvement of both kidneys throughout. The calcifications are small, round, and within the peak of the pyramid adjacent to the calyx. Medullary sponge kidney is also associated with nephrolithiasis, inasmuch as the small calculi in the distal collecting tubules may pass into the collecting systems and ureters, resulting in renal colic.[150]

The calcifications that occur in renal tuberculosis are typically medullary in location and may mimic other forms of nephrocalcinosis.[151] Renal tuberculosis begins in the renal cortex and progresses to the medulla. Invasion and erosion of the calyceal system subsequently occurs, resulting in spread of the tuberculous infection down the ureters and into the bladder. Calcification occurs in the pyramids as part of the healing process. With overwhelming involvement of the kidney, the entire kidney may be destroyed; this results in diffuse, heavy calcification throughout the entire kidney, which is small and scarred. Medullary calcifications are also visible in patients with renal papillary necrosis. With necrosis of the papilla, the material is sloughed into the calyces. Retained tissue fragments may calcify and have the appearance of medullary nephrocalcinosis.

Nephrolithiasis is a common clinical entity. The lifetime risk of developing renal calculi is 12%; the risk is two to three times higher in men than in women.[152] Most renal stones occur in individuals aged 30 to 60. Renal stone disease is a multifactorial problem with metabolic disorders, and other factors, such as geography, diet, family history, diabetes, sedentary lifestyle, and dehydration, contribute to the disorder.

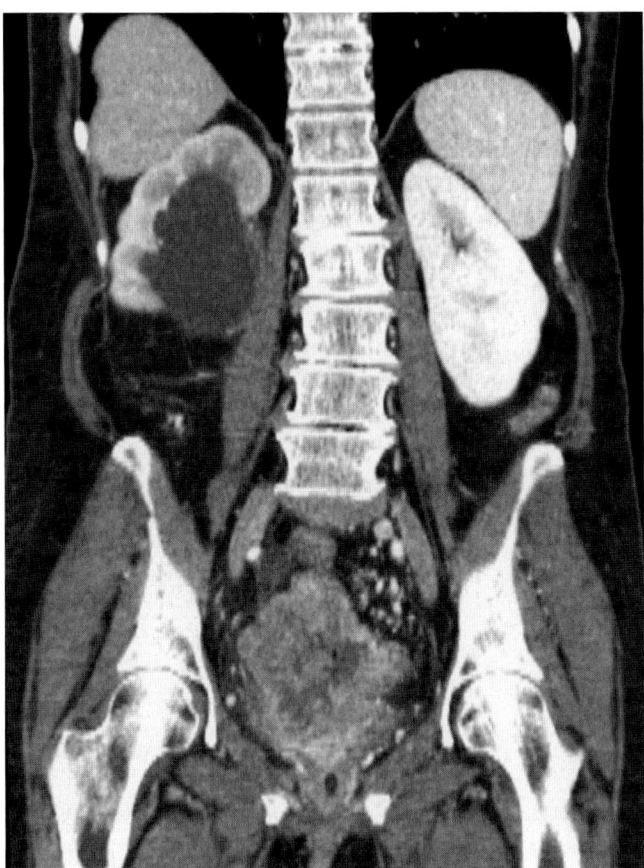

FIGURE 27-35 Unilateral obstruction: contrast material–enhanced computed tomographic scan. The coronal image demonstrates the difference in enhancement between the two kidneys, with the moderately dilated renal pelvis and calyces on the right. The large heterogeneous pelvis mass is the source of the obstruction: recurrent rectal carcinoma.

administration of ^{99m}Tc-MAG3. In this comparative study of 21 patients with dilation of the pelvicalyceal system, the F–15 protocol produced fewer equivocal results than did the F+20 method and therefore was considered the preferable protocol. Further experience is needed to determine the most optimal timing interval between furosemide and ^{99m}Tc-MAG3 injections in diuresis renography.

Renal Calcifications and Renal Stone Disease

Calcifications may occur in many regions of the kidney.[149] Nephrolithiasis or renal calculi are the most common and occur in the pelvicalyceal system. *Nephrocalcinosis* refers to renal parenchymal calcification occurring in either the medulla or cortex. These calcifications are usually associated with diseases in which patients have hypercalcemia or hypercalciuria or with conditions in which specific pathologic lesions are in the cortex or medulla. In nephrocalcinosis, calcifications may be diffuse or punctate and are usually bilateral. Some patients with nephrocalcinosis may also develop nephrolithiasis. Calcifications may also occur in vascular structures, particularly in patients with diabetes and advanced atherosclerotic disease. Rimlike calcifications may occur in simple renal cysts and polycystic disease. Patients with renal carcinomas may exhibit variable calcifications as well. Sloughed papilla may

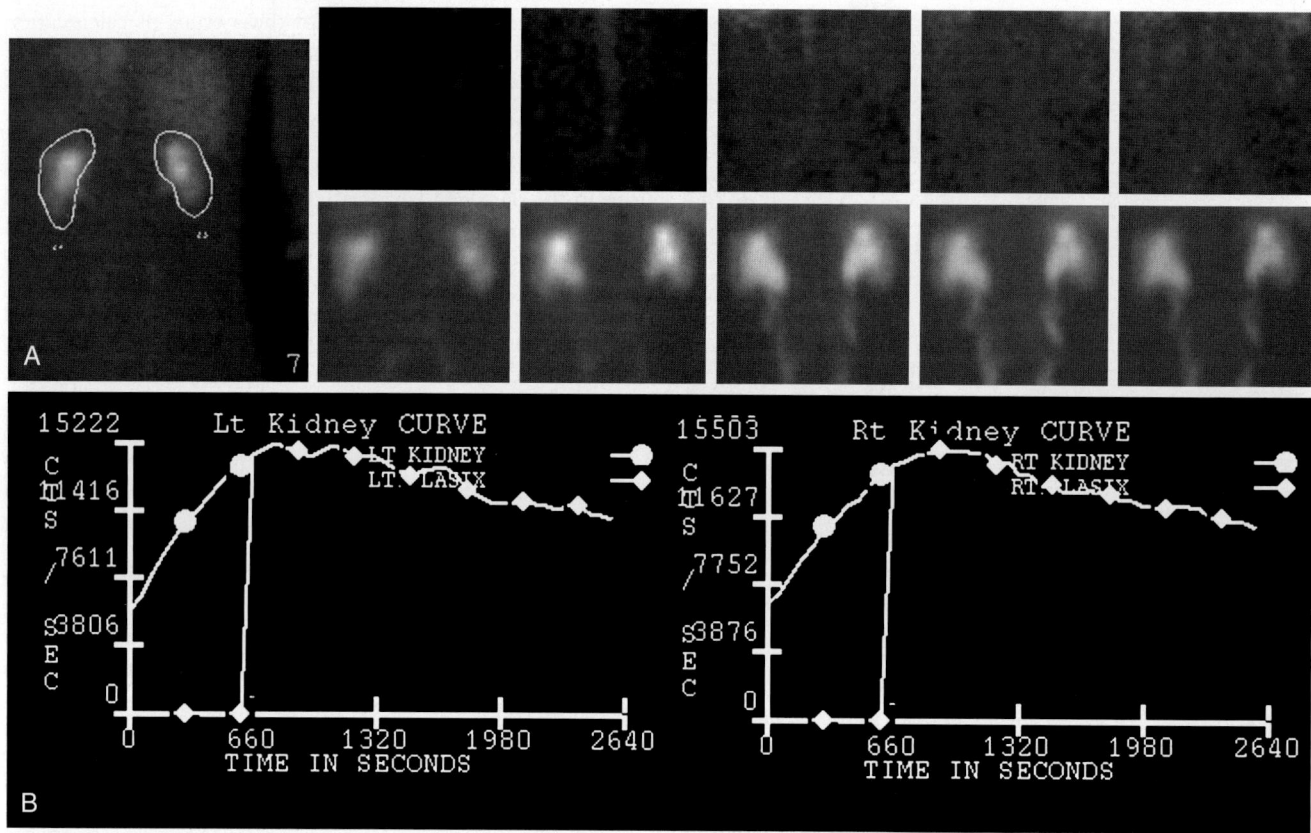

FIGURE 27-36 Abnormal findings on renogram with technetium 99m–labeled mercaptoacetyltriglycine, demonstrating obstructive urinary kinetics with a poor response to furosemide. **A,** Static and timed images. **B,** Individual curves for each kidney.

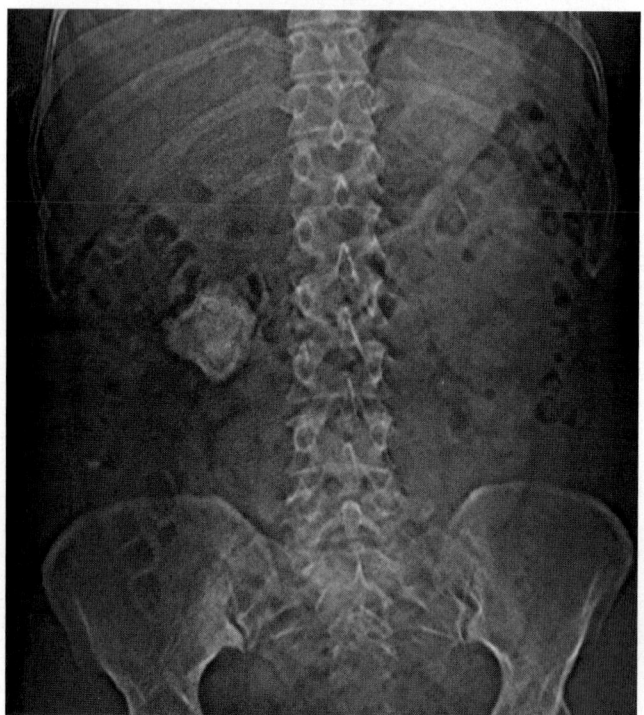

FIGURE 27-37 Renal stone: plain radiograph of the kidneys, ureters, and bladder (KUB). A large laminated stone is visible in the renal pelvis of the right kidney. The outline of the normal left kidney can be seen with no calcifications overlying it. The right kidney outline cannot be seen.

Most urinary tract stones are composed of calcium salts of either oxalate or phosphate or a combination of the two.[153-156] This composition accounts for the dense appearance on radiographs. Stasis contributes to the formation of stones in the urinary tract. Renal colic or flank pain is the most common presenting symptom. Most patients also have hematuria, although it may be absent if the ureters are completely obstructed by the stone. The pain that occurs with a passing renal stone is probably caused by the distension of the tubular system and renal capsule of the kidney and by the peristalsis associated with ureteral contractions as the stone moves distally.

Most urinary calculi that are 4 mm or smaller pass with conservative treatment.[157] The larger the stone, the more likely other measures will be necessary in order to treat the stone and associated obstruction. Extracorporal shock wave lithotripsy is the method of choice for treating larger stones. Success rates are best for stones in the renal pelvis and kidney.[158] Other methods, such as percutaneous or transureteral lithotripsy, may be necessary.

Plain radiographs of the abdomen are most useful when a stone is densely calcified and large enough to be visible (see Figure 27-37). Overlying bowel gas and feces frequently make visualization difficult. Costal cartilage calcifications in the upper abdomen may be confused with renal calculi, as may gallstones in the right upper quadrant. For years, IVU has been the method of choice for the assessment of patients with renal colic.[159,160] After the injection of intravenous contrast media, the nephrogram appears unequal, with a delayed appearance on the affected sides. Once the nephrogram

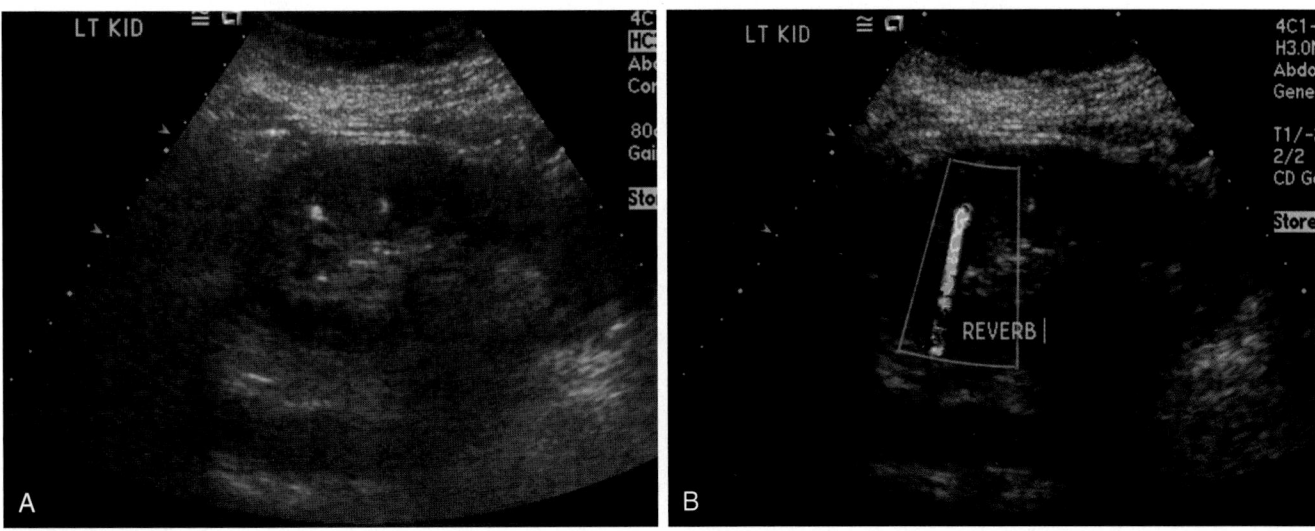

FIGURE 27-38 Renal stone: ultrasonography. Longitudinal image (**A**) and color Doppler image (**B**) demonstrate an echogenic focus at the corticomedullary junction. Not all stones show shadowing, but in this case, reverberation artifact is visible on the color Doppler image, which helps establish the diagnosis.

appears, it may also be prolonged and increase in density with time, specifically with complete obstruction caused by a ureteric stone. The excretion of contrast material into the collecting system is usually delayed, and the pelvicalyceal system is dilated. Delayed images up to 24 hours after injection are occasionally necessary to visualize the contrast material–filled dilated collecting systems, pelvis, and ureter to the point of obstruction by the calculus. When the pelvicalyceal system is filled with contrast material and the ureter is not, positioning the patient upright or prone for images may help fill the ureter with contrast material. The injection of contrast material, being a fluid load, may facilitate the stone's passage through the ureters into the bladder.

Ultrasound assessment has also been used in the evaluation of renal colic.[161] This examination is quick and usually performed easily. The clinician is looking for the effect of a passing renal stone, which is obstruction. Unilateral hydronephrosis may be observed, although the examination may yield normal results early in the passage of a renal stone. Renal stones may be visualized within the kidneys as hyperechoic foci with distal acoustic shadowing or reverberation artifacts (Figure 27-38).[161] Ureteric stones are rarely visible, because of overlying bowel gas and stone. Distal ureteral stones near the ureterovesical junction may be visualized through the urine-filled bladder transabdominally. Transvaginal and transperineal ultrasonography has also been suggested as a method for evaluating for distal ureteral stones. Ultrasonography may demonstrate absence of a ureteral jet in the bladder on the side in which a stone is being passed. Doppler ultrasonography and assessment of the peripheral vasculature resistance is occasionally helpful in pinpointing the affected kidney, but the study results have been variable.[137]

Noncontrast CT scanning of the abdomen and pelvis has emerged as the standard evaluation in patients with renal colic.[162-164] The sensitivities for CT are 96% to 100%; the specificities are 95% to 100%; and the accuracy rates are 96% to 98%; for this reason, nonenhanced CT has supplanted plain radiography, IVU, and ultrasonography.[163,165-167] In comparisons of nonenhanced CT and IVU, CT is much more useful, with 94% to 100% sensitivity and 92% to 100% specificity;

IVU has 64% to 97% sensitivity and 92% to 94% specificity.[163] Also, when noncontrast CT was used as the reference standard in comparison with ultrasonography, 24% sensitivity and 90% specificity were found for ultrasonography.[168,169] Because x-ray radiation is used in CT scanning, ultrasound examination should be reserved for the pediatric population and pregnant women. An alternative diagnosis is made in patients with "renal colic" in 9% to 29% of cases in which noncontrast CT is used for evaluation.[170]

Nonenhanced CT is performed from the top of the kidneys to below the pubic symphysis. No preparation is needed. Intravenous contrast material is rarely needed. The studies are performed with 3-mm collimation or less, and the slices are reconstructed to be contiguous or slightly overlapping.[171-173] The images should be viewed on a monitor as axial images, with multiplanar reconstructions used as adjunct views. Virtually all renal stones are denser than the adjacent soft tissues (Figure 27-39)[174]; exceptions are renal stones associated with indinavir (a protease inhibitor used in the management of acquired immunodeficiency syndrome [AIDS]) and very small uric acid stones (<1 to 2 mm in diameter).[175,176] As expected, calcium oxalate and calcium phosphate stones are the most dense.[154,155] Matrix stones, which are rare, may also be relatively low in density, but they usually contain calcium impurities that make them visible.[153,156]

For detecting stones, low-dose scanning has been shown to be as effective as CT with standard techniques.[177,178] The radiation dose is usually 20% to 25% of the standard dose. Dual-energy imaging with CT has demonstrated the ability to distinguish different types of stones into specific groups.[179,180]

Calculi appear as calcifications within the urinary tract. Renal calculi may be visible in all parts of the collecting systems and the urinary tract. Small punctuate calcifications (≈1 mm) are occasionally observed just at the tip of the renal pyramid. These may represent the calcification noted in Randall plaques.[181] Obstruction occurs most commonly at the ureteropelvic junction; at the pelvic brim, where the ureters cross over the iliac vessels; and at the ureterovesical junction. The diagnosis is made on the noncontrast CT scan by demonstrating the calcified stone within the urine-filled ureters

(Figure 27-40).[171] Secondary signs may be present to assist in the diagnosis.[165] Hydronephrosis and hydroureter to the point of the stone may be visible (see Figure 27-39). Asymmetric perinephric and periureteral stranding may also be related to forniceal rupture and urine leak (Figure 27-41).[182] The involved kidney may be less dense than the normal kidney because of increased interstitial fluid and edema.[183,184] The affected kidney may also be larger than the normal kidney. At the point of obstruction, the stone may be visible within the ureter, with soft tissue thickening of the ureteral wall at that level. This thickening is probably caused by edema and inflammation associated with the passage of the stone.

Noncontrast CT has the additional advantage of assessing the overall stone burden of the patient, not just the passing stone. Also, the size may be accurately measured, which enables clinicians to make treatment decisions.[157,185,186] Distal ureteral stones are occasionally confused with phleboliths,

which are common in the pelvis (see Figure 27-40). Images reconstructed in the coronal plane along the course of the ureters down to the level of the stone may be helpful.[187] Also, close inspection of phleboliths frequently reveals a small, soft tissue tag leading to the calcification: the "comet tail" sign.[188] Enhancement with contrast material is occasionally necessary in confusing or difficult cases. Also, it may be used in complicated cases in which the patient is febrile and pyelonephritis or pyohydronephrosis is suspected.

CT is more sensitive for the evaluation of renal and collecting system calcifications, especially in the absence of urinary tract obstruction. In the evaluation of acute stone disease, MRI is not the examination of first choice, but it is a suitable alternative for selected patients.[189] Stones are difficult to identify in nondilated systems, even in retrospect. When stones are observed on MRI, they are visible as black foci on both T1- and T2-weighted sequences. Stones become more

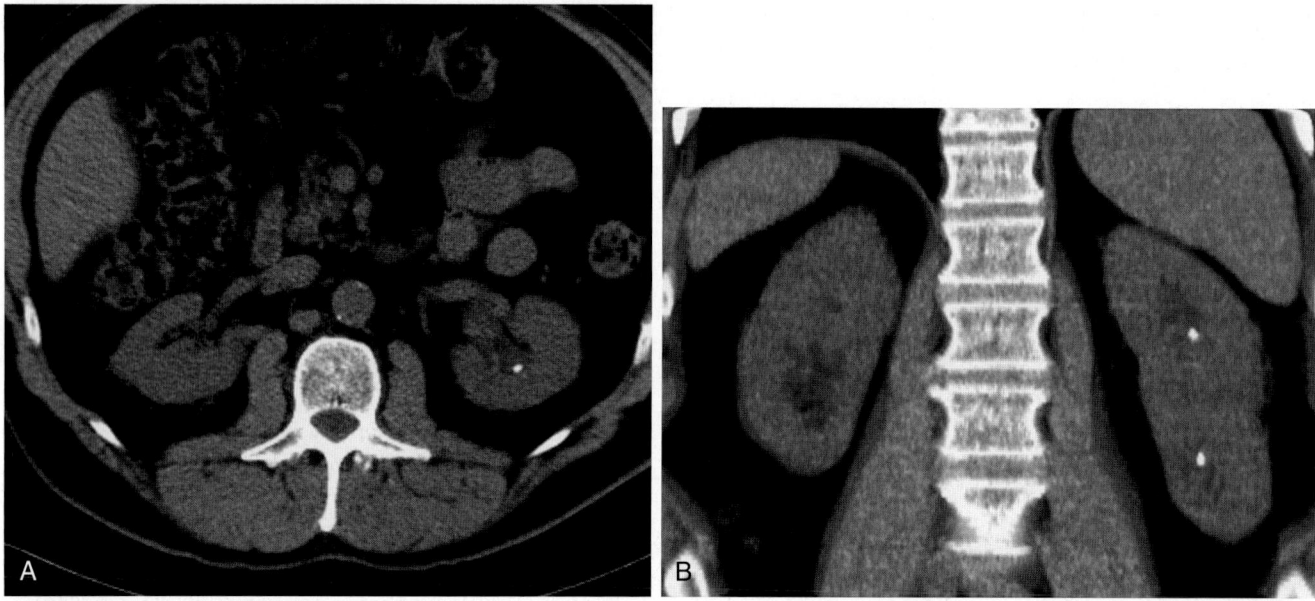

FIGURE 27-39 Renal stones: noncontrast computed tomographic scan. Axial image (**A**) and coronal image (**B**) demonstrate 4- to 5-mm stones in the upper and lower poles of the left kidney. There are no signs of obstruction.

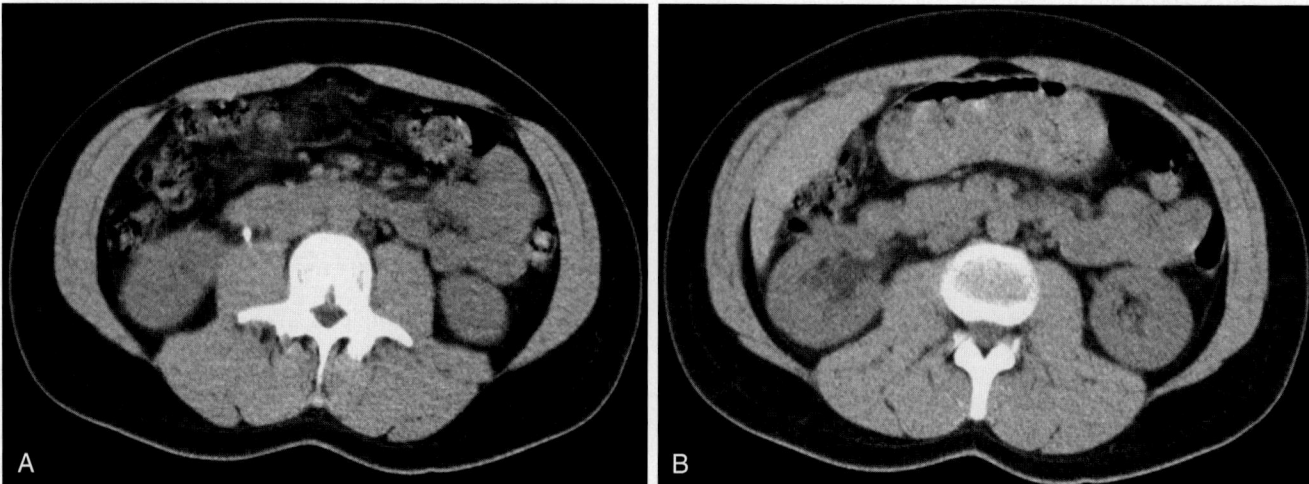

FIGURE 27-40 Ureteral stone: noncontrast computed tomographic scan. **A,** A 5- to 6-mm stone is noted in the midportion of the right ureter. **B,** Axial images of the midportion of the kidneys reveals the urine-filled right renal pelvis and a right kidney that is slightly less dense than the left. These are signs of obstruction.

conspicuous in a dilated collecting system (Figure 27-42); however, a nonenhanced filling defect is a nonspecific finding. Blood, air, or debris may have the same appearance. If stones or other calcifications are a concern, noncontrast CT is the examination of choice for improved conspicuity (Figure 27-43).

When the use of iodinated contrast material is contraindicated, or when reduction of radiation exposure is desired, MRU can be used to determine the cause and location of an obstructing process (Figure 27-44). MRU is highly accurate in demonstrating obstruction, regardless of whether the process is acute or chronic.[189] Acute obstruction may be associated with perinephric fluid, which is well demonstrated on T2-weighted sequences.[189,190] However, perinephric fluid is a nonspecific finding and can be found in association with other renal disease.

Although MRI is not the imaging modality of choice for evaluation of acute renal trauma, MRI is useful in evaluating the patient who has recently undergone surgery for renal stone disease. MRI has been reported as being more accurate than CT in differentiating perirenal and intrarenal hematomas (Figures 27-45 to 27-47).[191] With contrast material, MRI can also demonstrate damage to the collecting system and areas of ischemia without the risk of nephrotoxicity.

Renal Infection

Acute pyelonephritis is typically a clinical diagnosis based on signs and symptoms of flank pain, tenderness, and fever with accompanying laboratory findings of leukocytosis, pyuria, positive urine culture, and occasionally bacteremia and hematuria.[192] Most cases of acute pyelonephritis occur by the ascending route from the bladder and are caused by gram-negative bacteria.[192] Vesicoureteral reflux may contribute, although the ascent of the bacteria up the ureter also occurs in its absence. Vesicoureteral reflux is caused by the presence of adhesive P fimbria and powerful endotoxins that appear to inhibit ureteral peristalsis, thereby creating a functional obstruction.[193] The gram-negative bacteria, most commonly *Escherichia coli,* are transported to the renal pelvis, where intrarenal reflux occurs and the bacteria traverse the calyceal system to the ducts and tubules within the renal pyramid. When the bacteria are within the tubules, there is a leukocyte response. Enzyme release results in destruction of tubular cells with subsequent bacterial invasion of the interstitium.

The resultant inflammatory response involves both the interstitium and tubules. As the infection progresses, it spreads throughout the pyramid and to the adjacent parenchyma. The inflammatory response leads to focal or more diffuse swelling of the kidney. Vasoconstriction of the involved arteries and arterioles is noted. Without adequate treatment, necrosis of the involved regions and microabscess formation occur. These microabscesses may coalesce into larger macroabscesses, which tend to be surrounded by a rim of granulation tissue.[194] Perinephric abscess results from the rupture of an intrarenal abscess through the renal capsule or the leak from an infected and obstructed kidney (pyonephrosis). The overall distribution in the kidney is usually patchy or lobar, but sometimes it is diffuse.[192] Subsequent scarring of the kidney after treatment reflects the magnitude of the infection and tissue destruction that occurred. Vesicoureteral reflux is most common in childhood but may occur in adults with lower urinary tract infections or neurogenic bladders.

Hematogenous infection occurs initially in the cortex of the kidney. It eventually involves the medulla. It does not tend to be lobar or pyramidal in distribution. The areas of involvement are usually round, peripheral, and frequently multiple. These infections are usually caused by gram-positive bacteria, such as *Staphylococcus aureus* and *Streptococcus* species. Blood-borne infection is less common than

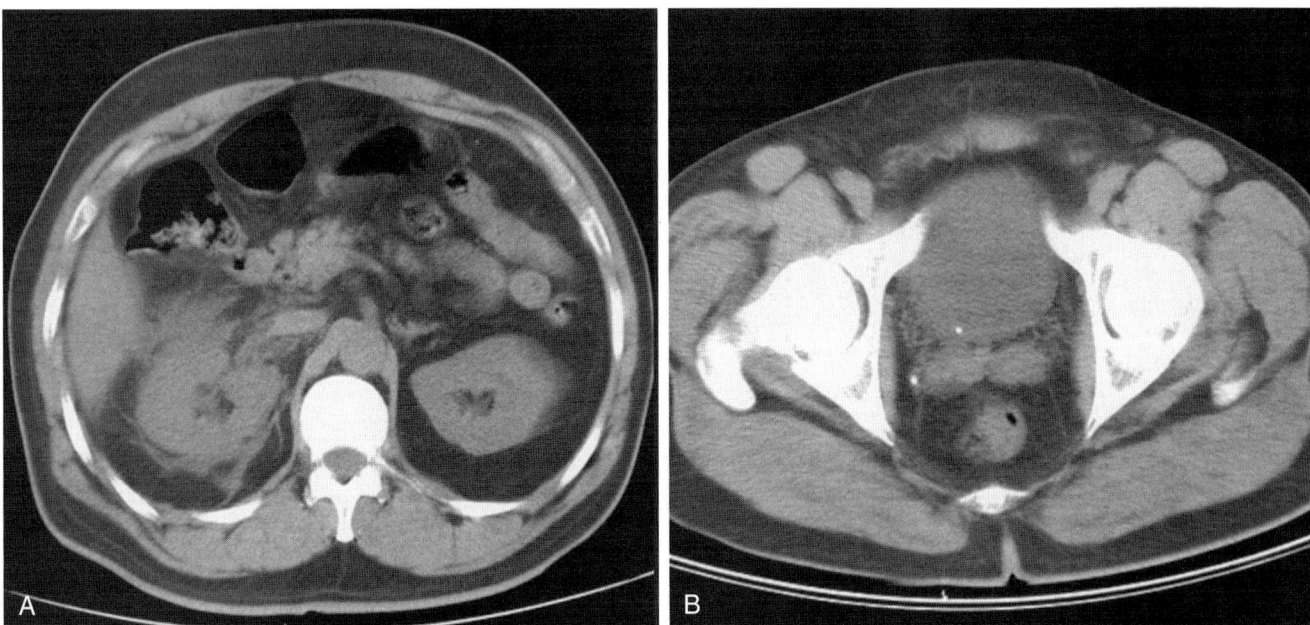

FIGURE 27-41 Ureteral stone: noncontrast computed tomographic scan. Axial images of the kidneys shows perinephric and peripelvic stranding and fluid on the right (**A**) caused by forniceal rupture and leakage of urine as a result of the distal obstructing stone at the right ureterovesical junction (**B**). Note the phlebolith on the right posterior to the bladder and lateral to the seminal vesicle; phleboliths are commonly confused with distal ureteral stones.

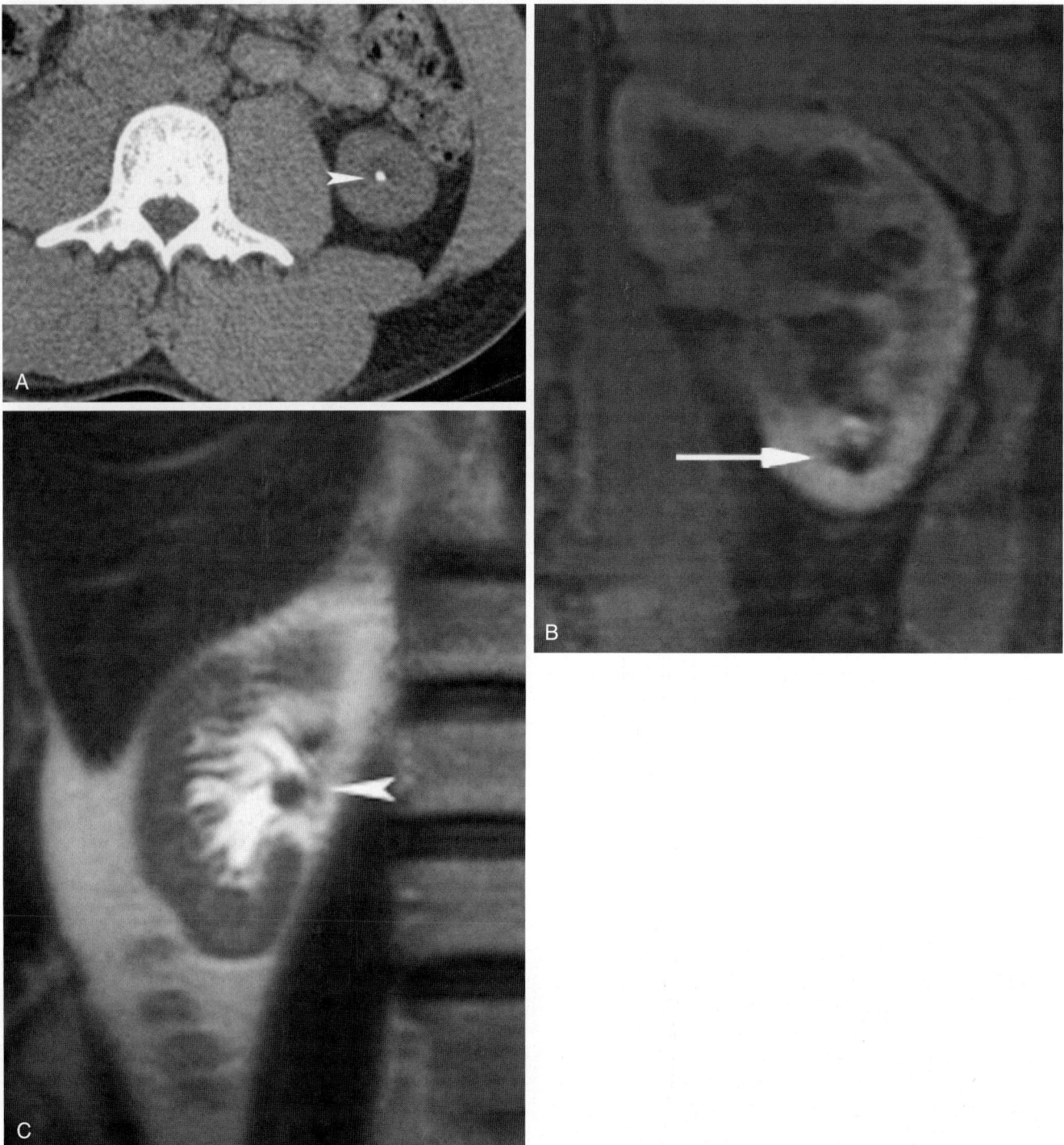

FIGURE 27-42 Renal stones. Calcification (*arrowhead*) well viewed on computed tomography (**A**) is difficult to demonstrate on magnetic resonance imaging (**B**) (*arrow*), even in retrospect. **C,** A stone (*arrowhead*) is more conspicuous when it is located within a mildly dilated collection system.

ascending infections and is usually observed in intravenous drug abusers, immunocompromised patients, or patients with a source of infection outside the kidney, such as heart valves or teeth.

In patients with AIDS, urinary tract infections are quite common.[195,196] The infections are frequently hematogenous with unusual organisms such as *Pneumocystis carinii*, cytomegalovirus, and *Mycobacterium avium–intracellulare*. The infections may also be apparent in other abdominal structures, such as the liver, spleen, and adrenal glands.[197,198]

Imaging is rarely used or needed in the uncomplicated case of acute pyelonephritis. It is reserved for patients who are not responding to conventional antibiotic treatment, patients with an unclear diagnosis, patients with coexisting stone disease and possible obstruction, patients with diabetes and poor antibiotic response, and immunocompromised patients. Imaging is used to assist in confirming the diagnosis and determining the extent of the disease. It is also used in assessing complications of acute pyelonephritis, including renal abscess, emphysematous pyelonephritis, and perinephric abscess.

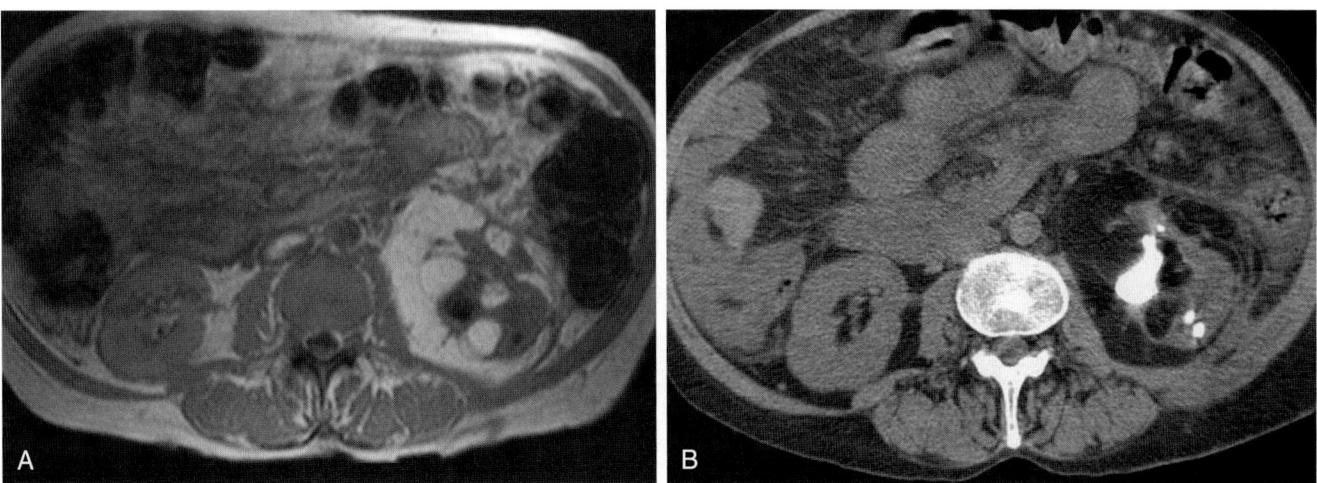

FIGURE 27-43 Staghorn calculus. Magnetic resonance imaging (MRI) **(A)** and computed tomography (CT) **(B)** demonstrate large pelvic calculus with associated left renal atrophy. Even large stones may be difficult to recognize on MRI. Calcifications are more conspicuous on CT.

Renal abscess formation is more common with hematogenous infection than with ascending infection.[192] Emphysematous pyelonephritis is a severe necrotizing infection of the renal parenchyma, usually caused by gram-negative bacteria (*E. coli, Klebsiella pneumoniae, Proteus mirabilis*).[199] Of patients with emphysematous pyelonephritis, 90% have uncontrolled diabetes.[200] Emphysematous pyelonephritis is characterized by severe acute pyelonephritis, urosepsis, and hypotension. The gas found in the renal parenchyma is believed to form as a result of the high levels of glucose in the tissue by fermentation with the production of CO_2. The gas may also be observed in the pelvicalyceal system or perinephric space (or both). Xanthogranulomatous pyelonephritis is a complication of long-standing obstruction and chronic infection, usually with *Proteus* species or *E. coli*.[201] The renal parenchyma is destroyed and replaced by vast amounts of lipid-laden macrophages. Staghorn calculi are commonly observed. The kidney is usually barely functional or nonfunctional. The destruction is typically global, but it may involve only a portion of the kidney.

Renal tuberculosis occurs by hematogenous spread of pulmonary infections. The genitourinary tract is the second most common site of involvement. Evidence of previous pulmonary tuberculosis is found in fewer than 50% of patients with genitourinary tuberculosis. Only 5% may have active tuberculosis. Renal involvement is bilateral; the findings are determined by the extent of the infection, the stage of the infection, and the host's response. Calcified granuloma may be found within the cortex or medulla, papillary necrosis may be visible (Figure 27-48), and hydrocalyx with infundibular strictures may develop (Figure 27-49). The kidney may become focally or globally scarred as the disease progresses. There may be areas of nonfunction with dystrophic calcifications. In the end stage, the kidney may be small and scarred with bizarre calcifications; this condition is the so-called autonephrectomy.[151,202] Malacoplakia is a rare inflammatory condition that most commonly involves the bladder but may also involve the ureter and kidney. It is believed to be caused by an altered intracellular response to ingested bacterial organisms by histiocytes. The presence of Michaelis-Gutmann bodies—large intracellular inclusion bodies within eosinophilic macrophages—is pathognomic for malacoplakia. Typically, the kidney is affected by obstruction from the lower urinary tract. When the kidney is directly involved, it is a multifocal process that may appear similar to xanthogranulomatous pyelonephritis on imaging.

In uncomplicated acute pyelonephritis, IVU findings may appear normal in up to 75% of cases.[194,203] When present, the findings are usually unilateral and may be segmental. The findings include renal enlargement, altered nephrogram, decreased concentration of contrast material, and delayed appearance of contrast material in the calyces. The calyces and renal pelvis may be narrowed or mildly dilated, as is the ureter. The kidney may be globally enlarged by edema or may have a contour bulge with more focal involvement. The nephrogram may be diminished in intensity in comparison with the opposite normal side, or even absent. Delayed images occasionally produce a prolonged nephrogram on the affected side. The appearance time of the excreted contrast material in the calyces may be delayed segmentally or globally, and the overall density of the contrast material may be diminished in comparison with the opposite side. In the affected region, calyces appear narrowed as a result of the edema, although on occasion the calyces may be dilated. Dilation of the pelvicalyceal system and ureter is caused by atony or poor peristalsis in the system. This is a form of nonobstructive dilation or hydronephrosis. The findings on IVU usually return to normal within 3 to 6 weeks after the episode of acute pyelonephritis.

The ultrasound appearance is normal in the majority of patients with acute pyelonephritis. When the appearance is abnormal, the findings are often nonspecific. Ultrasonography is performed to look for a cause for acute pyelonephritis, such as obstruction or renal calculi, and to search for complications. Altered parenchymal echogenicity is the most frequent finding, with loss of the normal corticomedullary differentiation. The echogenicity is usually decreased or heterogeneous in the affected area (Figure 27-50). There may be focal or generalized swelling of the kidney. Power Doppler imaging may improve sensitivity in demonstrating focal hypoperfusion, but this finding is nonspecific. Tissue harmonic ultrasound imaging may be more sensitive in demonstrating focal or segmental, patchy, hypoechoic areas extending from the medulla to the renal capsule.[204] In patients with AIDS, renal involvement is associated with increased cortical echogenicity and loss of the corticomedullary differentiation (Figure 27-51).[198] Renal size is also increased, and this is generally a bilateral process.

CT is the most sensitive and specific imaging study in the patient with acute pyelonephritis.[203] Although the study may yield normal results in mild, uncomplicated pyelonephritis, it is still the most effective imaging means of establishing the diagnosis, judging the extent of disease, and evaluating for complications. In general, noncontrast and postcontrast scans are used; the contrast material–enhanced study is the most effective. The nephrographic phase of CT is best for imaging in patients with acute pyelonephritis (Figure 27-52). Wedge-shaped areas of decreased density extending from the renal pyramid to the cortex are most characteristic.[203] The nephrogram may be streaky or striated in a focal

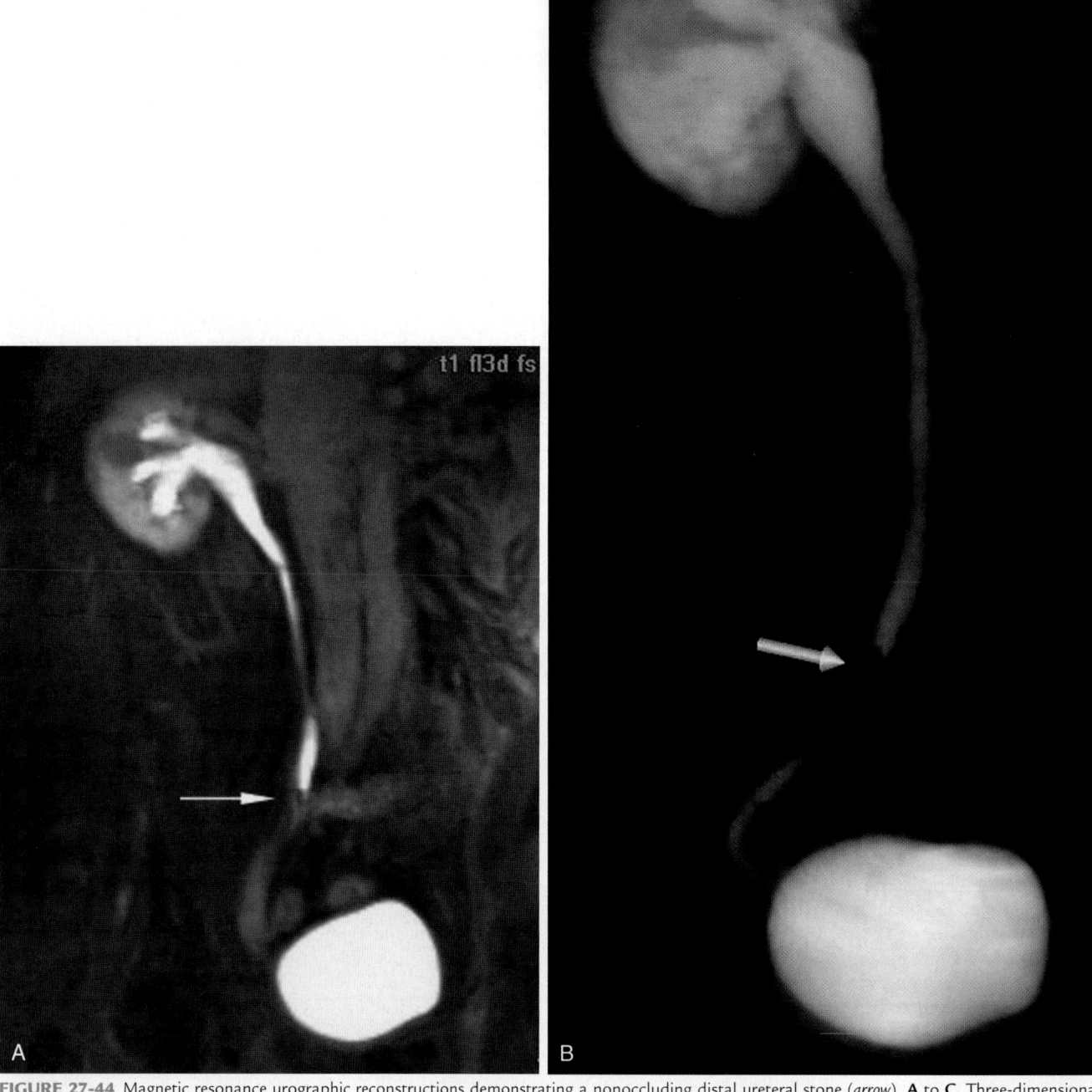

FIGURE 27-44 Magnetic resonance urographic reconstructions demonstrating a nonoccluding distal ureteral stone (*arrow*). **A** to **C,** Three-dimensional postrenal processing techniques are used to mimic intravenous urography. **D,** Postcontrast axial imaging demonstrates a stone within the lumen of the distal ureters.

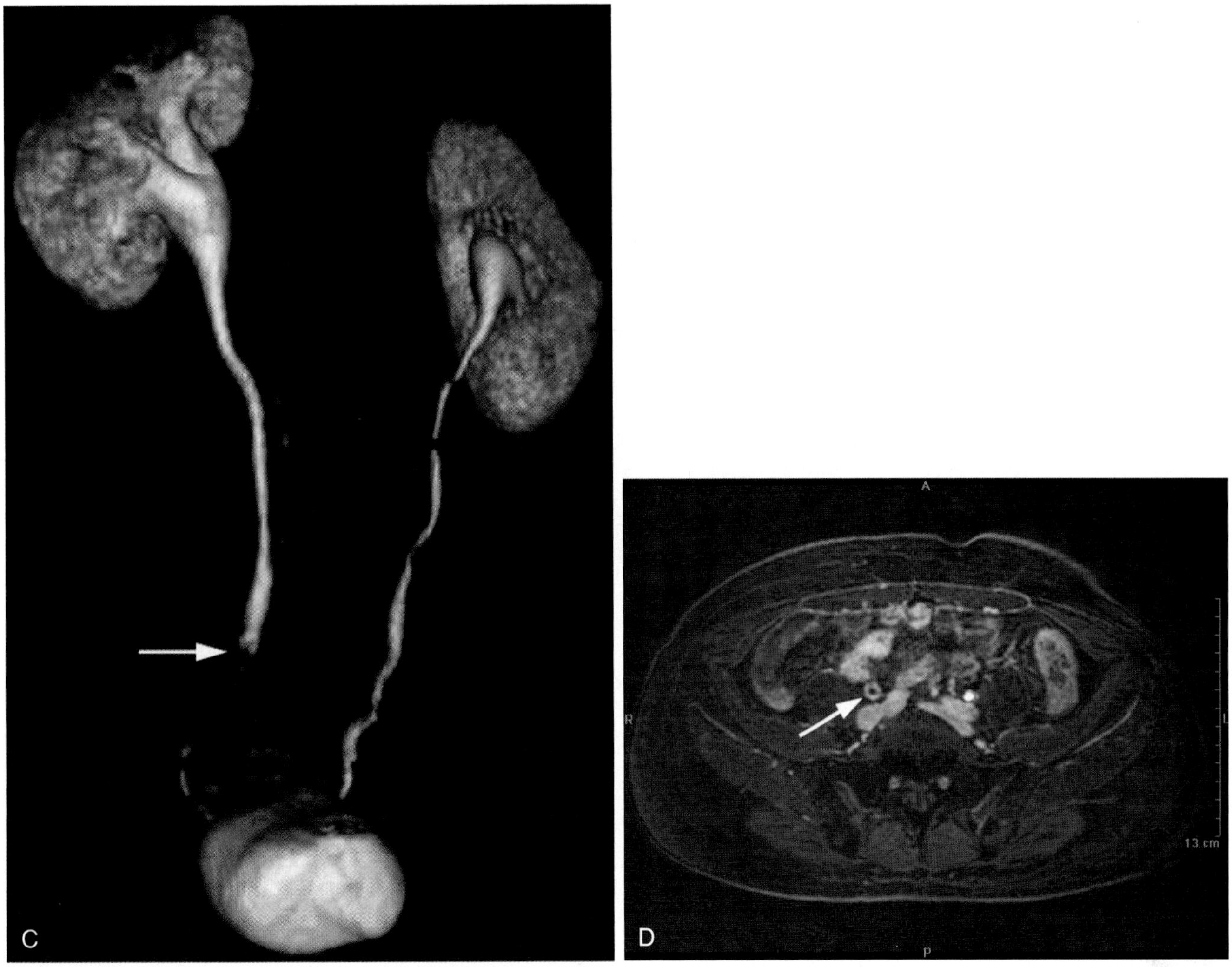

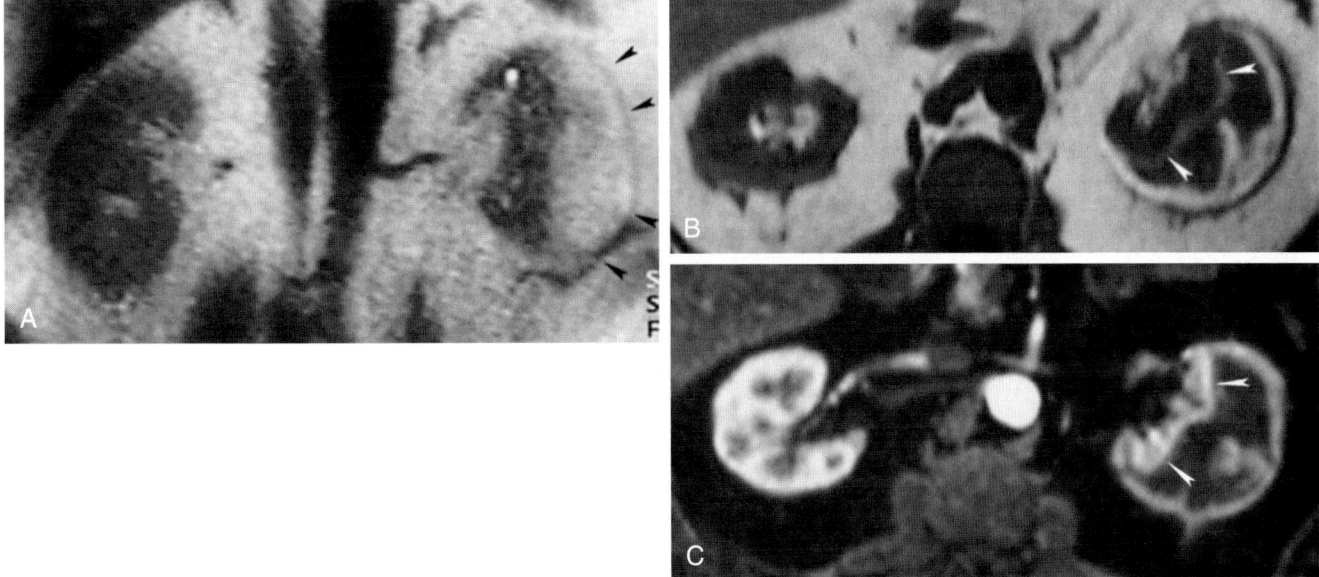

FIGURE 27-44, cont'd

FIGURE 27-45 Subcapsular hematoma after lithotripsy. Coronal T2-weighted sequence (**A**) demonstrates high–signal intensity blood contained by left renal capsule (*arrowheads*). Axial T1-weighted image (**B**) and gadolinium-enhanced T1-weighted image (**C**) show mass effect on left kidney (*arrowheads*) caused by a subcapsular hematoma. The signal intensity is consistent with the presence of intracellular methemoglobin.

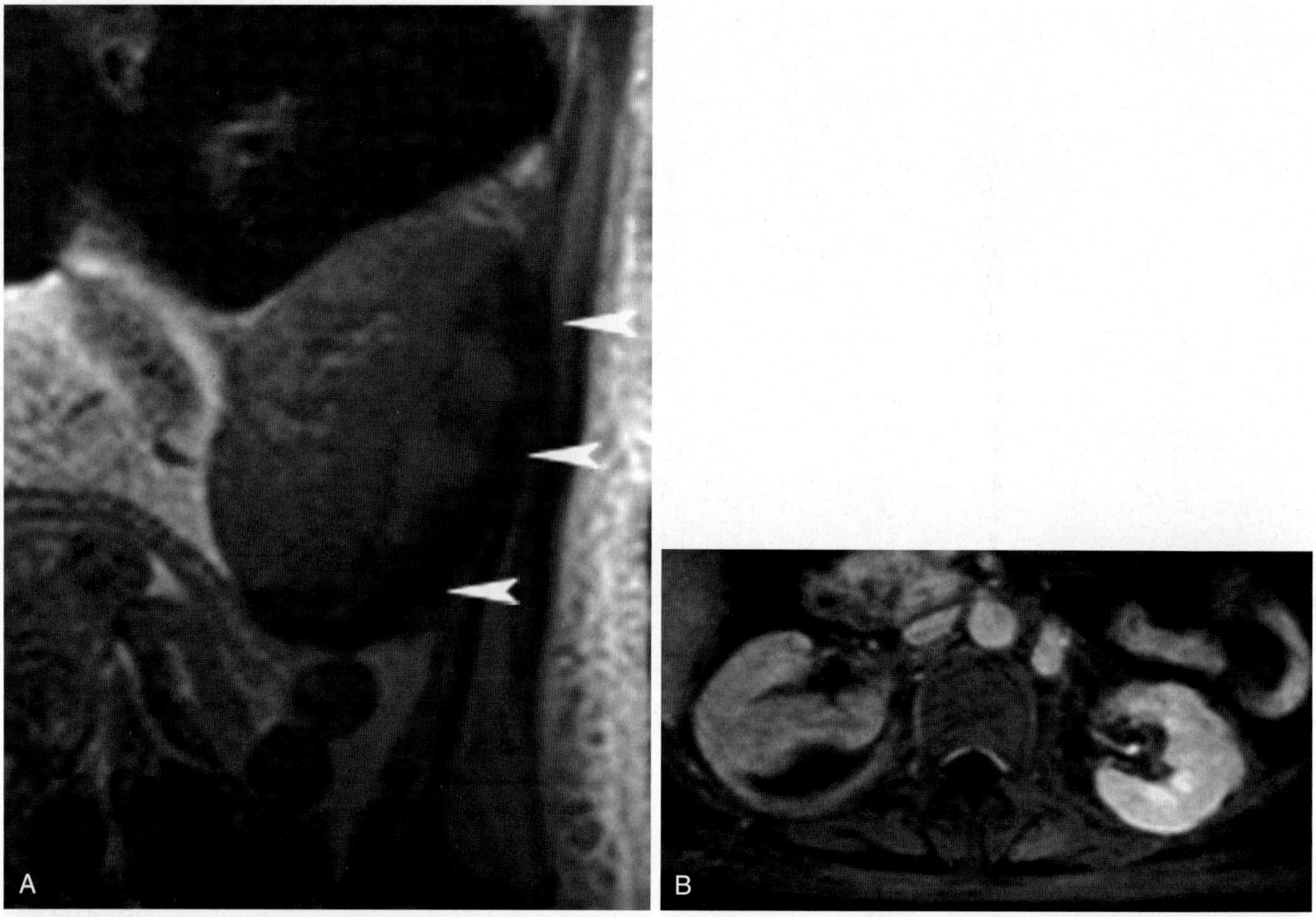

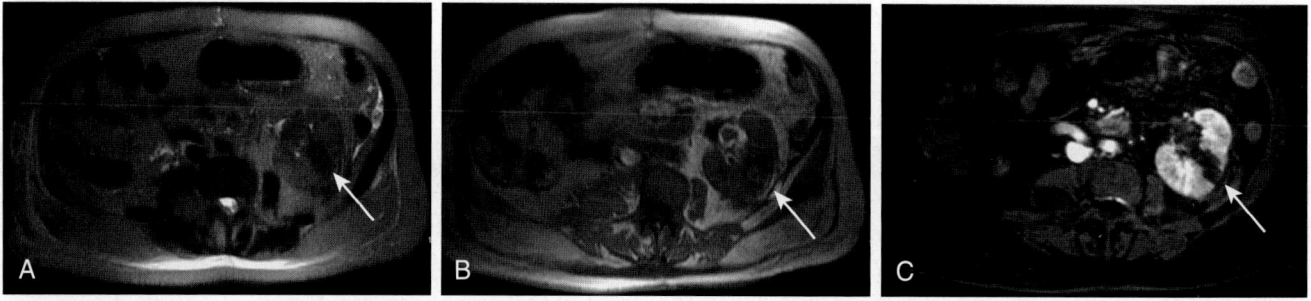

FIGURE 27-46 Posttraumatic subcapsular hematoma. Sagittal T2-weighted image (**A**) and postcontrast T1-weighted image (**B**) show a subcapsular hematoma (*arrowheads*) in which signal intensity is consistent with the presence of extracellular methemoglobin. This hematoma is older than the one shown in Figure 27-45.

FIGURE 27-47 Hematoma status after surgical removal of staghorn calculus. T2-weighted axial image (**A**), T1-weighted axial image (**B**), and postcontrast T1-weighted axial image (**C**) show an intrarenal hematoma (*arrows*) at the site of incision plane. This extends into the renal pelvis. No urine extravasation was demonstrated.

or global manner (Figure 27-53).[205] There may be focal or diffuse swelling of the kidney.[206] The areas of involvement may appear almost masslike (see Figure 27-52). The changes in the nephrogram are related to decreased concentration of contrast media in the tubules with focal ischemia. Tubular destruction and obstruction with debris are also present. There is usually a sharp demarcation between diseased tissue and the normal parenchyma, which continues to be enhanced normally in the nephrographic phase. Soft tissue stranding and thickening of Gerota's fascia are caused by the adjacent inflammatory process (see Figure 27-53).[194] The walls of the renal pelvis and proximal ureter may be thickened. The

calyces and renal pelvis may be effaced. Mild dilation is also occasionally noted. The kidney may have a single focal area of involvement or multiple areas with similar findings. With hematogenous-related pyelonephritis, the early findings tend to be multiple, round cortical regions of hypodensity that become more confluent and involve the medulla with time.[206] These findings persist for weeks despite successful treatment with antibiotics.

MRI is comparable with contrast material–enhanced CT for the evaluation of pyelonephritis.[207] The enhancement characteristics of acute pyelonephritis on MRI are similar to those on CT. On noncontrast sequences, the affected area has

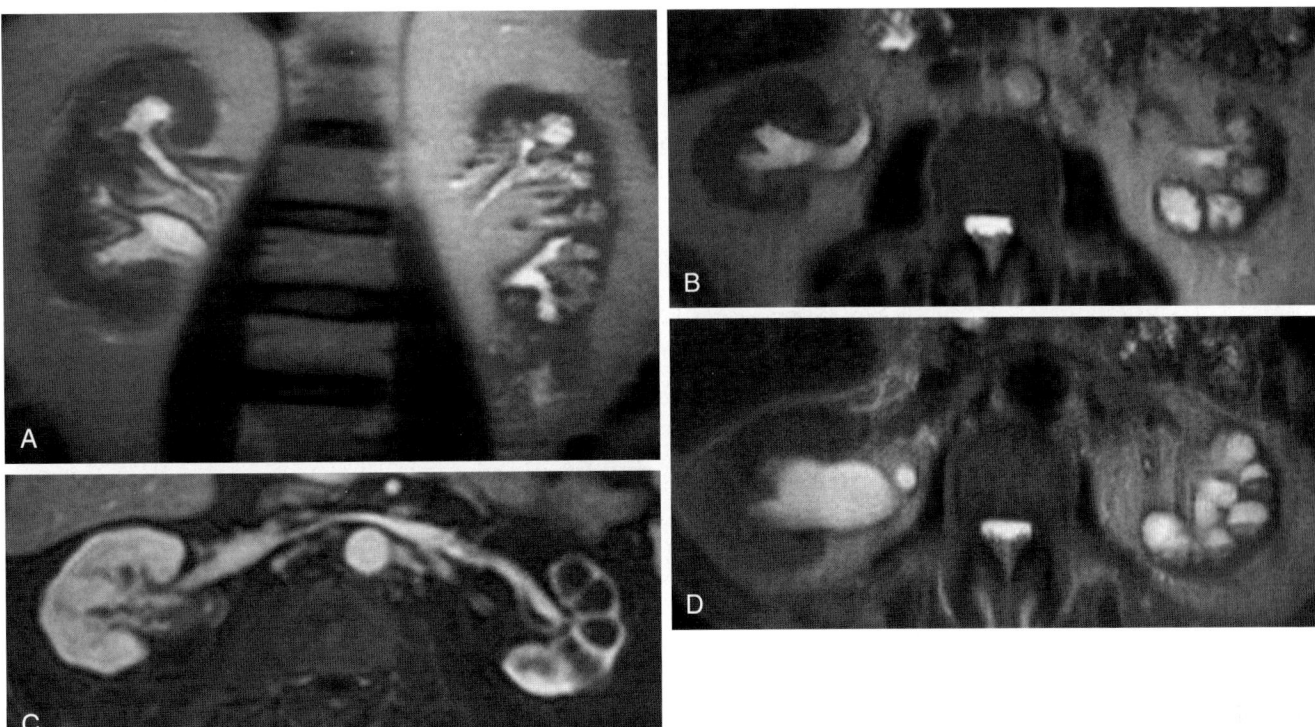

FIGURE 27-48 Renal tuberculosis. **A** and **B,** T2-weighted images demonstrate asymmetric cortical thinning and focal areas of increased signal intensity in the distribution of the medullary pyramids. **C,** Postcontrast T1-weighted image shows absence of enhancement, which is consistent with the presence of granulomas with caseous necrosis. **D,** T2-weighted image after treatment shows distorted, dilated calyces containing debris. Right-sided hydronephrosis is present as a result of a distal ureteral stricture.

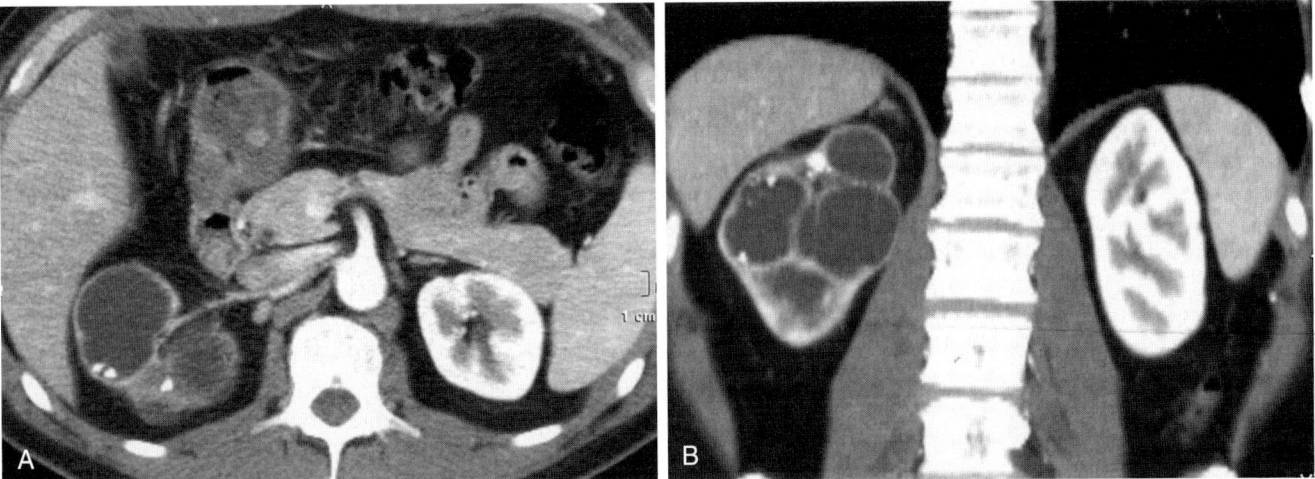

FIGURE 27-49 Renal tuberculosis: contrast material–enhanced computed tomographic scan. Axial (**A**) and coronal (**B**) images show the destruction of the right kidney as a result of renal tuberculosis. Parenchymal calcifications are present with dilated calyces as a result of the attenuation and truncation of the renal pelvis and ureter.

increased T2 signal intensity and decreased T1 signal intensity in relation to the normal renal parenchyma.

Complications of acute pyelonephritis include renal abscess, perinephric abscess, emphysematous pyelonephritis, and xanthogranulomatous pyelonephritis. All of these entities are imaged best with cross-sectional imaging techniques, specifically CT. Renal abscess results from severe pyelonephritis, with coalescence of necrotic regions and microabcesses. They occur two to three times more frequently in diabetic patients.[200] The findings on IVU are nonspecific; renal mass is suggested by the contour bulge of the kidney and the hypodense region in the nephrogram. Adjacent calyces are not visualized because of either edema or their destruction by the abscess cavity. Ultrasound assessment reveals an anechoic or hypoechoic mass with irregular walls. There is usually debris within the abscess, which causes to some low-level echoes. Through-transmission is usually poor. Highly echogenic foci within an abscess may represent microbubbles or gas. The wall may demonstrate increased vascular on color Doppler ultrasonography. CT findings in renal abscess include a reasonably well-defined mass with a low-density central region and a thick, irregular wall or pseudocapsule (Figure 27-54).[203] The enhancement in the

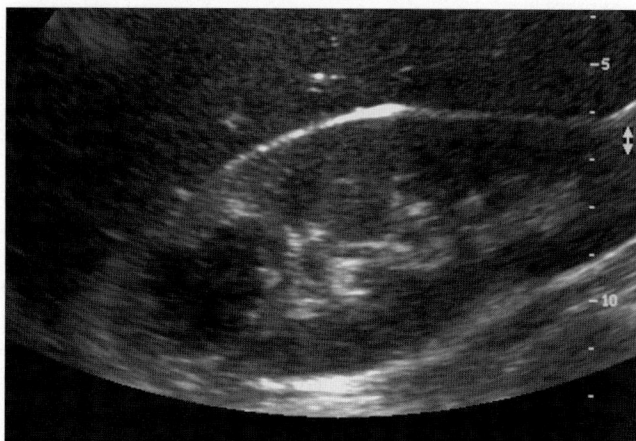

FIGURE 27-50 Acute pyelonephritis: renal ultrasonography. The hypoechoic region in the upper pole represents an area affected by acute pyelonephritis. The surrounding parenchyma is somewhat distorted, with loss of the normal corticomedullary junction.

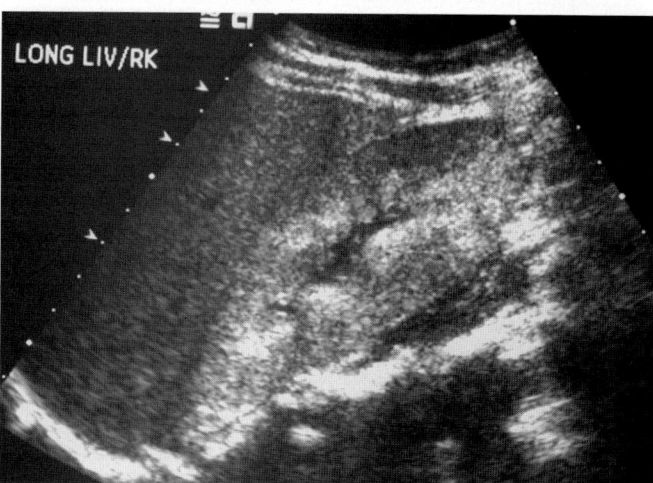

FIGURE 27-51 Acquired immunodeficiency syndrome (AIDS)-related nephropathy: ultrasonography. Longitudinal image of the right kidney. The size of the kidney is normal to slightly increased. The corticomedullary distinction is lost with diffuse increased cortical echogenicity.

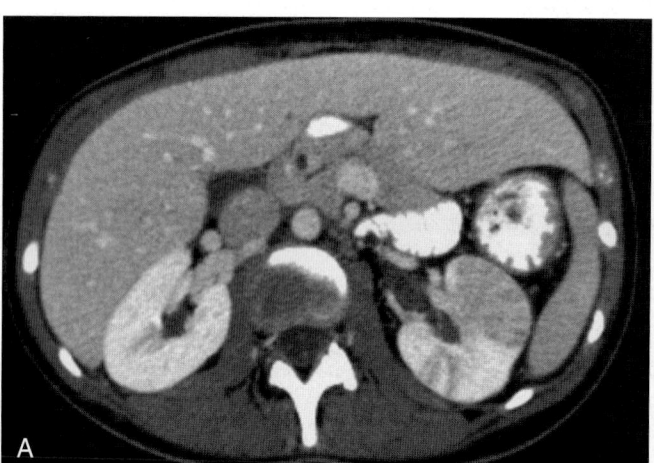

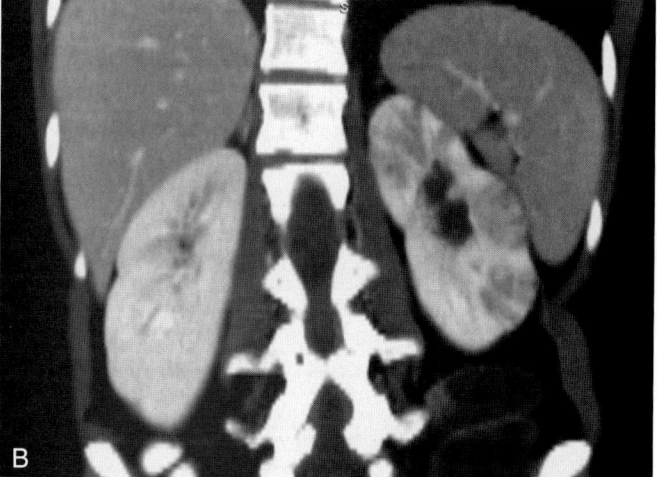

FIGURE 27-52 Acute pyelonephritis: contrast material–enhanced computed tomographic scan, axial (**A**) and coronal (**B**) images. The left kidney shows multiple areas of involvement. The hypodense region in the midportion of the kidney appears almost masslike (**A** and **B**). A nephrogram is striated in the region of involvement in the upper pole (**B**).

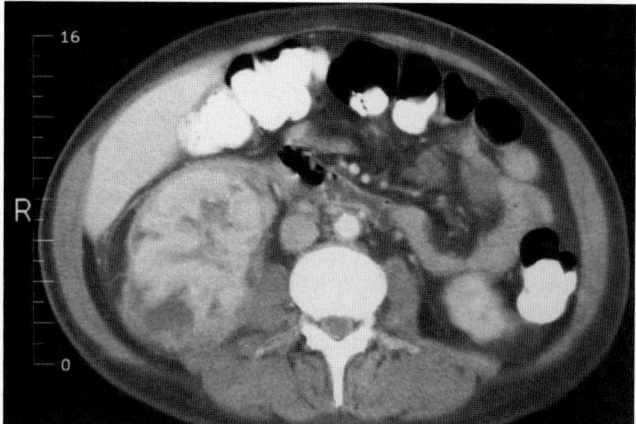

FIGURE 27-53 Acute pyelonephritis: contrast material–enhanced computed tomographic (CT) scan. The heterogeneous CT nephrogram shows the diffuse involvement of the right kidney. Stranding and some fluid are visible in the perinephritic space with thickening of Gerota's fascia.

region adjacent to the abscess is variable, depending on the amount of inflammation. Mature abscesses may demonstrate a more sharply demarcated border with peripheral rim enhancement. Gas may be visible within the abscess. MRI is comparable with contrast material–enhanced CT for the evaluation of renal abscess.[207] The central region of the abscess can have a variable appearance, but generally it is of decreased T1 and increased T2 signal intensity. The wall enhancement characteristics are also similar to those on CT (Figure 27-55).

Perinephric abscess formation results from rupture of renal abscesses through the renal capsule or from extension of emphysematous pyelonephritis through the capsule into the perinephric space.[206] On the nephrogram, IVU may demonstrate lucency around the kidney. The kidney is usually poorly functioning, and so complete assessment is difficult. Ultrasound assessment may show fluid or debris (or both) in a localized or generalized pattern around the kidney. CT and MRI may reveal the complete extent of perinephric involvement.

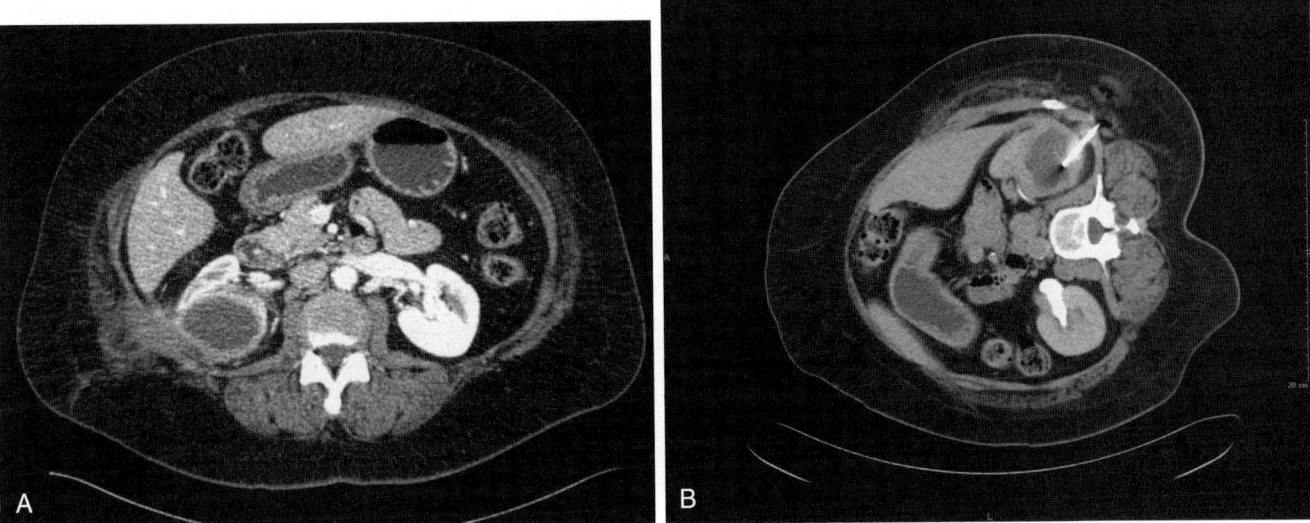

FIGURE 27-54 *Renal abscess: contrast material–enhanced computed tomographic scan.* **A,** *Axial image demonstrates the hypodense abscess in the right kidney with extension into the perinephritic space and the right flank.* **B,** *Axial image with the patient in the decubitus position reveals the method of diagnosis: needle aspiration. A drainage catheter was subsequently placed for treatment.*

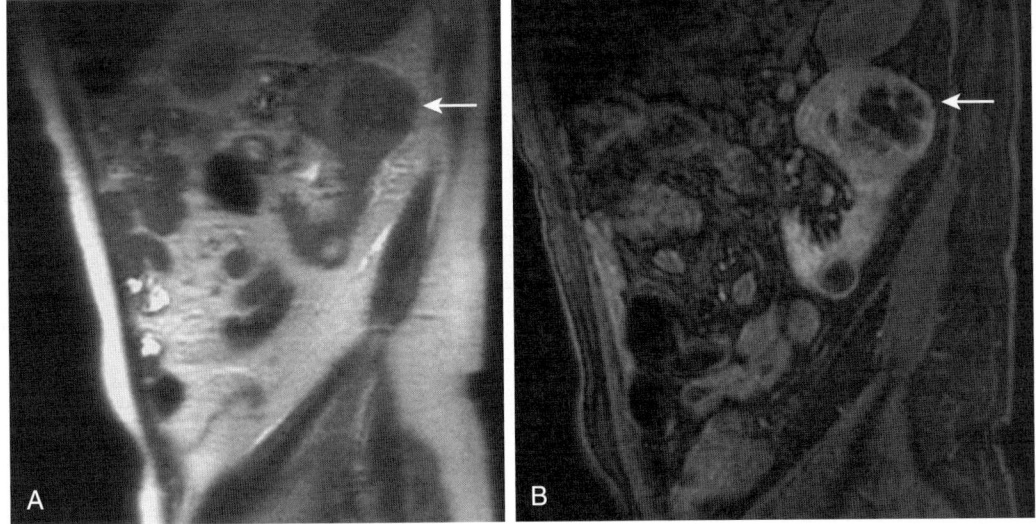

FIGURE 27-55 *Renal abscess. A mass in the upper pole of the left kidney demonstrates intermediate to low signal intensity on the sagittal T2-weighted image (**A**) and heterogeneous but predominantly peripheral enhancement (*arrow*) on the sagittal postcontrast T1-weighted image (**B**). On biopsy, this mass was found to be* Aspergillus *infection.*

Subcapsular extension may be distinguished from perinephric involvement. In general, heterogeneous fluid-density material is visible in the perinephric space. It may contain gas as well, which is best viewed on CT. Extension material within the retroperitoneum into the psoas muscle and adjacent structures is easily recognized (see Figure 27-52). With psoas involvement, it may extend into the pelvis and as far as the groin, following the course of the iliopsoas muscle.

With emphysematous pyelonephritis, gas is visible within the renal parenchyma.[199] If the gas is extensive enough, it may be visible on plain radiographs or KUB images. The gas is usually mottled, bubbly, or streaky in appearance and may be observed in the areas over the kidneys. Gas in the pelvicalyceal system may be visible as the gas-filled outline of the renal pelvis and collecting systems. IVU contributes little to the diagnosis, inasmuch as the involved kidney is usually nonfunctional. Nephrotomography may display the gas within the kidney to better advantage. Ultrasonography may suggest the diagnosis of emphysematous pyelonephritis by demonstrating gas within the kidney.[208] With gas present, there is acoustic shadowing in the involved region, with adjacent microbubbles that cause ring-down artifacts. CT is most specific in comparison with ultrasonography or MRI in that the gas may be visualized and the extent of involvement determined.[209] There is generally extensive parenchymal destruction with streaks of gas or mottled collections of gas within the kidney (Figure 27-56). Little or no fluid is seen. The gas is observed dissecting through the parenchyma in a linear focal or global manner. The gas usually radiates along the pyramid to the cortex. It may extend through into the perinephric space. Emphysematous pyelitis represents gas only in the pelvicalyceal system.[210] It is best diagnosed with CT, on which parenchymal gas is easily viewed. The diagnosis distinction is important because emphysematous pyelitis carries a less grave prognosis.

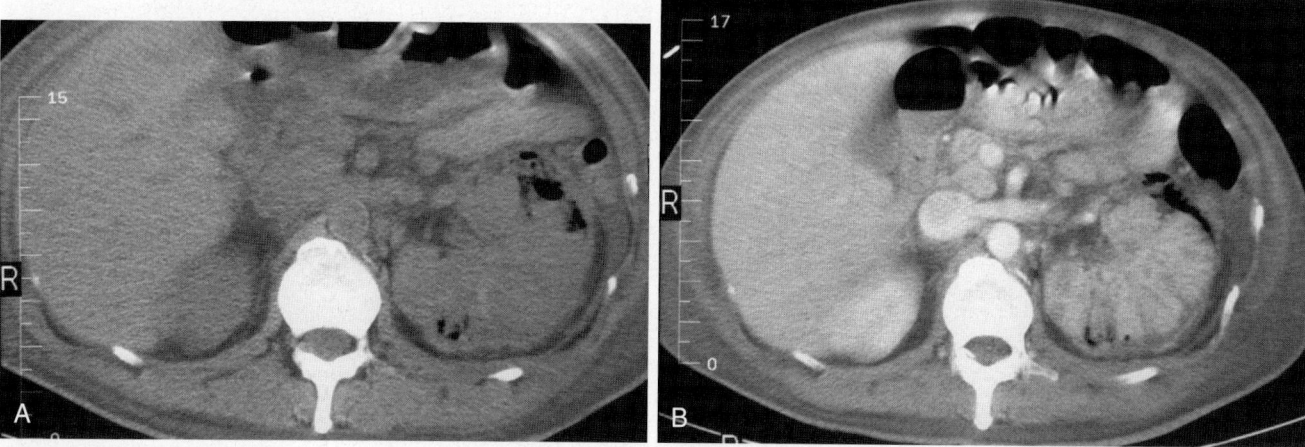

FIGURE 27-56 Emphysematous pyelonephritis: contrast material-enhanced computed tomographic scan. A noncontrast image (A) and a contrast material-enhanced image (B) demonstrate gas in the renal parenchyma with extension into the perinephritic space. The nephrogram is striated throughout. Global involvement of the kidney is frequent.

Xanthogranulomatous pyelonephritis is an end-stage condition resulting from chronic obstruction with long-standing infection.[201] The plain radiograph or KUB image shows a staghorn calculus or a large calcification overlying the region of the kidney, with a large mass filling the space. On ultrasonography, the kidney appears enlarged with loss of identifiable landmarks. The renal sinus echoes are lost. A large calculus or staghorn calculus usually fills the space, with debris filling adjacent hypoechoic regions (Figure 27-57). At times it appears as a large heterogeneous mass. CT defines the extent and adjacent organ involvement best in patients with xanthogranulomatous pyelonephritis. The findings on CT include an enlarged but generally reniform mass filling the perinephric space.[201,211] Calcification, specifically calculi and staghorn calculi, are found in 75% of cases. Excretion is absent or markedly decreased in 85% of cases, and the involved region appears as a mass in more than 85% of cases.[201] In fewer than 15% of cases, the process is focal, and normally functioning areas of the kidney remain. The kidney appears enlarged and usually nonfunctional with multiple round, hypoattenuating regions with adjacent calcification. There is frequent perinephric extension. Fistulas may occur in adjacent structures, with adenopathy noted in the retroperitoneum. Because CT is more sensitive for the evaluation of stones and gas, MRI is reserved for patients with contraindications to iodinated contrast material or radiation exposure (Figure 27-58).

Chronic pyelonephritis is usually associated with vesicoureteral reflux that occurs in childhood.[202] One or both kidneys may be involved. An affected kidney has focal scars that are associated with calyceal dilation. The scarring is often separated by normal regions of the kidney and normal-appearing calyces. When involvement is global, the kidney may be small. IVU demonstrates dilated or ballooned calyces that extend to the cortical surface, which is thinned. The outline of the affected kidney is distorted. With ultrasonography, the kidneys have irregular outlines with regions of cortical loss. Underlying dilated calyces may be visible. The regions of scarring may be echogenic in comparison with the adjacent normal kidney. CT demonstrates abnormal architecture within the affected kidney.[206] Nephrographic phase images reveal the regions of cortical loss; the involved dilated calyces extend to the capsular surface. Dilation of the calyces is variable. Again,

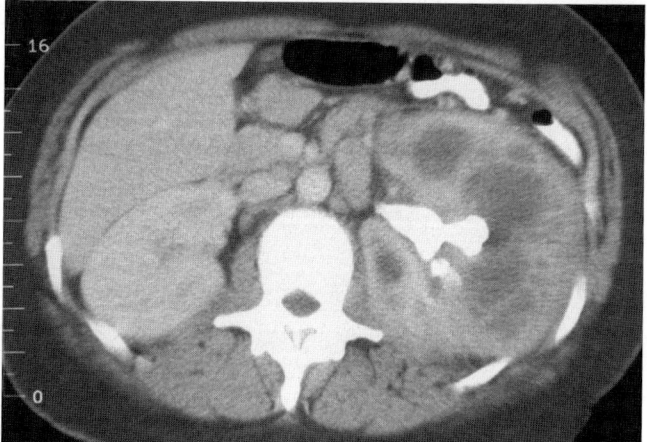

FIGURE 27-57 Xanthogranulomatous pyelonephritis: contrast material-enhanced computed tomographic scan. A large staghorn calculus fills the renal pelvis and collecting systems in the left kidney. Much of the remainder of the kidney is replaced by hypodense material—the xanthogranulomatous infection—within the calyces and parenchyma; some minimal enhancement of the cortex remains.

chronic may be unilateral or bilateral. Excretory phase images best delineate the extent of involvement, especially in the coronal format. MRI is comparable with contrast material–enhanced CT for the evaluation of chronic pyelonephritis and postinfectious scarring.[207]

Acute pyelonephritis is associated with fever, flank pain, leukocytosis, and pyuria. Radiolabeled leukocyte scans (e.g., indium 111–labeled white blood cells) and gallium 67 citrate scans can be helpful in identifying acute pyelonephritis. However, these methods have the drawbacks of extended imaging time (more than 24 hours) and higher radiation exposure. Cortical imaging with ^{99m}Tc-DMSA has been shown to be highly sensitive for detecting acute pyelonephritis in the appropriate clinical setting.[212,213] In acute pyelonephritis, segmental regions of decreased tracer uptake are demonstrated in oval, round, or wedge patterns. There may also be diffuse generalized decrease in renal uptake, which, in association with a normal or slightly enlarged kidney, is suspect for an acute infectious process. The pathophysiologic basis for decline in ^{99m}Tc-DMSA cortical uptake in infection is related to diminished delivery of the tracer to the infected area and to direct

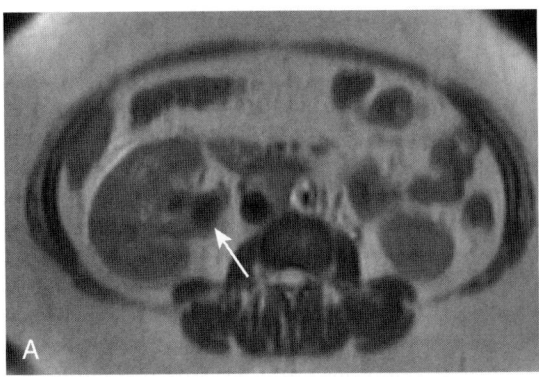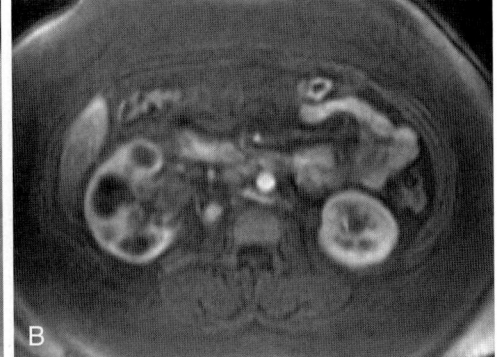

FIGURE 27-58 Xanthogranulomatous pyelonephritis with staghorn calculus. **A,** Axial T2-weighted image demonstrates a stone of low signal intensity within the right renal pelvis (*arrow*) that is associated with increased renal size and replacement of the medullary pyramids and calyces with material of high signal intensity. **B,** Axial postcontrast T1-weighted image demonstrates asymmetric enhancement and hydronephrosis.

infectious injury to the tubular cells, which compromises their function and tracer uptake. A wedge-shaped cortical defect with regional decrease in renal size is compatible with postinfectious scarring. Renal infarcts may also have similar appearance.[113,119] Attention to ^{99m}Tc-DMSA image processing and quality is paramount to achieve high interreader agreement.[214,215] There may also be a role for FDG PET-CT in the imaging evaluation of renal infection.[216]

Renal Mass: Cysts to Renal Cell Carcinoma

Renal masses are quite common; simple renal cysts are found in more than 50% of patients older than 50. Most renal masses are simple cysts; a minority are solid renal masses, such as renal cell carcinoma. Renal masses produce variable findings in the kidneys, depending on their location. The contour of the kidney may be deformed, the calyces displaced or splayed, the density of the kidney altered, or the axis of the kidney changed. For years, IVU was the method of choice for detection of renal masses. Studies have shown that it has low sensitivity for detection of renal masses, especially those smaller than 3 cm in diameter.[217] Normal IVU findings do not exclude a renal mass. With CT as the "gold standard," IVU detected 10% of masses smaller than 1 cm in diameter, 21% of masses 1 to 2 cm in diameter, 52% of masses 2 to 3 cm in diameter, and 85% of masses larger than 3 cm in diameter.[217] Ultrasonography fared better but nonetheless detected only 26% of masses smaller than 1 cm, 60% of those 1 to 2 cm, 82% of those 2 to 3 cm, and 85% of those larger than 3 cm.[217] The findings on IVU are frequently nonspecific, and further imaging is necessary to characterize the renal mass accurately. Ultrasonography, CT, and MRI are needed to differentiate solid from cystic renal masses.

Simple renal cysts are commonly encountered with all imaging studies today. They rarely occur in individuals younger than 25 but occur with great frequency in individuals older than 50. Typically, renal cysts are asymptomatic, cortical in location, and may be single or multiple. The cause is unknown, although tubular obstruction has been postulated to be a necessary element. The plain radiograph (KUB) is rarely helpful unless the cyst is quite large. A thin, curvilinear peripheral rim of calcification may be observed in 1% to 2% of cases. The findings on IVU depend on the size, the position in the kidney, associated deformity of the renal contour,

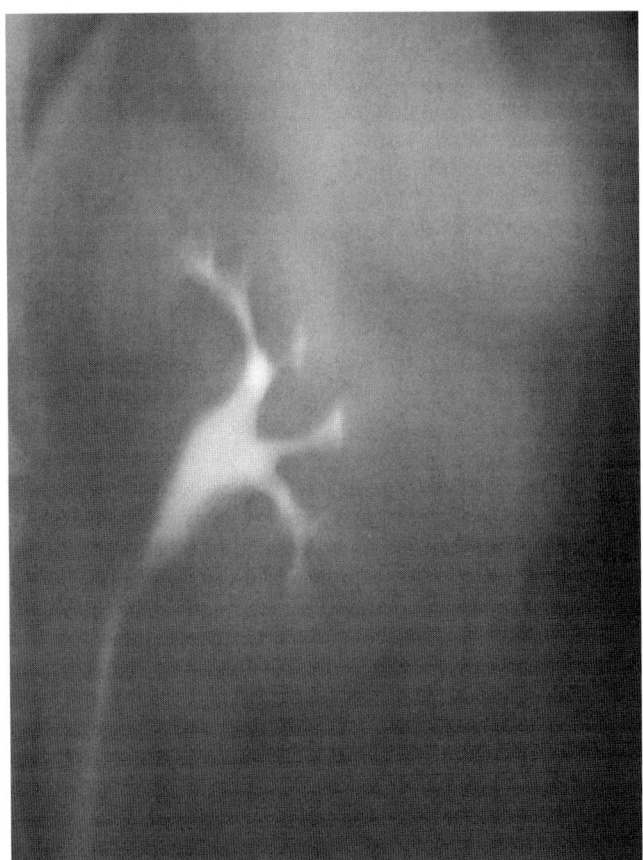

FIGURE 27-59 Renal mass: nephrotomogram. A slightly hypodense mass projects off the lateral border of the left kidney. Subsequent imaging proved this to be a renal cyst.

and splaying of the pelvicalyceal system. Nephrotomography yields a well-outlined, homogeneous lesion that is less dense than the surrounding kidney (Figure 27-59). The wall of the cyst is paper thin with a sharp, clear-cut demarcation with the adjacent kidney. The interface with the kidney when a cyst lies on the surface is beaklike. The calyces are displaced or splayed.

Ultrasonography is an excellent means of diagnosing a simple renal cyst if all imaging criteria are met.[48] The lesion in the kidney must be round or oval and must be anechoic (no echoes within) (Figure 27-60); it must be well circumscribed with a smooth wall; there must be enhanced through-transmission of the sound beyond the cyst with a sharp

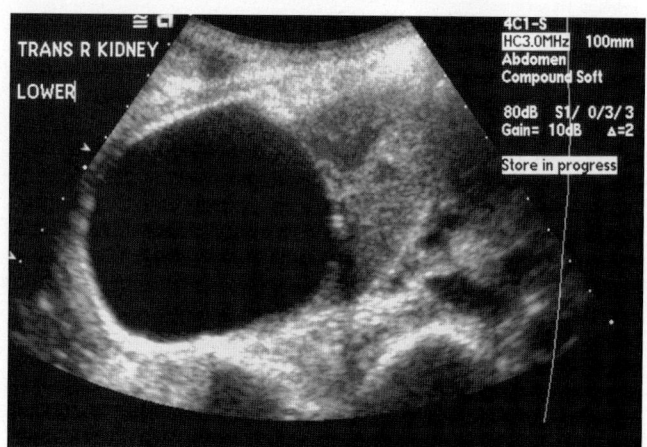

FIGURE 27-60 Renal cyst: ultrasonography. A large, anechoic renal mass projects off the lateral border of the right kidney. The cyst's features include a well-circumscribed lesion with a sharp back wall and increased through-transmission. There are no internal echoes or nodularity, and the wall is smooth. There is a clear interface with the kidney.

interface of the back wall with the renal parenchyma; and thin septa may be visible within the cyst, but no nodules are visible on the wall. If all these criteria are met, the diagnosis is established. If there is any deviation from these criteria, further imaging with CT or MRI is necessary.

CT is the method of choice for characterizing and differentiating renal masses.[218-220] A simple renal cyst appears as a well-circumscribed, round, water-density lesion within the kidney (Figure 27-61). The CT numbers of the cyst are near zero. The contents are not significantly enhanced after the injection of contrast media. The CT numbers may vary slightly from water density, but no more than 10 to 15 Hounsfield units. The cyst is uniform throughout with no measurable wall. The interface with the adjacent parenchyma is sharp. The margins are smooth with no perceptible nodules. Thin rimlike calcification may be visible. On occasion, "high-density" cysts may be encountered with CT numbers ranging from 50 to 80. These are cysts containing hemorrhagic or proteinaceous debris. They too demonstrate no wall nodularity and have no significant enhancement after injection of contrast material. They are common in polycystic kidneys.

Cysts are well demonstrated on MRI because of excellent soft tissue contrast. On MRI, simple cysts are well circumscribed, thin-walled structures containing fluid that appears dark on T1-weighted sequences and bright on T2-weighted sequences (Figure 27-62). Complex cysts are those that contain material of signal intensity that is not characteristic for simple fluid. Complex cysts contain proteinaceous or hemorrhagic fluid and may have septations and calcification. The T1 signal intensity of the fluid is higher than expected for simple fluid, ranging from isointense to hyperintense. T2 signal intensity is lower than expected for simple fluid and may be black, depending on the blood content. Cysts are not enhanced. In comparison with CT, MRI has been found to have higher contrast resolution, which allows for better visualization of septa.[221,222] MRI also better characterizes blood products. MRI is more sensitive to subtle enhancement, especially with subtraction techniques, which make MRI superior to CT in differentiating a complex cyst from a cystic neoplasm[221-223] (Figures 27-63 and 27-64).

Polycystic renal disease is classified as infantile, adult, or acquired. The infantile form is inherited as an autosomal recessive disorder.[224] It has a variable manifestation: Severe kidney injury is found in the neonatal period, and congenital hepatic fibrosis and hepatic failure manifest in older children. Organomegaly is common, with bilateral symmetric renal enlargement. IVU yields poor visualization of the kidneys because of renal impairment, and the nephrogram is prolonged and mottled with a striated or streaky appearance. Ultrasonography reveals enlarged, diffusely hyperechoic kidneys as a result of of dilated, ectatic collecting tubules.[225] There is loss of the corticomedullary differentiation as well. Because the diagnosis is made clinically with the associated ultrasound findings, CT and MRI are rarely used in this condition.

Autosomal dominant polycystic kidney disease is the adult form.[226] Plain radiographs appear normal early in the disease process, but as the cysts increase in size, so does the overall renal size. When the disease is advanced, large masses are present bilaterally, with occasional curvilinear calcifications in the wall of some of the cysts. IVU demonstrates multiple lucent areas throughout the kidneys, a Swiss-cheese appearance. When renal function is still normal, there is extensive splaying and distortion of the pelvicalyceal system. Ultrasonography reveals bilateral enlargement of the kidneys, which are markedly lobulated and contain multiple sonolucent areas of varying size throughout.[227]

CT and MRI in autosomal dominant polycystic kidney disease depict enlarged, lobulated kidneys with a myriad of cysts of varying size throughout (Figure 27-65). One kidney may be more involved than the other. The cysts may have calcifications with the wall. It is not uncommon to encounter cysts with varying density or signal intensity as a result of episodes of hemorrhage that occur within the cysts (Figure 27-66). A fluid level may be visible as a result of the presence of debris or hemorrhage within some of the cysts. In the excretory phase, there is marked distortion of the calyces. The extent of renal involvement by autosomal dominant polycystic kidney disease is better appreciated on CT and MRI than on ultrasonography or IVU. Cysts may be found in the liver, spleen, and pancreas as well.

Adult acquired polycystic kidney disease (AAPKD) occurs in patients with kidney injury who are undergoing continuous peritoneal dialysis or hemodialysis.[228] The longer the patient has undergone dialysis, the more likely the patient is to develop AAPKD.[229] Most patients will have undergone dialysis for several years before it is discovered.[230] The cysts are generally quite small (0.5 to 2 cm in most patients). Calcification may occur in the wall. Plain radiographs and IVU play no role in evaluation because renal function is impaired. Ultrasonography reveals small, shrunken kidneys with anechoic or hypoechoic regions that represent the cysts. The findings are usually bilateral. CT or MRI shows the small bilateral kidneys with cysts of size that varies but is usually in the range of 1 to 2 cm (Figure 27-67; see also Figure 27-29).[231,232] These cysts must be closely evaluated for solid components because carcinomas and adenomas occur with increased frequency in these patients. Solid lesions smaller than 3 cm in diameter may represent either adenomas or renal cell carcinomas, whereas most lesions larger than 3 cm are renal cell carcinomas.[233,234] Screening for AAPKD is usually done with ultrasonography every 6 months; CT or MRI is reserved for patients with questionable or solid lesions.[235]

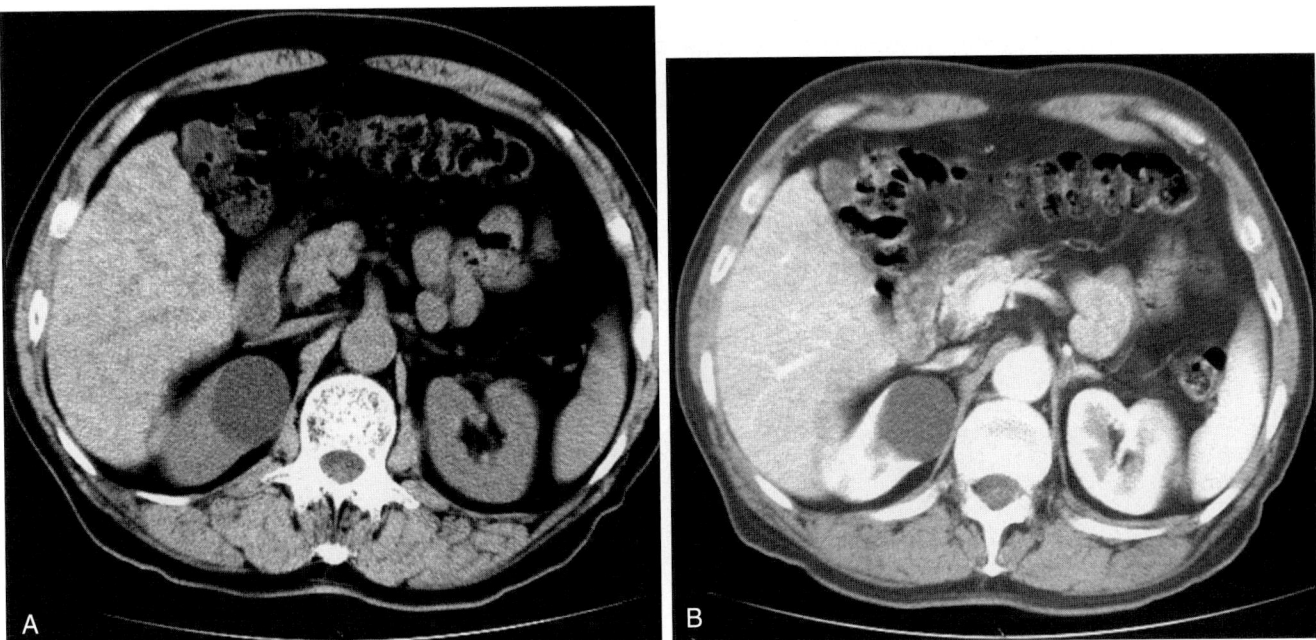

FIGURE 27-61 Renal cyst: computed tomographic (CT) scan. Noncontrast (**A**) and postcontrast (**B**) axial images. The cyst is well circumscribed with no enhancement. It displays water density with CT numbers of 0 to 5. There is a sharp interface with the kidney and no perceptible wall. No nodules are visible, and the cyst is uniform throughout.

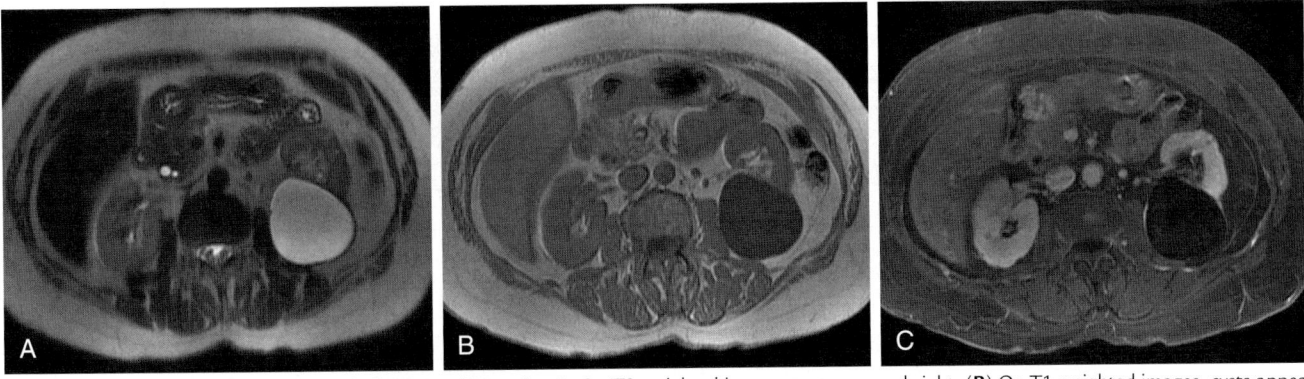

FIGURE 27-62 Simple cysts follow simple fluid signal intensity. **A,** On T2-weighted images, cysts appear bright. (**B**) On T1-weighted images, cysts appear dark. **C,** No enhancement is visible on gadolinium-enhanced T1-weighted images.

Medullary sponge kidney, or renal tubular ectasia, is a nonhereditary developmental disorder with ectasia and cystic dilation of the distal collecting tubules. The cystic spaces predispose to stasis, which leads to stone formation and potential infection. Involvement is usually bilateral, although not always symmetric, with as few as one calyx involved. The kidneys are typically normal sized with an appearance of medullary nephrocalcinosis when the small stones are present.[150] IVU reveals linear or round collections of contrast material extending from the calyceal border, forming parallel brushlike striations. With more severe involvement, the cystic dilations may appear grapelike or beadlike. CT is an excellent method for demonstrating the calculi, although the striations or cystic dilation may be difficult to visualize even with thin-section excretory phase imaging.

Multicystic dysplastic kidney is an uncommon, congenital, nonhereditary condition. It is usually unilateral and affects the entire kidney. In rare cases, only a portion of the kidney is involved. The affected kidney appears nonfunctional on IVU. Ultrasonography reveals multiple anechoic cystic structures of varying size replacing the kidney, with no normal parenchyma. Calcification in the wall of the cystic spaces may be visible. CT demonstrates multiple fluid-filled structures filling the renal fossa. Septa and some rimlike calcifications may be visible. The density of the fluid is usually the same as that of water ($\approx$0) or slightly higher. The injection of intravenous contrast material produces no enhancement. The renal artery to the affected side is not visible. It may be difficult to differentiate this condition from severe hydronephrosis if no cyst walls or septa are visible.

Small cortical cysts may occur in some hereditary syndromes (e.g., tuberous sclerosis) and in acquired conditions (e.g., lithium nephropathy; Figure 27-68). These cysts are typically multiple and very small (i.e., a few millimeters). They are viewed best with MRI but may also be viewed on CT if the cysts are slightly larger.[236] Pyelogenic cysts or calyceal diverticula are small cystic structures that connect with a portion of the pelvicalyceal system. On IVU, a calyceal diverticulum appears as a small round or oval collection of contrast material connected to the fornix of the calyx. As stasis occurs

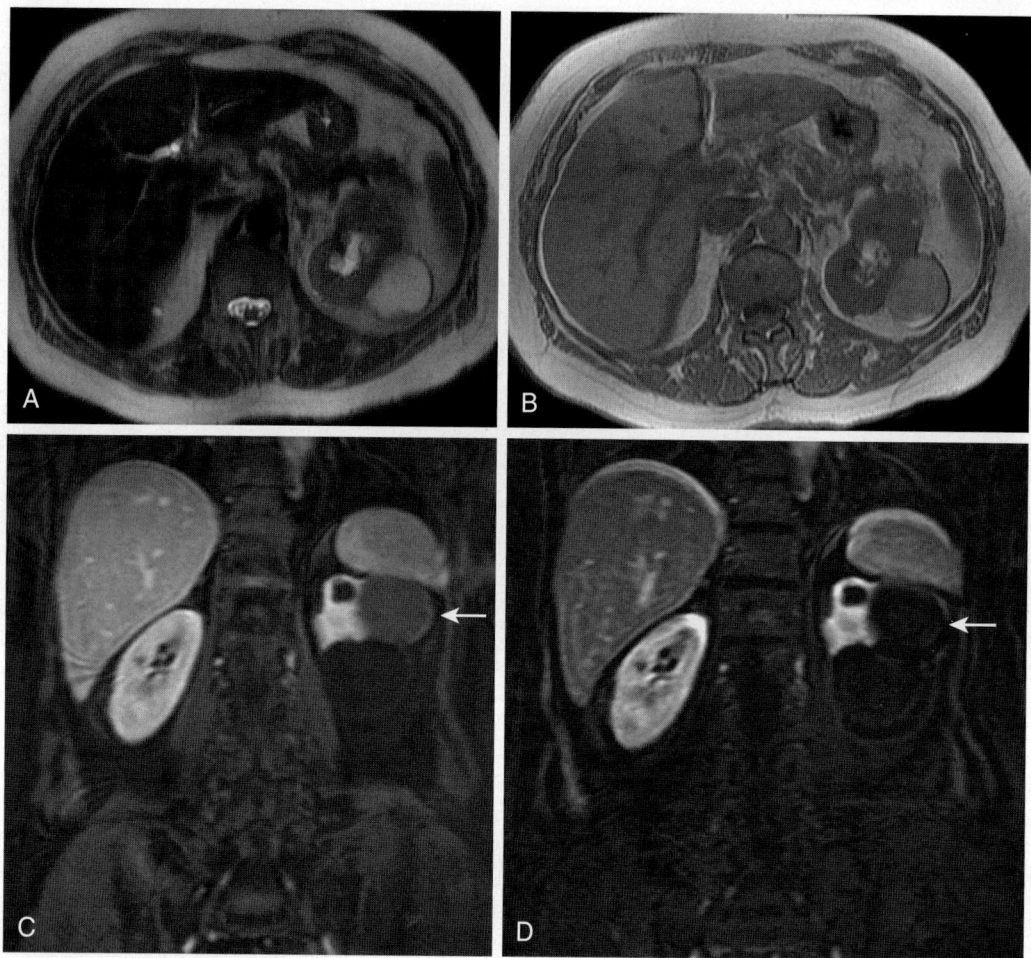

FIGURE 27-63 Complex cyst confirmed by computed tomography with image subtraction. **A,** T2-weighted axial image shows a bright left upper pole structure. **B,** T1-weighted axial image shows the same structure as intermediate in signal intensity. The cyst has internal debris that is visible on both sequences. Because the postcontrast T1 coronal image (**C**) shows higher signal intensity than expected for a cyst (*arrow*), postcontrast subtraction images (**D**) are needed to confirm absence of enhancement (*arrow*).

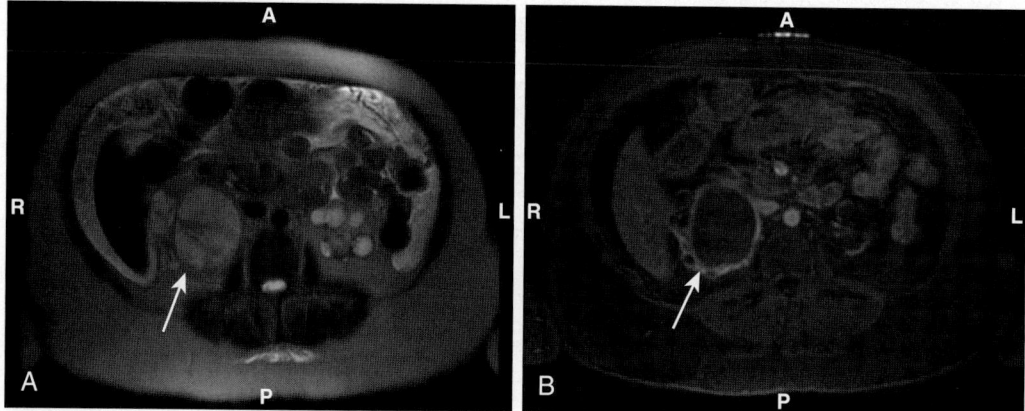

FIGURE 27-64 Complex hemorrhagic cyst. **A,** T1-weighted axial images show a complex right renal structure, bright on both sequences and with internal septations (*arrow*). **B,** Gadolinium on T1-weighted images produced no enhancement (*arrow*). This structure was diagnosed on fine needle aspiration as a hemorrhagic cyst.

within the diverticulum, renal stone formation may occur. Cortical cysts may be larger in hereditary disorders, such as von Hippel–Lindau disease (Figure 27-69).[237]

Parapelvic and peripelvic cysts are extraparenchymal cysts that occur in the region of the renal pelvis. They may be single or multiple, unilateral or bilateral. With the increased use of cross-sectional imaging techniques, they are observed with increased frequency. They may result from lymphangiectasia caused by prior insult to the kidney. Depending on the size and number, IVU reveals compression of the renal pelvis and infundibula but no calyceal dilation. The condition may be confused with renal sinus lipomatosis. Ultrasonography, CT, and MRI reveal the true nature of the process with the water-filled cystic structures in the renal sinus (Figure 27-70).

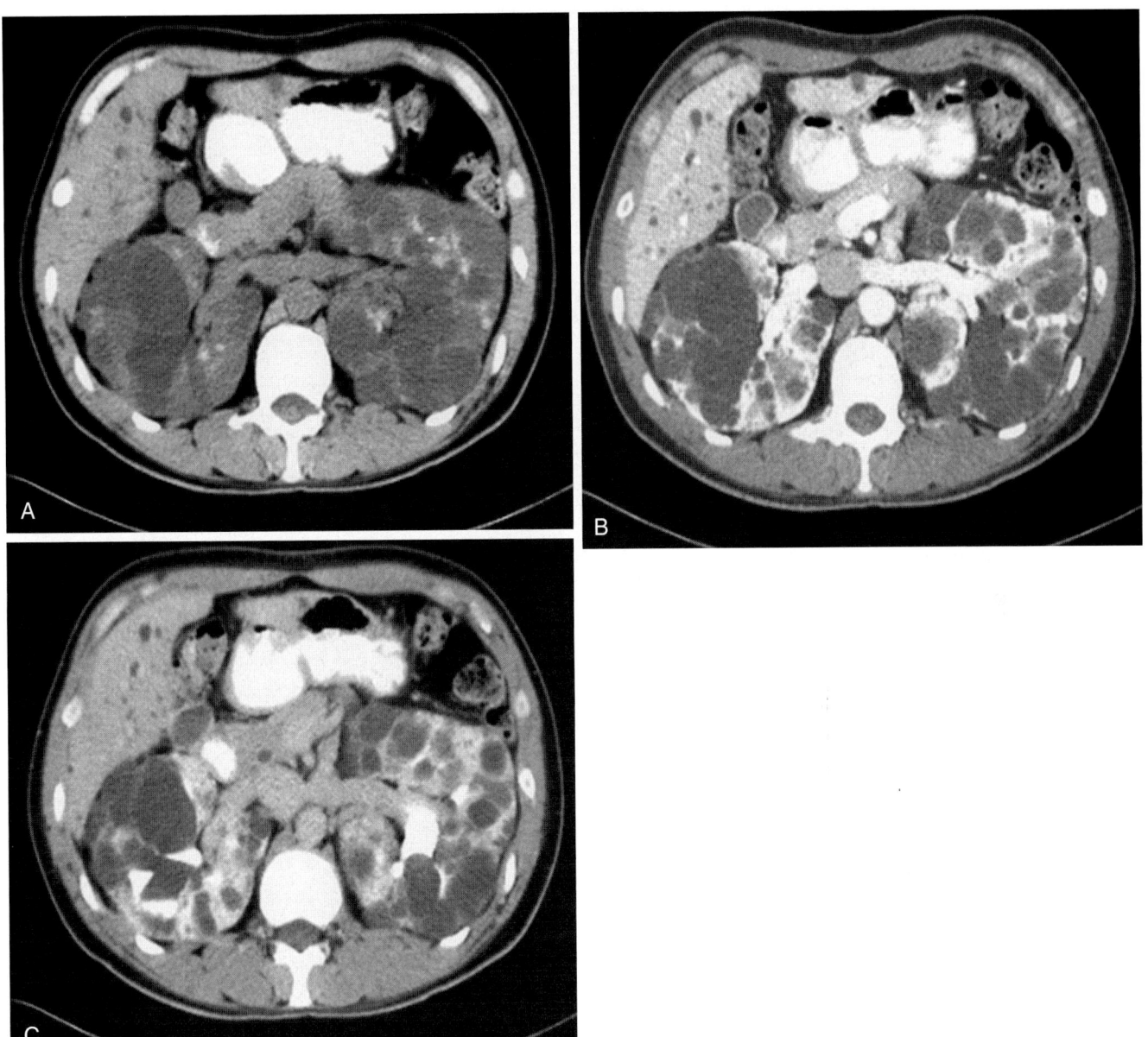

FIGURE 27-65 Autosomal dominant polycystic kidney disease: computed tomographic scan. Noncontrast (**A**), nephrographic phase (**B**), and excretory phase (**C**) axial images. The kidneys are equally enlarged, and the multiple various-sized cysts involve both kidneys. The calyces are splayed apart and appear distorted in the excretory phase image (**C**). Note the multiple small cysts also present in the involved liver.

All imaging modalities have been used to discover renal masses. The distinction between solid and cystic lesions is paramount as it guides differential diagnosis and subsequent treatment as needed. As discussed previously, this distinction is significantly limited with both IVU and ultrasonography in detecting renal masses less than 2 to 3 cm in size.[217] IVU also is very limited in differentiating cystic from solid lesions and should not be used for that purpose. Although less accurate than CT, ultrasonography provides a noninvasive means for differentiating solid from cystic renal masses. If all imaging criteria for a renal cyst are met on ultrasonography, an accurate diagnosis can be made. CT is the imaging modality of choice for the characterization of all solid mass, suspected solid masses, or masses that do not meet ultrasound criteria for a true renal cyst.[238-240] The advantage of CT lies in the multiphase manner in which studies can be performed. Noncontrast, arterial, corticomedullary, nephrographic, and

excretory phase imaging may all play a role in the accurate display and characterization of renal masses. MRI has sensitivities and specificities similar to those of CT but is generally reserved for cases in which the patient has a contraindication to iodinated contrast medium or in which radiation dose must be limited. MRI is technically more demanding but may be helpful in cases of renal masses for which CT yielded indeterminate findings, in cases with venous involvement, and in distinguishing vessels from retroperitoneal lymph nodes. The findings of any and all studies must be linked to the clinical history, especially in the case of complex or complicated cystic renal masses.

Renal neoplasms may arise from either the renal parenchyma or the urothelium of the pelvicalyceal system. Renal tumors have been reported during every decade of life, including the neonatal period.[241] Tumors within the kidney may be either benign or malignant.[242] Benign tumors of any significant

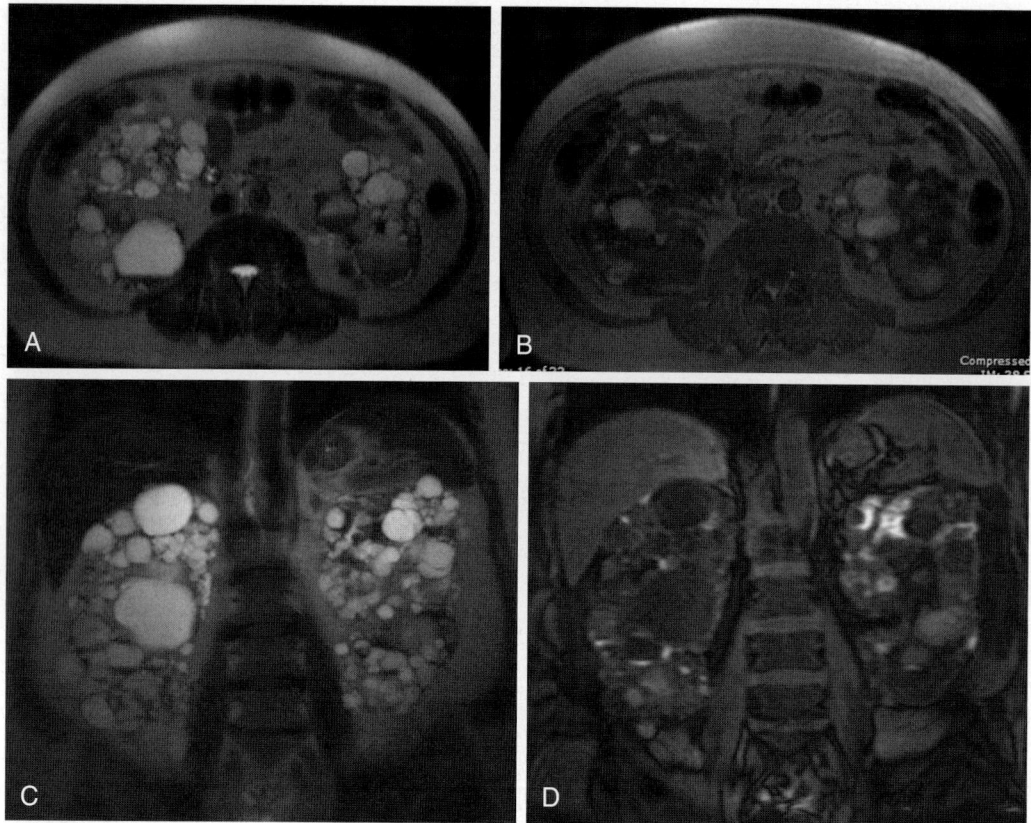

FIGURE 27-66 Autosomal dominant polycystic kidney disease. Axial (**A**) and coronal (**C**) T2-weighted images show bilateral renal cortical atrophy and multiple cysts, most of which are bright. Axial T1-weighted images (**B**) show multiple bright and dark structures that are not enhanced after gadolinium injection; this appearance was confirmed with subtraction images (**D**), and is therefore consistent with cysts.

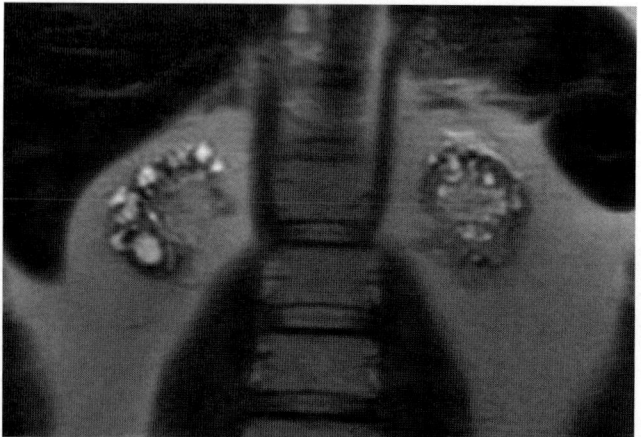

FIGURE 27-67 Chronic kidney injury. T2-weighted coronal image shows diffuse atrophy and multiple cysts in a patient on chronic dialysis.

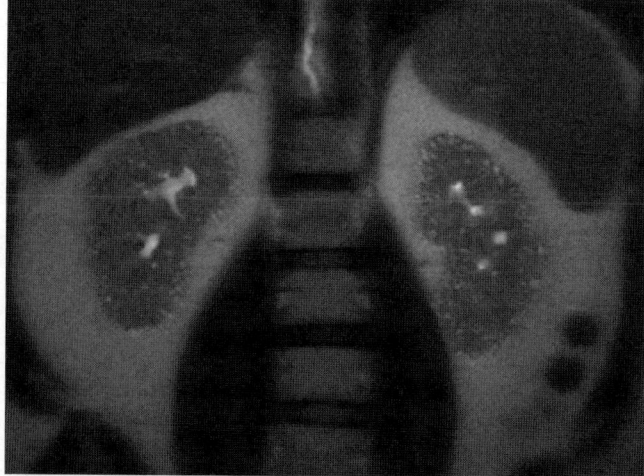

FIGURE 27-68 Lithium toxicity. Coronal T2-weighted image demonstrates innumerable small renal cortical cysts, characteristic of lithium toxicity.

size are extremely uncommon. The diagnosis is typically made at autopsy because they rarely cause symptoms. With the increased use of cross-sectional imaging techniques, more are being discovered. Renal adenoma is the most common benign neoplasm. Arising from mature renal tubular cells, it almost always is less than 2 to 3 cm in size. It has no characteristic radiologic features to distinguish it from other solid tumors. Typically, these renal adenomas are corticomedullary in location, appear solid on ultrasonography, and demonstrate uniform enhancement on CT. Other benign lesions—including hamartomas, oncocytomas, fibromas, myomas, lipomas, and hemangiomas—have been reported but uncommonly.

Hamartomas of the kidney, known as angiomyolipomas, are one group of benign renal tumors that are distinguishable radiologically.[243] Because angiomyolipomas are composed of different tissues, including fat, muscle, vascular elements, and even cartilage, the fat in particular may be detected radiographically.[244] Angiomyolipomas occur in two different populations of patients. A solitary unilateral form is most frequently found in women aged 30 to 50. These are usually discovered because of pain associated with hemorrhage. Multiple bilateral angiomyolipomas are found in patients with tuberous

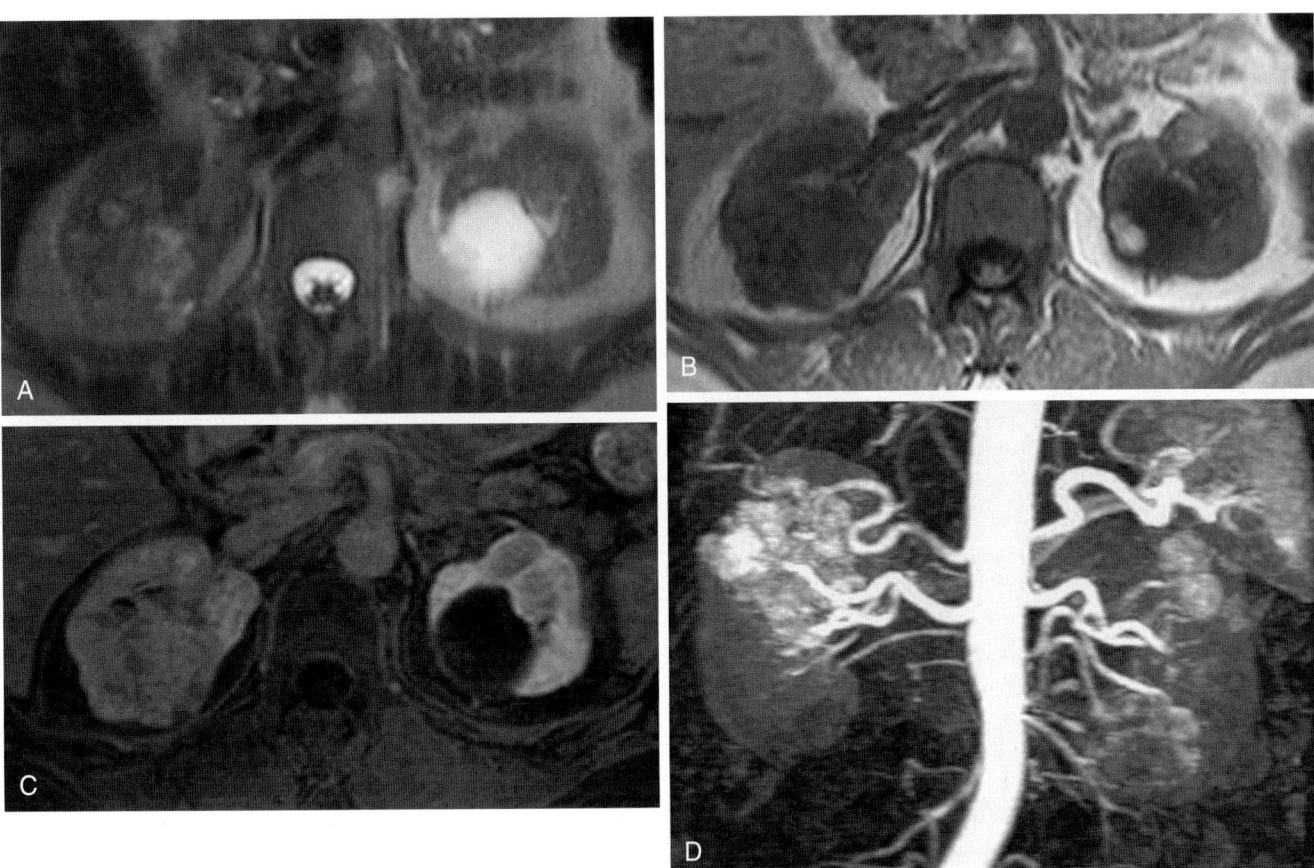

FIGURE 27-69 Bilateral clear cell carcinoma in von Hippel–Lindau syndrome. Bilateral heterogeneous renal masses and left renal cyst are visible on T2-weighted image (**A**) and T1-weighted image (**B**). **C,** The larger right renal mass demonstrates heterogeneous enhancement, and two smaller left renal masses demonstrate more homogeneous enhancement. **D,** Maximum-intensity projection depicts the multiple renal masses in angiographic format.

sclerosis. With marked involvement of the kidneys, multiple masses are found bilaterally with an appearance not unlike that of polycystic disease, except for the presence of fat in the masses. The solitary angiomyolipoma may be visible as a renal mass on conventional studies, KUB images, and IVU, if of sufficient size. Ultrasonography demonstrates the mass to be solid with increased echoes as a result of the presence of fat in the lesion.[245,246] CT is diagnostic in that fat is visible within the mass (Figure 27-71). Usually the CT numbers are –20 or lower.

Most angiomyolipomas have a large amount of fat, and the diagnosis can be made with ease. In uncommon cases, only a minimal amount of fat is present, and it must be searched for diligently on thin-section noncontrast CT or through histographic analysis.[247-250] Because angiomyolipomas contain macroscopic fat, MRI with fat-suppressed and opposed-phase chemical shift sequences can be used to make an accurate diagnosis.[251] Signal intensity of fat is high on both T1- and T2-weighted sequences. Macroscopic fat in angiomyolipomas has decreased signal intensity with fat-suppression sequences. Opposed-phase chemical shift sequences causes an "India ink" outline of the tumor at its interface with normal renal parenchyma. The enhancement pattern of angiomyolipomas may be variable, depending on the composition of the lesion. All solid lesions in the kidney should be searched for fat; if it is present, the diagnosis of angiomyolipoma is virtually ensured.[252-254] Most angiomyolipomas 4 cm in diameter or smaller are monitored; surgery is reserved for larger ones, especially with hemorrhage.[255,256]

Oncocytoma is another benign renal tumor whose presence is occasionally suggested preoperatively in a patient with a solid renal mass.[257] This uncommon benign tumor originates in the epithelium of the proximal collecting tubule. Radiologically, it is usually found incidentally in asymptomatic adults. Its features include a solid mass with homogeneous enhancement; a central stellate scar that may be visible on ultrasonography, CT, or MRI; and a spoked wheel pattern on angiography.[258-260] These findings are nonspecific, however, and histologic confirmation is needed.[261,262] Oncocytic renal cell carcinomas also occur, and surgery is generally needed for the correct diagnosis.

Renal cell carcinoma is the third most common tumor of the genitourinary tract after carcinoma of the prostate and bladder. This tumor constitutes 2% to 3% of all tumors in adults and is the most common retroperitoneal tumor. Clear cell renal carcinoma is the most common subtype, accounting for 70% of cases. In patients with this tumor, the average rate of 5-year survival is 55% to 60%. Papillary renal carcinoma represents 15% to 20% of cases, with a 5-year survival rate of 80% to 90%; 6% to 11% of renal cell carcinomas are of the chromophobe subtype, with a 5-year survival rate of 90%. Collecting duct renal cell carcinomas are the rarest, occurring in 1% of cases, and the 5-year survival rate is less than 5%. Chromophobe and papillary tumors tend to grow more slowly, are less aggressive, and are more likely to contain calcification.[263-265]

Imaging studies in renal cell carcinoma are used for initial detection, characterization, and staging. Accurate

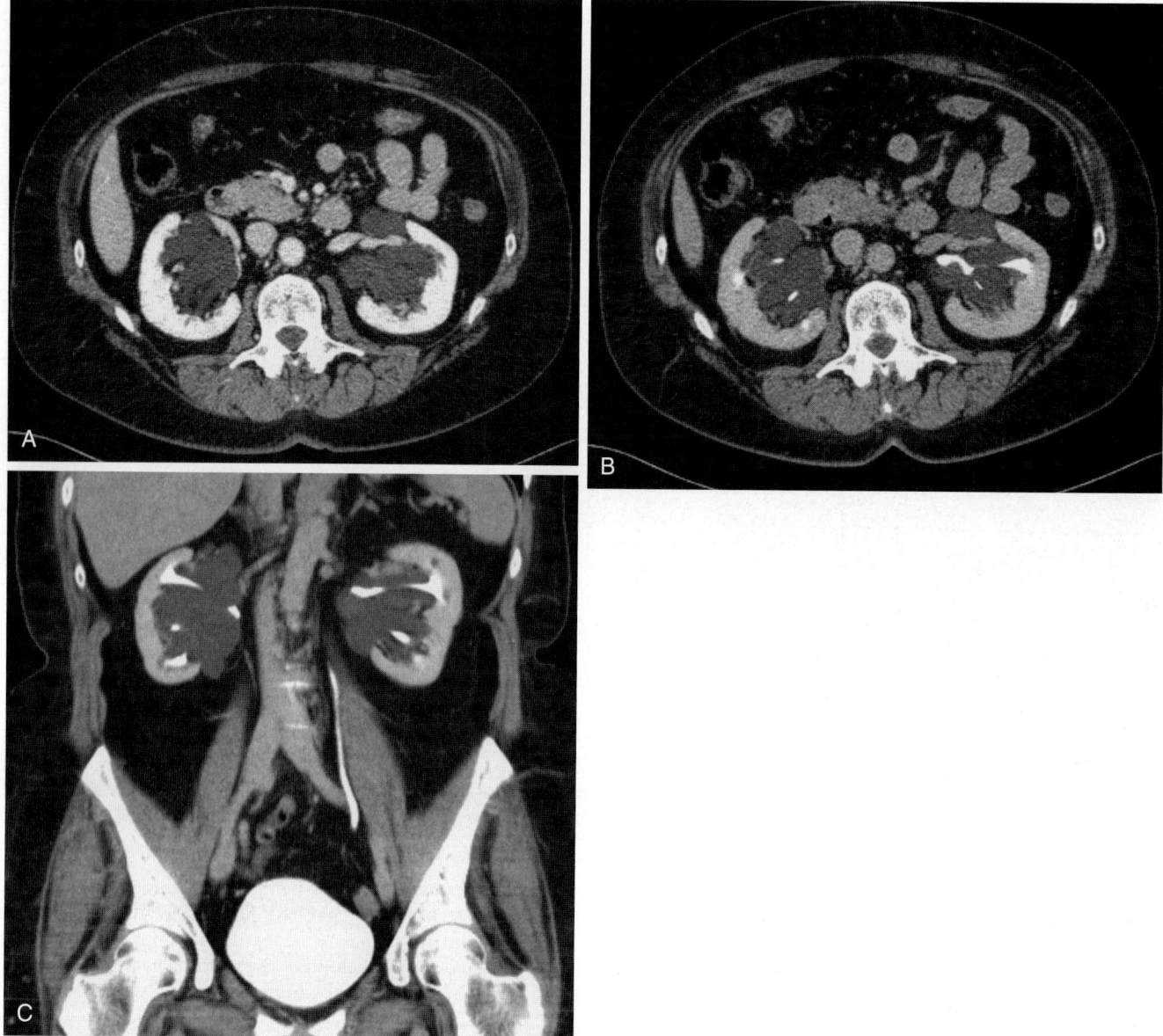

FIGURE 27-70 Peripelvic cysts: computed tomographic scan, axial nephrographic phase image (**A**), excretory phase image (**B**), and coronal excretory phase image (**C**) image. Multiple bilateral water-density cysts fill the renal hilum, displacing and splaying the collecting system and renal pelvis (**B** and **C**). The cortex is preserved, with no cysts visible.

staging is imperative for the treatment decision. Surgery is the primary means of treatment; radical nephrectomy, simple nephrectomy, or nephron-sparing partial nephrectomy are traditional options.[266,267] More recently, radiofrequency ablation and cryoablation have been used successfully in a limited population.[268-270] Immunotherapy for metastatic renal cell carcinoma has been delivered through CT guidance.[271]

The classic manifestation of a renal cell carcinoma in a patient with painless hematuria is that of a renal mass.[58,66] The plain radiograph may reveal an enlarged kidney or a mass in the region of the kidney; 10% to 20% of cases may demonstrate calcification on the KUB image. Calcification may be visible, however, in benign and malignant renal masses. Peripheral rimlike calcification on plain radiographs does not exclude malignancy. Most often, malignant lesions have central, punctate, or mottled calcification.

Most renal cell carcinomas today are found incidentally on CT or MRI being performed for other reasons. IVU was traditionally the standard examination performed in patients suspected of having a mass lesion in the kidney.[217] Renal cell carcinoma distorts the kidney outline or causes renal enlargement.[58] The mass has an irregular or indistinct junction with the normal renal parenchyma. The calyces are stretched, distorted, or obliterated by the tumor. When the neoplasm extends medially into the renal pelvis, it narrows or obliterates the renal pelvis or causes an irregular filling defect that represents either tumor or blood clot within the pelvis. A non-functioning kidney may be observed with renal vein occlusion, replacement of the majority of the kidney by tumor, or complete involvement of the renal pelvis. A mass lesion in the kidney necessitates further evaluation with cross-sectional imaging techniques. The ultrasound findings in a renal cell carcinoma include a mass with variable complex internal

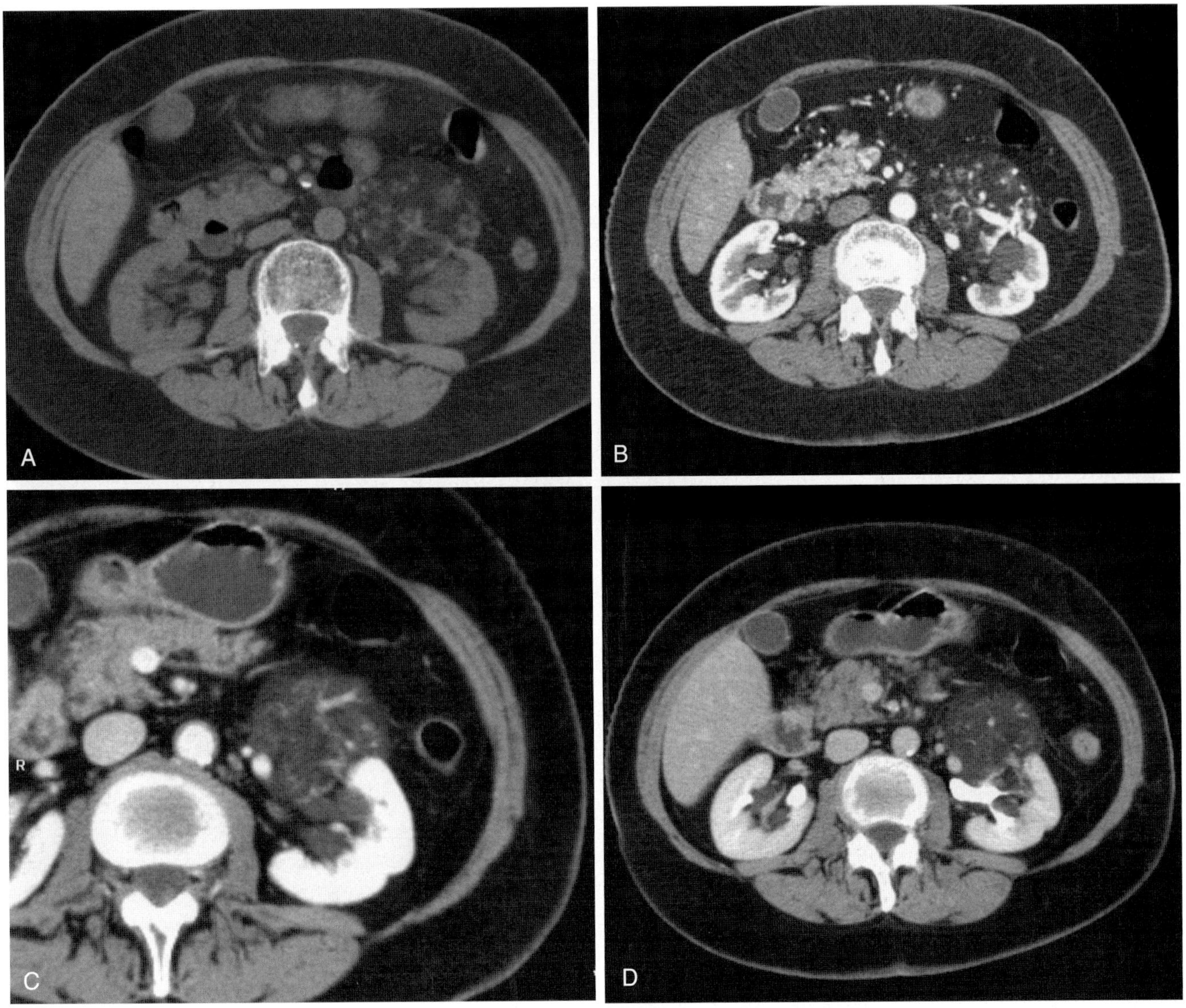

FIGURE 27-71 Angiomyolipoma: computed tomographic scan, noncontrast (**A**), corticomedullary phase (**B**), nephrographic phase (**C**), and excretory phase (**D**) axial images. The fat-containing mass is visible projecting anteriorly from the left kidney. The internal structure in this very vascular benign tumor demonstrates enhancement.

echoes, impaired through-transmission, and poor definition of the back wall or distal aspect of the lesion (Figure 27-72). Mural nodules may be visible in cystic lesions, and the internal wall may be thickened and irregular. Ultrasonography is less accurate than CT in revealing small renal masses. Normal findings on ultrasonography do not exclude a small renal mass. In one study of 205 lesions observed on CT, 79 were missed with ultrasonography.[272] Thirty of these lesions were solid renal masses. Power Doppler imaging, phase-inversion tissue harmonic imaging, and contrast material–enhanced harmonic imaging may improve the sensitivity of ultrasonography for the detection and characterization of solid renal masses.[273-276]

CT is the modality of choice for imaging renal cell carcinoma because it has proved to be effective in detection, diagnosis, characterization, and staging, with accuracy exceeding 90%.[266,277] On noncontrast CT, renal cell carcinoma appears as an ill-defined, irregular area in the kidney with CT numbers close to that of the renal parenchyma (Figure 27-73). After the injection of intravenous iodinated contrast material,

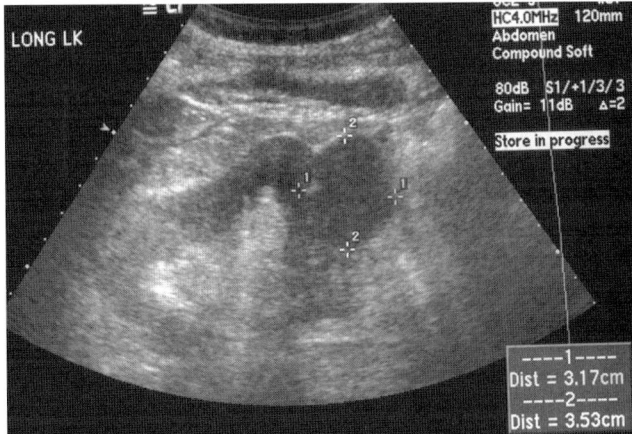

FIGURE 27-72 Renal cell carcinoma: ultrasonography. Longitudinal image reveals a solid mass projecting from the left kidney. The mass contains internal echoes and does not have any of the features of a renal cyst. It has an ill-defined interface with the kidney and no increased through-transmission.

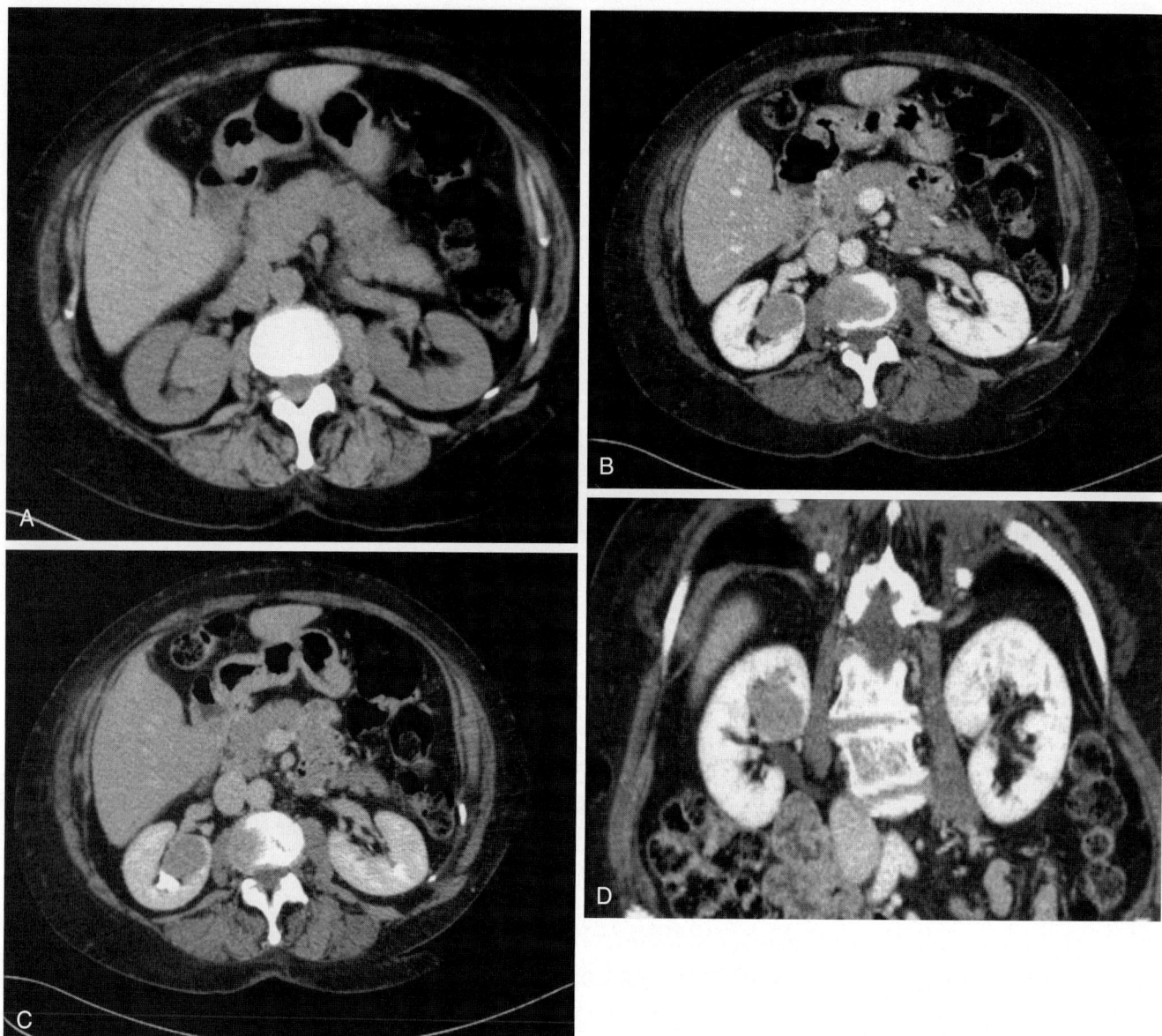

FIGURE 27-73 Renal cell carcinoma: computed tomographic scan. Noncontrast (**A**), nephrographic phase (**B**), and excretory phase (**C**) axial images combined with a coronal nephrographic phase image (**D**). On the noncontrast scan (**A**), the right renal mass appears slightly hyperdense in relation to the rest of the kidney. Contrast material–enhanced scans (**B, C,** and **D**) show the enhanced structure surrounded by the normal renal parenchyma. This proved to be a renal cell carcinoma, chromophobe type.

most renal cell carcinomas show significant enhancement. The best phase for depiction of the mass is the nephrographic phase, although lesions are certainly detectable in the corticomedullary and excretory phases as well (Figure 27-74; see also Figure 27-73).[278-280] In the corticomedullary phase, there is maximal enhancement of the arteries and veins that must be viewed for accurate staging and preoperative planning (see Figure 27-74).[281,282] The excretory phase is most helpful for showing the relationship of the tumor to the pelvicalyceal system and in preoperative planning for nephron-sparing partial nephrectomy (see Figure 27-73).[283,284] Clear cell renal cell carcinoma tends to have greater enhancement than the papillary or chromophobe types (see Figures 27-73 and 27-74).[285,286] Enhancement patterns for clear cell and papillary tumors appear more heterogeneous than those for the chromophobe tumor, which frequently has a homogeneous enhancement pattern (see Figure 27-73).[285] Chromophobe

and papillary types more often contain calcification than does the clear cell type, and they demonstrate only mild enhancement of 25 to 30 Hounsfield units.[287]

The appearance of renal cell carcinoma on MRI can vary with the histologic type. For example, the clear cell type tends to be larger and is associated more frequently with hemorrhage and necrosis (Figures 27-75 and 27-76) than is the papillary type (Figure 27-77) and chromophobe renal cell carcinoma. Differentiating histologic types is difficult because their imaging features overlap. The feasibility of renal cell carcinoma differentiation by means of advanced MRI techniques such as diffusion weighting is being evaluated, but further research is required.[288] Renal cell carcinoma most commonly is heterogeneously hyperintense on T2-weighted sequences and hypointense to isointense on T1-weighted sequences (Figure 27-78). Renal cell carcinoma is enhanced less than normal renal cortex tissue. The heterogeneity increases with increasing size as a

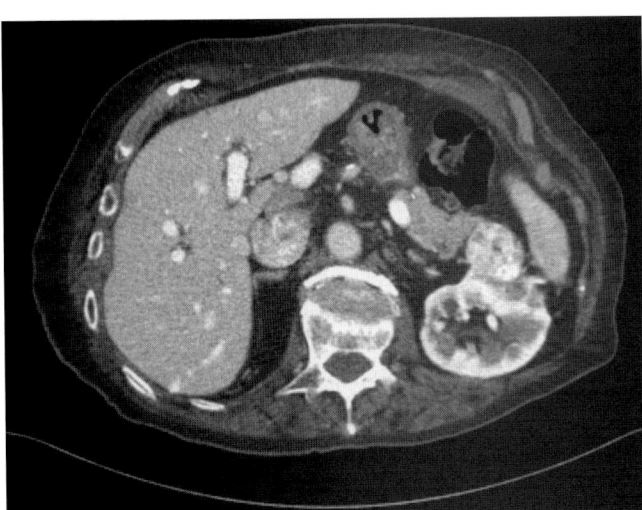

FIGURE 27-74 Renal cell carcinoma: computed tomographic scan. Contrast material–enhanced axial image in the corticomedullary phase. Note the heterogeneously enhanced mass in the anterior aspect of the left kidney. This is a stage II renal cell carcinoma, inasmuch as it has extended through the renal capsule into Gerota's fascia. This proved to be a renal cell carcinoma, clear cell type.

result of variable amounts of necrosis and intraluminal lipid. The intraluminal lipid may make areas of the mass drop in signal intensity on opposed-phase T1-weighted sequences.

The staging of renal cell carcinoma is important in predicting survival rates and planning the proper surgical approach to the mass. Both the World Health Organization and the Robson classifications are used in the staging of renal cell carcinoma.[266] In the Robson classification of renal cell carcinoma, a stage I tumor is confined to the renal parenchyma by the renal capsule (see Figure 27-73). In stage II renal cell carcinoma, the tumor extends through the renal capsule into the perinephric fat but is still within Gerota's fascia (see Figure 27-74). Stage III lesions are subdivided: IIIa tumors extend into the renal vein or IVC; IIIb tumors involve regional retroperitoneal lymph nodes; and IIIc tumors involve the veins and nodes (Figure 27-79). In atage IVa renal cell carcinoma, the tumor extends outside Gerota's fascia with involvement of adjacent organs or muscles other than the ipsilateral adrenal gland. Stage IVb renal cell carcinoma represents tumor with distant metastases, the most common sites being the lungs, mediastinum, liver, and bone.

Although MRI has been found to be highly accurate in staging renal cell carcinoma, the areas of greatest challenge remain the evaluation for local invasion of the perinephric fat and direct invasion of adjacent organs, especially with large tumors.[289] The presence of an intact pseudocapsule aids in ruling out local invasion. A pseudocapsule is a hypointense rim around the tumor, viewed best on T2-weighted images (see Figure 27-78). These are most frequently observed in association with small or slow-growing tumors. When the tumor extends beyond the confines of the kidney, the pseudocapsule is made of fibrous tissue; otherwise it is made up of compressed normal renal tissue.[290] If the pseudocapsule is intact, the perinephric fat is unlikely to have been invaded.[290]

Detecting and assessing vascular thrombosis in patients with renal cell carcinoma is highly accurate and reliable with contrast material–enhanced MRI.[289,291] Coronal imaging in the venous and delayed phases demonstrates the presence or absence of venous invasion; determines the extent of venous invasion, if present; and differentiates tumor thrombus, which is enhanced, from nonenhanced bland thrombus (Figure 27-80). Accurate determination of renal vein, IVC, and right atrial involvement is important for deciding the surgical approach.[292]

Although renal cell carcinoma is the most common primary malignancy in the kidney, transitional cell carcinoma also occurs within the kidneys.[293] Most transitional cell carcinomas involve the urothelium and project into the lumen of the renal pelvis or ureter. As a result, images show a filling defect within the renal pelvis or ureter that can be confused with a renal stone, blood clot, or debris (Figure 27-81). Transitional cell carcinoma of the bladder is much more common than that of the kidney or ureter.[294] The neoplasm may extend into the renal parenchyma and, on imaging, appears as a mass within the kidney. The imaging findings are similar to those of renal cell carcinoma, except the lesions tend not to be enhanced as much with injection of contrast material. Renal vein involvement is rare. Retrograde pyelography with ureteroscopy is a diagnostic tool. CTU and MRU probably show similar findings. Transitional cell carcinoma in the upper collecting system can be either a focal, irregularly enhanced mass within the collecting system (Figure 27-82) or an ill-defined mass infiltrating the renal parenchyma. When small, they may be difficult to identify on both CT and MRI. Evaluation of the entire collecting system is required because synchronous lesions may be present. Both CTU and MRU are valuable for complete evaluation of the collecting system.

Lymphoma may involve the kidney as part of multiorgan involvement or, in rare cases, as a primary neoplasm.[295] Lymphoma manifests with single or multiple masses within one or both kidneys. Perirenal extension may be visible as well. An infiltrative picture with lymphomatous replacement of the kidney may also be observed. This form is usually accompanied by adjacent retroperitoneal adenopathy. The imaging findings are representative of either the mass or infiltrative involvement. CT has usually been the imaging method of choice in these patients. Because MRI of lymphoma are similar to those in CT, MRI probably shows no additional findings that would affect treatment. Lymphoma typically appears hypointense on T1-weighted sequences and heterogeneous to slightly hypointense on T2-weighted sequences. Enhancement is minimal on postcontrast sequences[296] (Figure 27-83). Vessels are usually encased and are not invaded, and necrosis is usually not observed. Treated lymphoma may vary in signal intensity, as a result of the effects of therapy.[296]

Metastatic disease may also involve the kidney. Actually, it is quite often found at autopsy. Because individuals live longer with cancer and new drugs are being developed, the number of cases of visible renal metastases will probably rise. Metastases are most commonly hematogenous and usually result in multiple foci of involvement, although single lesions do occur (Figure 27-84). They are observed most frequently with CT, inasmuch as CT is used in the regular follow-up of most patients with cancer. Hypodense round masses, usually in the periphery, are the typical finding. When present as a single lesion, a metastasis cannot be differentiated from a primary renal neoplasm without biopsy.

Cystic renal masses present a vexing problem in that not all are benign.[297] Cystic renal cell carcinomas occur, as do tumors within the wall of benign cysts. In 1986, Bosniak[239]

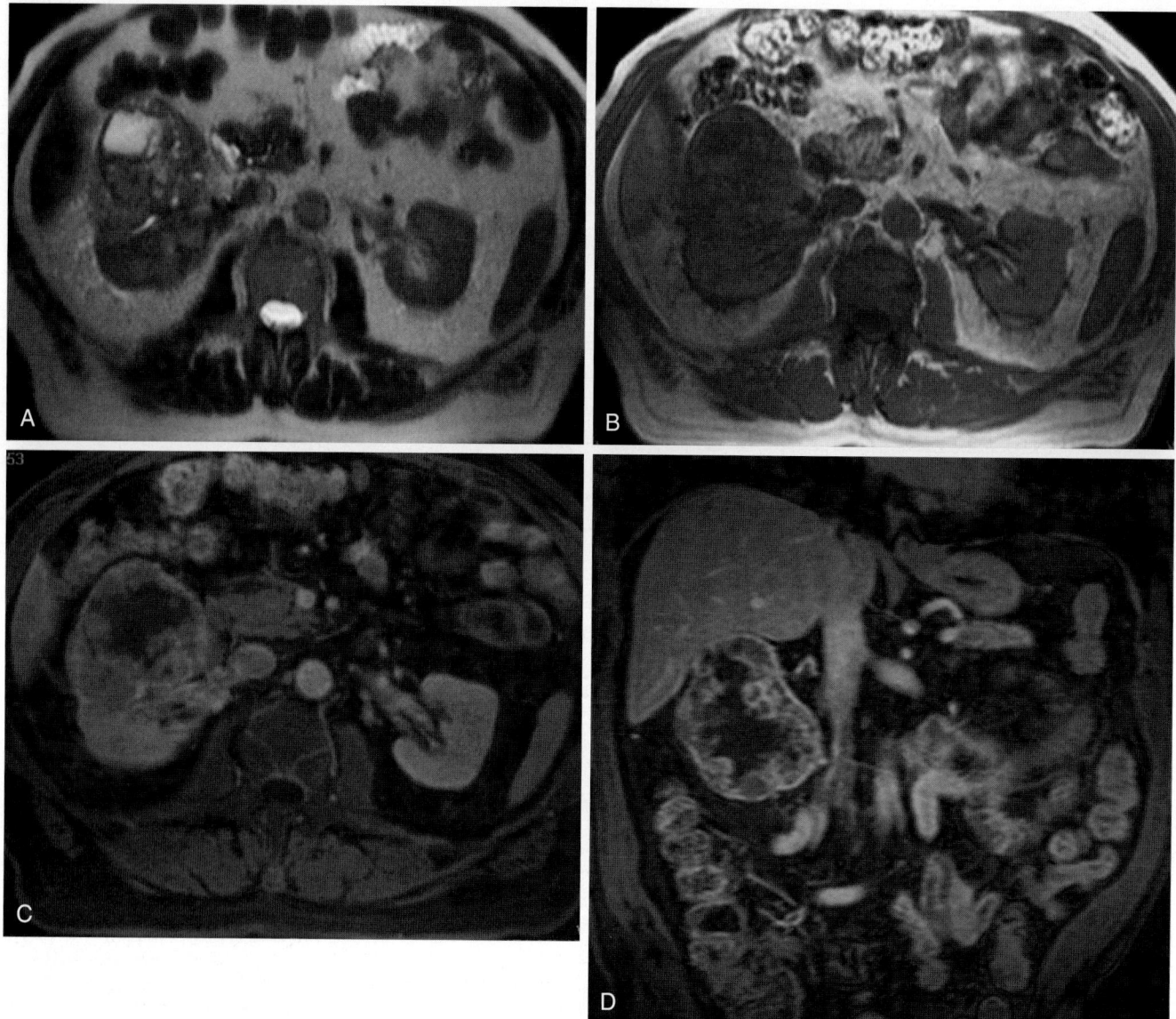

FIGURE 27-75 Clear cell renal cell carcinoma, stage IIIA. **A,** Axial T2-weighted image shows a 7.5-cm right renal mass with areas of high signal intensity, consistent with necrosis and cystic degeneration. **B,** Axial T1-weighted image shows a heterogeneous, isointense mass with increased perinephric fat stranding. Axial (**C**) and coronal (**D**) gadolinium-enhanced images confirm central areas of necrosis. No venous invasion is visible. Focal microinvasion of the perinephric fat was found at surgery.

developed a classification system for cystic masses that has stood the test of time.[298,299] It is not a pathologic classification system but actually an imaging and clinical management guide for handling the cystic renal mass. Category I lesions are simple benign cyst (see Figure 27-61). Category II cysts are benign with thin septa, fine rimlike calcification, or they are uniform high-density cysts less than 3 cm in diameter that are not enhanced by contrast material on CT (Figure 27-85). Category IIF represents lesions characteristic of categories II and III that necessitate follow-up, usually at 6 to 12 months, to prove benignity (Figure 27-86).[300] These cystic lesions may have multiple septa, or an area of thick or nodular calcification, or they may be high-density cysts larger than 3 cm in diameter. Category III cystic lesions have thickened, irregular walls, which demonstrate some enhancement with contrast material. Dense irregular calcification may also be visible. In these cases, clinical history may be helpful in determining whether they are renal abscesses or infected cysts. Although

many of these lesions are benign, surgery may be necessary for diagnosis and treatment.[301] Biopsy has been advocated by some authorities[302-305] (see Figure 27-54). Category IV cystic masses are clearly malignant and demonstrate distinct enhanced soft tissue masses or nodules within the cyst (Figure 27-87).[306] Nephrectomy is required for these lesions, although if they are not larger than 5 to 6 cm and are in proper locations, a nephron-sparing procedure may be performed.

Renal Cancer: Positron Emission Tomography and Positron Emission Tomography–Computed Tomography

Renal cell carcinoma arises from the renal tubular epithelium and accounts for the majority of kidney tumors in adults. The tumor is angioinvasive and is associated with widespread hematogenous and lymphatic metastases, especially to the

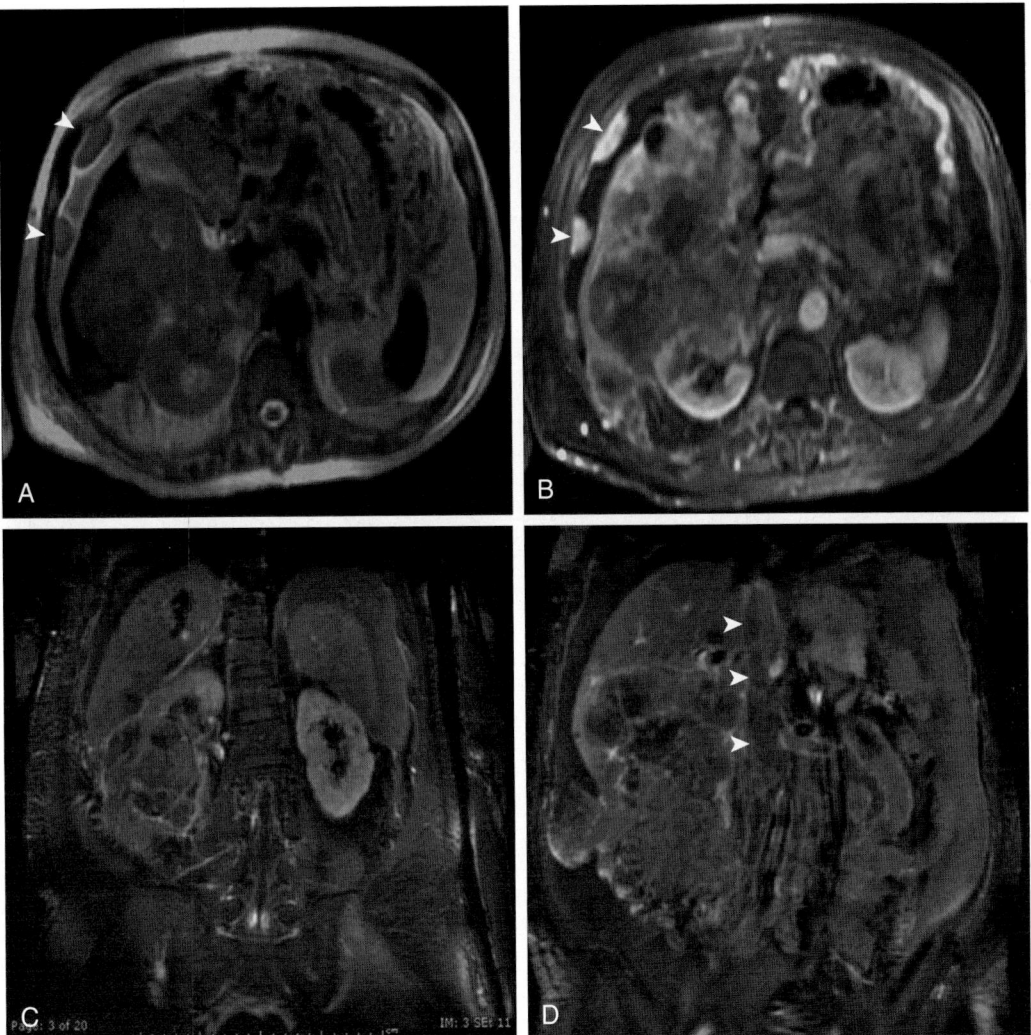

FIGURE 27-76 Metastatic clear cell renal cell carcinoma, stage IV. T2-weighted (**A**) and gadolinium-enhanced T1-weighted (**B**) axial images show a large, heterogeneous mass with invasion of the adjacent liver and peritoneal metastases (*arrowheads*). **C** and **D,** Coronal gadolinium-enhanced T1-weighted images show the large mass extending inferiorly and medially, with invasion of the inferior vena cava to the level of the hepatic veins (*arrowheads*).

lungs, liver, lymph nodes, bone, and brain. Metastases are present in about 50% of affected patients at initial presentation. Radical nephrectomy is the main treatment for the early stages of disease, although palliative nephrectomy may also be performed in advanced disease with intractable bleeding. Solitary metastasis may also be resected. Renal cell carcinoma responds poorly to chemotherapy. Radiation therapy for renal cell carcinoma is used for palliation of metastatic sites, specifically bone and brain. Immunotherapy with biologic response modifiers such as interleukin-2 and interferon-α has the most impact in the treatment of metastatic disease. The rate of 5-year survival may be as high as 80% to 90% among patients with early stages of disease, whereas advanced disease carries a poor prognosis.[307]

Preliminary studies of PET imaging of renal cell carcinoma with have revealed a promising role in the evaluation of indeterminate renal masses, in preoperative staging and assessment of tumor burden, in detection of osseous and nonosseous metastases (including tumor thrombus), in restaging after therapy, in treatment evaluation, and in the determination of effect of imaging findings on clinical management.[308-315] However, other PET studies have demonstrated less encouraging results and no advantage over standard imaging methods.[316-318]

A relatively high false-negative rate (23%) has been reported with FDG PET in the preoperative staging of renal cell carcinoma in comparison with histologic analysis of surgical specimens. In one study, PET exhibited 60% sensitivity of (vs. 91.7% for CT) and 100% specificity (vs. 100% for CT) for primary renal cell carcinoma tumors. For retroperitoneal lymph node metastases or renal bed recurrence, PET had 75.0% sensitivity (vs. 92.6% for CT) and 100.0% specificity (vs. 98.1% for CT). For metastases to the lung parenchyma, PET had 75.0% sensitivity of (vs. 91.1% for chest CT) and 97.1% specificity of (vs. 73.1% for chest CT). For bone metastases, PET had 77.3% sensitivity and 100.0% specificity (in comparison with 93.8% and 87.2% for combined CT and bone scan).[319] For restaging renal cell carcinoma, 87% sensitivity and 100% specificity of have been reported.[320] A comparative investigation of bone scan and FDG PET for detecting osseous metastases in renal cell carcinoma revealed that PET had 100% sensitivity (vs. 77.5% for bone scan) and 100% specificity (vs. 59.6% for bone scan).[313] Another report revealed a negative predictive value of 33% and a positive

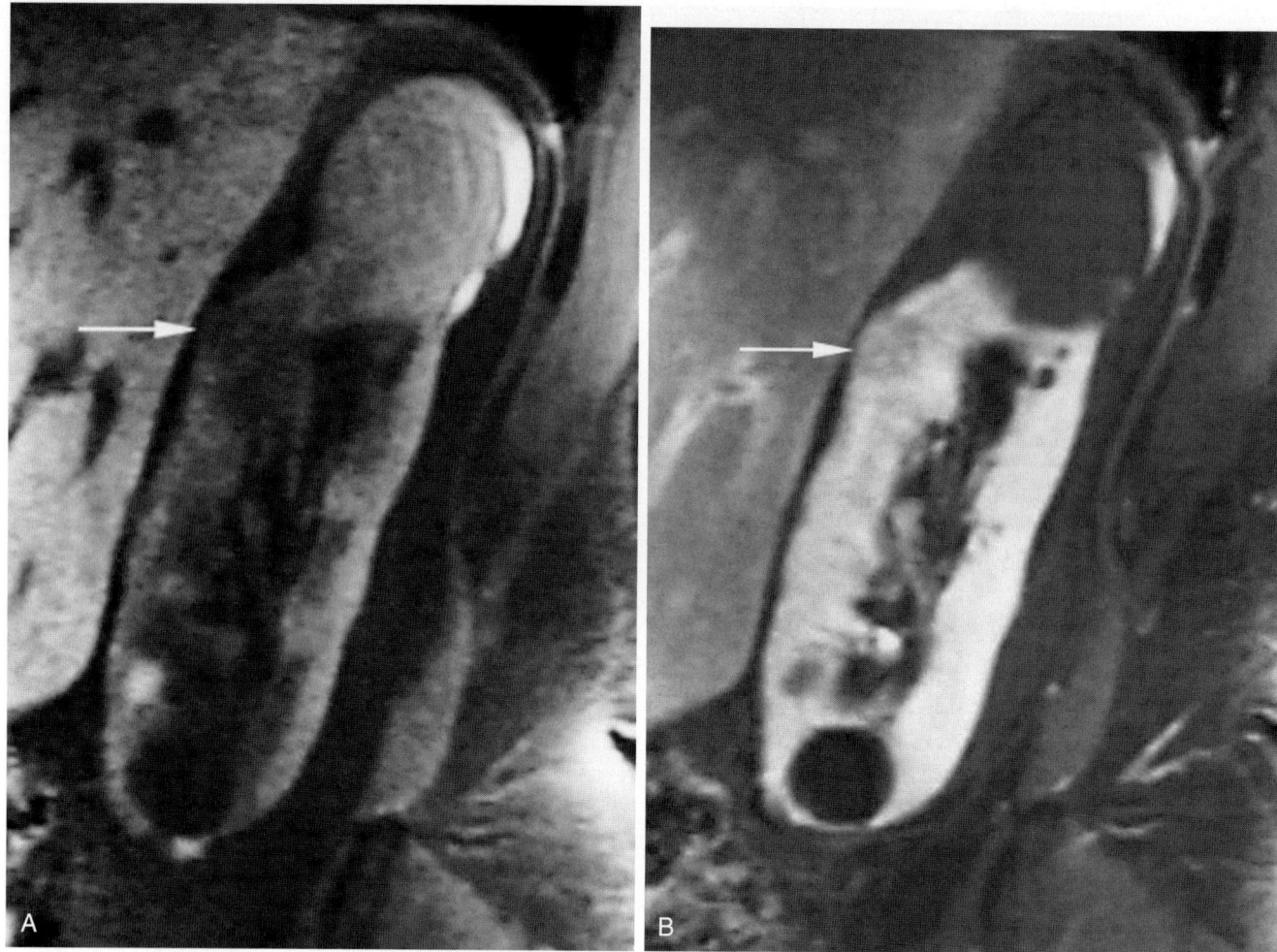

FIGURE 27-77 Papillary renal cell carcinoma, stage I. Sagittal T1-weighted images before (**A**) and after (**B**) the administration of gadolinium show a subtle mass (*arrow*) in the anterior cortex and multiple nonenhanced cysts. No perinephric invasion was found at surgery.

predictive value of 94% for restaging renal cell carcinoma.[309] Other studies have revealed high accuracy in characterizing indeterminate renal masses, with a mean tumor-to-kidney uptake ratio of 3.0 for malignancy.[308]

These mixed observations are probably related to the heterogeneous expression of glucose transporter-1 in renal cell carcinoma, which may not be correlated with the tumor grade or extent.[321,322] Negative study findings may not rule out disease, whereas a positive result is highly suspect for malignancy.[323] If the tumor binds FDG avidly, then PET can be a reasonable imaging modality for follow-up after treatment and for surveillance (Figure 27-88). In fact, it has been shown that FDG PET can alter clinical management in up to 40% of patients with suspected locally recurrent and metastatic renal cancer.[311]

The diagnostic accuracy of FDG PET appears not to be improved by semiquantitative image analysis, probably because of the fundamental variability of glucose metabolism in renal cell carcinoma.[318] In one study, the maximum and average standardized uptake values for FDG-positive primary renal malignant tumors were 7.9 ± 4.9 and 6.0 ± 3.6, respectively. The maximum and average standardized uptake values of metastatic renal masses were 6.1 ± 3.4 and 4.7 ± 2.8, respectively. Maximum and average standardized uptake values of primary and metastatic renal masses did not differ significantly.[324] Because FDG is excreted in the urine, the intense

urine activity may confound lesion detection in and near the renal bed. Intravenous administration of furosemide has been proposed to improve urine clearance from the renal collecting system, although the exact benefit of such intervention in improving lesion detection remains undefined.

Other tracers used in PET (e.g., carbon 11–labeled acetate [^{11}C-acetate], fluorine 18–labeled fluoromisonidazole, fluorine 18–labeled sodium fluoride) have been investigated in the imaging evaluation of patients with renal cell carcinoma, but further studies are needed to establish the exact role of these and other non-FDG tracers in this clinical setting.[325-328] For example, one study revealed high accumulation of ^{11}C-acetate in 70% of renal cell carcinoma's.[329] However, an earlier similar study had demonstrated that in most kidney tumors, accumulation of ^{11}C-acetate was not higher than in normal renal parenchyma.[330] Aside from renal cell carcinoma, ^{11}C-acetate has also been demonstrated to be useful in the imaging-based assessment of renal oxygen consumption and tubular sodium reabsorption.[331]

Moreover, many investigators since have reported on the diagnostic synergism of the combined PET-CT imaging systems.[332] In Park and colleagues' study in South Korea, 63 patients with renal cell carcinoma underwent both FDG PET-CT and conventional imaging evaluation during follow-up after surgical treatment.[333] FDG PET-CT demonstrated

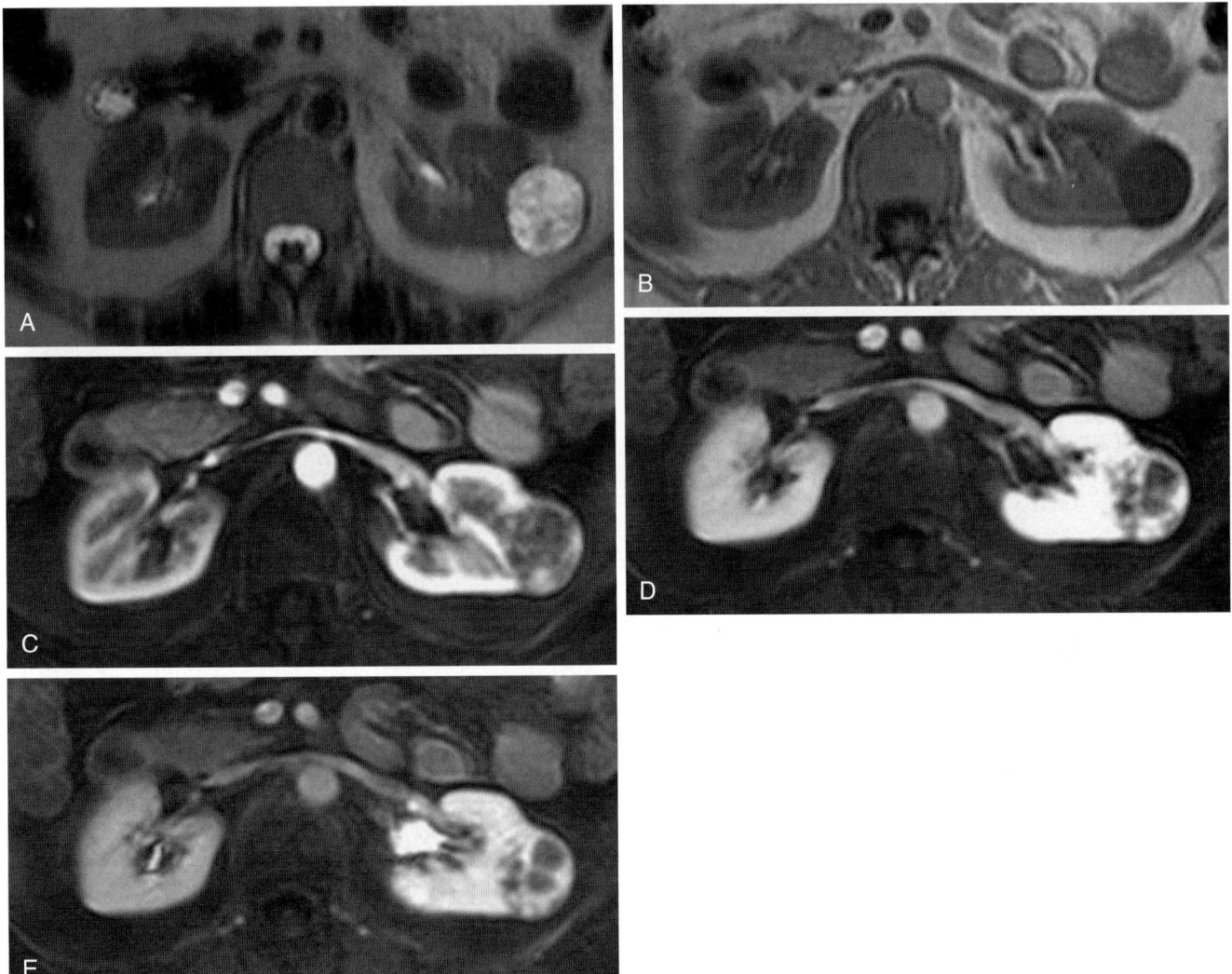

FIGURE 27-78 Renal cell carcinoma with pseudocapsule, stage I. **A,** T2-weighted image shows a heterogeneous, bright mass on the left with a well-defined pseudocapsule. **B,** T1-weighted image confirms a well-defined dark mass involving the left renal cortex. **C to E,** Axial gadolinium-enhanced T1-weighted images in the arterial, venous, and excretory phases demonstrate heterogeneous enhancement and no evidence of renal vein involvement. No perinephric invasion was found at surgery.

89.5% sensitivity, 83.3% specificity, a positive predictive value of 77.3%, and a negative predictive value of 92.6% in detecting recurrent and metastatic disease; these values were not significantly different from the diagnostic performance of conventional imaging studies. Park and colleagues concluded that FDG PET-CT can replace multiple conventional imaging studies without the need for contrast agents. The role of PET-CT in renal cancer imaging and its effect on both short- and long-term clinical management and decision making also must be investigated. Other uses of PET in the imaging evaluation of renal perfusion, function, and metabolism have also been investigated.[334] In addition, there is some effort for evaluating the role of radiolabeled antibodies as therapeutic agents in the treatment of renal cell carcinoma.[335]

Renal Vascular Disease

Renal artery stenosis is a potential treatable cause of hypertension but is found in less than 5% of the hypertensive population.[336] When the expected signs and symptoms are present,

the diagnosis may be made in 20% to 30% of patients.[337] Renal artery stenosis is usually defined as 50% or more stenosis of the renal artery.[338] Atherosclerosis is the most common cause, accounting for up to 70% of cases and is typically found in men older than 50 years. The stenosis is caused by an atherosclerotic plaque, with or without calcification, located in the proximal renal artery at or near the ostia (Figure 27-89).[339] It is bilateral in 30% of cases. Fibromuscular dysplasia is the second most common cause, accounting for approximately 25% of cases.[340] Fibromuscular dysplasia is subclassified by the location of the involvement within the vessel wall; medial fibroplasia is the most common. The classic finding in this form is the "string of beads" appearance in the distal main renal artery and segmental branches, caused by the alternating areas of stenosis and dilation.

IVU is of only historical note in the assessment of patients with renovascular hypertension. For renal hypertension, IVU was traditionally performed by obtaining a series of radiographs of the kidneys after the injection of contrast material at 1-minute intervals to evaluate for discrepancies in renal size, appearance of the nephrogram, prolongation of the

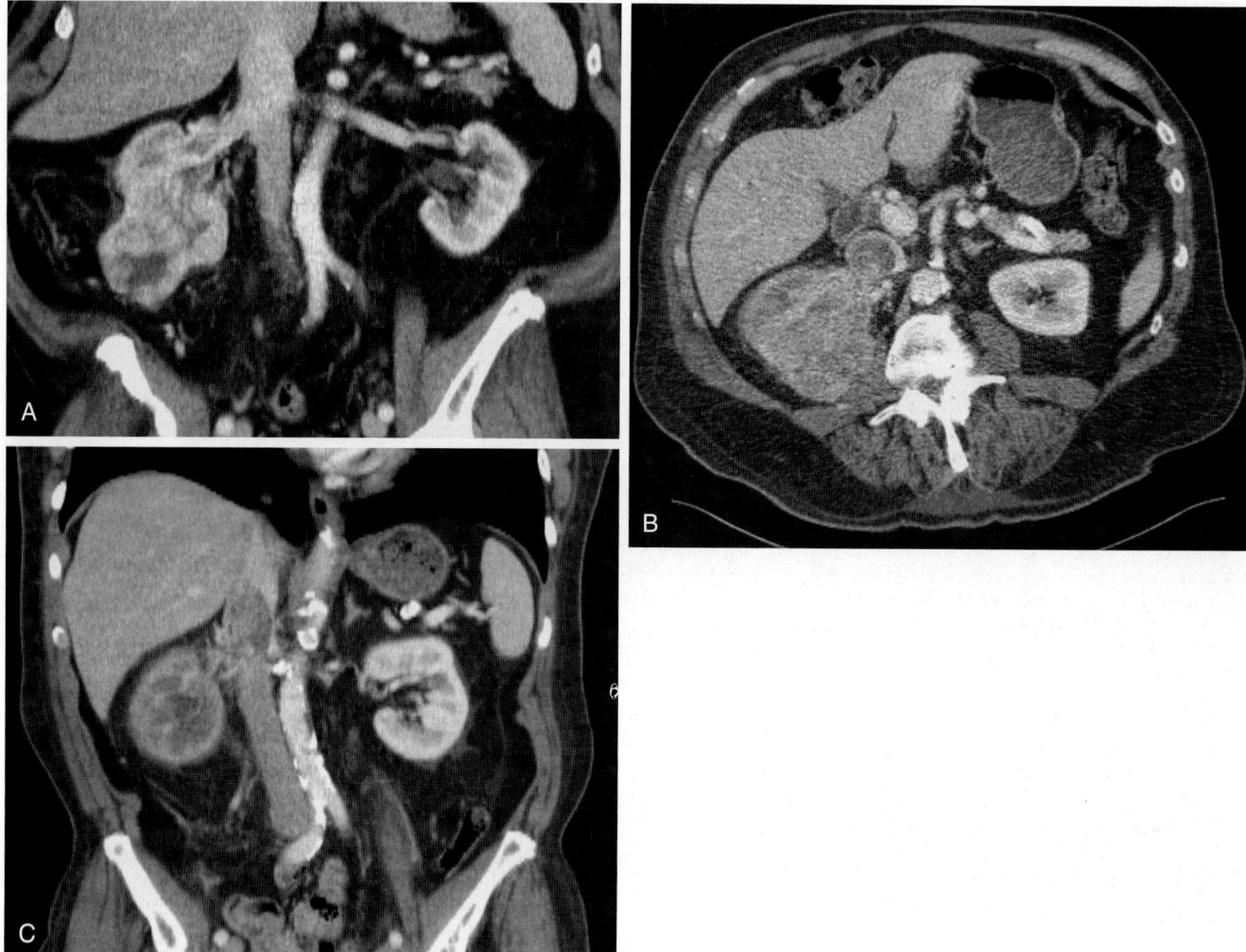

FIGURE 27-79 Renal cell carcinoma, stage IIIA: computed tomographic scan. Coronal contrast medium–enhanced image (**A**) shows a stage IIIA mass in the right kidney and a tumor thrombus extending into the right renal vein. In a different patient, axial (**B**) and coronal (**C**) contrast medium–enhanced images also show a right renal mass with a tumor thrombus, but the thrombus has extended into the inferior vena cava. Both these tumors proved to be of the clear cell type.

nephrogram, and excretion patterns. This study is no longer performed because it has been supplanted by Doppler ultrasonography, by CT and MRA, and by captopril-enhanced renography (described in the "Nuclear Imaging and Renovascular Disease" section).[341,342]

Conventional ultrasonography and Doppler ultrasonography have been used to assess patients with renovascular hypertension.[343] Renal size and the presence or absence of medical renal disease may be evaluated with gray-scale ultrasonography. Doppler ultrasonography has been used with variable success to assess the main renal arteries for renal artery stenosis and the intrarenal vasculature for secondary effects.[344,345] The success of Doppler ultrasonography is highly operator dependent, and results may be inadequate or incomplete because of overlying bowel gas, body habitus, or aortic pulsatility.[344] A stable Doppler signal may be difficult to reproduce in some patients with renovascular hypertension. A complete examination has been possible in 50% to 90% of affected patients. Accessory renal arteries, which occur in 15% to 20% of affected patients, may not be imaged.[346]

The criteria used for evaluation of the main renal artery include an increase in the peak systolic velocity to more than

185 cm/second, a renal/aortic ratio of peak systolic velocity of more than 3.0, and turbulent flow beyond the region of the stenosis.[347] Visualization of the main renal artery with no detectable Doppler signal is suggestive of renal artery occlusion. Intrarenal vascular assessment with Doppler ultrasonography has depicted the shape and character of the waveform. A dampened appearance of the waveform, with a slowed systolic upstroke and delay to peak velocity (tardus-parvus effect), has been shown in varying degrees in renal artery stenosis.[348] In the resistive indices, a difference between the kidneys of more than 5% has also been suggestive of renal artery stenosis. Sensitivity and specificity for the techniques have generally been in the range of 50% to 70%. Contrast material–enhanced ultrasonography has been suggested as a means of improving the accuracy of Doppler ultrasonography.[349,350]

CTA performed with MDCT has sensitivity and specificity at or near 100% (see Figure 27-85).[351-353] A normal result should rule out renal artery stenosis.[354] This study is performed with an injection of 4 to 5 mL of contrast material per second, volume of contrast material of 100 to 120 mL, and rapid scanning at 15 to 20 seconds for proper assessment of the renal arteries. The angiographic study takes less than

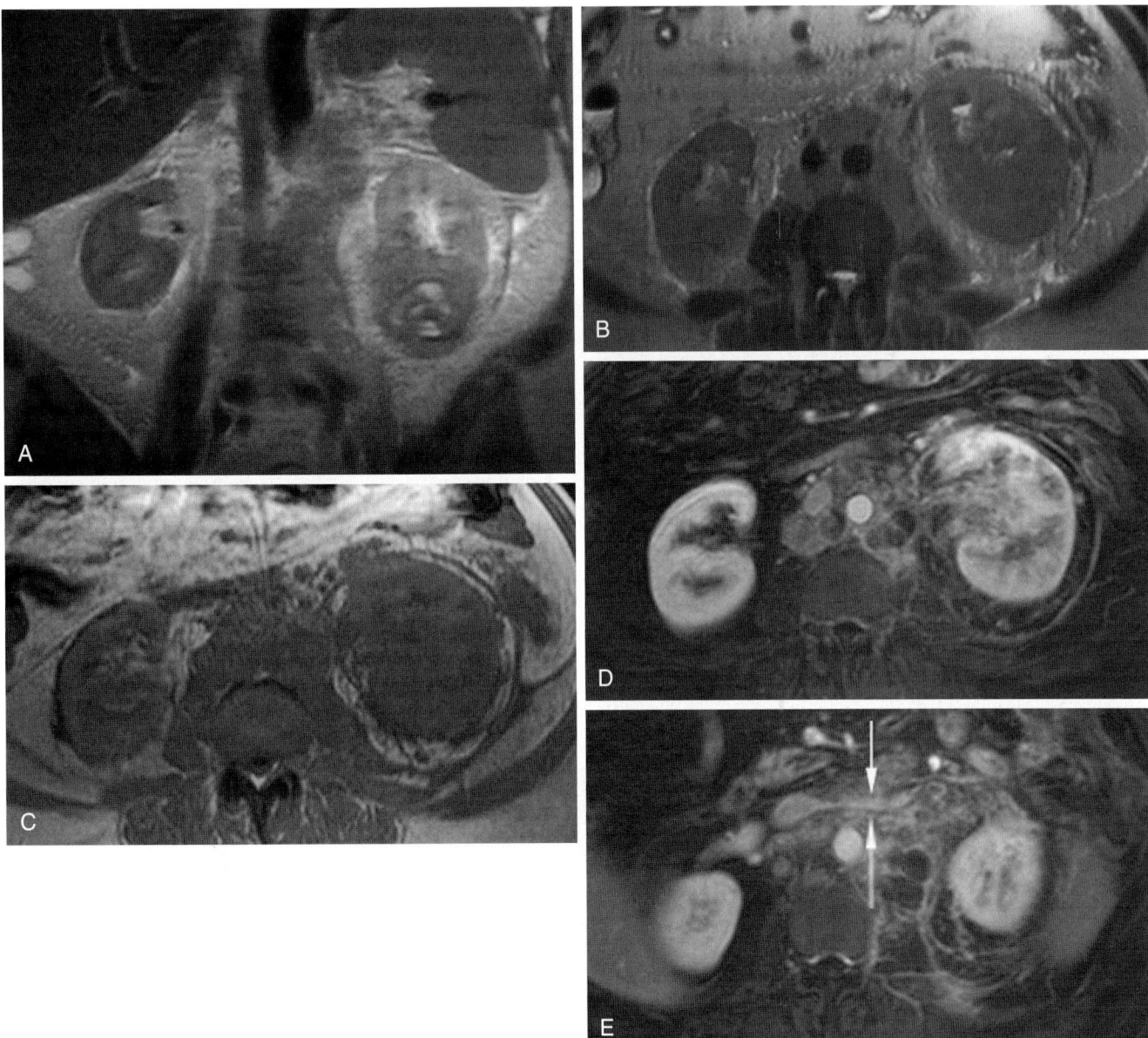

FIGURE 27-80 Poorly differentiated renal cell carcinoma, stage IV. Coronal (**A**) and axial (**B**) T2-weighted images show a heterogeneous mass in the lower pole of the left kidney with infiltration of the perinephric fat and extensive retroperitoneal lymphadenopathy. T1-weighted image (**C**) shows the masses to be intermediate in signal intensity. Gadolinium enhancement of axial T1-weighted images (**D** and **E**) make the local invasion and adenopathy more conspicuous and show that the left renal vein is encased, not invaded (*arrows*).

10 seconds to complete.[351] Computer processing of images with three-dimensional volume renderings and MIP images is imperative (Figures 27-90 and 27-91).[354-356] Assessment of the axial images alone is insufficient. The main renal artery, as well as its segmental branches, can be viewed and evaluated. Accessory renal arteries as small as 1 mm in diameter can be seen.[357] CTA may also demonstrate other findings in the patient with renal artery stenosis, including a smaller kidney with a smooth contour, thinning of the cortex, a delayed or prolonged nephrogram, all on the affected side. Patients with renal artery stents can be successfully imaged with CTA (Figure 27-92).[358,359] CTA and MRA are of equivalent quality in the detection of hemodynamically significant renal artery stenosis.[360] Patients with impaired renal function or allergy to contrast agents need evaluation with MRA, because they cannot tolerate the iodinated contrast material necessary with

CTA. Digital subtraction angiography should be reserved for patients who require an intervention (either angioplasty or angioplasty and stent placement). It is unnecessary for diagnosis today.

Ultrasonography, CTA, and MRA have been shown to be accurate alternatives to conventional angiography.[361,362] Because CTA is sensitive, accurate, fast, and reproducible, MRA is reserved for patients for whom iodinated contrast material is contraindicated. Renal insufficiency is not uncommon in the population clinically at high risk for renal artery stenosis. For this reason, CE-MRA has been widely accepted as a reliable and accurate examination in the evaluation of renal artery stenosis in this population.[100,360,363,364] Because the risk of NSF is higher in this population, however, CE-MRA is being used more selectively. Noncontrast MRA techniques are being used more frequently to reduce the amount of

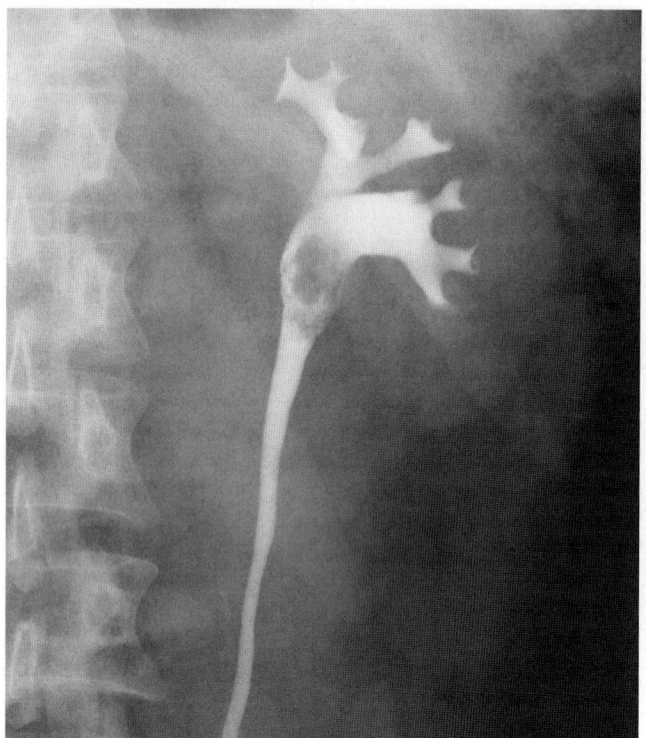

FIGURE 27-81 Transitional cell carcinoma: intravenous urogram. The irregular filling defect in the left renal pelvis represents a transitional cell carcinoma. Note that there is no significant obstruction of the left kidney, and the calyces appear normal.

Gd-C needed. Like CTA, MRA is noninvasive and provides excellent visualization of the aortoiliac and renal arteries.[360]

Contrast material–enhanced MRA is more than 95% sensitive in demonstrating the main renal arteries and has a high negative predictive value. A normal CE-MRA finding almost completely rules out a stenosis in the visualized vessels.[362] CE-MRA is a reliable examination but has been limited by incomplete visualization of segmental and small accessory vessels.[365] Whereas visualization of all accessory vessels is desired, Bude and colleagues[366] found isolated hemodynamically significant stenosis of an accessory artery in only 1 (1.5%) of their 68 patients. Bude and colleagues concluded that this limitation does not substantially reduce the rate of detection of renovascular hypertension by MRI. With the use of three-dimensional reconstruction, studies have demonstrated no significant difference between CE-MRA and MDCT in the detection of hemodynamically significant renal artery stenosis.[360] Volume rendering and multiplanar reformatting improve accuracy in depicting renal artery stenosis.[99] Volume rendering increases the positive predictive value of CE-MRA by reducing the overestimation of stenosis yielded by earlier reconstruction techniques (Figure 27-93).[100,362] Volume rendering has better correlation with digital subtraction angiography and improves delineation of the renal arteries.[100]

The usefulness of MRA is restricted in part by limitations in resolution and by motion artifacts.[361,367] Advancements in magnetic resonance gradient strengths and newer MRA techniques have improved image resolution and reduced motion

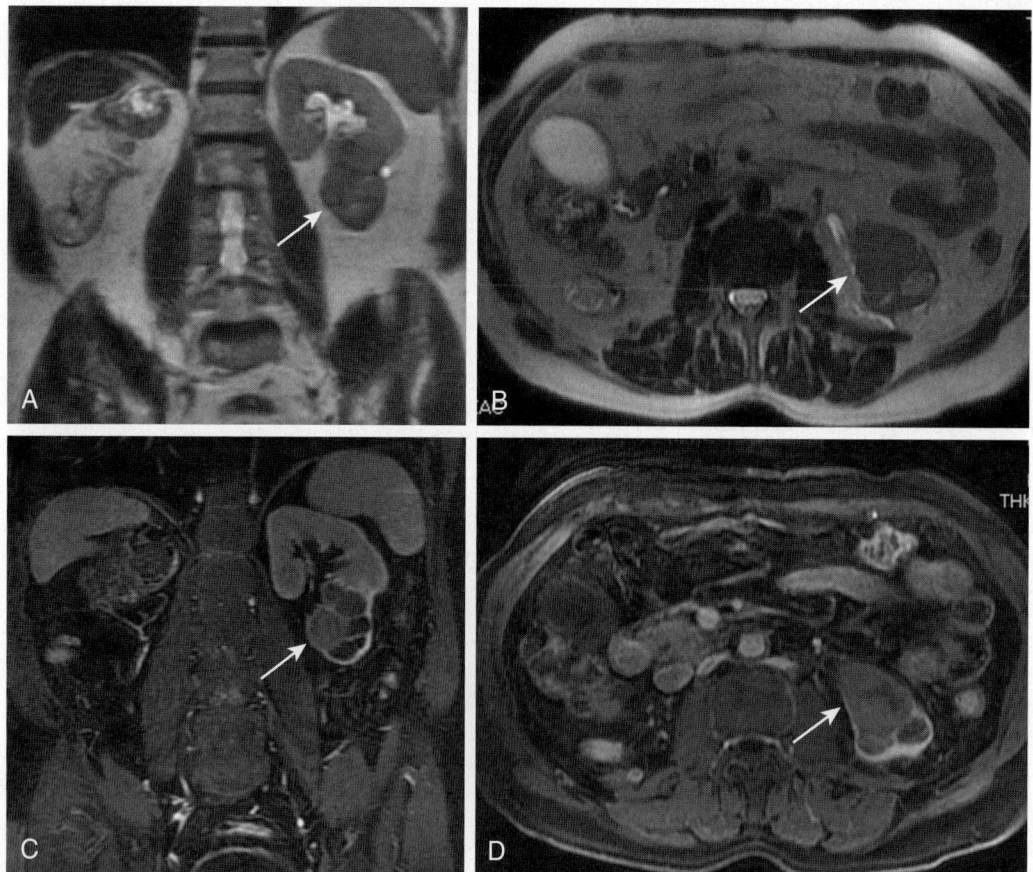

FIGURE 27-82 Transitional cell carcinoma. Coronal (**A**) and axial (**B**) T2-weighted images show intermediate signal intensity and an infiltrating mass (*arrow*) within the atrophic lower pole moiety of a duplicated left kidney. Coronal (**C**) and axial (**D**) gadolinium-enhanced T1-weighted images show enhancing material within dilated calyces and pelvis of the lower pole moiety (*arrow*). The cortical atrophy is well demonstrated.

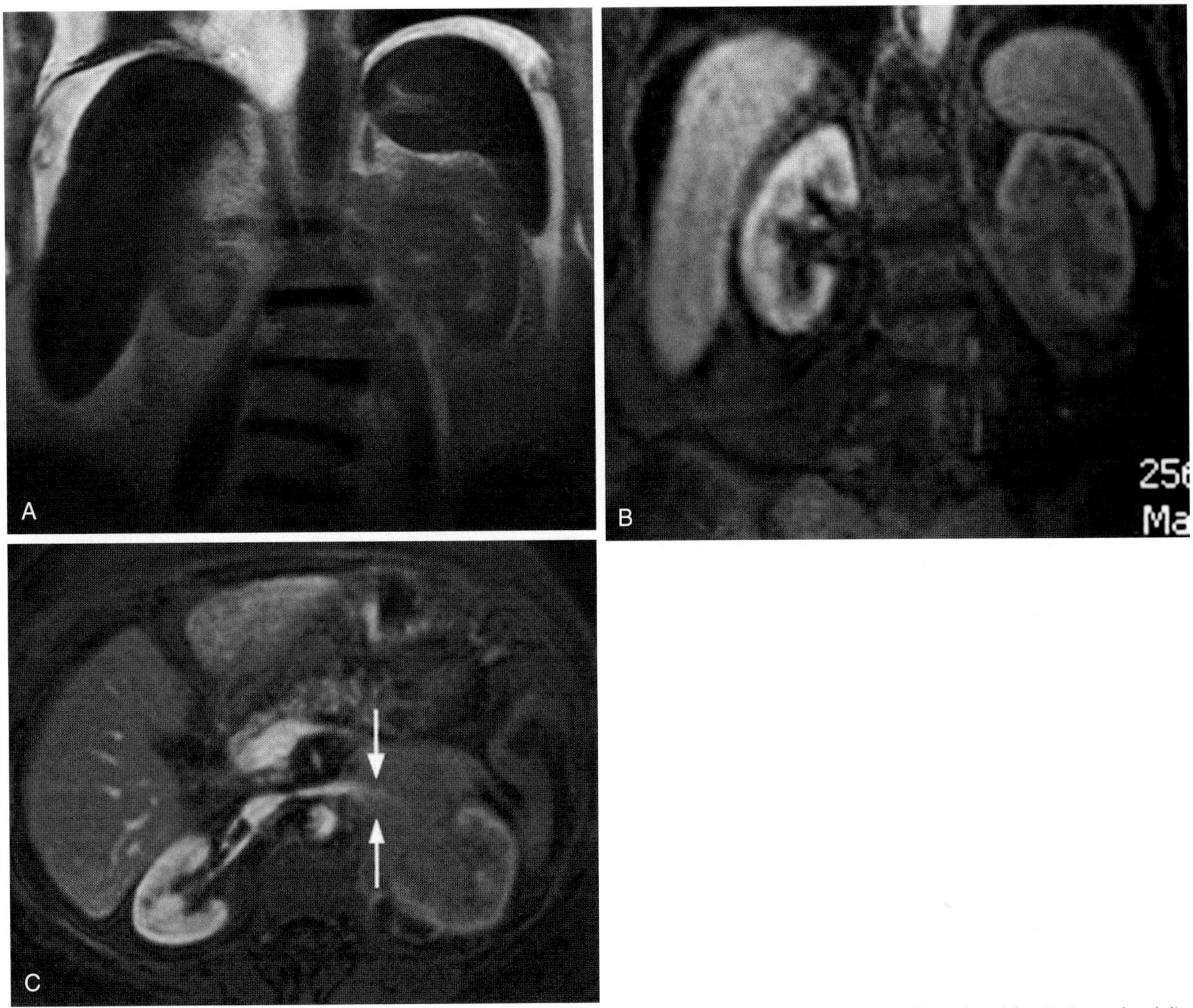

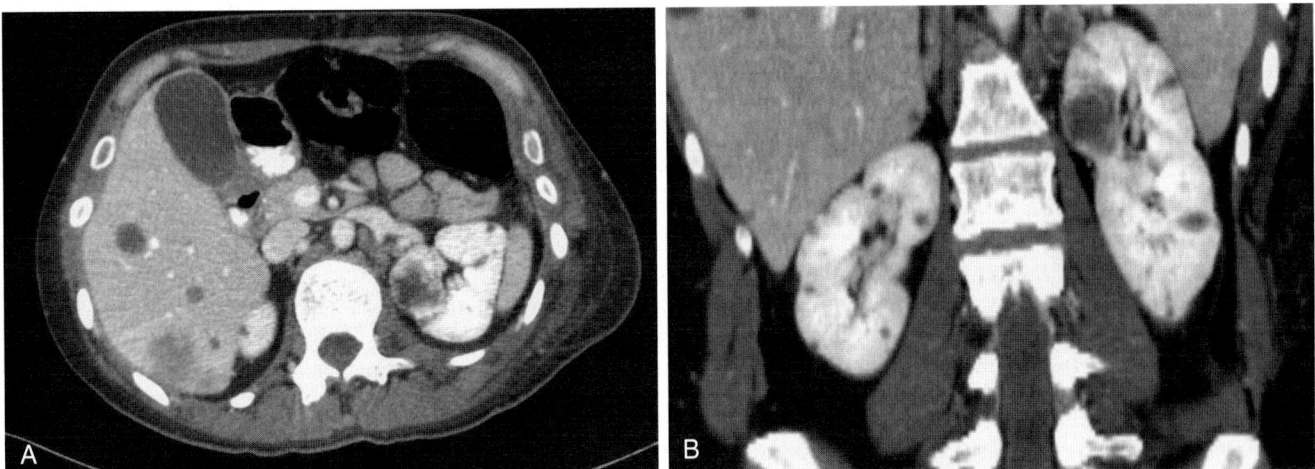

FIGURE 27-83 Lymphoma. **A,** Coronal T2-weighted image shows a large, infiltrating left renal mass extending into the perirenal fat. **B,** Coronal gadolinium-enhanced T1-weighted image better differentiates the mass from the renal cortex. **C,** Axial gadolinium-enhanced T1-weighted image shows encasement of the left renal vein (*arrows*).

FIGURE 27-84 Metastases to the kidney: computed tomographic scan, axial (**A**) and coronal (**B**) contrast material–enhanced images in the nephrographic phase. Multiple heterogeneous but hypodense lesions are visible in the kidneys bilaterally; the largest is in the left upper pole. These appeared in a 2-month period in a patient with metastatic lung carcinoma. Note the metastases also present in the liver.

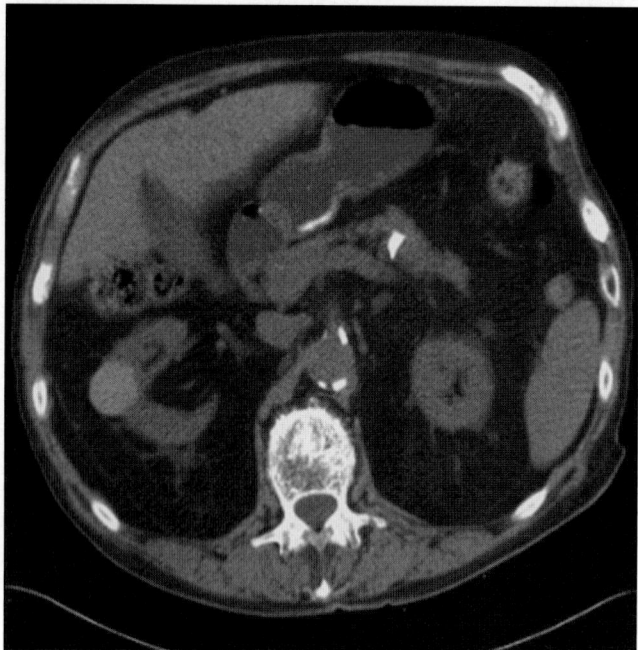

FIGURE 27-85 Hyperdense renal cyst: computed tomographic scan, axial noncontrast image. A single well-circumscribed hyperdense mass is visible in the right kidney. This represents a Bosniak category II renal cyst. It is sharply defined and less than 3 cm in diameter, and it will demonstrate no enhancement on the contrast material–enhanced scan.

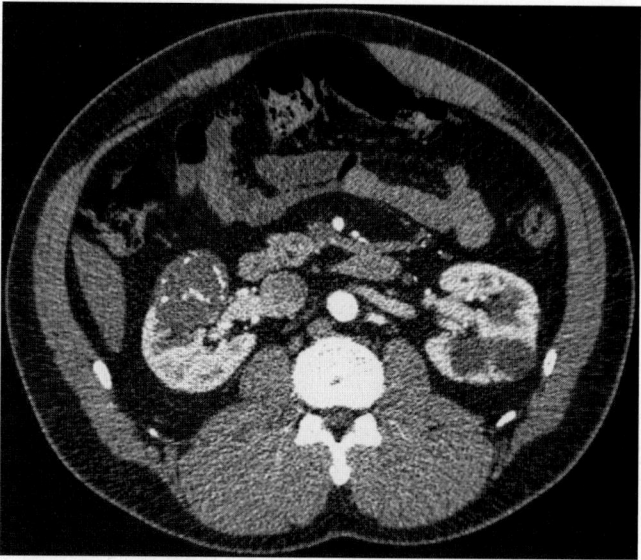

FIGURE 27-86 Bosniak category IIF renal cyst: computed tomographic (CT) scan, axial nephrographic phase image. A cystic lesion in the right kidney also demonstrates large clumps of calcification on the outer wall and on internal septa. There was no change in the CT numbers between the noncontrast scan and the enhanced images. This cyst necessitates follow-up. Note the Bosniak category I cysts in the left kidney.

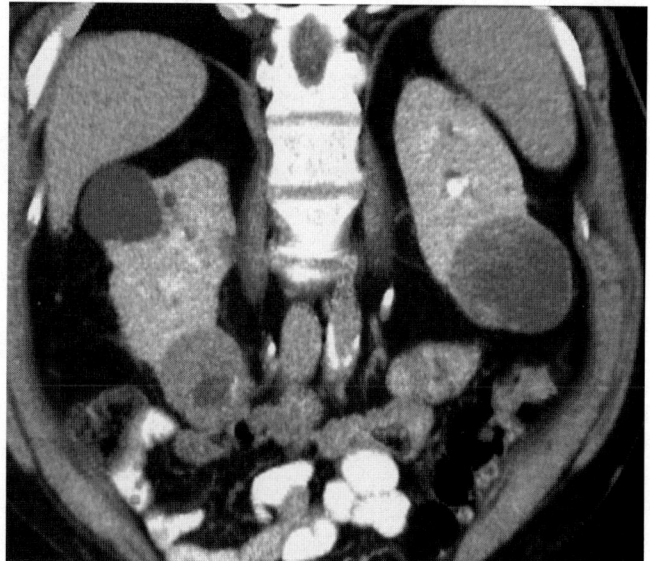

FIGURE 27-87 Bosniak category IV renal cyst: computed tomographic scan, coronal nephrographic phase image. A cystic mass is visible in the left kidney with an internal solid component in the lower pole. In the lower pole of the right kidney, there is a solid mass with central necrosis, which represents a renal cell carcinoma. Note the Bosniak category I cysts in the upper pole of the right kidney. A renal calculus is also present in the midportion of the left kidney. The left lower pole cystic lesion proved to be a renal cell carcinoma, papillary type.

artifacts, while reducing imaging times.[367] Work with cardiac imaging has demonstrated that imaging at 3 T can result in higher spatial and temporal resolution than does imaging at 1.5 T. This higher resolution was found to improve the evaluation of smaller structures of the heart.[368] Further evaluation is needed to determine how imaging at 3 T will affect MRA of the renal arteries.[369]

Phase-contrast MRA can be used to calculate blood flow through the renal artery.[370] Phase-contrast flow curves can be generated, and the severity of the hemodynamic abnormalities can be graded as normal, low-grade, moderate, and high-grade stenosis. This is similar to the Doppler ultrasound method. Grading can be used to evaluate the hemodynamic significance of a detected stenosis.[371] The significance of a stenosis on parenchymal function, however, is not currently evaluated by conventional MRA. Renal MRI perfusion studies are being performed to grade the effect of renal artery stenosis on parenchymal perfusion; initial results show that MRI perfusion measurements with high spatial and temporal resolution reflect renal function as measured with serum creatinine level.[372] Volumetric analysis of functional renal cortical tissue may also yield clinically useful information in patients with renal artery stenosis.[373] Further research is required before this will be known, however.

MRA is currently of limited value in the evaluation of restenosis in patients with renal artery stents. Although stent technology is rapidly changing, metal artifact still obscures the stent lumen to varying degrees as a result of susceptibility artifacts (Figure 27-94). Phase-contrast MRA may be used to measure velocities proximal and distal to the stent, but this is an indirect approach to evaluating for stenosis. Work is being done to develop a metallic renal artery stent that will allow for lumen visualization on MRI; however, this is not currently available clinically.[374]

Fibromuscular dysplasia has a characteristic appearance of focal narrowing and dilation ("string of beads"; Figure 27-95). Because fibromuscular dysplasia frequently involves the middle to distal portions of the renal artery and segmental branches, resolution limits MRA evaluation. For this reason, MRA is not as reliable for diagnosis of fibromuscular dysplasia as it is for atherosclerotic renal artery stenosis. Renal infarctions are well demonstrated on MRA as wedge-shaped areas of decreased parenchymal enhancement. These areas are

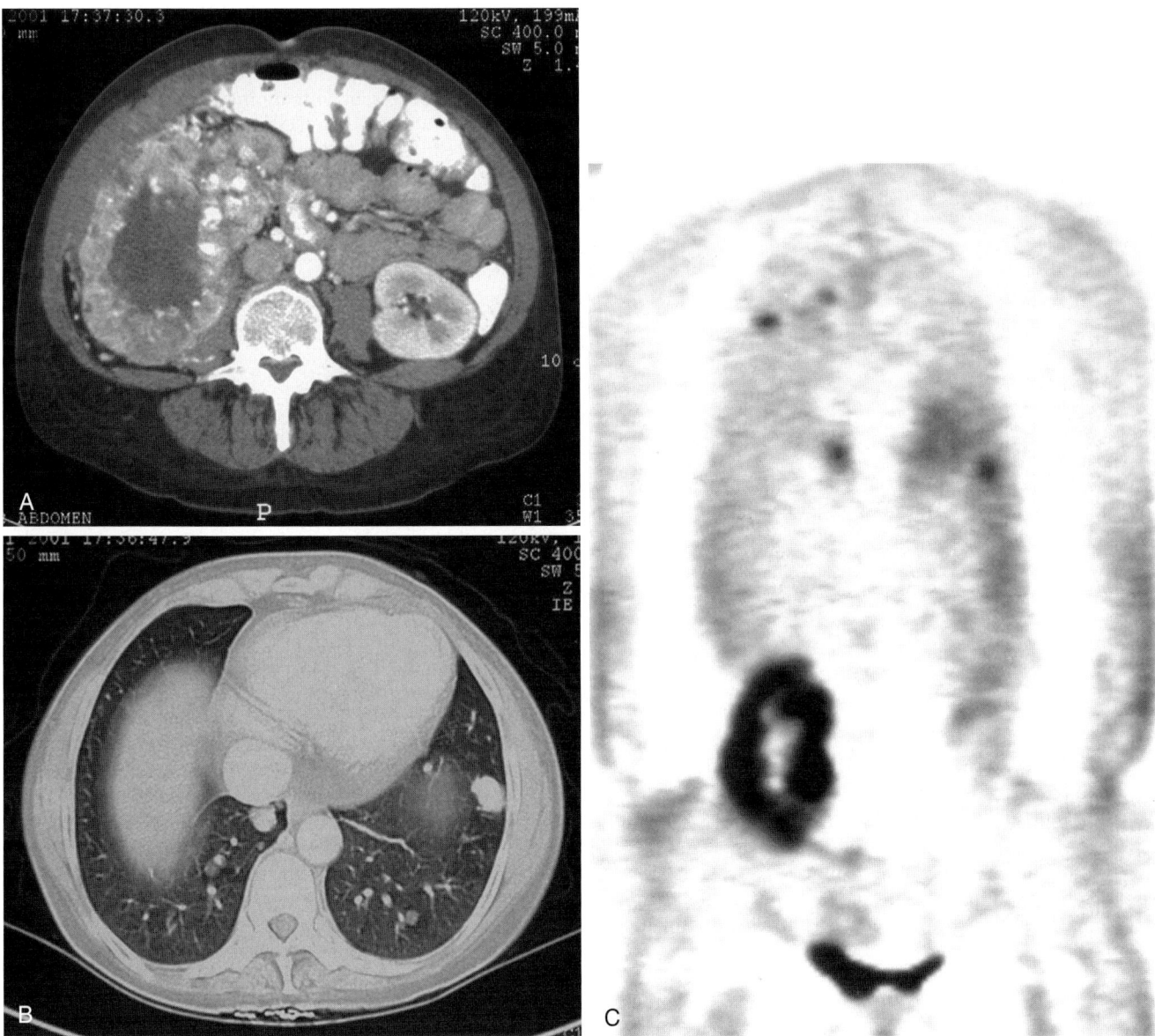

FIGURE 27-88 Renal cell carcinoma. Computed tomography shows a large necrotic renal mass (**A**) with several bilateral pulmonary nodules (**B**). The positron emission tomographic scan (**C**) shows hypermetabolism at the periphery of the large renal mass and within the pulmonary nodules. The interior hypometabolism of the renal mass is compatible with central tumor necrosis.

most conspicuous in the nephrographic phase. Evaluation of the arterial and venous structures may demonstrate the origin of the emboli or thrombosis (Figure 27-96).

Nuclear Imaging and Renovascular Disease

ACE inhibition prevents conversion of angiotensin I to angiotensin II. In renal artery stenosis, angiotensin II constricts the efferent arterioles as a compensatory mechanism to maintain GFR despite diminished afferent renal blood flow. Therefore, ACE inhibition in renal artery stenosis reduces GFR by interfering with the compensatory mechanism. Captopril-enhanced renography has been successful in evaluating patients with renal artery stenosis.

Before the study, the patient should be well hydrated, and ACE inhibitors should be discontinued (captopril for 2 days; enalapril or lisinopril for 4 to 5 days) because diagnostic

sensitivity may otherwise be reduced. Diuretics should also be discontinued before the study, preferably for 1 week. Dehydration resulting from diuretics may potentiate the effect of captopril and contribute to hypotension. Captopril (25 to 50 mg) crushed and dissolved in 250 mL water is administered orally, followed by blood pressure monitoring every 15 minutes for 1 hour. Alternatively, enalaprilat (40 μg/kg up to 2.5 mg) is administered intravenously over 3 to 5 minutes. A baseline scan can be performed before captopril-enhanced renography (1-day protocol) or the next day, only if captopril-enhanced study is abnormal (2-day protocol).

The affected kidney in renovascular hypertension often has a renogram curve with reduced initial slope, a delayed time to peak activity, prolonged cortical retention, and a slow downward slope after the peak (Figure 27-97). These findings are caused by the slowing of renal tracer transit as a result of increased retention of solute and water in response to ACE inhibition. Reduced urine flow causes delayed and decreased

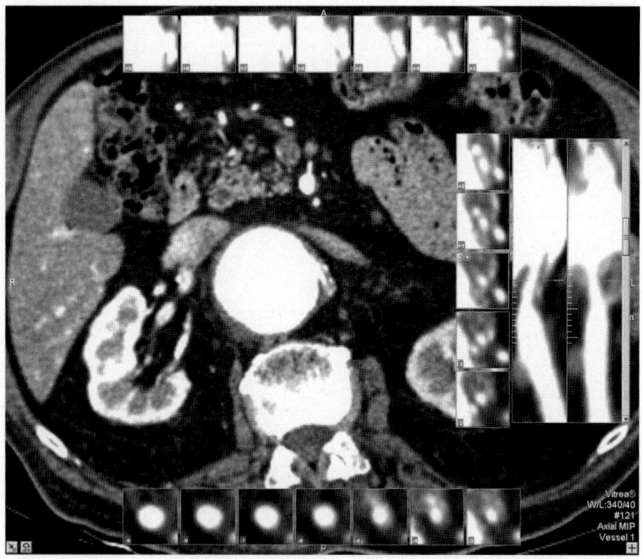

FIGURE 27-89 Renal artery stenosis: computed tomographic angiogram, axial image with vessel analysis. The origin of the left renal artery is markedly narrowed by calcified and noncalcified atherosclerotic plaque. The vessel analysis demonstrates the renal artery in cross section for accurate calculation of the degree of stenosis, which in this case was greater than 70%.

washout of tracer into the collecting system in ^{99m}Tc-MAG3 and ^{131}I-ortho-iodohippurate studies. ^{99m}Tc-DTPA demonstrates reduced uptake on the affected side.[375]

Consensus reports regarding methods and interpretation of ACE-enhanced renograms elaborate on a scoring system of renographic curves.[376-378] It has been recommended that high (>90%), intermediate (10% to 90%), and low (<10%) probability categories be applied to captopril-enhanced renography on the basis of the change of renographic curve score between baseline values and those after captopril-enhanced renograms. Among quantitative measurements, relative renal function, the time to peak activity, and the ratio of 20-minute renal activity to peak activity (20/peak) are used more commonly than other parameters. For ^{99m}Tc-MAG3 renal scintigraphy, a 10% change in relative renal function, peak activity increase of 2 minutes or more, and a parenchymal increase by 0.15 in 20/peak after captopril-enhanced study represent a high probability of renovascular hypertension.[379]

Captopril-enhanced renography has 80% to 95% sensitivity and 50% specificity for detecting impaired GFR; the detection of stenosis by captopril-enhanced renography may be more complicated.[375] With bilateral renovascular stenosis, it is more the exception than the rule for findings to be symmetric on captopril-enhanced renography. Studies in canine models with bilateral renal artery stenosis demonstrated that captopril produced striking changes in the time-activity curve of each kidney, which are even more pronounced in the more severely stenotic kidney.[375] In practice, captopril-enhanced renography has largely been replaced by CTA or MRA for the investigation of renovascular disease.

Renal Vein Thrombosis

Renal vein thrombosis is usually clinically unsuspected. It is found in patients with a hypercoagulable state, underlying renal disease, or both.[380] The classic manifestation of acute renal vein thrombosis with gross hematuria, flank pain, and decreasing renal function is uncommon.[381] Nephrotic syndrome is a common mode of manifestation.[382] Two thirds of affected patients present with minimal or no symptoms. In one study, 22% of patients with nephrotic syndrome were found to have renal vein thrombosis, usually chronic and asymptomatic; 60% of these patients had membranous glomerulonephritis.[382] Other causes include collagen vascular diseases, diabetic nephropathy, trauma, and tumor thrombus. Renal venography has been the definitive method of diagnosis, but it has been supplanted by other methods of evaluation, including Doppler ultrasonography, CT, and MRI.

IVU yields nonspecific findings in renal vein thrombosis and is no longer used for diagnosis. It may yield normal findings in more than 25% of cases. On gray-scale and Doppler ultrasonography, the involved kidney appears enlarged and swollen with relative hypoechogenicity in comparison with the normal kidney.[381] The finding of a filling defect in the renal vein is both sensitive and specific for diagnosis and is the only convincing sign of renal vein thrombosis. The lack of flow on Doppler ultrasonography, however, is a nonspecific finding and is frequently observed because of technical limitations of the study. Absence or reversal of the diastolic waveform on Doppler ultrasonography should not be interpreted to suggest renal vein thrombosis.

Contrast material–enhanced CT is needed to properly assess the patient with suspected renal vein thrombosis. If renal function is impaired, MRI must be used. Findings on CT include an enlarged renal vein with a low signal-attenuating filling defect that represents the clot within the renal vein.[383] Parenchymal enhancement may be abnormal, with prolonged corticomedullary differentiation and a delayed or persistent nephrogram. The kidney appears enlarged, with edema in the renal sinus. Stranding and thickening of Gerota's fascia may be observed. A nephrogram is occasionally striated. Attenuation of the pelvicalyceal system may occur as a result of edema. The appearance of the pelvicalyceal system may also be delayed or absent altogether. Within chronic renal vein thrombosis, the renal vein may be shortened or narrowed because of clot retraction, and pericapsular collateral veins may be noted. Affected patients have an increased risk of pulmonary emboli as well. With renal tumors and, in rare cases, adrenal tumors, thrombus may develop in the renal vein with extension to the IVC. Nonhomogeneous enhancement of the thrombus is suggestive of direct tumor involvement, not of a bland thrombus.

The appearance of renal vein thrombosis on noncontrast MRI is variable. If the thrombosis is acute, the renal vein appears distended, no normal flow void is visible, and the affected kidney appears enlarged. Renal infarction may also be present. If the thrombosis is chronic, the renal vein is small and difficult to see. A nonenhanced filling defect in the vein is visible on contrast material–enhanced magnetic resonance venography, which is consistent with thrombus. Enhancement of the thrombus is characteristic of tumor.

Assessment for Renal Transplantation

The treatment of choice for patients with end-stage renal disease is renal transplantation. Although there have been significant improvements in continuous peritoneal dialysis and

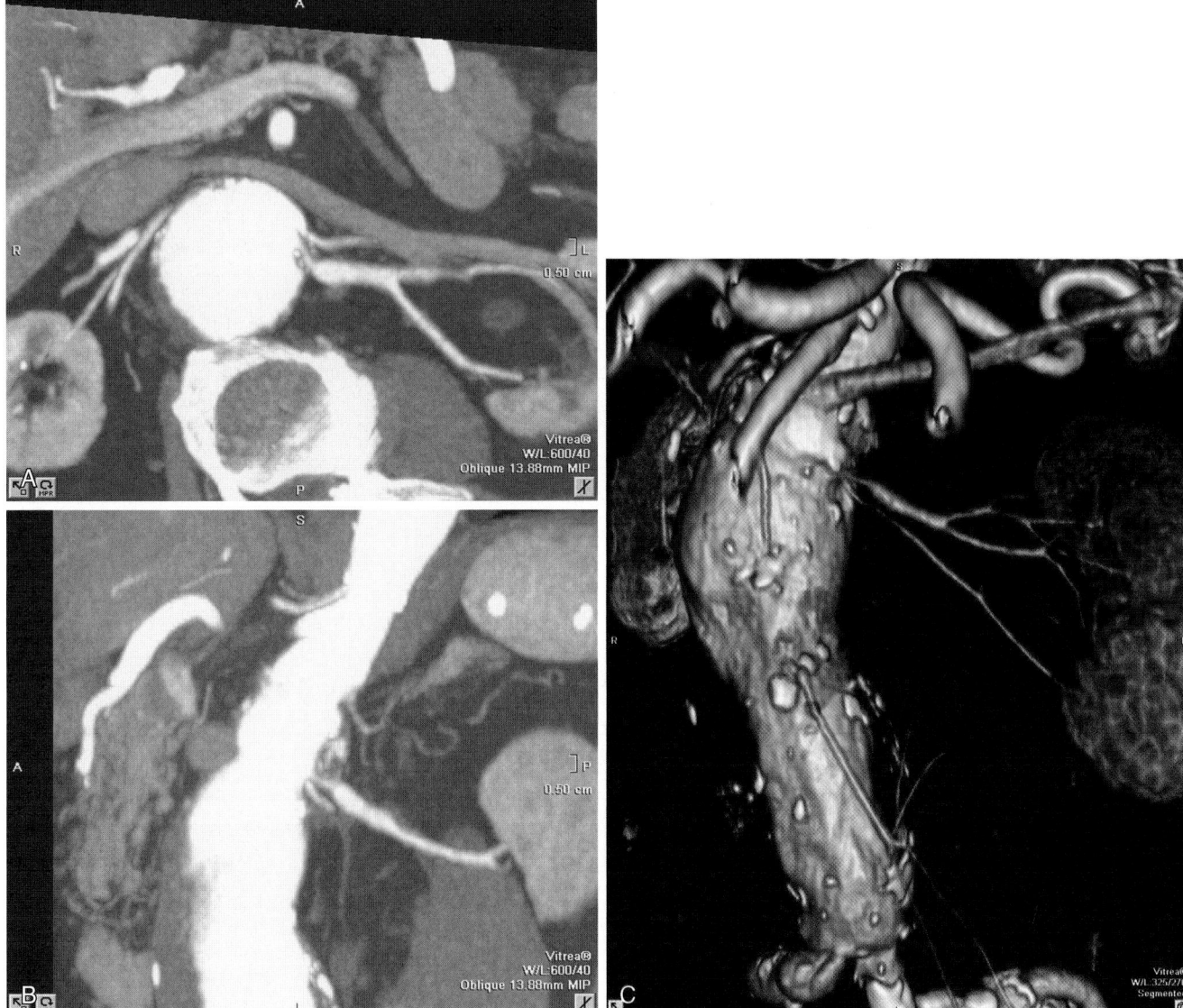

FIGURE 27-90 Renal artery stenosis: computed tomographic angiography (CTA). Image processing was applied to the case depicted in Figure 27-89. Axial (**A**) and coronal (**B**) slab maximum-intensity projection (MIP) images demonstrate the atherosclerotic stenosis of the proximal renal artery. Note the accessory renal artery arising adjacent to the left main renal artery. Volume rendering of the CTA produced a three-dimensional display (**C**), which may be rotated for best viewing and analysis.

hemodialysis, patient survival is longer and overall quality of life is better after renal transplantation. Radiologic evaluation is performed on the renal transplant donor and in the postoperative assessment of the transplant recipient. Although IVU and angiography were used in the past, ultrasonography, CT, MRI, and renal scintigraphy are the current methods used in evaluation of these patients (Figure 27-98).[384-386]

A comprehensive radiologic assessment of the living renal transplant donor is crucial.[387] The anatomic information that is necessary is vascular, parenchymal, and pelvicalyceal. The renal artery must be visualized for number, length, location, and branching pattern. The parenchyma must be evaluated for scars, overall volume, renal masses, and calculi. The venous anatomy must be viewed, and the number of veins, anatomic variants, and significant systemic tributaries noted. The pelvicalyceal system must be scrutinized for anomalies such as duplication and papillary necrosis. As a choice exists for the type of nephrectomy (laparoscopic or open), complete and

accurate information is necessary. The field of view is limited with laparoscopic nephrectomy, this information is necessary to ensure safety.[388-391]

With the development of MDCT, the complete evaluation of the living renal transplant donor is possible.[388,392,393] Noncontrast CT is performed with a low dose of radiation just to search for renal stones, locate the kidneys, and identify renal masses (see Figure 27-9). Arterial phase scanning is generally performed at 15 to 25 seconds to demonstrate the main renal artery, branching pattern of the artery, and abnormalities such as atherosclerotic plaques or fibromuscular dysplasia (see Figure 27-11); 25% to 40% of donors have accessory renal arteries, and 10% have early branching patterns in the main renal artery.[389,391] For transplantation, the main renal artery must be free of branching for the first 15 mm to 20 mm. Because of the rapid transit of contrast material through the kidney, most renal veins are also well viewed in this phase (see Figure 27-10). Venous variants occur in 15% to 28% of donors with multiple

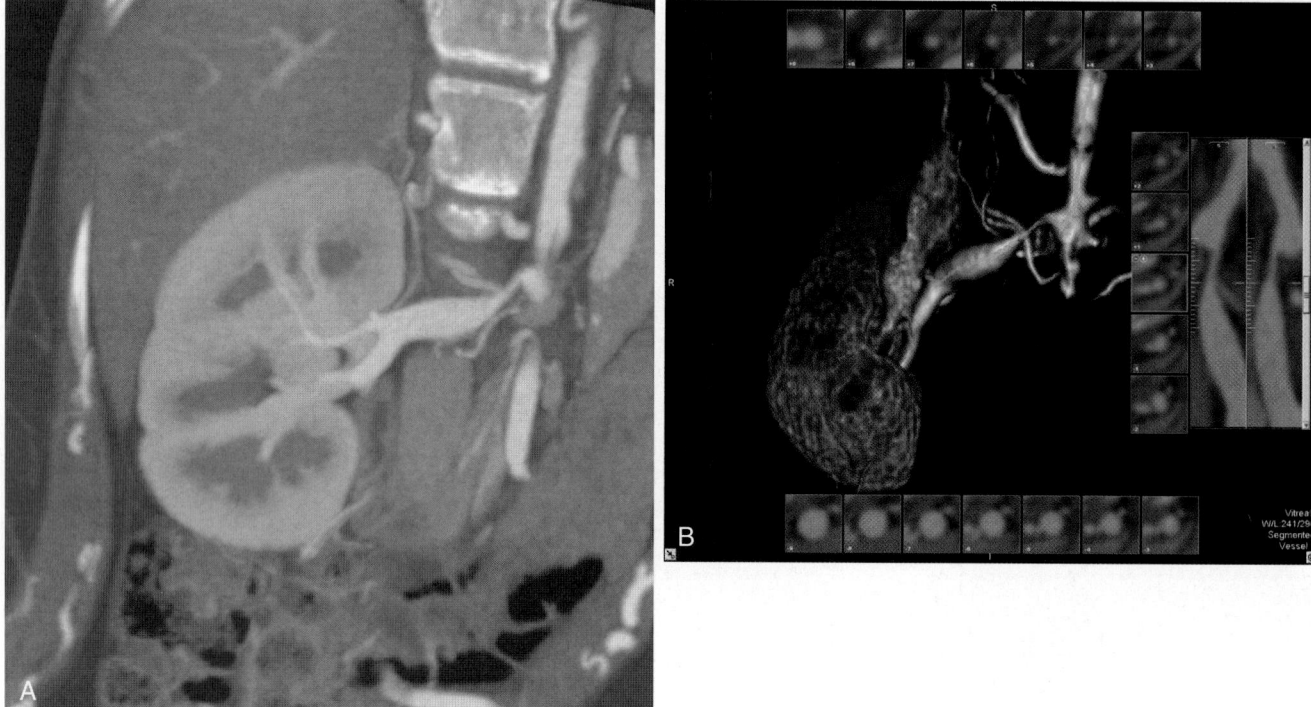

FIGURE 27-91 Renal artery stenosis: abdominal computed tomographic angiography (CTA) with image processing. **A,** Coronal slab maximum-intensity projection (MIP) demonstrates the smooth narrowing of the proximal right renal artery in a patient with Takayasu's arteritis. Note the markedly abnormal aorta with occlusion distal to the origin of the renal artery. **B,** Volume rendering of the CTA with vessel analysis reveals the 80% stenosis of the right renal artery. The left renal artery had been occluded previously, and the kidney was supplied by collateral vessels.

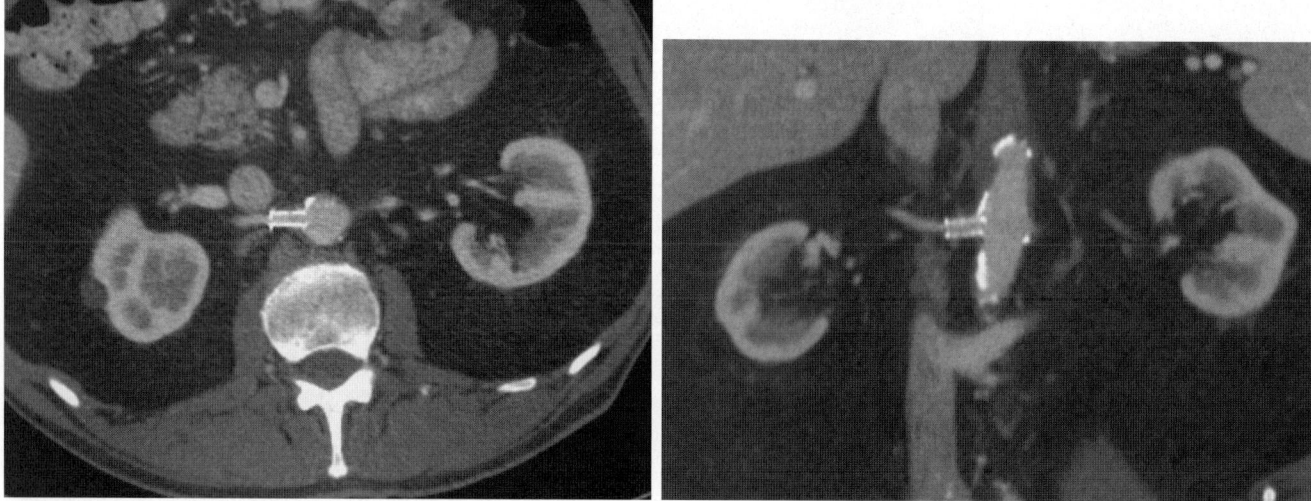

FIGURE 27-92 Renal artery stent: computed tomographic scan. Axial (**A**) and coronal (**B**) images of a contrast material–enhanced scan in the corticomedullary phase. The metallic stent is visible at the origin of the right renal artery. It had been placed for treatment of renal artery stenosis that was caused by atherosclerosis. Good flow through the stent is observed as contrast material fills the lumen.

renal veins being most common, especially on the right. On the left side, 8% to 15% have a circumaortic renal vein and 1% to 3% have a retroaortic vein.[391,394] It is also important to visualize venous tributaries, including the gonadal, left adrenal, and lumbar veins. These are best viewed on the nephrographic phase.[389,390] Imaging in this phase is performed 80 to 120 seconds after injection of contrast material and is used to evaluate the cortex and medulla for scars and masses (see Figure 27-12). Excretory phase imaging is performed with CT, CT digital radiography, or plain radiography to note anomalies or abnormalities in the pelvocalyceal system (see Figures 27-13 and 27-14). CT

has a demonstrated accuracy of 91% to 97% for arterial phase imaging, 93% to 100% for the venous phase, and 99% for the pelvicalyceal system.[393,395,396] Similar results have been noted for MRI; the biggest discrepancy is found in imaging accessory renal arteries.[397,398] The lack of ionizing radiation and iodinated contrast material makes MRI attractive for the future. Most centers today use CT in the evaluation of living renal transplant donors.

MRI, MRA, and MRU can be combined into one examination for the evaluation of the renal transplant donor.[399] MRI and CT are comparable for the evaluation of renal vasculature,

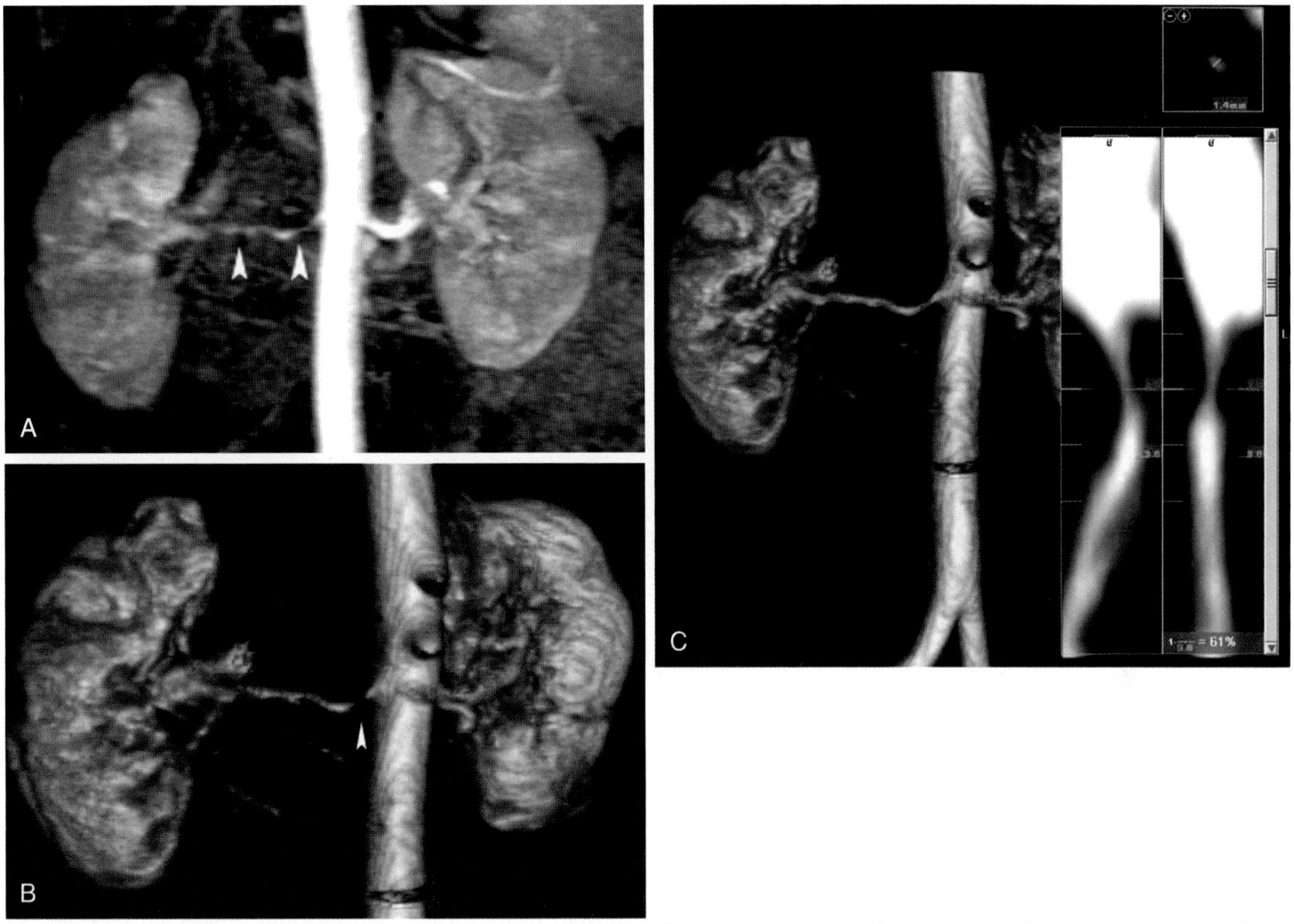

FIGURE 27-93 Renal artery stenosis. Advancements in postprocessing allow for more accurate evaluation of stenosis with magnetic resonance angiography. **A,** Maximum intensity projection displays a high-grade stenosis near the origin of the renal artery with areas of apparent narrowing in the midportion of the renal artery (*arrowheads*), mimicking fibromuscular dysplasia. **B,** Volume rendering shows the proximal stenosis (*arrowhead*), but the midportion of the artery is more normal in appearance. **C,** A view of the artery in two dimensions alloeds measurement of the proximal stenosis and demonstrated a normal midportion of the artery. This stenosis was confirmed with angiography.

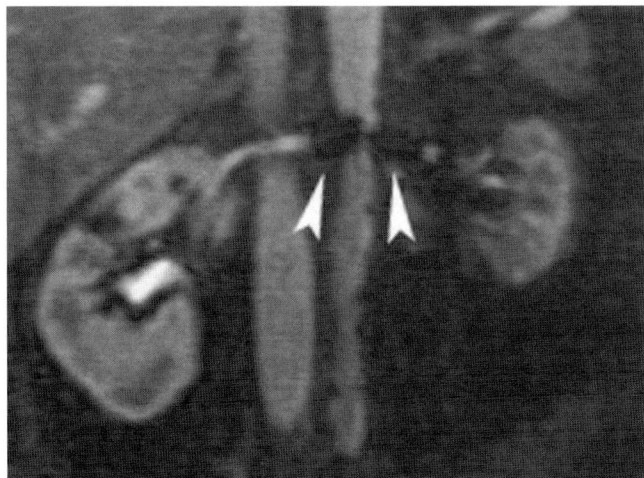

FIGURE 27-94 Magnetic resonance angiography in a patient with bilateral renal artery stents (*arrowheads*). The metal in the stent causes artifact that obscures the vessel lumen. Contrast material is visible beyond the stent, which indicates that no complete occlusion is present.

structure, and function. In order to avoid radiation exposure and nephrotoxicity, MRI may be preferred over CT for preoperative evaluation.

In healthy renal donors, it is possible to quantify functional renal volume with MRA by determining only the cortical volume. The hypothesis supported by Van den Dool and colleagues[400] was that glomerular filtration is an important component of renal function, and because the majority of glomeruli are in the cortex, renal function should be well correlated with cortical volume. Further research is needed to confirm Van den Dool and colleagues' findings, however.

After surgically successful renal transplantation, radiologic evaluation is frequently necessary. Conventional ultrasonography, Doppler ultrasonography, CT, MRI, and renal scintigraphy are used in various settings. Ultrasonography assumes the primary role for assessing patients with changes in serum creatinine level, urine output, pain, or hematuria.[401] It is also used to direct renal biopsy. Doppler ultrasonography is used to evaluate renal perfusion, the patency of the renal artery and vein, and the integrity of the vascular anastomoses.[402] CT, MRI, and renal scintigraphy are adjunctive studies.

Conventional gray-scale ultrasonography is essential in assessing for transplant obstruction and fluid collections around the transplanted kidney.[386] Conventional ultrasonography yields nonspecific findings in acute tubular necrosis and acute rejection, including obliteration of the corticomedullary junction, prominent swollen pyramids, and loss of the renal sinus echoes.[385,387] All these findings are indicative of edema of the transplanted kidney, which leads to increased peripheral vascular resistance, decreased diastolic perfusion, and elevation of the resistive index (>0.80) (Figure 27-99).[389] Chronic rejection may lead to diffusely increased echogenicity throughout the kidney.

Doppler ultrasonography adds valuable information pertaining to the integrity of the vascular elements. Despite early enthusiasm with the ability of Doppler ultrasonography to differentiate acute transplant rejection from acute tubular necrosis, it is now known that the findings are nonspecific

and cannot obviate the need for renal biopsy in these cases.[403] Both acute tubular necrosis and acute rejection can cause an increase in peripheral vascular resistance.[404,405] A significant number of patients with acute rejection have a normal resistive index (<0.80). It is now known that vascular rejection is no more likely to cause increases in peripheral vascular resistance than is cellular rejection.[403] Neither the timing nor clinical symptoms of the renal dysfunction can be used to differentiate acute rejection from acute tubular necrosis.[403] Doppler ultrasonography is most helpful in detecting acute arterial thrombosis when signal in the artery is absent or renal vein thrombosis when the waveform is plateau-like and diastolic flow is retrograde. An abnormal Doppler waveform in the

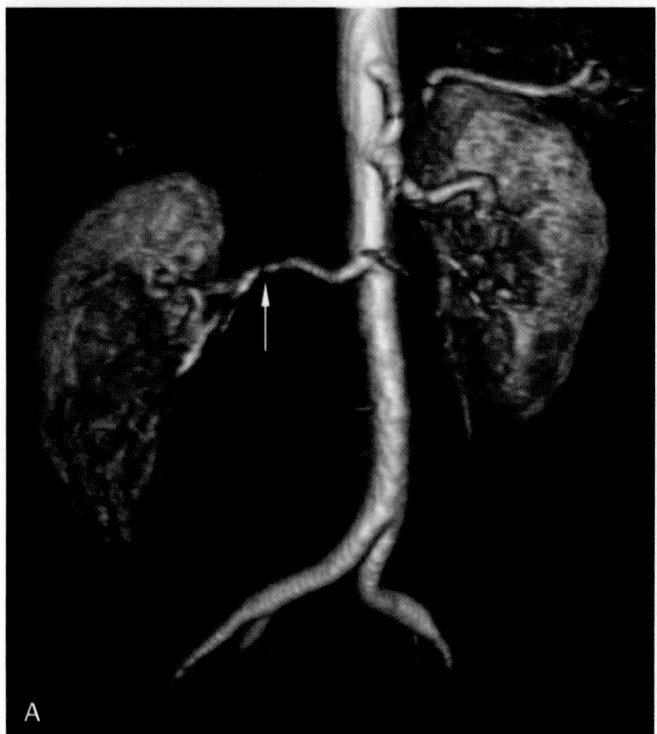
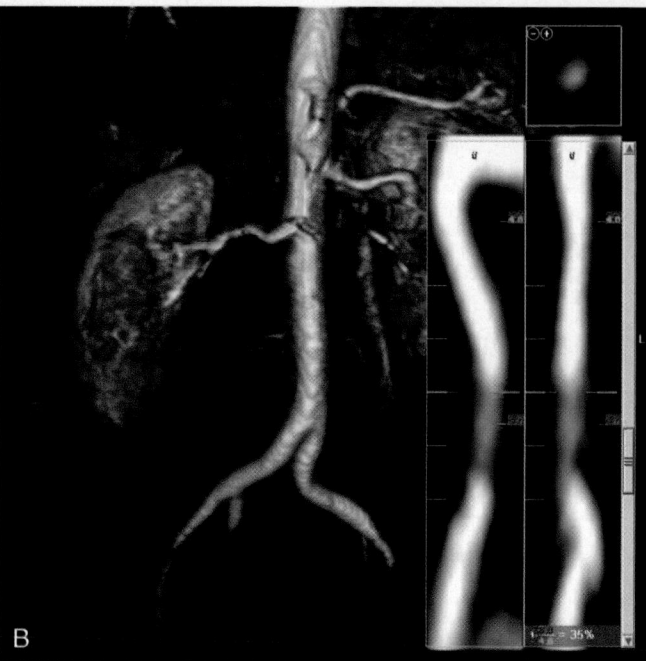

FIGURE 27-95 A and B, Magnetic resonance angiography with volume reconstruction demonstrates a subtle irregularity in the midportion of the right renal artery (arrow). Fibromuscular dysplasia was confirmed with conventional angiography.

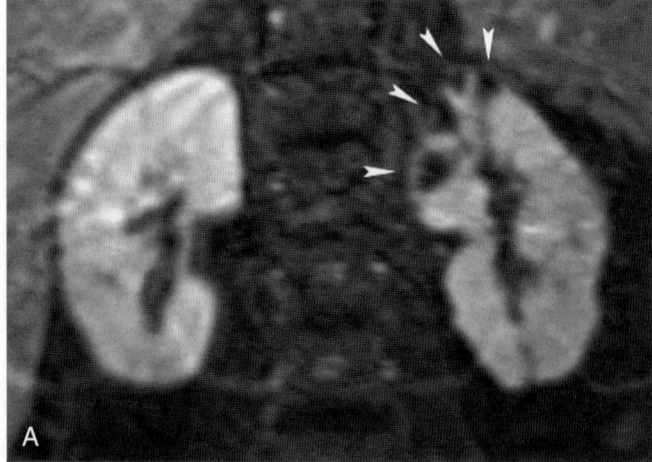
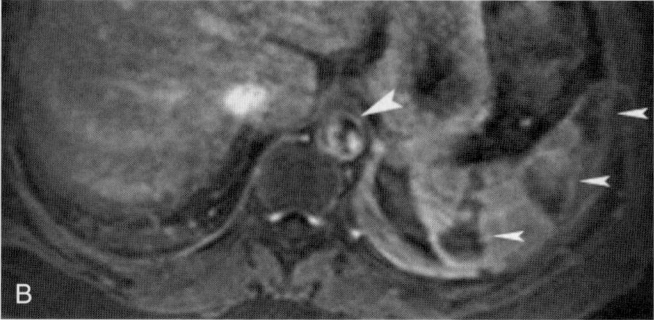

FIGURE 27-96 Renal infarcts caused by embolic disease. A, Coronal gadolinium-enhanced T1-weighted image shows wedge-shaped cortical areas without enhancement (arrowheads). B, Axial gadolinium-enhanced T1-weighted image shows an irregular filling defect in the aorta (large arrowhead), which is consistent with thrombus, and three focal defects in the spleen (small arrowheads), which are consistent with splenic infarcts.

allograft indicates compromise of the transplanted kidney.[406] Sequential examinations may be used to show improvement or deterioration in the condition affecting the kidney and to note the progress of treatment.

MRI and contrast material–enhanced CT are useful in patients in whom the transplanted kidney is obscured by overlying bowel gas or in patients with large body habitus in whom ultrasonography may be limited by the depth of the transplanted kidney. If any doubt exists after a thorough ultrasound evaluation, MRI or CT may be performed to clarify or confirm the ultrasound findings.

Fluid collections around a transplanted kidney are very common, occurring in up to 50% of cases.[401] These fluid collections may represent urinoma, hematoma, lymphocele, abscess, or seroma. The effects of the collection depend on the size and location. Urinomas and hematomas are found early, usually immediately after surgery. Lymphoceles generally are not found until 3 to 6 weeks after surgery. Abscesses are usually associated with transplant infection.

On ultrasound evaluation, extrarenal or subcapsular hematomas usually have a complex echogenic appearance, which becomes less echogenic with time (Figure 27-100).[401] On CT, they appear as high signal-attenuating fluid collections early. Such collections are usually too complex to be successfully drained percutaneously. Urine leaks and the associated urinoma

are also found in the immediate postoperative period (Figure 27-101).[401] On ultrasonography, these appear as anechoic fluid collection with no septations. They may rapidly increase in size. Drainage may be performed under guidance by either ultrasonography or CT.[407] Antegrade pyelography via a percutaneous nephrostomy is needed to detect the site of leak, usually the ureteral anastomoses. Stent placement for treatment is necessary.

Lymphoceles are recognized weeks to years after transplantation and occur in up to 20% of cases.[401] They form from the leakage of lymph fluid from the interrupted lymphatic vessels at surgery. Lymphoceles appear on ultrasonography as anechoic fluid collections with septations. The size and effect on the kidney determine the need for treatment. Because lymphoceles are frequently located medial and inferior to the kidney, they are a common cause of obstruction to the kidney. Ultrasound or CT guidance for drainage may be used. In a minority of cases, sclerotherapy may be needed to treat the lymphocele.[407]

Abscess near the transplanted kidney usually develops in association with renal infection or the infection of other fluid collections in the immunocompromised patient. On ultrasound examination, abscess appears as a complex fluid collection, possibly containing gas.[401] Fluid aspiration is usually necessary for the accurate characterization of fluid within a collection. Because blood products have characteristic signal intensities on T1- and T2-weighted sequences, MRI can

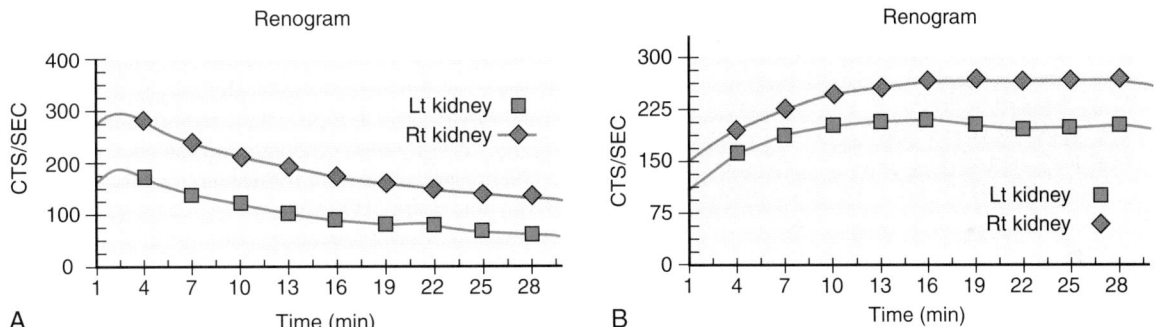

FIGURE 27-97 Technetium 99m–labeled mercaptoacetyltriglycine renograms before (**A**) and after (**B**) angiotensin converting enzyme (ACE) inhibition with captopril. Note the relatively normal renograms (**A**) and the reduced initial slope, delayed time to peak activity, and plateau compatible with captopril-induced cortical tracer retention (**B**). These findings suggest a high probability of hemodynamically significant bilateral renal artery stenosis that is more severe on the left side (*connected squares*) than the right side (*connected diamonds*). Bilateral renal artery stenosis was later confirmed with angiography. (Adapted from Saremi F, Jadvar H, Siegel M: Pharmacologic interventions in nuclear radiology: indications, imaging protocols, and clinical results, *Radio-Graphics* 22:447-490, 2002.)

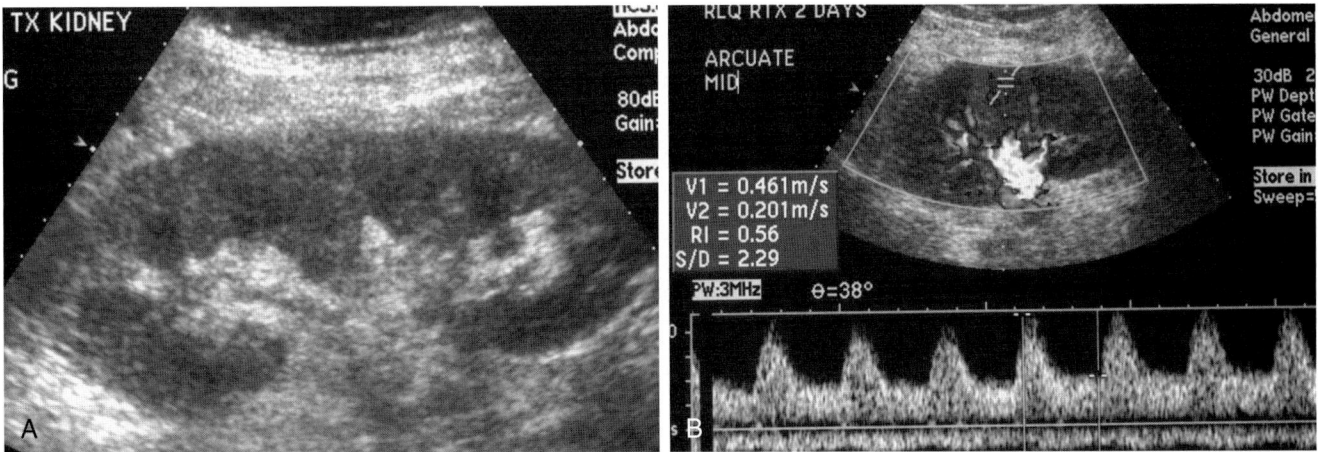

FIGURE 27-98 Normal renal transplant: ultrasonography. Coronal image (**A**) of a recently transplanted kidney in the right lower quadrant. The central echo complex, medullary pyramids, and cortex are well depicted. The duplex Doppler image (**B**) demonstrates normal flow to the transplanted kidney with a normal resistive index of 0.56.

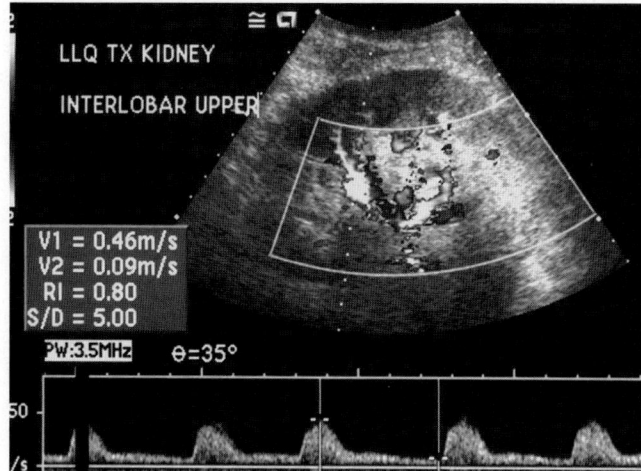

FIGURE 27-99 Renal transplant with acute tubular necrosis: ultrasonography. Duplex Doppler image of the transplanted kidney shows normal size and normal appearance with a high resistive index of 0.80 in the interlobar artery. The patient recovered with return of normal renal function in 5 days.

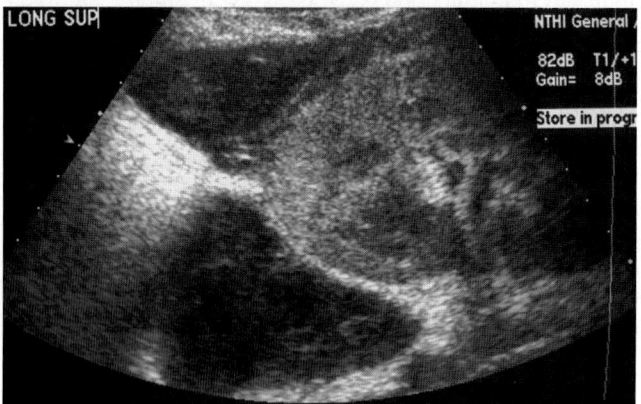

FIGURE 27-100 Renal transplant with hematoma: ultrasonography. Longitudinal image of the upper aspect of the transplanted kidney reveals two hypoechoic collections adjacent to the kidney. The heterogeneous hypoechoic nature of the collections suggests that they are hematomas, as opposed to urinomas or lymphoceles, which in general are anechoic.

provide specific diagnostic information that may help avoid an unnecessary interventional procedure, in cases of hematoma.

Renal obstruction or hydronephrosis may be observed in the transplanted kidney with renal dysfunction and is reversible. Ultrasonography is the best means for assessment.[402] In the immediate posttransplantation period, mild caliectasis is common as a result of edema at the ureteric anastomosis site. Obstruction may also be caused by fluid collections around the transplanted kidney that may be visible also with ultrasonography. Blood clots within the pelvicalyceal system may also lead to hydronephrosis. Later strictures may occur, primarily at the ureteral anastomosis site. Renal stones may also cause hydronephrosis during their passage to the bladder. A functional obstruction may be visible with an overdistended bladder. With bladder emptying, ultrasonography demonstrates a resolution of the hydronephrosis.

Hypertension with or without renal dysfunction may be observed in many transplant recipients.[401] Vascular and nonvascular causes must be differentiated. Doppler ultrasonography is the first step of evaluation. Renal artery stenosis may be found in up to 23% of patients.[408] The stenosis may occur before the anastomosis in the iliac artery, at the anastomosis site, or more distally. In more than half the cases, the stenosis is at the anastomotic site,

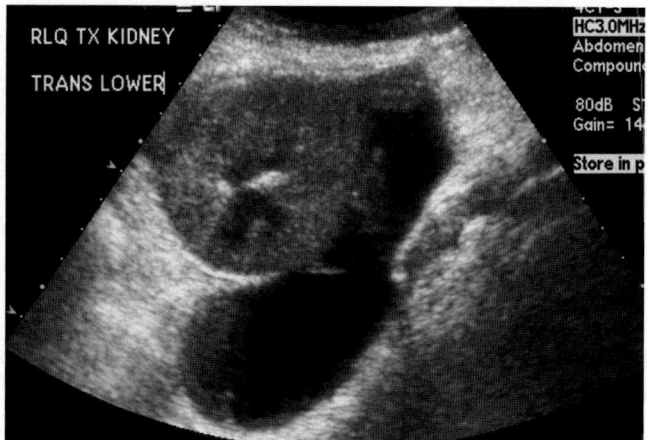

FIGURE 27-101 Renal transplant with urinoma: ultrasonography. Transverse image through the lower aspect of the transplanted kidney reveals a normal appearance with a large anechoic fluid collection adjacent to the kidney. This fluid was aspirated under ultrasound guidance, and the findings led to the diagnosis of urinoma. The patient was treated with catheter placement and drainage, also performed with ultrasound guidance.

and it is more common in end-to-end anastomosis. CT or MRA is used to determine the site and the degree of stenosis (Figure 27-102). Angioplasty is successful in managing most cases.[408]

Arteriovenous fistulas occur in transplant recipients after renal biopsy. Most close spontaneously within 4 to 6 weeks. Color and duplex Doppler imaging demonstrate high-velocity and turbulent flow localized to a single segmental or interlobar artery and the adjacent vein. Arterialized flow is noted in the draining vein. Gray-scale images demonstrate only a simple- or complex-appearing cystic structure. If the structure is large and growing, embolization may become necessary.

Neoplasm occurs in transplant recipients with increased frequency, up to 100 times more frequently than in the general population.[401] Neoplasms develop as a result of prolonged immunosuppression. Skin cancers and lymphoma are the most common neoplasms. The risk of renal cell carcinoma in the transplanted kidney may be increased. Posttransplantation lymphoproliferative disorder may also occur in renal transplant recipients.[409] Although the transplanted kidney may be involved, the most frequent sites are the brain, liver, lungs, and gastrointestinal tract. The appearance is similar to that of conventional lymphomas with mass lesions in the organs, with or without associated adenopathy.

The MRI findings of renal transplant rejection are nonspecific (Figure 27-103; see also Figures 27-31 and 27-32). More recently, Sadowski and colleagues demonstrated the feasibility of using BOLD MRI to evaluate the renal transplant oxygen status and presence of acute rejection.[110] The authors conclude that MRI may differentiate acute rejection from normal function and acute tubular necrosis, but further research is required. Animal research is being performed with the hope of using noninvasive diffusion MRI techniques as a tool for monitoring early renal graft rejection after transplantation.[109]

Nuclear medicine procedures are also employed in the renal transplant recipient and play a role in the assessment of the complications associated with transplantation. These include vascular compromise (arterial or venous thrombosis), lymphocele formation, urine extravasation, acute tubular necrosis, drug toxicity, and organ rejection. Scintigraphy provides important imaging information about these potential complications, which can then guide corrective intervention.[410]

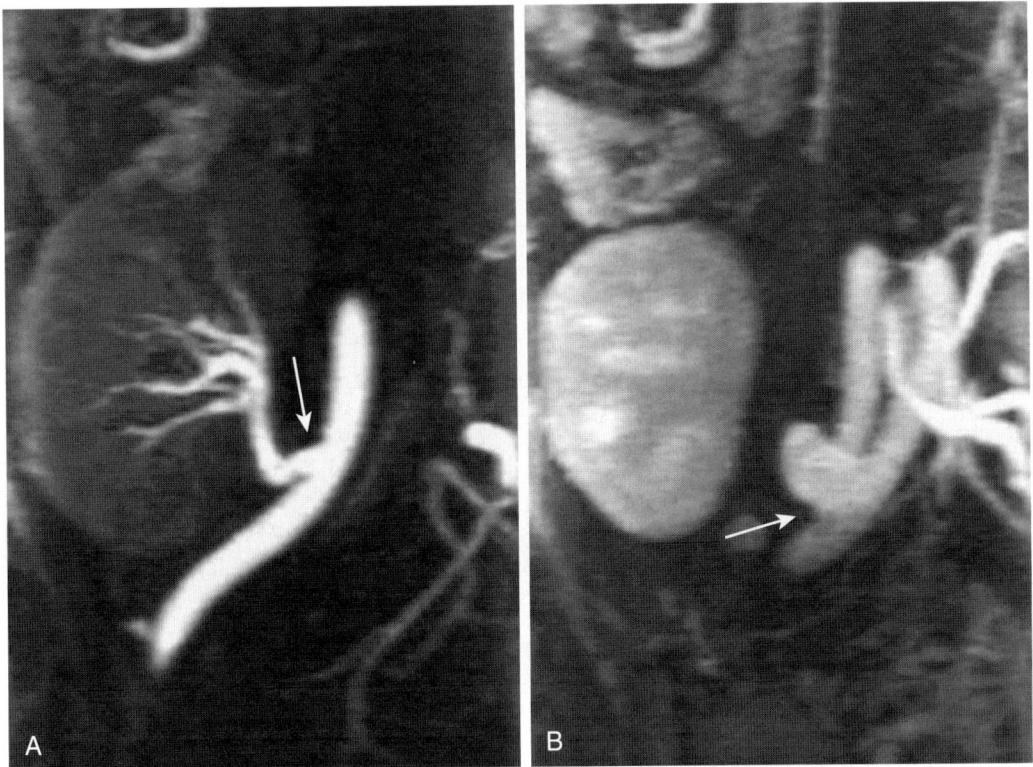

FIGURE 27-102 Renal transplant magnetic resonance angiogram, showing normal arterial (**A**) and normal venous (**B**) anastomoses.

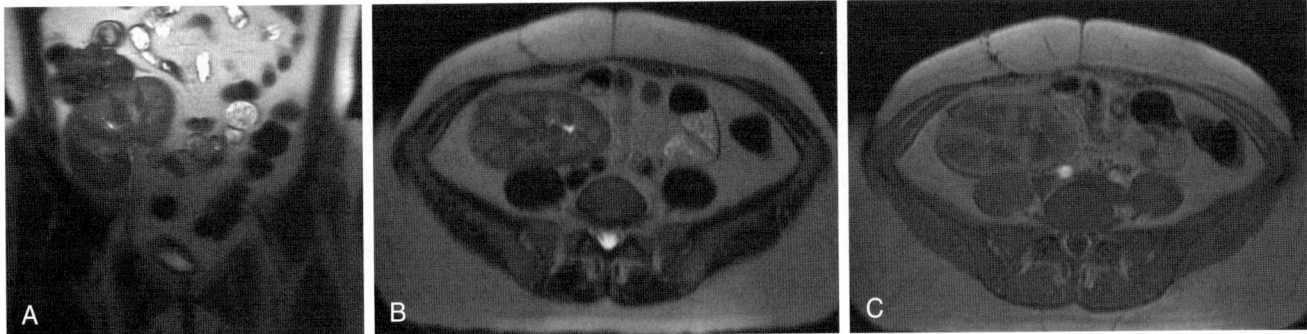

FIGURE 27-103 Renal transplant graft with normal function. **A**, Axial T2-weighted image; **B**, coronal T2-weighted image; **C**, axial T1-weighted image.

An early complication may be hyperacute rejection, which is often apparent immediately after transplantation and is caused by preformed cytotoxic antibodies. Other early complications include sudden decline in urine output and acute urinary obstruction. Scintigraphy with ^{99m}Tc-DTPA or ^{99m}Tc-MAG3 demonstrates absence of perfusion and function with complete thrombosis in the renal artery or renal vein. A sensitive but nonspecific sign of acute rejection is the finding of more than a 20% decline in the ratio of renal activity to the aortic activity.[411]

Renal scintigraphy performed a few days after the transplantation often reveals intact perfusion but delayed and decreased excretion of the tracer and some cortical retention of the tracer. These findings are typically caused by acute tubular necrosis and are more common with cadaveric grafts than with grafts from living related donors (Figure 27-104). If both perfusion and function continue to decline, then the possibility of rejection should be considered. However, acute tubular necrosis, obstruction, drug (cyclosporine) toxicity, and rejection can produce relatively similar scintigraphic appearances.

The differential diagnosis should be considered in the clinical context and with regard to the interval since transplantation, although two or more of these conditions may coexist. In one report, a nonascending second phase of ^{99m}Tc-MAG3 renogram curve was predictive of graft dysfunction. However, patients with acute tubular necrosis were not significantly more likely to have a nonascending curve than were those with acute rejection. An ascending curve was nonspecific and could be observed in both normally and poorly functioning grafts.[412]

Urine extravasation may be noted on the renal scans as collections of excreted radiotracer outside of the transplanted kidney and the urinary bladder. Because of small urine leaks and impaired renal transplant function, it may be difficult to identify a leak on scintigraphy. However, a cold-appearing defect that becomes warmer in appearance with time on the sequential images usually represents a urinoma or a urinary leak. If the activity declines with voiding, then the finding probably represents a urinoma. A chronic photopenic defect may represent a hematoma or a lymphocele (or both).[413] For

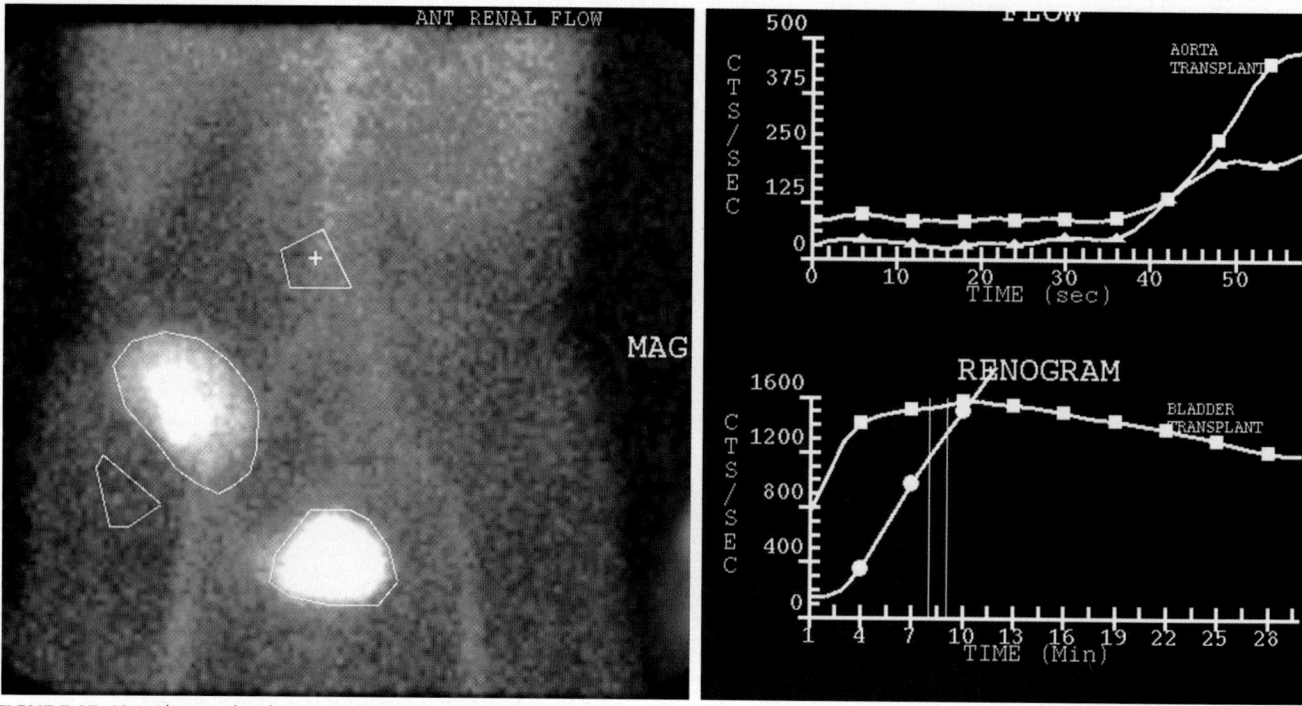

FIGURE 27-104 Abnormal technetium 99m–labeled mercaptoacetyltriglycine renogram. The pattern involving the right pelvic renal transplant from a living related donor is compatible with acute tubular necrosis.

assessing potential obstructive disease, scintigraphy with a diuretic may be considered, as previously discussed. Results of an animal-based study[414] also suggested that FDG PET may have a role in early detection of graft rejection by demonstrating significantly elevated graft tracer uptake induced by inflammatory infiltrates.

References

1. Amis ES. Epitaph for the urogram. *Radiology.* 1999;213:639-640:[editorial].
2. Pollack HM, Banner MP. Current status of excretory urography: a premature epitaph? *Urol Clin North Am.* 1985;12:585-601.
3. Dyer RB, Chen MYM, Zagoria RF. Intravenous urography: technique and interpretation. *Radiographics.* 2001;21:799-824.
4. Hattery RR, Williamson Jr B, Hartman GW, et al. Intravenous urographic technique. *Radiology.* 1988;167:593-599.
5. Saxton HM. Review article: urography. *Br J Radiol.* 1969;42:321-346.
6. Fry IK, Cattell WR. The nephrographic pattern during excretion urography. *Br Med Bull.* 1972;28:227-232.
7. Katzberg RW. Urography into the 21st century: new contrast media, renal handling, imaging characteristics and nephrotoxicity. *Radiology.* 1997;204:297-312.
8. Almén T. Contrast agent design: some aspects on the synthesis of water soluble contrast agents of low osmolality. *J Theor Biol.* 1969;24:216-226.
9. McClennan BL. Ionic and nonionic iodinated contrast media: evolution and strategies for use. *AJR Am J Roentgenol.* 1990;155:225-233.
10. Lasser EC. Etiology of anaphylactoid responses: the promise of nonionics. *Invest Radiol.* 1985;20:579-583.
11. Shehadi WH. Contrast media adverse reactions: occurrence, recurrence, and distribution patterns. *Radiology.* 1982;143:11-17.
12. Katayama H, Yamaguchi K, Kozuka T, et al. Adverse reactions to ionic and nonionic contrast media: a report from the Japanese Committee on the Safety of Contrast Media. *Radiology.* 1990;175:621-628.
13. Jacobsson BF, Jorulf H, Kalantar MS, et al. Nonionic versus ionic contrast media in intravenous urography: clinical trial in 1000 consecutive patients. *Radiology.* 1988;167:601-605.
14. Callahan MJ, Poznauskis L, Zurakowski D, et al. Nonionic iodinated intravenous contrast material-related reactions: incidence in large urban children's hospital—retrospective analysis of data in 12,494 patients. *Radiology.* 2009;250:674-681.
15. Brasch RC. Allergic reactions to contrast media: accumulated evidence. *AJR Am J Roentgenol.* 1980;134:797-801.
16. Lasser EC. Basic mechanisms of contrast media reactions: theoretical and experimental considerations. *Radiology.* 1968;91:63-65.
17. Lasser EC, Berry CC, Talner LB, et al. Pre-treatment with corticosteroids to alleviate reactions to intravenous contrast material. *N Engl J Med.* 1987;317:845-849.
18. Taliercio CP, Vietstra RE, Fisher LD, et al. Risks of renal dysfunction with cardiac angiography. *Ann Intern Med.* 1986;104:501-504.
19. Hou SS, Bushinsky DA, Wish JB, et al. Hospital-acquired renal insufficiency: a prospective study. *Am J Med.* 1983;74:243-248.
20. Tublin ME, Murphy ME, Tessler FN. Current concepts in contrast media–induced nephropathy. *AJR Am J Roentgenol.* 1998;171:933-939.
21. Bruce RJ, Djamali A, Shinki K, et al. Background fluctuation of kidney function versus contrast-induced nephrotoxicity. *AJR Am J Roentgenol.* 2009;192:711-718.
22. Newhouse JH, Kho D, Rao QA, et al. Frequency of serum creatinine changes in the absence of iodinated contrast material: implications for studies of contrast nephrotoxicity. *AJR Am J Roentgenol.* 2008;191:376-382.
23. Heinrich MC, Häberle L, Müller V, et al. Nephrotoxicity of iso-osmolar iodixanol compared with nonionic low-osmolar contrast media: meta-analysis of randomized controlled trials. *Radiology.* 2009;250:68-86.
24. Nguyen SA, Suranyi P, Ravenel JG, et al. Iso-osmolality versus low-osmolality iodinated contrast medium at intravenous contrast-enhanced CT: effect on kidney function. *Radiology.* 2008;248:97-105.
25. Herts BR, Schneider E, Poggio ED, et al. Identifying outpatients with renal insufficiency before contrast-enhanced CT by using estimated glomerular filtration rates versus serum creatinine levels. *Radiology.* 2008;248:106-113.
26. Barrett BJ, Carlisle EJ. Metaanalysis of the relative nephrotoxicity of high- and low-osmolality iodinated contrast media. *Radiology.* 1993;188:171-178.
27. Aspelin P, Aubry P, Fransson S-G, et al. Nephrotoxic effects in high-risk patients undergoing angiography. *N Engl J Med.* 2003;348:491-499.
28. Gleeson TG, Bulugahapitiya S. Contrast-induced nephropathy. *AJR Am J Roentgenol.* 2004;183:1673-1689.
29. Heinrich MC, Kuhlmann MK, Grgic A, et al. Cytotoxic effects of ionic high-osmolar, nonionic, monomeric, and nonionic iso-osmolar dimeric iodinated contrast media on renal tubular cells in vitro. *Radiology.* 2005;235:843-849.
30. Katzberg RW. Contrast medium-induced nephrotoxicity: which pathway? *Radiology.* 2005;235:752-755.
31. Cohan RH, Dunnick NR. Intravascular contrast media: adverse reactions. *AJR Am J Roentgenol.* 1987;149:665-670.
32. Thomsen HS. Guidelines for contrast media from the European Society of Urogenital Radiology. *AJR Am J Roentgenol.* 2003;181:1463-1471.
33. Bettmann MA, Heeren T, Greenfield A, et al. Adverse events with radiographic contrast agents: results of the SCVIR Contrast Agent Registry. *Radiology.* 1997;203:611-620.

34. Rudnick MR, Goldfarb S, Wexler L, et al. for the Iohexol Cooperative Study: Nephrotoxicity of ionic and nonionic contrast media in 1196 patients: a randomized trial. *Kidney Int.* 1995;47:254-261.
35. Ashley JB, Millward SF. Contrast agent-induced nephropathy: a simple way to identify patients with preexisting renal insufficiency. *AJR Am J Roentgenol.* 2003;181:451-454.
36. American College of Radiology Committee on Drugs and Contrast Media. *Manual on contrast media.* ed 5. Reston, Va: American College of Radiology; 2004.
37. Trivedi HS, Moore H, Nasr S, et al. A randomized prospective trial to assess the role of saline hydration on the development of contrast nephrotoxicity. *Nephron Clin Pract.* 2003;93(1):c29-c34.
38. Tepel M, Van Der Giet M, Schwarzfeld C, et al. Prevention of radiographic-contrast-agent–induced reductions in renal function by acetylcysteine. *N Engl J Med.* 2000;343:180-184.
39. Pannu N, Manns B, Lee H, et al. Systematic review of the impact of N-acetylcysteine on contrast nephropathy. *Kidney Int.* 2004;65:1366-1374.
40. Merten GJ, Burgess WP, Gray LV, et al. Prevention of contrast-induced nephropathy with sodium bicarbonate: a randomized controlled trial. *JAMA.* 2004;291:2328-2334.
41. Murphy SW, Barrett BJ, Parfrey PS. Contrast nephropathy. *J Am Soc Nephrol.* 2000;11:177-182.
42. Ellis JH, Cohan RH. Reducing the risk of contrast-induced nephropathy: a perspective on the controversies. *AJR Am J Roentgenol.* 2009;192:1544-1549:[review].
43. Poletti PA, Saudan P, Platon A, et al. N-acetylcysteine and emergency CT: use of serum creatinine and cystatin C as markers of radiocontrast nephrotoxicity. *AJR Am J Roentgenol.* 2007;189:687-692.
44. Morikawa S, Sone T, Tsuboi H, et al. Renal protective effects and the prevention of contrast-induced nephropathy by atrial natriuretic peptide. *J Am Coll Cardiol.* 2009;53:1040-1046.
44a. Amis ES, Hartman DS. Renal ultrasonography 1984: a practical overview. *Radiol Clin North Am.* 1984;22:315-332.
45. Chen P, Maklad N, Redwine M. Color and power Doppler imaging of the kidneys. *World J Urol.* 1998;16:41-45.
46. Jafri SZ, Madrazo BL, Miller JH. Color Doppler ultrasound of the genitourinary tract. *Curr Opin Radiol.* 1992;4:16-23.
47. Hricak H, Cruz C, Romanski R, et al. Renal parenchymal disease: sonographic-histologic correlation. *Radiology.* 1982;144:141-147.
48. Coleman BG. Ultrasonography of the upper genitourinary tract. *Urol Clin North Am.* 1985;12:633-644.
49. Wells PNT. Doppler ultrasound in medical diagnosis. *Br J Radiol.* 1989;62:399-420.
50. Tublin ME, Bude RO, Platt JF. Review—the resistive index in renal Doppler sonography: where do we stand? *AJR Am J Roentgenol.* 2003;180:885-892.
51. Keogan MT, Kliewer MA, Hertzberg BS, et al. Renal resistive indexes: variability in Doppler US measurements in a healthy population. *Radiology.* 1996;199:165-169.
52. Page JE, Morgan SH, Eastwood JB, et al. Ultrasound findings in renal parenchymal disease: comparison with histological appearances. *Clin Radiol.* 1994;49:867-870.
53. Hounsfield GN. Computerized transverse axial scanning (tomography): part I. Description of system. *Br J Radiol.* 1973;46:1016-1022.
54. Horton KM, Sheth S, Corl F, et al. Multidetector row CT: principles and clinical applications. *Crit Rev Comput Tomogr.* 2002;43:143-181.
55. Saunders HS, Dyer RB, Shifrin RY, et al. The CT nephrogram: implications for evaluation of urinary tract disease. *Radiographics.* 1995;15:1069-1085.
56. Perlman ES, Rosenfield AT, Wexler JS, et al. CT urography in the evaluation of urinary tract disease. *J Comput Assist Tomogr.* 1996;20:620-626.
57. Sudakoff GS, Dunn DP, Hellman RS, et al. Opacification of the genitourinary collecting system during MDCT urography with enhanced CT digital radiography: nonsaline versus saline bolus. *AJR Am J Roentgenol.* 2006;186:122-129.
58. Lang EK, Macchia RJ, Thomas R, et al. Improved detection of renal pathologic features on multiphasic helical CT compared with IVU in patients presenting with microscopic hematuria. *Urology.* 2003;61:528-532.
59. Kawashima A, Glockner JF, King BF. CT urography and MR urography. *Radiol Clin North Am.* 2003;41:945-961.
60. McTavish JD, Jinzaki M, Zou KH, et al. Multi-detector row CT urography: comparison of strategies for depicting the normal urinary collecting system. *Radiology.* 2002;225:783-790.
61. Engelstad BL, McClennan BL, Levitt RG, et al. The role of pre-contrast images in computed tomography of the kidney. *Radiology.* 1980;136:153-155.
62. McNicholas MM, Raptopoulos VD, Schwartz RK, et al. Excretory phase CT urography for opacification of the urinary collecting system. *AJR Am J Roentgenol.* 1998;170:1261-1267.
63. Caoili EM. Imaging of the urinary tract using multidetector computed tomography urography. *Semin Urol Oncol.* 2002;20:174-179.
64. Kocakoc E, Bhatt S, Dogra VS. Renal multidetector row CT. *Radiol Clin North Am.* 2005;43:1021-1047.
65. Caoili EM, Cohan RH, Korobkin M, et al. Urinary tract abnormalities: initial experience with multi-detector row CT urography. *Radiology.* 2002;222:353-360.
66. Joffe SA, Servaes S, Okon S, et al. Multi-detector row CT urography in the evaluation of hematuria. *Radiographics.* 2003;23:1441-1455.
67. Schild HH. *MRI made easy.* Wayne, NJ: Berlex Laboratories; 1999.
68. Hashemi RH, Bradley WG, Lisanti CJ. *MRI: the basics.* ed 2. Philadelphia: Lippincott Williams & Wilkins; 2004.
69. Mitchell DG, Cohen MS. *MRI principles.* ed 2. Philadelphia: WB Saunders; 2004.
70. Keogan MT, Edelman RR. Technologic advances in abdominal MR imaging. *Radiology.* 2001;220:310-320.
71. Shellock FG. *Reference manual for magnetic resonance safety, implants and devices.* ed 2006 Los Angeles: Biomedical Research Publishing Company; 2006.
72. Prince MR, Arnoldus C, Frisoli JK. Nephrotoxicity of high-dose gadolinium compared with iodinated contrast. *J Magn Reson Imaging.* 1996;6:162-166.
73. Rofsky NM, Weinreb JC, Bosniak MA, et al. Renal lesion characterization with gadolinium-enhanced MR imaging: efficacy and safety in patients with renal insufficiency. *Radiology.* 1991;180:85-89.
74. Townsend RR, Cohen DL, Katholi R, et al. Safety of intravenous gadolinium (Gd-BOPTA) infusion in patients with renal insufficiency. *Am J Kidney Dis.* 2000;36:1207-1212.
75. Cohen MD. Safe use of imaging contrast agents in children. *J Am Coll Radiol.* 2009;6:576-581.
76. Sam AD, Morasch MD, Collins J, et al. Safety of gadolinium contrast angiography in patients with chronic renal insufficiency. *J Vasc Surg.* 2003;38:313-318.
77. Ergün I, Keven K, Uruc I, et al. The safety of gadolinium in patients with stage 3 and 4 renal failure. *Nephrol Dial Transpl.* 2006;21:697-700.
78. Zhang HL, Ersoy H, Prince MR. Effects of gadopentetate dimeglumine and gadodiamide on serum calcium, magnesium, and creatinine measurements. *J Magn Reson Imaging.* 2006;23:383-387.
79. Choyke PL, Girton ME, Frank JA, et al. Clearance of gadolinium chelates by hemodialysis: an in vitro study. *J Magn Reson Imaging.* 2005;5:470-472.
80. Grobner T. Gadolinium: a specific trigger for the development of nephrogenic fibrosing dermopathy and nephrogenic systemic fibrosis? *Nephrol Dial Transplant.* 2006;21:1104-1108.
81. Marckmann P, Skov L, Rossen K, et al. Nephrogenic systemic fibrosis: suspected causative role of gadodiamide used for contrast-enhanced magnetic resonance imaging. *J Am Soc Nephrol.* 2006;17:2359-2362.
82. Maloo M, Abt P, Kashyap R, et al. Nephrogenic systemic fibrosis among liver transplant recipients: a single institution experience and topic update. *Am J Transplant.* 2006;6:2212-2217.
83. Sadowski EA, Bennett LK, Chan MR, et al. Nephrogenic systemic fibrosis: risk factors and incidence estimation. *Radiology.* 2007;243:148-157.
84. Broome DR, Girguis MS, Baron PW, et al. Gadodiamide-associated nephrogenic systemic fibrosis: why radiologists should be concerned. *Am J Radiol.* 2007;188:586-592.
85. U.S. Food and Drug Administration. *Information for healthcare professionals: gadolinium-based contrast agents for magnetic resonance imaging (marketed as Magnevist, MultiHance, Omniscan, OptiMARK, ProHance).* Available at http://www.fda.gov/Drugs/DrugSafety/PostmarketDrugSafety InformationforPatientsandProviders/ ucm142884.htm. Accessed June 14, 2011.
86. Kanal E, Barkovich AJ, Bell C, et al. ACR guidance document for safe MR practices:2007. *AJR Am J Roentgenol.* 2007;188:1447-1474.
87. Cowper SE. *The International Center for Nephrogenic Systemic Fibrosis Research (ICNSFR).* (website) http://www.icnfdr.org. Accessed August 27, 2011.
88. Cowper SE, Robin HS, Steinberg HM, et al. Scleromyxedema-like cutaneous disease in renal-dialysis patients. *Lancet.* 2000;356:1000-1001.
89. Juluru K, Vogel-Claussen J, Macura KJ, et al. MR imaging in patients at risk for developing nephrogenic systemic fibrosis: protocols, practices, and imaging techniques to maximize patient safety. *Radiographics.* 2009;29:9-22.
90. Thomsen HS. European Society of Urogenital Radiology guidelines on contrast media application. *Curr Opin Urol.* 2007;17:70-76.
91. Shellock FG, Spinazzi A. MRI safety update 2008: part 1, MRI contrast agents and nephrogenic systemic fibrosis. *AJR Am J Roentgenol.* 2008;191:1129-1139.
92. Thomsen HS, Marckmann P, Logager VB. Update on nephrogenic systemic fibrosis. *Magn Reson Imaging Clin North Am.* 2008;16:551-560:vii.
93. Chung JJ, Semelka RC, Martin DR. Acute renal failure: common occurrence of preservation of corticomedullary differentiation on MR images. *Magn Reson Imaging.* 2001;19:789-793.

94. Semelka RC, Corrigan K, Ascher SM, et al. renal corticomedullary differentiation: observation in patients with differing serum creatinine levels. *Radiology.* 1994;190:149-152.

95. Lee VS, Rofsky NM, Krinsky GA, et al. Single-dose breath-hold gadolinium-enhanced three-dimensional MR angiography of the renal arteries. *Radiology.* 1999;211:69-78.

96. Kopka L, Vosshenrich R, Rodenwaldt J, et al. Differences in injection rates on contrast-enhanced breath-hold three-dimensional MR angiography. *AJR Am J Roentgenol.* 1998;170:345-348.

97. Mitsuzaki K, Yamashita Y, Ogata I, et al. Optimal protocol for injection of contrast material at MR angiography: study of healthy volunteers. *Radiology.* 1999;213:913-918.

98. Alley MT, Shifrin RY, Pelc NJ, et al. Ultrafast contrast-enhanced three-dimensional MR angiography: state of the art. *Radiographics.* 1998;18:273-285.

99. Baskaran V, Pereles FS, Nemcek AA, et al. Gadolinium-enhanced 3D MR angiography of renal artery stenosis: a pilot comparison of maximum intensity projection, multiplanar reformatting, and 3D volume-rendering postprocessing algorithms. *Acad Radiol.* 2002;9:50-59.

100. Prince MR, Schoenberg SO, Ward JS, et al. Hemodynamically significant atherosclerotic renal artery stenosis: MR angiographic features. *Radiology.* 1997;205:128-136.

101. Willmann JK, Wildermuth S, Pfammatter T, et al. Aortoiliac and renal arteries: prospective intraindividual comparison of contrast-enhanced three-dimensional MR angiography and multi-detector row CT angiography. *Radiology.* 2003;226:798-811.

102. Jara H, Barish MA, Yucel EK, et al. MR hydrography: theory and practice of static fluid imaging. *AJR Am J Roentgenol.* 1998;170:873-882.

103. Nolte-Ernsting CCA, Bücker A, Adam GB, et al. Gadolinium-enhanced excretory MR urography after low-dose diuretic injection: comparison with conventional excretory urography. *Radiology.* 1998;209:147-157.

104. Sudah M, Vanninen RL, Partanen K, et al. Patients with acute flank pain: comparison of MR urography with unenhanced helical CT. *Radiology.* 2002;223:98-105.

105. Nolte-Ernsting CCA, Staatz G, Tacke J, et al. MR urography today. *Abdom Imaging.* 2003;28:191-209.

106. El-Diasty T, Mansour O, Farouk A. Diuretic contrast-enhanced magnetic resonance urography versus intravenous urography for depiction of nondilated urinary tracts. *Abdom Imaging.* 2003;28:135-145.

107. Chandarana H, Lee VS. Renal functional MRI: are we ready for clinical application? *AJR Am J Roentgenol.* 2009;192:1550-1557.

108. Thoeny HC, De Keyzer F, Oyen RH, et al. Diffusion-weighted MR imaging of kidneys in healthy volunteers and patients with parenchymal diseases: initial experience. *Radiology.* 2005;235:911-917.

109. Yang D, Ye Q, Williams DS, et al. Normal and transplanted rat kidneys: diffusion MR imaging at 7 T. *Radiology.* 2004;231:702-709.

110. Sadowski EA, Fain SB, Alford SK, et al. Assessment of acute renal transplant rejection with blood oxygen level–dependent MR imaging: initial experience. *Radiology.* 2005;236:911-919.

111. He W, Fischman AJ. Nuclear imaging in the genitourinary tract: recent advances and future directions. *Radiol Clin North Am.* 2008;46:25-43.

112. Szabo Z, Xia J, Mathews WB. Radiopharmaceuticals for renal positron emission tomography imaging. *Semin Nucl Med.* 2008;38:20-31.

113. Perlman SB, Bushnell DL, Barnes WE. Genitourinary system. In: Wilson MA, ed. *Textbook of nuclear medicine.* Philadelphia: Lippincott-Raven; 1998:117-136.

114. Mejia AA, Nakamura T, Masatoshi I, et al. Estimation of absorbed doses in humans due to intravenous administration of fluorine-18–fluorode-oxyglucose in PET studies. *J Nucl Med.* 1991;32:699-706.

115. Hays MT, Watson EE, Thomas SR, et al. MIRD dose estimate report no. 19: radiation absorbed dose estimates from ^{18}F-FDG. *J Nucl Med.* 2002;43:210-214.

116. Jones SC, Alavi A, Christman D, et al. The radiation dosimetry of 2[F-18] fluoro-2-deoxy-D-glucose in man. *J Nucl Med.* 1982;23:613-617.

117. Laffon E, Cazeau AL, Monet A, et al. The effect of renal failure on ^{18}F-FDG uptake: a theoretic assessment. *J Nucl Med.* 2008;36:200-202.

118. Minamimoto R, Takahashi N, Inoue T. FDG PET of patients with suspected renal failure: standardized uptake values in normal tissues. *Ann Nucl Med.* 2007;21:217-222.

119. Kuni CC, duCret RP. *Genitourinary system, in Manual of nuclear medicine imaging.* New York: Thieme; 1997:106-128.

120. Bagni B, Portaluppi F, Montanari L, et al. ^{99m}Tc-MAG3 versus ^{131}I-orthoiodohippurate in the routine determination of effective renal plasma flow. *J Nucl Med Allied Sci.* 1990;34:67-70.

121. Caglar M, Gedik GK, Karabulut E. Differential renal function estimation by dynamic renal scintigraphy: influence of background definition and radiopharmaceutical. *Nucl Med Commun.* 2008;29:1002-1005.

122. Lezaic L, Hodolic M, Fettich J, et al. Reproducibility of ^{99m}Tc-mercaptoacetyltriglycine renography: population comparison. *Nucl Med Commun.* 2008;29:695-704.

123. Schwartz BF, Dykes TE, Rubenstein JN, et al. Effect of position on renal parenchyma perfusion as measured by nuclear scintigraphy. *Urology.* 2007;70:227-229.

124. Esteves FP, Taylor A, Manatunga A, et al. ^{99m}Tc-MAG3 renography: normal values for MAG3 clearance and curve parameters, excretory parameters, and residual urine volume. *AJR Am J Roentgenol.* 2006;187:W610-W617.

125. Ritchie WW, Vick CW, Glocheski SK, et al. Evaluation of azotemic patients: diagnostic yield of initial US examination. *Radiology.* 1988;167:245-247.

126. Yassa NA, Peng M, Ralls PW. Perirenal lucency ("kidney sweat"): a new sign of renal failure. *AJR Am J Roentgenol.* 1999;173:1075-1077.

127. Lee JKT, Baron RL, Melson GL, et al. Can real-time ultrasonography replace static B-scanning in the diagnosis of renal obstruction? *Radiology.* 1981;139:161-165.

128. Ellenbogen PH, Schieble FW, Talner LB, et al. Sensitivity of gray scale US in detecting urinary tract obstruction. *AJR Am J Roentgenol.* 1978;130:731-733.

129. Stuck KJ, White GM, Granke DS, et al. Urinary obstruction in azotemic patients: detection by sonography. *AJR Am J Roentgenol.* 1987;149:1191-1193.

130. Platt JF. Advances in ultrasonography of urinary tract obstruction. *Abdom Imaging.* 1998;23:3-9.

131. Platt JF. Urinary obstruction. *Radiol Clin North Am.* 1996;34:1113-1129.

132. Kamholtz RG, Cronan JJ, Dorfman GS. Obstruction and the minimally dilated renal collecting system: US evaluation. *Radiology.* 1989;170:51-53.

133. Cronan JJ. Contemporary concepts in imaging urinary tract obstruction. *Radiol Clin North Am.* 1991;29:527-542.

134. Mallek R, Bankier AA, Etele-Hainz A, et al. Distinction between obstructive and nonobstructive hydronephrosis: value of diuresis duplex Doppler sonography. *AJR Am J Roentgenol.* 1996;166:113-117.

135. Scola FH, Cronan JJ, Schepps B. Grade I hydronephrosis: pulsed Doppler US evaluation. *Radiology.* 1989;171:519-520.

136. Platt JF, Rubin JM, Ellis JH, et al. Duplex Doppler US of the kidneys: differentiation of obstructive from nonobstructive dilatation. *Radiology.* 1989;171:515-517.

137. Cronan JJ, Tublin ME. Role of the resistive index in the evaluation of acute renal obstruction. *AJR Am J Roentgenol.* 1995;164:377-378.

138. Platt JF, Ellis JH, Rubin JM. Role of renal Doppler imaging in the evaluation of acute renal obstruction. *AJR Am J Roentgenol.* 1995;164:379-380.

139. Platt JF. Looking for renal obstruction: the view from renal Doppler US. *Radiology.* 1994;193:610-612.

140. Platt JF, Rubin JM, Bowerman RA, et al. The inability to detect kidney disease on the basis of echogenicity. *AJR Am J Roentgenol.* 1988;151:317-319.

141. Gourtsoyiannis N, Prassopoulos P, Cavouras D, et al. The thickness of the renal parenchyma decreases with age: a CT study of 360 patients. *AJR Am J Roentgenol.* 1990;155:541-544.

142. Marotti M, Hricak H, Terrier F, et al. MR in renal disease: importance of cortical-medullary distinction. *Magn Reson Med.* 1987;5:160-172.

143. Kim S, Naik M, Sigmund E, et al. Diffusion-weighted MR imaging of the kidneys and the urinary tract. *Magn Reson Imaging Clin North Am.* 2008;16:585-596:vii-viii.

144. Lin EC, Gellens ME, Goodgold HM. Prognostic value of renal scintigraphy with Tc-99m MAG3 in patients with acute renal failure. *J Nucl Med.* 1995;36:232P-233P.

145. Saremi F, Jadvar H, Siegel M. Pharmacologic interventions in nuclear radiology: indications, imaging protocols, and clinical results. *Radiographics.* 2002;22:477-490.

146. Kuni CC, duCret RP. *Genitourinary system, in Manual of nuclear medicine imaging.* New York: Thieme; 1997:106-128.

147. Sfakianakis GN, Sfakianaki F, Georgiou M, et al. A renal protocol for all ages and all indications: mercapto-acetyl-triglycine (MAG3) with simultaneous injection of furosemide (MAG3-F0): a 17-year experience. *Sem Nucl Med.* 2009;39:156-173.

148. Taghavi R, Ariana K, Arab D. Diuresis renography for differentiation of upper urinary tract dilatation from obstruction: F+20 and F-15 methods. *Urol J.* 2007;4:36-40.

149. Dyer RB, Chen MYM, Zagoria RJ. Abnormal calcifications in the urinary tract. *Radiographics.* 1998;18:1405-1424.

150. Ginalski JM, Portmann L, Jaeger PH. Does medullary sponge kidney cause nephrolithiasis? *AJR Am J Roentgenol.* 1990;155:299-302.

151. Gibson MS, Puckett ML, Shelly ME. Renal tuberculosis. *Radiographics.* 2004;24:251-256.

152. Clark JY, Thompson IM, Optenberg SA. Economic impact of urolithiasis in the United States. *J Urol.* 1995;154:2020-2042.

153. Tublin ME, Murphy ME, Delong DM, et al. Conspicuity of renal calculi at unenhanced CT: effects of calculus composition and size and CT technique. *Radiology.* 2002;225:91-96.

154. Newhouse JH, Prien EL, Amis ES, et al. Computed tomographic analysis of urinary calculi. *AJR Am J Roentgenol.* 1984;142:545-548.
155. Hillman BJ, Drach GW, Tracey P, et al. Computed tomographic analysis of renal calculi. *AJR Am J Roentgenol.* 1984;142:549-552.
156. Mostafavi MR, Ernst RD, Saltzman B. Accurate determination of chemical composition of urinary calculi by spiral computerized tomography. *J Urol.* 1998;159:673-675.
157. Coll DM, Varanelli MJ, Smith RC. Relationship of spontaneous passage of ureteral calculi to stone size and location as revealed by unenhanced helical CT. *AJR Am J Roentgenol.* 2002;178:101-103.
158. Smith RC, Varanelli M. Diagnosis and management of acute ureterolithiasis. *AJR Am J Roentgenol.* 2000;175:3-6.
159. Smith RC, Rosenfield AT, Choe KA, et al. Acute flank pain: comparison of non–contrast-enhanced CT and intravenous urography. *Radiology.* 1995;194:789-794.
160. Haddad MC, Sharif HS, Abomelha MS, et al. Management of renal colic: redefining the role of the urogram. *Radiology.* 1992;184:35-36.
161. Middleton WD, Dodds WJ, Lawson TL, et al. Renal calculi: sensitivity for detection with US. *Radiology.* 1988;167:239-244.
162. Gottlieb RH, La TC, Erturk EN, et al. CT in detecting urinary tract calculi: influence on patient imaging and clinical outcomes. *Radiology.* 2002;225:441-449.
163. Sourtzis S, Thibeau JF, Damry N, et al. Radiologic investigation of renal colic: unenhanced helical CT compared with excretory urography. *AJR Am J Roentgenol.* 1999;172:1491-1494.
164. Boulay I, Holtz P, Foley WD, et al. Ureteral calculi: diagnostic efficacy of helical CT and implications for treatment of patients. *AJR Am J Roentgenol.* 1999;172:1485-1490.
165. Katz DS, Hines J, Rausch DR, et al. Unenhanced helical CT for suspected renal colic. *AJR Am J Roentgenol.* 1999;173:425-430.
166. Haddad MC, Sharif HS, Shahed MS, et al. Renal colic: diagnosis and outcome. *Radiology.* 1992;184:83-88.
167. Smith RC, Rosenfield AT, Choe KA, et al. Acute flank pain: comparison of non–contrast-enhanced CT and intravenous urography. *Radiology.* 1995;194:789-794.
168. Flowler KAB, Locken JA, Duchesne JH, et al. US for detecting renal calculi with nonenhanced CT as a reference standard. *Radiology.* 2002;222:109-113.
169. Catalano O, Nunziata A, Altei F, et al. Suspected ureteral colic: primary helical CT versus selective helical CT after unenhanced radiography and sonography. *AJR Am J Roentgenol.* 2002;178:379-387.
170. Rucker CM, Menias CO, Bhalla S. Mimics of renal colic: alternative diagnoses at unenhanced helical CT. *Radiographics.* 2004;24:S11-S33.
171. Tamm EP, Silverman PM, Shuman WP. Evaluation of the patient with flank pain and possible ureteral calculus. *Radiology.* 2003;228:319-329.
172. Diel J, Perlmutter S, Venkataramanan, et al. Unenhanced helical CT using increased pitch for suspected renal colic: an effective technique for radiation dose reduction? *J Computer Assist Tomogr.* 2000;24:795-801.
173. Katz DS, Venkataramanan Napel S, et al. Can low-dose unenhanced multidetector CT be used for routine evaluation of suspected renal colic? *AJR Am J Roentgenol.* 2003;180:313-315.
174. Saw KC, McAteer JA, Monga AG, et al. Helical CT of urinary calculi: effect of stone composition, stone size, and scan collimation. *AJR Am J Roentgenol.* 2000;175:329-332.
175. Nadler RB, Rubenstein JN, Eggener SE, et al. The etiology of urolithiasis in HIV infected patients. *J Urol.* 2003;169:475-477.
176. Blake SP, McNicholas MMJ, Raptopoulos V. Nonopaque crystal deposition causing ureteric obstruction in patients with HIV undergoing indinavir therapy. *AJR Am J Roentgenol.* 1998;171:717-720.
177. Ciaschini MW, Remer EM, Baker ME, et al. Urinary calculi: radiation dose reduction of 50% and 75% at CT—effect on sensitivity. *Radiology.* 2009;251:105-111.
178. Paulson EK, Weaver C, Ho LM, et al. Conventional and reduced radiation dose of 16-MDCT for detection of nephrolithiasis and ureterolithiasis. *AJR Am J Roentgenol.* 2008;190:151-157.
179. Grosjean R, Sauer B, Guerra RM, et al. Characterization of human renal stones with MDCT: advantage of dual energy and limitations due to respiratory motion. *AJR Am J Roentgenol 190.* 2008:720-728.
180. Boll DT, Patil NA, Paulson EK, et al. Renal stone assessment with dual-energy multidetector CT and advanced postprocessing techniques: improved characterization of renal stone composition—pilot study. *Radiology.* 2009;250:813-820.
181. Miller NL, Evan AP, Lingeman JE. Pathogenesis of renal calculi. *Urol Clin North Am.* 2007;34:295-313.
182. Boridy IC, Kawashima A, Goldman SM, et al. Acute uroterolithiasis: nonenhanced helical CT findings of perinephric edema for prediction of degree of ureteral obstruction. *Radiology.* 1999;213:663-667.
183. Georgiades CS, Moore CJ, Smith DP. Differences of renal parenchymal attenuation for acutely obstructed and unobstructed kidneys on unenhanced helical CT: a useful secondary sign? *AJR Am J Roentgenol.* 2001;176:965-968.
184. Goldman SM, Faintuch S, Ajzen SA, et al. Diagnostic value of attenuation measurements of the kidney on unenhanced helical CT of obstructive ureterolithiasis. *AJR Am J Roentgenol.* 2004;182:1251-1254.
185. Narepalem N, Sundaram CP, Boridy IC, et al. Comparison of helical computerized tomography and plain radiography for estimating urinary stone size. *J Urol.* 2002;167:1235-1238.
186. Takahashi N, Kawashima A, Ernst RD, et al. Ureterolithiasis: can clinical outcome be predicted with unenhanced helical CT? *Radiology.* 1998;208:97-102.
187. Metser U, Ghai S, Ong YY, et al. Assessment of urinary tract calculi with 64-MDCT: the axial versus coronal plane. *AJR Am J Roentgenol.* 2009;192:1509-1513.
188. Dalrymple NC, Casford B, Raiken DP, et al. Pearls and pitfalls in the diagnosis of ureterolithiasis with unenhanced helical CT. *Radiographics.* 2000;20:439-447.
189. Sudah M, Vanninen RL, Partanen K, et al. Patients with acute flank pain: comparison of MR urography with unenhanced helical CT. *Radiology.* 2002;223:98-105.
190. Regan F, Bohlman ME, Khazan R, et al. MR urography using HASTE imaging in the assessment of ureteric obstruction. *AJR Am J Roentgenol.* 1996;167:1115-1120.
191. Ku JH, Jeon YS, Kim ME, et al. Is there a role for magnetic resonance imaging in renal trauma? *Int J Urol.* 2001;8:261-267.
192. Talner LB, Davidson AJ, Lebowitz RL, et al. Acute pyelonephritis: can we agree on terminology? *Radiology.* 1994;192:297-305.
193. Craig WD, Wagner BJ, Travis MD. Pyelonephritis: radiologic-pathologic review. *Radiographics.* 2008;28:255-277.
194. Papanicolaou N, Pfister RC. Acute renal infections. *Radiol Clin North Am.* 1996;34:965-995.
195. Hamper UM, Goldblum LE, Hutchins GM, et al. Renal involvement in AIDS: sonographic-pathologic correlation. *AJR Am J Roentgenol.* 1988;150:1321-1325.
196. Symeonidou C, Standish R, Sahdev A, et al. Imaging and histopathologic features of HIV-related renal disease. *Radiographics.* 2008;28:1339-1354.
197. Koh DM, Langroudi B. Padley SPG: Abdominal CT in patients with AIDS. *Imaging.* 2002;14:24-34.
198. Kay CJ. Renal diseases in patients with AIDS: sonographic findings. *AJR Am J Roentgenol.* 1992;159:551-554.
199. Grayson DE, Abbott RM, Levy AD, et al. Emphysematous infections of the abdomen and pelvis: a pictorial review. *Radiographics.* 2002;22:543-561.
200. Rodriguez-de-Velasquez A, Yoder IC, Velasquez PA, et al. Imaging the effects of diabetes on the genitourinary system. *Radiographics.* 1995;15:1051-1068.
201. Hayes WS, Hartman DS, Sesterbenn I. From the archives of the AFIP. Xanthogranulomatous pyelonephritis. *Radiographics.* 1991;11:485-498.
202. Kenney PJ. Imaging of chronic renal infections. *AJR Am J Roentgenol.* 1990;155:485-494.
203. Soulen MC, Fishman EK, Goldman SM, et al. Bacterial renal infection: role of CT. *Radiology.* 1989;171:703-707.
204. Kim B, Lim HK, Choi MH, et al. Detection of parenchymal abnormalities in acute pyelonephritis by pulse inversion harmonic imaging with or without microbubble ultrasonographic contrast agent: correlation with computed tomography. *J Ultrasound Med.* 2001;20:5-14.
205. Sheth S, Fishman EK. Multi-detector row CT of the kidneys and urinary tract: techniques and applications in the diagnosis of benign diseases. *Radiographics.* 2004;24:e20.
206. Kawashima A, Sandler CM, Goldman SM, et al. CT of renal inflammatory disease. *Radiographics.* 1997;17:851-866.
207. Majd M, Blask ARN, Markle BM, et al. Acute pyelonephritis: comparison of diagnosis with ^{99m}Tc-DMSA SPECT, spiral CT, MR imaging, and power Doppler US in an experimental pig model. *Radiology.* 2001;218:101-108.
208. Gervais DA, Shitman GJ. Emphysematous pyelonephritis. *AJR Am J Roentgenol.* 1994;162:348.
209. Wan Y-L, Lee T-Y, Bullard MJ, et al. Acute gas-producing bacterial renal infection: correlation between imaging findings and clinical outcome. *Radiology.* 1996;198:433-438.
210. Roy C, Pfleger DD, Tuchmann CM, et al. Emphysematous pyelitis: findings in five patients. *Radiology.* 2001;218:647-650.
211. Fan CM, Whitman GJ, Chew FS. Xanthogranulomatous pyelonephritis. *AJR Am J Roentgenol.* 1995;165:862.
212. Bjorgvinsson E, Majd M, Eggli KD. Diagnosis of acute pyelonephritis in children: comparison of sonography and ^{99m}Tc-DMSA scintigraphy. *AJR Am J Roentgenol.* 1991;157:539-543.
213. Rossleigh MA. Scintigraphic imaging in renal infections. *Q J Nucl Med Mol Imaging.* 2009;53:72-77.
214. Ziessman HA, Majd M. Importance of methodology on (99m)technetium dimercapto-succinic acid scintigraphic image quality: imaging pilot study for RIVUR (Randomized Intervention for Children With Vesicoureteral Reflux) multicenter investigation. *J Urol.* 2009;182:272-279.

215. Sheehy N, Tetrault TA, Zurakowski D, et al. Pediatric 99m-Tc-DMSA SPECT performed by using iterative reconstruction with isotropic resolution recovery: improved image quality and reduced radiopharmaceutical activity. *Radiology.* 2009;251:511-516.

216. Soussan M, Sberro R, Wartski M, et al. Diagnosis and localization of renal cyst infection by 18F-fluorodeoxyglucose PET/CT in polycystic kidney disease. *Ann Nucl Med.* 2008;22:529-531.

217. Warshauer DM, McCarthy SM, Street L, et al. Detection of renal masses: sensitivities and specificities of excretory urography/linear tomography, US, and CT. *Radiology.* 1988;169:363-365.

218. Bosniak Morton. A: The use of the Bosniak classification system for renal cysts and cystic tumors. *J Urol.* 1997;157:1852-1853.

219. Jinzaki M, McTavish JD, Zou KH, et al. Evaluation of small (≤3 cm) renal masses with MDCT: Benefits of thin overlapping reconstructions. *AJR Am J Roentgenol.* 2004;183:223-228.

220. Silverman SG, Lee BY, Seltzer SE, et al. Small (≤3 cm) renal masses: correlation of spiral CT features and pathologic findings. *AJR Am J Roentgenol.* 1994;163:597-605.

221. Israel GM, Hindman N, Bosniak MA. Evaluation of cystic renal masses: comparison of CT and MR imaging by using the Bosniak classification system. *Radiology.* 2004;231:365-371.

222. Semelka RC, Shoenut JP, Kroeker MA, et al. Renal lesions: controlled comparison between CT and 1.5-T MR imaging with nonenhanced and gadolinium-enhanced fat-suppressed spin-echo and breath-hold FLASH techniques. *Radiology.* 1992;182:425-430.

223. Hecht EM, Israel GM, Krinsky GA, et al. Renal masses: quantitative analysis of enhancement with signal intensity measurements versus qualitative analysis of enhancement with image subtraction for diagnosing malignancy at MR imaging. *Radiology.* 2004;232:373-378.

224. Hayden CK, Swischuk LE, Smith TH, et al. Renal cystic disease in childhood. *Radiographics.* 1986;6:97-116.

225. Lonergan GF, Rice RR, Suarez ES. Autosomal recessive polycystic kidney disease: radiologic-pathologic correlation. *Radiographics.* 2000;20:837-855.

226. Walker FC, Loney LC, Root ER, et al. Diagnostic evaluation of adult polycystic kidney disease in childhood. *AJR Am J Roentgenol.* 1984;142:1273-1277.

227. Nicolau C, Torra R, Badenas C, et al. Autosomal dominant polycystic kidney disease types 1 and 2: assessment of US sensitivity for diagnosis. *Radiology.* 1999;213:273-276.

228. Heinz-Peer G, Schoder M, Rand T, et al. Prevalence of acquired cystic kidney disease and tumors in native kidneys of renal transplant recipients: a prospective US study. *Radiology.* 1995;195:667-671.

229. Levine E. Acquired cystic kidney disease. *Radiol Clin North Am.* 1996;34:947-964.

230. Levine E, Slusher SL, Grantham JJ, et al. Natural history of acquired renal cystic disease in dialysis patients: a prospective longitudinal CT study. *AJR Am J Roentgenol.* 1991;156:501-506.

231. Takebayashi S, Hidai H, Chiba T, et al. Using helical CT to evaluate renal cell carcinoma in patients undergoing hemodialysis: value of early enhanced images. *AJR Am J Roentgenol.* 1999;172:429-433.

232. Taylor AJ, Cohen EP, Erickson SJ, et al. Renal imaging in long-term dialysis patients: a comparison of CT and sonography. *AJR Am J Roentgenol.* 1989;153:765-767.

233. Takase K, Takahashi S, Tazawa S, et al. Renal cell carcinoma associated with chronic renal failure: evaluation with sonographic angiography. *Radiology.* 1994;192:787-792.

234. Siegel SC, Sandler MA, Alpern MB, et al. CT of renal cell carcinoma in patients on chronic hemodialysis. *AJR Am J Roentgenol.* 1988;150:583-585.

235. Matson MA, Cohen EP. Acquired cystic kidney disease: occurrence, prevalence, and renal cancers. *Medicine.* 1990;69:217-226.

236. Farres MT, Ronco P, Saadoun D, et al. Chronic lithium nephropathy: MR imaging for diagnosis. *Radiology.* 2003;229:570-574.

237. Leung RS, Biswas SV, Duncan M, et al. Imaging features of von Hippel–Lindau disease. *Radiographics.* 2008;28:65-79.

238. Choyke PL, Glenn GM, Walther MM, et al. Hereditary renal cancers. *Radiology.* 2003;226:33-46.

239. Bosniak MA. State of the art. The current radiological approach to renal cysts. *Radiology.* 1986;158:1-10.

240. Zagoria RJ. Imaging of small renal masses: a medical success story. *AJR Am J Roentgenol.* 2000;175:945-955.

241. Lowe LH, Isuani BH, Heller RM, et al. Pediatric renal masses: Wilms tumor and beyond. *Radiographics.* 2000;20:1585-1603.

242. Prasad SR, Surabhi VR, Menias CO, et al. Benign renal neoplasms in adults: cross-sectional imaging findings. *AJR Am J Roentgenol.* 2008;190:158-164:Review.

243. Wagner BJ, Maj MC, Wong-You-Cheong JJ, et al. Adult renal hamartomas. *Radiographics.* 1997;17:155-169.

244. Bosniak MA, Megibow AJ, Hulnick DH, et al. CT diagnosis of renal angiomyolipoma: the importance of detecting small amounts of fat. *AJR Am J Roentgenol.* 1988;151:497-501.

245. Silverman SG, Pearson GDN, Seltzer SE, et al. Small (≤3 cm) hyperechoic renal masses: comparison of helical and conventional CT for diagnosing angiomyolipoma. *AJR Am J Roentgenol.* 1996;167:877-881.

246. Siegel CL, Middleton WD, Teefey SA, et al. Angiomyolipoma and renal cell carcinoma: US differentiation. *Radiology.* 1996;198:789-793.

247. Kim JK, Park SY, Shon JH, et al. Angiomyolipoma with minimal fat: differentiation from renal cell carcinoma at biphasic helical CT. *Radiology.* 2004;230:677-684.

248. Jinzaki M, Tanimoto A, Narimatsu Y, et al. Angiomyolipoma: imaging findings in lesions with minimal fat. *Radiology.* 1997;205:497-502.

249. Catalano OA, Samir AE, Sahani DV, et al. Pixel distribution analysis: can it be used to distinguish clear cell carcinomas from angiomyolipomas with minimal fat? *Radiology.* 2008;247:738-746.

250. Kim JY, Kim JK, Kim N, et al. CT histogram analysis: differentiation of angiomyolipoma without visible fat from renal cell carcinoma at CT imaging. *Radiology.* 2008;246:472-479.

251. Israel GM, Hindman N, Hecht E, et al. The use of opposed-phase chemical shift MRI in the diagnosis of renal angiomyolipomas. *AJR Am J Roentgenol.* 2005;184:1868-1872.

252. Lesavre A, Correas JM, Merran S, et al. CT of papillary renal cell carcinomas with cholesterol necrosis mimicking angiomyolipomas. *AJR Am J Roentgenol.* 2003;181:143-145.

253. Israel GM, Bosniak MA, Slywotzky CM, et al. CT differentiation of large exophytic renal angiomyolipomas and perirenal liposarcomas. *AJR Am J Roentgenol.* 2002;179:769-773.

254. Bosniak M, Megibow AJ, Hulnick DH, et al. CT diagnosis of renal angiomyolipoma: the importance of detecting small amounts of fat. *AJR Am J Roentgenol.* 1988;151:497-501.

255. Lemaitre L, Robert Y, Dubrulle F, et al. Renal angiomyolipoma: growth followed up with CT and/or US. *Radiology.* 1995;197:598-602.

256. Yamakado K, Tanaka N, Nakagawa T, et al. Renal angiomyolipoma: relationships between tumor size, aneurysm formation, and rupture. *Radiology.* 2002;225:78-82.

257. Palmer WE, Chew FS. Renal oncocytoma. *AJR Am J Roentgenol.* 1991;156:1144.

258. Levine E, Huntrakoon M. Computed tomography of renal oncocytoma. *AJR Am J Roentgenol.* 1983;141:741-746.

259. Blake MA, McKernan M, Setty B, et al. Renal oncocytoma displaying intense activity on 18F-FDG PET. *AJR Am J Roentgenol.* 2006;186:269-271.

260. Neisius D, Braedel HU, Schindler E, et al. Computed tomographic and angiographic findings in renal oncocytoma. *Br J Radiol.* 1988;61:1019-1025.

261. Davidson AJ, Hayes WS, Hartman DS, et al. Renal oncocytoma and carcinoma: failure of differentiation with CT. *Radiology.* 1993;186:693-696.

262. Curry NS, Schabel SI, Garvin AJ, et al. Case report. Intratumoral fat in a renal oncocytoma mimicking angiomyolipoma. *AJR Am J Roentgenol.* 1990;154:307-308.

263. Bostwick DG, Eble JN, Murphy GP. Conference summary. Diagnosis and prognosis of renal cell carcinoma: 1997 workshop, Rochester, Minnesota, March 21-22, 1997. *Cancer.* 1997;80:975-976.

264. Bonsib SM. Risk and prognosis in renal neoplasms. A pathologist's prospective. *Urol Clin North Am.* 1999;26:643-660.

265. Russo P. Renal cell carcinoma: presentation, staging, and surgical treatment. *Semin Oncol.* 2000;27:160-176.

266. Sheth S, Scatarige JC, Horton KM, et al. Current concepts in the diagnosis and management of renal cell carcinoma: role of multidetector CT and three-dimensional CT. *Radiographics.* 2001;21:S237-S254.

267. Coll DM, Herts BR, Davros WJ, et al. Preoperative use of 3D volume rendering to demonstrate renal tumors and renal anatomy. *Radiographics.* 2000;20:431-438.

268. Gervais DA, McGovern FJ, Arellano RS, et al. Renal cell carcinoma: clinical experience and technical success with radio-frequency ablation of 42 tumors. *Radiology.* 2003;226:417-424.

269. Mayo-Smith WW, Dupuy DE, Parikh PM, et al. Imaging-guided percutaneous radiofrequency ablation of solid renal masses: techniques and outcomes of 38 treatment sessions in 32 consecutive patients. *AJR Am J Roentgenol.* 2003;180:1503-1508.

270. Zagoria RF. Imaging-guided radio-frequency ablation of renal masses. *Radiographics.* 2004;24:S59-S71.

271. Suh RD, Goldin JG, Wallace AB, et al. Metastatic renal cell carcinoma: CT-guided immunotherapy as a technically feasible and safe approach to delivery of gene therapy for treatment. *Radiology.* 2004;231:359-364.

272. Jamis-Dow CA, Choyke PL, Jennings SB, et al. Small (<3-cm) renal masses: detection with CT versus US and pathologic correlation. *Radiology.* 1996;198:785-788.

273. Jinzaki M, Ohkuma K, Tanimoto A, et al. Small solid renal lesions: usefulness of power Doppler US. *Radiology.* 1998;209:543-550.

274. Forman HP, Middleton WD, Melson GL, et al. Hyperechoic renal cell carcinomas: increase in detection at US. *Radiology.* 1993;188:431-434.

275. Ascenti G, Gaeta M, Magno C, et al. Contrast-enhanced second-harmonic sonography in the detection of pseudocapsule in renal cell carcinoma. *AJR Am J Roentgenol.* 2004;182:1525-1530.
276. Schmidt T, Hohl C, Haage P, et al. Diagnostic accuracy of phase-inversion tissue harmonic imaging versus fundamental B-mode sonography in the evaluation of focal lesions of the kidney. *AJR Am J Roentgenol.* 2003;180:1639-1647.
277. Davidson AJ, Hartman DS, Choyke PL, et al. Radiologic assessment of renal masses: implications for patient care. *Radiology.* 1997;202:297-305.
278. Yuh BI, Cohan RH. Different phases of renal enhancement: role in detecting and characterizing renal masses during helical CT. *AJR Am J Roentgenol.* 1999;173:747-755.
279. Cohan RH, Sherman LS, Korobkin M, et al. Renal masses: assessment of corticomedullary-phase and nephrographic-phase CT scans. *Radiology.* 1995;196:445-451.
280. Suh M, Coakley FV, Qayyum A, et al. Distinction of renal cell carcinomas from high-attenuation renal cysts at portal venous phase contrast–enhanced CT. *Radiology.* 2003;228:330-334.
281. Birnbaum BA, Jacobs JE, Ramchandani P. Multiphasic renal CT: comparison of renal mass enhancement during the corticomedullary and nephrographic phases. *Radiology.* 1996;200:753-758.
282. Kopka L, Fischer U, Zoeller G, et al. Dual-phase helical CT of the kidney: value of the corticomedullary and nephrographic phase for evaluation of renal lesions and preoperative staging of renal cell carcinoma. *AJR Am J Roentgenol.* 1997;169:1573-1578.
283. Macari M, Bosniak MA. Delayed CT to evaluate renal masses incidentally discovered at contrast-enhanced CT: demonstration of vascularity with deenhancement. *Radiology.* 1999;213:674-680.
284. Zeman RK, Zeiberg A, Hayes WS, et al. Helical CT of renal masses: the value of delayed scans. *AJR Am J Roentgenol.* 1996;167:771-776.
285. Benjaminov O, Atri M, O'Malley M, et al. Enhancing component on CT to predict malignancy in cystic renal masses and interobserver agreement of different CT features. *AJR Am J Roentgenol.* 2006;186:665-672.
286. Ruppert-Kohlmayr AJ, Uggowitzer M, Meissnitzer T, et al. Differentiation of renal clear cell carcinoma and renal papillary carcinoma using quantitative CT enhancement parameters. *AJR Am J Roentgenol.* 2004;183:1387-1391.
287. Kim JK, Kim TK, Ahn HJ, et al. Differentiation of subtypes of renal cell carcinoma on helical CT scans. *AJR Am J Roentgenol.* 2002;178:1499-1506.
288. Yoshimitsu K, Kakihara D, Irie H, et al. Papillary renal carcinoma: diagnostic approach by chemical shift gradient-echo and echo-planar MR imaging. *J Magn Reson Imaging.* 2006;23:339-344.
289. Ergen FB, Hussain HK, Caoili EM, et al. MRI for preoperative staging of renal cell carcinoma using the 1997 TNM classification: comparison with surgical and pathologic staging. *AJR Am J Roentgenol.* 2004;182:217-225.
290. Roy C, El Ghali S, Buy X, et al. Significance of the pseudocapsule on MRI of renal neoplasms and its potential application for local staging: a retrospective study. *AJR Am J Roentgenol.* 2005;184:113-120.
291. Choyke PL, Walther MM, Wagner JR. Renal cancer: preoperative evaluation with dual-phase three-dimensional MR angiography. *Radiology.* 1997;205:767-771.
292. El-Galley R. Surgical management of renal tumors. *Radiol Clin North Am.* 2003;41:1053-1065.
293. Browne RFJ, Meehan CP, Colville J, et al. Transitional cell carcinoma of the upper urinary tract: spectrum of imaging findings. *Radiographics.* 2005;25:1609-1627.
294. Pickhardt PF, Lonergan GF, Davis CF, et al. From the archives of the AFIP. Infiltrative renal lesions: radiologic-pathologic correlation. *Radiographics.* 2000;20:215-243.
295. Urban BA, Fishman EK. Renal lymphoma: CT patterns with emphasis on helical CT. *Radiographics.* 2000;20:197-212.
296. Semelka RC, Kelekis NL, Burdeny DA, et al. Renal lymphoma: demonstration by MR imaging. *AJR Am J Roentgenol.* 1996;166:823-827.
297. Hartman DS, Choyke PL, Hartman MS. From the RSNA refresher courses. A practical approach to the cystic renal mass. *Radiographics.* 2004;24:S101-S115.
298. Israel GM, Hindman N, Bosniak MA. Evaluation of cystic renal masses: comparison of CT and MR imaging by using the Bosniak classification system. *Radiology.* 2004;231:365-371.
299. Siegel CL, McFarland EG, Brink JA, et al. CT of cystic renal masses: analysis of diagnostic performance and interobserver variation. *AJR Am J Roentgenol.* 1997;169:813-818.
300. Israel GM, Bosniak MA. Follow-up CT of moderately complex cystic lesions of the kidney (Bosniak category IIF). *AJR Am J Roentgenol.* 2003;181:627-633.
301. Curry NS, Cochran ST, Bissada NK. Cystic renal masses: accurate Bosniak classification requires adequate renal CT. *AJR Am J Roentgenol.* 2000;175:339-342.
302. Harisinghani MG, Maher MM, Gervais DA, et al. Incidence of malignancy in complex cystic renal masses (Bosniak category III): should imaging-guided biopsy precede surgery? *AJR Am J Roentgenol.* 2003;180:755-758.
303. Dechet CB, Sebo T, Farrow G, et al. Prospective analysis of intraoperative frozen needle biopsy of solid renal masses in adults. *J Urol.* 1999;162:1282-1285.
304. Wood BJ, Khan MA, McGovern F, et al. Imaging guided biopsy of renal masses: indications, accuracy and impact on clinical management. *J Urol.* 1999;161:1470-1474.
305. Rybicki FJ, Shu KM, Cibas ES, et al. Percutaneous biopsy of renal masses: sensitivity and negative predictive value stratified by clinical setting and size of masses. *AJR Am J Roentgenol.* 2003;180:1281-1287.
306. Freire M, Remer EM. Clinical and radiologic features of cystic renal masses. *AJR Am J Roentgenol.* 2009;192:1367-1372.
307. Frank IN, Graham Jr S, Nabors WL. Urologic and male genital cancers. In: Holleb AI, Fink DJ, Murphy GP, eds. *American Cancer Society textbook of clinical oncology.* Atlanta: American Cancer Society; 1991:272-274.
308. Goldberg MA, Mayo-Smith WW, Papanicolaou N, et al. FDG PET characterization of renal masses: preliminary experience. *Clin Radiol.* 1997;52:510-515.
309. Jadvar H, Kherbache HM, Pinski JK, et al. Diagnostic role of [F-18]-FDG positron emission tomography in restaging renal cell carcinoma. *Clin Nephrol.* 2003;60:395-400.
310. Mankoff DA, Thompson JA, Gold P, et al. Identification of interleukin-2–induced complete response in metastatic renal cell carcinoma by FDG PET despite radiographic evidence suggesting persistent tumor. *AJR Am J Roentgenol.* 1997;169:1049-1050.
311. Ramdave S, Thomas GW, Berlangieri SU, et al. Clinical role of F-18 fluorodeoxyglucose positron emission tomography for detection and management of renal cell carcinoma. *J Urol.* 2001;166:825-830.
312. Wahl RL, Harney J, Hutchins G, et al. Imaging of renal cancer using positron emission tomography with 2-deoxy-2-(^{18}F)-fluoro-D-glucose: pilot animal and human studies. *J Urol.* 1991;146:1470-1474.
313. Wu HC, Yen RF, Shen YY, et al. Comparing whole body ^{18}F-2-deoxyglucose positron emission tomography and technetium-99m methylene diphosphate bone scan to detect bone metastases in patients with renal cell carcinomas—a preliminary report. *J Cancer Res Clin Oncol.* 2002;128:503-506.
314. Vercellino L, Bousquet G, Baillet G, et al. ^{18}F-FDG PET/CT imaging for an early assessment of response to sunitinib in metastatic renal carcinoma: preliminary study. *Cancer Biother Radiopharm.* 2009;24:137-144.
315. Snow D, Cohen D, Chapman WC, et al. Positron emission tomography enhancing tumor thrombus in patient with renal cell carcinoma. *Urology.* 2009;73:270-271.
316. Majhail NS, Urbain JL, Albani JM, et al. F-18 Fluorodeoxyglucose positron emission tomography in the evaluation of distant metastases from renal cell carcinoma. *J Clin Oncol.* 2003;21:3995-4000.
317. Seto E, Segall GM, Terris MK. Positron emission tomography detection of osseous metastases of renal cell carcinoma not identified on bone scan. *Urology.* 2000;55:286.
318. Zhuang H, Duarte PS, Pourdehand M, et al. Standardized uptake value as an unreliable index of renal disease on fluorodeoxyglucose PET imaging. *Clin Nucl Med.* 2000;25:358-360.
319. Kang DE, White Jr RL, Zuger JH, et al. Clinical use of fluorodeoxyglucose F 18 positron emission tomography for detection of renal cell carcinoma. *J Urol.* 2004;171:1806-1809.
320. Safaei A, Figlin R, Hoh CK, et al. The usefulness of F-18 deoxyglucose whole-body positron emission tomography (PET) for re-staging of renal cell cancer. *Clin Nephrol.* 2002;57:56-62.
321. Miyakita H, Tokunaga M, Onda H, et al. Significance of ^{18}F-fluorodeoxyglucose positron emission tomography (FDG-PET) for detection of renal cell carcinoma and immunohistochemical glucose transporter 1 (GLUT-1) expression in the cancer. *Int J Urol.* 2002;9:15-18.
322. Nagase Y, Takata K, Moriyama N, et al. Immunohistochemical localization of glucose transporters in human renal cell carcinoma. *J Urol.* 1995;153(3 pt 1):798-801.
323. Dilhuydy MS, Durieux A, Pariente A, et al. PET scans for decision-making in metastatic renal cell carcinoma: a single institution evaluation. *Oncology.* 2006;70:339-344.
324. Kumar R, Chauhan A, Lakhani P, et al. 2-Deoxy-2-[F-18]fluoro-D-glucose–positron emission tomography in characterization of solid renal masses. *Mol Imaging Biol.* 2005;7:431-439.
325. Shreve P, Chiao PC, Humes HD, et al. Carbon-11–acetate PET imaging in renal disease. *J Nucl Med.* 1995;36:1595-1601.
326. Lawrentschuk N, Poon AM, Foo SS, et al. Assessing regional hypoxia in human renal tumors using 18F-fluoromisonidazole positron emission tomography. *BJU Int.* 2005;96:540-546.
327. Bhargava P, Hanif M, Nash C. Whole-body F-18 sodium fluoride PET-CT in a patient with renal cell carcinoma. *Clin Nucl Med.* 2008;33:894-895.

328. Perini R, Pryma D, Divgi C. Molecular imaging of renal cell carcinoma. *Urol Clin North Am.* 2008;35:605-611.

329. Oyama N, Okazawa H, Kusukawa N, et al. ¹¹C-Acetate PET imaging for renal cell carcinomas. *Eur J Nucl Med Mol Imaging.* 2009;36:422-427.

330. Kotzerke J, Linne C, Meinhardt M, et al. [1-(11)C] Acetate uptake is not increased in renal cell carcinoma. *Eur J Nucl Med Mol Imaging.* 2007;34:884-888.

331. Juillard L, Lemoine S, Janier MF, et al. Validation of renal oxidative metabolism measurement by positron emission tomography. *Hypertension.* 2007;50:242-247.

332. Hyodo T, Sugawara Y, Tsuda T, et al. Widespread metastases from sarcomatoid renal cell carcinoma detected by (18)F-FDG positron emission tomography/computed tomography. *Jpn J Radiol.* 2009;27:111-114.

333. Park JW, Jo MK, Lee HM. Significance of ¹⁸F-fluorodeoxyglucose positron emission tomography/computed tomography for the postoperative surveillance of advanced renal cell carcinoma. *BJU Int.* 2009;103:615-619.

334. Kudomi N, Koivuviita N, Liukko KE, et al. Parametric renal blood flow imaging using [¹⁵O]H₂O and PET. *Eur J Nucl Med Mol Imaging.* 2009;36:683-691.

335. Stillebroer AB, Oosterwijk E, Oyen WJ, et al. Radiolabeled antibodies in renal cell carcinoma. *Cancer Imaging.* 2007;7:179-188.

336. Hillman BJ. Imaging advances in the diagnosis of renovascular hypertension. *AJR Am J Roentgenol.* 1989;153:5-14.

337. Albers FJ. Clinical characteristics of atherosclerotic renovascular disease. *Am J Kidney Dis.* 1994;24:636-641.

338. Ota H, Takase K, Rikimaru H, et al. Quantitative vascular measurements in arterial occlusive disease. *Radiographics.* 2005;25:1141-1158.

339. Siegel CL, Ellis JH, Korobkin M, Dunnick NR. CT-Detected renal arterial calcification: Correlation with renal artery stenosis on angiography. *AJR Am J Roentgenol.* 1994;163:867-872.

340. Beregi JP, Louvegny S, Gautier C, et al. Fibromuscular dysplasia of the renal arteries: comparison of helical CT angiography and arteriography. *AJR Am J Roentgenol.* 1999;172:27-34.

341. Bolduc JP, Oliva VL, Therasse E, et al. Diagnosis and treatment of renovascular hypertension: a cost-benefit analysis. *AJR Am J Roentgenol.* 2005;184:931-937.

342. Soulez G, Oliva VL, Turpin S, et al. Imaging of renovascular hypertension: respective values of renal scintigraphy, renal Doppler US, and MR angiography. *Radiographics.* 2000;20:1355-1368.

343. Desberg AL, Paushter DM, Lammert GK, et al. Renal artery stenosis: evaluation with color Doppler flow imaging. *Radiology.* 1990;177:749-753.

344. Hamper UM, DeJong MR, Caskey CI, et al. Power Doppler imaging: clinical experience and correlation with color Doppler US and other imaging modalities. *Radiographics.* 1977;17:499-513.

345. Helenon O, El Rody F, Correas JM, et al. Color Doppler US of renovascular disease in native kidneys. *Radiographics.* 1995;15:833-854.

346. Halpern EJ, Needleman L, Nack TL, et al. Renal artery stenosis: should we study the main renal artery or segmental vessels? *Radiology.* 1995;195:799-804.

347. House MK, Dowling RJ, King P, et al. Using Doppler sonography to reveal renal artery stenosis: an evaluation of optimal imaging parameters. *AJR Am J Roentgenol.* 1999;173:761-765.

348. Kliewer MA, Tupler RH, Carroll BA, et al. Renal artery stenosis: analysis of Doppler waveform parameters and tardus-parvus pattern. *Radiology.* 1993;189:779-787.

349. Melany ML, Grant EG, Duerinckx AJ, et al. Ability of a phase shift US contrast agent to improve imaging of the main renal arteries. *Radiology.* 1997;205:147-152.

350. Claudon M, Plouin PF, Baxter GM, et al. Renal arteries in patients at risk of renal arterial stenosis: multicenter evaluation of the echo-enhancer SH U 508A at color and spectral Doppler US. Levovist Renal Artery Stenosis Study Group. *Radiology.* 2000;214:739-746.

351. Urban BA, Ratner LE, Fishman EK. Three-dimensional volume-rendered CT angiography of the renal arteries and veins: normal anatomy, variants, and clinical applications. *Radiographics.* 2001;21:373-386.

352. Kaatee R, Beek FJA, DeLange EE, et al. Renal artery stenosis: detection and quantification with spiral CT angiography versus optimized digital subtraction angiography. *Radiology.* 1997;205:121-127.

353. Beregi JP, Elkohen M, Deklunder G, et al. Helical CT angiography compared with arteriography in the detection of renal artery stenosis. *AJR Am J Roentgenol.* 1996;167:495-501.

354. Kawashima A, Sandler CM, Ernst RD, et al. CT evaluation of renovascular disease. *Radiographics.* 2000;20:1321-1340.

355. Rubin GD, Dake MD, Napel S, et al. Spiral CT of renal artery stenosis: comparison of three-dimensional rendering techniques. *Radiology.* 1994;190:181-189.

356. Brink JA, Lim JT, Wang G, et al. Technical optimization of spiral CT for depiction of renal artery stenosis: in vitro analysis. *Radiology.* 1995;194:157-163.

357. Bude RO, Forauer AR, Caoili EM, et al. Is it necessary to study accessory arteries when screening the renal arteries for renovascular hypertension? *Radiology.* 2003;226:411-416.

358. Mallouhi A, Rieger M, Czermak B, et al. Volume-rendered multidetector CT angiography: noninvasive follow-up of patients treated with renal artery stents. *AJR Am J Roentgenol.* 2003;180:233-239.

359. Behar JV, Nelson RC, Zidar JP, et al. Thin-section multidetector CT angiography of renal artery stents. *AJR Am J Roentgenol.* 2002;178:1155-1159.

360. Willmann J, Wildermuth S, Pfammatter T, et al. Aortoiliac and renal arteries: prospective intraindividual comparison of contrast-enhanced three-dimensional MR angiography and multi-detector row CT angiography. *Radiology.* 2003;226:798-811.

361. Thornton MJ, Thornton F, O'Callaghan J, et al. Evaluation of dynamic gadolinium-enhanced breath-hold MR angiography in the diagnosis of renal artery stenosis. *AJR Am J Roentgenol.* 1999;173:1279-1283.

362. Qanadli SD, Soulez G, Therasse E, et al. Detection of renal artery stenosis: prospective comparison of captopril-enhanced Doppler sonography, captopril-enhanced scintigraphy, and MR angiography. *AJR Am J Roentgenol.* 2001;177:1123-1129.

363. Mallouhi A, Schocke M, Judmaier W, et al. 3D MR angiography of renal arteries: comparison of volume rendering and maximum intensity projection algorithms. *Radiology.* 2002;223:509-516.

364. Schoenberg SO, Knopp MV, Londy F, et al. Morphologic and functional magnetic resonance imaging of renal artery stenosis: a multireader tricenter study. *J Am Soc Nephrol.* 2002;13:158-169.

365. Soulez G, Oliva VL, Turpin S, et al. Imaging of renovascular hypertension: respective values of renal scintigraphy, renal Doppler US, and MR angiography. *Radiographics.* 2000;20:1355-1368.

366. Bude RO, Forauer AR, Caoili EM, et al. Is it necessary to study accessory arteries when screening the renal arteries for renovascular hypertension? *Radiology.* 2003;226:411-416.

367. Wilson GJ, Hoogeveen RM, Willinek WA, et al. Parellel imaging in MR angiography. *Top Magn Reson Imaging.* 2004;15:169-185.

368. Gutberlet M, Noeske R, Schwinge K, et al. Comprehensive cardiac magnetic resonance imaging at 3.0 tesla: feasibility and implications for clinical applications. *Invest Radiol.* 2006;41:154-167.

369. Chen Q, Quijano CV, Mai VM, et al. On improving temporal and spatial resolution of 3D contrast-enhanced body MR angiography with parallel imaging. *Radiology.* 2004;231:893-899.

370. de Haan MW, van Engelshoven JMA, Houben AJHM, et al. Phase-contrast magnetic resonance flow quantification in renal arteries comparison with 133 xenon washout measurements. *Hypertension.* 2003;41:114-118.

371. Schoenberg SO, Knopp MV, Londy F, et al. Morphologic and functional magnetic resonance imaging of renal artery stenosis: a multireader tricenter study. *J Am Soc Nephrol.* 2002;13:158-169.

372. Michaely HJ, Schoenberg SO, Oesingmann N, et al. Renal artery stenosis: functional assessment with dynamic MR perfusion measurements—feasibility study. *Radiology.* 2006;238:586-596.

373. van den Dool SW, Wasser MN, de Fijter JW, et al. Functional renal volume: quantitative analysis at gadolinium-enhanced MR angiography—feasibility study in healthy potential kidney donors. *Radiology.* 2005;236:189-195.

374. Spuentrup E, Ruebben A, Stuber M, et al. Metallic renal artery MR imaging stent: artifact-free lumen visualization with projection and standard renal MR angiography. *Radiology.* 2003;227:897-902.

375. Nally Jr JV, Black HR. State-of-the-art review: captopril renography—pathophysiological considerations and clinical observations. *Semin Nucl Med.* 1992;22:85-97.

376. Taylor A, Nally J, Aurell M, et al. Consensus report on ACE inhibitor renography for detecting renovascular hypertension. Radionuclides in Nephrourology Group. Consensus Group on ACEI Renography. *J Nucl Med.* 1996;37:1876-1882.

377. Taylor Jr AT, Fletcher JW, Nally Jr JV, et al. Procedure guideline for diagnosis of renovascular hypertension. Society of Nuclear Medicine. *J Nucl Med.* 1998;39:1297-1302.

378. Nally Jr JV, Chen C, Fine E, et al. Diagnostic criteria of renovascular hypertension with captopril renography: a consensus statement. *Am J Hypertens.* 1991;4:749S-752S.

379. Fine EJ. Interventions in renal scintigraphy. *Semin Nucl Med.* 1999;29:128-145.

380. Llach F, Papper S, Massey SG. The clinical spectrum of renal vein thrombosis: acute and chronic. *Am J Med.* 1980;69:819-827.

381. Witz M, Kantarovsky A, Baruch M, et al. Renal vein occlusion: a review. *J Urol.* 1996;155:1173-1179.

382. Llach F, Koffler A, Finck E, et al. On the incidence of renal vein thrombosis in the nephrotic syndrome. *Arch Intern Med.* 1977;137:333-336.

383. Gatewood OMB, Fishman EK, Burrow CR, et al. Renal vein thrombosis in patients with nephrotic syndrome: CT diagnosis. *Radiology.* 1986;159:117-122.

384. Sebastia C, Quiroga S, Boye R, et al. Helical CT in renal transplantation: normal findings and early and late complications. *Radiographics.* 2001;21:1103-1117.

385. Brown ED, Chen MYM, Wolfman NT, et al. Complications of renal transplantation: evaluation with US and radionuclide imaging. *Radiographics.* 2000;20:607-622.

386. Letourneau JG, Day DL, Ascher NL, et al. Perspective. Imaging of renal transplants. *AJR Am J Roentgenol.* 1988;150:833-838.

387. Kelcz F, Pozniak MA, Pirsch JD, et al. Pyramidal appearance and resistive index: insensitive and nonspecific sonographic indicators of renal transplant rejection. *AJR Am J Roentgenol.* 1990;155:531-535.

388. Smith PA, Ratner LE, Lynch FC, et al. Role of CT angiography in the preoperative evaluation for laparoscopic nephrectomy. *Radiographics.* 1998;18:589-601.

389. Holden A, Smith A, Dukes P, et al. Assessment of 100 live potential renal donors for laparoscopic nephrectomy with multi-detector row helical CT. *Radiology.* 2005;237:973-980.

390. Rydberg J, Kopecky KK, Tann M, et al. Evaluation of prospective living renal donors for laparoscopic nephrectomy with multisection CT: the marriage of minimally invasive imaging with minimally invasive surgery. *Radiographics.* 2001;21:S223-S236.

391. Kawamoto S, Montgomery R, Lawler LP, et al. Multi-detector row CT evaluation of living renal donors prior to laparoscopic nephrectomy. *Radiographics.* 2003;24:1513-1514.

392. Hofmann LV, Smith PA, Kuszyk BS, et al. Original report. Three-dimensional helical CT angiography in renal transplant recipients: a new problem-solving tool. *AJR Am J Roentgenol.* 1999;173:1085-1089.

393. Pozniak MA, Balison DJ, Lee FT, et al. CT angiography of potential renal transplant donors. *Radiographics.* 1998;18:565-587.

394. Kawamoto S, Lawler LP, Fishman EK. Evaluation of the renal venous system on late arterial and venous phase images with MDCT angiography in potential living laparoscopic renal donors. *AJR Am J Roentgenol.* 2005;184:539-545.

395. Sahani DV, Rastogi N, Greenfield AC, et al. Multi-detector row CT in evaluation of 94 living renal donors by readers with varied experience. *Radiology.* 2005;235:905-910.

396. Rubin GD. Invited commentary. Helical CT of potential living renal donors: toward a greater understanding. *Radiographics.* 1998;18:601-604.

397. Hohenwalter MD, Skowlund CJ, Erickson SJ, et al. Renal transplant evaluation with MR angiography and MR imaging. *Radiographics.* 2001;21:1505-1517.

398. Hussain SM, Kock MCJM, Ifzermans JNM, et al. MR imaging: A "one-stop shop" modality for preoperative evaluation of potential living kidney donors. *Radiographics.* 2003;23:505-520.

399. Israel GM, Lee VS, Edye M, et al. Comprehensive MR imaging in the preoperative evaluation of living donor candidates for laparoscopic nephrectomy: initial experience. *Radiology.* 2002;225:427-432.

400. Van den Dool SW, Wasser MN, de Fijter JW, et al. Functional renal volume: quantitative analysis at gadolinium-enhanced MR angiography—feasibility study in healthy potential kidney donors. *Radiology.* 2005;236:189-195.

401. Akbar SA, Jafri ZH, Amendola MA, et al. Complications of renal transplantation. *Radiographics.* 2005;25:1335-1356.

402. Allen KS, Jorkasky DK, Arger PH, et al. Renal allografts: prospective analysis of Doppler sonography. *Radiology.* 1998;169:371-376.

403. Grant EG, Perrella RR. Commentary. Wishing won't make it so: duplex Doppler sonography in the evaluation of renal transplant dysfunction. *AJR Am J Roentgenol.* 1990;155:538-539.

404. Reuther G, Wanjura D, Bauer H. Acute renal vein thrombosis in renal allografts: detection with duplex Doppler US. *Radiology.* 1989;170:557-558.

405. Buckley AR, Cooperberg PL, Reeve CE, et al. The distinction between acute renal transplant rejection and cyclosporine nephrotoxicity: value of duplex sonography. *AJR Am J Roentgenol.* 1987;149:521-525.

406. Kaveggia LP, Perrella RR, Grant EG, et al. Duplex Doppler sonography in renal allografts: the significance of reversed flow in diastole. *AJR Am J Roentgenol.* 1990;155:295-298.

407. Voegeli DR, Crummy AB, McDermott JC, et al. Percutaneous management of the urological complications of renal transplantation. *Radiographics.* 1986;6:1007-1022.

408. Patel NH, Jindal RM, Wilkin T, et al. Renal arterial stenosis in renal allografts: retrospective study of predisposing factors and outcome after percutaneous transluminal angioplasty. *Radiology.* 2001;219:663-667.

409. Vrachliotis TG, Vaswani KK, Davies EA, et al. Pictorial essay. CT findings in posttransplantation lymphoproliferative disorder of renal transplants. *AJR Am J Roentgenol.* 2000;175:183-188.

410. Dubovsky EV, Russell CD, Erbas B. Radionuclide evaluation of renal transplants. *Semin Nucl Med.* 1995;25:49-59.

411. Dunagin P, Alijani M, Atkins F, et al. Application of the kidney to aortic blood flow index to renal transplants. *Clin Nucl Med.* 1983;8:360-364.

412. Lin E, Alavi A. Significance of early tubular extraction in the first minute of Tc-99m MAG3 renal transplant scintigraphy. *Clin Nucl Med.* 1998;23:217-222.

413. Fortenbery EJ, Blue PW, Van Nostrand D, et al. Lymphocele: The spectrum of scintigraphic findings in lymphoceles associated with renal transplant. *J Nucl Med.* 1990;31:1627-1631.

414. Reuter S, Schnockel U, Schroter O, et al. Noninvasive imaging of acute renal allograft rejection in rats using small FDG PET. *PLoS One.* 2009;4:e5296.

The Renal Biopsy

Alan D. Salama and H. Terence Cook

The renal biopsy has become a fundamental component in the management of renal disease. Prior to its routine use, only autopsy material was available to investigate the pathophysiology of kidney disease, which limited antemortem diagnosis. However, its development and refinement since the late 1950s has been fundamental for the diagnosis and definition of clinical syndromes and the discovery of new pathologic entities.[1] Through the critical analysis of renal biopsy specimens taken at different disease time points, key pathophysiologic features of kidney disease have been discovered, which have in turn helped to establish new paradigms in nephrology, and have led to considerable alterations in patient management. This is true for biopsies of both native kidneys and renal transplants.[2] In addition, much is still being learned regarding disease pathogenesis through the study of renal biopsy material, which not only remains a gold standard for disease diagnosis, but has allowed the development of novel biopsy markers, which have revolutionized our concepts of pathologic mechanisms.

The first percutaneous kidney biopsies were performed over 50 years ago using a liver biopsy needle and intravenous pyelograms for screening, with the patient either sitting or supine. The success of these biopsies in obtaining renal tissue and in aiding management confirmed the benefit of the procedure.[1] Many innovations, including the use of real-time ultrasonography that allows visualization of the needle entering the kidney, spring-loaded needles[3] or needle holders, and careful preoperative evaluation of the patient, have improved the success rate in obtaining renal tissue while minimizing the risks of the procedure.[4] As a result, percutaneous renal biopsy has been placed at the very center of modern clinical nephrology.

There are numerous indications for renal biopsy (Table 28-1), but the threshold for acting on these indications varies among individual centers. For example, if all cases of microscopic hematuria are investigated, a large number of cases of immunoglobulin A (IgA) nephropathy and thin basement membrane lesion are likely to be diagnosed, and the threshold for performing biopsy in patients with diabetes influences the number of biopsy specimens demonstrating diabetic nephropathy. The range of diagnoses for a group of 1666 native kidney biopsies and 1458 transplant biopsies performed at the authors' institution over the last 4 years is shown in Figure 28-1.

Safety and Complications of Biopsies

Although renal biopsy is generally considered safe, there is morbidity and a measurable mortality associated with the procedure, and therefore it is imperative to subject to the procedure only those patients who will derive a potential benefit that offsets those risks. The significant complications related to the procedure are hemorrhage, development of arteriovenous fistulas, and to a lesser extent sepsis.[5-7] Bleeding with macroscopic hematuria and the development of perinephric hematomas may be minor and self-resolving or major and require intervention in the form of blood transfusions, embolization, or rarely surgery. Arteriovenous fistulas may be asymptomatic and resolve spontaneously or may lead to a significant vascular steal syndrome that compromises the rest of the kidney through ischemia. Finally, there is a risk of sepsis following the procedure through the introduction of a septic focus or its dissemination.

Overall, the risks of complication vary from center to center, but can be estimated to be between 3.5% and 13%; the majority (approximately 3% to 9%) are minor complications.[5-7] In addition, there is the chance that an inadequate core will be obtained for diagnosis, containing too few glomeruli or insufficient cortical material, and this is reported in 1% and 5% of cases. The specimen size requirements for accurate diagnosis are discussed later.

Mortality from the procedure is generally a result of undiagnosed bleeding with significant hematoma formation and was reported in up to 0.2% of cases in some of the larger biopsy series,[6,7] although recent studies suggest that it is an extremely rare adverse event.[4] Some degree of bleeding is common, with approximately half of patients showing a drop in hemoglobin level after biopsy and a third developing some hematoma, but bleeding is significant and requires intervention in only a minority (up to 7%).[4,7,8]

Complications appear to be more common in biopsies of native than of transplant kidneys, and in patients with more advanced renal impairment, prolonged bleeding times, or lower hemoglobin levels (11 ± 2 vs. 12 ± 2 g/dL).[6,7] One prospective study identified the only risk factors for bleeding complications as female gender, younger age (35 ± 14.5 years vs. 40.3 ± 15.4 years), and prolonged partial thromboplastin time.[9] Interestingly, in another investigation needle size, number of passes, blood pressure, and renal impairment did not differ for those with bleeding complications and those without. In this study, however, all patients with prolonged bleeding times received desmopressin (DDAVP) to correct the abnormality, and 75% of patients had serum creatinine values of less than 132 μmol. Conversely, other investigators using retrospective

TABLE 28-1 Indications for Renal Biopsy

Significant proteinuria (>1 g/day or equivalent spot protein/creatinine ratio)

Microscopic hematuria with any degree of proteinuria

Unexplained renal impairment (native or transplanted kidney)

Renal manifestations of systemic disease

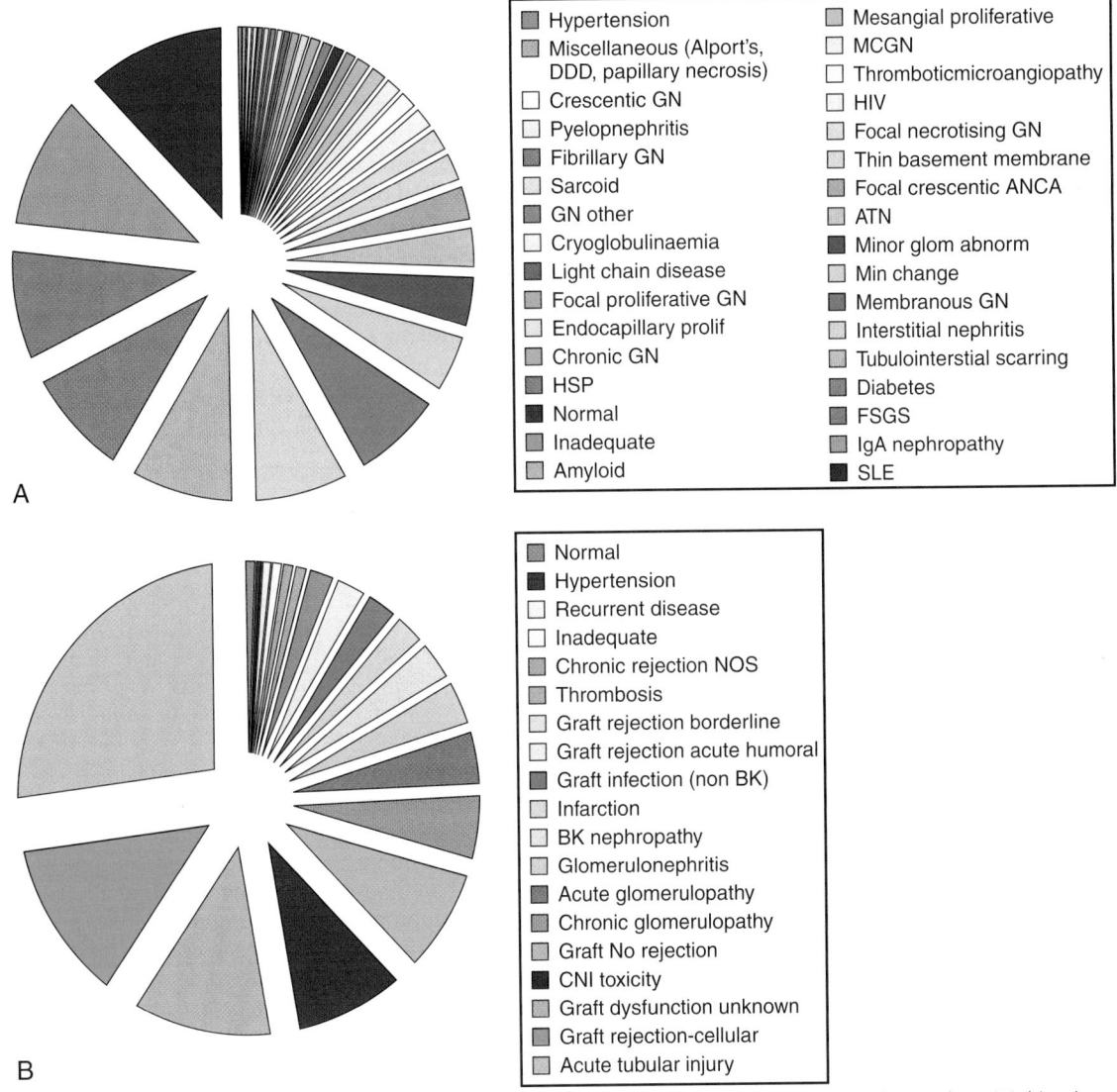

FIGURE 28-1 Proportion of various diagnoses for specimens from 1666 native kidney (**A**) and 1458 renal transplant (**B**) biopsies performed at Hammersmith Hospital over a 4-year period. BK, BK virus infection; CNI, calcineurin inhibitor damage; DDD, dense deposit disease; HSP, Henoch-Schönlein purpura; NOS, not otherwise specified.

univariate analysis have reported that a blood pressure higher than 160/100 mm Hg or a serum creatinine level of more than 2 mg/dL more than doubled the risk of bleeding.[7,10]

Overall, no effective means has been established to identify those individuals at risk of developing clinically significant complications. In one small series, however, the results of ultrasonography performed within an hour after biopsy had a 95% negative predictive value for predicting clinically significant hemorrhagic complications,[8] so that the absence of a hematoma on the postbiopsy scan was very suggestive of an uncomplicated clinical course. Debate continues regarding the benefit of estimation of bleeding time or the routine use of DDAVP to improve uremic bleeding tendencies, and many units have abandoned these practices. In part this is because studies have suggested that complication rates are no different when bleeding time estimation is omitted from the preoperative assessment,[11,12] that when it is measured it does not predict clinical complications,[9] and that DDAVP should be reserved only for those patients with prolonged bleeding times.

There are certain absolute contraindications that preclude percutaneous biopsy, whereas there are a number of relative contraindications (Table 28-2) that may be circumvented depending on the importance of the biopsy, the operator's experience, and the supportive facilities available. Ideally, all efforts should be made to deal with the relative contraindications; however, in the context of acute renal failure this may not always be possible. The critical preoperative steps are to ensure that blood pressure is controlled, that the patient does not have a bleeding diathesis or a urinary tract infection, and that the kidneys are suitably imaged and show no evidence of obstruction, widespread cystic disease, or malignancy (although percutaneous biopsy is increasingly used to determine the nature of renal masses).

Preoperative assessment should allow those patients unsuitable for percutaneous biopsy to be referred for an alternative approach (Figure 28-2). For these patients, there are other means of obtaining renal tissue, including open biopsy,[13] laparoscopic biopsy, or transjugular biopsy.[14] Each is associated with certain complications and has particular merits depending on the clinical situation (Table 28-3). Overall, these approaches are generally required for only a minority of potential biopsy patients.

The safe duration of observation following renal biopsy has been investigated in a number of studies. Findings suggest that early discharge (after only 4 hours of observation) will result in a number of missed complications, with many more occurring between 8 and 24 hours after the procedure. Even after 8 hours of observation, 23% to 33% of complications will be missed. However, an overnight stay will allow an extra 20% of complications to be identified before discharge,

with between 85% and 95% of complications being identified at 12 hours and 89% to 98% after 24-hour observation.[7,15] Some units practice a policy of performing day biopsies with a minimum 6-hour bed rest period, which is extended only if there is evidence of bleeding. Vigilant observation of blood pressure and pulse rate, and monitoring for evidence of hematuria is required in all cases.

Performing the Biopsy

After informed consent is obtained, the patient is positioned prone for biopsy of a native kidney and supine for biopsy of a renal transplant. A posterolateral approach is used for biopsies of native kidneys. The procedure is performed under sterile conditions with disposable sterile ultrasonic probe covers allowing real-time ultrasonographic visualization of the kidneys. The procedure is generally performed with the patient under light sedation and with local anesthesia. The lower pole of the left kidney is commonly the biopsy site, but the kidney that is best visualized and most accessible is preferable.

A small incision is made in the skin to accommodate the biopsy needle, which is advanced until it reaches the renal capsule. The patient is asked to hold the breath, and the needle mechanism is engaged. Most operators now prefer to use spring-loaded Tru-Cut needles or Biopty guns. Needle size varies from 14 gauge to 18 gauge, with many using 16 gauge as a compromise between obtaining a larger core and increasing the risk of bleeding. Two cores are taken, which should be divided for different assessments as outlined later. In high-risk patients the needle track may be plugged following the procedure with appropriate material such as Gelfoam. In such cases, the biopsy is performed using a coaxial introducer needle, and after biopsy the track is plugged during removal of the coaxial introducer needle.

After the procedure vital signs are monitored carefully to detect early signs of bleeding, and all urine is dipstick tested for blood.

Biopsy Specimen Handling

Detailed descriptions of methods of handling biopsy specimens can be found in a number of publications, including Churg and colleagues,[16] Furness,[17] and Walker and colleagues.[18] A full assessment of the renal biopsy specimen requires examination by light microscopy, immunohistochemical methods, and electron microscopy (EM), and other tests are used in some circumstances. Therefore it is necessary for the biopsy specimen to be divided to provide material for each of these methods of examination. During this process it is extremely important that the biopsy specimen not be damaged by handling or by drying, and that the tissue be fixed using an appropriate fixative as quickly as possible, ideally within minutes. This is best achieved by dividing the biopsy specimen at the bedside.

Examination of the biopsy specimen with a dissecting microscope allows cortex, containing glomeruli, to be distinguished from medulla and thus facilitates assessment of the adequacy of the cores and division of the biopsy material so that glomeruli are present in the samples for each modality of examination. If a dissecting microscope is not available then a

TABLE 28-2 Contraindications to Percutaneous Renal Biopsy	
ABSOLUTE CONTRAINDICATIONS	**RELATIVE CONTRAINDICATIONS**
Uncontrolled hypertension	Single kidney
Bleeding diathesis	Antiplatelet or anticoagulant therapy
Widespread cystic disease or renal malignancy	Anatomic abnormalities
Hydronephrosis	Small kidneys
Uncooperative patient	Active urinary or skin sepsis
	Obesity

standard light microscope can be used with the biopsy specimen placed in a drop of normal saline on a microscope slide. If it is not possible to examine the biopsy specimen in this way, then a standard approach to obtain material for EM is to take small fragments (approximately 1 mm in length) from each end of each core. In that way if there is cortex in the core glomeruli should be sampled. The remainder of the cores can then be divided for light microscopy and for immunofluorescent testing. The part of the biopsy specimen for light microscopy is then placed in appropriate fixative and that for immunofluorescent testing is either snap frozen or transported to the laboratory in a suitable transport medium such as that described by Michel and colleagues[19]; tissue placed in this medium can remain at room temperature for several days without loss of antigens.

During division of the biopsy specimen it is important not to introduce artifacts due to crushing or stretching. Forceps should not be used to pick up the specimen; this can be done

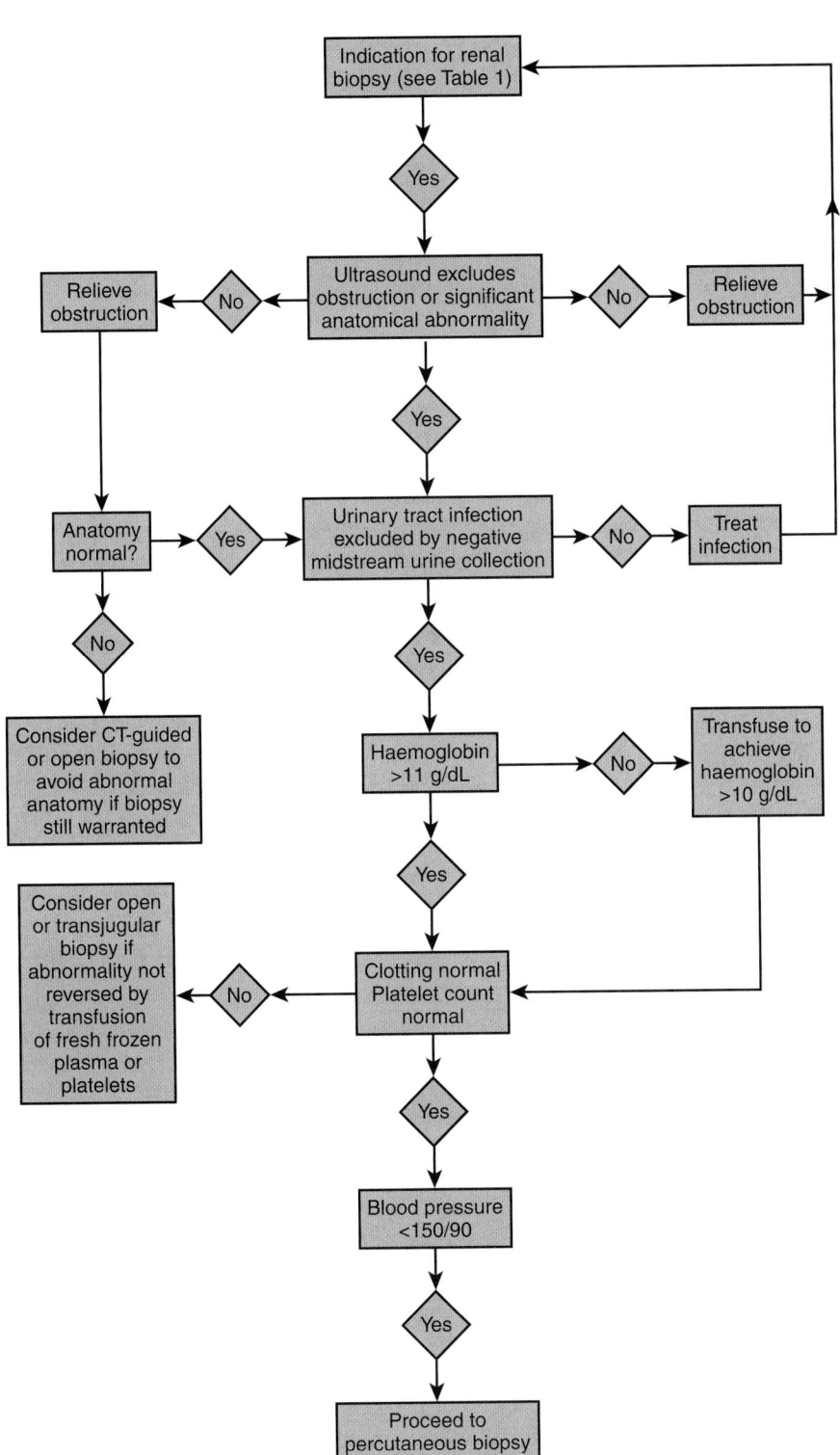

FIGURE 28-2 Indication for renal biopsy (see Table 28-1).

TABLE 28-3 Alternative Methods for Obtaining Renal Tissue and Their Risks and Benefits Compared with a Percutaneous Approach

METHOD	ADVANTAGES	DISADVANTAGES
Transjugular approach	Can be useful in those with a bleeding diathesis and in patients receiving artificial ventilation or if combined liver and renal biopsy is required	Carries risk of capsular perforation Inadequate material retrieved in up to 24%
Open approach	Provides high yield of adequate tissue Hemostasis is more secure	Requires general or spinal anaesthesia; recovery period is longer
Laparoscopic approach	Provides high yield of adequate tissue Hemostasis is more secure	Requires general or spinal anaesthesia; recovery period is longer

using either a needle or a small wooden stick such as a toothpick. The biopsy material should be cut using a fresh scalpel. If the biopsy specimen has to be taken to the histology laboratory for division, this should be done as quickly as possible with the specimen wrapped in saline-moistened gauze or in tissue culture medium. Artifacts may be produced if the biopsy material is placed on dry gauze or gauze moistened with water, or if it is placed in ice-cold saline.

If the amount of material obtained at biopsy is limited then it may be necessary to adapt the way in which it is divided, and the decision as to how this is done must depend on the clinical question. In most cases it is possible to omit frozen material for immunofluorescent testing and instead perform immunohistochemical analysis on paraffin sections. If there is suspicion of crescentic glomerulonephritis due to anti–glomerular basement membrane (anti-GBM) disease, however, immunofluorescence is more reliable for detecting the linear capillary wall staining. It may be possible to omit EM and perform it if necessary on material reprocessed from the paraffin block, but if this is done it is not possible to obtain accurate measurements of glomerular capillary membrane thickness.[20]

Light Microscopy

The most commonly used fixative for light microscopy is buffered 10% aqueous formaldehyde solution. This is actually a 10% solution of the 37% commercially available concentrated solution of formaldehyde, which gives a final concentration of about 4%. This fixative is generally available in all histology laboratories, provides adequate fixation for light microscopy, and also allows the tissue to be used for immunohistochemical assay and EM.

Some more specialized fixatives such as Bouin's or Zenker's fixative provide better preservation of certain morphologic details, but in general the problems with handling these fixatives and the difficulties of subsequently using the material for immunohistochemical assay or EM outweigh the advantages. For example, Bouin's fixative contains picric acid, which is explosive when dry. However, Bouin's fixative is commonly

used for examination of mouse kidneys, for which the improvement in glomerular morphology is significant. Methacarn, a modified Carnoy's fixative, also provides good fixation for light microscopy and EM and may allow the immunohistochemical detection of antigens that are not detected in formalin-fixed tissue.

Details of the preparation of various fixatives can be found in the appendix of Churg and colleagues.[16] The standard method of processing tissue for light microscopy is by dehydrating in graded alcohols, transferring to a clearing agent such as xylene, and embedding in paraffin wax. This is usually performed by an automated instrument but can be done by hand. Rapid processing schedules allow for same-day processing, and it is possible to obtain stained slides within 3 to 4 hours of receipt of the specimen in the laboratory.

It is important to have thin, uniform sections for light microscopy. These should be cut as thin as possible—no more than 3 μm. It is often stated that renal biopsy sections should be cut at 2 μm, but this may lead to problems in cutting with damage to the tissue. Because many pathologic lesions may be focal within glomeruli, interstitium, or vessels, it is essential that the biopsy specimen be examined at multiple levels, and each laboratory will have its preferred way to achieve that. In general, serial sections should be cut with at least two placed on each slide. Multiple slides can then be stained with each stain, with some intervening unstained sections kept either for potential immunohistochemical examination or for staining with other special stains as necessary.

Staining for Light Microscopy

Most renal pathologists employ a number of stains for light microscopy. The commonly used stains are hematoxylin and eosin (H&E), periodic acid–Schiff (PAS), silver methenamine, and a trichrome stain. The H&E stain is a good general histologic stain for studying the overall architecture of the kidney. It is good for studying the morphology of tubular cells and the morphology of interstitial infiltrates. With experience the different staining characteristics of hyaline, fibrin and amyloid, all of which are eosinophilic, can usually be distinguished. However, the H&E stain does not distinguish glomerular matrix and basement membrane from cell cytoplasm, and therefore it is less useful for the assessment of glomerular architecture.

In the PAS reaction the mesangial matrix and basement membrane are stained purple, and this allows a good assessment of the amount of matrix and the thickness of the GBM. PAS also stains the tubular basement membranes and hyaline deposits. The silver methenamine stain is the best stain for studying the detailed morphology of the GBM and for highlighting the membrane spikes seen in membranous glomerulonephritis and the double contours seen in membranoproliferative glomerulonephritis. Its only drawback is that obtaining a satisfactory result is more technically demanding than the other stains. A trichrome stain, such as Masson's trichrome, stains the glomerular mesangial matrix and basement membrane and may also help in highlighting fibrin and immune complex deposits.

Other stains are a matter of personal preference. The authors always use an elastin stain to demonstrate the elastic laminae of vessels, and this preparation is counterstained with picrosirius red to stain fibrillar collagen in the interstitium. Amyloid is most specifically detected using a Congo red stain, and the authors feel it is prudent to perform this staining for all native kidney biopsy specimens. This is the exception to the requirement for thin sections; because the Congo red stain is relatively insensitive, a section cut at 10 μm should be used. Details of staining methods are given in the appendix of Churg and colleagues.[16] Other stains that may be employed when necessary include von Kossa's stain, which demonstrates calcium deposition, and Perl's Prussian blue stain for iron.

Examination of the Biopsy Specimen by Light Microscopy

It is important to approach the examination of the biopsy specimen systematically. Sections should first be assessed at low power to determine what parts of the kidney (or other structures in some cases) they contain, including whether there is cortex and/or medulla. A low-power view will also allow an assessment of the amount of chronic nephron damage, as demonstrated by tubular atrophy and interstitial fibrosis, and the presence of interstitial inflammatory infiltrates. It will also allow an assessment of interstitial expansion, most commonly caused by either edema or fibrosis, but occasionally due to infiltration by, for example, amyloid. Examination should then proceed by studying the glomeruli, tubules, interstitium, and vessels, including arteries, arterioles, and veins, in more detail. Features that should be looked for in glomeruli and tubules are detailed in Tables 28-4 and 28-5 respectively. Arterioles should be examined for the presence of hyalinosis, thrombosis, and necrosis. Arteries should be assessed to determine whether intimal thickening is present and whether it is accompanied by reduplication of the internal elastic lamina, thrombosis, necrosis, inflammation, and cholesterol emboli.

Terminology for Description of Glomerular Disease

The involvement of glomeruli by a pathologic process can be described in terms of what percentage of glomeruli are involved by a lesion and whether the lesion involves all or only part of any individual glomerulus. A lesion that involves all or nearly all glomeruli is described as *diffuse*, whereas one that involves some but not all glomeruli is described as *focal*. In the definitions given in the World Health Organization atlas of glomerular diseases it was suggested that the cutoff for focal versus diffuse should be 80% of glomerular involvement. In recent classifications of lupus glomerulonephritis[21] and IgA nephropathy,[22] however, the cutoff is specified as 50%.

If a lesion involves only part of a glomerulus (i.e., some capillary lumens remain uninvolved), it is called *segmental*, whereas if it involves the whole glomerulus it is called *global*. In the classifications of lupus glomerulonephritis[21] and IgA nephropathy,[22] the cutoff is set at 50% glomerular tuft involvement except for segmental sclerosis in IgA nephropathy, in which any area of sclerosis that leaves some of the glomerulus unaffected is defined as segmental.

A number of other terms, such as *sclerosis* and *hyalinosis*, have specific definitions with regard to the glomerulus, and these are listed in Table 28-6.

TABLE 28-4 Features to Be Assessed by Light Microscopy in Glomeruli

Size

Cellularity: If increased, then are the extra cells mesangial, in capillary lumens (endocapillary), or in Bowman's space? (Normal mesangial areas contain two or three cells.)

Capillary wall thickness (use periodic acid–Schiff or silver stain): If thickened, are double contours or spikes seen on the silver-stain section?

Is the mesangium expanded? If so, are there nodules?

Is there deposition of abnormal material (e.g., amyloid)?

Is there segmental sclerosis?

Is there thrombosis?

Is there necrosis?

TABLE 28-5 Features to Be Assessed by Light Microscopy in Tubules

Percentage of atrophy

Signs of acute damage (e.g., dilatation, epithelial flattening, granular casts, mitoses)

Tubulitis

Casts: granular casts suggest acute tubular injury; eosinophilic fractured casts suggest myeloma; neutrophil casts suggest acute pyelonephritis

Crystals (e.g., oxalate)

Viral inclusions (e.g., BK virus)

TABLE 28-6 Definitions of Terms Used in Describing Glomerular Lesions

Sclerosis: lesion resulting from an increase in mesangial matrix and/or collapse and condensation of the basement membranes; the sclerotic material stains with eosin, PAS, and silver stains.

Hyalinosis: lesion containing an acellular structureless material consisting of glycoproteins and sometimes lipids; stains intensely with eosin and PAS but not with silver stains.

Fibrosis: lesion consisting of collagen fibers, which may be differentiated from sclerosis by failure to stain with PAS reagent or silver stains.

Necrosis: lesion characterized by fragmentation of nuclei and/or disruption of the basement membrane, often associated with the presence of fibrin-rich material.

Extracapillary proliferation or cellular crescent: extracapillary cell proliferation of more than two cell layers with >50% of the lesion occupied by cells.

Extracapillary fibrocellular proliferation or fibrocellular crescent: extracapillary lesion composed of cells and extracellular matrix, with <50% cells and <90% matrix.

Extracapillary fibrosis or fibrous crescent: >10% of the circumference of Bowman's capsule covered by a lesion composed of >90% matrix.

PAS, Periodic acid–Schiff stain.

Immunohistochemical Assay

The understanding of renal pathology was transformed in the 1960s by the use of immunofluorescence microscopy. This allowed the detection and localization of immunoglobulins and complement components in glomeruli, and the identification of new entities such as IgA nephropathy. It is mandatory to perform immunohistochemical testing for a full assessment of glomerular pathology in biopsy specimens from native kidneys. The use of immunohistochemical testing in transplant biopsy specimens is discussed further later.

There are a number of diagnoses that cannot be made without immunohistochemical assay, including IgA nephropathy, C1q nephropathy, anti–GBM disease, and light-chain deposition disease. In native kidneys a minimum panel of immunohistochemical stains would include antibodies for IgA, IgG, IgM, C3c, and κ and λ light chains. Light-chain immunohistochemical assay is very important if diagnoses such as light-chain deposition disease and monoclonal immunoglobulin deposition disease are not to be missed. Many pathologists would add antibodies for C1q, C4c, and fibrinogen to this routine panel. In transplant kidney biopsy specimens staining for C4d is invaluable in assessing the activation of the classical pathway of complement by antibody and hence in the diagnosis of antibody-mediated rejection.

There are a number of other antigens whose detection may be useful in particular circumstances. These include the following:

1. Microorganisms, including BK virus, cytomegalovirus, and Epstein-Barr virus.
2. Amyloid proteins. Antibodies are available to AA amyloid and many of the rarer inherited forms of amyloid.
3. α-Chains of type IV collagen. In suspected hereditary nephropathy of the Alport type it may be helpful to stain for the α3 and α5 chains of type IV collagen
4. IgG subclasses in cases of suspected monoclonal immunoglobulin deposition.
5. Myoglobin in suspected myoglobinuria.
6. Lymphocyte surface antigens, particularly in cases of suspected lymphoid neoplasia.
7. Type III collagen in collagenofibrotic glomerulopathy.
8. Fibronectin in fibronectin glomerulopathy.

Immunohistochemical testing is performed either on cryostat sections of a piece of snap-frozen tissue or on paraffin sections. Antigen detection on frozen sections is usually performed using an antibody labeled with a fluorochrome, and this preparation is then viewed using a fluorescence microscope—a technique commonly referred to as *immunofluorescence* or *IF*. The use of fluorescence-labeled antibodies on frozen sections is technically straightforward and very sensitive since the antigens have not been altered by fixation. There are some drawbacks, however. First, a separate piece of tissue must be obtained at the time of biopsy. Second, the morphology of frozen sections is never as good as that of paraffin sections, and so it may be more difficult to define the site of the antigen within the glomerulus. In addition immunofluorescent sections fade over time, but if they are appropriately mounted and refrigerated in the dark they will retain the staining for weeks to months.

If paraffin sections are used, then some form of antigen retrieval is essential for most antigens, because they become masked during fixation and processing. For the detection of immunoglobulins and complement the antigen retrieval method that works best is some form of protease digestion. The length of time required for protease digestion is critically dependent on a number of factors such as the length of time the biopsy specimen has been in fixative and the particular processing schedule used. Some of these factors may be difficult to control. This variability of the antigen retrieval process is the major drawback of immunohistochemical analysis of paraffin sections and means that results are highly dependent on the skills of the technician performing the staining.

After the antigen retrieval step, antigens are generally detected using a primary antibody followed by a detection system that leads to the deposition of a colored reaction product that is visible by light microscopy. Commonly this product is developed by a reaction that utilizes the enzyme horseradish peroxidase, and hence this method is often referred to as *immunoperoxidase staining*. However, it is also possible to use fluorescent antibody staining on paraffin sections after antigen retrieval.[23]

The major advantage of performing immunohistochemical analysis on paraffin sections is that it is not necessary to take a separate piece of tissue for frozen section. In addition it is possible to specifically localize antigens and compare these sections with adjacent sections examined by light microscopy. However, the procedure is technically demanding and also is significantly less sensitive for some antigens. The authors' experience is that it is extremely difficult to obtain satisfactory staining for light chains using peroxidase techniques on paraffin sections (although fluorescence techniques on paraffin sections may be more successful) and that detection of the linear capillary wall staining of anti-GBM antibodies is more difficult in paraffin sections. It may also be more difficult to detect very early deposits in membranous glomerulonephritis in paraffin sections than in frozen tissue.

In the authors' experience most renal pathologists find immunofluorescent testing on frozen sections to be the most satisfactory way to detect immunoglobulins and complement, but regardless of preference, there will always be cases in which no material is available for frozen section or the material is inadequate, and so laboratories should also be competent to carry out immunohistochemical analysis on paraffin sections. In reporting immunohistochemical staining for immunoglobulins and complement it is important to describe the site of staining in the glomerulus (e.g., mesangial or capillary wall), its nature (e.g., whether linear, finely or coarsely granular), and its intensity. For estimation of intensity most pathologists rely on a semiquantitative subjective scale ranging from 0 to 3+, but formal quantitation by image analysis may be useful for research. Staining should be assessed not only in the glomerulus but also in the tubules, particularly the tubular basement membrane, interstitium, and vessels.

Electron Microscopy

EM is invaluable for assessing structural changes in the glomerulus and for identifying immune complexes, which are seen as areas of electron density. Although the importance of EM has become much reduced in other areas of surgical pathology, because of the development of immunohistochemical assays, it remains an invaluable technique for the examination of glomeruli in biopsy specimens from in native kidneys and, increasingly, for the determination of causes of dysfunction in transplanted kidneys.

The part of the renal biopsy specimen on which EM is to be performed is usually placed in separate fixative, although entirely satisfactory results can be obtained using material fixed in formalin. Most laboratories prefer either ice-cold glutaraldehyde or paraformaldehyde. The material is then exposed to osmium tetroxide and processed into resin blocks. To select the areas to be studied, "semithin" 0.5 μm sections are first screened by light microscopy to select areas of interest that can then be examined further using the electron microscope. An ultramicrotome is then used to obtain the very thin sections required for the electron microscope. A permanent record of the electron microscopic images is kept either as photographs or, increasingly, as digital files.

As with light microscopy, examination of the biopsy specimen by EM should be systematic, with assessment of the glomerular capillary basement membrane and its thickness; the endothelium, with note of any thickening or loss of fenestrations; the capillary lumen, and particularly any narrowing by cells or other material; and the podocytes, with particular attention to the preservation of the foot processes and any vacuolation or microvillous change in the cell bodies. The presence of any electron-dense deposits—most commonly due to immune complex deposition—should be noted, together with their distribution—mesangial, subendothelial, or subepithelial. EM may also demonstrate a number of other structures, such as fibrils in amyloidosis or fibrillary glomerulonephritis, tubules in immunotactoid glomerulopathy, or the characteristic inclusion bodies of various storage diseases.

Although EM is most useful in the assessment of glomerular morphology it may also be very helpful in demonstrating ultrastructural changes in other parts of the kidney. For example, it may help in demonstrating tubular basement membrane immune complexes, in elucidating the nature of tubular epithelial cell inclusions, and in examining the morphology of mitochondria in tubular epithelial cells, which may show abnormalities in inherited conditions or as a result of drugs.

Several studies have assessed the utility of EM in the assessment of native kidney biopsy specimens. Most studies suggest that EM provides useful information in about half of all native kidney biopsy specimens and is essential for diagnosis in about 20%.[24] Because it is impossible to know which cases these are at the time of biopsy it is prudent always to have material available for EM even if, in some cases, it is not processed further after light microscopy and immunohistochemical assay. Table 28-7 shows some conditions for which EM is essential for the diagnosis and others for which it is helpful. Also listed are some conditions in which the diagnosis may be reached without EM, but even in these cases it is important to remember that EM may allow a more detailed description of the morphology of these conditions or may even reveal a totally unrelated pathology.

Morphometric analysis using EM is mainly of importance for research. However, the microscopist should be able to measure the thickness of the GBM to quantitate the thinning that may be seen in a thin basement membrane lesion or the thickening commonly seen in diabetic glomerulosclerosis. Accurate, unbiased measurement of GBM thickness requires the use of complex morphometric techniques to avoid the bias introduced by tangential sectioning of capillary loops. In practice, however, it is satisfactory to directly measure GBM thickness (distance from endothelial to podocyte plasma membrane) and to calculate the arithmetic mean of such measurements. Das and colleagues[25] found that if 16 measurements from each of two glomeruli were made using this direct

TABLE 28-7 Examples of the Use of Electron Microscopy (EM) in Diagnosing Disease in Kidney Biopsy Specimens
EM Essential for Diagnosis
Thin membrane lesion
Fibrillary glomerulopathy
Immunotactoid glomerulopathy
Alport's syndrome
Fabry's disease
Lecithin-cholesterol acetyltransferase deficiency
Nail-patella syndrome
EM Very Helpful for Diagnosis
Dense deposit disease
Minimal change disease
Early diabetic glomerulopathy
Early membranous glomerulonephritis (particularly if only paraffin sections are available for immunohistochemical analysis)
Causes of secondary membranous glomerulonephritis
Membranoproliferative glomerulonephritis
Postinfectious glomerulonephritis
Human immunodeficiency virus–associated nephropathy
Lipoprotein glomerulopathy
Collagenofibrotic glomerulopathy
Diagnosis May Be Made without EM
Immunoglobulin A nephropathy
Acute tubulointerstitial nephritis
Myeloma cast nephropathy
Pauci-immune crescentic glomerulonephritis
Amyloid disorder (although amyloid fibrils may be detected by EM when it has been missed on light microscopy)

method, the results were reproducible. Ideally each laboratory should define a normal range using this method.

Other Studies Performed on the Renal Biopsy Specimen

In addition to examination by light microscopy, immunohistochemical analysis, and EM, it may also be appropriate to consider other methods for studying the tissue. In cases of suspected infection part of the biopsy specimen may be sent for culture or for polymerase chain reaction testing for infective organisms. In biopsy specimens with lymphoid infiltrates immunoglobulin gene rearrangement studies may allow the confirmation of clonality. The chemical composition of material in the biopsy specimen—for example, crystalline material—may be determined by energy-dispersive x-ray spectroscopy.

There has been considerable interest in the possibility of extracting messenger RNA from biopsy specimens to study differences in gene expression in various pathologic conditions,[26] and to study the range of proteins in the biopsy specimen—the proteome.[27] These techniques have been applied to whole biopsy specimens or to parts of the biopsy specimen—for example, glomeruli isolated either by simple dissection under a dissecting microscope or by laser capture microdissection. At present these remain promising research techniques and do not have a clear place in routine diagnostic practice, although in the future microarray data may provide additional diagnostic information.[28] For instance, recent results from a group in Edmonton have suggested that transcript analysis of transplant kidney biopsy specimens could play a role in diagnosis of acute antibody-mediated rejection.[29]

Biopsy Specimens from Transplanted Kidneys

The handling of transplant biopsy specimens differs in some respects from that of native kidney specimens. For biopsy specimens taken to assess the cause of kidney dysfunction in the first few months after transplantation it may not be necessary to carry out immunohistochemical analysis with a full panel of antibodies to immunoglobulins and complement, or to perform EM, unless there is a clinical suspicion of glomerular disease. However, immunohistochemical assay for C4d is always helpful to assess antibody binding and complement activation on peritubular capillary endothelium. In later biopsy specimens EM is very useful in the diagnosis of chronic allograft glomerulopathy and its differentiation from recurrence of de novo glomerulonephritis. It is also helpful in identifying chronic rejection involving peritubular capillaries, which is associated with multilayering of the peritubular capillary basement membranes.[30]

Size of the Biopsy Specimen

The renal biopsy specimen is only a small sample of the renal parenchyma, and this must always be kept in mind when making inferences about the state of the whole kidney from changes seen in the biopsy specimen. Some diseases may affect the kidney only focally and therefore may be missed on biopsy (e.g., reflux nephropathy or arterial cholesterol emboli). Others may be segmental at the level of the glomerulus (e.g., focal and segmental glomerulosclerosis or pauci-immune necrotizing glomerulonephritis) and therefore the chance of detecting them will depend on how many glomeruli are present in the biopsy specimen and how many sections are examined.

Sampling is also a problem when extrapolating from the amount of disease seen in the biopsy specimen to the amount that affects the kidney. For example, if 20% of the glomeruli in a biopsy specimen have crescents, the examiner tends to assume that this is the percentage of the glomeruli in the kidney that have crescents. Because of the small size of most biopsy specimens, however, the confidence limits that can be placed on estimates of the true involvement of glomeruli are usually very wide.

An elegant mathematical description of the problems of glomerular sampling has been published by Corwin and colleagues.[31] It shows, for example, that to confidently exclude a segmental glomerular disease that is affecting about 5% of the glomeruli a biopsy specimen containing 20 glomeruli is needed. The situation is worse when one considers the problem of comparing the amount of glomerular involvement in two different biopsy specimens, a question that often arises,

for example, in patients with lupus glomerulonephritis who undergo repeat biopsies. In such a case, to confidently detect a 10% difference in glomerular involvement between two biopsy specimens would require over 100 glomeruli in each biopsy specimen. To detect differences of 25% to 40% glomerular involvement the minimum specimen size is 20 to 25 glomeruli.

For some diseases classification schemes have defined minimum sizes for biopsy specimen adequacy. Thus for lupus glomerulonephritis it is suggested that a biopsy specimen contain a minimum of 10 glomeruli.[21] In transplant biopsies a group in Banff has suggested that the requirements for biopsy specimen adequacy are 10 or more glomeruli and at least two arteries.[32] It has been shown that examining two rather than one core of tissue increases the sensitivity for the diagnosis of acute rejection from 91% to 99%.[33] In acute cellular rejection, examining slides taken at only one level rather than at three levels misses 33% of cases of intimal arteritis.[34]

Biopsy Report

The biopsy report should include a morphologic description of the biopsy specimen and an interpretation of its appearance in light of the clinical presentation. The changes seen on light microscopy, immunohistochemical assay, and EM must be integrated, and this is best done if a single person examines the biopsy specimen using each modality. The description of the light microscopic findings should include the number of glomeruli present and the number that show global or segmental sclerosis.

It is essential to provide a quantitative estimate of the amount of irreversible nephron damage in the biopsy specimen and, where appropriate, the severity of any active inflammatory process. The best way to estimate the irreversible damage is by specifying the number of globally sclerosed glomeruli and the amount of tubular atrophy and interstitial fibrosis. The estimate of activity will depend on the particular disease process but should include an indication of the proportion of glomeruli involved by crescents, necrosis, and endocapillary hypercellularity. For some diagnoses there are established classification schemes that should be applied to the biopsy specimen, for example, the International Society of Nephrology/Renal Pathology Society classification of lupus nephritis and the Banff classification of allograft pathology.

The interpretation of renal biopsy findings requires the pathologist to integrate the biopsy specimen characteristics with detailed clinical information and therefore requires a thorough understanding of renal disease and the therapeutic implications of the biopsy diagnosis. Close communication between the clinician and pathologist is essential, and it is generally very helpful for the biopsy specimen to be viewed and discussed at a clinicopathologic conference so that the implications of the biopsy specimen appearance for patient management can be considered fully.

Conclusions

Percutaneous renal biopsy is generally safe if care is taken to select and prepare the patients beforehand. It has become a cornerstone of nephrologic practice, and the handling and interpretation of the biopsy specimen should be done by those experienced in renal pathology. The interpretation of the biopsy specimen should be carried out with adequate clinical information to allow integrated clinicopathologic conclusions to be drawn.

References

1. Cameron JS, Hicks J. The introduction of renal biopsy into nephrology from 1901 to 1961: a paradigm of the forming of nephrology by technology. *Am J Nephrol*. 1997;17:347-358.
2. Pascual M, Vallhonrat H, Cosimi AB, et al. The clinical usefulness of the renal allograft biopsy in the cyclosporine era: a prospective study. *Transplantation*. 1999;67:737-741.
3. Kim D, Kim H, Shin G, et al. A randomized, prospective, comparative study of manual and automated renal biopsies. *Am J Kidney Dis*. 1998;32:426-431.
4. Korbet SM. Percutaneous renal biopsy. *Semin Nephrol*. 2002;22:254-267.
5. Hergesell O, Felten H, Andrassy K, et al. Safety of ultrasound-guided percutaneous renal biopsy—retrospective analysis of 1090 consecutive cases. *Nephrol Dial Transplant*. 1998;13:975-977.
6. Preda A, Van Dijk LC, Van Oostaijen JA, et al. Complication rate and diagnostic yield of 515 consecutive ultrasound-guided biopsies of renal allografts and native kidneys using a 14-gauge Biopty gun. *Eur Radiol*. 2003;13:527-530.
7. Whittier WL, Korbet SM. Timing of complications in percutaneous renal biopsy. *J Am Soc Nephrol*. 2004;15:142-147.
8. Waldo B, Korbet SM, Freimanis MG, et al. The value of post-biopsy ultrasound in predicting complications after percutaneous renal biopsy of native kidneys. *Nephrol Dial Transplant*. 2009;24:2433-2439.
9. Manno C, Strippoli GF, Arnesano L, et al. Predictors of bleeding complications in percutaneous ultrasound-guided renal biopsy. *Kidney Int*. 2004;66:1570-1577.
10. Shidham GB, Siddiqi N, Beres JA, et al. Clinical risk factors associated with bleeding after native kidney biopsy. *Nephrology (Carlton)*. 2005;10:305-310.
11. Stiles KP, Hill C, LeBrun CJ, et al. The impact of bleeding times on major complication rates after percutaneous real-time ultrasound-guided renal biopsies. *J Nephrol*. 2001;14:275-279.
12. Lehman CM, Blaylock RC, Alexander DP, et al. Discontinuation of the bleeding time test without detectable adverse clinical impact. *Clin Chem*. 2001;47:1204-1211.
13. Nomoto Y, Tomino Y, Endoh M, et al. Modified open renal biopsy: results in 934 patients. *Nephron*. 1987;45:224-228.
14. Mal F, Meyrier A, Callard P, et al. Transjugular renal biopsy. *Lancet*. 1990;335:1512-1513.
15. Marwah DS, Korbet SM. Timing of complications in percutaneous renal biopsy: what is the optimal period of observation? *Am J Kidney Dis*. 1996;28:47-52.
16. Churg J, Bernstein J, Glassock RJ. *Renal disease: classification and atlas of glomerular diseases*. New York: Igaku-Shoin Medical Publishers; 1995.
17. Furness PN. Acp. Best practice no 160. Renal biopsy specimens. *J Clin Pathol*. 2000;53:433-438.
18. Walker PD, Cavallo T, Bonsib SM. Practice guidelines for the renal biopsy. *Mod Pathol*. 2004;17:1555-1563.
19. Michel B, Milner Y, David K. Preservation of tissue-fixed immunoglobulins in skin biopsies of patients with lupus erythematosus and bullous diseases—preliminary report. *J Invest Dermatol*. 1972;59:449-452.
20. Nasr SH, Markowitz GS, Valeri AM, et al. Thin basement membrane nephropathy cannot be diagnosed reliably in deparaffinized, formalin-fixed tissue. *Nephrol Dial Transplant*. 2007;22:1228-1232.
21. Weening JJ, D'Agati VD, Schwartz MM, et al. The classification of glomerulonephritis in systemic lupus erythematosus revisited. *J Am Soc Nephrol*. 2004;15:241-250.
22. Roberts IS, Cook HT, Troyanov S, et al. The Oxford classification of IgA nephropathy: pathology definitions, correlations, and reproducibility. *Kidney Int*. 2009;76:546-556.
23. Nasr SH, Galgano SJ, Markowitz GS, et al. Immunofluorescence on pronase-digested paraffin sections: a valuable salvage technique for renal biopsies. *Kidney Int*. 2006;70:2148-2151.
24. Haas M. A reevaluation of routine electron microscopy in the examination of native renal biopsies. *J Am Soc Nephrol*. 1997;8:70-76.
25. Das AK, Pickett TM, Tungekar MF. Glomerular basement membrane thickness—a comparison of two methods of measurement in patients with unexplained haematuria. *Nephrol Dial Transplant*. 1996;11:1256-1260.
26. Neusser MA, Lindenmeyer MT, Kretzler M, et al. Genomic analysis in nephrology—towards systems biology and systematic medicine? *Nephrol Ther*. 2008;4:306-311.
27. Sedor JR. Tissue proteomics: a new investigative tool for renal biopsy analysis. *Kidney Int*. 2009;75:876-879.
28. Colvin RB. Getting out of flatland: into the third dimension of microarrays. *Am J Transplant*. 2007;7:2650-2651.
29. Sis B, Halloran PF. Endothelial transcripts uncover a previously unknown phenotype: C4d-negative antibody-mediated rejection. *Curr Opin Organ Transplant*. 2010;15:42-48.
30. Ivanyi B, Fahmy H, Brown H, et al. Peritubular capillaries in chronic renal allograft rejection: a quantitative ultrastructural study. *Hum Pathol*. 2000;31:1129-1138.
31. Corwin HL, Schwartz MM, Lewis EJ. The importance of sample size in the interpretation of the renal biopsy. *Am J Nephrol*. 1988;8:85-89.
32. Racusen LC, Solez K, Colvin RB, et al. The Banff 97 working classification of renal allograft pathology. *Kidney Int*. 1999;55:713-723.
33. Colvin RB, Cohen AH, Saiontz C, et al. Evaluation of pathologic criteria for acute renal allograft rejection: reproducibility, sensitivity, and clinical correlation. *J Am Soc Nephrol*. 1997;8:1930-1941.
34. McCarthy GP, Roberts IS. Diagnosis of acute renal allograft rejection: evaluation of the Banff 97 Guidelines for Slide Preparation. *Transplantation*. 2002;73:1518-1521.

Biomarkers in Acute and Chronic Kidney Diseases

Venkata Sabbisetti and Joseph V. Bonventre

Kidney disease is a global health problem. Acute kidney injury (AKI) and chronic kidney disease (CKD) are increasing in incidence.[1] In the United States, it is clear that the incidence of AKI has been steadily increasing at a rate that is disturbingly high, and it is increasingly recognized that AKI predisposes to the progression of CKD toward end-stage renal disease (ESRD), which ultimately requires dialysis or kidney transplantation.[2] According to the World Health Organization, approximately 850,000 patients develop kidney disease every year.[2-5] Across the globe, treatment of ESRD poses a major challenge for health care systems and the global economy. The burden of kidney disease is most significant in developing countries and is adversely influenced by inadequate socioeconomic and health care infrastructures.[4,6,7] Importantly, kidney disease progression can often be curtailed if the disease is diagnosed early, especially if the disease process is secondary to pharmacologic agents or environmental toxins. Hence detection and management of kidney diseases in the early, reversible, and potentially treatable stages is of paramount importance. Biomarkers that will help diagnose kidney injury, predict progression of kidney disease, and provide information regarding the effectiveness of therapeutic intervention will be important adjuncts to our standard management strategies.

Recently, many novel high-throughput technologies in the fields of genomics, proteomics, and metabolomics have made it easier to interrogate hundreds or even thousands of potential biomarkers at once, without prior knowledge of the underlying biology or pathophysiology of the system being studied.[8-11] As a result, there is a renewed interest in discovering novel biomarkers for use in drug development and patient care. Despite notable achievements, however, only a few biomarkers—blood urea nitrogen (BUN) level, creatinine concentration, and urinalysis results—are routinely used to diagnose and monitor kidney injury. These commonly used "gold standard" biomarkers of kidney function are not optimal to detect injury or dysfunction early enough to allow prompt therapeutic intervention. Although additional candidate biomarkers have been reported, none have been adequately validated to justify their use in making patient care decisions, but a few look quite promising.

Biomarker Definition

When the term *biologic marker* (biomarker) was introduced in 1989 as a term in the U.S. National Library of Medicine's controlled vocabulary thesaurus Medical Subject Headings (MeSH), it was defined as "measurable and quantifiable biological parameters (e.g., specific enzyme concentration, hormone concentration, and gene phenotype distribution in a population; presence of biological substances) which serve as indices for health- and physiology-related assessments, such as disease risk, psychiatric disorders, environmental exposure and its effects, disease diagnosis, metabolic processes, substance abuse, pregnancy, cell line development, epidemiologic studies, etc." In 2001, the U.S. Food and Drug Administration (FDA) standardized the definition of a biomarker as "a characteristic that is objectively measured and evaluated as an indicator of normal biologic processes, pathogenic processes, or pharmacologic responses to therapeutic intervention."[12] The National Institutes of Health further classified biomarkers based on their utility (Table 29-1).[12]

Biomarkers can potentially serve a wide range of functions in drug development, clinical trials, and therapeutic management strategies. There are many different types of biomarkers: disease biomarkers, toxicity biomarkers, mechanistic biomarkers, efficacy biomarkers, predictive biomarkers, and biomarkers of drug-target interaction. Examples of biomarkers are proteins, lipids, genomic or proteomic patterns, imaging determinations, electrical signals, and cells present in urine. Some biomarkers also serve as surrogate endpoints. A surrogate endpoint is a biomarker intended to substitute for a clinical endpoint. Furthermore, a surrogate endpoint biomarker is expected to predict clinical benefit (harm or lack of benefit) based on epidemiologic, therapeutic, pathophysiologic, or other scientific evidence.[13] An ideal biomarker is easily measurable, reproducible, sensitive, cost effective, easily interpretable, and present in readily available specimens (blood and urine).

TABLE 29-1 Biomarker Definitions

Biomarker: A characteristic that is objectively measured and evaluated as an indicator of normal biologic process, pathogenic processes, or pharmacologic responses to therapeutic intervention.

Type 0 biomarker: A marker of the natural history of a disease that correlates longitudinally with known clinical indices, such as symptoms over the full range of disease states.

Type 1 biomarker: A marker that captures the effects of an intervention in accordance with the mechanism of action of the drug, even though the mechanism might not be known to be associated with clinical outcome.

Clinical endpoint: A characteristic or variable that reflects how a patient fares or functions, or how long a patient survives.

Surrogate endpoint biomarker (type 2 biomarker): A marker that is intended to substitute for clinical endpoint. A surrogate endpoint is expected to predict clinical benefit, harm, lack of benefit, or lack of harm on the basis of epidemiologic, therapeutic, pathophysiologic, or other scientific evidence.

Process of Biomarker Discovery, Assay Validation, and Qualification in a Clinical Context

Primary challenges to the development of biomarkers for kidney injury and toxicity are discovery of candidate markers, design of an assay, validation of the assay, and qualification of the biomarker for use in specific clinical contexts. The process of biomarker identification and development is arduous and involves several phases.[14,15] For the purpose of simplicity this process can be divided into the following five phases (adapted and modified from Pepe and colleagues[14]).

Phase 1: Discovery of Potential Biomarkers though Hypothesis-Generating Exploratory Studies

The primary goal of phase 1 is to identify potential leads using various technologies and to confirm and prioritize the identified leads. The search for biomarkers often begins with preclinical studies that compare either tissue or biologic fluids in diseased animals (e.g., animals with kidney injury) with those in healthy animals to identify genes or proteins that appear to be upregulated or decreased in diseased tissue relative to control tissue. When biologic samples, such as blood and urine, are readily available from humans it is possible to forgo the animal model stage. Innovative discovery technologies include microarray-based gene expression profiling that provides information regarding expression of genes, microRNA-based expression, and proteomic as well as metabolomic profiling of biologic fluids based on mass spectrophotometry and other technologies. The candidate marker approach, especially when informed by the pathophysiology of the disease for which the biomarker is being evaluated, should not be ignored.

Once the lead biomarker is discovered, the validation process begins. An assay has to be developed and validated. The validation process is laborious and expensive, often requiring access to many patient samples with complete clinical annotation and long-term follow-up, as described in the following section on phase 2. In addition, each biomarker must be qualified for specific application. This is especially true in the case of kidney diseases, for which one biomarker alone may not satisfy the requirements of an ideal biomarker. This is described in the section on phase 4 later. Incorporation of several of these novel biomarkers into a biomarker panel may enable simultaneous assessment of site-specific kidney injury with an indication of the degree of damage.

Phase 2: Development and Validation of an Assay for the Measurement or Identification of the Biomarker in Clinical Samples

The primary goals of phase 2 are (1) to develop and validate a clinically useful assay that has the ability to distinguish a person with kidney disease from persons with healthy kidneys in high-throughput fashion, and (2) to evaluate the performance of the biomarker in clinical samples obtained from patients with kidney injury. This phase involves development of an assay, optimization of assay performance, and evaluation of the reproducibility of the assay results within and among laboratories. Defining reference ranges of biomarker values is a crucial step before the biomarker can be used clinically.[16,17] It is important to characterize how the levels of these markers vary with patient age, sex, and race or ethnicity, and how biomarker values are related to known risk factors.[18]

Phase 3: Demonstration of the Biomarker's Potential Clinical Utility in Retrospective Studies

In phase 3 the primary objectives are to (1) evaluate the biomarker potential in samples obtained from a completed clinical study, (2) test the diagnostic potential of the biomarker for early detection, and (3) determine the sensitivity and specificity of the biomarker using defined threshold values of the biomarker for utility in prospective studies. For instance, if the levels of biomarker differ significantly between cases (those with acute or chronic kidney injury) and control subjects only at the time of clinical diagnosis, then the biomarker shows little promise for population screening or early detection. In contrast, if levels differ significantly hours, days, or years before clinical symptoms appear, then the biomarker's potential for early detection is increased. This phase also involves comparing the biomarker with several other novel biomarkers or existing gold standard biomarkers and defining the biomarkers' performance characteristics (i.e., sensitivity, specificity, positive and negative predictive values) using receiver operating characteristic curve analysis. This latter process is particularly challenging in kidney disease given uncertainties in the sensitivity and specificity of the gold standard used.[19]

Phase 4: Performance of Prospective Screening Studies

The primary aim of phase 4 studies is to determine the operating characteristics of the biomarker in a relevant population by measuring detection rate and false referral rate. In contrast to phase 1, 2, and 3 studies, which are based primarily on stored specimens, studies in phase 4 involve screening subjects prospectively and demonstrating that clinical care is changed as a result of the information provided by the biomarker analysis.

Biomarker Qualification Process

The application for FDA qualification of novel biomarkers requires the intended use of the biomarker in nonclinical and clinical contexts and collection of evidence supporting qualification. This can be a joint and collaborative effort among regulatory agencies, pharmaceutical companies, and academic scientists.

Steps involved in the biomarker qualification pilot process as described by Dr. Federico Goodsaid when he was at the FDA include the following[20]: (1) submission to an FDA interdisciplinary pharmacogenomic review group of a request to qualify the biomarker for a specific use; (2) recruitment of a biomarker qualification review team (containing both nonclinical and clinical members); (3) assessment of the biomarker context and available data in a voluntary data submission; (4) evaluation of the qualification study strategy; (5) review of the qualification study results; and (6) acceptance or rejection of the biomarker for the suggested use.

Data are shared between the FDA and pharmaceutical industry or academic laboratories through voluntary exploratory data submissions (VXDSs).[20] Submission of exploratory biomarker data through VXDSs allows interaction between reviewers at the FDA and researchers in industry or academia regarding study designs, sample collection and storage protocols, technology platforms, and data analysis. This pilot process for biomarker qualification allowed the Predictive Safety Testing Consortium to apply to both U.S. and European drug authorities simultaneously for qualification of new nephrotoxic biomarkers (kidney injury molecule-1, albumin, total protein, cystatin C, clusterin, trefoil factor 3, and α_2-microglobulin) as predictors of drug-mediated nephrotoxicity.[20-22] The FDA and the corresponding European authority (European Medicines Agency, or EMA) reviewed the application separately and made decisions as to whether each would allow the new biomarkers to be used as "fit for purpose" in preclinical research.[21,22] Some of these markers were proposed to be qualified as biomarkers for clinical drug–induced nephrotoxicity once further supportive human data are submitted.

Phase 5: Continued Assessment of the Validity of the Biomarker in Routine Clinical Practice

Phase 5 addresses whether measurement of the biomarker alters physician decision making and/or reduces mortality or morbidity associated with the given disease in the population.

Analysis of Biomarker Performance

The widely accepted measure of biomarker sensitivity and specificity is the receiver operating characteristic (ROC) curve.[23] ROC curves display the proportion of subjects both with and without disease correctly identified at various cutoff points. An ROC curve is a graphic display of trade-offs between the true-positive rate (sensitivity) and the false-positive rate (1 – specificity, where specificity is expressed as a value from 0 to 1) when the biomarker is a continuous variable (Figure 29-1).[24,25] Sensitivity is plotted along the ordinate and the value of (1 – specificity) is plotted on the abscissa. Each point on the curve represents the true-positive rate and false-positive rate associated with a particular test value. The diagonal, represented by the equation true-positive rate (sensitivity) = false-positive rate (1 – specificity), corresponds to the set of points for which there is no selectivity in predicting disease. The area under this line of "unity" is 0.5, which indicates no advantage relative to the flip of a coin. The performance of a biomarker can be quantified by calculating the area under the ROC curve (AUC). The ROC curve of the ideal biomarker would start at the origin (0,0), move vertically up the y-axis to (0,1), and then go horizontally across to (1,1), which corresponds to an AUC of 1.0 for the biomarker.[25]

Other important parameters related to biomarker performance, primarily with respect to the testing of larger or specific populations, are positive and negative predictive values. The positive predictive value is the proportion of persons who test positive for a disease and truly have the disease, whereas negative predictive value represents the proportion of persons who test negative and do not have the disease. There is considerable interest in developing algorithms that use a composite of values of several biomarkers that are measured in parallel

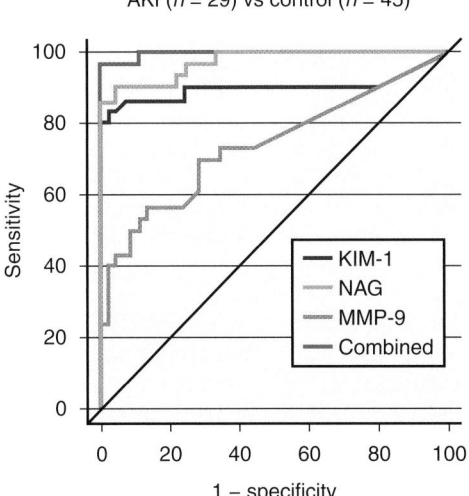

AKI (*n* = 29) vs control (*n* = 45)

FIGURE 29-1 Receiver operating characteristic (ROC) analysis for normalized urinary biomarkers in a cross-sectional study. ROC curves for normalized matrix metalloproteinase-9 (MMP-9), *N*-acetyl-β-D-glucosaminidase (NAG), and kidney injury molecule-1 (KIM-1) as single tests and in combination are plotted. The greater the displacement above and to the left of the line of identity, the greater the likelihood that increased values of the biomarkers will identify AKI. (From Han WK, Waikar SS, Johnson A, et al: Urinary biomarkers in the early diagnosis of acute kidney injury, *Kidney Int* 73:863-869, 2008.)

for the purpose of increasing diagnostic potential or predicting disease course and patient outcomes.

Characteristics of an Ideal Biomarker for Kidney Disease

Characteristics of an ideal biomarker for kidney disease are described in Table 29-2. For AKI the biomarker should (1) be organ specific and allow differentiation between intrarenal, prerenal, and postrenal causes of AKI as well as acute glomerular injury; (2) be able to detect AKI early in the course and be able to predict the course of AKI and potentially the future implications of AKI; (3) be able to identify the cause of AKI; (4) be site specific and able to inform pathologic changes in various segments of renal tubules during AKI as well as correlate with the histologic findings in kidney biopsy specimens; (5) be easily and reliably measured in a noninvasive or minimally invasive manner; (6) be stable in its matrix; (7) be rapidly and reliably measurable at the bedside; and (8) be inexpensive to measure.

In CKD (unlike AKI), the timing and nature of the insult is very hard to estimate, and this makes the search for early biomarkers for CKD very difficult. An ideal biomarker for CKD shares many of the same requirements described earlier for AKI biomarkers, including providing insight into (1) the location of the injury (e.g., glomerular, interstitial, tubular), (2) the disease mechanism, (3) the progressive course of the disease, and (4) the risk of complications from comorbid conditions such as cardiovascular disease and diabetes.

Acute Kidney Injury Markers

In the cardiac sciences, the discovery of biomarkers such as troponins that reflect early cardiomyocyte damage rather than decreased cardiac function has enabled the development and

TABLE 29-2 Characteristics of an Ideal Kidney Biomarker

FUNCTIONAL PROPERTIES	PHYSIOCHEMICAL PROPERTIES
Rapid and reliable increase in response to kidney diseases Highly sensitive and specific for acute and/or chronic kidney disease Shows good correlation with degree of renal injury Provides risk stratification and prognostic information (severity of kidney disease, need for dialysis, length of hospital stay, and mortality) Site specific to detect early injury (proximal, distal, interstitium or vasculature) and identify pathologic changes in specific segments of renal tubules Applicable across different races and age groups Allows recognition of the cause of kidney injury or disease (e.g., ischemia, toxins, sepsis, cardiovascular disease, diabetic nephropathy, lupus, or combinations) Organ specific and allows differentiation among intrarenal, prerenal, and extrarenal causes of kidney injury Noninvasive Identifies the duration of kidney failure (acute kidney injury, chronic kidney injury) Useful to monitor the response to therapeutic interventions Provides information on the risk of complications from comorbid conditions (especially in chronic kidney disease)	Stable over time across different temperature and pH conditions, with clinically relevant storage conditions Rapidly and easily measurable Not subject to interference by drugs and endogenous substances

implementation of novel therapeutic strategies to reduce coronary insufficiency and associated morbidity and mortality.[26,27] By contrast, the delay in diagnosis that is associated with the use of kidney biomarkers such as serum creatinine concentration has impaired the ability of nephrologists to conduct interventional studies in which the intervention can be done early in the course of the disease process. The utility of diagnostic criteria such as the RIFLE (*R*isk, *I*njury, *F*ailure, *L*oss, End-stage kidney disease) classification (Table 29-3) and the Acute Kidney Injury Network (AKIN) definition of AKI (Table 29-4) is limited by the fact that they rely on the serum creatinine concentration, which can increase in cases of prerenal azotemia when there is no tubular injury and can be unchanged under conditions of significant tubular injury, particularly when patients have good underlying kidney function and significant kidney reserve.

Furthermore, the application of early biomarkers to drug discovery and development has the potential of improving the efficacy and speed of bringing more effective and safe new drugs to market. A good predictive biomarker for AKI will be very useful in evaluation of potential therapies, because it will enable the identification of subgroups of patients who would be expected to have a high incidence of kidney injury. This will not only reduce the number of patients who are needed in studies to test potential therapeutic strategies, but also aid in better clinical trial design. Kidney toxicity noted late in the clinical development of new drugs is very costly given the exposure of patients to risk and the large amount of money, time, and effort that have been invested up to that point. The

TABLE 29-3 RIFLE Serum Creatinine and Glomerular Filtration Rate (GFR) Criteria for Severity of Acute Kidney Injury

RIFLE STAGE	SERUM CREATININE* AND GFR CRITERIA
R (risk)	≥150% of baseline serum creatinine level, or >25% decrease in GFR
I (injury)	>200% of baseline serum creatinine level, or >50% decrease in GFR
F (failure)	>300% of baseline serum creatinine level, or serum creatinine level of ≥4 mg/dL (acute rise of ≥0.5 mg/dL) or >75% decrease in GFR
L (loss)	Persistent acute renal failure (complete loss of renal function for >4 wk)
E (end-stage renal disease)	End-stage renal disease (complete loss of renal function for >3 mo)

*Serum creatinine increases are all relative to baseline values for the individual patient.

TABLE 29-4 Acute Kidney Injury Network (AKIN) Serum Creatinine and Urine Output Criteria for Severity of Acute Kidney Disease

AKIN STAGE	SERUM CREATININE CRITERIA*	URINE OUTPUT CRITERIA
1	≥50% or ≥0.3 mg/dL increase in serum creatinine	<0.5 mL/kg/hr for >6 hr
2	>100% increase in serum creatinine	<0.5 mL/kg/hr for >12 hr
3	>200% or 4.0 mg/dL increase in serum creatinine, with an acute rise of ≥5 mg/dL	<0.3 mL/kg/hr for 24 hr or anuria for 12 hr

*Serum creatinine increases are all relative to baseline values for the individual patient.

use of specific and sensitive biomarkers in drug development strategy would help implement the principle of "fail fast, fail early." Information yielded by biomarkers can greatly influence the go/no-go decision with regard to a new therapeutic entity. The challenge is to identify biomarkers that are capable of providing the accurate data that are essential in making these go/no-go decisions.

Hence it is very important to the clinical, pharmaceutical, and regulatory communities to develop better biomarkers for kidney diseases. Recently, several new putative biomarkers have been developed and translated into clinical settings. It is likely that some biomarkers of AKI will also be useful for monitoring the severity and progression of tubular interstitial disease in patients with CKD. Identification of patients at risk for or in the early stages of CKD may translate into more favorable outcomes, since therapeutic interventions can be started at an earlier stage of kidney disease. This chapter summarizes current and promising biomarkers for both acute and chronic kidney diseases.

Urine and serum biomarkers each have advantages and disadvantages. Serum biomarkers are often not stable and are difficult to measure because of interference with several serum proteins. By contrast, urinary biomarkers are relatively stable and easy to assess; however, their concentrations are greatly influenced by the volume status of the patient and other conditions that affect urinary volume. To deal with this challenge, urinary biomarker concentrations have often been normalized to urinary creatinine concentrations to eliminate the influence of urinary volume, on the assumption that urinary creatinine

excretion rate is constant over time and that biomarker production or excretion has a linear relationship with urinary creatinine excretion rate. Recently, the authors' group has challenged this assumption, especially in AKI settings, when urine creatinine excretion rate is not constant and changes over time, greatly influencing the normalized value of a putative urinary biomarker after normalization.[28] We have suggested that the most accurate method to quantify biomarkers is the timed collection of urine samples to estimate the renal excretion rate[28]; however, this approach is not practical for routine clinical care. The normalization process will often amplify the signal. For example, when glomerular filtration rate (GFR) is reduced in immediate response to a tubular injury the amount of biomarker produced will increase and urinary creatinine level will decrease. The normalized value will therefore increase by a greater amount in the short term than can be explained by the increase in the absolute level of biomarker production.

Because AKI and CKD share functional and structural aspects, there are overlapping as well as distinct classes of functional and structural biomarkers. Among the functional markers, GFR is often used as the gold standard. Although true GFR, as determined by agents that are freely filtered and undergo minimal handling by the tubule (iothalamate, iohexol, inulin), represents a sensitive measure for determining changes in kidney function, these tests are invasive and laborious to perform. Moreover, because of the renal reserve, changes in GFR may not indicate structural injury until significant injury has occurred. On the other hand, structural markers of tubular injury are expressed by tubular cells, and subtle changes in epithelial cells lead to release of these markers into the urine. Some of these biomarkers serve as markers for both acute and chronic kidney disease and also can be used to monitor progression from AKI to CKD. A challenge is to define at what level of release of these markers the injury is clinically significant.

Glomerular Injury Markers

Serum Glomerular Filtration Markers

During the course of injury, kidney function may be impaired with reduction in GFR and accumulation of several nitrogenous compounds in the blood. Serum creatinine and BUN concentrations are routinely used as markers of kidney injury, but it is important to recognize these parameters as markers for kidney dysfunction, rather than direct markers of injury.

The estimated GFR (eGFR), using creatinine as a biomarker, is most reliable for CKD under steady-state conditions. In the acute setting its use is more problematic for reasons that have already been discussed. In healthy persons, GFR is in the range of 90 to 130 mL/min/1.73 m². By definition, patients with stage 4 or 5 CKD have GFRs that are below 30 mL/min/1.73 m².[29] Complications of CKD are more pronounced at lower GFRs, and mild to moderate CKD may progress to ESRD.

In AKI the GFR is only indirectly linked to kidney injury, and changes in the GFR reflect a late consequence in a sequence of events associated with a primary insult to the kidney. Furthermore, because of renal reserve, a large amount of functioning renal tissue can be lost without significant changes in the GFR.[30,31] The functional effects of renal reserve on GFR can be demonstrated in kidney donors, who often have only modest changes in serum creatinine level and GFR after donating one kidney, even though half of the renal mass is lost.[32]

Ideally, a serum GFR marker should be freely filtered with no reabsorption in the kidney and should maintain a constant plasma level when kidney function is stable. GFR can be determined using exogenous and endogenous markers of filtration. Evaluation of GFR using the exogenous markers sucrose iothalamate or iohexol provides reliable results and represents the gold standard; however, the process is time consuming and expensive, and can be performed only in specialized settings.[29] Once the GFR level falls below 60 mL/min/1.73 m², renal functional impairment can be estimated adequately by serum creatinine using various equations to calculate the eGFR. These equations are less accurate at higher GFRs.

Creatinine

Determination of eGFR using endogenous creatinine is cost effective but can be problematic. Creatinine is a breakdown product of creatine and phosphocreatine, which are involved in the energy metabolism of skeletal muscle. Creatinine is freely filtered by the glomerulus, but is also to a lesser degree (10% to 30%) secreted by the proximal tubule. Under normal conditions the daily synthesis of creatinine of approximately 20 mg/kg of body weight reflects muscle mass and varies little.[33]

Accumulated data from various studies indicates that the creatinine concentration is not an ideal marker for diagnosing AKI for a variety of reasons, including the folllowing[34-36]:
1. Creatinine production and its release into the circulation varies greatly with age, gender, muscle mass, certain disease states, and, to a lesser extent, diet. For example, in rhabdomyolysis, serum creatinine concentrations may rise more rapidly, due to the release of preformed creatinine from the damaged muscle. Also, body creatinine production, as measured by 24-hour urinary excretion, decreases with older age, falling from a mean of 23.8 mg/kg of body weight in men aged 20 to 29 years to 9.8 mg/kg of body weight in men aged 90 to 99 years, largely because of the reduction in muscle mass.[37]
2. Serum creatinine concentrations are not specific for renal tubular injury. For example, prerenal factors (severe dehydration, blood volume loss, altered vasomotor tone, or age-related decrease in renal blood flow) and postrenal factors (obstruction or extravasation of urine into the peritoneal cavity) may falsely elevate serum concentrations in the absence of parenchymal damage. Thus, a decrease in eGFR inferred from an increase in serum creatinine level may not distinguish between prerenal, intrinsic renal, and postrenal causes of impaired kidney function. Even in cases in which serum creatinine is elevated as a consequence of direct renal injury, it cannot be used to determine the location of the injury (glomerular vs. tubular, or proximal tubular vs. distal tubular).
3. Static measurement of serum creatinine level does not reflect the real-time changes in GFR resulting from acute changes in kidney function as creatinine accumulates over time. Given the large amounts of functional kidney reserve in healthy persons and the variable amounts of kidney reserve in patients with mild to moderate disease, creatinine is not a sensitive marker.[38]
4. Drug-induced reduction in tubular secretion of creatinine might result in underestimation of kidney function. Medications such as cimetidine and trimethoprim inhibit creatinine secretion and increase the serum creatinine concentration without affecting true GFR.[39,40]
5. The creatinine assay is subject to interference by intake of certain drugs or due to certain pathophysiologic states, including hyperbilirubinemia and diabetic ketoacidosis.[39]

Similarly, the use of serum creatinine level in CKD is also limited by several patient-dependent and independent variables. Serum creatinine concentration can significantly decrease in advanced kidney disease, unrelated to its renal clearance.[41] The sensitivity of serum creatinine level in determining kidney function can be improved by serial measurements of timed creatinine clearance (usually, but not always, 24-hour collections). However, many individuals find this collection cumbersome, and errors (e.g., skipped voids) typically lead to underestimation of function.

Serum creatinine is stable during long-term storage, after repeated thawing and refreezing,[42] and for up to 24 hours in clotted whole blood at room temperature.[43] The Jaffé reaction–based assay (alkaline picrate assay) is routinely used in clinical laboratories to assess creatinine levels. However, Jaffé methods overestimate serum creatinine concentration by approximately 25% due to the interference of noncreatinine chromogens, particularly proteins. Interference from glucose[44,45] and acetoacetate[46] are particularly important, because diabetic patients are particularly prone to develop CKD. As a result, eGFRs are higher when Jaffé methods are used than when other approaches are employed. Expert professional bodies have recommended that all methods of creatinine measurement should become traceable to a reference method based on isotope dilution mass spectrometry.[47] Several modifications of the Jaffé method have been made to increase the specificity by decreasing the influence of interfering substances.[48,49] Enzymatic methods of measuring creatinine are widely adopted by clinical laboratories as an alternative to alkaline picrate assays. Although various substances do interfere with enzymatic assays, the assays are reported to be subject to less interference than Jaffé methods.[50-52] The high-performance liquid chromatography (HPLC)–based assay has evolved as a potential alternative approach for the measurement of serum creatinine level.[53,54] Several studies have demonstrated that HPLC methods have greater analytical specificity than conventional methods.[55-57] This approach clearly has severe limitations with respect to throughput, however.

Blood Urea Nitrogen

Blood urea is a low-molecular-weight waste product derived from dietary protein catabolism and tissue protein turnover, and its levels are inversely correlated with decline in GFR.[58] Urea is filtered freely, and a variable amount (approximately 30% to 70%) is reabsorbed by the tubule, with recycling between tubule and interstitium in the kidney medulla. The normal range of urea nitrogen in blood or serum is 5 to 20 mg/dL (1.8 to 7.2 mmol urea per liter).[58] The wide reference range reflects the influence on BUN of nonrenal factors, including dietary protein intake, endogenous protein catabolism, fluid intake, and hepatic urea synthesis.[58,59] BUN concentrations also increase with excessive tissue catabolism, especially in cases of fever, severe burns, high corticosteroid dosage, chronic liver disease, and sepsis.[58] In addition, any factor that increases the tubular reabsorption of urea, including decreased effective arterial volume (i.e., impaired renal perfusion) and/or obstruction of urinary drainage, will increase the BUN concentration.[58,60,61] Because of these limitations, BUN is a not sensitive and specific marker for acute or chronic kidney disease. BUN is measured by spectrophotometry. Because of all these undesirable limitations of creatinine and BUN as markers, there has been a great deal of interest in the identification of improved biomarkers for kidney injury.

Cystatin C

Recently, a large body of evidence suggests that serum cystatin C is a more sensitive biomarker to detect changes in GFR since it is less subject to extrarenal factors than serum creatinine and may be superior to serum creatinine in both acute and chronic kidney diseases.[62] Whereas serum cystatin C level has been touted as a good GFR marker, urinary cystatin C excretion has been proposed as a tubular injury marker. In 1961, Butler and Flynn studied the urine proteins of 223 individuals by starch gel electrophoresis and found a new urine protein fraction in the post–gamma globulin fraction.[63] They named this protein fraction *cystatin C*. Cystatin C is a low-molecular-weight protein produced at a constant rate by all nucleated cells and eliminated exclusively by glomerular filtration. It has a small size (13 kDa) and a positive charge at physiologic pH. It is neither secreted nor reabsorbed by renal tubules but undergoes almost complete catabolism by proximal tubular cells, and thus little, if any, appears in the urine under normal circumstances. Any impairment of reabsorption in proximal tubules can lead to marked increases in urinary levels of cystatin C in humans and animals. There have been a number of studies on the diagnostic potential of both serum and urinary cystatin C level in acute and chronic kidney disease in humans.

Because of its short half-life (approximately 2 hours) and other properties described earlier, serum cystatin C level reflects GFR better than creatinine concentration. For example, in a study of 164 patients with stage 2 or 3 CKD (GFR of 30 to 89 mL/min/1.73 m^2), serum cystatin C had significantly higher diagnostic accuracy in detecting a GFR of less than 60 mL/min/1.73 m^2 than serum creatinine, but only in women.[64] In patients with cardiovascular disease, cystatin C level showed a stronger risk relationship with mortality than creatinine concentration or eGFR.[65] In the Cardiovascular Health Study cohort of community-dwelling elderly, higher serum cystatin C concentrations were associated with a higher risk of mortality and cardiovascular disease outcomes. Furthermore, a study in the general population suggests that cystatin C level has a stronger association with cardiovascular disease outcomes than does creatinine concentration or estimated GFR, especially among the elderly.[62,66,67] Thus, serum cystatin C level may be a better marker of kidney function than serum creatinine concentration, especially in elderly persons and in the setting of mild (in contrast to moderate or advanced) kidney dysfunction. However, there are no data demonstrating that knowledge of serum cystatin C level would materially alter clinical practice compared with data on serum creatinine concentration alone or eGFR.

Although cystatin C level is increasingly reported as an endpoint in studies, the diagnostic and prognostic characteristics of this marker for AKI are yet to be defined. In a mixed critical care population, determination of serum cystatin C level enabled a diagnosis of AKI 1.5 days earlier than plasma creatinine concentration and had moderate ability to predict dialysis requirement. Similarly, in a study of 202 diverse intensive care unit (ICU) patients, of whom 49 developed AKI based on urine output and/or serum creatinine RIFLE F criteria, serum cystatin C levels showed excellent predictive value for AKI. However, serum cystatin C concentration did not rise earlier than serum creatinine concentration.[68] Cystatin C level was shown to be capable of detecting a decrease in GFR earlier after contrast agent administration than the serum creatinine value in adult patients who underwent coronary angiography.[69] In a prospective study of 87 patients who underwent elective catheterization, contrast medium–induced nephropathy occurred in 18 patients, and ROC analysis showed a higher AUC for cystatin C level than for serum creatinine concentration (0.933 vs. 0.832; $P = 0.012$). When a cutoff value of more than 1.2 mg/L was used, cystatin C level before catheterization exhibited 94.7% sensitivity and 84.8% specificity for predicting contrast medium–induced nephropathy.[70]

β-Trace Protein

β-Trace protein (BTP), also referred as *prostaglandin D synthase*, has emerged as another promising biomarker for GFR. BTP is a small protein with a molecular weight of 23 to 29 kDa depending on the size of the glycosyl moiety. BTP belongs to the lipocalin protein family, whose members are primarily involved in the binding and transport of small hydrophobic ligands. It is primary produced in the cerebral fluid, where its concentrations are more than 40-fold higher than in serum. BTP is primarily eliminated by glomerular filtration, and its concentrations in urine range from 600 to 1200 μg/L.[71]

The first observation of elevated BTP levels in association with impaired kidney function was reported by Hoffman and associates in 1997.[72] Since then several research studies have been conducted to evaluate the sensitivity and specificity of BTP as a marker of GFR and to compare it with serum creatinine in patients with CKD[73] and in kidney transplant recipients. Woitas and colleagues compared the diagnostic performance of serum cystatin C, BTP, β$_2$-microglobulin, and creatinine in relation to inulin clearance.[74] They reported that the performance of cystatin C concentration was better than β$_2$-microglobulin level and BTP level as an indicator of reduced GFR and was a possible replacement for creatinine concentration in clinical practice.[74]

In another similar study, Filler and associates compared the diagnostic accuracy of cystatin C, BTP, and eGFR for the detection of impaired GFR in serum samples from 225 children with various renal pathologies. ROC analysis showed a significantly higher diagnostic accuracy of BTP and cystatin C compared with serum creatinine for the detection of impaired GFR, but BTP was not more sensitive than cystatin C or the Schwartz GFR estimate.[75] Another study by Donadio and colleagues evaluated the relations among serum concentrations of BTP and GFR compared with cystatin C level. Serum concentrations of BTP progressively increased with reduced GFR, and strong direct correlations were found between GFR and serum concentrations of BTP ($r = 0.918$) and cystatin C ($r = 0.937$). Importantly, no statistically significant difference was found between BTP and cystatin C as indicators of a moderate degree of impaired kidney function.[76]

The Mild and Moderate Kidney Disease (MMKD) Study Group evaluated GFR and the serum markers cystatin C and

BTP for diagnostic accuracy in defining stage of kidney disease and as predictors of risk of CKD progression.[77] They measured serum marker concentrations in 227 patients with primary nondiabetic CKD and various degrees of impaired kidney function and followed 177 patients prospectively for up to 7 years to assess progression of CKD. At baseline, cystatin C and BTP levels were strongly correlated with GFR as measured by iohexol clearance. Sixty-five patients experienced progression of CKD, defined as doubling of baseline serum creatinine concentration and/or ESRD during follow-up. Patients who progressed were older and had lower GFR and higher cystatin C and BTP concentrations at baseline compared with patients who did not reach the predefined renal endpoint. Proportional hazards (Cox) regression analysis showed that both BTP and cystatin C were equally strong predictors of CKD progression, even after adjustment for age, sex, iohexol GFR, and proteinuria.

Concentrations of BTP are not affected by commonly used immunosuppressive medications such as prednisone, mycophenolate mofetil, and cyclosporine.[78] This is especially useful when evaluating kidney function in kidney transplant recipients, in whom cystatin C concentrations may be falsely elevated due to steroid treatment.[79] Unlike for serum creatinine values, age and race were not associated with BTP concentrations. Several new GFR estimation equations based on BTP have recently been developed for use in kidney transplant recipients[78,79] However, these equations will require external validation in larger and more diverse patient groups. In contrast to creatinine, one limitation of using BTP is lack of widespread availability and standardization of the assay.

Urinary Glomerular Cell Injury Markers

Defects in podocyte structure have been reported in many glomerular diseases, which have been classified as "podocytopathies."[80,81] Injured podocytes have been reported in immunologic and nonimmunologic forms of human glomerular disease, including hemodynamic injury, protein overload states, injury from environmental toxins, minimal change disease, focal segmental glomerulosclerosis, membranous glomerulopathy, diabetic nephropathy, and lupus nephritis.[82-87] Podocytes may be injured in many forms of human and experimental primary glomerular disease and in secondary forms of focal segmental glomerulosclerosis, including that caused by hypertension, diabetes, and tubulointerstitial disease.[88-90] Before detachment from the glomerular basement membrane, podocytes undergo structural changes, including effacement of foot processes and microvillous transformation.[80,81,91,92]

Podocyte Count

After undergoing the aforementioned structural changes, podocytes detach from glomerular basement membrane and are excreted into the urine. Urinary levels of viable podocytes have been extensively studied in several renal diseases.[93-96] Numerous studies have reported that the number of podocytes shed in patients with active glomerular disease is significantly higher than in healthy controls and in patients with inactive disease. Importantly, podocyte number in urine correlates with disease activity (assessed by renal biopsy) and has been shown to decline with treatment. For example, Nakamura and colleagues found podocytes in the urine of

type 2 diabetic patients with microalbuminuria and macroalbuminuria, but patients with chronic renal failure failed to show urinary podocytes, which suggests that urinary podocytes may represent the active phase of diabetic nephropathy.[97] Numerous studies have linked podocytopenia and disease severity in immunoglobulin (IgA) nephropathy[93,94] and diabetic nephropathy.[95,96] Thus, urinary levels of podocytes may reflect real-time changes in disease activity. The methods used to count urinary podocytes, however, are limited by several factors: (1) cytologists are needed to perform the counting, (2) the process is very time consuming, and (3) urine sediments contain whole viable podocytes as well as cell debris, and the latter may not necessarily reflect disease status. An improved and standardized laboratory method is urgently needed to facilitate measurement of urinary podocyte number. Nevertheless, the podocyte number may still be useful as a marker for glomerular disease. Alternative methods that indirectly assess the number of podocytes in urine include detection of messenger RNA (mRNA) and protein levels of podocyte-specific proteins by polymerase chain reaction (PCR) and enzyme-linked immunosorbent assay (ELISA), respectively.

Podocalyxin

Podocalyxin is the most commonly used marker protein for detecting podocytes in urine.[98] It is a highly *O*-glycosylated and sialylated type I transmembrane protein of approximately 140 kDa and is expressed in podocytes, hematopoietic progenitor cells, vascular endothelial cells, and a subset of neurons.[98] Podocalyxin participates in a number of cellular functions through its association with the actin cytoskeleton, ezrin, and Na$^+$/H$^+$ exchanger regulatory factor 1 and 2 (NHERF1 and NHERF2) proteins. Urinary podocalyxin has been reported as a marker of activity in a number of diseases, including IgA nephropathy, Henoch-Schönlein purpura, diabetic nephropathy, lupus nephritis, poststreptococcal glomerulonephritis, focal segmental glomerulosclerosis, and preeclampsia.[99,100,100a,100b,100c] Podocalyxin has been reported to be the most reproducible marker for podocyte injury in the urine. Measurements of podocalyxin protein in the urine by ELISA also correlated with histologic changes and disease activity in children with IgA nephropathy, Henoch-Schönlein purpura, lupus nephritis, membranoproliferative glomerulonephritis, and poststreptococcal glomerulonephritis.[99,101,102] Several studies have also shown that the number of podocalyxin-positive cells in the urine falls after various therapeutic interventions in patients with focal segmental glomerulosclerosis, lupus nephritis, Henoch-Schönlein purpura, IgA nephropathy, poststreptococcal glomerulonephritis, and diabetic nephropathy.[96,99,101,102] Unfortunately, because podocalyxin is expressed on a number of cell types, the presence of podocalyxin in the urine is not always reflective of urinary podocytes.

Nephrin

Nephrin, a transmembrane protein of the immunoglobulin superfamily, is a component of the filtration slit diaphragm between neighboring podocytes.[103,104] Immunohistochemical analysis and in situ hybridization have shown that nephrin is primarily expressed in glomerular podocytes.[105] Based on these observations, it has been proposed that nephrin is a key component of the glomerular filtration barrier, which plays a pivotal role in preventing protein leakage. Various experimental models of diabetes and hypertension show alterations in nephrin mRNA or protein levels in glomeruli. In experimental models of diabetes, glomerular nephrin mRNA expression was reduced, but treatment with an angiotensin converting enzyme (ACE) inhibitor or angiotensin II antagonist was able to abrogate this reduced expression.[110,111] In line with this, nephrin protein expression seems to be altered in various human proteinuric kidney diseases.[108,109] Langham and associates examined renal biopsy specimens from 14 patients with type 2 diabetes and nephropathy who had been randomly assigned to receive treatment with either the ACE inhibitor perindopril (4 mg/day) or placebo for the preceding 2 years.[112] They reported that glomeruli from placebo-treated patients with diabetic nephropathy showed a significant reduction in nephrin expression compared with those from control subjects. On the other hand, nephrin RNA in glomeruli from ACE inhibitor–treated patients was no different from that in the nondiabetic control group. In both placebo- and perindopril-treated patients, a close inverse correlation was observed between the magnitude of nephrin gene expression and the degree of proteinuria.[112]

In line with these observations, nephrin has been reported in urine (nephrinuria) in several experimental and human proteinuric diseases.[106,107] Because nephrin is known to be expressed in pancreatic β-cells, there was speculation that β-cells may release nephrin into the serum, which ultimately is excreted in the urine. However, Patari and colleagues demonstrated that nephrin was absent in the sera of nephrinuric patients.[113] Thus, urinary nephrin most likely is produced by the kidneys.

Urinary Tubular Injury Markers

Microscopic examination of the urine has been used for many years to gain insight into the degree of glomerular and tubular injury. Other components of the urine have been used to quantitate tubular cell injury in a more specific and sensitive fashion. These markers have been demonstrated to be extremely valuable in detecting kidney injury in the setting of AKI. Moreover, some of these biomarkers, such as, kidney injury molecule-1, neutrophil gelatinase–associated lipocalin (NGAL), and liver-type fatty acid–binding protein, have been shown to be potentially useful in a variety of contexts in both acute and chronic kidney injury. Here, the utility of urine microscopy is described briefly and some of the emerging biomarkers of tubular injury are discussed.

Urine Microscopy

Urine microscopy with sediment examination is a time-honored test that is routinely used to assist in the diagnosis of kidney injury.[114-116] The urine from patients with tubular injury typically contains proximal tubular epithelial cells, proximal tubule epithelial cells casts, granular casts, and mixed cellular casts. Patients with predominantly prerenal azotemia occasionally have hyaline or fine granular casts in their urine.[117-119] Several studies have shown that the increase in urinary cast excretion correlates well with AKI.[119-121] Marcussen and associates demonstrated that patients with tubular injury had a high number of granular casts compared with those with prerenal

azotemia.[120] Furthermore, Perazella and colleagues developed a sediment scoring system for the diagnosis of AKI. They concluded that a score of 2 or higher according to their system is an extremely strong predictor of acute tubular necrosis.[118] Nevertheless, the sensitivity of this test as an early indicator of tubular injury in the kidney remains controversial.[118,122]

α₁-Microglobulin

$α_1$-Microglobulin is a low-molecular-weight glycoprotein of approximately 27 to 30 kDa and a member of the lipocalin superfamily. $α_1$-Microglobulin is primarily synthesized by the liver and is available both in free form and as a complex with IgA.[123] $α_1$-Microglobulin has been detected in human serum, urine, and cerebrospinal fluid. Urine and serum levels have been found to be elevated in patients with renal tubular diseases. $α_1$-Microglobulin is freely filtered at the glomerulus and completely reabsorbed and catabolized by the normal proximal tubule. Megalin mediates the uptake of this protein in the proximal tubule. Therefore, an increase in the urinary concentration of $α_1$-microglobulin indicates proximal tubular injury or dysfunction. The urinary levels of $α_1$-microglobulin are influenced by age. The normal range in populations younger than 50 years is less than 13 mg/g of creatinine and in those 50 years or older is less than 20 mg/g of creatinine.[123] Unlike $β_2$-microglobulin, $α_1$-microglobulin is more stable over a range of pH levels in the urine,[124] which makes it a more acceptable urinary biomarker.

$α_1$-Microglobulin quantitation in the urine has been reported as a sensitive biomarker for proximal tubule dysfunction in both adults and children.[123,125] In a small cohort of 73 patients, of whom 26 required renal replacement therapy, Herget-Rosenthal and colleagues compared levels of $α_1$-microglobulin, $β_2$-microglobulin, cystatin C, retinol-binding protein, α-glutathione S-transferase, lactate dehydrogenase, and N-acetyl-β-D-glucosaminidase (NAG) early in the course of AKI. They found that urinary cystatin C and $α_1$-microglobulin had the highest ability to predict the need for renal replacement therapy.[126] In this study, urinary $α_1$-microglobulin had an AUC of 0.86 for prediction of the need for renal replacement therapy. In addition, $α_1$-microglobulin has also been reported as a useful marker for proximal tubular damage and recovery in early infancy.[127]

Limitations associated with the use of $α_1$-microglobulin level include the variation in serum levels with age, gender,[128] and clinical conditions, including liver diseases,[123] ulcerative colitis,[129] human immunodeficiency virus (HIV) infection, and mood disorders,[123] as well as the lack of international standardization. Urinary $α_1$-microglobulin is measured by an immunonephelometric assay.

β₂-Microglobulin

$β_2$-Microglobulin is a low-molecular-weight polypeptide with a molecular weight of 11.8 kDa. $β_2$-Microglobulin is present on the cell surface of all nucleated cells and in most biologic fluids, including serum, urine, and synovial fluid. $β_2$-Microglobulin is normally excreted by glomerular filtration, reabsorbed almost completely (approximately 99%), and catabolized by the normal proximal tubule in humans.[130,131]

Megalin mediates the uptake of this protein in the proximal tubule.[131] In healthy individuals, approximately 150 to 200 mg of β_2-microglobulin is synthesized daily with a normal concentration of 1.5 to 3 mg/L. Any pathologic state that affects kidney function will result in an increase in β_2-microglobulin levels in the urine because of the impeded uptake of β_2-microglobulin by renal tubular cells. For spot urine collections, the concentration of β_2-microglobulin in healthy individuals is typically 160 μg/L or less or 300 μg/g of creatinine or less. Unlike urea, its serum levels are not influenced by food intake, which makes it an attractive marker for malnourished patients with low serum urea levels. In patients with CKD, increases in serum β_2-microglobulin levels reflect the decrease in glomerular function. In ESRD patients, serum levels of β_2-microglobulin are usually in the range of 20 to 50 mg/L. β_2-Microglobulin accumulation is linked to toxicity, because the molecule precipitates and forms fibrillary structures and amyloid deposits, particularly in bone and periarticular tissue, which leads to the development of carpal tunnel syndrome and erosive arthritis.[131,132] Elevated levels of β_2-microglobulin have been reported in several AKI and CKD clinical settings, including cadmium toxicity,[133] cardiac surgery,[134] and renal transplantation.[135] In idiopathic membranous nephropathy, β_2-microglobulin level was identified as a superior independent predictor of the development of renal insufficiency.[136] Another study reported that β_2-microglobulin and cystatin C outperformed serum creatinine for the detection of acute kidney injury in critically ill children.[137]

A review of urinary AKI biomarkers in patients with sepsis reported that β_2-microglobulin level is correlated with changes in serum creatinine concentration, has the potential to distinguish prerenal azotemia from acute tubular necrosis, and can detect subclinical AKI or predict AKI.[138] In a study in patients with peripheral arterial disease and stage 1 or 2 CKD, serum β_2-microglobulin concentrations were elevated and correlated with the severity of disease, independent of other risk factors.

Serum concentrations of β_2-microglobulin should be interpreted cautiously because they are altered significantly in various diseases, including rheumatoid disorders and several types of cancers.[139,140] Initially, it was believed that the increase in β_2-microglobulin levels in CKD is solely due to declines in kidney function, but recent studies have shown that other factors, including increased synthesis of β_2-microglobulin, may contribute in patients with ESRD.[141] Another significant drawback associated with the use of urinary β_2-microglobulin as a marker of injury is its instability in the urine at room temperature, particularly when the pH is less than 5.5; because of this, the urine should be alkalinized and frozen at −80° C immediately after collection.[132,142]

Glutathione S-Transferase

Primarily two subtypes of glutathione S-transferase (GST) enzymes are found in the kidney. α-GST is found mainly in the proximal tubular cells, whereas π-GST is found predominantly in the distal tubular epithelial cells. Elevation of urinary α-GST has been reported in several animal models treated with nephrotoxic drugs or after ischemic renal injury.[143,144] In a prospective study of patients with sepsis admitted to the ICU, α-GST levels were no different in

patients who developed AKI and in patients without AKI. π-GST levels were elevated in all patients with sepsis compared with healthy volunteers; however, π-GST levels were not predictive of AKI as defined by the AKIN criteria.[145] In kidney transplant patients, increased levels of α-GST were associated with cyclosporine A toxicity, whereas π-GST elevation was associated with acute allograft rejection.[146] In a cross-sectional study of patients with diabetes, the relationships between urine albumin/creatinine ratio and urinary levels of collagen IV, α-GST, and π-GST were assessed. Levels of all three markers were directly (albeit weakly) correlated with urine albumin/creatinine ratio, but a progressive increase in the proportion of patients with abnormal biomarker levels in those with normal urine albumin levels, microalbuminuria, and macroalbuminuria was observed only for collagen IV and π-GST.[147] In another study of patients undergoing cardiac surgery, levels of both α-GST and π-GST were elevated in those developing AKI as defined by the AKIN criteria.[148] In one prospective study, the value of tubular enzyme levels in predicting AKI was assessed in 26 critically ill adult patients admitted to the ICU. Four patients developed AKI, and ROC analysis showed that γ-glutamyl transpeptidase, π-GST, α-GST, alkaline phosphatase, and NAG had excellent discriminating power for AKI (AUC = 0.950, 0.929, 0.893, 0.863, and 0.845, respectively).[149]

Interleukin-18

Interleukin-18 (IL-18) is an 18-kDa proinflammatory cytokine produced by renal tubule cells and macrophages. Animal studies indicate that IL-18 is a mediator of acute tubular injury, including both neutrophil and monocyte infiltration of the renal parenchyma.[150,151] In the kidney, IL-18 is induced and cleaved mainly in the proximal tubules and released into the urine. IL-18 has been shown to participate in a variety of renal disease processes, including ischemia-reperfusion injury, allograft rejection, infection, autoimmune conditions, and malignancy. Several studies have demonstrated the usefulness of IL-18 as a biomarker for detection of AKI. Parikh and associates studied a group of 72 patients and reported urinary IL-18 levels significantly higher in patients diagnosed with acute tubular necrosis than in patients with prerenal azotemia or urinary infection or in healthy control subjects with normal renal function.[152] At kidney transplantation, IL-18 level accurately identified delayed graft function (AUC = 0.90) and predicted the rate of decline in serum creatinine concentration.[153] In patients with diabetic kidney disease and proteinuria, IL-18 levels in renal tubular cells are higher than in patients with nondiabetic proteinuric disease.[153a]

Increased urinary concentrations of IL-18 in AKI and CKD have been reported by several groups. In a pediatric critical care population, elevated urinary IL-18 concentrations were associated with an increased risk of developing AKI during the subsequent 48 hours (odds ratio = 3.5) but with poor discrimination (AUC = 0.54) and a sensitivity of less than 40%.[154] In multiple studies of patients undergoing cardiac surgery, urinary IL-18 concentrations alone showed at best a modest predictive performance (AUC = 0.53 to 0.66).[155,156] In a single-center, prospective, observational cohort study of adults undergoing cardiac surgery, Haase and associates reported that urinary IL-18 concentrations were directly correlated with the duration of cardiopulmonary bypass but did not predict AKI after bypass.[156] Similarly, in a prospective study of 451 critically ill adult patients admitted to the ICU, urinary IL-18 concentrations did not predict the development of AKI (AUC = 0.62) but did predict poor clinical outcomes, including death and the need for short-term dialysis.[157]

To understand the utility of IL-18 and urinary NGAL in predicting graft recovery after kidney transplantation, Hall and colleagues conducted a prospective, multicenter, observational cohort study of recipients of deceased-donor kidney transplants.[158] They collected serial urine samples from 91 patients for 3 days after transplantation. After adjustment for recipient and donor age, cold ischemia time, urine output, and serum creatinine concentration, NGAL and IL-18 concentrations accurately predicted the need for dialysis in transplant recipients. Furthermore, NGAL and IL-18 concentrations also predicted graft recovery up to 3 months later.[158] In a study by Ling and associates involving patients who underwent coronary angiography, urinary IL-18 and NGAL concentrations were significantly increased at 24 hours after the procedure in those who developed contrast medium–induced nephropathy, but not in the control group. ROC curve analysis demonstrated that both IL-18 and NGAL showed better performance in early diagnosis of contrast nephropathy than serum creatinine ($P < 0.05$). Importantly, elevated urinary IL-18 concentrations 24 hours after contrast administration were also found to be an independent predictive marker for later major cardiac events (relative risk = 2.1).[159]

The clinical utility of IL-18 as a biomarker to predict or diagnose AKI in other settings, such as drug-induced kidney injury, has not been evaluated. Although IL-18 is easily and reliably measured in the urine by commercially available ELISA and microbead-based assays, the pathophysiology of IL-18 is not well elucidated, and its role may be as a mediator of specific injury subtypes rather than as a marker of injury. Further studies are required to demonstrate the usefulness of IL-18 as biomarker in AKI and CKD.

Kidney Injury Molecule-1

Kidney injury molecule-1 (KIM-1 in humans, Kim-1 in rodents), which is also referred as *T cell immunoglobulin and mucin domains–containing protein-1* (TIM-1) and *hepatitis A virus cellular receptor-1* (HAVCR-1), is a type I transmembrane glycoprotein with an ectodomain containing a six-cysteine immunoglobulin-like domain, two *N*-glycosylation sites, and a mucin domain. In an effort to identify molecules involved in kidney injury, the authors' laboratory originally discovered Kim-1 using representational difference analysis (a PCR-based technique) in rat models of acute ischemic kidney injury.[160,161] Importantly, KIM-1 was shown to be significantly expressed in kidneys specifically in proximal tubular cells of humans after ischemia injury, whereas it was virtually absent or present at low levels in healthy kidneys. The ectodomain of KIM-1 (approximately 90 kDa) is cleaved by metalloproteinases and sheds from cells both in vitro[162] and in vivo into the urine in rodents and humans after proximal tubular kidney injury.[163,164] The full-length form of KIM-1 is 104 kDa, whereas the molecular weight of the shed form of KIM-1 ectodomain is approximately 90 kDa. The selective KIM-1 expression by injured proximal tubular cells and the shedding of its ectodomain into

urine provided a strong impetus for testing KIM-1 as a biomarker of kidney damage. Importantly, KIM-1 mRNA levels are highly correlated with urinary KIM-1 excretion in rats exposed to ischemia for various periods, which indicates that the kidney is the only source of KIM-1 production following a renal insult.[163,165] Since that observation, KIM-1 has evolved as a marker of proximal tubular injury, the hallmark of virtually all proteinuric, toxic, and ischemic renal diseases. KIM-1 orthologs are present in many species besides rodents and man, including zebrafish, monkeys, and dogs. Kim-1 has been shown to be a highly sensitive and specific marker of kidney injury in several rodent models, including models of injury due to ischemia,[160,164] cisplatin, folic acid, gentamicin, mercury, chromium,[164,166] cadmium,[167] contrast agents,[168] cyclosporine,[169] ochratoxin A, aristolochic acid, d-serine, and protein overload.[170] Furthermore, Kim-1 expression was upregulated in a model of aging-induced nephropathy[171] and in angiotensin-mediated injury in Ren2 rats (a strain with overexpression of a mouse renin transgene).[172] The finding that Kim-1 protein was easily detected in the urine soon after AKI in animal studies has motivated a number of translational studies to evaluate KIM-1 as a noninvasive biomarker for human AKI.

Favorable characteristics of KIM-1 as a biomarker include much higher expression in the proximal tubular cell of the kidney than in any other cell of the kidney or any other organ, stability of the soluble ectodomain in the urine over a broad range of pH, sustained expression in proximal tubular epithelial cells until complete recovery, and undetectable levels in the healthy kidney, which provides a high signal-to-noise ratio with injury.

In the first clinical study linking urinary levels of KIM-1 with AKI, the author's laboratory demonstrated that tissue expression of KIM-1 is correlated with the severity of acute tubular necrosis and corresponding levels of KIM-1 ectodomain in the urine of patients with clinically significant AKI.[165] Since then, numerous other studies have been published demonstrating the potential utility of KIM-1 as a biomarker of AKI and CKD. In a study of 201 patients with clinically established AKI, Liangos and colleagues evaluated the ability of urinary KIM-1 and NAG concentrations to predict adverse clinical outcomes and reported that elevated levels of urinary KIM-1 and NAG were significantly associated with the composite endpoint of death or the need for dialysis, even after adjustment for disease severity and comorbid conditions.[173] Recently, the same group studied the performance of six candidate urinary biomarkers—KIM-1, NAG, NGAL, IL-18, cystatin C, and α_1-microglobulin—in 103 patients undergoing cardiac surgery.[174] Urinary KIM-1 concentration 2 hours postoperatively achieved the highest AUC (0.78; 95% confidence interval [CI] = 0.64 to 0.91), followed by IL-18 and NAG. Only urinary KIM-1 remained independently associated with AKI after adjustment for a preoperative AKI prediction score (Cleveland Clinic Foundation score; $P = 0.02$) and cardiopulmonary bypass perfusion time ($P = 0.006$), and it performed best as an early biomarker of AKI.[174]

The usefulness of KIM-1 has been demonstrated not only as a urinary marker but also as a tool for evaluating kidney injury in kidney biopsy specimens by immunohistochemical methods. For example, Van Timmeren and associates found that the level of KIM-1 protein expression in proximal tubule cells correlated with tubulointerstitial fibrosis and inflammation in kidney tissue specimens from 102 patients who underwent kidney biopsy for a variety of kidney diseases.[175] In a subset of patients whose urine was collected near the time of biopsy, urinary KIM-1 levels correlated with tissue KIM-1 expression in 100% of biopsy samples from patients with deterioration in kidney function and histologic changes indicative of tubular damage. In biopsy specimens from transplanted kidneys, increased KIM-1 staining was detected in 100% of patients with a deterioration of kidney function and pathologic changes indicating tubular injury, in 92% of patients with acute cellular rejection, and in 28% of patients with normal biopsy findings.[176] Moreover, KIM-1 levels showed a positive correlation with serum creatinine and BUN levels, and an inverse correlation with eGFR. Focal positive KIM-1 expression was found in 28% of protocol biopsy specimens in the presence of no detectable tubular injury on histologic examination. This observation demonstrates the superior sensitivity of KIM-1 expression in detecting proximal tubule injury compared with morphologic features alone. Van Timmeren and colleagues also found that occurrence of renal allograft loss over time increased with increasing levels of KIM-1 excretion measured at baseline. High KIM-1 levels were associated with lower creatinine clearance, proteinuria, and higher donor age. KIM-1 levels predicted graft loss independent of creatinine clearance, proteinuria, and donor age.[177]

In a cross-sectional study of 29 patients with AKI of various causes, including sepsis and hypoperfusion, nephrotoxins, and contrast agent toxicity, and 40 control subjects (healthy volunteers and patients with CKD or urinary tract infection) the diagnostic utility of urinary levels of matrix metalloproteinase 9, NAG, and KIM-1 was determined.[178] The AUC showed lowest performance for matrix metalloproteinase 9, followed by KIM-1 and NAG. Combining all three biomarkers achieved a perfect score in diagnosing AKI. A case-control study of children undergoing cardiopulmonary bypass surgery included urine specimens from each of 20 patients with and without AKI. In this study, KIM-1 performed better than NAG at all time points. Combining both was no better than KIM-1 alone.[178]

Urinary concentrations of KIM-1 have been demonstrated to be predictive of AKI in prospective studies of patients undergoing cardiopulmonary bypass. In a study of 40 children undergoing cardiac surgery, urinary KIM-1 levels could diagnose AKI at 12 hours after surgery with an ROC AUC of 0.81, whereas elevation of serum creatinine concentration was noted only at 24 to 72 hours. In a prospective study of 90 adults undergoing cardiac surgery, urinary KIM-1 levels were significantly higher immediately postoperatively and for up to 24 hours after surgery in those who developed AKI compared with levels in patients who did not develop AKI. The AUCs for KIM-1, NAG, and NGAL for prediction of AKI immediately and 3 hours after operation were 0.68 and 0.65, 0.61 and 0.63, and 0.59 and 0.65, respectively. The specificity of KIM-1 varied from 78% to 89% for 0 hours and from 90% to 96% for 3 hours.[181] In another prospective cohort study of hospitalized patients who developed AKI from a variety of causes, patients with the highest quartile of urinary KIM-1 concentrations were statistically more likely to have higher peak serum creatinine concentrations, multiorgan failure, and oliguria. The AUC of KIM-1 for prediction of need for dialysis or death was 0.61, but increased to 0.80 when combined with the Acute Physiology and Chronic Health Evaluation II (APACHE II) score.[173]

KIM-1 also shows promise as a useful biomarker in CKD. In patients with IgA nephropathy, urinary KIM-1 levels were significantly higher than in healthy controls. Furthermore, the levels of urinary KIM-1 correlated positively with serum creatinine concentration and proteinuria and correlated inversely with creatinine clearance. Similar to the authors' observations, tubular KIM-1 expression as determined by immunohistochemical analysis correlated closely with urinary levels ($r = 0.553$; $P = 0.032$).[179] Recently, Sundaram and associates evaluated the potential of KIM-1, liver-type fatty acid–binding protein, NAG, NGAL, and transforming growth factor-β1 (TGF-β1), together with conventional renal biomarkers (urine albumin level, serum creatinine concentration, and serum cystatin C–estimated GFR) to detect nephropathy early in patients with sickle cell anemia. Only KIM-1 and NAG showed a strong correlation with albuminuria; other markers did not show any association with albuminuria.[180]

In an effort to investigate the early pathophysiology of diabetic nephropathy, the authors evaluated the association between kidney tubular injury biomarkers and changes in albuminuria in patients with type 1 diabetes mellitus.[182] Urine levels of KIM-1, NAG, interferon-γ–inducible protein 10 (IP-10), IL-6, IL-8, and monocyte chemoattractant protein-1 were measured in 38 healthy individuals and 659 patients with type 1 diabetes mellitus who had varying degrees of albuminuria.[182] Urinary levels of IL-6, IP-10, NAG, and KIM-1 were low in healthy individuals, were increased in patients with type 1 diabetes patients with normal urine albumin levels, and were highest in patients with diabetes and microalbuminuria. In this study lower urinary KIM-1 and NAG levels were found to be associated with regression of microalbuminuria, whereas progression or regression of microalbuminuria was unrelated to urinary levels of the other biomarkers assessed.

Because of its ability to predict clinical outcomes, KIM-1 is emerging as a useful biomarker in clinical trials. For example, a reduction in urinary KIM-1 level has been employed as an outcome variable in clinical trials demonstrating the efficacy of benfotiamine in patients with type 2 diabetes and nephropathy.[185] Similarly, in a randomized, double-blind, placebo-controlled crossover trial, Waanders and colleagues tested the hypothesis that a reduction in proteinuria by therapeutic interventions is associated with decreased urinary KIM-1 level. In 34 patients without diabetes and with proteinuric CKD, the authors found that the urinary excretion of KIM-1 was significantly reduced by antiproteinuric regimens, including losartan alone or in combination with hydrochlorothiazide.[186] Reduction in urinary KIM-1 levels paralleled the decline in proteinuria, but not in blood pressure. In contrast, changes in urinary levels of NAG were not closely related to proteinuria.

The authors' group devised an ELISA-based immunoassay to measure urinary KIM-1 levels in human and rodent samples and subsequently developed a microbead-based assay that is more sensitive, has very good dynamic range, is rapid, requires a smaller urine volume (30 μL), and offers multiplexing capabilities.[183] The majority of KIM-1 results described in the literature have been obtained using these ELISA assays. The assays are accurate, but are not practical to use at point of care in a clinical setting. In an effort to develop a rapid and user-friendly urine KIM-1 assay, the authors' laboratory also developed a dipstick test[184] that achieves sensitive and accurate detection of Kim-1/KIM-1, thereby facilitating the rapid detection of kidney injury in preclinical and clinical studies. We have studied the stability of KIM-1 under several conditions, including long-term storage, multiple freeze-thaw cycles, fresh versus frozen specimens, and changes in urinary pH. We and other groups found that KIM-1 is very stable at different pH values (pH of 6, 7, and 8) and after prolonged storage (2 years) at -80° C (data not published).

In summary, the utility of KIM-1 as a biomarker in humans is based on the following characteristics: (1) Its expression is not measurable in normal proximal tubule cells, but is markedly upregulated with injury or dedifferentiation. KIM-1 is highly expressed on the apical membrane of the injured proximal tubule cells, and its ectodomain is cleaved and excreted in the urine, which reflects kidney injury.[160,163] Importantly, KIM-1 excretion in the urine is highly specific for kidney injury because no other organs have been shown to express KIM-1 to a degree that would modulate its urinary concentrations. (2) Its measurement, like that of other urinary markers, is noninvasive and can be performed using readily available techniques. (3) Urinary KIM-1 level has been found to be much more sensitive than BUN and creatinine concentrations as a marker of injury in a large number of preclinical studies involving a wide variety of kidney insults, including exposure to various toxins. (4) Urinary KIM-1 is stable over time of storage across different pH conditions. (5) KIM-1 concentration can be used to monitor the response to therapeutic interventions. (6) KIM-1 is a translational biomarker, because its behavior in humans mirrors its behavior in animals. Hence it is likely to be very useful in safety monitoring and drug development, particularly under conditions in which toxicity is noted in preclinical studies and a toxicity monitoring system must be put in place to advance the drug into clinical studies. Recently, the FDA and the EMA have included KIM-1 in the small list of kidney injury biomarkers that they will now consider in the evaluation of kidney damage in animal studies of new drugs as part of their respective drug review processes.

The authors' recent studies in animals have demonstrated that Kim-1 acts as a scavenger receptor on renal epithelial cells; this converts the normal proximal tubule cell into a phagocyte, facilitates the clearance of dead cells in the lumen, takes up oxidized lipids, and likely plays an important role in the innate immune response after injury.[187] This finding suggests new avenues to develop novel therapeutics to protect the kidney from acute injury and/or to monitor its repair.

Liver-Type Fatty Acid–Binding Protein

Urinary fatty acid–binding protein 1 (FABP1) has been proposed to be a useful biomarker for early detection of AKI and monitoring of CKD. Also known as *L-type* or *liver-type fatty acid–binding protein* (L-FABP), FABP1 was first isolated in the liver as a binding protein for oleic acid and bilirubin. FABP1 binds selectively to free fatty acids and transports them to mitochondria or peroxisomes, where free fatty acids are β-oxidized and participate in intracellular fatty acid homeostasis. There are several different types of FABP, which are ubiquitously expressed in a variety of tissues. At this time, nine different FABPs have been reported: liver (L), intestinal (I), muscle and heart (H), epidermal (E), ileal (I1), myelin (M), adipocyte (A), brain (B), and testis (T). L-FABP is expressed in proximal tubules of the human kidney and localized in the cytoplasm. Increased cytosolic L-FABP in proximal tubular epithelial cells may derive not only from endogenous expression but also from circulating L-FABP that might be filtered at the glomeruli and reabsorbed by tubular cells.

Recently, a number of clinical studies have explored the potential utility of urinary L-FABP as a biomarker for the early diagnosis of AKI. Yamamoto and associates reported that urinary L-FABP levels correlated well with the ischemic time of the transplanted kidney and the length of hospital stay in human recipients of living related donor renal transplants.[188] Portilla and colleagues demonstrated that L-FABP predicts the development of AKI in children undergoing cardiac surgery.[189] This group reported that L-FABP was elevated within 4 hours after cardiac surgery, and these elevated levels anticipated the subsequent development of AKI with an accuracy of 81%.

In a study of a cohort of 40 patients with sepsis, the urinary L-FABP levels were greatly reduced with treatment in the 28 patients who survived but not the 12 patients who died.[190] These results suggest that urinary L-FABP concentrations might reflect the severity of sepsis and response to treatment.

In a cross-sectional study of 92 patients with AKI and 68 control subjects consisting of 26 healthy volunteers and 42 hospitalized patients (29 patients about to undergo coronary catheterization and 13 patients in the ICU), the authors' laboratory demonstrated that urinary levels of L-FABP were significantly higher in those with AKI than in hospitalized control patients without AKI, with an AUC of 0.93 (95% CI = 0.88 to 0.97; sensitivity = 83% and specificity = 90% at a cutoff value of 47.1 ng/mg of creatinine).[191] When healthy volunteers were used as controls, sensitivity and AUC improved to 95% and 0.96 respectively. In the same study, the authors compared the diagnostic performance of urinary L-FABP with that of other biomarkers of AKI, including NGAL, KIM-1, NAG, and IL-18, and reported that L-FABP performance was comparable to that of NGAL (AUC = 0.92), KIM-1 (AUC = 0.89), and NAG (AUC = 0.89), but better than that of IL-18 (AUC = 0.83).[191,192] These observations are in concordance with the results of prior studies using mice transgenic for human L-FABP that were exposed to ischemia-reperfusion injury.[192] As determined by ROC analysis, urinary L-FABP performance was superior to that of BUN and NAG for the detection of significant histologic injuries and functional declines.[193] Furthermore, age-adjusted logistic regression analysis showed that urinary L-FABP levels are predictive of the need for short-term renal replacement therapy and the composite endpoint of death or need for renal replacement therapy, but not of in-hospital mortality.[191] Because L-FABP is also expressed by the liver, liver injury can be a potential contributor to increased urinary levels of L-FABP during AKI. However, previous studies in patients with CKD, AKI, and sepsis have shown that serum L-FABP levels do not have an influence on urinary levels and that urinary L-FABP levels are not significantly higher in patients with liver disease than in healthy subjects.[189,190,194]

Urinary L-FABP level has been investigated as an early diagnostic and predictive marker for contrast medium–induced nephropathy.[195,196] In a study of adult patients with normal serum creatinine concentrations who underwent percutaneous coronary intervention, serum NGAL level rose at 2 and 4 hours, whereas urinary NGAL and urinary L-FABP increased significantly after 4 hours and remained elevated up to 48 hours after cardiac catheterization.[195] Nakamura and associates demonstrated that baseline urinary L-FABP levels were significantly higher in those patients who developed contrast medium–induced nephropathy after coronary angiography; however, the authors did not evaluate the diagnostic performance of urinary L-FABP in predicting AKI.[196]

Thus, current data from several clinical studies suggest a potential role for urinary L-FABP in the clinical evaluation of AKI. Larger multicenter studies that include early serial urine samples and larger patient cohorts are required for further evaluation of this promising biomarker.

Netrin-1

Netrin-1 is a 50- to 75-kDa laminin-like protein, initially recognized as a chemotropic factor that plays an essential role in guiding neurons and axons to their targets. Recent studies have revealed diverse roles of netrin-1 beyond axonal guidance, including development of various organs, angiogenesis, adhesion, tissue morphogenesis, inflammation, and tumorigenic processes.[197,198] Netrin-1 is expressed in several tissue types, including brain, lung, heart, liver, intestine, and kidney.[199]

A study by Wang and colleagues showed a rapid induction of netrin-1 in tubular epithelial cells in response to ischemia-reperfusion injury of the kidney in animal models.[200] In this study, netrin-1 was excreted in the urine as early as 1 hour after a kidney insult, increased over 40-fold by 3 hours, and reached its peak levels (approximately 50-fold) before the elevation of blood creatinine and BUN concentrations.[201] Importantly, this rapid increase in netrin-1 expression appeared to be regulated at the translational level, because netrin-1 gene transcription was actually decreased after ischemia-reperfusion injury.[201] The authors also tested the sensitivity and specificity of netrin-1 in animal models of toxin-induced kidney injury, using cisplatin, folic acid, and endotoxin (lipopolysaccharide). These kidney insults resulted in increases in the excretion of netrin-1 in urine, which supports a potential role as an early biomarker for hypoxic and toxic renal injuries.

Ramesh and colleagues also demonstrated a significant increase in urine levels of netrin-1 in patients with established AKI due to various causes (n = 16) compared with healthy volunteers. Very recently, the same group of scientists evaluated the potential of netrin-1 to predict AKI in patients undergoing cardiopulmonary bypass.[202] They included serial urine samples that were collected from 26 patients who developed AKI and 36 patients who did not develop AKI after cardiopulmonary bypass. By ROC analysis, the authors demonstrated that netrin-1 could predict AKI at 2 hours, 6 hours, and 12 hours, with an AUC of 0.74, 0.86, and 0.89, respectively. The levels of urinary netrin-1 6 hours after cardiopulmonary bypass correlated with the severity of AKI as well as the length of hospital stay, and remained a powerful independent predictor of AKI.[203]

Netrin-1 seems to be a promising early biomarker for AKI, but additional studies need to be done in larger cohorts with AKI due to various causes to further evaluate its potential.

Neutrophil Gelatinase–Associated Lipocalin

Neutrophil gelatinase–associated lipocalin (NGAL; also known as *lipocalin 2* or *lcn2*) is one of the new biomarkers for kidney injury that has been studied extensively. NGAL has many characteristics required for a good biomarker for AKI compared with serum creatinine measurement or urine output.[204] It is a 25-kDa protein with 178 amino acids belonging to the lipocalin superfamily. Lipocalins are extracellular proteins with diverse functions involving transport of hydrophilic substances through the membrane, thereby maintaining cell homeostasis.[205] NGAL is a glycoprotein bound to matrix metalloproteinase-9 in human neutrophils. It is expressed in various tissues in the body, such as salivary glands, prostate, uterus, trachea, lung, stomach, and kidney,[206] and its expression is markedly induced in injured epithelial cells, including those in the kidney, colon, liver, and lung.

Transcriptome profiling studies in rodent models identified NGAL as one of the most upregulated genes in the kidney very early after tubular injury.[207,208] Mishra and associates demonstrated that NGAL level was significantly elevated within 2 hours after injury in mouse models of renal ischemia-reperfusion.[209] In addition, urinary NGAL was detectable after 1 day of cisplatin administration, which suggests its sensitivity in other models of tubular injury.[209]

Many clinical studies followed these important observations in animals. Mishra and associates first demonstrated the value of NGAL as a clinical marker in a prospective study of 71 children undergoing cardiopulmonary bypass. In this study, both serum and urinary NGAL levels were upregulated within 2 hours in patients who developed AKI. A cutoff value of 50 µg/L was 100% sensitive and 98% specific in predicting AKI.[210] A larger follow-up study of 120 children by Dent and colleagues (with similar exclusion criteria used) showed that 2-hour postoperative serum NGAL level was predictive of AKI (AUC = 0.96) and correlated with postoperative change in serum creatinine concentration, duration of AKI, and length of hospital stay.[211] NGAL level at 12 hours was strongly correlated with mortality. In a subsequent study, Zapitelli and associates evaluated the predictive utility of urinary NGAL concentration in 140 critically ill children undergoing mechanical ventilation. Urinary NGAL levels increased significantly (by more than sixfold) 2 days earlier than a 50% increase in serum creatinine levels was reached.[212] Unlike in Mishra's study, however, in Zapitelli's study the AKI population was more heterogeneous with the timing of AKI unknown, and the AUCs of urinary NGAL level for prediction of AKI were lower than those reported by Mishra and colleagues.[210] The authors concluded that urinary NGAL is neither sensitive nor specific for predicting the course of AKI once it is established. Furthermore, in a cohort of 143 critically ill children with systemic inflammatory response syndrome, serum NGAL concentrations were measured during the first 24 hours of admission to the pediatric ICU and found to be a sensitive but nonspecific biomarker of AKI (sensitivity = 84%; specificity = 39%).[213]

In a study involving adults, Wagener and colleagues found that the best AUC for urinary NGAL concentration for prediction of AKI was 0.80 at 18 hours after cardiac surgery.[214] The same group reported that, in a cohort of 426 adult patients, NGAL had limited diagnostic accuracy in predicting AKI immediately after and at 3, 18, and 24 hours after cardiac surgery, with AUCs of 0.573, 0.603, 0.611, and 0.584, respectively.[214a] In another study, urinary NGAL level, but not serum creatinine concentrations, correlated with cardiopulmonary bypass time and aortic cross-clamp time.[215] APACHE II scores along with NGAL have been shown to be sensitive in predicting AKI in patients after liver transplantation.[216]

The function of NGAL as a diagnostic marker of contrast agent–induced nephropathy has also been evaluated. In a prospective study of 91 children undergoing coronary angiography, both urine and plasma NGAL levels were found to be significantly increased within 2 hours of contrast agent administration in the group that developed contrast medium–induced nephropathy, but not in the control group. By comparison, AKI detection using increases in serum creatinine concentration was possible only 6 to 24 hours after contrast agent administration. When a cutoff value of 100 ng/mL was used, both urine and serum NGAL levels at 2 hours predicted contrast medium–induced nephropathy, with AUCs of 0.91 and 0.92, respectively.[223] In several studies of adults undergoing procedures requiring contrast media, an early rise in both urine (4-hour) and plasma (2-hour) NGAL levels were documented, compared with a much later increase in plasma cystatin C levels, which provides support for the use of NGAL as an early biomarker for contrast medium–induced nephropathy.[159,224] A recent meta-analysis revealed an overall AUC of 0.894 for prediction of AKI when NGAL was measured within 6 hours after contrast agent administration when AKI was defined as a 25% or greater increase in serum creatinine concentration.[225]

NGAL has been investigated as a biomarker in CKD. In a 4-year follow-up study of 78 patients with type 1 diabetes conducted to evaluate the potential of urinary NGAL level to predict progression to diabetic nephropathy, NGAL levels were not associated with decline in GFR or development of ESRD and death after adjustment for known progression promoters.[217]

As discussed earlier, NGAL level has been evaluated in a variety of patient groups. Studies have reported different cutoff levels for NGAL to predict AKI, probably because of the heterogeneity among studies. Therefore, it seems that each clinical setting requires the determination of a normal range and cutoff value. Mishra and associates reported that serum NGAL values above a cutoff of 24 ng/mL predicted the development of AKI with a sensitivity of 1.00 and a specificity of 0.98.[210] Dent and colleagues reported that plasma NGAL values above 150 ng/mL in specimens collected 2 hours after cardiopulmonary bypass predicted the development of AKI with an AUC of 0.96 (sensitivity = 0.84; specificity = 0.94).[211] Aghel and associates recently reported that an elevated serum NGAL concentration on hospital admission was associated with a heightened risk of subsequent development of worsening kidney function in 91 patients admitted with acute heart failure.[218] In patients with chronic heart failure, Damman and colleagues suggested that impaired kidney function is not only characterized by decreased eGFR and increased urinary albumin excretion, but also by increased urinary NGAL concentration.[219] Poniatowski and colleagues found serum and urine NGAL levels to be sensitive early markers of impaired kidney function in patients with chronic heart failure who had normal serum creatinine concentrations but reduced eGFR.[220] In a recent study of 374 children undergoing cardiopulmonary bypass, both plasma and urine NGAL thresholds were found to be early predictive biomarkers for AKI and its clinical outcomes after cardiopulmonary bypass. In neonates, a 2-hour plasma NGAL threshold of 100 ng/mL and a 2-hour urine NGAL threshold of 185 ng/mL was recommended for the diagnosis of AKI.[221] Similarly, in an adult population of 100 patients undergoing cardiopulmonary bypass, a plasma NGAL level above 150 ng/mL in a sample taken on arrival to the ICU was again highly predictive of AKI (AUC = 0.8; sensitivity = 79%; specificity = 78%).[222] The predictive performance of NGAL in the adult population is not as striking as its performance in pediatric population.

NGAL has also been employed as a biomarker in interventional trials. A reduction in urine NGAL level has been used as an outcome variable in clinical investigations demonstrating the improved efficacy of a modern hydroxyethyl starch preparation compared with albumin or gelatin in maintaining kidney function in patients undergoing cardiac surgery.[226] NGAL in both serum and urine can be measured using commercially available ELISA kits. Recently an NGAL assay has been developed by Abbott Laboratories (Abbott Park, Illinois) for use in their ARCHITECT platform in clinical laboratories. A major advance has been the development of a point-of-care kit for the clinical measurement of plasma NGAL (Triage NGAL Test, Biosite Inc., San Diego, California).

The origin of plasma and urinary NGAL after AKI requires further clarification. Gene expression and transgenic animal studies have demonstrated an upregulation of NGAL in the distal nephron segments, specifically in the thick ascending limb of Henle and the collecting ducts; however, most of the injury in AKI occurs in the proximal tubules.[226,227] On the other hand, the source of plasma NGAL in AKI is not well defined. For instance, in animal studies, direct ipsilateral renal vein sampling after unilateral ischemia indicates that NGAL synthesized in the kidney does not enter the circulation.[227] The systemic pool in AKI may derive from the fact that NGAL is an acute phase reactant and may be released from neutrophils, macrophages, and other immune cells. Yndestad and colleagues reported strong immunostaining in cardiomyocytes within the failing myocardium in experimental and clinical heart failure.[228] Furthermore, any impairment in GFR resulting from AKI would be expected to decrease renal clearance of NGAL, with subsequent accumulation in the systemic circulation. However, the contribution of these mechanisms to the rise in plasma NGAL concentration after AKI has yet to be investigated. NGAL levels are also influenced by various medical conditions such as CKD, hypertension, anemia, systemic infections, hypoxia, inflammatory conditions, and cancers, which makes it relatively less specific for kidney injury.[229] Nevertheless, NGAL represents a very promising candidate as a biomarker for early diagnosis of AKI and potential prediction of outcome.

N-Acetyl-β-D-Glucosaminidase

N-Acetyl-β-D-glucosaminidase (NAG) is a lysosomal brush border enzyme that resides in the microvilli of tubular epithelial cells. Damage to these cells results in shedding of this enzyme into the urine. NAG has a high molecular weight of 130 kDa, and hence plasma NAG is not filtered by the glomeruli. Its excretion into urine correlates with tubular lysosomal activity. Increased urinary concentrations of NAG have been found in patients with AKI, chronic glomerular disease, diabetic nephropathy, exposure to nephrotoxic drugs, delayed renal allograft function, environmental exposure, contrast medium–induced nephropathy, and sepsis, and following cardiopulmonary bypass.[149,173,230-235] In a prospective study involving 201 hospitalized patients with AKI, patients with higher concentrations of urinary NAG and KIM-1 were more likely to die or require dialysis. This study suggests the utility of NAG in combination with KIM-1 in predicting adverse clinical outcomes in patients with AKI.[173] Urinary NAG concentrations were significantly higher in patients with contrast medium–induced nephropathy than in patients without such nephropathy within

24 hours after the administration of a contrast agent.[234] In a recent study of patients with type 1 diabetes and nephropathy, we have shown that lower levels of urinary KIM-1 and NAG were associated with the regression of microalbuminuria.[182]

There are some limitations in the use of NAG as a marker of kidney injury. Inhibition of NAG enzyme activity has been reported in the presence of metal ions and at higher urea concentrations in the urine. Moreover, increased urinary levels of NAG have been reported in several nonrenal diseases, including rheumatoid arthritis and hyperthyroidism, as well as in conditions with increased lysosomal activity without cellular damage.[236,237] Because of concerns about its specificity, the clinical utility of NAG as a biomarker has been limited.

Proteinuria

In a healthy person, urinary protein excretion is less than 150 mg/day and consists mainly of filtered plasma proteins (60%) and tubular Tamm-Horsfall proteins (40%).[237a,237b] Proteinuria can result from at least three different pathophysiologic mechanisms, including glomerular (increased permeability of glomerular filtration barrier to protein due to glomerulopathy, raised glomerular capillary hydrostatic pressure, or altered glomerular filtration coefficient), overflow (due to increased production of low molecular weight proteins, e.g., immunoglobulin light chains in myeloma), and tubular processes (decreased tubular absorption of filtered proteins or increased production of tubular proteins by damaged tubules). Proteinuria mechanisms and consequences are discussed in Chapter 52.

Proteinuria is diagnosed when total urinary protein is greater than 300 mg/24 hour. Methods for detecting and monitoring proteinuria are discussed in Chapter 25.

Recent publications highlight the diagnostic power of total protein for AKI in various drug-induced nephrotoxicities, including cisplatin and nonsteroidal antiinflammatory drugs.[237c,237d] Low eGFR is widely recognized as a risk factor for AKI, but the utility of proteinuria in combination with eGFR to predict the risk of this disease is now being investigated.[237e] Recently, in a large cohort of nearly 1 million adult Canadians, James and colleagues demonstrated an independent association between eGFR, proteinuria, and incidence of AKI.[237f] This group reported that patients with normal eGFR levels (≥60 ml/min per 1.73m²) and mild proteinuria (urine dipstick trace to 1+) have 2.5 times more risk of admission to hospital with AKI than do patients with no proteinuria. The risk was increased to 4.4-fold when they included patients with heavy proteinuria (urine dipstick ≥ 2+). Adjusted rates of admission with AKI and kidney injury requiring dialysis remained high in patients with heavy dipstick proteinuria independent of eGFR.[16] These findings confirm previous reports suggesting that eGFR and albuminuria are potent risk factors for subsequent AKI.[237g,237h]

Albuminuria

Albuminuria is recognized as one the most important risk factors for progression of kidney diseases. Albumin is a major serum protein with a size larger than the pores of the glomerular filtration membrane, so albuminiuria is best known as a biomarker of glomerular dysfunction; its appearance in large amounts in urine represents compromised integrity of the glomerular basement membrane.[237i] In smaller amounts, however, the presence of albumin in the urine may reflect tubular injury. Albuminuria is classified as microalbuminuria (UAE 30-300 mg/day or uACR=30-300 mg/g creatinine) and macroalbuminuria (UAE >300 mg/day or uACR >300 mg/g creatinine). In a number of clinical studies, albuminiuria has been shown to be a sensitive biomarker of drug-induced tubular injury.[237j,237k] It is routinely used as a marker of kidney damage for making a CKD diagnosis at eGFR levels above 60 ml/min per 1.73m².[237b] Guidelines of the National Kidney Foundation (NKF) and of the American Heart Association (AHA) included microalbuminuria as well as an increase in the urinary total protein excretion as a risk factor for renal and cardiovascular disease. Both NFK and AHA guidelines suggest measurement of uACR in an untimed spot urine sample. Ideally uACR should be assessed in at least three different samples to decrease the intra-individual variation.[237l] Albuminuria is a continuous risk factor for ESRD and cardiovascular mortality with no lower limit, even after adjustment for eGFR and other established risk factors.[237m,237n,237o] Urinary albumin has been in use as a biomarker for monitoring CKD progression and to monitor potential therapeutic efficacy, although the FDA does not accept albuminuria as a surrogate marker. Using microalbuminuria as a marker, Levin and colleagues demonstrated that N-acetylcysteine may attenuate contrast-induced glomerular and tubular injury.[237p]

Urinary Cystatin C

Any damage to proximal tubular cells can impede the reabsorption and enhance the urinary excretion of cystatin C. Several clinical studies sought to understand the potential of urinary levels for prediction of kidney injury and its prognosis. Herget-Rosenthal and associates analyzed data for 85 patients in the ICU who were at high risk of developing AKI and used the RIFLE classification to define AKI. In that study, the authors reported that serum cystatin C level detected AKI 1 to 2 days before changes in serum creatinine level, with an AUC of 0.82 and 0.97 on day 2 and day 1, respectively.[238] Urinary cystatin C/urinary creatinine ratios of more than 11.3 mg/mmol were significantly associated with proteinuria. In contrast to these findings, Royakkers and colleagues reported that both serum and urine cystatin C were poor predictors of AKI in a multicenter, prospective, observational cohort study of 151 patients (of whom 60 did not have AKI, 35 developed AKI after admission, and 56 had AKI at admission).[238a] The authors reported that the diagnostic performance of serum cystatin C level was fair on day 2 (AUC = 0.72) and poor on day 1 (AUC = 0.62). Furthermore, urinary cystatin C level had no diagnostic value on either of the 2 days before the development of AKI (AUC < 0.50). The small number of study subjects and methodologic limitations probably explain these discrepant findings.

A number of studies have reported increased urinary cystatin C levels in patients with proteinuria, which suggests the possibility of tubular damage as a consequence of protein overload.[238b,238c,238d] Currently, cystatin C level has several disadvantages as a biomarker, including lack of international standardization and expense of the assay. Furthermore, cystatin C is not always a reliable marker of renal function because its synthesis is increased in smokers, patients with hyperthyroidism, those receiving glucocorticoid therapy, and those with elevated levels of inflammatory markers such as white blood cell count and C-reactive protein level.[239,240] All of these factors are common in critically ill patients and could affect the reference value. Furthermore, different assays are available to measure cystatin C, and several different regression equations have been proposed to measure GFR. Advantages are that the commercially available immunonephelometric assay provides rapid, automated measurement of cystatin C and results are available in minutes.[241] In addition, preanalytic factors such as routine clinical storage conditions, freezing and thawing cycles, and interfering substances such as bilirubin or triglycerides do not affect cystatin C measurement.[241,242]

Chronic Kidney Disease Markers

Currently, eGFR and proteinuria are used as markers of CKD progression because of the widespread availability and ease of performing the tests. All forms of CKD are associated with tubulointerstitial injury. As described previously, markers of tubular injury, including KIM-1, NGAL, and L-FABP, have been shown to predict outcomes in CKD associated with a variety of causes. In addition, elevated systemic levels of molecules that have impaired kidney clearance or increased production in CKD (e.g., asymmetric dimethylarginine, fibroblast growth factor 23) as well as chemokines (e.g., monocyte chemoattractant protein-1) and fibrotic markers (connective tissue growth factor, TGF-β1, and collagen IV) are discussed here.

Plasma Asymmetric Dimethylarginine

Nitric oxide is synthesized by oxidation of the terminal guanidine nitrogen of L-arginine by nitric oxide synthase (NOS). This process can be reversibly inhibited by guanidine-substituted analogs of L-arginine, such as in asymmetric dimethylarginine (ADMA).[243,244] Three types of methylated arginines have been described in vivo: ADMA, N^G-monomethyl-L-arginine, and symmetric dimethylarginine, an inert isomer of ADMA. Of these, ADMA is the major type of endogenously generated methylated arginine that displays inhibitor activity of NOS. However, administration of ADMA to endothelial NOS knockout mice also induces vascular lesions, which suggests that ADMA may have actions independent of nitric oxide and NOS in vivo.[245] Vallance and associates first reported that plasma levels of ADMA are elevated in patients with renal failure[246] and hypothesized that impaired renal clearance of ADMA may account for the rise in plasma levels. This assumption has been challenged by follow-up studies in animal models demonstrating that only a small portion of circulating ADMA is excreted in the urine.[247] Moreover, elevated plasma ADMA levels are also reported in patients with incipient renal disease but normal renal function.[248]

Elevated plasma levels of ADMA have been reported in patients with a variety of cardiovascular risk factors, such as hypertension, diabetes, and hyperlipidemia.[249-251] Among these groups, plasma ADMA levels are particularly high in patients with CKD,[246,252,253] patients with ESRD undergoing hemodialysis or peritoneal dialysis, and kidney transplant recipients. Plasma levels of ADMA are strongly associated with carotid intima-media thickness, left ventricular hypertrophy, cardiovascular complications, and mortality in patients

with ESRD.[254-256] Furthermore, plasma ADMA levels predict the progression of renal injury in patients with CKD. Large longitudinal studies are needed to demonstrate the ability of ADMA to identify CKD and predict its progression in cohorts with CKD due to multiple causes.

Fibroblast Growth Factor 23

CKD is generally known to cause imbalance in mineral metabolism because of phosphate retention and decrease in serum calcium and activated vitamin D levels. A large body of evidence has demonstrated significant associations between increased levels of serum phosphate and adverse clinical outcomes, including more rapid progression of kidney disease, cardiovascular disease, and death.[257-259] Although all these studies reported disordered phosphorus metabolism, the changes in serum phosphate level within the normal range were very small. Hence, a more sensitive biomarker of disordered phosphorus metabolism with greater resolution in defining risk for adverse outcomes than serum phosphate concentration is needed, especially when the latter is normal as it usually is in CKD before dialysis is required. On the basis of a large set of studies, fibroblast growth factor 23 (FGF-23) has emerged as a candidate to fill this gap.

FGF-23 is a 32-kDa protein consisting of 251 amino acids coded by the FGF gene located on chromosome 12 in the human genome. It belongs to the FGF family of proteins secreted by bone cells, primarily osteoblasts, and is involved in phosphate metabolism, which in turn affects the levels of parathyroid hormone and calcitriol. FGF-23 is thought to play a vital role in regulating serum phosphate concentrations through direct and indirect effects on kidney, intestines, and bone.

FGF-23 is principally expressed in the ventrolateral thalamic nucleus in mice and is also known be secreted in minimal amounts in liver, heart, thymus, and lymph node. Maintenance of phosphate homeostasis is carried out by the sodium-dependent phosphate cotransporters NaPi-IIa and NaPi-IIc at the brush border membrane of proximal tubule cells in kidney, and FGF-23 has been shown to regulate the activity of these transporters.[260,261]

FGF-23 is increased in CKD and is a prognostic indicator for cardiovascular disease in patients with CKD. Recent studies have shown that elevated plasma FGF-23 concentrations are associated with cardiovascular events in patients not requiring dialysis and with mortality in patients receiving hemodialysis. It has been reported that serum FGF-23 concentrations may be a useful marker for predicting future development of refractory hyperparathyroidism and the response to vitamin D therapy in patients receiving dialysis.[262] Similarly, FGF-23 may be useful in the evaluation of calcium, phosphate, and vitamin D disorders in early-stage CKD in pediatric as well as adult patients.[264,265] Lowering FGF-23 levels (e.g., with oral phosphate binders) may reduce cardiovascular morbidity in CKD patients.[263] For further discussion of FGF-23, see Chapter 54.

Urinary Monocyte Chemoattractant Protein-1

Monocyte chemoattractant protein-1 (MCP-1) is a chemotactic protein secreted by a variety of cells that attracts blood monocytes and tissue macrophages through interaction with the cell surface receptor CCR2 (chemokine C-C motif receptor 2).[266,267] Induction of MCP-1 at the transcript or protein level has been demonstrated in a variety of human cell types, including fibroblasts, endothelial cells, peripheral blood mononuclear cells, and epithelial cells, on proinflammatory stimuli.[267-271] Kidney cells also produce MCP-1 in response to proinflammatory cytokines, including tumor necrosis factor-α and IL-1β.[272] Expression of MCP-1 is induced in kidney diseases with significant inflammation, such as diabetic nephropathy.[273,274] In particular, podocytes and tubular cells produce MCP-1 in response to high levels of glucose and advanced glycosylation end products.[275] Furthermore, urine levels of MCP-1 are significantly elevated in patients with diabetic nephropathy, and its levels correlate significantly with albuminuria and NAG levels in human as well as experimental diabetic nephropathy.[276-279] In a prospective observational study[280] of patients with diabetic nephropathy, urinary levels of connective tissue growth factor (CTGF) were elevated in patients with microalbuminuria and macroalbuminuria, but urinary MCP-1 level was elevated only in those with macroalbuminuria. Urinary CTGF levels correlated with progression to macroalbuminuria, whereas urinary MCP-1 levels (but not CTGF levels) correlated with the subsequent rate of eGFR decline (at a median follow-up of 6 years). The authors concluded that increased urinary CTGF level is associated with early progression of diabetic nephropathy, whereas MCP-1 level is associated with later-stage disease.[280]

Elevated levels of urinary MCP-1 were also reported in patients with lupus nephritis, and the presence of MCP-1 in urine reflected its intrarenal expression.[281,282] Serum concentrations of MCP-1 were also shown to be elevated in patients with diabetic nephropathy and lupus nephritis, but the serum levels did not correlate with disease progression.[281-283] Moreover, the lack of correlation between urinary and serum MCP-1 levels suggests that urinary MCP-1 is the result of local production of MCP-1 by the kidney rather than simply filtration of serum MCP-1. Munshi and associates demonstrated that urinary levels of both MCP-1 transcripts and protein were elevated in patients with AKI as well as in experimental models of AKI.[284]

Urinary Renal Fibrosis Markers

Excessive production of extracellular matrix (collagen IV) and profibrotic growth factors contributes to renal fibrosis, and CTGF as well as TGF-β1 are growth factors implicated in the progression of renal fibrosis.

Connective Tissue Growth Factor

Connective tissue growth factor (CTGF; also known as *CCN2*), a member of CCN family of matricellular proteins, was first discovered by Bradham and colleagues in 1991 as a secreted protein in the conditioned media of human umbilical vascular endothelial cells.[285] CTGF has been implicated in a variety of cellular functions, including proliferation, cell adhesion, angiogenesis, and wound healing.[254,286,287] Accumulated evidence on CTFG in the last few years indicates that CTGF is both a marker and a mediator of tissue fibrosis.[288] CTGF is an immediate-early gene potently induced by TGF-β and shown to promote fibrosis primarily through TGF-β.[289] CTGF is overexpressed in several fibrotic diseases,

such as scleroderma and lung and hepatic fibrosis.[290-292] In the kidney, CTGF expression has been shown to be upregulated in various forms of renal disease, including IgA nephropathy, focal and segmental glomerulosclerosis, and diabetic nephropathy.[291] CTGF has been found to be elevated in the glomeruli at early and late stages of diabetic nephropathy.[293] Riser and associates first reported that CTGF is elevated in the urine of diabetic rats and in diabetic patients.[294] Subsequently several groups reported higher urinary levels of CTGF in diabetic patients than in healthy individuals,[295,296] which indicates its potential as a marker for diabetic nephropathy. In patients with diabetes, plasma CTGF level was shown to be higher in those with macroalbuminuria than in those with a normal urine albumin level. CTGF was an independent predictor of ESRD and correlated with the rate of decline in GFR.[297] In another study, both blood and urine levels of whole molecules of CTGF and the N-terminal fragment were measured in 1050 patients with type 1 diabetes.[298] Patients with macroalbuminuria had higher levels of CTGF N-terminal fragment than diabetic patients with or without microalbuminuria.

Transforming Growth Factor-β₁

Transforming growth factor-β (TGF-β) is essential for the development and differentiation of various tissues.[299] Three isoforms of TGF-β have been identified in mammalian species: TGF-β1, TGF-β2, and TGF-β3. TGF-β1 is the predominant isoform in humans.[300] It is mainly secreted as high-molecular-weight inactive complex and undergoes a cleavage process for its activation.[301] Several studies have demonstrated the association of urine levels of TGF-β1 with the progression of CKD. Elevated urinary TGF-β1 levels were found in patients with glomerulonephritis and diabetic nephropathy, as well as in renal allograft recipients.[301-304] In addition, some of the profibrotic molecules induced by TGF-β1, including TGF-β–inducible gene H3 (βig-H3) and plasminogen activator inhibitor-1 (PAI-1), were also detected at high levels in the urine.[305,306] Because TGF-β1 is mostly secreted as an inactive complex that requires chemical modification for its activation, βig-H3 and PAI-1 can be used as surrogate markers for TGF-β1 activity. Urinary levels of both βig-H3 and PAI-1 have been shown to correlate with renal injury and fibrosis in patients with diabetic nephropathy.[305,306]

Collagen IV

Collagen IV is a component of the extracellular matrix, and excess deposition of collagen IV is present in renal fibrosis. Furthermore, elevation of urinary collagen IV has been reported in patients with IgA nephropathy as well as in those with diabetic nephropathy and has been correlated with declining renal function.[307,308]

Combinations of Multiple Biomarkers

In the classical biomarker paradigm one biomarker detects one disease. However, acute and chronic kidney diseases are complex with multiple underlying causes. A single biomarker may not be optimal to make an early diagnosis and predict the longer-term outcome of the disease process. Different biomarkers provide different information. Thus, it is important to consider the clinical utility of a panel of biomarkers for acute and chronic kidney diseases.

To this end, in a cross-sectional study, the authors' laboratory evaluated the diagnostic performance of nine urinary biomarkers of AKI—KIM-1, NGAL, IL-18, hepatocyte growth factor (HGF), cystatin C, NAG, vascular endothelial growth factor (VEGF), interferon-γ–inducible protein 10 (IP-10; also known as *C-X-C motif chemokine 10*, or *CXCL10*), and total protein—in 102 patients with AKI of various causes and 102 individuals without clinically documented AKI[183] (Figure 29-2). The control group included healthy volunteers, patients scheduled for cardiac catheterization, and patients who were in the ICU but were not diagnosed with AKI. For each of the urinary proteins, median concentrations were significantly higher in patients with AKI than in those without AKI. The AUC for KIM-1 was 0.95 when patients with AKI were compared to healthy controls. When the authors took a nonbiased logistic regression model approach to optimize the combination of biomarkers so as to yield an algorithm that could best fit the data and be prospectively tested, the following was obtained: risk score = $2.93 \times$ [NGAL(ng/mg.uCr) >5.72 and HGF(ng/mg uCr) >0.17] + 2.93[protein(mg/mg.–uCr) >0.22] – $2 \times$ [KIM-1(ng/mg uCr) <0.58]. This combination of four biomarkers yielded an AUC (0.94) that was significantly higher than the AUCs for individual biomarkers when a number of hospitalized control groups were included (even though some of these "controls" likely had clinically silent AKI). It is particularly interesting to examine the scatter plots of urinary biomarkers across the four groups (see Figure 29-2). It is clear that there was a little overlap between the AKI group and the healthy controls for KIM-1, total protein, NGAL, NAG, and HGF. The overlap may be due to misdiagnosis due to an incorrect diagnosis of AKI clinically, because creatinine concentration can be elevated in the absence of kidney injury in patients with prerenal azotemia. Alternatively, in this cross-sectional analysis a few patients may already have been in a postinjury or tissue repair state with lower biomarker levels despite the fact that serum creatinine concentration had not yet fallen completely back to normal. NAG was the best performer when patients with AKI were compared with healthy volunteers, but its performance deteriorated when other control groups were included, especially the ICU patients with no clinical or laboratory diagnosis of AKI. In this latter group, NAG level was elevated in 13 of 13 patients, which suggests that it may be a nonspecific marker of critical illness. Age-adjusted levels of urinary KIM-1, NAG, HGF, VEGF, and total protein were significantly higher in patients who died or required renal replacement therapy than in those who survived and did not require renal replacement therapy.[183]

Triple Biomarker Approach for Detection of Chronic Kidney Disease

David Warnock's group studied the potential benefits of adding a cystatin C–based measure of eGFR ($GFR_{cystatin}$) and albumin/creatinine ratio to the current standard eGFR based on serum creatinine concentration ($GFR_{creatinine}$) in a prospective cohort study involving 26,643 U.S. adults enrolled in the Reasons for Geographic and Racial Differences in Stroke (REGARDS) study. The authors found that the adjusted risk of mortality was threefold higher in patients with CKD defined by both $GFR_{cystatin}$ and $GFR_{creatinine}$ than in those with CKD defined by $GFR_{creatinine}$ alone and approximately sixfold higher in patients with CKD identified by all three markers. Furthermore, the risk of ESRD was highest among patients with CKD defined by all three markers.[309]

Assays and Technologies

The methods traditionally used to quantitate tubular urinary enzymes are typically enzyme substrate–based spectrophotometric assays. With the recent emergence of urinary and serum proteins as biomarkers, ELISA assays have become the workhorses for accurate quantification. Although reliable ELISA assays exist for most of the described renal biomarkers in serum and urine, this technique is very limited due to the fact that it allows measurement of only one biomarker per assay. This makes assessment of multiple biomarkers time consuming and expensive. Moreover, measurement of several biomarkers requires larger quantities of specimens. To overcome these limitations, kidney biomarker multiplex assays have been developed on two automated, user-friendly, high-throughput technologies: the platforms developed by Luminex (Austin, Texas) and Meso Scale Discover (Gaithersburg, Maryland).

The authors have developed multiplex assays for renal biomarkers on the Luminex platform. This technology uses principles of both ELISA and flow cytometry to simultaneously quantitate multiple analytes in biologic fluids. The Luminex xMAP technology relies on capture antibodies conjugated to the surface of color-coded microbeads that react with specific antigens present in the sample, as in sandwich assays. Quantification is achieved by addition of a biotinylated secondary antibody and streptavidin coupled to fluorochrome. The signal is directly proportional to the amount of antigen bound at the microbead surface. This technique is theoretically capable of assessing up to 100 different antigens and requires only small volumes of biologic fluid (25 to 30 μL).

Meso Scale Discovery assays are electrochemiluminescence assays based on the sandwich ELISA assay format. Unlike the Luminex instrument, in which microbeads loaded with antibodies are in suspension, in the Meso Scale Discovery device, antibodies are immobilized in planar arrays in microplate format and the readout is the light signal emitted by an electrochemiluminescence reaction. The manufacturers of the Meso Scale Discovery platform claim to allow testing of up to 10 different analytes in a 96-well format and up to 100 assays in a 24-well format.

Although both the Luminex and Meso Scale Discovery platforms offer advantages, these instruments may not be available in all clinical laboratories. Recently, some of the biomarker assays have been made available on clinical analyzer platforms to ensure the broader availability of the assays in clinical units. For instance, an NGAL assay has been developed on the Abbott Diagnostics ARCHITECT clinical analyzer.[310]

There has been growing interest in developing point-of-care testing tools that will facilitate the timely testing of renal biomarkers in small hospitals and health care centers. For example, the transfer of an NGAL assay onto Biosite's Triage NGAL device enables the measurement of NGAL at the bedside in approximately 15 minutes.[310,311] The authors'

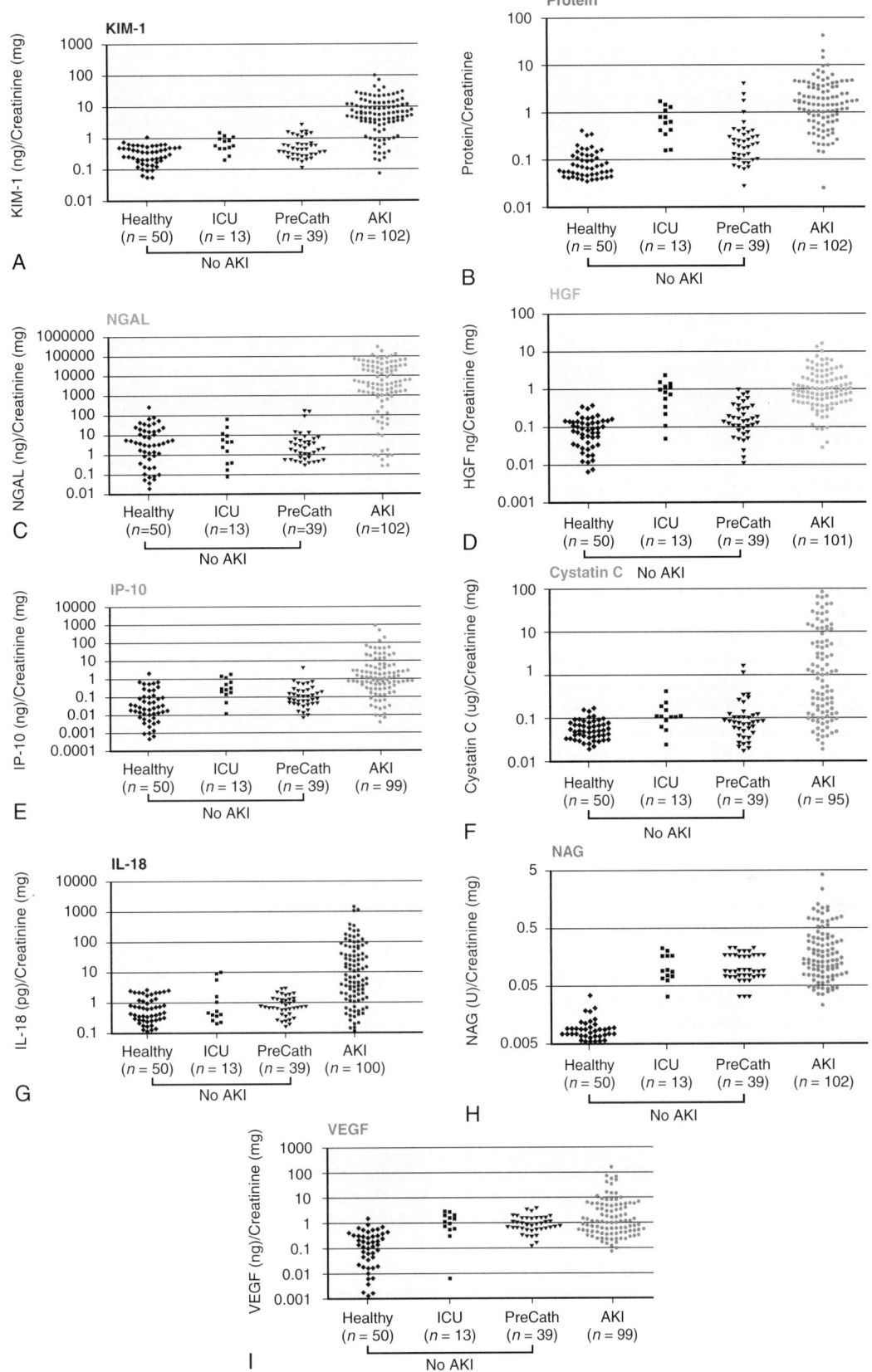

FIGURE 29-2 Urinary biomarker levels in patients with a diagnosis of AKI compared with levels in three control groups without this diagnosis. Patients with documented AKI as defined by the RIFLE criteria[316] (increase in peak serum creatinine level of 50% or more over admission value or known baseline) were recruited. Clinical causes of AKI were identified by chart review and evaluation of laboratory data. Individuals without AKI were categorized into distinct populations: healthy volunteers, patients undergoing cardiac catheterization, and patients admitted to the intensive care unit. Patients undergoing cardiac catheterization and those admitted to the intensive care unit were included in the non-AKI cohort if they had normal urine output (>0.5 mL/kg/hr), stable serum creatinine level during hospitalization (<0.3 mg/dL change from baseline), and an estimated glomerular filtration rate (GFR) of more than 50 mL/min. Urine samples were obtained from cardiac catheterization patients before administration of an intravenous contrast medium. Some patients in the non-AKI groups had elevated biomarker levels, likely due to the fact that they had subclinical kidney injury. Each point represents one subject. (From Vaidya VS, Waikar SS, Ferguson MA, et al: Urinary biomarkers for sensitive and specific detection of acute kidney injury in humans, *Clin Transl Sci* 1:200-208, 2008.)

laboratory has developed a rapid KIM-1 assay on a diagnostic dipstick. The dipstick test allows a visual readout within 15 minutes and can be used at the bedside without additional equipment.[184] With the use of a hand-held lateral flow reader one can obtain absolute quantification of KIM-1 in urine using dipsticks.

FDA Critical Path Initiative

The Critical Path Initiative was launched in March 2004 by the FDA as a strategy for modernizing the sciences through which FDA-regulated products are developed, evaluated, manufactured, and used. The 2006 report of the Critical Path Initiative outlined specific key areas of Critical Path focus identified by FDA experts and the public. Commenting on a major initiative of the FDA that focuses on biomarkers, Janet Woodcock, MD, deputy commissioner for operations and head of the FDA's Critical Path Initiative, stated: "Most researchers agree that a new generation of predictive biomarkers would dramatically improve the efficiency of product development, help identify safety problems before a product is on the market (and even before it is tested in humans), and facilitate the development of new types of clinical trials that will produce better data faster."[312] The Critical Path Initiative is the FDA's attempt to stimulate and facilitate a national effort to modernize the scientific process through which a potential human drug, biologic product, or medical device progresses from the discovery or "proof of concept" stage into a medical product.[313] The FDA has provided guidelines stating that a biomarker can be considered "valid" only if (1) it is measured in an analytical test system with well-established performance characteristics, and (2) there is an established scientific framework or body of evidence that elucidates the physiologic, pharmacologic, toxicologic, or clinical significance of the test result.

The initial project hosted by Critical Path Institute, the Predictive Safety Testing Consortium (PSTC), brought together 16 pharmaceutical and biotechnology companies, one nonprofit patient organization, and advisors from academic institutions, the FDA, and the EMA to exchange data and methodologies with the goal of qualifying organ safety biomarkers for regulatory decision making in preclinical, translational, and clinical contexts.[21,22] Seven urinary proteins (KIM-1, albumin, total protein, β_2-microglobulin, cystatin C, clusterin, and trefoil factor 3) were evaluated for their utility to outperform current tests, including serum creatinine concentration and BUN concentration, in the detection of drug-induced kidney injury. The Predictive Safety Testing Consortium submitted the data to the FDA, EMA, and Japanese Pharmaceutical and Medical Devices Agency for evaluation.[21] In 2010, the FDA and EMA reached the formal conclusion that these biomarkers are considered qualified for use in regulatory decision making for drug safety to detect acute drug-induced kidney injury in preclinical studies and, on a case-by-case basis, in early clinical studies in combination with standard biomarkers.[21,22,314,315]

Future of Biomarkers

Recent advances in molecular analysis and proteomics have resulted in the identification of a wide range of potential serum and urine biomarkers for assessing renal function and injury as well as predicting the development of kidney disease. Not only are many of these biomarkers sensitive, but some are site specific. A number of them have been reported to be predictive of an adverse outcome. A great deal of additional work is still needed, however, to bring these biomarkers successfully to clinical practice for kidney diseases.

Because kidney disease is complex with multiple causes and often presents in the setting of systemic diseases, a single biomarker may be insufficient for early diagnosis, insight into pathophysiology, and prediction of clinical course and outcome. Different biomarkers will be useful in different contexts. In some circumstances a single biomarker may suffice, but in others benefit will come from the use of multiple biomarkers in plasma, urine, or both to provide early evidence of risk and injury, and to distinguish between various types of kidney diseases. Many of these biomarkers can be grouped according to their association with a particular type of injury (e.g., podocyte or tubular injury) or mechanism of damage (e.g., oxidative stress, inflammation, fibrosis). Understanding the relationships between these different biomarker categories may help us to better understand disease processes.

These biomarkers not only are useful for accessing kidney injury in humans in early stages and predicting progression of disease but also are crucial for translating novel therapeutic compounds from preclinical animal models to first human trials. Until recently, the use of newly emerged biomarkers in preclinical and clinical studies and drug development has been hindered by lack of regulatory acceptance. Hopefully in the future, biomarker measurements obtained using biomarker test panels will not only be used to diagnose kidney injury and predict outcome but will also be used as surrogate endpoints in clinical trials, which might speed up clinical evaluation of desperately needed therapies for kidney diseases.

Acknowledgement

Dr. Bonventre's laboratory is supported by National Institutes of Health grants DK39773, DK72831, and DK85660.

Disclosure

Dr. Bonventre is listed as coinventor on KIM-1 patents that have been licensed by Partners HealthCare to a number of companies, including Johnson & Johnson, Sekisui, Biogen Idec, R and D, Rules Based Medicine, and BioAssay Works. He has received royalty income from Partners HealthCare and grant funding from Johnson & Johnson and BASF. Dr. Bonventre or members of his family have received income for consulting from Genzyme Corporation, Dicerna Pharmaceuticals, Celgene Corporation, AstraZeneca, and PTC Therapeutics, and have stock ownership in AMAG Pharmaceuticals, Theravance, PatientKeeper, and Pacific Biosciences.

References

1. Uchino S, Kellum JA, Bellomo R, et al. Acute renal failure in critically ill patients: a multinational, multicenter study. *JAMA*. 2005;294:813-818.
2. Collins AJ, Foley RN, Herzog C, et al. US Renal Data System 2010 annual data report. *Am J Kidney Dis*. 2011;57:A28, e1-526.

3. Sanoff S, Okusa MD. Impact of acute kidney injury on chronic kidney disease and its progression. *Contrib Nephrol.* 2011;171:213-217.
4. Nugent RA, Fathima SF, Feigl AB, et al. The burden of chronic kidney disease on developing nations: a 21st century challenge in global health. *Nephron Clin Pract.* 2011;118:c269-c277.
5. Schieppati A, Remuzzi G. Chronic renal diseases as a public health problem: epidemiology, social, and economic implications. *Kidney Int Suppl.* 2005, (98):S7-S10.
6. Blagg CR. Chronic kidney disease is but one of the many global threats to health. *Hemodial Int.* 2010;14:345.
7. Saran R, Hedgeman E, Huseini M, et al. Surveillance of chronic kidney disease around the world: tracking and reining in a global problem. *Adv Chronic Kidney Dis.* 2010;17:271-281.
8. Zurbig P, Dihazi H, Metzger J, et al. Urine proteomics in kidney and urogenital diseases: moving towards clinical applications. *Proteomics Clin Appl.* 2011;5:256-268.
9. Shao C, Wang Y, Gao Y. Applications of urinary proteomics in biomarker discovery. *Sci China Life Sci.* 2001;54:409-417.
10. Boudonck KJ, Rose DJ, Karoly ED, et al. Metabolomics for early detection of drug-induced kidney injury: review of the current status. *Bioanalysis.* 2009;1:1645-1663.
11. Prunotto M, Ghiggeri GM, Candiano G, et al. Urinary proteomics and drug discovery in chronic kidney disease: a new perspective. *J Proteome Res.* 2011;10:126-132.
12. Group BW. Biomarkers and surrogate endpoints: preferred definitions and conceptual framework. *Clin Pharmacol Ther.* 2001;69:89-95.
13. Biomarkers and surrogate endpoints. preferred definitions and conceptual framework. *Clin Pharmacol Ther.* 2001;69:89-95.
14. Pepe MS, Etzioni R, Feng Z, et al. Phases of biomarker development for early detection of cancer. *J Natl Cancer Inst.* 2001;93:1054-1061.
15. Srivastava S, Gopal-Srivastava R. Biomarkers in cancer screening: a public health perspective. *J Nutr.* 2002;132:2471S-2475S.
16. Solberg HE. International Federation of Clinical Chemistry. Scientific committee, Clinical Section. Expert Panel on Theory of Reference Values and International Committee for Standardization in Haematology Standing Committee on Reference Values. Approved recommendation (1986) on the theory of reference values. Part 1. The concept of reference values. *Clin Chim Acta.* 1987;165:111-118.
17. Solberg HE, Petitclerc C. International Federation of Clinical Chemistry (IFCC), Scientific Committee, Clinical Section, Expert Panel on Theory of Reference Values. Approved recommendation (1988) on the theory of reference values. Part 3. Preparation of individuals and collection of specimens for the production of reference values. *J Clin Chem Clin Biochem.* 1988;26:593-598.
18. Labaer J. So, you want to look for biomarkers (introduction to the special biomarkers issue). *J Proteome Res.* 2005;4:1053-1059.
19. Waikar SS, Betensky RA, Emerson SC, et al. Imperfect gold standards for kidney injury biomarker evaluation. *J Am Soc Nephrol.* 2011. (In press).
20. Goodsaid F, Frueh F. Biomarker qualification pilot process at the US Food and Drug Administration. *AAPS J.* 2007;9:E105-108.
21. Dieterle F, Sistare F, Goodsaid F, et al. Renal biomarker qualification submission: a dialog between the FDA-EMEA and Predictive Safety Testing Consortium. *Nat Biotechnol.* 2010;28:455-462.
22. Sistare FD, Dieterle F, Troth S, et al. Towards consensus practices to qualify safety biomarkers for use in early drug development. *Nat Biotechnol.* 2010;28:446-454.
23. Zweig MH, Campbell G. Receiver-operating characteristic (ROC) plots: a fundamental evaluation tool in clinical medicine. *Clin Chem.* 1993;39:561-577.
24. Soreide K. Receiver-operating characteristic curve analysis in diagnostic, prognostic and predictive biomarker research. *J Clin Pathol.* 2009;62:1-5.
25. Bharti B, Bharti S. Receiver-operating characteristic curve analysis in diagnostic, prognostic and predictive biomarker research: trade-off between sensitivity and specificity with change of test cut-offs. *J Clin Pathol.* 2009;62:1051.
26. Defilippi CR, De Lemos JA, Christenson RH, et al. Association of serial measures of cardiac troponin T using a sensitive assay with incident heart failure and cardiovascular mortality in older adults. *JAMA.* 2010;304:2494-2502.
27. Gomes S, Pereira D, Oliveira R, et al. New diagnostic criteria for acute myocardial infarction and in-hospital mortality. *Rev Port Cardiol.* 2005;24:231-237.
28. Waikar SS, Sabbisetti VS, Bonventre JV. Normalization of urinary biomarkers to creatinine during changes in glomerular filtration rate. *Kidney Int.* 2010;78:486-494.
29. Coresh J, Byrd-Holt D, Astor BC, et al. Chronic kidney disease awareness, prevalence, and trends among U.S. adults, 1999 to 2000. *J Am Soc Nephrol.* 2005;16:180-188.
30. Bosch JP. Renal reserve: a functional view of glomerular filtration rate. *Semin Nephrol.* 1995;15:381-385.
31. Herrera J, Rodriguez-Iturbe B. Stimulation of tubular secretion of creatinine in health and in conditions associated with reduced nephron mass. Evidence for a tubular functional reserve. *Nephrol Dial Transplant.* 1998;13:623-629.
32. Fehrman-Ekholm I, Duner F, Brink B, et al. No evidence of accelerated loss of kidney function in living kidney donors: results from a cross-sectional follow-up. *Transplantation.* 2001;72:444-449.
33. Baum N, Dichoso CC, Carlton CE. Blood urea nitrogen and serum creatinine. Physiology and interpretations. *Urology.* 1975;5:583-588.
34. Schrier RW, Wang W, Poole B, et al. Acute renal failure: definitions, diagnosis, pathogenesis, and therapy. *J Clin Invest.* 2004;114:5-14.
35. Endre ZH, Pickering JW. New markers of acute kidney injury: giant leaps and baby steps. *Clin Biochem Rev.* 2011;32:121-124.
36. Soni SS, Ronco C, Katz N, et al. Early diagnosis of acute kidney injury: the promise of novel biomarkers. *Blood Purif.* 2009;28:165-174.
37. Kampmann J, Siersbaek-Nielsen K, Kristensen M, et al. Rapid evaluation of creatinine clearance. *Acta Med Scand.* 1974;196:517-520.
38. Wu I, Parikh CR. Screening for kidney diseases: older measures versus novel biomarkers. *Clin J Am Soc Nephrol.* 2008;3:1895-1901.
39. Ducharme MP, Smythe M, Strohs G. Drug-induced alterations in serum creatinine concentrations. *Ann Pharmacother.* 1993;27:622-633.
40. Rocci Jr ML, Vlasses PH, Ferguson RK. Creatinine serum concentrations and H_2-receptor antagonists. *Clin Nephrol.* 1984;22:214-215.
41. Nickolas TL, Barasch J, Devarajan P. Biomarkers in acute and chronic kidney disease. *Curr Opin Nephrol Hypertens.* 2008;17:127-132.
42. Dimagno EP, Corle D, O'Brien JF, et al. Effect of long-term freezer storage, thawing, and refreezing on selected constituents of serum. *Mayo Clin Proc.* 1989;64:1226-1234.
43. Zhang DJ, Elswick RK, Miller WG, et al. Effect of serum-clot contact time on clinical chemistry laboratory results. *Clin Chem.* 1998;44:1325-1333.
44. Da Rin G, Amici G, Virga G, et al. Correction of glucose concentration interference on Jaffé kinetic creatinine assay in peritoneal dialysis. *Am J Nephrol.* 1995;15:480-487.
45. Lo SC, Tsai KS. Glucose interference in Jaffé creatinine method: effect of calcium from peritoneal dialysate. *Clin Chem.* 1994;40:2326-2327.
46. Koumantakis G, Wyndham L. Fluorescein interference with urinary creatinine and protein measurements. *Clin Chem.* 1991;37:1799.
47. Myers GL, Miller WG, Coresh J, et al. Recommendations for improving serum creatinine measurement: a report from the Laboratory Working Group of the National Kidney Disease Education Program. *Clin Chem.* 2006;52:5-18.
48. Fabiny DL, Ertingshausen G. Automated reaction-rate method for determination of serum creatinine with the CentrifiChem. *Clin Chem.* 1971;17:696-700.
49. Swain RR, Briggs SL. Positive interference with the Jaffé reaction by cephalosporin antibiotics. *Clin Chem.* 1977;23:1340-1342.
50. Bagnoud MA, Reymond JP. Interference of metamizol (dipyrone) on the determination of creatinine with the Kodak dry chemistry slide: comparison with the enzymatic method from Boehringer. *Eur J Clin Chem Clin Biochem.* 1993;31:753-757.
51. Ali AC, Mihas CC, Campbell JA. Interferences of o-raffinose cross-linked hemoglobin in three methods for serum creatinine. *Clin Chem.* 1997;43:1738-1743.
52. Hummel KM, Von Ahsen N, Kuhn RB, et al. Pseudohypercreatininemia due to positive interference in enzymatic creatinine measurements caused by monoclonal IgM in patients with Waldenström's macroglobulinemia. *Nephron.* 2000;86:188-189.
53. Lim CK, Richmond W, Robinson DP, et al. Towards a definitive assay of creatinine in serum and in urine: separation by high-performance liquid chromatography. *J Chromatogr.* 1978;145:41-49.
54. Brown ND, Sing HC, Neeley WE, et al. Determination of "true" serum creatinine by high-performance liquid chromatography combined with a continuous-flow microanalyzer. *Clin Chem.* 1977;23:1281-1283.
55. Chiou WL, Peng GW, Gadalla MA, et al. Comparison of plasma creatinine levels in patients determined by high-pressure liquid chromatography, automated analysis, and boiling alkaline picrate method. *J Pharm Sci.* 1978;67:292-293.
56. Ambrose RT, Ketchum DF, Smith JW. Creatinine determined by "high-performance" liquid chromatography. *Clin Chem.* 1983;29:256-259.
57. Maruyama Y, Kusaka M, Mori J, et al. Simple method for the determination of choline and acetylcholine by prolysis gas chromatography. *J Chromatogr.* 1979;164:121-127.
58. Dossetor JB. Creatininemia versus uremia. The relative significance of blood urea nitrogen and serum creatinine concentrations in azotemia. *Ann Intern Med.* 1966;65:1287-1299.
59. Winkler AW, Parra J. The measurement of glomerular filtration. the creatinine, sucrose and urea clearances in subjects with renal disease. *J Clin Invest.* 1937;16:869-877.
60. Baldus WP, Feichter RN, Summerskill WH. The kidney in cirrhosis. I. Clinical and biochemical features of azotemia in hepatic failure. *Ann Intern Med.* 1964;60:353-365.
61. Marshall S. Urea-creatinine ratio in obstructive uropathy and renal hypertension. *JAMA.* 1964;190:719-720.
62. Shlipak MG, Sarnak MJ, Katz R, et al. Cystatin C and the risk of death and cardiovascular events among elderly persons. *N Engl J Med.* 2005;352:2049-2060.

63. Butler EA, Flynn FV. The occurrence of post-gamma protein in urine: a new protein abnormality. *J Clin Pathol*. 1961;14:172-178.

64. Hojs R, Bevc S, Ekart R, et al. Serum cystatin C as an endogenous marker of renal function in patients with mild to moderate impairment of kidney function. *Nephrol Dial Transplant*. 2006;21:1855-1862.

65. Koenig W, Twardella D, Brenner H, et al. Plasma concentrations of cystatin C in patients with coronary heart disease and risk for secondary cardiovascular events: more than simply a marker of glomerular filtration rate. *Clin Chem*. 2005;51:321-327.

66. Sarnak MJ, Katz R, Stehman-Breen CO, et al. Cystatin C concentration as a risk factor for heart failure in older adults. *Ann Intern Med*. 2005;142:497-505.

67. Shlipak MG, Wassel Fyr CL, Chertow GM, et al. Cystatin C and mortality risk in the elderly: the health, aging, and body composition study. *J Am Soc Nephrol*. 2006;17:254-261.

68. Ahlstrom A, Tallgren M, Peltonen S, et al. Evolution and predictive power of serum cystatin C in acute renal failure. *Clin Nephrol*. 2004;62:344-350.

69. Rickli H, Benou K, Ammann P, et al. Time course of serial cystatin C levels in comparison with serum creatinine after application of radiocontrast media. *Clin Nephrol*. 2004;61:98-102.

70. Kato K, Sato N, Yamamoto T, et al. Valuable markers for contrast-induced nephropathy in patients undergoing cardiac catheterization. *Circ J*. 2008;72:1499-1505.

71. Melegos DN, Diamandis EP, Oda H, et al. Immunofluorometric assay of prostaglandin D synthase in human tissue extracts and fluids. *Clin Chem*. 1996;42:1984-1991.

72. Hoffmann A, Nimtz M, Conradt HS. Molecular characterization of beta-trace protein in human serum and urine: a potential diagnostic marker for renal diseases. *Glycobiology*. 1997;7:499-506.

73. Priem F, Althaus H, Birnbaum M, et al. Beta-trace protein in serum: a new marker of glomerular filtration rate in the creatinine-blind range. *Clin Chem*. 1999;45:567-568.

74. Woitas RP, Stoffel-Wagner B, Poege U, et al. Low-molecular weight proteins as markers for glomerular filtration rate. *Clin Chem*. 2001;47:2179-2180.

75. Filler G, Priem F, Lepage N, et al. Beta-trace protein, cystatin C, β_2-microglobulin, and creatinine compared for detecting impaired glomerular filtration rates in children. *Clin Chem*. 2002;48:729-736.

76. Donadio C, Lucchesi A, Ardini M, et al. Serum levels of beta-trace protein and glomerular filtration rate—preliminary results. *J Pharm Biomed Anal*. 2003;32:1099-1104.

77. Spanaus KS, Kollerits B, Ritz E, et al. Serum creatinine, cystatin C, and beta-trace protein in diagnostic staging and predicting progression of primary nondiabetic chronic kidney disease. *Clin Chem*. 2010;56:740-749.

78. Poge U, Gerhardt T, Stoffel-Wagner B, et al. Beta-trace protein-based equations for calculation of GFR in renal transplant recipients. *Am J Transplant*. 2008;8:608-615.

79. White CA, Akbari A, Doucette S, et al. Estimating GFR using serum beta trace protein: accuracy and validation in kidney transplant and pediatric populations. *Kidney Int*. 2009;76:784-791.

80. Barisoni L, Mundel P. Podocyte biology and the emerging understanding of podocyte diseases. *Am J Nephrol*. 2003;23:353-360.

81. Camici M. Urinary detection of podocyte injury. *Biomed Pharmacother*. 2007;61:245-249.

82. Schwartz MM, Evans J, Bain R, et al. Focal segmental glomerulosclerosis: prognostic implications of the cellular lesion. *J Am Soc Nephrol*. 1999;10:1900-1907.

83. Couser WG, Abrass CK. Pathogenesis of membranous nephropathy. *Annu Rev Med*. 1988;39:517-530.

84. Eddy AA. Interstitial nephritis induced by protein-overload proteinuria. *Am J Pathol*. 1989;135:719-733.

85. Brenner BM. Nephron adaptation to renal injury or ablation. *Am J Physiol*. 1985;249:F324-F337.

86. Whiteside C, Prutis K, Cameron R, et al. Glomerular epithelial detachment, not reduced charge density, correlates with proteinuria in Adriamycin and puromycin nephrosis. *Lab Invest*. 1989;61:650-660.

87. Ross MJ, Klotman PE. Recent progress in HIV-associated nephropathy. *J Am Soc Nephrol*. 2002;13:2997-3004.

88. Schwartz MM, Bidani AK, Lewis EJ. Glomerular epithelial cell function and pathology following extreme ablation of renal mass. *Am J Pathol*. 1987;126:315-324.

89. Lemley KV, Lafayette RA, Safai M, et al. Podocytopenia and disease severity in IgA nephropathy. *Kidney Int*. 2002;61:1475-1485.

90. Steffes MW, Schmidt D, McCrery R, et al. Glomerular cell number in normal subjects and in type 1 diabetic patients. *Kidney Int*. 2001;59:2104-2113.

91. Somlo S, Mundel P. Getting a foothold in nephrotic syndrome. *Nat Genet*. 2000;24:333-335.

92. Smoyer WE, Mundel P. Regulation of podocyte structure during the development of nephrotic syndrome. *J Mol Med*. 1998;76:172-183.

93. Choi SY, Suh KS, Choi DE, et al: Morphometric analysis of podocyte foot process effacement in IgA nephropathy and its association with proteinuria. Ultrastruct Pathol 34: 195-198.

94. Xu L, Yang HC, Hao CM, et al. Podocyte number predicts progression of proteinuria in IgA nephropathy. *Mod Pathol*. 2010;23:1241-1250.

95. Rask-Madsen C, King GL. Diabetes: podocytes lose their footing. *Nature*. 2010;468:42-44.

96. Busch M, Franke S, Ruster C, et al. Advanced glycation end-products and the kidney. *Eur J Clin Invest*. 2010;40:742-755.

97. Nakamura T, Ushiyama C, Suzuki S, et al. Urinary excretion of podocytes in patients with diabetic nephropathy. *Nephrol Dial Transplant*. 2000;15:1379-1383.

98. Kerjaschki D, Sharkey DJ, Farquhar MG. Identification and characterization of podocalyxin—the major sialoprotein of the renal glomerular epithelial cell. *J Cell Biol*. 1984;98:1591-1596.

99. Hara M, Yanagihara T, Kihara I. Cumulative excretion of urinary podocytes reflects disease progression in IgA nephropathy and Schönlein-Henoch purpura nephritis. *Clin J Am Soc Nephrol*. 2007;2:231-238.

100. Garovic VD, Wagner SJ, Turner ST, et al. Urinary podocyte excretion as a marker for preeclampsia. *Am J Obstet Gynecol*. 2007;196(320):e321-e327.

100a. Hara M, Yangihara T, Kihara I, et al. Apical cell membranes are shed into urine from injured podocytes: a novel phenomenon of podocyte injury. *J Am Soc Nephrol*. 2005;16:408-416.

100b. Zheng M, Lv L, Ni J, et al. Urinary podocyte-associated mRNA profile in various stages of diabetic nephropathy. *PloS One*. 2011;6:e20431.

100c. Koop K, Eikmans M, Baelde H, et al. Expression of podocyte-associated molecules in acquired human kidney diseases. *J Am Soc Nephrol*. 2003;14:2063-2071.

101. Achenbach J, Mengel M, Tossidou I, et al. Parietal epithelia cells in the urine as a marker of disease activity in glomerular diseases. *Nephrol Dial Transplant*. 2008;23:3138-3145.

102. Kanno K, Kawachi H, Uchida Y, et al. Urinary sediment podocalyxin in children with glomerular diseases. *Nephron Clin Pract*. 2003;95:c91-c99.

103. Ruotsalainen V, Ljungberg P, Wartiovaara J, et al. Nephrin is specifically located at the slit diaphragm of glomerular podocytes. *Proc Natl Acad Sci U S A*. 1999;96:7962-7967.

104. Kuusniemi AM, Kestila M, Patrakka J, et al. Tissue expression of nephrin in human and pig. *Pediatr Res*. 2004;55:774-781.

105. Kestila M, Lenkkeri U, Mannikko M, et al. Positionally cloned gene for a novel glomerular protein—nephrin—is mutated in congenital nephrotic syndrome. *Mol Cell*. 1998;1:575-582.

106. Bonnet F, Cooper ME, Kawachi H, et al. Irbesartan normalises the deficiency in glomerular nephrin expression in a model of diabetes and hypertension. *Diabetologia*. 2001;44:874-877.

107. Forbes JM, Bonnet F, Russo LM, et al. Modulation of nephrin in the diabetic kidney: association with systemic hypertension and increasing albuminuria. *J Hypertens*. 2002;20:985-992.

108. Wang SX, Rastaldi MP, Patari A, et al. Patterns of nephrin and a new proteinuria-associated protein expression in human renal diseases. *Kidney Int*. 2002;61:141-147.

109. Huh W, Kim DJ, Kim MK, et al. Expression of nephrin in acquired human glomerular disease. *Nephrol Dial Transplant*. 2002;17:478-484.

110. Davis BJ, Cao Z, De Gasparo M, et al. Disparate effects of angiotensin II antagonists and calcium channel blockers on albuminuria in experimental diabetes and hypertension: potential role of nephrin. *J Hypertens*. 2003;21:209-216.

111. Kelly DJ, Aaltonen P, Cox AJ, et al. Expression of the slit-diaphragm protein, nephrin, in experimental diabetic nephropathy: differing effects of anti-proteinuric therapies. *Nephrol Dial Transplant*. 2002;17:1327-1332.

112. Langham RG, Kelly DJ, Cox AJ, et al. Proteinuria and the expression of the podocyte slit diaphragm protein, nephrin, in diabetic nephropathy: effects of angiotensin converting enzyme inhibition. *Diabetologia*. 2002;45:1572-1576.

113. Patari A, Forsblom C, Havana M, et al. Nephrinuria in diabetic nephropathy of type 1 diabetes. *Diabetes*. 2003;52:2969-2974.

114. Miller TR, Anderson RJ, Linas SL, et al. Urinary diagnostic indices in acute renal failure: a prospective study. *Ann Intern Med*. 1978;89:47-50.

115. Espinel CH, Gregory AW. Differential diagnosis of acute renal failure. *Clin Nephrol*. 1980;13:73-77.

116. Bock HA. Pathophysiology of acute renal failure in septic shock: from prerenal to renal failure. *Kidney Int Suppl*. 1998;64:S15-S18.

117. Perazella MA, Coca SG, Hall IE, et al. Urine microscopy is associated with severity and worsening of acute kidney injury in hospitalized patients. *Clin J Am Soc Nephrol*. 2010;5:402-408.

118. Perazella MA, Coca SG, Kanbay M, et al. Diagnostic value of urine microscopy for differential diagnosis of acute kidney injury in hospitalized patients. *Clin J Am Soc Nephrol*. 2008;3:1615-1619.

119. Esson ML, Schrier RW. Diagnosis and treatment of acute tubular necrosis. *Ann Intern Med*. 2002;137:744-752.

120. Marcussen N, Schumann J, Campbell P, et al. Cytodiagnostic urinalysis is very useful in the differential diagnosis of acute renal failure and can predict the severity. *Ren Fail*. 1995;17:721-729.

121. Rabb H. Evaluation of urinary markers in acute renal failure. *Curr Opin Nephrol Hypertens*. 1998;7:681-685.

122. Bagshaw SM, Langenberg C, Bellomo R. Urinary biochemistry and microscopy in septic acute renal failure: a systematic review. *Am J Kidney Dis.* 2006;48:695-705.

123. Penders J, Delanghe Jr . Alpha 1-microglobulin: clinical laboratory aspects and applications. *Clin Chim Acta.* 2004;346:107-118.

124. Itoh Y, Kawai T. Human alpha 1-microglobulin: its measurement and clinical significance. *J Clin Lab Anal.* 1990;4:376-384.

125. Guder WG, Hofmann W. Clinical role of urinary low molecular weight proteins: their diagnostic and prognostic implications. *Scand J Clin Lab Invest Suppl.* 2008;241:95-98.

126. Herget-Rosenthal S, Poppen D, Husing J, et al. Prognostic value of tubular proteinuria and enzymuria in nonoliguric acute tubular necrosis. *Clin Chem.* 2004;50:552-558.

127. Tsukahara H, Hiraoka M, Kuriyama M, et al. Urinary alpha 1-microglobulin as an index of proximal tubular function in early infancy. *Pediatr Nephrol.* 1993;7:199-201.

128. Takagi K, Kin K, Itoh Y, et al. Human alpha 1-microglobulin levels in various body fluids. *J Clin Pathol.* 1980;33:786-791.

129. Derici U, Tuncer C, Ebinc FA, et al. Does the urinary excretion of α_1-microglobulin and albumin predict clinical disease activity in ulcerative colitis? *Adv Ther.* 2008;25:1342-1352.

130. Tolkoff-Rubin NE, Rubin RH, et al. Noninvasive renal diagnostic studies. *Clin Lab Med.* 1988;8:507-526.

131. Miyata T, Jadoul M, Kurokawa K, et al. Beta-2 microglobulin in renal disease. *J Am Soc Nephrol.* 1998;9:1723-1735.

132. Davey PG, Gosling P. Beta 2-microglobulin instability in pathological urine. *Clin Chem.* 1982;28:1330-1333.

133. Kobayashi E, Suwazono Y, Honda R, et al. Serial changes in urinary cadmium concentrations and degree of renal tubular injury after soil replacement in cadmium-polluted rice paddies. *Toxicol Lett.* 2008;176:124-130.

134. Yavuz S, Ayabakan N, Dilek K, et al. Renal dose dopamine in open heart surgery. Does it protect renal tubular function? *J Cardiovasc Surg (Torino).* 2002;43:25-30.

135. Christopher K, Liang Y, Mueller TF, et al. Analysis of the major histocompatibility complex in graft rejection revisited by gene expression profiles. *Transplantation.* 2004;78:788-798.

136. Hofstra JM, Deegens JK, Willems HL, et al. Beta-2-microglobulin is superior to *N*-acetyl-beta-glucosaminidase in predicting prognosis in idiopathic membranous nephropathy. *Nephrol Dial Transplant.* 2008;23:2546-2551.

137. Herrero-Morin JD, Malaga S, Fernandez N, et al. Cystatin C and β_2-microglobulin: markers of glomerular filtration in critically ill children. *Crit Care.* 2007;11:R59.

138. Bagshaw SM, Langenberg C, Haase M, et al. Urinary biomarkers in septic acute kidney injury. *Intensive Care Med.* 2007;33:1285-1296.

139. Onishi S, Ikenoya K, Matsumoto K, et al. Urinary β_2-microglobulin as a sensitive marker for haemophagocytic syndrome associated with collagen vascular diseases. *Rheumatology (Oxford).* 2008;47:1730-1732.

140. Josson S, Nomura T, Lin JT, et al. β_2-Microglobulin induces epithelial to mesenchymal transition and confers cancer lethality and bone metastasis in human cancer cells. *Cancer Res.* 2011;71(7):2600-2610.

141. Mumtaz A, Anees M, Bilal M, et al. Beta-2 microglobulin levels in hemodialysis patients. *Saudi J Kidney Dis Transpl.* 2010;21:701-706.

142. Schardijn GH. Statius Van Eps LW: Beta 2-microglobulin: its significance in the evaluation of renal function. *Kidney Int.* 1987;32:635-641.

143. Hoffmann D, Fuchs TC, Henzler T, et al. Evaluation of a urinary kidney biomarker panel in rat models of acute and subchronic nephrotoxicity. *Toxicology.* 2010;277:49-58.

144. Gautier JC, Riefke B, Walter J, et al. Evaluation of novel biomarkers of nephrotoxicity in two strains of rat treated with cisplatin. *Toxicol Pathol.* 2010;38:943-956.

145. Walshe CM, Odejayi F, Ng S, et al. Urinary glutathione S-transferase as an early marker for renal dysfunction in patients admitted to intensive care with sepsis. *Crit Care Resusc.* 2009;11:204-209.

146. Sundberg AG, Appelkvist EL, Backman L, et al. Urinary pi-class glutathione transferase as an indicator of tubular damage in the human kidney. *Nephron.* 1994;67:308-316.

147. Cawood TJ, Bashir M, Brady J, et al. Urinary collagen IV and πGST: potential biomarkers for detecting localized kidney injury in diabetes—a pilot study. *Am J Nephrol.* 2010;32:219-225.

148. McMahon BA, Blaithin A, Koyner JL, et al. Urinary glutathione S-transferases in the pathogenesis and diagnostic evaluation of acute kidney injury following cardiac surgery: a critical review. *Curr Opin Crit Care.* 2010;16(6):550-555.

149. Westhuyzen J, Endre ZH, Reece G, et al. Measurement of tubular enzymuria facilitates early detection of acute renal impairment in the intensive care unit. *Nephrol Dial Transplant.* 2003;18:543-551.

150. Edelstein CL, Hoke TS, Somerset H, et al. Proximal tubules from caspase-1–deficient mice are protected against hypoxia-induced membrane injury. *Nephrol Dial Transplant.* 2007;22:1052-1061.

151. Melnikov VY, Ecder T, Fantuzzi G, et al. Impaired IL-18 processing protects caspase-1–deficient mice from ischemic acute renal failure. *J Clin Invest.* 2001;107:1145-1152.

152. Parikh CR, Jani A, Melnikov VY, et al. Urinary interleukin-18 is a marker of human acute tubular necrosis. *Am J Kidney Dis.* 2004;43:405-414.

153. Parikh CR, Jani A, Mishra J, et al. Urine NGAL and IL-18 are predictive biomarkers for delayed graft function following kidney transplantation. *Am J Transplant.* 2006;6:1639-1645.

153a. Miyauchi K, Takiyama Y, Honjyo J, et al. Upregulated IL-18 expression in type 2 diabetic subjects with nephropathy: TGF-beta1 enhanced IL-18 expression in human renal proximal tubular epithelial cells. *Diabetes Res Clin Pract.* 2009;83:190-199.

154. Washburn KK, Zappitelli M, Arikan AA, et al. Urinary interleukin-18 is an acute kidney injury biomarker in critically ill children. *Nephrol Dial Transplant.* 2008;23:566-572.

155. Liangos O, Tighiouart H, Perianayagam MC, et al. Comparative analysis of urinary biomarkers for early detection of acute kidney injury following cardiopulmonary bypass. *Biomarkers.* 2009;14:423-431.

156. Haase M, Bellomo R, Story D, et al. Urinary interleukin-18 does not predict acute kidney injury after adult cardiac surgery: a prospective observational cohort study. *Crit Care.* 2008;12:R96.

157. Siew ED, Ikizler TA, Gebretsadik T, et al. Elevated urinary IL-18 levels at the time of ICU admission predict adverse clinical outcomes. *Clin J Am Soc Nephrol.* 2010;5:1497-1505.

158. Hall IE, Yarlagadda SG, Coca SG, et al. IL-18 and urinary NGAL predict dialysis and graft recovery after kidney transplantation. *J Am Soc Nephrol.* 2010;21:189-197.

159. Ling W, Zhaohui N, Ben H, et al. Urinary IL-18 and NGAL as early predictive biomarkers in contrast-induced nephropathy after coronary angiography. *Nephron Clin Pract.* 2008;108:c176-181.

160. Ichimura T, Bonventre JV, Bailly V, et al. Kidney injury molecule-1 (KIM-1), a putative epithelial cell adhesion molecule containing a novel immunoglobulin domain, is up-regulated in renal cells after injury. *J Biol Chem.* 1998;273:4135-4142.

161. Hubank M, Schatz DG. Identifying differences in mRNA expression by representational difference analysis of cDNA. *Nucl Acid Res.* 1994;22:5640-5648.

162. Bailly V, Zhang Z, Meier W, et al. Shedding of kidney injury molecule-1, a putative adhesion protein involved in renal regeneration. *J Biol Chem.* 2002;277:39739-39748.

163. Ichimura T, Hung CC, Yang SA, et al. Kidney injury molecule-1: a tissue and urinary biomarker for nephrotoxicant-induced renal injury. *Am J Physiol Renal Physiol.* 2004;286:F552-563.

164. Vaidya VS, Ramirez V, Ichimura T, et al. Urinary kidney injury molecule-1: a sensitive quantitative biomarker for early detection of kidney tubular injury. *Am J Physiol Renal Physiol.* 2006;290:F517-F529.

165. Han WK, Bailly V, Abichandani R, et al. Kidney injury molecule-1 (KIM-1): a novel biomarker for human renal proximal tubule injury. *Kidney Int.* 2002;62:237-244.

166. Zhou Y, Vaidya VS, Brown RP, et al. Comparison of kidney injury molecule-1 and other nephrotoxicity biomarkers in urine and kidney following acute exposure to gentamicin, mercury, and chromium. *Toxicol Sci.* 2008;101:159-170.

167. Prozialeck WC, Vaidya VS, Liu J, et al. Kidney injury molecule-1 is an early biomarker of cadmium nephrotoxicity. *Kidney Int.* 2007;72:985-993.

168. Jost G, Pietsch H, Sommer J, et al. Retention of iodine and expression of biomarkers for renal damage in the kidney after application of iodinated contrast media in rats. *Invest Radiol.* 2009;44(2):114-123.

169. Perez-Rojas J, Blanco JA, Cruz C, et al. Mineralocorticoid receptor blockade confers renoprotection in preexisting chronic cyclosporine nephrotoxicity. *Am J Physiol Renal Physiol.* 2007;292:F131-F139.

170. Van Timmeren MM, Bakker SJ, Vaidya VS, et al. Tubular kidney injury molecule-1 in protein-overload nephropathy. *Am J Physiol Renal Physiol.* 2006;291:F456-F464.

171. Chen G, Bridenbaugh EA, Akintola AD, et al. Increased susceptibility of aging kidney to ischemic injury: identification of candidate genes changed during aging, but corrected by caloric restriction. *Am J Physiol Renal Physiol.* 2007;293:F1272-F1281.

172. De Borst MH, Van Timmeren MM, Vaidya VS, et al. Induction of kidney injury molecule-1 in homozygous Ren2 rats is attenuated by blockade of the renin-angiotensin system or p38 MAP kinase. *Am J Physiol Renal Physiol.* 2007;292:F313-F320.

173. Liangos O, Perianayagam MC, Vaidya VS, et al. Urinary *N*-acetyl-beta-(D)-glucosaminidase activity and kidney injury molecule-1 level are associated with adverse outcomes in acute renal failure. *J Am Soc Nephrol.* 2007;18:904-912.

174. Liangos O, Addabbo F, Tighiouart H, et al. Exploration of disease mechanism in acute kidney injury using a multiplex bead array assay: a nested case-control pilot study. *Biomarkers.* 2010;15:436-445.

175. Van Timmeren MM, Van Den Heuvel MC, Bailly V, et al. Tubular kidney injury molecule-1 (KIM-1) in human renal disease. *J Pathol.* 2007;212:209-217.

176. Zhang PL, Rothblum LI, Han WK, et al. Kidney injury molecule-1 expression in transplant biopsies is a sensitive measure of cell injury. *Kidney Int.* 2008;73:608-614.

177. Van Timmeren MM, Vaidya VS, Van Ree RM, et al. High urinary excretion of kidney injury molecule-1 is an independent predictor of graft loss in renal transplant recipients. *Transplantation.* 2007;84:1625-1630.

178. Han WK, Waikar SS, Johnson A, et al. Urinary biomarkers in the early diagnosis of acute kidney injury. *Kidney Int.* 2008;73:863-869.

179. Xu PC, Zhang JJ, Chen M, et-al. Urinary kidney injury molecule-1 in patients with IgA nephropathy is closely associated with disease severity. *Nephrol Dial Transplant.* Epub March 14, 2011.

180. Sundaram N, Bennett M, Wilhelm J, et al. Biomarkers for early detection of sickle nephropathy. *Am J Hematol.* 2011;86(7):559-566.

181. Han WK, Wagener G, Zhu Y, et al. Urinary biomarkers in the early detection of acute kidney injury after cardiac surgery. *Clin J Am Soc Nephrol.* 2009;4:873-882.

182. Vaidya VS, Niewczas MA, Ficociello LH, et al. Regression of microalbuminuria in type 1 diabetes is associated with lower levels of urinary tubular injury biomarkers, kidney injury molecule-1, and N-acetyl-β-D-glucosaminidase. *Kidney Int.* 2011;79:464-470.

183. Vaidya VS, Waikar SS, Ferguson MA, et al. Urinary biomarkers for sensitive and specific detection of acute kidney injury in humans. *Clin Transl Sci.* 2008;1:200-208.

184. Vaidya VS, Ford GM, Waikar SS, et al. A rapid urine test for early detection of kidney injury. *Kidney Int.* 2009;76:108-114.

185. Alkhalaf A, Klooster A, Van Oeveren W, et al. A double-blind, randomized, placebo-controlled clinical trial on benfotiamine treatment in patients with diabetic nephropathy. *Diabetes Care.* 2010;33:1598-1601.

186. Waanders F, Vaidya VS, Van Goor H, et al. Effect of renin-angiotensin-aldosterone system inhibition, dietary sodium restriction, and/or diuretics on urinary kidney injury molecule 1 excretion in nondiabetic proteinuric kidney disease: a post hoc analysis of a randomized controlled trial. *Am J Kidney Dis.* 2009;53:16-25.

187. Ichimura T, Asseldonk EJ, Humphreys BD, et al. Kidney injury molecule-1 is a phosphatidylserine receptor that confers a phagocytic phenotype on epithelial cells. *J Clin Invest.* 2008;118:1657-1668.

188. Yamamoto T, Noiri E, Ono Y, et al. Renal L-type fatty acid–binding protein in acute ischemic injury. *J Am Soc Nephrol.* 2007;18:2894-2902.

189. Portilla D, Dent C, Sugaya T, et al. Liver fatty acid–binding protein as a biomarker of acute kidney injury after cardiac surgery. *Kidney Int.* 2008;73:465-472.

190. Nakamura T, Sugaya T, Koide H. Urinary liver-type fatty acid–binding protein in septic shock: effect of polymyxin B–immobilized fiber hemoperfusion. *Shock.* 2009;31:454-459.

191. Ferguson MA, Vaidya VS, Waikar SS, et al. Urinary liver-type fatty acid–binding protein predicts adverse outcomes in acute kidney injury. *Kidney Int.* 2010;77:708-714.

192. Doi K, Noiri E, Sugaya T. Urinary L-type fatty acid–binding protein as a new renal biomarker in critical care. *Curr Opin Crit Care.* 2010;16(6):545-549:Epub August 21, 2010.

193. Negishi K, Noiri E, Doi K, et al. Monitoring of urinary L-type fatty acid–binding protein predicts histological severity of acute kidney injury. *Am J Pathol.* 2009;174:1154-1159.

194. Kamijo A, Sugaya T, Hikawa A, et al. Urinary liver-type fatty acid binding protein as a useful biomarker in chronic kidney disease. *Mol Cell Biochem.* 2006;284:175-182.

195. Bachorzewska-Gajewska H, Poniatowski B, Dobrzycki S. NGAL (neutrophil gelatinase-associated lipocalin) and L-FABP after percutaneous coronary interventions due to unstable angina in patients with normal serum creatinine. *Adv Med Sci.* 2009;54:221-224.

196. Nakamura T, Sugaya T, Node K, et al. Urinary excretion of liver-type fatty acid-binding protein in contrast medium-induced nephropathy. *Am J Kidney Dis.* 2006;47:439-444.

197. Masuda T, Sakuma C, Yaginuma H. Role for netrin-1 in sensory axonal guidance in higher vertebrates. *Fukushima J Med Sci.* 2009;55:1-6.

198. Rajasekharan S, Kennedy TE. The netrin protein family. *Genome Biol.* 2009;10:239.

199. Ly NP, Komatsuzaki K, Fraser IP, et al. Netrin-1 inhibits leukocyte migration in vitro and in vivo. *Proc Natl Acad Sci U S A.* 2005;102:14729-14734.

200. Wang W, Reeves WB, Ramesh G. Netrin-1 and kidney injury. I. Netrin-1 protects against ischemia-reperfusion injury of the kidney. *Am J Physiol Renal Physiol.* 2008;294:F739-F747.

201. Reeves WB, Kwon O, Ramesh G. Netrin-1 and kidney injury. II. Netrin-1 is an early biomarker of acute kidney injury. *Am J Physiol Renal Physiol.* 2008;294:F731-F738.

202. Ramesh G, Kwon O, Ahn K. Netrin-1: a novel universal biomarker of human kidney injury. *Transplant Proc.* 2010;42:1519-1522.

203. Ramesh G, Krawczeski CD, Woo JG, et al. Urinary netrin-1 is an early predictive biomarker of acute kidney injury after cardiac surgery. *Clin J Am Soc Nephrol.* 2010;5:395-401.

204. Haase M, Haase-Fielitz A, Bellomo R, et al. Neutrophil gelatinase–associated lipocalin as a marker of acute renal disease. *Curr Opin Hematol.* 2011;18(1):11-18.

205. Flower DR. The lipocalin protein family: structure and function. *Biochem J.* 1996;318(pt 1):1-14.

206. Soni SS, Cruz D, Bobek I, et al. NGAL: a biomarker of acute kidney injury and other systemic conditions. *Int Urol Nephrol.* 2010;42:141-150.

207. Supavekin S, Zhang W, Kucherlapati R, et al. Differential gene expression following early renal ischemia/reperfusion. *Kidney Int.* 2003;63:1714-1724.

208. Yuen PS, Jo SK, Holly MK, et al. Ischemic and nephrotoxic acute renal failure are distinguished by their broad transcriptomic responses. *Physiol Genomics.* 2006;25:375-386.

209. Mishra J, Ma Q, Prada A, et al. Identification of neutrophil gelatinase–associated lipocalin as a novel early urinary biomarker for ischemic renal injury. *J Am Soc Nephrol.* 2003;14:2534-2543.

210. Mishra J, Dent C, Tarabishi R, et al. Neutrophil gelatinase–associated lipocalin (NGAL) as a biomarker for acute renal injury after cardiac surgery. *Lancet.* 2005;365:1231-1238.

211. Dent CL, Ma Q, Dastrala S, et al. Plasma neutrophil gelatinase–associated lipocalin predicts acute kidney injury, morbidity and mortality after pediatric cardiac surgery: a prospective uncontrolled cohort study. *Crit Care.* 2007;11:R127.

212. Zappitelli M, Washburn KK, Arikan AA, et al. Urine neutrophil gelatinase–associated lipocalin is an early marker of acute kidney injury in critically ill children: a prospective cohort study. *Crit Care.* 2007;11:R84.

213. Wheeler DS, Devarajan P, Ma Q, et al. Serum neutrophil gelatinase–associated lipocalin (NGAL) as a marker of acute kidney injury in critically ill children with septic shock. *Crit Care Med.* 2008;36:1297-1303.

214. Wagener G, Jan M, Kim M, et al. Association between increases in urinary neutrophil gelatinase–associated lipocalin and acute renal dysfunction after adult cardiac surgery. *Anesthesiology.* 2006;105:485-491.

214a. Mcilroy D, Wagener G, Lee H. Neutrophil gelatinase-associated lipocalin and acute kidney injury after cardiac surgery: the effect of baseline renal function on diagnostic performance. *Clin J Am Sco Nephrol.* 2010;5:211-219.

215. Shavit L, Dolgoker I, Ivgi H, et al. Neutrophil gelatinase–associated lipocalin as a predictor of complications and mortality in patients undergoing non-cardiac major surgery. *Kidney Blood Press Res.* 2011;34:116-124.

216. Portal AJ, McPhail MJ, Bruce M, et al. Neutrophil gelatinase–associated lipocalin predicts acute kidney injury in patients undergoing liver transplantation. *Liver Transpl.* 2010;16:1257-1266.

217. Nielsen SE, Hansen HP, Br Jensen, et al. Urinary neutrophil gelatinase–associated lipocalin and progression of diabetic nephropathy in type 1 diabetic patients in a four-year follow-up study. *Nephron Clin Pract.* 2011;118:c130-c135.

218. Aghel A, Shrestha K, Mullens W, et al. Serum neutrophil gelatinase–associated lipocalin (NGAL) in predicting worsening renal function in acute decompensated heart failure. *J Card Fail.* 2010;16:49-54.

219. Damman K, Van Veldhuisen DJ, Navis G, et al. Urinary neutrophil gelatinase associated lipocalin (NGAL), a marker of tubular damage, is increased in patients with chronic heart failure. *Eur J Heart Fail.* 2008;10:997-1000.

220. Poniatowski B, Malyszko J, Bachorzewska-Gajewska H, et al. Serum neutrophil gelatinase–associated lipocalin as a marker of renal function in patients with chronic heart failure and coronary artery disease. *Kidney Blood Press Res.* 2009;32:77-80.

221. Krawczeski CD, Woo JG, Wang Y, et al. Neutrophil gelatinase–associated lipocalin concentrations predict development of acute kidney injury in neonates and children after cardiopulmonary bypass. *J Pediatr.* 2011;158(6):1009–1015.e1.

222. Haase-Fielitz A, Bellomo R, Devarajan P, et al. Novel and conventional serum biomarkers predicting acute kidney injury in adult cardiac surgery—a prospective cohort study. *Crit Care Med.* 2009;37:553-560.

223. Hirsch R, Dent C, Pfriem H, et al. NGAL is an early predictive biomarker of contrast-induced nephropathy in children. *Pediatr Nephrol.* 2007;22:2089-2095.

224. Bachorzewska-Gajewska H, Malyszko J, Sitniewska E, et al. Neutrophil-gelatinase–associated lipocalin and renal function after percutaneous coronary interventions. *Am J Nephrol.* 2006;26:287-292.

225. Haase M, Bellomo R, Devarajan P, et al. Accuracy of neutrophil gelatinase–associated lipocalin (NGAL) in diagnosis and prognosis in acute kidney injury: a systematic review and meta-analysis. *Am J Kidney Dis.* 2009;54:1012-1024.

226. Boldt J, Brosch C, Ducke M, et al. Influence of volume therapy with a modern hydroxyethylstarch preparation on kidney function in cardiac surgery patients with compromised renal function: a comparison with human albumin. *Crit Care Med.* 2007;35:2740-2746.

227. Schmidt-Ott KM, Mori K, Li JY, et al. Dual action of neutrophil gelatinase–associated lipocalin. *J Am Soc Nephrol*. 2007;18:407-413.

228. Yndestad A, Landro L, Ueland T, et al. Increased systemic and myocardial expression of neutrophil gelatinase–associated lipocalin in clinical and experimental heart failure. *Eur Heart J*. 2009;30:1229-1236.

229. Devarajan P. Review: neutrophil gelatinase–associated lipocalin: a troponin-like biomarker for human acute kidney injury. *Nephrology (Carlton)*. 2010;15:419-428.

230. Price RG. The role of NAG (N-acetyl-β-D-glucosaminidase) in the diagnosis of kidney disease including the monitoring of nephrotoxicity. *Clin Nephrol*. 1992;38(suppl 1):S14-S19.

231. Ida S, Yokota M, Ueoka M, et al. Mild to severe lithium-induced nephropathy models and urine N-acetyl-β-D-glucosaminidase in rats. *Methods Find Exp Clin Pharmacol*. 2001;23:445-448.

232. Wellwood JM, Ellis BG, Price RG, et al. Urinary *N*-acetyl-β-D-glucosaminidase activities in patients with renal disease. *Br Med J*. 1975;3:408-411.

233. Nauta FL, Bakker SJ, Van Oeveren W, et al. Albuminuria, proteinuria, and novel urine biomarkers as predictors of long-term allograft outcomes in kidney transplant recipients. *Am J Kidney Dis*. 2011;57:733-743.

234. Ren L, Ji J, Fang Y, et al. Assessment of urinary N-acetyl-β-glucosaminidase as an early marker of contrast-induced nephropathy. *J Int Med Res*. 2011;39:647-653.

235. Abdel-Hady E, El Hamamsy M, Hedaya M, et al. The efficacy and toxicity of two dosing-regimens of amikacin in neonates with sepsis. *J Clin Pharm Ther*. 2011;36:45-52.

236. Bondiou MT, Bourbouze R, Bernard M, et al. Inhibition of A and B *N*-acetyl-β-D-glucosaminidase urinary isoenzymes by urea. *Clin Chim Acta*. 1985;149:67-73.

237. Wiley RA, Choo HY, Traiger GJ. The effect of nephrotoxic furans on urinary *N*-acetylglucosaminidase levels in mice. *Toxicol Lett*. 1982;14:93-96.

237a. Venkat K. Proteinuria and microalbuminuria in adults: significance, evaluation, and treatment. *South Med J*. 2004;97:969-979.

237b. K/DOQI clinical practice guidelines for chronic kidney disease: evaluation, classification, and stratification. *Am J Kidney Dis*. 2002;39:S1-266.

237c. Perazella M, Moeckel G. Nephrotoxicity from chemotherapeutic agents: clinical manifestations, pathobiology, and prevention/therapy. *Semin Nephrol*. 2010;30:570-581.

237d. Guo X, Nzerue C. How to prevent, recognize, and treat drug-induced nephrotoxicity. *Cleve Clin J Med*. 2002;69:289-290, 293-284, 296-287 passim.

237e. Hsu R, Hsu C. Proteinuria and reduced glomerular filtration rate as risk factors for acute kidney injury. *Curr Opin Nephrol Hypertens*.1011; 20:211-217.

237f. James M, Hemmelgarn B, Wiebe N, et al. Glomerular filtration rate, proteinuria, and the incidence and consequences of acute kidney injury: a cohort study. *Lancet*. 2010;376:2096-2103.

237g. Hsu C, Ordonez J, Chertow G, et al. The risk of acute renal failure in patients with chronic kidney disease. *Kidney Int*. 2008;74:101-107.

237h. Hallan Si, Ritz E, Lydersen S, et al. Combining GFR and albuminuria to classify CKD improves prediction of ESRD. *J Am Soc Nephrol*. 2009;20:1069-1077.

237i. Gekle M. Renal albumin handling: a look at the dark side of the filter. *Kidney Int*. 2007;71:479-481.

237j. Pfaller W, Thorwartl U, Nevinny-Stickel M, et al. Clinical value of fructose 1,6 bisphosphatase in monitoring renal proximal tubular injury. *Kidney Int Suppl*. 1994;47:S68-75.

237k. Metz-Kurschel U, Kurschel E, Niederle N, et al. Investigations on the acute and chronic nephrotoxicity of the new platinum analogue carboplatin. *J Cancer Res Clin Oncol*. 1990;116:203-206.

237l. De Jong P, Curhan G. Screening, monitoring, and treatment of albuminuria: Public health perspectives. *J Am Soc Nephrol*. 2006;17:2120-2126.

237m. Verhave J, Gansevoort R, Hillege H, et al. An elevated urinary albumin excretion predicts de novo development of renal function impairment in the general population. *Kidney Int Suppl*. 2004;92:S18-21.

237n. Hillege H, Janssen W, Bak A, et al. Microalbuminuria is common, also in a nondiabetic, nonhypertensive population, and an independent indicator of cardiovascular risk factors and cardiovascular morbidity. *J Intern Med*. 2001;249:519-526.

237o. Astor B, Hallan S, Miller 3rd E, et al. Glomerular filtration rate, albuminuria, and risk of cardiovascular and all-cause mortality in the US population. *Am J Epidemiol*. 2008;167:1226-1234.

237p. Levin A, Pate Ge, Shalansky S, et al. N-acetylcysteine reduces urinary albumin excretion following contrast administration: evidence of biological effect. *Nephrol Dial Transplant*. 2007;22:2520-2524.

238. Herget-Rosenthal S, Marggraf G, Husing J, et al. Early detection of acute renal failure by serum cystatin C. *Kidney Int*. 2004;66:1115-1122.

238a. Royakkers A, Korevaar J, Van Suijlen J, et al. Serum and urine cystatin C are poor biomarkers for acute kidney injury and renal replacement therapy. *Intensive Care Med*. 2011;37:493-501.

238b. Nauta F, Boertien W, Bakker S, et al. Glomerular and tubular damage markers are elevated in patients with diabetes. *Diabetes Care*. 2011;34:975-981.

238c. Jeon Y, Kim M, Huh J, et al. Cystatin C as an early biomarker of nephropathy in patients with type 2 diabetes. *J Korean Med Sci*. 2011; 26:258-263.

238d. Herget-Rosenthal S, Van Wijk J, Brocker-Preuss M, et al. Increased urinary cystatin C reflects structural and functional renal tubular impairment independent of glomerular filtration rate. *Clin Biochem*. 2007;40:946-951.

239. Stevens LA, Schmid CH, Greene T, et al. Factors other than glomerular filtration rate affect serum cystatin C levels. *Kidney Int*. 2009;75:652-660.

240. Ichihara K, Saito K, Itoh Y. Sources of variation and reference intervals for serum cystatin C in a healthy Japanese adult population. *Clin Chem Lab Med*. 2007;45:1232-1236.

241. Finney H, Newman DJ, Gruber W, et al. Initial evaluation of cystatin C measurement by particle-enhanced immunonephelometry on the Behring nephelometer systems (BNA, BN II). *Clin Chem*. 1997;43:1016-1022.

242. Newman DJ. Cystatin C. *Ann Clin Biochem*. 2002;39:89-104.

243. Ueda S, Yamagishi S, Kaida Y, et al. Asymmetric dimethylarginine may be a missing link between cardiovascular disease and chronic kidney disease. *Nephrology (Carlton)*. 2007;12:582-590.

244. Ueda S, Yamagishi S, Okuda S. New pathways to renal damage: role of ADMA in retarding renal disease progression. *J Nephrol*. 2010;23:377-386.

245. Suda O, Tsutsui M, Morishita T, et al. Asymmetric dimethylarginine produces vascular lesions in endothelial nitric oxide synthase-deficient mice: involvement of renin-angiotensin system and oxidative stress. *Arterioscler Thromb Vasc Biol*. 2004;24:1682-1688.

246. Vallance P, Leone A, Calver A, et al. Accumulation of an endogenous inhibitor of nitric oxide synthesis in chronic renal failure. *Lancet*. 1992;339:572-575.

247. McDermott JR. Studies on the catabolism of Ng-methylarginine, Ng, Ng-dimethylarginine and Ng, Ng-dimethylarginine in the rabbit. *Biochem J*. 1976;154:179-184.

248. Kielstein JT, Boger RH, Bode-Boger SM, et al. Marked increase of asymmetric dimethylarginine in patients with incipient primary chronic renal disease. *J Am Soc Nephrol*. 2002;13:170-176.

249. Miyazaki H, Matsuoka H, Cooke JP, et al. Endogenous nitric oxide synthase inhibitor: a novel marker of atherosclerosis. *Circulation*. 1999;99:1141-1146.

250. Tarnow L, Hovind P, Teerlink T, et al. Elevated plasma asymmetric dimethylarginine as a marker of cardiovascular morbidity in early diabetic nephropathy in type 1 diabetes. *Diabetes Care*. 2004;27:765-769.

251. Boger RH, Bode-Boger SM, Szuba A, et al. Asymmetric dimethylarginine (ADMA): a novel risk factor for endothelial dysfunction: its role in hypercholesterolemia. *Circulation*. 1998;98:1842-1847.

252. Lu TM, Chung MY, Lin CC, et al. Asymmetric dimethylarginine and clinical outcomes in chronic kidney disease. *Clin J Am Soc Nephrol*. 2011;6(7):1566-1572.

253. Caglar K, Yilmaz MI, Sonmez A, et al. ADMA, proteinuria, and insulin resistance in non-diabetic stage I chronic kidney disease. *Kidney Int*. 2006;70:781-787.

254. Schober JM, Chen N, Grzeszkiewicz TM, et al. Identification of integrin $\alpha_M\beta_2$ as an adhesion receptor on peripheral blood monocytes for Cyr61 (CCN1) and connective tissue growth factor (CCN2): immediate-early gene products expressed in atherosclerotic lesions. *Blood*. 2002;99:4457-4465.

255. Zoccali C, Mallamaci F, Maas R, et al. Left ventricular hypertrophy, cardiac remodeling and asymmetric dimethylarginine (ADMA) in hemodialysis patients. *Kidney Int*. 2002;62:339-345.

256. Cross JM, Donald A, Vallance PJ, et al. Dialysis improves endothelial function in humans. *Nephrol Dial Transplant*. 2001;16:1823-1829.

257. Kestenbaum B, Sampson JN, Rudser KD, et al. Serum phosphate levels and mortality risk among people with chronic kidney disease. *J Am Soc Nephrol*. 2005;16:520-528.

258. Dhingra R, Sullivan LM, Fox CS, et al. Relations of serum phosphorus and calcium levels to the incidence of cardiovascular disease in the community. *Arch Intern Med*. 2007;167:879-885.

259. Norris KC, Greene T, Kopple J, et al. Baseline predictors of renal disease progression in the African American Study of Hypertension and Kidney Disease. *J Am Soc Nephrol*. 2006;17:2928-2936.

260. Amatschek S, Haller M, Oberbauer R. Renal phosphate handling in humans—what can we learn from hereditary hypophosphataemias? *Eur J Clin Invest*. 2010;40:552-560.

261. Fukumoto S. Disorders of phosphate metabolism. *Rinsho Byori*. 2010;58:225-231.

262. Fukagawa M, Kazama JJ. FGF23: its role in renal bone disease. *Pediatr Nephrol*. 2006;21:1802-1806.

263. Seiler S, Reichart B, Roth D, et al: FGF-23 and future cardiovascular events in patients with chronic kidney disease before initiation of dialysis treatment. Nephrol Dial Transplant 25: 3983-3989.

264. Fitzpatrick RE, Ruiz-Esparza J, Goldman MP. The depth of thermal necrosis using the CO_2 laser: a comparison of the superpulsed mode and conventional mode. *J Dermatol Surg Oncol*. 1991;17:340-344.

265. Isakova T, Xie H, Yang W, et al. Fibroblast growth factor 23 and risks of mortality and end-stage renal disease in patients with chronic kidney disease. *JAMA*. 2011;305:2432-2439.
266. Boring L, Gosling J, Chensue SW, et al. Impaired monocyte migration and reduced type 1 (Th1) cytokine responses in C-C chemokine receptor 2 knockout mice. *J Clin Invest*. 1997;100:2552-2561.
267. Leonard EJ, Yoshimura T. Human monocyte chemoattractant protein-1 (MCP-1). *Immunol Today*. 1990;11:97-101.
268. Yoshimura T, Leonard EJ. Secretion by human fibroblasts of monocyte chemoattractant protein-1, the product of gene JE. *J Immunol*. 1990;144:2377-2383.
269. Yoshimura T, Robinson EA, Tanaka S, et al. Purification and amino acid analysis of two human monocyte chemoattractants produced by phytohemagglutinin-stimulated human blood mononuclear leukocytes. *J Immunol*. 1989;142:1956-1962.
270. Cushing SD, Berliner JA, Valente AJ, et al. Minimally modified low density lipoprotein induces monocyte chemotactic protein 1 in human endothelial cells and smooth muscle cells. *Proc Natl Acad Sci U S A*. 1990;87:5134-5138.
271. Elner SG, Strieter RM, Elner VM, et al. Monocyte chemotactic protein gene expression by cytokine-treated human retinal pigment epithelial cells. *Lab Invest*. 1991;64:819-825.
272. Rovin BH, Yoshiumura T, Tan L. Cytokine-induced production of monocyte chemoattractant protein-1 by cultured human mesangial cells. *J Immunol*. 1992;148:2148-2153.
273. Wada T, Furuichi K, Sakai N, et al. Up-regulation of monocyte chemoattractant protein-1 in tubulointerstitial lesions of human diabetic nephropathy. *Kidney Int*. 2000;58:1492-1499.
274. Amann B, Tinzmann R, Angelkort B. ACE inhibitors improve diabetic nephropathy through suppression of renal MCP-1. *Diabetes Care*. 2003;26:2421-2425.
275. Han SY, So GA, Jee YH, et al. Effect of retinoic acid in experimental diabetic nephropathy. *Immunol Cell Biol*. 2004;82:568-576.
276. Banba N, Nakamura T, Matsumura M, et al. Possible relationship of monocyte chemoattractant protein-1 with diabetic nephropathy. *Kidney Int*. 2000;58:684-690.
277. Chow FY, Nikolic-Paterson DJ, Ozols E, et al. Monocyte chemoattractant protein-1 promotes the development of diabetic renal injury in streptozotocin-treated mice. *Kidney Int*. 2006;69:73-80.
278. Morii T, Fujita H, Narita T, et al. Association of monocyte chemoattractant protein-1 with renal tubular damage in diabetic nephropathy. *J Diabetes Complications*. 2003;17:11-15.
279. Takebayashi K, Matsumoto S, Aso Y, et al. Aldosterone blockade attenuates urinary monocyte chemoattractant protein-1 and oxidative stress in patients with type 2 diabetes complicated by diabetic nephropathy. *J Clin Endocrinol Metab*. 2006;91:2214-2217.
280. Tam FW, Riser BL, Meeran K, et al. Urinary monocyte chemoattractant protein-1 (MCP-1) and connective tissue growth factor (CCN2) as prognostic markers for progression of diabetic nephropathy. *Cytokine*. 2009;47:37-42.
281. Wada T, Yokoyama H, Su SB, et al. Monitoring urinary levels of monocyte chemotactic and activating factor reflects disease activity of lupus nephritis. *Kidney Int*. 1996;49:761-767.
282. Noris M, Bernasconi S, Casiraghi F, et al. Monocyte chemoattractant protein-1 is excreted in excessive amounts in the urine of patients with lupus nephritis. *Lab Invest*. 1995;73:804-809.
283. Kiyici S, Erturk E, Budak F, et al. Serum monocyte chemoattractant protein-1 and monocyte adhesion molecules in type 1 diabetic patients with nephropathy. *Arch Med Res*. 2006;37:998-1003.
284. Munshi R, Johnson A, Siew ED, et al. MCP-1 gene activation marks acute kidney injury. *J Am Soc Nephrol*. 2011;22:165-175.
285. Bradham DM, Igarashi A, Potter RL, et al. Connective tissue growth factor: a cysteine-rich mitogen secreted by human vascular endothelial cells is related to the SRC-induced immediate early gene product CEF-10. *J Cell Biol*. 1991;114:1285-1294.
286. Leask A, Abraham DJ. The role of connective tissue growth factor, a multifunctional matricellular protein, in fibroblast biology. *Biochem Cell Biol*. 2003;81:355-363.
287. Chien W, O'Kelly J, Lu D, et al. Expression of connective tissue growth factor (CTGF/CCN2) in breast cancer cells is associated with increased migration and angiogenesis. *Int J Oncol*. 2011;38:1741-1747.
288. Phanish MK, Winn SK, Dockrell ME. Connective tissue growth factor-(CTGF, CCN2)—a marker, mediator and therapeutic target for renal fibrosis. *Nephron Exp Nephrol*. 2011;114:e83-e92.
289. Grotendorst GR. Connective tissue growth factor: a mediator of TGF-β action on fibroblasts. *Cytokine Growth Factor Rev*. 1997;8:171-179.
290. Gupta S, Clarkson MR, Duggan J, et al. Connective tissue growth factor: potential role in glomerulosclerosis and tubulointerstitial fibrosis. *Kidney Int*. 2000;58:1389-1399.
291. Ito Y, Aten J, Bende RJ, et al. Expression of connective tissue growth factor in human renal fibrosis. *Kidney Int*. 1998;53:853-861.
292. Paradis V, Dargere D, Vidaud M, et al. Expression of connective tissue growth factor in experimental rat and human liver fibrosis. *Hepatology*. 1999;30:968-976.
293. Robinson HC, Brett MJ, Tralaggan PJ, et al. The effect of D-xylose, β-D-xylosides and β-D-galactosides on chondroitin sulphate biosynthesis in embryonic chicken cartilage. *Biochem J*. 1975;148:25-34.
294. Riser BL, Cortes P, Denichilo M, et al. Urinary CCN2 (CTGF) as a possible predictor of diabetic nephropathy: preliminary report. *Kidney Int*. 2003;64:451-458.
295. Gilbert RE, Akdeniz A, Weitz S, et al. Urinary connective tissue growth factor excretion in patients with type 1 diabetes and nephropathy. *Diabetes Care*. 2003;26:2632-2636.
296. Nguyen TQ, Tarnow L, Andersen S, et al. Urinary connective tissue growth factor excretion correlates with clinical markers of renal disease in a large population of type 1 diabetic patients with diabetic nephropathy. *Diabetes Care*. 2006;29:83-88.
297. Nguyen TQ, Tarnow L, Jorsal A, et al. Plasma connective tissue growth factor is an independent predictor of end-stage renal disease and mortality in type 1 diabetic nephropathy. *Diabetes Care*. 2008;31:1177-1182.
298. Jaffa AA, Usinger WR, McHenry MB, et al. Connective tissue growth factor and susceptibility to renal and vascular disease risk in type 1 diabetes. *J Clin Endocrinol Metab*. 2008;93:1893-1900.
299. Border WA, Noble NA. Transforming growth factor β in tissue fibrosis. *N Engl J Med*. 1994;331:1286-1292.
300. Lawrence DA. Transforming growth factor-β: an overview. *Kidney Int Suppl*. 1995;49:S19-S23.
301. Tsakas S, Goumenos DS. Accurate measurement and clinical significance of urinary transforming growth factor-β1. *Am J Nephrol*. 2006;26:186-193.
302. Goumenos DS, Tsakas S, El Nahas AM, et al. Transforming growth factor-β1 in the kidney and urine of patients with glomerular disease and proteinuria. *Nephrol Dial Transplant*. 2002;17:2145-2152.
303. Haramaki R, Tamaki K, Fujisawa M, et al. Steroid therapy and urinary transforming growth factor-β1 in IgA nephropathy. *Am J Kidney Dis*. 2001;38:1191-1198.
304. Honkanen E, Teppo AM, Tornroth T, et al. Urinary transforming growth factor-β1 in membranous glomerulonephritis. *Nephrol Dial Transplant*. 1997;12:2562-2568.
305. Cha DR, Kim IS, Kang YS, et al. Urinary concentration of transforming growth factor-β–inducible gene-h3(β ig-h3) in patients with type 2 diabetes mellitus. *Diabet Med*. 2005;22:14-20.
306. Grandaliano G, Di Paolo S, Monno R, et al. Protease-activated receptor 1 and plasminogen activator inhibitor 1 expression in chronic allograft nephropathy: the role of coagulation and fibrinolysis in renal graft fibrosis. *Transplantation*. 2001;72:1437-1443.
307. Io H, Hamada C, Fukui M, et al. Relationship between levels of urinary type IV collagen and renal injuries in patients with IgA nephropathy. *J Clin Lab Anal*. 2004;18:14-18.
308. Cohen MP, Lautenslager GT, Shearman CW. Increased urinary type IV collagen marks the development of glomerular pathology in diabetic d/db mice. *Metabolism*. 2001;50:1435-1440.
309. Peralta CA, Shlipak MG, Judd S, et al. Detection of chronic kidney disease with creatinine, cystatin C, and urine albumin-to-creatinine ratio and association with progression to end-stage renal disease and mortality. *JAMA*. 2011;305:1545-1552.
310. Cavalier E, Bekaert AC, Carlisi A, et al. Neutrophil gelatinase–associated lipocalin (NGAL) determined in urine with the Abbott Architect or in plasma with the Biosite Triage? The laboratory's point of view. *Clin Chem Lab Med*. 2011;49:339-341.
311. De Geus HR, Bakker J, Lesaffre EM, et al. Neutrophil gelatinase–associated lipocalin at ICU admission predicts for acute kidney injury in adult patients. *Am J Respir Crit Care Med*. 2011;183:907-914.
312. US Food and Drug Administration. *FDA unveils critical path opportunities list outlining blueprint to modernizing medical product development by 2010. Biomarker development and clinical trial design greatest areas for impact*. FDA news release, Silver Spring, Md: The Administration; March 16, 2006.
313. US Food and Drug Administration. *Challenge and opportunity on the critical path to new medical products*. The Administration: Silver Spring, MD; 2004.
314. Bonventre JV, Vaidya VS, Schmouder R, et al. Next-generation biomarkers for detecting kidney toxicity. *Nat Biotechnol*. 2010;28:436-440.
315. US Food and Drug Administration. *FDA, European Medicines Agency to consider additional test results when assessing new drug safety. Collaborative effort by FDA and EMEA expected to yield additional safety data*. FDA news release, Silver Spring, Md: The Administration; June 12, 2008.
316. Bellomo R, Ronco C, Kellum JA, et al. Acute renal failure—definition, outcome measures, animal models, fluid therapy and information technology needs: the Second International Consensus Conference of the Acute Dialysis Quality Initiative (ADQI) Group. *Crit Care*. 2004;8:R204-R212.

Disorders of Kidney Structure and Function

Acute Kidney Injury

Asif A. Sharfuddin, Steven D. Weisbord, Paul M. Palevsky, and
Bruce A. Molitoris

Definition of Acute Kidney Injury

Acute kidney injury (AKI) is a heterogenous syndrome defined by a rapid (over hours to days) decline in the glomerular filtration rate (GFR) resulting in the retention of metabolic waste products, including urea and creatinine, and dysregulation of fluid, electrolyte, and acid-base homeostasis.[1] Although often considered a discrete syndrome, AKI represents a broad constellation of pathophysiologic processes of varied severity and etiology. These include decreases in GFR as a result of hemodynamic perturbations that disrupt normal renal perfusion without causing parenchymal injury; partial or complete obstruction to urinary flow; and a spectrum of processes with characteristic patterns of glomerular, interstitial, tubular, or vascular parenchymal injury.

Over the past decade, the term *acute kidney injury* has largely supplanted the older term *acute renal failure* (ARF).

This change reflects the recognition of serious shortcomings in the older terminology. The term *acute renal failure* suggested a dichotomous relationship between normal kidney function and overt organ failure; in contrast, the term *acute kidney injury* attempts to capture the growing body of data associating small acute and transient decrements in kidney function with serious adverse outcomes. Although the newer terminology does emphasize the graded aspect of acute kidney disease, it should be recognized that this terminology is also imperfect. Implicit in the word *injury* is the presence of parenchymal organ damage, which may be absent in a variety of settings associated with an acute decline in kidney function, such as early obstructive disease and prerenal azotemia related to volume depletion. Although the term *acute kidney dysfunction* might better characterize the entire spectrum of the syndrome, *acute kidney injury* is the term that has been adopted by consensus and is now increasingly used in the medical literature. In this chapter, the term *AKI* will be used to describe the entire spectrum of the syndrome, whereas *ARF* will be restricted to situations of organ failure requiring renal replacement therapy. Although in clinical practice the term *acute tubular necrosis* (ATN) is often used synonymously with AKI, these terms should not be used interchangeably. Although ATN is the most common form of intrinsic AKI, particularly in critically ill patients, it represents only one of multiple causes of AKI.

Decreased urine output is often a cardinal manifestation of AKI, and patients are frequently classified based on urine flow rates as nonoliguric (urine output >400 mL/day), oliguric (urine output <400 mL/day), or anuric (urine output <100 mL/day).[2] Transient oliguria may occur in the absence of significant decrements in kidney function, because increased tubular salt and water reabsorption is a normal physiologic response to volume depletion. In contradistinction, persistent oliguria despite the presence of adequate intravascular volume is virtually always a manifestation of AKI, with lower levels of urine output typically associated with more severe initial renal injury. The categorization of AKI based on urine volume has clinical implications for the development of volume overload, severity of electrolyte disturbances, and overall prognosis; greater mortality risk is associated with oliguric than with nonoliguric AKI.[3] However, therapeutic interventions to augment urine output have not been shown to improve outcomes.

AKI can develop de novo in the setting of intact kidney function or can be superimposed on underlying CKD (acute on chronic kidney injury). In fact, the presence of underlying renal impairment has been shown to be one of the most important risk factors for the development of AKI.[4,5] Multiple mechanisms may contribute to this increased susceptibility, including diminished renal functional reserve, impaired salt and water conservation predisposing to intravascular volume contraction, decreased activity of detoxification mechanisms increasing susceptibility to cytotoxic injury, impaired clearance of potential nephrotoxins increasing the risk and/or duration of exposure, and associated macrovascular and microvascular disease increasing the risk of ischemic injury.

AKI is usually divided into three broad pathophysiologic categories based on cause:
1. Prerenal AKI—diseases characterized by effective hypoperfusion of the kidneys in which there is no parenchymal damage to the kidney (Table 30-1)
2. Intrinsic AKI—diseases involving the renal parenchyma (Table 30-2)
3. Postrenal (obstructive) AKI—diseases associated with acute obstruction of the urinary tract (Table 30-3)

Although these categories are useful for didactic purposes and help to inform the initial clinical assessment of patients with AKI, there is often a degree of overlap between these categories. For example, renal hypoperfusion may cause a spectrum of renal injury ranging from prerenal azotemia to overt ATN depending on its severity and duration. As a result, precise categorization of the cause of AKI into one of these three groups may not always be possible, and transitions between etiologic categories may occur.

The absence of a uniform operational definition of AKI has impeded studies of its epidemiology and hampered clinical evaluations of preventative and therapeutic interventions. A review of the literature demonstrates a plethora of definitions based on varying absolute and/or relative changes in the

TABLE 30-1 Causes of Prerenal Acute Kidney Injury

Intravascular Volume Depletion
Hemorrhage—trauma, surgery, postpartum, gastrointestinal
Gastrointestinal losses—diarrhea, vomiting, nasogastric tube loss
Renal losses—diuretic use, osmotic diuresis, diabetes insipidus
Skin and mucous membrane losses—burns, hyperthermia
Nephrotic syndrome
Cirrhosis
Capillary leak

Reduced Cardiac Output
Cardiogenic shock
Pericardial diseases—restrictive, constrictive, tamponade
Congestive heart failure
Valvular diseases
Pulmonary diseases—pulmonary hypertension, pulmonary embolism
Sepsis

Systemic Vasodilation
Sepsis
Cirrhosis
Anaphylaxis
Drugs

Renal Vasoconstriction
Early sepsis
Hepatorenal syndrome
Acute hypercalcemia
Drugs—norepinephrine, vasopressin, nonsteroidal antiinflammatory drugs, angiotensin-converting enzyme inhibitors, calcineurin inhibitors
Iodinated contrast agents

Increased Intraabdominal Pressure
Abdominal compartment syndrome

serum creatinine concentration with or without associated decrements in urine output. This lack of standardization has made it difficult to compare findings across epidemiologic studies and has led to a series of attempts to formulate a consensus definition.

In 2002, the Acute Dialysis Quality Initiative (ADQI) Group proposed the first consensus definition of AKI. The ADQI work group proposed a classification scheme with three strata based on the magnitude of the increase in serum creatinine level and/or the duration of oliguria. Conceptually, the first stratum would provide the greatest sensitivity for diagnosing AKI, whereas the higher strata would provide increasing specificity of diagnosis. These three strata were combined with two outcome stages defined by the need for and duration of renal replacement therapy, which resulted in the five-tiered RIFLE classification (*R*isk of renal dysfunction, *I*njury to the kidney, and *F*ailure of kidney function, as well as the two outcome stages, *L*oss of kidney function and *E*nd-stage kidney disease).[6] More recently, the Acute Kidney Injury Network (AKIN) proposed a modification of the RIFLE classification that includes the Risk, Injury, and Failure criteria with the addition of a 0.3 mg/dL or higher increase in the serum creatinine level to the criterion that define Risk (Table 30-4).[7]

Although the RIFLE and AKIN criteria have introduced a degree of uniformity to clinical studies of AKI, several limitations to both of these sets of criteria have been recognized. First, although validation studies have demonstrated that AKI stage correlates with increasing mortality risk, it is not clear that this is the appropriate metric for assessing the validity of the criteria. Second, concordance between the serum creatinine level and urine output criterion has not been established, even with regard to mortality risk. Third, there is poor correlation between AKI stage and GFR. Since the magnitude of

TABLE 30-2 Major Causes of Intrinsic Acute Kidney Injury

Tubular Injury

Ischemia due to hypoperfusion	Hypovolemia, sepsis, hemorrhage, cirrhosis, congestive heart failure; see Table 30-1
Endogenous toxins	Myoglobin, hemoglobin, paraproteinemia, uric acid; see Table 30-5
Exogenous toxins	Antibiotics, chemotherapy agents, radiocontrast agents, phosphate preparations

Tubulointerstitial Injury

Acute allergic interstitial nephritis	Nonsteroidal antiinflammatory drugs, antibiotics
Infections	Viral, bacterial, and fungal infections
Infiltration	Lymphoma, leukemia, sarcoid
Allograft rejection	

Glomerular Injury

Inflammation	Anti–glomerular basement membrane disease, antineutrophil cytoplasmic autoantibody disease, infection, cryoglobulinemia, membranoproliferative glomerulonephritis, Immunoglobulin A nephropathy, systemic lupus erythematosus, Henoch-Schönlein purpura, polyarteritis nodosa
Hematologic disorders	Hemolytic uremic syndrome, thrombotic thrombocytopenic purpura, drugs

Renal Microvasculature

	Malignant hypertension, toxemia of pregnancy, hypercalcemia, radiocontrast agents, scleroderma, drugs

Large Vessels

Arteries	Thrombosis, vasculitis, dissection, thromboembolism, atheroembolism, trauma
Veins	Thrombosis, compression, trauma

TABLE 30-3 Causes of Postrenal Acute Kidney Injury

Upper Urinary Tract Extrinsic Causes
Retroperitoneal space—lymph nodes, tumors
Pelvic or intraabdominal tumors—cervix, uterus, ovary, prostate
Fibrosis—radiation, drugs, inflammatory conditions
Ureteral ligation or surgical trauma
Granulomatosis diseases
Hematoma

Lower Urinary Tract Causes
Prostate—benign prostatic hypertrophy, carcinoma, infection
Bladder—neck obstruction, calculi, carcinoma, infection (schistosomiasis)
Functional—neurogenic bladder secondary to spinal cord injury, diabetes, multiple sclerosis, stroke, pharmacologic side effects of drugs (anticholinergics, antidepressants)
Urethral—posterior urethral valves, strictures, trauma, infections, tuberculosis, tumors

Upper Urinary Tract Intrinsic Causes
Nephrolithiasis
Strictures
Edema
Debris, blood clots, sloughed papillae, fungal ball
Malignancy

TABLE 30-4 RIFLE and Acute Kidney Injury Network (AKIN) Definition and Staging of Acute Kidney Injury

DEFINITION

RIFLE	AKIN
An increase in serum creatinine of ≥50% developing over <7 days *or* A urine output of <0.5 mL/kg/hr for >6 hr	An increase in serum creatinine of ≥0.3 mg/dL or ≥50% developing over <48 hr *or* A urine output of <0.5 mL/kg/hr for >6 hr

STAGING CRITERIA

RIFLE STAGE	INCREASE IN SERUM CREATININE	URINE OUTPUT CRITERIA	INCREASE IN SERUM CREATININE	AKIN STAGE
Risk	≥50%	<0.5 mL/kg/hr for >6 hr	≥0.3 mg/dL; or ≥50%	Stage 1
Injury	≥100%	<0.5 mL/kg/hr for >12 hr	≥100%	Stage 2
Failure	≥200%	<0.5 mL/kg/hr for >24 hr or anuria for >12 hr	≥200%	Stage 3
Loss	Need for renal replacement therapy for >4 wk			
End stage	Need for renal replacement therapy for >3 mo			

stage AKI. Analysis of creatinine kinetics demonstrates that the time required to attain a fixed percentage change in serum creatinine concentration in the setting of severe AKI depends upon the baseline level of kidney function, whereas the initial rate of change in serum creatinine level is relatively independent of kidney function. Thus, early in the course of AKI, absolute changes in serum creatinine level may be detected more readily than relative changes. Finally, it must be remembered that these classification systems are independent of the various causes of AKI (i.e., prerenal, intrinsic, obstructive). Despite these shortcomings, the use of standardized classification schemes has enhanced interpretation of epidemiologic studies and design of clinical trials.

Conceptually, AKI comprises a spectrum of structural and functional kidney disease in which there may be an evolution from injury to organ dysfunction and finally to overt organ failure (Figure 30-1). Reliance solely on changes in serum creatinine level and/or urine output to diagnose AKI[8] has resulted in the inability to identify the incipient stages of intrinsic kidney injury, which may be the most opportune time for pharmacologic intervention. To facilitate the early diagnosis of intrinsic injury, multiple biomarkers of tubular injury have been evaluated.[9,10] Biomarkers for AKI include N-acetyl-β-D-glucosaminidase (NAG), kidney injury molecule 1 (KIM-1), neutrophil gelatinase–associated lipocalin (NGAL), and interleukin 18 (IL-18), among others.[9,10] In addition, serum cystatin C has been proposed as more sensitive than serum

change in serum creatinine concentration is time dependent, a patient with a GFR that is essentially zero may only fulfill the RIFLE stage R or AKIN stage 1 criteria, but may later meet the criteria for RIFLE stage F or AKIN stage 3 despite an increasing GFR. Fourth, the definition of AKI by serum creatinine criteria in both schemes relies on a referent baseline serum creatinine level, which is often unavailable. Variations in the definitions used for this referent value can alter the classification of patients. Fifth, both the RIFLE and AKIN classifications employ relative changes in serum creatinine level to

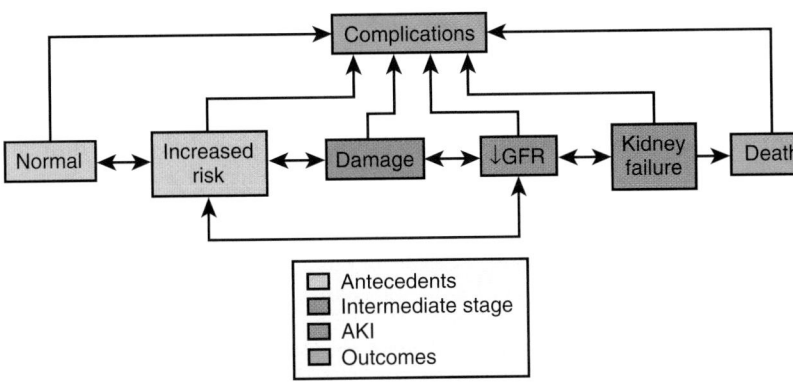

FIGURE 30-1 Conceptual model depicting stages in the development of (*left to right*) and recovery from (*right to left*) acute kidney injury (AKI). (From Murray PT, Devarajan P, Levey AS, et al: A framework and key research questions in AKI diagnosis and staging in different environments, *Clin J Am Soc Nephrol* 3:865, 2008, Figure 1.)

creatinine for detecting changes in GFR, and urinary cystatin C has been proposed as a marker of tubular injury.[9,11,12] Although none of these biomarkers has yet been adequately validated for routine clinical use, they have the potential to provide an early diagnosis of intrinsic AKI, to differentiate volume-responsive (prerenal) AKI from intrinsic disease, and to provide prognostic information regarding the clinical course of an episode of AKI. One or more of these biomarkers may provide a means by which patients can be identified at the incipient stage of AKI to guide the implementation of specific therapy to ameliorate kidney damage or promote recovery of kidney function.

Incidence of Acute Kidney Injury

The precise incidence of AKI has been difficult to estimate because of the absence, until recently, of a standard definition. It has been estimated that 3% to 7% of hospitalized patients and 25% to 30% of patients in the intensive care unit (ICU) develop AKI, with 5% to 6% of the ICU population requiring renal replacement therapy after developing AKI.[13-16] However, estimates of the incidence of AKI are highly dependent on the definition employed, with rates among hospitalized patients ranging from as high as 44% when the definition is based on a change in serum creatinine level of at least 0.3 mg/dL to as low as 1% when the required increase is at least 2.0 mg/dL. In a single-center analysis at an urban tertiary care hospital conducted in 1996 that defined AKI as an increase in serum creatinine concentration of 0.5 mg/dL for patients with a baseline serum creatinine level of 1.9 mg/dL or less, an increase of 1.0 mg/dL for patients with a baseline serum creatinine level of 2.0 to 4.9 mg/dL, and an increase of 1.5 mg/dL for patients with a baseline serum creatinine level greater than 5 mg/dL, AKI was found to develop in 7.2% of 4622 consecutively treated patients.[13] This rate was higher than the 4.9% rate the investigators had observed in a similar study in 1979.[17] The most frequent type was AKI caused by decreased renal perfusion, observed in 39% of episodes of AKI, followed by medication-associated AKI (16%), radiocontrast agent–induced AKI (11%), postoperative AKI (9%), and sepsis-associated AKI (6.5%). Overall mortality was 19.4%, with higher mortality rates associated with greater increases in serum creatinine concentration.

Although definition is less of an issue with regard to rates of AKI requiring renal replacement therapy, reported rates vary considerably because of differences in the characteristics of patient populations and variability in the criteria for the initiation of renal replacement therapy. In a multinational, multicenter observational study of 29,269 critically ill patients, 5.7% developed severe AKI and 4.3% received renal replacement therapy.[18]

Many epidemiologic studies of AKI have relied on data from large administrative databases. These data need to be interpreted with caution, however, because administrative coding for AKI is incomplete and may only capture 20% to 30% of all episodes of AKI. Identification of AKI requiring renal replacement therapy using administrative data is substantially more complete. In an analysis of data from the National Hospital Discharge Survey in the United States, the Centers for Disease Control and Prevention observed an increase in hospital discharges with a diagnosis of AKI from 18 per 100,000 population in 1980 to 365 per 100,000 in 2005.[19] Similar trends have been observed in analyses of the U.S. Nationwide Inpatient Sample (NIS) and a 5% sample of U.S. hospitalized Medicare beneficiaries. In an analysis that combined administrative and clinical data from a single integrated health care delivery system, the incidence of AKI that did not require the use of renal replacement therapy was found to increase from 322.7 to 522.4 per 100,000 person-years from 1996 to 2003.[20] Over the same period, AKI requiring renal replacement therapy increased from 19.5 to 29.5 per 100,000 person-years.[20] AKI was more common in men and in the elderly. In a subsequent analysis, preexisting kidney disease was demonstrated to be an important risk factor for the development of AKI requiring dialysis. Increasing levels of risk were associated with more severe baseline chronic kidney disease (CKD). Compared with patients with a baseline estimated GFR (eGFR) of more than 60 mL/min/1.73 m^2, those with eGFR values of 45 to 59 mL/min/1.73 m^2 had a nearly twofold increased risk of developing dialysis-requiring AKI. This risk increased to more than 40-fold among patients with baseline eGFR values of less than 15 mL/min/1.73 m^2. Underlying diabetes mellitus, hypertension, and the presence of proteinuria were also associated with increased risk of hospital-acquired AKI.

Etiologies of Acute Kidney Injury

Although in the clinical setting AKI is quite often multifactorial, it should always be approached diagnostically by keeping in mind the three major functional causes: namely, prerenal, intrinsic, and postrenal.

Prerenal Acute Kidney Injury

Prerenal azotemia is the most common cause of AKI and accounts for about 40% to 55% of all cases.[13,15,21] It results from kidney hypoperfusion owing to a reduced effective arterial blood volume. Effective arterial blood volume is the volume of blood effectively perfusing the body organs. Common conditions causing hypovolemia-mediated reduced effective arterial blood volume include hemorrhage (traumatic, gastrointestinal, surgical), gastrointestinal losses (vomiting, diarrhea, nasogastric suction), renal losses (overdiuresis, diabetes insipidus), and third spacing (pancreatitis, hypoalbuminemia). In addition, cardiogenic shock, septic shock, cirrhosis, hypoalbuminemia, and anaphylaxis all are pathophysiologic conditions that decrease effective arterial circulating volume, independent of total body volume status, and result in reduced kidney blood flow. Prerenal azotemia reverses rapidly if kidney perfusion is restored, because by definition the integrity of the renal parenchyma has remained intact. However, severe and prolonged hypoperfusion may result in tissue ischemia leading to ATN. Therefore, prerenal azotemia and ischemic ATN are part of a continuous spectrum of manifestations of renal hypoperfusion.

Prerenal azotemia has also been divided into volume responsive and volume nonresponsive types. The former is easy to comprehend, but the latter is less straightforward. In volume-nonresponsive forms, additional intravenous volume is of no help in restoring kidney perfusion and function. Disease processes such as congestive heart failure and sepsis may not respond to intravenous fluids because markedly reduced cardiac output or total vascular resistance, respectively, prevent improved kidney function (see Table 30-1).

Hypovolemia causes a decrease in mean arterial pressure that activates baroreceptors and initiates a cascade of neural and humoral responses, which leads to activation of the sympathetic nervous system and increases production of catecholamines, especially norepinephrine. There is increased release of antidiuretic hormone mediated both by hypovolemia and by a rise in extracellular osmolality, resulting in vasoconstriction, water retention, and urea back diffusion into the papillary interstitium. In response to volume depletion or states of decreased effective arterial blood volume, there is increased intrarenal angiotensin II activity via activation of the renin-angiotensin-aldosterone system. Angiotensin II is a very potent vasoconstrictor, increasing proximal tubule sodium absorption through a complex effect in the glomerulus by preferentially increasing efferent arteriolar resistance. GFR is preserved overall by the resulting increase in glomerular hydrostatic pressure. During severe volume depletion, angiotensin II activity is even greater, leading to afferent arteriolar constriction that reduces renal plasma flow, GFR, and the filtration fraction, and markedly augments proximal tubular sodium reabsorption in an effort to restore plasma volume.[22] Angiotensin II has also been shown to have direct effects on transport in the proximal tubule through receptors located in the tubule. It has also been postulated that the proximal tubule can locally produce angiotensin II. Hence, under conditions of volume depletion, angiotensin II stimulates a larger fraction of the transport, whereas volume expansion blunts this response.[23-27]

Renal sympathetic nerve activity is significantly increased in prerenal azotemia. Studies have shown that in the setting of hypovolemia, adrenergic activity independently constricts the afferent arteriole as well as changing the efferent arteriolar resistance through angiotensin II. α-Adrenergic activity primarily influences kidney vascular resistance, whereas renal nerve activity is linked to renin release through β-adrenergic receptors on renin-containing cells. In contrast, α2-adrenergic agonists primarily decrease the glomerular ultrafiltration coefficient via angiotensin II. Although vasodilation might be expected as a result of acute removal of adrenergic activity, a transient increase in angiotensin II is actually seen, along with constancy in GFR and renal blood flow. Even after subacute renal denervation, renal vascular sensitivity to angiotensin II increases as a result of major upregulation of angiotensin II receptors. Hence, complex effects on renin-angiotensin activity occur within the kidney secondary to increased renal adrenergic activity during prerenal azotemia.[28]

All of these systems work together and stimulate vasoconstriction in musculocutaneous and splanchnic circulations, inhibit salt loss through sweat, and stimulate thirst, thereby causing retention of salt and water to maintain blood pressure and preserve cardiac output and cerebral perfusion. Concomitantly, there are various compensatory mechanisms to preserve glomerular perfusion.[29] Autoregulation is achieved by stretch receptors in afferent arterioles that cause vasodilation in response to reduced perfusion pressure. Under physiologic conditions autoregulation works until a mean systemic arterial blood pressure of 75 to 80 mm Hg is reached. Below this, the glomerular ultrafiltration pressure and GRF decline abruptly. Renal production of prostaglandins, kallikrein, and kinins, as well as nitric oxide, is increased, which contributes to the vasodilation.[30,31] Nonsteroidal antiinflammatory drugs (NSAIDs), by inhibiting prostaglandin production, worsen kidney perfusion in patients with hypoperfusion. Selective efferent arteriolar constriction, a result of angiotensin II, helps preserve the intraglomerular pressure and hence GFR. Angiotensin converting enzyme (ACE) inhibitors inhibit synthesis of angiotensin II and so disturb this delicate balance in patients with severe reductions in effective arterial blood volume such as severe congestive heart failure or bilateral renal artery stenosis and thus can worsen prerenal azotemia. On the other hand, very high levels of angiotensin II, as seen in circulatory shock, cause constriction of both afferent and efferent arterioles, which negates its protective effect.

Although these compensatory mechanisms minimize the progression toward AKI, they too are overcome in states of severe hypoperfusion. Renovascular disease, hypertensive nephrosclerosis, and diabetic nephropathy, as well as older age, predispose patients to prerenal azotemia[32] at lesser degrees of hypotension.[32] Prerenal azotemia predisposes patients to ischemic ATN or nephrotoxic AKI. Superimposition of events such as anesthesia and surgery that are known to result in further decreases in renal blood flow and that would not normally result in kidney injury may precipitate ischemic ATN in the setting of prerenal azotemia. Similarly, prerenal azotemia also predisposes patients to radiocontrast agent-induced AKI and to other forms of nephrotoxic AKI. Therefore it is imperative to diagnose prerenal azotemia promptly and initiate effective treatment, because it is a potentially reversible condition that can lead to ischemic ATN or nephrotoxic AKI if therapy is delayed or its severity is increased.

Abdominal Compartment Syndrome

AKI can result from elevations in intraabdominal pressure, which leads to a clinical presentation with features similar to those of prerenal AKI. Abdominal compartment syndrome (ACS) is defined by an intraabdominal pressure of 20 mm Hg or more associated with dysfunction of one or more organ systems.[33] However, intraabdominal pressures lower than 20 mm Hg may be associated with ACS, and values higher than this threshold do not universally lead to ACS.[34-37] ACS typically develops in critically ill patients, most commonly in the setting of trauma with abdominal hemorrhage, abdominal surgery, massive fluid resuscitation, liver transplantation, and gastrointestinal conditions, including peritonitis and pancreatitis. Mechanisms underlying the development of AKI in ACS are believed to involve renal vein compression and constriction of the renal artery from sympathetic and renin-angiotensin system activation and reduced cardiac output.[38-40] Oliguria, which can lead to anuria, often develops, and as is true in other forms of AKI associated with impaired renal perfusion, urine sodium concentration is commonly reduced.

Intrinsic Acute Kidney Injury

Diseases of Large Vessels and Microvasculature

Total occlusion of the renal artery or vein is an uncommon event, but can be seen in certain scenarios such as trauma, instrumentation, thromboemboli, thrombosis, and dissection of an aortic aneurysm. Stenosis of the renal artery is a slow chronic process with or without evidence of declining GFR and rarely presents as an acute event. Renal vein thrombosis has classically and frequently been associated with hypercoagulable states such as nephrotic syndrome, particularly when associated with membranous nephropathy. An atheroembolic source should be considered in patients who have AKI after instrumentation with angiography, arteriography, or aortic surgery.[41] There can be dislodgement of cholesterol fragments from plaques in the aortic or other larger arteries that settle into smaller renal arteries, leading to hypoperfusion and an intense inflammatory reaction, akin to a vasculitis. Other organs may also be affected in this condition, resulting in gastrointestinal ischemia, peripheral gangrene, livedo reticularis, or acute pancreatitis. Patients frequently develop fevers and exhibit eosinophilia, elevated erythrocyte sedimentation rate, and hypocomplementemia, which sometimes help in differentiating this condition from other simultaneous insults (e.g., administration of a contrast agent). Renal artery thrombosis is usually a posttraumatic or postsurgical complication, especially in the transplant setting, but can also occur in other hypercoagable states such as antiphospholipid antibody syndrome.[42-44]

Diseases affecting the small vessels, generally termed *vasculitides*, including polyarteritis nodosa, necrotizing granulomatous vasculitis, hemolytic uremic syndrome (HUS), thrombotic thrombocytopenic purpura (TTP), and malignant hypertension, usually tend to occlude the vessels by deposition of fibrin along with platelets. Endothelial cell damage leads to an inflammatory response in the renal microvasculature (and in other organs), which results in reduced microvascular blood flow and tissue ischemia giving rise to superimposed ATN. One should keep in mind the intricate relationship between these inflammatory vasculitides and subsequent ischemic injury, because even though the origin of these disease processes is located at a site distant from the tubules, the final result is quite often ATN if the disorder is not treated early. Hence virtually any disease that compromises blood flow within the renal microvasculature can induce AKI (see Table 30-2).

Diseases of the Tubulointerstitium

Ischemic and septic ATN are the most common causes of intrinsic AKI. These are discussed extensively in later sections of the chapter dealing with ATN. Other disorders of the tubulointerstitium causing AKI, such as acute allergic interstitial nephritis, drug-induced tubular toxicity, and endogenous toxins, are described in the following sections.

INTERSTITIAL DISEASE

Acute interstitial nephritis results from an idiosyncratic allergic response to different pharmacologic agents, most commonly to antibiotics (e.g., methicillin and other penicillins, cephalosporins, sulfonamides, and quinolones) or to NSAIDs (e.g., ibuprofen).[45] Other conditions such as leukemia, lymphoma, sarcoidosis, bacterial infections (e.g., *Escherichia coli*), and viral infections (e.g., cytomegalovirus) can also cause acute interstitial nephritis leading to AKI. Systemic allergic signs such as fever, rash, and eosinophilia are often present in antibiotic-associated acute interstitial nephritis, but are not usually present in NSAID-related acute interstitial nephritis, in which lymphocytes tend to predominate.[46] The presence of inflammatory infiltrates within the interstitium is the hallmark of acute interstitial nephritis. These are often patchy and are present most commonly in the deep cortex and outer medulla. Interstitial edema is typically seen with the infiltrates, and sometimes patchy tubular necrosis may be present in close proximity to areas with extensive inflammatory infiltrates.[45] The majority of cases of acute interstitial nephritis are probably caused by extrarenal antigens produced by drugs or infectious agents that may be able to induce acute interstitial nephritis by (1) binding to kidney structures, (2) modifying the immunogenetics of native renal proteins, (3) mimicking renal antigens, or (4) precipitating as immune complexes and hence serving as the site of antibody- or cell-mediated injury.[47] This reaction is triggered by many events, including activation of complements and release of inflammatory cytokines by T cells and phagocytes. Acute allograft rejection in the transplant recipient is by far the most common immunologic cause of acute interstitial nephritis.

TUBULAR DISEASE—EXOGENOUS NEPHROTOXINS

Nephrotoxic ATN is the second most common cause of intrinsic AKI. The following sections briefly review the common drug nephrotoxicities in the context of AKI (Table 30-5). The kidneys are vulnerable to toxicity due to their high blood flow, and they are the major route for metabolizing and eliminating many of these substances. Furthermore, concentration of drugs within the tubular lumen and the interstitium leads to higher exposure rates.

Radiocontrast Medium–Induced Nephropathy. Iodinated radiocontrast agent–induced nephropathy is a common complication of radiologic or angiographic procedures. The incidence varies from 3% to 7% in patients without any risk factors, but can be as high as 50% in patients with moderate to advanced CKD. Other risk factors include diabetes, intravascular volume depletion, use of high-osmolal contrast, advanced age, proteinuria, and anemia.[48,49] Unlike most other forms of intrinsic tubular injury, contrast medium–induced AKI is usually associated with urinary sodium retention and a fractional excretion of sodium of less than 1%. AKI resulting from iodinated contrast agents is typically nonoliguric and rarely requires dialysis. However, requirement for renal support, prolonged hospitalization, and increased mortality are associated with this condition.

The pathophysiology of radiocontrast medium–induced nephropathy likely consists of combined hypoxic and toxic renal tubular damage associated with renal endothelial dysfunction and altered microcirculation.[50,51] The administration of radiocontrast agents mediates vasoconstriction and markedly affects renal parenchymal oxygenation, especially in the outer medulla, as documented in various studies in which the cortical oxygen pressure (Po_2) declined from 40 to 25 mm Hg, and the medullary Po_2 fell from 30 to 26 mm Hg to 9 to 15 mm Hg.[51-53] Radiocontrast injection leads to an abrupt but transient increase in renal plasma flow, GFR, and urinary output.[54] This mannitol-like effect occurs because the hyperosmolar radiocontrast agent enhances solute delivery to the distal nephron, which leads to higher oxygen consumption owing to increased tubular sodium reabsorption. It has also

been documented using video microscopy that radiocontrast agents markedly reduced inner medullary papillary blood flow, even to the extent of near cessation of red blood cell (RBC) movement in papillary vessels, associated with RBC aggregation within the papillary vasa recta.[55] However, it should be noted that there may be different patterns of response possibly related to the type, volume, and route of radiocontrast administration. Numerous neurohumoral mediators may contribute to the changes in renal microcirculation caused by radiocontrast injection. Intrarenal nitric oxide synthase activity, nitric oxide concentration, plasma endothelin, adenosine, prostaglandins, and vasopressin are all thought to play a role in altering the cortical and medullary microcirculation after radiocontrast injection. Mechanical factors may also play a role, because radiocontrast agents do increase blood viscosity and may affect flow in the low-pressure complex medullary microcirculation.[53] An increase in plasma viscosity after radiocontrast administration can interfere with blood flow, particularly under the hypertonic conditions of the (inner) renal medulla where the plasma viscosity is already increased as a result of hemoconcentration. Indeed, several animal studies have shown a correlation between experimental contrast medium–induced nephropathy and the viscosity of the radiopaque compound.[56,57]

Evidence also suggests direct tubular toxicity from radiocontrast agents. Early studies of isolated renal tubules in vitro have shown direct toxic effects of radiocontrast agents on proximal tubular cells.[58] Radiocontrast agents (diatrizoate, iopamidol) induced a decline in tubule K^+, adenosine triphosphate (ATP), and total adenine nucleotide contents. At the same time, there was a decrease in rate of tubular respiration and an increase of Ca^{2+} content. These changes were more pronounced with the ionic compound diatrizoate than with the nonionic iopamidol. Importantly, the cytotoxic effects were aggravated by hypoxia, which indicates interactions between direct cellular mechanisms and vasoconstriction-mediated hypoxia.[59] Andersen and colleagues have demonstrated the concentration-dependent radiocontrast-mediated release of tubular marker enzymes, ultrastructural changes, and cell death in both Madin-Darby canine kidney cells and LLC-PK$_1$ cells (a strain of epithelial-like pig kidney cells).[60] Radiocontrast medium–induced critical medullary hypoxia may lead to the formation of reactive oxygen species with subsequent membrane and DNA damage. A vicious cycle of hypoxia, free radical formation, and further hypoxic injury may be activated after radiocontrast exposure. Clinically, radiocontrast medium–induced nephropathy presents with an acute decline in GFR within 24 to 48 hours of administration, with a peak serum creatinine concentration in 3 to 5 days and a return to baseline within 1 week. Preexisting CKD, diabetic nephropathy, advanced age, congestive heart failure, volume depletion, and coincident use of NSAIDs increase the risk of contrast agent–induced nephropathy. Although numerous agents have been shown to be protective in the experimental setting, only volume expansion with isotonic crystalloid is of proven clinical benefit, with possible benefits associated with the use of bicarbonate-containing fluids and administration of N-acetylcysteine.

Recent data suggest that the renoprotective effects of acetylcysteine may be related to improved nitric oxide–dependent vasodilation and medullary oxygenation in addition to scavenging of free radicals.[50]

TABLE 30-5 Major Sources of Endogenous and Exogenous Toxins Causing Acute Tubular Injury	
ENDOGENOUS TOXINS	**EXOGENOUS TOXINS**
Myoglobulinuria	Antibiotics
Muscle breakdown—trauma, compression, electric shock, hypothermia, hyperthermia, seizures, exercise, burns	Aminoglycosides
	Amphotericin B
Metabolic disorders—hypokalemia, hypophosphatemia	Antiviral agents—acyclovir, cidofovir, indinavir, foscarnet, tenofovir
Infections—tetanus, influenza	Pentamidine
Toxins—isopropyl alcohol, ethanol, ethylene glycol, toluene, snake and insect bites, cocaine, heroin	Chemotherapeutic Agents
	Ifosfamide
Drugs—hydroxymethylglutaryl–coenzyme A reductase inhibitors, amphetamines, fibrates	Cisplatin
	Plicamycin
	5-Fluorouracil
Inherited diseases—deficiency of myophosphorylase, phosphofructokinase, carnitine palmityltransferase	Cytarabine
	6-Thioguanine
Autoimmune disorders—polymyositis, dermatomyositis	Calcineurin Inhibitors
	Cyclosporin
Hemoglobinuria	Tacrolimus
Mechanical causes—prosthetic valves, microangiopathic hemolytic anemia, extracorporeal circulation	Organic Solvents
	Toluene
	Ethylene glycol
Drugs—hydralazine, methyldopa	Poisons
Chemicals—benzene, arsine, fava beans, glycerol, phenol	Snake venom
	Paraquat
Immunologic disorders—transfusion reaction	Miscellaneous
	Radiocontrast agents
Genetic disorders—glucose-6-phosphate dehydrogenase deficiency, paroxysmal nocturnal hemoglobinuria	Intravenous immune globulin
	Nonsteroidal antiinflammatory drugs
Hyperuricemia with Hyperuricosuria	Oral phosphate bowel preparations
Tumor lysis syndrome	
Hypoxanthine-guanine phosphoribosyltransferase deficiency	
Myeloma (light-chain production)	
Oxalate crystalluria (ethylene glycol)	

Aminoglycoside Nephrotoxicity. The nephrotoxicity of aminoglycosides has been best characterized for gentamicin, a polar drug excreted by glomerular filtration. It is thought that cationic amino groups (NH_3^+) on the drug bind to anionic phospholipid residues on the brush border of proximal tubule cells and are then internalized by endocytosis. Although precise subcellular mechanisms of the pathologic insult of aminoglycosides have not been fully elucidated, binding at the apical surface of proximal tubule cells is now known to involve megalin.[61,62] Once aminoglycosides undergo endocytosis, the drugs inhibit endosomal fusion. They are also directly trafficked to the Golgi apparatus and through retrograde movement to the endoplasmic reticulum. From the endoplasmic reticulum, gentamicin moves into the cytosol in a size- and charge-dependent manner.[63] Once in the cytosol, either from the endoplasmic reticulum[63] or via lysosomal rupture, aminoglycosides distribute to various intracellular organelles and mediate organelle-specific toxicity such as mitochondrial dysfunction.[63,64] Also, delivery to the endoplasmic reticulum via retrograde transport from the Golgi apparatus allows for binding of aminoglycosides to the 16S (16-Svedberg-unit) ribosomal RNA subunit,[65] which results in a reduction of protein synthesis. The number of cationic groups on the molecules determines the facility with which these drugs are transported across the cell membrane and is an important determinant of toxicity.[66,67] Neomycin is associated with the most nephrotoxicity; gentamicin, tobramycin, and amikacin are intermediate; and streptomycin is the least nephrotoxic. Risk factors for aminoglycoside nephrotoxicity include the use of high or repeated doses or prolonged therapy, CKD, volume depletion, diabetes, advanced age, and the presence of renal ischemia or other nephrotoxins[68-70] (Figure 30-2).

Cisplatin Nephrotoxicity. Cisplatin (cisplatinum), a platinum-based compound widely used for chemotherapy, is commonly associated with nephrotoxicity. Its active metabolites can cause mitochondrial damage, cell cycle arrest, inhibition of ATP activity, alterations of cell transport, and, ultimately, apoptosis or necrosis. The S3 segment of the proximal tubule in the corticomedullary region is the most common site of cisplatin nephrotoxicity in rats.

More distal sites may be affected in humans, but glomeruli remain unaffected. Cisplatin causes a decrease in kidney function in a dose-dependant fashion, and effects are usually reversible after cessation of the drug[71] (Tables 30-5 and 30-6).

Acute Phosphate Nephropathy. AKI has been described as a complication following the administration of oral sodium phosphate solution as a bowel cathartic in preparation for colonoscopy and bowel surgery.[72-74] Although the mechanism linking oral sodium phosphate administration with AKI remains incompletely understood, the pathogenesis likely relates to a transient and significant rise in serum phosphate concentration that occurs simultaneously with intravascular volume depletion. This may lead to intratubular precipitation of calcium phosphate salts that obstruct the tubular lumen and cause direct tubular damage. Risk factors for acute phosphate nephropathy include preexisting volume depletion, the use of ACE inhibitors and angiotensin receptor blockers, CKD, older age, female sex, and higher dose of oral sodium phosphate.[73,74] Patients who develop acute phosphate nephropathy typically show elevated serum creatinine concentrations days to months after the administration of oral sodium solution and can experience progression to chronic and end-stage kidney disease.

Tubular Disease—Endogenous Nephrotoxins

Myoglobin and hemoglobin are endogenous toxins most commonly associated with ATN. Myoglobin, a 17.8-kDa hemoprotein released during muscle injury, is freely filtered and causes red-brown urine with a dipstick result positive for heme but with a relative absence of RBCs. Intravascular hemolysis results in circulating free hemoglobin, which when excessive is filtered, leading to hemoglobinuria, hemoglobin cast formation, and heme uptake by proximal tubule cells. The renal injury is due to a combination of factors, including volume depletion, renal vasoconstriction, direct heme protein–mediated cytotoxicity, and intraluminal cast formation. The heme center of myoglobin may directly induce lipid peroxidation and liberation of free iron. Iron is an intermediate accelerator in the generation of free radicals. Evidence suggests that there is increased formation of hydrogen peroxide in a

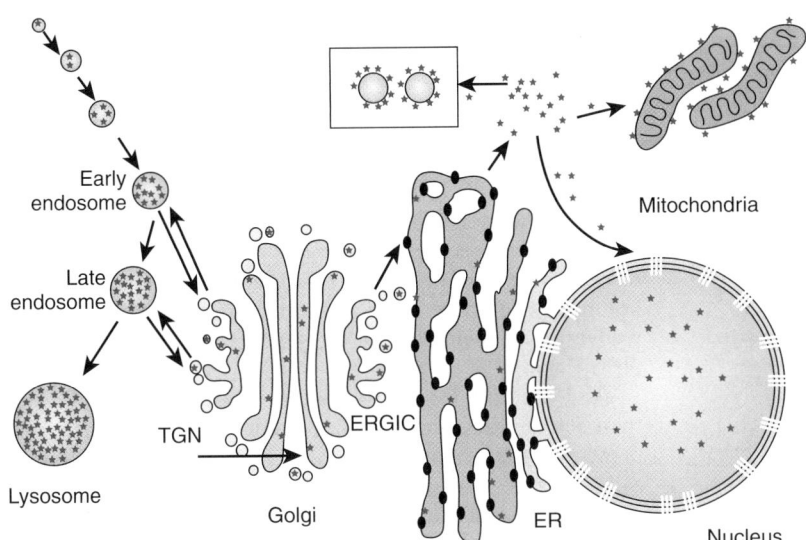

FIGURE 30-2 Retrograde trafficking of gentamicin along the endocytic pathway in LLC-PK cells. Internalization occurs via receptor-mediated endocytosis with approximately 90% of the internalized material accumulating within lysosomes. However approximately 10% is shuttled to the Golgi complex and is transported past the endoplasmic reticulum (ER)–Golgi intermediate compartment (ERGIC) to the ER. From there, translocation to the cytosol occurs. Once the drug is in the cytosol, association with various organelles such as the mitochondrial membranes and nuclei can initiate an additional cascade of events leading to renal proximal tubule injury. (From Sandoval RM, Molitoris BA: Gentamicin traffics retrograde through the secretory pathway and is released in the cytosol via the endoplasmic reticulum, *Am J Physiol Renal Physiol* 286:F617-F624, 2004.)

Early endosome
Late endosome
Lysosome
TGN
Golgi
ERGIC
ER
Nucleus
Mitochondria

rat kidney model of myohemoglobinuria.[75] The subsequent hydroxyl (OH−) radical plays a vital role in oxidative stress–induced AKI through mechanisms discussed in detail later in the chapter. Various iron chelators such as deferoxamine and other scavengers of reactive oxygen species such as glutathione have been shown to provide protection against myohemoglobinuric AKI.[76] Similarly, endothelin antagonists have been shown to prevent hypofiltration and proteinuria in rats that underwent glycerol-induced rhabdomyolysis.[77] Others have shown that nitric oxide supplementation might be beneficial by preventing heme-induced renal vasoconstriction, because heme proteins scavenge nitric oxide.[78,79]

Finally, precipitation of myoglobin with Tamm-Horsfall protein and shed proximal tubule cells leads to cast formation and tubular obstruction, which is enhanced in acidic urine.[80] In human studies, volume expansion and perhaps alkalinization of urine to limit cast formation are the preventive measures generally employed, because none of the experimental agents used in animal studies have been convincingly beneficial. This is again a reminder of the multifactorial nature of this condition and the fact that a single agent is unlikely to be beneficial in this setting.[81]

Other endogenous nephrotoxins include uric acid and light chains. Excessive light chains, produced in diseases such as multiple myeloma, are filtered, absorbed, and then catabolized in proximal tubule cells. The concentration of light chains leaving the proximal portion of the nephron depends on the capacity of the proximal tubule to reabsorb and catabolize them as well as the filtrate volume and concentration. Certain light chains can be directly toxic to the proximal tubules themselves.[82] Light chain–induced cytokine release has been associated with nuclear translocation of nuclear factor κB (NF-κB), which suggests that light-chain endocytosis leads to production of inflammatory cytokines through activation of NF-κB.[83] Once the capacity for proximal tubule uptake is overwhelmed, a light-chain load is presented to the distal tubule where, upon reaching a critical concentration, the light chains aggregate and co-precipitate with Tamm-Horsfall protein and form characteristic light-chain casts.[84] Recent studies have also shown that light chains, in the amount seen in patients with plasma cell dyscrasia, are capable of catalyzing the formation of hydrogen peroxide in cultured HK-2 cells (a proximal tubule epithelial cell line from human kidney). Hydrogen peroxide stimulates the production of monocyte chemoattractant protein-1 (MCP-1), a key chemokine involved in recruitment of monocytes/macrophages to proximal tubule cells.[85]

Any process reducing GFR, such as volume depletion, hypercalcemia, or NSAID use, will accelerate and aggravate this cast formation. It has been proposed that short-term reduction of the presented light-chain load by plasmapheresis might be beneficial in limiting cast formation and reducing the extent of AKI in certain select patients, so that chemotherapy can be initiated to decrease bone marrow–dependent light-chain formation.[86] Tumor cell necrosis following chemotherapy can release large amounts of intracellular contents such as uric acid, phosphate, and xanthine into the circulation, which can potentially lead to AKI. Acute uric acid nephropathy with intratubular crystallization leading to obstruction and interstitial nephritis is not seen as commonly as it was in the past, mainly due to prophylactic use of allopurinol or rasburicase before chemotherapy to provide short-term reduction of serum uric acid levels. Several other well-known therapeutic agents such as amphotericin B, acyclovir, indinavir, cidofovir, foscarnet, pentamidine, and ifosfamide can all directly cause tubular injury.

Postrenal Acute Kidney Injury

Postrenal azotemia is caused by either ureteric obstruction or bladder or urethral obstruction. AKI due to ureteric obstruction requires that the blockage occur either bilaterally at any level of the ureters or unilaterally in a patient with a solitary functioning kidney or CKD. Ureteric obstruction can be either intraluminal or external. Bilateral ureteric calculi, blood clots, and sloughed renal papillae can obstruct the lumen. External compression from tumor or hemorrhage can block the ureters as well. Fibrosis of the ureters intrinsically or from the retroperitoneum can narrow the lumen to the point of complete luminal obstruction. The most common cause of postrenal azotemia is structural or functional obstruction of the bladder neck. Prostatic conditions, therapy with anticholinergic agents, and a neurogenic bladder can all cause postrenal AKI. Relief of the obstruction usually leads to prompt return of GFR if the duration of obstruction has not been excessive. The rate and magnitude of functional recovery is dependent on the extent and duration of the obstruction.[87]

AKI resulting from obstruction usually accounts for fewer than 5% of cases, although in certain settings such as transplantation the proportion can be as high as 6% to 10%. Clinically the patient can have pain and oliguria at presentation, although these are nonspecific. Because of the ease of ultrasonography, the diagnosis is usually straightforward, although

---

TABLE 30-6 Classification of Various Common Drugs Based on Pathophysiologic Categories of Acute Kidney Injury

1. Vasoconstriction/Impaired Microvasculature Hemodynamics (Prerenal)
Nonsteroidal antiinflammatory drugs (NSAIDs), angiotensin converting enzyme inhibitors, angiotensin receptor blockers, norepinephrine, tacrolimus, cyclosporine, diuretics, cocaine, mitomycin C, estrogen, quinine, interleukin-2, cyclooxygenase-2 inhibitors

2. Tubular Cell Toxicity
Antibiotics—aminoglycosides, amphotericin B, vancomycin, rifampicin, foscarnet, pentamidine, cephaloridine, cephalothin
Radiocontrast agents, NSAIDs, acetaminophen, cyclosporine, cisplatin, mannitol, heavy metals, intravenous immune globulin (IVIG), ifosfamide, tenofovir

3. Acute Interstitial Nephritis
Antibiotics—ampicillin, penicillin G, methicillin, oxacillin, rifampicin, ciprofloxacin, cephalothin, sulfonamides
NSAIDs, aspirin, fenoprofen, naproxen, piroxicam, phenylbutazone, radiocontrast agents, thiazide diuretics, phenytoin, furosemide, allopurinol, cimetidine, omeprazole

4. Tubular Lumen Obstruction
Sulfonamides, acyclovir, cidofovir, methotrexate, triamterene, methoxyflurane, protease inhibitors, ethylene glycol, indinavir, oral sodium phosphate bowel preparations

5. Thrombotic Microangiopathy
Clopidogrel, cocaine, ticlopidine, cyclosporine, tacrolimus, mitomycin C, oral contraceptives, gemcitabine, bevacizumab

6. Osmotic Nephrosis
IVIG, mannitol, dextrans, hetastarch

on occasion a patient with volume depletion or severe reduction in GFR may not show hydronephrosis on radiologic assessment. Since initially during the course of the disease GFR is not affected, volume repletion can help with the diagnosis by increasing GFR and urine production into the ureter, which leads to dilation of the ureter proximal to the obstruction and enhances ultrasonographic visualization. Early diagnosis and prompt relief of obstruction remain key goals in preventing long-term parenchymal damage, because the shorter the period of obstruction, the better the chances for recovery and good long-term outcomes. The pathophysiology and treatment of obstructive uropathy are discussed extensively in Chapter 37 (see Table 30-3).

Pathophysiology of Acute Kidney Injury

Experimental Models

A variety of animal and cell culture models of AKI exist that are designed to improve understanding of the pathophysiology of AKI and to investigate the use of novel therapeutic agents. However, there remains a need to develop in vivo experimental models of AKI that more closely resemble clinical AKI for the development of effective therapies.[88,89] Some of the important principles in studying the pathophysiology of AKI in various models include assessment of outcome measures at multiple time points and the ability to control physiologic functions known to affect kidney function (e.g., temperature, blood pressure, anesthesia, fluid status). Another limitation of most experimental models is the lack of comorbid conditions such as older animal age, impaired kidney function, multiorgan failure, preexisting vascular changes, or multiple renal insults, which quite often coexist in human AKI. The pros and cons of using presently characterized experimental models are discussed briefly (Table 30-7).

The warm ischemia–reperfusion renal pedicle clamp model is one of the most widely used experimental models in rats and mice because of its simplicity and reproducibility. However, the inflammatory response differs greatly between mice and rats. Furthermore, tubular injury and repair and medullary congestion are difficult to compare with human ischemic ATN. In human AKI, "pure" ischemia alone is seen in a minority of cases, and there is usually not complete cessation of blood flow to the kidneys. Delivery of preventive therapeutic agents, which might be beneficial during the peak ischemic insult, is not possible in models of complete occlusion. Since oxygen and metabolic substrates are totally stopped from flowing into the kidney, generation of reactive oxygen species and peroxynitrite species, considered to be an important mediator of injury, might have a different or delayed role compared with low-oxygen states in hypoperfusion models. Total blood flow cessation also prevents the degradative products of the ischemic kidney from being washed out. Other factors playing a role in the pathophysiology of AKI such as inflammatory mediators released from ischemic gut, endothelium, and vascular smooth muscle cells need to be taken into consideration in any experimental model. Bowel proteins released into the circulation can act as inflammatory mediators and increase the susceptibility to AKI.[90] The S3 segment of the proximal tubule undergoes almost complete necrosis in clamp models, a finding not seen very frequently in human AKI. Unlike in

animal models, human AKI histologic biopsy data are lacking at early time intervals from the onset of insult.[89] This has made comparison between animal models and human AKI of limited value.

The cold ischemia–warm reperfusion model resembles the human transplant scenario but is inadequately studied and difficult experimentally. In the isolated perfused kidney model, the kidney is perfused ex vivo using perfusates with and without erythrocytes, and either ischemia (stopping perfusate) or hypoxia (reduced oxygen tension of erythrocytes) is used to induce functional impairment. The morphologic patterns are different with erythrocyte-free and erythrocyte-rich perfusates. The latter system is more comparable to what is observed histologically in animal models. In addition, limitations include exclusion of various inflammatory mediators, neuroendocrine hemodynamic regulation, and systemic cytokine and growth factor interactions known to be present and to play a pathophysiologic role in animal models and likely in human ischemia.

Cardiac arrest is a common scenario leading to human AKI. Rabb's group[91] described a whole-body ischemia-reperfusion injury model in which AKI was induced by 10 minutes of cardiac arrest followed by cardiac compression resuscitation, ventilation, epinephrine, and fluids that led to a significant rise in serum creatinine level and renal tubular injury at 24 hours. One of the unique advantages of this model is that it permits crosstalk between vital organs such as the brain, heart, and lung and the renal hemodynamics.[92] A hypoperfusion model of AKI using partial aortic clamping, first described by Zager,[93] may be more representative of human AKI, reflecting a state of reduced blood flow to the kidney with systolic blood pressure around 20 mm Hg and resulting in reproducible AKI.[93,94] This method was recently adapted and refined in a study by Sharfuddin and associates in which a novel compound, soluble thrombomodulin, was used to minimize ischemic injury in a partial aortic clamp AKI model.[95]

Models of toxicity-induced renal failure employ various known toxins, such as radiocontrast agents, gentamicin, cis-platinum, glycerol, and pigments, including myoglobin and hemoglobin. Models for the study of sepsis-associated AKI utilize cecal ligation and puncture (CLP), endotoxin infusion, and bacterial infusion into the peritoneal cavity. The endotoxin model is simple, inexpensive, and suitable for the study of new pharmacologic agents, but it has certain drawbacks as well. There is variability in the lipopolysaccharide endotoxin from different sources, the rates and methods of administration vary, and the experiment is usually of short duration due to the high mortality associated with the doses required to induce AKI. The model also tends to be a vasoconstrictive one and does not recapitulate the early hemodynamics or inflammation of human sepsis.[96] Wichterman and colleagues were the first to describe a sepsis model in the early 1980s utilizing the CLP laboratory method.[97] In the CLP model, there is considerable similarity with sepsis in humans with acute lung injury, metabolic derangement, and systemic vasodilation, accompanied by increased cardiac output initially. However, some variability is seen depending on the mode and size of cecal perforation. Star's laboratory has developed a new sepsis model with consideration of the following facts: (1) animals should received the same supportive therapy that is standard for ICU patients (i.e., fluid resuscitation and antibiotics); (2) age, chronic comorbid conditions, and genetic heterogeneity

TABLE 30-7 Comparison of Models for Studying Acute Kidney Injury

| | HUMANS | ANIMALS | | | | | | | | CELLS | |
| | | ISCHEMIC | | | | SEPTIC | | | TOXIC | | |
		WARM-ISCHEMIA–REPERFUSION	COLD-ISCHEMIA–REPERFUSION	HYPOPERFUSION/CARDIAC ARREST	ISOLATED PERFUSED KIDNEYS	ENDOTOXIN	CECAL LIGATION & PUNCTURE	BACTERIAL INFUSION	CONTRAST AGENT/PIGMENT/GLYCEROL/DRUG	ISOLATED PROXIMAL TUBULE CELLS	CULTURED TUBULAR CELLS
Simplicity	+	++++	++	++	++	++++	+++	+++	++++	+++	++++
Reproducibility	++	++++	+++	+++	+++	+++	++	+++	+++	+++	++
Clinical relevance	++++	++	+++	++++	++	++	++++	+++	+++	+	+
Therapeutic value	+++	++	++	++++	++	++	+++	+++	+++	+	+
Study of mechanisms	++	++	++	+++	++	++	+++	+++	+++	+++	+++
Control of extrinsic factors	+	+	++	++	+++	++	++	++	++	++++	++++
Isolation of single variables	++	+	++	+	+++	+++	++	++	+++	++++	++++
Standardization value	+	++++	+++	++	+++	+++	++	+++	++	++	+++
Experimental limitation	++++	+++	+++	+++	++	++	+++	++	++	+	+

Ratings are on a scale from "+," minimally applicable to "++++," very applicable.

vary.[98] Complex animal models of human sepsis that introduce these disease-modifying factors are likely more relevant and may be more pharmacologically applicable than simple animal models.[98] However, do such models replicate the early, clinically silent phase of sepsis? Another toxic nephropathy model is the zebrafish model studied by Bonventre's group. The zebrafish has the advantages of markedly improved accessibility of the kidney, feasibility of knockdown and upregulation of genes using morpholinos, and a short phenotypic readout time, while at the same time possessing the complexity of an organism necessary to study kidney injury. These properties may make it a useful and inexpensive tool to screen therapeutic agents in the future.[99]

The foregoing description was intended to remind the reader of the potential pitfalls associated with each model when evaluating experimental studies or therapeutic interventions based on these models. The failure to demonstrate the effectiveness of an agent in humans that has been shown to be efficacious in animal models does not necessarily reflect a flaw in the model or in the agent in question. Most often, the agent is administered very late in the course of the human disease, and patient heterogeneity and the inability to stratify patients by severity of injury makes it even more difficult to establish true efficacy.[100] It is also important to remember that experimental models of hypoxic acute kidney damage differ both conceptually and morphologically in the distribution of tubular cell injury. Tubular segment types differ in their capacity to undergo anaerobic metabolism and to mount hypoxia-adaptive responses mediated by hypoxia-inducible factors, as well as in the cell type-specific molecules shed into the urine, which may serve as early biomarkers of kidney damage.[101]

Acute Tubular Necrosis

Epithelial Cell Injury

Although all segments of the nephron may undergo injury during an ischemic insult, the major and most commonly injured epithelial cell involved in AKI from ischemia, sepsis, or other nephrotoxins is the proximal tubular cell. Of the three segments (S1 to S3), the S3 segment of the proximal tubule in the outer stripe of the medulla is the most damaged cell during ischemic injury for several reasons.[102] First, it has limited capacity to undergo anaerobic glycolysis. Second, because of its unique primarily venous capillary regional blood flow, there is marked hypoperfusion and congestion in this medullary region after injury that persists even though cortical blood flow may have returned to near-normal levels following ischemic injury. Endothelial cell injury and dysfunction are primarily responsible for this phenomenon, known now as the *extension phase* of AKI.[103] The other major epithelial cells of the nephron involved are those of the medullary thick ascending limb located more distally. The S1 and S2 segments are most commonly involved in toxic nephropathy because of their high rates of endocytosis, which leads to increased cellular uptake of the toxin.

Proximal tubule cell injury and dysfunction during ischemia or sepsis lead to a profound drop in GFR through afferent arteriolar vasoconstriction, mediated by tubular glomerular feedback and proximal tubular obstruction. This, along with tubular backleakage, leads to a fall in effective GFR[104,105] (Figure 30-3).

MORPHOLOGIC CHANGES

On histologic examination, the classical hallmark of ATN is the loss of the apical brush border of the proximal tubular cells. Disruption and detachment of microvilli from the apical cell surface forming membrane-bound blebs occurs early with release into the tubular lumen. Patchy detachment and subsequent loss of tubular cells exposing areas of denuded tubular basement and focal areas of proximal tubular dilatation along with the presence of distal tubular casts are also major pathologic findings in ATN.[106] The sloughed tubule cells, brush border vesicle remnants, and cellular debris in combination with Tamm-Horsfall glycoprotein form the classical muddy-brown granular casts.[107] These distal casts have the potential to obstruct the tubular lumen. Necrosis itself is inconspicuous and restricted to the highly susceptible outer medullary regions. On the other hand, features of apoptosis are more

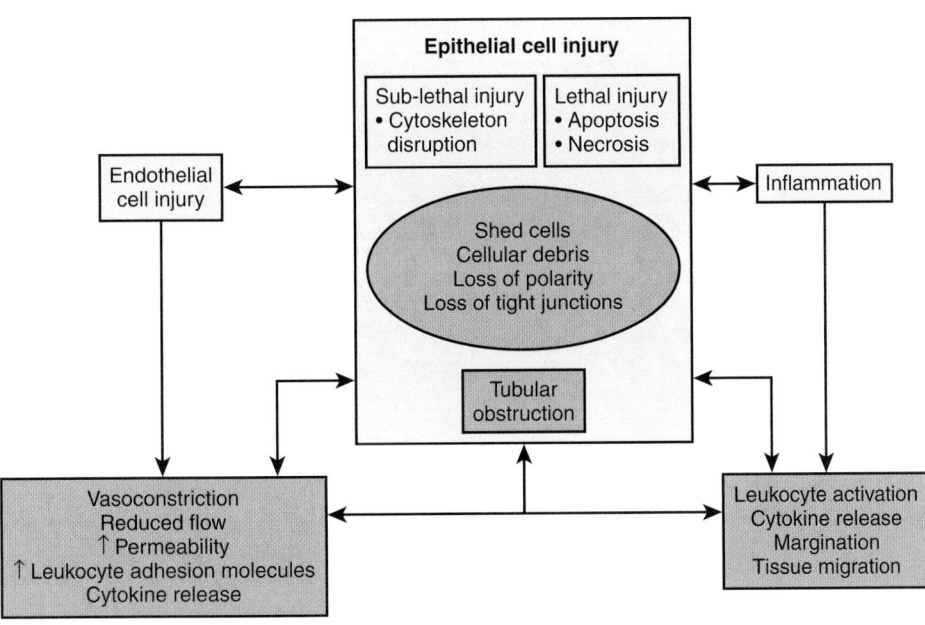

FIGURE 30-3 Overview of pathogenesis in acute kidney injury showing the major pathways of impairment of glomerular filtration rate (GFR) in ischemic acute tubular necrosis as a result of vascular and tubular injury (see text for details). (From Sharfuddin A, Molitoris B: Epithelial cell injury, in Vincent JL, Hall JB [editors]: *Encyclopedia of intensive care medicine,* New York, 2012, Springer.)

commonly seen in both proximal and distal tubule cells. Glomerular epithelial cell injury in ischemic, septic, or nephrotoxic injury is not classically seen, although some studies have shown thickening and coarsening of foot processes, and recently Wagner and colleagues have shown podocyte-specific molecular and cellular changes.[108] The future morphologic course of the tubular cell alterations varies according to the type and extent of injury as discussed later (Figure 30-4).

CYTOSKELETAL AND INTRACELLULAR STRUCTURAL CHANGES

Epithelial cell structure and function are mediated in part by the actin cytoskeleton, which plays an integral role in surface membrane structure and function, cell polarity, endocytosis, cell motility, movement of organelles, exocytosis, cell division,

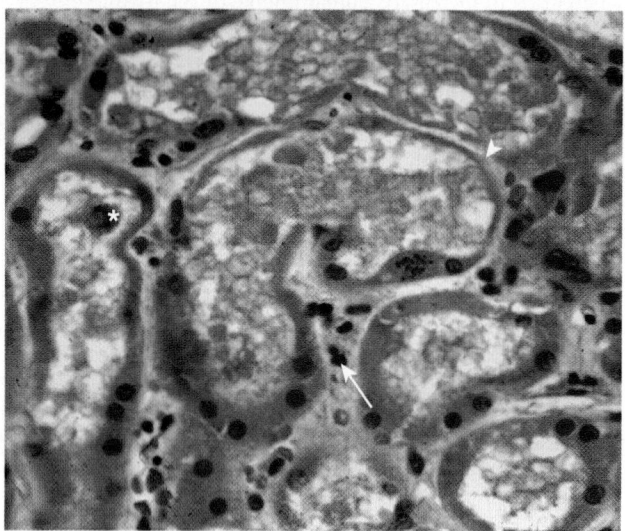

FIGURE 30-4 Morphology of acute tubular necrosis in human biopsy specimen. The biopsy sample, obtained within 24 hours from a patient with exercise-induced rhabdomyolysis, revealed significant proximal tubule cell damage with intraluminal accumulation of apical membrane fragments and detached cell (*), thinning of proximal tubular cells to maintain monolayer tubule integrity (*arrowhead*), and dividing cells and accumulation of white cells within the microvascular space in the peritubular area (*arrow*). The patient required renal replacement therapy but did regain complete renal function eventually. (From Molitoris BA: Actin cytoskeleton in ischemic acute renal failure, *Kidney Int* 66:874, 2004.)

cell migration, barrier function of the junctional complexes, cell matrix adhesion, and last, but not least, signal transduction.[109] Based on its role in this multitude of processes, any disruption of the actin cytoskeleton results in changes in and/or disruption of the aforementioned functions. This is especially important for proximal tubular cells, in which amplification of the apical membrane by microvilli is essential for normal cell function.

Actin microfilaments are formed by self-assembly of globular or G-actin into filamentous F-actin. In proximal tubule cells the actin cytoskeleton forms a terminal web layer just below the apical plasma membrane, and a core of F-actin filaments extends from the terminal web into the tips of the microvilli to maintain the architectural integrity of the brush border. Ischemic insult results in cellular ATP depletion, which in turn leads to a rapid disruption of the apical actin and disruption and redistribution of the cytoskeleton F-actin core, resulting in formation of membrane-bound extracellular vesicles or blebs.[110] These can be either exfoliated into the tubular lumen or internalized with the capability of being recycled. The core mechanism of disruption is the depolymerization mediated by the actin-binding protein known as *actin depolymerizing factor* (ADF) or *cofilin*.[111] This protein family is normally maintained in the inactive phosphorylated form in which it cannot bind to actin. Ischemia results in ATP depletion, which has been shown to cause Rho guanosine triphosphatase inactivation.[112] This can lead to activation and relocalization of ADF/cofilin to the apical membranes, where it can mediate different effects, including depolymerization, severing, capping, and nucleation of F-actin. This destroys the actin filament core structure of microvilli and results in surface membrane instability and blebbing[113,114] (Figure 30-5).

Concomitantly, the concentration of F-actin in the cell increases with the formation of large cytosolic aggregates in the perinuclear region and near the junctional complexes of the basolateral membranes. Other proteins involved in the depolymerization process are tropomyosin and ezrin. Specifically, it has been shown that during ischemia ezrin, an actin-binding phosphorylated protein, becomes dephosphorlylated, and the attachment between the microvillar F-actin core and the plasma membrane is lost. Similarly, tropomyosins physiologically bind to and stabilize the F-actin microfilament

FIGURE 30-5 Overview of sublethally injured tubular cells. Na+-K+-adenosine triphosphatase (Na+-K+-ATPase) pumps are normally located at the basolateral membrane. In sublethal ischemia the pumps redistribute to the apical membrane of the proximal tubule. Upon reperfusion, the pumps reverse back to their basolateral location. (From Sharfuddin A, Molitoris B: Epithelial cell injury, in Vincent JL, Hall JB [editors]: *Encyclopedia of intensive care medicine*, New York, 2012, Springer.)

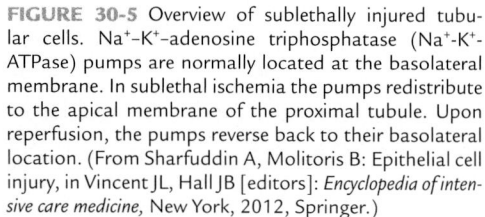
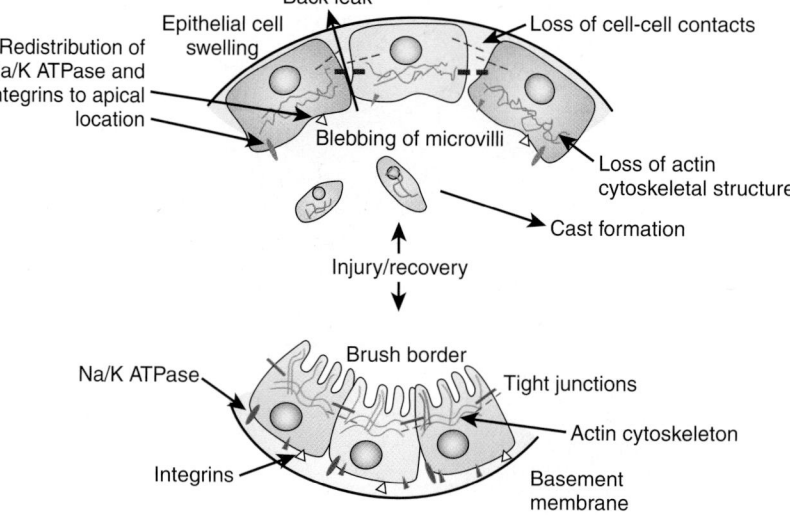

core in the terminal web by preventing access to ADF/cofilin. After ischemia, there is dissociation of tropomyosins from the microfilament core, resulting in access of the microfilaments in the terminal web to the binding, severing, and depolymerizing actions of ADF/cofilin.[115,116]

Another important consequence of disruption of the actin cytoskeleton is the loss of tight junctions and adherens junctions. These junctional complexes actively participate in numerous functions, including paracellular transport, cell polarity, and cellular shape. The tight junctions, also known as *zonula occludens,* are composed of a growing number of proteins such as occludin, claudin, zonula occludens 1 (ZO-1), and protein kinase C with numerous barrier functions, including adhesion, permeability, and transport. The actin present in the terminal web is linked to zonula occludens, and hence any disruption of the terminal web results in disruption of the tight junctions. Early ischemic injury causes opening of these tight junctions, which leads to increased paracellular permeability producing further backleak of the glomerular filtrate into the interstitium.[109] Only recently it has been shown that in the glomerulus ischemia also induces rapid loss of interaction between slit diaphragm junctional proteins Neph1 and ZO-1,[108] leading to podocyte damage and effacement, and proteinuria.

During ischemia, epithelial cells also lose their attachment to the underlying extracellular matrix due to disruption of integrins. Integrins are transmembrane proteins normally responsible for the anchoring of epithelial cells to the substrate matrix via the actin cytoskeleton. It has been shown that ATP depletion results in relocalization of β-integrins from the basal membrane to the apical membrane, with subsequent detachment of the viable cells from the tubular basement membrane. The exfoliated cells can then exhibit abnormal adhesions among themselves within the tubular lumen, forming cellular casts within the tubular lumen as mentioned earlier.

Actin cytoskeleton alterations and dysfunction during ischemia result in changes in cell polarity and function. Normally, Na$^+$-K$^+$-ATPase pumps reside in the basolateral membrane of the tubular epithelial cell, but under conditions of ischemia, they redistribute to the apical membrane as early as within 10 minutes.[117] This occurs due to the disruption of the pumps' attachment to the membrane via the spectrin/actin cytoskeleton. Postulated mediating mechanisms include hyperphosphorylation of the protein ankyrin, with consequent loss of the binding protein spectrin, and cleavage of spectrin by activation of proteases such as calpain. This redistribution of the Na$^+$-K$^+$-ATPase pump results in bidirectional transport of Na and water across the epithelial cell apical membrane as well as the basolateral membrane; this results in the transport of cellular Na back into the tubular lumen—one of the major mechanisms of the high fractional excretion of Na seen in patients with ATN[118]—and in the inefficient use of cellular ATP, because it uncouples ATP use and effective Na transport.

APOPTOSIS AND NECROSIS

The fate of the epithelial cell after an injury ultimately depends on the extent of the injury. Cells undergoing sublethal or less severe injury have the capability of functional and structural recovery if the insult is interrupted. Cells that experience a more severe or lethal injury undergo apoptosis or necrosis. Apoptosis is an energy-dependent, programmed cell death after injury that results in condensation of nuclear and cytoplasmic material, and formation of apoptotic bodies. These apoptotic bodies, which are plasma membrane bound, undergo rapid phagocytosis by macrophages and neighboring viable epithelial cells. In necrosis, there is cellular and organelle swelling, with loss of plasma membrane integrity, and release of cytoplasmic and nuclear material into the lumen or interstitium.[119]

Apoptotic mechanisms are complex, with various interplaying and counteracting factors affecting a number of pathways. The caspase family of proteases has now been identified to be an important initiator as well as an effector of apoptosis.[120,121] Both the intrinsic (mitochondrial) and extrinsic (death receptor) apoptotic pathways are activated in human AKI. Specifically, activation of procaspase-9 primarily depends on intrinsic mitochondrial pathways regulated by the Bcl-2 family of proteins, whereas that of procaspase-8 results from extrinsic signaling via cell surface death receptors such as Fas and their ligand FADD (Fas-associated protein with death domain). There also exists considerable crosstalk between the intrinsic and extrinsic pathways. The other group of caspases, 3, 6, and 7, are effector caspases that are more abundant and catalytically robust, cleaving many cellular proteins and resulting in the classical apoptotic phenotype. Caspase activation in epithelial cells occurs due to ischemic and other cytotoxic insults, whereas inhibition of caspase activity has been shown to be protective against such injury in renal epithelial tubular AKI in cultures and in vivo[122,123] (Figures 30-6 and 30-7).

Several pathways, including the intrinsic (Bcl-2 family, cytochrome c, caspase-9), extrinsic (Fas, FADD, caspase-8), and regulatory (p53 and NF-κB), appear to be activated during ischemic renal tubular cell injury. It has also been shown that the balance between cell survival and cell death depends on the relative concentrations of the proapoptotic members (Bax, Bad, and Bid) and antiapoptotic members (Bcl-2 and Bcl-xL) of the Bcl-2 family of proteins. Overexpression of proapoptotic or relative deficiency of antiapoptotic proteins may lead to formation of mitochondrial pores. Conversely, the inhibition of such pore formation may occur with the opposite imbalance.[124-126]

Other important proteins that have been shown to play a significant role in the apoptotic pathways are NF-κB and p53.[127,128] The central proapoptotic transcription factor p53 can be activated by hypoxia, via hypoxia-inducible factor-1α, as well as by other noxious stimuli such as certain drugs (e.g., cisplatin). The kinase-mediated pathways such as extracellular signal–regulated kinases and c-Jun N-terminal kinases are responsible for mediating cellular responses involved in apoptosis, survival, and repair through their interaction with other signals from growth factors such as hepatocyte growth factor, insulin-like growth factor-1, epidermal growth factor, and vascular endothelial growth factor (VEGF).[129,130] These independent mechanisms can inhibit proapoptotic proteins such as Bad and activate the antiapoptotic transcription of CREB (cyclic adenosine monophosphate response element-binding) factors. More recent data indicate that there is rapid delivery of small interfering RNA (siRNA) to proximal tubule cells in AKI, and targeting siRNA to minimize p53 production leads to a dose-dependent attenuation of apoptotic signaling and kidney function, which suggests potential therapeutic benefit for ischemic and nephrotoxic kidney injury.[131]

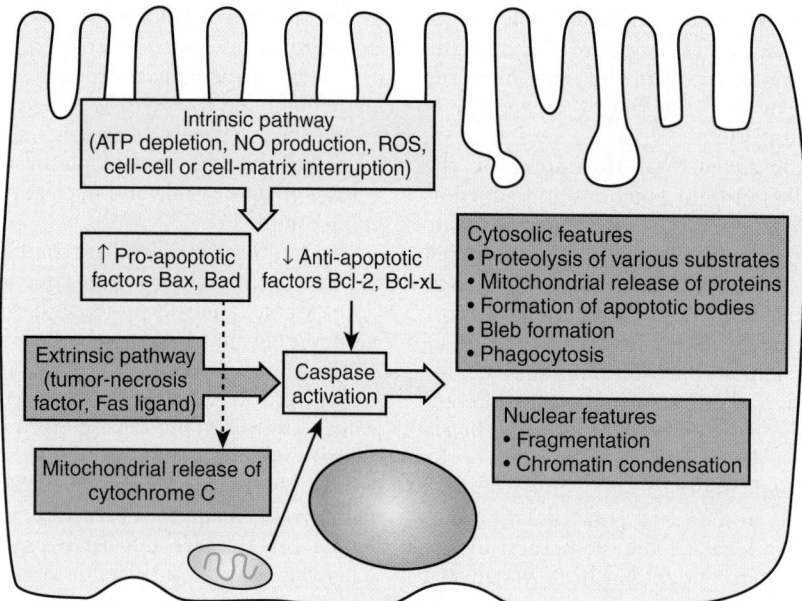

FIGURE 30-6 Overview of apoptosis in epithelial cell injury. The cell injury or intrinsic pathway leads to the translocation of Bax and other proapoptotic proteins from the cytosol to the mitochondria, forming pores and causing the release of cytochrome c. Apoptosis-activating factor (APAF) is activated by cytochrome c, which binds to and activates procaspase-9. Caspase-3 is activated by activated caspase-9, which along with other downstream caspases induces proteolysis of various cytosolic and nuclear proteins. The death receptor or extrinsic pathway functions primarily by the binding of death ligands such as Fas or tumor necrosis factor-α (TNF-α) to their cell surface receptor, which results in the conversion of procaspase-8 to its active form. This occurs through mediation with adaptor proteins such as FADD (Fas-associated protein with death domain) and TRADD (TNF receptor 1–associated death domain). Active caspase-8 activates caspase-3 and also cleaves proapoptotic protein Bid to its truncated form tBid, which acts via Bax to induce cytochrome c from the mitochondria. Hence the extrinsic pathway also amplifies the events induced by the intrinsic pathway. (Adapted from Levine JS, Lieberthal W: Terminal pathways to cell death, in Molitoris BA, Finn WF [editors]: *Acute renal failure: a companion to Brenner & Rector's the kidney,* Philadelphia, 2001, Saunders, p 43; and Sharfuddin A, Molitoris B: Epithelial cell injury, in Vincent JL, Hall JB [editors]: *Encyclopedia of intensive care medicine,* New York, 2012, Springer.)

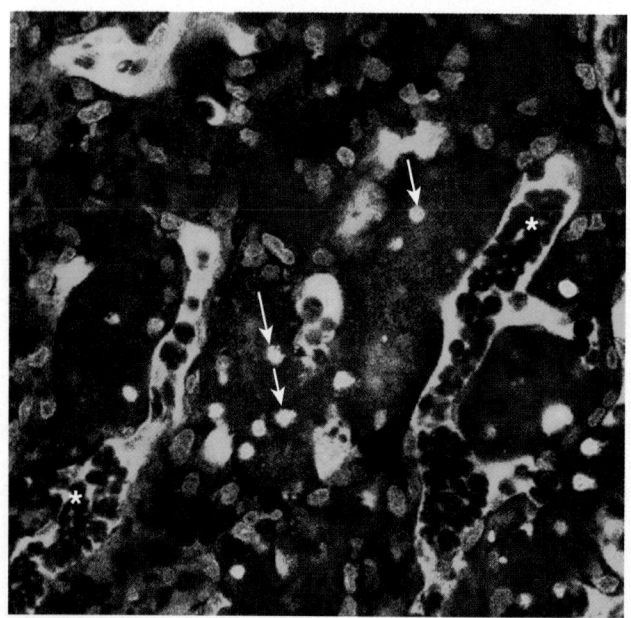

FIGURE 30-7 Live two-photon image of a Sprague-Dawley rat kidney 24 hours after cecal ligation and puncture. Nuclei are labeled *blue* with Hoechst stain. *Green* represents 500-kDa fluorescein isothiocyanate (FITC) dextran, which labels the vasculature. *Red* represents 3-kDa Texas Red dextran, which is filtered and labels the tubular lumens. Note apoptotic nuclei, which show intense Hoechst staining along with condensation and fragmentation (*arrows*). Many of these apoptotic nuclei are shed into the lumens of tubules with compromised urine flow. Also shown are the rouleaux formation and congestion in a peritubular capillary with lack of blood flow (*). (Courtesy of Pierre Dagher, MD, Division of Nephrology, Indiana University School of Medicine.)

Overall, the therapeutic implications of apoptosis in preventing epithelial cell injury are significant considering that various targets are available for blockade or modulation. It is also possible that the window for preventing lethal injury and blocking cells from progressing to necrosis is in the early initiating apoptotic phases. Epithelial cell necrosis, on the other hand, is a passive, non–energy dependent process that occurs secondary to severe ATP depletion from toxic or ischemic insult. It is not dependent on caspase activation, but rather results from a rise in intracellular calcium and the activation of membrane phospholipases.[132,133] Hence morphologically, necrotic cells do not exhibit the nuclear fragmentation or chromatin condensation seen in apoptosis, and neither do they form apoptotic bodies.

Functionally, severe ATP depletion results first in mitochondrial injury, with subsequent arrest of oxidative phosphorylation causing further depletion of energy stores and robust formation of reactive oxygen species that in turn mediate further cellular injury. Second, numerous studies have shown that ATP depletion leads to a rise in intracellular calcium through impairment of calcium ATPases, while inhibition of the Na^+-K^+-ATPase activity potentiates calcium entry into the cell via the sodium–calcium exchanger. Increased cytosolic calcium causes further mitochondrial injury and cytoskeletal alterations.[134] This results in downstream activation of proteases such as calpain and phospholipases. Phospholipases such as phospholipase A_2 cause direct hydrolytic damage to membranes and also release toxic free fatty acids. They also cause release of eicosanoids that have vasoactive and hemokinetic activities, which results in an intense surrounding inflammatory response. Calpain mediates plasma membrane permeability as well as hydrolysis of the cytoskeleton proteins.[135,136] Finally, there is also release of lysosomal enzymes and proteases that degrade histones, which results in accessibility of the endonucleases to the entire segment; this is classically seen as the "smear" pattern on gel electrophoresis, in contrast to the typical "ladder" pattern seen in apoptosis.[137]

PARENCHYMAL INFLAMMATION

Inflammation and recruitment of leukocytes during epithelial injury are now recognized as major mediators of all phases of endothelial and tubular cell injury. Early inflammation is classically characterized by margination of leukocytes to the activated vascular endothelium, via interactions between selectins and ligands that allows firm adhesion, followed by transmigration. A number of potent mediators are generated by the injured proximal epithelial tubular cell, including proinflammatory cytokines such as tumor necrosis factor-α (TNF-α), IL-6, IL-1β, MCP-1, IL-8, transforming growth factor-β, and RANTES (regulated on activation, normal T expressed, and secreted).[138] Toll-like receptor 2 (TLR2) has been shown to be an important mediator of endothelial ischemic injury, whereas TLR4 has been shown to play a similar role in animal models of both ischemic and septic injury,[139] especially in proximal tubular cell.[140]

Neutrophils are the earliest to accumulate in ischemic injury in animal models but are rarely seen in human ATN. Blockade of neutrophil function or neutrophil depletion has been shown to provide only partial protection against injury. Hence other leukocytes also play an important role. These include macrophages, B lymphocytes, and T lymphocytes.[141] Animal experiments employing selective deletion, knockout mice, and specific blockade have shown that all these cells do mediate tubular injury at various phases and that these are synergistic interactions among different cellular types.[142] It is also known that during ischemic injury complement receptor C5a expression is markedly upregulated on proximal tubule epithelial cells as well as interstitial macrophages. C5a is a powerful chemoattractant that recruits these inflammatory cells. Complement cascades are activated during sepsis, and C5a, a potent complement component with procoagulant properties, has been found to be elevated in rodent models of sepsis. Blocking C5a or its receptor has shown some promise in improving survival with sepsis.[143] Whether released from the endothelium or from the epithelial cell, numerous cytokines exert a concerted effort to augment the inflammatory response seen as a result of ischemic or septic injury.[144] Furthermore it has been shown that mouse tubular cells, when stimulated with lipopolysaccharide in culture, upregulate TLR2, TLR3, and TLR4 and secrete chemokines such as CC motif chemokine ligand 2 (CCL2)/MCP-1 and CCL5/RANTES. These data suggest that tubular TLR expression might be involved in mediating interstitial leukocyte infiltration and tubular injury during bacterial sepsis.[145]

TLR2 and TLR4 are constitutively expressed on renal epithelium, and their expression is enhanced after renal ischemia-reperfusion injury. El-Achkar and associates have shown that in the CLP rat model of sepsis, TLR4 expression increases markedly in all tubules (proximal and distal), glomeruli, and the renal vasculature.[146] Furthermore they demonstrated that in sepsis there is a TLR4-dependent increase in expression of the proinflammatory mediator cyclooxygenase-2 that was mostly restricted to cortical and medullary thick ascending loops of Henle, which characteristically express and secrete Tamm-Horsfall protein.[147] Tamm-Horsfall protein may stabilize the outer medulla in the face of injury by decreasing inflammation, possibly through an effect on TLR4.[148] Genetic deletion of either TLR2 or TLR4 protects from renal ischemia-reperfusion injury,[140,149] which indicates the prominent role TLR plays in AKI.

Macrophages produce proinflammatory cytokines that can stimulate the activity of other leukocytes. Okusa's group has shown that depletion of kidney and spleen macrophages using liposomal clodronate before renal ischemia-reperfusion injury prevented AKI, and adoptive transfer of macrophages reconstituted AKI.[150] Dendritic cells are also thought to play an important role in AKI as shown by the work of Dong and colleagues, who demonstrated that after AKI, renal dendritic cells produced the proinflammatory cytokines TNF, IL-6, MCP-1, and RANTES, and that depletion of dendritic cells before ischemia significantly reduced the kidney levels of TNF produced.[151] These studies suggest that both macrophages and dendritic cells play a role in ischemic injury and that additional studies will further determine their effects and exact mechanisms.

Regulatory T (T_reg) cells have also recently been demonstrated to play a role in ischemic AKI. Rabb's group has shown that in a murine model of ischemic AKI there was a significant trafficking of T_reg cells into the kidneys after 3 and 10 days. Postischemic kidneys had increased numbers of T cell receptor β-chain (TCR-β)⁺CD4⁺ and TCR-β⁺CD8⁺ T cells with enhanced proinflammatory cytokine production. They also noted that depletion of T_reg cells starting 1 day after ischemic injury by means of anti-CD25 antibodies increased renal tubular damage, reduced tubular proliferation at days 3 and 10, infiltrating T lymphocyte cytokine production at 3 days, and increased TNF-α generation by TCR-β⁺CD4⁺ T cells at 10 days. In separate mice studies, infusion of CD4⁺CD25⁺ T_reg cells 1 day after initial injury reduced interferon-γ production by TCR-β⁺CD4⁺ T cells at 3 days, improved repair, and reduced cytokine generation at 10 days. These studies demonstrate that T_reg cells infiltrate ischemic-reperfused kidneys during the healing process promoting repair, likely through modulation of proinflammatory cytokine production by other T cell subsets.[152]

Knowledge of the role of T_reg cells has been further extended by Okusa's group, which has shown that partial depletion of T_reg cells with an anti-CD25 monoclonal antibody potentiated kidney damage induced by ischemia-reperfusion injury and that reducing the number of T_reg cells resulted in more neutrophils, macrophages, and innate cytokine transcription in the kidney after the injury.[153] Furthermore, mice deficient in FoxP3 (forkhead box P3)⁺ T_reg cells accumulated a greater number of inflammatory leukocytes after renal ischemia-reperfusion injury than mice containing T_reg cells, and co-transfer of lymph node cells from FoxP3-deficient Scurfy mice and isolated T_reg cells significantly attenuated ischemia-reperfusion–induced renal injury and leukocyte accumulation.[154]

Finally, it has been shown that the anticoagulant function of activated protein C is responsible for suppressing lipopolysaccharide-induced stimulation of the proinflammatory mediators ACE-1, IL-6, and IL-18, which perhaps accounts for its ability to modulate renal hemodynamics and protect against septic AKI.[155] Taken together, these findings show that suppression of inflammation could be a fruitful target in efforts to prevent and/or limit AKI.

INTRACELLULAR MECHANISMS—ROLE OF REACTIVE OXYGEN SPECIES, HEME OXYGENASE, AND HEAT SHOCK PROTEINS

Reactive oxygen species such as the hydroxyl radical (HO^-), peroxynitrite ($ONOO^-$), and hyperchlorous acid (OCl^-) are generated in epithelial cells during ischemic injury by catalytic conversion. These reactive oxygen species can damage cells in a variety of ways, such as by peroxidation of lipids in plasma and intracellular membranes. They can also destabilize the cytoskeletal proteins and integrins required to maintain adhesion of cells to other cells as well as to extracellular matrix. These reactive oxygen species can also have vasoconstrictive effects due to their capacity to scavenge nitric oxide.[156] Much of the earlier discussion has been about proteins or mechanisms that promote injury. However, there are protective mechanisms that allow cells to defend against numerous stresses. The complex heat shock protein (hsp) system is induced to exceptionally high levels during stress conditions. These proteins are believed to facilitate the restoration of normal function by assisting in the refolding of denatured proteins, along with aiding the appropriate folding of newly synthesized proteins. They also help in degradation of irreparable proteins and toxins to limit their accumulation. Thus, their role has been studied, and overexpression before injury has been found to have protective effects.[157-159] The proteins hsp90, hsp72, and hsp25 in particular have been extensively studied (e.g., overexpression of hsp25 has been shown to be protective against actin-cytoskeleton disruption).[160] After in vivo renal ischemia, hsp90 has been shown to be rapidly induced in cytosolic proximal tubular epithelial cells, particularly in the late stages, which leads to the conclusion that hsp90 may be crucial for the disposition of damaged proteins and the assembly of newly formed peptides. In nephrotoxic models, hsp72 has been shown to limit apoptosis through an increase in Bcl-2/Bax ratio, which indicates a role of hsp72 in cell death as well.[160]

The enzyme heme oxygenase 1 (HO-1) has also emerged as a prominent constituent in epithelial cell injury. Numerous observations have shown that the biologic actions of HO-1 include antiinflammatory, vasodilatory, cytoprotective, antiapoptotic, and cellular proliferative effects in the setting of AKI. Its gene is arguably one of the most readily inducible genes responding to numerous stressors including, but not limited to, hypoxia, hyperthermia, oxidative stress, and exposure to lipopolysaccharide. Consequently, induction of HO has been described in various forms of AKI, including ischemic, endotoxin, and nephrotoxic models. A number of studies indicate a protective effect of induction of HO-1 in AKI.[161,162] Prior induction of HO-1 by hemoglobin can reduce endotoxemia-induced renal dysfunction and mortality. Inhibition of HO activity in the intact, disease-free kidney reduces medullary blood flow without exerting any effect on cortical blood flow. Overexpression of HO-1 by hemin results in a significant reduction in cisplatin-induced cytotoxicity.[163] TNF-α–induced apoptosis in endothelial cells is also attenuated by induction of HO-1. These findings have been supported by studies in which mice deficient in HO-1, after glycerol-induced AKI, exhibited marked exacerbation of renal insufficiency and mortality.[164]

The protective mechanisms of HO-1 have been extensively studied by Nath's group, which showed that overexpression of HO-1 in cultured renal epithelial cells induces upregulation of the cell cycle inhibitory protein p21 and confers resistance to apoptosis.[165] Thus the biologic actions of HO-1 that appear particularly relevant to AKI include vasodilatory effects, cytoprotective effects, antiinflammatory actions, antiapoptotic effects, and cellular proliferative effects, which makes it a potentially exploitable expressive enzyme in the prevention and reduction of AKI. Perhaps more importantly, HO-1 might also be of benefit in the repair and regeneration of tubular cells.[78,162] Hence, upregulation or overexpression of HO-1 is an attractive protective strategy and therapeutic target against cellular injury.

REPAIR, REGENERATION, AND ROLE OF STEM CELLS

The renal tubular epithelial cells have the remarkable potential to regenerate functionally and structurally after ischemic or toxic insults. Once the insulting factors have been removed (e.g., reperfusion, cessation of toxic drugs, treatment of sepsis), minimally injured cells repair themselves without going through a dedifferentiated stage. More severely injured cells, however, can undergo this stage, in which they appear morphologically as flattened cells with an ill-defined brush border. Essentially, there is proliferation of the viable cells, which spread across the denuded basement membrane, after which they regain their differential character by converting back into normal tubular epithelial cells.

Functionally, there is reassembly of the cytoskeletal structure once ATP repletion occurs. It has been shown that the apical microvilli can be restored by as early as 24 hours after ATP depletion following mild injury. Similarly, Na^+-K^+-ATPase is lost from the apical location and relocates to the basolateral membranes within 24 hours. Finally, although lipid polarity is eventually reestablished, its restoration can lag behind reestablishment of protein polarity and is completed by about 10 days after injury.[166,167]

Growth factors and signals from injured cells are crucial at this stage to promote timely and appropriate regeneration of the viable cells. In animal models, administration of exogenous growth factors has been shown to accelerate renal recovery from injury. These include epidermal growth factor, insulin-like growth factor-1, α-melanocyte–stimulating hormone, erythropoietin, hepatocyte growth factor, and bone morphogenic protein 7.[168-172] These effects have not yet been validated in human clinical trials investigating ATN.[173,174] They all likely increase GFR through direct hemodynamic effects and hasten tubular epithelial cell recovery.

More recently, there has been major interest in studying the roles of progenitor/stem cells and mesenchymal stem cells in tubular epithelial cell injury. Investigators have now shown that different types of stems cells may reside in the renal architecture. In the human kidney, CD133+ progenitor/stem cells with regenerative potential have been identified.[175] These cells were able to differentiate in vitro toward renal epithelium and endothelium. When injected into mice with glycerol-induced AKI, they enhanced recovery from tubular damage, possibly by integrating into the proximal and distal tubules.[176] Mesenchymal stem cells are also present in the kidney and may have been derived from the embryonic tissue or bone marrow. Bone marrow cells are known to migrate to the kidney and participate in normal tubular epithelial cell turnover and repair after AKI.[177] Evidence of the kidney engraftment capacity of cells derived from male bone marrow is based on the presence of cells positive for the Y chromosome with epithelial cell markers in the tubules of kidneys of female recipient mice.[178,179] Although the data are not yet conclusive, there is early evidence that stem cells as well as bone marrow–derived mesenchymal stem cells may contribute to structural and functional renal repair.

Westenfelder and colleagues have demonstrated in a series of experiments the role of mesenchymal stem cells in AKI. They have shown that infusion of mesenchymal stem cells enhances recovery of kidney function, and the cells were found to be located in the kidney cortex after injection, as demonstrated by magnetic resonance imaging. Mesenchymal stem cell–treated animals had both significantly better kidney function on days 2 and 3 and better injury scores at day 3 after AKI. Histologically, mesenchymal stem cells were predominantly located in glomerular capillaries, whereas tubules showed no iron labeling, which indicates absent tubular transdifferentiation.[180] This group has also shown that knockdown of vascular endothelial growth factor by siRNA reduced effectiveness of mesenchymal stem cells in the treatment of ischemic AKI in a rat model. Animals treated with mesenchymal stem cells had increased renal microvessel density compared with VEGF knockdown mesenchymal stem cell–treated and vehicle-treated animals. These results show that VEGF is an important mediator of the early and late phase of renoprotective action after AKI in the context of stem cell treatment.[181] Using genetic fate–mapping techniques in chimeric mice undergoing ischemic AKI, Bonventre's group has shown that the predominant mechanism of tubular repair is regeneration of surviving epithelial cells rather than actual engraftment of bone marrow stem cells.[182,183]

Although the protective mechanisms of stem cells have not yet been completely elucidated, they have been postulated to relate less to direct differentiation of stem cells into renal epithelial cells and more to paracrine effects such as supplying growth factors that stimulate the regeneration of tubular and resident stem cells. The "renotropism" exhibited by these cells may have a huge impact on therapeutic options in the future once their roles have been more fully defined.[184]

Endothelial Dysfunction

Endothelial cells control vascular tone, regulation of blood flow to local tissue beds, modulation of coagulation and inflammation, and lastly permeability. Both ischemia and sepsis have profound effects on the endothelium. The renal vasculature and endothelium are particularly sensitive to these insults. When such an insult occurs, the endothelial bed becomes ineffective in performing its function, and the ensuing vascular dysregulation leads to continued ischemic conditions and further injury following the initial insult. As noted earlier, this is termed the *extension phase* of AKI.[103] Histopathologically this is seen as vascular congestion, edema formation, diminished microvascular blood flow, and margination and adherence of inflammatory cells to endothelial cells.

Vascular Tone

Conger and associates were among the first to demonstrate that postischemic rat kidneys manifest vasoconstriction in response to decreased renal perfusion pressure and hence cannot autoregulate blood flow, even when total renal blood flow has returned to baseline values up to 1 week after injury.[185,186] Goligorsky and his group have extensively studied this increased constrictor response and found that it could be blocked by Ca^{2+} antagonists. They also demonstrated that the phenomenon loss of normal endothelial nitric oxide synthase

(NOS) function was due to a loss of vasodilator responses to acetylcholine and bradykinin. Selective inhibition, depletion, and deletion of inducible NOS (iNOS) have clearly shown renoprotective effects during ischemia.[187,188] Although it is still unclear, nitric oxide production from the endothelium (eNOS) may be impaired at the level of enzyme activity or modified by reactive oxygen species to impair normal vasodilatory activity.[189] Hence overall, in ischemic AKI, *there is an imbalance of eNOS and iNOS.* Thus it is also proposed that because of a relative decrease in eNOS, secondary to endothelial dysfunction and damage, there is a loss of antithrombogenic properties of the endothelium, which leads to increased susceptibility to microvascular thrombosis.[190]

Administration of L-arginine, nitric oxide–donor molsidomine, or the eNOS cofactor tetrahydrobiopterin can preserve medullary perfusion and attenuate AKI induced by ischemia-reperfusion; conversely, the administration of N^{ω}-nitro-L-arginine methyl ester, a nitric oxide blocker, has been reported to aggravate the course of AKI following ischemia-reperfusion injury. Although these pharmacologic studies are clearly important, the contribution of eNOS impairment in the overall course of reduced renal function after ischemia-reperfusion continues to be assessed.[191,192]

Cytoskeleton

The cytoskeletal structure of endothelial cells includes actin filament bundles that form a supportive ring around the periphery, along with the adhesion complexes that provide the integrity of the endothelial layer. The assembly and disassembly of actin filaments is regulated by a large family of actin-binding proteins, including ADF/cofilin. With ischemic injury, the normal architecture of the actin cytoskeleton is markedly changed along with endothelial cell swelling, impaired cell-cell and cell-substrate adhesion, and loss of tight junction barrier functions. ATP depletion in cultured endothelial cells has been shown to induce dephosphorylation and activation of ADF/cofilin in a direct and concentration-dependant fashion. This results in depolymerized and severed actin filaments, seen as filamentous (F) actin aggregates at the basolateral aspects of the cell.[193]

Recent studies also show a role for the sphingosine-1 phosphate receptor (S1PR) in maintaining structural integrity after AKI. Okusa's laboratory has shown that S1PRs in the proximal tubule are necessary for stress-induced cell survival, and S1PR type 1 agonists are renoprotective via direct effects on tubular cells.[194]

Permeability

The endothelial barrier serves to separate the inner space of the blood vessel from the surrounding tissue and to control the exchange of cells and fluids between the two. It is defined by a combination of transcellular and paracellular pathways, the latter being a major contributor to inflammation-induced barrier dysfunction.

Sutton and colleagues have studied the role of endothelial cells in AKI in a series of experiments utilizing florescent dextrans and two-photon intravital imaging. The increased microvascular permeability observed in AKI is likely a combination of numerous factors, such as loss of endothelial monolayer, breakdown of perivascular matrix, alterations of endothelial cell contacts, and upregulated leukocyte-endothelial interactions. They have shown that 24 hours after ischemic injury there was loss of localization in vascular endothelial cadherin immunostaining, which suggests severe alterations in the integrity of the adherens junctions of the renal microvasculature.[195] In vivo two-photon imaging demonstrated a loss of capillary barrier function within 2 hours of reperfusion as evidenced by the leakiness of high-molecular-weight dextrans (>300,000 Da) into the interstitial space.

Critical constituents of the perivascular matrix, including collagen IV, are known to be substrates of matrix metalloproteinase 2 (MMP-2) and MMP-9, which are collectively known as *gelatinases*. Breakdown of barrier function may also be due to MMP-2 or MMP-9 activation, and this upregulation is temporally correlated with an increase in microvascular permeability.[103,196] In addition, minocycline, a broad-based MMP inhibitor, and the gelatinase-specific inhibitor ABT-518 both ameliorated the increase in microvascular permeability in this model. Taken together, many findings indicate that the loss of endothelial cells following ischemic injury is not a major contributor to altered microvascular permeability, although renal microvascular endothelial cells are vulnerable to the initiation of apoptotic mechanisms after ischemic injury that can ultimately impact microvascular density[197] (Figure 30-8).

COAGULATION

The endothelial cell plays a central role in coagulation via its interaction with protein C through the endothelial cell protein C receptor (EPCR) and thrombomodulin. The protein C pathway helps to maintain normal homeostasis and limits inflammatory responses. Protein C is activated by thrombin-mediated cleavage, and the rate of this reaction is further augmented 1000-fold when thrombin binds to the endothelial cell surface receptor protein thrombomodulin. The activation rate of protein C is further increased by approximately 10-fold when EPCR binds protein C and presents it to the thrombin-thrombomodulin complex. Activated protein C essentially then has antithrombotic actions, shows profibrinolytic properties, and participates in numerous antiinflammatory and cytoprotective pathways to restore normal homeostasis.[198] It has also been shown to be an agonist of protease-activated receptor 1.[199] Based on these properties, the endothelial cell plays an absolutely essential and critical role in maintaining a normal and healthy vasculature and endothelial bed. During an inflammatory response, many of the natural anticoagulants, including protein C, are consumed along with downregulation of EPCR and thrombomodulin expression, which decreases the anticoagulant and antiinflammatory effects of the protein C pathway. Damaged endothelial cells undergo apoptosis, and this further contributes to amplifying the coagulation cascade, because the disrupted endothelium provides a procoagulant surface.[200] Activation of inflammation and coagulation pathways continues to proceed without effective counterregulatory mechanisms, which leads to enhanced microvascular coagulation and endothelial cell dysfunction. Ultimately, microvascular function is compromised, which results in disseminated

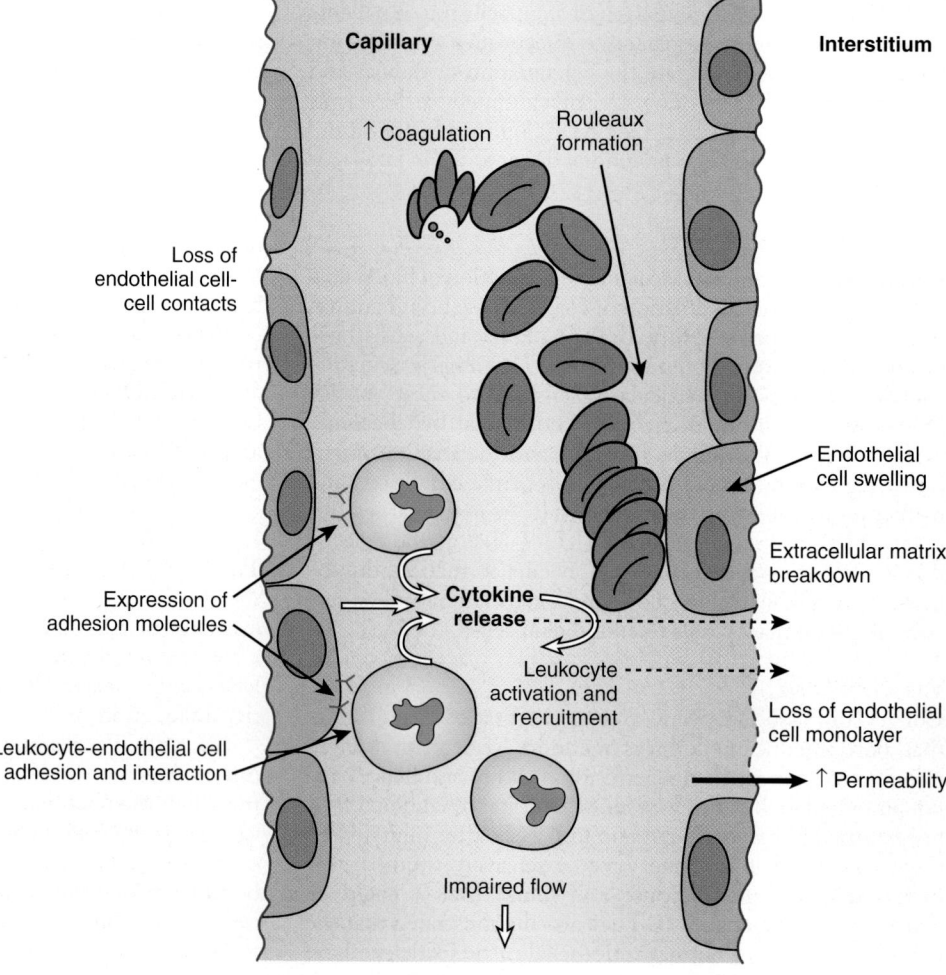

FIGURE 30-8 Key events in endothelial cell activation and injury. Ischemia causes upregulation and expression of genes coding for various cell surface proteins such as E (endothelial)–selectin and P (platelet)–selectin, vascular cell adhesion molecule-1 (VCAM-1), intercellular adhesion molecule-1 (ICAM-1), and reduced thrombomodulin (TM). Activated leukocytes adhere to endothelial cells through these adhesion molecules. Endothelial injury increases the production of endothelin-1 and decreases endothelial-derived nitric oxide synthase (eNOS), which induces vasoconstriction and platelet aggregation. The combination of leukocyte adhesion and activation, platelet aggregation, and endothelial injury serves as the platform for vascular congestion of the medullary microvasculature. There are permeability defects between endothelial cells as a result of alterations in tight junctions and adherens junctions. (From Sharfuddin A, Molitoris B: Epithelial cell injury, in Vincent JL, Hall JB [editors]: *Encyclopedia of intensive care medicine*, New York, 2012, Springer.)

intravascular coagulation and microvascular thrombosis, decreased tissue perfusion, and hypoxemia, leading to organ dysfunction and failure. It has been shown that both pretreatment and postinjury treatment with soluble thrombomodulin attenuate renal injury, minimizing vascular permeability defects and improving capillary renal blood flow.[95]

The leukocytes as well as the endothelial cells are dynamically involved in the process of adherence of leukocytes to the vascular endothelium. Leukocyte activation and leukocyte release of cytokines require signals through chemokines circulating in the bloodstream or through direct contact with the endothelium. Rolling leukocytes can be activated by chemoattractants such as complement C5a and platelet-activating factor. Once activated, leukocyte integrins bind to endothelial ligands to promote firm adhesion. β2 Integrin (CD18) seems to be most important for neutrophil adherence. These interactions with the endothelium are mediated through endothelial adhesion molecules that are upregulated under ischemic conditions.[201]

The initial phase starts with slow neutrophil migration mediated by tethering interactions between selectins and their endothelial cell ligands. Singbartl and Ley found that platelet P-selectin and not endothelial P-selectin was the main determinant in neutrophil-mediated ischemic renal injury.[201] Significant protection from both ischemic injury and mortality is also afforded by blockade of the shared ligand to all three selectins (E-selectin, P-selectin, and L-selectin), which seems to be dependent on the presence of a key fucosyl sugar on the selectin ligand.[202,203] In a CLP model of septic azotemia, mice gene-deficient for E-selectin or P-selectin or both were completely protected. Furthermore, selectin-deficient mice demonstrated similar intraperitoneal leukocyte recruitment but altered cytokine levels compared with wild-type mice.[204] Therefore, it is possible that selectins exert their effects through modulation of systemic cytokine profiles rather than through engagement in leukocyte–endothelial cell interactions.[205]

INFLAMMATION

Altered endothelial cell function also mediates inflammation, a hallmark of ischemic injury that has been the subject of numerous recent studies. Ischemia induces the increased expression of a number of leukocyte adhesion molecules such as P-selectin, E-selectin, intercellular adhesion molecule (ICAM), and B7-1. It has been shown that strategies to pharmacologically block or genetically ablate the expression of these molecules are protective against ischemic or septic AKI.[206] Investigators have also shown that T cells play a major role in vascular permeability during ischemic injury. Gene microarray analysis showed that production of TNF-α and interferon-γ protein was increased in CD3 and CD4 T cells from the blood and kidney after ischemia. Furthermore, it has also been demonstrated that in CD3, CD4, and CD8 T cell–deficient mice, there is a significantly attenuated rise in renal vascular permeability after ischemic injury. Hence T cells directly contribute to the increased vascular permeability, potentially through T cell cytokine production.[207,208] Another feature noted during inflammation and endothelial cell injury is the phenomenon of erythrocyte trapping with rouleaux formation, which prolongs the reduction in renal blood flow and exacerbates tubular injury.[209]

LONG-TERM EFFECTS OF ENDOTHELIAL CELL INJURY

Recent evidence demonstrates that acute injury to endothelial cells may have long-term implications, as shown in a series of publications by Basile and colleagues in which the investigators found significant reduction in blood vessel density following ischemic injury, which led to the phenomenon of vascular dropout.[210] Vascular dropout was verified by Sutton and his group, who found that vascular density had dropped by almost 45% at 4 weeks after an ischemic insult.[197] This suggests that, unlike the renal epithelial tubular cells, the renal vascular system lacks regenerative potential. It is not clear yet whether apoptosis and/or necrosis play a major role in endothelial cell dropout. Ischemia has been shown to inhibit the angiogenic protein VEGF while inducing ADAMTS1 (a disintegrin-like and metalloproteinase with thrombospondin type 1 repeats 1), thought to be a VEGF inhibitor.[211] It was then postulated that the lack of vascular repair could be due to lack of VEGF, as shown by experiments in which administration of VEGF-121 preserved the microvascular density.[212] Reduction of the microvasculature density increases hypoxia-mediated fibrosis and alters the usual hemodynamics, which may lead to hypertension. Thus, loss of microvasculature density and its consequent effects may play a critical role in the progression of CKD after initial recovery from ischemia-reperfusion–induced AKI.[210]

TARGETS OF THERAPY—ROLE OF ENDOTHELIAL PROGENITOR CELLS

Due to the numerous mechanisms involved in initiating endothelial cell injury as well as continuing existing injury, several targets are available to reduce the effect of endothelial cell injury as well as potentially to minimize actual endothelial cell damage itself. The concept of restoration of vascular supply to damaged or ischemic organs to accelerate their regeneration is well established. One therapeutic strategy based on this concept is the delivery of angiogenic factors. The current view is that endothelial progenitor cells are a heterogeneous group, which by latest count originate from hematopoietic stem cells or their angioblastic subpopulation and mesenchymal stem cells. In the bone marrow these cells are characterized by the combination of surface markers such as CD34, VEGF receptor 2 (Flk-1), and an early marker CD133; moreover, in the blood they may express markers of hematopoietic stem cells, c-kit, and Sca-1. Upon further differentiation, these cells lose CD133 and acquire vascular endothelial cadherin and von Willebrand factor.[213]

There is a growing body of evidence that endothelial progenitor cells may improve vascular regeneration in different ischemic organs. Recent data also suggest that endothelial progenitor cells are mobilized after acute ischemic injury and are recruited in the ischemic kidney, where they can ameliorate AKI through both paracrine effects and repair of the injured renal microvasculature.[214] Transplanting intact endothelial cells into injured ischemic vasculature has also shown promise in reducing ischemic injury. Although the underlying mechanisms are not fully understood, replacements for damaged cells are mainly generated by neighboring cells or cells recruited from the circulation.[214]

In summary, the endothelial cell is now recognized as a major contributor to the initiation and extension of AKI, and targeting the mechanisms that can block these dysfunctional intracellular processes may be of key therapeutic value in the field of intensive care medicine (see Figure 30-8).

Some authors consider AKI a systemic event that can potentially cause alterations in other organs of the body. Kelly has demonstrated the effects of renal ischemia on cardiac tissues.[92] Induction of IL-1, TNF-α, and ICAM-1 messenger RNA was seen in cardiac tissues as early as 6 hours after renal ischemic injury, and levels remained elevated up to 48 hours following renal ischemic injury. There was also a significant increase in myeloperoxidase activity in the heart and liver, apart from the kidneys. The increase in cardiac myeloperoxidase activity could be prevented by administration of anti–ICAM-1 antibody at the time of renal ischemia. At 48 hours, cardiac function evaluation by echocardiography also revealed increases in left ventricular end-systolic and diastolic diameter and decreased fractional shortening. As little as 15 minutes of ischemia also resulted in significantly more apoptosis in cardiac tissue.[92] Rabb and associates have shown that renal ischemic injury leads to an increase in pulmonary vascular permeability defects that are mediated by macrophages.[215] Furthermore, they showed that there was downregulation of lung epithelial Na channel, Na⁺-K⁺-ATPase, and aquaporin-5 expression in a rat model of bilateral renal ischemic injury or nephrectomy, but not in unilateral ischemic models, which suggests a role for uremic toxins in modulating these effects in the lung.[216] Finally, Rabb's laboratory has also shown an effect of AKI on functional changes in the brain. Mice with AKI had increased neuronal pyknosis and microgliosis in the brain, with increased levels of the proinflammatory chemokines keratinocyte-derived chemoattractant and granulocyte colony-stimulating factor in the cerebral cortex and hippocampus, and increased expression of glial fibrillary acidic protein in astrocytes in the cortex and corpus callosum. In addition, extravasation of Evans blue dye into the brain suggested that the blood-brain barrier was disrupted in mice with AKI.[217]

Conversely, other organs also regulate ischemic renal injury. Slutsky and his group have demonstrated the role of lung injury in inducing renal damage. They found that in rabbits, injurious lung ventilatory strategies (high tidal volume and low peak end-expiratory pressure) alone were sufficient to induce renal epithelial cell apoptosis. This was further substantiated by the fact that plasma obtained from rabbits that underwent the injurious ventilation strategy induced greater apoptosis in cultured LLC-RK₁ cells (a rabbit kidney epithelial cell line) in vitro, which suggests that circulating soluble factors associated with the injurious mechanical ventilation might be involved in this process.[218]

Another example of regulation of ischemic AKI by extrarenal organs is the effect of brain death on renal transplants. Traumatic brain injury elicits a cytokine and inflammatory response. These cytokines lead to renal inflammation in renal transplants from brain-dead donors that does not occur in transplants from living donors.[219] The absence of such inflammation may contribute to the success of renal transplants from living unrelated donors compared with cadaveric transplants that are better immunologic matches.[220] Since AKI is associated with a high mortality and morbidity, these studies indicate that multiorgan crosstalk that occurs in the setting of AKI is a major and likely contributor to nonrenal organ dysfunction that may mediate clinically observable effects such as cardiac, pulmonary, and central nervous system events.

Evaluation of Acute Kidney Injury

In addition to a comprehensive review of previous medical records, the assessment of patients with AKI requires a meticulous history taking and physical examination; evaluation of urinary findings, including the urinary sediment; review of laboratory test results; renal imaging; and, when appropriate, renal biopsy.[221] Analysis of serum creatinine concentration over time is invaluable for differentiating acute from chronic kidney disease and identifying the timing of events that precipitated the acute decline in kidney function. An acute process is easily established if review of laboratory records reveals a sudden rise in blood urea nitrogen (BUN) and serum creatinine concentrations from previously stable baseline values. Spurious causes of elevated BUN and serum creatinine levels should be excluded before a diagnosis of AKI is made. When prior BUN and serum creatinine measurements are not available, key findings that indicate a chronic process include physical manifestations of hyperparathyroidism (resorption of distal phalangeal tufts or the lateral aspect of clavicles), band keratopathy, half-and-half nails, and small echogenic kidneys on radiographic imaging. Enlarged kidneys do not necessarily rule out a chronic cause for renal impairment, because diabetic nephropathy, human immunodeficiency virus–associated nephropathy, amyloidosis, and polycystic kidney disease are characterized by increased kidney size even with moderate to advanced CKD. Anemia is a less useful differentiating feature because it can complicate both AKI and CKD. Once the presence of AKI has been confirmed, attention should focus on patient, urine, laboratory, and radiographic assessments to help differentiate among prerenal, intrinsic, and postrenal processes in order to identify the cause of AKI and guide treatment.

Clinical Assessment of the Patient

Prerenal AKI should be suspected in clinical settings associated with intravascular volume depletion, including hemorrhage and excessive gastrointestinal (e.g., vomiting or diarrhea), urinary, or insensible fluid losses as well as severe burns, or with effective intravascular volume depletion due to congestive heart failure, liver disease, or nephrotic syndrome (Table 30-8). The risk of intravascular volume depletion is increased in comatose, sedated, or obtunded patients and in patients with restricted access to salt and water. Clinical clues to a prerenal cause of AKI in the history include a patient report of excessive thirst, orthostatic lightheadedness or dizziness, significant diarrhea and/or vomiting, diuretic use, and recent use of medications that alter intrarenal hemodynamics, including NSAIDs, ACE inhibitors, and/or angiotensin receptor blockers. Findings suggestive of volume depletion on physical examination may include orthostatic hypotension (postural drop in diastolic blood pressure of >10 mm Hg) and tachycardia (postural increase in heart rate of >10 beats/min), reduced jugular venous pressure, diminished skin turgor, dry mucous membranes, and the absence of axillary sweat. However, overt signs and symptoms of hypovolemia are usually not manifest until extracellular fluid volume has fallen by more than 10% to 20%. In addition, in patients with heart failure or liver disease, renal hypoperfusion may occur despite total body volume overload. Findings on physical examination

TABLE 30-8 Useful Clinical Features, Urinary Findings, and Confirmatory Tests in the Differential Diagnosis of Acute Kidney Injury (AKI)

CAUSE OF AKI	SOME SUGGESTIVE CLINICAL FEATURES	TYPICAL URINALYSIS RESULTS	SOME CONFIRMATORY TESTS/FINDINGS
Prerenal Azotemia	Evidence of true volume depletion (thirst, postural or absolute hypotension and tachycardia, low jugular venous pressure, dry mucous membranes and axillae, weight loss, fluid output greater than input) or decreased effective circulatory volume (e.g., heart failure, liver failure), treatment with NSAID, diuretic, or ACE inhibitor/ARB	Hyaline casts $FE_{Na} < 1\%$ $U_{Na} < 10$ mEq/L $SG > 1.018$	Occasionally requires invasive hemodynamic monitoring Rapid resolution of AKI with restoration of renal perfusion
Diseases Involving Large Renal Vessels			
Renal artery thrombosis	History of atrial fibrillation or recent myocardial infarction, nausea, vomiting, flank or abdominal pain	Mild proteinuria, occasionally RBCs	Elevated LDH with normal transaminase levels Renal arteriogram, MAG3 renal scan, MRA[*]
Atheroembolism	Usually age >50 yr, recent manipulation of aorta, retinal plaques, subcutaneous nodules, palpable purpura, livedo reticularis	Often normal, eosinophiluria, rarely casts	Eosinophilia, hypocomplementemia Skin biopsy, renal biopsy
Renal vein thrombosis	Evidence of nephrotic syndrome or pulmonary embolism, flank pain	Proteinuria, hematuria	Inferior venacavogram, Doppler flow studies, MRV[*]
Diseases of Small Renal Vessels and Glomeruli			
Glomerulonephritis or vasculitis	Compatible clinical history (e.g., recent infection), sinusitis, lung hemorrhage, rash or skin ulcers, arthralgias, hypertension, edema	RBC or granular casts, RBCs, WBCs, proteinuria	Low complement levels; positive antineutrophil cytoplasmic antibodies, antiglomerular basement membrane antibodies, anti–streptolysin O antibodies, antideoxyribonuclease, cryoglobulins Renal biopsy
HUS/TTP	Compatible clinical history (e.g., recent gastrointestinal infection, treatment with cyclosporine or anovulants), pallor, ecchymoses, neurologic findings	May be normal, RBCs, mild proteinuria, rarely RBC or granular casts	Anemia, thrombocytopenia, schistocytes on peripheral blood smear, low haptoglobin level, increased LDH Renal biopsy
Malignant hypertension	Severe hypertension with headaches, cardiac failure, retinopathy, neurologic dysfunction, papilledema	May be normal, RBCs, mild proteinuria, rarely RBC casts	LVH by echocardiography or electrocardiography, resolution of AKI with blood pressure control
Ischemic or Nephrotoxic Acute Tubular Necrosis			
Ischemia	Recent hemorrhage; hypotension; surgery, often in combination with vasoactive medication (e.g., ACE inhibitor, NSAID)	Muddy brown granular or tubular epithelial cell casts $FE_{Na} > 1\%$, $U_{Na} > 20$ mEq/L $SG \sim 1.010$	Clinical assessment and urinalysis usually inform diagnosis
Exogenous toxin	Recent procedure requiring contrast agent; nephrotoxic medications; certain chemotherapeutic agents often with coexistent volume depletion; sepsis or chronic kidney disease	Muddy brown granular or tubular epithelial cell cases $FE_{Na} > 1\%$, $U_{Na} > 20$ mEq/L $SG \sim 1.010$	Clinical assessment and urinalysis usually inform diagnosis
Endogenous toxin	History suggestive of rhabdomyolysis (coma, seizures, drug abuse, trauma)	Urine supernatant tests positive for heme in absence of RBCs	Hyperkalemia, hyperphosphatemia, hypocalcemia, increased creatine kinase, myoglobin
	History suggestive of hemolysis (recent blood transfusion)	Urine supernatant pink and tests positive for heme in absence of RBCs	Hyperkalemia, hyperphosphatemia, hypocalcemia, hyperuricemia, and free circulating hemoglobin
	History suggestive of tumor lysis (recent chemotherapy), myeloma (bone pain), or ethylene glycol ingestion	Urate crystals (tumor lysis), dipstick test negative for proteinuria (myeloma), oxalate crystals (ethylene glycol)	Hyperuricemia, hyperkalemia, hyperphosphatemia (tumor lysis); circulating or urinary monoclonal protein (myeloma); toxicology screen, acidosis, osmolal gap (ethylene glycol)
Diseases of the Tubulointerstitium			
Allergic interstitial nephritis	Recent ingestion of drug and fever, rash, loin pain, or arthralgia	WBC casts, WBCs (frequently eosinophiluria), RBCs, rarely RBC casts, proteinuria (occasionally nephritic)	Systemic eosinophilia, renal biopsy
Acute bilateral pyelonephritis	Fever, flank pain and tenderness, toxic state	Leukocytes, occasionally WBCs, RBCs, bacteria	Urine and blood cultures
Postrenal AKI	Abdominal and flank pain, palpable bladder	Frequently normal, hematuria if stones, prostatic hypertrophy	Plain abdominal radiography, renal ultrasonography, postvoid residual bladder volume, computed tomography, retrograde or antegrade pyelography

[*]Contrast medium–enhanced MRA and MRV should be used with extreme caution in patients with AKI.

ACE, Angiotensin converting enzyme; *ARB,* angiotensin receptor blocker; FE_{Na}, fractional excretion of sodium; *HUS,* hemolytic uremic syndrome; *LDH,* lactate dehydrogenase; *LVH,* left ventricular hypertrophy; *MAG3,* mercaptoacetyltriglycine; *MRA,* magnetic resonance angiography; *MRV,* magnetic resonance venography; *NSAID,* nonsteroidal antiinflammatory drug; *RBC,* red blood cell; *SG,* specific gravity; *TTP,* thrombotic thrombocytopenic purpura; U_{Na}, urine sodium concentration; *WBC,* white blood cell.

of peripheral edema, pulmonary vascular congestion, pleural effusion, cardiomegaly, gallop rhythms, elevated jugular venous pressure, or hepatic congestion may point to a state of reduced cardiac output. The presence of acute or chronic liver disease is suggested by evidence of icterus, ascites, splenomegaly, palmar erythema, telangiectasia, and caput medusa. In select critically ill patients, invasive hemodynamic monitoring using central venous or pulmonary artery catheters may assist in assessing intravascular volume status. Definitive diagnosis of prerenal AKI is usually based on prompt resolution of AKI after restoration of renal perfusion. In patients with underlying systolic heart failure, restoration of renal perfusion may be difficult and may require the use of inotropic support.

There is a high likelihood of ischemic ATN if AKI follows a period of severe renal hypoperfusion and the impairment in kidney function persists or worsens despite restoration of renal perfusion. It should be noted, however, that significant hypotension is evident in fewer than 50% of patients with postsurgical ATN. The diagnosis of nephrotoxic ATN requires a comprehensive review of all clinical, pharmacy, nursing, radiographic, and procedural notes for evidence of administration of nephrotoxic agents. Pigment-induced ATN may be suspected if the clinical assessment reveals risk factors for rhabdomyolysis (e.g., seizures, excessive exercise, alcohol or drug abuse, treatment with statins, prolonged immobilization, limb ischemia, crush injury) or hemolysis, as well as selected signs and symptoms of the former (e.g., muscle tenderness, weakness, evidence of trauma, or prolonged immobilization).[222-225]

Although most AKI is prerenal or ischemic or nephrotoxic ATN, patients should be carefully evaluated for other intrinsic renal parenchymal processes, because their management and prognosis may differ substantially. Flank pain may be a prominent symptom of acute renal artery or renal vein occlusion, acute pyelonephritis, and rarely necrotizing glomerulonephritis.[226-228] Interstitial edema leading to distension of the renal capsule and flank pain may be seen in up to one third of patients with acute interstitial nephritis.[229] Dermatologic examination is also important, because a maculopapular rash may accompany allergic interstitial nephritis; subcutaneous nodules, livedo reticularis, digital ischemia, and palpable purpura may suggest atheroembolism or vasculitis; a malar butterfly rash may be associated with systemic lupus erythematosus; and impetigo or needle tracks from intravenous drug use may underlie infection-associated glomerulonephritis.

Ophthalmologic examination is useful to assess for signs of atheroembolism; hypertensive or diabetic retinopathy; the keratitis, uveitis, and iritis of autoimmune vasculitides; icterus; and the rare but nevertheless pathognomonic band keratopathy of hypercalcemia and flecked retina of hyperoxalemia. Uveitis may also be an indicator of coexistent allergic interstitial nephritis, sarcoidosis, and tubulointerstitial nephritis and uveitis syndrome.[230] Examination of the ears, nose and throat may reveal conductive deafness and mucosal inflammation or ulceration suggestive of necrotizing granulomatous vasculitis or neural deafness caused by aminoglycoside toxicity.

Respiratory failure, particularly if associated with hemoptysis, suggests the presence of a pulmonary-renal syndrome, and the stigmata of chronic liver disease suggest the possibility of hepatorenal syndrome. Cardiovascular assessment may reveal marked elevation in systemic blood pressure suggesting malignant hypertension or scleroderma, or demonstrate a new arrhythmia or murmur suggesting a potential source of

thromboemboli or subacute bacterial endocarditis (acute glomerulonephritis), respectively. Chest or abdominal pain and reduced pulses in the lower limbs suggest aortic dissection or, rarely, Takayasu's arteritis. Abdominal pain and nausea are frequent clinical correlates of atheroembolic disease, commonly in patients who have recently undergone angiographic evaluation, particularly in the presence of widespread atheromatous disease. A tensely distended abdomen may indicate the presence of abdominal compartment syndrome. Pallor and recent bruising are important clues to the thrombotic microangiopathies, and the combination of bleeding and fever should raise the possibility of AKI resulting from viral hemorrhagic fever. A recent jejunoileal bypass may be a vital clue to oxalosis, a rare but reversible cause of AKI following bariatric surgery.[231] Hyperreflexia and asterixis often portend the development of uremic encephalopathy or may, in the presence of focal neurologic signs, suggest a diagnosis of thrombotic microangiopathy (i.e., HUS or TTP; see Chapter 34).

Postrenal AKI may be asymptomatic if obstruction of urine drainage develops gradually. Although anuria will be seen in complete obstruction, urine volume may be normal or even increased in the setting of partial obstruction. A pattern of fluctuating urine output may also be seen in some patients with partial obstruction. Suprapubic or flank pain may be the presenting complaint if there is acute distention of the bladder or renal collecting system and capsule, respectively. Colicky flank pain radiating to the groin suggests acute ureteral obstruction, most commonly from renal stone disease. Prostatic disease should be suspected in older men with a history of nocturia; urinary frequency, urgency, or hesitancy; and an enlarged prostate on rectal examination. Urinary retention may be exacerbated acutely in such patients by medications with anticholinergic properties, such as antihistamine agents and antidepressants. Rectal or pelvic examination may reveal obstructing tumors in female patients. Neurogenic bladder is a likely diagnosis in patients with spinal cord injury or autonomic insufficiency, and should be suspected in patients with long-standing diabetes mellitus. Bladder distension may be evident on abdominal percussion and palpation in patients with bladder neck or urethral obstruction. Definitive diagnosis of postrenal AKI usually relies on examination of the postvoid bladder volume and radiographic evaluation of the upper urinary tract, and is confirmed by improvement in renal function following relief of the obstruction.

Urine Assessment

Urine volume is a relatively unhelpful parameter in differentiating the various forms and causes of AKI. Anuria can be seen with complete urinary tract obstruction, but can also occur with severe prerenal or intrinsic renal disease (e.g., renal artery occlusion, severe proliferative glomerulonephritis or vasculitis, bilateral cortical necrosis). Wide fluctuation in urine output may be suggestive of intermittent obstruction. Patients with partial urinary tract obstruction may have polyuria caused by secondary impairment of urinary concentrating mechanisms.

Assessment of the urine is essential in patients with AKI and is an inexpensive and useful diagnostic tool.[232] The initial step is examination of the urine using dipstick testing. A urine specific gravity above 1.015 to 1.020 often accompanies prerenal AKI, although impaired urinary concentration may be present due to underlying CKD or as a result of diuretic therapy. Acute glomerulonephritis may also present with concentrated urine. Isosthenuria (a urine specific gravity of 1.010, similar to that of plasma) is characteristic of ATN. Hematuria may result from urologic trauma from catheterization, urologic disease, interstitial nephritis, acute glomerulonephritis, atheroembolic disease, renal infarction, or pigment (hemoglobinuric or myoglobinuric) nephropathy. The latter are suggested when the dipstick test for blood is positive but no RBCs are seen on microscopic examination of the sediment.

Examination of the urine sediment and supernatant of a centrifuged urine specimen complements the dipstick analysis and is highly valuable for distinguishing among the various forms of AKI. The urine sediment should be inspected for the presence of cells, casts, and crystals (Table 30-9). In prerenal AKI, the urine sediment is typically bland (i.e., devoid of cells or casts) but may contain transparent hyaline casts. Hyaline casts are formed in concentrated urine from normal urinary constituents, principally Tamm-Horsfall protein secreted by epithelial cells of the loop of Henle. Postrenal AKI may also present with a bland urine sediment, although hematuria is common in patients with intraluminal obstruction (e.g., stones, sloughed papilla, blood clot) or prostatic disease. Pigmented muddy brown granular casts and tubule epithelial cell casts are characteristic of ischemic or nephrotoxic ATN. They may be found in association with microscopic hematuria and mild tubular proteinuria (<1 g/day). Casts may be absent, however, in approximately 20% to 30% of patients with ischemic or nephrotoxic ATN and are not a requisite for diagnosis.[232,233] In general, there is poor correlation between the severity of AKI and the amount of debris in the urine sediment in these conditions (see the section "Acute Tubular Necrosis" earlier). RBC casts almost always indicate acute glomerular disease but in rare cases may be observed in acute interstitial nephritis. Dysmorphic RBCs, best seen using phase-contrast microscopy, are a more common urinary finding in patients with glomerular injury but are a less specific finding than RBC casts.

Urine sediment abnormalities vary in diseases involving preglomerular blood vessels, such as HUS, TTP, atheroembolic disease, and vasculitis involving medium-sized or large vessels, and range from benign to overtly nephritic. White blood cell casts and nonpigmented granular casts suggest interstitial nephritis, whereas broad granular casts are characteristic of CKD and probably reflect interstitial fibrosis and dilatation of tubules. Eosinophiluria (between 1% and 50% of urine leukocytes) is a common finding in drug-induced allergic interstitial nephritis (90% of cases).[234,235] However, eosinophiluria is only 85% specific for allergic interstitial nephritis, and eosinophiluria of 1% to 5% can occur in a variety of other diseases, including atheroembolization, ischemic and nephrotoxic AKI, proliferative glomerulonephritis, pyelonephritis, cystitis, and prostatitis. Uric acid crystals (pleomorphic) may be seen in the urine in prerenal AKI but should raise the possibility of acute urate nephropathy if seen in abundance. Oxalate crystalluria (either needle- or dumbbell-shaped monohydrate crystals or envelope-shaped dihydrate crystals) may suggest a diagnosis of ethylene glycol toxicity.[236]

Increased urinary protein excretion, characteristically less than 1 g/day, is a common finding in ischemic or nephrotoxic ATN and reflects both failure of injured proximal tubule cells to reabsorb normally filtered protein and excretion of cellular debris (tubular proteinuria). Proteinuria of more than 1 g protein per day suggests injury to the glomerular ultrafiltration barrier (glomerular proteinuria) or excretion of light chains.[82,237] The latter are not detected by conventional dipstick tests (which detect albumin) and must be sought by other means (e.g., sulfosalicylic acid test). Heavy proteinuria is also a frequent finding in patients with allergic interstitial nephritis triggered by NSAIDs (80% of cases). In addition to acute interstitial inflammation, these patients have a glomerular lesion that is almost identical to that of minimal-change disease.[238] A similar syndrome has been reported in patients receiving other agents such as ampicillin, rifampin, and interferon alfa.[239,240] Hemolysis and rhabdomyolysis may often be differentiated by inspection of plasma, which is characteristically pink in hemolysis, but clear in rhabdomyolysis.

Analysis of urine biochemical parameters is often helpful in differentiating between prerenal and intrinsic ischemic or nephrotoxic AKI. Sodium is usually avidly reabsorbed from the glomerular filtrate in patients with prerenal AKI as a consequence of renal adrenergic activation, stimulation of the renin-angiotensin-aldosterone axis, suppression of atrial natriuretic peptide secretion and local changes in peritubular hemodynamics. In contrast, sodium reabsorption is impaired in ATN as a result of injury to the renal tubular epithelium. Renal sodium handling can be assessed based on the urinary sodium concentration (U_{Na}) with values of less than 10 mEq/L commonly seen in prerenal disease compared with more than 20 mEq/L in ATN (Table 30-10). Normalizing sodium excretion to creatinine provides a more sensitive index.

TABLE 30-9 Characteristics of Urine Sediment in the Differential Diagnosis of Acute Kidney Injury

Normal or Few Red Blood Cells or White Blood Cells
Prerenal azotemia
Arterial thrombosis or embolism
Preglomerular vasculitis
Hemolytic uremic syndrome/thrombotic thrombocytopenic purpura
Scleroderma crisis
Postrenal acute kidney injury

Granular Casts
Acute tubular necrosis
Glomerulonephritis or vasculitis
Interstitial nephritis

Red Blood Cell Casts
Glomerulonephritis or vasculitis
Malignant hypertension
Rarely interstitial nephritis

White Blood Cell Casts
Acute interstitial nephritis or exudative glomerulonephritis
Severe pyelonephritis
Marked leukemic or lymphomatous infiltration

Eosinophiluria (>5% Eosinophils)
Allergic interstitial nephritis (antibiotics much more frequently than nonsteroidal antiinflammatory drugs)
Atheroembolism

Crystalluria
Acute urate nephropathy
Calcium oxalate (ethylene glycol intoxication)
Acyclovir
Indinavir
Sulfonamides
Radiocontrast agents

TABLE 30-10 Urine Indices Used in the Differential Diagnosis of Prerenal Acute Kidney Injury and Acute Tubular Necrosis

DIAGNOSTIC INDEX	PRERENAL ACUTE KIDNEY INJURY	ACUTE TUBULAR NECROSIS
Fractional excretion of sodium (%)	<1*	>2*
Urine sodium concentration (mEq/L)	<20	>40
Urine creatinine/plasma creatinine ratio	>40	<20
Urine urea nitrogen/plasma urea nitrogen ratio	>8	<3
Urine specific gravity	>1.018	~1.010
Urine osmolality (mOsm/kg H$_2$O)	>500	~300
Plasma blood urea nitrogen/creatinine ratio	>20	<10-15
Renal failure index, $U_{Na}/(U_{Cr}/P_{Cr})$	<1	>1
Urine sediment	Hyaline casts	Muddy brown granular casts

*Fractional excretion of sodium (FE$_{Na}$) may be >1% in prerenal acute kidney injury associated with diuretic use and/or in the setting of bicarbonaturia or chronic kidney disease; FE$_{Na}$ is often <1% in acute tubular necrosis caused by radiocontrast agents or rhabdomyolysis.

P_{Cr}, Plasma creatinine concentration; U_{Cr}, urine creatinine concentration; U_{Na}, urine sodium concentration.

The fractional excretion of sodium (FE$_{Na}$) is the ratio between urine sodium excretion (U$_{Na}$ × V, where V is the urine volume) and the filtered load of sodium (calculated as P$_{Na}$ × [U$_{Cr}$ × V/P$_{Cr}$], where P$_{Na}$ is the plasma sodium concentration and [U$_{Cr}$ × V/P$_{Cr}$] is the creatinine clearance calculated from the urine volume and the urine and plasma creatinine concentrations [U$_{Cr}$ and P$_{Cr}$, respectively]). The FE$_{Na}$, calculated as [(U$_{Na}$ ÷ P$_{Na}$)/(U$_{Cr}$ ÷ P$_{Cr}$)] × 100, is usually less than 1% (frequently <0.5%), in the setting of prerenal azotemia, whereas it is typically more than 2% in patients with ischemic or nephrotoxic AKI. The usefulness of the FE$_{Na}$ value is limited in a variety of clinical settings. Values greater than 1% are not uncommon in the setting of prerenal AKI in patients receiving diuretics, those with metabolic alkalosis and bicarbonaturia (in whom Na$^+$ is excreted with HCO$_3^-$ to maintain electroneutrality), those with adrenal insufficiency, and those with underlying CKD.[241-243] On the other hand, a FE$_{Na}$ of less than 1% is often observed in the setting of ATN. Although this is most common following radiocontrast administration and in the setting of rhabdomyolysis, it has been reported in approximately 15% of patients with ATN owing to a variety of other causes, including ischemia, burns, and sepsis. It has been postulated that this reflects a milder degree of intrinsic renal injury in which epithelial cell damage is probably localized to the corticomedullary junction and outer medulla with relative preservation of function in other Na$^+$-transporting segments and may represent a transition state between prerenal azotemia and ATN. It should be recognized that a FE$_{Na}$ of less than 1% is not abnormal and reflects normal sodium homeostasis in patients consuming a moderate- or low-sodium diet. The FE$_{Na}$ is also often less than 1% in AKI caused by urinary tract obstruction, glomerulonephritis, and diseases of the renal vasculature; other parameters must be used to distinguish these conditions from prerenal AKI.

A variety of other indices have also been proposed to differentiate among the causes of AKI. The renal failure index, calculated as $U_{Na}/(U_{Cr} \div P_{Cr})$, provides information comparable to that of the FE$_{Na}$, because clinical variations in serum Na$^+$ concentration are relatively small. The fractional excretion of urea (FE$_{urea}$), calculated as ([U$_{urea}$ ÷ P$_{urea}$]/[U$_{Cr}$ ÷ P$_{Cr}$] × 100), has been proposed as an alternative to the FE$_{Na}$, with particular usefulness in patients receiving diuretic therapy. Values of FE$_{urea}$ of less than 35% are suggestive of a prerenal disease state. Similarly, indices of urinary concentrating ability such as urine specific gravity, urine osmolality, urine/plasma creatinine or urea ratios, and serum urea nitrogen/creatinine ratio are of limited value in differentiating between prerenal and intrinsic AKI. This is particularly true for elderly individuals, in whom urine concentrating mechanisms are frequently impaired whereas mechanisms for Na$^+$ reabsorption are typically preserved.

Laboratory Evaluation

The pattern and timing of change in BUN and serum creatinine concentrations often provide clues to the cause of AKI. Enhanced tubular reabsorption of filtered urea in parallel with sodium and water reabsorption in prerenal states commonly leads to a disproportionate elevation in BUN compared with serum creatinine (ratio of >20:1). Conversely, with intrinsic AKI, the increase in BUN usually parallels the rise in serum creatinine, so that a ratio of approximately 10:1 is maintained (see Table 30-10). However, severe malnutrition and low dietary protein intake blunt the rise in BUN and creatinine, whereas gastrointestinal bleeding, steroid therapy, and hypercatabolic states may lead to increases in BUN that do not reflect prerenal physiology. The serum creatinine concentration typically begins to rise within 24 to 48 hours when ATN results from an ischemic insult. Although the clinical course can be highly variable, the serum creatinine level will generally peak within 7 to 10 days, and depending on the severity of the insult and underlying comorbid illnesses, the AKI will resolve over the ensuing 1 to 2 weeks. After exposure to an iodinated contrast agent the peak in serum creatinine level is generally within 5 to 7 days. The time course of nephrotoxic ATN caused by aminoglycoside antibiotics or cisplatin is more variable, often with delayed onset of AKI (7 to 10 days).

Additional clues to the diagnosis can be obtained from biochemical and hematologic tests. The presence of marked hyperkalemia, hyperuricemia, and hyperphosphatemia point to cell lysis, which in the setting of elevated creatine kinase levels and hypocalcemia strongly suggests rhabdomyolysis.[244,245] Biochemical signs of cell lysis with very high levels of uric acid, normal or mildly elevated creatine kinase levels, and a urine uric acid/creatinine ratio greater than 1.0 are suggestive of acute urate nephropathy and tumor lysis syndrome.[246,247] Severe hypercalcemia can precipitate AKI, commonly in the form of prerenal AKI from concomitant hypovolemia. AKI associated with widening of both the serum anion gaps (Na$^+$ − [HCO$_3^-$ + Cl$^-$]) and osmolal gap (measured serum osmolality minus calculated osmolality) suggests a diagnosis of ethylene glycol toxicity and should prompt a search for urine oxalate crystals. Severe anemia in the absence of hemorrhage may reflect the presence of hemolysis, multiple myeloma, or thrombotic microangiopathy (e.g., HUS, TTP, toxemia, disseminated intravascular coagulation, accelerated hypertension, systemic lupus erythematosus, scleroderma, radiation injury). Other laboratory findings suggestive of thrombotic microangiopathy include thrombocytopenia, dysmorphic RBCs on peripheral blood smear, a low circulating haptoglobin level, and elevated circulating levels of lactate dehydrogenase. Systemic eosinophilia suggests allergic interstitial nephritis but may also be a prominent feature in other diseases such as atheroembolic disease and polyarteritis nodosa, particularly the Churg-Strauss variant. Tests to detect depressed complement levels and high titers of anti–glomerular basement membrane antibodies, antineutrophil cytoplasmic antibodies, antinuclear antibodies, circulating immune complexes, or cryoglobulins are useful diagnostic tools when glomerulonephritis or vasculitis is suspected (see Table 30-8).

Radiologic Evaluation

Imaging of the abdomen is a highly useful adjunct to laboratory testing to determine the cause of AKI. In cases of suspected obstructive uropathy, postvoid residual volumes of more than 100 to 150 mL suggest a diagnosis of bladder outlet obstruction. Although plain radiographs rarely provide definitive evidence of postrenal AKI, they may identify the presence of calcium-containing stones that can cause obstructive disease. Renal ultrasonography is the screening test of choice to assess cortical thickness, differences in cortical and medullary density, the integrity of the collecting system, and kidney size. Although pelvicaliceal dilatation is usual in cases of urinary tract obstruction (98% sensitivity), dilatation may not be observed when the patient is volume depleted, during the initial 1 to 3 days after obstruction, when the collecting system is relatively noncompliant, or when obstruction is caused by ureteric encasement or infiltration (e.g., retroperitoneal fibrosis, neoplasia).[248] Alternatively, computed tomography (CT) may be used to visualize the kidneys and collecting system, although radiocontrast agent administration should be avoided in patients with AKI. Visualization of the collecting system may be suboptimal in the absence of contrast agent enhancement; however unenhanced CT scans are useful for the identification of obstructing ureteral stones. Ultrasonography and CT have essentially replaced the use of intravenous pyelography, which now has little role in the evaluation of AKI. Cystoscopic retrograde or percutaneous anterograde pyelography is useful for precise localization of the site of obstruction and can be combined with placement of ureteral stents or percutaneous nephrostomy tubes to allow therapeutic decompression of the urinary tract. Radionuclide scans have been proposed as useful for assessing renal blood flow, glomerular filtration, tubule function, and infiltration by inflammatory cells in AKI; however, these tests generally lack specificity or yield conflicting or poor results in controlled studies.[249,250] Magnetic resonance angiography (MRA) of the kidneys is extremely useful for detecting renal artery stenosis and has been used in the evaluation of acute renovascular crises.[251] However, given the association of gadolinium-based contrast agent administration with the development of nephrogenic systemic fibrosis, contrast medium–enhanced MRA is relatively contraindicated in the majority of patients with AKI.[252,253] Doppler ultrasonography and spiral CT are also useful in patients with suspected vascular obstruction; however, contrast angiography remains the gold standard for definitive diagnosis.

Renal Biopsy

Renal biopsy is usually reserved for patients in whom prerenal and postrenal AKI have been excluded and the cause of intrinsic AKI is unclear.[254] Renal biopsy is particularly useful when clinical assessment, urinalysis, and laboratory investigation suggest diagnoses other than ischemic or nephrotoxic injury that may respond to specific therapy. Examples include anti–glomerular basement membrane disease and other forms of necrotizing glomerulonephritis, vasculitis, HUS and TTP, allergic interstitial nephritis, and myeloma cast nephropathy.

Differential Diagnosis of Acute Kidney Injury in Specific Clinical Settings

The differential diagnosis of AKI in several common clinical settings warrants special mention (Table 30-11).

Acute Kidney Injury in the Setting of Cancer

There are several potential causes of AKI in a patient with cancer. Prerenal AKI is common in the setting of underlying malignancy and may be related to tumor- or chemotherapy-induced vomiting or diarrhea, reduced oral intake secondary to anorexia, the use of NSAIDs for pain management, and malignancy-associated hypercalcemia.[255,256] Intrinsic AKI can be triggered by a variety of chemotherapeutic agents. Cisplatin is the chemotherapeutic medication classically associated with AKI.[257,258] The principal site of renal damage due to cisplatin is the proximal tubule. The nephrotoxicity of cisplatin is dose dependent, yet AKI can result from a single exposure. Electrolyte disturbances, including hypomagnesemia and hypokalemia, are not uncommon. Iphosphamide, which has been used to treat germ cell tumors and pediatric sarcomas, is also associated with AKI in a dose-dependent fashion.[259-261] Renal parenchymal invasion by solid and hematologic cancers is reported in 5% to 10% of autopsy studies but is an uncommon cause of AKI.[262,263] Infiltration of leukemic cells into the renal parenchyma can precipitate AKI and typically presents with hematuria, proteinuria, and enlarged kidneys on ultrasonographic imaging. Prompt diagnosis is important, because the AKI may respond to chemotherapeutic intervention.

Tumor lysis syndrome, which is associated with hyperuricemia, hyperphosphatemia, and hypocalcemia, is a well-recognized cause of AKI in patients with cancer.[264,265] Tumor lysis syndrome occurs most commonly after initiation of chemotherapy in patients with poorly differentiated lymphoproliferative malignancies (e.g., Burkitt's lymphoma or acute lymphoblastic or promyelocytic leukemia), but it can occur spontaneously and in the setting of certain solid tumors that are highly sensitive to radiation therapy and/or chemotherapy (e.g., testicular carcinoma). AKI associated with tumor lysis syndrome is triggered by direct tubular injury and luminal obstruction by uric acid and calcium phosphate crystals. Prophylactic therapy with aggressive volume administration and either inhibition of uric acid synthesis using xanthine oxidase

TABLE 30-11 Major Causes of Acute Kidney Injury (AKI) in Specific Clinical Settings

AKI in the Cancer Patient
Prerenal azotemia
    Hypovolemia (e.g., poor intake, vomiting, diarrhea)
Intrinsic AKI
    Exogenous nephrotoxins: chemotherapy, antibiotics, contrast agents
    Endogenous toxins: hyperuricemia, hypercalcemia, tumor lysis, paraproteins
    Other: radiation therapy, HUS/TTP, glomerulonephritis, amyloidosis, malignant infiltration
Postrenal AKI
    Ureteric or bladder neck obstruction

AKI after Cardiac Surgery
Prerenal azotemia
    Hypovolemia (surgical losses, diuretics), cardiac failure, vasodilators
Intrinsic AKI
    Ischemic ATN (even in absence of hypotension)
    Atheroembolic disease after aortic manipulation/intraaortic balloon pump placement
    Preoperative or perioperative administration of contrast agent
    Allergic interstitial nephritis induced by perioperative antibiotics
Postrenal AKI
    Obstructed urinary catheter, exacerbation of voiding dysfunction

AKI in Pregnancy
Prerenal azotemia
    Acute fatty liver of pregnancy with fulminate hepatic failure
Intrinsic AKI
    Preeclampsia or eclampsia
    Postpartum HUS/TTP
    HELLP syndrome
    Ischemia—postpartum hemorrhage, abruptio placentae, amniotic fluid embolus
    Direct toxicity of illegal abortifacients
Postrenal AKI
    Obstruction with pyelonephritis

AKI after Solid Organ or Bone Marrow Transplantation
Prerenal azotemia
    Intravascular volume depletion (e.g., diuretic therapy)
    Vasoactive drugs (e.g., calcineurin inhibitors, amphotericin B)
    Hepatorenal syndrome, venoocclusive disease of liver (bone marrow transplantation)
Intrinsic AKI
    Postoperative ischemic ATN (even in absence of hypotension)
    Sepsis
    Exogenous nephrotoxins—aminoglycosides, amphotericin B, radiocontrast agents
    HUS/TTP (e.g., cyclosporine or myeloablative radiotherapy related)
    Allergic tubulointerstitial nephritis
Postrenal AKI
    Obstructed urinary catheter

AKI and Pulmonary Disease (Pulmonary-Renal Syndrome)
Prerenal azotemia
    Diminished cardiac output complicating pulmonary embolism, severe pulmonary hypertension, or positive
pressure mechanical ventilation
    Intrinsic AKI
    Vasculitis
        Goodpasture's syndrome, ANCA-associated vasculitis, SLE, Churg-Strauss syndrome, polyarteritis nodosa, cryoglobulinemia, right-sided
        endocarditis, lymphomatoid granulomatosis, sarcoidosis, scleroderma
    Toxins
        Ingestion of paraquat or diquat
    Infections
        Legionnaires' disease, *Mycoplasma* infection, tuberculosis, disseminated viral or fungal infection
AKI from any cause with hypervolemia and pulmonary edema
Lung cancer with hypercalcemia, tumor lysis, or glomerulonephritis

AKI and Liver Disease
Prerenal azotemia
    Reduced true circulatory volume (GI hemorrhage, GI losses from lactulose, diuretics, large-volume paracentesis) or effective circulatory volume (hypoal-
buminemia, splanchnic vasodilatation)
    Hepatorenal syndrome type 1 or 2
    Tense ascites with abdominal compartment syndrome
Intrinsic AKI
    Ischemic (severe hypoperfusion—see earlier) or direct nephrotoxicity and hepatotoxicity of drugs or toxins (e.g., carbon tetrachloride, acetaminophen,
tetracyclines, methoxyflurane)
    Tubulointerstitial nephritis plus hepatitis caused by drugs (e.g., sulfonamides, rifampin, phenytoin, allopurinol, phenindione), infections (leptospirosis,
brucellosis, Epstein-Barr virus infection, cytomegalovirus infection), malignant infiltration (leukemia, lymphoma) or sarcoidosis
    Glomerulonephritis or vasculitis (e.g., polyarteritis nodosa, ANCA-associated glomerulonephritis, cryoglobulinemia, SLE, postinfectious hepatitis or
liver abscess)

TABLE 30-11 Major Causes of Acute Kidney Injury (AKI) in Specific Clinical Settings—cont'd

AKI and Nephrotic Syndrome
Prerenal azotemia
   Intravascular volume depletion (diuretic therapy, hypoalbuminemia)
   Intravascular volume depletion (diuretic therapy, hypoalbuminemia)
Intrinsic AKI
   Manifestation of primary glomerular disease
   Collapsing glomerulopathy (e.g., human immunodeficiency virus infection, pamidronate)
   Associated ATN (elderly hypertensive males)
   Associated interstitial nephritis (nonsteroidal antiinflammatory drugs, rifampin, interferon alfa)
Other—amyloid or light-chain deposition disease, renal vein thrombosis, severe interstitial edema

ANCA, Antineutrophil cytoplasmic antibodies; *ATN,* acute tubular necrosis; *GI,* gastrointestinal; *HELLP,* hemolysis, elevated liver enzymes, low platelets; *HUS,* hemolytic uremic syndrome; *SLE,* systemic lupus erythematosus; *TTP,* thrombotic thrombocytopenic purpura.

inhibitors or, more recently, conversion of uric acid to allantoin using recombinant uricase has markedly reduced the incidence of this form of AKI.[266-268]

Less common causes of AKI include tumor-associated glomerulonephritis and thrombotic microangiopathy induced by medications or irradiation. Chemotherapy-associated thrombotic microangiopathy is a well-recognized complication of several agents, including mitomycin C and gemcitabine.[269-271]

AKI is a common complication of multiple myeloma.[237,272] Causes of AKI in this setting include intravascular volume depletion, myeloma cast nephropathy, sepsis, hypercalcemia, ATN induced by drugs or tumor lysis during therapy, light-chain deposition disease, cryoglobulinemia, hyperviscosity syndrome, plasma cell infiltration, and amyloidosis. Myeloma cast nephropathy results from the binding of filtered immunoglobulin Bence Jones proteins to Tamm-Horsfall glycoprotein, forming casts that obstruct the tubular lumen. Higher excretion rates of free light chains, volume depletion, and hypercalcemia are associated with greater risk of development of myeloma cast nephropathy. Prompt treatment to lower free light-chain burden may result in recovery of kidney function. Studies of the effectiveness of plasmapheresis in the treatment of myeloma cast nephropathy have yielded conflicting results.[273-275]

Acute Kidney Injury in Pregnancy

In the industrialized world, the incidence of dialysis-requiring AKI in the setting of pregnancy is approximately 1 in 20,000 births.[276,277] The marked decline in this complication over the past 50 years is a result of improved prenatal care and advancements in obstetrics practice. In early pregnancy, ATN induced by nephrotoxic abortifacients remains a relatively common cause of AKI in developing countries, but is rare in the developed world. Ischemic ATN, severe toxemia of pregnancy, and postpartum HUS and TTP are the most common causes of AKI in late-term pregnancy.[276,278,279] Ischemic ATN is usually precipitated by abruptio placentae or postpartum hemorrhage and, less commonly, by amniotic fluid embolism or sepsis. Glomerular filtration is usually normal in mild or moderate preeclampsia; however, AKI may complicate severe preeclampsia.[279,280] In this setting, AKI is typically transient and found in association with intrarenal vasospasm, marked hypertension, and neurologic abnormalities. A variant of preeclampsia, the HELLP syndrome (hemolysis, elevated liver enzymes, low platelets), is characterized by a benign initial course that can rapidly deteriorate with the development of thrombotic microangiopathy with hemolysis, coagulation

abnormalities, derangement in hepatic function, and AKI.[280-282] Immediate delivery of the fetus is indicated in this setting. Thrombotic microangiopathy can also develop in the postpartum setting and typically occurs in patients who have had a normal pregnancy.[283] Postpartum thrombotic microangiopathy is characterized by thrombocytopenia, microangiopathic anemia, and normal prothrombin and partial thromboplastin times and frequently results in long-term impairment of renal function.

Acute fatty liver of pregnancy occurs in approximately 1 in 7000 pregnancies and is associated with AKI, likely as a result of intrarenal vasoconstriction as occurs in hepatorenal syndrome. Although the exact origin of acute fatty liver of pregnancy is unknown, the incidence is increased in women who carry a fetus with a defect in fatty acid oxidation and who are themselves carriers of a genetic mutation that compromises intramitochondrial fatty acid oxidation.[282] Acute bilateral pyelonephritis may also precipitate AKI in pregnancy and should be obvious from the patient's signs and symptoms (fever, flank pain), findings on urinalysis (bacteria, leukocytes), and laboratory test results (leukocytosis, elevated serum creatinine concentration).[278,281,284,285] The diagnosis of postrenal AKI in the pregnant patient is particularly challenging due to the physiologic dilatation of the collecting system that normally occurs in the second and third trimesters. As a result, determining the presence of abnormal findings on renal ultrasonography is more difficult.

Acute Kidney Injury Following Cardiac Surgery

An acute deterioration in renal function is a common complication following cardiac surgery, with an incidence of 7.7% to 42% depending on the criteria used to define AKI.[286-290] AKI requiring dialytic support occurs in up to 5% of patients after cardiac surgery.[286-290] AKI in the perioperative period is most commonly attributed to prerenal azotemia associated with decreased cardiac function or to ATN. Risk factors for cardiac surgery–associated AKI can be broadly categorized into presurgical patient-related factors; surgical factors; and postoperative events. The principal patient-related risk factors include underlying CKD, advanced age, left ventricular dysfunction, previous myocardial revascularization, diabetes mellitus, and peripheral vascular disease.[289-292] Operative factors include the need for emergent surgery, prolonged time on cardiopulmonary bypass, insertion of an intraaortic balloon pump, the performance of concomitant valvular surgery, and repeated coronary artery bypass grafting (CABG). Several studies have compared the incidence of AKI following on-pump versus off-pump CABG, with some data suggesting that off-pump CABG is associated with a lower incidence of AKI.[293-296] Postoperative factors associated with an increased risk for AKI include reduced cardiac output, bleeding, vasodilatory shock, and the overzealous use of diuretics and afterload-reducing agents.

Additional potential causes of AKI following CABG include the administration of an iodinated contrast agent in the preoperative, perioperative, and/or postoperative period; antibiotic-associated acute interstitial nephritis; and atheroembolic disease.[41] Whereas prerenal azotemia and ATN typically occur within days of the surgical procedure, atheroembolic AKI may take longer to develop and can be distinguished by the characteristic clinical features of livedo reticularis, cyanosis, and gangrenous digital lesions, as well as the findings of eosinophilia, eosinophiluria, and hypocomplementemia.

Acute Kidney Injury after Solid Organ or Bone Marrow Transplantation

Nonrenal solid organ transplant recipients have a particularly high risk of AKI from cardiopulmonary and hepatic failure, sepsis, and the nephrotoxic effects of antimicrobial and immunosuppressive agents. In a large retrospective multicenter study, 25% of all nonrenal solid organ transplant recipients developed AKI, with 8% requiring renal replacement therapy.[297] The development of AKI requiring dialysis was associated with a 9- to 12-fold increase in mortality. AKI developed in 35% of heart transplant recipients and 15% of lung transplant recipients. As many as 30% of liver transplant recipients developed AKI, many of whom had CKD before transplantation.[298,299] Data are conflicting as to whether impaired kidney function before transplantation predicts outcomes in patients undergoing orthotopic liver transplantation; however, patients with impaired kidney function preoperatively have longer hospital and ICU stays and are more likely to need dialysis than patients with intact kidney function before transplantation.[300-302]

AKI is a well-recognized complication of hematopoietic cell transplantation (HCT).[255,303,304] The three types of HCT are myeloablative autologous, myeloablative allogeneic, and nonmyeloablative allogeneic, and the incidence, severity, and outcomes of AKI following these forms of HCT vary considerably.[303,305,306] In a study of 272 patients who underwent myeloablative HCT (predominantly allogeneic), 53% developed AKI and 24% required dialysis.[307] Among patients with AKI who required dialysis, the mortality rate was 84%. One study found an incidence of severe AKI in this patient population of 73%.[308] AKI following nonmyeloablative allogeneic HCT is less common.[308,309] A study of 253 patients found an incidence of AKI within 3 months of HCT of 40.4%, with just 4.4% of patients requiring dialysis.[309] The incidence of AKI after myeloablative autologous HCT is considerably lower.[310,311] A study of 173 patients who underwent autologous HCT reported an incidence of AKI of 21%, with 5% of patients requiring dialysis.[311] The absence of graft-versus-host disease and more rapid engraftment likely account for the lower incidence of AKI in this setting. Causes of HCT-associated AKI include hypovolemia, sepsis, tumor lysis syndrome, direct tubular toxicity from cytoreductive therapy, thrombotic microangiopathy, graft-versus-host disease, antibiotics,

immunosuppressive agents, and hepatic venoocclusive disease. Venoocclusive disease results from acute radiochemotherapy-induced endothelial cell injury of hepatic venules.[307,312-314] This occurs most commonly in conditioning regimens that include total-body irradiation and cyclophosphamide and/or busulphan administration and in the setting of myeloablative allogeneic HCT. The syndrome is characterized clinically by profound jaundice and avid salt retention with edema and ascites within the first month after engraftment, and subsequent development of AKI. Oliguric AKI is common in moderate venoocclusive disease and certain in severe cases. The mortality rate for patients with severe venoocclusive disease approaches 100%.

Acute Kidney Injury Associated with Pulmonary Disease

The coexistence of AKI and pulmonary disease (pulmonary-renal syndrome) classically suggests the presence of Goodpasture's syndrome, antineutrophil cytoplasmic antibody–associated vasculitis, or other vasculitides.[315-317] The detection of anti–glomerular basement membrane antibodies, antineutrophil cytoplasmic antibodies, or low serum complement concentrations can be helpful in differentiating among the various causes of pulmonary-renal syndrome, although the urgent need for definitive diagnosis and treatment may mandate lung or renal biopsy. Several toxic ingestions and infections may also precipitate simultaneous pulmonary and kidney injury that mimics vasculitis-associated pulmonary-renal syndrome. Furthermore, AKI of any cause may be complicated by secondary hypervolemia and pulmonary edema. Severe lung disease and ventilator support with increased intrathoracic pressure may compromise cardiac output and induce prerenal AKI.

Acute Kidney Injury Associated with Liver Disease

The differential diagnosis of AKI in patients with liver disease is broad. Common causes of AKI in this setting include intravascular volume depletion, gastrointestinal bleeding, sepsis, and nephrotoxins. Most cases of AKI in advanced liver disease are due to prerenal azotemia, ATN, or hepatorenal syndrome, and differentiating these conditions can be clinically challenging.[318-320] Although a U_{Na} of less than 20 mEq/L and an FE_{Na} of less than 1% are typical of prerenal AKI and hepatorenal syndrome, high dosages of diuretics, which are commonly prescribed in patients with advanced liver disease, may lead to higher sodium excretion rates. Differentiating ATN from other forms of AKI is further confounded by the fact that bile-stained casts, which can be seen in prerenal AKI and hepatorenal syndrome, have an appearance similar to that of the classical muddy brown granular casts of ATN. Kidney disease in patients with liver disease may also result from acute glomerular disease, including immunoglobulin A nephropathy, hepatitis B virus–associated membranous nephropathy, and hepatitis C virus–associated membranoproliferative glomerulonephritis and cryoglobulinemia. Acetaminophen toxicity may cause nephrotoxic ATN and is also one of the most common causes of acute hepatotoxicity.

The term *hepatorenal syndrome* is typically reserved for a clinical syndrome marked by irreversible AKI that develops in patients with advanced cirrhosis, although it has been described in the setting of fulminant viral and alcoholic hepatitis. Hepatorenal syndrome almost certainly represents the terminal stage of a state of hypoperfusion that begins early in the course of chronic liver disease. The precise pathophysiologic mechanisms underlying the hemodynamic alterations in hepatorenal syndrome are incompletely understood. In the early stages of the syndrome, increased vascular capacitance as a result of splanchnic and systemic vasodilation is thought to trigger activation of the renin-angiotensin and sympathetic nervous systems.[318] Renal perfusion is preserved in this stage by the local release of renal vasodilatory factors; however, these compensatory mechanisms are eventually overwhelmed, and progressive renal hypoperfusion ensues. An inadequate increase in cardiac output relative to the fall in vascular resistance is thought also to contribute to the development of hepatorenal syndrome.

Clinically, the presentation of hepatorenal syndrome closely resembles that of prerenal AKI. Unlike prerenal AKI, however, hepatorenal syndrome does not improve with aggressive expansion of the intravascular space. Criteria for the diagnosis of hepatorenal syndrome include an increase in serum creatinine concentration above 1.5 mg/dL in the setting of cirrhosis with ascites; failure of kidney function to improve after at least 2 days of diuretic withdrawal and volume expansion with albumin; and the absence of shock, concurrent or recent treatment with nephrotoxic drugs, or parenchymal kidney disease (defined by proteinuria of >500 mg of protein per day), hematuria of >50 RBCs per high-power field, and/or abnormal renal ultrasonographic findings).[321]

Two subtypes of hepatorenal syndrome have been described. Type 1 hepatorenal syndrome is characterized by a rapid onset of AKI defined by at least a doubling of the serum creatinine concentration to a level of at least 2.5 mg/dL, or a reduction in glomerular filtration of 50% or more to a level of less than 20 mL/min over a 2-week period.[322,323] Type 1 hepatorenal syndrome typically develops in hospitalized patients and may be precipitated by variceal bleeding, overly rapid diuresis, the performance of paracentesis, or, most commonly, the development of spontaneous bacterial peritonitis. Other postulated triggers include infections, minor surgery, or the use of NSAIDs or other drugs. However, caution must be used in these cases to exclude reversible causes of AKI. Type 1 hepatorenal syndrome is generally characterized by a fulminant course with oliguria, encephalopathy, marked hyperbilirubinemia, and death within 1 month of clinical presentation. However, recent advances in the management of hepatorenal syndrome as discussed later suggest that there may be a trend toward better survival in those patients who respond to therapy.[324,325]

Type 2 hepatorenal syndrome is typified by a more gradual decline in renal function that develops in the setting of diuretic-resistant ascites and avid sodium retention. The prognosis of type 2 hepatorenal syndrome is considerably better than that of type 1 hepatorenal syndrome, with a reported median survival of 6 months and a 1-year survival as high as 30%.[326,327] The development of a sudden deterioration in renal function after a prolonged period of more stable renal impairment may occur in patients with type 2 hepatorenal syndrome, leading to outcomes similar to those in type 1 hepatorenal syndrome.

Definitive treatment of hepatorenal syndrome is dependent upon recovery of hepatic function or successful liver transplantation. However, the use of vasoconstrictive agents combined with volume expansion with colloid has shown promise for improving kidney function.[328,329] It is postulated that by reversal of the splanchnic and peripheral vasodilatation, more normal renal perfusion can be restored. Vasoconstrictive regimens that have been used include norepinephrine, combination therapy with midodrine and octreotide, and the vasopressin agonist terlipressin.[330-333] Although vasoconstrictive therapy is associated with improvement in kidney function and short-term outcomes are better in patients who show a response, the use of vasoconstrictive therapy has not been shown to improve overall prognosis in patients with AKI, which suggests that survival remains limited by the underlying severity of liver disease.

Acute Kidney Injury and Nephrotic Syndrome

AKI in the context of nephrotic syndrome presents a unique array of potential diagnoses. Epithelial injury, if severe, can trigger both nephrotic-range proteinuria and acute or subacute kidney injury.[334,335] The epithelial injury typically occurs as a manifestation of primary glomerular diseases such as collapsing glomerulopathy or crescentic membranous nephropathy. Less dramatic visceral epithelial cell injury, in combination with proximal tubular injury (e.g., pan–epithelial cell injury induced by NSAIDs or possible undiagnosed viral illness) or interstitial nephritis (e.g., rifampicin induced) can also present as AKI complicating nephrotic syndrome.[336-338] Massive excretion of light-chain proteins in patients with multiple myeloma may also present in this fashion.[339,340] ATN in association with nephrotic syndrome is seen in a subpopulation of older patients with minimal change disease and in other patients with nephrosis and hypoalbuminemia who have been treated with overzealous diuresis. On average, patients with AKI complicating nephrotic syndrome have higher urinary protein excretion than patients without AKI.[334] The higher incidence of arteriosclerosis in biopsy samples from these patients may point to preexisting hypertensive nephrosclerosis as a risk factor for the development of this complication. Renal vein thrombosis must always be considered in the differential diagnosis of nephrotic syndrome and AKI, particularly in the pediatric population and in adults with membranous nephropathy as a cause of nephrosis.

Complications of Acute Kidney Injury

The acute loss of kidney function in AKI results in multiple derangements in fluid, electrolyte, and acid-base homeostasis and in hematologic, gastroenterologic, and immunologic function (Table 30-12).

Complications of Potassium Homeostasis

Hyperkalemia is a common and potentially life-threatening complication of AKI.[341,342] Serum K^+ typically rises by 0.5 mEq/L/day in oligoanuric patients and reflects impaired excretion of K^+ derived from the patient's diet,

			TABLE 30-12 Common Complications of Acute Kidney Injury			
METABOLIC	**CARDIOVASCULAR**	**GASTROINTESTINAL**	**NEUROLOGIC**	**HEMATOLOGIC**	**INFECTIOUS**	**OTHER**
Hyperkalemia	Pulmonary edema	Nausea	Neuromuscular irritability	Anemia	Pneumonia	Hiccups
Metabolic acidosis	Arrhythmias	Vomiting	Asterixis	Bleeding	Septicemia	Elevated parathyroid hormone level
Hyponatremia	Pericarditis	Malnutrition	Seizures		Urinary tract infection	Low total triiodothyronine and thyroxine levels
Hypocalcemia	Pericardial effusion	Hemorrhage	Mental status changes			
Hyperphosphatemia	Pulmonary embolism					
Hypermagnesemia	Hypertension					
Hyperuricemia	Myocardial infarction					

the administration of K^+-containing solutions and drugs administered as potassium salts, as well as the release of K^+ from the injured tubular epithelium. Hyperkalemia may be compounded by coexistent metabolic acidosis and/or hyperglycemia or other hyperosmolar states that promotes K^+ efflux from cells. Severe hyperkalemia or hyperkalemia present at the time of diagnosis of AKI suggests massive tissue destruction such as rhabdomyolysis, hemolysis, or tumor lysis.[222,244,343] Hyperuricemia and hyperphosphatemia may accompany hyperkalemia in these settings. Mild hyperkalemia (<6.0 mEq/L) is usually asymptomatic. Higher levels are frequently associated with electrocardiographic abnormalities, including peaked T waves, prolongation of the PR interval, flattening of P waves, widening of the QRS complex, and left axis deviation.[344-346] These electrocardiographic findings may precede the onset of life-threatening cardiac arrhythmias such as bradycardia, heart block, ventricular tachycardia or fibrillation, and asystole. In addition, hyperkalemia may induce neuromuscular abnormalities such as paresthesias, hyporeflexia, weakness, ascending flaccid paralysis, and respiratory failure.

*Hypo*kalemia is unusual in AKI but may complicate nonoliguric ATN caused by aminoglycosides, cisplatin, or amphotericin B, presumably because of impaired K^+ reabsorption resulting from epithelial cell injury in the thick ascending limb of the loop of Henle.[347,348]

Complications of Acid-Base Homeostasis

Normal metabolism of dietary protein yields between 50 and 100 mmol/day of fixed nonvolatile acids (principally sulfuric and phosphoric acid), which must be excreted by the kidneys for preservation of acid-base homeostasis. Predictably, AKI is commonly complicated by metabolic acidosis, typically with a widening of the serum anion gap.[349] Acidosis may be severe (daily fall in plasma HCO_3^- of >2 mEq/L) when the generation of H^+ is increased by additional mechanisms (e.g., diabetic or fasting ketoacidosis; lactic acidosis complicating generalized tissue hypoperfusion, liver disease, or sepsis; metabolism of ethylene glycol).[236,320,350] In contrast, metabolic alkalosis is an infrequent finding but may complicate overzealous

correction of acidosis with HCO_3^- or loss of gastric acid by vomiting or nasogastric aspiration.

Complications of Mineral and Uric Acid Homeostasis

Mild hyperphosphatemia (5 to 10 mg/dL) is a common consequence of AKI, and hyperphosphatemia may be severe (10 to 20 mg/dL) in patients with high catabolism or with AKI associated with rapid cell death, as in rhabdomyolysis, severe burns, hemolysis, or tumor lysis.[351-354]

Factors that potentially contribute to hypocalcemia include skeletal resistance to the actions of parathyroid hormone, reduced levels of 1,25-dihydroxyvitamin D, Ca^{2+} sequestration in injured tissues such as muscle in the setting of rhabdomyolysis, and metastatic deposition of calcium phosphate in the setting of severe hyperphosphatemia.[355-357] Hypocalcemia is usually asymptomatic, possibly because of the counterbalancing effects of acidosis on neuromuscular excitability. However, symptomatic hypocalcemia can occur in patients with rhabdomyolysis or acute pancreatitis or after treatment of acidosis with HCO_3^-.[355] Clinical manifestations of hypocalcemia include perioral paresthesias, muscle cramps, seizures, hallucinations, and confusion, as well as prolongation of the QT interval and nonspecific T wave changes on electrocardiogram. Chvostek's sign (contraction of facial muscles on tapping of the jaw over the facial nerve) and Trousseau's sign (carpopedal spasm after occlusion of the arterial blood supply to the arm for 3 minutes with a blood pressure cuff) are useful indicators of latent tetany in high-risk patients.

Mild asymptomatic hypermagnesemia is common in oliguric AKI and reflects impaired excretion of ingested magnesium (dietary magnesium, magnesium-containing laxatives, or antacids).[358,359] More significant hypermagnesemia is usually the result of overzealous parenteral magnesium administration, as in the management of AKI associated with preeclampsia. Hypomagnesemia occasionally complicates nonoliguric ATN associated with cisplatin or amphotericin B administration and, as with hypokalemia, likely reflects injury to the thick ascending limb of the loop of Henle, a principal site for Mg^{2+} reabsorption.[348,360,361] Hypomagnesemia is usually asymptomatic but may occasionally manifest as neuro-muscular instability, cramps, seizures, cardiac arrhythmias, or resistant hypokalemia or hypocalcemia.[358,362]

Uric acid is cleared from the blood by glomerular filtration and secretion by proximal tubule cells, and mild asymptomatic hyperuricemia (12 to 15 mg/dL) is typical in established AKI. Higher levels suggest increased production of uric acid and may point to a diagnosis of acute urate nephropathy.[363-365] In borderline cases, measurement of the urinary uric acid/creatinine ratio in a random urine specimen may help to distinguish between hyperuricemia caused by overproduction and impaired excretion. This ratio is typically greater than 1.0 when uric acid production is increased and less than 0.75 in normal individuals and in patients with impaired kidney function.[366]

Volume Overload and Cardiac Complications

Intravascular volume overload is an almost inevitable consequence of diminished salt and water excretion in AKI and may present clinically as mild hypertension, increased jugular venous pressure, pulmonary vascular congestion, pleural effusion, ascites, peripheral edema, increased body weight, and life-threatening pulmonary edema. Hypervolemia may be particularly troublesome in patients receiving multiple intravenous medications, high volumes of enteral or parenteral nutrition, or excessive volumes of maintenance IV fluids. Moderate or severe hypertension is unusual in ATN and should suggest other diagnoses such as hypertensive nephrosclerosis, glomerulonephritis, renal artery stenosis, and other diseases of the renal vasculature.[278,367-369] Excessive water ingestion or administration of hypotonic saline or dextrose solutions can trigger hyponatremia, which, if severe, may cause cerebral edema, seizures, and other neurologic abnormalities.[370] Cardiac complications include arrhythmias, myocardial infarction, and pulmonary embolism. Although these events may reflect primary cardiac disease, abnormalities in myocardial contractility and excitability may be triggered or compounded by hypervolemia, acidosis, hyperkalemia, and other metabolic sequelae of AKI.[371]

Hematologic Complications

Anemia develops rapidly in AKI and is usually mild and multifactorial in origin. Contributing factors include inhibition of erythropoiesis, hemolysis, bleeding, hemodilution, and reduced RBC survival time.[372-374] Prolongation of the bleeding time is also common, resulting from mild thrombocytopenia, platelet dysfunction, and clotting factor abnormalities (e.g., factor VIII dysfunction).

Nutritional and Gastrointestinal Complications

Malnutrition remains one of the most frustrating and troublesome complications of AKI. The majority of patients have net protein breakdown, which may exceed 200 g/day in individuals with catabolism.[375-377] Malnutrition is usually multifactorial and may reflect inability to eat, loss of appetite, and/or inadequate nutritional support; the catabolic nature of the underlying medical disorder (e.g., sepsis, rhabdomyolysis, trauma); nutrient losses in drainage fluids or dialysate; and increased breakdown as well as reduced synthesis of muscle protein and increased hepatic gluconeogenesis, probably through the actions of toxins, hormones (e.g., glucagon, parathyroid hormone), or other substances (e.g., proteases) that accumulate in AKI.[378-382] Nutrition may also be compromised by acute gastrointestinal hemorrhage, which complicates up to 15% of cases of AKI. Mild gastrointestinal bleeding is common (10% to 30%) and is usually due to stress ulceration of gastric or small intestinal mucosa.[383,384]

Infectious Complications

Infection is the most common and serious complication of AKI, occurring in 50% to 90% of cases and accounting for up to 75% of deaths.[13,341,385-387] It is unclear whether this high incidence of infection is due to a defect in host immune responses or repeated breaches of mucocutaneous barriers (e.g., intravenous cannulae, mechanical ventilation, bladder catheterization) resulting from therapeutic interventions.

Other Sequelae of Acute Kidney Injury

Protracted periods of severe AKI or short intervals of catabolic, anuric AKI often lead to the development of uremic syndrome. Clinical manifestations of uremic syndrome, in addition to those already listed, include pericarditis, pericardial effusion, and cardiac tamponade; gastrointestinal complications such as anorexia, nausea, vomiting, and ileus; and neuropsychiatric disturbances including lethargy, confusion, stupor, coma, agitation, psychosis, asterixis, myoclonus, hyperreflexia, restless leg syndrome, focal neurologic deficit, or seizures (see Table 30-12). The uremic toxin responsible for this syndrome has yet to be defined. Candidate molecules include urea, other products of nitrogen metabolism such as guanidine compounds, products of bacterial metabolism such as aromatic amines and skatoles, and other compounds that are inappropriately retained in the circulation in AKI or are underproduced, such as nitric oxide.[388]

Complications during Recovery from Acute Kidney Injury

A vigorous diuresis may complicate the recovery phase of AKI and precipitate intravascular volume depletion that results in a delay in recovery of renal function. This diuretic response probably reflects the combined effects of an osmotic diuresis induced by retained urea and other waste products, excretion of retained salt and water accumulated during AKI, and delayed recovery of tubular reabsorptive function relative to glomerular filtration, which leads to salt wasting.[389-392] Hypernatremia may also complicate this recovery phase if free water losses are not replenished or are inappropriately replaced by relatively hypertonic saline solutions. Hypokalemia, hypomagnesemia, hypophosphatemia, and hypocalcemia are rarer metabolic complications during recovery from AKI. Mild transient hypercalcemia is relatively frequent during recovery and appears to be a consequence of delayed resolution of secondary hyperparathyroidism. In addition, hypercalcemia may complicate recovery from rhabdomyolysis because of mobilization of sequestered Ca^{2+} from injured muscle.[393]

Prevention and Management of Acute Kidney Injury

Specific treatment is not available for the majority of forms of AKI. As a result, management focuses on interventions to prevent the development of AKI when possible and on provision of supportive therapy to ameliorate derangements of fluid and electrolyte homeostasis and prevent uremic complications. In advanced AKI, renal replacement therapy is often required. The ultimate goals of management are to prevent death, facilitate recovery of kidney function, and minimize the risk of CKD.

Prerenal Acute Kidney Injury

Prerenal AKI is defined as hemodynamically mediated kidney dysfunction that is rapidly reversible following normalization of renal perfusion.[28] In patients in whom prerenal AKI develops as the result of intravascular volume depletion, treatment consists of restoration of normal circulating blood volume. The optimal composition of administered fluids in patients with hypovolemic prerenal AKI depends on the source of fluid loss and associated electrolyte and acid-base disturbances. The initial management usually consists of volume resuscitation with an isotonic electrolyte solution such as 0.9% saline. RBC transfusion should be used for hemorrhagic hypovolemia if there is ongoing bleeding, if the patient is in hemodynamically unstable condition, or if the blood hemoglobin concentration is dangerously low.

The relative merits of colloid and crystalloid resuscitation fluids in the management of nonhemorrhagic renal, extrarenal, and third-space fluid losses are controversial, with advocates of the use of colloids positing that they are more effective at restoring circulating blood volume due to greater retention in the intravascular compartment. However, randomized controlled trials and meta-analyses comparing crystalloid with colloid replacement for resuscitation in critically ill patients have not confirmed this theoretical benefit and have suggested an increased risk of adverse outcomes with the use of some colloid formulations.[394-399] In a meta-analysis of 55 trials involving 3504 patients randomly assigned to treatment with albumin or crystalloid, there was no evidence of either improved outcomes or increased mortality or other complications associated with albumin administration.[400] These results were subsequently confirmed in a multicenter randomized controlled trial involving nearly 7000 patients that investigated fluid resuscitation in hypovolemic medical and surgical ICU patients; 28-day survival, development of single- or multiple-organ failure, and duration of hospitalization were similar in the group receiving albumin and the group receiving saline.[401] Although specific data on the development of AKI were not provided, the need for renal replacement therapy was similar in the patients receiving saline and those given albumin. However, in a post hoc analysis of the data for patients with traumatic brain injury, albumin resuscitation was associated with increased mortality risk.[402]

The use of synthetic colloid solutions has been proposed as an alternative to albumin administration; however, the use of hydroxyethyl starch preparations has been associated with an increased risk of AKI. In a multicenter randomized controlled trial comparing fluid resuscitation with hydroxyethyl starch and with a 3% gelatin solution in 129 patients with sepsis, the use of hydroxyethyl starch was associated with a more than twofold increased risk of AKI.[397] A subsequent meta-analysis confirmed the increased risk of AKI associated with hydroxyethyl starch across 34 studies that encompassed 2604 individuals.[398] Based on these data demonstrating no benefit and a potential increased risk of AKI with colloid use, along with the greater cost of these solutions, their routine use for volume resuscitation in patients with hypovolemia and sepsis is not advisable. In particular, hydroxyethyl starch solutions should be used only sparingly, with regular monitoring of renal function, and the risk of hyperoncotic renal failure should be minimized by the concomitant use of appropriate crystalloid solutions.[397,398]

After initial volume resuscitation, replacement of ongoing urine and gastrointestinal fluid losses should generally be accomplished using hypotonic crystalloid solutions (e.g., 0.45% saline); even though urinary and gastrointestinal losses may vary greatly in composition, they are usually hypotonic to plasma. The volume and electrolyte content of replacement solutions, as well as patient serum electrolyte levels and acid-base status, should be closely monitored to guide adjustments in the composition of the replacement fluids. Although the potassium content of gastric juices tends to be low, concomitant urinary potassium losses may be quite high as the result of metabolic alkalosis.

Heart Failure

The management of prerenal AKI in the setting of heart failure depends on the clinical setting and cause of the heart failure. In patients with congestive heart failure in whom AKI has developed as a result of excessive diuresis, withholding of diuretics and cautious volume replacement may be sufficient to restore kidney function. In acute decompensated heart failure (ADHF), AKI may develop despite worsening volume overload; intensification of diuretic therapy is often required for treatment of pulmonary vascular congestion. Although diuretic therapy may exacerbate prerenal AKI, it can also result in improvement in kidney function via several postulated mechanisms: (1) by decreasing ventricular distension, which results in a shift from the descending limb to the ascending limb of the Starling curve and improvement in myocardial contractility; (2) by decreasing venous congestion[403-406]; and (3) by diminishing intraabdominal pressure.[407,408] Additional therapies for ADHF in the setting of AKI include inotropic support, administration of vasodilators for afterload reduction, and mechanical support, including intraaortic balloon pumps and ventricular assist devices. The use of invasive hemodynamic monitoring in ADHF has been controversial; although it is often employed to guide pharmacologic management, clinical data have not demonstrated improved renal outcomes when treatment is based on readings from pulmonary artery catheters.[409] The role of isolated ultrafiltration in ADHF is also controversial. Although negative fluid balance can be achieved more readily using extracorporeal ultrafiltration than conventional diuretic therapy, studies have not demonstrated differences in kidney function or survival.[410,411]

Liver Failure and Hepatorenal Syndrome

Although volume-responsive prerenal azotemia is common in patients with advanced liver disease, differentiation from hepatorenal syndrome and intrinsic AKI may be difficult.[320,327,412-414] Patients with liver failure typically have total-body sodium overload, with peripheral edema and ascites; however, true hypovolemia or reduced effective systemic arterial blood volume is often an important contributory factor in the development AKI. The underlying pathophysiology of salt and water retention in cirrhosis involves multiple pathways. Portal hypertension leads directly to ascites formation, whereas splanchnic and peripheral vasodilatation result in a state of relative arterial underfilling, which activates neurohumoral vasoconstrictors that produce intrarenal vasoconstriction, salt and water retention, and decreased GFR.[415,416] Volume-responsive AKI may develop in the setting of excessive diuresis, increased gastrointestinal losses (often as a result of therapy for hepatic encephalopathy), rapid drainage of ascites, or spontaneous bacterial peritonitis. Worsening hepatic function is often associated with diuretic resistance and progressive or precipitous worsening of kidney function. It has been postulated that an inadequate increase in cardiac output in response to the fall in peripheral vascular resistance may be central to the development of hepatorenal syndrome.[417]

Differentiation between volume-responsive prerenal AKI and hepatorenal syndrome is based on the clinical response to volume loading. The optimal fluid for volume expansion in this setting has been controversial. Recent expert opinion has advocated the use of hyperoncotic (20% or 25%) albumin at a dosage of 1 g/kg/day[321,418]; however, there are no rigorously collected data supporting this regimen compared with volume expansion with isotonic crystalloid solutions. More data are available regarding the use of albumin infusion to prevent renal dysfunction in patients undergoing large-volume (>5 L) paracentesis[327,419,420] and in the treatment of spontaneous bacterial peritonitis.[421] In a randomized controlled trial, patients who received infusion of 10 g of albumin per liter of drained ascites experienced less activation of the renin-angiotensin system and a significantly lower rate of worsening of kidney function than patients who did not receive albumin infusion.[419] In a subsequent study, albumin infusion was superior to administration of either dextran or gelatin solutions in preventing renal dysfunction after large-volume paracentesis.[420] Current recommendations are to infuse 6 to 8 g of albumin per liter of ascites drained when paracentesis volume exceeds 5 L. In a randomized controlled trial comparing antibiotics alone with antibiotics plus albumin in patients with spontaneous bacterial peritonitis, infusion of 1.5 g/kg of albumin at initiation of treatment and an additional 1 g/kg on the third day of treatment was associated with reduced rates of both AKI and mortality,[421] although the benefit appears to be restricted to patients in whom the serum creatinine concentration is more than 1 mg/dL, the blood urea nitrogen level is above 30 mg/dL, or the total bilirubin level is more than 4 mg/dL.[422]

Definitive treatment of hepatorenal syndrome requires restoration of hepatic function, usually achieved through liver transplantation.[320,418] The role of peritoneovenous shunting (e.g., LeVeen and Denver shunts) in hepatorenal syndrome

has been inadequately studied. In a subset of 33 patients with hepatorenal syndrome included in a randomized trial comparing placement of peritoneovenous shunts with medical therapy, shunting was not associated with improved survival.[423] These data need to be interpreted with caution because of the small sample size and because data on improvement in kidney function were not reported. In addition, due to poor long-term patency rates and high rates of complications, particularly encephalopathy, peritoneovenous shunts have largely been supplanted by transjugular portosystemic shunts. Transjugular portosystemic shunts have been demonstrated to provide better control of ascites than sequential paracentesis[424-427] and, in one series, lower rates of hepatorenal syndrome,[425] albeit with a higher risk of encephalopathy.[428] In a small case series, transjugular portosystemic shunting has been reported to be effective as primary therapy for hepatorenal syndrome,[429] but it has not been evaluated in a randomized trial.[418]

Pharmacologic therapy with vasoconstrictors, when combined with albumin infusion, has been associated with improvement in kidney function in patients with hepatorenal syndrome.[418,430] Agents that have shown benefit include norepinephrine,[431] a combination of octreotide and midodrine,[432-435] and the V_1 vasopressin receptor agonist terlipressin,[328,329,436] although only terlipressin has been evaluated in randomized controlled trials. In a meta-analysis of five published randomized trials, treatment with terlipressin was associated with an odds ratio for reversal of hepatorenal syndrome of 8.1 (95% confidence interval = 3.5 to 18.6) compared with treatment with albumin infusion alone, but did not significantly improve survival.[437]

Intrinsic Acute Kidney Injury

General Principles

Strategies to prevent intrinsic AKI vary based on the specific cause of kidney injury. Optimization of cardiovascular function and restoration of intravascular volume status are key interventions to minimize the risk that prerenal AKI will evolve into ischemic ATN. There is compelling evidence that aggressive intravascular volume expansion dramatically reduces the incidence of ATN after major surgery or trauma, in burns, and in cholera.[225,394,438,439] AKI due to sepsis is common and is associated with mortality rates as high as 80%.[18,387,440] Recent studies have emphasized two salient features of successful management of sepsis that may be of importance in the prevention of AKI. First, early goal-directed resuscitation to defined hemodynamic targets (mean arterial pressure of >65 mm Hg, central venous pressure of 10 to 12 mm Hg, urine output of >0.5 mL/kg/hr, central venous oxygen saturation of >70%) using a combination of crystalloid solutions, RBC transfusion, and vasopressors resulted in a significant reduction in organ dysfunction and mortality in patients with sepsis syndrome.[441] Although the therapeutic goals chosen in this study were to a degree arbitrary, these findings emphasize the imperative for early and aggressive volume resuscitation and hemodynamic stabilization in the management of patients with sepsis syndrome. Second, in another study of critically ill patients, intensive insulin therapy to maintain a glucose level of 80 to 110 mg/dL, compared with conventional management to maintain the glucose concentration between 180 and 220 mg/dL, resulted in decreases in AKI, defined based on either the change in serum creatinine concentration or the need for renal replacement therapy.[442,443] Although these strategies have been incorporated into the Surviving Sepsis Campaign,[444,445] it should be recognized that the data supporting both early goal-directed therapy and intensive glycemic control are derived primarily from single-center clinical trials. Early goal-directed therapy has not been evaluated in a multicenter trial; the benefit of tight glycemic control was not confirmed in a multicenter trial of intensive therapy to achieve a target glucose level of approximately 80 to 110 mg/dL compared with more conventional therapy designed to maintain the blood glucose level below 180 mg/dL.[446]

Intravascular volume depletion has been identified as a risk factor for ATN resulting from exposure to iodinated contrast material, rhabdomyolysis, hemolysis, cisplatin, amphotericin B, multiple myeloma, aminoglycosides, and other nephrotoxins; crystal-associated AKI related to acyclovir and acute urate nephropathy; and AKI stemming from hypercalcemia.[82,237,265,273,343,365,439,447-449] Restoration of intravascular volume status prevents the development of experimental and human ATN in many of these clinical settings.

Avoidance of potentially nephrotoxic medications or insults in high-risk patients and settings is also important to reduce the risk for ATN. Specifically, in patients with advanced cardiac and/or liver disease, in whom renal perfusion may be diminished, use of selective or nonselective NSAIDs that inhibit the production of vasodilatory prostaglandins may exacerbate intrarenal vasoconstriction and precipitate AKI.[450-454] Diuretics, NSAIDs (including selective cyclooxygenase-2 inhibitors), ACE inhibitors, angiotensin receptor blockers, and other inhibitors of the renin-angiotensin-aldosterone system should be used with caution in patients with suspected absolute or effective hypovolemia or in patients with renovascular disease, because they may convert reversible prerenal AKI to intrinsic ischemic ATN. The combined use of agents that block the renin-angiotensin-aldosterone system, diuretics, and NSAIDs has been identified as a risk factor for AKI, particularly in patients with heart failure, liver failure, or other causes of reduced baseline renal perfusion.[455,456]

Careful monitoring of circulating drug levels appears to reduce the incidence of AKI associated with aminoglycoside antibiotics and calcineurin inhibitors.[457-459] The observation that the antimicrobial efficacy of aminoglycosides persists in tissues even after the drug has been cleared from the circulation (postantibiotic killing) has led to the use of once-daily dosing with these agents. Dosing regimens that provide higher peak drug levels but less-frequent administration appear to produce comparable antimicrobial activity and less nephrotoxicity than older conventional dosing regimens.[70,459-461] Nephrotoxicity of drugs may also be reduced through changes in formulation. For example, the use of lipid-encapsulated formulations of amphotericin B may decrease the risk of amphotericin-induced AKI.[462]

Prevention of Contrast Medium–Induced Acute Kidney Injury

The preventive role of intravascular volume resuscitation has been best demonstrated in the setting of AKI caused by administration iodinated contrast agents. A series of clinical trials have established that the provision of intravenous fluids before and after the administration of iodinated contrast

media in high-risk patients diminishes the risk of contrast medium–induced AKI.[463,464] Multiple studies have sought to identify the optimal intravenous fluid regimen. Prophylactic infusion of half-normal saline (1 mL/kg for 12 hours before and after the procedure requiring the contrast agent) is more effective in preventing AKI than either mannitol or furosemide, both of which should be avoided in this setting.[465,466] In a large randomized trial, administration of isotonic saline significantly reduced the incidence of contrast nephropathy following coronary angiography compared with use of half-normal saline, with a particular benefit noted in diabetic patients and those receiving large volumes of contrast agent.[463] More recently, clinical trials have compared isotonic sodium bicarbonate with isotonic sodium chloride, and results have been conflicting.[467-470] As a result, isotonic fluid comprised of either sodium bicarbonate or sodium chloride is considered the standard of care for the prevention of contrast agent–induced AKI. For hospitalized patients, a regimen of isotonic saline or sodium bicarbonate at 1 mL/kg/hr administered for 12 hours before and 12 hours after the procedure requiring the contrast agent is recommended. An alternative regimen that may be more feasible in the outpatient setting is 3 mL/kg/hr for 1 hour before the procedure followed by 1 to 1.5 mL/kg/hr for 6 hours after the procedure.

N-Acetylcysteine is an antioxidant with vasodilatory properties that has been investigated in numerous clinical trials for the prevention of contrast medium–induced AKI. The rationale for the use of N-acetylcysteine in this setting relates to its capacity to scavenge reactive oxygen species, reduce the depletion of glutathione, and stimulate the production of vasodilatory mediators, including nitric oxide.[471,472] Clinical trials of oral and intravenous N-acetylcysteine have yielded conflicting findings.[473-478] N-Acetylcysteine was initially administered at a dosage of 600 mg twice daily,[479] but studies have suggested greater efficacy with higher dosages of up to 1200 mg twice daily.[480,481] Although N-acetylcysteine should not be used in lieu of intravenous fluids for the prevention of contrast medium–induced AKI, it is safe and inexpensive in its oral form and therefore can be employed until further studies clarify its role.

Trials of other pharmacologic interventions, including furosemide, dopamine, fenoldopam, calcium channel blockers, and mannitol, have failed to demonstrate significant benefit and, in some cases, have found such drugs to be associated with an increased risk of contrast medium–induced AKI.[482-487] Studies of the benefit of natriuretic peptides, aminophylline, theophylline, statins, and ascorbic acid have also yielded conflicting results.[488-497] Given the absence of convincing data as to the efficacy of these interventions as well as potential safety concerns with the use of natriuretic peptides, aminophylline, and theophylline in patients with cardiovascular disease, their routine use is not recommended.[496]

Renal replacement therapies for the prevention of contrast agent–induced AKI have been largely ineffective, and in some instances the use of prophylactic hemodialysis has been associated with harm.[498-500] Interpretation of the results of studies of hemofiltration for prevention of contrast medium–induced AKI are confounded by their consideration of change in serum creatinine level as an endpoint, since hemofiltration lowers serum creatinine concentrations.[501,502] Given the risks associated with intravenous line placement and the procedures themselves, along with lack of definitive demonstration of benefit, use of dialysis or hemofiltration to prevent contrast medium–induced AKI is not currently recommended.[503]

Over the past 25 years, there has been considerable progress in the development of less nephrotoxic contrast agents.[504] The use of lower-osmolality contrast agents in place of the older and more nephrotoxic high-osmolality agents has resulted in a decreased incidence of contrast medium–induced AKI.[505,506] Data regarding the added benefit associated with the isoosmolal radiocontrast agent iodixanol has been less consistent.[507-513] Until more definitive trials are available, the use of either lower-osmolality or isoosmolal contrast media in the lowest possible dose in patients at increased risk is advised.

Prevention of Other Forms of Intrinsic Acute Kidney Injury

Allopurinol (10 mg/kg/day in three divided doses, to a maximum of 800 mg/day) is useful for limiting uric acid generation in patients at high risk for acute urate nephropathy; however, AKI can develop despite the use of allopurinol, probably through the toxic actions of hypoxanthine crystals on tubule function.[265,343,363,365,514,515] In settings in which rates of uric acid generation are high, such as tumor lysis syndrome, the use of recombinant urate oxidase (rasburicase, 0.05 to 0.2 mg/kg) may be more effective. Rasburicase catalyzes the degradation of uric acid to allantoin and has been shown to be effective both as prophylaxis and as treatment for acute uric acid–mediated tumor lysis syndrome and to prevent the development of AKI due to tumor lysis syndrome–associated hyperuricemia.[343,515-518] In oligoanuric patients, prophylactic hemodialysis may be used for short-term reduction of uric acid levels.

Amifostine, an organic thiophosphate, has been demonstrated to ameliorate cisplatin nephrotoxicity in patients with solid organ or hematologic malignancies.[519-522] *N*-Acetylcysteine limits acetaminophen-induced renal injury if given within 24 hours of ingestion, and dimercaprol, a chelating agent, may prevent heavy metal nephrotoxicity.[523,524] Ethanol inhibits the metabolism of ethylene glycol to oxalic acid and other toxic metabolites, but it has been largely replaced by fomepizole, an inhibitor of alcohol dehydrogenase that decreases production of ethylene glycol metabolites and prevents the development of AKI.[525-528]

Pharmacologic Therapy for Acute Tubular Necrosis

During the past two decades there has been extensive investigation into the pathogenesis of AKI using experimental animal models and cultured cells. These studies have resulted in substantial advances in our understanding of the pathophysiology of ATN in humans and have led to the discovery of an array of potentially novel targets for the treatment of this common and serious disease. However, several interventions shown to ameliorate AKI in animals have failed to prove effective in humans with ATN. There are many possible reasons for the lack of success in translating effective therapies for AKI from animal models to clinical practice. A principal obstacle is the difficulty in identifying the incipient stage of ATN before elevations in the serum creatinine concentration or clinical evidence of decreased urine output. Over the past decade, several serum and urinary biomarkers have been investigated for their ability to identify AKI in its earliest stages and differentiate ATN from volume-responsive

AKI.[9,10] Work in this area may facilitate the identification of those patients most likely to respond to treatments that have been found to be effective in animal models.

DOPAMINE

Low-dose dopamine (1 to 3 mg/kg/min) had been widely advocated for the management of oliguric AKI.[529-531] In experimental animals and healthy human volunteers, low-dose dopamine increases renal blood flow and, to a lesser extent, GFR. However, low-dose dopamine has not been demonstrated to prevent or alter the course of ischemic or nephrotoxic ATN in prospective clinical trials.[532-536] This absence of clinical benefit may relate to differences in the hemodynamic response to low-dose dopamine in patients with renal disease compared with healthy individuals. In contrast to the reduction in renal resistive index associated with low-dose dopamine in critically ill patients without kidney disease, dopamine infusion is associated with an increase in renal resistance in patients with AKI.[537] Moreover, dopamine, even at low dosages, is potentially toxic in critically ill patients and can induce tachyarrhythmias, myocardial ischemia, and extravasation necrosis.[537] Thus, the routine administration of low-dose dopamine to ameliorate or reverse the course of AKI is not justified based on the balance of experimental and clinical evidence.[538,539]

FENOLDOPAM

Fenoldopam is a selective postsynaptic dopamine agonist that acts on dopamine D_1 receptors and mediates more potent renal vasodilatation and natriuresis than dopamine.[540] However, fenoldopam is a potent antihypertensive agent and causes hypotension by decreasing peripheral vascular resistance. Several small studies suggested that fenoldopam might reduce the incidence of AKI in high-risk clinical situations[541,542]; however, a subsequent larger randomized trial comparing fenoldopam with standard hydration in patients undergoing invasive angiographic procedures found no benefit with regard to decreasing the incidence of contrast medium–induced AKI.[485] In another large randomized controlled trial, fenoldopam administration failed to reduce mortality or the need for renal replacement therapy in ICU patients with early ATN.[543] Therefore, there is currently no clinical role for fenoldopam in the prevention or treatment of AKI.

NATRIURETIC PEPTIDES

Atrial natriuretic peptide (ANP) is a 28–amino-acid polypeptide synthesized in cardiac atrial muscle.[544,545] ANP augments GFR by triggering afferent arteriolar vasodilatation and constriction of the efferent arteriole.[546,547] In addition, ANP inhibits sodium transport and lowers oxygen requirements in several nephron segments.[548,549] Synthetic analogs of ANP showed promise in the management of ATN in the laboratory setting; however, these benefits in animal models of AKI have failed to translate into clinical benefit in humans. A large multicenter, prospective, randomized, placebo-controlled trial of anaritide, a synthetic analog of ANP, in patients with ATN failed to show clinically significant improvement in dialysis-free survival or overall mortality,[550] although there was an improvement in dialysis-free survival in oliguric patients. This benefit in oliguric patients was not confirmed in a subsequent prospective study.[551] It has been suggested that the absence of benefit may be related both to the relatively late initiation of therapy and to the effect of ANP on systemic blood pressure. In a subsequent pilot study, low-dose recombinant ANP administration in high-risk cardiac surgery patients was associated with a reduction in the requirement for postoperative renal replacement therapy.[552] Until these results are confirmed in a larger multicenter trial, the use of ANP in this setting cannot be recommended. Trials of ANP for the prevention of contrast medium–induced AKI have generated mixed results.[493,494] Urodilatin (Ularitide) is a natriuretic pro-ANP fragment produced within the kidney. In a small randomized trial, urodilatin did not reduce the need for dialysis in patients with AKI.[553] A recent meta-analysis of studies investigating the use of ANP for the treatment of AKI concluded that the paucity of high-quality studies precluded a determination of the effects of this therapy.[554]

LOOP DIURETICS

High-dose intravenous diuretics to increase urine output are commonly prescribed for patients with oliguric AKI. Although this strategy assists in volume management and minimizes the risk of progressive volume overload, there is no evidence that diuretic therapy alters the natural history of AKI or improves mortality or dialysis-free survival. In a retrospective analysis, diuretic therapy was associated with an increased risk of death and nonrecovery of renal function.[555] These risks, however, were restricted to patients who did not respond to diuretic administration with increased urine volume; in diuretic-responsive patients, outcomes were similar to those in untreated patients. In a prospective randomized trial, high-dose intravenous furosemide augmented urine output but did not alter the outcome of established AKI.[556] In a post hoc analysis of data from the Fluid and Catheter Treatment Trial, a positive fluid balance after AKI in patients with acute lung injury was strongly associated with mortality, whereas diuretic therapy was associated with improved 60-day patient survival.[557] Given the risks of loop diuretic use in AKI, including irreversible ototoxicity and exacerbation of prerenal AKI, these agents should be used solely to facilitate the management of extracellular volume overload.[558]

MANNITOL

The osmotic diuretic mannitol, which also has renal vasodilatory and oxygen free radical–scavenging properties, has been investigated as a preventive treatment for AKI.[465,559] No adequate data exist to support the routine administration of mannitol to oliguric patients. Moreover, when administered to severely oliguric or anuric patients, mannitol may trigger expansion of intravascular volume and pulmonary edema, as well as severe hyponatremia due to an osmotic shift of water from the intracellular to the intravascular space.[465,560-563]

Management of Other Causes of Intrinsic Acute Kidney Injury

ACUTE VASCULITIS AND ACUTE GLOMERULAR DISEASE

The management of acute vasculitis involving the kidney and acute glomerular disease is covered in detail in Chapters 31 though 33. AKI caused by acute glomerulonephritis or vasculitis may respond to corticosteroids, alkylating agents, and plasmapheresis depending on the primary cause of the disease. Plasma exchange is useful in the treatment of sporadic TTP and possibly sporadic HUS in adults.[564,565] The role of plasmapheresis in treatment of the drug-induced thrombotic microangiopathies is less certain, and removal of the offending agent is the most important initial therapeutic maneuver.[255,566,567] Postdiarrheal HUS in children is usually managed conservatively, because evidence suggests that early antibiotic therapy may actually promote the development of HUS.[568] Hypertension and AKI associated with scleroderma may be exquisitely sensitive to treatment with ACE inhibitors.[569-571]

ACUTE KIDNEY INJURY IN MULTIPLE MYELOMA

Early studies suggested that plasmapheresis may be of benefit in AKI due to myeloma cast nephropathy.[572,273] Clearance of circulating light chains with concomitant chemotherapy to decrease the rate of production had been postulated to reverse renal injury in patients with circulating light chains, heavy Bence Jones proteinuria, and AKI. A recent relatively large randomized controlled trial compared plasma exchange and standard chemotherapy with chemotherapy alone. Although the study did not demonstrate improvement with plasma exchange with regard to a composite outcome of death, dialysis dependence, or GFR less than 30 mL/min at 6 months, the study was inadequately powered to definitively exclude a clinical benefit, and there was a trend toward improved outcomes with plasmapheresis.[573]

ACUTE INTERSTITIAL NEPHRITIS

Acute interstitial nephritis is a relatively common cause of AKI and in the majority of cases is due to an allergic response to a medication.[574] The initial therapeutic step in acute interstitial nephritis is discontinuation of the offending medication or treatment of the probable inciting factor if not drug induced. Data on the efficacy of corticosteroids derive from small observational studies that have yielded highly discordant results. Although some studies suggest that early use of corticosteroids (i.e., before significant renal damage and within 7 to 14 days of discontinuation of the offending medication)[575] may be beneficial, other studies demonstrate no clear evidence of efficacy.[229] There have been no large prospective randomized clinical trials to date investigating the role of corticosteroids in the treatment of acute interstitial nephritis. Because corticosteroids are associated with a series of potentially serious side effects, their use should be considered on a case-by-case basis. If corticosteroid therapy is being considered and no patient-related contraindications exist, one potential regimen is that used in a recent study consisting of the intravenous administration of methylprednisolone (250 to 500 mg/day) for 3 to 4 days followed by oral prednisone at a dosage of 1 mg/kg/day tapered over 8 to 12 weeks.[575] However, there are no data supporting the superiority of this specific approach over others. Mycophenolate mofetil has also been investigated as a therapeutic agent for acute interstitial nephritis. In a study of eight patients with acute interstitial nephritis, six experienced improvement in renal function with mycophenolate mofetil therapy, whereas two showed stabilization of renal function.[576] Although this small case series suggests a possible role for mycophenolate mofetil in the treatment of acute interstitial nephritis, additional data are needed to confirm its efficacy for this indication.

Postrenal Acute Kidney Injury

The principle underlying the management of postrenal AKI is the prompt relief of urinary tract obstruction. This topic is reviewed extensively in Chapter 37. Urethral or bladder neck obstruction may be relieved with transurethral or suprapubic placement of a bladder catheter. Similarly, ureteric obstruction may be relieved in the short term by placement of percutaneous nephrostomy tubes or by cystoscopic placement of ureteral stents. Following the initial relief of obstruction most patients experience a physiologic diuresis, caused by the excretion of volume and solutes retained during the period of renal obstruction, that resolves after several days; however, approximately 5% of patients have a more prolonged diuretic phase because of delayed recovery of tubule function relative to GFR, which results in a salt-wasting syndrome, and intravenous fluid replacement may be required to maintain blood pressure.[391,392,577] Following initial relief of obstruction, urologic evaluation is required for definitive evaluation and management of the underlying cause of obstruction.

Nondialytic Supportive Management of Acute Kidney Injury

Metabolic complications such as intravascular volume overload, hyperkalemia, hyperphosphatemia, and metabolic acidosis are common in oliguric AKI, and preventive measures should be implemented beginning at initial diagnosis (Table 30-13). Adequate nutrition should be provided to meet caloric requirements and minimize catabolism. In addition, all medications that are normally excreted by the kidney need to be adjusted based on the severity of renal impairment.

After correction of intravascular volume deficits, salt and water intake should be adjusted to match ongoing losses (urinary and gastrointestinal losses, losses from drainage sites, insensible losses). Intravascular volume overload can usually be managed by restriction of salt and water intake and by judicious use of diuretics. High doses of loop diuretics (e.g., the equivalent of 200 mg of furosemide administered as an intravenous bolus infusion or 20 mg/hr as a continuous infusion) or combination therapy with both thiazide and loop diuretics may be required. If an adequate diuresis cannot be attained, further use of diuretics should be discontinued to minimize the risk of complications such as ototoxicity. Fluid administration should be closely monitored to avoid progressive volume overload. Although there is a strong association between progressive fluid overload and mortality risk in patients with AKI,[578-580] a causal relationship has not been definitively established, and volume overload may be a surrogate for hemodynamic instability and capillary leak. Conservative fluid management has, however, been demonstrated to result in improved outcomes in critically ill patients with lung failure.[581] Ultrafiltration or dialysis may be required for volume management when conservative measures fail.

Hyponatremia associated with a fall in effective serum osmolality can usually be corrected by restriction of water intake. Conversely, hypernatremia is treated by administration of water, hypotonic saline solutions, or hypotonic dextrose-containing solutions (the latter are effectively hypotonic because dextrose is rapidly metabolized).

Mild hyperkalemia (<5.5 mEq/L of potassium) should be managed initially by restriction of dietary potassium intake

TABLE 30-13 Supportive Management of Acute Kidney Injury	
MANAGEMENT ISSUE	**TREATMENT**
Intravascular volume overload	Restriction of salt (<1-1.5 g/day) and water (<1 L/day) Consideration of diuretic therapy Ultrafiltration
Hyponatremia	Restriction of oral and intravenous free water
Hyperkalemia	Restriction of dietary potassium Discontinuation of K^+ supplements or K^+-sparing diuretics K^+-binding resin Loop diuretics Glucose (50 mL of 50%) + insulin (10-15 units regular) intravenously Sodium bicarbonate (50-100 mEq intravenously) Calcium gluconate (10 mL of 10% solution over 5 min) Renal replacement therapy
Metabolic acidosis	Restriction of dietary protein Sodium bicarbonate (if HCO_3^- <15 mEq/L) Renal replacement therapy
Hyperphosphatemia	Restriction of dietary phosphate intake Phosphate-binding agents (calcium carbonate, calcium acetate, sevelamer, lanthanum)
Hypocalcemia	Calcium carbonate (if symptomatic or sodium bicarbonate to be administered)
Hypermagnesemia	Discontinuation of magnesium-containing antacids
Nutrition	Restriction of dietary protein (<0.8g/kg/day up to 1.5 g/kg/day for patients undergoing continuous renal replacement therapy) Provision of 25-30 kcal/day Enteral route of nutrition preferred
Drug dosage	Adjustment of all dosages for glomerular filtration rate and renal replacement modality

and elimination of potassium supplements and potassium-sparing diuretics. More severe degrees of hyperkalemia (5.5 to 6.5 mEq/L of potassium) can usually be controlled with administration of sodium polystyrene sulfonate, a potassium-binding resin, to enhance gastrointestinal potassium losses. Although this resin has been widely used for decades, concerns have been raised regarding its safety, particularly when it is administered in 70% sorbitol, due to reports of bowel necrosis.[582,583] Loop diuretics can also increase potassium excretion in diuretic-responsive patients. Emergency measures must be employed in patients with more severe hyperkalemia and in patients with electrocardiographic manifestations of hyperkalemia. Intravenous insulin (10 to 20 units of regular insulin) promotes potassium entry into cells and lowers extracellular potassium concentration within 15 to 30 minutes, with an effect that lasts for several hours.[584,585] Concomitant administration of intravenous dextrose (25 to 50 g over 30 to 60 minutes) is required to prevent hypoglycemia in patients who do not have hyperglycemia. Administration of β-adrenergic agonists, such as inhaled albuterol (10 to 20 mg by nebulizer), also promotes rapid potassium uptake into the intracellular compartment.[584] Although sodium bicarbonate also stimulates potassium uptake into the intracellular compartment, this effect is not sufficiently rapid for sodium bicarbonate to be clinically useful for the emergent management of hyperkalemia.[585] In patients with severe hyperkalemia with concomitant electrocardiographic manifestations the intravenous administration of calcium will antagonize the cardiac and neuromuscular effects of hyperkalemia and is a valuable emergency temporizing measure. Intravenous calcium must be used with caution, however, if there is concomitant severe hyperphosphatemia or evidence of digitalis toxicity. Emergent dialysis is indicated if hyperkalemia is resistant to these measures.

The treatment of metabolic acidosis is dependent upon the clinical setting and cause. As a general rule, metabolic acidosis does not require treatment unless the serum HCO_3 concentration falls below 15 mEq/L or the pH is lower than 7.15 to 7.20. In patients with AKI in whom metabolic acidosis is due to the underlying renal failure, more severe acidosis can be corrected by either oral or intravenous bicarbonate administration. Initial rates of replacement should be based on estimates of HCO_3 deficit and adjusted thereafter according to serum levels. In patients with underlying lactic acidosis, the role of bicarbonate therapy is controversial, and the primary focus of therapy should be on correction of the underlying cause.[586-589] Patients treated with intravenous bicarbonate need to be monitored for complications of therapy, including metabolic alkalosis, hypocalcemia, hypokalemia, hypernatremia, and volume overload.

Hyperphosphatemia can usually be controlled by restricting dietary phosphate intake and administering gastrointestinal phosphate binders (e.g., aluminum hydroxide, calcium salts, sevelamer carbonate, or lanthanum carbonate). Hypocalcemia does not usually require treatment unless it is severe, as may occur in patients with rhabdomyolysis or pancreatitis or after administration of bicarbonate. Hyperuricemia is usually mild in acute renal failure (<15 mg/dL) and does not require specific intervention. Severe hyperuricemia secondary to cell lysis may be managed by blocking xanthine oxidase with allopurinol or by enhancing degradation with recombinant uricase.

Patients with AKI represent a heterogenous group, and individualized nutritional management is required, especially in critically ill patients receiving renal replacement therapy in whom protein catabolic rates can exceed 1.5 g/kg body weight per day day.[376,377,379,380,590,591] The objective of nutritional management in AKI is to provide sufficient calories to preserve lean body mass, avoid starvation ketoacidosis, and promote healing and tissue repair while minimizing production of nitrogenous waste. If the duration of renal insufficiency is likely to be short and the patient is not extremely catabolic, then dietary protein should be restricted to approximately 0.8 g/kg body weight per day. Protein intake should not be restricted in patients in whom AKI is likely to be prolonged, who are in a hypercatabolic state, or who are receiving renal replacement therapy. Protein intake in these patients should be at least 1.4 to 1.5 g/kg body weight per day.[376,377,590,591] Total caloric intake should not exceed 35 kcal/kg body weight per day and will typically be in the range of 25 to 30 kcal/kg body weight per day.[376,377,590,591] Management of nutrition is easier in nonoliguric patients and after institution of dialysis. Vigorous parenteral hyperalimentation has been claimed to improve prognosis in AKI; however, a consistent benefit has yet to be demonstrated. The enteral route of nutrition is preferred, because it avoids the morbidity associated with parenteral nutrition while providing support to intestinal function.[379]

Water-soluble vitamins and trace elements should be supplemented in patients receiving renal replacement therapy.[590,591]

Severe anemia is generally managed with blood transfusion. Transfusion is usually not required for patients with a hemoglobin level above 7 g/dL.[592] The role of erythropoiesis-stimulating agents in AKI has not been well studied.[593] Patients with AKI or other acute illness are relatively resistant to the effect of these agents. In randomized controlled trials involving critically ill patients, recombinant human erythropoietin decreased transfusion requirement but had no effect on other outcomes.[594,595] Uremic bleeding usually responds to desmopressin, correction of anemia, estrogens, or dialysis.

Dosages of drugs that are excreted by the kidney must be adjusted for renal impairment and the use of renal replacement therapy.[596-599] Whenever possible pharmacokinetic monitoring should be employed to ensure appropriate drug dosing, especially for agents with narrow therapeutic windows (see Chapter 63). In addition to careful monitoring for toxicity of agents that are normally excreted by the kidney, careful attention must be paid to dosing of antibiotics and other drugs removed by renal replacement therapy to ensure that therapeutic drug levels are achieved, particularly in patients receiving renal replacement therapy of augmented intensity.

Renal Replacement Therapy in Acute Kidney Injury

Renal replacement therapy (RRT) is the generic term for the multiple modalities of dialysis and hemofiltration employed in the management of kidney failure. Although kidney transplantation is also a form of RRT for end-stage renal disease (ESRD), transplantation does not play a role in the management of AKI given the potential for recovery of kidney function. RRT facilitates the management of patients with AKI, allowing correction of acid-base and electrolyte disturbances, amelioration of volume overload, and removal of uremic waste products. Although RRT can forestall or reverse the life-threatening complications of uremia associated with severe and prolonged AKI, it does not hasten and can potentially delay the recovery of kidney function in patients with AKI[600] and can be associated with potentially life-threatening complications.[601] Despite more than 60 years of research and clinical experience,[602,603] numerous questions regarding the optimal application of RRT in AKI remain.[604-608]

Indications for Renal Replacement Therapy

In clinical practice there are wide variations in the timing of initiation of RRT for patients with AKI.[609] Widely accepted indications for initiation of RRT include volume overload unresponsive to diuretic therapy, severe metabolic acidosis or hyperkalemia despite appropriate medical therapy, and overt manifestations of uremia, including encephalopathy, pericarditis, or uremic bleeding diathesis (Table 30-14); however, even these indications are subject to substantial clinical interpretation. In many patients RRT is initiated in the absence of these specific indications in response to a clinical course marked by progressive azotemia or sustained oliguria. A precise correlation does not exist between the blood urea concentration and the onset of uremic symptoms, although the longer the duration and the greater the severity of azotemia,

TABLE 30-14 Indications for Renal Replacement Therapy	
Absolute indications	Volume overload unresponsive to diuretic therapy
	Hyperkalemia despite medical treatment
	Persistent metabolic acidosis
	Overt uremic symptoms
	Encephalopathy
	Pericarditis
	Uremic bleeding diathesis
Relative indications	Progressive azotemia without uremic manifestations
	Persistent oliguria

the more likely that overt symptoms will develop. Observational series and small clinical trials dating from the 1950s through the 1980s suggested that initiating RRT when the BUN concentration approached 90 to 100 mg/dL was associated with improved survival compared with more delayed initiation of therapy.[610-614] More recent observational studies have suggested that initiation of RRT at even less severe degrees of azotemia may further improve survival.[615-618] The results of these studies need to be interpreted with caution, however, because the outcomes associated with earlier initiation of RRT may reflect differences in the reasons for initiation of therapy (e.g., volume overload or hyperkalemia versus progressive azotemia) rather than a benefit due to the earlier therapy per se. In addition, these observational series included only patients in whom RRT was actually initiated rather than the broader population of patients with AKI, including patients who either recovered kidney function or died without receiving RRT. In the single randomized controlled trial in which patients were randomly assigned to immediate or delayed initiation of RRT no benefit was associated with earlier initiation of treatment, although the strength of this finding is limited by the small size of the clinical trial.[619]

Although volume overload unresponsive to diuretic therapy is a widely accepted indication for initiation of RRT, wide variations exist in the degree of volume overload at initiation of therapy.[579,620,621] Observational studies have demonstrated a strong association between the degree of volume overload and mortality risk, which suggests that RRT should be initiated early, before the development of progressive volume overload.[578,622] It should be recognized, however, that the association between volume overload and mortality risk does not establish a causal relationship; diseases processes that contribute to the development of volume overload may independently contribute to mortality risk in these patients. Prospective studies will therefore be required to demonstrate that preemptive RRT, before the development of more severe degrees of volume overload, decreases morbidity and mortality.

Modalities of Renal Replacement Therapy

Multiple modalities of RRT are available for the management of patients with AKI, including conventional intermittent hemodialysis (IHD), peritoneal dialysis, multiple forms of continuous renal replacement therapy (CRRT), and "hybrid" therapies such as sustained low-efficiency dialysis (SLED; also known as *extended duration dialysis,* or EDD). Detailed descriptions of the technical aspects of these modalities are provided in Chapters 64 through 66. Objective data to guide the selection of modality for individual patients are limited, and the choice of modality is often based on the resources of

the health care institution and the technical expertise of the physician and nursing staff.

INTERMITTENT HEMODIALYSIS

Short-term IHD has been the mainstay of RRT in AKI for more than five decades. Patients typically undergo dialysis treatments for 3 to 5 hours on a thrice-weekly, alternate-day, or daily schedule depending on catabolic demands, electrolyte disturbances, and volume status. As with the timing of initiation of dialysis, the most appropriate dosing strategy for IHD in patients with AKI has been the subject of considerable investigation. The dose of IHD may be adjusted by altering the intensity of each individual dialysis session, usually quantified as the product of urea clearance and dialysis duration normalized to volume of distribution of urea (Kt/V), or by changing the frequency of the dialysis sessions.

In an observational study, Paganini and colleagues demonstrated a survival benefit in patients with intermediate severity of illness scores when the delivered Kt/V was more than 1.0 per treatment compared with a delivered Kt/V of less than 1.0 per treatment.[623] However, there have been no prospective clinical trials evaluating the relationship between outcomes and the delivered Kt/V when dialysis is provided on a constant treatment schedule.

Schiffl and colleagues reported on a prospective trial of 160 patients with AKI assigned in an alternating fashion to alternate-day or daily IHD.[624] The more frequent treatment schedule was associated with a reduction in mortality at 14 days after the last dialysis session from 46% in the alternate-day dialysis arm to 28% in the daily treatment arm ($P = 0.01$). Duration of renal failure declined from 16 ± 6 days to 9 ± 2 days ($P = 0.001$). This study has been criticized, however, because the delivered dose of therapy per session was low in both treatment arms (Kt/V of <0.95), which resulted in a high rate of symptoms in the alternate-day dialysis arm that may have been associated with overtly inadequate dialysis.[625]

The impact of frequency of IHD was also evaluated in the Veterans Affairs/National Institutes of Health (VA/NIH) Acute Renal Failure Trial Network study.[626] In this study, 1124 critically ill patients were randomly assigned to an intensive or less-intensive strategy for the management of RRT. When patients were in hemodynamically stable condition, they received IHD, and when they were in hemodynamically unstable condition they were treated with CRRT or SLED, regardless of treatment arm. Patients randomly assigned to the less-intensive treatment arm received hemodialysis on a thrice-weekly schedule (alternate days except Sunday), whereas patients randomly assigned to the intensive treatment arm received hemodialysis six times per week (daily except Sunday). Sixty-day all-cause mortality was 53.6% in the intensive treatment arm compared with 51.5% in the less-intensive arm ($P = 0.47$).[626] The mean delivered Kt/V was 1.3 per treatment after the first IHD session. Although the study was not designed to evaluate outcomes by individual modality of RRT, there were no differences in mortality between groups when evaluated in terms of percentage of time treated using IHD.[627] Based on these results, it does not appear that there is further benefit to routinely increasing the frequency of IHD treatments beyond three times per week as long as the delivered Kt/V is at least 1.2 per treatment. More frequent treatments may be necessary in patients in whom the target dose per treatment cannot be achieved, in patients in a hypercatabolic state, in patients with severe hyperkalemia or metabolic acidosis, and in patients with problems related to volume management.

The selection of IHD dialyzer membrane may also impact clinical outcomes. Exposure to cellulosic membranes results in greater leukocyte and complement activation and delayed recovery of kidney function in experimental models of AKI compared with exposure to more biocompatible synthetic membranes.[628,629] Clinical trials have yielded conflicting results. Although some studies demonstrated delayed recovery of kidney function with cellulosic membranes,[630-632] other studies observed no benefit with synthetic membranes.[633-637] When these data have been aggregated in systematic reviews a benefit of the synthetic membranes is not convincingly demonstrated.[638,639] Although the effect of membrane type on humoral and cellular activation may still influence recovery of kidney function in AKI, the clinical impact of this issue has diminished as the cost differential between synthetic and cellulosic membranes has narrowed and the use of unsubstituted cellulosic membranes has decreased.

The major complications associated with acute dialysis are related to the need to access the vasculature, the need for anticoagulation to maintain patency of the extracorporeal circuit, and intradialytic hypotension primarily resulting from shifts in solute and volume.[624,626,640] Many of these issues, particularly the need for vascular access and anticoagulation, are similar for IHD, CRRT, and SLED.

Vascular access is usually obtained through insertion of a double-lumen catheter into a large-caliber central (internal jugular or subclavian) or femoral vein.[641] The major complications associated with vascular access include vascular and organ trauma during insertion; bleeding; catheter malfunction and thrombosis; and infection.[641] Although femoral catheters are generally associated with a greater risk of infection than catheters in the subclavian or internal jugular veins, an increased risk of infection was observed only when femoral vein catheters were used in patients with a high body mass index in a randomized controlled trial involving patients undergoing acute RRT.[642] The use of tunneled dialysis catheters has been proposed as a means of decreasing the risk of infection in patients undergoing acute dialysis[643,644]; however, this strategy has not been rigorously evaluated in prospective clinical trials.

Anticoagulation is used to help maintain patency of the extracorporeal dialysis circuit in IHD, CRRT, and SLED.[645,646] The most commonly used anticoagulant for dialysis is unfractionated heparin, with multiple protocols used to attain sufficient anticoagulation of the dialysis circuit while minimizing systemic effects.[645,646] Regional heparinization can be used, in which heparin is infused proximal to the dialyzer and protamine is infused into the return line to reverse its effect,[647] but this method has generally been supplanted by the use of low-dose heparin protocols.[648] Low-molecular-weight heparin may be used as an alternative to unfractionated heparin; however, the benefits of this approach are unclear, because low-molecular-weight heparin is not associated with enhanced efficacy, drug half-life is variably prolonged in renal failure, and monitoring of the anticoagulant effect is more difficult.[645] In patients with heparin-induced thrombocytopenia, heparin administration is contraindicated. Alternative anticoagulant agents include regional citrate,[645,649-651] the serine protease inhibitor nafamostat,[652] the direct thrombin

inhibitors hirudin lepirudin and argatroban,[653-658] and, rarely, the prostanoids epoprostenol and iloprost.[645,646] In many patients, particularly those with underlying coagulopathy or thrombocytopenia, and in patients with active hemorrhage or recent postoperative status, acute RRT can be provided in the absence of anticoagulation.[626,659,660]

Intradialytic hypotension is common in patients undergoing acute IHD.[600,626,627,640,661] Episodes of hypotension may impair solute clearance and the efficiency of dialysis and can further compromise renal perfusion and delay recovery of kidney function.[600,662-664] Intradialytic hypotension is typically triggered by intercompartmental fluid shifts or excessive fluid removal, which leads to decreased intravascular volume, and may be exacerbated by altered vascular responsiveness related to the underlying acute process.[640,665] Hypotension may be particularly problematic in critically ill patients, in whom sepsis, cardiac dysfunction, hypoalbuminemia, malnutrition, or large third-space losses may accompany the development of AKI. Prevention of intradialytic hypotension requires careful assessment of intravascular volume; prescription of realistic ultrafiltration targets; extension of treatment time to minimize the ultrafiltration rate; increase of the dialysate sodium concentration; and reduction of the dialysate temperature.[661,665,666] Although there is a tendency to reduce the extracorporeal blood flow in patients prone to hypotension, there is little evidence that this provides any benefit. Although reducing blood flow decreased the volume of the extracorporeal circuit in the past when parallel plate and coil dialyzers were used, there is little change in the volume of the extracorporeal circuit in response to changes in blood flow when hollow fiber dialyzers are employed. Reducing blood flow may, however, result in reduction of the delivered dose of dialysis.

CONTINUOUS RENAL REPLACEMENT THERAPY

The CRRTs represent a spectrum of treatment modalities. Initially, CRRT was provided using an arteriovenous extracorporeal circuit.[667-671] Although this approach offered technical simplicity, blood flow was dependent upon the gradient between mean arterial and central venous pressure, and there was an increased risk of complications from prolonged arterial cannulation.[672] As a result, the continuous arteriovenous therapies have largely been supplanted by pump-driven, venovenous CRRT.[673-676] The modalities of venovenous CRRT vary primarily in their mechanism of solute removal: in continuous venovenous hemofiltration (CVVH), solute transport occurs by convection; in continuous venovenous hemodialysis (CVVHD), it occurs by diffusion; and in continuous venovenous hemodiafiltration (CVVHDF), it occurs by a combination of the two.[676-678] Although, at the same level of urea clearance, convective therapies provide enhanced clearance of higher-molecular-weight solutes than diffusive therapies, no clear clinical benefit has been demonstrated for CVVH or CVVHDF compared with CVVHD.

The clearance of urea and other small solutes during CRRT is proportional to the total effluent flow rate (the sum of ultrafiltrate and dialysate flow rates),[671,676,677] and dose of therapy is usually expressed as the effluent volume indexed to body weight. Several single-center randomized controlled trials demonstrated an improvement in survival when doses of CVVH were increased from 20 to 25 mL/kg/hr to more than 35 to 45 mL/kg/hr[679,680]; however, other small studies did not find a similar benefit.[619,681] Two large multicenter randomized controlled trials also failed to find a survival benefit associated with more intensive CRRT.[626,682] As described earlier, in the VA/NIH Acute Renal Failure Trial Network study, 1124 patients were randomly assigned to two intensities of RRT.[626] In both treatment arms, patients received IHD when in hemodynamically stable condition and CVVHDF or SLED when in hemodynamically unstable condition. CVVHDF was provided at an effluent flow rate of 20 mL/kg/hr in the less-intensive treatment arm and at 35 mL/kg/hr in the more-intensive arm. Sixty-day all-cause mortality was 51.5% in the less-intensive arm and 53.6% in the more-intensive arm ($P = 0.47$).[626] In the Randomized Evaluation of Normal versus Augmented Level (RENAL) Replacement Therapy Study, 1508 patients were randomly assigned to CVVHDF at either 25 mL/kg/hr or 40 mL/kg/hr.[682] Ninety-day all-cause mortality was 44.7% in both treatment arms ($P = 0.99$).[682] Based on these two studies, there does not appear to be a need to establish a routine target dose of CRRT of more than 20 to 25 mL/kg/hr, although a slightly higher dose may have to be prescribed to achieve the target delivered dose to compensate for interruptions in treatment.

Given the greater hemodynamic tolerance of CRRT compared with IHD, particularly in patients with underlying hemodynamic instability, it has been postulated that CRRT should be associated with improved clinical outcomes. Results of five randomized controlled trials comparing outcomes with CRRT and IHD have been published. In a multicenter randomized controlled trial of 166 patients with AKI, Mehta and colleagues observed ICU and hospital mortality rates of 59.5% and 65.5%, respectively, in patients randomly assigned to undergo CRRT compared with 41.5% and 47.6%, respectively, in patients randomly assigned to receive IHD ($P < 0.02$).[683] As a result of an imbalance in randomization, patients in the CRRT arm had greater severity of illness as measured by Acute Physiology and Chronic Health Evaluation III (APACHE III) score and a higher rate of liver failure. After adjusting for the imbalanced randomization in a post hoc analysis, the investigators found no difference in mortality attributable to modality of RRT. In a single-center randomized trial involving 80 patients, Augustine and colleagues reported more effective fluid removal and greater hemodynamic stability with CVVHD than with IHD but observed no difference in survival.[684] Similarly, in another single-center randomized controlled trial in Switzerland, Uehlinger and colleagues observed no difference in survival in 70 patients randomly assigned to CVVHDF and in 55 patients assigned to IHD.[685] In the Hemodiafe study, a multicenter randomized controlled trial conducted in 21 ICUs in France, Vinsonneau and colleagues reported 60-day survival rates of 31.5% in 184 patients randomly assigned to receive IHD compared with 32.6% in 175 patients randomly assigned to undergo CVVHDF ($P = 0.98$).[661] Similarly, Lins and colleagues observed hospital morality rates of 62.5% in 144 patients randomly assigned to receive IHD and 58.1% in 172 patients randomly assigned undergo to CRRT ($P = 0.43$).[686]

Multiple meta-analyses have concluded that there is no association between survival and use of either of these modalities of RRT.[687-689] Although several studies have suggested that CRRT is associated with higher rates of recovery of kidney function than IHD in surviving patients,[683,690-692] all of these studies are notable for having higher morality rates in the CRRT group. When data are analyzed across studies in which there were no differences in mortality, rates of recovery of kidney function do not appear to be impacted by modality of RRT.[600,687,689]

HYBRID THERAPIES

The hybrid modalities of RRT represent therapies in which conventional hemodialysis equipment is modified to provide extended-duration dialysis using lower blood flow rates and dialysate flow rates.[693] A variety of terms have been used to describe these therapies, including *sustained low-efficiency dialysis* (SLED),[694,695] *extended daily dialysis* (EDD),[696] and *sustained low-efficiency daily diafiltration* (SLEDD-f).[697] Because these therapies extend the duration of the dialysis treatment while providing slower ultrafiltration and solute clearance, they are associated with enhanced hemodynamic tolerability compared with IHD. The degree of metabolic control attained with these treatments is comparable to that observed with CRRT[698]; however, there has been an absence of studies evaluating clinical outcomes.

PERITONEAL DIALYSIS

The use of peritoneal dialysis in the management of AKI has diminished as the use of continuous and hybrid therapies has increased.[699-701] Peritoneal dialysis has the advantage of requiring minimal technology, which facilitates its use in remote or resource-constrained areas.[702] As a result, it is still used in the treatment of AKI in regions without access to IHD or CRRT. Access for short-term peritoneal dialysis can be obtained either by percutaneous placement of an uncuffed temporary peritoneal catheter or through surgical placement of a tunneled cuffed catheter. Peritoneal dialysis has the advantage of avoiding the need for vascular access or anticoagulation. Solute clearance and control of metabolic parameters may be inferior to that achieved with other modalities of RRT.[703] Although systemic hypotension is less of an issue than with other modalities of RRT, ultrafiltration cannot be as tightly controlled. Other limitations include the relative contraindication in patients with acute abdominal processes or recent abdominal surgery, the risk of visceral organ injury during catheter placement, the risk of peritoneal dialysis–associated peritonitis, and an increased tendency toward hyperglycemia, which is associated with adverse outcomes in acute illness, due to the high glucose concentrations in peritoneal dialysate.

Two trials have compared outcomes with peritoneal dialysis to outcomes with other modalities of RRT in AKI.[703,704] In a study of 70 patients with infection-associated AKI in Vietnam, 58 of whom had severe *Plasmodium falciparum* malaria, peritoneal dialysis was associated with less adequate metabolic control and higher mortality than continuous hemofiltration.[703] In contrast, in a study of 120 patients in Brazil who were randomly assigned to undergo high-volume peritoneal dialysis or daily hemodialysis, indices of metabolic control, recovery of kidney function, and survival were similar for both modalities of therapy.[704]

Outcomes of Acute Kidney Injury

The crude short-term mortality rate among patients with intrinsic AKI approximates 50% and has changed little over the past three decades.[13,14,16,18,341,386,387,624,705-713] This lack of improvement in survival despite significant advances in supportive care may reflect a decrease in the proportion of patients with isolated AKI and a corresponding increase in the number of patients with AKI complicating multiorgan dysfunction syndrome.[16,18,714,715] The risk of death differs considerably depending on the cause of AKI and the clinical setting, with mortality estimates of approximately 15% in obstetric patients with AKI, 30% in those with toxin-related AKI, and 60% to 90% in patients with sepsis.[13,14,278,714,716,717] In the recently completed VA/NIH Acute Renal Failure Trial Network study comparing intensive with less-intensive renal support in critically ill patients with AKI due to ATN in the United States, the overall 60-day mortality rate was 52.6%,[626] whereas in the RENAL Replacement Therapy Study, which compared two intensities of CVVHDF in critically ill patients with AKI in Australia and New Zealand the 90-day mortality rate was 44.7%.[682]

Factors that have been found to predict poor outcomes in AKI include male sex, advanced age, oliguria (<400 mL/day), a rise in the serum creatinine value of greater than 3 mg/dL, and coexistent sepsis or nonrenal organ failure—factors that reflect more severe renal injury and overall severity of illness. However, even mild decrements in renal function that do not necessitate dialytic support are recognized as being associated with poor patient outcomes. Lassnigg and colleagues demonstrated that increases in serum creatinine concentration of less than 0.6 mg/dL after cardiothoracic surgery were independently associated with a nearly twofold increase in 30-day mortality (hazard ratio [HR] = 1.92; 95% CI = 1.34 to 2.77).[718] Furthermore, several studies of contrast agent–induced AKI have demonstrated that small increments in serum creatinine level, even if transient, are associated with increased short and long-term mortality.[719-722] Whether such transient increases in serum creatinine concentration directly mediate adverse long-term outcomes or represent a biochemical marker in patients at higher risk of such outcomes remains unclear.[723]

Not only is the development of AKI associated with remarkably high short-term mortality rates, surviving an episode of AKI is also associated with an increased risk of serious longer-term morbidity and mortality. Although older data suggested that complete recovery of kidney function was common in patients surviving an episode of AKI, with only 5% of patients experiencing no recovery of kidney function and an additional 5% manifesting progressive deterioration in kidney function after an initial recovery phase, more recent data have challenged this view. Rates of recovery of kidney function in recent clinical trials of renal replacement therapy in AKI have been highly variable, with fewer than 10% of surviving patients remaining dialysis dependent in the RENAL Replacement Therapy Study[682] compared with approximately 25% of surviving patients in the VA/NIH Acute Renal Failure Trial Network study[626] and approximately 40% in the Hanover Dialysis Outcome study.[724] The reason for this wide variation in recovery of kidney function across studies is not known.

Among patients who recovery kidney function, approximately half have subclinical functional defects in glomerular filtration, tubular solute transport, H^+ secretion, and urinary concentrating mechanisms or have tubulointerstitial scarring on kidney biopsy specimens.[725-728] More recent epidemiologic studies have demonstrated that patients who recover from AKI are at increased risk of progressive CKD and development of

ESRD. Using data from a 5% representative sample of elderly Medicare beneficiaries, Ishani and associates recently reported that AKI in the absence of underlying CKD was independently associated with a markedly increased risk of the development of ESRD at 2 years of follow-up (HR = 13.0; 95% CI = 10.6 to 16).[729] AKI that developed in the setting of preexistent CKD was associated with an even higher risk of ESRD (HR = 41.2; 95% CI = 34.6 to 49.1). Thus, elderly patients who develop AKI, particularly with underlying CKD, are at markedly increased risk for the development of ESRD.

Wald and colleagues conducted a population-based cohort study comparing long-term outcomes for 3769 patients who developed AKI that required temporary dialysis with outcomes for 13,598 matched control patients who were hospitalized but did not develop AKI.[730] At a median of 3 years of follow-up, the risk of ESRD was more than threefold higher among patients who required acute transient dialysis than among control patients with equal severity of illness (adjusted HR = 3.23; 95% CI = 2.70 to 3.86). Lo and colleagues examined the association between AKI that required transient dialysis and long-term mortality.[731] Among 562,799 hospitalized patients who had a baseline eGFR 45 mL/min/1.73 m^2 or more, 703 sustained dialysis-requiring AKI, of whom 295 (42%) died, 65 (9%) remained dependent on long-term dialysis, and 343 (49%) recovered sufficient kidney function to be able to discontinue dialysis by the time of hospital discharge. In multivariable analyses, AKI requiring transient dialysis was associated with a twofold increased risk of death over 6 years of follow-up.[731] In a study of over 87,000 patients, Newsome and colleagues demonstrated that increases in serum creatinine concentration of 0.3 to 0.5 mg/dL after acute myocardial infarction were independently associated with an increased risk of ESRD (HR = 2.36; $P < 0.05$) and long-term mortality (HR = 1.26; $P < 0.05$).[732] Thus, small changes in serum creatinine level as well as AKI that requires transient renal support are associated with an increased risk for development of ESRD and mortality.

CKD is now recognized as a principal risk factor for the development of AKI. Recent data support a robust association between AKI and the subsequent development and progression of CKD. In the aforementioned large epidemiologic study by Lo and associates,[731] AKI requiring transient dialysis was associated with a 28-fold increased risk of developing progressive CKD, defined as a decline in kidney function to an eGFR of less than 30 mL/min/1.73 m^2. As part of an epidemiologic study of 11,249 patients in Alberta, Canada, James and colleagues demonstrated that mild AKI following coronary angiography, defined as an increase in serum creatinine level of 50% to 99% or 0.3 mg/dL or more was associated with a nearly fivefold increased risk of experiencing a sustained reduction in kidney function at 90 days (adjusted odds ratio [OR] = 4.74; 95% CI = 3.92 to 5.74).[733] Patients who developed more severe AKI, defined as an increase in serum creatinine level of 100% or more, had a greater than 17-fold increased risk of persistent renal injury at 90 days after angiography (adjusted OR = 17.3; 95% CI = 12.0 to 24.9), a finding that supports a graded relationship between the severity of AKI and risk of sustained renal damage at 90 days. AKI was also associated with an increased risk of accelerated decline in kidney function, defined as a loss of eGFR of more than 4 mL/min/1.73 m^2 per year over 2 to 3 years of follow-up (OR = 2.9; 95% CI = 2.2 to 3.7), as well as with a markedly increased risk of ESRD over this same period of follow-up (OR = 13.8; 95% CI = 7.4 to 25.9).[733] Thus the development of AKI appears to accelerate the progression of CKD and development of ESRD.

AKI also extends the length of hospitalization and is associated with substantial health resource utilization.[341,690,734-736] The U.S. cost of treating AKI was estimated in 1999 to be $50,000 per quality-adjusted life-year, a level that is important to consider in terms of the cost-benefit assessment of potential interventions for this condition.[737] In a more recent analysis of long-term outcomes of 153 ICU survivors who had recovered from AKI, quality-adjusted survival was poor in comparison with an age- and gender-matched community population.[738] Quality-adjusted survival in this cohort was poor (15 quality-adjusted years per 100 patient-years in the first year after discharge); however, despite the low health-related quality of life, the subjects' self-perceived health satisfaction was not significantly different from that of the general population.[738] Similarly poor health-related quality of life was also observed in follow-up of 415 individuals who participated in the VA/NIH Acute Renal Failure Trial Network study and survived at least 60 days, with 27% of respondents' health states corresponding to levels considered by the general population to be equivalent to or worse than death.[739]

The design of many of the clinical studies that have examined the efficacy of therapeutic interventions on hard outcomes of AKI has been problematic. Measurement of the benefit of interventions for the treatment AKI have been confounded by the difficulty in accurately defining the onset and resolution of this condition. Furthermore, many human studies of AKI suffer from a lack of well-defined endpoints.[6] For example, although the need for dialysis has been used as an endpoint in many trials of AKI, uniform criteria for the initiation and discontinuation of dialysis often have not been established before the study, and among studies that do define specific criteria for dialysis, such criteria may differ across trials and study populations. Finally, the necessary duration of follow-up to fully capture the sequelae of AKI remains uncertain. The assessment of outcomes clearly needs to extend beyond ICU and hospital discharge, because accumulating data associate AKI with longer-term morbidity and mortality.[729,731,740]

References

1. Lameire N, Van Biesen W, Vanholder R. Acute renal failure. *Lancet.* 2005;365:417-430.
2. Klahr S, Miller SB. Acute oliguria. *N Engl J Med.* 1998;338:671-675.
3. Morgan DJ, Ho KM. A comparison of nonoliguric and oliguric severe acute kidney injury according to the risk injury failure loss end-stage (RIFLE) criteria. *Nephron.* 115:c59-c65.
4. McCullough PA, Adam A, Becker CR, et al. Risk prediction of contrast-induced nephropathy. *Am J Cardiol.* 2006;98:27K-36K.
5. Mehta RH, Grab JD, O'Brien SM, et al. Bedside tool for predicting the risk of postoperative dialysis in patients undergoing cardiac surgery. *Circulation.* 2006;114:2208-2216.
6. Bellomo R, Ronco C, Kellum JA, et al. Acute renal failure—definition, outcome measures, animal models, fluid therapy and information technology needs: the Second International Consensus Conference of the Acute Dialysis Quality Initiative (ADQI) Group. *Critical Care.* 2004;8:R204-R212.
7. Mehta RL, Kellum JA, Shah SV, et al. Acute Kidney Injury Network: report of an initiative to improve outcomes in acute kidney injury. *Critical Care.* 2007;11:R31.
8. Murray PT, Devarajan P, Levey AS, et al. A framework and key research questions in AKI diagnosis and staging in different environments. *Clin J Am Soc Nephrol.* 2008;3:864-868.
9. Coca SG, Parikh CR. Urinary biomarkers for acute kidney injury: perspectives on translation. *Clin J Am Soc Nephrol.* 2008;3:481-490.
10. Coca SG, Yalavarthy R, Concato J, et al. Biomarkers for the diagnosis and risk stratification of acute kidney injury: a systematic review. *Kidney Int.* 2008;73:1008-1016.
11. Herget-Rosenthal S, Pietruck F, Volbracht L, et al. Serum cystatin C—a superior marker of rapidly reduced glomerular filtration after uninephrectomy in kidney donors compared to creatinine. *Clin Nephrol.* 2005;64:41-46.
12. Dharnidharka VR, Kwon C, Stevens G. Serum cystatin C is superior to serum creatinine as a marker of kidney function: a meta-analysis. *Am J Kidney Dis.* 2002;40:221-226.
13. Nash K, Hafeez A, Hou S. Hospital-acquired renal insufficiency. *Am J Kidney Dis.* 2002;39:930-936.
14. Soubrier S, Leroy O, Devos P, et al. Epidemiology and prognostic factors of critically ill patients treated with hemodiafiltration. *J Crit Care.* 2006;21:66-72.
15. Liano F, Pascual J. Epidemiology of acute renal failure: a prospective, multicenter, community-based study. Madrid Acute Renal Failure Study Group. *Kidney Int.* 1996;50:811-818.
16. Mehta RL, Pascual MT, Soroko S, et al. Spectrum of acute renal failure in the intensive care unit: the PICARD experience. *Kidney Int.* 2004;66:1613-1621.
17. Hou SH, Bushinsky DA, Wish JB, et al. Hospital-acquired renal insufficiency: a prospective study. *Am J Med.* 1983;74:243-248.
18. Uchino S, Kellum JA, Bellomo R, et al. Acute renal failure in critically ill patients: a multinational, multicenter study. *JAMA.* 2005;294:813-818.
19. Hospitalization discharge diagnoses for kidney disease—United States, 1980-2005. *MMWR Morb Mortal Wkly Rep.* 2008;57:309-312.
20. Hsu CY, McCulloch CE, Fan D, et al. Community-based incidence of acute renal failure. *Kidney Int.* 2007;72:208-212.
21. Sesso R, Roque A, Vicioso B, et al. Prognosis of ARF in hospitalized elderly patients. *Am J Kidney Dis.* 2004;44:410-419.
22. Kastner PR, Hall JE, Guyton AC. Control of glomerular filtration rate: role of intrarenally formed angiotensin II. *Am J Physiol.* 1984;246:F897-F906.
23. Cogan MG. Angiotensin II: a powerful controller of sodium transport in the early proximal tubule. *Hypertension.* 1990;15:451-458.
24. Quan A, Baum M. Regulation of proximal tubule transport by endogenously produced angiotensin II. *Nephron.* 2000;84:103-110.
25. Liu FY, Cogan MG. Angiotensin II stimulation of hydrogen ion secretion in the rat early proximal tubule. Modes of action, mechanism, and kinetics. *J Clin Invest.* 1988;82:601-607.
26. Liu FY, Cogan MG. Angiotensin II stimulates early proximal bicarbonate absorption in the rat by decreasing cyclic adenosine monophosphate. *J Clin Invest.* 1989;84:83-91.
27. Schuster VL, Kokko JP, Jacobson HR. Angiotensin II directly stimulates sodium transport in rabbit proximal convoluted tubules. *J Clin Invest.* 1984;73:507-515.
28. Blantz RC. Pathophysiology of pre-renal azotemia. *Kidney Int.* 1998;53:512-523.
29. Badr KF, Ichikawa I. Prerenal failure: a deleterious shift from renal compensation to decompensation. *N Engl J Med.* 1988;319:623-629.
30. Yared A, Kon V, Ichikawa I. Mechanism of preservation of glomerular perfusion and filtration during acute extracellular fluid volume depletion. Importance of intrarenal vasopressin-prostaglandin interaction for protecting kidneys from constrictor action of vasopressin. *J Clin Invest.* 1985;75:1477-1487.
31. Oliver JA, Sciacca RR, Cannon PJ. Renal vasodilation by converting enzyme inhibition. Role of renal prostaglandins. *Hypertension.* 1983;5:166-171.
32. Pascual J, Liano F, Ortuno J. The elderly patient with acute renal failure. *J Am Soc Nephrol.* 1995;6:144-153.
33. Malbrain ML, Cheatham ML, Kirkpatrick A, et al. Results from the International Conference of Experts on Intra-abdominal Hypertension and Abdominal Compartment Syndrome. I. Definitions. *Intensive Care Med.* 2006;32:1722-1732.
34. Sugrue M. Abdominal compartment syndrome. *Curr Opin Crit Care.* 2005;11:333-338.
35. Malbrain ML, Chiumello D, Pelosi P, et al. Incidence and prognosis of intraabdominal hypertension in a mixed population of critically ill patients: a multiple-center epidemiological study. *Crit Care Med.* 2005;33:315-322.
36. Cheatham ML, White MW, Sagraves SG, et al. Abdominal perfusion pressure: a superior parameter in the assessment of intra-abdominal hypertension. *J Trauma.* 2000;49:621-626:discussion, 6-7.
37. Moore AF, Hargest R, Martin M, et al. Intra-abdominal hypertension and the abdominal compartment syndrome. *Br J Surg.* 2004;91:1102-1110.
38. Doty JM, Saggi BH, Blocher CR, et al. Effects of increased renal parenchymal pressure on renal function. *J Trauma.* 2000;48:874-877.
39. Doty JM, Saggi BH, Sugerman HJ, et al. Effect of increased renal venous pressure on renal function. *J Trauma.* 1999;47:1000-1003.

40. Shenasky 2nd JH. The renal hemodynamic and functional effects of external counterpressure. *Surg Gynecol Obstet*. 1972;134:253-258.
41. Thadhani RI, Camargo Jr CA, Xavier RJ, et al. Atheroembolic renal failure after invasive procedures. Natural history based on 52 histologically proven cases. *Medicine (Baltimore)*. 1995;74:350-358.
42. van der Wal MA, Wisselink W, Rauwerda JA. Traumatic bilateral renal artery thrombosis: case report and review of the literature. *Cardiovasc Surg*. 2003;11:527-529.
43. Dinchman KH, Spirnak JP. Traumatic renal artery thrombosis: evaluation and treatment. *Semin Urol*. 1995;13:90-93.
44. Piette JC, Cacoub P, Wechsler B. Renal manifestations of the antiphospholipid syndrome. *Semin Arthritis Rheum*. 1994;23:357-366.
45. Kodner CM, Kudrimoti A. Diagnosis and management of acute interstitial nephritis. *Am Fam Physician*. 2003;67:2527-2534.
46. Sturmer T, Elseviers MM, De Broe ME. Nonsteroidal anti-inflammatory drugs and the kidney. *Curr Opin Nephrol Hypertens*. 2001;10:161-163.
47. Michel DM, Kelly CJ. Acute interstitial nephritis. *J Am Soc Nephrol*. 1998;9:506-515.
48. Persson PB, Hansell P, Liss P. Pathophysiology of contrast medium-induced nephropathy. *Kidney Int*. 2005;68:14-22.
49. Bettmann MA. Contrast medium-induced nephropathy: critical review of the existing clinical evidence. *Nephrol Dial Transplant*. 2005;20(suppl 1):i12-i17.
50. McCullough PA. Radiocontrast-induced acute kidney injury. *Nephron Physiol*. 2008;109:p61-p72.
51. Liss P, Carlsson PO, Nygren A, et al. Et-A receptor antagonist BQ123 prevents radiocontrast media-induced renal medullary hypoxia. *Acta Radiol*. 2003;44:111-117.
52. Heyman SN, Reichman J, Brezis M. Pathophysiology of radiocontrast nephropathy: a role for medullary hypoxia. *Invest Radiol*. 1999;34:685-691.
53. Liss P, Nygren A, Hansell P. Hypoperfusion in the renal outer medulla after injection of contrast media in rats. *Acta Radiol*. 1999;40:521-527.
54. Nygren A, Ulfendahl HR. Effects of high- and low-osmolar contrast media on renal plasma flow and glomerular filtration rate in euvolaemic and dehydrated rats. A comparison between ioxithalamate, iopamidol, iohexol and ioxaglate. *Acta Radiol*. 1989;30:383-389.
55. Nygren A, Ulfendahl HR, Hansell P, et al. Effects of intravenous contrast media on cortical and medullary blood flow in the rat kidney. *Invest Radiol*. 1988;23:753-761.
56. Ueda J, Nygren A, Sjoquist M, et al. Iodine concentrations in the rat kidney measured by X-ray microanalysis. Comparison of concentrations and viscosities in the proximal tubules and renal pelvis after intravenous injections of contrast media. *Acta Radiol*. 1998;39:90-95.
57. Lancelot E, Idee JM, Couturier V, et al. Influence of the viscosity of iodixanol on medullary and cortical blood flow in the rat kidney: a potential cause of nephrotoxicity. *J Appl Toxicol*. 1999;19:341-346.
58. Humes HD, Hunt DA, White MD. Direct toxic effect of the radio-contrast agent diatrizoate on renal proximal tubule cells. *Am J Physiol*. 1987;252:F246-F255.
59. Messana JM, Cieslinski DA, Nguyen VD, et al. Comparison of the toxicity of the radiocontrast agents, iopamidol and diatrizoate, to rabbit renal proximal tubule cells in vitro. *J Pharmacol Exp Ther*. 1988;244:1139-1144.
60. Andersen KJ, Christensen EI, Vik H. Effects of iodinated x-ray contrast media on renal epithelial cells in culture. *Invest Radiol*. 1994;29:955-962.
61. Nagai J, Tanaka H, Nakanishi N, et al. Role of megalin in renal handling of aminoglycosides. *Am J Physiol Renal Physiol*. 2001;281:F337-F344.
62. Schmitz C, Hilpert J, Jacobsen C, et al. Megalin deficiency offers protection from renal aminoglycoside accumulation. *J Biol Chem*. 2002;277:618-622.
63. Sandoval RM, Molitoris BA. Gentamicin traffics retrograde through the secretory pathway and is released in the cytosol via the endoplasmic reticulum. *Am J Physiol Renal Physiol*. 2004;286:F617-F624.
64. Sandoval RM, Dunn KW, Molitoris BA. Gentamicin traffics rapidly and directly to the Golgi complex in LLC-PK$_1$ cells. *Am J Physiol Renal Physiol*. 2000;279:F884-F890.
65. Zingman LV, Park S, Olson TM, et al. Aminoglycoside-induced translational read-through in disease: overcoming nonsense mutations by pharmacogenetic therapy. *Clin Pharmacol Ther*. 2007;81:99-103.
66. Humes HD. Aminoglycoside nephrotoxicity. *Kidney Int*. 1988;33:900-911.
67. Bennett WM. Mechanisms of aminoglycoside nephrotoxicity. *Clin Exp Pharmacol Physiol*. 1989;16:1-6.
68. Rea RS, Capitano B. Optimizing use of aminoglycosides in the critically ill. *Semin Respir Crit Care Med*. 2007;28:596-603.
69. Rougier F, Claude D, Maurin M, et al. Aminoglycoside nephrotoxicity. *Curr Drug Targets Infect Disord*. 2004;4:153-162.
70. Hatala R, Dinh T, Cook DJ. Once-daily aminoglycoside dosing in immunocompetent adults: a meta-analysis. *Ann Intern Med*. 1996;124:717-725.
71. Arany I, Safirstein RL. Cisplatin nephrotoxicity. *Semin Nephrol*. 2003;23:460-464.
72. Hurst FP, Abbott KC. Acute phosphate nephropathy. *Curr Opin Nephrol Hypertens*. 2009;18:513-518.
73. Markowitz GS, Perazella MA. Acute phosphate nephropathy. *Kidney Int*. 2009;76:1027-1034.
74. Markowitz GS, Stokes MB, Radhakrishnan J, et al. Acute phosphate nephropathy following oral sodium phosphate bowel purgative: an underrecognized cause of chronic renal failure. *J Am Soc Nephrol*. 2005;16:3389-3396.
75. Holt S, Moore K. Pathogenesis of renal failure in rhabdomyolysis: the role of myoglobin. *Exp Nephrol*. 2000;8:72-76.
76. Zager RA, Burkhart KM. Differential effects of glutathione and cysteine on Fe^{2+}, Fe^{3+}, H$_2$O$_2$ and myoglobin-induced proximal tubular cell attack. *Kidney Int*. 1998;53:1661-1672.
77. Karam H, Bruneval P, Clozel JP, et al. Role of endothelin in acute renal failure due to rhabdomyolysis in rats. *J Pharmacol Exp Ther*. 1995;274:481-486.
78. Hill-Kapturczak N, Chang SH, Agarwal A. Heme oxygenase and the kidney. *DNA Cell Biol*. 2002;21:307-321.
79. Ogawa T, Nussler AK, Tuzuner E, et al. Contribution of nitric oxide to the protective effects of ischemic preconditioning in ischemia-reperfused rat kidneys. *J Lab Clin Med*. 2001;138:50-58.
80. Sanders PW, Booker BB, Bishop JB, et al. Mechanisms of intranephronal proteinaceous cast formation by low molecular weight proteins. *J Clin Invest*. 1990;85:570-576.
81. Bosch X, Poch E, Grau JM. Rhabdomyolysis and acute kidney injury. *N Engl J Med*. 2009;361:62-72.
82. Winearls CG. Acute myeloma kidney. *Kidney Int*. 1995;48:1347-1361.
83. Sengul S, Zwizinski C, Simon EE, et al. Endocytosis of light chains induces cytokines through activation of NF-κB in human proximal tubule cells. *Kidney Int*. 2002;62:1977-1988.
84. Chauveau D, Choukroun G. Bence Jones proteinuria and myeloma kidney. *Nephrol Dial Transplant*. 1996;11:413-415.
85. Wang PX, Sanders PW. Immunoglobulin light chains generate hydrogen peroxide. *J Am Soc Nephrol*. 2007;18:1239-1245.
86. Kaplan AA. Therapeutic apheresis for the renal complications of multiple myeloma and the dysglobulinemias. *Ther Apher*. 2001;5:171-175.
87. Mustonen S, Ala-Houhala IO, Tammela TL. Long-term renal dysfunction in patients with acute urinary retention. *Scand J Urol Nephrol*. 2001;35:44-48.
88. Lieberthal W, Nigam SK. Acute renal failure. II. Experimental models of acute renal failure: imperfect but indispensable. *Am J Physiol Renal Physiol*. 2000;278:F1-F12.
89. Rosen S, Heyman SN. Difficulties in understanding human "acute tubular necrosis": limited data and flawed animal models. *Kidney Int*. 2001;60:1220-1224.
90. Adrie C, Adib-Conquy M, Laurent I, et al. Successful cardiopulmonary resuscitation after cardiac arrest as a "sepsis-like" syndrome. *Circulation*. 2002;106:562-568.
91. Burne-Taney MJ, Kofler J, Yokota N, et al. Acute renal failure after whole body ischemia is characterized by inflammation and T cell-mediated injury. *Am J Physiol Renal Physiol*. 2003;285:F87-F94.
92. Kelly KJ. Distant effects of experimental renal ischemia/reperfusion injury. *J Am Soc Nephrol*. 2003;14:1549-1558.
93. Zager RA. Partial aortic ligation: a hypoperfusion model of ischemic acute renal failure and a comparison with renal artery occlusion. *J Lab Clin Med*. 1987;110:396-405.
94. McDougal G, Compos S, Molitoris BA. *Hypotensive ischemic nephropathy. The rat partial aortic clamp.* San Diego, California F-PO-979.5: American Society of Nephrology Annual Meeting; November 12-17, 2003. Published *J Am Soc Nephrol*. 2003;4:S277-S278.
95. Sharfuddin AA, Sandoval RM, Berg DT, et al. Soluble thrombomodulin protects ischemic kidneys. *J Am Soc Nephrol*. 2009;20:524-534.
96. Kikeri D, Pennell JP, Hwang KH, et al. Endotoxemic acute renal failure in awake rats. *Am J Physiol*. 1986;250:F1098-F1106.
97. Wichterman KA, Baue AE, Chaudry IH. Sepsis and septic shock—a review of laboratory models and a proposal. *J Surg Res*. 1980;29:189-201.
98. Doi K, Leelahavanichkul A, Yuen PS, et al. Animal models of sepsis and sepsis-induced kidney injury. *J Clin Invest*. 2009;119:2868-2878.
99. Hentschel DM, Park KM, Cilenti L, et al. Acute renal failure in zebrafish—a novel system to study a complex disease. *Am J Physiol Renal Physiol*. 2005;288:F923-F929.
100. Heyman SN, Lieberthal W, Rogiers P, et al. Animal models of acute tubular necrosis. *Curr Opin Crit Care*. 2002;8:526-534.
101. Heyman SN, Rosenberger C, Rosen S. Experimental ischemia-reperfusion: biases and myths—the proximal vs. distal hypoxic tubular injury debate revisited. *Kidney Int*. 2010;77:9-16.
102. Venkatachalam MA, Bernard DB, Donohoe JF, et al. Ischemic damage and repair in the rat proximal tubule: differences among the S1, S2, and S3 segments. *Kidney Int*. 1978;14:31-49.
103. Molitoris BA, Sutton TA. Endothelial injury and dysfunction: role in the extension phase of acute renal failure. *Kidney Int*. 2004;66:496-499.

104. Alejandro V, Scandling Jr JD, Sibley RK, et al. Mechanisms of filtration failure during postischemic injury of the human kidney. A study of the reperfused renal allograft. *J Clin Invest.* 1995;95:820-831.

105. Ramaswamy D, Corrigan G, Polhemus C, et al. Maintenance and recovery stages of postischemic acute renal failure in humans. *Am J Physiol Renal Physiol.* 2002;282:F271-F280.

106. Solez K, Morel-Maroger L, Sraer JD. The morphology of "acute tubular necrosis" in man: analysis of 57 renal biopsies and a comparison with the glycerol model. *Medicine (Baltimore).* 1979;58:362-376.

107. Racusen L. *The morphologic basis of acute renal failure.* Philadelphia: Saunders; 2001.

108. Wagner MC, Rhodes G, Wang E, et al. Ischemic injury to kidney induces glomerular podocyte effacement and dissociation of slit diaphragm proteins Neph1 and ZO-1. *J Biol Chem.* 2008;283:35579-35589.

109. Molitoris BA. Actin cytoskeleton in ischemic acute renal failure. *Kidney Int.* 2004;66:871-883.

110. Molitoris BA, Dahl R, Hosford M. Cellular ATP depletion induces disruption of the spectrin cytoskeletal network. *Am J Physiol.* 1996;271: F790-F798.

111. Atkinson SJ, Hosford MA, Molitoris BA. Mechanism of actin polymerization in cellular ATP depletion. *J Biol Chem.* 2004;279:5194-5199.

112. Raman N, Atkinson SJ. Rho controls actin cytoskeletal assembly in renal epithelial cells during ATP depletion and recovery. *Am J Physiol.* 1999;276:C1312-C1324.

113. Ashworth SL, Sandoval RM, Hosford M, et al. Ischemic injury induces ADF relocation to the apical domain of rat proximal tubule cells. *Am J Physiol Renal Physiol.* 2001;280:F886-F894.

114. Ashworth SL, Southgate EL, Sandoval RM, et al. ADF/cofilin mediates actin cytoskeletal alterations in LLC-PK cells during ATP depletion. *Am J Physiol Renal Physiol.* 2003;284:F852-F862.

115. Suurna MV, Ashworth SL, Hosford M, et al. Cofilin mediates ATP depletion-induced endothelial cell actin alterations. *Am J Physiol Renal Physiol.* 2006;290:F1398-F1407.

116. Ashworth SL, Wean SE, Campos SB, et al. Renal ischemia induces tropomyosin dissociation–destabilizing microvilli microfilaments. *Am J Physiol Renal Physiol.* 2004;286:F988-F996.

117. Molitoris BA, Geerdes A, McIntosh JR. Dissociation and redistribution of Na$^+$, K$^+$-ATPase from its surface membrane actin cytoskeletal complex during cellular ATP depletion. *J Clin Invest.* 1991;88:462-469.

118. Molitoris BA. Na$^+$-K$^+$-ATPase that redistributes to apical membrane during ATP depletion remains functional. *Am J Physiol.* 1993;265:F693-F697.

119. Lieberthal W, Koh JS, Levine JS. Necrosis and apoptosis in acute renal failure. *Semin Nephrol.* 1998;18:505-518.

120. Bonegio R, Lieberthal W. Role of apoptosis in the pathogenesis of acute renal failure. *Curr Opin Nephrol Hypertens.* 2002;11:301-308.

121. Guo R, Wang Y, Minto AW, et al. Acute renal failure in endotoxemia is dependent on caspase activation. *J Am Soc Nephrol.* 2004;15:3093-3102.

122. Safirstein RL. Acute renal failure: from renal physiology to the renal transcriptome. *Kidney Int Suppl.* 2004:S62-S66.

123. Nicholson DW. From bench to clinic with apoptosis-based therapeutic agents. *Nature.* 2000;407:810-816.

124. Kaufmann SH, Hengartner MO. Programmed cell death: alive and well in the new millennium. *Trends Cell Biol.* 2001;11:526-534.

125. Lee RH, Song JM, Park MY, et al. Cisplatin-induced apoptosis by translocation of endogenous Bax in mouse collecting duct cells. *Biochem Pharmacol.* 2001;62:1013-1023.

126. Peherstorfer E, Mayer B, Boehm S, et al. Effects of microinjection of synthetic Bcl-2 domain peptides on apoptosis of renal tubular epithelial cells. *Am J Physiol Renal Physiol.* 2002;283:F190-F196.

127. Edelstein LC, Lagos L, Simmons M, et al. NF-κB–dependent assembly of an enhanceosome-like complex on the promoter region of apoptosis inhibitor Bfl-1/A1. *Mol Cell Biol.* 2003;23:2749-2761.

128. Kelly KJ, Plotkin Z, Vulgamott SL, et al. P53 mediates the apoptotic response to GTP depletion after renal ischemia-reperfusion: protective role of a p53 inhibitor. *J Am Soc Nephrol.* 2003;14:128-138.

129. Park KM, Chen A, Bonventre JV. Prevention of kidney ischemia/reperfusion-induced functional injury and JNK, p38, and MAPK kinase activation by remote ischemic pretreatment. *J Biol Chem.* 2001;276:11870-11876.

130. Scheid MP, Schubert KM, Duronio V. Regulation of bad phosphorylation and association with Bcl-x(L) by the MAPK/Erk kinase. *J Biol Chem.* 1999;274:31108-31113.

131. Molitoris BA, Dagher PC, Sandoval RM, et al. siRNA targeted to p53 attenuates ischemic and cisplatin-induced acute kidney injury. *J Am Soc Nephrol.* 2009;20:1754-1764.

132. Sogabe K, Roeser NF, Davis JA, et al. Calcium dependence of integrity of the actin cytoskeleton of proximal tubule cell microvilli. *Am J Physiol.* 1996;271:F292-F303.

133. Portilla D. Role of fatty acid beta-oxidation and calcium-independent phospholipase A$_2$ in ischemic acute renal failure. *Curr Opin Nephrol Hypertens.* 1999;8:473-477.

134. Edelstein CL. Calcium-mediated proximal tubular injury—what is the role of cysteine proteases? *Nephrol Dial Transplant.* 2000;15:141-144.

135. Liu X, Van Vleet T, Schnellmann RG. The role of calpain in oncotic cell death. *Annu Rev Pharmacol Toxicol.* 2004;44:349-370.

136. Liu X, Schnellmann RG. Calpain mediates progressive plasma membrane permeability and proteolysis of cytoskeleton-associated paxillin, talin, and vinculin during renal cell death. *J Pharmacol Exp Ther.* 2003;304: 63-70.

137. Devarajan P. Cellular and molecular derangements in acute tubular necrosis. *Curr Opin Pediatr.* 2005;17:193-199.

138. Akcay A, Nguyen Q, Edelstein CL. Mediators of inflammation in acute kidney injury. *Mediators Inflamm.* 2009;2009:137072.

139. Gluba A, Banach M, Hannam S, et al. The role of Toll-like receptors in renal diseases. *Nat Rev Nephrol.* 2010;6:224-235.

140. Wu H, Chen G, Wyburn KR, et al. TLR4 activation mediates kidney ischemia/reperfusion injury. *J Clin Invest.* 2007;117:2847-2859.

141. Burne-Taney MJ, Rabb H. The role of adhesion molecules and T cells in ischemic renal injury. *Curr Opin Nephrol Hypertens.* 2003;12:85-90.

142. Burne-Taney MJ, Ascon DB, Daniels F, et al. B cell deficiency confers protection from renal ischemia reperfusion injury. *J Immunol.* 2003;171: 3210-3215.

143. Riedemann NC, Guo RF, Ward PA. The enigma of sepsis. *J Clin Invest.* 2003;112:460-467.

144. Kinsey GR, Li L, Okusa MD. Inflammation in acute kidney injury. *Nephron Exp Nephrol.* 2008;109:e102-e107.

145. Tsuboi N, Yoshikai Y, Matsuo S, et al. Roles of toll-like receptors in C-C chemokine production by renal tubular epithelial cells. *J Immunol.* 2002;169:2026-2033.

146. El-Achkar TM, Huang X, Plotkin Z, et al. Sepsis induces changes in the expression and distribution of Toll-like receptor 4 in the rat kidney. *Am J Physiol Renal Physiol.* 2006;290:F1034-F1043.

147. El-Achkar TM, Plotkin Z, Marcic B, et al. Sepsis induces an increase in thick ascending limb Cox-2 that is TLR4 dependent. *Am J Physiol Renal Physiol.* 2007;293:F1187-F1196.

148. El-Achkar TM, Wu XR, Rauchman M, et al. Tamm-Horsfall protein protects the kidney from ischemic injury by decreasing inflammation and altering TLR4 expression. *Am J Physiol Renal Physiol.* 2008;295: F534-F544.

149. Rusai K, Sollinger D, Baumann M, et al. Toll-like receptors 2 and 4 in renal ischemia/reperfusion injury. *Pediatr Nephrol.* 25:853-860.

150. Day YJ, Huang L, Ye H, et al. Renal ischemia-reperfusion injury and adenosine 2A receptor-mediated tissue protection: role of macrophages. *Am J Physiol Renal Physiol.* 2005;288:F722-F731.

151. Dong X, Swaminathan S, Bachman LA, et al. Resident dendritic cells are the predominant TNF-secreting cell in early renal ischemia-reperfusion injury. *Kidney Int.* 2007;71:619-628.

152. Gandolfo MT, Jang HR, Bagnasco SM, et al. Foxp3$^+$ regulatory T cells participate in repair of ischemic acute kidney injury. *Kidney Int.* 2009;76:717-729.

153. Kinsey GR, Huang L, Vergis AL, et al. D. Regulatory T cells contribute to the protective effect of ischemic preconditioning in the kidney. *Kidney Int.* 2010 May;77(9):771–180.

154. Kinsey GR, Sharma R, Huang L, et al. Regulatory T cells suppress innate immunity in kidney ischemia-reperfusion injury. *J Am Soc Nephrol.* 2009;20:1744-1753.

155. Gupta A, Gerlitz B, Richardson MA, et al. Distinct functions of activated protein C differentially attenuate acute kidney injury. *J Am Soc Nephrol.* 2009;20:267-277.

156. Galli F, Piroddi M, Annetti C, et al. Oxidative stress and reactive oxygen species. *Contrib Nephrol.* 2005;149:240-260.

157. Pinsky MR. Pathophysiology of sepsis and multiple organ failure: pro-versus anti-inflammatory aspects. *Contrib Nephrol.* 2004;144:31-43.

158. Kelly KJ. Stress response proteins and renal ischemia. *Minerva Urol Nefrol.* 2002;54:81-91.

159. Paller MS, Weber K, Patten M. Nitric oxide–mediated renal epithelial cell injury during hypoxia and reoxygenation. *Ren Fail.* 1998;20:459-469.

160. Bidmon B, Endemann M, Muller T, et al. HSP-25 and HSP-90 stabilize Na, K-ATPase in cytoskeletal fractions of ischemic rat renal cortex. *Kidney Int.* 2002;62:1620-1627.

161. Kanakiriya S, Nath KA. *Heme oxygenase and acute renal injury.* ed 1. Philadelphia: Saunders; 2001.

162. Kapturczak MH, Wasserfall C, Brusko T, et al. Heme oxygenase-1 modulates early inflammatory responses: evidence from the heme oxygenase-1-deficient mouse. *Am J Pathol.* 2004;165:1045-1053.

163. Shiraishi F, Curtis LM, Truong L, et al. Heme oxygenase-1 gene ablation or expression modulates cisplatin-induced renal tubular apoptosis. *Am J Physiol Renal Physiol.* 2000;278:F726-F736.

164. Nath KA, Haggard JJ, Croatt AJ, et al. The indispensability of heme oxygenase-1 in protecting against acute heme protein–induced toxicity in vivo. *Am J Pathol.* 2000;156:1527-1535.

165. Inguaggiato P, Gonzalez-Michaca L, Croatt AJ, et al. Cellular overexpression of heme oxygenase-1 up-regulates p21 and confers resistance to apoptosis. *Kidney Int.* 2001;60:2181-2191.
166. Stromski ME, Cooper K, Thulin G, et al. Chemical and functional correlates of postischemic renal ATP levels. *Proc Natl Acad Sci U S A.* 1986;83:6142-6145.
167. Spiegel DM, Wilson PD, Molitoris BA. Epithelial polarity following ischemia: a requirement for normal cell function. *Am J Physiol.* 1989;256:F430-F436.
168. Ichimura T, Bonventre JV. *Growth factors, signaling, and renal injury and repair.* ed 1. Philadelphia: Saunders; 2001.
169. Hammerman MR. Growth factors and apoptosis in acute renal injury. *Curr Opin Nephrol Hypertens.* 1998;7:419-424.
170. Fiaschi-Taesch NM, Santos S, Reddy V, et al. Prevention of acute ischemic renal failure by targeted delivery of growth factors to the proximal tubule in transgenic mice: the efficacy of parathyroid hormone-related protein and hepatocyte growth factor. *J Am Soc Nephrol.* 2004;15:112-125.
171. Matsumoto M, Makino Y, Tanaka T, et al. Induction of renoprotective gene expression by cobalt ameliorates ischemic injury of the kidney in rats. *J Am Soc Nephrol.* 2003;14:1825-1832.
172. Vannay A, Fekete A, Adori C, et al. Divergence of renal vascular endothelial growth factor mRNA expression and protein level in post-ischaemic rat kidneys. *Exp Physiol.* 2004;89:435-444.
173. Hladunewich MA, Corrigan G, Derby GC, et al. A randomized, placebo-controlled trial of IGF-1 for delayed graft function: a human model to study postischemic ARF. *Kidney Int.* 2003;64:593-602.
174. Hirschberg R, Kopple J, Lipsett P, et al. Multicenter clinical trial of recombinant human insulin-like growth factor I in patients with acute renal failure. *Kidney Int.* 1999;55:2423-2432.
175. Gupta S, Verfaillie C, Chmielewski D, et al. Isolation and characterization of kidney-derived stem cells. *J Am Soc Nephrol.* 2006;17:3028-3040.
176. Bussolati B, Bruno S, Grange C, et al. Isolation of renal progenitor cells from adult human kidney. *Am J Pathol.* 2005;166:545-555.
177. De Broe ME. Tubular regeneration and the role of bone marrow cells: "stem cell therapy"—a panacea? *Nephrol Dial Transplant.* 2005;20:2318-2320.
178. Fang TC, Alison MR, Cook HT, et al. Proliferation of bone marrow–derived cells contributes to regeneration after folic acid-induced acute tubular injury. *J Am Soc Nephrol.* 2005;16:1723-1732.
179. Poulsom R, Forbes SJ, Hodivala-Dilke K, et al. Bone marrow contributes to renal parenchymal turnover and regeneration. *J Pathol.* 2001;195:229-235.
180. Lange C, Togel F, Ittrich H, et al. Administered mesenchymal stem cells enhance recovery from ischemia/reperfusion-induced acute renal failure in rats. *Kidney Int.* 2005;68:1613-1617.
181. Togel F, Zhang P, Hu Z, et al. VEGF is a mediator of the renoprotective effects of multipotent marrow stromal cells in acute kidney injury. *J Cell Mol Med.* 2009;13:2109-2114.
182. Humphreys BD, Bonventre JV. Mesenchymal stem cells in acute kidney injury. *Annu Rev Med.* 2008;59:311-325.
183. Humphreys BD, Valerius MT, Kobayashi A, et al. Intrinsic epithelial cells repair the kidney after injury. *Cell Stem Cell.* 2008;2:284-291.
184. Cantley LG. Adult stem cells in the repair of the injured renal tubule. *Nat Clin Pract Nephrol.* 2005;1:22-32.
185. Conger JD, Schrier RW. Renal hemodynamics in acute renal failure. *Annu Rev Physiol.* 1980;42:603-614.
186. Conger JD, Robinette JB, Hammond WS. Differences in vascular reactivity in models of ischemic acute renal failure. *Kidney Int.* 1991;39:1087-1097.
187. Noiri E, Nakao A, Uchida K, et al. Oxidative and nitrosative stress in acute renal ischemia. *Am J Physiol Renal Physiol.* 2001;281:F948-F957.
188. Ling H, Edelstein C, Gengaro P, et al. Attenuation of renal ischemia-reperfusion injury in inducible nitric oxide synthase knockout mice. *Am J Physiol.* 1999;277:F383-F390.
189. Goligorsky MS, Noiri E. Duality of nitric oxide in acute renal injury. *Semin Nephrol.* 1999;19:263-271.
190. Goligorsky MS, Brodsky SV, Noiri E. NO bioavailability, endothelial dysfunction, and acute renal failure: new insights into pathophysiology. *Semin Nephrol.* 2004;24:316-323.
191. Mattson DL, Wu F. Control of arterial blood pressure and renal sodium excretion by nitric oxide synthase in the renal medulla. *Acta Physiol Scand.* 2000;168:149-154.
192. Chander V, Chopra K. Renal protective effect of molsidomine and L-arginine in ischemia-reperfusion induced injury in rats. *J Surg Res.* 2005;128:132-139.
193. Bogatcheva NV, Verin AD. The role of cytoskeleton in the regulation of vascular endothelial barrier function. *Microvasc Res.* 2008;76:202-207.
194. Bajwa A, Jo SK, Ye H, et al. Activation of sphingosine-1-phosphate 1 receptor in the proximal tubule protects against ischemia-reperfusion injury. *J Am Soc Nephrol.* 2010;21(6):955-965.
195. Sutton TA, Mang HE, Campos SB, et al. Injury of the renal microvascular endothelium alters barrier function after ischemia. *Am J Physiol Renal Physiol.* 2003;285:F191-F198.
196. Sutton TA, Kelly KJ, Mang HE, et al. Minocycline reduces renal microvascular leakage in a rat model of ischemic renal injury. *Am J Physiol Renal Physiol.* 2005;288:F91-F97.
197. Horbelt M, Lee SY, Mang HE, et al. Acute and chronic microvascular alterations in a mouse model of ischemic acute kidney injury. *Am J Physiol Renal Physiol.* 2007;293:F688-F695.
198. Gupta A, Rhodes GJ, Berg DT, et al. Activated protein C ameliorates LPS-induced acute kidney injury and downregulates renal INOS and angiotensin 2. *Am J Physiol Renal Physiol.* 2007;293:F245-F254.
199. Gupta A, Williams MD, Macias WL, et al. Activated protein C and acute kidney injury: selective targeting of PAR-1. *Curr Drug Targets.* 2009;10:1212-1226.
200. Mizutani A, Okajima K, Uchiba M, et al. Activated protein C reduces ischemia/reperfusion-induced renal injury in rats by inhibiting leukocyte activation. *Blood.* 2000;95:3781-3787.
201. Singbartl K, Ley K. Leukocyte recruitment and acute renal failure. *J Mol Med.* 2004;82:91-101.
202. Burne MJ, Rabb H. Pathophysiological contributions of fucosyltransferases in renal ischemia reperfusion injury. *J Immunol.* 2002;169:2648-2652.
203. Nemoto T, Burne MJ, Daniels F, et al. Small molecule selectin ligand inhibition improves outcome in ischemic acute renal failure. *Kidney Int.* 2001;60:2205-2214.
204. Singbartl K, Forlow SB, Ley K. Platelet, but not endothelial, P-selectin is critical for neutrophil-mediated acute postischemic renal failure. *FASEB J.* 2001;15:2337-2344.
205. Matsukawa A, Lukacs NW, Hogaboam CM, et al. Mice genetically lacking endothelial selectins are resistant to the lethality in septic peritonitis. *Exp Mol Pathol.* 2002;72:68-76.
206. Kelly KJ, Williams Jr WW, Colvin RB, et al. Intercellular adhesion molecule-1–deficient mice are protected against ischemic renal injury. *J Clin Invest.* 1996;97:1056-1063.
207. Liu M, Chien CC, Grigoryev DN, et al. Effect of T cells on vascular permeability in early ischemic acute kidney injury in mice. *Microvasc Res.* 2009;77:340-347.
208. Savransky V, Molls RR, Burne-Taney M, et al. Role of the T-cell receptor in kidney ischemia-reperfusion injury. *Kidney Int.* 2006;69:233-238.
209. Ashworth SL, Sandoval RM, Tanner GA, et al. Two-photon microscopy: visualization of kidney dynamics. *Kidney Int.* 2007;72:416-421.
210. Basile DP. The endothelial cell in ischemic acute kidney injury: implications for acute and chronic function. *Kidney Int.* 2007;72:151-156.
211. Basile DP, Fredrich K, Chelladurai B, et al. Renal ischemia reperfusion inhibits VEGF expression and induces ADAMTS-1, a novel VEGF inhibitor. *Am J Physiol Renal Physiol.* 2008;294:F928-F936.
212. Leonard EC, Friedrich JL, Basile DP. VEGF-121 preserves renal microvessel structure and ameliorates secondary renal disease following acute kidney injury. *Am J Physiol Renal Physiol.* 2008;295:F1648-F1657.
213. Tongers J, Losordo DW. Frontiers in nephrology: the evolving therapeutic applications of endothelial progenitor cells. *J Am Soc Nephrol.* 2007;18:2843-2852.
214. Becherucci F, Mazzinghi B, Ronconi E, et al. The role of endothelial progenitor cells in acute kidney injury. *Blood Purif.* 2009;27:261-270.
215. Kramer AA, Postler G, Salhab KF, et al. Renal ischemia/reperfusion leads to macrophage-mediated increase in pulmonary vascular permeability. *Kidney Int.* 1999;55:2362-2367.
216. Rabb H, Wang Z, Nemoto T, et al. Acute renal failure leads to dysregulation of lung salt and water channels. *Kidney Int.* 2003;63:600-606.
217. Liu M, Liang Y, Chigurupati S, et al. Acute kidney injury leads to inflammation and functional changes in the brain. *J Am Soc Nephrol.* 2008;19:1360-1370.
218. Imai Y, Parodo J, Kajikawa O, et al. Injurious mechanical ventilation and end-organ epithelial cell apoptosis and organ dysfunction in an experimental model of acute respiratory distress syndrome. *JAMA.* 2003;289:2104-2112.
219. Pratschke J, Wilhelm MJ, Laskowski I, et al. Influence of donor brain death on chronic rejection of renal transplants in rats. *J Am Soc Nephrol.* 2001;12:2474-2481.
220. Kielar ML, Rohan Jeyarajah D, Lu CY. The regulation of ischemic acute renal failure by extrarenal organs. *Curr Opin Nephrol Hypertens.* 2002;11:451-457.
221. Thadhani R, Pascual M, Bonventre JV. Acute renal failure. *N Engl J Med.* 1996;334:1448-1460.
222. Abernethy VE, Lieberthal W. Acute renal failure in the critically ill patient. *Crit Care Clin.* 2002;18:203-222, v.
223. Abassi ZA, Hoffman A, Better OS. Acute renal failure complicating muscle crush injury. *Semin Nephrol.* 1998;18:558-565.
224. Zager RA. Rhabdomyolysis and myohemoglobinuric acute renal failure. *Kidney Int.* 1996;49:314-326.
225. Sever MS, Vanholder R, Lameire N. Management of crush-related injuries after disasters. *N Engl J Med.* 2006;354:1052-1063.

226. Pontremoli R, Rampoldi V, Morbidelli A, et al. Acute renal failure due to acute bilateral renal artery thrombosis: successful surgical revascularization after prolonged anuria. *Nephron*. 1990;56:322-324.

227. Delans RJ, Ramirez G, Farber MS, et al. Renal artery thrombosis: a cause of reversible acute renal failure. *J Urol*. 1982;128:1287-1289.

228. Nahar A, Akom M, Hanes D, et al. Pyelonephritis and acute renal failure. *Am J Med Sci*. 2004;328:121-123.

229. Clarkson MR, Giblin L, O'Connell FP, et al. Acute interstitial nephritis: clinical features and response to corticosteroid therapy. *Nephrol Dial Transplant*. 2004;19:2778-2783.

230. Sessa A, Meroni M, Battini G, et al. Acute renal failure due to idiopathic tubulo-intestinal nephritis and uveitis: "TINU syndrome." Case report and review of the literature. *J Nephrol*. 2000;13:377-380.

231. Ehlers SM, Posalaky Z, Strate RG, et al. Acute reversible renal failure following jejunoileal bypass for morbid obesity: a clinical and pathological (EM) study of a case. *Surgery*. 1977;82:629-634.

232. Szwed JJ. Urinalysis and clinical renal disease. *Am J Med Technol*. 1980;46:720-725.

233. Tsai JJ, Yeun JY, Kumar VA, et al. Comparison and interpretation of urinalysis performed by a nephrologist versus a hospital-based clinical laboratory. *Am J Kidney Dis*. 2005;46:820-829.

234. Nolan 3rd CR, Anger MS, Kelleher SP. Eosinophiluria—a new method of detection and definition of the clinical spectrum. *N Engl J Med*. 1986;315:1516-1519.

235. Corwin HL, Korbet SM, Schwartz MM. Clinical correlates of eosinophiluria. *Arch Intern Med*. 1985;145:1097-1099.

236. Meier M, Nitschke M, Perras B, et al. Ethylene glycol intoxication and xylitol infusion—metabolic steps of oxalate-induced acute renal failure. *Clin Nephrol*. 2005;63:225-228.

237. Cohen DJ, Sherman WH, Osserman EF, et al. Acute renal failure in patients with multiple myeloma. *Am J Med*. 1984;76:247-256.

238. Revai T, Harmos G. Nephrotic syndrome and acute interstitial nephritis associated with the use of diclofenac. *Wien Klin Wochenschr*. 1999;111:523-524.

239. Averbuch SD, Austin 3rd HA, Sherwin SA, et al. Acute interstitial nephritis with the nephrotic syndrome following recombinant leukocyte a interferon therapy for mycosis fungoides. *N Engl J Med*. 1984;310:32-35.

240. Neugarten J, Gallo GR, Baldwin DS. Rifampin-induced nephrotic syndrome and acute interstitial nephritis. *Am J Nephrol*. 1983;3:38-42.

241. Zarich S, Fang LS, Diamond JR. Fractional excretion of sodium. Exceptions to its diagnostic value. *Arch Intern Med*. 1985;145:108-112.

242. Diamond JR, Yoburn DC. Nonoliguric acute renal failure associated with a low fractional excretion of sodium. *Ann Intern Med*. 1982;96:597-600.

243. Espinel CH. The FENa test. Use in the differential diagnosis of acute renal failure. *JAMA*. 1976;236:579-581.

244. Vanholder R, Sever MS, Erek E, et al. Rhabdomyolysis. *J Am Soc Nephrol*. 2000;11:1553-1561.

245. Honda N. Acute renal failure and rhabdomyolysis. *Kidney Int*. 1983;23:888-898.

246. Boles JM, Dutel JL, Briere J, et al. Acute renal failure caused by extreme hyperphosphatemia after chemotherapy of an acute lymphoblastic leukemia. *Cancer*. 1984;53:2425-2429.

247. Razis E, Arlin ZA, Ahmed T, et al. Incidence and treatment of tumor lysis syndrome in patients with acute leukemia. *Acta Haematol*. 1994;91:171-174.

248. Bhandari S. The patient with acute renal failure and non-dilated urinary tract. *Nephrol Dial Transplant*. 1998;13:1888.

249. Pozzi Mucelli R, Bertolotto M, Quaia E. Imaging techniques in acute renal failure. *Contrib Nephrol*. 2001:76-91.

250. Mucelli RP, Bertolotto M. Imaging techniques in acute renal failure. *Kidney Int Suppl*. 1998;66:S102-S105.

251. Marcos HB, Choyke PL. Magnetic resonance angiography of the kidney. *Semin Nephrol*. 2000;20:450-455.

252. Cowper SE. Nephrogenic systemic fibrosis: a review and exploration of the role of gadolinium. *Adv Dermatol*. 2007;23:131-154.

253. Cowper SE. Nephrogenic systemic fibrosis: an overview. *J Am Coll Radiol*. 2008;5:23-28.

254. Solez K, Racusen LC. Role of the renal biopsy in acute renal failure. *Contrib Nephrol*. 2001:68-75.

255. Humphreys BD, Soiffer RJ, Magee CC. Renal failure associated with cancer and its treatment: an update. *J Am Soc Nephrol*. 2005;16:151-161.

256. Finkel KW, Foringer JR. Renal disease in patients with cancer. *Nat Clin Pract*. 2007;3:669-678.

257. Daugaard G. Cisplatin nephrotoxicity: experimental and clinical studies. *Dan Med Bull*. 1990;37:1-12.

258. Daugaard G, Abildgaard U. Cisplatin nephrotoxicity. A review. *Cancer Chemother Pharmacol*. 1989;25:1-9.

259. Lee BS, Lee JH, Kang HG, et al. Ifosfamide nephrotoxicity in pediatric cancer patients. *Pediatr Nephrol*. 2001;16:796-799.

260. Nissim I, Horyn O, Daikhin Y, et al. Ifosfamide-induced nephrotoxicity: mechanism and prevention. *Cancer Res*. 2006;66:7824-7831.

261. Rossi R. Nephrotoxicity of ifosfamide—moving towards understanding the molecular mechanisms. *Nephrol Dial Transplant*. 1997;12:1091-1092.

262. Lundberg WB, Cadman ED, Finch SC, et al. Renal failure secondary to leukemic infiltration of the kidneys. *Am J Med*. 1977;62:636-642.

263. Srinivasa NS, McGovern CH, Solez K, et al. Progressive renal failure due to renal invasion and parenchymal destruction by adult T-cell lymphoma. *Am J Kidney Dis*. 1990;16:70-72.

264. Jeha S. Tumor lysis syndrome. *Semin Hematol*. 2001;38:4-8.

265. Cairo MS, Bishop M. Tumour lysis syndrome: new therapeutic strategies and classification. *Br J Haematol*. 2004;127:3-11.

266. Cammalleri L, Malaguarnera M. Rasburicase represents a new tool for hyperuricemia in tumor lysis syndrome and in gout. *Int J Med Sci*. 2007;4:83-93.

267. Coiffier B, Riouffol C. Management of tumor lysis syndrome in adults. *Expert Rev Anticancer Ther*. 2007;7:233-239.

268. Wang LY, Shih LY, Chang H, et al. Recombinant urate oxidase (rasburicase) for the prevention and treatment of tumor lysis syndrome in patients with hematologic malignancies. *Acta Haematol*. 2006;115:35-38.

269. Giroux L, Bettez P, Giroux L. Mitomycin-C nephrotoxicity: a clinico-pathologic study of 17 cases. *Am J Kidney Dis*. 1985;6:28-39.

270. Jolivet J, Giroux L, Laurin S, et al. Microangiopathic hemolytic anemia, renal failure, and noncardiogenic pulmonary edema: a chemotherapy-induced syndrome. *Cancer Treat Rep*. 1983;67:429-434.

271. Medina PJ, Sipols JM, George JN. Drug-associated thrombotic thrombocytopenic purpura-hemolytic uremic syndrome. *Curr Opin Hematol*. 2001;8:286-293.

272. Siami GA, Siami FS. Plasmapheresis and paraproteinemia: cryoprotein-induced diseases, monoclonal gammopathy, Waldenström's macroglobulinemia, hyperviscosity syndrome, multiple myeloma, light chain disease, and amyloidosis. *Ther Apher*. 1999;3:8-19.

273. Johnson WJ, Kyle RA, Pineda AA, et al. Treatment of renal failure associated with multiple myeloma. Plasmapheresis, hemodialysis, and chemotherapy. *Arch Intern Med*. 1990;150:863-869.

274. Madore F. Does plasmapheresis have a role in the management of myeloma cast nephropathy? *Nat Clin Pract*. 2006;2:406-407.

275. Pillon L, Sweeting RS, Arora A, et al. Approach to acute renal failure in biopsy proven myeloma cast nephropathy: is there still a role for plasmapheresis? *Kidney Int*. 2008;74:956-961.

276. Prakash J, Kumar H, Sinha DK, et al. Acute renal failure in pregnancy in a developing country: twenty years of experience. *Ren Fail*. 2006;28:309-313.

277. Gammill HS, Jeyabalan A. Acute renal failure in pregnancy. *Crit Care Med*. 2005;33:S372-S384.

278. Ventura JE, Villa M, Mizraji R, et al. Acute renal failure in pregnancy. *Ren Fail*. 1997;19:217-220.

279. Alexopoulos E, Tambakoudis P, Bili H, et al. Acute renal failure in pregnancy. *Ren Fail*. 1993;15:609-613.

280. Sibai BM, Kustermann L, Velasco J. Current understanding of severe preeclampsia, pregnancy-associated hemolytic uremic syndrome, thrombotic thrombocytopenic purpura, hemolysis, elevated liver enzymes, and low platelet syndrome, and postpartum acute renal failure: different clinical syndromes or just different names? *Curr Opin Nephrol Hypertens*. 1994;3:436-445.

281. Pertuiset N, Grunfeld JP. Acute renal failure in pregnancy. *Baillieres Clin Obstet Gynaecol*. 1994;8:333-351.

282. Treem WR. Mitochondrial fatty acid oxidation and acute fatty liver of pregnancy. *Semin Gastrointest Dis*. 2002;13:55-66.

283. Weiner CP. Thrombotic microangiopathy in pregnancy and the postpartum period. *Semin Hematol*. 1987;24:119-129.

284. Grunfeld JP, Ganeval D, Bournerias F. Acute renal failure in pregnancy. *Kidney Int*. 1980;18:179-191.

285. Davies MH, Wilkinson SP, Hanid MA, et al. Acute liver disease with encephalopathy and renal failure in late pregnancy and the early puerperium—a study of fourteen patients. *Br J Obstet Gynaecol*. 1980;87:1005-1014.

286. Thakar CV, Worley S, Arrigain S, et al. Influence of renal dysfunction on mortality after cardiac surgery: modifying effect of preoperative renal function. *Kidney Int*. 2005;67:1112-1119.

287. Fortescue EB, Bates DW, Chertow GM. Predicting acute renal failure after coronary bypass surgery: cross-validation of two risk-stratification algorithms. *Kidney Int*. 2000;57:2594-2602.

288. Bahar I, Akgul A, Ozatik MA, et al. Acute renal failure following open heart surgery: risk factors and prognosis. *Perfusion*. 2005;20:317-322.

289. Mangos GJ, Brown MA, Chan WY, et al. Acute renal failure following cardiac surgery: incidence, outcomes and risk factors. *Aust N Z J Med*. 1995;25:284-289.

290. Conlon PJ, Stafford-Smith M, White WD, et al. Acute renal failure following cardiac surgery. *Nephrol Dial Transplant*. 1999;14:1158-1162.

291. Chertow GM, Lazarus JM, Christiansen CL, et al. Preoperative renal risk stratification. *Circulation*. 1997;95:878-884.

292. Thakar CV, Arrigain S, Worley S, et al. A clinical score to predict acute renal failure after cardiac surgery. *J Am Soc Nephrol.* 2005;16:162-168.
293. Wijeysundera DN, Beattie WS, Djaiani G, et al. Off-pump coronary artery surgery for reducing mortality and morbidity: meta-analysis of randomized and observational studies. *J Am Coll Cardiol.* 2005;46:872-882.
294. Nathoe HM, van Dijk D, Jansen EW, et al. A comparison of on-pump and off-pump coronary bypass surgery in low-risk patients. *N Engl J Med.* 2003;348:394-402.
295. Hix JK, Thakar CV, Katz EM, et al. Effect of off-pump coronary artery bypass graft surgery on postoperative acute kidney injury and mortality. *Crit Care Med.* 2006;34:2979-2983.
296. Nigwekar SU, Kandula P, Hix JK, et al. Off-pump coronary artery bypass surgery and acute kidney injury: a meta-analysis of randomized and observational studies. *Am J Kidney Dis.* 2009;54:413-423.
297. Wyatt CM, Arons RR. The burden of acute renal failure in nonrenal solid organ transplantation. *Transplantation.* 2004;78:1351-1355.
298. Bilbao I, Charco R, Balsells J, et al. Risk factors for acute renal failure requiring dialysis after liver transplantation. *Clin Transplant.* 1998;12:123-129.
299. Brown Jr RS, Lombardero M, Lake JR. Outcome of patients with renal insufficiency undergoing liver or liver-kidney transplantation. *Transplantation.* 1996;62:1788-1793.
300. Nair S, Verma S, Thuluvath PJ. Pretransplant renal function predicts survival in patients undergoing orthotopic liver transplantation. *Hepatology.* 2002;35:1179-1185.
301. Lafayette RA, Pare G, Schmid CH, et al. Pretransplant renal dysfunction predicts poorer outcome in liver transplantation. *Clin Nephrol.* 1997;48:159-164.
302. Gonwa TA, Klintmalm GB, Levy M, et al. Impact of pretransplant renal function on survival after liver transplantation. *Transplantation.* 1995;59:361-365.
303. Parikh CR, McSweeney PA, Korular D, et al. Renal dysfunction in allogeneic hematopoietic cell transplantation. *Kidney Int.* 2002;62:566-573.
304. Hingorani SR, Guthrie K, Batchelder A, et al. Acute renal failure after myeloablative hematopoietic cell transplant: incidence and risk factors. *Kidney Int.* 2005;67:272-277.
305. Parikh CR, Coca SG. Acute renal failure in hematopoietic cell transplantation. *Kidney Int.* 2006;69:430-435.
306. Schrier RW, Parikh CR. Comparison of renal injury in myeloablative autologous, myeloablative allogeneic and non-myeloablative allogeneic haematopoietic cell transplantation. *Nephrol Dial Transplant.* 2005;20:678-683.
307. Zager RA, O'Quigley J, Zager BK, et al. Acute renal failure following bone marrow transplantation: a retrospective study of 272 patients. *Am J Kidney Dis.* 1989;13:210-216.
308. Parikh CR, Schrier RW, Storer B, et al. Comparison of ARF after myeloablative and nonmyeloablative hematopoietic cell transplantation. *Am J Kidney Dis.* 2005;45:502-509.
309. Parikh CR, Sandmaier BM, Storb RF, et al. Acute renal failure after nonmyeloablative hematopoietic cell transplantation. *J Am Soc Nephrol.* 2004;15:1868-1876.
310. Merouani A, Shpall EJ, Jones RB, et al. Renal function in high dose chemotherapy and autologous hematopoietic cell support treatment for breast cancer. *Kidney Int.* 1996;50:1026-1031.
311. Fadia A, Casserly LF, Sanchorawala V, et al. Incidence and outcome of acute renal failure complicating autologous stem cell transplantation for AL amyloidosis. *Kidney Int.* 2003;63:1868-1873.
312. McDonald GB, Hinds MS, Fisher LD, et al. Veno-occlusive disease of the liver and multiorgan failure after bone marrow transplantation: a cohort study of 355 patients. *Ann Intern Med.* 1993;118:255-267.
313. Shulman HM, Fisher LB, Schoch HG, et al. Veno-occlusive disease of the liver after marrow transplantation: histological correlates of clinical signs and symptoms. *Hepatology.* 1994;19:1171-1181.
314. Jones RJ, Lee KS, Beschorner WE, et al. Venoocclusive disease of the liver following bone marrow transplantation. *Transplantation.* 1987;44:778-783.
315. Dalpiaz G, Nassetti C, Stasi G. Diffuse alveolar haemorrhage from a rare primary renal-pulmonary syndrome: micropolyangiitis. Case report and differential diagnosis. *Radiol Med.* 2003;106:114-119.
316. Gallagher H, Kwan JT, Jayne DR. Pulmonary renal syndrome: a 4-year, single-center experience. *Am J Kidney Dis.* 2002;39:42-47.
317. Bonsib SM, Walker WP. Pulmonary-renal syndrome: clinical similarity amidst etiologic diversity. *Mod Pathol.* 1989;2:129-137.
318. Wadei HM, Mai ML, Ahsan N, et al. Hepatorenal syndrome: pathophysiology and management. *Clin J Am Soc Nephrol.* 2006;1:1066-1079.
319. Arroyo V, Guevara M, Gines P. Hepatorenal syndrome in cirrhosis: pathogenesis and treatment. *Gastroenterology.* 2002;122:1658-1676.
320. Gines P, Guevara M, Arroyo V, et al. Hepatorenal syndrome. *Lancet.* 2003;362:1819-1827.
321. Salerno F, Gerbes A, Gines P, et al. Diagnosis, prevention and treatment of hepatorenal syndrome in cirrhosis. *Gut.* 2007;56:1310-1318.
322. Gines P, Arroyo V. Hepatorenal syndrome. *J Am Soc Nephrol.* 1999;10:1833-1839.
323. Arroyo V, Gines P, Gerbes AL, et al. Definition and diagnostic criteria of refractory ascites and hepatorenal syndrome in cirrhosis. International Ascites Club. *Hepatology.* 1996;23:164-176.
324. Esrailian E, Pantangco ER, Kyulo NL, et al. Octreotide/midodrine therapy significantly improves renal function and 30-day survival in patients with type 1 hepatorenal syndrome. *Dig Dis Sci.* 2007;52:742-748.
325. Esrailian E, Runyon BA. Alcoholic cirrhosis–associated hepatorenal syndrome treated with vasoactive agents. *Nat Clin Pract.* 2006;2:169-172.
326. Cardenas A. Hepatorenal syndrome: a dreaded complication of end-stage liver disease. *Am J Gastroenterol.* 2005;100:460-467.
327. Gines P, Cardenas A, Arroyo V, et al. Management of cirrhosis and ascites. *N Engl J Med.* 2004;350:1646-1654.
328. Sanyal AJ, Boyer T, Garcia-Tsao G, et al. A randomized, prospective, double-blind, placebo-controlled trial of terlipressin for type 1 hepatorenal syndrome. *Gastroenterology.* 2008;134:1360-1368.
329. Martin-Llahi M, Pepin MN, Guevara M, et al. Terlipressin and albumin vs albumin in patients with cirrhosis and hepatorenal syndrome: a randomized study. *Gastroenterology.* 2008;134:1352-1359.
330. Kiser TH, Fish DN, Obritsch MD, et al. Vasopressin, not octreotide, may be beneficial in the treatment of hepatorenal syndrome: a retrospective study. *Nephrol Dial Transplant.* 2005;20:1813-1820.
331. Gluud LL, Kjaer MS, Christensen E. Terlipressin for hepatorenal syndrome. *Cochrane Database Syst Rev.* 2006;(4):CD005162.
332. Alessandria C, Ottobrelli A, Debernardi-Venon W, et al. Noradrenalin vs terlipressin in patients with hepatorenal syndrome: a prospective, randomized, unblinded, pilot study. *J Hepatol.* 2007;47:499-505.
333. Lim JK, Groszmann RJ. Vasoconstrictor therapy for the hepatorenal syndrome. *Gastroenterology.* 2008;134:1608-1611.
334. Loghman-Adham M, Siegler RL, Pysher TJ. Acute renal failure in idiopathic nephrotic syndrome. *Clin Nephrol.* 1997;47:76-80.
335. James SH, Lien YH, Ruffenach SJ, et al. Acute renal failure in membranous glomerulonephropathy: a result of superimposed crescentic glomerulonephritis. *J Am Soc Nephrol.* 1995;6:1541-1546.
336. Blackshear JL, Davidman M, Stillman MT. Identification of risk for renal insufficiency from nonsteroidal anti-inflammatory drugs. *Arch Intern Med.* 1983;143:1130-1134.
337. Clive DM, Stoff JS. Renal syndromes associated with nonsteroidal antiinflammatory drugs. *N Engl J Med.* 1984;310:563-572.
338. Brezin JH, Katz SM, Schwartz AB, et al. Reversible renal failure and nephrotic syndrome associated with nonsteroidal anti-inflammatory drugs. *N Engl J Med.* 1979;301:1271-1273.
339. Booth LJ, Minielly JA, Smith EK. Acute renal failure in multiple myeloma. *CMAJ.* 1974;111:334-335.
340. Kjeldsberg CR, Holman RE. Acute renal failure in multiple myeloma. *J Urol.* 1971;105:21-23.
341. Chertow GM, Burdick E, Honour M, et al. Acute kidney injury, mortality, length of stay, and costs in hospitalized patients. *J Am Soc Nephrol.* 2005;16:3365-3370.
342. Kellum JA, Angus DC. Patients are dying of acute renal failure. *Crit Care Med.* 2002;30:2156-2157.
343. Del Toro G, Morris E, Cairo MS. Tumor lysis syndrome: pathophysiology, definition, and alternative treatment approaches. *Clin Adv Hematol Oncol.* 2005;3:54-61.
344. Esposito C, Bellotti N, Fasoli G, et al. A. Hyperkalemia-induced ECG abnormalities in patients with reduced renal function. *Clin Nephrol.* 2004;62:465-468.
345. Mattu A, Brady WJ, Robinson DA. Electrocardiographic manifestations of hyperkalemia. *Am J Emerg Med.* 2000;18:721-729.
346. Arnsdorf MF. Electrocardiogram in hyperkalemia: electrocardiographic pattern of anteroseptal myocardial infarction mimicked by hyperkalemia-induced disturbance of impulse conduction. *Arch Intern Med.* 1976;136:1161-1163.
347. Cronin RE, Bulger RE, Southern P, et al. Natural history of aminoglycoside nephrotoxicity in the dog. *J Lab Clin Med.* 1980;95:463-474.
348. Patel R, Savage A. Symptomatic hypomagnesemia associated with gentamicin therapy. *Nephron.* 1979;23:50-52.
349. Miltenyi M, Tulassay T, Korner A, et al. Tubular dysfunction in metabolic acidosis. First step to acute renal failure. *Contrib Nephrol.* 1988;67:58-66.
350. Frommer JP, Ayus JC. Acute ethylene glycol intoxication. *Am J Nephrol.* 1982;2:1-5.
351. Kaplan BS, Hebert D, Morrell RE. Acute renal failure induced by hyperphosphatemia in acute lymphoblastic leukemia. *CMAJ.* 1981;124:429-431.
352. Singhal PC, Kumar A, Desroches L, et al. Prevalence and predictors of rhabdomyolysis in patients with hypophosphatemia. *Am J Med.* 1992;92:458-464.
353. Tsokos GC, Balow JE, Spiegel RJ, et al. Renal and metabolic complications of undifferentiated and lymphoblastic lymphomas. *Medicine.* 1981;60:218-229.

354. Ettinger DS, Harker WG, Gerry HW, et al. Hyperphosphatemia, hypocalcemia, and transient renal failure. Results of cytotoxic treatment of acute lymphoblastic leukemia. *JAMA*. 1978;239:2472-2474.

355. May R, Stivelman JC, Maroni BJ. Metabolic and electrolyte disturbances in acute renal failure. In: Lazarus JM, Brenner BM, eds. *Acute renal failure*. ed 3. New York: Churchill Livingston; 1993:107-117.

356. Pietrek J, Kokot F, Kuska J. Serum 25-hydroxyvitamin D and parathyroid hormone in patients with acute renal failure. *Kidney Int*. 1978;13:178-185.

357. Arieff AI, Massry SG. Calcium metabolism of brain in acute renal failure. Effects of uremia, hemodialysis, and parathyroid hormone. *J Clin Invest*. 1974;53:387-392.

358. Zaman F, Abreo K. Severe hypermagnesemia as a result of laxative use in renal insufficiency. *South Med J*. 2003;96:102-103.

359. Massry SG, Seelig MS. Hypomagnesemia and hypermagnesemia. *Clin Nephrol*. 1977;7:147-153.

360. Schilsky RL, Anderson T. Hypomagnesemia and renal magnesium wasting in patients receiving cisplatin. *Ann Intern Med*. 1979;90:929-931.

361. Blachley JD, Hill JB. Renal and electrolyte disturbances associated with cisplatin. *Ann Intern Med*. 1981;95:628-632.

362. Schelling JR. Fatal hypermagnesemia. *Clin Nephrol*. 2000;53:61-65.

363. Conger JD. Acute uric acid nephropathy. *Med Clin North Am*. 1990;74:859-871.

364. Conger JD, Falk SA. Intrarenal dynamics in the pathogenesis and prevention of acute urate nephropathy. *J Clin Invest*. 1977;59:786-793.

365. Cairo MS. Prevention and treatment of hyperuricemia in hematological malignancies. *Clin Lymphoma*. 2002;3(suppl 1):S26-S31.

366. Tungsanga K, Boonwichit D, Lekhakula A, et al. Urine uric acid and urine creatine ratio in acute renal failure. *Arch Intern Med*. 1984;144:934-937.

367. Sanchez M, Bosch X, Martinez C, et al. Idiopathic pulmonary-renal syndrome with antiproteinase 3 antibodies. *Respiration*. 1994;61:295-299.

368. Mattern WD, Sommers SC, Kassirer JP. Oliguric acute renal failure in malignant hypertension. *Am J Med*. 1972;52:187-197.

369. Rasmussen HH, Ibels LS. Acute renal failure. Multivariate analysis of causes and risk factors. *Am J Med*. 1982;73:211-218.

370. Anderson RJ, Chung HM, Kluge R, et al. Hyponatremia: a prospective analysis of its epidemiology and the pathogenetic role of vasopressin. *Ann Intern Med*. 1985;102:164-168.

371. Acker CG, Johnson JP, Palevsky PM, et al. Hyperkalemia in hospitalized patients: causes, adequacy of treatment, and results of an attempt to improve physician compliance with published therapy guidelines. *Arch Intern Med*. 1998;158:917-924.

372. du Cheyron D, Parienti JJ, Fekih-Hassen M, et al. Impact of anemia on outcome in critically ill patients with severe acute renal failure. *Intensive Care Med*. 2005;31:1529-1536.

373. Lipkin GW, Kendall RG, Russon LJ, et al. Erythropoietin deficiency in acute renal failure. *Nephrol Dial Transplant*. 1990;5:920-922.

374. Radtke HW, Claussner A, Erbes PM, et al. Serum erythropoietin concentration in chronic renal failure: relationship to degree of anemia and excretory renal function. *Blood*. 1979;54:877-884.

375. Fiaccadori E, Lombardi M, Leonardi S, et al. Prevalence and clinical outcome associated with preexisting malnutrition in acute renal failure: a prospective cohort study. *J Am Soc Nephrol*. 1999;10:581-593.

376. Druml W. Nutritional management of acute renal failure. *Am J Kidney Dis*. 2001;37:S89-S94.

377. Druml W. Nutritional management of acute renal failure. *J Ren Nutr*. 2005;15:63-70.

378. Riella MC. Nutrition in acute renal failure. *Ren Fail*. 1997;19:237-252.

379. Fiaccadori E, Maggiore U, Giacosa R, et al. Enteral nutrition in patients with acute renal failure. *Kidney Int*. 2004;65:999-1008.

380. Chima CS, Meyer L, Hummell AC, et al. Protein catabolic rate in patients with acute renal failure on continuous arteriovenous hemofiltration and total parenteral nutrition. *J Am Soc Nephrol*. 1993;3:1516-1521.

381. Sponsel H, Conger JD. Is parenteral nutrition therapy of value in acute renal failure patients? *Am J Kidney Dis*. 1995;25:96-102.

382. Mitch WE. Mechanisms causing loss of muscle in acute uremia. *Ren Fail*. 1996;18:389-394.

383. Priebe HJ, Skillman JJ, Bushnell LS, et al. Antacid versus cimetidine in preventing acute gastrointestinal bleeding. A randomized trial in 75 critically ill patients. *N Engl J Med*. 1980;302:426-430.

384. Fiaccadori E, Maggiore U, Clima B, et al. Incidence, risk factors, and prognosis of gastrointestinal hemorrhage complicating acute renal failure. *Kidney Int*. 2001;59:1510-1519.

385. Metcalfe W, Simpson M, Khan IH, et al. Acute renal failure requiring renal replacement therapy: incidence and outcome. *QJM*. 2002;95:579-583.

386. Silvester W, Bellomo R, Cole L. Epidemiology, management, and outcome of severe acute renal failure of critical illness in Australia. *Crit Care Med*. 2001;29:1910-1915.

387. Brivet FG, Kleinknecht DJ, Loirat P, et al. Acute renal failure in intensive care units—causes, outcome, and prognostic factors of hospital mortality; a prospective, multicenter study. French Study Group on Acute Renal Failure. *Crit Care Med*. 1996;24:192-198.

388. Brenner BM, Yu AS. Uremic syndrome revisited: a pathogenetic role for retained endogenous inhibitors of nitric oxide synthesis. *Curr Opin Nephrol Hypertens*. 1992;1:3-7.

389. Finn WF. Diagnosis and management of acute tubular necrosis. *Med Clin North Am*. 1990;74:873-891.

390. Belizon IJ, Chou S, Porush JG. Recovery without a diuresis after protracted acute tubular necrosis. *Arch Intern Med*. 1980;140:133-134.

391. Jones BF, Nanra RS. Post-obstructive diuresis. *Aust N Z J Med*. 1983;13:519-521.

392. Wahlberg J. The renal response to ureteral obstruction. *Scand J Urol Nephrol*. 1983;73:1-30.

393. Meneghini LF, Oster JR, Camacho JR, et al. Hypercalcemia in association with acute renal failure and rhabdomyolysis. Case report and literature review. *Miner Electrolyte Metab*. 1993;19:1-16.

394. Alderson P, Schierhout G, Roberts I, et al. Colloids versus crystalloids for fluid resuscitation in critically ill patients. *Cochrane Database Syst Rev*. 2000;(2):CD000567.

395. Waikar SS, Chertow GM. Crystalloids versus colloids for resuscitation in shock. *Curr Opin Nephrol Hypertens*. 2000;9:501-504.

396. Ragaller MJ, Theilen H, Koch T. Volume replacement in critically ill patients with acute renal failure. *J Am Soc Nephrol*. 2001;12(Suppl 17):S33-S39.

397. Schortgen F, Lacherade JC, Bruneel F, et al. Effects of hydroxyethylstarch and gelatin on renal function in severe sepsis: a multicentre randomised study. *Lancet*. 2001;357:911-916.

398. Dart AB, Mutter TC, Ruth CA, et al. Hydroxyethyl starch (HES) versus other fluid therapies: effects on kidney function. *Cochrane Database Syst Rev*. 2010;20:CD007594.

399. Schierhout G, Roberts I. Fluid resuscitation with colloid or crystalloid solutions in critically ill patients: a systematic review of randomised trials. *BMJ*. 1998;316:961-964.

400. Wilkes MM, Navickis RJ. Patient survival after human albumin administration. A meta-analysis of randomized, controlled trials. *Ann Intern Med*. 2001;135:149-164.

401. Finfer S, Bellomo R, Boyce N, et al. A comparison of albumin and saline for fluid resuscitation in the intensive care unit. *N Engl J Med*. 2004;350:2247-2256.

402. Myburgh J, Cooper DJ, Finfer S, et al. Saline or albumin for fluid resuscitation in patients with traumatic brain injury. *N Engl J Med*. 2007;357:874-884.

403. Firth JD, Raine AE, Ledingham JG. Raised venous pressure: a direct cause of renal sodium retention in oedema? *Lancet*. 1988;1:1033-1035.

404. Winton FR. The influence of venous pressure on the isolated mammalian kidney. *J Physiol*. 1931;72:49-61.

405. Mullens W, Abrahams Z, Francis GS, et al. Importance of venous congestion for worsening of renal function in advanced decompensated heart failure. *J Am Coll Cardiol*. 2009;53:589-596.

406. Damman K, van Deursen VM, Navis G, et al. Increased central venous pressure is associated with impaired renal function and mortality in a broad spectrum of patients with cardiovascular disease. *J Am Coll Cardiol*. 2009;53:582-588.

407. Mullens W, Abrahams Z, Francis GS, et al. Prompt reduction in intra-abdominal pressure following large-volume mechanical fluid removal improves renal insufficiency in refractory decompensated heart failure. *J Card Fail*. 2008;14:508-514.

408. Mullens W, Abrahams Z, Skouri HN, et al. Elevated intra-abdominal pressure in acute decompensated heart failure: a potential contributor to worsening renal function? *J Am Coll Cardiol*. 2008;51:300-306.

409. Nohria A, Hasselblad V, Stebbins A, et al. Cardiorenal interactions: insights from the ESCAPE trial. *J Am Coll Cardiol*. 2008;51:1268-1274.

410. Bart BA, Boyle A, Bank AJ, et al. Ultrafiltration versus usual care for hospitalized patients with heart failure: the Relief for Acutely Fluid-Overloaded Patients With Decompensated Congestive Heart Failure (RAPID-CHF) trial. *J Am Coll Cardiol*. 2005;46:2043-2046.

411. Costanzo MR, Guglin ME, Saltzberg MT, et al. Ultrafiltration versus intravenous diuretics for patients hospitalized for acute decompensated heart failure. *J Am Coll Cardiol*. 2007;49:675-683.

412. Guevara M, Gines P. Hepatorenal syndrome. *Dig Dis*. 2005;23:47-55.

413. Moreau R, Lebrec D. Diagnosis and treatment of acute renal failure in patients with cirrhosis. *Best Pract Res Clin Gastroenterol*. 2007;21:111-123.

414. Wadei HM, Mai ML, Ahsan N, et al. Hepatorenal syndrome: pathophysiology and management. *Clin J Am Soc Nephrol*. 2006;1:1066-1079.

415. Arroyo V, Bernardi M, Epstein M, et al. Pathophysiology of ascites and functional renal failure in cirrhosis. *J Hepatol*. 1988;6:239-257.

416. Schrier RW, Arroyo V, Bernardi M, et al. Peripheral arterial vasodilation hypothesis: a proposal for the initiation of renal sodium and water retention in cirrhosis. *Hepatology*. 1988;8:1151-1157.

417. Ruiz-del-Arbol L, Monescillo A, Arocena C, et al. Circulatory function and hepatorenal syndrome in cirrhosis. *Hepatology*. 2005;42:439-447.

418. Runyon BA. Management of adult patients with ascites due to cirrhosis: an update. *Hepatology.* 2009;49:2087-2107.

419. Gines P, Tito L, Arroyo V, et al. Randomized comparative study of therapeutic paracentesis with and without intravenous albumin in cirrhosis. *Gastroenterology.* 1988;94:1493-1502.

420. Gines A, Fernandez-Esparrach G, Monescillo A, et al. Randomized trial comparing albumin, dextran 70, and polygeline in cirrhotic patients with ascites treated by paracentesis. *Gastroenterology.* 1996;111:1002-1010.

421. Sort P, Navasa M, Arroyo V, et al. Effect of intravenous albumin on renal impairment and mortality in patients with cirrhosis and spontaneous bacterial peritonitis. *N Engl J Med.* 1999;341:403-409.

422. Sigal SH, Stanca CM, Fernandez J, et al. Restricted use of albumin for spontaneous bacterial peritonitis. *Gut.* 2007;56:597-599.

423. Stanley MM, Ochi S, Lee KK, et al. Peritoneovenous shunting as compared with medical treatment in patients with alcoholic cirrhosis and massive ascites. Veterans Administration Cooperative Study on Treatment of Alcoholic Cirrhosis with Ascites. *N Engl J Med.* 1989;321:1632-1638.

424. Rossle M, Ochs A, Gulberg V, et al. A comparison of paracentesis and transjugular intrahepatic portosystemic shunting in patients with ascites. *N Engl J Med.* 2000;342:1701-1707.

425. Gines P, Uriz J, Calahorra B, et al. Transjugular intrahepatic portosystemic shunting versus paracentesis plus albumin for refractory ascites in cirrhosis. *Gastroenterology.* 2002;123:1839-1847.

426. Sanyal AJ, Genning C, Reddy KR, et al. The North American Study for the Treatment of Refractory Ascites. *Gastroenterology.* 2003;124:634-641.

427. Salerno F, Merli M, Riggio O, et al. Randomized controlled study of TIPS versus paracentesis plus albumin in cirrhosis with severe ascites. *Hepatology.* 2004;40:629-635.

428. Salerno F, Camma C, Enea M, et al. Transjugular intrahepatic porto-systemic shunt for refractory ascites: a meta-analysis of individual patient data. *Gastroenterology.* 2007;133:825-834.

429. Guevara M, Gines P, Bandi JC, et al. Transjugular intrahepatic porto-systemic shunt in hepatorenal syndrome: effects on renal function and vasoactive systems. *Hepatology.* 1998;28:416-422.

430. Gines P, Torre A, Terra C, et al. Review article: pharmacological treatment of hepatorenal syndrome. *Aliment Pharmacol Ther.* 2004;20(suppl 3):57-62:discussion, 3-4.

431. Duvoux C, Zanditenas D, Hezode C, et al. Effects of noradrenalin and albumin in patients with type I hepatorenal syndrome: a pilot study. *Hepatology.* 2002;36:374-380.

432. Angeli P, Volpin R, Gerunda G, et al. Reversal of type 1 hepatorenal syndrome with the administration of midodrine and octreotide. *Hepatology.* 1999;29:1690-1697.

433. Esrailian E, Pantangco ER, Kyulo NL, et al. Octreotide/midodrine therapy significantly improves renal function and 30-day survival in patients with type 1 hepatorenal syndrome. *Dig Dis Sci.* 2007;52:742-748.

434. Wong F, Pantea L, Sniderman K. Midodrine, octreotide, albumin, and TIPS in selected patients with cirrhosis and type 1 hepatorenal syndrome. *Hepatology.* 2004;40:55-64.

435. Skagen C, Einstein M, Lucey MR, et al. Combination treatment with octreotide, midodrine, and albumin improves survival in patients with type 1 and type 2 hepatorenal syndrome. *J Clin Gastroenterol.* 2009;43:680-685.

436. Moreau R, Durand F, Poynard T, et al. Terlipressin in patients with cirrhosis and type 1 hepatorenal syndrome: a retrospective multicenter study. *Gastroenterology.* 2002;122:923-930.

437. Fabrizi F, Dixit V, Messa P, et al. Terlipressin for hepatorenal syndrome: a meta-analysis of randomized trials. *Int J Artif Organs.* 2009;32:133-140.

438. Alderson P, Bunn F, Lefebvre C, et al. Human albumin solution for resuscitation and volume expansion in critically ill patients. *Cochrane Database Syst Rev.* 2004;(4):CD001208.

439. Gunal AI, Celiker H, Dogukan A, et al. Early and vigorous fluid resuscitation prevents acute renal failure in the crush victims of catastrophic earthquakes. *J Am Soc Nephrol.* 2004;15:1862-1867.

440. Bagshaw SM, Uchino S, Bellomo R, et al. Septic acute kidney injury in critically ill patients: clinical characteristics and outcomes. *Clin J Am Soc Nephrol.* 2007;2:431-439.

441. Rivers E, Nguyen B, Havstad S, et al. Early goal-directed therapy in the treatment of severe sepsis and septic shock. *N Engl J Med.* 2001;345:1368-1377.

442. Schetz M, Vanhorebeek I, Wouters PJ, et al. Tight blood glucose control is renoprotective in critically ill patients. *J Am Soc Nephrol.* 2008;19:571-578.

443. van den Berghe G, Wouters P, Weekers F, et al. Intensive insulin therapy in critically ill patients. *N Engl J Med.* 2001;345:1359-1367.

444. Dellinger RP, Carlet JM, Masur H, et al. Surviving Sepsis Campaign guidelines for management of severe sepsis and septic shock. *Crit Care Med.* 2004;32:858-873.

445. Townsend SR, Schorr C, Levy MM, et al. Reducing mortality in severe sepsis: the Surviving Sepsis Campaign. *Clin Chest Med.* 2008;29:721-733, x.

446. Finfer S, Chittock DR, Su SY, et al. Intensive versus conventional glucose control in critically ill patients. *N Engl J Med.* 2009;360:1283-1297.

447. Ozols RF, Corden BJ, Jacob J, et al. C. High-dose cisplatin in hypertonic saline. *Ann Intern Med.* 1984;100:19-24.

448. Heyman SN, Rosen S, Silva P, et al. Protective action of glycine in cisplatin nephrotoxicity. *Kidney Int.* 1991;40:273-279.

449. Bush Jr HL, Huse JB, Johnson WC, et al. Prevention of renal insufficiency after abdominal aortic aneurysm resection by optimal volume loading. *Arch Surg.* 1981;116:1517-1524.

450. Braden GL, O'Shea MH, Mulhern JG, et al. Acute renal failure and hyperkalaemia associated with cyclooxygenase-2 inhibitors. *Nephrol Dial Transplant.* 2004;19:1149-1153.

451. Griffin MR, Yared A, Ray WA. Nonsteroidal antiinflammatory drugs and acute renal failure in elderly persons. *Am J Epidemiol.* 2000;151:488-496.

452. Zipser RD, Hoefs JC, Speckart PF, et al. Prostaglandins: modulators of renal function and pressor resistance in chronic liver disease. *J Clin Endocrinol Metab.* 1979;48:895-900.

453. Huerta C, Castellsague J, Varas-Lorenzo C, et al. Nonsteroidal anti-inflammatory drugs and risk of ARF in the general population. *Am J Kidney Dis.* 2005;45:531-539.

454. Murray MD, Brater DC. Renal toxicity of the nonsteroidal anti-inflammatory drugs. *Ann Rev Pharmacol Toxicol.* 1993;33:435-465.

455. Palmer BF, Henrich WL. Clinical acute renal failure with nonsteroidal anti-inflammatory drugs. *Semin Nephrol.* 1995;15:214-227.

456. Thomas MC. Diuretics, ACE inhibitors and NSAIDs—the triple whammy. *Med J Aust.* 2000;172:184-185.

457. Appel GB. Aminoglycoside nephrotoxicity. *Am J Med.* 1990;88:16S-20S: discussion, 38S-42S.

458. Moore RD, Smith CR, Lipsky JJ, et al. Risk factors for nephrotoxicity in patients treated with aminoglycosides. *Ann Intern Med.* 1984;100:352-357.

459. Blaser J, Konig C. Once-daily dosing of aminoglycosides. *Eur J Clin Microbiol Infect Dis.* 1995;14:1029-1038.

460. Craig WA. Once-daily versus multiple-daily dosing of aminoglycosides. *J Chemother.* 1995;7(suppl 2):47-52.

461. Gilbert DN. Once-daily aminoglycoside therapy. *Antimicrob Agents Chemother.* 1991;35:399-405.

462. Deray G. Amphotericin B nephrotoxicity. *J Antimicrob Chemother.* 2002;49(suppl 1):37-41.

463. Mueller C, Buerkle G, Buettner HJ, et al. Prevention of contrast media–associated nephropathy: randomized comparison of 2 hydration regimens in 1620 patients undergoing coronary angioplasty. *Arch Intern Med.* 2002;162:329-336.

464. Trivedi HS, Moore H, Nasr S, et al. A randomized prospective trial to assess the role of saline hydration on the development of contrast nephrotoxicity. *Nephron Clin Pract.* 2003;93:C29-C34.

465. Solomon R, Werner C, Mann D, et al. Effects of saline, mannitol, and furosemide to prevent acute decreases in renal function induced by radiocontrast agents. *N Engl J Med.* 1994;331:1416-1420.

466. Majumdar SR, Kjellstrand CM, Tymchak WJ, et al. Forced euvolemic diuresis with mannitol and furosemide for prevention of contrast-induced nephropathy in patients with CKD undergoing coronary angiography: a randomized controlled trial. *Am J Kidney Dis.* 2009;54:602-609.

467. Brar SS, Shen AY, Jorgensen MB, et al. Sodium bicarbonate vs sodium chloride for the prevention of contrast medium-induced nephropathy in patients undergoing coronary angiography: a randomized trial. *JAMA.* 2008;300:1038-1046.

468. Maioli M, Toso A, Leoncini M, et al. Sodium bicarbonate versus saline for the prevention of contrast-induced nephropathy in patients with renal dysfunction undergoing coronary angiography or intervention. *J Am Coll Cardiol.* 2008;52:599-604.

469. Merten GJ, Burgess WP, Gray LV, et al. Prevention of contrast-induced nephropathy with sodium bicarbonate: a randomized controlled trial. *JAMA.* 2004;291:2328-2334.

470. Vasheghani-Farahani A, Sadigh G, Kassaian SE, et al. Sodium bicarbonate in preventing contrast nephropathy in patients at risk for volume overload: a randomized controlled trial. *J Nephrol.* 2010;23:216-223.

471. DiMari J, Megyesi J, Udvarhelyi N, et al. N-Acetyl cysteine ameliorates ischemic renal failure. *Am J Physiol.* 1997;272:F292-F298.

472. Fishbane S. N-Acetylcysteine in the prevention of contrast-induced nephropathy. *Clin J Am Soc Nephrol.* 2008;3:281-287.

473. Carbonell N, Blasco M, Sanjuan R, et al. Intravenous N-acetylcysteine for preventing contrast-induced nephropathy: a randomised trial. *Int J Cardiol.* 2007;115:57-62.

474. Durham JD, Caputo C, Dokko J, et al. A randomized controlled trial of N-acetylcysteine to prevent contrast nephropathy in cardiac angiography. *Kidney Int.* 2002;62:2202-2207.

475. Fung JW, Szeto CC, Chan WW, et al. Effect of N-acetylcysteine for prevention of contrast nephropathy in patients with moderate to severe renal insufficiency: a randomized trial. *Am J Kidney Dis.* 2004;43:801-808.

476. Gomes VO, Poli de Figueredo CE, Caramori P, et al. *N*-Acetylcysteine does not prevent contrast induced nephropathy after cardiac catheterisation with an ionic low osmolality contrast medium: a multicentre clinical trial. *Heart.* 2005;91:774-778.

477. Rashid ST, Salman M, Myint F, et al. Prevention of contrast-induced nephropathy in vascular patients undergoing angiography: a randomized controlled trial of intravenous *N*-acetylcysteine. *J Vasc Surg.* 2004;40: 1136-1141.

478. Webb JG, Pate GE, Humphries KH, et al. A randomized controlled trial of intravenous *N*-acetylcysteine for the prevention of contrast-induced nephropathy after cardiac catheterization: lack of effect. *Am Heart J.* 2004;148:422-429.

479. Tepel M, van der Giet M, Schwarzfeld C, et al. Prevention of radiographic-contrast-agent-induced reductions in renal function by acetylcysteine. *N Engl J Med.* 2000;343:180-184.

480. Marenzi G, Assanelli E, Marana I, et al. *N*-Acetylcysteine and contrast-induced nephropathy in primary angioplasty. *N Engl J Med.* 2006;354: 2773-2782.

481. Trivedi H, Daram S, Szabo A, et al. High-dose *N*-acetylcysteine for the prevention of contrast-induced nephropathy. *Am J Med.* 2009;122:874:e9-15.

482. Cacoub P, Deray G, Baumelou A, et al. No evidence for protective effects of nifedipine against radiocontrast-induced acute renal failure. *Clin Nephrol.* 1988;29:215-216.

483. Kellum JA. The use of diuretics and dopamine in acute renal failure: a systematic review of the evidence. *Crit Care.* 1997;1:53-59.

484. Khoury Z, Schlicht JR, Como J, et al. The effect of prophylactic nifedipine on renal function in patients administered contrast media. *Pharmacotherapy.* 1995;15:59-65.

485. Stone GW, McCullough PA, Tumlin JA, et al. Fenoldopam mesylate for the prevention of contrast-induced nephropathy: a randomized controlled trial. *JAMA.* 2003;290:2284-2291.

486. Solomon R, Werner C, Mann D, et al. Effects of saline, mannitol, and furosemide to prevent acute decreases in renal function induced by radiocontrast agents. *N Engl J Med.* 1994;331:1416-1420 [see comments].

487. Weinstein JM, Heyman S, Brezis M. Potential deleterious effect of furosemide in radiocontrast nephropathy. *Nephron.* 1992;62:413-415.

488. Jo SH, Koo BK, Park JS, et al. Prevention of radiocontrast medium–induced nephropathy using short-term high-dose simvastatin in patients with renal insufficiency undergoing coronary angiography (PROMISS) trial—a randomized controlled study. *Am Heart J.* 2008;155:499:e1-8.

489. Spargias K, Alexopoulos E, Kyrzopoulos S, et al. Ascorbic acid prevents contrast-mediated nephropathy in patients with renal dysfunction undergoing coronary angiography or intervention. *Circulation.* 2004;110: 2837-2842.

490. Boscheri A, Weinbrenner C, Botzek B, et al. Failure of ascorbic acid to prevent contrast-media induced nephropathy in patients with renal dysfunction. *Clin Nephrol.* 2007;68:279-286.

491. Spargias K, Adreanides E, Demerouti E, et al. Iloprost prevents contrast-induced nephropathy in patients with renal dysfunction undergoing coronary angiography or intervention. *Circulation.* 2009;120:1793-1799.

492. Spargias K, Adreanides E, Giamouzis G, et al. Iloprost for prevention of contrast-mediated nephropathy in high-risk patients undergoing a coronary procedure. Results of a randomized pilot study. *Eur J Clin Pharmacol.* 2006;62:589-595.

493. Kurnik BR, Allgren RL, Genter FC, et al. Prospective study of atrial natriuretic peptide for the prevention of radiocontrast-induced nephropathy. *Am J Kidney Dis.* 1998;31:674-680.

494. Morikawa S, Sone T, Tsuboi H, et al. Renal protective effects and the prevention of contrast-induced nephropathy by atrial natriuretic peptide. *J Am Coll Cardiol.* 2009;53:1040-1046.

495. Ix JH, McCulloch CE, Chertow GM. Theophylline for the prevention of radiocontrast nephropathy: a meta-analysis. *Nephrol Dial Transplant.* 2004;19:2747-2753.

496. Shammas NW, Kapalis MJ, Harris M, et al. Aminophylline does not protect against radiocontrast nephropathy in patients undergoing percutaneous angiographic procedures. *J Invasive Cardiol.* 2001;13:738-740.

497. Erley CM, Duda SH, Rehfuss D, et al. Prevention of radiocontrast-media–induced nephropathy in patients with pre-existing renal insufficiency by hydration in combination with the adenosine antagonist theophylline. *Nephrol Dial Transplant.* 1999;14:1146-1149.

498. Cruz DN, Perazella MA, Bellomo R, et al. Extracorporeal blood purification therapies for prevention of radiocontrast-induced nephropathy: a systematic review. *Am J Kidney Dis.* 2006;48:361-371.

499. Reinecke H, Fobker M, Wellmann J, et al. A randomized controlled trial comparing hydration therapy to additional hemodialysis or *N*-acetylcysteine for the prevention of contrast medium–induced nephropathy: the Dialysis-versus-Diuresis (DVD) Trial. *Clin Res Cardiol.* 2007;96:130-139.

500. Lehnert T, Keller E, Gondolf K, et al. Effect of haemodialysis after contrast medium administration in patients with renal insufficiency. *Nephrol Dial Transplant.* 1998;13:358-362.

501. Marenzi G, Lauri G, Campodonico J, et al. Comparison of two hemofiltration protocols for prevention of contrast-induced nephropathy in high-risk patients. *Am J Med.* 2006;119:155-162.

502. Marenzi G, Marana I, Lauri G, et al. The prevention of radiocontrast-agent-induced nephropathy by hemofiltration. *N Engl J Med.* 2003;349: 1333-1340.

503. Stacul F, Adam A, Becker CR, et al. Strategies to reduce the risk of contrast-induced nephropathy. *Am J Cardiol.* 2006;98:59K-77K.

504. Weisbord SD. Iodinated contrast media and the kidney. *Rev Cardiovasc Med.* 2008;9(suppl 1):S14-S23.

505. Rudnick MR, Goldfarb S, Wexler L, et al. Nephrotoxicity of ionic and nonionic contrast media in 1196 patients: a randomized trial. The Iohexol Cooperative Study. *Kidney Int.* 1995;47:254-261.

506. Barrett BJ, Carlisle EJ. Metaanalysis of the relative nephrotoxicity of high- and low-osmolality iodinated contrast media. *Radiology.* 1993;188:171-178.

507. Aspelin P, Aubry P, Fransson SG, et al. Nephrotoxic effects in high-risk patients undergoing angiography. *N Engl J Med.* 2003;348:491-499.

508. Solomon RJ, Natarajan MK, Doucet S, et al. Cardiac Angiography in Renally Impaired Patients (CARE) study: a randomized double-blind trial of contrast-induced nephropathy in patients with chronic kidney disease. *Circulation.* 2007;115:3189-3196.

509. McCullough PA, Bertrand ME, Brinker JA, et al. A meta-analysis of the renal safety of isosmolar iodixanol compared with low-osmolar contrast media. *J Am Coll Cardiol.* 2006;48:692-699.

510. Reed M, Meier P, Tamhane UU, et al. The relative renal safety of iodixanol compared with low-osmolar contrast media: a meta-analysis of randomized controlled trials. *J Am Coll Cardiol.* 2009;2:645-654.

511. Jo SH, Youn TJ, Koo BK, et al. Renal toxicity evaluation and comparison between Visipaque (iodixanol) and Hexabrix (ioxaglate) in patients with renal insufficiency undergoing coronary angiography: the RECOVER study: a randomized controlled trial. *J Am Coll Cardiol.* 2006;48:924-930.

512. Juergens CP, Winter JP, Nguyen-Do P, et al. Nephrotoxic effects of iodixanol and iopromide in patients with abnormal renal function receiving *N*-acetylcysteine and hydration before coronary angiography and intervention: a randomized trial. *Intern med j.* 2009;39:25-31.

513. Laskey W, Aspelin P, Davidson C, et al. Nephrotoxicity of iodixanol versus iopamidol in patients with chronic kidney disease and diabetes mellitus undergoing coronary angiographic procedures. *Am Heart J.* 2009;158: 822-828.e3.

514. Andreoli SP, Clark JH, McGuire WA, et al. Purine excretion during tumor lysis in children with acute lymphocytic leukemia receiving allopurinol: relationship to acute renal failure. *J Pediatr.* 1986;109:292-298.

515. Goldman SC, Holcenberg JS, Finklestein JZ, et al. A randomized comparison between rasburicase and allopurinol in children with lymphoma or leukemia at high risk for tumor lysis. *Blood.* 2001;97:2998-3003.

516. Bessmertny O, Robitaille LM, Cairo MS. Rasburicase: a new approach for preventing and/or treating tumor lysis syndrome. *Curr Pharm Des.* 2005;11:4177-4185.

517. Navolanic PM, Pui CH, Larson RA, et al. Elitek-rasburicase: an effective means to prevent and treat hyperuricemia associated with tumor lysis syndrome, a Meeting Report, Dallas, Texas, January 2002. *Leukemia.* 2003;17:499-514.

518. Cairo MS. Recombinant urate oxidase (rasburicase): a new targeted therapy for prophylaxis and treatment of patients with hematologic malignancies at risk of tumor lysis syndrome. *Clin Lymphoma.* 2003;3:233-234.

519. Santini V. Amifostine: chemotherapeutic and radiotherapeutic protective effects. *Expert Opin Pharmacother.* 2001;2:479-489.

520. Hartmann JT, von Vangerow A, Fels LM, et al. A randomized trial of amifostine in patients with high-dose VIC chemotherapy plus autologous blood stem cell transplantation. *Br J Cancer.* 2001;84:313-320.

521. Koukourakis MI. Amifostine in clinical oncology: current use and future applications. *Anticancer Drugs.* 2002;13:181-209.

522. Vaira M, Barone R, Aghemo B, et al. [Renal protection with amifostine during intraoperative peritoneal chemohyperthermia (IPCH) with cisplatin (CDDP) for peritoneal carcinosis. Phase 1 study]. *Minerva Med.* 2001;92:207-211.

523. Morgan JM. Chelation therapy in lead nephropathy. *South Med J.* 1975;68:1001-1006.

524. Murray KM, Hedgepeth JC. Intravenous self-administration of elemental mercury: efficacy of dimercaprol therapy. *Drug Intell Clin Pharm.* 1988;22:972-975.

525. Brent J, McMartin K, Phillips S, et al. Fomepizole for the treatment of ethylene glycol poisoning. Methylpyrazole for Toxic Alcohols Study Group. *N Engl J Med.* 1999;340:832-838.

526. Goldfarb DS. Fomepizole for ethylene-glycol poisoning. *Lancet.* 1999;354:1646.

527. Najafi CC, Hertko LJ, Leikin JB, et al. Fomepizole in ethylene glycol intoxication. *Ann Emerg Med.* 2001;37:358-359.

528. Battistella M. Fomepizole as an antidote for ethylene glycol poisoning. *Ann Pharmacother.* 2002;36:1085-1089.

529. Graziani G, Cantaluppi A, Casati S, et al. Dopamine and furosemide in oliguric acute renal failure. *Nephron.* 1984;37:39-42.
530. Conger JD, Falk SA, Hammond WS. Atrial natriuretic peptide and dopamine in established acute renal failure in the rat. *Kidney Int.* 1991;40:21-28.
531. Parker S, Carlon GC, Isaacs M, et al. Dopamine administration in oliguria and oliguric renal failure. *Crit Care Med.* 1981;9:630-632.
532. Kellum JA, Decker JM. Use of dopamine in acute renal failure: a meta-analysis. *Crit Care Med.* 2001;29:1526-1531.
533. Denton MD, Chertow GM, Brady HR. "Renal-dose" dopamine for the treatment of acute renal failure: scientific rationale, experimental studies and clinical trials. *Kidney Int.* 1996;50:4-14.
534. Marik PE, Iglesias J. Low-dose dopamine does not prevent acute renal failure in patients with septic shock and oliguria. NORASEPT II Study Investigators. *Am J Med.* 1999;107:387-390.
535. Friedrich JO, Adhikari N, Herridge MS, et al. Meta-analysis: low-dose dopamine increases urine output but does not prevent renal dysfunction or death. *Ann Intern Med.* 2005;142:510-524.
536. Bellomo R, Chapman M, Finfer S, et al. Low-dose dopamine in patients with early renal dysfunction: a placebo-controlled randomised trial. Australian and New Zealand Intensive Care Society (ANZICS) Clinical Trials Group. *Lancet.* 2000;356:2139-2143.
537. Lauschke A, Teichgraber UK, Frei U, et al. "Low-dose" dopamine worsens renal perfusion in patients with acute renal failure. *Kidney Int.* 2006;69:1669-1674.
538. Jones D, Bellomo R. Renal-dose dopamine: from hypothesis to paradigm to dogma to myth and, finally, superstition? *J Intensive Care Med.* 2005;20:199-211.
539. Bellomo R. Has renal-dose dopamine finally been relegated to join the long list of medical myths? *Crit Care Resusc.* 2001;3:7-10.
540. Singer I, Epstein M. Potential of dopamine A-1 agonists in the management of acute renal failure. *Am J Kidney Dis.* 1998;31:743-755.
541. Tumlin JA, Wang A, Murray PT, et al. Fenoldopam mesylate blocks reductions in renal plasma flow after radiocontrast dye infusion: a pilot trial in the prevention of contrast nephropathy. *Am Heart J.* 2002;143:894-903.
542. Caimmi PP, Pagani L, Micalizzi E, et al. Fenoldopam for renal protection in patients undergoing cardiopulmonary bypass. *J Cardiothorac Vasc Anesth.* 2003;17:491-494.
543. Tumlin JA, Finkel KW, Murray PT, et al. Fenoldopam mesylate in early acute tubular necrosis: a randomized, double-blind, placebo-controlled clinical trial. *Am J Kidney Dis.* 2005;46:26-34.
544. Goetz KL. Atrial receptors, natriuretic peptides, and the kidney—current understanding. *Mayo Clin Proc.* 1986;61:600-603.
545. Goetz KL. Physiology and pathophysiology of atrial peptides. *Am J Physiol.* 1988;254:E1-E15.
546. Margulies KB, Burnett Jr JC. Atrial natriuretic factor modulates whole kidney tubuloglomerular feedback. *Am J Physiol.* 1990;259:R97-R101.
547. Lanese DM, Yuan BH, Falk SA, et al. Effects of atriopeptin III on isolated rat afferent and efferent arterioles. *Am J Physiol.* 1991;261:F1102-F1109.
548. Roy DR. Effect of synthetic ANP on renal and loop of Henle functions in the young rat. *Am J Physiol.* 1986;251:F220-F225.
549. Zeidel ML, Seifter JL, Lear S, et al. Atrial peptides inhibit oxygen consumption in kidney medullary collecting duct cells. *Am J Physiol.* 1986;251:F379-F383.
550. Allgren RL, Marbury TC, Rahman SN, et al. Anaritide in acute tubular necrosis. Auriculin Anaritide Acute Renal Failure Study Group. *N Engl J Med.* 1997;336:828-834.
551. Lewis J, Salem MM, Chertow GM, et al. Atrial natriuretic factor in oliguric acute renal failure. Anaritide Acute Renal Failure Study Group. *Am J Kidney Dis.* 2000;36:767-774.
552. Sward K, Valsson F, Odencrants P, et al. Recombinant human atrial natriuretic peptide in ischemic acute renal failure: a randomized placebo-controlled trial. *Crit Care Med.* 2004;32:1310-1315.
553. Meyer M, Pfarr E, Schirmer G, et al. Therapeutic use of the natriuretic peptide ularitide in acute renal failure. *Ren Fail.* 1999;21:85-100.
554. Nigwekar SU, Navaneethan SD, Parikh CR, et al. Atrial natriuretic peptide for management of acute kidney injury: a systematic review and meta-analysis. *Clin J Am Soc Nephrol.* 2009;4:261-272.
555. Mehta RL, Pascual MT, Soroko S, et al. Diuretics, mortality, and nonrecovery of renal function in acute renal failure. *JAMA.* 2002;288:2547-2553.
556. Cantarovich F, Rangoonwala B, Lorenz H, et al. High-dose furosemide for established ARF: a prospective, randomized, double-blind, placebo-controlled, multicenter trial. *Am J Kidney Dis.* 2004;44:402-409.
557. Grams ME, Estrella MM, Coresh J, et al. D. Fluid balance, diuretic use, and mortality in acute kidney injury. *Clin J Am Soc Nephrol.* 2011;6:966-973.
558. Ikeda K, Oshima T, Hidaka H, et al. Molecular and clinical implications of loop diuretic ototoxicity. *Hearing Res.* 1997;107:1-8.
559. Better OS, Rubinstein I, Winaver JM, et al. Mannitol therapy revisited (1940-1997). *Kidney Int.* 1997;52:886-894.
560. Hanley MJ, Davidson K. Prior mannitol and furosemide infusion in a model of ischemic acute renal failure. *Am J Physiol.* 1981;241:F556-F564.
561. Vanholder R, Leusen I, Lameire N. Comparison between mannitol and saline infusion in HgCl$_2$-induced acute renal failure. *Nephron.* 1984;38:193-201.
562. Grino JM, Miravitlles R, Castelao AM, et al. Flush solution with mannitol in the prevention of post-transplant renal failure. *Transplant Proc.* 1987;19:4140-4142.
563. Zager RA, Mahan J, Merola AJ. Effects of mannitol on the postischemic kidney. Biochemical, functional, and morphologic assessments. *Lab Invest.* 1985;53:433-442.
564. von Baeyer H. Plasmapheresis in thrombotic microangiopathy–associated syndromes: review of outcome data derived from clinical trials and open studies. *Ther Apher.* 2002;6:320-328.
565. Madore F, Lazarus JM, Brady HR. Therapeutic plasma exchange in renal diseases. *J Am Soc Nephrol.* 1996;7:367-386.
566. Humphreys BD, Sharman JP, Henderson JM, et al. Gemcitabine-associated thrombotic microangiopathy. *Cancer.* 2004;100:2664-2670.
567. Magee CC. Renal thrombotic microangiopathy induced by interferon-alpha. *Nephrol Dial Transplant.* 2001;16:2111-2112.
568. Wong CS, Jelacic S, Habeeb RL, et al. The risk of the hemolytic-uremic syndrome after antibiotic treatment of *Escherichia coli* O157:H7 infections. *N Engl J Med.* 2000;342:1930-1936.
569. Beckett VL, Donadio Jr JV, Brennan Jr LA, et al. Use of captopril as early therapy for renal scleroderma: a prospective study. *Mayo Clin Proc.* 1985;60:763-771.
570. Lopez-Ovejero JA, Saal SD, D'Angelo WA, et al. Reversal of vascular and renal crises of scleroderma by oral angiotensin-converting-enzyme blockade. *N Engl J Med.* 1979;300:1417-1419.
571. Traub YM, Shapiro AP, Rodnan GP, et al. Hypertension and renal failure (scleroderma renal crisis) in progressive systemic sclerosis. Review of a 25-year experience with 68 cases. *Medicine.* 1983;62:335-352.
572. Zucchelli P, Pasquali S, Cagnoli L, et al. Controlled plasma exchange trial in acute renal failure due to multiple myeloma. *Kidney Int.* 1988;33:1175-1180.
573. Clark WF, Stewart AK, Rock GA, et al. Plasma exchange when myeloma presents as acute renal failure: a randomized, controlled trial. *Ann Intern Med.* 2005;143:777-784.
574. Perazella MA, Markowitz GS. Drug-induced acute interstitial nephritis. *Nat Rev Nephrol.* 2010;6:461-470.
575. Gonzalez E, Gutierrez E, Galeano C, et al. Early steroid treatment improves the recovery of renal function in patients with drug-induced acute interstitial nephritis. *Kidney Int.* 2008;73:940-946.
576. Preddie DC, Markowitz GS, Radhakrishnan J, et al. Mycophenolate mofetil for the treatment of interstitial nephritis. *Clin J Am Soc Nephrol.* 2006;1:718-722.
577. Coar D. Obstructive nephropathy. *Del Med J.* 1991;63:743-749.
578. Bouchard J, Mehta RL. Fluid accumulation and acute kidney injury: consequence or cause. *Curr Opin Crit Care.* 2009;15:509-513.
579. Sutherland SM, Zappitelli M, Alexander SR, et al. Fluid overload and mortality in children receiving continuous renal replacement therapy: the prospective pediatric continuous renal replacement therapy registry. *Am J Kidney Dis.* 2010;55:316-325.
580. Payen D, de Pont AC, Sakr Y, et al. A positive fluid balance is associated with a worse outcome in patients with acute renal failure. *Crit Care.* 2008;12:R74.
581. Wiedemann HP, Wheeler AP, Bernard GR, et al. Comparison of two fluid-management strategies in acute lung injury. *N Engl J Med.* 2006;354:2564-2575.
582. Watson M, Abbott KC, Yuan CM. Damned if you do, damned if you don't: potassium binding resins in hyperkalemia. *Clin J Am Soc Nephrol.* 5:1723-1726.
583. Sterns RH, Rojas M, Bernstein P, et al. Ion-exchange resins for the treatment of hyperkalemia: are they safe and effective? *J Am Soc Nephrol.* 2010;21:733-735.
584. Allon M, Copkney C. Albuterol and insulin for treatment of hyperkalemia in hemodialysis patients. *Kidney Int.* 1990;38:869-872.
585. Blumberg A, Weidmann P, Shaw S, et al. Effect of various therapeutic approaches on plasma potassium and major regulating factors in terminal renal failure. *Am J Med.* 1988;85:507-512.
586. Stacpoole PW. Lactic acidosis: the case against bicarbonate therapy. *Ann Intern Med.* 1986;105:276-279.
587. Narins RG, Cohen JJ. Bicarbonate therapy for organic acidosis: the case for its continued use. *Ann Intern Med.* 1987;106:615-618.
588. Cooper DJ, Walley KR, Wiggs BR, et al. Bicarbonate does not improve hemodynamics in critically ill patients who have lactic acidosis. A prospective, controlled clinical study. *Ann Intern Med.* 1990;112:492-498.
589. Forsythe SM, Schmidt GA. Sodium bicarbonate for the treatment of lactic acidosis. *Chest.* 2000;117:260-267.
590. Fiaccadori E, Parenti E, Maggiore U. Nutritional support in acute kidney injury. *J Nephrol.* 2008;21:645-656.

591. Fiaccadori E, Cremaschi E. Nutritional assessment and support in acute kidney injury. *Curr Opin Crit Care.* 2009;15:474-480.
592. Hebert PC, Wells G, Blajchman MA, et al. A multicenter, randomized, controlled clinical trial of transfusion requirements in critical care. Transfusion Requirements in Critical Care Investigators, Canadian Critical Care Trials Group. *N Engl J Med.* 1999;340:409-417.
593. Park J, Gage BF, Vijayan A. Use of EPO in critically ill patients with acute renal failure requiring renal replacement therapy. *Am J Kidney Dis.* 2005;46:791-798.
594. Corwin HL, Gettinger A, Rodriguez RM, et al. Efficacy of recombinant human erythropoietin in the critically ill patient: a randomized, double-blind, placebo-controlled trial. *Crit Care Med.* 1999;27:2346-2350.
595. Corwin HL, Gettinger A, Pearl RG, et al. Efficacy of recombinant human erythropoietin in critically ill patients: a randomized controlled trial. *JAMA.* 2002;288:2827-2835.
596. Churchwell MD, Mueller BA. Drug dosing during continuous renal replacement therapy. *Semin Dial.* 2009;22:185-188.
597. Mueller BA, Pasko DA, Sowinski KM. Higher renal replacement therapy dose delivery influences on drug therapy. *Artif Organs.* 2003;27:808-814.
598. Mueller BA, Smoyer WE. Challenges in developing evidence-based drug dosing guidelines for adults and children receiving renal replacement therapy. *Clin Pharmacol Ther.* 2009;86:479-482.
599. Vilay AM, Churchwell MD, Mueller BA. Clinical review: drug metabolism and nonrenal clearance in acute kidney injury. *Crit Care.* 2008;12:235.
600. Palevsky PM, Baldwin I, Davenport A, et al. Renal replacement therapy and the kidney: minimizing the impact of renal replacement therapy on recovery of acute renal failure. *Curr Opin Crit Care.* 2005;11:548-554.
601. Finkel KW, Podoll AS. Complications of continuous renal replacement therapy. *Semin Dial.* 2009;22:155-159.
602. Kolff WJ. First clinical experience with the artificial kidney. *Ann Intern Med.* 1965;62:608-619.
603. Teschan PE, Baxter CR, O'Brien TF, et al. Prophylactic hemodialysis in the treatment of acute renal failure. *Ann Intern Med.* 1960;53:992-1016.
604. Davenport A, Bouman C, Kirpalani A, et al. Delivery of renal replacement therapy in acute kidney injury: what are the key issues? *Clin J Am Soc Nephrol.* 2008;3:869-875.
605. Kellum JA, Mehta RL, Angus DC, et al. The first international consensus conference on continuous renal replacement therapy. *Kidney Int.* 2002;62:1855-1863.
606. Palevsky PM. Renal replacement therapy I: indications and timing. *Crit Care Clin.* 2005;21:347-356.
607. Palevsky PM. Clinical review: timing and dose of continuous renal replacement therapy in acute kidney injury. *Crit Care.* 2007;11:232.
608. Rondon-Berrios H, Palevsky PM. Treatment of acute kidney injury: an update on the management of renal replacement therapy. *Curr Opin Nephrol Hypertens.* 2007;16:64-70.
609. Gibney N, Hoste E, Burdmann EA, et al. Timing of initiation and discontinuation of renal replacement therapy in AKI: unanswered key questions. *Clin J Am Soc Nephrol.* 2008;3:876-880.
610. Fischer RP, Griffen Jr WO, Reiser M, et al. Early dialysis in the treatment of acute renal failure. *Surg Gynecol Obstet.* 1966;123:1019-1023.
611. Parsons FM, Hobson SM, Blagg CR, et al. Optimum time for dialysis in acute reversible renal failure. Description and value of an improved dialyser with large surface area. *Lancet.* 1961;1:129-134.
612. Kleinknecht D, Jungers P, Chanard J, et al. Uremic and non-uremic complications in acute renal failure: Evaluation of early and frequent dialysis on prognosis. *Kidney Int.* 1972;1:190-196.
613. Conger JD. A controlled evaluation of prophylactic dialysis in post-traumatic acute renal failure. *J Trauma.* 1975;15:1056-1063.
614. Gillum DM, Dixon BS, Yanover MJ, et al. The role of intensive dialysis in acute renal failure. *Clin Nephrol.* 1986;25:249-255.
615. Gettings LG, Reynolds HN, Scalea T. Outcome in post-traumatic acute renal failure when continuous renal replacement therapy is applied early vs. late. *Intensive Care Med.* 1999;25:805-813.
616. Demirkilic U, Kuralay E, Yenicesu M, et al. Timing of replacement therapy for acute renal failure after cardiac surgery. *J Card Surg.* 2004;19:17-20.
617. Elahi M, Asopa S, Pflueger A, et al. Acute kidney injury following cardiac surgery: impact of early versus late haemofiltration on morbidity and mortality. *Eur J Cardiothorac Surg.* 2009;35:854-863.
618. Liu KD, Himmelfarb J, Paganini E, et al. Timing of initiation of dialysis in critically ill patients with acute kidney injury. *Clin J Am Soc Nephrol.* 2006;1:915-919.
619. Bouman CS, Oudemans-Van Straaten HM, Tijssen JG, et al. Effects of early high-volume continuous venovenous hemofiltration on survival and recovery of renal function in intensive care patients with acute renal failure: a prospective, randomized trial. *Crit Care Med.* 2002;30:2205-2211.
620. Goldstein SL, Somers MJ, Baum MA, et al. Pediatric patients with multi-organ dysfunction syndrome receiving continuous renal replacement therapy. *Kidney Int.* 2005;67:653-658.
621. Bouchard J, Soroko SB, Chertow GM, et al. Fluid accumulation, survival and recovery of kidney function in critically ill patients with acute kidney injury. *Kidney Int.* 2009;76:422-427.
622. Prowle JR, Echeverri JE, Ligabo EV, et al. Fluid balance and acute kidney injury. *Nat Rev Nephrol.* 2010;6:107-115.
623. Paganini E, Tapolyai M, Goormastic M, et al. Establishing a dialysis therapy/patient outcome link in intensive care unit acute dialysis for patients with acute renal failure. *Am J Kidney Dis.* 1996;28:S81-S89.
624. Schiffl H, Lang SM, Fischer R. Daily hemodialysis and the outcome of acute renal failure. *N Engl J Med.* 2002;346:305-310.
625. Bonventre JV. Daily hemodialysis—will treatment each day improve the outcome in patients with acute renal failure? *N Engl J Med.* 2002;346:362-364.
626. Palevsky PM, Zhang JH, O'Connor TZ, et al. Intensity of renal support in critically ill patients with acute kidney injury. *N Engl J Med.* 2008;359:7-20.
627. Palevsky PM, O'Connor TZ, Chertow GM, et al. Intensity of renal replacement therapy in acute kidney injury: perspective from within the Acute Renal Failure Trial Network Study. *Crit Care.* 2009;13:310.
628. Schulman G, Fogo A, Gung A, et al. Complement activation retards resolution of acute ischemic renal failure in the rat. *Kidney Int.* 1991;40:1069-1074.
629. Schulman G, Hakim R. Hemodialysis membrane biocompatibility in acute renal failure. *Adv Ren Replace Ther.* 1994;1:75-82.
630. Hakim RM, Wingard RL, Parker RA. Effect of the dialysis membrane in the treatment of patients with acute renal failure. *N Engl J Med.* 1994;331:1338-1342.
631. Himmelfarb J, Tolkoff Rubin N, Chandran P, et al. A multicenter comparison of dialysis membranes in the treatment of acute renal failure requiring dialysis. *J Am Soc Nephrol.* 1998;9:257-266.
632. Schiffl H, Lang SM, Konig A, et al. Biocompatible membranes in acute renal failure: prospective case-controlled study. *Lancet.* 1994;344:570-572.
633. Kurtal H, von Herrath D, Schaefer K. Is the choice of membrane important for patients with acute renal failure requiring hemodialysis? *Artif Organs.* 1995;19:391-394.
634. Jorres A, Gahl GM, Dobis C, et al. Haemodialysis-membrane biocompatibility and mortality of patients with dialysis-dependent acute renal failure: a prospective randomised multicentre trial. International Multicentre Study Group. *Lancet.* 1999;354:1337-1341.
635. Gastaldello K, Melot C, Kahn RJ, et al. Comparison of cellulose diacetate and polysulfone membranes in the outcome of acute renal failure. A prospective randomized study. *Nephrol Dial Transplant.* 2000;15:224-230.
636. Albright Jr RC, Smelser JM, McCarthy JT, et al. Patient survival and renal recovery in acute renal failure: randomized comparison of cellulose acetate and polysulfone membrane dialyzers. *Mayo Clin Proc.* 2000;75:1141-1147.
637. Jaber BL, Cendoroglo M, Balakrishnan VS, et al. Impact of dialyzer membrane selection on cellular responses in acute renal failure: a crossover study. *Kidney Int.* 2000;57:2107-2116.
638. Jaber BL, Lau J, Schmid CH, et al. Effect of biocompatibility of hemodialysis membranes on mortality in acute renal failure: a meta-analysis. *Clin Nephrol.* 2002;57:274-282.
639. Alonso A, Lau J, Jaber BL. Biocompatible hemodialysis membranes for acute renal failure. *Cochrane Database Syst Rev.* 2005;(2):CD005283.
640. Schortgen F, Soubrier N, Delclaux C, et al. Hemodynamic tolerance of intermittent hemodialysis in critically ill patients: usefulness of practice guidelines. *Am J Respir Crit Care Med.* 2000;162:197-202.
641. Vijayan A. Vascular access for continuous renal replacement therapy. *Semin Dial.* 2009;22:133-136.
642. Parienti JJ, Thirion M, Megarbane B, et al. Femoral vs jugular venous catheterization and risk of nosocomial events in adults requiring acute renal replacement therapy: a randomized controlled trial. *JAMA.* 2008;299:2413-2422.
643. Schetz M. Vascular access for HD and CRRT. *Contrib Nephrol.* 2007;156:275-286.
644. Coryell L, Lott JP, Stavropoulos SW, et al. The case for primary placement of tunneled hemodialysis catheters in acute kidney injury. *J Vasc Interv Radiol.* 2009;20:1578-1581;quiz, 82.
645. Ward D. Anticoagulation in patients on hemodialysis. In: Nissenson A, Fine R, eds. *Clinical dialysis.* ed 4. New York: McGraw-Hill; 2005:127-152.
646. Tolwani AJ, Wille KM. Anticoagulation for continuous renal replacement therapy. *Semin Dial.* 2009;22:141-145.
647. Maher J, Lapierre L, Schriner G, et al. Regional heparinization for hemodialysis—technic and clinical experiences. *N Engl J Med.* 1963;268:451-456.
648. Swartz RD, Port FK. Preventing hemorrhage in high-risk hemodialysis: regional versus low-dose heparin. *Kidney Int.* 1979;16:513-518.
649. Morita Y, Johnson RW, Dorn RE, et al. Regional anticoagulation during hemodialysis using citrate. *Am J Med Sci.* 1961;242:32-43.
650. Mehta RL, McDonald BR, Aguilar MM, et al. Regional citrate anticoagulation for continuous arteriovenous hemodialysis in critically ill patients. *Kidney Int.* 1990;38:976-981.

651. Tolwani AJ, Prendergast MB, Speer RR, et al. A practical citrate anticoagulation continuous venovenous hemodiafiltration protocol for metabolic control and high solute clearance. *Clin J Am Soc Nephrol.* 2006;1:79-87.

652. Matsuo T, Matsuo M, Kario K, et al. Effect of an anticoagulant (heparin versus nafamostat mesilate) on the extrinsic coagulation pathway in chronic hemodialysis. *Blood Coagul Fibrinolysis.* 1998;9:391-393.

653. Fischer KG, van de Loo A, Bohler J. Recombinant hirudin (lepirudin) as anticoagulant in intensive care patients treated with continuous hemodialysis. *Kidney Int.* 1999:S46-S50.

654. Vargas Hein O, von Heymann C, Lipps M, et al. Hirudin versus heparin for anticoagulation in continuous renal replacement therapy. *Intensive Care Med.* 2001;27:673-679.

655. Hein OV, von Heymann C, Diehl T, et al. Intermittent hirudin versus continuous heparin for anticoagulation in continuous renal replacement therapy. *Ren Fail.* 2004;26:297-303.

656. Murray PT, Reddy BV, Grossman EJ, et al. A prospective comparison of three argatroban treatment regimens during hemodialysis in end-stage renal disease. *Kidney Int.* 2004;66:2446-2453.

657. Reddy BV, Grossman EJ, Trevino SA, et al. Argatroban anticoagulation in patients with heparin-induced thrombocytopenia requiring renal replacement therapy. *Ann Pharmacother.* 2005;39:1601-1605.

658. Tang IY, Cox DS, Patel K, et al. Argatroban and renal replacement therapy in patients with heparin-induced thrombocytopenia. *Ann Pharmacother.* 2005;39:231-236.

659. Sanders PW, Taylor H, Curtis JJ. Hemodialysis without anticoagulation. *Am J Kidney Dis.* 1985;5:32-35.

660. Schwab SJ, Onorato JJ, Sharar LR, et al. Hemodialysis without anticoagulation. One-year prospective trial in hospitalized patients at risk for bleeding. *Am J Med.* 1987;83:405-410.

661. Vinsonneau C, Camus C, Combes A, et al. Continuous venovenous haemodiafiltration versus intermittent haemodialysis for acute renal failure in patients with multiple-organ dysfunction syndrome: a multicentre randomised trial. *Lancet.* 2006;368:379-385.

662. Conger JD, Schultz MF, Miller F, et al. Responses to hemorrhagic arterial pressure reduction in different ischemic renal failure models. *Kidney Int.* 1994;46:318-323.

663. Conger JD. Interventions in clinical acute renal failure: what are the data? *Am J Kidney Dis.* 1995;26:565-576.

664. Conger J. Hemodynamic factors in acute renal failure. *Advances in renal replacement therapy.* 1997;4:25-37.

665. Doshi M, Murray PT. Approach to intradialytic hypotension in intensive care unit patients with acute renal failure. *Artif Organs.* 2003;27:772-780.

666. Darmon M, Schortgen F, Vargas F, et-al. Diagnostic accuracy of Doppler renal resistive index for reversibility of acute kidney injury in critically ill patients. *Intensive Care Med.* 2011;37:68-76.

667. Kramer P, Schrader J, Bohnsack W, et al. Continuous arteriovenous haemofiltration. A new kidney replacement therapy. *Proc Eur Dial Transplant Assoc.* 1981;18:743-749.

668. Paganini EP, Nakamoto S. Continuous slow ultrafiltration in oliguric acute renal failure. *Trans Am Soc Artif Intern Organs.* 1980;26:201-204.

669. Golper TA. Continuous arteriovenous hemofiltration in acute renal failure. *Am J Kidney Dis.* 1985;6:373-386.

670. Kaplan AA, Longnecker RE, Folkert VW. Continuous arteriovenous hemofiltration. A report of six months' experience. *Ann Intern Med.* 1984;100:358-367.

671. Sigler MH, Teehan BP. Solute transport in continuous hemodialysis: a new treatment for acute renal failure. *Kidney Int.* 1987;32:562-571.

672. Bellomo R, Parkin G, Love J, et al. A prospective comparative study of continuous arteriovenous hemodiafiltration and continuous venovenous hemodiafiltration in critically ill patients. *Am J Kidney Dis.* 1993;21:400-404.

673. Wendon J, Smithies M, Sheppard M, et al. Continuous high volume venous-venous haemofiltration in acute renal failure. *Intensive Care Med.* 1989;15:358-363.

674. Macias WL, Mueller BA, Scarim SK, et al. Continuous venovenous hemofiltration: an alternative to continuous arteriovenous hemofiltration and hemodiafiltration in acute renal failure. *Am J Kidney Dis.* 1991;18:451-458.

675. Manns M, Sigler MH, Teehan BP. Continuous renal replacement therapies: an update. *Am J Kidney Dis.* 1998;32:185-207.

676. Cerda J, Ronco C. Modalities of continuous renal replacement therapy: technical and clinical considerations. *Semin Dial.* 2009;22:114-122.

677. Ronco C, Bellomo R. Basic mechanisms and definitions for continuous renal replacement therapies. *Int J Artif Organs.* 1996;19:95-99.

678. Ronco C, Bellomo R. Continuous renal replacement therapies: the need for a standard nomenclature. *Contrib Nephrol.* 1995;116:28-33.

679. Ronco C, Bellomo R, Homel P, et al. Effects of different doses in continuous veno-venous haemofiltration on outcomes of acute renal failure: a prospective randomised trial. *Lancet.* 2000;356:26-30.

680. Saudan P, Niederberger M, De Seigneux S, et al. Adding a dialysis dose to continuous hemofiltration increases survival in patients with acute renal failure. *Kidney Int.* 2006;70:1312-1317.

681. Tolwani AJ, Campbell RC, Stofan BS, et al. Standard versus high-dose CVVHDF for ICU-related acute renal failure. *J Am Soc Nephrol.* 2008;19:1233-1238.

682. Bellomo R, Cass A, Cole L, et al. Intensity of continuous renal-replacement therapy in critically ill patients. *N Engl J Med.* 2009;361:1627-1638.

683. Mehta RL, McDonald B, Gabbai FB, et al. A randomized clinical trial of continuous versus intermittent dialysis for acute renal failure. *Kidney Int.* 2001;60:1154-1163.

684. Augustine JJ, Sandy D, Seifert TH, et al. A randomized controlled trial comparing intermittent with continuous dialysis in patients with ARF. *Am J Kidney Dis.* 2004;44:1000-1007.

685. Uehlinger DE, Jakob SM, Ferrari P, et al. Comparison of continuous and intermittent renal replacement therapy for acute renal failure. *Nephrol Dial Transplant.* 2005;20:1630-1637.

686. Lins RL, Elseviers MM, Van der Niepen P, et al. Intermittent versus continuous renal replacement therapy for acute kidney injury patients admitted to the intensive care unit: results of a randomized clinical trial. *Nephrol Dial Transplant.* 2009;24:512-518.

687. Rabindranath K, Adams J, Macleod AM, et al. Intermittent versus continuous renal replacement therapy for acute renal failure in adults. *Cochrane Database Syst Rev.* 2007:CD003773.

688. Bagshaw SM, Berthiaume LR, Delaney A, et al. Continuous versus intermittent renal replacement therapy for critically ill patients with acute kidney injury: a meta-analysis. *Crit Care Med.* 2008;36:610-617.

689. Pannu N, Klarenbach S, Wiebe N, et al. Renal replacement therapy in patients with acute renal failure: a systematic review. *JAMA.* 2008;299:793-805.

690. Manns B, Doig CJ, Lee H, et al. Cost of acute renal failure requiring dialysis in the intensive care unit: clinical and resource implications of renal recovery. *Crit Care Med.* 2003;31:449-455.

691. Jacka MJ, Ivancinova X, Gibney RT. Continuous renal replacement therapy improves renal recovery from acute renal failure. *Can J Anaesth.* 2005;52:327-332.

692. Uchino S, Bellomo R, Kellum JA, et al. Patient and kidney survival by dialysis modality in critically ill patients with acute kidney injury. *Int J Artif Organs.* 2007;30:281-292.

693. Tolwani AJ, Wheeler TS, Wille KM. Sustained low-efficiency dialysis. *Contrib Nephrol.* 2007;156:320-324.

694. Marshall MR, Golper TA, Shaver MJ, et al. Sustained low-efficiency dialysis for critically ill patients requiring renal replacement therapy. *Kidney Int.* 2001;60:777-785.

695. Marshall MR, Golper TA, Shaver MJ, et al. Urea kinetics during sustained low-efficiency dialysis in critically ill patients requiring renal replacement therapy. *Am J Kidney Dis.* 2002;39:556-570.

696. Kumar VA, Craig M, Depner TA, et al. Extended daily dialysis: a new approach to renal replacement for acute renal failure in the intensive care unit. *Am J Kidney Dis.* 2000;36:294-300.

697. Marshall MR, Ma T, Galler D, et al. Sustained low-efficiency daily diafiltration (SLEDD-f) for critically ill patients requiring renal replacement therapy: towards an adequate therapy. *Nephrol Dial Transplant.* 2004;19:877-884.

698. Kielstein JT, Kretschmer U, Ernst T, et al. Efficacy and cardiovascular tolerability of extended dialysis in critically ill patients: a randomized controlled study. *Am J Kidney Dis.* 2004;43:342-349.

699. Ash SR. Peritoneal dialysis in acute renal failure of adults: the under-utilized modality. *Contrib Nephrol.* 2004;144:239-254.

700. Davenport A. Peritoneal dialysis in acute kidney injury. *Perit Dial Int.* 2008;28:423-424 [author reply, 4-5].

701. Passadakis PS, Oreopoulos DG. Peritoneal dialysis in patients with acute renal failure. *Adv Perit Dial.* 2007;23:7-16.

702. Perkins R, Simon J, Jayakumar A, et al. Renal replacement therapy in support of Operation Iraqi Freedom: a tri-service perspective. *Mil Med.* 2008;173:1115-1121.

703. Phu NH, Hien TT, Mai NT, et al. Hemofiltration and peritoneal dialysis in infection-associated acute renal failure in Vietnam. *N Engl J Med.* 2002;347:895-902.

704. Gabriel DP, Caramori JT, Martim LC, et al. High volume peritoneal dialysis vs daily hemodialysis: a randomized, controlled trial in patients with acute kidney injury. *Kidney Int Suppl.* 2008:S87-S93.

705. Abosaif NY, Tolba YA, Heap M, et al. The outcome of acute renal failure in the intensive care unit according to RIFLE: model application, sensitivity, and predictability. *Am J Kidney Dis.* 2005;46:1038-1048.

706. Clermont G, Acker CG, Angus DC, et al. Renal failure in the ICU: comparison of the impact of acute renal failure and end-stage renal disease on ICU outcomes. *Kidney Int.* 2002;62:986-996.

707. Metnitz PG, Krenn CG, Steltzer H, et al. Effect of acute renal failure requiring renal replacement therapy on outcome in critically ill patients. *Crit Care Med.* 2002;30:2051-2058.

708. Benoit DD, Hoste EA, Depuydt PO, et al. Outcome in critically ill medical patients treated with renal replacement therapy for acute renal failure: comparison between patients with and those without haematological malignancies. *Nephrol Dial Transplant.* 2005;20:552-558.

709. Ympa YP, Sakr Y, Reinhart K, et al. Has mortality from acute renal failure decreased? A systematic review of the literature. *Am J Med.* 2005;118:827-832.

710. Tonelli M, Manns B, Feller-Kopman D. Acute renal failure in the intensive care unit: a systematic review of the impact of dialytic modality on mortality and renal recovery. *Am J Kidney Dis.* 2002;40:875-885.

711. Palevsky PM, Metnitz PG, Piccinni P, et al. Selection of endpoints for clinical trials of acute renal failure in critically ill patients. *Curr Opin Crit Care.* 2002;8:515-518.

712. Chertow GM, Lazarus JM, Paganini EP, et al. Predictors of mortality and the provision of dialysis in patients with acute tubular necrosis. The Auriculin Anaritide Acute Renal Failure Study Group. *J Am Soc Nephrol.* 1998;9:692-698.

713. Rasmussen HH, Pitt EA, Ibels LS, et al. Prediction of outcome in acute renal failure by discriminant analysis of clinical variables. *Arch Intern Med.* 1985;145:2015-2018.

714. Turney JH, Marshall DH, Brownjohn AM, et al. The evolution of acute renal failure, 1956-1988. *Q J Med.* 1990;74:83-104.

715. Biesenbach G, Zazgornik J, Kaiser W, et al. Improvement in prognosis of patients with acute renal failure over a period of 15 years: an analysis of 710 cases in a dialysis center. *Am J Nephrol.* 1992;12:319-325.

716. Schrier RW, Wang W. Acute renal failure and sepsis. *N Engl J Med.* 2004;351:159-169.

717. Frankel MC, Weinstein AM, Stenzel KH. Prognostic patterns in acute renal failure: the New York Hospital, 1981-1982. *Clin Exp Dial Apheresis.* 1983;7:145-167.

718. Lassnigg A, Schmid ER, Hiesmayr M, et al. Impact of minimal increases in serum creatinine on outcome in patients after cardiothoracic surgery: do we have to revise current definitions of acute renal failure? *Crit Care Med.* 2008;36:1129-1137.

719. Levy EM, Viscoli CM, Horwitz RI. The effect of acute renal failure on mortality. A cohort analysis. *JAMA.* 1996;275:1489-1494.

720. Goldenberg I, Chonchol M, Guetta V. Reversible acute kidney injury following contrast exposure and the risk of long-term mortality. *Am J Nephrol.* 2009;29:136-144.

721. Gruberg L, Mintz GS, Mehran R, et al. The prognostic implications of further renal function deterioration within 48 h of interventional coronary procedures in patients with pre-existent chronic renal insufficiency. *J Am Coll Cardiol.* 2000;36:1542-1548.

722. Bartholomew BA, Harjai KJ, Dukkipati S, et al. Impact of nephropathy after percutaneous coronary intervention and a method for risk stratification. *Am J Cardiol.* 2004;93:1515-1519.

723. Weisbord SD, Palevsky PM. Acute kidney injury: kidney injury after contrast media: marker or mediator? *Nat Rev Nephrol.* 2010;6:634-636.

724. Faulhaber-Walter R, Hafer C, Jahr N, et al. The Hannover Dialysis Outcome study: comparison of standard versus intensified extended dialysis for treatment of patients with acute kidney injury in the intensive care unit. *Nephrol Dial Transplant.* 2009;24:2179-2186.

725. Edwards KD. Recovery of renal function after acute renal failure. *Australas Ann Med.* 1959;8:195-199.

726. Price JD, Palmer RA. A functional and morphological follow-up study of acute renal failure. *Arch Intern Med.* 1960;105:90-98.

727. Briggs JD, Kennedy AC, Young LN, et al. Renal function after acute tubular necrosis. *Br Med J.* 1967;3:513-516.

728. Lewers DT, Mathew TH, Maher JF, et al. Long-term follow-up of renal function and histology after acute tubular necrosis. *Ann Intern Med.* 1970;73:523-529.

729. Ishani A, Xue JL, Himmelfarb J, et al. Acute kidney injury increases risk of ESRD among elderly. *J Am Soc Nephrol.* 2009;20:223-228.

730. Wald R, Quinn RR, Luo J, et al. Chronic dialysis and death among survivors of acute kidney injury requiring dialysis. *JAMA.* 2009;302:1179-1185.

731. Lo LJ, Go AS, Chertow GM, et al. Dialysis-requiring acute renal failure increases the risk of progressive chronic kidney disease. *Kidney Int.* 2009;76:893-899.

732. Newsome BB, Warnock DG, McClellan WM, et al. Long-term risk of mortality and end-stage renal disease among the elderly after small increases in serum creatinine level during hospitalization for acute myocardial infarction. *Arch Intern Med.* 2008;168:609-616.

733. James MT, Ghali WA, Tonelli M, et al. Acute kidney injury following coronary angiography is associated with a long-term decline in kidney function. *Kidney Int.* 2010;78:803-809.

734. Hoste EA, Kellum JA. Acute renal failure in the critically ill: impact on morbidity and mortality. *Contrib Nephrol.* 2004;144:1-11.

735. Bates DW, Su L, Yu DT, et al. Mortality and costs of acute renal failure associated with amphotericin B therapy. *Clin Infect Dis.* 2001;32:686-693.

736. Fischer MJ, Brimhall BB, Lezotte DC, et al. Uncomplicated acute renal failure and hospital resource utilization: a retrospective multicenter analysis. *Am J Kidney Dis.* 2005;46:1049-1057.

737. Hamel MB, Phillips RS, Davis RB, et al. Outcomes and cost-effectiveness of initiating dialysis and continuing aggressive care in seriously ill hospitalized adults. SUPPORT Investigators. Study to Understand Prognoses and Preferences for Outcomes and Risks of Treatments. *Ann Intern Med.* 1997;127:195-202.

738. Ahlstrom A, Tallgren M, Peltonen S, et al. Survival and quality of life of patients requiring acute renal replacement therapy. *Intensive Care Med.* 2005;31:1222-1228.

739. Johansen KL, Smith MW, Unruh ML, et al. Predictors of health utility among 60-day survivors of acute kidney injury in the Veterans Affairs/National Institutes of Health Acute Renal Failure Trial Network Study. *Clin J Am Soc Nephrol.* 2010;5:1366-1372.

740. Bell M, Liljestam E, Granath F, et al. Optimal follow-up time after continuous renal replacement therapy in actual renal failure patients stratified with the RIFLE criteria. *Nephrol Dial Transplant.* 2005;20:354-360.

Primary Glomerular Disease

Patrick H. Nachman, J. Charles Jennette, and Ronald J. Falk

The underlying cause of most glomerular diseases remains an enigma, although important discoveries have been made since the last edition of this book that substantially increase our understanding of the etiology and pathogenesis of a number of glomerular diseases—for example, membranous glomerulopathy (membranous nephropathy), focal segmental glomerulosclerosis, immunoglobulin A (IgA) nephropathy, antineutrophil cytoplasmic antibody (ANCA)–associated glomerulonephritis, and dense deposit disease. Infectious agents, autoimmunity, drugs, inherited disorders, and environmental agents have been implicated as causes of certain glomerular diseases. Until the precise etiology and pathogenesis of glomerular disorders is unraveled, we continue in the tradition of Richard Bright—studying the relationship of clinical, pathologic, and laboratory signs and symptoms of disease, and basing our diagnostic categorization on these features rather than on etiology.

Glomerular diseases may be categorized into those that primarily involve the kidney (primary glomerular diseases), and those in which kidney involvement is part of a systemic disorder (secondary glomerular diseases). This chapter focuses on primary glomerular diseases. Chapter 32 concentrates on secondary glomerular diseases. Chapter 33 is new to this edition and focuses on therapy for glomerular disease. The separation of glomerular diseases into primary and secondary is somewhat problematic, because in some instances what are considered primary glomerular diseases are similar, if not identical, to secondary glomerular diseases. For example, IgA

nephropathy, pauci-immune necrotizing and crescentic glomerulonephritis, antiglomerular basement membrane (anti-GBM) glomerulonephritis, membranous glomerulopathy, and type I membranoproliferative glomerulonephritis can occur as primary renal diseases or as components of the systemic diseases Henoch-Schönlein purpura, pauci-immune small vessel vasculitis, Goodpasture's syndrome, systemic lupus erythematosus, and cryoglobulinemic vasculitis, respectively. This chapter focuses on the diagnosis and management of glomerular diseases that do not appear to be a component of a systemic disease.

When a patient has glomerular disease, the clinician not only must evaluate the clinical signs and symptoms, but also must be vigilant for evidence of a systemic process or disease that could be causing the renal disease. Clinical evaluation includes assessment of proteinuria, hematuria, the presence or absence of renal insufficiency, and the presence or absence of hypertension. Some glomerular diseases cause isolated proteinuria or isolated hematuria with no other signs or symptoms of disease. More severe glomerular disease often results in nephrotic syndrome or nephritic (glomerulonephritic) syndrome. Glomerular disease may have an indolent course or begin abruptly, leading to acute or rapidly progressive glomerulonephritis. Although some glomerular disorders consistently cause a specific syndrome (e.g., minimal change glomerulopathy results in nephrotic syndrome), most disorders are capable of causing features of both nephrosis and nephritis (Table 31-1). This sharing and variability of clinical

TABLE 31-1 Manifestations of Nephrotic and Nephritic Features by Glomerular Diseases

	NEPHROTIC FEATURES	NEPHRITIC FEATURES
Minimal change glomerulopathy	++++	–
Membranous glomerulopathy	++++	+
Focal segmental glomerulosclerosis	+++	++
Fibrillary glomerulonephritis	+++	++
Mesangioproliferative glomerulopathy*	++	++
Membranoproliferative glomerulonephritis†	++	+++
Proliferative glomerulonephritis*	++	+++
Acute diffuse proliferative glomerulonephritis‡	+	++++
Crescentic glomerulonephritis§	+	++++

*Mesangioproliferative and proliferative glomerulonephritis (focal or diffuse) are structural manifestations of a number of glomerulonephritides, including immunoglobulin A nephropathy and lupus nephritis.

†Both type I (mesangiocapillary) and type II (dense deposit disease).

‡Often a structural manifestation of acute poststreptococcal glomerulonephritis.

§Can be immune complex mediated, anti–glomerular basement membrane antibody mediated, or associated with antineutrophil cytoplasmic autoantibodies.

Modified from Jennette JC, Mandal AK: The nephrotic syndrome, in Mandal AK, Jennette JC (editors): *Diagnosis and management of renal disease and hypertension*, Durham NC, 1994, Carolina Academic Press, pp 235-272.

manifestations among different glomerular diseases confounds determination of an accurate diagnosis based on clinical features alone. Therefore, renal biopsy has an important role to play in the evaluation of glomerular disease in many patients and remains the gold standard.

This chapter describes the clinical syndromes caused by glomerular diseases, including isolated proteinuria, isolated hematuria, and specific forms of primary glomerular disease that cause nephrotic or nephritic syndrome.

General Description of Glomerular Syndromes

Isolated Proteinuria

Proteinuria can be caused by systemic overproduction (e.g., multiple myeloma with Bence Jones proteinuria), tubular dysfunction (e.g., Fanconi's syndrome), or glomerular dysfunction. It is important to differentiate patients in whom proteinuria is a manifestation of substantial glomerular disease from patients who have benign functional, transient, postural (orthostatic), or intermittent proteinuria.

Plasma proteins larger than 70 kDa cross the basement membrane in a manner normally restricted by both size-selective and charge-selective barriers.[1,2] The functional characteristics of the glomerular capillary filter have been extensively studied by the evaluation of the fractional clearance of molecules of different size and charge.[3] The size-selective barrier is most likely a consequence of functional pores within the GBM that restrict the filtration of plasma proteins of more than 150 kDa. There is also a shape restriction of molecules that allows elongated molecules to cross the glomerular capillary wall more readily than globular molecules of the same molecular weight.

Furthermore, there is a charge-selective feature of the barrier, which is largely a consequence of the presence of glycosaminoglycans arranged along the capillary wall. Loss of charge selectivity may be the defect in minimal change glomerulopathy, whereas a loss of size selectivity may be the cause of proteinuria in, for instance, membranous glomerulopathy.[2]

A number of factors have proved to be important in the disruption of the glomerular capillary wall as a consequence of tissue-degrading enzymes, complement components that assemble upon it, and oxygen radicals that target both the GBM and the slit diaphragm. Heparinase- and hyaluronidase-mediated alterations in the aminoglycan content of the glomerular capillary wall may play a role in increased protein excretion.[4,5] Genetic studies have provided exciting clues to the specific components of the glomerular capillary wall, including mutations in the podocyte or proteins in the slit diaphragm, that result in proteinuria (recently reviewed by Tryggvason and colleagues[6]).

Another major mechanism resulting in proteinuria is impaired reabsorption of plasma proteins by proximal tubular epithelial cells. A number of low-molecular-weight proteins, including β_1-, β_2-, and α_1-microglobulins, are filtered by the glomerulus and absorbed by tubular epithelial cells. When tubular epithelial cells are damaged, these proteins are excreted. The critical importance of tubular absorption of proteins has been recently studied.[7] The glomerular capillary sieving coefficient for albumin was examined in normal and nephrotic rats by two-photon (laser) intravital microscopy. The glomerular capillary sieving coefficient for albumin was 3.4×10^{-2} rather than 6.2×10^{-4} as found by earlier micropuncture studies in rats.

Several important observations were made in this study. First, a large amount of albumin is filtered across the glomerular capillary bed daily in the normal rat. Second, no evidence was found for a charge-based restriction to the passage of albumin through the glomerular filter. Third, in normal and nephrotic animals, the vast majority of the filtered albumin was "reclaimed" from the filtrate by a high-capacity transcytotic pathway in the proximal tubule, which returns intact (unaltered) albumin to the peritubular capillary circulation. These are important new concepts, because most nephrologists view albuminuria as resulting solely from enhanced glomerular permeability.

The term *isolated proteinuria* is used in several conditions, including mild transient proteinuria of less than 1 g protein per day that typically accompanies physiologically stressful conditions such as fever in hospitalized patients, exercise, and congestive heart failure.[8] In other patients, transient proteinuria is a consequence of the overflow of proteins of low molecular weight due to overproduction of light chains, heavy chains, or other fragments of immunoglobulins. The differential diagnosis of overproduction of proteinuria includes multiple myeloma, Bence Jones proteinuria, β_2-microglobinuria, and hemoglobinuria.

The term *orthostatic proteinuria* is defined by the absence of proteinuria while the patient is in a recumbent posture and its appearance during upright posture, especially during ambulation or exercise.[9] The total amount of protein excreted in a 24-hour period is generally less than 1 g, but may be as much as 2 g. Orthostatic proteinuria is more common in adolescents and is uncommon in individuals older than age 30.[9,10] Some 2% to 5% of adolescents have orthostatic proteinuria. When patients with orthostatic proteinuria underwent renal biopsy 47% were found to have normal glomeruli by light microscopy,

45% to have minimal to moderate glomerular abnormalities of a nonspecific nature, and the remainder to have evidence of a primary glomerular disease.[11]

Why is proteinuria increased during upright posture in individuals who have normal glomeruli by light microscopy? Although the answer to this question remains an enigma, there are several likely possibilities. Orthostatic proteinuria may occur as a consequence of alterations in glomerular hemodynamics. It is possible that even in histologically "normal" glomeruli, in which there are no specific lesions, there are subtle glomerular abnormalities, including abnormal basement membranes or focal changes of the mesangium.[12] Alternatively, orthostatic proteinuria has been demonstrated with entrapment of the left renal vein by the aorta and superior mesenteric artery. Thirteen of 15 children with orthostatic proteinuria were found to have venous entrapment, compared with 9 of 80 children with normal protein excretion.[13] In addition, the observation that surgical correction of a kink in an allograft renal vein resulted in the disappearance of orthostatic proteinuria gives credence to venous entrapment as a cause of orthostatic proteinuria.[12]

There are several approaches to the diagnosis of orthostatic proteinuria. These include comparison of protein excretion in two 12-hour urine collections, one during recumbency and one during ambulation. Another approach is to compare protein level in a split collection of 16 hours during ambulation and 8 hours of overnight collection. It is important that patients be recumbent for at least 2 hours before their ambulatory collection is completed to avoid the possibility of contamination of the recumbent collection by urine formed during ambulation. The diagnosis of orthostatic proteinuria requires that protein excretion during recumbency be less than 50 mg during those 8 hours. Few convincing data exist on the usefulness of comparing urinary protein/creatinine ratio measurements during recumbency with those during ambulation as a diagnostic test for orthostatic proteinuria.

Twenty-year follow-up of patients with orthostatic proteinuria suggests a benign long-term course.[10] Orthostatic proteinuria resolves in most patients. It is present in one half of patients after 10 years and only 17% of patients after 20 years.[10] In the absence of a kidney biopsy, an underlying glomerulopathy cannot be completely excluded, and an orthostatic component of proteinuria may be found in early glomerular disease. Thus, it is important to reassess patients after an interval of about 1 year to be certain that the degree or pattern of proteinuria has not changed.

Fixed proteinuria is present whether the patient is upright or recumbent. The proteinuria disappears in some patients, whereas others have a more ominous glomerular lesion that portends an adverse long-term outcome. The prognosis depends on the persistence and severity of the proteinuria. If proteinuria disappears, it is less likely that the patient will develop hypertension or reduced glomerular filtration rate (GFR). These patients must be evaluated periodically for as long as proteinuria persists.

Recurrent or Persistent Hematuria

Hematuria is the presence of an excessive number of red blood cells in the urine and is categorized as either microscopic (visible only with the aid of a microscope) or macroscopic (the urine is tea-colored or cola-colored, pink, or even red).

Hematuria can result from injury to the kidney or to another site in the urinary tract.

Healthy individuals may excrete as many as 10^5 red cells in the urine in a 12-hour period. An acceptable definition of hematuria is more than two red cells per high-power field in centrifuged urine.[14] The approach to processing urine varies from laboratory to laboratory, however; thus the number of red cells per high-power field that is an accurate indicator of hematuria may vary slightly among different laboratories. The urinary dipstick test detects one to two red cells per high-power field and is a very sensitive test. A negative result on dipstick examination virtually excludes hematuria.[15]

Hematuria is present in about 5% to 6% of the general population[16] and 4% of schoolchildren. In the majority of children, results of follow-up urinalyses are normal.[17] In most people, the hematuria emanates from the lower urinary tract, especially in conditions affecting the urethra, bladder, and prostate. Fewer than 10% of cases of hematuria are caused by glomerular bleeding.[14] Persistent hematuria, especially in older individuals, should raise the possibility of malignancy. The incidence of malignancy, especially of the bladder, ranges from 5% in individuals with persistent microscopic hematuria to over 20% in individuals with gross hematuria.[18] Other causes of nonglomerular hematuria include neoplasms, trauma, metabolic defects such as hypercalciuria, vascular diseases including renal infarctions and renal vein thrombosis, cystic diseases of the kidney including polycystic kidney disease, medullary cystic disease and medullary sponge kidney, and interstitial kidney disease such as papillary necrosis, hydronephrosis, and drug-induced interstitial nephritis. In children with asymptomatic hematuria, hypercalciuria is the cause in 15% of cases, and 10% to 15% have IgA nephropathy. In up to 80% of children and 15% to 20% of adults with hematuria no cause can be identified.[19]

Transient hematuria has been found in a number of settings. Transient hematuria is present in 13% of postmenopausal women.[20] Episodic hematuria in a cyclical pattern during a menstrual cycle is most likely a consequence of the invasion of the urinary tract by endometrial implants.[21] In 1000 males between the ages of 18 and 33, hematuria was present at least once in 39%, and on two or more occasions in 16%. In patients with isolated asymptomatic hematuria without proteinuria or renal insufficiency, the hematuria resolves in 20% of cases; however, even some of these patients will develop hypertension and proteinuria.[22] In older individuals, transient hematuria should raise a concern for malignancy.[14,23,24] In some individuals, transient hematuria may be a consequence of exercise.

Glomerular hematuria, in contrast to hematuria caused by injury elsewhere in the urinary tract, is characterized by misshapen red cells that have been distorted by osmotic and chemical stress the cells pass through the nephron. Hematuria with dysmorphic cells, especially cells that have membrane blebs producing the picture of acanthocyturia, is strong evidence for glomerular bleeding.[18] The finding of protein (especially >2 g/day), hemoglobin, or red cell casts in the urine enhances the possibility that hematuria is of glomerular origin. Although brown or cola-colored urine is most commonly associated with glomerular hematuria, its absence does not exclude glomerular disease. Interestingly, clots do not occur in the urine with glomerular bleeding.

The differential pathologic diagnosis of glomerular hematuria without proteinuria, renal insufficiency, or red blood

TABLE 31-2 Frequency of Renal Disease in Patients with Hematuria Undergoing Renal Biopsy (in Percent)*

BIOPSY FINDINGS	HEMATURIA, URINARY PROTEIN <1 g/day, CREATININE <1.5 mg/dL	HEMATURIA, URINARY PROTEIN 1-3 g/day, CREATININE <1.5 mg/dL	HEMATURIA, CREATININE >3 mg/dL
No abnormality	30	2	0
Thin basement nephropathy	26	4	0
Immunoglobulin A nephropathy	28	24	8
Glomerulonephritis without crescents[†]	9	26	23
Glomerulonephritis with crescents[†]	2	24	44
Other renal disease[‡]	5	20	25
Total	100 (*n* = 43)	100 (*n* = 123)	100 (*n* = 255)

*Based on an analysis of renal biopsy specimens evaluated at the University of North Carolina Nephropathology Laboratory. Specimens from patients with systemic lupus erythematosus were excluded from the analysis.

†Proliferative or necrotizing glomerulonephritis other than immunoglobulin A nephropathy or lupus nephritis.

‡Includes causes of nephrotic syndrome, such as membranous glomerulopathy and focal segmental glomerulosclerosis.

Data from Caldas ML, Charles LA, Falk RJ, et al. Immunoelectron microscopic documentation of the translocation of proteins reactive with ANCA to neutrophil cell surfaces during neutrophil activation. [Abstract]. Third International Workshop on ANCA, 1990.

cell casts is IgA nephropathy, thin basement membrane nephropathy, hereditary nephritis, and histologically normal glomeruli.[25] In a study in Europe,[26] 80 normotensive adults underwent renal biopsy for evaluation of recurrent macroscopic hematuria or persistent microscopic hematuria. Approximately 30% of these patients had IgA nephropathy, 20% had thin basement membrane nephropathy, and 30% had no discernible lesion. Hematuria disappeared in 13 of the latter patients. The remaining patients had mesangioproliferative glomerulonephritis, interstitial nephritis, or focal glomerulosclerosis. In contrast, 216 Chinese adults with isolated hematuria who underwent renal biopsy were much more likely to have IgA nephropathy than any other lesion.[27]

Table 31-2 provides data from an analysis of native kidney biopsy specimens from patients with hematuria performed by the University of North Carolina (UNC) Nephropathology Laboratory. Patients with systemic lupus erythematosus were excluded from the study. The patients selected for the study had a serum creatinine level of less than 1.5 mg/dL or more than 3 mg/dL. The patients with a serum creatinine level of less than 1.5 mg/dL were further divided into those with proteinuria of less than 1 g protein per day and those with proteinuria of 1 to 3 g protein per day. The data showed that patients with a relatively normal serum creatinine level, hematuria, and proteinuria of less than 1 g protein per day were most likely to have thin basement membrane nephropathy, IgA nephropathy, or no identifiable renal lesion. When hematuria was accompanied by proteinuria of 1 to 3 g protein per day but no significant renal insufficiency, IgA nephropathy was the most likely specific cause. Patients with hematuria and a serum creatinine level of more than 3 mg/dL most often had aggressive glomerulonephritis with crescents.

Despite these overall tendencies, it is not possible to definitively determine the cause of asymptomatic hematuria without renal biopsy, and even renal biopsy specimen evaluation fails to reveal a cause in a minority of patients. Certain rules generally apply to the clinical prediction of the most likely cause. Gross hematuria is most commonly found in IgA nephropathy or hereditary nephritis. Patients with thin basement membrane nephropathy typically do not have substantial proteinuria.

The potential benefits of renal biopsy in patients with isolated hematuria include reduction of patient and physician uncertainty by confirmation of a specific diagnosis. Nonetheless, the role of renal biopsy in the evaluation of asymptomatic hematuria in patients without proteinuria, hypertension, or kidney insufficiency remains unclear. In biopsy series involving patients in whom asymptomatic hematuria is accompanied by low-grade proteinuria, specific glomerular diseases including IgA nephropathy and membranoproliferative glomerular disease may be discovered when there is no proteinuria, and IgA nephropathy and thin basement membrane disease or nondiagnostic minor changes remain the most common findings.[28,29] Confirmation of a glomerular cause eliminates the need for repeated urologic studies, and a more accurate long-term prognosis can be made (e.g., thin basement membrane nephropathy is less likely to progress than IgA nephropathy). However, isolated glomerular hematuria without proteinuria or renal insufficiency may not warrant a renal biopsy, because the findings often will not affect management. In one study of patients with isolated hematuria, the biopsy results altered patient management in only 1of 36 patients.[30]

Glomerular Diseases That Cause Nephrotic Syndrome

Nephrotic syndrome results from proteinuria of more than 3.5 g protein per day and is characterized by edema, hyperlipidemia, hypoproteinemia, and other metabolic disorders (described in detail later). Nephrotic syndrome not only may be caused by primary (idiopathic) glomerular diseases but also may be secondary to a large number of identifiable disease states (Table 31-3). Despite the differences in these causes, the loss of substantial amounts of protein in the urine results in a shared set of abnormalities that comprise nephrotic syndrome (Tables 31-4, 31-5, and 31-6).

Minimal Change Glomerulopathy

Epidemiology

Minimal change glomerulopathy, also known as *minimal change disease*, was first described in 1913 by Munk, who called it *lipoid nephrosis* because of the presence of lipid in

TABLE 31-3 Classification of the Disease States Associated with the Development of Nephrotic Syndrome

Idiopathic Nephrotic Syndrome due to Primary Glomerular Disease

Nephrotic Syndrome Associated with Specific Etiologic Events or in Which Glomerular Disease Arises as a Complication of Other Diseases

1. *Medications and other chemicals*
   Organic, inorganic, elemental mercury*
   Organic gold
   Penicillamine, bucillamine
   Street heroin
   Probenecid
   Captopril
   Nonsteroidal antiinflammatory drugs
   Lithium
   Interferon-α
   Chlorpropamide
   Rifampin
   Pamidronate
   Paramethadione (Paradione), trimethadione (Tridione)
   Mephenytoin (Mesantoin)
   Tolbutamide†
   Phenindione†
   Warfarin
   Clonidine†
   Perchlorate†
   Bismuth†
   Trichloroethylene†
   Silver†
   Insect repellent†
   Contrast media

2. *Allergens, venoms, immunizing agents*
   Bee sting
   Pollens
   Poison ivy and poison oak
   Antitoxins (serum sickness)
   Snake venom
   Diphtheria, pertussis, tetanus toxoid
   Vaccines

3. *Infections*
   Bacterial: *poststreptococcal glomerulonephritis*, infective endocarditis, *shunt nephritis*, leprosy, syphilis (congenital and secondary), *Mycoplasma* infection, tuberculosis,† chronic bacterial pyelonephritis with vesicoureteral reflux
   Viral: hepatitis B, hepatitis C, cytomegalovirus infection, infectious mononucleosis (Epstein-Barr virus infection), herpes zoster, vaccinia, infection with human immunodeficiency virus type 1
   Protozoal: *malaria* (especially quartan malaria), toxoplasmosis
   Helminthic: *schistosomiasis*, trypanosomiasis, filariasis

4. *Neoplasms*
   Solid tumors (carcinoma and sarcoma): tumors of the *lung, colon, stomach, breast*, cervix, kidney, thyroid, ovary, prostate, adrenal, oropharynx, carotid body†; melanoma, pheochromocytoma, Wilms' tumor, mesothelioma, oncocytoma
   Leukemia and lymphoma: *Hodgkin's disease,* chronic lymphocytic leukemia, multiple myeloma (amyloidosis), Waldenström's macroglobulinemia, lymphoma
   Graft-versus-host disease after bone marrow transplantation

5. *Multisystem disease‡*
   Systemic lupus erythematosus
   Mixed connective tissue disease
   Dermatomyositis
   Rheumatoid arthritis
   Goodpasture's syndrome
   Henoch-Schönlein purpura (see also immunoglobulin A nephropathy, Berger's disease)
   Systemic vasculitis (including Wegener's granulomatosis)
   Takayasu's arteritis
   Mixed cryoglobulinemia
   Light- and heavy-chain disease (Randall type)
   Partial lipodystrophy
   Sjögren's syndrome
   Toxic epidermolysis
   Dermatitis herpetiformis
   Sarcoidosis
   Ulcerative colitis
   Amyloidosis (primary and secondary)

6. *Hereditary-familial and metabolic disease‡*
   Diabetes mellitus
   Hypothyroidism (myxedema)
   Graves' disease
   Amyloidosis (familial Mediterranean fever and other hereditary forms, Muckle-Wells syndrome)
   Alport's syndrome
   Fabry's disease
   Nail-patella syndrome
   Lipoprotein glomerulopathy
   Sickle cell disease
   α$_1$-Antitrypsin deficiency
   Asphyxiating thoracic dystrophy (Jeune's syndrome)
   Von Gierke's disease
   Podocyte/slit diaphragm mutation
   Nephrin mutation
   FAT2 mutation
   Podocin mutation
   CD2AP mutation
   Denys-Drash syndrome (*WT1* mutation)
   ACTN4 mutation
   Charcot-Marie-Tooth syndrome
   Congenital nephrotic syndrome (Finnish type)
   Cystinosis (adult)
   Galloway-Mowat syndrome
   Hurler's syndrome
   Familial dysautonomia

7. *Miscellaneous‡*
   Pregnancy associated (preeclampsia, recurrent, transient)
   Chronic renal allograft failure
   Accelerated or malignant nephrosclerosis
   Unilateral renal arterial hypertension
   Intestinal lymphangiectasia
   Chronic jejunoileitis†
   Spherocytosis†
   Renal artery stenosis
   Congenital heart disease† (cyanotic)
   Severe congestive heart failure†
   Constrictive pericarditis†
   Tricuspid insufficiency†
   Massive obesity
   Vesicoureteric reflux nephropathy
   Papillary necrosis
   Gardner-Diamond syndrome
   Castleman's disease
   Kartagener's syndrome
   Buckley's syndrome
   Kimura's disease
   Silica exposure

*Diseases and other agents in italics are the more commonly encountered causes of nephrotic syndrome.
†Based on single case reports or small series in which cause-and-effect relationship cannot be established. Other factors (e.g., use of mercurial diuretics in heart failure) may have been the true inciting event.
‡See Chapter 32 for detailed discussion of the secondary forms of nephrotic syndrome.
ACTN4, α-Actinin-4; *CD2AP*, CD2-associated protein; *FAT2*, FAT tumor suppressor homolog 2 (*Drosophila*); *WT1*, Wilms' tumor 1.

TABLE 31-4 Alterations of Plasma Proteins in Nephrotic Syndrome

Immunoglobulins (Ig)
Decreased IgG
Normal or increased IgA, IgM, or IgE
Increased $\alpha_2 k$- and β-globulins
Decreased α_1-globulin

Metal-Binding Proteins
Loss of metal binding proteins
   Iron
   Copper
   Zinc
Loss of erythropoietin
Depletion of transferrin

Complement
Decreased factor B
Decreased C3
Decreased C1q, C2, C8, Ci
Increased C3, C4bp
Normal levels of C1s, C4, and C1 inhibitor

Coagulation Components
Decreased factors XI, XII, kallikrein inhibitor
Decreased factors IX, XII
Decreased alpha2-antiplasmin and alpha1-antitrypsin
Increased tissue type plasminogen activator and plasminogen
Increased tissue factor and tissue factor pathway indicator
Elevated β-thromboglobulin

Data from references 388, 1238-1254.

TABLE 31-5 Coagulation Abnormalities in Nephrotic Syndrome

Increased blood viscosity
Hemoconcentration
Increased plasma fibrinogen
Increased intravascular fibrin formation
Increased α_2-macroglobulins
Increased tissue plasminogen activator
Increased factors II, V, VII, VIII, X, XIII
Decreased factors IX, XI, XII
Decreased α_1-antitrypsin
Decreased fibrinolytic activity
Decreased plasma plasminogen
Decreased antithrombin III
Decreased protein S
Thrombocytosis
Increased platelet aggregability

Data from references 439, 1253, 1255-1269.

TABLE 31-6 Diseases That Cause Nephrotic Syndrome

GLOMERULAR LESION	N	MALE/FEMALE RATIO	WHITE/AFRICAN AMERICAN RATIO
Minimal change glomerulopathy	522	1.1:1.0	1.9:1.0
Focal segmental glomerulosclerosis (FSGS) (typical)	1103	1.4:1.0	1.0:1.0
Collapsing variant of FSGS	135	1.2:1.0	1.0:7.8
Glomerular tip lesion variant of FSGS	94	1.0:1.0	4.7:1.0
Membranous glomerulopathy	1120	1.4:1.0	1.9:1.0
C1q nephropathy	114	1.0:1.0	1.0:4.8
Fibrillary glomerulonephritis	76	1.0:1.2	14.3:1.0

Data are derived from analysis of 9605 native kidney biopsy specimens evaluated at the University of North Carolina Nephropathology Laboratory. This laboratory evaluates kidney biopsy specimens from a base population of approximately 10 million throughout the southeastern United States and centered in North Carolina. The expected white/African American ratio in this renal biopsy population is approximately 2:1.

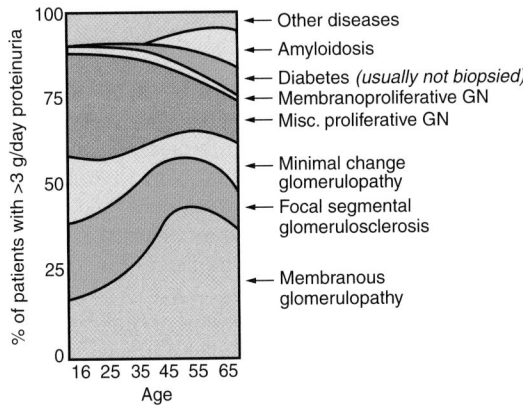

FIGURE 31-1 Graph depicting the frequencies of different forms of glomerular disease identified in renal biopsy specimens from patients with proteinuria of more than 3 g of protein per day evaluated at the University of North Carolina Nephropathology Laboratory. Some diseases that cause proteinuria are underrepresented because they are not always evaluated by renal biopsy. For example, in many patients steroid-responsive proteinuria is given a presumptive diagnosis of minimal change glomerulopathy and patients do not undergo biopsy, and most patients with diabetes and proteinuria are presumed to have diabetic glomerulosclerosis and do not undergo biopsy.

the tubular epithelial cells and urine.[31] Minimal change glomerulopathy is most common in children, accounting for 70% to 90% of nephrotic syndrome in children under age 10 and 50% in older children. Minimal change glomerulopathy also causes 10% to 15% of primary nephrotic syndrome in adults (Figure 31-1).

The incidence of minimal change glomerulopathy has geographic variations. Minimal change glomerulopathy is more common in Asia than in North America or Europe.[32] This may be a consequence of differences in renal biopsy practices, or of differences in environmental or genetic influences. The disease may also affect elderly patients, in whom there is a higher propensity for the clinical syndrome of minimal change glomerulopathy and acute renal failure (discussed later). There appears to be a male preponderance of this process in some series, especially in children, in whom the male/female ratio is 2:1 to 3:1[33]; however, data from the authors' institution do not support this.

Pathology

The effacement of podocyte foot processes is accompanied by increased density of the cytoskeleton, including actin filaments, in clumps near the basement membrane surface of the

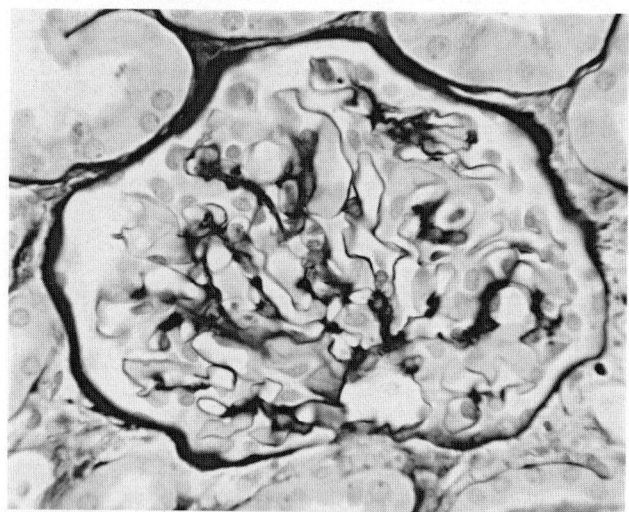

FIGURE 31-2 Unremarkable light microscopic appearance of a biopsy specimen from a patient with minimal change glomerulopathy. Glomerular basement membranes are thin, and there is no glomerular hypercellularity or mesangial matrix expansion. (Jones' methenamine silver stain, ×300.)

visceral epithelial cells. However, the extent of effacement appears to correlate more with the duration of active nephrotic syndrome than with the magnitude of proteinuria.[34]

LIGHT MICROSCOPY

In minimal change glomerulopathy no glomerular lesions are seen by light microscopy (Figure 31-2) or only a minimal focal segmental mesangial prominence is noted.[35] This mesangial prominence should have no more than three or four cells embedded in the matrix of a segment, and the matrix should not be expanded to the extent that capillary lumens are compromised. Capillary walls should be thin and capillary lumens patent.

The most consistent tubular lesion is increased protein and lipid resorption droplets in tubular epithelial cells. These droplets stain with periodic acid–Schiff stain. Conspicuous resorbed lipid in epithelial cells prompted the designation *lipoid nephrosis* for this disease prior to the recognition of the ultrastructural glomerular lesion. Interstitial edema is rare, even in patients with severe nephrotic syndrome and anasarca. Focal proximal tubular epithelial flattening (simplification), which is histologically identical to that seen with ischemic acute renal failure, occurs in patients who have the syndrome of minimal change glomerulopathy with acute renal failure.[36]

Focal areas of interstitial fibrosis and tubular atrophy in a specimen that otherwise looks like minimal change glomerulopathy, especially in a young person, should raise the possibility of FSGS that was not sampled in the biopsy specimen. Examination of additional levels of section may reveal a sclerotic glomerulus.

IMMUNOFLUORESCENCE MICROSCOPY

Glomeruli usually show no staining with antisera specific for IgG, IgA, IgM, C3, C4, or C1q. The most frequent positive finding is low-level mesangial staining for IgM, sometimes accompanied by low-level staining for C3. If the IgM staining is not accompanied by mesangial electron-dense deposits by electron microscopy, it is consistent with a diagnosis of minimal change glomerulopathy. Patients whose specimens show mesangial IgM staining by immunofluorescence microscopy

(in the absence of dense deposits by electron microscopy) do not have a worse prognosis than patients whose specimens are without IgM staining.[37,38] The presence of mesangial dense deposits identified by electron microscopy worsens the prognosis and thus justifies altering the diagnosis, for example to IgM mesangial nephropathy.[39] Anything more than trace staining for IgG or IgA casts substantial doubt on a diagnosis of minimal change glomerulopathy. Even when no sclerotic glomerular lesions are seen by light microscopy, well-defined irregular focal segmental staining for C3 and IgM should raise the possibility of FSGS, because sclerotic lesions can be enriched for C3 and IgM. Glomerular and tubular epithelial cell cytoplasmic droplets and tubular casts may stain positively for immunoglobulins and other plasma proteins when there is substantial proteinuria.

ELECTRON MICROSCOPY

The pathologic sine qua non of minimal change glomerulopathy is effacement of visceral epithelial cell foot processes observed by electron microscopy (Figures 31-3 and 31-4). However, this is not a specific feature, because it occurs in the glomeruli of patients with severe proteinuria due to any cause. During active nephrosis, the effacement often is very extensive, with only a few scattered intact foot processes. As the disease enters remission, the extent of foot process effacement diminishes. The effacement usually is accompanied by microvillous transformation, which is the development of numerous villous projections from the epithelial surface into the urinary space. These intracytoplasmic densities should not be confused with subepithelial immune complex dense deposits. Glomerular and proximal tubular epithelial cells have increased clear and dense cytoplasmic droplets.

All of these ultrastructural glomerular changes occur in other glomerular disease when there is nephrotic-range proteinuria. Therefore, minimal change glomerulopathy is a diagnosis by exclusion that is made only when there is no evidence by light, immunofluorescence, and electron microscopy of any other glomerular disease.

Pathogenesis

Although the pathogenesis of minimal change glomerulopathy remains unclear, this disorder is most likely a consequence of abnormal regulation of a T cell subset[40-44] and pathologic elaboration of one or more circulating permeability factors. Specifically, corticosteroids and alkylating drugs cause a remission of minimal change glomerulopathy, there is an association of minimal change glomerulopathy with Hodgkin's disease,[45,46] and remissions are associated with depression of cell-mediated immunity during viral infections such as measles. Specific evidence stems from the finding that a glomerular permeability factor is produced by human T cell hybridomas obtained from a patient with minimal change nephrosis. When this factor was injected into rodents, proteinuria occurred with partial fusion of glomerular epithelial cell foot processes.[47] Although there are no observable abnormalities in T or B cell populations in patients with relapsing or quiescent minimal change glomerulopathy,[48-51] lymphocytes have depressed reactivity when challenged with mitogens.[52-60] T cells apparently produce a product, most likely a lymphokine, that increases glomerular permeability to protein. When the glomerular permeability factor is removed from the

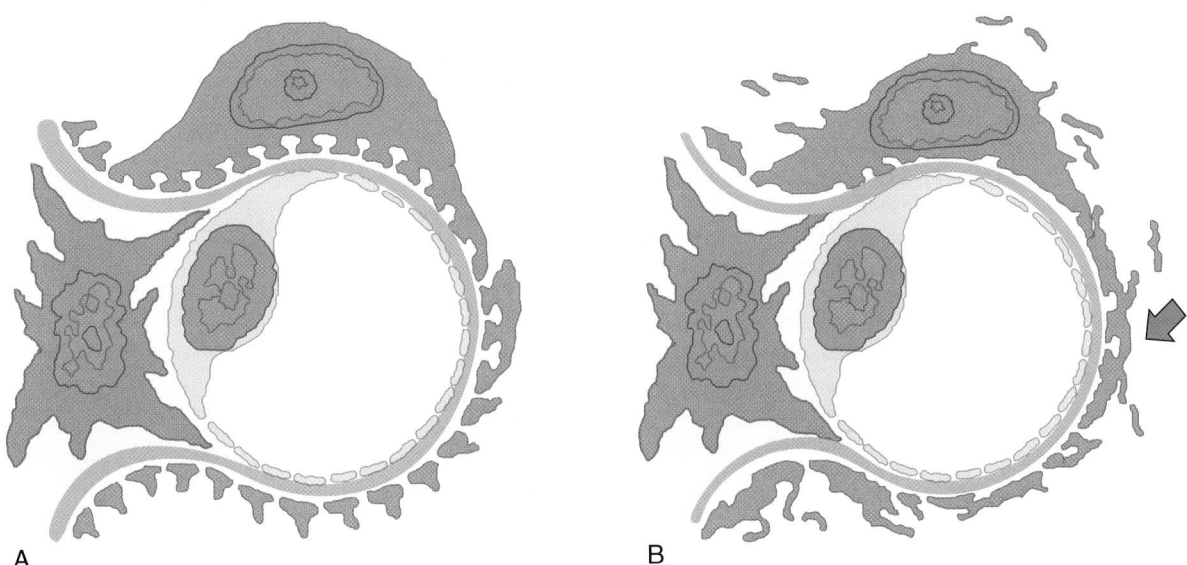

A   B

FIGURE 31-3 Diagrams depicting the ultrastructural features of a normal glomerular capillary loop (**A**) and a capillary loop with features of minimal change glomerulopathy (**B**). The latter has effacement of epithelial foot processes (*arrow*) and microvillous projections of epithelial cytoplasm. (Courtesy of J.C. Jennette.)

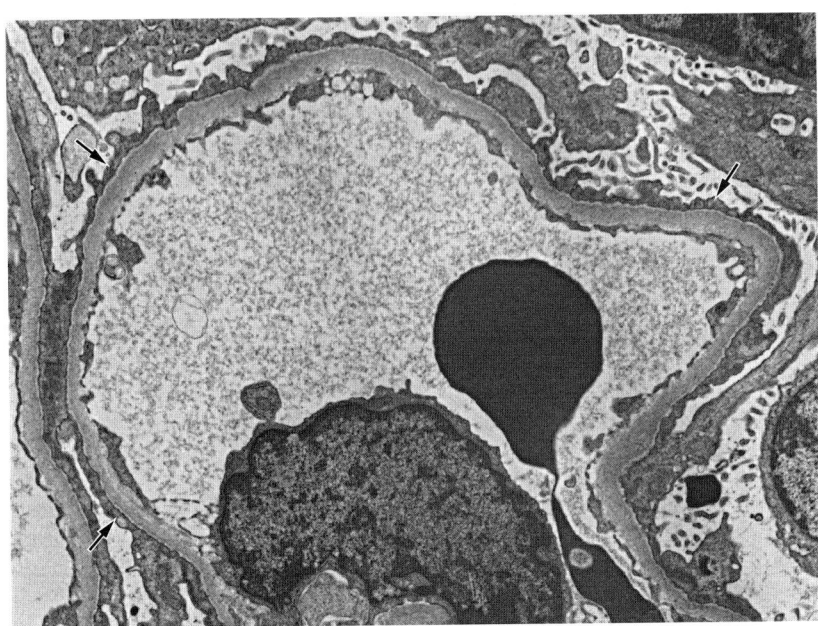

FIGURE 31-4 Electron micrograph of a glomerular capillary wall from a patient with minimal change glomerulopathy showing extensive foot process effacement (*arrows*) and microvillous transformation. (×5000.)

kidney, it functions normally. This is supported by the intriguing observation that transplantation of a kidney from a patient with refractory minimal change glomerulopathy resulted in rapid disappearance of proteinuria.[61]

It is generally agreed that the target of the pathogenetic vector of the lesion is the podocyte, most likely a constituent of the slit pore membrane. Attention has focused on the role of plasma hemopexin in minimal change disease.[62,63] Hemopexin is present in normal plasma, but an active isoform of the protein has been suggested to cause increased glomerular permeability due to enhanced protease activity.[62] Patients with minimal change disease in relapse demonstrate altered isoforms of plasma hemopexin with increased protease activity compared with patients with minimal change disease in remission, other forms of nephrotic syndrome, and normal

individuals.[63] It is not understood how and why the plasma hemopexin is altered in minimal change disease or how the enhanced protease activity results in alterations in glomerular permeability.

New data using differential gene expression techniques have also suggested an alteration in tumor necrosis factor (TNF)–related apoptosis-inducing ligand (TRAIL) in peripheral blood mononuclear cells in minimal change disease during relapse compared with remission.[64] Many additional genes (at least 15 of the more than 20,000 examined) were upregulated during relapse, which demonstrates the complexity of the events occurring in minimal change disease. Included among these is the IgE-dependent histamine-releasing factor gene.[65] The well-known association of minimal change disease with atopic allergic states could be the reason for this finding.

This factor may have specificity for glomerular epithelial cells that results in loss of the charge-selective barrier of the GBM. The loss of charge selectivity has been assessed by dextran studies.[66,67] In these studies, there is less evidence for a defect in the size-selective barrier and more of an alteration of the basement membrane electrostatic charge. The glomerular negative charge is reduced in relapse.[68]

The genetic aspects of minimal change disease have also attracted recent attention. Familial clustering of minimal change disease has not generally been observed.[69] Heterozygous amino acid changes in nephrin and podocin are seen in about one third of patients with typical minimal change disease, but no amino acid changes were observed for *NEPH1* and *CD2AP* in a study involving 104 adults who had childhood-onset minimal change disease.[69] Thus the genotype in minimal change disease may be quite variable.

Polymorphisms in the genes encoding interleukins 4 and 13 (IL-4 and IL-13), activating transcription factor 6, and macrophage migration inhibitory factor have been described in minimal change disease.[70-72] The polymorphisms in IL-13 may relate to phenotype, because they have been associated with relapsing forms of minimal change disease.[9] IL-13 has also been suggested as a potential permeability factor in minimal change disease. The implication of IL-13 in the pathogenesis of minimal change disease is further suggested by the rat model of Lai and collegus,[73] in which IL-13 was exogenously overexpressed through transfection of a heterologous mammalian expression vector containing the rat IL-13 gene. The IL-13–transfected Wistar rats ($n = 41$) showed significant albuminuria, hypoalbuminemia, and hypercholesterolemia compared with control rats ($n = 17$). No significant histologic changes were seen in glomeruli of IL-13–transfected rats; however, electron microscopy revealed up to 80% effacement of podocyte foot processes.

Clinical Features and Natural History

The cardinal clinical feature of minimal change glomerulopathy in children is the relatively abrupt onset of proteinuria and the development of nephrotic syndrome with heavy proteinuria, hypoalbuminemia, and hyperlipidemia.[35] The edematous picture is typically what prompts the parents of these children to seek medical attention. Hematuria is distinctly unusual, and in children, hypertension is uncommon. The clinical features of minimal change glomerulopathy in adults tend to be somewhat different. In a group of 89 adults older than age 60, hypertension, sometimes severe, as well as renal insufficiency were more common.[74] Because individuals older than age 60 account for almost one quarter of adult patients with minimal change glomerulopathy, this presentation must be considered.

Minimal change glomerulopathy has been associated with several other conditions, including viral infections, use of certain pharmaceutical agents, malignancy, and allergy (Table 31-7). In some patients, there is a history of a drug reaction before the onset of minimal change glomerulopathy. The use of nonsteroidal antiinflammatory drugs, and in particular fenoprofen, has been associated with and may cause minimal change glomerulopathy.[75] In this setting, most patients have not only proteinuria, but also pyuria and renal insufficiency as a consequence of the simultaneous development of acute tubulointerstitial nephritis. This same process

TABLE 31-7 Common Associations with Minimal Change Glomerulopathy

Infections
Viral
Parasitic

Pharmaceutical Agents
Nonsteroidal antiinflammatory drugs
Gold
Lithium
Interferon
Ampicillin
Rifampin
Trimethadione
Tiopronin

Tumors
Hodgkin's disease
Lymphoma/leukemia
Solid tumors

Allergies
Food
Dust
Bee stings
Pollen
Poison ivy and poison oak
Dermatitis herpetiformis

Diseases and Other Associations
Systemic lupus erythematosus
Following allogeneic stem cell transplantation for leukemia
Following hematopoietic cell transplantation

Data from references 76, 93, 121-123, 811, 1270-1277.

has also been described in connection with other compounds, including interferon,[76] penicillins, and rifampin. In most of these patients, discontinuation of the offending drug leads to resolution of the proteinuria, but it may take weeks to months for complete amelioration of pyuria and renal insufficiency.

Minimal change glomerulopathy has been associated with lymphoid malignancy, usually Hodgkin's disease. In a retrospective study of adult patients,[77] minimal change disease was associated with classic Hodgkin's lymphoma of the nodular sclerosis type. Minimal change disease appeared before the diagnosis of lymphoma in 40% of patients.

Minimal change disease has also been associated with a variety of underlying exposures such as use of nonsteroidal antiinflammatory drugs[78] (as mentioned earlier) and with syndromes such as systemic lupus erythematosus[79,80]; it has also occurred after allogeneic stem cell transplantation for leukemia[81] and after hematopoietic cell transplantation.

There is an association of glomerular disease with simultaneous graft-versus-host disease. Nephrotic syndrome generally follows graft-versus-host disease within 5 months in approximately 60% of patients with either minimal change disease or membranous glomerulopathy. Compared with membranous glomerulopathy, minimal change disease occurred earlier after hematopoietic cell transplantation, was diagnosed soon after medication change, and exhibited a better prognosis, because 90% of patients attained complete remission (versus 27% of patients with membranous glomerulopathy).

Minimal change glomerulopathy is also associated with food allergy. This is an important association, because in some patients, removal of the allergen has resulted in resolution of the proteinuria. Of 42 patients with idiopathic nephrotic syndrome who did not undergo biopsy, 16 had positive results on skin tests for food allergy. For 13 of 42 a minimally antigenic diet was prescribed that resulted in a significant reduction in proteinuria.[82] Thus, it is important to ask patients about potential allergens, especially those found in food.

A syndrome of minimal change glomerulopathy accompanied by a reversible acute renal failure occurs at a higher incidence in adults than in children.[74,83,84] This syndrome of adult minimal change glomerulopathy with acute renal failure was studied in 21 patients who, on presentation, had a serum creatinine level of more than 177 μmol/L and who were compared with 50 adult patients with minimal change glomerulopathy who had a serum creatinine level of less than 133 μmol/L. Patients who had acute renal failure were older (59 years versus 40 years), had a higher systolic blood pressure (158 mm Hg versus 138 mm Hg), and had more proteinuria (13.5 versus 7.9 g of protein per 24 hours). Importantly, renal biopsy specimens showed evidence of atherosclerosis and focal tubular epithelial simplification compatible with ischemic acute renal failure. Of the 18 patients with renal failure for whom follow-up data were available, all showed recovery of renal function, but only after prolonged periods of dialytic renal replacement therapy.[36]

The complications of nephrotic syndrome in minimal change disease have been well described. The development of acute renal failure during the course of minimal change disease, mostly in adults older than age 40, has been well recognized, but the underlying mechanisms are debated. Explanations for this phenomenon include marked decrease in glomerular permeability due to extensive foot process effacement, tubular obstruction from proteinaceous casts, and intrarenal hemodynamic changes. Increased endothelin-1 expression in the kidneys of patients with minimal change disease and acute renal failure could indicate a hemodynamic change that underlies the pathogenesis of renal failure in these circumstances,[85] but the true cause of acute renal failure in minimal change disease remains uncertain and is probably multifactorial.

Another complication of minimal change disease with nephrotic syndrome is the development of reduced bone mineral density, possibly due to the effects of glucocorticoids and/or vitamin D deficiency.[86] Statins may have a beneficial effect on bone mineral density, but one study reported no beneficial effect of fluvastatin on the bone mineral density of children with minimal change disease, although it did have some effect in lowering proteinuria.[87]

Laboratory Findings

The ubiquitous laboratory feature of minimal change glomerulopathy is severe proteinuria.[35] Microscopic hematuria is seen in fewer than 15% of patients, with only rare cases of macroscopic hematuria. The rapidity of the development of proteinuria in some patients is associated with evidence of volume contraction with increased hematocrit and hemoglobin level. The erythrocyte sedimentation rate is increased as a consequence of the hyperfibrinogenemia as well as hypoalbuminemia. The serum albumin concentration is usually depressed, whereas the total cholesterol, low-density lipoprotein (LDL), and triglyceride levels are increased. Total serum protein concentration is usually reduced to between 4.5 and 5.5 g/dL with a serum albumin concentration of generally less than 2 g/dL and, in more severe cases, less than 1 g/dL. Pseudohyponatremia has been observed in the setting of marked hyperlipidemia. Serum calcium level may be low, largely due to hypoproteinemia.

Several abnormalities that promote thrombosis are frequent in patients with severe nephrosis, including increased plasma viscosity, increased red cell aggregation, low plasminogen levels, and low levels of antithrombin III.[88] Renal function is usually normal, although the serum creatinine level may be slightly increased at the time of presentation. A minority of patients (usually older adults) have substantial acute renal failure, as discussed earlier.

The loss of albumin into the urine is largely a function of a loss of charge-selective permselectivity.[66,67,89,90] Consequently, the fractional excretion of albumin is proportionately greater than the fractional excretion of IgG. IgG levels may be profoundly decreased, however—a condition that occurs most notably during episodes of relapse. This low level of immunoglobulin may result in susceptibility to infections. IgM levels may be elevated after a remission.[91] Mean serum IgA levels may be substantially higher in patients with minimal change glomerulopathy than in those with other renal disease[92] and are also elevated in association with relapse in children.[93] Among adult patients with minimal change glomerulopathy, over half have elevated levels of serum IgE and two thirds of patients have evidence of some allergic symptoms.[94] Elevation of IgE suggests a relationship between minimal change glomerulopathy and allergy. Complement levels are typically normal in patients with minimal change glomerulopathy.

Treatment

The general approach to treatment of patients with minimal change glomerulopathy has been to institute corticosteroid therapy. For children, the dosage of prednisone is 60 mg/m²/day. For adults, the dosage of prednisone is 1 mg/kg of body weight, not to exceed 80 mg/day. In children, this form of therapy results in a complete remission with disappearance of proteinuria in over 90% of patients within 4 to 6 weeks of initiation of therapy. A response to prednisone therapy is considered to have occurred if the patient has had no proteinuria as measured by dipstick analysis for at least 3 days. It should be noted that the serum albumin and serum lipid levels might not return to normal for prolonged periods following resolution of the proteinuria.[95]

Treatment is generally continued for 6 weeks after there is complete remission of proteinuria. During those 6 weeks, the dosage should be changed to alternate-day administration of prednisone or to a stepwise reduction in the daily dose of prednisone. If the dosing is changed to alternate-day dosing when remission has occurred, the dosage may be decreased in children from 60 mg/m²/day to 40 mg/m²/day.[44,96-100]

In adult patients with minimal change glomerulopathy, a response to corticosteroid treatment may take up to 15 weeks.[74] In a study of 89 adult patients given prednisolone, remission occurred in 60% after 8 weeks, in 76% after 16 weeks, and in 81% over the course of the study. Of the 58 treated patients who showed a response, 24% never experienced relapse, 56% experienced relapse on a single occasion or infrequently, and only 21% had frequent relapses. Of these 89 patients, only 4 remained nephrotic, and 2 of these presented with acute renal failure. Cyclophosphamide therapy was administered to 36 of the 89 patients, and in 66% of these patients the disease was in remission at 5 years.

In a large retrospective analysis of 95 patients with primary adult-onset minimal change disease, acute renal failure complicated the nephrotic syndrome in 20% of patients.[101] The cohort was largely middle-aged with a substantial prevalence of hypertension (45%) and microscopic hematuria (30%). Ninety-two percent of patients were initially treated with oral corticosteroids; two thirds were on a daily regimen and one third were on an alternate-day regimen. The initial steroid dose was approximately 1 mg/kg on the daily regimen and approximately 2 mg/kg on the alternate-day regimen, so that cumulative doses were similar in the two groups. There were no significant differences in demographic features between the two groups, but patients treated with the alternate-day steroid regimen tended to have a lower serum albumin level at presentation than those treated with the daily regimen (1.91 ± 0.14 g/dL vs. 2.31 ± 0.1 g/dL, respectively; $P = 0.055$). No significant differences were seen between the daily and alternate-day treatment groups in the percentage of patients experiencing complete or partial remission (remissions in 76.8% and 73.9% of patients, respectively) or in the time to remission. It is interesting to note that the rate of relapse of nephrotic syndrome was quite elevated at 73% of those who showed an initial response. Of the patients who were treated with at least one additional course of corticosteroids, 92% achieved a remission (complete remission in 84.4%). This nonrandomized, uncontrolled study does suggest that alternate-day and daily steroid regimens are of equivalent efficacy and safety in the treatment of minimal change disease.

One of the most controversial issues with respect to treatment pertains to the regimen for tapering the prednisone after the initial response. Sudden withdrawal of corticosteroids, or a rapid taper of prednisone immediately following complete remission, may prompt a relapse. Whether this is a consequence of adrenal insufficiency or depression of the hypothalamic-pituitary-adrenal axis has been a matter of debate.[100,102,103] At least in children, the likelihood of relapse is decreased with prolonged administration of corticosteroids over a 10- to 12-week period.[98,104,105] Once remission has been obtained, an alternate-day schedule should begin within at least 4 weeks of the response to decrease steroid-induced side effects.

In children who have not undergone biopsy prior to treatment, a renal biopsy is usually appropriate if there is failure to respond to a 4- to 6-week course of prednisone, particularly if changes have occurred in the clinical course during this period of time suggestive of another glomerular disease. Many pediatricians advocate performing a biopsy at the onset of the disease if there are clinical features suggesting a diagnosis other than minimal change glomerulopathy (e.g., hypertension, red blood cell casts in the urine, or hypocomplementemia) or if the nephrotic syndrome begins in the first year of life or after 6 years of age.

After the clinical response to initial treatment, as few as 25% experience a long-term remission,[84] 25% to 30% have infrequent relapses (no more than one a year), and the remainder experience frequent relapses, steroid dependence, or steroid resistance (Table 31-8). Nephrotic patients who are steroid dependent or experience frequent relapses require additional forms of therapy. The treatment is aimed at minimizing the complications of corticosteroid therapy. In general, induction of a remission with prednisone therapy followed by the institution of cyclophosphamide treatment results in higher urine

TABLE 31-8 Patterns of Response of Minimal Change Glomerulopathy to Corticosteroid Treatment

Primary response, no relapse

Primary response with only one relapse in the first 6 months after an initial response

Initial steroid response with two or more relapses within 6 months (frequent relapse)

Initial steroid-induced remission with relapses during tapering of corticosteroid therapy or within 2 weeks after their withdrawal (steroid dependency)

Steroid-induced remission, but no response to steroids during a subsequent relapse

No response to treatment (steroid resistance)

Data from Nephrotic syndrome in children: a randomized trial comparing two prednisone regimens in steroid-responsive patients who relapse early. Report of the International Study of Kidney Disease in Children, *J Pediatr* 95:239-243, 1979; from Alternate-day versus intermittent prednisone in frequently relapsing nephrotic syndrome. A report of "Arbetsgemeinschaft für Pädiatrische Nephrologie," *Lancet* 1:401-403, 1979; from Primary nephrotic syndrome in children: clinical significance of histopathologic variants of minimal change and of diffuse mesangial hypercellularity. A Report of the International Study of Kidney Disease in Children, *Kidney Int* 20:765-771, 1981; and from The primary nephrotic syndrome in children. Identification of patients with minimal change nephrotic syndrome from initial response to prednisone. A report of the International Study of Kidney Disease in Children, *J Pediatr* 98:561-564, 1981.

flow rates and reduced risk of hemorrhagic cystitis. When cyclophosphamide is given in dosages of 2 mg/kg for 8 to 12 weeks, 75% of patients remain free of proteinuria for at least 2 years.[74,106-108] The response to cyclophosphamide may be predicted from the response to corticosteroids. Patients who have experienced an immediate relapse after the cessation of corticosteroid therapy have a greater chance of experiencing relapse immediately after the cessation of cyclophosphamide treatment. Those who have had longer remissions after corticosteroid therapy have a decreased risk of relapse after cyclophosphamide thereapy.[109] In one study, in patients who were steroid dependent, the response to cyclophosphamide was improved by increasing the duration of therapy to up to 12 weeks.[106] In at least one other investigation, however, a 12-week course of cyclophosphamide did not prove efficacious.[110]

Cyclosporine is emerging as a reasonable alternative to cyclophosphamide.[111,112] Based on uncontrolled observations, complete remissions are common (over 80%), and cyclosporine resistance is seen in only about 10% to 15% of patients. Side effects such as a rise in serum creatinine level, hypertrichosis, and gingival hyperplasia are quite common. Relapses are very common after cessation of cyclosporine treatment. The best method of monitoring cyclosporine levels is not agreed upon. Measurement of trough blood levels with twice-daily dosing, measurement of cyclosporine level 1 to 2 hours after a once-daily dose (C1 – C2), and abbreviated under-the-curve monitoring of cyclosporine have all been recommended.[112-114] Cyclosporine may be an acceptable alternative to cyclophosphamide therapy for relapsing or steroid-dependent minimal change disease.

Steroid-Resistant Minimal Change Glomerulopathy

Approximately 5% of children with minimal change glomerulopathy appear to be steroid resistant. In those patients who never underwent renal biopsy, resistance to corticosteroid therapy is an indication for renal biopsy. Often, evaluation of the renal biopsy specimen will demonstrate FSGS or forms of glomerular injury other than minimal change glomerulopathy.[115]

If the diagnosis remains minimal change glomerulopathy after renal biopsy specimen evaluation, there may be several reasons for steroid resistance. Some patients, especially those for whom corticosteroid therapy is overly toxic, may skip doses or not fully adhere to the therapy regimen. For other patients, especially some adults, alternate-day therapy may not provide sufficient amounts of corticosteroid to induce clinical remission. In very edematous patients, oral corticosteroids may not be well absorbed, and intravenous administration of a dose of methylprednisolone may provide a more reliable route. Available data suggest that pulse methylprednisolone may induce remission in some corticosteroid-resistant children. In one study, five of eight corticosteroid-resistant children experienced remission with pulse methylprednisolone therapy,[116] although this experience is not universal.[117]

Patients with minimal change disease may have an unrecognized lesion of focal and segmental glomerulosclerosis that requires longer courses of steroid therapy (usually >4 months) to achieve a lasting remission. A regimen of calcineurin inhibitor (cyclosporine or tacrolimus) followed by mycophenolate mofetil and monthly intravenous pulse cyclophosphamide therapy was demonstrated in an uncontrolled study to result in a high frequency of complete remission.[118] There are anecdotal reports of the use of combinations of sirolimus and tacrolimus to treat steroid-resistant minimal change disease,[119] but the overall safety and efficacy of this regimen is unknown. In a small nonrandomized trial, use of cyclosporine with steroids was associated with better outcomes in steroid-resistant minimal change disease.[120]

Cyclosporine can be administered at a dose of approximately 5 mg/kg. Up to 90% of patients may experience either a partial or complete remission with cyclosporine.[93,98,121-123] Unfortunately, only rarely do patients experience long-term remission once cyclosporine is discontinued.[99] Two trials examined the use of cyclosporine in the treatment of steroid-resistant nephrosis. A study conducted by the French Society of Pediatric Nephrology combined cyclosporine with prednisone. Prednisone was given at a dosage of 30 mg/m²/day for the first month and then changed to alternate-day dosing for 5 months. Cyclosporine was administered at a dosage of 150 to 200 mg/m²/day.[124] In this study, 48% of patients with minimal change glomerulopathy experienced complete remission, some within the first month of therapy. A minority of those who showed a response became steroid sensitive when they later experienced relapse. In a study by Ponticelli and colleagues,[125] 13 of 45 patients had minimal change glomerulopathy and were treated with cyclosporine. In those patients with minimal change glomerulopathy, partial or complete remission occurred within 2 months of initiation of therapy. Unfortunately, in spite of the early positive results of this study, relapses occurred in all patients after cyclosporine was stopped.

In a summary of nine studies,[126] only 20% of children were reported to experience complete remission with cyclosporine treatment, and many, if not most, experienced relapse with cessation of therapy. Moreover, although cyclosporine and cyclophosphamide appear to have a similar degree of efficacy with respect to controlling nephrotic syndrome, one study

found that cyclophosphamide-treated patients experience a more stable long-term remission.[127] In this study, the likelihood of a long-term remission was 63% in patients treated with cyclophosphamide, but was only 25% in those treated with cyclosporine.

To counteract the usual relapse of nephrosis when cyclosporine has been used for 6 months, an alternative approach to cyclosporine treatment relies on a long-term course of this drug, using gradually lower doses to maintain the patient in remission. In one study,[128] patients who had been in complete remission for longer than 1 year while taking cyclosporine remained in remission if the cyclosporine was gradually tapered and then stopped. Serial biopsy specimens from patients treated for as long as 20 months showed no overt sign of nephrotoxicity.

Focal Segmental Glomerulosclerosis

Focal segmental glomerulosclerosis (FSGS) is not a single disease but rather a diagnostic term for a clinical-pathologic syndrome that has multiple causes and pathogenic mechanisms.[129,130] The ubiquitous clinical feature of the syndrome is proteinuria, which may be nephrotic or nonnephrotic, and the ubiquitous pathologic feature is focal segmental glomerular consolidation or scarring, which may have several distinctive patterns (Figure 31-5). These patterns can be classified as collapsing FSGS, tip lesion FSGS, cellular FSGS, perihilar FSGS, and FSGS not otherwise specified (NOS).[129,130] The collapsing variant of FSGS is a clinically aggressive variant that is much more common in African American than in white populations and is characterized pathologically by segmental collapse of capillaries accompanied by hypertrophy and hyperplasia of epithelial cells, and accumulation of prominent protein resorption droplets in podocytes. The glomerular tip lesion variant of FSGS, which typically presents with marked nephrosis but often has a good outcome, is characterized by consolidation and sclerosis in the glomerular segment that is adjacent to the origin of the proximal tubule.[130] The term *cellular FSGS* has been used in a number of ways in the literature. For example, this term has been used to describe the collapsing variant and the tip lesion variant of FSGS. Thus care must be taken when reading the literature to determine if the term is being used as defined by the Columbia classification system in some other way.[129] The perihilar variant of FSGS is characterized pathologically by sclerosis at the hilum of the glomerulus that typically contains foci of hyalinosis.[129]

As shown in Table 31-9, FSGS may appear to be a primary renal disease or it may be associated with, and possibly caused by, a variety of other conditions. When FSGS is secondary to obesity or reduced numbers of nephrons, it often has a perihilar pattern and is accompanied by glomerular enlargement. FSGS that is associated with human immunodeficiency virus (HIV) infection has a collapsing pattern.

Epidemiology

Over the past two decades, the incidence of FSGS has increased, whether expressed as an absolute number of patients or as a proportion of the total incident population of patients with ESRD.[131] This trend appears to hold true

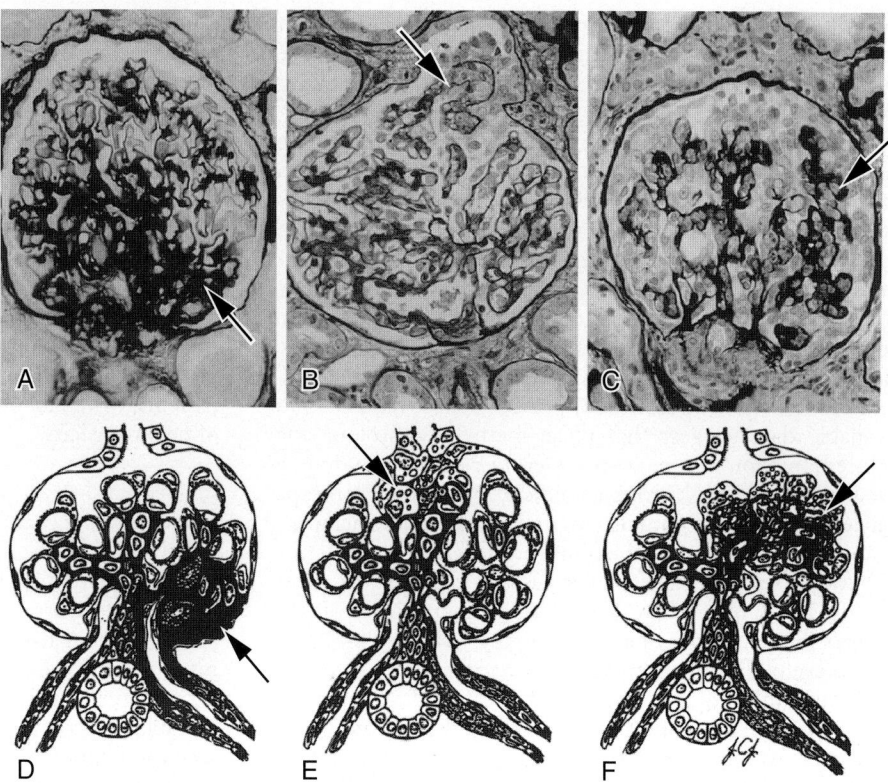

FIGURE 31-5 Light micrographs and diagrams depicting patterns of focal segmental glomerulosclerosis. One pattern has a predilection for sclerosis in the perihilar regions of the glomeruli (**A** and **D**). The glomerular tip lesion variant has segmental consolidation confined to the segment adjacent to the origin of the proximal tubule (**B** and **E**). The collapsing glomerulopathy variant has segmental collapse of capillaries with hypertrophy and hyperplasia of overlying epithelial cells (**C** and **F**). (Jones' methenamine silver stain, ×100.)

TABLE 31-9 Classification of Focal Segmental Glomerulosclerosis (FSGS)
Primary (Idiopathic) FSGS
FSGS not otherwise specified (NOS)
Glomerular tip lesion variant of FSGS
Collapsing variant of FSGS
Perihilar variant of FSGS
Cellular variant of FSGS
Secondary FSGS
With human immunodeficiency virus infection
With intravenous drug abuse
With exposure to other drugs (e.g., pamidronate, interferon)
With identified genetic abnormalities (e.g., mutations in podocin, α-actinin-4, *TRPC6*)
With glomerulomegaly
Morbid obesity
Sickle cell disease
Cyanotic congenital heart disease
Hypoxic pulmonary disease
With reduced nephron numbers
Unilateral renal agenesis
Oligomeganephronia
Reflux-interstitial nephritis
After focal cortical necrosis
After nephrectomy

TRPC6, Transient receptor potential cation channel, subfamily C, member 6.

even when one accounts for a possible increase in the rate of diagnosis resulting from an increase in the frequency of renal biopsies. Although this trend was previously reported to be most significant among African Americans, it has now been confirmed among whites as well. In a review of the findings of renal biopsies performed between 1974 and 2003 in Olmstead County, Minnesota, in which 90% of the population are whites of northern European extraction, FSGS was found to account for 17% of glomerulonephritides, second only to IgA

nephropathy (22%), and was more frequent than membranous glomerulopathy (10%).[132] Over that period of time, the incidence of FSGS increased by 13-fold (*P* < 0.001), compared with a 2-fold increase in the incidence of all glomerular diseases (*P* < 0.001) and a 2.5- to 3-fold increase in membranous glomerulopathy and IgA nephropathy, respectively.

Pathology

LIGHT MICROSCOPY

FSGS is characterized by focal and segmental glomerular sclerosis.[129,130] The sclerosis may begin as segmental consolidation caused by insudation of plasma proteins causing hyalinosis, by accumulation of foam cells, by swelling of epithelial cells, and by collapse of capillaries resulting in obliteration of capillary lumens. These events are accompanied by an increase in extracellular matrix material that ultimately accounts for the sclerosis component of the lesion.

FSGS is, by definition, a focal process, and the limited number of glomeruli in a renal biopsy specimen may not include any of the segmentally sclerotic glomeruli that are present in the kidney. In this instance, focal tubulointerstitial injury or glomerular enlargement, which often accompanies FSGS, can be used as a surrogate marker. For example, FSGS should be considered in renal biopsy specimens of patients with nephrotic syndrome when there is relatively well-circumscribed focal tubular atrophy and interstitial fibrosis with slight chronic inflammation, even when there are no light microscopic glomerular lesions, no immune deposits, and no ultrastructural changes other than foot process effacement. Segmental sclerosis that is adequate for diagnosis may be present only in the tissue examined by immunofluorescence or electron microscopy.

The focal segmental glomerular scarring is not specific. Many injurious processes can cause focal glomerular scarring and must be ruled out before making a diagnosis of FSGS. For example, hereditary nephritis causes progressive glomerular scarring that can mimic FSGS. This is revealed by identification of the ultrastructural changes that are characteristic of hereditary nephritis. Focal segmental glomerulonephritis, for example caused by IgA nephropathy, lupus nephritis, or ANCA-associated glomerulonephritis, can result in focal segmental glomerular scarring that is histologically indistinguishable from that caused by FSGS. Findings by immunofluorescence and electron microscopy, and by serologic testing, can reveal a glomerulonephritic basis for focal glomerular scarring.

Based on the character and glomerular distribution of lesions, five major structural variants of FSGS can be recognized that correlate, at least in part, with outcome (prognosis) and that may have different causes and pathogenic mechanisms.[129,130] As mentioned earlier, these five pathologic variants are collapsing FSGS, tip lesion FSGS, cellular FSGS, perihilar FSGS, and FSGS NOS.[129,130]

The characteristic feature of the collapsing variant of FSGS is focal segmental or global collapse of glomerular capillaries with obliteration of capillary lumens. Podocytes overlying collapsed segments are usually enlarged and contain conspicuous resorption droplets. Hyperplasia of podocytes raises the possibility of crescentic glomerulonephritis. The convention among most renal pathologists is not to refer to the epithelial hyperplasia of collapsing glomerulopathy as crescent formation. The degree of adhesion formation relative to the extent of glomerular sclerosis is much less in collapsing glomerulopathy than in typical FSGS. This may result in contracted (collapsed) tuft basement membranes and sclerotic matrix separated from Bowman's capsule by hypertrophied and hyperplastic epithelial cells. The collapsing glomerulopathy variant of FSGS is the major pathologic expression of HIV nephropathy[35,133-135] and also occurs with intravenous drug abuse and as an idiopathic process.[136,137] In renal transplants, this phenotype of FSGS occurs as both recurrent and de novo disease.[138,139]

Relative to the extent of glomerular sclerosis, tubulointerstitial injury is more severe in collapsing glomerulopathy than in typical FSGS. Tubular epithelial cells have larger resorption droplets, extensive proteinaceous casts, and marked focal dilation of lumens (microcystic change). There also is more extensive interstitial infiltration by mononuclear leukocytes. Immunofluorescence microscopic findings are similar to those observed in typical FSGS except for the usual finding of larger resorption droplets in glomerular visceral epithelial cells and tubular epithelial cells. Electron microscopy reveals the same structural changes seen by light microscopy. In a specimen with the collapsing glomerulopathy variant of FSGS, the most important ultrastructural assessment is for the presence or absence of endothelial tuboreticular inclusions. Endothelial tuboreticular inclusions are identified in over 90% of patients with HIV infection and collapsing glomerulopathy, but in fewer than 10% of patients with idiopathic collapsing glomerulopathy or collapsing glomerulopathy associated with intravenous drug abuse. The only other settings in which endothelial tuboreticular inclusions are numerous are in patients with systemic lupus erythematosus and in patients treated with interferon-α.

The tip lesion variant of FSGS is characterized by consolidation of segments contiguous with the proximal tubule. These lesions may be sclerotic or cellular. However, the increased cellularity is predominantly within the tuft, unlike the extracapillary hypercellularity of collapsing FSGS. Foam cells often contribute to this endocapillary hypercellularity.

The glomerular tip lesion variant of FSGS was first described by Howie and colleagues and is characterized by consolidation of the glomerular segment that is adjacent to the origin of the proximal tubule and thus opposite the hilum (Figure 31-5B and E).[140-145] The initial consolidation usually has obliteration of capillary lumens by foam cells, swollen endothelial cells, and an increase in collagenous matrix material (sclerosis). Hyalinosis is seen less often than with typical FSGS. Podocytes adjacent to the consolidated segment are enlarged and contain clear vacuoles and hyaline droplets. These altered podocytes often are contiguous to, if not attached to, adjacent parietal epithelial cells and tubular epithelial cells at the origin of the proximal tubule, which also have irregular enlargement and vacuolation. The tip lesion may project into the lumen of the proximal tubule. Some lesions are less cellular with a predominance of matrix and collagenous adhesions to Bowman's capsule at the origin of the proximal tubule.

The cellular variant of FSGS as defined by D'Agati and colleagues has lesions that resemble the cellular lesion for the tip variant, but they are distributed throughout the glomerular tuft.[129] Perihilar FSGS is characterized by the perihilar predilection of lesions and the presence of hyalinosis. The FSGS NOS category is a nonspecific category that is used when the lesions do not have the distinctive features of any of the other four specific variants.

As is discussed later, different pathologic variants of FSGS have distinctive demographic characteristics, clinical presentations, and outcomes.

IMMUNOFLUORESCENCE MICROSCOPY

In all of the histologic variants, nonsclerotic glomeruli and segments usually show no staining for immunoglobulins or complement. As in patients with minimal change glomerulopathy as well as individuals with no renal dysfunction, a minority of patients with FSGS have low-level mesangial staining for IgM in nonsclerotic glomeruli. Low-level mesangial C3 staining is less frequent, and low-level IgG and IgA staining is rare. The presence of substantial staining of nonsclerotic glomeruli for immunoglobulins, especially if immune complex–type electron-dense deposits are present, points toward the sclerotic phase of a focal immune complex glomerulonephritis rather than FSGS.

Sclerotic segments typically show irregular staining for C3, C1q, and IgM (Figure 31-6). Other plasma constituents are less frequently identified in the sclerotic areas. Epithelial resorption droplets stain for plasma proteins.

ELECTRON MICROSCOPY

The ultrastructural features of FSGS are nonspecific. Electron microscopy plays an important role in the diagnosis of FSGS by helping to identify other causes for glomerular scarring that can be mistaken for FSGS by light microscopy alone.

Foot process effacement in FSGS affects sclerotic and nonsclerotic glomeruli, and usually is more focal than in minimal change glomerulopathy. Foot process effacement is less extensive in some forms of secondary FSGS than in idiopathic

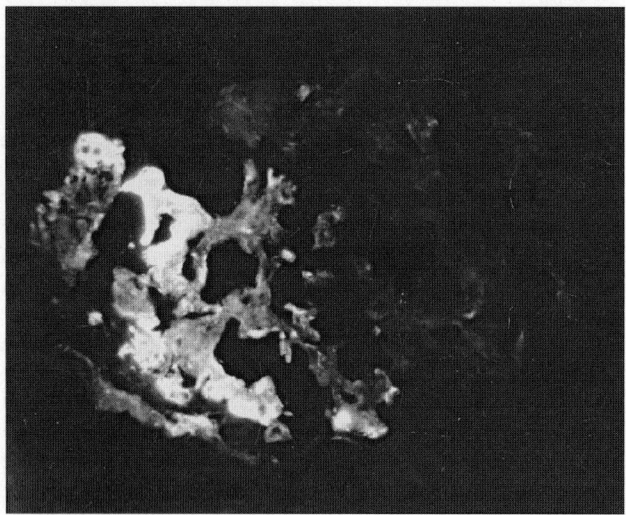

FIGURE 31-6 Immunofluorescence micrograph showing irregular segmental staining for C3 corresponding to a site of segmental sclerosis. (Fluorescein isothiocyanate anti-C3 stain, ×3000.)

TABLE 31-10 Gene Mutations Causally Linked to Focal Segmental Glomerulosclerosis		
GENE	**PROTEIN**	**MODE OF INHERITANCE**
NPHS1	Nephrin	Autosomal recessive
NPHS2	Podocin	Autosomal recessive
PLCE1	Phospholipase Cε	Autosomal recessive
CD2AP	CD2-associated protein	Autosomal recessive
TRPC6	Transient receptor potential cation channel, subfamily C, member 6	Autosomal dominant
ACTN4	α-Actinin-4	Autosomal dominant
MYH9	Nonmuscle myosin heavy chain A (NMMHC-A)	Autosomal dominant, de novo mutation
COQ2	Coenzyme Q_2 homolog, prenyl transferase	Autosomal recessive
ITGB4	β4 Integrin	Autosomal recessive
WT1	Wilms' tumor suppressor protein	Autosomal dominant, de novo mutation

FSGS. Occasionally, glomerular capillaries have focal denudation of foot processes. Podocytes adjacent to collapsed segments in collapsing FSGS are cuboidal and appear dedifferentiated. Nonsclerotic glomeruli and segments should have no immune complex–type electron-dense deposits. One must be careful not to confuse electron-dense "insudative" lesions with immune complex deposits. These lesions correspond to the hyalinosis seen by light microscopy and result from the accumulation of plasma proteins within sclerotic areas. Thus, if the electron-dense material is present in sclerotic but not in nonsclerotic glomerular segments, it should not be considered to be evidence for immune complex–mediated glomerular disease. On the other hand, well-defined mesangial or capillary wall electron-dense deposits in nonsclerotic segments indicate immune complex–mediated glomerulonephritis with secondary scarring, which should be confirmed and further characterized by immunofluorescence microscopy.

Pathogenesis

The last 20 years have witnessed an explosion of interest in the role of the podocyte in FSGS. Podocytes are highly differentiated postmitotic cells whose function is based on their architecture. Tremendous interest has centered on the genetics of familial FSGS, and defects in the podocyte have taken center stage (reviewed by Tryggvason and colleagues[6] and Woroniecki and Kopp[146]). This has led to the identification of several proteins important to the normal function of podocytes and the development of proteinuria. Mutations in several genes have been identified and linked to familial and sporadic cases of FSGS. These include genes coding for podocin (*NPHS2*),[147] nephrin (*NPHS1*),[148] α-actinin-4 (*ACTN4*),[149,150] transient receptor potential cation channel, subfamily C, member 6 (*TRPC6*),[151-153] and phospholipase Cε$_1$ (*PLCE1*).[154] In addition to mutations in genes encoding podocyte-specific proteins, mutations in other genes are associated with syndromes of which FSGS is often a part.[146] These include the *COQ2* gene,[155] Wilms' tumor gene (*WT1*), and gene for LIM homeobox transcription factor 1β (*LMX1B*), which is a transcription factor required for the expression of

CD2AP and *NPHS2*, associated with nail-patella syndrome. The genes implicated in the pathogenesis of FGS are listed in Table 31-10.

Whereas these genetic mutations were primarily identified based on cases of familial forms of FSGS, their implication in sporadic FSGS in children and adults, and their impact on treatment and outcome and recurrence after transplantation, have been the focus of several recent investigations.

Mutations in *NPHS2*, the gene encoding podocin, are the most frequent genetic cause of steroid-resistant nephrotic syndrome and were initially described in early-onset disease. In a study of a large cohort of 430 patients from 404 different families with steroid-resistant nephrotic syndrome, recessive podocin mutations were found in 18.1%.[156] The R138Q mutation (a single nucleotide substitution of G to A at position 413 in the third exon of podocine gene) was found in 57% of families with two disease-causing mutations on each of the parental gene copies. Seventy percent of podocin mutations were nonsense, frameshift, or homozygous R138Q mutations. Patients with these mutations manifested symptoms at a significantly earlier age (mean onset of <1.75 years) than any other patient group, with or without podocin mutations (mean onset of >4.17 years). The sequence variant R229Q was found in 9% of families as a heterozygous mutation and in 0.5% as a homozygous mutation.

The significance of this sequence variant as a cause of nephrotic syndrome was addressed in a study of 546 patients (from 455 families) with familial or sporadic FSGS, only 24% of whom developed nephrotic syndrome after age 18.[156a] The R229Q allele frequency was significantly higher among European and South American patients than among control individuals (0.089 for European patients vs. 0.026 for controls, $P = 0.00001$; and 0.17 for South American patients vs. 0.007 for controls, $P = 0.000002$). Compared with individuals without a p.R229Q allele, those with a p.R229Q allele had a significantly higher likelihood of having a single pathogenic *NPHS2* mutation, which strongly suggests a pathogenic role of p.R229Q in the compound heterozygous state with an *NPHS2* mutation. Patients carrying p.R229Q and one *NPHS2* mutation developed nephrotic syndrome significantly later than those carrying two pathogenic mutations (median of 19.0 vs. 1.1 years, $P < 0.01$). This study therefore suggests that compound heterozygosity for p.R229Q is associated with adult-onset, steroid-resistant nephrotic syndrome. The frequency of *NPHS2* mutations in adults with treatment-resistant nephrotic syndrome was 11% in sporadic cases and 25% in familial cases.

The role of *NPHS2* polymorphisms in sporadic cases of late-onset idiopathic or HIV-associated FSGS was also studied in 377 biopsy-confirmed FSGS cases and 919 controls without known kidney disease.[157] No homozygotes or compound heterozygotes were observed for any of five missense mutations identified on gene sequencing. R138Q carriers were five times more frequent among FSGS cases than among controls ($P = 0.06$), but heterozygosity for the other four missense mutations (including R229Q) was equally distributed among FSGS cases and controls. Genetic variation or mutation of *NPHS2* may therefore play a role in late-onset sporadic FSGS. However, given the very low frequency of the R138Q mutation (4 to 8 per 1000) and the lack of involvement of other mutations, the attributable risk of *NPHS2* for adult sporadic or HIV-associated FSGS is extremely small. The presence of the nonsynonymous variants of *NPHS2* (p.R229Q and p.A242V) did not significantly alter the risk of albuminuria in the Nurses' Health Study participants.[158]

In summary, mutations of the *NPHS2* gene are associated with familial and childhood-onset steroid-resistant nephrotic syndrome, but do not contribute significantly to adult-onset sporadic FSGS. Heterozygosity for R138Q is associated with a fivefold increased risk of FSGS in adults. When combined with other pathogenic mutations of *NPHS2*, the R229Q variant appears to be associated with disease with onset at an older age.

Classically, mutations in NPHS1, which encodes nephrin, are associated with congenital nephrotic syndrome of the Finnish type presenting within the first 3 months of life. A study of 160 patients from 142 unrelated families who developed nephrotic syndrome at least 3 months after birth identified *NPHS1* mutations in one familial case and in nine sporadic cases.[159] Renal biopsy specimens at presentation revealed mesangioproliferative lesions in one patient, minimal change disease in six patients, and FSGS in three patients. This study broadens the spectrum of renal disease related to nephrin mutations and raises the possibility that mutations in NPHS1 may contribute to sporadic nephrotic syndrome in combination with mutations in other genes associated with this syndrome.[159,160]

Mutations in *ACTN4*, the gene encoding the actin-binding protein α-actinin-4, are a cause of familial FSGS with an autosomal dominant pattern of inheritance and may be associated with a distinctive ultrastructural feature of podocyte injury consisting of cytoplasmic electron-dense aggregates.[161] On indirect immunofluorescence microscopy using antibodies to a conserved domain of α-actinin-4, a segmental and irregular granular staining pattern can be seen in the capillary walls of specimens from patients with *ACTN4* mutations, as opposed to a global linear staining pattern for α-actinin-4 in specimens from patients with other podocyte diseases. These characteristics may aid in identifying patients with *ACTN4* mutations.

African Americans have a disproportionate risk for several forms of kidney disease, including a fourfold increased risk for FSGS and an 18- to 50-fold increased risk for HIV-associated FSGS. The basis for that susceptibility is thought to be multifactorial, with a suspected genetic component. Two landmark studies, both of which used genome-wide mapping by admixture linkage disequilibrium, identified a chromosome 22 region that was associated with kidney disease in subjects of African ancestry[162,162a] Initial efforts focused on *MYH9*, which encodes a nonmuscle myosin heavy-chain type IIA expressed in kidney podocytes and possibly mesangial cells, where it binds to actin to perform intracellular motor functions. Multiple *MYH9* single-nucleotide polymorphisms (SNPs) and haplotypes were recessively associated with FSGS, most strongly a haplotype spanning exons 14 through 23 (odds ratio [OR] = 5.0, 95% confidence interval [CI] = 3.5 to 7.1, $P = 4 \times 10^{-23}$, n = 852). This haplotype has a frequency of 60% in African Americans but of only 4% in European Americans. Nine *MYH9* SNPs and the same haplotype as for FSGS were associated with hypertensive end-stage renal disease (ESRD) (OR = 2.2, 95% CI = 1.5 to 3.4; n = 433), but not ESRD associated with type 2 diabetes.[162]

Unlike other mutations directly linked to the development of FSGS, the association of *MYH9* does not establish direct causality. Although genetic variation at the *MYH9* locus substantially explains the increased burden of FSGS and hypertensive ESRD among African Americans, the absolute risk for an individual with this disease-associated haplotype is quite low. Which other genetic or environmental factors trigger disease among carriers of the *MYH9* polymorphism or haplotype is unknown.[163] Despite intensive efforts, including resequencing of the *MYH9* gene, no functional mutation was identified.

In more recent work, two groups have identified sequence variants in the apolipoprotein L-I (*APOL1*) gene that may explain the genetic association of kidney disease in patients of African ancestry.[163a,163b] Reexamination of the interval surrounding *MYH9* led to these newer findings. Genovese and colleagues[163a] and Tzur and colleagues[163b] both used data from the 1000 Genomes Project—which conducts the sequencing of genomic DNA derived from subjects around the globe, especially the Yoruba tribe of Western Africa—and identified sequence variants in the *APOL1* gene that were associated with kidney disease. These variants were more strongly associated with ESRD than previously reported *MYH9* variants.

In African Americans, Genovese and colleagues found that FSGS and hypertension-attributed ESRD were associated with two independent sequence variants in the *APOL1* gene on chromosome 22 (FSGS OR = 10.5, 95% CI = 6.0 to 18.4; hypertension-attributed ESRD OR = 7.3, 95% CI = 5.6 to 9.5). The two *APOL1* variants were common in African chromosomes but absent from European chromosomes, and both reside within haplotypes that harbor signatures of positive selection. The *APOL1* gene product, apolipoprotein L-I, has been studied for its roles in trypanosomal lysis, autophagic cell death, and lipid metabolism, as well as for its vascular effects.

Apolipoprotein L-I is a serum factor that lyses trypanosomes. Of interest, it was hypothesized that *APOL1* variants protect patients against *Trypanosoma brucei*, the parasite that causes sleeping sickness in thousands of people in Africa. Conversely, and with great irony, these same sequences are associated with kidney disease. In vitro assays revealed that only the kidney disease–associated apolipoprotein L-I variants lysed *Trypanosoma brucei rhodesiense,* a particularly aggressive newer subspecies. Carrying two copies of the haplotype carried significantly more risk of kidney disease than carrying one copy. In some respects, therefore, kidney disease–associated *APOL1* variants and protection from tsetse flies mirrors sickle cell anemia and protection from malaria.

Risk variants in *MYH9* and *APOL1* are in strong linkage dysequilibrium. Therefore, the genetic risk that was previously attributed to *MYH9* may reside in *APOL1.* However, future studies will be required to test whether more complex models of risk are operative. In summary, this genetic association on chromosome 22 explains, at least in part, racial disparities in nondiabetic ESRD and HIV-associated kidney disease because of the high prevalence of these haplotypes in individuals of African ancestry.

In addition to being the site of genetic anomalies, the podocyte may be the target of injury through several mechanisms.[164] These mechanisms include antibodies (e.g., antibodies to the phospholipase A_2 receptor) or immune complexes, infection (e.g., HIV infection), exposure to certain drugs (e.g., pamidronate or interferon), metabolic disorders (e.g., diabetes), and deposition of abnormal protein (e.g., amyloid). Podocyte injury can lead to proteinuria through abnormalities of the slit diaphragm (e.g., due to genetic mutations); podocyte loss; loss of negative charges from either loss of podocyte proteins (decreased podocalyxin or glomerular epithelial protein), decreased production of these proteins (decreased heparin sulfates), or destruction of the GBM (e.g., proteases); or podocyte-related endothelial cell dysfunction (e.g., decrease in vascular endothelial growth factor).[164] In addition, the response of the podocyte to injury may be expressed differently depending on the nature of the insult and result in different clinical syndromes. Thus, it has been proposed that various clinical and histologic variants of nephrotic syndromes depend on whether the podocyte injury results in apoptosis, podocyte loss, or podocyte dedifferentiation and reentry into the cell cycle and proliferation.[165] Indeed, this concept led to proposals to change the classification of nephrotic syndromes based on the understanding of the pathogenetic mechanisms of disease in addition to a description of histologic variants.[166]

In collapsing forms of FSGS, podocytes undergo irreversible ultrastructural changes in which mature podocyte markers disappear, which suggests a dysregulated podocyte phenotype in these diseases.[167-169] In fact, podocyte proliferation is seen in some examples of FSGS, which may be a consequence of the decrease in cyclin-dependent kinase inhibitors P27 and P57.[170] This has led to the concept that in collapsing FSGS, podocytes become dysregulated and proliferate.[171] However, the concept that the podocyte is a proliferating cell in collapsing FSGS has been challenged. In a mouse model of focal sclerosis, parietal epithelial and not visceral epithelial cells were involved in the proliferative event.[172] This challenge is also supported by the findings of a study of two patients with HIV- and pamidronate-associated collapsing FSGS.[173]

The effacement of foot processes may be a consequence of the overproduction of oxygen radicals and accumulation of lipid peroxidase.[174] In theory, the loss of podocytes could result in focal areas of GBM denudation with diminished barrier function. Podocyte dropout may be a major factor in the development of glomerulosclerosis in general and specifically in the development of collapsing FSGS.[175-178]

Some of the same pathogenic events that result in segmental scarring secondary to focal glomerular injury caused by a proliferative or necrotizing glomerulonephritis are probably operative in producing the sclerosis of FSGS. In this regard, the overproduction of transforming growth factor-β_1 (TGF-β_1) in glomeruli due to acute inflammatory lesions may cause glomerular sclerosis.[179] In experimental models of glomerular inflammation, the administration of antibodies to TGF-β or other inhibitors of TGF-β resulted in a decrease in matrix accumulation and a reduction in the severity of glomerular scarring.[180] Several mechanisms are associated with the fibrosis of renal disease. Extracellular matrix, and proteoglycans such as decorin and biglycan, may have a pathogenic role in fibrosing diseases through regulation of TGF-β.[181]

FSGS also results from the loss of nephrons, which causes compensatory intraglomerular hypertension and hypertrophy in the remaining glomeruli. The compensatory capillary hypertension results in podocytes and endothelial cell injury, as well as mesangial alterations that lead to progressive focal and segmental sclerosis.[182-188] This process, at least in experimental animals, is made worse by increased dietary protein intake and is ameliorated by both protein restriction and antihypertensive therapy.

A permeability factor has been described in some patients with FSGS. In a seminal study, 33 patients with FSGS that recurred after renal transplantation had a higher mean value for permeability to albumin than did normal subjects.[189] After plasmapheresis, the level of permeability factor in six patients was reduced, and proteinuria significantly decreased. The nature of the FSGS permeability factor continues to elude research efforts at identifying it. It is hypothesized to consist of low-molecular-weight anionic proteins or proteins that alter phosphorylation of glomerular proteins.[190] Recent data suggest a high affinity of the FSGS permeability factor to galactose, which appears to inhibit its activity in vitro.[191] Treatment with oral galactose is anecdotally reported to afford remission of nephrotic syndrome[192] and is the subject of a pilot study (National Clinical Trial [NCT] 01113385 at http://ClinicalTrials.gov). In a minority of patients with steroid-resistant FSGS in native kidneys, plasmapheresis may diminish proteinuria and stabilize renal function. In most patients, however, there is no improvement in proteinuria despite loss of the permeability factor after plasmapheresis.[193]

Glomerular enlargement accompanied by the development of FSGS occurs in the setting of hypoxemia, for example in patients with sickle cell anemia, congenital pulmonary disease, or cyanotic congenital heart disease. Obesity appears to predispose to FSGS.[194,195] Weight loss and the administration of an angiotensin-converting enzyme (ACE) inhibitor decreased protein excretion by 80% to 85%.[196,197] Patients with sleep apnea may have proteinuria that is more functional in nature, but with little or no evidence of glomerular scarring or epithelial injury observed in biopsy specimens.[198,199] The association between sleep apnea and proteinuria was questioned by an analysis of 148 patients referred for polysomnography who were not diabetic and had not been treated previously for obstructive sleep apnea.[200] In this patient population, clinically significant proteinuria was uncommon; it was found to be associated with older age, hypertension, coronary artery disease, and arousal index by univariate analysis, but only with age and hypertension by multiple regression analysis. Body mass index and apnea-hypopnea index were not associated with urine protein/creatinine ratio. The authors concluded that nephrotic-range proteinuria should not be ascribed to sleep apnea and deserves a thorough renal evaluation.

A number of infections cause FSGS. HIV-associated FSGS is pathologically identical to idiopathic collapsing FSGS, except that endothelial tubuloreticular inclusions are present in the former but not the latter. This close association of HIV infection with collapsing FSGS, as well as experimental evidence of focal glomerular sclerosis in mice transgenic for HIV type 1 genes,[133,179,201-206] raise the possibility that the HIV virus can be an etiologic agent of FSGS in infected patients. Whether other viral diseases, including parvovirus B19 infection, cause the idiopathic collapsing variant of FSGS remains to be elucidated.[207,208] Parvovirus B19 has been found with greater frequency in patients with idiopathic and collapsing FSGS than in patients with other diagnoses.[207] The polyomavirus SV40 may also play a role.[209]

Focal sclerosis is associated with a number of malignant conditions that have been linked to lymphoproliferative disease. In one study,[210] an association of FSGS was found with monoclonal gammopathies of undetermined significance (MGUS) and multiple myeloma. When the lymphoproliferative disease was treated, the renal lesion improved.

Finally, FSGS has been linked to exposure to a number of medications, including pamidronate[172,211] and interferon,[212] and with the use of anabolic steroids.[213] Like pamidronate and interferon therapy, the latter may also be associated with collapsing FSGS. Discontinuation of the anabolic steroids may lead to reduction of proteinuria.

Clinical Features and Natural History

Proteinuria is the hallmark feature of all forms of primary FSGS. The degree of proteinuria varies from nonnephrotic (1 to 2 g of protein per day) to over 10 g of protein per day, associated with all of the morbid features of nephrotic syndrome. Hematuria occurs in over half of FSGS patients, and approximately one third of patients have some degree of renal insufficiency at presentation. Gross hematuria is more commonly seen in FSGS than in minimal change glomerulopathy.[214] Hypertension is a presenting feature in one third of patients. There are differences in the presentation of FSGS in adults and children.[215-218] Children tend to have more proteinuria, whereas hypertension is more common in adults.

Differences in clinical manifestations correlate with different pathologic phenotypes of FSGS.[214] Patients with perihilar FSGS accompanied by glomerular hypertrophy more commonly have nonnephrotic-range proteinuria than do FSGS patients who do not have glomerular hypertrophy. In addition there are differences in the clinical presentation of the collapsing variant of FSGS and the glomerular tip lesion variant of FSGS.

Patients with collapsing FSGS have substantially more proteinuria, a lower serum albumin level, and a higher serum creatinine level than patients with perihilar FSGS.[136,137,219] The development of proteinuria, edema, or hypoalbuminemia may occur rapidly over the course of days to weeks, in contrast to the more indolent development of proteinuria in most patients with typical FSGS. Moreover, patients with collapsing FSGS more frequently have extrarenal manifestations of disease a few weeks prior to onset of the nephrosis, such as episodes of diarrhea, upper respiratory tract infections, or lower respiratory tract–like symptoms that are usually ascribed

to viral or other infectious processes. However, the systemic symptoms of fever, malaise, and anorexia occur in fewer than 20% of patients at the time of onset of nephrosis. Pamidronate, a bisphosphonate that prevents bone disease in patients with myeloma and metastatic tumors, has been reported to be associated with collapsing FSGS in a number of series.[172,211] After discontinuation of the drug, kidney function stabilized in all patients except those with collapsing FSGS. Recently, treatment with interferon has also been reported to be associated with the development of collapsing FSGS.[212]

The clinical presentation of glomerular tip lesion differs from that of both perihilar FSGS and collapsing FSGS.[214] Patients with glomerular tip lesion tend to be older white males, in sharp contrast to the younger black male prevalence in collapsing FSGS. The proteinuria in these patients usually is severe and the onset is abrupt, with sudden development of edema and hypoalbuminemia. The rapidity of onset of the disease process is similar to the clinical presentation of minimal change glomerulopathy.[143,220,221] Patients with glomerular tip lesion may develop reversible acute renal failure, especially at the time of initial presentation when the degree of proteinuria, edema, and hypoalbuminemia are at their peak. This also is similar to the presentation of minimal change glomerulopathy but rarely occurs with other variants of FSGS.

Several studies addressed the clinical applicability and implications of distinguishing the variants of FSGS. An analysis of data for 197 patients followed within the Glomerular Disease Collaborative Network between 1982 and 2001 found the FSGS NOS variant in 42% of cases, the perihilar variant in 26%, the tip lesion in 17%, the collapsing lesion in 11%, and the cellular variant in 3% of patients.[221a] African Americans accounted for 91% of patients with collapsing FSGS, but only 15% of patients with the tip lesion variant. Both collapsing and tip variants were associated with significantly greater amounts of proteinuria (10.0 ± 5.3 g protein per day and 9.7 ± 7.0 g protein per day, respectively) than perihilar or NOS variants of FSGS (4.4 ± 3.3 g protein per day and 5.5 ± 4.6 g protein per day, respectively; $P < 0.001$). In this retrospective, uncontrolled analysis, patients with the tip lesion variant of FSGS were significantly more likely to attain a complete remission even after adjustment for corticosteroid exposure ($P < 0.001$). Collapsing FSGS had the worst 1-year (74%) and 3-year renal survival rates of all variants, regardless of differences in the histologic severity of injury, which suggests the possibility that the nature of the injury was inherently different.

Similarly, an analysis of data for 225 patients studied at Columbia University[222] confirmed the predilection of the tip lesion variant of FSGS for whites (86.2%), although the predominance of African Americans among patients with collapsing FSGS was less pronounced (53.6%). In this large cohort, 10% of patients had the cellular variant, of whom 32% were African American. The mean proteinuria (9.5 ± 1.2 g of protein per day) in these patients was comparable to that in patients with the collapsing or tip variants (8.8 ± 1.3 g of protein per day and 7.8 ± 0.6 g of protein per day, respectively). Patients with cellular FSGS showed intermediate rates of remission (44.5%) and ESRD (27.8%) compared with patients with collapsing FSGS (remission rate = 13.2%, ESRD rate = 65.3%) and tip FSGS (remission rate = 75.8% and ESRD rate = 5.7%).

A retrospective analysis of data for a cohort of 93 adult patients in the Netherlands confirms the improved renal survival of patients with the tip variant compared with patients with the other variants (5-year survival of 78% for tip vs. 63% for FSGS NOS and 55% for perihilar FSGS, $P = 0.02$).[223]

The degree of proteinuria is a predictor of the long-term clinical outcome. Nonnephrotic-range proteinuria correlates with a more favorable renal survival of over 80% after 10 years of follow-up.[224,225] In contrast, patients who have proteinuria of more than 10 g of protein per day have very poor long-term renal survival, with the majority of patients reaching ESRD within 3 years.[226,227] Patients with FSGS and protein excretion that measures between nonnephrotic range and massive proteinuria have variable long-term renal outcomes. In general, these patients have a relatively poor outcome, with half reaching ESRD by 10 years.[217,218,228]

One of the most useful prognostic indicators for patients with FSGS is whether remission of nephrotic syndrome is achieved.[216] Patients who experience remission of nephrosis have a substantially greater renal survival rate than those who do not.[216,224,225,229,230] According to Korbet and colleagues,[217,218] fewer than 15% of patients who achieve complete or partial remission progress to ESRD within 5 years of follow-up. Up to 50% of patients who do not experience remission progress to end-stage disease within 6 years of follow-up.

As in other forms of glomerular injury, entry serum creatinine level correlates with long-term renal survival.[224,226,231,232] Patients with a serum creatinine level of over 1.3 mg/dL have poorer renal survival than those with lower serum creatinine concentrations, irrespective of the level of proteinuria (10-year renal survival of 27% vs. 100%).[218] Multivariate analysis indicates that entry serum creatinine level may be more important than proteinuria as a predictor of progression to ESRD.[224,225,227,228,231,232]

Controversy abounds regarding whether long-term prognosis is poorer in black patients than in white patients. In children, Ingulli and Tejani noted that within 8.5 years of follow-up, 78% of black patients but only 33% of white patients progressed to ESRD.[232] The racial predilection for poor long-term prognosis has not been corroborated in studies of adult patients with nephrosis.[224,225]

Laboratory Findings

Hypoproteinemia is common in patients with FSGS, with total serum protein concentration reduced to varying extents. The serum albumin concentration may fall to below 2 g/dL, especially in patients with the collapsing and glomerular tip variants of FSGS. As in other forms of nephrotic syndrome, levels of immunoglobulins are typically depressed, and levels of lipids are increased, especially serum cholesterol level. Serum levels of complement components are generally in the normal range in FSGS. Circulating immune complexes have been detected in patients with FSGS,[233,234] although their pathogenic significance has not been determined. Serologic testing for HIV infection should be performed for patients with FSGS, especially those with the collapsing pattern.

Treatment

Angiotensin Inhibitors
ACE inhibitors and angiotensin II receptor blockers (ARBs) have been evaluated in the treatment of FSGS. ACE inhibitors have been shown to decrease proteinuria and the rate of

progression to ESRD.[235-238] These results have been obtained not only in the presence of diabetes, but also in cases of nondiabetic renal disease. In patients with sickle cell disease, glomerulomegaly, and FSGS, ACE inhibitors decreased proteinuria acutely while maintaining GFR and renal plasma flow.[239] In general, these studies suggest that ACE inhibitors, and perhaps ARBs, would provide a substantial effect in ameliorating the nephrotic symptoms of FSGS. A systematic review of studies reveals that ACE inhibitors significantly reduce proteinuria in children with steroid-resistant nephrotic syndrome.[240] In a randomized controlled trial involving normotensive children with steroid-resistant nephrotic syndrome, the addition of fosinopril to prednisone resulted in a greater reduction in proteinuria than prednisone alone.[241]

In patients with glomerulomegaly and resultant nonnephrotic-range proteinuria, an ACE inhibitor or angiotensin II receptor antagonist sufficiently decreases proteinuria and potentially decreases hyperlipidemia, edema, and other manifestations of persistent loss of protein in the urine with excellent long-term prognosis. Regardless of what other forms of antiinflammatory or immunosuppressive therapy are employed, the beneficial effects of these agents indicates that they should be added, despite the well-known side effects of hyperkalemia and reduction in GFR, especially in patients with serum creatinine levels of over 3 mg/dL.

Before immunomodulatory or immunosuppressive therapy is initiated in a patient with FSGS, a careful evaluation should be undertaken to exclude the possibility of an underlying cause as described in the section on pathogenesis. Patients with secondary FSGS are unlikely to benefit from immunosuppressive therapy and may be at particularly high risk of complications. In addition, an assessment of the risk and benefit of immunosuppressive therapy should be undertaken for each patient. Patients with subnephrotic-range proteinuria have a generally good prognosis, and the initial therapy should be focused on blood pressure control, preferentially using maximal tolerated dosages of renin-angiotensin-aldosterone system (RAAS) blockers. Glucocorticoids or immunosuppressive therapy should be targeted to patients with idiopathic FSGS and nephrotic syndrome.

Glucocorticoids
No randomized placebo-controlled trial has been conducted to formally assess the role of glucocorticoids in the treatment of FSGS. The available data are based on case series using different treatment protocols; different definitions of remission, response, relapse, and resistance; and different lengths of therapy.[216,224,229,242] One review of studies suggested that only 15% of patients with FSGS responded to treatment, in sharp contrast to those with minimal change glomerulopathy.[243] More optimistic reports have been published by groups in Toronto and Chicago[216,217] that suggest that 30% to 40% of adult patients may achieve some form of remission with corticosteroid treatment. A compilation of these studies by Korbet and colleagues[218] suggests that of 177 patients who received a variety of different forms of therapy, 45% experienced complete remission, 10% experienced partial remission, and 45% showed no response.[216,224,229,242,244]

In children, the initial treatment of FSGS is similar to the treatment of minimal change glomerulopathy, because therapy is typically initiated without histologic confirmation of the disease process. Thus, the International Study of Kidney

Diseases in Children recommended using an initial course of prednisone of 60 mg/day/m^2, up to 80 mg/day, for 4 weeks. This is followed with 40 mg/day/m^2, up to 60 mg/day, administered in divided doses for 3 consecutive days out of 7, for 4 weeks, and then tapered off for 4 more weeks. As in adult patients with minimal change glomerulopathy, a longer course of therapy at higher dosages of prednisone may be necessary to induce remission. Thus, in those series and retrospective analyses that showed an increased remission rate,[125,216,224,229,242,245,246] prednisone treatment was continued for 16 weeks to achieve remission. In adult patients, median time for complete remission was 3 to 4 months.[128]

Of patients who showed a positive response to corticosteroid treatment, a portion will experience relapse. Guidelines for retreatment of this group of patients are similar to those for treatment of patients with relapsing minimal change glomerulopathy. In patients whose remission prior to relapse was prolonged (over 6 months), a repeat course of corticosteroid therapy may again induce a remission. In steroid-dependent patients who experience frequent relapses, repeated rounds of high-dose corticosteroid therapy result in unacceptable cumulative toxicity. Thus, alternative strategies such as the addition of cyclosporine may be useful. In patients with the glomerular tip lesion variant of FSGS, a trial of corticosteroids is appropriate, because many patients experience a decline in protein excretion.[141,221,247]

The practice of using higher dosages of corticosteroids to produce remission has resulted in the use of alternative therapeutic approaches.

The use of very high dosages of corticosteroids in children, and continuation of daily prednisone therapy for up to 6 to 9 months in adults, is not without enormous short- and long-term side effects. In studies in which long-term, high-dose corticosteroid therapy is administered, few analyses have been undertaken of the development of osteoporosis, short- and long-term risk of infection, and the development of cataracts, diabetes, or other long-term sequelae. Thus, the available data do not allow for a careful understanding of the risk/benefit ratios. Until the use of high doses of methylprednisolone has been studied in controlled clinical trials, this potentially useful yet dangerous approach must be viewed with caution.

Attempts at alternate-day steroid therapy have not been successful except in elderly populations. The Toronto group[248] demonstrated that a 40% remission rate could be achieved in patients older than age 60 by administering up to 100 mg of prednisone on alternate days for 3 to 5 months. This therapy was well tolerated in this population, with not obvious side effects during the study period. Alternate-day prednisone therapy most likely works in this population because of an increased susceptibility to the immunosuppressive effects of corticosteroids and altered glucocorticoid kinetics in the elderly.

The benefit of corticosteroid therapy may differ among whites and African Americans. In a retrospective analysis[249] of renal survival in predominantly African American individuals with FSGS, renal survival was found to be higher when the initial serum creatinine level was lower and blood pressure was well controlled, but treatment with steroids had no affect on renal survival.

CYCLOPHOSPHAMIDE
Several studies have failed to document the effectiveness of cytotoxic drugs in the treatment of FSGS.[229,250] In one review, only 23% of 247 children with FSGS showed a response to

steroid therapy, and 70 patients were treated with cytotoxic drugs. Of these, 30% showed a response. In the final analysis, the disease was in remission in fewer than 20% of the 247 children. The use of cytotoxic drugs has been evaluated in only one series of adults.[229] Although their use correlated with longer remissions and fewer relapses, no other study has corroborated these results.

The International Study of Kidney Disease in Children carefully examined the role of cyclophosphamide in the treatment of children with FSGS.[251] Daily oral cyclophosphamide (2.5 mg/kg) was administered in addition to prednisone (40 mg/m^2 every other day) for 12 months, and results were compared with those for prednisone alone. The addition of cyclophosphamide had no effect on the change in proteinuria or the likelihood of achieving complete resolution of proteinuria.[251] Similarly, in a nonrandomized comparative study involving children with FSGS or steroid-resistant or frequently relapsing nephrotic syndrome, the addition of oral cyclophosphamide to prednisone for 3 months had no statistically significant effect on the rate of complete or partial remission or progression to ESRD.[252] In summary, the limited currently available data do not support the use of cyclophosphamide in patients with FSGS.

CYCLOSPORINE
FSGS that is resistant to prednisone may be induced into remission by cyclosporine. The effectiveness of cyclosporine in inducing remission of proteinuria in patients with FSGS has been demonstrated in two randomized controlled trials. In a study by Ponticelli and colleagues, 45 patients with steroid-resistant nephrotic syndrome were randomly assigned to receive supportive therapy or cyclosporine (5 mg/kg/day for adults, 6 mg/kg/day for children) for 6 months, with the drug then tapered off by 25% every 2 months.[125] Remission occurred in 13 of 22 patients receiving cyclosporine, compared with 3 of 19 patients in the control group ($P < 0.001$). Unfortunately relapses occurred in 69% of patients after withdrawal of cyclosporine.

In the North America Nephrotic Syndrome Study Group trial, 49 patients were randomly assigned to treatment with low doses of prednisone alone or in combination with oral cyclosporine for 26 weeks.[253] At the end of 26 weeks of therapy, partial or complete remission of proteinuria occurred in 70% of patients in the cyclosporine-treated group compared with only 4% in the control group ($P < 0.001$); however, relapses occurred by 52 weeks in 40% of those experiencing remission. Treatment with cyclosporine was also associated with a 70% reduction in the risk that GFR would decline by 50%.[253]

How long should patients be treated with cyclosporine? In a study by Meyrier and colleagues,[128] when patients remained in remission for longer than 12 months, cyclosporine was slowly tapered and eventually removed without subsequent relapse.[128] Unfortunately, long-term treatment with cyclosporine was associated with increases in tubular atrophy and interstitial fibrosis, the degree of which was positively correlated with the initial serum creatinine level, the number of segmental scars on initial biopsy specimens, and a cyclosporine dosage of more than 5.5 mg/kg/day. Thus, there is a clear trade-off, with the use of cyclosporine over the long term well established to lead to the development of interstitial fibrosis and tubular atrophy.

A randomized controlled trial compared the efficacy of cyclosporine to intravenous cyclophosphamide in the initial treatment of 22 children with steroid-resistant nephrotic syndrome related to minimal change glomerulopathy, FSGS, or mesangial hypercellularity.[254] All patients were also receiving alternate-day prednisone therapy. Treatment with cyclosporine afforded a statistically significantly higher rate of partial remission of proteinuria at both 12 weeks (60% of cyclosporine-treated patients vs. 17% in the cyclophosphamide group, $P < 0.05$) and 24 weeks (46% vs. 11%, $P < 0.05$). By study's end, 12 of the 14 patients who showed no response to cyclophosphamide were patients with FSGS. Of note, all six patients who were heterozygous for the NPHS2 R229Q variant or the R6Q(h) mutation were assigned to the cyclophosphamide group, and only one of those showed a response to treatment. These results support the use of cyclosporine over cyclophosphamide in children with steroid-resistant nephrotic syndrome.

MYCOPHENOLATE MOFETIL

The data regarding the use of mycophenolate mofetil (MMF) in the treatment of FSGS remain largely anecdotal, with one small case series reporting transient improvement in proteinuria in 8 of 18 patients. A recent randomized controlled trial compared the efficacy of an MMF-based regimen to treatment with corticosteroids with or without cyclophosphamide in adult patients with idiopathic membranous glomerulopathy ($n = 21$) or FSGS ($n = 33$).[255] MMF was given at a dosage of 2 g/day for 6 months along with prednisolone at 0.5 mg/kg/day for 2 to 3 months. Patients with FSGS in the comparison group received prednisolone 1 mg/kg/day for 3 to 6 months. There was no difference between the two groups with respect to the proportion of complete or partial remissions (70% vs. 69%) or the time to remission or proteinuria at any point. Remission was achieved faster in the MMF-treated FSGS patients than in the corticosteroid-only group (5.6 months vs. 10.2 months, respectively), and cumulative steroid dose was lower (1.9 ± 0.3 g vs. 7.3 ± 0.9 g, respectively). Although limited to a small number of patients and relatively short follow-up, this first controlled study suggests that the addition of MMF is steroid sparing and achieves rates of remission comparable to those for corticosteroids alone in patients with FSGS.

Further controlled trials are required to evaluate the role of MMF in the treatment of FSGS, especially in comparison to cyclosporine. This issue is being addressed, in part, by the large Focal Segmental Glomerulosclerosis Clinical Trial (NCT00135811) sponsored by the National Institutes of Health that compares cyclosporine to MMF combined with dexamethasone. All patients will also receive treatment with an angiotensin II inhibitor and alternate-day, low-dose prednisone. The primary objective of the trial is to determine whether treatment with MMF plus pulse steroids is superior to treatment with cyclosporine in inducing remission from proteinuria over 12 months. The secondary objective is to determine whether treatment with MMF plus pulse steroids is superior to treatment with cyclosporine in inducing remissions persisting for at least 6 months after withdrawal of immunosuppressive therapy. This trial has enrolled 138 patients, of whom 38% were African American and 36% were older than 18 years at enrollment. The results of this trial have not yet been published.

OTHER THERAPIES

The use of sirolimus in the management of FSGS is poorly supported. Several reports have emerged of new-onset proteinuria in kidney transplant recipients who were switched from calcineurin inhibitor–based therapy to sirolimus.[256-260] In a study of 78 solid organ transplant recipients treated with sirolimus, 18 patients (23.1%) developed proteinuria in an average of 11.2 ± 2.1 months after starting sirolimus therapy.[261] Renal biopsy specimens obtained after the onset of proteinuria revealed various degrees of mesangial proliferation and mesangial expansion commonly seen in patients who previously had a diagnosis of chronic allograft nephropathy, but showed FSGS in only two patients (14.3%). There was no correlation between proteinuria levels and sirolimus dose or trough blood levels. In the six patients in whom sirolimus treatment was withdrawn, a complete reversal of proteinuria and edema was observed. This study certainly raises significant concern about the induction of proteinuria by sirolimus in transplant recipients.

The data pertaining to the use of sirolimus in the management of FSGS in native kidneys is rather conflicting. In a prospective open-label trial of sirolimus in 21 patients with steroid-resistant FSGS, at 6 months 4 patients (19%) had achieved a complete remission, 8 (38%) had experienced a partial remission, and 1 patient had experienced a rapid decline in renal function.[262] Sirolimus therapy was associated with a substantial number of adverse events, including hyperlipidemia and anemia in 43% of patients. In patients who showed no response to sirolimus, the mean serum creatinine level increased from 1.66 mg/dL at baseline to 2.2 mg/dL at 6 months and 3.24 mg/dL at 12 months (significantly different from baseline at the $P = 0.028$ level). In patients who did show a response to sirolimus, the mean serum creatinine level increased from 1.76 mg/dL at baseline to 1.91 mg/dL at 12 months.

In contrast, a phase II open-label clinical trial of sirolimus had to be interrupted for safety reasons after five out of six patients enrolled experienced a sharp decrease in GFR, and none achieved a complete remission.[263] Three patients had a more than twofold increase in proteinuria during sirolimus therapy. Similar deleterious effects were reported in a cohort of 11 patients with a variety of glomerular diseases.[264] Although inconclusive, the bulk of the data currently available suggest that sirolimus has a deleterious effect in FSGS and should be avoided.

Future approaches to the treatment of FSGS may come from the treatment of recurrent FSGS following transplantation. Intriguing cases of recurrent FSGS after transplantation have been published in which the proteinuria resolved after treatment with rituximab.[265] Interestingly, in one case[266] the diagnosis of posttransplant lymphoproliferative disease was established 5 months after the transplantation, even though recurrent nephrotic syndrome occurred within 2 weeks postoperatively. In addition, there are a few reports of recurrent FSGS after transplantation that responded to rituximab (after plasmapheresis or immunoadsorption) that are not related to posttransplant lymphoproliferative disease.[267-270] These patients may represent a specific category, and the lessons learned from their treatment may not necessarily apply to the general population of patients with FSGS. Anecdotal reports are emerging of treatment of primary and recurrent FSGS with rituximab, usually in combination with other immunomodulating therapies, but results show a mixed response to this treatment,[271,272] with several reports of failures.[273] In the largest case series, five of eight adult patients with resistant FSGS failed to show a response to a course of rituximab, and two patients suffered a rapid deterioration of renal function.[274] Only two patients had a clear and sustained improvement of renal function and proteinuria. The use of rituximab for the treatment of FSGS clearly requires further evaluation in the setting of a randomized controlled trial.

Another potential future approach targets renal fibrosis, which represents a common final pathway of FSGS and other chronic kidney diseases.[275] The orally available antifibrotic agent pirfenidone was evaluated in an open-label pilot study to determine its effect on the rate of decline in GFR in 18 patients with FSGS selected for having a monthly rate of decline in estimated GFR of more than 0.35 mL/min/1.73 m^2.[276] The monthly change in GFR improved from a median of −0.61 mL/min/1.73 m^2 during the baseline period to −0.45 mL/min/1.73 m^2 with pirfenidone therapy, which represented a median of 25% improvement in the rate of decline ($P < 0.01$). Pirfenidone had no effect on blood pressure or proteinuria and was associated with frequent dyspepsia, sedation, and photosensitive dermatitis. These enticing results provide a strong rationale for a larger placebo-controlled trial in patients with progressive chronic kidney disease.

Other forms of treatment have been used. Plasmapheresis and protein absorption strategies to remove circulating factors responsible for FSGS have led to remission of recurrent FSGS, but do not appear to be beneficial in treating the primary disease.[193,277]

In summary, patients with primary FSGS remain frustrating patients to treat. Enthusiasm for the use of high-dose, prolonged corticosteroid therapy in adults and children has prompted the use of this therapy in many FSGS patients. Only a prospective randomized trial that carefully evaluates this approach will determine its effectiveness. The first step in therapy should be geared toward achieving excellent blood pressure control using RAAS blockers. In those patients who have nephrotic-range proteinuria, careful supportive care and consideration of a trial of oral corticosteroids in adult patients may be an acceptable approach after patients are carefully informed about the risks and potential benefits of 12 to 16 weeks of daily corticosteroid therapy. Alternatively a trial of cyclosporine may be warranted for patients who have contraindications to corticosteroid therapy or in whom corticosteroid therapy fails to produce improvement.

C1q Nephropathy

C1q nephropathy is a relatively rare cause of proteinuria and nephrotic syndrome that can mimic FSGS clinically and histologically, although the clinical and pathologic presentations are quite variable.[278,279] In a single-center retrospective analysis of renal biopsy specimens from children and adolescents, C1q nephropathy was found in 6.6% of native kidney biopsy specimens.[280] In the largest case series, which was conducted at the University of Ljubljana, Slovenia, and included both children and adults, C1q nephropathy was identified in 1.9% of native kidney biopsy specimens.[281] There appears to be a slight male predominance (56% to 68%).[281,282] Depending on the case series, there may be an association with African American or Hispanic ethnicity.[282] Patients of all ages with C1q nephropathy have been described.

The diagnosis is based on the presence of mesangial immune complex deposits that show conspicuous staining for C1q in a patient with no evidence of systemic lupus erythematosus. The C1q staining usually is accompanied by staining for IgG, IgM, and C3. Electron microscopy demonstrates well-defined mesangial immune complex–type dense deposits. Light microscopic findings vary from no lesion (mimicking minimal change glomerulopathy), to focal glomerular hypercellularity, to proliferative glomerulonephritis with mesangial hypercellularity, to focal segmental sclerosing lesions that may be indistinguishable histologically from those of FSGS. Anecdotal case reports have described C1q nephropathy associated with a collapsing FSGS lesion.[283,284] The findings by immunofluorescence microscopy and electron microscopy, however, readily differentiate C1q nephropathy from minimal change glomerulopathy and FSGS. The pathologic features suggest an immune complex pathogenesis, but the details of the pathogenic mechanism and the etiology are unknown.

Patients with C1q nephropathy generally have proteinuria, which may or may not be associated with nephrotic syndrome. Hematuria is present in at least 50% of patients and is more common among patients with a mesangial proliferative lesion on light microscopy.[281] Likewise, hypertension affects a minority of patients with no discernible lesions on light microscopy (similar to minimal change disease) but is much more prevalent among those patients with mesangial proliferation (55%).[281] Interestingly, many patients are relatively asymptomatic, and proteinuria may first be detected at the time of a physical examination in connection with sports participation or induction into the armed forces. These patients, by definition, have no clinical or serologic evidence of systemic lupus erythematosus, despite the presence of C1q in the renal biopsy specimen. C1q nephropathy may show spontaneous improvement.[285]

The renal outcome of patients with C1q nephropathy appears generally favorable,[280] especially in patients whose biopsy specimens show minimal change–like histologic features.[281,286] Studies suggest, however, that they may experience more frequent relapses and require additional immunosuppressants more often than patients with "pure" minimal change disease.[280,281,286] Patients whose biopsy specimens show FSGS-like or mesangial proliferative lesions on histologic analysis may show a less favorable response to immunosuppressive therapy although the data are rather limited.

Membranous Glomerulopathy

Epidemiology

Membranous glomerulopathy (also known as *membranous nephropathy*, or *MN*) is one of the most common causes of nephrotic syndrome in adults.[137,141,142,145,185,216,219,221,225,287-300,300a] MN occurs as an idiopathic (primary) or secondary disease. Secondary MN is caused by autoimmune diseases (e.g., systemic lupus erythematosus, autoimmune thyroiditis), infection (e.g., hepatitis B, hepatitis C, malaria), drugs (e.g., penicillamine, gold), and malignancies (e.g., colon or lung cancer). Secondary MN, especially that caused by hepatitis B[296,297,301-305] and lupus, is more frequent in children than in adults. In patients older than age 60, MN is associated with a malignancy in 20% to 30% of cases.[295]

MN is the cause of nephrotic syndrome in approximately 25% of adults with the syndrome.[306-315] A study of patients who had urinary excretion of more than 1 g of protein per 24 hours, conducted by the Medical Research Council in the United Kingdom from 1978 to 1990, determined that 20% had MN. The peak incidence of MN is in the fourth to fifth decade of life.[309,316-320] A pooled analysis of studies of patients with idiopathic MN found a 2:1 predominance of males (1190 males and 598 females).[321] The adult/child ratio was 26:1 (1734 adults and 67 children); however, this low proportion of children among MN patients was biased by the exclusion of children from some of the studies included in the analysis. MN affects all races.

Although most patients with MN present with nephrotic syndrome, 10% to 20% of patients have proteinuria that remains at less than 2 g of protein per day.[322] It is thus likely that the frequency of MN in the general population is underestimated, because asymptomatic individuals with subclinical proteinuria often do not come to diagnosis or undergo renal biopsy.

There are geographic variations in the clinical manifestations of MN. In studies in Australia and Japan lower percentages of patients have nephrotic syndrome at entry than in Europe and North America. The geographic differences may be related to difference in the prevalence of underlying causes of secondary MN, such as hepatitis B, malaria, and other infections.[297,303]

The association of MN with underlying malignancy is well recognized. In a large cohort study of 240 patients in France,[323] the incidence of cancer was significantly higher in patients with MN than in the general population (standardized incidence ratio = 9.8 [5.5 to 16.2] for men and 12.3 [4.5 to 26.9] for women). In almost half the patients the tumor was asymptomatic and was detected only because of diagnostic procedures prompted by the diagnosis of MN. The most common malignancies were cancers of the lung and prostate. The frequency of malignancy increased with age. In a separate cohort study in Norway,[324] the incidence of cancer in 161 patients with MN was significantly higher compared with the age- and sex-adjusted general Norwegian population, corresponding to a standardized incidence ratio of 2.25 (95% CI = 1.44 to 3.35). The median time from diagnosis of MN to diagnosis of cancer was 60 months. Patients with MN who developed cancer were older (65 years vs. 52 years, $P < 0.001$).[324]

Risk factors for malignancy in patients with MN include older age and a history of smoking, although the clinical presentation does not differ between patients with cancer-associated MN and those with idiopathic MN.[323] In patients with cancer-associated MN, clinical remission of the cancer is associated with a reduction of proteinuria.[323] These studies highlight the importance of thorough cancer screening among older patients with MN, not only at the time of first diagnosis, but also during subsequent long-term follow up.[325]

Pathology

ELECTRON MICROSCOPY

The pathologic sine qua non of MN is the presence of subepithelial immune complex deposits or their structural consequences.[326] Electron microscopy provides the most definitive

diagnosis of MN, although a relatively confident diagnosis can be made based on typical light microscopic and immunofluorescence microscopic findings.

Figure 31-7 depicts the four ultrastructural stages of MN as described by Ehrenreich and Churg.[316] The earliest ultrastructural manifestation, stage I, is characterized by the presence of scattered or more regularly distributed small immune complex–type electron-dense deposits in the subepithelial zone between the basement membrane and the podocyte. Podocyte process effacement and microvillous transformation occur in all stages of MN when there is substantial proteinuria. Stage II is characterized by projections of basement membrane material around the subepithelial deposits. In three dimensions, these projections surround the sides of the deposits, but when observed in cross section, they appear as spikes extending between the deposits (Figures 31-7 and 31-8). In stage III, the new basement membrane material surrounds the deposits, and thus in cross section there is basement membrane material between the deposits and the epithelial cytoplasm. At this point the deposits are in essence intramembranous rather than subepithelial; however, the ultrastructural appearance allows the inference that they once were subepithelial and thus indicative of MN. Stage IV is characterized by loss of the electron density of the deposits, which often results in irregular electron-lucent zones within an irregularly thickened basement membrane. Although not described by Ehrenreich and Churg, some nephropathologists recognize stage V, which is characterized by a repaired outer basement membrane zone with the only residual basement membrane disturbance in the inner aspect of the basement membrane. At the time of renal biopsy, most patients in the United States have stage I or II disease (Table 31-11).

Mesangial dense deposits are rare in idiopathic MN but are more frequent in secondary MN (see Table 31-11). This suggests, but does not prove, that idiopathic MN is caused by subepithelial in situ immune complex formation with antibodies from the circulation complexing with antigens derived from the podocyte. Immune complexes formed only at this site could not go against the direction of filtration to reach the mesangium. Secondary forms of MN usually are caused by immune complexes that contain antigens that are in the circulation, such as antigens derived from infections (e.g., hepatitis B), tumor antigens (e.g., colon cancer), or autoantigens (e.g., thyroglobulin). With both the antigens and antibodies in the systemic circulation, it is likely that some immune complexes would form that would localize not only in the subepithelial zone but also in the mesangium or subendothelial zone. This is demonstrated in the secondary form of MN that occurs in patients with systemic lupus erythematosus. In over 90% of lupus MN specimens mesangial dense deposits are identified by electron microscopy.[328] Therefore, the presence of mesangial dense deposits should raise the index of suspicion for secondary rather than primary MN.

IMMUNOFLUORESCENCE MICROSCOPY

The characteristic immunofluorescence microscopic finding in MN is diffuse global granular capillary wall staining for immunoglobulin and complement (Figure 31-9).[326] IgG is the most frequent and usually the most intensely staining immunoglobulin, although less pronounced staining for IgA and IgM is common (see Table 31-11). C3 staining is present over 95% of the time but typically is relatively low in intensity.

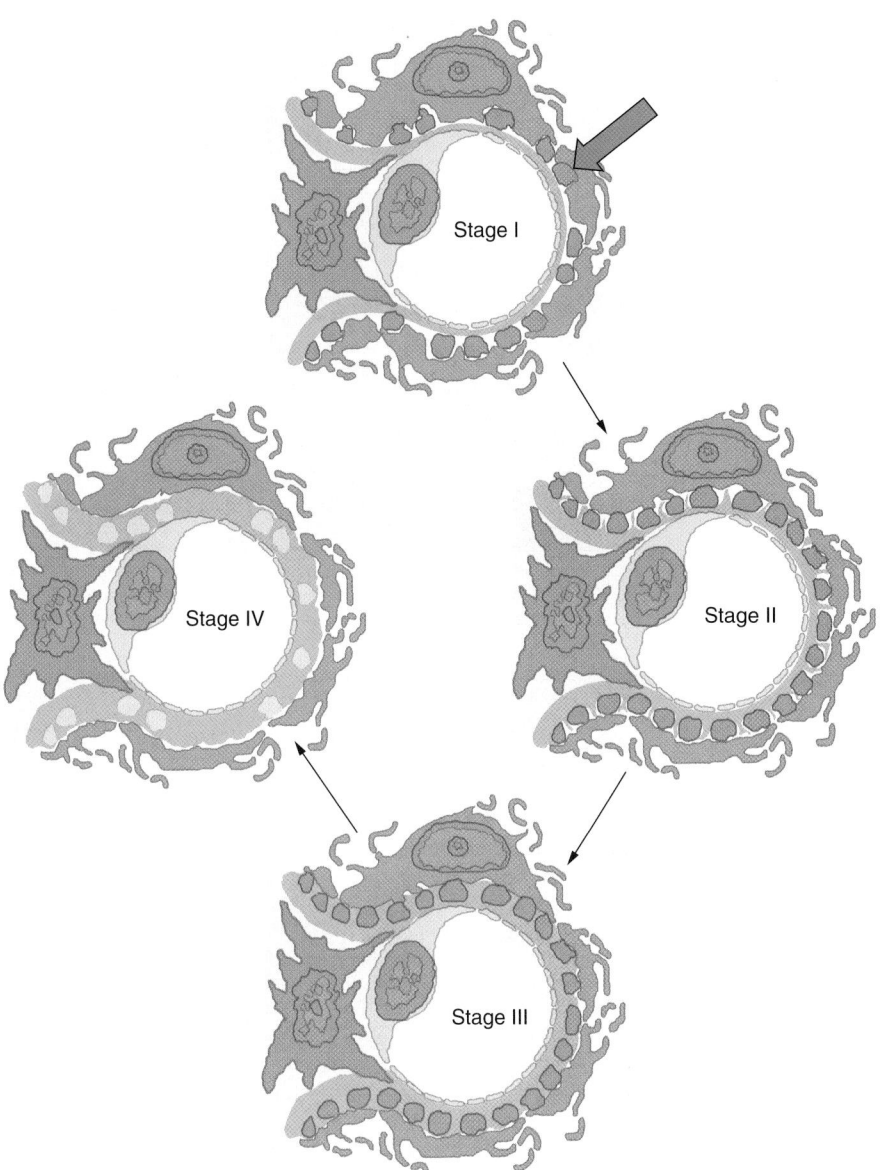

FIGURE 31-7 Diagram depicting the four ultrastructural stages of membranous glomerulopathy. Stage I has subepithelial dense deposits (*arrow*) without adjacent basement membrane reaction. Stage II has projections of basement membrane adjacent to deposits. Stage III has deposits surrounded by basement membrane. Stage IV has thickened basement membrane with irregular lucent zones. (Courtesy of J.C. Jennette.)

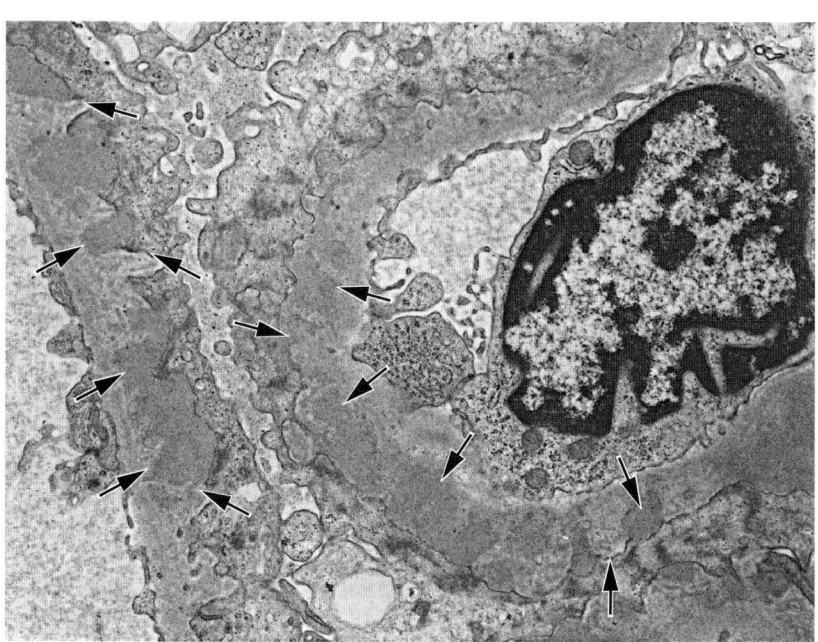

FIGURE 31-8 Electron micrograph showing features of stage II membranous glomerulopathy with numerous subepithelial dense deposits (*straight arrows*) and adjacent projections of basement membrane material. (*curved arrows*). (×100.)

TABLE 31-11   Pathologic Features of Nonlupus Membranous Glomerulopathy*

	FEATURE PRESENT %
Immunofluorescence Microscopy	
Immunoglobulin G	99 (3.5+)†
Immunoglobulin M	95 (1.2+)
Immunoglobulin A	84 (1.1+)
C3	97 (1.6+)
C1q	34 (1.1+)
κ light chains	98 (3.1+)
λ light chains	98 (2.8+)
Electron Microscopy	
Subepithelial electron-dense deposits	99
Mesangial electron-dense deposits	16
Subendothelial electron-dense deposits	7
Endothelial tubuloreticular inclusions	3
Stage I	38
Stage II	32
Stage III	6
Stage IV	5
Stage V	1
Mixed stage	20

*Based on an analysis of 350 consecutive renal biopsy specimens from patients with nonlupus membranous glomerulopathy evaluated at the University of North Carolina Nephropathology Laboratory.

†Values in parentheses indicate mean intensity of positive staining on a scale of 0 to 4+.

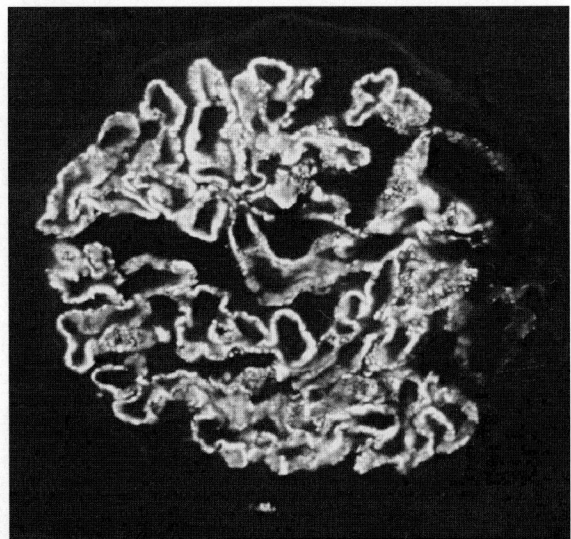

FIGURE 31-9 Immunofluorescence micrograph showing global granular capillary wall staining for immunoglobulin G (IgG) in a glomerulus with membranous glomerulopathy. (Fluorescein isothiocyanate anti-IgG stain, ×300.)

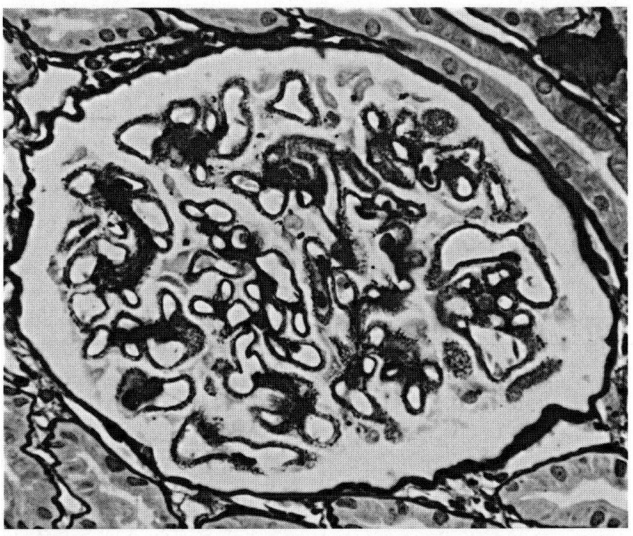

FIGURE 31-10 Light micrograph of a glomerulus with features of stage II membranous glomerulopathy demonstrating spikes along the outer aspects of the glomerular basement membrane (see Figure 31-2). These correspond to the projections of basement membrane material between the immune deposits. (Jones' methenamine silver stain, ×300.)

C1q staining is uncommon and of low intensity in idiopathic MN but is frequent and of high intensity in lupus MN.[328] Although terminal complement components (i.e., components of the membrane attack complex) are not usually evaluated in routine diagnostic preparations, there is very intense staining of the capillary walls for these components. In the rare patients who have concurrent anti-GBM glomerulonephritis and MN, linear staining for IgG can be discerned just below the granular staining.[329]

Tubular basement membrane staining for immunoglobulins or complement is rare in idiopathic MN, but is common in secondary MN, especially lupus MN.[328]

LIGHT MICROSCOPY

The characteristic histologic abnormality by light microscopy is diffuse global capillary wall thickening in the absence of significant glomerular hypercellularity.[330] The light microscopic features of MN, however, vary with the stage of the disease and with the degree of secondary chronic sclerosing glomerular and tubulointerstitial injury. Mild stage I lesions may not be discernible by light microscopy, especially when only a hematoxylin and eosin stain is used. Stage II, III and IV lesions usually have readily discernible thickening of the capillary walls.

Masson trichrome stains may demonstrate the subepithelial immune complex deposits as tiny fuchsinophilic (red) grains along the outer aspect of the GBM. However, this is not a sensitive, specific, or technically reliable method for detecting glomerular immune complex deposits. Special stains that accentuate basement membrane material, such as Jones' silver methenamine stain, may reveal the basement membrane changes that are induced by the subepithelial immune deposits. Spikes along the outer aspect of the GBM usually are seen in stage II lesions (Figure 31-10). Stage III and IV lesions have irregularly thickened and trabeculated basement membranes, which resemble changes that occur with membranoproliferative glomerulonephritis and chronic thrombotic microangiopathy.

Overt mesangial hypercellularity is uncommon in idiopathic MN, although it is more frequent in secondary MN.[328] Crescent formation is rare unless there is concurrent anti-GBM disease or ANCA disease.[331-337]

With disease progression, chronic sclerosing glomerular and tubulointerstitial lesions develop. Glomeruli become segmentally and globally sclerotic, and develop adhesions to Bowman's capsule. Worsening tubular atrophy, interstitial fibrosis, and interstitial infiltration by mononuclear leukocytes parallels progressive loss of renal function.[338]

Pathogenesis

MN is caused by immune complex localization in the subepithelial zone of glomerular capillaries. The nephritogenic antigens can be endogenous to the glomerulus itself (e.g., podocyte autoantigens) or can be exogenous (e.g., hepatitis B antigens). In the latter case, the antigen may be deposited in the subepithelial zone as part of preformed, circulating immune complexes or can be produced in or planted in the subepithelial zone as free antigen to which antibodies bind to form immune complexes in situ. In rat Heymann's nephritis, an animal model that closely resembles human idiopathic MN, there is convincing evidence that the subepithelial immune deposits form in situ as a result of the binding of antibodies to glycoproteins produced by visceral epithelial cells followed by accumulation of masses of the immune complexes in the subepithelial zone.[339-341]

The search for the antigens targeted in a substantial proportion of patients with MN has recently witnessed significant breakthroughs. The podocyte neutral endopeptidase was identified as the endogenous target of autoantibodies in a neonate with nephrotic syndrome. This antibody crossed the placenta and was induced in the mother, who lacked the neutral endopeptidase epitope because of a mutational deletion. Sensitization to the nascent antigen was induced during a previous pregnancy.[342-344] Although this target antigen does not account for a significant proportion of MN cases, these findings provide direct support for the paradigm of in situ immune complex formation in the pathogenesis of human idiopathic MN and constitute an example of alloimmunization leading to the generation of immune complex–mediated glomerulopathy.[325,345]

The team of Salant and Beck recently identified the M-type phospholipase A_2 receptor (PLA_2R) as a target antigen common to about 70% of patients with idiopathic MN.[346] In contrast, none of the sera from normal control subjects, patients with MN secondary to systemic lupus erythematosus or hepatitis B, patients with proteinuric conditions other than MN, or patients with other autoimmune disorders ($n = 7$) reacted with this antigen. Anti-PLA_2R autoantibodies in serum samples from patients with idiopathic MN were predominantly of the IgG4 subclass, which is the predominant immunoglobulin subclass seen in glomerular deposits of patients with this disease. PLA_2R expression in podocytes was confirmed by immunofluorescence microscopy and in cultured immortalized human podocytes, which indicates that this target antigen is intrinsic to the glomeruli rather than deposited from the sera of patients with idiopathic MN. Analysis of serial samples from patients with MN suggests a decline or disappearance of anti-PLA_2R antibodies with the remission of proteinuria.

In a separate set of experiments, the team led by Ghiggeri detected specific anti–aldose reductase (AR) and anti–manganese superoxide dismutase (SOD2) IgG4 in sera of patients with MN.[347] Anti-AR IgG4 and anti-SOD2 IgG4 were also eluted from microdissected glomeruli of patients with MN but not from biopsy specimens of patients with lupus nephritis or membranoproliferative glomerulonephritis. Anti-AR and anti-SOD2 co-localized with IgG4 and C5b9 in electron-dense immune deposits. Interestingly these antigens were detected in glomeruli of patients with MN but not in those of patients with minimal change disease or in normal kidneys. AR was minimally detected in biopsy specimens from patients with IgA nephropathy and type 2 diabetes mellitus, whereas SOD2 was not detected in these patients. The mechanism and trigger for the "neo-expression" of these antigens in podocytes in unknown, and it may be a result of

an initial injury mediated by pathogenic antibody deposition such as anti-PLA_2R, possibly driven by oxidative stress. These important breakthroughs in identifying target antigens in human MN open the door to understanding the role of these autoantibodies in the pathogenesis of primary MN. Their role in the diagnosis, management, and monitoring of patients with MN remains to be established.

Although the nature of the immune complex deposits in MN requires further study, the mechanisms leading to the proteinuric and nephrotic state are better understood. The current understanding of these mechanisms is largely based on data emerging from studies of passive Heymann's nephritis.[341,348] In this model, immune complex formation in the subepithelial zone initiates activation of the complement pathway leading to the formation of the C5b9 membrane attack complex. This results in complement-mediated injury to the epithelial cells.[349-351] The proposed sequence of events includes complement activation and sublytic complement C5b9 attack on podocytes resulting in upregulated expression of genes for the production of oxidants, proteases, prostanoids, growth factors, connective tissue growth factor, TGF, and TGF receptors leading to overproduction of extracellular matrix.[343,345,352] C5b9 also causes alterations of the cytoskeleton that lead to abnormal distribution of slit diaphragm proteins and detachment of viable podocytes. These events result in disruption of the functional integrity of the GBM and the protein filtration barrier of podocytes.

The characteristic findings of a predominance of IgG4 with less IgG3 and no IgG1 in subepithelial deposits,[353,354] and the paucity of C1q and C4 in these deposits,[355] argues against a predominant role for the classical pathway of complement activation in MN, and rather points to a role of the alternative pathway.[356] The fact that the alternative pathway is spontaneously active in turn indicates the likely importance of the complement-regulatory proteins. Podocytes primarily rely on membrane complement receptor 1 (CR1; Crry in rodents) and decay-accelerating factor, and have the capability to make their own factor H. The importance of complement-mediated injury (at least in passive Heymann's nephritis) comes from evidence that nephritogenic serum contains antibodies to membrane complement-regulatory proteins (Crry).[357,358] In a model of active Heymann's nephritis, immunization with fraction 1A (Fx1A) lacking Crry leads to the formation of anti-Fx1A antibodies and subepithelial immune complex deposits, but no complement activation or development of proteinuria.[359] Conversely, the overexpression of Crry or treatment with exogenous Crry has a salutary effect on immune complex–mediated glomerulonephritis.[360,361] Subsequent injury to the epithelial cell membrane and to the GBM is hypothesized to be mediated at least in part by the production of reactive oxygen species and lipid peroxidation of cell membrane proteins and of type IV collagen.[362]

Proteinuria may also be mediated by mechanisms independent of the formation of the C5b9 membrane attack complex, as is suggested by the generation of proteinuria in passive Heymann's nephritis in PVG rats that are deficient in complement factor 6 (PVG/C6− rats). These rats are incapable of generating the membrane attack complex. In this study, PVG/C6− and normal PVG rats developed similar levels of proteinuria after injection of Fx1a antisera. Isolated glomeruli showed similar deposition of rat Ig and C3 staining in both groups of rats, but C9 deposition was not detected in the glomeruli of C6-deficient rats, which indicates that the C5b9 membrane attack complex had not formed.[363] Furthermore, the alteration in the glomerular extracellular matrix seen in MN may be caused, at least in part, by a decrease in fibrinolytic activity, due to the stabilization of active plasminogen activator inhibitor 1 in conjunction with vitronectin in the subepithelial deposits.[364]

Complement activation also results in tubular epithelial cell injury and mediates progressive interstitial disease in MN.[365-367] Proteinuria itself may lead to tubulointerstitial damage through activation of the alternative complement pathway. Strong staining for properdin, a soluble complement regulator also known as *complement factor P*, on the luminal surface of the tubules was observed in kidney biopsy specimens from patients with idiopathic MN, but not in those from healthy kidney donors.[368] After spontaneous hydrolysis of C3, properdin binds to C3b and enhances complement activation by stabilizing C3 convertase. Target-bound properdin may serve as a focal point for amplification of C3 activation. Properdin was shown in vitro to bind proximal tubular epithelial cells. Exposure of proximal tubular epithelial cells to normal human serum as a source of complement, but not to properdin-depleted serum, resulted in complement activation with deposition of C3 and generation of C5b9. This led to the hypothesis that in proteinuric renal disease, filtered properdin may bind to proximal tubular epithelial cells and act as a focal point for alternative pathway activation.

The HLA class II antigen DR3 has been linked with MN,[369-371] and its presence is associated with a relative risk of 12.[369] In a Japanese population, there is an increased frequency of HLA-DR2[372,373] and HLA-Dqw1[374] in patients with MN. It is possible that a haplotype containing HLA-DR3 and specific HLA class I antigens may be common in these patients as well.[369] For instance, HLA-B18 and HLA-DR3 haplotype may confer an even greater risk of the development of MN.[375] Also associated with an increased susceptibility to MN are polymorphisms of the TNF-α gene.[376,377] C4-null alleles are more frequently found in patients with MN, especially in white populations.[378] Whether or not these immunogenetic markers confer a worse prognosis has been controversial.[301] Despite the relative risk associated with some of these immunogenetic markers, there are relatively few examples of familial MN.[379-384]

Clinical Features and Natural History

Patients with MN usually have nephrotic syndrome with hypoalbuminemia, hyperlipidemia, peripheral edema, and lipiduria. This presentation occurs in 70% to 80% of patients.[318,385] The onset of nephrotic syndrome is usually not associated with any prodromal disease process or antecedent infections. Hypertension is present at the outset of disease in 13% to 55% of patients.[320] Most patients have normal or slightly decreased renal function at presentation.

If progressive renal insufficiency develops, it is usually relatively indolent. An abrupt change to more acute renal insufficiency should prompt investigation of a superimposed condition, such as a crescentic glomerulonephritis,[386] which is idiopathic in most cases. One third of these patients have anti-GBM antibodies, and some may have ANCAs.

Other causes of sudden deterioration of renal function include acute bilateral renal vein thrombosis, and hypovolemia

in the setting of massive nephrosis. The incidence of renal vein thrombosis in MN varies from 4% to 52%.[387,388] The diagnosis of renal vein thrombosis may be clinically apparent based on the sudden development of macroscopic hematuria, flank pain, and reduction in renal function, but a more insidious development is also common.[91,389] Although ultrasonography with Doppler studies may demonstrate the renal thrombus,[390] venography with contrast remains the gold standard. Spiral computerized tomography[391] and magnetic resonance imaging with contrast have also been used.

Drug-induced renal injury is another reason for sudden deterioration in renal function in a patient with MN. The use of nonsteroidal antiinflammatory drugs, diuretics, and antimicrobials has been linked to the occurrence of acute interstitial nephritis or acute tubular necrosis.

An estimate of renal survival in patients with MN can be obtained from a pooled analysis of outcomes in clinical studies.[321] In this pooled analysis encompassing 1189 patients,[309,310,319,392-404] the probability of renal survival was 86% at 5 years, 65% at 10 years, and 59% at 15 years. Although 35% of patients may progress to ESRD by 10 years, 25% may experience a complete spontaneous remission of proteinuria within 5 years.[405] In a study in Italy of 100 untreated patients with MN who were followed for 10 years, 30% had progressive renal impairment after 8 years of follow-up. On the other hand, of the 62% who had nephrotic-range proteinuria at presentation, 50% underwent spontaneous remission in 5 years.[399]

In a recent retrospective study of 328 patients with MN who were not treated with immunosuppressive agents, spontaneous remission of proteinuria occurred in 32% of patients: partial remission (proteinuria of ≤3.5 g of protein per day) occurred in a mean of 14.7 ± 11.4 months, and the mean time to complete remission was 38.0 ± 25.2 months.[406] Importantly, severe proteinuria at the onset of disease does not preclude the possibility of spontaneous remission, because it occurred in 26% of patients with baseline proteinuria of 8 to 12 g of protein per day and 21% of patients with baseline proteinuria of more than 12 g of protein per day. On multivariate analysis, the best predictor of spontaneous remission was a decrease in proteinuria of more than 50% in the first year of follow-up (hazard ratio [HR] = 12.6, 95% CI = 5.2 to 30.5, $P < 0.0001$). Other predictors were the baseline serum creatinine level, baseline proteinuria, and the use of angiotensin II inhibitors.[406]

Persistent proteinuria is more predictive of renal insufficiency than proteinuria at a single time point. Thus, persistent proteinuria of ≥8 g protein per day for ≥6 months was associated with a 66% probability of progression to chronic renal failure; patients excreting at least 6 g of protein per day for 9 months or longer had a 55% probability of developing chronic renal insufficiency, and persistent proteinuria of ≥4 g protein per day for longer than 18 months was associated with an even greater increased risk of chronic renal insufficiency.[407] Patients with overtly declining renal function are at higher risk for progressive renal deterioration.[405]

In addition to renal insufficiency and proteinuria, other factors may be associated with an increased risk of progressive renal failure. Male sex, advanced age (older than age 50), poorly controlled hypertension, and reduced GFR at the outset of presentation have been reported as risk factors for progressive decline in renal function.[317,399,403,405,407-411] In addition to the clinical prognostic features, the presence of advanced MN on renal biopsy specimens (stage III or IV), tubular atrophy, and interstitial fibrosis can also be associated with increased risk. In fact, chronic interstitial fibrosis and tubular atrophy have been shown to be independent predictors of progressive renal failure in idiopathic MN.[398,412-414] The presence of crescents on renal biopsy specimens may also portend a poor long-term prognosis. The stage of glomerular lesions detected by electron microscopy has also been suggested as a risk factor for poor prognosis in some[415-417] but not all studies.[306,403,412,418] Similarly, FSGS superimposed on MN may have a worse long-term renal prognosis than MN without sclerosis.[419,420] However, the importance of these demographic and histologic risk factors was not substantiated in a retrospective analysis of a large cohort of patients conducted at the University of Toronto that examined the *rate* of progression (slope).[421] Of the histologic variables, only a greater degree of complement deposition appeared to be associated with a more rapid decline in GFR.[422]

In a prospective study, a urinary β_2-microglobulin level of more than 0.5 µg/min and a urinary IgG level of more than 250 mg/24 hr, assessed in a timed urine sample, were found to predict progressive loss of GFR in a cohort of 57 patients with idiopathic MN and normal kidney function.[423] In a multivariate analysis, urine β_2-microglobulin excretion was the strongest independent predictor of the development of renal insufficiency, with a sensitivity and specificity of 88% and 91%, respectively. Unfortunately, the measurement of urine β_2-microglobulin is cumbersome because it is unstable in urine and requires alkalinization of the urine prior to collection.

In summary, the strongest indicator of progressive disease appears to be *persistence* of moderate proteinuria.[410] Impaired renal function, severe proteinuria at presentation, the presence of substantial interstitial infiltrates on a biopsy specimen, superimposed crescentic glomerulonephritis, and segmental sclerosis also portended a poorer outcome.

Laboratory Findings

Proteinuria is the hallmark of MN. Well over 80% of MN patients excrete more than 3 g of protein per 24 hours. In some patients, the amount of urinary protein may exceed 20 g/day. A Medical Research Council study reported that 30% of patients with MN excreted more than 10 g of protein per day at the time of presentation.[322] Microscopic hematuria is present in 30% to 50% of patients at the time of presentation.[318,424,425] Macroscopic hematuria, on the other hand, is distinctly uncommon and occurs in fewer than 4% of adult patients,[426,427] although it may be common in children.[428] Most patients have either normal or only slightly decreased renal function. In fact, impaired renal function is found in fewer than 10% of patients at the time of presentation.[424,429]

In patients with severe nephrosis, hypoalbuminemia is common, as is the loss of other serum proteins, including IgG. Serum lipoprotein levels are characteristically elevated, as they are in other forms of nephrotic syndrome. Elevated levels of low-density and very low-density lipoproteins are common in MN. In one study, elevated levels of lipoprotein (a) normalized in patients whose disease was in remission.[430]

Levels of complement components C3 and C4 are typically normal in patients with MN. The complex of terminal complement components known as *C5b9* is found in the urine of some patients with active MN. There is increased excretion of this complex in patients with active immune complex formation. The excretion may decrease during disease inactivity.[349-351,431-436]

To exclude common causes of secondary MN, one should order serologic tests for nephritogenic infections such as hepatitis B, hepatitis C, and syphilis, as well as tests for immunologic disorders such as lupus, mixed connective tissue disease, and cryoglobulinemia. MN has been associated with graft-versus-host disease following allogenic stem cell transplantation, and this should be considered as well.[437]

Although hypercoagulability appears to be present in patients with nephrosis in general, this tendency may be enhanced in patients with MN.[387,388,438] The exact mechanisms leading to thrombophilia in this group of patients are poorly understood. Patients with MN have hyperfibrinogenemia with increased levels of circulating procoagulants and decreased levels of anticoagulant factors such as antithrombin III.[439] The thrombotic tendency may be increased by the erythrocytosis that occurs in some patients, as well as by the effect of lipoprotein (a) to retard thrombolysis. Other possible contributors to the thrombophilic state include volume depletion, diuretic and/or steroid use, venous stasis, immobilization, and immune complex activation of the clotting cascade and anti–α-enolase antibodies.[440-442] Renal vein thrombosis is reported more frequently in patients with MN than in those with nephrotic syndrome due to other causes.[387,443-446] The prevalence of renal vein thrombosis in patients with MN ranges from approximately 5% to 63%, depending what mode of diagnosis is used and whether or not systematic screening is performed. The prevalence of all forms of deep vein thrombosis in patients with MN ranges from 9% to 44%. The combined burden of deep vein and renal vein thrombosis has been estimated to be as high as 45%.[442] Renal vein thrombosis is often silent, with pulmonary embolism being the first presenting sign. The risk of venous thromboembolic events appears to be higher when the serum albumin concentration is less than 2.5 g/dL, and such events occur in as many as 40% of these patients.[442,447]

It is the concern for the morbidity and, at times, mortality associated with pulmonary embolism that has led to the use of prophylactic anticoagulation for patients with severe nephrotic syndrome and MN. A decision analysis suggests that the risk of life-threatening complications of pulmonary embolism outweighs the risks associated with anticoagulant therapy.[448] However, this analysis may be based on an overestimation of the true incidence of thromboses among patients with MN. No direct controlled data are available to support or refute such a contention. There is no direct support for the routine use of prophylactic anticoagulation in patients with idiopathic MN. The case could be made for the judicious use of warfarin in patients with severe nephrotic syndrome who have a profoundly decreased serum albumin level (probably <2 mg/dL) if no contraindications are present.[325]

Treatment

CORTICOSTEROIDS

Despite numerous studies, the optimal treatment of MN remains incompletely defined. The difficulty in treating MN is a consequence of the chronic nature of the disease, the tendency for spontaneous remission and relapse, the variability of clinical severity, and the only partial efficacy of existing treatment protocols. The role of corticosteroids and alkylating agents in the treatment of this disease has been debated for decades. The common therapeutic approaches for new-onset disease include (1) conservative therapy with RAAS blockade, (2) corticosteroid therapy (usually prednisone or methylprednisolone), and (3) administration of alkylating agents, such as chlorambucil or cyclophosphamide, with or without concurrent corticosteroid treatment.

Numerous studies providing corticosteroid treatment have demonstrated different outcomes.[308-310,319,392-399,402-405,418,449,450] In a pooled analysis of these studies, corticosteroid therapy was found to have no beneficial effect on renal survival.[321] Three large prospective randomized trials examined the efficacy of oral corticosteroid therapy in adult patients with MN with different results.[394,395,451] Findings of the U.S. Collaborative Study[308] suggested that 8 weeks of treatment with 100 to 150 mg of prednisone given on alternate days resulted in a transient decrease in urinary protein excretion to less than 2 g of protein compared with placebo. Prednisone was discontinued after 3 months unless proteinuria recurred after either a partial or complete remission. Relapses were treated by reinstitution of high-dose prednisone therapy for 1 month followed by a taper. The results of this study suggested that patients treated with prednisone were less likely to experience a doubling of their entry serum creatinine level and were more likely to experience a transient decrease in proteinuria to less than 2 g of protein per day, and that even a partial remission of proteinuria was associated with well-preserved, long-term renal function. This seminal study was criticized because the control group faired substantially worse than did nontreated patients in several other studies.

A British Medical Research Council study[394] utilized a similar regimen except that prednisolone was discontinued after 8 weeks without tapering and without treatment of any relapse of proteinuria. Patients with lower creatinine clearance (≤30 mL/min) were included in the study. Three to nine months after study entry, patients showed no improvement in renal function, and urine protein excretion and albumin levels improved only transiently.

A third prospective randomized study of corticosteroid therapy reported by Cattran and colleagues[395] included patients with relatively low levels of proteinuria (≤0.3 g of protein per day). In this study, alternate-day treatment with prednisone (45 mg/m² of body surface area) afforded no benefit with regard to either proteinuria or renal function.

In a meta-analysis[321] of the U.S. Collaborative Study[308] and the studies by Cameron and colleagues,[394] Cattran and colleagues,[395] and Kobayashi and colleagues[396] comparing glucocorticoid treatment with supportive therapy, corticosteroid therapy was associated with a trend toward achievement of complete remission at 24 to 36 months, but this result did not reach statistical significance. A pooled analysis of randomized trials and prospective studies again demonstrated a lack of benefit of corticosteroid therapy in inducing a remission of nephrotic syndrome or preserving renal function.

An alternative to oral glucocorticoid therapy has been treatment with pulse methylprednisolone, largely in patients with deteriorating renal function. Treatment of patients with renal insufficiency using pulse methylprednisolone at 1 g/day for 5 days followed by oral prednisone was associated with an improvement in renal function for 6 months and a reduction in proteinuria.[452] The long-term outcomes for over half of these patients were discouraging: one third experienced renal failure, and 13% developed myocardial infarction with renal dysfunction. A similar study[453] combined pulse methylprednisolone with azathioprine or cyclophosphamide. Although there may have been some improvement in proteinuria and renal function in a minority of patients, substantial side effects were experienced by almost the entire study population. The evidence to date does not support the use of oral corticosteroids alone for the treatment of idiopathic MN.

CYCLOPHOSPHAMIDE OR CHLORAMBUCIL

Cytotoxic drugs, including cyclophosphamide and chlorambucil, have been used for the treatment of idiopathic MN in conjunction with intravenous and oral corticosteroids. In a number of studies, Ponticelli and colleagues demonstrated that chlorambucil has a beneficial effect in the treatment of MN.[398,416,418,454] In these studies, patients with idiopathic MN were treated initially with intravenous pulse methylprednisolone at 1 g/day for the first 3 days of each month, with daily oral glucocorticoid therapy (methylprednisolone at 0.4 mg/kg/day or prednisone at 0.5 mg/kg/day), given on an alternating monthly schedule with chlorambucil at a dose of 0.2 mg/kg/day. In patients randomly assigned to the treatment group, nephrotic syndrome lasted for a significantly shorter duration and a complete or partial remission of proteinuria occurred in 83% of MN patients compared with 38% of control patients.[454] The slope of the mean reciprocal plasma creatinine level remained stable in the treatment group, but declined in the untreated patients beginning at 12 months. At 10-year follow-up, the probability of having a functioning kidney was 92% in the treated patients and 60% in the control patients. In only 10% of patients was therapy discontinued because of side effects. Compared to treatment with glucocorticoids alone, treatment with a combination of chlorambucil and methylprednisolone was associated with an earlier remission of nephrotic syndrome and a greater stability of complete or partial remission of proteinuria.[418] Interestingly, the overall decline in renal function was no different in the two treatment groups. Unfortunately, although a difference in favor of the chlorambucil-treated patients persisted for the first 3 years of follow-up, it was no longer statistically significant by 4 years (62% without nephrotic syndrome in the group receiving combination therapy vs. 42% in the steroid-only group, $P = 0.102$). In a study comparing cyclophosphamide with chlorambucil, cyclophosphamide was found to be at least as effective as chlorambucil when used in a similar dosing protocol and appeared to have somewhat fewer side effects.[455]

Despite these reported benefits, the salutary effects of alkylating agents combined with prednisone or other agents have not been confirmed in other trials.[397,401,404,456] These conflicting results prompted two meta-analyses of controlled trials of either cyclophosphamide or chlorambucil treatment of MN.[321,457] Both meta-analyses suggested that use of cytotoxic agents improves the chance of a complete remission of proteinuria by fourfold to fivefold, but has no long-term protective effect on renal survival.

A new prospective, open-label, randomized study in India[458] involving 93 patients followed for a median of 11 years (range = 10.5 to 12 years) compared supportive therapy (dietary sodium restriction, diuretics, and antihypertensive agents) with a 6-month course of alternate months of steroid and cyclophosphamide treatment similar to the Ponticelli protocol.[459] Unfortunately, angiotensin II blockade was withheld in all patients for at least 1 year. Study endpoints were doubling of serum creatinine level, development of ESRD, or patient death. Of the 47 patients who received the immunosuppressive protocol, 34 experienced remission compared with 16 of 46 in the control group ($P < 0.0001$). The 10-year dialysis-free survival was 89% in the immunosuppression group and 65% in the supportive treatment group ($P = 0.016$) and the likelihood of survival without death, dialysis, or doubling of serum creatinine level was 79% and 44% ($P = 0.0006$), respectively. A significant divergence between the two groups in terms of proteinuria became apparent within the first year, and the estimated GFR was significantly lower in the control group than in the cyclophosphamide-treated group from 4 years onward. This study confirms, in a different patient population, the short- and long-term benefits associated with treatment with cyclophosphamide and corticosteroids according to the Ponticelli protocol.[454,459]

CALCINEURIN INHIBITORS
There has been substantial interest in the use of cyclosporine, which has resulted in improvement in proteinuria and stability of renal function in many patients.[460-462] In a randomized, controlled trial comparing 26 weeks of treatment with cyclosporine plus low-dose prednisone to treatment with placebo plus prednisone, 75% of the cyclosporine group but only 22% of the control group ($P < 0.001$) experienced a partial or complete remission of proteinuria by 26 weeks. Relapse occurred in about 40% of patients achieving remission in both treatment groups. The fraction of patients achieving sustained remission remained significantly different between the two groups until the end of the study (cyclosporine treatment 39% vs. placebo 13%, $P = 0.007$). Renal function was unchanged and equal in the two groups over the test medication period.[463] This study was criticized for the rapid discontinuation of cyclosporine over 4 weeks at the end of the 26-week treatment period.

In a prospective study, treatment with cyclosporine alone (2 to 3 mg/kg/day) was compared to treatment with a combination of cyclosporine and oral prednisolone in 51 patients.[464] Prednisolone was started at 0.6 mg/kg/day then gradually tapered to 10 to 15 mg/day at 6 months and continued to 12 months. Patients who experienced complete or partial remission then received long-term treatment with lower dosages of cyclosporine (1 to 1.5 mg/kg/day) plus prednisolone (0.1 mg/kg/day) or cyclosporine alone. This study did not have a randomized design because patients with contraindications to corticosteroid use were assigned to the cyclosporine-only group. During the follow-up phase of the study, relapses were more common in patients treated with cyclosporine alone than in patients receiving cyclosporine plus oral prednisolone (47% vs. 15%, respectively; $P < 0.05$). However, the results suggests that the risk of relapse may be determined by the levels of cyclosporine, because patients in both groups who experienced relapse had lower cyclosporine trough levels than those who did not experience nonrelapse (72 ± 48 ng/mL vs. 194 ± 80 ng/mL, respectively; $P < 0.03$).

A prospective randomized controlled trial was undertaken to evaluate monotherapy with tacrolimus versus supportive therapy alone in 48 patients with MN who had preserved renal function and had had persistent nephrotic syndrome for longer than 9 months despite treatment with an ACE inhibitor or ARB.[465] Treatment with tacrolimus consisted of 0.05 mg/kg/day divided into two daily doses and adjusted to achieve a whole-blood 12-hour trough level between 3 and 5 ng/mL. The target trough level was increased to between 5 and 8 ng/mL if a remission was not obtained after the first 2 months of treatment. Tacrolimus was continued for a total of 12 months followed by a 6-month taper. The probability of remission in the treatment group was 58%, 82%, and 94% after 6, 12, and 18 months, but was only 10%, 24%, and 35%, respectively, in the control group. The decrease in proteinuria was significantly greater in the treatment group. Notably, six patients in the control group and only one in the treatment group reached the secondary endpoint of a 50% increase in serum creatinine level. Unfortunately, as in the previously published study of cyclosporine, almost half of the patients who had achieved remission experienced a recurrence of nephrotic syndrome by the eighteenth month after tacrolimus withdrawal.

An interesting pilot study in Spain[466] looked at combination therapy with corticosteroids, MMF, and tacrolimus in patients who had persistent nephrotic syndrome after 6 months of treatment with full-dose RAAS blockers and a creatinine clearance of more than 60 mL/min/1.73 m². The initial dosage of prednisone was 0.5 mg/kg/day for the first month, and the drug was then tapered to 7.5 mg/day at month 6. The starting dosage of tacrolimus was 0.05 mg/kg/day to achieve target whole-blood trough levels of 7 to 9 ng/mL. If the level of proteinuria was less than 1 g of protein per day at the end of 3 months of this therapy, the tacrolimus dosage was reduced to maintain blood levels between 5 and 7 ng/mL and continued for a period of 9 more months. If, however, the level of proteinuria was greater than 1 g of protein per day, the dose of tacrolimus was reduced and MMF was added at a dosage of 0.5 g twice daily and adjusted to achieve a target whole-blood trough level of 2 to 4 mg/L. Triple therapy was then maintained for 9 additional months, after which immunosuppressants were tapered off over 3 months in all patients. Of the 21 adult patients enrolled, 11 had proteinuria of less than 1 g of protein per day in at the end of 3 months and then received maintenance dosages of prednisone plus tacrolimus. MMF was added after the third month in nine patients and was associated with complete or partial remission in five. Unfortunately, the relapse rate was very high in all groups of patients, whether treated with double or triple therapy. Clearly, additional controlled trials are required to determine the optimal duration of treatment and the benefit of adding MMF in patients who show only partial response to treatment with calcineurin inhibitors alone.

OTHER FORMS OF IMMUNOSUPPRESSIVE THERAPY
The use of synthetic adrenocorticotropic hormone (ACTH) has been assessed in patients with nephrotic syndrome, including those with MN.[467] In one randomized controlled trial,[468] 32 patients were treated with either corticosteroids and chlorambucil or cyclophosphamide administered according to the Ponticelli protocol, or with ACTH (tetracosactide) administered intramuscularly twice weekly for a year. Eighty-seven percent of patients in the ACTH arm experienced complete or partial remission with a dramatic reduction in proteinuria and mean serum cholesterol level at almost 3 years.[468] Few patients developed symptoms and signs of excess glucocorticoids. The

long-acting synthetic ACTH formulation used in this study is not available in the United States, but is available in Europe. The mechanism responsible for the beneficial effect of ACTH is unknown. Recent evidence points to the expression of the melanocortin 1 receptor on podocytes, which suggests a possible direct effect of ACTH on these cells.[469]

In the last few years, interest has arisen in the use of MMF and rituximab for the management of MN. The use of MMF to treat MN has been the focus of a few small studies yielding disparate results. In an open-label study in the Netherlands 32 patients with idiopathic MN treated with MMF were compared with a historical matched control group treated with oral cyclophosphamide for 12 months.[470] Both groups received intermittent methylprednisolone and alternate-day prednisone. Although on average the degree of proteinuria decreased similarly in the MMF-treated group and in the cyclophosphamide-treated group, and although the cumulative incidence of remission of proteinuria at 12 months was comparable in the two groups, the percentage of patients who showed no response to therapy was statistically significantly higher in the MMF-treated group, as was the proportion of patients who experienced a relapse.

In a 1-year randomized controlled trial of 36 patients, treatment with MMF (target dose of 2 g/day) for 12 months was compared with conservative care alone.[471] The change in mean urine protein/creatinine ratio from baseline to month 12 was measured; the ratio decreased by 1834 mg/g in the control group, and increased by 213 mg/g in the MMF group ($P = 0.3$). Complete or partial remission at month 12 was observed in 37% of patients in the MMF group and 41% in the control group.

In a separate prospective, randomized, controlled, open-label study involving 20 patients in Hong Kong and Shanghai,[472] treatment with MMF and prednisolone given for 6 months was compared with treatment that followed a modified Ponticelli regime.[455] Over a total follow-up of 15 months, proteinuria decreased to a similar extent in both groups. The rates of complete and partial remission were 27.3% and 36.4%, respectively, in the MMF group, and 33.3% and 33.3% in the control group. These results are in marked distinction to those of the previously described study comparing MMF with conservative therapy.[471] These two studies differ in the makeup of the patient populations (whites versus Asians) and in the concomitant use of prednisolone in the Hong Kong/Shanghai study. Overall, the results of studies of MMF have been disappointing with a notable exception of that involving Chinese patients.

Recent years have seen great interest in the use of the anti-CD20 monoclonal antibody rituximab for the treatment of a number of antibody-mediated autoimmune diseases, including MN. In an initial report of eight patients, treatment with rituximab (4 weekly doses of 375 mg/m² body surface area) was associated with prompt and sustained reduction in proteinuria.[473,474] There have since been additional open-label studies,[475-478] but no controlled trial of this agent has been undertaken yet, and its effects on long-term renal outcome are unproven. The available uncontrolled data suggest that rituximab, dosed either at 375 mg/m² once weekly for 4 weeks or at 1 g on days 1 and 15, achieves a 15% to 20% rate of complete remission and a 40% to 45% rate of partial remission.[479]

A recent cohort study reported on the effect of rituximab therapy in 13 patients with MN deemed to be calcineurin

inhibitor dependent (defined as the occurrence of at least four calcineurin inhibitor–responsive relapses of nephrotic proteinuria while the patient was being weaned off these drugs).[480] After rituximab therapy (375 mg/m² weekly for 4 weeks, with each dose preceded by 125 mg of methylprednisolone), proteinuria decreased significantly, and calcineurin inhibitors and other immunosuppressant drugs could be withdrawn in all patients.

Although the aggregate of these uncontrolled case series suggests a beneficial effect of rituximab in the management of MN, whether, when, and how (and how long) to use rituximab in treating MN remain to be determined, and a randomized controlled study comparing rituximab with either cyclophosphamide and corticosteroids, or calcineurin inhibitor therapy is needed.

Other forms of therapy have been tried in idiopathic MN, with varying results. These include the use of azathioprine,[449,450] which demonstrated no positive effect either alone or in combination with prednisone. The use of pooled intravenous immunoglobulin has been evaluated only in a small case series[481] and a retrospective study.[482]

Based on the greater appreciation of the role of complement activation and especially that of complement-regulatory proteins in the pathogenesis of MN, a great deal of interest exists in targeting this pathway for therapy. Several compounds are under development. To date, human trials have been conducted only for eculizumab, a monoclonal antibody directed against the fifth component of complement (C5). In a randomized trial involving patients with de novo MN, treatment with eculizumab was not associated with a statistically significant improvement in proteinuria or preservation of renal function. These disappointing results were likely due to insufficient dosing, because consistent inhibition of complement was achieved in only a minority of patients.[483] Nevertheless, this general approach is thought to hold a great deal of promise based on early animal studies.

In the absence of a full understanding of the pathogenesis of MN, and thus an effective targeted therapy, the current approach to the treatment of MN must rely on risk stratification. The indolent disease process that results in spontaneous remissions in one quarter of patients, coupled with the known adverse consequences of long-term treatment with oral glucocorticoids, alkylating agents, and calcineurin inhibitors, should prompt a careful analysis of the risk/benefit ratio in the treatment of any given patient. All patients should receive excellent supportive care, including treatment with RAAS blockers[235,484-487] and lipid-lowering agents. Most patients should be observed for the development of adverse prognostic factors or the occurrence of spontaneous remissions. Adult patients with good prognostic features should be managed conservatively without the use of immunomodulatory or immunosuppressive agents.

Patients at moderate risk (persistent proteinuria of between 4 and 6 g of protein per day despite RAAS blockade and normal renal function) or at high risk of progression (persistent proteinuria of more than 8 g of protein per day with or without renal insufficiency) should be considered for immunosuppressive therapy with either a combination of glucocorticoids and cyclophosphamide (or chlorambucil) in alternating monthly pulses (Ponticelli protocol), or a calcineurin inhibitor with low-dose glucocorticoids. A current recommendation gives preference to the use of a cytotoxic treatment approach in patients with moderate risk of progression and to the use of cyclosporine in patients at high risk of progression.[488] This decision must be individualized to each patient with consideration of the patient's comorbidities and assessment of the risk associated with each kind of therapy. Whenever a calcineurin inhibitor is used, close attention must be given to the consistent use of the same formulation over time, and therapy should be initiated at a low to moderate dosage, followed by a dosage adjustment with careful evaluation of changes in blood pressure and creatinine clearance. The data currently available do not suggest that MMF alone is effective. Whether ACTH and rituximab are viable effective alternatives awaits further confirmation.

Individuals who have advanced chronic renal failure are best managed by supportive care while awaiting dialysis and renal transplantation. Acute renal insufficiency in this population should prompt evaluation for interstitial nephritis, crescentic nephritis, and renal vein thrombosis.

Membranoproliferative Glomerulonephritis (Mesangial Capillary Glomerulonephritis)

Membranoproliferative glomerulonephritis (MPGN) is a collection of morphologically related but pathogenetically distinct disorders that have traditionally been classified into three subtypes, MPGN types I, II, and III. The primary basis for this classification is histologic, namely, the appearance of the capillary wall by electron microscopy and the location of electron-dense deposits. MPGN types I and II (dense deposit disease) form the major subtypes of this rare form of glomerular disease. MPGN is identified in approximately 10% of renal biopsy specimens[489,490] and appears to be decreasing in frequency.[491] Recent advances in the understanding of the different pathogeneses of these subtypes and the diverse morphologic findings in MPGN type II have raised the question as to whether these disease entities should be completely separated rather than grouped under the umbrella of MPGN. They are described separately in this section.

Membranoproliferative Glomerulonephritis Type I

EPIDEMIOLOGY
The majority of patients with MPGN are children between the ages of 8 and 16 years,[492] who account for 90% of the cases of MPGN type I. The proportions of males and females with the disorder are nearly equal.[489,490,493-501]

PATHOLOGY
Light Microscopy. The most common histologic features of type I MPGN are diffuse global capillary wall thickening, increased mesangial matrix, and endocapillary hypercellularity.[493,502] Infiltrating mononuclear leukocytes and neutrophils also contribute to the glomerular hypercellularity. The consolidation of glomerular segments that results from these changes often causes an accentuation of the segmentation referred to as *hypersegmentation* or *lobulation*. As a consequence, an earlier name for this phenotype of glomerular injury was *lobular glomerulonephritis*. Markedly expanded mesangial regions may develop a nodular appearance with a central zone of sclerosis that may resemble that of diabetic glomerulosclerosis or monoclonal immunoglobulin deposition disease. However,

the integration of light, immunofluorescence, and electron microscopic findings differentiates type I MPGN from other diseases that can mimic it by light microscopy.

A distinctive but not completely specific feature of type I MPGN is a doubling or more complex replication of GBMs that can be seen with stains that highlight basement membranes, such as Jones' silver methenamine stain or periodic acid–Schiff stain (Figure 31-11). This change is caused by the production of basement membrane material between and around projections of mesangial cytoplasm that extend into an expanded subendothelial zone, probably in response to the presence of subendothelial immune complex deposits (Figure 31-12). The presence of "hyaline thrombi" within capillary lumens should raise the possibility of cryoglobulinemia or lupus as the cause for the MPGN. Hyaline thrombi are not true thrombi but rather are aggregates of immune complexes

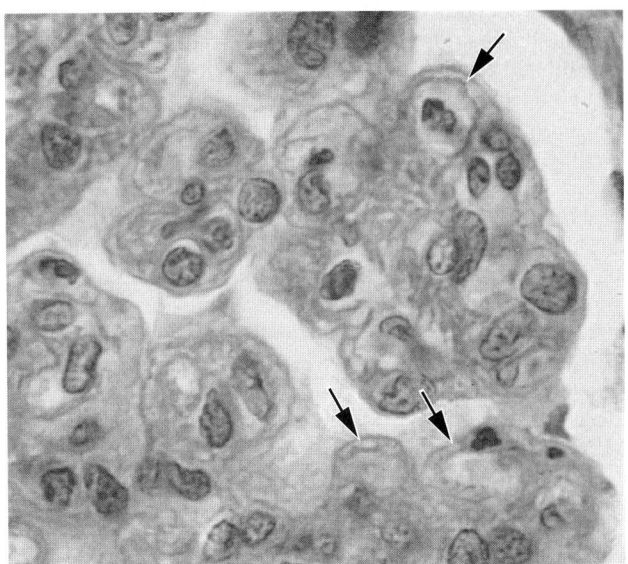

FIGURE 31-11 Light micrograph of a glomerular segment from a patient with type I membranoproliferative glomerulonephritis (MPGN) demonstrating doubling (*arrows*) and more complex replication of glomerular basement membranes. (Periodic acid–Schiff stain, ×1000.)

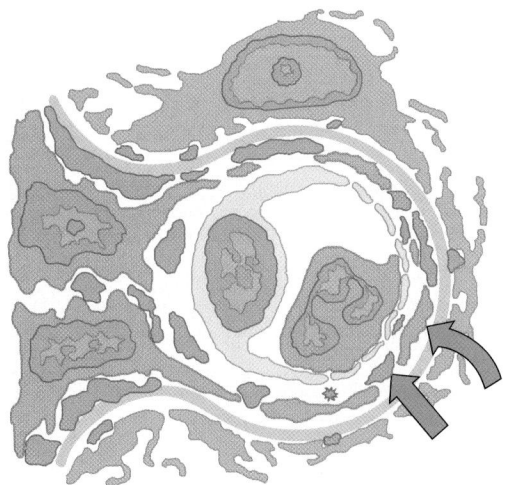

FIGURE 31-12 Diagram depicting the ultrastructural features of type I membranoproliferative glomerulonephritis (MPGN). Note the subendothelial dense deposits (*straight arrow*), subendothelial mesangial cytoplasm interposition (*curved arrow*), and production of new basement material (*asterisk*). (Courtesy of J.C. Jennette.)

filling capillary lumens. A minority of patients with type I MPGN have crescents, but these rarely involve more than 50% of glomeruli.[503,504] As with other types of glomerulonephritis, substantial crescent formation correlates with a more rapid progression of disease.[502]

Immunofluorescence Microscopy. The characteristic pattern of immunofluorescence staining is peripheral granular to bandlike staining for complement, especially C3, and usually immunoglobulins (Figure 31-13). This corresponds to the prominent subendothelial immune complex localization seen by electron microscopy. The staining pattern is less granular and less symmetrical than that usually seen in MN. Mesangial granular staining may be conspicuous or inconspicuous. The hypersegmentation or lobulation that is seen by light microscopy often can be discerned by immunofluorescence microscopy. A minority of patients with type I MPGN have staining of immune complexes along tubular basement membranes or in extraglomerular vessels, or both.

The composition of the immune deposits is variable, which probably reflects the many different causes of type I MPGN. Most specimens have more intense staining for C3 than for any immunoglobulin, but some specimens have more intense staining for IgG or IgM. Rare specimens have a predominance of IgA and can be considered an MPGN expression of IgA nephropathy. Even when C3 is the most intensely staining immune determinant, most specimens have clear-cut staining for IgG or IgM or both. Intracapillary globular structures that stain intensely for immunoglobulin and complement correspond to the hyaline thrombi seen by light microscopy and raise the possibility of MPGN caused by lupus or cryoglobulinemia.

Electron Microscopy. The ultrastructural hallmark of type I MPGN is mesangial interposition into an expanded subendothelial zone that contains electron-dense immune complex deposits (Figures 31-12 and 31-14). This distinct pattern of mesangial and capillary involvement has prompted a synonym for type I MPGN, *mesangiocapillary glomerulonephritis.* New

basement membrane material is formed around the subendothelial deposits and around the projections of mesangial cytoplasm, which is the basis for the basement membrane replication seen by light microscopy (see Figure 31-11). Scattered mesangial dense deposits are usually found in association with mesangial hypercellularity and mesangial matrix expansion. Variable numbers of subepithelial electron-dense deposits occur. When they are numerous enough to resemble MN, some nephropathologists apply the diagnosis "mixed membranous and proliferative glomerulonephritis" or "type III MPGN" as proposed by Burkholder and colleagues.[505] The term *type III MPGN* also has been applied to a very rare pattern of glomerular injury that resembles type I MPGN by light

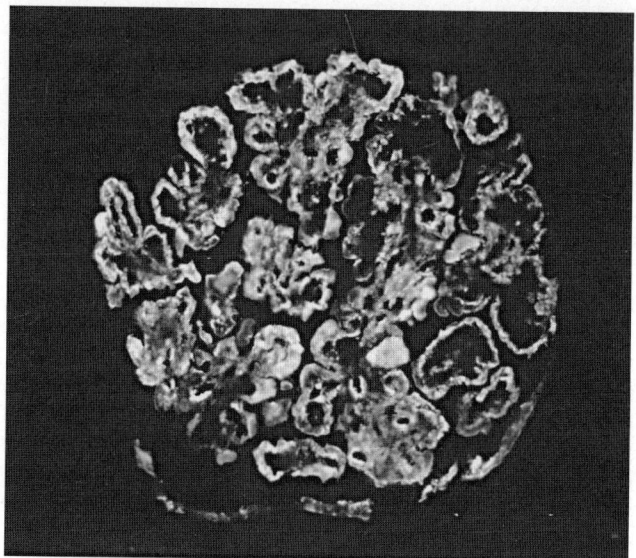

FIGURE 31-13 Immunofluorescence micrograph of a glomerulus with features of type I membranoproliferative glomerulonephritis (MPGN) showing global bandlike capillary wall staining for C3, as well as irregular mesangial staining. (Fluorescein isothiocyanate anti-C3 stain, ×300.)

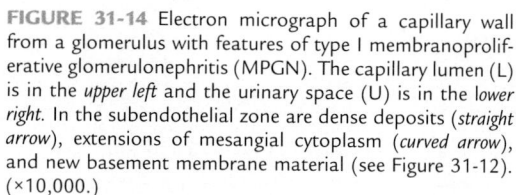

FIGURE 31-14 Electron micrograph of a capillary wall from a glomerulus with features of type I membranoproliferative glomerulonephritis (MPGN). The capillary lumen (L) is in the *upper left* and the urinary space (U) is in the *lower right.* In the subendothelial zone are dense deposits (*straight arrow*), extensions of mesangial cytoplasm (*curved arrow*), and new basement membrane material (see Figure 31-12). (×10,000.)

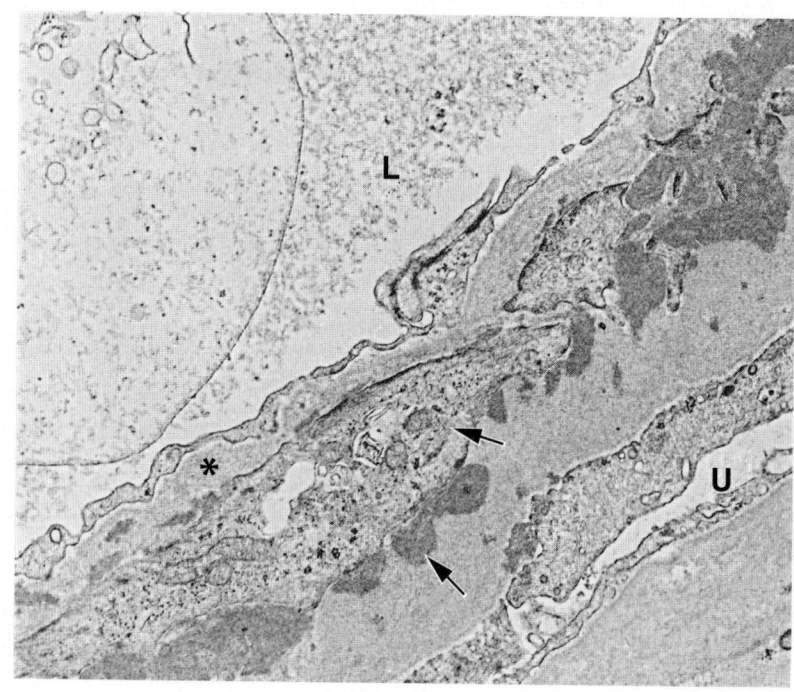

microscopy and immunofluorescence microscopy, but is characterized ultrastructurally by irregularly thickened GBMs with numerous intramembranous deposits of variable density.[497,506]

The hyaline thrombi seen by light microscopy appear as intraluminal spherical densities. When these structures, or any of the other electron-dense deposits, have a microtubular substructure, the possibility of cryoglobulinemic glomerulonephritis or immunotactoid glomerulopathy should be considered.

PATHOGENESIS

Although the pathologic findings indicate that type I MPGN is an immune complex disease, the identity of the nephritogenic antigen is unknown in most patients. In the minority of patients in whom the nature of the antigen has been identified, the sources have included infections, neoplasms, hereditary diseases, and autoimmune diseases (Table 31-12). The pathologic finding of intense immune complex deposition with hypercellularity suggests that the inflammation caused by the immune complexes has resulted in both proliferation of mesangial and endothelial cells, and the recruitment of inflammatory cells, including neutrophils and monocytes. These leukocytes are attracted to the glomerulus by activation of multiple mediator systems, including the complement system, cytokines, and chemokines.

Type I MGPN often is secondary to recognizable causes, such as cryoglobulinemia, hepatitis C, hepatitis B, osteomyelitis, subacute bacterial endocarditis, infected ventriculoatrial shunt, malignancies,[507–509] autoimmune diseases (systemic lupus erythematosus or autoimmune thyroiditis[510]), light-chain nephropathy,[511] and celiac sprue.[512] Serologic and clinical evidence of these processes should be sought. The precise percentage of patients with MPGN due to hepatitis C may vary according to geographic area and cultural factors. The observation that upper respiratory tract infections precede the onset of what is considered idiopathic MPGN in as many as one half of patients[492] raises the possibility that infectious agents contribute to the pathogenesis of many cases of idiopathic type I MPGN.

When type I MPGN is secondary to other disease processes such as malignancy or a rheumatic condition, the laboratory results associated with the systemic disease (e.g., systemic lupus erythematosus) are positive (e.g., antibodies to double-stranded DNA). (See Chapter 32.)

One of the hallmarks of the laboratory abnormalities in types I and II MPGN is alteration in the complement cascade (Table 31-13). C3 level is persistently depressed in approximately 75% of MPGN patients.[489,493,513-515] This is in contrast to poststreptococcal glomerulonephritis, in

TABLE 31-12 Classification of Membranoproliferative Glomerulonephritis (MPGN)

Primary (Idiopathic) MPGN
Type I
Type II
Type III

Secondary MPGN
Associated with Infection
Hepatitis C and B
Visceral abscesses
Infective endocarditis
Shunt nephritis
Quartan malaria
Schistosoma nephropathy
Mycoplasma infection

Associated with Rheumatologic Disease
Systemic lupus erythematosus
Scleroderma
Sjögren's syndrome
Sarcoidosis
Mixed essential cryoglobulinemia with or without hepatitis C infection
Anti–smooth muscle syndrome

Associated with Malignancy
Carcinoma
Lymphoma
Leukemia

Associated with an Inherited Disorder
α_1-Antitrypsin deficiency
Complement deficiency (C2 or C3), with or without partial lipodystrophy

From references 971, 1279-1287.

TABLE 31-13 Selected Serologic Findings in Patients with Primary Glomerular Disease

DISEASE	C4	C3	ASO, ADNase B	cryo Ig	ANTI-GBM	ANCA
Minimal change glomerulopathy	N	N	-	-	-	-
Focal glomerulosclerosis	N	N	-	-	-	-
Membranous GN	N	N	-	-	-	-
Membranoproliferative GN						
Type I	N or ⇊	⇊	+	++	-	-
Type II	N	⇊⇊⇊	+		-	-
Fibrillary GN	N	N	-	-	-	-
Immunoglobulin A nephropathy	N	N	-	-	-	-
Acute poststreptococcal GN	N or ↓	⇊	+++	++	-	-
Crescentic GN						
Anti-GBM	N	N	-	-	+++	±
Immune complex	N or ↓	N or ⇊	-	N/++	-	±
ANCA small vessel vasculitis	N	N	-	-	±	+++

ANCA, Antineutrophil cytoplasmic antibody; *ASO*, anti–streptolysin O; *ADNase B*, antideoxyribonuclease B; *cryo Ig*, cryoglobulins; *GBM*, glomerular basement membrane; *GN*, glomerulonephritis; *N*, normal levels.

which depressed C3 levels typically return to normal within 2 months.[516-518] The persistent depression of C3 levels and the presence of nephritic syndrome should suggest type I MPGN. The depression of C3 levels is a consequence of both the activation of the alternative complement pathway and low synthetic levels. Activation of the alternative pathway is suggested by the observation that in type I MPGN, C3 levels are depressed, whereas levels of the classical pathway activators C1q and C4 are usually normal. When MPGN is caused by cryoglobulinemia, however, there may be more depression of C4 than of C3.[519]

Type I MPGN is also associated with underlying complement deficiency, notably of C2 and C3,[520] as well as deficiency in α_1-antitrypsin.

CLINICAL FEATURES

Type I MPGN (characterized by deposits of electron-dense material in the subendothelial zones of glomeruli) is a very heterogeneous disorder. Some combination of proteinuria (often nephrotic range), hematuria, hypertension, and renal failure are usually present.

TREATMENT

The prognosis of type I MPGN has been reviewed and described in several reports.[489,493,521,522] The 10-year renal survival rate appears to be between 40% in persistently nephrotic patients[493] and 65%.[489] Nonnephrotic patients have an improved 10-year renal survival of 85%.[493] A minority of patients may experience spontaneous remission.[489] The features suggestive of poor prognosis in idiopathic type I MPGN include hypertension,[501,523] impaired GFR,[501,523-525] the presence of nephrotic syndrome,[493,523,524,526] and the appearance of cellular crescents in biopsy specimens.[493,525,527]

The treatment of type I MPGN is based on the underlying cause of the disease process. Thus, the therapy for MPGN associated with cryoglobulinemia and hepatitis C should be aimed at treating hepatitis C virus infection, whereas the treatment of MPGN associated with lupus or scleroderma should be based on the principles of care for those rheumatologic conditions. Most recommendations for the treatment of type I MPGN are derived from studies involving children.[528-535] West touted the benefits of continuous prednisone therapy for improved renal survival.[530] Whether the benefit of low-dose prednisone therapy is seen only in children or whether similar effects can be achieved in adults has never been investigated in a prospective randomized trial. However, low-dose, alternate-day prednisone therapy may improve renal function.[533,534]

In addition to glucocorticoids, a number of other immunosuppressive and anticoagulant agents have been used in the treatment of type I MPGN. Initial reports indicated that treatment with aspirin and dipyridamole had a positive effect in renal survival.[490] This approach was widely accepted; however, statistical design flaws led to a reanalysis of the data, which revealed no difference in the treatment and control groups with respect to long-term outcome.[513] A subsequent study using aspirin with dipyridamole demonstrated a slight decrease in urine protein excretion by 3 years but no effect on renal function.[536] Treatment with dipyridamole, aspirin, and warfarin, with and without cyclophosphamide, was examined in both controlled and uncontrolled studies.[397,490,535-540] A regimen of warfarin, dipyridamole, and cyclophosphamide[535] was suggested to improve long-term renal survival based on

a retrospective analysis; however, a controlled trial in Canada demonstrated no benefit of this approach.[395]

The use of MMF and corticosteroids has been suggested based on uncontrolled and anecdotal observations.[541] In patients with a defined underlying disease (e.g., neoplasia or hepatitis B or C), treatment should be directed at the underlying condition.[542,543]

Type I MPGN is significantly ameliorated by the use of cyclosporine in the very rare condition known as *Buckley's syndrome*.[96,97,544]

Membranoproliferative Glomerulonephritis Type III

Type III MPGN occurs in a very small number of children and young adults. Regardless of the pathologic distinctions of MPGN type III made by Burkholder and colleagues[505] and Strife and colleagues,[506] few distinguishing clinical characteristics are noted in these patients. These patients may have clinical features of disease quite similar to those of type I MPGN, and the long-term clinical course is quite similar as well. Patients with MPGN described by Strife and colleagues[497] had low C3 levels in the absence of C3 nephritic factor. Patients with nonnephrotic proteinuria do better than patients who have nephrotic syndrome. In the authors' own experience, progression to ESRD is quite variable, but it appears that in some patients the disease stabilizes or even improves with long-term renal survival.

Dense Deposit Disease (Membranoproliferative Glomerulonephritis Type II)

EPIDEMIOLOGY

Dense deposit disease (also known as *type II MPGN*) accounts for about 25% of MPGN in children but is much less common in adults. The large majority of patients are children between the ages of 8 and 16 years,[492] who account for about 70% of cases. It is estimated to affect 2 to 3 persons per million. Males and females were reported to be similarly affected in some studies,[545] whereas others reported a female predominance.[493,546,547] A recent retrospective of 32 cases identified through the nephropathology laboratory at Columbia University between 1977 and 2007 reported that 43% of patients were children, of whom 65% were between the ages of 5 and 10 years, and 22% of patients were adults older than 60 years. The female/male ratio was 1.9, and 85% of patients were white.[548] It is unclear whether the unexpectedly high representation of older adults in this cohort reflects a change in the demographics of the disease or a change in biopsy practices, or selection or referral bias in this or the older studies.

PATHOLOGY

The term *dense deposit disease* emphasizes the pathognomonic feature of discontinuous electron-dense bands within the GBM[502] (Figures 31-15 and 31-16). These are accompanied by spherical to irregular mesangial dense deposits and occasional subendothelial and subepithelial deposits, some of which may resemble the "humps" seen in postinfectious glomerulonephritis.

Immunofluorescence microscopy demonstrates intense capillary wall linear to bandlike staining for C3 (Figure 31-17), with little or no staining for immunoglobulin.[549,550] The capillary wall staining may have a fine double contour

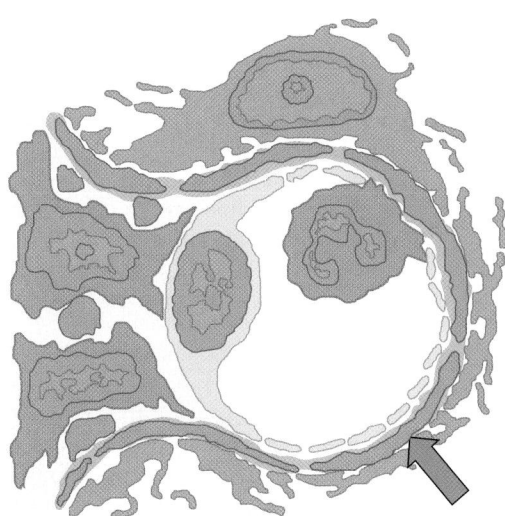

FIGURE 31-15 Diagram depicting a glomerular capillary loop with features of membranoproliferative glomerulonephritis (MPGN) type II (dense deposit disease) with bandlike intramembranous dense deposits (*arrow*) and spherical mesangial dense deposits. (Courtesy of J.C. Jennette.)

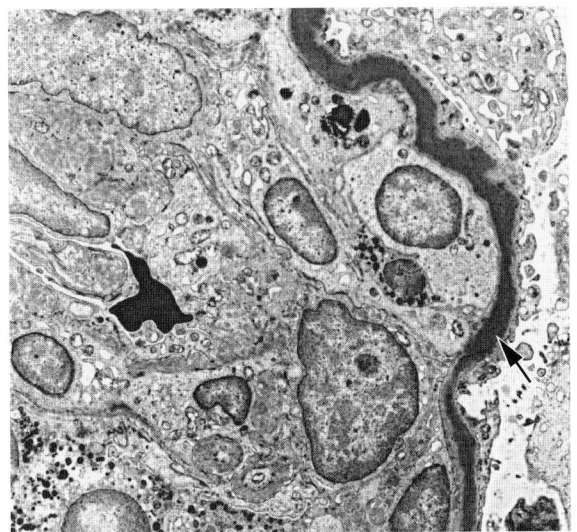

FIGURE 31-16 Electron micrograph of a glomerular capillary from a patient with membranoproliferative glomerulonephritis (MPGN) type II (dense deposit disease) showing a bandlike intramembranous dense deposit that has essentially replaced the normal glomerular basement membrane. Also note the endocapillary hypercellularity. (×5000.)

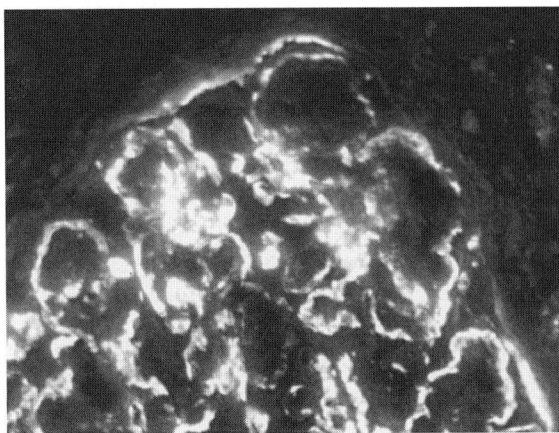

FIGURE 31-17 Immunofluorescence micrograph of a portion of a glomerulus with features of membranoproliferative glomerulonephritis (dense deposit disease (MPGN) type II (dense deposit disease) demonstrating discontinuous bandlike capillary wall staining and granular mesangial staining for C3. (Fluorescein isothiocyanate anti-C3 stain, ×600.)

with outlining of the outer and inner aspects of the dense deposits. The mesangial deposits usually appear as scattered spherules or rings, with the latter resulting from staining of the outer surface but not the interior of the spherical deposits.

The light microscopic appearance of type II MPGN is much more variable than that of type I MPGN, and often does not have a membranoproliferative appearance. Thus the term *dense deposit disease* is preferable to *type II MPGN*.[550,551] In a review of a large number of renal biopsy specimens obtained in North America, Europe, and Japan from patients with dense deposit disease, the light microscopic findings could be classified into five distinct patterns: (1) membranoproliferative pattern, (2) mesangioproliferative pattern, (3) crescentic pattern, (4) acute proliferative and exudative pattern, and (5) unclassified dense deposit disease. Of these, the mesangioproliferative lesion characterized by focal segmental and mesangial

hypercellularity accounted for about 50% of the cases reviewed, with 28% presenting with a membranoproliferative pattern (type I) and 20% with a crescentic lesion. Although the patients' ages ranged from 3 to 67 years, nearly 75% of the patients were younger than 20 years of age, and all patients with either crescentic dense deposit disease or acute proliferative dense deposit disease were between the ages of 3 and 18 years.[551] Therefore, the histologic appearance of type II MPGN (dense deposit disease) can mimic many other categories of glomerulonephritis, and the findings by immunofluorescence and especially electron microscopy are required for accurate diagnosis.

PATHOGENESIS

Dense deposit disease is characterized by deposits of dense material within the basement membranes of glomeruli, Bowman's capsule, and tubules. Interestingly, these deposits do not appear to contain immunoglobulins, but seem to activate the alternative pathway of complement. A porcine model of MPGN (porcine dense deposit disease) suggests that there is massive deposition of C3 and the terminal C5b9 complement complex (the membrane attack complex). In the circulation, there is extensive complement activation with very low C3 levels and high levels of circulating terminal complement components. No immune complex deposits were detected in renal tissue. At least in this animal model of dense deposit disease, the pathogenetic mechanism does not appear to involve immune complexes, but rather utilizes some other mechanism for the activation of complement and the trapping of activating complement components within the GBM.[552]

The hypocomplementemia in dense deposit disease reflects activation of the alternative complement pathway. Three distinct mechanisms result in uncontrolled activation of C3 convertase: (1) the development of an autoantibody, the C3 nephritic factor (C3NeF); (2) the absence of circulating factor H; and (3) the presence of a circulating inhibitor of factor H.[553] The most common of these is the presence of the autoantibody C3NeF. C3NeF is an antibody that protects C3 convertase (C3bBb) from dissociation by factor H and thus prolongs its half-life by 10-fold.[554] It does so in one of two ways—by binding either to C3bBb or to IgG-C3b-C3bBb of the assembled convertase. The stabilization of this complex results in perpetual C3 breakdown. It is tempting to impugn this factor as central to the pathogenesis of MPGN. However, C3NeF does not always correlate with disease activity, and more importantly, progressive renal damage still occurs in patients who have normal levels of complement.[555-557]

Normal protective, or regulatory, mechanisms control C3bBb levels and complement deposition, of which factor H is one of the most important. Factor H is a soluble glycoprotein that regulates complement in the fluid phase and on cell surfaces by binding to C3b.[553] Some mutations in factor H result in MPGN-like diseases.[558,559]

The genetics of dense deposit disease are complex. Only a few families have been identified with more than one affected member, although families exist with one patient with dense deposit disease and others members affected by other autoimmune diseases. The most robust genetic association with dense deposit disease is a deficiency of factor H, associated with a mutation of the complement factor H (*CFH*) gene. Affected children with dense deposit disease were homozygous for the deletion of a lysine residue at position 224.[560]

CLINICAL FEATURES
Patients with dense deposit disease may have hematuria, proteinuria, or both. They may have a nephrotic or acute nephritic syndrome. At least a third of patients have all of the components of nephrotic syndrome on presentation. Microhematuria is present in the overwhelming majority of patients, whereas gross hematuria occurs only in about 15%.[548] Finally, one quarter of patients have acute nephritic syndrome associated with red cells and red cell casts in the urine, hypertension, and renal insufficiency.[489,493,513,514] Hypertension is typically mild, but may be severe in some cases. Renal dysfunction occurs in at least half of cases and is more common in adults than in children.[548] When present at the outset of disease, renal dysfunction portends a poor prognosis.

Hypocomplementemia of the C3 factor is present in 80% to 90% of patients with dense deposit disease. In the recent retrospective review from Columbia University depressed C3 levels occurred in 100% of children, but in only 41% of adults (*P* = 0.001).[548] Depressed C4 levels were very uncommon in both age groups. C3 hypocomplementemia is prolonged in patients with dense deposit disease[403] and is associated with decrements in terminal complement components C5b9. C3NeF is present in more than 80% of patients.

Respiratory tract infections precede cases of MPGN in half of patients, especially in children.[548] On rare occasions, the onset can be triggered by a streptococcal infection, so that the disease mimics acute poststreptococcal glomerulonephritis except for the persistence of C3 hypocomplementemia beyond 8 weeks from onset.[561] Comorbid conditions may be seen in adult patients with dense deposit disease, including plasma cell dyscrasias, which were noted in 4 of 18 patients (22%) in the Columbia University review.[548]

Patients with dense deposit disease may have deposits in the retina, along Bruch's membrane, that are similar in structure and composition to the deposits in the GBM. These whitish yellow drusen develop at an early age. Initially, the drusen have little impact on visual acuity, but visual loss can occur in about 10% of patients.[562] A careful retinal examination is therefore indicated in all patients with proven dense deposit disease. There is no correlation between the severity of kidney and ocular involvement.[563]

Dense deposit disease may be associated with the syndrome of acquired partial lipodystrophy.[557] About 80% of patients with this syndrome have low C3 levels and C3NeF. About 20% of patients develop MPGN, although the lipodystrophy and glomerular disease may occur several years apart.[564] The link between acquired partial lipodystrophy and MPGN stems from the production by adipocytes of C3, factor B, and factor D (adipsin), whose function is the cleavage of factor B. In the presence of C3NeF, the alternative pathway of complement activation is dysregulated, which leads to the destruction of adipocytes.[564]

TREATMENT
The prognosis for type II disease is worse than that for type I. The less favorable prognosis is probably because dense deposit disease is frequently associated with crescentic glomerulonephritis and chronic tubulointerstitial nephritis at the time of biopsy.[523,565,566] In dense deposit disease, clinical remissions are rare,[493,494] occurring in fewer than 5% of children. Patients generally reach ESRD in 8 to 12 years from the onset of disease. In dense deposit disease, the prognosis is worse in adults than in children.[548]

There is currently no established treatment for dense deposit disease, and the available information is based on small case series. Inhibition of angiotensin II may be helpful, but has not been formally tested.[548] The use of corticosteroid therapy is probably not effective.[560] Immunosuppressive therapy with such agents as MMF and rituximab aimed at reducing C3NeF in dense deposit disease has been suggested.[567] It is not likely that immunosuppression with or without plasma exchange will be beneficial, except perhaps if an inhibitory autoantibody to complement factor H is present. There are reports of effective treatment of patients with defined deficiency of complement factor H with infusion of fresh frozen plasma every 14 days to provide functionally intact factor H.[568-572] In a proof-of-concept study in mice genetically deficient in complement factor H, treatment with purified human complement factor H resulted in rapid normalization of plasma C3 levels and resolution of the GBM C3 deposition.[573] Based on the current understanding of the pathogenesis of dense deposit disease, inhibition of C5 activation and formation of the terminal component of complement activation (C5b9) with the monoclonal antibody eculizumab would be theoretically beneficial, but evidence for this approach is lacking.[570]

Recurrences in renal transplants of dense deposit disease are common (80% or higher),[494,574-576] especially in the presence of C3NeF or *CFH* mutations.[577] Prophylactic plasma infusions or simultaneous liver transplantation can be beneficial in the latter cases.[568,569] Levels of C3 in the serum do not seem to predict recurrences.[577]

Acute Poststreptococcal Glomerulonephritis

Epidemiology

Acute poststreptococcal glomerulonephritis (PSGN) is a disease that affects primarily children, with a peak incidence between the ages of 2 and 6 years. Children younger than age 2 and adults older than age 40 account for only about 15% of patients with acute PSGN. Subclinical microscopic hematuria may be four times more common than overt acute PSGN, as documented in studies of family members of affected patients.[578-580] Only rarely do PSGN and rheumatic fever occur concomitantly.[581] Males are more likely than females to have overt nephritis.

Acute PSGN may occur as part of an epidemic or as sporadic disease. During epidemic infections of streptococci of proven nephrogenicity, the clinical attack rate appears to be about 12%,[582-584] but has been reported to be 25%[585] or even as high as 38% in certain affected families.[580]

Differences in incidence rates among different families argue for the existence of host genetic susceptibility factors affecting the propensity for overt nephritis.[586] An association was found between PSGN and HLA-DRW4,[586] HLA-DPA*02-022 and DPB1*05-01,[587] and, more recently, DRB1*03011.[588]

The rate of acute PSGN after sporadic infections with group A streptococci of potentially nephritogenic types is quite variable,[589,590] which again points to an effect of ill-defined host factors. A minority of streptococcal infections lead to nephritic syndrome, which argues for the presence of certain nephritogenic characteristics in the offending agent. Indeed, in the 1950s Rammelkamp and colleagues[589,590] identified certain strains of streptococci within Lancefield group A, in particular type XII, that are capable of leading to acute glomerulonephritis. Other nephritogenic serotypes include M types 1, 2, 3, 4, 18, 25, 31, 49, 52, 55, 56, 57, 59, 60, and 61. There are differences among these serotypes in their propensity to be associated with nephritis depending on the site of infection. Certain strains, such as types 2, 49, 55, 57, and 60, are usually associated with nephritis after pyoderma,[591,592] whereas M type 49 can lead to nephritis after either pharyngitis or pyoderma. In addition to occurring after infection with group A β-hemolytic streptococci, acute PSGN has also been described after infection with group C streptococci and possibly group G streptococci.[593,594]

Acute PSGN is on the decline in developed countries, but it continues to occur in developing communities.[595,596] Epidemic PSGN is frequently associated with skin infections, whereas pharyngitides are associated with sporadic PSGN in developed countries. Overt glomerulonephritis is found in about 10% of children at risk, but when one includes subclinical disease as evidenced by microscopic hematuria, about 25% of children at risk are found to be affected.[597,598] In some developing countries, acute PSGN remains the most common form of acute nephritic syndrome among children. The incidence rate appears to follow a cyclical pattern, with outbreaks occurring every 10 years or so.[599] A review of 11 published population-based studies estimated the median incidence of PSGN in children to be 24 cases per 100,000 person-years, based on studies that examined populations in less developed countries or included substantial minority populations in more developed countries; the incidence in adults was conservatively estimated to be 2 cases per 100,000 person-years in less developed countries and 0.3 cases per 100,000 person-years in more developed countries.[600] The review authors estimated that over 470,000 cases of acute PSGN occur annually, leading to approximately 5000 deaths (1% of total cases), 97% of which occur in less developed countries.

Interestingly, the epidemiology of PSGN in Florida appears to have changed in the last two decades, compared with the 1960s and 1970s: pharyngitis has replaced impetigo as the predominant underlying infection, a shift has occurred in racial distribution (now predominantly whites are affected) and in seasonal variation, and the severity of disease has decreased. These changes are thought to reflect a change in the causal agent of impetigo.[601]

Pathology

LIGHT MICROSCOPY

The pathologic appearance of acute PSGN varies during the course of the disease. The acute histologic change is influx of neutrophils, which results in diffuse global hypercellularity (Figure 31-18).[602-606] Endocapillary proliferation of mesangial cells and endothelial cells also contributes to the hypercellularity. The hypercellularity often is very marked and results in enlarged consolidated glomeruli. The description *acute diffuse proliferative glomerulonephritis* often is used as a pathologic designation for this stage of acute PSGN. A minority of patients have crescent formation, which usually affects only a small proportion of glomeruli.[607] Extensive crescent formation is rare.[608,609] Special stains that have differential reactions with immune deposits may demonstrate subepithelial deposits. For example, the subepithelial deposits may stain red (fuchsinophilic) with Masson trichrome stain.

Interstitial edema and interstitial infiltration of predominantly mononuclear leukocytes usually are present and occasionally are pronounced, especially with unusually severe disease associated with crescents. Focal tubular epithelial cell simplification (flattening) also may accompany severe disease. Arteries and arterioles typically have no acute changes, although preexisting sclerotic changes may be present in older patients.

During the resolving phase of self-limited PSGN, which usually begins within several weeks of onset, the infiltrating neutrophils disappear and endothelial hypercellularity resolves, leaving behind only mesangial hypercellularity.[602,610] This mesangioproliferative stage often is present in patients with acute PSGN who have had resolution of nephritis but have persistent isolated proteinuria, and it may persist for several months in patients who have complete clinical resolution. There may be focal segmental glomerular scarring as sequelae of particularly injurious inflammation, but this is seldom extensive except in the rare patients with crescentic acute PSGN. Ultimately, the pathologic changes of acute PSGN can resolve completely.[610,611]

IMMUNOFLUORESCENCE MICROSCOPY

Immunofluorescence microscopy demonstrates glomerular immune complex deposits in PSGN.[603,605,606,612] The pattern and composition of deposits change during the course of PSGN. During the acute diffuse proliferative phase of the disease there is diffuse global coarsely granular capillary wall and mesangial staining that usually is very intense for C3 and of varying levels for IgG from intense to absent (Figure 31-19). Staining for IgM and IgA is less frequent and usually less intense. In self-limited disease, biopsy should be performed later in the disease course, because it is more likely that the staining will be predominantly or exclusively for C3 with little or no immunoglobulin staining. Because most patients with uncomplicated new-onset acute PSGN do not undergo renal biopsy, most biopsy specimens are obtained later in the course when there is diagnostic uncertainty due to equivocal serologic confirmation or unusually aggressive or persistent clinical features. At this time, the immunofluorescence microscopy

LIGHT MICROSCOPIC MORPHOLOGY

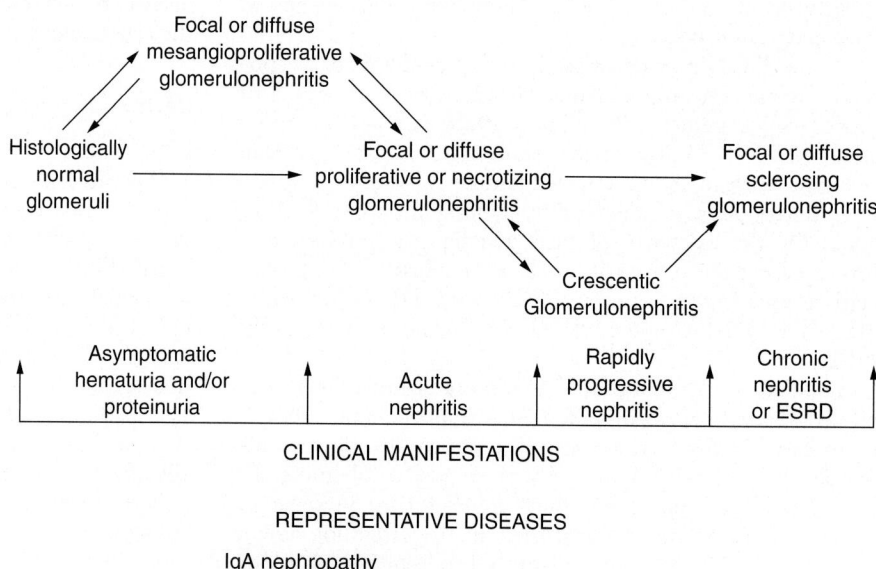

FIGURE 31-18 Diagram depicting the continuum of structural changes that can be caused by glomerular inflammation (*top*), the usual clinical syndromes that are caused by each expression of glomerular injury (*middle*), and the portion of the continuum that most often corresponds to several specific categories of glomerular disease (*bottom*). ANCA, Antineutrophil cytoplasmic antibody; ESRD, end-stage renal disease; GBM, glomerular basement membrane; IgA, immunoglobulin A. (From Ferrario F, Kourilsky O, Morel-Maroger L: Acute endocapillary glomerulonephritis in adults: a histologic and clinical comparison between patients with and without initial acute renal failure, *Clin Nephrol* 19:17-23, 1983.)

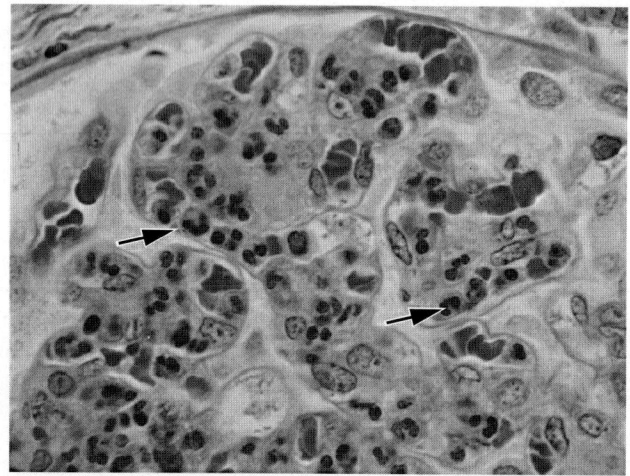

FIGURE 31-19 Light micrograph of a glomerulus with features of acute poststreptococcal glomerulonephritis demonstrating marked influx of neutrophils (*arrows*). (Masson trichrome stain, ×700.)

staining is usually predominantly for C3. This may reflect termination of nephritogenic immune complex localization in the kidney with masking of residual complexes by complement. The continued presence of intense staining for IgG a month or more into the course of what otherwise looks like pathologically typical PSGN is cause for concern that the process will not be self-limited.

Several patterns of immune staining have been described but are of limited prognostic value.[603,606,613] The garland pattern is characterized by numerous large, closely apposed granular deposits along the capillary walls. Patients with this pattern usually have nephrotic-range proteinuria as a component of

their disease. The starry sky pattern has more scattered granular staining, which corresponds somewhat to less severe disease. The mesangial pattern, especially when it is predominantly C3 staining, corresponds to the resolving phase with a mesangioproliferative light microscopic appearance.

ELECTRON MICROSCOPY
The hallmark ultrastructural feature of PSGN is the subepithelial humplike dense deposits (Figures 31-20 and 31-21).[605,610-612,614] However, small subendothelial and mesangial dense deposits can usually be identified with careful observation and theoretically may be more important in the pathogenesis of the disease, especially the neutrophilic influx and endocapillary proliferative response, than are the subepithelial humps. The subepithelial humps are covered by effaced epithelial foot processes, which usually contain condensed cytoskeletal filaments (including actin) that form a corona around the immune deposits (see Figure 31-21). During the acute phase, capillary lumens often contain marginated neutrophils, some of which are in direct contact with GBMs (see Figure 31-21). Lesser numbers of monocytes and macrophages contribute to the leukocyte influx. Mesangial regions are expanded by increased numbers of mesangial cells and leukocytes as well as increased matrix material and varying amounts of electron-dense material.

During the resolution phase, usually 6 to 8 weeks into the course, the subepithelial humps disappear, leaving behind only mesangial and sometimes a few scattered subendothelial and intramembranous dense deposits. The subepithelial deposits first become electron lucent and then disappear completely. The humps in peripheral capillary loops disappear before the humps in the subepithelial zone adjacent to the perimesangial basement membrane.

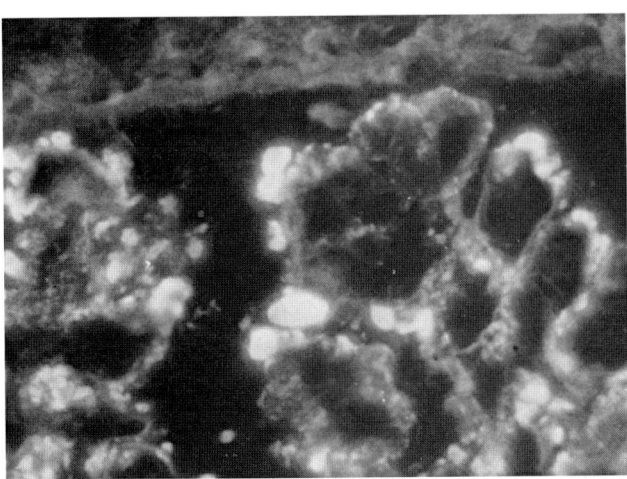

FIGURE 31-20 Immunofluorescence micrograph of a glomerular segment from a patient with acute poststreptococcal glomerulonephritis (PSGN) showing coarsely granular capillary wall staining for C3. Compare this to the finely granular capillary wall staining of membranous glomerulopathy in Figure 31-9. (Fluorescein isothiocyanateanti-C3 stain, ×800.)

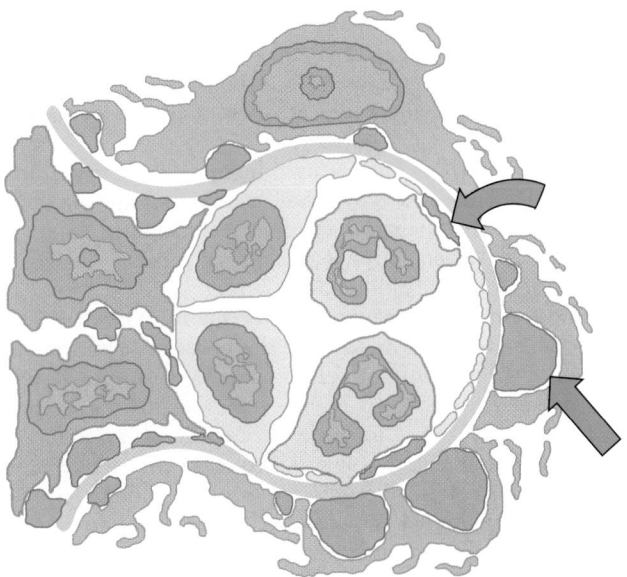

FIGURE 31-21 Diagram of the ultrastructural features of acute post-streptococcal glomerulonephritis (PSGN). Note the subepithelial humplike dense deposits (*straight arrow*), subendothelial deposits (*curved arrow*), and mesangial deposits. There is endocapillary hypercellularity caused by neutrophil infiltration, and endothelial and mesangial proliferation. (Courtesy of J.C. Jennette.)

Pathogenesis

Acute PSGN is the prototype disease of acute glomerulonephritis associated with an infectious cause. The first description of this link dates back to the early nineteenth century after scarlet fever epidemics in Florence and Vienna. Richard Bright first described the association in 1836, reporting that scarlet fever was sometimes followed by hematuria and kidney disease.[615] In 1907, Schick described an asymptomatic interval of 12 days to 7 weeks between the onset of streptococcal infection and the onset of nephritis.[616] In the early 1950s, Rammelkamp and Weaver further defined the association of PSGN with specific serotypes of streptococci.[589,617]

Despite the early recognition of an association between streptococcal infection and acute glomerulonephritis, the pathogenic mechanism of disease remains incompletely understood. Conceptually, either acute PSGN could be secondary to a direct toxic effect on the glomerulus of a streptococcal protein, or the streptococcal product could induce an immune complex–mediated injury. This could occur by a number of different mechanisms: (1) by introduction of an antigen into the glomerulus (planted antigen), (2) by the deposition of circulating immune complexes, (3) by alteration of a normal renal antigen that causes it to become a self-antigen, or (4) by induction of an autoimmune response to a self-antigen by way of antigenic mimicry. It is conceivable that more than one streptococcal antigen may be involved in the pathogenesis of acute PSGN, and more than one pathogenic mechanism may be at play simultaneously.

Several streptococcal proteins have been implicated in the pathogenesis of acute PSGN.[618] M protein molecules protruding from the surface of group A streptococci contain epitopes that cross-react with glomerular antigens. Shared sequences of M protein types 5, 6, and 19 have been shown to elicit antibodies that react with several myocardial and skeletal muscle proteins.[619] Conversely, monoclonal antibodies raised against human renal cortex have been shown to cross-react with type 6 and 12 M proteins, which provides evidence that certain M proteins may share antigenic determinants in all glomeruli.[620] The renal glomerular cross reactivity of the amino-terminal region of type 1 M protein was further localized

to a tetrapeptide sequence at position 23-26.[621] Antibodies raised against the amino-terminal of type 1 M protein was shown to cross-react with the cytoskeletal protein of glomerular mesangial cells, namely, the filament protein vimentin.[619] More recently, two antigens have been found within the glomerular deposits in renal biopsy specimens from patients with PSGN and have been reported to induce an antibody response characteristic for nephritogenic streptococcal infections: streptococcal proteinase exotoxin B (zymogen)[622] and the glycolytic enzyme glyceraldehyde phosphate dehydrogenase.[623] In a study that tested antigen deposition in 17 renal biopsy specimens and circulating antibodies in sera from 53 patients, response to streptococcal proteinase exotoxin B was more consistently found than deposits and antibody response to glyceraldehyde phosphate dehydrogenase.[624]

Currently, the spectrum of infectious agents associated with postinfectious or peri-infectious glomerulonephritis includes many more bacterial pathogens than streptococci. Other agents include staphylococci, gram-negative rods, and intracellular bacteria.[625] Likewise, the population at risk for peri-infectious glomerulonephritis has changed to include alcoholic individuals, intravenous drug users, and patients with ventricular atrial shunts. However, PSGN remains the most extensively studied and documented infection-associated glomerulonephritis.

Clinical Features and Natural History

Classically, the syndrome of acute PSGN presents abruptly with hematuria, proteinuria, hypertension, and azotemia. This syndrome can show a wide spectrum of severity from asymptomatic disease to oliguric acute renal failure.[626] A latent period occurs from the onset of pharyngitis to the onset of nephritis. In postpharyngitic cases, the latent period averages 10 days with a range of 7 to 21 days. The latent period may be longer after a skin infection (from 14 to 21 days), although this period is harder to define after impetigo.[627] The latency period can exceed 3 weeks.[628] Short latency periods of less than 1 week are suggestive of a "synpharyngitic" syndrome corresponding typically to exacerbation of an underlying IgA nephropathy.

The hematuria is microscopic in more than two thirds of cases. Patients presenting with macroscopic anemia commonly report gross hematuria and transient oliguria. Anuria is infrequent, however, and if persistent may indicate the development of crescentic glomerulonephritis.

Mild to moderate hypertension occurs in more than 75% of patients. It is most evident at the onset of nephritis and typically subsides promptly after diuresis.[581] Antihypertensive treatment is necessary in only about one half of patients. Signs and symptoms of congestive heart failure may occur and indeed may dominate the clinical picture. These include jugular venous distention, the presence of an S_3 gallop, dyspnea, and signs of pulmonary congestion.[628-631] Frank heart failure may be a complication in as many of 40% of elderly patients with PSGN.

Edema is the presenting symptom in two thirds of patients and is present in as many as 90% of cases.[578] The presence of edema is caused by primary renal sodium and fluid retention. The edema typically appears in the face and upper extremities. Ascites and anasarca may occur in children.

Encephalopathy presenting as confusion, headache, somnolence, or even convulsion is not common and may affect children more frequently than adults. The encephalopathy is not always attributable to severe hypertension, but may be the result of central nervous system vasculitis instead.[628,630-632]

The clinical manifestations of acute PSGN typically resolve in 1 to 2 weeks as the edema and hypertension disappear after diuresis, and the patient typically remains asymptomatic. Both the hematuria and proteinuria may persist for several months, but are usually resolved within a year. However, proteinuria may persist in those patients who initially had nephrotic syndrome.[578] The long-term persistence of proteinuria, and especially albuminuria, may be an indication of persistence of proliferative glomerulonephritis.[584]

The differential diagnosis of acute PSGN includes (1) IgA nephropathy[633] and Henoch-Schönlein purpura (especially when the acute nephritic syndrome is associated with gross or rusty hematuria), (2) MPGN, and (3) acute crescentic glomerulonephritis (rapidly progressive glomerulonephritis immune complex mediated, anti-GBM mediated, or pauci-immune). The occurrence of acute nephritis in the setting of persistent fever should raise the suspicion of a peri-infectious glomerulonephritis, especially with persistence of an infection such as an occult abscess or infective endocarditis.

Although rheumatic fever and PSGN rarely occur together, their co-occurrence has been described.[634]

Laboratory Findings

Hematuria, microscopic or gross, is nearly always present in acute PSGN. There are, however, rare cases of documented acute PSGN with no associated hematuria.[580,635] Microscopic examination of urine typically reveals the presence of dysmorphic red blood cells[636] or red blood cell casts. Other findings on microscopy are leukocytes, renal tubule epithelial cells, and hyaline and granular casts.[581] When the hematuria is macroscopic, the urine typically has a rusty or tea color.

Proteinuria is nearly always present but is typically in the subnephrotic range. In half of patients, it may be less than 500 mg of protein per day.[637,638] Nephrotic-range proteinuria may occur in as many as 20% of patients and is more frequent in adults than in children.[578] The excreted proteins may include large amounts of fibrin degradation products and fibrinopeptides.[635,639]

A pronounced decline in urine GFR is common in elderly patients with acute PSGN, affecting nearly 60% of patients 55 years of age and older.[630] This profound decrease in GFR is uncommon in patients from childhood to middle age. Indeed, because of the accompanying fluid retention and increase in circulatory volumes, a mild decrease in GFR may not be accompanied by an increase in serum creatinine concentration above laboratory limits of normal. Renal plasma flow, tubular reabsorptive capacity, and concentrating ability are typically not affected. On the other hand, urinary sodium excretion and calcium excretion are greatly reduced.[640]

A transient hyporeninemic hypoaldosteronism may lead to mild to moderate hyperkalemia. This may be exacerbated by a concomitant decrease in GFR and reduced distal delivery of solute. This type 4 renal tubular acidosis may resolve with the resolution of nephritis in the event of diuresis, but may be persistent beyond that point in some patients.[641] The suppressed plasma renin activity may be a consequence of the volume expansion present in those patients.[642]

Cultures of throat or skin samples frequently reveal group A streptococci.[581,643] The sensitivity and specificity of these tests are likely affected by the method of obtaining a culture specimen and the test used.[644] Such cultures may be less satisfactory than serologic studies to evaluate for the presence of recent streptococcal infection in patients suspected of having PSGN.[585] The antibodies most commonly studied for the detection of a recent streptococcal infection are anti–streptolysin O, antistreptokinase, antihyaluronidase, antideoxyribonuclease B, and anti–nicotinamide adenine dinucleotidase.[645] Of these, the most commonly used is the anti–streptolysin O test. An anti–streptolysin O titer above 200 units may be found in 90% of patients with pharyngeal infection.[581] In the diagnosis of acute PSGN, however, a rise in titer is more specific than the absolute level of the titer. The latter is likely affected by the geographic and socioeconomic prevalence of pharyngeal infections with group A streptococci. Increased anti–streptolysin O titers are present in about two thirds of patients with upper respiratory tract infection, but in only about one third of patients following streptococcal impetigo.[578] Serial anti–streptolysin O titer determinations with a twofold or greater rise in titer are highly indicative of a recent infection.[578,581]

The streptozyme test combines several antistreptococcal antibody assays and may be a useful screening test.[646] Since certain strains of type 12 group A streptococci do not produce streptolysin S or O, and in patients in whom impetigo-associated PSGN is suspected, testing for anti-deoxyribonuclease B and antihyaluronidase is a useful procedure.[591] Antibodies to other streptococcal cell wall glycoproteins may also increase, including those for endostreptosin.[581,647-650] On occasion, autoantibodies to collagen and laminin may be detected.[581,651] Cultures of throat or skin specimens may yield positive results in as few as one fourth of patients.

The serial measurement of complement component levels is important in the diagnosis of PSGN. Early in the acute phase, the levels of hemolytic complement activity (CH-50 and C3) are reduced. These levels usually return to normal within 8 weeks.[581,628,652-657] The reduction in serum C3 levels is especially marked in patients with C3NeF, which is capable of cleaving native C3.[516-518] The finding of low properdin and C3 levels, and concomitant normal to modestly reduced levels of C1q, C2, and C4[652,653,658] all point to the importance of the activation of the alternative pathway of the complement cascade.[652] Immunohistochemical analysis of mannose-binding protein and mannose-binding protein–associated serine proteinase 1 suggests that the lectin pathway of complement activation is engaged in about a third of patients.[659] There is some evidence as well for activation via the classical pathway.[660] Another other complement level abnormality is a mild depression of C5 levels, whereas levels of C6 and C7 are most often normal.[516,581,658] The plasma level of soluble terminal complement components (C5b9) rises acutely and then falls to normal.[653] Because complement levels typically return to normal within 8 weeks, the presence of persistent depression of C3 levels may be indicative of another diagnosis, such as MPGN, endocarditis, occult sepsis, systemic lupus erythematosus, atheromatous emboli, or congenital chronic complement deficiency.[652]

Circulating cryoglobulins[661,662] as well as circulating immune complexes[663-666] may be detected in some patients with PSGN. The pathophysiologic importance of these circulating immune complexes for the development of acute nephritis is unclear.[665-667]

Abnormalities in blood coagulation systems may be detected in acute PSGN; thus thrombocytopenia may be seen.[668] Elevated levels of fibrinogen, factor VIII, plasmin activity, and circulating high-molecular-weight fibrinogen complexes may be seen and correlate with disease activity and an unfavorable prognosis.[669-673]

Although complement studies suggest that the alternative pathways are primarily involved in acute PSGN, there is some evidence also for activation via the classical pathway.[660]

Treatment

Treatment of acute PSGN is largely supportive care. Children almost invariably recover from the initial episode.[585,674,675] Of concern to clinicians are those patients who have acute renal failure at presentation. An initial episode of acute renal failure is not necessarily associated with a bad prognosis.[626] In a study of 20 adult patients with diffuse proliferative glomerulonephritis, 11 had acute renal failure and 9 had normal or mild renal insufficiency. There were no differences between these groups in clinical, immunologic, or histologic features. After 18 months of follow-up, outcome was similar in the two groups. Thus, there is little evidence to suggest the need for any form of immunosuppressive therapy. Because of the profound salt and water retention observed in these patients—and, in some, pulmonary congestion—it is important to use loop diuretics such as furosemide to avoid volume expansion and hypertension. When volume expansion does occur, antihypertensive agents are frequently useful to ameliorate the hypertension. Interestingly, plasma renin levels are reduced; yet captopril has been shown to lower blood pressure and improve GFR in patients with PSGN.[676]

Some patients with substantial volume expansion and marked pulmonary congestion show no response to diuretic therapy. In those individuals, dialytic support is appropriate, either hemodialysis or continuous venovenous hemofiltration in adults or peritoneal dialysis in children. Some patients develop substantial hyperkalemia. In those patients, treatment with exchange resins or dialysis may be useful. Importantly, so-called potassium-sparing agents, including triamterene, spironolactone, and amiloride, should not be used in this disease state. Usually, patients undergo spontaneous diuresis within 7 to 10 days after the onset of their illness and no longer require supportive care.[626,677] There is no evidence to date that early treatment of streptococcal disease, either pharyngitic or cellulitic, will alter the risk of PSGN. It has long been speculated that treatment with penicillin might control the spread of outbreaks of epidemic PSGN. In studies of aboriginal communities in Australia, the use of benzathine penicillin prevented new cases of PSGN, especially in children with skin sores and household contact with affected individuals.[678]

The long-term prognosis of PSGN is not as benign as previously thought. Widespread crescentic glomerulonephritis results in an increased number of obsolescent glomeruli associated with tubulointerstitial disease that leads to progressive reduction of the renal mass over time.[679] A proportion of patients with streptococcal glomerulonephritis develop hypertension, proteinuria, and renal insufficiency between 10 and 40 years after the illness.[679-681] Nonetheless, it is most common that the long-term disease process is marked only by mild hypertension.

In some patients, there is evidence to suggest that the original diagnosis of PSGN may have been in error. This is especially true for in individuals in whom a renal biopsy was never performed. For instance, a patient who has an upper respiratory tract infection and then develops glomerulonephritis may be considered to have PSGN when in fact the patient has another proliferative form of glomerulonephritis. In these patients, lack of resolution of the renal disease should prompt a renal biopsy to elucidate the underlying cause of the glomerular injury.

Immunoglobulin A Nephropathy

Epidemiology

IgA nephropathy remains one of, if not the, most common glomerular lesion of all of forms of glomerulonephritis. Initially described in the late 1960s by Berger and Hinglais,[682,683] the disorder is characterized by the deposition predominantly of IgA (and, to a lesser extent, of other immunoglobulins) in the mesangium with mesangial proliferation and with clinical features that span the spectrum from asymptomatic hematuria to rapidly progressive glomerulonephritis. Although it was previously considered a benign disease, it is now clear that up to 40% of patients may progress to ESRD. Moreover, it has become recognized that, in addition to an idiopathic form of the disorder, IgA nephropathy is also associated with a variety of disease processes (Table 31-14).

IgA nephropathy occurs in individuals of all ages, but it is still most common in the second and third decades of life, and it is much more common in males than in females (Table 31-15). IgA nephropathy is uncommon in children younger

TABLE 31-14 Classification of Immunoglobulin A (IgA) Nephropathy

Primary IgA Nephropathy

Secondary IgA Nephropathy
Associated Disorders
Henoch-Schönlein purpura
Human immunodeficiency virus infection
Toxoplasmosis
Seronegative spondyloarthropathy
Celiac disease
Dermatitis herpetiformis
Crohn's disease
Liver disease
Alcoholic cirrhosis
Ankylosing spondylitis
Reiter's syndrome
Neoplasia
   Mycosi fungoides
   Lung carcinoma
   Mucin-secreting carcinoma
Cyclic neutropenia
Immunothrombocytopenia
Gluten-sensitive enteropathy
Scleritis
Sicca syndrome
Mastitis
Pulmonary hemosiderosis
Berger's disease
Leprosy

Familial IgA Nephropathy

Data from references 731, 748, 760, 864, 865, 1288-1315.

TABLE 31-15 Diseases That Cause Glomerulonephritis

GLOMERULAR LESION	N	MALE/FEMALE RATIO	WHITE/AFRICAN AMERICAN RATIO
Immunoglobulin A nephropathy	693	2.0:1.0	14.0:1.0
Membranoproliferative glomerulonephritis type I	248	1.2:1.0	3.3:1.0
Anti–glomerular basement membrane glomerulonephritis	82	1.1:1.0	7.9:1.0
Antineutrophil cytoplasmic antibody–associated glomerulonephritis	257	1.0:1.0	6.7:1.0
Fibrillary glomerulonephritis	76	1.0:1.2	14.3:1.0

Based on the analysis of 9605 native kidney biopsy specimens evaluated at the University of North Carolina Nephropathology Laboratory. This laboratory evaluates kidney biopsy specimens from a base population of approximately 10 million throughout the southeastern United States and centered in North Carolina. The expected white/African American ratio in this renal biopsy population is approximately 2:1.

than 10 years of age. In fact, 80% of patients are between the ages of 16 and 35 at the time of renal biopsy.[684-689] The male/female ratio has been described as anywhere from 2:1 to 6:1.[684-689]

The distribution of IgA nephropathy varies in different geographic regions throughout the world.[690] It is the most common form of primary glomerular disease in Asia, accounting for up to 30% to 40% of all biopsies performed for glomerular disease, and it accounts for 20% of all biopsies in Europe and 10% of all biopsies in North America.[690] This wide variation in incidence is partly attributable to the differing indications for renal biopsy in Asia compared with those in North America. In Asia, urinalyses are performed routinely in school-aged children. Those with asymptomatic hematuria typically undergo biopsy, which may lead to an increased number of diagnoses of IgA nephropathy. Genetic issues may also be important in the geographic differences. A Japanese study of biopsy specimens obtained from kidney donors immediately before transplantation showed that 16% of donors had covert mesangial deposition of IgA.[691] IgA nephropathy has been reported to be rare in African Americans,[692,693] although population-based incidence rates of newly diagnosed IgA nephropathy have been found to be similar in African American and white populations.[694] IgA nephropathy is quite common in Native Americans of the Zuni and Navajo tribes.[695] The prevalence of IgA in the general population has been estimated to be between 25 and 50 cases per 100,000,[690,696] although notably, almost 5% of all patients undergoing biopsy have at least some IgA deposits in their glomeruli.[697] Population studies in Germany and France calculated an incidence of 2 cases per 10,000,[698-701] but autopsy studies performed in Singapore[702] suggested that 2.0% to 4.8% of the population had IgA deposition in their glomeruli.

Genetics

IgA nephropathy is a histologically based diagnosis; it is unlikely to be related to a single genetic locus, but rather is probably due to the interactions of multiple susceptibility and progression genes in combination with environmental factors.[703] A number of studies suggest that there are genes that render an individual susceptible to IgA nephropathy and genes that portend a more rapid progression of IgA nephropathy. Polymorphism in a number of genes, including those coding for ACE, angiotensinogen, angiotensin II receptor, T cell receptor, IL-1 and IL-6, interleukin receptor antagonist, TGF, mannose-binding lectin, uteroglobin, nitric oxide synthase, and TNF, as well as major histocompatibility loci, have been evaluated as possibly affecting both the susceptibility to and progression of disease.[704-710] A number of studies have examined the role of the ACE gene in IgA nephropathy with or without progressive disease. The D allele of the ACE gene may be associated with susceptibility to IgA nephropathy in Asians but not in whites.[711] The Polymorphism Research to Distinguish Genetic Factors Contributing to Progression of IgA Nephropathy (PREDICT-IgAN) study, which investigated associations between progression of IgA nephropathy and 100 atherosclerotic disease–related gene polymorphisms using a retrospective candidate gene approach, found significant associations between polymorphisms in the glycoprotein Ia and intercellular adhesion molecule-1 genes and progression of disease.[712] In this study, the association between the ACE I/D polymorphism and progression of disease was not found to be significant after adjustment for multiple comparisons.

Familial IgA nephropathy has been reported in multiple ethnic groups around the world, including in Africa and Central America. Indeed, some studies suggest that 4% to 14% of patients with IgA nephropathy may have a family history of renal disease,[698,713,714] and systematic screening of asymptomatic first-degree relatives has detected hematuria in more than 25% of them.[715] Disease findings in most pedigrees are consistent with autosomal dominant transmission with incomplete

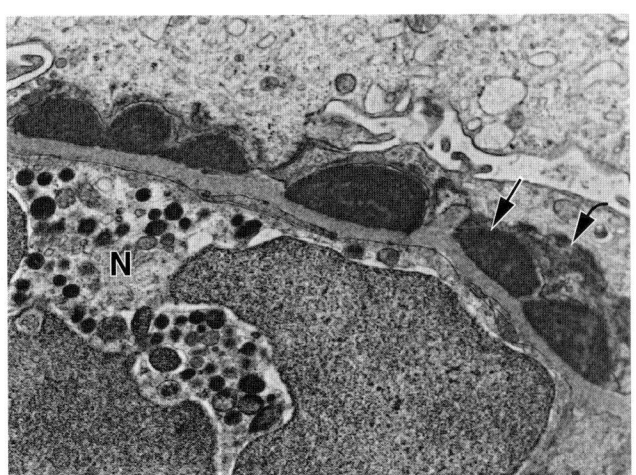

FIGURE 31-22 Electron micrograph of a portion of a glomerular capillary from a patient with acute poststreptococcal glomerulonephritis (PSGN) showing subepithelial dense deposits (*straight arrow*), condensation of cytoskeleton in adjacent epithelial cytoplasm (*small curved arrow*), and a neutrophil (N) marginated against the basement membrane with no intervening endothelial cytoplasm. (×5000.)

penetrance.[713] However, in some families, IgA nephropathy may aggregate with other glomerular diseases.[713,716]

Genomewide association studies are underway to identify candidate genes and SNPs that may correlate with susceptibility to or protection against IgA nephropathy. Linkage studies have suggested an association of IgA nephropathy with genes at several loci.[713] Based on a genomewide linkage study of 30 kindreds with IgA nephropathy, a locus on chromosome bands 6q22-23 was identified with a logarithm of odds (LOD) score of 5.6,[717] and was named *IGAN1* (a LOD score ≥3 signifies odds ≥1000:1 in favor of linkage).[713] Linkages to other loci were also detected, albeit with lower LOD scores, namely, 2q36 (LOD = 3.47),[718] 3p24-23 (LOD = 2.8),[717] 4q26-31 (LOD = 1.8), and 17q12-22 (LOD = 2.6).[719] However, the disease-causing DNA variant or haplotype at these loci has not yet been identified.

The prevailing hypothesis regarding the pathogenesis of IgA nephropathy focuses on defects in protein glycosylation, particularly in B cells secreting IgA1. Studies measuring the serum levels of galactose-deficient IgA1 in a cohort of patients with IgA nephropathy, their relatives, and unrelated controls found a higher level of the aberrantly glycosylated IgA1 in patients with familial or sporadic IgA nephropathy and in their at-risk relatives than in unrelated individuals or control subjects.[720,721] This finding suggests that abnormal IgA1 glycosylation is an inherited rather than an acquired trait. Polymorphisms of the genes for the enzymes responsible for glycosylation of IgA1 may thus be associated with increased susceptibility to IgA nephropathy.

Such genes include the core 1 β-galactosyltransferase gene (*C1GALT1*)[722,723] and the molecular chaperone COSMC (*C1GALT1C1*), although the findings are inconsistent across studies.[724] In a Chinese population, SNPs of *C1GALT1* were reported in association with IgA nephropathy,[723] this finding was but not confirmed in a French population.[725] The activity of the α2,6-sialyltransferase enzyme and gene expression (*ST6GALNAC2*) are also altered in IgA nephropathy,[726] and variants of the gene promoter were linked to susceptibility to IgA nephropathy.[723] In addition, interactions between certain

C1GALT1C1 and *ST6GALNAC2* haplotypes were associated with susceptibility to IgA nephropathy, a greater likelihood of disease progression, and greater exposure of *N*-acetylgalactosamine residues on serum IgA1.[727]

Other genetic variants may affect the risk of susceptibility to IgA nephropathy.[728] A genomewide screen comparing SNPs in patients with IgA nephropathy with sequences in healthy controls suggested possible associations with 42 genes, one of which, triadin, mapped within the *IGAN1* locus (6q22.31).[729] The most comprehensive candidate gene identified by association studies is the selectin gene cluster on chromosome 1.[730]

Pathology

IMMUNOFLUORESCENCE MICROSCOPY

IgA nephropathy can be definitively diagnosed only by the immunohistologic demonstration of glomerular immune deposits that stain dominantly or codominantly for IgA compared with IgG and IgM (Figure 31-22).[731-734] The staining is usually exclusively or predominantly mesangial, although a minority of specimens, especially from patients with severe disease, have substantial capillary wall staining. By definition, 100% of IgA nephropathy specimens stain for IgA. On a scale of 0 to 4+, the mean intensity of IgA staining is approximately 3+.[733] IgM staining is observed in 84% of specimens with a mean intensity (when present) of only approximately 1+. IgG staining is observed in 62% of specimens, also with a mean intensity (when present) of approximately 1+. Early studies of IgA nephropathy described more frequent and more intense IgG staining than is seen today, but this probably was caused by the use of less specific antibodies that cross-reacted between IgA and IgG. Almost all IgA nephropathy specimens have substantial staining for C3. In contrast, staining for C1q is rare and weak if present. If there is intense staining in a specimen that shows substantial IgA and IgG, the possibility of lupus nephritis rather than IgA nephropathy should be considered.[733] An additional relatively distinctive feature of IgA nephropathy is that, unlike any other glomerular immune complex disease, the immune deposits usually have more intense staining for λ light chains than for κ light chains.[731,733]

ELECTRON MICROSCOPY

The ubiquitous ultrastructural finding is mesangial electron-dense deposits that correspond to the immune deposits seen by immunohistologic analysis (Figures 31-23 and 31-24).[732] The mesangial deposits often are immediately beneath the perimesangial basement membrane. They are accompanied by varying degrees of mesangial matrix expansion and hypercellularity. Most specimens do not have capillary wall deposits, but a minority, especially from patients with more severe disease, show scattered subendothelial dense deposits or subepithelial dense deposits or both. The extent of endocapillary proliferation and leukocyte infiltration parallel the pattern of injury observed by light microscopy. Epithelial foot process effacement is observed in those patients with substantial proteinuria.

LIGHT MICROSCOPY

IgA nephropathy can cause any of the light microscopic phenotypes of proliferative glomerulonephritis (Figure 31-25) or may cause no discernible histologic changes.[732-739]

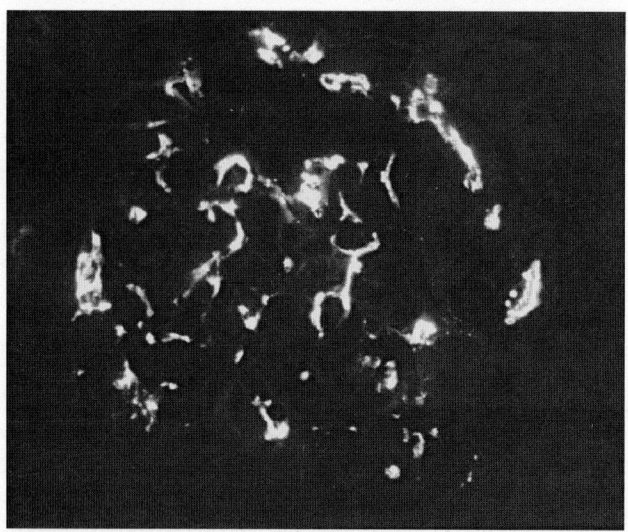

FIGURE 31-23 Immunofluorescence micrograph of a glomerulus with features of immunoglobulin A (IgA) nephropathy showing intense mesangial staining for IgA. (Fluorescein isothiocyanate anti-IgA stain, ×300.)

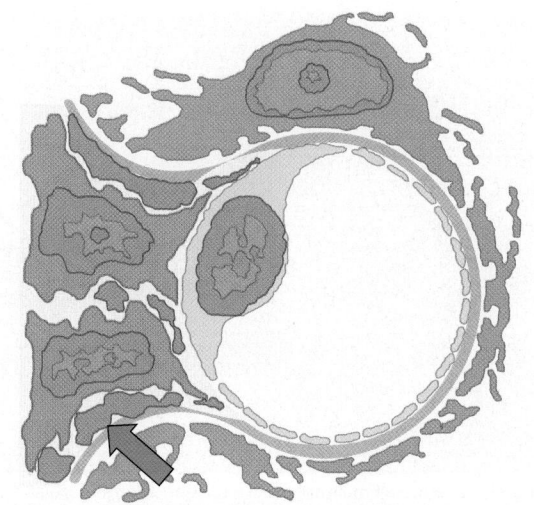

FIGURE 31-24 Diagram depicting the ultrastructural features of immunoglobulin A (IgA) nephropathy. Note the mesangial dense deposits (*straight arrow*) and mesangial hypercellularity. (Courtesy of J.C. Jennette.)

FIGURE 31-25 Electron micrograph of a capillary and adjacent mesangium from a patient with immunoglobulin A (IgA) nephropathy showing mesangial dense deposits immediately beneath the paramesangial basement membrane. (×7000.)

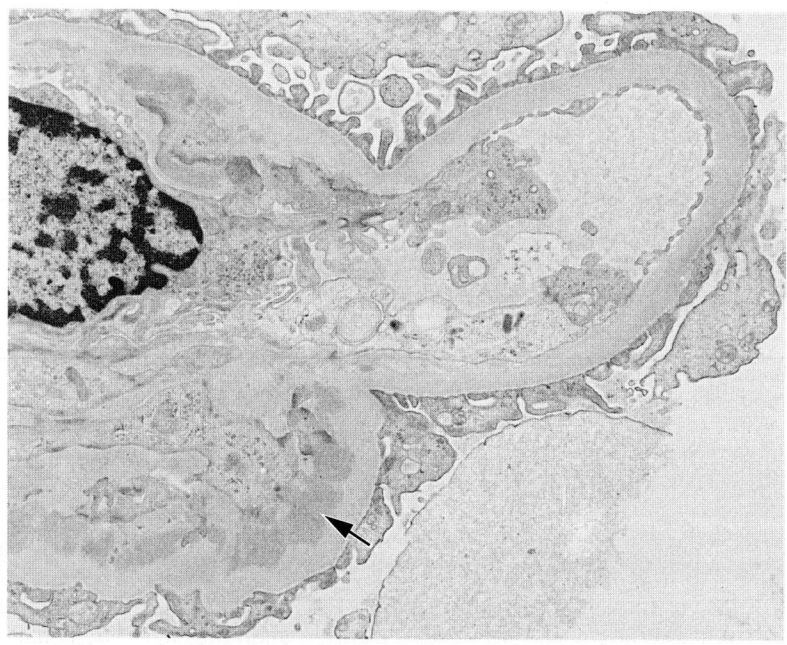

As depicted in Figure 31-26, this spectrum of glomerular inflammatory responses is shared by a variety of glomerulonephritides that have different etiologies but induce similar or identical light microscopic alterations in glomeruli. Figure 31-18 also depicts the most frequent clinical manifestations at the time of biopsy of the different histologic phenotypes of glomerulonephritis, all of which can be caused by IgA nephropathy. At the time of biopsy, IgA nephropathy usually manifests as a focal or diffuse mesangioproliferative or proliferative glomerulonephritis, although specimens from a few patients will have no lesion by light microscopy, those from a few will show aggressive disease with crescents, and occasional specimens will already demonstrate chronic sclerosing disease. Different criteria for performing renal biopsy result in different frequencies of the various phenotypes of IgA nephropathy among distinct populations of patients. Of

668 consecutive native kidney IgA nephropathy specimens diagnosed in the UNC Nephropathology Laboratory, 4% showed no lesion by light microscopy, 13% had exclusively mesangioproliferative glomerulonephritis, 37% had focal proliferative glomerulonephritis (25% of these had <50% crescents), 28% had diffuse proliferative glomerulonephritis (45% of these had <50% crescents), 4% had crescentic glomerulonephritis (50% or more crescents), 6% had focal sclerosing glomerulonephritis without residual proliferative activity, 6% had diffuse chronic sclerosing glomerulonephritis, and 2% had lesions that did not fall into any of these categories.

The mildest light microscopic expression of IgA nephropathy, other than no discernible lesion, is focal or diffuse mesangial hypercellularity without more complex endocapillary hypercellularity, such as endothelial proliferation or influx

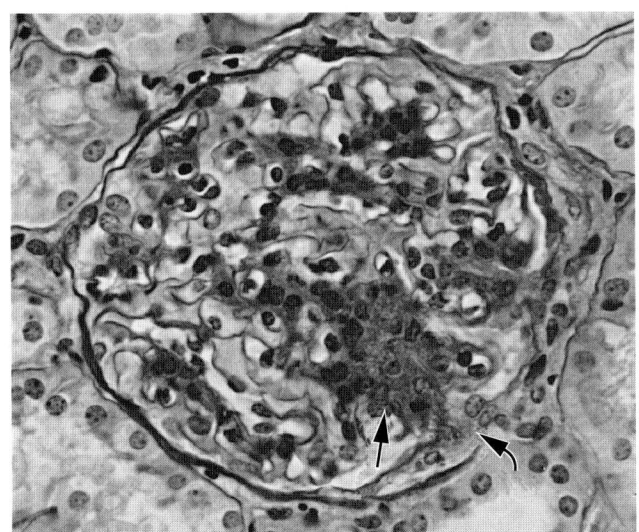

FIGURE 31-26 Light micrograph of a glomerulus with features of immunoglobulin A (IgA) nephropathy showing segmental mesangial matrix expansion and hypercellularity (*straight arrow*) and an adhesion to Bowman's capsule (*curved arrow*). (Periodic acid–Schiff stain, ×300.)

of leukocytes. This is analogous to the International Society of Nephrology/Renal Pathology Society (ISN/RPS) class II lupus nephritis. More severe inflammatory injury causes focal (involving fewer than 50% of glomeruli) or diffuse proliferative glomerulonephritis as the pathologic expression of IgA nephropathy, which is pathologically analogous to class III and class IV lupus nephritis. The lesions are characterized by not only mesangial hypercellularity but also some degree of endothelial proliferation or leukocyte infiltration that distorts or obliterates some capillary lumens. Extensive necrosis is rare in IgA nephropathy, although slight focal segmental necrosis with karyorrhexis can occur in severely inflamed glomeruli. With time, destructive glomerular inflammatory lesions progress to sclerotic lesions that may form adhesions to Bowman's capsule. Occasional patients with IgA nephropathy will have focal glomerular sclerosis by light microscopy that is indistinguishable from FSGS until the immunofluorescence microscopic findings are taken into consideration. Because of the episodic nature of IgA nephropathy, many patients have combinations of focal sclerotic lesions and focal active proliferative lesions. Patients with the most severe IgA nephropathy have crescent formation because of extensive disruption of capillaries.[739] Advanced chronic disease is characterized by extensive glomerular sclerosis associated with marked tubular atrophy, interstitial fibrosis, and interstitial infiltration by mononuclear leukocytes.

Whether histologic features detected on renal biopsy can be used to predict the progression of IgA nephropathy has been studied over many years. Renal pathologic findings have previously provided limited prognostic value over and above that of simple clinical parameters such as blood pressure, serum creatinine level, and the degree of proteinuria. The Oxford classification of IgA nephropathy study is a landmark investigation that assessed the value of specific pathologic features in predicting the risk of progression of renal disease in IgA nephropathy.[740,741] The study population was a multiethnic cohort of patients with IgA nephropathy that included children (n = 59) and adults (n = 206) who were followed for a mean of 69 months. By an iterative

process, pathologic variables selected based on reproducibility, least susceptibility to sampling error, ease of scoring, and independent association with outcome were then correlated through multivariate analysis with three clinical outcomes: the rate of renal function decline, survival from a 50% decline in renal function or ESRD, and proteinuria during follow-up.[740]

Four parameters emerged as independently predictive of clinical outcomes: mesangial hypercellularity, endocapillary hypercellularity, segmental glomerulosclerosis, and tubular atrophy/interstitial fibrosis. Of these, mesangial hypercellularity was significantly associated with ESRD or 50% reduction in GFR, segmental sclerosis was associated with the rate of decline in renal function, and tubular atrophy/interstitial fibrosis was statistically associated with both the rate of decline and ESRD, or 50% decline in renal function. Endocapillary hypercellularity was not significantly predictive of the rate of decline of renal function or survival from ESRD or 50% reduction in renal function. However, patients with endocapillary (or extracapillary) hypercellularity were more likely to receive immunosuppressive therapy, and the relationship between this pathologic variable and the rate of decline in renal function may have been influenced by the use of immunosuppression. This latter finding suggests, indirectly, that patients with this type of lesion are responsive to immunosuppressive therapy.

The results of the study led to a proposal to incorporate the following scoring of the four identified parameters (known as the *Oxford-MEST score*) into the pathology report for IgA nephropathy[740]:

Mesangial hypercellularity: score ≤0.5 = 0, or score >0.5 = 1
Endocapillary hypercellularity: absent = 0 or present = 1
Segmental glomerulosclerosis: absent = 0 or present = 1
Tubular atrophy/interstitial fibrosis: percentage of cortical area ≤25% = 0, 26% to 50% = 1, or >50% = 2

The usefulness of this classification system will need to be prospectively validated in separate cohorts, especially in comparison with clinical features such as serum creatinine level and proteinuria.[742]

Pathogenesis

The last decade has witnessed a great deal of progress in our understanding of the pathogenesis of IgA nephropathy. The characteristic pathologic finding by immunofluorescence microscopy of granular deposits of IgA and C3 in the glomerular mesangium, as well as in the dermal capillaries in Henoch-Schönlein purpura, suggests that this disease is the result of the deposition of circulating immune complexes leading to the activation of the complement cascade via the alternative pathway. The deposited IgA is predominantly polymeric IgA1.[743-746] The fact that polymeric IgA1 is usually derived mainly from the mucosal immune system, as well as the association of clinical flare-ups in some cases of IgA nephropathy with syndromes that affect the respiratory tract or gastrointestinal tract, has led to the suggestion that IgA nephropathy is a consequence of defective mucosal immunity.[747] This concept was supported by the finding in some patients with IgA nephropathy of antibodies to dietary antigens or various infectious agents, both viral and bacterial,[748-761] and the clinical observation that hematuria increases acutely in some patients at the time of upper respiratory tract or gastrointestinal tract infections. However, it has now been determined that the elevation in polymeric IgA1 antibody synthesis does not occur in the mucosa, and polymeric IgA levels are increased after systemic immunization with tetanus toxoid.[744,762,763] In addition, an increase in IgA-secreting B cells was documented in both the peripheral blood[764] and the bone marrow[765] of patients.

Serum levels of IgA do not correlate with either disease activity or mesangial deposits; therefore, it is unlikely that the pathogenesis of IgA nephropathy is related to a quantitative increase in serum levels of polymeric IgA1. Rather, it relates to an anomaly in the IgA molecule itself, namely, in its glycosylation.[766] This is best exemplified in patients with IgA-secreting multiple myeloma, among whom only those patients with aberrant IgA glycosylation develop glomerulonephritis.

In humans, the heavy chain of IgA1, but not that of IgA2, contains an 18–amino acid hinge region that is rich in proline, serine, and threonine residues. O-linked monosaccharides or oligosaccharides consisting of N-acetylgalactosamine can be posttranslationally added to these amino acid residues. This N-acetylgalactosamine is usually substituted with a terminal galactose.[767] Lectin-binding studies and carbohydrate composition analysis have demonstrated that the IgA1 in patients with IgA nephropathy contains less terminal galactose than that of healthy control subjects.[744,768] It has been recently determined that the addition of a galactose residue to the glycosyl side chain is blocked by premature sialylation of the N-acetylgalactosamine residues on the hinge region of IgA1. The precise cause of this has not been fully elucidated. Three mechanisms have been postulated: excessive activity of $\alpha 2,6$-sialyltransferase, decreased activity of $\beta 1,3$-galactosyltransferase, and decreased stability of $\beta 1,3$-galactosyltransferase due to decreased activity of its chaperone (Cosmc).[769,770] Whether these abnormalities are acquired or genetically determined remains unclear.[723,724,771] IgA glycosylation may also be influenced by acquired abnormalities such as the polarity of the T cell cytokine milieu.[772]

Abnormally galactosylated IgA1 molecules are the target of IgG autoantibodies as demonstrated in studies of immortalized B cells from patients with IgA nephropathy,[770,773] and IgG antibodies specific for these galactose-deficient IgA1 molecules are found in the circulation of such patients.[774] These autoantibodies were found to be of highly restricted heterogeneity directed at the unique epitopes present on the abnormally glycosylated IgA1.[773] The autoantibodies and target IgA1 form circulating immune complexes[775,776] that escape removal by the reticuloendothelial system and deposit in glomeruli via an interaction with a mesangial IgA receptor, possibly the transferrin receptor.[777-780] Once deposited in the glomerular mesangium, these immune complexes provoke mesangial proliferation.[781] The deposition of IgA in glomeruli may also occur independently of immune complex formation,[782] because abnormally glycosylated IgA1 also leads to an increased binding in the kidney.[766,776,783] However, aberrantly glycosylated IgA in isolation does not cause mesangial proliferation in tissue culture.[773] Mesangial galactose-deficient IgA1 molecules induce a variety of phlogistic mediators, including cytokines, chemokines, and growth factors, as well as complement activation through the mannose-binding lectin pathway.[784-786]

Another component of the pathogenesis of IgA nephropathy pertains to direct cytokine- or chemokine-induced podocyte injury, which is reflected by increased podocyturia. Podocyte damage may be the result of local complement activation and elevated levels of platelet-derived growth factor or TNF-α.[787-789]

It is hypothesized that a subsequent autoantibody response may be triggered by an environmental cross-reacting antigen and lead to in situ immune complex formation by interaction of circulating autoantibodies to the "planted" autoantigen. Formation of circulating immune complexes with abnormally glycosylated IgA and circulating IgA receptor molecules could also be involved.[790] Because IgA1 is normally cleared from the circulation by the liver via the asialoglycoprotein receptor,[791-793] it is thought that the defective galactosylation of the hinge region in IgA1 may lead to decreased clearance of IgA1 molecules in patients with IgA nephropathy.[783,794]

The existence, nature, and role of other autoantibodies in IgA nephropathy is also under investigation. A number of autoantibodies to various putative autoantigens have been described in IgA nephropathy.[795] Such autoantigens include a mesangial cell membrane antigen,[796] endothelial cells (human umbilical vein endothelial cells),[749,795] single-stranded DNA,[749] and cardiolipin.[749,797] Most of these autoantibodies were found in subsets of patients that rarely exceeded 3% of patients with IgA nephropathy and may sometimes be the result of high circulating levels of IgA in these patients.[797] The presence of IgG ANCAs has been described to occur in a minority of patients with IgA nephropathy.[798] In addition, IgA ANCAs have been rarely associated with a systemic vasculitis of the Henoch-Schönlein purpura type.[799-801] In the setting of IgA ANCA, the autoantigen seems to be different from the major ANCA autoantigens, namely, myeloperoxidase (MPO) and proteinase 3 (PR3). Circulating IgA-fibronectin complexes have also been described in the circulation of patients with IgA nephropathy and HIV infection.[802] These complexes may not be true immune complexes, however, and may be directly related to increased IgA levels in patients with IgA nephropathy.[803] A special form of IgA-dominant immune complex glomerulonephritis that resembles postinfectious glomerulonephritis occurs secondary to staphylococcal infection, especially but not exclusively in patients with diabetes.[804]

Clinical Features and Natural History

Approximately 40% to 50% of patients have macroscopic hematuria at the time of their initial presentation. The episodes tend to occur in close temporal relationship to upper respiratory tract infection, including tonsillitis or pharyngitis. This synchronous association of pharyngitis and macroscopic hematuria has been give the name *synpharyngitic nephritis*. Much less commonly, episodes of macroscopic hematuria follow infections that involve the urinary tract or gastroenteritis. Macroscopic hematuria may be entirely asymptomatic, but more often is associated with dysuria that may prompt the treating physician to consider bacterial cystitis. Systemic symptoms are frequently found, including nonspecific symptoms such as malaise, fatigue, myalgia, and fever. Some patients have abdominal or flank pain.[805,806] In a minority of patients (fewer than 5%), malignant hypertension may be an associated presenting feature.[807] In the most severe cases (fewer than 10%), acute glomerulonephritis results in acute renal insufficiency and failure.[808,809] Recovery typically occurs with resolution of symptoms, even in those patients who have been temporarily dialysis dependent.[809]

Macroscopic hematuria due to IgA nephropathy occurs more often in children than in young adults. When it occurs in older individuals, it should raise the possibility of the more common causes of urinary tract bleeding, such as stones or malignancy.

A presentation with asymptomatic microscopic hematuria, with or without proteinuria, occurs in 30% to 40% of patients. Patients with IgA nephropathy come for evaluation of asymptomatic hematuria with or without the presence of proteinuria. In addition to glomerulonephritis, these patients may commonly have hypertension. In fact, in white patients with hypertension and hematuria, IgA nephropathy is the most common cause of hematuria.[810] Intermittent macroscopic hematuria occurs in 25% of these patients. Microscopic hematuria and proteinuria persist between episodes of macroscopic hematuria.

Patients with nephrotic syndrome at presentation may have widespread proliferative glomerulonephritis or coexisting IgA nephropathy and minimal change glomerulopathies.[811] Finally, some patients with IgA nephropathy have reached ESRD at the time of their initial presentation. These individuals typically have had asymptomatic microscopic hematuria and proteinuria that has remained undetected.[808]

In addition to idiopathic IgA nephropathy, there is secondary IgA nephropathy that is the glomerular expression of a systemic disease (see Table 31-14). For example, patients with Henoch-Schönlein purpura have abdominal pain, arthritis, a vasculitic rash, and a glomerulonephritis that is indistinguishable from that of primary IgA nephropathy. This condition is discussed more fully in Chapter 32.

Although IgA nephropathy was earlier thought to carry a relatively benign prognosis, it is estimated that, measured from the time of diagnosis, 1% to 2% of all patients with IgA nephropathy develop end-stage renal failure each year. In a review encompassing 1900 patients in 11 separate series, long-term renal survival was estimated to be 78% to 87% at a decade after presentation.[812] Similarly, European studies have suggested that renal insufficiency may occur in 20% to 30% of patients within two decades of initial presentation.[688] In a study of the natural history of IgA nephropathy and "isolated" microscopic hematuria in 135 Chinese children,[27] spontaneous clinical remission occurred in 12%, whereas 88% had persisting hematuria. Almost 30% developed new onset of proteinuria, and hypertension developed in 32%. Eventually, 20% developed renal insufficiency of varying severity. A poor outcome was associated with persistent hematuria, microalbuminuria, and tubulointerstitial changes on the renal biopsy specimen. This study clearly demonstrates that careful follow-up is required for all patients given the diagnosis of IgA nephropathy.

Overall, about 25% of patients develop ESRD within 10 to 25 years from diagnosis, depending on the initial severity of disease. Patients with episodes of gross (macroscopic) hematuria generally have a more favorable prognosis than those with persisting microhematuria; however, after an episode of microhematuria associated with acute renal failure a portion of patients (about 25%) do not recover normal renal function.[813]

The proliferative forms of IgA nephropathy seem to be associated with better outcomes in children than in adults.[814] It is unclear whether sex affects the prognosis of IgA nephropathy,[815] with some studies suggesting that prognosis may be worse for males. Older age at disease onset may also connote a poor prognosis.[812,816-820]

Several studies have assessed features that predict a poor prognosis. Sustained hypertension, persistent proteinuria (especially proteinuria of >1 g protein per 24 hours), impaired renal function, and nephrotic syndrome are markers of poor prognosis.[714,734,816] Controversy persists with respect to the issue of recurring bouts of macroscopic hematuria.[821] It is possible that macroscopic hematuria is an overt manifestation of disease and therefore identifies patients earlier in the course of their disease. Alternatively, macroscopic hematuria may represent an episodic process that results in self-limited inflammation, in contrast to persistent hematuria that represents ongoing, low-grade inflammation. In general, persistent microscopic hematuria is associated with a poor prognosis.[822] It is important to note that acute renal failure associated with macroscopic hematuria does not affect long-term prognosis. The fact that acute renal failure does occur during gross episodes of hematuria has been confirmed.[823-825] In these patients, the acute renal failure is most likely associated with acute tubular damage and not true crescentic disease. After the episodes of gross hematuria, renal function typically returns to baseline, and the long-term prognosis is good.

The degree of proteinuria is more than likely an additional marker of glomerular disease. Whether this is a consequence of the relationship between proteinuria and the tubular dysfunction found in many forms of glomerular disease or is specific to IgA nephropathy is not clear. In a study by Chen and colleagues,[826] mice that had been made proteinuric by various methods had enhanced deposition of administered IgA immune complexes. This suggests that these complexes might be more easily deposited in proteinuric states. More importantly, the amount of protein excretion 1 year after diagnosis was found to be highly predictive of the development of ESRD within 7 years of subsequent follow-up. Individuals with protein excretion of less than 500 mg/dL/24 hr had no renal failure within 7 years, whereas those with over 3 g had an approximately 60% chance of ESRD.[827]

Many formulas have been advanced to predict progression of IgA nephropathy in individual patients that yield different results for a same patient. The Toronto formula based on average mean arterial pressure and proteinuria during the first 2 years of observation is the best-validated in white American and European subjects,[828] but a large fraction of the variation in progression remains unexplained by these two factors. Risk stratification for progression can be aided by algorithms employing a small set of variables (age, sex, family history of chronic kidney disease, reduced estimated GFR at diagnosis, proteinuria, serum albumin and total serum protein levels, hematuria, systolic or diastolic blood pressure, and histologic variables).[829-831] Treatment has also favorably influenced the long-term trends of progression in IgA nephropathy,[832] and a postdiagnosis *decline* in the level of protein excretion to less than 1.0 gm/day is a very reliable surrogate measure of a more favorable long-term prognosis.[833]

A large number of factors other than simple clinical assessment have been examined for their ability to predict outcomes.

Some have been independently correlated with outcomes, whereas others have failed to demonstrate any added value in prognostication or therapeutic decision making.[834] Some of the more recently described factors include autophagy in podocytes,[835] the presence of CD19+CD5+ B cells in kidney biopsy specimens and in blood,[836] C5b9 glomerular deposition,[837] extensive C4d deposition in the mesangium,[838] tubular α3β1 integrin expression,[837] granule membrane protein of 17 kDa (GMP-17)–positive T cells in renal tubules,[839] glomerular density and size,[840] urinary epidermal growth factor/monocyte chemoattractant protein-1 ratios,[841,842] urinary growth arrest and DNA damage-45γ (GADD45γ) expression,[843] analysis of the urinary proteome (kininogen, inter-alpha-trypsin-inhibitor heavy chain 4, transthyretin),[844] and the fractional urinary excretion of IgG (in combination with assessment of nephron loss) in crescentic IgA nephropathy.[845] Likewise, hematuria associated with podocyturia may be associated with a poorer prognosis.[846] The clinical utility and applicability of these assays in prognostication and treatment decision making remains to be established.

In addition to these variables, obesity,[847] elevated nocturnal blood pressure,[848] increased uric acid levels,[848] and elevated levels of C4-binding protein[849] have been associated with a poorer prognosis. Moderate alcohol consumption is associated with an improved prognosis in IgA nephropathy.[850] A mildly elevated serum bilirubin level (>0.6 mg/dL) was associated with an *improved* long-term outcome in Korean patients with IgA nephropathy,[851] a finding that has not been confirmed in a non-Asian population. Prolonged high-level exposure to organic solvents may also confer a worse prognosis in IgA nephropathy.[852]

Women with IgA tolerate pregnancy well. Only those women with uncontrolled hypertension, a GFR of less than 70 mL/min, or severe arteriolar or interstitial damage on renal biopsy are at risk for renal dysfunction.[853,854] Women with creatinine levels higher than 1.4 mg/dL have a greater propensity for hypertension and a progressive increase in creatinine level during the course of pregnancy, and pregnancy-related loss of maternal renal function occurs in 43% of these patients. The infant survival rate was 93% in this study; preterm delivery occurred in almost two thirds and growth retardation in one third of infants.[855]

Laboratory Findings

To date, there are no specific serologic or laboratory tests diagnostic of IgA nephropathy or Henoch-Schönlein purpura. The identification of abnormally galactosylated IgA1 has led to the development of a potential diagnostic test based on the detection of increased lectin binding in patients with IgA nephropathy.[856]

Although the serum IgA levels are elevated in up to 50% of patients, the presence of elevated IgA in the circulation is not specific for IgA nephropathy. The detection of IgA-fibronectin complexes was initially thought to be a marker in patients with IgA nephropathy, but has not proven to be a useful clinical test.[857,858] As noted earlier, polymeric IgA also appears to be found in some patients with IgA nephropathy.[743,859-863] The polymeric IgA itself is of the IgA1 subclass. IgA may also be contained in circulating immune complexes that are not complement binding. Similar immune complexes have been described in Henoch-Schönlein purpura.[864-881]

The levels of circulating immune complexes wax and wane and may sometimes correlate with episodes of macroscopic hematuria. In one interesting study, the level of circulating immune complexes was increased after patients drank cow's milk. This phenomenon occurred in 10% to 15% of patients and possibly suggests sensitivity to bovine serum albumin. Unfortunately, none of these findings is pathognomonic of IgA nephropathy.

Antibodies to the GBM,[882] the mesangium,[883,884] glomerular endothelial cells,[748] neutrophil cytoplasmic constituents,[750,751] IgA rheumatoid factor,[885,886] and a number of infectious agents, bovine serum proteins, and soy proteins[753-760,887,888] have been found in patients with IgA nephropathy. Until studies demonstrate that certain patients have sensitivity to a particular pathogen or food allergen, it is difficult to know whether to perform antibody testing to identify certain foods that should be eliminated from the patient's diet. None of these antibody tests has been standardized in large patient populations. Therefore their applicability for all patients with IgA nephropathy is not known. Levels of complements, such as C3 and C4, are typically normal and, in some patients, even elevated,[889] as are complement components C1q, C2-C9.[686,864,865,889,890] The fact that these complement levels are normal may belie the fact that either the alternative or the classical pathway of complement may be activated. In this regard, C3 fragments are increased in 50% to 75% of patients,[891,892] and C4-binding protein concentrations are also increased.[890] It has been suggested that an elevated IgA/C3 ratio may have diagnostic utility in IgA nephropathy[27] and may be associated with a higher risk of progression.[893]

A typical finding is microscopic hematuria on urinalysis that may persist even at very low levels of macroscopic hematuria. The finding of dysmorphic erythrocytes in the urine is typical.[894] Proteinuria is found in many patients with IgA nephropathy, although in the majority protein excretion is less than 1 g/day. Mesangial and endocapillary hypercellularity, segmental glomerulosclerosis, and extracapillary proliferation on the biopsy specimen are strongly associated with proteinuria.[740]

Although older studies suggested that the detection of dermal capillary IgA deposits in the skin may be of diagnostic utility in IgA nephropathy,[895] this test has not gained widespread acceptance, largely because of the substantial variation in sensitivity and specificity of skin biopsy findings in identifying IgA in patients with nephropathy.[896]

Treatment

In part because of the outcome variability of patients with IgA nephropathy, the best approach to therapy remains incompletely established.[897-899] Treatment is indicated for patients with proteinuria of more than 0.5 g of protein per day.[900] Three major approaches have emerged and are supported by substantial direct evidence: (1) RAAS blockade, (2) oral and/or intravenous glucocorticoids, and (3) combined immunosuppressive (cytotoxic) therapy. The latter is usually reserved for those patients with documented progressive disease. Combinations of these approaches are under intense evaluation, including in the Supportive versus Immunosuppressive Therapy of Progressive IgA Nephropathy (STOP-IgAN) trial (NCT00554502).[901]

ANGIOTENSIN II INHIBITION

In retrospective studies, angiotensin II inhibition has been associated with a slower rate of loss of renal function and a higher frequency of remission of proteinuria compared with either no therapy[902] or the use of β-blockers.[903] Several randomized controlled trials of angiotensin II inhibition in patients with IgA nephropathy have been undertaken.[905-910]

A meta-analysis of 11 studies (totaling 585 subjects) revealed that the use of angiotensin II inhibition is associated with a reduction in proteinuria and preservation of GFR.[911] The antiproteinuric effects of the ACE inhibitor appear to be more profound in patients with the ACE gene DD genotype.[912] Observational studies of patients with IgA nephropathy suggest that an elevated fractional excretion of IgG is a powerful predictor of the renoprotective response to angiotensin II inhibition.[913] Higher dosages of angiotensin II inhibitors may afford additional renoprotective effect. In a randomized controlled trial involving 207 patients, a high-dose ARB (losartan 200 mg/day) was compared with an ARB given at the usual dose (losartan 100 mg/day) as well as with a usual-dose ACE inhibitor and a low-dose ACE inhibitor (equivalent to enalapril 20 mg/day and 10 mg/day, respectively).[914] High-dose ARB therapy was most efficacious in reducing proteinuria and slowing the rate of decline in estimated GFR. At the present time, administration of escalating doses of an ARB to achieve a target urinary protein excretion of less than 1 g/day, along with dietary sodium restriction, appears to be the first line of treatment for patients of any age with IgA nephropathy and proteinuria of more than 500 mg of protein per day.

GLUCOCORTICOIDS

Studies of glucocorticoid therapy for IgA nephropathy have been inconclusive. Although prednisone was initially considered to be without effect,[812] some cohort studies have suggested that corticosteroid therapy may afford some benefit.[915,916] For instance, a randomized controlled trial demonstrated that a 6-month course of intravenous plus oral glucocorticoids may be useful in patients with IgA nephropathy who have well-preserved renal function (serum creatinine level of <1.5 mg/dL and proteinuria of 1 to 3.5 g of protein per day).[917] After a 5-year follow-up, the risk of a doubling in plasma creatinine concentration was significantly lower in the corticosteroid-treated patients, who also showed a significant decrease in mean urinary protein excretion after 1 year that persisted throughout the follow-up.[917] This beneficial effect was maintained after 10 years of follow-up as reflected by a rate of renal survival (failure to double the serum creatinine level) of 97% in the treated group compared with 53% in the placebo group (log rank test, *P* = 0.0003).[918] On the other hand, no benefit of corticosteroids over placebo could be demonstrated in the multicenter randomized controlled trial conducted by the Southwest Pediatric Nephrology Study Group,[919] although this negative result is mitigated by a statistically significant lower degree of proteinuria at baseline among placebo-treated patients. A recent meta-analysis of seven randomized controlled trials encompassing 366 patients suggested that glucocorticoid therapy was effective in reducing proteinuria and preventing loss of renal function.[920]

Another circumstance in which prednisone has a demonstrated substantial beneficial effect is in the treatment of patients with IgA nephropathy and concurrent minimal change glomerulopathy. These patients have nephrotic-range proteinuria and diffuse foot process effacement. They respond to prednisone in a manner very similar to that of patients with minimal change glomerulopathy.[121,811,921,922] Low doses of prednisone (20 to 30 mg/day tapered to 5 to 10 mg/day over 2 years) may also be effective in lowering proteinuria in patients with mild inflammatory glomerular lesions.[923] Conversely, poor response to glucocorticoids can be predicted in patients with extensive glomerular obsolescence, tuft adhesions, severe interstitial fibrosis, low serum albumin, low estimated GFR, and marked proteinuria.[924] A high number of fibroblast-specific protein 1 (FSP1)–positive cells in the interstitium (>33 FSP-1+ cells per high-power field) is highly predictive of a poor response to steroids.[925]

In summary, glucocorticoid therapy is a reasonable option for treatment of patients with adverse prognostic features with well-preserved renal function (GFR >60 mL/min/1.73m²) who remain proteinuric despite a 3- to 6-month trial of angiotensin II inhibitors or patients with features of minimal change disease and nephrotic syndrome.[926]

COMBINATIONS OF ANGIOTENSIN II INHIBITION AND GLUCOCORTICOID THERAPY

Two recent randomized controlled trials in patient with IgA nephropathy have compared the combined use of glucocorticoids and angiotensin II inhibitors with the use of angiotensin II inhibitors alone, but not with glucocorticoid therapy alone.[927,928] In the larger of the two studies[928] (97 subjects with IgA nephropathy and urinary protein excretion of >1.0 g/day and estimated GFR of >50 mL/min/1.73 m²), 27% of the subjects receiving ramipril alone developed a doubling of baseline serum creatinine level or ESRD, whereas only 4% of subjects in the ramipril plus steroid group reached these endpoints (*P* = 0.003) after a follow-up of 8 years. These studies demonstrate an added benefit of glucocorticoids over angiotensin II inhibitors alone. Whether such combined therapy should be instituted as initial therapy or only after a trial of angiotensin II inhibition alone remains to be investigated.

More aggressive treatment may be appropriate in patients with severe crescentic or progressive IgA nephropathy.[929-931] In a randomized controlled trial, patients with a serum creatinine concentration of more than 1.5 mg/dL and a GFR declining at a rate of more than 15% per year either received no immunosuppression or were treated with oral prednisolone (initially at 40 mg/day) and cyclophosphamide (at 1.5 mg/kg/day) for 3 months followed by 2 years of treatment with azathioprine (1.5 mg/kg/day).[932] Follow-up lasted 2 to 6 years. Renal survival, assessed by Kaplan-Meier analysis annually to 5 years, showed preservation of renal function from 3 years in the treatment group and 82%, 82%, 72%, and 72% for 2, 3, 4, and 5 years respectively, compared with 68%, 47%, 26%, and 6% in controls.[932] This approach of prednisone coupled with oral azathioprine for 2 years in patients with proteinuria of over 2.5 g of protein per day was also observed in a retrospective survey.[933,934]

The use of pulse methylprednisolone, oral prednisone, and/or cyclophosphamide to treat patients who have rapidly progressive glomerulonephritis with widespread crescentic transformation has been reported.[935-937] It is reasonable to treat crescentic disease in IgA nephropathy in a manner similar to other forms of crescentic glomerulonephritis (e.g., ANCA glomerulonephritis). Of concern, however, was the finding in 12 patients of the persistence of crescents on repeat biopsy, despite early and aggressive treatment with pulse methylprednisolone and oral prednisone and a short-term reversal of the acute crescentic glomerulonephritis.[937] This study suggests that there was only a diminution in the rate of progression to ESRD.

OTHER MODALITIES

It is reasonably clear that treatment with the combination of oral cyclophosphamide, dipyridamole, and low-dose warfarin[938] has very little long-term benefit in patients with IgA nephropathy. Five years after the end of a small controlled trial (total of 48 patients), there was no significant difference in the rate of ESRD between patients previously treated with cyclophospamide, dipyridamole and warfarin (22%) and the control group (33%).

Whether MMF is useful in the treatment of IgA nephropathy is currently unknown. Three randomized trials of MMF have shown conflicting results.[939-942] The studies based in China and Hong Kong reported a beneficial effect of MMF on proteinuria and hyperlipidemia[939,940] but no effect on renal function in the short term.[939] Long-term follow-up of this cohort suggested better preservation of renal function in the MMF-treated group.[943] On the other hand, the two placebo-controlled studies of MMF in white populations of 32 and 34 patients failed to demonstrate a benefit of MMF on proteinuria or the preservation of renal function.[941,942] It is noteworthy that in one study,[941] patients had relatively advanced renal insufficiency (mean serum creatinine level of 2.4 mg/dL). Collectively, these underpowered studies fail to establish a role for MMF in the treatment of IgA nephropathy and raise the question of whether certain ethnic groups (Asians) may be more responsive to this form of therapy.

There has been much discussion in the literature about the use of tonsillectomy in IgA nephropathy. The results of the retrospective trials are inconsistent.[944-946] Based on a retrospective multivariate analysis[945] of a large cohort of 329 patients in Japan, treatment with tonsillectomy and pulse glucocorticoid therapy (methylprednisolone 0.5 g/day for 3 days for three courses, followed by oral prednisolone at an initial dose of 0.6 mg/kg on alternate days, with a decrease of 0.1 mg/kg every 2 months) was associated with clinical remission. Similarly, in a multivariate analysis[947] focusing on the subgroup of 70 patients from the same cohort with a baseline serum creatinine concentration of more than 1.5 mg/dL, treatment with the combination of tonsillectomy and pulse glucocorticoids was associated with improved long-term renal survival. Another retrospective analysis,[944] however, showed no benefit of tonsillectomy on the clinical course of IgA nephropathy. No study has yet demonstrated a superiority for tonsillectomy alone, or a superiority of tonsillectomy plus pulse glucocorticoids over a similar course of pulse glucocorticoids alone on the preservation of renal function. In a controlled nonrandomized trial, tonsillectomy plus pulse glucocorticoids was associated with a higher rate of remission of proteinuria and hematuria (but not renal function) than pulse glucocorticoids alone.[947a]

ω-3 Fatty Acids. Despite a great deal of interest in the past decade, the value of treatment with ω-3 long-chain polyunsaturated fatty acids (eicosapentaenoic and docosahexanoic acids) in IgA nephropathy remains unproven. In a study by the Mayo Clinic,[948] 106 patients were randomly assigned to receive either 12 g of ω-3 fatty acids or olive oil for 2 years. Only 6% of patients treated with fish oil experienced a doubling of their plasma creatinine concentration, compared with 33% of those treated with olive oil. In the fish oil–treated patients, only 14% excreted over 3.5 g of protein per day, in contrast to 65% of those treated with olive oil. The enthusiasm for this approach, however, was tempered by subsequent studies that showed no benefit of fish oil therapy.[949,950]

A recent meta-analysis of published trials of ω-3 fatty acids encompassing 17 trials and 626 patients with a variety of renal diseases, including 5 trials in patients with IgA nephropathy,[951] revealed no beneficial effects on proteinuria or slowing in the rate of GFR decline. In a recent randomized controlled trial involving 30 patients the addition of ω-3 fatty acids to angiotensin II inhibition was more effective than angiotensin II inhibition alone in decreasing proteinuria and erythrocyturia over 6 months.[952]

In summary, if ω-3 fatty acids should be used at all in the treatment of IgA nephropathy, they should be used in combination with angiotensin II inhibition and not as monotherapy.

Summary of Recommended Treatment

In summary, patients with IgA nephropathy should be treated with maximally tolerated angiotensin II inhibition to a target protein excretion of less than 500 mg/day.[904,959-961] Should proteinuria persist despite angiotensin II inhibition, the addition of glucocorticoids (oral or intravenous plus oral) should be considered for patients with well-preserved renal function (GFR of ≥60 mL/min/1.73 m^2). In those patients with progressive renal insufficiency, the use of prednisone and cyclophosphamide followed by azathioprine should be considered.[932] This approach to therapy is the subject of an ongoing large multicenter randomized controlled trial in Germany, the STOP-IgAN study.[901] High-dose corticosteroids and/or cyclophosphamide should also be considered for patients with widespread crescentic glomerulonephritis, whereas patients with acute renal failure associated with tubular necrosis and little glomerular damage should be treated conservatively, because these individuals have an excellent long-term response. Although there is no conclusive evidence of efficacy, the relatively benign side effect profile of ω-3 fatty acid therapy permits its use in patients who have an unfavorable prognosis. Those patients with nephrotic syndrome and minimal change glomerulopathy may benefit from oral glucocorticoids.

Immunoglobulin A Nephropathy and Kidney Transplantation

The recurrence of IgA deposits after renal transplantation is common, and the rate may reach 75% to 80% with long-term (>20-year) survival of the patient and graft.[953] Fortunately, most of these recurrences are clinically mild or are discovered incidentally at the time of an allograft biopsy to assess for possible rejection. Although graft loss due to recurrent IgA nephropathy is quite uncommon (<5%),[954] a recurrence of IgA nephropathy does worsen the overall prognosis for long-term survival of an allograft,[955,956] especially if crescentic disease is present. Nevertheless, overall graft survival in patients with IgA nephropathy is similar to that in patients with ESRD due to other causes.[954] Suggested risk factors for recurrent IgA nephropathy after transplantation include a rapid course of the original disease due to crescentic glomerulonephritis, younger age, IgA deposits in the donor kidney at the time of grafting, and living related or "zero-mismatched" kidney donor.[956,957] Induction therapy with antithymocyte globulin appears to decrease the incidence of recurrent disease.[958]

Fibrillary Glomerulonephritis and Immunotactoid Glomerulopathy

Nomenclature

Fibrillary glomerulonephritis and immunotactoid glomerulopathy are glomerular diseases that are characterized by patterned deposits seen by electron microscopy (Figures 31-27 and 31-28).[962-969] Most renal pathologists prefer to distinguish fibrillary glomerulonephritis from immunotactoid glomerulopathy based on the presence of fibrils of approximately 20 nm in diameter in the former and larger 30- to 40-nm–diameter microtubular structures in the latter[962,964-967] (see Figures 31-27 and 31-28). A minority of pathologists, however, advocate grouping glomerular diseases with either fibrillary deposits or microtubular deposits under the term *immunotactoid glomerulopathy*.[966,969]

Fibrillary Glomerulonephritis Pathology

ELECTRON MICROSCOPY

The diagnosis of fibrillary glomerulonephritis requires the identification by electron microscopy of irregular accumulations of randomly arranged nonbranching fibrils of approximately 20-nm diameter in glomerular mesangium or capillary walls or both[962-968,970] (see Figure 31-27A). In capillary walls, the fibrillary deposits can be subepithelial, subendothelial, or intramembranous. The fibrillary deposits often contain blotchy electron-dense material, but only rarely have associated well-defined electron-dense deposits. The fibrils are distinctly larger than the actin filaments in adjacent cells, which is a useful observation that helps distinguish the fibrils of fibrillary glomerulonephritis from those of amyloidosis, which are only slightly larger than actin. The fibrils of fibrillary glomerulonephritis are not as large

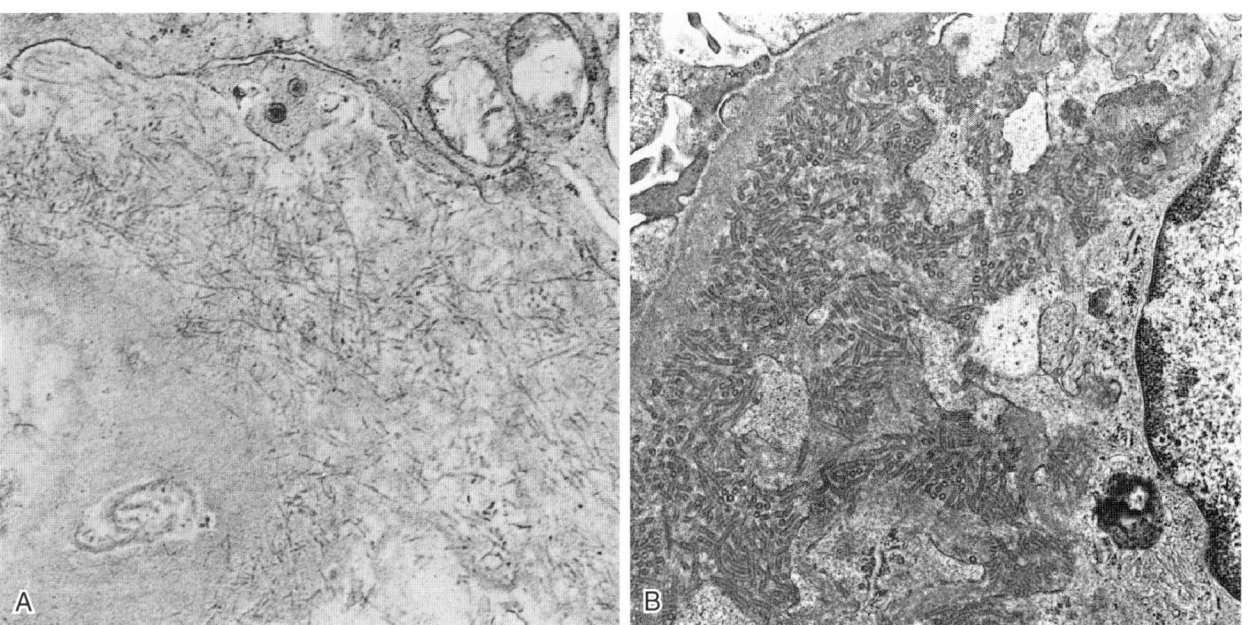

FIGURE 31-27 Electron micrographs showing the glomerular deposits of fibrillary glomerulonephritis (**A**) and immunotactoid glomerulopathy (**B**). Note the random orientation of the former and the microtubular appearance and greater organization of the latter. (×20,000.)

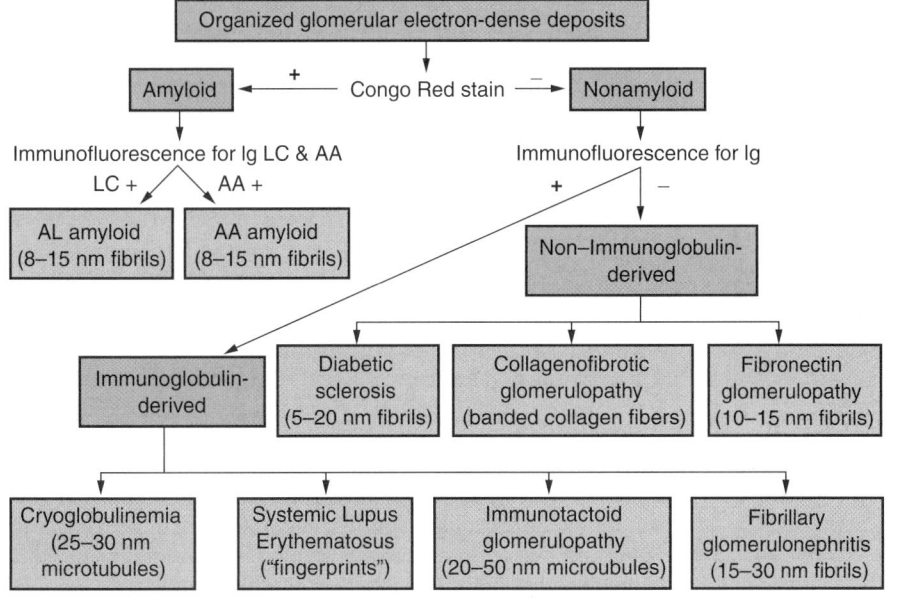

FIGURE 31-28 Algorithm for the pathologic categorization of glomerular diseases with patterned or organized deposits. The first division is into amyloid versus nonamyloid disease, and the second is into diseases that are caused by immunoglobulin molecule deposition and those that are not. By the approach illustrated, fibrillary glomerulonephritis is distinguished from immunotactoid glomerulopathy based on the ultrastructural characteristics of the deposits.

as the microtubular deposits of immunotactoid glomerulopathy or cryoglobulinemia, and they do not have the "fingerprint" configuration occasionally observed in lupus nephritis dense deposits. Most patients with fibrillary glomerulonephritis have substantial proteinuria, and therefore there usually is extensive effacement of visceral epithelial foot processes.

LIGHT MICROSCOPY

In fibrillary glomerulonephritis, extensive localization of fibrils in capillary walls causes capillary wall thickening. Mesangial localization causes increased mesangial matrix and usually stimulates mesangial hypercellularity. Varying distribution of the fibrillary deposits causes the light microscopic appearance of fibrillary glomerulonephritis to be extremely variable.[962-968] Therefore, fibrillary glomerulonephritis can mimic the light microscopic appearance of MPGN, proliferative glomerulonephritis, or MN. Crescents occur in the most aggressive phenotypes. Of 74 sequential fibrillary glomerulonephritis specimens evaluated at UNC, 28% had crescents with an average involvement of 29% of glomeruli (range = 5% to 80%). The fibrillary deposits typically have a moth-eaten appearance when stained with Jones' silver methenamine stain. They do not show Congo red staining, which distinguishes them from amyloid deposits.

IMMUNOFLUORESCENCE MICROSCOPY

The deposits of fibrillary glomerulonephritis almost always stain more intensely for IgG than for IgM or IgA, and many specimens have little or no staining for IgM and IgA.[962-968] IgG4 is the dominant subclass. Only rare specimens have staining for only one light-chain type. C3 staining usually is intense. The immunofluorescence staining pattern of fibrillary glomerulonephritis is relatively distinctive (Figure 31-29). It is not granular or linear, but rather has an irregular bandlike appearance in capillary walls and an irregular shaggy appearance in the mesangium.

Immunotactoid Glomerulopathy Pathology

ELECTRON MICROSCOPY

The tubular substructure of the deposits of immunotactoid glomerulopathy is readily discerned at 5000 to 10,000 magnification (see Figure 31-27B). At this magnification, the

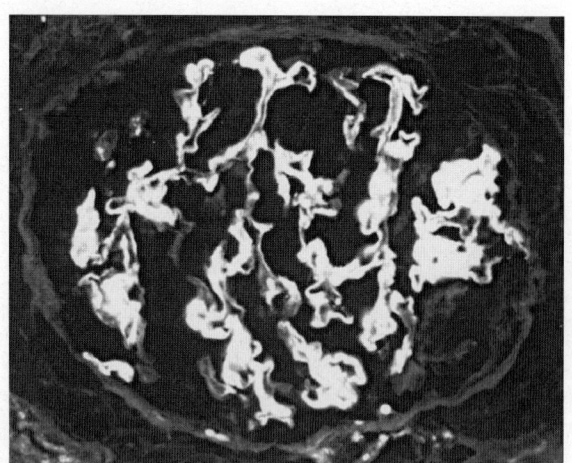

FIGURE 31-29 Immunofluorescence micrograph of a glomerulus with features of fibrillary glomerulonephritis showing mesangial and bandlike capillary wall staining for immunoglobulin G (IgG). (Fluorescein isothiocyanate anti-IgG stain, ×300.)

deposits of fibrillary glomerulonephritis have no tubular structure. The microtubules of immunotactoid glomerulopathy also have a greater tendency to align in parallel arrays, whereas the fibrils of fibrillary glomerulonephritis always are randomly distributed.[970] The ultrastructural deposits of immunotactoid glomerulonephritis resemble those seen in cryoglobulinemic glomerulonephritis, and thus the latter must be ruled out before making a diagnosis of immunotactoid glomerulopathy. However, cryoglobulinemic microtubules typically are shorter and less well designed than immunotactoid microtubules.

LIGHT MICROSCOPY

Immunotactoid glomerulopathy has a varied light microscopic appearance. Combined capillary wall thickening and mesangial expansion are most common, which often gives a membranoproliferative appearance. Immunotactoid deposits may be massive, resulting in nodular mesangial expansion in some specimens.

IMMUNOFLUORESCENCE MICROSCOPY

The deposits of immunotactoid glomerulopathy usually are IgG dominant with staining for both κ and λ light chains; however, the immunoglobulin in the deposits of immunotactoid glomerulopathy is more often monoclonal than in fibrillary glomerulonephritis.[964] Monoclonality warrants clinical workup for a B cell dyscrasia.

Pathogenesis

The etiology and pathogenesis of fibrillary glomerulonephritis and immunotactoid glomerulopathy are not known. Fibrillary glomerulonephritis and immunotactoid glomerulonephritis have been associated with lymphoproliferative disease (e.g., chronic lymphocytic leukemia or B cell lymphomas).[964,970,971] Immunotactoid glomerulonephritis is more frequently associated with a monoclonal gammopathy.[972] On rare occasions, fibrillary glomerulonephritis can also be associated with a monoclonal gammopathy.[973,974] The possible oligoclonal character of the deposits of fibrillary glomerulonephritis may facilitate self-association and fibrillar organization in a fashion analogous to that of the monoclonal light chains in immunoglobulin light chain (AL) amyloidosis.[967] The resemblance of immunotactoid deposits to those of cryoglobulinemia, which often contain a monoclonal component, also raises the possibility that the presence of some type of uniformity of the immunoglobulin in the deposits may be causing the patterned organization in immunotactoid glomerulopathy. Rarely, fibrillary glomerulonephritis may be associated with concomitant hepatitis C virus infection[975] or an unusual IgM glomerular deposition disease.[976]

Epidemiology and Clinical Features

An analysis of 9085 consecutive native kidney biopsy specimens evaluated by the UNC Nephropathology Laboratory revealed a frequency of 0.8% for fibrillary glomerulonephritis and 0.1% for immunotactoid glomerulonephritis, compared with 14.5% for MN, 7.5% for IgA nephropathy, 2.6% for type I MPGN, 1.5% for amyloidosis, and 0.8% for anti-GBM glomerulonephritis. Thus, fibrillary glomerulonephritis is about as common as anti-GBM glomerulonephritis and much more frequent than immunotactoid glomerulopathy.

Patients with fibrillary glomerulonephritis present with a mixture of nephrotic and nephritic syndrome features.[965,967,970] Patients may have microscopic or macroscopic hematuria, renal insufficiency (including rapidly progressive glomerulonephritis in a few patients), hypertension, and proteinuria, which may be in the nephrotic range. In a series of 28 patients with fibrillary glomerulonephritis, the mean age was 49 years (range = 21 to 75 years); the ratio of males to females was 1:1.8, and the ratio of whites to blacks was 8.3:1.[967] After 24 months of follow-up, renal survival was only 48%.[967] Renal insufficiency is common at the time of presentation, as are hematuria and hypertension. In patients in whom these disorders are diagnosed, cryoglobulinemia and systemic lupus erythematosus must be ruled out. Such patients have progressive renal failure in fewer than 5 years, although long-term patient survival is more than 80% at 5 years.[972,977]

In a group of six patients with immunotactoid glomerulopathy, the mean age was 62.[965] At presentation, the clinical features in these patients looked very much like those in patients with fibrillary glomerulonephritis and included proteinuria, hematuria, and renal insufficiency. Importantly, patients with immunotactoid glomerular disease are more likely to have an associated hematopoietic process and poor long-term survival.[965] In a review study of 67 patients presenting with fibrillary glomerulopathy (n = 61) or immunotactoid glomerulopathy (n = 6), all patients had proteinuria and half had nephrotic syndrome, whereas hematuria occurred in approximately two thirds of patients and hypertension in about 75% of patients.[978] Renal insufficiency was discovered in half the patient population. There were no statistically significant differences in clinical presentation between patients with fibrillary glomerulonephritis and those with immunotactoid glomerulonephritis. Etiologically, patients with immunotactoid glomerulonephritis were statistically more likely to have an underlying lymphoproliferative disease, a monoclonal spike on serum protein electrophoresis, and hypocomplementemia.[978]

Fibrillary glomerulonephritis with associated pulmonary hemorrhage has been reported anecdotally.[979] One patient with immunotactoid glomerulopathy also had extrarenal deposits in both the liver and bone.[980]

Treatment

At this time, there is no convincingly effective form of treatment for patients with either fibrillary glomerulonephritis or immunotactoid glomerulopathy.[970] The dismal prognosis in patients with either of these diseases has prompted physicians to search for some immunosuppressive form of treatment. Fully 40% to 50% of patients with these diseases develop ESRD within 6 years of presentation.[962,963,965,967] Efforts at treatment with either glucocorticoids or alkylating agents such as cyclophosphamide have typically shown either no response or, at best, some amelioration of proteinuria.[981] In the authors' own experience, prednisone therapy alone has had no benefit. One small case series (three patients) reported significant improvement in proteinuria in response to rituximab, either alone or in combination with corticosteroids, or tacrolimus.[982] In fibrillary glomerulonephritis and other forms of glomerulonephritis associated with chronic lymphocytic leukemia or other forms of lymphocytic lymphoma, there is a report of improvement in a minority of patients treated with chlorambucil. Thus, it is possible that the treatment of the underlying malignancy, if present, may improve the glomerulonephritis.[971]

The recurrence rate of fibrillary glomerulonephritis after renal transplantation is unclear. One report describes recurrent disease in three of four patients who had received five transplants.[983] In a larger case series, recurrent disease occurred in none of five patients with fibrillary glomerulonephritis, but in five of seven patients with monoclonal gammopathy and fibrillary deposits.[984]

Rapidly Progressive Glomerulonephritis and Crescentic Glomerulonephritis

Nomenclature and Categorization

The term *rapidly progressive glomerulonephritis* (RPGN) refers to a clinical syndrome characterized by a rapid loss of renal function, often accompanied by oliguria or anuria, by features of glomerulonephritis, including dysmorphic erythrocyturia, erythrocyte cylindruria, and glomerular proteinuria.[985] Aggressive glomerulonephritis that causes RPGN usually has extensive crescent formation.[986] For this reason, the clinical term *rapidly progressive glomerulonephritis* is sometimes used interchangeably with the pathologic term *crescentic glomerulonephritis*. Crescentic glomerulonephritis is the most aggressive structural phenotype in the continuum of injury that results from glomerular inflammation (see Figure 31-18). This pathologic feature can be seen on light and electron microscopy.[986-988] It is the result of focal rupture of glomerular capillary walls that allows inflammatory mediators and leukocytes to enter Bowman's space, where they induce epithelial cell proliferation and macrophage maturation that together produce cellular crescents (Figure 31-30).[989-991]

Renal diseases other than crescentic glomerulonephritis can cause the signs and symptoms of RPGN. Two examples are acute thrombotic microangiopathy and atheroembolic

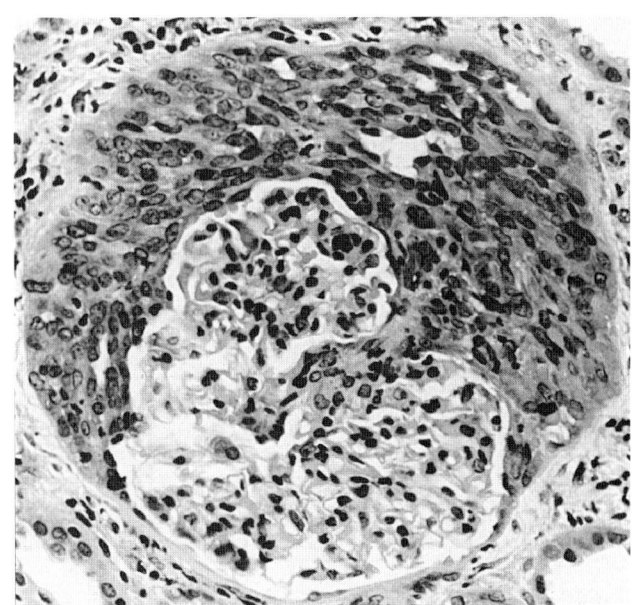

FIGURE 31-30 Light micrograph showing a large cellular crescent. (×500.)

renal disease. Although acute tubular necrosis and acute tubulointerstitial nephritis may cause rapid loss of renal function and oliguria, these processes typically do not cause dysmorphic erythrocyturia, erythrocyte cylindruria, or substantial proteinuria.

A small minority of all patients with glomerulonephritis develop RPGN. The incidence of the clinical syndrome has been estimated to be as low as 7 cases per million population per year.[581,992] The three major immunopathologic categories of crescentic glomerulonephritis have different frequencies in different age groups (Table 31-16).[985-987,993] In a patient who has RPGN clinically and in whom crescentic glomerulonephritis is identified by light microscopy in a renal biopsy specimen, the precise diagnostic categorization of the disease requires integration of clinical, serologic, immunohistologic, and electron microscopic data (Figure 31-31).

Immune complex crescentic glomerulonephritis is caused by immune complex localization within glomeruli. It is the most common cause of RPGN in children (see Table 31-16).[986] The major clinical differential diagnosis in children is hemolytic uremic syndrome, which also can cause rapid loss of renal function, hypertension, hematuria, and proteinuria. The presence of microangiopathic hemolytic anemia and thrombocytopenia are indicators that the rapid loss of renal function is more

TABLE 31-16 Relative Frequency of Immunopathologic Categories of Crescentic Glomerulonephritis (CGN) in Different Age Groups (in Percent)*

IMMUNO-PATHOLOGIC CATEGORY	AGE IN YEARS			
	ALL AGES (n = 632)	1-20 (n = 73)	21-60 (n = 303)	>60 (n = 256)
Anti–glomerular basement membrane CGN	15	12	15	15
Immune complex CGN	24	45	35	6
Pauci-immune CGN†	60	42	48	79
Other	1	0	3	0

*CGN is defined as the presence of crescents in >50% of glomeruli. Frequency is determined with respect to age in patients whose renal biopsy specimens were evaluated at the University of North Carolina Nephropathology Laboratory. Notice the very high frequency of pauci-immune disease (usually antineutrophil cytoplasmic antibody [ANCA] associated) in the elderly.

†Approximately 90% associated with ANCA.

Data from Jennette JC, Nickeleit V: Anti-glomerular basement membrane glomerulonephritis and Goodpasture's syndrome. In Jennette JC, Olson JL, Schwartz MM, et al (editors): *Heptinstall's pathology of the kidney,* ed 6, Philadelphia, 2006, Lippincott Williams & Wilkins, Table 13.1.

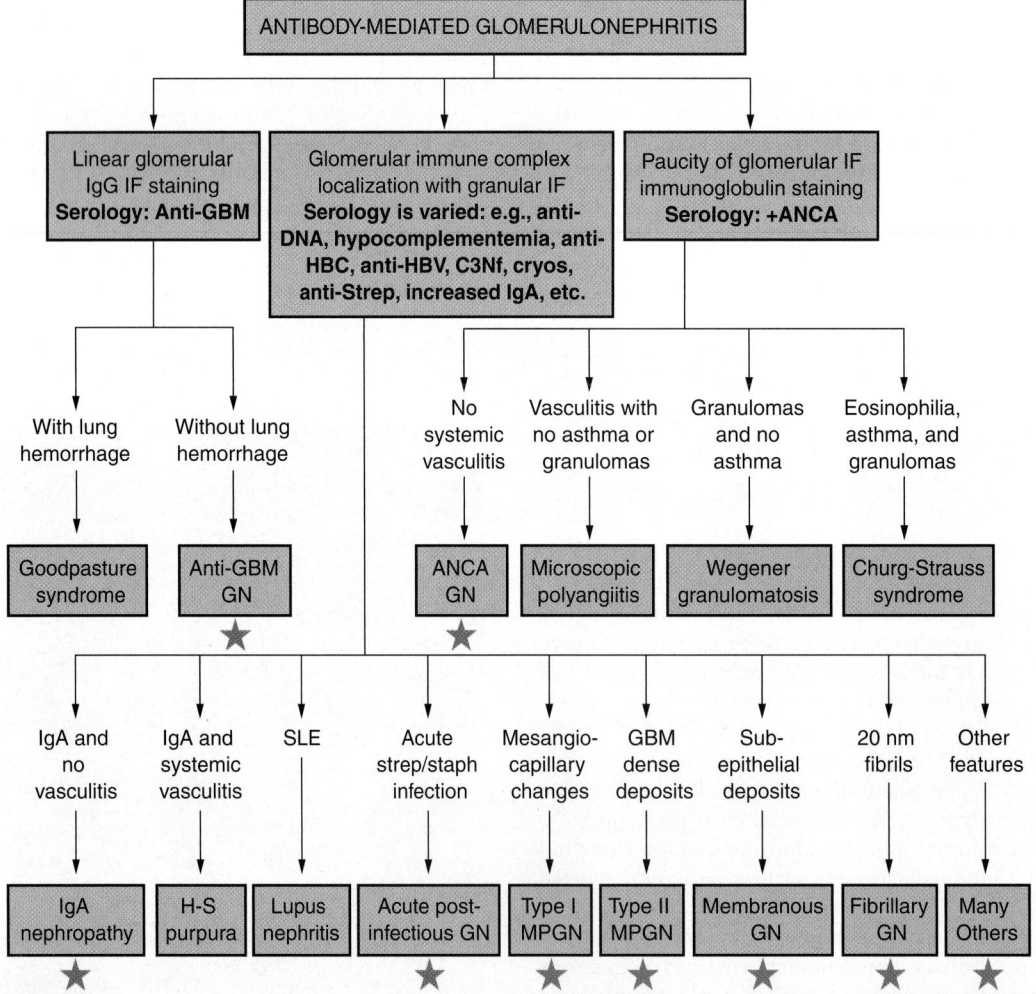

FIGURE 31-31 Algorithm for categorizing glomerulonephritis that is known or suspected of being mediated by antibodies. This categorization applies to glomerulonephritis with crescents as well as to glomerulonephritis without crescents. The diseases with stars beneath them can be considered primary glomerular diseases, whereas those without stars are secondary to (components of) systemic diseases.

likely caused by hemolytic uremic syndrome than by crescentic glomerulonephritis. Pauci-immune crescentic glomerulonephritis, which shows no evidence of localization of immune complex or anti-GBM antibodies in glomeruli, is usually associated with the present of ANCAs and is the most common cause of RPGN and crescentic glomerulonephritis in adults, especially older adults (Tables 31-16 and 31-17).[985,993-995] In most patients, pauci-immune crescentic glomerulonephritis is a component of a systemic small vessel vasculitis, such as Wegener's granulomatosis or microscopic polyangiitis; however, some patients have renal-limited (primary) disease.[986,996] Anti-GBM disease is the least frequent cause of crescentic glomerulonephritis (see Tables 31-16 and 31-17).[985,986,993,994]

Immune Complex–Mediated Crescentic Glomerulonephritis

Epidemiology

Most patients with immune complex–mediated crescentic glomerulonephritis have clinical or pathologic evidence of a specific category of primary glomerulonephritis, such as IgA nephropathy, postinfectious glomerulonephritis, or MPGN, or they have glomerulonephritis that is a component of a systemic immune complex disease, such as systemic lupus erythematosus, cryoglobulinemia, or Henoch-Schönlein purpura. A minority of patients with immune complex crescentic glomerulonephritis, however, do not have patterns of immune complex localization that readily fit into these specific categories of immune complex glomerulonephritis.[997] This rare entity is sometimes called *idiopathic crescentic immune complex glomerulonephritis.*

Immune complex crescentic glomerulonephritis accounts for the majority of crescentic glomerulonephritis in children, but for only a minority of crescentic glomerulonephritis in the elderly (see Table 31-16). The higher frequency in children and young adults reflects a similar trend in other types of immune complex glomerulonephritis such as IgA nephropathy, PSGN, MPGN types I and II, and lupus nephritis.

Pathology

LIGHT MICROSCOPY
The light microscopic appearance of crescentic immune complex glomerulonephritis depends on the underlying category of glomerulonephritis; for example, in their most aggressive expressions, MPGN, MN, acute postinfectious glomerulonephritis, and proliferative glomerulonephritis, including IgA nephropathy, can all have crescent formation.[331-335,603,609,736,937,992,998] This underlying phenotype of immune complex glomerulonephritis is recognized best in the intact glomeruli or glomerular segments. There usually are varying combinations of capillary wall thickening and endocapillary hypercellularity in the intact glomeruli. This is in contrast to anti-GBM glomerulonephritis and ANCA glomerulonephritis, which tend to have surprisingly little alteration in intact glomeruli and segments in spite of the severe necrotizing injury in involved glomeruli and segments. In glomerular segments adjacent to crescents in immune complex glomerulonephritis, there usually is some degree of necrosis with karyorrhexis; however, the necrosis rarely is as extensive as that typically seen with anti-GBM or ANCA glomerulonephritis. In addition, there is less destruction of Bowman's capsule associated with crescents in immune complex glomerulonephritis, as well as less pronounced periglomerular tubulointerstitial inflammation. Crescents in immune complex glomerulonephritis have a higher proportion of epithelial cells to macrophages than crescents in anti-GBM or ANCA glomerulonephritis, which may be related to the less severe disruption of Bowman's capsule and thus less opportunity for macrophages to migrate in from the interstitium.[997]

IMMUNOFLUORESCENCE MICROSCOPY
Immunofluorescence microscopy, as well as electron microscopy, provides the evidence that crescentic glomerulonephritis is immune complex mediated versus anti-GBM antibody mediated or ANCA associated. The pattern and composition of immunoglobulin and complement staining depends on the underlying category of immune complex glomerulonephritis that has induced crescent formation.[332,608,999] For example, crescentic glomerulonephritis with predominantly mesangial IgA-dominant deposits is indicative of crescentic IgA nephropathy; C3-dominant deposits with peripheral bandlike configurations suggest crescentic MPGN; coarsely granular capillary wall deposits raise the possibility of crescentic postinfectious glomerulonephritis; and finely granular IgG-dominant capillary wall deposits suggest crescentic MN. The latter may be a result of concurrent anti-GBM disease, which also causes linear GBM staining beneath the granular staining, or concurrent ANCA disease, which can be documented serologically. About a quarter of all patients with

TABLE 31-17 Frequency of Immunopathologic Categories of Glomerulonephritis (GN) in Renal Biopsy Specimens Evaluated by Immunofluorescence Microscopy*

IMMUNOHISTOLOGIC CATEGORY	ALL PROLIFERATIVE GN (n = 1093)	ANY CRESCENTS (n = 540)	>50% CRESCENTS (n = 195)	ARTERITIS IN SPECIMEN (n = 37)
Pauci-immune GN (<2+ immunoglobulin staining)	45% (496/1093)	51% (227/540)	61% (118/195)[†]	84% (31/37)
Immune complex GN (≥2+ immunoglobulin staining)	52% (570/1093)	44% (238/540)	29% (56/195)	14% (5/37)[‡]
Anti–glomerular basement membrane GN	3% (27/1093)	5% (25/540)[§]	11% (21/195)	3% (1/37)[¶]

*Based on the analysis of over 3000 consecutive nontransplant renal biopsy specimens evaluated at the University of North Carolina Nephropathology Laboratory.
†Seventy of 77 patients (91%) tested positive for antineutrophil cytoplasmic antibody (ANCA) (44 for perinuclear ANCA [P-ANCA] and 26 cytoplasmic ANCA [C-ANCA]).
‡Four patients had lupus and one had poststreptococcal glomerulonephritis.
§Three of 19 patients (16%) tested positive for ANCA (2 for P-ANCA and 1 for C-ANCA).
¶This patient also tested positive for P-ANCA (myeloperoxidase ANCA).
Data from Jennette JC, Falk RJ: The pathology of vasculitis involving the kidney, *Am J Kidney Dis* 24:130-141, 1994.

crescentic immune complex glomerulonephritis are ANCA positive, whereas fewer than 5% of patients with noncrescentic immune complex glomerulonephritis are ANCA positive. This suggests that the presence of ANCAs in patients with immune complex glomerulonephritis may predispose to a disease that is more aggressive.

ELECTRON MICROSCOPY

As with the findings by immunofluorescence microscopy, the findings by electron microscopy in patients with crescentic immune complex glomerulonephritis depend on the type of immune complex disease that has induced crescent formation. The hallmark ultrastructural finding is immune complex–type electron-dense deposits. These can be mesangial, subendothelial, intramembranous, subepithelial, or any combinations of these. The pattern and distribution of deposits may indicate a particular phenotype of primary crescentic immune complex glomerulonephritis, such as postinfectious, membranous, or membranoproliferative type I or II.[332,608,999] Ultrastructural findings also may suggest that the disease is secondary to some unrecognized systemic process. For example, endothelial tubuloreticular inclusions suggest lupus nephritis, and microtubular configurations in immune deposits suggest cryoglobulinemia.

As with all types of crescentic glomerulonephritis, breaks in GBMs usually can be identified if looked for carefully, especially in glomerular segments adjacent to crescents. Dense fibrin tactoids occur in thrombosed capillaries, in sites of fibrinoid necrosis, and in the interstices between the cells in crescents. In general, the extent of fibrin tactoid formation in areas of fibrinoid necrosis is less conspicuous in crescentic immune complex glomerulonephritis than in crescentic anti-GBM or ANCA glomerulonephritis.

Pathogenesis

Crescentic glomerulonephritis is the result of a final common pathway of glomerular injury that results in crescent formation. Multiple causes and pathogenic mechanisms can lead to the final common pathway, including many types of immune complex disease. The general dogma is that immune complex localization in glomerular capillary walls and mesangium, by either deposition or in situ formation or both, activates multiple inflammatory mediator systems.[188,985,986] This includes humoral mediator systems, such as the coagulation system, kinin system, and complement system, as well as phlogogenic cells, such as neutrophils, monocytes/macrophages, platelets, lymphocytes, endothelial cells, and mesangial cells. The activated cells also release soluble mediators, such as cytokines and chemokines. If the resultant inflammation is contained within the GBM, a proliferative or membranoproliferative phenotype of injury ensues with only endocapillary hypercellularity. However, if the inflammation breaks through capillary walls into Bowman's space, extracapillary hypercellularity (crescent formation) results.

Complement activation has often been considered a major mediator of injury in immune complex glomerulonephritis; however, experimental data also indicate the importance of Fc receptors in immune complex–mediated injury.[1000,1001] For example, mice deficient for the FcγRI and FcγRIII receptors have a markedly reduced tendency to develop immune complex glomerulonephritis.[1002,1003]

Treatment

The therapy for crescentic immune complex glomerulonephritis is influenced by the nature of the underlying category of immune complex glomerulonephritis. For example, acute PSGN with 50% crescents might not prompt the same therapy as IgA nephropathy with 50% crescents. However, there is an inadequate number of controlled prospective studies to guide therapy for most forms of crescentic immune complex glomerulonephritis. Some nephrologists extrapolate from the lupus nephritis experience and choose to treat patients with crescentic immune complex disease with immunosuppressive drugs that they would not use if the glomerular lesions appeared less aggressive. For the minority of patients who have idiopathic immune complex crescentic glomerulonephritis, the most common treatment is immunosuppressive therapy with pulse methylprednisolone, followed by prednisone at a dosage of 1 mg/kg daily tapered over the second to third month to an alternate-day regimen until completely discontinued.[581,1004-1006] In patients with a rapid decline in renal function, cytotoxic agents in addition to corticosteroids may be considered. As with anti-GBM and ANCA disease, immunotherapy should be initiated as early as possible during the course of crescentic immune complex glomerulonephritis to reduce the likelihood of reaching the irreversible stage of advanced scarring. There is evidence, however, that crescentic glomerulonephritis with an underlying immune complex proliferative glomerulonephritis is less responsive to aggressive immunosuppressive therapy than is anti-GBM or ANCA crescentic glomerulonephritis.[937,997]

Anti–Glomerular Basement Membrane Glomerulonephritis

Epidemiology

Anti-GBM disease accounts for about 10% to 20% of crescentic glomerulonephritis.[581] This disease is characterized by circulating antibodies to the GBM (anti-GBM) and deposition of IgG or, rarely, IgA along the GBM.[581,997,1007-1019] Anti-GBM antibodies may be eluted from renal tissue samples from patients with anti-GBM disease, which allows verification that the antibodies are specific to the GBM.[581,1013,1017] The antibodies eluted from renal tissue bind to the same epitope of type IV collagen as the circulating anti-GBM antibodies from the same patient.[1020]

Anti-GBM disease occurs as a renal-limited disease (anti-GBM glomerulonephritis) and as a pulmonary-renal vasculitic syndrome (Goodpasture's syndrome).[581,997,1007-1019,1021] The incidence of anti-GBM disease has two peaks with respect to age. The first peak is in the second and third decades of life, and anti-GBM disease in this age group shows a male preponderance and a higher frequency of pulmonary hemorrhage (Goodpasture's syndrome). The second peak is in the sixth and seventh decades, and this later-onset disease is more common in women, who more often have renal-limited disease.

Genetic susceptibility to anti-GBM disease is associated with HLA-DR2 specificity.[1022] More detailed analysis of the association with HLA-DR2 revealed a link with the DRB1 alleles DRB1*1501 and DQB*0602.[1023-1027] Further refinement of this association showed that polymorphic residues in the second peptide-binding region of the HLA class II antigen segregated with disease, which supports the hypothesis that the HLA association in anti-GBM disease reflects the ability of certain class II molecules to bind and present anti-GBM peptides to helper T (T_H) cells.[1023]

This concept is further supported by mouse models of anti-GBM disease in which crescentic glomerulonephritis and lung hemorrhage are restricted to only certain major histocompatibility complex (MHC) haplotypes, despite the ability of mice of all haplotypes to produce antibodies to the $\alpha 3$ NC1 ("noncollagenous") domain of type IV collagen.[1028] Analysis of gene expression in the kidneys of mouse strains susceptible to anti-GBM antibody–induced nephritis, compared with those of control strains, revealed that one fifth of the underexpressed genes in these mice belonged to the kallikrein gene family, which encodes serine esterases implicated in the regulation of inflammation, apoptosis, redox balance, and fibrosis.[1029] Antagonizing the kallikrein pathway by blocking the bradykinin receptors B1 and B2 augmented disease, whereas bradykinin administration reduced the severity of anti-GBM antibody–induced nephritis in a susceptible mouse strain. Nephritis-sensitive mouse strains had kallikrein haplotypes that were distinct from those of control strains, including several regulatory polymorphisms. These results suggest that kallikreins are protective disease-associated genes in anti-GBM antibody–induced nephritis.[1029] Whether these findings pertain to susceptibility to or severity of anti-GBM disease in humans is unknown.

Pathology

IMMUNOFLUORESCENCE MICROSCOPY

The pathologic finding of linear staining of the GBMs for immunoglobulin is indicative of anti-GBM glomerulonephritis (Figure 31-32).[1014,1017,1018,1030-1033] The immunoglobulin is predominantly IgG; however, rare patients with IgA-dominant anti-GBM glomerulonephritis have also been reported.[1015,1034] Linear staining for both κ and λ light chains typically accompanies the staining for γ heavy chains. Linear staining for γ heavy chains alone indicates γ heavy-chain deposition disease. Most specimens with anti-GBM glomerulonephritis have discontinuous linear to granular capillary wall staining for C3, but a minority show little or no C3 staining. Linear staining for IgG may also occur along tubular basement membranes.[1018]

The linear IgG staining of GBMs frequently seen in patients with diabetic glomerulosclerosis and the less intense linear staining seen in older patients with hypertensive vascular disease must not be confused with that in anti-GBM disease. The clinical data and light microscopic findings should help make this distinction. Serologic confirmation should always be obtained to substantiate the diagnosis of anti-GBM disease.

Serologic testing for ANCAs should be ordered simultaneously, because a quarter to a third of patients with anti-GBM disease are also ANCA positive, and this may modify the prognosis and the likelihood of systemic small vessel vasculitis.[1035,1036]

LIGHT MICROSCOPY

At the time of biopsy, 97% of patients have some degree of crescent formation and 85% have crescents in 50% or more of glomeruli (Tables 31-17 and 31-18).[986,1030] On average, 77%

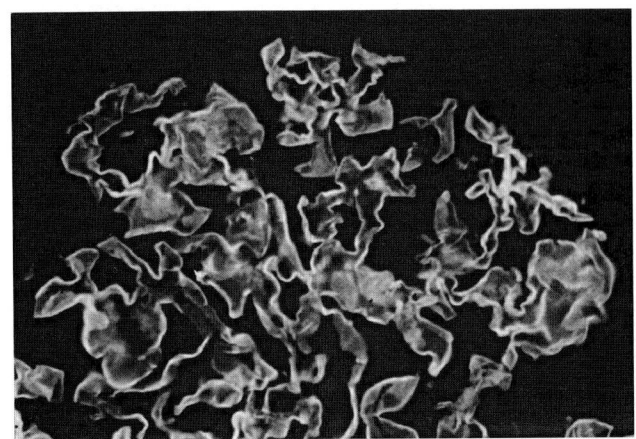

FIGURE 31-32 Immunofluorescence micrograph of a portion of a glomerulus with features of anti-glomerular basement membrane (anti-GBM) glomerulonephritis showing linear staining of GBMs for immunoglobulin G (IgG). (Fluorescein isothiocyanate anti-IgG stain, ×600.) (Modified from Ferrario F, Kourilsky O, Morel-Maroger L: Acute endocapillary glomerulonephritis in adults: a histologic and clinical comparison between patients with and without initial acute renal failure, *Clin Nephrol* 19:17-23, 1983.)

of glomeruli have crescents. Glomeruli with crescents typically have fibrinoid necrosis in adjacent glomerular segments. Nonnecrotic segments may look entirely normal by light microscopy or may have slight infiltration by neutrophils or mononuclear leukocytes. This differs from crescentic immune complex glomerulonephritis, which typically has capillary wall thickening and endocapillary hypercellularity in the intact glomeruli. Special stains that outline basement membranes, such Jones' silver methenamine or periodic acid–Schiff stains, often demonstrate focal breaks in GBMs in areas of necrosis and also show focal breaks in Bowman's capsule. The most severely injured glomeruli have global glomerular necrosis, circumferential cellular crescents, and extensive disruption of Bowman's capsule.

The acute necrotizing glomerular lesions and the cellular crescents evolve into glomerular sclerosis and fibrotic crescents, respectively.[1030] If the renal biopsy specimen is obtained several weeks into the course of anti-GBM disease, the only lesions may be these chronic sclerotic lesions. There may be a mixture of acute and chronic lesions; however, the glomerular lesions of anti-GBM glomerulonephritis tend to be more in synchrony than those of ANCA glomerulonephritis, which more often show admixtures of acute and chronic injury.

Tubulointerstitial changes are commensurate with the degree of glomerular injury. Glomeruli with extensive necrosis and disruption of Bowman's capsule typically have intense periglomerular inflammation, including occasional multinucleated giant cells. There also is focal tubular epithelial acute simplification or atrophy, focal interstitial edema and fibrosis, and focal interstitial infiltration of predominantly mononuclear leukocytes. There are no specific changes in arteries or arterioles. If necrotizing inflammation is observed in arteries or arterioles, the possibility of concurrent anti-GBM and ANCA disease should be considered.

ELECTRON MICROSCOPY

The findings by electron microscopy reflect those seen by light microscopy.[1030,1037] In acute disease, there is focal glomerular necrosis with disruption of capillary walls. Bowman's capsule also may have focal gaps. Leukocytes, including neutrophils

TABLE 31-18 Frequency of Crescent Formation in Various Glomerular Diseases*

DISEASE	PATIENTS WITH CRESCENTS (%)	PATIENTS WITH CRESCENTS IN ≥50% OF GLOMERULI (%)	AVERAGE % OF GLOMERULI WITH CRESCENTS
Anti–glomerular basement membrane GN	97	85	77
Antineutrophil cytoplasmic antibody–associated GN	90	50	49
Immune complex–mediated GN			
Lupus GN (classes III and IV)	56	13	27
Henoch-Schönlein purpura GN†	61	10	27
Immunoglobulin A nephropathy†	32	4	21
Acute postinfectious GN†	33	3	19
Fibrillary GN	23	5	26
Membranoproliferative GN type I	24	5	25
Membranous lupus GN (class V)	12	1	17
Membranous GN (nonlupus)	3	0	15

*Based on analysis of over 6000 native kidney biopsy specimens evaluated at the University of North Carolina Nephropathology Laboratory. In general, diseases in which crescents are most often seen also have the largest percentage of glomeruli involved by crescents when they are present.

†Because more severe cases of immunoglobulin A nephropathy and postinfectious glomerulonephritis are more often evaluated by renal biopsy, the extent of crescent formation is higher in the patients included in this table than in the general group of patients with these diseases.

GN, Glomerulonephritis.

Adapted from Jennette JC: Rapidly progressive and crescentic glomerulonephritis, *Kidney Int* 63:1164-1172, 2003.

and monocytes, often are present at sites of necrosis, but are uncommon in intact glomerular segments. Fibrin tactoids, which are electron-dense curvilinear accumulations of polymerized fibrin, accumulate at sites of coagulation system activation, including sites of capillary thrombosis, fibrinoid necrosis, and fibrin formation in Bowman's space (Figure 31-33). Cellular crescents contain cells with ultrastructural features of macrophages and epithelial cells. An important negative observation is the absence of immune complex–type electron-dense deposits. These occur only in specimens from patients with anti-GBM disease who have concurrent immune complex disease. Glomerular segments that do not have necrosis may appear remarkably normal, with only focal effacement of visceral epithelial foot processes. There may be slight lucent expansion of the lamina rara interna, but this is an inconstant and nonspecific feature. In chronic lesions, amorphous and banded collagen deposition distorts or replaces the normal architecture.

Pathogenesis

The landmark studies opening the way to an understanding of the pathogenesis of anti-GBM disease were those of Lerner, Glassock, and Dixon.[1013] In these studies, antibodies eluted from the kidneys of patients with Goodpasture's syndrome and injected into monkeys led to the induction of fulminant glomerulonephritis, proteinuria, renal failure, and pulmonary hemorrhage along with intense staining of the GBM for human IgG.

The antigen to which anti-GBM antibodies react was initially found to be in the collagenase-resistant part of type IV collagen, the "noncollagenous" or NC1 domain.[1038-1040] The antigenic epitopes found in the NC1 domain are in a cryptic form, as evidenced by the fact that little reactivity is found against the native hexameric structure of the NC1 domain. However, when the hexameric NC1 domain is denatured and dissociates into dimers and monomers, the reactivity of antibodies increases 15-fold.[1040] About 90% of anti–type IV

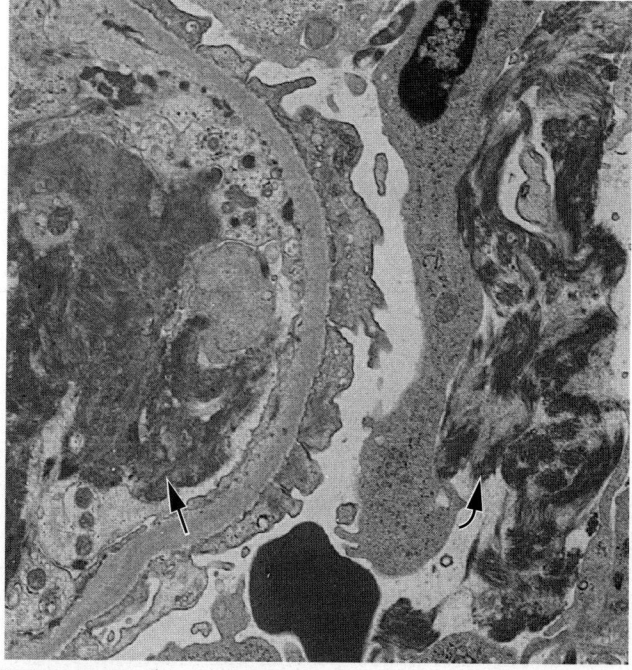

FIGURE 31-33 Electron micrograph of a portion of a glomerular capillary wall and adjacent urinary space from a patient with anti–glomerular basement membrane (anti-GBM) glomerulonephritis. Note the fibrin tactoids within a capillary thrombus (*straight arrow*) and in Bowman's space (*curved arrow*) between the cells of a crescent. Also note the absence of immune complex-type electron-dense deposits in the capillary wall. (×6000.)

collagen antibodies are directed against the α3 chain of type IV collagen.[1005,1041] The Goodpasture epitopes in the native autoantigen are sequestered within the NC1 hexamers of the α3α4α5(IV) collagen network and are a feature of the quaternary structure of two distinct subsets of α3α4α5(IV) NC1 hexamers. Goodpasture antibodies breach only the quaternary structure of hexamers containing only monomer subunits, whereas hexamers composed of both dimer and monomer subunits (D-hexamers) are resistant to autoantibodies under native conditions.[1042,1043] The epitopes of D-hexamers are structurally sequestered by dimer reinforcement of the quaternary complex.[1043] It is presumed that environmental factors, such as exposure to hydrocarbons,[1044] tobacco smoke,[1045] and endogenous oxidants,[1046] can also expose the cryptic Goodpasture epitopes. In patients with anti-GBM disease who do not have antibodies to the classical epitope on the α3 chain, antibodies to entactin have been detected.[1047] A small percentage of patients with anti-GBM disease may in addition have limited reactivity with the NC1 domains of the α1 or α4 chains of type IV collagen. These additional reactivities seem to be more frequent in patients with anti-GBM–mediated glomerulonephritis alone.[1048]

The majority of patients with anti-GBM disease express antibodies to two major conformational epitopes (E_A and E_B) located within the carboxy-terminal noncollagenous (NC1) domain of the α3 chain of type IV collagen.[1049-1052] The immunodominant target epitope, E_A, is encompassed by α3 NC1 residues 17 to 31. A homologous region at α3 NC1 residues 127 to 141 encompasses the E_B epitope, recognized by the autoantibodies of only a small number of patients.[1053] In a large cohort of Chinese patients,[1054] the levels of antibody against E_A and E_B were strongly correlated with each other. Antibody levels against α3, E_A, and E_B correlated with serum creatinine level and with death or ESRD at 1 year, but not with sex, age, presence of ANCAs, or hemoptysis. The stimuli and mechanism(s) leading to the formation of autoantibodies remain unclear; as is the mechanism by which the normally hidden target epitopes become accessible to circulating autoantibodies.

About one third of patients with anti-GBM/Goodpasture's disease also have circulating ANCAs, the majority being to MPO (MPO-ANCA).[1036,1048,1051,1055,1056] In a study of a large cohort of Chinese patients with Goodpasture's disease, with or without ANCAs, no differences in reactivity to the E_A, E_B, and S2 epitopes (a recombinant construct expressing the nine amino acid residues critical for the Goodpasture's epitope)[1057] was detected between patients with anti-GBM antibodies plus ANCAs and with anti-GBM antibodies alone.[1058] The mechanism by which some patients develop both anti-GBM antibodies and ANCAs is unknown. It is speculated that in such patients ANCAs may appear first and cause damage to the GBM, thus exposing the normally hidden target epitopes of anti-GBM antibodies. Coexistence of ANCAs in patients with anti-GBM antibodies is associated with small vessel vasculitis in organs in addition to lung and kidney. In experimental models, the presence of antibodies to MPO aggravate experimental anti-GBM disease.[1036,1059]

Unlike the anti-GBM autoantibodies seen in Goodpasture's disease, which are directed at the NC1 domain of the α3 chain of type IV collagen, the anti-GBM alloantibodies that cause posttransplant nephritis in some patients with X-linked Alport's syndrome are directed against conformational epitopes in the NC1 domain of α5(IV) collagen only.[1060] Allograft-eluted alloantibodies mainly targeted two epitopes accessible in the α3α4α5 NC1 hexamers of human GBM, unlike the sequestered α3 NC1 epitopes of anti-GBM autoantibodies.

A number of animal models of anti-GBM disease have been developed over the years, based on the immunization of animals with heterologous or homologous GBM.[1061]

Alternatively, anti-GBM antibody–induced injury can be produced passively by the intravenous injection of heterologous anti-GBM antibodies. This leads to two phases of injury. The first, or so-called heterologous, phase occurs in the first 24 hours and is mediated by the direct deposition of the heterologous antibodies on the GBM with subsequent recruitment of neutrophils. This is usually followed by an autologous phase, depending on the host's immune response to the heterologous immunoglobulin bound to the GBM.[1061]

The rat model of anti-GBM disease induced by injection of heterologous anti-GBM antibodies has permitted the study of the roles of various inflammatory mediators in the development of anti-GBM disease.[1063-1065] Thus, in Wistar-Kyoto (WKY) rats injected with a rabbit antiserum to rat GBM, impairing leukocyte recruitment and monocyte/macrophage glomerular infiltrate by blocking the chemokine C-X-C motif ligand 16 (CXCL16) with a polyclonal anti-CXCL16 antiserum in the acute inflammatory phase or progressive phase of established glomerulonephritis significantly attenuated glomerular injury and improved proteinuria.[1066] Similarly, the depletion of CD8+ cells prevented the initiation and progression of anti-GBM crescentic glomerulonephritis. In the same animal model, treatment with an antibody to perforin resulted in a significant reduction in the amount of proteinuria, frequency of glomerular crescents, and number of glomerular monocytes and macrophages, although the number of glomerular CD8+ cells was not changed.[1067] These results suggest that CD8+ cells play a role in glomerular injury as effector cells, in part through a perforin/granzyme-mediated pathway.

The more recent development of analogous murine models of anti-GBM disease opens the way for more specific evaluations of the inflammatory processes with the use of strains of mice with specific gene knockouts.[1028] For example, the role of protease-activated receptor 2 (PAR-2) in renal inflammation was studied using PAR-2–deficient (PAR-2$^{-/-}$) mice.[1068] PAR-2 is a cellular receptor expressed predominantly on epithelial, mesangial, and endothelial cells in the kidney and on macrophages. PAR-2 is activated by serine proteases and coagulation factors VIIa and Xa. In the kidney, PAR-2 induces both endothelium-dependent and -independent vasodilatation of afferent renal arteries and renal mesangial cells proliferation in vitro. Glomerulonephritis was induced in mice by intravenous injection of sheep antimouse GBM globulin. In this model, PAR-2–deficient mice had reduced crescent formation, proteinuria, and serum creatinine level compared with wild-type mice, but this was not associated with a difference in glomerular accumulation of CD4+ T cells or macrophages, or with the number of proliferating cells in glomeruli. These results demonstrate a proinflammatory role for PAR-2 in crescentic glomerulonephritis that is independent of effects on glomerular leukocyte recruitment and mesangial cell proliferation.

Although anti-GBM disease is considered a prototypical antibody-mediated glomerulonephritis, several lines of evidence point to an important role for T cells in the initiation or pathogenesis of this disease. A role of T cells is suggested by the increased susceptibility to the disease associated with the presence of HLA class II antigens DRB1*1501 and DQB*0602.[1023-1027] Further evidence of the involvement of T cell activation in the development of the autoimmune response to the NC1 domain of the α3 chain of type IV collagen comes from studies of T cell proliferation in response to other monomeric components of the GBM[1069] and synthetic oligopeptides.[1070] The transfer of CD4+ T cells specific to a recombinant GBM antigen into syngeneic rats resulted in a crescentic glomerulonephritis without linear anti-GBM IgG deposition.[1071] Furthermore a single nephritogenic T cell epitope of type IV collagen α3 NC1 was demonstrated to induce glomerulonephritis in Wistar-Kyoto rats.[1072] Interestingly, cross-reactive peptides from human infection-related microbes could be identified that also induced severe proteinuria and modest to severe glomerulonephritis in immunized rats.[1073] One peptide derived from *Clostridium botulinum* also induced pulmonary hemorrhage.[1073]

After immunization of mice with α3 NC1 domains of type IV collagen, the development of glomerulonephritis and lung hemorrhage depends on certain MHC haplotypes and the ability of mice to mount a T_H1 response.[1028] The role of T cells in this model was further documented by the fact that the passive transfer of lymphocytes or antibodies from nephritogenic strains to syngenetic recipients led to the development of nephritis, whereas the passive transfer of antibodies to T cell receptor–deficient mice failed to do so.[1028]

Conversely, CD4+CD25+ regulatory T cells may play an important role in regulating the immune response in anti-GBM disease. Thus, the transfer of regulatory T cells into mice that were previously immunized with rabbit IgG, and before an injection of anti-GBM rabbit serum, significantly attenuated the development of proteinuria and dramatically decreased glomerular damage. On histologic analysis there was reduced infiltration of CD4+ T cells, CD8+ T cells, and macrophages, but the deposition of immune complexes was not prevented.[1074] In humans, the action of regulatory T cells may explain, in part, the uncommon occurrence of disease relapses and the eventual disappearance of anti-GBM antibodies in patients even without the use of immunosuppressant medications.[1075] Thus, analysis of peripheral blood mononuclear cells from patients with Goodpasture's disease revealed the emergence of GBM-specific CD25+ regulatory T cells in the convalescent period, whereas they were undetected at the time of acute presentation.[1076]

The role of complement in the pathogenesis of anti-GBM disease is evidenced by the deposition of C3 along the GBM. The role of complement activation has been examined largely in studies of passive injection of heterologous antibodies to GBM. Investigations using this model suggest that the terminal components of the complement system are not involved in the pathogenesis of disease.[1077] Results of further studies in rabbits that are congenitally deficient in the sixth component of complement also suggested that the terminal components of complement do not play a major part in the pathogenesis of the disease except in leucocyte-depleted animals.[1078,1079] The study of complement cascade activation in a murine model of heterologous anti-GBM nephritis previously led to conflicting results as to the role of complement activation in this model.[1080] More recent studies involving the same murine model, using mice completely deficient of complement components C3 or C4, revealed a greater protective effect of C3 deficiency than of C4 deficiency. Both protective effects could be overcome if the dose of nephritogenic antibodies was increased.[1081]

To further evaluate the role of complement activation and of Fcγ receptors, an "attenuated" mouse model of anti-GBM disease was developed by using a subnephritogenic dose of rabbit anti-mouse GBM antibody followed 1 week later with an injection of mouse monoclonal antibody against rabbit IgG, which resulted in albuminuria.[1082] In this model, albuminuria was absent in Fcγ chain–deficient mice and reduced in C3–deficient mice, which indicates a role for both Fcγ receptors and complement. C1q and C4 deficient mice did develop proteinuria, which is suggestive of involvement of the alternative complement pathway.[1082] The role of Fcγ receptors is also evidenced by the occurrence of severe lung hemorrhage in mice deficient in the inhibitory Fcγ 2b receptor that were treated with bovine type IV collagen.[1083]

Conclusions about the pathogenesis of human anti-GBM disease from animal models must be tempered, because the animal models may not replicate human disease.

Clinical Features and Natural History

The onset of renal anti-GBM disease is typically characterized by an abrupt, acute glomerulonephritis with severe oliguria or anuria. There is a high risk of progression to ESRD if appropriate therapy is not instituted immediately. Prompt treatment with plasmapheresis, corticosteroids, and cyclophosphamide results in patient survival of approximately 85% and renal survival of approximately 60%.[1004,1084-1088]

Rarely, the disorder has a more insidious onset, and patients remain essentially asymptomatic until the development of uremic symptoms and fluid retention.[581,1021,1033,1089] The onset of disease may be associated with arthralgias, fever, myalgias, and abdominal pain; however, gastrointestinal complaints or neurologic disturbances are rare.

Goodpasture's syndrome is characterized by the presence of pulmonary hemorrhage concurrent with glomerulonephritis. The usual pulmonary manifestation is severe pulmonary hemorrhage, which may be life threatening; however, patients may have milder disease that can be focal. The absence of hemoptysis does not rule out diffuse alveolar hemorrhage. For patients with early or focal disease, a high level of suspicion is necessary to establish the diagnosis, especially in the presence of unexplained anemia. The diagnosis may be aided by measurements showing an increased diffusing capacity of carbon monoxide and by findings on computed tomographic images of the chest. Ultimately the diagnostic evaluation of alveolar hemorrhage usually includes bronchoscopic examination and bronchoalveolar lavage.[1090] This approach also allows exclusion of airway sources of bleeding and possible associated infections. In patients with anti-GBM disease, the occurrence of pulmonary hemorrhage is far more common in smokers than nonsmokers,[1091] and may be associated with environmental exposures to hydrocarbons[1091-1094] or upper respiratory tract infections.[1095] Occupational exposure to petroleum-based mineral oils is a risk factor for the development of anti-GBM antibodies per se.[1096] The association of pulmonary hemorrhage with environmental toxins and infection raises the theoretical possibility that they expose the cryptic antigen in the alveolar basement membrane and thus allow its recognition by circulating anti–GBM antibodies.

Laboratory Findings

Renal involvement by anti-GBM disease typically causes an acute nephritic syndrome with hematuria that includes dysmorphic erythrocytes and red blood cells casts. Although nephrotic-range proteinuria may occur, full nephrotic syndrome is rarely seen.[1018,1021,1030,1033,1089]

The diagnostic laboratory finding in anti-GBM disease is detection of circulating antibodies to GBM, and specifically to the α3 chain of type IV collagen. These antibodies are detected in approximately 95% of patients by immunoassays using various forms of purified or recombinant substrates.[1098] The anti-GBM antibodies are most often of the IgG1 subclass, but may also be of the IgG4 subclass, with the latter being seen more often in females.[1099]

Treatment

The standard treatment for anti-GBM disease is intensive plasmapheresis combined with corticosteroids and cyclophosphamide.[1004,1085,1100-1103] Plasmapheresis consists of removal of 2 to 4 L of plasma and their replacement with a 5% albumin solution continued on a daily basis until circulating antibody levels become undetectable. In those patients with pulmonary hemorrhage, clotting factors should be replaced by administering fresh-frozen plasma at the end of each treatment. Prednisone should be administered starting at a dose of 1 mg/kg of body weight for at least the first month and then should be tapered to alternate-day therapy during the second and third months of treatment. Cyclophosphamide is administered orally (at a dosage of 2 mg/kg/day, adjusted with consideration of the degree of impairment of renal function and the white blood cell count) for 8 to 12 weeks. The role of high-dose intravenous methylprednisolone pulses remains unproven in the treatment of anti-GBM disease.[1104-1108] Nonetheless, the urgent nature of the clinical process prompts some nephrologists to administer methylprednisolone (7 mg/kg daily for 3 consecutive days) as part of induction therapy in this and other forms of crescentic glomerulonephritis.

When the regimen of aggressive plasmapheresis with corticosteroids and cyclophosphamide is used, patient survival is approximately 85%, with 40% progression to ESRD.[1004,1084-1089] These results are better than those achieved before the introduction of plasmapheresis, when patient survival was less than 50% with a near 90% rate of ESRD. In a study at the Hammersmith Hospital in the United Kingdom, Gaskin and Pusey demonstrated that aggressive plasmapheresis, even in patients with severe renal insufficiency, may have an ameliorative effect and provide improved long-term patient and renal survival.[1109] In that cohort, among patients who had a creatinine concentration of 500 μmol/L or more (>5.7 mg/dL) at presentation but did not require immediate dialysis, patient and renal survival were 83% and 82% at 1 year and 62% and 69% at last follow-up, respectively. The renal prognosis of patients who presented with dialysis-dependent renal failure was poor—92% of patients had at ESRD at 1 year. All patients who required immediate dialysis and whose renal biopsy specimens had crescents involving 100% of glomeruli remained dialysis dependent.[1110]

The major prognostic marker for progression to ESRD is the serum creatinine level at the time of initiation of treatment. Patients with a serum creatinine concentration above 7 mg/dL are unlikely to recover sufficient renal function to discontinue renal replacement therapy.[1016] At issue is whether and for how long aggressive immunosuppression should persist in dialysis-dependent patients. Aggressive immunosuppression and plasmapheresis are warranted in patients with pulmonary hemorrhage. Aggressive immunosuppression should be withheld in patients with disease limited to the kidney whose renal biopsy specimens show widespread glomerular and interstitial scarring and who have a serum creatinine concentration of more than 7 mg/dL at presentation. In such patients, the risks of therapy outweigh the potential benefits. In patients who have an elevated serum creatinine level, yet whose biopsy specimens show active crescentic glomerulonephritis, aggressive treatment should continue for at least 4 weeks. If there is no restoration of renal function by 4 to 8 weeks, and in the absence of pulmonary bleeding, immunosuppression should be discontinued.

Patients who have both circulating anti-GBM antibodies and ANCAs, may have a better chance of recovery of renal function than do patients with anti-GBM antibodies alone. In these patients, immunosuppressive therapy should not be withheld, even when serum creatinine levels are above 7 mg/dL, because the concomitant presence of ANCAs has been associated with a more favorable renal outcome in some studies,[1108,1111] though not in all.[1097] In a retrospective analysis comparing patients with anti-GBM antibodies, MPO-ANCAs, and both, "double-positive" patients and those with anti-GBM autoantibodies had significantly higher serum creatinine levels at presentation (10.3 ± 5.6 and 9.6 ± 8.1 mg/dL, respectively) than did patients with MPO-ANCAs alone (5.0 ± 2.9 mg/dL). One-year renal survival was better in patients with MPO-ANCAs alone (63%) than in the double-positive group (10.0%, $P = 0.01$) and the anti-GBM group (15.4%, $P = 0.17$).[1097]

Once remission of anti-GBM disease is achieved with immunosuppressive therapy, recurrent disease occurs only rarely.[1112-1115] Similarly, the recurrence of anti-GBM disease after renal transplantation is also rare, especially when transplantation is delayed until after the disappearance or substantial diminution of anti-GBM antibodies in the circulation.[1116]

Pauci-Immune Crescentic Glomerulonephritis

Epidemiology

In pauci-immune crescentic glomerulonephritis, the characteristic feature of the glomerular lesion is focal necrotizing and crescentic glomerulonephritis with little or no glomerular staining for immunoglobulins by immunofluorescence microscopy.[986,1008,1030,1101,1103] Pauci-immune crescentic glomerulonephritis usually is a component of a systemic small vessel vasculitis; however, some patients have renal-limited (primary) pauci-immune crescentic glomerulonephritis.[986,996,1035] ANCA-associated small vessel vasculitis is discussed in more detail in Chapter 32. Pauci-immune crescentic glomerulonephritis, including that accompanying small vessel vasculitis, is the most common category of RPGN in adults, especially older adults (see Table 31-16). The disease has a predilection for whites compared with blacks (see Table 31-15). There are no sex differences (see Table 31-15).

Pathology

LIGHT MICROSCOPY

The light microscopic appearance of ANCA-associated pauci-immune crescentic glomerulonephritis is indistinguishable from that of anti-GBM crescentic glomerulonephritis.[332,607,987,997,1117-1120] Renal-limited (primary) pauci-immune crescentic glomerulonephritis also is indistinguishable from pauci-immune crescentic glomerulonephritis that occurs as a component of a systemic small vessel vasculitis such as Wegener's granulomatosis, microscopic polyangiitis, or Churg-Strauss syndrome. As illustrated in Figure 31-18, ANCA glomerulonephritis and anti-GBM glomerulonephritis most often manifest as crescentic glomerulonephritis.

At the time of biopsy, approximately 90% of renal biopsy specimens showing ANCA-associated pauci-immune glomerulonephritis have some degree of crescent formation, and approximately half of the specimens have crescents involving 50% or more of glomeruli (Tables 31-17 and 31-18). Over 90% of specimens have focal segmental to global fibrinoid necrosis (Figure 31-34). As with anti-GBM disease, the intact glomerular segments often have no light microscopic abnormalities. The most severely injured glomeruli have not only extensive necrosis of glomerular tufts but also extensive lysis of Bowman's capsule with resultant periglomerular inflammation. The periglomerular inflammatory area contains varying mixtures of neutrophils, eosinophils, lymphocytes, monocytes, and macrophages, including occasional multinucleated giant cells. This periglomerular inflammatory area may have a granulomatous appearance, especially when the glomerulus that was the nidus of inflammation has been destroyed or is not in the plane of section. This granulomatous appearance is a result of the periglomerular reaction to extensive glomerular necrosis and is not specific for a particular category of necrotizing glomerulonephritis.

This pattern of injury can be seen with anti-GBM glomerulonephritis, renal-limited pauci-immune crescentic glomerulonephritis, and crescentic glomerulonephritis secondary to microscopic polyangiitis, Wegener's granulomatosis, and Churg-Strauss syndrome. Necrotizing granulomatous inflammation that is not centered on a glomerulus, but rather is in the interstitium or centered on an artery, raises the possibility of Wegener's granulomatosis or Churg-Strauss syndrome. The presence of arteritis in a biopsy specimen that has pauci-immune crescentic glomerulonephritis indicates that the glomerulonephritis is a component of a more widespread vasculitis, such as microscopic polyangiitis, Wegener's granulomatosis, or Churg-Strauss syndrome.

The acute necrotizing glomerular lesions evolve into sclerotic lesions. During completely quiescent phases, a renal biopsy specimen may have only focal sclerotic lesions that may mimic FSGS. ANCA-associated glomerulonephritis is often characterized by many recurrent bouts of exacerbation. Therefore, combinations of active acute necrotizing glomerular lesions and chronic sclerotic lesions often occur in the same renal biopsy specimen.

IMMUNOFLUORESCENCE MICROSCOPY

By definition, the distinguishing pathologic difference between pauci-immune crescentic glomerulonephritis and anti-GBM and immune complex crescentic glomerulonephritis is the absence or paucity of glomerular staining for immunoglobulins. How pauci-immune is pauci-immune crescentic glomerulonephritis? One basis for categorizing the glomerular disorder as pauci-immune crescentic glomerulonephritis is to determine whether the patient is likely to be ANCA positive, which increases the likelihood of certain systemic small vessel vasculitides.[337,1117,1121,1122] The likelihood of positivity for ANCA is inversely proportional to the intensity of glomerular immunoglobulin staining by immunofluorescence microscopy in a specimen with crescentic glomerulonephritis.[1120] The likelihood of a positive result on an ANCA serologic assay is approximately 90% if there is no staining for immunoglobulin, approximately 80% if there is trace to 1+ staining (on a scale of 0 to 4+), approximately 50% if there is 2+ staining, approximately 30% if there is 3+ staining, and less than 10% if there is 4+ staining. Thus, even patients with definite evidence of immune complex–mediated glomerulonephritis have a higher than expected frequency of ANCAs, but the highest frequency is in those patients who have little or no evidence of immune complex– or anti-GBM–mediated disease.

The presence of ANCAs at a higher than expected frequency in immune complex disease is intriguing and raises the possibility that ANCAs are contributing to the pathogenesis of not only pauci-immune crescentic glomerulonephritis but also the most severe examples of immune complex disease.[337] Looking at this issue from a different perspective, approximately 25% of patients with idiopathic immune complex crescentic glomerulonephritis (i.e., immune complex glomerulonephritis that does not fit well into one of the categories of primary or secondary immune complex disease) are ANCA positive, compared with fewer than 5% of patients who have idiopathic immune complex glomerulonephritis with no crescents.[337]

Glomerular capillary wall or mesangial staining usually accompanies immunoglobulin staining and is present in occasional specimens that do not have immunoglobulin staining. There is irregular staining for fibrin at sites of intraglomerular fibrinoid necrosis and capillary thrombosis, and in the interstices of crescents. Foci of glomerular necrosis and sclerosis also may have irregular staining for C3 and IgM.

ELECTRON MICROSCOPY

The findings by electron microscopy are indistinguishable from those described earlier for anti-GBM glomerulonephritis.[1037] Specimens with pure pauci-immune crescentic glomerulonephritis have no or only a few immune complex–type electron-dense deposits. Foci of glomerular necrosis have

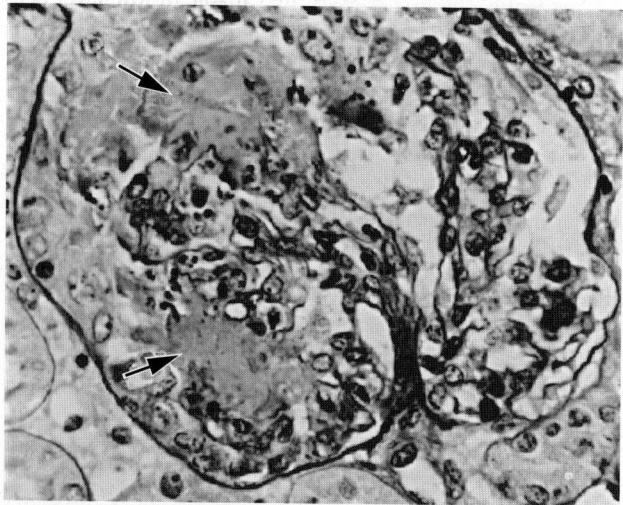

FIGURE 31-34 Light micrograph showing segmental fibrinoid necrosis in a glomerulus from a patient with antineutrophil cytoplasmic antibody–associated pauci-immune crescentic glomerulonephritis. (Periodic acid–Schiff stain, ×300.)

leukocyte influx, breaks in GBMs, and fibrin tactoids in capillary thrombi and sites of fibrinoid necrosis.

Pathogenesis

The pathogenesis of pauci-immune crescentic glomerulonephritis is currently not fully understood.[1123,1124] In the absence or paucity of immune complex deposition within glomeruli or other vessels, it is difficult to implicate classical mechanisms of immune complex–mediated damage in the pathogenesis of pauci-immune crescentic glomerulonephritis. On the other hand, the substantial accumulation of polymorphonuclear leukocytes at the sites of vascular necrosis has led to examination of the role of neutrophil activation in this disease. There is now convincing evidence that ANCAs are directly involved in the pathogenesis of pauci-immune small vessel vasculitis or glomerulonephritis. Substantial in vitro data implicates a pathogenic role for ANCAs based on the demonstration that these autoantibodies activate normal human polymorphonuclear leukocytes.[1120,1123,1125]

For anti-MPO antibodies, anti-PR3 antibodies, or autoantibodies to other neutrophil antigens contained in the azurophilic granules to interact with their corresponding antigens, either the antibodies must penetrate the cell or, alternatively, those antigens must translocate to the cell surface. Indeed, small amounts of cytokine (e.g., TNF-α and IL-1) at concentrations too low to cause full neutrophil activation are capable of inducing such a translocation of ANCA antigens to the cell surface.[1126] This translocation of ANCA antigens to the cell surface has been demonstrated in vivo on the neutrophils of patients with Wegener's granulomatosis and in patients with sepsis.[1127-1129] Patients with ANCA disease aberrantly express PR3 and MPO genes, and this expression correlates with disease activity.[1130] Despite the fact that these genes exist on different chromosomes, their expression appears coordinately upregulated during disease activity and downregulated during remission. Epigenetic changes occur as a result of loss of recruitment by histone demethylase PRC2 (polycomb recessive complex 2) by RUNX3 (Runt-related transcription factor 3) in both MPO and PR3 genes with depressed gene transcription. Not only is there loss of histone demethylase, but jumonji D3 appears to be expressed in these patients, which further diminishes methylation status.[1131]

Regardless of whether the antigen is expressed on the surface of the cell as a consequence of cytokine stimulation or gene expression, in the presence of circulating ANCAs the interaction of the autoantibody with its externalized antigen results in full activation of the neutrophil, which leads to the respiratory burst and degranulation of primary and secondary granule constituents.[1129,1132] The current hypothesis stipulates that ANCAs induce a premature degranulation and activation of neutrophils at the time of their margination and diapedesis, which leads to the release of lytic enzymes and toxic oxygen metabolites at the site of the vessel wall and thus produces a necrotizing inflammatory injury. This view is supported by in vitro studies demonstrating that neutrophils activated by ANCAs lead to the damage and destruction of human umbilical vein endothelial cells in culture.[1133,1134]

Not only does neutrophil degranulation cause direct damage of the endothelium, but ANCA antigens released from neutrophils and monocytes enter endothelial cells and cause cell damage. PR3 can enter the endothelial cells by a receptor-mediated process[1135-1137] and result in the production of IL-8[1138] and chemoattractant protein-1. PR3 also induces an apoptotic event through both proteolytic and nonproteolytic mechanisms.[1139,1140] Similarly, MPO enters endothelial cells by an energy-dependent process[1141] and transcytoses intact endothelium to localize within the extracellular matrix. There, in the presence of the substrates H_2O_2 and NO_2^-, MPO catalyzes nitration of tyrosine residues on extracellular matrix proteins,[1142] which results in the fragmentation of extracellular matrix proteins.[1143] However, a recent study suggests that endothelial cells inhibit superoxide generation by ANCA-activated neutrophils and that serine proteases may play a more important role than reactive oxygen species as mediators of endothelial injury during ANCA-associated systemic vasculitis.[1144]

Neutrophil activation by ANCAs is likely mediated by both the antigen-binding portion of the autoantibodies (F[ab′]2) and by the engagement of their Fc fraction to Fcγ receptors on the surface of neutrophils.[996,1134,1145,1146] Human neutrophils constitutively express the IgG receptors FcγRIIa and FcγRIIIb.[1147] Engagement of the Fc receptors results in a number of neutrophil-activation events, including respiratory burst, degranulation, phagocytosis, cytokine production, and upregulation of adhesion molecules. ANCAs have been shown to engage both types of receptors.[1134,1148] In particular, FcγRIIa engagement by ANCAs appears to increase actin polymerization in neutrophils, which leads to distortion in their shape and possibly decreases their ability to pass through capillaries (the primary site of injury in ANCA vasculitis).[1149] Furthermore, polymorphisms of the FcγRIIIb receptors[1150,1151] (but not of FcγRIIa[1152,1153]) appear to influence the severity of ANCA vasculitis.

In addition to the Fc receptor–mediated mechanism, substantial data support a role for the F(ab′)2 portion of the antibody molecule in leukocyte activation. ANCA F(ab′)2 portions induce oxygen radical production[1146] and the transcription of cytokine genes in normal human neutrophils and monocytes. Microarray gene chip analysis showed that ANCA IgG and ANCA F(ab′)2 stimulate transcription of a distinct subset of genes, some unique to whole IgG, some unique to F(ab′)2 fragments, and some common to both.[1154] It is most likely that F(ab′)2 portions of ANCA are capable of low-level neutrophil and monocyte activation.[1146] The Fc portion of the molecule almost certainly causes leukocyte activation once the F(ab′)2 portion of the immunoglobulin has interacted with the antigen, either on the cell surface or in the microenvironment.[1134] The signal transduction pathways of F(ab′)2 and Fc receptor activation through a specific p21ras (Kirsten-ras) pathway have now been elucidated.[1155]

The role of T cells in the pathogenesis of pauci-immune necrotizing small vessel vasculitis or glomerulonephritis, although suspected,[1156,1157] is less well defined. Such a role is suggested by the presence of CD4+ T cells in granulomatous[1158] and active vasculitic lesions[1159-1163] and by some correlation of the levels of soluble markers of T cell activation with disease activity,[1158,1164] specifically, soluble interleukin-2 receptor and sCD3.[1165,1166] Much is known about T cell responsivity in ANCA disease, including the recognition of PR3 or MPO by T cells.[1167,1168] The proportion of regulatory T cells in ANCA patients increases, although these regulatory T cells seem defective in their inability to suppress proliferation of effector cells in cytokine production. In addition, the percentage of T cells secreting IL-17 increases in the periphery, and serum levels of T_H17-associated cytokine IL-23 correlate with the propensity for disease activity.[1169]

Further establishment of a pathogenetic link between ANCAs and the development of pauci-immune necrotizing glomerulonephritis and small vessel vasculitis greatly benefited from the development of animal models of this disease.

Early models of disease were based on the finding of circulating anti-MPO antibodies in 20% of female MRL/lpr/lpr mice[1170] and in an inbred strain of mice, SCG/Kj, derived from the MRL/lpr mice and BXSB strains that develop a severe form of crescentic glomerulonephritis and systemic necrotizing vasculitis.[1171] Anti-MPO antibodies have been isolated from these strains of mice. Treatment of rats with mercuric chloride led to the development of widespread inflammation, including necrotizing vasculitis in the presence of anti-MPO antibodies and anti-GBM antibodies.[1172] A more convincing model points to a pathogenetic role for ANCAs. Aggravation of a mild anti-GBM–mediated glomerulonephritis in rats when the animals were previously immunized with MPO[1059] suggests that minor proinflammatory events could be driven to severe necrotizing processes in the presence of ANCAs.

Compelling models for ANCA small vessel vasculitis were recently described. MPO knockout mice were immunized with murine MPO. Splenocytes from these mice were transferred to immunoincompetent recombination-activating gene 2 (Rag2)–deficient mice, which resulted in the development of anti-MPO antibodies, severe necrotizing and crescentic glomerulonephritis, and, in some animals, vasculitis in the lung and other organ systems. In a separate but similar set of experiments, anti-MPO antibodies alone were transferred into Rag2$^{-/-}$ mice and induced pauci-immune necrotizing and crescentic glomerulonephritis.[1173] These studies indicate that anti-MPO antibodies cause pauci-immune necrotizing disease. The glomerulonephritis induced by anti-MPO antibodies is aggravated by the administration of lipopolysaccharide.[1174] Conversely, the disease is abrogated when the neutrophils of anti-MPO–recipient mice are depleted by a selective antineutrophil monoclonal antibody.[1175] In experiments to assess the role of T cells using this animal model, the transfer of T cell–enriched splenocytes (>99% T cells) did not cause glomerular crescent formation or vascular necrosis. These data do not support a pathogenic role for anti-MPO T cells in the induction of acute injury.[1176]

Using this same model, a previously unsuspected role of complement activation was demonstrated. Glomerulonephritis and vasculitis were abolished with administration of cobra venom factor and failed to develop in mice deficient in complement factors C5 and B, whereas C4-deficient mice developed disease comparable with that in wild-type mice.[1177] These results indicate that the alternative complement pathway is required for disease induction, but not the classical or lectin pathways. Using this same mouse model, glomerulonephritis was completely abolished or markedly ameliorated by treating the mice with a C5-inhibiting monoclonal antibody either 8 hours before or 1 day after disease induction with anti-MPO IgG and lipopolysaccharide.[1178] Thus, anti-C5 had a dramatic therapeutic effect in this mouse model of ANCA vasculitis. These results are corroborated by in vitro experiments which demonstrate that blockade of the C5a receptor on human neutrophils abolished their stimulation.[1179] In aggregate, these results suggest an important role of complement activation in

the pathogenesis of ANCA vasculitis and have implications for possible future therapeutic interventions using blockers of the complement cascade.

The pathogenic role of anti-MPO antibodies has also been documented in a second animal model in which rats immunized with human MPO developed anti–rat MPO antibodies and necrotizing and crescentic glomerulonephritis, as well as pulmonary capillaritis.[1180] Using intravital microscopy, elegant studies have shown that anti-MPO–activated neutrophils undergo margination and diapedesis along the vascular wall.[1180,1181] These two animal models document that anti-MPO antibodies are capable of causing necrotizing and crescentic glomerulonephritis and widespread systemic vasculitis.

A model of anti-PR3–induced vascular injury was developed in PR3/neutrophil elastase–deficient mice in which the passive transfer of murine anti–mouse PR3 was associated with a stronger localized cutaneous inflammation, and perivascular infiltrates were observed around cutaneous vessels at the sites of intradermal injection of TNF-α.[1176,1182] In summary, these animal studies document that both anti-MPO and PR3 antibodies are capable of causing disease.

As is true for most autoimmune responses, the inciting events in the breakdown of tolerance and the generation of anti-MPO or anti-PR3 antibodies are not known. Although genetic predispositions[1183] and environmental exposure to foreign pathogens,[1184] notably silica,[1185,1186] have been implicated, no direct link between these exposures and the formation of ANCAs has been established. A serendipitous finding in ANCA vasculitis has spawned a theory of autoantigen complementarity.[1187,1188] This theory rests on evidence that proteins transcribed and translated from the sense strand of DNA bind to proteins that are transcribed and translated from the antisense strand of DNA. It has been demonstrated that some patients with PR3-ANCAs harbor antibodies to an antigen complementary to the middle portion of PR3. These anticomplementary PR3 antibodies form an antiidiotypic pair with PR3-ANCAs. Moreover, cloned complementary PR3 proteins bind to PR3 and function as a serine proteinase inhibitor. Preliminary data suggest that the complementary PR3 antigens are found on a variety of microbes, some of which have been associated with ANCA vasculitis and have also been found in the genome of some patients with both PR3-ANCAs and MPO-ANCAs.[1188] Although these studies need to be confirmed and expanded to determine the source of the complementary PR3 antigens and their role (if any) in inducing vasculitis, these observations may provide a promising avenue for detection of the proximate cause of the ANCA autoimmune response.

Clinical Features and Natural History

The majority of patients with pauci-immune necrotizing crescentic glomerulonephritis and ANCAs have glomerular disease as part of a systemic small vessel vasculitis. The disease is clinically limited to the kidney in about one third of patients.[1189] When both renal-limited and vasculitis-associated pauci-immune crescentic glomerulonephritis are considered, this category of crescentic glomerulonephritis is the most common cause of RPGN in adults.[986,992,1035,1189,1190] When the disorder is part of a systemic vasculitis, patients have pulmonary-renal, dermal-renal, or a multisystem disease. Frequent sites of involvement are the lungs, upper airways, sinuses, ears, eyes, gastrointestinal tract, skin, peripheral nerves, joints, and central nervous system. The three major ANCA-associated syndromes are microscopic polyangiitis, Wegener's granulomatosis, and Churg-Strauss syndrome (discussed more fully in Chapter 32).[1118,1191,1192] Even when patients have no clinical evidence of extrarenal manifestation of active vasculitis, systemic symptoms consisting of fever, fatigue, myalgias, and arthralgias are common.

Although most patients with ANCA-associated pauci-immune necrotizing glomerulonephritis have RPGN with rapid loss of renal function associated with hematuria, proteinuria, and hypertension, in some patients the disease follows a more indolent course of slow decline in function and less active urine sediment. In the latter group of patients, episodes of focal necrosis and hematuria resolve with focal glomerular scarring. Subsequent relapses result in cumulative damage to glomeruli.

It is important to note that patients who have only pauci-immune crescentic glomerulonephritis at presentation may later develop signs and symptoms of systemic disease with involvement of extrarenal organ systems.[1193] An autopsy study was conducted in deceased patients with ANCA-associated vasculitis. This study revealed the widespread presence of glomerulonephritis, but also demonstrated the finding of clinically silent extrarenal vasculitis. Eight percent of patients died either from septic infections or from progressive recurrent vasculitis.[1193]

No studies currently available specifically examine the prognostic factors of pauci-immune crescentic glomerulonephritis in the absence of extrarenal manifestations of disease. In studies addressing the question of prognosis of patients with ANCA-related small vessel vasculitis in general,[1121,1193,1194] the presence of pulmonary hemorrhage was found to be the most important determinant of patient survival. With respect to the risk of ESRD, the most important predictor of outcome is the entry serum creatinine level at the time of initiation of treatment.[1194] This parameter remained the most important predictive factor for renal outcome in a multivariate analysis that corrected for variables such as the presence or absence of extrarenal disease. Treatment resistance and progression to ESRD is also predicted by longer disease duration and vascular sclerosis on renal biopsy specimens (presence of glomerular sclerosis, interstitial infiltrates, tubular necrosis, and atrophy),[1195] and the presence of clinical markers of chronic disease, including cumulative organ damage (measured by the Vasculitis Damage Index).[1196] A finding of vascular sclerosis on the biopsy specimen was also found to be an independent predictor of treatment resistance[1197] and may be a reflection of chronic renal damage due to hypertension or other atherosclerotic processes, with ANCA-associated nephritis providing an additional insult.

The impact of renal damage as a predictor of resistance emphasizes the importance of early diagnosis and prompt initiation of therapy. It is important to note that although the entry serum creatinine level is the most important predictor of renal outcome, there is no threshold of renal dysfunction beyond which treatment is deemed futile, because more than half of patients who have a GFR of less than 10 mL/min at presentation reach a remission and experience a substantial improvement in renal function. Therefore, aggressive immunosuppressive therapy is warranted in all patients with newly diagnosed disease.[1197] However, the risk of progression to ESRD is also determined by the change in GFR within the first 4 months of treatment. In the absence of other disease manifestations, the decision to continue immunosuppressive therapy in patients with a sharply declining GFR should be weighed against the diminishing chance of renal recovery.[1197]

Relapses of ANCA small vessel vasculitis occur in up to 40% of patients. Based on a large cohort study, the risk of relapse appears to be predicted by the presence of PR3-ANCAs (as opposed to MPO-ANCAs) and the presence of upper respiratory tract or lung involvement.[1197] Patients with glomerulonephritis alone who predominantly have MPO-ANCAs belong to the subgroup of patients with a relatively low risk of relapse, with a relapse rate of around 25% at a median of 62 months.

Pauci-immune necrotizing glomerulonephritis and small vessel vasculitis may recur after renal transplantation.[1198,1199] The rate of recurrence of ANCA small vessel vasculitis in general, including pauci-immune necrotizing glomerulonephritis alone, is about 20%.[1200] The rate of recurrence in the subset of patients who have pauci-immune necrotizing glomerulonephritis alone without systemic vasculitis is unknown, but may be lower than 20%. A positive ANCA test result at the time of transplantation does not seem to be associated with an increased risk of recurrent disease.

Laboratory Findings

Approximately 80% to 90% of patients with pauci-immune necrotizing and crescentic glomerulonephritis have circulating ANCAs.[337,1121,1124,1191,1201-1203] On indirect immunofluorescence microscopy of alcohol-fixed neutrophils, ANCAs cause two patterns of staining: perinuclear (P-ANCA) and cytoplasmic (C-ANCA).[1124,1203] The two major antigen specificities for ANCA are MPO and PR3.[1117,1203-1207] Both proteins are found in the primary granules of neutrophils and the lysosomes of monocytes. With rare exceptions, anti-MPO antibodies produce a P-ANCA pattern of staining on indirect immunofluorescence microscopy, whereas anti-PR3 antibodies cause a C-ANCA pattern of staining. About two thirds of patients with pauci-immune necrotizing crescentic glomerulonephritis without clinical evidence of systemic vasculitis have MPO-ANCAs or P-ANCAs, and approximately 30% have PR3-ANCAs or C-ANCAs.[1118,1208] The relative frequency of MPO-ANCAs to PR3-ANCAs is higher in patients with renal-limited disease than in patients with microscopic polyangiitis or Wegener's granulomatosis.[1118]

As mentioned previously, about one third of patients with anti-GBM disease and approximately a quarter of patients with idiopathic immune complex crescent glomerulonephritis test positive for ANCAs; therefore, ANCA positivity is not completely specific for pauci-immune crescentic glomerulonephritis.[337] Maximal sensitivity and specificity with ANCA testing is achieved when both immunofluorescence and antigen-specific assays are performed. Antigen-specific assays may be either enzyme-linked immunosorbent assays or radioimmunoassays. A variety of commercial tests are now available; their diagnostic specificity ranges from 70% to 90%, and sensitivity ranges from 81% to 91%.[337,1209] Tests still do not provide the necessary sensitivity, specificity, and predictive power to allow their use as the basis for initiating or altering cytotoxic therapy.

The positive predictive value (PPV) of a positive ANCA test result (i.e., the percentage of patients with a positive result who have pauci-immune crescentic glomerulonephritis) depends on the signs and symptoms of disease in the patient who is being tested. The signs and symptoms indicate the pretest likelihood of pauci-immune crescentic glomerulonephritis (predicted prevalence), which greatly influences predictive value. The PPV of a positive ANCA result in a patient with classic features of RPGN is 95%.[337] In patients with hematuria and proteinuria, the PPV of a positive ANCA result is 84% if the serum creatinine level is more than 3 mg/dL, 60% if the serum creatinine level is 1.5 to 3.0 mg/dL, and only 29% if the serum creatinine level is less than 1 mg/dL.[1210] Although the PPV is not good in this last setting, the negative predictive value is greater than 95%, and thus a negative result can allay any concerns that the patient has early or mild pauci-immune necrotizing glomerulonephritis.

Urinalysis findings in pauci-immune crescentic glomerulonephritis include hematuria with dysmorphic red blood cells, with or without red cell casts, and proteinuria. The proteinuria ranges from 1 g of protein per 24 hours to as much as 16 g of protein per 24 hours.[1193,1211] Serum creatinine concentration usually is elevated at the time of diagnosis and rising, although a minority of patients have relatively indolent disease. Erythrocyte sedimentation rate and C-reactive protein level are elevated during active disease. Serum complement component levels are typically within normal limits.

Whether a renal biopsy is essential for the management of ANCA-associated pauci-immune glomerulonephritis depends on a number of factors, including the diagnostic accuracy of ANCA testing, the pretest probability of finding pauci-immune glomerulonephritis, the value of knowing the activity and chronicity of the renal lesions, and the risk associated with immunotherapy for ANCA-associated pauci-immune necrotizing glomerulonephritis. Based on a study of 1000 patients with proliferative and/or necrotizing glomerulonephritis and a positive test result for either PR3-ANCA or MPO-ANCA, the PPV of ANCA testing was found to be 86% with a false-positive rate of 14% and a false-negative rate of 16%. Considering the serious risks inherent in treatment with high-dose corticosteroids and cytotoxic agents, it is prudent to confirm the diagnosis and characterize the activity and chronicity of ANCA-associated pauci-immune crescentic glomerulonephritis by renal biopsy unless the patient is too ill to tolerate the procedure.[1210]

Treatment

Data on the treatment of ANCA-positive pauci-immune necrotizing and crescentic glomerulonephritis are derived from studies of ANCA-associated small vessel vasculitis, including Wegener's granulomatosis and microscopic polyangiitis. There are scant data specifically addressing the treatment of patients with renal-limited pauci-immune necrotizing glomerulonephritis. The treatment of pauci-immune crescentic glomerulonephritis (with or without systemic vasculitis) remains based primarily on varying regimens of corticosteroids and cyclophosphamide.[1194,1212,1213]

In view of the potential explosive and fulminant nature of this disease, induction therapy should be instituted using pulse methylprednisolone at a dosage of 7 mg/kg/day for three consecutive days in an attempt to halt the aggressive, destructive inflammatory process. This is followed by the institution of daily oral prednisone, as well as cyclophosphamide, either orally or intravenously. Prednisone is usually started at a dosage of 1 mg/kg/day for the first month, then tapered to an alternate-day regimen, and then discontinued by the end of the fourth to fifth month. When a regimen of monthly intravenous doses of cyclophosphamide is used, the starting dose should be about 0.5 g/m^2 and should be adjusted upward to 1 g/m^2 based on the 2-week leukocyte count nadir.[1213,1214] A regimen based on daily oral cyclophosphamide should begin at a dosage of 2 mg/kg/day[1212] and should be adjusted downward as needed to keep the nadir leukocyte count above 3000 cells/mm^3.

The optimal form of cyclophosphamide therapy (daily oral vs. intravenous pulse) has been the subject of investigation. In general, the intravenous regimen allows for an approximately twofold lower cumulative dose of cyclophosphamide than the oral regimen and is associated with a significant decrease in the rate of clinically significant neutropenia and other complications. In a meta-analysis of three randomized controlled trials, the rate of relapse associated with pulse cyclophosphamide was not statistically higher than the rate with a daily oral regimen, but the intravenous pulse regimen was associated with a statistically higher rate of remission and lower rates of leucopenia and infections.[1215] The final outcomes (death or ESRD) were no different for the two dosing regimen.

A large randomized controlled trial of pulse versus daily oral cyclophosphamide for induction of remission was recently conducted that included 149 patients with newly diagnosed generalized ANCA vasculitis with renal involvement.[1215a] Patients were randomly assigned to receive either pulse cyclophosphamide, 15 mg/kg every 2 weeks × 3 then every 3 weeks, or daily oral cyclophosphamide, 2 mg/kg/day. Cyclophosphamide therapy was continued for 3 months beyond the time of remission. All patients were then switched to azathioprine (2 mg/kg/day orally) until month 18. All patients received prednisolone starting at 1 mg/kg orally, followed by a taper. Patients with a serum creatinine level of more than 500 μmol/L (5.7 mg/dL) were excluded from the study. Seventy-nine percent of patients achieved remission by 9 months (median time to remission was 3 months for both groups). The two treatment groups did not differ in time to remission or proportion of patients who achieved remission at 9 months (88.1% in the pulse group vs. 87.7% in the daily oral group). GFR did not differ between the two groups at any time point. By 18 months, 13 patients in the pulse group and 6 in the daily oral group had experienced a relapse (HR = 2.01, CI = 0.77 to 5.30). Absolute cumulative cyclophosphamide dose in the daily oral group was almost twice that in the pulse group (15.9 g vs. 8.2 g, respectively; $P < 0.001$). The pulse group had a lower rate of leukopenia (HR = 0.41, CI = 0.23 to 0.71), but the frequency of serious infections was not statistically different between the two treatment groups.

This randomized controlled trial confirms that the two cyclophosphamide regimens are associated with similar remission rates and time to remission, with the pulse cyclophosphamide regimen resulting in about one half the cumulative medication dose of the oral regimen and a significantly lower rate of leucopenia. The trend toward a higher rate of relapse in the pulse group appears late (after 15 to 18 months) and is of unclear clinical significance for the long-term outcome of patients. In the absence of a clear advantage for daily oral cyclophosphamide, the pulse regimen can be favored as first-line induction therapy because it is associated with a lower cumulative dose and lower risks from severe leukopenia.

The length of cyclophosphamide therapy has changed significantly in recent years, largely based on the results of a large controlled trial in which patients who attained a complete remission after 3 months of cyclophosphamide therapy were randomly assigned to switch to azathioprine or to continue taking cyclophosphamide for a total of 12 months. After 12 months, both groups received azathioprine maintenance therapy for an additional year.[1062] Changing to azathioprine after 3 months of cyclophosphamide treatment appears as effective as receiving oral cyclophosphamide for 12 months followed by 12 months of azathioprine based on renal function and the frequency of relapse. It is noteworthy that patients whose PR3-ANCA titers remained positive at the time of the switch had about a twofold increased risk of subsequent relapse compared with patients whose ANCA titers had reverted to negative.[1216]

In three relatively small randomized controlled trials addressing the role of plasmapheresis in the treatment of ANCA-associated small vessel vasculitis and glomerulonephritis,[1217-1219] plasmapheresis was not found to provide any added benefit over immunosuppressive treatment alone in patients with renal-limited disease or in patients with mild to moderate renal dysfunction. However, the use of plasmapheresis in addition to immunosuppressive therapy appears to be beneficial in the subset of patients who require dialysis at the time of presentation.[1219,1220] In a study performed by a European vasculitis study group, the use of plasma exchange was found to be superior to pulse methylprednisolone in producing recovery of renal function in patients with severe renal dysfunction at the time of entry into the study (serum creatinine level of >5.7 mg/dL).[1221] Because of the clinically observed increased risk of severe bone marrow suppression with the use of cyclophosphamide in patients receiving dialysis, such treatment should be pursued with extreme caution.

Patients who eventually are able to discontinue dialysis usually do so within 12 weeks of initiation of therapy.[1214] For this reason, continuing immunosuppressive therapy beyond 12 weeks in patients who are still receiving dialysis is unlikely to be of added benefit (unless they continue to have extrarenal manifestations of vasculitis). In a retrospective analysis of 523 patients with ANCA vasculitis followed over a median of 40 months, 136 patients reached ESRD.[1222] Relapse rates of vasculitis were significantly lower in patients on long-term dialysis (0.08 episodes per person-year) than in the same patients before they reached ESRD (0.20 episodes per person-year) and in patients with preserved renal function (0.16 episodes per person year). Infections were almost twice as frequent among patients with ESRD receiving maintenance immunosuppressants and were an important cause of death. Given the lower risk of relapse with hemodialysis and the higher risk of infection and death with long-term immunosuppression, the risk/benefit ratio does not support the routine use of maintenance immunosuppression therapy in patients with ANCA small vessel vasculitis who are on long-term dialysis.

Although high-dose intravenous pooled immunoglobulin has been used in the treatment of systemic vasculitis resistant to the usual immunosuppressive treatment,[1223-1228] there are no published reports of its use in patients with pauci-immune crescentic glomerulonephritis alone without systemic involvement.

Trimethoprim-sulfamethoxazole has been suggested to be of benefit in the treatment of patients with Wegener's granulomatosis.[1229,1230] Such beneficial effects, if any, seem to be limited to the upper respiratory tract, and this antibiotic is unlikely to have a role in the treatment of pauci-immune crescentic glomerulonephritis alone. Induction therapy with methotrexate has been compared with cyclophosphamide treatment in patients with "early" limited Wegener's granulomatosis and mild renal disease.[1231-1235] The rate of remission at 6 months was comparable in the two treatment groups.[1233] However, the onset of remission was delayed in methotrexate-treated patients with more extensive disease or pulmonary involvement. Methotrexate was also associated with a significantly higher rate of relapse than cyclophosphamide (69.5% vs. 46.5%, respectively), and 45% of relapses occurred while patients were receiving methotrexate. The dose of methotrexate must be reduced in patients whose creatinine clearance is less than 80 mL/min, and its use is contraindicated when creatinine clearance is less than 10 mL/min. Moreover, in the authors' experience there are patients taking methotrexate who have progressive glomerulonephritis. Methotrexate is therefore unlikely to have any role in the treatment of pauci-immune crescentic glomerulonephritis alone.

Whether the use of cyclophosphamide can be reduced or avoided completely by the use of rituximab has been the subject of two randomized controlled trials. In the RITUXI-VAS trial, 44 patients with newly diagnosed ANCA vasculitis were randomly assigned in a ratio of 3:1 to receive either rituximab (375 mg/m² weekly × 4) in addition to cyclophosphamide (15 mg/kg intravenously × 2, 2 weeks apart), or to cyclophosphamide (15 mg/kg intravenously every 2 weeks × 3 then every 3 weeks for a maximum total of 10 doses).[1236] Both groups received the same intravenous and oral prednisolone regimen. Patients in the rituximab group did not receive maintenance therapy, whereas those in the cyclophosphamide group were switched to azathioprine until the end of the trial. Minimum follow-up was 12 months. The rate of sustained remission was similar in the two treatment groups (76% in the rituximab group vs. 82% in the cyclophosphamide group, P = 0.67). Severe adverse events were common in both groups, affecting 45% of patients in the rituximab group and 36% in the cyclophosphamide group (P = 0.60). This study suggests that a combination of rituximab and reduced-dose cyclophosphamide may be no less effective than a traditional cyclophosphamide regimen, but it did not demonstrate a safety benefit of a rituximab-based approach. This study was not powered to establish either equivalence or noninferiority.

In a large controlled trial designed to assess the noninferiority of rituximab compared with cyclophosphamide (http://www.immunetolerance.org/studies/rituximab-treatment-wegeners-granulomatosis-and-microscopic-polyangiitis-rave [NCT00104299]), 197 patients were randomly assigned to treatment with either rituximab (375 mg/m² infusions once weekly × 4) or cyclophosphamide (2 mg/kg/day orally) for months 1 to 3 followed by azathioprine (2 mg/kg/day orally) for months 4 to 6. All patients received methylprednisolone (1 g/day intravenously for up to 3 days) followed by prednisone (1 mg/kg/day, tapered off completely by 6 months). The induction phase of this trial revealed similar rates between the two treatment groups in complete remission at 6 months

(64% in the rituximab group vs. 55% in the cyclophosphamide group, P = 0.21).[1237] No differences were observed between the groups in the rates of disease flares. The evaluation of rituximab compared with cyclophosphamide awaits completion of the trial and analysis of the long-term outcomes (sustained remission, rate of relapses) and safety data.

These studies suggest that the substitution of cyclophosphamide with rituximab may be effective in patients with ANCA vasculitis. Rituximab has not been formally evaluated in patients with severe renal failure requiring dialysis.

The studies examining maintenance immunosuppression for the prevention of relapse are primarily geared to patients with Wegener's granulomatosis or microscopic polyangiitis. Current data suggest that patients with pauci-immune glomerulonephritis alone and MPO-ANCAs are at a relatively low risk of relapse.[1197] The value of prolonged maintenance immunosuppression in this group of patients is unknown, and any benefit in preventing a relapse would have to be weighed against the potential toxicity of immunosuppressive agents and the risks associated with their use. The diagnosis and management of ANCA-associated small vessel vasculitis is discussed in more detail in Chapter 32.

References

1. Brenner BM, Hostetter TH, Humes HD. Glomerular permselectivity: barrier function based on discrimination of molecular size and charge. *Am J Physiol.* 1978;234:F455-F460.
2. Shemesh O, Deen WM, Brenner BM, et al. Effect of colloid volume expansion on glomerular barrier size-selectivity in humans. *Kidney Int.* 1986;29:916-923.
3. Brenner BM, Bohrer MP, Baylis C, et al. Determinants of glomerular permselectivity: insights derived from observations in vivo. *Kidney Int.* 1977;12:229-237.
4. Levidiotis V, Freeman C, Tikellis C, et al. Heparanase is involved in the pathogenesis of proteinuria as a result of glomerulonephritis. *J Am Soc Nephrol.* 2004;15:68-78.
5. Jeansson M, Haraldsson B. Glomerular size and charge selectivity in the mouse after exposure to glucosaminoglycan-degrading enzymes. *J Am Soc Nephrol.* 2003;14:1756-1765.
6. Tryggvason K, Patrakka J, Wartiovaara J. Hereditary proteinuria syndromes and mechanisms of proteinuria. *N Engl J Med.* 2006;354:1387-1401.
7. Russo LM, Sandoval RM, Campos SB, et al. Impaired tubular uptake explains albuminuria in early diabetic nephropathy. *J Am Soc Nephrol.* 2009;20:489-494.
8. Albright R, Brensilver J, Cortell S. Proteinuria in congestive heart failure. *Am J Nephrol.* 1983;3:272-275.
9. Wingo CS, Clapp WL. Proteinuria: potential causes and approach to evaluation. *Am J Med Sci.* 2000;320:188-194.
10. Springberg PD, Garrett Jr LE, Thompson Jr AL, et al. Fixed and reproducible orthostatic proteinuria: results of a 20-year follow-up study. *Ann Intern Med.* 1982;97:516-519.
11. Robinson RR, Ashworth CT, Glover SN, et al. Fixed and reproducible orthostatic proteinuria. II. Electron microscopy of renal biopsy specimens from five cases. *Am J Pathol.* 1961;39:405-417.
12. Devarajan P. Mechanisms of orthostatic proteinuria: lessons from a transplant donor. *J Am Soc Nephrol.* 1993;4:36-39.
13. Shintaku N, Takahashi Y, Akaishi K, et al. Entrapment of left renal vein in children with orthostatic proteinuria. *Pediatr Nephrol.* 1990;4:324-327.
14. Mariani AJ, Mariani MC, Macchioni C, et al. The significance of adult hematuria: 1,000 hematuria evaluations including a risk-benefit and cost-effectiveness analysis. *J Urol.* 1989;141:350-355.
15. Schroder FH. Microscopic haematuria. *BMJ.* 1994;309:70-72.
16. Kincaid-Smith P, Fairley K. The investigation of hematuria. *Semin Nephrol.* 2005;25:127-135.
17. Meyers KE. Evaluation of hematuria in children. *Urol Clin North Am.* 2004;31:559-573.
18. Schramek P, Schuster FX, Georgopoulos M, et al. Value of urinary erythrocyte morphology in assessment of symptomless microhaematuria. *Lancet.* 1989;2:1316-1319.
19. Mazhari R, Kimmel PL. Hematuria: an algorithmic approach to finding the cause. *Cleve Clin J Med.* 2002;870, 872-874, 876.
20. Mohr DN, Offord KP, Owen RA, et al. Asymptomatic microhematuria and urologic disease. A population-based study. *JAMA.* 1986;256:224-229.
21. Case records of the Massachusetts General Hospital. Weekly clinicopathological exercises. Case 33-1992. A 34-year-old woman with endometriosis and bilateral hydronephrosis. *N Engl J Med.* 1992;327:481-485.
22. Chow KM, Kwan BC, Li PK, et al. Asymptomatic isolated microscopic haematuria: long-term follow-up. *QJM.* 2004;97:739-745.
23. Murakami S, Igarashi T, Hara S, et al. Strategies for asymptomatic microscopic hematuria: a prospective study of 1,034 patients. *J Urol.* 1990;144:99-101.
24. Britton JP, Dowell AC, Whelan P. Dipstick haematuria and bladder cancer in men over 60: results of a community study. *BMJ.* 1989;299:1010-1012.
25. Topham PS, Harper SJ, Furness PN, et al. Glomerular disease as a cause of isolated microscopic haematuria. *Q J Med.* 1994;87:329-335.
26. Tiebosch AT, Frederik PM, Breda Vriesman PJ, et al. Thin-basement-membrane nephropathy in adults with persistent hematuria. *N Engl J Med.* 1989;320:14-18.
27. Shen P, He L, Jiang Y, et al. Useful indicators for performing renal biopsy in adult patients with isolated microscopic haematuria. *Int J Clin Pract.* 2007;61:789-794.
28. Assadi FK. Value of urinary excretion of microalbumin in predicting glomerular lesions in children with isolated microscopic hematuria. *Pediatr Nephrol.* 2005;20:1131-1135.
29. Eardley KS, Ferreira MA, Howie AJ, et al. Urinary albumin excretion: a predictor of glomerular findings in adults with microscopic haematuria. *QJM.* 2004;97:297-301.
30. Richards NT, Darby S, Howie AJ, et al. Knowledge of renal histology alters patient management in over 40% of cases. *Nephrol Dial Transplant.* 1994;9:1255-1259.
31. Munk F. Klinische diagnostik der degenerativen nierenerkrankungen. *Z Klin Med.* 1913;78:1.
32. Sharples PM, Poulton J, White RH. Steroid responsive nephrotic syndrome is more common in Asians. *Arch Dis Child.* 1985;60:1014-1017.
33. Wyatt RJ, Marx MB, Kazee M, et al. Current estimates of the incidence of steroid responsive idiopathic nephrosis in Kentucky children 1-9 years of age. *Int J Pediatr Nephrol.* 1982;3:63-65.
34. van den Berg JG, van den Bergh Weerman MA, Assmann KJ, et al. Podocyte foot process effacement is not correlated with the level of proteinuria in human glomerulopathies. *Kidney Int.* 2004;66:1901-1906.
35. Olson JL. The nephrotic syndrome and minimal change disease. In: Jennette JC, Olson JL, Schwartz MM, et al, eds. *Heptinstall's pathology of the kidney.* 6th ed. Philadelphia: Lippincott Williams & Wilkins; 2006:125-154.
36. Jennette JC, Falk RJ. Adult minimal change glomerulopathy with acute renal failure. *Am J Kidney Dis.* 1990;16:432-437.
37. Murphy MJ, Bailey RR, McGiven AR. Is there an IgM nephropathy? *Aust N Z J Med.* 1983;13:35-38.
38. Pardo V, Riesgo I, Zilleruelo G, et al. The clinical significance of mesangial IgM deposits and mesangial hypercellularity in minimal change nephrotic syndrome. *Am J Kidney Dis.* 1984;3:264-269.
39. Cohen AH, Border WA, Glassock RJ. Nephrotic syndrome with glomerular mesangial IgM deposits. *Lab Invest.* 1978;38:610-619.
40. Shalhoub RJ. Pathogenesis of lipoid nephrosis: a disorder of T-cell function. *Lancet.* 1974;2:556-560.
41. Schnaper HW, Aune TM. Identification of the lymphokine soluble immune response suppressor in urine of nephrotic children. *J Clin Invest.* 1985;76:341-349.
42. Mallick NP. The pathogenesis of minimal change nephropathy. *Clin Nephrol.* 1977;7:87-95.
43. Fujimoto S, Yamamoto Y, Hisanaga S, et al. Minimal change nephrotic syndrome in adults: response to corticosteroid therapy and frequency of relapse. *Am J Kidney Dis.* 1991;17:687-692.
44. Mendoza SA, Tune BM. Treatment of childhood nephrotic syndrome. *J Am Soc Nephrol.* 1992;3:889-894.
45. Branten AJ, Wetzels JF. Immunosuppressive treatment of patients with a nephrotic syndrome due to minimal change glomerulopathy. *Ned Tijdschr Geneeskd.* 1998;142:2832-2838.
46. Walker F, Neill S, Carmody M, et al. Nephrotic syndrome in Hodgkin's disease. *Int J Pediatr Nephrol.* 1983;4:39-41.
47. Koyama A, Fujisaki M, Kobayashi M, et al. A glomerular permeability factor produced by human T cell hybridomas. *Kidney Int.* 1991;40:453-460.
48. Kobayashi K, Yoshikawa N, Nakamura H. T-cell subpopulations in childhood nephrotic syndrome. *Clin Nephrol.* 1994;41:253-258.
49. Fiser RT, Arnold WC, Charlton RK, et al. T-lymphocyte subsets in nephrotic syndrome. *Kidney Int.* 1991;40:913-916.
50. Sasdelli M, Rovinetti C, Cagnoli L, et al. Lymphocyte subpopulations in minimal-change nephropathy. *Nephron.* 1980;25:72-76.

51. Kerpen HO, Bhat JG, Kantor R, et al. Lymphocyte subpopulations in minimal change nephrotic syndrome. *Clin Immunol Immunopathol.* 1979;14:130-136.

52. Lagrue G, Branellec A, Blanc C, et al. A vascular permeability factor in lymphocyte culture supernatants from patients with nephrotic syndrome. II. Pharmacological and physicochemical properties. *Biomedicine.* 1975;23:73-75.

53. Savin VJ. Mechanisms of proteinuria in noninflammatory glomerular diseases. *Am J Kidney Dis.* 1993;21:347-362.

54. Boulton J, Tulloch I, Dore B, et al. Changes in the glomerular capillary wall induced by lymphocyte products and serum of nephrotic patients. *Clin Nephrol.* 1983;20:72-77.

55. Sewell RF, Short CD. Minimal-change nephropathy: how does the immune system affect the glomerulus? *Nephrol Dial Transplant.* 1993;8:108-112.

56. Bakker WW, van Luijik WH, Hené RJ, et al. Loss of glomerular polyanion in vitro induced by mononuclear blood cells from patients with minimal-change nephrotic syndrome. *Am J Nephrol.* 1986;6:107-111.

57. Maruyama K, Tomizawa S, Seki Y, et al. Inhibition of vascular permeability factor production by ciclosporin in minimal change nephrotic syndrome. *Nephron.* 1992;62:27-30.

58. Tomizawa S, Maruyama K, Nagasawa N, et al. Studies of vascular permeability factor derived from T lymphocytes and inhibitory effect of plasma on its production in minimal change nephrotic syndrome. *Nephron.* 1985;41:157-160.

59. Trompeter RS, Barratt TM, Layward L. Vascular permeability factor and nephrotic syndrome. *Lancet.* 1978;2:900.

60. Lagrue G, Xheneumont S, Branellec A, et al. A vascular permeability factor elaborated from lymphocytes. I. Demonstration in patients with nephrotic syndrome. *Biomedicine.* 1975;23:37-40.

61. Pru C, Kjellstrand CM, Cohn RA, et al. Late recurrence of minimal lesion nephrotic syndrome. *Ann Intern Med.* 1984;100:69-72.

62. Bakker WW, Borghuis T, Harmsen MC, et al. Protease activity of plasma hemopexin. *Kidney Int.* 2005;68:603-610.

63. Bakker WW, van Dael CM, Pierik LJ, et al. Altered activity of plasma hemopexin in patients with minimal change disease in relapse. *Pediatr Nephrol.* 2005;20:1410-1415.

64. Okuyama S, Komatsuda A, Wakui H, et al. Up-regulation of TRAIL mRNA expression in peripheral blood mononuclear cells from patients with minimal-change nephrotic syndrome. *Nephrol Dial Transplant.* 2005;20:539-544.

65. Toyabe S, Kaneko U, Hara M, et al. Expression of immunoglobulin E–dependent histamine-releasing factor in idiopathic nephrotic syndrome of childhood. *Clin Exp Immunol.* 2005;142:162-166.

66. Winetz JA, Robertson CR, Golbetz HV, et al. The nature of the glomerular injury in minimal change and focal sclerosing glomerulopathies. *Am J Kidney Dis.* 1981;1:91-98.

67. Carrie BJ, Salyer WR, Myers BD. Minimal change nephropathy: an electrochemical disorder of the glomerular membrane. *Am J Med.* 1981;70:262-268.

68. Kitano Y, Yoshikawa N, Nakamura H. Glomerular anionic sites in minimal change nephrotic syndrome and focal segmental glomerulosclerosis. *Clin Nephrol.* 1993;40:199-204.

69. Lahdenkari AT, Suvanto M, Kajantie E, et al. Clinical features and outcome of childhood minimal change nephrotic syndrome: is genetics involved? *Pediatr Nephrol.* 2005;20:1073-1080.

70. Acharya B, Shirakawa T, Pungky A, et al. Polymorphism of the interleukin-4, interleukin-13, and signal transducer and activator of transcription 6 genes in Indonesian children with minimal change nephrotic syndrome. *Am J Nephrol.* 2005;25:30-35.

71. Wei CL, Cheung W, Heng CK, et al. Interleukin-13 genetic polymorphisms in Singapore Chinese children correlate with long-term outcome of minimal-change disease. *Nephrol Dial Transplant.* 2005;20:728-734.

72. Berdeli A, Mir S, Ozkayin N, et al. Association of macrophage migration inhibitory factor-173C allele polymorphism with steroid resistance in children with nephrotic syndrome. *Pediatr Nephrol.* 2005;20:1566-1571.

73. Lai KW, Wei CL, Tan LK, et al. Overexpression of interleukin-13 induces minimal-change-like nephropathy in rats. *J Am Soc Nephrol.* 2007;18:1476-1485.

74. Nolasco F, Cameron JS, Heywood EF, et al. Adult-onset minimal change nephrotic syndrome: a long-term follow-up. *Kidney Int.* 1986;29:1215-1223.

75. Artinano M, Etheridge WB, Stroehlein KB, et al. Progression of minimal-change glomerulopathy to focal glomerulosclerosis in a patient with fenoprofen nephropathy. *Am J Nephrol.* 1986;6:353-357.

76. Averbuch SD, Austin HA, Sherwin SA, et al. Acute interstitial nephritis with the nephrotic syndrome following recombinant leukocyte A interferon therapy for mycosis fungoides. *N Engl J Med.* 1984;310:32-35.

77. Audard V, Larousserie F, Grimbert P, et al. Minimal change nephrotic syndrome and classical Hodgkin's lymphoma: report of 21 cases and review of the literature. *Kidney Int.* 2006;69:2251-2260.

78. Sekhon I, Munjal S, Croker B, et al. Glomerular tip lesion associated with nonsteroidal anti-inflammatory drug–induced nephrotic syndrome. *Am J Kidney Dis.* 2005;46:e55-e58.

79. Kraft SW, Schwartz MM, Korbet SM, et al. Glomerular podocytopathy in patients with systemic lupus erythematosus. *J Am Soc Nephrol.* 2005;16:175-179.

80. Horino T, Takao T, Morita T, et al. Minimal change nephrotic syndrome associated with systemic lupus erythematosus. *Nephrol Dial Transplant.* 2006;21:230.

81. Stevenson WS, Nankivell BJ, Hertzberg MS. Nephrotic syndrome after stem cell transplantation. *Clin Transplant.* 2005;19:141-144.

82. Laurent J, Rostoker G, Robeva R, et al. Is adult idiopathic nephrotic syndrome food allergy? Value of oligoantigenic diets. *Nephron.* 1987;47:7-11.

83. Smith JD, Hayslett JP. Reversible renal failure in the nephrotic syndrome. *Am J Kidney Dis.* 1992;19:201-213.

84. Grupe WE. Childhood nephrotic syndrome: clinical associations and response to therapy. *Postgrad Med.* 1979;65:229-231.

85. Chen CL, Fang HC, Chou KJ, et al. Increased endothelin 1 expression in adult-onset minimal change nephropathy with acute renal failure. *Am J Kidney Dis.* 2005;45:818-825.

86. Hegarty J, Mughal MZ, Adams J, et al. Reduced bone mineral density in adults treated with high-dose corticosteroids for childhood nephrotic syndrome. *Kidney Int.* 2005;68:2304-2309.

87. Kano K, Nishikura K, Yamada Y, et al. No effect of fluvastatin on the bone mineral density of children with minimal change glomerulonephritis and some focal mesangial cell proliferation, other than an ameliorating effect on their proteinuria. *Clin Nephrol.* 2005;63:74-79.

88. Ueda N. Effect of corticosteroids on some hemostatic parameters in children with minimal change nephrotic syndrome. *Nephron.* 1990;56:374-378.

89. Bridges CR, Myers BD, Brenner BM, et al. Glomerular charge alterations in human minimal change nephropathy. *Kidney Int.* 1982;22:677-684.

90. Ghiggeri GM, Candiano G, Ginevri F, et al. Renal selectivity properties towards endogenous albumin in minimal change nephropathy. *Kidney Int.* 1987;32:69-77.

91. Giangiacomo J, Cleary TG, Cole BR, et al. Serum immunoglobulins in the nephrotic syndrome. A possible cause of minimal-change nephrotic syndrome. *N Engl J Med.* 1975;293:8-12.

92. Groshong T, Mendelson L, Mendoza S, et al. Serum IgE in patients with minimal-change nephrotic syndrome. *J Pediatr.* 1973;83:767-771.

93. Meadow SR, Sarsfield JK. Steroid-responsive and nephrotic syndrome and allergy: clinical studies. *Arch Dis Child.* 1981;56:509-516.

94. Lagrue G, Laurent J, Hirbec G, et al. Serum IgE in primary glomerular diseases. *Nephron.* 1984;36:5-9.

95. Zilleruelo G, Hsia SL, Freundlich M, et al. Persistence of serum lipid abnormalities in children with idiopathic nephrotic syndrome. *J Pediatr.* 1984;104:61-64.

96. Glassock RJ. Therapy of idiopathic nephrotic syndrome in adults. A conservative or aggressive therapeutic approach? *Am J Nephrol.* 1993;13:422-428.

97. Ponticelli C, Passerini P. Treatment of the nephrotic syndrome associated with primary glomerulonephritis. *Kidney Int.* 1994;46:595-604.

98. Nephrotic syndrome in children. a randomized trial comparing two prednisone regimens in steroid-responsive patients who relapse early. Report of the international study of kidney disease in children. *J Pediatr.* 1979;95:239-243.

99. Alternate-day versus intermittent prednisone in frequently relapsing nephrotic syndrome. A report of "Arbetsgemeinschaft für Pädiatrische Nephrologie." *Lancet.* 1979;1:401-403.

100. Leisti S, Hallman N, Koskimies O, et al. Association of postmedication hypocortisolism with early first relapse of idiopathic nephrotic syndrome. *Lancet.* 1977;2:795-796.

101. Waldman M, Crew RJ, Valeri A, et al. Adult minimal-change disease: clinical characteristics, treatment, and outcomes. *Clin J Am Soc Nephrol.* 2007;2:445-453.

102. Leisti S, Koskimies O, Perheentupa J, et al. Idiopathic nephrotic syndrome: prevention of early relapse. *Br Med J.* 1978;1:892.

103. Leisti S, Koskimies O. Risk of relapse in steroid-sensitive nephrotic syndrome: effect of stage of post-prednisone adrenocortical suppression. *J Pediatr.* 1983;103:553-557.

104. Ehrich JH, Brodehl J. Long versus standard prednisone therapy for initial treatment of idiopathic nephrotic syndrome in children. Arbeitsgemeinschaft für Pädiatrische Nephrologie. *Eur J Pediatr.* 1993;152:357-361.

105. Short versus standard prednisone therapy for initial treatment of idiopathic nephrotic syndrome in children. Arbeitsgemeinschaft für Pädiatrische Nephrologie. *Lancet.* 1988;1:380-383.

106. Cyclophosphamide treatment of steroid dependent nephrotic syndrome. comparison of eight week with 12 week course. Report of Arbeitsgemeinschaft für Pädiatrische Nephrologie. *Arch Dis Child.* 1987;62:1102-1106.

107. Berns JS, Gaudio KM, Krassner LS, et al. Steroid-responsive nephrotic syndrome of childhood: a long-term study of clinical course, histopathology, efficacy of cyclophosphamide therapy, and effects on growth. *Am J Kidney Dis.* 1987;9:108-114.

108. Schulman SL, Kaiser BA, Polinsky MS, et al. Predicting the response to cytotoxic therapy for childhood nephrotic syndrome: superiority of response to corticosteroid therapy over histopathologic patterns. *J Pediatr.* 1988;113:996-1001.

109. Effect of cytotoxic drugs in frequently relapsing nephrotic syndrome with and without steroid dependence. *N Engl J Med.* 1982;306:451-454.

110. Ueda N, Kuno K, Ito S. Eight and 12 week courses of cyclophosphamide in nephrotic syndrome. *Arch Dis Child.* 1990;65:1147-1150.

111. El-Husseini A, El-Basuony F, Mahmoud I, et al. Long-term effects of cyclosporine in children with idiopathic nephrotic syndrome: a single-centre experience. *Nephrol Dial Transplant.* 2005;20:2433-2438.

112. Iyengar A, Karthik S, Kumar A, et al. Cyclosporine in steroid dependent and resistant childhood nephrotic syndrome. *Indian Pediatr.* 2006;43:14-19.

113. Nakahata T, Tanaka H, Tsugawa K, et al. C1-C2 point monitoring of low-dose cyclosporin a given as a single daily dose in children with steroid-dependent relapsing nephrotic syndrome. *Clin Nephrol.* 2005;64:258-263.

114. Rinaldi S, Sesto A, Barsotti P, et al. Cyclosporine therapy monitored with abbreviated area under curve in nephrotic syndrome. *Pediatr Nephrol.* 2005;20:25-29.

115. Primary nephrotic syndrome in children: clinical significance of histopathologic variants of minimal change and of diffuse mesangial hypercellularity. A Report of the International Study of Kidney Disease in Children. *Kidney Int.* 1981;20:765-771.

116. Murnaghan K, Vasmant D, Bensman A. Pulse methylprednisolone therapy in severe idiopathic childhood nephrotic syndrome. *Acta Paediatr Scand.* 1984;73:733-739.

117. Rose GM, Cole BR, Robson AM. The treatment of severe glomerulopathies in children using high dose intravenous methylprednisolone pulses. *Am J Kidney Dis.* 1981;1:148-156.

118. El-Reshaid K, El-Reshaid W, Madda J. Combination of immunosuppressive agents in treatment of steroid-resistant minimal change disease and primary focal segmental glomerulosclerosis. *Ren Fail.* 2005;27:523-530.

119. Patel P, Pal S, Ashley C, et al. Combination therapy with sirolimus (rapamycin) and tacrolimus (FK-506) in treatment of refractory minimal change nephropathy, a clinical case report. *Nephrol Dial Transplant.* 2005;20:985-987.

120. Hafeez F, Ahmad TM, Anwar S. Efficacy of steroids, cyclosporin and cyclophosphamide in steroid resistant idiopathic nephrotic syndrome. *J Coll Physicians Surg Pak.* 2005;15:329-332.

121. Cheng IK, Chan KW, Chan MK. Mesangial IgA nephropathy with steroid-responsive nephrotic syndrome: disappearance of mesangial IgA deposits following steroid-induced remission. *Am J Kidney Dis.* 1989;14:361-364.

122. Lagrue G, Laurent J. Allergy and lipoid nephrosis. *Adv Nephrol Necker Hosp.* 1983;12:151-175.

123. Lagrue G, Laurent J. Is lipoid nephrosis an "allergic" disease? *Transplant Proc.* 1982;14:485-488.

124. Niaudet P, Drachman R, Gagnadoux MF, et al. Treatment of idiopathic nephrotic syndrome with levamisole. *Acta Paediatr Scand.* 1984;73:637-641.

125. Ponticelli C, Rizzoni G, Edefonti A, et al. A randomized trial of cyclosporine in steroid-resistant idiopathic nephrotic syndrome. *Kidney Int.* 1993;43:1377-1384.

126. Niaudet P, Habib R. Cyclosporine in the treatment of idiopathic nephrosis. *J Am Soc Nephrol.* 1994;5:1049-1056.

127. Ponticelli C, Edefonti A, Ghio L, et al. Cyclosporin versus cyclophosphamide for patients with steroid-dependent and frequently relapsing idiopathic nephrotic syndrome: a multicentre randomized controlled trial. *Nephrol Dial Transplant.* 1993;8:1326-1332.

128. Meyrier A, Noel LH, Auriche P, et al. Long-term renal tolerance of cyclosporin A treatment in adult idiopathic nephrotic syndrome. Collaborative Group of the Société de Néphrologie. *Kidney Int.* 1994;45:1446-1456.

129. D'Agati VD, Fogo AB, Bruijn JA, et al. Pathologic classification of focal segmental glomerulosclerosis: a working proposal. *Am J Kidney Dis.* 2004;43:368-382.

130. Thomas DB, Franceschini N, Hogan SL, et al. Clinical and pathologic characteristics of focal segmental glomerulosclerosis pathologic variants. *Kidney Int.* 2006;69:920-926.

131. Kitiyakara C, Eggers P, Kopp JB. Twenty-one-year trend in ESRD due to focal segmental glomerulosclerosis in the United States. *Am J Kidney Dis.* 2004;44:815-825.

132. Swaminathan S, Leung N, Lager DJ, et al. Changing incidence of glomerular disease in Olmsted County, Minnesota: a 30-year renal biopsy study. *Clin J Am Soc Nephrol.* 2006;1:483-487.

133. D'Agati V. The many masks of focal segmental glomerulosclerosis. *Kidney Int.* 1994;46:1223-1241.

134. Cohen AH, Nast CC. HIV-associated nephropathy. A unique combined glomerular, tubular, and interstitial lesion. *Mod Pathol.* 1988;1:87-97.

135. D'Agati V, Suh JI, Carbone L, et al. Pathology of HIV-associated nephropathy: a detailed morphologic and comparative study. *Kidney Int.* 1989;35:1358-1370.

136. Valeri A, Barisoni L, Appel GB, et al. Idiopathic collapsing focal segmental glomerulosclerosis: a clinicopathologic study. *Kidney Int.* 1996;50:1734-1746.

137. Detwiler RK, Falk RJ, Hogan SL, et al. Collapsing glomerulopathy: a clinically and pathologically distinct variant of focal segmental glomerulosclerosis. *Kidney Int.* 1994;45:1416-1424.

138. Clarkson MR, Meara YM, Murphy B, et al. Collapsing glomerulopathy—recurrence in a renal allograft. *Nephrol Dial Transplant.* 1998;13:503-506.

139. Meehan SM, Pascual M, Williams WW, et al. De novo collapsing glomerulopathy in renal allografts. *Transplantation.* 1998;65:1192-1197.

140. Howie AJ, Lee SJ, Green NJ, et al. Different clinicopathological types of segmental sclerosing glomerular lesions in adults. *Nephrol Dial Transplant.* 1993;8:590-599.

141. Beaman M, Howie AJ, Hardwicke J, et al. The glomerular tip lesion: a steroid responsive nephrotic syndrome. *Clin Nephrol.* 1987;27:217-221.

142. Howie AJ. Changes at the glomerular tip: a feature of membranous nephropathy and other disorders associated with proteinuria. *J Pathol.* 1986;150:13-20.

143. Howie AJ, Brewer DB. The glomerular tip lesion: a previously undescribed type of segmental glomerular abnormality. *J Pathol.* 1984;142:205-220.

144. Howie AJ, Brewer DB. Further studies on the glomerular tip lesion: early and late stages and life table analysis. *J Pathol.* 1985;147:245-255.

145. Yoshikawa N, Ito H, Akamatsu R, et al. Focal segmental glomerulosclerosis with and without nephrotic syndrome in children. *J Pediatr.* 1986;109:65-70.

146. Woroniecki RP, Kopp JB. Genetics of focal segmental glomerulosclerosis. *Pediatr Nephrol.* 2007;22:638-644.

147. Franceschini N, North KE, Kopp JB, et al. NPHS2 gene, nephrotic syndrome and focal segmental glomerulosclerosis: a HuGE review. *Genet Med.* 2006;8:63-75.

148. Koziell A, Grech V, Hussain S, et al. Genotype/phenotype correlations of NPHS1 and NPHS2 mutations in nephrotic syndrome advocate a functional inter-relationship in glomerular filtration. *Hum Mol Genet.* 2002;11:379-388.

149. Weins A, Kenlan P, Herbert S, et al. Mutational and biological analysis of α-actinin-4 in focal segmental glomerulosclerosis. *J Am Soc Nephrol.* 2005;16:3694-3701.

150. Aucella F, De Bonis P, Gatta G, et al. Molecular analysis of NPHS2 and ACTN4 genes in a series of 33 Italian patients affected by adult-onset nonfamilial focal segmental glomerulosclerosis. *Nephron Clin Pract.* 2005;99:c31-c36.

151. Winn MP, Conlon PJ, Lynn KL, et al. A mutation in the TRPC6 cation channel causes familial focal segmental glomerulosclerosis. *Science.* 2005;308:1801-1804.

152. Pollak MR. The genetic basis of FSGS and steroid-resistant nephrosis. *Semin Nephrol.* 2003;23:141-146.

153. Reiser J, Polu KR, Moller CC, et al. TRPC6 is a glomerular slit diaphragm–associated channel required for normal renal function. *Nat Genet.* 2005;37:739-744.

154. Hinkes B, Wiggins RC, Gbadegesin R, et al. Positional cloning uncovers mutations in PLCE1 responsible for a nephrotic syndrome variant that may be reversible. *Nat Genet.* 2006;38:1397-1405.

155. Diomedi-Camassei F, Di Giandomenico S, Santorelli FM, et al. COQ2 nephropathy: a newly described inherited mitochondriopathy with primary renal involvement. *J Am Soc Nephrol.* 2007;18:2773-2780.

156. Hinkes B, Vlangos C, Heeringa S, et al. Specific podocin mutations correlate with age of onset in steroid-resistant nephrotic syndrome. *J Am Soc Nephrol.* 2008;19:365-371.

156a. Machuca E, Hummel A, Nevo F, et al. Clinical and epidemiological assessment of steroid-resistant nephrotic syndrome associated with the *NPHS2* R229Q variant. *Kidney Int.* 2009;75:727-735.

157. McKenzie LM, Hendrickson SL, Briggs WA, et al. NPHS2 variation in sporadic focal segmental glomerulosclerosis. *J Am Soc Nephrol.* 2007;18:2987-2995.

158. Tonna S, Dandapani SV, Uscinski A, et al. Functional genetic variation in aminopeptidase A (ENPEP): lack of clear association with focal and segmental glomerulosclerosis (FSGS). *Gene.* 2008;410:44-52.

159. Philippe A, Nevo F, Esquivel EL, et al. Nephrin mutations can cause childhood-onset steroid-resistant nephrotic syndrome. *J Am Soc Nephrol.* 2008;19:1871-1878.

160. Lemley KV. Yet more ways to skin a cat: nephrin mutations outside the neonatal period. *J Am Soc Nephrol.* 2008;19:1837-1838.

161. Henderson JM, Alexander MP, Pollak MR. Patients with ACTN4 mutations demonstrate distinctive features of glomerular injury. *J Am Soc Nephrol.* 2009;20:961-968.

162. Kopp JB, Smith MW, Nelson GW, et al. MYH9 is a major-effect risk gene for focal segmental glomerulosclerosis. *Nat Genet.* 2008;40:1175-1184.

162a. Kao WH, Klag MJ, Meoni LA, et al. Family Investigation of Nephropathy and Diabetes Research Group: MYH9 is associated with nondiabetic end-stage renal disease in African Americans. *Nat Genet.* 2008;10:1185-1192.

163. Pollak MR. Kidney disease and African ancestry. *Nat Genet.* 2008;40:1145-1146.

163a. Genovese G, Friedman DJ, Ross MD, et al. Association of trypanolytic ApoL1 variants with kidney disease in African Americans. *Science.* 2010;329:841-845.

163b. Tzur S, Rosset S, Shemer R, et al. Missense mutations in the APOL1 gene are highly associated with end stage kidney disease risk previously attributed to the MYH9 gene. *Hum Genet.* 2010;128:345-350.

164. Shankland SJ. The podocyte's response to injury: role in proteinuria and glomerulosclerosis. *Kidney Int.* 2006;69:2131-2147.

165. Meyrier A. Mechanisms of disease: focal segmental glomerulosclerosis. *Nat Clin Pract Nephrol.* 2005;1:44-54.

166. Barisoni L, Schnaper HW, Kopp JB. A proposed taxonomy for the podocytopathies: a reassessment of the primary nephrotic diseases. *Clin J Am Soc Nephrol.* 2007;2:529-542.

167. Yang Y, Gubler MC, Beaufils H. Dysregulation of podocyte phenotype in idiopathic collapsing glomerulopathy and HIV-associated nephropathy. *Nephron.* 2002;91:416-423.

168. Schmid H, Henger A, Cohen CD, et al. Gene expression profiles of podocyte-associated molecules as diagnostic markers in acquired proteinuric diseases. *J Am Soc Nephrol.* 2003;14:2958-2966.

169. Ohtaka A, Ootaka T, Sato H, et al. Phenotypic change of glomerular podocytes in primary focal segmental glomerulosclerosis: developmental paradigm? *Nephrol Dial Transplant.* 2002;17(suppl 9):11-15.

170. Shankland SJ, Eitner F, Hudkins KL, et al. Differential expression of cyclin-dependent kinase inhibitors in human glomerular disease: role in podocyte proliferation and maturation. *Kidney Int.* 2000;58:674-683.

171. Wiggins JE, Goyal M, Sanden SK, et al. Podocyte hypertrophy, "adaptation," and "decompensation" associated with glomerular enlargement and glomerulosclerosis in the aging rat: prevention by calorie restriction. *J Am Soc Nephrol.* 2005;16:2953-2966.

172. Dijkman H, Smeets B, van der Laak J, et al. The parietal epithelial cell is crucially involved in human idiopathic focal segmental glomerulosclerosis. *Kidney Int.* 2005;68:1562-1572.

173. Dijkman HB, Weening JJ, Smeets B, et al. Proliferating cells in HIV and pamidronate-associated collapsing focal segmental glomerulosclerosis are parietal epithelial cells. *Kidney Int.* 2006;70:338-344.

174. Binder CJ, Weiher H, Exner M, et al. Glomerular overproduction of oxygen radicals in Mpv17 gene–inactivated mice causes podocyte foot process flattening and proteinuria: a model of steroid-resistant nephrosis sensitive to radical scavenger therapy. *Am J Pathol.* 1999;154:1067-1075.

175. Kretzler M. Role of podocytes in focal sclerosis: defining the point of no return. *J Am Soc Nephrol.* 2005;16:2830-2832.

176. Johnstone DB, Holzman LB. Clinical impact of research on the podocyte slit diaphragm. *Nat Clin Pract Nephrol.* 2006;2:271-282.

177. Kriz W, LeHir M. Pathways to nephron loss starting from glomerular diseases-insights from animal models. *Kidney Int.* 2005;67:404-419.

178. Barisoni L, Kopp JB. Update in podocyte biology: putting one's best foot forward. *Curr Opin Nephrol Hypertens.* 2003;12:251-258.

179. Sharma K, Ziyadeh FN. The emerging role of transforming growth factor-beta in kidney diseases. *Am J Physiol.* 1994;266:F829-F842.

180. Border WA, Okuda S, Languino LR, et al. Suppression of experimental glomerulonephritis by antiserum against transforming growth factor beta 1. *Nature.* 1990;346:371-374.

181. Stokes MB, Holler S, Cui Y, et al. Expression of decorin, biglycan, and collagen type I in human renal fibrosing disease. *Kidney Int.* 2000;57:487-498.

182. Eagen JW. Glomerulopathies of neoplasia. *Kidney Int.* 1977;11:297-303.

183. Olson JL, Hostetter TH, Rennke HG, et al. Altered glomerular permselectivity and progressive sclerosis following extreme ablation of renal mass. *Kidney Int.* 1982;22:112-126.

184. Brenner BM, Meyer TW, Hostetter TH. Dietary protein intake and the progressive nature of kidney disease: the role of hemodynamically mediated glomerular injury in the pathogenesis of progressive glomerular sclerosis in aging, renal ablation, and intrinsic renal disease. *N Engl J Med.* 1982;307:652-659.

185. Brenner BM. Hemodynamically mediated glomerular injury and the progressive nature of kidney disease. *Kidney Int.* 1983;23:647-655.

186. Simons JL, Provoost AP, Anderson S, et al. Modulation of glomerular hypertension defines susceptibility to progressive glomerular injury. *Kidney Int.* 1994;46:396-404.

187. Johnson RJ. The glomerular response to injury: progression or resolution? *Kidney Int.* 1994;45:1769-1782.

188. Couser WG. Mechanisms of glomerular injury: an overview. *Semin Nephrol.* 1991;11:254-258.

189. Savin VJ, Sharma R, Sharma M, et al. Circulating factor associated with increased glomerular permeability to albumin in recurrent focal segmental glomerulosclerosis. *N Engl J Med.* 1996;334:878-883.

190. Sharma M, Sharma R, McCarthy ET, et al. The focal segmental glomerulosclerosis permeability factor: biochemical characteristics and biological effects. *Exp Biol Med (Maywood).* 2004;229:85-98.

191. Savin VJ, McCarthy ET, Sharma R, et al. Galactose binds to focal segmental glomerulosclerosis permeability factor and inhibits its activity. *Transl Res.* 2008;151:288-292.

192. De Smet E, Rioux JP, Ammann H, et al. FSGS permeability factor-associated nephrotic syndrome: remission after oral galactose therapy. *Nephrol Dial Transplant.* 2009;24:2938-2940.

193. Feld SM, Figueroa P, Savin V, et al. Plasmapheresis in the treatment of steroid-resistant focal segmental glomerulosclerosis in native kidneys. *Am J Kidney Dis.* 1998;32:230-237.

194. Verani RR. Obesity-associated focal segmental glomerulosclerosis: pathological features of the lesion and relationship with cardiomegaly and hyperlipidemia. *Am J Kidney Dis.* 1992;20:629-634.

195. Kambham N, Markowitz GS, Valeri AM, et al. Obesity-related glomerulopathy: an emerging epidemic. *Kidney Int.* 2001;59:1498-1509.

196. Praga M, Hernandez E, Andres A, et al. Effects of body-weight loss and captopril treatment on proteinuria associated with obesity. *Nephron.* 1995;70:35-41.

197. Huan Y, Tomaszewski JE, Cohen DL. Resolution of nephrotic syndrome after successful bariatric surgery in patient with biopsy-proven FSGS. *Clin Nephrol.* 2009;71:69-73.

198. Chaudhary BA, Sklar AH, Chaudhary TK, et al. Sleep apnea, proteinuria, and nephrotic syndrome. *Sleep.* 1988;11:69-74.

199. Sklar AH, Chaudhary BA. Reversible proteinuria in obstructive sleep apnea syndrome. *Arch Intern Med.* 1988;148:87-89.

200. Casserly LF, Chow N, Ali S, et al. Proteinuria in obstructive sleep apnea. *Kidney Int.* 2001;60:1484-1489.

201. Haas M, Meehan SM, Karrison TG, et al. Changing etiologies of unexplained adult nephrotic syndrome: a comparison of renal biopsy findings from 1976-1979 and 1995-1997. *Am J Kidney Dis.* 1997;30:621-631.

202. Yoshioka K, Takemura T, Murakami K, et al. Transforming growth factor-beta protein and mRNA in glomeruli in normal and diseased human kidneys. *Lab Invest.* 1993;68:154-163.

203. Novick AC, Gephardt G, Guz B, et al. Long-term follow-up after partial removal of a solitary kidney. *N Engl J Med.* 1991;325:1058-1062.

204. Rennke HG, Klein PS. Pathogenesis and significance of nonprimary focal and segmental glomerulosclerosis. *Am J Kidney Dis.* 1989;13:443-456.

205. Fogo A, Glick AD, Horn SL, et al. Is focal segmental glomerulosclerosis really focal? Distribution of lesions in adults and children. *Kidney Int.* 1995;47:1690-1696.

206. Border WA, Noble NA, Yamamoto T, et al. Natural inhibitor of transforming growth factor-beta protects against scarring in experimental kidney disease. *Nature.* 1992;360:361-364.

207. Tanawattanacharoen S, Falk RJ, Jennette JC, et al. Parvovirus B19 DNA in kidney tissue of patients with focal segmental glomerulosclerosis. *Am J Kidney Dis.* 2000;35:1166-1174.

208. Moudgil A, Nast CC, Bagga A, et al. Association of parvovirus B19 infection with idiopathic collapsing glomerulopathy. *Kidney Int.* 2001;59:2126-2133.

209. Li RM, Branton MH, Tanawattanacharoen S, et al. Molecular identification of SV40 infection in human subjects and possible association with kidney disease. *J Am Soc Nephrol.* 2002;13:2320-2330.

210. Dingli D, Larson DR, Plevak MF, et al. Focal and segmental glomerulosclerosis and plasma cell proliferative disorders. *Am J Kidney Dis.* 2005;46:278-282.

211. Barri YM, Munshi NC, Sukumalchantra S, et al. Podocyte injury associated glomerulopathies induced by pamidronate. *Kidney Int.* 2004;65:634-641.

212. Markowitz GS, Nasr SH, Stokes MB, et al. Treatment with IFN-α, -β, or -γ is associated with collapsing focal segmental glomerulosclerosis. *Clin J Am Soc Nephrol.* 2010;5:607-615.

213. Herlitz LC, Markowitz GS, Farris AB, et al. Development of focal segmental glomerulosclerosis after anabolic steroid abuse. *J Am Soc Nephrol.* 2010;21:163-172.

214. Focal segmental glomerulosclerosis in children with idiopathic nephrotic syndrome. A report of the Southwest Pediatric Nephrology Study Group. *Kidney Int.* 1985;27:442-449.

215. Newman WJ, Tisher CC, McCoy RC, et al. Focal glomerular sclerosis: contrasting clinical patterns in children and adults. *Medicine (Baltimore)*. 1976;55:67-87.

216. Pei Y, Cattran D, Delmore T, et al. Evidence suggesting under-treatment in adults with idiopathic focal segmental glomerulosclerosis. Regional Glomerulonephritis Registry Study. *Am J Med*. 1987;82:938-944.

217. Korbet SM, Schwartz MM, Lewis EJ. Primary focal segmental glomerulosclerosis: clinical course and response to therapy. *Am J Kidney Dis*. 1994;23:773-783.

218. Korbet SM. Primary focal segmental glomerulosclerosis. *J Am Soc Nephrol*. 1998;9:1333-1340.

219. Weiss MA, Daquioag E, Margolin EG, et al. Nephrotic syndrome, progressive irreversible renal failure, and glomerular "collapse": a new clinicopathologic entity? *Am J Kidney Dis*. 1986;7:20-28.

220. Schwartz MM, Korbet SM. Primary focal segmental glomerulosclerosis: pathology, histological variants, and pathogenesis. *Am J Kidney Dis*. 1993;22:874-883.

221. Ito H, Yoshikawa N, Aozai F, et al. Twenty-seven children with focal segmental glomerulosclerosis: correlation between the segmental location of the glomerular lesions and prognosis. *Clin Nephrol*. 1984;22:9-14.

221a. Thomas DB, Franceschini N, Hogan SL, et al. Clinical and pathologic characteristics of focal segmental glomerulosclerosis pathological variants. *Kidney Int*. 2006;69:920-926.

222. Stokes MB, Valeri AM, Markowitz GS, et al. Cellular focal segmental glomerulosclerosis: clinical and pathologic features. *Kidney Int*. 2006;70:1783-1792.

223. Deegens JK, Steenbergen EJ, Borm GF, et al. Pathological variants of focal segmental glomerulosclerosis in an adult Dutch population—epidemiology and outcome. *Nephrol Dial Transplant*. 2008;23:186-192.

224. Rydel JJ, Korbet SM, Borok RZ, et al. Focal segmental glomerular sclerosis in adults: presentation, course, and response to treatment. *Am J Kidney Dis*. 1995;25:534-542.

225. Korbet SM, Schwartz MM, Lewis EJ. The prognosis of focal segmental glomerular sclerosis of adulthood. *Medicine (Baltimore)*. 1986;65:304-311.

226. Velosa JA, Holley KE, Torres VE, et al. Significance of proteinuria on the outcome of renal function in patients with focal segmental glomerulosclerosis. *Mayo Clin Proc*. 1983;58:568-577.

227. Brown CB, Cameron JS, Turner DR, et al. Focal segmental glomerulosclerosis with rapid decline in renal function ("malignant FSGS"). *Clin Nephrol*. 1978;10:51-61.

228. Korbet SM. Clinical picture and outcome of primary focal segmental glomerulosclerosis. *Nephrol Dial Transplant*. 1999;14(suppl 3):68-73.

229. Banfi G, Moriggi M, Sabadini E, et al. The impact of prolonged immunosuppression on the outcome of idiopathic focal-segmental glomerulosclerosis with nephrotic syndrome in adults. A collaborative retrospective study. *Clin Nephrol*. 1991;36:53-59.

230. Arbus GS, Poucell S, Bacheyie GS, et al. Focal segmental glomerulosclerosis with idiopathic nephrotic syndrome: three types of clinical response. *J Pediatr*. 1982;101:40-45.

231. Wehrmann M, Bohle A, Held H, et al. Long-term prognosis of focal sclerosing glomerulonephritis. An analysis of 250 cases with particular regard to tubulointerstitial changes. *Clin Nephrol*. 1990;33:115-122.

232. Ingulli E, Tejani A. Racial differences in the incidence and renal outcome of idiopathic focal segmental glomerulosclerosis in children. *Pediatr Nephrol*. 1991;5:393-397.

233. Levinsky RJ, Malleson PN, Barratt TM, et al. Circulating immune complexes in steroid-responsive nephrotic syndrome. *N Engl J Med*. 1978;298:126-129.

234. Cairns SA, London RA, Mallick NP. Circulating immune complexes in idiopathic glomerular disease. *Kidney Int*. 1982;21:507-512.

235. Praga M, Hernandez E, Montoyo C, et al. Long-term beneficial effects of angiotensin-converting enzyme inhibition in patients with nephrotic proteinuria. *Am J Kidney Dis*. 1992;20:240-248.

236. Huissoon AP, Meehan S, Keogh JA. Reduction of proteinuria with captopril therapy in patients with focal segmental glomerulosclerosis and IgA nephropathy. *Ir J Med Sci*. 1991;160:319-321.

237. Bedogna V, Valvo E, Casagrande P, et al. Effects of ACE inhibition in normotensive patients with chronic glomerular disease and normal renal function. *Kidney Int*. 1990;38:101-107.

238. Maschio G, Alberti D, Janin G, et al. Effect of the angiotensin-converting-enzyme inhibitor benazepril on the progression of chronic renal insufficiency. The Angiotensin-Converting-Enzyme Inhibition in Progressive Renal Insufficiency Study Group. *N Engl J Med*. 1996;334:939-945.

239. Falk RJ, Becker M, Terrell R, et al. Anti-myeloperoxidase autoantibodies react with native but not denatured myeloperoxidase. *Clin Exp Immunol*. 1992;89:274-278.

240. Hodson EM, Willis NS, Craig JC. Interventions for idiopathic steroid-resistant nephrotic syndrome in children. *Cochrane Database Syst Rev*. 2010;11:DC003594.

241. Yi Z, Li Z, Wu XC, et al. Effect of fosinopril in children with steroid-resistant idiopathic nephrotic syndrome. *Pediatr Nephrol*. 2006;21:967-972.

242. Agarwal SK, Dash SC, Tiwari SC, et al. Idiopathic adult focal segmental glomerulosclerosis: a clinicopathological study and response to steroid. *Nephron*. 1993;63:168-171.

243. Meyrier A, Simon P. Treatment of corticoresistant idiopathic nephrotic syndrome in the adult: minimal change disease and focal segmental glomerulosclerosis. *Adv Nephrol Necker Hosp*. 1988;17:127-150.

244. Miyata J, Takebayashi S, Taguchi T, et al. Evaluation and correlation of clinical and histological features of focal segmental glomerulosclerosis. *Nephron*. 1986;44:115-120.

245. Schwartz MM, Evans J, Bain R, et al. Focal segmental glomerulosclerosis: prognostic implications of the cellular lesion. *J Am Soc Nephrol*. 1999;10:1900-1907.

246. Ponticelli C, Villa M, Banfi G, et al. Can prolonged treatment improve the prognosis in adults with focal segmental glomerulosclerosis? *Am J Kidney Dis*. 1999;34:618-625.

247. Schwartz MM, Korbet SM, Rydel J, et al. Primary focal segmental glomerular sclerosis in adults: prognostic value of histologic variants. *Am J Kidney Dis*. 1995;25:845-852.

248. Nagai R, Cattran DC, Pei Y. Steroid therapy and prognosis of focal segmental glomerulosclerosis in the elderly. *Clin Nephrol*. 1994;42:18-21.

249. Crook ED, Habeeb D, Gowdy O, et al. Effects of steroids in focal segmental glomerulosclerosis in a predominantly African-American population. *Am J Med Sci*. 2005;330:19-24.

250. Melvin T, Bennett W. Management of nephrotic syndrome in childhood. *Drugs*. 1991;42:30-51.

251. Tarshish P, Tobin JN, Bernstein J, et al. Cyclophosphamide does not benefit patients with focal segmental glomerulosclerosis. A report of the International Study of Kidney Disease in Children. *Pediatr Nephrol*. 1996;10:590-593.

252. Martinelli R, Pereira LJ, Silva OM, et al. Cyclophosphamide in the treatment of focal segmental glomerulosclerosis. *Braz J Med Biol Res*. 2004;37:1365-1372.

253. Cattran DC, Appel GB, Hebert LA, et al. A randomized trial of cyclosporine in patients with steroid-resistant focal segmental glomerulosclerosis. North America Nephrotic Syndrome Study Group. *Kidney Int*. 1999;56:2220-2226.

254. Plank C, Kalb V, Hinkes B, et al. Cyclosporin A is superior to cyclophosphamide in children with steroid-resistant nephrotic syndrome—a randomized controlled multicentre trial by the Arbeitsgemeinschaft für Pädiatrische Nephrologie. *Pediatr Nephrol*. 2008;23:1483-1493.

255. Senthil NL, Ganguli A, Rathi M, et al. Mycophenolate mofetil or standard therapy for membranous nephropathy and focal segmental glomerulosclerosis: a pilot study. *Nephrol Dial Transplant*. 2008;23:1926-1930.

256. Dervaux T, Caillard S, Meyer C, et al. Is sirolimus responsible for proteinuria? *Transplant Proc*. 2005;37:2828-2829.

257. Ruiz JC, Diekmann F, Campistol JM, et al. Evolution of proteinuria after conversion from calcineurin inhibitors (CNI) to sirolimus (SRL) in renal transplant patients: a multicenter study. *Transplant Proc*. 2005;37:3833-3835.

258. Letavernier E, Pe'raldi MN, Pariente A, et al. Proteinuria following a switch from calcineurin inhibitors to sirolimus. *Transplantation*. 2005;80:1198-1203.

259. Saurina A, Campistol JM, Piera C, et al. Conversion from calcineurin inhibitors to sirolimus in chronic allograft dysfunction: changes in glomerular haemodynamics and proteinuria. *Nephrol Dial Transplant*. 2006;21:488-493.

260. Boratynska M, Banasik M, Watorek E, et al. Conversion to sirolimus from cyclosporine may induce nephrotic proteinuria and progressive deterioration of renal function in chronic allograft nephropathy patients. *Transplant Proc*. 2006;38:101-104.

261. Franco AF, Martini D, Abensur H, et al. Proteinuria in transplant patients associated with sirolimus. *Transplant Proc*. 2007;39:449-452.

262. Tumlin JA, Miller D, Near M, et al. A prospective, open-label trial of sirolimus in the treatment of focal segmental glomerulosclerosis. *Clin J Am Soc Nephrol*. 2006;1:109-116.

263. Cho ME, Hurley JK, Kopp JB. Sirolimus therapy of focal segmental glomerulosclerosis is associated with nephrotoxicity. *Am J Kidney Dis*. 2007;49:310-317.

264. Fervenza FC, Fitzpatrick PM, Mertz J, et al. Acute rapamycin nephrotoxicity in native kidneys of patients with chronic glomerulopathies. *Nephrol Dial Transplant*. 2004;19:1288-1292.

265. Nozu K, Iijima K, Fujisawa M, et al. Rituximab treatment for posttransplant lymphoproliferative disorder (PTLD) induces complete remission of recurrent nephrotic syndrome. *Pediatr Nephrol*. 2005;20:1660-1663.

266. Pescovitz MD, Book BK, Sidner RA. Resolution of recurrent focal segmental glomerulosclerosis proteinuria after rituximab treatment. *N Engl J Med*. 2006;354:1961-1963.

267. Meyer TN, Thaiss F, Stahl RA. Immunoadsorption and rituximab therapy in a second living-related kidney transplant patient with recurrent focal segmental glomerulosclerosis. *Transpl Int*. 2007;20:1066-1071.

268. Kamar N, Faguer S, Esposito L, et al. Treatment of focal segmental glomerular sclerosis with rituximab: 2 case reports. *Clin Nephrol.* 2007;67:250-254.

269. Gossmann J, Scheuermann EH, Porubsky S, et al. Abrogation of nephrotic proteinuria by rituximab treatment in a renal transplant patient with relapsed focal segmental glomerulosclerosis. *Transpl Int.* 2007;20:558-562.

270. Hristea D, Hadaya K, Marangon N, et al. Successful treatment of recurrent focal segmental glomerulosclerosis after kidney transplantation by plasmapheresis and rituximab. *Transpl Int.* 2007;20:102-105.

271. Kaito H, Kamei K, Kikuchi E, et al. Successful treatment of collapsing focal segmental glomerulosclerosis with a combination of rituximab, steroids and ciclosporin. *Pediatr Nephrol.* 2010;25:957-959.

272. Peters HP, van de Kar NC, Wetzels JF. Rituximab in minimal change nephropathy and focal segmental glomerulosclerosis: report of four cases and review of the literature. *Neth J Med.* 2008;66:408-415.

273. Yabu JM, Ho B, Scandling JD, et al. Rituximab failed to improve nephrotic syndrome in renal transplant patients with recurrent focal segmental glomerulosclerosis. *Am J Transplant.* 2008;8:222-227.

274. Fernandez-Fresnedo G, Segarra A, Gonzalez E, et al. Rituximab treatment of adult patients with steroid-resistant focal segmental glomerulosclerosis. *Clin J Am Soc Nephrol.* 2009;4:1317-1323.

275. Shihab FS. Do we have a pill for renal fibrosis? *Clin J Am Soc Nephrol.* 2007;2:876-878.

276. Cho ME, Smith DC, Branton MH, et al. Pirfenidone slows renal function decline in patients with focal segmental glomerulosclerosis. *Clin J Am Soc Nephrol.* 2007;2:906-913.

277. Haas M, Godfrin Y, Oberbauer R, et al. Plasma immunadsorption treatment in patients with primary focal and segmental glomerulosclerosis. *Nephrol Dial Transplant.* 1998;13:2013-2016.

278. Reddick RL, Jennette JC, Askin FB. Squamous metaplasia of the breast. An ultrastructural and immunologic evaluation. *Am J Clin Pathol.* 1985;84:530-533.

279. Jennette JC, Falk RJ. C1q nephropathy. In: Massry S, Glassock R, eds. *Textbook of nephrology.* 3rd ed. Baltimore: Williams & Wilkins; 1995:749-752.

280. Roberti I, Baqi N, Vyas S, et al. A single-center study of C1q nephropathy in children. *Pediatr Nephrol.* 2009;24:77-82.

281. Vizjak A, Ferluga D, Rozic M, et al. Pathology, clinical presentations, and outcomes of C1q nephropathy. *J Am Soc Nephrol.* 2008;19:2237-2244.

282. Wong CS, Fink CA, Baechle J, et al. C1q nephropathy and minimal change nephrotic syndrome. *Pediatr Nephrol.* 2009;24:761-767.

283. Reeves-Daniel AM, Iskandar SS, Bowden DW, et al. Is collapsing C1q nephropathy another MYH9-associated kidney disease? A case report. *Am J Kidney Dis.* 2010;55:e21-e24.

284. Bitzan M, Ouahed JD, Krishnamoorthy P, et al. Rituximab treatment of collapsing C1q glomerulopathy: clinical and histopathological evolution. *Pediatr Nephrol.* 2008;23:1355-1361.

285. Nishida M, Kawakatsu H, Komatsu H, et al. Spontaneous improvement in a case of C1q nephropathy. *Am J Kidney Dis.* 2000;35:E22.

286. Hisano S, Fukuma Y, Segawa Y, et al. Clinicopathologic correlation and outcome of C1q nephropathy. *Clin J Am Soc Nephrol.* 2008;3:1637-1643.

287. Yamamoto T, Noble NA, Miller DE, et al. Sustained expression of TGF-beta 1 underlies development of progressive kidney fibrosis. *Kidney Int.* 1994;45:916-927.

288. Remuzzi G, Bertani T. Is glomerulosclerosis a consequence of altered glomerular permeability to macromolecules? *Kidney Int.* 1990;38:384-394.

289. Thomas ME, Schreiner GF. Contribution of proteinuria to progressive renal injury: consequences of tubular uptake of fatty acid bearing albumin. *Am J Nephrol.* 1993;13:385-398.

290. Agarwal A, Nath KA. Effect of proteinuria on renal interstitium: effect of products of nitrogen metabolism. *Am J Nephrol.* 1993;13:376-384.

291. Ramirez F, Travis LB, Cunningham RJ, et al. Focal segmental glomerulosclerosis, crescent, and rapidly progressive renal failure. *Int J Pediatr Nephrol.* 1982;3:175-178.

292. Packham DK, North RA, Fairley KF, et al. Pregnancy in women with primary focal and segmental hyalinosis and sclerosis. *Clin Nephrol.* 1988;29:185-192.

293. Muso E, Yashiro M, Matsushima M, et al. Does LDL-apheresis in steroid-resistant nephrotic syndrome affect prognosis? *Nephrol Dial Transplant.* 1994;9:257-264.

294. Coggins CH. Is membranous nephropathy treatable? *Am J Nephrol.* 1981;1:219-221.

295. Glassock RJ. Secondary membranous glomerulonephritis. *Nephrol Dial Transplant.* 1992;7(suppl 1):64-71.

296. Kleinknecht C, Levy M, Gagnadoux MF, et al. Membranous glomerulonephritis with extra-renal disorders in children. *Medicine (Baltimore).* 1979;58:219-228.

297. Takekoshi Y, Tanaka M, Shida N, et al. Strong association between membranous nephropathy and hepatitis-B surface antigenaemia in Japanese children. *Lancet.* 1978;2:1065-1068.

298. Weetman AP, Pinching AJ, Pussel BA, et al. Membranous glomerulonephritis and autoimmune thyroid disease. *Clin Nephrol.* 1981;15:50-51.

299. Kobayashi K, Harada A, Onoyama K, et al. Idiopathic membranous glomerulonephritis associated with diabetes mellitus: light, immunofluorescence and electron microscopic study. *Nephron.* 1981;28:163-168.

300. Burstein DM, Korbet SM, Schwartz MM. Membranous glomerulonephritis and malignancy. *Am J Kidney Dis.* 1993;22:5-10.

300a. Swaminathan S, Leung N, Lager DJ, et al. Changing incidence of glomerular disease in Olmstead County, Minnesota: a 30-year renal biopsy study. *Clin J Am Soc Nephrol.* 2006;1(3):483-487.

301. Hsu HC, Lin GH, Chang MH, et al. Association of hepatitis B surface (HBs) antigenemia and membranous nephropathy in children in Taiwan. *Clin Nephrol.* 1983;20:121-129.

302. Kirdpon S, Vuttivirojana A, Kovitangkoon K, et al. The primary nephrotic syndrome in children and histopathologic study. *J Med Assoc Thai.* 1989;72(suppl 1):26-31.

303. Yoshikawa N, Ito H, Yamada Y, et al. Membranous glomerulonephritis associated with hepatitis B antigen in children: a comparison with idiopathic membranous glomerulonephritis. *Clin Nephrol.* 1985;23:28-34.

304. Del Vecchio-Blanco C, Polito C, Caporaso N, et al. Membranous glomerulopathy and hepatitis B virus (HBV) infection in children. *Int J Pediatr Nephrol.* 1983;4:235-238.

305. Slusarczyk J, Michalak T, Nazarewicz D, et al. Membranous glomerulopathy associated with hepatitis B core antigen immune complexes in children. *Am J Pathol.* 1980;98:29-43.

306. Black DA, Rose G, Brewer DB. Controlled trial of prednisone in adult patients with the nephrotic syndrome. *Br Med J.* 1970;3:421-426.

307. Bolton WK, Atuk NO, Sturgill BC, et al. Therapy of the idiopathic nephrotic syndrome with alternate day steroids. *Am J Med.* 1977;62:60-70.

308. A controlled study of short-term prednisone treatment in adults with membranous nephropathy. Collaborative Study of the Adult Idiopathic Nephrotic Syndrome. *N Engl J Med.* 1979;301:1301-1306.

309. Forland M, Spargo BH. Clinicopathological correlations in idiopathic nephrotic syndrome with membranous nephropathy. *Nephron.* 1969;6:498-525.

310. Hayslett JP, Kashgarian M, Bensch KG, et al. Clinicopathological correlations in the nephrotic syndrome due to primary renal disease. *Medicine (Baltimore).* 1973;52:93-120.

311. Miller RB, Harrington JT, Ramos CP, et al. Long-term results of steroid therapy in adults with idiopathic nephrotic syndrome. *Am J Med.* 1969;46:919-929.

312. Nyberg M, Petterson E, Tallqvist G, et al. Survival in idiopathic glomerulonephritis. *Acta Pathol Microbiol Scand A.* 1980;88:319-325.

313. Comparison of idiopathic and systemic lupus erythematosus–associated membranous glomerulonephropathy in children. The Southwest Pediatric Nephrology Study Group. *Am J Kidney Dis.* 1986;7:115-124.

314. Pierides AM, Malasit P, Morley AR, et al. Idiopathic membranous nephropathy. *Q J Med.* 1977;46:163-177.

315. Medawar W, Green A, Campbell E, et al. Clinical and histopathologic findings in adults with the nephrotic syndrome. *Ir J Med Sci.* 1990;159:137-140.

316. Churg J, Ehrenreich T. Membranous nephropathy. *Perspect Nephrol Hypertens.* 1973;1(pt 1):443-448.

317. Hopper J, Trew PA, Biava CG. Membranous nephropathy: its relative benignity in women. *Nephron.* 1981;29:18-24.

318. Noel LH, Zanetti M, Droz D, et al. Long-term prognosis of idiopathic membranous glomerulonephritis. Study of 116 untreated patients. *Am J Med.* 1979;66:82-90.

319. Ehrenreich T, Porush JG, Churg J, et al. Treatment of idiopathic membranous nephropathy. *N Engl J Med.* 1976;295:741-746.

320. Honkanen E, Tornroth T, Gronhagen R. Natural history, clinical course and morphological evolution of membranous nephropathy. *Nephrol Dial Transplant.* 1992;7(suppl 1):35-41.

321. Hogan SL, Muller KE, Jennette JC, et al. A review of therapeutic studies of idiopathic membranous glomerulopathy. *Am J Kidney Dis.* 1995;25:862-875.

322. Mallick NP, Short CD, Manos J. Clinical membranous nephropathy. *Nephron.* 1983;34:209-219.

323. Lefaucheur C, Stengel B, Nochy D, et al. Membranous nephropathy and cancer: epidemiologic evidence and determinants of high-risk cancer association. *Kidney Int.* 2006;70:1510-1517.

324. Bjorneklett R, Vikse BE, Svarstad E, et al. Long-term risk of cancer in membranous nephropathy patients. *Am J Kidney Dis.* 2007;50:396-403.

325. Nachman PH, Glassock RJ. Glomerular, vascular, and tubulointerstitial diseases. *NephSAP.* 2008;7:185-189.

326. Schwartz MM. Membranous glomerulonephritis. In: Jennette JC, Olson JL, Schwartz MM, et al, eds. *Heptinstall's pathology of the kidney.* 6th ed. Philadelphia: Lippincott Williams & Wilkins; 2006:205-252.

327. Magori A, Sonkodi S, Szabo E, et al. Clinical pathology of membranous nephropathy based on kidney biopsy studies. *Orv Hetil.* 1977;118: 2013-2020.

328. Jennette JC, Iskandar SS, Dalldorf FG. Pathologic differentiation between lupus and nonlupus membranous glomerulopathy. *Kidney Int.* 1983;24:377-385.

329. Jennette JC, Lamanna RW, Burnette JP, et al. Concurrent antiglomerular basement membrane antibody and immune complex mediated glomerulonephritis. *Am J Clin Pathol.* 1982;78:381-386.

330. Silva FG. Membranoproliferative glomerulonephritis. In: Jennette JC, Olson JL, Schwartz MM, et al, eds. *Heptinstall's pathology of the kidney.* 5th ed. Philadelphia: Lippincott-Raven Publishers; 1998:309-368.

331. Abreo K, Abreo F, Mitchell B, et al. Idiopathic crescentic membranous glomerulonephritis. *Am J Kidney Dis.* 1986;8:257-261.

332. Jennette JC, Falk RJ. Nephritic syndrome and glomerulonephritis. In: Silva FG, D'Agati VD, Nadasdy R, eds. *Renal biopsy interpretation.* New York: Churchill Livingstone; 1996:71-114.

333. Klassen J, Elwood C, Grossberg AL, et al. Evolution of membranous nephropathy into anti-glomerular-basement-membrane glomerulonephritis. *N Engl J Med.* 1974;290:1340-1344.

334. Kurki P, Helve T, von Bonsdorff M, et al. Transformation of membranous glomerulonephritis into crescentic glomerulonephritis with glomerular basement membrane antibodies. Serial determinations of anti-GBM before the transformation. *Nephron.* 1984;38:134-137.

335. Mathieson PW, Peat DS, Short A, et al. Coexistent membranous nephropathy and ANCA-positive crescentic glomerulonephritis in association with penicillamine. *Nephrol Dial Transplant.* 1996;11: 863-866.

336. Mitas JA, Frank LR, Swerdlin AR, et al. Crescentic glomerulonephritis complicating idiopathic membranous glomerulonephropathy. *South Med J.* 1983;76:664-667.

337. Lim LC, Taylor III JG, Schmitz JL, et al. Diagnostic usefulness of antineutrophil cytoplasmic autoantibody serology. Comparative evaluation of commercial indirect fluorescent antibody kits and enzyme immunoassay kits. *Am J Clin Pathol.* 1999;111:363-369.

338. Schwartz MM. Membranous glomerulonephritis. In: Jennette JC, Olson JL, Schwartz MM, et al, eds. *Heptinstall's pathology of the kidney.* 5th ed. Philadelphia: Lippincott-Raven Publishers; 1998:259-308.

339. Camussi G, Noble B, Van L, et al. Pathogenesis of passive Heymann glomerulonephritis: chlorpromazine inhibits antibody-mediated redistribution of cell surface antigens and prevents development of the disease. *J Immunol.* 1986;136:2127-2135.

340. Kerjaschki D, Farquhar MG. Immunocytochemical localization of the Heymann nephritis antigen (GP330) in glomerular epithelial cells of normal Lewis rats. *J Exp Med.* 1983;157:667-686.

341. Cavallo T. Membranous nephropathy. Insights from Heymann nephritis. *Am J Pathol.* 1994;144:651-658.

342. Debiec H, Guigonis V, Mougenot B, et al. Antenatal membranous glomerulonephritis due to anti-neutral endopeptidase antibodies. *N Engl J Med.* 2002;346:2053-2060.

343. Kerjaschki D. Pathomechanisms and molecular basis of membranous glomerulopathy. *Lancet.* 2004;364:1194-1196.

344. Ronco P, Debiec H. Molecular pathomechanisms of membranous nephropathy: from Heymann nephritis to alloimmunization. *J Am Soc Nephrol.* 2005;16:1205-1213.

345. Ronco P, Debiec H. New insights into the pathogenesis of membranous glomerulonephritis. *Curr Opin Nephrol Hypertens.* 2006;15:258-263.

346. Beck Jr LH, Bonegio RG, Lambeau G, et al. M-type phospholipase A₂ receptor as target antigen in idiopathic membranous nephropathy. *N Engl J Med.* 2009;361:11-21.

347. Prunotto M, Carnevali ML, Candiano G, et al. Autoimmunity in membranous nephropathy targets aldose reductase and SOD2. *J Am Soc Nephrol.* 2010;21:507-519.

348. Kerjaschki D. Molecular pathogenesis of membranous nephropathy. *Kidney Int.* 1992;41:1090-1105.

349. Cybulsky AV, Rennke HG, Feintzeig ID, et al. Complement-induced glomerular epithelial cell injury. Role of the membrane attack complex in rat membranous nephropathy. *J Clin Invest.* 1986;77:1096-1107.

350. Couser WG, Schulze M, Pruchno CJ. Role of C5b-9 in experimental membranous nephropathy. *Nephrol Dial Transplant.* 1992;7(suppl 1): 25-31.

351. Coupes B, Brenchley PE, Short CD, et al. Clinical aspects of C3dg and C5b-9 in human membranous nephropathy. *Nephrol Dial Transplant.* 1992;7(suppl 1):32-34.

352. Couser WG, Nangaku M. Cellular and molecular biology of membranous nephropathy. *J Nephrol.* 2006;19:699-705.

353. Doi T, Mayumi M, Kanatsu K, et al. Distribution of IgG subclasses in membranous nephropathy. *Clin Exp Immunol.* 1984;58:57-62.

354. Haas M. IgG subclass deposits in glomeruli of lupus and nonlupus membranous nephropathies. *Am J Kidney Dis.* 1994;23:358-364.

355. Doi T, Kanatsu K, Nagai H, et al. Demonstration of C3d deposits in membranous nephropathy. *Nephron.* 1984;37:232-235.

356. Cunningham PN, Quigg RJ. Contrasting roles of complement activation and its regulation in membranous nephropathy. *J Am Soc Nephrol.* 2005;16:1214-1222.

357. Quigg RJ, Holers VM, Morgan BP, et al. Crry and CD59 regulate complement in rat glomerular epithelial cells and are inhibited by the nephritogenic antibody of passive Heymann nephritis. *J Immunol.* 1995;154:3437-3443.

358. Salant DJ, Belok S, Madaio MP, et al. A new role for complement in experimental membranous nephropathy in rats. *J Clin Invest.* 1980;66:1339-1350.

359. Schiller B, He C, Salant DJ, et al. Inhibition of complement regulation is key to the pathogenesis of active Heymann nephritis. *J Exp Med.* 1998;188:1353-1358.

360. Nangaku M, Quigg RJ, Shankland SJ, et al. Overexpression of Crry protects mesangial cells from complement-mediated injury. *J Am Soc Nephrol.* 1997;8:223-233.

361. Quigg RJ, Kozono Y, Berthiaume D, et al. Blockade of antibody-induced glomerulonephritis with Crry-Ig, a soluble murine complement inhibitor. *J Immunol.* 1998;160:4553-4560.

362. Neale TJ, Ojha PP, Exner M, et al. Proteinuria in passive Heymann nephritis is associated with lipid peroxidation and formation of adducts on type IV collagen. *J Clin Invest.* 1994;94:1577-1584.

363. Spicer ST, Tran GT, Killingsworth MC, et al. Induction of passive Heymann nephritis in complement component 6–deficient PVG rats. *J Immunol.* 2007;179:172-178.

364. Nakamura T, Tanaka N, Higuma N, et al. The localization of plasminogen activator inhibitor-1 in glomerular subepithelial deposits in membranous nephropathy. *J Am Soc Nephrol.* 1996;7:2434-2444.

365. Nangaku M, Shankland SJ, Couser WG. Cellular response to injury in membranous nephropathy. *J Am Soc Nephrol.* 2005;16:1195-1204.

366. Hsu SI, Couser WG. Chronic progression of tubulointerstitial damage in proteinuric renal disease is mediated by complement activation: a therapeutic role for complement inhibitors? *J Am Soc Nephrol.* 2003;14:S186-S191.

367. Tang S, Lai KN, Sacks SH. Role of complement in tubulointerstitial injury from proteinuria. *Kidney Blood Press Res.* 2002;25:120-126.

368. Gaarkeuken H, Siezenga MA, Zuidwijk K, et al. Complement activation by tubular cells is mediated by properdin binding. *Am J Physiol Renal Physiol.* 2008;295:F1397-F1403.

369. Klouda PT, Manos J, Acheson EJ, et al. Strong association between idiopathic membranous nephropathy and HLA-DRW3. *Lancet.* 1979;2:770-771.

370. Laurent B, Berthoux FC, Le Petit JC, et al. Immunogenetics and immunopathology of human membranous glomerulonephritis. *Proc Eur Dial Transplant Assoc.* 1983;19:629-634.

371. Le Petit JC, Laurent B, Berthoux FC. HLA-DR3 and idiopathic membranous nephritis (IMN) association. *Tissue Antigens.* 1982;20: 227-228.

372. Hiki Y, Kobayashi Y, Itoh I, et al. Strong association of HLA-DR2 and MT1 with idiopathic membranous nephropathy in Japan. *Kidney Int.* 1984;25:953-957.

373. Tomura S, Kashiwabara H, Tuchida H, et al. Strong association of idiopathic membranous nephropathy with HLA-DR2 and MT1 in Japanese. *Nephron.* 1984;36:242-245.

374. Ogahara S, Naito S, Abe K, et al. Analysis of HLA class II genes in Japanese patients with idiopathic membranous glomerulonephritis. *Kidney Int.* 1992;41:175-182.

375. Dyer PA, Klouda PT, Harris R, et al. Properdin factor B alleles in patients with idiopathic membranous nephropathy. *Tissue Antigens.* 1980;15: 505-507.

376. Bantis C, Heering PJ, Aker S, et al. Tumor necrosis factor-alpha gene G-308A polymorphism is a risk factor for the development of membranous glomerulonephritis. *Am J Nephrol.* 2006;26:12-15.

377. Thibaudin D, Thibaudin L, Berthoux P, et al. TNFA2 and d2 alleles of the tumor necrosis factor alpha gene polymorphism are associated with onset/occurrence of idiopathic membranous nephropathy. *Kidney Int.* 2007;71(5):431-437.

378. Sacks SH, Nomura S, Warner C, et al. Analysis of complement C4 loci in Caucasoids and Japanese with idiopathic membranous nephropathy. *Kidney Int.* 1992;42:882-887.

379. Short CD, Feehally J, Gokal R, et al. Familial membranous nephropathy. *Br Med J (Clin Res Ed).* 1984;289:1500.

380. Sato K, Oguchi H, Hora K, et al. Idiopathic membranous nephropathy in two brothers. *Nephron.* 1987;46:174-178.

381. Dumas R, Dumas ML, Baldet P, et al. [Membranous glomerulonephritis in two brothers associated in one with tubulo-interstitial disease, Fanconi syndrome and anti-TBM antibodies]. *Arch Fr Pediatr.* 1982;39:75-78.

382. Elshihabi I, Kaye CI, Brzowski A. Membranous nephropathy in two human leukocyte antigen–identical brothers. *J Pediatr.* 1993;123:940-942.

383. Vangelista A, Tazzari R, Bonomini V. Idiopathic membranous nephropathy in two twin brothers. *Nephron.* 1988;50:79-80.

384. Bockenhauer D, Debiec H, Sebire N, et al. Familial membranous nephropathy: an X-linked genetic susceptibility? *Nephron Clin Pract.* 2008;108:c10-c15.

385. Sherman RA, Dodelson R, Gary NE, et al. Membranous nephropathy. *J Med Soc N J.* 1980;77:649-652.

386. James SH, Lien YH, Ruffenach SJ, et al. Acute renal failure in membranous glomerulonephropathy: a result of superimposed crescentic glomerulonephritis. *J Am Soc Nephrol.* 1995;6:1541-1546.

387. Wagoner RD, Stanson AW, Holley KE, et al. Renal vein thrombosis in idiopathic membranous glomerulopathy and nephrotic syndrome: incidence and significance. *Kidney Int.* 1983;23:368-374.

388. Llach F. Hypercoagulability, renal vein thrombosis, and other thrombotic complications of nephrotic syndrome. *Kidney Int.* 1985;28:429-439.

389. Kanwar YS, Farquhar MG. Anionic sites in the glomerular basement membrane. In vivo and in vitro localization to the laminae rarae by cationic probes. *J Cell Biol.* 1979;81:137-153.

390. Cai S, Zhong GX, Li JC, et al. Color Doppler ultrasonography appearances of renal vein thrombosis and its diagnostic value. *Chin Med Sci J.* 2007;22:17-21.

391. Wei LQ, Rong ZK, Gui L, et al. CT diagnosis of renal vein thrombosis in nephrotic syndrome. *J Comput Assist Tomogr.* 1991;15:454-457.

392. Pollak VE, Rosen S, Pirani CL, et al. Natural history of lipoid nephrosis and of membranous glomerulonephritis. *Ann Intern Med.* 1968;69:1171-1196.

393. Row PG, Cameron JS, Turner DR, et al. Membranous nephropathy. Long-term follow-up and association with neoplasia. *Q J Med.* 1975;44:207-239.

394. Cameron JS, Healy MJ, Adu D. The Medical Research Council trial of short-term high-dose alternate day prednisolone in idiopathic membranous nephropathy with nephrotic syndrome in adults. The MRC Glomerulonephritis Working Party. *Q J Med.* 1990;74:133-156.

395. Cattran DC, Delmore T, Roscoe J, et al. A randomized controlled trial of prednisone in patients with idiopathic membranous nephropathy. *N Engl J Med.* 1989;320:210-215.

396. Kobayashi Y, Tateno S, Shigematsu H, et al. Prednisone treatment of non-nephrotic patients with idiopathic membranous nephropathy. A prospective study. *Nephron.* 1982;30:210-219.

397. Donadio JV, Holley KE, Anderson CF, et al. Controlled trial of cyclophosphamide in idiopathic membranous nephropathy. *Kidney Int.* 1974;6:431-439.

398. Ponticelli C, Zucchelli P, Passerini P, et al. A randomized trial of methylprednisolone and chlorambucil in idiopathic membranous nephropathy. *N Engl J Med.* 1989;320:8-13.

399. Schieppati A, Mosconi L, Perna A, et al. Prognosis of untreated patients with idiopathic membranous nephropathy. *N Engl J Med.* 1993;329:85-89.

400. Franklin WA, Jennings RB, Earle DP. Membranous glomerulonephritis: long-term serial observations on clinical course and morphology. *Kidney Int.* 1973;4:36-56.

401. Suki WN, Chavez A. Membranous nephropathy: response to steroids and immunosuppression. *Am J Nephrol.* 1981;1:11-16.

402. Harrison DJ, Thomson D, MacDonald MK. Membranous glomerulonephritis. *J Clin Pathol.* 1986;39:167.

403. Donadio JV, Torres VE, Velosa JA, et al. Idiopathic membranous nephropathy: the natural history of untreated patients. *Kidney Int.* 1988;33:708-715.

404. Alexopoulos E, Sakellariou G, Memmos D, et al. Cyclophosphamide provides no additional benefit to steroid therapy in the treatment of idiopathic membranous nephropathy. *Am J Kidney Dis.* 1993;21:497-503.

405. Davison AM, Cameron JS, Kerr DN, et al. The natural history of renal function in untreated idiopathic membranous glomerulonephritis in adults. *Clin Nephrol.* 1984;22:61-67.

406. Polanco N, Gutierrez E, Covarsi A, et al. Spontaneous remission of nephrotic syndrome in idiopathic membranous nephropathy. *J Am Soc Nephrol.* 2010;21:697-704.

407. Pei Y, Cattran D, Greenwood C. Predicting chronic renal insufficiency in idiopathic membranous glomerulonephritis. *Kidney Int.* 1992;42:960-966.

408. MacTier R, Boulton J, Payton CD, et al. The natural history of membranous nephropathy in the West of Scotland. *Q J Med.* 1986;60:793-802.

409. Tu WH, Petitti DB, Biava CG, Tulunay O, Hopper J. Membranous nephropathy: predictors of terminal renal failure. *Nephron.* 1984;36:118-124.

410. Cattran DC, Pei Y, Greenwood C. Predicting progression in membranous glomerulonephritis. *Nephrol Dial Transplant.* 1992;7(suppl 1):48-52.

411. Honkanen E, Tornroth T, Gronhagen R, et al. Long-term survival in idiopathic membranous glomerulonephritis: can the course be clinically predicted? *Clin Nephrol.* 1994;41:127-134.

412. Ramzy MH, Cameron JS, Turner DR, et al. The long-term outcome of idiopathic membranous nephropathy. *Clin Nephrol.* 1981;16:13-19.

413. Wehrmann M, Bohle A, Bogenschutz O, et al. Long-term prognosis of chronic idiopathic membranous glomerulonephritis. An analysis of 334 cases with particular regard to tubulo-interstitial changes. *Clin Nephrol.* 1989;31:67-76.

414. Austin HA, Boumpas DT, Vaughan EM, et al. High-risk features of lupus nephritis: importance of race and clinical and histological factors in 166 patients. *Nephrol Dial Transplant.* 1995;10:1620-1628.

415. Abe S, Amagasaki Y, Konishi K, et al. Idiopathic membranous glomerulonephritis: aspects of geographical differences. *J Clin Pathol.* 1986;39:1193-1198.

416. Ponticelli C, Zucchelli P, Imbasciati E, et al. Controlled trial of methylprednisolone and chlorambucil in idiopathic membranous nephropathy. *N Engl J Med.* 1984;310:946-950.

417. Zucchelli P, Cagnoli L, Pasquali S, et al. Clinical and morphologic evolution of idiopathic membranous nephropathy. *Clin Nephrol.* 1986;25:282-288.

418. Ponticelli C, Zucchelli P, Passerini P, et al. Methylprednisolone plus chlorambucil as compared with methylprednisolone alone for the treatment of idiopathic membranous nephropathy. The Italian Idiopathic Membranous Nephropathy Treatment Study Group. *N Engl J Med.* 1992;327:599-603.

419. Wakai S, Magil AB. Focal glomerulosclerosis in idiopathic membranous glomerulonephritis. *Kidney Int.* 1992;41:428-434.

420. Lee HS, Koh HI. Nature of progressive glomerulosclerosis in human membranous nephropathy. *Clin Nephrol.* 1993;39:7-16.

421. Troyanov S, Roasio L, Pandes M, et al. Renal pathology in idiopathic membranous nephropathy: a new perspective. *Kidney Int.* 2006;64(9):164-168.

422. Hoshino J, Hara S, Ubara Y, et al. Distribution of IgG subclasses in a biopsy specimen showing membranous nephropathy with anti-glomerular basement membrane glomerulonephritis: an uncharacteristically good outcome with corticosteroid therapy. *Am J Kidney Dis.* 2005;45:e67-e72.

423. Branten AJ, du Buf-Vereijken PW, Klasen IS, et al. Urinary excretion of β_2-microglobulin and IgG predict prognosis in idiopathic membranous nephropathy: a validation study. *J Am Soc Nephrol.* 2005;16:169-174.

424. Murphy BF, Fairley KF, Kincaid S. Idiopathic membranous glomerulonephritis: long-term follow-up in 139 cases. *Clin Nephrol.* 1988;30:175-181.

425. Zucchelli P, Pasquali S. Membranous nephropathy. In: Cameron JS, ed. *Oxford textbook of clinical nephrology.* Oxford, UK: Oxford University Press; 1992.

426. Pruchno CJ, Burns MW, Schulze M, et al. Urinary excretion of C5b-9 reflects disease activity in passive Heymann nephritis. *Kidney Int.* 1989;36:65-71.

427. Rosen S, Tornroth T, Bernard DB. Membranous glomerulonephritis. In: Tisher CC, Brenner BM, eds. *Renal pathology with clinical and functional correlations.* Philadelphia: JB Lippincott; 1989.

428. Habib R, Kleinknecht C, Gubler MC. Extramembranous glomerulonephritis in children: report of 50 cases. *J Pediatr.* 1973;82:754-766.

429. Honkanen E. Survival in idiopathic membranous glomerulonephritis. *Clin Nephrol.* 1986;25:122-128.

430. Short CD, Durrington PN, Mallick NP, et al. Serum lipoprotein (a) in men with proteinuria due to idiopathic membranous nephropathy. *Nephrol Dial Transplant.* 1992;7(suppl 1):109-113.

431. Schulze M, Donadio JV, Pruchno CJ, et al. Elevated urinary excretion of the C5b-9 complex in membranous nephropathy. *Kidney Int.* 1991;40:533-538.

432. Ogrodowski JL, Hebert LA, Sedmak D, et al. Measurement of SC5b-9 in urine in patients with the nephrotic syndrome. *Kidney Int.* 1991;40:1141-1147.

433. Brenchley PE, Coupes B, Short CD, et al. Urinary C3dg and C5b-9 indicate active immune disease in human membranous nephropathy. *Kidney Int.* 1992;41:933-937.

434. Coupes BM, Kon SP, Brenchley PE, et al. The temporal relationship between urinary C5b-9 and C3dg and clinical parameters in human membranous nephropathy. *Nephrol Dial Transplant.* 1993;8:397-401.

435. Savin VJ, Johnson RJ, Couser WG. C5b-9 increases albumin permeability of isolated glomeruli in vitro. *Kidney Int.* 1994;46:382-387.

436. Kusunoki Y, Akutsu Y, Itami N, et al. Urinary excretion of terminal complement complexes in glomerular disease. *Nephron.* 1991;59:27-32.

437. Lin J, Markowitz GS, Nicolaides M, et al. Membranous glomerulopathy associated with graft-versus-host disease following allogeneic stem cell transplantation. Report of 2 cases and review of the literature. *Am J Nephrol.* 2001;21:351-356.

438. Llach F. Thromboembolic complications in nephrotic syndrome. Coagulation abnormalities, renal vein thrombosis, and other conditions. *Postgrad Med.* 1984;76(121):111-118.

439. Kauffmann RH, Veltkamp JJ, Van T, et al. Acquired antithrombin III deficiency and thrombosis in the nephrotic syndrome. *Am J Med.* 1978;65:607-613.

440. Wakui H, Imai H, Komatsuda A, et al. Circulating antibodies against alpha-enolase in patients with primary membranous nephropathy (MN). *Clin Exp Immunol.* 1999;118:445-450.

441. Lopez-Alemany R, Longstaff C, Hawley S, et al. Inhibition of cell surface mediated plasminogen activation by a monoclonal antibody against alpha-enolase. *Am J Hematol.* 2003;72:234-242.

442. Glassock RJ. Prophylactic anticoagulation in nephrotic syndrome: a clinical conundrum. *J Am Soc Nephrol.* 2007;18:2221-2225.

443. Velasquez F, Garcia P, Ruiz M. Idiopathic nephrotic syndrome of the adult with asymptomatic thrombosis of the renal vein. *Am J Nephrol.* 1988;8:457-462.

444. Llach F, Koffler A, Finck E, et al. On the incidence of renal vein thrombosis in the nephrotic syndrome. *Arch Intern Med.* 1977;137:333-336.

445. Llach F, Arieff AI, Massry SG. Renal vein thrombosis and nephrotic syndrome. A prospective study of 36 adult patients. *Ann Intern Med.* 1975;83:8-14.

446. Trew PA, Biava CG, Jacobs RP, et al. Renal vein thrombosis in membranous glomerulonephropathy: incidence and association. *Medicine (Baltimore).* 1978;57:69-82.

447. Bellomo R, Atkins RC. Membranous nephropathy and thromboembolism: is prophylactic anticoagulation warranted? *Nephron.* 1993;63:249-254.

448. Sarasin FP, Schifferli JA. Prophylactic oral anticoagulation in nephrotic patients with idiopathic membranous nephropathy. *Kidney Int.* 1994;45:578-585.

449. Controlled trial of azathioprine and prednisone in chronic renal disease. Report by Medical Research Council Working Party. *Br Med J.* 1971;2:239-241.

450. Controlled trial of azathioprine in the nephrotic syndrome secondary to idiopathic membranous glomerulonephritis. *Can Med Assoc J.* 1976;115:1209-1210.

451. Saag KG, Koehnke R, Caldwell JR, et al. Low dose long-term corticosteroid therapy in rheumatoid arthritis: an analysis of serious adverse events. *Am J Med.* 1994;96:115-123.

452. Short CD, Solomon LR, Gokal R, et al. Methylprednisolone in patients with membranous nephropathy and declining renal function. *Q J Med.* 1987;65:929-940.

453. Williams PS, Bone JM. Immunosuppression can arrest progressive renal failure due to idiopathic membranous glomerulonephritis. *Nephrol Dial Transplant.* 1989;4:181-186.

454. Ponticelli C, Zucchelli P, Passerini P, et al. A 10-year follow-up of a randomized study with methylprednisolone and chlorambucil in membranous nephropathy. *Kidney Int.* 1995;48:1600-1604.

455. Branten AJ, Reichert LJ, Koene RA, et al. Oral cyclophosphamide versus chlorambucil in the treatment of patients with membranous nephropathy and renal insufficiency. *QJM.* 1998;91:359-366.

456. Murphy BF, McDonald I, Fairley KF, et al. Randomized controlled trial of cyclophosphamide, warfarin and dipyridamole in idiopathic membranous glomerulonephritis. *Clin Nephrol.* 1992;37:229-234.

457. Imperiale TF, Goldfarb S, Berns JS. Are cytotoxic agents beneficial in idiopathic membranous nephropathy? A meta-analysis of the controlled trials. *J Am Soc Nephrol.* 1995;5:1553-1558.

458. Jha V, Ganguli A, Saha TK, et al. A randomized, controlled trial of steroids and cyclophosphamide in adults with nephrotic syndrome caused by idiopathic membranous nephropathy. *J Am Soc Nephrol.* 2007;18:1899-1904.

459. Ponticelli C, Altieri P, Scolari F, et al. A randomized study comparing methylprednisolone plus chlorambucil versus methylprednisolone plus cyclophosphamide in idiopathic membranous nephropathy. *J Am Soc Nephrol.* 1998;9:444-450.

460. Meyrier A. Treatment of idiopathic nephrotic syndrome with cyclosporine A. *J Nephrol.* 1997;10:14-24.

461. Guasch A, Suranyi M, Newton L, et al. Short-term responsiveness of membranous glomerulopathy to cyclosporine. *Am J Kidney Dis.* 1992;20:472-481.

462. Rostoker G, Belghiti D, Ben M, et al. Long-term cyclosporin A therapy for severe idiopathic membranous nephropathy. *Nephron.* 1993;63:335-341.

463. Cattran DC, Appel GB, Hebert LA, et al. Cyclosporine in patients with steroid-resistant membranous nephropathy: a randomized trial. *Kidney Int.* 2001;59:1484-1490.

464. Alexopoulos E, Papagianni A, Tsamelashvili M, et al. Induction and long-term treatment with cyclosporine in membranous nephropathy with the nephrotic syndrome. *Nephrol Dial Transplant.* 2006;21:3127-3132.

465. Praga M, Barrio V, Juarez GF, et al. Tacrolimus monotherapy in membranous nephropathy: a randomized controlled trial. *Kidney Int.* 2007;71:924-930.

466. Ballarin J, Poveda R, Ara J, et al. Treatment of idiopathic membranous nephropathy with the combination of steroids, tacrolimus and mycophenolate mofetil: results of a pilot study. *Nephrol Dial Transplant.* 2007;22:3196-3201.

467. Berg AL, Arnadottir M. ACTH-induced improvement in the nephrotic syndrome in patients with a variety of diagnoses. *Nephrol Dial Transplant.* 2004;19:1305-1307.

468. Ponticelli C, Passerini P, Salvadori M, et al. A randomized pilot trial comparing methylprednisolone plus a cytotoxic agent versus synthetic adrenocorticotropic hormone in idiopathic membranous nephropathy. *Am J Kidney Dis.* 2006;47:233-240.

469. Lindskog A, Ebefors K, Johansson ME, et al. Melanocortin 1 receptor agonists reduce proteinuria. *J Am Soc Nephrol.* 2010;121(8):1290-1298.

470. Branten AJ, du Buf-Vereijken PW, Vervloet M, et al. Mycophenolate mofetil in idiopathic membranous nephropathy: a clinical trial with comparison to a historic control group treated with cyclophosphamide. *Am J Kidney Dis.* 2007;50:248-256.

471. Dussol B, Morange S, Burtey S, et al. Mycophenolate mofetil monotherapy in membranous nephropathy: a 1-year randomized controlled trial. *Am J Kidney Dis.* 2008;52:699-705.

472. Chan TM, Lin AW, Tang SC, et al. Prospective controlled study on mycophenolate mofetil and prednisolone in the treatment of membranous nephropathy with nephrotic syndrome. *Nephrology (Carlton).* 2007;12:576-581.

473. Remuzzi G, Chiurchiu C, Abbate M, et al. Rituximab for idiopathic membranous nephropathy. *Lancet.* 2002;360:923-924.

474. Ruggenenti P, Chiurchiu C, Brusegan V, et al. Rituximab in idiopathic membranous nephropathy: a one-year prospective study. *J Am Soc Nephrol.* 2003;14:1851-1857.

475. Ruggenenti P, Chiurchiu C, Abbate M, et al. Rituximab for idiopathic membranous nephropathy: who can benefit? *Clin J Am Soc Nephrol.* 2006;1:738-748.

476. Ruggenenti P, Cravedi P, Sghirlanzoni MC, et al. Effects of rituximab on morphofunctional abnormalities of membranous glomerulopathy. *Clin J Am Soc Nephrol.* 2008;3:1652-1659.

477. Fervenza FC, Sethi S, Specks U. Idiopathic membranous nephropathy: diagnosis and treatment. *Clin J Am Soc Nephrol.* 2008;3:905-919.

478. Cravedi P, Ruggenenti P, Sghirlanzoni MC, et al. Titrating rituximab to circulating B cells to optimize lymphocytolytic therapy in idiopathic membranous nephropathy. *Clin J Am Soc Nephrol.* 2007;2:932-937.

479. Bomback AS, Derebail VK, McGregor JG, et al. Rituximab therapy for membranous nephropathy: a systematic review. *Clin J Am Soc Nephrol.* 2009;4(4):734-744.

480. Segarra A, Praga M, Ramos N, et al. Successful treatment of membranous glomerulonephritis with rituximab in calcineurin inhibitor–dependent patients. *Clin J Am Soc Nephrol.* 2009;4:1083-1088.

481. Palla R, Cirami C, Panichi V, et al. Intravenous immunoglobulin therapy of membranous nephropathy: efficacy and safety. *Clin Nephrol.* 1991;35:98-104.

482. Yokoyama H, Goshima S, Wada T, et al. The short- and long-term outcomes of membranous nephropathy treated with intravenous immune globulin therapy. Kanazawa Study Group for Renal Diseases and Hypertension. *Nephrol Dial Transplant.* 1999;14:2379-2386.

483. Appel GB, Nachman PH, Hogan SL, et al. Eculizumab (c5 complement inhibitor) in the treatment of idiopathic membranous nephropathy. *J Am Soc Nephrol.* 2002;13:[abstract].

484. Rostoker G, Ben M, Remy P, et al. Low-dose angiotensin-converting-enzyme inhibitor captopril to reduce proteinuria in adult idiopathic membranous nephropathy: a prospective study of long-term treatment. *Nephrol Dial Transplant.* 1995;10:25-29.

485. Thomas DM, Hillis AN, Coles GA, et al. Enalapril can treat the proteinuria of membranous glomerulonephritis without detriment to systemic or renal hemodynamics. *Am J Kidney Dis.* 1991;18:38-43.

486. Gansevoort RT, Heeg JE, Vriesendorp R, et al. Antiproteinuric drugs in patients with idiopathic membranous glomerulopathy. *Nephrol Dial Transplant.* 1992;7(suppl 1):91-96.

487. Ruilope LM, Casal MC, Praga M, et al. Additive antiproteinuric effect of converting enzyme inhibition and a low protein intake. *J Am Soc Nephrol.* 1992;3:1307-1311.

488. Cattran D. Management of membranous nephropathy: when and what for treatment. *J Am Soc Nephrol.* 2005;15:1188-1194.

489. D'Amico G, Ferrario F. Mesangiocapillary glomerulonephritis. *J Am Soc Nephrol.* 1992;2:S159-S166.

490. Donadio Jr JV, Anderson CF, Mitchell III JC, et al. Membranoproliferative glomerulonephritis. A prospective clinical trial of platelet-inhibitor therapy. *N Engl J Med.* 1984;310:1421-1426.

491. Barbiano D, Baroni M, Pagliari B, et al. Is membranoproliferative glomerulonephritis really decreasing? A multicentre study of 1,548 cases of primary glomerulonephritis. *Nephron.* 1985;40:380-381.

492. Levy M, Gubler MC, Habib R. New concepts in membranoproliferative glomerulonephritis. In: Kincaid-Smith P, d'Apice AJF, Atkins RC, eds. *Progress in glomerulonephritis.* New York: Wiley; 1979:177.

493. Cameron JS, Turner DR, Heaton J, et al. Idiopathic mesangiocapillary glomerulonephritis. Comparison of types I and II in children and adults and long-term prognosis. *Am J Med.* 1983;74:175-192.
494. Habib R, Gubler MC, Loirat C, et al. Dense deposit disease: a variant of membranoproliferative glomerulonephritis. *Kidney Int.* 1975;7:204-215.
495. Davis AE, Schneeberger EE, McCluskey RT, et al. Mesangial proliferative glomerulonephritis with irregular intramembranous deposits. Another variant of hypocomplementemic nephritis. *Am J Med.* 1977;63:481-487.
496. King JT, Valenzuela R, McCormack LJ, et al. Granular dense deposit disease. *Lab Invest.* 1978;39:591-596.
497. Strife CF, Jackson EC, McAdams AJ. Type III membranoproliferative glomerulonephritis: long-term clinical and morphologic evaluation. *Clin Nephrol.* 1984;21:323-334.
498. Klein M, Poucell S, Arbus GS, et al. Characteristics of a benign subtype of dense deposit disease: comparison with the progressive form of this disease. *Clin Nephrol.* 1983;20:163-171.
499. Sasdelli M, Santoro A, Cagnoli L, et al. [Membranoproliferative glomerulonephritis. Clinical, biological and histological study of 31 cases]. *Minerva Nefrol.* 1975;22:229-238.
500. Vargas R, Thomson KJ, Wilson D, et al. Mesangiocapillary glomerulonephritis with dense "deposits" in the basement membranes of the kidney. *Clin Nephrol.* 1976;5:73-82.
501. Donadio Jr JV, Slack TK, Holley KE, et al. Idiopathic membranoproliferative (mesangiocapillary) glomerulonephritis: a clinicopathologic study. *Mayo Clin Proc.* 1979;54:141-150.
502. Zhou XJ, Silva FG. Membranoproliferative glomerulonephritis. In: Jennette JC, Olson JL, Schwartz MM, et al, eds. *Heptinstall's pathology of the kidney.* 6th ed. Philadelphia: Lippincott Williams & Wilkins; 2006:253-320.
503. Korzets Z, Bernheim J, Bernheim J. Rapidly progressive glomerulonephritis (crescentic glomerulonephritis) in the course of type I idiopathic membranoproliferative glomerulonephritis. *Am J Kidney Dis.* 1987;10:56-61.
504. McCoy R, Clapp J, Seigler HF. Membranoproliferative glomerulonephritis. Progression from the pure form to the crescentic form with recurrence after transplantation. *Am J Med.* 1975;59:288-292.
505. Burkholder PM, Marchand A, Krueger RP. Mixed membranous and proliferative glomerulonephritis. A correlative light, immunofluorescence, and electron microscopic study. *Lab Invest.* 1970;23:459-479.
506. Strife CF, McEnery PT, McAdams AJ, et al. Membranoproliferative glomerulonephritis with disruption of the glomerular basement membrane. *Clin Nephrol.* 1977;7:65-72.
507. Ahmed MS, Wong CF, Abraham KA. Membrano-proliferative glomerulonephritis associated with metastatic prostate carcinoma—should immunosuppressive therapy be considered? *Nephrol Dial Transplant.* 2008;23:777.
508. Bockenhauer D, van't Hoff W, Chernin G, et al. Membranoproliferative glomerulonephritis associated with a mutation in Wilms' tumour suppressor gene 1. *Pediatr Nephrol.* 2009;24:1399-1401.
509. Favre G, Courtellemont C, Callard P, et al. Membranoproliferative glomerulonephritis, chronic lymphocytic leukemia, and cryoglobulinemia. *Am J Kidney Dis.* 2009;55(2):391-394.
510. Gurkan S, Dikman S, Saland MJ. A case of autoimmune thyroiditis and membranoproliferative glomerulonephritis. *Pediatr Nephrol.* 2009;24:193-197.
511. Mutluay R, Aki SZ, Erten Y, et al. Membranoproliferative glomerulonephritis and light-chain nephropathy in association with chronic lymphocytic leukemia. *Clin Nephrol.* 2008;70:527-531.
512. Jhaveri KD, D'Agati VD, Pursell R, et al. Coeliac sprue–associated membranoproliferative glomerulonephritis (MPGN). *Nephrol Dial Transplant.* 2009;24:3545-3548.
513. Donadio Jr JV, Offord KP. Reassessment of treatment results in membranoproliferative glomerulonephritis, with emphasis on life-table analysis. *Am J Kidney Dis.* 1989;14:445-451.
514. Holley KE, Donadio JV. Mesangioproliferative glomerulonephritis. In: Tisher CC, Brenner BM, eds. *Renal pathology with clinical and functional correlations.* Philadelphia: JB Lippincott; 1994:294-329.
515. Varade WS, Forristal J, West CD. Patterns of complement activation in idiopathic membranoproliferative glomerulonephritis, types I, II, and III. *Am J Kidney Dis.* 1990;16:196-206.
516. Williams DG, Peters DK, Fallows J, et al. Studies of serum complement in the hypocomplementaemic nephritides. *Clin Exp Immunol.* 1974;18:391-405.
517. Pickering RJ, Gewurz H, Good RA. Complement inactivation by serum from patients with acute and hypocomplementemic chronic glomerulonephritis. *J Lab Clin Med.* 1968;72:298-307.
518. Halbwachs L, Leveille M, Lesavre P, et al. Nephritic factor of the classical pathway of complement: immunoglobulin G autoantibody directed against the classical pathway C3 convertase enzyme. *J Clin Invest.* 1980;65:1249-1256.
519. Misiani R, Bellavita P, Fenili D, et al. Hepatitis C virus infection in patients with essential mixed cryoglobulinemia. *Ann Intern Med.* 1992;117:573-577.
520. Coleman TH, Forristal J, Kosaka T, et al. Inherited complement component deficiencies in membranoproliferative glomerulonephritis. *Kidney Int.* 1983;24:681-690.
521. Schmitt H, Bohle A, Reineke T, et al. Long-term prognosis of membranoproliferative glomerulonephritis type I. Significance of clinical and morphological parameters: an investigation of 220 cases. *Nephron.* 1990;55:242-250.
522. Garcia-de la Puente S, Orozco-Loza IL, Zaltzman-Girshevich S, et al. Prognostic factors in children with membranoproliferative glomerulonephritis type I. *Pediatr Nephrol.* 2008;23:929-935.
523. di Belgiojoso B, Tarantino A, Colasanti G, et al. The prognostic value of some clinical and histological parameters in membranoproliferative glomerulonephritis (MPGN): report of 112 cases. *Nephron.* 1977;19:250-258.
524. Habib R, Kleinknecht C, Gubler MC, et al. Idiopathic membranoproliferative glomerulonephritis in children. Report of 105 cases. *Clin Nephrol.* 1973;1:194-214.
525. Swainson CP, Robson JS, Thomson D, et al. Mesangiocapillary glomerulonephritis: a long-term study of 40 cases. *J Pathol.* 1983;141:449-468.
526. Antoine B, Faye C. The clinical course associated with dense deposits in the kidney basement membranes. *Kidney Int.* 1972;1:420-427.
527. Miller MN, Baumal R, Poucell S, et al. Incidence and prognostic importance of glomerular crescents in renal diseases of childhood. *Am J Nephrol.* 1984;4:244-247.
528. McAdams AJ, McEnery PT, West CD. Mesangiocapillary glomerulonephritis: changes in glomerular morphology with long-term alternate-day prednisone therapy. *J Pediatr.* 1975;86:23-31.
529. McEnery PT, McAdams AJ, West CD. Membranoproliferative glomerulonephritis: improved survival with alternate day prednisone therapy. *Clin Nephrol.* 1980;13:117-124.
530. West CD. Childhood membranoproliferative glomerulonephritis: an approach to management. *Kidney Int.* 1986;29:1077-1093.
531. McEnery PT, McAdams AJ, West CD. The effect of prednisone in a high-dose, alternate-day regimen on the natural history of idiopathic membranoproliferative glomerulonephritis. *Medicine (Baltimore).* 1985;64:401-424.
532. McEnery PT, McAdams AJ. Regression of membranoproliferative glomerulonephritis type II (dense deposit disease): observations in six children. *Am J Kidney Dis.* 1988;12:138-146.
533. Ford DM, Briscoe DM, Shanley PF, et al. Childhood membranoproliferative glomerulonephritis type I: limited steroid therapy. *Kidney Int.* 1992;41:1606-1612.
534. Warady BA, Guggenheim SJ, Sedman A, et al. Prednisone therapy of membranoproliferative glomerulonephritis in children. *J Pediatr.* 1985;107:702-707.
535. Kincaid-Smith P. The natural history and treatment of mesangiocapillary glomerulonephritis. *Perspect Nephrol Hypertens.* 1973;1(pt 1):591-609.
536. Zauner I, Bohler J, Braun N, et al. Effect of aspirin and dipyridamole on proteinuria in idiopathic membranoproliferative glomerulonephritis: a multicentre prospective clinical trial. Collaborative Glomerulonephritis Therapy Study Group (CGTS). *Nephrol Dial Transplant.* 1994;9:619-622.
537. Kher KK, Makker SP, Aikawa M, et al. Regression of dense deposits in type II membranoproliferative glomerulonephritis: case report of clinical course in a child. *Clin Nephrol.* 1982;17:100-103.
538. Chapman SJ, Cameron JS, Chantler C, et al. Treatment of mesangiocapillary glomerulonephritis in children with combined immunosuppression and anticoagulation. *Arch Dis Child.* 1980;55:446-451.
539. Zimmerman SW, Moorthy AV, Dreher WH, et al. Prospective trial of warfarin and dipyridamole in patients with membranoproliferative glomerulonephritis. *Am J Med.* 1983;75:920-927.
540. Cattran DC, Cardella CJ, Roscoe JM, et al. Results of a controlled drug trial in membranoproliferative glomerulonephritis. *Kidney Int.* 1985;27:436-441.
541. De S, Al-Nabhani D, Thorner P, et al. Remission of resistant MPGN type I with mycophenolate mofetil and steroids. *Pediatr Nephrol.* 2009;24:597-600.
542. Mak SK, Lo KY, Lo MW, et al. Refractory thrombotic thrombocytopenic purpura and membranoproliferative glomerulonephritis successfully treated with rituximab: a case associated with hepatitis C virus infection. *Hong Kong Med J.* 2009;15:201-208.
543. Bartel C, Oberma LN, Rummel MJ, et al. Remission of a B cell CLL-associated membranoproliferative glomerulonephritis type I with rituximab and bendamustine. *Clin Nephrol.* 2008;69:285-289.
544. Glassock RJ. Role of cyclosporine in glomerular diseases. *Cleve Clin J Med.* 1994;61:363-369.

545. Walker PD, Ferrario F, Joh K, et al. Dense deposit disease is not a membranoproliferative glomerulonephritis. *Mod Pathol.* 2007;20:605-616.

546. Bennett WM, Fassett RG, Walker RG, et al. Mesangiocapillary glomerulonephritis type II (dense-deposit disease): clinical features of progressive disease. *Am J Kidney Dis.* 1989;13:469-476.

547. Little MA, Bhangal G, Smyth CL, et al. Therapeutic effect of anti-TNF-alpha antibodies in an experimental model of anti-neutrophil cytoplasm antibody–associated systemic vasculitis. *J Am Soc Nephrol.* 2006;17:160-169.

548. Nasr SH, Valeri AM, Appel GB, et al. Dense deposit disease: clinicopathologic study of 32 pediatric and adult patients. *Clin J Am Soc Nephrol.* 2009;4:22-32.

549. Jennette JC. Immunohistology of renal disease. In: Jennette JC, ed. *Immunohistopathology in diagnostic pathology.* Boca Raton, FL: CRC Press; 1989:29-84.

550. Sibley RK, Kim Y. Dense intramembranous deposit disease: new pathologic features. *Kidney Int.* 1984;25:660-670.

551. Walker PD. Dense deposit disease: new insights. *Curr Opin Nephrol Hypertens.* 2007;16:204-212.

552. Jansen JH, Hogasen K, Mollnes TE. Extensive complement activation in hereditary porcine membranoproliferative glomerulonephritis type II (porcine dense deposit disease). *Am J Pathol.* 1993;143:1356-1365.

553. Appel GB, Cook HT, Hageman G, et al. Membranoproliferative glomerulonephritis type II (dense deposit disease): an update. *J Am Soc Nephrol.* 2005;16:1392-1403.

554. Daha MR, Fearon DT, Austen KF. C3 nephritic factor (C3NeF): stabilization of fluid phase and cell-bound alternative pathway convertase. *J Immunol.* 1976;116:1-7.

555. Mathieson PW, Peters K. Are nephritic factors nephritogenic? *Am J Kidney Dis.* 1994;24:964-966.

556. Droz D, Nabarra B, Noel LH, et al. Recurrence of dense deposits in transplanted kidneys: I. Sequential survey of the lesions. *Kidney Int.* 1979;15:386-395.

557. Eisinger AJ, Shortland JR, Moorhead PJ. Renal disease in partial lipodystrophy. *Q J Med.* 1972;41:343-354.

558. Dragon-Durey MA, Fremeaux-Bacchi V, Loirat C, et al. Heterozygous and homozygous factor H deficiencies associated with hemolytic uremic syndrome or membranoproliferative glomerulonephritis: report and genetic analysis of 16 cases. *J Am Soc Nephrol.* 2004;15:787-795.

559. Ault BH, Schmidt BZ, Fowler NL, et al. Human factor H deficiency. Mutations in framework cysteine residues and block in H protein secretion and intracellular catabolism. *J Biol Chem.* 1997;272:25168-25175.

560. Smith RJ, Alexander J, Barlow PN, et al. New approaches to the treatment of dense deposit disease. *J Am Soc Nephrol.* 2007;18:2447-2456.

561. Sawanobori E, Umino A, Kanai H, et al. A prolonged course of group A streptococcus–associated nephritis: a mild case of dense deposit disease (DDD)? *Clin Nephrol.* 2009;71:703-707.

562. D'souza Y, Short CD, McLeod D, et al. Long-term follow-up of drusen-like lesions in patients with type II mesangiocapillary glomerulonephritis. *Br J Ophthalmol.* 2008;92:950-953.

563. McAvoy CE, Best J, Sharkey JA. Extensive peripapillary exudation secondary to cat-scratch disease. *Eye (Lond).* 2004;18:331-332.

564. Mathieson PW, Peters DK. Lipodystrophy in MCGN type II: the clue to links between the adipocyte and the complement system. *Nephrol Dial Transplant.* 1997;12:1804-1806.

565. Kashtan CE, Burke B, Burch G, et al. Dense intramembranous deposit disease: a clinical comparison of histological subtypes. *Clin Nephrol.* 1990;33:1-6.

566. Dense deposit disease in children. prognostic value of clinical and pathologic indicators. The Southwest Pediatric Nephrology Study Group. *Am J Kidney Dis.* 1985;6:161-169.

567. Salama AD, Pusey CD. Drug insight: rituximab in renal disease and transplantation. *Nat Clin Pract Nephrol.* 2006;2:221-230.

568. Pickering MC, Cook HT. Translational mini-review series on complement factor H: renal diseases associated with complement factor H: novel insights from humans and animals. *Clin Exp Immunol.* 2008;151:210-230.

569. Noris M, Remuzzi G. Translational mini-review series on complement factor H: therapies of renal diseases associated with complement factor H abnormalities: atypical haemolytic uraemic syndrome and membranoproliferative glomerulonephritis. *Clin Exp Immunol.* 2008;151:199-209.

570. Andresdottir MB. Recommendations for the diagnosis and treatment of dense deposit disease. *Nat Clin Pract Nephrol.* 2008;4:68-69.

571. Habbig S, Mihatsch MJ, Heinen S, et al. C3 deposition glomerulopathy due to a functional factor H defect. *Kidney Int.* 2009;75:1230-1234.

572. Jozsi M, Heinen S, Hartmann A, et al. Factor H and atypical hemolytic uremic syndrome: mutations in the C-terminus cause structural changes and defective recognition functions. *J Am Soc Nephrol.* 2006;17:170-177.

573. Fakhouri F, de Jorge EG, Brune F, et al. Treatment with human complement factor H rapidly reverses renal complement deposition in factor H–deficient mice. *Kidney Int.* 2010;78(3):279-286.

574. Cameron JS. Glomerulonephritis in renal transplants. *Transplantation.* 1982;34:237-245.

575. Cameron JS, Turner DR. Recurrent glomerulonephritis in allografted kidneys. *Clin Nephrol.* 1977;7:47-54.

576. Curtis JJ, Wyatt RJ, Bhathena D, et al. Renal transplantation for patients with type I and type II membranoproliferative glomerulonephritis: serial complement and nephritic factor measurements and the problem of recurrence of disease. *Am J Med.* 1979;66:216-225.

577. West CD, Bissler JJ. Nephritic factor and recurrence in the renal transplant of membranoproliferative glomerulonephritis type II. *Pediatr Nephrol.* 2008;23:1867-1876.

578. Rodriguez-Iturbe B. Poststreptococcal glomerulonephritis. In: Glassock RJ, ed. *Current therapy in nephrology and hypertension.* 4th ed. St. Louis: Mosby–Year Book; 1998:141-145.

579. Ginsburg BE, Wasserman J, Huldt G, et al. Case of glomerulonephritis associated with acute toxoplasmosis. *Br Med J.* 1974;3:664-665.

580. Rodriguez-Iturbe B, Rubio L, Garcia R. Attack rate of poststreptococcal nephritis in families. A prospective study. *Lancet.* 1981;1:401-403.

581. Glassock RJ, Adler SG, Ward HJ, et al. Primary glomerular diseases. In: Brenner BM, Rector Jr FC, eds. *The kidney.* 4th ed. Philadelphia: Saunders; 1991:1182-1279.

582. Mota-Hernandez F, Briseno-Mondragon E, Gordillo-Paniagua G. Glomerular lesions and final outcome in children with glomerulonephritis of acute onset. *Nephron.* 1976;16:272-281.

583. Popovic-Rolovic M, Kostic M, Antic-Peco A, et al. Medium- and long-term prognosis of patients with acute poststreptococcal glomerulonephritis. *Nephron.* 1991;58:393-399.

584. Buzio C, Allegri L, Mutti A, et al. Significance of albuminuria in the follow-up of acute poststreptococcal glomerulonephritis. *Clin Nephrol.* 1994;41:259-264.

585. Tejani A, Ingulli E. Poststreptococcal glomerulonephritis. Current clinical and pathologic concepts. *Nephron.* 1990;55:1-5.

586. Layrisse Z, Rodriguez-Iturbe B, Garcia-Ramirez R, et al. Family studies of the HLA system in acute post-streptococcal glomerulonephritis. *Hum Immunol.* 1983;7:177-185.

587. Mori K, Sasazuki T, Kimura A, et al. HLA-DP antigens and post-streptococcal acute glomerulonephritis. *Acta Paediatr.* 1996;85:916-918.

588. Bakr A, Mahmoud LA, Al-Chenawi F, et al. HLA-DRB1* alleles in Egyptian children with post-streptococcal acute glomerulonephritis. *Pediatr Nephrol.* 2007;22:376-379.

589. Rammelkamp CH, Weaver RS. Acute glomerulonephritis. The significance of the variations in the incidence of the disease. *J Clin Invest.* 1953;32:345-358.

590. Stetson CA, Rammelkamp CH, Krause RM. Epidemic acute nephritis: studies on etiology, natural history, and prevention. *Medicine (Baltimore).* 1955;34:431-450.

591. Dillon Jr HC. The treatment of streptococcal skin infections. *J Pediatr.* 1970;76:676-684.

592. Dillon Jr HC, Reeves MS. Streptococcal immune responses in nephritis after skin infections. *Am J Med.* 1974;56:333-346.

593. Reid HF, Bassett DC, Poon-King T, et al. Group G streptococci in healthy school-children and in patients with glomerulonephritis in Trinidad. *J Hyg (Lond).* 1985;94:61-68.

594. Svartman M, Finklea JF, Earle DP, et al. Epidemic scabies and acute glomerulonephritis in Trinidad. *Lancet.* 1972;1:249-251.

595. Oner A, Demircin G, Bulbul M. Post-streptococcal acute glomerulonephritis in Turkey. *Acta Paediatr.* 1995;84:817-819.

596. Becquet O, Pasche J, Gatti H, et al. Acute post-streptococcal glomerulonephritis in children of French Polynesia: a 3-year retrospective study. *Pediatr Nephrol.* 2010;25:275-280.

597. Streeton CL, Hanna JN, Messer RD, et al. An epidemic of acute post-streptococcal glomerulonephritis among aboriginal children. *J Paediatr Child Health.* 1995;31:245-248.

598. Thomson PD. Renal problems in black South African children. *Pediatr Nephrol.* 1997;11:508-512.

599. Zoric D, Kelmendi M, Shehu B, et al. Acute poststreptococcal glomerulonephritis in children. *Adv Exp Med Biol.* 1997;418:125-127.

600. Carapetis JR, Steer AC, Mulholland EK, et al. The global burden of group A streptococcal diseases. *Lancet Infect Dis.* 2005;5:685-694.

601. Ilyas M, Tolaymat A. Changing epidemiology of acute post-streptococcal glomerulonephritis in Northeast Florida: a comparative study. *Pediatr Nephrol.* 2008;23(7):1101-1106.

602. Rosenberg HG, Vial SU, Pomeroy J, et al. Acute glomerulonephritis in children. An evolutive morphologic and immunologic study of the glomerular inflammation. *Pathol Res Pract.* 1985;180:633-643.

603. Edelstein CL, Bates WD. Subtypes of acute postinfectious glomerulonephritis: a clinico-pathological correlation. *Clin Nephrol.* 1992;38:311-317.

604. Feldman JD, Mardiney MR, Shuler SE. Immunology and morphology of acute post-streptococcal glomerulonephritis. *Lab Invest.* 1966;15:283-301.

605. Fish AJ, Herdman RC, Michael AF, et al. Epidemic acute glomerulonephritis associated with type 49 streptococcal pyoderma. II. Correlative study of light, immunofluorescent and electron microscopic findings. *Am J Med.* 1970;48:28-39.

606. Nadasdy T, Silva FG. Acute postinfectious glomerulonephritis. In: Jennette JC, Olson JL, Schwartz MM, et al, eds. *Heptinstall's pathology of the kidney.* 6th ed. Philadelphia: Lippincott Williams & Wilkins; 2006:321-396.

607. Jennette JC, Thomas DB. Crescentic glomerulonephritis. *Nephrol Dial Transplant.* 2001;16(suppl 6):80-82.

608. Modai D, Pik A, Behar M, et al. Biopsy proven evolution of post streptococcal glomerulonephritis to rapidly progressive glomerulonephritis of a post infectious type. *Clin Nephrol.* 1985;23:198-202.

609. Montseny JJ, Kleinknecht D, Meyrier A. [Rapidly progressive glomerulonephritis of infectious origin]. *Ann Med Interne (Paris).* 1993;144:308-310.

610. Velhote V, Saldanha LB, Malheiro PS, et al. Acute glomerulonephritis: three episodes demonstrated by light and electron microscopy, and immunofluorescence studies—a case report. *Clin Nephrol.* 1986;26:307-310.

611. Rosenberg HG, Donoso PL, Vial SU, et al. Clinical and morphological recovery between two episodes of acute glomerulonephritis: a light and electron microscopic study with immunofluorescence. *Clin Nephrol.* 1984;21:350-354.

612. Michael Jr AF, Drummond KN, Good RA, et al. Acute poststreptococcal glomerulonephritis: immune deposit disease. *J Clin Invest.* 1966;45:237-248.

613. Sorger K, Gessler M, Hubner FK, et al. Follow-up studies of three subtypes of acute postinfectious glomerulonephritis ascertained by renal biopsy. *Clin Nephrol.* 1987;27:111-124.

614. Jennings RB, Earle DP. Poststreptococcal glomerulonephritis: histopathologic and clinical studies on the acute, subsiding acute and early chronic latent phases. *J Clin Invest.* 1961;40:1525-1595.

615. Bright R. Cases and observations, illustrative of renal disease accompanied with the secretion of albuminous urine. *Guys Hosp Rep.* 1836;1:338-400.

616. Schick B. Die nachkrankheiten des scharlachs. *Jahrb Kinderheilkd.* 1907;65(suppl):132-173.

617. Rammelkamp CH, Weaver RS, Dingle JH. Significance of the epidemiological differences between acute nephritis and acute rheumatic fever. *Trans Assoc Am Physicians.* 1952;65:168.

618. Holm SE. The pathogenesis of acute post-streptococcal glomerulonephritis in new lights. Review article. *APMIS.* 1988;96:189-193.

619. Kraus W, Ohyama K, Snyder DS, et al. Autoimmune sequence of streptococcal M protein shared with the intermediate filament protein, vimentin. *J Exp Med.* 1989;169:481-492.

620. Goroncy-Bermes P, Dale JB, Beachey EH, et al. Monoclonal antibody to human renal glomeruli cross-reacts with streptococcal M protein. *Infect Immun.* 1987;55:2416-2419.

621. Kraus W, Beachey EH. Renal autoimmune epitope of group A streptococci specified by M protein tetrapeptide Ile-Arg-Leu-Arg. *Proc Natl Acad Sci U S A.* 1988;85:4516-4520.

622. Parra EJ, Marcini A, Akey J, et al. Estimating African American admixture proportions by use of population-specific alleles. *Am J Hum Genet.* 1998;63:1839-1851.

623. Yoshizawa N, Yamakami K, Fujino M, et al. Nephritis-associated plasmin receptor and acute poststreptococcal glomerulonephritis: characterization of the antigen and associated immune response. *J Am Soc Nephrol.* 2004;15:1785-1793.

624. Batsford SR, Mezzano S, Mihatsch M, et al. Is the nephritogenic antigen in post-streptococcal glomerulonephritis pyrogenic exotoxin B (SPE B) or GAPDH? *Kidney Int.* 2005;68:1120-1129.

625. Montseny JJ, Meyrier A, Kleinknecht D, et al. The current spectrum of infectious glomerulonephritis. Experience with 76 patients and review of the literature. *Medicine (Baltimore).* 1995;74:63-73.

626. Ferrario F, Kourilsky O, Morel-Maroger L. Acute endocapillary glomerulonephritis in adults: a histologic and clinical comparison between patients with and without initial acute renal failure. *Clin Nephrol.* 1983;19:17-23.

627. Richards J. Acute post-streptococcal glomerulonephritis. *W V Med J.* 1991;87:61-65.

628. Madaio MP, Harrington JT. Current concepts. The diagnosis of acute glomerulonephritis. *N Engl J Med.* 1983;309:1299-1302.

629. Lee HA, Stirling G, Sharpstone P. Acute glomerulonephritis in middle-aged and elderly patients. *Br Med J.* 1966;2:1361-1363.

630. Washio M, Oh Y, Okuda S, et al. Clinicopathological study of poststreptococcal glomerulonephritis in the elderly. *Clin Nephrol.* 1994;41:265-270.

631. Rovang RD, Zawada Jr ET, Santella RN, et al. Cerebral vasculitis associated with acute post-streptococcal glomerulonephritis. *Am J Nephrol.* 1997;17:89-92.

632. Kaplan RA, Zwick DL, Hellerstein S, et al. Cerebral vasculitis in acute post-streptococcal glomerulonephritis. *Pediatr Nephrol.* 1993;7:194-195.

633. Okada K, Saitoh S, Sakaguchi Z, et al. IgA nephropathy presenting clinicopathological features of acute post-streptococcal glomerulonephritis. *Eur J Pediatr.* 1996;155:327-330.

634. Akasheh MS, al-Lozi M, Affarah HB, et al. Rapidly progressive glomerulonephritis complicating acute rheumatic fever. *Postgrad Med J.* 1995;71:553-554.

635. Dodge WF, Spargo BH, Travis LB, et al. Poststreptococcal glomerulonephritis. A prospective study in children. *N Engl J Med.* 1972;286:273-278.

636. Fairley KF, Birch DF. Hematuria: a simple method for identifying glomerular bleeding. *Kidney Int.* 1982;21:105-108.

637. Baldwin DS, Gluck MC, Schacht RG, et al. The long-term course of poststreptococcal glomerulonephritis. *Ann Intern Med.* 1974;80:342-358.

638. Hinglais N, Garcia T, Kleinknecht D. Long-term prognosis in acute glomerulonephritis. The predictive value of early clinical and pathological features observed in 65 patients. *Am J Med.* 1974;56:52-60.

639. Cortes P, Potter EV, Kwaan HC. Characterization and significance of urinary fibrin degradation products. *J Lab Clin Med.* 1973;82:377-389.

640. Wilson RJ. Renal excretion of calcium and sodium in acute nephritis. *Br Med J.* 1969;4:713-715.

641. Don BR, Schambelan M. Hyperkalemia in acute glomerulonephritis due to transient hyporeninemic hypoaldosteronism. *Kidney Int.* 1990;38:1159-1163.

642. Martin DR. Rheumatogenic and nephritogenic group A streptococci. Myth or reality? An opening lecture. *Adv Exp Med Biol.* 1997;418:21-27.

643. Rodriguez-Iturbe B. Epidemic poststreptococcal glomerulonephritis. *Kidney Int.* 1984;25:129-136.

644. Tanz RR, Gerber MA, Shulman ST. What is a throat culture? *Adv Exp Med Biol.* 1997;418:29-33.

645. Peter G, Smith AL. Group A streptococcal infections of the skin and pharynx (first of two parts). *N Engl J Med.* 1977;297:311-317.

646. Bergner R, Fleiderman S, Ferne M, et al. The new streptozyme test for streptococcal antibodies. Studies in the value of this multiple antigen test in glomerulonephritis, acute pharyngitis, and acute rheumatic fever. *Clin Pediatr (Phila).* 1975;14:804-809.

647. Lange K, Seligson G, Cronin W. Evidence for the in situ origin of poststreptococcal glomerulonephritis: glomerular localization of endostreptosin and the clinical significance of the subsequent antibody response. *Clin Nephrol.* 1983;19:3-10.

648. Lange K, Ahmed U, Kleinberger H, et al. A hitherto unknown streptococcal antigen and its probable relation to acute poststreptococcal glomerulonephritis. *Clin Nephrol.* 1976;5:207-215.

649. Cronin WJ, Lange K. Immunologic evidence for the in situ deposition of a cytoplasmic streptococcal antigen (endostreptosin) on the glomerular basement membrane in rats. *Clin Nephrol.* 1990;34:143-146.

650. Yoshimoto M, Hosoi S, Fujisawa S, et al. High levels of antibodies to streptococcal cell membrane antigens specifically bound to monoclonal antibodies in acute poststreptococcal glomerulonephritis. *J Clin Microbiol.* 1987;25:680-684.

651. Kefalides NA, Pegg MT, Ohno N, et al. Antibodies to basement membrane collagen and to laminin are present in sera from patients with poststreptococcal glomerulonephritis. *J Exp Med.* 1986;163:588-602.

652. Hebert LA, Cosio FG, Neff JC. Diagnostic significance of hypocomplementemia. *Kidney Int.* 1991;39:811-821.

653. Matsell DG, Roy S, Tamerius JD, et al. Plasma terminal complement complexes in acute poststreptococcal glomerulonephritis. *Am J Kidney Dis.* 1991;17:311-316.

654. McLean RH, Schrager MA, Rothfield NF, et al. Normal complement in early poststreptococcal glomerulonephritis. *Br Med J.* 1977;1:1326.

655. Lewis EJ, Carpenter CB, Schur PH. Serum complement component levels in human glomerulonephritis. *Ann Intern Med.* 1971;75:555-560.

656. Cameron JS, Vick RM, Ogg CS, et al. Plasma C3 and C4 concentrations in management of glomerulonephritis. *Br Med J.* 1973;3:668-672.

657. Sjoholm AG. Complement components and complement activation in acute poststreptococcal glomerulonephritis. *Int Arch Allergy Appl Immunol.* 1979;58:274-284.

658. Schreiber RD, Muller-Eberhard HJ. Complement and renal disease. In: Wilson CB, Brenner BM, Stein JH, eds. *Contemporary issues in nephrology.* New York: Churchill Livingstone; 1979:67.

659. Hisano S, Matsushita M, Fujita T, et al. Activation of the lectin complement pathway in post-streptococcal acute glomerulonephritis. *Pathol Int.* 2007;57:351-357.

660. Wyatt RJ, Forristal J, West CD, et al. Complement profiles in acute post-streptococcal glomerulonephritis. *Pediatr Nephrol.* 1988;2:219-223.
661. McIntosh RM, Kulvinskas C, Kaufman DB. Cryoglobulins. II. The biological and chemical properties of cryoproteins in acute post-streptococcal glomerulonephritis. *Int Arch Allergy Appl Immunol.* 1971;41:700-715.
662. McIntosh RM, Griswold WR, Chernack WB, et al. Cryoglobulins. III. Further studies on the nature, incidence, clinical, diagnostic, prognostic, and immunopathologic significance of cryoproteins in renal disease. *Q J Med.* 1975;44:285-307.
663. Rodriguez-Iturbe B, Carr RI, Garcia R, et al. Circulating immune complexes and serum immunoglobulins in acute poststreptococcal glomerulonephritis. *Clin Nephrol.* 1980;13:1-4.
664. Yoshizawa N, Treser G, McClung JA, et al. Circulating immune complexes in patients with uncomplicated group A streptococcal pharyngitis and patients with acute poststreptococcal glomerulonephritis. *Am J Nephrol.* 1983;3:23-29.
665. Mezzano S, Olavarria F, Ardiles L, et al. Incidence of circulating immune complexes in patients with acute poststreptococcal glomerulonephritis and in patients with streptococcal impetigo. *Clin Nephrol.* 1986;26:61-65.
666. Sesso RC, Ramos OL, Pereira AB. Detection of IgG-rheumatoid factor in sera of patients with acute poststreptococcal glomerulonephritis and its relationship with circulating immune complexes. *Clin Nephrol.* 1986;26:55-60.
667. Villarreal Jr H, Fischetti VA, van de Rijn I, et al. The occurrence of a protein in the extracellular products of streptococci isolated from patients with acute glomerulonephritis. *J Exp Med.* 1979;149:459-472.
668. Kaplan BS, Esseltine D. Thrombocytopenia in patients with acute post-streptococcal glomerulonephritis. *J Pediatr.* 1978;93:974-976.
669. Ekert H, Powell H, Muntz R. Hypercoagulability in acute glomerulonephritis. *Lancet.* 1972;1:965-966.
670. Ekberg M, Nilsson IM. Factor VIII and glomerulonephritis. *Lancet.* 1975;1:1111-1113.
671. Alkjaersig NK, Fletcher AP, Lewis ML, et al. Pathophysiological response of the blood coagulation system in acute glomerulonephritis. *Kidney Int.* 1976;10:319-328.
672. Adhikari M, Coovadia HM, Greig HB, et al. Factor VIII procoagulant activity in children with nephrotic syndrome and post-streptococcal glomerulonephritis. *Nephron.* 1978;22:301-305.
673. Mezzano S, Kunick M, Olavarria F, et al. Detection of platelet-activating factor in plasma of patients with streptococcal nephritis. *J Am Soc Nephrol.* 1993;4:235-242.
674. Lewy JE, Salinas M, Herdson PB, et al. Clinico-pathologic correlations in acute poststreptococcal glomerulonephritis. A correlation between renal functions, morphologic damage and clinical course of 46 children with acute poststreptococcal glomerulonephritis. *Medicine (Baltimore).* 1971;50:453-501.
675. Potter EV, Lipschultz SA, Abidh S, et al. Twelve- to seventeen-year follow-up of patients with poststreptococcal acute glomerulonephritis in Trinidad. *N Engl J Med.* 1982;307:725-729.
676. Parra G, Rodriguez-Iturbe B, Colina-Chourio J, et al. Short-term treatment with captopril in hypertension due to acute glomerulonephritis. *Clin Nephrol.* 1988;29:58-62.
677. Leonard CD, Nagle RB, Striker GE, et al. Acute glomerulonephritis with prolonged oliguria. An analysis of 29 cases. *Ann Intern Med.* 1970;73:703-711.
678. Johnston F, Carapetis J, Patel MS, et al. Evaluating the use of penicillin to control outbreaks of acute poststreptococcal glomerulonephritis. *Pediatr Infect Dis J.* 1999;18:327-332.
679. Baldwin DS. Chronic glomerulonephritis: nonimmunologic mechanisms of progressive glomerular damage. *Kidney Int.* 1982;21:109-120.
680. Baldwin DS. Poststreptococcal glomerulonephritis. A progressive disease? *Am J Med.* 1977;62:1-11.
681. Lien JW, Mathew TH, Meadows R. Acute post-streptococcal glomerulonephritis in adults: a long-term study. *Q J Med.* 1979;48:99-111.
682. Berger J. IgA glomerular deposits in renal disease. *Transplant Proc.* 1969;1:939-944.
683. Berger J, Hinglais N. Intercapillary deposits of IgA-IgG. *J Urol Nephrol (Paris).* 1968;74:694-695.
684. Niaudet P, Murcia I, Beaufils H, et al. Primary IgA nephropathies in children: prognosis and treatment. *Adv Nephrol Necker Hosp.* 1993;22:121-140.
685. Schena FP. A retrospective analysis of the natural history of primary IgA nephropathy worldwide. *Am J Med.* 1990;89:209-215.
686. Clarkson AR, Seymour AE, Thompson AJ, et al. IgA nephropathy: a syndrome of uniform morphology, diverse clinical features and uncertain prognosis. *Clin Nephrol.* 1977;8:459-471.
687. Colasanti G, Banfi G, di Belgiojoso GB, et al. Idiopathic IgA mesangial nephropathy: clinical features. *Contrib Nephrol.* 1984;40:147-155.
688. Clarkson AR, Woodroffe AJ, Bannister KM, et al. The syndrome of IgA nephropathy. *Clin Nephrol.* 1984;21:7-14.
689. Schena FP, Gesualdo L, Montinaro V. Immunopathological aspects of immunoglobulin A nephropathy and other mesangial proliferative glomerulonephritides. *J Am Soc Nephrol.* 1992;2:S167-S172.
690. D'Amico G. The commonest glomerulonephritis in the world: IgA nephropathy. *Q J Med.* 1987;64:709-727.
691. Suzuki K, Honda K, Tanabe K, et al. Incidence of latent mesangial IgA deposition in renal allograft donors in Japan. *Kidney Int.* 2003;63(6):2286-2294.
692. Crowley-Nowick PA, Julian BA, Wyatt RJ, et al. IgA nephropathy in blacks: studies of IgA2 allotypes and clinical course. *Kidney Int.* 1991;39:1218-1224.
693. Jennette JC, Wall SD, Wilkman AS. Low incidence of IgA nephropathy in blacks. *Kidney Int.* 1985;28:944-950.
694. Wyatt RJ, Julian BA, Baehler RW, et al. Epidemiology of IgA nephropathy in central and eastern Kentucky for the period 1975 through 1994. Central Kentucky Region of the Southeastern United States IgA Nephropathy DATABANK Project. *J Am Soc Nephrol.* 1998;9:853-858.
695. Hoy WE, Hughson MD, Smith SM, et al. Mesangial proliferative glomerulonephritis in southwestern American Indians. *Am J Kidney Dis.* 1993;21:486-496.
696. Power DA, Muirhead N, Simpson JG, et al. IgA nephropathy is not a rare disease in the United Kingdom. *Nephron.* 1985;40:180-184.
697. Waldherr R, Rambausek M, Duncker WD, et al. Frequency of mesangial IgA deposits in a non-selected autopsy series. *Nephrol Dial Transplant.* 1989;4:943-946.
698. Rambausek M, Rauterberg EW, Waldherr R, et al. Evolution of IgA glomerulonephritis: relation to morphology, immunogenetics, and BP. *Semin Nephrol.* 1987;7:370-373.
699. Simon P, Ang KS, Bavay P, et al. Immunoglobulin A glomerulonephritis. Epidemiology in a population of 250 000 inhabitants. *Presse Med.* 1984;13:257-260.
700. Simon P, Ramee MP, Ang KS, et al. Course of the annual incidence of primary glomerulopathies in a population of 400,000 inhabitants over a 10-year period (1976-1985). *Nephrologie.* 1986;7:185-189.
701. Simon P, Ramee MP, Autuly V, et al. Epidemiology of primary glomerular diseases in a French region. Variations according to period and age. *Kidney Int.* 1994;46:1192-1198.
702. Levy M, Berger J. Worldwide perspective of IgA nephropathy. *Am J Kidney Dis.* 1988;12:340-347.
703. Frimat L, Kessler M. Controversies concerning the importance of genetic polymorphism in IgA nephropathy. *Nephrol Dial Transplant.* 2002;17:542-545.
704. Frimat L, Philippe C, Maghakian MN, et al. Polymorphism of angiotensin converting enzyme, angiotensinogen, and angiotensin II type 1 receptor genes and end-stage renal failure in IgA nephropathy: IGARAS—a study of 274 men. *J Am Soc Nephrol.* 2000;11:2062-2067.
705. Gong R, Liu Z, Li L. Mannose-binding lectin gene polymorphism associated with the patterns of glomerular immune deposition in IgA nephropathy. *Scand J Urol Nephrol.* 2001;35:228-232.
706. Kim W, Kang SK, Lee DY, et al. Endothelial nitric oxide synthase gene polymorphism in patients with IgA nephropathy. *Nephron.* 2000;86:232-233.
707. Matsunaga A, Numakura C, Kawakami T, et al. Association of the uteroglobin gene polymorphism with IgA nephropathy. *Am J Kidney Dis.* 2002;39:36-41.
708. Lee EY, Yang DH, Hwang KY, et al. Is tumor necrosis factor genotype (TNFA2/TNFA2) a genetic prognostic factor of an unfavorable outcome in IgA nephropathy? *J Korean Med Sci.* 2001;16:751-755.
709. Schroeder Jr HW. Genetics of IgA deficiency and common variable immunodeficiency. *Clin Rev Allergy Immunol.* 2000;19:127-140.
710. Niemir ZI, Stein H, Noronha IL, et al. PDGF and TGF-beta contribute to the natural course of human IgA glomerulonephritis. *Kidney Int.* 1995;48:1530-1541.
711. Yong D, Qing WQ, Hua L, et al. Association of angiotensin I–converting enzyme gene insertion/deletion polymorphism and IgA nephropathy: a meta-analysis. *Am J Nephrol.* 2006;26:511-518.
712. Yamamoto R, Nagasawa Y, Shoji T, et al. A candidate gene approach to genetic prognostic factors of IgA nephropathy—a result of Polymorphism REsearch to DIstinguish genetic factors Contributing To progression of IgA Nephropathy (PREDICT-IgAN). *Nephrol Dial Transplant.* 2009;24:3686-3694.
713. Beerman I, Novak J, Wyatt RJ, et al. The genetics of IgA nephropathy. *Nat Clin Pract Nephrol.* 2007;3:325-338.
714. Johnston PA, Brown JS, Braumholtz DA, et al. Clinico-pathological correlations and long-term follow-up of 253 United Kingdom patients with IgA nephropathy. A report from the MRC Glomerulonephritis Registry. *Q J Med.* 1992;84:619-627.

715. Schena FP, Scivittaro V, Ranieri E. IgA nephropathy: pros and cons for a familial disease. *Contrib Nephrol*. 1993;104:36-45.
716. Scolari F, Amoroso A, Savoldi S, et al. Familial occurrence of primary glomerulonephritis: evidence for a role of genetic factors. *Nephrol Dial Transplant*. 1992;7:587-596.
717. Gharavi AG, Yan Y, Scolari F, et al. IgA nephropathy, the most common cause of glomerulonephritis, is linked to 6q22-23. *Nat Genet*. 2000;26:354-357.
718. Paterson AD, Liu XQ, Wang K, et al. Genome-wide linkage scan of a large family with IgA nephropathy localizes a novel susceptibility locus to chromosome 2q36. *J Am Soc Nephrol*. 2007;18:2408-2415.
719. Bisceglia M, Galliani CA, Senger C, et al. Renal cystic diseases: a review. *Adv Anat Pathol*. 2006;13:26-56.
720. Gharavi AG, Moldoveanu Z, Wyatt RJ, et al. Aberrant IgA1 glycosylation is inherited in familial and sporadic IgA nephropathy. *J Am Soc Nephrol*. 2008;19:1008-1014.
721. Lin X, Ding J, Zhu L, et al. Aberrant galactosylation of IgA1 is involved in the genetic susceptibility of Chinese patients with IgA nephropathy. *Nephrol Dial Transplant*. 2009;24:3372-3375.
722. Pirulli D, Crovella S, Ulivi S, et al. Genetic variant of C1GalT1 contributes to the susceptibility to IgA nephropathy. *J Nephrol*. 2009;22:152-159.
723. Li GS, Zhang H, Lv JC, et al. Variants of C1GALT1 gene are associated with the genetic susceptibility to IgA nephropathy. *Kidney Int*. 2007;71:448-453.
724. Malycha F, Eggermann T, Hristov M, et al. No evidence for a role of cosmc-chaperone mutations in European IgA nephropathy patients. *Nephrol Dial Transplant*. 2009;24:321-324.
725. Coppo R, Feehally J, Glassock RJ. IgA nephropathy at two score and one. *Kidney Int*. 2010;77:181-186.
726. Ding JX, Xu LX, Zhu L, et al. Activity of α2,6-sialyltransferase and its gene expression in peripheral B lymphocytes in patients with IgA nephropathy. *Scand J Immunol*. 2009;69:174-180.
727. Zhu L, Tang W, Li G, et al. Interaction between variants of two glycosyltransferase genes in IgA nephropathy. *Kidney Int*. 2009;76:190-198.
728. Li R, Xue C, Li C, et al. TRAC variants associate with IgA nephropathy. *J Am Soc Nephrol*. 2009;20:1359-1367.
729. Woo KT, Lau YK, Wong KS, et al. Parallel genotyping of 10,204 single nucleotide polymorphisms to screen for susceptible genes for IgA nephropathy. *Ann Acad Med Singapore*. 2009;38:894-899.
730. Takei T, Iida A, Nitta K, et al. Association between single-nucleotide polymorphisms in selectin genes and immunoglobulin A nephropathy. *Am J Hum Genet*. 2002;70:781-786.
731. Lai KN, Chan KW, Mac-Moune F, et al. The immunochemical characterization of the light chains in the mesangial IgA deposits in IgA nephropathy. *Am J Clin Pathol*. 1986;85:548-551.
732. Emancipator SN. IgA nephropathy and Henoch-Schönlein purpura. In: Jennette JC, Olson JL, Schwartz MM, et al, eds. *Heptinstall's pathology of the kidney*. 5th ed. Philadelphia: Lippincott-Raven; 1998pp 479-450.
733. Willoughby PB, Jennette JC, Haughton G. Analysis of a murine B cell lymphoma, CH44, with an associated non- neoplastic T cell population. I. Proliferation of normal T lymphocytes is induced by a secreted product of the malignant B cells. *Am J Pathol*. 1988;133:507-515.
734. Haas M. Histologic subclassification of IgA nephropathy: a clinicopathologic study of 244 cases. *Am J Kidney Dis*. 1997;29:829-842.
735. Lee SM, Rao VM, Franklin WA, et al. IgA nephropathy: morphologic predictors of progressive renal disease. *Hum Pathol*. 1982;13:314-322.
736. Abuelo JG, Esparza AR, Matarese RA, et al. Crescentic IgA nephropathy. *Medicine (Baltimore)*. 1984;63:396-406.
737. Hogg RJ, Silva FG, Wyatt RJ, et al. Prognostic indicators in children with IgA nephropathy—report of the Southwest Pediatric Nephrology Study Group. *Pediatr Nephrol*. 1994;8:15-20.
738. Croker BP, Dawson DV, Sanfilippo F. IgA nephropathy. Correlation of clinical and histologic features. *Lab Invest*. 1983;48:19-24.
739. Streather CP, Scoble JE. Recurrent IgA nephropathy in a renal allograft presenting as crescentic glomerulonephritis. *Nephron*. 1994;66:113-114.
740. Cattran DC, Coppo R, Cook HT, et al. The Oxford classification of IgA nephropathy: rationale, clinicopathological correlations, and classification. *Kidney Int*. 2009;76:534-545.
741. Roberts IS, Cook HT, Troyanov S, et al. The Oxford classification of IgA nephropathy: pathology definitions, correlations, and reproducibility. *Kidney Int*. 2009;76:546-556.
742. Yamamoto R, Imai E. A novel classification for IgA nephropathy. *Kidney Int*. 2009;76:477-480.
743. Egido J, Sancho J, Blasco R, et al. Immunopathogenetic aspects of IgA nephropathy. *Adv Nephrol Necker Hosp*. 1983;12:103-137.
744. Allen A, Feehally J. IgA glycosylation in IgA nephropathy. *Adv Exp Med Biol*. 1995;435:175-183.
745. Feehally J. Immune mechanisms in glomerular IgA deposition. *Nephrol Dial Transplant*. 1988;3:361-378.
746. Conley ME, Cooper MD, Michael AF. Selective deposition of immunoglobulin A1 in immunoglobulin A nephropathy, anaphylactoid purpura nephritis, and systemic lupus erythematosus. *J Clin Invest*. 1980;66.
747. Bene MC, Hurault DL, Kessler M, et al. Confirmation of tonsillar anomalies in IgA nephropathy: a multicenter study. *Nephron*. 1991;58:425-428.
748. Wang MX, Walker RG, Kincaid-Smith P. Endothelial cell antigens recognized by IgA autoantibodies in patients with IgA nephropathy: partial characterization. *Nephrol Dial Transplant*. 1992;7:805-810.
749. Frampton G, Walker RG, Perry GJ, et al. IgA affinity to ssDNA or endothelial cells and its deposition in glomerular capillary walls in IgA nephropathy. *Nephrol Dial Transplant*. 1990;5:841-846.
750. Saulsbury FT, Kirkpatrick PR, Bolton WK. IgA antineutrophil cytoplasmic antibody in Henoch-Schönlein purpura. *Am J Nephrol*. 1991;11:295-300.
751. Savige JA, Gallicchio M. IgA antimyeloperoxidase antibodies associated with crescentic IgA glomerulonephritis. *Nephrol Dial Transplant*. 1992;7:952-955.
752. O'Donoghue DJ, Feehally J. Autoantibodies in IgA nephropathy. *Contrib Nephrol*. 1995;111:93-103.
753. Fornasieri A, Sinico RA, Maldifassi P, et al. IgA-antigliadin antibodies in IgA mesangial nephropathy (Berger's disease). *Br Med J (Clin Res Ed)*. 1987;295:78-80.
754. Laurent J, Branellec A, Heslan JM, et al. An increase in circulating IgA antibodies to gliadin in IgA mesangial glomerulonephritis. *Am J Nephrol*. 1987;7:178-183.
755. Yagame M, Tomino Y, Eguchi K, et al. Levels of circulating IgA immune complexes after gluten-rich diet in patients with IgA nephropathy. *Nephron*. 1988;49:104-106.
756. Nagy J, Scott H, Brandtzaeg P. Antibodies to dietary antigens in IgA nephropathy. *Clin Nephrol*. 1988;29:275-279.
757. Rostoker G, Andre C, Branellec A, et al. Lack of antireticulin and IgA antiendomysium antibodies in sera of patients with primary IgA nephropathy associated with circulating IgA antibodies to gliadin. *Nephron*. 1988;48:81.
758. Davin JC, Malaise M, Foidart J, et al. Anti-alpha-galactosyl antibodies and immune complexes in children with Henoch-Schönlein purpura or IgA nephropathy. *Kidney Int*. 1987;31:1132-1139.
759. Yap HK, Sakai RS, Woo KT, et al. Detection of bovine serum albumin in the circulating IgA immune complexes of patients with IgA nephropathy. *Clin Immunol Immunopathol*. 1987;43:395-402.
760. Suzuki S, Nakatomi Y, Sato H, et al. *Haemophilus parainfluenzae* antigen and antibody in renal biopsy samples and serum of patients with IgA nephropathy. *Lancet*. 1994;343:12-16.
761. Drew PA, Nieuwhof WN, Clarkson AR, et al. Increased concentration of serum IgA antibody to pneumococcal polysaccharides in patients with IgA nephropathy. *Clin Exp Immunol*. 1987;67:124-129.
762. Layward L, Allen AC, Hattersley JM, et al. Elevation of IgA in IgA nephropathy is localized in the serum and not saliva and is restricted to the IgA1 subclass. *Nephrol Dial Transplant*. 1993;8:25-28.
763. Layward L, Allen AC, Harper SJ, et al. Increased and prolonged production of specific polymeric IgA after systemic immunization with tetanus toxoid in IgA nephropathy. *Clin Exp Immunol*. 1992;88:394-398.
764. Schena FP, Mastrolitti G, Fracasso AR, et al. Increased immunoglobulin-secreting cells in the blood of patients with active idiopathic IgA nephropathy. *Clin Nephrol*. 1986;26:163-168.
765. Harper SJ, Allen AC, Pringle JH, et al. Increased dimeric IgA producing B cells in the bone marrow in IgA nephropathy determined by in situ hybridisation for J chain mRNA. *J Clin Pathol*. 1996;49:38-42.
766. Mestecky J, Hashim OH, Tomana M. Alterations in the IgA carbohydrate chains influence the cellular distribution of IgA1. *Contrib Nephrol*. 1995;111:66-71.
767. Baenziger J, Kornfeld S. Structure of the carbohydrate units of IgA1 immunoglobulin. II. Structure of the O-glycosidically linked oligosaccharide units. *J Biol Chem*. 1974;249:7270-7281.
768. Mestecky J, Tomana M, Crowley-Nowick PA, et al. Defective galactosylation and clearance of IgA1 molecules as a possible etiopathogenic factor in IgA nephropathy. *Contrib Nephrol*. 1993;104:172-182.
769. Smith A, Molyneux K, Feehally J, et al. Is sialylation of IgA the agent provocateur of IgA nephropathy? *Nephrol Dial Transplant*. 2008;23:2176-2178.
770. Suzuki H, Moldoveanu Z, Hall S, et al. IgA1-secreting cell lines from patients with IgA nephropathy produce aberrantly glycosylated IgA1. *J Clin Invest*. 2008;118:629-639.
771. Qin W, Zhong X, Fan JM, et al. External suppression causes the low expression of the Cosmc gene in IgA nephropathy. *Nephrol Dial Transplant*. 2008;23:1608-1614.

772. Chintalacharuvu SR, Yamashita M, Bagheri N, et al. T cell cytokine polarity as a determinant of immunoglobulin A (IgA) glycosylation and the severity of experimental IgA nephropathy. *Clin Exp Immunol.* 2008;153:456-462.

773. Suzuki H, Fan R, Zhang Z, et al. Aberrantly glycosylated IgA1 in IgA nephropathy patients is recognized by IgG antibodies with restricted heterogeneity. *J Clin Invest.* 2009;119:1668-1677.

774. Suzuki H, Moldoveanu Z, Hall S, et al. IgA nephropathy: characterization of IgG antibodies specific for galactose-deficient IgA1. *Contrib Nephrol.* 2007;157:129-133.

775. Tomana M, Novak J, Julian BA, et al. Circulating immune complexes in IgA nephropathy consist of IgA1 with galactose-deficient hinge region and antiglycan antibodies. *J Clin Invest.* 1999;104:73-81.

776. Tomana M, Matousovic K, Julian BA, et al. Galactose-deficient IgA1 in sera of IgA nephropathy patients is present in complexes with IgG. *Kidney Int.* 1997;52:509-516.

777. Novak J, Julian BA, Tomana M, et al. IgA glycosylation and IgA immune complexes in the pathogenesis of IgA nephropathy. *Semin Nephrol.* 2008;28:78-87.

778. Barratt J, Eitner F. Glomerular disease: sugars and immune complex formation in IgA nephropathy. *Nat Rev Nephrol.* 2009;5:612-614.

779. Hiki Y. O-linked oligosaccharides of the IgA1 hinge region: roles of its aberrant structure in the occurrence and/or progression of IgA nephropathy. *Clin Exp Nephrol.* 2009;13:415-423.

780. Barratt J, Eitner F, Feehally J, et al. Immune complex formation in IgA nephropathy: a case of the "right" antibodies in the "wrong" place at the "wrong" time? *Nephrol Dial Transplant.* 2009;24:3620-3623.

781. Novak J, Tomana M, Matousovic K, et al. IgA1-containing immune complexes in IgA nephropathy differentially affect proliferation of mesangial cells. *Kidney Int.* 2005;67:504-513.

782. Glassock RJ. Analyzing antibody activity in IgA nephropathy. *J Clin Invest.* 2009;119:1450-1452.

783. Hiki Y, Iwase H, Saitoh M, et al. Reactivity of glomerular and serum IgA1 to jacalin in IgA nephropathy. *Nephron.* 1996;72:429-435.

784. Kokubo T, Hashizume K, Iwase H, et al. Humoral immunity against the proline-rich peptide epitope of the IgA1 hinge region in IgA nephropathy. *Nephrol Dial Transplant.* 2000;15:28-33.

785. Hiki Y, Odani H, Takahashi M, et al. Mass spectrometry proves under-O-glycosylation of glomerular IgA1 in IgA nephropathy. *Kidney Int.* 2001;59:1077-1085.

786. Leung JC, Tang SC, Lam MF, et al. Charge-dependent binding of polymeric IgA1 to human mesangial cells in IgA nephropathy. *Kidney Int.* 2001;59:277-285.

787. Lai KN, Leung JC, Chan LY, et al. C: Activation of podocytes by mesangial-derived TNF-α: glomerulo-podocytic communication in IgA nephropathy. *Am J Physiol Renal Physiol.* 2008;294:F945-F955.

788. Boor P, Eitner F, Cohen CD, et al. Patients with IgA nephropathy exhibit high systemic PDGF-DD levels. *Nephrol Dial Transplant.* 2009;24: 2755-2762.

789. Oortwijn BD, Eijgenraam JW, Rastaldi MP, et al. The role of secretory IgA and complement in IgA nephropathy. *Semin Nephrol.* 2008;28:58-65.

790. Moura IC, Benhamou M, Launay P, et al. The glomerular response to IgA deposition in IgA nephropathy. *Semin Nephrol.* 2008;28:88-95.

791. Stockert RJ, Kressner MS, Collins JC, et al. IgA interaction with the asialoglycoprotein receptor. *Proc Natl Acad Sci U S A.* 1982;79:6229-6231.

792. Moldoveanu Z, Moro I, Radl J, et al. Site of catabolism of autologous and heterologous IgA in non-human primates. *Scand J Immunol.* 1990;32: 577-583.

793. Tomana M, Kulhavy R, Mestecky J. Receptor-mediated binding and uptake of immunoglobulin A by human liver. *Gastroenterology.* 1988;94:762-770.

794. Andre PM, Le Pogamp P, Chevet D. Impairment of jacalin binding to serum IgA in IgA nephropathy. *J Clin Lab Anal.* 1990;4:115-119.

795. O'Donoghue DJ, Darvill A, Ballardie FW. Mesangial cell autoantigens in immunoglobulin A nephropathy and Henoch-Schönlein purpura. *J Clin Invest.* 1991;88:1522-1530.

796. Ballardie FW, Brenchley PE, Williams S, et al. Autoimmunity in IgA nephropathy. *Lancet.* 1988;2:588-592.

797. Goshen E, Livne A, Nagy J, et al. Antinuclear autoantibodies in sera of patients with IgA nephropathy. *Nephron.* 1990;55:33-36.

798. O'Donoghue DJ, Nusbaum P, Noel LH, et al. Antineutrophil cytoplasmic antibodies in IgA nephropathy and Henoch-Schönlein purpura. *Nephrol Dial Transplant.* 1992;7:534-538.

799. Esnault VL, Ronda N, Jayne DR, et al. Association of ANCA isotype and affinity with disease expression. *J Autoimmun.* 1993;6:197-205.

800. Ramirez SB, Rosen S, Niles J, et al. IgG antineutrophil cytoplasmic antibodies in IgA nephropathy: a clinical variant? *Am J Kidney Dis.* 1998;31:341-344.

801. Martin SJ, Audrain MA, Baranger T, et al. Recurrence of immunoglobulin A nephropathy with immunoglobulin A antineutrophil cytoplasmic antibodies following renal transplantation. *Am J Kidney Dis.* 1997;29:125-131.

802. van den Wall Bake AW, Kirk KA, Gay RE, et al. Binding of serum immunoglobulins to collagens in IgA nephropathy and HIV infection. *Kidney Int.* 1992;42:374-382.

803. Eitner F, Schulze M, Brunkhorst R, et al. On the specificity of assays to detect circulating immunoglobulin A–fibronectin complexes: implications for the study of serologic phenomena in patients with immunoglobulin A nephropathy. *J Am Soc Nephrol.* 1994;5:1400-1406.

804. Nasr SH, Markowitz GS, Whelan JD, et al. IgA-dominant acute poststaphylococcal glomerulonephritis complicating diabetic nephropathy. *Hum Pathol.* 2003;34:1235-1241.

805. Walshe JJ, Brentjens JR, Costa GG, et al. Abdominal pain associated with IgA nephropathy. Possible mechanism. *Am J Med.* 1984;77:765-767.

806. MacDonald IM, Fairley KF, Hobbs JB, et al. Loin pain as a presenting symptom in idiopathic glomerulonephritis. *Clin Nephrol.* 1975;3:129-133.

807. Perez-Fontan M, Miguel JL, Picazo ML, et al. Idiopathic IgA nephropathy presenting as malignant hypertension. *Am J Nephrol.* 1986;6:482-486.

808. Kincaid-Smith P, Bennett WM, Dowling JP, et al. Acute renal failure and tubular necrosis associated with hematuria due to glomerulonephritis. *Clin Nephrol.* 1983;19:206-210.

809. Delclaux C, Jacquot C, Callard P, et al. Acute reversible renal failure with macroscopic haematuria in IgA nephropathy. *Nephrol Dial Transplant.* 1993;8:195-199.

810. Kapoor A, Mowbray JF, Porter KA, et al. Significance of haematuria in hypertensive patients. *Lancet.* 1980;1:231-232.

811. Mustonen J, Pasternack A, Rantala I. The nephrotic syndrome in IgA glomerulonephritis: response to corticosteroid therapy. *Clin Nephrol.* 1983;20:172-176.

812. D'Amico G. Influence of clinical and histological features on actuarial renal survival in adult patients with idiopathic IgA nephropathy, membranous nephropathy, and membranoproliferative glomerulonephritis: survey of the recent literature. *Am J Kidney Dis.* 1992;20:315-323.

813. Gutierrez E, Gonzalez E, Hernandez E, et al. Factors that determine an incomplete recovery of renal function in macrohematuria-induced acute renal failure of IgA nephropathy. *Clin J Am Soc Nephrol.* 2007;2:51-57.

814. Haas M, Rahman MH, Cohn RA, et al. IgA nephropathy in children and adults: comparison of histologic features and clinical outcomes. *Nephrol Dial Transplant.* 2008;23:2537-2545.

815. Cattran DC, Reich HN, Beanlands HJ, et al. The impact of sex in primary glomerulonephritis. *Nephrol Dial Transplant.* 2008;23(7):2247-2253.

816. Alamartine E, Sabatier JC, Guerin C, et al. Prognostic factors in mesangial IgA glomerulonephritis: an extensive study with univariate and multivariate analyses. *Am J Kidney Dis.* 1991;18:12-19.

817. Bogenschutz O, Bohle A, Batz C, et al. IgA nephritis: on the importance of morphological and clinical parameters in the long-term prognosis of 239 patients. *Am J Nephrol.* 1990;10:137-147.

818. Donadio JV, Bergstralh EJ, Offord KP, et al. Clinical and histopathologic associations with impaired renal function in IgA nephropathy. Mayo Nephrology Collaborative Group. *Clin Nephrol.* 1994;41:65-71.

819. Katafuchi R, Oh Y, Hori K, et al. An important role of glomerular segmental lesions on progression of IgA nephropathy: a multivariate analysis. *Clin Nephrol.* 1994;41:191-198.

820. Clarkson AR, Woodroffe AJ. Therapeutic perspectives in mesangial IgA nephropathy. *Contrib Nephrol.* 1984;40:187-194.

821. Bennett WM, Kincaid-Smith P. Macroscopic hematuria in mesangial IgA nephropathy: correlation with glomerular crescents and renal dysfunction. *Kidney Int.* 1983;23:393-400.

822. Bradford WD, Croker BP, Tisher CC. Kidney lesions in Rocky Mountain spotted fever: a light-, immunofluorescence-, and electron-microscopic study. *Am J Pathol.* 1979;97:381-392.

823. Packham DK, Hewitson TD, Yan HD, et al. Acute renal failure in IgA nephropathy. *Clin Nephrol.* 1994;42:349-353.

824. Praga M, Gutierrez-Millet V, Navas JJ, et al. Acute worsening of renal function during episodes of macroscopic hematuria in IgA nephropathy. *Kidney Int.* 1985;28:69-74.

825. Fogazzi GB, Imbasciati E, Moroni G, et al. Reversible acute renal failure from gross haematuria due to glomerulonephritis: not only in IgA nephropathy and not associated with intratubular obstruction. *Nephrol Dial Transplant.* 1995;10:624-629.

826. Chen A, Ding SL, Sheu LF, et al. Experimental IgA nephropathy. Enhanced deposition of glomerular IgA immune complex in proteinuric states. *Lab Invest.* 1994;70:639-647.

827. Donadio JV, Bergstralh EJ, Grande JP, et al. Proteinuria patterns and their association with subsequent end-stage renal disease in IgA nephropathy. *Nephrol Dial Transplant.* 2002;17:1197-1203.

828. Mackinnon B, Fraser EP, Cattran DC, et al. Validation of the Toronto formula to predict progression in IgA nephropathy. *Nephron Clin Pract.* 2008;109:c148-c153.

829. Goto M, Wakai K, Kawamura T, et al. A scoring system to predict renal outcome in IgA nephropathy: a nationwide 10-year prospective cohort study. *Nephrol Dial Transplant.* 2009;24:3068-3074.

830. Goto M, Kawamura T, Wakai K, et al. Risk stratification for progression of IgA nephropathy using a decision tree induction algorithm. *Nephrol Dial Transplant.* 2009;24:1242-1247.

831. Roufosse CA, Cook HT. Pathological predictors of prognosis in immunoglobulin A nephropathy: a review. *Curr Opin Nephrol Hypertens.* 2009;18:212-219.

832. Asaba K, Tojo A, Onozato ML, et al. Long-term renal prognosis of IgA nephropathy with therapeutic trend shifts. *Intern Med.* 2009;48:883-890.

833. Reich HN, Troyanov S, Scholey JW, et al. Remission of proteinuria improves prognosis in IgA nephropathy. *J Am Soc Nephrol.* 2007;18:3177-3183.

834. Ito K, Hirooka Y, Sunagawa K. Acquisition of brain Na sensitivity contributes to salt-induced sympathoexcitation and cardiac dysfunction in mice with pressure overload. *Circ Res.* 2009;104:1004-1011.

835. Sato S, Yanagihara T, Ghazizadeh M, et al. Correlation of autophagy type in podocytes with histopathological diagnosis of IgA nephropathy. *Pathobiology.* 2009;76:221-226.

836. Yuling H, Ruijing X, Xiang J, et al. CD19⁺CD5⁺ B cells in primary IgA nephropathy. *J Am Soc Nephrol.* 2008;19:2130-2139.

837. Stangou M, Alexopoulos E, Pantzaki A, et al. C5b-9 glomerular deposition and tubular α3β1-integrin expression are implicated in the development of chronic lesions and predict renal function outcome in immunoglobulin A nephropathy. *Scand J Urol Nephrol.* 2008;42:373-380.

838. Espinosa M, Ortega R, Gomez-Carrasco JM, et al. Mesangial C4d deposition: a new prognostic factor in IgA nephropathy. *Nephrol Dial Transplant.* 2009;24:886-891.

839. van Es LA, de Heer E, Vleming LJ, et al. GMP-17-positive T-lymphocytes in renal tubules predict progression in early stages of IgA nephropathy. *Kidney Int.* 2008;73:1426-1433.

840. Tsuboi N, Kawamura T, Ishii T, et al. Changes in the glomerular density and size in serial renal biopsies during the progression of IgA nephropathy. *Nephrol Dial Transplant.* 2009;24:892-899.

841. Torres DD, Rossini M, Manno C, et al. The ratio of epidermal growth factor to monocyte chemotactic peptide-1 in the urine predicts renal prognosis in IgA nephropathy. *Kidney Int.* 2008;73:327-333.

842. Wada T. Predicting outcome of IgA nephropathy by use of urinary epidermal growth factor: monocyte chemotactic peptide 1 ratio. *Nat Clin Pract Nephrol.* 2008;4:184-185.

843. Yu S, Cho J, Park I, et al. Urinary GADD45γ expression is associated with progression of IgA nephropathy. *Am J Nephrol.* 2009;30:133-139.

844. Rocchetti MT, Centra M, Papale M, et al. Urine protein profile of IgA nephropathy patients may predict the response to ACE-inhibitor therapy. *Proteomics.* 2008;8:206-216.

845. Bazzi C, Rizza V, Raimondi S, et al. In crescentic IgA nephropathy, fractional excretion of IgG in combination with nephron loss is the best predictor of progression and responsiveness to immunosuppression. *Clin J Am Soc Nephrol.* 2009;4:929-935.

846. Hara M, Yanagihara T, Kihara I. Cumulative excretion of urinary podocytes reflects disease progression in IgA nephropathy and Schönlein-Henoch purpura nephritis. *Clin J Am Soc Nephrol.* 2007;2:231-238.

847. Tanaka M, Yamada S, Iwasaki Y, et al. Impact of obesity on IgA nephropathy: comparative ultrastructural study between obese and non-obese patients. *Nephron Clin Pract.* 2009;112:c71-c78.

848. Seeman T, Pohl M, John U, et al. Ambulatory blood pressure, proteinuria and uric acid in children with IgA nephropathy and their correlation with histopathological findings. *Kidney Blood Press Res.* 2008;31:337-342.

849. Onda K, Ohi H, Tamano M, et al. Hypercomplementemia in adult patients with IgA nephropathy. *J Clin Lab Anal.* 2007;21:77-84.

850. Kaartinen K, Niemela O, Syrjanen J, et al. Alcohol consumption and kidney function in IgA glomerulonephritis. *Nephron Clin Pract.* 2009;112:c86-c93.

851. Chin HJ, Cho HJ, Lee TW, et al. The mildly elevated serum bilirubin level is negatively associated with the incidence of end stage renal disease in patients with IgA nephropathy. *J Korean Med Sci.* 2009;24(suppl):S22-S29.

852. Jacob S, Hery M, Protois JC, et al. Effect of organic solvent exposure on chronic kidney disease progression: the GN-PROGRESS cohort study. *J Am Soc Nephrol.* 2007;18:274-281.

853. Abe S. Pregnancy in IgA nephropathy. *Kidney Int.* 1991;40:1098-1102.

854. Abe S. The influence of pregnancy on the long-term renal prognosis of IgA nephropathy. *Clin Nephrol.* 1994;41:61-64.

855. Jones DC, Hayslett JP. Outcome of pregnancy in women with moderate or severe renal insufficiency. *N Engl J Med.* 1996;335:226-232.

856. Moldoveanu Z, Wyatt RJ, Lee JY, et al. Patients with IgA nephropathy have increased serum galactose-deficient IgA1 levels. *Kidney Int.* 2007;71:1148-1154.

857. Cederholm B, Wieslander J, Bygren P, et al. Circulating complexes containing IgA and fibronectin in patients with primary IgA nephropathy. *Proc Natl Acad Sci U S A.* 1988;85:4865-4868.

858. Davin JC, Li VM, Nagy J, et al. Evidence that the interaction between circulating IgA and fibronectin is a normal process enhanced in primary IgA nephropathy. *J Clin Immunol.* 1991;11:78-94.

859. Jones CL, Powell HR, Kincaid-Smith P, et al. Polymeric IgA and immune complex concentrations in IgA-related renal disease. *Kidney Int.* 1990;38:323-331.

860. Cosio FG, Lam S, Folami AO, et al. Immune regulation of immunoglobulin production in IgA-nephropathy. *Clin Immunol Immunopathol.* 1982;23:430-436.

861. Trascasa ML, Egido J, Sancho J, et al. Evidence of high polymeric IgA levels in serum of patients with Berger's disease and its modification with phenytoin treatment. *Proc Eur Dial Transplant Assoc.* 1979;16:513-519.

862. Newkirk MM, Klein MH, Katz A, et al. Estimation of polymeric IgA in human serum: an assay based on binding of radiolabeled human secretory component with applications in the study of IgA nephropathy, IgA monoclonal gammopathy, and liver disease. *J Immunol.* 1983;130:1176-1181.

863. Sancho J, Egido J, Sanchez-Crespo M, et al. Detection of monomeric and polymeric IgA containing immune complexes in serum and kidney from patients with alcoholic liver disease. *Clin Exp Immunol.* 1982;47:327-335.

864. Evans DJ, Williams DG, Peters DK, et al. Glomerular deposition of properdin in Henoch-Schönlein syndrome and idiopathic focal nephritis. *Br Med J.* 1973;3:326-328.

865. Gluckman JC, Jacob N, Beaufils H, et al. Clinical significance of circulating immune complexes detection in chronic glomerulonephritis. *Nephron.* 1978;22:138-145.

866. Coppo R, Basolo B, Martina G, et al. Circulating immune complexes containing IgA, IgG and IgM in patients with primary IgA nephropathy and with Henoch-Schoenlein nephritis. Correlation with clinical and histologic signs of activity. *Clin Nephrol.* 1982;18:230-239.

867. Danielsen H, Eriksen EF, Johansen A, et al. Serum immunoglobulin sedimentation patterns and circulating immune complexes in IgA glomerulonephritis and Schönlein-Henoch nephritis. *Acta Med Scand.* 1984;215:435-441.

868. Doi T, Kanatsu K, Sekita K, et al. Detection of IgA class circulating immune complexes bound to anti-C3d antibody in patients with IgA nephropathy. *J Immunol Methods.* 1984;69:95-104.

869. Hall RP, Stachura I, Cason J, et al. IgA-containing circulating immune complexes in patients with IgA nephropathy. *Am J Med.* 1983;74:56-63.

870. Lesavre P, Digeon M, Bach JF. Analysis of circulating IgA and detection of immune complexes in primary IgA nephropathy. *Clin Exp Immunol.* 1982;48:61-69.

871. Mustonen J, Pasternack A, Helin H, et al. Circulating immune complexes, the concentration of serum IgA and the distribution of HLA antigens in IgA nephropathy. *Nephron.* 1981;29:170-175.

872. Sancho J, Egido J, Rivera F, et al. Immune complexes in IgA nephropathy: presence of antibodies against diet antigens and delayed clearance of specific polymeric IgA immune complexes. *Clin Exp Immunol.* 1983;54:194-202.

873. Tomino Y, Miura M, Suga T, et al. Detection of IgA1-dominant immune complexes in peripheral blood polymorphonuclear leukocytes by double immunofluorescence in patients with IgA nephropathy. *Nephron.* 1984;37:137-139.

874. Tomino Y, Sakai H, Endoh M, et al. Detection of immune complexes in polymorphonuclear leukocytes by double immunofluorescence in patients with IgA nephropathy. *Clin Immunol Immunopathol.* 1982;24:63-71.

875. Woodroffe AJ, Gormly AA, McKenzie PE, et al. Immunologic studies in IgA nephropathy. *Kidney Int.* 1980;18:366-374.

876. Doi T, Kanatsu K, Sekita K, et al. Circulating immune complexes of IgG, IgA, and IgM classes in various glomerular diseases. *Nephron.* 1982;32:335-341.

877. Nagy J, Fust G, Ambrus M, et al. Circulating immune complexes in patients with IgA glomerulonephritis. *Acta Med Acad Sci Hung.* 1982;39:211-218.

878. Ooi YM, Ooi BS, Pollak VE. Relationship of levels of circulating immune complexes to histologic patterns of nephritis: a comparative study of membranous glomerulonephropathy and diffuse proliferative glomerulonephritis. *J Lab Clin Med.* 1977;90:891-898.

879. Valentijn RM, Kauffmann RH, de la Riviere GB, et al. Presence of circulating macromolecular IgA in patients with hematuria due to primary IgA nephropathy. *Am J Med.* 1983;74:375-381.

880. Kauffmann RH, Herrmann WA, Meyer CJ, et al. Circulating IgA-immune complexes in Henoch-Schönlein purpura. A longitudinal study of their relationship to disease activity and vascular deposition of IgA. *Am J Med.* 1980;69:859-866.

881. Levinsky RJ, Barratt TM. IgA immune complexes in Henoch-Schönlein purpura. *Lancet.* 1979;2:1100-1103.

882. Cederholm B, Wieslander J, Bygren P, et al. Patients with IgA nephropathy have circulating anti-basement membrane antibodies reacting with structures common to collagen I, II, and IV. *Proc Natl Acad Sci U S A.* 1986;83:6151-6155.

883. Tomino Y, Sakai H, Endoh M, et al. Cross-reactivity of eluted antibodies from renal tissues of patients with Henoch-Schönlein purpura nephritis and IgA nephropathy. *Am J Nephrol.* 1983;3:315-318.

884. Tomino Y, Sakai H, Miura M, et al. Specific binding of circulating IgA antibodies in patients with IgA nephropathy. *Am J Kidney Dis.* 1985;6:149-153.

885. Czerkinsky C, Koopman WJ, Jackson S, et al. Circulating immune complexes and immunoglobulin A rheumatoid factor in patients with mesangial immunoglobulin A nephropathies. *J Clin Invest.* 1986;77: 1931-1938.

886. Sinico RA, Fornasieri A, Oreni N, et al. Polymeric IgA rheumatoid factor in idiopathic IgA mesangial nephropathy (Berger's disease). *J Immunol.* 1986;137:536-541.

887. Nagy J, Uj M, Szucs G, et al. Herpes virus antigens and antibodies in kidney biopsies and sera of IgA glomerulonephritic patients. *Clin Nephrol.* 1984;21:259-262.

888. Tomino Y, Yagame M, Omata F, et al. A case of IgA nephropathy associated with adeno- and herpes simplex viruses. *Nephron.* 1987;47: 258-261.

889. Julian BA, Wyatt RJ, McMorrow RG, et al. Serum complement proteins in IgA nephropathy. *Clin Nephrol.* 1983;20:251-258.

890. Miyazaki R, Kuroda M, Akiyama T, et al. Glomerular deposition and serum levels of complement control proteins in patients with IgA nephropathy. *Clin Nephrol.* 1984;21:335-340.

891. Geiger H, Good RA, Day NK. A study of complement components C3, C5, C6, C7, C8 and C9 in chronic membranoproliferative glomerulonephritis, systemic lupus erythematosus, poststreptococcal nephritis, idiopathic nephrotic syndrome and anaphylactoid purpura. *Z Kinderheilkd.* 1975;119:269-278.

892. Wyatt RJ, Kanayama Y, Julian BA, et al. Complement activation in IgA nephropathy. *Kidney Int.* 1987;31:1019-1023.

893. Komatsu H, Fujimoto S, Hara S, et al. Relationship between serum IgA/C3 ratio and progression of IgA nephropathy. *Intern Med.* 2004;43: 1023-1028.

894. Birch DF, Fairley KF, Whitworth JA, et al. Urinary erythrocyte morphology in the diagnosis of glomerular hematuria. *Clin Nephrol.* 1983;20:78-84.

895. Hene RJ, Velthuis P, van de WA, et al. The relevance of IgA deposits in vessel walls of clinically normal skin. A prospective study. *Arch Intern Med.* 1986;146:745-749.

896. Hasbargen JA, Copley JB. Utility of skin biopsy in the diagnosis of IgA nephropathy. *Am J Kidney Dis.* 1985;6:100-102.

897. Ballardie FW, Cowley RD. Prognostic indices and therapy in IgA nephropathy: toward a solution. *Kidney Int.* 2008;73:249-251.

898. Strippoli GF, Maione A, Schena FP, et al. IgA nephropathy: a disease in search of a large-scale clinical trial to reliably inform practice. *Am J Kidney Dis.* 2009;53:5-8.

899. Floege J, Eitner F. Immune modulating therapy for IgA nephropathy: rationale and evidence. *Semin Nephrol.* 2008;28:38-47.

900. Woo KT, Lau YK. Proteinuria: clinical significance and basis for therapy. *Singapore Med J.* 2001;42:385-389.

901. Eitner F, Ackermann D, Hilgers RD, et al. Supportive versus immunosuppressive therapy of progressive IgA nephropathy (STOP) IgAN trial: rationale and study protocol. *J Nephrol.* 2008;21:284-289.

902. Cattran DC, Greenwood C, Ritchie S. Long-term benefits of angiotensin-converting enzyme inhibitor therapy in patients with severe immunoglobulin A nephropathy: a comparison to patients receiving treatment with other antihypertensive agents and to patients receiving no therapy. *Am J Kidney Dis.* 1994;23:247-254.

903. Rekola S, Bergstrand A, Bucht H. Deterioration rate in hypertensive IgA nephropathy: comparison of a converting enzyme inhibitor and beta-blocking agents. *Nephron.* 1991;59:57-60.

904. Nakao N, Yoshimura A, Morita H, et al. Combination treatment of angiotensin-II receptor blocker and angiotensin-converting-enzyme inhibitor in non-diabetic renal disease (COOPERATE): a randomised controlled trial. *Lancet.* 2003;361:117-124.

905. Ruggenenti P, Perna A, Gherardi G, et al. Chronic proteinuric nephropathies: outcomes and response to treatment in a prospective cohort of 352 patients with different patterns of renal injury. *Am J Kidney Dis.* 2000;35:1155-1165.

906. Kanno Y, Okada H, Yamaji Y, et al. Angiotensin-converting-enzyme inhibitors slow renal decline in IgA nephropathy, independent of tubulointerstitial fibrosis at presentation. *QJM.* 2005;98:199-203.

907. Maschio G, Cagnoli L, Claroni F, et al. ACE inhibition reduces proteinuria in normotensive patients with IgA nephropathy: a multicentre, randomized, placebo-controlled study. *Nephrol Dial Transplant.* 1994;9:265-269.

908. Woo KT, Lau YK, Wong KS, et al. ACEI/ATRA therapy decreases proteinuria by improving glomerular permselectivity in IgA nephritis. *Kidney Int.* 2000;58:2485-2491.

909. Praga M, Gutierrez E, Gonzalez E, et al. Treatment of IgA nephropathy with ACE inhibitors: a randomized and controlled trial. *J Am Soc Nephrol.* 2003;14:1578-1583.

910. Coppo R, Peruzzi L, Amore A, et al. IgACE: a placebo-controlled, randomized trial of angiotensin-converting enzyme inhibitors in children and young people with IgA nephropathy and moderate proteinuria. *J Am Soc Nephrol.* 2007;18:1880-1888.

911. Cheng J, Zhang W, Zhang XH, et al. ACEI/ARB therapy for IgA nephropathy: a meta analysis of randomised controlled trials. *Int J Clin Pract.* 2009;63:880-888.

912. Yoshida H, Mitarai T, Kawamura T, et al. Role of the deletion of polymorphism of the angiotensin converting enzyme gene in the progression and therapeutic responsiveness of IgA nephropathy. *J Clin Invest.* 1995;96:2162-2169.

913. Bazzi C, Rizza V, Paparella M, et al. G: Fractional urinary excretion of IgG is the most powerful predictor of renoprotection by ACE inhibitors in IgA nephropathy. *J Nephrol.* 2009;22:387-396.

914. Woo KT, Chan CM, Tan HK, et al. Beneficial effects of high-dose losartan in IgA nephritis. *Clin Nephrol.* 2009;71:617-624.

915. Galla JH. IgA nephropathy. *Kidney Int.* 1995;47:377-387.

916. Kobayashi Y, Hiki Y, Fujii K, et al. Moderately proteinuric IgA nephropathy: prognostic prediction of individual clinical courses and steroid therapy in progressive cases. *Nephron.* 1989;53:250-256.

917. Pozzi C, Bolasco PG, Fogazzi GB, et al. Corticosteroids in IgA nephropathy: a randomised controlled trial. *Lancet.* 1999;353:883-887.

918. Pozzi C, Andrulli S, Del VL, et al. Corticosteroid effectiveness in IgA nephropathy: long-term results of a randomized, controlled trial. *J Am Soc Nephrol.* 2004;15:157-163.

919. Hogg RJ, Lee J, Nardelli N, et al. Clinical trial to evaluate omega-3 fatty acids and alternate day prednisone in patients with IgA nephropathy: report from the Southwest Pediatric Nephrology Study Group. *Clin J Am Soc Nephrol.* 2006;1:467-474.

920. Cheng J, Zhang X, Zhang W, et al. Efficacy and safety of glucocorticoids therapy for IgA nephropathy: a meta-analysis of randomized controlled trials. *Am J Nephrol.* 2009;30:315-322.

921. Lai KN, Lai FM, Ho CP, et al. Corticosteroid therapy in IgA nephropathy with nephrotic syndrome: a long-term controlled trial. *Clin Nephrol.* 1986;26:174-180.

922. Kim SM, Moon KC, Oh KH, et al. Clinicopathologic characteristics of IgA nephropathy with steroid-responsive nephrotic syndrome. *J Korean Med Sci.* 2009;24(suppl):S44-S49.

923. Koike M, Takei T, Uchida K, et al. Clinical assessment of low-dose steroid therapy for patients with IgA nephropathy: a prospective study in a single center. *Clin Exp Nephrol.* 2008;12(4):250-255.

924. Shimizu A, Takei T, Uchida K, et al. Predictors of poor outcomes in steroid therapy for immunoglobulin A nephropathy. *Nephrology (Carlton).* 2009;14:521-526.

925. Harada K, Akai Y, Yamaguchi Y, et al. Prediction of corticosteroid responsiveness based on fibroblast-specific protein 1 (FSP1) in patients with IgA nephropathy. *Nephrol Dial Transplant.* 2008;23:3152-3159.

926. Nachman PH, Glassock RJ. Glomerular, vascular and tubulointerstitial diseases. *NephSAP.* 2010;9:140-149.

927. Lv J, Zhang H, Chen Y, et al. Combination therapy of prednisone and ACE inhibitor versus ACE-inhibitor therapy alone in patients with IgA nephropathy: a randomized controlled trial. *Am J Kidney Dis.* 2009;53: 26-32.

928. Manno C, Torres DD, Rossini M, et al. Randomized controlled clinical trial of corticosteroids plus ACE-inhibitors with long-term follow-up in proteinuric IgA nephropathy. *Nephrol Dial Transplant.* 2009;24:3694-3701.

929. Jiang XY, Mo Y, Sun LZ, et al. Efficacy of methylprednisolone, cyclophosphamide in pediatric IgA nephropathy assessed by renal biopsy. *Clin Nephrol.* 2009;71:625-631.

930. Mitsuiki K, Harada A, Okura T, et al. Histologically advanced IgA nephropathy treated successfully with prednisolone and cyclophosphamide. *Clin Exp Nephrol.* 2007;11:297-303.

931. Oshima S, Kawamura O. Long-term follow-up of patients with IgA nephropathy treated with prednisolone and cyclophosphamide therapy. *Clin Exp Nephrol.* 2008;12(4):264-269.

932. Ballardie FW, Roberts IS. Controlled prospective trial of prednisolone and cytotoxics in progressive IgA nephropathy. *J Am Soc Nephrol.* 2002;13: 142-148.

933. Goumenos D, Ahuja M, Shortland JR, et al. Can immunosuppressive drugs slow the progression of IgA nephropathy? *Nephrol Dial Transplant.* 1995;10:1173-1181.

934. Ahuja M, Goumenos D, Shortland JR, et al. Does immunosuppression with prednisolone and azathioprine alter the progression of idiopathic membranous nephropathy? *Am J Kidney Dis.* 1999;34:521-529.

935. Welch TR, McAdams AJ, Berry A. Rapidly progressive IgA nephropathy. *Am J Dis Child.* 1988;142:789-793.

936. Lai KN, Lai FM, Leung AC, et al. Plasma exchange in patients with rapidly progressive idiopathic IgA nephropathy: a report of two cases and review of literature. *Am J Kidney Dis.* 1987;10:66-70.

937. Roccatello D, Ferro M, Coppo R, et al. Report on intensive treatment of extracapillary glomerulonephritis with focus on crescentic IgA nephropathy. *Nephrol Dial Transplant.* 1995;10:2054-2059.

938. Woo KT, Lee GS, Lau YK, et al. Effects of triple therapy in IgA nephritis: a follow-up study 5 years later. *Clin Nephrol.* 1991;36:60-66.

939. Tang S, Leung JC, Chan LY, et al. Mycophenolate mofetil alleviates persistent proteinuria in IgA nephropathy. *Kidney Int.* 2005;68:802-812.

940. Chen X, Chen P, Cai G, et al. [A randomized control trial of mycophenolate mofetil treatment in severe IgA nephropathy]. *Zhonghua Yi Xue Za Zhi.* 2002;82:796-801.

941. Frisch G, Lin J, Rosenstock J, et al. Mycophenolate mofetil (MMF) vs placebo in patients with moderately advanced IgA nephropathy: a double-blind randomized controlled trial. *Nephrol Dial Transplant.* 2005;20:2139-2145.

942. Maes BD, Oyen R, Claes K, et al. Mycophenolate mofetil in IgA nephropathy: results of a 3-year prospective placebo-controlled randomized study. *Kidney Int.* 2004;65:1842-1849.

943. Tang SC, Tang AW, Wong SS, et al. Long-term study of mycophenolate mofetil treatment in IgA nephropathy. *Kidney Int.* 2010;77:543-549.

944. Rasche FM, Schwarz A, Keller F. Tonsillectomy does not prevent a progressive course in IgA nephropathy. *Clin Nephrol.* 1999;51:147-152.

945. Hotta O, Miyazaki M, Furuta T, et al. Tonsillectomy and steroid pulse therapy significantly impact on clinical remission in patients with IgA nephropathy. *Am J Kidney Dis.* 2001;38:736-743.

946. Xie Y, Nishi S, Ueno M, et al. The efficacy of tonsillectomy on long-term renal survival in patients with IgA nephropathy. *Kidney Int.* 2003;63:1861-1867.

947. Sato M, Hotta O, Tomioka S, et al. Cohort study of advanced IgA nephropathy: efficacy and limitations of corticosteroids with tonsillectomy. *Nephron Clin Pract.* 2003;93:c137-c145.

947a. Komatsu H, Fujimoto S, Hara S, et al. Effect of tonsillectomy plus steroid pulse therapy on clinical remission of IgA nephropathy: a controlled study. *Clin J Am Soc Nephrol.* 2008;3(5):1301-1307.

948. Donadio Jr JV, Bergstralh EJ, Offord KP, et al. A controlled trial of fish oil in IgA nephropathy. Mayo Nephrology Collaborative Group. *N Engl J Med.* 1994;331:1194-1199.

949. Pettersson EE, Rekola S, Berglund L, et al. Treatment of IgA nephropathy with omega-3-polyunsaturated fatty acids: a prospective, double-blind, randomized study. *Clin Nephrol.* 1994;41:183-190.

950. Bennett WM, Walker RG, Kincaid-Smith P. Treatment of IgA nephropathy with eicosapentaenoic acid (EPA): a two-year prospective trial. *Clin Nephrol.* 1989;31:128-131.

951. Miller III ER, Juraschek SP, Appel LJ, et al. The effect of n-3 long-chain polyunsaturated fatty acid supplementation on urine protein excretion and kidney function: meta-analysis of clinical trials. *Am J Clin Nutr.* 2009;89:1937-1945.

952. Ferraro PM, Ferraccioli GF, Gambaro G, et al. Combined treatment with renin-angiotensin system blockers and polyunsaturated fatty acids in proteinuric IgA nephropathy: a randomized controlled trial. *Nephrol Dial Transplant.* 2009;24:156-160.

953. Ivanyi B. A primer on recurrent and de novo glomerulonephritis in renal allografts. *Nat Clin Pract Nephrol.* 2008;4:446-457.

954. Ng YS, Vathsala A, Chew ST, et al. Long term outcome of renal allografts in patients with immunoglobulin A nephropathy. *Med J Malaysia.* 2007;62:109-113.

955. Kiattisunthorn K, Premasathian N, Wongwiwatana A, et al. Evaluating the clinical course and prognostic factors of posttransplantation immunoglobulin A nephropathy. *Transplant Proc.* 2008;40:2349-2354.

956. Han SS, Huh W, Park SK, et al. Impact of recurrent disease and chronic allograft nephropathy on the long-term allograft outcome in patients with IgA nephropathy. *Transpl Int.* 2010;23(2):169-175. Epub September 16, 2009.

957. Coppo R, Amore A, Chiesa M, et al. Serological and genetic factors in early recurrence of IgA nephropathy after renal transplantation. *Clin Transplant.* 2007;21:728-737.

958. Berthoux F, El Deeb S, Mariat C, et al. Antithymocyte globulin (ATG) induction therapy and disease recurrence in renal transplant recipients with primary IgA nephropathy. *Transplantation.* 2008;85:1505-1507.

959. Nolin L, Courteau M. Management of IgA nephropathy: evidence-based recommendations. *Kidney Int Suppl.* 1999;70:S56-S62.

960. Kincaid-Smith P, Fairley K, Packham D. Randomized controlled crossover study of the effect on proteinuria and blood pressure of adding an angiotensin II receptor antagonist to an angiotensin converting enzyme inhibitor in normotensive patients with chronic renal disease and proteinuria. *Nephrol Dial Transplant.* 2002;17:597-601.

961. Laverman GD, Navis G, Henning RH, et al. Dual renin-angiotensin system blockade at optimal doses for proteinuria. *Kidney Int.* 2002;62:1020-1025.

962. Alpers CE, Rennke HG, Hopper Jr J, et al. Fibrillary glomerulonephritis: an entity with unusual immunofluorescence features. *Kidney Int.* 1987;31:781-789.

963. Korbet SM, Schwartz MM, Lewis EJ. Immunotactoid glomerulopathy. *Am J Kidney Dis.* 1991;17:247-257.

964. Alpers CE. Immunotactoid (microtubular) glomerulopathy: an entity distinct from fibrillary glomerulonephritis? *Am J Kidney Dis.* 1992;19:185-191.

965. Fogo A, Qureshi N, Horn RG. Morphologic and clinical features of fibrillary glomerulonephritis versus immunotactoid glomerulopathy. *Am J Kidney Dis.* 1993;22:367-377.

966. Korbet SM, Schwartz MM, Lewis EJ. The fibrillary glomerulopathies. *Am J Kidney Dis.* 1994;23:751-765.

967. Iskandar SS, Falk RJ, Jennette JC. Clinical and pathologic features of fibrillary glomerulonephritis. *Kidney Int.* 1992;42:1401-1407.

968. Jennette JC, Falk RJ. Fibrillary glomerulonephritis. In: Tisher CC, Brenner BM, eds. *Renal pathology with clinical and functional correlations.* Philadelphia: JB Lippincott; 1994:553-563.

969. D'Agati V, Jennette JC, Silva FG. *Non-neoplastic kidney diseases.* Washington, D.C.: American Registry of Pathology; 2005:199-238.

970. Schwartz MM. Glomerular diseases with organized deposits. In: Jennette JC, Olson JL, Schwartz MM, et al, eds. *Heptinstall's pathology of the kidney.* 5th ed. Philadelphia: Lippincott-Raven; 1998:369-388.

971. Moulin B, Ronco PM, Mougenot B, et al. Glomerulonephritis in chronic lymphocytic leukemia and related B-cell lymphomas. *Kidney Int.* 1992;42:127-135.

972. Bridoux F, Hugue V, Coldefy O, et al. Fibrillary glomerulonephritis and immunotactoid (microtubular) glomerulopathy are associated with distinct immunologic features. *Kidney Int.* 2002;62:1764-1775.

973. Sundaram S, Mainali R, Norfolk ER, et al. Fibrillary glomerulopathy secondary to light chain deposition disease in a patient with monoclonal gammopathy. *Ann Clin Lab Sci.* 2007;37:370-374.

974. Joh K. Pathology of glomerular deposition diseases and fibrillary glomerulopathies associated with paraproteinemia and haematopoietic disorder. *Nephrology (Carlton).* 2007;12(suppl 3):S21-S24.

975. Ray S, Rouse K, Appis A, et al. Fibrillary glomerulonephritis with hepatitis C viral infection and hypocomplementemia. *Ren Fail.* 2008;30:759-762.

976. Shim YH, Lee SJ, Sung SH. A case of fibrillary glomerulonephritis with unusual IgM deposits and hypocomplementemia. *Pediatr Nephrol.* 2008;23:1163-1166.

977. Schwartz MM, Korbet SM, Lewis EJ. Immunotactoid glomerulopathy. *J Am Soc Nephrol.* 2002;13:1390-1397.

978. Rosenstock JL, Markowitz GS, Valeri AM, et al. Fibrillary and immunotactoid glomerulonephritis: distinct entities with different clinical and pathologic features. *Kidney Int.* 2003;63:1450-1461.

979. Masson RG, Rennke HG, Gottlieb MN. Pulmonary hemorrhage in a patient with fibrillary glomerulonephritis. *N Engl J Med.* 1992;326:36-39.

980. Wallner M, Prischl FC, Hobling W, et al. Immunotactoid glomerulopathy with extrarenal deposits in the bone, and chronic cholestatic liver disease. *Nephrol Dial Transplant.* 1996;11:1619-1624.

981. D'Agati V, Sacchi G, Truong L. Fibrillary glomerulopathy: defining the disease spectrum. *J Am Soc Nephrol.* 1991;2:591:[abstract].

982. Collins M, Navaneethan SD, Chung M, et al. Rituximab treatment of fibrillary glomerulonephritis. *Am J Kidney Dis.* 2008;52:1158-1162.

983. Pronovost PH, Brady HR, Gunning ME, et al. Clinical features, predictors of disease progression and results of renal transplantation in fibrillary/immunotactoid glomerulopathy. *Nephrol Dial Transplant.* 1996;11:837-842.

984. Czarnecki PG, Lager DJ, Leung N, et al. Long-term outcome of kidney transplantation in patients with fibrillary glomerulonephritis or monoclonal gammopathy with fibrillary deposits. *Kidney Int.* 2009;75:420-427.

985. Couser WG. Rapidly progressive glomerulonephritis: classification, pathogenetic mechanisms, and therapy. *Am J Kidney Dis.* 1988;11:449-464.

986. Jennette JC. Rapidly progressive crescentic glomerulonephritis. *Kidney Int.* 2003;63:1164-1177.

987. Jennette JC. Crescentic glomerulonephritis. In: Jennette JC, Olson JL, Schwartz MM, et al, eds. *Heptinstall's pathology of the kidney.* 5th ed. Philadelphia: Lippincott-Raven; 1998:625-656.

988. Bonsib SM. Glomerular basement membrane necrosis and crescent organization. *Kidney Int.* 1988;33:966-974.

989. Jennette JC, Hipp CG. The epithelial antigen phenotype of glomerular crescent cells. *Am J Clin Pathol.* 1986;86:274-280.

990. Hancock WW, Atkins RC. Cellular composition of crescents in human rapidly progressive glomerulonephritis identified using monoclonal antibodies. *Am J Nephrol.* 1984;4:177-181.

991. Guettier C, Nochy D, Jacquot C, et al. Immunohistochemical demonstration of parietal epithelial cells and macrophages in human proliferative extra-capillary lesions. *Virchows Arch A Pathol Anat Histopathol.* 1986;409:739-748.

992. Andrassy K, Kuster S, Waldherr R, et al. Rapidly progressive glomerulonephritis: analysis of prevalence and clinical course. *Nephron.* 1991;59:206-212.

993. Stilmant MM, Bolton WK, Sturgill BC, et al. Crescentic glomerulonephritis without immune deposits: clinicopathologic features. *Kidney Int.* 1979;15:184-195.

994. Prasad AN, Kapoor KK, Katarya S, et al. Periarteritis nodosa in a child. *Indian Pediatr.* 1983;20:57-61.

995. Moutzouris DA, Herlitz L, Appel GB, et al. Renal biopsy in the very elderly. *Clin J Am Soc Nephrol.* 2009;4:1073-1082.

996. Falk RJ, Terrell RS, Charles LA, et al. Anti-neutrophil cytoplasmic autoantibodies induce neutrophils to degranulate and produce oxygen radicals in vitro. *Proc Natl Acad Sci U S A.* 1990;87:4115-4119.

997. Ferrario F, Tadros MT, Napodano P, et al. Critical re-evaluation of 41 cases of "idiopathic" crescentic glomerulonephritis. *Clin Nephrol.* 1994;41:1-9.

998. Chugh KS, Gupta VK, Singhal PC, et al. Case report: poststreptococcal crescentic glomerulonephritis and pulmonary hemorrhage simulating Goodpasture's syndrome. *Ann Allergy.* 1981;47:104-106.

999. Moorthy AV, Zimmerman SW, Burkholder PM, et al. Association of crescentic glomerulonephritis with membranous glomerulonephropathy: a report of three cases. *Clin Nephrol.* 1976;6:319-325.

1000. Hazenbos WL, Gessner JE, Hofhuis FM, et al. Impaired IgG-dependent anaphylaxis and Arthus reaction in Fc gamma RIII (CD16) deficient mice. *Immunity.* 1996;5:181-188.

1001. Sylvestre DL, Ravetch JV. Fc receptors initiate the Arthus reaction: redefining the inflammatory cascade. *Science.* 1994;265:1095-1098.

1002. Clynes R, Dumitru C, Ravetch JV. Uncoupling of immune complex formation and kidney damage in autoimmune glomerulonephritis. *Science.* 1998;279:1052-1054.

1003. Park SY, Ueda S, Ohno H, et al. Resistance of Fc receptor-deficient mice to fatal glomerulonephritis. *J Clin Invest.* 1998;102:1229-1238.

1004. Lockwood CM, Rees AJ, Pearson TA, et al. Immunosuppression and plasma-exchange in the treatment of Goodpasture's syndrome. *Lancet.* 1976;1:711-715.

1005. Hellmark T, Johansson C, Wieslander J. Characterization of anti-GBM antibodies involved in Goodpasture's syndrome. *Kidney Int.* 1994;46:823-829.

1006. O'Neill Jr WM, Etheridge WB, Bloomer HA. High-dose corticosteroids: their use in treating idiopathic rapidly progressive glomerulonephritis. *Arch Intern Med.* 1979;139:514-518.

1007. Salant DJ. Immunopathogenesis of crescentic glomerulonephritis and lung purpura. *Kidney Int.* 1987;32:408-425.

1008. Glassock RJ. A clinical and immunopathologic dissection of rapidly progressive glomerulonephritis. *Nephron.* 1978;22:253-264.

1009. Angangco R, Thiru S, Esnault VL, et al. Does truly "idiopathic" crescentic glomerulonephritis exist? *Nephrol Dial Transplant.* 1994;9:630-636.

1010. Couser WG. Idiopathic rapidly progressive glomerulonephritis. *Am J Nephrol.* 1982;2:57-69.

1011. Beirne GJ, Wagnild JP, Zimmerman SW, et al. Idiopathic crescentic glomerulonephritis. *Medicine (Baltimore).* 1977;56:349-381.

1012. Neild GH, Cameron JS, Ogg CS, et al. Rapidly progressive glomerulonephritis with extensive glomerular crescent formation. *Q J Med.* 1983;52:395-416.

1013. Lerner RA, Glassock RJ, Dixon FJ. The role of anti-glomerular basement membrane antibody in the pathogenesis of human glomerulonephritis. *J Exp Med.* 1967;126:989-1004.

1014. Briggs WA, Johnson JP, Teichman S, et al. Antiglomerular basement membrane antibody-mediated glomerulonephritis and Goodpasture's syndrome. *Medicine (Baltimore).* 1979;58:348-361.

1015. Border WA, Baehler RW, Bhathena D, et al. IgA antibasement membrane nephritis with pulmonary hemorrhage. *Ann Intern Med.* 1979;91:21-25.

1016. Savage CO, Pusey CD, Bowman C, et al. Antiglomerular basement membrane antibody mediated disease in the British Isles 1980-4. *Br Med J (Clin Res Ed).* 1986;292:301-304.

1017. Senekjian HO, Knight TF, Weinman EJ. The spectrum of renal diseases associated with anti-basement membrane antibodies. *Arch Intern Med.* 1980;140:79-81.

1018. Conlon Jr PJ, Walshe JJ, Daly C, et al. Antiglomerular basement membrane disease: the long-term pulmonary outcome. *Am J Kidney Dis.* 1994;23:794-796.

1019. Savige JA, Kincaid-Smith P. Antiglomerular basement membrane (GBM) antibody-mediated disease. *Am J Kidney Dis.* 1989;13:355-356.

1020. Kalluri R, Melendez E, Rumpf KW, et al. Specificity of circulating and tissue-bound autoantibodies in Goodpasture syndrome. *Proc Assoc Am Physicians.* 1996;108:134-139.

1021. Kelly PT, Haponik EF. Goodpasture syndrome: molecular and clinical advances. *Medicine (Baltimore).* 1994;73:171-185.

1022. Rees AJ, Peters DK, Compston DA, et al. Strong association between HLA-DRW2 and antibody-mediated Goodpasture's syndrome. *Lancet.* 1978;1:966-968.

1023. Fisher M, Pusey CD, Vaughan RW, et al. Susceptibility to anti-glomerular basement membrane disease is strongly associated with HLA-DRB1 genes. *Kidney Int.* 1997;51:222-229.

1024. Huey B, McCormick K, Capper J, et al. Associations of HLA-DR and HLA-DQ types with anti-GBM nephritis by sequence-specific oligonucleotide probe hybridization. *Kidney Int.* 1993;44:307-312.

1025. Dunckley H, Chapman JR, Burke J, et al. HLA-DR and -DQ genotyping in anti-GBM disease. *Dis Markers.* 1991;9:249-256.

1026. Burns AP, Fisher M, Li P, et al. Molecular analysis of HLA class II genes in Goodpasture's disease. *QJM.* 1995;88:93-100.

1027. Kitagawa W, Imai H, Komatsuda A, et al. The HLA-DRB1*1501 allele is prevalent among Japanese patients with anti-glomerular basement membrane antibody–mediated disease. *Nephrol Dial Transplant.* 2008;23:3126-3129.

1028. Kalluri R, Danoff TM, Okada H, et al. Susceptibility to anti-glomerular basement membrane disease and Goodpasture syndrome is linked to MHC class II genes and the emergence of T cell–mediated immunity in mice. *J Clin Invest.* 1997;100:2263-2275.

1029. Liu K, Li QZ, Delgado-Vega AM, et al. Kallikrein genes are associated with lupus and glomerular basement membrane–specific antibody–induced nephritis in mice and humans. *J Clin Invest.* 2009;119:911-923.

1030. Jennette JC, Thomas DB. Pauci-immune and antineutrophil cytoplasmic autoantibody glomerulonephritis and vasculitis. In: Jennette JC, Olson JL, Schwartz MM, et al, eds. *Heptinstall's pathology of the kidney.* 6th ed. Philadelphia: Lippincott Williams & Wilkins; 2006:643-674.

1031. Germuth Jr FG, Choi IJ, Taylor JJ, et al. Antibasement membrane disease. I. The glomerular lesions of Goodpasture's disease and experimental disease in sheep. *Johns Hopkins Med J.* 1972;131:367-384.

1032. McPhaul Jr JJ, Mullins JD. Glomerulonephritis mediated by antibody to glomerular basement membrane. Immunological, clinical, and histopathological characteristics. *J Clin Invest.* 1976;57:351-361.

1033. Walker RG, Scheinkestel C, Becker GJ, et al. Clinical and morphological aspects of the management of crescentic anti-glomerular basement membrane antibody (anti-GBM) nephritis/Goodpasture's syndrome. *Q J Med.* 1985;54:75-89.

1034. Fivush B, Melvin T, Solez K, et al. Idiopathic linear glomerular IgA deposition. *Arch Pathol Lab Med.* 1986;110:1189-1191.

1035. Jennette JC, Falk RJ, Milling DM. Pathogenesis of vasculitis. *Semin Neurol.* 1994;14:291-299.

1036. Short AK, Esnault VL, Lockwood CM. Anti-neutrophil cytoplasm antibodies and anti-glomerular basement membrane antibodies: two coexisting distinct autoreactivities detectable in patients with rapidly progressive glomerulonephritis. *Am J Kidney Dis.* 1995;26:439-445.

1037. Poskitt TR. Immunologic and electron microscopic studies in Goodpasture's syndrome. *Am J Med.* 1970;49:250-257.

1038. Wieslander J, Barr JF, Butkowski RJ, et al. Goodpasture antigen of the glomerular basement membrane: localization to noncollagenous regions of type IV collagen. *Proc Natl Acad Sci U S A.* 1984;81:3838-3842.

1039. Wieslander J, Langeveld J, Butkowski R, et al. Physical and immunochemical studies of the globular domain of type IV collagen. Cryptic properties of the Goodpasture antigen. *J Biol Chem.* 1985;260:8564-8570.

1040. Hellmark T, Segelmark M, Wieslander J. Anti-GBM antibodies in Goodpasture syndrome; anatomy of an epitope. *Nephrol Dial Transplant.* 1997;12:646-648.

1041. Kalluri R, Sun MJ, Hudson BG, et al. The Goodpasture autoantigen. Structural delineation of two immunologically privileged epitopes on α3(IV) chain of type IV collagen. *J Biol Chem.* 1996;271:9062-9068.

1042. Calvete JJ, Revert F, Blanco M, et al. Conformational diversity of the Goodpasture antigen, the noncollagenous-1 domain of the α3 chain of collagen IV. *Proteomics suppl.* 2006;1:S237-S244.

1043. Borza DB, Bondar O, Colon S, et al. Goodpasture autoantibodies unmask cryptic epitopes by selectively dissociating autoantigen complexes lacking structural reinforcement: novel mechanisms for immune privilege and autoimmune pathogenesis. *J Biol Chem.* 2005;280:27147-27154.

1044. Stevenson A, Yaqoob M, Mason H, et al. Biochemical markers of basement membrane disturbances and occupational exposure to hydrocarbons and mixed solvents. *QJM.* 1995;88:23-28.

1045. Donaghy M, Rees AJ. Cigarette smoking and lung haemorrhage in glomerulonephritis caused by autoantibodies to glomerular basement membrane. *Lancet.* 1983;2:1390-1393.

1046. Kalluri R, Cantley LG, Kerjaschki D, et al. Reactive oxygen species expose cryptic epitopes associated with autoimmune Goodpasture syndrome. *J Biol Chem.* 2000;275:20027-20032.

1047. Saxena R, Bygren P, Butkowski R, et al. Entactin: a possible auto-antigen in the pathogenesis of non-Goodpasture anti-GBM nephritis. *Kidney Int.* 1990;38:263-272.

1048. Kalluri R, Danoff T, Neilson EG. Murine anti-α3(IV) collagen disease: a model of human Goodpasture syndrome and anti-GBM nephritis. *J Am Soc Nephrol.* 1995;6:833.

1049. Netzer KO, Leinonen A, Boutaud A, et al. The Goodpasture autoantigen. Mapping the major conformational epitope(s) of α3(IV) collagen to residues 17-31 and 127-141 of the NC1 domain. *J Biol Chem.* 1999;274:11267-11274.

1050. Hellmark T, Segelmark M, Unger C, et al. Identification of a clinically relevant immunodominant region of collagen IV in Goodpasture disease. *Kidney Int.* 1999;55:936-944.

1051. Hellmark T, Niles JL, Collins AB, et al. Comparison of anti-GBM antibodies in sera with or without ANCA. *J Am Soc Nephrol.* 1997;8:376-385.

1052. Meyers KE, Kinniry PA, Kalluri R, et al. Human Goodpasture anti-α3(IV)NC1 autoantibodies share structural determinants. *Kidney Int.* 1998;53:402-407.

1053. Borza DB. Autoepitopes and alloepitopes of type IV collagen: role in the molecular pathogenesis of anti-GBM antibody glomerulonephritis. *Nephron Exp Nephrol.* 2007;106:e37-e43.

1054. Yang R, Hellmark T, Zhao J, et al. Levels of epitope-specific autoantibodies correlate with renal damage in anti-GBM disease. *Nephrol Dial Transplant.* 2009;24:1838-1844.

1055. Kalluri R, Meyers K, Mogyorosi A, et al. Goodpasture syndrome involving overlap with Wegener's granulomatosis and anti-glomerular basement membrane disease. *J Am Soc Nephrol.* 1997;8:1795-1800.

1056. Savage CO, Lockwood CM. Antineutrophil antibodies in vasculitis. *Adv Nephrol Necker Hosp.* 1990;19:225-236.

1057. Hellmark T, Burkhardt H, Wieslander J. Goodpasture disease. Characterization of a single conformational epitope as the target of pathogenic autoantibodies. *J Biol Chem.* 1999;274:25862-25868.

1058. Yang R, Cui Z, Hellmark T, et al. Natural anti-GBM antibodies from normal human sera recognize α3(IV)NC1 restrictively and recognize the same epitopes as anti-GBM antibodies from patients with anti-GBM disease. *Clin Immunol.* 2007;124:207-212.

1059. Heeringa P, Brouwer E, Klok PA, et al. Autoantibodies to myeloperoxidase aggravate mild anti-glomerular-basement-membrane–mediated glomerular injury in the rat. *Am J Pathol.* 1996;149:1695-1706.

1060. Kang JS, Kashtan CE, Turner AN, et al. The alloantigenic sites of α3α4α5(IV) collagen: pathogenic X-linked Alport alloantibodies target two accessible conformational epitopes in the α5NC1 domain. *J Biol Chem.* 2007;282:10670-10677.

1061. Wilson CB. Immunologic aspects of renal diseases. *JAMA.* 1992;268:2904-2909.

1062. Jayne D, Rasmussen N, Andrassy K, et al. European Vasculitis Study Group. A randomized trial of maintenance therapy for vasculitis associated with antineutrophil cytoplasmic autoantibodies. *N Engl J Med.* 2003;349(1):36-44.

1063. Sado Y, Naito I. Experimental autoimmune glomerulonephritis in rats by soluble isologous or homologous antigens from glomerular and tubular basement membranes. *Br J Exp Pathol.* 1987;68:695-704.

1064. Sado Y, Naito I, Okigaki T. Transfer of anti-glomerular basement membrane antibody-induced glomerulonephritis in inbred rats with isologous antibodies from the urine of nephritic rats. *J Pathol.* 1989;158:325-332.

1065. Bolton WK, May WJ, Sturgill BC. Proliferative autoimmune glomerulonephritis in rats: a model for autoimmune glomerulonephritis in humans. *Kidney Int.* 1993;44:294-306.

1066. Garcia GE, Truong LD, Li P, et al. Inhibition of CXCL16 attenuates inflammatory and progressive phases of anti-glomerular basement membrane antibody-associated glomerulonephritis. *Am J Pathol.* 2007;170:1485-1496.

1067. Fujinaka H, Yamamoto T, Feng L, et al. Anti-perforin antibody treatment ameliorates experimental crescentic glomerulonephritis in WKY rats. *Kidney Int.* 2007;72(7):P823-830.

1068. Moussa L, Apostolopoulos J, Davenport P, et al. Protease-activated receptor-2 augments experimental crescentic glomerulonephritis. *Am J Pathol.* 2007;171:800-808.

1069. Derry CJ, Ross CN, Lombardi G, et al. Analysis of T cell responses to the autoantigen in Goodpasture's disease. *Clin Exp Immunol.* 1995;100:262-268.

1070. Steblay RW, Rudofsky U. Autoimmune glomerulonephritis induced in sheep by injections of human lung and Freund's adjuvant. *Science.* 1968;160:204-206.

1071. Wu J, Hicks J, Borillo J, et al. CD4+ T cells specific to a glomerular basement membrane antigen mediate glomerulonephritis. *J Clin Invest.* 2002;109:517-524.

1072. Wu J, Borillo J, Glass WF, et al. T-cell epitope of α3 chain of type IV collagen induces severe glomerulonephritis. *Kidney Int.* 2003;64:1292-1301.

1073. Arends J, Wu J, Borillo J, et al. T cell epitope mimicry in antiglomerular basement membrane disease. *J Immunol.* 2006;176:1252-1258.

1074. Wolf D, Hochegger K, Wolf AM, et al. CD4+CD25+ regulatory T cells inhibit experimental anti-glomerular basement membrane glomerulonephritis in mice. *J Am Soc Nephrol.* 2005;16:1360-1370.

1075. Ooi JD, Holdsworth SR, Kitching AR. Advances in the pathogenesis of Goodpasture's disease: from epitopes to autoantibodies to effector T cells. *J Autoimmun.* 2008;31:295-300.

1076. Salama AD, Chaudhry AN, Holthaus KA, et al. Regulation by CD25+ lymphocytes of autoantigen-specific T-cell responses in Goodpasture's (anti-GBM) disease. *Kidney Int.* 2003;64:1685-1694.

1077. Adler S, Baker PJ, Pritzl P, et al. Detection of terminal complement components in experimental immune glomerular injury. *Kidney Int.* 1984;26:830-837.

1078. Groggel GC, Salant DJ, Darby C, et al. Role of terminal complement pathway in the heterologous phase of antiglomerular basement membrane nephritis. *Kidney Int.* 1985;27:643-651.

1079. Tipping PG, Boyce NW, Holdsworth SR. Relative contributions of chemo-attractant and terminal components of complement to anti-glomerular basement membrane (GBM) glomerulonephritis. *Clin Exp Immunol.* 1989;78:444-448.

1080. Schrijver G, Assmann KJ, Bogman MJ, et al. Antiglomerular basement membrane nephritis in the mouse. Study on the role of complement in the heterologous phase. *Lab Invest.* 1988;59:484-491.

1081. Sheerin NS, Springall T, Carroll MC, et al. Protection against anti-glomerular basement membrane (GBM)–mediated nephritis in C3- and C4-deficient mice. *Clin Exp Immunol.* 1997;110:403-409.

1082. Otten MA, Groeneveld TW, Flierman R, et al. Both complement and IgG Fc receptors are required for development of attenuated antiglomerular basement membrane nephritis in mice. *J Immunol.* 2009;183:3980-3988.

1083. Nakamura A, Yuasa T, Ujike A, et al. Fcγ receptor IIB–deficient mice develop Goodpasture's syndrome upon immunization with type IV collagen: a novel murine model for autoimmune glomerular basement membrane disease. *J Exp Med.* 2000;191:899-906.

1084. Lockwood CM, Boulton-Jones JM, Lowenthal RM, et al. Recovery from Goodpasture's syndrome after immunosuppressive treatment and plasmapheresis. *Br Med J.* 1975;2:252-254.

1085. Pusey CD. Plasma exchange in immunological disease. *Prog Clin Biol Res.* 1990;337:419-424.

1086. Peters DK, Rees AJ, Lockwood CM, et al. Treatment and prognosis in antibasement membrane antibody–mediated nephritis. *Transplant Proc.* 1982;14:513-521.

1087. Pusey CD, Lockwood CM, Peters DK. Plasma exchange and immunosuppressive drugs in the treatment of glomerulonephritis due to antibodies to the glomerular basement membrane. *Int J Artif Organs.* 1983;6(suppl 1):15-18.

1088. Madore F, Lazarus JM, Brady HR. Therapeutic plasma exchange in renal diseases. *J Am Soc Nephrol.* 1996;7:367-386.

1089. Wilson CB, Dixon FJ. Anti-glomerular basement membrane antibody–induced glomerulonephritis. *Kidney Int.* 1973;3:74-89.

1090. Ioachimescu OC, Stoller JK. Diffuse alveolar hemorrhage: diagnosing it and finding the cause. *Cleve Clin J Med.* 2008;75:258, 260, 264-258, 260, 265.

1091. Zimmerman SW, Groehler K, Beirne GJ. Hydrocarbon exposure and chronic glomerulonephritis. *Lancet.* 1975;2:199-201.

1092. Churchill DN, Fine A, Gault MH. Association between hydrocarbon exposure and glomerulonephritis. An appraisal of the evidence. *Nephron.* 1983;33:169-172.

1093. Ravnskov U, Lundstrom S, Norden A. Hydrocarbon exposure and glomerulonephritis: evidence from patients' occupations. *Lancet.* 1983;2:1214-1216.

1094. Daniell WE, Couser WG, Rosenstock L. Occupational solvent exposure and glomerulonephritis. A case report and review of the literature. *JAMA.* 1988;259:2280-2283.

1095. Rees AJ, Lockwood CM, Peters DK. Enhanced allergic tissue injury in Goodpasture's syndrome by intercurrent bacterial infection. *Br Med J.* 1977;2:723-726.

1096. Merkel F, Kalluri R, Marx M, et al. Autoreactive T-cells in Goodpasture's syndrome recognize the N-terminal NC1 domain on alpha 3 type IV collagen. *Kidney Int.* 1996;49:1127-1133.

1097. Rutgers A, Slot M, van Paassen P, et al. Coexistence of anti-glomerular basement membrane antibodies and myeloperoxidase-ANCAs in crescentic glomerulonephritis. *Am J Kidney Dis.* 2005;46:253-262.

1098. Sinico RA, Radice A, Corace C, et al. Anti-glomerular basement membrane antibodies in the diagnosis of Goodpasture syndrome: a comparison of different assays. *Nephrol Dial Transplant.* 2006;21:397-401.

1099. Segelmark M, Butkowski R, Wieslander J. Antigen restriction and IgG subclasses among anti-GBM autoantibodies. *Nephrol Dial Transplant.* 1990;5:991-996.

1100. Strauch BS, Charney A, Doctorouff S, et al. Goodpasture syndrome with recovery after renal failure. *JAMA.* 1974;229:444.

1101. Lang CH, Brown DC, Staley N, et al. Goodpasture syndrome treated with immunosuppression and plasma exchange. *Arch Intern Med.* 1977;137:1076-1078.
1102. Johnson JP, Whitman W, Briggs WA, et al. Plasmapheresis and immunosuppressive agents in antibasement membrane antibody–induced Goodpasture's syndrome. *Am J Med.* 1978;64:354-359.
1103. Smith PK, d'Apice JF. Plasmapheresis in rapidly progressive glomerulonephritis. *Am J Med.* 1978;65:564-566.
1104. Thysell H, Bygren P, Bengtsson U, et al. Immunosuppression and the additive effect of plasma exchange in treatment of rapidly progressive glomerulonephritis. *Acta Med Scand.* 1982;212:107-114.
1105. Glassock RJ. The role of high-dose steroids in nephritic syndromes: the case for a conservative approach. In: Narins R, ed. *Controversies in nephrology and hypertension.* New York: Churchill Livingstone; 1984:421.
1106. Bolton WK. The role of high-dose steroids in nephritic syndromes: the case for aggressive use. In: Narins R, ed. *Controversies in nephrology and hypertension.* New York: Churchill Livingstone; 1984:421.
1107. Adler S, Bruns FJ, Fraley DS, et al. Rapid progressive glomerulonephritis: relapse after prolonged remission. *Arch Intern Med.* 1981;141:852-854.
1108. Jayne DR, Marshall PD, Jones SJ, et al. Autoantibodies to GBM and neutrophil cytoplasm in rapidly progressive glomerulonephritis. *Kidney Int.* 1990;37:965-970.
1109. Gaskin G, Pusey CD. Plasmapheresis in antineutrophil cytoplasmic antibody–associated systemic vasculitis. *Ther Apher.* 2001;5:176-181.
1110. Levy JB, Turner AN, Rees AJ, et al. Long-term outcome of anti-glomerular basement membrane antibody disease treated with plasma exchange and immunosuppression. *Ann Intern Med.* 2001;134:1033-1042.
1111. O'Donoghue DJ, Short CD, Brenchley PE, et al. Sequential development of systemic vasculitis with anti-neutrophil cytoplasmic antibodies complicating anti-glomerular basement membrane disease. *Clin Nephrol.* 1989;32:251-255.
1112. Dahlberg PJ, Kurtz SB, Donadio JV, et al. Recurrent Goodpasture's syndrome. *Mayo Clin Proc.* 1978;53:533-537.
1113. Klasa RJ, Abboud RT, Ballon HS, et al. Goodpasture's syndrome: recurrence after a five-year remission. Case report and review of the literature. *Am J Med.* 1988;84:751-755.
1114. Wu MJ, Moorthy AV, Beirne GJ. Relapse in anti glomerular basement membrane antibody mediated crescentic glomerulonephritis. *Clin Nephrol.* 1980;13:97-102.
1115. Hind CR, Bowman C, Winearls CG, et al. Recurrence of circulating anti-glomerular basement membrane antibody three years after immunosuppressive treatment and plasma exchange. *Clin Nephrol.* 1984;21:244-246.
1116. Almkuist RD, Buckalew Jr VM, Hirszel P, et al. Recurrence of anti-glomerular basement membrane antibody mediated glomerulonephritis in an isograft. *Clin Immunol Immunopathol.* 1981;18:54-60.
1117. Deleted in page proofs.
1118. Jennette JC, Wilkman AS, Falk RJ. Anti-neutrophil cytoplasmic autoantibody–associated glomerulonephritis and vasculitis. *Am J Pathol.* 1989;135:921-930.
1119. Jennette JC, Falk RJ. Diagnostic classification of antineutrophil cytoplasmic autoantibody–associated vasculitides. *Am J Kidney Dis.* 1991;18:184-187.
1120. Harris AA, Falk RJ, Jennette JC. Crescentic glomerulonephritis with a paucity of glomerular immunoglobulin localization. *Am J Kidney Dis.* 1998;32:179-184.
1121. Jennette JC, Falk RJ. Antineutrophil cytoplasmic autoantibodies and associated diseases: a review. *Am J Kidney Dis.* 1990;15:517-529.
1122. Yang JJ, Jennette JC, Falk RJ. Immune complex glomerulonephritis is induced in rats immunized with heterologous myeloperoxidase. *Clin Exp Immunol.* 1994;97:466-473.
1123. Jennette JC, Falk RJ. Pathogenic potential of anti-neutrophil cytoplasmic autoantibodies. *Adv Exp Med Biol.* 1993;336:7-15.
1124. Kallenberg CG, Brouwer E, Weening JJ, et al. Anti-neutrophil cytoplasmic antibodies: current diagnostic and pathophysiological potential. *Kidney Int.* 1994;46:1-15.
1125. Keogan MT, Esnault VL, Green AJ, et al. Activation of normal neutrophils by anti-neutrophil cytoplasm antibodies. *Clin Exp Immunol.* 1992;90:228-234.
1126. Charles LA, Caldas ML, Falk RJ, et al. Antibodies against granule proteins activate neutrophils in vitro. *J Leukoc Biol.* 1991;50:539-546.
1127. Braun MG, Csernok E, Muller-Hermelink HK, et al. Distribution pattern of proteinase 3 in Wegener's granulomatosis and other vasculitic diseases. *Immun Infekt.* 1991;19:23-24.
1128. Brouwer E, Huitema MG, Mulder AH, et al. Neutrophil activation in vitro and in vivo in Wegener's granulomatosis. *Kidney Int.* 1994;45:1120-1131.
1129. Ewert BH, Jennette JC. Anti-myeloperoxidase antibodies (aMPO) stimulate neutrophils to adhere to cultured human endothelial cells utilizing the beta-2-integrin CD11/18. *J Am Soc Nephrol.* 1992;3:585:[abstract].
1130. Yang JJ, Pendergraft WF, Alcorta DA, et al. Circumvention of normal constraints on granule protein gene expression in peripheral blood neutrophils and monocytes of patients with antineutrophil cytoplasmic autoantibody–associated glomerulonephritis. *J Am Soc Nephrol.* 2004;15:2103-2114.
1131. Ciavatta D, Preston GA, Yang JJ, et al. Epigenetic basis for aberrant upregulation of autoantigen genes in ANCA vasculitis patients. *J Clin Invest.* 2010;120(9):3209-3219.
1132. Braun MG, Csernok E, Gross WL, et al. Proteinase 3, the target antigen of anticytoplasmic antibodies circulating in Wegener's granulomatosis. Immunolocalization in normal and pathologic tissues. *Am J Pathol.* 1991;139:831-838.
1133. Savage CO, Pottinger BE, Gaskin G, et al. Autoantibodies developing to myeloperoxidase and proteinase 3 in systemic vasculitis stimulate neutrophil cytotoxicity toward cultured endothelial cells. *Am J Pathol.* 1992;141:335-342.
1134. Porges AJ, Redecha PB, Kimberly WT, et al. Anti-neutrophil cytoplasmic antibodies engage and activate human neutrophils via Fc gamma RIIa. *J Immunol.* 1994;153:1271-1280.
1135. Taekema-Roelvink ME, van Kooten C, Heemskerk E, et al. Proteinase 3 interacts with a 111-kD membrane molecule of human umbilical vein endothelial cells. *J Am Soc Nephrol.* 2000;11:640-648.
1136. Kurosawa S, Esmon CT, Stearns-Kurosawa DJ. The soluble endothelial protein C receptor binds to activated neutrophils: involvement of proteinase-3 and CD11b/CD18. *J Immunol.* 2000;165:4697-4703.
1137. Esmon CT. Structure and functions of the endothelial cell protein C receptor. *Crit Care Med.* 2004;32:S298-S301.
1138. Ballieux BE, Hiemstra PS, Klar-Mohamad N, et al. Detachment and cytolysis of human endothelial cells by proteinase 3. *Eur J Immunol.* 1994;24:3211-3215.
1139. Yang JJ, Kettritz R, Falk RJ, et al. Apoptosis of endothelial cells induced by the neutrophil serine proteases proteinase 3 and elastase. *Am J Pathol.* 1996;149:1617-1626.
1140. Taekema-Roelvink ME, van Kooten C, Janssens MC, et al. Effect of anti-neutrophil cytoplasmic antibodies on proteinase 3-induced apoptosis of human endothelial cells. *Scand J Immunol.* 1998;48:37-43.
1141. Baldus S, Eiserich JP, Mani A, et al. Endothelial transcytosis of myeloperoxidase confers specificity to vascular ECM proteins as targets of tyrosine nitration. *J Clin Invest.* 2001;108:1759-1770.
1142. Brennan ML, Wu W, Fu X, et al. A tale of two controversies: defining both the role of peroxidases in nitrotyrosine formation in vivo using eosinophil peroxidase and myeloperoxidase-deficient mice, and the nature of peroxidase-generated reactive nitrogen species. *J Biol Chem.* 2002;277:17415-17427.
1143. Woods AA, Linton SM, Davies MJ. Detection of HOCl-mediated protein oxidation products in the extracellular matrix of human atherosclerotic plaques. *Biochem J.* 2003;370:729-735.
1144. Lu X, Garfield A, Rainger GE, et al. Mediation of endothelial cell damage by serine proteases, but not superoxide, released from antineutrophil cytoplasmic antibody–stimulated neutrophils. *Arthritis Rheum.* 2006;54:1619-1628.
1145. Mulder AH, Broekroelofs J, Horst G, et al. Anti-neutrophil cytoplasmic antibodies (ANCA) in inflammatory bowel disease: characterization and clinical correlates. *Clin Exp Immunol.* 1994;95:490-497.
1146. Kettritz R, Jennette JC, Falk RJ. Crosslinking of ANCA-antigens stimulates superoxide release by human neutrophils. *J Am Soc Nephrol.* 1997;8:386-394.
1147. Kimberly RP. Fcγ receptors and neutrophil activation. *Clin Exp Immunol.* 2000;120(suppl 1):18-19.
1148. Kocher M, Edberg JC, Fleit HB, et al. Antineutrophil cytoplasmic antibodies preferentially engage FcγRIIIb on human neutrophils. *J Immunol.* 1998;161:6909-6914.
1149. Tse WY, Nash GB, Hewins P, et al. ANCA-induced neutrophil F-actin polymerization: implications for microvascular inflammation. *Kidney Int.* 2005;67:130-139.
1150. Wainstein E, Edberg J, Csernok E, et al. FcγRIIIb alleles predict renal dysfunction in Wegener's granulomatosis (WG). *Arthritis Rheum.* 1995;39:210.
1151. Dijstelbloem HM, Scheepers RH, Oost WW, et al. Fcγ receptor polymorphisms in Wegener's granulomatosis: risk factors for disease relapse. *Arthritis Rheum.* 1999;42:1823-1827.
1152. Edberg JC, Wainstein E, Wu J, et al. Analysis of FcγRII gene polymorphisms in Wegener's granulomatosis. *Exp Clin Immunogenet.* 1997;14:183-195.
1153. Tse WY, Abadeh S, McTiernan A, et al. No association between neutrophil FcγRIIa allelic polymorphism and anti-neutrophil cytoplasmic antibody (ANCA)–positive systemic vasculitis. *Clin Exp Immunol.* 1999;117:198-205.
1154. Yang JJ, Alcorta DA, Preston GA, et al. Genes activated by ANCA IgG and ANCA F(ab')2 fragments. *J Am Soc Nephrol.* 2000;11:485A:[abstract].

1155. Williams JM, Savage COS. Characterization of the regulation and functional consequences of p21ras activation in neutrophils by antineutrophil cytoplasm antibodies. *J Am Soc Nephrol.* 2005;16:90-96.

1156. Franssen CF, Stegeman CA, Kallenberg CG, et al. Antiproteinase 3- and antimyeloperoxidase-associated vasculitis. *Kidney Int.* 2000;57:2195-2206.

1157. Harper L, Savage CO. Pathogenesis of ANCA-associated systemic vasculitis. *J Pathol.* 2000;190:349-359.

1158. Schmitt WH, Heesen C, Csernok E, et al. Elevated serum levels of soluble interleukin-2 receptor in patients with Wegener's granulomatosis. Association with disease activity. *Arthritis Rheum.* 1992;35:1088-1096.

1159. Bolton WK, Innes Jr DJ, Sturgill BC, et al. T-cells and macrophages in rapidly progressive glomerulonephritis: clinicopathologic correlations. *Kidney Int.* 1987;32:869-876.

1160. Csernok E, Trabandt A, Muller A, et al. Cytokine profiles in Wegener's granulomatosis: predominance of type 1 (Th1) in the granulomatous inflammation. *Arthritis Rheum.* 1999;42:742-750.

1161. Balding CE, Howie AJ, Drake-Lee AB, et al. Th2 dominance in nasal mucosa in patients with Wegener's granulomatosis. *Clin Exp Immunol.* 2001;125:332-339.

1162. Komocsi A, Lamprecht P, Csernok E, et al. Peripheral blood and granuloma CD4+CD28- T cells are a major source of interferon-gamma and tumor necrosis factor-alpha in Wegener's granulomatosis. *Am J Pathol.* 2002;160:1717-1724.

1163. Cunningham MA, Huang XR, Dowling JP, et al. Prominence of cell-mediated immunity effectors in "pauci-immune" glomerulonephritis. *J Am Soc Nephrol.* 1999;10:499-506:[see comments].

1164. Wang G, Hansen H, Tatsis E, et al. High plasma levels of the soluble form of CD30 activation molecule reflect disease activity in patients with Wegener's granulomatosis. *Am J Med.* 1997;102:517-523.

1165. Stegeman CA, Tervaert JW, Huitema MG, et al. Serum markers of T cell activation in relapses of Wegener's granulomatosis. *Clin Exp Immunol.* 1993;91:415-420.

1166. Van Der Woude FJ, van Es LA, Daha MR. The role of the c-ANCA antigen in the pathogenesis of Wegener's granulomatosis. A hypothesis based on both humoral and cellular mechanisms. *Neth J Med.* 1990;36:169-171.

1167. Abdulahad WH, Stegeman CA, Kallenberg CG. Review article: the role of CD4+ T cells in ANCA-associated systemic vasculitis. *Nephrology (Carlton).* 2009;14:26-32.

1168. Yang J, Bautz DJ, Lionaki S, et al. ANCA patients have T cells responsive to complementary PR-3 antigen. *Kidney Int.* 2008;74:1159-1169.

1169. Nogueira E, Hamour S, Sawant D, et al. Serum IL-17 and IL-23 levels and autoantigen-specific Th17 cells are elevated in patients with ANCA-associated vasculitis. *Nephrol Dial Transplant.* 2010;25(7):2209-2217.

1170. Esnault VL, Mathieson PW, Thiru S, et al. Autoantibodies to myeloperoxidase in brown Norway rats treated with mercuric chloride. *Lab Invest.* 1992;67:114-120.

1171. Harper MC, Milstein C, Cooke A. Pathogenic anti-MPO antibody in MRL/lpr mice. *Clin Exp Immunol.* 1995;101:54:[abstract].

1172. Nachman PH, Reisner HM, Yang JJ, et al. Shared idiotypy among patients with myeloperoxidase-anti-neutrophil cytoplasmic autoantibody associated glomerulonephritis and vasculitis. *Lab Invest.* 1996;74:519-527.

1173. Xiao H, Heeringa P, Hu P, et al. Antineutrophil cytoplasmic autoantibodies specific for myeloperoxidase cause glomerulonephritis and vasculitis in mice. *J Clin Invest.* 2002;110:955-963.

1174. Huugen D, Xiao H, van Esch A, et al. Aggravation of anti-myeloperoxidase antibody-induced glomerulonephritis by bacterial lipopolysaccharide: role of tumor necrosis factor-alpha. *Am J Pathol.* 2005;167:47-58.

1175. Xiao H, Heeringa P, Liu Z, et al. The role of neutrophils in the induction of glomerulonephritis by anti-myeloperoxidase antibodies. *Am J Pathol.* 2005;167:39-45.

1176. Jennette JC, Xiao H, Falk RJ. Pathogenesis of vascular inflammation by anti-neutrophil cytoplasmic antibodies. *J Am Soc Nephrol.* 2006;17:1235-1242.

1177. Xiao H, Schreiber A, Heeringa P, et al. Alternative complement pathway in the pathogenesis of disease mediated by anti-neutrophil cytoplasmic autoantibodies. *Am J Pathol.* 2007;170:52-64.

1178. Huugen D, van Esch A, Xiao H, et al. Inhibition of complement factor C5 protects against anti-myeloperoxidase antibody-mediated glomerulonephritis in mice. *Kidney Int.* 2007;71:646-654.

1179. Schreiber A, Xiao H, Jennette JC, et al. C5a receptor mediates neutrophil activation and ANCA-induced glomerulonephritis. *J Am Soc Nephrol.* 2009;20:289-298.

1180. Little MA, Smyth CL, Yadav R, et al. Antineutrophil cytoplasm antibodies directed against myeloperoxidase augment leukocyte-microvascular interactions in vivo. *Blood.* 2005;106:2050-2058.

1181. Savage CO. Vascular biology and vasculitis. *APMIS Suppl.* 2009(127):37-40.

1182. Pfister H, Ollert M, Froehlich LF, et al. Anti-neutrophil cytoplasmic autoantibodies (ANCA) against the murine homolog of proteinase 3 (Wegener's autoantigen) are pathogenic in vivo. *Blood.* 2004;104(5):1411-1418.

1183. Spencer SJ, Burns A, Gaskin G, et al. HLA class II specificities in vasculitis with antibodies to neutrophil cytoplasmic antigens. *Kidney Int.* 1992;41:1059-1063.

1184. Stegeman CA, Tervaert JW, Sluiter WJ, et al. Association of chronic nasal carriage of *Staphylococcus aureus* and higher relapse rates in Wegener granulomatosis. *Ann Intern Med.* 1994;120:12-17:[see comments].

1185. Gregorini G, Ferioli A, Donato F, et al. Association between silica exposure and necrotizing crescentic glomerulonephritis with p-ANCA and anti-MPO antibodies: a hospital-based case-control study. *Adv Exp Med Biol.* 1993;336:435-440.

1186. Hogan SL, Satterly KK, Dooley MA, et al. Silica exposure in anti-neutrophil cytoplasmic autoantibody-associated glomerulonephritis and lupus nephritis. *J Am Soc Nephrol.* 2001;12:134-142.

1187. Pendergraft III WF, Pressler BM, Jennette JC, et al. Autoantigen complementarity: a new theory implicating complementary proteins as initiators of autoimmune disease. *J Mol Med.* 2005;83:12-25.

1188. Pendergraft WF, Preston GA, Shah RR, et al. Autoimmunity is triggered by cPR-3(105-201), a protein complementary to human autoantigen proteinase-3. *Nat Med.* 2004;10:72-79.

1189. Bonsib SM, Walker WP. Pulmonary-renal syndrome: clinical similarity amidst etiologic diversity. *Mod Pathol.* 1989;2:129-137.

1190. Niles JL, Bottinger EP, Saurina GR, et al. The syndrome of lung hemorrhage and nephritis is usually an ANCA-associated condition. *Arch Intern Med.* 1996;156:440-445.

1191. Lai FM, Li PK, Suen MW, et al. Crescentic glomerulonephritis related to hepatitis B virus. *Mod Pathol.* 1992;5:262-267.

1192. Jennette JC, Falk RJ, Andrassy K, et al. Nomenclature of systemic vasculitides. Proposal of an international consensus conference. *Arthritis Rheum.* 1994;37:187-192.

1193. Savage CO, Winearls CG, Evans DJ, et al. Microscopic polyarteritis: presentation, pathology and prognosis. *Q J Med.* 1985;56:467-483.

1194. Hogan SL, Nachman PH, Wilkman AS, et al. Prognostic markers in patients with antineutrophil cytoplasmic autoantibody-associated microscopic polyangiitis and glomerulonephritis. *J Am Soc Nephrol.* 1996;7:23-32.

1195. Bajema IM, Hagen EC, Hermans J, et al. Kidney biopsy as a predictor for renal outcome in ANCA-associated necrotizing glomerulonephritis. *Kidney Int.* 1999;56:1751-1758.

1196. Koldingsnes W, Nossent JC. Baseline features and initial treatment as predictors of remission and relapse in Wegener's granulomatosis. *J Rheumatol.* 2003;30:80-88.

1197. Hogan SL, Falk RJ, Chin H, et al. Predictors of relapse and treatment resistance in antineutrophil cytoplasmic antibody-associated small-vessel vasculitis. *Ann Intern Med.* 2005;143:621-631.

1198. Frasca GM, Neri L, Martello M, et al. Renal transplantation in patients with microscopic polyarteritis and antimyeloperoxidase antibodies: report of three cases. *Nephron.* 1996;72:82-85.

1199. Rosenstein ED, Ribot S, Ventresca E, et al. Recurrence of Wegener's granulomatosis following renal transplantation. *Br J Rheumatol.* 1994;33:869-871.

1200. Nachman PH, Segelmark M, Westman K, et al. Recurrent ANCA-associated small vessel vasculitis after transplantation: a pooled analysis. *Kidney Int.* 1999;56:1544-1550.

1201. Geffriaud-Ricouard C, Noel LH, Chauveau D, et al. Clinical spectrum associated with ANCA of defined antigen specificities in 98 selected patients. *Clin Nephrol.* 1993;39:125-136.

1202. Kallenberg CG, Mulder AH, Tervaert JW. Antineutrophil cytoplasmic antibodies: a still-growing class of autoantibodies in inflammatory disorders. *Am J Med.* 1992;93:675-682.

1203. Falk RJ, Jennette JC. Anti-neutrophil cytoplasmic autoantibodies with specificity for myeloperoxidase in patients with systemic vasculitis and idiopathic necrotizing and crescentic glomerulonephritis. *N Engl J Med.* 1988;318:1651-1657.

1204. Ludemann J, Utecht B, Gross WL. Anti-neutrophil cytoplasm antibodies in Wegener's granulomatosis recognize an elastinolytic enzyme. *J Exp Med.* 1990;171:357-362.

1205. Goldschmeding R, van der Schoot CE, ten Bokkel HD, et al. Wegener's granulomatosis autoantibodies identify a novel diisopropylfluorophosphate-binding protein in the lysosomes of normal human neutrophils. *J Clin Invest.* 1989;84:1577-1587.

1206. Jennette JC, Hoidal JR, Falk RJ. Specificity of anti-neutrophil cytoplasmic autoantibodies for proteinase 3. *Blood.* 1990;75:2263-2264.

1207. Niles JL, McCluskey RT, Ahmad MF, et al. Wegener's granulomatosis autoantigen is a novel neutrophil serine proteinase. *Blood.* 1989;74:1888-1893.

1208. Bosch X, Mirapeix E, Font J, et al. Anti-myeloperoxidase autoantibodies in patients with necrotizing glomerular and alveolar capillaritis. *Am J Kidney Dis.* 1992;20:231-239.

1209. Choi HK, Liu S, Merkel PA, et al. Diagnostic performance of antineutrophil cytoplasmic antibody tests for idiopathic vasculitides: metaanalysis with a focus on antimyeloperoxidase antibodies. *J Rheumatol.* 2001;28:1584-1590.

1210. Falk RJ, Moore DT, Hogan SL, et al. A renal biopsy is essential for the management of ANCA-positive patients with glomerulonephritis. *Sarcoidosis Vasc Diffuse Lung Dis.* 1996;13:230-231.

1211. Savage CO, Harper L, Adu D. Primary systemic vasculitis. *Lancet.* 1997;349:553-558.

1212. Fauci AS, Katz P, Haynes BF, et al. Cyclophosphamide therapy of severe systemic necrotizing vasculitis. *N Engl J Med.* 1979;301:235-238.

1213. Falk RJ, Hogan S, Carey TS, et al. Clinical course of anti-neutrophil cytoplasmic autoantibody–associated glomerulonephritis and systemic vasculitis. The Glomerular Disease Collaborative Network. *Ann Intern Med.* 1990;113:656-663.

1214. Nachman PH, Hogan SL, Jennette JC, et al. Treatment response and relapse in antineutrophil cytoplasmic autoantibody–associated microscopic polyangiitis and glomerulonephritis. *J Am Soc Nephrol.* 1996;7:33-39.

1215. de Groot K, Adu D, Savage CO. The value of pulse cyclophosphamide in ANCA-associated vasculitis: meta-analysis and critical review. *Nephrol Dial Transplant.* 2001;16:2018-2027

1215a. de Groot K, Harper L, Jayne DR, et al., for EUVAS (European Vasculitis Study Group). Pulse versus daily oral cyclophosphamide for induction of remission in antineutrophil cytoplasmic antibody-associated vasculitis: a randomized trial. *Ann Intern Med.* 2009;150(10):670-680.

1216. Sanders JS, Huitma MG, Kallenberg CG, et al. Prediction of relapses in PR3-ANCA–associated vasculitis by assessing responses of ANCA titres to treatment. *Rheumatology (Oxford).* 2006;45:724-729.

1217. Glockner WM, Sieberth HG, Wichmann HE, et al. Plasma exchange and immunosuppression in rapidly progressive glomerulonephritis: a controlled, multi-center study. *Clin Nephrol.* 1988;29:1-8.

1218. Cole E, Cattran D, Magil A, et al. A prospective randomized trial of plasma exchange as additive therapy in idiopathic crescentic glomerulonephritis. The Canadian Apheresis Study Group. *Am J Kidney Dis.* 1992;20:261-269.

1219. Pusey CD, Rees AJ, Evans DJ, et al. Plasma exchange in focal necrotizing glomerulonephritis without anti-GBM antibodies. *Kidney Int.* 1991;40:757-763.

1220. Levy JB, Pusey CD. Still a role for plasma exchange in rapidly progressive glomerulonephritis? *J Nephrol.* 1997;10:7-13.

1221. Gaskin G, Jayne DR. European Vasculitis Study Group. Adjunctive plasma exchange is superior to methylprednisolone in acute renal failure due to ANCA-associated glomerulonephritis. *J Am Soc Nephrol.* 2002;13:2A-3A.

1222. Lionaki S, Hogan SL, Jennette CE, et al. The clinical course of ANCA small-vessel vasculitis on chronic dialysis. *Kidney Int.* 2009;76:644-651.

1223. Jayne DR, Davies MJ, Fox CJ, et al. Treatment of systemic vasculitis with pooled intravenous immunoglobulin. *Lancet.* 1991;337: 1137-1139.

1224. Tuso P, Moudgil A, Hay J, et al. Treatment of antineutrophil cytoplasmic autoantibody-positive systemic vasculitis and glomerulonephritis with pooled intravenous gammaglobulin. *Am J Kidney Dis.* 1992;20:504-508.

1225. Jayne DR, Lockwood CM. Pooled intravenous immunoglobulin in the management of systemic vasculitis. *Adv Exp Med Biol.* 1993;336: 469-472.

1226. Richter C, Schnabel A, Csernok E, et al. Treatment of anti-neutrophil cytoplasmic antibody (ANCA)–associated systemic vasculitis with high-dose intravenous immunoglobulin. *Clin Exp Immunol.* 1995;101:2-7.

1227. Richter C, Schnabel A, Csernok E, et al. Treatment of Wegener's granulomatosis with intravenous immunoglobulin. *Adv Exp Med Biol.* 1993;336:487-489.

1228. Jayne DR, Chapel H, Adu D, et al. Intravenous immunoglobulin for ANCA-associated systemic vasculitis with persistent disease activity. *QJM.* 2000;93:433-439.

1229. DeRemee RA, McDonald TJ, Weiland LH. Wegener's granulomatosis: observations on treatment with antimicrobial agents. *Mayo Clin Proc.* 1985;60:27-32.

1230. Stegeman CA, Tervaert JW, De Jong PE, et al. Trimethoprim-sulfamethoxazole (co-trimoxazole) for the prevention of relapses of Wegener's granulomatosis. Dutch Co-Trimoxazole Wegener Study Group. *N Engl J Med.* 1996;335:16-20.

1231. Langford CA, Talar W, Sneller MC. Use of methotrexate and glucocorticoids in the treatment of Wegener's granulomatosis. Long-term renal outcome in patients with glomerulonephritis. *Arthritis Rheum.* 2000;43:1836-1840.

1232. Specks U. Methotrexate for Wegener's granulomatosis: what is the evidence? *Arthritis Rheum.* 2005;52:2237-2242.

1233. de Groot K, Rasmussen N, Bacon PA, et al. Randomized trial of cyclophosphamide versus methotrexate for induction of remission in early systemic antineutrophil cytoplasmic antibody–associated vasculitis. *Arthritis Rheum.* 2005;52:2461-2469.

1234. Villa-Forte A, Clark TM, Gomes M, et al. Substitution of methotrexate for cyclophosphamide in Wegener granulomatosis: a 12-year single-practice experience. *Medicine (Baltimore).* 2007;86:269-277.

1235. Mukhtyar C, Guillevin L, Cid MC, et al. EULAR recommendations for the management of primary small and medium vessel vasculitis. *Ann Rheum Dis.* 2009;68:310-317.

1236. Jones R, Walsh M, Jayne DR. European Vasculitis Study Group: Randomised trial of rituximab versus cyclophosphamide for ANCA-associated renal vasculitis: RITUXVAS. *J Am Soc Nephrol.* 2008;19:61A: [abstract].

1237. Stone JH, Merkel PA, Spiera R, et al. Rituximab versus cyclophosphamide for ANCA-associated vasculitis. *N Engl J Med.* 2010;363(3):221-231.

1238. Vaziri ND, Gonzales EC, Shayestehfar B, et al. Plasma levels and urinary excretion of fibrinolytic and protease inhibitory proteins in nephrotic syndrome. *J Lab Clin Med.* 1994;124(1):118-124.

1239. Lizakowski S, Zdrojewski Z, Jagodzinski P, et al. Plasma tissue factor and tissue factory pathway inhibitor in patients with primary glomerulonephritis. *Scand J Urol Nephrol.* 2007;41(3):237-242.

1240. Ellis D. Anemia in the course of the nephrotic syndrome secondary to transferrin depletion. *J Pediatr.* 1977;90:953-955.

1241. Harris RC, Ismail N. Extrarenal complications of the nephrotic syndrome. *Am J Kidney Dis.* 1994;23:477-497.

1242. Howard RL, Buddington B, Alfrey AC. Urinary albumin, transferrin and iron excretion in diabetic patients. *Kidney Int.* 1991;40:923-926.

1243. Cartwright GE, Gubler CJ, Wintrobe MM. Studies on copper metabolism. XI. Copper and iron metabolism in the nephrotic syndrome. *J Clin Invest.* 1954;33:685-698.

1244. Pedraza C, Torres R, Cruz C, et al. Copper and zinc metabolism in aminonucleoside-induced nephrotic syndrome. *Nephron.* 1994;66:87-92.

1245. Freeman RM, Richards CJ, Rames LK. Zinc metabolism in aminonucleoside-induced nephrosis. *Am J Clin Nutr.* 1975;28:699-703.

1246. Hancock DE, Onstad JW, Wolf PL. Transferrin loss into the urine with hypochromic, microcytic anemia. *Am J Clin Pathol.* 1976;65:73-78.

1247. Bergrem H. Pharmacokinetics and protein binding of prednisolone in patients with nephrotic syndrome and patients undergoing hemodialysis. *Kidney Int.* 1983;23:876-881.

1248. Frey FJ, Frey BM. Altered prednisolone kinetics in patients with the nephrotic syndrome. *Nephron.* 1982;32:45-48.

1249. Strife CF, Jackson EC, Forristal J, et al. Effect of the nephrotic syndrome on the concentration of serum complement components. *Am J Kidney Dis.* 1986;8:37-42.

1250. Kaysen GA, Gambertoglio J, Jimenez I, et al. Effect of dietary protein intake on albumin homeostasis in nephrotic patients. *Kidney Int.* 1986;29:572-577.

1251. Cameron JS. Coagulation and thromboembolic complications in the nephrotic syndrome. *Adv Nephrol Necker Hosp.* 1984;13:75-114.

1252. Panicucci F, Sagripanti A, Vispi M, et al. Comprehensive study of haemostasis in nephrotic syndrome. *Nephron.* 1983;33:9-13.

1253. Adler AJ, Lundin AP, Feinroth MV, et al. Beta-thromboglobulin levels in the nephrotic syndrome. *Am J Med.* 1980;69:551-554.

1254. Kuhlmann U, Steurer J, Rhyner K, et al. Platelet aggregation and beta-thromboglobulin levels in nephrotic patients with and without thrombosis. *Clin Nephrol.* 1981;15:229-235.

1255. Alkjaersig N, Fletcher AP, Narayanan M, et al. Course and resolution of the coagulopathy in nephrotic children. *Kidney Int.* 1987;31:772-780.

1256. Kendall AG, Lohmann RC, Dossetor JB. Nephrotic syndrome. A hypercoagulable state. *Arch Intern Med.* 1971;127:1021-1027.

1257. Coppola R, Guerra L, Ruggeri ZM, et al. Factor VIII/von Willebrand factor in glomerular nephropathies. *Clin Nephrol.* 1981;16:217-222.

1258. Thomson C, Forbes CD, Prentice CR, et al. Changes in blood coagulation and fibrinolysis in the nephrotic syndrome. *Q J Med.* 1974;43:399-407.

1259. Vaziri ND, Ngo JL, Ibsen KH, et al. Deficiency and urinary losses of factor XII in adult nephrotic syndrome. *Nephron.* 1982;32:342-346.

1260. Kanfer A. Coagulation factors in nephrotic syndrome. *Am J Nephrol.* 1990;10(suppl 1):63-68.

1261. Lau SO, Tkachuck JY, Hasegawa DK, et al. Plasminogen and antithrombin III deficiencies in the childhood nephrotic syndrome associated with plasminogenuria and antithrombinuria. *J Pediatr.* 1980;96:390-392.

1262. Shimamatsu K, Onoyama K, Maeda T, et al. Massive pulmonary embolism occurring with corticosteroid and diuretics therapy in a minimal-change nephrotic patient. *Nephron.* 1982;32:78-79.

1263. Vaziri ND, Gonzales EC, Shayestehfar B, et al. Plasma levels and urinary excretion of fibrinolytic and protease inhibitory proteins in nephrotic syndrome. *J Lab Clin Med.* 1994;124:118-124.

1264. Ozanne P, Francis RB, Meiselman HJ. Red blood cell aggregation in nephrotic syndrome. *Kidney Int.* 1983;23:519-525.

1265. Boneu B, Bouissou F, Abbal M, et al. Comparison of progressive antithrombin activity and the concentration of three thrombin inhibitors in nephrotic syndrome. *Thromb Haemost.* 1981;46:623-625.

1266. Jorgensen KA, Stoffersen E. Antithrombin III and the nephrotic syndrome. *Scand J Haematol*. 1979;22:442-448.
1267. Thaler E, Balzar E, Kopsa H, et al. Acquired antithrombin III deficiency in patients with glomerular proteinuria. *Haemostasis*. 1978;7:257-272.
1268. Vigano D, Angelo A, Kaufman CE, et al. Protein S deficiency occurs in the nephrotic syndrome. *Ann Intern Med*. 1987;107:42-47.
1269. Mehls O, Andrassy K, Koderisch J, et al. Hemostasis and thromboembolism in children with nephrotic syndrome: differences from adults. *J Pediatr*. 1987;110:862-867.
1270. Warren GV, Korbet SM, Schwartz MM, et al. Minimal change glomerulopathy associated with nonsteroidal antiinflammatory drugs. *Am J Kidney Dis*. 1989;13:127-130.
1271. Tornroth T, Skrifvars B. The development and resolution of glomerular basement membrane changes associated with subepithelial immune deposits. *Am J Pathol*. 1975;79:219-236.
1272. Criteria for diagnosis of Behçet's disease. International Study Group for Behçet's Disease. *Lancet*. 1990;335:1078-1080.
1273. Korzets Z, Golan E, Manor Y, et al. Spontaneously remitting minimal change nephropathy preceding a relapse of Hodgkin's disease by 19 months. *Clin Nephrol*. 1992;38:125-127.
1274. Dabbs DJ, Striker LM, Mignon F, et al. Glomerular lesions in lymphomas and leukemias. *Am J Med*. 1986;80:63-70.
1275. Alpers CE, Cotran RS. Neoplasia and glomerular injury. *Kidney Int*. 1986;30:465-473.
1276. Meyrier A, Delahousse M, Callard P, et al. Minimal change nephrotic syndrome revealing solid tumors. *Nephron*. 1992;61:220-223.
1277. Lagrue G, Laurent J, Rostoker G. Food allergy and idiopathic nephrotic syndrome. *Kidney Int Suppl*. 1989;27:S147-S151.
1278. Deleted in page proofs
1279. Rennke HG. Secondary membranoproliferative glomerulonephritis. *Kidney Int*. 1995;47:643-656.
1280. Beaufils M, Morel-Maroger L, Sraer JD, et al. Acute renal failure of glomerular origin during visceral abscesses. *N Engl J Med*. 1976;295:185-189.
1281. Martinelli R, Noblat AC, Brito E, et al. *Schistosoma mansoni*–induced mesangiocapillary glomerulonephritis: influence of therapy. *Kidney Int*. 1989;35:1227-1233.
1282. Sissons JG, West RJ, Fallows J, et al. The complement abnormalities of lipodystrophy. *N Engl J Med*. 1976;294:461-465.
1283. Molle D, Baumelou A, Beaufils H, et al. Membranoproliferative glomerulonephritis associated with pulmonary sarcoidosis. *Am J Nephrol*. 1986;6:386-387.
1284. Zell SC, Duxbury G, Shankel SW. Alveolar hemorrhage associated with a membranoproliferative glomerulonephritis and smooth muscle antibody. *Am J Med*. 1987;82:1073-1076.
1285. Strife CF, Hug G, Chuck G, et al. Membranoproliferative glomerulonephritis and α$_1$-antitrypsin deficiency in children. *Pediatrics*. 1983;71:88-92.
1286. Lagrue G, Laurent J, Dubertret L, et al. Buckley's syndrome and membranoproliferative glomerulonephritis. *Nephron*. 1982;31:279-280.
1287. Swarbrick ET, Fairclough PD, Campbell PJ, et al. Coeliac disease, chronic active hepatitis, and mesangiocapillary glomerulonephritis in the same patient. *Lancet*. 1980;2:1084-1085.
1288. Katz A, Dyck RF, Bear RA. Celiac disease associated with immune complex glomerulonephritis. *Clin Nephrol*. 1979;11:39-44.
1289. Pasternack A, Collin P, Mustonen J, et al. Glomerular IgA deposits in patients with celiac disease. *Clin Nephrol*. 1990;34:56-60.
1290. Iskandar SS, Jennette JC, Wilkman AS, et al. Interstrain variations in nephritogenicity of heterologous protein in mice. *Lab Invest*. 1982;46:344-351.
1291. Woodroffe AJ. IgA, glomerulonephritis and liver disease. *Aust N Z J Med*. 1981;11:109-111.
1292. Hirsch DJ, Jindal KK, Trillo A, et al. Acute renal failure in Crohn's disease due to IgA nephropathy. *Am J Kidney Dis*. 1992;20:189-190.
1293. Kalsi J, Delacroix DL, Hodgson HJ. IgA in alcoholic cirrhosis. *Clin Exp Immunol*. 1983;52:499-504.
1294. Ramirez G, Stinson JB, Zawada ET, et al. IgA nephritis associated with mycosis fungoides. Report of two cases. *Arch Intern Med*. 1981;141:1287-1291.
1295. Sinniah R. Mucin secreting cancer with mesangial IgA deposits. *Pathology*. 1982;14:303-308.
1296. Monteiro GE, Lillicrap CA. Case of mumps nephritis. *Br Med J*. 1967;4:721-722.
1297. Spichtin HP, Truniger B, Mihatsch MJ, et al. Immunothrombocytopenia and IgA nephritis. *Clin Nephrol*. 1980;14:304-308.
1298. Woodrow G, Innes A, Boyd SM, et al. A case of IgA nephropathy with coeliac disease responding to a gluten-free diet. *Nephrol Dial Transplant*. 1993;8:1382-1383.
1299. Nomoto Y, Sakai H, Endoh M, et al. Scleritis and IgA nephropathy. *Arch Intern Med*. 1980;140:783-785.
1300. Andrassy K, Lichtenberg G, Rambausek M. Sicca syndrome in mesangial IgA glomerulonephritis. *Clin Nephrol*. 1985;24:60-62.
1301. Thomas M, Ibels LS, Abbot N. IgA nephropathy associated with mastitis and haematuria. *Br Med J (Clin Res Ed)*. 1985;291:867-868.
1302. Yum MN, Lampton LM, Bloom PM, et al. Asymptomatic IgA nephropathy associated with pulmonary hemosiderosis. *Am J Med*. 1978;64:1056-1060.
1303. Remy P, Jacquot C, Nochy D, et al. Buerger's disease associated with IgA nephropathy: report of two cases. *Br Med J (Clin Res Ed)*. 1988;296:683-684.
1304. Kimmel PL, Phillips TM, Ferreira-Centeno A, et al. Brief report: idiotypic IgA nephropathy in patients with human immunodeficiency virus infection. *N Engl J Med*. 1992;327:702-706.
1305. Newell GC. Cirrhotic glomerulonephritis: incidence, morphology, clinical features, and pathogenesis. *Am J Kidney Dis*. 1987;9:183-190.
1306. Beaufils H, Jouanneau C, Katlama C, et al. HIV-associated IgA nephropathy—a post-mortem study. *Nephrol Dial Transplant*. 1995;10:35-38.
1307. van de Wiel A, Valentijn RM, Schuurman HJ, et al. Circulating IgA immune complexes and skin IgA deposits in liver disease. Relation to liver histopathology. *Dig Dis Sci*. 1988;33:679-684.
1308. Druet P, Bariety J, Bernard D, et al. [Primary glomerulopathy with IgA and IgG mesangial deposits. Clinical and morphological study of 52 cases]. *Presse Med*. 1970;78:583-587.
1309. Garcia-Fuentes M, Martin A, Chantler C, et al. Serum complement components in Henoch-Schönlein purpura. *Arch Dis Child*. 1978;53:417-419.
1310. Gartner HV, Honlein F, Traub U, et al. IgA-nephropathy (IgA-IgG-nephropathy/IgA-nephritis)—a disease entity? *Virchows Arch A Pathol Anat Histol*. 1979;385:1-27.
1311. Frasca GM, Vangelista A, Biagini G, et al. Immunological tubulo-interstitial deposits in IgA nephropathy. *Kidney Int*. 1982;22:184-191.
1312. Gutierrez M, Navas P, Ortega R, et al. [Familial and hereditary mesangial glomerulonephritis with IgA deposits]. *Med Clin (Barc)*. 1981;76:1-7.
1313. Garcia-Fuentes M, Chantler C, Williams DG. Cryoglobulinaemia in Henoch-Schönlein purpura. *Br Med J*. 1977;2:163-165.
1314. Galla JH, Kohaut EC, Alexander R, et al. Racial difference in the prevalence of IgA-associated nephropathies. *Lancet*. 1984;2:522.
1315. Lagrue G, Sadreux T, Laurent J, et al. Is there a treatment of mesangial IgA glomerulonephritis? *Clin Nephrol*. 1981;16:161.

Secondary Glomerular Disease

Gerald B. Appel, Jai Radhakrishnan, and Vivette D. D'Agati

Systemic Lupus Erythematosus

Lupus nephritis (LN) is a frequent and potentially serious complication of systemic lupus erythematosus (SLE).[1-6] Kidney disease influences morbidity and mortality, both directly and indirectly, through complications of therapy. Recent studies have more clearly defined the spectrum of clinical, prognostic, and renal histopathologic findings in SLE. Controlled, randomized trials of induction therapy for both severe proliferative LN and membranous LN have focused on achieving remissions of renal disease while minimizing adverse reactions to therapy. Maintenance trials have attempted to compare the efficacy of therapeutic agents in preventing renal flares and the progression of renal disease over the long term. Because some patients fail to respond to modern treatment regimens, a number of newer immunomodulatory agents are being studied in resistant or relapsing patients.

Epidemiology

The incidence and prevalence of SLE depend on the population studied and the diagnostic criteria for defining SLE.[3,6-8] Females outnumber males by about 10 to one. However, males with SLE have the same incidence of renal disease as females. The onset of disease peaks between 15 and 45 years of age, and more than 85% of patients are younger than 55 years of age. SLE is more likely to be associated with severe nephritis in children and in males and is less likely in elderly individuals.[2-4,7,8] SLE and LN are more common and certainly are associated with more severe renal involvement in the African-American population, although the precise roles of biologic-genetic versus socioeconomic factors have not been defined.[7-12] Worldwide certain other populations, including Afro-Caribbeans, Asians, and Hispanics, have an increased incidence of SLE and LN.[3] The overall incidence of SLE ranges from 1.8 to 7.6 cases per 100,000 with a prevalence of from 40 to 200 cases per 100,000.[3,6,7] The incidence of renal involvement varies depending on the populations studied, the diagnostic criteria for kidney disease, and whether involvement is defined by renal biopsy or clinical findings. Approximately 25% to 50% of unselected lupus patients have clinical renal disease at onset, and as many as 60% of adults with SLE develop renal disease during their course.[3-5,7,8]

Although the etiology of SLE remains unknown, certain genetic, hormonal, and environmental factors clearly influence the course and severity of disease expression.[3,6-8,13,14]

A multiplicity of genes are involved in both SLE and LN. Almost 20 different genetic loci have been associated with an increased risk of SLE, including genes involved in B-cell signaling, neutrophil function, and toll-like receptors.[3,13,14] A genetic predisposition is supported by a higher concordance rate in monozygotic twins (25%) than fraternal, dizygotic twins (<5%); the greater risk of developing SLE or other autoimmune disease among relatives of SLE patients; the association with certain HLA genotypes (e.g., HLA-B8, DR2, and DR3); inherited deficiencies in complement components (e.g., C1q, C2, and C4 deficiencies); and Fc receptor polymorphisms.[3,15] Genome-wide analyses have identified candidate susceptibility genes for SLE that regulate diverse immune functions such as T-cell activation and signal transduction, B-cell signaling, and interferon (INF) production.[16] Inbred genetic murine models of SLE and LN include the NZB B/W F1 hybrid, the BXSB/yaa, and the MRL/lpr mouse. Evidence for hormonal factors includes the strong predominance of SLE in women of childbearing age, the increased incidence of SLE in postmenopausal women given estrogen replacement, and the increased incidence of SLE flares during or shortly after pregnancy.[3,6-8,13] In murine models of SLE (F1 NZB/NZW), females have more severe disease than males, and disease severity in females is ameliorated by oophorectomy or androgen therapy. Environmental factors other than estrogens also may modulate disease expression, including immune responses to viral or bacterial antigens, exposure to sunlight, ultraviolet radiation, and certain medications.[3,6,13,14]

The diagnosis of SLE can be established by the presence of certain clinical and laboratory features defined by the 1997 modified American Rheumatism Association (ARA) criteria.[5] Development of any four of the 11 criteria over a lifetime gives a 96% sensitivity and specificity for SLE. The criteria include malar rash, discoid rash, photosensitivity, oral ulcerations, nondeforming arthritis, serositis (including pleuritis or pericarditis), central nervous system (CNS) disorder (e.g., seizures or psychoses), hematologic disorder (including immune-mediated hemolytic anemia, leukopenia, lymphopenia, or thrombocytopenia), immunologic disorder (including anti-DNA antibody, anti-Sm antibody, lupus anticoagulant, or antiphospholipid [APL] antibody), and antinuclear antibody (ANA). The last remaining criterion is renal involvement, which is defined as persistent proteinuria exceeding 500 mg/day (or 3+ on the dipstick) or the presence of cellular urinary casts. Because some patients, especially those with mesangial or membranous LN, present with clinical renal disease before they have fulfilled ARA criteria for SLE, the diagnosis of SLE remains a clinical diagnosis with histopathologic findings supporting or confirming the presumed diagnosis.[3]

Pathogenesis

SLE is a disease in which abnormalities of immune regulation lead to a loss of self-tolerance and subsequent autoimmune responses.[6-8,13,18-20] SLE has been associated with a decreased number of cytotoxic and suppressor T cells; increased helper (CD4+) T cells; polyclonal activation of B cells; defective B-cell tolerance; dysfunctional T-cell signaling; and abnormal Th1, Th2, and Th17 cytokine production.[6,8,18-23] The failure of apoptotic mechanisms to delete autoreactive B- and T-cell clones may promote their expansion and autoantibody production. Exposure to viral or bacterial peptides containing sequences similar to native antigens may lead to "antigen mimicry" and stimulation of autoantibody production. Defective clearance of apoptotic cells and prolonged exposure to nuclear antigens may trigger immune responses through interactions with toll-like receptors. Regardless of the specific mechanism(s), autoantibody production is directed against such nuclear antigens as ds-DNA, Sm, RNA, Ro, La, and histones, among others.[3,6,14,22,23] The formation of circulating immune complexes (CICs) and their deposition in tissues followed by complement activation is important for certain patterns of glomerular damage.[2,8,24] Immune complexes are also detectable in the skin at the dermal–epidermal junction and in the choroid plexus, pericardium, and pleural spaces. Renal involvement in SLE has been considered a human prototype of classic experimental chronic immune complex–induced glomerulonephritis (GN).[24] The chronic deposition of CICs plays a major role in the mesangial and the endocapillary proliferative patterns of LN. Immune complex size, charge, avidity, local hemodynamic factors, and the clearing ability of the mesangium all influence the localization of CICs within the glomerulus.[6,19,24,25] In diffuse proliferative LN, the deposited complexes consist of nuclear antigens (e.g., DNA) and high-affinity complement–fixing immunoglobulin G (IgG) antibodies.[8,24] In other SLE patients, rather than deposition of CICs, the initiating event may be the local binding of cationic nuclear antigens such as histones to the subepithelial region of the glomerular capillary wall followed by in situ immune complex formation. After immune deposits form in the glomerulus, the complement cascade is activated, leading to complement-mediated damage, activation of procoagulant factors, leukocyte infiltration, release of proteolytic enzymes, and production of various cytokines regulating glomerular cellular proliferation and matrix synthesis. Glomerular damage may be potentiated by hypertension and coagulation abnormalities. Recent studies have documented focal segmental necrotizing glomerular lesions without significant immune complex deposition, resembling a "pauci-immune" pattern, with or without antineutrophil cytoplasmic antibodies (ANCAs).[26] This may be an independent mechanism of glomerular and vascular damage in some patients with LN.[27] The presence of APL antibodies directed against a phospholipid-β2 glycoprotein complex and their attendant alterations in endothelial and platelet function, including reduced production of prostacyclin and other endothelial anticoagulant factors, activation of plasminogen, inhibition of protein C or S, and enhanced platelet aggregation, can also potentiate glomerular and vascular lesions.

Pathology of Lupus Nephritis

The histopathology of LN is extremely pleomorphic.[1-4,8,24] This diversity is evident when comparing the biopsy findings from different patients or even comparing adjacent glomeruli in a single biopsy specimen. Moreover, the lesions have the capacity to transform from one pattern to another spontaneously or after treatment. Early classifications of LN simply divided glomerular changes into mild and severe forms.[2,24] The World Health Organization (WHO) Classification, widely used for almost 30 years,[17,28] classified LN by combining glomerular light microscopic (LM) findings with the immunofluorescence (IF) and electron microscopic (EM) findings. Nevertheless, this classification still had major shortcomings. The 2003 International Society of Nephrology (ISN)/Renal Pathology Society (RPS) classification of LN formulated by a joint working group of the ISN and the RPS addressed these limitations and is now widely accepted by nephrologists, pathologists, and rheumatologists[29] (Table 32-1). It has proven more reproducible and provides more standardized definitions for precise clinical pathologic correlations.[30,31]

ISN/RPS class I denotes normal-appearing glomeruli by LM but with mesangial immune deposits by IF and EM. Even patients without clinical renal disease often have mesangial immune deposits when studied carefully by the more sensitive techniques of IF and EM.[29]

ISN/RPS class II is defined on LM by pure mesangial hypercellularity of any degree, with mesangial immune deposits on IF and EM (Figures 32-1 to 32-3).[29] Mesangial hypercellularity is defined as greater than three cells in mesangial regions distant from the vascular pole in 3-μm–thick sections.

TABLE 32-1 International Society of Nephrology/Renal Pathology Society (2003) Classification of Lupus Nephritis (LN)

CLASS	DESCRIPTION
I	Minimal mesangial LN
II	Mesangial proliferative LN
III	Focal LN* (<50% of glomeruli)
III (A)	Active lesions
III (A/C)	Active and chronic lesions
III (C)	Chronic lesions
IV	Diffuse LN* (≥50% of glomeruli) Diffuse segmental (IV-S) or global (IV-G) LN
IV (A)	Active lesions
IV (A/C)	Active and chronic lesions
IV (C)	Chronic lesions
V	Membranous LN
VI	Advanced sclerosing LN (≥90% globally sclerosed glomeruli without residual activity)

*Indicate the proportion of glomeruli with active and with sclerotic lesions.
Indicate the proportion of glomeruli with fibrinoid necrosis and with cellular crescents.
Indicate and grade (mild, moderate, severe) tubular atrophy, interstitial inflammation and fibrosis, the severity of arteriosclerosis, or other vascular lesions.
Class V may occur in combination with III or IV, in which case both will be diagnosed.

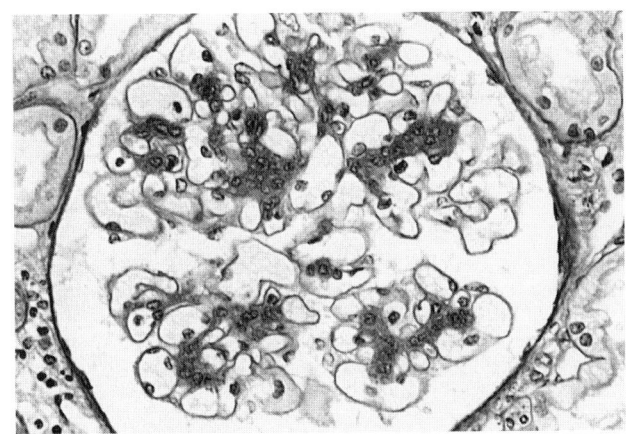

FIGURE 32-1 Lupus nephritis class II. There is mild global mesangial hypercellularity (periodic acid–Schiff, ×400).

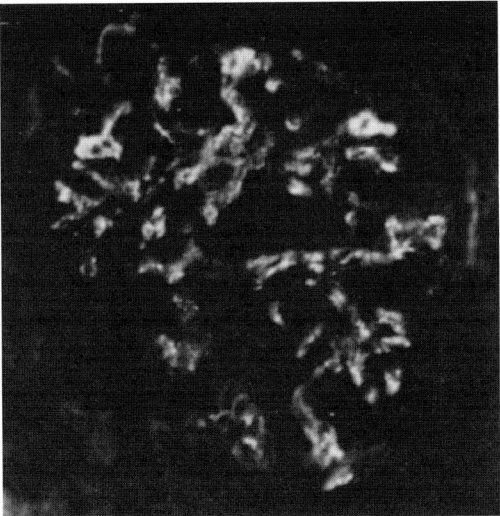

FIGURE 32-2 Lupus nephritis class II. Immunofluorescence photomicrograph showing deposits of C3 restricted to the glomerular mesangium (×400).

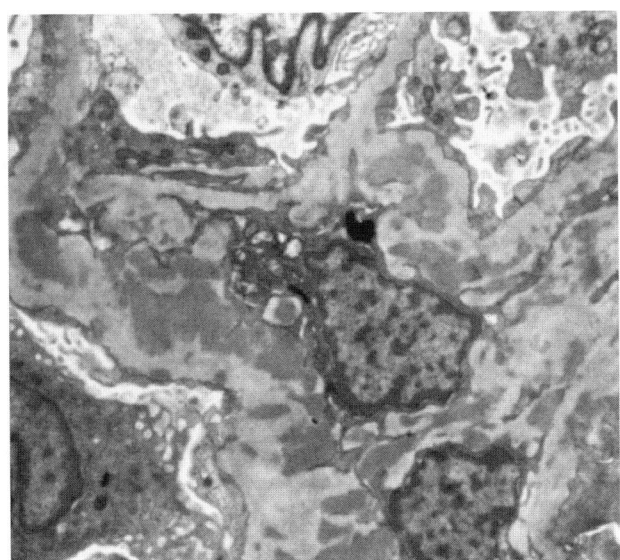

FIGURE 32-3 Lupus nephritis class II. Electron micrograph showing abundant mesangial electron-dense deposits (×12,000).

There may be rare minute subendothelial or subepithelial deposits visible by IF or EM but not by LM.

ISN/RPS class III, focal LN, is defined as focal segmental or global endocapillary or extracapillary GN affecting less than 50% of the total glomeruli sampled. There is usually focal segmental endocapillary proliferation, including mesangial cells and endothelial cells, with infiltrating mononuclear and polymorphonuclear leukocytes (Figures 32-4 to 32-6).[29] Class III biopsies may have active (proliferative), inactive (sclerosing), or active and inactive lesions subclassified as A, C, or A/C, respectively. Active lesions may display cellular crescents, fibrinoid necrosis, nuclear pyknosis or karyorrhexis, and rupture of the glomerular basement membrane (GBM). Hematoxylin bodies, swollen basophilic nuclear material acted upon by antinuclear antibodies, are occasionally found within the necrotizing lesions. Subendothelial immune deposits may be visible by LM as "wire loop" thickenings of the glomerular capillary walls or large intraluminal masses known as "hyaline thrombi." Segmental scarring involving less than 50% of the glomeruli qualifies for an ISN/RPS class III (C) lesion.[29] In class III biopsies, glomeruli adjacent to those with severe histologic changes may show only mesangial abnormalities by LM. In class III, diffuse mesangial and focal and segmental subendothelial immune deposits are typically identified by IF and EM. The segmental subendothelial deposits are usually

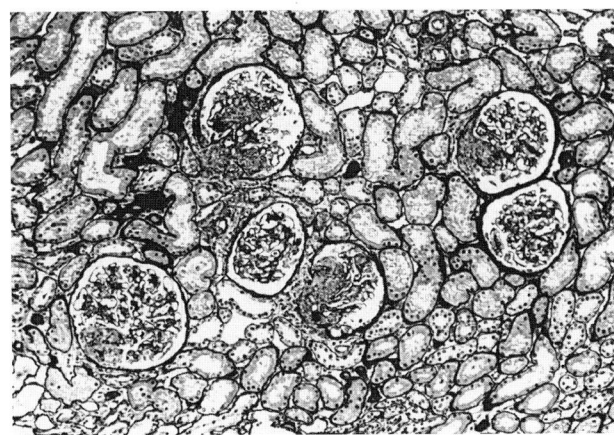

FIGURE 32-4 Lupus nephritis class III. There is focal segmental endocapillary proliferation (Jones methenamine silver, ×100).

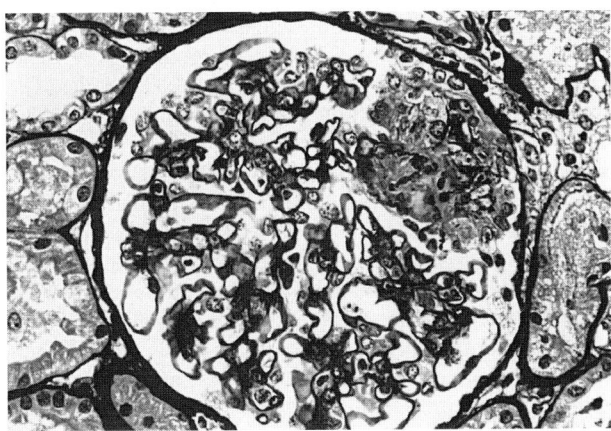

FIGURE 32-5 Lupus nephritis class III. The glomerular endocapillary proliferation is discretely segmental with necrotizing features and an early cellular crescent (Jones methenamine silver, ×400).

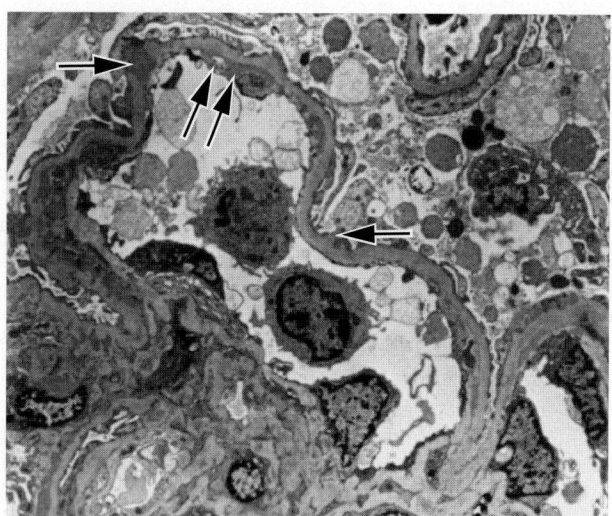

FIGURE 32-6 Lupus nephritis class III. Electron micrograph showing deposits in the mesangium as well as involving the peripheral capillary wall in subendothelial (*double arrow*) and subepithelial (*single arrow*) locations. (×4900).

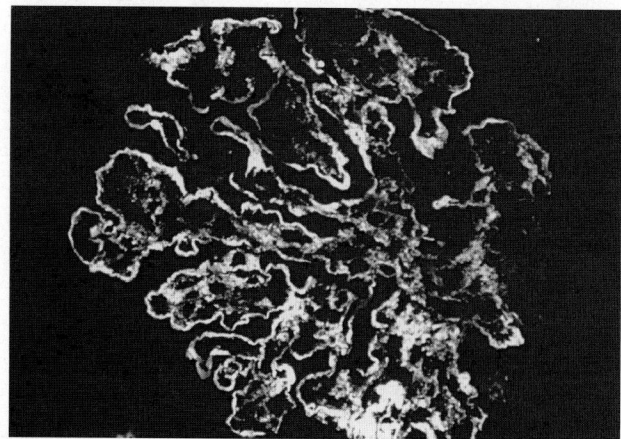

FIGURE 32-8 Lupus nephritis class IV. Immunofluorescence photomicrograph showing global deposits of immunoglobulin G in the mesangial regions and outlining the subendothelial aspect of the peripheral glomerular capillary walls (×600).

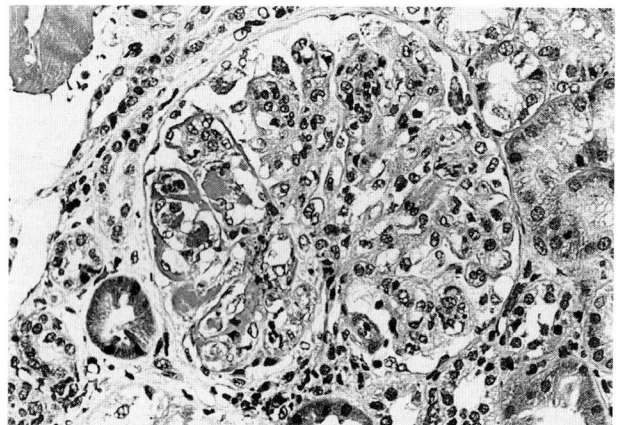

FIGURE 32-7 Lupus nephritis class IV. There is global endocapillary proliferation with infiltrating neutrophils and segmental wire loop deposits (hematoxylin and eosin, ×320).

present in the distribution of the segmental endocapillary proliferative lesions

ISN/RPS class IV, diffuse proliferative LN, has qualitatively similar glomerular endocapillary proliferation as class III, but the proliferation involves more than 50% of the glomeruli (Figures 32-7 to 32-9).[29,32-34] ISN/RPS class IV is subdivided into diffuse segmental proliferation, class IV-S in which more than 50% of affected glomeruli have segmental lesions, and diffuse global proliferation, class IV-G in which more than 50% of affected glomeruli have global lesions. All of the active features described above for class III (including fibrinoid necrosis, leukocyte infiltration, wire loop deposits, hyaline thrombi, hematoxylin bodies, and crescents) may be encountered in ISN/RPS class IV LN. In general, there is more extensive peripheral capillary wall subendothelial immune deposition in class IV biopsies, and extracapillary proliferation in the form of crescents is common. Class IV lesions may have features similar to primary membranoproliferative (mesangiocapillary GN) with mesangial interposition along the peripheral capillary walls and double contours of

the GBMs. Some class III and IV biopsies have focal necrotizing and crescentic lesions akin to those seen in small vessel vasculitides. Some of these patients have had circulating ANCAs.[26,35]

ISN/RPS class V is defined by regular subepithelial immune deposits producing a membranous pattern (Figures 32-10 to 32-12).[29,36-38] The coexistence of mesangial immune deposits and mesangial hypercellularity in most cases helps to distinguish membranous LN from primary membranous glomerulopathy.[39] Early membranous LN class V may have no identifiable abnormalities by LM, but subepithelial deposits are detectable by IF. In well-developed membranous lesions, there is typically thickening of the glomerular capillary walls and "spike" formation between the subepithelial deposits. When the membranous alterations are accompanied by focal or diffuse endocapillary proliferative lesions and subendothelial immune complex deposition, they are classified as class V + III and V + IV, respectively. Because sparse subepithelial deposits may also be encountered in other classes (III or IV) of LN, a diagnosis of pure lupus membranous LN should be reserved only for cases in which the membranous pattern predominates.

ISN/RPS class VI, advanced sclerosing LN or end-stage LN, is reserved for biopsies with more than 90% of the glomeruli sclerotic.[29] There are no active lesions, and it may be difficult to even establish the diagnosis of LN without the identification of residual glomerular immune deposits by IF and EM.

Immunofluorescence

In LN, immune deposits can be found in the glomeruli, tubules, interstitium, and blood vessels.[2-4,24,39] IgG is almost universal, with co-deposits of IgM and IgA in most specimens. Both C3 and C1q are commonly identified.[2-4,24] The presence of all three immunoglobulins, IgG, IgA, and IgM, along with the two complement components, C1q and C3, is known as "full house" staining and is highly suggestive of LN. Staining for fibrin-fibrinogen is common in the distribution of crescents and segmental necrotizing lesions. The "tissue ANA,"[39] nuclear staining of renal epithelial cells in

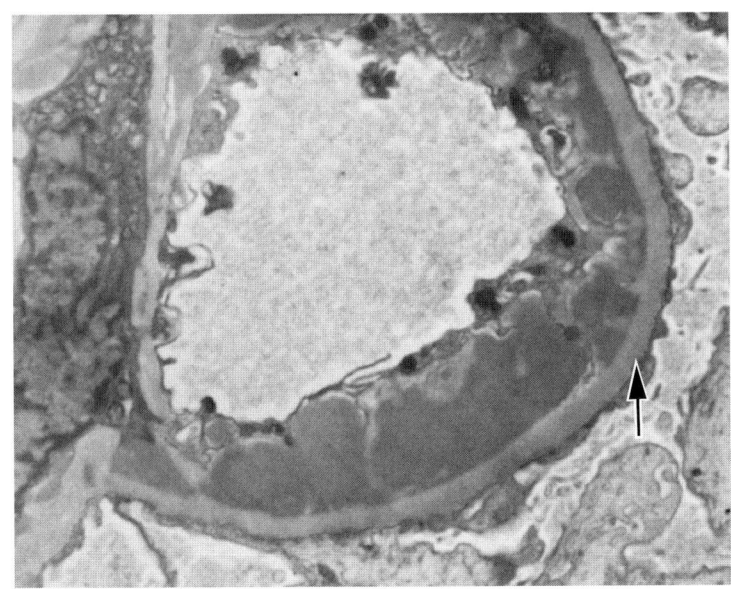

FIGURE 32-9 Lupus nephritis class IV. Electron micrograph showing a large subendothelial electron-dense deposit as well as a few small subepithelial deposits (*arrow*) (×1200).

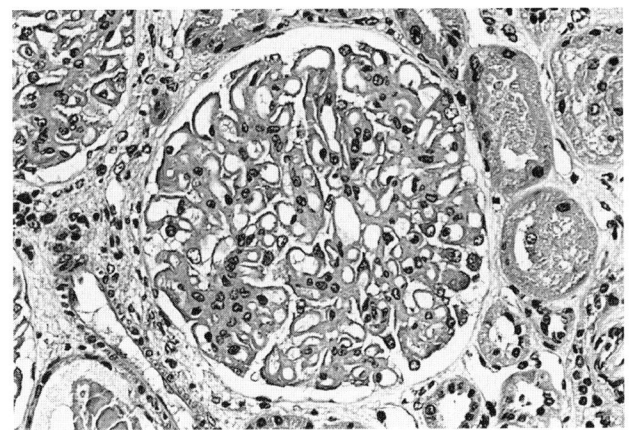

FIGURE 32-10 Lupus nephritis class V. There is diffuse uniform thickening of glomerular basement membranes accompanied by mild segmental mesangial hypercellularity (hematoxylin and eosin, ×320).

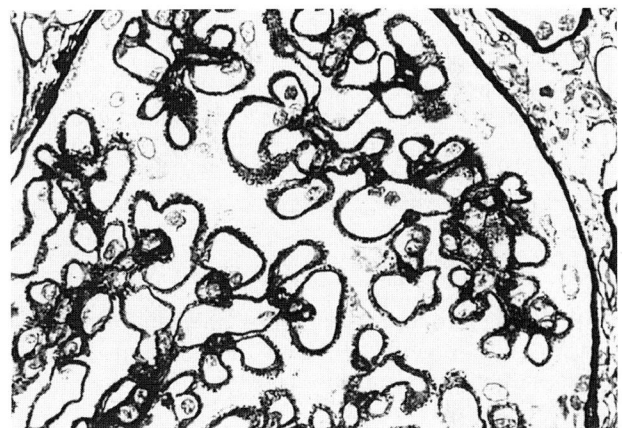

FIGURE 32-11 Lupus nephritis class V. Silver stain highlights glomerular basement membrane spikes projecting outward from the glomerular basement membranes toward the urinary space (Jones methenamine silver, ×800).

sections stained with fluoresceinated antisera to human IgG, is a frequent finding in any class. It results from the binding of patient's own ANA to nuclei exposed in the course of cryostat sectioning.

Electron Microscopy

The distribution of glomerular, tubulointerstitial, and vascular deposits seen by EM correlates closely with that observed by IF.[2-6,24] Deposits are typically electron dense and granular. Some exhibit focal organization with a "fingerprint" substructure composed of curvilinear parallel arrays measuring 10 to 15 nm in diameter.[2,4,24] Tubuloreticular inclusions (TRIs), intracellular branching tubular structures measuring 24 nm in diameter located within dilated cisternae of the endoplasmic reticulum of glomerular and vascular endothelial cells, are commonly observed in SLE biopsies.[2,4,24] TRIs are inducible upon exposure to INF-α (so-called "INF footprints") and are also present in biopsies of HIV-infected patients and those with some other viral infections.[40]

Activity and Chronicity

Some investigators have also found it useful to grade biopsies for features of activity (potentially reversible lesions) and chronicity (irreversible lesions). In the widely used National Institutes of Health (NIH) system, for an activity index, the biopsy is graded on a scale of 0 to 3+ for each of six histologic features including endocapillary proliferation, glomerular leukocyte infiltration, wire loop deposits, fibrinoid necrosis and karyorrhexis, cellular crescents, and interstitial inflammation.[41] The severe lesions of crescents, and fibrinoid necrosis are assigned double weight. The sum of the individual components yields a total histologic activity index score of from 0 to 24. Likewise, a chronicity index of 0 to 12 is derived from the sum of glomerulosclerosis, fibrous crescents, tubular atrophy, and interstitial fibrosis, each graded on a scale of 0 to 3+. Studies at the NIH correlated both a high activity index (>12) and especially a high chronicity index (>4) with a poor 10-year renal survival.[41] However, in several other large studies, neither the activity index nor the chronicity index correlated well with long-term prognosis.[17,42,43] Other NIH

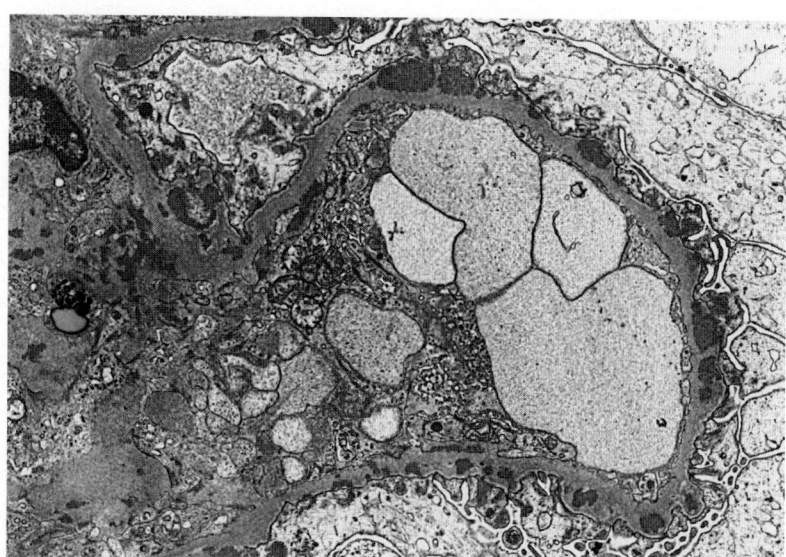

FIGURE 32-12 Lupus nephritis class V. Electron micrograph showing numerous subepithelial electron-dense deposits as well as mesangial deposits (×5000).

studies concluded that a combination of an elevated activity index (>7) and chronicity index (>3) predicts a poor long-term outcome.[41] A major value of calculating the activity and chronicity indices is in the comparison of sequential biopsies in individual patients. This provides useful information about the efficacy of therapy and the relative degree of reversible versus irreversible lesions.[2-4,24,44,45]

Tubulointerstitial Disease

Some patients with SLE have major changes in the tubulointerstitial compartment.[46-50] Active tubulointerstitial lesions include edema and inflammatory infiltrates, including T lymphocytes (both CD4 and CD8 positive cells), monocytes, and plasma cells.[50] Tubulointerstitial immune deposits of immunoglobulin or complement may be present along the basement membranes of tubules and interstitial capillaries. Severe acute interstitial changes and tubulointerstitial immune deposits are most commonly found in patients with active proliferative class III and IV LN. The degree of interstitial inflammation does not correlate well with the presence or quantity of tubulointerstitial immune deposits.[46,48] Interstitial fibrosis or tubular atrophy are commonly encountered in the more chronic phases of LN. One study documented a strong inverse correlation between the degree of tubular damage and renal survival.[47] In addition, renal survival was higher for patients with less expression on their renal biopsy of the adhesion molecule intercellular adhesion molecule 1 (ICAM-1).[49]

Vascular lesions are not included in either the ISN/RPS classification or in the NIH activity and chronicity indices despite their frequent occurrence and clinical significance.[27,51-53] The most frequent vascular lesion is simple vascular immune deposition, which is most common in patients with active class III and IV biopsies. The vessels may show no abnormalities by LM, but by IF and EM, there are granular immune deposits in the media and intima of small arteries and arterioles. Noninflammatory necrotizing vasculopathy, most common in arterioles in active class IV LN, is a fibrinoid necrotizing lesion without leukocyte infiltration that severely narrows or occludes the arteriolar lumen. True

inflammatory vasculitis resembling polyangiitis is extremely rare in biopsies from SLE patients. It may be limited to the kidney or be part of a more generalized systemic vasculitis.[27,52,53] Thrombotic microangiopathy involving vessels and glomeruli may be associated with anticardiolipin (ACLN) or APL antibody or hemolytic-uremic syndrome (HUS) and thrombotic thrombocytopenic purpura (TTP)–like syndrome caused by autoantibody to the von Willebrand's factor cleaving protease.[27,52-53]

A number of other renal diseases have been documented on biopsy in SLE patients, including podocytopathies with features of minimal change disease, focal segmental glomerulosclerosis (FSGS), or collapsing glomerulopathy.[54-56] In some, the relationship between SLE and the podocytopathy suggests this is not a coincidental occurrence but is related to SLE-induced cytokine effects on podocyte function.

Clinical Manifestations

Although SLE predominantly affects young females, the clinical manifestations are similar in both sexes and in adults and children.[5-8] Organ systems commonly affected include the kidneys; joints; serosal surfaces, including pleura and pericardium; CNS; and skin. In addition, cardiac, hepatic, pulmonary, hematopoietic, and gastrointestinal (GI) involvement is not infrequent.

Renal involvement often develops concurrently or shortly after the onset of SLE and may follow a protracted course with periods of remissions and exacerbations. Clinical renal involvement usually correlates well with the degree of glomerular involvement in SLE. However, some patients may have disproportionately severe vascular or tubulointerstitial lesions that dominate the clinical course.[27,46,53]

Patients with ISN/RPS class I biopsies often have no, or at most mild, evidence of clinical renal disease. Likewise, most patients with disease confined to the mesangial regions of the glomeruli (ISN/RPS class II) have mild or minimal clinical renal findings.[1-4,8,32] They may have a high anti-DNA antibody titer and low serum complement, but the urinary sediment is inactive, hypertension is infrequent, proteinuria is usually less than 1 g/day, and the serum creatinine and glomerular filtration rate (GFR) are usually normal. Nephrotic range proteinuria is extremely rare unless there is a superimposed podocytopathy.[54,55]

Class III, focal proliferative LN, is often associated with active lupus serologies, although the degree of serologic activity does not necessarily correlate with the histologic severity.[17,33] Hypertension and active urinary sediment are commonly present. Proteinuria is often more than 1 g/day, and one-fourth to one-third of patients with focal LN have the nephrotic syndrome at presentation. Many patients have an elevated serum creatinine at presentation. Patients with less extensive glomerular proliferation, fewer necrotizing features, and no crescents are more likely to be normotensive and have preserved renal function.

Patients with ISN/RPS class IV, diffuse proliferative LN, typically present with the most active and severe clinical features. These patients often have high anti-DNA antibody titers, low serum complement levels, and very active urinary sediment with erythrocytes and cellular casts on urinalysis.[1-4,8,9,17,31,34,35] Virtually all have proteinuria, and as many as half of the patients will have the nephrotic syndrome. Likewise, hypertension and renal dysfunction are typical. Even when the serum creatinine is in the "normal range," the GFR is usually depressed.

Patients with membranous LN, ISN/RPS class V typically present with proteinuria, edema, and other manifestations of the nephrotic syndrome.[1-4,8,17,36-38] However, as many as 40% will have proteinuria of less than 3 g/day and 16% to 20% have less than 1 g/day. Only about 60% of membranous LN patients have a low serum complement and an elevated anti-DNA antibody titer at presentation.[17] However, hypertension and renal dysfunction may occur without superimposed proliferative lesions. Patients with membranous LN may present with apparently idiopathic nephrotic syndrome before developing other clinical and laboratory manifestations of SLE.[8,17,36-38] In addition, they are predisposed to thrombotic complications such as renal vein thrombosis and pulmonary emboli.[27,52,53] Patients with mixed membranous and proliferative patterns on biopsy have clinical features that reflect both disease components.

End-stage LN, ISN/RPS class VI, is usually the result of "burnt-out" LN of long duration.[8,9,24] It typically develops after years of lupus flares alternating with periods of inactivity. Some of the renal histologic damage may represent nonimmunologic progression of sclerosis mediated by hyperfiltration in remnant nephrons. Although the lesions are sclerosing and inactive, some class VI patients still manifest microhematuria and proteinuria. Virtually all patients have both hypertension and a decreased GFR. Levels of anti-DNA antibodies and serum complement levels often normalize at this late stage of disease.

"Silent LN"[3,57] has been described in patients without clinical evidence of renal involvement despite biopsy evidence of active proliferative LN. Some define "silent LN" as active biopsy lesions without active urinary sediment, proteinuria, or a depressed GFR, and others require negative lupus serologies as well. Although silent LN is well described in some studies, others have been unable to find even isolated examples.[3,17] It appears to be a rare phenomenon, and it is highly likely that even patients with true "silent disease" will manifest clinical renal involvement shortly into their course.

Serologic Tests

The presence of antibodies directed against nuclear antigens (ANA) and especially against DNA (anti-DNA) antibodies are included in the ARA criteria for SLE, and are commonly used to monitor the disease course.[1,3,6,8,14] ANA's are a highly sensitive screen for SLE, being found in more than 90% of untreated patients, but they are not specific for SLE and occur in many other rheumatologic and non-rheumatologic conditions.[3,6,7,24] Neither the particular pattern of ANA fluorescence (homogeneous, speckled, nucleolar, rim) nor the titer of the ANA correlates well with the presence or the severity of renal involvement in SLE.

Autoantibodies directed against double-stranded DNA (ant-dsDNA) are a more specific but less sensitive marker of SLE and are found in almost three-fourths of untreated active SLE patients.[3,6,14] These antibodies may be detected by the Farr radioimmunoassay, by an IF test directed against the DNA in the kinetoplast of the single-celled organism *Crithidia luciliae*, and by enzyme-linked immunosorbent assay (ELISA).[14,22] Anti-ds DNA IgG antibodies of high avidity that fix complement have correlated best with the presence of renal disease,[3,6,8] and such anti-dsDNA antibodies have been found in the glomerular immune deposits of murine and human LN.[3,14,58,59,63] High anti-dsDNA antibody titers correlate well with clinical activity.[3,6,14,23] Anti–single-stranded DNA antibodies (anti-ssDNA), commonly found in SLE and other collagen vascular diseases, do not correlate with clinical lupus activity.

Autoantibodies directed against ribonuclear antigens are commonly present in lupus patients and include anti-Sm and anti-nRNP against extracted nuclear antigen (ENA).[6,14,22,23] Anti-Sm antibodies, although very specific for SLE, are found in only about 25% of lupus patients and are of unclear prognostic value. Anti-nRNP antibodies, found in over one-third of SLE patients, are also present in many rheumatologic diseases, particularly mixed connective tissue disease (MCTD).[14,22,60] Anti-Ro/SSA antibodies are directed against the protein complex of a cytoplasmic RNA and are present in 25% to 30% of SLE patients. Anti-La/SSB autoantibodies, directed against a nuclear RNP antigen, are present in from 5% to 15% of lupus patients. Neither of the latter two antibodies is specific for SLE and both are found in other collagen vascular diseases, especially Sjögren's syndrome. Maternal anti-Ro antibodies are important in the pathogenesis of neonatal lupus and the development of cardiac conduction abnormalities in newborns.[61] Anti-Ro antibodies are also associated with a unique dermal form of lupus manifesting psoriaform features, with SLE patients who are homozygous C2 deficient, and with a vasculitic disease associated with CNS involvement and cutaneous ulcers.[62] In addition, lupus patients may develop antibodies directed against histones, endothelial cells, phospholipids, the N-methyl D aspartate receptor (associated with CNS disease in SLE), and ANCAs.[64-67]

Levels of total hemolytic complement (CH50) and complement components are usually decreased during active SLE and especially active LN.[1-4,6,8] Levels of C4 and C3 often decline before a clinical flare of SLE. Serial monitoring of complement levels, with a decline in levels predicting a flare, is considered more useful clinically than an isolated depressed C3 or C4 value.[3,8] Likewise, normalization of depressed serum complement levels is often associated with improved renal outcome.[68] Levels of total complement and C3 may be decreased in the absence of active systemic or renal disease in patients with extensive dermatologic involvement by SLE. Several heritable complement deficiency states (including C1r, C1s, C2, C4, C5, and C8) have been associated with SLE, and such patients may have depressed total complement levels despite inactive disease.[69]

Other immunologic tests commonly found in lupus patients include elevated levels of CICs, a positive lupus band test result, and the presence of cryoglobulins. None correlates well with SLE or LN activity.[8,70,71,72] In both SLE and isolated discoid lupus, immune complex deposits containing IgG antibody and complement are found along the dermal–epidermal junction of involved skin lesions.[3,8,71] The presence of granular deposits in clinically unaffected skin (the lupus band test) is usually found only in patients with systemic disease. However, the specificity and sensitivity of this test is debated, and it requires IF of the dermal biopsy.[3] Mixed IgG–IgM cryoglobulins containing anti-DNA antibodies, DNA, and fibronectin may be found in patients with SLE and active renal disease. Patients with SLE commonly have a false-positive Venereal Disease Research Laboratory (VDRL) test result because of the presence of APL antibodies.[3]

Monitoring Clinical Disease

It is important to be able to predict systemic and renal relapses and prevent their occurrence through the judicious use of immunosuppressive agents. Serial measurements of many serologic tests (including complement components; autoantibodies; erythrocyte sedimentation rate [ESR]; C-reactive protein [CRP]; CICs; and recently, levels of cytokines and interleukins [ILs]) have been used to predict flares of lupus activity. Although there is controversy regarding the value of serum C3 and C4 levels and anti-DNA antibody titers in predicting a clinical flare of SLE or active renal disease, these have yet to be replaced by new biomarkers of activity.[3,8,72] Serum levels of anti-ds DNA typically increase, and serum complement levels typically decrease as the clinical activity of SLE increases, typically preceding clinical renal deterioration. In patients with active renal involvement, the urinalysis frequently reveals dysmorphic erythrocytes, red blood cell (RBC) casts, and other formed elements. An increase in proteinuria from levels of less than 1 g/day to over this amount and certainly from low levels to nephrotic levels is a clear indication of either increased activity or a change in renal histologic class.[3,17]

Drug-Induced Lupus

A variety of medications may induce a lupus-like syndrome or exacerbate an underlying predisposition to SLE. Those metabolized by acetylation such as procainamide and hydralazine have been common causes.[73,74] This occurs more commonly in patients who are slow acetylators because of a genetic decrease in hepatic N-acyltransferase.[75] Diltiazem, minocycline, penicillamine, isoniazid, methyldopa, chlorpromazine, and practolol are other potential causes of drug-induced lupus.[73,74,76,77] A number of other drugs that have been associated less frequently with this syndrome include phenytoin, quinidine, propylthiouracil (PTU), sulfonamides, lithium, β-blockers, nitrofurantoin, periodic acid-Schiff (PAS), captopril, glyburide, hydrochlorothiazide, INF-α, carbamazepine, sulfasalazine, rifampin, and tumor necrosis factor-α (TNF-α) blockers.[78,79] Clinical manifestations of drug-induced lupus include fever, rash, myalgias, arthralgias and arthritis, and serositis. CNS and renal involvement are relatively uncommon.[73,80,81] Although elevated anti-DNA antibodies and depressed serum complement levels are unusual in drug-induced lupus, antihistone autoantibodies are present in more than 95% of patients.[73] These are usually formed against a complex of the histone dimer H2A-H2B and DNA and other histone components.[73,82] Antihistone antibodies are also present in the vast majority of idiopathic, non–drug-related SLE patients, but they are directed primarily against different histone antigens (H1 and H2B).[73] The presence of antihistone antibodies in the absence of anti-DNA antibodies and other serologic markers for SLE is also indicative of drug-induced disease.[73] The diagnosis of drug-induced lupus depends on documenting the offending agent and achieving a remission after withdrawal of the drug. The primary treatment consists of discontinuing the offending drug, although nonsteroidal antiinflammatory drugs (NSAIDs) and corticosteroids may be effective in suppressing the serositis and constitutional symptoms.

Pregnancy and Systemic Lupus Erythematosus

Because SLE occurs so commonly in women of childbearing age, the issue of pregnancy arises often in the care of this population. Independent but related issues are the health of the mother both in terms of flares of lupus activity and progression of renal disease and the fate of the fetus. It is unclear whether flares of lupus activity occur more commonly during pregnancy or shortly after delivery.[83-86] Some controlled studies found no increase in lupus flares in pregnant patients versus nonpregnant lupus control participants.[83-86] Patients with quiescent lupus at the time of pregnancy are less likely to experience exacerbations of SLE. However, in two small retrospective studies, flares of lupus activity, including renal involvement, occurred in more than 50% of the pregnancies.[85,86] This was significantly greater than the rate of flare after delivery and in nonpregnant lupus patients.

Pregnancy in patients with preexisting LN has also been associated with worsening of renal function.[87,88] This is less likely to occur in patients who have been in remission for at least 6 months. Patients with hypertension are likely to develop higher blood pressure levels, and those with proteinuria are likely to have increased levels during pregnancy. Patients with elevated serum creatinine levels are most likely to experience worsening of renal function and to be at highest risk for fetal loss. Although high-dose corticosteroids, cyclosporine, and azathioprine have all been used in pregnant lupus patients, their safety is unclear. Cyclophosphamide is contraindicated because of its teratogenicity, and newer agents such as mycophenolate and rituximab are not recommended, making the treatment of patients with severe LN difficult.

The rate of fetal loss in all SLE patients in most series is 20% to 40% and may approach 50% in some series.[84-88] Although fetal mortality is increased in SLE patients with renal disease, it may be decreasing in the modern treatment era.[84,85,87-90] Patients with ACLN or APL antibodies, hypertension, or heavy proteinuria are at higher risk for fetal loss.[84] One review of 10 studies in more than 550 women with SLE found that fetal death occurred in 38% to 59% of all pregnant SLE patients with antiphospholipid antibodies compared with 16% to 20% of those without these antibodies.[91]

Dialysis and Transplantation

The percentage of patients with severe LN who progress to dialysis or transplantation varies from 5% to 50% depending on the population studied, the length of follow-up, and the response to therapy.[3-5,17,92-95] Many patients with progressive renal failure have a resolution of their extrarenal manifestations of disease and serologic activity.[96,97] With more prolonged time on dialysis, the incidence of clinically active patients declines further, decreasing in one study from 55% at the onset of dialysis to less than 10% by the fifth year and 0% by the tenth year of dialysis.[97] Patients with end-stage renal disease (ESRD) caused by LN have increased mortality during the early months of dialysis because of infectious complications of immunosuppressive therapy.[96,97] Long-term survival for SLE patients on chronic hemodialysis or continuous ambulatory peritoneal dialysis is similar to that of other patients with chronic kidney disease (CKD) stage V, with the most common cause of death being cardiovascular.[66,97]

Most renal transplant programs allow patients with active SLE to undergo a period of dialysis for 3 to 12 months to allow clinical and serologic disease activity to become quiescent.[97] Allograft survival rates in patients with LN are comparable to those of the rest of the transplant population.[3,98-102] The rate of recurrent SLE in the allograft has been low—less than 4% in most series[98-102]—although in several recent reports, a higher recurrence rate has been noted.[100] The prevalence of recurrent LN was only 2.44% in a 20-year study of nearly 7000 lupus transplant recipients and was more common in black, female, and younger patients.[101] When surveillance biopsies are used, however, recurrences could be detected in as many as 54% of a small cohort of lupus transplant recipients, although this was mostly subclinical mild mesangial LN, class I or II.[102] The low rate of clinically important recurrence may be partly attributable to the immunosuppressive action of the renal failure before transplantation and partly to the immunosuppressive regimens used to prevent allograft rejection. Lupus patients with an APL antibody may benefit from anticoagulation therapy during the posttransplant period.[103,104]

Course and Prognosis of Lupus Nephritis

The course of patients with LN is extremely varied with from less than 5% to more than 60% of patients developing progressive renal failure.[1,5,3,17,33,44,92-95,105] This course is defined by the initial pattern and severity of renal involvement as modified by therapy, exacerbations of the disease, and complications of treatment. The prognosis has clearly improved in recent decades with wider and more judicious use of new immunosuppressives. Most studies have found additional prognostic value of renal biopsy over clinical data in patients with LN.[106-109]

Patients with lesions limited to the renal mesangium generally have an excellent course and prognosis.[1-4,24] Those who do not transform into other patterns are unlikely to develop progressive renal failure, and mortality is attributable to extrarenal manifestations and complications of therapy. Patients with focal proliferative disease have an extremely varied course. Those with mild proliferation in a small percentage of glomeruli respond well to therapy, and fewer than 5% progress to renal failure over 5 years.[1-6,8,17,109,110] Patients with more proliferation, necrotizing features, or crescent formation have a prognosis more akin to patients with class IV diffuse proliferative disease. Class III patients may transform into class IV over time. Some patients with very active segmental proliferative and necrotizing lesions resembling ANCA-associated small vessel vasculitis have a worse renal prognosis than other patients with focal proliferative lesions.[26,35,111]

Patients with diffuse proliferative disease have the least favorable prognosis in most older series.[1-4,8,17,24,33,34] Nevertheless, the prognosis for this group has markedly improved, with renal survivals now exceeding 90% in some series of patients treated with modern immunosuppressive agents.[3,34,35,110,112] In recent trials from the NIH, the risk of doubling the serum creatinine, a surrogate marker for progressive renal disease, at 5 years in diffuse proliferative lupus treated with cyclophosphamide-containing regimens ranged from 35% to less than 5%.[93,94,112] In an Italian study of diffuse proliferative LN, survival was 77% at 10 years and above 90% if extrarenal deaths were excluded.[34] In a U.S. study of 89 patients with diffuse proliferative LN, renal survival was 89% at 1 year and 71% at 5 years.[10] It is unclear whether the improved survival in these recent series is largely attributable to improved immunosuppression or better supportive care and clinical use of these medications.

In the past, some studies have found age, gender, and race to be as important prognostic variables as clinical features in patient and renal survival in SLE.[1,3,4,10-12,16,108,113-115] However, a consistent finding is that African Americans have a greater frequency of LN and a worse renal and overall prognosis.[1,3,4,10-12,113-115] This worse prognosis appears to relate to both biologic or genetic factors and to socioeconomic ones.[11,12] In a study from the NIH of 65 patients with severe LN, clinical features at study entry associated with progressive renal failure included age, black race, hematocrit less than 26%, and serum creatinine greater than 2.4 mg/dL.[41] Patients with combined activity index (>7) plus chronicity index (>3) on renal biopsy, as well as those with the combination of cellular crescents and interstitial fibrosis also had a worse prognosis.

In another U.S. study of 89 patients with diffuse proliferative LN, none of the following features impacted on renal survival: age, gender, SLE duration, uncontrolled hypertension, or any individual histologic variable.[10] Entry serum creatinine over 3.0 mg/dL, combined activity and chronicity indices on biopsy, and black race did predict a poor outcome. Five-year renal survival was 95% for the white patients but only 58% for the black patients. In a study of more than 125 LN patients with WHO class III or IV from New York, both racial and socioeconomic factors influenced the poor outcomes in African Americans and Hispanics.[11] An evaluation of 203 patients from the Miami area confirmed worse renal outcomes in African Americans and Hispanics related to both biologic and economic factors.[12]

More rapid and more complete renal remissions are associated with improved long-term prognosis.[116,117] Renal flares during the course of SLE also may predict a poor renal outcome.[105,118,119] Relapses of severe LN over 5 to 10 years of follow-up occur in up to 50% of patients and usually respond less well and more slowly to repeated courses of therapy.[3,105,120-122] A retrospective analysis of 70 Italian patients in which more than half had diffuse proliferative disease found an excellent patient survival (100% at 10 years and 86% at 20 years) as well as preserved renal function with a probability of not doubling the serum creatinine to be 85% at 10 years and 72% at 20 years.[105] Most patients in this study were white, which likely influenced the excellent long-term prognosis. Multivariable analysis in the Italian study showed men, those who were more anemic, and especially those with flare-ups of disease to have a worse outcome. Patients with renal flares of any type had seven times the risk of renal failure, and those with rapid rises in creatinine had 27 times the chance of doubling their serum creatinine. Another Italian study of 91 patients with diffuse proliferative LN showed more than 50% having a renal flare, which correlated with a younger age at biopsy (younger than 30 years old), higher activity index, and karyorrhexis on biopsy.[118] The number of flares, nephritic flares, and flares with increased proteinuria correlated with a doubling of the serum creatinine. The role of relapses in predicting progressive disease has been documented by others as well, although relapse does not invariably predict a bad outcome.[123]

Although an elevated anti-DNA antibody titer and low serum complement levels have correlated with active renal involvement, they have not correlated with long-term prognosis.[3,10,17,92,105] In several studies, anemia has been a poor prognostic finding regardless of the underlying etiology.[41,105] Severe hypertension has also been related to renal prognosis in some studies but not others.[17] Renal dysfunction as noted by an elevated serum creatinine or decreased GFR or by heavy proteinuria and the nephrotic syndrome are indicative of a poor renal prognosis in the vast majority of series.[1-4,7,8,116] However, not all studies have found an elevation of the initial serum creatinine to predict a poor long-term prognosis, and in some, the initial serum creatinine only predicted short-term renal survival.[10] Other renal features such as duration of nephritis and rate of decline of GFR may also predict prognosis.[92,110]

Finally, histologic features such as the class, the degree of activity and chronicity, and the severity of tubulointerstitial damage have also predicted prognosis. In a number of studies, the pattern of renal involvement, especially when using the ISN/RPS or older WHO classification, has been a useful guide to prognosis.[1-4,8,17,30,31] In NIH trials, patients with severe proliferative LN with a higher activity index or chronicity index were more likely to have progressive renal failure.[110] Other studies with different referral populations could not confirm this.[2,4,8,17,24,42,43] Regardless, the contribution of chronic renal scarring to a poor long-term outcome has been confirmed by many studies.[49,92,118,123,124] Some studies have found the initial renal biopsy to have little predictive value but rather certain features on a repeat biopsy at 6 months to be strong predictors of doubling the serum creatinine or progression to renal failure.[47,125] These include ongoing inflammation with cellular crescents, macrophages in the tubular lumens, persistent immune deposits (especially C3) on IF, and persistent subendothelial and mesangial deposits. More recent studies by this group suggest that reversal of interstitial fibrosis and glomerular segmental scarring along with remission

of initial inflammation and immune deposition is an important favorable prognostic finding on the 6-month biopsy.[123] Thus, chronic changes on biopsy are not always cumulative and immutable, and their reversal may be crucial in preventing ultimate renal failure when new acute lesions develop.

The natural history of membranous LN is less clear. In early studies with short follow-up periods, the course of membranous LN appeared far better than that of patients with active proliferative lesions.[32] Subsequent studies with longer follow-up periods suggested a worse outcome for those with membranous LN with persistent nephrotic syndrome.[17] Recent retrospective studies with long-term follow-up show that 5-year renal survival rates largely depend upon whether patients have pure membranous lesions (class V) or superimposed proliferative lesions in a focal (class III + V) or diffuse (IV + V) distribution.[37,38] One U.S. study found that the 10-year survival rate was 72% for patients with pure membranous lesions but only 20% to 48% for those with superimposed proliferative lesions.[37] Black race, elevated serum creatinine, higher degrees of proteinuria, hypertension, and transformation to another WHO pattern all portended a worse outcome.[1,4] The poor survival in blacks with membranous LN may explain the excellent results in retrospective Italian studies, which include mostly whites. One such Italian study found the 10-year survival of membranous LN patients to be 93%.[38] Even in this Italian population, survival was far better than in patients with superimposed proliferative lesions classes III + V or IV + V. Thus, at least in part, the variability of prognosis in older studies can be explained by the differences in racial background, histology, and therapy.

Treatment of Lupus Nephritis

The treatment of many patients with severe LN remains controversial.[1,3,8] Although recent controlled randomized studies have better defined the course and therapy for this group, the most effective and least toxic regimen for any given patient is often less clear. Effective therapy in severe LN has been available since the widespread use of cyclophosphamide. Newer regimens have been developed with the hope of attaining equal or greater efficacy with less toxicity. The concept of more vigorous initial therapy during the "induction" treatment phase followed by more prolonged lower dose therapy as a "maintenance phase" is now widely accepted.[1,3,8]

Patients with ISN/RPS class I and II biopsies have an excellent renal prognosis and need no therapy directed to the kidney. Transformation to another histologic class is usually heralded by increasing proteinuria and activity of the urinary sediment. At this point, repeat renal biopsy may serve as a guide to therapy.[8] ISN/RPS class III patients with only few mild proliferative lesions and no necrotizing features or crescent formation have a good prognosis and often respond to a short course of high-dose corticosteroid therapy or a brief course of other immunosuppressive agents. Patients with greater numbers of affected glomeruli, and those with necrotizing features and crescents usually require more vigorous therapy similar to patients with diffuse proliferative LN.

Patients with diffuse proliferative disease, ISN/RPS class IV lesions, require aggressive treatment to avoid irreversible renal damage and progression to ESRD.[1-4,8,34,35,110,112,116] The ideal immunosuppressive regimen should be individualized and based on the patient's prior therapy, risk and concern over side effects (e.g., cyclophosphamide-induced alopecia and infertility), compliance, and tolerability. Regimens may include daily or alternate-day corticosteroids, azathioprine, intravenous (IV) pulse methylprednisolone, oral or IV cyclophosphamide, cyclosporine, tacrolimus, mycophenolate mofetil (MMF), or rituximab. Although a number of other treatments have been studied, they have proven less effective or too toxic or have not yet been proven comparable to these agents in controlled randomized trials. Because no current regimen of immunosuppressives is universally effective or without the risk of major side effects, newer therapeutic agents are being developed to treat active disease, prevent flares, and minimize the side effects of current regimens.

Prednisone has been used for more than 50 years to treat LN. Despite the lack of controlled trials, higher doses of corticosteroids appeared more effective than low-dose therapy (<30 mg/day of prednisone) in retrospective studies.[1,3-4,8] Initial use of high dose corticosteroid treatment for severe LN, reserving other immunosuppressive agents for patients who fail to respond to several months of therapy, is still used by some clinicians for limited focal proliferative disease. However, for severe proliferative LN, either class III or class IV, most clinicians institute corticosteroids along with other immunosuppressives.[3] Some have used regimens of 1 mg/kg/day of prednisone, converting to 2 mg/kg/day on alternate days after 4 to 6 weeks of treatment. Others prefer to start with pulses of IV methylprednisolone.

There have been few randomized trials using pulse IV methylprednisolone therapy versus other immunosuppressives for severe LN.[93,94] Initial trials of pulse methylprednisolone in diffuse proliferative disease showed favorable results using three consecutive daily 1-g pulses.[1,3] Subsequent uncontrolled trials using a variety of immunosuppressives with the pulse steroids gave favorable results. Two NIH trials have found pulse corticosteroids to be less effective than IV cyclophosphamide in preventing progressive renal failure.[93,94,130] In one trial, 48% of the patients treated with pulse steroids doubled their serum creatinine at 5 years compared with only 25% of the cyclophosphamide-treated group.[94]

Controlled randomized trials at the NIH and elsewhere have helped clarify the role of cyclophosphamide in the treatment of patients with severe LN.[44,93,94,112,126-128] In one seminal trial, patients were randomly assigned to regimens of high-dose corticosteroids for 6 months or oral cyclophosphamide, oral azathioprine, combined oral azathioprine plus cyclophosphamide, or IV cyclophosphamide every third month, all given with low-dose corticosteroids.[112] Evaluation at 120 months showed superior renal survival in the IV cyclophosphamide group versus the steroid group. At longer follow-up to 200 months, the renal survival of the azathioprine group was statistically no better than that of the corticosteroid group.[112] A subsequent Dutch collaborative trial found remission rates comparable between oral azathioprine and cyclophosphamide but more relapses and worse long-term outcome with the azathioprine.[129] Thus, for a number of years, cyclophosphamide was the most effective immunosuppressive agent for LN. Because side effects in the NIH trial appeared least severe in the IV cyclophosphamide group, subsequent protocols at the NIH used the drug IV. Subsequent trials at the NIH and elsewhere have also used monthly pulses

of IV cyclophosphamide for 6 consecutive months as opposed to every third monthly regimens.[120,126-128]

Other groups have confirmed the benefits and response rate of IV cyclophosphamide regimens in patients with severe LN.[9,44,120,126,127] In most patients treated with IV cyclophosphamide, side effects such as hemorrhagic cystitis, alopecia, and neoplasms have been infrequent.[1,3-6,8] Exceptions are menstrual irregularities and premature menopause, which are most common in women older than 25 years of age who have received IV cyclophosphamide for more than 6 months.[130] The dose of IV cyclophosphamide must be reduced in patients with significant renal impairment and adjusted for some removal by hemodialysis in ESRD patients. Mercaptoethane sulfonate (MESNA) therapy has been beneficial in reducing bladder complications from cyclophosphamide.[131]

A three-armed, controlled, randomized trial at NIH of 1 year of monthly doses of IV methylprednisolone versus monthly IV cyclophosphamide for 6 months and then every third month versus the combination of both therapies found the remission rate was highest with the combined treatment regimen (85%) as opposed to cyclophosphamide alone (62%) and methylprednisolone alone (29%).[93] Mortality was low and similar in all groups. Long follow-up indicated that drug toxicity was not different between the cyclophosphamide group and the combined cyclophosphamide–methylprednisolone group.[128] It is likely that through higher sustained remissions and fewer relapses, fewer patients required repeated treatments in the combined cyclophosphamide–steroid treated group. Moreover, the long-term efficacy, especially in terms of renal outcomes, was greatest for the combination therapy group. Thus, combined treatment with solumedrol pulses and IV cyclophosphamide pulses became a standard therapy for patients with severe LN despite problems with side effects. However, it should be noted that some groups have achieved equal efficacy and few side effects using short courses of oral cyclophosphamide[72,132] followed by other immunosuppressives.

MMF has proven to be an effective immunosuppressive in transplant patients and patients with a variety of other immunologic diseases.[133,134] It is a reversible inhibitor of inosine monophosphate dehydrogenase required for purine synthesis and blocks B- and T-cell proliferation, inhibits antibody formation, and decreases expression of adhesion molecules, among other effects. MMF is effective in treating murine LN.[133] MMF was shown to have efficacy and reduced complications compared with standard treatment regimens in a number of uncontrolled trials in LN.[135-137] In one 6-month trial of Chinese patients randomized to either MMF or IV pulse cyclophosphamide for induction therapy of severe LN,[138] proteinuria and microhematuria decreased more in the MMF-treated patients than in the cytotoxic group, with renal impairment before and after therapy, activity index on biopsy before and after therapy, and serologic improvement being equivalent. MMF was better tolerated with fewer GI side effects and fewer infections.

In another randomized controlled trial of patients given either a regimen of prednisone plus oral MMF or a regimen of prednisone plus cyclophosphamide orally for 6 months followed by oral azathioprine for another 6 months, both regimens proved similar in efficacy.[139] Of the MMF group, 81% achieved complete and 14% partial remission versus 76% complete and 14% partial remission for the cyclophosphamide–azathioprine group. Treatment failures, relapses after therapy, discontinuations of therapy, mortality, and time to remission were similar. Longer follow-up at 4 years with the addition of more patients showed MMF to have comparable efficacy to cyclophosphamide with no significant difference in complete or partial remissions, doubling of baseline creatinine, or relapses. Significantly fewer MMF-treated patients developed severe infections, leukopenia, or amenorrhea, and all deaths and renal failure were in the cyclophosphamide group.[140]

A multicenter U.S. study compared induction therapy in 140 patients with severe class III and IV LN, including more than 50% blacks, most with heavy proteinuria and active urinary sediment.[141] Patients were randomized to receive either standard monthly pulses of 0.5 to 1 g/m^2 of IV cyclophosphamide for 6 months or 2 to 3 g/day of oral MMF. Although this was designed as an equivalency study, the MMF proved superior in attaining both complete remissions and complete and partial remissions. The side effect profile also appeared better with MMF. At 3-year follow–up, there was a trend to less renal failure and mortality with MMF. Thus, in a patient population at high risk for poor renal outcomes, MMF proved superior to IV cyclophosphamide.

A subsequent international multicenter randomized controlled trial compared similar regimens of MMF with IV cyclophosphamide for induction therapy in 370 LN patients with ISN/RPS classes III, IV, or V.[142] This study found virtually identical rates of complete and partial remission (>50%) improvement of renal function and proteinuria and mortality rates between the two regimens. Diarrhea and GI side effects were most common in the MMF group, and nausea, vomiting and alopecia were more common in the cyclophosphamide group. In the small group of about 30 patients with a greatly reduced GFR (<30 mL/min), MMF proved at least as effective, if not more so, than IV cyclophosphamide. In an analysis of different geographic and ethnic backgrounds, MMF proved more uniformly effective across different groups.[143] Thus, taken together, these two large, randomized, controlled trials support the use of MMF as a first-line regimen for the treatment of patients with severe LN.

Another approach to obtain efficacy with cyclophosphamide while reducing toxic side effects is to use lower induction doses of the cytotoxic agent. The Euro Lupus Nephritis Trial, a multicenter, prospective trial of 90 patients with severe LN, compared low-dose versus "conventional" high-dose IV cyclophosphamide.[144] Patients were randomized to either six monthly IV pulses of 0.5 to 1 g/m^2 cyclophosphamide followed by two quarterly pulses or only 500 mg IV every 2 weeks for a total of six doses, both followed by oral azathioprine as maintenance therapy. At 40 months follow-up, there were no statistically significant differences in treatment failures, renal remissions, or renal flares, but twice as many infections occurred in the high dose group. Although this trial may have included some patients with milder renal disease (mean creatinine, 1.0–1.3 mg/dL; mean proteinuria, 2.5–3.5 g/day for both groups) and contained a predominantly white patient population, it supports the use of shorter duration and lower total dose cyclophosphamide for induction therapy. A longer follow-up period of the same population confirms these data and suggests that early response to therapy is predictive of a good long-term outcome and that the long-term results are excellent.[145]

A number of studies have focused on the optimal maintenance therapy for patients with LN. The goal here is to avoid relapse and flares of disease while minimizing the long-term toxicity of the immunosuppressive regimens. A randomized controlled trial from Miami examined LN patients who had successfully completed induction of remission with four to seven monthly pulses of IV cyclophosphamide and were then randomized to either continued every third month IV cyclophosphamide, oral azathioprine, or oral MMF.[1,3,146] The 54 LN patients randomized were largely composed of blacks (50%) and Hispanics and included many patients with the nephrotic syndrome (64%), reduced GFR, and severe proliferative LN on biopsy. Fewer patients in the azathioprine and the MMF groups reached the primary endpoints of death and chronic renal failure compared with the cyclophosphamide group. The cumulative probability of remaining relapse free was higher with MMF (78%) and azathioprine (58%) compared with cyclophosphamide (43%), and there was increased mortality in patients given continued cyclophosphamide. Complications of therapy, including days of hospitalization, amenorrhea, and infections, were also reduced in the MMF and azathioprine groups. Thus, maintenance therapy with either MMF or azathioprine was superior to IV cyclophosphamide with less toxicity.

The results of two large randomized trials further delineate the role of these oral agents in the maintenance of patients with proliferative LN.[147,148] In the European MAINTAIN trial, 105 patients were randomized to either azathioprine or MMF for at least 3 years of maintenance (mean, 53 months).[147] There were no differences between these medications in time to renal flares or to renal remission. In the worldwide ALMS Maintenance Trial, 227 patients who were initially in remission after induction therapy with either IV cyclophosphamide or MMF were rerandomized to either MMF or azathioprine maintenance for 3 years.[148] MMF proved superior to azathioprine with respect to the primary endpoint of time to treatment failure (death, ESRD, doubling of serum creatinine, LN flare, or requirement for rescue therapy).[148] At present, it is thus unclear whether one agent is truly superior to the other. Differences may depend on disease severity, racial or geographic location of the patients, or other standard of care differences between these two studies.

A number of other immunosuppressive agents have been used in smaller studies in LN patients. Low-dose cyclosporine (4–6 mg/kg/day) has been used usually in combination with other immunosuppressive agents for LN.[1,8] Some groups treating resistant LN patients found those who received cyclosporine plus tapering corticosteroids experienced improvement. Other investigators have found that cyclosporine is unsatisfactory monotherapy for severe proliferative disease because flares of disease activity usually occur after reductions in the dose of cyclosporine (e.g., for increases in the serum creatinine). Tacrolimus has been compared successfully with standard IV cyclophosphamide therapy in a number of small trials. It has also been used as part of a multidrug regimen for patients with severe LN with combined ISN/RPS class IV and V lesions.[149] IV cyclophosphamide resulted in complete remission in 5% and partial remissions in 40% at 6 months versus a "multi-targeted regimen" of tacrolimus, MMF, and corticosteroids, which led to a 50% complete and 40% partial remission rate in this time period.[152]

Rituximab, a chimeric monoclonal antibody targeting CD20 positive B cells, depletes them through multiple mechanisms, including complement-dependent cell lysis; FcRγ-dependent, antibody-dependent, cell-mediated cytotoxicity; and induction of apoptosis. Rituximab, which is approved by the U.S. Food and Drug Administration (FDA) for the treatment of rheumatoid arthritis, has been used with varying success in many immunologic and autoimmune diseases, including a variety of primary glomerular diseases.[1,3,150] In LN, it has been used in more than 300 patients, mostly in case reports and open-label, uncontrolled trials.[1,3] It clearly has been successful in some patients with both severe and refractory LN. Two recent randomized controlled trials have given disappointing results.[1,3] In one randomized trial of 257 SLE patients without severe renal disease, patients received rituximab (1 g for four doses over 182 days) or placebo.[151] Although subgroup analyses suggested a beneficial effect in the African American and Hispanic subgroups, there were no significant differences between the placebo arm and the rituximab arms of therapy.[151] In the Lupus Nephritis Assessment with Rituximab (LUNAR) trial, 140 patients with class III and IV LN were randomized to rituximab or placebo in addition to an induction regimen of MMF (goal, 3 g/day) and tapering corticosteroids.[1,8,152] Although the rituximab group had a greater decrease in anti-DNA antibody titers and increase in serum complement levels, there was no statistically significant difference in the primary renal response between treatment groups at 1 year.[152] At present, rituximab is not a first-line agent for induction therapy of most patients with severe LN. It continues to be used in patients resistant to other treatments and in those who do not tolerate conventional treatment, but its true value in induction and maintenance therapy remains to be defined.[153,154]

Other monoclonal antibodies directed at B cells are being studied. Ocrelizumab, a fully humanized anti-CD20 monoclonal antibody, had the advantages of avoiding first dose infusion reactions and the development of HACAs (human antichimeric antibodies) that were potential problems with rituximab therapy.[1] A controlled randomized trial, the Study to Evaluate Ocrelizumab in Patients with Nephritis Due to SLE, was terminated early because of adverse events. Epratuzumab, a humanized monoclonal antibody against CD22, a marker of mature B-cells but not plasma cells, is currently being studied.[1]

T-lymphocyte activation requires two signals.[155] The first occurs when the antigen is presented to the T-cell receptor in the context of MHC class II molecules on antigen presenting cells and the second by the interaction of co-stimulatory molecules on T lymphocytes and antigen presenting cells. Disruption of costimulatory signals interrupts the (auto)immune response. Two clinical trials using different humanized antiCD40L monoclonal antibodies in LN patients to block B- and T-cell co-stimulation have not been successful.[156,157] One study was terminated prematurely because of thromboembolic complications, and the second trial, although showing no major safety concerns, did not prove to have clinical efficacy. Another costimulatory pathway is mediated through the interaction of CD28-CD80/86.[1] CTLA-4 Ig, a fusion molecule that combines the extracellular domain of human CTLA4 with the constant region (Fc) of the human IgG$_1$ heavy chain, interrupts the CD28-CD80/86 interaction. It is FDA approved for the treatment of rheumatoid arthritis. Two

major randomized controlled trials are ongoing comparing the role of this form of costimulatory blockade in severe LN treated with IV cyclophosphamide and steroids.

Other therapies used in LN have included plasmapheresis, IV γ-globulin administration, total lymphoid irradiation, thromboxane antagonists, a monoclonal C5 inhibitor, marrow ablation with stem cell rescue, laquinimod therapy, and use of tolerance molecules.[3,95,158-166] All are still experimental because none has yet undergone large successful controlled clinical trials.[158-166] Inhibition of the B-cell stimulating cytokine (BLyS) by a monoclonal antibody belimumab has been evaluated with success in a large controlled population with SLE but has not yet been evaluated in patients with LN.[168] One new agent, abetimus (Riquent), evaluated in large multicenter blinded trials, is a designer molecule directed at inducing tolerance, preventing anti-DNA antibody formation, and preventing flares of disease.[167] Despite efficacy in animal models and encouraging early controlled trials in hundreds of LN patients, in the largest controlled randomized trial the drug failed to produce a significant reduction in renal flares. Other agents under preliminary investigation that have successfully been used in lupus-prone animal models or small numbers of patients include an antibody directed against the fifth component of complement to block the membrane attack complex (anti-C5 antibody),[164] adrenocorticotropic hormone, and blockers of inflammatory mediators such as INF-γ.[169] Immunoablative therapy with high-dose cyclophosphamide with and without stem cell transplantation has been used successfully in a limited number of SLE patients with only a short period of follow-up.[165,166]

Plasmapheresis was studied in multicenter controlled trial of 86 patients with severe LN. This study found no benefit in terms of clinical remission, progression to renal failure, or patient survival beyond a more rapid lowering of anti-DNA antibody titers.[158] Likewise, plasmapheresis synchronized to IV cyclophosphamide pulse therapy has not proven effective.[159] At present, plasmapheresis should be reserved for only certain LN patients (e.g., those with severe pulmonary hemorrhage, patients with a TTP-like syndrome, patients with ACLN antibodies and a clotting episode who cannot be anticoagulated because of hemorrhage).[160]

IV immunoglobulin (IVIG) has been used successfully in a number of SLE patients to treat thrombocytopenia as well as LN, leading to clinical and histologic improvement in some patients.[161,162] One controlled trial included only 14 patients but did show stabilization of the plasma creatinine, creatinine clearance, and proteinuria when IVIG was used as maintenance therapy after successful induction of remission with IV cyclophosphamide.[162]

For patients with class V membranous LN, there have been conflicting data regarding the course, prognosis, and response to treatment.[8,13] The degree of superimposed proliferative lesions greatly influences outcome in class V patients, and it is unclear if older trials included only pure membranous LN patients. Thus, early trials reported low and inconsistent response rates with oral corticosteroids.[36] Excellent long-term results with intensive immunosuppressive regimens from Italian studies and others raise questions of whether the results are related to the therapeutic intervention or to the population studied and better supportive treatments.[38] A retrospective Italian trial found better remission with a regimen of chlorambucil and methylprednisolone over that with corticosteroids alone.[170] In a small nonrandomized trial of cyclosporine in membranous LN, there was an excellent remission rate of the nephrotic syndrome with mean proteinuria decreasing from 6 to 1 to 2 g/day by 6 months.[45] At long-term follow-up and rebiopsy, there was no evidence of cyclosporine-induced renal damage, but two patients had developed superimposed proliferative lesions over time. An NIH trial of 42 nephrotic patients with membranous LN compared cyclosporine, prednisone, and IV cyclophosphamide and found superior remission rates for the cyclosporine and cyclophosphamide regimens but a trend toward more relapses when the cyclosporine was withdrawn.[171] Tacrolimus has also been used for class V LN with good results. A study of 38 patients with pure membranous LN evaluated long-term treatment with prednisone plus azathioprine.[172] At 12 months, 67% of the patients had experienced a complete remission and 22% a partial remission. At 3 years, only 12% had relapsed; at 5 years, only 16% had relapsed; and at 90 months, only 19% had relapsed. At the end of follow-up period, no patient had doubled the serum creatinine. Clearly, in this population, a regimen of steroids plus azathioprine was highly effective. The response of patients with membranous LN to MMF has been varied.[173-175] Eighty-four patients with pure ISN class V membranous LN included among the 510 patients enrolled in two similarly designed randomized controlled trials comparing MMF and IV cyclophosphamide induction thrapy.[175] Rates of remissions, relapse, and course were similar in both treatment groups. Thus, MMF can also be considered a first-line therapy for certain patients with membranous LN.

Given limited data, the treatment of membranous LN should be individualized. Patients with pure membranous LN and a good renal prognosis (subnephrotic levels of proteinuria and preserved GFR) may benefit from a short course of cyclosporine with low-dose corticosteroids along with inhibitors of the renin–angiotensin system and statins. For those at higher risk of progressive disease (African Americans, those who are fully nephrotic), options include cyclosporine, monthly IV pulses of cyclophosphamide, MMF, or azathioprine plus corticosteroids. Patients with mixed membranous and proliferative LN are treated in the same way as those with proliferative disease alone.

As effective and safer therapies for LN have evolved, greater attention has been directed to other causes of morbidity and mortality in the SLE population. Patients with lupus have accelerated atherogenesis and a disproportionate rate of coronary vascular disease, leading to a high mortality many years after the onset of their LN.[176] The high cardiovascular risk rate has been attributed to concurrent hypertension; hyperlipidemia; nephrotic syndrome; prolonged corticosteroid use; APL antibody syndrome; and in some, the added vascular risks of CKD.[177,178] Despite limited data on therapeutic interventions in this population, aggressive management of modifiable cardiovascular risk factors may alter the morbidity and mortality of this population. Extrapolating from other proteinuric CKD populations, closely monitored blood pressure control (<130/80), the use of angiotensin-converting enzyme (ACE) inhibitors or angiotensin receptor blockers, and correction of dyslipidemia with statins are reasonable in all LN patients. In addition, use of calcium, vitamin D supplements, and bisphosphonates to prevent glucocorticoid-induced osteoporosis may be useful.

Some form of APL antibodies is present in 40% to 75% of patients with lupus.[179-182] Because most do not experience thrombotic complications, they require no special treatment. However, some recommend low-dose aspirin and hydroxychloroquine for prophylaxis of asymptomatic patients with APL antibodies (see later discussion). In patients with evidence of a clinical thrombotic event, most investigators use chronic anticoagulation with Coumadin as long as the antibody persists. Although the standard practice has been not to anticoagulate other patients, in one recent series of more than 100 SLE patients, more than one-fourth had APL antibodies, of whom almost 80% had a thrombotic event. The antibody-positive patients also had a greater incidence of chronic renal failure than the antibody-negative patients.[181] (See discussion of ACLN antibodies and GN in following section.)

Antiphospholipid Antibody Syndrome

APL syndrome (APLS) may be associated with glomerular disease, small and large vessel renal involvement, and coagulation problems in dialysis and renal transplant patients.[179-182] Patients with the APLS have autoantibodies directed against plasma proteins bound to phospholipids. They may include immunoglobulin G (IgG) or IgM ACLN antibodies in moderate or high titer by ELISA, antibodies to ß2-glycoprotein 1 of IgG or IgM isotype at high titer by ELISA, or lupus anticoagulant activity.[183-185] In some studies, the presence of specific ß2-glycoprotein 1 antibodies has been correlated with an increased risk of thrombotic events in patients with APLS.[186] APL antibodies may cause a false-positive VDRL test result. In addition to having one of these autoantibodies, patients with APLS must have at least one of the following clinical criteria: one or more episodes of venous, arterial, or small vessel thrombosis; fetal morbidity; and thrombocytopenia. The presence of APL antibodies should be documented on two or more occasions at least 12 weeks apart and within 5 years of clinical manifestations.

The pathogenesis of the APLS remains unclear.[187-191] Susceptible individuals may develop APL antibodies after exposure to infectious or other noxious agents. SLE patients appear to be predisposed to this autoantibody production. However, after the APL antibodies are present, a "second hit" (e.g., pregnancy, contraceptive use, nephrotic syndrome, hyperlipidemia) may be necessary for them to produce thrombotic events and the APLS. The mechanism(s) of the procoagulant effect is likely to be multifactorial. APL antibodies exert procoagulant effects at multiple sites in the clotting cascade, including prothrombin, protein C, annexin V, coagulation factors VII and XII, platelets, serum proteases, and tissue factor procoagulant. They may also impair fibrinolysis through inhibition of such factors as tissue-type plasminogen activator. The result is endothelial damage and intravascular coagulation.

A total of 30% to 50% of patients with APL antibodies have the primary APL syndrome in which there is no associated autoimmune disease.[178-185] APL antibodies are found in from 25% to 75% of SLE patients, although most patients never experience clinical features of APLS.[178-185] In an analysis of 29 published series with more than 1000 SLE patients, 34% were positive for the lupus anticoagulant and 44% for ACLN antibodies.[192] Most studies have found a higher incidence of thrombotic events in SLE patients positive for APL antibodies.[181,193,194] A recent European study of almost 575 SLE patients found the prevalence of IgG ACLN antibodies to be 23% and of IgM 14%.[195] Patients with IgG antibodies had a clear association with thrombocytopenia and thromboses. A multicenter European analysis of 1000 SLE patients found thromboses in 7% of patients over 5 years. Patients with IgG ACLN antibodies again had a higher incidence of thromboses, as did those with a lupus anticoagulant.[196] APL antibodies are also found in up to 2% of normal individuals and in those with a variety of infections (commonly in HIV- and in hepatitis C virus [HCV]–infected patients) and drug reactions, but these are not usually associated with the clinical features of the APL syndrome.[197-199]

The clinical features of the APL syndrome relate to thrombotic events and consequent ischemia. In 1000 APL syndrome patients, the most common features were deep vein thrombosis (32%), thrombocytopenia (22%), livedo reticularis (20%), stroke (13%), pulmonary embolism (9%), and fetal loss (9%).[196] Patients may also experience pulmonary hypertension, memory impairment and other neurologic manifestations, fever, malaise, and constitutional symptoms.[179-182] Catastrophic APLS, a rare event (occurring in 0.8% of APLS patients), is associated with rapid thromboses in multiple organ systems and has a high fatality rate.[200]

Renal involvement, so-called APL nephropathy, occurs in as many as 25% of patients with primary APLS and is characterized by thrombosis of blood vessels ranging from the glomerular capillaries to the main renal artery and vein.[179-182,201,202] Lesions involving the arteries and arterioles often have both a thrombotic component and a reactive or proliferative one with intimal mucoid thickening, subendothelial fibrosis, and medial hyperplasia (Figure 32-13).[201,202] Inflammatory vasculitis has been identified rarely. Interstitial fibrosis and cortical atrophy may occur because of tissue ischemia. Glomerular lesions include glomerular capillary thrombosis with associated mesangiolysis; mesangial interposition and duplication of GBMs; and electron-lucent, flocculent subendothelial material resembling other forms of glomerular thrombotic microangiopathies such as HUS and TTP.

One retrospective renal biopsy study found that APL nephropathy existed in almost 40% of APL-positive patients versus only 4% of patients without APL antibody and was associated with both lupus anticoagulant and ACLN antibodies.[203] Among APL-positive SLE patients, APL nephropathy was found in two-thirds of those with APLS and in

one-third of those without APLS. Although patients with APL nephropathy had a higher frequency of hypertension and elevated serum creatinine levels at biopsy in this series, they did not have a higher frequency of progressive renal insufficiency, ESRD, or death at follow-up.[203] This is in contrast to another series of more than 100 SLE patients, which found the presence of APL antibodies to be associated with both thrombotic events and a greater progression to renal failure.[181] In patients with APL nephropathy, renal biopsies have been misclassified as focal segmental glomerulosclerosis, membranous nephropathy, and membranoproliferative GN when they truly display a thrombotic microangiopathy.[204] However, a recent study reports patients with a number of glomerular histologic patterns on LM, including membranous nephropathy, minimal change or focal sclerosis, mesangial proliferative GN, and pauci-immune rapidly progressive GN, to actually have classic APL syndrome.[205]

The most frequent clinical renal findings are proteinuria, at times in the nephrotic range; active urinary sediment; hypertension; and progressive renal dysfunction.[179,180,201-205] Some patients present with an acute deterioration in renal function.[204] With major renal arterial involvement, there may be renal infarction, and renal vein thrombosis may be silent or present with sudden flank pain and a decrease in renal function. Renal artery stenosis has been reported with and without malignant hypertension.[206-208]

About 10% of biopsied lupus patients have glomerular microthromboses as a major histopathologic finding. Therapy of this glomerular lesion clearly differs from that of immune complex–mediated GN.[52] One study of 114 biopsied SLE patients found vaso-occlusive lesions in one-third of biopsies, which both correlated with hypertension and an increased serum creatinine level.[209] In SLE, features that correlate well with high titers of IgG APL antibodies are thrombocytopenia, the presence of a false-positive VDRL test result for syphilis (fluorescent treponemal antibody negative), and a prolonged activated partial thromboplastin time.[179,180,182,209] Neither the titer of anti-DNA antibodies nor the serum complement levels correlate well with the APL antibody levels. In SLE, high titers of IgG ACLN antibody usually correlate well with the risk of thromboses. However, in one study of 114 biopsied SLE patients, renal thrombi were related to lupus anticoagulant but not ACLN antibodies.[209] The clinical features of APLS in SLE patients are identical to those of primary APLS. An important study documents the prevalence of APL antibodies in 26% of 111 LN patients followed for a mean of 173 months.[181] Of the APL antibody–positive patients, 79% developed a thrombotic event or fetal loss, and the presence of antibodies was strongly correlated with the developed of progressive CKD.

There is a high prevalence of APL antibodies (10%–30%) in hemodialysis patients not associated with patient age, gender, or duration of the dialysis.[210,211] In contrast, patients with renal insufficiency and those on peritoneal dialysis have a much lower incidence of APL antibodies.[179] One hemodialysis study found more patients with arteriovenous grafts than native fistulas to have a raised titer of IgG ACLN antibody.[211] There was a significant increase in the odds of having two or more episodes of hemodialysis graft thrombosis in patients with raised ACLN titers. Whether hemodialysis grafts induce ACLN antibodies or whether patients with ACLN antibodies require AV grafts remains unclear.[179] In another study of 230 hemodialyzed

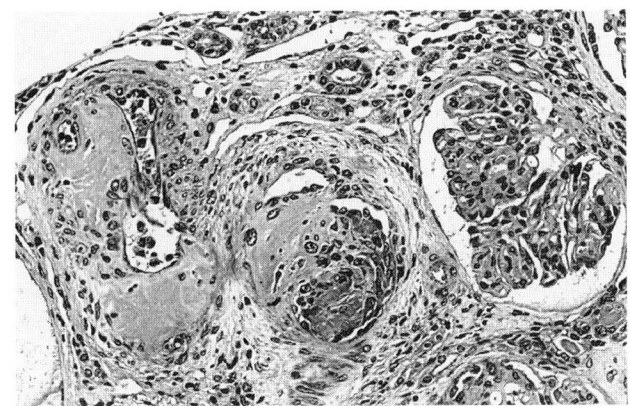

FIGURE 32-13 Antiphospholipid antibody syndrome. Organizing recanalized thrombi narrow the lumens of two interlobular arteries. The adjacent glomerulus displays ischemic-type retraction of its tuft (hematoxylin and eosin, ×200).

patients, titers of IgG ACLN antibodies were elevated in 26% of the patients as opposed to elevated titers of IgM antibodies in only 4%.[212] The mean time to AV graft failure was significantly shorter in the group with elevated IgG antibodies, and the use of Coumadin increased graft survival in these patients.

The presence of APL antibodies may also damage the renal allograft. In several studies 20% to 60% of SLE patients with APL antibodies who received renal transplants had evidence of related problems with venous thromboses, pulmonary emboli, or persistent thrombocytopenia.[103,104,213,214] In one large study of non-SLE patients, 28% of 178 transplant patients had APL antibodies that were associated with a three- to fourfold increased risk of arterial and venous thromboses.[213] However, another study of 337 renal transplant recipients found the 18% who were IgG or IgM ACLN antibody positive (even after correction for the effects of anticoagulation) had no greater allograft loss or reduction in GFR over time than did patients who were ACLN antibody negative.[215] Although most HCV-positive patients with APL antibodies do not have evidence of increased thromboses and APLS, when transplanted, they appear to have a higher risk of allograft thrombotic microangiopathy.[216] In many of these transplant studies, treatment with anticoagulation has proven successful in preventing recurrent thromboses and graft loss.[103,104,214]

Treatment

The optimal treatment of patients with APL antibodies and APLS remains to be defined.[179,180,217,218] Many patients with APL antibodies do not experience thrombotic events. In asymptomatic patients with APL antibodies but no evidence of thrombotic events or APLS, low-dose aspirin may be beneficial based on limited data.[219]

Because patients with higher titers of IgG APL antibodies have a greater incidence of thrombotic events, they may benefit from anticoagulation.[195,196] In patients with the full APLS, either primary or secondary to SLE, anticoagulation with heparin followed by warfarin has proven more effective than either no therapy, aspirin, or low-dose anticoagulation in preventing recurrent thromboses.[21,179,182] A retrospective analysis of 147 APLS patients (including 62 with primary disease, 66 with SLE, and 19 with lupus-like syndrome) reported 186 recurrent thrombotic events in 69% of the patients.[217] The median time between the initial thrombosis and the first recurrence was 12 months but with a broad range (0.5–144 months). Treatment with warfarin to produce an international normalized ratio (INR) greater than 3 was significantly more effective than treatment with low-dose warfarin (INR <3) or treatment with aspirin alone. The highest rate of thrombosis (1.3 per patient-year) occurred in patients within 6 months after discontinuing anticoagulation. Bleeding complications occurred in 29 of the 147 patients but were severe in only seven patients. The role of immunosuppressives has been uncertain in APLS.[179,182,197,218] Thus, in SLE patients, the anti-DNA antibody titer and the serum complement may normalize with immunosuppressives without a significant change in a high titer of IgG APL antibody.[218] In pregnant patients with APLS, heparin and low-dose aspirin have been successful in several studies, but prednisone therapy has not.[219-221] In rare patients who cannot tolerate anticoagulation because of recent bleeding, who have thromboembolic events despite adequate

anticoagulation, or who are pregnant, plasmapheresis with corticosteroids and other immunosuppressives have been used with some success.[222,223] Success with other treatments such as IVIG and hydroxychloroquine remains anecdotal.[221,224,225]

Mixed Connective Tissue Disease

MCTD, which was first described in 1972, is defined by a combination of clinical and serologic features.[226-228] Patients with MCTD share many overlapping features with patients with SLE, scleroderma, and polymyositis.[227-230] They also typically have distinct serologic findings with very high ANA titers, often with a speckled pattern, and antibodies directed against a specific ribonuclease sensitive ENA, U1 RNP.[227-230] MCTD has a 16 to one female-to-male sex ratio and has been linked to HLA-DR4 and DR2 genotypes.[231] Not all patients with clinical features of the syndrome have a positive ENA, and not all patients with a positive ENA have the clinical features of MCTD.[230] Because some patients fulfill diagnostic criteria for other connective tissue diseases, investigators have questioned whether MCTD is a distinct syndrome. The terms *undifferentiated autoimmune rheumatic and connective tissue disorder* and *overlap syndrome* are sometimes used because many patients with features of MCTD eventually develop SLE, scleroderma, or rheumatoid arthritis.[229-232]

In the early stages of MCTD, patients usually manifest only nonspecific symptoms such as malaise, fatigue, myalgias, arthralgias, and low-grade fever. Over time, systemic clinical features similar to other rheumatologic connective tissue diseases appear. These include arthralgias and in some deforming arthritis, myalgias and myositis, Raynaud's phenomenon, swollen hands and fingers, restrictive pulmonary disease and pulmonary hypertension, esophageal dysmotility, pericarditis and myocarditis, serositis, oral and nasal ulcers, digital ulcers and gangrene, discoid lupus-like lesions, malar rash, alopecia, photosensitivity, and lymphadenopathy.[228-230,232-235] However, patients with MCTD, especially those documented to have anti-U1RNP antibodies, infrequently have major CNS disease or severe proliferative GN.[228-230,232-235] Low-grade anemia, lymphocytopenia, and hypergammaglobulinemia are all common in MCTD.

The most widely used serologic test to confirm a diagnosis of MCTD is the ENA with anti-U1RNP antibodies.[229,230,236] The diagnosis of MCTD is even firmer in patients with IgG antibodies against an antigenic component of U1RNP, the 68kD protein.[236,237] Antibodies to other nuclear antigens have been found in MCTD, and some correlate better with clinical features of specific rheumatologic diseases.[228,229,232] Antibodies against dsDNA, Sm antigen, and Ro are infrequently positive in those with MCTD, but up to 70% of patients have a positive rheumatoid factor. APL antibodies are found less frequently than in SLE.

The incidence of renal involvement has varied from 10% to 26% of adults and from 33% to 50% of children with MCTD.[229,230,232,237] Many patients may have mild or minimal clinical manifestations with only microhematuria and less than 500 mg/day of proteinuria. However, heavier proteinuria, severe hypertension, and acute renal failure reminiscent of a "scleroderma renal crisis" may occur.[234,238,239] Although the titer of anti-RNP does not correlate with renal involvement, the presence of serologic markers of active SLE (e.g., high anti-dsDNA antibody titers, anti-Sm antibody) are more common with renal disease.[229,230] Low serum complement levels have not always correlated with the presence of renal involvement.[234] Children with MCTD more often have glomerular involvement with few clinical or urinary findings.[240]

The pathology of MCTD is diverse with the glomerular lesions resembling the spectrum found in SLE and the vascular lesions resembling those in scleroderma. Glomerular disease is most common and is usually superimposed on a background of mesangial deposits and mesangial hypercellularity as in SLE.[234,238,240-244] As many as 30% of biopsied patients have mesangial deposits of IgG and C3. Other patients have focal proliferative GN with both mesangial and subendothelial deposits, but fibrinoid necrosis and crescent formation are rare. The most common pattern of glomerular involvement is membranous nephropathy, which is reported in up to 35% of cases[234,238,240-243] with typical peripheral capillary wall granular IF staining for IgG, C3, and at times IgA and IgM. Some patients, especially children, have a mixed pattern of membranous plus mesangial proliferative GN.[240] Renal biopsy findings may transform over time from one pattern of glomerular involvement to another in a fashion similar to SLE patients. By ultrastructural analysis, findings such as those in SLE have been reported, including endothelial TRIs, deposits with "fingerprint" substructure, and tubular basement membrane deposits.[234,243] In one review of 100 biopsied patients with MCTD, 12% had normal biopsies, 35% had mesangial lesions, 10% had proliferative lesions, and 36% had membranous nephropathy.[243] In addition, 15% to 25% of patients had interstitial disease and vascular lesions. In autopsy series, in which two-thirds of patients had clinical renal disease, a similar distribution of glomerular lesions with a predominance of membranous features was found.[244] Other renal pathology findings in MCTD include secondary renal amyloidosis,[245] vascular sclerosis ranging from intimal sclerosis to medial hyperplasia,[234] and vascular lesions resembling those in scleroderma kidney with involvement of the interlobular arteries by intimal mucoid edema and fibrous sclerosis.

Therapy of MCTD with corticosteroids is effective in treating the inflammatory features of joint disease and serositis.[229,230,234] There have been no controlled treatment trials in patients with MCTD. Steroids are less effective in treating sclerodermatous features such as cutaneous disease, esophageal involvement, Raynaud's phenomenon, and especially pulmonary hypertension, which has been treated with calcium channel blockers, ACE inhibitors, prolonged immunosuppression, or IV prostacyclin.[246] IVIG has been used as in SLE patients with decreased platelets and hemolytic anemia.[247] Treatment of the glomerular lesions is similar to that for LN.

Originally, MCTD was believed to have a good prognosis with low mortality and few patients developing other distinct connective tissue disorders. The longer patients with MCTD are followed, the greater percentage who evolve more clearly into a specific connective tissue disorder.[229,230,232] In some series, almost half of the patients with a short duration of follow-up were still believed to have true MCTD, but in those with longer follow-up periods, the percentage had dropped to 15% or less.[229,230,232,234] Most patients evolve toward a picture of either SLE or systemic sclerosis, but some develop prominent features of rheumatoid arthritis.[234] Mortally rates have been found to range from 15% to 30% at 10 to 12 years with

patients with more clinical features of scleroderma and polymyositis faring worse.[229,230,234] The leading causes of mortality in MCTD are pulmonary hypertension, myocarditis, and renovascular hypertension with cerebral hemorrhage.[229,230] Other causes include vascular lesions of the coronary and other vessels, hypertensive scleroderma crisis, and chronic renal failure. Clearly, MCTD is not a benign disorder but rather a disease with significant morbidity and mortality.

Small Vessel Vasculitis

A number of diseases, including Wegener's granulomatosis (WG), microscopic polyangiitis, and Churg-Strauss syndrome, are usually classified together as small vessel vasculitides.[248-257] There is considerable overlap in the clinical, histologic, and laboratory features of these entities. Moreover, all may be associated with a positive serologic test for ANCAs, and the treatment for many patients includes potent immunosuppressives.

Wegener's Granulomatosis

WG has been traditionally defined by the triad of systemic vasculitis associated with necrotizing, granulomatous inflammation of the upper and lower respiratory tracts and GN.[249] Subsequent descriptions of "limited" upper respiratory tract disease, of multiorgan system involvement, and of the nature and pathogenesis of the serologic marker ANCA have enhanced our understanding of this disease.[250-254] Even in the pre-ANCA era, these criteria yielded a sensitivity of 88% and a specificity of 92% for the diagnosis of WG. Clearly, adding ANCA to the diagnostic criteria increases these percentages.[255-257]

WG has a slight male predominance and a peak incidence in the fourth to sixth decades of life.[249,253,258,259] Pauci-immune rapidly progressive GN (including WG and microscopic polyangiitis) are the most common forms of crescentic GN at all ages, especially in elderly individuals.[256,257] Most reported patients have been white, but with use of newer serologic tests such as the ANCA, patients of all races are being diagnosed.[260] The occurrence of WG in more than one family member has rarely been noted.[261] Although certain HLA frequencies such as HLA DR2, HLA B7, and HLA DR1 and DR1-DQW1 have been reported more commonly in WG patients, no clear genetic profile has emerged.[262]

Pathology

The classic histopathologic finding in WG is a focal segmental necrotizing and crescentic GN (Figure 32-14).[253,258,263] Although the percentage of affected glomeruli can vary widely, the necrotizing changes are usually segmental in distribution.[253,263,264] Unaffected glomeruli typically appear normal. Global proliferation and necrotizing glomerular tuft involvement are more common in the more severe cases. The earliest lesions are "intracapillary thrombosis" with deposition of eosinophilic "fibrinoid" material associated with endothelial cell swelling, infiltration by polymorphonuclear leukocytes, and pyknosis or karyorrhexis.[253,263,264] In areas of

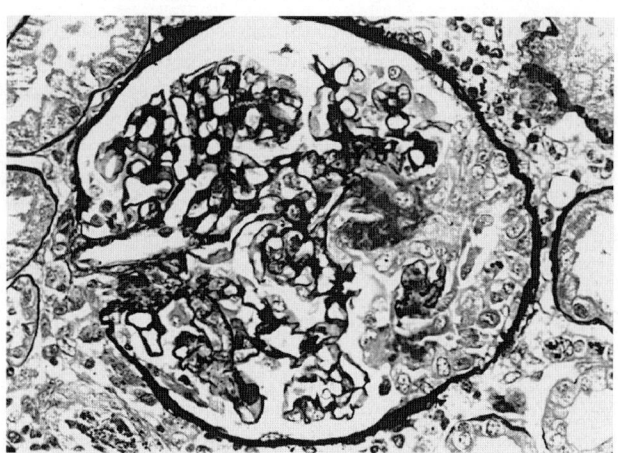

FIGURE 32-14 Wegener granulomatosis. A representative glomerulus displays segmental fibrinoid necrosis with rupture of glomerular basement membrane, fibrin extravasation into the urinary space, and an overlying segmental cellular crescent (Jones methenamine silver, ×500).

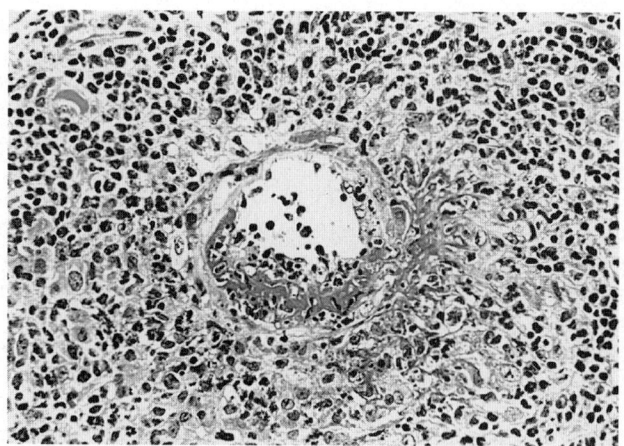

FIGURE 32-15 Wegener granulomatosis. An interlobular artery displays necrotizing vasculitis with intimal fibrin deposition and transmural inflammation by neutrophils and lymphocytes (hematoxylin and eosin, ×375).

active necrotizing glomerular lesions, there are ruptures in the GBM and formation of overlying cellular crescents that range from segmental to circumferential. Crescents are frequently associated with breaks in or broad destruction of Bowman's capsule.[265] Granulomatous crescents containing epithelioid histiocytes and giant cells may involve from fewer than 15% to more than 50% of cases, and the finding of large numbers of them is more typical of WG and cytoplasmic ANCA (C-ANCA) positivity than other vasculitides. Chronic segmental or global glomerulosclerosis with fibrous crescents often occur side by side with more active glomerular lesions. Although there is much overlap in the histologic findings between microscopic polyangiitis and WG, some differences have been noted. Patients with microscopic polyangiitis and those who have anti-myeloperoxidase (anti-MPO) ANCA are more likely to have a greater degree and severity of glomerulosclerosis, interstitial fibrosis, and tubular atrophy on initial biopsy.[266]

The vasculitis in WG may affect small- and medium-sized renal arteries, veins, and capillaries.[253,263,264] It is focal in nature and has been reported in 5% to 10% of biopsies of WG patients.[249,252,253,267] It is more commonly found at autopsy, with larger tissue samples and where serial sectioning and a directed search for the lesions have been performed. The necrotizing arteritis consists of endothelial cell swelling and denudation, intimal fibrin deposition, and mononuclear and polymorphonuclear leukocyte infiltration of the vessel wall with mural necrosis (Figure 32-15). The vasculitis may have granulomatous features. Tubules show focal degenerative and regenerative changes, and cortical infarcts may occur.[248,253] Interstitial inflammatory infiltrates of lymphocytes, monocytes, plasma cells, and polymorphonuclear leukocytes associated with edema are common. Granulomas containing giant cells may form in the interstitium of the cortex and medulla in from 3% to 20% of cases.[258] Some of these cortical granulomas represent foci of glomerular destruction by granulomatous crescents. Papillary necrosis, which is usually bilateral and affects most papillae, has been reported is as many as one-fifth of WG patients, usually in those with necrotizing interstitial capillaritis affecting the vasa recta of the medulla. Biopsy of extrarenal tissue may show necrotizing and granulomatous inflammation or evidence of vasculitis.[252,253,263]

There is no specific glomerular immune staining in most cases of WG. Low-level staining for immunoglobulins and complement components in the glomerular tuft and vasculature are likely to represent non-immunologic trapping in areas of necrosis and sclerosis. This negative or only focal low-intensity IF staining pattern is referred to as "pauci-immune."[249-253,263] Positivity for fibrin or fibrinogen is common in the distribution of the necrotizing glomerular lesions, crescents, and vasculitic lesions. By EM, the glomeruli affected by necrotizing lesions often show areas of intraluminal and subendothelial fibrin deposition associated with endothelial necrosis and gaps in the GBM through which fibrin and leukocytes extravasate into Bowman's space.[249-253,263] There may be subendothelial accumulation of electron-lucent flocculent material associated with intravascular coagulation. True electron-dense immune type deposits are not usually identified and when present are sparse and ill defined.[249-253,263] EM of the vessels in WG may show swelling and denudation of endothelial cells and subendothelial accumulation of fibrin, platelets, and amorphous electron-dense material but no typical immune-type electron-dense deposits.

Pathogenesis

Although the pathogenesis of WG remains unknown, abnormalities of both humoral and cell-mediated immunity have been noted.[250-253] Recent in vitro and animal experiments strongly support a role for ANCA in the pathogenesis of the disease.[268-271] ANCA production may relate to infectious, genetic, environmental, and other risk factors.[268] Both molecular mimicry to infectious antigens and formation of antibody to antisense peptide have been proposed in the development of ANCA. Patients with proteinase-3 (PR3)–positive ANCA have been shown to have antibodies to complementary PR3, a protein encoded by the antisense RNA of the PR3 gene, and CD4-positive TH1 memory cells responsive to the complementary PR3 peptide.[269] In RAG-2 mice, transfer of anti-MPO IgG causes GN with necrosis and crescent formation that appears identical to human ANCA-associated GN by LM and IF.[271] This can occur in the absence of antigen-specific T lymphocytes, strongly suggesting a pathogenetic role for the antibodies themselves. In humans, neonatal microscopic polyangiitis with pulmonary hemorrhage and renal disease has occurred secondary to the transfer of maternal MPO-ANCA.[272] At least one study has found a unique subgroup of ANCA directed against lysosomal-associated membrane protein 2 (LAMP-2) as opposed to MPO or serine PR3 to be present in more than 90% of ANCA-positive pauci-immune necrotizing GN.[273] These anti–LAMP-2 antibodies, produced through mimicry with bacterial antigens, can also activate neutrophils and injure the vascular endothelium. Others have not been able to confirm a high incidence of anti–LAMP-2 antibodies in this population.

Cell-mediated mechanisms of tissue injury in WG are supported by a predominance of CD4-positive T lymphocytes and monocytes in the inflammatory respiratory tract infiltrates, high levels of Th1 cytokines, defects in delayed hypersensitivity, an increase in soluble markers of T-cell activation as soluble IL-2 receptor and CD30, impaired lymphocyte blastogenesis, and T-cell response to PR3.[254,274-276] Despite prominent respiratory tract involvement, no inhaled pathogen or environmental allergen has been identified as the initiator of the disease process. However, respiratory infections may allow the release of cytokines such as TNF from cells that can "prime" neutrophils to express PR3 and other antigens on their cell surfaces. The expression of granule proteins on the surface of neutrophils and monocytes allows for the interaction with circulating ANCA, leading to a respiratory burst in the cell, degranulation and local release of damaging proteases and reactive oxygen species, release of chemoattractant products, and neutrophil apoptosis.[252-254,277-279] Endothelial injury, fibrinoid necrosis, and inflammation ensue. In the presence of ANCA, neutrophils exhibit exaggerated adhesion and transmigration through endothelium.[279]

A spectrum of glomerular and vascular disease reaction is seen depending on antigen expression, host leukocyte activation, circulating and local cytokines and chemokines, the condition of the endothelium, and the nature of T- and B-cell interactions.[252-254,277-279] The membranes of leukocytes from WG patients may be primed to express PR3 molecules on their surfaces, making them ripe for activation of the disease process.[254,278,280,281] This priming phenomenon might explain the exacerbations of disease activity associated with respiratory infections as well as the potential benefits of prophylaxis with trimethoprim–sulfamethoxazole.[281,282]

Clinical and Laboratory Features

Patients with WG may present with an indolent, slowly progressive involvement of the respiratory tract and mild renal findings or with fulminant acute GN. In the past, there was often a delay between the onset of symptoms and diagnosis.[249,258] Despite greater awareness of the disease, more extensive use of renal biopsy, and the widespread availability of ANCA serologic testing, diagnosis is still often delayed. Most patients have constitutional symptoms, including fever, weakness, and malaise, at presentation.[249-253,258,283,284] From 70% to 80% of patients have upper respiratory findings at presentation, and even more develop these findings over time.[249-253,258,283,284] There may be rhinitis; purulent or bloody nasal discharge and crusting; and sinusitis typically involving the maxillary sinus and less commonly the sphenoid, ethmoid,

and frontal sinuses.[249,253,258,283] Radiographs show opacification, air fluid levels, mass lesion, or rarely bony erosions. Upper respiratory tract involvement can also be manifest by tinnitus and hearing loss, otic discharge and earache, perforation of the tympanic membrane, hoarseness, and throat pain.[249-253,258] Chronic sequelae include deafness, chronic sinusitis, and nasal septal collapse with saddle nose deformity.

Lower respiratory tract disease, found at presentation in up to 75% of patients, eventually develops in most of the remainder.[249-253,258] Symptoms include cough, often with sputum production; dyspnea on exertion and shortness of breath; alveolar hemorrhage and hemoptysis; and pleuritic pain.[285,286] Chest radiographs and computed tomography (CT) scans may reveal single or multiple nodules some with areas of cavitation, alveolar infiltrates and interstitial changes, and less commonly small pleural effusions and atelectatic areas. Radiologic findings may occur in the absence of pulmonary symptoms or clinical findings.[258]

WG is a multisystem disease with many organs involved by the vasculitic process and its sequelae.[249-253,258] Cutaneous involvement, present in 15% to 50% of patients, occurs with a variety of macular lesions, papules, nodules, or purpura, usually on the lower extremities. Patients with rheumatologic involvement have arthralgias of large and small joints and nondeforming arthritis of the knees and ankles or more rarely a myopathy or myositis. Up to 65% of patients have ophthalmologic disease with conjunctivitis, episcleritis and uveitis, optic nerve vasculitis, or proptosis caused by retro-orbital inflammation. Nervous system involvement is most typically manifested as a mononeuritis multiplex but may involve cranial nerves or the CNS. Other organs involved include the liver, parotids, thyroid, gallbladder, and heart.[249-253,258] Recent reports have emphasized the risks of thromboembolism, especially during active disease, perhaps related to endothelial injury and hypercoagulability induced by the vasculitis and its treatment.[287]

Abnormal laboratory test results in WG include a normochromic, normocytic anemia and mild leukocytosis and thrombocytosis.[249,253,258] Eosinophilia is uncommon, and there have been no abnormalities of circulating lymphocytes subsets in the disease.[259] Nonspecific markers of an inflammatory disease process, such as an elevated ESR, CRP levels, and rheumatoid factor test results, are often positive and correlate with the general disease activity. Other serologic test results, including those for ANA, serum complement levels, and cryoglobulins, are normal or negative.[249]

ANCA has been detected by a variety of assays in from 85% to 96% of patients with WG.[250-255] Patients with granulomatous lesions are more likely to be C-ANCA positive with antibody directed against PR3, a 228–amino acid serine proteinase found in the azurophilic granules of neutrophils and the lysosomes of monocytes.[248-254,257] However, many patients fitting the clinical and histologic definition of WG are perinuclear ANCA (P-ANCA) positive with antibodies directed against MPO, a highly cationic 140-kDa dimer located in a similar cellular distribution to PR3.[248-254] ANCA may also be directed to other antigens (e.g., lactoferrin, cathepsin, elastase), but these antibodies are not usually associated with vasculitis and are usually found in other immune-mediated diseases. In a study of 89 patients from China who fulfilled clinical and histopathologic criteria for WG, 61% were MPO-ANCA positive, and only 38%

were PR3-ANCA positive.[260] Although the specificity of C-ANCA for WG has been as high as 98% to 99% by different assays, the sensitivity may be low in certain populations with inactive or limited disease.[250-255,288] Some patients with pauci-immune crescentic GN are ANCA negative and may have a distinct disease from the more common ANCA-positive patients.[289] Other patients with crescentic GN are positive for both ANCA and anti-GBM antibodies (see section on anti-GBM disease).

"False-positive" C-ANCA test results have been reported in patients with certain infections (e.g., HIV, tuberculosis, subacute bacterial endocarditis) and neoplastic diseases. A number of medications have also been associated with ANCA, usually anti-MPO, and at very high titers. The strongest association is with the antithyroid drugs, including PTU, methimazole, and carbimazole. Hydralazine, minocycline, penicillamine, allopurinol, clozapine, rifampin, cefotaxime, isoniazid, and a number of other drugs have also been associated with ANCA-positive vasculitis.[290] Although there has been debate whether the ANCA levels parallel the clinical and histologic activity in WG, many patients normalize their ANCA titers during periods of quiescence.[257,288,291-295] Nevertheless, some patients in remission still have positive test results for C-ANCA. A subsequent increase in ANCA titer from low titer has been suggested to be predictive of renal and systemic flares.[250-254,291,293-295] Most clinicians prefer to use the ANCA level in the context of other clinical findings and often with other markers of active inflammation such as ESR and CRP. At times, renal biopsy is the only way to be certain of the clinical significance of a change in ANCA titer.

Renal Findings

Renal findings in WG are extremely variable and usually occur together with other systemic manifestations.[249-254,258,284] Most patients have evidence of renal disease at presentation, and from 50% to 95% eventually develop clinical evidence of renal involvement. There is typically mild proteinuria and urinary sediment abnormalities, including microscopic hematuria and RBC casts. Patients with more severe glomerular involvement often have a decrease in GFR and greater levels of proteinuria, but the nephrotic syndrome is uncommon. The level of proteinuria may be high in those without severe renal insufficiency and may actually increase during therapy as the GFR improves.[258,284] The degree of renal failure and serum creatinine do not always correlate well with the percent of glomerular necrotizing lesions, the percent of glomerular crescent formation, or the presence of interstitial granulomas or vasculitis. The incidence of both acute oliguric renal failure and significant hypertension varies among reports but is higher in reports from renal centers. IV pyelogram results are typically normal, and by angiography, vascular aneurysms are not usually present.[249-254]

In addition to glomerular and vascular lesions, other renal conditions associated with WG have included pyelonephritis and hydronephrosis caused by vasculitis causing ureteral stenosis, papillary necrosis, perirenal hematoma from arterial aneurysm rupture, and lymphoid malignancies with neoplastic infiltration of the renal parenchyma in patients treated with immunosuppression.[296]

Course and Treatment

The course of the active GN is typical of rapidly progressive GN with progression to renal failure over days to months.[249-254,258] Patients with severe necrotizing, granulomatous GN are more likely to develop renal failure, and patients with more global glomerulosclerosis are more likely to develop ESRD.[297] One study found greater glomerulosclerosis and interstitial fibrosis to predict a poor renal outcome.[298] Even with immunosuppressive therapy, a significant number of patients eventually progress over the long term to renal failure.[298]

The introduction of effective cytotoxic immunosuppressive therapy dramatically changed the course of WG. Initial studies of untreated patients and even those using corticosteroids alone documented survivals of 20% to 60% at 1 year.[243] There may be progression of both renal and extrarenal lesions during corticosteroid therapy.[249-254] Cyclophosphamide became the treatment of choice for WG and other pauci-immune rapidly progressive glomerulonephritides. Long-term survival with cyclophosphamide-based regimens ranges from 87% at 8 years to 64% at 10 years.[249-254,299,300] Using a regimen of combined cyclophosphamide (1.5–2 mg/kg/day) and corticosteroids, investigators at the NIH achieved remissions in 85% to 90% of 133 WG patients.[249] Most patients were converted to every-other-day steroid usage in several months and were able to discontinue steroid use by 1 year. Although half of the patients eventually relapsed, many patients remained in long-term remission off immunosuppressives. Similar results have been found by other investigators.[251-254,290,299,300] Complete remissions of renal and extrarenal symptoms, including severe pulmonary disease and renal failure requiring dialysis, have been well described.[251-254,299,301] More than 50% of dialysis-dependent patients are able to discontinue dialysis and remain stable for years. Although resistance to therapy is well documented, some patients are treatment failures because of noncompliance, intercurrent infection requiring decreased treatment, or inadequate duration of therapy. Until recent controlled trials using rituximab and MMF, other immunosuppressives were less effective at inducing an initial remission.

The optimal dose, duration of treatment, route of administration, and concomitant therapy to be given with cyclophosphamide are still debated for patients with ANCA-positive small vessel vasculitis.[250-254] Cyclophosphamide is usually administered with corticosteroids initially, with the dose of the steroids tapered or changed to alternate-day therapy. Some regimens include IV high-dose "pulse" corticosteroids initially, and others have used plasmapheresis in critically ill patients. A typical regimen for induction therapy of severe WG or other ANCA-positive rapidly progressive GN might include IV pulse methylprednisolone (7 mg/kg, to a maximum dose of 500–1000 mg) for 3 consecutive days followed by daily oral prednisone 1 mg/kg (to a maximum of 60–80 mg/day) for the first month with subsequent tapering of the dose along with either IV or oral cyclophosphamide given for approximately 6 months.[250-254] Doses are adjusted for leukopenia and other side effects as well as for treatment response. Several studies have evaluated the role of pulse IV cyclophosphamide versus oral cyclophosphamide in ANCA-positive small vessel vasculitis.[250,301-306] In one study of 50 WG patients randomly assigned to either 2 years of IV or oral cyclophosphamide, remissions at 6 months occurred in 89% or the IV group versus 78% of the oral group.[302] At the end of the study, remissions occurred in 67% of the IV group and 57% of the oral group, but relapses were more common in the IV group (60% vs. 13%). In a meta-analysis of 11 non-randomized studies including more than 200 ANCA-associated vasculitis patients, complete remissions occurred in more than 60% of patients and partial remissions in another 15%.[303] IV pulse cyclophosphamide was more likely to induce remission and less likely to cause infection than oral cyclophosphamide. However, relapses may be more frequent with IV use of the drug. This is clarified by a recent large multicenter trial that randomized 149 ANCA-positive vasculitis patients to either solumedrol plus pulsed IV cyclophosphamide (15 mg/kg every 2–3 weeks) or plus daily oral cyclophosphamide 2 mg/kg/day.[304] There was no difference in time to remission or the percentage of patients who achieved remission by 9 months (88% of both groups) and no difference in improvement of GFR over time. Although there were more relapses in the IV group, this was not statistically significant. The total dose of cyclophosphamide was approximately half as much in the IV group versus the oral group, and infections were more common with oral cyclophosphamide. Thus, both regimens are effective and relapses appear more common with IV therapy, but total dose and adverse effects of the cytotoxic agent are reduced by IV usage. It is unclear how frequently the initial IV "pulses" of cyclophosphamide should be given, with some investigators using monthly doses and others starting with smaller doses every 2 to 3 weeks. It is clear that early application of an intensive immunosuppressive regimen helps prevent long-term morbidity and end-organ damage. Because the total dose of the cyclophosphamide is far less in patients receiving pulsed IV therapy, many prefer to use it as a less toxic regimen and try to enhance maintenance therapy to avoid relapse.

Methotrexate has been used for both induction and maintenance therapy in patients with WG and other ANCA-associated vasculitides.[305-308] The largest trial, the NORAM trial, compared methotrexate (20–25 mg per week orally) to oral cyclophosphamide (2 mg/kg/day) both for 1 year with corticosteroids in 95 ANCA-positive vasculitis patients (89 with WG; six with microscopic polyangiitis).[305]Although an equal percent of both groups achieved remission, the time to remission was longer in the methotrexate group and the relapse rate much higher (70% vs. 47%). Given these data, methotrexate is rarely used for induction therapy in ANCA-positive vasculitis unless the disease is very mild and rapidly controllable.

Although the role of the addition of plasmapheresis in WG was debated in the past, it appears to benefit certain patients with severe renal failure, those with pulmonary hemorrhage, those with coexistent anti-GBM antibodies, and those failing all other therapeutic agents.[298,301,309] In one study of 20 ANCA-positive small vessel vasculitis, patients with massive pulmonary hemorrhage treated with methylprednisolone, IV cyclophosphamide, and plasmapheresis, all 20 patients had resolution of their pulmonary hemorrhage with this regimen.[310] Likewise, a review of 88 patients with ANCA-positive renal vasculitis in seven series in the literature showed a benefit in renal survival with plasmapheresis added (67%) over standard steroid and cyclophosphamide therapy (40%). A trial of 137 patients with ANCA-positive GN, the Methylprednisolone versus Plasma Exchange (MEPEX) trial, evaluated patients with a marked elevation of the serum creatinine (>500 μm/L or 5.7 mg/dL) treated with induction therapy with either plasma exchange versus IV pulsed methylprednisolone, both with oral corticosteroids and cyclophosphamide.[311] Although both groups had an equal and high 1-year mortality rate, the plasma exchange group had an improved short-term patient survival and a greater likelihood of not reaching renal failure at 1 year (19 vs. 43%). The addition of etanercept, a TNF-α blocker, to a standard induction regimen for WG was evaluated in 174 patients and provided no additional benefit in terms of sustained remissions or time to achieve remission.[312] Disease flares and adverse events were common in both treatment groups, and solid tumors developed in six of the etanercept group. The use of infliximab, a TNF-α blocker, in four uncontrolled trials was associated with an 80% remission rate but a high rate of infectious complications.[313] Likewise, a study of alemtuzumab, an anti-CD52 monoclonal antibody, in 70 patients gave a remission rate of 83% but was associated with high rates of relapse, infection, and mortality.[314]

Small uncontrolled trials initially found a role for rituximab in ANCA-positive vasculitis, with sustained remissions in many of the patients studied.[315,316] Two controlled randomized studies support the use of rituximab as a first-line therapy comparable in efficacy to cyclophosphamide for the treatment of ANCA-associated vasculitis.[317-319] In the Rituxivas Study, 44 patients (mean age, 68 years) were randomized, with two-thirds receiving four doses of IV rituximab and only two doses of IV cyclophosphamide and one of IV pulse solumedrol versus the remaining one-third of patients who received six to 10 pulses of IV cyclophosphamide.[317] Both groups received steroids in tapering doses. The number of remissions, time to remission, and side effects were similar in the two groups. Mortality and morbidity were high in both groups because of the age of the patients and their renal dysfunction. In the Rituximab in ANCA Associated Vasculitis (RAVE) trial, 197 patients with severe ANCA-associated vasculitis (75% with WG) were randomized to steroids plus either four weekly doses (375 mg/m²) of rituximab or oral cyclophosphamide (2 mg/kg/day) with replacement by azathioprine maintenance in both groups.[318] Sixty-four percent of the rituximab group reached remission, but only 53% of the cyclophosphamide group did. More patients in the rituximab arm had resolution of active vasculitis by activity scores. Adverse events were similar in both arms of the study. The subgroups with renal involvement and pulmonary hemorrhage also fared the same. Although this does not mean that rituximab will replace cyclophosphamide as standard treatment for patients with WG or ANCA-positive vasculitis, it does allow it to be used as an initial treatment option for many patients.[319]

Relapse rates from 20% to 50% have been reported often when infectious complications have led to a discontinuation of immunosuppressive therapy.[291,294,299,320,321] Predictors of relapse in a cohort of 350 patients with ANCA-positive vasculitis included C-ANCA or PR3 positivity, lung involvement, and upper respiratory involvement as opposed to factors not predicting relapse such as age, gender, race, and a clinical diagnosis of WG rather than microscopic polyangiitis or renal-limited vasculitis.[316] Most patients respond to another course of cyclophosphamide therapy.[299] In patients whose ANCA levels have declined during remission, a major increase in titer may predict a relapse, although ANCA levels and clinical disease activity do not always correlate.[291-295]

Because of the potential for severe complications with cyclophosphamide therapy (infections, infertility, hemorrhagic cystitis, and an increased risk of long-term malignancy), after an initial remission has been achieved, patients have usually been switched to less toxic immunosuppressive agents such as azathioprine, low-dose methotrexate, or MMF.[320-325] A study of 155 patients with ANCA-positive vasculitis treated patients with cyclophosphamide and steroids to induce a remission and then randomized patients to either oral azathioprine or continued cyclophosphamide maintenance therapy.[325] Of the 155 patients, 144 entered remission and were randomized. There was no difference in the relapse rate in the two groups or in the adverse event rate. Relapse rates were lower in patients with microscopic polyangiitis than in the WG group. Cyclosporine has also been used successfully as maintenance therapy in small numbers of patients.[326] Because respiratory infections, perhaps through priming of neutrophils or activation of ANCA, may be associated with flares of disease activity, prophylactic use of trimethoprim–sulfamethoxazole has been advocated.[327] Methotrexate has also been used as maintenance therapy in WG.[307,308] Other agents evaluated in WG include IVIG, 15-deoxyspergualin, and humanized monoclonal antibodies directed at T cells.[328-330] Supportive measures such as sinus drainage procedures, hearing aids, and corrective surgery for nasal septal collapse may be helpful in individuals with chronic sequelae of upper respiratory involvement.[249-253]

Dialysis and transplantation have been performed in increasing numbers of WG patients.[331-337] Many patients' disease activity diminishes with the onset of renal failure.[335] Some patients still require intensive immunosuppression after reaching renal failure, and relapses have been reported well after the onset of ESRD. Fatality rates may be high in some ESRD populations because of slow recognition of relapses of the vasculitic process in the presence of dialysis. Most patients receiving allografts have been maintained on prednisone and cyclosporine or tacrolimus with or without mycophenolate with very good patient and allograft survival rates.[331-337] Recurrent active GN in the allograft occurs in 15% to 37% of patients and may respond to cyclophosphamide therapy or other more intensive therapies.[332-337] There is no evidence that regimens, including MMF or tacrolimus, have advantages over older immunosuppressive regimens in preventing recurrences of WG activity.[333,336] There is only limited experience with sirolimus and other newer transplant immunosuppressive agents.[338]

Microscopic Polyangiitis and Polyarteritis Nodosa

Polyarteritis nodosa (PAN) was first described by Rokitansky in 1852, and the term *periarteritis nodosa* was first used by Kussmaul and Maier in 1866.[339] The disease had been divided into a "classic" pattern with a systemic necrotizing vasculitis primarily affecting muscular arteries, often at branch points, producing lesions of varying ages with focal aneurysm formation and a "microscopic" polyangiitis with a necrotizing inflammation of small arteries, veins, and capillaries involving multiple viscera, including lung and dermis and producing lesions of similar age, usually without aneurysms. Although there are some overlapping features between these diseases and some patients with both presentations may be ANCA positive and have a pauci-immune crescentic GN, it is best to consider these entities separately because the

pathology in most is distinct and the etiologies are likely to be different.[248,250-254] ANCA-positive microscopic polyangiitis should clearly be considered as part of the spectrum of ANCA-associated small vessel vasculitis ranging from renal-limited rapidly progressive glomerulonephritis (RPGN) to multisystem diseases, including WG and Churg-Strauss syndrome.[248,250-254]

Classic Macroscopic Polyarteritis Nodosa

PAN is more common in males than females (sex ratio, 2.5:1) and occurs most often in the fifth and sixth decades of life. Clinically, the prevalence of renal disease in PAN varies from 64% to 76% in unselected series and virtually 100% in nephrology-based series.[340-343] The prevalence of pathologic renal involvement may exceed that of clinically evident renal disease. True idiopathic polyarteritis is a primary vasculitis. Classic polyarteritis has been associated with drug abuse with amphetamines and other illicit drugs, but it is unclear how many of these patients had associated viral infectious hepatitis.[344] The most common associated illness found in patients with classic PAN is hepatitis B infection. The incidence ranges from 0% to 55% of different series but is probably less than 10% of all cases.[345] It is unclear how many of these patients have had concomitant hepatitis C infection. Hairy cell leukemia has also been reported in association with PAN.[346]

Pathology

In classic PAN, the glomeruli are usually unaffected. Some glomeruli may show ischemic retraction of the tuft and sclerosis of Bowman's capsule. Some patients with large vessel vasculitis may also have a focal necrotizing GN with or without crescents identical to that seen in microscopic polyarteritis and idiopathic pauci-immune RPGN.[263,340] The vasculitis in classic PAN affects the medium-sized to large arteries (i.e., those of subarcuate, arcuate, and interlobar caliber) in a segmental distribution, often producing lesions of different ages, including acute, healing, and chronic lesions.[263,340] Segments of arterial involvement are interspersed with normal areas producing "skip lesions" and often have eccentric inflammation of the vessel wall. In areas of active vasculitis, there is inflammation of the vessel wall with infiltrates composed of lymphocytes, polymorphonuclear leukocytes, monocytes, and occasionally eosinophils that may involve the intima alone, the intima and media, or all three layers of the vessel wall. Lesions are often necrotizing with mural fibrin deposition and rupture of the elastic membranes. Areas of necrosis may lead to aneurysm formation, particularly in larger arteries (i.e., arcuate, interlobar), which can be associated with rupture and hemorrhage into the renal parenchyma. Superimposed thrombosis with luminal occlusion is common. In the healing phase, the vascular inflammation subsides, and the vessel wall is thickened by concentric cellular proliferation of myointimal cells separated by a loose, ground substance. Localized destruction of elastic lamellae is demonstrable with elastic stains. Eventually, the media is replaced by areas of broad fibrous scars. There may be almost total occlusion of the vessel lumen by intimal fibroplasia with areas of concentric reduplication and discontinuity of the internal elastic membrane. Wedge-shaped, macroscopic cortical infarcts are common in "classic" polyarteritis and are usually caused by thrombotic occlusion of the vasculitic lesions.[340] In more chronic phases, tubular atrophy and interstitial fibrosis develop.

Autopsy studies in PAN describe the kidneys as being the most commonly affected organ (65%) followed by the liver (54%); periadrenal tissue (41%); pancreas (39%); and less commonly, the muscle and brain.[340-342] Other tissues giving high yields when biopsied for diagnostic vasculitic lesions include the testes, sural nerve, skin, rectum, and skeletal muscle.

Pathogenesis of Polyarteritis Nodosa

The vasculitis of PAN may be mediated by diverse pathogenetic factors, including humoral vascular immune deposits, cellular immunity, endothelial cytopathic factors, and ANCA. An immune complex pathogenesis of vasculitis is suggested by experiments of acute serum sickness in which an acute GN is produced along with a systemic vasculitis resembling PAN.[340] The vasculitis can be largely prevented by complement or neutrophil depletion. The experimental Arthus reaction can also induce a vasculitis resulting from in situ vascular immune complex formation with vessel injury preventable by neutrophil or complement depletion.[347] MRL-1 mice develop an immune complex GN with necrotizing vasculitis similar to PAN[348] in association with high levels of CICs, predominantly with autoantibodies containing anti-DNA. Viral infection of the muscle cells of the vessel media by murine leukemia virus is also associated with a necrotizing vasculitis and lupus-like syndrome with vascular deposits of immunoglobulin and complement.[348,349] However, glomerular and vascular immune deposits are rarely found in human PAN despite significant levels of CICs.

Two models of cell-mediated vasculitis have been produced experimentally in mice.[350] There is no evidence in these models for vascular immune deposits, and some have a granulomatous form of vasculitis similar to that of PAN in multiple organs. In Kawasaki vasculitis, IgM anti-endothelial antibodies directed against endothelial surface antigens inducible by cytokines have been found.[351] Likewise, several viral infections in humans are capable of inducing direct cytopathic injury to arterial endothelium.[340]

Clinical Features of Polyarteritis Nodosa

The clinical features of PAN are quite variable. In the past, many patients with ANCA-positive idiopathic pauci-immune rapidly progressive GN with evidence of extrarenal symptoms were included in the spectrum of polyarteritis.[352] The most common clinical findings of true PAN relate to constitutional symptoms of fever, weight loss, and malaise. GI involvement may include nausea, vomiting, abdominal pain, GI bleeding, bowel infarcts, and perforations.[340,353] Liver involvement may be associated with hepatitis B or C, and vasculitis of the mesenteric vessels, hepatic arteries, and gallbladder leading to cholecystitis have all been found.[345,354] Patients may develop heart failure; coronary artery ischemia with angina or myocardial infarction; and less commonly, pericarditis and conduction abnormalities.[340] Disease of the nervous system may be central, with seizures and cerebrovascular accidents or related to peripheral nerves, with mononeuritis multiple and peripheral neuropathies.[340,355-357]

Patients may develop muscle weakness, myalgias or myositis, and arthralgias, but frank arthritis is less common.[340,358] Other clinical findings relate to disease in the gonads, salivary glands, pancreas, adrenal, ureter, breast, and eyes.[340,359] In general, with the exception of liver manifestations and arthralgias, there is little difference between the clinical findings of patients who are hepatitis B positive or negative. Cutaneous disease may present with "palpable purpura" with a leukocytoclastic angiitis or with petechiae, nodules, papules, livedo reticularis, and skin ulcerations. Pulmonary involvement is variable depending on the criteria for classification of PAN and whether patients with small vessel ANCA-positive vasculitis such as WG and Churg-Strauss syndrome have been excluded.[340] In classic PAN, patients typically have findings related to visceral organ infarction and ischemia, and abdominal, cardiac, and neurologic findings are prominent. This is in distinction to ANCA-positive microscopic polyangiitis, in which cutaneous disease and pulmonary findings are more frequent.[250-254]

Laboratory Tests

Laboratory tests in patients with PAN include an elevated ESR and anemia, leukocytosis, and thrombocytosis.[340,352] Eosinophilia is found in from 10% to 40% of patients with PAN. Patients with classic PAN are usually ANCA negative. Most patients have negative test results for ANA and normal serum complement values. Test results for CICs and rheumatoid factor are often positive.[360] Although cryoglobulin results have often been reported to be positive, it is unclear what percent have had associated viral hepatitis.[340] The incidence of hepatitis B antigenemia has been variable, ranging form 0% to as many as 40%. It is usually positive in fewer than 10% of unselected patients.[340,360]

Renal Findings in Polyarteritis Nodosa

The renal manifestations in classic PAN reflect renal ischemia and infarction because of predominant involvement of the larger vessels. Hypertension is common and is found initially in up to half of patients.[340] Hypertension may be mild or severe, and if not present initially, it can develop at any time during the course of the disease.[341,342,352,353,361] Presenting symptoms related to kidney disease are uncommon in PAN but may include hemorrhage from a renal artery aneurysm, flank pain, and gross hematuria. Oliguric acute renal failure is uncommon, as are symptoms related to the nephrotic syndrome.

Angiographic examination of the vasculature in PAN often reveals evidence of vasculitis. Angiograms reveal multiple rounded, saccular aneurysms of medium-sized vessels in about 70% of cases as well as thromboses, stenoses, and other luminal irregularities.[340,362] Aneurysms most commonly involve the hepatic, splanchnic and renal vessels, are usually bilateral, multiple, and vary in size from 1 to 12 mm.[362] There is no way to clinically predict the presence of aneurysms.[379] Vasculitic changes and even aneurysms can heal over time as documented by angiography, usually correlating with the clinical response of the patient.[361,362] Similar aneurysms have been documented in patients with WG, SLE, TTP, bacterial endocarditis, and Churg-Strauss syndrome.[340]

Prognosis and Treatment of Polyarteritis Nodosa

In retrospective studies, untreated patients with PAN had a dismal survival.[340] Many patients had a fulminant course with a high early mortality because of acute vasculitis. A poor prognosis was found in elderly patients, those with a delay in diagnosis, those with GI tract catastrophes such as bowel infarction and hemorrhage, and those with severe renal disease. The presence of hypertension has affected the prognosis only in some studies. Renal prognosis has also been reported to be adversely affected by increased activity on the biopsy, more crescents, severity of endocapillary proliferation, and glomerulosclerosis.[340] Early mortality in PAN relates to the active vasculitis leading to renal failure, GI hemorrhage, or acute cardiovascular events, but late mortality has been attributed to chronic vascular changes with chronic renal failure and heart disease with congestive heart failure.[341] Survival has not been different in a series of more than 150 patients with focal segmental necrotizing GN, either alone or with associated arteritis.[363]

Corticosteroid use improved the survival of PAN patients significantly, with 5-year survival rates of approximately 50%.[341] Nevertheless, some patients achieved only partial remissions of the disease with continued activity leading to long-term morbidity and mortality. The use of cytotoxic immunosuppressives has greatly improved the survival with 5-year survival rate well over 80%.[364-366] Although a number of immunosuppressives, including azathioprine, busulfan, methotrexate, 6-mercaptopurine, and antithymocyte globulin, have all been used, cyclophosphamide is widely accepted as the most effective agent.[364-366] The initial therapy of patients with PAN usually consists of high doses of cyclophosphamide (e.g., 2 mg/kg/day), commonly given along with high doses of corticosteroids (e.g., 1 mg/kg/day of prednisone), which are then tapered over time. Successful treatment can lead to complete inactivity of the vasculitic process and even reversal of severe renal failure. INF-α and other antiviral agents have been used in the treatment of PAN associated with hepatitis B infection and hairy cell leukemia.[367,368] For patients with ESRD, immunosuppressive therapy should be continued for 6 months to 1 year after the disease appears inactive. Transplantation has been performed in only a limited number of patients with PAN.

Microscopic Polyangiitis

The incidence of renal disease associated with this ANCA-positive small vessel vasculitis appears to be increasing.[250-254] Although this may be because of wider use of ANCA testing and renal biopsy, many investigators believe the absolute incidence has increased. In one large series, ANCA-associated crescentic GN made up almost 10% of all glomerular diseases diagnosed by renal biopsy in a 2-year period. In very elderly patients, this was the most common etiologic diagnosis.[255,256] Vasculitis and GN similar to those seen in microscopic polyarteritis have been noted in relapsing polychondritis[369,370] and ANCA-positive polyangiitis induced by use of a number of medications, most notably the antithyroid medication PTU.[371]

Pathology of Microscopic Polyangiitis

Patients with microscopic polyangiitis infrequently have a true arteritis identified on renal biopsy. The frequency ranges from 11% to 22% with predominant involvement of interlobular arteries and arterioles rather than larger vessels as in "classic" PAN.[340] In contrast to PAN, involvement is circumferential, lesions are generally of the same age, and aneurysm formation is rare. The acute vasculitis is usually necrotizing with fibrinoid necrosis of the vessel wall and infiltration by neutrophils and mononuclear leukocytes. Vasculitis with granulomatous features is relatively uncommon. In later stages of the disease, there may be narrowing of the lumens of small arteries caused by concentric intimal fibroplasia and elastic reduplication, but medial scarring is less frequent and severe than in PAN. In microscopic polyangiitis, there is often a diffuse interstitial inflammatory cell infiltrate with plasma cells, lymphocytes, and polymorphonuclear leukocytes, especially around glomeruli and vessels. In some biopsies, the interstitial infiltrate also contains prominent eosinophils. Interstitial inflammatory cells may penetrate the tubular basement membrane, causing tubulitis.[340] In more chronic stages, patchy tubular atrophy with interstitial fibrosis parallels the distribution of the glomerular and vascular damage.

In microscopic polyangiitis, the most typical histologic finding is focal segmental necrotizing GN with crescents affecting from few to many glomeruli (Figure 32-16).[250-254,263,340] There is segmental rupture of the GBM associated with polymorphonuclear infiltration, karyorrhexis, and fibrin deposition within the glomerular tuft and the adjacent Bowman's space. Crescents characteristically overlie areas of segmental tuft necrosis and may be segmental or circumferential. Both cellular and fibrous crescents often coexist in the same biopsy. Some crescents are voluminous with a "sunburst" appearance caused by massive circumferential destruction of Bowman's capsule. Uninvolved glomeruli are typically normocellular. In the chronic or healing phase of the disease, there is segmental and global glomerulosclerosis with focal fibrous crescents. Although there are many similarities, one study documents differences between biopsies of patients with microscopic polyangiitis and WG. Biopsies from patients with polygiitis and patients who are MPO and ANCA positive were more likely to show glomerulosclerosis, interstitial fibrosis, and tubular atrophy. This suggests a more prolonged, less

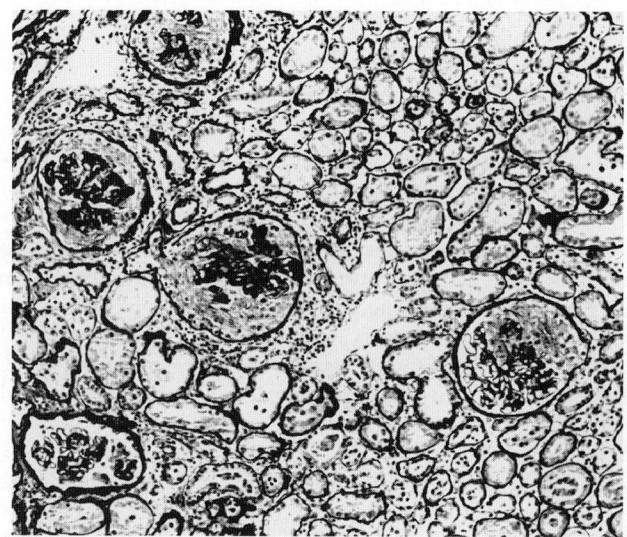

FIGURE 32-16 Microscopic polyangiitis. There are diffuse crescents with focal segmental necrosis of the glomerular tuft (Jones methenamine silver, ×125).

fulminant course in patients with microscopic polyangiitis compared to those with WG. A new international classification differentiates glomerular lesions depending on whether they are focal, crescentic, mixed, or sclerotic and found correlates with clinical outcome.[372]

Immunofluorescence and Electron Microscopic Findings

In most cases, the glomeruli show no or only weak IF staining consistent with the designation "pauci-immune" GN.[340,372] A review of a number of large series reported positivity for one or more immunoglobulins in from 3% to 35% of cases, with variability of intensity.[340] Fibrin or fibrinogen was the most common and intensely staining reactant identified in the glomeruli followed by C3 with relatively sparse IgG and Clq.[371] The pattern is believed to be consistent with "nonspecific trapping" in areas of glomerular necrosis and sclerosis rather than immune complex deposition. Vascular staining is similar.

By EM, the glomeruli in most patients with microscopic polyangiitis have no or rarely sparse irregular, glomerular electron-dense deposits.[263,340,372] Glomeruli may show endothelial swelling, subendothelial accumulation of "fluffy" electron-lucent material, and subendothelial and intracapillary fibrin deposition. Through gaps in the GBM, fibrin tactoids and neutrophils exude into Bowman's space associated with epithelial crescents. In the chronic phase, glomeruli develop segmental or global glomerulosclerosis with fibrous crescents. Vascular changes have included swelling and focal degeneration of the endothelium; separation of the endothelium from its basement membrane with subendothelial fibrin deposition; and with severe damage intraluminal and intramural fibrin deposition, edema and inflammatory infiltration of the intima and media by leukocytes.[340,372] As in the glomeruli, no discrete electron-dense deposits are found in the vessels, although there may be plasmatic insudation. In biopsies with chronic changes, there may be expansion of the vessel intima by concentric layers of elastic tissue, fibrillar collagen, and nonfibrillar basement membrane material with focal scarring of the media.

Pathogenesis of Microscopic Polyangiitis

ANCA may play a pathogenetic role in ANCA-associated microscopic polyangiitis and GN in a manner similar to WG[283-293] (see section on WG). There is initial priming of the neutrophil with cytokines and other mediators of inflammation, perhaps in response to infection, leading to expression of MPO ANCA antigens on the surface of the neutrophil. These exposed antigens are then poised to react with circulating ANCAs. Neutrophils become activated and undergo a respiratory burst, with degranulation and release of reactive oxygen species onto endothelial surfaces. In drug-induced microscopic polyangiitis, although ANCA develop in relation to many different antigens (e.g., elastase, cathepsin G, lactoferrin), only patients with high titers of high avidity and complement binding anti-MPO antibodies develop the disease.[290,371]

Clinical Features of Microscopic Polyangiitis

Patients with idiopathic ANCA-negative pauci-immune focal segmental necrotizing GN and ANCA-positive rapidly progressive GN have similar clinical findings and presentations regardless of whether vasculitis has been documented on renal biopsy.[250-254] Likewise the extrarenal findings in patients with ANCA-positive, rapidly progressive GN have been similar whether the patients are P-ANCA or C-ANCA positive.[250-254] Because microscopic polyangiitis is a multisystem disease with multiple organs involved, many of the clinical findings are similar to those of ANCA-positive WG. Cutaneous disease occurs commonly with macular lesions, papules, and purpura of the lower extremities. Rheumatologic involvement is seen with arthralgias, myalgias, and nondeforming arthritis of the large and small joints. Neurologic disease may present as mononeuritis multiplex or peripheral or central nervous system involvement. Pulmonary disease is quite common and presents with shortness of breath, dyspnea, cough, and wheezing.[250-254]

Laboratory Tests in Microscopic Polyangiitis

Abnormal laboratory test results may include a normochromic, normocytic anemia, and a mild leukocytosis and thrombocytosis.[250-254] Eosinophilia is found in a significant number of patients. Nonspecific inflammatory markers such as the ESR and CRP are often elevated. ANA, serum complement levels, and cryoglobulins are normal or negative.

The widespread use of accurate assays for ANCA has facilitated the clinical diagnosis of microscopic polyangiitis.[250-254] There is considerable clinical overlap between patients with microscopic polyangiitis, WG, and Churg-Strauss syndrome, and all have high rates of ANCA positivity. Although C-ANCA–positive patients are more likely to have biopsy-proven necrotizing vasculitis or granulomatous inflammation of the sinuses or lower respiratory tract, there is a large overlap in the clinical manifestations between C-ANCA–positive and P-ANCA–positive patients. ANCA titers vary considerably among patients with similar clinical manifestations, and the role of the titer in predicting flares of the disease is not fully defined (see section on WG). Some patients retain high ANCA levels despite clinical remission, and some patients are positive for anti-GBM antibodies as well as ANCA (see section on anti-GBM disease).

Renal Findings

In microscopic polyangiitis, most patients have laboratory evidence of their renal involvement at presentation. The majority of patients have urinary sediment changes with microscopic hematuria and often RBC casts.[250-254] Proteinuria is common, but the nephrotic syndrome is rare. A decreased GFR is present in up to half of the patients in unselected series and more in those selected for renal involvement. Severe renal insufficiency may be found at presentation. These renal findings are similar in patients with ANCA-positive RPGN, whether or not it is associated with systemic involvement.[250-254,266,352] In microscopic polyangiitis, the severity of the clinical renal findings generally correlates with the degree of glomerular involvement, as for patients with WG. Whereas patients with normal serum creatinines or creatinine clearances are likely to have greater numbers of normal glomeruli on biopsy, patients with reduced or deteriorating renal function are more likely to exhibit more glomeruli with severe segmental necrotizing GN or diffuse proliferative features.[340,343] Extensive crescent formation correlates with oliguria, severe renal failure, and a residual decrease in GFR after therapy.

Prognosis and Treatment

Standard treatment of patients with microscopic polyangiitis has included cyclophosphamide and corticosteroids in a fashion similar to the treatment of patients with WG.[250-254] Controlled trials of the use of IV versus oral cyclophosphamide, anti–TNF-α agents, methotrexate, and rituximab have all been examined in populations of ANCA-positive vasculitis patients, including those with WG, microscopic polyangiitis, and isolated renal vasculitis combined.[303-305,310-312,317-319] These regimens are discussed extensively in the section on WG. In most studies, both MPO- and PR3 ANCA-positive patients have responded equally. Likewise, the presence or absence of systemic symptoms has not dictated the response. However, even patients with a good initial response to therapy may experience residual glomerular damage and progress to ESRD.[365] Thus, aggressive, vigorous early therapy to turn off the disease process is believed to be crucial in preventing residual organ damage.[250-254] Therapeutic intervention in addition to immunosuppressive therapy includes measures to prevent non-immunologic glomerular disease progression such as the use of renin–angiotensin blockade, hyperlipidemia control, and low-protein diets in some patients.

Churg-Strauss Syndrome (Allergic Granulomatosis)

Churg-Strauss syndrome, or allergic granulomatosis and angiitis, is an uncommon systemic disease characterized by vasculitis, asthma, organ infiltration by eosinophils, and peripheral eosinophilia.[373-376] Churg and Strauss first fully described the syndrome in 1951.[340] Although there may be some overlap with other vasculitic and allergic processes such as PAN, WG, and microscopic polyangiitis, Loeffler syndrome, and chronic eosinophilic pneumonitis, the clinical and pathologic features of Churg-Strauss syndrome are distinct.[373-376]

Churg-Strauss syndrome is uncommon, with only several hundred cases reported.[373-378] In a review of almost 185,000 asthmatic patients taking medications, only 21 cases of Churg-Strauss syndrome were identified.[379] The low incidence may reflect underrecognition. There might also be a higher incidence if a looser definition was applied requiring only some of the clinical and histopathologic features. A more inclusive definition requires (1) asthma, (2) peripheral blood eosinophilia, and (3) systemic vasculitis involving two or more extrapulmonary organs. Using this definition, many cases described as other vasculitic syndromes in patients with asthma would fit the definition of Churg-Strauss syndrome.

There is no gender predominance in Churg-Strauss syndrome, and although the disease has been reported at all ages, the mean age at diagnosis is around 50 years old.[373-378] Clinical renal involvement is clearly less prevalent than morphologic renal involvement. However, a recent series reports a high incidence of clinical renal disease.[380] In autopsy series, the kidney is affected in more than half of patients, but clinical renal disease has been described in from 25% to more than 90% of patients.[374-378,380]

A number of studies document the rare occurrence of Churg-Strauss syndrome in steroid-dependent patients with asthma taking leukotriene receptor antagonists (e.g., montelukast, zafirlukast, pranlukast).[381-386] Although not all have investigators have been able to document an association between leukotriene receptor antagonists and the development of the disease, analysis of all cases in the literature does support this association.[387,388] This may occur via unmasking of the vasculitic syndrome because the leukotriene receptor antagonist permits steroid withdrawal, as similar cases have been reported in patients with asthma after a change from oral to inhaled steroids.[403,404] Rarely, substitution of a leukotriene receptor antagonist for inhaled steroids has also led to Churg-Strauss syndrome.[386,387]

Pathology

Renal biopsies in Churg-Strauss syndrome vary from normal kidney tissue to severe GN, vasculitis, and interstitial inflammation.[340,373-376,380,389,390] There may be a focal segmental necrotizing GN, sometimes with small crescents. In most cases, the GN is mild, affects only a minority of glomeruli, and involves the tuft segmentally. The GN may rarely be diffuse and global with severe necrotizing features and crescents. In some cases, there is only mesangial hypercellularity without endocapillary proliferation or necrosis. In the original autopsy studies by Churg and Strauss, vasculitis was found in the kidney in more than half of cases, and it has been noted on renal biopsy as well.[340] It may involve any level of the renal arterial tree from arterioles to large arcuate or interlobar arteries and may vary from fibrinoid necrotizing to granulomatous. Although resembling other forms of vasculitis, the arteritis is characterized by eosinophilic granulocytes within the arterial wall and in the surrounding connective tissue (Figure 32-17). Destruction of elastic membrane, aneurysms, and luminal thrombosis with recanalization, as well as epithelioid cells and multinucleated giant cells in the media, adventitia, and perivascular connective tissue, may occur. Active and healed lesions may coexist. Less commonly, venules and small veins of interlobular size may be affected, often with granulomatous features. The tubulointerstitial region is involved by an

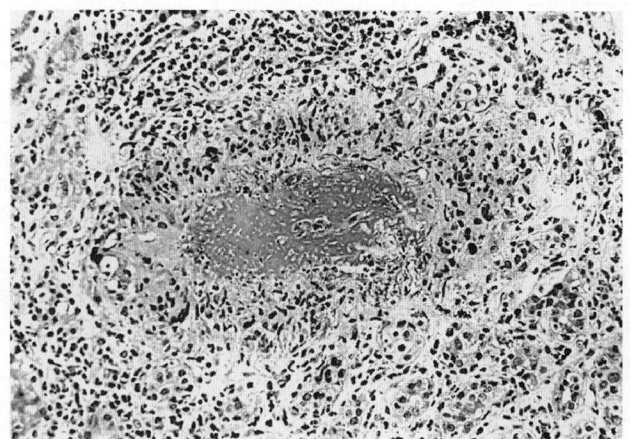

FIGURE 32-17 Churg-Strauss syndrome. Granulomatous vasculitis involves an arcuate artery. There is granulomatous transmural inflammation with focal giant cells and superimposed luminal thrombosis (hematoxylin and eosin, ×125).

inflammatory infiltrate containing many eosinophils and some lymphocytes, plasma cells, and polymorphonuclear leukocytes in association with interstitial edema.[340,380] In some cases, interstitial granulomas are present composed of a core of eosinophilic or basophilic necrotic material surrounded by a rim of radially oriented macrophages, giant cells of the Langhans type, and numerous eosinophils. Interstitial nephritis may be present without glomerular pathology.

By IF, areas of segmental necrosis in the glomeruli may contain IgM, C_3, and fibrinogen.[340,380] The presence of IgE in renal or other tissues has not been adequately investigated.[391] EM of the glomeruli, pulmonary granulomas, venules, and capillaries reveals no electron-dense deposits.[340,374-376]

Pathogenesis

Although the pathogenesis of Churg-Strauss syndrome remains unclear, allergic or hypersensitivity mechanisms are supported by the presence of asthma, hypereosinophilia, and elevated plasma levels of IgE.[373-376,388,391] Eosinophils in patients with Churg-Strauss syndrome have prolonged survival because of inhibition of CD95-mediated apoptosis and T-cell secretion of eosinophil-activating cytokines. Human eosinophil cationic proteins (ECPs), which are capable of tissue destruction in a variety of hypereosinophilic syndromes, have been found in granulomatous tissue from patients with Churg-Strauss syndrome.[392,393] Higher serum levels of ECP, soluble IL-2 receptor, and soluble thrombomodulin levels have been associated with disease activity.[393] Hypocomplementemia and CICs have rarely been observed, and the negative IF and EM findings do not support an immune complex mechanism. Cell-mediated immunity is likely involved, and high helper-to-suppressor ratios in the peripheral blood during active disease as well as a preponderance of helper T cells in the granulomas of skin biopsies have been reported.[340] In patients with positive ANCA, the ANCA antibody may play a pathogenic role akin to WG and microscopic polyangiitis.[277-282]

Clinical and Laboratory Features

Patients may have initial constitutional symptoms such as weight loss, fatigue, malaise, and fever.[340,373-376] Characteristic extrarenal features include asthma (present in >95% of cases), an allergic diathesis, allergic rhinitis, and peripheral eosinophilia.[373,378] Asthmatic disease typically precedes the onset of the vasculitis by years, but it may occur simultaneously. The severity of the asthma does not necessarily parallel the severity of the vasculitis. Many patients subsequently develop eosinophilia in the blood along with eosinophilic infiltrates in multiple organs. This is followed by vasculitis in some patients. Disease often involves the heart with pericarditis, heart failure, or ischemic disease; the GI tract with abdominal pain, ulceration, diarrhea, or bowel perforation; and the skin with subcutaneous nodules, petechiae, or purpuric lesions.[373-376,394,395] Peripheral neuropathy with mononeuritis multiplex is common, but migrating polyarthralgias and arthritis occur less frequently.[396] The eye, prostate, and genitourinary tract may be involved. Some patients with Churg-Strauss syndrome have overlapping features with PAN or the other ANCA-positive vasculitides.[373-376]

Laboratory evaluation typically reveals anemia, leukocytosis, and an elevated ESR and CRP level.[373-376] Eosinophilia is universally present and may reach 50% of the total peripheral leukocyte count. The degree of eosinophilia and the ESR may correlate with disease activity as may the level of ECP, soluble IL-2 receptor, and soluble thrombomodulin levels.[393] Rheumatoid factor is often positive, but serum complement, hepatitis markers, CICs, ANA, and cryoglobulins are usually negative or normal.[373-376] Elevated serum IgE levels and IgE-containing CICs are frequently found.[393-396,409] Chest radiography may show patchy infiltrates, nodules, diffuse interstitial disease, and pleural effusion.[373-376,397-399] Pleural effusions may be exudative and contain large numbers of eosinophils.[399] On angiography, visceral aneurysms may be present in patients with both PAN overlap syndromes and classic Churg-Strauss syndrome.

ANCA levels are elevated in 40% to 80% of Churg-Strauss patients.[373-376,400-402] Most are P-ANCA and anti-MPO positive, but some are C-ANCA and anti-PR3 positive. In one analysis of almost 100 patients, 35% were ANCA positive by indirect IF with a perinuclear pattern and anti-MPO specificity in about 75%.[401] Some investigators have found a good correlation between ANCA positivity and ANCA titers and clinical activity, but others have not.[394,401] Clearly, in some, ANCA titers may remain positive despite clinical remissions. In patients with Churg-Strauss syndrome, ANCA positivity has often correlated with active GN, pulmonary hemorrhage, neuropathy, and the presence of small vessel vasculitis.[375,376,400,401]

Although the clinical renal findings in Churg-Strauss syndrome are diverse, the kidney is rarely the major organ system involved. Microscopic hematuria and mild proteinuria are common, but nephrotic range proteinuria is infrequent. Hypertension is found in up to 75% of patients. In the past, renal failure has been uncommon. Recent reports, however, suggest a higher incidence of renal involvement and renal failure.[377,378,389] In one study of more than 100 patients, signs of renal involvement were present in 25%, with rapidly progressive renal failure in 14%.[389] Of the 16 patients undergoing renal biopsy, 11 had a necrotizing crescentic GN, and others had an eosinophilic interstitial nephritis. ANCA was positive in 75% of the patients with nephropathy as opposed to 25% of patients without nephropathy.

Prognosis, Course, and Treatment

Patients may have several phases of the syndrome over many years.[373-378] There may be a prodromal phase of asthma or allergic rhinitis followed by a phase of peripheral blood and tissue eosinophilia that is remitting and relapsing over months to years before the development of systemic vasculitis. A shorter duration of asthma before the onset of vasculitis has been associated with a worse prognosis. The correlation between ANCA levels and disease activity has been variable. In general, renal disease is mild with only 7% of patients in one large literature review having renal failure as a cause of death, even including untreated patients.[340,380] However, cases progressing to severe renal failure and dialysis have certainly been reported.[378] Most patients surviving the initial insult usually fare well with survival rates in treated patients of approximately 90% at 1 year and 70% at 5 years.[373-378,394]

Patients with significant cardiac, CNS, and GI involvement and those with greater degrees of renal damage have a poorer long-term survival.[394]

Corticosteroid therapy is successful in many patents with Churg-Strauss syndrome with mild disease and those with interstitial disease.[373-378] Patients may respond rapidly to high daily oral prednisone therapy, and even those with relapses respond to retreatment. Those with extrarenal disease often respond as well. In patients with multisystem disease with necrotizing GN and other signs of severe organ involvement, cyclophosphamide and corticosteroids have generally been used together.[403] Patients with resistant cases and those who require maintenance treatment may benefit from treatment with other immunosuppressive agents such as azathioprine, methotrexate, MMF, rituximab, or plasma exchange.[373-378,404] IVIG, INF-α, TNF blocking agents, mepolizumab (a humanized monoclonal antibody to IL-5), and omalizumab (a monoclonal anti-IgE) have all also been used successfully in a few resistant patients.[405-407] The prognosis for recovery is good, but some patients progress to dialysis and others relapse or have chronic sequelae such as permanent peripheral neuropathy, chronic pulmonary changes, and hypertension.[394]

Glomerular Involvement in Other Vasculitides (Temporal Arteritis, Takayasu Disease)

Temporal Arteritis

Temporal arteritis or giant cell arteritis is a systemic vasculitis with a characteristic giant cell vasculitis of medium and large arteries.[408-410] The disease is the most common form of arteritis in Western countries.[408-412] Temporal arteritis is primarily a disease of elderly individuals, the average age being 72 years, with more than 95% of patients exceeding 50 years of age.[411,412] Extracranial vascular involvement occurs in 10% to 15% of patients with giant cell arteritis.[408,410] Temporal arteritis should be suspected in older individuals who present with persistent headaches, abrupt visual disturbances, jaw claudication, symptoms of polymyalgia rheumatica, or unexplained fevers and malaise along with anemia and elevated levels of ESR and CRP level. Renal manifestations are rare and generally mild.[408-413]

There have been several reports of renal involvement occurring in association with temporal arteritis or polymyalgia rheumatica.[414] Some patients may be P-ANCA positive or less commonly C-ANCA positive.[415] The renal pathology has been described as a focal segmental necrotizing GN with focal crescents and vasculitis, primarily affecting small arteries and arterioles. Rarely, visceral aneurysms are demonstrable angiographically. Whether these cases represent true manifestations of temporal arteritis or forms of "overlap" with small vessel vasculitis is not clear. There also have been reports of LN, membranous nephropathy, and renal amyloidosis in patients with temporal arteritis.[416,417]

The most common renal manifestations of mild proteinuria and microhematuria are present in fewer than 10% of patients. Renal insufficiency is uncommon. Hypertension is infrequent and most often mild to moderate when present. Rare cases of renal failure have been attributed to renal arteritis affecting the main renal artery or its major intraparenchymal branches.[414,415] In some cases, the pathology has been inadequate to diagnose the precise etiology of the renal failure. The nephrotic syndrome has been reported in a patient with temporal arteritis and membranous glomerulopathy, with steroid therapy producing a reduction in proteinuria from 6.8 to 1.3 g/day.[417]

The vasculitis seen in temporal arteritis is characterized by segmental transmural inflammation of medium and large elastic arteries by a mixed infiltrate of lymphocytes, monocytes, polymorphonuclear leukocytes, scattered eosinophiles, and giant cells.[408-410]

The treatment of temporal arteritis with corticosteroids usually causes rapid and dramatic improvements in general well-being, specific symptomatology, and laboratory abnormalities.[408-413] IV pulse steroids and a number of corticosteroid-sparing and secondary immunosuppressives have been used successfully.[413,418,419] However, there are conflicting results as to whether any agent such as methotrexate is equivalent to corticosteroids in efficacy, and some agents such as infliximab do not appear useful.[409-412,418,419] With corticosteroid use, abnormalities of the urinary sediment disappear, and there is resolution of extracranial large vessel involvement.[410,412] However, after being established, visual loss is often permanent despite resolution of the active disease process. Exacerbation of systemic vasculitis may occur if corticosteroids are tapered too rapidly.

Takayasu Arteritis

Takayasu arteritis is a rare vasculitic disease of unknown pathogenesis characterized by inflammation and stenosis of medium and large arteries, with a predilection for the aortic arch and its branches.[421,422] The disease most commonly affects young women between the ages of 10 and 40 years, and Asians are much more commonly affected.[421,422] Although findings are typically confined to the aortic arch (including the subclavian, carotid, and pulmonary arteries), the abdominal aorta and its branches may be affected in some cases.[420] The histopathologic findings of the vessels include arteritis with transmural infiltration by lymphocytes; monocytes; polymorphonuclear leukocytes; and, in some cases Langhans giant cells. In the chronic phase of the disease, intimal fibroplasia and medial scarring may result in severe vascular stenoses or total luminal obliteration.

Although in the past renal disease was believed to be uncommon, it is now reported more frequently.[422-427] This is usually caused by an obliterative arteritis of the main renal artery or narrowing of the renal ostia by abdominal aortitis, leading to renovascular hypertension. Arteriography is usually used to make the diagnosis of Takayasu arteritis, although CT, magnetic resonance imaging, and positron emission tomography scanning also have been used.[420,428,429] Laboratory abnormalities reveal mild anemia, elevated ESR, increased levels of CRP, and elevated gamma globulin levels, but other serologic tests such as ANA, VDRL, anti-streptolysin O (ASLO), and serum complement levels are normal. Some patients have antiendothelial cell antibodies.[430] Hypertension, which may be severe, occurs in 40% to 60% of patients and has been attributed to decreased elasticity of the aorta, increased renin secretion caused by stenosis of major renal arteries, and other mechanisms.[424,426,431] Although mild proteinuria and hematuria are found in some patients, nephrotic range proteinuria is uncommon.[432]

The serum creatinine is usually normal, but may be mildly elevated or associated with a high ratio of blood urea nitrogen to creatinine suggestive of "prerenal" azotemia. Progressive renal failure is uncommon.[421,424,433]

A mild mesangial proliferative GN may occur in patients with Takayasu arteritis.[423,425] Mesangial deposits of IgG, IgM, IgA, C_3, and C_4 have been reported, and mesangial electron-dense deposits are found on EM. Most patients have normal renal function and only mild hematuria and proteinuria. Some patients have had glomerular involvement typical of IgA nephropathy.[425] Whether this is coincidental or part of the disease process is unclear. One series of patients with Takayasu arteritis had unusual glomerular histopathology with mesangial sclerosis and nodules, as well as mesangiolysis and glomerular microaneurysms resembling a chronic thrombotic microangiopathy or diabetic glomerulosclerosis.[423] IF and EM in these cases of "centrolobular mesangiopathy" did not support an immune pathogenesis. There have also been rare reports of renal amyloidosis and cases of membranoproliferative GN, crescentic GN, and proliferative GN.[434,435]

Treatment

In the majority of patients, corticosteroids are effective therapy for the vasculitis and systemic symptoms.[420,421,433] Other medications, including azathioprine, methotrexate, leflunomide, cyclophosphamide, MMF, and anti-TNF therapy, have also been used successfully in some individuals, as have anticoagulants, vasodilators, and acetyl salicylic acid.[436-440] Residual morbidity and mortality may result from the progressive fibrosis and stenosis of previously inflamed arteries.[441]

Henoch-Schonlein Purpura

Henoch-Schonlein purpura (HSP) is a systemic vasculitic syndrome with involvement of the skin and GI tract and joints in association with a characteristic GN.[442-444] In HSP, IgA-containing immune complexes deposit in association with an inflammatory reaction of the vessels. In the skin, this leads to a leukocytoclastic angiitis with petechiae and purpura. In the GI tract, there may be ulcerations, pain, and bleeding. In the kidney, an immune complex–mediated GN is found.[442-444]

Males are slightly more commonly affected than females, and children are far more frequently affected than adults, although the disease can occur at any age.[442,445-449] The peak age of patients with HSP is approximately 5 years old as opposed to IgA nephropathy, which has a broad age distribution.[442-448] HSP may account for up to 15% of all GN in young children. More severe renal disease occurs in older children and adults.[449] HSP is uncommon in blacks. Familial occurrence has rarely been reported, and the frequency of HLA-Bw35 is increased in some series.[450-451] About one-fourth of patients have a history of allergy, but exacerbations related to a specific allergen are rare. Relapses of the syndrome have occurred after exposure to allergens or the cold, and seasonal variations show peak occurrence in the winter months.

HSP may be confused with systemic illnesses such as SLE and PAN, with ongoing infections such as meningococcemia, gonococcemia, and *Yersinia* enterocolitis; with certain medications and vaccination related hypersensitivity; and with some postinfectious glomerulonephritides associated with systemic manifestations. Although an upper respiratory infection precedes HSP in 30% to 50% of patients, serologic evidence of streptococcal infection is often lacking. Abdominal pains may be mistaken for appendicitis, cholecystitis, or surgical emergencies, leading to exploratory laparotomy.

Clinical Findings

The classic tetrad of findings in HSP includes dermal involvement, GI disease, joint involvement, and GN, but not all patients have all organ systems involved clinically.[442-447] Constitutional symptoms may include fever, malaise, fatigue, and weakness. Skin lesions are almost universal with HSP and are commonly found on the lower and upper extremities but may also be on the buttocks or elsewhere.[442,444,452] They are characterized by urticarial macular and papular reddish-violaceous lesions that do not blanch. Lesions may be discrete or may coalesce into palpable purpuric lesions associated with lower extremity edema. New crops of lesions may recur over weeks or months. On skin biopsy, there is a leukocytoclastic angiitis with evidence of IgA containing immune complexes along with IgG, C3, and properdin but not C4 or C1q. GI manifestations are present in from 25% to 90% of patients and may include colicky pain, nausea and vomiting, melena, and hematochezia.[442-444,452-454] One study of more than 260 patients found that 58% had abdominal pain and 18% had evidence of GI bleeding.[454] Endoscopy may reveal purpuric lesions, and rarely, patients may develop areas of intussusception or perforation. Rheumatologic disease involves the larger joints, usually the ankles and knees, and less commonly the elbows and wrists. There may be arthralgias or frank arthritis with painful, tender effusions, but patients do not develop joint deformities or erosive arthritis.[442-444] Rarely, patients have evidence involvement of other organs (e.g., lungs, CNS, ureteritis).[442-444,455]

Renal involvement varies from 20% to 100% of patients with HSP.[442-444,449,452,456] In one series of more than 260 patients, 20% developed renal disease.[456] In studies routinely examining the urine, renal involvement ranges from 40% to 60% of patients.[457] In a series of 250 adults with HSP, 32% had renal insufficiency, usually with proteinuria (97%) and hematuria (93%).[452] The onset of active renal disease usually follows the onset of the systemic manifestations by days to weeks and is characterized by microscopic hematuria, active urinary sediment, and proteinuria.[442,444,452] Some patients develop the nephrotic syndrome, and some have a nephritic picture. There is no relationship between the severity of extrarenal organ involvement and the severity of the renal lesions.

Laboratory Features

In HSP, platelet counts and serum complement levels and other serologic test results are all usually normal.[442-444] Serum IgA levels are elevated in up to half of patients during active illness but do not correlate well with the severity of clinical manifestations or the course of the disease.[442-444,448] Patients with both IgA nephropathy and HSP have high levels of galactose-deficient IgA in their circulations.[458] A number of abnormal IgA antibodies have been noted, including IgA rheumatoid factor, CICs with IgA and IgG, IgA ACLN antibodies, IgA fibronectin aggregates, IgA anti–α-galactosyl antibodies, and IgA ANCA.[459-464] The relationship of these to active renal or systemic disease remains unclear, but concentrations of IgA and IgG immune complexes, IgA rheumatoid factor, and IgA anti-galactosyl antibodies have been correlated with clinical renal disease manifestations.[459-461,463]

Pathology

Although by LM the renal biopsy findings of HSP resemble those of IgA nephropathy, there are some histopathologic differences. The typical glomerular pathology of HSP is a mesangial and endocapillary proliferative GN with variable crescent formation.[442-445,465] The mesangial changes include both increased mesangial cellularity and matrix expansion that may be focal or diffuse (Figure 32-18). In severe cases, polymorphonuclear cells and mononuclear cells may also infiltrate the glomerular tufts, and there may be necrotizing features. Increased numbers of monocytes or macrophages and CD4 and CD8 T cells are found.[466,467] Some cases have a well-developed membranoproliferative pattern with double contours of the GBM. Crescents vary from segmental to circumferential and are initially cellular but later fibrotic in nature (Figure 32-19). Tubulointerstitial changes of atrophy and interstitial fibrosis are consistent with the degree of glomerular damage. In general, endocapillary and extracapillary proliferation as well as glomerular fibrin deposition are more frequent and severe in HSP than in IgA nephropathy. The histopathologic classification system proposed by the International Study of Kidney Disease of Childhood correlates the glomerular lesions with clinical manifestations as well as prognosis.[449,468] These categories include class I with minimal glomerular alterations; class II with mesangial proliferation only; class III with either focal (a) or diffuse (b) mesangial proliferation but less than 50% of glomeruli containing crescents or segmental lesions of thrombosis, necrosis, or sclerosis; class IV with similar mesangial proliferation as IIIa and IIIb but 50% to 75% of glomeruli with crescents; class V with similar changes and more than 75% crescents; and class VI with a "pseudo" membranoproliferative pattern. Although hematuria is common to all groups and proteinuria of some degree may be found in all, the nephrotic syndrome is present in only 25% of groups I, II, and III. Likewise, groups IIIb, IV, and V tend to have a more progressive course toward renal failure.[469] Even by LM, deposits may be seen in the mesangial regions and rarely along the capillary walls. It is unusual to find the presence of a vasculitis on renal biopsy.

By IF, IgA is the dominant or co-dominant immunoglobulin. Co-deposits of IgG and IgM, C3, and properdin are common. Deposits are typically found in the mesangium, especially involving the paramesangial regions, and may extend into the subendothelial areas (Figure 32-20).[442-445] Early classical complement components of C1q and C4 are rarely present. These findings contrast with LN in which IgG usually predominates and C1q is almost always present. The deposited IgA is usually IgA1 subclass and may have the J chain indicating its polymeric nature, but a secretory piece is not found.[442-445,470,471] Fibrin-related antigens are also commonly present. IgA may be deposited along with C3 and C5 in both involved and uninvolved skin in the small vessels similar to the findings in IgA nephropathy.[472,473] Similar IgA deposits may also occur in the skin in dermatitis herpetiformis and in SLE along with early and late complement components. IgA is also found in vasculitic lesions in the intestinal tract.[453,454]

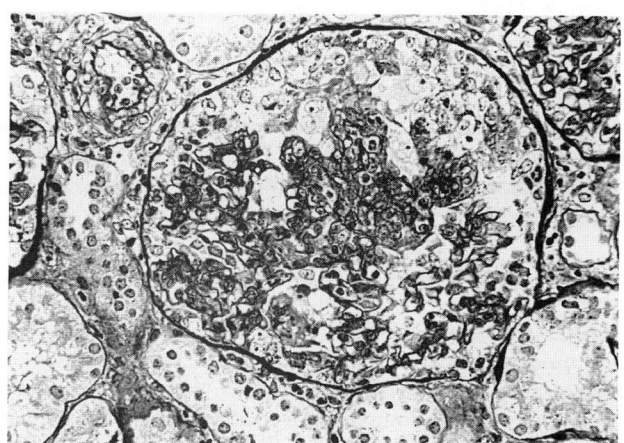

FIGURE 32-19 Henoch Schonlein purpura nephritis. There is segmental endocapillary proliferation with an overlying segmental cellular crescent (periodic acid–Schiff f, ×475).

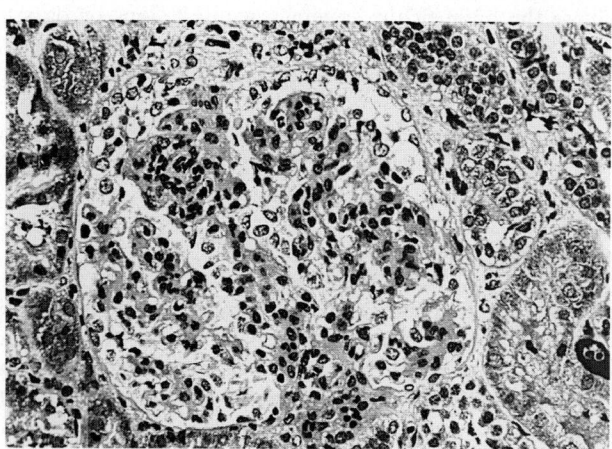

FIGURE 32-18 Henoch Schonlein purpura nephritis. An example with global mesangial proliferation and focal infiltrating neutrophils (hematoxylin and eosin, ×500).

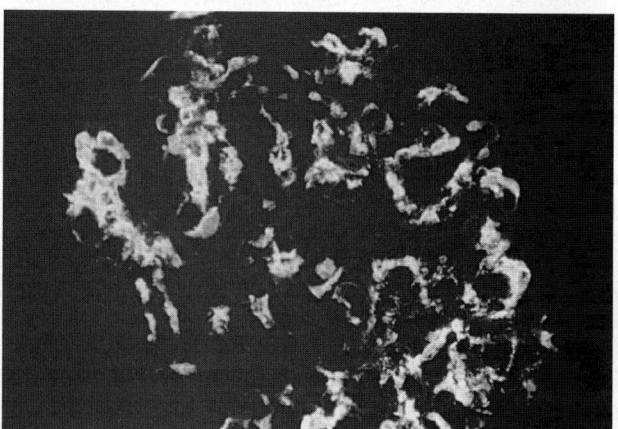

FIGURE 32-20 Henoch Schonlein purpura nephritis. Immunofluorescence photomicrograph showing intense deposits of immunoglobulin A distributed throughout the mesangium and also extending into a few peripheral glomerular capillary walls (×600).

By EM, characteristic immune-type electron-dense deposits are found predominantly in the mesangial regions accompanied by increase in mesangial cellularity and matrix.[442-445,468] In some capillaries, the deposits extend subendothelially from the adjacent mesangial regions. Occasionally, scattered subepithelial deposits are also present and may resemble the humps of poststreptococcal disease. Evidence of coagulation with fibrin and platelets thrombi may be found in capillary lumina. In cases with severe crescent involvement, there may be focal rupture of the GBMs. Immunoelectron microscopy has confirmed the predominance of IgA in association with some C3 and IgG in the deposits.[465]

Pathogenesis

The pathogenesis of HSP remains unknown. Patients with HSP, similar to those with IgA nephropathy, have high circulating levels of galactose deficient IgA.[458] HSP is clearly a systemic immune complex disease with IgA-containing deposits that are associated with a small vessel vasculitis and capillary damage. The deposits contain polymeric IgA of the IgA1 subclass and late-acting complement components. This composition suggests alternative pathway complement activation. Whether IgA immune complexes trigger complement activation and the ultimate role of complement participation are unclear. The presence of circulating polymeric IgA complexes; the deposition of IgA in the kidney as well as the skin, intestines, and other organs; and recurrence of disease in the allograft all point to the systemic nature of the disease process.[472-476] The precise mechanism(s) whereby IgA deposition causes tissue injury is unclear because IgA is deposited in some diseases such as celiac disease and chronic liver disease without causing major clinical glomerular damage.[477] Complement activation, platelet activation and coagulation, vasoactive prostanoids, cytokines, and growth factors are thought to play roles. Impaired T-cell activity has also been implicated in the pathogenesis of HSP.[478] HSP has also been reported in rare patients with IgA monoclonal gammopathy.[479] The relationship of HSP to IgA nephropathy is obscure with some investigators considering the diseases separate entities and others describing them as opposite ends of a pathogenetic spectrum encompassing systemic to renal limited disease.[480] Similar renal histologic findings and similar immunologic abnormalities such as elevated circulating galactose deficient IgA levels, IgA fibronectin aggregates, and antimesangial cell antibodies suggest a common mechanism of renal injury. IgG autoantibodies against mesangial cells parallel the course of the renal disease. Both IgA nephropathy and HSP have occurred in different members of the same families and in monozygotic twins after adenovirus infection.[480,481] Infectious agents associated with the occurrence of HSP have included varicella, measles, adenovirus, hepatitis A and B, *Yersinia* spp., *Shigella* spp., mycoplasma, HIV infection, and staphylococci (including methicillin-resistant organisms), but none has been proven to be etiologic.[443,444,480-484] Likewise, HSP has been reported to occur in association with vaccinations, insect bites, cold exposure, and trauma, although an etiologic relationship again is unproven.[485]

Course, Prognosis, and Treatment

In most patients, HSP is a self-limited disease with a good long-term outcome.[442-444] Patients may have recurrences of the rash, joint symptoms, and GI symptoms for months or years, but most patients have benign short- and long-term renal courses. In general, there is a good correlation between the clinical renal presentation and the ultimate prognosis.[442-444,453] Patients with focal mesangial involvement and only hematuria and mild proteinuria tend to have an excellent prognosis. In one recent large pediatric study, renal survival was 100%.[456] In another series of 150 patients with 50% renal involvement, only two patients had residual hematuria, and no patient had abnormal renal function at 2.5 years.[442] In most series, by several years from presentation, more than half of the patients had no renal abnormalities, fewer than 25% have sediment abnormalities or proteinuria, and only 10% have decreased GFR. Fewer than 10% of patients with severe clinical renal involvement at onset had persistent hypertension or declining GFR over a long period of time. A review of more than 50 patients followed over 24 years after childhood-onset HSP found seven of 20 with severe HSP at onset with residual renal impairment as adults as opposed to only two of 27 patients with mild initial renal disease.[486] In large series unselected for renal involvement, only 2% to 5% of patients developed ESRD. Long-term renal function may not be as good in adults with HSP.[452,486-488] In a series of more than 250 adults with HSP followed almost 15 years, 11% developed ESRD, 13% developed severe renal impairment with a clearance less than 30 mL/min, and 15% developed moderate renal insufficiency.[452] A poor renal prognosis is predicted by an acute nephritic presentation and older age and especially by larger amounts of proteinuria and more severe nephrotic syndrome.[487-489] On renal biopsy, a poor prognosis is predicted by IgA deposits extending from the mesangium into the peripheral capillary walls, increased interstitial fibrosis, glomerular fibrinoid necrosis, and especially the presence of greater percentage of crescents on renal biopsy.[452,488,489] In one study of more than 150 children with HSP, those with greater than 50% of glomeruli-containing crescents had progression to ESRD in more than one-third of cases and the development of chronic renal insufficiency in another 18%. Repeat biopsies in patients with HSP who have clinically improved show decreased mesangial deposits and hypercellularity. Although complete clinical recovery occurs in 95% of affected children and many adults with HSP, more than one-third of HSP patients who become pregnant have associated hypertension or proteinuria. The mortality rate in HSP is less than 10% at 10 years.

Therapy for the majority of patients with HSP remains supportive.[442-444] Most fare well despite the lack of any immunosuppressive intervention. The use of corticosteroids is controversial, and although associated with decreased abdominal and rheumatologic symptoms, they have not clearly been proven to ameliorate the renal lesions in any controlled fashion.[490-492] Patients with more severe clinical features, especially those with more crescents on biopsy, have been also been treated with anticoagulants, azathioprine, cyclophosphamide, chlorambucil and other immunosuppressives, and even plasma exchange.[490-499] Although these reports have shown anecdotal success in reversing the renal progression, controlled trials have not yet shown benefits of using cytotoxic immunosuppressive therapy.[489] IVIG has been used in several patients with the nephrotic syndrome and decreased GFR in an uncontrolled nonrandomized but apparently successful fashion.[497]

Renal disease caused by HSP has infrequently been reported to recur in the renal allograft.[474-476] However, as in IgA nephropathy, histologic recurrence is more common than clinical recurrence. This may be more common in patients who are transplanted either with living related donors or while still active clinically within the first few years of developing ESRD. Graft survival is similar to patients with IgA nephropathy and other disease leading to transplantation.[474]

Anti–Glomerular Basement Membrane Disease and Goodpasture's Syndrome

Anti-GBM disease is caused by circulating antibodies directed against an antigenic site on type IV collagen in the GBM.[500-503] In 1919, Goodpasture described the case of an 18-year-old man who died with an influenza like illness characterized by pulmonary hemorrhage and a proliferative GN. However, pulmonary hemorrhage can be associated with GN in many diseases.[504] True Goodpasture's syndrome should consist of the triad of (1) proliferative, usually crescentic, GN; (2) pulmonary hemorrhage; (3) and the presence of anti-GBM antibodies.[500-503] In anti-GBM disease the pulmonary hemorrhage may precede, occur concurrently with, or follow the glomerular involvement.[502,505,506] Some patients with anti-GBM antibodies and GN and hence "anti-GBM" disease never experience pulmonary involvement and thus do not have true "Goodpasture's syndrome." Documentation of anti-GBM antibody-induced disease may be via renal biopsy or by establishing the presence of circulating anti-GBM antibodies.[506,507] Indirect IF, although highly specific and positive in more than three-fourths of patients, requires an experienced pathologist.[507] Radioimmunoassay, ELISA, and immunoblotting for the antibodies are highly specific, sensitive, and readily available.[502,507]

Pathogenesis

Anti-GBM autoantibodies react with epitopes on the noncollagenous domain of the α-3 and -5 chains of type IV collagen.[500-503,508] The antigenic epitope has been localized between amino acids 198 and 237 of the terminal region of the α-3 chain.[509] The α-3 chain of type IV collagen is found predominantly in the GBM and alveolar capillary basement membranes, which correlates with the limited distribution of disease involvement in Goodpasture's syndrome.[522-524,531]. Goodpasture's syndrome is now considered an autoimmune "conformeropathy" involving perturbation of the quaternary structure of the α 345NC1 hexamer of type IV collagen.[540] In Goodpasture's disease, autoantibodies to both the α 3NC1 and the α 5NC1 domains bind to the kidneys and lungs. These autoantibodies bind to epitopes encompassing the Ea region in the α 5NC1 domain and the Ea and Eb region of the α 3NC1 domain, but they do not bind to nondenatured native cross-linked α 345 NC1 hexamers.[510] The epitope is identical in the glomeruli and the alveolar basement membranes and may require partial denaturation for full autoantigen exposure. Eluates of antibody from lung and kidney of patients with Goodpasture's syndrome cross-react with GBM

and the alveolar basement membrane and can produce disease in animal models.[511] Antibody reacting with autoantigen(s) and perhaps aided by autoreactive T cells leads to an inflammatory response, the formation of proliferative GN, breaks in the GBM, and the subsequent extracapillary proliferation with exuberant crescent formation.[502] A role for T cells in Goodpasture's syndrome is supported by the T-cell infiltrates on biopsy, patient T-cell proliferation in response to α 3 (IV) NC1 domain, the correlation of autoreactive T cells with disease activity, the role of CD4+CD25+ regulatory cells controlling the autoreactive T-cell response, and a role for T-cell epitope mimicry in disease induction.[502,512,513] When the anti-GBM antibodies cross-react with and cause damage to the basement membrane of pulmonary capillaries, the patient develops pulmonary hemorrhage and hemoptysis. An initial insult to the pulmonary vascular integrity may be required because alveolar capillaries are not normally permeable to passage of anti-GBM antibodies.[514-516] Exacerbations of disease, especially pulmonary disease with hemoptysis, have been related to exposure to hydrocarbon fumes, cigarette smoking, hair dyes, metallic dust, D-penicillamine, and cocaine inhalation.[514-517] Although smokers with anti-GBM disease have a higher incidence of pulmonary hemorrhage, circulating anti-GBM antibody levels are no higher than in nonsmokers with the disease.[514,515] Goodpasture's syndrome has occasionally been reported in more than one family member and has rarely occurred in clusters of unrelated patients occasionally at a particular season of the year.[502,505] HLA-DR15 and DR4 may predispose to the syndrome and perhaps more severe disease. Influenza A2 infection has also been associated with Goodpasture's syndrome. Anti-GBM disease can also occur in patients with typical membranous nephropathy and in 5% to 10% of patients with Alport's syndrome receiving allografts.[518,519] However, in patients with Alport's syndrome, posttransplantation the alloantibodies, in contrast to those in anti-GBM disease, bind to the Ea region of the α 5NC1 domain of the intact α345NC1 hexamer (rather than to denatured hexamer).[510]

Clinical Features

GN mediated by anti-GBM antibodies is an infrequent pattern of glomerular injury.[500-503,505]Although some studies suggested estimates of occurrence as high as 3% to 5% of all glomerular diseases, most studies reduce this to 1% to 2%. The disease has two peaks of occurrence, the first in younger men and the second in elderly women, but it can occur at any age and in either sex.[500-502,505,515,520] Anti-GBM disease limited to the kidney may be more common in older patients. Goodpasture's syndrome is less common in blacks perhaps because of less frequent occurrence of certain predisposing HLA antigens in this population. An upper respiratory infection precedes the onset of disease in 20% to 60% of cases.[500-502,515]

The most common extrarenal findings are pulmonary, including cough, dyspnea, and shortness of breath, and hemoptysis, which may vary from trivial amounts to life-threatening amounts associated with exsanguination and suffocation.[500-502,515,520] In almost three-fourths of cases, pulmonary hemorrhage precedes or is coincident with the glomerular disease.[500-502] Some patients may have constitutional symptoms of weakness, fatigue, weight loss, chills, and fevers, although this is less prominent than in other systemic vasculitides. Others may have skin rash, hepatosplenomegaly, nausea and vomiting, and arthralgias at onset.[502]

The clinical renal presentation is usually an acute nephritic picture with hypertension, edema, hematuria and active urinary sediment, and reduced renal function; however, only 20% of patients have hypertension at onset.[500-502,520] Renal function is usually already reduced at presentation and may deteriorate from normal to dialysis requiring levels in a matter of days to weeks.[500-502,520] However, one recent study found more than one-third of patients to have normal GFRs.[521] There is a good correlation between the serum creatinine level and the percentage of glomeruli involved by severe crescent formation.

Laboratory Findings

Laboratory evaluation typically shows active urinary sediment with RBCs and RBCs casts.[502,520] Proteinuria, although common, is usually not in the nephrotic range. Serologic test results such as ASLO, ANA, serum complement levels, rheumatoid factor, cryoglobulins, and CICs are all either negative or normal.[502,520] Circulating anti-GBM antibodies are present in more than 90% of patients, although the antibody titer does not always correlate well with the manifestations or course of either the pulmonary or renal disease.[502,522] Most patients have a decrease in serum antibody titer with time. From 10% to 38% of patients have both positive anti-GBM antibodies and ANCA usually directed against MPO but occasionally against PR3.[502,523,524] The anti-GBM antibodies in patients who are ANCA positive have the same antigenic specificity as in patients who are ANCA negative.[525] Some studies suggest that the course of patients double positive for anti-GBM antibodies and ANCA parallels that of patients with anti-GBM antibody disease, such that these patients are more likely to develop severe renal failure than those with purely ANCA-positive vasculitis.[526] Some patients have a clinical systemic vasculitis with purpura and arthralgias and arthritis, findings that are rarely seen in isolated Goodpasture's syndrome without coexistent ANCA.[523,524] In Goodpasture's syndrome, a microcytic, hypochromic anemia is common even without overt pulmonary hemorrhage. Other patients may have a leukocytosis. Iron deposition in the lungs may be documented by Fe59 scanning, bronchopulmonary lavage, or expectorated sputum showing hemosiderin-laden macrophages.[520] In patients with pulmonary involvement, chest radiography is abnormal in more than 75% and typically shows infiltrates corresponding to areas of pulmonary hemorrhage. It may also demonstrate atelectasis, pulmonary edema, and areas of coexistent pneumonia.[502-504] Lung function discloses restrictive ventilatory defects and hypoxemia, and an increased arterial alveolar gradient is present in severe cases.[520]

Pathology

By LM, patients with mild clinical involvement often have a focal, segmental proliferative GN associated with areas of segmental necrosis and overlying small crescents.[502-504,522] However, the most common biopsy picture is diffuse crescentic

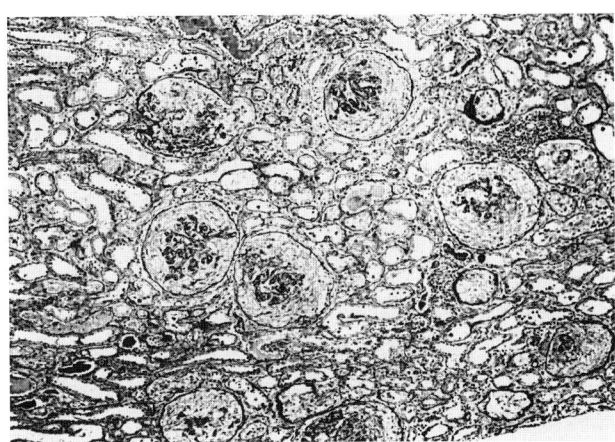

FIGURE 32-21 Anti–glomerular basement membrane disease (Goodpasture's syndrome). There is diffuse crescentic glomerulonephritis with large circumferential cellular crescents and severe compression of the glomerular tuft (periodic acid–Schiff, ×80).

GN involving more than 50% of glomeruli, with exuberant, predominantly circumferential crescents (Figure 32-21).[504,527] The underlying tuft is compressed but displays focal necrotizing features. Disruption and destruction of large portions of the GBM and the basal lamina of Bowman's capsule may be seen on silver stain.[527] Early crescents are formed by proliferating glomerular epithelial cells and infiltrating T lymphocytes, monocytes, and polymorphonuclear leukocytes, but older ones are composed predominantly of spindled fibroblast-like cells, with few, if any, infiltrating leukocytes.[527] An associated tubulointerstitial nephritis with inflammatory cells and edema is common. Multinucleated giant cells may be present in the crescents or tubulointerstitial regions. Some patients, especially those who are ANCA positive, have necrotizing vasculitis of small arteries and arterioles. In biopsies taken later in the disease, there are progressive global and segmental glomerulosclerosis and interstitial fibrosis. Pulmonary histology reveals intraalveolar hemorrhage with widening and disruption of the alveolar septa and accumulations of hemosiderin laden macrophages.[500-502]

The IF findings define the disease process in Goodpasture's syndrome and differentiate it from both pauci-immune and immune complex–mediated forms of crescentic GN that may share similar LM features. The diagnostic finding is an intense and diffuse linear staining for IgG, especially IgG1 and IgG4, involving the GBMs (Figure 32-22).[528,529] Rarely has IgM or IgA been identified in a linear distribution. C3 deposits are found in a more finely granular GBM distribution in many patients. C1q is typically absent. Linear IF staining for IgG may also be found along some tubular basement membranes, particularly of distal tubules. Fibrin-related antigens are commonly present within the crescents and segmental necrotizing lesions. In the lungs, similar linear deposition of IgG occurs along the alveolar capillary walls.[502]

EM typically does not reveal immune-type electron-dense deposits. There may be widening of the subendothelial space by fibrin-like material, and gaps in the GBM and in Bowman's capsule are commonly present.[527] Rare patients have coexistent membranous glomerulopathy with typical findings by LM, IF, and EM.[541] EM of pulmonary tissue may demonstrate hyperplasia of pneumocytes and alveolar basement membrane thickening.

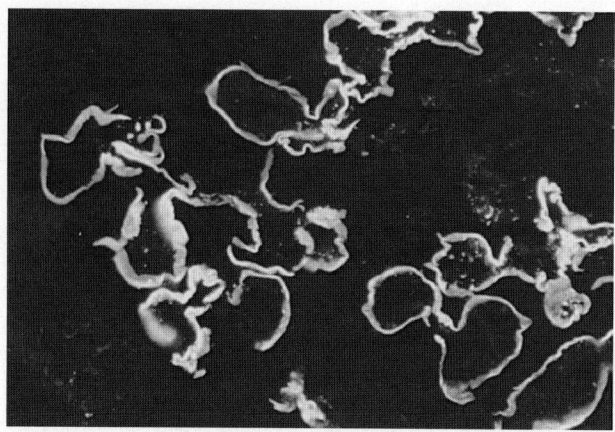

FIGURE 32-22 Anti–glomerular basement membrane disease (Goodpasture's syndrome). Immunofluorescence photomicrograph showing linear glomerular basement membrane deposits of immunoglobulin G. Some of the glomerular basement membranes are discontinuous, indicating sites of rupture (×800).

Course, Treatment, and Prognosis

The course of untreated Goodpasture's syndrome is one of progressive renal dysfunction leading to uremia.[502-504,520] In early studies, almost all patients died from either pulmonary hemorrhage or progressive renal failure. In recent studies, mortality is less than 10%, probably related to improved supportive care and more rapid diagnosis and treatment.[504,529,530] Infrequent patients have one or more relapses of the pulmonary disease. Spontaneous remission of the renal disease is rare, although with therapy, many patients have a stable course and some dramatic improvement.[502-504,529,530] If treatment is started early, patients may regain considerable kidney function. The plasma creatinine correlates fairly well with the degree of crescentic involvement, and if the plasma creatinine is markedly elevated and the patient requires dialysis, most such patients will develop ESRD.[502] A recent study from China in more than 100 patients with anti-GBM antibodies noted a poorer prognosis in patients with creatinines over 600 μm/L, oligoanuria at presentation, more than 85% crescents on biopsy, and renal involvement before pulmonary hemorrhage.[529] Anti-GBM autoantibodies against different target antigens may influence the disease severity.

There have been no large randomized studies defining the benefits of any given therapy for anti-GBM disease. Although pulmonary hemorrhage and even renal disease have abated in some patients with high-dose oral or IV corticosteroid therapy, combination therapy with steroids, cyclophosphamide, and plasmapheresis is now standard.[502,530] A typical treatment regimen might include a combination of prednisone (1 mg/kg/day) or IV pulse methylprednisolone (30 mg/kg/day or 1000 mg/day) for several days followed by high-dose oral therapy along with cyclophosphamide (2 mg/kg/day) and plasmapheresis. Plasmapheresis may have a dramatic effect in reversing pulmonary hemorrhage and renal disease when used early in the course in combination with immunosuppressants.[502,529,531] Plasmapheresis removes the circulating anti-GBM antibodies, and immunosuppressive therapy prevents new antibody formation and controls the ongoing inflammatory response. One review of uncontrolled trials found that 40% of patients had stabilized or improved renal function with plasmapheresis.[531] Patients with severe renal failure who are already on dialysis or who have serum creatinines greater than 5 to 8 mg/dL are less likely to respond to therapy, but some have recovered.[504,520,529,531] In one series, patients who were positive for both anti-GBM antibodies and ANCA behaved similarly to those with anti-GBM antibodies alone with a 1-year renal survival of 73% in those with a plasma creatinine below 500 μm/L and 0% in those on dialysis.[526]

In other series, dialysis-dependent patients who are both anti-GBM antibody and ANCA positive are still more likely to recover than patients who are dialysis dependent with only anti-GBM antibody positivity.[523,524] Although daily plasmapheresis is often maintained for weeks, its frequency can be determined by the rapidity of clinical response. Exacerbations of disease may occur with intercurrent infections. Immunosuppressive therapy is usually continued for 6 months with a tapering regimen to allow spontaneous cessation of autoantibody production. Some patients with early disappearance of circulating anti-GBM antibodies may respond to shorter therapy or tolerate change to less toxic maintenance immunosuppressives such as azathioprine.[502,520] There are limited data on other immunosuppressive regimens in Goodpasture's syndrome.[531-533] Immunoadsorption has also been used to remove the anti-GBM antibodies in Goodpasture's syndrome.[534] Even in patients with initial improvement of renal function, some with severe crescentic glomerular involvement progress to renal failure over time, perhaps related to non-immunologic progression of disease. The incidence of ESRD in patients with significant glomerular involvement is more than 50%, and the renal outcome is usually progressively downhill unless vigorous prompt therapy is instituted.

Anti-GBM–mediated renal disease may recur in the renal allograft.[535-537] As with a number of other forms of GN, evidence of histologic recurrence (i.e., linear staining for IgG along GBMs) is far higher than clinical involvement and may be as high as 50%. The low recurrence rate recently reported in transplants probably reflects a combination of waiting sufficient time to document the absence of anti-GBM antibodies, the use of immunosuppressives and plasmapheresis to remove current antibody, and the "one-shot" nature of the disease.[536,537] Graft loss secondary to recurrent disease is rare. Patients should not undergo transplantation during the acute phase of their illness when autoantibody levels are high, and prophylactic pretransplant immunosuppression has been recommended for those receiving allografts from living related donors. Although patients with resolving pulmonary disease may have residual diminished gas exchange, most pulmonary function test results return to normal and do not limit the renal transplant process.[538]

Sjögren's Syndrome

Sjögren's syndrome is characterized by a chronic inflammatory cell infiltration of the exocrine salivary and lacrimal glands and is associated with the "sicca complex" of xerostomia and xerophthalmia.[539-541] Some patients may have involvement by a systemic inflammatory disease of the kidneys, lungs, esophagus, thyroid, stomach, and pancreas.[539-541] Others have manifestations of a collagen vascular disease, most commonly rheumatoid arthritis, and less frequently SLE, scleroderma, polymyositis, or MCTD. Still other patients have different immunologic disorders such as chronic active hepatitis, primary biliary cirrhosis, Crohn's disease, and fibrosing alveolitis or develop lymphoma or Waldenström's macroglobulinemia. Serologic abnormalities in Sjögren's syndrome include hypergammaglobulinemia, rheumatoid factor, cryoglobulins, a homogeneous or speckled pattern ANA, anti-Ro/SSA and anti-La/SSB, but serum complement levels are generally normal unless the patient has associated SLE.[539-541]

The major clinical renal manifestations of patients with Sjögren's syndrome usually relate to tubulointerstitial involvement of the kidneys with tubular defects such as a distal renal tubular acidosis (RTA), impaired concentrating ability, hypercalciuria, and (less frequently) proximal tubular defects.[539-543] Most patients have no evidence of glomerular disease and a relatively bland urinalysis with only mild elevations of the serum creatinine. In one recent analysis of more than 470 patients with primary Sjögren's syndrome followed for a mean of 10 years, only 20 patients (4%) developed overt renal disease.[540] Ten patients had interstitial nephritis on biopsy, eight patients had glomerular lesions, and two patient had both lesions. In the infrequent patients with glomerular lesions hematuria, proteinuria, the nephrotic syndrome, and renal insufficiency are found. Others may develop renal vasculitis with hypertension and renal insufficiency.

In most cases, the renal pathology shows prominent tubulointerstitial nephritis with sparing of the glomeruli.[539-543] There is a chronic active interstitial inflammation by a predominantly lymphocytic infiltrate admixed with plasma cells, with variable interstitial fibrosis and tubular atrophy. By IF, there are usually no detectable deposits, but in some cases, tubular basement membrane deposits of IgG and C3 have been described. A nonspecific glomerulosclerosis with mesangial sclerosis and GBM thickening and wrinkling is found in those with chronic and severe tubulointerstitial damage. Infrequent patients have immune complex–mediated glomerular involvement.[540,541-548] In one series of biopsied patients with primary Sjögren syndrome, patients had either mesangial proliferative GN or membranoproliferative GN.[540] Other series have had SLE features with the similar spectrum of glomerular involvement ranging from mesangial proliferative to focal proliferative, diffuse proliferative and membranous GN.[544-548] A membranoproliferative pattern of GN has been reported in patients with associated cryoglobulinemia.[540,546-548] By IF and EM, immune deposits have been localized in the various patterns to the mesangial region or the subendothelial or subepithelial aspect of the GBM as in SLE. Some patients with Sjögren's syndrome have a necrotizing arteritis of the kidney, occasionally with extrarenal involvement.[549] Most patients with Sjögren's syndrome with severe tubulointerstitial disease respond to treatment with corticosteroids.[539-541,543] Patients with immune complex GN and Sjögren's syndrome are generally treated in a similar fashion to those with SLE, and those with vasculitis generally receive cytotoxic therapy similar to those with other necrotizing vasculitides.[540]

Sarcoidosis

Most manifestations of sarcoidosis are not related to the kidneys.[550] The most common renal findings are granulomatous interstitial nephritis, nephrolithiasis, and tubular functional abnormalities.[551,552] Glomerular disease is infrequent and

may be coincidental. A variety of glomerular lesions have been described, including minimal change disease, FSGS, membranous nephropathy, IgA nephropathy, membranoproliferative GN, and proliferative and crescentic GN with and without a positive ANCA serology.[551-561] The IF and EM features conform to the various histologic patterns. Some patients have granulomatous renal interstitial nephritis in addition to the glomerular lesions. The clinical presentation of glomerular disease in sarcoidosis is usually that of proteinuria; active urinary sediment at times; and most commonly, the nephrotic syndrome. Patients have been treated with various forms of immunosuppression, including steroids, depending on their glomerular lesions.[553-561]

Amyloidosis

Amyloidosis comprises a diverse group of systemic and local diseases characterized by the extracellular deposition of fibrils in various organs.[562-564] Although the precursor proteins vary, all share an antiparallel β-pleated sheet configuration on x-ray diffraction, leading to their amyloidogenic properties. All amyloid fibrils bind Congo red (leading to diagnostic applegreen birefringence under polarized light) and thioflavin T and have a characteristic ultrastructural appearance. All types of amyloid contain a 25-kDa glycoprotein, serum amyloid P component (SAP) a member of the pentraxin family that includes CRP. Amyloid deposits may also contain restricted sulfated glycosaminoglycans and proteoglycans noncovalently linked to the amyloid fibrils.[562-565] Only some amyloid proteins deposit in the kidney. The vast majority of cases of renal amyloidosis are caused either by AL amyloidosis (formerly called primary amyloidosis) and AA amyloidosis (formerly called secondary amyloidosis). In AL amyloidosis, the deposited fibrils are derived from the variable portion of immunoglobulin light chains produced by a clonal population of plasma cells or B cells. AA amyloid results from the deposition of serum amyloid A (SAA) protein in chronic inflammatory states.[562] Only a small fraction of cases of renal amyloidosis are caused by much rarer hereditary forms of amyloidosis, such as those caused by inherited mutations in genes encoding transthyretin, fibrinogen Aa, apolipoprotein A-I or A-II, lysozyme, cystatin C, and gelsolin.[564,566-568] A newly recognized form of renal amyloidosis is caused by deposition of leukocyte chemotactic factor 2 (LECT2) peptide encoded by a distinct genetic polymorphism more common in Mexican Americans.[569]

It is unclear what factors confer the propensity for certain amyloidogenic proteins to fold into amyloid fibrils.[570-573] Cofactors such as amyloid P component may have important roles in the pathogenesis of tissue deposition. These may act by promoting fibrillogenesis, stabilization of the fibrils, binding to matrix proteins, or inhibiting denaturation and proteolysis. It is also possible that stabilizing cofactors are deposited after fibrillogenesis.[564,568-573] Amyloid fibrils generally resist biodegradation and accumulate in the tissues, resulting in organ dysfunction. However, amyloid deposits do exist in a dynamic state and have been shown to regress by radiolabeled SAP scintigraphy.[574] In SAA amyloid, the SAA concentration has correlated with amyloid burden and reduction in circulating SAA with regression of amyloid deposits. Patients with secondary amyloidosis have levels of circulating SAA protein that are no greater than in patients with inflammatory diseases who do not have amyloid deposition. Therefore, some additional unknown stimulus is required for amyloid fibrils to form and precipitate. In AL amyloid, biochemical characteristics of the light chain, such as an aberrant amino acid composition at certain sites, appear important in determining amyloid formation.[573] This may account for the reproducibility of a given form of renal disease (cast nephropathy vs. amyloid) in animal models infused with monoclonal light chains from affected patients.[575] Certain light chains may also form high-molecular-weight aggregates in vitro.[576] Macrophage-dependent generation of preamyloid fragments with chemical properties, allowing aggregation may also play a role.[599] Amyloid P component may prevent degradation of amyloid fibrils after being formed.[577]

AL and AA Amyloidosis

In AL amyloidosis, fibrils are composed of the N-terminal amino acid residues of the variable region of an immunoglobulin light chain. λ Light chains predominate over κ, and there is an increased incidence of monoclonal λ subtype VI.[567,578] Although the diagnosis of AL amyloidosis may be suspected on clinical grounds, confirmation requires biopsy documentation. Organ involvement is quite variable, and the absence of other organ involvement does not exclude amyloidosis as a cause of major renal disease.[562,563] The kidneys are the most common major organ involved by AL amyloid, and most patients eventually have renal amyloid on autopsy.[578] As many as 10% to 20% of patients older than age 60 years with presumed idiopathic nephrotic syndrome have amyloidosis on renal biopsy.[579] Multiple myeloma occurs in up to 20% of patients with primary amyloidosis. Amyloidosis should be suspected in all patients with circulating serum monoclonal M proteins, and approximately 90% of primary amyloid patients have a paraprotein spike in the serum or urine by immunofixation.[562,563,578]

The incidence of AL amyloid is about 8 per million annually but varies greatly in different locations.[580] Most patients with AL amyloidosis are older than 50 years old (median age, 59–63 years), and fewer than 1% are younger than 40 years old. Men are affected twice as often as women.[562,563,578] Presenting symptoms include weight loss, fatigue, lightheadedness, shortness of breath, peripheral edema, pain caused by peripheral neuropathy, and orthostatic hypotension. Patients may have cardiomyopathy, hepatosplenomegaly, macroglossia, or rarely enlarged lymph nodes. Multisystem organ involvement is typical with the most commonly affected organs being the kidney (50%), heart (40%), and peripheral nerves (≤25%).[562,563,578]

AA amyloidosis occurs in chronic inflammatory diseases and is composed of the amino terminal end of the acute phase reactant SAA protein.[562,564,572,581,582] SAA is produced in the liver and circulates in association with high-density lipoprotein (HDL). AA amyloid is commonly found in patients with rheumatoid arthritis and other inflammatory arthritides, inflammatory bowel disease, familial Mediterranean fever, quadriplegia with chronic urinary infections and decubitus ulcers, bronchiectasis, poorly treated osteomyelitis, and chronic heroin addicts who inject drugs subcutaneously.[562,564,572,582-586] In an autopsy study of 150 addicts 14%

of subcutaneous and 26% of those with chronic suppurative infections had renal amyloidosis.[585] AA amyloid typically occurs in older addicts with a long history of substance abuse who have exhausted sites of IV access and resorted to "skin popping."[586]

The diagnosis of amyloid is usually established by tissue biopsy of an affected organ.[562-564] Liver and kidney biopsy results are positive in as many as 90% of clinically affected cases. A diagnosis may be made less invasively with fat pad aspirate (60%–90%), rectal biopsy (50%–80%), bone marrow aspirate (30%–50%), gingival biopsy (60%), or dermal biopsy (50%).[587-589] SAP whole-body scintigraphy after injection of radiolabeled SAP allows the noninvasive diagnosis of amyloidosis as well as allowing a quantification of the extent of organ system involvement and assessment of the response to treatment.[590] This test result may be positive even when tissue biopsy results have been negative and may be more accurate in AA than in AL amyloidosis. In AL amyloidosis, detection of an abnormal ratio of free κ to λ light chains in the serum is a technique to detect plasma cell dyscrasias that has a higher sensitivity then either serum or urinary electropheresis.[590] It also allows assessment of response to therapy by following the level of abnormal free light chin in the serum.[591] Patients with hereditary amyloidosis caused by deposition of abnormal transthyretin, apolipoproteins, lysozyme, or fibrinogen AA may present in a fashion similar to those with AL amyloid. In one series, 10% of 350 patients with hereditary amyloidosis were misdiagnosed as having AL amyloid.[568] Hereditary amyloidoses may present at any age from the second to eighth decade of life. Although their course is often more prolonged and more benign than that of AL amyloid, presentation can be identical. Establishing the correct diagnosis is crucial because the treatment of patients with hereditary amyloid may include liver transplantation rather than chemotherapy or stem cell transplantation as in AL amyloid.[566]

Clinical manifestations of renal disease depend on the location and extent of amyloid deposition. Renal involvement predominates in AL amyloidosis with one-third to half of patients having renal manifestations at presentation.[562-564] Most patients have proteinuria, approximately 25% have the nephrotic syndrome at diagnosis, and others present with varying degrees of azotemia.[562-564,578,580] Over time, as many as 40% develop the nephrotic syndrome; others will have lesser degrees of proteinuria or azotemia. Urinalysis is typically bland, but microhematuria and cellular casts have been reported. Proteinuria is typically nonselective, and almost 90% of patients with greater than 1 g/day urinary protein have a monoclonal protein in the urine. Hypercholesterolemia is less common than in other forms of the nephrotic syndrome. The amount of glomerular amyloid deposition does not correlate well with the degree of renal dysfunction.[562,563] Despite the literature's suggestion of enlarged kidneys in AL amyloid, by ultrasonography, most patients have normal-sized kidneys.[562] Hypertension is found in 20% to 50% of patients, but many have orthostatic hypotension because of peripheral neuropathy, autonomic neuropathy, or the nephrotic syndrome. Patients with predominantly vascular involvement may have little proteinuria but rather renal insufficiency caused by decreased renal blood flow. Infrequently, patients have predominantly tubulointerstitial deposition of amyloid with renal insufficiency and tubular defects such as distal RTA and nephrogenic diabetes insipidus.[562,563,578]

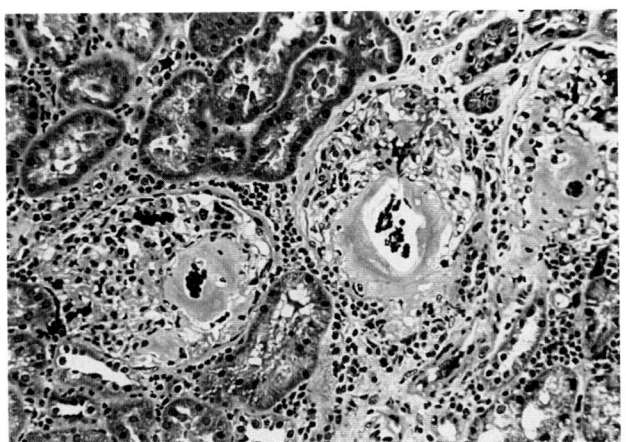

FIGURE 32-23 Amyloidosis. The glomerular tuft contains segmental deposits of amorphous eosinophilic hyaline material involving the vascular pole and some mesangial regions (hematoxylin and eosin, ×375).

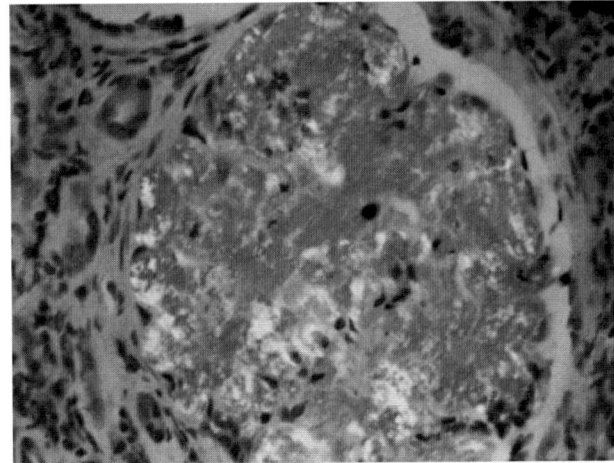

FIGURE 32-25 Amyloidosis. Congo red stain of a glomerulus that is largely replaced by amyloid demonstrates the characteristic birefringence under polarized light (×450).

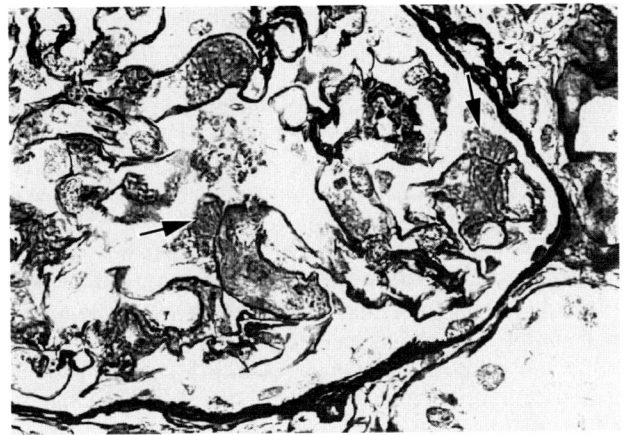

FIGURE 32-24 Amyloidosis. The amyloid deposits expand the mesangium and form focal spicular projections through the glomerular capillary walls, resembling spikes (*arrows*) (Jones methenamine silver, ×800).

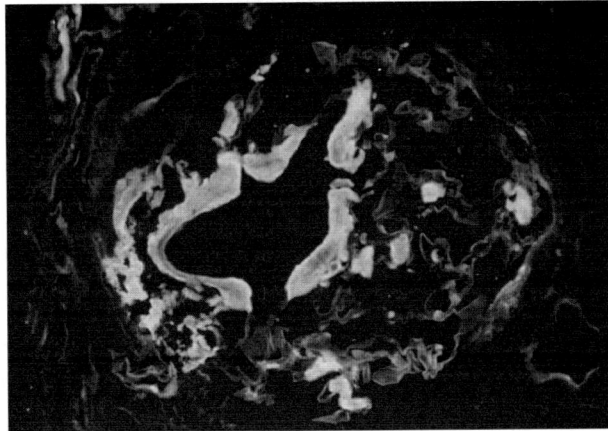

FIGURE 32-26 Amyloidosis. Immunofluorescence photomicrograph showing glomerular staining for λ light chain in the distribution of the glomerular amyloid deposits in a patient with AL amyloidosis and plasma cell dyscrasia (×600).

Pathology

In patients with clinical renal disease, the sensitivity of renal biopsy with adequate tissue sampling approaches 100%.[563,591-595] Renal biopsy distinguishes primary AL amyloid from AA amyloid and excludes involvement by other renal disease in patients with known amyloidosis of other organs.

By LM, there is glomerular deposition of amorphous hyaline material that usually begins in the mesangium and extends into the peripheral capillary walls (Figure 32-23). The deposited material is eosinophilic, weakly periodic acid–Schiff positive (PAS), and nonargyrophilic. In trichrome-stained sections, it may appear lavender or grayblue. Affected glomeruli appear hypocellular and may have a nodular aspect. In the peripheral GBM, amyloid deposits form spicular hairlike projections (Figure 32-24). Congo red stain gives an orange staining reaction and the diagnostic apple-green birefringence under polarized light (Figure 32-25). Amyloid deposits stain metachromatically with crystal or methyl violet and fluoresce under ultraviolet light after thioflavin T staining. Amyloid deposition may be confined to the glomeruli or involve tubular basement membranes, interstitium, and blood vessels as well. The IF in AL amyloidosis gives strong staining with antisera to the pathogenic light chain, usually λ (Figure 32-26). In AA amyloidosis, immunostaining results for immunoglobulins and complement components are usually negative or give a generalized weak reactivity because of nonspecific trapping. Diagnosis depends on the demonstration of strong reactivity for SAA protein by IF or immunoperoxidase staining (Figure 32-27). Hereditary amyloidoses neither stain selectively for a single light chain nor for AA protein, but stain with antisera to the particular precursor protein. In difficult cases, mass spectrometry-based proteomic analysis of the amyloid deposits extracted by laser capture microdissection from renal biopsy sections may be required to identify the etiology of the amyloidosis.[596] By EM, in all glomerular amyloidosis, typical nonbranching 8- to 12-nm-wide fibrils are randomly distributed in the mesangium and frequently along the GBM in the subepithelial, intramembranous, and subendothelial locations (Figure 32-28). Mild cases may have deposition limited to the mesangium. More severe cases usually have more extensive deposition in the peripheral capillary walls and obliterating the lumina. By EM, glomerular capillary wall infiltration by amyloid may form characteristic spicular projections along the subepithelial aspect of the GBMs.

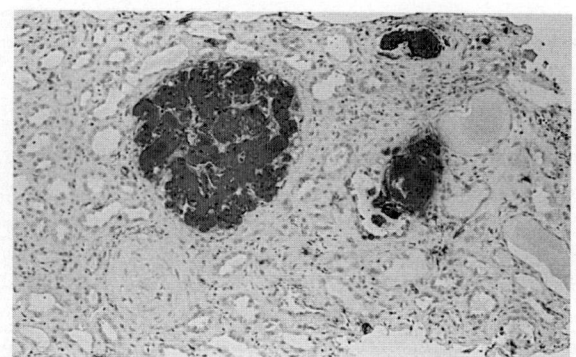

FIGURE 32-27 Amyloidosis. Immunoperoxidase staining for serum amyloid A protein stains the amyloid deposits in the glomeruli and arteries of a patient with secondary (AA) amyloidosis caused by rheumatoid arthritis (×125).

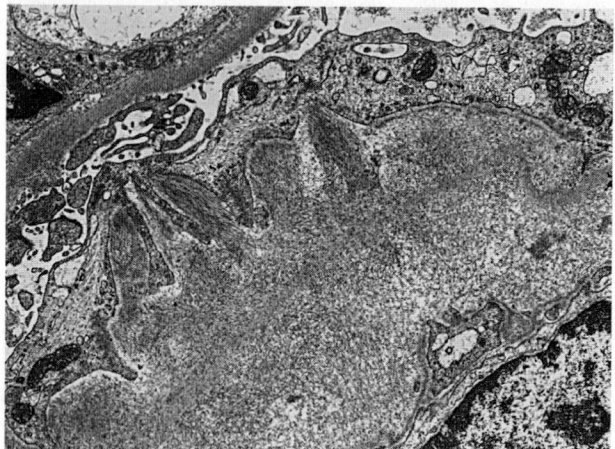

FIGURE 32-28 Amyloidosis. Electron micrograph showing extensive infiltration of the glomerular basement membrane by 10-nm fibrils that project toward the urinary space (×8000).

Course, Prognosis, and Treatment

The prognosis of patients with AL amyloidosis in the past has been poor with some series having a median survival of less than 2 years.[562,563,578] The baseline serum creatinine at diagnosis and the degree of proteinuria are predictive of the progression to ESRD. In older series, the median time from diagnosis to dialysis was 14 months and from dialysis to death was only 8 months.[563,578] Recent data suggest improved survival. Factors associated with decreased patient survival include evidence of cardiac involvement, renal dysfunction, and interstitial fibrosis on renal biopsy.[562,578] Cardiac involvement with associated heart failure and arrhythmias is the primary cause of death in amyloidosis followed by renal disease.[562,578,597]

The course of AA amyloidosis has recently been defined in a study of 374 patients followed for a median time of more than 7 years.[582] Therapy to suppress the inflammatory disease was used whenever possible. The predominant manifestation and influence on the course of the disease was renal dysfunction, and the median survival time was more than 10 years. The SAA concentration correlated with overall mortality, amyloid burden, and renal prognosis. Amyloid deposits regressed (as assessed by SAP scans) in patients whose SAA concentration was kept low.

The optimal treatment for patients with AL amyloid differs depending on the age, organ systems involved, and overall health of the patient.[562,563,598] Treatment strategies focus on methods to decrease the production of monoclonal light chains, akin to myeloma therapy, using chemotherapeutic drugs such as melphalan and corticosteroids, cyclophosphamide, or vincristine, doxorubicin, and dexamethasone (VAD) therapy. In some patients, there has been evidence of resolution of proteinuria, stabilization of renal function, improvement of symptoms, and occasionally evidence of decreased organ involvement such as reduced hepatosplenomegaly.[599] In a review of 153 AL amyloid patients treated with melphalan and prednisone only, 18% of the patients had a regression of organ manifestations of amyloidosis with responders having a 5-year survival rate of 78% versus only 7% in the nonresponders.[600] Patients with renal amyloidosis fared best with 25% having a 50% reduction in nephrotic range proteinuria and stable or improved GFR. Colchicine, used to treat AL amyloidosis in the past, has proved to be inferior to chemotherapeutic options and adds no benefit as a supplement to these regimens.[601,602] A prospective trial in more than 100 patients compared an intensive regimen with five agents (vincristine, BCNU [carmustine], melphalan, cyclophosphamide, and prednisone) with melphalan and prednisone alone and showed no survival advantage for the intensive treatment group.[603] Promising chemotherapeutic agents used in conjunction with dexamethasone successfully in amyloid include a number of agents used in myeloma, including lenalidomide, thalidomide, bortezomib, and cyclophosphamide.[603-606] Other therapies for AL amyloid used experimentally to treat small numbers of patients include dimethyl sulfoxide, 4'-iodo-4'-deoxydoxorubicin, fludarabine, vitamin E, high-dose dexamethasone monotherapy, and INF-α2.[562,607,608] None has proven efficacy at this time.

Recent reports using high-dose melphalan followed by allogeneic bone marrow transplant or stem cell transplant have given promising results.[609,610] Such regimens have led to resolution of the nephrotic syndrome and biopsy-proven improvement of amyloid organ involvement in some cases. Although there was a high mortality in early reports (20% in the first 3 months), many survivors had a complete hematologic response, and many with renal involvement survived with a major decrease in proteinuria without a worsening of GFR. One retrospective study analyzed 65 AL amyloid patients with more than 1 g/day of proteinuria treated with dose-intensive ablative chemotherapy followed by autologous blood stem cell transplantation.[611] Three-fourths of the patients survived the first year, and among those, a good renal response was found in 36% at 1 year and 52% at 2 years. Patients with a complete hematologic response were more likely to have a good renal response, and patient survival was superior in younger patients with fewer than three organ systems involved and those able to tolerate higher doses of the ablative therapy. Toxicities included mucositis; edema; elevated liver function test results; pulmonary edema; GI bleeding; and in 23%, transient acute renal failure. Thus, for some younger patients with predominantly renal involvement, stem cell transplantation is currently a reasonable alternative therapy. Some studies have supported stem cell transplantation as a beneficial therapy for some AL amyloid patients.[612] Even patients with ESRD caused by amyloidosis may undergo this form of therapy with results no different from non-ESRD patients with AL amyloidosis.[613] However, the only large randomized trial of stem cell transplantation for amyloid found this treatment to be inferior to standard chemotherapy.[614] In this multicenter French trial, 100 patients were randomized to hematopoietic cell transplantation or melphalan plus dexamethasone. The chemotherapeutic group had a better overall survival. Although this study has been criticized for patient selection and the high subsequent mortality, it is the only large randomized trial.

Regardless of whether chemotherapy or marrow transplant is used, the treatment of nephrotic amyloid patients requires supportive care. This may include judicious use of diuretics and salt restriction in those with edema and treatment of orthostatic hypotension with compression stockings; fludrocortisone; and in some, midodrine, an oral α-adrenergic agonist.

The treatment of AA amyloid focuses on the treatment of the underlying inflammatory disease process.[582,615] This has included surgical debridement of inflammatory tissue, antibiotic therapy of infectious processes, and antiinflammatory medications and immunosuppressive agents in rheumatoid arthritis and inflammatory bowel disease. Therapy may lead to stabilization of renal function, reduction in proteinuria, and resolution of amyloid deposits.[582] The prognosis may be good if the underlying disease can be controlled and there is not already extensive amyloid deposition. Immunosuppressive and antiinflammatory agents have been used in rheumatologic diseases, with evidence of increased GFR and decreased proteinuria, with prolonged renal survival, and in several cases with regression of renal amyloid deposits.[562,615,616]

In familial Mediterranean fever, an autosomal recessive disease primarily found in Sephardic Jews, Turks, Armenians, and Arabs, there are recurrent attacks of fever and serositis associated with the development of AA amyloidosis in up to 90% of untreated patients.[582,617] Colchicine has long been used successfully to prevent the febrile attacks and is effective in preventing the development of proteinuria and stabilizing proteinuria. However, renal function did deteriorate in patients with the nephrotic syndrome at presentation. A retrospective analysis of FMF patients with milder renal clinical involvement and at least 5 years follow-up concluded that high doses of colchicine were more effective in preventing renal dysfunction and that patients with lower levels of serum creatinine at presentation responded better to therapy.[612] After the serum creatinine level was elevated, however, increasing the dose of colchicine did not seem to prevent progression. AA amyloidosis seen in drug abusers has occasionally responded to colchicine therapy, although most investigators believe the key to improvement appears to be treatment of the underlying infections and cessation of skin popping.[585,586]

A recent multicenter, randomized, controlled trial compared a glycosaminoglycan (GAG) mimetic (used to block fibrillogenesis) to placebo in 183 patients with AA amyloid. Although the specified endpoint of the study, preventing progression to ESRD, was not achieved, the GAG mimetic did reduce the risk of rate of progression of the renal disease.[618] This study clearly shows the need for newer therapies for amyloidosis and the value of controlled trials in studying these agents. Several promising experimental therapies for treating amyloid include the use of anti-amyloid antibodies and the use of an inhibitor of the binding of amyloid P component to amyloid fibrils.[615]

End-Stage Renal Disease in Amyloidosis

In most series, the median survival of amyloid patients with ESRD is less than 1 year with the primary cause of death being complications of cardiac amyloid.[619,620] However, for patients who survive the first month of ESRD replacement therapy, the survival rate is more than 50% at 2 years and 30% at 5 years.[620] This is still 20% lower than an age-matched general ESRD population. There is no survival difference between peritoneal dialysis or hemodialysis.[620] Experience with renal transplantation is largely in patients with AA amyloid and is limited in AL amyloid.[621,622] One series on transplantation in amyloid included 45 patients (42 with AA amyloid) and found an overall low patient survival, particularly in the early posttransplant period in older patients because of infectious and cardiovascular complications.[621] Graft survival, however, was not decreased despite rates of recurrence of amyloidosis in the allograft as high as 20% to 33%.[621,622]

Fibrillary Glomerulonephritis and Immunotactoid Glomerulonephritis

Some glomerular lesions have fibrillar deposits differing in size from that of amyloid and without the typical staining properties of amyloid.[562,623,624] In the past, they were reported as being Congo red–negative amyloid, amyloid-like glomerulopathy, and non-amyloidotic fibrillary glomerulopathy. Many investigators subdivide these patients into two major groups depending on clinical associations and fibril size.[562,623,625-627] In fibrillary GN, the fibrils are approximately 16 to 24 nm (mean, 20 nm) in diameter, and in immunotactoid GN, the deposits form larger hollow microtubules of 30 to 50 nm in diameter. It has been suggested that the organized deposits represent a slow acting cryoprecipitate of polyclonal or monoclonal immunoglobulin. A third rare form of fibrillary renal disease is fibronectin glomerulopathy in which the glomeruli are infiltrated by massive deposits of fibronectin.[628-630]

Although some classify both fibrillary GN and immunotactoid GN as a single disease entity, most clinicians and nephropathologists divide them into distinct disorders.[623-626] Almost 90% of cases have the smaller 20-nm fibrils of fibrillary GN. Fibrillary GN occurs mostly in adults, in both sexes, in all age groups, and most commonly in whites. It is usually an isolated renal entity of unknown etiology. Patients with immunotactoid GN tend to be older; may have a less rapidly progressive course; and in all series are more likely to have underlying lymphoproliferative disease, often with a circulating paraprotein and sometimes with hypocomplementemia.[623-626] Patients with both diseases usually have proteinuria, and most have hypertension and hematuria. About 70% have the nephrotic syndrome at biopsy. At presentation, renal insufficiency is common, and most patients progress to ESRD. Both fibrillary GN and immunotactoid GN may be associated with HCV infection.[627] The course to ESRD appears to be more rapid in older patients, those with an elevated serum creatinine, and those with crescentic lesions on biopsy.

Fibronectin glomerulopathy is a familial disease with autosomal dominant inheritance that presents with proteinuria and hematuria, usually in adolescence, and eventually progresses to the nephrotic syndrome and slowly deteriorating renal function.[628-630] It is caused by an inherited mutation in the gene

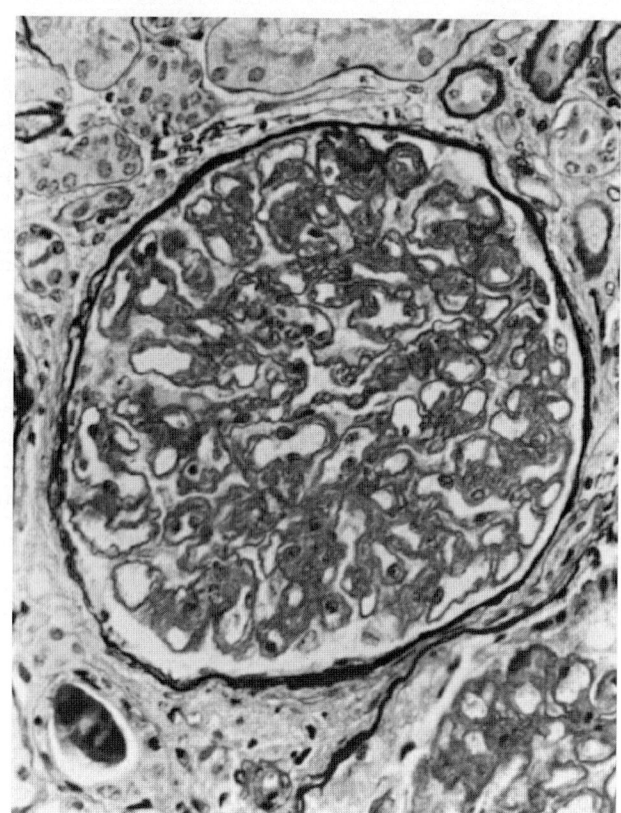

FIGURE 32-29 Fibrillary glomerulonephritis. The mesangium is mildly expanded, and the glomerular capillary walls appear thickened with segmental double contours (periodic acid–Schiff, ×300).

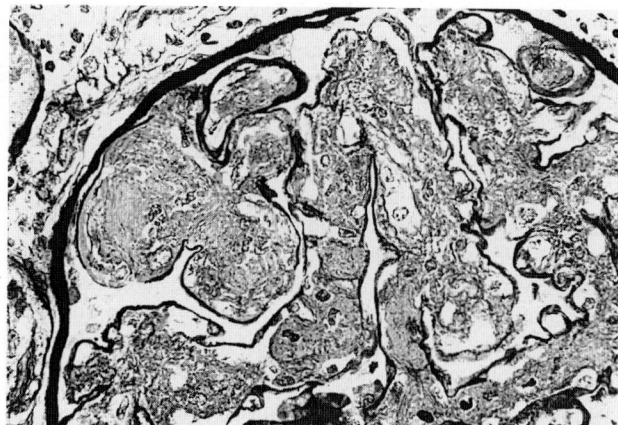

FIGURE 32-30 Immunotactoid glomerulonephritis. There is lobular expansion of the glomerular tuft by abundant mesangial deposits of silver-negative material. Segmental extension of deposits into the subendothelial aspect of some glomerular capillaries is also seen (Jones methenamine silver, ×500).

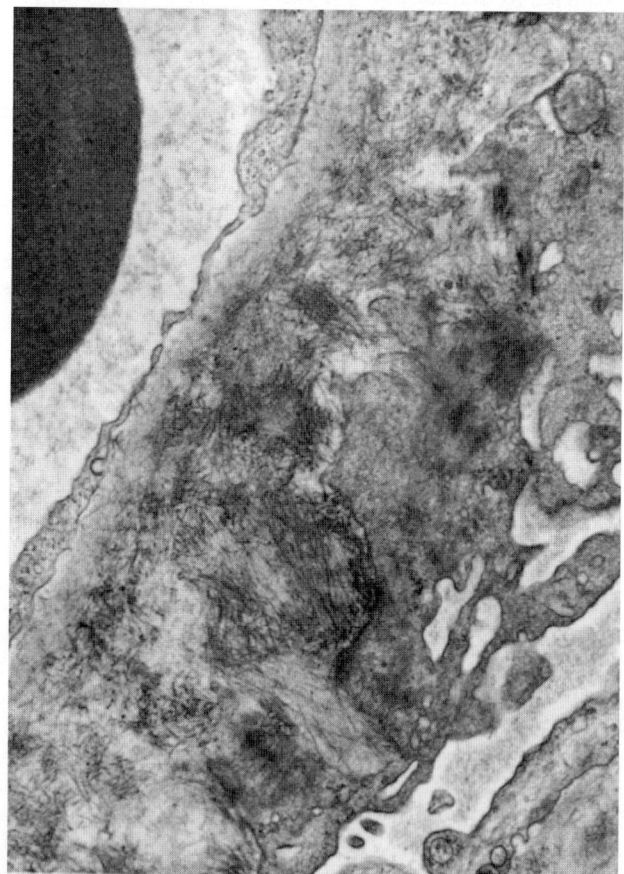

FIGURE 32-31 Fibrillary glomerulonephritis. Electron micrograph showing the characteristic randomly oriented fibrils, measuring 16 to 20 nm within the glomerular basement membrane. The foot processes are effaced (×8000).

encoding fibronectin-1.[630] Patients who progress to ESRD may develop recurrent fibronectin glomerulopathy in the allograft.

The diagnosis of all of these fibrillary disorders requires renal biopsy to demonstrate the defining ultrastructural features.[562,623-626] LM findings in fibrillary GN are highly variable and include mesangial proliferation; mesangial expansion by amorphous amyloid-like material; and membranous, membranoproliferative, and crescentic GN (Figure 32-29).[623] In immunotactoid GN, glomerular lesions are often nodular and sclerosing, but others are proliferative or membranous (Figure 32-30). The pathognomonic findings are seen on EM and consist of nonbranching fibrils of 16 to 24 nm diameter in fibrillary GN (as opposed to 8–12 nm for amyloid) (Figure 32-31) and hollow microtubules of 30 to 50 nm in immunotactoid GN (Figure 32-32). In fibrillary GN, fibrils are arranged randomly in the mesangial matrix and GBMs. By contrast, the microtubules of immunotactoid GN are often arranged in parallel stacks in the mesangium, subendothelial, or subepithelial regions. The fibrils and microtubules do not stain with Congo red or thioflavin T. In fibrillary GN, IF is almost always positive for IgG (Figure 32-33) (especially subclasses IgG1 and IgG4), C3, and both κ and λ chains, indicating polyclonal deposits.[623-626] Staining for IgM, IgA, and C1 has been reported in a minority of cases. In immunotactoid GN, the immunoglobulin deposits are often monoclonal, consisting of IgG with a restricted light chain isotype (either κ or λ). IgG subtypes IgG1 and IgG3 are most common and have the capacity to fix complement, leading to glomerular co-deposits of C1q and C3. In both diseases, the deposits are usually limited to the kidney. In fibrillary GN, the fibrils may be focally admixed with more granular immune type electron-dense deposits.[628-630] Rare patients with fibrillary GN have been reported to have extrarenal deposits involving alveolar capillaries, and in the case of immunotactoid GN, the bone marrow.[631,632]

Although there is no proven therapy for fibrillary GN, some clinicians choose to treat the LM pattern observed on renal

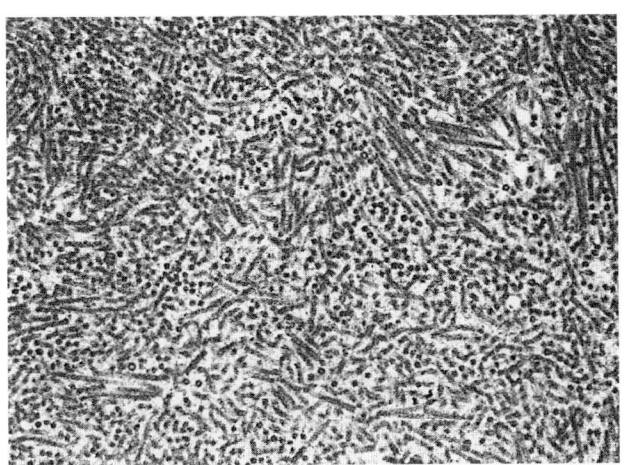

FIGURE 32-32 Immunotactoid glomerulonephritis. Electron micrograph showing abundant mesangial deposits of microtubular structures measuring approximately 35 nm in diameter (×10,000).

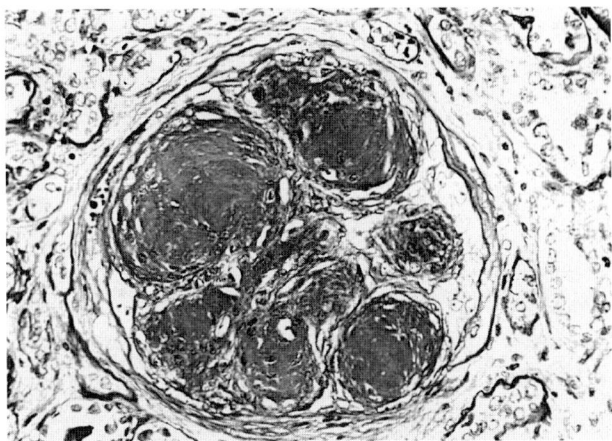

FIGURE 32-34 Light chain deposition disease. There is nodular glomerulosclerosis with marked global expansion of the mesangium by intensely periodic acid–Schiff–positive material but without appreciable thickening of the glomerular capillary walls (periodic acid–Schiff, ×375).

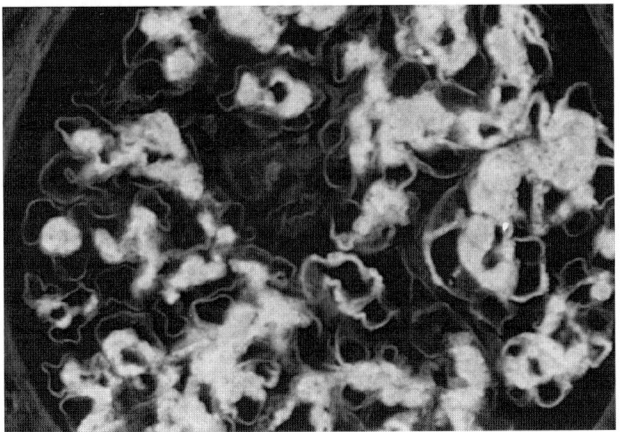

FIGURE 32-33 Fibrillary glomerulonephritis. Immunofluorescence photomicrograph showing smudgy deposits of immunoglobulin G throughout the mesangium with segmental extension into the peripheral glomerular capillary walls (×800).

biopsy (e.g., membranous, membranoproliferative, crescentic).[562,623] Prednisone, cyclophosphamide, and colchicine have not led to consistent benefit in most patients.[562,623] However, in some with crescentic GN, cyclophosphamide and corticosteroid therapy has led to a dramatic improvement in GFR and proteinuria with some patients being able to discontinue dialytic support.[586,643] Cyclosporine has also been used successfully in some patients with fibrillary GN and a membranous pattern on LM, and rituximab has been used in those with an MPGN pattern.[562,623] In patients with associated chronic lymphocytic leukemia (CLL), treatment with chemotherapy has been associated with improved renal function and decreased proteinuria.[562,623,633] Dialysis and transplantation have been performed in fibrillary GN, but there is a recurrence of disease in half of patients.[623,634,635]

Monoclonal Immunoglobulin Deposition Disease

Monoclonal immunoglobulin deposition disease (MIDD), which includes light chain deposition disease (LCDD), combined light and heavy chain deposition disease (LHCDD), and heavy chain deposition disease (HCDD), is a systemic disease caused by the overproduction and extracellular deposition of a fragment of monoclonal immunoglobulins.[636-638] LCDD is by far the most common pattern. As opposed to amyloidosis, in LCDD, the deposits in approximately 80% of cases are composed of κ rather than λ light chains.[636-640] The deposits are also granular in nature, do not form fibrils or beta pleated sheets, do not bind Congo red stain or thioflavine-T, and are not associated with amyloid P protein.[636-640] In amyloid, the fibrils are usually derived primarily from the variable region of the light chains, but in LCDD, the deposits are predominantly composed of the constant region of the light chain. This may explain the far brighter IF staining for light chains found in LCDD as opposed to amyloidosis. The pathogenesis of the glomerulosclerosis in LCDD is not entirely clear, but mesangial cells from patients with LCDD produce transforming growth factor-β, which acting as an autacoid, in turn promotes these cells to produce matrix proteins such as type IV collagen, laminin, and fibronectin.[641]

Patients with LCDD are generally older than 45 years old.[636-640] Many such patients develop frank myeloma, and others clearly have a lymphoplasmacytic B-cell disease such as lymphoma or Waldenström's macroglobulinemia.[636,638,640] As in amyloidosis, the clinical features vary with the location and extent of organ deposition of the monoclonal protein. Patients typically have cardiac, neural, hepatic, and renal involvement, but other organs such as the skin, spleen, thyroid, adrenal gland, and GI tract may be involved.[636-640] Patients with renal disease usually have significant glomerular involvement and present with proteinuria, with the nephrotic syndrome, hypertension, and renal insufficiency. Some patients may have greater tubulointerstitial involvement and less proteinuria along with renal insufficiency.[640]

The glomerular pattern by LM is usually nodular sclerosing with mesangial nodules of acellular eosinophilic material resembling the nodular glomerulosclerosis seen in patients with diabetes (Figure 32-34).[636-640] Glomerular capillary microaneurysms may also be found.[642] Some glomeruli have associated membranoproliferative features. In LCDD, the nodules are more strongly PAS positive and less argyrophilic than in diabetes.[636,643] Unlike diabetic glomerulosclerosis, the GBMs in LCDD are not usually visibly thickened by LM. Other glomeruli may be entirely normal or have only mild

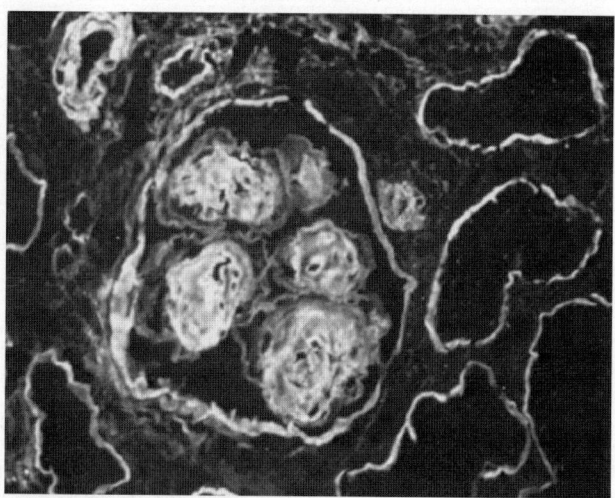

FIGURE 32-35 Light chain deposition disease. Immunofluorescence photomicrograph showing linear staining for κ light chain involving glomerular and tubular basement membranes, the mesangial nodules, Bowman's capsule, and vessel walls (×250).

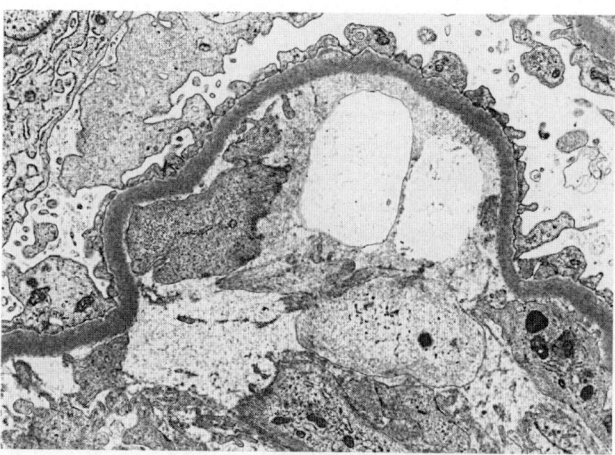

FIGURE 32-36 Heavy chain deposition disease. Electron micrograph showing bandlike finely granular electron-dense deposits involving the glomerular basement membrane, with greatest concentration along the inner aspect (×5000).

mesangial sclerosis. IF is usually diagnostic with a monoclonal light chain (κ in 80%) staining in a diffuse linear pattern along the GBMs, in the nodules, and along the tubular basement membranes as well as vessel walls (Figure 32-35).[636,640] Staining results for complement components are usually negative. By EM, deposition of a finely granular punctate highly electron-dense material occurs along the lamina rara interna of the GBM, in the mesangium, and along tubular and vascular basement membranes.[636-640,643]

The prognosis for patients with LCDD is variable. Death is often attributed to heart failure, infectious complications, or the development of frank myeloma and renal failure.[636-640,644] In one series of 63 patients, 65% of patients developed myeloma.[638] Of all 63 patients, 36 developed uremia, and 37 died. Predictors of worse renal outcome included increased age and elevated serum creatinine at presentation. Predictors of worse patient survival included increased age, occurrence of myeloma, and extrarenal deposition of light chains. Treatment with melphalan and corticosteroids, as in amyloid, has led to stabilized or improved renal function in LCDD. However, this therapy is not successful in patients with significant renal dysfunction and a plasma creatinine above 4 mg/dL at initiation of treatment.[644] Patient survival is about 90% at 1 year and 70% at 5 years, with renal survival 67% and 37% at 1 and 5 years.[644] Patients with LCDD and associated cast nephropathy have a worse renal and patient survival. Marrow or stem cell transplantation is a therapeutic option for some patients with LCDD.[636,638] Although there are few data on dialysis and transplantation in LCDD, patients appear to fare as well as those with amyloidosis. Recurrences in the renal transplant have been reported,[636,640,644,645] and one recent trial of seven patients with LCDD who received renal transplants found recurrences in five of seven in a mean time of less than 1 year.[646] Thus, suppression of the abnormal paraprotein producing cell clone is crucial prior to renal transplantation.

In some patients with a plasma cell dyscrasia, monoclonal light and heavy immunoglobulin chains combined (LHCDD) or monoclonal truncated heavy chains alone (HCDD) are deposited in the tissue (Figure 32-36).[636,637,639,647,648] The clinical features are similar to those of LCDD and amyloidosis.[648]

Most patients are middle age or older, although at least one patient was 35 years of age. They present with renal insufficiency, proteinuria, hypertension, and often the nephrotic syndrome. In most patients, a monoclonal protein is detected in the serum or urine. In contrast to amyloid and LCDD, HCDD may be associated with hypocomplementemia if the heavy chain avidly binds complement (especially γ heavy chain subtypes G1 and G3).[648] All patients with HCDD have a deletion of the CH1 domain of the heavy chain, which causes it to be secreted prematurely by the plasma cell.[648-650] The characteristic LM finding in HCDD is a nodular sclerosing glomerulopathy at times with crescents.[636,648] The diagnosis is made by IF with linear positivity for the heavy chain of immunoglobulin (usually γ) and negativity for both κ and λ light chains.[648] The distribution is diffuse involving glomerular, tubular, and vascular basement membranes. Treatment has been similar to that for LCDD, and many patients have progressed to renal failure.[648,651] Recurrence in the renal transplant has been documented with eventual loss of the allograft.[636]

Other Glomerular Diseases in Plasma Cell Dyscrasias

Patients with plasma cell dyscrasia may develop pathology in the tubulointerstitial, glomerular, and vascular compartments.[752] Glomerular and vascular lesions are usually restricted to patients with associated AL amyloidosis or monoclonal light or heavy chain deposition disease (see discussion of amyloid and MIDD). Recently, patients with a proliferative GN resembling immune complex GN have been described in association with plasma cell disorders.[652,653] These patients presented with renal insufficiency and proteinuria with many having the nephrotic syndrome but no evidence of cryoglobulinemia. On biopsy, all had granular non-organized electron-dense deposits in the mesangial, subendothelial, and subepithelial sites, but by IF, these were restricted to a single monoclonal γ subclass and light chain isotype (e.g., IgG1κ, IgG2λ, or IgG3κ). M spike was identified in the serum in 30% of cases, but no patient developed overt myeloma or lymphoma during the follow-up period. Other rare patients with

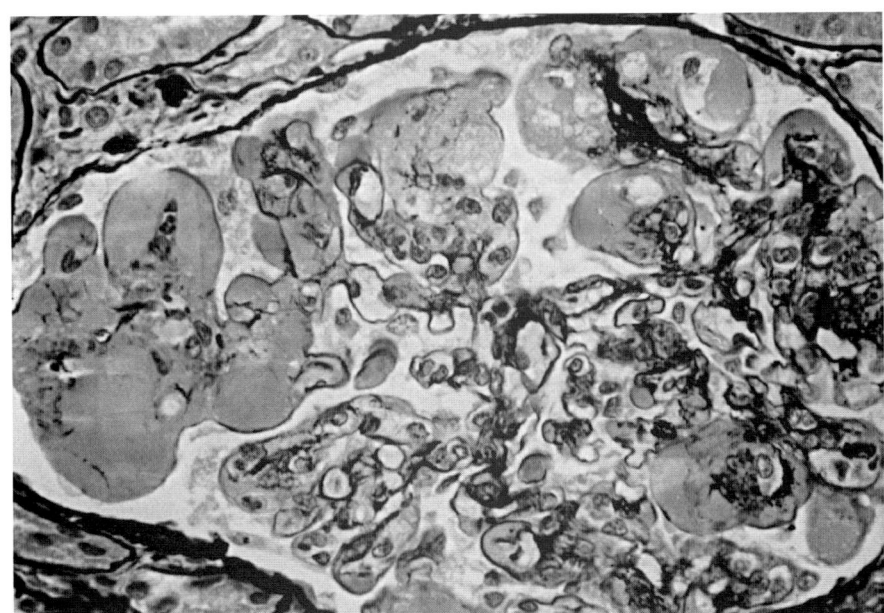

FIGURE 32-37 Waldenström's macroglobulinemia. Large "protein thrombi" corresponding to the monoclonal immunoglobulin M deposits fill the glomerular capillary lumina with minimal associated glomerular hypercellularity (Jones methenamine silver, ×600).

plasma cell dyscrasias have had intracellular glomerular crystals within the podocytes, sometimes in association with tubular epithelial crystalline deposits.[654] Pamidronate-induced collapsing focal sclerosis has been noted in myeloma[655] as has crescentic GN. Membranoproliferative GN has been reported rarely, particularly in patients with associated cryoglobulinemia (see section on cryoglobulinemia).

Waldenström's Macroglobulinemia

Waldenström's macroglobulinemia is a syndrome in which patients have abnormal circulating monoclonal IgM protein in association with a B-cell lymphoproliferative disorder involving small lymphocytes.[656-658] This slowly progressive disorder occurs in older patients (median age, 60 years with a slight male predominance) who present with fatigue, weight loss, bleeding, visual disturbances, peripheral neuropathy, hepatosplenomegaly, lymphadenopathy, anemia, and often hyperviscosity syndrome.[656-658] Renal involvement is uncommon, but glomerular lesions are found in some patients.[659,660] Renal involvement is usually manifested by microscopic hematuria and proteinuria, which may be nephrotic or at lower levels. In some cases, it is attributable to excreted light chains. Patients may have enlarged kidneys. The renal pathology in Waldenström's macroglobulinemia is varied.[659] Some patients have invasion of the renal parenchyma by neoplastic lymphoplasmacytic cells. Acute renal failure associated with intraglomerular occlusive thrombi of the IgM paraprotein has also been reported. These cases have large eosinophilic, amorphous, PAS-positive deposits occluding the glomerular capillary loops with little or no glomerular hypercellularity (Figure 32-37). By IF, these glomerular "thrombi" stain for IgM and a single light chain isotype, consistent with monoclonal IgM deposits, but complement component results are usually negative. By EM, the deposits contain non-amyloid fibrillar or amorphous electron-dense material. Some patients develop membranoproliferative GN with an associated type 1 or type 2 cryoglobulinemia (Figure 32-38). Cases of LCDD

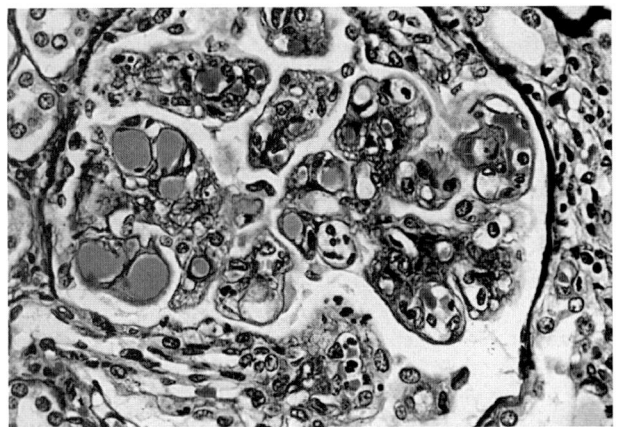

FIGURE 32-38 Waldenström's macroglobulinemia. An example with cryoglobulinemic glomerulonephritis showing the characteristic intraluminal deposits, infiltrating leukocytes, and double-contoured glomerular basement membranes (Jones methenamine silver, ×600).

have also been reported. At times, intratubular casts similar to those of myeloma cast nephropathy are present. Amyloid has been found in a number of patients with Waldenström's macroglobulinemia. Treatment of patients with Waldenström's macroglobulinemia is directed against the lymphoproliferative disease with alkylating agents, melphalan, and corticosteroids and at times plasmapheresis for hyperviscosity signs and symptoms. Newer therapies include fludarabine, cladribine, INF-α, and rituximab, and marrow transplantation.[661-663]

Mixed Cryoglobulinemia

Cryoglobulinemia is caused circulating immunoglobulins that precipitate upon cooling and resolubilize on warming.[664] Cryoglobulinemia is associated with a variety of infections, especially HCV (see below) as well as collagen vascular disease and lymphoproliferative diseases. Cryoglobulins have been divided into three major groups based on the nature of the circulating immunoglobulins.[664,665] In type I cryoglobuline-mia, the cryoglobulin is a single monoclonal immunoglobulin often found associated with Waldenström's macroglobulin-emia or myeloma. Both type II and III cryoglobulinemia are defined as mixed cryoglobulins, containing a least two immu-noglobulins. In type II, a monoclonal immunoglobulin (IgM κ in >90%) is directed against polyclonal IgG and has rheu-matoid factor activity.[666] In type III, the antiglobulin is poly-clonal in nature with both polyclonal IgG and IgM in most cases. The majority of patients with type II and III mixed cryoglobulins have now been clearly shown to have HCV infection.[667-669] To establish a diagnosis of cryoglobulinemia, the offending cryoglobulins or the characteristic renal tissue involvement must be demonstrated.

In the past, there was often no obvious etiology for cryo-globulinemia, and the name *essential mixed cryoglobulinemia* was appropriate.[664,665,668] It is now clear that many such patients had HCV-related disease. Systemic manifestation of mixed cryoglobulinemia include weakness, malaise, Raynaud's phenomena, arthralgias-arthritis, hepatosplenomegaly with abnormal liver function test results in two-thirds to three-fourths of patients, peripheral neuropathy, and purpuric–vas-culitic skin lesions.[664,665,668] Hypocomplementemia, especially of the early components (low C4 level) is a characteristic and often helpful finding. Renal disease occurs at presentation in fewer than one-fourth of patients but develops in as many as 50% over time.[664,665,667-669] In many, an acute nephritic picture with hematuria, hypertension, proteinuria, and pro-gressive renal insufficiency develops. An oliguric rapidly pro-gressive GN picture is present only rarely, and about 20% of patients present with the nephrotic syndrome. The majority of patients with renal disease have a slow, indolent renal course characterized by proteinuria, hypertension, hematuria, and renal insufficiency.

Many studies of type II cryoglobulinemia have shown evi-dence of hepatitis B infection or other viral infections (e.g., Epstein-Barr virus [EBV]).[670] However, recent studies have clearly documented HCV as a major cause of cryoglobulin production in most patients previously believed to have essen-tial mixed cryoglobulinemia.[670-672] Antibodies to HCV anti-gens have been documented in the serum and HCV RNA, and anti-HCV antibodies are enriched in the cryoglobulins of these patients.[667,671-674] This is true even for patients with normal levels of aminotransferases and no clinical evidence of hepatitis. HCV antigens have also been localized by immuno-histochemistry to the glomerular deposits.[672]

In cryoglobulinemia, immunoglobulin complexes deposit in the glomeruli and small- and medium-sized arteries, bind-ing complement and inciting a proliferative response.[667,669] The serum cryoglobulin participates in the formation of the glomerular immune complex. in vitro studies have shown that IgM-κ rheumatoid factor from patients with type II cryoglob-ulinemia are much more likely to bind to cellular fibronectin (a component of the glomerular mesangium) than IgM from normal control participants or IgM containing rheumatoid factor from patients with rheumatoid arthritis.[675,676] The par-ticular physicochemical characteristics of the variable region of the immunoglobulin cryoglobulin may be important in the localization of the renal deposits.

Although by LM, the glomerular lesions of cryoglobuli-nemia may show a variety of proliferative and sclerosing fea-tures (Figure 32-39), certain features help to distinguish the

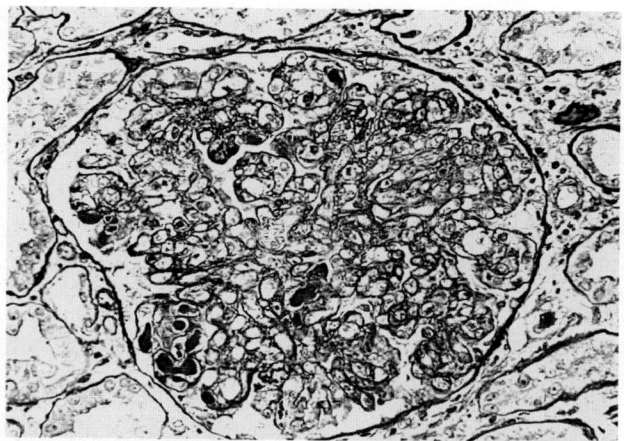

FIGURE 32-39 Cryoglobulinemic glomerulonephritis. There is global endocapillary proliferative glomerulonephritis with membranoproliferative features and focal intraluminal cryoglobulin deposits, forming "immune thrombi" (periodic acid–Schiff, ×375).

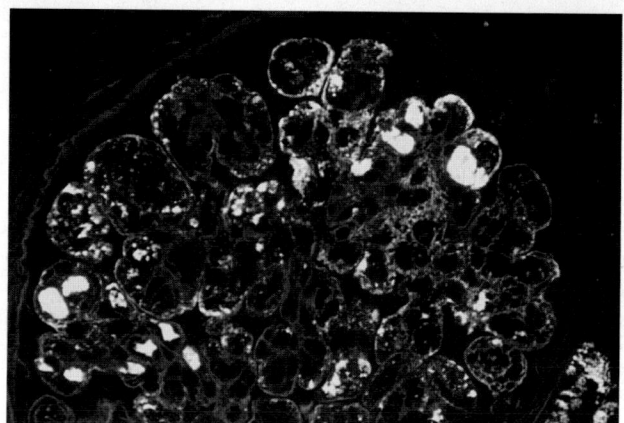

FIGURE 32-40 Cryoglobulinemic glomerulonephritis. Immunofluores-cence photomicrograph showing deposits of immunoglobulin M corre-sponding to the large glomerular intracapillary deposits with more finely granular subendothelial deposits outlining the glomerular capillary walls (×900).

proliferative GN of essential mixed cryoglobulinemia from other proliferative glomerulonephriti   des.[664,666,667] These include massive exudation of monocytes and to a lesser degree polymorphonuclear leukocytes; amorphous eosino-philic PAS-positive, Congo red negative deposits on the inner side of the glomerular capillary wall and sometimes filling the capillary lumens; membranoproliferative features with double-contoured GBMs and interposition of deposits, mesangial cells, and monocytes; and the rarity of extracapil-lary proliferation (crescents) despite the intense intracapillary proliferation. The glomerular lesions may be accompanied by an acute vasculitis of small- or medium-sized vessels. The monocytes of patients with active cryoglobulinemia and asso-ciated nephritis have been shown to phagocytose cryoglobu-lins but to be unable to catabolize them. By IF (Figure 32-40), the glomeruli in type 2 or 3 cryoglobulinemia contain depos-its of both IgM as well as IgG with C3 and frequently C1q in the distribution of subendothelial and mesangial deposits and the intracapillary "thrombi." By EM (Figure 32-41), depos-its present in the subendothelial position or filling the capil-lary lumens often appear as either amorphous electron-dense deposits or organized deposits of curvilinear parallel fibrils

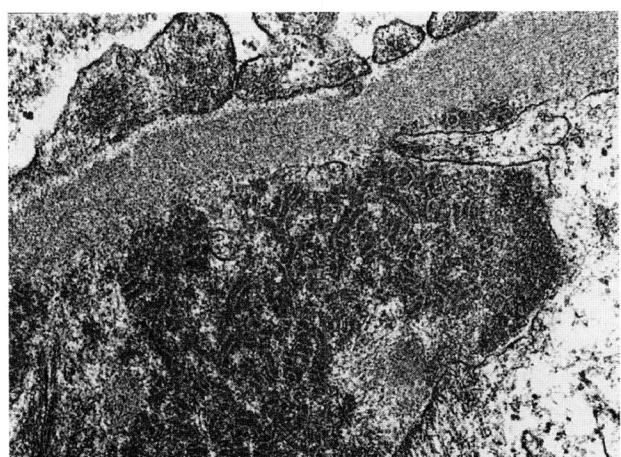

FIGURE 32-41 Cryoglobulinemic glomerulonephritis. Electron micrograph showing organized subendothelial deposits with an annular–tubular substructure. These curvilinear tubular structures measure approximately 30 nm in diameter (×30,000).

that appear tubular in cross-section and have a diameter of 20 to 35 nm.[664,666,667]

Some patients with mixed cryoglobulinemia have a partial or total remission of their disease, but most have episodic exacerbations of their systemic and renal disease.[664,671] Before the association of mixed cryoglobulinemia and HCV was discovered, many patients were treated successfully with prednisone and cytotoxic agents such as cyclophosphamide and chlorambucil.[664,665] None was used in a controlled fashion. In patients with severe renal disease, those with digital necrosis from the cryoglobulins, and those with life-threatening organ involvement, plasmapheresis has also been used in combination with steroids and cytotoxics.[671,677,678] Currently, most patients with HCV-associated cryoglobulinemia are treated with antiviral agents[679] (see section on HCV). Aggressive immunosuppressive therapy carries the risk of promoting HCV replication in HCV-infected patients and of lymphoma in others. Most patients with cryoglobulinemia in the past did not die of renal disease but rather of cardiac or other systemic disease and infectious complications.[678] Rituximab has recently been used successfully for treatment of type II mixed cryoglobulinemia in patients with or without evidence of HCV infection.[680] Dialysis and transplantation in cryoglobulinemia have been used, but recurrences in the allograft have been reported.[681]

Hereditary Nephritis, Including Alport's Syndrome

Alport's syndrome is an inherited (usually X-linked) disorder with characteristic glomerular pathology, frequently associated with hearing loss and ocular abnormalities. Guthrie first reported a family with recurrent hematuria.[682] Alport reported additional observations on this family, the occurrence of deafness associated with hematuria, and the observation that affected males died of uremia but affected females lived to an old age.[683] Since then, several hundred unrelated kindreds exhibiting hereditary nephritis, with and without deafness, have been described, representing a wide variety of geographic and ethnic groups.[684-690] Alport's syndrome and

other hereditary and familial disease accounts for 0.4% of adults with ESRD in the United States.[691]

Clinical Features

The disease usually manifests in children or young adults.[688,689,692] Males have persistent microscopic hematuria with episodic gross hematuria that may be exacerbated by respiratory infections or exercise. Flank pain or abdominal discomfort may accompany these episodes. Proteinuria is usually mild at first and increases progressively with age. The nephrotic syndrome has also been described.[693] Hypertension is a late manifestation. Slowly progressive renal failure is common in males. ESRD usually occurs in boys and men between the ages of 16 and 35 years. In some kindreds, the course may be more delayed with renal failure occurring between 45 and 65 years of age. In most females, the disease is mild and only partially expressed; however, some females have experienced renal failure.[694] In the European Community Alport Syndrome Concerted Action (ECASCA) cohort, hematuria was observed in 95% of carriers and consistently absent in the others. Proteinuria, hearing loss, and ocular defects developed in 75%, 28%, and 15%, respectively.[695] This variability in disease severity in females can be explained by the degree of random inactivation of the mutated versus wild-type X chromosome during lyonization.

High-frequency sensorineural deafness occurs in 30% to 50% of patients. Hearing impairment is always accompanied by renal involvement. The severity of hearing loss is variable, and there is no relationship between the severity of hearing loss and of the renal disease. Based on brainstem auditory evoked responses, the site of the aural lesion is in the cochlea.[696,697] Families with hereditary nephritis but without sensorineural hearing loss have been described.[697,698]

Ocular abnormalities occur in 15% to 30% of patients.[699] Anterior lenticonus, which is the protrusion of the central portion of the lens into the anterior capsule, is virtually pathognomonic of Alport's syndrome. Other ocular abnormalities include keratoconus, spherophakia, myopia, retinal flecks, cataracts, retinitis pigmentosa, and amaurosis.[688,689,700]

Aortic disease, including dissections, aneurysms, dilation, and aortic insufficiency, may be an unusual feature in some patients.[701]

Other variants of Alport's syndrome, now known to be distinct entities, include the association of hereditary nephritis with thrombocytopathia (megathrombocytopenia) so-called Epstein syndrome,[702,703] diffuse leiomyomatosis,[704] ichthyosis and hyperprolinuria,[705] and Fechtner syndrome (nephritis, macrothrombocytopenia, Döhle-like leukocyte inclusions, deafness, and cataract).[706]

Pathology

The LM appearance of biopsies is nonspecific.[707] The diagnosis rests on the EM findings. By LM, most biopsies have glomerular and tubulointerstitial lesions. In the early stages (<5 years of age), the kidney biopsy may be normal or nearly normal.[708] The only abnormality may be the presence of superficially located fetal glomeruli involving 5% to 30% of the glomeruli or interstitial foam cells.[709,710] In older children

(5–10 years of age), mesangial and capillary wall lesions may be visible. These consist of segmental to diffuse mesangial cell proliferation, matrix increase, and thickening of the glomerular capillary wall.[711] Special stains such as Jones methenamine silver or PAS may reveal thickening and lamellation of the GBM. Segmentally or globally sclerosed glomeruli may be present. Tubulointerstitial changes may include interstitial fibrosis, tubular atrophy, focal tubular basement membrane thickening, and interstitial foam cells. The glomerular and tubular lesions progress over time. A pattern of focal segmental and global glomerulosclerosis with hyalinosis is common in advanced cases, especially those with nephrotic-range proteinuria. Tubulointerstitial lesions progress from focal to diffuse involvement.[709,712]

By IF, many specimen results are negative,[709,713] but some may have nonspecific granular deposits of C3 and IgM within the mesangium and vascular pole and along the glomerular capillary wall in a segmental or global distribution.[689,697] The finding in rare cases of nonspecifically trapped immune deposits within the lamellated GBMs may lead to an erroneous diagnosis of immune complex GN.[714] With segmental sclerosis, subendothelial deposits of IgM, C3, properdin, and C4 are found.[689,709] The GBM of males with Alport's syndrome frequently lacks reactivity with sera from patients with anti-GBM antibody disease or with monoclonal antibodies directed against the Goodpasture epitope.[715,716] This abnormality can help in diagnosing equivocal cases in which the EM findings are not specific.[707]

In the mature kidney, collagen IV is composed of heterotrimers made up of six possible α chains. Chains composed of $\alpha1$, $\alpha1$, and $\alpha2$ are distributed in all renal basement membranes. Collagen IV chains composed of $\alpha3$, $\alpha4$, and $\alpha5$ are present in mature GBM and some distal TBM. Chains of $\alpha5$, $\alpha5$, and $\alpha6$ are distributed in Bowman's capsule and collecting duct TBM, as well as in epidermal basement membrane. Commercially available antisera to the subunits of collagen IV reveal preservation of the α_1 and α_2 subunits but loss of immunoreactivity for the α_3, α_4 and α_5-subunits from the GBM of affected males with X-linked disease. In addition, there is loss of α_5 staining from Bowman's capsule, distal tubular basement membranes, and skin in affected males with X-linked disease. Females are chimeras with segmental loss of α_5 in glomerular and epidermal basement membranes because of random inactivation of the mutated X chromosome in podocytes and basal keratinocytes. Patients with autosomal recessive forms of Alport disease typically lack the α_3-, α_4, and α_5 subunits in GBM but retain α_5 immunoreactivity in Bowman's capsule, collecting ducts, and skin (where $\alpha5$ forms a heterotrimer with $\alpha6$). Thus, absence of α_5 staining in skin biopsies is highly specific for the diagnosis of X-linked Alport's syndrome.[717]

On EM, the earliest change in young males is thinning of the GBM (which is not specific for hereditary nephritis and can occur in thin basement membrane disease).[718] The cardinal ultrastructural abnormality is the variable thickening, thinning, basket weaving, and lamellation of the GBM (Figure 32-42). These abnormalities may also be seen in some patients without a family history of nephritis.[719] These patients may be offspring of asymptomatic carriers or may represent new mutations. The endothelial cells are intact, and foot process effacement may be seen overlying the altered capillary walls. The mesangium may be normal in early cases, but with time, matrix and cells increase, and mesangial interposition into

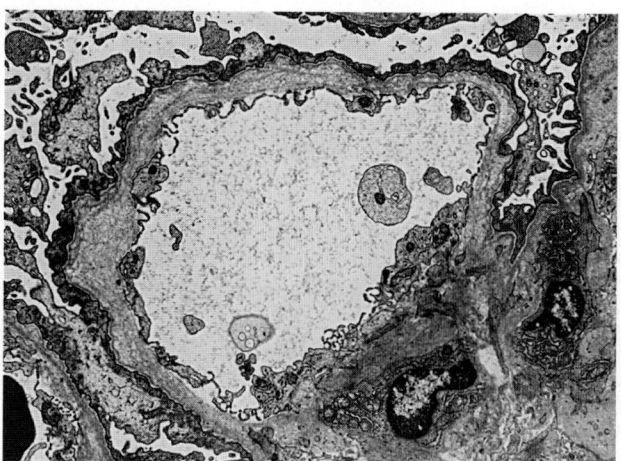

FIGURE 32-42 Alport's syndrome. Electron micrograph showing a thickened, lamellated glomerular basement membrane with the characteristic "split and splintered" appearance (×4000).

the capillary wall may be observed.[689,713] In males, the number of glomeruli showing lamellation increases from about 30% by age 10 years to more than 90% by age 30 years. In females with mild disease, less than 30% of the glomeruli may be affected.[720] Some affected females have a predominantly thin basement membrane phenotype with only rare segmental areas of lamellation.

The specificity of the GBM findings has been questioned.[721] Foci of lamina densa lamellation and splitting have been seen in 6% to 15% of unselected renal biopsies. These changes also may be seen focally in other glomerulopathies. Thus, clinical correlation and IF examination are essential when the ultrastructural features suggest Alport's syndrome. Although diffuse thickening and splitting of the GBM strongly suggests Alport's syndrome, not all Alport kindreds show these characteristic features. Thick, thin, normal, and nonspecific changes have also been described.

Pathogenesis and Genetics of Hereditary Nephritis

There are three genetic forms of hereditary nephritis (see Table 32-1). In the majority of cases, the disease is transmitted via an X-linked inheritance (i.e., father to son transmission does not occur), and women tend to be carriers because of lyonization. Autosomal dominant and recessive inheritance have also been described, as has sporadic occurrence.[686,688,722] The frequency of the Alport gene has been estimated to be 1 in 5000 in Utah[723] and 1 in 10,000 in the United States.[724]

Hereditary nephritis is caused by defects in type IV collagen. Six genes for type IV collagen have been characterized. Mutations in the *COL4A5* gene (encoding the α-$_5$ subunit of collagen type IV) on the X chromosome are responsible for the more frequent X-linked form of hereditary nephritis.[725] The identified mutations include deletions, insertions, substitutions, and duplications.[725-729] However, other abnormalities are not encoded by the *COL4A5* gene. Other type IV collagen peptides are abnormally distributed. The α_1 and α_2 peptides that are normally confined to the mesangial and subendothelial regions of the mature glomerulus become distributed throughout the full thickness of the GBM in hereditary nephritis. With progressive glomerular obsolescence, these peptide chains disappear, with an increase in collagen V and VI.[730] Moreover, the basement membranes of these patients do not react with anti-GBM antibodies. This implies that the NC1 domain of the α_3 subunit of type IV collagen is not incorporated normally into the GBM, probably because the α_5 subunit is required for normal assembly of the minor α chains of collagen IV into heterotrimers.[731] Cationic antigenic components are also absent.[732] The reason why these GBM abnormalities occur in not known but may be because of alteration in the incorporation of other collagens into the GBM.[733] Genetic screening is difficult because of the large number of mutations and the lack of hot spots on the genomic sequence involved.[734] Autosomal recessive and autosomal dominant hereditary nephritis have been shown to involve the α_3 or α_4 chains. The genes for these proteins are encoded on chromosome 2. An abnormality of any of these chains could impair the integrity of the basement membranes in the glomerulus and cochlea, leading to similar clinical findings.

Recently, the minor causes of familial hematuria, the Fechtner and Epstein syndromes, along with two other genetic conditions featuring macrothrombocytes (Sebastian's syndrome and May-Hegglin's anomaly), were shown to result from heterozygous mutations in the gene *MYH9*, which encodes nonmuscle myosin heavy chain IIA (NMMHC-IIA).[735]

Course and Treatment

Recurrent hematuria and proteinuria may be present for many years followed by the insidious onset of renal failure. Virtually all affected males reach ESRD, but there is considerable interkindred variability in the rate of progression. The rate of progression within male members of an affected family is usually but not always relatively constant.[689,736,737] The presence of gross hematuria in childhood, nephrotic syndrome, sensorineural deafness, anterior lenticonus, and diffuse GBM thickening are indicative of an unfavorable outcome in females.[694] ECASCA has been established to define the AS phenotype and to determine genotype–phenotype correlations. A report on 401 male patients belonging to the 195 families with *COL4A5* mutation showed a 90% probability rate of progression to end-stage renal failure by age 30 years in patients with large deletions, nonsense mutations, or frameshift mutations. The same risk was 50% and 70%, respectively, in patients with missense or splice site mutations. The risk of developing hearing loss before 30 years of age was approximately 60% in patients with missense mutations compared with 90% for the other types of mutations.[690] Female carriers with the *COL4A5* mutation generally have less severe disease. In the ECASCA cohort described above, the probability of developing ESRD before the age of 40 years was 12% in females versus 90% in males. The risk of progression to ESRD appears to increase after the age of 60 years in women. Risk factors for renal failure in women included the development and progressive increase in proteinuria and the occurrence of a hearing defect.[695]

There is no proven therapy for Alport's syndrome. Proteinuria-reduction strategies, such as aggressive control of hypertension and use of ACE inhibitors, might slow the rate of progression in patients with hereditary nephritis.[738] The addition of an aldosterone antagonist may further reduce proteinuria.[739] A small number of patients showed apparent stabilization when treated long term with cyclosporine,[740] but calcineurin inhibitor toxicity can occur with long-term use.[741]

Renal replacement therapy (either dialysis or transplantation) may be performed in patients with hereditary nephritis. Allograft and patient survival were comparable to survival rates in the United Network for Organ Sharing (UNOS) database.[742] In approximately 2% to 4% of male patients receiving a renal transplant, anti-GBM antibody disease may develop.[743] These antibodies are directed against the α-5 noncollagenous (NC1) subunit of the intact α345 hexamer of collagen IV.[744] This antigen, which presumably does not exist in the kidneys in patients with hereditary nephritis, is present in normal kidneys and is thus recognized as foreign.[745,746] A profile of these patients has been compiled.[707] The patients are usually male, always deaf, and likely to have reached ESRD before the age of 30 years. There is a suggestion that certain mutations in the *COL4A5* gene, such as deletions (which account for 11%–12% of Alport's cases), may predispose patients to the development of allograft anti-GBM nephritis.[746] In 75% of cases, the onset of anti-GBM nephritis occurs within the first year after transplantation, and 76% of the allografts were lost.

Thin Basement Membrane Nephropathy

Thin basement membrane nephropathy (TBMN) (also known as benign familial hematuria and thin GBM nephropathy) describes a condition that differs from Alport disease in its generally benign course and lack of progression. The typical finding on renal pathology is diffuse thinning of the GBM. However, thin GBM may be found in other conditions as well (including early Alport's disease and IgA nephropathy).[747] The true incidence of TBMN disease is unknown but may approach 5% of the population; reports evaluating patients with isolated hematuria suggest that 20% to 25% of such patients have thin GBM disease.[748-750]

Clinical Features

Patients usually present in childhood with microhematuria. Hematuria is usually persistent but may be intermittent in some patients. Episodic gross hematuria may occur, particularly with upper respiratory infections.[751,752] Patients do not typically have overt proteinuria, but when present, this may suggest progression of disease.[748,753]

Pathology

Renal biopsies typically show no histologic abnormalities with the exception of focal erythrocyte casts. By IF, no glomerular deposits of immunoglobulins or complement are found. By EM, there is diffuse and relatively uniform thinning of the GBM (Figure 32-43). The normal thickness of the GBM is age and gender dependent. Vogler and colleagues[754] have defined normal ranges for children at birth as 169 + 30 nm; at 2 years of age as 245 + 49 nm; and at 11 years as 285 + 39 nm. Steffes and colleagues[755] have defined normal ranges for adults 373 + 42 (men) and 326 + 45 nm (women). Each laboratory should attempt to establish its own normal ranges for GBM thickness. A cutoff value of 250 nm has been reported by some authors,[756-758] but other groups have used a cutoff of 330 nm.[753] There is often accentuation of the lamina rara interna and externa. Focal GBM gaps may be identified ultrastructurally. Immunostaining for the α subunits of collagen IV reveals a normal distribution in the GBM.

Pathogenesis

About 40% of TBMN disease has been linked to mutations of the *COL4A3* and *COL4A4* genes.[759] In most kindreds with TBMN, the disorder appears to be transmitted in an autosomal dominant pattern. The existence of a few families with several affected children and apparently unaffected parents suggests a recessive mode of inheritance or that one parent was an asymptomatic carrier.[750,751,760] There appears to be a reduction or loss of the subepithelial portion of the basement membrane, which apparently contains normal amounts of type IV collagen.[761] The degree of GBM thinning does not appear to affect the clinical presentation or outcome.[762]

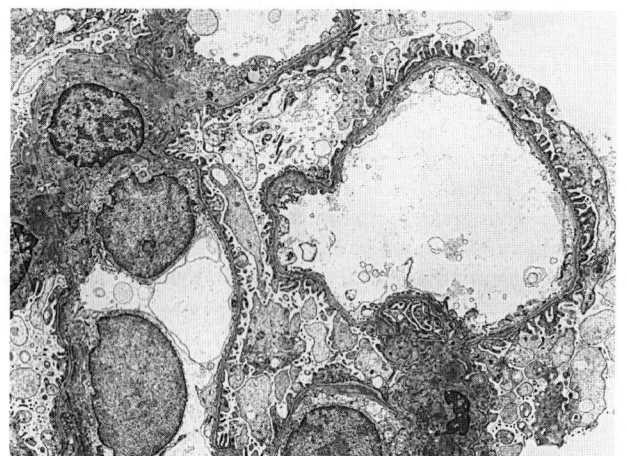

FIGURE 32-43 Thin basement membrane disease. By electron microscopy, the glomerular basement membranes are diffusely and uniformly thinned, measuring less than 200 nm in thickness (×2500).

Differential Diagnosis of Familial Hematurias

Type IV collagen defects can cause both TBMN and Alport's syndrome. Patients with TBMN can be considered carriers of autosomal recessive Alport's syndrome.[763,764] With advances in molecular biology and immunopathology, hereditary forms of hematuria have been better characterized. Table 32-2 shows a summary of the clinical, pathologic, and genetics of the various forms of hereditary nephritis.[765] Because GBM thinning may be seen in early cases of Alport's syndrome, immunohistochemical analysis of α_3, α_4, and α_5-subunits should be undertaken (because genetic tests are not always practical). Table 32-3 shows the typical immunostaining patterns in the kidney and skin basement membranes.

NAIL–PATELLA SYNDROME (HEREDITARY OSTEO-ONYCHODYSPLASIA)

Nail-patella syndrome (NPS) is an autosomal dominant condition affecting tissues of both ectodermal and mesodermal origin, manifested as symmetric nail, skeletal, ocular, and renal anomalies.

Clinical Features. The classical tetrad of anomalies of the nails, elbows and knees, and iliac horns was described by Mino and colleagues in 1948.[766] Nail dysplasia and patellar aplasia or hypoplasia are essential features for the diagnosis of NPS. The presence of triangular nail lunulae is a pathognomonic sign for NPS. Other skeletal abnormalities include dysplasia of the elbow joints, posterior iliac horns, and foot deformities. Various ocular anomalies have sporadically been found in NPS patients, including microcornea, sclerocornea, congenital cataract, iris processes, pigmentation of the inner margin of the iris, and congenital glaucoma.[767]

Renal involvement is variable, being present in up to 38% of patients. Renal manifestations first appear in children and young adults and may include proteinuria, hematuria, hypertension, or edema. The nephrotic syndrome and progressive renal failure may occasionally occur. The course is generally benign with renal failure being a late feature.[768,769] Congenital malformations of the urinary tract and nephrolithiasis are also more frequent in these patients.

	LOCUS	PROGRESSIVE NEPHROPATHY	DEAFNESS	OCULAR CHANGES	GBM CHANGES	HEMATOLOGIC CHANGES
TABLE 32-2 Classification of the Familial Hematurias						
Type IV Collagen Disorders						
Alport syndrome						
X-linked	COL4A5	+	+	+	Thickening	–
X-linked + diffuse leiomyomatosis	COL4A5 + COL4A6	+	+	+	Thickening	–
Autosomal recessive	COL4A3 or COL4A4	+	+	+	Thickening	–
Autosomal dominant	COL4A3 or COL4A4	+	+	–	Thickening	–
Thin basement membrane nephropathy*	COL4A3 or COL4A4	–	–	–	Thinning	
Noncollagen Disorders						
Fechtner syndrome	MYH9	+	+	+	Thickening	Thrombocytopenia May-Hegglin
Epstein syndrome	MYH9	+	+	+	Thickening	Thrombocytopenia

*Some families with thing basement membrane disease have mutations at loci other than the type IV collagen genes.
From Kasthan CE: Familial hematurias: what we know and what we don't. *Pediatr Nephrol* 20(8):1027-1035, 2005.

Pathology. The findings on LM are nonspecific and include focal and segmental glomerular sclerosis, segmental thickening of the glomerular capillary wall, and mild mesangial hypercellularity.[770] IF microscopy is nonspecific, and IgM and C3 have been observed in sclerosed segments. Ultrastructural studies show a thickened basement membrane that contains irregular lucencies, imparting a "moth-eaten" appearance (Figure 32-44*A*). The presence of intramembranous fibrils with the periodicity of collagen is revealed by phosphotungstic acid stains in EM sections, corresponding to the distribution of the intramembranous lucencies (Figure 32-44*B*). These must be distinguished from the occasional collagen fibrils that can accumulate nonspecifically in the sclerotic mesangium in a variety of sclerosing glomerular conditions.[770]

Pathogenesis. The genetic locus for this syndrome appears to be on chromosome 9 and results from mutations in the LIM—homeodomain protein *Lmx1b* gene and is transmitted in an autosomal dominant pattern. Lmx1b plays a central role in dorsoventral patterning of the vertebrate limb.[771,772]

Treatment. There is no treatment for this condition; occasional patients with renal failure have successfully undergone transplantation.[773]

Fabry's Disease (Angiokeratoma Corporis Diffusum Universale)

Fabry's disease[774] is an X-linked inborn error of glycosphingolipid metabolism involving a lysosomal enzyme, α-galactosidase A (also known as ceramide trihexosidase). The enzyme deficiency leads to the accumulation of globotriaosylceramide (ceramide trihexoside) and related neutral glycosphingolipids leading to multisystem involvement and dysfunction. Clinical guidelines for the diagnosis and treatment of Fabry's disease have been published.[775]

Clinical Features

Fabry's disease has been reported in all ethnic groups, and the estimated incidence in males is 1 in 40,000 to 1 in 60,000. In male hemizygotes, the initial clinical presentation usually begins in childhood with episodic pain in the extremities and acroparesthesias. Renal involvement is common in male hemizygotes and is occasional in female heterozygotes. The disease presents with hematuria and proteinuria, which often progresses to nephrotic levels. In men, progressive renal failure generally develops by the fifth decade of life. Data from the Fabry Registry suggest that proteinuria is a strong determinant of renal outcome.[776] In the United States, Fabry's disease accounted for 0.02% of patients who began renal replacement therapy between 1995 and 1998.[777]

The skin is commonly involved with reddish-purple macules (angiokeratomas), typically found "below the belt" on the abdomen, buttocks, hips, genitalia, and upper thighs. Other findings include palmar erythema, conjunctival and oral mucous membrane telangiectasia, and subungual splinter hemorrhages. The nervous system is involved with peripheral and autonomic neuropathy. Premature arterial disease of coronary vessels leads to myocardial ischemia and arrhythmias at a young age. Similarly, cerebrovascular involvement leads to an early onset of strokes. In the heart, valvular disease and hypertrophic cardiomyopathy have also been reported. Corneal opacities are seen in virtually all hemizygotes and most heterozygotes. Posterior capsular cataracts, edema of retina and eyelids, and tortuous retinal and conjunctival vessels may also been seen in the eye. Generalized lymphadenopathy, hepatosplenomegaly, aseptic necrosis of the femoral and humeral

TABLE 32-3 Immunostaining Patterns for α$_5$ in Kidney and Epidermal Basement Membranes			
	GLOMERULAR BASEMENT MEMBRANE	**BOWMAN'S CAPSULE**	**EPIDERMAL BASEMENT MEMBRANE**
Normal	Present/normal	Present/normal	Present/normal
X-linked Alport males	Absent	Absent	Absent
X-linked Alport female carriers	Present segmentally/mosaic	Present segmentally/mosaic	Present focally/mosaic
Autosomal recessive Alport's	Absent	Present/normal	Present/normal
Thin basement membrane disease	Present/normal	Present/normal	Present/normal

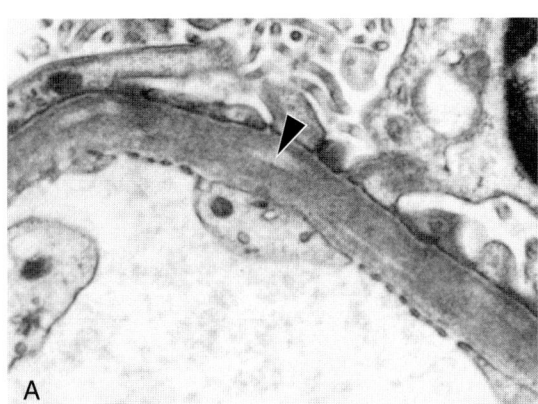
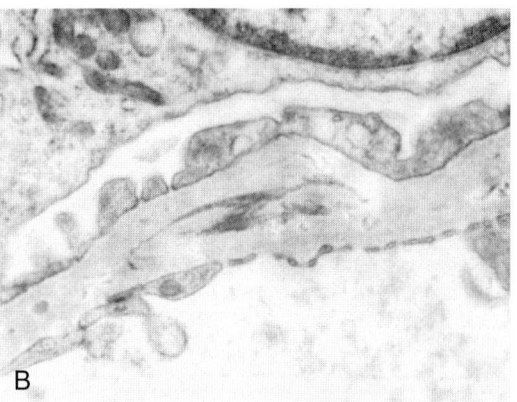

FIGURE 32-44 Nail–patella syndrome. **A.** Routine electron micrograph showing thickening of a glomerular basement membrane with focal irregular internal lucencies (×15,000). **B.** Phosphotungstic acid–stained electron micrograph demonstrating the characteristic banded collagen fibrils within the rarefied segments of glomerular basement membrane (×15,000).

heads, myopathy, hypoalbuminemia, and hypogammaglobulinemia have been reported.

In carrier females, clinical manifestations may range from asymptomatic to severe disease similar to male hemizygotes. Up to one-third of female carriers have been reported to have significant disease manifestations.[778]

Pathology

Glycosphingolipid accumulation begins early in life,[779] and the major renal site of accumulation is the podocyte (visceral epithelial cells). By LM, these cells are enlarged with numerous clear, uniform vacuoles in the cytoplasm, causing a foamy appearance (Figure 32-45). These vacuoles can be shown to contain lipids when fat stains (e.g., Oil Red O) are used or when viewed under the polarizing microscope, where they exhibit a double refractile appearance before being processed with lipid solvents. All renal cells may accumulate the lipid. These include (in addition to podocytes) parietal epithelial cells, glomerular endothelial cells, mesangial cells, interstitial capillary endothelial cells, distal convoluted tubule cells, and to a lesser extent, cells of the loops of Henle, and proximal tubular cells. Indeed, vascular endothelial cells are involved in virtually every organ and tissue.[780] In the kidney, the myocytes and endothelial cells of arteries are commonly involved. In heterozygotes, similar changes are present but with less severity.[781] Characteristic findings are noted on EM (Figure 32-46). The major finding is large numbers of "myelin figures" or "zebra bodies" within the cytoplasm of the podocytes, and to a variable extent, in other renal cell types. These intracytoplasmic vacuoles consist of single membrane-bound dense bodies with a concentric whorled or multilamellar appearance. Glomerular podocytes exhibit variable foot process effacement. The GBMs are initially normal, but with progression of disease, there may be thickening and collapse of the GBM and focal and segmental glomerular sclerosis with accompanying tubular atrophy and interstitial fibrosis.[782] Findings on IF microscopy are usually negative except in areas of segmental sclerosis, in which IgM and complement may be demonstrated. Orange autofluorescence corresponding to the lipid inclusions may be found in podocytes and other renal cells.

Pathogenesis

The mutations in the GLA gene generally are "private" with specific molecular defects that vary from family to family and include rearrangements, deletions, and point mutations.[783] Deficiency of the enzyme leads to accumulation of globotriaosylceramide, especially in the vascular endothelium, with subsequent ischemic organ dysfunction. Patients with blood groups B and AB have earlier and more severe symptoms, likely related to accumulation of the terminal α-galactose substance occurring during the synthesis of the B antigen on RBC membranes.[784] Globotriaosylceramide accumulation in podocytes may lead to proteinuria and renal dysfunction, but functional abnormalities are not always noted, especially in female heterozygotes. A gene-knockout mouse model of Fabry's disease has been produced, which shows the characteristic changes.[785,786]

Diagnosis

The diagnosis in affected males can be established by measuring levels of α-galactosidase-A in plasma or peripheral blood leukocytes. Hemizygotes have almost no measurable enzyme activity. Female carriers may have enzyme levels in the low to normal range; to diagnose female carriers, the specific mutation in the family must be demonstrated.[775] The measurement of urinary ceramide digalactoside and trihexoside levels may also be of use to identify the carrier state. Prenatal diagnosis can be made by measuring amniocyte enzyme levels in amniotic fluid. Screening dialysis and renal transplant patients with undiagnosed renal failure, patients with hypertrophic cardiomyopathy, and patients with strokes have yielded the diagnosis of Fabry's disease in 1% to 5%.[786]

Treatment

Recombinant enzyme replacement therapy is available as agalsidase-α (from human cell line) and agalsidase-β (from Chinese hamster ovary cells) and are administered IV

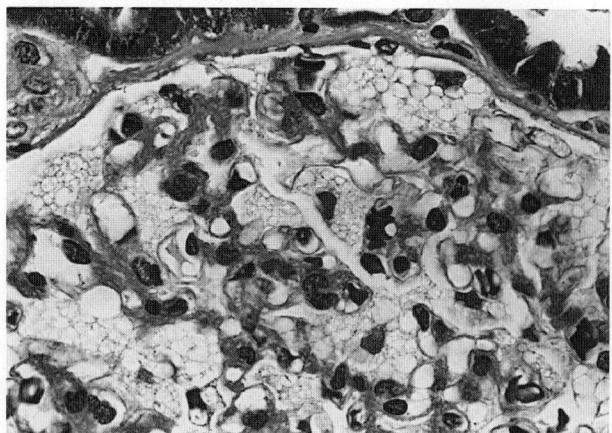

FIGURE 32-45 Fabry's disease. By light microscopy, the visceral epithelial cells (podocytes) are markedly enlarged with foamy-appearing cytoplasm (trichrome, ×800).

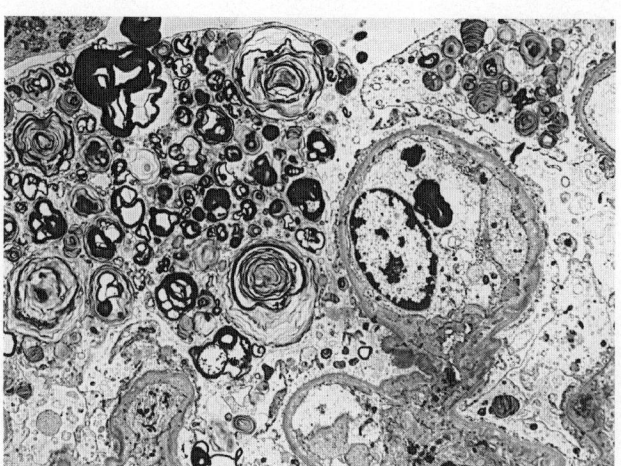

FIGURE 32-46 Fabry's disease. Electron micrograph showing abundant whorled myelin figures within the cytoplasm of the podocytes. A few similar inclusions are also identified within the glomerular endothelial cells (×2000).

indefinitely every 2 weeks. Two pivotal randomized, controlled trials have shown that recombinant human α-galactosidase-A enzyme replacement therapy (ERT) is safe and can improve clinical parameters. In one short-term study, α-galactosidase-A treatment was associated with improved neuropathic pain, decreased mesangial widening, and improved creatinine clearance.[787] In the second study, repeat renal biopsies showed decreased microvascular endothelial deposits of globotriaosylceramide.[780,788] The use of ERT appears to be firmly established, and long-term open-label study data and registry data have shown improvements in clinical parameters tested.[789] However, a systematic review that included 5 small trials and 187 patients did not provide robust evidence for the use of ERT.[790] From a renal standpoint, open-label extension studies showed that renal function remained stable in the long term in most patients with normal renal function at baseline.[791,792] However, patients with impaired baseline renal function may show continued decline despite ERT.[792] The experience with ERT in female carriers is limited. Clinical recommendations for the treatment of Fabry's disease have been published.[775,789]

The ERA-EDTA Registry in Europe has reported outcomes on patients with Fabry's disease. Since 1985, 4 to 13 new patients per year have commenced renal replacement therapy in Europe. Patient survival on dialysis was 41% at 5 years; cardiovascular complications (48%) and cachexia (17%) were the main causes of death. Graft survival at 3 years in 33 patients was not inferior to that of other nephropathies (72% vs. 69%), and patient survival after transplantation was comparable to that of patients younger than 55 years of age.[793] In the U.S. population, survival of patients with Fabry's disease was lower than for nondiabetic renal failure patients.[777] Long-term allograft function in patients with Fabry's disease has been reported. Glycosphingolipid deposits do recur in allografts but have not been reported to cause graft failure.[794]

Sickle Cell Nephropathy

Renal disease associated with sickle cell disease includes gross hematuria, papillary necrosis, nephrotic syndrome, renal infarction, an inability to concentrate urine, renal medullary carcinoma, and pyelonephritis.[795,796] Microscopic or gross hematuria is likely the result of microinfarcts in the renal medulla.[797] Glomerular lesions however, are less commonly encountered and may be seen in patients with sickle cell hemoglobin (HbSS), sickle–hemoglobin C disease (HbSC), and sickle cell thalassemia.[798]

Clinical Features

In one study, the prevalence of proteinuria (>1+ on a dipstick) in HbSS disease was 26%.[798] The majority of proteinuric patients had less than 3 g/day, and elevated serum creatinine levels were present in 7% of patients. In another study, 4.2% with HbSS disease and 2.4% with sickle cell disease developed renal failure. The median age of disease onset for these patients was 23.1 and 49.9 years, respectively. Survival time for patients with HbSS anemia after the diagnosis of renal failure, despite dialysis, was 4 years, and the median age at the time of death was 27 years. The risk for renal failure was increased in patients with the Central African Republic β S-gene cluster haplotype, hypertension, proteinuria, and severe anemia.[799] The course of HbSS renal disease is progressive; in one series, 18% of patients with HbSS disease progressed to ESRD.[800]

Pathology

Early glomerular lesions may be seen in patients with HbSS, including enlarged glomeruli and dilated and congested capillaries (some of these patients may have nephrotic proteinuria).[801] Heterogeneous patterns of glomerular injury have been reported. A membranoproliferative pattern exhibits mesangial proliferation with mild to moderate capillary wall thickening caused by GBM reduplication and mesangial interposition (Figure 32-47). Some of these patients also exhibit features of chronic thrombotic microangiopathy with narrow double contours of the GBM and mesangiolysis. A pattern of membranous GN has also been described. On IF microscopy, a few patients may show irregular granular deposits of IgG and C3 have been reported in association with membranous or mesangiocapillary findings on LM.[801,802] Ultrastructural studies show granular dense deposits in the mesangial and subepithelial area. Some cases have no detectable deposits but exhibit subendothelial accumulation of electron-lucent "fluff" resembling the changes in chronic thrombotic microangiopathies. Mild mesangial proliferation and peripheral mesangial interposition are frequently seen. Sickled erythrocytes containing paracrystalline inclusions may be identified within glomerular capillaries.[802-806]

In the second form of sickle glomerulopathy, focal and segmental glomerulosclerosis is seen associated with glomerulomegaly (Figure 32-48). Two patterns of FSGS may be observed: a "collapsing" pattern and an "expansive" pattern.[795,798,807-809] Using the modern classification of FSGS, collapsing, perihilar, tip, and not otherwise specified variants have been reported.[801] On IF, nonspecific IgM and C3 are seen in sclerosed segments. In all of these forms, there may be prominent intracapillary erythrocyte sickling and congestion.

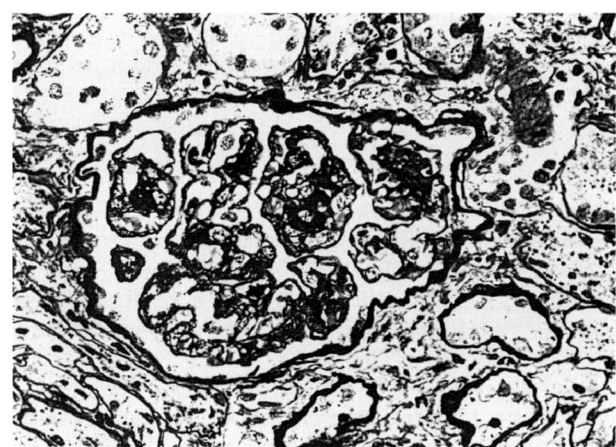

FIGURE 32-47 Sickle cell disease. An example of sickle cell glomerulopathy with membranoproliferative features. There are double contours of the glomerular basement membrane associated with segmental mesangiolysis (Jones methenamine silver, ×500).

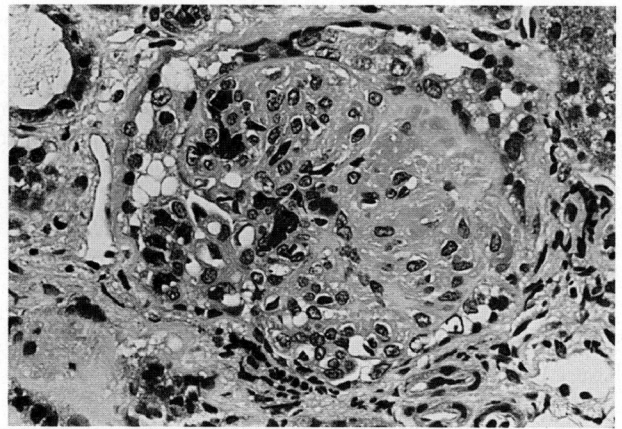

FIGURE 32-48 Sickle cell disease. An example with focal segmental glomerulosclerosis. The nonsclerotic glomerular capillaries are congested with sickled erythrocytes (hematoxylin and eosin, ×500).

Pathogenesis

The mechanism(s) for glomerular abnormalities in HbSS patients is not fully understood. One theory proposes that mesangial cells are activated by the presence of fragmented RBCs in glomerular capillaries. This activation of mesangial cells promotes synthesis of matrix proteins and GBM reduplication.[810] In another study, renal tubular epithelial antigens and complement components were detected in a granular pattern along the GBM, leading the authors to hypothesize that GN was mediated by glomerular deposition of immune complexes containing renal tubular epithelial antigen and antibody to renal tubular epithelial antigen (the antigen possibly released after tubular damage secondary to decreased oxygenation and hemodynamic alterations related to SS disease).[802]

In patients with the FSGS pattern, it is proposed that the there is an initial but progressive obliteration of the glomerular capillary bed by RBC sickling that cannot be compensated by further glomerular hypertrophy. Hemodynamic glomerular injury then ensues from the sustained or increasing hyperfiltration in a diminishing capillary bed, manifesting morphologically as the expansive pattern of sclerosis.[798,807] According to one report, the hyperfiltration observed in 51% of SS patients correlated positively with lower hemoglobin levels and reticulocyte counts, implying that the hemolysis-related vasculopathy may be contributing.[811] The role of reactive oxygen species in producing chronic vascular endothelial injury has also been suggested.[812]

Treatment

The treatment of patients with renal disease has generally not been satisfactory. Treatment of patients with sickle cell nephropathy with ACE inhibitors reduces the degree of proteinuria.[798,813] However, their effectiveness in preserving renal function remains to be established.

SS nephropathy accounts for 0.1% of ESRD patients in the United States.[814] Renal transplantation has been performed in SS patients. One-year graft survival in SS patients was similar to that for other transplanted patients; however, long-term renal outcome was worse, as were short- and long-term mortality.[815] Transplanted SS patients commonly experience sickle cell crises.[816,817] Recurrent sickle cell nephropathy has been reported in the transplanted kidney.[808,818]

Lipodystrophy

Lipodystrophies are rare diseases associated with insulin resistance in which there is loss of fat, which may be localized to the upper part of the body in partial lipodystrophy (PLD) or more diffuse in generalized lipodystrophy (GLD).[819,820] Despite diabetes being common, diabetic nephropathy is surprisingly rare in these patients; other glomerular disease predominate, and a renal biopsy is thus recommended in these patients.[821] PLD is commonly associated with type II mesangiocapillary (membranoproliferative GN).

PLD most often presents in girls between ages 5 and 15 years. In addition to the loss of fat, the lipodystrophies are associated with a wide variety of metabolic and systemic abnormalities. Hyperinsulinism, insulin resistance, and diabetes are common. Other metabolic abnormalities include hyperlipidemia, hyperproteinemia, and euthyroid hypermetabolism. Clinical findings may include tall stature, muscular hypertrophy, hirsutism, macroglossia, abdominal distension, subcutaneous nodules, acanthosis nigricans, hepatomegaly, cirrhosis, clitoral or penile enlargement, febrile adenopathy, cerebral atrophy, cerebral ventricular dilatation, hemiplegia, mental retardation and cardiomegaly.[819,820] Renal disease occurs in 20% to 50% of patients with PLD,[819,820] and PLD occurs in 10% of patients with MPGN type II.[822,823] Patients are noted to have asymptomatic proteinuria and microhematuria, but the nephrotic syndrome is occasionally present.[824,825] Diminished C3 levels in association with the C3 nephritic (C3NeF) is the most prominent serologic abnormality. The course of glomerular disease is fairly rapid progression to ESRD, and the prognosis of PLD is determined mainly by renal disease.[820]

In GLD, the nephrotic syndrome, non-nephrotic proteinuria, and hypertension have been reported.[819] A total of 88% of these patients had albumin excretion greater than 30 mg/24 hours, 60% had macroalbuminuria (>300 mg/24 hr), and 20% had nephrotic-range proteinuria greater than 3500 mg/24 hours.[826]

Pathology

PLD is frequently associated with mesangiocapillary (membranoproliferative) GN type II or dense deposit disease.[824,825,827,828] Patients with type III MPGN[829] and minimal change disease[830] have also been reported. Conversely, in GLD, focal and segmental glomerulosclerosis, membranoproliferative GN, and diabetic glomerulosclerosis have been reported.[826]

Pathogenesis and Treatment

The pathogenesis of PLD and GLD is poorly understood. It is unlikely that one unifying link will be found given the differences in epidemiology, genetics, and clinical features. Acquired forms of lipodystrophy are believed to be autoimmune disorders. Most patients with PLD possess an IgG autoantibody,

C3 nephritic factor (C3NeF), which binds to and stabilizes the alternate pathway convertase C3 convertase-C3bBb. In the presence of C3NeF, C3bBb becomes resistant to its regulatory proteins, H and I. Although the majority of patients with partial dystrophy have low serum C3, not all patients will exhibit nephritis.[828] Recombinant leptin appears to decrease the proteinuria in some patients with GLD.[826] There is no effective therapy for PLD, and although renal transplantation is the treatment of choice when ESRD ensues, recurrence in transplants has been reported.[820,827,831] In GLD, leptin therapy has been associated with improvement of renal parameters.[832] A single GLD patient has undergone renal transplantation.[833]

Lecithin–Cholesterol Acyltransferase Deficiency

Gjone and Norum reported a familial disorder characterized by proteinuria, anemia, hyperlipidemia, and corneal opacity.[834,835] Most of the initial patients were of Scandinavian origin; subsequent the disease has also been reported from other countries.[836,837]

Clinical Features

The triad of anemia, nephrotic syndrome, and corneal opacities suggests this disorder. Renal disease is a universal finding with albuminuria noted early in life. Proteinuria increases in severity during the fourth and fifth decades of life, often with development of the nephrotic syndrome. The latter is accompanied by hypertension and progressive renal failure. Most patients are mildly anemic with target cells and poikilocytes on the peripheral smear. There is evidence of low-grade hemolysis. During childhood, corneal opacities appear as grayish spots over the cornea accompanied by a lipoid arcus. Visual acuity is unimpaired. Fish eye disease results from a partial deficiency of lecithin–cholesterol acyltransferase (LCAT) and presents with corneal disease and without renal manifestations. Patients have reduced plasma HDL cholesterol concentrations (usually <0.3 mmol/L; 11.6 mg/dL) and plasma levels of apolipoprotein AI (apo-AI) below 50 mg/dL. Premature atherosclerosis is unusual in complete LCAT deficiency but may occur from unknown reasons in fish eye disease.[838]

Pathology

Abnormalities are found mainly in the glomeruli, but the arteries and arterioles may also be affected.[834,835,839,840] By LM (Figure 32-49), the glomerular capillary walls are thickened, and there is mesangial expansion. Basement membranes are irregular and often appear to contain vacuoles, resembling stage 3 membranous alterations. Double contouring of capillary walls is occasionally present. Similar vacuoles in the mesangium impart a honeycomb appearance. There is no associated glomerular hypercellularity. By IF microscopy, there is typically negative staining for all immunoglobulin and complement components. On EM (Figure 32-50), the vacuolated areas seen by LM correspond to extracellular irregular lucent zones (lacunae) in the mesangial matrix and

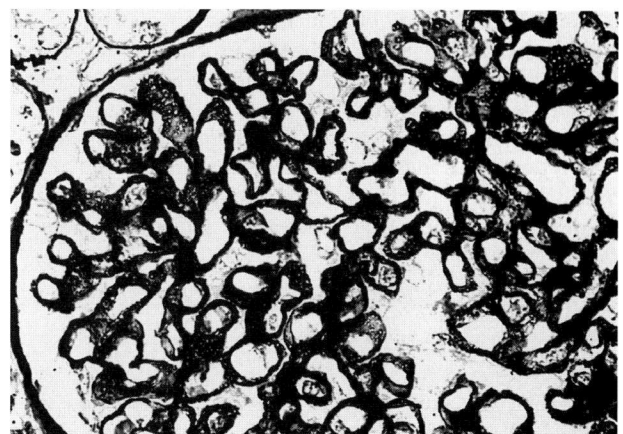

FIGURE 32-49 Lecithin–cholesterol acyltransferase deficiency. The glomerular basement membranes and mesangium have a vacuolated appearance, resembling stage 3 membranous glomerulopathy (Jones methenamine silver, ×800).

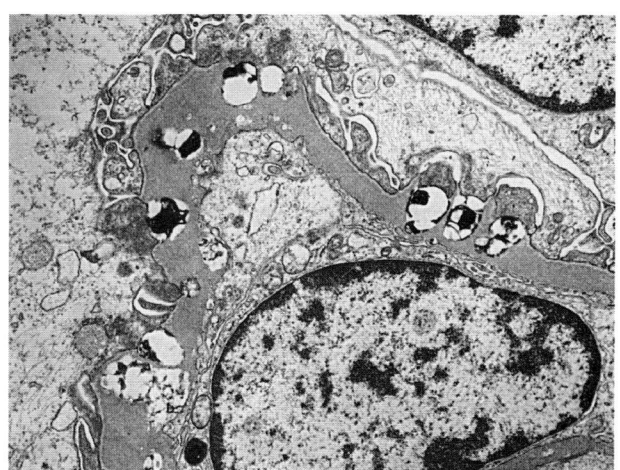

FIGURE 32-50 Lecithin–cholesterol acyltransferase deficiency. Electron micrograph showing intramembranous lacunae with rounded structures containing an electron-dense membranous core and electron-lucent periphery (×5000).

GBM containing lipid inclusions. These inclusions contain rounded, small, dense structures, either solid or with a lamellar substructure.

Pathogenesis

The disorder is inherited in an autosomal recessive pattern. Patients have little or no LCAT activity in their blood circulation because of mutations in the *LCAT* gene.[841,842] LCAT is an enzyme that circulates in the blood primarily bound to HDL and catalyzes the formation of cholesteryl esters via the hydrolysis and transfer of the sn-2 fatty acid from phosphatidylcholine to the 3-hydroxyl group of cholesterol. Thus, patients with LCAT deficiency have high levels of phosphatidylcholine and unesterified cholesterol with corresponding low levels of lysophosphatidylcholine and cholesteryl ester in the blood. An abnormal lipoprotein, lipoprotein-X (Lp-X) is present in patients' plasma. Lp-X is thought to arise from the surface of chylomicron remnants that are not further metabolized because of the absence of active LCAT.

Accumulation of lipid component occurs in both intra- and extracellular sites. Damage to the GBM occurs from these lipids, resulting in proteinuria. Endothelial damage and resulting vascular insufficiency may contribute to renal insufficiency. It has been proposed that Lp-X stimulates mesangial cells, leading to the production of monocyte chemoattractant protein-1, promoting monocyte infiltration, foam cell formation, and progressive glomerulosclerosis in a manner similar to atherosclerosis.[843]

Diagnosis

In patients suspected of having LCAT deficiency, measurements of plasma enzyme should be performed. The enzyme levels and activity vary among kindreds[844]; thus, enzyme measurements should include activity as well as mass.

Treatment

A low-lipid diet or lipid-lowering drugs have not shown to be of benefit.[839] Plasma infusions may provide reversal of erythrocytic abnormalities, but long-term benefits have yet to be demonstrated.[845] The lesions may recur in the allograft, but renal function is adequately preserved.[846]

Lipoprotein Glomerulopathy

Lipoprotein glomerulopathy (LPG) is a characterized by dysbetalipoproteinemia and lipid deposition in the kidney, leading to glomerulosclerosis and renal failure. The majority of patients have been from Japan.[847,848]

The histologic hallmark of LPG is the presence of laminated thrombi consisting of lipids within the lumina of dilated glomerular capillaries. The pathogenesis of LPG is unknown, but the presence of thrombi consisting of lipoproteins raised the possibility that LPG might be related to a primary abnormality in lipid metabolism.[849] Indeed, type III hyperlipidemia (elevated low-density lipoprotein and high apo-E levels) have been reported in Japanese patients associated with apo-E variants (commonly apo-E2 as opposed to apo-E3).[848,850-854] Furthermore, LPG-like deposits were detected in apo-E–deficient mice transfected with apo-E (Sendai), one of the apo-E variants associated with LPG.

There is no uniformly effective therapy for patients with LPG; however, intensive lipid-lowering therapy was reported to be effective in one patient with LPG.[855] Recurrence of lesions of LPG have occurred in renal allografts.[856,857]

Glomerular Involvement with Bacterial Infections

Infective Endocarditis

The natural history of endocarditis-associated GN has changed significantly in parallel with the changing epidemiology of infective endocarditis (IE) and the advent of antibiotics. In the pre-antibiotic era, *Streptococcus viridans* was the most common organism, and GN occurred in between 50% and 80% of cases.[858] During that era, GN was less common in association with acute endocarditis.[859,860] With the use of prophylactic antibiotics in patients with valvular heart disease and an increase in IV drug use, *Staphylococcus aureus* has replaced *S. viridans* as the primary pathogen. GN in these patients with acute IE occurs as commonly as in subacute endocarditis.[858,861-863] The incidence of GN with endocarditis with *S. aureus* ranges from 22% to 78%[861,864] and is higher in series consisting predominantly of IV drug users.[864,865]

Clinical Features

Renal complications of IE include infarcts, abscesses, and GN (all of which may coexist). In focal GN, mild asymptomatic urinary abnormalities, including hematuria, pyuria, and albuminuria, may be noted. Infrequently, with severe focal GN, renal insufficiency or uremia may be present. Renal dysfunction, micro or gross hematuria, and nephrotic-range proteinuria may be present with diffuse GN.[858,861,866] Rapidly progressive renal failure with crescents has been reported.[858,867] Rarely, patients may present with vasculitic features (including purpura).[868] Although hypocomplementemia is frequent, it is neither invariable (occurring in 60% to 90% of patients with GN) nor specific for renal involvement.[863,864] The majority of patients demonstrate activation of the classical pathway.[864,869] Alternate pathway activation has been described in some cases of *S. aureus* endocarditis.[864] The degree of complement activation correlates with the severity of renal impairment,[864] and the complement levels normalize with successful therapy of the infection. CICs have been found in the serum in up to 90% of patients.[869,870] Mixed cryoglobulins and rheumatoid factor may also be present in the serum of patients.[863,871] ANCA positivity has been occasionally reported in patients with biopsy-proven immune complex GN associated with IE.[872] Anti-GBM antibody in eluates from diseased glomeruli has been reported.[873]

Pathology

On LM, focal and segmental endocapillary proliferative GN with focal crescents is the most typical finding. Some patients may exhibit a more diffuse proliferative GN lesion with or without crescents.[858,859,861,874,875] IF reveals granular capillary and mesangial deposits of IgG, IgM, and C3.[858,861,874] EM shows electron-dense deposits in mesangial, subendothelial, and occasionally subepithelial locations, with varying degrees of mesangial and endocapillary proliferation.[858,861,874,876]

Pathogenesis

The diffuse deposition of immunoglobulin, the depression of complement, and electron-dense deposits supports an immune complex mechanism for the production of this form of GN. The demonstration of specific antibody in kidney eluates and the detection of bacterial antigen in the deposits further supported this view. Both *S. aureus*[877] and hemolytic *Streptococcus*[878] antigens have been identified.

Treatment

With the initiation of antibiotic therapy, the manifestations of GN begin to subside. Rarely, microhematuria and proteinuria may persist for years.[858] Plasmapheresis and corticosteroids have been reported to promote renal recovery in some patients with renal failure.[867,879] However, this approach should be taken cautiously because of the risk of promoting infectious aspects of the disease while ameliorating the immunologic manifestations.

Shunt Nephritis

Ventriculovascular (ventriculoatrial, ventriculojugular) shunts used for the treatment of hydrocephalus used to be colonized commonly with microorganisms, particularly *Staphylococcus albus* (75%).[880] Less often, other bacteria (e.g., *Propionibacterium acnes*) have been implicated.[881,882] Ventriculoperitoneal shunts are more resistant to infection. However, GN has been reported with these shunts as well.[883] Infected peritoneovenous (LeVeen) shunts also have been associated occasionally with GN.[884]

Patients commonly present with fever. Anemia, hepatosplenomegaly, purpura, arthralgias, and lymphadenopathy are found on examination. Renal manifestations include hematuria (microscopic or gross), proteinuria (nephrotic syndrome in 30% of patients), azotemia, and hypertension. Laboratory abnormalities include the presence of rheumatoid factor, cryoimmunoglobulins, elevated ESR and CRP levels, hypocomplementemia, and the presence of CICs.[885,886] Shunt nephritis usually presents within a few months of shunt placement, but delayed manifestations, as late as 17 years, have been reported.[887] By LM, glomeruli exhibit mesangial proliferation or membranoproliferative changes. IF reveals diffuse granular deposits of IgG, IgM, and C3. Electron-dense mesangial and subendothelial deposits are found by EM.[882,888] Antibiotic therapy and prompt removal of the infected catheter usually lead to remission of the GN.[889] However, cases progressing to chronic renal failure have been reported.[890] Rarely, patients have elevated PR3-specific ANCA titers, which also improved after removal of the infected shunt with or without corticosteroid therapy.[891]

Visceral Infection

Visceral infections in the form of abdominal, pulmonary, and retroperitoneal abscesses are known to be associated with GN.[892] The clinical and pathologic syndrome resembles IE. Beaufils and colleagues[893] reported on 11 patients who had visceral abscesses and in whom acute renal failure developed. Circulating cryoglobulins, decreased serum complement levels, and CICs were found in some of these patients. All renal biopsies showed a diffuse proliferative and crescentic GN. The evolution of the GN, documented by serial biopsies, closely paralleled the course of the infection. A complete recovery of renal function occurred in patients in whom a rapid and complete cure of the infection was obtained. For patients in whom the infection was not cured or in whom therapy was delayed, chronic renal failure also developed.[893] Outcome is worse in elderly patients and in individuals with diabetes.[893a]

Other Bacterial Infections and Fungal Infections

Congenital, secondary, and latent forms of syphilis rarely may be complicated by glomerular involvement. Patients are typically nephrotic, and proteinuria usually responds to penicillin therapy.[894-898] Membranous nephropathy with varying degrees of proliferation and with granular IgG and C3 deposits is the commonest finding on biopsies. Treponemal antigen and antibody have been eluted from deposits. Rarely, minimal change lesions[899] and crescentic GN[900] or amyloidosis may be seen.

Bartonella henselae is the organism responsible for bartonellosis (cat scratch disease), which typically manifests as a skin papule followed by regional lymphadenopathy. Rarely, endocarditis, CNS involvement (encephalopathy), generalized skin rash, and the Parinaud oculoglandular syndrome (fever, regional lymphadenopathy, and follicular conjunctivitis) may be seen. Renal manifestations are rare and can include IgA nephropathy,[901] postinfectious GN,[902] or necrotizing GN.[903] In general, spontaneous recovery may occur with control of infection; however, end-stage renal failure has been reported with aggressive renal disease.[903]

Renal involvement, including azotemia, proteinuria, nephrotic syndrome, renal tubular defects, and hematuria, is common in leprosy, especially with the lepra reaction.[904-909] Rarely, presentation with RPGN[910] and ESRD[911] can occur. Mesangial proliferation, diffuse proliferative GN, crescentic GN, membranous nephropathy, membranoproliferative GN, microscopic angiitis, and amyloidosis may all be seen in kidney biopsies. Organisms consistent with *Mycobacterium leprae* have been found in glomeruli.

Aspergillosis has been associated with immune complex–mediated GN.[912] Membranous nephropathy, membranoproliferative GN, crescentic GN, and amyloidosis have been associated with *Mycobacterium tuberculosis* infection.[913-916] *Mycoplasma* spp. has been reported to be associated with nephrotic syndrome and rapidly progressive GN. Antibiotics do not seem to alter the course of the disease. Mycoplasmal antigen has been reported to be present in glomerular lesions.[917-921] Acute GN with hypocomplementemia has been reported with pneumococcal infections. Proliferative GN with deposition of IgG; IgM; complements C1q, C3, and C4; and pneumococcal antigens have been observed in renal biopsies.[922,923] Nocardiosis has been associated with mesangiocapillary GN.[924] In infections with *Brucella* spp., patients may present with hematuria, proteinuria (usually nephrotic), and varying degrees of renal functional impairment. There usually is improvement after antibiotics, but histologic abnormalities, proteinuria, and hypertension may persist. Glomerular mesangial proliferation, focal and segmental endocapillary proliferation, diffuse proliferation, and crescents may be found in renal biopsies. IF may show no deposits, IgG, or occasionally IgA.[925-929] Asymptomatic urinary abnormalities may be seen in up to 80% of patients infected with *Leptospira* spp. Patients usual present with acute renal failure caused by tubulointerstial nephritis. Rarely, mesangial or diffuse proliferative GN may be seen.[930,931] From 1% to 4% of patients with typhoid fever secondary to *Salmonella* infection experience GN. Asymptomatic urinary abnormalities may be more frequent. Renal manifestations are usually transient and resolve within 2 to 3 weeks. Serum C3 may be depressed. Mesangial proliferation with deposits of IgG, C3, and C4 is the commonest finding. IgA nephropathy has also been reported.[932-934]

Glomerular Involvement with Parasitic Diseases

Four strains of malaria parasite cause human disease: *Plasmodium vivax*, *Plasmodium falciparum*, *Plasmodium malariae* (causing quartan malaria), and *Plasmodium ovale*. Of these, renal involvement has been extensively documented and studied in *P. malariae* and *P. falciparum*. In *P. falciparum* malaria, clinically overt glomerular disease is uncommon. Asymptomatic urinary abnormalities may occur with subnephrotic proteinuria and hematuria or pyuria. Renal function is usually normal. Renal biopsies show mesangial proliferation or membranoproliferative lesions.[935] Severe malaria may be manifest with hemoglobinuric acute renal failure.[936] In initial reports, quartan malaria was strongly associated with nephrotic syndrome in children. There was progression to end-stage renal failure within 3 to 5 years with no improvement with antimalarial treatment or steroids.[937] Renal biopsies in Ugandan adults and children with quartan malaria showed some form of proliferative GN (diffuse, focal, lobular, or minimal). Membranous nephropathy had also been described in these patients.[938] However, in Nigerian children, the most common lesion was a localized or diffuse thickening of glomerular capillary walls with focal or generalized double contouring and segmental sclerosis of the tuft.[939] IF examination revealed deposits of IgG, IgM, C3, and *P. malariae* antigen in the glomeruli. By EM, electron-dense material had been observed within the irregularly thickened GBM.[940] Of note, a recent report from endemic areas in Nigeria has not shown any cases of childhood nephrotic syndrome associated with quartan malaria.[941]

Schistosomiasis is a visceral parasitic disease caused by the blood flukes of the genus Schistosoma. *Schistosoma mansoni* and *Schistosoma japonicum* cause cirrhosis of the liver, and *Schistosoma hematobium* causes cystitis. Glomerular involvement in *S. mansoni* includes mesangial proliferation, focal sclerosis, membranoproliferative lesions, crescentic changes, membranous nephropathy, amyloidosis, and eventually ESRD.[942-944] Schistosomal antigens have been demonstrated in renal biopsies is such patients.[945] Treatment with antiparasitic agents does not appear to influence the progression of renal disease.[946] *S. hematobium* is occasionally associated with the nephrotic syndrome, which may respond to treatment of the parasite.[942] In some patients with schistosomiasis, renal involvement may be related to concomitant *Salmonella* infection.[947]

Leishmaniasis also known as kala azar is caused by *Leishmania donovani*. Renal involvement in kala azar appears to be mild and reverts with anti-leishmanial treatment. Renal biopsies show glomerular mesangial proliferation or focal endocapillary proliferation. IgG, IgM, and C3 may be observed in areas of proliferation. Amyloidosis may also complicate kala azar.[948,949] In trypanosomiasis, *Trypanosome brucei*, *Trypanosome gambiense*, and *Trypanosome rhodesiense* cause African sleeping sickness and have rarely been associated with proteinuria.[950] Filariasis caused by organisms in the genus *Onchocerca*, *Brugia*, *Loa loa*, and *Wuchereria*. Hematuria and proteinuria (including nephrotic syndrome) have been described. Renal manifestations may appear with treatment of infection. Renal biopsy findings have included mesangial proliferative GN with C3 deposition, diffuse proliferative GN, and collapsing glomerulopathy with loiasis.[951-956] In patients with lymphatic filariasis of the renal hilus, chyluria (the passage of milky white urine containing lymphatic fluid) may mimic nephrotic syndrome by producing nephrotic-range proteinuria but is distinguished by the absence of hypoalbuminemia or glomerular disease on biopsy.[956a] Trichinosis is caused by *Trichinella spiralis* and may be associated with proteinuria and hematuria that abates after specific treatment. Renal biopsies in patients with loiasis have shown mesangial proliferative GN with C3 deposition.[957,958] *Echinococcus granulosus* and *Echinococcus multilocularis* cause hydatid disease or echinococcosis in humans. Mesangiocapillary GN and membranous nephropathy have occasionally been associated with hepatic hydatid cysts.[959,960] Toxoplasmosis may be associated with nephrotic syndrome in infants and rarely in adults. Mesangial and endothelial proliferation may be found, with deposition of IgG, IgA, IgM, C3, and fibrinogen in areas of proliferation.[961-963]

Glomerular Involvement with Viral Infections

Viruses have been postulated to cause glomerular injury by various mechanisms, including direct cytopathic effects, the deposition of immune complexes, or by initiation of autoimmune mechanisms.

In a study of previously healthy people with nonstreptococcal upper respiratory infections, 4% had erythrocyte casts and GN on biopsy. A reduction in serum complement and serologic evidence of infection with adenovirus, influenza A, or influenza B were observed in some. Initial renal biopsy showed either focal or diffuse mesangial proliferation in all nine, with mesangial C3 deposits in six specimens. Sequential creatinine clearances were reduced in about half of these patients during follow-up.[964]

The nephrotic syndrome has been described with EBV infections.[965] Renal biopsies in patients with urinary abnormalities have included immune complex–mediated GN with tubulointerstitial nephritis,[966] minimal glomerular lesions with IgM deposition,[967] membranous nephropathy,[968] and widespread glomerular mesangiolysis sometimes admixed with segmental mesangial sclerosis.[969] In addition, the presence of EBV DNA in the glomerulus is thought to worsen glomerular damage in chronic glomerulopathies.[970] Other viruses have rarely been associated with GN, including herpes zoster, mumps, adenovirus, echovirus, Coxsackie virus, and influenza A and B.[971]

HIV-Related Glomerulopathies

More than 33 million people have been infected with the human immunodeficiency virus (HIV) worldwide, with more than 2 million new infections each year.[972] A variety of glomerular lesions, particularly, a unique form of glomerular damage, HIV-associated nephropathy (HIVAN), are associated with HIV-infected patients.[973,974]

HIV-Associated Nephropathy

Clinical Features

In 1984, the first detailed report of a new pattern of sclerosing glomerulopathy in HIV-infected patients was published.[975] Subsequent studies, largely from large urban centers, confirmed the occurrence and described the features of HIVAN.[975-980-985] In these largely urban East Coast centers, the prevalence of HIVAN approached 90% in nephrotic HIV-positive patients in contrast to a prevalence of only 2% in San Francisco, where most seropositive patients were white homosexuals.[986-988]

There is a strong predilection for HIVAN among black HIV-infected patients. The black:white ratio among patients with HIVAN is 12:1.[989] HIVAN is the third leading cause of ESRD among black Americans ages 20 to 64 years, following only diabetes and hypertension.[982,990] Of HIV-infected adults who do not use IV drugs with glomerular lesions, 17% of whites had very mild FSGS, 75% diffuse mesangial hyperplasia (DMH), and none severe FSGS in contrast to blacks, in whom only 27% had DMH but in whom 55% had severe FSGS. Blacks were also more likely to have more severe clinical renal disease with heavier proteinuria, a higher incidence of the nephrotic syndrome, and greater renal insufficiency. A similar presentation has been found in Los Angeles and Europe.[991,992] Racial factors are important in mutations of HIV receptors, which may in part explain some differences in the racial predisposition to HIV infection and HIVAN.[993-995] Mapping by admixture linkage disequilibrium has linked HIVAN and sporadic FSGS to variants in the myosin heavy chain-9 gene and the closely linked *APOL1* gene on chromosome 22, which may explain the strong black racial predominance in these conditions.[996,997]

Although IV drug use has been the most common risk factor for the HIVAN, the disease has been seen in all groups at risk for AIDS, including homosexuals, perinatally acquired disease, heterosexual transmission, and exposure to contaminated blood products.[973] HIVAN usually occurs in patients with low CD4 counts, but full-blown AIDS is certainly not a prerequisite for the disease. In one New York study, the onset of HIVAN was most common in otherwise asymptomatic HIV-infected patients (i.e., 12 of 26 were asymptomatic patients).[975,979] There is no relationship between the development of HIVAN and patient age and duration of HIV infection or types of opportunistic infections or malignancies.[973] The prevalence of HIVAN in patients who test positive for HIV is reported to be 3.5% in patients screened in the clinic setting[998]; the same group reported that HIVAN was found in 6.9% of autopsies in HIV-infected patients.[999]

The clinical features of HIVAN include presenting features of proteinuria, typically in the nephrotic range (and often massive), and renal insufficiency. Other manifestation of the nephrotic syndrome, including edema, hypoalbuminemia, and hypercholesterolemia, have been common in some series but less so in others despite the heavy proteinuria.[973,975,978,979,983,985,1000] Likewise, the incidence of hypertension has been variable even in patients with severe renal failure. Some patients, however, present with subnephrotic-range proteinuria and urinary sediment findings of microhematuria and sterile pyuria.[1001] Renal ultrasounds in patients with HIVAN show echogenic kidneys with preserved or enlarged size with an average of more than 12 cm despite the severe renal insufficiency.[979,983] Echogenicity may correlate with the histopathologic tubulointerstitial changes better than the glomerular changes.[983]

Pathology

The term *HIVAN* is reserved for the characteristic LM pattern of FSGS of the "collapsing" type with retraction of the glomerular capillary walls and luminal occlusion either in a

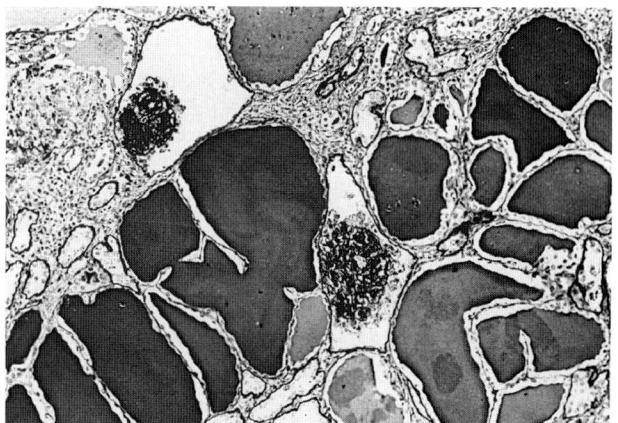

FIGURE 32-51 HIV-associated nephropathy. Glomeruli have collapsed tufts with capping of the overlying podocytes and dilatation of the urinary space. The tubules are dilated forming microcysts with abundant proteinaceous casts (periodic acid–Schiff, ×125)

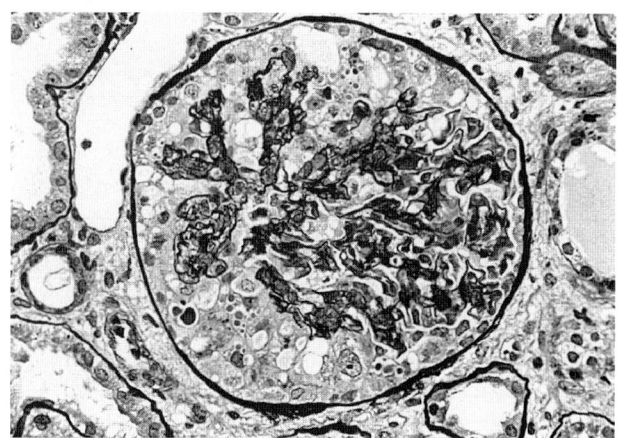

FIGURE 32-52 HIV-associated nephropathy. The characteristic pattern of collapsing glomerular sclerosis is depicted. Glomerular capillary lumina are occluded by wrinkling and retraction of the glomerular capillary walls associated with marked hypertrophy and hyperplasia of the visceral epithelial cells, forming a pseudocrescent (periodic acid–Schiff, ×325)

segmental or global distribution[974,977,1002] (Figure 32-51). In the acute phase, this occurs without a substantial increase in matrix or hyalinosis. There is striking hypertrophy and hyperplasia of the visceral epithelial cells, which form a cellular crown over the collapsed glomerular lobules (Figure 32-52). In one study analyzing the expression pattern of podocyte differentiation and proliferation markers, there was disappearance of all podocyte differentiation markers from collapsed glomeruli, associated with cell proliferation, suggesting that the podocyte phenotype is dysregulated.[1003] Patients with HIVAN have a higher percentage of glomerular collapse, less hyalinosis, and greater visceral cell swelling than patients with classic idiopathic FSGS or heroin nephropathy even when matched for serum creatinine and degree of proteinuria.[977] The tubulointerstitial disease is also more severe in HIVAN with tubular degenerative changes and regenerative features, interstitial edema, fibrosis, and inflammation.[974,977] Tubules are often greatly dilated into microcysts containing proteinaceous casts (see Figure 32-51). By IF, IgM and C3 are present; however, by EM, immune deposits are not detected (Figure 32-53). In almost all biopsies of HIVAN, there are numerous TRIs within the cytoplasm of glomerular and

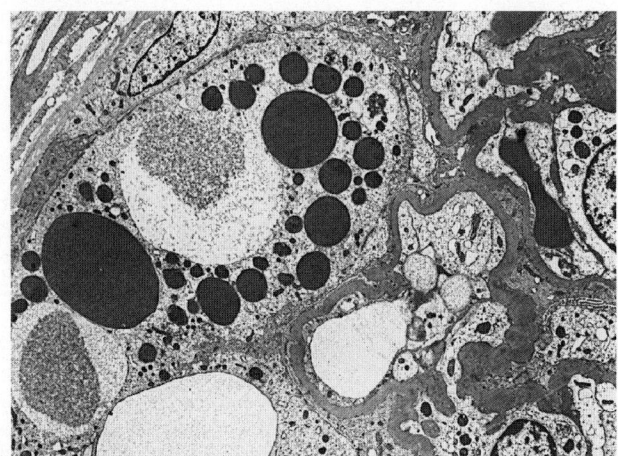

FIGURE 32-53 HIV-associated nephropathy. Electron micrograph showing wrinkling of glomerular basement membranes with marked podocyte hypertrophy, complete foot process effacement, and numerous intracytoplasmic protein resorption droplets (×2500).

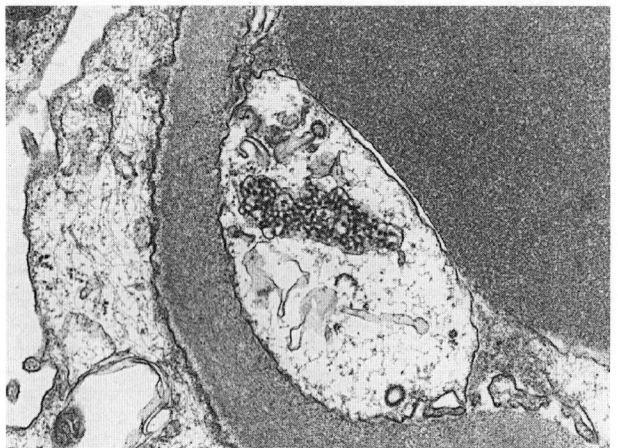

FIGURE 32-54 HIV-associated nephropathy. Electron micrograph showing a typical tubuloreticular inclusion within the endoplasmic reticulum of a glomerular endothelial cell (×6000).

vascular endothelial cells (Figure 32-54).[973,974,977,1002] These 24-nm interanastomosing tubular structures, known as "INF footprints," are located within dilated cisternae of the endoplasmic reticulum.

Pathogenesis

Experimental evidence strongly supports a role for direct HIV-1 infection of renal parenchymal cells. By in situ hybridization, HIV-1 RNA was detected in renal tubular epithelial cells, glomerular epithelial cells (visceral and parietal), and interstitial leukocytes.[1004] Renal epithelial cells may be an important reservoir for HIV because HIV RNA was found in the kidneys of patients with undetectable viral loads in peripheral blood.[1004] Moreover, HIV-infected tubular epithelium can support viral replication, as evidenced by the detection of HIV quasispecies separate from those found in peripheral blood of the same patient.[1005]

A replicative-deficient transgenic mouse model of HIVAN has been developed with lesions identical to HIV nephropathy,[1006-1008] suggesting that expression of viral gene products in renal epithelium underlies the development of nephropathy.

The lesions of collapsing glomerulopathy are associated with podocyte proliferation and de-differentiation.[1003] The expression of two cyclin-dependent kinase inhibitors (which regulate cell cycle) p27 and p57 were decreased in podocytes from HIVAN biopsies, but expression of another CDK inhibitor, p21, was increased.[1009] The specific HIV gene(s) required to produce these changes have been investigated. The *nef* gene (which is thought to act by activation of tyrosine kinases) was found to be essential in producing HIV-induced changes in podocyte cultures,[1010] and in one murine model of HIVAN,[1011] there appears to be a synergistic role for *nef* and *vpr* on podocyte dysfunction and progressive glomerulosclerosis.[1012] *Vpr* has a role in G2 cell cycle arrest and possibly the induction of apoptosis.[1013]

Course and Treatment

The natural history of HIVAN during the early part of the AIDS epidemic was characterized by rapid progression to ESRD. Case series from the United States that were published during the years that HIVAN was first described demonstrated an almost universal requirement for dialysis within less than 1 year of diagnosis.[975] The role of combined antiviral therapies and the use of newer agents in the treatment of patients with HIVAN have been associated with beneficial effects.[1014-1017] The development of HIVAN is now considered an indication for antiretroviral therapy. Corresponding to the introduction of highly active antiretroviral therapy (HAART), the increase in new cases of ESRD caused by HIVAN slowed markedly.[1018]

There have been a few studies using corticosteroids in patients with HIVAN. In an early study, prednisone was not associated with improvement in children with HIVAN.[1019,1020] Remissions in HIV-infected children with the minimal change pattern on biopsy treated with steroids have been noted but not in children with sclerosing or collapsing lesions.[973] In adults, however, several retrospective studies have shown short-term improvement in clinical parameters.[1021-1023]

Three pediatric patients with HIVAN on biopsy had sustained remissions of the nephrotic syndrome when treated with cyclosporine.[1019] They eventually developed opportunistic infections, requiring cyclosporine to be discontinued, and subsequently experienced relapses of the nephrotic proteinuria and renal failure.

In isolated patients and in several small trials, the use of ACE inhibitors has been shown to decrease proteinuria in patients with HIVAN and to slow the progression to renal failure.[1024-1026] Serum ACE levels are elevated in patients with HIV, and ACE inhibitors may prevent proteinuria and glomerulosclerosis by hemodynamic mechanisms, through modulation of matrix production and mesangial cell proliferation, or even by affecting HIV protease activity.[1024-1026] Although some of these studies used control groups of untreated HIV patients of similar age, sex, race, and degree of renal insufficiency and proteinuria, the studies were not randomized, blinded trials. Nevertheless, in each study, the ACE inhibitor–treated group had less proteinuria, less increase in serum creatinine, and less progression to ESRD.

At present, the therapy of patients with HIVAN should include use of multiple antiviral agents as in HIV-infected patients without nephropathy. Use of ACE inhibitors or perhaps angiotensin II receptor blockers, with careful attention to hyperkalemia and acute increases in the serum creatinine, may be beneficial. Immunosuppressive therapy with steroids or cyclosporine should be used only in certain patients in whom the potential benefits of therapy outweigh the risks of further immunulocompromise and opportunistic infections.

Several studies have documented favorable outcomes in patients with HIVAN who received renal transplants.[1027-1029] The current opinion is that renal transplantation is no longer a contraindication in HIV-positive patients who have undetectable viral loads and CD4 greater than 200 cells/µL for at least 6 months.[1030]

Other Glomerular Lesions in Patients with HIV Infection

In the pre-HAART era, HIVAN was the most common form of glomerulopathy found in HIV-infected patients, but other lesions had been reported as well. In one series of more than 100 biopsies for glomerular disease in HIV-positive patients, 73% were classic HIVAN, but other lesions included MPGN in 10%; minimal change disease in 6%; amyloid in 3%; lupuslike nephritis in 3%; acute postinfectious GN in 2%; membranous nephropathy in 2%; and 1% each of focal and segmental necrotizing GN, thrombotic microangiopathy, IgA nephropathy, and immunotactoid nephropathy.[974] Whereas collapsing FSGS is most common in urban centers with large black populations, higher rates of immune complex GN are found in other cities, especially in European white populations.[991,992] In a study from Paris, immune complex GN was found in more than 50% of the white HIV-seropositive patients but only 21% of the blacks.[991,992] Likewise, in a study from northern Italy of 26 biopsies in HIV-infected patients, most cases were of immune complex GN but none of classic HIVAN.[1031] In the present era with the availability of HAART, a renal biopsy in an HIV-positive patient with viral loads below 400 copies/mL are more likely to show hypertensive nephrosclerosis[1032] or diabetic nephropathy.[1033]

IgA nephropathy has been reported in a number of series of HIV-infected patients.[1034-1038] This has occurred in both whites and blacks despite the rarity of typical IgA nephropathy in black populations. The clinical features usually include hematuria, proteinuria, and some renal insufficiency. Cases with leukocytoclastic angiitis of the skin (consistent with HSP) have also been noted. The histology shows a variety of changes from mesangial proliferative GN to collapsing glomerulosclerosis with mesangial IgA deposits. IgA anti-HIV immune complexes have been eluted from the kidneys of several such patients, and several patients have had CICs containing IgA idiotypic antibodies directed against viral proteins, either anti-HIV p24 or HIV gp41.[1037]

Membranoproliferative GN may be the most common pattern of immune complex–mediated GN seen in HIV-infected patients. Two series document a high occurrence in IV drug abusers coinfected with HIV and hepatitis C.[1039,1040] Most patients have had microscopic hematuria, nephrotic-range proteinuria, and renal insufficiency at biopsy. Cryoglobulin results are commonly positive, as are results for hypocomplementemia, and some have had both hepatitis B and C infection. The pathology of the glomerulopathy may be similar to idiopathic MPGN type 1 or type 3, although some patients also have features of segmental membranous or mesangioproliferative features.

A lupus-like immune complex GN has been reported in a number of patients.[982,1041-1044] Most of these patients have had positive serology for SLE with positive ANA, anti-DNA, and low complement levels. This contrasts with a low incidence of ANA positivity and almost no anti-DNA positivity in the general HIV-infected population.[1045] These patients are generally treated with corticosteroids with or without mycophenolate and concomitant HAART therapy. The results have been variable.[1044]

A not-infrequent association in both white and black HIV-infected patients has been TTP. Most have been in an advanced stage of HIV infection and had renal involvement with hematuria, proteinuria, and variable renal insufficiency. Other typical findings of TTP, such as fever, neurologic symptoms, thrombocytopenia, and microangiopathic hemolytic anemia, are often present. Mortality can be high even if the patient is treated with vigorous therapy (plasmapheresis, fresh-frozen plasma infusion, and corticosteroids).[1046] The role of ADAMTS13 in diagnosing HIV-associated TTP is uncertain. Other entities such as malignant hypertension, angioinvasive infections such as Kaposi's sarcoma, and direct HIV-associated HUS need to be excluded.[1047]

Glomerular Manifestations of Liver Disease

Hepatitis B

Hepatitis B antigenemia has been associated with GN for more than 30 years. Hepatitis B has a worldwide distribution. In countries where the virus is endemic (sub-Saharan Africa, Southeast Asia, Eastern Europe), there is vertical transmission from mother to infant and horizontal transmission between siblings. Hepatitis B–associated nephropathy occurs in these children with a 4:1 male preponderance.[1048-1050] In the United States and Western Europe, where hepatitis B is acquired by parenteral routes or sexually, the nephropathy affects mainly adults and has a different clinical course from the endemic form.[1051-1053] However, hepatitis B–associated nephropathy is rare in hepatitis B carriers.[1054] PAN has also been associated with hepatitis B.[1055]

Clinical Features

Most patients present with proteinuria or the nephrotic syndrome. In endemic areas, there may not be a preceding history of hepatitis. The majority of patients have normal renal function at the time of presentation. There may be urinary erythrocytes, but the majority have a bland sediment. Liver disease may be absent (carrier state) or chronic and clinically mild. Serum aminotransferases may be normal or modestly elevated (100–200 IU/L). Liver biopsies in these patients often show chronic active hepatitis. Some patients ultimately develop cirrhosis in their biopsies. There is often a spontaneous resolution of the carrier state with resolution of renal abnormalities. Spontaneous resolution of HBV-associated nephropathy is particularly common in children from endemic areas. The probability of a spontaneous remission may be as high as 80% after 10 years.[1056,1057]

Pathology

Most cases of hepatitis B–associated nephropathy manifest membranous nephropathy, although mesangial proliferation and sclerosis have also been seen.[1048,1049,1051-1053,1058,1059] In a cohort of Chinese patients with membranous nephropathy, HBV was found in 12%. There are fewer reports of membranoproliferative GN with mesangial cell interposition, reduplication of the GBM, and subendothelial glomerular deposits.[1051,1053,1058] In a few series, type III MPGN has been reported in which there are electron-dense subepithelial deposits in addition to the changes seen in type I MPGN.[1053] Crescentic GN in association with membranous changes and primary crescentic GN have also been described.[1060,1061]

The glomerular lesions appear to be immune complex mediated. Hepatitis B surface antigen (HBsAg), hepatitis B core antigen (HBcAg), and HBeAg[1062] have all been demonstrated in glomerular lesions, as has HBV DNA.[1050,1063]

Treatment

In children with a mild endemic form of hepatitis B–associated nephropathy, no treatment other than supportive care is advocated. In patients with progressive renal dysfunction, INF has been used with mixed results.[1064-1067] Steroids do not significantly improve proteinuria and may potentially enhance viral replication.[1068,1069] Nucleoside analogs, including lamivudine, telbivudine, adefovir, entecavir, and tenofovir, suppress HBV replication by inhibiting viral DNA polymerase and have demonstrated clinical utility in treating hepatitis B infection. Lamivudine was shown to reduce proteinuria and lead to a lesser incidence of ESRD in 10 patients with hepatitis B–associated nephropathy.[1070] Preemptive lamivudine therapy in renal transplant recipients has shown improved survival compared with historical control participants.[1071,1072]

Hepatitis C

Renal disease associated with HCV infection includes membranoproliferative GN with or without associated mixed cryoglobulinemia and membranous glomerulopathy. The membranoproliferative GN is most often type 1, with fewer cases of type 3.[1073-1075] Rare cases of diffuse proliferative and exudative GN, polyarteritis, and fibrillary and immunotactoid glomerulopathy have also been described in association with HCV.[1076,1077] Most patients have evidence of liver disease as reflected by elevated plasma transaminase levels. However, transaminase levels are normal in some cases, and a history of acute hepatitis is often absent.

Pathogenesis

The pathogenesis of HCV-related nephropathies is immune complex mediated. A clonal expansion of B cells secreting IgM rheumatoid factors has been seen with chronic HCV infection. HCV-specific proteins have been isolated from glomerular lesions.[1078] The disappearance of viremia in response to INF (see below) is associated with a diminution of proteinuria; a relapse of viremia is accompanied by increasing proteinuria.

Clinical and Pathologic Features

Mixed cryoglobulinemia is associated with HCV and may cause a systemic vasculitis. Patients may exhibit constitutional systemic symptoms, palpable purpura, peripheral neuropathy, and hypocomplementemia. The renal manifestations include hematuria, proteinuria (often in the nephrotic range), and renal insufficiency. The histologic findings resemble those in idiopathic MPGN type 1 or type 3 (Figures 32-55 and 32-56) except for intraluminal protein "thrombi" on LM and the organized annular–tubular substructure of the electron-dense deposits on EM. Before the advent of hepatitis C serologic tests, mixed cryoglobulinemia had been considered an idiopathic disease ("essential" mixed cryoglobulinemia). Up to 95% of these patients show signs of HCV infection.[1079] Few patients with thrombotic microangiopathy associated with cryoglobulinemia have been described.[1080] Membranoproliferative GN without associated cryoglobulinemia may occur but is much less common.[1074]

Rarely, membranous nephropathy may be associated with HCV infection. Patients present with the nephrotic syndrome

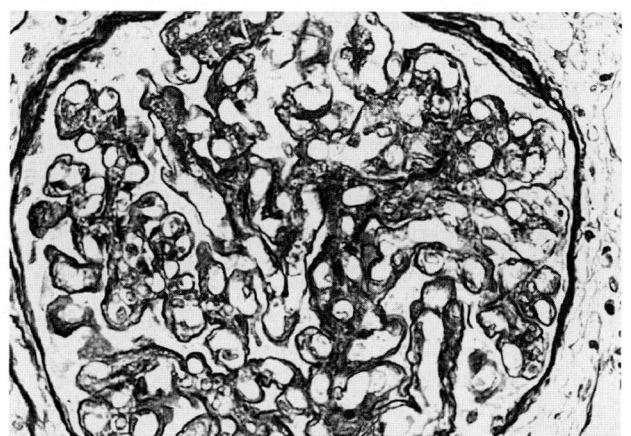

FIGURE 32-55 Hepatitis C–associated membranoproliferative glomerulonephritis type 1. The mesangium is expanded by global mesangial hypercellularity associated with numerous double contours of the glomerular basement membranes (periodic acid–Schiff, ×500).

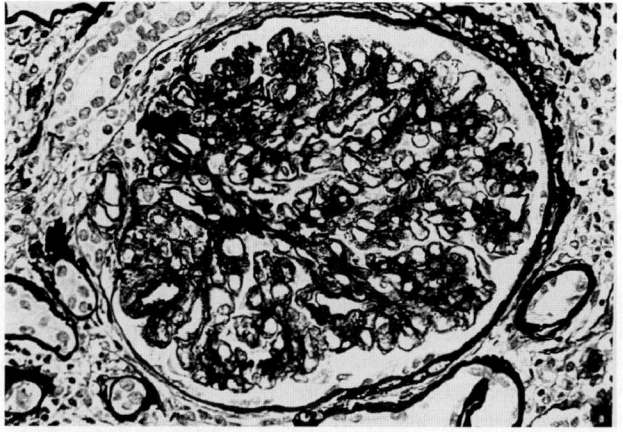

FIGURE 32-56 Hepatitis C–associated membranoproliferative glomerulonephritis type 3. There are mixed features of membranoproliferative glomerulonephritis type 1 (with mesangial proliferation and duplication of glomerular basement membrane) and membranous glomerulopathy (with basement membrane spikes) (Jones methenamine silver, ×325).

or proteinuria. Complement levels tend to normal, and neither cryoglobulins nor rheumatoid factors are present in HCV-associated membranous nephropathy.[1081]

Both type I MPGN (with and without cryoglobulinemia) and membranous nephropathy may recur in the allograft after renal transplantation, sometimes leading to graft loss.[1082-1085] Similar lesions have occurred in native kidneys after liver transplantation in HCV-positive patients.[1086,1087]

Treatment

The treatment of patients with HCV-associated renal disease is limited to case reports and small randomized trials.[1088] Although a number of early reports demonstrated a beneficial response to INF-α therapy,[1081,1089,1090] cessation of INF therapy was associated with a recurrence of viremia and cryoglobulinemia in a majority of patients in these studies. INF therapy may paradoxically exacerbate proteinuria and hematuria that appears to be unrelated to viral antigenic effects.[1091] Currently, combination therapy with ribavirin and pegylated INF is considered to be standard therapy for HCV.[1092] Combination therapy appeared to improve biochemical parameters of renal dysfunction in 20 HCV-GN patients, which was not accompanied by a significant virologic response.[1093] Another report on 18 patients showed sustained virologic responses in two-thirds of patients that was associated with improvement in renal parameters.[1094] Combination therapy (especially ribavirin) may not be well tolerated in the presence of significant renal dysfunction. In patients with severe disease, immunosuppressive agents have been used.[1095] INF-α treatment of renal transplant patients with HCV has been associated with acute renal failure[1096] and acute humoral rejection.[1097]

In patients with symptomatic cryoglobulinemia, immunosuppressive therapy may provide symptomatic relief before the use of antiviral therapy. Cyclophosphamide treatment has been used successfully in patients with HCV-GN[1098] even if they are INF resistant.[1099] Cyclophosphamide treatment may be associated with a temporary, reversible increase in viral load and a change of quasispecies.[1100] Fludarabine has been reported to decrease proteinuria in HCV-associated cryoglobulinemic MPGN.[1101] Recently, there have been reports of rituximab-induced remissions of proteinuria in HCV-GN.[1102-1104] In renal transplant patients with HCV-GN, similar improvement in renal parameters have been reported, albeit with a higher incidence of infectious complications.[1105] It has been suggested that in patients with moderate proteinuria and slowly progressive renal dysfunction, INF with or without ribavirin should be considered. When there is an acute flare of disease with nephrotic proteinuria or rapidly progressive GN, treatment with plasma exchange and immunosuppressive drugs (rituximab or cyclophosphamide with corticosteroids) followed by antiviral therapy be considered.[1088]

Autoimmune Chronic Active Hepatitis

Autoimmune chronic hepatitis is a distinctive progressive necrotic and fibrotic disorder of the liver with clinical or serologic evidence of a generalized autoimmune disorder.[1106] Two distinct clinical lesions have been associated with this disorder: GN and interstitial nephritis. Patients with the glomerular lesion present with nephrotic syndrome or renal insufficiency.

On renal biopsy, they have membranous or membranoproliferative GN. In two patients with membranous nephropathy, CICs containing U1-RNP (ribonucleoprotein) and IgG have been reported. Eluates from the kidney tissue revealed higher concentrations of anti U1-RNP antibody. It is not known whether immunosuppressive therapy ameliorates the renal disorder.[1106] It is unclear if coexistent HCV infection had been present in many of these patients.

Liver Cirrhosis

GN is a rare manifestation of liver cirrhosis. Glomerular morphologic abnormalities with IgA deposition have been noted in more than 50% of patients with cirrhosis at both necropsy and biopsy,[1107,1108] although this has also been found in some autopsies of noncirrhotic kidneys.[1109] Clinically, there may be mild proteinuria, hematuria, or both. There are two patterns on histology: a mesangial sclerosis ("cirrhotic glomerular sclerosis") and membranoproliferative GN. The latter may be associated with more severe renal symptoms and a depression of serum complement C3 levels.[1110] Again, it is unclear if some patients had coexistent HCV infection. Rarely, HSP with rapidly progressive GN has been described in association with cirrhosis.[1111]

Renal biopsies of patients with cirrhosis on LM show an increase in mesangial matrix with little on no increase in mesangial cellularity, a lesion known as "hepatic glomerulopathy." Less commonly, the distinctive pathologic findings consist of mesangial proliferative GN with mesangial IgA deposits usually accompanied by complement deposition and less intense IgG or IgM.[1107,1112,1113] By EM, the mesangium and subendothelial regions contain lucencies with dense, granular, and rounded membranous structures consistent with lipid inclusions (Figure 32-57). Increased serum IgA levels are found in more than 90% of cirrhotic patients with glomerular IgA deposition. Other authors have reported IgM as the dominant immunoglobulin.[1108] Cirrhotic GN is usually a clinically silent disease; however, the diagnosis can be suspected by finding proteinuria or abnormalities of the urine

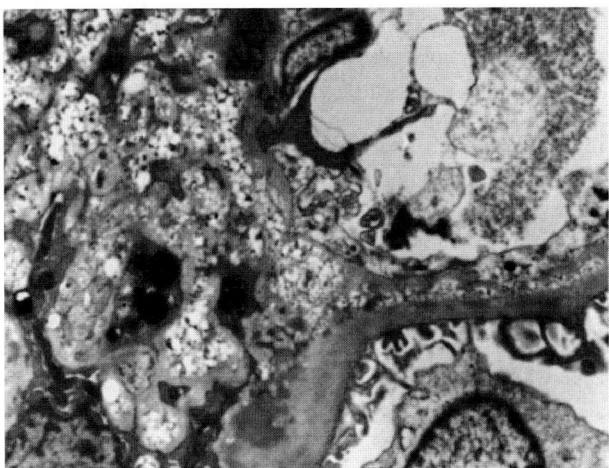

FIGURE 32-57 Hepatic glomerulopathy. A paramesangial electron-dense deposit corresponding to immune staining for IgA is seen. In addition, there are irregular lucencies containing dense granular and rounded membranous structures within the mesangial matrix and extending into the subendothelial space (×6000).

sediment. The pathogenesis may relate to defective hepatic clearance of IgA as well as altered processing or portacaval shunting of CICs.[1114] This theory is bolstered by the finding of increased deposits of IgA in the skin and hepatic sinusoids in patients with cirrhosis.[1115] Moreover, in patients with noncirrhotic portal fibrosis who underwent portal-systemic bypass procedures, there was an increase in the incidence of clinically overt GN (from 78% to 32%) associated with deposition of IgA after the procedure. In the latter group, there was also a significant incidence of renal failure (50% after 5 years).[1116] Similar findings were noted in children with end-stage liver disease from α-1 antitrypsin deficiency or biliary atresia, which resolved after liver transplantation.[1117]

Glomerular Lesions Associated with Neoplasia

The occurrence of glomerular syndromes, both nephrotic and nephritic, may be associated with malignancy but is rare (<1%). Glomerular disease may be seen with a wide variety of malignancies. Carcinomas of the lung, stomach, breast, and colon are most frequently associated with glomerular lesions. Membranous nephropathy is the commonest lesion associated with carcinoma.[1118-1120] Patients older than the age of 50 years presenting with nephrotic syndrome should be reviewed for the presence of a malignancy.[1121,1122]

Clinical and Pathologic Features

Clinically, the glomerulopathy of neoplasia may be manifested by proteinuria or the nephrotic syndrome, an active urine sediment, or diminished glomerular filtration. Significant renal impairment is uncommon and is usually associated with the proliferative forms of GN. In evaluating an ESR in patients with nephrotic syndrome, it should be noted that most such patients have an ESR above 60 mm/hr, with roughly 20% being above 100 mm/hr. As a result, an elevated ESR alone in a patient with the nephrotic syndrome (or with ESRD) is not an indication to evaluate the patient for an occult malignancy or underlying inflammatory disease.[1123,1124]

Membranous Nephropathy

Membranous nephropathy may be associated with malignancies in 10% to 40% of cases.[1122,1125] These include carcinoma of bronchus,[1126] breast,[1127] colon,[1128,1129] stomach, ovary,[1130] kidney,[1131] pancreas,[1132] and prostate[1133,1134] as well as testicular seminoma,[1135] parotid adenolymphoma, carcinoid tumor,[1136,1137] Hodgkin's disease, and carotid body tumor.[1138] In some cases of membranous nephropathy associated with malignancy, tumor antigens have been detected within the glomeruli. It is postulated that tumor antigen deposition in the glomerulus is followed by antibody deposition, causing "in situ" immune complex formation and subsequent complement activation.[1139,1140] Immune complexes and complement have been found in cancer patients without overt renal disease.[1139] Antibody to phospholipase A2 receptor (PLA2R), the target antigen in primary membranous nephropathy, has not been identified in the sera of patients with membranous

nephropathy secondary to malignancy. Removal of the tumor may lead to remission of the nephrotic syndrome, which may then recur after the development of metastasis. In many instances, successful treatment of the neoplasm has induced a partial or complete remission of the associated glomerulopathy.

Minimal Change Disease or Focal Glomerulosclerosis

Minimal change disease or focal glomerulosclerosis may occur in association with Hodgkin's disease[1141-1143]; less often, non-Hodgkin's lymphoma or leukemia[1142]; and rarely thymoma,[1144] mycosis fungoides,[1145] renal cell carcinoma,[1146] and other solid tumors.[1147-1149] Secretion of a lymphokine by abnormal T cells may underlie glomerular injury in these disorders.[1150,1151]

Secondary Amyloidosis

Secondary amyloidosis has been described with a number of malignancies, particularly renal cell carcinoma, Hodgkin's disease, and chronic lymphocytic leukemia.[1,2,4] In Hodgkin's disease, for example, renal amyloidosis is generally a late event resulting from a chronic inflammatory state; by comparison, minimal change disease most often occurs at the time of initial presentation.[5]

Proliferative Glomerulonephritides and Vasculitides

Both membranoproliferative and rapidly progressive GN have been described in patients with solid tumors and lymphomas, although the etiologic relationship between these conditions is not proven.[1149,1152] The association is probably strongest for membranoproliferative GN and chronic lymphocytic leukemia and may be associated with circulating cryoglobulins.[1153,1154] Mesangial proliferation with IgA deposition has been associated with mucosa-associated lymphoid tissue lymphoma that resolved after treatment of the malignancy with chlorambucil.[1155] Although the association between crescentic GN and vasculitis with tumors may be coincidental, it has been suggested that the malignancy may act as a trigger for the vasculitis.[1156-1158] In contrast to the nephrotic states described above in which renal function is generally well preserved at presentation and the urine sediment is usually benign, patients with proliferative GN often have an acute decline in renal function and an active urine sediment.

Thrombotic Microangiopathy

Both the HUS and the related disorder TTP can occur in patients with malignancy. An underlying carcinoma of the stomach, pancreas, or prostate may be associated with HUS. More commonly, however, antitumor therapy is implicated: mitomycin, gemcitabine, the combination of bleomycin and cisplatin, and radiation plus high-dose cyclophosphamide before bone marrow transplantation all can lead to the HUS, which may first become apparent months after therapy has been discontinued.[1159] Anti–vascular endothelial growth factor agents are newly identified causes of glomerular thrombotic microangiopathy, leading to proteinuria, renal insufficiency, and hypertension.[1159a] This topic is reviewed further in Chapter 34. For further discussion of kidney disease in patients with malignancy, see Chapter 41.

Glomerular Disease Associated with Drugs

Heroin Nephropathy

In the 1970s, reports began to appear linking heroin abuse to the nephrotic syndrome and renal biopsy findings of appearing with lesions of focal and segmental glomerulosclerosis. This syndrome was referred to as heroin-associated nephropathy (HAN).[1160-1165] Similar lesions were seen in users of IV pentazocine (Talwin) and tripelennamine (pyribenzamine), so-called Ts and Blues.[1166] This syndrome occurred almost exclusively in blacks; it has been suggested that blacks may have a genetic predisposition for developing HAN.[1167,1168] The mean age was younger than 30 years old with 90% of the patients being males. The duration of drug abuse varied from 6 months to 30 years (mean, 6 years) before the onset of renal disease. Most patients presented with the nephrotic syndrome. The course of HAN was relentless progression to ESRD over many years in addicts who continued to use heroin; a regression of abnormalities was seen in patients that were able to stop using the drug. Kidney biopsies of these patients showed lesions of focal segmental and global sclerosis. Nonspecific trapping leads to the deposition of IgM and C3 in areas of sclerosis. There was usually significant interstitial inflammation associated with the glomerular lesion. The pathogenesis of HAN is unknown. Abnormalities of cellular and humoral immunity have been well described in heroin addicts.[1169] It has been suggested that morphine itself could act as an antigen and that contaminants used to "cut" the heroin could contribute to the pathogenesis. Morphine (the active metabolite of heroin) has been shown to stimulate proliferation and sclerosis of mesangial cells and fibroblasts.[1170,1171] The syndrome of HAN has almost disappeared among drug addicts presenting with renal failure; for example, there has been a sharp decline in incident case of HAN, and there have been no reported cases of HAN-associated ESRD from Brooklyn, New York, during the period from 1991 to 1993.[1172,1173] In part, this trend coincides with the increase of HIV infection and HIVAN.

Nonsteroidal Antiinflammatory Drug-Induced Nephropathy

NSAIDs are being used by approximately 50 million of the general public in the United States at any point in time. Approximately 1% to 3% of patients exposed to NSAIDs will manifest one of the renal abnormalities associated with its use, including fluid and electrolyte disturbances, acute renal failure, and nephrotic syndrome with interstitial nephritis and papillary necrosis.[1174] The combination of acute interstitial nephritis and nephrotic syndrome is characteristic of this group of compounds. Essentially all NSAIDS can cause this type of renal disease,[1175-1177] including the cyclooxygenase-2 (COX-2) inhibitors.[1178,1179]

Clinical and Pathologic Features

MINIMAL CHANGE DISEASE WITH INTERSTITIAL NEPHRITIS

The onset of NSAID-induced nephrotic syndrome is usually delayed, with a mean time of onset of 5.4 months (range, 2 weeks–18 months) after initiation of NSAID therapy. Patients may present with edema and oliguria. Systemic signs of allergic interstitial nephritis are usually absent. The urine exhibits microhematuria and pyuria. Proteinuria is usually in the nephrotic range. The extent of renal dysfunction may be mild to severe. On LM, the findings consist of minimal change disease with interstitial nephritis. A focal or diffuse interstitial infiltrate consists predominantly of cytotoxic T lymphocytes (also other T-cell subsets, B cells, and plasma cells).[1180,1181] The syndrome usually reverses after discontinuing therapy, and the time to recovery may be between 1 month and 1 year.[1177] Complete remission is usually seen.[1182] Relapse of proteinuria has been reported.[1183] Treatment of patients with the nephrotic syndrome is usually unnecessary because the disorder is self-limiting. However, a short course of corticosteroids may be beneficial in patients in whom no response is seen after several weeks of discontinuation of the drug.[1184] Plasma exchange was reported with being associated with rapid recovery of renal function in two patients.[1185]

OTHER PATTERNS

Minimal change nephrotic syndrome without interstitial disease has been occasionally reported.[1186] Granulomatous interstitial disease without glomerular changes has also been described.[1187] Membranous nephropathy has also been reported in association with NSAID use,[1188] including the newer COX-2 inhibitors.[1179] As in minimal change nephrotic syndrome, there is rapid recovery after drug withdrawal in NSAID-induced membranous nephropathy.

Pathogenesis

The mechanism of NSAID-induced nephrotic syndrome has not been defined. It has been proposed that inhibition of COX by NSAID inhibits prostaglandin synthesis and shunts arachidonic acid pathways toward the production of leukotrienes. These byproducts of arachidonic acid metabolism may promote T-lymphocyte activation and enhanced vascular permeability, leading to minimal change disease.[1175-1177]

Antirheumatoid Arthritis Therapy–Induced Glomerulopathy

Gold Salts

Proteinuria and nephrotic syndrome have been reported to occur in association with both oral and parenteral gold.[1189,1190] Dermatitis may occur concurrently. Membranous nephropathy and rarely minimal change disease have been reported.[1191] A higher incidence of nephropathy has been reported in patients with HLA B8/DR3.[1192,1193]

D-Penicillamine

Proteinuria in association with membranous nephropathy is the commonest lesion reported. Less commonly, minimal change disease and mesangial proliferative lesions have been reported.[1193] Goodpasture-like syndrome,[1194] minimal change nephrotic syndrome,[1195] and membranous nephropathy concurrently with vasculitis[1196] have been described rarely. HLA B8/DR3 haplotypes are also associated with penicillamine nephropathy.[1197] Tiopronin and bucillamine (a penicillamine-like compound) have also been associated with the same renal lesions described for penicillamine.[1198,1199] The onset of proteinuria with gold or penicillamine therapy is usually between 6 and 12 months after starting therapy. Proteinuria usually resolves after withdrawing the offending agent; persistent renal dysfunction is uncommon.[1193,1197,1200] Under close supervision, gold and penicillamine have been continued in patients with nephropathy with no obvious adverse effect on renal function.[1201] Anti–TNF-α agents have been reported to promote the development of lupus-like nephritis and ANCA-associated GN in patients with rheumatoid arthritis.[1202]

Other Medications

Organic mercurial exposure can occur with diuretics, skin-lightening creams, gold refining, and industrial exposure. Proteinuria and nephrotic syndrome have been reported.[1203-1205] Renal biopsy in such patients has shown membranous nephropathy[1206,1207] or minimal change disease.[1208] The nephrotic syndrome has been associated with the anticonvulsants ethosuccimide,[1209] trimethadione,[1210] and paradione.[1211] Diffuse proliferative GN may be seen with mephenytoin.[1212] ANCA-associated vasculitis as well as a lupus-like nephritis has been reported with PTU.[1213-1216] Captopril has been associated with the development of proteinuria and the nephrotic syndrome because of membranous nephropathy.[1217] Substituting enalapril for captopril has been reported to ameliorate the nephrotic syndrome.[1218] INF-α has been associated with interstitial nephritis, minimal change disease, focal and segmental glomerulosclerosis, and acute renal failure.[1219,1220] In patients with collapsing FSGS caused by INF therapy, discontinuation of therapy usually leads to improvement in renal function and proteinuria.[1221] Cases of thrombotic microangiopathy[1222] and crescentic GN[1224] have also been reported. Mercaptopropionyl glycine (2-MPG) used in the treatment of cystinuria has been associated with membranous glomerulopathy.[1225] Lithium use has been associated with minimal change disease,[1226,1227] membranous nephropathy,[1228] and focal and segmental glomerulosclerosis.[1229,1230] The use of high-dose pamidronate in patients with malignancies has been associated with HIV-negative collapsing focal and segmental glomerulosclerosis.[1231]

Miscellaneous Diseases Associated with Glomerular Lesions

Well-documented cases exist of nephrotic syndrome associated with unilateral renal artery stenosis, which improved after correction of the stenosis. The mechanism of proteinuria presumably relates to high levels of angiotensin II.[1232-1234]

Acute silicosis has been associated with a proliferative GN with IgM and C3 deposits, leading to renal failure.[1235] A patient with dense lamellar inclusions in swollen glomerular epithelial cells, similar to those seen in Fabry's disease, has also been described.[1236]

Membranous nephropathy and membranoproliferative GN[1237] have been described in association with ulcerative colitis.[1238]

Kimura disease and angiolymphoid hyperplasia with eosinophilia (ALHE) produce skin lesions that appear as single or multiple red-brown papules or as subcutaneous nodules with a predilection for the head and neck region. Other associated features include eosinophilia and elevated IgE levels. Both Kimura disease and the similar ALHE are frequently associated with glomerular disease. Mesangial proliferative GN[1239] and minimal change disease[1240] have been described.

Renal complications of Castleman's disease (angiofollicular lymph node hyperplasia) are uncommon. The reported cases are very heterogeneous, and their renal pathology includes minimal change disease, mesangial proliferative GN,[1241] membranous nephropathy,[1242] membranoproliferative GN,[1243] crescentic GN,[1244] fibrillary GN,[1245] and amyloidosis.[1246] Serum IL-6 levels appear to be elevated and decline with corticosteroid therapy.[1241] Removal of tumor mass or treatment with steroids appears to ameliorate the renal manifestations in some cases.

Angioimmunoblastic lymphadenopathy has been associated with diffuse proliferative GN with necrotizing arteritis and minimal change disease.[1142,1247] Hemophagocytic syndrome related to infections or lymphoproliferative disease has been associated with collapsing FSGS.[1248]

References

1. Bomback AS, Appel GB. Update on the treatment of lupus nephritis. *J Am Soc Nephrol.* 2010;21:2028-2033.
2. Appel GB, D'Agati VD: Lupus nephritis—pathology and pathogenesis. In Wallace DJ, Hahn BH, eds. *Dubois' Lupus Erythematosus.* 7th ed. Philadelphia: Lippincott Williams & Wilkins; 2007:1094-1112.
3. Appel GB, Jayne D. Lupus nephritis. In: Johnson R, Floege J, Feehaly J, eds. *Comprehensive Clinical Nephrology.* St. Louis: Elsevier; 2010.
4. Appel GB, D'Agati V. Renal involvement in systemic lupus erythematosus. In: Massary S, Glassock R, eds. *Text of Kidney Disease.* St. Louis: Williams & Wilkins; 2000:787-797.
5. Tutuncu ZN, Kalunian KC: The definition and classification of SLE. In Wallace DJ, Hahn BH, eds. *Dubois' Lupus Erythematosus.* 7th ed. Philadelphia: Lippincott Williams & Wilkins; 2007:16-21.
6. Rahman A, Isenberg DA. Systemic lupus erythematosus. *N Engl J Med.* 2008;358:929-939.
7. Rus V, Maury EE, Hochberg MC: The epidemiology of SLE. In Wallace DJ, Hahn BH, eds. *Dubois' Lupus Erythematosus.* 7th ed. Philadelphia: Lippincott Williams & Wilkins; 2007:34-43.
8. Waldman M, Appel GB. Update on the treatment of lupus nephritis. *Kidney Int.* 2006;70:1403-1412.
9. Appel GB. Cyclophosphamide therapy of severe lupus nephritis. *Am J Kidney Dis.* 1997;30:872-878.
10. Dooly MA, Hogan S, Jenette C, et al., for the Glomerulonephritis Disease Collaborative Network. Cyclophosphamide therapy for lupus nephritis: poor survival in black Americans. *Kidney Int.* 1997;51:1188-1195.
11. Barr RG, Seliger S, Appel GB, et al. Prognosis in proliferative lupus nephritis: role of socioeconomic status and race/ethnicity. *Nephrol Dial Transplant.* 2003;18:2039-2046.
12. Contreras G, Lenz O, Pardo V, et al. Outcome in African Americans and Hispanics with lupus nephritis. *Kidney Int.* 2006;69:1846-1851.
13. Hahn BH: Over-view of the pathogenesis of SLE. In Wallace DJ, Hahn BH, eds. *Dubois' Lupus Erythematosus.* 7th ed. Philadelphia: Lippincott Williams & Wilkins; 2007:46-53.
14. Waldman M, Madaio MP. Pathogenic autoantibodies in lupus nephritis. *Lupus.* 2005;14:19-24.
15. Salmon J, Millard S, Schacter L, et al. FcgammaRIIA alleles are heritable risk factors for lupus nephritis in African-Americans. *J Clin Invest.* 1996;97:1348-1354.
16. Hom G, Graham RR, Modrek B, et al. Association of SLE with C8orf13-BLK and ITGAM–ITGAY. *N Engl J Med.* 2008;358:900-909.
17. Appel GB, Cohen DJ, Pirani CL, et al. Long term follow-up of lupus nephritis: a study based on the WHO classification. *Am J Med.* 1987;83:877.

18. Crow MK. Developments in the clinical understanding of lupus. *Arthritis Res Therapy*. 2009;11:245-264.

19. Crispin JC, Liossis SN, Kis-Toth K, et al. Pathogenesis of human SLE: recent advances. *Trends Mol Med*. 2010;16:47-57.

20. Berden JH, Licht R, van Bruggen MC, et al. Role of nucleosomes for induction and glomerular binding of autoantibodies in lupus nephritis. *Curr Opin Nephrol Hypertension*. 1999;8:299-301.

21. Bhatt P, Radhakrishnan J. B lymphocytes and lupus nephritis: new insights into pathogenesis and targeted therapies. *Kidney Int*. 2008;73:261-268.

22. Hahn BH. Antibodies to DNA. *N Engl J Med*. 1998;338:1359-1368.

23 Ng KP, Manson JJ, Rahman A, et al. Association of anti-nucleosome antibodies with disease flare in serologically active clinically quiescent SLE. *Rheumatology*. 2006;55:900-904.

24. D'Agati VD. Renal disease in systemic lupus erythematosus, mixed connective tissue disease, Sjogren's syndrome, and rheumatoid arthritis. In: Jennette CJ, Olson L, Schwartz MM, et al., eds. *Pathology of the Kidney*. 5th ed. Philadelphia: Lippincott-Raven; 1998.

25. Mortensen ES, Fentor KA, Rekvig O. Lupus nephritis: the central role of nucleosomes. *Am J Pathol*. 2008;172:275-283.

26. Behara VY, Whittier WL, Korbet SM, et al. Pathogenetic features of severe segmental lupus nephritis. *Nephrol Dial Transplant*. 2010;25:153-159.

27. Sprangers B, Appel GB. Renal vascular involvement in SLE. In: Lewis EJ, Schwartz M, Korbet SM, eds. *Lupus Nephritis*. Oxford: Oxford Press; 2010.

28. Churg J, Bernstien J, Glassock R. *Renal Disease: Classification and Atlas of Glomerular Diseases*. 2nd ed. New York: Igaku-Shoin; 1995:152.

29. Weening JJ, D'Agati VD, Appel GB, et al. The classification of glomerulonephritis systemic lupus nephritis revisited. *Kidney Int*. 2004;65:521-530.

30. Markowitz GS, D'Agati VD. The ISN/RPS 2003 classification of lupus nephritis: an assessment at 3 years. *Kidney Int*. 2007;71:491–195.

31. Markowitz GS, D'Agati VD. Classification of lupus nephritis. *Curr Opin Nephrol Hypertens*. 2009;18:220-225.

32. Appel GB, Silva FG, Pirani CL, et al. Renal involvement in systemic lupus erythematosus: a study involving 56 patients emphasizing histologic classification. *Medicine*. 1978;57:371-410.

33. Magil AB, Puterman ML, Ballon HS, et al. Prognostic factors in diffuse proliferative lupus glomerulonephritis. *Kidney Int*. 1988;34:511-517.

34. Ponticelli C, Zucchelli P, Moroni G, et al. Long-term prognosis of diffuse lupus nephritis. *Clin Nephrol*. 1987;28:263.

35 Nasr SH, D'Agati VD, Park HR, et al. Necrotizing and crescentic lupus nephritis with antineutrophil cytoplasmic antibody seropositivity. *Clin J Am Soc Nephrol*. 2008;3:682-690.

36. Donadio Jr JV, Burgess JK, Holley KE. Membranous lupus nephropathy: a clinicopathologic study. *Medicine*. 1977;56:527.

37. Sloane RP, Schwartz MM, Korbet SM, et al. Long-term outcome in systemic lupus erythematosus membranous glomerulonephritis. *J Am Soc Nephrol*. 1996;7:299-305.

38. Pasquali S, Banfi G, Zucchelli A, et al. Lupus membranous nephropathy: long-term outcome. *Clin Nephrol*. 1993;39:175-182.

39. Jennette JC, Iskander SS, Dalldorf FG. Pathologic differentiation between lupus and nonlupus membranous glomerulopathy. *Kidney Int*. 1983;24:377.

40. D'Agati VD, Appel GB. Renal pathology of HIV infection. *Semin Nephrol*. 1998;18:406-421.

41. Austin HA, Boumpas DT, Vaughan EM, et al. Predicting renal outcomes in severe lupus nephritis: contributions of clinical and histologic data. *Kidney Int*. 1994;43:544-550.

42. Schwartz M, Berstein J, Hill GS, et al. Predictive value of renal pathology in diffuse proliferative lupus glomerulonephritis. *Kidney Int*. 1989;36:891-896.

43. Schwartz MM. The holy grail: pathological indices in LN. *Kidney Int*. 2000;58:1354-1355.

44. Valeri A, Rhadhakrishnan J, D'Agati V, et al. IV pulse Cytoxan treatment of severe lupus nephritis. *Clin Nephrol*. 1994;42:71-78.

45. Radharkrishnan J, Kunis CL, D'Agati V, et al. Cyclosporin treatment of membranous lupus nephropathy. *Clin Nephrol*. 1994;42:147-154.

46. Park MH, D'Agati VD, Appel GB, et al. Tubulointerstitial disease in lupus nephritis: relationship to immune deposits, interstitial inflammation, glomerular changes, renal function, and prognosis. *Nephron*. 1986;44:309-319.

47. Hill G, Delahousse M, Nochy D, et al. A new index for evaluation of renal biopsies in lupus nephritis. *Kidney Int*. 2000;58:11600–1173.

48. Hill GS, Delahousse M, Nochy D, et al. Proteinuria and tubulointerstitial lesions in LN. *Kidney Int*. 2001;60:1893-1903.

49. Daniel L, Sichez H, Giorgi R, et al. Tubular lesions and tubular cell adhesion molecules for the prognosis of lupus nephritis. *Kidney Int*. 2001;60:2215-2221.

50. D'Agati V, Appel GB, Knowles D, et al. Monoclonal antibody identification of mononuclear cells in renal biopsies of lupus nephritis. *Kidney Int*. 1986;30:573.

51. Banfi G, Bertani T, Boeri V, et al. Renal vascular lesions as a marker of a poor prognosis in patients with lupus nephritis. *Am J Kidney Dis*. 1991;18:240.

52. Appel GB, Pirani CL, D'Agati VD. Renal vascular complications of systemic lupus erythematosus. *J Am Soc Nephrol*. 1994;4:1499.

53. Abdellatif AA, Waris J, Lakhani A, et al. True vasculitis in lupus nephritis. *Clin Nephrol*. 2010;74:106-112.

54. Hertig A, Droz D, Lesavre P, et al. SLE and idiopathic nephrotic syndrome: coincidence or not? *Am J Kidney Dis*. 2002;40:1179-1184.

55. Dube GK, Markowitz GS, Radhakrishnan J, et al. Minimal change disease in SLE. *Clin Nephrol*. 2002;57:120-126.

56. Chang BG, Markowitz GS, Seshan SV, et al. Renal manifestations of concurrent SLE and HIV infection. *Am J Kidney Dis*. 1999;33:441-449.

57. Font J, Torras A, Cervera R, et al. Silent renal disease in systemic lupus erythematosus. *Clin Nephrol*. 27(6):283-288.

58. Mannik M, Merrill CE, Stamps LD, et al. Multiple autoantibodies form the glomerular immune deposits in patients with SLE. *J Rheum*. 2003;30:1495-1504.

59. Foster MH, Cizman B, Madaio MP. Nephritogenic autoantibodies in systemic lupus erythematosus: immunochemical properties, mechanisms of immune deposition, and genetic origins. *Lab Invest*. 1993;69:494.

60. Sharp GC, Irvin WS, Tan EJ, et al. Mixed connective tissue disease: an apparently distinct rheumatic disease syndrome associated with a specific antibody to an extractable nuclear antigen (ENA). *Am J Med*. 1972;52:148.

61 Buyon JD, Clancy RM. Maternal autoantibodies and congenital heart block: mediators, markers, and therapeutic approach. *Semin Arthritis Rheum*. 2003;33:140-154.

62. Reichlin M. Clinical and immunologic significance of antibodies to Ro and La in systemic lupus erythematosus. *Arthritis Rheum*. 1982;25:767.

63. Termaat RM, Assmann KJM, Dijkman HBPM, et al. Anti-DNA antibodies can bind to the glomerulus via two distinct mechanisms. *Kidney Int*. 1992;43:1363.

64. Morioka T, Woitas R, Fujigaki Y, et al. Histone mediates glomerular deposition of small size DNA anti-DNA complex. *Kidney Int*. 1994;45:991.

65. D'Cruz DP, Houssiau FA, Ramirez G, et al. Antibodies to endothelial cells in systemic lupus erythematosus: a potential marker for nephritis and vasculitis. *Clin Exp Immunol*. 1991;85:254.

66. Kowal C, Degiorgio LA, Lee JY, et al. Human lupus autoantibodies against NMDA receptors mediate cognitive impairment. *Proc Nat Acad Sci*. 2000;103:19854.

67. Frampton G, Hicks J, Cameron JS. Significance of anti-phospholipid antibodies in patients with lupus nephritis. *Kidney Int*. 1991;39:1225.

68. Laitman RS, Glicklich D, Sablay L, et al. Effect of long-term normalization of serum complement levels on the course of lupus nephritis. *Am J Med*. 1989;87:132.

69. Walport MJ. Complement. *N Engl J Med*. 2001;344:1058-1060, 1140–1144.

70. Greisman SG, Redecha PB, Kimberly RP, et al. Differences among immune complexes: association of C1q in SLE immune complexes with renal disease. *J Immunol*. 1987;138:739.

71. Noel L-H, Droz D, Rothfield NF. Clinical and serologic significance of cutaneous deposits of immunoglobulins, C3 and C1q, in SLE patients with nephritis. *Clin Immunol Immunopathol*. 1978;10:318.

72. Rovin B. Biomarkers for lupus nephritis. *Clin J Am Soc Nephrol*. 2009;4:1858-1865.

73. Rubin RL: Drug induced lupus. In Wallace DJ, Hahn BH, eds. *Dubois' Lupus Erythematosus*. 7th ed. Philadelphia: Lippincott Williams & Wilkins; 2007:870-900.

74. Yung RL, Johnson KJ, Richardson BC. New concepts in the pathogenesis of drug-induced lupus. *Lab Invest*. 1995;73:746.

75. Reidenberg MM, Drayer DE, Lorenzo B, et al. Acetylation phenotypes and environmental chemical exposure of people with idiopathic systemic lupus erythematosus. *Arthritis Rheum 3*. 1992;36(7):971-973.

76. Crowson AN, Magro CM. Diltiazem and subacute cutaneous lupus erythematosus-like lesions [letter]. *N Engl J Med*. 1995;333:1429.

77. Gordon MM, Porter D. Minocycline induced lupus, case series in the west of Scotland. *J Rheumatol*. 2001;28:1004-1006.

78. Debandt M, Vittecq O, Descamps V, et al. Anti-TNF alpha induced SLE. *Clin Rheumatol*. 2003;22:56-61.

79. Shakoor N, Michalska M, Harris CD, et al. Drug induced SLE associated with etanercept therapy. *Lancet*. 2002;359:579-580.

80. Shapiro KS, Pinn VW, Harrington JT, et al. Immune complex glomerulonephritis in hydralazine-induced SLE. *Am J Kidney Dis*. 1984;3:270.

81. Short AK, Lockwood CM. Antigen specificity in hydralazine associated ANCA positive vasculitis. *Q J Med*. 1995;88:775.

82. Burlingame RW, Rubin RL. Drug-induced anti-histone autoantibodies display two patterns of reactivity with substructures of chromatin. *J Clin Invest*. 1991;88:680.

83. Urowitz MIB, Gladman DD, Farewell VT, et al. Lupus and pregnancy studies. *Arthritis Rheum*. 1993;36:1392.

84. Moroni G, Quaglini S, Banfi G, et al. Pregnancy in LN. *Am J Kidney Dis.* 2002;40:713-720.

85. Ruiz-Irastorza G, Lima F, Alves J, et al. Increased rate of lupus flare during pregnancy and the puerperium: a prospective study of 78 pregnancies. *Br J Rheumatol.* 1996;35:133.

86. Petri M, Howard D, Repke J. Frequency of lupus flare in pregnancy: the Hopkins lupus pregnancy center experience. *Arthritis Rheum.* 1991;34:1358.

87. Hayslett JP. Maternal and fetal complications in pregnant women with systemic lupus erythematosus. *Am J Kidney Dis.* 1991;17:123.

88. Julkunen K, Kaaja R, Palosuo T, et al. Pregnancy in lupus nephropathy. *Acta Obstet Gynecol Scand.* 1993;72:258.

89. Julkunen EL, Jouhaikainen T, Kaaja R, et al. Fetal outcome in lupus pregnancy: a retrospective case-control study of 242 pregnancies in 112 patients. *Lupus.* 1993;2:125.

90. Petri M, Albritton J. Fetal outcome of lupus pregnancy: a retrospective case-control study of the Hopkins lupus cohort. *J Rheumatol.* 1993;20:650.

91. McNeil HP, Chesterman CN, Krilis SA. Immunology and clinical importance of antiphospholipid antibodies. *Adv Immunol.* 1991;49:193.

92. Conlon PJ, Fischer CA, Levesqu MC, et al. Clinical, biochemical, and pathological predictors of poor response to IV cyclophosphamide in DPLN. *Clin Nephrol.* 1996;46:170-175.

93. Gourley MF, Austin HA, Scott D, et al. Methylprednisolone and cyclophosphamide, alone or in combination, in patients with lupus nephritis. *Ann Intern Med.* 1996;125:549-557.

94. Boumpas DT, Austin HA, Vaughn EM, et al. Controlled trial of pulse methylprednisolone versus two regimens of cyclophosphamide in severe lupus nephritis. *Lancet.* 1992;340:741-745.

95. Chagnac A, Kiberd BA, Farinas MC, et al. Outcome of the acute glomerular injury in proliferative lupus nephritis. *J Clin Invest.* 1989;84:922-930.

96. Ward MM. Cardiovascular and cerebrovascular morbidity and mortality among women with ESRD attributed to LN. *Am J Kidney Dis.* 2000;36:516-525.

97. Cheigh JS, Stenzel KH. End-stage renal disease in SLE. *Am J Kidney Dis.* 1993;21:2.

98. Ward MM. Outcomes of renal transplantation among patients with end-stage renal disease caused by lupus nephritis. *Kidney Int.* 2000;57:2136-2143.

99. Lochhead KM, Pirsch JD, D'Alessandro AK, et al. Risk factors for renal allograft loss in patients with systemic lupus erythematosus. *Kidney Int.* 1996;49:512.

100. Stone JH, Millwood CL, Olson JL, et al. Frequency of recurrent lupus nephritis among 97 renal transplant patients during the cyclophosphamide era. *Arthritis Rheum.* 1998;41:678-686.

101. Contreras G, Mattiazzi A, Guerra G, et al. Recurrence of lupus nephritis after kidney transplantation. *J Am Soc Nephrol.* 2010;21:1200-1207.

102. Norby GE, Strom EH, Midtvedt K, et al. Recurrent lupus nephritis after kidney transplantation: a surveillance biopsy study. *Ann Rheum Dis.* 2010;69:1484-1487.

103. Radhakrishnan J, Williams GS, Appel GB, et al. Renal transplantation in anticardiolipin positive lupus erythematosus patients. *Am J Kidney Dis.* 1994;23:286.

104. Stone JH, Amend WJ, Criswell LA. Antiphospholipid antibody syndrome in renal transplantation: occurrence of clinical events in 96 consecutive patients with systemic lupus erythematosus. *Am J Kidney Dis.* 1999;34:1040.

105. Moroni G, Qualini S, Maccario M, et al. "Nephritic flares" are predictors of bad long-term renal outcome in lupus nephritis. *Kidney Int.* 1996;50:2047-2053.

106. Magil AB, Puterman ML, Ballon HS, et al. Prognostic factors in diffuse proliferative lupus glomerulonephritis. *Kidney Int.* 1988;34:511.

107. Nossent HC, Henzen-Logmans SC, Vroom TM, et al. Contribution of renal biopsy data in predicting outcome in lupus nephritis. Analysis of 116 patients. *Arthritis Rheum.* 1990;33:970.

108. Esdaile JM, Federgreen W, Quintal H, et al. Predictors of one year out-come in lupus nephritis: the importance of renal biopsy. *Q J Med.* 1991;81:907.

109. Schwartz MM, Lan S-P, Bernstain J, et al. Role of pathology indices in the management of severe lupus glomerulonephritis. *Kidney Int.* 1992;42:743-748.

110. Balow JE, Boumpas DT, Fessler BJ, et al. Management of lupus nephritis. *Kidney Int.* 1996;49(suppl):S88-S92.

111. Najafi CC, Korbet SM, Lewis EJ, et al. Significance of histologic patterns of glomerular injury upon long-term prognosis in severe lupus glomerulonephritis. *Kidney Int.* 2001;59:2156-2163.

112. Steinberg AD, Steinberg SC. Long-term preservation of renal function in patients with lupus nephritis receiving treatment that includes cyclophosphamide versus those treated with prednisone only. *Arthritis Rheum.* 1991;34:945-950.

113. Bakir AA, Levy PS, Dunea G. The prognosis of lupus nephritis in African-Americans: a retrospective analysis. *Am J Kidney Dis.* 1994;24:159.

114. Tejani A, Nicastri AD, Chen C-K, et al. Lupus nephritis in Black and Hispanic children. *Am J Dis Child.* 1983;137:481-483.

115. Austin HA, Boumpas DT, Vaughan EM, et al. Predicting renal outcomes in severe lupus nephritis: contributions of clinical and histologic data. *Kidney Int.* 1994;43:544-550.

116. Houssieau FA, Vasconcelos C, D'Cruz D, et al. Early response to immunosuppressive therapy predicts good renal outcome in lupus nephritis: lessons from long-term follow of patients in the Euro-Lupus Nephritis Trial. *Arthritis Rheum.* 2004;50:3934-3940.

117. Korbet SM, Lewsi EJ, Schwartz MM, et al. Factors predictive of outcome in severe lupus nephritis. *Am J Kidney Dis.* 2000;35:904-914.

118. Mosca M, Bencivelli W, Neri R, et al. Renal flares in 91 SLE patients with diffuse proliferative glomerulonephritis. *Kidney Int.* 2002;61:1502-1509.

119. Ponticelli C, Moroni G. Flares in lupus nephritis: incidence, impact on renal survival and management. *Lupus.* 1998;7:635-638.

120. Ioannidis JPA, Boki KA, Katsorida ME, et al. Remission, relapse, and re-remission of LN treated with cyclophosphamide. *Kidney Int.* 2000;57:258-264.

121. Pablos JL, Gutierrez-Millet V, Gomez-Reino JJ. Remission of LN with cyclophosphamide and late relapse following therapy withdrawal. *Scand J Rheumatol.* 1994;23:142-144.

122. Ciruelo E, DelaCruz J, Lopez I, et al. Cumulative rate of relapse of LN after successful treatment with cyclophosphamide. *Arthritis Rheum.* 1996;12:2028-2034.

123. Hill GS, Delahousse M, Nochy D, et al. Outcome of relapse in lupus nephritis: roles of reverse of renal fibrosis and response of inflammation therapy. *Kidney Int.* 2002;61:2176-2186.

124. Martins L, Rocha G, Rodriguez A, et al. LN: a retrospective review of 78 cases from a single center. *Clin Nephrol.* 2002;57:114-119.

125. Hill GS, Delahousse M, Nochy D, et al. Predictive power of the second renal biopsy in lupus nephritis: significance of macrophages. *Kidney Int.* 2001;59:304-316.

126. McCune WJ, Golbus J, Zeldes W, et al. Clinical and immunologic effects of monthly administration of intravenous cyclophosphamide in severe lupus erythematosus. *N Engl J Med.* 1988;318:1423-1431.

127. Lehman TJA, Sherry DD, Wagner-Weiner L, et al. Intermittent intravenous cyclophosphamide therapy for lupus nephritis. *J Pediatr.* 1989;114:1055-1060.

128. Illei GG, Austin HA, Crane M, et al. Combination therapy with pulse cyclophosphamide plus pulse methylprednisolone improves long-term renal outcome without adding toxicity in patients with LN. *Ann Intern Med.* 2001;21:248-257.

129. Grootscholten C, Ligtenberg G, Hagen EC, et al. Azathioprine/methylprednisolone versus cyclophosphamide in proliferative lupus nephritis. A randomized controlled trial. *Kidney Int.* 2006;70:732-742.

130. Boumpas DT, Austin HA, Vaughn EM, et al. Risk for sustained amenorrhea in patients with SLE receiving intermittent pulse cyclophosphamide therapy. *Ann Intern Med.* 1993;119:366-369.

131. Kleta R. Cyclophosphamide and mercaptoethane sulfonate (MESNA) therapy for minimal lesion glomerulonephritis. *Kidney Int.* 1999;56:2312-2313.

132. McKinley A, Park E, Spetie D, et al. Oral cyclophosphamide for lupus glomerulonephritis: an underused therapeutic option. *Clin J Am Soc Nephrol.* 2009;4:1754-1760.

133. Appel AS, Appel GB. An update on the use of mycophenolate in lupus nephritis and other primary glomerular diseases. *Nat Clin Pract Nephrol.* 2009;5:132-142.

134. Appel GB, Waldman M, Radhakrishnan J. New approaches to the treatment of glomerular disease. *Kidney Int.* 2006;70(suppl):S45-S50.

135. Dooley MA, Cosio FG, Nachman PH, et al. MMF therapy in LN: clinical observations. *J Am Soc Nephrol.* 1999;10:833-839.

136. Kingdon EJ, McLean AG, Psimerrou E, et al. The safety and efficacy of MMF in lupus nephritis: a pilot study. *Lupus.* 2001;10:606-611.

137. Mok CC, Lai KN. Mycophenolate mofetil in lupus glomerulonephritis. *Am J Kidney Dis.* 2002;40:447-457.

138. Li LS, Hu WX, Chen HP, Liu ZH. Comparison of MMF versus cyclophosphamide pulse therapy in the induction treatment of severe diffuse proliferative LN in Chinese population. *J Am Nephrol.* 2000;11(suppl A):486A.

139. Chan TM, Li FK, Tang CS, et al. Efficacy of mycophenolate mofetil in patients with diffuse proliferative LN. *N Engl J Med.* 2000;343:1156-1162.

140. Chan TM, Tse KC, Tang CS, et al. Hong Kong Nephrology Study Group. Long-term study of mycophenolate mofetil as continuous induction and maintenance treatment of diffuse proliferative lupus nephritis. *J Am Soc Nephrol.* 2005;16:1076-1084.

141. Ginzler E, Dooley MA, Aranow C, et al. Mycophenolate mofetil or intravenous cyclophosphamide for lupus nephritis. *N Engl J Med.* 2005;353:2219-2228.

142. Appel GB, Contreras G, Dooley MA, et al and the Aspreva Lupus Management Study Group: Mycophenolate mofetil compared with intravenous cyclophosphamide as induction treatment for lupus nephritis. *J Am Soc Nephrol.* 2009;20:1103-1113.

143. Isenberg D, Appel G, Contreras G, et al. Influence of race/ethnicity on response to lupus nephritis treatment: the ALMS study. *Rheumatology.* 2009;49:128-140.

144. Houssiau FA, Vasconcelos C, D'Cruz D, et al. Immunosuppressive therapy in lupus nephritis, Euro-Lupus Trial. A randomized trial of low dose versus high dose intravenous cyclophosphamide. *Arthritis Rheum.* 2002;46:2121-2131.

145. Houssieau FA, Vasconcelos C, D'Cruz D, et al. Early response to immunosuppressive therapy predicts good renal outcome in lupus nephritis: lessons from long-term follow of patients in the Euro-Lupus Nephritis Trial. *Arthritis Rheum.* 2004;50:3934-3940.

146. Contreras G, Pardo V, Leclercq B, et al. Sequential therapies for proliferative lupus nephritis. *N Engl J Med.* 2004;350:971-980.

147. Houssiau FA, D'Cruz D, Sangle S, et al., for the MAINTAIN Nephritis Trial Group. Azathioprine versus mycophenolate mofetil for long-term immunosuppression in lupus nephritis: results from the MAINTAIN Nephritis Trial. *Ann Rheum Dis.* 2010;9(12):2083-2089.

148. Jayne DRW, Appel GB, Dooley MA, et al. Results of Aspreva Lupus Management Study (ALMS) Maintenance Phase (abstr). *J Am Soc Nephrol.* 2010;21:25A.

149. Bao H, Liu Z-H, Xie H-L, et al. Successful treatment of class V+IV lupus nephritis with multitarget therapy. *J Am Soc Nephrol.* 2008;19:2001-2010.

150. Vincenti F, Cohen SD, Appel G. Novel B cell therapeutic targets in transplantation and immune mediated glomerular diseases. *Clin J Am Soc Nephrol.* 2010;5(1):142-151.

151. Merrill JT, Neuwelt CM, Wallace DJ, et al. Efficacy and safety of rituximab in moderately-to-severely active systemic lupus erythematosus: the randomized, double-blind, phase II/III systemic lupus erythematosus evaluation of rituximab trial. *Arthritis Rheum.* 2010;62(1):222-233.

152. Bao H, Liu ZH, Xie HL, et al. Successful treatment of class V+IV lupus nephritis with multitarget therapy. *J Am Soc Nephrol.* 2008;19(10):2001-2010.

153. Ng KP, Leandro MJ, Edwards JC, et al. Repeated B cell depletion in treatment of refractory SLE. *Ann Rheum Dis.* 2006;65:942-945.

154. Terrier B, Amoura Z, Ravaud P, et al. Club Rhumatismes et Inflammation: Safety and efficacy of rituximab in systemic lupus erythematosus: results from 136 patients from the French AutoImmunity and Rituximab registry. *Arthritis Rheum.* 2010;62(8):2458-2466.

155. Sharpe AH, Abbas AK. T-cell costimulation: biology, therapeutic potential, and challenges. *N Engl J Med.* 2006;355:973-975.

156. Davis J, Totositis M, Rosenberg J, et al. Phase I clinical trial of AntiCD40 ligand (IDEC 131) in patients with SLE. *J Rheum.* 2001;28:95-101.

157. Kawai T, Andrews D, Colvin RB, et al. Thromboembolitic complications after treatment with antiCD40 ligand. *Nature Med.* 2000;6:114.

158. Lewis EJ, Hunsicker LG, Lau SP, et al. For the Lupus Collaboration Study Group. A controlled trial of plasmapheresis in severe lupus nephritis. *N Engl J Med.* 1992;326:1373-1379.

159. Euler HH, Schroeder JO, Marten P, et al. Treatment free remission in sever SLE following synchronization of plasmapheresis with subsequent pulse cyclophosphamide. *Arthritis Rheum.* 1994;37:1784-1794.

160 Gelfand J, Truong L, Stern L, et al. Thrombotic thrombocytopenic purpura syndrome in SLE: treatment with plasma infusion. *Am J Kidney Dis.* 1985;6:154-160.

161. Lin C-Y, Hsu H-C, Chiang H. Improvement of histological and immunological change in steroid and immunosuppressive drug-resistant lupus nephritis by high-dose intravenous gamma globulin. *Nephron.* 1989;53:303-310.

162. Boletis JN, Ioannidis JPA, Boki KA, et al. Intravenous immunoglobulin compared with cyclophosphamide for proliferative LN. *Lancet.* 1999;354:569.

163. Pierucci A, Simonetti BM, Pecci G, et al. Improvement of renal function with selective thromboxane antagonism in lupus nephritis. *N Engl J Med.* 1989;320:421-425.

164. Wang Y, Hu Q, Madri JA, et al. Amelioration of lupus-like autoimmune disease in NZB/NZW F1 mice after treatment with a blocking monoclonal antibody specific for complement component 5. *Proc Nat Acad Sci.* 1996;93:8563-8568.

165. Brodsky R, Petri M, Smith D, et al. Immunoablative high dose cyclophosphamide without stem cell rescue for refractory severe autoimmune disease. *Ann Intern Med.* 1998;129:1031-1035.

166. Traynor AE, Schroeder J, Rosa RM, et al. Stem cell transplantation for resistant lupus. *Arthritis Rheum.* 1999;42:5170.

167. Alarcon-Segovia D, Tumlin JA, Furie RA, et al. LJP 394 for the prevention of renal flare in patients with SLE. *Arthritis Rheum.* 2003;48:442-454.

168. Navarra SV, Guzmán RM, Gallacher AE, et al., for the BLISS-52 Study Group. Efficacy and safety of belimumab in patients with active systemic lupus erythematosus: a randomised, placebo-controlled, phase 3 trial. *Lancet.* 2011;377(9767):721-731.

169. Lawson BR, Prud'homme GJ, Chang Y, et al. Treatment of murine lupus with cDNA encoding IFN gamma receptor/Fc. *J Clin Invest.* 2000;106(2):207-215.

170. Moroni G, Moccario M, Banfi G, et al. Treatment of membranous lupus nephritis. *Am J Kidney Dis.* 1998;31:681-686.

171. Austin HA, Vaughn EK, Boumpas DT, et al. Lupus membranous nephropathy: controlled trial of prednisone, pulse cyclophosphamide and cyclosporine. *J Am Soc Nephrol.* 2009;90:901-911.

172. Mok CC, Ying KY, Lau CS, et al. Treatment of membranous lupus with azathioprine and prednisone. *Am J Kidney Dis.* 2004;43:269.

173. Spetie DN, Tang Y, Rovin BH, et al. Mycophenolate mofetil therapy of SLE membranous nephropathy. *Kidney Int.* 2004;66:2411-2415.

174. Kavim MY, Pisoni CN, Ferro L, et al. Reduction of proteinuria with mycophenolate mofetil in predominantly membranous lupus nephropathy. *Rheumatology (Oxford).* 2005;44:1317-1321.

175. Radhakrishnan J, Moutzouris D-A, Ginzler E, et al. Mycophenolate mofetil and intravenous cyclophosphamide are similar as induction therapy for class V lupus nephritis. *Kidney Int.* 2010;77:152-160.

176. Uramoto KM, Michet Jr CJ, Thumboo J, et al. Trends in the incidence and mortality of systemic lupus erythematosus, 1950-1992. *Arthritis Rheum.* 1999;42(1):46-50.

177. Roman MJ, Shanker BA, Davis A, et al. Prevalence and correlates of accelerated atherosclerosis in SLE. *N Engl J Med.* 2003;349:2399-2406.

178. Bruce IN, Urowitz MB, Gladman DD, et al. Risk factors for coronary heart disease in women with SLE the Toronto Risk Factor Study. *Arthritis Rheum.* 2003;48:3159-3167.

179. Joseph RE, Radhakrishnan J, Appel GB. Antiphospholipid antibody syndrome and renal disease. *Curr Opin Nephrol Hypertens.* 2001;10:175-181.

180. Nzerue CM, Hewann-Lowe K, Pierangeli S, et al. "Black swan in the kidney." Renal involvement in the antiphospholipid antibody syndrome. *Kidney Int.* 2002;62:733-734.

181. Moroni G, Ventura D, Riva P, et al. Antiphospholipid antibodies are associated with an increased risk for chronic renal insufficiency in patients with lupus nephritis. *Am J Kidney Dis.* 2004;43:28.

182. Levine JS, Brauch DW, Rauch J. The antiphospholipid syndrome. *N Engl J Med.* 2002;346:752-763.

183. Giannakopoulos B, Passam F, Ioaanou Y, et al. How do we diagnose the antiphospholipid syndrome. *Blood.* 2009;113:985-994.

184. Miyakis S, Lockshin MD, Atsumi T, et al. International consensus statement on an update of the classification criteria for definite antiphospholipid syndrome (APS). *J Thromb Haemost.* 2006;4:295.

185. Kaul M, Erkan D, Sammaritano L, et al. Assessment of the 2006 revised antiphospholipid syndrome classification criteria. *Ann Rheum Dis.* 2007;66:927-930.

186. Detkova D, Gil-Aguado A, Lavilla P, et al. Do antibodies to beta2-glycoprotein I contribute to the better characterization of the antiphospholipid syndrome?. *Lupus.* 1999;6:430-436.

187. Forastiero R, Martinuzzo M. Prothrombotic mechanisms based on the impairment of fibrinolysis in the antiphospholipid syndrome. *Lupus.* 2008;10:872-877.

188. Urbanus RT, Derksen RH, de Groot PG. Platelets and the antiphospholipid syndrome. *Lupus.* 2008;17(10):888-894.

189. Raschi E, Borghi MO, Grossi C, et al. Toll-like receptors: another player in the pathogenesis of the anti-phospholipid syndrome. *Lupus.* 2008;17(10):937-942.

190. Rand JH, Wu XX, Quinn AS, et al. Resistance to annexin A5 anticoagulant activity: a thrombogenic mechanism for the antiphospholipid syndrome. *Lupus.* 2008;17(10):922-930.

191. Kaplanski G, Cacoub P, Farnarier C, et al. Increased soluble vascular cell adhesion molecule 1 concentrations in patients with primary or systemic lupus erythematosus-related antiphospholipid syndrome. Correlations with severity of thrombosis. *Arthritis Rheum.* 2000;43:55-64.

192. Love PE, Santoro SA. Antiphospholipid antibodies: Anticardiolipin and the lupus anticoagulant in SLE and in SLE disorders. *Ann Intern Med.* 1990;112:682-698.

193. de Bandt M, Benali K, Guillevin L, et al. Longitudinal determination of antiphospholipid antibodies in lupus patients without previous manifestations of antiphospholipid syndrome. A prospective study. *J Rheumatol.* 1999;26:91-96.

194. Shah NM, Khamashta MA, Alsumi T, et al. Outcome of patients with anticardiolipin antibodies: a 10 year follow-up of 52 patients. *Lupus.* 1998;7:3-6.

195. Sebastiani GD, Galeazzi M, Tincani A, et al. Anticardiolipin and antibetaGP1 antibodies in a large series of European patients with systemic lupus erythematosus. Prevalence and clinical associations. *Scand J Rheumatol.* 1999;28:344-351.

196. Cervera R, Piette JC, Font J, et al. Antiphospholipid syndrome: Clinical and immunologic manifestations and patterns of disease expression in a cohort of 1000 patients. *Arthritis Rheum.* 2002;46:1019-1027.

197. Lockshin MD. Answers to the Antiphospholipid antibody syndrome. *N Engl J Med.* 1995;332:1025-1027.

198. Harada M, Fujisawa Y, Sakisaka S, et al. High prevalence of anticardiolipin antibodies in hepatitis C virus infection: lack of effects on thrombocytopenia and thrombotic complications. *J Gastroenterol.* 2000;35:272-277.

199. Ankri A, Bonmarchand M, Coutellier A, et al. Antiphospholipid antibodies are an epiphenomenon in HIV-infected patients [letter]. *AIDS.* 1999;13:1282-1283.

200. Asherson RA, Espinosa G, Cervera R, et al. Disseminated intravascular coagulation in catastrophic antiphospholipid syndrome: clinical and haematological characteristics of 23 patients. *Ann Rheum Dis.* 2005;64:943.

201. Venkataseshan S, Barisoni L, Smith S, et al. Renal disease in antiphospholipid antibody syndrome (a study of 26 biopsied patients). *J Am Soc Nephrol.* 1996;7:1343.

202. Nochy D, Daugas E, Droz D, et al. The intrarenal vascular lesions associated with primary antiphospholipid syndrome. *J Am Soc Nephrol.* 1999;10:507-518.

203. Tektonidou MG, Sotsiou F, Nakopoulou L, et al. Antiphospholipid syndrome nephropathy in patients with systemic lupus erythematosus and antiphospholipid antibodies: prevalence, clinical associations, and long-term outcome. *Arthritis Rheum.* 2004;50:2569.

204. Saracino A, Ramunni A, Pannarale G, et al. Kidney disease associated with primary antiphospholipid syndrome: clinical signs and histopathological features in an case experience of five cases. *Clin Nephrol.* 2005;63:471.

205. Fakhouri F, Noel LH, Zuber J, et al. The expanding spectrum of renal diseases associated with antiphospholipid syndrome. *Am J Kidney Dis.* 2003;41:1205.

206. Godfrey T, Khamsahta MA, Hughes GRV. Antiphospholipid syndrome and renal artery stenosis. *Q J Med.* 2000;93:127-129.

207. Remondino GI, Mysler E, Pissano MN, et al. A reversible bilateral renal artery stenosis in association with the antiphospholipid syndrome. *Lupus.* 2000;9:65-67.

208. Riccialdelli L, Arnaldi G, Giacchetti G, et al. Hypertension due to renal artery occlusion in a patient with the antiphospholipid syndrome. *Am J Hypertens.* 2001;14:62-65.

209. Daugas E, Nochy D, Huong DL, et al. Anti-phospholipid syndrome nephropathy in SLE. *J Am Soc Nephrol.* 2002;13:42.

210. Prakash R, Miller CC, Suki WN. Anticardiolipin antibody in patients on maintenance hemodialysis and its association with recurrent AV graft thrombosis. *Am J Kidney Dis.* 1995;26:347-352.

211. Brunet P, Aillaud MF, SanMarco M, et al. Antiphospholipids in hemodialysis patients relationships between lupus anticoagulant and thrombosis. *Kidney Int.* 1995;48:794-800.

212. Valeri A, Radhakrishnan J. Anti-cardiolipin antibodies (ACLA) in hemodialysis patients: a prospective study of 230 patients. *J Am Soc Nephrol.* 1996;7:1423.

213. Ducloux D, Pettetm E, Fournier V, et al. Prevalence and clinical significance of antiphospholipid antibodies in renal transplant recipients. *Transplantation.* 1999;67:90.

214. Friedman GS, Meier-Kriesche HU, Kaplan B, et al. Hypercoagulable states in renal transplantation candidates: impact of anticoagulation upon incidence of renal allograft thrombosis. *Transplantation.* 2001;72:1073.

215. Forman JP, Lin J, Pascual M, et al. Significance of anticardiolipin antibodies on short and long-term allograft survival and function following kidney transplantation. *Am J Transplant.* 2004;11:1786-1791.

216. Baid S, Pascual M, Williams Jr WW, et al. Renal thrombotic microangiopathy associated with anticardiolipin antibodies in hepatitis C-positive renal allograft recipients. *J Am Soc Nephrol.* 1999;10:146-153.

217. Khamashta MA, Cuadrado MJ, Mujic F, et al. The management of thrombosis in the antiphospholipid-antibody syndrome. *N Engl J Med.* 1995;332:993-997.

218. Joseph RE, Valeri A, Radhakrishnan J, et al. Anticardiolipin antibody levels in lupus nephritis: effects of immunosuppression. *J Am Soc Nephrol.* 1997;8:89.

219. Alarcon-Segovia D, Boffa MC, Branch W, et al. Prophylaxis of the antiphospholipid syndrome: a consensus report. *Lupus.* 2003;12:499-503.

220. Kutteh WH. Antiphospholipid antibody-associated recurrent pregnancy: treatment with heparin and low dose aspirin is superior to low dose aspirin alone. *Am J Obstet Gynecol.* 1996;174:1584-1589.

221. Kobayashi S, Tamura N, Tsuda H, et al. Immunoadsorbent plasmapheresis for a patient with antiphospholipid syndrome during pregnancy. *Ann Rheum Dis.* 1992;51(3):399-401.

222. Faria MS, Mota C, Barbot J, et al. Haemolytic uraemic syndrome, cardiomyopathy, cutaneous vasculopathy and anti-phospholipid activity. *Nephrol Dial Transplant.* 2000;15:1891-1892.

223. Takeshita Y, Turumi Y, Touma S, et al. Successful delivery in a pregnant woman with lupus anticoagulant positive systemic lupus erythematosus treated with double plasmapheresis. *Ther Apher.* 2001;5:22-24.

224. Piette JC, Le Tiu Huong D, Wechsler B. Therapeutic use of intravenous immunoglobulins in the antiphospholipid syndrome. *Ann Med Intern.* 2000;151(suppl 1):1551-1554.

225. Nasai R, Janicinova V, Petrikova ML. Chloroquine inhibits stimulated platelets at the arachidonic acid pathway. *Thromb Res.* 1995;77:531-542.

226. Sharp GC, Irvin WS, Tan EM, et al. Mixed connective tissue disease: an apparently distinct rheumatic disease syndrome associated with a specific antibody to an extractable nuclear antigen (ENA). *Am J Med.* 1972;52:148.

227. Alarcon-Segovia D, Cardiel MH. Comparison between 3 diagnostic criteria for mixed connective tissue disease. Study of 593 patients. *J Rheumatol.* 1989;16:328.

228. Maldonandado ME, Perez M, Pignac-Kobinger J, et al. Clinical and immunologic manifestations of mixed connective tissue disease in a Miami population compared to a Midwestern US Caucasian population. *J Rheumatol.* 2008;35:429.

229. Kasukawa R. Mixed connective tissue disease. *Intern Med.* 1999;38:386.

230. Hoffman RW, Greidinger EL. Mixed connective tissue disease. *Curr Opin Rheumatol.* 2000;12:386.

231. Gendi NS, Welsh KI, van Venrooij WJ, et al. HLA type as a predictor of MCTD differentiation. Ten year clinical and immunogenetic follow-up of 46 patients. *Arthritis Rheum.* 1995;38:259.

232. Burdt MA, Hoffman RW, Deutscher SL, et al. Long-term outcome in MCTD. Longitudinal clinical and serologic findings. *Arthritis Rheum.* 1999;42:899.

233. Piirainen HI, Kurki PT. Clinical and serologic follow-up of patients with polyarthritis, Raynaud's phenomenon, and circulating RNP antibodies. *Scand J Rheumatol.* 1990;19:51.

234. Kitridou RC, Akmal M, Turkel SB, et al. Renal involvement in MCTD a longitudinal clinicopathologic study. *Semin Arthritis Rheum.* 1986;16:135.

235. Bennett RM. Scleroderma overlap syndromes. *Rheum Dis Clin North Am.* 1990;16:185.

236. Hoffman RW, Cassidy JT, Takeda Y, et al. U1-70kd autoantibody positive MCTD in children. A longitudinal clinical and serologic analysis. *Arthritis Rheum.* 1993;36:1599.

237. Appelboom T, Kahn MF, Mairesse N. Antibodies to small ribonucleoprotein and to 73 KD heat shock protein: two distinct markers of MCTD. *Clin Exp Immunol.* 1995;100:486.

238. Fuller TJ, Richman AV, Auerbach D, et al. Immune complex glomerulonephritis in a patient with MCTD. *Am J Med.* 1977;62:761.

239. Celikbilek M, Elsurer R, Afsar B, et al. Mixed connective tissue disease: a case with scleroderma renal crisis following abortion. *Clin Rheumatol.* 2007;26:1545-1547.

240. Ito S, Nakamura T, Kurosawa R, et al. Glomerulonephritis in children with mixed connective tissue disease. *Clin Nephrol.* 2006;66:160-165.

241. Pelferman TG, McIntosh CS, Kershaw M. MCTD associated with glomerulonephritis and hypocomplementemia. *Postgrad Med J.* 1980;56:177.

242. Kobayashi S, Nagase M, Kimura M, et al. Renal involvement in MCTD. *Am J Nephrol.* 1985;5:282.

243. Bennett RM. MCTD. In: Grishman E, Churg J, Needle MA, Venkataseshan VS, eds. *The Kidney in Collagen Vascular Diseases.* New York: Raven Press; 1993:167.

244. Sawait, Murakami K, Kurasano Y. Morphometric analysis of the kidney lesions in MCTD. *Tohoku J Exp Med.* 1994;174:141.

245. Kessler E, Halpern M, Chagnac A, et al. Unusual renal deposits in MCTD. *Arch Pathol Lab Med.* 1992;116:261.

246. McLaughlin VV, Genthner DE, Pannella MM, et al. Compassionate use of continuous prostacyclin in the management of secondary pulmonary hypertension: a case series. *Ann Intern Med.* 1999;130:740.

247. Ulmer A, Kotter I, Pfaff A, et al. Efficacy of pulsed IV immunoglobulin therapy in MCTD. *J Am Acad Dermatol.* 2002;46:123.

248. Watts R, Lane S, Hanslik T, et al. Development and validation of a consensus methodology for the classification of the ANCA-associated vasculitides and polyarteritis nodosa for epidemiologic studies. *Ann Rheum Dis.* 2007;66:222-227.

249. Hoffman GS, Kerr GS, Leavitt RY, et al. Wegener's granulomatosis: an analysis of 158 patients. *Ann Interm Med.* 1992;116:488-498.

250. Falk RJ, Nachman PH, Hogan SL, et al. ANCA Glomerulonephritis and vasculitis: a Chapel Hill perspective. *Semin Nephrol.* 2000;20:233-242.

251. Savage J, Davies D, Falk RJ, et al. Antineutrophil cytoplasmic antibodies and associated diseases: a review of the clinical and laboratory features. *Kidney Int.* 2000;57:846.

252. Savage CO. ANCA-associated renal vasculitis: Nephrology Forum. *Kidney Int.* 2001;60:1614-1627.

253. Jennette JC, Falk RJ. Small-vessel vasculitis. *N Engl J Med.* 1997;337:1512-1523.

254. Franssen CF, Stegman CA, Kellenberg CGM, et al. Antiproteinase 3 and antimyeloperoxidase associated vasculitis. *Kidney Int.* 2000;57:2195-2206.

255. Moutsakis D-A, Herlitz L, Appel GB, et al. Renal biopsy in the very elderly. *Clin J Am Soc Nephrol.* 2009;4:1073-1082.

256. Kallenberg CG, Brouwer E, Weening JJ, et al. Anti-neutrophil cytoplasmic antibodies: current diagnostic and pathophysiological potential. *Kidney Int.* 1994;46:1.
257. Bomback AS, Appel GB, Radhakrishnan J, et al. ANCA-associated glomerulonephritis in the very elderly. *Kidney Int.* 2011;79(7):757-764.
258. Appel GB, Gee B, Kashgarian M, et al. Wegener's granulomatosis clinical-pathologic correlations and longterm course. *Am J Kidney Dis.* 1981;1:27-37.
259. ten Berge IJM, Wilmink JM, Meyer CJLM, et al. Clinical and immunological follow-up of patients with severe renal disease in Wegener's granulomatosis. *Am J Nephrol.* 1985;5:21-29.
260. Chen M, Yu F, Zhang Y, et al. Characteristics of Chinese patients with Wegener's granulomatosis with anti MPO antibodies. *Kidney Int.* 2005;68:2225-2229.
261. Muniain MA, Moreno JC, Gonzalez Campora R. Wegener's granulomatosis in two sisters. *J Rheum Dis.* 1986;45:417-421.
262. Papiha SS, Murty GE, Ad Hia A, et al. Association of Wegener's granulomatosis with HLA antigens and other genetic markers. *Ann Rheum Dis.* 1992;51:246-248.
263. Jennette JC, Falk RJ. The pathology of vasculitis involving the kidney. *Am J Kidney Dis.* 1994;24:130.
264. Ronco P, Mougenot B, Bindi P, et al. Clinicohistological features and long-term outcome of Wegener's granulomatosis in: renal involvement in systemic vasculitis. *Contrib Nephrol.* 1991;94:47-57.
265. Boucher A, Droz D, Adafer E, et al. Relationship between the integrity of Bowman's capsule and the composition of cellular crescents in human crescentic glomerulonephritis. *Lab Invest.* 1987;56:526-533.
266. Hauer HA, Bajema IM, Van Houwelingen HC, et al., for the European Vasculitis Study Group (EUVAS). Renal histology in ANCA-associated vasculitis: differences between diagnosis and serologic subgroups. *Kidney Int.* 2002;61:80-89.
267. Grotz W, Wanner C, Keller E, et al. Crescentic glomerulonephritis in Wegener's granulomatosis: morphology, therapy, and outcome. *Clin Nephrol.* 1991;35:243-251.
268. de Lind van Wijngaarden RA, van Rijn L, Hagen EC, et al. Hypotheses on the etiology of antineutrophil cytoplasmic autoantibody associated vasculitis: the cause is hidden, but the result is known. *Clin J Am Soc Nephrol.* 2008;3:237-252.
269. Yang J, Bautz DJ, Lionaki S, et al. ANCA patients have T cells responsive to complementary PR-3 antigen. *Kidney Int.* 2008;74:1159-1169.
270. Jennette JC, Xiao H, Falk RJ. The pathogenesis of vascular inflammation by antineutrophil cytoplasmic antibodies. *J Am Soc Nephrol.* 2006;17:1236-1242.
271. Xiao H, Heeringa P, Hu P, et al. Antineutrophil cytoplasmic autoantibodies specific for myeloperoxidase causes glomerulonephritis and vasculitis in mice. *J Clin Invest.* 2002;110:955-963.
272. Schlieben DJ, Korbet SM, Kimura RE, et al. Pulmonary-renal syndrome in a newborn with placental transmission of ANCAs. *Am J Kidney Dis.* 2003;45:758-761.
273. Salama AD, Pusey CD. Shining a LAMP on pauci-immune focal segmental glomerulonephritis. *Kidney Int.* 2009;76:15-17.
274. Marinaki S, Kalsch AI, Grimminger P, et al. Persistent T-cell activation and clinical correlations in patients with ANCA-associated systemic vasculitis. *Nephrol Dial Transplant.* 2006;21:1825-1832.
275. King WJ, Brooks CJ, Holder R, et al. T lymphocytes response to ANCA antigens are present in patients with ANCA-associated systemic vasculitis. *Clin Exp Immunol.* 1998;112:539-546.
276. Griffith ME, Coulhart A, Pusey CD. T cell responses to myeloperoxidase and proteinase 3 in patients with systemic vasculitis. *Clin Exp Immunol.* 1996;103:253-258.
277. Preston GA, Falk RJ. ANCA signaling is not just a matter of respiratory burst. *Kidney Int.* 2001;59:1981-1982.
278. Harper L, Crockwell P, Dwoma A, et al. Neutrophil priming and apoptosis in ANCA-associated vasculitis. *Kidney Int.* 2001;59:1729-1738.
279. Little MA, Pusey CD. Glomerulonephritis due to ANCA- associated vasculitis: An update on approaches to management. *Nephrology.* 2005;10:368-376.
280. Witko-Sarsat V, Lesavre P, Lopez S, et al. A large subset of neutrophils expressing membrane proteinase 3 is a risk factor for vasculitis and rheumatoid arthritis. *J Am Soc Nephrol.* 1995;10:1224-1233.
281. Franseen CF, Huitema MG, Kobold AC, et al. In vitro neutrophil activation by antibodies to proteinase 3 and myeloperoxidase from patients with crescentic glomerulonephritis. *J Am Soc Nephrol.* 1999;10:1506-1515.
282. Rarok AA, Stegman CA, Limburg PG, et al. Neutrophil membrane expression of proteinase 3 is related to relapse in PR3-ANCA-associated vasculitis. *J Am Soc Nephrol.* 2002;13:2232-2238.
283. Cannady SB, Batra PS, Koening C, et al. Sinonasal Wegener granulomatosis: a single-institution experience with 120 cases. *Laryngoscope.* 2009;119:757-761.
284. Andrassy K, Erb A, Koderisch J, et al. Wegener's granulomatosis with renal involvement: patient survival and correlations between initial renal function, renal histology, therapy, and renal outcome. *Clin Nephrol.* 1991;35:139-147.
285. Cordier JF, Valeyre D, Guillevin L, et al. Pulmonary Wegener's granulomatosis. A clinical and imaging study of 77 cases. *Chest.* 1990;97:906.
286. Gaudin PB, Askin FB, Falk RJ, et al. The pathologic spectrum of pulmonary lesions in patients with anti-neutrophil cytoplasmic autoantibodies specific for anti-proteinase 3 and anti-myeloperoxidase. *Am J Clin Pathol.* 1995;104:7.
287. Stassen PM, Derks RP, Kallenberg CG, et al. Venous thromboembolism in ANCA-associated vasculitis—incidence and risk factors. *Rheumatology (Oxford).* 2008;47(4):530-534.
288. Rao JK, Allen NB, Feussner JR, et al. A prospective study of c-ANCA and clinical criteria in diagnosing Wegener's granulomatosis. *Lancet.* 1995;346:926.
289. Chen M, Yu F, Wang SX, et al. Antineutrophil cytoplasmic autoantibody-negative Pauci-immune crescentic glomerulonephritis. *J Am Soc Nephrol.* 2007;18:599-605.
290. Slot MC, Links TP, Stegeman CA, et al. Occurrence of antineutrophil cytoplasmic antibodies and associated vasculitis in patients with hyperthyroidism treated with antithyroid drugs: a long-term followup study. *Arthritis Rheum.* 2005;53:108-113.
291. Finkelman JD, Merkel PA, Schroeder D, et al. Antiproteinase 3 antineutrophil cytoplasmic antibodies and disease activity in Wegener granulomatosis. *Ann Intern Med.* 2007;147:611-619.
292. Boomsma MM, Stegeman CA, van der Leij MJ, et al. Prediction of relapses in Wegener's granulomatosis by measurement of antineutrophil cytoplasmic antibody levels: a prospective study. *Arthritis Rheum.* 2000;43:2025-2033.
293. Han WK, Choi HK, Roth RM, et al. Serial ANCA titers: useful tool for prevention of relapses in ANCA-associated vasculitis. *Kidney Int.* 2003;63:1079-1085.
294. Birck R, Schmitt WH, Kaelsch IA, et al. Serial ANCA determinations for monitoring disease activity in patients with ANCA-associated vasculitis: systematic review. *Am J Kidney Dis.* 2006;47:15-23.
295. Kyndt X, Renmanx D, Bridoux F, et al. Serial measurements of ANCA in patients with systemic vasculitis. *Am J Med.* 1999;106:527.
296. Rich LM, Piering WF. Ureteral stenosis due to recurrent Wegener's granulomatosis after kidney transplantation. *J Am Soc Nephrol.* 1994;4:1516.
297. Jennette JC, Hogan SL, Wilkman AS, et al. Pathologic features of antineutrophil cytoplasmic autoantibody-associated renal disease as predictors of long-term loss of renal function. *Mod Pathol.* 1992;5 (suppl):102A.
298. Zauner I, Bach D, Braun N, et al. Predictive value of initial histology and effect of plasmapheresis on long-term prognosis of rapidly progressive glomerulonephritis. *Am J Kidney Dis.* 2002;39:28-35.
299. Nachman PH, Hogan SL, Jennette JC, et al. Treatment response and relapse in antineutrophil cytoplasmic antibody-associated microscopic polyangiitis and glomerulonephritis. *J Am Soc Nephrol.* 1996;7:33.
300. Matteson EL, Gold KN, Bloch DA, et al. Long-term survival of patients with Wegener's granulomatosis from the American College of Rheumatology Wegener's Granulomatosis Classification Criteria Cohort. *Am J Med.* 1996;101(2):129-134.
301. Gallagher H, Kwan JT, Jayne DR. Pulmonary renal syndrome: a 4 year single center experience. *Am J Kidney Dis.* 2002;39:42-47.
302. Guillevin L, Cordier J-F, Lhote F, et al. A prospective multicenter randomized trial comparing steroids and pulse cyclophosphamide versus steroids and oral cyclophosphamide in the treatment of generalized Wegener's granulomatosis. *Arthritis Rheum.* 1997;40:2187.
303. de Groot K, Adu D, Savage CO. The value of pulse cyclophosphamide in ANCA-associated vasculitis: meta-analysis and critical review. *Nephrol Dial Transplant.* 2001;16:2018.
304. de Groot K, Harper L, Jayne DR, et al. Pulse versus daily oral cyclophosphamide for induction of remission in antineutrophil cytoplasmic antibody-associated vasculitis: a randomized trial. *Ann Intern Med.* 2009;150:670-680.
305. De Groot K, Rasmussen N, Bacon PA, et al. Randomized trial of cyclophosphamide versus methotrexate for induction of remission in early systemic antineutrophil cytoplasmic antibody-associated vasculitis. *Arthritis Rheum.* 2005;52:2461-2469.
306. Specks U. Methotrexate for Wegener's granulomatosis: what is the evidence? *Arthritis Rheum.* 2005;52:2237.
307. Sneller MC, Hoffinan GS, Tular-Williams C, et al. An analysis of 42 Wegener's granulomatosis patients treated with methotrexate and prednisone. *Arthritis Rheum.* 1995;38:608.

308. Langford CA, Tular-Williams C, Sneller MC. Use of methotrexate and glucocorticoids in the treatment of Wegener's granulomatosis. Long-term renal outcome in patients with glomerulonephritis. *Arthritis Rheum.* 2000;43:1836.

309. Cole E, Cattran D, Magil A, et al. A prospective randomized trial of plasma exchange as additive therapy in idiopathic crescentic glomerulonephritis. *Am J Kidney Dis.* 1992;20:261-265.

310. Klemmer PJ, Chalermskulrat W, Reif MS, et al. Plasmapheresis therapy for diffuse alveolar hemorrhage in patients with small-vessel vasculitis. *Am J Kidney Dis.* 2003;42:1149-1153.

311. Jayne DR, Gaskin G, Rasmussen N, et al. Randomized trial of plasma exchange or high-dosage methylprednisolone as adjunctive therapy for severe renal vasculitis. *J Am Soc Nephrol.* 2007;18:2180-2188.

312. Etanercept plus standard therapy for Wegener's granulomatosis. *N Engl J Med.* 2005;352:351-361.

313. Booth A, Harper L, Hammad T, et al. Prospective study of TNFalpha blockade with infliximab in anti-neutrophil cytoplasmic antibody-associated systemic vasculitis. *J Am Soc Nephrol.* 2004;15:717-721.

314. Walsh M, Chaudhry A, Jayne D. Long-term follow-up of relapsing/refractory anti-neutrophil cytoplasm antibody associated vasculitis treated with the lymphocyte depleting antibody alemtuzumab (CAMPATH-1H). *Ann Rheum Dis.* 2008;67(9):1322-1327.

315. Keogh KA, Wylam ME, Stone JH, et al. Induction of remission by B lymphocyte depletion in eleven patients with antineutrophil cytoplasmic antibody associated vasculitis. *Arthritis Rheum.* 2005;52:262-268.

316. Ferraro AJ, Day CJ, Drayson MT, et al. Effective therapeutic use of rituximab in refractory Wegener's granulomatosis. *Nephrol Dial Transplant.* 2005;20:622.

317. Jones RB, Tervaert JW, Hauser T, et al. Rituximab versus cyclophosphamide in ANCA-associated renal vasculitis. *N Engl J Med.* 2010;363:211-220.

318. Stone JH, Merkel PA, Spiera R, et al. Rituximab versus cyclophosphamide for ANCA-associated vasculitis. *N Engl J Med.* 2010;363:221-232.

319. Falk RJ, Jennette JC. Rituximab in ANCA-associated disease. *N Engl J Med.* 2010;363:285.

320. Westman KW, Bygren PG, Olsson H, et al. Relapse rate, renal survival, and cancer morbidity in patients with Wegener's granulomatosis or microscopic polyangiitis with renal involvement. *J Am Soc Nephrol.* 1998;9:842.

321. Hogan SL, Falk RJ, Chin H, et al. Predictors of relapse and treatment resistance in antineutrophil cytoplasmic antibody associated small vessel vasculitis. *Ann Intern Med.* 2005;143:621-631.

322. de Groot K, Reinhold-Keller E, Tatsis E, et al. Therapy for the maintenance of remission in 65 patients with generalized Wegener's granulomatosis. *Arthritis Rheum.* 1996;39:2052.

323. Langford CA, Talar-Williams C, Barron KS, et al. Use of a cyclophosphamide induction: methotrexate maintenance regimen for the treatment of Wegener's granulomatosis. *Arthritis Rheum.* 2001;44:271.

324. Luqmani R, Jane D. EUVAS. European Vasculitis Study Group: A multicenter randomized trial of cyclophosphamide versus azathioprine during remission in ANCA-associated vasculitis. *Arthritis Rheum.* 1995;42:225.

325. Jayne D, Rasmussen N, Andrassy K, et al. A randomized trial for maintenance therapy for vasculitis associated with antineutrophil cytoplasmic antibodies. *N Engl J Med.* 2003;349:36-44.

326. Haubitz M, Koch KM, Brunkhorst R. Cyclosporin for the prevention of disease reactivation in relapsing ANCA-associated vasculitis. *Nephrol Dial Transplant.* 1998;13:2074.

327. Stegman CA, Cohen Tervaert JW, de Jong PE, et al. Trimethoprim-sulfamethoxazole (co-trimoxazole) for the prevention of relapses of Wegener's granulomatosis. *N Engl J Med.* 1996;335:16.

328. Jayne DR, Davies MJ, Fox CJ, et al. Treatment of systemic vasculitis with pooled intravenous immunoglobulin. *Lancet.* 1991;337:1137.

329. Richter C, Schnabel A, Csemok E, et al. Treatment of antineutrophil cytoplasmic antibody (ANCA)-associated systemic vasculitis with high dose intravenous immunoglobulin. *Clin Exp Immunol.* 1995;101:2.

330. Birck R, Warnatz K, Lorenz HM, et al. 15-Deoxyspergualin in patients with refractory ANCA-associated systemic vasculitis: a six-month open-label trial to evaluate safety and efficacy. *J Am Soc Nephrol.* 2003;14(2):440-447.

331. Mekhail TM, Hoffman GS. Long-term outcome of Wegener's granulomatosis in patients with renal disease requiring dialysis. *J Rheumatol.* 2000;27:1237.

332. Nachman PH, Segelmark M, Westman K, et al. Recurrent ANCA associated small vessel vasculitis after transplantation. A pooled analysis. *Kidney Int.* 1999;56:1544.

333. Moroni G, Torri A, Gallelli B, et al. The long-term prognosis of renal transplant in patients with systemic disease. *Am J Transplant.* 2007;7:2133-2139.

334. Allen A, Pusey C, Gaskin G. Outcome of renal replacement therapy in ANCA associated systemic vasculitis. *J Am Soc Nephrol.* 1998;9:1258.

335. Lionaki S, Hogan SL, Jennette CE, et al. The clinical course of ANCA small-vessel vasculitis on chronic dialysis. *Kidney Int.* 2009;76:644-651.

336. Gera M, Griffin MD, Specks U, et al. Recurrence of ANCA-associated vasculitis following renal transplantation in the modern era of immunosuppression. *Kidney Int.* 2007;71:1296-1301.

337. Haubitz M, Kliem V, Koch KM, et al. Renal transplantation for patients with autoimmune diseases: single-center experience with 42 patients. *Transplantation.* 1997;63:1251.

338. Constantinescu A, Liang M, Laskow DA. Sirolimus lowers myeloperoxidase and p-ANCA titers in a pediatric patient before kidney transplantation. *Am J Kidney Dis.* 2002;40:407-410.

339. Churg J. Nomenclature of vasculitic syndrome: a historical perspective. *Am J Kidney Dis.* 1991;18:148-153.

340. D'Agati V, Appel GB. Polyarteritis, Wegener's granulomatosis, Churg-Strauss syndrome. In: Brenner B, Tischer C, eds. *Renal Pathology.* 2nd ed. Philadelphia: J.B. Lippincott; 1994.

341. Leib SS, Restivo C, Paulus HE. Immunosuppressive and corticosteroid therapy of polyarteritis nodosa. *Am J Med.* 1979;67:941-947.

342. Scott DGI, Bacon PA, Elliott PJ, et al. Systemic vasculitis in a district general hospital, 1972-1980: clinical and laboratory features, classification and prognosis of 80 cases. *Q J Med.* 1982;51(203):292-311.

343. Serra A, Cameron JS, Turner DR, et al. Vasculitis affecting the kidney: presentation, histopathology and long-term outcome. *Q J Med.* 1984;53:181-208.

344. Citron BP, Halpern M, McCarron M, et al. Necrotizing angiitis associated with drug abuse. *N Engl J Med.* 1970;283:1003-1011.

345. Guillevin L, Lhote F, Cohen P, et al. Polyarteritis nodosa related hepatitis B virus. A prospective study with long-terms observation of 41 patients. *Medicine (Baltimore).* 1995;74:238.

346. Carpenter MT, West SG. Polyarteritis nodosa in hairy cell leukemia: treatment with interferon-alpha. *J Rheumatol.* 1994;21:1150.

347. Crawford JP, Movat HZ, Ranadive NS, Hay JB. Pathways to inflammation induced by immune complexes: development of the Arthus reaction. *Fed Proc.* 1982;41:2583-2587.

348. Berden JHM, Hang L, McConahey PJ, et al. Analysis of vascular lesions in murine SLE. I. Association with serologic abnormalities. *J Immunol.* 1983;130:1699-1705.

349. Yoshiki T, Hayasaka T, Fukatso R, et al. The structural proteins of murine leukemia virus and the pathogenesis of necrotizing arteritis and glomerulonephritis in SL/Ni mice. *J Immunol.* 1979;122:1812-1820.

350. Hart MN, Tassell SK, Sadewasser KL, et al. Autoimmune vasculitis resulting from in vitro immunization of lymphocytes to smooth muscle. *Am J Pathol.* 1985;119:448-455.

351. Leung DYM, Geha RS, Newberger JW, et al. Two monokines, interlukin-1 and tumor necrosis factor, render cultured vascular endothelial cells susceptible to lysis by antibodies circulating during Kawasaki syndrome. *J Exp Med.* 1988;164:1958-1972.

352. Serra A, Cameron JS. Clinical and pathologic aspects of renal vasculitis. *Semin Nephrol.* 1985;5:15-33.

353. Travers RL, Allison DJ, Brettle RP, et al. Polyarteritis nodosa: a clinical and angiographic analysis of 17 cases. *Semin Arthritis Rheum.* 1979;8:184-199.

354. Guillevin L, Lhote L, Gallais V, et al. Gastrointestinal involvement in periarteritis nodosa and Churg-Strauss syndrome. *Ann Med Intern.* 1995;146:260.

355. Ohkoshi N, Mgusama K, Oguni E, et al. Sural nerve biopsy in vasculitic neuropathies: morphometric analysis of the caliber of involved vessels. *J Med.* 1996;27:153.

356. Cohen Tervaret JW, Kallenberg C. Neurologic manifestations of systemic vasculitides. *Rheum Dis Clin North Am.* 1993;19:913.

357. Moore PM. Neurologic manifestations of vasculitis: Update on immunopathogenic mechanisms and clinical features. *Ann Neurol.* 1995;37(suppl 1):S131-S141.

358. Plumley SG, Rubio R, Alasfar S, et al. Polyarteritis nodosa presenting as polymyositis. *Semin Arthritis Rheum.* 2002;31:377.

359. Ng WF, Chow LT, Lam PW. Localized polyarteritis of the breast: report of two cases and a review of the literature. *Histopathology.* 1993;23:535.

360. Guillevin L, Ronco P, Verroust P. Circulating immune complexes in systemic necrotizing vasculitis of the polyarteritis nodosa group. Comparison of HBV-related polyarteritis nodosa and Churg-Strauss angiitis. *J Autoimmunity.* 1990;3:789-792.

361. O'Connell MT, Kubrusly DB, Fournier AM. Systemic necrotizing vasculitis seen initially as hypertensive crisis. *Arch Intern Med.* 1985;145:265-267.

362. Vazquez JJ, San Martin P, Barbado FJ, et al. Angiographic findings in systemic necrotizing vasculitis. *Angiology.* 1981;32:773-779.

363. Wilkowski MJ, Velosa JA, Holley KE, et al. Risk factors in idiopathic renal vasculitis and glomerulonephritis. *Kidney Intern.* 1989;36:1133-1141.

364. Fauci A, Doppman JL, Wilf SM. Cyclophosphamide-induced remissions in advance polyarteritis nodosa. *Am J Med.* 1978;64:890-894.

365. Gayraud M, Guillevin L, Le Toumelin P, et al. Long-term follow up of polyarteritis nodosa, microscopic polyangiitis, and Churg-Strauss syndrome. *Arthritis Rheum.* 2001;44:666.

366. Guillevin L. Treatment of classic polyarteritis nodosa in 1999. *Nephrol Dial Transplant.* 1999;14:2077.

367. Kruger K, Boker KK, Zeidler K, et al. Treatment of hepatitis B-related polyarteritis nodosa with famciclovir and interferon alfa-2b. *J Hepatol.* 1997;26:935.

368. Guillevin L, Lhote F, Cohen P, et al. Polyarteritis nodosa related hepatitis B virus. A prospective study with long-term observation of 41 patients. *Medicine (Baltimore).* 1995;74:238.

369. Chang-Miller A, Okamura M, Torres VE, et al. Renal involvement in relapsing polychondritis. *Medicine.* 1987;66:202-217.

370. Espinoza LR, Richman A, Bocanegra T, et al. Immune complex-mediated renal involvement in relapsing polychondritis. *Am J Med.* 1983;71:181183.

371. Zhao MH, Chen M, Gao Y, et al. Propylthiouracil-induced ANCA-associated vasculitis. *Kidney Int.* 2006;69:1477-1481.

372. Berden AE, Ferrario F, Hagen EC, et al. Histopathologic classification of ANCA-associated glomerulonephritis. *J Am Soc Nephrol.* 2010;10:1628-1636.

373. Keogh KA, Specks U. Churg-Strauss syndrome. *Semin Respir Crit Care Med.* 2006;27(2):148-157.

374. Hellmich B, Ehlers S, Csernok E, et al. Update on the pathogenesis of Churg-Strauss syndrome. *Clin Exp Rheumatol.* 2003;21(suppl):S69-S77.

375. Sinico RA, Bottero P. Churg-Strauss angiitis. *Best Pract Res Clin Rheumatol.* 2009;23(3):355-366.

376. Pagnoux C, Guillevin L. Churg-Strauss syndrome: evidence for disease subtypes?. *Curr Opin Rheumatol.* 2010;22(1):21-28.

377. Reid AJC, Harrison BDW, Watts RH, et al. Churg-Strauss syndrome in a district hospital. *Q J Med.* 1998;91:219.

378. Guillerin L, Cohen P, Gayrand, et al. Churg-Strauss syndrome. Clinical study and long-term follow-up of 96 patients. *Medicine.* 1999;78:26.

379. Harold LR, Andrade SE, Go AS, et al. The incidence of Churg Strauss syndrome in asthma drug users: a population-based prospective. *J Rheumatol.* 2005;32:1076-1080.

380. Clutterbuck EJ, Evans DJ, Pusey CD. Renal Involvement in Churg-Strauss syndrome. *Nephrol Dial Transplant.* 1990;5:161-167.

381. Wechsler ME, Garpestad E, Flier SF, et al. Pulmonary infiltrates, eosinophilia, and cardiomyopathy following corticosteroid withdrawal in patients with asthma receiving zafirlukast. *JAMA.* 1998;279:455.

382. Green RI, Vayonis AG. Churg-Strauss syndrome after zafirlukast in two patients not receiving systemic steroid treatment. *Lancet.* 1999;353:725.

383. Kinoshita M, Shiraishi T, Koga T, et al. Churg-Strauss syndrome after corticosteroid withdrawal in an asthmatic patient treated with pranlikast. *J Allergy Clin Immunol.* 1999;103:534.

384. Martin RM, Wilton LV, Mann RDL. Prevalence of Churg-Strauss syndrome, vasculitis, eosinophilia and associated condition: Retrospective analysis of 58 prescription-event monitoring cohort studies. *Pharmacoepidemiol Drug Safety.* 1999;8:179.

385. Wechsler M, Finn D, Gunawardena D, et al. Churg-Strauss syndrome in patients receiving montelukast as treatment for asthma. *Chest.* 2000;117:708.

386. Le Gall C, Pham S, Vignes S, et al. Inhaled corticosteroids and Churg-Strauss syndrome: a report of five cases. *Eur Respir J.* 2000;15:978.

387. Keogh KA, Specks U. Churg-Strauss syndrome: clinical presentation, antineutrophil cytoplasmic antibodies, and leukotriene receptor antagonists. *Am J Med.* 2003;115:284-290.

388. Nathani N, Little MA, Kunst H, et al. Churg-Strauss syndrome and leukotriene antagonist use: a respiratory perspective. *Thorax.* 2008;63(10):883-888.

389. Sinico RA, Di Toma L, Maggiore U, et al. Renal involvement in Churg-Strauss syndrome. *Am J Kidney Dis.* 2006;47(5):770-779.

390. Antiga G, Volpi A, Battini G, et al. Acute renal failure in a patient affected with Churg and Strauss syndrome. *Nephron.* 1991;57:113-114.

391. Manger BJ, Krapf FE, Gramatzi M, et al. IgE-containing circulating immune complexes in Churg-Strauss vasculitis. *Scand J Immunol.* 1985;21:369.

392. Tai PC, Kolt ME, Denny P, et al. Deposition of eosinophil cationic protein in granulomas in allergic granulomatosis and vasculitis: the Churg-Strauss syndrome. *Br Med J.* 1984;289:400.

393. Schmitt WH, Csernock E, Kobayashi S. Churg-Strauss syndrome markers of lymphocyte activation and endothelial damage. *Arthritis Rheum.* 1998;41:445.

394. Solans R, Bosch JA, Perez-Bocanegra C, et al. Churg-Strauss syndrome: outcome and long-term follow-up of 32 patients. *Rheumatology.* 2001;40:763-771.

395. Neumann T, Manger B, Schmid M, et al. Cardiac involvement in Churg-Strauss syndrome: impact of endomyocarditis. *Medicine (Baltimore).* 2009;88(4):236-243.

396. Wolf J, Bergner R, Mutallib S, et al. Neurologic complications of Churg-Strauss syndrome—a prospective monocentric study. *Eur J Neurol.* 2010;17(4):582-588.

397. Choi YH, Im JG, Han BK, et al. Thoracic manifestation of Churg-Strauss syndrome: radiologic and clinical findings. *Chest.* 2000;117:117.

398. Buschman DL, Waldron JA, King Jr TE. Churg-Straus pulmonary vasculitis. High resolution CT scanning and pathologic findings. *Am Rev Respir Dis.* 1990;142:458.

399. Erzurum SC, Underwood GA, Hamilos DL, et al. Pleural effusion in Churg-Strauss syndrome. *Chest.* 1989;95:1357.

400. Hellmich B, Goss WL. Recent progress in the pharmacotherapy of Churg-Strauss syndrome. *Exp Opin Pharmacother.* 2004;5:25-35.

401. Sinico RA, DiToma L, Maggiore U, et al. Prevalence and clinical significance of antineutrophil cytoplasmic antibodies in Churg-Strauss syndrome. *Arthritis Rheum.* 2005;52:2926-2935.

402. Sable-Fourtassou R, Cohen P, Mahr A, et al. Antineutrophil cytoplasmic antibodies and the Churg-Strauss syndrome. *Ann Intern Med.* 2005;143:632-638.

403. Cohen P, Pagnoux C, Mahr A, et al. Churg-Strauss syndrome with poor-prognosis factors: a prospective multicenter trial comparing glucocorticoids and six or twelve cyclophosphamide pulses in forty-eight patients. *Arthritis Rheum.* 2007;57(4):686-693.

404. Pepper RJ, Fabre MA, Pavesio C, et al. Rituximab is effective in the treatment of refractory Churg-Strauss syndrome and is associated with diminished T-cell interleukin-5 production. *Rheumatology (Oxford).* 2008;47:1104.

405. Danielli MG, Cappelli M, Malcangi G, et al. Long term effectiveness of intravenous immunoglobulin in Churg-Strauss syndrome. *Ann Rheum Dis.* 2004;63:1649-1654.

406. Assaf C, Mewis G, Orfanos CE, et al. Churg-Strauss syndrome: successful treatment with mycophenolate mofetil. *Br J Dermatol.* 2004;150:598.

407. Pabst S, Tiyerili V, Grohe C. Apparent response to anti-IgE therapy in two patients with refractory "forme fruste" of Churg-Strauss syndrome. *Thorax.* 2008;63(8):747-748.

408. Gonzalez-Gay MA, Barros S, Lopez-Diaz MJ, et al. Giant cell arteritis: disease patterns of clinical presentation in a series of 240 patients. *Medicine.* 2005;84:269-276, 277-290.

409. Hoffman GS, Cid MC, Rendt-Zagar KE, et al. Infliximab for maintenance of glucocorticosteroid-induced remission of giant cell arteritis: a randomized trial. *Ann Intern Med.* 2007;146(9):621-630.

410. Levine SM, Hellmann DB. Giant cell arteritis. *Curr Opin Rheumatol.* 2002;14:3-10.

411. Mazlumzadeh M, Hunder GG, Easley KA, et al. Treatment of giant cell arteritis using induction therapy with high-dose glucocorticoids: a double-blind, placebo-controlled, randomized prospective clinical trial. *Arthritis Rheum.* 2006;54(10):3310-3318.

412. Hoffman GS, Cid MC, Hellmann DB, et al. A multicenter, randomized, double-blind, placebo-controlled trial of adjuvant methotrexate treatment for giant cell arteritis. *Arthritis Rheum.* 2002;46(5):1309-1318.

413. Lie JT. Aortic and extracranial large vessel giant cell arteritis: a review of 72 cases with histopathologic documentation. *Semin Arthritis Rheum.* 1995;24:422-431.

414. Highton J, Anderson KR. Concurrent polyarteritis nodosa and temporal arteritis. *N Z Med J.* 1984;14:766.

415. Bosch X, Mirapeix E, Font J, et al. Antimyeloperoxidase autoantibodies in patients with necrotizing glomerular and alveolar capillaritis. *Am J Kidney Dis.* 1992;20:231-239.

416. Fauchald P, Rygvold O, Oystese B. Temporal arteritis and polymyalgia rheumatica. *Ann Intern Med.* 1972;77:845.

417. Truong L, Kopelman RG, Williams GS, et al. Temporal arteritis and renal disease. *Am J Med.* 1985;78:171.

418. Jover JA, Hernandez-Garcia C, Murado IC, et al. Combined treatment of giant cell arteritis with methotrexate and prednisone. *Ann Intern Med.* 2001;134:106-114.

419. Wilke WS, Hoffman GS. Treatment of corticosteroid resistant giant cell arteritis. *Rheum Dis Clin North Am.* 1995;21:59-71.

420. Weyand CM, Goronzy JJ. Medium- and large-vessel vasculitis. *N Engl J Med.* 2003;349:160.

421. Cid MC, Font C, Coll-Vincent B, et al. Large vessel vasculitides. *Curr Opin Rheumatol.* 1998;10:18.

422. Sharma BK, Jain S, Sagar S. Systemic manifestations of Takayasu arteritis: the expanding spectrum. *Int J Cardiol.* 1997;54(suppl):149.

423. Yoshimura M, Kida H, Saito Y, et al. Peculiar glomerular lesions in Takayasu's arteritis. *Clin Nephrol.* 1985;24:120.

424. Weiss RA, Jodorkovsky R, Weiner S, et al. Chronic renal failure due to Takayasu's arteritis: recovery of renal function after nine months of dialysis. *Clin Nephrol.* 1982;17:104.

425. Takagi M, Ikeda T, Kimura K, et al. Renal histological studies in patients with Takayasu's arteritis. *Nephron.* 1984;36:68.

426. Lagneau P, Michel JB. Renovascular hypertension and Takayasu's disease. *J Urol.* 1985;134:876.

427. Greene NB, Baughman RP, Kim CK. Takayasu's arteritis associated with interstitial lung disease and glomerulonephritis. *Chest.* 1986;89:605.

428. Andrews J, Al-Nahhas A, Pennell DJ, et al. Non-invasive imaging in the diagnosis and management of Takayasu's arteritis. *Ann Rheum Dis.* 2004;63:995-1000.

429. Keenan NG, Mason JC, Maceira A, et al. Integrated cardiac and vascular assessment in Takayasu arteritis by cardiovascular magnetic resonance. *Arthritis Rheum.* 2009;60(11):3501-3509.

430. Eichorn J, Sima D, Thiele B, et al. Anti-endothelial cell antibodies in Takayasu's arteritis. *Circulation.* 1996;94:2396.

431. Yoneda S, Nukada T, Imaizumi M, et al. Hemodynamic and volume characteristics and peripheral plasma renin activity in Takayasu's arteritis. *Jpn Circ J.* 1980;44:951.

432. Kurihara S, Fukuda Y, Saito Y, et al. Three cases of "IgA nephritis" associated with other disease. *J Kanazawa Med Univ.* 1982;7:51.

433. Hall S, Barr W, Lie JT, et al. Takayasu arteritis. A study of 32 North American patients. *Medicine.* 1985;64:89.

434. Graham AN, Delahunt B, Renouf JJ, et al. Takayasu's disease associated with generalized amyloidosis. *Aus N Z J Med.* 1985;15:343.

435. Yoshikawa Y, Truong LD, Mattioli CA, et al. Membranoproliferative glomerulonephritis in Takayasu's arteritis. *Am J Nephrol.* 1988;8:240-244.

436. Hoffman GS, Leavitt RY, Kerr GS, et al. Treatment of glucocorticoid resistant or relapsing Takayasu arteritis with methotrexate. *Arthritis Rheum.* 1994;37:578.

437. Haberhauer G, Kittl EM, Dunky A, et al. Beneficial effects of leflunomide in glucocorticoid- and methotrexate-resistant Takayasu's arteritis. *Clin Exp Rheumatol.* 2001;19:477.

438. Daino E, Schieppati A, Remuzzi G. Mycophenolate mofetil for the treatment of Takayasu's arteritis: report of three cases. *Ann Intern Med.* 1999;130:422.

439. Valsakumar AK, Valappil UC, Jorapur V, et al. Role of immunosuppressive therapy on clinical, immunological, and angiographic outcome in active Takayasu's arteritis. *J Rheumatol.* 2003;30:1793-1798.

440. Hoffman GS, Merkel PA, Brasington RD, et al. Anti-tumor necrosis factor therapy in patients with difficult to treat Takayasu's arteritis. *Arthritis Rheum.* 2004;50:2296-2304.

441. Ishikawa K, Martani S. Long-term outcome for 120 Japanese patients with Takayasu's Disease. *Circulation.* 1853;90:1994.

442. Trapani S, Micheli A, Grisolia F, et al. Henoch Schonlein purpura in childhood: epidemiological and clinical analysis of 150 cases over a 5 year period and review of the literature. *Semin Arthritis Rheum.* 2005;35: 143-153.

443. Rai A, Nast C, Adler S. Henoch-Schonlein purpura nephritis. *J Am Soc Nephrol.* 1999;10:2637.

444. Saulsbury FT. Henoch-Schoenlein purpura in children. Report of 100 patients and review of the literature. *Medicine.* 1999;78:395.

445. Yang YH, Hung CF, Hsu CR, et al. A nationwide survey on epidemiologic characteristics of childhood HSP in Taiwan. *Rheumatology.* 2005;44:618-622.

446. Yoshikawa N, Ito H, Yoshiya K, et al. Henoch-Schonlein nephritis and IgA nephropathy in children: a comparison clinical course. *Clin Nephrol.* 1987;27:233.

447. Gardner-Medwin JM, Dolezalova P, Cummins C, et al. Incidence of Henoch-Schonlein purpura, Kawasaki disease, and rare vasculitides in children of different ethnic origins. *Lancet.* 2002;360:1197-1202.

448. Davin JC, Ten Berge IJ, Weening JJ. What is the difference between IgA nephropathy and Henoch-Schönlein purpura nephritis? *Kidney Int.* 2001;59(3):823-834.

449. Blanco R, Martinez-Taboada VK, Rodriguez-Valverde V, et al. Henoch-Schonlein purpura in adulthood and childhood: Two different expressions of the same syndrome. *Arthritis Rheum.* 1997;40:859.

450. Ostergaard JR, Storm K, Lamm LU. Lack of association between HLA and Schonlein-Henoch purpura. *Tissue Antigens.* 1990;35:234.

451. Farley TA, Gillespie S, Rasoulpour M, et al. Epidemiology of a cluster of Henoch-Schonlein purpura. *Am J Dis Child.* 1989;143:798.

452. Pillebout E, Thervet E, Hill G, et al. Henoch-Schonlein purpura in adults: outcome and prognostic factors. *J Am Soc Nephrol.* 2002;13: 1271-1278.

453. Nakasone H, Hokama A, Fukuch J, et al. Colonoscopic findings in an adult patient with HSP. *Gastrointest Endosc.* 2000;52:392.

454. Chang WL, Yang YH, Lin YT, et al. Gastrointestinal manifestations in Henoch-Schonlein purpura: a review of 261 patients. *Acta Paediatr.* 2004;93:142-1431.

455. Payton CD, Allison MEM, Boulton-Jones JM. Henoch-Schonlein purpura presenting with pulmonary hemorrhage. *Scott Med J.* 1987;32: 26.

456. Chang WL, Yang YH, Wang LC, et al. Renal manifestations of Henoch-Schonlein purpura: a 10 year clinical study. *Pediatr Nephrol.* 2005;20: 1269-1272.

457. Martini A, Ravelli A, Beluffi G. Urinary microscopy in the diagnosis of hematuria in Henoch-Schonlein purpura. *Eur J Pediatr.* 1986;144:591.

458. Lau KK, Wyatt RJ, Moldoveanu Z, et al. Serum levels of galactose-deficient IgA in children with IgA nephropathy and Henoch-Schonlein purpura. *Pediatr Nephrol.* 2007;22(12):2067-2072.

459. Coppo R, Basolo B, Martina G, et al. Circulating immune complexes containing IgA, IgM, and IgG in patients with primary IgA nephropathy and Henoch-Schonlein mephitis; correlation with clinical and histologic signs of activity. *Clin Nephrol.* 1982;18:230.

460. Shaw G, Ronda N, Bevan JS, et al. ANCA of IgA class correlate with disease activity in adult Henoch-Schonlein purpura. *Nephrol Dial transplant.* 1992;7:1238.

461. Darvin J-C, Malaise M, Foidart J, et al. Anti-alpha- galactosyl antibodies and immune complexes in children with Henoch-Schonlein purpura or IgA nephropathy. *Kidney Int.* 1987;31:1132.

462. Ronda N, Esnault VL, Layward L, et al. ANCA of IgA isotype in adult Henoch-Schonlein purpura. *Clin Exp Immunol.* 1994;95:49.

463. Burden A, Gibson I, Roger R, et al. IgA anticardiolipin antibodies associated with Henoch-Schoenlein purpura. *Am Acad Dermatol.* 1994;31:857-860.

464. Jennette JC, Wieslander J, Tuttle R, et al. Serum IgA fibronectin aggregates in patients with IgA nephropathy and Henoch-Schonlein purpura. *Am J Kidney Dis.* 1991;18:466.

465. Yoshiara S, Yoshikawa N, Matsuo T. Immunoelectronmicroscopic study of childhood IgA nephropathy and Henoch-Schonlein nephritis. *Virchows Arch.* 1987;412:95.

466. Nolasco F, Cameron J, Hartley B. Intraglomerular T cells and monocytes in nephritis: study with monoclonal antibodies. *Kidney Int.* 1987;31:1160.

467. Yoshioka K, Takemura T, Aya N, et al. Monocyte infiltration and cross-linked fibrin deposition in IgA nephritis and Henoch-Schonlein purpura nephritis. *Clin Nephrol.* 1989;32:107.

468. Yoshikawa N, White RK, Cameron AH. Prognostic significance of the glomerular changes in Henoch-Schonlein nephritis. *Clin Nephrol.* 1981;16:223.

469. Bergstein J, Leiser J, Andreoli SP. Response of crescentic Henoch-Schoenlein purpura nephritis to corticosteroid and azathioprine therapy. *Clin Nephrol.* 1998;49:9.

470. Rajaraman S, Goldblum RM, Cavallo T. IgA-associated glomerulo-nephritides: a study with monoclonal antibodies. *Clin Immunol Immunopathol.* 1986;39:514.

471. Russel MW, Mestecky J, Julian BA, et al. IgA-associated renal diseases: antibodies to environmental antigens in sera and deposition of immunoglobulins and antigens in glomeruli. *J Clin Immunol.* 1986;6:74.

472. Hene RJ, Velthuis P, van de Wiel A, et al. The relevance of IgA deposits in vessel walls of clinically normal skin. *Arch Intern Med.* 1986;146:745.

473. Kawana S, Nishiyama S. Serum SC5-9 (terminal complement complex), a sensitive indicator of disease activity in patients with Henoch-Schonlein purpura. *Dermatology.* 1992;184(3):171-176.

474. Han SS, Sun HK, Lee JP, et al. Outcome of renal allograft in patients with Henoch-Schonlein nephritis: single-center experience and systematic review. *Transplantation.* 2010;89(6):721-726.

475. Hasegawa A, Kawamura T, Ito FL, et al. Fate of renal grafts with recurrent Henoch Schonlein purpura nephritis in children. *Transplant Proc.* 1989;21:2130.

476. Meulders Q, Pirson Y, Cosyns JP, et al. Course of Henoch-Schonlein nephritis after renal transplantation. Report of ten patients and review of the literature. *Transplantation.* 1994;58:1179.

477. Pasternack A, Collin P, Mustonen J, et al. Glomerular IgA deposits in patients with celiac disease. *Clin Nephrol.* 1990;34:56.

478. Cassaneuva B, Rodriguez VV, Farinas MC, et al. Autologous mixed lymphocyte reaction and T-cell suppressor activity in patients with Henoch-Schonlein purpura and IgA nephropathy. *Nephron.* 1990;54:224.

479. Dosa S, Cairns SA, Mallick NP, et al. Relapsing Henoch-Schonlein syndrome with renal involvement in a patient with an IgA monoclonal gammopathy: a study of the result of immunosuppressant and cytotoxic therapy. *Nephron.* 1980;26:145.

480. Davin JC, Ten Berge IJ, Weening JJ. What is the difference between IgA nephropathy and Henoch-Schönlein purpura nephritis? *Kidney Int.* 2001;59(3):823-834.

481. Montoliu J, Lens XM, Torra A, et al. Henoch-Schonlein purpura and IgA nephropathy in a father and son. *Nephron.* 1990;54:77.

482. Garty BZ, Danon YL, Nitzan M. Schonlein-Henoch purpura associated with hepatitis A infection. *Am J Dis Child.* 1985;135.

483. Maggiore G, Martini A, Grifeo S, et al. Hepatitis B infection and Henoch-Schonlein purpura. *Am J Dis Child.* 1984;138:681.

484. Eftychiou C, Samarkos M, Golfinopoulou S, et al. Henoch-Schonlein purpura associated with methicillin-resistant Staphylococcus aureus infection. *Am J Med.* 2006;119:85-86.

485. Patel U, Bradley JR, Hamilton DV. Henoch-Schonlein purpura after influenza vaccination. *Br Med J Clin Res Educ.* 1988;296:1800.

486. Ronkainen J, Nuutinen M, Koskimies O. The adult kidney 24 years after childhood Henoch-Schonlein purpura: a retrospective cohort study. *Lancet*. 2002;360:666-670.

487. Rauta V, Tonroth T, Gronhagen-Riska C. Henoch-Schonlein nephritis in adults—clinical features and outcomes in Finnish patients. *Clin Nephrol*. 2002;58:1-8.

488. Shrestha S, Sumingan N, Tan J, et al. Henoch Schonlein purpura with nephritis in adults: adverse prognostic indicators in a UK population. *Q J Med*. 2006;99:253-265.

489. Tarshish P, Bernstein J, Edelman Jr CM. Henoch-Schonlein purpura nephritis: course of disease and efficacy of cyclophosphamide. *Pediatr Nephrol*. 2004;19:51-56.

490. Weiss PF, Feinstein JA, Luan X, et al. Effects of corticosteroid on Henoch-Schonlein purpura: a systematic review. *Pediatrics*. 2007;120(5):1079-1087.

491. Chartapisak W, Opastirakul S, Hodson EM, et al. Interventions for preventing and treating kidney disease in Henoch-Schonlein Purpura (HSP). *Cochrane Database Syst Rev*. 2009;(3):CD005128.

492. Huber AM, King J, McLaine P, et al. A randomized, placebo-controlled trial of prednisone in early Henoch Schonlein purpura. *BMC Med*. 2004;2:7.

493. Niaudet P, Habib R. Methylprednisolone pulse therapy in the treatment of severe forms of Schoenlein-Henoch purpura nephritis. *Pediatr Nephrol*. 1998;12:238.

494. Kauffman RK, Honwert DA. Plasmapheresis in rapidly progressive Henoch-Schonlein glomerulonephritis and the effect on circulating IgA immune complexes. *Clin Nephrol*. 1981;16:155.

495. Kunis CL, Kiss B, Williams G, et al. Treatment of rapidly progressive glomerulonephritis with IV pulse cyclophosphamide. *Clin Nephrol*. 1992;37:1.

496. Coppo R, Basolo B, Roccatello D, et al. Plasma exchange in primary IgA nephropathy and Henoch-Schonlein syndrome nephritis. *Plasma Ther*. 1985;6:705.

497. Rostoker G, Desvaux-Belghiti D, Pilatte Y, et al. High dose immunoglobulin therapy for severe IgA nephropathy and Henoch-Schonlein purpura. *Ann Intern Med*. 1994;120:476.

498. Iijima K, Ito-Kariya S, Nakamura H, et al. Multiple combined therapy for severe Henoch-Schoenlein nephritis in children. *Pediatr Nephrol*. 1998;12:244.

499. Shin JI, Park JM, Kim JH, et al. Factors affecting histological regression of crescentic Henoch-Schonlein nephritis in children. *Pediatr Nephrol*. 2005;20.

500. Hudson BG. The molecular basis of Goodpasture and Alport's syndromes: beacon for the discovery of the collagen IV family. *J Am Soc Nephrol*. 2004;15:2514-2527.

501. Wang XP, Fogo AB, Colon S, et al. Distinct epitopes for anti–glomerular basement membrane Alport alloantibodies and Goodpasture autoantibodies within the noncollagenous domain of α3(IV) collagen: a Janus-faced antigen. *J Am Soc Nephrol*. 2005;16(12):3563-3571.

502. Pusey C. Anti-glomerular basement membrane disease. *Kidney Int*. 2003;64:1535-1550.

503. Hudson BG, Tryggvason K, Sundaramoorthy M, et al. Alport's syndrome, Goodpasture's syndrome, and type IV collagen. *N Engl J Med*. 2003;348:2543.

504. Niles JL, Bottinger EP, Saurina GR, et al. The syndrome of lung hemorrhage and nephritis is usually an ANCA-associated condition. *Arch Intern Med*. 1996;156:440.

505. Kelly PT, Haponick EF. Goodpasture's syndrome: molecular and clinical advances. *Medicine*. 1994;73:171.

506. Salama AD, Dougan T, Levy JB, et al. Goodpasture's disease in the absence of circulating anti-GBM antibodies as detected by standard techniques. *Am J Kidney Dis*. 2002;39:1162.

507. Sinico RA, Radice A, Corace C, et al. Anti-glomerular basement membrane antibodies in the diagnosis of Goodpasture syndrome: a comparison of different assays. *Nephrol Dial Transplant*. 2006;21(2):397-401.

508. Kalluri R, Wilson CB, Weber K, et al. Identification of the alpha-3 chain of type IV collagen as the common autoantigen in antibasement membrane disease and Goodpasture syndrome. *J Am Soc Nephrol*. 1995;6:1178.

509. Leinonen A, Netzer KO, Bontaud A, et al. Goodpasture antigen: expression of the full-length alpha 3 (IV) chain of collagen IV and localization of epitopes exclusively to the noncollagenous domain. *Kidney Int*. 1999;55:926.

510. Pedchenko V, Bondar O, Fogo A, et al. Molecular Architecture of the Goodpasture autoantigen in the anti-GBM nephritis. *N Engl J Med*. 2010:343-354.

511. Rutgers A, Meyers KE, Canziani G, et al. High affinity og anti-GBM antibodies from Goodpasture and transplanted Alport patients to alpha3 (IV) NC I collagen. *Kidney Int*. 2000;58:115.

512. Arends J, Wu J, Borillo J, et al. T cell epitope mimicry in antiglomerular basement membrane disease. *J Immunol*. 2006;176(2):1252-1258.

513. Pusey CD. Anti-glomerular basement membrane disease. *Kidney Int*. 2003;64:1535-1550.

514. Stevenson A, Yaqoob M, Mason H, et al. Biochemical markers of basement membrane disturbances and occupational exposure to hydrocarbons and mixed solvents. *Q J Med*. 1995;88:23.

515. Herody M, Bobrie G, Gouarin C, et al. Anti-GBM disease: predictive value of clinical, histological, and serological data. *Clin Nephrol*. 1993;40:249.

516. Donaghy K, Rees AJ. Cigarette smoking and lung hemorrhage in glomerulonephritis caused by antibodies to glomerular basement membrane. *Lancet*. 1983;2:1390.

517. Lechleitner P, DeFregger M, Lhotta K, et al. Goodpasture's syndrome. Unusual presentation after exposure to hard metal dust. *Chest*. 1993;103:956.

518. Petterson E, Tonroth T, Miettinen A. Simultaneous anti-GBM and membranous glomerulonephritis: case report and literature review. *Clin Immunol Immunopathol*. 1984;31:171.

519. Kalluri R, Weber M, Netzer KO, et al. COL4A5 gene deletion and production of posttransplant anti-a3(IV) collagen alloantibodies in Alport syndrome. *Kidney Int*. 1994;45:721.

520. Lazor R, Bigay-Game L, Cottin V, et al. Alveolar hemorrhage in anti-basement membrane antibody disease: a series of 28 cases. *Medicine (Baltimore)*. 2007;86(3):181-193.

521. Ang C, Savige J, Dawborn J, et al. Antiglomerular basement membrane antibody mediated disease with normal renal function. *Nephrol Dial Transplant*. 1998;13:935.

522. Merkel R, Pullin O, Marx M, et al. Course and prognosis of anti-basement membrane antibody-mediated disease: report of 35 cases. *Nephrol Dial Transplant*. 1994;9:372.

523. Rutgers A, Slot M, van Paassen P, et al. Coexistence of anti-glomerular basement membrane antibodies and myeloperoxidase-ANCAs in crescentic glomerulonephritis. *Am J Kidney Dis*. 2005;46(2):253-262.

524. Yang R, Hellmark T, Zhao J, et al. Antigen and epitope specificity of anti-glomerular basement membrane antibodies in patients with Goodpasture disease with or without anti-neutrophil cytoplasmic antibodies. *J Am Soc Nephrol*. 2007;8(4):1338-1343.

525. Hellmark T, Niles JL, Collins AB, et al. A comparison of anti-GBM antibodies in sera with and without ANCA. *J Am Soc Nephrol*. 1997;8:376.

526. Levy JB, Hammad T, Coulhart A, et al. Clinical features and outcomes of patients with both ANCA and anti-GBM antibodies. *Kidney Int*. 2004;66:1535-1540.

527. Boucher A, Droz D, Adafer E, et al. Relationship between the integrity of Bowman's capsule and the composition of cellular crescents in human crescentic glomerulonephritis. *Lab Invest*. 1987;56:526.

528. Segelmark M, Butkowski R, Wieslander J. Antigen restrictions and IgG subclasses among anti-GBM antibodies. *Nephrol Dial Transplant*. 1990;5:991.

529. Cui Z, Zhao MH, Xin G, et al. Characteristics and prognosis of Chinese patients with anti-glomerular basement membrane disease. *Nephron Clin Pract*. 2005;99(2):c49-c55.

530. Jindal KK. Management of idiopathic crescentic and diffuse proliferative glomerulonephritis: evidence-based recommendations. *Kidney Int*. 1999;55(suppl):S33-S40.

531. Levy JB, Turner AN, Rees AJ, et al. Long term outcome of anti-GBM antibody disease treated with plasma exchange and immunosuppression. *Ann Intern Med*. 2001;134:1033-1042.

532. Querin S, Schurch W, Beaulieu R. Cyclosporin in Goodpasture's syndrome. *Nephron*. 1992;60:355.

533. Reynolds J, Tam FW, Chandraker A, et al. CD28-B7 blockade prevents the development of experimental autoimmune glomerulonephritis. *J Clin Invest*. 2000;105:643.

534. Laczika K, Knapp S, Derflerk K, et al. Immunoadsorption in Goodpasture's syndrome. *Am J Kidney Dis*. 2000;36:392.

535. Denton MD, Singh AK. Recurrent and de novo glomerulonephritis in the renal allograft. *Semin Nephrol*. 2000;20:164.

536. Netzer KO, Merkel F, Weber M. Goodpasture's Syndrome and ESRD – to transplant or not to transplant? *Nephrol Dial Transpl*. 1998;13:1346.

537. Floege J. Recurrent glomerulonephritis following renal transplantation: an update. *Nephrol Dial Transplant*. 2003;18:1260-1263.

538. Knoll G, Cockfield S, Blydt-Hansen T, et al. Canadian Society of Transplantation consensus guidelines on eligibility for kidney transplantation. *Can Med Assoc J*. 2005;173:1181-1190.

539. Ramos-Casals M, Tzioufas AG, Font J. Primary Sjogren's syndrome: new clinical and therapeutic concepts. *Ann Rheum Dis*. 2005;64:347-354.

540. Goulos A, Masouridi S, Tzionfas AG, et al. Clinically significant and biopsy documented renal involvement in primary Sjogren syndrome. *Medicine*. 2000;79:241-249.

541. Bossini N, Savoldi S, Franceschin F, et al. Clinical and morphological features of kidney involvement in primary Sjogren's syndrome. *Nephrol Dial Transplant.* 2001;16:2328.

542. Pertovaarc M, Korpels M, Pasternack A. Factors predictive of renal involvement in patients with primary Sjogren's syndrome. *Clin Nephrol.* 2001;56:10.

543. Maripuri S, Grande JP, Osborn T, et al. Renal involvement in primary Sjögren's Syndrome: a clinicopathologic study. *Clin J Am Soc Nephrol.* 2009;4(9):1423-1431.

544. Font J, Cervera R, Lopez-Soto A, et al. Mixed membranous and proliferative glomerulonephritis in primary Sjogren's syndrome. *Br J Rheumatol.* 1989;28:548.

545. Khan MA, Akhtar M, Taher SM. Membranoproliferative glomerulonephritis in a patient with primary Sjogren's syndrome. *Am J Nephrol.* 1988;8:235.

546. Palcoux JB, Janin-Mercier A, Campagne D, et al. Sjogren's syndrome and lupus erythematosus nephritis. *Arch Dis Child.* 1984;59:175.

547. Schlesinger I, Carlson TS, Nelson D. Type III membranoproliferative glomerulonephritis in primary Sjogren's syndrome. *Conn Med J.* 1989;53:629.

548. Cortez MS, Sturgil BC, Bolton WK. Membranoproliferative glomerulonephritis with primary Sjogren's syndrome. *Am J Kidney Dis.* 1995;25:632.

549. Molina R, Provost TT, Alexander EL. Two types of inflammatory vascular disease in Sjogren's syndrome. *Arthritis Rheum.* 1985;28:1251.

550. Baughman RP, Lowere EE, du Bois RM. Sarcoidosis. *Lancet.* 2003;361:1111-1118.

551. Gobel U, Kettritz R, Schneider W, Luft FC. The protean face of renal sarcoidosis. *J Am Soc Nephrol.* 2001;12:616-623.

552. Brause M, Magnusson K, Degenhardt S, et al. Renal involvement in sarcoidosis—a report of 6 cases. *Clin Nephrol.* 2002;57:142-148.

553. Mundlein E, Greter T, Ritz E. Grave's disease, sarcoidosis in a patient with minimal change disease. *Nephrol Dial Transplant.* 1996;11:860-862.

554. Parry RG, Falk C. Minimal change disease in association with sarcoidosis. *Nephrol Dial Transplant.* 1997;12:2159-2160.

555. Veronese FS, Henn L, Faccin C, et al. Pulmonary sarcoidosis and focal segmental glomerulosclerosis: case report and renal transplant follow up. *Nephrol Dial Transplant.* 1998;13:493-495.

556. Toda T, Kimoto S, Nishio Y, et al. Sarcoidosis with membranous nephropathy and granulomatous nephritis. *Intern Med.* 1999;38:882-886.

557. Dimitriades C, Shetty AK, Vehaskari M, et al. Membranous nephropathy associated with childhood sarcoid. *Pediatr Nephrol.* 1999;13:444-447.

558. Paydas S, Abayli B, Kocabas A, et al. Membranoproliferative glomerulonephritis associated pulmonary sarcoidosis. *Nephrol Dial Transplant.* 1998;13:228-229.

559. Nishiki M, Murakami Y, Yamane Y, et al. Steroid sensitive nephrotic syndrome, sarcoidosis, and thyroiditis. *Nephrol Dial Transplant.* 1999;14:2008-2010.

560. van Uum SH, Coorman MP, Assman WJ, et al. A 58 year old man with sarcoidosis complicated by focal crescentic glomerulonephritis. *Nephrol Dial Transplant.* 1997;12:2703.

561. Auinger M, Irsigler K, Breiteneder S, et al. Normocalcemic hepatorenal sarcoidosis with crescentic glomerulonephritis. *Nephrol Dial Transplant.* 1997;12:1474.

562. Schwimmer JA, Joseph RE, Appel GB. Amyloid, fibrillary, and other glomerular deposition diseases. In: Wilcox HR, Brady CS, eds. *Therapy in Nephrology and Hypertension.* 2nd ed. Philadelphia: Saunders; 2003:253-260.

563. Gertz MA, Lacy MQ, Dispenzier A. Immunoglobulin light chain amyloidosis and the kidney. *Kidney Int.* 2002;61:1-9.

564. Picken MM. New insights into systemic amyloidosis: the importance of diagnosis of specific type. *Curr Opin Nephrol Hypertens.* 2007;16(3):196-203.

565. Gillmore JD, Hawkins PN. Drug insight: emerging therapies for amyloidosis. *Nature Clin Pract Nephrol.* 2006;2:263-270.

566. Sekijima Y, Kelly JW, Ikeda S. Pathogenesis of and therapeutic strategies to ameliorate the transthyretin amyloidoses. *Curr Pharm Des.* 2008;14(30):3219-3230.

567. Valleix S, Drunat S, Philit J-B, et al. Hereditary renal amyloidosis caused by a new variant lysozyme WG4R in a French family. *Kidney Int.* 2002;61:907-912.

568. Lachmann HJ, Booth DR, Booth SE, et al. Misdiagnosis or hereditary amyloidosis as primary AL amyloidosis. *N Engl J Med.* 2002;346:1786-1791.

569. Murphy CL, Wang S, Kestler D, et al. Leukocyte chemotactic factor 2 (LECT2)-associated renal amyloidosis: a case series. *Am J Kidney Dis.* 2010;56:1100-1107.

570. Bellotti V, Nuvolone M, Giorgetti S, et al. The workings of the amyloid diseases. *Ann Med.* 2007;39(3):200-207.

571. Husby G, Stenstad T, Magnus JH, et al. Interaction between circulating amyloid fibril protein precursors and extracellular matrix components in the pathogenesis of systemic amyloidosis. *Clin Immunol Immunopathol.* 1994;70:2.

572. Cunnane G. Amyloid proteins in the pathogenesis of AA amyloidosis. *Lancet.* 2001;358:4-5.

573. Jahn TR, Radford SE. Folding versus aggregation: polypeptide conformations on competing pathways. *Arch Biochem Biophys.* 2008;469(1):100-117.

574. Gillmore JD, Lovat LB, Persey MR, et al. Amyloid load and clinical outcome in AA amyloidosis in relation to circulating concentration of serum amyloid A protein. *Lancet.* 2001;358:24-29.

575. Solomon A, Weiss DT, Kattine AA. Nephrotoxic potential of Bence Jones proteins. *N Engl J Med.* 1845;324:1991.

576. Myat EA, Westholm FA, Weiss DT, et al. Pathogenic potential of human monoclonal immunoglobulin fight chains: relationship between in vitro aggregation and in vivo organ deposition. *Proc Natl Acad Sci U S A.* 1994;91:3034.

577. Pepys MB, Herbert J, Hutchinson WL, et al. Targeted pharmacological depletion of serum amyloid P component for treatment of human amyloidosis. *Nature.* 2002;417:254-259.

578. Kyle RA, Gertz MA. Primary systemic amyloidosis: clinical and laboratory features in 474 cases. *Semin Hematol.* 1995;32:45-59.

579. Kunis CL, Teng SN. Treatment of glomerulonephritis in the elderly. *Semin Nephrol.* 2000;20:256-264.

580. Kyle RA, Linos A, Beard CM, et al. Incidence and natural history of primary systemic amyloidosis in Olmstead County Minnesota. *Blood.* 1992;79:1817-1822.

581. Gillmore J, Lovat L, Pearsey M, et al. Amyloid load and clinical outcome in AA amyloidosis in relation to circulating concentrations of serum amyloid A protein. *Lancet.* 2001;358:24-29.

582. Lachmann HJ, Goodman HJ, Gilbertson JA, et al. Natural history and outcome in systemic AA amyloidosis. *N Engl J Med.* 2007;356(23):2361-2371.

583. Said R, Hamzeh Y, Said S, et al. Spectrum of renal involvement in familial Mediterranean fever. *Kidney Int.* 1992;41:414.

584. Agha I, Mahoney R, Beardslee M, et al. Systemic amyloidosis associated with pleomorphic sarcoma of the spleen and remission of nephrotic syndrome after removal. *Am J Kidney Dis.* 2002;40:411-415.

585. Kunis CL, Aggarwal N, Appel GB. Illicit drug use and renal disease. In: Debroe M, Porter G, eds. *Nephrotoxicity in Clinical Medicine: Renal Injury from Drugs and Chemicals.* New York: Springer Press; 2008:595-617.

586. Manner I, Sagedal S, Roger M, et al. Renal amyloidosis in intravenous heroin addicts with nephrotic syndrome and renal failure. *Clin Nephrol.* 2009;72(3):224-228.

587. van Gameren II, Hazenberg BP, Bijzet J, et al. Diagnostic accuracy of subcutaneous abdominal fat tissue aspiration for detecting systemic amyloidosis and its utility in clinical practice. *Arthritis Rheum.* 2006;54(6):2015-2021.

588. Delgado WA, Arana-Chavez VE. Amyloid deposits in labial, salivary glands identified by electron microscopy. *J Oral Pathol Med.* 1997;26:51-52.

589. Hawkins PN, Lavender JP, Pepys MB. Evaluation of systemic amyloid by scintigraphy with I[123]-labeled serum amyloid P component. *N Engl J Med.* 1990;323:508-513.

590. Drayson M, Tang LX, Drew R, et al. Serum free light chain measurements for identifying and monitoring patients with nonsecretory multiple myeloma. *Blood.* 2001;97:2900-2902.

591. Lachman HJ, Gallimore R, Gillmore JD, et al. Outcome in systemic AL amyloidosis in relationship to changing serum concentrations of circulating free immunoglobulin light chains following chemotherapy. *Br J Hematol.* 2003;122:78-84.

592. Piken MM, Pelton K, Frangione B, et al. Primary amyloidosis A: immunohistochemical and biochemical characterization. *Am J Pathol.* 1987;129:536.

593. Herrera G. Renal disease associated with plasma cell dyscrasias, amyloidosis, Waldenstrom's macroglobulinemia, and cryoglobulinemia. In: Jennette JC, Olson JL, Schwartz MM, eds. *Heptinstall's Pathology of the Kidney,* 6th ed. Philadelphia: Lippincott Williams & Wilkins; 2006:853-910.

594. Picken MM. The changing concepts of amyloid. *Arch Pathol Lab Med.* 2001;25:38-46.

595. Markowitz GS. Dysproteinemias and the kidney. *Adv Anatomic Pathol.* 2004;11:49-63.

596. Sethi S, Theis JD, Leung N, et al. Mass spectrometry-based proteomic diagnosis of renal immunoglobulin heavy chain amyloidosis. *Clin J Am Soc Nephrol.* 2010;5(12):2180-2187.

597. Dubrey SW, Cha K, Anderson J, et al. The clinical features of immunoglobulin light-chain (AL) amyloidosis with heart involvement. *Q J Med.* 1998;91:141-157.

598. Dember LM. Modern treatment of amyloidosis: unresolved questions. *J Am Soc Nephrol.* 2009;20(3):469-472.

599. Kyle RA, Wagoner RD, Holley KE. Primary systemic amyloidosis, resolution of the nephrotic syndrome with melphalan and prednisone. *Arch Intern Med.* 1982;142:1445.

600. Gertz MA, Kyle RA, Greipp PR. Response rates and survival in primary systemic amyloidosis. *Blood.* 1991;77(2):257.

601. Skinner M, Anderson J, Simms R, et al. Treatment of 100 patients with primary amyloidosis: a randomized trial of melphalan, prednisone, and colchicine versus colchicine only. *Am J Med.* 1996;100:290.

602. Kyle RA, Gertz MA, Greipp PR, et al. A trial of those three regimens for primary amyloidosis: colchicine alone, melphalan and prednisone, and melphalan, prednisone and colchicine. *N Engl J Med.* 1997;336:1202-1207.

603. Gertz MA, Lacy MQ, Lust JA, et al. Prospective randomized trial of melphalan and prednisone versus vincristine, carmustine, melphalan, cyclophosphamide, and prednisone in the treatment of primary amyloidosis. *J Clin Oncol.* 1999;17:262-267.

604. Wang WJ, Lin CD, Wong CK, et al. Response of systemic amyloidosis to dimethyl sulfoxide. *J Am Acad Dermatol.* 1986;15:402.

605. Wechalekar AD, Goodman HJ, Lachmann HJ, et al. Safety and efficacy of risk-adapted cyclophosphamide, thalidomide, and dexamethasone in systemic AL amyloidosis. *Blood.* 2007;109(2):457-464.

606. Sanchorawala V, Wright DG, Rosenzweig M, et al. Lenalidomide and dexamethasone in the treatment of AL amyloidosis: results of a phase 2 trial. *Blood.* 2007;109(2):492-496.

607. Gertz MA, Kyle RA. Phase II trial of recombinant interferon alfa-2 in the treatment of primary systemic amyloidosis. *Am J Hematol.* 1993;44:125.

608. Gertz MA, Lacy MQ, Lust JA, et al. Phase II trial of high dose dexamethasone for untreated patients with primary systemic amyloidosis. *Am J Hematol.* 1999;61:115-119.

609. Gertz MA, Lacy MQ, Dispenzieri A. Myeloablative chemotherapy with stem cell rescue for the treatment of primary systemic amyloidosis: a status report. *Bone Marrow Transplant.* 2000;25:465-470.

610. Comenzo RL. Hematopoietic cell transplantation for primary systemic amyloidosis: what have we learned? *Leuk Lymphoma.* 2000;37:245-258.

611. Dember LM, Sanchorawala V, Seldin DC, et al. Effect of dose-intensive intravenous melphalan and autologous blood stem-cell transplantation on AL amyloidosis-associated renal disease. *Ann Intern Med.* 2001;134:746-753.

612. Leung N, Dispenzierri A, Fervenza F, et al. Renal response after high dose melphalan and stem cell transplantation is a favorable marker in patients with primary systemic amyloid. *Am J Kidney Dis.* 2005;46:270-277.

613. Casserly LF, Fadia A, Sanchorawala V, et al. High dose intravenous melphalan with autologous stem cell transplantation in AL amyloid associated end stage renal disease. *Kidney Int.* 2003;63:11051-11057.

614. Jaccard A, Moreau P, Leblond V, et al., for Myélome Autogreffe (MAG) and Intergroupe Francophone du Myélome (IFM) Intergroup. Autologous stem cell transplantation (ASCT) versus chemotherapy in AL amyloidosis. *N Engl J Med.* 2007;357:1083-1093.

615. Pettersson T, Konttinen YT, Maury CP. Treatment strategies for amyloid A amyloidosis. *Exp Opin Pharmacother.* 2008;9(12):2117-2128.

616. Chevrel G, Jenvrin C, McGregoe B, et al. Renal type AA amyloidosis associated with rheumatoid arthritis: a cohort study showing improved survival on treatment with pulse cyclophosphamide. *Rheumatology (Oxford).* 2001;40:821-825.

617. Livneh A, Zemer D, Langevitz P, et al. Colchicine in the treatment of AA amyloidosis of familial Mediterranean fever. *Arthritis Rheum.* 1994;37(12):1804.

618. Dember LM, Hawkins PN, Hazenberg BP, et al. Eprodisate for the treatment of renal disease in AA amyloidosis. *N Engl J Med.* 2007;356(23):2349-2360.

619. Gertz MA, Kyle RA, O'Fallon WM. Dialysis support of patients with primary systemic amyloidosis, a study of 211 patients. *Arch Intern Med.* 1992;152:2245.

620. Moroni G, Banfi G, Montoli A, et al. Chronic dialysis in patients with systemic amyloidosis: the experience in Northern Italy. *Clin Nephrol.* 1992;38(2):81.

621. Pasternack A, Ahonen J, Kuhlback B. Renal transplantation in 45 patients with amyloidosis. *Transplantation.* 1986;42(6):598.

622. Sobh K, Refaie A, Moustafa F, et al. Study of live donor kidney transplantation outcome in recipients with renal amyloidosis. *Nephrol Dial Transplant.* 1994;9:704.

623. Rosenstock J, Valeri A, Appel GB, et al. Fibrillary glomerulonephritis. Defining the disease spectrum. *Kidney Int.* 2003;63:1450-1462.

624. Schwartz MM, Korbet SM, Lewis EJ. Immunotactoid glomerulopathy. *J Am Soc Nephrol.* 2002;13:1390-1397.

625. Bridoux F, Hugue V, Coldefy O, et al. Fibrillary glomerulonephritis and immunotactoid (microtubular) glomerulopathy are associated with distinct immunologic features. *Kidney Int.* 2002;62(5):1764-1775.

626. Fogo A, Nauman Q, Horn RG. Morphological and clinical features of fibrillary glomerulonephritis versus immunotactoid glomerulopathy. *Am J Kidney Dis.* 1993;22(3):367.

627. Markowitz GS, Cheng JT, Colvin RB, et al. Hepatitis C viral infection is associated with fibrillary glomerulonephritis and immunotactoid glomerulopathy. *J Am Soc Nephrol.* 1998;9(12):2244-2252.

628. Strom EH, Banfi G, Krapf R, et al. Glomerulopathy associated with predominant fibronectin deposits: a newly recognized hereditary disease. *Kidney Int.* 1995;48:163.

629. Assmann KJ, Koene RA, Wetzels JF. Familial glomerulonephritis characterized by massive deposits of fibronectin. *Am J Kidney Dis.* 1995;25:781.

630. Castelletti F, Donadelli R, Banteria F, et al. Mutations in FN1 cause glomerulopathy with fibronectin deposits. *Proc Nat Acad Sci.* 2008;105:2538-2543.

631. Masson RG, Rennke HG, Gottlieb MN. Pulmonary hemorrhage in a patient with fibrillary glomerulonephritis. *N Engl J Med.* 1992;326:36.

632. Wallner K, Prischl FC, Hobling W, et al. Immunotactoid glomerulopathy with extrarenal deposits in the bone, and chronic cholestatic liver disease. *Nephrol Dial Transplant.* 1996;1:1619.

633. Collins M, Navaneethan SD, Chung M, et al. Rituximab treatment of fibrillary glomerulonephritis. *Am J Kidney Dis.* 2008;52(6):1158-1162.

634. Samaniego M, Nadasdy GM, Laszik Z, et al. Outcome of renal transplantation in fibrillary glomerulonephritis. *Clin Nephrol.* 2001;55:159-166.

635. Pronovost PK, Brady HR, Gunning ME, et al. Clinical features, predictors of disease progression and results of renal transplantation in fibrillary/immunotactoid glomerulopathy. *Nephrol Dial Transplant.* 1996;11(5):83-87.

636. Lin J, Markowitz GS, Valeri AM, et al. Renal monoclonal immunoglobulin deposition disease: the disease spectrum. *Am J Soc Nephrol.* 2001;12:1482-1492.

637. Buxbaum J, Gallo G. Nonamyloidotic monoclonal immunoglobulin deposition disease. Light-chain, heavy-chain, and light- and heavy-chain deposition diseases. *Hematol Oncol Clin North Am.* 1999;13:1235-1248.

638. Pozzi C, D'Amico M, Fogazzi GB, et al. Light chain deposition disease with renal involvement: clinical characteristics and prognostic factors. *Am J Kidney Dis.* 2003;42:1154-1163.

639. Preud'Homme JL, Aucouturier P, Touchard G, et al. Monoclonal immunoglobulin deposition disease (Randall type). Relationship with structural abnormalities of immunoglobulin chains. *Kidney Int.* 1994;46:965-972.

640. Buxbaum JN, Chuba JV, Hellman GC, et al. Monoclonal immunoglobulin deposition disease: light chain and light and heavy chain deposition diseases and their relation to light chain amyloidosis. *Ann Intern Med.* 1990;12:455-464.

641. Zhu L, Herrera GA, Murphy-Ullrich JE, et al. Pathogenesis of glomerulosclerosis in LCDD: role of TGF-beta. *Am J Pathol.* 1995;147:375-385.

642. Sinniah R, Cohen AH. Glomerular capillary aneurysms in light chain nephropathy: an ultrastructural proposal of morphogenesis. *Am J Pathol.* 1985;118:298.

643. Noel LH, Droz D, Ganeval D, et al. Renal granular monoclonal light chain deposits: Morphological aspects in 11 cases. *Clin Nephrol.* 1984;21:263.

644. Heilman RL, Velosa JA, Holley KE, et al. Long-term follow-up and response to chemotherapy in patients with LCDD. *Am J Kidney Dis.* 1992;20:34-41.

645. Lin JJ, Miller F, Waltzer W, et al. Recurrence of immunoglobulin A-kappa crystalline deposition disease after kidney transplantation. *Am J Kidney Dis.* 1995;25:75-78.

646. Leung N, Lager DJ, Gertz MA, et al. Long-term outcome of renal transplantation in light-chain deposition disease. *Am J Kidney Dis.* 2004;43:147-153.

647. Aucouturier P, Khamlichi AA, Touchard G, et al. Brief report: heavy chain deposition disease. *N Engl J Med.* 1993;329:1389.

648. Kambham N, Markowitz GS, Appel GB, et al. Heavy chain deposition disease: the disease spectrum. *Am J Kidney Dis.* 1999;33:954-962.

649. Cheng IKP, Ho SKN, Chan DMT, et al. Crescenteric nodular glomerulosclerosis secondary to truncated immunoglobulin a heavy chain deposition. *Am J Kidney Dis.* 1996;28:283-288.

650. Khamlichi AA, Aucouturier P, Preud'homme JL, et al. Structure of abnormal heavy chains in human heavy-chain deposition disease. *Eur J Biochem.* 1995;229:54-60.

651. Royer B, Arnulf B, Martinez F, et al. High dose chemotherapy in light chain or light and heavy chain deposition disease. *Kidney Int.* 2004;65(2):642-648.

652. Nasr SH, Markowitz GS, Stokes B, et al. Proliferative glomerulonephritis with monoclonal IgG deposits: a distinct entity mimicking immune-complex glomerulonephritis. *Kidney Int.* 2004;65:85-96.

653. Nasr S, Satoskar A, Markowitz GS, et al. Proliferative glomerulonephritis with monoclonal IgG deposits: a report of 37 cases. *J Am Soc Nephrol.* 2009;20:2055-2064.

654. Nasr SH, Preddie DC, Markowitz GS, et al. Multiple myeloma, nephritic syndrome and crystalloid inclusions in podocytes. *Kidney Int.* 2006;69:616-620.

655. Markowitz G, Appel GB, Fine P, et al. Collapsing FSGS following treatment with high dose pamidronate. *J Am Soc Nephrol.* 2001;12:1164-1172.

656. Fonseca R, Hayman S. Waldenstrom macroglobulinaemia. *Br J Haematol.* 2007;138(6):700-720.
657. Garcia Suz R, Mantoto S, Torrequebrada A, et al. Waldenstrom's macroglobulinemia: presenting features and outcomes in a series with 217 cases. *Br J Haematol.* 2001;115:575.
658. Dimopoulos MA, Panayiotidis P, Moupoulos LA, et al. Waldenstrom's urinemia: clinical features, complications and management. *J Clin Oncol.* 2000;18:214-226.
659. Veltman GA, van Veen S, Kluin-Nelemans JC, et al. Renal disease in Waldenström's macroglobulinemia. *Nephrol Dial Transplant.* 1997;12(6):1256.
660. Tsuji M, Ochiai S, Taka T, et al. Non-amyloidogenic nephrotic syndrome in Waldenstrom's macroglobulinemia. *Nephron.* 1990;54:176.
661. Treon SP, Gertz MA, Dimopouols M, et al. Update on treatment recommendations from the Third International Workshop on Waldenstrom's macroglobulinemia. *Blood.* 2006;107:3442-3446.
662. Annibali O, Petrucci MT, Martini V, et al. Treatment of 72 newly diagnosed Waldenstrom macroglobulinemia cases with oral melphalan, cyclophosphamide, and prednisone: results and cost analysis. *Cancer.* 2005;103:582-587.
663. Gertz MA, Rue M, Blood E, et al. Multicenter phase 2 trial of rituximab for Waldenström macroglobulinemia (WM): an Eastern Cooperative Oncology Group Study (E3A98). *Leuk Lymphoma.* 2004;45(10):2047-2055.
664. D'Amico G, Colasanti G, Ferrario F, et al. Renal involvement in essential mixed cryoglobulinemia. *Kidney Int.* 1989;35:1004.
665. Tarantino A, de Vecchi A, Montaguino G, et al. Renal disease in essential mixed cryoglobulinemia: long-term follow-up of 44 patients. *Q J Med.* 1981;50:1.
666. Frankel AK, Singer DR, Winearls CG, et al. Type 11 essential mixed cryoglobulinemia: Presentation, treatment and outcome in 13 patients. *Q J Med.* 1992;82(298):101-124.
667. Agnello V, Chung RT, Kaplan LM. A role for hepatitis C virus infection in type II cryoglobulinemia. *N Engl J Med.* 1992;327:1490-1495.
668. Cordonnier D, Vialfel P, Renversy J, et al. Renal disease in 18 patients with mixed type II IgM-IgG cryoglobulinemia: monoclonal lymphoid infiltration and membranoproliferative glomerulonephritis (14 cases). *Adv Nephrol.* 1983;12:177.
669. Appel GB. Immune-complex glomerulonephritis—deposits plus interest. *N Engl J Med.* 1993;328:505-506.
670. Galli M, Monti G, Invernizzi F, et al. Hepatitis B virus-related markers in secondary and essential mixed cryoglobulinemias: a multicenter study of 596 cases. *Ann Ital Med Intern.* 1992;7:209-214.
671. D'Amico G, Ferrario F. Cryoglobulinemic glomerulonephritis: a MPGN induced by hepatitis C virus. *Am J Kidney Dis.* 1995;25:361-369.
672. Sansonno D, Gesualdo L, Manno C, et al. Hepatitis C virus-related proteins in kidney tissue from hepatitis C virus-infected patients with cryoglobulinemic membranoproliferative glomerulonephritis. *Hepatology.* 1997;25:1237.
673. Bichard P, Ounanian A, Girard M, et al. High prevalence of HCV RNA in the supernatant and the cryoprecipitate of patients with essential and secondary type II mixed cryoglobulinemia. *J Hepatol.* 1994;21:58-63.
674. Johnson RJ, Willson R, Yamabe K, et al. Renal manifestations of hepatitis C virus infection. *Kidney Int.* 1994;46:1255.
675. Fornasieri A, Armelloni S, Bernasconi P, et al. High binding of IgMk rheumatoid factor from type II cryoglobulins to cellular fibronectin. *Am J Kidney Dis.* 1996;27:476-483.
676. Sinico RA, Winearls CG, Sabadini E, et al. Identification of glomerular immune complexes in cryoglobulinemia glomerulonephritis. *Kidney Int.* 1988;34:109.
677. Madore F, Lazarus JK, Brady HR. Therapeutic plasma exchange in renal diseases. *J Am Soc Nephrol.* 1996;7:367.
678. Tarantino A, Carnpise K, Banfi G, et al. Long-term predictors of survival in essential mixed cryoglobulinemic glomerulonephritis. *Kidney Int.* 1995;47:618.
679. Iannuzzella F, Vaglio A, Garini G. Management of hepatitis C virus-related mixed cryoglobulinemia. *Am J Med.* 2010;123(5):400-408.
680. Zaja F, De Vita S, Mazzaro C, et al. Efficacy and safety of rituximab in type II mixed cryoglobulinemia. *Blood.* 2003;101:3827-3834.
681. Tarantino A, Moroni G, Banfi G, et al. Renal replacement therapy in cryoglobulinemic nephritis. *Nephrol Dial Transplant.* 1994;9:1426.
682. Guthrie LB. Idiopathic or congenital hereditary and family haematuria. *Lancet.* 1902;1:1243-1246.
683. Alport AC. Hereditary familial congenital hemorrhagic nephritis. *Br Med J.* 1927;1:504-506.
684. Kendall G, Hertz AF. Hereditary familial congenital hemorrhagic nephritis. *Guys Hosp Rep.* 1912;66:137.
685. Crawfurd MD, Toghill PJ. Alport's syndrome of hereditary chronic nephritis and deafness. *Q J Med.* 1968;37:563-576.
686. Gubler M-C, Antignac C, Deschenes G. Genetic, clinical and morphologic heterogeneity in Alport's syndrome. *Adv Nephrol.* 1993;22:15-35.
687. Chazan JA, Zacks J, Cohen JJ, et al. Hereditary nephritis: clinical spectrum and mode of inheritance in five new kindreds. *Am J Med.* 1971;50:764-771.
688. Chugh KS, Sakhuja V, Agarwal A. Hereditary nephritis Alport's syndrome: clinical profile and inheritance in 28 kindreds. *Nephrol Dial Transplant.* 1993;8:690-695.
689. Gubler M, Levy M, Broyer M, et al. Alport's syndrome: a report of 58 cases and a review of the literature. *Am J Med.* 1981;70:493-505.
690. Jais JP, Knebelmann B, Giatras I, et al. X-linked Alport syndrome: natural history in 195 families and genotype-phenotype correlations in males. *J Am Soc Nephrol.* 2000;11:649-657.
691. U.S. Renal Data System. *USRDS 2009 Annual Data Report: Atlas of Chronic Kidney Disease and End-Stage Renal Disease in the United States.* Washington, DC: National Institutes of Health, National Institute of Diabetes and Digestive and Kidney Diseases; 2009.
692. O'Neill WM, Atkin CL, Bloomer HA. Hereditary nephritis: a re-examination of its clinical and genetic features. *Ann Intern Med.* 1978;88:176-182.
693. Knepshield JH, Roberts PL, Davis CJ, et al. Hereditary chronic nephritis complicated by nephrotic syndrome. *Arch Intern Med.* 1968;122:156-158.
694. Grunfeld J-P, Noel LH, Hafex S, et al. Renal prognosis in women with hereditary nephritis. *Clin Nephrol.* 1985;23:267-271.
695. Jais JP, Knebelmann B, Giatras I, et al. X-linked Alport syndrome: Natural history and genotype-phenotype correlations in girls and women belonging to 195 families: a "European community Alport syndrome concerted action" study. *J Am Soc Nephrol.* 2003;14:2603-2610.
696. Gleeson MJ. Alport's syndrome: audiological manifestations and implications. *J Laryngol Otol.* 1984;98:449-465.
697. Yoshikawa N, White RHR, Cameron AH. Familial hematuria: clinicopathological correlations. *Clin Nephrol.* 1982;17:172-182.
698. Grunfeld J-P, Bois EP, Hinglais N. Progressive and non-progressive hereditary nephritis. *Kidney Int.* 1973;4:216-228.
699. Chance JK, Stanley JA. Alport's syndrome: case report and review of ocular manifestations. *Ann Ophthalmol.* 1977;9:1527-1530.
700. Thompson SM, Deady JP, Willshaw HR, et al. Ocular signs in Alport's syndrome. *Eye.* 1987;1:146-153.
701. Kashtan CE, Segal Y, Flinter F, et al. Aortic abnormalities in males with Alport syndrome. *Nephrol Dial Transplant.* 2010;25(11):3554-3360.
702. Epstein CJ, Sahud MA, Piel CF, et al. Hereditary macrothombocytopenia, nephritis and deafness. *Am J Med.* 1972;52:299-310.
703. Parsa KP, Lee DBN, Zamboni L, et al. Hereditary nephritis, deafness and abnormal thrombopoiesis: study of a new kindred. *Am J Med.* 1976;60:665-671.
704. Antignac C, Zhou J, Sanak M, et al. Alport syndrome and diffuse leiomyomatosis: deletions in the 5' end of the COL4A5 collagen gene. *Kidney Int.* 1992;42:1178-1183.
705. Goyer RA, Reynolds Jr J, Burke J, et al. Hereditary renal disease with neurosensory hearing loss, prolinuria and ichthyosis. *Am J Med Sci.* 1968;256:166-179.
706. Ghiggeri GM, Caridi G, Magrini U, et al. Genetics, clinical and pathological features of glomerulonephritis associated with mutations of nonmuscle myosin IIA Fechtner syndrome. *Am J Kidney Dis.* 2003;41:95-104.
707. Kashtan CE, Michael AF, Sibley RK, et al. Hereditary nephritis: Alport syndrome and thin glomerular basement membrane disease. In: Craig Tisher C, Brenner BM, eds. *Renal Pathology: With Clinical and Functional Correlation.* 2nd ed. Philadelphia: J.B. Lippincott; 1994:1239-166.
708. Rumpelt HJ. Hereditary nephropathy Alport's syndrome: spectrum and development of glomerular lesions. In: Rosen S, ed. *Pathology of Glomerular Disease.* New York: Churchill Livingstone; 1983:225.
709. Gaboardi R, Edefonti A, Imbasciati E, et al. Alport's syndrome progressive hereditary nephritis. *Clin Nephrol.* 1974;2:143-156.
710. Langer KH, Theones W. Alport syndrome: licht und electronen-mikroskopische nierenefunde im fruhstadium. *Verh D Dtsch Ges Pathol.* 1971;55:497-502.
711. Krickstein HI, Gloor FJ, Balogh K. Renal pathology in hereditary nephritis with nerve deafness. *Arch Pathol.* 1966;82:506-517.
712. Habib R, Gubler M-C, Hinglais N, et al. Alport's syndrome: experience at Hopital Necker. *Kidney Int.* 1982;21(suppl):S20-S28.
713. Hinglais N, Grunfeld J-P, Bois LE. Characteristic ultrastructural lesion of the glomerular basement membrane in progressive hereditary nephritis Alport's syndrome. *Lab Invest.* 1972;27:473-487.
714. Nasr SH, Markowitz GS, Goldstein CS, et al. Hereditary nephritis mimicking immune complex-mediated glomerulonephritis. *Hum Pathol.* 2006;37:547-554.

715. Olson FL, Anand SK, Landing BH, et al. Diagnosis of hereditary nephritis by failure of glomeruli to bind anti-glomerular basement membrane antibodies. *J Pediatr.* 1980;96:697-699.

716. Savage COS, Kershaw M, Pusey CD, et al. Use of a monoclonal antibody in differential diagnosis of children with hematuria and hereditary nephritis. *Lancet.* 1986;1:1459-1461.

717. Grunfeld JP. Contemporary diagnostic approach in Alport's syndrome. *Renal Failure.* 2000;22:759-763.

718. Kashtan CE, Michael AF. Alport syndrome. *Kidney Int.* 1996;2750: 1445-1463.

719. Reznick VM, Griswold WR, Vazquez MD, et al. Glomerulonephritis with absent glomerular basement membrane antigens. *Am J Nephrol.* 1984;4: 296-298.

720. Rumpelt HJ. Hereditary nephropathy Alport's syndrome: correlation of clinical data with glomerular basement membrane alterations. *Clin Nephrol.* 1980;13:203-207.

721. Hill GS, Jenis EH, Goodloe SG. The nonspecificity of the ultrastructural alterations in hereditary nephritis. *Lab Invest.* 1974;31:516-532.

722. Tryggvasson K, Zhou J, Hostikka SL, et al. Molecular genetics of Alport syndrome. *Kidney Int.* 1993;43:38-44.

723. Hasstedt SJ, Atkin CL. X-linked inheritance of Alport syndrome: family P revisited. *Am J Hum Gen.* 1983;35:1241-1251.

724. Shaw RF, Kallen RJ. Population genetics of Alport's syndrome: hypothesis of abnormal segregation and the necessary existence of mutation. *Nephrology.* 1976;16:427-432.

725. Barker DF, Hostikka SL, Zhou J. Identification of mutations in the COL4A5 collagen gene in Alport syndrome. *Science.* 1990;248:1224-1227.

726. Kleppel MM, Kashtan C, Santi PA. Distribution of familial nephritis antigen in normal tissue and renal basement membranes of patients with homozygous and heterozygous Alport familial nephritis: relationships of familial nephritis and Goodpasture antigens to novel collagen chains and type IV collagen. *Lab Invest.* 1989;61:278-289.

727. Hostikka SL, Eddy RL, Byers MG. Identification of a distinct type IV collagen a chain with restricted kidney distribution and assignment of its gene to the locus of X-chromosome-linked Alport syndrome. *Proc Natl Acad Sci.* 1990;87:1606-1610.

728. Knebelman B, Antignac C, Gubler M-C, et al. Molecular genetics of Alport's syndrome: the clinical consequences. *Nephrol Dial Transplant.* 1993;8:677-679.

729. Netzer KO, Renders L, Zhou J. Deletions of the COL4A5 gene in patients with Alport syndrome. *Kidney Int.* 1992;42:1336-1344.

730. Kashtan C, Kim Y. Distribution of the a1_and a2 chains of collagen IV and of collagens V and VI in Alport syndrome. *Kidney Int.* 1992;42: 115-126.

731. Kalluri R, Weber M, Netzer K. COL4A5 gene deletion and production of post-transplant anti-a3IV. collagen alloantibodies in Alport syndrome. *Kidney Int.* 1994;45:721-726.

732. Van den Heuvel LPWJ, Savage COS, et al. The glomerular basement membrane defect in Alport-type hereditary nephritis: absence of cationic antigenic components. *Nephrol Dial Transplant.* 1989;4:770-775.

733. Nakanishi K, Yolhikawa N, Iijima K, et al. Expression of type IV collagen alpha-3 and alpha-4 chain mRNA in X-linked Alport syndrome. *J Am Soc Nephrol.* 1996;7:938-945.

734. Kashtan CE, Michael AF. Alport syndrome: from bedside to genome to bedside. *Am J Kidney Dis.* 1993;22:627-640.

735. Seri M, Pecci A, Di Bari F, et al. MYH9-related disease—May-Hegglin anomaly, Sebastian syndrome, Fechtner syndrome, and Epstein syndrome are not distinct entities but represent a variable expression of a single illness. *Medicine.* 2003;82:203-215.

736. Tishler PV, Rosner B. The genetics of the Alport syndrome. *Birth Defects.* 1979;10:93-99.

737. Hasstedt SJ, Atkin CL, San Juan AC: Genetic heterogeneity among kindreds with Alport syndrome. *Am J Hum Gen.* 1986;38:940-953.

738. Cohen EP, Lemann Jr J. In hereditary nephritis, angiotensin converting enzyme inhibition decreases proteinuria and may slow the rate of progression. *Am J Kidney Dis.* 1996;27:199-203.

739. Kaito H, Nozu K, Iijima K, et al. The effect of aldosterone blockade in patients with Alport syndrome. *Pediatr Nephrol.* 2006;21:1824-1829.

740. Callis L, Vila A, Carrera M, et al. Long-term effects of cyclosporine A in Alport's syndrome. *Kidney Int.* 1999;55:1051-1056.

741. Charbit M, Gubler MC, Dechaux M, et al. Cyclosporin therapy in patients with Alport syndrome. *Pediatr Nephrol.* 2007;22:57-63.

742. Byrne MC, Budisavljevic MN, Fan Z, et al. Renal transplant in patients with Alport's syndrome. *Am J Kidney Dis.* 2002;39:769-775.

743. Goldman M, Depierreux M, De Pauw L, et al. Failure of two subsequent renal grafts by anti-GBM glomerulonephritis in Alport's syndrome: case report and review of literature. *Transplant Int.* 1990;3:82-85.

744. Pedchenko V, Bondar O, Fogo AB, et al. Molecular architecture of the Goodpasture autoantigen in anti-GBM nephritis. *N Engl J Med.* 2010;363:343-354.

745. Hudson BG, Kalluri R, Gunwar R, et al. The pathogenesis of Alport syndrome involves type IV collagen molecules containing the a3IV. chain: evidence from anti-GBM nephritis after renal transplantation. *Kidney Int.* 1992;42:179-187.

746. Ding J, Zhou J, Tryggvasson K, et al. COL4A5 deletions in three patients with Alport syndrome and posttransplant antiglomerular basement membrane nephritis. *J Am Soc Nephrol.* 1994;5:161-168.

747. Cosio FG, Falkenhain ME, Sedmak DD. Association of thin glomerular basement membrane with other glomerulopathies. *Kidney Int.* 1994;46: 471-474.

748. Perry GJ, George CRP, Field MJ, et al. Thin-membrane nephropathy: A common cause of glomerular haematuria. *Med J Aust.* 1989;151:638-642.

749. Lang S, Stevenson B, Risdon RA. Thin basement membrane nephropathy as a cause for recurrent haematuria in childhood. *Histopathology.* 1990;16:331-337.

750. Schroder CH, Bontemps CM, Assman KJM, et al. Renal biopsy and family studies in 65 children with isolated hematuria. *Acta Pediatr Scand.* 1990;79:630-636.

751. McConville JM, West CD, McAdams AJ. Familial and nonfamilial benign hematuria. *J Pediatr.* 1966;69:207-214.

752. Pardo V, Berian MG, Levi DF, et al. Benign primary hematuria: clinicopathologic study of 65 patients. *Am J Med.* 1979;67:817-822.

753. Dische FE, Anderson VER, Keane SJ, et al. Incidence of thin membrane nephropathy: morphometric investigation o a population sample. *J Clin Pathol.* 1990;43:457-460.

754. Vogler C, McAdams AJ, Homan SM. Glomerular basement membrane and lamina densa in infants and children: an ultrastructural evaluation. *Pediatr Pathol.* 1987;7:527-534.

755. Steffes MW, Barbosa J, Basgen JM, et al. Quantitative glomerular morphology of the normal human kidney. *Lab Invest.* 1983;49:82-86.

756. Tiebosch ATMG, Frederik PM, van Breda Vriesman PJC, et al. Thin-basement-membrane nephropathy in adults with persistent hematuria. *N Engl J Med.* 1989;320:14-18.

757. Basta-Jovanovic G, Venkataseshan VS, Gil J, et al. Morphometric analysis of glomerular basement membranes GBM in thin basement membrane disease TBMD. *Clin Nephrol.* 1990;33:110-114.

758. Abe S, Amagasaki Y, Iyori S, et al. Thin basement membrane syndrome in adults. *J Clin Pathol.* 1987;40:318-322.

759. Badenas C, Praga M, Tazon B, et al. Mutations in the COL4A4 and COL4A3 genes cause familial benign hematuria. *J Am Soc Nephrol.* 2002;13:1248-1254.

760. Eisenstein B, Stark H, Goodman RM. Benign familial hematuria in children from Jewish communities. *J Med Genet.* 1979;16:369-372.

761. Aarons I, Smith PS, Davies RA, et al. Thin membrane nephropathy: a clinico-pathological study. *Clin Nephrol.* 1989;32:151-158.

762. Szeto CC, Mac-Moune LF, Kwan BC, et al. The width of the basement membrane does not influence clinical presentation or outcome of thin glomerular basement membrane disease with persistent hematuria. *Kidney Int.* 2010;78(10):1041-1046.

763. Lemmink HH, Nillesen WN, Mochizuki T, et al. Benign familial hematuria due to mutation of the type IV collagen alpha4 gene. *J Clin Invest.* 1996;98:1114-1118.

764. Longo I, Porcedda P, Mari F, et al. COL4A3/COL4A4 mutations: From familial hematuria to autosomal-dominant or recessive Alport syndrome. *Kidney Int.* 2002;61:1947-1956.

765. Kashtan CE. Familial hematurias: what we know and what we don't. *Pediatr Nephrol.* 2005;20:1027-1035.

766. Mino RA, Mino VH, Livingstone RG. Osseous dysplasia and dystrophy of the nail: review of literature and report of a case. *Am J Roentgenol Radium Ther.* 1948;60:633-641.

767. Bongers EM, Gubler MC, Knoers NV. Nail-patella syndrome. Overview on clinical and molecular findings. *Pediatr Nephrol.* 2002;17:703-712.

768. Hoyer JR, Michael AF, Vernier RL, et al. Renal disease in nail-patella syndrome: clinical and morphologic studies. *Kidney Int.* 1972;2:231.

769. Bennett WM, Musgrave JE, Campbell RA, et al. The nephropathy of the nail-patella syndrome: clinicopathologic analysis of 11 kindreds. *Am J Med.* 1973;54:304.

770. Morita T, Laughlin LO, Kawano K, et al. Nail-patella syndrome: light and electron microscopic studies of the kidney. *Arch Intern Med.* 1973;131:217.

771. Dreyer SD, Zhou G, Baldini A, et al. Mutations in LMX1B cause abnormal skeletal patterning and renal dysplasia in nail patella syndrome. *Nat Genet.* 1998;19:47-50.

772. Vollrath D, Jaramillo-Babb VL, Clough MV, et al. Loss-of-function mutations in the LIM-homeodomain gene, LMX1B, in nail- patella syndrome. *Hum Mol Genet.* 1998;7:1091-1098.

773. Chan PCK, Chan KW, Cheng KP, et al. Living related renal transplantation in a patient with nail-patella syndrome. *Nephrology.* 1988;50:164-166.

774. Fabry J. Ein beitrag zur kenntnis der purpura hemorrhagica nodularis purpura papulosa hemorrhagica hebrae. *Arch Derm.* 1898;43:187.

775. Desnick RJ, Brady R, Barranger J, et al. Fabry disease, an under-recognized multisystemic disorder: expert recommendations for diagnosis, management, and enzyme replacement therapy. *Ann Intern Med.* 2003;138:338-346.

776. Wanner C, Oliveira JP, Ortiz A, et al. Prognostic indicators of renal disease progression in adults with Fabry disease: natural history data from the Fabry Registry. *Clin J Am Soc Nephrol.* 2010;5(12):2220-2228.

777. Obrador GT, Ojo A, Thadhani R. End-stage renal disease in patients with Fabry disease. *J Am Soc Nephrol.* 2002;13(suppl 2):S144-S146.

778. Whybra C, Kampmann C, Willers I, et al. Anderson-Fabry disease: clinical manifestations of disease in female heterozygotes. *J Inherit Metab Dis.* 2001;24:715-724.

779. Gubler MC, Lenoir G, Grunfeld J-P, et al. Early renal changes in homozygous and heterozygous patients with Fabry's disease. *Kidney Int.* 1978;13:223.

780. Thurberg BL, Rennke H, Colvin RB, et al. Globotriaosylceramide accumulation in the Fabry kidney is cleared from multiple cell types after enzyme replacement therapy. *Kidney Int.* 2002;62:1933-1946.

781. Farge D, Nadler S, Wolfe LS. Diagnostic value of kidney biopsy in heterozygous Fabry's disease. *Arch Pathol Lab Med.* 1985;109:85.

782. Ferraggiana T, Churg J, Grishman E, et al. Light- and electron-microscopic histochemistry of Fabry's disease. *Am J Pathol.* 1981;103:247.

783. Bernstein HS, Bishop DF, Astrin KH, et al. Fabry disease: six gene rearrangements and an exonic point mutation in the alpha galactosidase gene. *J Clin Invest.* 1989;83:1390.

784. Wherret JR, Hakomori S. Characterization of blood group B glycolipid, accumulating in the pancreas of a patient with Fabry's disease. *J Biol Chem.* 1973;218:3046.

785. Ohshima T, Murray GJ, Swaim WD, et al. Alpha-galactosidase A deficient mice: a model of Fabry disease. *Proc Natl Acad Sci U S A.* 1997;94: 2540-2544.

786. Hoffmann B. Fabry disease: recent advances in pathology, diagnosis, treatment and monitoring. *Orphanet J Rare Dis.* 2009;4:21.

787. Schiffmann R, Kopp JB, Austin III HA, et al. Enzyme replacement therapy in Fabry disease: a randomized controlled trial. *JAMA.* 2001;285: 2743-2749.

788. Eng CM, Guffon N, Wilcox WR, et al. Safety and efficacy of recombinant human alpha-galactosidase A—replacement therapy in Fabry's disease. *N Engl J Med.* 2001;345:9-16.

789. Mehta A, Beck M, Eyskens F, et al. Fabry disease: a review of current management strategies. *Q J Med.* 2010;103:641-659.

790. El Dib RP, Pastores GM. Enzyme replacement therapy for Anderson-Fabry disease. *Cochrane Database Syst Rev.* 2010;(5):CD006663.

791. Germain DP, Waldek S, Banikazemi M, et al. Sustained, long-term renal stabilization after 54 months of agalsidase beta therapy in patients with Fabry disease. *J Am Soc Nephrol.* 2007;18:1547-1557.

792. Schiffmann R, Ries M, Timmons M, et al. Long-term therapy with agalsidase alfa for Fabry disease: safety and effects on renal function in a home infusion setting. *Nephrol Dial Transplant.* 2006;21:345-354.

793. Tsakiris D, Simpson HK, Jones EH, et al. Report on management of renal failure in Europe, XXVI, 1995. Rare diseases in renal replacement therapy in the ERA-EDTA registry. *Nephrol Dial Transplant.* 1996;11(suppl 7): 4-20.

794. Helin I. Fabry's disease: a brief review in connection with a Scandinavian survey. *Scand J Urol Nephrol.* 1979;13:335.

795. Falk RJ, Jennette JC. Sickle cell nephropathy. *Adv Nephrol.* 1994;23:133-147.

796. Davis Jr CJ, Mostofi FK, Sesterhenn IA. Renal medullary carcinoma. The seventh sickle cell nephropathy. *Am J Surg Pathol.* 1995;19:1-11.

797. Kiryluk K, Jadoon A, Gupta M, et al. Sickle cell trait and gross hematuria. *Kidney Int.* 2007;71:706-710.

798. Falk RJ, Scheinman J, Phillips G, et al. Prevalence and pathologic features of sickle cell nephropathy and response to inhibition of angiotensin-converting enzyme. *N Engl J Med.* 1992;326:910-915.

799. Powars DR, Elliott-Mills DD, Chan L, et al. Chronic renal failure in sickle cell disease: risk factors, clinical course, and mortality. *Ann Intern Med.* 1991;115:614-620.

800. Thomas AN, Pattison C, Serjeant GR. Causes of death in sickle-cell disease in Jamaica. *Br Med J.* 1982;285:633-635.

801. Maigne G, Ferlicot S, Galacteros F, et al. Glomerular lesions in patients with sickle cell disease. *Medicine (Baltimore).* 2010;89:18-27.

802. Pardo V, Strauss J, Kramer H, et al. Nephropathy associated with sickle cell anemia: an autologous immune complex nephritis. II. Clinicopathologic study of seven patients. *Am J Med.* 1975;59(5):650-659.

803. Ozawa T, Mass M, Guggenheim S, et al. Autologous immune complex nephritis associated with sickle cell trait: diagnosis of the haemoglobinpathy after renal structural and immunological studies. *Br Med J.* 1976;1:369-371.

804. Effenbeing IB, Patchefsky A, Schwartz W, et al. Pathology of the glomerulus in sickle cell anemia with and without nephrotic syndrome. *Am J Pathol.* 1974;77:357.

805. McCoy RC. Ultrastructural alterations in the kidney of patients with sickle cell disease and the nephrotic syndrome. *Lab Invest.* 1969;21:85.

806. Walker BR, Alexander F, Birdsall TR, et al. Glomerular lesions in sickle cell nephropathy. *JAMA.* 1971;215:437-440.

807. Bhatena DB, Sondheimer JH. The glomerulopathy of homozygous sickle hemoglobin SS. disease: morphology and pathogenesis. *J Am Soc Nephrol.* 1991;1:1241-1252.

808. Tejani A, Phadke K, Adamson O, et al. Renal lesions in sickle cell nephropathy in children. *Nephrology.* 1985;39:352-355.

809. Nasr SH, Markowitz GS, Sentman RL, et al. Sickle cell disease, nephrotic syndrome, and renal failure. *Kidney Int.* 2006;69:1276-1280.

810. Elfenbein IB, Patchefsky A, Schwartz W, et al. Pathology of glomerulus in sickle-cell anemia with and without nephrotic syndrome. *Am J Pathol.* 1974;77:357.

811. Haymann JP, Stankovic K, Levy P, et al. Glomerular hyperfiltration in adult sickle cell anemia: a frequent hemolysis associated feature. *Clin J Am Soc Nephrol.* 2010;5:756-761.

812. Wesson DE. The initiation and progression of sickle cell nephropathy. *Kidney Int.* 2002;61:2277-2286.

813. Foucan L, Bourhis V, Bangou J, et al. A randomized trial of captopril for microalbuminuria in normotensive adults with sickle cell anemia. *Am J Med.* 1998;104:339-342.

814. Abbott KC, Hypolite IO, Agodoa LY. Sickle cell nephropathy at end-stage renal disease in the United States: patient characteristics and survival. *Clin Nephrol.* 2002;58:9-15.

815. Ojo AO, Govaerts TC, Schmouder RL, et al. Renal transplantation in end-stage sickle cell nephropathy. *Transplantation.* 1999;67:291-295.

816. Chatterjee SN. National study on natural history of renal allografts in sickle cell disease or trait. *Nephrology.* 1980;25:199-201.

817. Chatterjee SN. National study in natural history of renal allografts in sickle cell disease or trait: a second report. *Transplant Proc.* 1987;192 (suppl 2):33-35.

818. Miner DJ, Jorkasky DK, Perloff LJ, et al. Recurrent sickle cell nephropathy in a transplanted kidney. *Am J Kidney Dis.* 1987;10:306-313.

819. Senior B, Gellis SS. The syndromes of total lipodystrophy and partial lipodystrophy. *Pediatrics.* 1964;33:593-612.

820. Misra A, Peethambaram A, Garg A. Clinical features and metabolic and autoimmune derangements in acquired partial lipodystrophy: report of 35 cases and review of the literature. *Medicine.* 2004;83:18-34.

821. Musso C, Javor E, Cochran E, et al. Spectrum of renal diseases associated with extreme forms of insulin resistance. *Clin J Am Soc Nephrol.* 2006;1: 616-622.

822. Habib R, Gubler MC, Loirat C, et al. Dense deposit disease: a variant of membranoproliferative glomerulonephritis. *Kidney Int.* 1975;7:204-215.

823. Vargas RA, Thomson KJ, Wilson D, et al. Mesangiocapillary glomerulonephritis with "dense deposits" in the basement membranes of the kidney. *Clin Nephrol.* 1976;5:73-82.

824. Eisinger AJ, Shortland JR, Moorhead PJ. Renal disease in partial lipodystrophy. *Q J Med.* 1972;41:343-354.

825. Peters DK, Williams DG, Charlesworth JA, et al. Mesangiocapillary nephritis, partial lipodystrophy and hypocomplementaemia. *Lancet.* 1973;2:535-538.

826. Javor ED, Moran SA, Young JR, et al. Proteinuric nephropathy in acquired and congenital generalized lipodystrophy: baseline characteristics and course during recombinant leptin therapy. *J Clin Endocrinol Metab.* 2004;89:3199-3207.

827. Cahill J, Waldron S, O'Neill G, et al. Partial lipodystrophy and renal disease. *Ir J Med Sci.* 1983;152:451-453.

828. Sissons JGP, West RJ, Fallows J, et al. The complement abnormalities of lipodystrophy. *N Engl J Med.* 1976;294:461-465.

829. Chartier S, Buzzanga JB, Paquin F. Partial lipodystrophy associated with a type 3 form of membranoproliferative glomerulonephritis. *J Am Acad Dermatol.* 1987;16:201-205.

830. Jacob DK, Date A, Shastry JCM. Minimal change disease with partial lipodystrophy. *Child Nephrol Urol.* 1988;9:116-117.

831. Schmidt P, Kerjaschki D, Syre G, et al. Recurrence of intramembranous glomerulonephritis in 2 consecutive kidney transplantations. *Schweiz Med Wochenschr.* 1998;108:781-788.

832. Javor ED, Cochran EK, Musso C, et al. Long-term efficacy of leptin replacement in patients with generalized lipodystrophy. *Diabetes.* 2005;54:1994-2002.

833. McNally M, Mannon RB, Javor ED, et al. Successful renal transplantation in a patient with congenital generalized lipodystrophy: a case report. *Am J Transplant.* 2004;4:447-449.

834. Norum KR, Gjone E. Familial plasma lecithin-cholesterol acyltransferase deficiency: Biochemical study of a new inborn error of metabolism. *Scand J Clin Lab Invest.* 1967;20:231-243.

835. Gjone E, Norum KR. Familial serum cholesterol ester deficiency: Clinical study of a patient with a new syndrome. *Acta Med Scand.* 1968;183: 107-112.

836. Albers JJ, Chan C-H, Adolphson J, et al. Familial lecithin-cholesterol acyltransferase deficiency in a Japanese family: Evidence for functionally defective enzyme in homozygotes and obligate heterozygotes. *Hum Genet.* 1982;62:82-85.

837. Vergani C, Cataparo AL, Roma P, et al. A new case of familial LCAT deficiency. *Acta Med Scand.* 1983;214:173-176.

838. Ayyobi AF, McGladdery SH, Chan S, et al. Lecithin: cholesterol acyltransferase LCAT. deficiency and risk of vascular disease: 25 year follow-up. *Atherosclerosis.* 2004;177:361-366.

839. Gjone E. Familial lecithin-cholesterol acyl transferase deficiency: a new metabolic disease with renal involvement. *Adv Nephrol.* 1981;10:167-185.

840. Magil A, Chase W, Frohlich J. Unusual renal biopsy findings in a patient with lecithin-cholesterol acyltransferase deficiency. *Hum Pathol.* 1982;13:283-285.

841. McLean G, Wion K, Drayna D, et al. Human lecithin-cholesterol acyltransferase gene: complete gene sequence and sites of expression. *Nucleic Acids Res.* 1986;14:9397-9406.

842. McLean J, Fielding C, Drayna D, et al. Cloning and expression of human lecithin-cholesterol acyltransferase cDNA. *Proc Natl Acad Sci U S A.* 1986;83:2335-2339.

843. Lynn EG, Siow YL, Frohlich J, et al. Lipoprotein-X stimulates monocyte chemoattractant protein-1 expression in mesangial cells via nuclear factor-kappa B. *Kidney Int.* 2001;60:520-532.

844. Borysiewicz LK, Soutar AK, Evans DJ, et al. Renal failure in lecithin-cholesterol acyltransferase deficiency. *Q J Med.* 1982;51:411-426.

845. Murayama N, Asano Y, Kato K, et al. Effects of plasma infusion on plasma lipids, apoproteins and plasma enzyme activities in familial lecithin-cholesterol acyltransferase deficiency. *Eur J Clin Invest.* 1984;12:122-129.

846. Flatmark A, Hovig T, Mythre E, et al. Renal transplantation in patients with familial lecithin-cholesterol acyltransferase deficiency. *Transplant Proc.* 1977;9:1665-1671.

847. Saito T, Sato H, Kudo K, et al. Lipoprotein glomerulopathy: glomerular lipoprotein thrombi in a patient with hyperlipoproteinemia. *Am J Kidney Dis.* 1989;13:148-153.

848. Saito T, Oikawa S, Sato H, et al. Lipoprotein glomerulopathy: renal lipidosis induced by novel apolipoprotein E variants. *Nephrology.* 1999;83:193-201.

849. Karet FE, Lifton RP. Lipoprotein glomerulopathy: a new role for apolipoprotein E? *J Am Soc Nephrol.* 1997;8:840-842.

850. Oikawa S, Matsunaga A, Saito T, et al. Apolipoprotein E Sendai arginine 145->proline: a new variant associated with lipoprotein glomerulopathy. *J Am Soc Nephrol.* 1997;8:820-823.

851. Konishi K, Saruta T, Kuramochi S, et al. Association of a novel 3-amino acid deletion mutation of apolipoprotein E Apo E Tokyo with lipoprotein glomerulopathy. *Nephrology.* 1999;83:214-218.

852. Matsunaga A, Sasaki J, Komatsu T, et al. A novel apolipoprotein E mutation, E2 Arg25Cys., in lipoprotein glomerulopathy. *Kidney Int.* 1999;56:421-427.

853. Ando M, Sasaki J, Hua H, et al. A novel 18-amino acid deletion in apolipoprotein E associated with lipoprotein glomerulopathy. *Kidney Int.* 1999;56:1317-1323.

854. Ogawa T, Maruyama K, Hattori H, et al. A new variant of apolipoprotein E apo E Maebashi. in lipoprotein glomerulopathy. *Pediatr Nephrol.* 2000;14:149-151.

855. Ieiri N, Hotta O, Taguma Y. Resolution of typical lipoprotein glomerulopathy by intensive lipid-lowering therapy. *Am J Kidney Dis.* 2003;41:244-249.

856. Andrews PA. Lipoprotein glomerulopathy: a new cause of nephrotic syndrome after renal transplantation. Implications for renal transplantation. *Nephrol Dial Transplant.* 1999;14:239-240.

857. Miyata T, Sugiyama S, Nangaku M, et al. Apolipoprotein E2/E5 variants in lipoprotein glomerulopathy recurred in transplanted kidney. *J Am Soc Nephrol.* 1999;10:1590-1595.

858. Neugarten J, Baldwin DS. Glomerulonephritis in bacterial endocarditis. *Am J Med.* 1984;77:297-304.

859. Baehr G. Glomerular lesions of subacute bacterial endocarditis. *J Exp Med.* 1912;15:330-347.

860. Libman E. Characterization of the various forms of endocarditis. *JAMA.* 1923;80:813-818.

861. Neugarten J, Gallo GR, Baldwin DS. Glomerulonephritis in bacterial endocarditis. *Am J Kidney Dis.* 1984;35:371-379.

862. Garvey GJ, Neu HC. Infective endocarditis-and evolving disease. A review of endocarditis at the Columbia-Presbyterian Medical Center. *Medicine (Baltimore).* 1978;57:105-127.

863. Pelletier Jr LL, Petersdorf RG. Infective endocarditis: a review of 125 cases from the University of Washington Hospitals, 1962-1972. *Medicine (Baltimore).* 1977;56:287-313.

864. O'Connor DT, Weisman MH, Fierer J. Activation of the alternate complement pathway in *Staph. aureus* infective endocarditis and its relationship to thrombocytopenia, coagulation abnormalities, and acute glomerulonephritis. *Clin Exp Immunol.* 1978;19:131-141.

865. Levine DP, Cushing RD, Jui J, et al. Community-acquired methicillin-resistant *Staphylococcus aureus* endocarditis in the Detroit Medical Center. *Ann Intern Med.* 1982;97:330-338.

866. Gutman RA, Striker GE, Gilliland BC, et al. The immune complex glomerulonephritis of bacterial endocarditis. *Medicine (Baltimore).* 1972;51:1-25.

867. Daimon S, Mizuno Y, Fujii S, et al. Infective endocarditis-induced crescentic glomerulonephritis dramatically improved by plasmapheresis. *Am J Kidney Dis.* 1998;32:309-313.

868. Kodo K, Hida M, Omori S, et al. Vasculitis associated with septicemia: case report and review of the literature. *Pediatr Nephrol.* 2001;16:1089-1092.

869. Kauffman RH, Thompson J, Valentijn RM, et al. The clinical implications and the pathogenetic significance of circulating immune complexes in infective endocarditis. *Am J Med.* 1981;71:17-25.

870. Cabane J, Godeau P, Herreman G, et al. Fate of circulating immune complexes in infective endocarditis. *Am J Med.* 1979;66:277-282.

871. Hurwitz D, Quismorio FP, Friou GJ. Cryoglobulinemia in patients with infectious endocarditis. *Clin Exp Immunol.* 1975;19:131-141.

872. Subra JJ, Michelet C, Laporte J, et al. The presence of cytoplasmic antineutrophil cytoplasmic antibodies C-ANCA. in the course of subacute bacterial endocarditis with glomerular involvement, coincidence or association? *Clin Nephrol.* 1998;49:15-18.

873. Levy RL, Hong R. The immune nature of subacute bacterial endocarditis SBE nephritis. *Am J Med.* 1973;54:645-652.

874. Morel-Maroger L, Sraer JD, Herreman G, et al. Kidney in subacute endocarditis: Pathological and immunofluorescent findings. *Arch Pathol.* 1972;94:205-213.

875. Boulton JJM, Sissons JG, Evans DJ, et al. Renal lesions in subacute bacterial endocarditis. *Br Med J.* 1974;2:11-14.

876. Nasr SH, Markowitz GS, Stokes MB, et al. Acute postinfectious glomerulonephritis in the modern era: experience with 86 adults and review of the literature. *Medicine (Baltimore).* 2008;87:21-32.

877. Yum M, Wheat LJ, Maxwell D, et al. Immunofluorescent localization of Staphylococcus aureus antigen in acute bacterial endocarditis nephritis. *Am J Clin Pathol.* 1978;70:832-835.

878. Perez GO, Rothfield N, Williams Jr RC. Immune-complex nephritis in bacterial endocarditis. *Arch Intern Med.* 1976;136:334-336.

879. McKinsey DS, McMurray TI, Flynn JM. Immunosuppressive therapy and plasmapheresis in rapidly progressive glomerulonephritis associated with glomerulonephritis. *Rev Infect Dis.* 1990;12:125-127.

880. Schoenbaum SC, Gardner P, Shillito J. Infections of cerebrospinal fluid shunts: epidemiology, clinical manifestations, and therapy. *J Infect Dis.* 1975;131:543-552.

881. Balogun RA, Palmisano J, Kaplan AA, et al. Shunt nephritis from *Propionibacterium acnes* in a solitary kidney. *Am J Kidney Dis.* 2001;38:E18.

882. Kiryluk K, Preddie D, D'Agati VD, et al. A young man with *Propionibacterium acnes*-induced shunt nephritis. *Kidney Int.* 2008;73:1434-1440.

883. Rifkinson-Mann S, Rifkinson N, Leong T. Shunt nephritis. Case report. *J Neurosurg.* 1991;74:656-659.

884. Salcedo JR, Sorkin L. Nephritis associated with an infected peritoneovenous LeVeen shunt. *J Pediatr Gastroenterol Nutr.* 1985;4:842-844.

885. Black JA, Challacombe DN, Ockenden BG. Nephrotic syndrome associated with bacteraemia after shunt operations for hydrocephalus. *Lancet.* 1965;2:921-924.

886. Stickler GB, Shin MH, Burke EC, et al. Diffuse glomerulonephritis associated with infected ventriculoatrial shunt. *N Engl J Med.* 1968;279:1077-1082.

887. Kubota M, Sakata Y, Saeki N, et al. A case of shunt nephritis diagnosed 17 years after ventriculoatrial shunt implantation. *Clin Neurol Neurosurg.* 2001;103:245-246.

888. McKenzie SA, Hayden K. Two cases of "shunt nephritis." *Pediatrics.* 1974;54:806-808.

889. Vella J, Carmody M, Campbell E, et al. Glomerulonephritis after ventriculo-atrial shunt. *Q J Med.* 1995;88:911-918.

890. Schoeneman M, Bennett B, Greifer I. Shunt nephritis progressing to chronic renal failure. *Am J Kidney Dis.* 1982;2:375-377.

891. Iwata Y, Ohta S, Kawai K, et al. Shunt nephritis with positive titers for ANCA specific for proteinase 3. *Am J Kidney Dis.* 2004;43(5):e11-e16.

892. Danovitch GM, Nord EP, Barki Y, et al. Staphylococcal lung abscess and acute glomerulonephritis. *Isr J Med Sci.* 1979;15:840-843.

893. Beaufils M, Morel-Maroger L, Sraer JD, et al. Acute renal failure of glomerular origin during visceral abscesses. *N Engl J Med.* 1976;295:185-189.

893a. Nasr SH, Fidler ME, Valeri AM, et al. Postinfectious glomerulonephritis in the elderly. *J Am Soc Nephrol.* 2011;22(1):187-195.

894. Yuceoglu AM, Sagel I, Tresser G, et al. The glomerulopathy of congenital syphilis. A curable immune- deposit disease. *JAMA.* 1974;229:1085-1089.

895. Hunte W, al-Ghraoui F, Cohen RJ. Secondary syphilis and the nephrotic syndrome. *J Am Soc Nephrol.* 1993;3:1351-1355.

896. Sanchez-Bayle M, Ecija JL, Estepa R, et al. Incidence of glomerulonephritis in congenital syphilis. *Clin Nephrol.* 1983;20:27-31.

897. Hruby Z, Kuzniar J, Rabczynski J, et al. The variety of clinical and histopathologic presentations of glomerulonephritis associated with latent syphilis. *Int Urol Nephrol.* 1992;24:541-547.

898. Gamble CN, Reardan JB. Immunopathogenesis of syphilitic glomerulonephritis. Elution of antitreponemal antibody from glomerular immune-complex deposits. *N Engl J Med.* 1975;292:449-454.

899. Krane NK, Espenan P, Walker PD, et al. Renal disease and syphilis: a report of nephrotic syndrome with minimal change disease. *Am J Kidney Dis.* 1987;9:176-179.

900. Walker PD, Deeves EC, Sahba G, et al. Rapidly progressive glomerulo-nephritis in a patient with syphilis. Identification of antitreponemal antibody and treponemal antigen in renal tissue. *Am J Med.* 1984;76: 1106-1112.

901. Hopp L, Eppes SC. Development of IgA nephritis following cat scratch disease in a 13-year-old boy. *Pediatr Nephrol.* 2004;19:682-684.

902. D'Agati V, McEachrane S, Dicker R, et al. Cat scratch disease and glomerulonephritis. *Nephrology.* 1990;56:431-435.

903. Bookman I, Scholey JW, Jassal SV, et al. Necrotizing glomerulonephritis caused by Bartonella henselae endocarditis. *Am J Kidney Dis.* 2004;43: e25-e30.

904. Ponce P, Ramos A, Ferreira ML, et al. Renal involvement in leprosy. *Nephrol Dial Transplant.* 1989;4:81-84.

905. Ahsan N, Wheeler DE, Palmer BF. Leprosy-associated renal disease: case report and review of the literature. *J Am Soc Nephrol.* 1995;5:1546-1552.

906. Matsuo E, Furuno Y, Komatsu A, et al. Hansen's disease and nephropathy as its sequence. *Nihon Hansenbyo Gakkai Zasshi.* 1997;66:103-108.

907. Chugh KS, Damle PB, Kaur S, et al. Renal lesions in leprosy amongst north Indian patients. *Postgrad Med J.* 1983;59:707-711.

908. Grover S, Bobhate SK, Chaubey BS. Renal abnormality in leprosy. *Lepr India.* 1983;55:286-291.

909. Nakayama EE, Ura S, Fleury RN, Soares V. Renal lesions in leprosy: a retrospective study of 199 autopsies. *Am J Kidney Dis.* 2001;38:26-30.

910. Nigam P, Pant KC, Mukhija RD, et al. Rapidly progressive crescentic glomerulonephritis in erythema nodosum leprosum: case report. *Hansenol Int.* 1986;11:1-6.

911. Chugh KS, Sakhuja V. End stage renal disease in leprosy. *Int J Artif Organs.* 1986;9:9-10.

912. Slater DN, Brown CB, Ward AM, et al. Immune complex crescentic glomerulonephritis associated with pulmonary aspergillosis. *Histopathology.* 1983;7:957-966.

913. Pecchini F, Bufano G, Ghiringhelli P. Membranoproliferative glomerulonephritis secondary to tuberculosis. *Clin Nephrol.* 1997;47:63-64.

914. O'Brien AA, Kelly P, Gaffney EF, et al. Immune complex glomerulonephritis secondary to tuberculosis. *Ir J Med Sci.* 1990;159:187.

915. Rodriguez-Garcia JL, Fraile G, Mampaso F, et al. Pulmonary tuberculosis associated with membranous nephropathy. *Nephrology.* 1990;55:218-219.

916. Somvanshi PP, Patni PD, Khan MA. Renal involvement in chronic pulmonary tuberculosis. *Indian J Med Sci.* 1989;43:55-58.

917. Campbell JH, Warwick G, Boulton-Jones M, et al. Rapidly progressive glomerulonephritis and nephrotic syndrome associated with *Mycoplasma pneumoniae* pneumonia. *Nephrol Dial Transplant.* 1991;6:518-520.

918. Cochat P, Colon S, Bosshard S, et al. Membranoproliferative glomerulonephritis and *Mycoplasma pneumoniae* infection. *Arch Fr Pediatr.* 1985;42:29-31.

919. Von Bonsdorff M, Ponka A, Tornroth T. Mycoplasmal pneumonia associated with mesangiocapillary glomerulonephritis type II dense deposit disease. *Acta Med Scand.* 1984;216:427-429.

920. Vitullo BB, O'Regan S, de Chadarevian JP, et al. Mycoplasma pneumonia associated with acute glomerulonephritis. *Nephrology.* 1978;21:284-288.

921. Said MH, Layani MP, Colon S, et al. Mycoplasma pneumoniae-associated nephritis in children. *Pediatr Nephrol.* 1999;13:39-44.

922. Kaehny WD, Ozawa T, Schwarz MI, et al. Acute nephritis and pulmonary alveolitis following pneumococcal pneumonia. *Arch Intern Med.* 1978;138:806-808.

923. Schachter J, Pomeranz A, Berger I, et al. Acute glomerulonephritis secondary to lobar pneumonia. *Int J Pediatr Nephrol.* 1987;8:211-214.

924. Jose MD, Bannister KM, Clarkson AR, et al. Mesangiocapillary glomerulonephritis in a patient with Nocardia pneumonia. *Nephrol Dial Transplant.* 1998;13:2628-2629.

925. Dunea G, Kark RM, Lannigan R, et al. Brucella nephritis. *Ann Intern Med.* 1969;70:783-790.

926. Volpi A, Doregatti C, Tarelli T, et al. Acute glomerulonephritis in human brucellosis. Report of a case. *Pathologica.* 1985;77:519-524.

927. Elzouki AY, Akthar M, Mirza K. Brucella endocarditis associated with glomerulonephritis and renal vasculitis. *Pediatr Nephrol.* 1996;10:748-751.

928. Siegelmann N, Abraham AS, Rudensky B, et al. Brucellosis with nephrotic syndrome, nephritis and IgA nephropathy. *Postgrad Med J.* 1992;68:834-836.

929. Nunan TO, Eykyn SJ, Jones NF. Brucellosis with mesangial IgA nephropathy: successful treatment with doxycycline and rifampicin. *Br Med J Clin Res Ed.* 1984;288:1802.

930. Sitprija V, Pipatanagul V, Mertowidjojo K, et al. Pathogenesis of renal disease in leptospirosis: clinical and experimental studies. *Kidney Int.* 1980;17:827-836.

931. Lai KN, Aarons I, Woodroffe AJ, et al. Renal lesions in leptospirosis. *Aust N Z J Med.* 1982;12:276-279.

932. Sitprija V, Pipantanagul V, Boonpucknavig V, et al. Glomerulitis in typhoid fever. *Ann Intern Med.* 1974;81:210-213.

933. Lambertucci JR, Godoy P, Neves J, et al. Glomerulonephritis in *Salmonella-Schistosoma mansoni* association. *Am J Trop Med Hyg.* 1988;38:97-102.

934. Indraprasit S, Boonpucknavig V, Boonpucknavig S. IgA nephropathy associated with enteric fever. *Nephrology.* 1985;40:219-222.

935. Bhamarapravati N, Boonpucknavig S, Boonpucknavig V, et al. Glomerular changes in acute *Plasmodium falciparum* infection. An immunopathologic study. *Arch Pathol.* 1973;96:289-293.

936. Eiam-Ong S, Sitprija V. Falciparum malaria and the kidney: a model of inflammation. *Am J Kidney Dis.* 1998;32:361-375.

937. Hendrickse RG, Adeniyi A. Quartan malarial nephrotic syndrome in children. *Kidney Int.* 1979;16:64-74.

938. Kibukamusoke JW, Hutt MS. Histological features of the nephrotic syndrome associated with quartan malaria. *J Clin Pathol.* 1967;20:117-123.

939. Hendrickse RG, Adeniyi A, Edington GM, et al. Quartan malarial nephrotic syndrome. Collaborative clinicopathological study in Nigerian children. *Lancet.* 1972;1:1143-1149.

940. Houba V. Immunopathology of nephropathies associated with malaria. *Bull World Health Organ.* 1975;52:199-207.

941. Olowu WA, Adelusola KA, Adefehinti O, et al. Quartan malaria-associated childhood nephrotic syndrome: now a rare clinical entity in malaria endemic Nigeria. *Nephrol Dial Transplant.* 2010;25:794-801.

942. Greenham R, Cameron AH. Schistosoma haematobium and the nephrotic syndrome. *Trans R Soc Trop Med Hyg.* 1980;74:609-613.

943. Rocha H, Cruz T, Brito E, et al. Renal involvement in patients with hepatosplenic Schistosomiasis mansoni. *Am J Trop Med Hyg.* 1976;25: 108-115.

944. Barsoum RS. Schistosomiasis and the kidney. *Semin Nephrol.* 2003;23: 34-41.

945. Sobh MA, Moustafa FE, Sally SM, et al. Characterisation of kidney lesions in early schistosomal-specific nephropathy. *Nephrol Dial Transplant.* 1988;3:392-398.

946. Martinelli R, Noblat AC, Brito E, et al. Schistosoma mansoni-induced mesangiocapillary glomerulonephritis: influence of therapy. *Kidney Int.* 1989;35:1227-1233.

947. Barsoum RS. Schistosomal glomerulopathy: selection factors. *Nephrol Dial Transplant.* 1987;2:488-497.

948. Dutra M, Martinelli R, de Carvalho EM, et al. Renal involvement in visceral leishmaniasis. *Am J Kidney Dis.* 1985;6:22-27.

949. DE Brito T, Hoshino-Shimizu S, Neto VA, et al. Glomerular involvement in human kala-azar. A light, immunofluorescent, and electron microscopic study based on kidney biopsies. *Am J Trop Med Hyg.* 1975;24:9-18.

950. Basson W, Page ML, Myburgh DP. Human trypanosomiasis in Southern Africa. *S Afr Med J.* 1977;51:453-457.

951. Greene BM, Taylor HR, Brown EJ, et al. Ocular and systemic complications of diethylcarbamazine therapy for onchocerciasis: association with circulating immune complexes. *J Infect Dis.* 1983;147: 890-897.

952. Cruel T, Arborio M, Schill H, et al. Nephropathy and filariasis from Loa loa. Apropos of 1 case of adverse reaction to a dose of ivermectin. *Bull Soc Pathol Exot.* 1997;90:179-181.

953. Pakasa NM, Nseka NM, Nyimi LM. Secondary collapsing glomerulopathy associated with Loa loa filariasis. *Am J Kidney Dis.* 1997;30:836-839.

954. Yap HK, Woo KT, Yeo PP, et al. The nephrotic syndrome associated with filariasis. *Ann Acad Med Singapore.* 1982;11:60-63.

955. Date A, Gunasekaran V, Kirubakaran MG, et al. Acute eosinophilic glomerulonephritis with Bancroftian filariasis. *Postgrad Med J.* 1979;55: 905-907.

956. Chugh KS, Sakhuja V. Glomerular diseases in the tropics editorial. *Am J Nephrol.* 1990;10:437-450.

956a. Cheng JT, Mohan S, Nasr SH, et al. Chyluria presenting as milky urine and nephrotic range proteinuria. *Kidney Int.* 2006;70:1518-1522.

957. Sitprija V, Keoplung M, Boonpucknavig V, et al. Renal involvement in human trichinosis. *Arch Intern Med.* 1980;140:544-546.

958. Trandafirescu V, Georgescu L, Schwarzkopf A, et al. Trichinous nephropathy. *Morphol Embryol Bucur.* 1979;25:133-137.

959. Covic A, Mititiuc I, Caruntu L, et al. Reversible nephrotic syndrome due to mesangiocapillary glomerulonephritis secondary to hepatic hydatid disease. *Nephrol Dial Transplant.* 1996;11:2074-2076.

960. Vialtel P, Chenais F, Desgeorges P, et al. Membranous nephropathy associated with hydatid disease. *N Engl J Med.* 1981;304:610-611.

961. Oseroff A. Toxoplasmosis associated with nephrotic syndrome in an adult. *South Med J.* 1988;81:95-96.

962. Wickbom B, Winberg J. Coincidence of congenital toxoplasmosis and acute nephritis with nephrotic syndrome. *Acta Paediatr Scand.* 1972;61:470-472.

963. Ginsburg BE, Wasserman J, Huldt G, et al. Case of glomerulonephritis associated with acute toxoplasmosis. *Br Med J.* 1974;3:664-665.

964. Smith MC, Cooke JH, Zimmerman DM, et al. Asymptomatic glomerulonephritis after nonstreptococcal upper respiratory infections. *Ann Intern Med.* 1979;91:697-702.

965. Blowey DL. Nephrotic syndrome associated with an Epstein-Barr virus infection. *Pediatr Nephrol.* 1996;10:507-508.

966. Joh K, Kanetsuna Y, Ishikawa Y, et al. Epstein-Barr virus genome-positive tubulointerstitial nephritis associated with immune complex-mediated glomerulonephritis in chronic active EB virus infection. *Virchows Arch.* 1998;432:567-573.

967. Gilboa N, Wong W, Largent JA, et al. Association of infectious mononucleosis with nephrotic syndrome. *Arch Pathol Lab Med.* 1981;105:259-262.

968. Araya CE, Gonzalez-Peralta RP, Skoda-Smith S, et al. Systemic Epstein-Barr virus infection associated with membranous nephropathy in children. *Clin Nephrol.* 2006;65:160-164.

969. Nadasdy T, Park CS, Peiper SC, et al. Epstein-Barr virus infection-associated renal disease: diagnostic use of molecular hybridization technology in patients with negative serology. *J Am Soc Nephrol.* 1992;2:1734-1742.

970. Iwama H, Horikoshi S, Shirato I, et al. Epstein-Barr virus detection in kidney biopsy specimens correlates with glomerular mesangial injury. *Am J Kidney Dis.* 1998;32:785-793.

971. Gallo G, Neugarten J, Baldwin DS. Glomerulonephritis associated with systemic bacterial and viral infections. In: Tisher CC, Brenner BM, eds. *Renal Pathology: With Clinical and Functional Correlations.* 2nd ed. Philadelphia: J.B. Lippincott; 1994:564-595.

972. UNAIDS. *Annual Report 2009.* Geneva, Joint United Nations Programme on HIV/AIDS UNAIDS; 2009.

973. D'Agati V, Appel GB. HIV infection and the kidney. *J Am Soc Nephrol.* 1997;8:138-152.

974. D'Agati V, Appel GB. Renal pathology of human immunodeficiency virus infection. *Semin Nephrol.* 1998;18:406-421.

975. Rao TK, Filippone EJ, Nicastri AD, et al. Associated focal and segmental glomerulosclerosis in the acquired immunodeficiency syndrome. *N Engl J Med.* 1984;310:669-673.

976. Gardenswartz MH, Lerner CW, Seligson GR, et al. Renal disease in patients with AIDS: a clinicopathologic study. *Clin Nephrol.* 1984;21:197-204.

977. D'Agati V, Suh JI, Carbone L, et al. Pathology of HIV-associated nephropathy: a detailed morphologic and comparative study. *Kidney Int.* 1989;35:1358-1370.

978. Rao TK, Friedman EA, Nicastri AD. The types of renal disease in the acquired immunodeficiency syndrome. *N Engl J Med.* 1987;316:1062-1068.

979. Carbone L, D'Agati V, Cheng JT, et al. Course and prognosis of human immunodeficiency virus-associated nephropathy. *Am J Med.* 1989;87:389-395.

980. Langs C, Gallo GR, Schacht RG, et al. Rapid renal failure in AIDS-associated focal glomerulosclerosis. *Arch Intern Med.* 1990;150:287-292.

981. Pardo V, Meneses R, Ossa L, et al. AIDS-related glomerulopathy: occurrence in specific risk groups. *Kidney Int.* 1987;31:1167-1173.

982. Strauss J, Abitbol C, Zilleruelo G, et al. Renal disease in children with the acquired immunodeficiency syndrome. *N Engl J Med.* 1989;321:625-630.

983. Bourgoignie JJ, Meneses R, Ortiz C, et al. The clinical spectrum of renal disease associated with human immunodeficiency virus. *Am J Kidney Dis.* 1988;12:131-137.

984. Seney FDJ, Burns DK, Silva FG. Acquired immunodeficiency syndrome and the kidney. *Am J Kidney Dis.* 1990;16:1-13.

985. Glassock RJ, Cohen AH, Danovitch G, et al. Human immunodeficiency virus HIV. infection and the kidney. *Ann Intern Med.* 1990;112:35-49.

986. Humphreys MH. Human immunodeficiency virus-associated glomerulosclerosis. *Kidney Int.* 1995;48:311-320.

987. Mazbar SA, Schoenfeld PY, Humphreys MH. Renal involvement in patients infected with HIV: experience at San Francisco General Hospital. *Kidney Int.* 1990;37:1325-1332.

988. Ross MJ, Klotman PE. Recent progress in HIV-associated nephropathy. *J Am Soc Nephrol.* 2002;13:2997-3004.

989. Bourgoignie JJ, Ortiz-Interian C, Green DF. The human immunodeficiency virus epidemic and HIV associated nephropathy. In: Hatano M, ed. *Nephrology.* Tokyo: Springer Verlag; 1990:484-492.

990. Winston JA, Burns GC, Klotman PE. The human immunodeficiency virus HIV. Epidemic and HIV-associated nephropathy. *Semin Nephrol.* 1998;18:373-377.

991. Nochy D, Glotz D, Dosquet P, et al. Renal disease associated with HIV infection: a multicentric study of 60 patients from Paris hospitals. *Nephrol Dial Transplant.* 1993;8:11-19.

992. Nochy D, Glotz D, Dosquet P, et al. Renal lesions associated with human immunodeficiency virus infection: North American vs. European experience. *Adv Nephrol Necker Hosp.* 1993;22:269-286.

993. Liu R, Paxton WA, Choe S, et al. Homozygous defect in HIV-1 coreceptor accounts for resistance of some multiply-exposed individuals to HIV-1 infection. *Cell.* 1996;86:367-377.

994. Smith MW, Dean M, Carrington M, et al. Contrasting genetic influence of CCR2 and CCR5 variants on HIV-1 infection and disease progression. Hemophilia Growth and Development Study HGDS., Multicenter AIDS Cohort Study MACS., Multicenter Hemophilia Cohort Study MHCS., San Francisco City Cohort SFCC., ALIVE Study. *Science.* 1997;277:959-965.

995. Winkler C, Modi W, Smith MW, et al. Genetic restriction of AIDS pathogenesis by an SDF-1 chemokine gene variant. ALIVE Study, Hemophilia Growth and Development Study HGDS., Multicenter AIDS Cohort Study MACS. Multicenter Hemophilia Cohort Study MHCS., San Francisco City Cohort SFCC. *Science.* 1998;279:389-393.

996. Kopp JB, Smith MW, Nelson GW, et al. MYH9 is a major-effect risk gene for focal segmental glomerulosclerosis. *Nat Genet.* 2008;40:1175-1184.

997. Genovese G, Friedman DJ, Ross MD, et al. Association of trypanolytic ApoL1 variants with kidney disease in African Americans. *Science.* 2010;329:841-845.

998. Ahuja TS, Borucki M, Funtanilla M, et al. Is the prevalence of HIV-associated nephropathy decreasing? *Am J Nephrol.* 1999;19:655-659.

999. Shahinian V, Rajaraman S, Borucki M, et al. Prevalence of HIV-associated nephropathy in autopsies of HIV-infected patients. *Am J Kidney Dis.* 2000;35:884-888.

1000. Bourgoignie JJ. Renal complications of human immunodeficiency virus type 1. *Kidney Int.* 1990;37:1571-1584.

1001. Valeri A, Neusy AJ. Acute and chronic renal disease in hospitalized AIDS patients. *Clin Nephrol.* 1991;35:110-118.

1002. Chander P, Soni A, Suri A, et al. Renal ultrastructural markers in AIDS-associated nephropathy. *Am J Pathol.* 1987;126:513-526.

1003. Barisoni L, Kriz W, Mundel P, et al. The dysregulated podocyte phenotype: a novel concept in the pathogenesis of collapsing idiopathic focal segmental glomerulosclerosis and HIV-associated nephropathy. *J Am Soc Nephrol.* 1999;10:51-61.

1004. Bruggeman LA, Ross MD, Tanji N, et al. Renal epithelium is a previously unrecognized site of HIV-1 infection. *J Am Soc Nephrol.* 2000;11:2079-2087.

1005. Marras D, Bruggeman LA, Gao F, et al. Replication and compartmentalization of HIV-1 in kidney epithelium of patients with HIV-associated nephropathy. *Nat Med.* 2002;8:522-526.

1006. Dickie P, Felser J, Eckhaus M, et al. HIV-associated nephropathy in transgenic mice expressing HIV-1 genes. *Virology.* 1991;185:109-119.

1007. Kopp JB, Klotman ME, Adler SH, et al. Progressive glomerulosclerosis and enhanced renal accumulation of basement membrane components in mice transgenic for human immunodeficiency virus type 1 genes. *Proc Natl Acad Sci U S A.* 1992;89:1577-1581.

1008. Kopp JB, Ray PE, Adler SH, et al. Nephropathy in HIV-transgenic mice. *Contrib Nephrol.* 1994;107:194-204.

1009. Shankland SJ, Eitner F, Hudkins KL, et al. Differential expression of cyclin-dependent kinase inhibitors in human glomerular disease: role in podocyte proliferation and maturation. *Kidney Int.* 2000;58:674-683.

1010. Husain M, Gusella GL, Klotman ME, et al. HIV-1 nef induces proliferation and anchorage-independent growth in podocytes. *J Am Soc Nephrol.* 2002;13:1806-1815.

1011. Hanna Z, Weng XD, Kay DG, et al. The pathogenicity of human immunodeficiency virus HIV. type 1 Nef in CD4C/HIV transgenic mice is abolished by mutation of its SH3-binding domain, and disease development is delayed in the absence of Hck. *J Virol.* 2001;75:9378-9392.

1012. Zuo Y, Matsusaka T, Zhong J, et al. HIV-1 genes vpr and nef synergistically damage podocytes, leading to glomerulosclerosis. *J Am Soc Nephrol.* 2006;17:2832-2843.

1013. Rosenstiel PE, Gruosso T, Letourneau AM, et al. HIV-1 Vpr inhibits cytokinesis in human proximal tubule cells. *Kidney Int.* 2008;74:1049-1058.

1014. Wali RK, Drachenberg CI, Papadimitriou JC, et al. HIV-1-associated nephropathy and response to highly-active antiretroviral therapy. *Lancet.* 1998;352:783-784.

1015. Kirchner JT. Resolution of renal failure after initiation of HAART: 3 cases and a discussion of the literature. *AIDS Read.* 2002;12(3):103-105: 110-112.

1016. Atta MG, Gallant JE, Rahman MH, et al. Antiretroviral therapy in the treatment of HIV-associated nephropathy. *Nephrol Dial Transplant.* 2006;21:2809-2813.

1017. Wyatt CM, Klotman PE, D'Agati VD. HIV-associated nephropathy: clinical presentation, pathology, and epidemiology in the era of antiretroviral therapy. *Semin Nephrol.* 2008;28:513-522.

1018. USRDS 2002. *US Renal Data System: USRDS 2002 Annual Data Report.* Bethesda, MD: National Institutes of Health, National Institute of Diabetes and Digestive and Kidney Diseases, Division of Kidney, Urologic, and Hematologic Diseases; 2002.

1019. Ingulli E, Tejani A, Fikrig S, et al. Nephrotic syndrome associated with acquired immunodeficiency syndrome in children. *J Pediatr.* 1991;119: 710-716.

1020. Strauss J, Zilleruelo G, Abitbol C, et al. Human immunodeficiency virus nephropathy. *Pediatr Nephrol.* 1993;7:220-225.

1021. Smith MC, Pawar R, Carey JT, et al. Effect of corticosteroid therapy on human immunodeficiency virus-associated nephropathy. *Am J Med.* 1994;97:145-151.

1022. Smith MC, Austen JL, Carey JT, et al. Prednisone improves renal function and proteinuria in human immunodeficiency virus-associated nephropathy. *Am J Med.* 1996;101:41-48.

1023. Eustace JA, Nuermberger E, Choi M, et al. Cohort study of the treatment of severe HIV-associated nephropathy with corticosteroids. *Kidney Int.* 2000;58:1253-1260.

1024. Klotman PE. Early treatment with ACE inhibition may benefit HIV-associated nephropathy patients. *Am J Kidney Dis.* 1998;31:719-720.

1025. Burns GC, Paul SK, Toth IR, et al. Effect of angiotensin-converting enzyme inhibition in HIV-associated nephropathy. *J Am Soc Nephrol.* 1997;8:1140-1146.

1026. Ouellette DR, Kelly JW, Anders GT. Serum angiotensin-converting enzyme level is elevated in patients with human immunodeficiency virus infection. *Arch Intern Med.* 1992;152:321-324.

1027. Kumar MSA, Sierka DR, Damask AM, et al. Safety and success of kidney transplantation and concomitant immunosuppression in HIV-positive patients. *Kidney Int.* 2005;67:1622-1629.

1028. Long-term patient and graft survival after kidney transplantation in HIV positive patients. *Transplantation.* 2006;82:121-122.

1029. Qiu J, Terasaki PI, Waki K, et al. HIV-positive renal recipients can achieve survival rates similar to those of HIV-negative patients. *Transplantation.* 2006;81:1658-1661.

1030. Bhagani S, Sweny P, Brook G. Guidelines for kidney transplantation in patients with HIV disease. *HIV Med.* 2006;7:133-139.

1031. Casanova S, Mazzucco G, Barbiano DB, et al. Pattern of glomerular involvement in human immunodeficiency virus-infected patients: an Italian study. *Am J Kidney Dis.* 1995;26:446-453.

1032. Estrella M, Fine DM, Gallant JE, et al. HIV type 1 RNA level as a clinical indicator of renal pathology in HIV-infected patients. *Clin Infect Dis.* 2006;43:377-380.

1033. Wyatt CM, Morgello S, Katz-Malamed R, et al. The spectrum of kidney disease in patients with AIDS in the era of antiretroviral therapy. *Kidney Int.* 2009;75:428-434.

1034. Kimmel PL, Phillips TM, Ferreira-Centeno A, et al. HIV-associated immune-mediated renal disease. *Kidney Int.* 1993;44:1327-1340.

1035. Beaufils H, Jouanneau C, Katlama C, et al. HIV-associated IgA nephropathy—a post-mortem study. *Nephrol Dial Transplant.* 1995;10: 35-38.

1036. Kenouch S, Delahousse M, Mery JP, et al. Mesangial IgA deposits in two patients with AIDS-related complex. *Nephrology.* 1990;54:338-340.

1037. Kimmel PL, Phillips TM, Ferreira-Centeno A, et al. Brief report: idiotypic IgA nephropathy in patients with human immunodeficiency virus infection. *N Engl J Med.* 1992;327:702-706.

1038. Katz A, Bargman JM, Miller DC, et al. IgA nephritis in HIV-positive patients: a new HIV-associated nephropathy? *Clin Nephrol.* 1992;38: 61-68.

1039. Stokes MB, Chawla H, Brody RI, et al. Immune complex glomerulo-nephritis in patients coinfected with human immunodeficiency virus and hepatitis C virus. *Am J Kidney Dis.* 1997;29:514-525.

1040. Cheng JT, Anderson HL, Markowitz GS, et al. Hepatitis C virus-associated glomerular disease in patients with HIV co-infection. *J Am Soc Nephr.* 1999;10(7):1566-1574.

1041. D'Agati V, Seigle R. Coexistence of AIDS and lupus nephritis: a case report. *Am J Nephrol.* 1990;10:243-247.

1042. Contreras G, Green DF, Pardo V, et al. Systemic lupus erythematosus in two adults with human immunodeficiency virus infection. *Am J Kidney Dis.* 1996;28:292-295.

1043. Faubert PF, Porush JG, Venkataseshan VS. Lupus like syndromes. In: Grishman E, Churg J, Needleman P, et al., eds. *The Kidneys in Collagen Vascular Disease.* New York: Raven Press; 1993:96-98.

1044. Gindea S, Schwartzman J, Herlitz LC, et al. Proliferative glomerulonephritis in lupus patients with human immunodeficiency virus infection: a difficult clinical challenge. *Semin Arthritis Rheum.* 2010;40(3):201-209.

1045. Kopelman RG, Zolla-Pazner S. Association of human immunodeficiency virus infection and autoimmune phenomena. *Am J Med.* 1988;84:82-88.

1046. Rarick MU, Espina B, Mocharnuk R, et al. Thrombotic thrombocytopenic purpura in patients with human immunodeficiency virus infection: a report of three cases and review of the literature. *Am J Hematol.* 1992;40:103-109.

1047. Benjamin M, Terrell DR, Vesely SK, et al. Frequency and significance of HIV infection among patients diagnosed with thrombotic thrombocytopenic purpura. *Clin Infect Dis.* 2009;48:1129-1137.

1048. Kleinknecht C, Levy M, Peix A, et al. Membranous glomerulonephritis and hepatitis B surface antigen in children. *J Pediatr.* 1979;95:946-952.

1049. Hsu HC, Wu CY, Lin CY, et al. Membranous nephropathy in 52 hepatitis B surface antigen HBsAg. carrier children in Taiwan. *Kidney Int.* 1989;36:1103-1107.

1050. Wrzolkowa T, Zurowska A, Uszycka-Karcz M, et al. Hepatitis B virus-associated glomerulonephritis: electron microscopic studies in 98 children. *Am J Kidney Dis.* 1991;18:306-312.

1051. Venkataseshan VS, Lieberman K, Kim DU, et al. Hepatitis-B-associated glomerulonephritis: pathology, pathogenesis, and clinical course. *Medicine (Baltimore).* 1990;69:200-216.

1052. Lai KN, Li PK, Lui SF, et al. Membranous nephropathy related to hepatitis B virus in adults. *N Engl J Med.* 1991;324:1457-1463.

1053. Johnson RJ, Couser WG. Hepatitis B infection and renal disease: clinical, immunopathogenetic and therapeutic considerations. *Kidney Int.* 1990;37:663-676.

1054. McMahon BJ, Alberts SR, Wainwright RB, et al. Hepatitis B-related sequelae. Prospective study in 1400 hepatitis B surface antigen-positive Alaska native carriers. *Arch Intern Med.* 1990;150:1051-1054.

1055. Guillevin L, Lhote F, Cohen P, et al. Polyarteritis nodosa related to hepatitis B virus. A prospective study with long-term observation of 41 patients. *Medicine (Baltimore).* 1995;74:238-253.

1056. Gilbert RD, Wigglelinkhuizen J. The clinical course of hepatitis B virus-associated nephropathy. *Pediatr Nephrol.* 1994;8:11-14.

1057. Levy M, Gagnadoux MF. Membranous nephropathy following perinatal transmission of hepatitis B virus infection—long-term follow-up study. *Pediatr Nephrol.* 1996;10:76-78.

1058. Ozdamar SO, Gucer S, Tinaztepe K. Hepatitis-B virus associated nephropathies: a clinicopathological study in 14 children. *Pediatr Nephrol.* 2003;18:23-28.

1059. Combes B, Shorey J, Barrera A, et al. Glomerulonephritis with deposition of Australia antigen-antibody complexes in glomerular basement membrane. *Lancet.* 1971;2:234-237.

1060. Lai FM, Li PK, Suen MW, et al. Crescentic glomerulonephritis related to hepatitis B virus. *Mod Pathol.* 1992;5:262-267.

1061. Li PK, Lai FM, Ho SS, et al. Acute renal failure in hepatitis B virus-related membranous nephropathy with mesangiocapillary transition and crescentic transformation. *Am J Kidney Dis.* 1992;19:76-80.

1062. Ohba S, Kimura K, Mise N, et al. Differential localization of s and e antigens in hepatitis B virus-associated glomerulonephritis. *Clin Nephrol.* 1997;48:44-47.

1063. Lai KN, Ho RT, Tam JS, et al. Detection of hepatitis B virus DNA and RNA in kidneys of HBV related glomerulonephritis. *Kidney Int.* 1996;50:1965-1977.

1064. Conjeevaram HS, Hoofnagle JH, Austin HA, et al. Long-term outcome of hepatitis B virus-related glomerulonephritis after therapy with interferon alfa. *Gastroenterology.* 1995;109:540-546.

1065. Lin CY. Treatment of hepatitis B virus-associated membranous nephropathy with recombinant alpha-interferon. *Kidney Int.* 1995;47: 225-230.

1066. Lisker-Melman M, Webb D, Di Bisceglie AM, et al. Glomerulonephritis caused by chronic hepatitis B virus infection: treatment with recombinant human alpha-interferon. *Ann Intern Med.* 1989;111:479-483.

1067. Bhimma R, Coovadia HM, Kramvis A, et al. Treatment of hepatitis B virus-associated nephropathy in black children. *Pediatr Nephrol.* 2002;17:393-399.

1068. Lin CY. Clinical features and natural course of HBV-related glomerulopathy in children. *Kidney Int Suppl.* 1991;35(suppl):S46-S53.

1069. Lai KN, Tam JS, Lin HJ, et al. The therapeutic dilemma of the usage of corticosteroid in patients with membranous nephropathy and persistent hepatitis B virus surface antigenaemia. *Nephrology.* 1990;54:12-17.

1070. Tang S, Lai FMM, Lui YH, et al. Lamivudine in hepatitis B-associated membranous nephropathy. *Kidney Int.* 2005;68:1750-1758.

1071. Chan TM, Fang GX, Tang CS, et al. Preemptive lamivudine therapy based on HBV DNA level in HBsAg-positive kidney allograft recipients. *Hepatology.* 2002;36:1246-1252.

1072. Lee WC, Wu MJ, Cheng CH, et al. Lamivudine is effective for the treatment of reactivation of hepatitis B virus and fulminant hepatic failure in renal transplant recipients. *Am J Kidney Dis.* 2001;38:1074-1081.

1073. Johnson RJ, Willson R, Yamabe H, et al. Renal manifestations of hepatitis C virus infection. *Kidney Int.* 1994;46:1255-1263.

1074. Johnson RJ, Gretch DR, Yamabe H, et al. Membranoproliferative glomerulonephritis associated with hepatitis C virus infection. *N Engl J Med.* 1993;328:465-470.

1075. D'Amico G. Renal involvement in hepatitis C infection: cryoglobulinemic glomerulonephritis. *Kidney Int.* 1998;54:650-671.

1076. Markowitz GS, Cheng JT, Colvin RB, et al. Hepatitis C viral infection is associated with fibrillary glomerulonephritis and immunotactoid glomerulopathy. *J Am Soc Nephrol.* 1998;9:2244-2252.

1077. Radhakrishnan J, Uppot RN, Colvin RB. Case records of the Massachusetts General Hospital. Case 5-2010. A 51-year-old man with HIV infection, proteinuria, and edema. *N Engl J Med.* 2010;362:636-646.

1078. Sansonno D, Gesualdo L, Manno C, et al. Hepatitis C virus-related proteins in kidney tissue from hepatitis C virus-infected patients with cryoglobulinemic membranoproliferative glomerulonephritis. *Hepatology.* 1997;25:1237-1244.

1079. Agnello V, Chung RT, Kaplan LM. A role for hepatitis C virus infection in type II cryoglobulinemia. *N Engl J Med.* 1992;327:1490-1495.

1080. Herzenberg AM, Telford JJ, De Luca LG, et al. Thrombotic microangiopathy associated with cryoglobulinemic membranoproliferative glomerulonephritis and hepatitis C. *Am J Kidney Dis.* 1998;31:521-526.

1081. Stehman-Breen C, Alpers CE, Couser WG, et al. Hepatitis C virus associated membranous glomerulonephritis. *Clin Nephrol.* 1995;44:141-147.

1082. Hammoud H, Haem J, Laurent B, et al. Glomerular disease during HCV infection in renal transplantation. *Nephrol Dial Transplant.* 1996;11(suppl 4):54-55.

1083. Morales JM, Campistol JM, Andres A, et al. Glomerular diseases in patients with hepatitis C virus infection after renal transplantation. *Curr Opin Nephrol Hypertens.* 1997;6:511-515.

1084. Morales JM, Pascual-Capdevila J, Campistol JM, et al. Membranous glomerulonephritis associated with hepatitis C virus infection in renal transplant patients. *Transplantation.* 1997;63:1634-1639.

1085. Cruzado JM, Gil-Vernet S, Ercilla G, et al. Hepatitis C virus-associated membranoproliferative glomerulonephritis in renal allografts. *J Am Soc Nephrol.* 1996;7:2469-2475.

1086. Davis CL, Gretch DR, Perkins JD, et al. Hepatitis C–associated glomerular disease in liver transplant recipients. *Liver Transpl Surg.* 1995;1:166-175.

1087. Kendrick EA, McVicar JP, Kowdley KV, et al. Renal disease in hepatitis C-positive liver transplant recipients. *Transplantation.* 1997;63:1287-1293.

1088. Kidney Disease. Improving Global Outcomes (KDIGO): KDIGO Clinical Practice Guidelines for the Prevention, Diagnosis, Evaluation, and Treatment of Hepatitis C in Chronic Kidney Disease. *Kidney Int Suppl.* 2008(109):S1-S99.

1089. Misiani R, Bellavita P, Fenili D, et al. Interferon alfa-2a therapy in cryoglobulinemia associated with hepatitis C virus. *N Engl J Med.* 1994;330:751-756.

1090. Johnson RJ, Gretch DR, Couser WG, et al. Hepatitis C virus-associated glomerulonephritis. Effect of alpha- interferon therapy. *Kidney Int.* 1994;46:1700-1704.

1091. Ohta S, Yokoyama H, Wada T, et al. Exacerbation of glomerulonephritis in subjects with chronic hepatitis C virus infection after interferon therapy. *Am J Kidney Dis.* 1999;33:1040-1048.

1092. Dienstag JL, McHutchison JG. American Gastroenterological Association technical review on the management of hepatitis C. *Gastroenterology.* 2006;130:231-264.

1093. Sabry AA, Sobh MA, Sheaashaa HA, et al. Effect of combination therapy ribavirin and interferon. in HCV-related glomerulopathy. *Nephrol Dial Transplant.* 2002;17:1924-1930.

1094. Alric L, Plaisier E, Theault S, et al. Influence of antiviral therapy in hepatitis C virus-associated cryoglobulinemic MPGN. *Am J Kidney Dis.* 2004;43:617-623.

1095. D'Amico G, Ferrario F, Colasanti G, et al. Glomerulonephritis in essential mixed cryoglobulinaemia. *Proc Eur Dial Transplant Assoc Eur Ren Assoc.* 1985;21:527-548.

1096. Rostaing L, Modesto A, Baron E, et al. Acute renal failure in kidney transplant patients treated with interferon alpha 2b for chronic hepatitis C. *Nephrology.* 1996;74:512-516.

1097. Baid S, Tolkoff-Rubin N, Saidman S, et al. Acute humoral rejection in hepatitis C-infected renal transplant recipients receiving antiviral therapy. *Am J Transplant.* 2003;3:74-78.

1098. Quigg RJ, Brathwaite M, Gardner DF, et al. Successful cyclophosphamide treatment of cryoglobulinemic membranoproliferative glomerulonephritis associated with hepatitis C virus infection. *Am J Kidney Dis.* 1995;25:798-800.

1099. Beddhu S, Bastacky S, Johnson JP. The clinical and morphologic spectrum of renal cryoglobulinemia. *Medicine (Baltimore).* 2002;81:398-409.

1100. Thiel J, Peters T, Mas MA, et al. Kinetics of hepatitis C HCV. viraemia and quasispecies during treatment of HCV associated cryoglobulinaemia with pulse cyclophosphamide. *Ann Rheum Dis.* 2002;61:838-841.

1101. Rosenstock JL, Stern L, Sherman WH, et al. Fludarabine treatment of cryoglobulinemic glomerulonephritis. *Am J Kidney Dis.* 2002;40:644-648.

1102. Quartuccio L, Soardo G, Romano G, et al. Treatment of glomerulonephritis in type II mixed cryoglobulinemia with rituximab. *Arthritis Rheum.* 2004;50(suppl):S235.

1103. Saadoun D, Resche-Rigon M, Sene D, et al. Rituximab combined with Peg-interferon-ribavirin in refractory hepatitis C virus-associated cryoglobulinaemia vasculitis. *Ann Rheum Dis.* 2008;67:1431-1436.

1104. Sansonno D, De RV, Lauletta G, et al. Monoclonal antibody treatment of mixed cryoglobulinemia resistant to interferon alpha with an anti-CD20. *Blood.* 2003;101:3818-3826.

1105. Basse G, Ribes D, Kamar N, et al. Rituximab therapy for de novo mixed cryoglobulinemia in renal transplant patients. *Transplantation.* 2005;80:1560-1564.

1106. Penner E. Nature of immune complexes in autoimmune chronic active hepatitis. *Gastroenterology.* 1987;92:304-308.

1107. Axelsen RA, Crawford DH, Endre ZH, et al. Renal glomerular lesions in unselected patients with cirrhosis undergoing orthotopic liver transplantation. *Pathology.* 1995;27:237-246.

1108. Kawaguchi K, Koike M. Glomerular lesions associated with liver cirrhosis: an immunohistochemical and clinicopathologic analysis. *Hum Pathol.* 1986;17:1137-1143.

1109. Bene MC, De Korwin JD, de Ligny BH, et al. IgA nephropathy and alcoholic liver cirrhosis. A prospective necropsy study. *Am J Clin Pathol.* 1988;89:769-773.

1110. Nochy D, Callard P, Bellon B, et al. Association of overt glomerulonephritis and liver disease: a study of 34 patients. *Clin Nephrol.* 1976;6:422-427.

1111. Aggarwal M, Manske CL, Lynch PJ, et al. Henoch-Schonlein vasculitis as a manifestation of IgA-associated disease in cirrhosis. *Am J Kidney Dis.* 1992;20:400-402.

1112. Berger J, Yaneva H, Nabarra B. Glomerular changes in patients with cirrhosis of the liver. *Adv Nephrol Necker Hosp.* 1977;7:3-14.

1113. Callard P, Feldmann G, Prandi D, et al. Immune complex type glomerulonephritis in cirrhosis of the liver. *Am J Pathol.* 1975;80:329-340.

1114. Newell GC. Cirrhotic glomerulonephritis: incidence, morphology, clinical features, and pathogenesis. *Am J Kidney Dis.* 1987;9:183-190.

1115. van de Wiel A, Valentijn RM, Schuurman HJ, et al. Circulating IgA immune complexes and skin IgA deposits in liver disease. Relation to liver histopathology. *Dig Dis Sci.* 1988;33:679-684.

1116. Dash SC, Bhuyan UN, Dinda AK, et al. Increased incidence of glomerulonephritis following spleno-renal shunt surgery in non-cirrhotic portal fibrosis. *Kidney Int.* 1997;52:482-485.

1117. Noble-Jamieson G, Thiru S, Johnston P, et al. Glomerulonephritis with end-stage liver disease in childhood. *Lancet.* 1992;339:706-707.

1118. Alpers CE, Cotran RS. Neoplasia and glomerular injury. *Kidney Int.* 1986;30:465-473.

1119. Norris SH. Paraneoplastic glomerulopathies. *Semin Nephrol.* 1993;13:258-272.

1120. Morel-Maroger Striker L, Striker GE. Glomerular lesions in malignancies. *Contrib Nephrol.* 1985;48:111-124.

1121. Brueggemeyer CD, Ramirez G. Membranous nephropathy: a concern for malignancy. *Am J Kidney Dis.* 1987;9:23-26.

1122. Zech P, Colon S, Pointet P, et al. The nephrotic syndrome in adults aged over 60: etiology, evolution and treatment of 76 cases. *Clin Nephrol.* 1982;17:232-236.

1123. Liverman PC, Tucker FL, Bolton WK. Erythrocyte sedimentation rate in glomerular disease: association with urinary protein. *Am J Nephrol.* 1988;8:363-367.

1124. Bathon J, Graves J, Jens P, et al. The erythrocyte sedimentation rate in end-stage renal failure. *Am J Kidney Dis.* 1987;10:34-40.

1125. Burstein DM, Korbet SM, Schwartz MM. Membranous glomerulonephritis and malignancy. *Am J Kidney Dis.* 1993;22:5-10.

1126. da Costa CR, Dupont E, Hamers R, et al. Nephrotic syndrome in bronchogenic carcinoma: report of two cases with immunochemical studies. *Clin Nephrol.* 1974;2:245-251.

1127. Barton CH, Vaziri ND, Spear GS. Nephrotic syndrome associated with adenocarcinoma of the breast. *Am J Med.* 1980;68:308-312.

1128. Couser WG, Wagonfeld JB, Spargo BH, Lewis EJ. Glomerular deposition of tumor antigen in membranous nephropathy associated with colonic carcinoma. *Am J Med.* 1974;57:962-970.

1129. Wakashin M, Wakashin Y, Iesato K, et al. Association of gastric cancer and nephrotic syndrome. An immunologic study in three patients. *Gastroenterology*. 1980;78:749-756.

1130. Beauvais P, Vaudour G, Boccon Gibod L, et al. Membranous nephropathy associated with ovarian tumour in a young girl: recovery after removal. *Eur J Pediatr*. 1989;148:624-625.

1131. Nishibara G, Sukemi T, Ikeda Y, et al. Nephrotic syndrome due to membranous nephropathy associated with renal cell carcinoma. *Clin Nephrol*. 1996;45:424.

1132. Helin K, Honkanen E, Metsaniitty J, et al. A case of membranous glomerulonephritis associated with adenocarcinoma of pancreas. *Nephrol Dial Transplant*. 1998;13:1049-1050.

1133. Stuart K, Fallon BG, Cardi MA. Development of the nephrotic syndrome in a patient with prostatic carcinoma. *Am J Med*. 1986;80:295-298.

1134. Kon SP, Fan SL, Kwan JT, et al. Membranous nephropathy complicating adenolymphoma of the parotid Warthin's tumour. *Nephrology*. 1996;73:692-694.

1135. Schneider BF, Glass WF, Brooks CH, et al. Membranous glomerulonephritis associated with testicular seminoma. *J Intern Med*. 1995;237:599-602.

1136. Becker BN, Goldin G, Santos R, et al. Carcinoid tumor and the nephrotic syndrome: a novel association between neoplasia and glomerular disease. *South Med J*. 1996;89:240-242.

1137. Hotta O, Taguma Y, Kurosawa K, et al. Membranous nephropathy associated with nodular sclerosing Hodgkin's disease. *Nephrology*. 1993;63:347-350.

1138. Lumeng J, Moran JF. Carotid body tumor associated with mild membranous glomerulonephritis. *Ann Intern Med*. 1966;65:1266-1270.

1139. Pascal RR, Iannaccone PM, Rollwagen FM, et al. Electron microscopy and immunofluorescence of glomerular immune complex deposits in cancer patients. *Cancer Res*. 1976;36:43-47.

1140. Helin H, Pasternack A, Hakala T, et al. Glomerular electron-dense deposits and circulating immune complexes in patients with malignant tumours. *Clin Nephrol*. 1980;14:23-30.

1141. Sherman RL, Susin M, Weksler ME, et al. Lipoid nephrosis in Hodgkin's disease. *Am J Med*. 1972;52:699-706.

1142. Dabbs DJ, Striker LM, Mignon F, et al. Glomerular lesions in lymphomas and leukemias. *Am J Med*. 1986;80:63-70.

1143. Watson A, Stachura I, Fragola J, et al. Focal segmental glomerulosclerosis in Hodgkin's disease. *Am J Nephrol*. 1983;3:228-232.

1144. Ishida I, Hirakata H, Kanai Y, et al. Steroid-resistant nephrotic syndrome associated with malignant thymoma. *Clin Nephrol*. 1996;46:340-346.

1145. Cather JC, Jackow C, Yegge J, et al. Mycosis fungoides with focal segmental glomerular sclerosis and nephrotic syndrome. *J Am Acad Dermatol*. 1998;38:301-305.

1146. Auguet T, Lorenzo A, Colomer E, et al. Recovery of minimal change nephrotic syndrome and acute renal failure in a patient with renal cell carcinoma. *Am J Nephrol*. 1998;18:433-435.

1147. Gandini E, Allaria P, Castiglioni A, et al. Minimal change nephrotic syndrome with cecum adenocarcinoma. *Clin Nephrol*. 1996;45:268-270.

1148. Singer CR, Boulton-Jones JM. Minimal change nephropathy associated with anaplastic carcinoma of bronchus. *Postgrad Med J*. 1986;62:213-217.

1149. Thorner P, McGraw M, Weitzman S, et al. Wilms' tumor and glomerular disease. Occurrence with features of membranoproliferative glomerulonephritis and secondary focal, segmental glomerulosclerosis. *Arch Pathol Lab Med*. 1984;108:141-146.

1150. Moorthy AV, Zimmerman SW, Burkholder PM. Nephrotic syndrome in Hodgkin's disease. Evidence for pathogenesis alternative to immune complex deposition. *Am J Med*. 1976;61:471-477.

1151. Shalhoub RJ. Pathogenesis of lipoid nephrosis: a disorder of T cell function. *Lancet*. 1974;ii:556-560.

1152. Walker JF, O'Neil S, Campbell E, et al. Carcinoma of the oesophagus associated with membrano-proliferative glomerulonephritis. *Postgrad Med J*. 1981;57:592-596.

1153. Moulin B, Ronco PM, Mougenot B, et al. Glomerulonephritis in chronic lymphocytic leukemia and related B-cell lymphomas. *Kidney Int*. 1992;42:127-135.

1154. Feehally J, Hutchinson RM, Mackay EH, et al. Recurrent proteinuria in chronic lymphocytic leukemia. *Clin Nephrol*. 1981;16:51-54.

1155. Mak SK, Wong PN, Lo KY, et al. Successful treatment of IgA nephropathy in association with low- grade B-cell lymphoma of the mucosa-associated lymphoid tissue type. *Am J Kidney Dis*. 1998;31:713-718.

1156. Edgar JD, Rooney DP, McNamee P, et al. An association between ANCA positive renal disease and malignancy. *Clin Nephrol*. 1993;40:22-25.

1157. Hruby Z, Bronowicz A, Rabczynski J, et al. A case of severe anti-neutrophil cytoplasmic antibody ANCA-positive crescentic glomerulonephritis and asymptomatic gastric cancer. *Int Urol Nephrol*. 1994;26:579-586.

1158. Biava CG, Gonwa TA, Naughton JL, et al. Crescentic glomerulonephritis associated with nonrenal malignancies. *Am J Nephrol*. 1984;4:208-214.

1159. Gordon LI, Kwaan HC. Cancer- and drug-associated thrombotic thrombocytopenic purpura and hemolytic uremic syndrome. *Semin Hematol*. 1997;34:140-147.

1159a. Eremina V, Jefferson JA, Kowalewska J, et al. VEGF inhibition and renal thrombotic microangiopathy. *N Engl J Med*. 2008;358:1129-1136.

1160. Kilcoyne MM, Gocke DJ, Meltzer JI, et al. Nephrotic syndrome in heroin addicts. *Lancet*. 1972;1:17-20.

1161. Rao TK, Nicastri AD, Friedman EA. Natural history of heroin-associated nephropathy. *N Engl J Med*. 1974;290:19-23.

1162. Cunningham EE, Brentjens JR, Zielezny MA, et al. Heroin nephropathy. A clinicopathologic and epidemiologic study. *Am J Med*. 1980;68:47-53.

1163. Llach F, Descoeudres C, Massry SG. Heroin associated nephropathy: clinical and histological studies in 19 patients. *Clin Nephrol*. 1979;11:7-12.

1164. Treser G, Cherubin C, Longergan ET, et al. Renal lesions in narcotic addicts. *Am J Med*. 1974;57:687-694.

1165. Eknoyan G, Gyorkey F, Dichoso C, et al. Renal involvement in drug abuse. *Arch Intern Med*. 1973;132:801-806.

1166. May DC, Helderman JH, Eigenbrodt EH, et al. Chronic sclerosing glomerulopathy heroin-associated nephropathy in intravenous T's and Blues abusers. *Am J Kidney Dis*. 1986;8:404-409.

1167. Friedman EA, Rao TK. Why does uremia in heroin abusers occur predominantly among blacks? *JAMA*. 1983;250:2965-2966.

1168. Haskell LP, Glicklich D, Senitzer D. HLA associations in heroin-associated nephropathy. *Am J Kidney Dis*. 1988;12:45-50.

1169. Brown SM, Stimmel B, Taub RN, et al. Immunologic dysfunction in heroin addicts. *Arch Intern Med*. 1974;134:1001-1006.

1170. Singhal PC, Sharma P, Sanwal V, et al. Morphine modulates proliferation of kidney fibroblasts. *Kidney Int*. 1998;53:350-357.

1171. Singhal PC, Gibbons N, Abramovici M. Long term effects of morphine on mesangial cell proliferation and matrix synthesis. *Kidney Int*. 1992;41:1560-1570.

1172. Friedman EA, Rao TK. Disappearance of uremia due to heroin-associated nephropathy. *Am J Kidney Dis*. 1995;25:689-693.

1173. D'Agati V. The many masks of focal segmental glomerulosclerosis. *Kidney Int*. 1994;46:1223-1241.

1174. Whelton A, Watson AJ. Nonsteroidal anti-inflammatory drugs: effects on kidney function. In: DeBroe ME, Porter GA, Bennett WM, et al., eds. *Clinical Nephrotoxins. Renal Injury from Drugs and Chemicals*. Dordrecht, The Netherlands: Kluwer Academic Publishers; 1998:203-216.

1175. Clive DM, Stoff JS. Renal syndromes associated with nonsteroidal anti-inflammatory drugs. *N Engl J Med*. 1984;310:563-572.

1176. Abraham PA, Keane WF. Glomerular and interstitial disease induced by nonsteroidal anti- inflammatory drugs. *Am J Nephrol*. 1984;4:1-6.

1177. Levin ML. Patterns of tubulo-interstitial damage associated with nonsteroidal antiinflammatory drugs. *Semin Nephrol*. 1988;8:55-61.

1178. Alper Jr AB, Meleg-Smith S, Krane NK. Nephrotic syndrome and interstitial nephritis associated with celecoxib. *Am J Kidney Dis*. 2002;40:1086-1090.

1179. Markowitz GS, Falkowitz DC, Isom R, et al. Membranous glomerulopathy and acute interstitial nephritis following treatment with celecoxib. *Clin Nephrol*. 2003;59:137-142.

1180. Stachura I, Jayakumar S, Bourke E. T and B lymphocyte subsets in fenoprofen nephropathy. *Am J Med*. 1983;75:9-16.

1181. Bender WL, Whelton A, Beschorner WE, et al. Interstitial nephritis, proteinuria, and renal failure caused by nonsteroidal anti-inflammatory drugs. Immunologic characterization of the inflammatory infiltrate. *Am J Med*. 1984;76:1006-1012.

1182. Warren GV, Korbet SM, Schwartz MM, et al. Minimal change glomerulopathy associated with nonsteroidal antiinflammatory drugs. *Am J Kidney Dis*. 1989;13:127-130.

1183. Schwartzman M, D'Agati V. Spontaneous relapse of naproxen-related nephrotic syndrome. *Am J Med*. 1987;82:329-332.

1184. Neilson EG. Pathogenesis and therapy of interstitial nephritis. *Kidney Int*. 1989;35:1257-1270.

1185. Thysell H, Brun C, Larsen S, et al. Plasma exchange in two cases of minimal change nephrotic syndrome with acute renal failure. *Int J Artif Organs*. 1983;6(suppl 1):75-78.

1186. Bander SJ. Reversible renal failure and nephrotic syndrome without interstitial nephritis from zomepirac. *Am J Kidney Dis*. 1985;6:233-236.

1187. Schwarz A, Krause PH, Keller F, et al. Granulomatous interstitial nephritis after nonsteroidal anti-inflammatory drugs. *Am J Nephrol*. 1988;8:410-416.

1188. Radford Jr MG, Holley KE, Grande JP, et al. Reversible membranous nephropathy associated with the use of nonsteroidal anti-inflammatory drugs. *JAMA*. 1996;276:466-469.

1189. Antonovych TT. Gold nephropathy. *Ann Clin Lab Sci*. 1981;11:386-391.

1190. Wilkinson R, Eccleston DW. Nephrotic syndrome induced by gold therapy. *Br Med J.* 1970;2:772.

1191. Francis KL, Jenis EH, Jensen GE, et al. Gold-associated nephropathy. *Arch Pathol Lab Med.* 1984;108:234-238.

1192. Speerstra F, Reekers P, van de Putte LB, et al. HLA-DR antigens and proteinuria induced by aurothioglucose and D-penicillamine in patients with rheumatoid arthritis. *J Rheumatol.* 1983;10:948-953.

1193. Hall CL. The natural course of gold and penicillamine nephropathy: a longterm study of 54 patients. *Adv Exp Med Biol.* 1989;252:247-256.

1194. Matloff DS, Kaplan MM. D-Penicillamine-induced Goodpasture's-like syndrome in primary biliary cirrhosis—successful treatment with plasma-pheresis and immunosuppressives. *Gastroenterology.* 1980;78:1046-1049.

1195. Falck HM, Tornroth T, Kock B, et al. Fatal renal vasculitis and minimal change glomerulonephritis complicating treatment with penicillamine. Report on two cases. *Acta Med Scand.* 1979;205:133-138.

1196. Mathieson PW, Peat DS, Short A, et al. Coexistent membranous nephropathy and ANCA-positive crescentic glomerulonephritis in association with penicillamine. *Nephrol Dial Transplant.* 1996;11:863-866.

1197. Moens HJ, Ament BJ, Feltkamp BW, et al. Longterm followup of treatment with D-penicillamine for rheumatoid arthritis: effectivity and toxicity in relation to HLA antigens. *J Rheumatol.* 1987;14:1115-1119.

1198. Ferraccioli GF, Peri F, Nervetti A, et al. Tiopronin-nephropathy: clinical, pathological, immunological and immunogenetic characteristics. *Clin Exp Rheumatol.* 1986;4:9-15.

1199. Yoshida A, Morozumi K, Suganuma T, et al. Clinicopathological findings of bucillamine-induced nephrotic syndrome in patients with rheumatoid arthritis. *Am J Nephrol.* 1991;11:284-288.

1200. Hall CL, Jawad S, Harrison PR, et al. Natural course of penicillamine nephropathy: a long term study of 33 patients. *Br Med J Clin Res Ed.* 1988;296:1083-1086.

1201. Hall CL, Tighe R. The effect of continuing penicillamine and gold treatment on the course of penicillamine and gold nephropathy. *Br J Rheumatol.* 1989;28:53-57.

1202. Stokes MB, Foster K, Markowitz GS, et al. Development of glomerulonephritis during anti-TNF-alpha therapy for rheumatoid arthritis. *Nephrol Dial Transplant.* 2005;20:1400-1406.

1203. Oliveira DB, Foster G, Savill J, et al. Membranous nephropathy caused by mercury-containing skin lightening cream. *Postgrad Med J.* 1987;63:303-304.

1204. Meeks A, Keith PR, Tanner MS. Nephrotic syndrome in two members of a family with mercury poisoning. *J Trace Elem Electrolytes Health Dis.* 1990;4:237-239.

1205. Hill GS. Drug-associated glomerulopathies. *Toxicol Pathol.* 1986;14:37-44.

1206. Kibukamusoke JW, Davies DR, Hutt MS. Membranous nephropathy due to skin-lightening cream. *Br Med J.* 1974;2:646-647.

1207. Tubbs RR, Gephardt GN, McMahon JT, et al. Membranous glomerulonephritis associated with industrial mercury exposure. Study of pathogenetic mechanisms. *Am J Clin Pathol.* 1982;77:409-413.

1208. Belghiti D, Patey O, Berry JP, et al. Lipoid nephrosis of toxic origin. 2 cases. *Presse Med.* 1986;15:1953-1955.

1209. Silverman SH, Gribetz D, Rausen AR. Nephrotic syndrome associated with ethosuccimide. *Am J Dis Child.* 1978;132:99.

1210. Bar-Khayim Y, Teplitz C, Garella S, et al. Trimethadione Tridione-induced nephrotic syndrome. A report of a case with unique ultrastructural renal pathology. *Am J Med.* 1973;54:272-280.

1211. Heymann W. Nephrotic syndrome after use of trimethadione and paramethadione in petit mal. *JAMA.* 1967;202:893-894.

1212. Snead C, Siegel N, Hayslett J. Generalized lymphadenopathy and nephrotic syndrome as a manifestation of mephenytoin Mesantoin toxicity. *Pediatrics.* 1976;57:98-101.

1213. Yuasa S, Hashimoto M, Yura T, et al. Antineutrophil cytoplasmic antibodies ANCA-associated crescentic glomerulonephritis and propylthiouracil therapy. *Nephrology.* 1996;73:701-703.

1214. Dolman KM, Gans RO, Vervaat TJ, et al. Vasculitis and antineutrophil cytoplasmic autoantibodies associated with propylthiouracil therapy. *Lancet.* 1993;342:651-652.

1215. Vogt BA, Kim Y, Jennette JC, et al. Antineutrophil cytoplasmic autoantibody-positive crescentic glomerulonephritis as a complication of treatment with propylthiouracil in children. *J Pediatr.* 1994;124:986-988.

1216. Prasad GV, Bastacky S, Johnson JP. Propylthiouracil-induced diffuse proliferative lupus nephritis: review of immunological complications. *J Am Soc Nephrol.* 1997;8:1205-1210.

1217. Hoorntje SJ, Kallenberg CG, Weening JJ, et al. Immune-complex glomerulopathy in patients treated with captopril. *Lancet.* 1980;1:1212-1215.

1218. Webb DJ, Atkinson AB. Enalapril following captopril-induced nephrotic syndrome. *Scott Med J.* 1986;31:30-32.

1219. Coroneos E, Petrusevska G, Varghese F, et al. Focal segmental glomerulosclerosis with acute renal failure associated with alpha-interferon therapy. *Am J Kidney Dis.* 1996;28:888-892.

1220. Shah M, Jenis EH, Mookerjee BK, et al. Interferon-alpha-associated focal segmental glomerulosclerosis with massive proteinuria in patients with chronic myeloid leukemia following high dose chemotherapy. *Cancer.* 1998;83:1938-1946.

1221. Markowitz GS, Nasr SH, Stokes MB, et al. Treatment with IFN-{alpha}, -{beta}, or -{gamma} is associated with collapsing focal segmental glomerulosclerosis. *Clin J Am Soc Nephrol.* 2010;5:607-615.

1222. Honda K, Ando A, Endo M, et al. Thrombotic microangiopathy associated with alpha-interferon therapy for chronic myelocytic leukemia. *Am J Kidney Dis.* 1997;30:123-130.

1223. Ohashi N, Yonemura K, Sugiura T, et al. Withdrawal of interferon-alpha results in prompt resolution of thrombocytopenia and hemolysis but not renal failure in hemolytic uremic syndrome caused by interferon-alpha. *Am J Kidney Dis.* 2003;41:E10.

1224. Parker MG, Atkins MB, Ucci AA, et al. Rapidly progressive glomerulonephritis after immunotherapy for cancer. *J Am Soc Nephrol.* 1995;5:1740-1744.

1225. Lindell A, Denneberg T, Enestrom S, et al. Membranous glomerulonephritis induced by 2-mercaptopropionylglycine 2-MPG. *Clin Nephrol.* 1990;34:108-115.

1226. Richman AV, Masco HL, Rifkin SI, et al. Minimal-change disease and the nephrotic syndrome associated with lithium therapy. *Ann Intern Med.* 1980;92:70-72.

1227. Tam VK, Green J, Schwieger J, et al. Nephrotic syndrome and renal insufficiency associated with lithium therapy. *Am J Kidney Dis.* 1996;27:715-720.

1228. Phan L, Coulomb F, Boudon M, et al. Extramembranous glomerulonephritis induced by lithium. *Nephrologie.* 1991;12:185-187.

1229. Santella RN, Rimmer JM, MacPherson BR. Focal segmental glomerulosclerosis in patients receiving lithium carbonate. *Am J Med.* 1988;84:951-954.

1230. Markowitz GS, Radhakrishnan J, Kambham N, et al. Lithium nephrotoxicity: a progressive combined glomerular and tubulointerstitial nephropathy. *J Am Soc Nephrol.* 2000;11:1439-1448.

1231. Markowitz GS, Appel GB, Fine PL, et al. Collapsing focal segmental glomerulosclerosis following treatment with high-dose pamidronate. *J Am Soc Nephrol.* 2001;12:1164-1172.

1232. Ie EH, Karschner JK, Shapiro AP. Reversible nephrotic syndrome due to high renin state in renovascular hypertension. *Neth J Med.* 1995;46:136-141.

1233. Chen R, Novick AC, Pohl M. Reversible renin mediated massive proteinuria successfully treated by nephrectomy. *J Urol.* 1995;153:133-134.

1234. Jardine DL, Pidgeon GB, Bailey RR. Renal artery stenosis as a cause of heavy albuminuria. *N Z Med J.* 1993;106:30-31.

1235. Giles RD, Sturgill BC, Suratt PM, et al. Massive proteinuria and acute renal failure in a patient with acute silicoproteinosis. *Am J Med.* 1978;64:336-342.

1236. Banks DE, Milutinovic J, Desnick RJ, et al. Silicon nephropathy mimicking Fabry's disease. *Am J Nephrol.* 1983;3:279-284.

1237. Moayyedi P, Fletcher S, Harnden P, et al. Mesangiocapillary glomerulonephritis associated with ulcerative colitis: case reports of two patients. *Nephrol Dial Transplant.* 1995;10:1923-1924.

1238. Dhiman RK, Poddar U, Sharma BC, et al. Membranous glomerulonephritis in association with ulcerative colitis. *Indian J Gastroenterol.* 1998;17:62.

1239. Whelan TV, Maher JF, Kragel P, et al. Nephrotic syndrome associated with Kimura's disease. *Am J Kidney Dis.* 1988;11:353-356.

1240. Sud K, Saha T, Das A, et al. Kimura's disease and minimal-change nephrotic syndrome. *Nephrol Dial Transplant.* 1996;11:1349-1351.

1241. Lui SL, Chan KW, Li FK, et al. Castleman's disease and mesangial proliferative glomerulonephritis: the role of interleukin-6. *Nephrology.* 1998;78:323-327.

1242. Ruggieri G, Barsotti P, Coppola G, et al. Membranous nephropathy associated with giant lymph node hyperplasia. A case report with histological and ultrastructural studies. *Am J Nephrol.* 1990;10:323-328.

1243. Said R, Tarawneh M. Membranoproliferative glomerulonephritis associated with multicentric angiofollicular lymph node hyperplasia. Case report and review of the literature. *Am J Nephrol.* 1992;12:466-470.

1244. Tsukamoto Y, Hanada N, Nomura Y, et al. Rapidly progressive renal failure associated with angiofollicular lymph node hyperplasia. *Am J Nephrol.* 1991;11:430-436.

1245. Miadonna A, Salmaso C, Palazzi P, et al. Fibrillary glomerulonephritis in Castleman's disease. *Leuk Lymphoma.* 1998;28:429-435.

1246. Ikeda S, Chisuwa H, Kawasaki S, et al. Systemic reactive amyloidosis associated with Castleman's disease: serial changes of the concentrations of acute phase serum amyloid A and interleukin 6 in serum. *J Clin Pathol.* 1997;50:965-967.

1247. Wood WG, Harkins MM. Nephropathy in angioimmunoblastic lymphadenopathy. *Am J Clin Pathol.* 1979;71:58-63.

1248. Thaunat O, Delahousse M, Fakhouri F, et al. Nephrotic syndrome associated with hemophagocytic syndrome. *Kidney Int.* 2006;69:1892-1898.

Overview of Therapy for Glomerular Disease

Daniel C. Cattran and Heather N. Reich

The previous two chapters have discussed the approach to the management of patients with primary and secondary glomerulonephritis (GN). Why do we need another chapter addressing treatment? There are several parts to the answer. First, we believe it is necessary to have a more comprehensive picture of the importance of these disorders in nephrology practice compared with what is provided in most standard nephrology texts. Next, we believe it is it is relevant to know the evidence that supports the benefits of disease control recognizing our current inability to cure most of the progressive GN variants. Last, we believe that nephrologists need to comprehensively understand both the mechanisms of action of the immunosuppressive medications used in the various GN treatment regimens and, in particular, their toxicities to better manage patients.

These are the essential components of risk-to-benefit analysis and are the focus of this chapter. The recognition that most of the progressive GN variants are chronic diseases has translated into extended treatment courses with the corollary of increased risk of drug toxicity. This has necessitated a heightened awareness of the adverse effects of these drugs and the requirement for constant surveillance to maintain the proper balance between their benefits and risks. In accordance with these concerns, this chapter focuses on establishing a better understanding of the scope of these diseases in nephrology practice, of the relevance and benefits of GN disease control, and the increased importance of risk-to-benefit analyses

profiling the drug regimens advocated in the treatment of patients with these disorders.

The Scope of the Problem

There are two nuances intrinsic to our evolving understanding the current scope of GN in clinical practice. The first relates to potential changes in the incidence rate of GN and the second to whether significant alteration within the histologic variants has occurred over time. Identifying shifts in the incidence and distribution of GN should be straightforward. Unfortunately, the lack of any coherent national or international registry of GN, even at the level of renal pathology, limits our ability to answer these questions. Reviewing dialysis or transplant end-stage renal disease (ESRD) registries and examining the numbers associated with either primary or secondary GN does not provide a clear view to the practicing nephrologist of either the extent of these disease processes or of variations within the diagnostic categories. This is related partly to major confounding effects of the varied diseases on overall patient survival and ESRD treatment choices.

There is a generally held belief that the overall frequency of GN as a cause of ESRD has declined.[1] A plausible alternative[2] is that there has been no change in the absolute numbers but only a relative percentage reduction (at least in North America) in proportion because of the increased numbers of ESRD cases attributable to other causes, particularly diabetes mellitus.[3] In addition, although the incidence rate may be decreasing, a significant proportion of prevalent patients in many ESRD registries are still secondary to progressive GN.[4,5]

According to the United States Renal Data System (USRDS), GN accounts for between 10% and 20% of the total incident cases of ESRD.[5] Very similar data have been reported from the Canadian Organ Replacement Registry (CORR).[6] In the latest CORR report, GN accounted for 11.2% of ESRD, ranking third among identifiable causes (diabetes, 35%; vascular disease, 18.1%). This is a decline from the 16% incidence rate reported previously.[7,8] These percentages are misleading because the absolute number of affected individuals has remained unchanged. A similar trend in the USRDS supports the contention that the absolute incidence of GN has not declined.[5] In contrast, in several countries belonging to the European Dialysis and Transplant Association ESRD Registry, GN remains the leading cause of kidney failure, representing up to 40% of incident cases.[9] Within the countries of the registry, however, significant variations are noted. In the United Kingdom, for instance, the data suggest similar causal percentages as those observed in North America compared with a much higher GN incidence rate from the Eastern European countries.[9] Another ESRD data system with an excellent data tracking record is the Australia and New Zealand Registry. Until recently, GN had dominated causation of ESRD, but current reports suggest the same trends as those observed in North American databases.[10] There are dramatic global variations in these trends. In Asian registries, GN continues to account for the majority of cases of incident ESRD.[4] This difference has been attributed to various factors, including genetic background and environmental and infectious exposures, but additional factors such as differences in health care policies and disparities in access to ESRD programs also exist.[11]

In contrast to data describing incident ESRD populations, if one examines prevalent patients on renal replacement therapy or registries that track functioning renal transplants, GN—either biopsy-proven or suspected—remains a leading cause of ESRD. These numbers, however, are also likely to be biased and reflect the younger age on average as well as the enhanced survival of the GN patient population compared with subjects who have diabetes.[4,12]

There are additional important considerations when using ESRD registries to estimate the incidence and prevalence of kidney failure attributable to GN. Even within the best renal replacement registries, the underlying etiology of kidney failure is poorly captured, and the incidence and prevalence of the cases attributed to GN are probably underestimated. A significant proportion of the "known" causes of ESRD, for instance, is allocated to the category of hypertensive nephrosclerosis based solely on the presence of hypertension at the time of initiation of renal replacement therapy. Given that, on a global basis, the most common biopsy-proven type of GN is immunoglobulin A (IgA) nephropathy and that IgA nephropathy (IgAN) is often asymptomatic throughout its course and almost universally associated with hypertension (particularly later in the course), one can surmise that many of the patients in the "hypertension" or "nephrosclerosis" diagnostic categories have this glomerular pathology underlying their renal failure.

Renal replacement registries should not be used to estimate the prevalence of GN because they do not capture patients with early disease or patients who do not ultimately progress to dialysis or die before reaching that stage. It is possible to better estimate the extent of these diseases by imputing incidence rates from countrywide renal pathology registry data. Such a registry from Finland, for example, reported an incidence of GN in the range of 18 per 100,000 population, acknowledging a relatively high center-specific biopsy rate.[2] However even using this relatively crude estimate of incidence, dramatic variations are seen throughout the world. Reported renal biopsy rates have varied from 48 per million population (pmp) in certain regions in Spain to as high as 261 pmp in Australia.[13] This variation is undoubtedly biased by biopsy practice patterns. In some countries—for instance, Finland—isolated hematuria found during routine screening obliges the patient to submit to a renal biopsy, but in North America, significant clinical indicators of underlying renal disease such as proteinuria over 1 g/day or systemic features of disease are the dominant indicators for a renal biopsy.[14] It is possible to extrapolate from these data the crude incidence of GN in the North American population. If we take the average of these incidence numbers to be between 100 and 200 pmp, this would indicate an annual incident rate of GN in North America (population, 400 million) of between 40,000 and 80,000 cases.

Pathology-based regional GN registries also offer information regarding potential shifts in the distribution of histologic subtypes of GN. Broadly inclusive local pathology-based registries (i.e., capturing all biopsies performed in a large and defined geographic region) provide important insights in this regard and, if they are linked to a clinical database, can also provide important information in regard to the natural history of these disorders. Our own linked clinical and pathology regional registry has captured all GN cases from the greater Toronto area since 1975[15]; our data indicate that the annual absolute number of biopsy-proven cases of GN has not substantially changed (Table 33-1), but shifts within the specific histologic groups have occurred. There have been two- to threefold increases in IgAN and focal segmental glomerulosclerosis (FSGS), a twofold reduction in idiopathic membranoproliferative GN (MPGN), and virtually no change in the incidence of membranous GN (MGN) over the past 3 decades. Although similar shifts over time have been reported from other large North American centers, it is not entirely clear if this represents true changes in incidence patterns, reporting biases created by highly specialized local clinical or renal pathology expertise, or variations in biopsy practice patterns. The changes in the absolute incidence of GN subtypes observed in the Toronto registry may also reflect the increasing rates of immigration to the Toronto region[16] as well as variation in the ethnic composition of the city. Geographic and ethnic variation clearly influences diagnostic patterns. In a recent large retrospective review of 600 biopsies from China, IgAN accounted for 40% of all diagnoses and was almost twice as common as the second leading type of biopsy-proven GN, which was vasculitis; three times more common than FSGS; and 30 times more common than membranous nephropathy.[1]

The recognition of "new" causative factors, such as hepatitis C virus producing the injury pattern of MPGN, is another possible explanation for variation and changes in histologic subtypes.[17] Many cases of previously diagnosed "idiopathic MPGN" were subsequently attributable to hepatitis C

TABLE 33-1 Trends in Selected Kidney Biopsy Diagnoses Captured in the Regional Toronto Glomerulonephritis Registry Between 1975 and 2005 (Total Number of Biopsies During This Period, 9256)*

	1975–1979	1980–1984	1985–1990	1990–1994	1995–1999	2000–2004	TOTAL
IgA	129 (18.6)	215 (24.6)	227 (27.9)	262 (26.8)	309 (31.0)	356 (36.7)	1498 (28.0)
FSGS	141 (20.3)	164 (18.7)	163 (20.0)	239 (24.4)	311 (31.2)	271 (28.0)	1289 (24.1)
Membranous	134 (19.3)	172 (19.7)	171 (21.0)	164 (16.8)	129 (12.9)	143 (14.8)	920 (17.2)
MPGN	90 (13.0)	67 (7.7)	33 (4.1)	46 (4.7)	37 (3.7)	31 (3.2)	304 (5.7)
Lupus	170 (24.5)	191 (21.8)	143 (17.6)	174 (17.8)	136 (13.6)	100 (10.3)	921 (17.2)
Vasculitis	29 (4.2)	66 (7.5)	76 (9.3)	93 (9.5)	76 (7.6)	68 (7.0)	411 (7.7)
Total	693	875	813	978	998	969	5343

*Data are n (%).

FSGS, Focal segmental glomerulosclerosis; *IgA*, immunoglobulin A; *MPGN*, membranoproliferative glomerulonephritis.

infection, so the incidence of idiopathic MPGN now appears to be decreasing. However, other registries have shown similar changes to our data regarding the increased frequency of IgAN and FSGS without any identified "new" secondary causes or dramatic shifts in the ethnic demographics of the region.[18,19] In contrast to these dramatic variations over time, are recent reports from Denmark, where standardized population-based epidemiologic data suggest that neither the number nor the distribution of GN diagnoses has altered substantially over the past 2 decades.[2] The changes in histologic subtypes of GN, if real, may reflect fundamental shifts in biologic and environmental factors underlying the pathogenesis of these diseases and is another substantive reason for the creation of national and international registries of GN.

In summary, most data suggest that the absolute incidence of GN is relatively constant, and its impact on nephrology practice is likely underestimated. The societal burden of GN—to both the individual and to the health care system—is also substantially discounted, especially if assessed solely from figures derived from ESRD registries. Strong indicators suggest that dramatic shifts in the histologic subtypes of GN have occurred; however, this is more difficult to confirm and is undoubtedly influenced by kidney biopsy practice patterns and by complex variables such as differences in population demographics and socioeconomic factors as well as genetics and environmental exposures.

Outcome Measures in Glomerulonephritis

Crude estimates of the population incidence of GN are not informative with respect to describing the natural history of these disorders over the critical period between biopsy and registration as an ESRD statistic. Despite this limitation, during the past decade, there have been important changes in our approach to the treatment of patients with GN driven by prospectively collected natural history data, therapeutic studies, and the evolution toward a more evidence-based approach to clinical care.

Assessment and follow-up of large cohorts of GN patients during the trajectory of their chronic kidney disease (CKD) has yielded new and important information that has influenced patient management and altered how we assess treatment benefit. These efforts (elaborated in the next section) have allowed a more accurate identification of modifiable predictors of clinical outcome, thus allowing physicians to alter

the course of the patient's disease. A significant contribution to this domain of practice has been a better understanding of the importance of proteinuria on renal injury and the recognition that its reduction has a substantial impact on both the rate of progression of kidney disease and ultimately on renal survival. Although this has significantly improved our capacity to assess the benefits of treatment, our evaluation of risks of therapy requires further refinement.

There has also been an important shift in the treatment of patients with GN to a more evidence-based approach, and clinical practice guidelines have been developed to help nephrologists in the management of patients with these disorders.[20] Currently, a new set of evidence-based recommendations for management of patients with GN is being developed under the auspices of KDIGO (Kidney Disease Improving Global Outcomes) with the expectation of publication in 2011.

The randomized controlled trial (RCT) remains the gold standard for the assessment of therapeutic efficacy. However, there are important limitations to both the execution and interpretation of such studies in patients with GN. RCTs in GN are not appealing to funding agencies (either in the private or public sector), as the target population is relatively small and the cost of such studies is high. Part of the financial burden relates to the size and duration of studies required to demonstrate "clinical benefit" in patients with GN. A major disincentive for the development of such studies is a lack of consensus regarding the clinical relevance of surrogate outcome measures. In general, only "hard outcomes" such as patient or renal survival are acceptable to granting agencies, government policy regulators, and the pharmaceutical industry.[21] Because the great majority of patients with GN, regardless of the specific subtype, will have slowly progressive disease, this limits the capacity to organize, fund, and properly interpret clinical trials.

Even the currently available clinical trials have limitations in regard to their generalizability. Whether the results of current studies can be applied to an individual patient remains a major concern of many physicians. To design statistically and financially viable studies, investigators must select a relatively homogeneous population to ensure that the required sample size is achievable and that the study can be completed within an acceptable time frame. A homogeneous population, by definition, excludes many patients such as those with atypical presentations and comorbid conditions, and often represents a skewed ethnic composition because of language fluency requirements for participation. Furthermore, major changes in nonspecific treatment (e.g., introduction of inhibitors of the renin–angiotensin system for blood pressure control) and in our understanding of the pathogenesis of these diseases (e.g., the recognition of the causal link between MPGN and hepatitis C) have reduced the external validity of previously completed trials, even though they may have been well-designed RCTs.[22,23]

All of these considerations are critical in GN management given that the majority of the specific immunomodulatory drugs used for treatment are potent and inherently dangerous. It is in large part the confluence of these issues that has been the impetus for the creation of this new chapter. The relative rarity of the disease, combined with the limitations of available trial data, especially given the hard endpoints listed above and the potential toxicity of our current therapy, evokes considerable concern in the minds of nephrologists when dealing with patients with GN. A consensus regarding acceptable surrogate markers of clinical benefit would thus be helpful for practicing physicians and be of considerable benefit in our efforts strengthen the evidence base in GN management.

The Current Status of Glomerulonephritis Surrogate Markers

Although renal and patient survival remains the gold standard of benefit in the treatment of patients with GN, surrogate markers of these endpoints have emerged during the past decade. It is generally accepted that complete remission of proteinuria does lead to significant improvement in quality of life (e.g., improvement of edema) as well as in renal survival.[21,24] A quantitative assessment of the value of proteinuria reduction is also emerging and will be a crucial element in the decision making of nephrologists in terms of balancing the risks and benefits of treatment. However, the quantitative impact of a partial remission in proteinuria, including its definition and duration on renal survival, requires further clarification before its universal acceptance as a surrogate indicator of long-term survival.

Recently, a series of publications in the most common primary and secondary progressive GNs has provided a more comprehensive framework focused on a more uniform definition and an improved estimate of the benefits of achieving a partial remission of proteinuria. This series should provide practicing nephrologists with a critical piece of information to assist them both in their therapeutic decisions and in patient counseling. The capacity to translate proteinuria reduction into a semiquantifiable estimate of improvement in long-term outcome provides an important element of the benefit in the benefit-to-risk equation not only in terms of whether to initiate treatment but more commonly today to provide help in the decision about prolonging treatment or retreating a patient to maintain or reestablish a partial remission.

Quantification of the Benefits of Proteinuria Reduction

Membranous Glomerulonephritis

Many natural history studies in MGN have demonstrated the value of complete remission of proteinuria and the unfavorable outcome in patients with persistent high-grade proteinuria.

However, neither the definition of partial remission nor its value on renal survival or rate of progression has been consistently shown.[25] A recent study examined a prospective cohort of 348 patients with the nephrotic syndrome with MGN to assess the benefit of a complete or partial remission of proteinuria on both renal survival and rate of decline in renal function. Although a variety of definitions of partial remission have been applied to membranous nephropathy over the past 25 years, the great majority have required reduction to subnephrotic range proteinuria (<3.5 g/day). The additional requirement in this study was a 50% decrease from peak proteinuria because this would mandate a substantial change in proteinuria in all patients, regardless of their initial value. Over a median follow-up of 60 months (range, 12–400 months), 30% had a complete remission, 40% had a partial remission, and the remaining 30% no remission. At 10 years, renal survival in those with a complete remission was 100% with little disease progression over the same time frame as measured by slope of the creatinine clearance (-1 mL/min/yr). Those achieving a partial remission had a 90% renal survival at 10 years and a more rapid rate of progression compared with complete remission, although still limited to a loss of -2 mL/min/yr of creatinine clearance. In comparison, those with no remission had a renal survival of only 50% at 10 years and a very significant increase in progression rate (-10 mL/min/yr) that was five times the rate seen in the partial remission group. By multivariate analysis, achieving a partial remission was an independent predictor of renal survival and rate of progression of this group. Survival from renal failure for partial remission was significantly improved (hazard ratio for ESRD compared with the reference group of no remission of 0.08, 95% confidence interval [CI] 0.03–0.19; $P < 0.001$). In addition, the value of a partial remission was also analyzed using time-dependent variables to ensure attribution of any benefit on survival to the time after partial remission has been achieved. Indeed, the adjusted hazard ratio for the risk of ESRD in patients achieving a partial remission (expressed as a time-dependent variable) was 0.17 compared with those not achieving a remission of proteinuria (95% CI 0.09–0.33; $P < 0.001$). Additional important information gleaned from the study included the observation that treatment-induced partial remissions had the same favorable long-term outcome as those acquired spontaneously, and although the rate of relapse was high (47%), the relapses were often reversible with repeat treatment. These data strongly support the contention that partial remission is an important therapeutic target in patients with membranous GN with measurable and clinically relevant benefits on both progression rate and renal survival. The findings allow a better assessment of treatment benefits by attributing a quantitative value to partial remission. This in turn facilitates the assessment of the balance between benefits and risk of treatment of patients with MGN.

Focal and Segmental Glomerulosclerosis

The same estimates of benefit of proteinuria reduction in regard to the long-term outcome in patients with FSGS are now available. It has been appreciated for some time that complete remission of proteinuria is the best long-term predictor of favorable renal survival.[26,27] However, a standardized definition of partial remission and an assessment of its benefit would improve the physician's ability to balance the benefits of intense immunosuppressive treatment versus the well-recognized risks of the current available treatment regimens for FSGS.[27,28] Factors that have been previously associated with a poor outcome in FSGS have included the severity of initial proteinuria, the initial creatinine clearance, and the extent of tubulointerstitial disease on histologic examination. Although these may be relevant factors, they all lack precision in terms of the benefits that would accrue if proteinuria was only partially reduced.[29,30]

These issues were recently addressed in a long-term cohort study of 281 patients with nephrotic syndrome with biopsy-proven primary FSGS followed over an average of 65 months (range, 12–346 months).[31] The authors found that defining partial remission by both a reduction of proteinuria to subnephrotic range (<3.5 g/day) and a 50% reduction from peak proteinuria provided the best discrimination among the patients in terms of both renal survival and progression rate. During the observation period, 55 patients had a complete remission, 117 patients achieved a partial remission, and 109 had no remission of proteinuria. Partial remission was independently predictive of both renal survival and rate of decline in renal function by multivariate analysis. Partial remission was associated with improved renal survival with a time-adjusted hazard ratio of 0.48 (CI 95% 0.24 to 0.96; $P = .04$). The 10-year renal survival rate was 75% in the partial remission group compared with 35% in those with no remission.[31] Additional important observations from the study included a significant relapse rate of close to 50% in patients who achieved a partial remission, and although relapse predicted both a lower renal survival and faster rate of disease progression than those with no relapse, patients with partial remissions overall still had a more favorable outcomes than those who never achieved a remission. Similar to MGN, this information on the quantitative benefits of partial remission is important in the assessment of patients with FSGS because it provides equipoise to the risks of treatment.

IgA Nephropathy

The importance of proteinuria in IgAN has been long recognized, but its relative value compared with FSGS and membranous nephropathy is quite distinct. In addition, until recently, the definition and incremental benefit of proteinuria reduction in IgAN was not well described. Furthermore, the widespread application of angiotensin-converting enzyme (ACE) inhibitors or angiotensin receptor blockade as therapy for IgAN[32,33] may have significantly altered the natural history of these patients' kidney disease, potentially complicating the assessment of the independent value of proteinuria reduction.

Analyzing patients with IgAN enrolled in a series of RCTs of fish oils, Donadio and associates[34] demonstrated an association between proteinuria reduction and both improved renal survival and prolonged time to doubling of serum creatinine. More recently, in a study by Reich and associates,[65] the definition of partial remission was further refined, and the incremental benefits that accrued by proteinuria reduction were documented. The authors studied a prospectively enrolled cohort of more than 500 patients with primary IgAN, followed for an average of 78 months (range, 12–315 months). They defined a partial remission as achieving a level

of proteinuria below 1 g/day. Multivariate analysis, using all of the clinical and laboratory parameters currently available, indicated that the level of proteinuria during the follow-up was the most important predictor of the rate of decline of glomerular filtration rate (GFR). In the almost 200 patients who achieved and sustained partial remission of proteinuria (either spontaneously or through treatment), the mean rate of decline in renal function was only 10% of those who did not. There was a clear gradation in the rate of decline of kidney function, such that those with sustained proteinuria levels greater than 3 g/day ($n = 121$) had a 25-fold faster decline in renal function that those with less than 1 g /day, and their hazard ratio for renal failure was almost 10 times greater (95% CI 5–18). An additional observation of equal importance was that regardless of the level of presenting proteinuria, those who attained a partial remission had the same long-term prognosis and slow rate of disease progression as those whose peak proteinuria levels never exceeded 1 g/day. Although there were other modifiable factors identified in the multivariate analysis associated with kidney function decline (time averaged mean arterial pressure and exposure to agents that blocked the renin–angiotensin system), the level of sustained proteinuria was the dominant modifiable risk. The differential in progression rate and renal failure risk was dramatic, and understanding the impact of even a small but sustained improvement in proteinuria is extremely valuable information for practicing physicians.

There are important quantitative differences in the impact of proteinuria in patients with IgAN compared with those with FSGS and MGN. This variation in the value of proteinuria reduction according to histologic diagnosis was recently demonstrated in a paper examining the impact of sex on kidney disease outcome. The study clearly illustrated that the quantitative impact of proteinuria is not uniform across GN subtypes (Figure 33-1); for example, 3 g/day of proteinuria has a vastly different implication in terms of both renal survival and the rate of deterioration in renal function in a patient with IgAN compared with a patient with MGN or FSGS.[35]

Systemic Lupus Erythematosus

An important secondary form of GN leading to CKD and kidney failure is systemic lupus erythematosus (SLE). Similar to the primary progressive variants of GN, complete absence of active renal disease has been associated with an excellent long-term renal survival, although even this status does not guarantee freedom from ever developing kidney disease.[36] Recently, quantitation of the effect of remission of proteinuria on long-term outcome has been estimated in a long-term observational study of 86 patients with biopsy-proven diffuse proliferative lupus nephritis followed for a decade.[37] The authors defined complete remission as absence of significant proteinuria and a serum creatinine of less than 1.5 mg/dL and a partial remission as a 50% reduction in baseline proteinuria with a nadir in proteinuria of less than 1.5 g/day and no more than a 25% increase in baseline serum creatinine. Patient and renal survival were strongly influenced by whether the patient achieved complete, partial, or no remission in proteinuria. At 10 years, the patient survival and renal survival rates in subjects achieving a complete remission were 95% and 94%, respectively; in those reaching a partial remission, they were 76% and 45%, respectively, and in those who

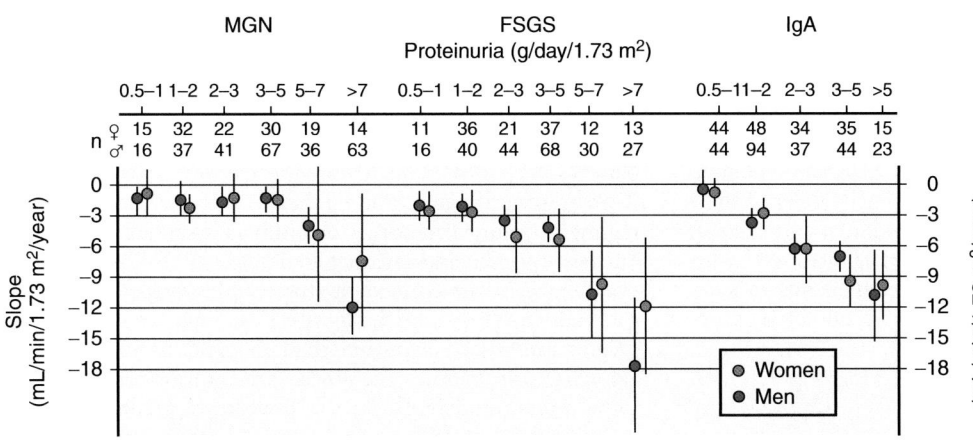

FIGURE 33-1 Differential impact of proteinuria according to sex and histologic subtype on the rate of renal function decline in membranous glomerulonephritis, focal segmental glomerulosclerosis, and immunoglobulin A nephropathy. (From Cattran DC, Reich HN, Beanlands HJ, et al: The impact of sex in primary glomerulonephritis. *Nephrol Dial Transplant* 23:2247-2253, 2008.)

never met criteria for a partial or complete remission, they were only 46% and 13%, respectively. The clinical value of a reduction in proteinuria in terms of amelioration of long-term outcome was confirmed in a 10-year follow-up of a clinical trial comparing immunosuppressive regimens.[38]

This provides strong evidence for clinicians that lowering of proteinuria, even without achieving complete remission status, is an important therapeutic goal in patients with SLE nephritis. This finding provides an important clinical tool for physicians that should help in the constant need to balance the risks of continuing or augmenting immunosuppressive therapy versus reducing or switching therapy to less potent but safer therapy, acknowledging the lesser but still substantial benefits of a partial remission.

Vasculitis

A rapid deterioration in renal function is a severe and relatively common manifestation of vasculitis, a systemic disorder that commonly terminates in ESRD or death of the patient. The rapidity of kidney disease progression and the significant risk of either disease-associated or drug-related mortality distinguish vasculitis from the previously described primary GNs and even from SLE nephritis. The significant benefits in terms of both kidney and patient survival with treatment compared with no treatment are countered by the current potent drug regimens required that have their own significant life-threatening consequences. Significant adverse effects have been described in up to 90% of treated patients.[39-43] This confluence of severe disease and toxic therapy is aggravated by the more advanced average age at presentation of patients with vasculitis compared with those who have other types of GN. This further emphasizes the importance of accurate and early assessment of the predictive markers of outcome for both patient and renal survival.[44] The need for considering both risk and benefits was demonstrated in a recent review of 100 patients with vasculitis whose presenting creatinine was greater than 500 μmol/L (5.6 mg/dL).[45] A total of 55% of the deaths were attributed to the adverse effects of treatment almost exclusively related to opportunistic infections, including *Pneumocystis jiroveci* (formerly *Pneumocystis carinii* pneumoniae) and cytomegalovirus (CMV) infections. In contrast, only 25% of the deaths were attributed to active uncontrolled vasculitic disease with the remaining 25% related to the underlying advanced age or comorbid conditions of the

patients, including myocardial infarctions and cerebrovascular accidents. The authors determined that in patients presenting with vasculitis and severe renal failure, predictors of the need for permanent renal replacement therapy were limited. The only indicators identified were age at onset of the disease and pathology, the degree of arteriosclerosis, and the presence of segmental crescents or eosinophilic infiltrates. Good prognostic indicators of kidney recovery were younger age at onset and on histology, a greater percentage of normal glomeruli and lower percentage of tubular atrophy, and interstitial infiltration. No clinical parameters were independently predictive of death. Even within these limited predictive indices, the variation was wide and the sensitivity low.[45]

In an earlier prospective study in vasculitic patients with mild to moderate renal involvement at presentation (i.e., serum creatinine <500 umol/L), the same authors noted that the level of renal function at onset and renal pathology lesions suggestive of chronicity were indicators of a poor prognosis. In contrast, active lesions such as crescents and necrosis were the only ones that predicted a treatment response and improved renal outcome at 18 months.[46] A semiquantitative assessment of prognosis based on any one individual factor or a combination of them has not been performed, likely related to the acuity of the condition and the wide deviations in these predictive indices. A recent systematic review of studies in vasculitis, including patients with minimal renal involvement, identified similar predictors of outcome in regards to remission, relapse, and renal and overall patient survival.[47]

Overview

On this background, a heightened awareness of the risks of our current therapies needs to be considered in every patient by practicing nephrologists. The real dangers associated with these therapies mandates repeated reviews of the patient, including a critical analysis of the response likelihood versus the accumulating risks of ongoing therapy. This assessment should include the possibility of a repeat renal biopsy to assess activity versus irreversible chronic damage. In addition, when evaluating the potential benefit of immunosuppressive therapy, an improvement in organ and patient survival should still be paramount, but the integration of the benefits of proteinuria reduction and improved quality of life should now also be counted. Often not considered in this balance of risks and benefits of treatment is the risk of inadequate treatment of

GN, forgetting that renal replacement modalities (i.e., dialysis and transplant) have their own attendant high rates of morbidity and mortality.

The purpose of this chapter is not to reiterate all of the specific regimens that have been used in the management of each of the specific types of GN. These treatment schemas have been presented in earlier chapters. The benefits of therapy have been described, and the remainder of this chapter focuses on the risks of the commonly used agents used in the treatment of patients with GN. It includes their mechanisms of action, their indications and toxicities, and potential strategies for minimizing adverse effects.

Corticosteroids

Glucocorticoids are the most common antiinflammatory and immunosuppressive drugs used in the treatment of both primary and secondary GN. They have protean effects on immune responses mediated by T and B cells, including reversibly blocking T-cell and antigen-presenting cell–derived cytokine and cytokine-receptor expression. Their hydrophobic structure permits corticosteroids to easily diffuse into cells and bind to specific cytoplasmic proteins, facilitating translocation of these proteins into the cell nucleus, where they bind to a highly conserved glucocorticoid receptor DNA-binding domain (the glucocorticoid response element) and modulate gene transcription.[48] Some of the downstream effects accounting for the antiinflammatory activity of glucocorticoids include the inhibition of synthesis of proinflammatory cytokines implicated in glomerular and tubulointerstitial injury, such as interleukin-2 (IL-2), -6, and -8 and tumor necrosis factor.[49,50] Glucocorticoids also exert a host of nontranscriptional immunomodulatory effects on immune effector cells, including alteration of leukocyte trafficking and chemotactic properties, and modulation of endothelial function, vasodilatation, and vascular permeability.[48]

Indications

Glucocorticoids, most commonly in the form of prednisone, remain a cornerstone of many forms of therapy in both primary and secondary GN today. As with virtually every one of the immunosuppressive agents used in the treatment of patients with GN, the risks of treatment versus potential benefits must be assessed on the basis of drug exposure (a composite of dose and duration) and individual patient factors, including age and comorbid conditions such as obesity, diabetes mellitus, and cardiac disease.

Minimal change disease in the pediatric population is most often responsive to a short, 4- to 8-week course of moderate dose daily prednisone. Under these conditions, the benefits of being relieved of the signs and symptoms of nephrotic range proteinuria and the permanent cure of the condition in approximately 50% of the these patients clearly weigh in favor of a course of treatment.[51] However, the 50% of pediatric patients who relapse and require multiple courses of treatment and other patient cohorts, including adult patients who often require a significantly longer course of corticosteroids and those with additional risk factors, including older adults, individuals with obesity, and those with a family history of diabetes, are at a substantially higher risk of adverse effects

from this drug. This does and should shift the risk-to-benefit balance of corticosteroid therapy and push physicians to consider alternative treatment for patients with minimal change disease.

Similar risk-to-benefit assessments must be made in patients with FSGS, in whom the current initial treatment is prednisone therapy. The application of this therapy in the regimens outlined in earlier chapters is based solely on large but retrospective and uncontrolled studies.[52,53] The most relevant issue in the context of this chapter is the recognition that these routines in patients with FSGS require substantially greater prednisone exposure than in patients with minimal change disease before reaching a remission or being deemed to be nonresponders. Instead of 8 weeks of prednisone therapy, patients with FSGS often require 3 to 6 months of high-dose daily treatment before they reach a complete or partial remission or before they can conclusively be labeled as "steroid resistant."[26] The adverse effects of these high-dose regimens are of particular concern given that the mean age of the adult FSGS patient at presentation has significantly changed over the past 2 decades, increasing from the 20s in the 1970s to the 50s today,[54] and age is a major risk factor for many steroid-related adverse effects such as osteoporosis, myopathy, and glucose intolerance. This aging of the FSGS population, combined with the pandemic of obesity and type 2 diabetes, makes the risk of this type of corticosteroid exposure to any individual patient daunting.

However, counterbalancing risk is that response to treatment offers substantial improvement in quality of life, such as relief of symptoms of the nephrotic syndrome as well as improved renal survival compared with no treatment.[55,56] In addition, we may now moderate our expectations in terms of the therapeutic response; achieving and maintaining a partial remission of proteinuria is associated with a doubling in the rate of renal survival—from 40% to 80%—at 10 years.[31] Although not as good a long-term renal outcome as with a complete remission, achieving a partial remission may be acceptable when balanced against the cumulative risks accrued with increased prednisone exposure. Given the availability of alternative agents, prolonged treatment before categorizing the patient as steroid resistant should be changed; if there is no evidence of improvement in proteinuria after 6 to 8 weeks of prednisone monotherapy, alternative treatment regimens could be considered.

Many of the multidrug protocols used in the management of patients with the nephrotic syndrome with membranous GN (MGN) require exposure to glucocorticoids. Although it has been shown that monotherapy with steroids in MGN is not superior to placebo,[57,58] they have been effective as part of a multidrug treatment regimen.[59] Although some of these strategies have used relatively modest steroid exposure (i.e., alternating corticosteroids monthly with an alkylating agent over a 6-month period[59-61]), others have used more prolonged and repeated steroid courses.[62,63] More prolonged or repeated courses, by definition, dramatically increase the exposure to corticosteroids and alter the balance between risks and benefits. An advantage of the calcineurin inhibitor (CNI)–based regimens in the treatment of patients with MGN is the lower or even absence of corticosteroid exposure.[20] The renal benefits derived by lowering proteinuria in those with MGN can be substantial but often require prolonged therapy, so the choice of which multidrug regimen and the cumulative risks of repeated courses are important considerations. As in FSGS, specific patient factors impact on these risks and are additional considerations.

Corticosteroid therapy for IgAN has also been advocated. The question of their efficacy has been discussed in earlier chapters, and we will only comment on the cumulative risks of steroid toxicity in this disease. The routine with the best evidence of efficacy requires a 6-month exposure to steroids but in relatively low dosage and given only on alternate days. However, in addition, it does require large pulses of Solu-Medrol at the beginning of months 1, 3, and 5.[23,64] Here again, it is vitally important that the individual patient is assessed in terms of both his or her risk of progressive disease and the potential benefits of treatment versus the risks of the drug even with this lower corticosteroid exposure. It is particularly important to assess risk of progression (see above section) given that the great majority of IgAN patients with only hematuria or low-level proteinuria will not progress and therefore do not need to steroid therapy.[65]

SLE and vasculitis share certain similarities in regard to corticosteroid exposure. This drug is almost universally used when either of these disorders has significant renal involvement, and multiple doses of intravenous corticosteroids in the form of Solu-Medrol followed by high doses of oral prednisone are commonly recommended. This exposure dramatically increases the acute risks of corticosteroid therapy, including infection with either bacterial or opportunistic organisms. These systemic diseases often also require long-term maintenance therapy, but typically, a second "steroid-sparing" immunosuppressive agent is added so that low-dose prednisone may be used.

Major Adverse Effects of Corticosteroids

Impaired glucose tolerance and overt diabetes are important potential metabolic adverse effects; glucocorticoids affect glucose metabolism by increasing hepatic gluconeogenesis and decreasing peripheral tissue insulin sensitivity.[66] These changes in glucose homeostasis may be ameliorated by dose reduction; it has been estimated that for each 1-mg reduction of the prednisone dose, there is an estimated decline in 2-hour blood glucose of 0.12 mmol/L.[67] However, the metabolic effects of these drugs may not be completely reversible, even when the dose is reduced to physiologic range or discontinued entirely.[68] Although higher doses of glucocorticoids are associated with a higher risk of hyperglycemia, additional risk factors for steroid-induced hyperglycemia include African American or Hispanic ancestry, obesity (defined as a body mass index >30 kg/m^2), age older than 40 years, family history of diabetes, and the presence of other components of the metabolic syndrome (e.g., hypertriglyceridemia, low high-density lipoprotein [HDL] defined as HDL<140 g/dL in men and <150 g/dL in women, hypertension, and hyperuricemia). Progression to overt diabetes is a well-established risk factor for subsequent cardiovascular disease.[69]

Glucocorticoids have important musculoskeletal effects. Muscle injury associated with chronic steroid treatment with glucocorticoid produces a pattern of proximal weakness, atrophy, and myalgia. The ideal management of patients with steroid myopathy includes discontinuation of steroid administration, although it must be recognized that recovery can take weeks or months. Steroid myopathy is more common when the patient has been exposed to the potent fluorinated steroids (dexamethasone, betamethasone, triamcinolone), but similar patterns of muscle injury have been described with nonfluorinated steroids such as prednisone.[70]

Osteopenia is commonly seen in patients with chronic, often low-dose, steroid exposure. In a recent retrospective cohort study, almost 25% of 1 million oral corticosteroids users older than 18 years were matched to an equal number of control patients matched by age, sex, and medical practice.[71] The relative rate of nonvertebral fracture during oral corticosteroid treatment was between 1.33 and 1.61 and that of vertebral fracture 2.60, with a strong dose dependency. When the daily dose was less than 2.5 mg, the relative risk compared with control participants was 0.99, rising to 1.77 at a daily dose of 2.5 to 7.5 mg and 2.27 at a daily dose of 7.5 mg or greater. All fracture risks rapidly declined toward baseline after stopping treatment. This study has obvious implications for the use of preventive agents against bone loss in patients at highest risk. Avascular necrosis is a different type of bone injury. It is a devastating condition associated with destruction of the head of the femur or other long bones. The relationship between development of avascular necrosis and dose of prednisone is less clear.[72]

Given the elevated risk of cardiovascular disease in patients with kidney disease, the known associated cardiovascular effects of glucocorticoids are also an important consideration. Doria and associates[73] demonstrated an association between the cumulative prednisolone dose and the presence of carotid plaque in a cohort of SLE patients, and others have found a higher cumulative steroid dose was predictive of symptomatic coronary artery disease.[74-77] Glucocorticoids also contribute to elevations in blood pressure by affecting both renal sodium handling and enhancing responsiveness to both angiotensin II and catecholamines.[48]

The gastrointestinal (GI) effects of glucocorticoids include induction of gastritis and GI bleeding. Vision may be affected by cataract formation and increased intraocular pressure. Thinning of the skin, easy bruising, development of striae, and impaired wound healing may also be potentiated by glucocorticoids. Mood lability and insomnia induced by glucocorticoids also contribute to their relatively poor patient tolerance.

Strategies for Modifying Adverse Effects

There are several strategies available for minimizing steroid exposure. These strategies vary according to the disease and the individual patient. In minimal change disease and some cases of FSGS, for instance, alternate-day prednisone therapy may be used in lieu of daily regimens. (See details in Chapters 31 and 32.) This alternate-day approach is associated with fewer features of steroid toxicity but does not eliminate their risk. When this routine is being considered, the physician should decide in advance on this option if the alternate-day strategy does not work because repeating an induction course with daily steroids if the patient fails the alternate-day regimen will negate the original goals of reducing drug exposure.

An alternate strategy is shortening the course or a more rapid taper of the prednisone (see Chapter 32), and this approach is currently being investigated in the context of vasculitis (PEXIVAS study; see www.clinicaltrials.gov). More commonly, a second nonglucocorticoid immunosuppressive agent is introduced for its "steroid-sparing" potential.

These agents include both intravenous and oral cyclophosphamide, azathioprine, and more recently mycophenolate mofetil (MMF). The introduction of these agents has allowed the total exposure to corticosteroids in many of these disorders to be limited by allowing a shorter initial total exposure to the drug, a lower maintenance dose, or a more rapid taper of the drug during the induction phase. Another potential advantage of the addition of a second drug is stabilization of the remission. Use of a short course of cyclophosphamide in children with frequently relapsing minimal change disease is a good example of this strategy.

Alternate strategies specifically focus on reducing or preventing the complications related to corticosteroid treatment. If daily corticosteroids (0.5–1 mg/kg) are expected to continue for longer than 8 to 12 weeks in adults, consideration should be given to adding vitamin D at 1000 international units/day and 1 g per day of calcium or consideration of the addition of bisphosphonate therapy while the patient is on the steroids. Other high risk indicators for fractures such as previous documented osteoporosis, age, or likelihood of inactivity or immobility during steroid use should also trigger preventive treatment. Additional prophylactic strategies include the use of antibiotics such as trimethoprim–sulfamethoxazole to prevent *P. jiroveci* pneumonia. Retrospective studies indicate that a corticosteroid dose equivalent to 16 mg/day of prednisone for a period of 8 weeks was associated with a significant risk of pneumocystis pneumonia.[78,79] In high-risk patients and when using multidrug immunosuppression, an antiviral agent such as valacyclovir may also be indicated to prevent CMV infection; this strategy has been effective in the field of solid organ transplantation.[80]

Alkylating Agents

Cyclophosphamide is the most common drug in this class used in the treatment of patients with GN. It is a cytotoxic agent that acts largely through the alkylation of purine bases. This DNA damage induces apoptosis or altered function of both B and T cells.[81] Chlorambucil is the other drug of this class that is used, although less commonly than cyclophosphamide because of some major differences in the adverse effect profile.

Indications

Cyclophosphamide has been used to prolong remission in both minimal change disease and FSGS. In the former, it is usually restricted to short periods of exposure, usually in the range of 8 to 12 weeks. However, significantly longer periods of treatment have been advocated by some authors in steroid-resistant minimal change disease or FSGS in the pediatric age group[82] and by others in the treatment of adults with FSGS.[28] In membranous nephropathy, prolonged cyclophosphamide treatment has been shown to be efficacious. Exposure to cyclophosphamide in these regimens varies from 3 to 12 months.[59,60,83] This produces a significantly different risk given the exposure is limited to 13 g with the shortest regimen but is 52 g with the 1-year regimen in the average 70-kg patient.

In IgAN, cyclophosphamide has been evaluated only in patients with clearly documented progressive renal failure.

However, even in this unusual circumstance, the authors limited cyclophosphamide exposure to the first 3 months followed by a switch to the less dangerous agent azathioprine.[84] Cyclophosphamide is an effective agent and is commonly recommended for the induction phase in both diffuse proliferative lupus nephritis and renal vasculitis. Intravenous and oral treatment regimens are effective (see Chapters 31 and 32). In lupus nephritis, a commonly used protocol involves cyclophosphamide both as an induction agent and as long-term maintenance therapy. The induction phase for vasculitis is often similar to lupus nephritis, but the duration of maintenance therapy has tended to be more limited and measured in months.

Major Adverse Effects

Infertility in both men and women has been reported with these agents, most commonly after cyclophosphamide. This effect is closely related to total exposure but is also strongly impacted as well by the age of the patient.[85] One early series indicated that the rate of permanent ovarian failure was 26% in those who received between 10 and 20 g of cyclophosphamide but was greater than 70% in those whose cumulative dose was more than 30 g.[86] This effect is of particular concern in women during the later part of their reproductive lives. It has been estimated that women who receive a single course of cyclophosphamide therapy (10–20 g exposure) before the age of 25 years are at significantly less risk of permanent sterility (0%–15% risk) compared with the same exposure after the age of 30 (30%–40% risk).[86-88] A higher risk was estimated by Ioannidis and associates,[89] who calculated the risk of permanent ovarian failure for a standard dose of 12 g/m^2 to be 90% in women when treated after the age of 3 years. This combination of age and exposure on fertility can be expressed as an odds ratio. These authors suggest an odds ratio for permanent ovarian failure of 1.48 per 100 mg/kg of cumulative dose and 1.07 per patient year of age.[90] Although more difficult to estimate, there is certainly a substantial risk of infertility in men as well. Studies have indicated that long-term gonadal toxicity was not evident until the cumulative exposure to cyclophosphamide was greater than 300 mg/kg, but more recent information suggests a substantial risk at a cumulative dose of greater than 168 mg/kg (equivalent to 12 g for a 70-kg patient).[91,92] Although the age effect has not been as clearly demonstrated as in women, gonadal toxicity as indicated by a reduction in sperm count has been documented with exposures as low as 100 mg/kg.[85]

The other major adverse effect is the risk of malignancy. It is suspected that this has been underestimated in the past at least in part because of the delay between exposure to the drug and the appearance of the cancer. This latent period may be many years. More recent data from an epidemiologic study of 293 Danish patients with antineutrophil cytoplasmic autoantibodies (ANCA)–associated Wegener' granulomatosis treated with cyclophosphamide suggested a much lower safety limit for exposure than previously indicated.[93] They concluded that patients who received a cumulative dose of more than 36 g of cyclophosphamide (equivalent to 2 mg/kg for 8 months in a 70-kg patient) had a substantial increase risk for the development of a malignancy compared with the normal age and sex population. Their standardized incidence ratio of acute myelocytic leukemia was 59.0, bladder cancer was

9.5, and nonmelanoma skin cancer was 5.2 above this cumulative cyclophosphamide exposure. They also confirmed the substantial delay between exposure and malignancies with a latent period of between 6.9 and 18.5 years. This exposure of 36 g is a much lower threshold for these serious complications than previous estimates and needs to be validated in an independent data set.[94,95] In the meantime, however, the potential for toxicity at much lower exposure limit should be kept in mind when considering the more prolonged course of cyclophosphamide as a treatment option in patients with membranous nephropathy, lupus nephritis, and vasculitis. This is particularly relevant given the knowledge that a number of treatment options are currently available and appear to be as efficacious as cyclophosphamide (see earlier chapters).

An additional well-recognized, short-term adverse effect of the alkylating agents is bone marrow suppression, particularly the white cell line. A recent meta-analysis reported significant leucopenia in 25% of patients with lupus nephritis who were treated with cyclophosphamide.[96] Another short-term adverse effect of cyclophosphamide is an increased susceptibility to infections. These infections can be severe and resistant to therapy, and in combination with leucopenia, they can be overwhelming. Additional less serious but disconcerting side effects that can impact on compliance include alopecia and hemorrhagic cystitis. This long list of potentially serious complications makes monitoring for both short- and long-term effects of these agents a critical and necessary component of management.

Chlorambucil is an alternative alkylating agent used in the treatment of patients with membranous nephropathy. The original regimen developed by Ponticelli and associates[24] with this agent cycled it monthly with corticosteroids over 6 months. The adverse effects of chlorambucil are similar to cyclophosphamide, although it has not been associated with bladder toxicity. Even so, recent reviews have suggested that chlorambucil is less well tolerated overall than cyclophosphamide and has the added associated risk of acute myelogenous leukemia.[24,83]

Strategies for Modifying Adverse Effects

Strategies to limit exposure most commonly focus on limiting duration of therapy rather than modifying the dose. The exception to this is the use of intravenous cyclophosphamide in vasculitis. A number of regimens had been compared (see earlier chapters), and less frequent and smaller doses of intravenous cyclophosphamide appeared to be as effective as the earlier higher dose regimens with fewer adverse events. A shorter duration regimen of exposure is also an established option in membranous nephropathy. The two published effective regimens differ very dramatically in terms of cyclophosphamide exposure (see earlier chapters). In the original classic 6-month regimen, for example, cyclophosphamide exposure is limited to 3 months compared with the later published routine that uses 1 full year of exposure.[24,83]

Substitution of other agents that may be less toxic than cyclophosphamide is another option. MMF or azathioprine for maintenance therapy in patients with lupus nephritis are well-established options and appear to have similar efficacy with significantly fewer adverse effects. Data from a recent RCT in patients with diffuse proliferative lupus nephritis confirmed that MMF (3 g/day) was associated with fewer pyogenic infections than a cyclophosphamide-based regimen (relative risk, 0.36).[97] Similarly, long-term therapy with azathioprine has been proved to be as efficacious as cyclophosphamide in the maintenance phase of vasculitis, with less toxicity.[98]

Similar results in terms of complete and partial remissions were obtained when MMF was substituted for the year of cyclophosphamide in membranous nephropathy, but a significantly lower incidence of serious side effects was observed. This study was not an RCT because the cyclophosphamide-treated patients represented a historical control group. Unfortunately, the relapse rate was very much higher in the MMF than in the cyclophosphamide group.[99]

Replacement of cyclophosphamide with a different class of agent such as a CNI is another option. Although still a potent immunosuppressive class, their adverse effect profile is remarkably different. This substitution strategy could be used when initial therapy with cyclophosphamide has failed, when the patient has relapsed, or when repeated exposure to alkylating agents is being considered. Such a strategy can be used in the management of membranous, lupus, or FSGS patients.

Monitoring the other potential adverse effects of cyclophosphamide by frequent blood counts and adjusting the dose relative to degree of renal impairment, age, and other comorbid conditions are additional tools to minimize cyclophosphamide toxicity. The likelihood of inducing opportunistic infections such as *P. jiroveci* pneumonia or CMV can also be reduced by the use of prophylactic antibiotics or antivirals as described above under corticosteroids.

Mycophenolate Mofetil

Mechanism of Action

MMF is a relatively new immunosuppressive agent. It is hydrolyzed into mycophenolic acid, the active moiety of the drug. Similar to azathioprine, MMF is a reversible inhibitor of inosine monophosphate dehydrogenase, a critical enzyme involved in de novo purine synthesis that is required for lymphocyte division.[100] Several factors contribute to the lymphocyte-specific effects of MMF on purine metabolism. First, unlike other cells, lymphocytes are uniquely dependent on de novo purine synthesis to generate RNA and DNA because they do not have a salvage pathway for purine generation. Inhibition of this pathway by MMF therefore predominantly affects lymphocyte metabolism. MMF also is a highly potent inhibitor of the isoform of inosine monophosphate dehydrogenase that is expressed in activated lymphocytes (the type II isoform), contributing to its specificity.[101-104] The selectivity of MMF for inhibiting lymphocyte proliferation is the concept that underlies the reduced toxicity of MMF compared with alkylating agents that affect all dividing cells. In addition to its effects on T and B cells, MMF may also affect fibroblast proliferation and activity[105] and endothelial function.[106]

Indications

MMF was first shown to reduce the rate of rejection in renal transplantation compared with azathioprine.[107,108] After its success in murine models of lupus nephritis, its use was extended to patients with a variety of primary and secondary glomerular diseases, including SLE.[109]

More RCTs have been undertaken examining the relative efficacy of MMF in lupus nephritis than in any other glomerular disease.[109] Overall, MMF appears to be both an effective induction and maintenance agent for lupus nephritis, and given the age and sex of the population at risk in lupus nephritis, is potentially of great value in reducing the risk of permanent sterility induced with cyclophosphamide. Recent literature suggests that ethnicity or geographic region may influence treatment response with a greater response in black and Hispanic patients with MMF compared with other agents.[110] There is still limited pharmacokinetic data to support this contention. Data regarding the efficacy of MMF for induction and maintenance of remission in ANCA-associated renal disease continue to emerge, and a randomized study supports a potential role for MMF as an induction agent.[111]

MMF has been primarily studied in idiopathic GN in limited series of high-risk or resistant patients, making its efficacy difficult to interpret compared with the average case. In IgAN, for example, an initial study comparing MMF therapy with daily oral prednisone in patients with proteinuria greater than 2 g/day found promising results.[112] However, randomized studies in both European and North American populations have not shown a similar benefit. This includes a recent Belgian IgA study of 34 patients with renal insufficiency randomized to receive either MMF at a dose of 2 g/day in combination with an ACE inhibitor or an ACE inhibitor alone; MMF was poorly tolerated, and there was no benefit observed after 3 years of treatment.[113] A U.S. study of similar size and design in IgA patients at high risk of progression[114] demonstrated no benefit compared with conservative therapy. The reason for this variation in outcome is currently unknown, although suggestions include a small sample size and lack of statistical power, ethnic differences in disease pathophysiology, or the need for earlier initiation of MMF therapy.

The efficacy of MMF in membranous nephropathy has not been studied in RCTs. Although nonrandomized pilot studies suggest a potential role in treatment-resistant disease, larger prospective controlled trials are required.[115] A similar role for MMF is suggested in FSGS from a small retrospective study[116] and a small uncontrolled prospective study[117] in steroid-dependent or -resistant disease. A beneficial effect of MMF was observed in these high-risk patients, including reduction in proteinuria and stabilization in renal function, but the data are limited, and interpretation of the results should be treated with caution. MMF may be steroid or CNI sparing, but studies need to be conducted before its widespread use even under these conditions. Even in minimal change disease, the role for MMF is not clear, at least in part because the studies have been limited to uncontrolled trials in patients with steroid-dependent or -resistant disease. One study of MCD in adults and several similar studies in the pediatric population have suggested a potential role for MMF as a second-line agent, but all of the studies are limited in terms of numbers, design, and duration.[118-120]

Major Adverse Effects

MMF was initially believed to have little effect on fertility compared with cyclophosphamide. More recent data suggest that it is teratogenic.[121] It does eliminate the risk of bladder toxicity because the causative metabolite, acrolein, is not generated by this drug.[122]

As with all antimetabolites, MMF can cause hematologic complications, including leucopenia, anemia, and rarely pure red cell aplasia.[123] The myelosuppressive effects of MMF contribute to the risk of infection associated with its use, and although some data suggest a lower infection risk than with cyclophosphamide in lupus nephritis, there are conflicting data,[96,124,125] and serious infections have been reported with its use.[98,126] Furthermore, the transplantation literature suggests an increased risk of viral infections with MMF but only in the context of multidrug regimens.[127] The risk of infection relative to that associated with azathioprine appears to be similar.[98] Whether there is a difference with respect to risks of late-onset malignancy with MMF when used for the treatment of lupus or other variants of GN is too early to determine.

Strategies for Modifying Adverse Effects

The principal adverse effects of MMF relate to GI symptoms, including both upper GI irritation with nausea and vomiting and lower GI tract involvement with diarrhea. This is more common with MMF than with cyclophosphamide.[128] These symptoms tend to occur early in the course of treatment and can improve with dosing adjustments. Unlike the transplantation context, the dose of MMF can frequently be titrated up over the course of days to weeks to minimize development of GI symptoms. Splitting the dosage into four times per day versus the standard two doses per day also reduces GI problems. Temporarily reducing the dose also may be tried. The predominant effect on the bone marrow is leucopenia and is usually corrected by a temporary dose reduction. If the full dose is still not tolerated, the addition of MMF-sparing agents such as a low dose of steroid or a CNI may be considered.

Calcineurin Inhibitors

Cyclosporine and tacrolimus are CNIs that suppress the immune response by downregulating T-cell activation. They specifically block calcium-dependent T-cell receptor signaling transduction, thereby inhibiting the transcription of IL-2 as well as other proinflammatory cytokines, in both T cells and antigen-presenting cells.[129,130] IL-2 serves as the major activation factor for T cells and a key modulator of both T- and B-cell activity in numerous immunologic processes.[130] Tacrolimus and cyclosporine have a common mechanism of action (i.e., inhibition of calcineurin phosphatase), although they bind different intracellular proteins. These intracellular proteins belong to the immunophilin family with cyclosporin binding cyclophilin and tacrolimus binding FKBP12.[131] The role of immunophilin binding in the mechanism of toxicity is not clear, but it may allow for the different side effect profile of these drugs.[132] More recently an alternative mechanism of action of these agents has been suggested relating to their capacity to stabilize the internal cytoskeletal structure of the glomerular podocyte.[133] This is a fascinating possibility and may help explain its efficacy in some of the glomerular-based diseases at lower drug levels compared with those required in solid organ transplantation.[134]

Indications

RCTs using CNIs have demonstrated clinical benefit in patients with idiopathic membranous nephropathy.[135,136] The larger study in this category had additional low-dose prednisone, but a recent trial with tacrolimus monotherapy showed comparable efficacy to the dual regimen in patients with idiopathic MGN.[137] CNIs have also been studied in lupus-associated MGN; cyclosporine in an RCT setting was found to have comparative efficacy, at least in the short term, to cytotoxic therapy and to be superior to steroids alone.[138] Tacrolimus has also been shown to have similar short-term efficacy in terms of its proteinuric response compared with a cyclophosphamide-treated historical control group.[139] RCTs carried out in pediatric patients with minimal change disease have indicated that the addition of cyclosporine to prednisone improved the short-term rate of remission compared with high-dose prednisone alone[140] and when combined with a standard prednisone regimen showed a lower relapse rate, at least in the short term, compared with the steroid treatment alone group.[141] Cyclosporine also offers comparable remission rates to cytotoxic therapy in patients with steroid-resistant idiopathic nephrotic syndrome, although late relapse was higher in the cyclosporine-treated group.[142] In the context of FSGS, RCTs indicate that cyclosporine therapy is superior to symptomatic management[143] and that short-term remission of proteinuria and preservation of renal function with cyclosporine are superior to placebo in adults with steroid-resistant disease.[144] Nonrandomized longer term studies in membranous nephropathy and minimal change disease and its variants and even small studies in IgAN have been published and suggest a potential role for CNIs in these disorders (reviewed by Cattran et al[20] and Lim et al[145]).

Major Adverse Effects

The CNI class of agents have significant adverse effects with the most concerning being its nephrotoxicity. This is particularly relevant when prolonged therapy is being contemplated. These longer treatment courses are usually given to prevent or modify the well-recognized risk of relapse of nephrotic syndrome that occurs upon withdrawal of these drugs. CNI-associated nephrotoxicity can be severe, and reports indicate a significant risk of CKD if the drug is given in high doses for prolonged periods, such as occurred in early recipients of nonrenal solid organ transplants.[146] However, the cyclosporine dose and duration used in these studies are no longer considered appropriate,[147] and lower doses in the glomerular-based diseases versus solid organ transplant are currently advocated.[20] In addition, modifications have occurred in the drug formulation of cyclosporine, which has resulted in more consistent and predictable pharmacokinetics, allowing lower drug exposure regimens.[20]

One of the mechanisms of the nephrotoxicity that is attributable to these agents is its renal vasoconstrictive properties. This hemodynamic effect is both dose-dependent and reversible.[148] The more delayed chronic damage in the tubular interstitial compartment and the small arterioles is less well understood but may also be ameliorated at least in part by a dose reduction or discontinuation of the agent.[149]

New onset or worsening of hypertension is another important and common dose-dependent adverse effect of CNI use and likely contributes to their long-term nephrotoxic potential. The reported incidence of hypertension in patients with glomerular diseases treated with CNIs varies from 10% to 30%.[150] An additional significant adverse effect is the induction of glucose intolerance and even frank diabetes.[151]

This seems to be specific to CNIs and is somewhat more common with tacrolimus.[152]

As with all immunosuppressive agents, CNIs affect immune surveillance and are associated with an increased rate of infections and malignancy; the incidence of drug-associated malignancy specifically in the context of GN therapy is not well described but considered to be low.[144,153] The underlying risks of infection associated with untreated nephrotic syndrome and the potential for malignancy associated with membranous nephropathy further complicate the assessment of risk of these complications with CNI treatment.

Other common adverse effects of CNIs are cosmetic and include gum hypertrophy and hypertrichosis (less frequent with tacrolimus than cyclosporine). The excess hair growth can be severe and can contribute to poor drug adherence. A cohort of approximately 200 pediatric patients with nephrotic syndrome treated with cyclosporine for an average of 22 months[154] was recently reviewed; reported side effects of such prolonged therapy included hypertrichosis (52.3%), gum hyperplasia (25.4%), hypertension (18.8%), and renal impairment (9.1%). Close examination of the subgroup of patients with renal impairment in this study is revealing. In the small number ($n = 18$ patients) that demonstrated renal impairment, 12 recovered completely after the cyclosporine was stopped, three experienced stable but continued renal impairment, and only three (1.5% of the total number exposed) had slow progression of their renal disease. On multivariate analysis, resistance to the cyclosporine treatment was the only factor predictive of renal impairment

Strategies for Reducing Toxicity

In contrast to transplantation, long-term, low-dose therapy with cyclosporine (1.0–2 mg/kg/day) with or without low-dose steroids has been shown to be both safe and effective at maintaining remission. The lower toxicity of CNIs in patients with GN is at least in part related to the lower daily maintenance dose required and the capacity to gradually increase the dose over days or weeks to achieve a therapeutic effect versus the need for a much more rapid dose escalation after solid organ transplant.[20] Although higher doses of cyclosporine may be required for the induction phase in membranous nephropathy, the initial dose can usually be reduced during the maintenance phase.[155] In renal transplant patients, CNI dose has been safely reduced after the first year with renal function remaining stable even after 20 years of exposure to this agent.[156] Nevertheless, nephrotoxicity is a risk with this therapy and careful monitoring of drug levels, a constant awareness of drug interactions (that may either increase or decrease drug levels), and frequent monitoring of renal function are mandatory. CNI toxicity may be more evident when used in patients with more advanced renal impairment or those with significant tubular interstitial or vascular changes noted on histology. However, with careful monitoring and the slow escalation of dosage, even patients with significant renal dysfunction can be safely treated with CNIs.[135]

The hypertension that commonly accompanies treatment with CNIs is another adverse effect that requires attention. However, the adjustments in antihypertensive medication are usually straightforward, and its presence does not generally preclude or limit CNI usage. The vasoconstrictive effects of cyclosporine, in addition to their effects on renal potassium secretion, may limit the ability to use higher doses of inhibitors of the renin–angiotensin system to control blood pressure in patients taking cyclosporine.

The induction of biochemical diabetes or frank hyperglycemia requiring oral agents or even insulin is a significant issue, especially in light of the increasing frequency of obesity in the general population. Although the frequency of diabetes in the transplantation literature has decreased, this is more likely attributable to the smaller doses of corticosteroids used today than change in this aspect of CNI toxicity. Even when CNIs are used as monotherapy, the risk of new onset diabetes has been reported to be as high as 4%.[137] This risk therefore requires ongoing vigilance by the prescribing physician. Patients at highest risk for developing glucose intolerance include obese individuals and those with a strong family history of diabetes. Strategies for preventing this adverse effect include preferential use of cyclosporine over tacrolimus or the use of CNI monotherapy, thereby avoiding the additive risk of corticosteroid exposure.

The incidence of malignancy induced by CNIs in the glomerular diseases is very hard to determine from the literature. Very few of the GN treatment studies have been long enough to assess CNI exposure as independent risk factors. Cyclosporine, however, has been used in the long-term management of patients with other autoimmune diseases, including rheumatoid arthritis (RA) and psoriasis. When patients with RA treated with cyclosporine were compared with control patients (who received placebo, D-penicillamine, or chloroquine), an increased cancer risk was not seen.[157] A recent review of patients with psoriasis did find an increase in the standardized incidence ratio of cancer in patients treated with cyclosporine compared with the general population. However, when examined more closely and when skin malignancies, known to be more common in patients with psoriasis, were excluded, the incidence was not significantly higher in the CNI-treated patients.[158]

Rituximab and Ocrelizumab

Mechanism of Action

Rituximab is a genetically engineered chimeric murine/human monoclonal antibody directed against the CD20, an antigen found on the surface of normal pre-B and mature B cells. in vitro studies have demonstrated that the Fc portion of rituximab binds human complement and can lead to cell lysis of the targeted cell through complement-dependent cytotoxicity. Therapy with this agent results in highly effective depletion of CD20-positive B cells via inhibition of cell proliferation and direct induction of B-cell apoptosis,[159] prompting the highly successful introduction of this agent for treatment of non-Hodgkin lymphoma.[160] The CD20 antigen is not expressed on hematopoietic stem cells, pro-B cells, normal plasma cells, or other normal tissues. It has an impressive safety record compared with classic cytotoxic agents. Ocrelizumab is a genetically engineered fully humanized monoclonal antibody directed against the same CD20 antigen found on the surface of normal B cells, with the same mode of action as rituximab. Because of its fully humanized nature, this anti-CD20 antibody can be infused more rapidly and has less immediate infusion-related reactions than rituximab. In addition, because of the fully humanized construct, formation of

autoantibodies directed against the drug are unlikely, thereby decreasing the possibility of inducing resistance secondary to repeated treatments with the drug.

The precise mechanism of action of anti-CD20 antibodies in autoimmune disease and in particular GN is unclear. It is known that B cells play an important role as immunoregulatory cells by both antigen presentation and cytokine release. Their elimination could have dampening effects on other immune cells such as T lymphocytes, dendritic cells, and macrophages. This hypothesis is supported by an observed reduction in activated T cells and a decrease in T-cell–derived cytokines in patients with SLE and RA after treatment with rituximab.[161,162] The correlation between B-cell depletion and response as well as the timing of the return of B cells and relapse is quite variable in the autoimmune diseases.[163] This may be because the circulating B cells do not accurately reflect the B-cell components of the bone marrow, lymphoid tissues and other organs that are recognized to be more resistant to depletion.[164] This may help to explain the relatively poor relationship between peripheral B cells count and relapse. An additional possible explanation for this lack of association in proteinuric conditions is the potential loss of rituximab in the urine.[165] This has not been confirmed by direct measurements of urinary rituximab nor has there been any uniformity in terms of an early return of B cells in patients with nephrotic syndrome treated with this drug.[166]

Indications

Treatment with rituximab has been successful in patients with B-cell lymphomas and in patients with autoimmune diseases including RA. Although it has been shown in non randomized studies to be of benefit in SLE these results have not been confirmed in a recently completed randomized study of diffuse proliferative lupus nephritis.[163,167-169]

Its utility in other primary forms of GN such as membranous nephropathy, focal and segmental glomerulosclerosis, and minimal change disease has been reported, but this has come from pilot studies and case-based reports. The benefit has not yet been confirmed in RCTs in these GN types.[165,166,170]

Adverse Effects of Rituximab

Acute infusion-related reactions can vary from minor symptoms, such as skin rash, pruritus, flushing, nausea, vomiting, fatigue, headache, flulike symptoms, dizziness, hypertension, or runny nose in up to 10% of patients exposed, to severe reactions, including anaphylaxis and shock (<1%). Rare side effects that have been seen with the use of rituximab include anemia, cardiac arrhythmias, respiratory failure, and acute kidney injury (occurring in <0.1.%).[165-167,170-173] The latter severe reactions have been seen primarily with its use in the treatment of cancers in which the tumor cell burden is high and an acute tumor lysis syndrome can develop. More delayed adverse effects include serum sickness and an increased incidence of infection, including reactivation of latent viral infections. Given its impact on antibody formation, vaccinations that contain live organisms should be avoided during treatment with rituximab. There have been several isolated reports of the development of progressive multifocal leukoencephalopathy (PML) in patients treated with this agent; this devastating syndrome is attributable to the activation of latent

JC polyomavirus, is associated with progressive neurologic impairment, and ultimately leads to death within months of diagnosis.[174] In the majority of reported cases, PML developed when rituximab was used in combination with other chemotherapy,[175] particularly in patients also receiving purine analogs or alkylating agents.

The effects of rituximab on fetuses are unknown; therefore, its use during pregnancy should be avoided.

Formation of human antichimeric antibodies (HACAs) does occur, although their clinical significance is unclear. The reported incidence of HACAs development varies widely from less than 1% in cancer patients to as high as 50% in a small case series of SLE patients.[165,167] The appearance of this antibody would be expected to result in a decreased response to rituximab treatment related to the drug's inactivation and accelerated clearance. These antibodies may also contribute to the incidence of serum sickness. Despite the appearance of HACAs in patients treated with rituximab and their theoretical consequences, these sequelae have not been uniformly observed in the small studies in GN.[163,165,167] The new fully humanized version of the anti-CD20 agent should either ameliorate or eliminate the problem of HACA formation.

Strategies for Modifying Adverse Effects

The precise dose or regimen to use in patients with autoimmune disorders is unknown. Although the relationship between peripheral CD20 positive cell depletion and response is poor, it has been suggested that a single dose is adequate for both B-cell depletion in membranous nephropathy and provides a similar response in proteinuria as multiple doses.[176]

Therapeutic Apheresis

Apheresis techniques have been applied as a therapeutic modality in glomerular-based disease with a view to either remove putative pathogenic proteins or cell populations or replace deficient plasma factors. Data suggest that although measurable risks are associated with this treatment—most commonly, urticaria, pruritus, hypocalcemic symptoms, and mild hypotension—the occurrence of serious adverse events necessitating premature cessation of therapy is as low as 0.4%.[177,178] The role of therapeutic plasmapheresis for the treatment of vasculitis, anti–glomerular basement membrane disease, and thrombotic microangiopathy is reviewed in other chapters in detail. Here we provide only a brief overview of the rationale and newer indications for the use of plasmapheresis in GN. In general, plasmapheresis should be regarded as an adjunct to specific pharmacotherapy targeted at the underlying cause of the glomerular disease.

Focal Segmental Glomerulosclerosis

The use of plasmapheresis for recurrence of idiopathic FSGS after kidney transplantation has supported a possible role for this therapeutic modality in native kidney FSGS disease. Idiopathic FSGS recurs in approximately 30% of patients after transplantation.[179] Plasmapheresis is thought to remove a putative pathogenic circulating permeability factor[180,181] and has been used for both prevention and treatment of recurrent FSGS in this setting. Although no RCTs have supported this approach, uncontrolled series report important reductions in proteinuria in up to 70% of individuals treated with plasmapheresis in this setting,[182] particularly when initiated early in the course of recurrence.[183] However, proteinuria may recur or worsen after cessation of therapy, and the impact of preemptive strategies using plasmapheresis remain unclear. More recently, a small number of case series have suggested that combining plasmapheresis with a B-cell depleting agent (rituximab) may be more effective than plasmapheresis alone in this setting.[184,185]

The effectiveness of plasmapheresis for treatment of idiopathic FSGS in native kidneys is not well defined and has typically been reserved for steroid-resistant cases. With this therapy alone, only a minority of treatment-resistant native kidney FSGS patients have shown a reduction in proteinuria and stabilization of renal function.[186] Even in these cases, it is not clear whether this was because of removal of the putative permeability factor or replacement of a serum factor. The use of plasmapheresis is therefore generally reserved for rare situations when hypoalbuminemia produces refractory symptomatic edema or very low effective circulating volume that limits the ability to introduce additional agent such as a CNI. No controlled data are available to support this practice. One other mechanism of potential benefit is related to the hyperlipidemia associated with nephrotic syndrome. In particular, specific lipid moieties such as low-density lipoprotein (LDL) may contribute directly to proteinuria and may be removed by LDL apheresis in resistant cases of FSGS. This has been used in only a few isolated cases and has not been rigorously studied.[187,188]

Cryoglobulinemic Disease

Cryoglobulinemia-associated proliferative GN is now most commonly seen in the context of hepatitis C infection and rarely in relation to B-cell lymphomas.[189-191] In this context, plasmapheresis is thought to remove the circulating cryoglobulin and is used in conjunction with pharmacologic agents that address the underlying cause of the protein production. The use of plasmapheresis is usually reserved for rapidly progressive proliferative GN or severe extrarenal features of vasculitis. In the context of hepatitis C, especially in the transplant population, use of immunosuppressive agents carries the risks of increased viremia, bacterial infections, and mortality.[192,193] Plasmapheresis in this context is also regarded as an adjunct to specific therapy for the underlying viral infection.

IgA Nephropathy

Only a minority of patients with rapidly progressive IgAN or Henoch-Schönlein purpura have elevated serum IgA levels. Plasmapheresis has been used to treat patients with these disorders with the theory that it is capable of removing circulating IgA antibodies, IgA-containing immune complexes, or both. Only uncontrolled case series have been reported, indicating possible benefit for this therapy in severe disease.[194,195] It is suggested that plasmapheresis should be reserved for situations when circulating IgA immune complexes can be demonstrated, although this is supported by only small and older studies.[196] Whether this can be extended to rapidly progressive IgA cases associated with crescents and necrosis, with or without accompanying ANCA positivity, is unknown.

Eculizumab

Eculizumab is an anti–complement factor 5 (C5) monoclonal antibody designed for use in diseases characterized by functional impairment of endogenous inhibitors of the activation of the alternative complement pathway. It was originally developed for the treatment of paroxysmal nocturnal hemoglobinuria.[197] Eculizumab is a very expensive drug. The activation of this cascade has classically been implicated in type II MPGN[198] and atypical hemolytic uremic syndrome,[199] thus providing a potential rationale for this agent in these diseases.[200] Emerging evidence suggests that complement dysregulation may be a critical contributor to many forms of progressive glomerular injury traditionally attributed to classical or lectin-activated complement pathways. Activation of these pathways and their potential inhibition by eculizumab may have relevance in the context of SLE[201] as well as other forms of GN.[202]

Adrenocorticotrophic Hormone

The administration of synthetic forms of adrenocorticotrophic hormone (ACTH) has recently emerged as a potential therapeutic option for patients with nephrotic syndrome. Interest in the use of this agent in patients with kidney disease was first raised when it was noted that its exogenous administration ameliorated the lipid profile associated with nephrotic syndrome.[203] Experimental and clinical data suggest that lipid-lowering therapy may improve kidney injury in proteinuric kidney disease,[204] and this may be one mechanism of the effect of this drug. Specifically, the complement-mediated podocyte injury associated with membranous nephropathy may be associated with abnormal apolipoprotein J (clusterin) levels that could potentially be restored by ACTH therapy.[205] Alternatively the effects of ACTH may be attributable to a direct tissue or cellular action of the drug on the abnormal podocyte improving its stability and thereby reduced proteinuria with the improvement in lipid profile merely secondary to the improvement in the underlying GFR barrier.

In an early uncontrolled pilot study, 14 patients received ACTH intramuscularly at increasing doses over or a 56-day period, with ACTH continued at a dosage of 1 mg twice weekly in 5 of the patients for further 10 months. The patients were followed for a further 18 months off treatment.[206] At that dose, a marked improvements in lipid profile occurred (reductions by 30%–60% in the serum cholesterol and triglycerides). In addition, the urinary albumin excretion decreased by 90%, and the GFR increased by 25%. Deterioration in renal function was observed in all cases when ACTH was discontinued after the 56 days of treatment. However, the 5 patients in whom ACTH therapy was prolonged were still in remission 18 months after discontinuation the drug. Similarly, Picardi and associates[207] treated 7 patients with MN with the same schedule of ACTH; 5 patients entered complete remission of proteinuria within 6 months of treatment with ACTH, and two patients had to interrupt treatment because of side effects. More recently, Ponticelli and associates[208] conducted a randomized pilot study comparing methylprednisolone plus a cytotoxic agent versus synthetic ACTH in 32 patients with idiopathic MN. Patients were randomly assigned to receive either methylprednisolone plus chlorambucil or cyclophosphamide cycled over

6 months (group A) or to receive ACTH (group B) administered by injection (1 mg) for a total treatment period of 1 year. According to intention-to-treat analysis, complete or partial remission as a first event was attained by 93% of patients in group A (5 complete; 10 partial) and 87% in group B (10 complete; 4 partial); the difference between the two groups was not significant, although this study was not powered to indicate superiority of one therapy. Although these studies suggest that prolonged synthetic ACTH therapy may represent an effective therapy in patients with idiopathic MN, more extensive randomized studies with longer follow-up are needed before therapeutic recommendations can be made. At the present time, the synthetic formulation of ACTH used in the above studies is not available in the United States.

Reported side effects associated with the use of ACTH include dizziness, altered level of alertness, disturbed sleep, fluid retention, hypokalemia, glucose intolerance, and diarrhea, and there is an additional risk of infection. As in the case of endogenous ACTH excess, exogenous administration of ACTH can promote the development of bronze-colored skin, which generally resolves after the end of ACTH therapy.[208]

Conclusion

Despite challenges quantifying trends in the incidence and prevalence of GN, it remains a leading cause of chronic kidney disease and kidney failure. New data regarding clinically relevant surrogate endpoints and therapeutic goals will hopefully facilitate the development and study of novel agents to treat patients with GN and prevent loss of kidney function. The toxicity of immunotherapeutic agents requires careful consideration by clinicians; the risks of these drugs must always be weighed against the potential benefits in each individual patient, considering patient, disease, and drug-specific characteristics.

References

1. Li LS, Liu ZH. Epidemiologic data of renal diseases from a single unit in China: analysis based on 13,519 renal biopsies. *Kidney Int.* 2004;66:920-923.
2. Wirta O, Mustonen J, Helin H, Pasternack A. Incidence of biopsy-proven glomerulonephritis. *Nephrol Dial Transplant.* 2008;23:193-200.
3. Coresh J, Selvin E, Stevens LA, et al. Prevalence of chronic kidney disease in the United States. *JAMA.* 2007;298:2038-2047.
4. Yang WC, Hwang SJ. Incidence, prevalence and mortality trends of dialysis end-stage renal disease in Taiwan from 1990 to 2001: the impact of national health insurance. *Nephrol Dial Transplant.* 2008;23:3977-3982.
5. U.S. Renal Data System. *USRDS 2009 Annual Data Report: Atlas of Chronic Kidney Disease and End-Stage Renal Disease in the United States.* Bethesda, MD: National Institutes of Health, National Institute of Diabetes and Digestive and Kidney Diseases; 2009.
6. Canadian Institute for Health Information. *2008 Annual Report—Treatment of End-Stage Organ Failure in Canada, 1997 to 2006.* Ottawa, ON: Author; 2008.
7. Canadian Institute of Health Information. *2004 CORR Report.* Ottawa, ON: Author; 2004.
8. Canadian Institute of Health Information. *Treatment of End-Stage Organ Failure in Canada, 1995 to 2004. 2006 Annual Report of the Canadian Organ Replacement Registry.* Ottawa, ON: Author; 2007.
9. ERA-EDTA Registry. *ERA-EDTA Registry Annual Report, 2007.* Amsterdam: Academic Medical Center, Department of Medical Informatics, Amsterdam, The Netherlands; 2009.
10. ANZDATA Registry 2007 Report: *Trends in Kidney Disease Over Time.* 2007. Adelaide, Australia. Avilable at www.anzdata.org.au.
11. Prakash S, Kanjanabuch T, Austin PC, et al. Continental variations in IgA nephropathy among Asians. *Clin Nephrol.* 2008;70:377-384.

12. The Renal Association UK Renal Registry: *UK Renal Registry Report 2008.* 2008. Bristol, United Kingdom. Available at www.renalreg.com.
13. Rivera F, Lopez-Gomez JM, Perez-Garcia R. Frequency of renal pathology in Spain 1994-1999. *Nephrol Dial Transplant.* 2002;17:1594-1602.
14. Geddes CC, Rauta V, Gronhagen-Riska C, et al. A tricontinental view of IgA nephropathy. *Nephrol Dial Transplant.* 2003;18:1541-1548.
15. Regional program for the study of glomerulonephritis. Central Committee of the Toronto Glomerulonephritis Registry. *Can Med Assoc J.* 1981;124:158-161.
16. Statistics Canada: *Selected Trend Data for Toronto, 1996, 2001, 2006 Censuses.* Ottawa, Canada. Available at www.statcan.gc.ca.
17. Haas M, Meehan SM, Karrison TG, Spargo BH. Changing etiologies of unexplained adult nephrotic syndrome: a comparison of renal biopsy findings from 1976-1979 and 1995-1997. *Am J Kidney Dis.* 1997;30: 621-631.
18. Kambham N, Markowitz GS, Valeri AM, et al. Obesity-related glomerulopathy: an emerging epidemic. *Kidney Int.* 2001;59:1498-1509.
19. Swaminathan S, Leung N, Lager DJ, et al. Changing incidence of glomerular disease in Olmsted County, Minnesota: a 30-year renal biopsy study. *Clin J Am Soc Nephrol.* 2006;1:483-487.
20. Cattran DC, Alexopoulos E, Heering P, et al. Cyclosporin in idiopathic glomerular disease associated with the nephrotic syndrome: workshop recommendations. *Kidney Int.* 2007;72:1429-1447.
21. Levey AS, Cattran D, Friedman A, et al. Proteinuria as a surrogate outcome in CKD: report of a scientific workshop sponsored by the National Kidney Foundation and the US Food and Drug Administration. *Am J Kidney Dis.* 2009;54:205-226.
22. Cattran DC, Cardella CJ, Roscoe JM, et al. Results of a controlled drug trial in membranoproliferative glomerulonephritis. *Kidney Int.* 1985;27: 436-441.
23. Pozzi C, Andrulli S, Del Vecchio L, et al. Corticosteroid effectiveness in IgA nephropathy: long-term results of a randomized, controlled trial. *J Am Soc Nephrol.* 2004;15:157-163.
24. Ponticelli C, Zucchelli P, Passerini P, et al. A 10-year follow-up of a randomized study with methylprednisolone and chlorambucil in membranous nephropathy. *Kidney Int.* 1995;48:1600-1604.
25. Troyanov S, Wall CA, Miller JA, et al. Idiopathic membranous nephropathy: definition and relevance of a partial remission. *Kidney Int.* 2004;66:1199-1205.
26. Pei Y, Cattran D, Delmore T, et al. Evidence suggesting under-treatment in adults with idiopathic focal segmental glomerulosclerosis. Regional Glomerulonephritis Registry Study. *Am J Med.* 1987;82:938-944.
27. Korbet SM, Schwartz MM, Lewis EJ. Primary focal segmental glomerulosclerosis: clinical course and response to therapy. *Am J Kidney Dis.* 1994;23:773-783.
28. Banfi G, Moriggi M, Sabadini E, et al. The impact of prolonged immunosuppression on the outcome of idiopathic focal-segmental glomerulosclerosis with nephrotic syndrome in adults. A collaborative retrospective study. *Clin Nephrol.* 1991;36:53-59.
29. Velosa JA, Holley KE, Torres VE, Offord KP. Significance of proteinuria on the outcome of renal function in patients with focal segmental glomerulosclerosis. *Mayo Clin Proc.* 1983;58:568-577.
30. Chitalia VC, Wells JE, Robson RA, et al. Predicting renal survival in primary focal glomerulosclerosis from the time of presentation. *Kidney Int.* 1999;56:2236-2242.
31. Troyanov S, Wall CA, Miller JA, et al. Focal and segmental glomerulosclerosis: definition and relevance of a partial remission. *J Am Soc Nephrol.* 2005;16:1061-1068.
32. Donadio Jr JV, Bergstralh EJ, Offord KP, et al. A controlled trial of fish oil in IgA nephropathy. Mayo Nephrology Collaborative Group. *N Engl J Med.* 1994;331:1194-1199.
33. Li PK, Leung CB, Chow KM, et al. Hong Kong study using valsartan in IgA nephropathy (HKVIN): a double-blind, randomized, placebo-controlled study. *Am J Kidney Dis.* 2006;47:751-760.
34. Donadio JV, Bergstralh EJ, Grande JP, Rademcher DM. Proteinuria patterns and their association with subsequent end-stage renal disease in IgA nephropathy. *Nephrol Dial Transplant.* 2002;17:1197-1203.
35. Cattran DC, Reich HN, Beanlands HJ, et al. The impact of sex in primary glomerulonephritis. *Nephrol Dial Transplant.* 2008;23:2247-2253.
36. Contreras G, Pardo V, Cely C, et al. Factors associated with poor outcomes in patients with lupus nephritis. *Lupus.* 2005;14:890-895.
37. Chen YE, Korbet SM, Katz RS, et al. Value of a complete or partial remission in severe lupus nephritis. *Clin J Am Soc Nephrol.* 2008;3: 46-53.
38. Houssiau FA, Vasconcelos C, D'Cruz D, et al. The 10-year follow-up data of the Euro-Lupus Nephritis Trial comparing low-dose and high-dose intravenous cyclophosphamide. *Ann Rheum Dis.* 2010;69:61-64.
39. Talar-Williams C, Hijazi YM, et al. Cyclophosphamide-induced cystitis and bladder cancer in patients with Wegener granulomatosis. *Ann Intern Med.* 1996;124:477-484.
40. Guillevin L, Cordier JF, Lhote F, et al. A prospective, multicenter, randomized trial comparing steroids and pulse cyclophosphamide versus steroids and oral cyclophosphamide in the treatment of generalized Wegener's granulomatosis. *Arthritis Rheum.* 1997;40:2187-2198.
41. Etanercept plus standard therapy for Wegener's granulomatosis. *N Engl J Med.* 2005;352:351-361.
42. Jayne D, Rasmussen N, Andrassy K, et al. A randomized trial of maintenance therapy for vasculitis associated with antineutrophil cytoplasmic autoantibodies. *N Engl J Med.* 2003;349:36-44.
43. de GK, Harper L, Jayne DR, et al. Pulse versus daily oral cyclophosphamide for induction of remission in antineutrophil cytoplasmic antibody-associated vasculitis: a randomized trial. *Ann Intern Med.* 2009;150:670-680.
44. Walsh M, Tonelli M, Jayne D, Manns B. Surrogate end points in clinical trials: the case of anti-neutrophil cytoplasm antibody-associated vasculitis. *J Nephrol.* 2007;20:119-129.
45. de Lind van Wijngaarden RA, Hauer HA, et al. Clinical and histologic determinants of renal outcome in ANCA-associated vasculitis: a prospective analysis of 100 patients with severe renal involvement. *J Am Soc Nephrol.* 2006;17:2264-2274.
46. Hauer HA, Bajema IM, Van Houwelingen HC, et al. Determinants of outcome in ANCA-associated glomerulonephritis: a prospective clinico-histopathological analysis of 96 patients. *Kidney Int.* 2002;62:1732-1742.
47. Mukhtyar C, Flossmann O, Hellmich B, et al. Outcomes from studies of antineutrophil cytoplasm antibody associated vasculitis: a systematic review by the European League Against Rheumatism systemic vasculitis task force. *Ann Rheum Dis.* 2008;67:1004-1010.
48. Rhen T, Cidlowski JA. Antiinflammatory action of glucocorticoids—new mechanisms for old drugs. *N Engl J Med.* 2005;353:1711-1723.
49. Scheinman RI, Cogswell PC, Lofquist AK, Baldwin Jr AS. Role of transcriptional activation of I kappa B alpha in mediation of immunosuppression by glucocorticoids. *Science.* 1995;270:283-286.
50. Auphan N, DiDonato JA, Rosette C, et al. Immunosuppression by glucocorticoids: inhibition of NF-kappa B activity through induction of I kappa B synthesis. *Science.* 1995;270:286-290.
51. The primary nephrotic syndrome in children. Identification of patients with minimal change nephrotic syndrome from initial response to prednisone. A report of the International Study of Kidney Disease in Children. *J Pediatr.* 1981;98:561-564.
52. Rydel JJ, Korbet SM, Borok RZ, Schwartz MM. Focal segmental glomerular sclerosis in adults: presentation, course, and response to treatment. *Am J Kidney Dis.* 1995;25:534-542.
53. Cattran DC, Rao P. Long-term outcome in children and adults with classic focal segmental glomerulosclerosis. *Am J Kidney Dis.* 1998;32:72-79.
54. Kitiyakara C, Eggers P, Kopp JB. Twenty-one-year trend in ESRD due to focal segmental glomerulosclerosis in the United States. *Am J Kidney Dis.* 2004;44:815-825.
55. Heaf J, Lokkegaard H, Larsen S. The epidemiology and prognosis of glomerulonephritis in Denmark 1985-1997. *Nephrol Dial Transplant.* 1999;14:1889-1897.
56. Cattran DC. Outcomes research in glomerulonephritis. *Semin Nephrol.* 2003;23:340-354.
57. Cattran DC, Delmore T, Roscoe J, et al. A randomized controlled trial of prednisone in patients with idiopathic membranous nephropathy. *N Engl J Med.* 1989;320:210-215.
58. Cameron JS. Proteinuria and progression in human glomerular diseases. *Am J Nephrol.* 1990;10(suppl 1):81-87.
59. Ponticelli C, Zucchelli P, Passerini P, Cesana B. Methylprednisolone plus chlorambucil as compared with methylprednisolone alone for the treatment of idiopathic membranous nephropathy. The Italian Idiopathic Membranous Nephropathy Treatment Study Group. *N Engl J Med.* 1992;327:599-603.
60. Ponticelli C, Zucchelli P, Passerini P, et al. A randomized trial of methylprednisolone and chlorambucil in idiopathic membranous nephropathy. *N Engl J Med.* 1989;320:8-13.
61. Jha V, Ganguli A, Saha TK, et al. A randomized, controlled trial of steroids and cyclophosphamide in adults with nephrotic syndrome caused by idiopathic membranous nephropathy. *J Am Soc Nephrol.* 2007;18: 1899-1904.
62. du Buf-Vereijken PW, Branten AJ, Wetzels JF. Cytotoxic therapy for membranous nephropathy and renal insufficiency: improved renal survival but high relapse rate. *Nephrol Dial Transplant.* 2004;19:1142-1148.
63. du Buf-Vereijken PW, Wetzels JF: Efficacy of a second course of immunosuppressive therapy in patients with membranous nephropathy and persistent or relapsing disease activity. *Nephrol Dial Transplant.* 2004;19:2036-2043.
64. Pozzi C, Bolasco PG, Fogazzi GB, et al. Corticosteroids in IgA nephropathy: a randomised controlled trial. *Lancet.* 1999;353:883-887.
65. Reich HN, Troyanov S, Scholey JW, Cattran DC. Remission of proteinuria improves prognosis in IgA nephropathy. *J Am Soc Nephrol.* 2007;18: 3177-3183.

66. Olefsky JM. Effect of dexamethasone on insulin binding, glucose transport, and glucose oxidation of isolated rat adipocytes. *J Clin Invest.* 1975;56:1499-1508.

67. Pham PT, Pham PC, Lipshutz GS, Wilkinson AH. New onset diabetes mellitus after solid organ transplantation. *Endocrinol Metab Clin North Am.* 2007;36:873-890.

68. Crutchlow MF, Bloom RD. Transplant-associated hyperglycemia: a new look at an old problem. *Clin J Am Soc Nephrol.* 2007;2:343-355.

69. Report of the Expert Committee on the Diagnosis and Classification of Diabetes Mellitus. *Diabetes Care.* 2002;25(suppl):S5-S20.

70. Owczarek J, Jasinska M, Orszulak-Michalak D. Drug-induced myopathies. An overview of the possible mechanisms. *Pharmacol Rep.* 2005;57:23-34.

71. Van Staa TP, Leufkens HG, Abenhaim L, et al. Use of oral corticosteroids and risk of fractures. *J Bone Miner Res.* 2000;15:993-1000.

72. Abeles M, Urman JD, Rothfield NF. Aseptic necrosis of bone in systemic lupus erythematosus. Relationship to corticosteroid therapy. *Arch Intern Med.* 1978;138:750-754.

73. Doria A, Shoenfeld Y, Wu R, Gambari PF, et al. Risk factors for subclinical atherosclerosis in a prospective cohort of patients with systemic lupus erythematosus. *Ann Rheum Dis.* 2003;62:1071-1077.

74. Svenungsson E, Jensen-Urstad K, Heimburger M, et al. Risk factors for cardiovascular disease in systemic lupus erythematosus. *Circulation.* 2001;104:1887-1893.

75. Petri M, Perez-Gutthann S, Spence D, Hochberg MC. Risk factors for coronary artery disease in patients with systemic lupus erythematosus. *Am J Med.* 1992;93:513-519.

76. Gladman DD, Urowitz MB. Morbidity in systemic lupus erythematosus. *J Rheumatol Suppl.* 1987;14(suppl 13):223-226.

77. Manzi S, Meilahn EN, Rairie JE, et al. Age-specific incidence rates of myocardial infarction and angina in women with systemic lupus erythematosus: comparison with the Framingham Study. *Am J Epidemiol.* 1997;145:408-415.

78. Yale SH, Limper AH. Pneumocystis carinii pneumonia in patients without acquired immunodeficiency syndrome: associated illness and prior corticosteroid therapy. *Mayo Clin Proc.* 1996;71:5-13.

79. Sepkowitz KA, Brown AE, Telzak EE, et al. Pneumocystis carinii pneumonia among patients without AIDS at a cancer hospital. *JAMA.* 1992;267:832-837.

80. Lowance D, Neumayer HH, Legendre CM, et al. Valacyclovir for the prevention of cytomegalovirus disease after renal transplantation. International Valacyclovir Cytomegalovirus Prophylaxis Transplantation Study Group. *N Engl J Med.* 1999;340:1462-1470.

81. Houssiau FA. Cyclophosphamide in lupus nephritis. *Lupus.* 2005;14:53-58.

82. Tune BM, Kirpekar R, Sibley RK, et al. Intravenous methylprednisolone and oral alkylating agent therapy of prednisone-resistant pediatric focal segmental glomerulosclerosis: a long-term follow-up. *Clin Nephrol.* 1995;43:84-88.

83. Branten AJ, Reichert LJ, Koene RA, Wetzels JF. Oral cyclophosphamide versus chlorambucil in the treatment of patients with membranous nephropathy and renal insufficiency. *QJM.* 1998;91:359-366.

84. Ballardie FW, Roberts IS. Controlled prospective trial of prednisolone and cytotoxics in progressive IgA nephropathy. *J Am Soc Nephrol.* 2002;13:142-148.

85. Rivkees SA, Crawford JD. The relationship of gonadal activity and chemotherapy-induced gonadal damage. *JAMA.* 1988;259:2123-2125.

86. Mok CC, Lau CS, Wong RW. Risk factors for ovarian failure in patients with systemic lupus erythematosus receiving cyclophosphamide therapy. *Arthritis Rheum.* 1998;41:831-837.

87. Boumpas DT, Austin III HA, Vaughan EM, et al. Risk for sustained amenorrhea in patients with systemic lupus erythematosus receiving intermittent pulse cyclophosphamide therapy. *Ann Intern Med.* 1993;119:366-369.

88. Huong DL, Amoura Z, Duhaut P, et al. Risk of ovarian failure and fertility after intravenous cyclophosphamide. A study in 84 patients. *J Rheumatol.* 2002;29:2571-2576.

89. Ioannidis JP, Katsifis GE, Tzioufas AG, Moutsopoulos HM. Predictors of sustained amenorrhea from pulsed intravenous cyclophosphamide in premenopausal women with systemic lupus erythematosus. *J Rheumatol.* 2002;29:2129-2135.

90. Mok CC, Ying KY, Ng WL, et al. Long-term outcome of diffuse proliferative lupus glomerulonephritis treated with cyclophosphamide. *Am J Med.* 2006;119:355-33.

91. Wetzels JF. Cyclophosphamide-induced gonadal toxicity: a treatment dilemma in patients with lupus nephritis? *Neth J Med.* 2004;62:347-352.

92. Meistrich ML, Wilson G, Brown BW, et al. Impact of cyclophosphamide on long-term reduction in sperm count in men treated with combination chemotherapy for Ewing and soft tissue sarcomas. *Cancer.* 1992;70:2703-2712.

93. Faurschou M, Sorensen IJ, Mellemkjaer L, et al. Malignancies in Wegener's granulomatosis: incidence and relation to cyclophosphamide therapy in a cohort of 293 patients. *J Rheumatol.* 2008;35:100-105.

94. Reinhold-Keller E, Beuge N, Latza U, et al. An interdisciplinary approach to the care of patients with Wegener's granulomatosis: long-term outcome in 155 patients. *Arthritis Rheum.* 2000;43:1021-1032.

95. Westman KW, Bygren PG, Olsson H, et al. Relapse rate, renal survival, and cancer morbidity in patients with Wegener's granulomatosis or microscopic polyangiitis with renal involvement. *J Am Soc Nephrol.* 1998;9:842-852.

96. Moore RA, Derry S. Systematic review and meta-analysis of randomised trials and cohort studies of mycophenolate mofetil in lupus nephritis. *Arthritis Res Ther.* 2006;8:R182.

97. Ginzler EM, Dooley MA, Aranow C, et al. Mycophenolate mofetil or intravenous cyclophosphamide for lupus nephritis. *N Engl J Med.* 2005;353:2219-2228.

98. Contreras G, Pardo V, Leclercq B, et al. Sequential therapies for proliferative lupus nephritis. *N Engl J Med.* 2004;350:971-980.

99. Branten AJ, du Buf-Vereijken PW, Vervloet M, Wetzels JF. Mycophenolate mofetil in idiopathic membranous nephropathy: a clinical trial with comparison to a historic control group treated with cyclophosphamide. *Am J Kidney Dis.* 2007;50:248-256.

100. Morris RE, Hoyt EG, Murphy MP, et al. Mycophenolic acid morpholinoethylester (RS-61443) is a new immunosuppressant that prevents and halts heart allograft rejection by selective inhibition of T- and B-cell purine synthesis. *Transplant Proc.* 1990;22:1659-1662.

101. Eugui EM, Almquist SJ, Muller CD, Allison AC. Lymphocyte-selective cytostatic and immunosuppressive effects of mycophenolic acid in vitro: role of deoxyguanosine nucleotide depletion. *Scand J Immunol.* 1991;33:161-173.

102. Allison AC, Eugui EM. Preferential suppression of lymphocyte proliferation by mycophenolic acid and predicted long-term effects of mycophenolate mofetil in transplantation. *Transplant Proc.* 1994;26:3205-3210.

103. Carr SF, Papp E, Wu JC, Natsumeda Y. Characterization of human type I and type II IMP dehydrogenases. *J Biol Chem.* 1993;268:27286-27290.

104. Corna D, Morigi M, Facchinetti D, et al. Mycophenolate mofetil limits renal damage and prolongs life in murine lupus autoimmune disease. *Kidney Int.* 1997;51:1583-1589.

105. Morath C, Schwenger V, Beimler J, et al. Antifibrotic actions of mycophenolic acid. *Clin Transplant.* 2006;17(20 Suppl):25-29.

106. Lui SL, Tsang R, Wong D, et al. Effect of mycophenolate mofetil on severity of nephritis and nitric oxide production in lupus-prone MRL/lpr mice. *Lupus.* 2002;11:411-418.

107. Sollinger HW. Mycophenolate mofetil for the prevention of acute rejection in primary cadaveric renal allograft recipients. U.S. Renal Transplant Mycophenolate Mofetil Study Group. *Transplantation.* 1995;60:225-232.

108. Placebo-controlled study of mycophenolate mofetil combined with cyclosporin and corticosteroids for prevention of acute rejection. European Mycophenolate Mofetil Cooperative Study Group. *Lancet.* 1995;345:1321-1325.

109. Appel AS, Appel GB. An update on the use of mycophenolate mofetil in lupus nephritis and other primary glomerular diseases. *Nat Clin Pract Nephrol.* 2009;5:132-142.

110. Isenberg D, Appel GB, Contreras G, et al. Influence of race/ethnicity on response to lupus nephritis treatment: the ALMS study. *Rheumatology (Oxford).* 2010;49:128-140.

111. Hu W, Liu C, Xie H, et al. Mycophenolate mofetil versus cyclophosphamide for inducing remission of ANCA vasculitis with moderate renal involvement. *Nephrol Dial Transplant.* 2008;23:1307-1312.

112. Tang S, Leung JC, Chan LY, et al. Mycophenolate mofetil alleviates persistent proteinuria in IgA nephropathy. *Kidney Int.* 2005;68:802-812.

113. Maes BD, Oyen R, Claes K, et al. Mycophenolate mofetil in IgA nephropathy: results of a 3-year prospective placebo-controlled randomized study. *Kidney Int.* 2004;65:1842-1849.

114. Frisch G, Lin J, Rosenstock J, et al. Mycophenolate mofetil (MMF) vs placebo in patients with moderately advanced IgA nephropathy: a double-blind randomized controlled trial. *Nephrol Dial Transplant.* 2005;20:2139-2145.

115. Miller G, Zimmerman III R, Radhakrishnan J, Appel G. Use of mycophenolate mofetil in resistant membranous nephropathy. *Am J Kidney Dis.* 2000;36:250-256.

116. Choi MJ, Eustace JA, Gimenez LF, et al. Mycophenolate mofetil treatment for primary glomerular diseases. *Kidney Int.* 2002;61:1098-1114.

117. Cattran DC, Wang MM, Appel G, et al. Mycophenolate mofetil in the treatment of focal segmental glomerulosclerosis. *Clin Nephrol.* 2004;62:405-411.

118. Waldman M, Crew RJ, Valeri A, et al. Adult minimal-change disease: clinical characteristics, treatment, and outcomes. *Clin J Am Soc Nephrol.* 2007;2:445-453.

119. Gellermann J, Querfeld U. Frequently relapsing nephrotic syndrome: treatment with mycophenolate mofetil. *Pediatr Nephrol.* 2004;19:101-104.

120. Mendizabal S, Zamora I, Berbel O, et al. Mycophenolate mofetil in steroid/cyclosporine-dependent/resistant nephrotic syndrome. *Pediatr Nephrol.* 2005;20:914-919.

121. Anderka MT, Lin AE, Abuelo DN, et al. Reviewing the evidence for mycophenolate mofetil as a new teratogen: case report and review of the literature. *Am J Med Genet A*. 2009;149A:1241-1248.
122. Petri M. Cyclophosphamide: new approaches for systemic lupus erythematosus. *Lupus*. 2004;13:366-371.
123. Engelen W, Verpooten GA, Van der Planken M, et al. Four cases of red blood cell aplasia in association with the use of mycophenolate mofetil in renal transplant patients. *Clin Nephrol*. 2003;60:119-124.
124. Zhu B, Chen N, Lin Y, et al. Mycophenolate mofetil in induction and maintenance therapy of severe lupus nephritis: a meta-analysis of randomized controlled trials. *Nephrol Dial Transplant*. 2007;22: 1933-1942.
125. Walsh M, James M, Jayne D, et al. Mycophenolate mofetil for induction therapy of lupus nephritis: a systematic review and meta-analysis. et al. *Am Soc Nephrol*. 2007;2:968-975.
126. Chan TM, Li FK, Tang CS, et al. Efficacy of mycophenolate mofetil in patients with diffuse proliferative lupus nephritis. Hong Kong-Guangzhou Nephrology Study Group. *N Engl J Med*. 2000;343:1156-1162.
127. Wang K, Zhang H, Li Y, et al. Safety of mycophenolate mofetil versus azathioprine in renal transplantation: a systematic review. *Transplant Proc*. 2004;36:2068-2070.
128. Appel GB, Contreras G, Dooley MA, et al. Mycophenolate mofetil versus cyclophosphamide for induction treatment of lupus nephritis. *J Am Soc Nephrol*. 2009;20:1103-1112.
129. Kronke M, Leonard WJ, Depper JM, et al. Cyclosporin A inhibits T-cell growth factor gene expression at the level of mRNA transcription. *Proc Natl Acad Sci U S A*. 1984;81:5214-5218.
130. Wiederrecht G, Lam E, Hung S, et al. The mechanism of action of FK-506 and cyclosporin A. *Ann N Y Acad Sci*. 1993;696:9-19.
131. Siekierka JJ, Sigal NH. FK-506 and cyclosporin A: immunosuppressive mechanism of action and beyond. *Curr Opin Immunol*. 1992;4:548-552.
132. McAlister VC, Haddad E, Renouf E, et al. Cyclosporin versus tacrolimus as primary immunosuppressant after liver transplantation: a meta-analysis. *Am J Transplant*. 2006;6:1578-1585.
133. Faul C, Asanuma K, Yanagida-Asanuma E, et al. Actin up: regulation of podocyte structure and function by components of the actin cytoskeleton. *Trends Cell Biol*. 2007;17:428-437.
134. Cattran D. Management of membranous nephropathy: when and what for treatment. *J Am Soc Nephrol*. 2005;16:1188-1194.
135. Cattran DC, Greenwood C, Ritchie S, et al. A controlled trial of cyclosporine in patients with progressive membranous nephropathy. Canadian Glomerulonephritis Study Group. *Kidney Int*. 1995;47: 1130-1135.
136. Cattran DC, Appel GB, Hebert LA, et al. Cyclosporine in patients with steroid-resistant membranous nephropathy: a randomized trial. *Kidney Int*. 2001;59:1484-1490.
137. Praga M, Barrio V, Juarez GF, Luno J. Tacrolimus monotherapy in membranous nephropathy: a randomized controlled trial. *Kidney Int*. 2007;71:924-930.
138. Austin III HA, Illei GG, Braun MJ, Balow JE. Randomized, controlled trial of prednisone, cyclophosphamide, and cyclosporine in lupus membranous nephropathy. *J Am Soc Nephrol*. 2009;20:901-911.
139. Szeto CC, Kwan BC, Lai FM, et al. Tacrolimus for the treatment of systemic lupus erythematosus with pure class V nephritis. *Rheumatology (Oxford)*. 2008;47:1678-1681.
140. Tejani A, Suthanthiran M, Pomrantz A. A randomized controlled trial of low-dose prednisone and cyclosporin versus high-dose prednisone in nephrotic syndrome of children. *Nephron*. 1991;59:96-99.
141. Hoyer PF, Brodeh J. Initial treatment of idiopathic nephrotic syndrome in children: prednisone versus prednisone plus cyclosporine A: a prospective, randomized trial. *J Am Soc Nephrol*. 2006;17:1151-1157.
142. Ponticelli C, Edefonti A, Ghio L, et al. Cyclosporin versus cyclophosphamide for patients with steroid-dependent and frequently relapsing idiopathic nephrotic syndrome: a multicentre randomized controlled trial. *Nephrol Dial Transplant*. 1993;8:1326-1332.
143. Ponticelli C, Rizzoni G, Edefonti A, et al. A randomized trial of cyclosporine in steroid-resistant idiopathic nephrotic syndrome. *Kidney Int*. 1993;43:1377-1384.
144. Cattran DC, Appel GB, Hebert LA, et al. A randomized trial of cyclosporine in patients with steroid-resistant focal segmental glomerulosclerosis. North America Nephrotic Syndrome Study Group. *Kidney Int*. 1999;56:2220-2226.
145. Lim BJ, Kim JH, Hong SW, Jeong HJ. Expression of fibrosis-associated molecules in IgA nephropathy treated with cyclosporine. *Pediatr Nephrol*. 2009;24:513-519.
146. Ojo AO, Held PJ, Port FK, et al. Chronic renal failure after transplantation of a nonrenal organ. *N Engl J Med*. 2003;349:931-940.
147. Myers BD, Sibley R, Newton L, et al. The long-term course of cyclosporine-associated chronic nephropathy. *Kidney Int*. 1988;33: 590-600.
148. Pei Y, Chan C, Cattran D, et al. Sustained vasoconstriction associated with daily cyclosporine dose in heart and lung transplant recipients: potential pathophysiologic role of endothelin. *J Lab Clin Med*. 1995;125:113-119.
149. Lowe NJ, Wieder JM, Rosenbach A, et al. Long-term low-dose cyclosporine therapy for severe psoriasis: effects on renal function and structure. *J Am Acad Dermatol*. 1996;35:710-719.
150. Philibert D, Cattran D. Remission of proteinuria in primary glomerulonephritis: we know the goal but do we know the price? *Nat Clin Pract Nephrol*. 2008;4:550-559.
151. Kasiske BL, Snyder JJ, Gilbertson D, Matas AJ. Diabetes mellitus after kidney transplantation in the United States. *Am J Transplant*. 2003;3: 178-185.
152. Vincenti F, Friman S, Scheuermann E, et al. Results of an international, randomized trial comparing glucose metabolism disorders and outcome with cyclosporine versus tacrolimus. *Am J Transplant*. 2007;7:1506-1514.
153. Ponticelli C, Villa M, Banfi G, et al. Can prolonged treatment improve the prognosis in adults with focal segmental glomerulosclerosis? *Am J Kidney Dis*. 1999;34:618-625.
154. Sheashaa H, Mahmoud I, El Basuony F, et al. Does cyclosporine achieve a real advantage for treatment of idiopathic nephrotic syndrome in children? A long-term efficacy and safety study. *Int Urol Nephrol*. 2007;39:923-928.
155. Alexopoulos E, Papagianni A, Tsamelashvili M, et al. Induction and long-term treatment with cyclosporine in membranous nephropathy with the nephrotic syndrome. *Nephrol Dial Transplant*. 2006;21:3127-3132.
156. Kandaswamy R, Humar A, Casingal V, et al. Stable kidney function in the second decade after kidney transplantation while on cyclosporine-based immunosuppression. *Transplantation*. 2007;83:722-726.
157. van den Borne BE, Landewe RB, Houkes I, et al. No increased risk of malignancies and mortality in cyclosporin A-treated patients with rheumatoid arthritis. *Arthritis Rheum*. 1998;41:1930-1937.
158. Paul CF, Ho VC, McGeown C, et al. Risk of malignancies in psoriasis patients treated with cyclosporine: a 5 y cohort study. *J Invest Dermatol*. 2003;120:211-216.
159. Reff ME, Carner K, Chambers KS, et al. Depletion of B cells in vivo by a chimeric mouse human monoclonal antibody to CD20. *Blood*. 1994;83: 435-445.
160. Maloney DG, Grillo-Lopez AJ, White CA, et al. IDEC-C2B8 (Rituximab) anti-CD20 monoclonal antibody therapy in patients with relapsed low-grade non-Hodgkin's lymphoma. *Blood*. 1997;90:2188-2195.
161. Cohen SB, Emery P, Greenwald MW, et al. Rituximab for rheumatoid arthritis refractory to anti-tumor necrosis factor therapy: results of a multicenter, randomized, double-blind, placebo-controlled, phase III trial evaluating primary efficacy and safety at twenty-four weeks. *Arthritis Rheum*. 2006;54:2793-2806.
162. Takemura S, Klimiuk PA, Braun A, et al. T cell activation in rheumatoid synovium is B cell dependent. *J Immunol*. 2001;167:4710-4718.
163. Smith KG, Jones RB, Burns SM, Jayne DR. Long-term comparison of rituximab treatment for refractory systemic lupus erythematosus and vasculitis: Remission, relapse, and re-treatment. *Arthritis Rheum*. 2006;54:2970-2982.
164. Uchida J, Hamaguchi Y, Oliver JA, et al. The innate mononuclear phagocyte network depletes B lymphocytes through Fc receptor-dependent mechanisms during anti-CD20 antibody immunotherapy. *J Exp Med*. 2004;199:1659-1669.
165. Fervenza FC, Cosio FG, Erickson SB, et al. Rituximab treatment of idiopathic membranous nephropathy. *Kidney Int*. 2008;73:117-125.
166. Ruggenenti P, Chiurchiu C, Brusegan V, et al. Rituximab in idiopathic membranous nephropathy: a one-year prospective study. *J Am Soc Nephrol*. 2003;14:1851-1857.
167. Looney RJ, Anolik JH, Campbell D, et al. B cell depletion as a novel treatment for systemic lupus erythematosus: a phase I/II dose-escalation trial of rituximab. *Arthritis Rheum*. 2004;50:2580-2589.
168. Tanaka Y, Yamamoto K, Takeuchi T, et al. A multicenter phase I/II trial of rituximab for refractory systemic lupus erythematosus. *Mod Rheumatol*. 2007;17:191-197.
169. Furie R, Looney RJ, Rovin B, et al. *Efficacy and safety of rituximab in subjects with active proliferative lupus nephritis (LN): results from the randomized, double-blind phase 3 LUNAR study [abstract 1149]*. Philadelphia: American College of Rheumatology Conference; 2009.
170. Fernandez-Fresnedo G, Segarra A, et al. Rituximab treatment of adult patients with steroid-resistant focal segmental glomerulosclerosis. *Clin J Am Soc Nephrol*. 2009;4:1317-1323.
171. McLaughlin P, Grillo-Lopez AJ, Link BK, et al. Rituximab chimeric anti-CD20 monoclonal antibody therapy for relapsed indolent lymphoma: half of patients respond to a four-dose treatment program. *J Clin Oncol*. 1998;16:2825-2833.
172. Igarashi T, Kobayashi Y, Ogura M, et al. Factors affecting toxicity, response and progression-free survival in relapsed patients with indolent B-cell lymphoma and mantle cell lymphoma treated with rituximab: a Japanese phase II study. *Ann Oncol*. 2002;13:928-943.

173. Seror R, Sordet C, Guillevin L, et al. Tolerance and efficacy of rituximab and changes in serum B cell biomarkers in patients with systemic complications of primary Sjogren's syndrome. *Ann Rheum Dis.* 2007;66: 351-357.

174. Goldberg SL, Pecora AL, Alter RS, et al. Unusual viral infections (progressive multifocal leukoencephalopathy and cytomegalovirus disease) after high-dose chemotherapy with autologous blood stem cell rescue and peritransplantation rituximab. *Blood.* 2002;99:1486-1488.

175. Carson KR, Evens AM, Richey EA, et al. Progressive multifocal leukoencephalopathy after rituximab therapy in HIV-negative patients: a report of 57 cases from the Research on Adverse Drug Events and Reports project. *Blood.* 2009;113:4834-4840.

176. Cravedi P, Ruggenenti P, Sghirlanzoni MC, Remuzzi G. Titrating rituximab to circulating B cells to optimize lymphocytolytic therapy in idiopathic membranous nephropathy. *Clin J Am Soc Nephrol.* 2007;2: 932-937.

177. Rock G, Clark B, Sutton D. The Canadian apheresis registry. *Transfus Apher Sci.* 2003;29:167-177.

178. Shemin D, Briggs D, Greenan M. Complications of therapeutic plasma exchange: a prospective study of 1,727 procedures. *J Clin Apher.* 2007;22:270-276.

179. Vincenti F, Ghiggeri GM. New insights into the pathogenesis and the therapy of recurrent focal glomerulosclerosis. *Am J Transplant.* 2005;5: 1179-1185.

180. Savin VJ, Sharma R, Sharma M, et al. Circulating factor associated with increased glomerular permeability to albumin in recurrent focal segmental glomerulosclerosis. *N Engl J Med.* 1996;334:878-883.

181. Sharma M, Sharma R, Reddy SR, et al. Proteinuria after injection of human focal segmental glomerulosclerosis factor. *Transplantation.* 2002;73: 366-372.

182. Ponticelli C. Recurrence of focal segmental glomerular sclerosis (FSGS) after renal transplantation. *Nephrol Dial Transplant.* 2010;25:25-31.

183. Canaud G, Zuber J, Sberro R, et al. Intensive and prolonged treatment of focal and segmental glomerulosclerosis recurrence in adult kidney transplant recipients: a pilot study. *Am J Transplant.* 2009;9:1081-1086.

184. Hickson LJ, Gera M, Amer H, et al. Kidney transplantation for primary focal segmental glomerulosclerosis: outcomes and response to therapy for recurrence. *Transplantation.* 2009;87:1232-1239.

185. Pescovitz MD, Book BK, Sidner RA. Resolution of recurrent focal segmental glomerulosclerosis proteinuria after rituximab treatment. *N Engl J Med.* 2006;354:1961-1963.

186. Feld SM, Figueroa P, Savin V, et al. Plasmapheresis in the treatment of steroid-resistant focal segmental glomerulosclerosis in native kidneys. *Am J Kidney Dis.* 1998;32:230-237.

187. Muso E, Mune M, Fujii Y, et al. Significantly rapid relief from steroid-resistant nephrotic syndrome by LDL apheresis compared with steroid monotherapy. *Nephron.* 2001;89:408-415.

188. Muso E, Mune M, Yorioka N, et al. Beneficial effect of low-density lipoprotein apheresis (LDL-A) on refractory nephrotic syndrome (NS) due to focal glomerulosclerosis (FGS). *Clin Nephrol.* 2007;67:341-344.

189. Misiani R, Bellavita P, Fenili D, et al. Hepatitis C virus infection in patients with essential mixed cryoglobulinemia. *Ann Intern Med.* 1992;117:573-577.

190. Bryce AH, Kyle RA, Dispenzieri A, Gertz MA. Natural history and therapy of 66 patients with mixed cryoglobulinemia. *Am J Hematol.* 2006;81:511-518.

191. Moulin B, Ronco PM, Mougenot B, et al. Glomerulonephritis in chronic lymphocytic leukemia and related B-cell lymphomas. *Kidney Int.* 1992;42:127-135.

192. Fong TL, Valinluck B, Govindarajan S, et al. Short-term prednisone therapy affects aminotransferase activity and hepatitis C virus RNA levels in chronic hepatitis C. *Gastroenterology.* 1994;107:196-199.

193. Fabrizi F, Martin P, Ponticelli C. Hepatitis C virus infection and renal transplantation. *Am J Kidney Dis.* 2001;38:919-934.

194. Hattori M, Ito K, Konomoto T, et al. Plasmapheresis as the sole therapy for rapidly progressive Henoch-Schonlein purpura nephritis in children. *Am J Kidney Dis.* 1999;33:427-433.

195. Kawasaki Y, Suzuki J, Murai M, et al. Plasmapheresis therapy for rapidly progressive Henoch-Schonlein nephritis. *Pediatr Nephrol.* 2004;19:920-923.

196. Kauffmann RH, Houwert DA. Plasmapheresis in rapidly progressive Henoch-Schoenlein glomerulonephritis and the effect on circulating IgA immune complexes. *Clin Nephrol.* 1981;16:155-160.

197. Rother RP, Rollins SA, Mojcik CF, et al. Discovery and development of the complement inhibitor eculizumab for the treatment of paroxysmal nocturnal hemoglobinuria. *Nat Biotechnol.* 2007;25:1256-1264.

198. Walker PD. Dense deposit disease: new insights. *Curr Opin Nephrol Hypertens.* 2007;16:204-212.

199. Pickering MC, de Jorge EG, Martinez-Barricarte R, et al. Spontaneous hemolytic uremic syndrome triggered by complement factor H lacking surface recognition domains. *J Exp Med.* 2007;204:1249-1256.

200. Smith RJ, Alexander J, Barlow PN, et al. New approaches to the treatment of dense deposit disease. *J Am Soc Nephrol.* 2007;18:2447-2456.

201. Wang Y, Hu Q, Madri JA, Rollins SA, et al. Amelioration of lupus-like autoimmune disease in NZB/WF1 mice after treatment with a blocking monoclonal antibody specific for complement component C5. *Proc Natl Acad Sci U S A.* 1996;93:8563-8568.

202. Holers VM. The spectrum of complement alternative pathway-mediated diseases. *Immunol Rev.* 2008;223:300-316.

203. Berg AL, Nilsson-Ehle P. ACTH lowers serum lipids in steroid-treated hyperlipemic patients with kidney disease. *Kidney Int.* 1996;50:538-542.

204. Keane WF. Lipids and the kidney. *Kidney Int.* 1994;46:910-920.

205. Ghiggeri GM, Bruschi M, Candiano G, et al. Depletion of clusterin in renal diseases causing nephrotic syndrome. *Kidney Int.* 2002;62:2184-2194.

206. Berg AL, Nilsson-Ehle P, Arnadottir M. Beneficial effects of ACTH on the serum lipoprotein profile and glomerular function in patients with membranous nephropathy. *Kidney Int.* 1999;56:1534-1543.

207. Picardi L, Villa G, Galli F, et al. ACTH therapy in nephrotic syndrome induced by idiopathic membranous nephropathy. *Clin Nephrol.* 2004;62:403-404.

208. Ponticelli C, Passerini P, Salvadori M, et al. A randomized pilot trial comparing methylprednisolone plus a cytotoxic agent versus synthetic adrenocorticotropic hormone in idiopathic membranous nephropathy. *Am J Kidney Dis.* 2006;47:233-240.

Microvascular and Macrovascular Diseases of the Kidney

Piero Ruggenenti, Paolo Cravedi, and Giuseppe Remuzzi

Microvascular Diseases

Changes in endothelial phenotype is the primary event in many microvascular diseases of the kidney, including thrombotic microangiopathies, radiation nephropathy, scleroderma, and the antiphospholipid syndrome. In this regard, the kidney is perhaps the best example of a solid organ in which injury to endothelial cells contributes prominently to changes in organ function. The large number of discrete microvascular beds sets the stage for varied clinicopathologic manifestations. For example, in sickle cell disease, physiologic conditions in the medulla predispose to erythrocyte deformation and occlusion of the microvasculature. In atherosclerosis, in contrast, small renal arteries and arterioles can be injured and occluded by cholesterol-containing emboli dislodged from atherosclerotic plaques lining the main arteries. Independent of the initiating events, diseases that occlude the renal microvasculature invariably impair kidney perfusion and function. Early diagnosis and effective interventions to restore the integrity of the kidney microvasculature are instrumental in preventing irreversible tissue damage and kidney failure.

Thrombotic Microangiopathies: Hemolytic Uremic Syndrome and Thrombotic Thrombocytopenic Purpura

The term *thrombotic microangiopathy* is defined as a lesion of arteriolar and capillary vessel wall thickening with intraluminal platelet thrombosis and partial or complete obstruction of the vessel lumina. Depending on whether brain or renal lesions prevail, two entities—pathologically indistinguishable and yet clinically different—have been described: the hemolytic uremic syndrome (HUS) and thrombotic thrombocytopenic purpura (TTP). Because HUS can include extrarenal manifestations and TTP can sometimes include severe renal disease, the two can be difficult to distinguish on only clinical grounds.[1] Newly identified pathophysiologic mechanisms, however, have enabled researchers to differentiate the two syndromes on a molecular basis (Table 34-1). Regardless of the initial cause, all different forms of HUS and TTP share particular features: the propensity for circulating blood to clot in the microvasculature because of primary endothelial damage, as in Shiga toxin–associated HUS; uncontrolled complement activation, as in atypical HUS; or abnormal cleavage of von Willebrand factor (vWF), as in TTP (Figure 34-1).

Clinical Features

Hemolytic Uremic Syndrome

The term *hemolytic uremic syndrome* was introduced in 1955 by Gasser and colleagues[2] in their description of an acute fatal syndrome in children characterized by hemolytic anemia, thrombocytopenia, and severe renal failure. HUS occurs most frequently in children younger than 5 years (incidence = 6.1/100,000 children/year, in comparison with an overall incidence of 1 to 2 per 100,000 population per year). Most cases (>90% of those in children) are associated with infection by Shiga toxin (Stx)–producing *Escherichia coli*; the illness is referred to as Stx-HUS.[3] Shiga toxins, also known as *verotoxins*, are bacteria-derived exotoxins that catalytically target host ribosomes. In 90% of cases, Stx-HUS is preceded

TABLE 34-1 Classification of Hemolytic Uremic Syndrome and Thrombotic Thrombocytopenic Purpura According to Clinical Manifestation and Underlying Cause

CLINICAL PRESENTATION	CAUSE
Hemolytic Uremic Syndrome	
Stx-associated	Infections by Shiga toxin–producing bacteria
Neuraminidase associated	Infections by *Streptococcus pneumoniae*
Atypical: Familial	Mutations: CFH (40%-45%); CFI (5%-10%); C3 (8%-10%); membrane cofactor protein (7%-15%); THBD (9%); CFB (1-2%)
Atypical: Sporadic	
Idiopathic	Mutations: CFH (15%-20%); CFI (3%-6%); C3 (4%-6%); membrane cofactor protein (6%-10%); THBD (2%); CFB (2 cases) Anti-CFH autoantibodies (6%-10%)
Pregnancy-associated	Mutations: CFH (20%); CFI (15%)
HELLP syndrome	Mutations: CFH (10%); CFI (20%); membrane cofactor protein (10%)
Drugs	Mutations: rare CFH mutations, the large majority unknown
Transplantation (de novo aHUS)	Mutations: CFH (15%); CFI (16%)
HIV	Unknown*
Malignancy	Unknown*
Thrombotic Thrombocytopenic Purpura	
Congenital	Homozygous or compound heterozygous mutations in ADAMTS13 gene
Idiopathic	Anti-ADAMTS13 autoantibodies
Secondary	
Ticlopidine clopidogrel	Anti-ADAMTS13 autoantibodies (ticlopidine, 80%-90%; clopidogrel, 30%)
HSC transplantation	Unknown; in rare cases, low ADAMTS13 levels
Malignancies	Unknown; in rare cases, low ADAMTS13 levels
AIDS	HIV; in rare cases, low ADAMTS13 levels
SLE, APL, and other autoimmune disease	Depends on the specific primary diseases

*No published data on frequency of complement gene mutations or anti-CFH autoantibodies.

aHUS, Atypical hemolytic uremic syndrome; *AIDS,* acquired immunodeficiency syndrome; *APL,* antiphospholipid syndrome; *CFH,* complement factor H; *CFI,* complement factor I; *HELLP,* hemolytic anemia, elevated liver enzyme levels, and low platelet count; *HIV,* human immunodeficiency virus; *HSC,* hematopoietic stem cell transplantation; *SLE,* systemic lupus erythematosus; *THBD,* thrombomodulin.

by diarrhea, often bloody. Usually patients are afebrile. The disease is either endemic or epidemic in origin, the latter often traced back to contaminated water or food sources. *Streptococcus pneumoniae* causes a distinctive form of HUS that accounts for 40% of cases not associated with Stx-producing bacteria.[4] Approximately 10% of HUS cases are classified as atypical, caused neither by Stx-producing bacteria nor by *S. pneumoniae.*[5] Atypical HUS occurs at any age, can be familial or sporadic, and has a poor outcome; 50% of affected patients progress to end-stage renal disease (ESRD), and 25% may die

in the acute phase.[4,6] Neurologic symptoms and fever occur in 30% of patients. Pulmonary, cardiac, and gastrointestinal manifestations can also occur.[4,6]

THROMBOTIC THROMBOCYTOPENIC PURPURA

TTP is a rare disease, with an incidence of approximately 2 to 4 cases per 1 million person-years.[7,8] It is more common in women (female/male ratio, 3:2 to 5:2) and in white people (white/black ratio, 3:1). Although the incidence peaks in the third and fourth decades of life, TTP can affect any age group.[8,9] TTP classically manifests with the pentad of thrombocytopenia, microangiopathic hemolytic anemia, fever, neurologic dysfunction, and renal dysfunction.[10] The presence of thrombocytopenia is diagnostic; most patients present with values below 60,000/μL.[8,9] Purpura is minor and may be absent. Retinal hemorrhages may be present; however, bleeding is rare. Neurologic symptoms are observed in more than 90% of patients during the entire course of the disease. Central nervous system involvement represents mainly thromboocclusive disease of the gray matter but may also include headache, cranial nerve palsies, confusion, stupor, seizures, and coma. These features are transient but recurrent. In up to half of patients who present with neurologic involvement, sequelae may remain. Renal insufficiency may occur. One group[9] reported that 25% of patients had creatinine clearance of less than 40 mL/min. Low-grade fever is present in 25% of patients at diagnosis, but it is often a consequence of plasma exchange. Less common manifestations include acute abdominal pain, pancreatitis, and sudden death.

Laboratory Findings

Laboratory features of thrombocytopenia and microangiopathic hemolytic anemia are almost invariably present in patients with lesions of thrombotic microangiopathy; they reflect consumption and disruption of platelets and erythrocytes in the microvasculature.[5,9,11] Hemoglobin levels are low (less than 10 g/dL in more than 90% of patients). Reticulocyte counts are always elevated. The peripheral smear reveals increased numbers of fragmented erythrocytes (schistocytes; Figure 34-2), with polychromasia and, often, nucleated erythrocytes. The latter may represent not only a compensatory response but also damage to the bone marrow–blood barrier that results from intramedullary vascular occlusion. Detection of fragmented erythrocytes is crucial to confirm the microangiopathic nature of the hemolytic anemia, if heart valvular disease and other anatomic artery abnormalities that may cause erythrocyte fragmentation are ruled out. Other indicators of intravascular hemolysis include elevated lactate dehydrogenase level, increased bilirubin level, low haptoglobin level, and, in severe cases, free plasma hemoglobin.[5,9,11] The Coombs test yields negative results, which is indicative of a nonimmune process. Moderate leukocytosis may accompany the hemolytic anemia. Thrombocytopenia is uniformly present in HUS and TTP. It may be severe but is usually less so in patients with predominantly renal involvement.[12] The presence of giant platelets in the peripheral smear or reduced platelet survival time (or both) is consistent with peripheral consumption. In children with Stx-HUS, the duration of thrombocytopenia is variable and may not be correlated with the course of renal disease.[13] Bone marrow biopsy specimens

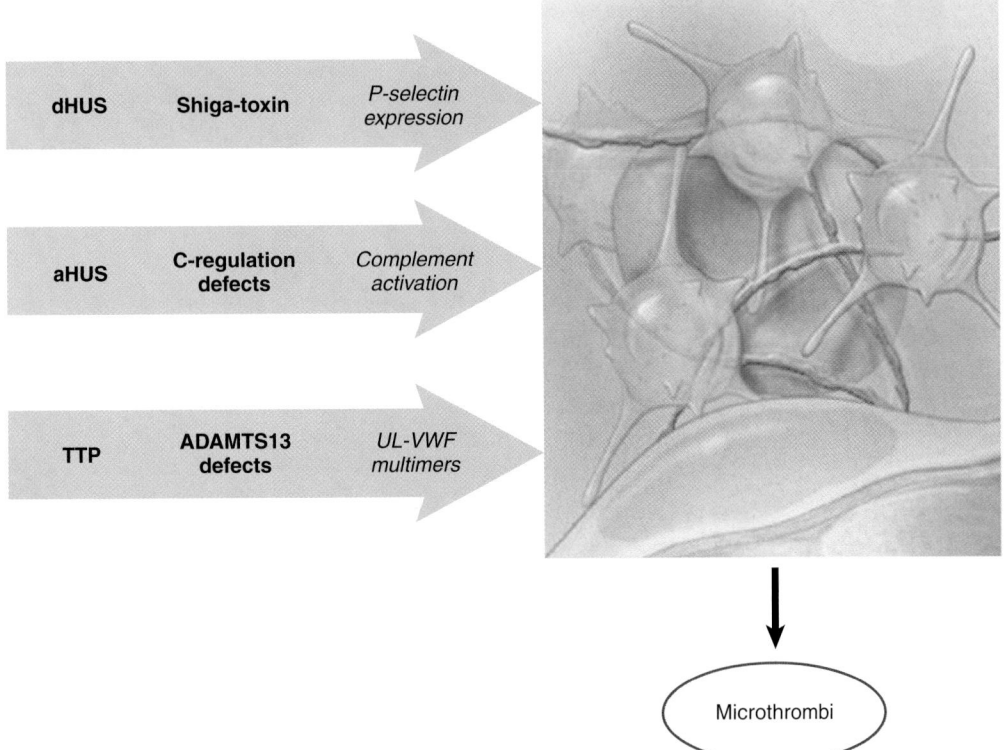

FIGURE 34-1 Pathways of thrombi formation in different forms of thrombotic microangiopathy. In diarrhea-associated hemolytic uremic syndrome (dHUS) the microangiopathic process is initiated by endothelial exposure to Shiga toxin (Stx) with consequent upregulation of P-selectin expression and other adhesion molecules. In atypical HUS (aHUS), the process is mediated by genetic or acquired defects in different modulators of the complement system with secondary uncontrolled complement activation. In thrombotic thrombocytopenic purpura (TTP), the process is mediated by genetic or acquired defects in ADAMTS13 activity with abnormal von Willebrand factor (vWF) cleavage and persistency in the circulation of ultralarge vWF multimers. Regardless of the initial event, microvascular occlusion by intravascular thrombi is the final event common to different forms of thrombotic microangiopathy.

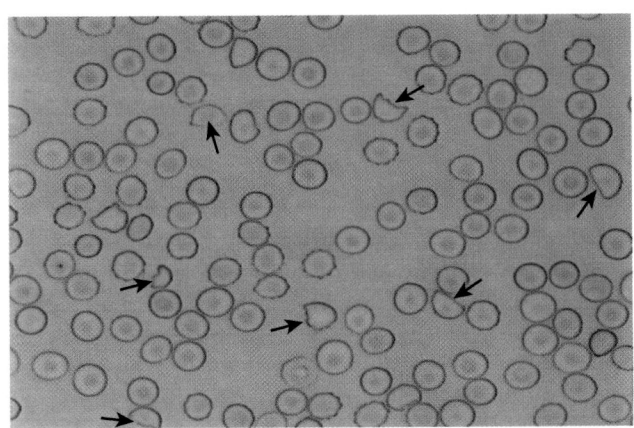

FIGURE 34-2 Peripheral blood smear from a patient with thrombotic microangiopathy. The presence of fragmented erythrocytes (schistocytes), which may assume the appearance of a helmet (*black arrows*), is pathognomonic for microangiopathic hemolysis in patients with no evidence of heart valvular disease.

usually show erythroid hyperplasia and an increased number of megakaryocytes. Prothrombin time, partial thromboplastin time, fibrinogen level, and levels of coagulation factors are normal, which differentiates HUS and TTP from disseminated intravascular coagulation (DIC). Mild fibrinolysis with elevation in amounts of fibrin degradation products, however, may be observed.

Evidence of renal involvement is present in all patients with HUS (by definition) and in about 25% of patients with TTP.[1,11,14] Microscopic hematuria and subnephrotic proteinuria are the most consistent findings. In a retrospective study of 216 patients with a clinical picture of TTP, hematuria was detected in 78% of cases and proteinuria in 75%.[14] Sterile pyuria and casts were present in 31% and 24% of cases, respectively. Gross hematuria was rare.[14]

Pathology

The histologic lesions that are diagnostic of thrombotic microangiopathy consist of widening of the subendothelial space and microvascular thrombosis (Figure 34-3). Electron microscopy best identifies the characteristic lesions of swelling and detachment of the endothelial cells from the basement membrane and the accumulation of "fluffy" material in the subendothelium (see Figure 34-3*A*), intraluminal platelet thrombi, and partial or complete obstruction of vessel lumina (see Figure 34-3*B, D,* and *E*).[15-17] These lesions are similar to those observed in other renal diseases such as scleroderma, malignant nephrosclerosis, chronic transplant rejection, and calcineurin inhibitor nephrotoxicity. In HUS, microthrombi are present primarily in the kidneys, whereas in TTP, they involve mainly the brain, where thrombi may repeatedly form and resolve, producing intermittent neurologic deficits. In pediatric patients, particularly in those

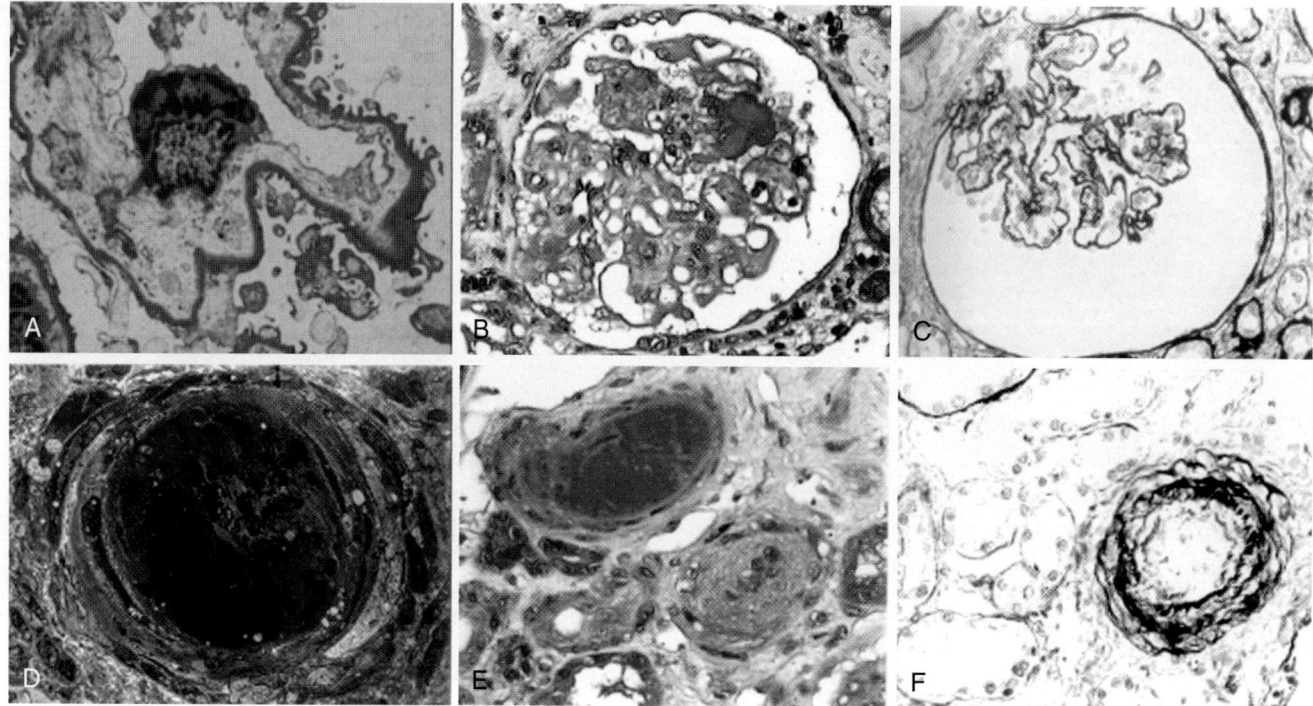

FIGURE 34-3 Micrographs of renal biopsy samples from patients with thrombotic microangiopathy. **A,** Electron micrograph of a glomerular capillary. The endothelium is detached from the glomerular basement membrane. Beneath the endothelium is a thin layer of newly formed glomerular basement membrane. The subendothelial space is widened and occupied by electron-lucent fluffy material and cell debris. **B,** Light microscopic image (periodic acid–Schiff stain) of a glomerular capillary with an intraluminal thrombus. **C,** Light micrograph (silver stain) of an ischemic and markedly retracted glomerulus with wrinkled capillary tuft. **D,** Electron micrograph of a renal arteriole. The vascular lumen is completely occluded by thrombotic material, and the wall contains several myointimal cells. **E,** Light micrograph (periodic acid–Schiff stain) showing one small renal artery that is occluded by a thrombus (*upper left*). A nearby arteriole (*middle right*) has an extremely narrowed lumen that appears surrounded by a swollen intimal layer. **F,** Light micrograph (silver stain) of an arteriole with intimal thickening and multilayering of the vascular wall. (**A** from Remuzzi G, Ruggenenti P, Bertani T: Thrombotic microangiopathy, in Tisher C, Brenner B [editors]: *Renal pathology with clinical and functional correlations*, ed 2, Philadelphia, 1994, J.B. Lippincott, pp 1154-1184; **D** from Pisoni R, Ruggenenti P, Remuzz G: Thrombotic microangiopathies including hemolytic-uremic syndrome, in Johnson R, Feehally J [editors]: *Comprehensive clinical nephrology*, ed 2, St. Louis, 2003, Mosby, pp 413-423).

younger than 2 years, and in patients with HUS secondary to gastrointestinal infection with Stx-producing strains of *E. coli,* the glomerular injury is predominant. Thrombi and infiltration by leukocytes are common in the early phases of the disease and usually resolve after 2 to 3 weeks. Patchy cortical necrosis may be present in severe cases; crescent formation is uncommon.

The presence of severe thrombocytopenia often precludes percutaneous renal biopsy for diagnosis. In idiopathic and familial forms and in adults, the injury mostly involves arteries and arterioles with thrombosis and intimal thickening (see Figure 34-3*F*), and secondary glomerular ischemia and retraction of the glomerular tuft (see Figure 34-3*C*). The prognosis is good when involvement is predominantly glomerular but worse when injury is predominantly preglomerular. Focal segmental glomerulosclerosis may be a long-term sequela of acute cases of HUS and is usually seen in children with long-lasting hypertension and progressive chronic deterioration of renal function.[15-17] The typical pathologic changes of TTP are the thrombi that occlude capillaries and arterioles in many organs and tissues. These thrombi consist of fibrin and platelets, and their distribution is widespread. Immunohistochemical stains for vWf may yield positive results. The thrombi are most commonly detected in the kidneys, pancreas, heart, adrenal glands, and brain. The pathologic changes of TTP, in comparison with those of HUS, are more extensively distributed, which probably reflects the more systemic nature of the disease.[15-17]

Mechanisms, Clinical Course, and Therapy According to Different Forms of Thrombotic Microangiopathy

HEMOLYTIC UREMIC SYNDROME
Shiga Toxin–Associated Hemolytic Uremic Syndrome
Mechanisms. Stx-HUS may follow infection with certain strains of *E. coli* or *Shigella dysenteriae,* which produce a powerful exotoxin (Stx, also known as verotoxin).[3] The term *Shiga toxin* was initially used to describe the exotoxin produced by *S. dysenteriae* type 1. Some strains of *E. coli* (mostly the serotype O157:H7 but also other serotypes such as O111:H8, O103:H2, O123, O26) isolated from human cases with diarrhea were subsequently found to produce a toxin similar to the one of *S. dysenteriae.* After food contaminated by Stx-producing *E. coli* or *S. dysenteriae* is ingested, the toxin is released in the gut and may cause watery or, most often, bloody diarrhea because of a direct effect on the intestinal mucosa. Stx-producing *E. coli* organisms closely adhere to the epithelial cells of the gastrointestinal mucosa, causing destruction of brush border villi.[18] The toxins are mobilized by polarized gastrointestinal cells via transcellular pathways that translocate the toxins into the circulation,[19] probably facilitated by the transmigration of polymorphonuclear neutrophils,[20]

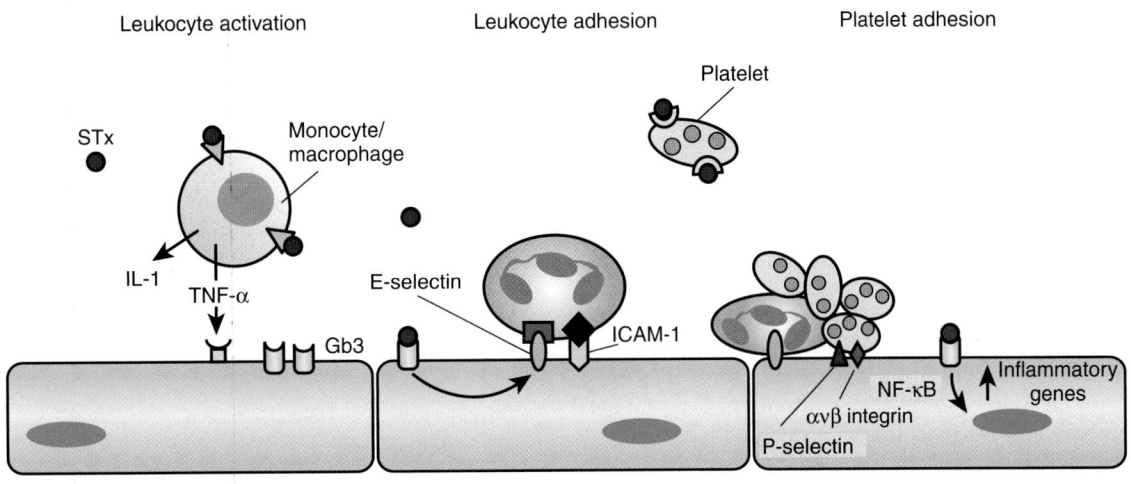

FIGURE 34-4 Pathways mediating microvascular thrombosis and inflammation upon Shiga toxin (Stx) exposure. Stx binds specific receptors on circulating leukocytes that are activated and release interleukin-1 and tumor necrosis factor-α (TNF-α), which enhance the expression of Stx receptors on endothelial cells. Stx binding enables upregulation of endothelial expression of E-selectin and intracellular adhesion molecule-1 (ICAM-1), which facilitates the adhesion of activated leukocytes to the endothelial cell. This further enhances the expression of P-selectin, with secondary adhesion of activated platelets and thrombi formation. Activated endothelial cells also express nuclear factor κ light-chain enhancer of activated B cells (NF-κB)-dependent inflammatory genes that sustain concomitant inflammation.

which increase paracellular permeability. Circulating human blood cells—such as erythrocytes,[21] platelets,[22,23] and monocytes[24]—express Stx receptors on their surface and have been suggested to serve as Stx carriers from the intestine to the kidney and other target organs (Figure 34-4).

Diagnosis depends on detection of *E. coli* O157:H7 and other Stx-producing bacteria in sorbitol-MacConkey stool cultures. Serologic tests for antibodies to Stx and *E. coli* O157:H7 lipopolysaccharide can be performed in research laboratories, and tests are being developed for rapid detection of *E. coli* O157:H7 and Stx in stools. Since 1990, *E. coli* O157:H7 and, less frequently, other Stx-producing *E. coli* strains have been responsible for multiple outbreaks of Stx-HUS throughout the world, becoming a public health problem in both developed and developing countries. Contaminated undercooked ground beef, meat patties, raw vegetables, fruit, milk, and recreational or drinking water have all been implicated in the transmission of *E. coli*. Differences in pathogen virulence account, in part, for the clinical phenotype. For example, a North American outbreak associated with spinach caused rates of both hospitalization (52%) and HUS (16%) that were dramatically higher than typical, because of the emergence of a new variant of *E. coli* O157:H7 serotype that has acquired several gene mutations that probably increased the severity of disease.[25]

Secondary person-to-person contact is a major route of spread in institutional centers, particularly daycare centers and nursing homes. To prevent further transmission, infected patients should stay away from daycare centers until stool cultures are shown to be negative for Stx-producing *E. coli*. However, the most important preventive measure in childcare centers is supervised handwashing.

Clinical Course. After exposure to Stx-producing *E. coli*, 38% to 61% of individuals develop hemorrhagic colitis, and 3% to 9% of cases (in sporadic infections) and 20% (in epidemic forms) progress to overt HUS.[26,27] Hemorrhagic colitis caused by Stx-producing *E. coli* that is not complicated by HUS is self-limiting and is not associated with an increased long-term

risk of high blood pressure or renal dysfunction, as shown by a 4-year follow-up study of 951 children who were exposed through drinking water to an outbreak of *E. coli* O157:H7.[28]

Stx-HUS is characterized by prodromal diarrhea, followed by acute renal failure. The average interval between *E. coli* exposure and illness is 3 days. Illness typically begins with abdominal cramps and nonbloody diarrhea; diarrhea becomes hemorrhagic in 70% of cases, usually within 1 or 2 days.[29] Vomiting occurs in 30% to 60% of cases and fever in 30%. The leukocyte count is usually elevated, and a barium enema may demonstrate "thumbprinting," suggestive of edema and submucosal hemorrhage, especially in the region of the ascending and transverse colon. HUS is usually diagnosed 6 days after the onset of diarrhea.[3] After symptoms resolve, Stx-producing *E. coli* may be shed in the stools for several weeks, particularly in children younger than 5 years.[3]

Bloody diarrhea, fever, vomiting, elevated leukocyte count, extremes of age, and female sex, as well as the use of antimotility agents,[30] have been associated with an increased risk of HUS after *E. coli* infection.[26] Stx-HUS is not a benign disease. Of patients who develop HUS, 70% require erythrocyte transfusions, 50% need dialysis, and 25% have neurologic involvement, including stroke, seizure, and coma.[26,31,32] Although rates of mortality among infants and young children in industrialized countries decreased when dialysis became available, as well as after the introduction of intensive care facilities, 3% to 5% of patients still die during the acute phase of Stx-HUS.[31] According to a meta-analysis of 49 published studies (accounting for 3476 patients; mean follow-up period, 4.4 years) describing the long-term prognosis of patients who survived an episode of Stx-HUS, death or permanent ESRD was reported in 12% of patients, and glomerular filtration rate (GFR) remained below 80 mL/min/1.73 m² in 25%.[32] The severity of acute illness—particularly central nervous system symptoms, the need for initial dialysis, and microalbuminuria in the first 6 to 8 months—was strongly associated with a worse long-term prognosis.[32-34] The extent to which interindividual differences in host genetic susceptibility predispose to HUS is not clear. Predisposing "at-risk" genetic features may explain variation in clinical phenotype after a common exposure to the pathogen.

Therapy. Typical treatment of Stx-HUS in children is based on supportive management of anemia, renal failure, hypertension, and electrolyte and water imbalance. Intravenous isotonic volume expansion as soon as an *E. coli* O157:H7 infection is suspected—that is, within the first 4 days of illness, even before culture results are available—may limit the severity of kidney dysfunction and the need for renal replacement therapy.[35] Indeed, a decrease in the effective arterial blood volume may mask recognition of early hemolytic anemia because of associated hemoconcentration that results from increases in vascular permeability. Bowel rest is important for patients with the enterohemorrhagic colitis associated with Stx-HUS. Antimotility agents should be avoided because they may prolong the persistency of *E. coli* in the intestinal lumen and therefore increase the patient's exposure to its toxin.

The use of antibiotics should be restricted to the very limited number of patients presenting with bacteremia[36] because in children with gastroenteritis, they may increase the risk of HUS by seventeenfold.[37] A possible explanation is that antibiotic-induced injury to the bacterial membrane might enable the acute release of large amounts of preformed toxin. Alternatively, antibiotic therapy might give *E. coli* O157:H7 a selective advantage if these organisms are not as readily eliminated from the bowel as are the normal intestinal flora. Moreover, several antimicrobial drugs, particularly the quinolones, trimethoprim, and furazolidone, are potent inducers of the expression of the Stx2 gene and may increase the level of toxin in the intestine. Although the possibility of a cause-and-effect relationship between antibiotic therapy and increased risk of HUS has been challenged by a meta-analysis of 26 reports,[38] there is no reason to prescribe antibiotics, because they do not improve the outcome of colitis, and bacteremia is found only rarely in Stx-associated HUS. However, when hemorrhagic colitis is caused by *S. dysenteriae* type 1, early and empirical antibiotic treatment shortens the duration of diarrhea, decreases the incidence of complications and reduces the risk of transmission by shortening the duration of bacterial shedding. Thus, in developing countries in which *S. dysenteriae* is the most frequent cause of hemorrhagic colitis, antibiotic therapy should be started early and even before the involved pathogen is identified.

Careful blood pressure control and renin-angiotensin system blockade may be particularly beneficial over the long term for patients who suffer chronic renal disease after an episode of Stx-HUS. In a study of 45 children with renal sequelae of HUS who were monitored for 9 to 11 years, investigators documented that early restriction of protein intake and use of angiotensin-converting enzyme (ACE) inhibitors may have had a beneficial effect on long-term renal outcome, as evidenced by a positive slope of inverse of serum creatinine values over time in treated patients.[39] In another study of patients who underwent 8- to 15-year treatment with ACE inhibitors after severe Stx-HUS, blood pressure was normalized, proteinuria was reduced, and GFR was improved.[40] An oral Stx-binding agent that may compete with endothelial and epithelial receptors for Stx in the gut (SYNSORB Pk) has been developed with the rationale of limiting exposure of target organs to the toxin (Table 34-2). However, a prospective, randomized, double blind, placebo-controlled clinical trial of

TABLE 34-2 Specific Therapies Used for Thrombotic Microangiopathy		
THERAPY	**DOSAGE**	**EFFICACY**
Antiplatelet		Anecdotal efficacy against TTP
Aspirin	325-1300 mg/day	
Dipyridamole	400-600 mg/day	
Dextran 70	500 mg twice/day	
Prostacyclin	4-20 mg/kg/min	
Antithrombotic		Anecdotal efficacy in HUS
Heparin	5000-U bolus followed by 750- to 1000-U/hr infusion	
Streptokinase	250,000-U bolus followed by 100,000-U/hr infusion	
Shiga toxin–binding (Synsorb)	500 mg/kg/day for 7 days	Not effective in preventing or treating STx-associated HUS
Antioxidant (vitamin E)	1000 mg/m²/day	Anecdotal efficacy in HUS
Immunosuppressive		Probably effective in addition to plasma exchange in patients with TTP and anti-ADAMTS13 autoantibodies or in atypical HUS with anti–factor H autoantibodies and in forms associated with autoimmune diseases Lack of evidence from controlled trials in immune-mediated HUS or TTP
Prednisone	200 mg/day, tapered to 60 mg/day, then 5-mg reduction per week	
Prednisolone	200 mg/day, tapered to 60 mg/day, then 5-mg reduction per week	
Immunoglobulins	400 mg/kg/day	
Vincristine	1.4 mg/m² followed by 1 mg every 4 days	
CD20 depletion (Rituximab)	375 mg/m² per week until CD20 depletion is achieved	Effective in treatment or prevention of TTP associated with immune-mediated ADAMTS13 deficiency resistant to, or relapsing after, immunosuppressive therapy
Fresh-frozen plasma		First-line therapy for atypical HUS and TTP; unproven efficacy in childhood Stx-HUS
Exchange	1-2 plasma volumes/day	
Infusion	20-30 mL/kg followed by 10-20 mL/kg/day	To be considered if plasma exchange is not available
Cryosupernatant	Same as for plasma infusion/exchanges	To replace whole plasma in case of plasma resistance or sensitization
Solvent detergent–treated plasma	Same as for plasma infusion/exchanges	To limit the risk of infections
Liver-kidney transplantation		To prevent FH-associated HUS recurrence after transplantation; risk for mortality, about 30%
Complement inhibition (Eculizumab)	600 mg weekly for the first 4 weeks 900 mg every 14 days for up to 6 months	Reported efficacy in FH-associated HUS

FH, Factor H; *HUS*, hemolytic uremic syndrome; *TTP*, thrombotic thrombocytopenic purpura.

145 children with diarrhea-associated HUS failed to demonstrate any beneficial effect of treatment on disease outcome.[41]

Heparin and antithrombotic agents may increase the risk of bleeding and should be avoided. Efficacy of specific treatments in adult patients is difficult to evaluate, inasmuch as most information is derived from uncontrolled series that may include cases of atypical HUS. In particular, no prospective, randomized trials have been conducted to establish definitely whether plasma infusion or plasma exchange offers some specific benefit in comparison with supportive treatment alone. However, comparative analyses of two large series of patients treated[42] or not treated[43] with plasma suggest that plasma therapy may dramatically decrease the overall rate of mortality from HUS associated with Stx-producing *E. coli* O157:H7. These findings, which need further study, may suggest that plasma infusion or exchange is suitable for adult patients, particularly those with severe renal insufficiency and central nervous system involvement. In these cases, the consideration of TTP in the differential diagnosis often confounds therapeutic decision making.

Kidney transplantation should be considered as an effective and safe treatment for pediatric patients who progress to ESRD. Indeed, recurrence rates range from 0% to 10%,[44,45] and graft survival at 10 years is even better in such patients than in control children with other diseases.[46]

Neuraminidase-Associated Hemolytic Uremic Syndrome

Mechanisms. Neuraminidase-associated HUS is a rare but potentially fatal disease that may be a complication of pneumonia or, less frequently, meningitis caused by *S. pneumoniae*.[47] Neuraminidase produced by *S. pneumoniae*, by removing sialic acid from the cell membranes, exposes the Thomsen-Friedenreich antigen (T-antigen).[48] T-antigen exposure on erythrocytes is detected through the use of the lectin *Arachis hypogaea*. T-antigen plays a leading role in docking cells onto endothelium by specifically interacting with galectin-3, an endothelium-expressed β-galactoside–binding protein. Moreover, an immunoglobulin M (IgM) cold antibody that is naturally present in human serum causes polyagglutination of erythrocytes in vitro. This may explain why, in contrast to other forms of HUS, Coomb's test yields positive results in neuraminidase-associated HUS. The interaction of T-antigen with anti-T-antigen on erythrocytes, platelets, and endothelium was thought to explain the pathogenesis, whereas the pathogenic role of the anti-T-antigen cold antibody in vivo is uncertain.[49]

Clinical Course. Affected patients, most of whom are younger than 2 years, present with severe microangiopathic hemolytic anemia. The clinical picture is acute, with respiratory distress, neurologic involvement, and coma. The rate of short-term mortality is about 25%.

Therapy. The outcome is strongly dependent on the effectiveness of antibiotic therapy. In theory, plasma, either infused or exchanged, is contraindicated because adult plasma contains antibodies against the T-antigen, which may accelerate polyagglutination and therefore enhance hemolysis.[48] Thus, patients should be treated only with antibiotics and washed erythrocytes. In some cases, however, plasma therapy, occasionally in combination with steroids, has been associated with recovery.

Atypical Hemolytic Uremic Syndrome.

Atypical HUS (aHUS) has a number of associations and manifestations. It can occur sporadically or within families. Research since 2000 has linked aHUS to uncontrolled activation of the complement system (Figure 34-5).[50]

Familial Atypical Hemolytic Uremic Syndrome. Fewer than 20% of aHUS cases are familial. Reports date back to 1965, when Campbell and Carre described hemolytic anemia and azotemia in concordant monozygotic twins.[51] Since this early description, familial aHUS has been reported in children and, less frequently, in adults. Some cases were identified in siblings whose parents were unaffected, which is suggestive of autosomal recessive transmission; other cases were identified across two to three family generations, which is suggestive of an autosomal dominant mode.[52,53] The prognosis is poor: The cumulative incidence of death or ESRD ranges from 50% to 80%.

Sporadic Atypical Hemolytic Uremic Syndrome. Sporadic aHUS encompasses cases without family history of the disease. Triggering conditions for sporadic aHUS[54] include human immunodeficiency virus (HIV) infection, treatment with anticancer drugs (e.g., mitomycin, cisplatin, bleomycin, gemcitabine), immunotherapeutic agents (e.g., cyclosporine, tacrolimus, OKT3, interferon, quinidine, anti–vascular endothelial growth factor [VEGF] therapy), antiplatelet agents (ticlopidine and clopidogrel), malignancies, transplantation, and pregnancy.[11,55]

De novo posttransplantation HUS has been reported in patients receiving renal transplants or other organ transplants, as a result of either treatment with calcineurin inhibitors or humoral rejection. It occurs in 5% to 15% of renal transplant recipients who receive cyclosporine and in approximately 1% of those who are given tacrolimus.[56-58] Dosage reduction or changing one calcineurin inhibitor for another sometimes results in recovery, which is suggestive of a causative role. In 10% to 15% of female patients, aHUS manifests during pregnancy or post partum[6,54]; aHUS may manifest at any time during pregnancy, but it occurs mostly in the last trimester and around the time of delivery. It is sometimes difficult to distinguish this clinical condition from preeclampsia. The syndrome of hemolytic anemia, elevated liver enzyme levels, and low platelets (HELPP) is a life-threatening disorder that occurs during either the last trimester or parturition, with severe thrombocytopenia, microangiopathic hemolytic anemia, renal failure, and liver involvement. These manifestations are always an indication for prompt delivery, which is usually followed by complete remission.[54] Postpartum HUS manifests within 3 months of delivery in most cases. The outcome is usually poor. In about 50% of sporadic aHUS cases, no trigger is clearly identified (idiopathic HUS).

Mechanisms

Complement Abnormalities. Reduced serum levels of C3 with normal levels of C4 in patients with aHUS have been known since 1974.[59,60] In cases of familial aHUS, serum C3 levels were low even during remission, hinting at genetic defects.[59,61] Low C3 levels reflected complement activation and consumption with high levels of activated products, C3b, C3c, and C3d.[62] The complement system is part of innate immunity and consists of numerous plasma and membrane-bound proteins protecting against invading organisms.[63] About half the factors are involved in activation of the complement cascade, whereas the remainder of soluble and membrane-bound complement regulatory proteins are inhibitory. Three activation pathways—classical, lectin, and alternative—produce protease complexes, termed C3 and

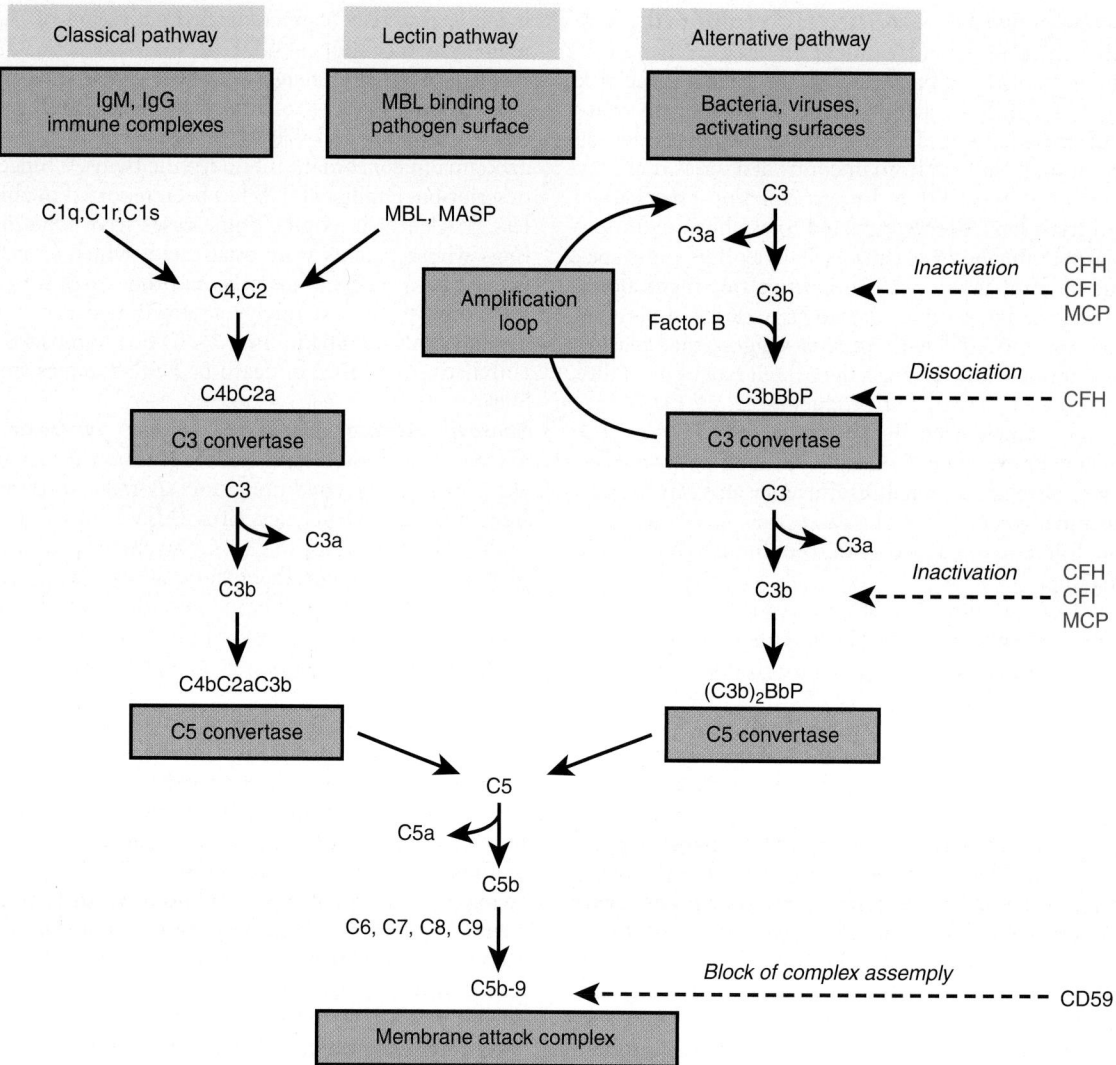

FIGURE 34-5 Complement activation pathways. The classical pathway is initiated by the binding of the C1 complex to antibodies bound to an antigen on the surface of a bacterial cell, which leads to the formation of a C4b2a enzyme complex, the C3 convertase of the classical pathway. The mannose-binding lectin pathway is initiated by binding of the complex of mannose-binding lectin (MBL) and of the mannose-binding lectin–associated proteases 1 and 2 (MASP1 and MASP2) to mannose residues on the surface of a bacterial cell; this, in turn, leads to the formation of C4bC2a, a C3 convertase enzyme. The alternative pathway is initiated by the covalent binding of a small amount of C3b generated by spontaneous hydrolysis in plasma to hydroxyl groups on cell-surface carbohydrates and proteins. This C3b binds factor B to form C3bBb, an alternative pathway C3 complex. The C3 convertase enzymes cleave many molecules of C3 to form C3a, an anaphylatoxin, and C3b, which binds covalently around the site of complement activation. Some of this C3b binds to C4b and C3b in the convertase enzymes of the classical and alternative pathways, respectively, forming C5 convertase enzymes that cleave C5 to form C5a, an anaphylatoxin, and C5b, which initiates the formation of the membrane-attack complex. The human complement system is highly regulated as to prevent nonspecific damage to host cells and limit the deposition of complement to the surface of pathogens. This fine regulation occurs through a number of membrane-anchored and fluid-phase (in *red*) regulators that inactivate complement products formed at various levels in the cascade and protect host tissues (the molecules involved in the regulation of the alternative pathway are shown in *red*). *CD59*, protectin (prevents the terminal polymerization of the membrane attack complex); *CFB*, complement factor B; *CFH*, complement factor H; *CFI*, complement factor I; *MCP*, membrane cofactor protein.

C5 convertases, that cleave C3 and C5, respectively, which eventually leads to the membrane attack lytic complex (see Figure 34-5). The alternative pathway is initiated spontaneously in plasma by C3 hydrolysis, which is responsible for covalent deposition of a low amount of C3b onto practically all plasma-exposed surfaces (see Figure 34-5). On bacterial surfaces, C3b leads to opsonization of phagocytosis by neutrophils and macrophages. Without regulation, a small initiating stimulus is quickly amplified to a self-harming response until consumption of complement components (see Figure 34-5). On host cells, such dangerous cascade is controlled by membrane-anchored and fluid-phase regulators (see Figure 34-5). Both favor the cleavage of C3b to inactive C3b by the plasma

serine protease complement factor I (CFI; cofactor activity) and dissociate the multicomponent C3- and C5-convertases (decay acceleration activity). Foreign targets and injured cells that either lack membrane-bound regulators or cannot bind soluble regulators are attacked by complement.

The C3 convertases of the classical and lectin pathways are formed by C2 and C4 fragments, whereas the alternative pathway convertase requires cleavage of C3 only[63] (see Figure 34-5). Thus, low serum C3 levels in aHUS with normal C4 levels are indicative of selective activation of the alternative pathway.[61]

Genetic Abnormalities. A variety of genetic abnormalities in members of the alternative pathway of complement have been

TABLE 34-3 Outcome of Atypical Hemolytic Uremic Syndrome According to the Associated Genetic Abnormality

AFFECTED GENE	AFFECTED PROTEIN AND MAIN EFFECT	FREQUENCY IN AHUS	RATE OF REMISSION WITH PLASMA EXCHANGE*	5- TO 10-YEAR RATE OF DEATH OR ESRD	RATE OF RECURRENCE AFTER KIDNEY TRANSPLANTATION
CFH	Complement factor H (no binding to endothelium)	20%-30%	60% (dose and timing dependent)	70%-80%	80%-90%†
CFHL1, CFHL3	Complement factors HR1, HR3 (anti–factor H antibodies)	6%	70%-80% (when plasma exchange is combined with immunosuppression)	30%-40%	20%†
MCP	Membrane cofactor protein (no surface expression)	10%-15%	No indication for plasma exchange	<20%	15%-20%‡
CFI	Complement factor I (low levels/ low cofactor act)	4%-10%	30%-40%	60%-70%	70%-80%
CFB	Complement factor B (C3 convertase stabilization)	1%-2%	30%	70%	One case reported
C3	Complement C3 (resistance to C3b inactivation)	5%-10%	40%-50%	60%	40%-50%
THBD	Thrombomodulin (reduced C3b inactivation)	5%	60%	60%	One case reported

*Complete remission or hematologic remission with renal sequelae.
†Kidney or combined liver and kidney transplantation.
‡Single kidney transplantation.
aHUS, Atypical hemolytic uremic syndrome; *ESRD*, end-stage renal disease.

described in aHUS; these abnormalities account for about 60% of cases (see Table 34-1). Of note, distinct genetic abnormalities account for different patterns of dysfunction of the complement system, with different clinical outcomes, different responses to therapy, and different risks of recurrence after kidney transplantation (Table 34-3).

Complement Factor H. Complement factor H (CFH) regulates the alternative pathway by competing with complement factor B (CFB) for C3b recognition, by acting as a cofactor for CFI, and by enhancing dissociation of C3 convertase.[64] In 1998, Warwicker and associates[65] demonstrated linkage of aHUS to the chromosome 1q32 locus, which contains genes for CFH and other complement regulators. Since then, more than 80 CFH gene mutations[65a] have been identified in patients with aHUS (mutation frequency: 40% to 45% in familial forms, 10% to 20% in sporadic forms).[66-72] Autoantibodies to CFH have been described, although the clinical relevance is not yet clear.

Membrane Cofactor Protein. Membrane cofactor protein blocks C3 activation on glomerular endothelium. Indeed, anti–membrane cofactor protein antibody completely blocked cofactor activity in cell extracts.[73] In 2003, two groups[74,75] described mutations in the membrane cofactor protein gene, encoding membrane cofactor protein, a widely expressed transmembrane regulator, in affected individuals of four families. Membrane cofactor protein serves as a cofactor for CFI to cleave C3b and C4b on cell surface.[76] Membrane cofactor protein gene mutations account for 10% to 15% of aHUS cases.[70] Most characterized genetic variations are heterozygous; about 25% are either homozygous or compound heterozygous.[65a] The majority of the mutations cluster in critical extracellular modules for regulation. Expression on blood leukocytes was reduced in about 75% of patients carrying the mutations, which caused a quantitative functional defect. Other affected patients have low C3b-binding capability and decreased cofactor activity.[70,77]

Complement Factor I. CFI is a plasma serine protease that regulates the three complement pathways by cleaving C3b and C4b in the presence of cofactor proteins. CFI gene mutations affect 4% to 10% of patients with aHUS.[70,78-80] All mutations are heterozygous; 80% cluster in the serine protease domain. Approximately 50% of mutations result in low CFI levels. Others disrupt C3b and C4b cleavage.[70,78-80]

Complement Factor B and C3. Gain-of-function mutations can affect genes encoding CFB and C3, two alternative pathway C3 convertase components.[81,82] CFB gene mutations are rare in aHUS (1% to 2%).[82] Affected patients have chronic alternative pathway activation with low C3 levels and, usually, normal C4 levels.[82] Patients carrying the CFB protein mutation have excess C3b affinity and form a hyperactive C3 convertase, which is resistant to dissociation. C3b formation is thereby enhanced in vivo.[82]

About 4% to 10% of patients with aHUS have heterozygous mutations in the C3 gene, usually in association with low C3 levels.[81] Most mutations reduce C3b binding to CFH and membrane cofactor protein, severely impairing the degradation and inactivation of mutant C3b.[81]

Thrombomodulin. Thrombomodulin is a membrane-bound glycoprotein with anticoagulant properties that modulates complement activation on cell surfaces. Mutations in the gene THBD, which encodes thrombomodulin, have been linked to aHUS.[83] Thrombomodulin also serves as a thrombin-binding molecule important for the activation of protein C. Therefore, thrombomodulin is an interesting molecule that sits at the interface of the coagulation system and the complement cascade. About 5% of patients with aHUS carry heterozygous THBD mutations. Cells expressing these variants inactivate C3b less efficiently than do cells expressing wild-type thrombomodulin.[83] The research data document a functional link between complement and coagulation, opening new perspectives for candidate gene research on aHUS.

Clinical Course. Of the patients with aHUS, irrespective of mutation type, 67% are affected during childhood,[70,84] and almost all patients with anti-CFH autoantibodies developed the disease before the age of 16 years.[85] Acute episodes manifest with severe hemolytic anemia, thrombocytopenia, and acute renal failure. Extrarenal involvement (central nervous system or multivisceral) occurs in 20% of cases.[5,70,84] Short- and long-term outcomes vary according to the underlying complement abnormality (see Table 34-3). About 60% to 70% of patients with CFH, CFI, and C3 gene mutations and 33% of children with anti-CFH autoantibodies lose renal function or die during the presenting episode or develop ESRD after relapses.[5,70,84] CFB gene mutations are associated with poor renal outcome (renal function loss in 87.5% of patients).[82] Chronic complement dysregulation may lead to atheroma-like lesions. About 20% of patients with CFH gene mutations have cardiovascular complications (coronary or cerebrovascular disease, myocardial infarction) and excess rates of mortality. The rate of long-term survival is worse in patients with CFH gene mutations (50% at 10 years) than in those with CFI and C3 gene mutations or anti-CFH autoantibodies (80% to 90% at 10 years).[5,70,84] Carriers of the membrane cofactor protein gene mutation have a good prognosis (complete remission: 80% to 90%): Recurrences are frequent, but long-term outcome is good, and 80% of patients remain dialysis free.[5,70,84] However, rare patients with membrane cofactor protein gene mutations have had severe disease, immediate ESRD, intractable hypertension, and coma,[70] possibly because of concurrent genetic abnormalities.

Therapy

Fresh-Frozen Plasma. According to current guidelines, plasma therapy (plasma exchange, 1 to 2 plasma volumes/day; plasma infusion, 20 to 30 mL/kg/day) should be started within 24 hours of diagnosis.[5] Plasma exchange allows supplying larger amounts of plasma than would be possible with infusion, while avoiding fluid overload (see Table 34-2). Trials of plasma therapy in HUS are scanty, and no clear-cut evidence exists on the impact and optimal implementation of this treatment. Two published trials involving patients with HUS,[86,87] in which supportive therapy alone was compared with supportive therapy plus plasma infusion, did not demonstrate significant benefit of plasma in inducing remission. However, in neither trial did the investigators examine outcomes separately for Stx-HUS versus aHUS; the lack of such data invariably weakened potential benefits of plasma in aHUS.[88,89] Because CFH is a plasma protein, plasma infusion or exchange offers the potential of providing normal CFH to patients carrying CFH gene mutations.[70,84,90,91] Long-term treatment, however, may fail because of the development of plasma resistance.[92] Heterozygous carriers of CFH gene mutations usually have normal levels of CFH, half of which is dysfunctional.

The beneficial effect of plasma is strongly dependent on amount, frequency, and modality of administration; plasma exchange is superior to plasma infusion in inducing remission and preventing recurrences by removal of mutant CFH that could antagonize the normal protein.[93,94] Overall published data[5,70,84] from patients with CFH gene mutations show remission—either complete or partial (hematologic normalization with renal sequelae)—after 60% of plasma-treated episodes (see Table 34-3). Plasma exchange is used to remove anti-CFH autoantibodies,[84,95] but the effect is usually transient. Immunosuppressants (corticosteroids and azathioprine

or mycophenolate-mofetil) and rituximab, an anti-CD20 antibody, in combination with plasma exchange allowed long-term dialysis-free survival in 60% to 70% of patients.[85,95-97]

Patients with CFI gene mutations show only a partial response, with remission after about 30% to 40% of plasma-treated episodes.[5,70,84,98] Because membrane cofactor protein is a cell-associated protein, effects of plasma are unlikely to occur in patients with membrane cofactor protein gene mutations. In fact, 80% to 90% of patients undergo remission independently of plasma treatment (see Table 34-3).[5,70,84,98] Thirty percent to 40% of patients with CFB gene mutations and 50% of those with C3 gene mutations responded to plasma infusion or exchange.[5,81,82] It is possible that these patients need abundant and frequent plasma exchanges to clear the hyperfunctional mutant CFB and C3.[5]

Transplantation. For patients with aHUS who have ESRD, the question of whether kidney transplantation is appropriate has been long debated. Disease recurred in around 50% of transplant recipients with CFH, CFI, CFB, and C3 gene mutations, and graft failure occurred in 80% to 90% of those recipients.[78,81,82,84,99-101] Transplantation from living related donors is contraindicated by a high risk of recurrences[101,102] and may be risky to donors; one male adult with a heterozygous CFH mutation developed de novo HUS after donating a kidney to his child.[102] Intensive chronic plasma prophylaxis prevented recurrence in one patient with a CFH gene mutation[103] but failed in another case.[104] Simultaneous kidney and liver transplantation was performed in two children with aHUS and CFH gene mutations with the rationale of providing a donor liver and thereby correcting the genetic defect and preventing recurrences.[105,106] However, both cases were complicated by premature liver failure. The first child recovered after a second liver transplantation. The child had no symptoms of HUS for 3 years but died from sequelae of hepatic encephalopathy.[105] This case offered the proof of concept that transplantation could cure HUS associated with CFH gene mutations by correcting the genetic defect. The second case was also complicated by liver failure with widespread microvascular thrombosis and complement deposition.[106] It was reasoned that the surgical stress, with ischemia and reperfusion, induced complement activation in the liver that could not be regulated because of functional CFH gene deficiency. A modified approach to the combined transplantation was applied to eight other cases,[107,108] including extensive plasma exchange before surgery to provide timely enough normal CFH until the liver graft recovered synthetic functions. This procedure was successful in seven patients; however, the eighth child[107] developed severe hepatic thrombosis and fatal encephalopathy. The risks of kidney and liver transplantation require a careful assessment of benefits for candidate patients.

The outcome of kidney transplantation is favorable in patients with membrane cofactor protein gene mutations. More than 80% of recipients did not experience HUS recurrence, and long-term graft survival was comparable with that in patients who received kidney transplants for other reasons.[5,84,99,100] The theoretical rationale is strong. Membrane cofactor protein is a transmembrane protein highly expressed in kidney. Not surprisingly, a donor kidney graft corrects the defect of recipients with membrane cofactor protein gene mutations. Combined liver and kidney transplantation is therefore not indicated. Screening for mutations should allow patients and clinicians to make informed decisions regarding

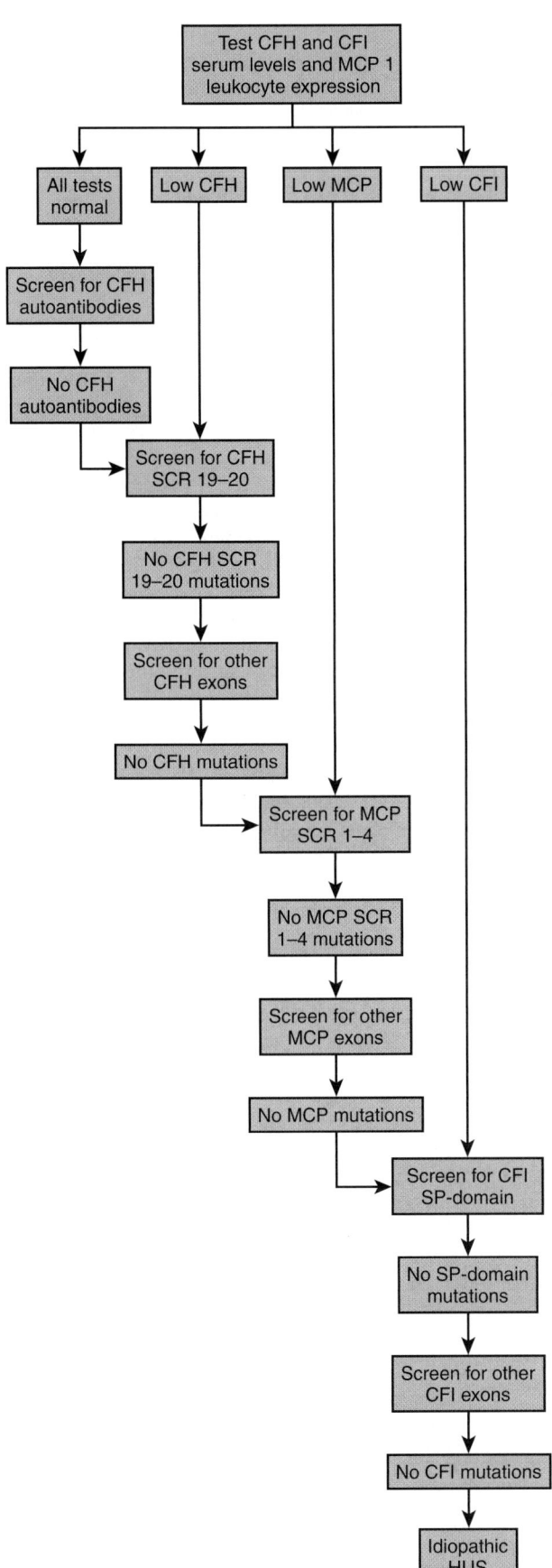

listing for transplantation on the basis of risk of recurrence (Figure 34-6). Algorithms have been developed to optimize the cost effectiveness of screening programs for genetic defects in patients with aHUS (see Figure 34-6). Jalanko and colleagues[107] defined the groups of patients in whom isolated kidney transplantation is extremely risky, whereas combined kidney-liver transplantation is recommended, and those eligible for isolated kidney transplantation.

Complement Inhibitors. Identifying complement genetic abnormalities has paved the way for treatments tailored specifically to reduce complement activation. A human plasma–derived CFH concentrate is being developed in accordance with the the European orphan drug designation.[108a] Numerous drug companies have complement inhibitors under preclinical and clinical development. Phase III clinical trials have demonstrated efficacy and tolerance of the humanized anti-C5 monoclonal antibody eculizumab in paroxysmal nocturnal hemoglobinuria.[109] The effectiveness of C5 blockade in aHUS has been documented.[110,111] However, results from single cases should be evaluated cautiously, and the efficacy of eculizumab in aHUS must be confirmed in controlled trials. Because eculizumab leaves upstream complement activation intact, high levels of C3-activated products might still trigger inflammation, leading to microangiopathic injury. Open-label controlled trials of eculizumab in patients with aHUS are ongoing.[111a]

Hemolytic Uremic Syndrome Associated with Inborn Abnormal Cobalamin C Metabolism

Mechanisms. A rare autosomal recessive form of HUS is associated with an inborn abnormality of cobalamin C metabolism.[112] The biochemical characteristics of cobalamin C deficiency are hyperhomocystinemia and methylmalonic aciduria.

Clinical Course. Patients with cobalamin C deficiency usually present in the early days and months of life with failure to thrive, poor feeding, and vomiting.[54,112] Metabolic acidosis, gastrointestinal bleeding, hemolytic anemia, thrombocytopenia, severe respiratory and hepatic failure, and renal insufficiency lead to rapid deterioration. Neurologic symptoms such as fatigue, delirium, psychosis, and seizures may be present. In cases of early onset, the disease has a fulminant evolution and occasionally involves the pulmonary vasculature. When the disease manifests later in childhood, it may follow a more chronic course. The hallmarks of defective cobalamin C metabolism are hyperhomocystinemia and methylmalonic aciduria, and the extremely high homocysteine levels (up to tenfold higher than normal) have been suggested to have a role in the pathogenesis of the vascular lesions. Without treatment, the disease is fatal. It is likely that in many children who die of the disease, the condition remains undiagnosed.

Therapy. Daily intramuscular administrations of hydroxycobalamin may reduce both homocysteine levels and methylmalonic aciduria, whereas oral hydroxycobalamin and cyanocobalamin are ineffective. Oral betaine helps further reduce serum homocysteine levels by activating betaine-homocysteine methyltransferase. Supplementation of folic acid to avoid folate deficiency induced by methyltetrahydrofolate trapping, and of L-carnitine to increase propionyl carnitine excretion have been suggested, but their role in improving disease outcome is unclear.[113] Despite treatment, the majority of children with early-onset disease die or have severe neurologic sequelae. Intensified treatment in older children with less acute disease may achieve remission of the microangiopathic process and amelioration of the other clinical manifestations of the metabolic disorder. The role of plasma therapy in improving disease outcome is unknown.

THROMBOTIC THROMBOCYTOPENIC PURPURA

In the microvasculature of patients with TTP, systemic platelet thrombi are formed, mainly by platelets and vWF. The large glycoprotein vWF plays a major role in primary hemostasis, forming platelet plugs at sites of vascular injury under high shear stress. It is synthesized in vascular endothelial cells and megakaryocytes. Upon stimulation, vWF is secreted by endothelial cells as ultra-large (UL) multimers that form stringlike structures attached to the endothelial cells, possibly through interaction with P-selectin.[114] Under fluid shear stress, the UL-vWF strings are cleaved to generate vWF multimers of various sizes ($\approx$500 kDa to 20 million Da) that normally circulate in the blood.[115] The proteolytic cleavage of vWF multimers appears to be critical in preventing thrombosis in the microvasculature (Figure 34-7, *right top*).

ADAMTS13 is the metalloprotease that cleaves UL-vWF. The enzyme is functionally deficient in the majority of patients with TTP, and this deficiency leads to the accumulation of UL-vWF multimers that are highly reactive with platelets (see Figure 34-7, *right bottom*).[116-118] ADAMTS13 is expressed predominantly in the liver. Two mechanisms for deficiency of the ADAMTS13 activity have been identified in patients with idiopathic TTP: an acquired deficiency resulting from the formation of anti-ADAMTS13 autoantibodies (acquired TTP) and a genetic deficiency resulting from homozygous or compound heterozygous mutations in the ADAMTS13 gene (congenital TTP; see Table 34-1).

Thrombotic Thrombocytopenic Purpura Associated with Immune-Mediated Deficiency of ADAMTS13

Mechanisms. This immune-mediated, nonfamilial form of TTP probably accounts for the majority of cases (from 60% to 90%) so far reported as acute idiopathic or sporadic TTP (see Table 34-2). The disease is characterized by a severe functional deficiency of ADAMTS13,[119] whose activity is inhibited by specific autoantibodies that develop transiently and tend to disappear during remission.[8,116,117,120] These inhibitory anti-ADAMTS13 autoantibodies are mainly immunoglobulin G (IgG),[116,117,121] although IgM and immunoglobulin A anti-ADAMTS13 autoantibodies have also been described.[121]

Patients with TTP secondary to hematopoietic stem cell transplantation, malignancies, or HIV infection rarely have severe ADAMTS13 deficiency and inhibitory IgG antibodies.[122-129] TTP associated with ticlopidine and clopidogrel

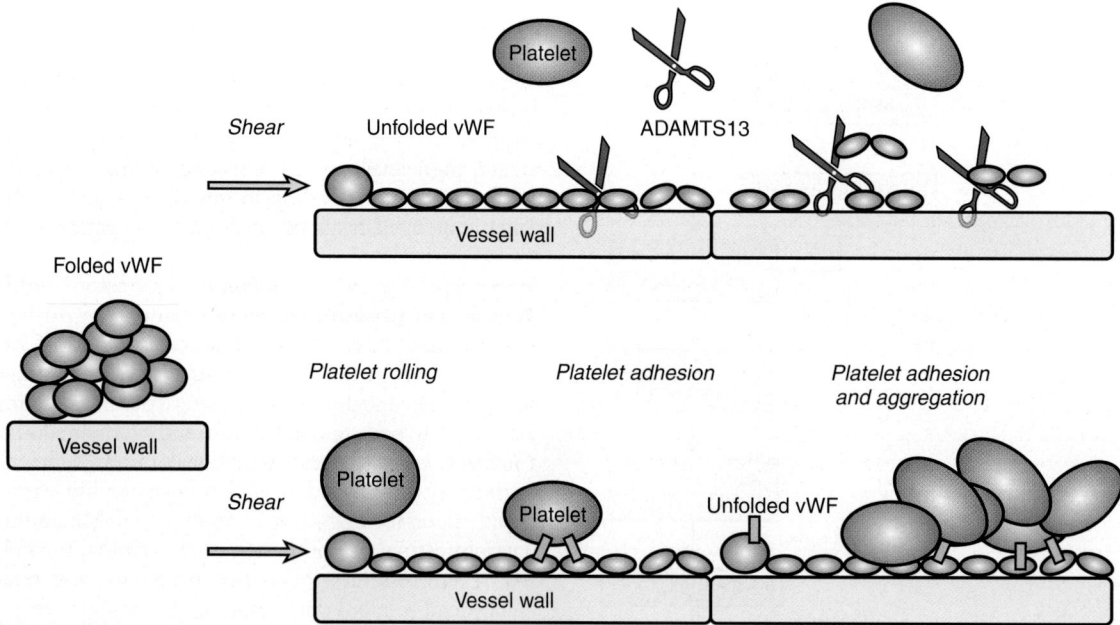

FIGURE 34-7 Pathophysiology of platelet aggregation in thrombotic thrombocytopenic purpura. von Willebrand factor (vWF) is synthesized and stored as ultra-large (UL) multimers in endothelial cells and megakaryocytes. Upon stimulation, UL-vWF multimers are secreted by endothelial cells into the circulation in a folded structure. Upon exposure to enhanced shear stress, UL multimers form stringlike structures that adhere to endothelial cells. Normally, UL-vWF strings are cleaved by the metalloprotease ADAMTS13 to generate vWF multimers ranging in size from 500 kDa to 20 million Da to prevent thrombosis in the microvasculature (**top**). When the ADAMTS13 proteolytic activity is defective because of the inhibitory effect of anti-ADAMTS13 autoantibodies or congenital defective synthesis of the protease, UL-vWF multimers accumulate and interact with activated platelet to facilitate platelet adhesion and aggregation, with thrombi formation and occlusion of the vascular lumen (**bottom**).

(thienopyridine drugs that inhibit platelet aggregation) represent interesting exceptions of secondary TTP that is consistent with a drug-induced autoimmune disorder. Severe ADAMTS13 deficiency and ADAMTS13 inhibitory antibodies were detected in 80% to 90% of patients with ticlopidine-associated TTP[130] and in two patients with clopidogrel-induced TTP.[130] The deficiency resolved after the drugs were discontinued.

Evidence of the pathogenic role of TTP-associated anti-ADAMTS13 autoantibodies is derived from the finding that they usually disappear from the circulation when remission is achieved by effective treatment, and this occurs in parallel with the normalization of ADAMTS13 activity. Of patients with acquired ADAMTS13 deficiency, 50% develop relapses.[131,132] Undetectable ADAMTS13 activity and persistence of anti-ADAMTS13 inhibitors during remission are predictive of recurrences.[121]

Clinical Course. Patients with TTP who have anti-ADAMTS13 inhibitors experience a more severe manifestation of the disease and have a higher mortality rate than do patients with TTP who do not have antibodies.[133] Neurologic symptoms usually dominate the clinical picture and may be fleeting and fluctuating, probably because of continuous thrombi formation and dispersion in the brain microcirculation. Coma and seizures complicate the most severe forms. The detection of high titers of anti-ADAMTS13 autoantibodies is correlated with relapsing disease and poor prognosis.

TTP has been reported in 1 per 1600 to 5000 patients treated with ticlopidine. Eleven cases have been reported during treatment with clopidogrel, a newer antiaggregating agent that has achieved widespread clinical use for its safety profile. Most affected patients had neurologic involvement. The overall survival rate is 67%, and survival is improved by early treatment withdrawal and plasma therapy.

Therapy. Plasma manipulation is a cornerstone in the therapy of an acute TTP episode (see Table 34-2). Plasma may induce remission of the disease by replacing defective protease activity. In theory, in comparison with infusion, exchange may offer the advantage of also rapidly removing anti-ADAMTS13 autoantibodies. This, however, needs to be proved in controlled trials. Corticosteroids might be of benefit in autoimmune forms of TTP by inhibiting the synthesis of anti-ADAMTS13 autoantibodies. In a series of 33 patients with undetectable ADAMTS-13 activity and anti-ADAMTS13 autoantibodies, combined treatment with plasma exchange and prednisone was associated with disease remission in approximately 90% of cases.[121] The rationale of combined treatment is that plasma exchange has only a temporary effect on the presumed autoimmune basis of the disease, and additional immunosuppressive treatment may cause a more durable response. Of 108 patients with either TTP or HUS, only 30 were reported to have recovered after treatment with corticosteroids alone. All 30, however, had mild forms of disease, and none of them were tested for ADAMTS13 activity.[134]

In prospective studies, researchers have successfully and safely used rituximab in patients who had failed to respond to standard daily plasma exchange and methylprednisolone and in patients with relapsed acute TTP who had previously demonstrated autoantibodies to ADAMTS13 (see Table 34-2).[135,136] Treatment was associated with clinical remission in all patients, disappearance of anti-ADAMTS13 autoantibodies, and increase of ADAMTS13 activity to levels higher than 10%

of the activity in patients with normal ADAMTS13 activity. Rituximab has been also used electively to prevent relapses in patients with autoantibodies and recurrent disease.[8,136-138] In one study, five patients with persistent undetectable ADMTS13 activity and high titers of autoantibody were treated with rituximab as preemptive therapy during remission. ADAMTS13 activity ranging from 15% to 75% and the disappearance of inhibitors were achieved after 3 months in all patients, and activity was still higher than 20% at 6 months. Three patients maintained disease-free status after 29, 24, and 6 months, respectively.[138,139] Relapses were documented at 13 and 51 months in the remaining two patients during follow-up. Longitudinal evaluation of ADAMTS13 activity and autoantibody levels may help in monitoring patients' response to treatment. If ADAMTS13 activity decreases and inhibitors reappear in the circulation, repeated treatment with rituximab should be considered, in order to prevent a relapse (see Table 34-2).

Thrombotic Thrombocytopenic Purpura Associated with Congenital Deficiency of ADAMTS13

Mechanisms. A rare form of TTP that is associated with a genetic defect of ADAMTS13 accounts for about 5% of all of cases of TTP (see Table 34-2).[116,119] Emerging data indicate that patients with a clinical diagnosis of HUS[105,120,140-142] may also lack ADAMTS13 activity completely, albeit less frequently. Thus, on clinical grounds, a possible congenital defect of ADAMTS13 cannot be ruled out only because disease manifestation is predominantly renal. TTP associated with congenital ADAMTS13 deficiency has occurred both in families and in patients with no familial history of the disease.[116,118-120] In both cases, the disease is inherited as a recessive trait, as documented by the fact that ADAMTS13 levels in unaffected relatives of patients exhibited a bimodal distribution: One group had half-normal levels, which was consistent with carrier status, and the other group had normal values. To date, more than 80 ADAMTS13 gene mutations have been identified in patients with TTP.[118,143] Most patients are carriers of compound heterozygous mutations; only 15 mutations have been observed in homozygous form. Studies on secretion and activity of the mutated forms of the protease revealed that most of these mutations led to impaired secretion from the cells, and, when the mutated protein is secreted, the proteolytic activity is greatly reduced.[144]

Clinical Course. Approximately 60% of patients with congenital deficiency of ADAMTS13 experience their first acute episode of disease in the neonatal period or during infancy; 10% to 20% manifest the disease after the third decade of life. TTP recurrences are common, but their frequency varies widely. Whereas some patients with congenital ADAMTS13 deficiency depend on frequent chronic plasma infusions to prevent recurrences, many patients who achieved clinical remission after plasma treatment remain in a disease-free state for long periods of time after plasma discontinuation, despite the absence of functional protease activity.[139]

Emerging data suggest that the type and location of ADAMTS13 gene mutations may influence the age at onset of TTP and the penetrance of the disease in mutation carriers.[139] One of the most frequently reported ADAMTS13 gene mutations is the 4143-4144insA in the second CUB (complement proteins C1r/C1s, uEGF, and BMP1) domain; this mutation leads to a frameshift and loss of the last 49 amino acids of the protein and is associated with neonatal and childhood onset. In fact, only 1 of 16 reported carriers, with either homozygous or compound heterozygous other ADAMTS13 gene mutations, reached adulthood without developing TTP.[139,145] In vitro expression studies revealed that the mutation causes a severe impairment of protein secretion, in combination with a strongly reduced specific protease activity. Other mutations—in the sixth and the seventh thrombospondin-1 (TSP1)–like domains,[139,146]—appear to cause TTP with an adulthood onset and a milder course. Expression studies revealed that these mutations result in severe defects in secretion of the metalloprotease, although a small fraction of the mutant protein is released in the supernatant, but carriers of the mutations maintain normal specific protease activity.[139,147] It is possible that in such carriers, ADAMTS13 activity may be present in the circulation in amounts that are limited but enough to prevent onset of the disease in childhood or even in adulthood. This possibility is supported by descriptions of asymptomatic carriers of such mutations who never developed TTP.[139,144,146]

Environmental factors may contribute to induce full-blown manifestation of the disease. According to this "two-hit model," a primary deficiency of ADAMTS13 predisposes to microvascular thrombosis and thrombotic microangiopathy that manifests after a secondary triggering event that activates microvascular endothelial cells and causes the secretion of UL-vWF multimers and P-selectin expression. Potential triggers of these phenomena include infections, possibly *E. coli* O157:H7 infection, and pregnancy. Six women with congenital ADAMTS13 deficiency developed late-onset TTP during pregnancy.[144,148] Genetic modifiers may also be implicated in the susceptibility to develop thrombotic microangiopathy in conditions of ADAMTS13 deficiency; these modifiers may include genes encoding proteins involved in the regulation of the coagulation cascade, vWF, or platelet function; components of the endothelial vessel surface; or components of the complement cascade.

Therapy. Therapy for TTP associated with congenital ADAMTS13 deficiency currently involves plasma infusion or exchange to replenish the active protease (see Table 34-2). Actually, providing just 5% normal enzymatic activity may be sufficient to degrade large vWF multimers—which may be relevant in inducing remission of the microangiopathic process—and this effect is sustained over time because of the relatively long half-life (2 to 4 days) of the protease. In two brothers with complete deficiency of the protease and relapsing TTP, disease remission was achieved by plasmapheresis and was concurrent with an almost full recovery of the ADAMTS13 activity. Both patients achieved a long-lasting remission, although protease activity decreased to less than 20% over 20 days after plasma therapy withdrawal.[149] Although individual attacks usually respond to treatment, long-term prognosis is invariably poor if therapy fails to achieve lasting remission.

Atheroembolic Renal Disease

Atheroembolic renal disease is part of a systemic syndrome of cholesterol crystal embolization. Renal damage results from embolization of cholesterol crystals traveling from atherosclerotic plaques present in large arteries, such as the aorta (see Figure 34-3), to small arteries in the renal vasculature. Calculations of prevalence appear to be dependent on sampling bias; they ranged from 0.8% in a series of 2126 autopsies in patients older than 60 years[150] to 36% in a cohort of patients undergoing surgical revascularization for atherosclerotic renal artery stenosis.[151]

Clinical Features

Atheroembolic renal disease may ensue suddenly, a few days after a precipitating factor, or insidiously, over weeks or months.[152] General systemic manifestations, which occur in fewer than half of the patients, include fever, myalgias, headaches, and weight loss.[153] The rate of cutaneous manifestations such as livedo reticularis, "purple" toes, and toe gangrene varies widely from 35% to 90%, in parallel with the heterogeneous accuracy of data reporting.[152,153] Cutaneous symptoms constitute the most common extrarenal findings and may herald renal involvement,[152] but other microvascular beds, such as the eyes, musculoskeletal system, nervous system, and abdominal organs, can be affected.[152] In an autopsy review of 121 cases of atheroembolic renal disease, the kidney was found to be the internal organ most commonly involved; 75% of the cases showed evidence of renal cholesterol emboli.[154] In other series, the kidneys have been affected in approximately 50% of patients.[155] Renal infarction, however, is rare. Almost half of patients manifest with mild or accelerated, and occasionally malignant, hypertension.[155] Renal function loss is most often progressive, but in a few cases, renal failure can be acute and oliguric.[152,155]

The proportion of patients who need dialysis varies from 30% to 40% in some series[155,156] to 61% in others.[157] Cholesterol emboli may also affect renal allografts[158] and can originate from both the donor and the recipient. In 10 of 15 cases of biopsy-proven cholesterol emboli to renal allografts, atheroemboli were believed to originate from the donor arteries, with poor prognosis for the graft.[152] The differential diagnosis includes systemic vasculitis, subacute bacterial endocarditis, polymyositis, myoglobinuric renal failure, drug-induced interstitial nephritis, and renal artery thrombosis or thromboembolism.[159] It is challenging to clinically distinguish acute kidney injury from atheroembolic renal disease in the early stages. Failure to recover from acute kidney injury after contrast exposure at the time of coronary angiography or after cardiac revascularization prompts clinical consideration of atheroembolic renal disease. The time course of renal dysfunction may help differentiating atheroembolic renal disease, which manifests more than 3 to 8 weeks after angiographic procedures, from radiocontrast-induced nephropathy, which manifests earlier and often resolves within 2 to 3 weeks after appropriate intervention.[160] Definitive diagnosis is based on histologic demonstration of cholesterol crystals in small arteries and arterioles of target organs.

Laboratory Findings

At the time of diagnosis, as many as 25% of patients have a serum creatinine concentration higher than 5 mg/dL, and in about 80%, it is higher than 2 mg/dL.[153] Changes in the urinary sediment are frequent but nonspecific.[152] Granular and hyaline casts occur in approximately 40% of cases, whereas microscopic hematuria or pyuria are observed in fewer than 30%.[153] Eosinophiluria was observed in 33% of patients with renal biopsy–proven atheroembolic renal disease. Proteinuria is present in more than 50% of patients, and values are occasionally in the nephrotic range.[152,153] Eosinophilia is reported in up to 60% to 80% of patients[152,153,157] and is usually transient.[155] Increased erythrocyte sedimentation rate, leukocytosis, and anemia are frequent, whereas hypocomplementemia is inconstant[155,152,161] and usually transient. Autoantibodies to neutrophil cytoplasmic antigens have been found in few cases[162] but not in large series,[152] and their relevance is uncertain.

Pathology

The histologic hallmark of atheroembolic renal disease is the presence of elongated, biconvex, transparent, needle-shaped clefts, which represent the cholesterol crystals that are dissolved during tissue processing. These crystals are usually small and may not completely occlude the vessel lumen; however, they frequently induce an endothelial inflammatory response, which leads to complete obstruction of the vessel within weeks or months (Figure 34-8). Cholesterol crystals are birefringent under polarized light. The subsequent intravascular inflammatory reaction has been studied in experimental models of atheroembolism and in human biopsy and autopsy samples.[152] The early phase is characterized by a variable polymorphonuclear neutrophil and eosinophil infiltrate, followed by the appearance of macrophages and multinucleated giant cells in the lumina of affected vessels within 24 to 48 hours after atheroembolism. In the chronic phase, tissue ischemia is perpetuated by marked endothelial proliferation, intimal thickening, concentric fibrosis of the vessel wall, and

persistence of cholesterol crystals and giant cells in the lumina of affected arteries. Hyalinization of glomeruli, atrophy of renal tubules, and multiple wedge-shaped infarcts in the kidney result in reduced kidney size.[152]

Mechanisms

Male gender, older age, hypertension, and diabetes mellitus are important predisposing factors.[161,163] Patients with atheroembolic renal disease often have a history of ischemic cardiovascular disease, aortic aneurysm, cerebrovascular disease, congestive heart failure, or renal insufficiency.[153,161] A significant association between renal artery stenosis and atheroembolic renal disease has also been reported.[152,161] At least one of the precipitating factors—which include vascular surgery, arteriography, angioplasty, anticoagulation, and thrombolytic therapy—can be identified in the majority of patients.[156,161,164] Arteriographic procedures constitute the most common intervention reported to incite cholesterol embolization.[153] The most common of these procedures is coronary angiography, for which the rate of cholesterol embolism is 0.1%[161] to 1.4%.[165] An estimated 15% of patients with atheroembolism do not have any of the known risk factors.[153]

Treatment

Various treatments have been attempted in order to improve the outcome of atheroembolic renal disease, but none has been found to be appreciably effective; the only exception

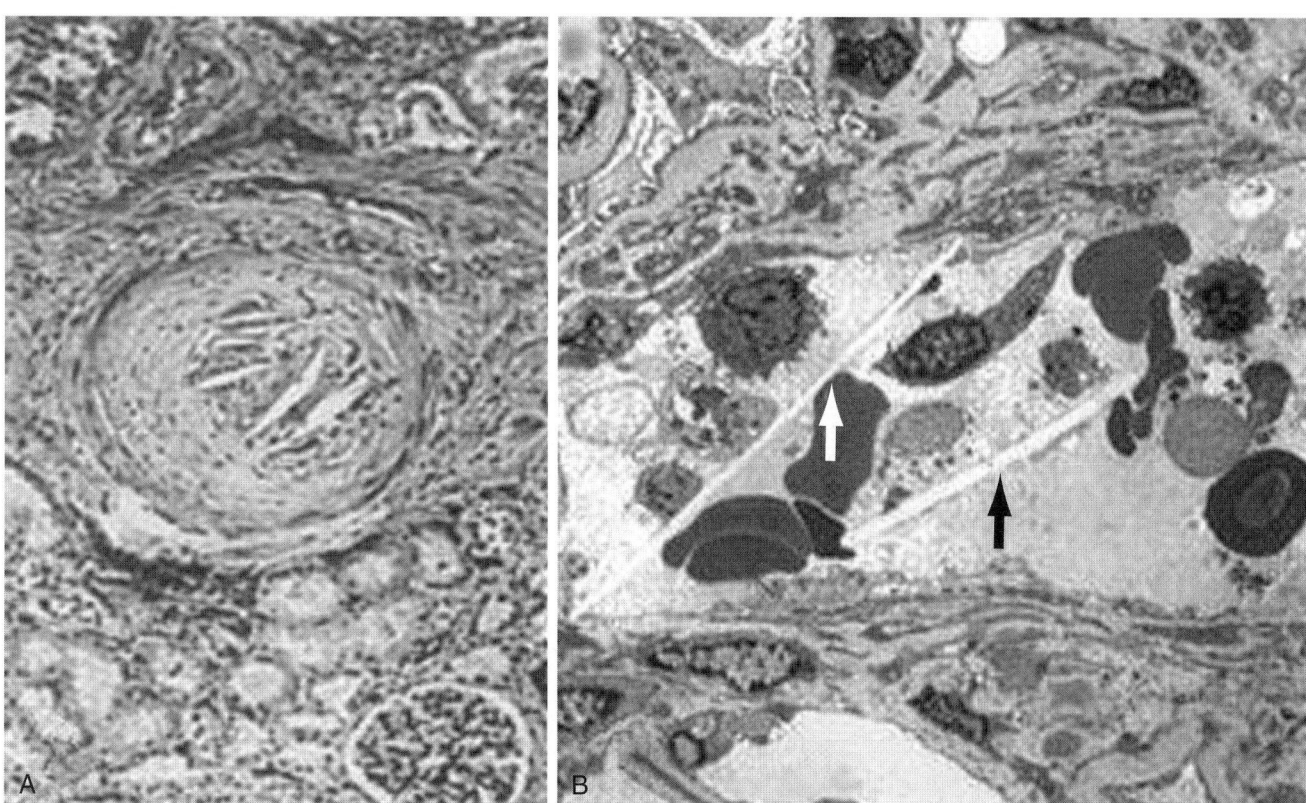

FIGURE 34-8 **A,** Atheroemboli lodged in an interlobular artery of a kidney obtained post mortem. The elongated clefts are actually voids where cholesterol crystals were located before fixation and staining. Note the exuberant intimal thickening and the cellular proliferation, which completely occlude the lumen. **B,** Electron microscopic view showing needle-like clefts from atheroemboli to afferent arterioles. (**A** courtesy of W. Margaretten. **B** from Polu KR, Wolf M: Clinical problem-solving. Needle in a haystack, *N Engl J Med* 354:68-73, 2006.)

may be chronic therapy with cholesterol-lowering agents.[156] A plausible explanation is that statins have a plaque-stabilizing effect, perhaps as a result of their cholesterol-lowering effect as well as antiinflammatory and immunomodulatory properties. The use of steroids is controversial[152]; in some series it has not appeared to be beneficial,[153,166] whereas in other series it has been associated with improved outcomes independent of the doses administered.[167-169] The therapeutic efficacy of low-density lipoprotein apheresis is also uncertain, whereas anticoagulants should be avoided because of the risk of precipitating more atheroembolization.[155] Surgical excision of atheromatous plaques in the suprarenal region of the aorta is not advocated because of significant postoperative mortality, worsening renal function, and lower limb loss.[170]

Altogether, improved outcomes appear to be attributable largely to better supportive therapy. Particular attention should be placed on immediate withdrawal of anticoagulants, postponement of aortic procedures, reduction of blood pressure to less than 140/80 mm Hg, careful treatment of heart failure, dialysis therapy, and adequate nutritional support.[152,157] On the other hand, the lack of effective specific treatments that are able to appreciably improve the outcome of the disease highlights the importance of preventive measures aimed at limiting the risk of arterial thromboembolism, particularly during angiographic studies. The brachial approach for aortography or coronary angiography appears to be burdened by less morbidity than does the femoral approach. The use of distal protection devices (DPDs) to prevent embolization of material during interventional procedures has attracted interest. They have been used most widely in the coronary and carotid vascular beds, in which they have demonstrated the capacity to trap embolic materials and, in some cases, to reduce complications. According to early experience with DPDs in the renal arteries of patients with suitable anatomy, embolic materials have been retrieved in approximately 70% of cases, and renal function has been improved or stabilized in 98%.[171] The combination of platelet inhibition and a DPD may provide even greater benefit.[171]

Radiation Nephropathy

After the original description in 1904 by Baerman and Linser,[172] extensive evidence demonstrated that external kidney irradiation causes progressive tissue injury that results in organ dysfunction and fibrosis. This process is an example of tissue response to radiation that may affect any organ exposed to therapeutic irradiation. Because kidney inflammation is minimal or absent upon radiation exposure, the term *radiation nephritis*, originally introduced to describe this clinical entity, has been progressively replaced with the more appropriate term *radiation nephropathy*. This is the term used throughout this section.

Clinical Features

ACUTE RADIATION NEPHROPATHY
Radiation nephropathy may ensue abruptly 6 to 12 months after exposure to ionizing radiation, manifesting with headache, vomiting, fatigue, hypertension, and edema. Arteriolarvenous nicking is visible on funduscopic examination, and normochromic normocytic anemia, microscopic hematuria, proteinuria, and urinary casts are present. Worsening of renal function may accompany these symptoms.[173] Outcome may range from complete or partial recovery of renal function to terminal kidney failure and can be complicated by malignant hypertension.[173] Acute bone marrow transplant nephropathy (BMTN) is one of the most frequent forms of acute radiation nephropathy and may follow total-body irradiation of candidates for bone marrow transplantation. Acute BMTN manifests with a HUS-like scenario, with severe hypertension, peripheral edema, microangiopathic hemolytic anemia, and thrombocytopenia. Renal function decreases progressively with significant proteinuria and microscopic hematuria, with or without casts. In a retrospective analysis of 363 recipients of allogeneic myeloablative bone marrow transplants, the incidence of severe renal failure (grades 2 and 3 combined) approximated 50%.[174] In this study, acute renal failure did not appear to affect patient survival,[174] but in another study, it was associated with increased mortality.[175]

CHRONIC RADIATION NEPHROPATHY
On occasion, radiation nephropathy manifests with hypertension, proteinuria, and gradual loss of renal function, with a latency period that varies between 18 months and years after the initial exposure.[173] Hypertension, isolated or occasionally in association with proteinuria, may ensue 2 to 5 years after exposure, and isolated low-level proteinuria may ensue 5 to 19 years after exposure. They are expressions of a mild disease with a benign outcome in most cases.[173] Chronic BMTN manifests with mild to moderate hypertension and mild hemolytic anemia. Kidney function decreases slowly in a biphasic pattern in most patients: persistent decline in the first 12 to 24 months, followed by a period of stabilization.[176] Also present is proteinuria, with values higher than 1 g/day, and microscopic hematuria, with or without casts. A period of 8 years is generally necessary for chronic renal failure to occur.[176] In a long-term study of 103 adult survivors of bone marrow transplantation, Lawton and colleagues[177] reported late renal dysfunction in 14 patients. All of them had received 1400 rads (equivalent to 14 Gy) before transplantation, whereas none of the patients receiving lower doses of radiation developed late hypertension or decreased GFR.

LATE MALIGNANT HYPERTENSION
This condition arises 18 months to 11 years after irradiation in patients with either chronic radiation nephropathy or benign hypertension.[173] High-renin hypertension resulting from irradiation of one kidney and recovery after removal of the affected kidney have been described.[173] Irradiation of one kidney and the ipsilateral renal artery may produce renovascular hypertension, mostly in infants and children.

Pathology

Early changes after renal irradiation include cellular atypia and endothelial microvascular damage, as observed on light microscopy, with mild endothelial cell swelling and basement membrane splitting in the glomerular capillaries. Electron microscopic examination reveals marked subendothelial expansion; deposition of basement membrane–like material adjacent to the endothelial cells is evident. The endothelial cell lining may be absent in some capillary loops.[173]

Immunofluorescence studies do not reveal specific staining patterns. Similar glomerular endothelial injury was observed in kidney biopsy specimens from patients who developed renal insufficiency and hypertension after total body irradiation and bone marrow transplantation.[178] In some cases, arteriolar intimal thickening and tubule atrophy were also evident. Glomerular capillary endothelial cell loss and mesangiolysis is observed within weeks after irradiation.[179]

After initial injury, the endothelial injury resolves, but mesangial lesions progress. Late changes include reduction in total renal mass, with prominent and sclerosed interlobar and arcuate arteries, glomerular capillary loop occlusion, and hyalinization, with progressive tubular atrophy,[173] increased mesangial matrix, mesangial sclerosis, and, finally, glomerulosclerosis.[179]

Mechanisms

Renal tissue damage and dysfunction are direct consequences of exposure to ionized radiation. The effect of radiation is dose dependent, and pathogenic doses exceed by at least 1000-fold the dose delivered by a standard radiologic examination, such as an abdominal computed tomographic (CT) scan. Irradiation for neoplastic diseases of the pelvis, particularly for the treatment of malignant seminomas, has historically been the major cause of radiation nephropathy. Because of the progressive replacement of irradiation with pharmacologic therapy for this disease, the incidence of radiation nephropathy has been declining. However, the incidence of the disease has started to increase again, in parallel with the rapidly increasing use of total body irradiation of candidates for bone marrow transplantation. It is suggested that chemotherapy administered as part of the preparative regimen could potentiate the effects of irradiation on the kidneys.[173] Actinomycin enhances the effects of irradiation on many tissues (gut, lung, and skin). Whether this applies also to the kidney is controversial. Cisplatin and carmustine are toxic mainly when irradiation precedes platinum administration. Most of the theories proposed to explain the pathogenesis of radiation nephropathy are based on results of murine studies.

These studies have consistently shown that endothelial, mesangial, and tubular cells are the major targets of radiation injury and that double-stranded DNA breaks are the initial cause of radiation-induced cell apoptosis and death.[180] Damage to the endothelial cell may impair the physiologic thromboresistance of the capillary vascular wall, which, in more severe cases, may cause intravascular clotting with pathologic patterns typical of thrombotic microangiopathy.[180] Impaired generation of prostacyclin by endothelial cells and increased production of plasminogen-activator inhibitor messenger RNA have been suggested to explain the microangiopathic process that often complicates radiation nephropathy.[180] On the other hand, mesangial cells may acquire a myofibroblast phenotype, which may further contribute to progressive fibrosis and scarring of the kidney tissue.

Diffuse apoptosis and lysis of tubular cells, with different degrees of proliferation of the residual ones, is another characteristic pattern of radiation nephropathy. In fact, after a 500-rad (5-Gy) single dose of total body irradiation, early apoptosis has been demonstrated in rats, followed by a late proliferative response.[180] The net balance between cell death

and replication eventually determines the extent of residual tubular atrophy and loss.

Activation of the renin-angiotensin system may also contribute to sustaining and amplifying the initial injury induced by radiation exposure. Indeed, angiotensin II infusion 4 to 8 weeks after total body irradiation caused greater azotemia than did irradiation alone. This effect was associated with the induction of arteriolar fibrinoid necrosis,[181] which, in combination with increased transforming growth factor-β (TGF-β) production and enhanced oxidative stress, may contribute to progressive tissue fibrosis and scarring. This sequence of events is attenuated by concomitant treatment with an inhibitor of the renin angiotensin system; that finding provided additional evidence of the central role of angiotensin II in the pathogenesis and progression of renal damage upon radiation injury.[180]

Therapy

No specific therapies are available for radiation nephropathy, and the disease often progresses independently of treatment. Thus measures to limit or prevent kidney sequelae must be observed during the administration of radiation therapy. These measures include selective shielding of the kidneys and the use of minimum effective doses of fractionated radiation when possible.[177] The use of radioprotectors such as glutathione or cysteine concomitantly with irradiation is still in the experimental phase.[182]

Treatment of hypertension may help slowing the progression of established nephropathy. As in chronic proteinuric nephropathies, ACE inhibitors appear to have a specific protective effect against progression of radiation nephropathy; this effect exceeds the benefit expected just on the basis of achieved blood pressure control.[177,183-185] Consistently, in a study in which 55 subjects exposed to total body irradiation were randomly assigned to receive ACE inhibitor therapy or placebo, ACE inhibition slowed serum creatinine increase over time; this finding was interpreted as indicating that blockade of the renin angiotensin system may be renoprotective in this population.[148,186] Radiation-induced renovascular hypertension may necessitate angioplasty or surgical repair.[173] In patients with radiation nephropathy who progress to ESRD, uncontrolled hypertension may warrant bilateral nephrectomy.

Renal Involvement in Systemic Diseases: Scleroderma, Sickle Cell Disease, and the Antiphospholipid Syndrome

Scleroderma

Scleroderma is a complex disease of extensive fibrosis, vascular changes, and autoantibodies against various cellular antigens. The reported incidence ranges from 2.3 to 22.8 cases per 1 million population[187]; the incidence is 3 to 14 four times higher among women than among men.[188]

CLINICAL FEATURES

The cutaneous involvement in scleroderma may range from limited to diffuse. In limited cutaneous scleroderma, fibrosis is restricted mainly to the hands, arms, and face. Raynaud's phenomenon affects approximately 95% of patients and usually is the first manifestation of the disease. Diffuse cutaneous scleroderma is a rapidly progressing disease that, in addition to affecting a large area of the skin, compromises one or more internal organs. Any internal organ can be involved; however, kidneys, along with the esophagus, heart, and lungs, are the most frequently targeted (Figure 34-9). In rare cases, skin may be spared in scleroderma. Systemic lupus erythematosus, rheumatoid arthritis, polymyositis, or Sjögren's syndrome may accompany scleroderma in the context of an overlap syndrome.[189]

Renal Involvement. Renal involvement in scleroderma typically manifests with malignant hypertension and acute renal failure (scleroderma renal crisis). The crisis may be a de novo event or may complicate a preexisting chronic kidney involvement. Renal involvement manifests less frequently with slowly progressing kidney dysfunction[189] and occasionally as rapidly progressive kidney disease.[190,191]

Renal Crisis. In adults, the incidence of renal crisis ranges from a minimum of 2% among patients with limited cutaneous involvement to a maximum of 12% among those with diffuse disease.[192,193] In juvenile-onset disease, the renal crisis is reported in fewer than 1% of cases.[130,192-194] Affected patients typically present with severe hypertension and acute renal impairment. Activation of the renin pathway and significant hypokalemia may be primary features. Hypertension, however, is not universal, and normotensive crises, usually with poor outcome, have been described.[195,196] Nonnephrotic proteinuria and hematuria, often with granular casts, are common findings. Oliguria is an ominous sign but is unusual when scleroderma is diagnosed and treated appropriately.[192,193] Other clinical features include hypertensive retinopathy and encephalopathy.[197] Evidence that retinal and central nervous system involvement may affect patients with seemingly mild hypertension, or even normal blood pressure, indicates that endothelial dysfunction may play a central role in the pathogenesis of vascular lesions of scleroderma, independent of blood pressure levels. Microangiopathic hemolytic anemia is common, although significant

coagulopathy is rare.[192,193] Pericarditis, myocarditis, and arrhythmias may supervene and are associated with a poorer prognosis.[198-200]

Chronic Kidney Disease. Kidney function can be decreased in patients with scleroderma even without renal crisis.[201] In these cases, decreased GFR reflects a chronic kidney disease that may also include chronic kidney hypoperfusion caused by concomitant cardiac and pulmonary arterial involvement or by concomitant treatment with nephrotoxic drugs; the decreased GFR is normally characterized by a benign prognosis.[200,202]

LABORATORY FINDINGS

Detection of autoantibodies against topoisomerase I (Scl-70), centromere-associated proteins, and nucleolar antigens is crucial for the diagnosis of scleroderma and may help predict clinical manifestations and prognosis. Autoantibodies against the centromere are associated with limited cutaneous involvement and risk for pulmonary hypertension, whereas autoantibodies targeting topoisomerase I are associated with diffuse progressive disease and severe interstitial lung disease. Patients with antibodies to Th/To ribonucleoprotein normally have limited skin involvement but are at high risk for lung fibrosis and pulmonary artery hypertension with severe involvement of kidneys and other internal organs, whereas those with anti–RNA polymerase I/III antibodies have predominantly renal involvement.[189]

PATHOLOGY

Renal Crisis. Biopsy samples from patients with scleroderma crisis show intimal and medial vessel proliferation with luminal narrowing that typically occur in arcuate arteries or interlobular arteries and are indistinguishable from changes of accelerated and malignant hypertension (Figure 34-10). Fibrinoid necrosis and thrombosis are also common. A study of 58 biopsy samples revealed that acute vascular changes, including mucoid intimal thickening and thrombosis, are invariably predictive of poor outcome; 50% of affected subjects progress to

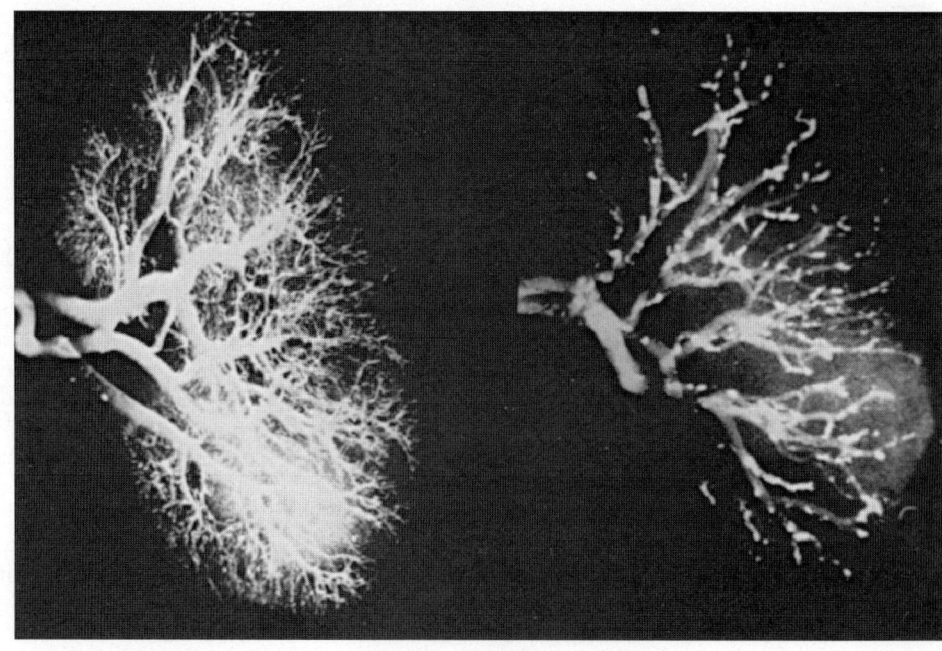

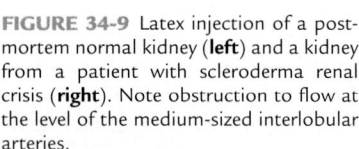

FIGURE 34-9 Latex injection of a postmortem normal kidney (**left**) and a kidney from a patient with scleroderma renal crisis (**right**). Note obstruction to flow at the level of the medium-sized interlobular arteries.

terminal kidney failure, in comparison with only 13% of those with predominantly chronic changes.[192,193]

Chronic Kidney Disease. As in other affected organs, the histologic pattern of chronic kidney involvement is characterized by extensive interstitial fibrosis that is invariably associated with glomerular sclerosis and tubular atrophy. Patterns of glomerulonephritis are occasionally reported but are rare, even in patients with concomitant connective diseases.[130,194]

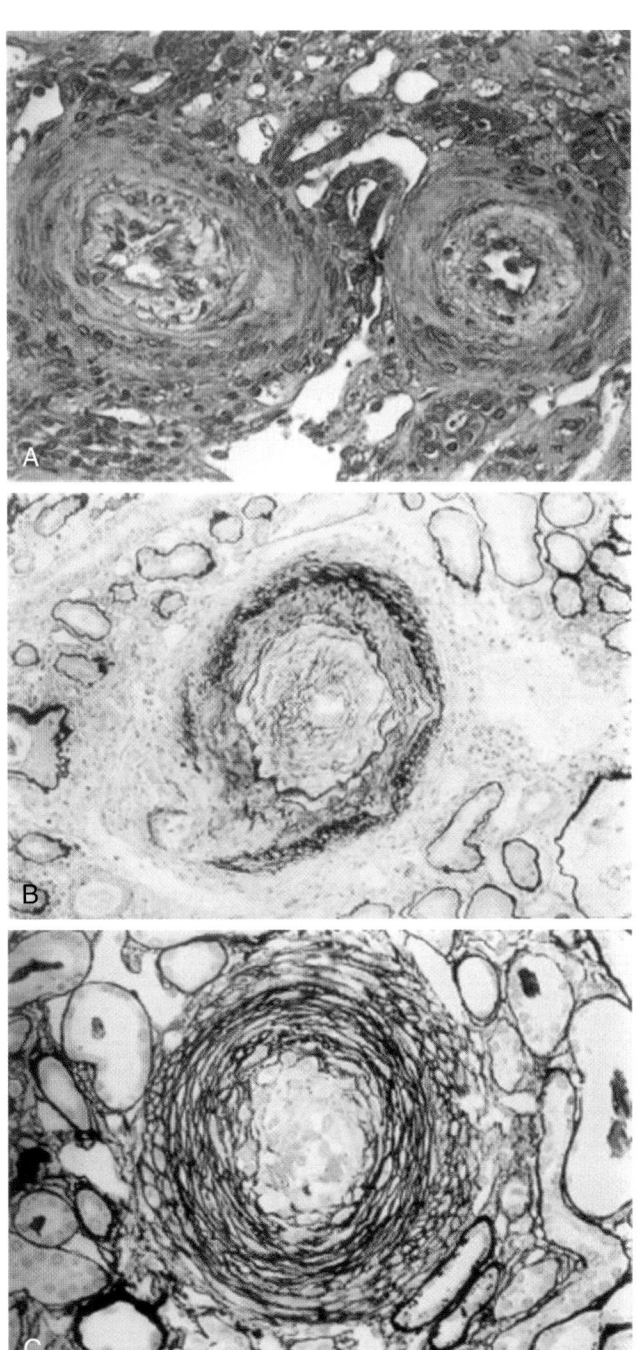

FIGURE 34-10 Micrographs of renal biopsy samples from patients with scleroderma renal crisis. **A,** Lumina of interlobular arteries are narrowed because of intimal thickening (trichrome stain). **B,** The thickened intima has mucoid appearance and is associated with severe luminal narrowing (silver stain). **C,** The arterial wall shows multilayering of the internal elastic lamina and medial hyperplasia (silver stain).

MECHANISMS

The pathogenesis of scleroderma is still unclear; multiple cells and mediators take part in the different phases of the microangiopathic process.[189] Microvascular injury is an early event that is probably initiated by endothelial cell damage with secondary proliferation of basal-laminal layers. Entrapment of peripheral blood mononuclear cells in the vessel wall, as well as perivascular mononuclear cell infiltrates, is occasionally observed. Activated endothelial cells, can release the potent endothelium-derived vasoconstrictor endothelin-1, which induces chemotaxis, proliferation, extracellular matrix production, and the release of cytokines and growth factors that amplify the inflammatory focus. The next phase is characterized by fibrosis, organ architecture disruption, rarefaction of blood vessels, and eventually hypoxia, which perpetuates fibrosis.[189]

Microvascular Injury. Patients with scleroderma often display early signs of vasculopathy; many experience Raynaud's phenomenon, often for many years before overt signs of skin fibrosis develop.[203] In keeping with this process, morphologic changes in capillaries are detectable before or at disease onset, which can be used for early diagnosis through nail fold capillaroscopy. Endothelial injury, whether caused by immunologic stimuli, ischemia-reperfusion injury, or other elements, results in increased production of endothelin-1.[204] Endothelin-1 is involved in the regulation of vascular function under normal physiologic conditions and plays a key role in vascular disease by promoting vasoconstriction, hypertrophy of vascular smooth muscle cells, enhanced vascular permeability, and activation of leukocytes through the induction of cytokine and adhesion molecule expression.[204] The effects of endothelin-1 are mediated upon binding to cognate endothelin types A and B (ET-A and ET-B) receptors. ET-A is expressed mainly on smooth muscle cells and fibroblasts,[203] whereas ET-B is expressed on endothelial cells. The finding that endothelial dysfunction is ameliorated by therapy with the endothelin-1 antagonist bosentan provides additional, although indirect, evidence of the pathogenic role of the endothelin system in the vascular damage of scleroderma.[203]

Increased Collagen Production. Fibroblast secretion of collagen, the main extracellular matrix component of connective tissue, is markedly increased in scleroderma.[205,206] Cytokines and growth factors—such as TGF-β, connective tissue growth factor, platelet-derived growth factor (PDGF), and endothelin-1—that are secreted in the skin and lungs activate resident fibroblasts, promoting accumulation of collagen, proteoglycans, fibronectin, tenascin, and elastin.[207,208] Furthermore, TGF-β induces the differentiati on of fibroblasts into smooth muscle cell–like myofibroblasts in situ. Myofibroblasts produce matrix molecules and profibrotic cytokines that increase the stiffness of the extracellular matrix. Moreover, they are relatively resistant to apoptosis, and they accumulate and persist in affected tissues, in which they contribute to further progression of the fibrosis. Bone marrow–derived mesenchymal progenitor cells fuel expansion of fibroblast population within affected tissue, which then further contributes to connective tissue accumulation. The signals that induce the bone marrow to mobilize progenitor cells and govern their homing and engraftment in lesional tissue remain largely unknown. An intriguing finding in patients with scleroderma is circulating antibodies directed against the PDGF receptor that activate fibroblasts.[209] Once collagen is secreted into the extracellular space, it undergoes cross-linking and maturation, which results in a highly stable matrix that accounts for the stiffness of fibrotic skin and other tissues. The stiff matrix may itself serve as a strong stimulus for integrin-mediated TGF-β activation and increasing fibrosis.[209]

Immunologic Mediators. Researchers have discovered a wide spectrum of autoantibodies that may have a major role in the pathogenesis of scleroderma—including autoantibodies against extracellular matrix components such as metalloproteinases and fibrillin-1, against fibroblasts and endothelial cells, and against the PDGF receptor—and have been associated with different clinical manifestations and outcomes. Thus, a careful evaluation of circulating autoantibodies is essential for predicting individual risk and to guide the treatment. Patients with anticentromere antibodies have limited cutaneous involvement and good outcome, provided that pulmonary hypertension is detected early and treated adequately.[210,211]

Cytokines. Beyond autoantibodies, the immune injury is sustained by the release of cytokines such as interleukins-1, -2, and -8 (IL-1, IL-2, and IL-8); tumor necrosis factor-α (TNF-α); PDGF; TGF-β; interferon-γ; and endothelin.[204] Moreover, intercellular adhesion molecules and soluble IL-2 receptors have been demonstrated in patients with scleroderma.[212-214] Skin fibroblasts from such patients produce much higher levels of interleukin-6 (IL-6) than do normal fibroblasts and may contribute to T cell activation.[215] IL-6 and PDGF-A were shown to be elevated through the action of endogenous IL-1α in fibroblasts from patients with scleroderma.[216]

Renal Crisis. The renal crisis appear to resemble a Raynaud-like phenomenon in the kidney.[217] Severe vasospasm leads to cortical ischemia and enhanced production of renin and angiotensin II, which in turn sustain renal vasoconstriction. Hormonal changes (as in pregnancy), physical and emotional stress, or cold temperature[205] may trigger the Raynaud-like arterial vasospasm. The role of the renin-angiotensin system in perpetuating renal ischemia is underscored by the significant benefit of ACE inhibitors in treating this potentially fatal complication.

THERAPY

Although there is no evidence of any effective strategy to prevent renal crises, it is a common practice to advise patients and local physicians of the risk of renal crisis in order to expedite rapid diagnosis and therapy. A major advancement in the treatment of scleroderma renal crises has been achieved with the introduction of ACE inhibitors in clinical practice (Table 34-4).[44,198,204,217] Before ACE inhibitors were available, the 1-year survival rate did not exceed 10%, whereas with the use of ACE inhibitors, up to 65% of patients survive the crisis.[44,198] In a prospective cohort study of the short- and long-term outcomes of 154 patients with renal crises treated with ACE inhibitors, researchers found that 61% of patients did not need chronic dialysis, and 80% to 85% were alive 8 years after the event; this survival rate was similar to that of patients with diffuse scleroderma without renal crises.[198-200]

Angiotensin II receptor blockers are less effective than ACE inhibitors and can be considered as add-on therapy when full-dose ACE inhibitor therapy is not sufficient to control the blood pressure.[218,219] α-Blockers and calcium antagonists are also helpful for refractory hypertension, whereas diuretics are best avoided because of their ability to stimulate renin

release.[220] Plasma exchange is also indicated when the renal crisis is accompanied by a microangiopathic process. With the approach described previously in this chapter, it is estimated that approximately two thirds of patients with renal crisis who present to an experienced center will require renal replacement therapy. However, approximately half of these patients eventually recover sufficiently to discontinue dialysis and to be maintained on conservative therapy, and they remain dialysis free. It is surprising but well documented that appropriately treated patients with scleroderma renal crisis may recover renal function even as late as 2 years after renal replacement therapy. This should be taken into consideration before patients join a waiting list for kidney transplantation.[192]

Renal transplant recipients who had progressed to end-stage renal disease because of renal crises have lower graft and patient survival rates than do transplant recipients with diabetic renal disease.[221] One of the causes of premature graft failure or patient mortality is the recurrence of the disease in the transplanted kidney, particularly in patients with more aggressive disease before transplantation.[222-224] New therapies for scleroderma include endothelin receptor blockers

TABLE 34-4	Therapies Used in Treatment of Scleroderma, Dosages, and Efficacy	
THERAPY	**DOSAGE**	**EFFICACY**
Antimetabolites: methotrexate	10-25 mg/week	Disappointing results, with only mild effect on skin disease
Antioxidants*	1 tablet/day	Not effective
Corticosteroids: dexamethasone	100 mg/month for 6 months	Improvement in skin scores
Endothelin receptor antagonists: bosentan	62.5 mg for 4 weeks, then 125 mg for 12 weeks	Improvement in pulmonary function
Hormones: relaxin	25/100 μg/kg/day (IV)	Improvement in skin scores
Immunosuppressive: cyclophosphamide	600 mg/m²	Significant, albeit modest, improvement in lung function
Interferons		Disappointing results with interferon-α, improved organ involvement with interferon-γ
Interferon-2α Interferon-γ	13.5 × 10⁶ units/week 300 mg/week	
RAS inhibitors ACE inhibitors Angiotensin II inhibitors	Up to maximal tolerated doses	Improved renal graft and patient survival in renal crisis, slowed progression in chronic renal involvement
Prostacyclin analogs		Improvement in pulmonary function
Iloprost Beraprost	960 ng/kg/day (IV) 60 μg three times daily	
Nonpharmacologic treatment: photopheresis		Not effective

*Selenium, β-carotene, vitamin E, vitamin C, and methionine.
ACE, Angiotensin converting enzyme; *IV,* intravenously; *RAS,* renin angiotensin system.
From Henness S, Wigley FM: Current drug therapy for scleroderma and secondary Raynaud's phenomenon: evidence-based review, *Curr Opin Rheumatol* 2007;19(6):611-618.

(bosentan), phosphodiesterase 5 inhibitors, prostanoids, antioxidants, and low-molecular-weight heparin. In patients with scleroderma and pulmonary hypertension, bosentan therapy prevented deterioration in exercise capacity and improved survival. Bosentan was also effective in reducing the number of new digital ulcers in patients with either a history of ulcers or an active ulcer, but it had no effect on promotion of healing of existing ulcers (see Table 34-4).[224] After initial encouraging results, studies failed to confirm any appreciable long-term benefit from prostacyclin analogues (iloprost and beraprost).[224]

Sickle Cell Disease

Sickle cell anemia, and occasionally the heterozygous forms of sickle cell disease, can lead to multiple renal abnormalities, which include hematuria, proteinuria, tubular dysfunction, or a combination of these, eventually resulting in renal function impairment.

CLINICAL FEATURES

Hematuria and Renal Papillary Necrosis. Gross and often painless hematuria is one of the most frequent features of sickle cell anemia (Hb-SS genotype), sickle cell trait (Hb-AS) disease, and sickle–hemoglobin C (Hb-SC) disease.[225] Hematuria in sickle cell disease can occur at any age and is reported most often with Hb-AS2.[226] A total of 15% to 36% of patients with sickle cell disease develop renal papillary necrosis,[225] which could manifest as an episode of gross hematuria or may be clinically silent. Papillary necrosis occurs in both the homozygous and the heterozygous forms of sickle cell disease and is best diagnosed through intravenous pyelography (Figure 34-11). Microscopic hematuria is present in most patients with sickle cell anemia. The origin of blood is more commonly the left kidney, but either kidney may be involved.[225]

Proteinuria. Proteinuria occurs in 20% to 30% of patients with sickle cell disease and more commonly in the homozygous Hb-SS state than in the heterozygous Hb-SA state; patients with with Hb-SC have an intermediate incidence.[226] Urine protein values can be in the nephrotic or nonnephrotic range. Patients with nephrotic values have a poorer prognosis and tend to progress to renal failure.[226]

Tubular Dysfunction. In patients with homozygous and heterozygous forms of sickle cell disease, the urine fails to concentrate maximally because of erythrocyte sickling in the medullary microcirculation, with secondary medullary ischemia and dysfunction. This abnormality is reversible with multiple transfusions for children younger than 15 years of age, but it becomes irreversible later in life.[227] Patients with sickle cell anemia are capable of diluting their urine normally. Another renal defect seen in patients with sickle cell disease, particularly those with the Hb-SS or Hb-SC genotype, is an incomplete form of distal renal tubule acidosis characterized by the inability to achieve minimal urinary pH during acid loading. This acidification defect, however, is usually not severe enough to cause systemic acidosis. Patients with sickle cell trait (Hb-AS) do not have evidence of impaired urinary acidification. Other tubule defects in sickle cell anemia include mild impairment of K^+ excretion that does not commonly lead to clinical hyperkalemia.[226] Fractional excretion of creatinine is increased, which necessitates the use of inulin clearance to measure GFR accurately.[227] However, Herrera and colleagues[228] demonstrated an impaired tubular secretion of creatinine in patients with sickle cell anemia who had normal GFR. In addition, phosphorus reabsorption in the proximal tubule is increased, which could account for the hyperphosphatemia observed in patients with sickle cell anemia.[227]

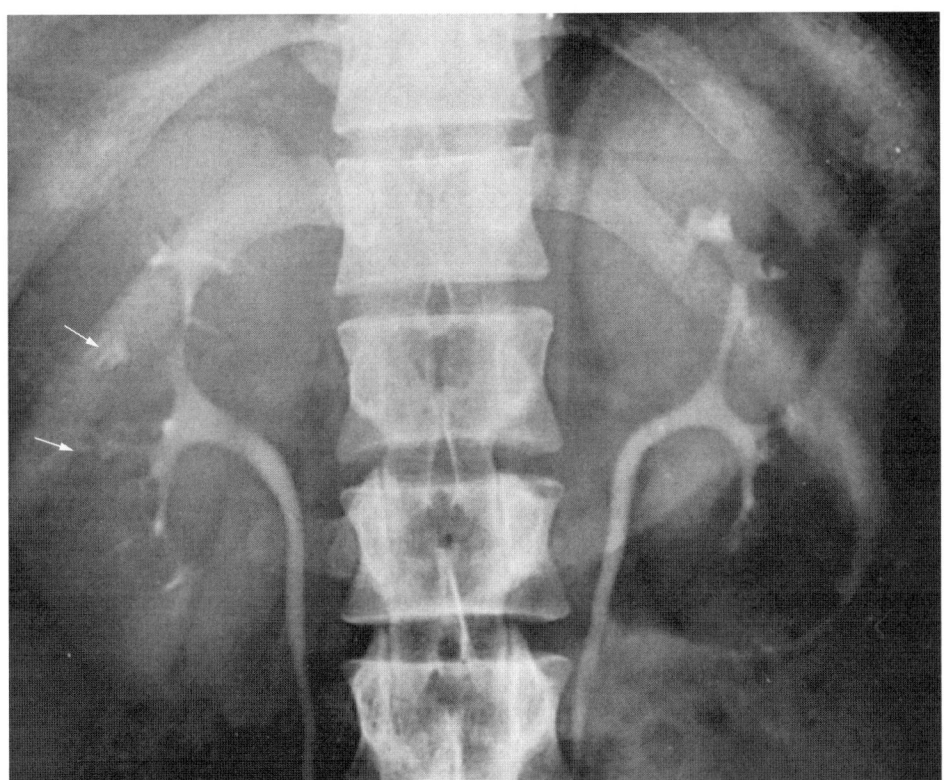

FIGURE 34-11 Renal papillary necrosis with various forms of cavitation in a 33-year-old man with sickle cell hemoglobinopathy and hematuria. Kidneys are normal size and smooth in contour. Central cavitation is present in many papillae, particularly in right interpolar areas (*arrows*). (From Davidson AJ, Hartman DS: *Radiology of the kidney and urinary tract,* ed 2, Philadelphia, 1994, W.B. Saunders, p 184.)

PATHOLOGY

In 1923, Sydenstricker and colleagues[229] described enlarged glomeruli distended with blood in the kidneys of patients with sickle cell disease. Necrosis and pigmentation of tubular cells were also observed.[225] Medullary lesions are the most prominent finding in the kidneys of these patients. Edema, focal scarring, interstitial fibrosis, and tubule atrophy are observed. Cortical infarction has also been reported in patients with sickle cell disease or sickle cell trait.[225] In Hb-SS patients without renal insufficiency, renal pathologic features include glomerular hypertrophy characterized by open, dilated glomerular capillary loops.[230] Enlarged glomeruli are most commonly found in the juxtamedullary region of the kidney. In patients with proteinuria and mild renal insufficiency, Falk and associates[231] reported glomerular hypertrophy and focal segmental glomerulosclerosis; the latter is thought to be the most common cause of renal failure in sickle cell disease.[232] In a study of 240 adult patients with sickle cell anemia and the nephrotic syndrome, Bakir and associates[233] reported the observation of mesangial expansion and glomerular basement membrane duplication on electron microscopic study, as well as effacement of epithelial cell foot processes. These changes are suggestive of hyperfiltration injury and often are referred to in these patients as *sickle cell glomerulopathy*. Membranoproliferative pathologic features were observed in some patients with sickle cell anemia, the majority of whom had no immune deposits.[225,232]

MECHANISMS

The underlying biologic defect in sickle cell disease is a single amino acid substitution of valine for glutamic acid at the sixth position in the hemoglobin β-chain. This alteration leads to aggregation of deoxygenated sickle cell hemoglobin (Hb-SS) tetramer molecules, resulting in deformation of the shape and decreased flexibility of erythrocytes.[234] Hb-SS polymer formation is promoted by higher degrees of deoxygenation, increased intracellular hemoglobin concentration, and the absence of fetal hemoglobin (Hb F).[234] As erythrocytes from sickle cell patients flow through arterioles and capillaries with decreasing oxygen content, Hb-SS polymerization may occur, increasing the adherence of Hb-SS erythrocytes to the vascular endothelium. Gee and Platt[235] and Wong and colleagues[236] found that sickle reticulocytes adhere to the endothelium via vascular cell adhesion molecule-1 (VCAM-1). Kumar and associates[237] reported that increased adherence of sickled erythrocytes to the endothelium involves α4β1 integrin receptors. α4β1 Integrins on the cell surface of erythrocytes bind to both fibronectin and VCAM-1 on endothelial cells. VCAM-1 expression is induced on the vascular endothelium by the presence of proinflammatory cytokines, such as TNF-α.[226] Platelet activation has also been suggested to play a role in sickle cell–mediated vasoocclusion.[238] Thrombospondin from activated platelets promotes adherence of sickled erythrocytes to the microvascular endothelium.[238] Increased concentration of intracellular hemoglobin of patients with sickle cell disease may promote polymerization and trigger the sickling process.

The pathogenesis of medullary renal lesions in sickle cell disease is the result of microvascular occlusion by erythrocytes that carry the mutant hemoglobin β-chain. Erythrocytes passing through the vessels of the inner renal medulla and the renal papillae are most vulnerable to sickling because of the decreasing oxygen content of the medulla and the high osmolality of the blood, which leads to cell shrinkage and increased hemoglobin concentration.

The pathogenesis of sickle cell glomerulopathy is generally attributed to hyperfiltration, which is common in children affected by the disease. Later in life, the GFR often declines, despite persistent high renal blood flow rates.[226] Guasch and associates[239,240] described a distinct pattern of glomerular dysfunction in patients with sickle cell anemia that consists of a generalized increase in permeability to dextrans that is secondary to increased pore radius in the glomerular basement membrane. With progression to chronic renal failure, the number of pores is reduced, and a size-selectivity defect occurs.[239] This abnormality may account for the proteinuria observed in patients with sickle cell glomerulopathy. Schmitt and colleagues[241] found that in early dysfunction, the ultrafiltration coefficient is increased. Hypoxia and decreased blood flow with a secondary increase in endothelin-1 secretion have been suggested in the pathogenesis of sickle cell nephropathy.[242,243] In addition, roles for nitric oxide and the activation of nitric oxide synthase have also been studied in the mechanism of glomerular hyperfiltration[244] and in ischemia- and reperfusion-mediated apoptosis of cells.[245]

THERAPY

The management of patients with sickle cell disease is targeted at limiting sickle cell crises and end-organ damage. Factors that trigger sickling, such as infection and dehydration, should be treated aggressively. Exposure to hypoxia, cold, or medications that may induce sickle cell crisis should be avoided. Treatment options include transfusion therapy and, more recently, bone marrow trasplantation.[246] Of interest is that multiple transfusions may restore urinary concentrating capacity in very young children with sickle cell anemia.[227] A conservative approach for hematuria is suggested, in view of its generally benign course. Maintaining high urinary flow through adequate fluid intake and use of diuretics is helpful in clearing clots from the bladder. Alternative approaches targeting pathogenic mechanisms have been proposed. The use of hydroxyurea in patients with sickle cell anemia aims at increasing the formation of Hb-F instead of Hb-SS. Studies in adults and children showed that Hb-F reduced the incidence of acute sickling episodes and allowed normal growth and development in children.[226] The use of ACE inhibitors significantly reduced proteinuria, and combined therapy with ACE inhibitor and hydroxyurea may prevent progression from microalbuminuria to frank proteinuaria,[226,227] but its effect on the rate of progression of sickle cell glomerulopathy remains to be studied.[225]

Patients with sickle cell disease who reach ESRD have a 60% survival rate at 2 years after the administration of renal replacement therapy. Dialysis is the most common form of renal replacement therapy employed. Kidney transplantation as a possible alternative to dialysis has been attempted with reported successes. However, most patients experience further episodes of painful sickle crises after renal transplantation.[225] Moreover, sickle cell nephropathy may recur after transplantation.[225] Follow-up studies of allograft recipients demonstrated lower rates of 3-year graft and patient survival in patients with sickle cell disease than in other patients with ESRD.[223,247] Nevertheless, an analysis of U.S. Renal Data System files for 2000 and earlier revealed that the rate of 10-year survival among patients who underwent renal transplantation was significantly higher than that of those who remained on chronic hemodialysis. These encouraging results should be taken into consideration when renal replacement therapy is offered to patients with end-stage sickle cell nephropathy.[166,248] There is no evidence supporting the use of nonsteroidal antiinflammatory drugs (NSAIDs) or steroids in the management or prevention of sickle cell nephropathy.[225]

Antiphospholipid Syndrome

The antiphospholipid syndrome (APS) is an autoimmune disorder characterized by hypercoagulability, arterial and venous thromboses, and pregnancy-related morbidity.[249] The diagnosis rests on the detection of lupus anticoagulant, anticardiolipin, or anti–β2-glycoprotein I antibodies persisting in the circulation for a minimum of 12 weeks. The cellular basis of APS-associated clinical manifestations is a variety of autoantibody effects on coagulation pathways—including the procoagulant actions of these antibodies on protein C, annexin V, and tissue factor—and impaired fibrinolysis. The interface between the endothelium and the fluid phase of blood is the major site of autoantibody-mediated injury. The syndrome may be an isolated, idiopathic entity or is found in subjects with other immune diseases, particularly systemic lupus erythematosus (SLE).[249] When APS is associated with SLE, rates of morbidity and mortality are markedly increased. Antiphospholipid antibodies are also found in otherwise healthy subjects (<1% in the general population and up to 5% of older persons). In those with SLE, the prevalence of antiphospholipid antibodies is much higher; IgG anticardiolipin, IgM anticardiolipin, and lupus anticoagulant have been observed in 24%, 13%, and 15% of patients, respectively.[250] Of note is that patients with persistently moderate to high anticardiolipin levels, lupus anticoagulant, or both who had sustained previous thrombotic events are at higher risk of future events than are patients with no history of thrombotic events.[251]

CLINICAL FEATURES

The most common manifestations of APS include deep vein thrombosis, pulmonary embolism, stroke, myocardial infarction, and renal macrovascular and microvascular thrombosis. Livedo reticularis is a hallmark of the disease that is almost invariably predictive of a poor outcome. Hypertension is frequent,[252] affecting more than 90% of patients with renal involvement,[253] and is often associated with vascular lesions, including arteriosclerosis, fibrous intimal hyperplasia, arterial and arteriolar fibrous and fibrocellular occlusions, and thrombotic microangiopathy. Poorly controlled hypertension often reflects renal artery stenosis, a disease that may affect up to 26% of hypertensive patients with antiphospholipid antibodies, in comparison with only 8% of young patients attending a hypertension clinic and 3% of live-related renal transplant donors with stenosis.[254] The stenotic lesions are generally smooth, noncritical stenoses in the midportion of the renal artery, quite distinct from either fibromuscular dysplasia or atherosclerosis. **Thrombotic Microangiopathy.** This is one of the more serious manifestations of APS. It may be isolated or may be a component of catastrophic APS, a rare but devastating disease that manifests in approximately 1% of patients with alternative pathway antibodies, in most cases triggered by an event such as infection, trauma, or surgery. Hypertension and proteinuria are almost invariable findings associated with renal impairment, even in the early phases of the disease. Proteinuria is

mild, and the sudden onset of nephrotic-range proteinuria may reflect a concomitant thrombosis of the renal veins and inferior vena cava. Outcome is poor, particularly when lupus nephritis and catastrophic APS are present.[255] In catastrophic APS, three or more target organs are involved, multiorgan failure is frequent, and the mortality rate approximates 50%.[256]

PATHOLOGY

Kidney biopsy samples from patients with APS-associated thrombotic microangiopathy show focal or diffuse microangiopathic changes affecting the whole intrarenal vascular tree and the glomerular tufts, with fresh as well as old and recanalizing thrombi.[257] Both acute and chronic microangiopathic abnormalities can coexist. Ultrastructural findings pathognomonic for APS nephropathy include a combination of wrinkling and reduplication of the glomerular basement membrane and redundant, wrinkled segments of basement membrane with straighter thin basement membrane sections adjacent to the endothelium.[257] Small arterioles can also be affected by a noninflammatory and frequently thrombotic vasculopathy. These changes, however, are less specific, inasmuch as they are observed in a wide variety of conditions, including TTP, HUS, scleroderma renal crisis, malignant hypertension, preeclampsia, postpartum renal failure, cyclosporine or chemotherapy toxicity, and renal transplant rejection.[249,257]

THERAPY

Risk factors for atherosclerosis and cardiovascular disease include obesity, smoking, hypertension, diabetes, and hyperlipidemia; these should be addressed with lifestyle measures and appropriate pharmacologic therapy. Oral contraceptives and estrogen replacement therapy are absolutely contraindicated because of their association with thromboembolic complications. Aspirin, heparin, warfarin, and immunosuppressive drugs are key elements of pharmacologic therapy for APS. Effective anticoagulation may help preventing worsening of hypertension, stent reocclusions, and progressive renal impairment, and it should be considered, even in the absence of previous thrombotic events.[258] Treatment with rituximab, an anti-CD20 monoclonal antibody, achieved persistent disappearance of alternative pathway antibodies from the circulation in isolated case reports.[259] However, whether this may translate into improvements in clinical outcomes remains to be addressed in adequately designed trials.[260] Thrombotic microangiopathy is an indication for plasmapheresis with fresh-frozen plasma. In secondary forms of APS, treatment is also be aimed at the underlying renal disease. Thus, steroids and immunosuppressants, including cyclophosphamide therapy, may be indicated in patients with SLE and renal involvement.[249] Recently, treatment with C5 inhibitor eculizumab was reported to safely prevant recurrence of catastrophic APS after renal transplantation.[260a] However, the potential role for complement inhibitors to enable transplantation in such patients will need large-scale investigation.

Macrovascular Diseases

Macrovascular diseases of the kidney include acute occlusion, aneurysms, and dissecting aneurysms and thrombosis of the renal artery. Stenosis of the renal artery is discussed in Chapter 47.

Acute Occlusion of the Renal Artery

Thromboembolism of the Renal Artery

Artery thrombi may form as a result of different conditions, including atherosclerosis, renal artery aneurysm (RAA), fibrinoid dysplasia, and aortic dissection,[261] or in the presence of endothelial injury and enhanced vascular tone secondary to use of vasoactive substances, such as cocaine.[262] Infectious and inflammatory states are also known to predispose to renal artery thrombosis; cases have been reported in patients with polyarteritis nodosa,[263] Takayasu's arteritis,[264] and Behçet's disease.[265] Although inherited hypercoagulable states are classically associated with venous rather than arterial thrombosis,[266] acquired hypercoagulable states—including heparin-induced thrombocytopenia, APS, factor V Leiden mutation, antithrombin, hyperhomocystinemia, and nephrotic syndrome—can lead to arterial thrombosis.[267-271]

CLINICAL FEATURES

The clinical manifestations of renal artery thromboembolism are variable and depend on the extent of renal injury and on the overall clinical picture.[272] Although anuria is characteristic of renal artery involvement in both kidneys and in a solitary kidney, it has been reported in unilateral renal artery thromboembolism, probably because of reflex vasospasm of the contralateral kidney.[273] Patients usually present with unexplained abdominal pain, gross hematuria, abdominal or flank tenderness, fever, and hypertension.[274] Patients may have signs of involvement of other end organs by thromboembolic events, or they may have suffered recent cardiac events, such as atrial fibrillation, endocarditis, or myocardial infarction. Most patients have an elevated serum level of lactate dehydrogenase, and hematuria and leukocytosis are common.[275] Doppler ultrasound examination with contrast agents may be the first-line investigation, although its accuracy is dependent on the operator's skill,[276] and false-negative results are possible.[277] In cases of high clinical suspicion (despite negative Doppler findings), contrast-enhanced CT scanning readily demonstrates the absence of enhancement in the affected renal tissue,[278] although there is concern about further damage to the kidney with the use of iodinated contrast material. Contrast-enhanced three-dimensional magnetic resonance angiography yields sharp images of the renal arteries and of perfusion abnormalities.[279] Isotopic flow scans show absence of or markedly reduced perfusion in the affected kidney.[276] Although angiography is considered the "gold standard" for diagnosis, its use is reserved for situations in which intervention is contemplated.

MECHANISMS

The heart is the main source of peripheral thromboemboli, including those that migrate to the renal arteries.[274] Men and women with atrial fibrillation have a fourfold and almost sevenfold risk, respectively, of developing peripheral thromboemboli in comparison with persons without atrial fibrillation, but only 2% of peripheral emboli secondary to atrial fibrillation target the kidney.[280] Myocardial infarction and heart failure may predispose to the formation of thromboemboli. Valvular heart disease, bacterial endocarditis, heart tumors, and dilated cardiomyopathy are other predisposing factors. The aorta can be a source of renal artery thromboemboli, especially after endovascular repair of aortic aneurysms.[281] The rate of renal infarctions after such a procedure is about 9%.[281] Endovascular revascularization of renal artery stenosis may be complicated by distal emboli as well.[282] However, the use of angioplasty and stents with distal protection baskets may decrease the rate of complications.[272]

THERAPY

The human kidney is believed to tolerate absence of blood flow for 60 to 90 minutes.[283] The presence of adequate collateral circulation from accessory renal arteries and from lumbar, suprarenal, or ureteral vessels may allow the kidney to tolerate longer periods of ischemia than do other organs.[284] The duration and the extent of ischemia are major determinants of the prognosis for an ischemic kidney.[276] Treatment options for an acutely occluded renal artery are surgical embolectomy, percutaneous interventional techniques, and intraarterial thrombolysis.[284] Of patients who undergo surgical interventions, up to 64% experience restored kidney function; however, the mortality rate ranges between 15% and 20%.[285] The outcome of surgical embolectomy has been reported to be worse with regard to kidney function.[286] The use of intraarterial thrombolytic agents has been associated with a high rate of renal artery recanalization[287]; however, the success of the procedure does not always translate into recovery of renal function.[287] Patients who sustain complete occlusions or in whom treatment is delayed have a generally worse prognosis. Nevertheless, several case reports have described favorable outcomes with intraarterial thrombolysis even in cases of prolonged ischemia (20 to 72 hours) and in renal transplant recipients.[276] Successful results have also been reported with the use of systemic thrombolysis. Percutaneous aspiration thrombolectomy and rheolytic thrombectomy have been performed with some success.[285]

Traumatic Thrombosis of the Renal Artery

Renal artery thrombosis is an uncommon sequela of blunt abdominal trauma. Motor vehicle accidents are the main cause of this injury.[288] Renal vessels can be affected by stretch injury, contusion, or avulsion, all of which may lead to thrombosis.[288] The left renal artery is slightly more affected than the right, but bilateral injury may be present as well.[288] Patients with traumatic renal artery thrombosis are usually critically ill and have other associated injuries, most commonly abdominal. The prognosis is poor: the mortality rate reaches 44%.[289]

CLINICAL FEATURES

Patients who have sustained major renal trauma have flank and abdominal pain, nausea, vomiting, and fever. They may develop severe hypertension. In patients with bilateral renal artery thrombosis or thrombosis of a solitary functioning kidney, anuria may develop.[276] Hematuria is present in about 75% of patients. Mild proteinuria is often present. Blood analyses show elevations of serum levels of lactate dehydrogenase, creatine phosphokinase, serum transaminases, and alkaline phosphatase.[276] CT scanning is the preferred diagnostic modality in patients with suspected renal artery thrombosis. It has the advantages of speed, accuracy, and the ability to detect other associated injuries.[288] In patients with renal artery thrombosis, parenchymal enhancement in the affected kidney is usually absent. CT scanning also displays abrupt termination of the renal artery just beyond its origin.[278] The cortex might be enhanced as a result of perfusion from peripheral and collateral arteries; such enhancement is referred to as the *rim sign* on CT scans.[290] The "gold standard" for diagnosis of renal artery injury is renal artery angiography, which shows intimal flaps with partial stenosis or complete occlusion.[288] Angiography has the advantage of detecting the location of the injury with high accuracy; however, angiography is associated with an increased risk of contrast-induced nephropathy and is not usually necessary for confirmation if the CT scan is diagnostic.[278] Ultrasonography is unreliable as a diagnostic evaluation.[291]

THERAPY

Ischemia time is a major determinant of the outcome of revascularization in patients with traumatic renal artery thrombosis; 80% of renal artery revascularizations performed within 12 hours are successful. The success rate decreases with time, reaching zero for revascularizations performed after more than 18 hours.[292] However, there have been case reports of late revascularizations that were successful.[293] Other determinants of the outcome are the extent of renal injury, the presence of collateral circulation, the technical difficulties of the surgical procedure, and the presence of injury to other organs.[276] A significant number of patients who underwent successful surgical revascularization develop hypertension. Many of them eventually require nephrectomy.[294] The outcome of surgical revascularization in patients with unilateral traumatic renal artery thrombosis may not be better than that of observation and medical management.[276] Nevertheless, revascularization is indicated in patients with bilateral renal artery thrombosis and in patients with a solitary kidney who had renal artery thrombosis.[294] Late revascularization may be considered if the kidney size appears normal on imaging studies and if preserved glomerular architecture is noted on renal biopsy.[295] Several surgical procedures can be performed for the repair of a renal pedicle injury: thrombectomy, resection of the injured arterial segment and replacement with a venous or graft bypass, and autotransplantation with ex vivo repair of the vascular lesions.[276] Endovascular stent placements for traumatic intimal tears have been described.[296] Nephrectomy is required at times to control renal hemorrhage.[276]

Aneurysms of the Renal Artery

Results of large autopsy studies suggest that the incidence of RAAs is 0.01% in the general population,[276] but among patients undergoing renal arteriography primarily for the evaluation of renovascular hypertension, the incidence is 1%.[276] Many RAAs remain asymptomatic. However, the clinical concerns with RAAs are their potential to rupture, to thrombose (causing distal embolization), or to lead to renovascular hypertension. Intrarenal aneurysms may erode into adjacent veins to produce arteriovenous fistulae.[276]

Clinical Features

RAAs are classified as saccular, fusiform, or intrarenal and may be located anywhere along the vascular tree, but most of them are found at the bifurcation of the renal artery or in the first-order branch arteries.[297] Saccular aneurysms, the most common type, constitute 60% to 90%. They are typically diagnosed at about 50 years of age but can be seen from 13 to 78 years of age.

Fusiform aneurysms are often seen in medial fibromuscular dysplasia and usually arise distal to a focal stenotic segment, giving the image of a poststenotic dilatation.[300] Occasionally, several small aneurysms in sequence give the "string of beads" appearance seen in fibromuscular dysplasia. Fusiform aneurysms are typically found in young hypertensive patients who undergo renal angiography for the evaluation of renovascular hypertension. As with fibromuscular dysplasia, fusiform aneurysms are more common in women. Fusiform aneurysms have been described in polyarteritis nodosa,[301] Takayasu's arteritis,[302] Behçet's disease,[265] Ehlers-Danlos syndrome,[302] and mycotic aneurysms.[303] Intrarenal aneurysms make up 10% to 15% of RAAs and are frequently multiple. They may be congenital, posttraumatic (e.g., occurring after renal biopsy), or associated with polyarteritis nodosa.

RAAs are sometimes attributed to atherosclerosis, but marked atherosclerotic changes are found in only 16% of cases, and may be secondary.[297] In approximately 20% of cases, RAAs are bilateral. Renal artery stenosis may be associated. RAAs that are asymptomatic are diagnosed as part of a workup for renovascular hypertension. On occasion, patients may complain of flank pain, which should raise the concern of an expanding aneurysm, rupture and hemorrhage, thrombosis or thromboemboli with impending renal infarction, or dissection.[276]

Rupture of RAA, a potentially catastrophic event, may manifest with vascular collapse and hemorrhagic shock. Aneurysm size is a factor in the potential for rupture. Rupture of RAAs less than 2.0 cm in diameter is unusual. Large aneurysms, however, especially those larger than 4.0 cm in diameter, have a greater tendency to rupture, and surgical intervention is usually required.[250] Pregnant women constitute a disproportionate number of cases of RAA rupture. In a review of 43 cases of rupture, 18 (42%) occurred in pregnant women.[298] Most of these occurred during the last trimester of pregnancy, but rupture and hemorrhage also occurred earlier in pregnancy in some cases and during the postpartum period in others.[297] Pathogenic factors include increased renal blood flow, particularly during the last trimester; the effect of female hormones on the vasculature; and increased intraabdominal pressure.[276] Emergency nephrectomy is usually required in this setting to control the hemorrhage. Since 1990, the rates of maternal mortality and fetal mortality have decreased to 6% and 25%, respectively, if the pregnancy reaches the third trimester.[299] If rupture occurs before the third trimester, the rate of fetal mortality approaches 100%. Rupture of RAAs manifests with flank pain, vascular collapse, and shock. Abdominal distension or a flank mass may be detected. Hematuria may be a helpful finding in some patients, but its absence does not rule out the diagnosis. Renal angiography and magnetic resonance angiography are used to diagnose RAA; CT scanning and radionuclide scanning may be useful screening techniques.

Therapy

Various authors have attempted to provide criteria for elective surgical intervention for RAAs.[276] Most agree that an aneurysm larger than 4.0 cm in diameter should be resected, and one less than 2.0 cm in diameter can be safely monitored with periodic imaging studies. There is uncertainty about the aneurysms between 2.1 and 4.0 cm in diameter. Repair of RAAs larger than 3.0 cm in diameter may be prudent in patients with surgical risks if there is reasonable certainty that nephrectomy will not be required.[276] In addition to the large size of the aneurysm, other factors to be considered in the choice for elective surgical intervention including the presence of lobulations, aneurysm expansion over time, presence of signs and symptoms, whether the patient is of childbearing age, localization in a solitary kidney with the potential for embolization or dissection, or presence of secondary renovascular hypertension.[276] Several surgical techniques for treatment of RAAs have been described, but the most commonly used approach is in situ aneurysmectomy and revascularization. When carefully performed, this surgery carries the lowest risk of damage to the kidney and ureter. However, even at experienced centers, almost 5% of patients eventually undergo unplanned nephrectomy because of technical complications encountered during attempted revascularization.[297]

Dissecting Aneurysms of the Renal Artery

Dissecting aneurysms of the renal artery are rare but severe disorders. Chronic dissection manifests most commonly as renovascular hypertension.[300] Acute dissections may manifest dramatically, with malignant hypertension, flank pain, and renal infarction; they can occur spontaneously and can be precipitated by strenuous physical activity or trauma.[304] Fibromuscular dysplasia and atherosclerosis are common predisposing factors that lead to intimal tears, medial necrosis of the artery wall, and dissection. Iatrogenic dissection that occurs after angiographic procedures may be caused by trauma induced by guide wires, catheters, or angioplasty balloons.[276] Dissections have also been found as incidental autopsy findings, apparently without clinical symptoms during life.[276] Renal artery dissections are about three times more common in men as in women, and there is a predilection toward involvement of the right side; however, approximately 20% to 30% are bilateral. Dissection is most common in the age range of 40 to 60 years, although younger patients with fibromuscular dysplasia may be affected. Patients with acute dissection may present with new-onset, accelerated, or worsening hypertension.[305] Flank pain is frequent, and headache may occur, perhaps as a result of hypertension. In some cases, especially with lesions that develop after an angiographic procedure, the patient may be asymptomatic except for worsening hypertension.

Selective angiography is necessary for the diagnosis.[276] The clinical picture is variable. Some patients have persistent severe renovascular hypertension that may be resistant to medical therapy. These patients may benefit from revascularization or nephrectomy if they suffered renal infarction, and many show improvement or complete resolution of hypertension after these procedures.[305] Endovascular interventions have also been reported.[306] Appropriate therapy depends on the severity of the hypertension and its response to therapy. Edwards and colleagues[304] noted adequate responses to medical management in the majority of patients. Other authors have emphasized the importance of vascular reconstruction, which may necessitate autotransplantation.[307]

Thrombosis of the Renal Vein

In adults, renal vein thrombosis (RVT) is associated most commonly with nephrotic syndrome, but it can also occur in a variety of other clinical settings such as tumors, aneurysm, or abscesses (resulting in direct compression) or in hypovolemic or hypercoagulable states.[308] The cumulative prevalence of RVT in nephrotic syndrome ranges from 5% to 62%[309] and is highest among patients affected with membranous nephropathy or membranoproliferative glomerulonephritis.[310]

Clinical Features

Rapidity of the venous occlusion and of the development of venous collateral circulation determines the clinical presentation and resultant renal function.

ACUTE RENAL VEIN THROMBOSIS

Acute presentation is observed most frequently in young patients with a short history of nephrotic syndrome. RVT manifests with acute flank pain, macroscopic hematuria, and loss of renal function[308] and may mimic renal colic or acute pyelonephritis.[311] It should be suspected strongly in such cases, especially in patients with predisposing risk factors for hypercoagulability. In these cases, imaging reveals an enlarged kidney and pyelocaliceal irregularities.[308]

CHRONIC RENAL VEIN THROMBOSIS

Chronic presentation is usually seen in older patients with the nephrotic syndrome[312] who have few or no accompanying symptoms except for peripheral edema, increase in proteinuria, and gradual decline in renal function.[312] Such patients also have a higher incidence of pulmonary emboli and other thromboembolic events.[308]

Diagnostic Procedures

Doppler ultrasonography can depict the actual venous flow, increased blood velocity, and turbulence in a narrowed vein or complete cessation of the flow if the lumen is totally occluded. Doppler color-flow ultrasonography should be the initial noninvasive diagnostic study. However, the accuracy of ultrasonography is highly dependent on the operator's skill, and results of the study have a low specificity (56%) despite a high sensitivity (85%) in experienced hands.[313]

A characteristic radiographic finding of RVT is notching of the ureter, which usually occurs when collateral veins in close relation to the ureters become tortuous as they dilate to form an alternative drainage route. This notching was originally interpreted as representing mucosal edema; however, more detailed radiographic studies revealed indentation of the ureters by the collateral venous circulation. Notching of the ureter is a very infrequent finding in nephrotic patients with RVT and usually occurs only in a minority of patients with chronic rather than acute RVT.[314]

Retrograde pyelography may demonstrate a rectangular, linear mucosal pattern with irregular renal pelvic outlines. Inferior venacavography with selective catheterization of the renal vein establishes the diagnosis of RVT. If the inferior vena cava is patent and free of filling defects, and if adequate streaming of unopacified renal blood is demonstrated to wash out contrast from the inferior vena cava, RVT is unlikely to be present. The Valsalva maneuver is useful during venacavography; when the intraabdominal pressure is increased, the transit of contrast agent and blood from the inferior vena cava is slowed, the proximal part of the main renal vein may be opacified, and the patency of the lumen and even the outline of the thrombus may be demonstrated.[276] The results of the inferior venacavogram are often not diagnostic, however, and selective catheterization of the renal vein must be performed.

A normal renal venogram demonstrates the entire intralobular venous system to the level of the arcuate vein. In general, the use of epinephrine for better visualization of the smaller vessels is not necessary. However, in the presence of normal renal blood flow, all contrast material is washed out of the renal vein within 3 seconds or less, and occasionally only the main renal vein and major branches are visualized. In this situation, the presence of thrombi in major or smaller branches may be uncertain. In that circumstance, the use of intrarenal arterial epinephrine, by decreasing blood flow, enhances retrograde venous filling and allows later visualization of the smaller intrarenal veins. An abnormal renal venogram usually demonstrates a thrombus within the lumen as a filling defect surrounded by contrast material. In the presence of partial thrombosis, extensive collateral circulation can be demonstrated. The presence of such collateral vessels usually reflects the chronicity of the RVT and may explain the lack of renal functional deterioration.[276]

Both contrast-enhanced CT scanning and magnetic resonance imaging (MRI) have been used for the diagnosis of RVT. Both are less invasive than venography; CT scanning entails the use of ionizing radiation and iodinated contrast agent, and hence MRI has significant advantages over CT scanning.[313] Because MRI produces highly contrasting images of flowing blood, vascular walls, and surrounding tissues, vascular patency may be determined by this technique best. However, low signal from the renal veins and pseudofilling defects due to slow flow in proximity of the thrombus makes interpretation of image difficult.[313] Gadolinium-enhanced MRI can overcome the limitation of poor signal from the renal vessels, and on a delayed second scan, the venous anatomy is well demonstrated, and occult renal artery stenosis can also be revealed.[313] Gadolinium, however, should not be used in patients with significant impairment of renal function because of the risk of nephrogenic systemic fibrosis.

Mechanisms

NEPHROTIC SYNDROME

Multiple hemostatic abnormalities have been described in patients with nephrotic syndrome. A systemic "thrombophilic state" is associated with the increased risk of RVT (Figure 34-12).[315] These abnormalities vary in intensity in proportion to the degree of albuminuria and hypoalbuminemia.[315]

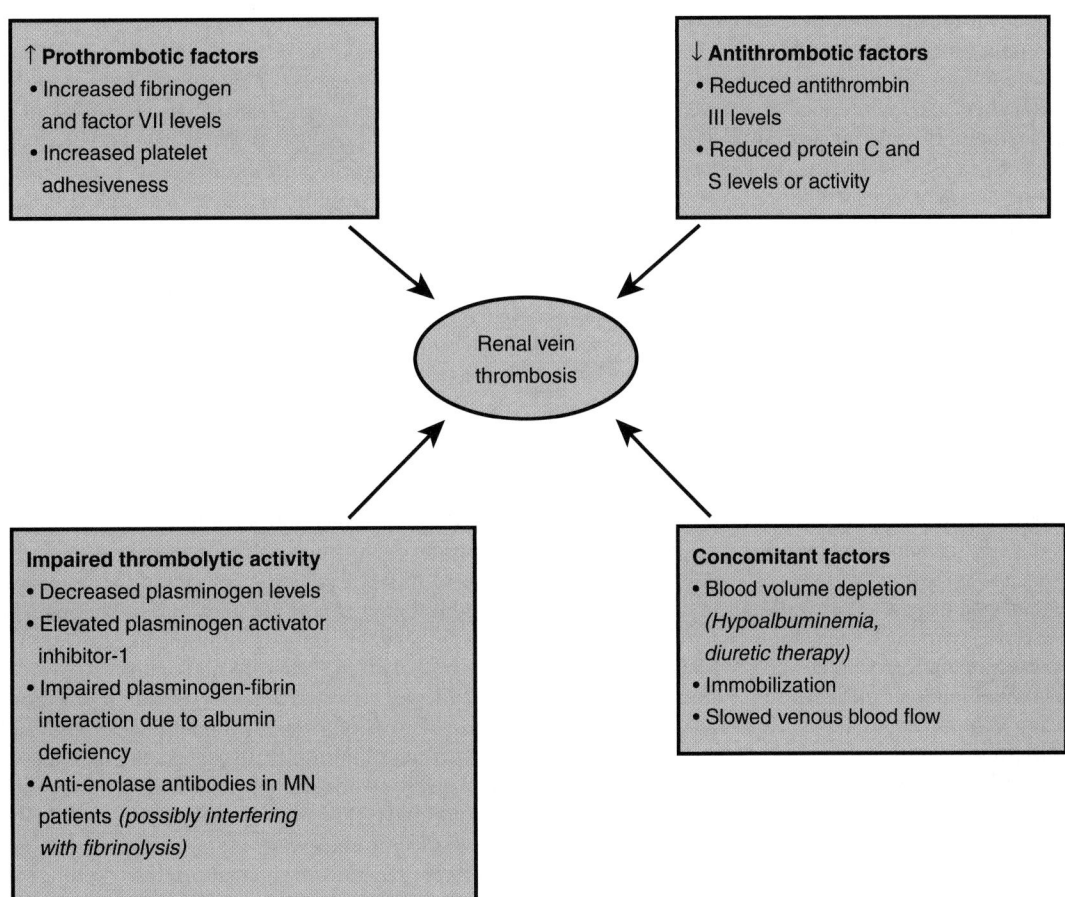

FIGURE 34-12 Pathogenic factors predisposing to renal vein thrombosis in patients with the nephrotic syndrome. If the bioavailability of prothrombotic and antithrombotic factors is imbalanced in favor of prothrombotic factors, the risk of intravascular clotting is higher. Impaired thrombolysis and concomitant factors such as volume depletion, hypoalbuminemia, impaired venous blood flow, and immobilization may contribute to precipitate renal vein thrombosis.

The underlying mechanisms of the "thrombophilia" of the nephrotic syndrome are essentially related to an imbalance of prothrombotic factors (e.g., increased fibrinogen levels, increased factor VIII levels, increased platelet adhesiveness) and antithrombotic factors (e.g., reduced antithrombin III levels and reduced protein C and S levels or activity) and impaired thrombolytic activity (decreased plasminogen levels, elevated plasminogen activator inhibitor-1 levels or albumin deficiency–related impairment of the interaction of plasminogen and fibrin).

An additional mechanism that sustains the procoagulant state is thrombocytosis, which has been found in a number of nephrotic adults and children. Moreover, platelets of nephrotic patients seem to display a tendency for hyperaggregability.[316] Hypoalbuminemia results in higher availability of arachidonic acid for the synthesis of the proaggregant thromboxane A_2 within platelets. Platelet activation may also be enhanced by high levels of cholesterol, fibrinogen, and vWF and by thrombin and immune complexes.[310] Volume depletion, diuretic or steroid therapy (or both), venous stasis, immobilization, or immune complex activation of the clotting cascade may also participate in the "thrombophilia" of the nephrotic syndrome. In nephrotic patients with edema and increases in total body salt content, the enhanced filtration fraction is also relevant inasmuch as efferent arteriolar hematocrit and oncotic pressure increase with increased filtrate removal within the glomerulus. It remains a mystery why only certain conditions have such a strong (but variable) association with RVT. The discovery of the association of antienolase autoantibodies with membranous nephropathy offers a tantalizing clue, because these autoantibodies could interfere with fibrinolysis.[317] The coexistence of another "thrombophilic" state, such as hereditary resistance to the activation of protein C (Leiden trait), with nephrotic syndrome could also be involved in the generation of thrombotic events in selected patients.[315,318]

OTHER PREDISPOSING FACTORS

In addition to the hemostatic abnormalities associated with the nephrotic syndrome, other etiologic factors include amyloidosis, oral contraceptives, steroid administration, and genetic procoagulant defects.[311] Thrombosis can occur secondary to trauma (blunt, surgical),[312] neoplasms (hypernephroma, Wilms' tumor), extrinsic compression (from retroperitoneal tumors, pregnancy, lymphoma), arterial diagnostic puncture,[312] placement of central catheters, and functional states of hypoperfusion such as congestive heart failure.[312] Hypovolemia, a cause of RVT in neonates, has also been reported in adults. Morrissey and colleagues[312] reported a case of bilateral RVT in a previously healthy 22-year-old man that resulted in moderate proteinuria without underlying glomerular disease and with a normal coagulation profile. The RVT was preceded by a 3-day history of nausea and vomiting, which were the only precipitating events. Treatment with fibrinolytic agents followed by heparin was successful.[312]

Other studies[316] have suggested that RVT may be triggered by hypovolemia. Steroids aggravate hypercoagulable states by increasing levels of factor VIII and other serum proteins and by decreasing fibrinolytic activity.[319] Historically, the advent of steroid therapy coincided with an increase in thromboembolic complications.[320] The use of oral contraceptives has been implicated as an additional cause of RVT and may unmask an underlying hypercoagulable disorder.[311]

TABLE 34-5   Maternal and Patient Risk Factors for Renal Vein Thrombosis

MATERNAL RISK FACTORS	PATIENT RISK FACTORS
Fetal distress: 26%	Respiratory distress: 30%
Diabetes, traumatic birth: 17%	Cardiac disease, diarrhea/dehydration, hypotension, polycythemia, factor V Leiden heterozygosity: 13%
Steroids, preeclampsia: 13%	Femoral/umbilical catheter, protein C deficiency, twin-twin transfusion: 4%
Polyhydramnios, amphetamine, protein C deficiency: 4%	No patient risk factors: 26%
No maternal risk factors: 35%	

From Zigman A, Yazbeck S, Emil S, et al: Renal vein thrombosis: a 10-year review, *J Pediatr Surg* 2000;35:1540-1542.

Acute RVT has been noted with increasing frequency in transplanted kidneys,[321] which, unlike native kidneys, have a single drainage system. In this setting, RVT may be accompanied by thrombosis of extrarenal sites.[271] RVT usually leads to permanent damage of the graft within hours. Predisposing factors are OKT3 and cyclosporine therapy.[321] Neonatal RVT accounts for 15% to 20% of systemic thromboembolic events in neonates and results in significant long-term morbidity.[322] Maternal and patient risk factors for RVT are presented in Table 34-5.

Therapy

TREATMENT OF OVERT THROMBOTIC OR EMBOLIC EVENTS

Treatment of established RVT can be categorized as measures targeting the specific cause of the occlusion (primary renal disease, tumors, systemic disease) and those aimed at the thrombus itself or its complications (or both). The latter include volume resuscitation, dialysis as necessary, and—first and foremost—anticoagulation. Current management of RVT has shifted from surgical to medical.[323]

Anticoagulation and Thrombolysis. Anticoagulation is the mainstay of therapy[308] and is intended both to prevent further propagation of the thrombus and thromboembolic complications and to enable recanalization of occluded vessels.[309] Thrombolytic agents provide the possibility of more rapid and complete resolution than do anticoagulants, at the expense of a higher risk of bleeding.[308] The efficacy of anticoagulants in relation to that of fibrinolytic agents in the treatment of RVT is not well defined.[308] Thrombolytic therapy is probably warranted in patients with bilateral RVT, extension into the inferior vena cava, pulmonary embolism, acute kidney injury or acute renal failure, or severe flank pain.[308]

Choice of systemic versus local administration depends on the evaluation of risk and benefit factors. Systemic administration is safe and effective if no obvious contraindications exist, and it avoids the need for invasive procedures.[324] Anticoagulation is indicated in nephrotic patients who experience a thromboembolic event. Heparin should be given, although its effect may be attenuated in the presence of low antithrombin III levels. It is rare for antithrombin III deficiency in nephrotic patients to cause heparin resistance.[319] If antithrombin III level are extremely low, fresh-frozen plasma or antithrombin III concentrates can be administered.[325] After heparin administration, oral vitamin K antagonists should be given. The optimal duration of warfarin therapy is unknown, but in view of the risk of recurrence, it is reasonable to maintain anticoagulation as long as the patient is nephrotic and has significant hypoalbuminemia. Treatment with heparin warrants monitoring of the anticoagulation response and is associated with some complications such as thrombocytopenia and osteoporosis.[326] Low-molecular-weight heparin has been suggested as an alternative in the treatment of RVT.[326]

Prophylactic Anticoagulation of Asymptomatic Patients with Nephrotic Syndrome. No randomized, controlled trials have been conducted to assess the risk/benefit profile of anticoagulation therapy in patients with nephrotic syndrome. However, a Markov-based decision analysis model[327] revealed that the number of fatal emboli prevented by prophylactic anticoagulation exceeds the number of episodes of fatal bleeding in nephrotic patients with idiopathic membranous nephropathy. Before formal evidence from a properly designed randomized trial is available, decision-making algorithms for initiation of anticoagulant therapy should be decided on an individual patient basis. Patients who have severe nephrotic syndrome, regardless of underlying cause and a history of a thromboembolic event (deep venous thrombosis or pulmonary embolus) should be offered prophylactic anticoagulants if no contraindications exist. Patients with severe nephrotic syndrome (serum albumin level <2.0 to 2.5 g/dL) should also be considered candidates for prophylactic anticoagulation if they have other risk factors for thrombosis (e.g., congestive heart failure; prolonged immobilization; morbid obesity; abdominal, orthopedic, or gynecologic surgery). Patients with a family history of "thrombophilia" might also be considered for prophylactic therapy. An alternative therapeutic approach is low-dose aspirin, in view of the increased platelet function in nephrotic patients.[328] In one retrospective study,[329] researchers assessed the influence of low-dose aspirin on the incidence of RVT in patients who received renal transplants from deceased and living-related donors and were being treated with cyclosporine-based triple immunosuppression; findings showed that the incidence of RVT, although not abolished, decreased significantly with the addition of low-dose aspirin to the therapeutic regimen.

Acknowledgments

The authors are grateful to Marina Noris for her invaluable contribution to the discussion of thrombotic microangiopathies and to Franco Marchetti and Mauro Abbate for their help in preparing the iconography of the chapter.

References

1. Remuzzi G. HUS and TTP: variable expression of a single entity. *Kidney Int.* 1987;32:292-308.
2. Gasser C, Gautier E, Steck A, et al. [Hemolytic-uremic syndrome: bilateral necrosis of the renal cortex in acute acquired hemolytic anemia]. *Schweiz Med Wochenschr.* 1955;85:905-909.
3. Ruggenenti P, Noris M, Remuzzi G. Thrombotic microangiopathy, hemolytic uremic syndrome, and thrombotic thrombocytopenic purpura. *Kidney Int.* 2001;60:831-846.
4. Constantinescu AR, Bitzan M, Weiss LS, et al. Non-enteropathic hemolytic uremic syndrome: causes and short-term course. *Am J Kidney Dis.* 2004;43:976-982.
5. Noris M, Remuzzi G. Atypical hemolytic-uremic syndrome. *N Engl J Med.* 2009;361:1676-1687.
6. Noris M, Remuzzi G. Hemolytic uremic syndrome. *J Am Soc Nephrol.* 2005;16:1035-1050.
7. Crowther MA, George JN. Thrombotic thrombocytopenic purpura: 2008 update. *Cleve Clin J Med.* 2008;75:369-375.
8. Galbusera M, Noris M, Remuzzi G. Thrombotic thrombocytopenic purpura—then and now. *Semin Thromb Hemost.* 2006;32:81-89.
9. George JN. Clinical practice. Thrombotic thrombocytopenic purpura. *N Engl J Med.* 2006;354:1927-1935.
10. Moschcowitz E. An acute febrile pleiochromic anemia with hyaline thrombosis of the terminal arterioles and capillaries: an undescribed disease. 1925. *Mt Sinai J Med.* 2003;70:352-355.
11. Ruggenenti P, Galli M, Remuzzi G. Hemolytic uremic syndrome, thrombotic thrombocytopenic purpura, and antiphospholipid antibody syndromes. In: Neilson EG, Couser WG, eds. *Immunologic renal diseases.* Philadelphia: Lippincott Williams & Wilkins; 2001:pp 1179-1208.
12. Rock G, Kelton JG, Shumak KH, et al. Laboratory abnormalities in thrombotic thrombocytopenic purpura. Canadian Apheresis Group. *Br J Haematol.* 1998;103:1031-1036.
13. Kaplan BS, Proesmans W. The hemolytic uremic syndrome of childhood and its variants. *Semin Hematol.* 1987;24:148-160.
14. Eknoyan G, Riggs SA. Renal involvement in patients with thrombotic thrombocytopenic purpura. *Am J Nephrol.* 1986;6:117-131.
15. Richardson SE, Karmali MA, Becker LE, et al. The histopathology of the hemolytic uremic syndrome associated with verocytotoxin-producing *Escherichia coli* infections. *Hum Pathol.* 1988;19:1102-1108.
16. Remuzzi G, Ruggenenti P. Thrombotic microangiopathies. In: Tisher C, Brenner B, eds. *Renal pathology.* Philadelphia: J.B. Lippincott; 1994:pp 1154-1184.
17. Remuzzi G, Ruggenenti P. The hemolytic uremic syndrome. *Kidney Int.* 1995;48:2-19.
18. Donnenberg MS, Tacket CO, James SP, et al. Role of the eaeA gene in experimental enteropathogenic *Escherichia coli* infection. *J Clin Invest.* 1993;92:1412-1417.
19. Acheson DW, Moore R, De Breucker S, et al. Translocation of Shiga toxin across polarized intestinal cells in tissue culture. *Infect Immun.* 1996;64:3294-3300.
20. Hurley BP, Thorpe CM, Acheson DW. Shiga toxin translocation across intestinal epithelial cells is enhanced by neutrophil transmigration. *Infect Immun.* 2001;69:6148-6155.
21. Bitzan M, Richardson S, Huang C, et al. Evidence that verotoxins (Shiga-like toxins) from *Escherichia coli* bind to P blood group antigens of human erythrocytes in vitro. *Infect Immun.* 1994;62:3337-3347.
22. Cooling LL, Walker KE, Gille T, et al. Shiga toxin binds human platelets via globotriaosylceramide (Pk antigen) and a novel platelet glycosphingolipid. *Infect Immun.* 1998;66:4355-4366.
23. Stahl AL, Svensson M, Morgelin M, et al. Lipopolysaccharide from enterohemorrhagic *Escherichia coli* binds to platelets through TLR4 and CD62 and is detected on circulating platelets in patients with hemolytic uremic syndrome. *Blood.* 2006;108:167-176.
24. van Setten PA, Monnens LA, Verstraten RG, van den Heuvel LP, van Hinsbergh VW. Effects of verocytotoxin-1 on nonadherent human monocytes: binding characteristics, protein synthesis, and induction of cytokine release. *Blood.* 1996;88:174-183.
25. Manning SD, Motiwala AS, Springman AC, et al. Variation in virulence among clades of *Escherichia coli* O157:H7 associated with disease outbreaks. *Proc Natl Acad Sci U S A.* 2008;105:4868-4873.
26. Mead PS, Griffin PM. *Escherichia coli* O157:H7. *Lancet.* 1998;352:1207-1212.
27. Banatvala N, Griffin PM, Greene KD, et al. The United States National Prospective Hemolytic Uremic Syndrome Study: microbiologic, serologic, clinical, and epidemiologic findings. *J Infect Dis.* 2001;183:1063-1070.
28. Garg AX, Clark WF, Salvadori M, et al. Absence of renal sequelae after childhood *Escherichia coli* O157:H7 gastroenteritis. *Kidney Int.* 2006;70:807-812.
29. Chandler WL, Jelacic S, Boster DR, et al. Prothrombotic coagulation abnormalities preceding the hemolytic-uremic syndrome. *N Engl J Med.* 2002;346:23-32.
30. Beatty ME, Griffin PM, Tulu AN, et al. Culturing practices and antibiotic use in children with diarrhea. *Pediatrics.* 2004;113:628-629.
31. Milford D. The hemolytic-uremic syndromes in the United Kingdom. In: Kaplan BS, Trompeter RS, Moake JL, eds. *Hemolytic-uremic syndrome and thrombotic thrombocytopenic purpura.* New York: Marcel Dekker; 1992:pp 39-59.
32. Garg AX, Suri RS, Barrowman N, et al. Long-term renal prognosis of diarrhea-associated hemolytic uremic syndrome: a systematic review, meta-analysis, and meta-regression. *JAMA.* 2003;290:1360-1370.
33. Tonshoff B, Sammet A, Sanden I, et al. Outcome and prognostic determinants in the hemolytic uremic syndrome of children. *Nephron.* 1994;68:63-70.

34. Lou-Meda R, Oakes RS, Gilstrap JN, et al. Prognostic significance of microalbuminuria in postdiarrheal hemolytic uremic syndrome. *Pediatr Nephrol.* 2007;22:117-120.

35. Ake JA, Jelacic S, Ciol MA, et al. Relative nephroprotection during *Escherichia coli* O157:H7 infections: association with intravenous volume expansion. *Pediatrics.* 2005;115:e673-e680.

36. Chiurchiu C, Firrincieli A, Santostefano M, et al. Adult nondiarrhea hemolytic uremic syndrome associated with Shiga toxin *Escherichia coli* O157:H7 bacteremia and urinary tract infection. *Am J Kidney Dis.* 2003;41:E4.

37. Wong CS, Jelacic S, Habeeb RL, et al. The risk of the hemolytic-uremic syndrome after antibiotic treatment of *Escherichia coli* O157:H7 infections. *N Engl J Med.* 2000;342:1930-1936.

38. Safdar N, Said A, Gangnon RE, et al. Risk of hemolytic uremic syndrome after antibiotic treatment of *Escherichia coli* O157:H7 enteritis: a meta-analysis. *JAMA.* 2002;288:996-1001.

39. Caletti MG, Lejarraga H, Kelmansky D, et al. Two different therapeutic regimens in patients with sequelae of hemolytic-uremic syndrome. *Pediatr Nephrol.* 2004;19:1148-1152.

40. Van Dyck M, Proesmans W. Renoprotection by ACE inhibitors after severe hemolytic uremic syndrome. *Pediatr Nephrol.* 2004;19:688-690.

41. Trachtman H, Cnaan A, Christen E, et al. Effect of an oral Shiga toxin–binding agent on diarrhea-associated hemolytic uremic syndrome in children: a randomized controlled trial. *JAMA.* 2003;290:1337-1344.

42. Dundas S, Murphy J, Soutar RL, et al. Effectiveness of therapeutic plasma exchange in the 1996 Lanarkshire *Escherichia coli* O157:H7 outbreak. *Lancet.* 1999;354:1327-1330.

43. Carter AO, Borczyk AA, Carlson JA, et al. A severe outbreak of *Escherichia coli* O157:H7–associated hemorrhagic colitis in a nursing home. *N Engl J Med.* 1987;317:1496-1500.

44. Artz MA, Steenbergen EJ, Hoitsma AJ, et al. Renal transplantation in patients with hemolytic uremic syndrome: high rate of recurrence and increased incidence of acute rejections. *Transplantation.* 2003;76:821-826.

45. Loirat C, Niaudet P. The risk of recurrence of hemolytic uremic syndrome after renal transplantation in children. *Pediatr Nephrol.* 2003;18:1095-1101.

46. Ferraris JR, Ramirez JA, Ruiz S, et al. Shiga toxin–associated hemolytic uremic syndrome: absence of recurrence after renal transplantation. *Pediatr Nephrol.* 2002;17:809-814.

47. Brandt J, Wong C, Mihm S, et al. Invasive pneumococcal disease and hemolytic uremic syndrome. *Pediatrics.* 2002;110:371-376.

48. McGraw ME, Lendon M, Stevens RF, et al. Haemolytic uraemic syndrome and the Thomsen Friedenreich antigen. *Pediatr Nephrol.* 1989;3:135-139.

49. Eder AF, Manno CS. Does red-cell T activation matter? *Br J Haematol.* 2001;114:25-30.

50. Noris M, Remuzzi G. Atypical hemolytic-uremic syndrome. *N Engl J Med.* 2009;361:1676-1687.

51. Campbell S, Carré IJ. Fatal haemolytic uraemic syndrome and idiopathic hyperlipaemia in monozygotic twins. *Arch Dis Child.* 1965;40:654-658.

52. Kaplan BS, Chesney RW, Drummond KN. Hemolytic uremic syndrome in families. *N Engl J Med.* 1975;292:1090-1093.

53. Kaplan BS, Leonard MB. Autosomal dominant hemolytic uremic syndrome: variable phenotypes and transplant results. *Pediatr Nephrol.* 2000;14:464-468.

54. Besbas N, Karpman D, Landau D, et al. A classification of hemolytic uremic syndrome and thrombotic thrombocytopenic purpura and related disorders. *Kidney Int.* 2006;70:423-431.

55. Zakarija A, Bennett C. Drug-induced thrombotic microangiopathy. *Semin Thromb Hemost.* 2005;31:681-690.

56. Ruggenenti P. Post-transplant hemolytic-uremic syndrome. *Kidney Int.* 2002;62:1093-1104.

57. Karthikeyan V, Parasuraman R, Shah V, et al. Outcome of plasma exchange therapy in thrombotic microangiopathy after renal transplantation. *Am J Transplant.* 2003;3:1289-1294.

58. Zarifian A, Meleg-Smith S, O'Donovan R, et al. Cyclosporine-associated thrombotic microangiopathy in renal allografts. *Kidney Int.* 1999;55:2457-2466.

59. Carreras L, Romero R, Requesens C, et al. Familial hypocomplementemic hemolytic uremic syndrome with HLA-A3, B7 haplotype. *JAMA.* 1981;245:602-604.

60. Stuhlinger W, Kourilsky O, Kanfer A, et al. Haemolytic-uraemic syndrome: evidence for intravascular C3 activation [Letter]. *Lancet.* 1974;2:788-789.

61. Noris M, Ruggenenti P, Perna A, et al. Hypocomplementemia discloses genetic predisposition to hemolytic uremic syndrome and thrombotic thrombocytopenic purpura: role of factor H abnormalities. Italian Registry of Familial and Recurrent Hemolytic Uremic Syndrome/Thrombotic Thrombocytopenic Purpura. *J Am Soc Nephrol.* 1999;10:281-293.

62. Kim Y, Miller K, Michael AF. Breakdown products of C3 and factor B in hemolytic-uremic syndrome. *J Lab Clin Med.* 1977;89:845-850.

63. Walport MJ. Complement. First of two parts. *N Engl J Med.* 2001;344:1058-1066.

64. Zipfel PF, Skerka C. Complement factor H and related proteins: an expanding family of complement-regulatory proteins? *Immunol Today.* 1994;15:121-126.

65. Warwicker P, Goodship TH, Donne RL, et al. Genetic studies into inherited and sporadic hemolytic uremic syndrome. *Kidney Int.* 1998;53:836-844.

65a. University College London. *FH aHUS mutation database.* Available at http://www.FH-HUS.org. Accessed December 29, 2010.

66. Richards A, Buddles MR, Donne RL, et al. Factor H mutations in hemolytic uremic syndrome cluster in exons 18-20, a domain important for host cell recognition. *Am J Hum Genet.* 2001;68:485-490.

67. Dragon-Durey MA, Fremeaux-Bacchi V, Loirat C, et al. Heterozygous and homozygous factor H deficiencies associated with hemolytic uremic syndrome or membranoproliferative glomerulonephritis: report and genetic analysis of 16 cases. *J Am Soc Nephrol.* 2004;15:787-795.

68. Caprioli J, Bettinaglio P, Zipfel PF, et al. The molecular basis of familial hemolytic uremic syndrome: mutation analysis of factor H gene reveals a hot spot in short consensus repeat 20. *J Am Soc Nephrol.* 2001;12:297-307.

69. Caprioli J, Castelletti F, Bucchioni S, et al. Complement factor H mutations and gene polymorphisms in haemolytic uraemic syndrome: the C-257T, the A2089G and the G2881T polymorphisms are strongly associated with the disease. *Hum Mol Genet.* 2003;12:3385-3395.

70. Caprioli J, Noris M, Brioschi S, et al. Genetics of HUS: the impact of MCP, CFH, and IF mutations on clinical presentation, response to treatment, and outcome. *Blood.* 2006;108:1267-1279.

71. Perez-Caballero D, Gonzalez-Rubio C, Gallardo ME, et al. Clustering of missense mutations in the C-terminal region of factor H in atypical hemolytic uremic syndrome. *Am J Hum Genet.* 2001;68:478-484.

72. Saunders RE, Abarrategui-Garrido C, Fremeaux-Bacchi V, et al. The interactive Factor H–Atypical Hemolytic Uremic Syndrome Mutation Database and website: update and integration of membrane cofactor protein and factor I mutations with structural models. *Hum Mutat.* 2007;28:222-234.

73. Nakanishi I, Moutabarrik A, Hara T, et al. Identification and characterization of membrane cofactor protein (CD46) in the human kidneys. *Eur J Immunol.* 1994;24:1529-1535.

74. Noris M, Brioschi S, Caprioli J, et al. Familial haemolytic uraemic syndrome and an MCP mutation. *Lancet.* 2003;362:1542-1547.

75. Richards A, Kemp EJ, Liszewski MK, et al. Mutations in human complement regulator, membrane cofactor protein (CD46), predispose to development of familial hemolytic uremic syndrome. *Proc Natl Acad Sci U S A.* 2003;100:12966-12971.

76. Liszewski MK, Leung M, Cui W, et al. Dissecting sites important for complement regulatory activity in membrane cofactor protein (MCP; CD46). *J Biol Chem.* 2000;275:37692-37701.

77. Fremeaux-Bacchi V, Moulton EA, Kavanagh D, et al. Genetic and functional analyses of membrane cofactor protein (CD46) mutations in atypical hemolytic uremic syndrome. *J Am Soc Nephrol.* 2006;17:2017-2025.

78. Kavanagh D, Kemp EJ, Mayland E, et al. Mutations in complement factor I predispose to development of atypical hemolytic uremic syndrome. *J Am Soc Nephrol.* 2005;16:2150-2155.

79. Kavanagh D, Richards A, Noris M, et al. Characterization of mutations in complement factor I (CFI) associated with hemolytic uremic syndrome. *Mol Immunol.* 2008;45:95-105.

80. Fremeaux-Bacchi V, Dragon-Durey MA, Blouin J, et al. Complement factor I: a susceptibility gene for atypical haemolytic uraemic syndrome. *J Med Genet.* 2004;41:e84.

81. Fremeaux-Bacchi V, Miller EC, Liszewski MK, et al. Mutations in complement C3 predispose to development of atypical hemolytic uremic syndrome. *Blood.* 2008;112:4948-4952.

82. Goicoechea de Jorge E, Harris CL, Esparza-Gordillo J, et al. Gain-of-function mutations in complement factor B are associated with atypical hemolytic uremic syndrome. *Proc Natl Acad Sci U S A.* 2007;104:240-245.

83. Delvaeye M, Noris M, DeVriese A, et al. Mutations in thrombomodulin in hemolytic-uremic syndrome. *N Engl J Med.* 2009;361:345-357.

84. Loirat C, Noris M, Fremeaux-Bacchi V. Complement and the atypical hemolytic uremic syndrome in children. *Pediatr Nephrol.* 2008;23:1957-1972.

85. Skerka C, Jozsi M, Zipfel PF, et al. Autoantibodies in haemolytic uraemic syndrome (HUS). *Thromb Haemost.* 2009;101:227-232.

86. Loirat C, Sonsino E, Hinglais N, et al. Treatment of the childhood haemolytic uraemic syndrome with plasma. A multicentre randomized controlled trial. The French Society of Paediatric Nephrology. *Pediatr Nephrol.* 1988;2:279-285.

87. Rizzoni G, Claris-Appiani A, Edefonti A, et al. Plasma infusion for hemolytic-uremic syndrome in children: results of a multicenter controlled trial. *J Pediatr.* 1988;112:284-290.

88. Noris M, Remuzzi G. Thrombotic microangiopathy: what not to learn from a meta-analysis. *Nat Rev Nephrol.* 2009;5:186-188.

89. Michael M, Elliott EJ, Craig JC, et al. Interventions for hemolytic uremic syndrome and thrombotic thrombocytopenic purpura: a systematic review of randomized controlled trials. *Am J Kidney Dis.* 2009;53:259-272.

90. Cho HY, Lee BS, Moon KC, et al. Complete factor H deficiency–associated atypical hemolytic uremic syndrome in a neonate. *Pediatr Nephrol.* 2007;22:874-880.
91. Licht C, Weyersberg A, Heinen S, et al. Successful plasma therapy for atypical hemolytic uremic syndrome caused by factor H deficiency owing to a novel mutation in the complement cofactor protein domain 15. *Am J Kidney Dis.* 2005;45:415-421.
92. Nathanson S, Fremeaux-Bacchi V, Deschenes G. Successful plasma therapy in hemolytic uremic syndrome with factor H deficiency. *Pediatr Nephrol.* 2001;16:554-556.
93. Davin JC, Strain L, Goodship TH. Plasma therapy in atypical haemolytic uremic syndrome: lessons from a family with a factor H mutation. *Pediatr Nephrol.* 2008;23:1517-1521.
94. Lapeyraque AL, Wagner E, Phan V, et al. Efficacy of plasma therapy in atypical hemolytic uremic syndrome with complement factor H mutations. *Pediatr Nephrol.* 2008;23:1363-1366.
95. Dragon-Durey MA, Loirat C, Cloarec S, et al. Anti–factor H autoantibodies associated with atypical hemolytic uremic syndrome. *J Am Soc Nephrol.* 2005;16:555-563.
96. Jozsi M, Strobel S, Dahse HM, et al. Anti factor H autoantibodies block C-terminal recognition function of factor H in hemolytic uremic syndrome. *Blood.* 2007;110:1516-1518.
97. Kwon T, Dragon-Durey MA, Macher MA, et al. Successful pre-transplant management of a patient with anti–factor H autoantibodies–associated haemolytic uraemic syndrome. *Nephrol Dial Transplant.* 2008;23:2088-2090.
98. Sellier-Leclerc AL, Fremeaux-Bacchi V, Dragon-Durey MA, et al. Differential impact of complement mutations on clinical characteristics in atypical hemolytic uremic syndrome. *J Am Soc Nephrol.* 2007;18:2392-2400.
99. Bresin E, Daina E, Noris M, et al. Outcome of renal transplantation in patients with non–Shiga toxin–associated haemolytic uremic syndrome: prognostic significance of genetic background. *Clin J Am Soc Nephrol.* 2006;1:88-99.
100. Loirat C, Fremeaux-Bacchi V. Hemolytic uremic syndrome recurrence after renal transplantation. *Pediatr Transplant.* 2008;12:619-629.
101. Chan MR, Thomas CP, Torrealba JR, et al. Recurrent atypical hemolytic uremic syndrome associated with factor I mutation in a living related renal transplant recipient. *Am J Kidney Dis.* 2009;53:321-326.
102. Donne RL, Abbs I, Barany P, et al. Recurrence of hemolytic uremic syndrome after live related renal transplantation associated with subsequent de novo disease in the donor. *Am J Kidney Dis.* 2002;40:E22.
103. Olie KH, Goodship TH, Verlaak R, et al. Posttransplantation cytomegalovirus-induced recurrence of atypical hemolytic uremic syndrome associated with a factor H mutation: successful treatment with intensive plasma exchanges and ganciclovir. *Am J Kidney Dis.* 2005;45:e12-e15.
104. Olie KH, Florquin S, Groothoff JW, et al. Atypical relapse of hemolytic uremic syndrome after transplantation. *Pediatr Nephrol.* 2004;19:1173-1176.
105. Remuzzi G, Ruggenenti P, Codazzi D, et al. Combined kidney and liver transplantation for familial haemolytic uraemic syndrome. *Lancet.* 2002;359:1671-1672.
106. Remuzzi G, Ruggenenti P, Colledan M, et al. Hemolytic uremic syndrome: a fatal outcome after kidney and liver transplantation performed to correct factor H gene mutation. *Am J Transplant.* 2005;5:1146-1150.
107. Jalanko H, Peltonen S, Koskinen A, et al. Successful liver-kidney transplantation in two children with aHUS caused by a mutation in complement factor H. *Am J Transplant.* 2008;8:216-221.
108. Saland JM, Emre SH, Shneider BL, et al. Favorable long-term outcome after liver-kidney transplant for recurrent hemolytic uremic syndrome associated with a factor H mutation. *Am J Transplant.* 2006;6:1948-1952.
108a. European Medicines Agency. *Public summary of positive opinion for orphan designation of complement factor H for the treatment of atypical haemolytic uraemic syndrome (aHUS) associated with an inherited abnormality of the complement system.* Available at http://www.emea.europa.eu/pdfs/human/comp/opinion/52123506en.pdf. Accessed December 30, 2010.
109. Brodsky RA, Young NS, Antonioli E, et al. Multicenter phase 3 study of the complement inhibitor eculizumab for the treatment of patients with paroxysmal nocturnal hemoglobinuria. *Blood.* 2008;111:1840-1847.
110. Gruppo RA, Rother RP. Eculizumab for congenital atypical hemolytic-uremic syndrome. *N Engl J Med.* 2009;360:544-546.
111. Nurnberger J, Witzke O, Saez AO, et al. Eculizumab for atypical hemolytic-uremic syndrome. *N Engl J Med.* 2009;360:542-544.
111a. National Institutes of Health. *ClinicalTrials.gov* [registry]. Available at www.clinicaltrials.gov. Accessed December 30, 2010.
112. Baumgartner ER, Wick H, Maurer R, et al. Congenital defect in intracellular cobalamin metabolism resulting in homocysteinuria and methylmalonic aciduria. I. Case report and histopathology. *Helv Paediatr Acta.* 1979;34:465-482.
113. Van Hove JL, Van Damme–Lombaerts R, Grunewald S, et al. Cobalamin disorder Cbl-C presenting with late-onset thrombotic microangiopathy. *Am J Med Genet.* 2002;111:195-201.
114. Padilla A, Moake JL, Bernardo A, et al. P-selectin anchors newly released ultralarge von Willebrand factor multimers to the endothelial cell surface. *Blood.* 2004;103:2150-2156.
115. Sadler JE. Von Willebrand factor, ADAMTS13, and thrombotic thrombocytopenic purpura. *Blood.* 2008;112:11-18.
116. Furlan M, Robles R, Galbusera M, et al. von Willebrand factor–cleaving protease in thrombotic thrombocytopenic purpura and the hemolytic-uremic syndrome. *N Engl J Med.* 1998;339:1578-1584.
117. Tsai HM, Lian EC. Antibodies to von Willebrand factor–cleaving protease in acute thrombotic thrombocytopenic purpura. *N Engl J Med.* 1998;339:1585-1594.
118. Levy GG, Nichols WC, Lian EC, et al. Mutations in a member of the ADAMTS gene family cause thrombotic thrombocytopenic purpura. *Nature.* 2001;413:488-494.
119. Furlan M, Robles R, Lamie B. Partial purification and characterization of a protease from human plasma cleaving von Willebrand factor to fragments produced by in vivo proteolysis. *Blood.* 1996;87:4223-4234.
120. Veyradier A, Obert B, Houllier A, et al. Specific von Willebrand factor–cleaving protease in thrombotic microangiopathies: a study of 111 cases. *Blood.* 2001;98:1765-1772.
121. Ferrari S, Scheiflinger F, Rieger M, et al. Prognostic value of anti–ADAMTS 13 antibody features (Ig isotype, titer, and inhibitory effect) in a cohort of 35 adult French patients undergoing a first episode of thrombotic microangiopathy with undetectable ADAMTS 13 activity. *Blood.* 2007;109:2815-2822.
122. Abroun S, Ishikawa H, Tsuyama N, et al. Receptor synergy of interleukin-6 (IL-6) and insulin-like growth factor-I in myeloma cells that highly express IL-6 receptor alpha [corrected]. *Blood.* 2004;103:2291-2298.
123. Guan YS, Zheng XH, Zhou XP, et al. Multidetector CT in evaluating blood supply of hepatocellular carcinoma after transcatheter arterial chemoembolization. *World J Gastroenterol.* 2004;10:2127-2129.
124. Li FJ, Tsuyama N, Ishikawa H, et al. A rapid translocation of CD45RO but not CD45RA to lipid rafts in IL-6–induced proliferation in myeloma. *Blood.* 2005;105:3295-3302.
125. Ma Z, Otsuyama K, Liu S, et al. Baicalein, a component of *Scutellaria radix* from Huang-Lian-Jie-Du-Tang (HLJDT), leads to suppression of proliferation and induction of apoptosis in human myeloma cells. *Blood.* 2005;105:3312-3318.
126. Zheng X, Beissert T, Kukoc-Zivojnov N, et al. Gamma-catenin contributes to leukemogenesis induced by AML-associated translocation products by increasing the self-renewal of very primitive progenitor cells. *Blood.* 2004;103:3535-3543.
127. Zheng XL, Kaufman RM, Goodnough LT, et al. Effect of plasma exchange on plasma ADAMTS13 metalloprotease activity, inhibitor level, and clinical outcome in patients with idiopathic and nonidiopathic thrombotic thrombocytopenic purpura. *Blood.* 2004;103:4043-4049.
128. Zhou ZG, Yan WW, Chen YQ, et al. Effect of inducible cyclooxygenase expression on local microvessel blood flow in acute interstitial pancreatitis. *Asian J Surg.* 2004;27:93-98.
129. Vesely SK, George JN, Lammle B, et al. ADAMTS13 activity in thrombotic thrombocytopenic purpura–hemolytic uremic syndrome: relation to presenting features and clinical outcomes in a prospective cohort of 142 patients. *Blood.* 2003;102:60-68.
130. Zheng XL, Sadler JE. Pathogenesis of thrombotic microangiopathies. *Annu Rev Pathol.* 2008;3:249-277.
131. Fremeaux-Bacchi V, Arzouk N, Ferlicot S, et al. Recurrence of HUS due to CD46/MCP mutation after renal transplantation: a role for endothelial microchimerism. *Am J Transplant.* 2007;7:2047-2051.
132. Fremeaux-Bacchi V, Sanlaville D, Menouer S, et al. Unusual clinical severity of complement membrane cofactor protein–associated hemolytic-uremic syndrome and uniparental isodisomy. *Am J Kidney Dis.* 2007;49:323-329.
133. Mannucci PM, Peyvandi F. TTP and ADAMTS13: when is testing appropriate? *Hematology Am Soc Hematol Educ Program.* 2007;121-126.
134. Ruggenenti P, Noris M, Remuzzi G. Thrombotic microangiopathies. In: Wilcox C, ed. *Therapy in nephrology & hypertension. A companion to Brenner & Rector's The Kidney.* Philadelphia: Elsevier; 2008:pp 294-312.
135. Scully M, Cohen H, Cavenagh J, et al. Remission in acute refractory and relapsing thrombotic thrombocytopenic purpura following rituximab is associated with a reduction in IgG antibodies to ADAMTS-13. *Br J Haematol.* 2007;136:451-461.
136. Fakhouri F, Vernant JP, Veyradier A, et al. Efficiency of curative and prophylactic treatment with rituximab in ADAMTS13-deficient thrombotic thrombocytopenic purpura: a study of 11 cases. *Blood.* 2005;106:1932-1937.
137. Galbusera M, Bresin E, Noris M, et al. Rituximab prevents recurrence of thrombotic thrombocytopenic purpura: a case report. *Blood.* 2005;106:925-928.
138. Bresin E, Gastoldi S, Daina E, et al. Rituximab as pre-emptive treatment in patients with thrombotic thrombocytopenic purpura and evidence of anti-ADAMTS13 autoantibodies. *Thromb Haemost.* 2009;101:233-238.

139. Galbusera M, Noris M, Remuzzi G. Inherited thrombotic thrombocytopenic purpura. *Haematologica*. 2009;94:166-170.

140. Remuzzi G, Chiurchiu C, Abbate M, et al. Rituximab for idiopathic membranous nephropathy. *Lancet*. 2002;360:923-924.

141. Remuzzi G, Galbusera M, Noris M, et al. von Willebrand factor cleaving protease (ADAMTS13) is deficient in recurrent and familial thrombotic thrombocytopenic purpura and hemolytic uremic syndrome. *Blood*. 2002;100:778-785.

142. Zoja C, Angioletti S, Donadelli R, et al. Shiga toxin-2 triggers endothelial leukocyte adhesion and transmigration via NF-kappaB dependent up-regulation of IL-8 and MCP-1. *Kidney Int*. 2002;62:846-856.

143. Fujikawa K, Suzuki H, McMullen B, et al. Purification of human von Willebrand factor–cleaving protease and its identification as a new member of the metalloproteinase family. *Blood*. 2001;98:1662-1666.

144. Donadelli R, Banterla F, Galbusera M, et al. In-vitro and in-vivo consequences of mutations in the von Willebrand factor cleaving protease ADAMTS13 in thrombotic thrombocytopenic purpura. *Thromb Haemost*. 2006;96:454-464.

145. Schneppenheim R, Kremer Hovinga JA, Becker T, et al. A common origin of the 4143insA ADAMTS13 mutation. *Thromb Haemost*. 2006;96:3-6.

146. Palla R, Lavoretano S, Lombardi R, et al. The first deletion mutation in the TSP1-6 repeat domain of ADAMTS13 in a family with inherited thrombotic thrombocytopenic purpura. *Haematologica*. 2009;94:289-293.

147. Tao Z, Anthony K, Peng Y, et al. Novel ADAMTS-13 mutations in an adult with delayed onset thrombotic thrombocytopenic purpura. *J Thromb Haemost*. 2006;4:1931-1935.

148. Camilleri RS, Cohen H, Mackie IJ, et al. Prevalence of the ADAMTS-13 missense mutation R1060W in late onset adult thrombotic thrombocytopenic purpura. *J Thromb Haemost*. 2008;6:331-338.

149. Furlan M, Robles R, Morselli B, et al. Recovery and half-life of von Willebrand factor–cleaving protease after plasma therapy in patients with thrombotic thrombocytopenic purpura. *Thromb Haemost*. 1999;81:8-13.

150. Kealy WF. Atheroembolism. *J Clin Pathol*. 1978;31:984-989.

151. Krishnamurthi V, Novick AC, Myles JL. Atheroembolic renal disease: effect on morbidity and survival after revascularization for atherosclerotic renal artery stenosis. *J Urol*. 1999;161:1093-1096.

152. Scolari F, Tardanico R, Zani R, et al. Cholesterol crystal embolism: a recognizable cause of renal disease. *Am J Kidney Dis*. 2000;36:1089-1109.

153. Fine MJ, Kapoor W, Falanga V. Cholesterol crystal embolization: a review of 221 cases in the English literature. *Angiology*. 1987;38:769-784.

154. Vitsky BH, Suzuki Y, Strauss L, et al. The hemolytic-uremic syndrome: a study of renal pathologic alterations. *Am J Pathol*. 1969;57:627-647.

155. Lye WC, Cheah JS, Sinniah R. Renal cholesterol embolic disease. Case report and review of the literature. *Am J Nephrol*. 1993;13:489-493.

156. Scolari F, Ravani P, Pola A, et al. Predictors of renal and patient outcomes in atheroembolic renal disease: a prospective study. *J Am Soc Nephrol*. 2003;14:1584-1590.

157. Belenfant X, Meyrier A, Jacquot C. Supportive treatment improves survival in multivisceral cholesterol crystal embolism. *Am J Kidney Dis*. 1999;33:840-850.

158. Singh I, Killen PD, Leichtman AB. Cholesterol emboli presenting as acute allograft dysfunction after renal transplantation. *J Am Soc Nephrol*. 1995;6:165-170.

159. Saleem S, Lakkis FG, Martinez-Maldonado M. Atheroembolic renal disease. *Semin Nephrol*. 1996;16:309-318.

160. Thadhani RI, Camargo Jr CA, Xavier RJ, et al. Atheroembolic renal failure after invasive procedures. Natural history based on 52 histologically proven cases. *Medicine (Baltimore)*. 1995;74:350-358.

161. Theriault J, Agharazzi M, Dumont M, et al. Atheroembolic renal failure requiring dialysis: potential for renal recovery? A review of 43 cases. *Nephron Clin Pract*. 2003;94:c11-c18.

162. Aviles B, Ubeda I, Blanco J, et al. Pauci-immune extracapillary glomerulonephritis and atheromatous embolization. *Am J Kidney Dis*. 2002;40:847-851.

163. Frock J, Bierman M, Hammeke M, et al. Atheroembolic renal disease: experience with 22 patients. *Nebr Med J*. 1994;79:317-321.

164. Polu KR, Wolf M. Clinical problem-solving. Needle in a haystack. *N Engl J Med*. 2006;354:68-73.

165. Hagiwara N, Toyoda K, Nakayama M, et al. Renal cholesterol embolism in patients with carotid stenosis: a severe and underdiagnosed complication following cerebrovascular procedures. *J Neurol Sci*. 2004;222:109-112.

166. Abbott KC, Hypolite IO, Agodoa LY. Sickle cell nephropathy at end-stage renal disease in the United States: patient characteristics and survival. *Clin Nephrol*. 2002;58:9-15.

167. Mann SJ, Sos TA. Treatment of atheroembolization with corticosteroids. *Am J Hypertens*. 2001;14:831-834.

168. Takahashi T, Konta T, Nishida W, et al. Renal cholesterol embolic disease effectively treated with steroid pulse therapy. *Intern Med*. 2003;42:1206-1209.

169. Stabellini N, Cerretani D, Russo G, et al. [Renal atheroembolic disease: evaluation of the efficacy of corticosteroid therapy]. *G Ital Nefrol*. 2002;19:18-21.

170. Keen RR, McCarthy WJ, Shireman PK, et al. Surgical management of atheroembolization. *J Vasc Surg*. 1995;21:773-780:discussion, *J Vasc Surg*. 1995; 21:780-781.

171. Dubel GJ, Murphy TP. The role of percutaneous revascularization for renal artery stenosis. *Vasc Med*. 2008;13:141-156.

172. Baermann G, Linser P. Über die lokale und allgemeine Wirkung der Röntgenstrahlen. *Münch Med Wschr*. 1904;51:996-999.

173. Cassady JR. Clinical radiation nephropathy. *Int J Radiat Oncol Biol Phys*. 1995;31:1249-1256.

174. Kersting S, Koomans HA, Hene RJ, et al. Acute renal failure after allogeneic myeloablative stem cell transplantation: retrospective analysis of incidence, risk factors and survival. *Bone Marrow Transplant*. 2007;39:359-365.

175. Kersting S, Dorp SV, Theobald M, et al. Acute renal failure after nonmyeloablative stem cell transplantation in adults. *Biol Blood Marrow Transplant*. 2008;14:125-131.

176. Cruz DN, Perazella MA, Mahnensmith RL. Bone marrow transplant nephropathy: a case report and review of the literature. *J Am Soc Nephrol*. 1997;8:166-173.

177. Lawton CA, Cohen EP, Murray KJ, et al. Long-term results of selective renal shielding in patients undergoing total body irradiation in preparation for bone marrow transplantation. *Bone Marrow Transplant*. 1997;20:1069-1074.

178. Lawton CA, Cohen EP, Barber-Derus SW, et al. Late renal dysfunction in adult survivors of bone marrow transplantation. *Cancer*. 1991;67:2795-2800.

179. Robbins ME, Bonsib SM. Radiation nephropathy: a review. *Scanning Microsc*. 1995;9:535-560.

180. Cohen EP. Radiation nephropathy after bone marrow transplantation. *Kidney Int*. 2000;58:903-918.

181. Cohen EP, Fish BL, Moulder JE. Angiotensin II infusion exacerbates radiation nephropathy. *J Lab Clin Med*. 1999;134:283-291.

182. Coia LR, Hanks GE. Complications from large field intermediate dose infradiaphragmatic radiation: an analysis of the patterns of care outcome studies for Hodgkin's disease and seminoma. *Int J Radiat Oncol Biol Phys*. 1988;15:29-35.

183. Juncos LI, Carrasco Duenas S, et al. Long-term enalapril and hydrochlorothiazide in radiation nephritis. *Nephron*. 1993;64:249-255.

184. Cohen EP, Fish BL, Moulder JE. Successful brief captopril treatment in experimental radiation nephropathy. *J Lab Clin Med*. 1997;129:536-547.

185. Cohen EP, Molteni A, Hill P, et al. Captopril preserves function and ultrastructure in experimental radiation nephropathy. *Lab Invest*. 1996;75:349-360.

186. Cohen EP, Irving AA, Drobyski WR, et al. Captopril to mitigate chronic renal failure after hematopoietic stem cell transplantation: a randomized controlled trial. *Int J Radiat Oncol Biol Phys*. 2008;70:1546-1551.

187. Chifflot H, Fautrel B, Sordet C, et al. Incidence and prevalence of systemic sclerosis: a systematic literature review. *Semin Arthritis Rheum*. 2008;37:223-235.

188. Mayes MD. Scleroderma epidemiology. *Rheum Dis Clin North Am*. 2003;29:239-254.

189. Gabrielli A, Avvedimento EV, Krieg T. Scleroderma. *N Engl J Med*. 2009;360:1989-2003.

190. Harashima S, Yoshizawa S, Horiuchi T, et al. [A case of systemic sclerosis with crescentic glomerulonephritis associated with perinuclear-antineutrophil cytoplasmic antibody (p-ANCA)]. *Nihon Rinsho Meneki Gakkai Kaishi*. 1999;22:86-92.

191. Kobayashi M, Saito M, Minoshima S, et al. [A case of progressive systemic sclerosis with crescentic glomerulonephritis associated with myeloperoxidase-antineutrophil cytoplasmic antibody (MPO-ANCA) and anti–glomerular basement membrane antibody (anti-GBM Ab)]. *Nippon Jinzo Gakkai Shi*. 1995;37:207-211.

192. Penn H, Howie AJ, Kingdon EJ, et al. Scleroderma renal crisis: patient characteristics and long-term outcomes. *Qjm*. 2007;100:485-494.

193. Ricklin D, Lambris JD. Complement-targeted therapeutics. *Nat Biotechnol*. 2007;25:1265-1275.

194. Penn H, Denton CP. Diagnosis, management and prevention of scleroderma renal disease. *Curr Opin Rheumatol*. 2008;20:692-696.

195. Bashandy HG, Javillo JS, Gambert SR. A case of early onset normotensive scleroderma renal crisis in a patient with diffuse cutaneous systemic sclerosis. *South Med J*. 2006;99:870-872.

196. Kohno K, Katayama T, Majima K, et al. A case of normotensive scleroderma renal crisis after high-dose methylprednisolone treatment. *Clin Nephrol*. 2000;53:479-482.

197. Teixeira L, Mahr A, Berezne A, et al. Scleroderma renal crisis, still a life-threatening complication. *Ann N Y Acad Sci*. 2007;1108:249-258.

198. Steen VD. Scleroderma renal crisis. *Rheum Dis Clin North Am*. 2003;29:315-333.

199. Steen VD, Medsger Jr TA. Long-term outcomes of scleroderma renal crisis. *Ann Intern Med.* 2000;133:600-603.
200. Steen VD, Syzd A, Johnson JP, et al. Kidney disease other than renal crisis in patients with diffuse scleroderma. *J Rheumatol.* 2005;32:649-655.
201. Kingdon EJ, Knight CJ, Dustan K, et al. Calculated glomerular filtration rate is a useful screening tool to identify scleroderma patients with renal impairment. *Rheumatology (Oxford).* 2003;42:26-33.
202. Uhlen M, Bjorling E, Agaton C, et al. A human protein atlas for normal and cancer tissues based on antibody proteomics. *Mol Cell Proteomics.* 2005;4:1920-1932.
203. Kahaleh B. The microvascular endothelium in scleroderma. *Rheumatology (Oxford).* 2008;47(Suppl 5):v14-v15.
204. Varga J. Systemic sclerosis: an update. *Bull NYU Hosp Jt Dis.* 2008;66: 198-202.
205. Cannon PJ, Hassar M, Case DB, et al. The relationship of hypertension and renal failure in scleroderma (progressive systemic sclerosis) to structural and functional abnormalities of the renal cortical circulation. *Medicine (Baltimore).* 1974;53:1-46.
206. LeRoy EC. Increased collagen synthesis by scleroderma skin fibroblasts in vitro: a possible defect in the regulation or activation of the scleroderma fibroblast. *J Clin Invest.* 1974;54:880-889.
207. Fonseca C, Lindahl GE, Ponticos M, et al. A polymorphism in the CTGF promoter region associated with systemic sclerosis. *N Engl J Med.* 2007;357:1210-1220.
208. Zhang R, Florman S, Devidoss S, et al. The long-term survival of simultaneous pancreas and kidney transplant with basiliximab induction therapy. *Clin Transplant.* 2007;21:583-589.
209. Baroni SS, Santillo M, Bevilacqua F, et al. Stimulatory autoantibodies to the PDGF receptor in systemic sclerosis. *N Engl J Med.* 2006;354:2667-2676.
210. Allanore Y, Avouac J, Wipff J, et al. New therapeutic strategies in the management of systemic sclerosis. *Expert Opin Pharmacother.* 2007;8:607-615.
211. Denton CP, Black CM. Targeted therapy comes of age in scleroderma. *Trends Immunol.* 2005;26:596-602.
212. Sfikakis PP, Tesar J, Baraf H, et al. Circulating intercellular adhesion molecule-1 in patients with systemic sclerosis. *Clin Immunol Immunopathol.* 1993;68:88-92.
213. Kahaleh MB, Yin TG. Enhanced expression of high-affinity interleukin-2 receptors in scleroderma: possible role for IL-6. *Clin Immunol Immunopathol.* 1992;62:97-102.
214. Needleman BW. Immunologic aspects of scleroderma. *Curr Opin Rheumatol.* 1992;4:862-868.
215. Feghali CA, Bost KL, Boulware DW, et al. Mechanisms of pathogenesis in scleroderma. I. Overproduction of interleukin 6 by fibroblasts cultured from affected skin sites of patients with scleroderma. *J Rheumatol.* 1992;19: 1207-1211.
216. Kawaguchi Y, Hara M, Wright TM. Endogenous IL-1α from systemic sclerosis fibroblasts induces IL-6 and PDGF-A. *J Clin Invest.* 1999;103:1253-1260.
217. Traub YM, Shapiro AP, Rodnan GP, et al. Hypertension and renal failure (scleroderma renal crisis) in progressive systemic sclerosis. Review of a 25-year experience with 68 cases. *Medicine (Baltimore).* 1983;62:335-352.
218. Caskey FJ, Thacker EJ, Johnston PA, et al. Failure of losartan to control blood pressure in scleroderma renal crisis. *Lancet.* 1997;349:620.
219. Cheung WY, Gibson IW, Rush D, et al. Late recurrence of scleroderma renal crisis in a renal transplant recipient despite angiotensin II blockade. *Am J Kidney Dis.* 2005;45:930-934.
220. Donohoe JF. Scleroderma and the kidney. *Kidney Int.* 1992;41:462-477.
221. Bleyer AJ, Donaldson LA, McIntosh M, et al. Relationship between underlying renal disease and renal transplantation outcome. *Am J Kidney Dis.* 2001;37:1152-1161.
222. Masutani K, Katafuchi R, Ikeda H, et al. Recurrent nephrotic syndrome after living-related renal transplantation resistant to plasma exchange: report of two cases. *Clin Transplant.* 2005;19(Suppl 14):59-64.
223. Pham PT, Pham PC, Danovitch GM, et al. Predictors and risk factors for recurrent scleroderma renal crisis in the kidney allograft: case report and review of the literature. *Am J Transplant.* 2005;5:2565-2569.
224. Zandman-Goddard G, Tweezer-Zaks N, Shoenfeld Y. New therapeutic strategies for systemic sclerosis—a critical analysis of the literature. *Clin Dev Immunol.* 2005;12:165-173.
225. Pham PT, Pham PC, Wilkinson AH, Lew SQ. Renal abnormalities in sickle cell disease. *Kidney Int.* 2000;57:1-8.
226. Scheinman JI. Sickle cell disease and the kidney. *Semin Nephrol.* 2003;23:66-76.
227. de Santis Feltran L, de Abreu Carvalhaes JT, Sesso R. Renal complications of sickle cell disease: managing for optimal outcomes. *Paediatr Drugs.* 2002;4:29-36.
228. Herrera J, Avila E, Marin C, et al. Impaired creatinine secretion after an intravenous creatinine load is an early characteristic of the nephropathy of sickle cell anaemia. *Nephrol Dial Transplant.* 2002;17:602-607.
229. Sydenstricker VP, Mulherin WA, Houseal RW. Sickle cell anemia, report of two cases in children, with necropsy in one case. *Am J Dis Child.* 1923;26:132.
230. Bhathena DB, Sondheimer JH. The glomerulopathy of homozygous sickle hemoglobin (SS) disease: morphology and pathogenesis. *J Am Soc Nephrol.* 1991;1:1241-1252.
231. Falk RJ, Scheinman J, Phillips G, et al. Prevalence and pathologic features of sickle cell nephropathy and response to inhibition of angiotensin-converting enzyme. *N Engl J Med.* 1992;326:910-915.
232. Wesson DE. The initiation and progression of sickle cell nephropathy. *Kidney Int.* 2002;61:2277-2286.
233. Bakir AA, Hathiwala SC, Ainis H, et al. Prognosis of the nephrotic syndrome in sickle glomerulopathy. A retrospective study. *Am J Nephrol.* 1987;7:110-115.
234. Bunn HF. Pathogenesis and treatment of sickle cell disease. *N Engl J Med.* 1997;337:762-769.
235. Gee BE, Platt OS. Sickle reticulocytes adhere to VCAM-1. *Blood.* 1995;85:268-274.
236. Wong CS, Hingorani S, Gillen DL, et al. Hypoalbuminemia and risk of death in pediatric patients with end-stage renal disease. *Kidney Int.* 2002;61:630-637.
237. Kumar A, Eckmam JR, Swerlick RA, et al. Phorbol ester stimulation increases sickle erythrocyte adherence to endothelium: a novel pathway involving alpha 4 beta 1 integrin receptors on sickle reticulocytes and fibronectin. *Blood.* 1996;88:4348-4358.
238. Sugihara K, Sugihara T, Mohandas N, et al. Thrombospondin mediates adherence of CD36⁺ sickle reticulocytes to endothelial cells. *Blood.* 1992;80:2634-2642.
239. Guasch A, Cua M, You W, et al. Sickle cell anemia causes a distinct pattern of glomerular dysfunction. *Kidney Int.* 1997;51:826-833.
240. Guasch A, Cua M, Mitch WE. Early detection and the course of glomerular injury in patients with sickle cell anemia. *Kidney Int.* 1996;49:786-791.
241. Schmitt F, Martinez F, Brillet G, et al. Early glomerular dysfunction in patients with sickle cell anemia. *Am J Kidney Dis.* 1998;32:208-214.
242. Tharaux PL, Hagege I, Placier S, et al. Urinary endothelin-1 as a marker of renal damage in sickle cell disease. *Nephrol Dial Transplant.* 2005;20: 2408-2413.
243. Guvenc B, Aikimbaev K, Unsal C, et al. Renal vascular resistance in sickle cell painful crisis. *Int J Hematol.* 2005;82:127-131.
244. Bank N, Aynedjian HS, Qiu JH, et al. Renal nitric oxide synthases in transgenic sickle cell mice. *Kidney Int.* 1996;50:184-189.
245. Bank N, Kiroycheva M, Ahmed F, et al. Peroxynitrite formation and apoptosis in transgenic sickle cell mouse kidneys. *Kidney Int.* 1998;54: 1520-1528.
246. Walters MC, Storb R, Patience M, et al. Impact of bone marrow transplantation for symptomatic sickle cell disease: an interim report. Multicenter investigation of bone marrow transplantation for sickle cell disease. *Blood.* 2000;95:1918-1924.
247. Ojo AO, Govaerts TC, Schmouder RL, et al. Renal transplantation in end-stage sickle cell nephropathy. *Transplantation.* 1999;67:291-295.
248. Saxena AK, Panhotra BR, Al-Ghamdi AM. Should early renal transplantation be deemed necessary among patients with end-stage sickle cell nephropathy who are receiving hemodialytic therapy? *Transplantation.* 2004;77:955-956.
249. Gigante A, Gasperini ML, Cianci R, et al. Antiphospholipid antibodies and renal involvement. *Am J Nephrol.* 2009;30:405-412.
250. Carreras LO, Forastiero RR, Martinuzzo ME. Which are the best biological markers of the antiphospholipid syndrome? *J Autoimmun.* 2000;15:163-172.
251. Wilson WA, Gharavi AE, Koike T, et al. International consensus statement on preliminary classification criteria for definite antiphospholipid syndrome: report of an international workshop. *Arthritis Rheum.* 1999;42: 1309-1311.
252. Hughes GR. The Prosser-White oration 1983. Connective tissue disease and the skin. *Clin Exp Dermatol.* 1984;9:535-544.
253. Nochy D, Daugas E, Droz D, et al. The intrarenal vascular lesions associated with primary antiphospholipid syndrome. *J Am Soc Nephrol.* 1999;10:507-518.
254. Sangle SR, D'Cruz DP. Renal artery stenosis: a new facet of the antiphospholipid (Hughes) syndrome. *Lupus.* 2003;12: 803-804.
255. Erkan D, Lockshin MD. New approaches for managing antiphospholipid syndrome. *Nat Clin Pract Rheumatol.* 2009;5:160-170.
256. Bucciarelli S, Erkan D, Espinosa G, et al. Catastrophic antiphospholipid syndrome: treatment, prognosis, and the risk of relapse. *Clin Rev Allergy Immunol.* 2009;36:80-84.
257. Fakhouri F, Noel LH, Zuber J, et al. The expanding spectrum of renal diseases associated with antiphospholipid syndrome. *Am J Kidney Dis.* 2003;41:1205-1211.

258. Gronhagen-Riska C, Teppo AM, Helantera A, et al. Raised concentrations of antibodies to cardiolipin in patients receiving dialysis. *BMJ.* 1990;300:1696-1697.

259. Erre GL, Pardini S, Faedda R, et al. Effect of rituximab on clinical and laboratory features of antiphospholipid syndrome: a case report and a review of literature. *Lupus.* 2008;17:50-55.

260. Edwards CJ, Hughes GR. Hughes syndrome (the antiphospholipid syndrome): 25 years old. *Mod Rheumatol.* 2008;18:119-124.

260a. Lonze BE, Singer AL, Montgomery RA. Eculizumab and renal transplantation in a patient with CAPS. *N Engl J Med.* 2010;362:1744-1745.

261. Bockler D, Allenberg JR, Schumacher H. Renal artery thrombosis in acute type B aortic dissection: what do you do? *Vasc Med.* 2005;10:237-238.

262. Goodman PE, Rennie WP. Renal infarction secondary to nasal insufflation of cocaine. *Am J Emerg Med.* 1995;13:421-423.

263. Templeton PA, Pais SO. Renal artery occlusion in PAN. *Radiology.* 1985;156:308.

264. Teoh MK. Takayasu's arteritis with renovascular hypertension: results of surgical treatment. *Cardiovasc Surg.* 1999;7:626-632.

265. Akpolat T, Akkoyunlu M, Akpolat I, et al. Renal Behçet's disease: a cumulative analysis. *Semin Arthritis Rheum.* 2002;31:317-337.

266. Thomas DP, Roberts HR. Hypercoagulability in venous and arterial thrombosis. *Ann Intern Med.* 1997;126:638-644.

267. Dasgupta B, Almond MK, Tanqueray A. Polyarteritis nodosa and the antiphospholipid syndrome. *Br J Rheumatol.* 1997;36:1210-1212.

268. Klein O, Bernheim J, Strahilevitz J, et al. Renal colic in a patient with anti-phospholipid antibodies and factor V Leiden mutation. *Nephrol Dial Transplant.* 1999;14:2502-2504.

269. Miura K, Takahashi T, Takahashi I, et al. Renovascular hypertension due to antithrombin deficiency in childhood. *Pediatr Nephrol.* 2004;19:1294-1296.

270. Queffeulou G, Michel C, Vrtovsnik F, et al. Hyperhomocysteinemia, low folate status, homozygous C677T mutation of the methylene tetrahydrofolate reductase and renal arterial thrombosis. *Clin Nephrol.* 2002;57:158-162.

271. Pochet JM, Bobrie G, Basile C, et al. [Renal arterial thrombosis complicating nephrotic syndrome]. *Presse Med.* 1988;17:2139.

272. Holden A, Hill A. Renal angioplasty and stenting with distal protection of the main renal artery in ischemic nephropathy: early experience. *J Vasc Surg.* 2003;38:962-968.

273. Levin M, Nakhoul F, Keidar Z, et al. Acute oliguric renal failure associated with unilateral renal embolism: a successful treatment with iloprost. *Am J Nephrol.* 1998;18:444-447.

274. Cheng KL, Tseng SS, Tarng DC. Acute renal failure caused by unilateral renal artery thromboembolism. *Nephrol Dial Transplant.* 2003;18:833-835.

275. Domanovits H, Paulis M, Nikfardjam M, et al. Acute renal infarction. Clinical characteristics of 17 patients. *Medicine (Baltimore).* 1999;78: 386-394.

276. Yudd M, Llach F. Disorders of renal arteries and veins. In: Brenner BM, ed. *Brenner & Rector's The Kidney.* Philadelphia: WB Saunders; 2004:pp 1571-1600.

277. Zubarev AV. Ultrasound of renal vessels. *Eur Radiol.* 2001;11:1902-1915.

278. Kawashima A, Sandler CM, Ernst RD, et al. CT evaluation of renovascular disease. *Radiographics.* 2000;20:1321-1340.

279. Vosshenrich R, Fischer U. Contrast-enhanced MR angiography of abdominal vessels: is there still a role for angiography? *Eur Radiol.* 2002;12:218-230.

280. Frost L, Engholm G, Johnsen S, et al. Incident thromboembolism in the aorta and the renal, mesenteric, pelvic, and extremity arteries after discharge from the hospital with a diagnosis of atrial fibrillation. *Arch Intern Med.* 2001;161:272-276.

281. Gorich J, Kramer S, Tomczak R, et al. Thromboembolic complications after endovascular aortic aneurysm repair. *J Endovasc Ther.* 2002;9:180-184.

282. Bush RL, Najibi S, MacDonald MJ, et al. Endovascular revascularization of renal artery stenosis: technical and clinical results. *J Vasc Surg.* 2001;33:1041-1049.

283. Yavuzgil O, Gurgun C, Zoghi M, et al. Bilateral renal arterial embolisation in a patient with mitral stenosis and atrial fibrillation: an uncommon reason of flank pain. *Anadolu Kardiyol Derg.* 2003;3:73-75.

284. Greenberg JM, Steiner MA, Marshall JJ. Acute renal artery thrombosis treated by percutaneous rheolytic thrombectomy. *Catheter Cardiovasc Interv.* 2002;56:66-68.

285. Gasparini M, Hofmann R, Stoller M. Renal artery embolism: clinical features and therapeutic options. *J Urol.* 1992;147:567-572.

286. Ouriel K, Andrus CH, Ricotta JJ, et al. Acute renal artery occlusion: when is revascularization justified? *J Vasc Surg.* 1987;5:348-355.

287. Blum U, Billmann P, Krause T, et al. Effect of local low-dose thrombolysis on clinical outcome in acute embolic renal artery occlusion. *Radiology.* 1993;189:549-554.

288. van der Wal MA, Wisselink W, Rauwerda JA. Traumatic bilateral renal artery thrombosis: case report and review of the literature. *Cardiovasc Surg.* 2003;11:527-529.

289. Cass AS. Renovascular injuries from external trauma. Diagnosis, treatment, and outcome. *Urol Clin North Am.* 1989;16:213-220.

290. Kamel IR, Berkowitz JF. Assessment of the cortical rim sign in posttraumatic renal infarction. *J Comput Assist Tomogr.* 1996;20:803-806.

291. McGahan JP, Richards JR, Jones CD, et al. Use of ultrasonography in the patient with acute renal trauma. *J Ultrasound Med.* 1999;18:207-213:quiz, *J Ultrasound Med.* 1999; 18:215-216.

292. Maggio Jr AJ, Brosman S. Renal artery trauma. *Urology.* 1978;11:125-130.

293. Fort J, Camps J, Ruiz P, et al. Renal artery embolism successfully revascularized by surgery after 5 days' anuria. Is it never too late? *Nephrol Dial Transplant.* 1996;11:1843-1845.

294. Haas CA, Spirnak JP. Traumatic renal artery occlusion: a review of the literature. *Tech Urol.* 1998;4:1-11.

295. Weimann S, Flora G, Dittrich P, et al. Traumatic renal artery occlusion: is late reconstruction advisable? *J Urol.* 1987;137:727-729.

296. Goodman DN, Saibil EA, Kodama RT. Traumatic intimal tear of the renal artery treated by insertion of a Palmaz stent. *Cardiovasc Intervent Radiol.* 1998;21:69-72.

297. Henke PK, Cardneau JD, Welling 3rd TH, et al. Renal artery aneurysms: a 35-year clinical experience with 252 aneurysms in 168 patients. *Ann Surg.* 2001;234:454-462:discussion, *Ann Surg.* 2001; 234:462-463.

298. Martin 3rd RS, Meacham PW, Ditesheim JA, et al. Renal artery aneurysm: selective treatment for hypertension and prevention of rupture. *J Vasc Surg.* 1989;9:26-34.

299. Cinat M, Yoon P, Wilson SE. Management of renal artery aneurysms. *Semin Vasc Surg.* 1996;9:236-244.

300. Barth RA. Fibromuscular dysplasia with clotted renal artery aneurysm. *Pediatr Radiol.* 1993;23:296-297.

301. Brogan PA, Davies R, Gordon I, et al. Renal angiography in children with polyarteritis nodosa. *Pediatr Nephrol.* 2002;17:277-283.

302. Millar AJ, Gilbert RD, Brown RA, et al. Abdominal aortic aneurysms in children. *J Pediatr Surg.* 1996;31:1624-1628.

303. Potti A, Danielson B, Sen K. "True" mycotic aneurysm of a renal artery allograft. *Am J Kidney Dis.* 1998;31:E3.

304. Edwards BS, Stanson AW, Holley KE, et al. Isolated renal artery dissection, presentation, evaluation, management, and pathology. *Mayo Clin Proc.* 1982;57:564-571.

305. Esayag-Tendler B, Yamase H, Ramsby G, et al. Accelerated hypertension with encephalopathy due to an isolated dissection of a renal artery branch vessel. *Am J Kidney Dis.* 1994;23:869-873.

306. Reilly LM, Cunningham CG, Maggisano R, et al. The role of arterial reconstruction in spontaneous renal artery dissection. *J Vasc Surg.* 1991;14:468-477:discussion, *J Vasc Surg.* 1991; 14:477-479.

307. Lauterbach SR, Cambria RP, Brewster DC, et al. Contemporary management of aortic branch compromise resulting from acute aortic dissection. *J Vasc Surg.* 2001;33:1185-1192.

308. Markowitz GS, Brignol F, Burns ER, et al. Renal vein thrombosis treated with thrombolytic therapy: case report and brief review. *Am J Kidney Dis.* 1995;25:801-806.

309. Jaar BG, Kim HS, Samaniego MD, et al. Percutaneous mechanical thrombectomy: a new approach in the treatment of acute renal-vein thrombosis. *Nephrol Dial Transplant.* 2002;17:1122-1125.

310. Sagripanti A, Barsotti G. Hypercoagulability, intraglomerular coagulation, and thromboembolism in nephrotic syndrome. *Nephron.* 1995;70:271-281.

311. Wolak T, Rogachev B, Tovbin D, et al. Renal vein thrombosis as a presenting symptom of multiple genetic pro-coagulant defects. *Nephrol Dial Transplant.* 2005;20:827-829.

312. Morrissey EC, McDonald BR, Rabetoy GM. Resolution of proteinuria secondary to bilateral renal vein thrombosis after treatment with systemic thrombolytic therapy. *Am J Kidney Dis.* 1997;29:615-619.

313. Kanagasundaram NS, Bandyopadhyay D, Brownjohn AM, et al. The diagnosis of renal vein thrombosis by magnetic resonance angiography. *Nephrol Dial Transplant.* 1998;13:200-202.

314. Llach F, Papper S, Massry SG. The clinical spectrum of renal vein thrombosis: acute and chronic. *Am J Med.* 1980;69:819-827.

315. Glassock RJ. Prophylactic anticoagulation in nephrotic syndrome: a clinical conundrum. *J Am Soc Nephrol.* 2007;18:2221-2225.

316. Robert A, Olmer M, Sampol J, et al. Clinical correlation between hypercoagulability and thrombo-embolic phenomena. *Kidney Int.* 1987;31:830-835.

317. Wakui H, Imai H, Komatsuda A, et al. Circulating antibodies against alpha-enolase in patients with primary membranous nephropathy (MN). *Clin Exp Immunol.* 1999;118:445-450.

318. Price DT, Ridker PM, Factor V. Leiden mutation and the risks for thromboembolic disease: a clinical perspective. *Ann Intern Med.* 1997;127:895-903.

319. Nishimura M, Shimada J, Ito K, et al. Acute arterial thrombosis with antithrombin III deficiency in nephrotic syndrome: report of a case. *Surg Today.* 2000;30:663-666.

320. Harms K, Speer CP. [Thrombosis: an underestimated complication of central catheters? Subclavian vein, vena cava and renal vein thrombosis after silastic catheters]. *Monatsschr Kinderheilkd.* 1993;141:21-25.
321. Hollenbeck M, Westhoff A, Bach D, et al. Doppler sonography and renal graft vessel thromboses after OKT3 treatment. *Lancet.* 1992;340:619-620.
322. Kuhle S, Massicotte P, Chan A, et al. A case series of 72 neonates with renal vein thrombosis. Data from the 1-800-NO-CLOTS Registry. *Thromb Haemost.* 2004;92:729-733.
323. Asghar M, Ahmed K, Shah SS, et al. Renal vein thrombosis. *Eur J Vasc Endovasc Surg.* 2007;34:217-223.
324. Hussein M, Mooij J, Khan H, et al. Renal vein thrombosis, diagnosis and treatment. *Nephrol Dial Transplant.* 1999;14:245-247.
325. Siddiqi FA, Tepler J, Fantini GA. Acquired protein S and antithrombin III deficiency caused by nephrotic syndrome: an unusual cause of graft thrombosis. *J Vasc Surg.* 1997;25:576-580.
326. Yang SH, Lee CH, Ko SF, et al. The successful treatment of renal-vein thrombosis by low-molecular-weight heparin in a steroid-sensitive nephrotic patient. *Nephrol Dial Transplant.* 2002;17:2017-2019.
327. Sarasin FP, Schifferli JA. Prophylactic oral anticoagulation in nephrotic patients with idiopathic membranous nephropathy. *Kidney Int.* 1994;45:578-585.
328. Orth SR, Ritz E. The nephrotic syndrome. *N Engl J Med.* 1998;338:1202-1211.
329. Robertson AJ, Nargund V, Gray DW, et al. Low dose aspirin as prophylaxis against renal-vein thrombosis in renal-transplant recipients. *Nephrol Dial Transplant.* 2000;15:1865-1868.

Tubulointerstitial Diseases

Carolyn J. Kelly and Eric G. Neilson

Tubulointerstitial injury is always present when kidney disease progresses clinically. Its presence is correlated with impaired renal function and the finding of renal fibrosis on biopsy.[1,2] Tubulointerstitial disease may be the primary inciting event or secondary to primary glomerular diseases such as glomerulonephritis and cystic renal diseases. Common systemic conditions such as hypertension, diabetes, and atherosclerosis probably damage both glomerular and interstitial compartments at the same time, and, of course, in the aging kidney, both glomerular and interstitial tissues are gradually altered, making the kidney even more sensitive to new injury in older individuals.[3]

Historical View, Including Structure-Function Relationships

In the middle of the nineteenth century, with Bowman's[4] description of the malpighian bodies connecting to tubules, the interstitial compartment was initially considered a separate anatomic region of the kidney.[5] In 1860, the finding of interstitial infiltrates at autopsy and the development of experimental models of interstitial injury[6] provided evidence that not only was the tubulointerstitium relevant in renal physiology but also tubulointerstitial disorders were a key feature of kidney disease. On the basis of previous observations of the presence of fibroblast-like cells in the renal interstitium,[7] Traube[8] hypothesized in 1870 that interstitial changes documented in Bright's disease were responsible for kidney scarring and shrinkage associated with renal failure.

In 1898, Councilman[9] observed cellular and fluid exudation in the interstitial tissue in the kidneys of patients dying of scarlet fever and diphtheria. In particular, the organs were sterile, which raises the possibility of an allergic-type phenomenon. This entity was termed *acute interstitial nephritis.* Councilman's report and insights from several models of tubulointerstitial injury developed across the century provided the rationale for Volhard and Fahr[10] to include interstitial nephritis in their 1914 classification of kidney diseases. Suggestions of an association between drugs and interstitial nephritis in humans emerged in the 1940s with the observation that antibiotics and analgesics could damage the interstitial compartment.[11] As a result, researchers began to consider the risk of interstitial nephritis with a variety other drugs. In 1913, injection of heterologous proteins into rabbits was found to lead to lymphocyte infiltration in the renal interstitium[12]; however, attention to the immunologic basis of interstitial injury was not renewed until 1971, when Steblay and Rudofsky[13] described a model of tubulointerstitial nephritis induced by antibodies reactive with tubular basement membrane (TBM) in guinea pigs. Since then, autoimmune tubulointerstitial disease has been observed in a number of species, including mice, rats, and rabbits, after immunization with heterologous TBM.[14]

Although all these models illustrated immune mechanisms that have been reported in humans with interstitial nephritis, none of them offered the intrinsic value of a spontaneously occurring renal lesion. In 1984, Neilson and associates[15] characterized a model of spontaneous interstitial nephritis in the kdkd strain of mice. In the absence of renal antibodies, they found that this inheritable model of interstitial nephritis, because of mutations in mitochondrial prenyltransferase,[16] involves the cellular and regulatory T cell limb of the immune system. In virtually all forms of progressive experimental and chronic human kidney disease, a prominent inflammatory infiltrate exists within the interstitial compartment. The extent of these infiltrates,[17] the number of fibroblasts present,[18] and the area of fibrosis are all correlated[16] with progressive decline in renal function.

The concept that tubulointerstitial damage mediates impaired renal function is not new.[11] Many investigators have pointed out the prognostic significance of severe injury of the tubulointerstitium in lupus nephritis[19] and membranous nephropathy.[20] In 1968, Risdon and colleagues[20] first described an association between the degree of renal impairment and the extent of tubulointerstitial damage in patients with glomerular disease. In 50 cases of persistent glomerular nephritis, the correlations between creatinine clearance, plasma creatinine concentration, ability of the kidney to concentrate the urine, and glomerular changes were less striking than those documented between the extent of tubular lesions and alterations in renal function. These findings suggested that in chronic glomerulonephritis, interstitial damage across multiple tubules has much more effect on the glomerular filtration rate (GFR) than does the structural injury in the glomeruli. Bohle and associates[21] also studied tubulointerstitial changes in a wide variety of glomerulopathies. As urine osmolality decreased, the renal function deteriorated. Conversely, decreasing maximal urine osmolality was correlated best with increasing interstitial volume, lowering the cross-sectional area of proximal tubular epithelium or epithelium from the thick segment of the loop of Henle. This was not a unique feature, because other key interstitial changes documented by light microscopy, immunofluorescence, or histochemistry—which include the presence of immune inflammatory cells, activated fibroblasts, extracellular matrix components, antibodies, and complement—are also predictive of the long-term prognosis in chronic glomerulonephritis.[21,22]

Several mechanisms may explain how tubulointerstitial disease affects renal function. The simplest explanation is that tubular obstruction from interstitial inflammation and fibrosis impedes urine flow, increases intratubular pressure, and eventually lowers GFR.[21] Although no direct measurements are available, tubular atrophy and cell debris within tubules would represent a hindrance to the draining of fluid.[23] A second possible mechanism implicates the reduction in the volume of peritubular capillaries,[24] and in this setting, the tubulointerstitial compartment becomes relatively avascular and ischemic. As a result of the increase in vascular resistance in the postglomerular region, the hydrostatic pressure in the glomerular capillaries also increases, impairing glomerular arteriolar outflow. A third explanation is that tubuloglomerular feedback is altered, which is perhaps more significant. The presence of edema and inflammation in the renal interstitium, by increasing the interstitial pressure, may lower the sensitivity of the feedback mechanism,[25] possibly through local control of production of vasoactive substances such as angiotensin II, nitric oxide, and prostaglandins.[26] When tubulointerstitial fibrosis develops, the autoregulation of renal blood flow is also disrupted permanently.[27] A fourth explanation is glomerular-tubular disconnection—the finding that atrophic tubules and glomeruli are no longer connected to each other—which is a well-recognized consequence of tubulointerstitial nephritis.[28] This is consistent with human data showing a positive correlation between the fractional volume of the interstitium, the percentage of proximal tubuli without connection to a glomerulus, and renal function decline in patients with chronic pyelonephritis.[29] Collectively, all of these pathophysiologic processes are interrelated and may apply in some combinatorial manner. It is difficult to make clean comparisons between experimental animals and humans because nearly all that is known about this process in humans comes from detailed work in experimental models.

Mechanisms of Tubulointerstitial Injury

Mechanisms of tubulointerstitial injury may have a glomerular component, depending on the development of interstitial cellular infiltrates. Such development always results in fibrosis.

Glomerular Disease–Related Events

Glomerular diseases incite tubulointerstitial injury through multiple pathways[30]: (1) Impaired glomerular permselectivity allows the escape into the urinary space of substances that are toxic to tubuli[2,30]; (2) altered glomerular hemodynamics can damage nephrons through intraglomerular hypertension[31] and, alternatively, glomerular hypoperfusion may diminish postglomerular blood flow that provokes tubular ischemia; (3) immunologic mechanisms in glomeruli may incur the loss of tolerance and thereby instigate tubulointerstitial injury[32]; and (4) inflammatory mediators may seep from glomeruli into the urinary space or into the interstitium through the juxtaglomerular apparatus.[33] In addition, leukocytes may migrate into the interstitium via the mesangial stalk and vascular pole of the glomerulus.[34] Nephron loss as a result of destruction of the glomeruli and attached tubules may instigate metabolic adaptations in surviving nephrons that induce tubulointerstitial injury through the renin-angiotensin system.[2]

Two additional hypotheses to explain the interstitial damage associated with chronic glomerular disease have been proposed[35]: misdirected filtration and crescentic cell proliferation. These hypothesized mechanisms are based on histologic studies of the development and progression in animal and human renal disease. According to the misdirection hypothesis, there is an extension of a proteinaceous crescent into the outer aspect of the proximal tubule. As a consequence of persistent misdirected filtration, the proteinaceous filtrate near the glomerulotubular junction expands in the space between the tubular epithelial membrane and the TBM and may spread within this space along the entire proximal convolution. This process is associated predominantly with degenerative glomerular disease[36] but may also be contributory along individual nephrons in inflammatory disease.[37] A more direct approach to the tubulointerstitial compartment, however, may simply be passage through the juxtaglomerular apparatus.[33] The other mechanism is the encroachment of a growing cellular crescent upon the glomerulotubular junction, where the initial segment of the proximal tubule is incorporated into the crescent. This process is more characteristic of the inflammatory models.[37,38] However, cellular proliferation is complemented frequently in inflammatory models by misdirected filtrate spreading, which leads to mixed crescents.

In both cases, the mechanism results in the loss of nephrons and subsequent fibrosis, which is, however, considered a reparative process important for the maintenance of renal structure rather than a determinant of further injury.[35] Although this theory does not exclude a direct effect of proteins filtered into the tubular lumen, it underlines the fact that therapeutic intervention to prevent disease progression should target these glomerular changes, as well as processes that activate proximal tubular cells. The loss of containment of injury within the confines of the glomerulus enables inflammation to spread to a very large tubulointerstitial compartment. Chronic injury and the accompanying fibrosis, driven by glomerular processes, provide a conduit for the easy transmission of more inflammation into areas previously uninvolved by original disease. Tubulointerstitial disease can thus bridge areas that separate injured and noninjured nephrons.

Proteinuria-Induced Tubular Cell Activation and Damage

One important mechanism of glomerular-tubulointerstitial interaction is through proteinuria. Although proteinuria has been considered historically as simply a surrogate marker of the severity of underlying glomerular damage, clinical and experimental data indicate that proteinuria is an independent risk factor and plays an important role in the progression of renal disease.[39] In 1932, Chanutin and Ferris[40] observed that removal of 75% of the total renal mass in rats led to a slowly progressive deterioration in the function of the remaining nephrons, with progressive azotemia and glomerulosclerosis. The glomerular lesions of the remnant kidneys were associated with abnormal glomerular permeability and proteinuria. At that time, proteinuria was considered a marker of the extent of the glomerular damage, despite the fact that Volhard and Fahr in 1914[10] and von Mollendorf and Stohr in 1924[41] had already found that renal damage was related to exuberant protein excretion in the urine. In 1954, Oliver and associates[42] recognized protein droplets in the cytoplasm of tubular cells, possibly the result of impaired reabsorption of plasma proteins that is normally carried out by renal tubules, and they proposed that proteinuria could damage nephrons.

The mechanisms by which increased urinary protein concentration leads to nephrotoxic injury are certainly multifactorial and involve numerous pathways of cellular damage. Obstruction of tubular lumen by casts and obliteration of the tubular neck by glomerular tuft adhesions may contribute to tubulointerstitial damage from proteinuria. However, accumulating evidence emphasizes direct effects of filtered macromolecules on tubular cells.[43] Proteins escaping into glomerular filtrate and reaching the tubular urine are largely reabsorbed in the proximal segments at the apical poles of tubular epithelium. This involves receptor-mediated endocytosis, followed by clustering of the ligand-receptor complex into clathrin-coated pits, which gives rise to endocytic vesicles. Upon endocytic uptake, progress to the lysosome requires endosomal acidification to dissociate proteins from the receptors, which enables their degradation in lysosomes by the action of specific enzymes. The tandem endocytic receptors megalin and cubilin, which are abundantly expressed at the brush border of proximal tubular cells, interact to mediate the reabsorption of

a large amount of proteins, including carrier proteins important for transport and cellular uptake of vitamins and lipids.[44]

Specific mechanisms linking the excess traffic of plasma proteins and tubulointerstitial injury have been described in in vitro studies in which polarized proximal tubular cells were used to assess the effect of apical exposure to proteins. Protein overload activates proximal tubular cells into acquiring a proinflammatory phenotype.[45] In fact, upregulation of inflammatory and fibrogenic genes and production of related proteins have been reported upon challenge of proximal tubular cells with plasma proteins. These entities include cytokines and chemokines such as monocyte chemoattractant protein-1, RANTES (regulated upon activation, normal T cell expressed, and secreted), interleukin-8,[46-48] and fractalkine.[49] Moreover, the profibrogenic cytokine transforming growth factor-β (TGF-β) and its type II receptor,[50] as well as tissue inhibitors of metalloproteinase-1 and -2, and membrane surface expression of the αvβ5 integrin[51] are also highly increased in vitro by plasma proteins. These events are triggered by protein kinase C–dependent generation of reactive oxygen species,[52] nuclear translocation of nuclear factor κ light-chain enhancer of activated B cells (NF-κB),[53] and the engagement of mitogen-activated protein kinase/extracellular signal–regulated kinase (MAPK/ERK).[49,54]

Extrapolation from such in vitro data to the in vivo situation in humans is difficult, in view of the somewhat conflicting data observed with different proteins in different cell systems,[55,56] as well as the reported changes in the expression of several genes of still-unknown function.[57] One issue concerns the possibility that in vitro evidence of the phenotypic changes induced in the proximal tubular cells by protein overload can adequately reflect the in vivo proteinuric conditions in animals and humans; the concentrations of albumin used to challenge proximal tubular cells in culture (≈10 mg/mL) may have been much higher than would be expected in human disease. The hypothesis of proteinuria-induced tubulointerstitial changes, however, is supported by attempts to interfere specifically with the cascade of events leading to renal damage, particularly by blocking the renin-angiotensin system.[58-62] Angiotensin-converting enzyme inhibitors given to animals with experimental chronic nephropathies markedly reduce urinary protein excretion and, at the same time, attenuate interstitial inflammation and fibrosis. Further evidence suggests that inhibition of renin-angiotensin system, in addition to reducing proteinuria, may also attenuate albumin-induced signaling in tubular cells.[63] Moreover, it has been shown that transfection with a monocyte chemotactic protein-1 antagonist or a truncated form of the α inhibitor of NF-κB (IκBα) inhibits albumin overload–induced tubulointerstitial injury.[1,53]

Proteinuria-Induced Tubular Cell Apoptosis

Apoptosis[64] and autophagy[65] are mechanisms that underlie protein-induced tubular cell injury. Protein overload causes a dose- and duration-dependent induction of apoptosis in cultured proximal tubular cells, as disclosed by evidence of internucleosomal DNA fragmentation, morphologic changes (including cell shrinkage and nuclear condensation), and plasma membrane alterations.[55] Apoptosis in this setting is associated with activation of the Fas-associated protein with death domain (FADD)–caspase 8 pathway.[64,65] Evidence of apoptotic responses to protein load is not confined to cultured tubular epithelial cells. In persistent proteinuria, the terminal deoxyuridine triphosphate (dUTP) nick-end labeling assay reveals increased numbers of positive apoptotic cells both in the tubulointerstitial compartment and in glomeruli in the rat model of albumin overload.[66] In tubuli, most of the positive cells belonged to rats expressing angiotensin II type 2 (AT_2) receptors. Findings of reduced phosphorylation of MAPK/ERK and the apoptosis regulator protein Bcl-2 reflect an AT_2 receptor–mediated mechanism underlying tubular cell apoptosis.[66] Apoptosis of proximal tubular cells, which may contribute to glomerular-tubular disconnection and atrophy,[28] was also found in response to proteinuria in passive Heymann's nephritis.[67] Apoptotic cells have been detected in both proximal and distal tubular profiles in biopsy specimens from patients with primary focal segmental glomerulosclerosis.[68] In support of the pathophysiologic significance of such observations, a strong positive correlation was found between proteinuria and the incidence of tubular cell apoptosis, which was identified as a strong predictor of outcome in these patients.

Glomerular Filtered Growth Factors and Cytokines

Plasma contains many growth factors and cytokines at considerable concentrations, usually in high-molecular-weight precursor forms or bound to specific binding proteins that regulate their biologic activity. They are present in nephrotic tubular fluid.[69]

Insulin-like growth factor-1 (IGF-1) is present in serum at levels of 20 to 40 nmol, which is more than 1000-fold of its biologic activity. Almost all of the circulating IGF-1 is present in complexes of higher molecular weight, about 50 and 150 kDa, which normally prevent glomerular ultrafiltration. However, in experimental proteinuria, this growth factor is translocated into tubular fluid (primarily as the 50-kDa complex), as shown by micropuncture collection of early proximal tubular fluid.[70] Tubular fluid from nephrotic rats activates IGF-1 receptors in cultured tubular cells that are expressed in both basolateral and apical membranes in some tubular segments.[70]

Hepatocyte growth factor (HGF) is largely of hepatic origin and is present in serum in an inactive, monomeric form (97 kDa) and in a heterodimeric form (80 to 92 kDa, depending on glycosylation). Its specific signaling receptor, the p190^MET protein, is expressed in apical membranes in proximal tubuli in normal rats and at increased levels in diabetic animals. HGF is present in early proximal tubular fluid from rats with streptozotocin-induced diabetic nephropathy and is excreted with urine in diabetic animals.[71] Circumstantial evidence suggests that HGF undergoes glomerular ultrafiltration in proteinuric states, probably as the mature, bioactive form of the molecule.

TGF-β is a pluripotent cytokine (25-kDa) that is also present in serum at considerable levels and in high concentrations in platelets. In these reservoirs, almost all of the peptide is maintained in inactive complexes by binding to latency-associated protein (LAP), which is further bound to latent TGF-β–binding protein (LTBP) forming an LAP-LTBP complex of high molecular weight (220 kDa). TGF-β is also associated in serum with α_2-macroglobulin (900 kDa). The high-molecular-weight TGF-β complexes prevent glomerular ultrafiltration under physiologic conditions. However, in proteinuric glomerular diseases, TGF-β is present in early proximal tubular fluid, and at least a portion is bioactive. The remainder is probably activated during downstream tubular flow by

acidification of tubular fluid, perhaps by increasing urea concentrations and through the presence of enzymes such as plasminogen activator inhibitor-1. The concentration of TGF-β in glomerular ultrafiltrate from rats with diabetic nephropathy is approximately 30 pmol, which is one to two orders of magnitude higher than required for biologic responses.[71]

TGF-β receptors are expressed in most tubular segments.[71,72] IGF-1, HGF, and TGF-β are also present in the urine of patients with proteinuric diseases.[73,74] Urinary excretion of these proteins, however, is not proof of glomerular ultrafiltration of IGF-1 and TGF-β, inasmuch as they are also expressed along tubular segments in some renal diseases; nevertheless, the presence of these cytokines in the urine of patients with proteinuric diseases is certainly compatible with their glomerular ultrafiltration. Ultrafiltered IGF-1, HGF, and TGF-β appear to act on tubular cells through their apical signaling receptors. There are several biochemical responses by tubular cells to these cytokines that, collectively, resemble activation and moderate change in phenotype. These responses includes a moderate increase in the production of collagen types I and IV in response to IGF-1.[70] Incubation of proximal tubular cells with pooled early proximal tubular fluid, collected by micropuncture specimens from rats with diabetic nephropathy, increases fibronectin expression.[71] TGF-β also increases the transcription of the genes encoding collagen α_1III and collagen α_2I, as well as fibronectin, in proximal tubular cells. Thus, ultrafiltered growth factors induce moderately increased expression of matrix proteins by tubular cells that probably contribute to interstitial fibrosis. HGF signals a mixed message by increasing the expression of fibronectin in tubular cells,[71] thereby blocking the expression of collagen α_1III,[71] which is consistent with an antifibrogenic role.

Glomerular Filtered Lipids

Beside proteins themselves, fatty acids carried by filtered proteins can trigger tubulointerstitial injury. In rats with overload proteinuria, a potent chemotactic lipid was isolated from the urine, which attracted monocytes but not neutrophils.[75] Similar results were observed in mice transgenic for human liver-type fatty acid–binding protein, which in human proximal tubular cells binds free fatty acids in the cytoplasm and carries them to mitochondria or peroxisomes for metabolism by β-oxidation.[76] Such mice develop less macrophage infiltration and a tendency towards reduced tubulointerstitial damage; thus, intracellular accumulation of free fatty acids may modulate proliferative activity. Attempts have also been made to differentiate the effects of individual fatty acids (palmitate, stearate, oleate, and linoleate) on cellular toxicity and fibronectin production in cultured proximal tubular cells.[77] Oleate and linoleate were identified as the most profibrogenic and tubulotoxic fatty acids.

An additional pathogenic pathway has been linked to a form of low-density lipoprotein (LDL) modified by hypochlorous acid that accumulates in tubular epithelial cells in settings of injury.[78] Hypochlorous acid (and hypochlorite, a salt of hypochlorous acid) is a major oxidant generated from hydrogen peroxide (H_2O_2) by myeloperoxidase during an oxidative burst. In the HK-2 proximal tubular cells, hypochlorite-modified LDL causes a rapid increase in the expression of several genes encoding for proteins that help control cellular proliferation and apoptosis (Gadd153), production of reactive oxygen species (hemeoxygenase 1, cytochrome b5 reductase), and tissue remodeling and inflammation (connective tissue growth factor, vascular cell adhesion molecule-1 (VCAM-1), interleukin-1β, matrix metalloproteinase-7, and vascular endothelial growth factor [VEGF]). Hypochlorite-modified LDL, but not nonmodified LDL, also had antiproliferative and proapoptotic effects in these cells. Comparable changes in gene expression were also found in renal biopsy samples microdissected from proteinuric patients with declining renal function. The presence of hypochlorite-modified LDL in damaged tubular cells was confirmed by immunohistochemistry profile.[78] These observations seem to mirror altered patterns of gene expression that occur selectively in response to oxidative LDL modifications and enhance inflammatory and fibrogenic processes in chronic proteinuric conditions.

Activation of Complement Components

Among specific components of proteinuria, serum-derived complement factors can be harmful, especially upon activation by the proximal tubules.[79] Renal tubular epithelial cells appear most susceptible to luminal attack by C5b-9 because of the relative lack of membrane-bound complement regulatory proteins such as membrane cofactor protein (CD46), decay-accelerating factor, or CD55 and CD59 on the apical surface,[80] as opposed to other cell types, such as endothelium or circulating cells that are routinely exposed to complement. C3 is an essential factor of both the classical and the alternative pathways of complement activation that lead to the formation of C5b-9 membrane attack complexes. In vitro, proximal tubular cells exposed to human serum activate complement by the alternative pathway, which leads to fixation of the C5b-9 membrane attack complex neoantigen on their cell surface.[81] These events are followed by marked cytoskeletal alterations with disruption of the network of actin stress fibers, formation of blebs, and cytolysis. Production of superoxide anion and H_2O_2 and synthesis of proinflammatory cytokines such as interleukin-6 and tumor necrosis factor-α are also increased.[82] Within the kidney, complement proteins form deposits along the luminal side and are internalized by proximal tubular cells in rats with protein overload proteinuria,[83] renal mass ablation,[84] and aminonucleoside nephrosis,[85] a pattern commonly observed in kidneys of patients with nonselective proteinuria. C6-deficient rats that underwent 5/6 nephrectomy show marked improvement in tubulointerstitial injury and function,[86] which suggests that treatments to reduce C5b-9 attack complexes on tubular cells may slow disease progression and facilitate functional recovery independent of initial incitement by glomerular injury.

Intracellular C3 staining is also evident in proximal tubules early after renal mass ablation in a stage closely preceding the appearance of inflammation. C3 co-localizes with immunoglobulin G (IgG) in the same tubules in adjacent sections. These accumulations in proximal tubular cells are followed by local recruitment of infiltrating mononuclear cells that concentrate almost exclusively in regions containing C3-positive proximal tubuli.[87] The amidation of C3 by ammonia in the presence of high protein catabolism may also contribute to luminal formation of C5b-9 complexes[88] and the generation of a monocyte-activating factor.[89] Treatment with an angiotensin-converting enzyme inhibitor, although preventing

proteinuria, simultaneously limited both the tubular accumulation of C3 and IgG and interstitial inflammation.[84] These results suggest that in order for complement to mediate progressive tubulointerstitial damage, an environment of protein-enriched ultrafiltrate is required; that theory has been substantiated by findings that, in the absence of proteinuria, C5b-9 does not exert significant pathogenic potential as a mediator of chronic tubulointerstitial disease.[90]

In three distinct models of nonproteinuric tubulointerstitial disease in PVG rats, an increase in deposition of C5b-9 at peritubular sites is associated with tubular and interstitial changes.[90] In each model, the severity of the disease is equivalent, regardless of whether the animals are from breeding pairs with normal complement activity or C6-deficiency. Finding that C6 deficiency does not alter the severity and progression of structural damage despite the upregulation of C5b-9 on basolateral membranes of tubuli also suggests, in contrast to proteinuric states, that C5b-9 does not have a significant effect on the progression of chronic nonglomerular kidney disease. Renal parenchymal tissues express a limited repertoire of complement receptors—including CR1, CR3, and CD88—that directly bind complement proteins present in the ultrafiltrate. Whether the stimulation of complement receptors on tubular cells has functional consequences in progressive renal disease is unknown.

In addition to activating exogenous complement, proximal tubular epithelial cells synthesize a number of complement components, including C3, C4, factor B, and C5.[91] As a result of exposure of cultured tubular epithelial cells to total serum proteins at the apical surface, messenger RNA encoding C3 and protein biosynthesis is upregulated.[92] The enhanced secretion of C3 is predominantly basolateral, which is in vitro evidence of roles for locally synthesized complement in the process of tubulointerstitial damage. Serum fractionation experiments identified one or more substances responsible for such effects in the molecular size range of 30 to 100 kDa. This fraction contains proteins that pass through the glomerular barrier in proteinuric states, including transferrin. After incubation with apical transferrin, C3 messenger RNA is overexpressed; as a result, both apical and basolateral secretion of C3 is increased.[93] A similar degree of C3 upregulation occurs when iron-poor transferrin, or apotransferrin, is used, which indicates that the synthesis of C3 in proximal tubular cells is upregulated by transferrin; thus, protein rather than the iron moiety probably accounts for the observed effects. These findings are indicative of the potential role of intrarenal C3 synthesis in progressive renal disease and the relative contribution of locally synthesized versus ultrafiltered complement components in promoting inflammation and fibrosis. C3-deficient mice significantly attenuate the interstitial accumulation of cells expressing the F4/80 marker of monocytes, macrophages, and dendritic cells in response to protein overload with serum albumin. The protein overload causes significant upregulation of messenger RNA encoding C3 throughout the kidney.[94]

Finally, complement activation may directly regulate the renal immunologic response. Of great interest is the observation that local synthesis of C3 stimulates the transmigration of T cells across tubular epithelial cell barriers.[95] This pathway involves the direct action of tissue C3 with infiltrating T cells expressing C3 receptors and is a potential target for lymphocyte inhibitor agents such as mycophenolate mofetil, which is effective, if combined with antiproteinuric therapy against primary nonimmune disease characterized by tubular deposition of complement.[84,96]

Tubulointerstitial Antigens

When the immune system targets the interstitial compartment of the kidney as a primary process, the targets are two types of antigens: (1) those derived from endogenous renal cells, from TBM, or from other extracellular matrix components or (2) exogenous antigens processed and presented by native renal cells or by minor populations of professional antigen-presenting cells (APCs), such as dendritic cells, within the interstitium. Drugs may also become nephritogenic antigens by acting as haptens.

Antigens from Renal Cells and Tubular Basement Membrane

The tubulointerstitial nephritis (TIN) antigen is the target of anti–TBM antibody–mediated tubulointerstitial nephritis in humans.[97] Immunofluorescent staining of sera from patients with anti-TBM nephritis or with monoclonal antibodies specific to TIN antigen reveals its localization in the basement membrane of the proximal and, to a lesser extent, distal tubules and Bowman's capsule in the kidney.[98] Glycoprotein isoforms with molecular weights of 54 to 58 and of 40 to 50 kDa have been identified as the TIN antigen recognized by anti-TBM antibodies.[97,98] These isoforms have affinity for both type IV collagen and laminin[99] and probably serve to stabilize the TBM. The human TIN antigen has been mapped to chromosome 6p11.2-12, and complement DNAs encoding rabbit TIN antigen and its human homolog have been cloned and sequenced.[98,100] The antigen of anti-TBM disease in rodent models has been named 3M-1.[101] Polymorphic expression of TIN antigen is observed in both humans and in inbred rat strains. The absence of TIN antigen does not appear to impair renal function. The absence of TIN antigen, however, may in rare cases result in anti-TBM disease after renal transplantation, and it is one reason for resistance to anti-TBM disease among inbred rat strains.[102]

Tamm-Horsfall glycoprotein, along with antibodies directed at this large glycoprotein, is frequently observed within the interstitium in a variety of renal diseases, including chronic interstitial nephritis and reflux nephropathy.[103] Such immune deposits can also be observed in experimental animal models when animals are immunized with this protein.[104] There is insufficient evidence, however, that abnormal deposits of Tamm-Horsfall glycoprotein in the kidney have a critical role in the inflammatory process.[104] Drugs, drug-hapten complexes, or both can also serve as nephritogenic antigens.[105,106] These antigens, along with antibodies recognizing them, can either form immune deposits in situ within the interstitium or precipitate as a circulating complex.[107] Examples of such drugs include members of the penicillin family, cephalosporins, and phenytoin. In some cases, antibodies directed against microorganisms may bind cross-reactive epitopes on interstitial components; for example, the antibodies to nephritogenic streptococci cross-react with type IV collagen. Some anti-DNA antibodies additionally react with laminin and heparin sulfate in the extracellular matrix.

Exogenous and Endogenous Antigen Presentation by Tubular Cells

T cells recognize foreign antigens only when they are properly digested into small fragments and presented on the surface of APCs bound to major histocompatibility complex (MHC) molecules.[108] The recognition of this bimolecular complex on the surface of APCs leads to activation of T cells. CD4+ T cells typically recognize antigens exogenous to an APC, after the processing and presentation of that antigen in conjunction with class II MHC molecules. In contrast, CD8+ T cells typically recognize antigens synthesized by the APC in conjunction with class I MHC molecules. Activation of T cells by APCs expressing processed antigen is additionally optimized by a number of cell-cell interactions involving cell surface costimulatory molecules and their ligands. In general, recognition of class II MHC molecules by CD4+ T cells results in proliferation and cytokine expression by these cells, whereas CD8+ T cells cause target cell death on encountering antigen–class I complex–bearing cells. Renal tubular epithelial cells in culture have the ability to process and present exogenous and self-proteins to T lymphocytes.[109-111]

In addition to processing multiple potentially immunogenic peptides, proximal tubular cells are also exposed to filtered low-molecular-weight proinflammatory cytokines such as interferon-γ, interleukin-1, and tumor necrosis factor-α. Such cells are also exposed to cytokines secreted by immune cells infiltrating the interstitium. Ultimately, the ability of renal epithelial cells to either present antigen or serve as a target for CD8+ T cells depends on the cytokine milieu and on whether the net effect of those mediators is proinflammatory or antiinflammatory. Proinflammatory cytokines would typically augment the expression of class II MHC molecules on epithelial cells. Expression of such molecules is typically observed in fewer than 5% of tubular epithelial cells in normal kidney, but it is markedly augmented in interstitial nephritis, as is the expression of adhesion molecules such as intracellular adhesion molecule-1 (ICAM-1).[112] In addition to requiring upregulation of class II MHC molecules, renal tubular cells require the augmented expression of costimulatory molecules, which are necessary for full activation of T cells.[113] The interaction of the costimulatory molecular pair (a T cell receptor and an APC ligand) can result either in activation or inhibition of the immune response. Many of the receptors on T cells are members of the immunoglobulin superfamily, including CD28, CTLA-4, inducible costimulator (ICOS), and programmed death-1 (PD-1). The ligands for these receptors are members of the B7 family. Proinflammatory cytokines can induce the expression of both B7.1 and B7.2 on tubular epithelial cells.[114] Tubular epithelial cells can also induce other accessory molecules, such as CD40, ICAM-1, VCAM-1, and ICOS-L, which are involved in T cell activation.[115,116] In the doxorubicin (Adriamycin) nephropathy model of chronic proteinuric renal disease, treatment of mice with a monoclonal antibody directed to the CD40 ligand protects against renal structural and functional injury.[117] On the other hand, renal tubular cell expression of PD-L1, the receptor for PD-1, may have inhibitory effects on T cell proliferation or effector functions, or both.[118,119] In renal biopsy samples from patients with immunoglobulin A (IgA) nephropathy, interstitial nephritis, or lupus nephritis, tubules exhibit significant staining for B7-H1 (PD-L1),[120] which suggests that the expression of this costimulatory molecule is also upregulated in vivo. Thus the number of receptor-ligand pairs that potentially regulate the outcome of renal tubule cell interactions with T cells is large, and the net effect of the interaction is difficult to predict without functional studies.

Cellular Infiltrates

Cell-mediated immune responses have historically been implicated in the pathogenesis of interstitial nephritis because of both in vivo (delayed-type hypersensitivity) and in vitro (lymphoblast transformation) evidence of hypersensitivity to specific inciting antigens. Tubulointerstitial inflammation may result from antigen-specific stimulation, but it may also occur in the absence of antigenic stimulation.[121] The interstitial infiltrate of most chronic renal diseases in humans consists of a number of different effector cells, including macrophages and CD4[+] and CD8[+] T cells. Researchers in most studies report that T cells predominate, and the majority of these are CD4[+] cells, although there is considerable variation among the analyses.[122]

Interstitial drug reactions are typically mediated as delayed-type hypersensitivity responses.[107,123] The predominant T cell population may also be altered by immunosuppressive therapy before biopsy or by the stage of disease at the time of biopsy. Corticosteroids can markedly deplete the number of lymphocytes observed in interstitial nephritis. Studies in animal models have revealed an important role for macrophages in the initiation and progression of injury in chronic renal disease. Direct damage to resident cells is caused through the generation by macrophages of reactive oxygen species, nitric oxide, complement factors, and proinflammatory cytokines.[121] Macrophages can also affect supporting matrix and vasculature through the expression of metalloproteinases and vasoactive peptides. In animals, treatment with a monoclonal antibody directed against the CD11b/CD18 integrin, which is expressed by macrophages, depleted renal cortical macrophages by almost 50% in Adriamycin nephropathy[124] and reduced structural and functional injury if animals were treated prophylactically before Adriamycin administration.[124] Macrophages can also play a beneficial role in interstitial injury. They may serve as markers of disease remission[125] or play an antifibrotic role, as documented in mice with unilateral ureteric obstruction reconstituted with bone marrow from angiotensin II type 1 receptor–null or wild-type mice.[126] Clearly, interstitial macrophages in numerous models of interstitial injury have phenotypic and functional heterogeneity.[127] In most cases, B and T lymphocytes are present with macrophages to varying degrees.

Idiopathic immune-mediated interstitial nephritis is probably an autoimmune disease.[128] In fact, the composition of the interstitial infiltrate is much the same whether the initiating cause of injury is chronic ischemia induced by unilateral renal artery stenosis,[129] autoimmune tubulointerstitial nephritis,[130] aminonucleoside nephrosis,[131] cyclosporine nephrotoxicity,[132] or protein overload proteinuria.[83] It is possible that immune responses to neoantigens expressed by interstitial cells damaged by ischemia or toxins are a final common pathway for such interstitial injury. This notion is supported by the known expression of neoantigens such as vimentin in animals with overload proteinuria.[83]

Heat shock proteins, which can be induced in response to a number of cellular stresses, may also be recognized by T cells. The heat shock protein Hsp70 is expressed in renal tubules after chronic exposure of mice to cadmium chloride. T cells infiltrating the interstitial compartment were reactive to Hsp70 and could induce interstitial nephritis in cadmium chloride-treated animals after adoptive transfer, which is suggestive of a general mechanism whereby a toxic nephropathy might induce chronic injury through an antigen-specific immune response.[133] In remnant kidney models, an infiltration of the interstitium with macrophages and lymphocytes is correlated with functional parameters of renal failure, and improvement in these parameters is obtained with immunosuppressive treatment[134]; this finding is indicative of the importance of immune-mediated injury in the progressive interstitial disease observed in nonimmune forms of primary injury.

The histologic appearance of human interstitial disease can vary from granulomatous interstitial nephritis with an intense cellular infiltrate to sparse infiltrates with striking microcystic change. Although this kind of variation may reflect different stages of an immune-mediated lesion or different target antigens, it may also reflect the biologic activity of discrete populations of activated T cells. Some experimental interstitial lesions are histologically analogous to a cutaneous delayed-type hypersensitivity reaction. This type of lesion is frequently observed in experimental anti-TBM disease, in which the interstitial compartment displays focal aggregates of mononuclear cells. In the murine form of this disease, this histologic appearance can be largely reproduced after adoptive transfer of a T cell clone, which mediates both delayed-type hypersensitivity to the target antigen and cytotoxic injury to renal tubular cells.[135] Although such interstitial injury can be induced by T cell clones, the resultant damage to interstitial and tubular cells is the end result of interactions between many cell types. The cytotoxic activity of renal antigen-reactive T cell clones may well account for tubular cell destruction and resultant tubular atrophy. Cultured cytotoxic T cell clones that express pore-forming proteins (such as perforin) and serine esterase granzymes elicit interstitial nephritis after adoptive transfer, and maneuvers that decrease the expression of these mediators abrogate the ability of the T cells to mediate interstitial inflammatory lesions.[136-138] The nature of the variable genes used to assemble T cell antigen receptors expressed on cells in interstitial nephritis has been examined both in human kidney tissue and in experimental models; results have varied from use of multiple V-regions[139] to an oligoclonal usage in a case of drug-associated interstitial nephritis.[123,140]

Finally, there is functional diversity among CD4[+] T cells, and it is clear that certain subpopulations suppress rather than initiate or augment immune responses. The most well-characterized example of an inhibitory subpopulation is the CD4[+]CD25[+] regulatory T cell, which plays an active role in downregulating pathogenic autoimmune responses.[141] Fontenot and associates[142] suggest that Foxp3 expression, regardless of CD25 expression, reflects the presence of regulatory T cells. CD4[+]CD25[+] T cells suppress T cell proliferation in vitro but also have the capacity to suppress immune responses to autoantigens and alloantigens, tumor antigens, and infectious antigens in vivo.[143] The regulatory activity of these cells has been examined in the Adriamycin nephropathy model, in which mice with severe combined immunodeficiency received reconstituted CD4+CD25+ T cells had significantly reduced glomerulosclerosis, tubular injury, and interstitial expansion.[124] In the same model, adoptive transfer of Foxp3-transduced T cells led to decreases in urine protein excretion, reduction in serum creatinine, less tubular and glomerular damage, and a diminution in the interstitial infiltrate.[144] Much of the earlier work with suppressor T cells conducted in rodent models of interstitial nephritis yielded results that probably represented the activity of cells, which are now defined by Foxp3 expression.[137,145-149]

Interstitial Fibrosis

Fibrosis is the final common pathway leading to end-stage renal disease, regardless of initiating events. The process of tubulointerstitial fibrosis involves the loss of renal tubules and the accumulation of fibroblasts and matrix proteins, such as collagen (types I, III, IV, V, and VII), fibronectin, and laminin.[150] Cells infiltrating the renal interstitium have long been thought to play a role in the initiation and progression of tubulointerstitial fibrosis.[151] This is because the degree to which a number of cell types, macrophages, lymphocytes, and fibroblasts accumulate in the renal interstitium parallels the extent of fibrogenesis.[1] Moreover, it has been difficult to distinguish harmful cells from beneficial cells without functional analyses.[152] Advances in molecular technology, however, have enabled investigators to analyze cell types separately, and fibroblasts have been identified as the principal effector mediating tubulointerstitial fibrosis.[153]

Since fibroblast-specific protein-1 was identified as a marker of tissue fibroblasts,[154] these fibroblasts have been found to originate or multiply from a variety of sources, including local epithelial/endothelial-to-mesenchymal transition (EMT), the bone marrow, resident fibroblasts, or myofibroblasts.[155] EMT is also now known to be a robust source of tissue fibroblasts.[156,157] Fibroblasts derived from EMT play a critical role in tubulointerstitial fibrosis.[158]

Epithelial-Mesenchymal Transitions in Fibrosis

Epithelial and endothelial cells that line tubes and ducts have plasticity.[159,160] Midway through development, these cells can become fibroblasts by EMT as part of organ growth.[158] Of 18 lineage tracing studies, all but 4 have confirmed these events in adult tissues.[1] Tubular epithelia[161] and endothelia[156] undergoing EMT during persistent injury are common in the kidney, and a healthy majority of renal fibroblasts are produced locally by this process, followed by proliferation. Approximately 12% to 14% of kidney fibroblasts are also derived from EMT events that occur in bone marrow,[161] and fibroblasts from this niche circulate to peripheral tissue. Some authorities have suggested that pericytes are also a source of fibroblasts,[162] but for this to happen, they too would have to undergo some sort of transition.

Persistent cytokine activity during renal inflammation and disruption of underlying basement membrane by local proteases initiates the process of EMT.[163] Rather than falling into the tubular lumen to be washed away, some epithelial cells transition into fibroblasts while translocating back into the interstitial space behind decondensing tubules through rents in the basement membrane.[1,64] WNT proteins, integrin-linked kinases, IGF-1 and insulin-like growth factor-2, epidermal growth factor (EGF), fibroblast growth factor-2 (FGF-2), and TGF-β are among the archetypal modulators of EMT by outside-inside signaling.[158] For example, FGF-2 promotes the transition of tubular epithelia by inducing the release of matrix metalloproteinases-2 and -9, which eventually damages the underlying basement membranes.[164,165] FGF-2 also synergizes with TGF-β and EGF in mediating EMT by reducing cytokeratin expression and stimulating the movement of transitioning cells across damaged basement membranes. Together, TGF-β and EGF provide the strongest stimulation for completion of epithelial transitions.[1]

During EMT, FGF-2 activates FGF-1 receptor on the cell surface. Together, these growth factors or their intermediates are imported into the nucleus, in which they engage a variety of sequence-specific transcription factors (CBF-A, Snail, Sma- and Mad-related protein 3 [SMAD3], and Twist).[166,167] The net result is the emergence of the EMT proteome that represses epithelial proteins.[163] Loss of E-cadherins and cytokeratins, rearrangement of actin stress fibers, and expression of fibroblast-specific protein-1, vimentin, interstitial collagens, and occasionally α-smooth muscle actin mark the morphologic transition of epithelial cells into fibroblasts. EMT also operates in human tubular cells[168,169] and pathologic renal tissues.[18,170,171] Of note, HGF and bone morphogenetic protein-7 antagonize the epithelial transitions driven by FGF-2 and TGF-β.[172,173] The stage at which antifibrotic modulators are most effective is not yet known. The transcriptional modulators for signaling in EMT or its reversal involve intracellular SMAD/β-catenin activity.[1,167]

EMT is also regulated by tumor necrosis factor–related activation protein (TRAP),[174] an accessory molecule that circulates in interstitial spaces as a soluble moiety to block receptor activation by free ligand.[175] This control mechanism favors a state of differentiation in epithelia, which preserves organ structure and function. What is becoming increasingly clear is that mature epithelial cells are in a dynamic but not terminal state of differentiation.[160] Morphogenic forces that normally maintain epithelial phenotypes are pitted against countervailing forces trying to weaken that stability. Chronic inflammation into the interstitium destabilizes epithelial tissues by favoring fibrogenesis.

Chronic Hypoxia in Fibrosis

One of the most important contributors to the development of tubulointerstitial fibrosis is chronic ischemia.[176,177] Production of angiotensin II and inhibition of production of nitric oxide underlie chronic vasoconstriction, which may contribute to tissue ischemia and hypoxia,[178] and hypoxia stimulates EMT.[176] In vitro, hypoxia induces fibroblast proliferation and matrix production by tubular epithelial cells.[179] Histologic studies of animal models and human kidneys have revealed that there is often a loss of peritubular capillaries in areas of tubulointerstitial fibrosis.[1,178] Downregulation of VEGF is implicated in the progressive rarefaction of peritubular capillaries.[180] Moreover, because the size of the interstitial compartment determines the diffusion distance between peritubular capillaries and tubular cells, interstitial fibrosis probably worsens tubular oxygen supply. This interstitial reduction of capillary blood flow, which leads to starvation of tubuli, may underlie tubular atrophy and loss. Under these conditions, the remaining tubules are subject to functional hypermetabolism, and increased oxygen consumption further exacerbates the hypoxic environment.

Acute Interstitial Nephritis

Acute interstitial nephritis (AIN) is a pattern of primary renal injury usually associated with an abrupt deterioration in renal function characterized histopathologically by inflammation and edema in the renal interstitium. The term was first used by Councilman[9] in 1898 to note the histopathologic changes in autopsy specimens from patients with diphtheria and scarlet fever. Although the term *acute interstitial nephritis* is more commonly used, *acute tubulointerstitial nephritis* more accurately describes the injury because lesions involve the tubules in addition to the interstitium. AIN is an important cause of acute renal failure, largely attributable to drug hypersensitivity reactions as a result of the increasing use of antibiotics and other medications that may induce an allergic response in the interstitium. AIN is found in approximately 1% of renal biopsy specimens during the evaluation of hematuria or proteinuria. In some studies of patients with acute renal failure, approximately 5% to 15% had AIN.[181]

Etiology

The most frequent cause of AIN is generally found in one of the three categories: drugs, infections, and autoimmune interstitial lesions (Table 35-1).

Drugs

The list of drugs implicated in causing AIN continues to expand. Drugs are more frequently recognized as etiologic in AIN as a result of the increased use of renal biopsy and because of the characteristic clinical presentation. Antibiotics have long been, and remain, a major cause of drug-related renal toxicity that produces both acute renal failure and tubulointerstitial disease, depending on the drug. Tubulointerstitial disease is more commonly observed with β-lactam antibiotics (including cephalosporins), but other antibiotics (sulfonamides, rifampin, vancomycin, ciprofloxacin) are also involved. Clarithromycin[182] (the newer ketolide semisynthetic erythromycin-A derivative) and telethromycin[183] are implicated in renal biopsy–proven AIN. Approximately a third of cases of drug-related AIN are attributable to antibiotics.[184]

Two complicating factors make the nephrotoxicity of antibiotics more common than that of drugs from other categories. First, many antibiotics are given in combination; consequently, the toxicity of one agent may be aggravated by another drug, as exemplified by the coadministration of aminoglycosides and nonsteroidal antiinflammatory drugs (NSAIDs). Second, many antimicrobial agents are removed from the body essentially, or at least predominantly, through a renal route. The serum levels of these drugs therefore increase as renal function declines, either as a consequence of drug toxicity itself or because of concomitant renal damage caused by another drug or by another cause of nephrotoxicity. β-Lactams produce interstitial nephritis because they behave like haptens, which may bind to serum or cellular proteins to be subsequently

TABLE 35-1 Acute Interstitial Nephritis: Causative Factors

CAUSE	SPECIFIC AGENT
Drugs	
Antibiotics	Cephalosporins, ciprofloxacin, ethambutol, isoniazid, macrolides, penicillins, rifampin, sulfonamides, tetracycline, vancomycin
Nonsteroidal antiinflammatory drugs (NSAIDs)	Almost all agents
Diuretics	Furosemide, thiazides, triamterene
Miscellaneous	Acyclovir, allopurinol, amlodipine, azathioprine, captopril, carbamazepine, clofibrate, cocaine, creatine, diltiazem, famotidine, indinavir, mesalazine, omeprazole, phentermine, phenytoin, pranlukast, propylthiouracil, quinine, ranitidine
Infectious Agents	
Bacteria	*Corynebacterium diphtheriae, Legionella* species, *Staphylococcus* species, *Streptococcus* species, *Yersinia* species, *Brucella* species, *Escherichia coli, Campylobacter* species
Viruses	Cytomegalovirus, Epstein-Barr virus, hantaviruses, hepatitis C, herpes simplex virus, human immunodeficiency virus, mumps, polyoma virus
Other agents	*Leptospira* species, *Mycobacterium* species, *Mycoplasma* species, *Rickettsia* species, *Treponema pallidum, Toxoplasma* species, *Chlamydia* species
Idiopathic	
Immune	Anti–tubular basement membrane disease, tubulointerstitial nephritis and uveitis (TINU) syndrome

processed and presented by MHC molecules as hapten-modified peptides.[185] The most common form of haptenization for penicillin is the penicilloyl configuration, which arises from the opening of a strained β-lactam ring, yielding an additional carboxylic function that allows the molecule to covalently bind to the lateral and terminal amino terminus of proteins. Serum molecules thus facilitate haptenization. This reaction occurs with the prototype benzylpenicillin and virtually all semisynthetic penicillins, but other derivatives (called *minor determinants*) can be formed in small quantities and stimulate variable immune responses. Because all β-lactams share the same basic structure, they are all conducive to haptenization. Variation in the side chains and the corresponding differences in the chemical nature of the haptens, however, explain why clinical consequences are variable among different classes of β-lactams. Cross-reactivity between penicillins and cephalosporins is, accordingly, rare.

Approximately 1% to 5% of patients exposed to NSAIDs develop a variety of nephrotoxic syndromes.[186] Although this relatively low prevalence is not alarming, the extensive use profile of analgesic, anti-inflammatory, and antipyretic agents suggests that an enormous number of individuals are at risk for kidney dysfunction. For instance, approximately 1 per 7 patients with rheumatologic disorders is likely to receive such a prescription, and approximately 1 per 5 (50 million) United States citizens report that they use an NSAID for other acute complaints.[187] Thus, it is possible to estimate that some type of renal abnormality is likely to develop among the 500,000 to 2.5 million individuals exposed to NSAIDs in the United States on a regular or intermittent basis per annum.[186] The problem takes on added dimensions in that 20% of patients taking NSAIDs are predisposed to the development of renal toxicity because of volume contraction, low cardiac output, or other conditions that compromise renal perfusion. The combination of AIN with moderate or severe proteinuria and minimal change glomerulopathy is characteristically observed in fewer than 0.2 per 1000 patients who take NSAIDs other than aspirin.[188] Preexisting renal impairment does not appear to be a factor. Advancing age is a risk factor, and this relationship may simply reflect the prevailing use of NSAIDs by elderly persons. Essentially all NSAIDs have been reported to cause the nephrotic syndrome. The onset of proteinuria in combination with interstitial nephritis occurs after several days or months of NSAID exposure (range, 0.5 to 18 months).[186] The AIN lesion may be the result of a toxic effect of NSAIDs on the immune system that results from blockade of cyclo-oxygenase, which causes arachidonic acid metabolism to favor the alternative lipoxygenase pathway, thus increasing production of proinflammatory leukotrienes, epoxyeicosanoids, and hydroxyeicosanoids.[188] However, some cases of NSAID-related interstitial disease may in fact be allergic reactions, which is suggested by the presence of tissue eosinophils or other manifestations of immunoglobulin E–mediated hypersensitivity. The risk factors for this latter form of NSAID-induced nephropathy are unknown.

Infections

AIN is associated with primary renal infections such as acute bacterial pyelonephritis, renal tuberculosis, and fungal nephritis. Streptococcal infection,[189] leptospirosis,[190] cryptococcosis,[191] legionellosis,[192] histoplasmosis,[193] and viruses such as cytomegalovirus,[190,194] hantavirus,[195,196] and Epstein-Barr virus[197,198] are classical risks for AIN. Pathologic processes in the kidney can be caused by systemic infections or can be associated with the medications used in the treatment of infection. Human immunodeficiency virus, for example, can underlie AIN as a result of opportunistic infections or the use of drugs such as indinavir, sulfonamide antibiotics, or perhaps the virus itself can cause AIN.[199,200] On the other hand, some authorities suggest that depressed cell-mediated immunity may minimize the development of AIN.

Idiopathic Autoimmune Conditions

Immunologic diseases such as Behçet's disease, Sjögren's syndrome, sarcoidosis, systemic lupus erythematosus, or vasculitides may also produce interstitial disease.[201] Anti-TBM nephritis occasionally manifests in association with membranous nephropathy.[202] The characteristics of this combination include a predominance of male patients, onset in early childhood, microscopic hematuria, and proteinuria with nephrotic-range values. In addition, patients show tubular dysfunction (complete or incomplete Fanconi's syndrome), circulating anti-TBM antibodies, and progression to end-stage renal disease.[202] Circulating anti-TBM antibodies from these patients react exclusively with the proximal TBM, not with the glomerular basement membrane (GBM), exhibiting binding to tubular antigen. The precise mechanism underlying combined immune

complex deposition in glomeruli and antibody formation against idiopathic tubulointerstitial antigens is unclear. Soluble tubulointerstitial antigen binding to its relevant antibody may participate in the formation of immune complexes in the glomerular lesions. However, tubulointerstitial antigens have not yet been detected within the immune complex deposits. The cases in which membranous nephropathy preceded anti-TBM nephritis suggest that anti-TBM antibodies are formed by tubulointerstitial antigens modified by certain components or exposed to enzymes present as a result of the massive proteinuria. The role of human leukocyte antigens (HLAs) in the evolution of these autoimmune disorders has also been suggested.

In 1975, Dobrin and associates[203] first described a syndrome characterized by anterior uveitis, bone marrow granulomas, hypergammaglobulinemia, increased erythrocyte sedimentation rate, and acute renal failure with renal histologic features of AIN caused by numerous interstitial inflammatory cells, including eosinophils. This entity—idiopathic tubulointerstitial nephritis in association with bilateral uveitis—that causes acute renal failure was thus termed *TINU syndrome*.[204] TINU syndrome among adults occurs predominantly in women (3:1). Familial occurrence has suggested that a genetic influence may play some role in pathogenesis.[205] A significant association has been reported in the frequency of HLA-DR6 and TINU syndrome. The anterior uveitis may precede, occur simultaneously with, or follow the nephropathy. Affected patients generally suffer from weight loss and anemia and have a raised erythrocyte sedimentation rate. Although associations with both *Chlamydia* and *Mycoplasma* infections have been suggested, the cause remains obscure.[206] The syndrome appears to be immune mediated with T cell proliferation in the kidney.[207] Moreover, the possibility of a delayed-type hypersensitivity reaction is also suggested on the basis of the 2:1 ratio of CD4+ to CD8+ interstitial lymphocytes. Prolonged steroid therapy usually leads to improvement in both renal function and uveitis, although the latter may relapse.[204]

Pathology

The hallmark of AIN is the infiltration of inflammatory cells with associated edema, which usually spares glomeruli and blood vessels.[181] The predominant pathologic process is interstitial and cortical more than medullary, and it comprises edema and inflammatory infiltrates, which may be sparse, focal, or intense. The most numerous cells are lymphocytes, with CD4+ T cells rather more frequent than CD8+ T cells, B lymphocytes, plasma cells, natural killer cells, or macrophages.[208] Polymorphonuclear granulocytes, usually eosinophils, are often present early in the course of disease. The inflammatory reaction may be concentrated around and observed invading the tubular epithelium (so-called tubulitis). In more severe cases, tubulitis is associated with epithelial cell degeneration resembling patchy tubular necrosis with some disruption of the TBM. Granulomas may occur in the interstitium, but vasculitis is uncommon. Increased matrix followed by destructive fibrogenesis may appear as early as the second week of acute inflammation.[208] Immunofluorescence microscopy or immunoperoxidase staining may show, in order of diminishing frequency, no complement or immunoglobulin; immune complexes, sometimes with complement along the TBM; or linear IgG and complement on the TBM.[208] Thus, the pathologic findings are indicative of a cell-mediated, delayed-type hypersensitivity reaction against tubular cells or nearby interstitial structures. However, dimethoxyphenyl-penicilloyl radicals may attach to TBM as hapten in β-lactam–associated nephritis,[185] and antibody to this combination is occasionally present. In AIN with minimal change glomerulopathy induced by NSAIDs, the interstitial inflammatory exudate resembles that of acute allergic interstitial nephritis except that cytotoxic T cells predominate and eosinophils are uncommon.[209] There is no evidence of antibody-mediated injury in this latter form of interstitial nephritis.

Clinical Features

The clinical presentation comprises both local and systemic manifestations of acute inflammation of the kidneys. Patients with AIN typically present with nonspecific symptoms of declining renal function, including oliguria, malaise, anorexia, or nausea and vomiting with acute or subacute onset.[210] The clinical features range from asymptomatic elevation in creatinine or blood urea nitrogen levels and an abnormal urinary sedimentation rate to generalized hypersensitivity syndrome with fever, rash, eosinophilia, and oliguric renal failure. The classic triad of low-grade fever, skin rash, and arthralgias was initially described with methicillin-induced AIN, but in only about a third of cases. More recently, three large series were conducted with a total of 128 patients with AIN (of whom 72 [56.3%] were men and the mean age was 46.6 years)[184,211,212] from 1968 to 2001. At presentation, rash was present in 14.8%, fever in 27.3%, and eosinophilia in 23.3%. The classic triad of fever, rash, and arthralgias was present in only 10% of patients for whom information was available. Nevertheless, this finding is in stark contrast to those of earlier series, in which allergic-type features were more robust.[184] Blood pressure is usually not high except with oliguric renal failure. Nonoliguric patients typically have a fractional sodium excretion higher than 1 g/day and usually have modest proteinuria (<1 g/day) but are not nephrotic unless injury is secondary to NSAIDs.

AIN should be considered in any patient with a rising serum creatinine level but little or no evidence of glomerular or arterial disease, no prerenal factors, and no dilation of the urinary collecting system visible on ultrasonography. The clinical history of exposure to a high-risk drug such as an NSAID or susceptibility to ascending urinary infection, in the absence of a recent or coexisting condition causing shock or associated exposure to contrast media, is usually suggestive of the diagnosis. Most difficulty in establishing the correct diagnosis is encountered with patients exposed to a nephritogenic or nephrotoxic agent at about the same time as a major operation, serious infection, or other significant illness that may itself have caused acute tubular necrosis. The presence of features such as a hypersensitivity reaction, significant eosinophiluria in the case of ingestion of β-lactam antibiotics, or moderate or severe albuminuria after exposure to NSAIDs is indicative of a drug-related cause. Urine eosinophils are often sought as confirmatory evidence of AIN. Early studies[213] revealed that Hansel's stain for eosinophils was more sensitive than Wright's stain but did not conclusively demonstrate that urinary eosinophils were diagnostically useful in confirming or excluding AIN. A more recent study[214] revealed a positive predictive value of 38% (95% confidence interval = 15% to 65%) and a negative predictive value of 74% (95% confidence interval = 57% to 88%) among 51 patients for whom urinary eosinophils were tested to help diagnose an acute renal disease; 15 of these patients were suspected of having AIN, although biopsies were not performed in all patients. Other conditions such as cystitis, prostatitis, and pyelonephritis can also be associated with eosinophiluria. Thus, the diagnostic value of urinary eosinophils remains unclear.

Renal ultrasonography may demonstrate kidneys that are normal to enlarged in size with increased cortical echogenicity, but no ultrasonographic findings reliably confirm or rule out AIN versus other causes of acute renal failure. Gallium 67 scanning has been proposed[215] as a useful test for diagnosing AIN. In one small series, nine patients with AIN had positive findings on gallium 67 scans, whereas six patients with acute tubulointerstitial nephritis had negative findings. Unfortunately, other renal disorders such as minimal-change glomerulonephritis and cortical necrosis have resulted in positive findings on gallium 67 scans. Nonrenal disorders such as iron overload or severe liver disease also can result in a positive finding. Likewise, patients with biopsy-proven acute tubulointerstitial disease have had negative findings on gallium 67 scans; therefore, the predictive value of this test remains limited. Renal biopsy is the "gold standard" for diagnosis of AIN; typical histopathologic findings are lymphocytic infiltrates in the peritubular areas of the interstitium, usually with interstitial edema. Renal biopsy, however, is not needed in all patients, for whom a probable precipitating drug can be easily withdrawn or whose condition improves readily after withdrawal of a potentially offending drug. Patients whose condition does not improve after withdrawal of potentially precipitating medications, who have no contraindications to renal biopsy, and who are being considered for steroid therapy are good candidates for renal biopsy.

Prognosis and Management

The detailed treatment of acute interstitial nephritis has been reviewed elsewhere.[216] Most patients with AIN in whom offending medications are withdrawn early can expect to recover normal or near-normal renal function within a few weeks. Patients who discontinue offending medications within 2 weeks of the onset of AIN (measured by increased serum creatinine levels) are more likely to recover nearly baseline renal function than are those who continue taking the precipitating medication for 3 weeks or longer. On the other hand, according to the three modern series of AIN, only 64.1% of patients made a full recovery (serum creatinine level <132 μmol/L), whereas 23.4% gained only a partial recovery (serum creatinine level >132 μmol/L), and 12.5% remained on renal replacement therapy.[184] This relatively poor outcome may reflect a different case-mix in more recent series, in which fewer patients had traditional allergic-type AIN.

Clearly, it would be useful to have prognostic indicators for AIN, and it has been suggested that the long-term outcome is worse if renal failure lasts for more than 3 weeks.[184] Two series demonstrated worse prognosis with increasing age, but there appears to be no correlation with peak creatinine concentration.[184] Attempts have also been made to gain prognostic information from the renal biopsy. Some authors have reported that the presence of patchy cellular infiltrates is predictive of a better outcome than is diffuse disease.[184] However, other studies have not supported a correlation between the degree of cellular infiltration or tubulitis and outcome.[217] The degree of interstitial fibrosis is correlated with outcome,[217] as is the number of interstitial fibroblasts.[18] These observations may conflict because of the patchy nature of the disease, random sampling on renal biopsy, and, of most importance, too few patients being studied.

Withdrawal of medications that are likely to cause AIN is the most significant step in early management of suspected or biopsy-proven AIN.[210] If multiple potentially precipitating medications are being used by a patient, it is reasonable to substitute other medications for as many of these as possible and to withdraw the most likely etiologic agent among medications that cannot be substituted. The majority of patients with early AIN improve spontaneously after the withdrawal of such medications. Other supportive care includes fluid and electrolyte management, maintenance of adequate extracellular volume, relief for fever and other systemic symptoms, and symptomatic relief for rash. Indications for dialysis in the management of acute renal failure include uncontrolled hyperkalemia, azotemia with changes in mental status, and other symptomatic fluid or electrolyte derangements.

The role of steroids in the treatment of AIN remains unclear. Some authorities continue to question the use of or indications for steroid therapy; no controlled, randomized trials have yielded evidence supporting its use.[184] However, small case reports and studies have demonstrated rapid diuresis, clinical improvement, and return of normal renal function within 72 hours after steroid treatment is started, although some case reports also indicate lack of efficacy, especially in NSAID-induced AIN.[218] The decision to use steroids should be guided by the clinical course after withdrawal of offending medications. Convincing clinical evidence for a role for steroid therapy, however, comes from studies of the idiopathic form of AIN, particularly TINU syndrome. Both the ocular and the renal changes of affected patients respond dramatically to a brief course of steroid therapy. Clearly, steroids are not to be used in cases caused by infectious agents, for which proper therapy is directed at eliminating infection. If steroid therapy is started, a reasonable regimen is prednisone, 1 mg/kg/day orally (or equivalent intravenous dose) for 2 or 3 weeks, followed by a gradually tapering dose over 3 to 4 weeks.[219]

The merits of immunosuppressive agents, specifically cyclophosphamide or cyclosporine, are even less certain. They can be used as steroid-sparing agents and should be considered for patients who fail to respond to a 2-week course of steroid therapy.[216] A 4-week course of cyclophosphamide (2 mg/kg of body weight per day) while renal function and white blood cell count are monitored should suffice to determine response. Therapy for longer than 4 to 6 weeks is not indicated. Plasmapheresis has been used in patients with circulating anti-TBM antibodies; this treatment is similar to that for anti-GBM disease.

Chronic Tubulointerstitial Nephritis

Pathology

The pathologic features of chronic tubulointerstitial nephritis are largely similar across a wide variety of distinct causes. These features include atrophy of tubular cells with flattened epithelial cells and tubule dilation, interstitial fibrosis, and areas of mononuclear cell infiltration within the interstitial compartment and between tubules. TBMs are frequently thickened. The cellular infiltrate in chronic interstitial disease is composed of lymphocytes, macrophages, and B cells with only occasional neutrophils, plasma cells, and eosinophils. This infiltrate is typically less conspicuous than that in acute interstitial nephritis. Immunofluorescent studies performed on biopsy specimens occasionally reveal immunoglobulin or C3 along the TBMs. Early in the course of chronic interstitial disease, the glomeruli may continue to appear remarkably normal on light microscopy, even when marked functional impairment is present. As chronic interstitial injury progresses, glomerular abnormalities are more evident and consist of periglomerular fibrosis, segmental sclerosis, and ultimately, global sclerosis. Small arteries and arterioles show fibrointimal thickening of variable severity, but vasculitis is not a feature of chronic interstitial disease.

Clinical Features

Unless a urinalysis result is found to be abnormal or a screening test reveals an elevated serum creatinine level, patients with chronic interstitial disease present either because of systemic symptoms of a primary disease or because of nonspecific symptoms of renal insufficiency. Such nonspecific symptoms depend on the severity of the renal insufficiency; they may include nocturia, lassitude, weakness, nausea, and sleep disturbances. In a series of patients with biopsy-documented chronic interstitial disease, the creatinine clearance at presentation was lower than 50 mL/min in 75% of cases and lower than 15 mL/min in approximately 33% of all cases. Typical laboratory findings in these patients included proteinuria with nonnephrotic values; microscopically documented hematuria and pyuria; glycosuria in 25% of cases; and, surprisingly, positive urine cultures in 28% of cases.[220]

Acidifying and concentrating defects are common. Chronic interstitial disease caused by certain entities manifests characteristic patterns of tubular dysfunction (proximal or distal renal tubular acidosis) or marked early concentrating defects (primary medullary dysfunction). More typically, the pattern of tubular dysfunction is not highly restricted. Serum uric acid levels are usually lower than expected for the degree of renal failure, presumably because of tubular defects in the reabsorption of uric acid. Anemia occurs relatively early in the course of certain forms of chronic interstitial disease, presumably because of early destruction of erythropoietin-producing interstitial cells. Approximately 50% of patients presenting with chronic interstitial disease have hypertension.[220]

Etiology

The pathologic and clinical scenarios outlined previously can occur in association with a number of diseases of presumably diverse causes. Distinguishing features of several of these are discussed individually in the following sections. For many of these entities, biopsies are performed only infrequently, which limits clinicopathologic correlations. Table 35-2 provides a more exhaustive list of common and rare causes of chronic interstitial disease.

TABLE 35-2 Causes of Chronic Interstitial Nephritis

CAUSE	EXAMPLE
Drugs and toxins	Combination analgesics 5-Aminosalicylic acid Nonsteroidal antiinflammatory drugs (NSAIDs) Chinese herbs Lithium Lead Cadmium Balkan endemic nephropathy Calcineurin inhibitors
Metabolic disorders	Abnormal uric acid metabolism Hypokalemia Hypercalcemia Hyperoxaluria Cystinosis
Immune mediated	Sarcoidosis Sjögren's syndrome Allograft rejection Systemic lupus erythematosus
Infection	Bacterial pyelonephritis Hantavirus Leptospirosis Xanthogranulomatous pyelonephritis
Hematologic disorders	Sickle cell disease Light chain nephropathy Amyloidosis Myeloma
Obstructive	Tumors Stones Outlet obstruction Vesicoureteral reflux
Miscellaneous	Radiation nephropathy Progressive glomerular disease Ischemia Hypertension

Analgesics

In epidemiologic studies, long-term ingestion of large quantities of analgesics has been associated with chronic interstitial nephritis and papillary necrosis.[221] The incidence of analgesic nephropathy varies among different countries and among different geographic areas of the United States. Before the removal of phenacetin from analgesic mixtures, it had been reported as a more common cause of chronic renal failure in Scotland, Belgium, and Australia, accounting for 10% to 20% of patients with end-stage renal disease in those countries.[222] In the United States, case control studies from the Philadelphia area did not reveal an excess risk of renal disease in daily users of analgesics, whereas such a risk was apparent in North Carolina. These two populations differed in the degree of regular analgesic use, which was consistent with previous suggestions that variations in the frequency of analgesic nephropathy are correlated with patterns of analgesic use. In the 1990s, there was a clear decrease in the prevalence and incidence of analgesic nephropathy among patients undergoing dialysis in several European countries and in Australia. Most authors associated this decrease with the removal of phenacetin from analgesic mixtures (Figure 35-1).[223]

The compounds implicated in analgesic nephropathy include aspirin or antipyrine in combination with phenacetin, paracetamol, or salicylamide and caffeine or codeine in over-the-counter proprietary mixtures.[224] Some generalities have emerged from epidemiologic studies: The development of analgesic nephropathy requires prolonged regular ingestion of combination analgesics (at least six tablets daily for more than 3 years). Most of the clinical features displayed by patients with analgesic nephropathy are consistent with the general features outlined previously. However, some distinctions are worth noting. This entity is recognized far more frequently (five to seven times) in women than in men. The patients typically

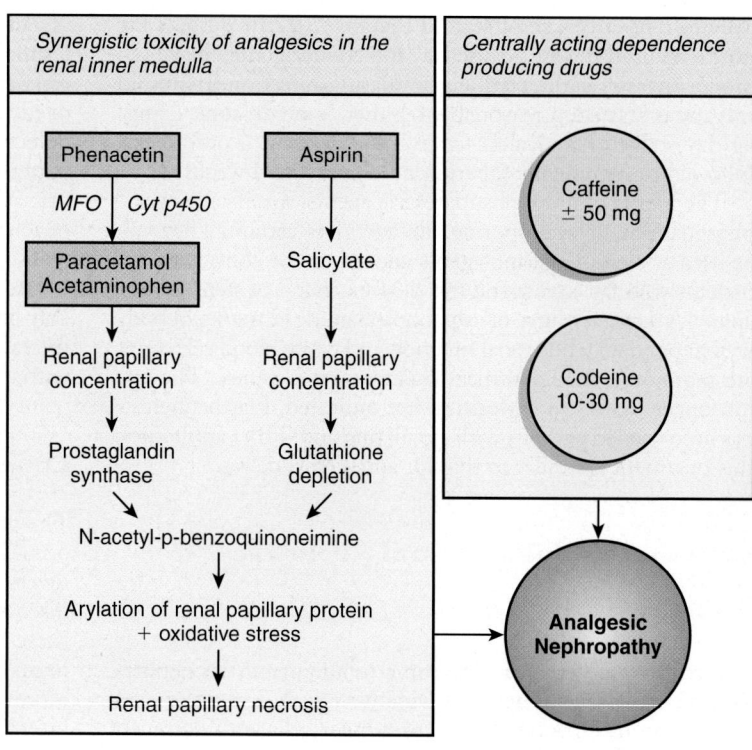

FIGURE 35-1 Synergistic toxicity of analgesics in the inner medulla and centrally acting dependence-producing drugs lead to analgesic nephropathy. Acetaminophen undergoes oxidative metabolism by prostaglandin H synthase to reactive quinone imine that is conjugated to glutathione. If acetaminophen is present alone, sufficient glutathione is generated in the papillae to detoxify the reactive intermediate. If the acetaminophen is ingested with aspirin, the aspirin is converted to salicylate, and salicylate becomes highly concentrated in both the cortex and the papillae of the kidney. Salicylate depletes stores of glutathione. With the cellular glutathione depleted, the reactive metabolite of acetaminophen then produces lipid peroxidases and arylation of tissue proteins, ultimately resulting in necrosis of the papillae. (Redrawn from Kincaid-Smith P, Nanra RS: Lithium-induced and analgesic-induced renal diseases, in Schrier RW, Gottschalk CW [editors]: *Diseases of the kidney*, ed 5, Boston, 1993, Little Brown, pp 1099-1129; Duggin GG: Combination analgesic-induced kidney disease: the Australian experience, *Am J Kidney Dis* 28[suppl 1]:S39-S47, 1996.)

give a history of chronic headaches, joint pain, or abdominal pain. Flank pain with or without associated hematuria may be indicative of a sloughed and potentially obstructing papilla. It is thought that the caffeine component of combination analgesics contributes to dependence on the drugs. Because these drugs are available over the counter, many patients may not seek attention of health care professionals until chronic kidney disease has reached an advanced stage. At that point, renal function abnormalities attributable to chronic interstitial nephritis—including nocturia, sterile pyuria, and azotemia—are nonspecific.[225] Anemia is common. Discontinuation of heavy use of analgesics can slow or arrest progression of the renal disease.[226]

The late stages of analgesic nephropathy may be complicated by urinary tract malignancy. The major presenting sign of this complication is microscopic or gross hematuria. New-onset hematuria should be evaluated with urinary cytologic study and, if indicated, cystoscopy with retrograde pyelography.[227] It is estimated that a urinary tract malignancy develops in as many as 8% to 10% of patients with analgesic nephropathy, typically after 15 to 25 years of heavy use of analgesics.[228] In some of these patients, analgesic nephropathy may not have been previously diagnosed.[229] Up to 50% of nephrectomy specimens from patients with analgesic nephropathy who eventually need transplantation show evidence of atypical uroepithelial cells within the renal pelvis.[227] Some authorities have proposed that such patients should have prophylactic nephrectomies of their native kidneys at the time of transplantation. The pathogenesis of these uroepithelial malignancies presumably relates to the concentration and accumulation of phenacetin metabolites with alkylating capabilities within the renal medulla and the lower urinary tract.[229] Nonsteroidal drugs and acetaminophen do not seem to be associated with these tumors.[226,230]

The likelihood that regular and sustained ingestion of single classes of nonnarcotic analgesics, as opposed to combination analgesics, can lead to chronic renal insufficiency has been the subject of a number of epidemiologic and case-control studies.[231-235] In a case-control study of the relative risk of end-stage renal failure after regular analgesic intake, the authors found increased risks varying from 2.6- to 4.8-fold for analgesic combination drugs, but no significant increased risk for single nonnarcotic analgesics.[236] They did identify increased risks for combination analgesics lacking phenacetin. Other researchers have also observed that classic analgesic nephropathy can occur in the absence of phenacetin, which was withdrawn from analgesic mixtures in the United States, Australia, and Western Europe in the early 1980s.[237] However, since about 2000, the results of a preponderance of epidemiologic studies have supported the conclusion that the classic form of analgesic nephropathy has greatly diminished, if not disappeared, after the removal of phenacetin from combination analgesics.[238-240] Such work does not directly address the issue as to whether nonphenacetin analgesics could contribute to progression of other forms of renal disease. In the classical analgesic nephropathy secondary to dose and time-dependent ingestion of combination analgesics containing phenacetin, most experimental findings have supported a mechanism of injury dependent on several drug components and their metabolites. Phenacetin and its metabolites, including acetaminophen, can injure cells through lipid peroxidation.[241] The highest concentrations of these drugs and metabolites are in the medulla and papillary tip, which are where the initial lesions of capillary sclerosis are observed.[242] Aspirin competes with glutathione within the cortex and papillae of the kidney. If cellular glutathione is depleted, the renal toxicity of phenacetin, acetaminophen, and their reactive metabolites may be potentiated.[222,242] In addition, because aspirin and other NSAIDs can suppress the production of vasodilatory prostaglandins, renal blood flow to the medulla may be compromised, which represents a hemodynamic contribution to injury.

In view of the high prevalence of analgesic nephropathy in Western Europe during the 1980s, attempts have been made to develop diagnostic criteria for the entity. Findings on noncontrast computed tomographic (CT) scans of small kidneys, with bumpy renal contours and papillary calcifications, were diagnostic of analgesic nephropathy with greater sensitivity and specific than were clinical signs and symptoms (Figure 35-2).[243,244] In a study from the United States, investigators found that these CT findings are infrequent in the population with end-stage renal disease. Because these findings do not occur frequently enough among patients with a history of heavy and sustained use of analgesics, CT scanning is not a sensitive tool in the United States to detect analgesic nephropathy.[245]

Chinese Herbs: Aristolochic Acid Nephropathy

In the early 1990s, there first appeared published reports from Belgium of patients, frequently women, presenting with an unusually rapidly progressive form of renal failure. Renal biopsy samples from these patients revealed findings consistent with chronic interstitial nephritis.[246] Initial reports noted that affected patients shared a history of chronic ingestion of the same preparation of slimming herbs from China as part of a weight loss regimen.[247] The number of case reports grew throughout the 1990s to more than 120 cases by early 2000. With growing numbers of case reports came the recognition that the spectrum and severity of the disease was heterogeneous, and the disease was more common but not consistently as severe as the initial reports had suggested.[248-250] Growing evidence from both clinical investigation as well as animal models suggests that this lesion is attributable, at least in part, to the presence of aristolochic acid in the slimming herb preparations.[251,252]

The diagnosis of chronic tubulointerstitial nephritis secondary to these slimming herbs relies on an accurate history. These patients typically present with mild to moderate renal insufficiency. As in many cases of chronic interstitial nephritis, hypertension is not a prominent finding. The urine sediment is typically bland, although evidence of tubular dysfunction may be present on chemical analysis, including low-grade proteinuria with nonnephrotic values (including both albumin and low-molecular-weight filtered proteins) and occasionally glycosuria.[253] CT scans of the retroperitoneum may reveal bilaterally small kidneys with irregular contours in the setting of advanced azotemia. The clinical course is variable. Some patients demonstrate a rapid progression over weeks to months to renal failure; others demonstrate either slowly progressive or relatively stable degrees of azotemia. Although there is no guarantee that discontinuation of ingestion of the slimming herbs will arrest disease progression, it is the prudent recommendation.

Analgesic nephropathy (AN)

Macroscopic aspect of an AN kidney

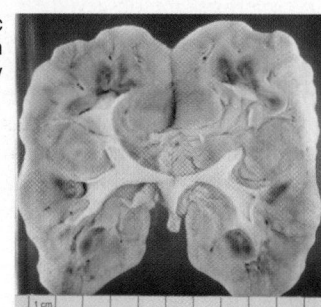

Measurement of diagnostic criteria

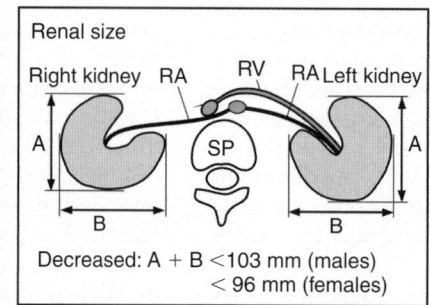

Renal size

Right kidney   RA   RV   RA Left kidney

Decreased: A + B <103 mm (males)
                     < 96 mm (females)

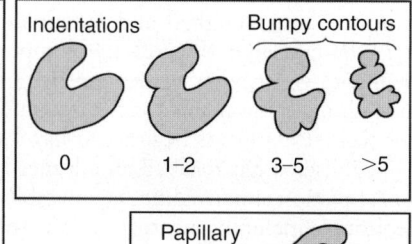

Indentations   Bumpy contours

0   1–2   3–5   >5

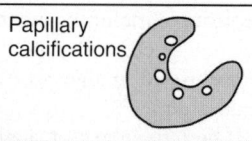

Papillary calcifications

CT scans without contrast material

Normal kidney

Analgesic abuse

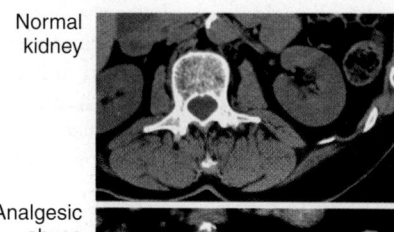

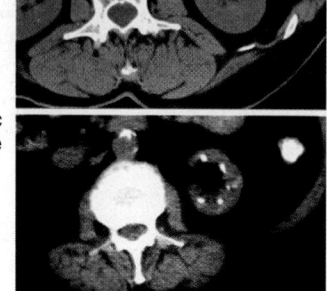

Moderate renal failure

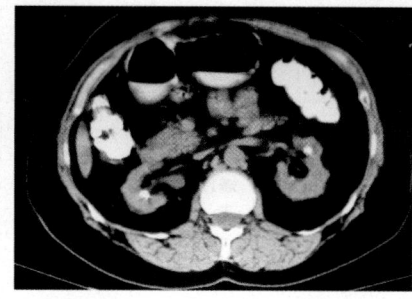

Belgian female, age 62 y, Scr 1.8 mg/dl.
Abuse: 20 y mixture of pyrazolone derivatives

End-stage renal failure

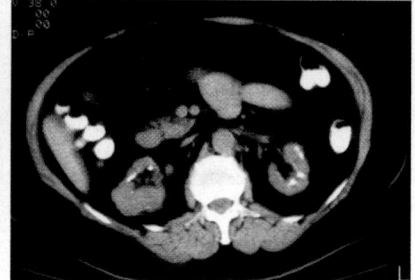

Belgian female, age 59 y, ESRF.
Abuse: 8 y mixture of pyrazolone derivatives 26 y mixture of aspirin + paracetamol

FIGURE 35-2 Renal imaging criteria of analgesic nephropathy as observed in a postmortem kidney and in computed tomographic (CT) scans without contrast material. These criteria include a decreased renal size, bumpy contours, and papillary calcifications. RA, renal artery; RV, renal vein; SP, spine. (Adapted from De Broe ME, Elseviers MM: Analgesic nephropathy, *N Engl J Med* 338:446-452, 1998.)

Other than the ingestion history, the clinical and laboratory findings are nonspecific. No specific therapies have been described to reliably arrest the progression of this disease process. The susceptibility of some but not all individuals exposed to the same herbal preparations is not well understood, although gender, dose, and toxin metabolism may all play a role.[248] Renal biopsy samples from these patients demonstrate significant cortical fibrosis with atrophy and dropout of tubules. Fibrosis has historically been reported as a far more dominant feature than has cellular infiltration (Figure 35-3).[249] Thickening of the interlobular arteriolar walls has been described. There are no immune deposits.[254] Research techniques may demonstrate aristolochic acid–related DNA adducts within the kidneys. One study demonstrated significant infiltration of the medullary rays and outer medulla by monocytes and macrophages, as well as T and B lymphocytes, even in kidneys removed from patients with end-stage renal disease.[252] The notion of a role of aristolochic acid in producing this lesion was supported by the creation of a similar renal lesion in rabbits and rats to which aristolochic acid was administered regularly over weeks to months.[255,256] Kidneys from these animals displayed interstitial fibrosis, tubular atrophy, and some cellular infiltration, along with atypical or malignant (or both) uroepithelial cells. Renal functional abnormalities, such as decreased GFR, may vary, depending on volume depletion or other exogenous factors. In genetically manipulated mice, the absence of the SMAD3 signaling system abrogates the expression of aristolochic acid nephropathy. In vitro, aristolochic acid elicits EMT and augments collagen

production, and these actions are dependent on both TGF-β/SMAD3 and c-Jun N-terminal kinase (JNK)/MAPK mechanisms.[257]

The potential for uroepithelial malignancies in patients exposed to aristolochic acid is well documented. For example, in a study of 39 patients with herbal substance–related nephropathy and end-stage renal disease who underwent removal of the native kidneys and ureters, 18 were found to have urothelial carcinoma and 19 to have mild-to-moderate urothelial dysplasia. Malignant transformation may relate to p53 mutations.[258] The occurrence of malignancy was correlated with the cumulative amount of Chinese herbs ingested. Such findings have led to recommendations that these patients undergo regular surveillance for abnormal urinary cytologic developments and perhaps, in patients at high risk, bilateral nephrectomies.[259]

Balkan Endemic Nephropathy

Balkan nephropathy is a chronic tubulointerstitial disease observed largely in families residing on the alluvial plains of the Danube River within Serbia, Bosnia, Herzegovina, Croatia, Romania, and Bulgaria. The prevalence is high in these populations, ranging from 0.5% to 5%.[260] Although historically both genetic and environmental factors have been suspected to play a role in its pathogenesis, current evidence suggests that environmental factors are dominant but may lead to disease only with certain genetic backgrounds.[261]

Patients with Balkan nephropathy share the clinical features common to many chronic tubulointerstitial diseases.

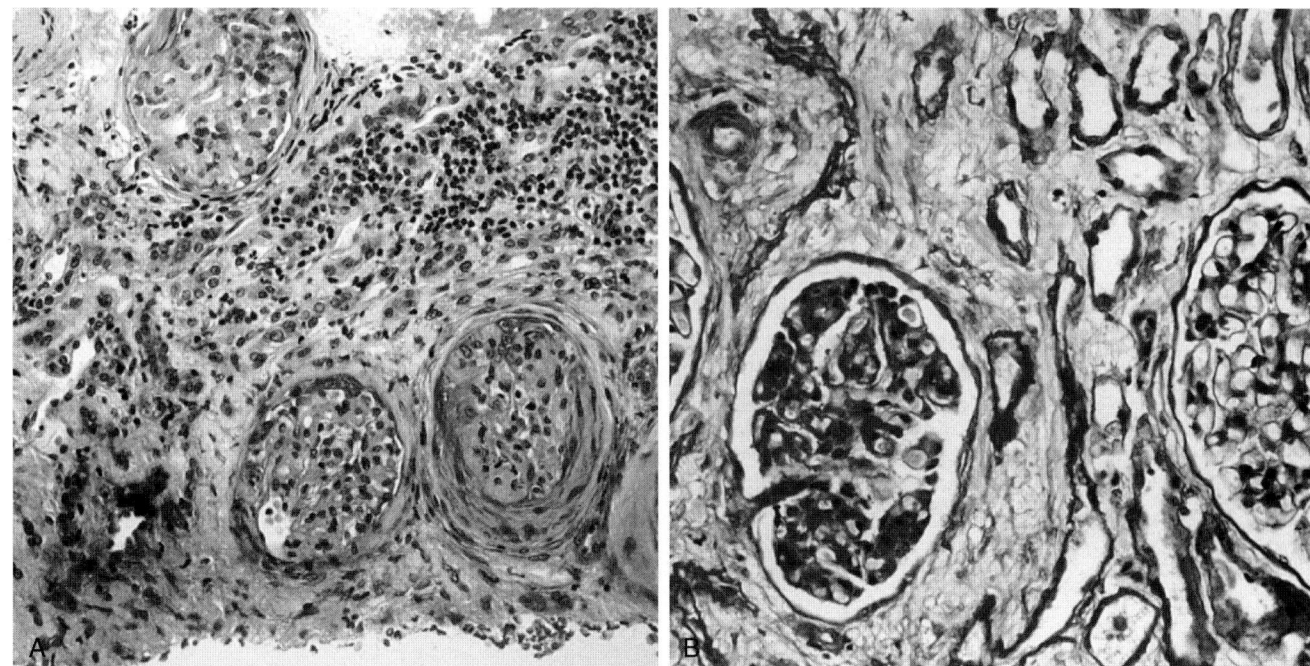

FIGURE 35-3 Case of Chinese herb nephropathy. Kidney biopsy shows tubular atrophy, widening of the interstitium, cellular infiltration, important fibrosis, and glomeruli surrounded by a fibrotic ring. **A,** Masson staining. **B,** Hematoxylin-eosin staining.

Renal and urinary abnormalities first appear after residence in an endemic area for at least 15 years. Affected individuals are not usually hypertensive. One initial renal abnormality is tubular dysfunction, characterized by tubular proteinuria, glycosuria, aminoaciduria, and impaired acid excretion. This is temporally followed by impairment in concentrating ability and slowly (over years) progressive azotemia, which can result in end-stage renal disease. Normochromic, normocytic anemia is typical as well. Kidneys are of normal size early in the course of the disease but diminish in size over time (Figure 35-4). The diagnosis is presumptive and based on renal abnormalities consistent with chronic interstitial disease in a patient residing in an endemic area.[262] There is no specific therapy for this form of interstitial disease. Renal pathologic evaluation demonstrates cortical tubular atrophy, interstitial fibrosis, and sparse mononuclear cell infiltrates. Glomerular sclerosis is observed in more advanced cases. The incidence of cellular atypia and urothelial carcinoma of the genitourinary tract is extremely high.[263] Like several other forms of chronic tubulointerstitial disease, Balkan nephropathy is also associated with uroepithelial malignancies, particularly transitional cell carcinoma of the renal pelvis or ureter.[260] Periodic screening of urine for abnormal cytologic developments is recommended.

Three major environmental factors are currently considered potential contributors to the pathogenesis of Balkan nephropathy.[264] Aristolochic acid has been proposed as a toxin underlying this disease, in addition to Chinese herb nephropathy.[265] The pathologic changes in the kidney are similar, and both are associated with a high prevalence of uroepithelial malignancies. Aristolochic acid DNA adducts are found in the kidneys of patients with Chinese herb nephropathy and those with Balkan nephropathy. The other environmental causes that have been considered include ochratoxin A, a mycotoxin, and polycyclic hydrocarbons, which leach into drinking water from low-rank coal present in endemic areas.[266] Exposure to the environmental factors has changed over the past several

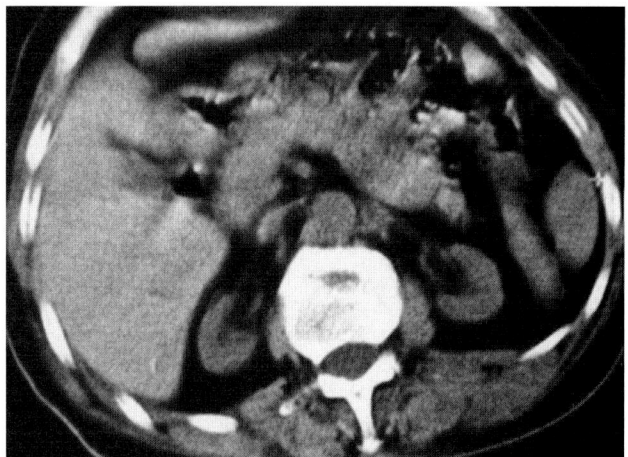

FIGURE 35-4 Computed tomographic (CT) scan without contrast media in a patient with Balkan endemic nephropathy, creatinine clearance of 15 mL/min, no hypertension, and proteinuria with values less than 1 g/24 hr. Of importance are the bilateral atrophy of the kidneys and absence of intrarenal calcifications.

decades in that the dominant population now affected by Balkan nephropathy are people older than 60.[261]

Lithium

Patients who take lithium for treatment of bipolar affective disorder commonly have a nephrogenic form of diabetes insipidus. This is a predictable side effect of therapeutic levels of the drug, and it is slowly reversible after discontinuation of the medication. The nephrogenic form of diabetes insipidus is reproducible in animals treated with lithium, in which it is associated with diminished expression of the vasopressin-regulated water channel aquaporin-2.[267] Hyperparathyroidism is also sometimes observed in patients treated with lithium,

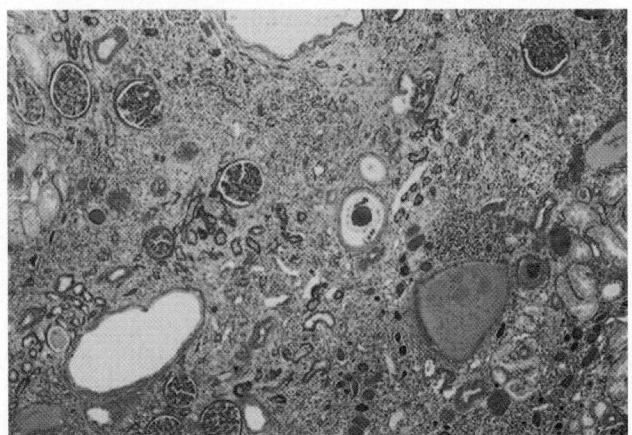

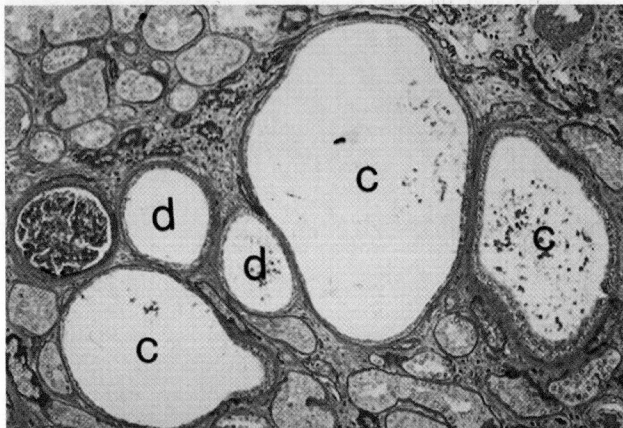

FIGURE 35-5 **Top,** Severe lithium-associated chronic tubulointerstitial nephropathy with the additional finding of focal tubular cysts arising in a background of severe interstitial fibrosis and tubular atrophy. (Periodic acid–Schiff [PAS] stain, ×40.) **Bottom,** High-power view of tubular cysts lined by simple cuboidal epithelium (c). Adjacent tubules show tubular dilatation (d). (PAS stain, ×100.) (From Markowitz GS, Radhakrishnan J, Kambham N, et al: Lithium nephrotoxicity: a progressive combined glomerular and tubulointerstitial nephropathy, *J Am Soc Nephrol* 11:1439-1448, 2000.)

and the associated hypercalcemia is an additional contributor to abnormalities in urinary concentration. Whether chronic ingestion of lithium is associated with a form of chronic tubulointerstitial nephritis and progressive azotemia has been more controversial.[268,269] Current prevailing views are that lithium is associated with the development of chronic tubulointerstitial nephritis (Figure 35-5). In some patients, focal segmental glomerular sclerosis has been reported as well.[270]

Support for the hypothesis that chronic lithium ingestion can lead to chronic interstitial nephritis and functional impairment was bolstered by the development of an animal model in rabbits. When the kidneys from rabbits fed lithium were examined over a 12-month period, clear differences were observed in comparison with kidneys from control rabbits. Epithelial cells lining the distal convoluted tubules and collecting ducts displayed cytoplasmic vacuolation, with accompanying histologic changes of focal interstitial nephritis, including tubular atrophy, interstitial fibrosis, and distal tubular dilation and microcyst formation. Glomerular sclerosis and azotemia occurred by 12 months as well.[271]

In a study of patients treated chronically with lithium (mean duration of therapy, >13 years), the authors examined renal biopsy specimens from 24 patients. Biopsies had been performed because of the presence of both azotemia and, in some of the patients, abnormal proteinuria with values exceeding 1.0 g/24 hr.[272] In this selected population, all the patients had findings consistent with chronic tubulointerstitial nephritis on biopsy. Tubular dilation and cysts were, in addition, present both in the cortex and medulla. A number of patients also had either focal or global glomerulosclerosis. A serum creatinine value higher than 2.5 mg/dL at the time of biopsy was the most powerful predictor of ultimate progression to end-stage renal disease, which occurred even if lithium was discontinued. Another epidemiologic study identified both the duration of lithium therapy and the cumulative dose as determinants of nephrotoxicity, and the prevalence of lithium-associated chronic tubulointerstitial nephritis in end-stage renal disease patients was estimated to be 0.22%.

In contrast, Lepkifker and colleagues[273] found that approximately 20% of long-term lithium patients demonstrate slowly rising serum creatinine values but also that this is not correlated with either duration of therapy or cumulative dose. The clinical management of patients taking long-term lithium who develop azotemia requires judgment and a risk/benefit analysis. The polyuria and polydipsia that are common in most patients on lithium, because of the nephrogenic form of diabetes insipidus, will cease if the drug is withdrawn, but these symptoms are frequently tolerated because of the efficacy of the drug in treating mania and bipolar disorder. Lithium levels should be carefully monitored and maintained at the lowest level that controls symptoms. In view of the more recent development and testing of a number of additional drugs—including olanzapine, quetiapine, and lamotrigine—for first-line treatment of bipolar disorder, it is reasonable to try these agents instead in patients with a stable elevated creatinine level, preferably before the onset of irreversible interstitial damage.

Lead

Epidemiologic studies have strongly implicated excessive exposure to lead as a cause of chronic tubulointerstitial nephritis that results in renal failure.[274] Despite restriction of occupational exposure to lead and the banning of lead-based paints, continuing exposure to low levels of lead occurs through old water pipes, pottery, crystal, and lead-based paint in older dwellings. The current focus is on whether low-level sustained exposure to lead contributes, either solely or in combination with other factors, to the development of end-stage renal disease. Part of the challenge in ascertaining this concerns the accurate measurement of body lead burden (ethylenediaminetetraacetic acid [EDTA] mobilization test), required because blood lead levels indicate only recent, not chronic, lead exposure.

Several studies have demonstrated correlations between elevated blood lead levels or body lead burden, or both, with the presence of kidney disease and accelerated rates of progression to chronic renal disease.[275,276] Using data from the Third National Health and Nutrition Examination Survey (NHANES III), Muntner and colleagues[276] concluded that among the adult population in the United States with hypertension, exposure to even low levels of lead is associated with chronic kidney disease. They also showed that in U.S. adolescents, higher blood lead levels were correlated with lower GFR.[277] Results of experimental studies in the rat remnant kidney model support the hypothesis that ingestion of lead can accelerate chronic kidney disease, in association with hypertension and accentuated vascular and interstitial injury.[278] The pathogenesis of lead nephropathy is related to reabsorption of filtered lead by the proximal tubule, with preferential deposition within the S3 segment of the proximal tubule. Lead exposure can thus lead to defects in proximal tubule function, especially in children, including aminoaciduria, glycosuria, and phosphaturia, all of which represent Fanconi's syndrome. These defects can also occur individually. Renal biopsies in adult patients with subclinical lead nephropathy and a mild-to-moderate decrease in GFR reveal primarily chronic interstitial nephritis, tubular atrophy, and interstitial fibrosis. Adults who develop chronic interstitial nephritis in association with lead exposure typically have hypertension and, frequently, gout as well.

Progression to end-stage renal disease develops slowly over years. Such slow progression has encouraged clinical investigators to examine whether chelation of lead might slow or reverse the progression of this disease. Results of early studies with small numbers of patients suggested that chronic injections of EDTA in patients with mild renal insufficiency and industrial exposure to lead could improve GFR.[279] More recently, in two larger prospective studies of patients with nondiabetic chronic renal disease, no lead exposure history, and normal or low-normal total body lead burdens, chronic EDTA chelation was shown to improve GFR over a 24-month period relative to the control group.[280,281] Although EDTA chelation may be exerting benefit through processes other than lead removal, it is intriguing to consider that lead may adversely affect the progression of other forms of renal disease and that this progression may be positively affected by EDTA chelation.

Cadmium

Cadmium accumulates in the body after inhalation or gastrointestinal absorption. Cadmium nephropathy can develop in individuals with prolonged low-level exposure to excess cadmium, such as zinc smelter workers, or in the setting of massive environmental contamination, as occurred in Japan in the early part of the twentieth century. In the latter case, water contaminated with cadmium from mining operations was used for drinking water and for irrigation of rice fields, thereby entering the food chain and leading to an epidemic of cadmium poisoning. Prominent features of this poisoning were bone pain ("Itai-Itai," or ouch-ouch, disease), osteopenia, and renal failure.[282] Cadmium is bound to metallothionein, and proximal tubular cells take up these complexes.

Cadmium induces a tubular proteinuria.[283] Other proximal tubule defects, including renal glycosuria, aminoaciduria, hypercalciuria, and phosphaturia. are also observed. The functional tubular defects that ensue may be related to apoptosis secondary to activation of both calpains and caspases.[284] Such renal damage uncommonly progresses to an irreversible reduction in glomerular filtration.[285] The high level of environmental contamination with cadmium related to mining in Japan was an unusual event. The extent to which chronic low-level environmental exposure to cadmium affects renal function is much less clear. In the CadmiBel study, more than 2000 adults were recruited from different areas of Belgium in an attempt to examine the relationships between hypertension, cardiovascular disease, and renal abnormalities in relation to urinary cadmium excretion. The results demonstrated that although hypertension and cardiovascular risk are not associated with urinary cadmium excretion, there is a direct correlation between alkaline phosphatase activity, urinary excretion of retinol-binding protein, N-acetyl-β-glucosaminidase, β₂-microglobulin, amino acids, and calcium with urinary cadmium excretion.[285] Interestingly, a 5-year follow-up study of subjects with the highest urinary levels of cadmium excretion did not demonstrate evidence of progressive renal damage or loss of function.[286] Although this is somewhat reassuring, it is still prudent to limit both nutritional and occupational exposure to cadmium.[287] The increased urinary calcium excretion observed in subjects exposed to cadmium is associated with an increased prevalence of calcium phosphate kidney stones.[288]

Hyperuricemia and Urate Nephropathy

As the major organ responsible for excretion of uric acid, the kidney can be affected in a number of ways by abnormal uric acid metabolism. In general, problems arise after the crystallization of uric acid within the tubules, collecting system, or outflow tract or after deposition of uric acid within the interstitium with attendant inflammation. Uric acid solubility is dependent on both pH and concentration. Thus, because uric acid within the tubular lumen is both concentrated and exposed to a lower pH in the distal nephron, the likelihood of precipitation increases. Uric acid stones are a well-recognized entity and discussed in Chapter 39. Acute uric acid nephropathy, typically observed as a phenotype of acute kidney injury after cell breakdown, is also a recognized entity for which prophylactic treatment can typically be given.

Whether sustained and chronic hyperuricemia leads to chronic interstitial nephritis has historically been a controversial issue. Claims in the 1970s that up to 11% of chronic interstitial disease could be attributed to disorders of uric acid metabolism[289] were challenged in the 1980s because of the difficulty in identifying effects of hyperuricemia that could not be attributed to hypertension, vascular disease, stones, or aging.[290] A subject of additional controversy is the possibility that in patients with coexisting gout and chronic interstitial nephritis, chronic lead intoxication might in fact be a cause of both disturbances. It is likely that only a minority of patients with sustained chronic hyperuricemia (with or without clinical gout) have chronic interstitial nephritis. Among such patients, men typically have serum urate levels higher than 13 mg/dL, and women have levels higher than 10 mg/dL. Clearly the coexistence of hypertension, diabetes mellitus, abnormal lipid metabolism, and nephrosclerosis are frequently confounding variables.[291]

An autosomal dominant disease in children, familial juvenile hyperuricemic nephropathy, is characterized by sustained hyperuricemia and chronic interstitial nephritis, which lead to progressive renal failure.[292] Sustained hyperuricemia could also contribute to progressive azotemia in a number of forms of chronic kidney disease. Thus it seems reasonable to recommend dietary restriction of protein and purines in either patients with gout and interstitial disease or patients with chronic kidney disease and a similarly elevated serum urate level.[293]

In seeking to understand how hyperuricemia may relate to progression of renal disease, researchers have shown that this abnormality induces endothelial dysfunction. Uric acid regulates critical proinflammatory pathways in vascular smooth muscle cells and thus potentially has a role in the vascular changes associated with hypertension and vascular disease.[294,295] Studies in rats in which hyperuricemia is induced by uricase inhibitor oxonic acid have demonstrated resultant hypertension, intrarenal vascular disease, and renal injury. Hyperuricemia accelerates renal progression in the remnant kidney model through a mechanism linked to high systemic blood pressure and cyclooxygenase-2–mediated, thromboxane-induced vascular disease.[296] Mice with systemic knockout of the Glut9 urate transporter (typically expressed in the liver and kidneys) have moderate hyperuricemia, significant hyperuricosuria, and renal injury with interstitial inflammation, uric acid stones, and progressive interstitial fibrosis.[297] In the aggregate, these studies provide strong evidence that uric acid may be a true mediator of renal disease and progression.

Sarcoidosis

Sarcoidosis most commonly affects the kidney through disordered calcium metabolism.[298] Of patients with sarcoidosis, 10% to 15% have hypercalcemia, and even more are affected by normocalcemic hypercalciuria. These abnormalities can lead to concentrating defects, depress glomerular filtration, and result in nephrocalcinosis or nephrolithiasis.[299] Nephrolithiasis occurs in approximately 1% to 14% of patients with sarcoidosis and may be the presenting feature. Nephrocalcinosis, observed in more than 50% of those with renal insufficiency, is the most common cause of chronic renal failure in sarcoidosis.[300] Less commonly, patients may develop granulomatous interstitial disease, glomerular disease, obstructive uropathy, and, very rarely, end-stage renal disease. In rare cases, renal disease can be the most prominent manifestation of the disease.[301,302]

Autopsy and renal biopsy series suggest that 15% to 30% of patients with sarcoidosis may have noncaseating granulomas within the renal interstitium. In many cases, these lesions are not clinically apparent. Typically, biopsy findings reveal interstitial noncaseating granulomas, composed of giant cells, histiocytes, and lymphocytes. The extent of these granulomas is variable, but they may replace the bulk of the cortical volume. Focal lymphocytic infiltrates and periglomerular fibrosis are commonly observed.[303] Immunofluorescent and electron microscopic studies typically reveal no immune deposits. Other diseases characterized by granuloma formation, including tuberculosis, silicosis, and histoplasmosis, can cause both hypercalcemia and renal insufficiency but are only rarely associated with granulomatous interstitial nephritis. Allergic interstitial nephritis related to drugs can result in a granulomatous interstitial nephritis. Glomerular abnormalities are unusual in sarcoidosis. Membranous nephropathy and focal glomerulosclerosis have been described, but they would be distinguishable clinically by severe proteinuria, which is not a feature in the granulomatous interstitial nephritis of sarcoidosis.

Affected patients often have an impressive therapeutic response to corticosteroid therapy, with improvement in glomerular filtration and, on repeat biopsy, loss of granulomas and lymphocytic infiltrates. Although this response has been documented in clinical experience, there are no controlled trials regarding such therapy. The often-concomitant hypercalcemia is also responsive to corticosteroid therapy and typically to lower doses. Healing of the granulomatous interstitial nephritis can lead to interstitial fibrosis. Ketoconazole, an inhibitor of steroidogenesis, has been used in a single patient who could not tolerate corticosteroids and was effective in decreasing the level of active vitamin D, as well as serum and urinary calcium levels.[304] According to one report, infliximab was used successfully in the treatment of interstitial nephritis in a patient with sarcoidosis.[302]

Acknowledgment

The authors would like to thank Giuseppe Remuzzi, Norberto Perico, and Marc E. De Broe for their work on this chapter in the previous edition of this book.

References

1. Zeisberg M, Neilson EG. Mechanisms of tubulointersitial fibrosis. *J Am Soc Nephrol.* 2010;21(11):1819-1834.
2. Harris RC, Neilson EG. Toward a unified theory of renal progression. *Annu Rev Med.* 2006;57:365-380.
3. Zhou XJ, Rakheja D, Yu X, et al. The aging kidney. *Kidney Int.* 2008;74:710-720.
4. Bowman W. On the structure and use of malpighian bodies of the kidney, with observations on the circulation through the gland. *Philos Trans R Soc Lond.* 1842;132:57-80.
5. Kolliker A. *Mikroskopische Anatomie oder Gewebelehre des Mensche.* Berlin: Wilhelm Engelmann; 1852, pp 347–365.
6. Taylor AS, Pavy FW. On poisoning by white precipitate. On the physiological effect of this substance on animals. *Guy's Hosp Rep Ser.* 1860;3(6):483-505:505-510.
7. Ponfick E. Studien über die Schicksale körniger Farbstoffe im Organismus. *Virchows Arch.* 1869;48:1-54.
8. Traube L, Zur Patholgie der Nierenkrankheiten, in Traube L. *Gessammelte Beiträge zur Pathologie und Physiologie.* Berlin: Verlag von August Hirschwald; 1870:966-975.
9. Councilman W. Acute interstitial nephritis. *J Exp Med.* 1898;3:393-420.
10. Volhard F, Fahr T. *Die Bright'sche Nierenkrankheiten.* Berlin: Springer; 1914.
11. Melnick P. Acute interstitial nephritis with uremia. *Arch Pathol.* 1943;36:499-504.
12. Longcope W. The production of experimental nephritis by repeated proteid intoxication. *J Exp Med.* 1913;18:678-703.
13. Steblay RW, Rudofsky U. Renal tubular disease and autoantibodies against tubular basement membrane induced in guinea pigs. *J Immunol.* 1971;107:589-594.
14. Wilson C. *The renal response to immunological injury.* 4th ed. Philadelphia: WB Saunders; 1991:1062-1181.
15. Neilson EG, McCafferty E, Feldman, et al. Spontaneous interstitial nephritis in kdkd mice. I. An experimental model of autoimmune renal disease. *J Immunol.* 1984;133:2560-2565.
16. Peng M, Jarett L, Meade R, et al. Mutant prenyltransferase-like mitochondrial protein (PLMP) and mitochondrial abnormalities in kd/kd mice. *Kidney Int.* 2004;66:20-28.
17. Jedlicka J, Soleiman A, Draganovici D, et al. Interstitial inflammation in Alport syndrome. *Hum Pathol.* 2010;41:582-593.
18. Nishitani Y, Iwano M, Yamaguchi Y, et al. Fibroblast-specific protein 1 is a specific prognostic marker for renal survival in patients with IgAN. *Kidney Int.* 2005;68:1078-1085.
19. Schwartz MM, Fennell JS, Lewis EJ. Pathologic changes in the renal tubule in systemic lupus erythematosus. *Hum Pathol.* 1982;13:534-547.
20. Risdon RA, Sloper JC, De Wardener HE. Relationship between renal function and histological changes found in renal-biopsy specimens from patients with persistent glomerular nephritis. *Lancet.* 1968;2:363-366.
21. Bohle A, Mackensen-Haen S, von Gise H. Significance of tubulointerstitial changes in the renal cortex for the excretory function and concentration ability of the kidney: a morphometric contribution. *Am J Nephrol.* 1987;7:421-433.
22. Bohle A, Mackensen-Haen S, von Gise H, et al. The consequences of tubulo-interstitial changes for renal function in glomerulopathies. A morphometric and cytological analysis. *Pathol Res Pract.* 1990;186:135-144.
23. Chevalier RL, Forbes MS, Thornhill BA. Ureteral obstruction as a model of renal interstitial fibrosis and obstructive nephropathy. *Kidney Int.* 2009;75:1145-1152.

24. Ljungquist A. The intrarenal arterial pattern in the normal and diseased human kidney. A micro-angiographic and histologic study. *Acta Med Scand.* 1963;174(suppl 401):1-38.
25. Persson AE, Boberg U, Hahne B, et al. Interstitial pressure as a modulator of tubuloglomerular feedback control. *Kidney Int Suppl.* 1982;12:S122-S128.
26. Thomson SC, Blantz RC. Glomerulotubular balance, tubuloglomerular feedback, and salt homeostasis. *J Am Soc Nephrol.* 2008;19:2272-2275.
27. Iversen BM, Ofstad J. Loss of renal blood flow autoregulation in chronic glomerulonephritic rats. *Am J Physiol.* 1988;254:F284-F290.
28. Chevalier RL, Forbes MS. Generation and evolution of atubular glomeruli in the progression of renal disorders. *J Am Soc Nephrol.* 2008;19:197-206.
29. Marcussen N, Olsen TS. Atubular glomeruli in patients with chronic pyelonephritis. *Lab Invest.* 1990;62:467-473.
30. Eddy AA. Proteinuria and interstitial injury. *Nephrol Dial Transplant.* 2004;19:277-281.
31. Brenner BM. Remission of renal disease: recounting the challenge, acquiring the goal. *J Clin Invest.* 2002;110:1753-1758.
32. Heeger PS, Neilson EG. Overcoming tolerance in autoimmune renal disease. *Curr Opin Nephrol Hypertens.* 1994;3:123-132.
33. Rosivall L, Mirzahosseini S, Toma I, et al. Fluid flow in the juxtaglomerular interstitium visualized in vivo. *Am J Physiol Renal Physiol.* 2006;291:F1241-F1247.
34. Wiggins RC. The spectrum of podocytopathies: a unifying view of glomerular diseases. *Kidney Int.* 2007;71:1205-1214.
35. Kriz W, LeHir M. Pathways to nephron loss starting from glomerular diseases—insights from animal models. *Kidney Int.* 2005;67:404-419.
36. Kriz W, Hartmann I, Hosser H, et al. Tracer studies in the rat demonstrate misdirected filtration and peritubular filtrate spreading in nephrons with segmental glomerulosclerosis. *J Am Soc Nephrol.* 2001;12:496-506.
37. Kriz W, Hahnel B, Hosser H, et al. Pathways to recovery and loss of nephrons in anti–Thy-1 nephritis. *J Am Soc Nephrol.* 2003;14:1904-1926.
38. Neumann I, Birck R, Newman M, et al. SCG/Kinjoh mice: a model of ANCA-associated crescentic glomerulonephritis with immune deposits. *Kidney Int.* 2003;64:140-148.
39. Abboud H, Henrich WL. Clinical practice. Stage IV chronic kidney disease. *N Engl J Med.* 2010;362:56-65.
40. Chanutin A, Ferris EB. Experimental renal insufficiency produced by partial nephrectomy 1. Control diet. *Arch Intern Med.* 1932:767-787.
41. von Mollendorf W, Stohr P. *Lehrbuch der histologie [in German].* Jena, Germany: Fischer; 1924, p 292.
42. Oliver J, Macdowell M, Lee YC. Cellular mechanisms of protein metabolism in the nephron. I. The structural aspects of proteinuria; tubular absorption, droplet formation, and the disposal of proteins. *J Exp Med.* 1954;99:589-604.
43. Zoja C, Benigni A, Remuzzi G. Cellular responses to protein overload: key event in renal disease progression. *Curr Opin Nephrol Hypertens.* 2004;13:31-37.
44. Birn H, Christensen EI. Renal albumin absorption in physiology and pathology. *Kidney Int.* 2006;69:440-449.
45. Abbate M, Zoja C, Remuzzi G. How does proteinuria cause progressive renal damage? *J Am Soc Nephrol.* 2006;17:2974-2984.
46. Tang S, Leung JC, Abe K, et al. Albumin stimulates interleukin-8 expression in proximal tubular epithelial cells in vitro and in vivo. *J Clin Invest.* 2003;111:515-527.
47. Wang Y, Chen J, Chen L, et al. Induction of monocyte chemoattractant protein-1 in proximal tubule cells by urinary protein. *J Am Soc Nephrol.* 1997;8:1537-1545.
48. Zoja C, Donadelli R, Colleoni S, et al. Protein overload stimulates RANTES production by proximal tubular cells depending on NF-kappa B activation. *Kidney Int.* 1998;53:1608-1615.
49. Donadelli R, Zanchi C, Morigi M, et al. Protein overload induces fractalkine upregulation in proximal tubular cells through nuclear factor kappaB– and p38 mitogen–activated protein kinase–dependent pathways. *J Am Soc Nephrol.* 2003;14:2436-2446.
50. Wolf G, Schroeder R, Ziyadeh FN, et al. Albumin up-regulates the type II transforming growth factor-beta receptor in cultured proximal tubular cells. *Kidney Int.* 2004;66:1849-1858.
51. Peruzzi L, Trusolino L, Amore A, et al. Tubulointerstitial responses in the progression of glomerular diseases: albuminuria modulates $\alpha_v\beta_5$ integrin. *Kidney Int.* 1996;50:1310-1320.
52. Morigi M, Macconi D, Zoja C, et al. Protein overload-induced NF-kappaB activation in proximal tubular cells requires H(2)O(2) through a PKC-dependent pathway. *J Am Soc Nephrol.* 2002;13:1179-1189.
53. Sanz AB, Sanchez-Niño MD, Ramos AM, et al. NF-κB in renal inflammation. *J Am Soc Nephrol.* 2010;21(8):1254-1262.
54. Takaya K, Koya D, Isono M, et al. Involvement of ERK pathway in albumin-induced MCP-1 expression in mouse proximal tubular cells. *Am J Physiol Renal Physiol.* 2003;284:F1037-F1045.
55. Erkan E, De Leon M, Devarajan P. Albumin overload induces apoptosis in LLC-PK(1) cells. *Am J Physiol Renal Physiol.* 2001;280:F1107-F1114.
56. Morais C, Westhuyzen J, Metharom P, et al. High molecular weight plasma proteins induce apoptosis and Fas/FasL expression in human proximal tubular cells. *Nephrol Dial Transplant.* 2005;20:50-58.
57. Nakajima H, Takenaka M, Kaimori JY, et al. Gene expression profile of renal proximal tubules regulated by proteinuria. *Kidney Int.* 2002;61:1577-1587.
58. Anderson S, Rennke HG, Brenner BM. Therapeutic advantage of converting enzyme inhibitors in arresting progressive renal disease associated with systemic hypertension in the rat. *J Clin Invest.* 1986;77:1993-2000.
59. Ruggenenti P. Angiotensin-converting enzyme inhibition and angiotensin II antagonism in nondiabetic chronic nephropathies. *Semin Nephrol.* 2004;24:158-167.
60. Ruggenenti P, Perna A, Gherardi G, et al. Renal function and requirement for dialysis in chronic nephropathy patients on long-term ramipril: REIN follow-up trial. Gruppo Italiano di Studi Epidemiologici in Nefrologia (GISEN). Ramipril Efficacy in Nephropathy. *Lancet.* 1998;352:1252-1256.
61. Ruiz-Ortega M, Gonzalez S, Seron D, et al. ACE inhibition reduces proteinuria, glomerular lesions and extracellular matrix production in a normotensive rat model of immune complex nephritis. *Kidney Int.* 1995;48:1778-1791.
62. Zoja C, Donadelli R, Corna D, et al. The renoprotective properties of angiotensin-converting enzyme inhibitors in a chronic model of membranous nephropathy are solely due to the inhibition of angiotensin II: evidence based on comparative studies with a receptor antagonist. *Am J Kidney Dis.* 1997;29:254-264.
63. Gomez-Garre D, Largo R, Tejera N, et al. Activation of NF-kappaB in tubular epithelial cells of rats with intense proteinuria: role of angiotensin II and endothelin-1. *Hypertension.* 2001;37:1171-1178.
64. Sanz AB, Santamaria B, Ruiz-Ortega M, et al. Mechanisms of renal apoptosis in health and disease. *J Am Soc Nephrol.* 2008;19:1634-1642.
65. Periyasamy-Thandavan S, Jiang M, Schoenlein P, et al. Autophagy: molecular machinery, regulation, and implications for renal pathophysiology. *Am J Physiol Renal Physiol.* 2009;297:F244-F256.
66. Tejera N, Gomez-Garre D, Lazaro A, et al. Persistent proteinuria up-regulates angiotensin II type 2 receptor and induces apoptosis in proximal tubular cells. *Am J Pathol.* 2004;164:1817-1826.
67. Benigni A, Gagliardini E, Remuzzi A, et al. Angiotensin-converting enzyme inhibition prevents glomerular-tubule disconnection and atrophy in passive Heymann nephritis, an effect not observed with a calcium antagonist. *Am J Pathol.* 2001;159:1743-1750.
68. Erkan E, Garcia CD, Patterson LT, et al. Induction of renal tubular cell apoptosis in focal segmental glomerulosclerosis: roles of proteinuria and Fas-dependent pathways. *J Am Soc Nephrol.* 2005;16:398-407.
69. Zoja C, Garcia PB, Remuzzi G. The role of chemokines in progressive renal disease. *Front Biosci.* 2009;14:1815-1822.
70. Hirschberg R. Bioactivity of glomerular ultrafiltrate during heavy proteinuria may contribute to renal tubulo-interstitial lesions: evidence for a role for insulin-like growth factor I. *J Clin Invest.* 1996;98:116-124.
71. Wang Y, Wang YP, Tay YC, et al. Progressive Adriamycin nephropathy in mice: sequence of histologic and immunohistochemical events. *Kidney Int.* 2000;58:1797-1804.
72. Ando T, Okuda S, Yanagida T, et al. Localization of TGF-beta and its receptors in the kidney. *Miner Electrolyte Metab.* 1998;24:149-153.
73. Sato H, Iwano M, Akai Y, et al. Increased excretion of urinary transforming growth factor beta 1 in patients with diabetic nephropathy. *Am J Nephrol.* 1998;18:490-494.
74. Song JH, Lee SW, Suh JH, et al. The effects of dual blockade of the renin-angiotensin system on urinary protein and transforming growth factor-beta excretion in 2 groups of patients with IgA and diabetic nephropathy. *Clin Nephrol.* 2003;60:318-326.
75. Kees-Folts D, Sadow JL, Schreiner GF. Tubular catabolism of albumin is associated with the release of an inflammatory lipid. *Kidney Int.* 1994;45:1697-1709.
76. Kamijo A, Sugaya T, Hikawa A, et al. Urinary excretion of fatty acid–binding protein reflects stress overload on the proximal tubules. *Am J Pathol.* 2004;165:1243-1255.
77. Arici M, Brown J, Williams M, et al. Fatty acids carried on albumin modulate proximal tubular cell fibronectin production: a role for protein kinase C. *Nephrol Dial Transplant.* 2002;17:1751-1757.
78. Porubsky S, Schmid H, Bonrouhi M, et al. Influence of native and hypochlorite-modified low-density lipoprotein on gene expression in human proximal tubular epithelium. *Am J Pathol.* 2004;164:2175-2187.
79. Hsu SI, Couser WG. Chronic progression of tubulointerstitial damage in proteinuric renal disease is mediated by complement activation: a therapeutic role for complement inhibitors? *J Am Soc Nephrol.* 2003;14:S186-S191.

80. Nangaku M. Complement regulatory proteins in glomerular diseases. *Kidney Int.* 1998;54:1419-1428.

81. Biancone L, David S, Della Pietra V, et al. Alternative pathway activation of complement by cultured human proximal tubular epithelial cells. *Kidney Int.* 1994;45:451-460.

82. David S, Biancone L, Caserta C, et al. Alternative pathway complement activation induces proinflammatory activity in human proximal tubular epithelial cells. *Nephrol Dial Transplant.* 1997;12:51-56.

83. Eddy AA. Interstitial nephritis induced by protein-overload proteinuria. *Am J Pathol.* 1989;135:719-733.

84. Abbate M, Zoja C, Rottoli D, et al. Antiproteinuric therapy while preventing the abnormal protein traffic in proximal tubule abrogates protein- and complement-dependent interstitial inflammation in experimental renal disease. *J Am Soc Nephrol.* 1999;10:804-813.

85. Nomura A, Morita Y, Maruyama S, et al. Role of complement in acute tubulointerstitial injury of rats with aminonucleoside nephrosis. *Am J Pathol.* 1997;151:539-547.

86. Nangaku M, Pippin J, Couser WG. C6 mediates chronic progression of tubulointerstitial damage in rats with remnant kidneys. *J Am Soc Nephrol.* 2002;13:928-936.

87. Abbate M, Zoja C, Rottoli D, et al. Proximal tubular cells promote fibrogenesis by TGF-beta1–mediated induction of peritubular myofibroblasts. *Kidney Int.* 2002;61:2066-2077.

88. Rangan GK, Pippin JW, Couser WG. C5b-9 regulates peritubular myofibroblast accumulation in experimental focal segmental glomerulosclerosis. *Kidney Int.* 2004;66:1838-1848.

89. Nath KA, Hostetter MK, Hostetter TH. Pathophysiology of chronic tubulo-interstitial disease in rats. Interactions of dietary acid load, ammonia, and complement component C3. *J Clin Invest.* 1985;76:667-675.

90. Rangan GK, Pippin JW, Coombes JD, et al. C5b-9 does not mediate chronic tubulointerstitial disease in the absence of proteinuria. *Kidney Int.* 2005;67:492-503.

91. Zhou W, Marsh JE, Sacks SH. Intrarenal synthesis of complement. *Kidney Int.* 2001;59:1227-1235.

92. Tang S, Sheerin NS, Zhou W, et al. Apical proteins stimulate complement synthesis by cultured human proximal tubular epithelial cells. *J Am Soc Nephrol.* 1999;10:69-76.

93. Tang S, Lai KN, Chan TM, et al. Transferrin but not albumin mediates stimulation of complement C3 biosynthesis in human proximal tubular epithelial cells. *Am J Kidney Dis.* 2001;37:94-103.

94. Abbate M, Corna D, Rottoli D, et al. An intact complement pathway is not dispensable for glomerular and tubulointerstitial injury induced by protein overload. *J Am Soc Nephrol.* 2004;15:479A.

95. Li K, Patel H, Farrar CA, et al. Complement activation regulates the capacity of proximal tubular epithelial cell to stimulate alloreactive T cell response. *J Am Soc Nephrol.* 2004;15:2414-2422.

96. Remuzzi G, Zoja C, Gagliardini E, et al. Combining an antiproteinuric approach with mycophenolate mofetil fully suppresses progressive nephropathy of experimental animals. *J Am Soc Nephrol.* 1999;10:1542-1549.

97. Butkowski RJ, Langeveld JP, Wieslander J, et al. Characterization of a tubular basement membrane component reactive with autoantibodies associated with tubulointerstitial nephritis. *J Biol Chem.* 1990;265:21091-21098.

98. Yoshioka K, Takemura T, Hattori S. Tubulointerstitial nephritis antigen: primary structure, expression and role in health and disease. *Nephron.* 2002;90:1-7.

99. Kalfa TA, Thull JD, Butkowski RJ, et al. Tubulointerstitial nephritis antigen interacts with laminin and type IV collagen and promotes cell adhesion. *J Biol Chem.* 1994;269:1654-1659.

100. Ikeda M, Takemura T, Hino S, et al. Molecular cloning, expression, and chromosomal localization of a human tubulointerstitial nephritis antigen. *Biochem Biophys Res Commun.* 2000;268:225-230.

101. Neilson EG, Sun MJ, Kelly CJ, et al. Molecular characterization of a major nephritogenic domain in the autoantigen of anti-tubular basement membrane disease. *Proc Natl Acad Sci U S A.* 1991;88:2006-2010.

102. Neilson EG, Gasser DL, McCafferty E, et al. Polymorphism of genes involved in anti–tubular basement membrane disease in rats. *Immunogenetics.* 1983;17:55-65.

103. Wilson CB. Nephritogenic tubulointerstitial antigens. *Kidney Int.* 1991;39:501-517.

104. Serafini-Cessi F, Malagolini N, Cavallone D. Tamm-Horsfall glycoprotein: biology and clinical relevance. *Am J Kidney Dis.* 2003;42:658-676.

105. Britschgi M, von Greyerz S, Burkhart C, et al. Molecular aspects of drug recognition by specific T cells. *Curr Drug Targets.* 2003;4:1-11.

106. Markowitz GS, Perazella MA. Drug-induced renal failure: a focus on tubulointerstitial disease. *Clin Chim Acta.* 2005;351:31-47.

107. Schnyder B, Pichler WJ. Mechanisms of drug-induced allergy. *Mayo Clin Proc.* 2009;84:268-272.

108. Schwartz RH. A cell culture model for T lymphocyte clonal anergy. *Science.* 1990;248:1349-1356.

109. Haverty TP, Kelly CJ, Hines WH, et al. Characterization of a renal tubular epithelial cell line which secretes the autologous target antigen of autoimmune experimental interstitial nephritis. *J Cell Biol.* 1988;107:1359-1368.

110. Rubin-Kelley VE, Jevnikar AM. Antigen presentation by renal tubular epithelial cells. *J Am Soc Nephrol.* 1991;2:13-26.

111. Hines WH, Haverty TP, Elias JA, et al. T cell recognition of epithelial self. *Autoimmunity.* 1989;5:37-47.

112. Cheng HF, Nolasco F, Cameron JS, et al. HLA-DR display by renal tubular epithelium and phenotype of infiltrate in interstitial nephritis. *Nephrol Dial Transplant.* 1989;4:205-215.

113. Frauwirth KA, Thompson CB. Activation and inhibition of lymphocytes by costimulation. *J Clin Invest.* 2002;109:295-299.

114. Niemann-Masanek U, Mueller A, Yard BA, et al. B7-1 (CD80) and B7-2 (CD 86) expression in human tubular epithelial cells in vivo and in vitro. *Nephron.* 2002;92:542-556.

115. van Kooten C, Gerritsma JS, Paape ME, et al. Possible role for CD40-CD40L in the regulation of interstitial infiltration in the kidney. *Kidney Int.* 1997;51:711-721.

116. de Haij S, Woltman AM, Trouw LA, et al. Renal tubular epithelial cells modulate T-cell responses via ICOS-L and B7-H1. *Kidney Int.* 2005;68:2091-2102.

117. Kairaitis L, Wang Y, Zheng L, et al. Blockade of CD40-CD40 ligand protects against renal injury in chronic proteinuric renal disease. *Kidney Int.* 2003;64:1265-1272.

118. Starke A, Lindenmeyer MT, Segerer S, et al. Renal tubular PD-L1 (CD274) suppresses alloreactive human T cell responses. *Kidney Int.* 2010;78(1):38-47.

119. Waeckerle-Men Y, Starke A, Wuthrich RP. PD-L1 partially protects renal tubular epithelial cells from the attack of CD8+ cytotoxic T cells. *Nephrol Dial Transplant.* 2007;22:1527-1536.

120. Chen Y, Zhang J, Li J, et al. Expression of B7-H1 in inflammatory renal tubular epithelial cells. *Nephron Exp Nephrol.* 2006;102:e81-e92.

121. Rodriguez-Iturbe B, Pons H, Herrera-Acosta J, et al. Role of immunocompetent cells in nonimmune renal diseases. *Kidney Int.* 2001;59:1626-1640.

122. Sean Eardley K, Cockwell P. Macrophages and progressive tubulointerstitial disease. *Kidney Int.* 2005;68:437-455.

123. Neilson EG. The downside of a drug-crazed world. *J Am Soc Nephrol.* 2006;17:2650-2651.

124. Zheng G, Wang Y, Mahajan D, et al. The role of tubulointerstitial inflammation. *Kidney Int Suppl.* 2005(94):S96-S100.

125. Schiffer L, Bethunaickan R, Ramanujam M, et al. Activated renal macrophages are markers of disease onset and disease remission in lupus nephritis. *J Immunol.* 2008;180:1938-1947.

126. Nishida M, Fujinaka H, Matsusaka T, et al. Absence of angiotensin II type 1 receptor in bone marrow–derived cells is detrimental in the evolution of renal fibrosis. *J Clin Invest.* 2002;110:1859-1868.

127. Rastaldi MP, Ferrario F, Crippa A, et al. Glomerular monocyte-macrophage features in ANCA-positive renal vasculitis and cryoglobulinemic nephritis. *J Am Soc Nephrol.* 2000;11:2036-2043.

128. Wuthrich RP, Sibalic V. Autoimmune tubulointerstitial nephritis: insight from experimental models. *Exp Nephrol.* 1998;6:288-293.

129. Truong LD, Farhood A, Tasby J, et al. Experimental chronic renal ischemia: morphologic and immunologic studies. *Kidney Int.* 1992;41:1676-1689.

130. Mampaso FM, Wilson CB. Characterization of inflammatory cells in autoimmune tubulointerstitial nephritis in rats. *Kidney Int.* 1983;23:448-457.

131. Eddy AA, Michael AF. Acute tubulointerstitial nephritis associated with aminonucleoside nephrosis. *Kidney Int.* 1988;33:14-23.

132. Gillum DM, Truong L, Tasby J. Characterization of the interstitial cellular infiltrate in experimental chronic cyclosporine nephropathy. *Transplantation.* 1990;49:793-797.

133. Weiss RA, Madaio MP, Tomaszewski JE, et al. T cells reactive to an inducible heat shock protein induce disease in toxin-induced interstitial nephritis. *J Exp Med.* 1994;180:2239-2250.

134. Romero F, Rodriguez-Iturbe B, Parra G, et al. Mycophenolate mofetil prevents the progressive renal failure induced by 5/6 renal ablation in rats. *Kidney Int.* 1999;55:945-955.

135. Meyers CM, Kelly CJ. Effector mechanisms in organ-specific autoimmunity. I. Characterization of a CD8+ T cell that mediates murine interstitial nephritis. *J Clin Invest.* 1991;88:408-416.

136. Bailey NC, Kelly CJ. Nephritogenic T cells use granzyme C as a cytotoxic mediator. *Eur J Immunol.* 1997;27:2302-2309.

137. Meyers CM, Kelly CJ. Inhibition of murine nephritogenic effector T cells by a clone-specific suppressor factor. *J Clin Invest.* 1994;94:2093-2104.

138. Meyers CM, Kelly CJ. Immunoregulation and TGF-beta 1. Suppression of a nephritogenic murine T cell clone. *Kidney Int.* 1994;46:1295-1301.

139. Heeger PS, Smoyer WE, Saad T, et al. Molecular analysis of the helper T cell response in murine interstitial nephritis. T cells recognizing an immunodominant epitope use multiple T cell receptor V beta genes with similarities across CDR3. *J Clin Invest.* 1994;94:2084-2092.

140. Spanou Z, Keller M, Britschgi M, et al. Involvement of drug-specific T cells in acute drug-induced interstitial nephritis. *J Am Soc Nephrol.* 2006;17:2919-2927.

141. Asano M, Toda M, Sakaguchi N, et al. Autoimmune disease as a consequence of developmental abnormality of a T cell subpopulation. *J Exp Med.* 1996;184:387-396.

142. Fontenot JD, Rasmussen JP, Williams LM, et al. Regulatory T cell lineage specification by the forkhead transcription factor foxp3. *Immunity.* 2005;22:329-341.

143. Thornton AM, Piccirillo CA, Shevach EM. Activation requirements for the induction of CD4+CD25+ T cell suppressor function. *Eur J Immunol.* 2004;34:366-376.

144. Wang YM, Zhang GY, Wang Y, et al. Foxp3-transduced polyclonal regulatory T cells protect against chronic renal injury from Adriamycin. *J Am Soc Nephrol.* 2006;17:697-706.

145. Bailey NC, Frishberg Y, Kelly CJ. Loss of high affinity transforming growth factor-beta 1 (TGF-beta 1) binding to a nephritogenic T cell results in absence of growth inhibition by TGF-beta 1 and augmented nephritogenicity. *J Immunol.* 1996;156:3009-3016.

146. Kelly CJ. T cell regulation of autoimmune interstitial nephritis. *J Am Soc Nephrol.* 1990;1:140-149.

147. Kelly CJ, Clayman MD, Neilson EG. Immunoregulation in experimental interstitial nephritis: immunization with renal tubular antigen in incomplete Freund's adjuvant induces major histocompatibility complex-restricted, OX8+ suppressor T cells which are antigen-specific and inhibit the expression of disease. *J Immunol.* 1986;136:903-907.

148. Kelly CJ, Silvers WK, Neilson EG. Tolerance to parenchymal self. Regulatory role of major histocompatibility complex-restricted, OX8+ suppressor T cells specific for autologous renal tubular antigen in experimental interstitial nephritis. *J Exp Med.* 1985;162:1892-1903.

149. Neilson EG, Kelly CJ, Clayman MD, et al. Murine interstitial nephritis. VII. Suppression of renal injury after treatment with soluble suppressor factor TsF1. *J Immunol.* 1987;139:1518-1524.

150. Eddy AA. Molecular insights into renal interstitial fibrosis. *J Am Soc Nephrol.* 1996;7:2495-2508.

151. Lange-Sperandio B, Trautmann A, Eickelberg O, et al. Leukocytes induce epithelial to mesenchymal transition after unilateral ureteral obstruction in neonatal mice. *Am J Pathol.* 2007;171:861-871.

152. Cao Q, Wang Y, Zheng D, et al. IL-10/TGF-β–modified macrophages induce regulatory T cells and protect against Adriamycin nephrosis. *J Am Soc Nephrol.* 2010;21(6):933-942.

153. Iwano M, Fischer A, Okada H, et al. Conditional abatement of tissue fibrosis using nucleoside analogs to selectively corrupt DNA replication in transgenic fibroblasts. *Mol Ther.* 2001;3:149-159.

154. Strutz F, Okada H, Lo CW, et al. Identification and characterization of a fibroblast marker: FSP1. *J Cell Biol.* 1995;130:393-405.

155. Iwano M, Neilson EG. Mechanisms of tubulointerstitial fibrosis. *Curr Opin Nephrol Hypertens.* 2004;13:279-284.

156. Zeisberg EM, Potenta SE, Sugimoto H, et al. Fibroblasts in kidney fibrosis emerge via endothelial-to-mesenchymal transition. *J Am Soc Nephrol.* 2008;19:2282-2287.

157. Zeisberg EM, Tarnavski O, Zeisberg M, et al. Endothelial-to-mesenchymal transition contributes to cardiac fibrosis. *Nat Med.* 2007;13:952-961.

158. Liu Y. New insights into epithelial-mesenchymal transition in kidney fibrosis. *J Am Soc Nephrol.* 2010;21:212-222.

159. Zeisberg M, Neilson EG. Biomarkers for epithelial-mesenchymal transitions. *J Clin Invest.* 2009;119:1429-1437.

160. Neilson EG. Plasticity, nuclear diapause, and a requiem for the terminal differentiation of epithelia. *J Am Soc Nephrol.* 2007;18:1995-1998.

161. Iwano M, Plieth D, Danoff TM, et al. Evidence that fibroblasts derive from epithelium during tissue fibrosis. *J Clin Invest.* 2002;110:341-350.

162. Humphreys BD, Lin SL, Kobayashi A, et al. Fate tracing reveals the pericyte and not epithelial origin of myofibroblasts in kidney fibrosis. *Am J Pathol.* 2010;176:85-97.

163. Kalluri R, Neilson EG. Epithelial-mesenchymal transition and its implications for fibrosis. *J Clin Invest.* 2003;112:1776-1784.

164. Cheng S, Lovett DH. Gelatinase A (MMP-2) is necessary and sufficient for renal tubular cell epithelial-mesenchymal transformation. *Am J Pathol.* 2003;162:1937-1949.

165. Strutz F, Zeisberg M, Ziyadeh FN, et al. Role of basic fibroblast growth factor-2 in epithelial-mesenchymal transformation. *Kidney Int.* 2002;61:1714-1728.

166. Venkov CD, Link AJ, Jennings JL, et al. A proximal activator of transcription in epithelial-mesenchymal transition. *J Clin Invest.* 2007;117:482-491.

167. Neilson EG. Mechanisms of disease: fibroblasts—a new look at an old problem. *Nat Clin Pract Nephrol.* 2006;2:101-108.

168. Huang WY, Li ZG, Rus H, et al. RGC-32 mediates transforming growth factor-beta–induced epithelial-mesenchymal transition in human renal proximal tubular cells. *J Biol Chem.* 2009;284:9426-9432.

169. Pollack V, Sarkozi R, Banki Z, et al. Oncostatin M–induced effects on EMT in human proximal tubular cells: differential role of ERK signaling. *Am J Physiol Renal Physiol.* 2007;293:F1714-F1726.

170. Chea SW, Lee KB. TGF-beta mediated epithelial-mesenchymal transition in autosomal dominant polycystic kidney disease. *Yonsei Med J.* 2009;50:105-111.

171. Rastaldi MP, Ferrario F, Giardino L, et al. Epithelial-mesenchymal transition of tubular epithelial cells in human renal biopsies. *Kidney Int.* 2002;62:137-146.

172. Zeisberg M, Hanai J, Sugimoto H, et al. BMP-7 counteracts TGF-beta1–induced epithelial-to-mesenchymal transition and reverses chronic renal injury. *Nat Med.* 2003;9:964-968.

173. Dworkin LD, Gong R, Tolbert E, et al. Hepatocyte growth factor ameliorates progression of interstitial fibrosis in rats with established renal injury. *Kidney Int.* 2004;65:409-419.

174. Lin J, Patel SR, Cheng X, et al. Kielin/chordin-like protein, a novel enhancer of BMP signaling, attenuates renal fibrotic disease. *Nat Med.* 2005;11:387-393.

175. Neilson EG. Setting a trap for tissue fibrosis. *Nat Med.* 2005;11:373-374.

176. Higgins DF, Kimura K, Bernhardt WM, et al. Hypoxia promotes fibrogenesis in vivo via HIF-1 stimulation of epithelial-to-mesenchymal transition. *J Clin Invest.* 2007;117:3810-3820.

177. Nangaku M. Mechanisms of tubulointerstitial injury in the kidney: final common pathways to end-stage renal failure. *Intern Med.* 2004;43:9-17.

178. Nakagawa T, Kang DH, Ohashi R, et al. Tubulointerstitial disease: role of ischemia and microvascular disease. *Curr Opin Nephrol Hypertens.* 2003;12:233-241.

179. Norman JT, Clark IM, Garcia PL. Hypoxia promotes fibrogenesis in human renal fibroblasts. *Kidney Int.* 2000;58:2351-2366.

180. Yuan HT, Li XZ, Pitera JE, et al. Peritubular capillary loss after mouse acute nephrotoxicity correlates with down-regulation of vascular endothelial growth factor-A and hypoxia-inducible factor-1 alpha. *Am J Pathol.* 2003;163:2289-2301.

181. Michel DM, Kelly CJ. Acute interstitial nephritis. *J Am Soc Nephrol.* 1998;9:506-515.

182. Baylor P, Williams K. Interstitial nephritis, thrombocytopenia, hepatitis, and elevated serum amylase levels in a patient receiving clarithromycin therapy. *Clin Infect Dis.* 1999;29:1350-1351.

183. Tintillier M, Kirch L, Almpanis C, et al. Telithromycin-induced acute interstitial nephritis: a first case report. *Am J Kidney Dis.* 2004;44:e25-e27.

184. Baker RJ, Pusey CD. The changing profile of acute tubulointerstitial nephritis. *Nephrol Dial Transplant.* 2004;19:8-11.

185. Zhao Z, Baldo BA, Rimmer J. β-Lactam allergenic determinants: fine structural recognition of a cross-reacting determinant on benzylpenicillin and cephalothin. *Clin Exp Allergy.* 2002;32:1644-1650.

186. Whelton A. Nephrotoxicity of nonsteroidal anti-inflammatory drugs: physiologic foundations and clinical implications. *Am J Med.* 1999;106:13S-24S.

187. Whelton A, Stout RL, Spilman PS, et al. Renal effects of ibuprofen, piroxicam, and sulindac in patients with asymptomatic renal failure. A prospective, randomized, crossover comparison. *Ann Intern Med.* 1990;112:568-576.

188. Murray MD, Brater DC. Renal toxicity of the nonsteroidal anti-inflammatory drugs. *Annu Rev Pharmacol Toxicol.* 1993;33:435-465.

189. Greenhill AH, Norman ME, Cornfeld D, et al. Acute renal failure secondary to acute pyelonephritis. *Clin Nephrol.* 1977;8:400-403.

190. Andrade L, de Francesco Daher E, Seguro AC. Leptospiral nephropathy. *Semin Nephrol.* 2008;28:383-394.

191. Chung S, Park CW, Chung HW, et al. Acute renal failure presenting as a granulomatous interstitial nephritis due to cryptococcal infection. *Kidney Int.* 2009;76:453-458.

192. Nishitarumizu K, Tokuda Y, Uehara H, et al. Tubulointerstitial nephritis associated with Legionnaires' disease. *Intern Med.* 2000;39:150-153.

193. Adams AL, Cook WJ. Granulomatous interstitial nephritis secondary to histoplasmosis. *Am J Kidney Dis.* 2007;50:681-685.

194. Matsukura H, Itoh Y, Kanegane H, et al. Acute tubulointerstitial nephritis: possible association with cytomegalovirus infection. *Pediatr Nephrol.* 2006;21:442-443.

195. Ferluga D, Vizjak A. Hantavirus nephropathy. *J Am Soc Nephrol.* 2008;19:1653-1658.

196. Miettinen MH, Makela SM, Ala-Houhala IO, et al. Ten-year prognosis of Puumala hantavirus–induced acute interstitial nephritis. *Kidney Int.* 2006;69:2043-2048.

197. Verma N, Arunabh S, Brady TM, et al. Acute interstitial nephritis secondary to infectious mononucleosis. *Clin Nephrol.* 2002;58:151-154.

198. Cataudella JA, Young ID, Iliescu EA. Epstein-Barr virus–associated acute interstitial nephritis: infection or immunologic phenomenon? *Nephron.* 2002;92:437-439.
199. Parkhie SM, Fine DM, Lucas GM, et al. Characteristics of patients with HIV and biopsy-proven acute interstitial nephritis. *Clin J Am Soc Nephrol.* 2010;5:798-804.
200. Jao J, Wyatt CM. Antiretroviral medications: adverse effects on the kidney. *Adv Chronic Kidney Dis.* 2010;17:72-82.
201. Neilson EG. Tubulointerstitial nephritis. In: Goldman L, Ausiello D, eds. *Cecil's textbook of medicine.* Philadelphia: Saunders; 2010.
202. Katz A, Fish AJ, Santamaria P, et al. Role of antibodies to tubulointerstitial nephritis antigen in human anti-tubular basement membrane nephritis associated with membranous nephropathy. *Am J Med.* 1992;93:691-698.
203. Dobrin RS, Vernier RL, Fish AL. Acute eosinophilic interstitial nephritis and renal failure with bone marrow–lymph node granulomas and anterior uveitis. A new syndrome. *Am J Med.* 1975;59:325-333.
204. Neilson EG, Farris AB. Case records of the Massachusetts General Hospital. Case 21-2009. A 61-year-old woman with abdominal pain, weight loss, and renal failure. *N Engl J Med.* 2009;361:179-187.
205. Morino M, Inami K, Kobayashi T, et al. Acute tubulointerstitial nephritis in two siblings and concomitant uveitis in one. *Acta Paediatr Jpn.* 1991;33:93-98.
206. Stupp R, Mihatsch MJ, Matter L, et al. Acute tubulo-interstitial nephritis with uveitis (TINU syndrome) in a patient with serologic evidence for *Chlamydia* infection. *Klin Wochenschr.* 1990;68:971-975.
207. Sessa A, Meroni M, Battini G, et al. Acute renal failure due to idiopathic tubulo-intestinal nephritis and uveitis: "TINU syndrome." Case report and review of the literature. *J Nephrol.* 2000;13:377-380.
208. Neilson EG. Pathogenesis and therapy of interstitial nephritis. *Kidney Int.* 1989;35:1257-1270.
209. Kleinknecht D. Interstitial nephritis, the nephrotic syndrome, and chronic renal failure secondary to nonsteroidal anti-inflammatory drugs. *Semin Nephrol.* 1995;15:228-235.
210. Cruz DN, Perazella MA. Drug-induced acute tubulointerstitial nephritis: the clinical spectrum. *Hosp Pract.* 1998;33:151-152:157-158, 161–164.
211. Buysen JG, Houthoff HJ, Krediet RT, et al. Acute interstitial nephritis: a clinical and morphological study in 27 patients. *Nephrol Dial Transplant.* 1990;5:94-99.
212. Schwarz A, Krause PH, Kunzendorf U, et al. The outcome of acute interstitial nephritis: risk factors for the transition from acute to chronic interstitial nephritis. *Clin Nephrol.* 2000;54:179-190.
213. Corwin HL, Bray RA, Haber MH. The detection and interpretation of urinary eosinophils. *Arch Pathol Lab Med.* 1989;113:1256-1258.
214. Ruffing KA, Hoppes P, Blend D, et al. Eosinophils in urine revisited. *Clin Nephrol.* 1994;41:163-166.
215. Shibasaki T, Ishimoto F, Sakai O, et al. Clinical characterization of drug-induced allergic nephritis. *Am J Nephrol.* 1991;11:174-180.
216. Smith J, Neilson EG. *Treatment of acute interstitial nephritis, in Wilcox CS (editor): Therapy in nephrology and hypertension.* 3rd ed. Philadelphia: Elsevier; 2008.
217. Ivanyi B, Hamilton-Dutoit SJ, Hansen HE, et al. Acute tubulointerstitial nephritis: phenotype of infiltrating cells and prognostic impact of tubulitis. *Virchows Arch.* 1996;428:5-12.
218. Pusey CD, Saltissi D, Bloodworth L, et al. Drug associated acute interstitial nephritis: clinical and pathological features and the response to high dose steroid therapy. *Q J Med.* 1983;52:194-211.
219. Eknoyan G. Acute hypersensitivity interstitial nephritis. In: Glassock RJ, ed. *Current therapy in nephrology and hypertension.* St. Louis: Mosby–Year Book; 1998:99-101.
220. Eknoyan G, McDonald MA, Appel D, et al. Chronic tubulo-interstitial nephritis: correlation between structural and functional findings. *Kidney Int.* 1990;38:736-743.
221. De Broe ME, Elseviers MM. Over-the-counter analgesic use. *J Am Soc Nephrol.* 2009;20:2098-2103.
222. Bennett WM, DeBroe ME. Analgesic nephropathy—a preventable renal disease. *N Engl J Med.* 1989;320:1269-1271.
223. Brunner FP, Selwood NH. End-stage renal failure due to analgesic nephropathy, its changing pattern and cardiovascular mortality. EDTA-ERA Registry Committee. *Nephrol Dial Transplant.* 1994;9:1371-1376.
224. Kincaid-Smith P, Nanra RS. Lithium-induced and analgesic-induced renal diseases. In: Schreier RW, Gottschalk CW, eds. *Diseases of the kidney.* Boston: Little, Brown; 1993:1099-1129.
225. Murray TG, Goldberg M. Analgesic-associated nephropathy in the U.S.A.: epidemiologic, clinical and pathogenetic features. *Kidney Int.* 1978;13:64-71.
226. Nanra RS. Analgesic nephropathy in the 1990s—an Australian perspective. *Kidney Int Suppl.* 1993;42:S86-S92.
227. Blohme I, Johansson S. Renal pelvic neoplasms and atypical urothelium in patients with end-stage analgesic nephropathy. *Kidney Int.* 1981;20:671-675.
228. Dubach UC, Rosner B, Sturmer T. An epidemiologic study of abuse of analgesic drugs. Effects of phenacetin and salicylate on mortality and cardiovascular morbidity (1968 to 1987). *N Engl J Med.* 1991;324:155-160.
229. McCredie M, Stewart JH, Carter JJ, et al. Phenacetin and papillary necrosis: independent risk factors for renal pelvic cancer. *Kidney Int.* 1986;30:81-84.
230. McCredie M, Stewart JH. Does paracetamol cause urothelial cancer or renal papillary necrosis? *Nephron.* 1988;49:296-300.
231. Fored CM, Ejerblad E, Lindblad P, et al. Acetaminophen, aspirin, and chronic renal failure. *N Engl J Med.* 2001;345:1801-1808.
232. Ibanez L, Morlans M, Vidal X, et al. Case-control study of regular analgesic and nonsteroidal anti-inflammatory use and end-stage renal disease. *Kidney Int.* 2005;67:2393-2398.
233. Morlans M, Laporte JR, Vidal X, et al. End-stage renal disease and non-narcotic analgesics: a case-control study. *Br J Clin Pharmacol.* 1990;30:717-723.
234. Perneger TV, Whelton PK, Klag MJ. Risk of kidney failure associated with the use of acetaminophen, aspirin, and nonsteroidal antiinflammatory drugs. *N Engl J Med.* 1994;331:1675-1679.
235. Sandler DP, Smith JC, Weinberg CR, et al. Analgesic use and chronic renal disease. *N Engl J Med.* 1989;320:1238-1243.
236. Pommer W, Bronder E, Greiser E, et al. Regular analgesic intake and the risk of end-stage renal failure. *Am J Nephrol.* 1989;9:403-412.
237. Elseviers MM, De Broe ME. Combination analgesic involvement in the pathogenesis of analgesic nephropathy: the European perspective. *Am J Kidney Dis.* 1996;28:S48-S55.
238. Mihatsch MJ, Khanlari B, Brunner FP. Obituary to analgesic nephropathy—an autopsy study. *Nephrol Dial Transplant.* 2006;21:3139-3145.
239. Michielsen P, Heinemann L, Mihatsch M, et al. Non-phenacetin analgesics and analgesic nephropathy: clinical assessment of high users from a case-control study. *Nephrol Dial Transplant.* 2009;24:1253-1259.
240. van der Woude FJ, Heinemann LA, Graf H, et al. Analgesics use and ESRD in younger age: a case-control study. *BMC Nephrol.* 2007;8:15.
241. Bach PH, Hardy TL. Relevance of animal models to analgesic-associated renal papillary necrosis in humans. *Kidney Int.* 1985;28:605-613.
242. Duggin GG. Combination analgesic-induced kidney disease: the Australian experience. *Am J Kidney Dis.* 1996;28:S39-S47.
243. Elseviers MM, De Schepper A, Corthouts R, et al. High diagnostic performance of CT scan for analgesic nephropathy in patients with incipient to severe renal failure. *Kidney Int.* 1995;48:1316-1323.
244. Elseviers MM, Waller I, Nenoy D, et al. Evaluation of diagnostic criteria for analgesic nephropathy in patients with end-stage renal failure: results of the ANNE study. Analgesic Nephropathy Network of Europe. *Nephrol Dial Transplant.* 1995;10:808-814.
245. Henrich WL, Clark RL, Kelly JP, et al. Non–contrast-enhanced computerized tomography and analgesic-related kidney disease: report of the National Analgesic Nephropathy Study. *J Am Soc Nephrol.* 2006;17:1472-1480.
246. Vanherweghem JL, Depierreux M, Tielemans C, et al. Rapidly progressive interstitial renal fibrosis in young women: association with slimming regimen including Chinese herbs. *Lancet.* 1993;341:387-391.
247. Vanherweghem JL, Abramowicz D, Tielemans C, et al. Effects of steroids on the progression of renal failure in chronic interstitial renal fibrosis: a pilot study in Chinese herbs nephropathy. *Am J Kidney Dis.* 1996;27:209-215.
248. Diamond JR, Pallone TL. Acute interstitial nephritis following use of tung shueh pills. *Am J Kidney Dis.* 1994;24:219-221.
249. Wu Y, Liu Z, Hu W, et al. Mast cell infiltration associated with tubulointerstitial fibrosis in chronic aristolochic acid nephropathy. *Hum Exp Toxicol.* 2005;24:41-47.
250. Yang CS, Lin CH, Chang SH, et al. Rapidly progressive fibrosing interstitial nephritis associated with Chinese herbal drugs. *Am J Kidney Dis.* 2000;35:313-318.
251. Cosyns JP, Jadoul M, Squifflet JP, et al. Chinese herbs nephropathy: a clue to Balkan endemic nephropathy? *Kidney Int.* 1994;45:1680-1688.
252. Pozdzik AA, Berton A, Schmeiser HH, et al. Aristolochic acid nephropathy revisited: a place for innate and adaptive immunity? *Histopathology.* 2010;56:449-463.
253. Kabanda A, Jadoul M, Lauwerys R, Bernard A, et al. Low molecular weight proteinuria in Chinese herbs nephropathy. *Kidney Int.* 1995;48:1571-1576.
254. Depierreux M, Van Damme B, Vanden Houte K, et al. Pathologic aspects of a newly described nephropathy related to the prolonged use of Chinese herbs. *Am J Kidney Dis.* 1994;24:172-180.
255. Cosyns JP, Dehoux JP, Guiot Y, et al. Chronic aristolochic acid toxicity in rabbits: a model of Chinese herbs nephropathy? *Kidney Int.* 2001;59:2164-2173.
256. Debelle FD, Nortier JL, De Prez EG, et al. Aristolochic acids induce chronic renal failure with interstitial fibrosis in salt-depleted rats. *J Am Soc Nephrol.* 2002;13:431-436.
257. Zhou L, Fu P, Huang XR, et al. Mechanism of chronic aristolochic acid nephropathy: role of SMAD3. *Am J Physiol Renal Physiol.* 2010;298:F1006-F1017.

258. Nortier JL, Martinez MC, Schmeiser HH, et al. Urothelial carcinoma associated with the use of a Chinese herb (*Aristolochia fangchi*). *N Engl J Med.* 2000;342:1686-1692.
259. Reginster F, Jadoul M, van Ypersele de Strihou C. Chinese herbs nephropathy presentation, natural history and fate after transplantation. *Nephrol Dial Transplant.* 1997;12:81-86.
260. Ceovic S, Hrabar A, Saric M. Epidemiology of Balkan endemic nephropathy. *Food Chem Toxicol.* 1992;30:183-188.
261. Stefanovic V, Cukuranovic R, Miljkovic S, et al. Fifty years of Balkan endemic nephropathy: challenges of study using epidemiological method. *Ren Fail.* 2009;31:409-418.
262. Djukanovic L, et al. Balkan endemic nephropathy. In: De Broe ME, Porter GA, Bennett WM, eds. *Clinical nephrotoxins—renal injury from drugs and chemicals.* Dordrecht, The Netherlands: Kluwer; 2003:587-602.
263. Petronic VJ, Bukurov NS, Djokic MR, et al. Balkan endemic nephropathy and papillary transitional cell tumors of the renal pelvis and ureters. *Kidney Int Suppl.* 1991;34:S77-S79.
264. Grollman AP, Jelakovic B, Role of environmental toxins in endemic (Balkan) nephropathy. October 2006, Zagreb, Croatia. *J Am Soc Nephrol.* 2007;18:2817-2823.
265. Grollman AP, Shibutani S, Moriya M, et al. Aristolochic acid and the etiology of endemic (Balkan) nephropathy. *Proc Natl Acad Sci U S A.* 2007;104:12129-12134.
266. Stefanovic V, Toncheva D, Atanasova S, et al. Etiology of Balkan endemic nephropathy and associated urothelial cancer. *Am J Nephrol.* 2006;26:1-11.
267. Marples D, Christensen S, Christensen EI, et al. Lithium-induced downregulation of aquaporin-2 water channel expression in rat kidney medulla. *J Clin Invest.* 1995;95:1838-1845.
268. Hestbech J, Hansen HE, Amdisen A, et al. Chronic renal lesions following long-term treatment with lithium. *Kidney Int.* 1977;12:205-213.
269. Walker RG, Bennett WM, Davies BM, et al. Structural and functional effects of long-term lithium therapy. *Kidney Int Suppl.* 1982;11:S13-S19.
270. Boton R, Gaviria M, Batlle DC. Prevalence, pathogenesis, and treatment of renal dysfunction associated with chronic lithium therapy. *Am J Kidney Dis.* 1987;10:329-345.
271. Walker RG, Escott M, Birchall I, et al. Chronic progressive renal lesions induced by lithium. *Kidney Int.* 1986;29:875-881.
272. Markowitz GS, Radhakrishnan J, Kambham N, et al. Lithium nephrotoxicity: a progressive combined glomerular and tubulointerstitial nephropathy. *J Am Soc Nephrol.* 2000;11:1439-1448.
273. Lepkifker E, Sverdlik A, Iancu I, et al. Renal insufficiency in long-term lithium treatment. *J Clin Psychiatry.* 2004;65:850-856.
274. Inglis JA, Henderson DA, Emmerson BT. The pathology and pathogenesis of chronic lead nephropathy occurring in Queensland. *J Pathol.* 1978;124:65-76.
275. Yu CC, Lin JL, Lin-Tan DT. Environmental exposure to lead and progression of chronic renal diseases: a four-year prospective longitudinal study. *J Am Soc Nephrol.* 2004;15:1016-1022.
276. Muntner P, He J, Vupputuri S, et al. Blood lead and chronic kidney disease in the general United States population: results from NHANES III. *Kidney Int.* 2003;63:1044-1050.
277. Fadrowski JJ, Navas-Acien A, Tellez-Plaza M, et al. Blood lead level and kidney function in US adolescents: The Third National Health and Nutrition Examination Survey. *Arch Intern Med.* 2010;170:75-82.
278. Roncal C, Mu W, Reungjui S, et al. Lead, at low levels, accelerates arteriolopathy and tubulointerstitial injury in chronic kidney disease. *Am J Physiol Renal Physiol.* 2007;293:F1391-F1396.
279. Wedeen RP, Malik DK, Batuman V. Detection and treatment of occupational lead nephropathy. *Arch Intern Med.* 1979;139:53-57.
280. Lin JL, Lin-Tan DT, Hsu KH, et al. Environmental lead exposure and progression of chronic renal diseases in patients without diabetes. *N Engl J Med.* 2003;348:277-286.
281. Lin JL, Lin-Tan DT, Yu CC, et al. Environmental exposure to lead and progressive diabetic nephropathy in patients with type II diabetes. *Kidney Int.* 2006;69:2049-2056.
282. Kido T, Nogawa K, Yamada Y, et al. Osteopenia in inhabitants with renal dysfunction induced by exposure to environmental cadmium. *Int Arch Occup Environ Health.* 1989;61:271-276.
283. Hellstrom L, Elinder CG, Dahlberg B, et al. Cadmium exposure and end-stage renal disease. *Am J Kidney Dis.* 2001;38:1001-1008.
284. Lee WK, Torchalski B, Thevenod F. Cadmium-induced ceramide formation triggers calpain-dependent apoptosis in cultured kidney proximal tubule cells. *Am J Physiol Cell Physiol.* 2007;293:C839-C847.
285. Staessen JA, Buchet JP, Ginucchio G, et al. Public health implications of environmental exposure to cadmium and lead: an overview of epidemiological studies in Belgium. Working Groups. *J Cardiovasc Risk.* 1996;3:26-41.
286. Hotz P, Buchet JP, Bernard A, et al. Renal effects of low-level environmental cadmium exposure: 5-year follow-up of a subcohort from the Cadmibel study. *Lancet.* 1999;354:1508-1513.
287. Satarug S, Haswell-Elkins MR, Moore MR. Safe levels of cadmium intake to prevent renal toxicity in human subjects. *Br J Nutr.* 2000;84:791-802.
288. Trevisan A, Gardin C. Nephrolithiasis in a worker with cadmium exposure in the past. *Int Arch Occup Environ Health.* 2005;78:670-672.
289. Murray T, Goldberg M. Chronic interstitial nephritis: etiologic factors. *Ann Intern Med.* 1975;82:453-459.
290. Yu TF, Berger L. Impaired renal function gout: its association with hypertensive vascular disease and intrinsic renal disease. *Am J Med.* 1982;72:95-100.
291. Messerli FH, Frohlich ED, Dreslinski GR, et al. Serum uric acid in essential hypertension: an indicator of renal vascular involvement. *Ann Intern Med.* 1980;93:817-821.
292. Dahan K, Fuchshuber A, Adamis S, et al. Familial juvenile hyperuricemic nephropathy and autosomal dominant medullary cystic kidney disease type 2: two facets of the same disease? *J Am Soc Nephrol.* 2001;12:2348-2357.
293. Duffy WB, Senekjian HO, Knight TF, et al. Management of asymptomatic hyperuricemia. *JAMA.* 1981;246:2215-2216.
294. Khosla UM, Zharikov S, Finch JL, et al. Hyperuricemia induces endothelial dysfunction. *Kidney Int.* 2005;67:1739-1742.
295. Kang DH, Park SK, Lee IK, et al. Uric acid–induced C-reactive protein expression: implication on cell proliferation and nitric oxide production of human vascular cells. *J Am Soc Nephrol.* 2005;16:3553-3562.
296. Kang DH, Nakagawa T, Feng L, et al. A role for uric acid in the progression of renal disease. *J Am Soc Nephrol.* 2002;13:2888-2897.
297. Preitner F, Bonny O, Laverriere A, et al. Glut9 is a major regulator of urate homeostasis and its genetic inactivation induces hyperuricosuria and urate nephropathy. *Proc Natl Acad Sci U S A.* 2009;106:15501-15506.
298. Muther RS, McCarron DA, Bennett WM. Renal manifestations of sarcoidosis. *Arch Intern Med.* 1981;141:643-645.
299. Casella FJ, Allon M. The kidney in sarcoidosis. *J Am Soc Nephrol.* 1993;3:1555-1562.
300. Darabi K, Torres G, Chewaproug D. Nephrolithiasis as primary symptom in sarcoidosis. *Scand J Urol Nephrol.* 2005;39:173-175.
301. Robson MG, Banerjee D, Hopster D, et al. Seven cases of granulomatous interstitial nephritis in the absence of extrarenal sarcoid. *Nephrol Dial Transplant.* 2003;18:280-284.
302. Thumfart J, Muller D, Rudolph B, et al. Isolated sarcoid granulomatous interstitial nephritis responding to infliximab therapy. *Am J Kidney Dis.* 2005;45:411-414.
303. Viero RM, Cavallo T. Granulomatous interstitial nephritis. *Hum Pathol.* 1995;26:1347-1353.
304. Bia MJ, Insogna K. Treatment of sarcoidosis-associated hypercalcemia with ketoconazole. *Am J Kidney Dis.* 1991;18:702-705.

Urinary Tract Infection in Adults

Lindsay E. Nicolle

Urinary tract infection of the bladder, kidney, or (in men) the prostate is one of the most common human infections. Infecting organisms are usually bacteria; fungi also contribute. Much less frequently, infection is caused by viruses or parasites. Other manifestations of genitourinary tract infection include renal and perinephric abscesses, emphysematous cystitis and pyelonephritis, xanthogranulomatous pyelonephritis, and pyocystitis. Disseminated viral infections (e.g., mumps, cytomegalovirus (CMV), and other herpesviruses) and fungal infections (e.g., blastomycosis, histoplasmosis) may also involve the urinary tract, but they are not discussed in this chapter. Polyomavirus BK infection in renal transplant recipients and urinary tract infection in children, including vesicoureteral reflux, are addressed in other chapters.

Definitions

Urinary tract infection is the presence of bacteria or other microorganisms in the urine or genitourinary tissues, which are normally sterile. The term *bacteriuria* describes identification of any bacteria in the urine, although in practice it usually refers to isolation of organisms in concentrations that meet standard quantitative criteria. Infection is asymptomatic when the urine culture meets quantitative criteria for bacteriuria without signs or symptoms attributable to infection. Symptomatic urinary tract infection may manifest as bladder infection (cystitis or lower tract infection), kidney infection (pyelonephritis or upper tract infection), or prostate infection (acute or chronic bacterial prostatitis). Acute uncomplicated urinary tract infection occurs in women with a normal genitourinary tract, usually manifesting as cystitis.[1,2] Pyelonephritis, also referred to as *acute nonobstructive* or *acute uncomplicated pyelonephritis,* also occurs in these women but much less frequently.[2] Complicated urinary tract infection occurs in individuals with functional or structural abnormalities of the genitourinary tract that are conducive to infection (Table 36-1).[3-5] In healthy postmenopausal women without genitourinary abnormalities and diabetic women without nephropathy or neurologic bladder impairment urinary tract infection is considered to be uncomplicated.

Acute uncomplicated urinary tract infection rarely occurs in men. A urinary tract infection in a man should be considered complicated until underlying abnormalities have been ruled out.

Urinary tract infection commonly recurs. *Reinfection* is infection that recurs after entry of an organism into the genitourinary tract, usually from the periurethral flora. Reinfection characteristically occurs with a different organism. However, when periurethral colonization with a potential uropathogen

TABLE 36-1 Abnormalities of the Urinary Tract That May Be Associated with Complicated Urinary Tract Infection

ABNORMALITY	EXAMPLE
Obstruction	Pelvicalyceal junction obstruction, ureteric or urethral strictures, prostate hypertrophy, urolithiasis, tumor, extrinsic compression
Neurologic impairment	Neurogenic bladder
Urologic devices	Indwelling catheter, ureteric stent, nephrostomy tube
Urologic abnormalities	Vesicoureteral reflux, bladder diverticuli, cystoceles, urologic procedures, ileal conduit, augmented bladder, neobladder
Metabolic/congenital diseases	Nephrocalcinosis, medullary sponge kidney, urethral valves, polycystic kidneys
Immunologic impairment	Renal transplantation

TABLE 36-2 Host Defenses Other Than Voiding That Contribute to Maintaining Sterility of Urine

DEFENSE	EXAMPLE
Urine characteristics	pH, osmolality, concentration of organic acids
Urine proteins	Tamm-Horsfall protein, secretory immunoglobulins, lactoferrin, lipocalin, cationic peptides (defensins, cathelicidins)
Inflammatory cells	Polymorphonuclear leukocytes
Uroepithelium	Mucopolysaccharide layer, cytokine production
Prostate secretions	Chemokines, immunoglobulins

persists, the same strain may be isolated from reinfection. Relapse occurs when an infecting organism persists in the urinary tract despite antimicrobial therapy; the same organism is isolated from recurrent infection after therapy.

General Concepts

Host Defenses of the Normal Urinary Tract

The urine and genitourinary tract are normally sterile, apart from the distal urethra. The normal flora of the distal urethra plays an important role in host defense by preventing colonization at this site by potential uropathogens. The flora includes aerobic bacteria that are common skin commensals, such as coagulase-negative staphylococci, viridans group streptococci, and *Corynebacterium* species.[6,7] There is also a large and complex anaerobic flora.[7] Molecular investigations have revealed that multiple additional, as yet unclassified bacteria are also present.[8] Urine is a good nutrient source for most bacterial species, and common uropathogens grow well in urine. The most important host defense that maintains sterility of the urine is normal, unobstructed voiding. An array of urine and uroepithelial cell components also contribute to maintaining sterile urine in the normal genitourinary tract (Table 36-2).[9,10] Inhibitors of bacterial adherence to uroepithelial cells prevent persistence of bacteria once they have entered the urinary tract. Tamm-Horsfall protein, the most abundant protein in the urine, appears to have an important role in this regard.[10] This protein prevents attachment of *Escherichia coli* to uroepithelial cell receptors by binding to the type 1 fimbria adhesin (FimH) and also removes other uropathogens such as *Klebsiella pneumoniae* and *Staphylococcus saprophyticus*.[11] It may have an immunomodulatory role through activation of the innate immune response by a Toll-like receptor-4–dependent mechanism.[10]

Adherence of bacteria to uroepitheal cells is also prevented by the surface mucopolysaccharide-glycosaminoglycan layer of the uroepithelium, by urine immunoglobulin G (IgG) and secretory immunoglobulin A (IgA), and by some low-molecular-weight oligosaccharides present in the urine. The relative importance of any of these specific components in vivo is not yet established. Despite this array of components contributing to sterility of the urine, bacteriuria is readily established once normal voiding is impaired. In the complicated urinary tract, infection occurs through increased entry of organisms into the bladder or kidney, which may be attributed to the use of urologic devices, turbulent urine flow, or reflux, and organisms then persist, despite other host defenses, when infected urine is retained if voiding is incomplete or in biofilm on urologic devices.

Immune and Inflammatory Response to Urinary Tract Infection

Urinary tract infection induces a wide spectrum of local and systemic inflammatory and immune responses. The intensity of response is determined by the interactions of microbial pathogenicity, individual genetic regulation, and the site of infection.[12] Unique *E. coli* strains have a variable capacity to stimulate or evade activation of the innate immune response. Uropathogenic strains that cause symptomatic infection induce a strong innate immune response, whereas strains isolated from asymptomatic bacteriuria evoke a limited response.[13,14] Strains that successfully evade immune activation probably have a pathogenetic advantage for establishing bladder colonization and persistent infection.[15]

Infecting organisms in the urinary tract activate uroepithelial cells through Toll-like receptors resulting in cytokine production, particularly interleukins-6 (IL-6) and -8 (CXCL8). These cytokines recruit neutrophils and other immunocompetent cells to the kidney and bladder.[10] Cytokine elaboration follows both direct stimulation of uroepithelial cells by bacterial lipopolysaccharide and bacterial adherence to epithelial cells. The chemotactic cytokine IL-8 is released at the mucosal site and recruits polymorphonuclear leukocytes, which results in pyuria. Urine and serum IL-6 concentrations are correlated with the severity of infection. The highest levels occur in patients with pyelonephritis. Systemic elaboration of interleukin-1β and IL-6 produces fever and activation of the acute phase response. The acute inflammatory infiltrate of polymorphonuclear leukocytes that develops in renal tissue during pyelonephritis limits bacterial spread and persistence within the kidney, but it also contributes to tissue damage and renal scarring.

Both IL-6 and IL-8 are also secreted by the bladder urothelium in direct response to bacterial antigens, including lipopolysaccharide.[16] IL-8 induces a rapid influx of neutrophils into the bladder, with subsequent phagocytosis and clearance of bacteria. This innate immune response rapidly clears most uropathogenic *E. coli* organisms from the bladder, but it does not produce a sterilizing immunity in murine models.[16] In humans, bacteriuria often persists despite marked pyuria. A vigorous local and systemic humoral immune response occurs in patients with pyelonephritis.[9,13] The antibody response is directed against surface antigens of the infecting bacteria, including O antigens and surface proteins such as the type 1 (Fim H) and P fimbriae, which are major adhesins of *E. coli*.[16,17] Immunoglobulin M antibodies dominate the systemic humoral response in the first episode of infection in the upper urinary tract, but subsequent episodes are characterized by an IgG response. In pyelonephritis, elevated levels of IgG antibodies to lipid A are correlated with severity of renal infection and parenchymal destruction. There is also a substantial urinary IgG and secretory IgA antibody response. Despite this robust response, the protective role, if any, of the antibody response in pyelonephritis is not clear. Bacteria often persist in the renal parenchyma despite very high levels of specific antibodies. In addition, in women who do not produce secretory IgA, the frequency of urinary tract infection is not increased.

IgA-producing plasma cells are found in higher numbers in the bladder submucosa of patients with bacterial cystitis than in that of healthy controls. However, acute cystitis is associated with a reduced or undetectable serologic response, which presumably reflects the superficial nature of the infection. The local immune response is of short duration and is reactivated for each infection. This limited immunologic response with bladder infection may explain why early reinfection with the same *E. coli* strain is observed in some women with acute cystitis. However, animal studies have demonstrated some protection against same-strain reinfection by systemic and local antibodies.[16]

Cell-mediated immunity appears to have a limited role in the host defense against urinary tract infection. A small number of mucosal T lymphocytes are present throughout the urinary tract, and both CD4+ and CD8+ T cells can be found in the submucosa and lamina propria of the bladder and urethra. Recruitment of B and T lymphocytes to the bladder wall is observed with secondary infections. T cell–derived proinflammatory cytokines also stimulate renal tubular epithelial cells to produce IL-6, which may increase IgA secretion of committed B cells.[16] However, women infected with human immunodeficiency virus (HIV) who have very low CD4 counts do not appear to have an increased susceptibility to or severity of urinary tract infection; this suggests that cell-mediated immunity is not an essential defense against such infection.

Urine Culture

The definitive diagnosis and appropriate management of urinary tract infection usually requires microbiologic confirmation by urine culture. Urine specimens for culture should always be obtained before antimicrobial therapy is initiated because urinary excretion of antimicrobial agents rapidly sterilizes urine. Once collected, the specimen should be forwarded promptly to the laboratory. Organisms present in small quantitative counts (i.e. contaminants) grow readily in urine at room temperature and reach high quantitative

counts within a few hours. If the specimen is delayed in reaching the laboratory, it should be refrigerated at 4° C until transported.

A urine specimen for culture must be collected using a method that minimizes contamination. For both men and women, a clean-catch voided specimen without additional periurethral cleaning is usually appropriate for obtaining a urine sample. For patients who cannot cooperate in the collection of a voided specimen, urine collected may be by an in-and-out catheter. For men, a specimen may be obtained in an external condom catheter after application of a clean condom catheter and collecting bag.[18] Urine samples may also be collected by suprapubic aspiration or directly from the renal pelvis when percutaneous drainage of an obstructed urinary tract is necessary. Specimens obtained from patients with short-term indwelling catheters should be collected by puncture of the catheter port. For a long-term indwelling catheter, two to five organisms are present in the catheter biofilm at any time, and urine collected through the catheter will contain both biofilm and bladder urine.[19] The chronic indwelling catheter should be removed and replaced by a new catheter with a specimen of bladder urine obtained through the newly placed catheter.[18,19]

The standard quantitative criteria for diagnosis of urinary tract infection with voided specimens is 10^5 colony-forming units (CFU) or more per milliliter. Women usually have low numbers of contaminating organisms from vaginal or periurethral flora isolated from voided specimens, and this quantitative criteria distinguishes bacteriuria from contamination. Application of this quantitative standard is always appropriate for the diagnosis of asymptomatic bacteriuria, but for symptomatic cases, the quantitative urine culture must be interpreted in the context of the clinical presentation and considering the method of specimen collection (Table 36-3). Bacteria require several hours of incubation in bladder urine to achieve a concentration of 10^5 CFU/mL or higher. Thus,

TABLE 36-3 Quantitative Counts of Bacteria in the Urine for Microbiologic Diagnosis of Urinary Tract Infection in Patients Not Receiving Antimicrobial Therapy

CONDITION	QUANTITATIVE CRITERIA
Voided	
Women: acute uncomplicated	
Cystitis	$\geq 10^3$ CFU/mL
Pyelonephritis	$\geq 10^4$ CFU/mL*
Asymptomatic	$\geq 10^5$ CFU/mL†
Men	$\geq 10^3$ CFU/mL
External condom collection	$\geq 10^5$ CFU/mL
Catheter	
In-and-out Indwelling‡	$\geq 10^2$ CFU/mL
Asymptomatic	$\geq 10^5$ CFU/mL
Symptomatic	$\geq 10^2$ CFU/mL
Suprapubic or percutaneous aspiration	Any growth

*In 95% of cases, values ≥ 10^5 colony-forming units (CFU) per milliliter.

†Two consecutive specimens are recommended.

‡A long-term catheters should be replaced and the specimen collected through a new catheter.

patients with frequency or diuresis may not retain urine in the bladder for a sufficient time to achieve the concentration of 10^5 CFU/mL or higher. Quantitative counts may also be lower when infection is caused by some fastidious organisms or if the patient is receiving a urinary antiseptic. For symptomatic men, a single urine specimen in which 10^3 CFU/mL or more of a uropathogen is isolated is diagnostic for bladder bacteriuria, according to studies with paired comparisons of voided specimens and suprapubic aspirates.

When a urine specimen is obtained by suprapubic aspiration or other percutaneous collection method, any quantitative count of an organism represents true bacteriuria, inasmuch as these methods yield samples only of bladder or renal pelvis urine. However, in specimens collected by an in-and-out catheter, contaminating organisms may be introduced from the periurethral area, and a quantitative criteria of 10^2 CFU/mL or higher is recommended. Other relevant considerations in interpreting a urine culture include the number and type of organisms isolated. A single infecting organism is usual, but in patients with complicated urinary tract infection, particularly those with indwelling urinary devices, more than one organism are frequently present. Commensal bacteria of the normal skin flora, such as diphtheroides and coagulase-negative staphylococci, usually represent contaminants when they are isolated from voided urine specimens. In young healthy women, group B streptococci and *Enterococcus* species are also usually contaminants.

Pharmacokinetic and Pharmacodynamic Considerations for Treatment

Therapeutic success in the treatment of cystitis is dependent on antimicrobial levels in the urine. Antimicrobial levels in renal tissue, which are correlated with serum levels, determine outcome for pyelonephritis.[20] Treatment of urinary tract infection is unique in some respects because of the exceptionally high urine concentrations achieved by many antimicrobial agents excreted into the urine (Table 36-4). The urine concentration is determined by the interplay of glomerular filtration, active tubular secretion, and tubular reabsorption, all influenced by pH, protein binding, and the molecular structure of the drug. Cystitis and pyelonephritis may be successfully treated with antimicrobial agents when the the infecting organism would not usually be considered susceptible on the basis of its minimal inhibitory concentration (MIC). The intermediate susceptibility designation reported by the clinical microbiology laboratory implies clinical efficacy in body sites where antimicrobial agents are physiologically concentrated, such as the urine, and is relevant to treatment of urinary tract infection. Thus, when an organism isolated from the urine is reported to have intermediate susceptibility to an antimicrobial agent, the drug is usually appropriate for treatment of urinary tract infection with that organism. The urine bactericidal activity of some antimicrobial agents is modified by the urine

ANTIMICROBIAL AGENT	% OF ABSORBED DRUG EXCRETED RENALLY AS PARENT METABOLITES (ACTIVE METABOLITES)*	USUAL DOSAGE FOR NORMAL RENAL FUNCTION†
Penicillins		
Penicillin G	80%	1-2 million U IV q4-6hr
Amoxicillin	90%	500 mg PO tid
Amoxicillin/clavulanic acid	Clavulanate: 20%-60%	500 mg PO tid or 875 mg PO bid
Ampicillin	90% (10%)	1-2 g IV q6hr
Cloxacillin	35%-50%	1-2 g IV q 4-6hr
Piperacillin	50%-80%	200-300 mg/kg/day IV qid
Piperacillin/tazobactam	Tazobactam: 60%-80%	3.375 g IV q6hr
Cephalosporins		
Cephalexin	>80% (18%)	500 mg PO qid
Cefazolin	>80%	1 g IV q8hr
Cefuroxime	>80%	250-500 mg PO bid
Cefotaxime	50%-60% (30%)	1 g IV q8hr
Ceftriaxone	50%	1-2 g IV q24hr
Cefepime	85%	1-2 g PO q12hr
Cefixime	15%-20%	400 mg PO od
Cefpodoxime	20%-35%	100-200 mg PO q12hr
Cefprozil	60%	250-500 mg PO q12hr
Ceftazidime	80%-90%	1-2g IV q8-12hr
Macrolides, Lincosamides		
Erythromycin	5%-15%	500 mg PO qid or 1g IV q6h
Clindamycin	≤6% (some active metabolites)	150-300 mg PO tid or 600-900 mg IV q6-8hr
Clarithromycin	20%-30% (10%-15%)	250-500 mg PO q12hr
Azithromycin	6%	500 mg PO od

TABLE 36-4 Urinary Excretion of Antimicrobial Agents in Persons with Normal Renal Function

Continued

TABLE 36-4	Urinary Excretion of Antimicrobial Agents in Persons with Normal Renal Function—cont'd	
ANTIMICROBIAL AGENT	**% OF ABSORBED DRUG EXCRETED RENALLY AS PARENT METABOLITES (ACTIVE METABOLITES)***	**USUAL DOSAGE FOR NORMAL RENAL FUNCTION†**
Aminoglycosides		
Gentamicin	99%	5 mg/kg/day IV in 1-3 divided doses
Tobramycin	99%	5 mg/kg/day IV in 1-3 divided doses
Amikacin	99%	15 mg/kg/day IV in 1-3 divided doses
Carbapenems		
Imipenem/cilastatin	70%-76%	500 mg IV q6hr
Meropenem	70%-80%	500 mg to 1 g IV q6-8hr
Ertapenem	40%	1g IV q24hr
Doripenem	70% (15%)	500 mg q8hr
Fluoroquinolones		
Norfloxacin	25%-40% (10%-20%)	400 mg bid
Ciprofloxacin	40% (10%-20%)	250-750 mg PO or 400 mg IV bid
Levofloxacin	70%-80%	250-750 mg PO or IV q24hr
Moxifloxacin	20%	400 mg PO or IV q24hr
Others		
Vancomycin	>90%	1 g IV q12hr
Teicoplanin	>90%	6-12 mg/kg IV q12hr
Daptomycin	54%	4 mg/kg IV q24hr
Linezolid	35%	600 mg PO or IV q12hr
Tigecycline	32%	250-500 mg IV q6hr
Trimethoprim	66%-95%	100 mg PO q12hr
Sulfamethoxazole	20%-40%	
Trimethoprim/sulfamethoxazole		180/800 mg PO bid
Nitrofurantoin monohydrate/macrocrystals	40%-60%	50-100 mg PO q6hr
Doxycycline	20%-30%	100 mg PO bid
Aztreonam	66%	1-2 g IV q6-8hr
Metronidazole	15% (30%-60%)	500 mg PO or IV tid
Rifampin	<10%/50%	600 mg PO od
Antifungals		
Amphotericin B deoxycholate	<10%	0.5-1 mg/kg IV od
Amphotericin B lipid formulations	<1%	1-5 mg/kg/day IV
5-Flucytosine	90%	100-150 mg/kg/day PO in 4 divided doses
Ketoconazole	<10%	400 mg PO od
Fluconazole	80%	100-400 mg PO or IV q24hr
Itraconazole	<1%	200 mg bid PO or IV × 2 days, then 200 mg PO od
Voriconazole	<1%	6 mg/kg IV × 1 dose, then 200 mg IV bid; 200-mg PO bid × 1 day, then 100 mg bid
Posaconazole	<1%	400 mg PO bid
Caspofungin	<1%	70-mg loading dose, then 50 mg IV q24hr
Micafungin	<1%	50-100 mg IV q24hr
Anidulafungin	<1%	100- to 200-mg IV loading dose, then 50-100 mg IV q24hr

*Except where noted, values are the proportion of dose renally excreted unchanged.
†Not all antimicrobial agents have an indication for urinary tract infection.
IV, Intravenously; *PO,* orally.

pH. Penicillins, tetracyclines, and nitrofurantoin are more active in acidic urine, and aminoglycosides, fluoroquinolones, and erythromycin are more active in alkaline urine. This pH variability has not been shown to be relevant for therapeutic outcomes, with the exception of methenamine salts, for which an acidic pH is necessary to release formaldehyde, the active component.

In the consideration of antimicrobial efficacy, the prostate is a unique compartment. The interior of the gland is an acidic environment. Drug entry and activity is dependent on lipid solubility, molecular size, local pH, and pKa of the antimicrobial agent.[21] Alkaline drugs such as trimethoprim diffuse into the prostate and are trapped, and high concentrations are thus achieved, but the drug remains in an inactive, ionized form. Fluoroquinolones and macrolides, however, penetrate well and remain active.

Current pharmacodynamic models for antimicrobial treatment of infection distinguish between time-dependent and concentration-dependent bacterial killing. The bacterial killing by β-Lactam antimicrobial agents is time dependent; the therapeutic efficacy depends on how long the concentration of the antimicrobial agent remains above the MIC of the infecting organism. The bacterial killing by fluoroquinolones and aminoglycosides is concentration dependent; the therapeutic efficacy is measured by the ratio of peak antimicrobial concentration to MIC, or the ratio of the area under the curve to MIC. The pharmacodynamic model in which the urine bactericidal titer replaces the MIC has been applied to predict optimal dosing regimens for antimicrobial treatment of urinary tract infection.[20,22] The validity of these models for urinary tract infection, however, still requires confirmation in clinical trials.[23,24] In particular, the relevance to treatment of complicated urinary tract infection is uncertain because impaired renal function and the presence of biofilms introduce variability that affects antimicrobial efficacy.[22]

Usual Presentations of Urinary Tract Infection

Acute Uncomplicated Urinary Tract Infection: Cystitis

Epidemiology

Acute uncomplicated urinary tract infection manifesting as acute cystitis is a common syndrome that affects otherwise healthy women.[1] About 10% of young, sexually active, premenopausal women experience a urinary tract infection each year, and 60% of all women have one or more such infections in their lifetime.[25] From 2% to 5% of women experience frequent recurrent infection for at least some period of time. After a first episode of cystitis, 21% of female college students reported a second infection within 6 months.[26] Among postmenopausal women aged 55 to 75 years who were enrolled in a Seattle health group, the incidence was 7 infections per 100 patient-years; in 24 months, 7% of women had one infection 1.6% had two infections, and 1% had three or more infections.[27] Acute cystitis is associated with considerable short-term morbidity in these women. Female college students reported that symptoms persisted for an average of 6.1 days.[1] In another survey of ambulatory women with cystitis, the mean duration of symptoms was reported to be 4.9 days, and for 63% of patients, their usual activities were compromised by the infection.[28] However, despite the large number of women affected, including many with frequent recurrence of infection, there is no long-term morbidity. Acute uncomplicated urinary tract infection is uncommon in healthy young men, with an estimated incidence of less than 0.1% per year.

Pathogenesis: Microbiology

Acute uncomplicated urinary tract infection is primarily a disease of extraintestinal pathogenic *E. coli*, also referred to as uropathogenic *E. coli*. These organisms are isolated in 80% to 85% of episodes of acute cystitis.[27,29] Infection occurs via the ascending route after bacterial strains that usually originate in the gut flora colonize the vagina or periurethral area.[7] Although urethral colonization with a potential uropathogen appears to be a prerequisite for infection, most women with periurethral colonization do not subsequently develop cystitis.[7] Strains of *E. coli* that colonize the periurethral area and subsequently cause urinary tract infection belong to a restricted number of phylogenetic *E. coli* groups and more frequently express diverse virulence factors than do periurethral strains that do not cause symptomatic infection.[30,31] A necessary characteristic for establishing bladder infection is production of the FimH, an adhesin attaching to receptors on uroepithelial cells.[32] This surface protein, however, is present on most *E. coli* strains, regardless of whether they cause infection. Other potential urovirulence characteristics include adhesins, iron sequestration systems, and toxins.[16] However, the putative virulence factors produced by strains isolated from symptomatic infection overlaps with those produced in asymptomatic infection, and no single characteristic is uniquely correlated with symptomatic infection.[33]

Uropathogenic *E. coli* strains are transmitted among household members and between sexual partners.[34,35] Clonal outbreaks may occur with transmission of a single strain within a community or larger geographic area.[36] *S. saprophyticus*, a coagulase-negative staphylococcal species, is an organism virtually unique to acute cystitis. It is the species second most frequently isolated (in 5% to 10% of episodes), and infections with it have a seasonal variation, whereby they occur most frequently in late summer or fall. Genetic elements described in the *S. saprophyticus* genome that may promote urovirulence include adhesins, transport systems to support growth in urine, and urease production.[37] Other Enterobacteriaceae, most commonly *K. pneumoniae*, are isolated in fewer than 5% of premenopausal women but in 10% to 15% of postmenopausal women.[27,38] Gram-positive organisms such as *Enterococcus* species and group B streptococci are uncommon pathogens in premenopausal women. *Salmonella* species and bacteria associated with sexually transmitted infections, such as *Ureaplasma urealyticum*, *Gardnerella vaginalis*, and *Mycoplasma hominis*, are occasionally isolated.[39]

Acute uncomplicated urinary tract infection recurs frequently and is characteristically reinfection. In as many as 30% of early reinfections, occurring within 1 month of treatment of an episode of acute cystitis, an *E. coli* strain similar to the pretherapy strain is isolated. This is assumed to be a consequence of failure of the antimicrobial therapy to eliminate organisms from the gut or vaginal flora reservoirs.[2] Intracellular persistence of *E. coli* in uroepithelial cells is an alternative mechanism proposed to explain same-strain recurrence, on the basis of observations in animal studies. However, prospective studies in women consistently document periurethral colonization before infection, and the existence of an intracellular reservoir for recurrent acute uncomplicated cystitis in humans has not yet been proved.[2]

Pathogenesis: Host Factors

Acute, uncomplicated urinary tract infection is a consequence of the interaction of a virulent organism with host genetic susceptibility and behavioral variables.[9,12] The notion of genetic propensity is supported by two consistent observations: (1) an increased frequency of urinary tract infection in first-degree female relatives of women with recurrent infection[1,40] and (2) the fact that infection at a younger age is a major risk factor for recurrent cystitis in women of any age.[27,41] One genetic characteristic that is well described is being a nonsecretor of the ABH blood-group antigens.[41,42] Women with recurrent urinary tract infection are at least three times more likely to be nonsecretors than are those without recurrent infection. Nonsecretors express cell-surface glycosphingolipids on the vaginal epithelium and, presumably, urethral mucosa that differ from those expressed by secretors and that bind uropathogenic *E. coli* more avidly.[12] Other potential genetic determinants include genetic polymorphisms of the IL-8 receptor CXCR1, Toll-like receptors, or the tumor necrosis factor promoter.[12]

The most important behavioral association of urinary tract infection in premenopausal women is sexual intercourse.[2] Of episodes of infection in young, sexually active women, 75% to 90% are attributable to intercourse, and there is a correlation between frequency of intercourse and infection.[42] Intercourse appears to promote infection by facilitating ascension of organisms from the periurethral area into the bladder, and the vaginal flora may also be altered. Spermicide use for birth control is another independent behavioral risk factor for acute cystitis in premenopausal women. The frequency of recurrent infection is at least twice as high among women who use spermicides as that among women who do not use these products.[42] Spermicides are bactericidal for the hydrogen peroxide–producing lactobacilli of the normal vaginal flora, which maintain the acidic pH. If these bacteria are not present, elevation of vaginal pH facilitates colonization with potential uropathogens, such as *E. coli*.

Case-control studies have consistently demonstrated that behavioral variables popularly identified as risks for cystitis—such as type of underwear, bathing rather than showering, postcoital voiding, frequency of voiding, perineal hygiene practices, vaginal douching, or tampon use—are not associated with an increased risk of infection.[43] A history of prior urinary tract infection at a younger age is the strongest association of recurrent acute cystitis in postmenopausal women.[44-46] Sexual intercourse is not an important contributor.[46,47] Estrogen deficiency has been proposed to promote recurrent urinary tract infection in these women through alterations in vaginal flora, including replacement of lactobacilli by potential uropathogens. However, prospective cohort studies and case-control studies uniformly demonstrate no association of oral or topical estrogen use with recurrent urinary tract infection, regardless of restoration of vaginal lactobacilli and acid pH.[48] Acute uncomplicated urinary tract infection in men is infrequent, but reported risk factors include intercourse with a female partner with recurrent urinary tract infection, not being circumcised, and anal intercourse.

Diagnosis

The classic clinical manifestation of symptomatic lower urinary tract infection is the acute onset of one or more irritative bladder symptoms such as urgency, frequency, dysuria, stranguria, or hesitancy. Gross hematuria is also common. The differential diagnosis includes sexually transmitted infections, vulvovaginal candidiasis, and noninfectious syndromes such as interstitial cystitis. The combination of new-onset frequency, dysuria, and urgency, together with the absence of vaginal discharge or pain, has a positive predictive value for acute cystitis of 90%.[49] Women who experience recurrent infection also have more than 90% accuracy in self-diagnosis on the basis of symptoms.[2]

A urine culture is not recommended routinely for women with a clinical presentation consistent with acute uncomplicated cystitis.[39,50] The utility of the urine culture is limited by the reliability of the clinical diagnosis, predictable microbiology, and prompt clinical response with short-course empirical antimicrobial therapy. Final culture results are not often available until therapy is completed, and quantitative counts of less than 10^5 CFU/mL are isolated in as many as 30% of women with acute cystitis. Therefore, interpretation of culture results may be problematic.[1,39,51] In fact, urine cultures are negative in 10% of women with a characteristic clinical presentation, and these women have a clinical response to antimicrobial therapy similar to that of women with positive cultures.[51] This high proportion of women who have low quantitative counts of organisms in the urine culture has been suggested to reflect urethritis, rather than cystitis. However, both urinary frequency and increased fluid intake are characteristic of patients with acute cystitis. Thus, the limited dwell time of urine in the bladder probably explains the observation of a high frequency of lower quantitative counts. Culture results may be negative because organisms are present in quantitative counts below the level of detection by standard laboratory procedures (usually $<10^3$ CFU/mL) or because fastidious organisms may not be identified by routine laboratory procedures recommended for processing of urine specimens.

A urine specimen for culture should be obtained, however, from some women with presumed acute uncomplicated urinary tract infection. If the clinical presentation is not characteristic, a urine culture may help confirm or exclude the diagnosis of urinary tract infection. Failure to respond to appropriate empirical antimicrobial therapy or an early (<1 month) symptomatic recurrence after therapy is suggestive of infection with a resistant organism. In these situations, a urine culture should be obtained to confirm whether antimicrobial resistance is present and to facilitate selection of an effective alternative regimen.

The presence of pyuria, identified by routine urinalysis or leukocyte esterase dipstick testing, is a consistent accompaniment of acute cystitis.[1,50] The absence of pyuria is suggestive of an alternative diagnosis but does not rule out urinary tract infection in women with a consistent clinical presentation.[1,52-54] Thus, routine screening for pyuria is not recommended in the management of women presenting with presumed acute cystitis.[1,48] A urine dipstick nitrite test screens for the presence of bacteria, rather than leukocytes, and results are usually positive in women with infection.[54] False-negative nitrite tests may yield negative results with infecting bacteria that do not reduce nitrate, such as *Enterococcus* species, or when urine has not been retained in the bladder a sufficient time to allow bacteria to convert nitrate to nitrite. Nitrite tests uncommonly yield false-positive results, but these may occur when blood, urobilinogen, or some dyes are present in the urine.

Treatment

For many women, the natural history of acute uncomplicated cystitis is spontaneous clinical and microbiologic resolution within a few days or weeks. In a clinical trial in which subjects were randomly assigned to receive antibiotic therapy or placebo, 28% of 277 women who received placebo were asymptomatic by 1 week, and 45% had negative culture results by 6 weeks.[55] In another study, 54% of women who received placebo were asymptomatic by 3 days and 52% at 7 days.[40] However, antimicrobial treatment is associated with a significantly shorter duration of symptoms. The rates of clinical cure were 77% with nitrofurantoin, in comparison with 54% with placebo at 3 days, and 88% and 52%, respectively, at 7 days.[40] After initiation of antimicrobial therapy, 54% of women reported symptom improvement by 6 hours, 87% by 24 hours, and 91% by 48 hours.[55] In another case series, 72% of women reported complete symptom resolution by the fourth day of effective treatment.[28]

Many antimicrobial agents are effective for treatment of acute cystitis (Table 36-5). The anticipated cure rates for recommended first-line empirical regimens is 80% to 95%.[56] Trimethoprim/sulfamethoxazole (TMP/SMX) has been a mainstay of empirical treatment of acute cystitis for decades and remains highly effective against susceptible organisms.[56,57] However, increasing rates of TMP/SMX resistance in community outbreaks of *E. coli* now compromise the use of this agent as first-line empirical therapy. Some antimicrobial agents—nitrofurantoin, pivmecillinam, and fosfomycin—have indications largely restricted to acute cystitis. These drugs do not induce cross-resistance with other classes of antimicrobial agents, and, to date, limited resistance has been observed in community uropathogens. Thus, they are ecologically attractive for treatment of acute cystitis. Fosfomycin and pivmecillinam, however, are not available in all countries, and results of clinical trials suggest that these agents may be 5% to 10% less effective than TMP/SMX or fluoroquinolones. The fluoroquinolones—norfloxacin, ciprofloxacin, and levofloxacin—are not generally recommended as first-line therapy because of concerns that widespread use will lead to the emergence of resistance. Fluoroquinolones with limited urinary excretion, such as moxifloxacin, should not be used for treatment of urinary tract infection.

β-Lactam antimicrobial agents, including amoxicillin, amoxicillin-clavulanic acid, and cephalosporins, are reported to be 10% to 15% less effective than first-line agents. These antimicrobial agents are useful, however, in treatment for pregnant women because they are safe for the fetus.[39] To limit adverse effects, cost, and emergence of bacterial resistance, the shortest effective duration of antimicrobial therapy should be prescribed. For TMP/SMX and the fluoroquinolones, 3 days is optimum.[56] The duration of nitrofurantoin therapy is 5 days.[58] For β-lactam antimicrobial

agents, 7 days is recommended; shorter courses are consistently less effective. Fosfomycin is given as a single dose; multiple doses of this antimicrobial are associated with rapid emergence of resistance. Single-dose therapy is not recommended for other agents because a single dose is generally 5% to 10% less effective than the recommended longer regimens.[39]

The antimicrobial susceptibility of uropathogenic *E. coli* strains acquired in the community evolves continually in response to antimicrobial pressure.[29,59] Resistance in community isolates has compromised the efficacy of ampicillin, cephalosporins, and TMP/SMX for use as empirical therapy, and increasing resistance to fluoroquinolones has been reported.[29] Recent prior antimicrobial therapy is most strongly associated with isolation of a resistant organism.[60] Treatment of cystitis with an antimicrobial agent to which the infecting organism is resistant is associated with a high failure rate, despite very high urinary levels of the drug.[61,62] In fact, cure rates when the organism is resistant to the antimicrobial agent are similar to those reported with placebo: about 50%. If the local prevalence of resistance to an antimicrobial agent in community *E. coli* strains exceeds 20%, that agent should not be used for first-line empirical therapy.[56] The current expansion of extended-spectrum β-lactamase (ESBL)–producing *E. coli* in community-acquired infections is of particular concern

TABLE 36-5 Preferred Antimicrobial Regimens for Treatment or Prevention of Acute Uncomplicated Urinary Cystitis in Women with Normal Renal Function

FIRST-LINE THERAPY	OTHER THERAPY
Acute Cystitis	
TMP/SMX, 160/800 mg bid × 3 days Nitrofurantoin, 50-100 mg qid, or monohydrate/macrocrystals, 100 mg bid × 5 days* Pivmecillinam, 400 mg bid × 5 days or 200 mg bid × 7 days* Fosfomycin trometanol, 3-g single dose*	Norfloxacin, 400 mg bid × 3 days Ciprofloxacin, 250 mg bid, or extended-release preparation, 500 mg od × 3 days Levofloxacin, 250-500 mg od × 3 days Trimethoprim, 100 mg bid × 3 days Amoxicillin 500 mg tid × 7 days* Amoxicillin/clavulanic acid, 500 mg tid or 875 mg bid × 7 days* Cephalexin, 250-500 mg qid × 7 days* Cefpodoxime proxetil, 100 mg bid × 3 days Cefuroxime axetil, 500 mg bid × 7 days* Cefixime, 400 mg od × 7 days* Doxycycline, 100 mg bid × 7 days
Prophylaxis	
Long-term low-dose regimens (at bedtime)	
Nitrofurantoin, 50 mg od, or monohydrate/macrocrystals, 100 mg od TMP/SMX, 40/200 mg od or every other day	Cephalexin, 500 mg od* Norfloxacin, 200 mg every other day Ciprofloxacin, 125 mg od Trimethoprim, 100 mg od
Postcoital (single-dose) regimen	
TMP/SMX, 40/200 mg or 80/400 mg Trimethoprim, 100 mg Nitrofurantoin, 50 or 100 mg*	Cephalexin, 250 mg* Norfloxacin, 200 mg Ciprofloxacin, 125 mg

*Recommended for pregnant women.
TMP/SMX, Trimethoprim/sulfamethoxazole.

because these strains are usually also resistant to TMP/SMX and fluoroquinolones.[63] Optimal treatment of infection with ESBL-producing *E. coli* is not yet well defined. Nitrofurantoin, fosfomycin trometamol, and pivmecillinam currently remain effective for many of these strains. Amoxicillin/clavulanic acid may also be effective, but clinical experience is limited.[64]

Other Investigations

Young women with a characteristic clinical presentation and prompt response to appropriate empirical therapy do not require further diagnostic imaging or urologic investigation.[65] Fewer than 5% of these women have urologic abnormalities, and the few women with abnormalities identified usually do not require further intervention. However, investigation may be appropriate to rule out alternative pathologic processes when the diagnosis is uncertain or to identify an underlying abnormality consistent with complicated urinary tract infection if the infecting organism is susceptible but responds inadequately to antimicrobial therapy.[66]

Recurrent Infection

Episodes of acute cystitis recur frequently in many women. Effective control can be achieved with low-dose prophylactic antimicrobial therapy given either daily or every other day at bedtime or after intercourse (see Table 36-5). This strategy is recommended for women who experience more than two episodes in 6 months. The initial course of prophylaxis lasts 6 or 12 months. Antimicrobial prophylactic therapy decreases recurrent symptomatic episodes by about 95% while the agent is being taken, but it does not alter the frequency of recurrent infection once prophylaxis is discontinued. About 50% of women experience reinfection within 3 months of discontinuing prophylaxis. Reinstitution of prophylaxis for as long as 2 years is appropriate for these women. Self-treatment is another effective strategy for managing recurrent infections, and this approach is often preferred by women who are traveling or who experience less frequent recurrences.[2] A 3-day course of TMP/SMX or ciprofloxacin has been shown to be effective for empirical self-treatment in clinical trials, but other regimens are also probably effective.

The only feasible behavioral intervention to prevent recurrent urinary tract infection is to avoid spermicide use. Other proposed nonantimicrobial approaches for prevention include daily intake of cranberry products, oral or vaginal probiotics to reestablish normal vaginal flora, estrogen replacement for postmenopausal women, and vaccines.[67] Daily intake of cranberry juice or tablets decreases episodes of recurrent cystitis by 30% in comparison with placebo.[68] The proposed mechanism is inhibition of the P fimbria–mediated adherence of *E. coli* to uroepithelial cells by the proanthocyanidins present in cranberry products and excreted in the urine. In clinical trials, oral or vaginal probiotics have not demonstrated convincing efficacy in preventing urinary tract infection, despite substantial popular interest in this approach.[69] The role of estrogen replacement to prevent urinary tract infection in postmenopausal women is controversial.[2] In prospective clinical trials of systemic estrogen therapy, researchers have uniformly reported no benefit of estrogen over placebo, despite restoration of an acidic vaginal pH and increased vaginal colonization

with lactobacilli in subjects who received estrogen.[48] Two small clinical trials of vaginal estrogen with placebo in postmenopausal women with frequent, recurrent infection demonstrated a decreased frequency of symptomatic episodes in women treated with topical estrogen therapy, but a comparative trial of an estrogen-containing pessary and nitrofurantoin prophylaxis revealed that the pessary was substantially less effective than the antimicrobial agent.[48,70] Currently, topical vaginal estrogen cannot be recommended solely for prevention of urinary tract infection.

Results both of animal studies and of some clinical trials in humans have suggested potential efficacy of vaccination in preventing recurrent cystitis or pyelonephritis.[71] However, the benefits reported, if any, are minimal, and the results of clinical trials in humans are conflicting. Vaccination would be expected to have limited efficacy because of the wide antigenic variation among uropathogenic *E. coli* strains and the limited serologic response observed in patients experiencing cystitis.

Acute Nonobstructive Pyelonephritis

Epidemiology

Pyelonephritis is a less common manifestation of acute uncomplicated urinary tract infection than is cystitis. The ratio of pyelonephritis to cystitis episodes is reported to be 18:1 and 29:1 in women with recurrent infection.[2] The highest incidence is among young women aged 20 to 30 years. Pyelonephritis is associated with substantially greater morbidity; hospitalization is required for as many as 20% of affected nonpregnant women.[72] Severe manifestations such as sepsis syndrome, are, however, uncommon. Acute pyelonephritis complicates 1% to 2% of pregnancies, often occurring at the end of the second trimester or early in the third trimester. Preterm labor and delivery may occur and lead to poor fetal outcomes, as with any febrile illness in later pregnancy.[73]

Acute nonobstructive pyelonephritis is rarely a direct cause of renal failure. In the few reports of renal failure attributed to pyelonephritis, patients were elderly[74] or had comorbid conditions such as diabetes or HIV infection.[75] Renal scarring is a complication of pyelonephritis in some women with more severe clinical manifestations. An Italian study reported renal scars identified by computed tomography (CT) or magnetic resonance imaging (MRI) at a 6-month follow-up in 29% of women who required hospitalization for pyelonephritis.[76] In an Israeli study, 30% of a cohort of 203 women admitted for acute pyelonephritis were reassessed 10 to 20 years after admission; renal scars were detected in 46% of these women on technetium 99m–labeled dimercaptosuccinic acid scanning. However, the renal scars were not associated with hypertension or renal impairment.[77] The histologic finding of "chronic pyelonephritis" in patients with renal failure was formerly attributed to infection. However, this is now recognized as an end stage of many chronic inflammatory conditions of the kidney, and it is attributable to infection in only a few patients in whom there is a clear history of renal infection.

Pathogenesis

E. coli is isolated in 85% to 90% of women who present with acute uncomplicated pyelonephritis.[78] Infecting strains are characterized by production of the P fimbria adhesin

Gal (α1-4) Galβ disaccharide galabiose. This surface protein appears to have a direct role in the pathogenesis of pyelonephritis through induction of mucosal inflammation.[31,33] A familial susceptibility to pyelonephritis has been reported and attributed to polymorphisms with decreased expression of CXCR1, an IL-8 receptor.[79] Other genetic and behavioral risk factors for pyelonephritis in healthy women are similar to those described for acute uncomplicated cystitis.[78] For premenopausal women, these associations are frequency of sexual intercourse, history of urinary tract infection, history of urinary tract infection in the patient's mother, a new sexual partner, and recent spermicide use. The strongest association is with recent sexual intercourse. Diabetes is also an independent risk factor for pyelonephritis. Young diabetic women are 15 times more likely to be hospitalized for pyelonephritis than age-matched nondiabetic women. Behavioral risk factors associated with pyelonephritis in postmenopausal women have not yet been described.

Diagnosis

The classic clinical manifestation of renal infection is costovertebral angle pain or tenderness, accompanied by variable fever and lower tract symptoms. There is a wide spectrum of severity, however, from mild irritative symptoms with minimal costovertebral angle tenderness to severe symptoms that may include high fever, nausea and vomiting, and severe pain. Acute cholecystitis, renal colic, or pelvic inflammatory disease is occasionally confused with pyelonephritis. When patients present with severe symptoms, underlying complicating factors such as obstruction or abscess must be excluded. A urine specimen for culture should be obtained before initiation of antimicrobial therapy in every case of suspected pyelonephritis. The culture will confirm the diagnosis of urinary tract infection and identify the specific infecting organism and susceptibilities so that antimicrobial therapy can be optimized. In more than 95% of women with pyelonephritis, 10^5 CFU/mL of organisms or more are isolated from the urine culture.

Bacteremia is identified in 10% to 25% of women presenting with acute pyelonephritis if blood cultures are collected routinely. However, the clinical utility of routine blood cultures is limited because bacteremia does not alter therapy, nor is it predictive of outcome.[80,81] Thus blood cultures should be obtained selectively, usually only if the diagnosis is uncertain or the clinical presentation is severe. Growth of the same organism from both blood and urine usually confirms a urinary source for the infection. However, bacteria isolated from the urine are occasionally attributable to bacteremia from a source outside the urinary tract. This may be a result of hematogenous seeding with development of renal microabscesses, which is well described for *Staphylococcus aureus* in particular. The proportion of cases in which *S. aureus* bacteriuria has a nonurinary source, however, is controversial.[81,82]

Additional investigations recommended for most patients presenting with acute pyelonephritis are measurements of peripheral leukocyte count and serum creatinine. The leukocyte count is usually elevated and may be useful as a parameter to monitor the response to therapy. C-reactive protein and procalcitonin levels are elevated in most women with acute pyelonephritis.[2,83,84] An elevated level of C-reactive protein at discharge has been associated with prolonged hospitalization and subsequent recurrence.[84] The serum procalcitonin level at presentation, however, is not predictive of outcome.[83]

Diagnostic Imaging

When the clinical presentation of pyelonephritis is mild or moderate and the clinical response after initiation of antimicrobial therapy is prompt, routine diagnostic imaging is not indicated.[39,66] Women whose clinical presentations are severe, who fail treatment, or who experience early posttreatment recurrent infection, should undergo prompt imaging to rule out obstruction or abscesses and to determine whether intervention is necessary. Ultrasonography is often the initial imaging modality because it is safe and widely accessible.[85] The ultrasound examination in women with uncomplicated pyelonephritis usually yields normal results, but enlargement and edema in one or both kidneys is observed in 20% of patients.[86] Ultrasonography is less sensitive or specific for pyelonephritis than is either CT or MRI.[86] Abnormalities observed on CT are characterized as unilateral or bilateral, focal or diffuse, focal swelling or no focal swelling, and renal enlargement or no renal enlargement.[85] In addition to renal enlargement and edema, dilation of the collecting system in the absence of obstruction, wedge-shaped areas of decreased attenuation, and rounded low-attenuation masses with delayed enhancement may be observed.

Obstruction of the renal tubules by inflammatory debris or impaired function with tubular ischemia may result in a "striated nephrogram."[85] Abnormalities within the renal cortex and medulla, inflammatory changes in Gerota's fascia or the renal sinuses, and thickening of the urothelium are sometimes observed. Acute focal pyelonephritis (or acute lobar nephronia) is infection confined to a single lobe and may be more common in women with diabetes or who are immunocompromised. The response to treatment is similar, however, for patients with or without this imaging finding.[86] The presence of a focal lesion characterized by peripheral ring enhancement without uptake of contrast material centrally on CT or MRI at presentation was the only imaging finding that was correlated with subsequent development of renal scars.[76]

Treatment

The majority of women with uncomplicated pyelonephritis can receive treatment as outpatients.[39] Indications for hospitalization include pregnancy, hemodynamic instability, uncertain gastrointestinal absorption or compliance with oral therapy, the need to exclude complicating factors such as obstruction or abscess, or the necessity of monitoring or treatment of associated medical illnesses. Appropriate supportive management for hypotension, nausea and vomiting, and pain control should be initiated promptly. When oral tolerance is uncertain because of nausea and vomiting, a strategy frequently used in emergency room management is to provide a single parenteral dose of ceftriaxone, 1 g, or of gentamicin, 120 mg, followed by oral therapy once gastrointestinal symptoms are controlled.

Many parenteral antimicrobial regimens are effective for pyelonephritis (Table 36-6). *E. coli* strains generally remain susceptible to aminoglycosides, and these agents are useful for empirical treatment. Aminoglycosides also have unique efficacy for the treatment of renal infection in that they are bound

TABLE 36-6 Antimicrobial Regimens for Treatment of Acute Uncomplicated Pyelonephritis in Women with Normal Renal Function and Susceptible Organisms

FIRST-LINE THERAPY	OTHER THERAPY
Oral	
Ciprofloxacin, 500 mg bid or 1000 mg extended-release preparation, od × 7 days Levofloxacin, 750 od × 5 days	TMP/SMX, 160/800 mg bid × 7-14 days Amoxicillin, 500 mg PO tid × 14 days* Amoxicillin/clavulanic acid, 500 mg tid or 875 mg PO bid × 14 days* Cephalexin, 500 mg qid × 14 days* Cefuroxime axetil, 500 mg bid × 14 days* Cefixime, 400 mg od × 14 days*
Parenteral†	
Ciprofloxacin, 400 mg q12h × 7 days Levofloxacin, 750 mg od × 5 days Gentamicin or tobramycin, 3-5 mg/kg od, ± ampicillin, 1 g q4-6hr Ceftriaxone, 1-2 g od* Cefotaxime, 1 g q8hr*	Ertapenem, 1 g od Meropenem, 500 mg q6h Piperacillin/tazobactam, 3.375 g q6hr

*Recommended for pregnant women.
†Change to oral therapy to complete course once condition is clinically stable.
TMP/SMX, Trimethoprim/sulfamethoxazole.

in high concentrations in the renal cortex.[18] Extended-spectrum cephalosporins, such as cefotaxime or ceftriaxone, and fluoroquinolones, such as ciprofloxacin and levofloxacin, are other options for parenteral therapy.[2] Ceftriaxone is the preferred empirical regimen for pregnant women. Although it is suggested that gentamicin be avoided in pregnancy because of potential fetal ototoxicity, excess otologic impairment has not been reported in large cohorts of newborn infants stratified by gentamicin exposure in utero.[87] Thus, when cephalosporins cannot be used because of antimicrobial resistance or patient intolerance, gentamicin remains an alternate antimicrobial for treatment of pregnant women.

A satisfactory clinical response is usually observed by 48 to 72 hours after initiation of antimicrobial therapy. Oral therapy selected on the basis of urine culture results can then be prescribed to complete the antimicrobial course. In most young, nonpregnant women, acute pyelonephritis is effectively managed with outpatient oral therapy (see Table 36-6).[39,56] The recommended empirical antimicrobial regimen is either ciprofloxacin or levofloxacin.[39] Oral TMP/SMX is effective, but because of the high prevalence of TMP/SMX resistant *E. coli* in many communities, it is recommended only when the infecting organism is known to be susceptible. Other oral regimens are also effective and may be appropriate, depending on organism susceptibility and the patient's tolerance. The usual duration of treatment is 10 to 14 days, but ciprofloxacin, 500 mg twice daily given for 7 days, is effective,[88] and levofloxacin 750 mg daily for 5 days.[89]

Women who receive effective antimicrobial therapy by 48 to 72 hours and have no underlying abnormalities are usually afebrile, with substantial improvement or resolution of other symptoms. Risk factors predictive of a poor outcome are hospitalization, isolation of a resistant organism, concurrent diabetes mellitus, and history of renal stones.[90] All these variables

are suggestive of greater severity of illness at presentation or of a complicated infection.[90] Prophylactic antimicrobial strategies similar to those for recurrent cystitis are effective for prevention of recurrent uncomplicated pyelonephritis.

Complicated Urinary Tract Infection

Epidemiology

The frequency of complicated urinary tract infection varies, depending on the underlying genitourinary abnormality (see Table 36-1).[3-5] Some individuals with a transient abnormality, such as pyelonephritis that complicates passage of a ureteric stone, may experience only a single infection. Other patients, including those with indwelling devices or persistent obstruction, may experience frequent recurrent infections. For instance, in men with spinal cord injury in whom voiding is managed with an indwelling catheter, the incidence is 2.72 infections/1000 days; when voiding is by intermittent catheterization, the incidence is 0.41/1000 days. In residents of long-term care facilities with chronic indwelling urethral catheters, the incidence of symptomatic infection is 3.2/1000 catheter days.[91,92]

Complicated urinary tract infection is a frequent cause of hospitalization. The urinary tract is the most common source of community-acquired bacteremia,[93,94] and most bacteremic episodes of urinary tract infection are attributable to complicated infection.[95] Patients with obstruction, with an indwelling catheter, or who have undergone recent manipulation of the urinary tract with mucosal bleeding are at greatest risk of bacteremia and severe sepsis. The genitourinary tract is the source of infection in 10% of patients admitted to critical care units with septic shock.[96]

These patients are also at risk for local suppurative complications, such as renal or perinephric abscesses, or metastatic infection after bacteremia, such as septic arthritis, osteomyelitis, or endocarditis. Serious complications are more frequent in patients who are diabetic, are immunocompromised, or have chronic urologic devices or obstruction. Renal functional impairment in patients with complicated urinary tract infection is usually attributable to the underlying abnormality or to organ failure complicating septic shock, rather than being a direct consequence of infection. For instance, introduction of voiding strategies to maintain low bladder pressure and to prevent reflux have almost eliminated the complication of chronic renal failure in persons with spinal cord injury, despite a continued high incidence of urinary tract infection in these patients.[97]

Pathogenesis: Microbiology

Host impairment rather than organism virulence is the major determinant of infection. *E. coli* remains the organism most frequently isolated in complicated urinary tract infection.[3,5] The *E. coli* strains are characterized by a low frequency of expression of virulence factors in comparison with strains isolated in acute uncomplicated infection.[33] Many other bacteria and yeast species are also isolated.[5,98,99] Enterobacteriaceae such as *Klebsiella* species, *Enterobacter* species, *Serratia* species, *Citrobacter* species, *Proteus mirabilis, Morganella morganii,* and *Providencia stuartii* are common. Other gram-negative organisms that may be isolated include *Pseudomonas aeruginosa,*

Stenotrophomonas maltophilia or *Acinetobacter* species. Gram-positive organisms are also frequently isolated, including group B streptococci, *Enterococcus* species, and coagulase-negative staphylococci. *S. aureus* is less commonly isolated. *Candida* species may be isolated, usually from patients with diabetes, with indwelling urologic devices, or receiving broad-spectrum antimicrobial therapy.[100]

Organisms isolated from patients with complicated urinary tract infection often have increased antimicrobial resistance.[101] Risk factors for isolation of a resistant organism include a history of recent antimicrobial therapy or of health care interventions, including an indwelling urethral catheter or an invasive urologic procedure. Uncommon bacteria are occasionally a cause of infection. Some of these organisms may not be identified with standard laboratory procedures for processing urine specimens. *Corynebacterium urealyticum* is a urease-producing gram-positive rod associated with the unique clinical manifestations of encrusted cystitis or pyelonephritis.[102] These chronic inflammatory conditions are characterized by ulcerative inflammation and struvite encrustations on the bladder or renal pelvis wall. Pyelitis, if untreated, may lead to destruction of the kidney. *U. urealyticum* is another urease-producing bacterium that may cause cystitis or pyelonephritis, often with urolithiasis. Healthy persons may become infected, but case reports suggest a predisposition in immunocompromised individuals, particularly those with hypogammaglobulinemia. *Aerococcus sanguinicola* is a rare cause of complicated urinary tract infection; the diagnosis is usually made by isolation of the organism in the blood culture.[103] *Aerococcus urinae* was isolated in 0.3% to 0.8% of urine specimens in one clinical microbiology laboratory, usually from older persons with underlying abnormalities and bacteremia.[104] Anaerobic organisms are seldom identified in the absence of suppurative complications such as abscesses.[105]

Pathogenesis: Host Factors

Genitourinary abnormalities facilitate infection through increased entry of organisms into the bladder (e.g., by intermittent catheterization, urologic procedures) and subsequent persistence because of incomplete voiding (e.g., as a result of obstruction, urolithiasis, diverticula, reflux).[3,4] Asymptomatic bacteriuria is the usual outcome in patients with persistent abnormalities.[106] The determinants that lead to symptomatic infection in chronically bacteriuric individuals are not well characterized. However, obstruction or mucosal trauma with bleeding are well-recognized risk factors for bacteremia and sepsis in patients with preexisting bacteriuria.

Clinical Presentations

Complicated urinary tract infection manifests across a wide clinical spectrum of signs and symptoms from mild, irritative symptoms of lower tract infection to pyelonephritis and bacteremia, including septic shock.[3-5] Localizing signs and symptoms consistent with cystitis or pyelonephritis are usually present. Patients with indwelling urethral catheters or other indwelling devices usually present with fever alone, although costovertebral angle pain or tenderness, hematuria, or catheter obstruction, if present, identify a genitourinary source. Patients with chronic neurologic impairment sometimes report symptoms that are not classical for urinary tract

infection. For instance, spinal cord–injured patients experience increased bladder and leg spasms or autonomic dysreflexia, whereas patients with multiple sclerosis may present with fatigue or deterioration in neurologic function.[5]

The clinical diagnosis of symptomatic infection is often problematic in older populations with cognitive impairment.[107] These patients frequently have chronic genitourinary symptoms and impaired communication, which limits the assessment of signs and symptoms. Because bacteriuria is very common in elderly individuals with functional impairment, nonlocalizing clinical deterioration is frequently attributed to urinary tract infection because the urine culture yields positive results.[108] However, nonlocalizing clinical manifestations, including fever, are unlikely to have a urinary source in persons without a chronic indwelling catheter.[18,108] Changes in character of the urine, such as cloudiness or odor, are also frequently interpreted as symptoms of urinary tract infection. Cloudiness may be attributed to pyuria, which usually accompanies bacteriuria, and an unpleasant odor is suggestive of production of polyamines by bacteria in the urine. However, alterations in characteristics of the urine are neither sensitive nor specific for the diagnosis of infection. They may be attributable to other causes such as precipitation of crystals or dehydration. Thus changes in character of the urine should not be interpreted as symptomatic urinary tract infection.

Laboratory Diagnosis

A urine specimen for culture should be obtained before initiation of antimicrobial therapy for every patient with suspected complicated urinary tract infection. Because of the wide variety of potential infecting organisms and increased likelihood of resistant strains, definitive microbiologic characterization is necessary to optimize antimicrobial management.

Interpretation of the urine culture is challenging in some patients with complicated infection. For patients with a chronic indwelling catheter, the catheter should be replaced, and the new catheter should be used to sample bladder urine and avoid contamination by organisms present in the biofilm.[18,19] When intestine is interposed into the urinary tract through creation of an ileal conduit, continent cutaneous diversion, or neobladder, urine collected through the conduit or reservoir is often bacteriuric, regardless of symptoms.[109] The organisms isolated represent mixed gram-positive flora, including streptococcal species and *Staphylococcus epidermidis*, but uropathogenic strains such as *E. coli, P. mirabilis, P. aeruginosa,* and *Enterococcus faecalis* may also be present. Similar urine culture findings are reported in 3% to 30% of patients with orthoptic bladder substitution or augmentation cystoplasty; individuals with these reservoirs who practice clean intermittent catheterization are more likely to have positive culture findings.[109] Thus, when symptomatic urinary tract infection is suspected, a urine culture obtained from these patients must be interpreted in the context of this usual bacteriuria.

Infection with a fastidious organism should be considered when the clinical manifestation is suggestive of symptomatic urinary tract infection but urine culture results are repeatedly negative, particularly when pyuria is present. These organisms may include *C. urealyticum, U. urealyticum,* or *Haemophilus* species. A persistently alkaline pH is indicative of a urease-producing organism such as *C. urealyticum* or *U. urealyticum*. The laboratory should be consulted if a fastidious organism is considered, and appropriate specimens should be collected for additional laboratory evaluation to maximize the likelihood of isolating potential infecting organisms.

Patients with genitourinary abnormalities frequently have pyuria, regardless of bacteriuria or symptomatic infection, and so pyuria by itself is not diagnostic for urinary tract infection.[5] The absence of pyuria, however, has a high negative predictive value for ruling out urinary tract infection in some populations, such as elderly patients.[18] The severity of clinical manifestations help determine whether additional investigations such as blood cultures or a peripheral leukocyte count are indicated. Renal function should be assessed in every patient with complicated urinary tract infection. A repeated urine culture after antimicrobial therapy is not recommended if the patient remains asymptomatic.

Antimicrobial Treatment

The principles of management for individuals with complicated urinary tract infection include prompt specimen collection to identify the specific infecting organism; characterization of renal function and underlying abnormalities; and early institution of appropriate antimicrobial therapy. The antimicrobial regimen selected is individualized on the basis of site of infection, severity of manifestations, known or presumed infecting organism and susceptibility, and the patient's tolerance.[3] When the presenting symptoms are mild, it is preferable to delay initiation of antimicrobial therapy until results of the urine culture are available. This allows selection of a narrow-spectrum agent specific for the infecting organism and minimizes antimicrobial pressure, which promotes resistance.

When patients present with severe symptoms, empirical antimicrobial therapy is initiated pending urine culture results. Previous urine culture results, if available, and recent antimicrobial therapy received by the patient should be considered when the empirical regimen is selected.[5] Parenteral therapy is indicated for patients who present with hemodynamic instability, who cannot tolerate or absorb oral medications, or who are known or suspected to have an infecting organism resistant to available oral options. Patients with presentations of sepsis, including septic shock, should receive initial empirical antimicrobial therapy that provides broad coverage for both gram-positive and gram-negative bacteria, including resistant organisms. Appropriate regimens for these patients may include an aminoglycoside, with or without ampicillin; piperacillin/tazobactam; piperacillin with an aminoglycoside; carbapenems (ertapenem, imipenem, meropenem); or extended-spectrum cephalosporins.

Fluoroquinolones with good urinary excretion and broad gram-negative coverage—norfloxacin, ciprofloxacin, and levofloxacin—are often used as empirical oral therapy.[5] Many other oral agents are effective and may be appropriate, depending on patient tolerance and the specific infecting organism.[5] These include TMP/SMX, amoxicillin, amoxicillin/clavulanic acid, oral cephalosporins, and doxycycline. Nitrofurantoin is effective for treatment of some episodes of bladder infection, but it is not effective for renal or prostate infection. It is contraindicated in treatment for patients with renal failure because peripheral neuropathy has been reported to occur with accumulation of toxic metabolites. *K. pneumoniae*, *P. aeruginosa*, or *P. mirabilis* strains are uniformly resistant. Nitrofurantoin remains effective, however, for some resistant organisms such as vancomycin-resistant *Enterococcus* and extended-spectrum β-lactamase–producing *E. coli*. Substantial clinical improvement is expected by 48 to 72 hours after initiation of effective antimicrobial therapy. Empirical therapy is reassessed at this time, considering the clinical response and urine culture results. Therapy is usually modified to an appropriate narrow-spectrum parenteral or oral agent to complete a 7- to 14 day course. If an organism isolated in the pretherapy urine culture is resistant to the empirical antimicrobial, therapy should be altered to include an antimicrobial agent to which the infecting organism is susceptible, even if clinical improvement has occurred.

Other Interventions

To manage complicated urinary tract infection optimally, the underlying genitourinary abnormality must be characterized and appropriate urologic or other interventions undertaken to manage the current infection and prevent subsequent infections. Urgent diagnostic imaging or urologic investigation is indicated for patients who have severe systemic symptoms or who do not respond to appropriate antimicrobial therapy. The goal of early imaging is to identify obstruction or abscesses, for which immediate drainage may be necessary for source control. When the underlying abnormality is already well characterized—as in the case of a patient with an indwelling catheter or a neurogenic bladder managed with intermittent catheterization—further investigations may still be appropriate if the patient has experienced a recent change in frequency or severity of infections. Such a patient remains at risk for development of urolithiasis, tumors, or suppurative complications.

The approach to diagnostic imaging and urologic investigation is determined by the clinical presentation and the patient's previous history. A plain radiograph of the abdomen may identify emphysematous infections and some stones. CT is the imaging modality of choice. It identifies calculi, gas, hemorrhage, calcification, obstruction, renal enlargement, and inflammatory masses. Contrast media–enhanced scans are recommended, with helical and multislice CT to study different phases of contrast excretion.[66,85,86] Ultrasound examination is less sensitive and specific than other imaging modalities such as spiral CT and MRI, but it may be more accessible.[86]

Appropriate supportive care must be initiated promptly. The removal and replacement of a chronic indwelling catheter before institution of antimicrobial therapy is associated with a more rapid defervescence and a lower risk of early relapse after therapy, as well as facilitating collection of a more valid urine culture.[30] The clinical benefits of catheter replacement are presumed to result from removal of the high concentration of organisms in the biofilm, which are often not eradicated by antimicrobial therapy and remain a source for relapse. Urologic investigations such as cystoscopy, retrograde pyelography, or urodynamic studies should be obtained as appropriate. If encrusted *C. urealyticum* infection is present, surgical resection of the encrustations is required, together with antimicrobial therapy. *C. urealyticum* strains are generally susceptible to vancomycin, tetracyclines, and fluoroquinolones.[102]

Management of Recurrent Infection

When symptoms recur early after antimicrobial treatment, the susceptibility of the pretherapy infecting organism should be reviewed to confirm that the antimicrobial agent prescribed is effective. If the organism is susceptible, underlying genitourinary abnormalities should be reviewed and further evaluation obtained, if appropriate, to identify abnormalities such as abscesses that may necessitate drainage. Even if the abnormalities cannot be fully corrected, interventions to improve urine drainage may decrease the frequency of episodes of symptomatic infection.[3,5] Indwelling devices should be removed whenever possible. Evidence-based infection control guidelines provide recommendations for prevention of catheter-acquired urinary tract infection.[110-112] Specific practices include appropriate catheter use, limiting duration of use, appropriate practices for catheter insertion and care, and selection of catheter size. Interventions shown not to be effective and that are not recommended include use of different catheter materials, antimicrobial coating of catheters, antiseptic or antimicrobial meatal care, or instillation of antiseptics into the drainage bag. Patients with chronic indwelling catheters and other indwelling devices experience infection because of biofilm formation on these devices; therefore, prevention of catheter-acquired infection ultimately requires development of biofilm-resistant biomaterials.

Prophylactic antimicrobial therapy is not recommended. When patients with impaired voiding or indwelling devices are given prophylactic antimicrobial agents, there is little, if any, decrease in symptomatic infection, but rapid reinfection with resistant organisms is uniformly observed.[5] For selected patients with a persistent abnormality and relapsing infection that cannot be eradicated, suppressive therapy may be considered. The goal of suppressive therapy is not to prevent reinfection but to control symptomatic episodes or prevent stone enlargement when inoperable infection stones are present. The antimicrobial regimen is selected on the basis of the infecting organism, and is prescribed initially at a full therapeutic dose. If the patient remains clinically stable and the urine is sterile, this dose is usually decreased to about half after 4 to 6 weeks. Suppressive therapy is not appropriate for patients with indwelling devices because biofilm formation facilitates rapid reinfection and emergence of resistant organisms. However, short-term use (several weeks or months) for patients with complex urologic abnormalities and indwelling devices may occasionally be considered as part of a palliative care strategy.

A novel approach currently being evaluated for control of recurrent infection in patients with impaired bladder emptying is "bacterial interference."[113] This strategy establishes asymptomatic bacteriuria with a nonpathogenic *E. coli* strain in patients with impaired voiding. The avirulent strain in the bladder then prevents infection by other, potentially more virulent strains. The proposed mechanisms for this protective effect include blocking of bacterial receptors present on uroepithelial cells, competition for nutrients in the urine, or toxin production. Preliminary clinical trials have revealed some efficacy of this approach in a small number of carefully selected patients.[114]

Asymptomatic Bacteriuria

Epidemiology

Asymptomatic bacteriuria is a common finding, particularly in women, older persons, and some patients with persistent genitourinary abnormalities (Table 36-7).[106] The prevalence of bacteriuria among sexually active young women ranges from 3% to 5% but is less than 1% among age-matched controls who are not sexually active. Bacteriuria is present in 5% to 10% of healthy postmenopausal women[106] and in 20% of women older than 80 years living in the community.[115] Asymptomatic bacteriuria is uncommon in younger men, but its prevalence increases in men older than 65 years, presumably concurrently with age-related prostate hypertrophy. Bacteriuria occurs in 10% of healthy men older than 80 years living in the community.[115] Among residents of nursing homes who do not have indwelling catheters, 20% to 50% of women and 15% to 40% of men are bacteriuric. The prevalence among persons with chronic indwelling catheters is 100%. Among spinal cord–injured patients with impaired voiding, the prevalence of bacteriuria is 50%, regardless of the method used for bladder emptying.

Patients with an increased prevalence of asymptomatic bacteriuria also have an increased incidence of symptomatic

TABLE 36-7 Asymptomatic Bacteriuria in Normal Populations and in Selected Patients with Underlying Genitourinary Abnormalities

	PREVALENCE OF BACTERIURIA
Healthy Women	
Aged 20-50 years	
Sexually active	3%-5%
Not sexually active	<1%
Aged 50-70 years	3%-9%
Aged ≥80 years	14%-22%
Healthy Men	
Aged <65 years	<1%
Aged ≥80 years	6%-10%
Patients with Complicated Genitourinary Abnormalities	
Spinal cord injury	
Bladder retrained	25%
Intermittent catheterization	23%-89%
Sphincterotomy/condom	58%
Residence in long-term care facility	
Women	25%-57%
Men	19%-37%
Indwelling urethral catheter	
Short term	5%-7% acquisition/day
Long term	100%
Urethral stents	
Temporary	45%
Permanent	100%

Data from Nicolle,[3] Nicolle et al,[106] and Rodhe et al.[115]

urinary tract infection. However, this increased frequency of symptomatic infection is not attributable to bacteriuria. The same biologic determinants promote both asymptomatic and symptomatic infection. Bacteriuria in healthy young women is usually transient, but up to 8% develop acute cystitis within 1 week of initial identification of a positive urine culture.[116] In women with diabetes and female or male residents of nursing homes, persistent bacteriuria for months or years, frequently with the same strain, is often observed. No long-term negative outcomes have been attributed to asymptomatic bacteriuria.[106,117] Bacteriuric individuals are not more likely to develop hypertension or chronic renal failure, and rates of survival are similar to those observed in persons without bacteriuria.

Harmful short-term outcomes attributable to asymptomatic bacteriuria are recognized in two different populations: pregnant women and patients who undergo traumatic genitourinary procedures.[106] The prevalence of bacteriuria during early pregnancy is 3% to 7%, similar to that among age-matched nonpregnant women. The physiologic changes of pregnancy that accompany increased progesterone levels include smooth muscle relaxation and decreased peristalsis, which result in dilation of the renal pelvis and ureters. In later pregnancy, ureteric obstruction may result from pressure of the uterus at the pelvic brim. For pregnant women with bacteriuria that is not treated, 20% to 35% develop acute pyelonephritis later in pregnancy, usually at the end of the second trimester or early in the third trimester. This incidence of pyelonephritis is 20- to 30-fold higher among untreated women with bacteriuria than among women whose initial screening urine cultures yielded negative results or in whom bacteriuria was treated. Acute pyelonephritis in later pregnancy is associated with premature delivery and poorer fetal outcomes. The second group of bacteriuric patients at risk are those who undergo traumatic urologic procedures. If bacteriuria remains untreated, as many as 60% develop bacteremia after the procedure, and 5% to 10% progress to severe sepsis or septic shock.

Pathogenesis: Microbiology

E. coli is isolated from 80% of healthy women with asymptomatic bacteriuria.[116] Most of the remaining bacterial strains comprise *K. pneumoniae*, *Enterococcus* species, and coagulase-negative staphylococci. For men older than 65 years, coagulase-negative staphylococci are isolated most frequently, followed by *E. coli* and *Enterococcus* species. In patients with underlying genitourinary abnormalities, a wider variety of organisms are isolated. *E. coli* and other organisms associated with asymptomatic bacteriuria are characterized by the absence of recognized virulence factors. These *E. coli* strains may originate from nonvirulent commensal strains or evolve from virulent strains by attenuation of virulence genes.[118,119] Other organisms that are frequently isolated, such as coagulase-negative staphylococci and *Enterococcus* species, are relatively nonpathogenic and seldom associated with symptomatic infection.

Biofilm formation is responsible for the universal development of bacteriuria in patients with indwelling urinary devices.[120] After insertion, a conditioning layer composed of proteins and other host components immediately coats the device. This provides a surface for subsequent attachment of bacteria or yeast that originate from drainage bags or the periurethral flora or are introduced after disruption of the closed drainage system. Organisms grow along the device, elaborating an extracellular polysaccharide substance, and colonies of microorganisms persist within this relatively protected environment. Urine components such as Tamm-Horsfall protein and magnesium or calcium ions are also incorporated into the biofilm. Organisms ascend in the biofilm along the interior and exterior surface of the device and reach the bladder within days. The initial infection is usually with a single organism, but a polymicrobial flora is invariably present on chronic devices.[19,121,122] Urease-producing organisms such as *P. mirabilis*, *K. pneumoniae*, *M. morganii*, and *P. stuartii* are isolated more frequently from individuals with chronic indwelling catheters and persist longer than do other organisms, such as *Enterococcus* species. Complications attributed to biofilm formation include development of renal or bladder stones and obstruction of the device. Although the most common device is the urethral catheter, the process of biofilm formation is similar with other indwelling devices such as ureteric stents or nephrostomy tubes.[121,122] From 34% to 42% of ureteral stents are found to be colonized with bacteria or yeast species at removal, often with multiple organisms. More than 50% of organisms present in the stent biofilm are not isolated from simultaneous urine cultures.

Pathogenesis: Host Factors

The genetic and behavioral risk factors and genitourinary abnormalities associated with asymptomatic bacteriuria are similar to those described for uncomplicated or complicated symptomatic urinary tract infection. For younger women, behavioral risks are sexual activity and spermicide use.[116] Bacteriuric women older than 80 years who reside in the community are characterized by reduced mobility, urinary incontinence, and receiving estrogen treatment, and men older than 80 years are characterized by prostate disease, history of stroke, and living in supervised housing.[115] Functional impairment is the major risk factor associated with asymptomatic bacteriuria in the long-term care facility population when an indwelling catheter is not present.[106] Increased residual urine volume is not associated with increased bacteriuria in elderly populations, but it has been associated with bacteriuria in patients referred to an ambulatory urology clinic.[123]

Diagnosis

The quantitative criterion for identification of asymptomatic bacteriuria is at least 10^5 CFU/mL of an organism. For women, two consecutive urine specimens with similar culture results are recommended, but a single specimen is sufficient for men.[106] When an initial urine culture in a young woman yields positive results, a second positive specimen obtained within 2 weeks confirms bacteriuria in 85% to 90% of women. When the second specimen is negative, the initial positive culture may have been contaminated; however, bacteriuria may also have resolved spontaneously. If a voided specimen has a low quantitative count of a single potential uropathogen, and if it is essential to rule out bacteriuria, a second urine specimen should be collected at the time of first morning void.

Pyuria accompanies bacteriuria in most patients, but there is variability in the frequency of pyuria observed in different populations. Pyuria is present in only 50% of bacteriuric pregnant women; therefore, screening for pyuria is not a reliable method to rule out bacteriuria in pregnancy.[124] Pyuria is present in about 75% of diabetic women with bacteriuria, in 90% of bacteriuric patients undergoing hemodialysis, and in more than 90% of elderly persons with bacteriuria.[106] Pyuria also occurs in 30% to 70% of bacteriuric patients with a short-term indwelling catheter and in 100% of those with a chronic indwelling catheter.

Treatment

Screening for and treatment of asymptomatic bacteriuria is recommended only for pregnant women or for patients who will undergo a traumatic genitourinary tract procedure.[103] For other patients, treatment does not improve short- or long-term clinical outcomes, but negative consequences, such as reinfection with organisms of increased antimicrobial resistance and adverse drug effects, do occur.[106,125] In girls and women, an increased frequency of symptomatic infection has been reported after treatment of asymptomatic bacteriuria.[106] This may be attributable to alteration of vaginal flora by antimicrobial therapy or replacement of a benign organism by a more virulent organism. The benefits, if any, of screening for or treatment of bacteriuria in immunocompromised patients, including those with neutropenia, have not been well characterized, and further clinical evaluation is required for these patients.

Identification and treatment of asymptomatic bacteriuria early in pregnancy reduces the risk of pyelonephritis from between 25% and 30% to between 1% and 2%.[106] All pregnant women should be screened for bacteriuria by urine culture at the end of the first trimester and treated if bacteriuria is present.[124] Recommended regimens include a 5-day course of nitrofurantoin[126] or a 7-day course of amoxicillin, amoxicillin/clavulanic acid, or a cephalosporin. The specific regimen is chosen on the basis of the organism isolated and the patient's tolerance. Shorter antimicrobial courses are sometimes prescribed, but these abbreviated courses have not yet been shown in clinical trials to be as effective as the recommended regimens. TMP/SMX should be avoided, especially in the first trimester, and fluoroquinolones are contraindicated during pregnancy. After treatment for asymptomatic or symptomatic urinary tract infection, urine cultures should be repeated at least monthly. If infection recurs, prophylactic antimicrobial therapy should be initiated and continued for the duration of the pregnancy. Nitrofurantoin and cephalexin are the preferred prophylactic regimens because both are safe for the fetus.

Initiation of effective antimicrobial treatment immediately before a traumatic urologic procedure prevents bacteremia and sepsis in a bacteriuric patient.[106,127] Conceptually, this is surgical prophylaxis rather than treatment of asymptomatic bacteriuria. A single dose of an antimicrobial agent is usually adequate, although some guidelines recommend that the antimicrobial agent be continued after transurethral resection of the prostate until the indwelling catheter is removed.[106] Antimicrobial agents are not recommended before replacement of a chronic urethral catheter because the risk of bacteremia and sepsis with this procedure is low, and clinical outcomes are not improved when antimicrobial agents are given for this intervention.[5,128]

Prostatitis

The development of the National Institutes of Health (NIH) classification of prostatitis syndromes (Table 36-8) and subsequent application of this classification in clinical trials and patient care has greatly advanced the understanding and appropriate management of this common problem.[129] Only acute bacterial and chronic bacterial prostatitis are considered attributable to infection and have indications for antimicrobial therapy.[21,130]

Acute bacterial prostatitis is a severe infection, which is a urologic emergency.[21] This syndrome is usually community acquired, although health care–associated infection may occur, particularly after prostate biopsy.[131] Affected patients present with severe systemic manifestations that include fever and marked urinary symptoms of dysuria and frequency. Urinary obstruction and intense suprapubic pain are often present. Bacteremia is reported in 27% of episodes. A digital rectal examination is not recommended because this may precipitate bacteremia.[21]

E. coli is isolated in 70% of episodes; *Proteus* species, *Klebsiella* species, *Enterococcus* species, *P. aeruginosa*, and *S. aureus* are isolated in fewer than 10%.[131] Management includes bladder drainage by insertion of a urethral or suprapubic catheter, blood and urine cultures to characterize the infecting organism, and initiation of empirical parenteral antimicrobial therapy. Most antimicrobial agents are active in the acutely inflamed prostate. A combination of a β-lactam and an aminoglycoside is considered first-line therapy, although other broad-spectrum parenteral antibiotics are also effective. After confirmation of the infecting organism and an adequate clinical response, antibiotic therapy is modified to oral therapy to complete a 6-week course. A fluoroquinolone, either ciprofloxacin or levofloxacin, is recommended as oral therapy if the infecting organism is susceptible. If the clinical response after bladder drainage and initiation of effective antimicrobial therapy is not prompt, CT or MRI is indicated to search for the uncommon complication of a prostate abscess. When an abscess is identified, transrectal ultrasonography-guided aspiration is usually effective for drainage.

Chronic bacterial prostatitis occurs in men with persistent prostate infection.[21,130] Bacteria enter the prostate from the urethra and persist because of limited antimicrobial diffusion or activity in the gland, as well as the frequent presence of infected prostate stones in older men. The most common manifestation is recurrent acute cystitis because bacteria in the

TABLE 36-8 National Institutes of Health Classification of Prostatitis Syndromes	
CLASS	**DESCRIPTION**
I	Acute bacterial prostatitis
II	Chronic bacterial prostatitis
III	Chronic pelvic pain syndrome (CPPS)
IIIa	Inflammatory CPPS Leukocytes present in semen, in urine after prostate massage, or in expressed prostate secretions
IIIb	Noninflammatory CPPS Absence of leukocytes in specimens
IV	Asymptomatic inflammatory prostatitis Leukocytes in specimens similar to those in inflammatory CPPS, but no symptoms

Data from Krieger JN, Nyberg L, Nickel JC: NIH consensus definition and classification of prostatitis, *JAMA* 281:236-237, 1999.

prostate intermittently enter the bladder. The same organism is often repeatedly isolated, but the intervals between symptomatic episodes may last months or even years. Other symptoms are generally mild, such as irritative voiding symptoms and discomfort localized to the testicles, lower back, or perineum. The prostate examination usually yields normal results, but tenderness may be elicited.

In about 10% of men who initially present with a clinical syndrome of chronic prostatitis or chronic pelvic pain syndrome, chronic bacterial prostatitis is subsequently documented microbiologically. The diagnosis requires paired cultures of midstream and post–prostatic massage urine specimens. The midstream specimen confirms negative results of a urine culture, and the post–prostatic massage specimen reveals pyuria and organisms of presumed prostate origin.[21] Gram-negative organisms, including Enterobacteriaceae and *P. aeruginosa*, and gram-positive *Enterococcus* species, *S. aureus*, coagulase-negative staphylococci, and group B streptococci are the bacteria most commonly isolated.[132] Sexually transmitted organisms such as *Chlamydia trachomatis*, *U. urealyticum*, *Mycoplasma genitalium*, and *Trichomonas vaginalis* are uncommon and, when present, usually identified in younger men. The clinical relevance of post–prostatic massage cultures, however, remains controversial. In one study of 463 patients and 121 age-matched controls, 70% were found to harbor at least one organism in a post–prostatic massage specimen, and uropathogens such as *E. coli* were isolated from 8% of patients and 8.3% of controls.[132] According to another study, 6% of 470 men had gram-positive organisms isolated after prostatic massage, but 97% of these organisms were not confirmed on repeat culture.[133]

Despite this uncertainty, chronic bacterial prostatitis does respond to appropriate antimicrobial treatment, although relapse after treatment is common. Ciprofloxacin and levofloxacin are the first choices for antimicrobial treatment of chronic bacterial prostatitis when susceptible organisms are isolated. These agents penetrate well into the prostate and seminal fluid, and they remain active in the acidic environment of the prostate. Cure rates at 6 months after a 4-week course are 75% to 89%,[130] although late relapses may occur after 6 months. Doxycycline and macrolides are considered second-line drugs. Men who present for the first time with chronic pelvic pain syndrome and whose culture findings are negative but who have evidence of inflammation (i.e., leukocytes) in expressed prostatic secretions should be prescribed a 4-week trial of antimicrobial therapy if they have not previously received a prolonged antimicrobial course.[130,134] In reported case series, as many as 10% of these men respond to antimicrobial therapy despite a negative culture finding; however, comparative clinical trials in treatment-naive men with negative culture findings have not been reported. If symptoms persist or recur after this 4-week antimicrobial trial, and if post–prostatic massage cultures remain negative, further antimicrobial therapy is not indicated.[135]

Urinary Tract Infection in Unique Patient Populations

Renal Transplant Recipients

Urinary tract infection accounts for 45% to 60% of infections that occur in patients after renal transplantation.[136-138] By 6 months after transplantation, 17% of recipients experience at least one urinary tract infection, and by 3 years, posttransplantation infection has occurred in 60% of female recipients and 47% of male recipients.[139] The incidence is highest in the first 3 months after transplantation, when infection is often attributable to surgical intervention and the use of urologic devices such as urinary catheters and ureteric stents.[140-143] The clinical manifestation may be either cystitis or pyelonephritis; 3% to 14% of episodes are with associated bacteremia.[137,141,144] Early posttransplantation infections tend to be more severe and manifest more frequently as pyelonephritis or with bacteremia.[145]

Risk factors for urinary tract infection are (1) patient specific, such as female gender, diabetes mellitus, pretransplantation urinary tract infections, prolonged prior dialysis, and polycystic kidney disease, or (2) transplant related, such as allograft trauma, microbial contamination of cadaveric kidneys, technical complications related to ureteral anastomosis, the presence of urinary catheters and ureteric stents, immunosuppression, reimplantation, and vesicoureteric reflux.[143,146,147] After transplantation, the risk of developing urinary tract infection is correlated with the duration of perioperative catheterization.[137,138,148] How routine use of ureteric stents at transplantation affects subsequent urinary tract infection is more controversial. The overall transplantation complication rate is decreased with routine stent implantation, but stent implantation is associated with a small, but significant, increased risk of urinary tract infection. The increased risk, however, was observed only in patients who did not receive posttransplantation prophylaxis with TMP/SMX.[149]

Asymptomatic bacteriuria is not a risk factor for impaired graft survival.[106] Transplant recipients with asymptomatic bacteriuria who progress to graft failure invariably also experience symptomatic infection. Graft failure in these patients is usually attributable to urologic abnormalities that promote infection, rather than a direct consequence of infection. In multivariate analyses, symptomatic urinary tract infection has also not been independently associated with graft survival.[144,150] However, case reports have described transplant recipients receiving stable immunosuppressive regimens who experience deterioration in graft function that is coincident with an episode of acute pyelonephritis.[151] This observation may be attributable to activation of the immune system by the infection.

The principles of management are similar to those for any patient with complicated urinary tract infection. These include prompt clinical diagnosis and antimicrobial initiation, obtaining appropriate specimens for culture, and evaluating for underlying genitourinary abnormalities that may promote infection. Enterobacteriaceae, particularly *E. coli*, are the most common infecting organisms, but a variety of other bacteria or yeast may be isolated. The choice of antimicrobial agent is determined by the susceptibility of the infecting organism and the patient's tolerance. A 2-week course of antimicrobial agents is recommended. The effect of type and intensity of immunosuppressive therapy on antimicrobial efficacy has not been reported. Treatment of asymptomatic bacteriuria, especially beyond the first 6 months after transplantation, is not recommended, because bacteriuria does not compromise renal function[147] and treatment probably does not prevent subsequent symptomatic episodes.[152] Whether screening for and treatment of bacteriuria in the first 6 months after transplantation is beneficial is not known, although some guidelines recommend this strategy.[106] Treatment of asymptomatic candiduria in renal transplant recipients has also not been shown to be beneficial, and is not recommended.[153]

Urinary tract infection can be prevented after transplantation by optimal surgical technique, which includes minimizing the perioperative duration of urethral catheterization. TMP/SMX prophylaxis given for the first 6 months after transplantation decreases the risk of both symptomatic and asymptomatic urinary tract infection, as well as other infections.[106] When urinary tract infection is diagnosed in patients receiving TMP/SMX prophylaxis, the organisms isolated are invariably resistant to TMP/SMX. Frequent recurrent symptomatic infection after transplantation may be attributable to an inadequate duration of antimicrobial treatment, resistance of the infecting organism, the presence of urologic abnormalities such as obstruction or stones, or infection of native kidneys. When infection recurs shortly after treatment, previous urine cultures should be reviewed to establish whether reinfection or relapse is occurring and determine whether the infecting organism is susceptible to the antimicrobial therapy given. If relapse with a susceptible organism occurs after a 2-week course of therapy, repeated treatment with a 4- to 6-week course is recommended, although the effectiveness of prolonged repeated treatment has not been critically evaluated.[144] Repeated relapse after prolonged antimicrobial therapy in a patient without identified urologic abnormalities is often caused by infection localized to the native kidneys. Such patients usually have a history of recurrent urinary tract infection before transplantation. The organisms frequently cannot be eradicated, presumably because of failure of antibiotics to achieve effective levels in the nonfunctioning kidney. Long-term suppressive therapy may be necessary to prevent further symptomatic episodes in these patients.

Urinary Tract Infection in Persons with Renal Failure

Patients with mild to moderate renal failure who experience urinary tract infection usually respond adequately to antimicrobial therapy.[154] When renal impairment is severe, however, adequate urine or renal levels of antimicrobial agents may not be achieved because of limited kidney perfusion. If renal failure occurs with acute pyelonephritis, the response following initiation of antimicrobial therapy may be delayed or the risk of relapse after therapy may be increased. Systematic evaluation of antimicrobial efficacy for treatment of urinary tract infection in patients with renal failure has been limited.[5] Aminoglycosides have little penetration into nonfunctioning kidneys and are not recommended for treatment. Fluoroquinolones, TMP/SMX, ampicillin, and cephalosporins have all been effective for treatment in individual case reports.

Another therapeutic problem arises when infection is localized to a unilateral nonfunctioning kidney. Antimicrobial therapy sterilizes the urine and often ameliorates symptoms because high urine levels are achieved by antimicrobial excretion through the functioning kidney. However, organisms persist in the kidney with impaired function because antimicrobial penetration to the site of infection is inadequate. When antimicrobial therapy is discontinued, a prompt relapse of infection occurs. Localization of infection to one kidney can be documented by culture of urine collected directly from the ureter when the patient is not receiving antibiotics and after bladder irrigation with normal saline to remove infected bladder urine before ureteric catheterization. For relapsing infection when a nonfunctioning kidney is known or suspected to be infected, management options include a trial of a more prolonged course of antimicrobial therapy, continuous suppressive therapy, or nephrectomy of the nonfunctioning kidney.

Urinary Stones

Urinary tract infection complicates urolithiasis through several different mechanisms; infection may be the cause of stone formation, noninfected stones may initially become colonized with bacteria, and obstructing noninfected stones may precipitate infection proximal to the obstruction. In any patient with urolithiasis and infection, the infection should be controlled with appropriate antimicrobial therapy before urologic manipulations.[155]

Infection stones, also called *struvite stones,* are a complication of infection with urease-producing organisms such as *P. mirabilis.* Urease catalyzes the hydrolysis of urea in the urine, producing ammonia and alkalinity of the urine. This condition favors precipitation of magnesium ammonium phosphate, carbonate apatite, and monoammonium urate.[156] These crystals are incorporated into bacterial biofilm, creating the infection stone.[120] Infection stones continue to enlarge, sometimes rapidly, and ultimately cause obstruction and renal failure if not adequately treated. Patients at increased risk for development of infection stones are those with long-term chronic indwelling catheters, urinary tract obstruction, neurogenic voiding dysfunction, distal renal tubular acidosis, and medullary sponge kidney.

Management of infection stones requires complete removal of the stone, together with sterilization of the urine.[155] Percutaneous shock wave lithotripsy is effective in removing 60% to 90% of these stones; in comparison, extracorporeal shock wave lithotripsy is only 30% to 60% effective. Multiple stone fragments are passed after lithotripsy. Antimicrobial therapy, selected on the basis of urine culture results, is continued until all fragments are passed. The optimal duration of antimicrobial therapy after lithotripsy is controversial. Currently, 4 weeks is recommended, although some authors suggest a shorter duration. When percutaneous lithotripsy is not effective or is contraindicated, open surgery or nephrectomy may be necessary for stone removal. For selected elderly or debilitated patients with complex urologic or medical problems, stone removal may not be possible. In such patients, continuous suppressive antimicrobial therapy is recommended to limit stone enlargement and preserve renal function. The antimicrobial agent is selected on the basis of urine culture results, and therapy is continued indefinitely if effective and tolerated. A stone that is not initially infected may have bacteria adhere to the surface and subsequently persist in biofilm.[120]

Culture of a voided urine specimen from these patients often does not reflect the bacteriologic features of a stone. A series of 75 patients with renal stones that were not infection stones revealed that 36 (49%) of the stones were colonized, but only 19 (53%) of these patients also had bacteriuria.[157] Organisms isolated from the colonized stones included *E. coli* (75%), *Enterococcus* species (100%), *P. aeruginosa* (19%), *Klebsiella* species (31%), *P. mirabilis* (8.3%), *Streptococcus* species (31%), *Citrobacter* species (8.3%), *S. saprophyticus* (19%), *M. morganii* (8.3%), and *Gemella* species (8.3%). Larger stones were more likely to be colonized.[158] Patients with stones colonized with bacteria are at increased risk for postprocedure sepsis, even when the voided urine culture yields negative results.[158]

Perioperative antimicrobial agents are recommended for all patients with stones who have indwelling catheters or stents, because these patients are at increased risk of stone colonization. A noninfected stone may cause ureteric obstruction complicated by infection of the undrained urine proximal to the stone. Complete obstruction is associated with a high risk for bacteremia and sepsis, and prompt drainage is essential. When the ureters are obstructed, the voided urine culture often does not accurately reflect the microbiology of urine obtained directly from the renal pelvis. Among patients with obstruction and a positive culture of urine from the renal pelvis, the voided urine culture yielded positive results in only 16.4% of cases in one report, and organisms isolated were concordant between the two specimens in only 23% of patients.[159] Thus, a urine specimen should be obtained for culture from the renal pelvis of patients with obstruction whenever possible.

Other Infections of the Urinary Tract

Renal and Perinephric Abscesses

Renal and perinephric abscesses are uncommon suppurative complications associated with substantial morbidity and mortality. Renal abscesses are located entirely within the renal parenchyma, whereas perinephric abscesses occupy the retroperitoneal fat and fascia surrounding the kidney. Abscesses may involve both the renal and perinephric tissues: 25% to 39% of abscesses are intranephric, 19% to 25% are both intranephric and perinephric, and 42% to 51% are perinephritic alone.[160,161] These abscesses develop after ascending urinary tract infection and pyelonephritis or after hematogenous spread to the renal cortex or retroperitoneum after bacteremia from another site. Single cortical abscesses that develop after hematogenous spread are usually unilateral, but multiple bilateral cortical microabscesses may also develop. Complicating factors such as diabetes, urolithiasis, or obstruction are present in most cases. The organisms most commonly isolated are *E. coli, K. pneumoniae, P. mirabilis, S. aureus,* and anaerobes. *S. aureus* abscesses are most likely to have originated with hematogenous spread from another site of infection. The clinical manifestation for both renal and perinephric abscesses mimics that of acute pyelonephritis. The characteristic findings are fever with costovertebral angle pain or tenderness. However, initiation of appropriate antimicrobial therapy usually results in clinical failure or delayed response.

CT is the preferred imaging modality for diagnosing the presence of an abscess; it also characterizes the extent of infection and identifies the potential source.[85] Ultrasonography identifies most perinephric abscesses, but it may not be able to distinguish an inflammatory lobar mass from a true renal abscess.[86]

The management goals for renal and perinephric abscesses include prompt diagnosis, early institution of effective antimicrobial therapy, and abscess drainage for both therapeutic and diagnostic purposes. Culture of the abscess fluid identifies the specific infecting organisms and directs antimicrobial choice.

If abscess fluid cannot be sampled for culture, organisms isolated from blood or urine culture should be considered in the selection of antimicrobial therapy. Initial antimicrobial administration is usually intravenous. Once the patient's condition is stabilized, therapy can be continued with an appropriate oral antimicrobial agent with good bioavailability. Small abscesses (1 to 3 cm in diameter) often respond to antimicrobial therapy without drainage, but for abscesses larger than 3 cm, drainage is usually required for resolution of infection.[160-163] Renal abscesses tend to be smaller, and 69% of these have been reported to resolve with medical therapy alone.[161] Perinephric or mixed abscesses are larger, and drainage is usually required. The current initial approach is to attempt percutaneous drainage and then, if percutaneous drainage is not effective, proceed to open drainage or even nephrectomy. Resolution of the abscess is monitored by repeated imaging studies. Antimicrobial therapy is continued until the abscess has completely resolved or until there is only a residual, stable scar.

Infected Renal Cysts

Infected cysts complicating polycystic kidney disease may be problematic to diagnose. The frequency of occurrence and risk factors for development of cyst infection are not well described. Fever with abdominal pain or tenderness, often with bacteremia, is the usual clinical manifestation. *E. coli, Enterococcus* species, and group B streptococci are the most common infecting organisms, but *P. aeruginosa, Clostridium* species, *Candida* species, and *Aspergillus* species have also been reported. In view of the wide spectrum of potential pathogens, the specific infecting organism should be confirmed by cyst aspiration whenever possible. Imaging studies are usually necessary to confirm the diagnosis and identify the implicated cyst. However, ultrasonography and CT are not useful.[164] MRI[164] and white blood cell–labeled scans[164,165] were successful in localizing the infected cyst in individual case reports. More recently, positron emission tomography with fludeoxyglucose F 18 has been reported to be effective in localizing the infected cyst, but access to this technology is limited.[166,167]

Once the potential infected cyst is identified, a cyst aspirate, if possible, can confirm the presence of infection and provide therapeutic drainage.[168] Antimicrobial penetration into the cyst is presumed to be transepithelial. Effective concentrations of TMP/SMX, chloramphenicol, and fluoroquinolones are achieved in the cyst.[154] Cyst and serum levels of levofloxacin are similar, whereas cyst levels reported with ciprofloxacin are only 40% of serum levels.[169] Therapeutic levels of the penicillins, cephalosporins, aminoglycosides,[154] and amphotericin B[170] are not achieved in cysts. Prolonged antimicrobial therapy for at least 4 weeks is recommended, although clinical trials defining the optimal duration of therapy have not been reported. Nephrectomy is occasionally necessary when cyst drainage and appropriate antimicrobial therapy are not successful in controlling the infection.

Emphysematous Cystitis and Pyelonephritis

Emphysematous cystitis and pyelonephritis are acute necrotizing infections characterized by gas formation. Gas within the urinary collecting system can be seen after many interventional procedures, but emphysematous infection is characterized by gas in the tissues.[86] Gas is localized to the bladder wall and lumen in cystitis[171] and in and around the kidney in pyelonephritis.[172] Emphysematous pyelitis is a gas-forming infection restricted to the collecting system; the renal parenchyma is spared. Affected patients usually have diabetes with poor glucose control. Obstruction is another common predisposing factor for emphysematous pyelonephritis. *E. coli* and *K. pneumoniae* are the organisms most commonly isolated. High levels of glucose in the urine serve as a substrate for these bacteria, and large amounts of gas are generated through natural fermentation. In affected patients who are not diabetic, protein fermentation is a proposed source of gas formation.[171]

CT is considered the optimal imaging technique for confirming emphysematous infection and characterizing the extent of involvement.[85,86] A review of 135 cases of emphysematous cystitis identified over a period of 50 years reported the median patient age was 66 years (range, <1 to 90 years), 64% of patients were women, and 67% had diabetes.[171] Presenting symptoms ranged from pneumaturia alone through irritative lower tract voiding symptoms to severe illness suggestive of acute abdominal disease or sepsis; 7% of cases were asymptomatic. *E. coli* was isolated from 58%, *K. pneumoniae* from 21%, and *Clostridium* species and *Enterobacter aerogenes* each from 7% of cases. The diagnosis was apparent on a plain radiograph of the abdomen in 84% of these cases. Medical management—including antimicrobial therapy, bladder drainage, and glycemic control—was usually effective. Surgical intervention, required in 10% of cases, included cystectomy, partial cystectomy, and surgical débridement if concomitant emphysematous pyelonephritis was present. The overall mortality rate was only 7%.

Emphysematous pyelonephritis is a more serious infection with a substantially higher mortality rate. Of 17 patients with emphysematous pyelonephritis identified at one center over an 18-year period, 70% were women and all were diabetic.[173] Initial serum glucose levels ranged from 270 to 658 mg/L, and the serum level of C-reactive protein ranged from 6.2 to 30.1 mg/L. *E. coli* was isolated in 52% of these patients and *K. pneumoniae* in 24%. Of 17 patients from whom blood cultures were obtained, 10 had bacteremia. The plain abdominal radiograph identified gas in the kidney in only 50% of cases. Ultrasonography of the kidneys usually showed some abnormalities but was less accurate than CT in identifying emphysematous infection. Management included antimicrobial therapy with percutaneous or open drainage of abscesses and correction of obstruction.[174] Aggressive glucose control and supportive care were also necessary. The rate of mortality ranged from 20% of patients with less severe manifestations to 70% of patients with a fulminant course characterized by necrosis, intravascular thrombosis, and microabscess formation.

Emergency nephrectomy was traditionally considered necessary for any patient presenting with emphysematous pyelonephritis. Currently, percutaneous drainage is the recommended initial approach because it is reported to be associated with lower mortality rates than is medical management alone or emergency nephrectomy.[174] In a retrospective case series with a relatively small number of patients, the mortality rates were 50% with medical management alone, 25% with medical management and emergency nephrectomy, and 13.5% with medical management combined with initial percutaneous drainage.[173] Delayed elective nephrectomy may subsequently be required for some patients.

Xanthogranulomatous Pyelonephritis

Xanthogranulomatous pyelonephritis is an uncommon, severe, subacute or chronic suppurative process characterized by destruction and replacement of the renal parenchyma by granulomatous tissue containing histocytes and foamy cells.[175,176] The inflammatory process may extend into such perinephric structures as Gerota's fascia, the posterior perirenal space, the psoas muscle, the diaphragm, or the spleen. Less than 1% to 8% of kidneys removed or sampled in biopsy for inflammatory conditions are reported to show evidence of xanthogranulomatous pyelonephritis.[176] The specific cause of this process is unknown, but potential contributing factors include chronic urinary tract infection, abnormal lipid metabolism, lymphatic obstruction, impaired leukocyte function, and vascular occlusion. The organisms most commonly isolated from renal tissue are *P. mirabilis* (38%), *E. coli* (33%), *Klebsiella/Enterobacter* species (8%), *P. aeruginosa* (8%), and *S. aureus* (10%).

In a single-center experience between 1994 and 2005, 35 (85%) of 41 cases occurred in women.[177] Xanthogranulomatous pyelonephritis was responsible for 19% of 214 nephrectomies performed at this facility during the review period. The most common presenting symptoms were fever, flank or abdominal pain, weight loss, lower urinary tract symptoms, and gross hematuria. All patients had renal calculi. In 17 cases in which urine cultures were obtained, 35% grew *E. coli*, 18% grew *P. mirabilis*, and 35% had no growth.

In a second single-center review from Greece of 39 cases occurring between 1980 and 1999, the female/male ratio was 2:1.[175] The presenting histories included urolithiasis or renal colic, recurrent urinary tract infections, and previous urologic procedures. All patients were symptomatic at presentation; symptoms included complaints of fever, flank or abdominal pain, chills, and malaise. Anorexia, weight loss, lower tract symptoms, and gross hematuria were also reported. *E. coli* organisms were isolated in 15 cases and *P. mirabilis* in 12. Plain radiographs or IVP showed a nonfunctioning kidney in 63% of cases, single or multiple calculi in 52%, staghorn calculus in 48%, calyceal deformity in 26%, and hydronephrosis in 23%.

CT is considered the optimal imaging modality; it identifies the abnormality in 74% to 90% of cases.[85,86,176] Because of the current widespread access to CT, the diagnosis is usually made preoperatively. Characteristic findings include an enlarged kidney, frequently with replacement of renal parenchyma and multiple fluid-filled cavities, together with urolithiasis. Ultrasonography identifies nonspecific abnormalities, including renal enlargement with relative preservation of renal contour and multiple hypoechoic round masses.[86] MRI shows abnormalities similar to those observed with CT.[178] The differential diagnosis includes malignancy and tuberculosis. The usual management is nephrectomy; antimicrobial therapy has only a secondary role.[176] If the diagnosis is made early, when there is only focal renal involvement, partial nephrectomy may be curative.

Pyocystis

Pyocystis, also called *vesical empyema,* is an infection characterized by a purulent fluid collection in the bladder of a patient with a nonfunctioning bladder. In effect, the bladder becomes an undrained abscess. This is a rare complication diagnosed in patients with anuric renal failure or surgically bypassed bladders. The clinical presentation includes suprapubic pain or distension, abdominal pain, foul-smelling urethral discharge, and fever or sepsis.[179,180] Organisms isolated have included *E. coli, P. mirabilis, P. aeruginosa, Serratia marcescens, Streptococcus* species, and *Enterococcus* species. Mixed cultures are common. It is not clear whether anaerobic organisms may also contribute.

When the condition is suspected, a specimen of bladder fluid should be obtained for diagnosis and culture. The laboratory should be requested to identify all organisms isolated, so that the specimen is processed as abscess fluid rather than urine. The treatment approach includes systemic antimicrobial agents and urethral catheterization for bladder drainage. Antimicrobial therapy is directed by the specific organisms isolated. Bladder irrigation with either saline or an antibiotic solution is sometimes recommended, but whether irrigation provides an additional therapeutic benefit is not clear.[181] Surgical intervention to achieve adequate drainage is necessary in rare recalcitrant cases.

Uncommon Organisms

Genitourinary Tuberculosis

Genitourinary tuberculosis is diagnosed in 1.1% to 1.5% of all tuberculosis cases, and 5% to 6% of cases of extrapulmonary tuberculosis.[182,183] This infection is a consequence of hematogenous dissemination of *Mycobacterium tuberculosis* to the renal cortex during primary pulmonary infection. The high oxygen tension of the renal cortex is favorable for renal localization. Men are infected twice as often as women. The latent period from the time of initial pulmonary infection to diagnosis of clinical urogenital tuberculosis is 22 years on average, with a range of 1 to 46 years.[184] Reactivation of tuberculosis usually occurs in only one kidney; thus disease is characteristically unilateral. Contiguous involvement of the collecting system leads to *M. tuberculosis* bacilluria with subsequent ureteric and bladder infection. Prostate and epididymis infection may result directly from hematogenous dissemination, rather than contiguous spread. The kidneys are affected in 60% to 100% of cases, the ureters in 19% to 41%, the bladder in 15% to 20%, and the prostate or epididymis in 20% to 50% of men.[184]

Substantial morbidity is attributed to urogenital tuberculosis. Severe calyceal clubbing and dilation of the renal pelvis and ureters, leading to total destruction of the kidney and autonephrectomy, occur in 23% to 33% of cases, and renal failure occurs in 1% to 10%.[184] A summary of cases reported worldwide noted 27% of patients had a nonfunctioning unilateral kidney at presentation, but this proportion varied from 8% to 72% in different countries, which presumably reflects the timeliness of diagnosis.[185]

Presenting genitourinary symptoms are often vague or nonspecific but may include back or flank pain, dysuria, and urinary frequency. As many as 50% of patients have no localizing genitourinary symptoms. About 25% to 33% of patients have systemic complaints, usually pulmonary symptoms, fever, and weight loss.[184,186] The subacute presentation and results of the initial evaluation can mimic those of xanthogranulomatous pyelonephritis. In men, additional features suggestive of tuberculosis include an enlarged, hard, and nontender epididymis; thickened or beaded vas deferens; indurated or nodular prostate; and nontender testicular mass.[183] Tuberculous

granulomatous prostatitis may manifest as a nodular prostate with an elevated level of prostate-specific antigen that is clinically indistinguishable from that of prostate carcinoma. Most patients with renal tuberculosis have evidence of concomitant extragenital disease. The most common site is the lungs, but pulmonary disease is usually inactive. The chest radiograph is abnormal in 67% to 75% of patients, and the tuberculin skin test yields positive results in 60% to 90%.

The urinalysis findings are abnormal in more than 90% of patients with genitourinary tuberculosis.[182] Sterile pyuria with hematuria is present in 51% of cases, sterile pyuria alone in 26%, and gross or microscopic hematuria alone in 13%. For patients with HIV infection, an algorithm that incorporates negative results of routine urine culture and the presence of pyuria, albuminuria, or hematuria has good predictive value for detecting genitourinary tuberculosis.[187,188] As many as half of patients, however, have concomitant bacteriuria with other organisms at presentation, and this finding may obscure the initial assessment of the urinalysis.

IVP was traditionally the standard imaging approach, but CT is now common.[184] Imaging studies identify unilateral disease in 75% of cases of renal tuberculosis (Figure 36-1). The characteristic early finding is erosions of the renal calyx; the erosions subsequently progress to papillary necrosis, hydronephrosis, renal parenchymal cavitation, and dilated calyces. Ureteric tuberculosis is characterized by a thickened ureteric wall and strictures. Lesions are most common in the distal third of the ureter. Bladder tuberculosis may manifest as reduced bladder volume with wall thickening, ulceration, and filling defects resulting from granulomatous involvement. In advanced disease, scarring results in permanent loss of volume and a residual small, irregular, calcified bladder. The most common finding on CT is renal calcification, present in 50% of cases.[189] Other characteristic findings include hydrocalyx secondary to infundibular stenosis and cavity formation. In advanced disease, cortical loss, uroepithelial thickening and dystrophic calcification are present.

The diagnosis is confirmed by growth of *M. tuberculosis* in urine or tissue. Appropriate specimens for mycobacterial culture should be obtained whenever this diagnosis is considered. Three sequential early morning urine specimens for mycobacterial culture are recommended. Urine cultures yield positive results in 75% to 90% of affected patients. A positive acid-fast bacillus smear of urine is usually *M. tuberculosis*, but culture confirmation is essential to rule out colonization with nonpathogenic mycobacteria and for susceptibility testing of the infecting isolate.[190,191] If a suggestive renal abnormality is present but urine culture results are negative, tissue biopsy may be necessary to confirm the diagnosis. Polymerase chain reaction (PCR) nucleic acid antigen testing of urine specimens has been reported to be more sensitive than culture and, if available, provides a more rapid diagnosis.[188] However, culture is still necessary to isolate the organism for susceptibility testing.

The treatment of genitourinary tuberculosis is similar to the treatment of extrapulmonary tuberculosis at other sites. The initial regimen consists of four drugs (isoniazid, rifampin, pyrazinamide, and ethambutol) for 2 months, followed by two drugs (isoniazid, rifampin) for 4 months if the isolate is susceptible to first-line therapy. Antimycobacterial treatment should be provided under the supervision of a physician with expertise in tuberculosis management. Follow-up intravenous urography (IVP) every 6 months has been recommended for

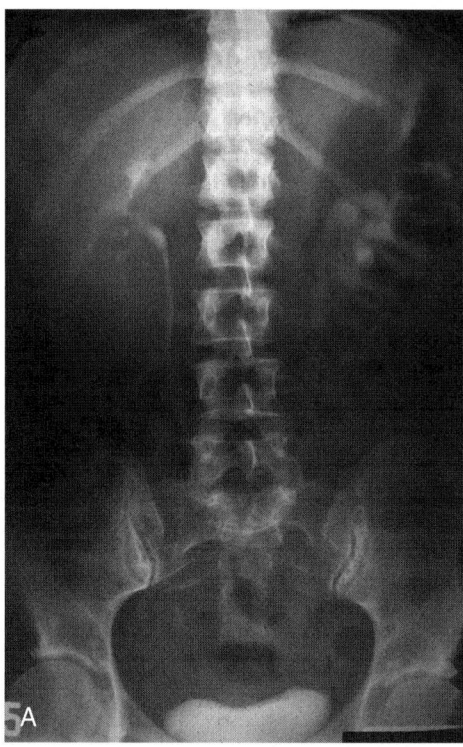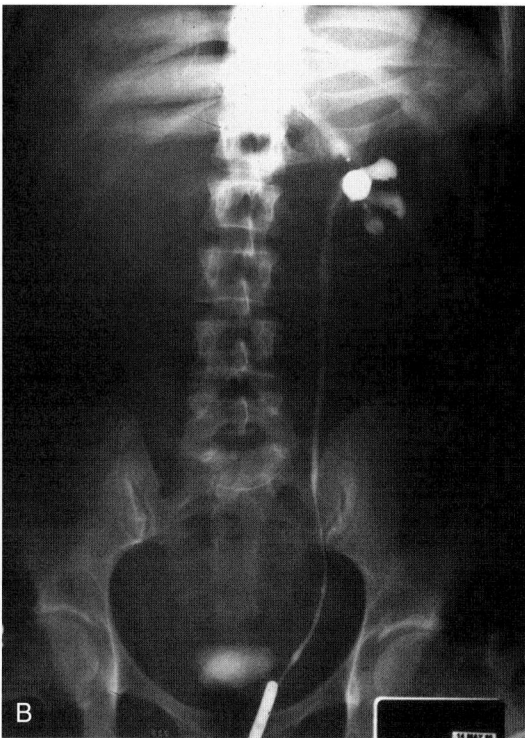

FIGURE 36-1 Renal tuberculosis. **A,** Intravenous pyelogram, showing unilateral hydronephrosis and calyceal distension. **B,** Retrograde pyelogram in the same patient, showing distal ureteric narrowing.

monitoring healing, because ureteral scarring and obstruction may develop or progress during therapy as part of the healing process. Corticosteroid therapy does not prevent this complication.[182] Ureteral reimplantation, endoscopic balloon dilatation, or implantation of ureteral stents may be necessary if progressive obstruction develops. Nephrectomy is rarely required but may be indicated for intractable pain, untreatable infection proximal to a stricture, uncontrollable hematuria or hypertension, or drug resistance. Bladder augmentation surgery may be required if the bladder is scarred and contracted after tuberculosis infection.[192]

Bacille de Calmette-Guérin Infection

Intravesical vaccine instillation of bacille de Calmette-Guérin (BCG) is considered first-line treatment for superficial bladder tumors and carcinoma in situ. Treatment with this biologic therapy may be complicated by systemic or local BCG infection.[193] BCG bladder instillation is followed by local irritative symptoms such as dysuria in 80% of cases, but these symptoms do not usually persist beyond 48 hours.[194] If symptoms do persist, isoniazid for 14 days is recommended, and if symptoms continue despite isoniazid therapy, a full course of antituberculous therapy is recommended.[195] Other less common genitourinary infections that accompany BCG instillation include prostatitis in 1% to 3% of patients, epididymitis in 0.2%, and, in rare cases, testicular abscesses, local skin infections, or renal infection. Reflux may be a risk factor for the rare complication of BCG pyelonephritis.[196] Localized genitourinary infection tends to have a delayed onset and is usually not apparent clinically until more than 3 months after BCG treatment.[193] BCG may not be isolated from urine or tissue cultures.[193] Tissue biopsy usually shows necrotizing granulomatous inflammation, and this finding in the context of prior BCG therapy is sufficient for diagnosis even if subsequent culture results are negative.

Fungal Urinary Tract Infection

Fungal urinary tract infection is usually caused by *Candida* species. It manifests as asymptomatic candiduria, cystitis, or pyelonephritis. Bladder or renal fungus balls and systemic fungemia are rare complications. *Candida albicans* is isolated from over 50% of episodes, followed by *Candida glabrata*, *Candida tropicalis* and *Candida parapsilosis*.[197] Candiduria is usually identified in patients who are seriously ill with multiple comorbid conditions, and most infections are asymptomatic. The most important risk factors for candiduria are the presence of an indwelling catheter or other indwelling urologic device, diabetes mellitus, and exposure to broad-spectrum antimicrobial agents.[197] Treatment of asymptomatic candiduria is not beneficial and is currently recommended only for selected patients with neutropenia or before a traumatic urologic procedure.[198,199] Indwelling devices should be removed whenever possible to facilitate resolution of candiduria. Imaging studies to exclude fungus balls should be considered when patients have recurrent symptomatic infection or urinary obstruction. If fungus balls are present, surgical removal is required for cure of the infection.

Fluconazole is the treatment of choice for *Candida* urinary tract infection because it is excreted in the urine in active form and high urinary levels are achieved.[199] A 2-week course of fluconazole, 200 to 400 mg daily, is recommended (Table 36-9). Amphotericin B deoxycholate, 0.3 to 0.6 mg/kg daily, is the alternative treatment recommended for fluconazole-resistant strains, including most *C. glabrata* organisms, as well as for patients allergic to fluconazole or in whom treatment fails despite optimal fluconazole therapy and urologic management.

TABLE 36-9 Recommended Treatment of Candiduria

	CYSTITIS	PYELONEPHRITIS
Fluconazole (if isolate is susceptible)	200-400 mg daily, 14 days	200-400 mg daily, 14 days
Amphotericin B deoxycholate	0.3-0.6 mg/kg daily, 1-7 days	0.5-0.7 mg/kg daily, 14 days
Amphotericin B* bladder irrigation	5-50 mg/L continuous irrigation for 2-7 days	Not indicated
Flucytosine	25 mg/kg qid; 7-10 days	25mg/kg qid, 14 days†

*Not generally recommended.
†May be used in combination with amphotericin B.
Data from Pappas PG, Kauffman CA, Andes D, et al. Clinical practice guidelines for the management of Candidiasis 2009: Update by the Infectious Diseases Society of America 48:503-535, 2009.

Treatment duration with amphotericin B is 1 to 7 days for cystitis and 2 weeks for pyelonephritis. Amphotericin B may also be effective for treatment of fungal cystitis when administered as a bladder washout, but this approach is not generally recommended because it requires several days of urethral catheterization and the optimal dose, frequency, and duration are not well established.[200] With lipid formulations of amphotericin B, low concentrations of active drug are achieved in renal tissue, and these formulations are thus not recommended.

The antifungal 5-flucytosine is excreted in the urine and is indicated for treatment of candidal urinary tract infection as a single agent or in combination with amphotericin B for renal infection. Resistance to 5-flucytosine develops rapidly when this drug is used as a single agent, and the frequent adverse effects of bone marrow suppression or enterocolitis also limit its use, particularly in patients with renal failure. Echinocandins such as caspofungin, micafungin, and anidulafungin and other azoles such as itraconazole, voriconazole, and posaconazole are not excreted into the urine and are not recommended for treatment of urinary tract infection. There are, however, case reports of successful treatment of *C. glabrata* urinary tract infection with caspofungin.[201]

Viral Infections

Viral urinary tract infections are uncommon in adults and occur largely in only immunocompromised patients.[202-205] The most common viruses are adenovirus, parvovirus B19, and CMV. More than one viral infection may coexist. Clinical manifestations of viral infection generally occur after reactivation of latent infection with immunosuppressive therapy, although de novo infection may occur. The usual clinical manifestation is hemorrhagic cystitis, but nephropathy has also been described.[202,206,207] Most adult cases occur in recipients of hematopoietic stem cell transplants, particularly those with severe graft-versus-host disease, and in renal transplant recipients. Infection has also been reported in other immunosuppressed individuals, including HIV-infected patients with low CD4 counts.[204]

Management of parvovirus B19 infection in the transplanted kidney is discussed elsewhere in the book. Adenovirus or CMV infection is diagnosed by viral culture or PCR of the urine. Management includes minimization of immunosuppressive therapy if possible. For HIV-infected patients, antiretroviral therapy should be initiated to increase the CD4

count. CMV infection responds to treatment with ganciclovir or foscarnet.[202] Treatment of adenovirus infection is with cidofovir, although some efficacy has been reported with vidarabine.[202] There have also been case reports of successful treatment of adenovirus with ganciclovir and ribavirin.[202,208]

Parasitic Infestations of the Urinary Tract

The most common and important parasitic infestation of the urinary tract is with *Schistosoma hematobium*.[209,210] This parasite is acquired after exposure to contaminated water. *Schistosoma* larvae penetrate the intact skin and migrate in the blood to the liver, where they transform into young worms (schistosomulae) that mature in 4 to 6 weeks and then further migrate to the perivesicle venules. The life span of the adult worm in the venule is usually 3 to 5 years but can be longer. Most eggs produced by the adult worms enter the bladder lumen and are removed in the urine. However, some eggs are retained locally in the bladder wall, where they incite an eosinophilic inflammatory and granulomatous immune response that causes progressive fibrosis.

The functional abnormality early in the disease is obstruction of the bladder neck. Late complications include recurrent bacterial urinary tract infection, bladder or ureteric stone formation, renal functional abnormalities, and, ultimately, kidney failure. *Schistosoma* infestation is also a risk factor for squamous cell carcinoma of the bladder. The relative risk of cancer for persons with schistosomiasis varies from 1.8 to 23.5; the incidence is highest in the 30- to 50-year age group.[211]

The prevalence of infection in endemic areas is high. Surveys from rural Zimbabwe revealed that 60% of women younger than 20 years of age and 29% of those aged 45 to 49 years have eggs in the urine. HIV-infected women older than 35 years had a significantly higher prevalence of infestation.[212] Travelers to endemic areas may become infested with only minimal exposure to contaminated water.[213,214]

Acute genitourinary symptoms occur in up to 50% of cases after infection and include hematuria, which is often terminal, together with dysuria and urinary frequency. Microhematuria is reported in 41% to 100% and gross hematuria in 0% to 97% of patients with chronic schistosomal infestation. Radiologic abnormalities are present in the upper urinary tract in 2% to 62% of chronic cases.[210] Ultrasonography of the urinary tract demonstrates thickening of the bladder wall, granulomatous changes, hydronephrosis, and, on occasion, bladder or ureteric calcification. The diagnosis is established by identification of parasite eggs in the urine or biopsy specimens or by serologic findings. Urine specimens collected for identification of eggs should be obtained on consecutive days between 1100 and 1300 hours because egg passage is maximal at this time. Sedimentation or filtration of the urine before examination increases the sensitivity of egg detection.[210,215]

Treatment with one dose of praziquantel, 40 mg/kg body weight, leads to cure in 80% of cases. Follow-up urine specimens for parasite egg identification are recommended 3 months after treatment to identify patients in whom treatment has failed and must be repeated. Bladder wall thickening and hydroureters may be reversed if treatment is given early in the course of infestation. However, when chronic disease is established with fibrotic lesions, changes may not be reversible, and corrective surgery or management of end-stage renal disease is required.[215]

Echinococcus granulosus infestation occasionally involves the kidneys.[209] Renal cysts are reported in 2% to 3% of cases of hydatid disease.[216,217] The diagnosis is usually made after incidental finding of a cyst in the kidneys, ureters, bladder, or testes. On occasion, flank pain or a mass is present. Hydatid cysts are not excreted in the urine. Treatment is surgical cyst removal or marsupialization; nephrectomy is occasionally necessary. Perioperative albendazole therapy is also usually recommended for patients with hydatid disease. A less common helminthic infestation is *Wucheria bancrofti* (filariasis), which may cause lymphatic obstruction and rupture into the urinary collecting system, producing chyluria.[209]

The protozoal parasite *T. vaginalis* is commonly transmitted sexually and is occasionally identified on microscopy with routine urinalysis. In women, the parasite may originate from contamination of the urine by vaginal secretions, but the organism is a well-described cause of urethritis for both men and women. Whenever *T. vaginalis* is identified, treatment of the patient and his or her sexual partners is indicated, regardless of symptoms. The recommended treatment is a single dose of metronidazole, 2 g, or tinidazole, 2 g.[218]

References

1. Fihn SD. Acute uncomplicated urinary tract infection in women. *N Engl J Med.* 2003;349:259-266.
2. Nicolle LE. Uncomplicated urinary tract infections in adults including uncomplicated pyelonephritis. *Urol Clin North Am.* 2008;35:1-12.
3. Nicolle LE. A practical approach to the management of complicated urinary tract infection. *Drugs Aging.* 2001;18:243-254.
4. Neal DE. Complicated urinary tract infections. *Urol Clin North Am.* 2008;35:13-22.
5. Nicolle LE. AMMI-Canada Guidelines Committee: Complicated urinary tract infection in adults. *Can J Infect Dis Med Microbiol.* 2005;16:349-360.
6. Montagnini Spaine D, Mamizuka EM, et al. Microbiology aerobic studies on normal male urethra. *Urology.* 2000;56:207-210.
7. Kunin CM, Evans C, Bartholomew D, et al. The antimicrobial defense mechanism of the female urethra: a reassessment. *J Urol.* 2002;168:413-419.
8. Riemersma WA, van der Schee CJ, van der Meijden W, et al. Microbial population diversity in the urethras of healthy males and males suffering from nonchlamydial, nongonococcal urethritis. *J Clin Microbiol.* 2003;41:1977-1986.
9. Sobel JD. Pathogenesis of urinary tract infection: role of host defenses. *Infect Dis Clin North Am.* 1997;3:531-549.
10. Weichhart T, Haidinger M, Horl WH, et al. Current concepts of molecular defense mechanisms operative during urinary tract infection. *Eur J Clin Invest.* 2008;38:29-38.
11. Raffi HS, Bates Jr JM, Laszik Z, et al. Tamm-Horsfall protein acts as a general host-defense factor against bacterial cystitis. *Am J Nephrol.* 2005;25:570-578.
12. Finer G, Landau D. Pathogenesis of urinary tract infections with normal female anatomy. *Lancet Infect Dis.* 2004;4:631-635.
13. Wullt B, Bergsten G, Fischer H, et al. The host response to urinary tract infection. *Infect Dis Clin North Am.* 2003;17:279-302.
14. Ragnarsdottir B, Fischer H, Godaly G, et al. TLR- and CXCR1-dependent innate immunity: insights into the genetics of urinary tract infections. *Eur J Clin Invest.* 2008;38:12-20.
15. Billips BK, Forrestal SG, Rycyk M, et al. Modulation of host innate immune response in the bladder by uropathogenic. *Escherichia coli. Infect Immun.* 2007;75:5353-5360.
16. Thumbikat P, Waltenbaugh C, Schaeffer AJ, et al. Antigen specific responses accelerate bacterial clearance in the bladder. *J Immunol.* 2006;176:3080-3086.
17. Kantek A, Mottonen T, Al-Kaila K, et al. P fimbria-s-ecific B cell responses in patients with urinary tract infection. *J Infect Dis.* 2003;188:1895-1891.
18. High KP, Bradley SF, Gravenstein S, et al. Clinical practice guideline for the evaluation of fever and infection in older adult residents of long term care facilities. *Clin Infect Dis.* 2009;48:149-171.
19. Raz R, Schiller D, Nicolle LE. Chronic indwelling catheter replacement before antimicrobial therapy for symptomatic urinary tract infection. *J Urol.* 2000;164:1254-1258.
20. Frimodt-Moller N. Correlation between pharmacokinetic/pharmacodynamic parameters and efficacy for antibiotics in the treatment of urinary tract infection. *Int J Antimicrob Agents.* 2002;19:546-553.
21. Benway BM, Moon TD. Bacterial prostatitis. *Urol Clin North Am.* 2008;35:23-32.
22. Wagenlehner FME, Weidner W, Naber KG. Pharmacokinetic characteristics of antimicrobials and optimal treatment of urosepsis. *Clin Pharmacokinet.* 2007;46:291-305.
23. Wagenlehner FME, Wagenlehner C, Redman R, et al. Urinary bactericidal activity of doripenem versus that of levofloxacin in patients with complicated urinary tract infections or pyelonephritis. *Antimicrob Agents Chemother.* 2009;53:1567-1573.
24. Nicolle L, Duckworth H, Sitar D, et al. Pharmacokinetics/pharmacodynamics of levofloxacin 750 mg once daily in young women with acute uncomplicated pyelonephritis. *Int J Antimicrob Agents.* 2008;31:287-289.
25. Foxman B, Barlow R, D'Arcy H, et al. Urinary tract infection: self-reported incidence and associated costs. *Ann Epidemiol.* 2000;10:509-515.
26. Foxman B, Gillespie B, Koopman J, et al. Risk factors for second urinary tract infection among college women. *Am J Epidemiol.* 2000;151:1194-1205.
27. Jackson SL, Boyko EJ, Scholes D, et al. Predictors of urinary tract infection after menopause. *Am J Med.* 2004;117:903-911.
28. Nickel JC, Lee JC, Grantmyre JE, et al. Natural history of urinary tract infection in a primary care environment in Canada. *Can J Urol.* 2005;12:2718-2737.
29. Kahlmeter G, ECO.SENS. An international survey of the antimicrobial susceptibility of pathogens from uncomplicated urinary tract infections: the ECO.SENS project. *J Antimicrob Chemother.* 2003;51:69-76.
30. Johnson JR, Owens K, Gajewski A, et al. Bacterial characteristics in relation to clinical source of *Escherichia coli* isolated from women with acute cystitis or pyelonephritis and uninfected women. *J Clin Microbiol.* 2005;43:6064-6072.
31. Johnson JR. Microbial virulence determinants and the pathogenesis of urinary tract infection. *Infect Dis Clin North Am.* 2003;17:261-278.
32. Gunther NW, Lockatell J, Johnson DE, et al. in vivo dynamics of type 1 fimbria regulation in uropathogenic *Escherichia coli* during experimental urinary tract infection. *Infect Immun.* 2001;69:2838-2846.
33. Takahashi A, Kanamaru S, Kurazono H, et al. *Escherichia coli* isolates associated with uncomplicated and complicated cystitis and asymptomatic bacteriuria possess similar phylogenies, virulence genes, and O-serogroup profiles. *J Clin Microbiol.* 2006;44:4589-4592.
34. Foxman B, Manning SD, Tallman P, et al. Uropathogenic *Escherichia coli* are more likely than commensal *E. coli* to be shared between heterosexual sex partners. *Am J Epidemiol.* 2002;156:1133-1140.
35. Johnson JR, Clabots C. Sharing of virulent *Escherichia coli* clones among household members of a woman with acute cystitis. *Clin Infect Dis.* 2006;43:c101-c108.
36. Manges AR, Johnson JR, Foxman B, et al. Widespread distribution of urinary tract infections caused by a multidrug-resistant *Escherichia coli* clonal group. *N Engl J Med.* 2001;345:1007-1013.
37. Kuroda M, Yamashita A, Hirakawa H, et al. Whole genome sequence of *Staphylococcus saprophyticus* reveals the pathogenesis of uncomplicated urinary tract infection. *Proc Natl Acad Sci U S A.* 2005;102:13272-13277.
38. Vogel T, Verreault R, Gourdeau M, et al. Optimal duration of antimicrobial therapy for uncomplicated urinary tract infection in older women: a double blind randomized controlled trial. *Can Med Assoc J.* 2004;170:469-473.
39. Hooton TM. The current management strategies for community-acquired urinary tract infection. *Infect Dis Clin North Am.* 2003;17:303-332.
40. Christiaens TC, DeMeyere M, Verschraegen G, et al. Randomized controlled trial of nitrofurantoin versus placebo in the treatment of uncomplicated urinary tract infection in adult women. *Br J Gen Pract.* 2002;52:729-734.
41. Raz R, Gennesin Y, Wasser J, et al. Recurrent urinary tract infections in postmenopausal women. *Clin Infect Dis.* 2000;30:152-156.
42. Scholes D, Hooton TM, Roberts PL, et al. Risk factors for recurrent urinary tract infection in young women. *J Infect Dis.* 2000;182:1177-1182.
43. Krieger JN. Urinary tract infections: what's new? *J Urol.* 2002;168:2351-2358.
44. Brown J, Vittinghoff E, Kanaya AM, et al. Urinary tract infections in post-menopausal women. Effects of hormone therapy and risk factors. *Obstet Gynecol.* 2001;98:1045-1052.
45. Foxman B, Somsel P, Tallman P, et al. Urinary tract infection among women aged 40 to 65: behavioral and sexual risk factors. *J Clin Epidemiol.* 2001;54:710-718.
46. Hu KK, Boyko EJ, Scholes D, et al. Risk factors for urinary tract infections in post-menopausal women. *Arch Intern Med.* 2004;164:989-993.
47. Moore EE, Howes SE, Scholes D, et al. Sexual intercourse and risk of symptomatic urinary tract infection in post-menopausal women. *J Gen Intern Med.* 2008;23:595-599.
48. Perrotta C, Aznar M, Mejia R, et al. Oestrogens for preventing recurrent urinary tract infection in postmenopausal women. *Cochrane Database Syst Rev.* 2008(2):CD005131.

49. Bent S, Nallamothu BK, Simel DL, et al. Does this women have an acute uncomplicated urinary tract infection? *JAMA*. 2002;287:2701-2710.

50. Bent S, Saint S. The optimal use of diagnostic testing in women with acute uncomplicated cystitis. *Am J Med*. 2002;113(suppl 1A):20S-28S.

51. Nicolle LE, Madsen KS, Debeeck GO, et al. Three days of pivmecillinam or norfloxacin for treatment of acute uncomplicated urinary infection in women. *Scand J Infect Dis*. 2002;34:487-492.

52. Saint S, Scholes D, Fihn SD, et al. The effectiveness of a clinical practice guideline for the management of presumed uncomplicated urinary tract infection in women. *Am J Med*. 1999;106:636-641.

53. Nys S, van Merode T, Bartelds AIM, et al. Urinary tract infection in general practice patients: diagnostic tests versus bacteriological culture. *J Antimicrob Chemother*. 2006;57:955-958.

54. St. John A, Boyd JC, Lowes AJ, et al. The use of urinary dipstick tests to exclude urinary tract infection. *Am J Clin Pathol*. 2006;126:428-436.

55. Ferry SA, Holm SE, Stenlund H, et al. The material course of uncomplicated lower urinary tract infection in women illustrated by a randomized placebo controlled study. *Scand J Infect Dis*. 2004;36:296-301.

56. Warren JW, Abrutyn E, Hebel JR, et al. Guidelines for antimicrobial treatment of uncomplicated acute bacterial cystitis and acute pyelonephritis in women. *Clin Infect Dis*. 1999;29:745-758.

57. Katchman EA, Milo G, Paul M, et al. Three day versus long duration of antibiotic treatment for cystitis in women: systematic review and meta-analysis. *Am J Med*. 2005;118:1196-1207.

58. Gupta K, Hooton TM, Roberts PL, et al. Short-course nitrofurantoin for the treatment of acute uncomplicated cystitis in women. *Arch Intern Med*. 2007;167:2207-2212.

59. Gupta K, Sahm DF, Mayfield D, et al. Antimicrobial resistance among uropathogens that cause community-acquired urinary tract infections in women: a nationwide analysis. *Clin Infect Dis*. 2001;33:89-94.

60. Gupta K. Addressing antibiotic resistance. *Am J Med*. 2002;113(1A): 29S-34S.

61. Raz R, Chazan B, Kennes Y, et al. Israel Urinary Tract Infection Group: Empiric use of trimethoprim-sulfamethoxazole in the treatment of women with uncomplicated urinary tract infections in a geographical area with a high prevalence of TMP-SMX resistant organisms. *Clin Infect Dis*. 2002;34:1165-1169.

62. McNulty CAM, Richards J, Livermore DM, et al. Clinical evidence of laboratory-reported antibiotic resistance in acute uncomplicated urinary tract infection in primary care. *J Antimicrob Chemother*. 2006;58:1000-1008.

63. Pitout JD, Gregson DB, Church PL, et al. Community-wide outbreaks of clonally related CTX-M-14 beta-lactamase–producing *Escherichia coli* strains in the Calgary health region. *J Clin Microbiol*. 2005;43:2844-2849.

64. Thomas K, Weinbren MJ, Warner M, et al. Activity of mecillinam against ESBL producers in vitro. *J Antimicrob Chemother*. 2006;57:367-368.

65. Lawrentschuk N, Ooi J, Pang A, et al. Cystoscopy in women with recurrent urinary tract infection. *Int J Urol*. 2006;13:350-353.

66. Stunell H, Buckley O, Feeney J, et al. Imaging of acute pyelonephritis in the adult. *Eur Radiol*. 2002;17:1820-1828.

67. Stapleton A. Novel approaches to prevention of urinary tract infection. *Infect Dis Clin North Am*. 2003;17:457-472.

68. Jepson RG, Craig JC. Cranberries for preventing urinary tract infections. *Cochrane Database Syst Rev*. 2008(1):CD001321.

69. Kontiokari T, Sundquist K, Nuutinen M, et al. Randomized trial of cranberry lingonberry juice or *Lactobacillus GG* drink for the prevention of urinary tract infections in women. *BMJ*. 2001;322(7302):1571.

70. Raz R, Colodner R, Rohana Y, et al. Effectiveness of estriol-containing vaginal pessaries and nitrofurantoin macrocrystal therapy in the prevention of recurrent urinary tract infection in postmenopausal women. *Clin infect Dis*. 2003;36:1362-1368.

71. Naber KG, Cho YH, Matsumoto T, et al. Immunoactive prophylaxis of recurrent urinary tract infections: a meta-analysis. *Int J Antimicrob Agents*. 2009;33:111-119.

72. Brown P, Ki M, Foxman B. Acute pyelonephritis among adults: cost of illness and considerations for the economic evaluation of therapy. *Pharmacoeconomics*. 2005;23:1123-1142.

73. Hill JB, Sheffield JS, McIntire DD, et al. Acute pyelonephritis in pregnancy. *Obstet Gynecol*. 2005;105:18-23.

74. Kooman JP, Barendregt JNM, van der Sande FM, et al. Acute pyelonephritis: a cause of renal failure? *Netherlands J Med*. 2000;57:185-189.

75. Nahar A, Akon M, Hanes D, et al. Pyelonephritis and acute renal failure. *Am J Med*. 2004;328:121-123.

76. Piccoli B, Colla L, Burdese M, et al. Development of kidney scars after acute uncomplicated pyelonephritis: relationship with clinical laboratory and imaging data at diagnosis. *World J Urol*. 2006;24:66-73.

77. Raz R, Sakran W, Chazan B, et al. Long-term follow-up of women hospitalized for acute pyelonephritis. *Clin Infect Dis*. 2003;37:1014-1020.

78. Scholes D, Hooton TM, Roberts PL, et al. Risk factors associated with acute pyelonephritis in healthy women. *Ann Intern Med*. 2005;142: 20-27.

79. Lundstedt A-C, Leijonhufuad I, Ragnarsdottir B, et al. Inherited susceptibility to acute pyelonephritis: a family study of urinary tract infection. *J Infect Dis*. 2007;195(8):1227-1234.

80. Velasco M, Martinez JA, Moreno-Martinez A, et al. Blood cultures for women with uncomplicated acute pyelonephritis: are they necessary? *Clin Infect Dis*. 2003;45:1127-1130.

81. Pasternack 3rd EL, Topinka MA. Blood cultures in pyelonephritis: do results change therapy? *Acad Emerg Med*. 2000;7:1170.

82. Huggan PJ, Murdoch DR, Gallagher K, et al. Concomitant *Staphylococcus aureus* bacteriuria is associated with poor clinical outcomes in adults with *S. aureus* bacteraemia. *J Hosp Infect*. 2008;69:345-349.

83. Lemiale V, Renaud B, Moutereau S, et al. A single procalcitonin level does not predict adverse outcomes of women with pyelonephritis. *Eur Urol*. 2007;51:1394-1401.

84. Yang WJ, Cho IR, Seong H, et al. Clinical implication of serum C reactive protein in patients with uncomplicated acute pyelonephritis as marker of prolonged hospitalization and recurrence. *Urology*. 2009;73:19-22.

85. Demetzis J, Menias CD. State of the art: imaging of renal infections. *Emerg Radiol*. 2007;14:13-22.

86. Vourganti S, Agarwal PK, Bodner DR, et al. Ultrasonographic evaluation of renal infections. *Radiol Clin North Am*. 2006;44:763-765.

87. Kirkwood A, Harris C, Timar N, et al. Is gentamicin ototoxic to the fetus? *J Obstet Gynaecol Can*. 2007;29:140-145.

88. Talan DA, Stamm WE, Hooton TM, et al. Comparison of ciprofloxacin (7 days) and trimethoprim/sulfamethoxazole (14 days) for acute uncomplicated pyelonephritis in women. *JAMA*. 2000;283:1583-1590.

89. Peterson J, Kaul S, Khashab M, et al. A double-blind randomized comparison of levofloxacin 750 mg once-daily for five days with ciprofloxacin 400/500mg twice daily for 10 days for the treatment of complicated urinary tract infections and acute pyelonephritis. *Urology*. 2008;71:17-22.

90. Pertel PE, Haverstock D. Risk factors for a poor outcome after therapy for acute pyelonephritis. *BJU Int*. 2006;98:141-147.

91. Stevenson KB, Moore J, Colwell H, et al. Standardized infection surveillance in long term care: interfacility surveillance from a regional cohort of facilities. *Infect Control Hosp Epidemiol*. 2005;26:231-238.

92. Esclarin De Ruz A, Garcia Leoni E, Herruzo Cabrera R. Epidemiology and risk factors for urinary tract infection in patients with spinal cord injury. *J Urol*. 2000;164:1285-1289.

93. Sogaard M, Schonheyder HC, Riis A, et al. Short-term mortality in relation to age and co-morbidity in older adults with community-acquired bacteremia: a population-based cohort study. *J Am Geriatr Soc*. 2008;56:1593-1600.

94. Lee C-C, Chen S-Y, Chaing I-J, et al. Comparison of clinical manifestations and outcome of community-acquired bloodstream infections among the oldest old, elderly, and adult patients. *Medicine*. 2007;86:138-144.

95. Bahagon Y, Rauch D, Schlesinger Y, et al. Prevalence and predictive features of bacteraemic urinary tract infection in emergency department patients. *Eur J Clin Microbiol*. 2007;26:349-352.

96. Kumar A, Roberts D, Wood KE, et al. Duration of hypotension before initiation of effective antimicrobial therapy is the critical determinant of survival in human septic shock. *Crit Care Med*. 2006;34:1589-1596.

97. Jamil F. Towards a catheter free status in neurogenic bladder dysfunction: a review of bladder management options in spinal cord injury. *Spinal Cord*. 2001;39:355-361.

98. Naber KG, Llorens L, Kaniga K, et al. Intravenous doripenem at 500 milligrams versus levofloxacin at 250 milligrams, with an option to switch to oral therapy, for treatment of complicated lower urinary tract infection and pyelonephritis. *Antimicrob Agents Chemother*. 2009;53:3782-3792.

99. Tabiban JH, Gornbein J, Heidari A, et al. Uropathogens and host characteristics. *J Clin Microbiol*. 2008;46:3980-3986.

100. Kauffman CA, Vazquez JA, Sobel JD, et al. National Institute for Allergy and Infectious Diseases Mycoses Study Group: prospective, multicenter surveillance study of funguria in hospitalized patients. *Clin Infect Dis*. 2000;30:14-18.

101. Gupta K. Emerging antibiotic resistance in urinary tract pathogens. *Infect Dis Clin North Am*. 2003;17:243-259.

102. Soriano F, Tauch A. Microbiological and clinical features of *Corynebacterium urealyticum*: urinary tract stones and genomics as the Rosetta stone. *Clin Microbiol Infect*. 2008;14:632-643.

103. Ibler K, Jensen KT, Ostergaard C, et al. Six cases of *Aerococcus sanguinicola* infection. Clinical relevance and bacterial identification. *Scand J Infect Dis*. 2008;40:761-765.

104. Christensen JJ, Kilian M, Fussing V, et al. *Aerococcus urinae*: polyphasic characterization of the species. *APMIS*. 2005;113:517-525.

105. Brook I. Urinary tract and genitourinary suppurative infections due to anaerobic bacteria. *Int J Urology*. 2004;11:133-141.

106. Nicolle LE, Bradley S, Colgan R, et al. IDSA guideline for the diagnosis and treatment of asymptomatic bacteriuria in adults. *Clin Infect Dis*. 2005;40:643-654.

107. Loeb M, Bentley DW, Bradley S, et al. Development of minimum criteria for the initiation of antibiotics in residents of long term care facilities: results of a consensus conference. *Infect Control Hosp Epidemiol.* 2001;22:120-124.

108. Juthani-Mehta M, Quagliariello V, Perrelli E, et al. Clinical features to identify urinary tract infection in nursing home residents: a cohort study. *J Am Geriat Soc.* 2009;57:963-970.

109. Wullt B, Agace W, Mansson W. Bladder, bowel and bugs—bacteriuria in patients with intestinal urinary diversion. *World J Urol.* 2004;22:186-195.

110. Lo E, Nicolle L, Classen D, et al. Strategies to prevent catheter-associated urinary tract infections in acute care hospitals. *Infect Control Hosp Epidemiol.* 2008;29(S1):S41-S50.

111. Hooton TM, Bradley SF, Cardenas DD, et al. Diagnosis, prevention, and treatment of catheter-associated urinary tract infections in adults: 2009 International Clinical practice Guidelines from the Infectious Diseases Society of America. *Clin Infect Dis.* 2010;50(5):625-663.

112. Gould CV, Umscheid CA, Agarwal RK, et al. Health Care Infection Control Practices Advisory Committee: Guideline for prevention of catheter-associated urinary tract infections 2009. *Infect Control Hosp Epidemiol.* 2010;31(4):319-326.

113. Sunden F, Hakansson L, Ljungren E, et al. Bacterial interference—is deliberate colonization with *Escherichia coli* 83972 an alternative treatment for patients with recurrent urinary tract infection? *Int J Antimicrob Agents.* 2006;28(suppl 1):S26-S29.

114. Prasad A, Cevallos ME, Riosa S, et al. A bacterial interference strategy for prevention of UTI in persons practicing intermittent catheterization. *Spinal Cord.* 2009;47(7):565-569.

115. Rodhe N, Mölstad S, Englund L, et al. Asymptomatic bacteriuria in a population of elderly residents living in a community setting: prevalence, characteristics, and associated factors. *Fam Pract.* 2006;23:303-307.

116. Hooton TM, Scholes D, Stapleton AE, et al. A prospective study of asymptomatic bacteriuria in sexually active young women. *New Engl J Med.* 2000;343:991-997.

117. Nicolle LE, Zhanel GG, Harding GK. Microbiological outcomes in women with diabetes and untreated asymptomatic bacteriuria. *World J Urol.* 2006;24:61-65.

118. Zdziarski J, Svanborg C, Wullt B, et al. Molecular basis of commensalism in the urinary tract: low virulence or virulence attenuation. *Infect Immun.* 2008;76:695-703.

119. Klemm P, Hancock V, Schembri MA. Mellowing out: adaptation to commensalism by *Escherichia coli* strain 83972. *Infect Immun.* 2007;75:3688-3695.

120. Marcus RJ, Post JC, Stoodley P, et al. Biofilms in nephrology. *Expert Opin Biol Ther.* 2008;8:1159-1166.

121. Akay AF, Aflay U, Gedik A, et al. Risk factors for lower urinary tract infection and bacterial stent colonization in patients with double J ureteral stent. *Int Urol Nephrol.* 2007;39:95-98.

122. Kehinde EO, Rotimi VO, Al-Hunayan A, et al. Bacteriology of urinary tract infection associated with indwelling J ureteral stents. *J Endourol.* 2004;18:891-896.

123 Nicolle LE: Urinary tract infections in the elderly. *Clin Geriatr Med.* 2009;259:423-436.

124. Mignini L, Carroli M, Abalos E, et al. World Health Organization Asymptomatic Bacteriuria Trial Group: accuracy of diagnostic tests to detect asymptomatic bacteriuria during pregnancy. *Obstet Gynecol.* 2009;113(2 pt 1):346-352.

125. Leone M, Perrin A-S, Granier I, et al. A randomized trial of catheter change and short course of antibiotics for asymptomatic bacteriuria in catheterized ICU patients. *Intens Care Med.* 2007;33:726-729.

126. Lumbiganon P, Villar J, Laopaiboon M, et al. One-day compared with 7-day nitrofurantoin for asymptomatic bacteriuria in pregnancy: a randomized controlled trial. *Obstet Gynecol.* 2009;113(2 pt 1):339-345.

127. Grabe M. Perioperative antibiotic prophylaxis in urology. *Curr Opin Urol.* 2001;11:81-85.

128. Hooton TM, Bradley SF, Cardenas DD, et al. Diagonsis, prevention, and treatment of catheter-associated urinary tract infection in adults: 2009 international clinical practice guidelines from the Infectious Diseases Society of America. *Clin Infect Dis.* 2010;50:625-663.

129. Krieger JN, Nyberg L, Nickel JC. NIH consensus definition and classification of prostatitis. *JAMA.* 1999;281:236-237.

130. Schaeffer AJ. Clinical practice: chronic prostatitis and the chronic pelvic pain syndrome. *New Engl J Med.* 2006;355:1690-1698.

131. Etienne M, Chavanet P, Sibert L, et al. Acute bacterial prostatitis: heterogenicity in diagnostic criteria and management. Retrospective multicentric analysis of 371 patients diagnosed with acute prostatitis. *BMC Infect Dis.* 2008;8:12.

132. Nickel JC, Alexaner RB, Schaeffer AJ, et al. Chronic Prostatitis Collaborative Research Network Study Group: Leukocytes and bacteria in men with chronic bacterial prostatitis/chronic pelvic pain syndrome compared to asymptomatic controls. *J Urol.* 2003;170:818-822.

133. Krieger JN, Ross SD, Limaye AP, et al. Inconsistent localization of gram positive bacteria to prostate specific specimens from patients with chronic prostatitis. *Urology.* 2005;66:721-725.

134. Pontari MA. Chronic prostatitis/chronic pelvic pain syndrome. *Urol Clin North Am.* 2008;35:81-89.

135. Alexander RB, Propert KJ, Schaeffer AJ, et al. Ciprofloxacin or tamsulosin in men with chronic prostatitis/chronic pelvic pain syndrome. *Ann Intern Med.* 2004;141:581-589.

136. de Souza RM, Olsburgh J. Urinary tract infection in the renal transplant patient. *Nature Clin Pract.* 2008;4:252-264.

137. Maraha B, Bonten H, van Hooff H, et al. Infectious complications and antibiotic use in renal transplant recipients during a 1-year follow-up. *Clin Microbiol Infect.* 2001;7:619-625.

138. Dantas SR, Kuboyama RH, Mazzali M, et al. Nosocomial infections in renal transplant patients: risk factors and treatment implications associated with urinary tract and surgical site infections. *J Hosp Infect.* 2006;63:117-123.

139. Abbott KC, Swanson SJ, Richter ER, et al. Late urinary tract infection after renal transplantation in the United States. *Am J Kidney Dis.* 2004;44:353-362.

140. Goya N, Tanabe K, Oshima T, et al. Prevalence of urinary tract infections during outpatient follow-up after renal transplantation. *Infection.* 1997;25:101-105.

141. Valera B, Gentil MA, Cabello V, et al. Epidemiology of urinary infections in renal transplant recipients. *Transplant Proc.* 2006;38:2414-2415.

142. Chan PC, Cheng IK, Wong KK, et al. Urinary tract infections in post–renal transplant patients. *Int Urol Nephrol.* 1990;22:389-396.

143. Schmaldienst S, Dittrich E, Horl WH. Urinary tract infections after renal transplantation. *Curr Opin Urol.* 2002;12:125-130.

144. Alangaden GJ, Thyagarajan R, Gruber SA, et al. Infectious complications after kidney transplantation: current epidemiology and associated risk factors. *Clin Transplant.* 2006;20:401-409.

145. Kamath NS, John GT, Neelakantan N, et al. Acute graft pyelonephritis following renal transplantation. *Transpl Infect Dis.* 2006;8:140-147.

146. Rubin RH. Infectious disease complications of renal transplantation. *Kidney Int.* 1993;44:221-236.

147. Munoz P. Management of urinary tract infection and lymphocele in renal transplant recipients. *Clin Infect Dis.* 2001;33:S53-S57.

148. Lapchik MS, Castelo Filho AC, Pestana JO, et al. Risk factors for nosocomial urinary tract and postoperative wound infections in renal transplant patients; a matched-pair case-control study. *J Urol.* 1992;147:994-998.

149. Wilson CH, Bhatti AA, Rix DA, et al. Routine intraoperative ureteric stenting for kidney transplant recipients. *Cochrane Database Syst Rev.* 2005(4):CD004925.

150. Valera B, Gentil MA, Cabello V, et al. Epidemiology of urinary infections in renal transplant recipients. *Transplant Proc.* 2006;38:2414-2415.

151. Audard V, Amor M, Desvaux D, et al. Acute graft pyelonephritis: a potential cause of acute rejection in renal transplant. *Transplantation.* 2005;80:1128-1130.

152. Moradi M, Abbasi M, Moradi A, et al. Effect of antibiotic therapy on asymptomatic bacteriuria in kidney transplant recipients. *Urol J.* 2005;2:32-35.

153. Safdar N, Slattery WR, Knasinski V, et al. Predictors and outcomes of candiduria in renal transplant recipients. *Clin Infect Dis.* 2005;40:1413.

154. Gilbert DN. Urinary tract infections in patients with chronic renal failure. *Clin J Am Soc Nephrol.* 2006;1:327-331.

155. Zanetta G, Paparella S, Trinchieri A, et al. Infections and urolithiasis: current clinical evidence in prophylaxis and antibiotic therapy. *Arch Ital di Urol Androl.* 2008;80:5-12.

156. Miano R, Germani S, Vespasiani G. Stones and urinary tract infections. *Urol Int.* 2007;79(suppl 1):32-36.

157. Margel D, Ehrlich Y, Brown N, et al. Clinical implications of routine stone culture in percutaneous nephrolithotomy—a prospective culture. *Urology.* 2006;67:26-29.

158. Mariappan P, Smith G, Baraol SV, et al. Stone and pelvic urine culture and sensitivity are better than bladder urine as predictors of urosepsis following percutaneous nephrolithotomy. A prospective clinical study. *J Urol.* 2005;173:1610-1614.

159. Mariappan P, Loong CW. Midstream urine culture and sensitivity test is a poor predictor of infected urine proximal to the obstructing ureteral stone or infected stones: a prospective clinical study. *J Urol.* 2004;171:2142-2145.

160. Meng MV, Mario LA, McAninch JW. Current treatment and outcomes of perinephric abscesses. *J Urol.* 2002;168:1337-1340.

161. Coelho RF, Schneider-Montero ED, Mesquita JLB, et al. Renal and perinephric abscess. Analysis of 65 consecutive cases. *World J Surg.* 2007;31:431-436.

162. Shu T, Green JM, Orihucla E. Renal and perirenal abscesses in patients with otherwise anatomically normal urinary tracts. *J Urol.* 2004;172:148-150.

163. Hung C-H, Liou J-D, Yan M-Y, et al. Immediate percutaneous drainage compared with surgical drainage of renal abscess. *Int Urol Nephrol.* 2007;39:51-55.

164. Chicoskie C, Chaoui A, Kuligowska E, et al. MRI isolation of infected renal cyst in autosomal dominant polycystic kidney disease. *J Clin Imag.* 2001;25:114-117.

165. Puliatti C, Stephens MR, Kenche J, et al. Cyst infection in renal allograft recipients with adult polycystic kidney disease. The diagnostic value of labeled leukocyte scanning. Case reports. *Transplant Proc.* 2007;39:1841-1842.

166. Bleeker-Rovers CP, de Sévaux RGL, van Hamersvelt HW, et al. Diagnosis of renal and hepatic cyst infections by 18-F-fluorodeoxyglucose positron emission tomography in autosomal dominant polycystic kidney disease. *Am J Kid Dis.* 2003;41(E22):1-4.

167. Soussan M, Sberro R, Wartski M, et al. Diagnosis and localization of renal cyst infection by 18F-fluorodeoxyglucose PET/CT in polycystic kidney disease. *Ann Nucl Med.* 2008;22:529-531.

168. Akinei D, Turkbey B, Yilmaz R, et al. Percutaneous treatment of pyocystitis in patients with autosomal dominant polycystic kidney disease. *Cardiovasc Intervent Radiol.* 2008;31:926-930.

169. Hiyama L, Tang A, Miller LG. Levofloxacin penetration into a renal cyst in a patient with autosomal dominant polycystic kidney disease. *Am J Kidney Dis.* 2006;47:E9-E12.

170. Hepburn MJ, Pennick GJ, Sutton DA, et al. *Candida krusei* renal cyst infection and measurement of amphotericin B levels in cystic fluid in a patient receiving AmBisome®. *Med Microbiol.* 2003;41:163-165.

171. Thomas AA, Lane BR, Thomas AZ, et al. Emphysematous cystitis: a review of 135 cases. *BJU Int.* 2007;100:17-20.

172. Mokabberi R, Ravakhab K. Emphysematous urinary tract infections: diagnosis, treatment and survival. *Am J Med Sci.* 2007;333:111-116.

173. Soo Park B, Lee SJ, Kim YW, et al. Outcome of nephrectomy and kidney-preserving procedure for the treatment of emphysematous pyelonephritis. *Scand J Urol Nephrol.* 2006;40:332-338.

174. Somani BK, Nabi G, Thorpe P, et al. Is percutaneous drainage the new gold standard in the management of emphysematous pyelonephritis? Evidence from a systematic review. *J Urol.* 2008;179:1844-1849.

175. Zorzos I, Moutzouris V, Korakianitis G, et al. Analysis of 39 cases of xanthogranulomatous pyelonephritis with emphasis on CT findings. *Scand J Urol Nephrol.* 2003;37:342-347.

176. Gregg CR, Rogers TE, Mumford RS. Xanthogranulomatous pyelonephritis. *Curr Clin Top Infect Dis.* 1999;19:287-304.

177. Korkes F, Favoretto RL, Broglio M, et al. Xanthogranulomatous pyelonephritis: clinical experience with 41 cases. *Urology.* 2008;71:178-180.

178. Loffroy R, Guiu B, Watfa J, et al. Xanthogranulomatous pyelonephritis in adults: clinical and radiological findings in diffuse and focal forms. *Clin Radiol.* 2007;62:884-890.

179. Remer EE, Peacock WF. Pyocystis; two case reports of patients in renal failure. *J Emerg Med.* 2000;19:131-133.

180. Bibb JL, Servilla KS, Gibel LJ, et al. Pyocystis in patients on chronic dialysis. A potentially misdiagnosed syndrome. *Int Urol Nephrol.* 2002;34:415-418.

181. Falagas ME, Vergidis PI. Irrigation with antibiotic containing solutions for the prevention and treatment of infection. *Clin Microbiol Infect.* 2005;11:862-867.

182. Wise GJ, Shteynshlyuger A. An update on lower urinary tract tuberculosis. *Curr Urol Rep.* 2008;9:305-313.

183. Jacob JT, Nguyen MLT, Ray SM. Male genital tuberculosis. *Lancet Infect Dis.* 2008;8:335-342.

184. Figuerido AA, Lucon AM. Urogenital tuberculosis: update and review of 8961 cases from the world literature. *Rev Urol.* 2008;10:207-217.

185. Figueiredo AA, Lucon AM, Júnior RF, et al. Epidemiology of urogenital tuberculosis worldwide. *Int J Urol.* 2008;15:827-832.

186. Altintepe L, Tonbul Z, Ozbey I, et al. Urinary tuberculosis: ten years' experience. *Ren Fail.* 2005;27:657-661.

187. Perez S, Andrade M, Bergel P, et al. A simple algorithm for the diagnosis of AIDS-associated genitourinary tuberculosis. *Clin Infect Dis.* 2006;42:1807-1808.

188. Hsieh HC, Lu PL, Chen YH, et al. Genitourinary tuberculosis in a medical center in southern Taiwan: an eleven year experience. *J Microbiol Immunol Infect.* 2006;39:408-413.

189. Burrill J, Williams CJ, Bain G, et al. Tuberculosis: a radiologic review. *Radiographics.* 2007;27:1255-1273.

190. Hillemann D, Richter E, Rusch-Gerdes S. Use of the BACTEC Mycobacteria Growth Indicates Tube 960 automated system for recovery of *Mycobacteria* from 9,558 extrapulmonary specimens, including urine samples. *J Clin Microbiol.* 2006;44:4014-4017.

191. Chan DSG, Choy MY, Wang S, et al. An evaluation of the recovery of *Mycobacteria* from urine specimens using the automated Mycobacteria Growth Indicator Tube System (BACTEC MGIT 960). *J Med Microbiol.* 2008;57:1220-1222.

192. Figucredo AA, Lucon AM, Srougi M. Bladder augmentation for the treatment of chronic tuberculosis cystitis. Clinical and urodynamic evaluation of 25 patients after long term followup. *Neurourol Urodynamics.* 2006;25:433-440.

193. Gonzalez DY, Musher DM, Brar I, et al. Spectrum of bacille Calmette-Guérin (BCG) infection after intravesical BCG immunotherapy. *Clin Infect Dis.* 2003;36:140-148.

194. Rischmannn P, Desgrandchamps F, Malavaud B, et al. BCG intravesical installations: recommendations for side-effects management. *Eur Urol.* 2000;37(suppl 1):33-36.

195. Nadasy KA, Patel RS, Emmett M, et al. Four cases of disseminated *Mycobacterium bovis* infection following intravesical BCG installation for treatment of bladder carcinoma. *South Med J.* 2008;101:91-95.

196. Garcia JE, Thiel DD, Broderick GA. BCG pyelonephritis following intravesical therapy for transitional cell carcinoma. *Can J Urol.* 2007;14:3523-3525.

197. Kauffman CA, Vazquez JA, Sobel JD, et al. Prospective multicenter surveillance study of funguria in hospitalized patients. *Clin Infect Dis.* 2000;30:14-18.

198. Sobel JD, Kauffman CA, McKinsey D, et al. Candiduria: a randomized double-blind study of treatment with fluconazole and placebo. *Clin Infect Dis.* 2000;30:19-24.

199. Pappas PG, Kauffman CA, Andes D, et al. Clinical practice guidelines for the management of candidiasis 2009: update by the Infectious Diseases Society of America. *Clin Infect Dis.* 2009;48:503-535.

200. Drew RH, Arthur RR, Perfect JR. Is it time to abandon the use of amphotericin B bladder irrigation? *Clin Infect Dis.* 2005;40:1465-1470.

201. Sobel JD, Bradshaw SK, Lipka CJ, et al. Caspofungin in the treatment of symptomatic candiduria. *Clin Infect Dis.* 2007;44:e46-e49.

202. Paduch DA. Viral lower urinary tract infections. *Curr Urol Rep.* 2007;8:324-335.

203. Runde V, Ross S, Trinschel R, et al. Adenoviral infection from allogeneic stem cell transplantation: report on 130 patients from 9 single SCT units involved in a prospective multicenter surveillance study. *Bone Marrow Transplant.* 2001;28:51-57.

204. Christensen LS, Madsen TV, Barfod T. Persistent erythrovirus B19 urinary tract infection in an HIV-positive patient. *Clin Microbiol Infect.* 2001;7(9):507-509.

205. Green WR, Greaves WL, Frederick WR, et al. Renal infection due to adenovirus in a patient with human immunodeficiency virus infection. *Clin Infect Dis.* 1994;18(6):989-991.

206. Bruno B, Zager RA, Boeckh MJ, et al. Adenovirus nephritis in hematopoietic stem-cell transplantation. *Transplant.* 2004;77:1049-1057.

207. Waldman M, Kopp JB. Parvovirus B19–associated complications in renal transplant recipients. *Nat Clin Pract Nephrol.* 2007;3:540-550.

208. Nakazawa Y, Suzuki T, Fukuyama T, et al. Urinary excretion of ganciclovir contributes to improvement of adenovirus-associated hemorrhagic cystitis after allogeneic bone marrow transplantation. *Pediatr Transplant.* 2009;13(5):632-635.

209. Kehinde ED, Anim JT, Hira PR. Parasites of urologic importance. *Urol Int.* 2008;81:1-13.

210. Gryseels B, Polman K, Clerinx J, et al. Human schistosomiasis. *Lancet.* 2006;368:1106-1118.

211. Parkin DM. The global health burden of infection-associated cancers in the year 2002. *Int J Cancer.* 2006;118:3030-3044.

212. Ndhlouu PD, Mduluza T, Kjetland EF, et al. Prevalence of urinary schistosomiasis and HIV in females living in a rural community of Zimbabwe: does age matter? *Trans Royal Soc Trop Med Hyg.* 2007;101:433-438.

213. Salvana EMT, King CH. Schistosomiasis in travelers and immigrants. *Curr Infect Dis Rep.* 2008;10:42-49.

214. Nicolls DJ, Weld LH, Schwartz E, et al. Characteristics of schistosomiasis in travelers reported to the Geo Sentinel Surveillance Network 1997-2008. *Am J Trop Med Hyg.* 2008;79:729-734.

215. Bichler K-H, Savatovsky I. UTI Working Group of the European Association of Urology: EAU guidelines for the management of urogenital schistosomiasis. *Eur Urol.* 2006;49:998-1003.

216. Biyabani SR, Abbas F, Ghaffer S, et al. Unusual presentations of hydatid disease of the urinary tract. *J Urol.* 2000;163:896-890.

217. Yilmaz Y, Kosem M, Ceylan K, et al. Our experience in eight cases with urinary hydatid disease. A series of 372 cases held in nine different clinics. *Int J Urol.* 2006;13:1162-1165.

218. Nanda N, Michel RG, Kurdgelashvili G, et al. Trichomoniasis and its treatment. *Expert Rev Anti Infect Ther.* 2006;4:125-135.

Urinary Tract Obstruction

Jørgen Frøkiaer and Mark L. Zeidel

In adults, 1.5 to 2.0 L of urine flows daily from the renal papillae through the ureter, bladder, and urethra in an uninterrupted, unidirectional flow. Any obstruction of urinary flow at any point along the urinary tract may cause retention of urine and increased retrograde hydrostatic pressure, leading to kidney damage and interference with waste and water excretion, as well as with fluid and electrolyte homeostasis. Because the extent of recovery of renal function in obstructive nephropathy is related inversely to the extent and duration of obstruction, prompt diagnosis and relief of obstruction are essential for effective management. Fortunately, urinary tract obstruction in most cases is a highly treatable form of kidney disease.

Several terms describe urinary tract obstruction, and definitions may vary.[1-3] In the following discussion *hydronephrosis* is defined as a dilation of the renal pelvis and calices proximal to the point of obstruction. *Obstructive uropathy* refers to blockage of urine flow due to a functional or structural derangement anywhere from the tip of the urethra back to the renal pelvis that increases pressure proximal to the site of obstruction. Obstructive uropathy may or may not result in renal parenchymal damage. Such functional or pathologic parenchymal damage is referred to as *obstructive nephropathy*. It should be noted that hydronephrosis and obstructive uropathy are not interchangeable terms—dilation of the renal pelvis and calices can occur without obstruction, and urinary tract obstruction may occur in the absence of hydronephrosis.

Prevalence and Incidence

The incidence of urinary tract obstruction varies widely among different populations and depends on concurrent medical conditions, sex, and age. Unfortunately, epidemiologic reports have been based on studies of selected "populations," such as women with high-risk pregnancies and autopsied cadavers. In the United States it has been estimated that 166 patients per 100,000 population had a presumptive diagnosis of obstructive uropathy on admission to hospitals in 1985.[4] With the increasing age of the population during the past 25 years this number may be expected to rise.

A review of 59,064 autopsies of individuals varying in age from birth to 80 years noted hydronephrosis as a finding in 3.1% (3.3% of males and 2.9% of females).[5] In individuals under age 10, representing 1.5% of all autopsies, the principal causes of urinary tract obstruction were ureteral or urethral strictures, or neurologic abnormalities. It is unclear how frequently these abnormalities represented incidental findings, as opposed to clinically recognized problems.

Until the age of 20, there was no substantial sex difference in frequency of abnormalities (for details, see Chapter 74). Between the ages of 20 and 60, urinary tract obstruction was more frequent among women than among men, mainly due to the effects of uterine cancer and pregnancy. Above the age of 60, prostatic disease raised the frequency of urinary tract obstruction in men above that observed in women.

In children younger than age 15, obstruction was found in 2% of autopsies. Hydronephrosis was found in 2.2% of boys and 1.5% of girls; 80% of the hydronephrosis found occurred in individuals younger than 1 year.[6] Consistent with these findings, another autopsy series of 3172 children identified urinary tract abnormalities in 2.5%. Hydroureter and hydronephrosis were the most common findings, representing 35.9% of all cases.[7] However, it was not clear what proportion of cases was diagnosed clinically before death.

Because a high proportion of these autopsy-identified cases of obstruction likely went undetected during life, the overall prevalence of urinary tract obstruction is very likely far greater than reports suggest. This conclusion is reinforced by the fact that there are several common but temporary causes of obstruction, such as pregnancy and renal calculi.

Classification

Urinary tract obstruction can be classified by its duration (acute or chronic[8]), by whether it is congenital or acquired, and by its location (upper or lower urinary tract; supravesical, vesical, or subvesical; and so on). Acute obstruction may be associated with sudden onset of symptoms. Upper urinary tract (ureter or ureteropelvic junction [UPJ]) obstruction may present with renal colic. Lower tract (bladder or urethra) obstruction may present with disorders of micturition. By contrast, chronic urinary tract obstruction may develop insidiously and present with few or only minor symptoms, and with more general manifestations. For example, recurrent urinary tract infections, bladder calculi, and progressive renal insufficiency all may result from chronic obstruction. Congenital obstruction arises from developmental abnormalities, whereas acquired lesions develop after birth, either due to disease processes or as a result of medical interventions.[9]

Etiology

Because congenital and acquired urinary tract obstructions differ greatly in cause and clinical course, they are described separately.

Congenital Obstruction

Congenital anomalies may obstruct the urinary tract at any level from the UPJ to the tip of urethra, and the obstruction may damage one or both kidneys (Table 37-1). Although some lesions occur only rarely, as a group they represent an important cause of urinary tract obstruction, because in younger patients they often lead to severe renal impairment and may result in catastrophic end-stage renal disease.[10] Thus, this condition is also considered in detail in Chapter 75.

The widespread use of fetal ultrasonography, and its increasing sensitivity, have led to early detection in an increasing number of cases. In cases of severe obstruction early detection may lead to termination of the pregnancy or attempts to ameliorate the obstruction in utero.[10-12] However, ultrasonography may detect mild obstruction of unknown clinical

TABLE 37-1 Causes of Congenital Urinary Tract Obstruction
Ureteropelvic Junction
Ureteropelvic junction obstruction
Proximal and Middle Ureter
Ureteral folds
Ureteral valves
Strictures
Benign fibroepithelial polyps
Retrocaval ureter
Distal Ureter
Ureterovesical junction obstruction
Vesicoureteral reflux
Prune-belly syndrome
Ureteroceles
Bladder
Bladder diverticula
Neurologic conditions (e.g., spina bifida)
Urethra
Posterior urethral valves
Urethral diverticula
Anterior urethral valves
Urethral atresia
Labial fusion

significance.[10,11] UPJ obstruction is the most common cause of hydronephrosis in fetuses[13] and young children,[14] with a reported incidence of 5 cases per 100,000 population per year,[15] and it may affect adults as well.[16] There is considerable controversy as to whether all cases of obstruction early in life are clinically significant. The extensive use of fetal ultrasonography has resulted in detection of many cases that remain asymptomatic and may resolve spontaneously with simple follow-up of the child.[3,17] Most cases of congenital UPJ obstruction are diagnosed prenatally by ultrasonography.[18] The most common neonatal clinical presentation is a flank or abdominal mass.[19] By contrast, adults generally present with flank pain.[16] Because intermittent obstruction may produce symptoms that mimic those of gastrointestinal disease, diagnosis may be delayed. At any age, UPJ obstruction may be associated with kidney stones, hematuria, hypertension, or recurrent urinary tract infection.[15,16]

A detailed description of the different causes of UPJ obstruction can be found in Chapter 75, which provides a thorough discussion of the pathophysiology of proximal and distal congenital ureter obstruction. Congenital bladder outlet obstruction may be caused by mechanical or functional factors and is also discussed thoroughly in Chapter 75.

Because operative complications may be high,[20] the use of fetal[12,21] or neonatal[21,22] surgery for the relief of obstruction remains controversial.[10-12] Although bilateral obstruction requires intervention, patients with unilateral hydronephrosis are often followed without surgery, but with aggressive observation to identify the approximately 20% of patients with congenital hydronephrosis who require pyeloplasty.[22,23]

Indications for surgery in unilateral hydronephrosis include symptoms of obstruction or impaired function in a presumably salvageable hydronephrotic kidney.

Acquired Obstruction

Intrinsic Causes

Acquired urinary tract obstruction may arise from causes intrinsic to the urinary tract (i.e., intraluminal or intramural processes) or from causes extrinsic to it (Table 37-2). Intrinsic causes of obstruction may be considered according to anatomic location. Intrinsic intraluminal causes of obstruction may be intrarenal or extrarenal. Intrarenal causes involve the formation of casts or crystals within the renal tubules. These include uric acid nephropathy[24]; deposition of crystals of drugs that precipitate in the urine, such as sulfonamides,[25] acyclovir,[26] indinavir,[27] and ciprofloxacin[28]; and multiple myeloma.[29]

Uric acid nephropathy usually results from the large uric acid load released when alkylating agents abruptly kill large numbers of tumor cells in the treatment of patients with malignant hematopoietic neoplasms. The risk of uric acid nephropathy relates directly to plasma uric acid concentrations.[24] Uric acid nephropathy may also occur in the setting of disseminated adenomatous carcinoma of the gastrointestinal tract.[30]

Sulfonamide crystal deposition, once a common occurrence, became rare with the introduction of sulfonamides that are more soluble in acid urine than earlier drugs. However, sulfadiazine enjoyed a recent resurgence in use prior to the widespread adoption of highly active antiretroviral therapy, because it is relatively lipophilic and penetrates the brain well, characteristics that make it an excellent treatment for toxoplasmosis in patients with acquired immunodeficiency syndrome (AIDS). The same lipophilicity makes the drug prone to forming intrarenal crystals, however, which can lead to acute renal failure when the drug is given in large doses.[25,31] Ciprofloxacin may also precipitate in the tubular fluid, leading to crystalluria with stone formation and urinary obstruction.[28]

In patients with multiple myeloma, casts composed of Bence Jones protein may obstruct tubules and exert toxic effects on tubular epithelium, which often leads to renal failure.[29,32] As a result of damage from Bence Jones protein and other abnormalities that frequently occur in patients with multiple myeloma (e.g., hypercalcemia and amyloidosis), renal failure is the second most common cause of death in this patient population.[29,32] In rare cases multiple myeloma may also cause proteinaceous precipitates in the renal pelvis, leading to obstructive uropathy.[33]

Several intrinsic intraluminal, extrarenal, or intraureteral processes may also cause obstruction. Nephrolithiasis represents the most common cause of ureteral obstruction in younger men.[34] In the U.S. population the prevalence of symptomatic kidney stones in adults aged 20 to 74 was estimated from self-reported incidents between 1988 and 1994 to be 5.2% (6.3% of men and 4.1% of women).[35] The significance of this number is also reinforced by the large number of hospital admissions caused by calculus of the kidney and ureters, amounting to 166,000 hospital stays in 2006.[36]

Calcium oxalate stones occur most commonly. Obstruction caused by such stones occurs sporadically, tends to be acute and unilateral, and usually has no long-term impact on renal function. Of course, when a stone obstructs a solitary kidney the result can be anuric or oliguric acute renal failure. Less common types of stones, such as struvite (magnesium ammonium phosphate) and cysteine stones, more frequently cause significant renal damage, because these substances accumulate over time and often form staghorn calculi. Stones tend to lodge and to obstruct urine flow at narrowings along the ureter, including the UPJ, the pelvic brim (where the ureter arches over the iliac vessels), and the ureterovesical junction.

Other processes that cause ureteral obstruction include papillary necrosis, blood clots, and cystic inflammation. Papillary necrosis[37] may result from sickle cell disease or trait, amyloidosis,[38] analgesic abuse, acute pyelonephritis, or diabetes mellitus. Renal allografts may develop papillary necrosis as well.[39] Acute obstruction may even require surgical intervention.[40] Blood clots secondary to a benign or malignant lesion of the urinary tract or cystic inflammation of the ureter (ureteritis cystica) can also lead to obstruction and hydronephrosis.[41]

Intrinsic intramural processes that cause obstruction include failure of micturition or more rarely of ureteral peristalsis. Bladder storage of urine and micturition require a complex interplay of spinal reflexes and midbrain and cortical function.[42] Neurologic dysfunction[43] occurring in diabetes mellitus, multiple sclerosis, spinal cord injury, cerebrovascular disease, and Parkinson's disease can result from upper motor neuron damage. This can produce a variety of forms of bladder dysfunction. If the bladder fails to empty properly, it can remain filled most of the time; this results in chronic increased intravesical pressure, which is transmitted retrograde into the ureters and to the renal pelvis and kidney. In addition, failure of coordination of bladder contraction with the opening of the urethral sphincter may lead to bladder hypertrophy. In this setting, bladder filling requires increased hydrostatic pressures to stretch the hypertrophic detrusor muscle. Again the increased pressure in the bladder is transmitted up the urinary tract to the ureters and renal pelvis. Lower spinal tract injury may result in a flaccid, atonic bladder and failure of micturition, as well as recurrent urinary tract infections.

Various drugs may cause intrinsic intramural obstruction by disrupting the normal function of the smooth muscle of the urinary tract. Anticholinergic agents[44] may interfere with bladder contraction, whereas levodopa[45] may mediate an α-adrenergic increase in urethral sphincter tone that results in increased bladder outlet resistance. Long-term use of tiaprofenic acid (Surgam) can cause severe cystitis with subsequent ureteral obstruction.[46] In all circumstances when the bladder does not void normally, renal damage may develop as a consequence of recurrent urinary tract infections and back pressure produced by the accumulation of residual urine.

Acquired anatomic abnormalities of the wall of the urinary tract include ureteral strictures and benign as well as malignant tumors of the urethra, bladder, ureter, or renal pelvis.[47] Ureteral strictures may result from radiation therapy in children[48] and in adults[49] treated for pelvic or lower abdominal cancers, such as cervical cancer, or these days from analgesic abuse in rare cases.[50] Strictures may also develop as a complication of ureteral instrumentation or surgery.

Infectious organisms may also produce intrinsic obstruction of the urinary tract. *Schistosoma haematobium* infects nearly 100 million people worldwide. Although active infection can be treated and obstructive uropathy may resolve, chronic

TABLE 37-2 Causes of Acquired Urinary Tract Obstruction	
Intrinsic processes	Males
Intraluminal	Benign prostatic hyperplasia
Intrarenal	Prostate cancer
Uric acid nephropathy	Malignant neoplasms
Sulfonamides	Genitourinary tract
Acyclovir	Tumors of the kidney, ureter, bladder, urethra
Indinavir	Other sites
Multiple myeloma	Metastatic spread
Intraureteral	Direct extension
Nephrolithiasis	Gastrointestinal system
Papillary necrosis	Crohn's disease
Blood clots	Appendicitis
Fungus balls	Diverticulosis
Intramural	Chronic pancreatitis with pseudocyst formation
Functional	Acute pancreatitis
Diseases	Vascular system
Diabetes mellitus	Arterial aneurysms
Multiple sclerosis	Abdominal aortic aneurysm
Cerebrovascular disease	Iliac artery aneurysm
Spinal cord injury	Venous
Parkinson's disease	Ovarian vein thrombophlebitis
Drugs	Vasculitides
Anticholinergic agents	Systemic lupus erythematosus
Levodopa (α-adrenergic properties)	Polyarteritis nodosa
Anatomic	Wegener's granulomatosis
Ureteral strictures	Henoch-Schönlein purpura
Schistosomiasis	Retroperitoneal processes
Tuberculosis	Fibrosis
Drugs (e.g., nonsteroidal antiinflammatory agents)	Idiopathic
Ureteral instrumentation	Drug induced
Urethral strictures	Inflammatory
Benign or malignant tumors of the renal pelvis, ureter, bladder	Ascending lymphangitis of the lower extremities
Extrinsic processes	Chronic urinary tract infection
Reproductive tract	Tuberculosis
Females	Sarcoidosis
Uterus	Iatrogenic (multiple abdominal surgical procedures)
Pregnancy	Enlarged retroperitoneal nodes
Tumor (fibroids, endometrial or cervical cancer)	Tumor invasion
Endometriosis	Tumor mass
Uterine prolapse	Hemorrhage
Ureteral ligation (surgical)	Urinoma
Ovary	Biologic agents
Tubo-ovarian abscess	Actinomycosis
Tumor	
Cyst	

schistosomiasis (bilharziasis) may develop in untreated cases, leading to irreversible ureteral or bladder fibrosis and obstruction.[51] As for other infections, 5% of patients with tuberculosis have genitourinary involvement,[52] predominantly unilateral tuberculous stricture of the ureter.[52] Mycoses such as *Candida albicans* or *Candida tropicalis* infection also may result in obstruction due to intraluminal obstruction (fungus ball) or invasion of the ureteral wall.[53]

Extrinsic Causes

Acquired extrinsic urinary tract obstruction occurs in a wide variety of settings. The relatively high frequency of obstructive uropathy caused by processes in the female reproductive tract such as pregnancy and pelvic neoplasms results in higher rates of urinary tract obstruction in younger women than in younger men.[2]

The advent of routine abdominal and fetal ultrasonography in pregnant women has revealed that more than two thirds of women entering their third trimester of pregnancy demonstrate some degree of dilation of the collecting system,[54] most often resulting from mechanical ureteral obstruction.[54] This temporary form of obstruction is usually observed above the point at which the ureter crosses the pelvic brim and affects the right ureter more often than the left.[54] The vast majority of these cases are subclinical and appear to resolve completely soon after delivery.[55]

Clinically significant obstructive uropathy in pregnancy almost always presents with flank pain.[56] In these cases, ultrasonography serves as a useful initial screening test,[19] and magnetic resonance imaging (MRI) can be used if the ultrasonographic study is not conclusive.[56] Of course, the diagnostic evaluation must be tailored to minimize fetal radiation exposure. If the obstruction is significant, a ureteral stent can be placed cystoscopically, and its efficacy can be monitored with repeated follow-up ultrasonography.[57] The stent can be left in place for the duration of pregnancy, if needed. Clinically significant ureteral obstruction is rare in pregnancy, and bilateral obstruction leading to acute renal failure is exceptionally rare.[56] Conditions in pregnancy that may predispose to obstructive uropathy and acute renal failure include multiple fetuses, polyhydramnios, an incarcerated gravid uterus, and a solitary kidney.[55]

Pelvic malignancies, especially cervical adenocarcinomas, represent the second most common cause of extrinsic obstructive uropathy in women.[58] In older women, uterine prolapse and other failures of normal pelvic floor tone may cause obstruction, with hydronephrosis developing in 5% of patients.[59] In this setting prolapse may lead to compression of the ureter by uterine blood vessels. In addition, prolapse has been associated with urinary tract infection, sepsis, pyonephrosis, and renal insufficiency. Prolapse of other pelvic organs due to weakening of the pelvic floor may also result in obstruction.[59]

Various benign pelvic abnormalities may cause ureter obstruction, including uterine tumors or cystic ovary and pelvic inflammatory disease, particularly a tubo-ovarian abscess. Pelvic lipomatosis, a disease with an unclear etiology that is seen more often in men, is another rare reason for compressive urinary tract obstruction.[60] Although endometriosis only rarely results in ureteral obstruction,[61] it should be included in the differential diagnosis any time a premenopausal woman experiences unilateral obstruction. The onset of obstruction may be insidious, and the process is usually confined to the pelvic portion of the ureter.[61] Ureteral involvement may be intrinsic or extrinsic, with extrinsic compression arising principally from adhesions associated with the endometriosis. Because ureteral involvement may come on slowly and may be unilateral, it is important to screen for obstructive uropathy in advanced cases of endometriosis,[61] preferably using computed tomography (CT), since ultrasonography may not reveal hydronephrosis if adhesions are preventing dilatation of the ureter above the site of obstruction.[62] When surgery of any kind is contemplated in patients with endometriosis, it is all the more important to image the ureters, because they cross the anticipated surgical field and may well be near, or attached to, adhesions.[61,62] It is important to note that 52% of inadvertent ligations of the ureter in abdominal and retroperitoneal operations occur in gynecologic procedures.[63]

Above age 60 obstructive uropathy occurs more commonly in men than in women. Benign prostatic hyperplasia, which is by far the most common cause of urinary tract obstruction in men, produces some symptoms of bladder outlet obstruction in 75% of men aged 50 years and older.[64,65] It is likely that the proportion of affected older men would be higher if physicians routinely took a detailed history seeking symptoms.[64,65] Presenting symptoms of bladder outlet obstruction include difficulty initiating micturition, weakened urinary stream, dribbling at the end of micturition, incomplete bladder emptying, and nocturia. The diagnosis may be established by history and urodynamic studies, as well as imaging in some cases.[64-66]

Malignant genitourinary tumors occasionally cause urinary tract obstruction. Bladder cancer is the second most common cause (after cervical cancer) of malignant obstruction of the ureter.[2] Prostate cancer may cause obstruction[67] by compression of the bladder neck, invasion of the ureteral orifices, or metastatic involvement of the ureter or pelvic nodes.[68] Although urothelial tumors of the renal pelvis, ureter, and urethra are very rare, they also may lead to urinary obstruction.[69]

Several gastrointestinal processes may rarely cause obstructive uropathy. Inflammation in Crohn's disease may extend into the retroperitoneum, leading to obstruction of the ureters,[70] usually on the right side.[71] In addition, several gastrointestinal diseases may cause oxalosis, which leads to nephrolithiasis.[72] Appendicitis may lead to retroperitoneal scarring or abscess formation in children and young adults,[73] resulting in obstruction of the right ureter. Diverticulitis in older patients[74] may rarely cause obstruction of the left ureter. Fecaloma is another rare cause of bilateral ureteral obstruction.[75] Chronic pancreatitis with pseudocyst formation sometimes causes left ureteral obstruction[76] and may very rarely cause bilateral obstruction.[77] Acute pancreatitis may result in right-sided obstruction.[78]

Vascular abnormalities or diseases may also lead to obstruction. Abdominal aortic aneurysm is the most common vascular cause of urinary obstruction,[79] which may be produced by direct pressure of the aneurysm on the ureter or associated retroperitoneal fibrosis. Aneurysms of the iliac vessels may also cause obstruction of the ureters as they cross over the vessels.[79] Rarely, the ovarian venous system may cause right ureteral obstruction.[80] In addition, and also rarely, vasculitis caused by systemic lupus erythematosus,[81] polyarteritis nodosa,[82] Wegener's granulomatosis,[83] and Henoch-Schönlein purpura[84,85] have been reported to cause obstruction.

Retroperitoneal processes, such as tumor invasion leading to compression, as well as retroperitoneal fibrosis, can result in obstruction. The major extrinsic causes of retroperitoneal obstruction, accounting for 70% of all cases, are tumors of the colon, bladder, prostate, ovary, uterus, or cervix.[2,86,87] When retroperitoneal fibrosis[86,87] is idiopathic, it usually involves the middle third of the ureter and affects men and women equally, predominantly those in the fifth and sixth decades of life.[87] Retroperitoneal fibrosis may also be induced by drugs (e.g., methysergide) or may occur as a consequence of scarring from multiple abdominal surgical procedures.[87] It may also be associated with conditions as varied as gonorrhea, sarcoidosis, chronic urinary tract infections, Henoch-Schönlein purpura, tuberculosis, biliary tract disease, and inflammatory processes of the lower extremities with ascending lymphangitis.[87]

Malignant neoplasms can obstruct the urinary tract by direct extension or by metastasis.[88] Such obstruction may be managed by retrograde stenting as a practical but conservative therapy, and treatment should be tailored to each patient.[88] As noted earlier, cervical cancer is the most common obstructing malignant neoplasm, followed by bladder cancer.[2,89,90] Rare childhood tumors such as pelvic neurofibromas can induce upper urinary tract obstruction in up to 60% of patients.[91] Wilms' tumor may obstruct via local compression of the renal pelvis.[92]

Miscellaneous inflammatory processes can also result in obstruction. These include granulomatous causes such as sarcoidosis[93] and chronic granulomatous disease of childhood.[94] Amyloid deposits may produce isolated involvement of the ureter. Furthermore, a pelvic mass or inflammatory process associated with actinomycosis may cause external ureteral compression.[95,96] Retrovesical echinococcal cyst can also impede urine flow.[97] Retroperitoneal malacoplakia is also a rare cause of urinary tract obstruction.[98] Polyarteritis nodosa associated with hepatitis B has also been reported to result in bilateral hydronephrosis.[99]

Hematologic abnormalities induce obstruction of the urinary tract by a variety of mechanisms. In the retroperitoneum, enlarged lymph nodes or a tumor mass may compress the ureter.[100] Alternatively, precipitation of cellular breakdown products such as uric acid (see earlier) and paraproteins, as in multiple myeloma, may cause intrinsic obstruction. In patients with clotting abnormalities, blood clots or hematomas may obstruct the urinary tract, as can sloughed papillae in patients with sickle cell disease or analgesic nephropathy (see earlier). Although leukemic infiltrates rarely cause obstruction in adults, in children they lead to obstruction in 5% of patients.[101] Lymphomatous infiltration of the kidney occurs relatively commonly, but obstruction related to ureteral involvement in lymphoma is rarer.[102]

Clinical Aspects

Urinary tract obstruction may cause symptoms referable to the urinary tract. However, even patients with severe obstruction may be asymptomatic, especially when the obstruction develops gradually or in patients with spinal cord injury.[103] The clinical presentation often depends on the rate of onset of the obstruction (acute or chronic), the degree of obstruction (partial or complete), whether the obstruction is unilateral or bilateral, and whether the obstruction is intrinsic or extrinsic.

Pain in obstructive uropathy is usually associated with obstruction of sudden onset, as from a kidney stone, blood clot, or sloughed papilla, and appears to result from abrupt stretching of the renal capsule or the wall of the collecting system, where C-type sensory fibers are located. The severity of the pain appears to correlate with the rate, rather than the degree, of distension. The pain may present as typical renal colic (sharp pain that may radiate toward the urethral orifice), or in patients with reflux, the pain may radiate to the flank only during micturition. With UPJ obstruction, flank pain may develop or worsen when the patient ingests large quantities of fluids or receives diuretics.[104]

Early satiety and weight loss may be another symptom.[105] Ileus or other gastrointestinal symptoms may be associated with the pain, especially in cases of renal colic, so that it can be difficult to differentiate obstruction from gastrointestinal disease. Sometimes, patients notice changes in urine output as obstruction sets in. Urinary tract obstruction is one of the few conditions that can result in anuria, usually because of bladder outlet obstruction or obstruction of a solitary kidney at any level. Obstruction may also occur with no change in urine output. Alternatively, episodes of polyuria may alternate with periods of oliguria. Recurrent urinary tract infections may be the only sign of obstruction, particularly in children. As mentioned earlier, prostatic disease with significant bladder outlet obstruction often presents as difficulty initiating urination, decreased size or force of the urine stream, postvoiding dribbling, and incomplete emptying.[106] Spastic bladder or irritative symptoms such as frequency, urgency, and dysuria may result from urinary tract infection. The appearance of obstructive symptoms synchronous with the menstrual cycle may also be a sign of endometriosis.[107]

On physical examination, several signs may suggest urinary obstruction. A palpable abdominal mass, especially in neonates, may represent hydronephrosis, and in all age groups, a palpable suprapubic mass may represent a distended bladder. On laboratory examination, proteinuria, if present, is generally less than 2 g/day. Microscopic hematuria is a common finding, but gross hematuria may develop occasionally such as, in rare cases, with appendiceal granuloma.[108] The urine sediment is often unremarkable. Less common manifestations of urinary tract obstruction include deterioration of renal function without apparent cause, hypertension,[109] polycythemia, and abnormal urine acidification and concentration.

Diagnosis

Careful history taking and physical examination represent the cornerstone of diagnosis, often leading to detection of urinary tract obstruction and suggesting the reason for it. The findings of the history and the physical examination focus the evaluation, so that minimal time and expense are incurred in determining the cause of the obstruction.

History and Physical Examination

Important information in the history includes the type and duration of symptoms (voiding difficulties, flank pain, decreased urine output), presence or absence of urinary tract infections and their number and frequency (especially in children), pattern of fluid intake and urine output, and any symptoms of chronic renal failure (such as fatigue, sleep disturbance, loss of appetite, pruritus). In addition, relevant earlier medical history should be reviewed in detail to look for predisposing causes, including stone disease, malignancies, gynecologic diseases, recent surgery, AIDS, and drug use.

The physical examination should focus first on vital signs, which may provide evidence of infection (fever, tachycardia) or of frank volume overload (hypertension). Evaluation of the patient's volume status will guide fluid therapy. The abdominal examination may reveal a flank mass, which may represent hydronephrosis (especially in children), or a suprapubic mass, which may represent a distended bladder. Features of chronic renal failure, such as pallor (anemia), drowsiness (uremia), neuromuscular irritability (metabolic abnormalities), or pericardial friction rub (uremic pericarditis), may also be noted. A thorough pelvic examination for women and a rectal examination for all patients are mandatory.

Careful history taking and a well-directed and complete physical examination often reveal the specific cause of urinary obstruction. Coexistence of obstruction and infection is a urologic emergency, and appropriate studies (ultrasonography, CT, MRI, or, less commonly today, intravenous urography) must be performed immediately, so that the obstruction can be relieved promptly.

Biochemical Evaluation

The laboratory evaluation includes urinalysis and examination of the sediment on a fresh specimen by an experienced observer. Unexplained renal failure with benign urinary sediment findings should suggest urinary tract obstruction. Microscopic hematuria without proteinuria may suggest calculus or tumor. Pyuria and bacteriuria may indicate pyelonephritis. Bacteriuria alone may suggest stasis. Crystals in a freshly voided specimen should lead to consideration of nephrolithiasis or intrarenal crystal deposition.

Hematologic evaluation includes hemoglobin level, hematocrit, and mean corpuscular volume (to identify anemia of chronic renal disease) and white blood cell count (to identify possible hematopoietic system neoplasm or infection). Serum electrolyte levels (Na^+, Cl^-, K^+, and HCO_3^-), blood urea nitrogen concentration, creatinine concentration, and levels of Ca^{2+}, phosphorus, Mg^{2+}, uric acid, and albumin should be measured. These will help identify disorders of distal nephron function (impaired acid excretion or osmoregulation) and uremia.

Urinary chemistry panels may also suggest distal tubular dysfunction (high urine pH, isosthenuric urine), inability to reabsorb sodium normally (urinary Na^+ > 20 mEq/L, fractional excretion of Na^+ [FE_{Na}] > 1%, and osmolality < 350 mOsm). Alternatively, in acute obstruction urinary chemistry values may be consistent with prerenal azotemia (urinary Na^+ < 20 mEq/L, FE_{Na} < 1%, and osmolality < 500 mOsm).[8]

Novel biomarkers relevant for functional as well as cellular and molecular changes are being developed to serve as an index of renal injury and to predict renal reserve or recovery after reconstruction. Attempts to predict the clinical outcome of congenital unilateral UPJ obstruction in newborns by urine proteome analysis is an example of this powerful new technology. Polypeptides in the urine were identified and enabled diagnosis of the severity of obstruction, and using this technique the clinical evolution was predicted with 94% precision in neonates with UPJ obstruction.[110]

Evaluation by Medical Imaging

The history, physical examination, and initial laboratory studies should guide the radiologic evaluation. Pain, degree of renal dysfunction, and presence or absence of infection dictate the speed and nature of the evaluation. Numerous imaging techniques are available. Each has advantages and disadvantages, including the ability to identify the site and cause of the obstruction and to separate functional obstruction from mere dilation of the urinary tract. Patient-specific factors, such as the risk of radiocontrast administration in the setting of renal insufficiency, or the risk of exposure to radiation in pregnant women, must also be weighed.[19]

Plain Radiography of the Abdomen

As noted earlier, acute abdominal or flank pain with normal or mildly impaired renal function suggests a renal calculus. In this setting, plain radiographs of the abdomen (kidney, ureter, and bladder) can provide information on the size and overall contour of the kidneys. Because 90% of calculi are radiopaque, they may be detected along the course of the ureter or even in the bladder (Figure 37-1). If necessary, plain radiographs can be taken in pregnant patients with appropriate shielding. In addition to calculi, the plain radiograph may reveal radiopaque foreign bodies such as stents (see Figure 37-1).

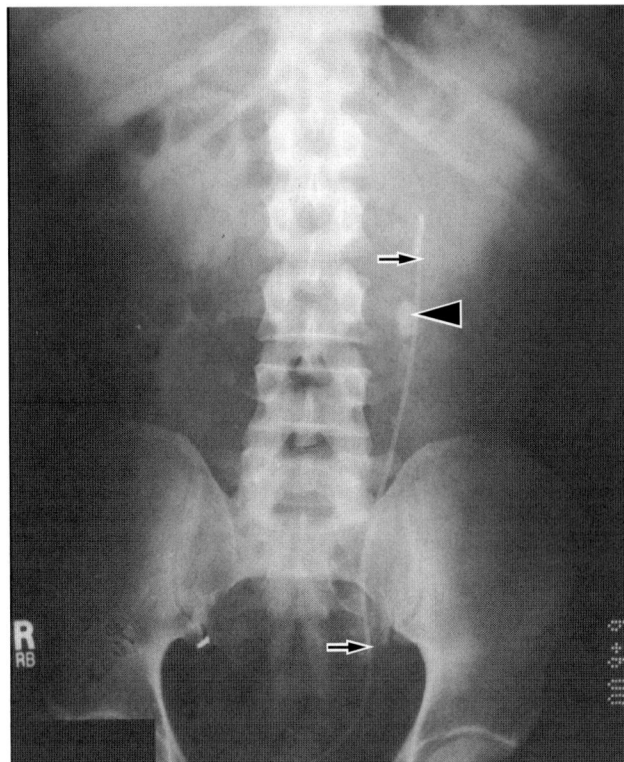

FIGURE 37-1 Plain radiograph of the abdomen. Calcifications are seen overlapping the left ureter (*arrowhead*). *Small arrows* indicate a stent inserted into the kidney to relieve the obstruction.

Ultrasonography

Ultrasonography is the preferred screening modality when obstruction is suspected[111,112] because it is highly sensitive for hydronephrosis,[111,112] it is safe and can be repeated frequently, it is low in cost, and it does not use ionizing radiation, which makes it ideal for pregnant patients,[19] infants, and children.[113] Moreover, because ultrasonography requires no radiographic contrast agent, it is well suited to rule out obstruction as a cause of renal insufficiency in patients in whom the use of contrast is contraindicated, including those with an elevated or rising serum creatinine level,[111,112] patients allergic to contrast material, and pediatric patients.

In addition to detecting hydronephrosis, ultrasonography can reveal dilatation of the renal pelvis and calices. It may also determine the size and shape of the kidney, and may demonstrate thinned cortex in the case of severe long-standing hydronephrosis (Figure 37-2). Finally, ultrasonography may detect perinephric abscesses, which may complicate some forms of obstructive nephropathy.

Ultrasonography is both highly sensitive and highly specific in detecting hydronephrosis, with the rates approaching 90%.[111,112,114,115] Importantly, ultrasonography works equally well in patients with azotemia, in whom radiocontrast studies are contraindicated.[115] Hydronephrosis is detected as a dilated collecting system—an anechoic central area surrounded by echogenic parenchyma. However, in some cases of acute urinary obstruction, ultrasonography may fail to detect pathology. During the first 48 hours of obstruction,[111,112,114,115] or when hydronephrosis is absent despite obstruction detected by CT, ultrasonography may reveal no abnormality.[116] False-negative results also occur in cases of dehydration, staghorn calculi,

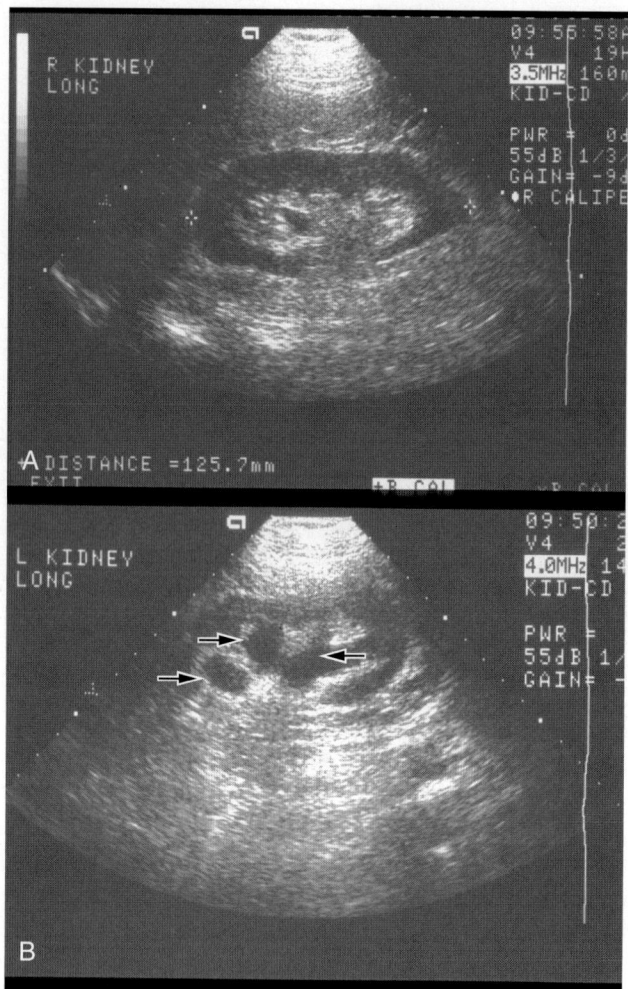

FIGURE 37-2 Renal ultrasonograms. **A,** Normal kidney. **B,** Hydronephrotic kidney with dilated calices and pelvis (*arrows*).

Antenatal Ultrasonography

Prenatal diagnosis of renal pathology was first described in the 1970s.[123] After that, routine maternal ultrasonography using devices of ever-increasing resolution resulted in a fourfold increase in antenatal detection of congenital urinary tract obstruction.[124] Prenatal hydronephrosis is diagnosed in between 1 in 100 and 1 in 500 maternal-fetal ultrasonography studies.[10,11,101]

Either obstructive or nonobstructive processes can cause dilation of the urinary tract. Overall, the causes of urinary tract obstruction are as follows: obstruction of the UPJ (44%) or the ureterovesical junction (21%); multicystic dysplastic kidney, ureterocele or ureteral ectopia, and duplex kidney (12%); posterior urethral valves (9%); urethral atresia; sacrococcygeal teratoma; and hydrometrocolpos (fluid distention of the uterus).[102,125-127] Nonobstructive causes of urinary tract dilation include vesicoureteral reflux (14%), physiologic dilation, prune-belly syndrome, renal cystic disease, and megacalycosis (massive dilatation of the renal calyces).[102,125-127]

Increased renal echogenicity and oligohydramnios (inadequate quantities of amniotic fluid) in the setting of bladder distention are highly predictive (87%) of an obstructive etiology. This finding is important in the prenatal counseling and treatment of boys with bilateral hydronephrosis and marked bladder dilation.[128]

Determining which cases require intervention and which can be treated conservatively remains a major issue in prenatal ultrasonographic diagnosis of urinary tract obstruction. Persistent postnatal renal abnormalities appear likely when the anteroposterior diameter of the fetal renal pelvis measures more than 6 mm at less than 20 weeks, more than 8 mm at 20 to 30 weeks, and more than 10 mm at more than 30 weeks of gestation.

The long-term morbidity of mild hydronephrosis (pelviectasis without caliceal dilation) is low.[10,11] Moderate hydronephrosis (dilated pelvis and calices without parenchymal thinning) may be associated with gradual improvement in severity of dilation, without loss of anticipated relative renal function. Cases of severe hydronephrosis (pelvicaliceal dilation with parenchymal thinning) may require surgical intervention to treat declining renal function, infection, or symptoms.

Overall, because approximately 5% to 25% of patients with antenatal hydronephrosis will ultimately require surgical intervention,[101,129] careful long-term follow-up of these patients is required throughout childhood and into adulthood. Almost all patients with antenatal hydronephrosis undergo postnatal ultrasonography in the first days of life, with recognition that most cases of mild hydronephrosis will resolve without intervention.[130]

Functional imaging is required to define residual renal function in patients with hydronephrosis and to monitor its course over postnatal life. However, in the absence of bilateral hydronephrosis, a solitary kidney, or suspected posterior urethral valve, functional imaging can be deferred until the first 4 to 6 weeks of life.[101] Otherwise, nuclear medicine examination with radioisotope renography should be performed. In the United States antibiotic prophylaxis is initiated for most infants with prenatally detected hydronephrosis that is confirmed by postnatal studies pending the outcome of further evaluation.[101] This is not the routine treatment in Europe. An infection in the setting of ureteral obstruction can cause significant morbidity, however, resulting in an infant with sepsis, and renal

nephrocalcinosis,[115] retroperitoneal fibrosis,[117] misinterpretation of caliectasis as cortical cysts,[118] and tumor encasement of the collecting system.[119] Dilatation of the collecting system without obstruction may be observed in up to 50% of patients with urinary diversion through ileal conduits.[120]

To enhance the sensitivity and specificity of ultrasonography, some investigators have developed special obstruction scoring systems, which grade increased echogenicity, parenchymal rims of more than 5 mm, contralateral hypertrophy, resistive index (RI) of 1.10 or more, and other features to differentiate between obstructing and nonobstructing hydronephrosis.[113] False-positive findings may result from a large extrarenal pelvis, parapelvic cysts,[121] vesicoureteral reflux, or high urine flow rate.[115] In addition, ultrasonography may only suggest, but not reveal, the presence or cause of the obstruction. Importantly, although ultrasonography is a useful screening test, it does not define renal function and cannot completely rule out obstruction, especially when prior clinical suspicion is high. Every experienced nephrologist has seen cases of obstruction with negative results on ultrasonography. Therefore, the diagnosis of obstruction must still be considered in patients with worsening renal function, chronic azotemia, or acute changes in renal function or urine output, even in the absence of hydronephrosis on the ultrasonogram.[122]

damage is a potential comorbidity. Oral amoxicillin (10 mg/kg/day) is the most commonly used prophylactic antibiotic.[101]

Duplex Doppler Ultrasonography

Ultrasonography has emerged as the primary imaging modality when either renal obstruction or renal medical disease is suspected on the basis of clinical and laboratory findings. In urinary tract obstruction, pathophysiologic changes affecting the pressure in the collecting system and kidney perfusion are well imaged, and form the basis for the correct interpretation of real-time ultrasonography and color duplex Doppler ultrasonography. As detailed earlier, ultrasonography is very sensitive in the detection of collecting system dilatation ("hydronephrosis"); however, obstruction is not synonymous with dilatation, because either obstructive or nonobstructive dilatation may be present. To differentiate these conditions, color duplex Doppler ultrasonography with measurement of the RI in the intrarenal arteries may be helpful, because obstruction (except in the acute and subacute stages) leads to intrarenal vasoconstriction with a consecutive increase in the RI above the upper limit of 0.7, whereas nonobstructive dilatation does not.[102,125] Diuretic challenge to the kidney may further enhance these differences in RI between obstruction and dilatation.[126]

Intravenous Urography

Intravenous urography (IVU), also known as *intravenous pyelography* (IVP), may be useful when history, physical examination, or ultrasonography findings suggest upper urinary tract obstruction in nonpregnant patients with normal renal function and no allergies to contrast material (Figure 37-3). Urography may provide data on the relative function of each kidney and anatomic information, particularly for the ureter, as well as the location of the obstruction. Until recently IVU was the gold standard for imaging in acute renal colic,[131] although recent data have questioned its diagnostic efficacy.[131]

The procedure has drawbacks. Contrast nephrotoxicity may be significant in any patient with obstruction and impaired renal function, but especially in high-risk patients such as those with diabetes and prior chronic renal insufficiency.[132] Kidneys may not be well visualized in patients with low glomerular filtration rate (GFR) because of delayed excretion of the contrast agent, or, in cases of severe obstruction, too little contrast material may be excreted on the affected side to allow adequate identification of the site of obstruction. All these concerns have led to replacement of IVU with CT, ultrasonography, and MRI in many cases. Nevertheless, because it is readily available, well known to most physicians, capable of identifying the site of obstruction in a significant portion of cases (especially in cases of intraluminal noncalculous obstruction), and able to depict the anatomy of the urinary tract, IVU may be a useful and informative diagnostic tool in selected cases.[133] In children, magnetic resonance (MR) urography and ultrasonography have replaced IVU in most cases (see later).

Computed Tomography

CT was initially used mainly in cases with a high index of clinical suspicion in which ultrasonography or IVU had failed to identify obstruction.[134] Given the higher resolution of

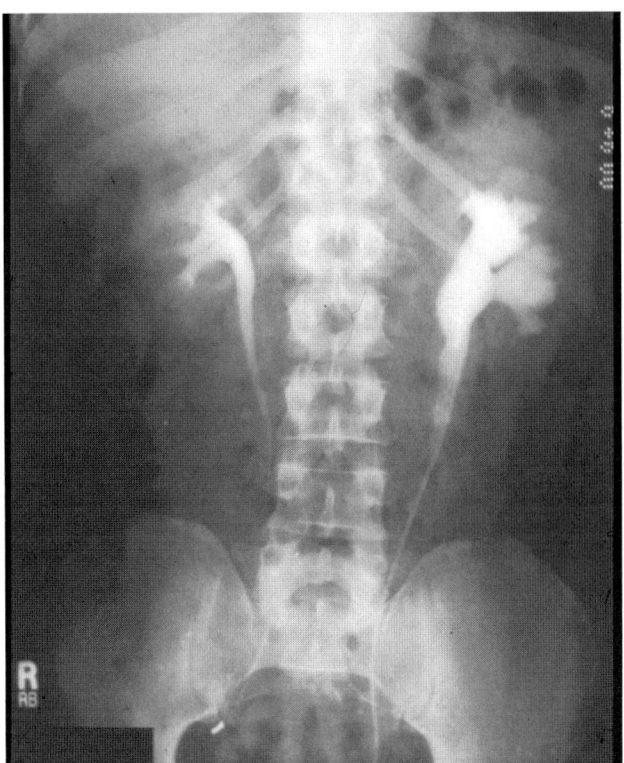

FIGURE 37-3 Intravenous pyelogram shows normal (right) kidney and dilated collecting system (left). The dilatation (obstruction) was relieved with placement of a stent.

multidetector row CT scanners, this approach is rapidly supplanting IVU for evaluation of the upper urinary tract.[134,135] CT has a particular advantage because it can visualize a dilated collecting system even without contrast enhancement. It can also be performed much more quickly than IVU, especially in cases in which renal impairment or obstruction would delay contrast excretion by the affected kidney in IVU (Figure 37-4). Non–contrast-enhanced CT identifies ureteral stones more effectively than IVU and detects the presence or absence of ureteral obstruction as effectively as IVU.[136,137]

Because of its exquisite sensitivity to density, CT can identify even radiolucent stones, because even uric acid stone density is at least 100 Hounsfield units, which is higher than soft tissue density on CT (usually 10 to 70 Hounsfield units). CT is especially effective in identifying extrinsic causes of obstruction (e.g., retroperitoneal fibrosis, lymphadenopathy, hematoma).

Helical CT has also proven to be an accurate and noninvasive method of demonstrating crossing vessels in UPJ obstruction.[138] CT can detect extraurinary pathology and can establish nonurogenital causes of pain. All of these advantages establish non–contrast-enhanced helical CT as the diagnostic study of choice for the evaluation of patients with acute flank pain.[116]

CT is very useful in delineating the pelvic organs, such as the bladder and prostate, and may demonstrate abnormalities such as an obstructed and distended bladder (Figure 37-5) secondary to an enlarged prostate. Ultrasonography may be the first method of diagnosis in this setting (Figure 37-6), but CT resolution and depiction of details are usually superior to those of ultrasonography.[134]

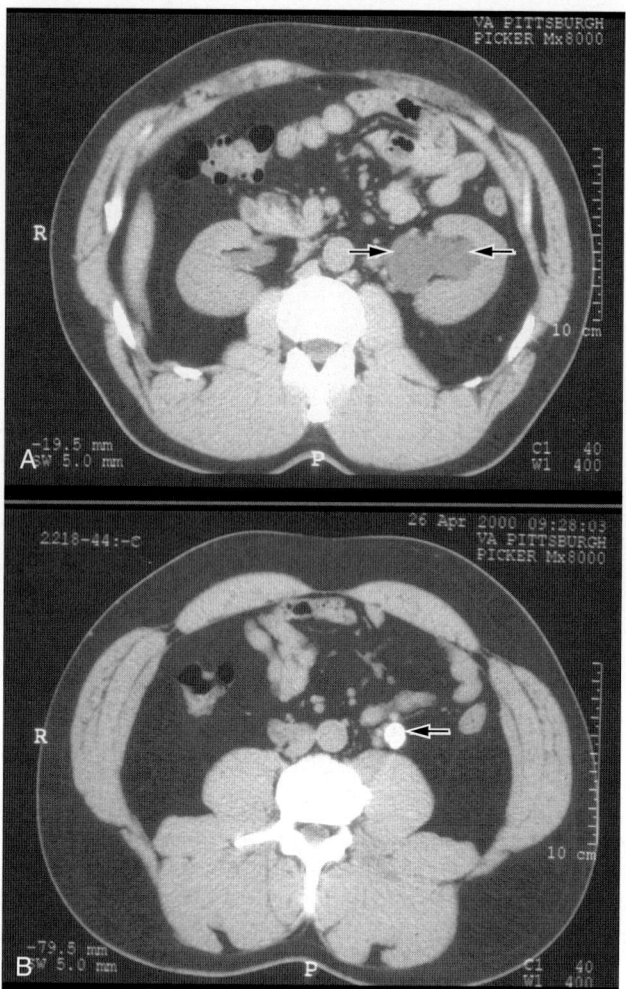

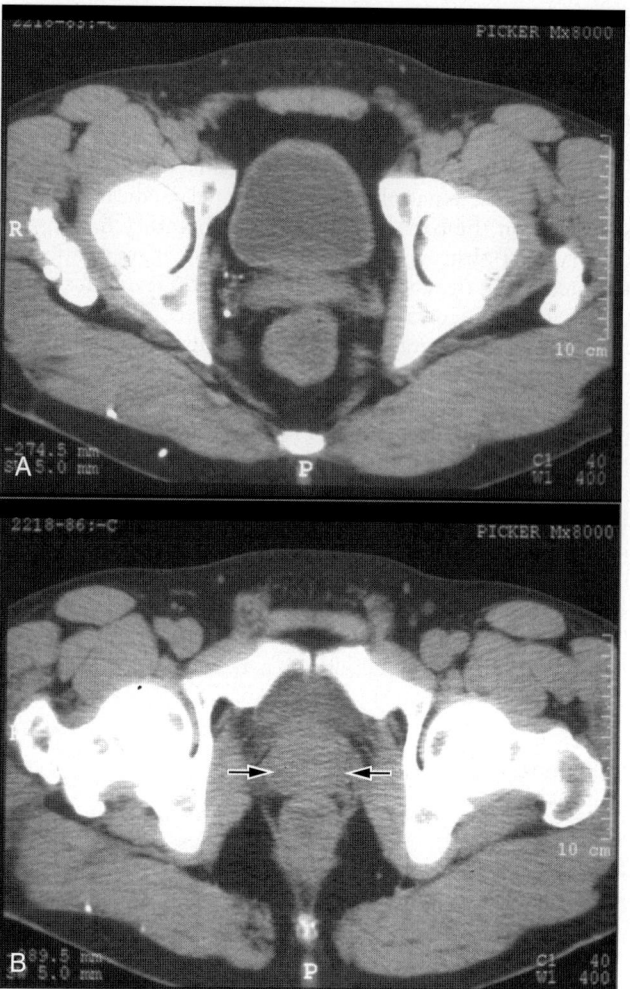

FIGURE 37-4 Computed tomographic noncontrast study. **A,** Left hydronephrosis with dilated renal pelvis (*arrows*); with normal kidney on right. **B,** Reason for obstruction: left midureteral stone (*arrow*).

FIGURE 37-5 Computed tomographic scan of the pelvis. **A,** Large amount of postvoiding residual urine in the bladder. **B,** Enlarged prostate (*arrows*), leading to urinary retention.

Isotopic Renography

Isotopic renography, or renal scintigraphy, is helpful in diagnosing upper urinary tract obstruction and provides information on the differential renal function (DRF) of the two kidneys while avoiding the risk of radiocontrast agents.[139,140] Radioisotope is injected intravenously, and its dynamic uptake and excretion by the kidneys is followed using imaging with a gamma camera. Although this method gives a functional assessment of the obstructed kidney, anatomic definition is poor. Isotopic renography is typically used to estimate the fractional contribution of each kidney to overall renal function.

The noninvasive character of this examination and the high reproducibility of results make it excellent for monitoring patients, and the findings help the urologist to decide whether to perform surgical intervention or watchful waiting.[22] In addition, the test can be repeated after the relief of obstruction to gauge the extent to which removal of the obstruction has restored renal function.

Diuretic renography was introduced into clinical practice in 1978[141] and may be used to distinguish between hydronephrosis or pelvic dilation with obstruction and dilation without obstruction. The method was developed, applied, and validated in adults.[141] This is particularly important when using diuretic renography in children and infants, in whom it

is not always easy to distinguish between dilation and obstruction. After administration of radioisotope, when the isotope appears in the renal pelvis, a loop diuretic such as furosemide is given intravenously. If stasis is causing the dilation, the induced diuresis may result in prompt washout of the tracer from the renal pelvis. By contrast, when dilation is caused by obstruction, the washout does not occur.[142]

Data should be interpreted visually and by quantitative measurement, including determination of the half-life ($t_{1/2}$) for the excretion of the tracer from the collecting system.[143] It is generally accepted that clearance of the isotope from the collecting system with a $t_{1/2}$ of less than 15 minutes is normal and that a $t_{1/2}$ of more than 20 minutes usually indicates obstruction in adults. Renal excretion of the tracer with a $t_{1/2}$ between 15 and 20 minutes is considered equivocal. An absent or blunted diuretic response resulting from decreased renal function or grossly dilated pelvis makes interpretation of the test difficult and limits its usefulness and may require the use of support tools to increase the diagnostic performance.[144]

In children diuretic renography is also a very important method for guiding the management of asymptomatic congenital hydronephrosis. From this examination one can obtain the DRF, which is a robust measure provided there is adequate background subtraction.

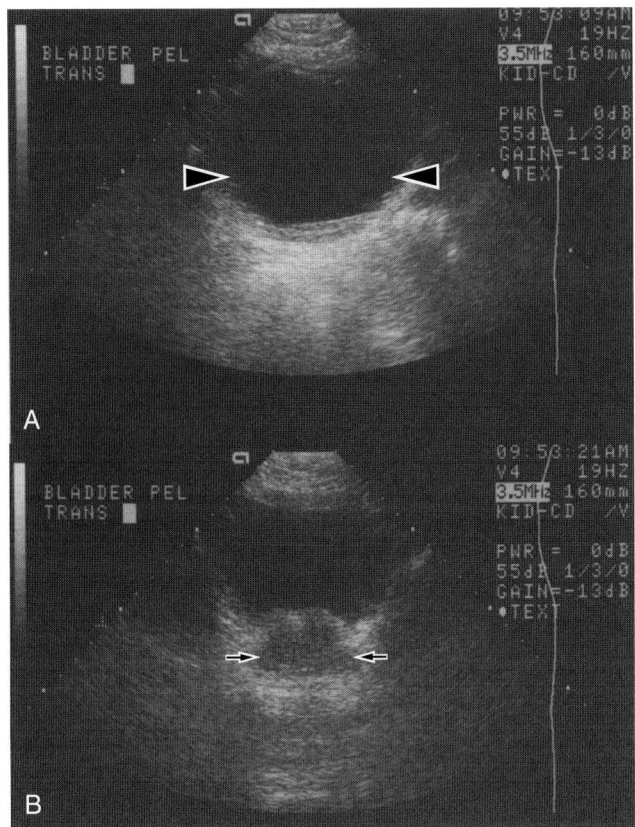

FIGURE 37-6 Pelvic ultrasonogram. **A,** Distended bladder (*arrowheads*). **B,** Enlarged prostate (*arrows*), causing infravesical urinary obstruction.

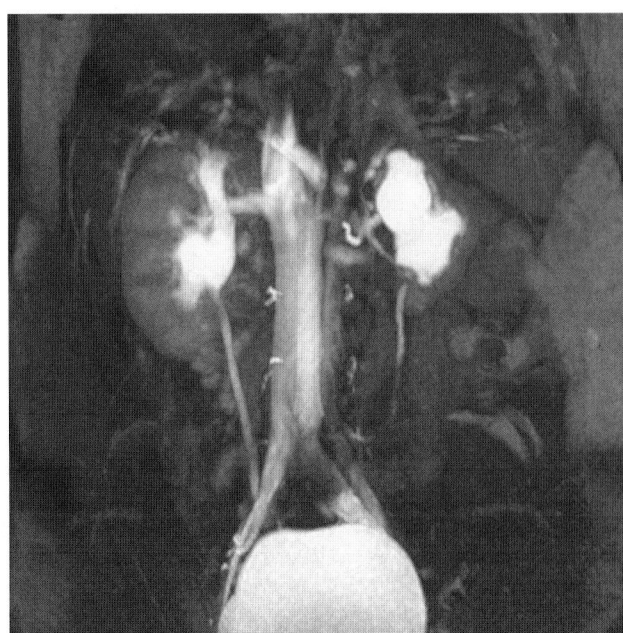

FIGURE 37-7 Magnetic resonance urographic scan of left-sided hydronephrosis with parenchymal thinning. Image shows large dilatation of the right pelvicaliceal system and narrowing of the left ureteropelvic junction (UPJ) segment.

Pitfalls are related to drawing the regions of interest, particularly in infants; to estimating the interval during which DRF is calculated; and to ensuring an adequate signal-to-noise ratio. There is no definition of a "significant" reduction in DRF. The classical variables of the diuretic renogram may not allow an estimate of the best drainage. Poor pelvic empty-ing may be observed because the bladder is full and because the effect of gravity on drainage is incomplete. Estimating the drainage as residual activity rather than as any parameter on the slope might be more adequate, especially if the time of furosemide administration is changed. Renal function and pelvic volume can influence the quality of drainage. Drainage may be better estimated using new tools.[145]

Magnetic Resonance Imaging

New MRI systems and specific MRI contrast agents have provided significant advances in the evaluation of renal per-formance (GFR measurement), in the search for prognos-tic factors (hypoxia, inflammation, reduced cell viability, decreased tubular function, and interstitial fibrosis), and in the monitoring of new therapies.[135,146] New developments that have provided a higher signal-to-noise ratio and higher spa-tial and/or temporal resolutions have the potential to direct new opportunities for obtaining morphologic and functional information on tissue characteristics relevant to various renal diseases, including urinary tract obstruction, that can aid diag-nosis, prognosis, and treatment follow-up.[135,146]

MRI can be used to explore the urinary tract when obstruc-tion is suspected. MRI provides improved spatial resolution,

and it is superior to IVU in detecting obstruction in the pres-ence of severe renal failure.[135] MRI has very limited appli-cation for the evaluation of stone disease because it cannot directly detect calcifications or stone material.[147] Depending on local conditions, MRI may be more expensive than other modalities. In children, MR urography (Figure 37-7) may replace conventional uroradiologic methods, and a recent study suggests that functional MRI may play an important potential role in identifying those who will benefit most from pyelo-plasty and those for whom observation is probably best.[148]

Promising experimental studies have recently demon-strated that MRI may provide valuable information regard-ing renal function, including energy consumption determined using blood oxygen level–dependent (BOLD) imaging. This kind of data may be helpful in the future in predicting the level of return of renal function after obstruction.[149,150]

Recently concerns regarding the use of MRI in renal patients were highlighted by the finding that patients with severely impaired renal function have increased risk of devel-oping nephrogenic systemic fibrosis induced by the toxicity of gadolinium; patients with normal renal function or mod-erate renal impairment do not develop nephrogenic systemic fibrosis.[151]

Whitaker's Test

Whitaker's test traditionally defines the functional effect of upper urinary tract dilatation by measuring the hydrostatic pressures in the renal pelvis and bladder during infusion of a saline and contrast mixture into the renal pelvis via catheter.[152] With a bladder catheter in place, the patient is placed in the prone position on a fluoroscopic table and a cannula is inserted percutaneously into the renal pelvis and connected to a pres-sure transducer. A mixture of saline and contrast material is infused through the renal cannula at a rate of 10 mL/min, and pressures are monitored. The urinary tract is considered nonobstructed if renal pelvic pressure is less than 15 cm H_2O, equivocal at a pressure between 15 and 22 cm H_2O, and obstructed if pressure exceeds 22 cm H_2O.[152]

Now that noninvasive imaging techniques are available, the test should be reserved for assessing potential upper urinary tract obstruction only in the following circumstances: equivocal results from less invasive tests; suspected obstruction with poor kidney function; loin pain with negative findings on diuresis renogram; suspected intermittent obstruction; and gross dilatation with positive findings on diuresis renogram.[153]

Retrograde and Antegrade Pyelography

When other tests do not provide adequate anatomic detail, or when obstruction must be relieved (e.g., obstruction of a solitary kidney, bilateral obstruction, or symptomatic infection in the obstructed system), more invasive investigation, with a combination of treatments, may be necessary. Retrograde pyelography is performed during cystoscopy by cannulating the ureteral orifice and injecting a contrast agent.[60,154,155] In some cases of complete obstruction, contrast may not reach the kidney, but the procedure will define the lower level of the obstruction.

Retrograde pyelography can be combined with placement of a ureteral stent to relieve an obstruction or with possible stone extraction. Because the procedure involves passage through the bladder to reach the upper urinary tract, the risk of introducing infection proximal to the obstruction must be kept in mind, and the obstruction should be relieved immediately after retrograde pyelography.

Antegrade pyelography is performed by percutaneous cannulation of the renal pelvis and injection of contrast material into the kidney and ureter.[154,155] This procedure should establish the proximal level of obstruction and may also serve as a first step in relieving obstruction by means of percutaneous nephrostomy (Figure 37-8).

Pathophysiology of Obstructive Nephropathy

Despite the fact that acquired obstructive nephropathy in humans usually results from partial urinary tract obstruction and is generally prolonged in its time course, most mechanistic studies of renal dysfunction in acquired obstruction use models of acute complete obstruction, usually for 24 hours. In these animal models, the extent of obstruction is clear and reproducible, and if the kidneys are studied soon after the obstruction is performed or released, the results are not confounded by changes in renal structure brought on by inflammation or fibrosis. Complete obstruction of short duration strikingly alters renal blood flow, glomerular filtration, and tubular function, while producing minimal anatomic changes in blood vessels, glomeruli, and tubules.[2]

Effects of Obstruction on Renal Blood Flow and Glomerular Filtration

Obstruction profoundly alters all components of glomerular function. The extent of the disturbance in GFR depends on how severe the obstruction is and how long it lasts, whether it

is unilateral or bilateral, and to what extent the obstruction has been relieved or persists.[2]

A description of the effects of obstruction on glomerular filtration requires a review of aspects of normal GFR. Whole-kidney GFR depends on the filtration rate of all functioning glomeruli and the proportion of glomeruli actually filtering. As detailed in Chapter 3, single-nephron GFR (SNGFR) is determined by the blood flow in the glomerulus, the net ultrafiltration pressure across the glomerular capillary, and the

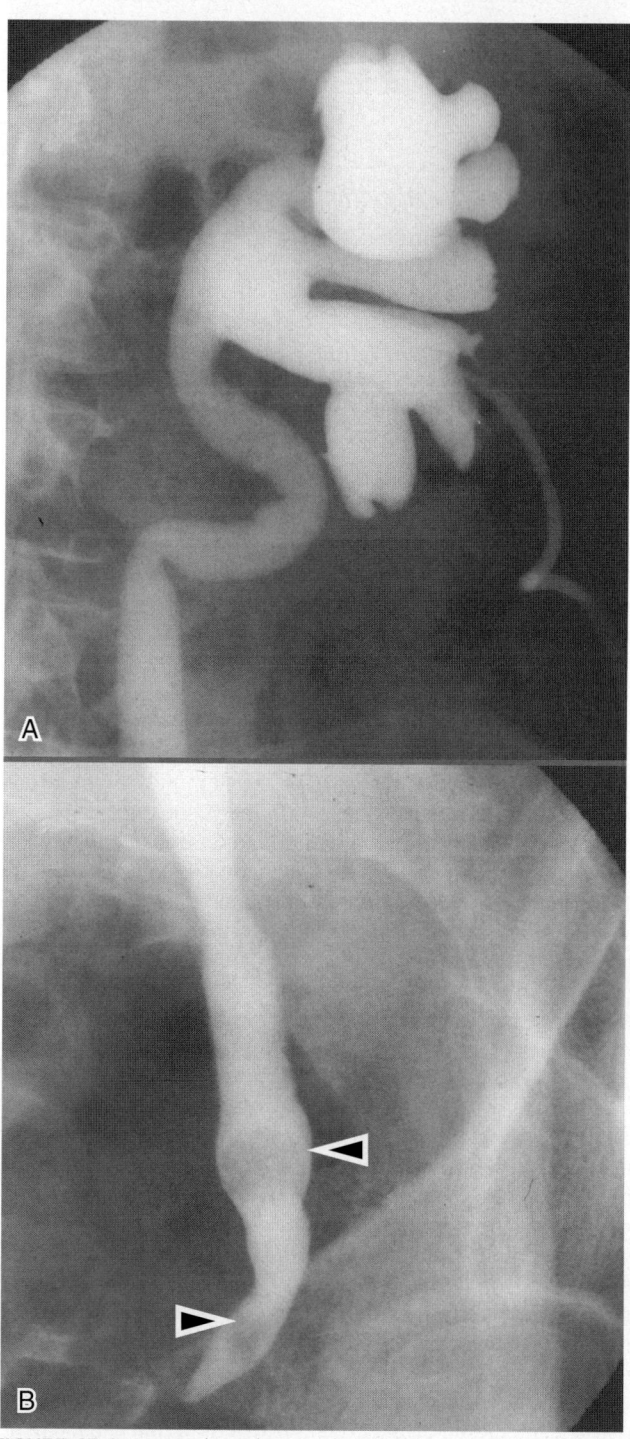

FIGURE 37-8 Antegrade pyelogram. **A,** Dilated renal pelvis and calices on *left.* **B,** Stones (*arrowheads*) appear as filling defects in the distal ureter (not seen on plain radiograph). Intravenous pyelography was unsuccessful owing to the obstructed and malfunctioning kidney.

ultrafiltration coefficient (K_f). Glomerular blood flow and the hydraulic pressure in the glomerular capillary (P_{GC}) are determined by the resistances of the afferent (R_A) and efferent (R_E) arterioles. Net ultrafiltration pressure is determined by P_{GC}, the hydraulic pressure of Bowman's space (which equals the proximal tubule hydraulic pressure, P_T), and the differences in oncotic pressure between the glomerular capillary and Bowman's space. K_f is determined by the permeability properties of the filtering surface and the surface area available for filtration. Obstruction can alter one or all of these determinants of GFR.

Early, Hyperemic Phase

In the 2 to 3 hours immediately following the onset of unilateral ureteral obstruction, blockade of antegrade urine flow markedly increases P_T. This increase in pressure in Bowman's space would be expected to halt GFR immediately.[156-158] However, during this early phase of obstruction, the afferent arterioles dilate, which decreases R_A, increases P_{GC}, and counteracts the increase in P_T.[156,157] Because this vasodilator or "hyperemic" response occurs in denervated kidneys in situ and in isolated perfused kidneys,[159,160] it must result from intrarenal mechanisms. In fact, glomeruli of individual nephrons exhibit the same response in in vivo micropuncture experiments when antegrade urine flow is blocked by placement of a wax block in the tubule of the nephron.[161]

Many mechanisms may mediate this afferent vasodilation, including increases in vasodilator hormones such as prostaglandins, regulation by the macula densa, and a direct myogenic reflex. This hyperemic response is not attenuated by renal nerve stimulation or infusion of catecholamines,[162] and it may be linked to changes in interstitial pressure.[160]

In the tubuloglomerular feedback response, reduced distal tubular flow past the macula densa induces reductions in R_A and increases in P_{GC}, so that SNGFR rises. Similarly, because obstruction reduces urine flow past the macula densa, this structure induces afferent vasodilation.[161] However, micropuncture studies have separated the stoppage in flow from increases in P_T by placing an additional puncture in the tubule that was proximal to the blockage of flow to the macula densa. In this setting, flow past the macula densa was halted, but P_T remained normal, because accumulating tubular fluid was permitted to leak out.[157] In such nephrons the increase in P_{GC} observed in obstructed tubules did not occur, which indicates that the obstruction itself, and not the macula densa, stimulates afferent vasodilation.[157]

Renal prostaglandins and renal nerves play important roles in the hyperemic response. Indomethacin blocks the hyperemic response, which indicates that vasodilator prostaglandins are critical to afferent vasodilation.[158,163] A renorenal reflex mechanism in the hemodynamic response to obstruction can be discerned from studies in bilateral obstruction, in which the afferent vasodilation response is absent or markedly attenuated.[2,160] Obstruction of the left kidney augments afferent renal nerve activity from the left kidney and efferent nerve activity to the right kidney. Increased efferent nerve activity to the right kidney was accompanied by reduced blood flow to that kidney. This vasoconstrictor response was ablated by denervation of either the left or right kidney before induction of left ureteral obstruction, which suggests that increased afferent renal nerve traffic triggers vasoconstrictive renorenal reflex activity that counteracts the early intrinsic renal vasodilator effects of obstruction in bilateral ureteral obstruction.[160]

Late, Vasoconstrictive Phase

Because obstruction results in cessation of glomerular filtration, efforts to study the regulation of SNGFR later in obstruction have measured determinants of GFR immediately after release of obstruction.[2,164] Using this approach, investigators have shown that renal blood flow declines progressively after 3 hours of unilateral obstruction and through 12 to 24 hours of obstruction.[165,166] Interestingly, although tubular pressures rise initially after obstruction, they then decline, so that by 24 hours renal plasma flow, GFR, and intratubular pressures have all dropped below normal values.[156,158,166,167]

At 24 hours into the obstruction, examination of regional blood flow in the kidney by injections of silicone rubber reveal large areas of the cortical vascular bed that are either underperfused or not perfused at all.[2,158,166] Depending on the species, the different vascular beds in the outer and juxtamedullary cortex receive differing proportions of the renal blood flow under basal conditions and following obstruction. However, it is clear that at 24 hours of obstruction, reduced whole-kidney GFR is due in large part to nonperfusion of many glomeruli.

Beyond 24 hours of obstruction, SNGFR of glomeruli that remain perfused is decreased markedly, both because of reduced blood flow to the afferent arteriole and because of afferent vasoconstriction, which in turn reduces P_{GC}.[167,168] Because, P_{GC} responds in the same manner when the individual nephron is blocked with oil for 24 hours before micropuncture measurements are performed, it is clear that afferent arteriolar vasoconstriction plays an important role in attenuating SNGFR during the established phase of obstruction.[169]

These results indicate that, as with the early hyperemic response, intrarenal mechanisms play the major role in the late vasoconstrictive response to unilateral obstruction. In bilateral obstruction, renal blood flow is reduced to levels 30% to 60% below normal[167,168,170] (Table 37-3). In both unilateral and bilateral obstruction, SNGFR falls to a similar degree. However, the mechanisms involved are different in the two conditions. In unilateral obstruction, reduced P_{GC} lowers the driving pressure for filtration when set against a nearly normal P_T. By contrast, in bilateral obstruction, P_{GC} remains normal and GFR is halted by a highly elevated P_T.[167] These results suggest that systemic factors, such as accumulation of extracellular fluid volume and urea, increases in natriuretic substances, and alterations in renal nerve activity modulate the vasoconstrictive effect of obstruction on the affected kidney.[170]

TABLE 37-3 Glomerular Hemodynamics in Ureteral Obstruction				
STAGE OF OBSTRUCTION	**P_T**	**R_A**	**P_{GC}**	**SNGFR**
1-2 hr unilateral	↑↑	↓	↑	=
24 hr unilateral	=	↑↑	↓	↓↓
24 hr bilateral	↑↑	=	=	↓↓
After release: 24 hr unilateral	↓	↑↑	↓↓	↓↓
After release: 24 hr bilateral	=	↑↑	↓	↓↓

See text for discussion and references.

=, Unchanged; ↑, increased; ↑↑, markedly increased; ↓, reduced; ↓↓, markedly reduced; P_T, proximal tubule hydraulic pressure; R_A, afferent arteriole resistance; P_{GC}, hydraulic pressure of Bowman's space; *SNGFR*, single-nephron glomerular filtration rate.

Regulation of the Glomerular Filtration Rate in Response to Obstruction

The level to which renal blood flow and GFR are reduced after release of obstruction varies with the species studied and the duration of obstruction.[2] After release of a 24-hour complete unilateral obstruction the GFR remains below 50% of normal in dogs and 25% of normal in rats; renal blood flow remains markedly reduced in both species.[2] After release of bilateral ureteral obstruction, renal blood flow reaches levels higher than that observed following unilateral obstruction, likely due to systemic natriuretic influences such as volume accumulation, reduced sympathetic tone, or increased circulating atrial natriuretic peptide (ANP). However, the GFR remains markedly attenuated. Despite the fact that renal blood flow is increased, GFR remains low in part because of nonperfusion or underperfusion of many glomeruli, as shown by experiments using silicone rubber injections.[158,166] Where glomeruli remain perfused, intense afferent vasoconstriction reduces P_{GC}, so that even though P_T also falls with release of the obstruction, the driving force for glomerular filtration remains low.[167,168] In addition, a sharp reduction in K_f also augments the fall in GFR at this point following release of unilateral and bilateral obstruction.[167,168]

Several mechanisms contribute to afferent vasoconstriction and a reduced K_f. First, release of obstruction strikingly augments the flow of tubular fluid past the macula densa. Although the absolute rate of flow is still far below normal, the macula densa likely senses the dramatic change in the rate of flow, and this may lead to intense vasoconstriction.[2] In support of this view, the sensitivity of the tubuloglomerular feedback mechanism is enhanced in unilateral obstruction compared with bilateral obstruction, which suggests that the ability of the mechanism to regulate afferent arteriolar tone is modulated by the extrarenal hormonal milieu.[171]

There is now substantial evidence that increased intrarenal secretion of angiotensin II participates actively in afferent vasoconstriction and reduced K_f following release of ureteral obstruction. Ureteral obstruction rapidly increases renal vein renin levels at a time when renal blood flow is normal or elevated, but at later time points, renal vein renin levels return to normal.[172-174] In addition, infusion of captopril attenuated the declines in renal blood flow and GFR observed in both unilateral and bilateral obstruction.[172,174] Because inhibition of angiotensin converting enzyme can also increase kinin activity, infusions of either carboxypeptidase B, which destroys kinins, or aprotinin, which blocks kinin generation, were used to eliminate the kinin effect. Captopril remained equally effective in the presence of either agent, which indicates that captopril reduced R_A primarily by blocking generation of angiotensin II.[2]

The significance of the renin-angiotensin system as an important contributor to the vasoconstriction has recently been highlighted in studies in which treatment with an angiotensin II type 1 (AT$_1$) receptor antagonist attenuated the reduction in GFR in the postobstructive period in both adult rats[175] and rats with neonatally induced unilateral partial obstruction in response to long-term AT$_1$ receptor antagonist treatment.[176]

There is substantial evidence that thromboxane A$_2$ (TXA$_2$) plays a major role in obstruction-induced vasoconstriction.[172,177] Chronically hydronephrotic kidneys exhibit increased TXA$_2$ accumulation, as measured by accumulation of its more stable metabolite, TXB$_2$.[177] Furthermore, whole-kidney GFR and renal blood flow were increased in response to thromboxane synthase inhibitor treatment,[172,178] likely due to a reduction in afferent arteriolar resistance and thus an increase in K_f.[179] Based on these results, TXA$_2$ appears to be generated in the kidney following release of obstruction and to mediate afferent vasoconstriction and reductions in K_f.

Although the source of TXA$_2$ generation remains unclear, in some cases[180] but not all[181] glomeruli isolated from obstructed kidneys have shown increased ability to synthesize TXA$_2$. Other studies have suggested that inflammatory cells are the source of TXA$_2$. This is consistent with the observations that suppressor T cells and macrophages migrate to the renal cortex and medulla during the first 24 hours of obstruction, reaching levels 15-fold higher than those observed in normal kidneys,[182] a migration paralleled by a rise in TXA$_2$ release and a fall in GFR.[182] These changes can be attenuated by renal irradiation, which indicates that obstruction stimulates immigration of inflammatory leukocytes that, in turn, generate vasoconstrictors such as TXA$_2$.[183]

The role of angiotensin II for this is highlighted, because glomeruli isolated from obstructed kidneys showed increased eicosanoid synthesis after angiotensin II stimulation, and treatment of obstructed animals with converting enzyme inhibitors enhanced GFR and reduced generation of TXA$_2$ by glomeruli isolated from these animals.[184] Thus, these vasoconstrictors may contribute to regulation of R_A and GFR following the release of obstruction.

Because vasoconstriction is less severe in animals with bilateral ureteral obstruction, as noted earlier, it is likely that extrarenal factors play a major role in modulating the hemodynamic response of the kidney to obstruction and release of obstruction. In addition to the renorenal reflexes already mentioned, various other factors, including accumulation of volume and solutes such as urea, ANP and its congeners, and other natriuretic substances, may ameliorate the vasoconstrictive effects of obstruction when both ureters are ligated.[185,186] Following 24 hours of obstruction, GFR is preserved to some degree if the contralateral kidney is also obstructed or removed.[185] In addition, following release of 24 hours of unilateral obstruction in animals, if the urea, salt, and water content of the urine from the contralateral kidney is reinfused into the animal, a striking increase in GFR is observed over that seen in standard unilateral obstruction.[185,187] This suggests that ANP, urea, and other excreted urine solutes have a protective effect and can ameliorate vasoconstriction following release of ureteral obstruction by direct vasodilation of afferent arterioles, constriction of efferent arterioles, and an increase in K_f.

Additional studies in dogs and rats have implicated endothelins as contributors to reduced GFR in obstruction and have suggested that prostaglandin E$_2$ (PGE$_2$) and nitric oxide (NO) may play an ameliorating role in glomerular vasoconstriction in obstructed kidneys.[188,189] Renal PGE$_2$ levels increase markedly in obstruction (see later) and in states of extracellular volume expansion, as occurs in bilateral ureteral obstruction. Given the vasodilator effects of PGE$_2$, it appears likely that increased levels could ameliorate falls in GFR in obstruction. Bilateral obstruction may reduce generation of NO, leading to a net vasoconstrictive effect.[184]

In summary, both intrarenal and extrarenal factors combine to decrease GFR profoundly during and immediately after release of obstruction. The decrease in GFR is caused by a sharp reduction in the number of perfused glomeruli and by a reduction in the SNGFR of functioning nephrons. Decreased K_f and increased R_A reduce SNGFR. Increases in angiotensin II and TXA_2 as well as in other vasoconstrictors, some coming from inflammatory cells, augment these hemodynamic effects. In the setting of bilateral obstruction, retention of urea and other solutes, as well as volume expansion and increases in circulating levels of vasodilators such as ANP, help to offset these vasoconstrictive effects, but only partially.

Recovery of Glomerular Function after Relief of Obstruction

The extent of recovery of glomerular filtration following release of obstruction depends on several factors, including the duration and extent of obstruction, the presence or absence of a functioning contralateral kidney, the presence or absence of associated infection, and the level of preobstruction renal blood flow.[2,190]

In a classic experiment in dogs subjected to a 1-week period of complete unilateral ureteral obstruction, GFR fell to 25% of normal on release of the obstruction and recovered gradually to 50% of normal levels 2 years later, which indicates persisting irreversible changes.[191]

In rats, release of unilateral ureteral obstruction of 7 and 14 days' duration left residual GFR at 17% and 9% of control levels, respectively, when the contralateral kidney remained in place, and 31% and 14% when the animals underwent contralateral nephrectomy at the time of release of the obstruction.[192] A similar beneficial effect on the obstructed kidney of contralateral nephrectomy was observed in rats subjected to chronic partial obstruction.[192] As discussed earlier, this beneficial effect likely results from the accumulation of urea and other solutes and increased levels of ANP when the functioning contralateral kidney is absent.

The partial recovery of total renal GFR following release of obstruction masks a very uneven distribution of blood flow and nephron function. In micropuncture studies, some nephrons never regain filtration function, whereas others reveal striking hyperfiltration.[190] It appeared in some studies that surface nephrons exhibited normal SNGFR, whereas the whole-kidney GFR was reduced to 18% of normal.[193] These results suggest that long-term partial obstruction causes selective damage to juxtamedullary and deep cortical nephrons.[166,190,193] Similarly, studies of the long-term outcome of complete 24-hour ureteral obstruction revealed that total renal GFR recovered to normal levels by 14 and 60 days after release of obstruction. However, 15% of the glomeruli were not filtering in recovered kidneys, and other nephrons were hyperfiltering. In this model of complete obstruction, there appeared to be no selective advantage for surface glomeruli over deep cortical and juxtamedullary glomeruli.[190]

Similarly, in the developing kidney, the duration of obstruction and timing of release have a striking impact on long-term renal function. Release after 1 week of obstruction completely prevented development of hydronephrosis, reduction in renal blood flow, and reduction in GFR in rats subjected to partial unilateral ureteral obstruction at birth, whereas release after 4 weeks resulted in little or no renal function in the obstructed kidney—results demonstrating that early release of neonatal obstruction provides dramatically better protection of renal function than release of obstruction after the maturation process is completed.[194]

Effects of Obstruction on Tubule Function

Obstruction severely impairs the ability of renal tubules to transport Na^+, K^+, and H^+, and reduces their ability to concentrate and dilute the urine (Table 37-4).[2,195-201] The resulting inability to reabsorb water and solutes facilitates postobstructive diuresis and natriuresis. As is the case with glomerular filtration, the extent of disruption of tubular transport depends directly on the duration and severity of the obstruction.

TABLE 37-4 Segmental Reabsorption in Superficial and Juxtamedullary Nephrons and in Collecting Ducts in Normal Rats after Release of Bilateral or Unilateral Obstruction

SITE	NORMAL WATER REMAINING (%)	Na+ REMAINING (%)	AFTER UNILATERAL OBSTRUCTION WATER REMAINING (%)	Na+ REMAINING (%)	AFTER BILATERAL OBSTRUCTION WATER REMAINING (%)	Na+ REMAINING (%)
S_1	100	100	100	100	100	100
S_2	44	44	26	26	45	45
S_3	26	14	21	12	40	22
S_4	9.4	5	3.2	1.9	25	7
J_1	100	100	100	100	100	100
J_2	12	40	42	52	42	62
CD_1	3.3	2	4.2	3.8	8	6
CD_2	0.4	0.6	2.9	2.5	16.7	12

S_1 to S_4 are values found in superficial nephrons: S_1, Bowman's space; S_2, end of proximal convoluted tubule; S_3, earliest portion of distal tubule; S_4, end of distal tubule/beginning of collecting duct. J_1 and J_2 are values found in juxtamedullary nephrons: J_1, Bowman's space; J_2, tip of the loop of Henle. CD_1 and CD_2 are values found in the collecting duct: CD_1, collecting duct at the base of the papilla, the first accessible portion of the inner medullary collecting duct; CD_2, end of collecting duct as it opens into the renal pelvis.
In obstruction, increased proportions of filtered salt and water were delivered to the loop of Henle in the juxtamedullary nephrons (J_1 and J_2), which indicates decreased reabsorption. Delivery of salt and water to the first accessible portion of the inner medullary collecting duct (CD_1) was also increased, and net salt and water reabsorption along the inner medullary collecting duct (between CD_1 and CD_2) was diminished in both bilateral and unilateral obstruction. In bilateral obstruction, there was net addition or secretion of salt and water into the lumen of the inner medullary collecting duct, which suggests that in this setting the inner medullary collecting duct secretes salt and water.[195]

Pathologically, prolonged obstruction leads to profound tubular atrophy and chronic interstitial inflammation and fibrosis (see later), whereas at early time points following the onset of obstruction, such as at 24 hours, there are only slight structural and ultrastructural changes, including mitochondrial swelling, modest blunting of basolateral interdigitations in the thick ascending limb and proximal tubule epithelial cells, and flattening of the epithelium and some widening of the intercellular spaces in the collecting ducts.[2,202,203] The only cell death at early time points is observed at the very tip of the papilla, where focal necrosis may be observed.[202]

Because there is so little cell damage, and because of the simplicity of the model, most investigators have examined the effect of 24 hours of complete ureteral obstruction on tubular function. As discussed later, regulation of tubular transport is complex, and the effects of obstruction are due both to direct damage of epithelial cells and the action of extratubular mediators arising both from the kidney and extrarenal sources.

Effects of Obstruction on Tubular Sodium Reabsorption

Following release of 24 hours of unilateral ureteral obstruction, volume excretion from the postobstructed kidney is normal or slightly increased[2,170,185,204] (see Table 37-4). However, as discussed earlier, normal volume excretion occurs in the setting of a markedly reduced (20% of normal) GFR. Consequently, fractional excretion of sodium, or FE_{Na}, is markedly elevated in the postobstructed kidney. After release of bilateral obstruction, salt and water excretion jumps to five to nine times normal.[2,170,195,196] Because GFR is also decreased in this setting, FE_{Na} may be 20-fold higher than normal. The micropuncture studies summarized in Table 37-4 demonstrate that the reabsorption defect following release of obstruction is localized similarly in both unilateral and bilateral ureteral obstruction. Obstruction reduces net salt and water reabsorption in the medullary thick ascending limb (MTAL), the distal convoluted tubule, and the entire length of the collecting duct, including its cortical, outer medullary, and inner medullary segments.[195]

These studies in whole animals were confirmed and extended by a series of studies in multiple laboratories using isolated perfused tubule and cell suspension preparations (Table 37-5). As shown in the table, the segments, including proximal straight tubule, MTAL, and cortical collecting duct isolated from unilaterally or bilaterally obstructed animals, exhibited profound impairment of reabsorptive capacity.[196,197] This finding was confirmed in studies of freshly prepared suspensions of MTAL cells from obstructed kidneys, in which transport-dependent oxygen consumption, a measure of salt reabsorptive capacity, was markedly reduced.[198] Given the major regulatory role of mineralocorticoid in the collecting duct, it is important to note that these decreases in collecting duct reabsorptive capacity occurred in tubules taken from obstructed kidneys, whether or not the animal had been pretreated with mineralocorticoid.[197,199,200]

Because the inner medullary collecting duct is highly branched and difficult to perfuse reliably in vitro, transport in this segment has been studied in cell suspensions. In these preparations, transport-dependent oxygen consumption was markedly reduced in cells isolated from animals with bilateral obstruction.[201]

TABLE 37-5 Function of Isolated Perfused Tubules in Obstructive Nephropathy

	J_v SPCT (nL/mm/min)	J_v PST (nL/mm/min)	ΔCL^- MTAL (mEq/L)	J_v CCT (ADH) (nL/mm/min)
Control	0.75 ± 0.08	0.25 ± 0.02	−37 ± 3	0.90 ± 0.08
Unilateral obstruction	0.73 ± 0.11	0.12 ± 0.03	−9 ± 1	0.22 ± 0.04
Bilateral obstruction	0.80 ± 0.08	0.16 ± 0.02	−10 ± 1	0.23 ± 0.04

The J_v in the SPCT was not affected by ureteral obstruction, whereas the J_v in the PST decreased by 52% in unilateral obstruction (0.12 ± 0.03 vs. 0.25 ± 0.02 nL/mm/min) and similarly in response to bilateral obstruction. In the MTAL the ability to lower the perfusate Cl^- concentration was reduced by 76% (−9 ± 1 vs. −37 ± 3 mEq/L) in unilateral obstruction and similarly in response to bilateral obstruction. The ability of the CCT to respond to ADH after relief of unilateral obstruction was reduced by 76% (0.22 ± 0.04 vs. 0.90 ± 0.08 nL/mm/min), and a similar reduction followed relief of bilateral obstruction.

ADH, Antidiuretic hormone; *CCT,* cortical collecting tubule; ΔCl^- *MTAL,* change in Cl^- concentration per length of the medullary thick ascending limb; J_v, net fluid reabsorption rate per length of the tubule segment; *PST,* cortical proximal straight tubule; *SPCT,* superficial proximal convoluted tubule.

Data from Buerkert J, Martin D, Head M, et al: Deep nephron function after release of acute unilateral ureteral obstruction in the young rat, *J Clin Invest* 62:1228-1239, 1978; and from Hanley MJ, Davidson K: Isolated nephron segments from rabbit models of obstructive nephropathy, *J Clin Invest* 69:165-174, 1982.

Taken together, the data derived from micropuncture, tubule perfusion, and cell suspension studies reveal a striking impairment of volume reabsorption in the proximal straight tubule, the MTAL, and the entire collecting duct. Since these functional derangements occur in the absence of clear-cut ultrastructural damage to the epithelial cells, obstruction likely induces a selective impairment in the regulation of active cellular transport mechanisms. Unlike the situation with glomerular filtration, the functional impairment is similar in both unilateral and bilateral obstruction.[197,200,201] Thus, it appears that a major component of impaired active transport is likely due to direct tubular cell injury, rather than to the continuous action of natriuretic substances. In addition to this intrinsic injury, natriuretic substances may be responsible for the apparent secretion of salt and water in the inner medullary collecting duct of animals following release of bilateral obstruction (see Table 37-4).

Studies of cell suspensions, combined with antibody-based targeted proteomics that permits the examination of long-term regulation by renal transporters and channels in intact animals to elucidate the integrated response to obstruction, have improved the molecular understanding of the mechanisms by which tubular epithelial cell salt reabsorption is impaired in the setting of obstruction. Active tubular Na^+ transport requires an apical entry step (e.g., Na-K-2Cl type 2 cotransporter [NKCC2] in MTAL or epithelial Na^+ channels [ENaCs] in the collecting duct) coupled to the basolateral Na^+–K^+–adenosine triphosphatase (ATPase). In addition, the cell must generate sufficient adenosine triphosphate (ATP) to fuel active transport by the ATPase.

Suspensions of MTAL cells from obstructed kidneys exhibited markedly reduced furosemide-sensitive oxygen consumption,[198] which indicates a striking decreases in apical NKCC2 cotransporter activity in these cells. Isotopic bumetanide binding revealed a marked reduction in the number of cotransporter protein molecules available for binding on the membrane, with no change in affinity of binding, a finding which indicates that obstruction downregulates the expression of the cotransporter protein on the membrane surface.[198]

More recent studies using antibody-based targeted approaches clearly showed that obstruction diminishes expression of the cotransporter protein on the MTAL cell apical membrane.[205] Similar approaches demonstrated downregulation of both α- and β-subunits of Na+-K+-ATPase at the transcriptional and posttranscriptional level.[205,206] Similar studies demonstrated downregulation of ENaC in the inner medullary collecting duct.[207] Consistent with these findings, suspensions from obstructed kidneys showed marked decreases in amiloride-sensitive oxygen consumption as well as amiloride-sensitive isotopic sodium entry into hyperpolarized cells.[201] As occurred in MTAL cells, the rates of ouabain-sensitive oxygen consumption and of ouabain-sensitive ATPase were markedly diminished in inner medullary collecting duct cells from obstructed animals, and the levels of both pump subunits were also reduced in these preparations.[201] Patterns of messenger RNA (mRNA) expression were also similar to those in MTAL, which indicates transcriptional and posttranscriptional downregulation of pump subunit expression.

Studies using the antibody-based targeted approach demonstrated that in both unilateral and bilateral ureteral obstruction, expression of the Na+/H+ exchanger NHE3 and the Na+/PO₄³⁻ exchanger NaPi-2 was strikingly decreased in the proximal tubule.[205,208] These changes in sodium transporter expression occurred in both the proximal convoluted and proximal straight tubule, even though the micropuncture and tubule perfusion studies cited earlier revealed preserved proximal convoluted tubule salt reabsorption and inhibition of proximal straight tubule reabsorption.[208,209] The same studies demonstrated significant downregulation of total transporter protein and apical membrane expression of the distal convoluted tubule Na-Cl cotransporter, which indicates that obstruction likely reduces distal convoluted tubule Na+ reabsorption by mechanisms similar to those observed in the MTAL and collecting duct.[205,208]

Taken together, these results demonstrate that obstruction downregulates membrane expression of transporter proteins responsible for apical sodium entry and basolateral sodium exit. Interestingly, metabolic studies reveal that obstruction reduces the activities of several enzymes of the oxidative and glycolytic pathways as well, consistent with a downregulation of metabolic capacity for energy generation in these cells. This may also be enhanced by the observed reductions in the extent of basolateral infolding and in the density of mitochondria in tubules of obstructed kidneys.[202]

Interestingly, in MTAL and collecting duct suspensions, obstruction reduces transport-dependent but not transport-independent oxygen consumption, which indicates that the rate of ATP generation (oxygen consumption) is not rate limiting for active transport in these cells. On this basis, it appears more likely that obstruction-induced reduction of epithelial sodium transport is a regulated process as a result of reduced metabolic demands during obstruction.

The mechanisms and pathways responsible for downregulation of transport proteins in tubular epithelial cells by obstruction remain to a large extent incompletely understood. Possible signals include the halting of urine flow, increased hydrostatic pressure on tubular epithelial cells, changes in

blood flow to the tubules or in interstitial pressure, and generation of natriuretic substances in the kidney that result in long-term inhibition of transporter function.

Obstruction impairs glomerular filtration, and urine production is dramatically reduced (stopped in occlusion). Consequently sodium delivery to each tubular segment is reduced, and apical membrane Na+ entry slows dramatically because the electrochemical gradients for Na+ entry between the stationary apical fluid and the cell interior become increasingly unfavorable for continued sodium transport. Reduced Na++ entry might then directly stimulate downregulation of transporter activity and expression.

Blocking Na+ entry into MTAL and inner medullary collecting duct cells by furosemide or amiloride, respectively, promptly reduces ouabain-sensitive oxygen consumption,[198,210] which indicates acute downregulation of Na+-K+-ATPase. In addition, in mineralocorticoid-clamped animals, long-term blockade of Na+ entry at the MTAL or cortical collecting duct by administration of furosemide or amiloride, respectively, reduces the levels of ouabain-sensitive ATPase in microdissected tubule segments.[211,212] These results suggest that the halt in urine flow might represent a major signaling mechanism by which obstruction downregulates Na+ transport.[210]

To test this hypothesis, apical Na+ entry was inhibited for 24 hours in a cell line that mimics cortical collecting duct cells, A6 cells, grown on permeable supports. When apical Na+ entry was blocked either by substituting another cation for sodium in the apical solution or by adding amiloride to the apical solution, apical sodium entry was markedly reduced for some hours after the blockade was removed.[213] This downregulation is accompanied by selective reduction in the levels of expression of the β-subunits of ENaC (but not the α- or γ-subunits) in the apical membranes of the A6 cells, but not in the whole-cell levels of these subunits.[214]

At the integrated level rats with urinary tract obstruction demonstrated downregulation of α-, β-, and γ-subunits of EnaC, which indicates that downregulation of all three subunits may play a role in the impaired sodium reabsorption in obstruction.[207] Interestingly, and in contrast to the results in cell suspensions or whole kidney,[198,201,205,208] inhibition of apical sodium entry had no effect on expression of either subunit of Na+-K+-ATPase.[214] These results provide direct evidence that reductions in the rate of Na+ entry, which may occur when urine flow is blocked, can directly downregulate Na+ transport in renal epithelial cells.

In addition to the direct effects of halting urine flow, changes in intrarenal mediators and subcellular pathways likely play a critical role in the reduction of salt transport observed with obstruction. Obstruction markedly accelerates the already rapid generation of PGE₂ in the renal medulla.[177,178,181,215] The molecular basis for this is a dramatic medullary cyclooxygenase-2 (COX-2) induction (Figure 37-9).[215,216] Consistent with the known effect of PGE₂ to markedly inhibit Na+ reabsorption in the MTAL as well as in the cortical and inner medullary collecting ducts,[217-219] COX-2 inhibition in rats with obstruction and release of obstruction attenuated the downregulation of NHE2, NKCC2, and Na+-K+-ATPase.[216,220] Given these results, obstruction likely reduces apically localized sodium cotransport proteins in the tubular epithelium and sodium pump activity in tubular epithelia in part by increasing renal levels of PGE₂.

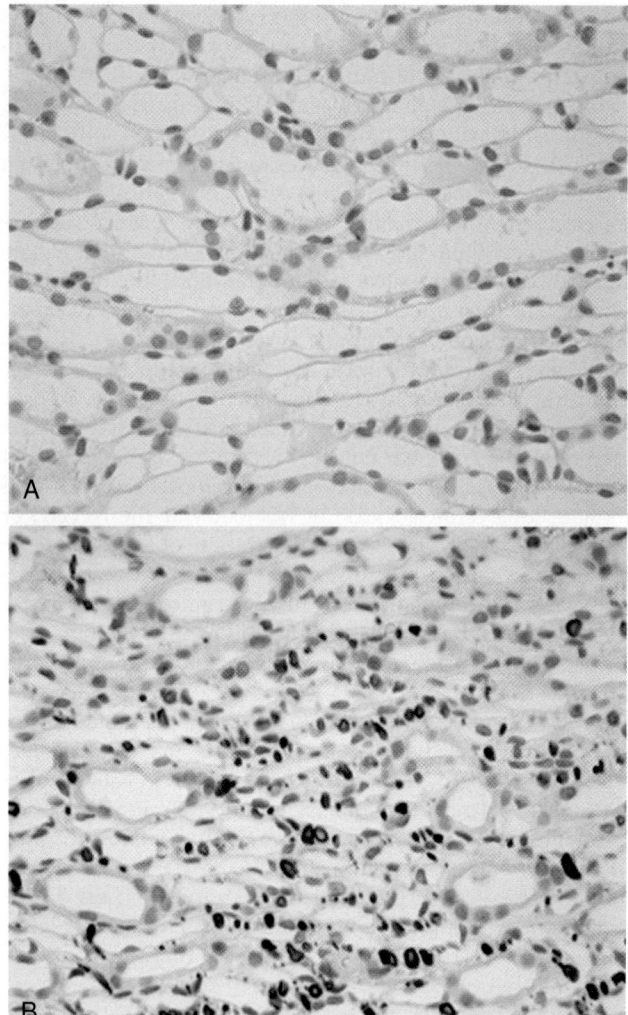

FIGURE 37-9 Immunohistochemical assay for cyclooxygenase-2 (COX-2) in kidney inner medulla (IM) of sham-operated rats (**A**) and rats subjected to 24 hours of bilateral ureteral obstruction (**B**). There is a strong labeling at the base of the IM in obstructed kidneys located exclusively in the interstitial cells (**B**). Labeling is not detectable in sham-operated kidneys (**A**).

As discussed earlier, obstruction brings on a monocellular infiltrate in the kidney,[182] and this infiltrate tends to follow a peritubular distribution.[182] When obstructed kidneys were irradiated, the level of medullary inflammation was diminished, and there was a modest decrease in the fractional excretion of sodium.[183] In addition, it has been shown that obstruction causes enhanced renal angiotensin II generation. This may have important implications for regulation of renal sodium handling. Blockade of the angiotensin II receptor AT_1 was associated with a marked attenuation of downregulation of NHE3 and NKCC2, which was paralleled by a reduction in renal sodium loss.[56]

In summary, obstruction reduces net reabsorption of salt in several nephron segments, including the proximal straight tubule, the MTAL, and the cortical and inner medullary collecting ducts, by downregulating the expression and activities of specific transporter proteins. Several signals mediate this downregulation, including the cessation of urine flow with its attendant reduction of the rate of Na^+ entry across the apical membrane, increased levels of natriuretic substances such

as PGE_2, and infiltration of the obstructed kidney by mononuclear cells.

When both ureters are obstructed, extrarenal factors markedly enhance the sodium wasting tendency already present in the obstructed kidney. One mechanism is the volume expansion that occurs when bilateral obstruction ablates all renal function. Volume expansion impairs activity in the sympathetic nervous system, reduces circulating levels of aldosterone, and, along with reduced renal clearance, increases levels of ANP. Reduced sympathetic tone and aldosterone levels, coupled with increased ANP, markedly stimulate sodium excretion.

ANP likely represents a particularly important mediator of salt wasting in bilateral obstruction. Levels of ANP are markedly elevated in bilateral but not unilateral obstruction.[221] ANP enhances salt wasting at several nephron segments. By blocking renin release in the macula densa and angiotensin action in the proximal tubule, ANP reduces proximal tubule sodium reabsorption.[186,221,222] ANP also reduces aldosterone release and directly inhibits sodium reabsorption in the collecting ducts.[186,221,222] In support of this mechanism, infusion of ANP into animals in which obstruction had just been released led to marked increases in sodium and water excretion.[221] Moreover, efforts to reduce circulating ANP levels following bilateral obstruction attenuated sodium excretion somewhat.[221]

Accumulation of urea and other solutes also enhances sodium wasting by obstructed kidneys. Following release after 24 hours of unilateral obstruction, removal or obstruction of the contralateral kidney markedly enhances salt wasting by the obstructed kidney.[185] If the contralateral kidney is left in place but amounts of urea, salt, and water equivalent to what the contralateral kidney is excreting are infused into the animal, there is a striking increase in sodium excretion by both the obstructed and the contralateral kidney.[185,187] These findings indicate that bilateral obstruction induces hormonal changes and promotes accumulation of solutes and volume that together enhance natriuresis from the obstructed kidney.

Effects of Obstruction on Urinary Concentration and Dilution

Because obstruction eliminates the ability of the renal tubules to concentrate and dilute the urine, urine osmolality after release of obstruction in humans and experimental animals approaches that of plasma.[2,223,224] Dilution of the urine requires that the thick ascending limb reabsorb sodium without water and that the collecting duct maintain the dilute urine by not reabsorbing water along its length, despite the presence of a concentrated medullary interstitium.[225]

Concentration of the urine requires active sodium reabsorption in the thick limb and the action of the countercurrent multiplier to generate a concentrated medullary interstitium, as well as the ability of the collecting duct to insert the vasopressin-regulated water channel aquaporin-2 (AQP2) into the apical membrane.[226,227]

Obstructive nephropathy disrupts several of these mechanisms.[208,223,224,228] As noted earlier, obstruction also markedly reduces MTAL sodium reabsorption, which limits the ability of this segment to dilute the urine and to generate a high medullary interstitial osmolality. Indeed, interstitial osmolality has been shown to be reduced in obstructed kidneys.[2]

In addition, collecting ducts isolated from obstructed kidneys reveal normal basal water permeabilities, but a marked reduction in their ability to increase water permeability in response to antidiuretic hormone or other stimulants of cyclic adenosine monophosphate (cAMP) accumulation in the cells. As was the case with sodium transport, the effects were similar with unilateral and bilateral obstruction.[223,228]

Detailed mechanistic studies show that obstruction markedly reduces transcription of mRNA encoding AQP2 as well as synthesis of AQP2 protein, and that collecting duct cells in obstructed kidneys do not traffic AQP2-containing vesicles effectively to the apical surface in response to vasopressin or increased cAMP.[223,227-229] Part of this failure in trafficking results from a decrease in phosphorylation of AQP2 in obstructed kidneys,[208] and the fact that vasopressin type 2 (V_2) receptor protein expression is downregulated likely also contributes.[230]

In addition, unilateral ureteral obstruction markedly decreases synthesis and deployment to the basolateral membrane of AQP3 and AQP4. When AQP2 is in the apical membrane, these aquaporins mediate the water flux across the basolateral membrane.[208] Providing support for a causal relationship between the changes in aquaporin activity and the ability to concentrate the urine, expression of AQP2 remains suppressed for 7 days after relief of the obstruction, and the rise in urinary concentration parallels the recovery in AQP2 expression.[208,223,224,228]

The fact that collecting ducts from obstructed kidneys do not respond to cAMP indicates that the lesion also involve sites beyond the receptor for antidiuretic hormone.[230] Consistent with the idea that PGE_2-mediated inhibition of collecting duct water permeability does not affect cAMP levels directly but may have post-cAMP effects rather than act via cAMP regulation,[231] recent experiments have shown that COX-2 inhibition prevented dysregulation of AQP2 in obstructed kidneys in which COX-2 protein expression was markedly increased (see Figure 37-9).[216,232]

Based on these results, the defect in urinary dilution in obstruction seems to be due to reduced ability of the thick ascending limb to dilute the urine by transporting salt from the lumen of the tubule to its basolateral side. The collecting duct in obstructed kidneys maintains its low water permeability in the absence of antidiuretic hormone, so that the failure to dilute the urine is not due to collapse of osmotic gradients in the collecting duct. The inability to concentrate the urine results from the failure of the thick limb to generate a concentrated interstitium, as well as the inability of the collecting duct to synthesize and to traffic AQP2 and other water channels in response to antidiuretic hormone.

Effects of Relief of Obstruction on Urinary Acidification

Obstruction dramatically reduces urinary acidification in both experimental animals and humans. In humans, release of obstruction does not lead to bicarbonate wasting, which indicates that proximal tubular bicarbonate reclamation is maintained. By contrast, in both experimental animals and patients following release of obstruction, the urine pH does not decrease in response to an acid load, which indicates that obstruction impairs the ability of the distal nephron to acidify the urine.[233-235] This defect likely involves proton transport

proteins both in the collecting duct[233,234] and in the proximal tubule and thick ascending limb of Henle.[235,236]

Reduced collecting duct acid secretion could result from defects in H^+ (H^+-ATPase or H^+-K^+-ATPase) or HCO_3^- (e.g., Cl^-/HCO_3^- exchange) transport pathways, backleak of protons down their electrochemical gradient from the lumen to the basolateral side of the tubule, or, in the cortical collecting duct, the failure to generate a sufficiently lumen-negative transepithelial voltage.[233,234,237] As described in detail earlier, obstruction reduces the activity of apical ENaC in the cortical collecting duct; the resulting loss of luminal negativity may attenuate acid secretion in these segments.[233,234]

In the rat inner medullary collecting duct (studied by micropuncture) and in isolated perfused rat and rabbit outer medullary collecting duct, obstruction markedly reduces luminal acidification rates.[233] Because sodium$^+$ transport does not play a major role in acidification in these segments, the defect must be due to direct inhibition of acid or HCO_3^- transport pathways, or backleak of protons from lumen to interstitium.[237] At low perfusion rates, outer medullary collecting ducts from obstructed animals maintained the ability to generate steep pH gradients,[233] which indicates that obstruction does not block the ability of the tubule to prevent back flux of protons. By contrast, at high perfusion rates, acidification was markedly lower in tubules from obstructed than from normal kidneys,[233] which demonstrates that obstruction inhibits activity or expression of H^+ or HCO_3^- transport pathways.

Antibody-based targeted studies examining the Cl^-/HCO_3^- exchanger and subunits of H^+-ATPase revealed reduced expression of these transporters in collecting ducts of unilaterally obstructed kidneys compared with contralateral and control kidneys.[235,237] Two possible mechanisms of reduced acid secretion were explored.[237] One was that the intercalated cells in obstructed kidneys would exhibit a high proportion of "reverse" orientation, with the proton pump in the basolateral membrane and the $Cl^-/HCO3^-$ exchanger in the apical membrane. The other possibility was that the orientation of intercalated cells would not change, but there would be reduced expression of the H^+ or HCO_3^- transporter. The orientation of the intercalated cells was not altered by obstruction. However, obstruction did reduce the appearance of H^+-ATPase along the apical membranes of intercalated cells in extracts of renal cortex or medulla from unilaterally obstructed kidneys compared with contralateral kidneys, although the total content of H^+-ATPase was not altered.[237]

In obstructed kidneys, fewer intercalated cells exhibited an apical labeling pattern, and many that did showed discontinuities or gaps in apical membrane labeling,[237] which suggests that obstruction inhibits trafficking of H^+-ATPase to the apical membranes of intercalated cells. However, this disorder alone cannot account for the entire acidification defect in obstructive nephropathy, because the labeling pattern returns to control levels as the obstruction persists, whereas the acidification defect remains.[237] In addition, the extent of the decrease in labeling appears to be too small to account for the profound defect in acidification.

In addition to defective collecting duct H^{++} transport, reduced generation of the main buffer that carries acid equivalents in the urine, ammonia, has been observed in kidneys released from obstruction. Cortical slices of obstructed kidneys exhibit reduced glutamine uptake and oxidation, reduced gluconeogenesis, and reduced total oxygen consumption, all of which add up to a reduced ability to generate ammonia from glutamine.[238,239]

Effects of Relief of Obstruction on Excretion of Potassium

As with sodium excretion, potassium excretion increases markedly following release of bilateral obstruction.[240,241] Micropuncture and microcatheterization studies show that proximal potassium reabsorption is unchanged by obstruction, whereas potassium is more rapidly secreted in the collecting duct, likely due to increased distal delivery and therefore more rapid distal luminal flux of sodium and volume following release of obstruction.[195,240] By contrast, following release of unilateral obstruction, potassium excretion falls roughly in proportion to the reduction in GFR,[242] an effect that may be related to reduced distal delivery of sodium. However, administration of sodium sulfate in this state does not stimulate potassium excretion in obstructed kidneys as it does in controls, which suggests that collecting ducts in unilaterally obstructed kidneys have an intrinsic defect in potassium secretion.[243] This intrinsic defect may represent a response similar to the downregulation of sodium transporters in obstructed kidneys described in detail earlier. The kaliuretic effect observed in bilateral obstruction may well be due also to the influence of the elevation in ANP, which, at high levels, can stimulate potassium secretion in the distal nephron.

Effects of Relief of Obstruction on Excretion of Phosphate and Divalent Cations

When bilateral ureteral obstruction is released, phosphate excretion rises in proportion to sodium excretion.[205,208,244,245] Phosphate restriction before the release of the obstruction prevents phosphate accumulation during bilateral obstruction and thereby blocks the increase in phosphate excretion.[244] This can also be achieved by blockade of angiotensin II–mediated effects, which highlights the importance of enhanced renal angiotensin II levels in the obstructed kidney.[56] In addition, phosphate wasting of similar magnitude to that observed after release of bilateral obstruction can be produced by phosphate loading of normal animals.[244] In contrast, release of unilateral obstruction results in phosphate retention, which is likely due to reduced GFR and avid proximal phosphate reabsorption.[246]

Calcium excretion may be increased or decreased, depending on whether the obstruction is unilateral or bilateral, and depending on the species studied.[244,246] Magnesium excretion is markedly increased following release of either bilateral or unilateral obstruction. This magnesium wasting probably occurs because both forms of obstruction markedly attenuate thick ascending limb sodium reabsorption, which leads to reduced positive luminal transepithelial voltages and therefore a reduced driving force for lumen to basolateral magnesium flux across the paracellular pathway.[247]

Effects of Obstruction on Metabolic Pathways and Gene Expression

Obstruction inhibits oxidative metabolism and promotes anaerobic respiration, which leads to decreased ATP levels and increased levels of adenosine diphosphate (ADP) and AMP.[239,248,249] In addition, obstruction alters a wide variety of metabolic enzymes as well as the expression of many different gene products.[239,249-251] These changes are summarized in Table 37-6. Many of these changes are difficult to link mechanistically with the changes in GFR or tubular transport function observed in obstruction. It is possible, however, that reduced ability to generate ATP, along with reductions in Na^+-K^+-ATPase expression, contributes to the natriuresis observed after release of obstruction (see earlier discussion).

Pathophysiology of Recovery of Tubular Epithelial Cells from Obstruction or Tubulointerstitial Fibrosis

An important focus of many experimental studies in obstructive nephropathy has been the renal effects of longer-term obstruction.[252] In part these studies use unilateral ureteral obstruction as a convenient model for chronic renal damage, because the timing of the injury is clear and because the extent of injury should be reproducible from animal to animal.[252] These studies, which have been conducted almost entirely in rodents, have elucidated an overall pathway for renal tubular epithelial damage and have identified several potential targets for intervention.

It is thought that chronic obstruction damages tubular epithelial cells by increasing hydrostatic pressure, reducing blood flow (due to the renal vasoconstriction that occurs in obstruction; see earlier), and increasing oxidative stress.[252] In response, tubular epithelial cells release a number of autocrine factors and cytokines, including angiotensin II,[252,253] transforming growth factor-β (TGF-β),[253,254] platelet activator inhibitor,[255] and tumor necrosis factor (TNF).[256] These factors, along with the presence and increase in levels of adhesion factors, lead to the infiltration of the renal interstitium with inflammatory cells, including macrophages. These in turn release additional cytokines.

All these factors accelerate the development of interstitial fibrosis by increased extracellular matrix, cell infiltration, apoptosis, and accumulation of activated myofibroblasts.[257] This process can become amplified by epithelial-mesenchymal transition (EMT),[258] which is characterized by downregulation of epithelial marker proteins such as E-cadherin, zonula occludens 1, and cytokeratin; loss of cell-to-cell adhesion; upregulation of mesenchymal markers, including vimentin, α-smooth muscle actin, and fibroblast-specific protein 1; basement membrane degradation; and migration to the interstitial compartment.[258] The entire cascade leads to tubulointerstitial fibrosis and permanent loss of renal function, which may continue to progress after the obstruction has been relieved (Figure 37-10).

Recently it has been hypothesized that changes in the intratubular dynamic forces—so-called tubular stretch—in urinary tract obstruction also is an important determinant of the development of tubulointerstitial fibrosis in the kidney.[259] Thus, both in vivo[254] and in vitro models[260,261] of obstructive uropathy demonstrate that tubular stretch induces robust expression of TGF-$β_1$, activation of tubular apoptosis, and induction of nuclear factor-κB signaling, which contribute to the inflammatory and fibrotic milieu.[259,262] Based on these findings, it has been suggested that mechanical stress leads to activation of stretch- and swelling-activated cation channels

TABLE 37-6 Effects of Urinary Tract Obstruction on Renal Enzymes and Renal Gene Expression

Changes in Energy and Substrate Metabolism

Decreased oxygen consumption
Decreased substrate uptake
Increased anaerobic glycolysis
Decreased ATP/(ADP + AMP)
Decreased ammoniagenesis

Changes in Enzyme Activity
Decreased
  Alkaline phosphatase
  Na^+-K^+-ATPase
  Glucose-6-phosphatase
  Succinate dehydrogenase
  NADH/NADPH dehydrogenase
Increased
  Glucose-6-phosphate dehydrogenase
  Phosphogluconate dehydrogenase

Changes in Gene Expression
Reduction in glomerular Gαs and Gαq/11 proteins
Reduction in preproepidermal growth factor and Tamm-Horsfall protein
Transient induction of growth factors FOS and MYC
Striking induction of cellular damage (TRPM2) genes

ADP, Adenosine diphosphate; *AMP,* adenosine monophosphate; *ATP,* adenosine triphosphate; *ATPase,* adenosine triphosphatase; *FOS,* FBJ murine osteosarcoma viral oncogene homolog; *MYC,* myelocytomatosis viral oncogene homolog; *NADH,* reduced form of nicotinamide adenine dinucleotide; *NADPH,* reduced form of nicotinamide adenine dinucleotide phosphate; *TRPM2,* transient receptor potential cation channel, subfamily M, member 2.

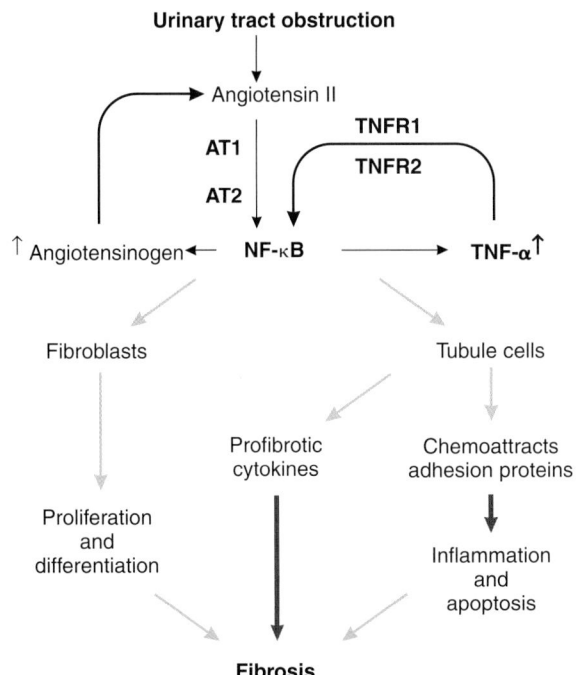

FIGURE 37-10 Urinary tract obstruction causes an enhanced expression of angiotensin II (ANG II). The regulation of gene expression by ANG II occurs through specific receptors that are ultimately linked to changes in the activity of transcription factors within the nucleus of target cells. In particular, members of the nuclear factor-κB (NF-κB) family of transcription factors are activated, which in turn fuels at least two autocrine-reinforcing loops that amplify ANG II and tumor necrosis factor-α (TNF-α) formation. TNFR1, TNFR2, Tumor necrosis factor-α receptor types 1 and 2.

within focal adhesions of the epithelial cells, causing subsequent influx of Ca^{2+}.[262]

Several studies have shown that antagonism of angiotensin II, TGF-β, TNF, or factors that attract inflammatory cells may ameliorate postobstructive renal damage.[252-257,263-265]

Similarly, augmentation of expression of factors that favor epithelial growth and differentiation, such as hepatocyte growth factor,[266] insulin-like growth factor, or bone morphogenetic protein 7 (BMP7)[252] may also have a protective effect. Given species differences and the fact that obstruction in humans is often partial, the animal models may not predict entirely the behavior of postobstructive kidneys in humans. However, if the studies are relevant to human obstructive nephropathy, they suggest that patients undergoing release of obstruction may benefit from therapies that block proapoptotic, proinflammatory, or profibrotic mediators, or from treatments that stimulate epithelial cell growth and differentiation.[252-257,263-265]

Experimentally, protection from obstruction-induced detrimental effects on renal function can also be achieved by NO supplementation. This can be accomplished either by angiotensin converting enzyme inhibition, which increases kinin levels and subsequently increases NO formation, or by stimulation of endogenous NO synthase (NOS) with L-arginine.[267] L-arginine is a semi-essential amino acid and is also substrate and the main source for the generation of nitric oxide via NOS.

Importantly, chronic unilateral obstruction in mice leads to significant reduction in inducible NOS (iNOS) activity, and the obstructed kidney of iNOS knockout mice exhibited significantly more apoptotic renal tubules than controls, results that underscore the important role NO plays in protecting cellular functions in the obstructed kidney.[268]

In a recent study it was demonstrated that dietary L-arginine supplementation attenuated renal damage associated with a 3-day unilateral ureteral obstruction in rats, which indicates that L-arginine treatment may be a pharmacologically useful avenue in obstructive nephropathy.[252] It was also shown recently that several of the detrimental effects of obstruction can be attenuated by treatment with α-melanocyte–stimulating-hormone (α-MSH), which is a potent antiinflammatory hormone.[269] These results support the view that inflammation is a crucial determinant of the onset of renal deterioration in urinary tract obstruction. Interestingly, it was recently demonstrated that treatment with recombinant human erythropoietin (rhEPO) inhibits the progression of renal fibrosis in the obstructed kidney and attenuates TGF-β₁–induced EMT, which suggests that the renoprotective effects of rhEPO could be mediated at least partly by inhibition of TGF-β₁–induced EMT.[270]

Fetal Urinary Tract Obstruction

Obstructive uropathy comprises the largest fraction of identifiable causes of renal insufficiency and renal failure in infants and children. Compared with adult obstructive nephropathy, fetal obstructive nephropathy is particularly devastating, because renal growth and continued nephron development are impaired by the progression of fibrosis.

Several studies have examined aspects of obstructive nephropathy in the newborn using a neonatal rat model of unilateral obstruction. The pathophysiology of fetal urinary tract obstruction is discussed in Chapter 75. Briefly, fetal urinary obstruction may lead to changes in tissue differentiation. At the time of birth, the rodent kidney is not fully developed and is representative of human renal development at about the midtrimester, and animal models reveal that fetal obstruction causes aberrations of morphogenesis, gene expression, cell turnover, and urine composition.[271,272] The earlier the kidney is obstructed in utero, the greater will be the changes in renal tissue.[271,272] After birth, obstruction may affect renal growth, especially in neonates and during the first year of life, but the obstruction will not cause tissue dedifferentiation.

Studies have demonstrated the upregulation of the renin-angiotensin system, as well as involvement of other substrates (TGF-β_1, endothelin-1) and many other mediators in obstructed kidneys.[271-274] The exact mechanisms of action of these molecules in the alteration of renal morphogenesis are not fully understood.

Whether obstruction alone is enough to induce renal dysplasia[271,272] or whether the latter results from secondary obstruction-induced mesenchymal disruption is not well understood. Knowledge of the exact role of obstruction in the kidney malformation is very important clinically, because, as mentioned earlier, it is now possible to detect and potentially relieve obstruction in utero. If urinary obstruction is not the cause of subsequent renal impairment, then some may question whether it is worthwhile to relieve the obstruction in utero. In experimental models, however, obstruction in utero can cause pulmonary hyperplasia and renal impairment directly or indirectly, which leads to significant morbidity and mortality.[271,272,275] In addition, shunting of urinary outflow from obstructed kidneys in animals before the end of nephrogenesis may allow reversal of the arrest of glomerulogenesis seen in this setting,[276] which favors early intervention.[275-278] The changes in renal gene expression and protein production afford many potential biomarkers of disease progression and targets for therapeutic manipulation.[279]

Treatment of Urinary Tract Obstruction and Recovery of Renal Function

Once the presence of obstruction is established, intervention is usually strongly indicated to relieve it. The type of intervention depends on the location of the obstruction, the degree of obstruction, and the cause, as well as the presence or absence of concomitant diseases and complications, and the general condition of the patient.[280] The initial emphasis is on prompt relief of the obstruction, followed by the definitive treatment of its cause.

Obstruction below the bladder (e.g., benign prostatic hyperplasia or urethral stricture) is easily relieved with placement of a urethral catheter. If the urethra is impassable, suprapubic cystostomy may be needed. For obstruction above the bladder, insertion of a nephrostomy tube or ureteral stent may be indicated. The urgency of the intervention depends on the degree of renal function, the presence or absence of infection, and the overall risk of the procedure.[271]

The presence of infection in an obstructed urinary tract, or urosepsis, is a urologic emergency that requires immediate relief of the obstruction, in addition to antibiotic treatment. Acute renal failure associated with bilateral ureteral obstruction or with the obstruction of single functioning kidney also calls for emergent intervention.

Calculi, the most common cause of acute unilateral urinary obstruction, can usually be managed conservatively with analgesics to control the exquisite pain that they cause and intravenous fluids to increase urine flow. Ninety percent of stones

smaller than 5 mm pass spontaneously, but as stones get larger, it becomes progressively less likely that they will pass without intervention. Active efforts to fragment or remove the stone are indicated for persistent obstruction, uncontrollable pain, or urinary tract infection.

Current possibilities for treatment include extracorporeal shock wave lithotripsy (which many require ureteral stent placement if the patient is symptomatic),[281] ureteroscopy with stone fragmentation (usually with laser lithotripsy), and, in rare cases, open excision of the stone.[154,155,282] In general, a combination of lithotripsy and endourologic procedures will succeed in removing the stone.

In the past, complex stones high up in the ureter or in the renal pelvis have been difficult to remove without open surgery. However, improved methods of lithotripsy, including the use of laser lithotripsy through the ureteroscope, has made more stones amenable to fragmentation, and miniaturization of flexible ureteroscopes has made the entire upper urinary tract accessible in nearly all patients except those with severe anatomic abnormalities.[154,155] Once the stone has been removed, of course, appropriate medical therapy is needed to prevent recurrence.[155]

Intramural or extrinsic ureteral obstruction may be relieved by placement of a ureteral stent through a cystoscope.[281] If this cannot be accomplished or is ineffective (especially in cases of extrinsic ureteral compression by tumors), then nephrostomy tubes must be inserted to effect prompt relief of the obstruction.[281]

For infravesical obstruction due to benign prostatic hyperplasia, surgery can be safely delayed or completely avoided in patients with minimal symptoms, absence of infection, and an anatomically normal upper urinary tract.[283] If needed, transurethral resection of the prostate, laser ablation, or other techniques can be used for definitive treatment.

Internal urethrotomy with direct visualization may be effective in the treatment of urethral strictures, because dilation usually has only a temporary effect. Suprapubic cystostomy may be necessary in patients with impassable urethral strictures, followed by open urethroplasty to restore urinary tract continuity, when possible.

Patients with neurogenic bladder require a variety of approaches, including frequent voiding, often by external compression or Credé methods; medications to stimulate bladder activity or relax the urethral sphincter; and intermittent catheterization using meticulous technique to avoid infection.[43,284] Long-term use of indwelling bladder catheters should be avoided, because they increase the risk of infection and renal damage. If more conservative measures such as frequent voiding or intermittent catheterization are not effective, ileovesicostomy or other forms of urinary diversion should be considered. Electrical stimulation has also been attempted with varying degrees of success.[285]

In many forms of obstruction, initial stabilization of the patient's condition is followed by a decision as to whether to continue observation or to move on to definitive surgery or nephrectomy. The actual course chosen depends on the likelihood that renal function will improve with the relief of obstruction. Factors that help in deciding whether to operate and what form of surgical intervention to use include the age and general condition of the patient, the appearance and function of the obstructed kidney and the contralateral one, the cause of the obstruction, and the absence or presence of infection.[286] As noted earlier, the extent of recovery of renal function depends on the extent and duration of the obstruction. A detailed discussion of the indications and surgical techniques for intervention to treat urinary tract obstruction is beyond the scope of this chapter and may be found in other sources.[280,287]

Estimation of Renal Damage and Potential for Recovery

As noted earlier, when deciding whether to bypass or reconstruct drainage of an obstructed kidney rather than excise it, the potential for meaningful recovery of function in the affected kidney is a critical issue. In many cases, obstruction may be partial, so that it is difficult on the basis of the history alone to predict the outcome. In addition, imaging studies that reveal both anatomy and function of the obstructed kidney predict the extent of functional recovery poorly (see earlier), because the extent of anatomic distortion during obstruction correlates poorly with the extent of recovery once the obstruction is relieved.[288]

Isotopic renography with a variety of isotopes can be used to examine renal function, as outlined earlier. This approach is a far more reliable indicator of potential renal function when applied well after temporary drainage of the obstructed kidney has been achieved (e.g., by nephrostomy tubes) than if it is performed while the obstruction is still present.[288] Imaging of the anatomy provides information about the size and volume of the kidney, but does not yield reliable information of kidney function.

All of these considerations figure into the clinical judgment as to whether attempts should be made to salvage the kidney. However, there are presently no methods available to predict reliably the functional potential recovery of an obstructed kidney. In cases of prenatal urinary tract obstruction, clinical decision making is complex because the risks of not intervening can be very high, as can the risks of prenatal surgery. Because prenatal intervention can be associated with frequent complications and a high rate of fetal wastage, patients undergoing the intervention should be carefully chosen. Fetal renal biopsy, which has a 50% to 60% success rate, produces findings that correlate well with outcome and is associated with few maternal complications.[10-12,271,277] It may be used as one of the methods to determine treatment strategy. Studies demonstrate that antenatal intervention may help fetuses with the most severe forms of obstructive uropathy, which are otherwise usually associated with a fatal neonatal course.[10-12,275]

Recovery of Renal Function after Prolonged Obstruction

In patients the potential for renal recovery depends primarily on the extent and duration of the obstruction. However, other factors, such as the presence of other illnesses and the presence or absence of urinary tract infection, play an important role as well. In dogs subjected to 40 days of ureteral ligation, release of the obstruction led to no recovery of renal function. However, recovery of renal function in humans has been documented following release of obstruction of 69 days' duration or longer.[289,290]

Because it is difficult to predict whether renal function will recover when temporary relief of obstruction has been achieved, it makes sense to measure function repeatedly with isotopic renography over time before deciding on a definitive surgical course. Chronic bilateral obstruction, as seen in benign prostatic hyperplasia, can cause chronic renal failure, especially when the obstruction is prolonged and when it is accompanied by urinary tract infections.[290,291] Progressive loss of renal function can be slowed or halted by relieving the obstruction and treating the infection. When obstruction has been relieved and there is poor return of renal function, interstitial fibrosis and inflammation may have supervened. To ensure that there is no other process hampering recovery of renal function, renal biopsy may be indicated.

As noted earlier, studies in experimental animals have implicated a variety of factors in chronic renal failure due to prolonged obstruction, including excessive production of renal vasoconstrictors such as renin and angiotensin, growth factors that may enhance fibrosis. Based on these findings, inhibitors like captopril[281] and angiotensin receptor antagonists[273] as well as NO,[267] α-MSH,[269] and rhEPO[270] have been shown to ameliorate to some degree the long-term damage observed after prolonged obstruction, but further clinical trials are required to evaluate their potential role.

Postobstructive Diuresis

Release of obstruction can lead to marked natriuresis and diuresis with the wasting of potassium, phosphate, and divalent cations. It is notable that clinically significant postobstructive diuresis usually occurs only in the setting of prior bilateral obstruction or unilateral obstruction of a solitary functioning kidney. The mechanisms involved have been described in detail earlier and include the combination of intrinsic damage to tubular salt, solute, and water reabsorption, as well as the effects of volume expansion, accumulation of solutes (e.g., urea), and attendant increases in natriuretic substances such as ANP. When the obstruction is unilateral and there is a functioning contralateral kidney, the volume expansion, solute accumulation, and increases in natriuretic substances do not occur, and the contralateral kidney may retain salt and water, which compensates somewhat for the natriuresis and diuresis occurring in the postobstructive kidney.

Management of the patient with postobstructive diuresis focuses on avoiding severe volume depletion due to salt wasting as well as other electrolyte imbalances such as hypokalemia, hyponatremia, hypernatremia, and hypomagnesemia. Postobstructive diuresis is usually self-limited. It generally lasts for several days to a week, but may persist for months in rare cases. Acute massive polyuria or prolonged postobstructive diuresis may deplete the patient of Na^+, K^+, Cl^-, HCO_3^-, and water, as well as divalent cations and phosphate.

Volume or free water replacement is appropriate only when the salt and water losses result in volume depletion or a disturbance of osmolality. In many cases, excessive volume or fluid replacement prolongs the diuresis and natriuresis. Because the initial urine is isosthenuric, with an initial Na^+ of approximately 80 mEq/L, an appropriate starting fluid for replacement may be 0.45% saline, given at a rate somewhat slower than the rate of urine output. During this period, meticulous monitoring of vital signs, volume status, urine output, and serum and urine chemistry and osmolality is imperative. This will determine the need for ongoing replacement of salt, free water, and other electrolytes. With massive diuresis, these measurements will need to be repeated frequently, up to four times daily, with frequent adjustment of replacement fluids as needed.

References

1. Bricker NS, Klahr S. Obstructive nephropathy. In: Strauss MB, Welt LG, eds. *Diseases of the kidney*. Boston: Little, Brown; 1971:997-1037.
2. Yarger WE. Urinary tract obstruction. In: Brenner BM, Rector FC, eds. *The Kidney*. Philadelphia: Saunders; 1991:1768-1808.
3. Peters CA. Urinary tract obstruction in children. *J Urol*. 1995;154:1874-1884.
4. Klahr S. Obstructive nephropathy. *Intern Med*. 2000;39:355-361.
5. Bell ET. Obstruction of the urinary tract—hydronephrosis. In: Bell ET, ed. *Renal diseases*. Philadelphia: Lea & Febiger; 1947:113-139.
6. Campbell MF. Urinary obstruction. In: Campbell MF, Harrison JH, eds. *Urology*. Philadelphia: Saunders; 1970:1772-1793.
7. Tan PH, Chiang GS, Tay AH. Pathology of urinary tract malformations in a paediatric autopsy series. *Ann Acad Med Singapore*. 1994;23:838-843.
8. Klahr S, Buerkert J, Morrison AR. Urinary tract obstruction. In: Brenner BM, Rector FC, eds. *The Kidney*. 3rd ed. Philadelphia: Saunders; 1986:1443-1490.
9. Chevalier RL, Klahr S. Therapeutic approaches in obstructive uropathy. *Semin Nephrol*. 1998;18:652-658.
10. Becker A, Baum M. Obstructive uropathy. *Early Hum Dev*. 2006;82:15-22.
11. Thomas DF. Prenatal diagnosis: does it alter outcome? *Prenat Diagn*. 2001;21:1004-1011.
12. Kilby MD, Daniels JP, Khan K. Congenital lower urinary tract obstruction: to shunt or not to shunt? *BJU Int*. 2006;97:6-8.
13. Snyder III HM, Lebowitz RL, Colodny AH, et al. Ureteropelvic junction obstruction in children. *Urol Clin North Am*. 1980;7:273-290.
14. Fefer S, Ellsworth P. Prenatal hydronephrosis. *Pediatr Clin North Am*. 2006;53:429-447:vii.
15. Graversen HP, Tofte T, Genster HG. Uretero-pelvic stenosis. *Int Urol Nephrol*. 1987;19:245-251.
16. Clark WR, Malek RS. Ureteropelvic junction obstruction. I. Observations on the classic type in adults. *J Urol*. 1987;138:276-279.
17. Rickwood AM, Godiwalla SY. The natural history of pelvi-ureteric junction obstruction in children presenting clinically with the complaint. *Br J Urol*. 1997;80:793-796.
18. Elder JS, Duckett JW: Perinatal urology. In: Gillenwater JY, Grayhack J, Howards S, et al, eds. *Adult and pediatric urology*, 1991:1711-1810.
19. Murthy LN. Urinary tract obstruction during pregnancy: recent developments in imaging. *Br J Urol*. 1997;80(suppl 1):1-3.
20. Thorup J, Mortensen T, Diemer H, et al. The prognosis of surgically treated congenital hydronephrosis after diagnosis in utero. *J Urol*. 1985;134:914-917.
21. Crombleholme TM, Harrison MR, Longaker MT, et al. Prenatal diagnosis and management of bilateral hydronephrosis. *Pediatr Nephrol*. 1988;2:334-342.
22. Ulman I, Jayanthi VR, Koff SA. The long-term followup of newborns with severe unilateral hydronephrosis initially treated nonoperatively. *J Urol*. 2000;164:1101-1105.
23. Belarmino JM, Kogan BA. Management of neonatal hydronephrosis. *Early Hum Dev*. 2006;82:9-14.
24. Conger JD. Acute uric acid nephropathy. *Med Clin North Am*. 1990;74(4):859-871.
25. Simon DI, Brosius III FC, Rothstein DM. Sulfadiazine crystalluria revisited. The treatment of *Toxoplasma* encephalitis in patients with acquired immunodeficiency syndrome. *Arch Intern Med*. 1990;150:2379-2384.
26. Sawyer MH, Webb DE, Balow JE, et al. Acyclovir-induced renal failure. Clinical course and histology. *Am J Med*. 1988;84:1067-1071.
27. Deeks SG, Smith M, Holodniy M, et al. HIV-1 protease inhibitors. A review for clinicians. *JAMA*. 1997;277:145-153.
28. Chopra N, Fine PL, Price B, et al. Bilateral hydronephrosis from ciprofloxacin induced crystalluria and stone formation. *J Urol*. 2000;164:438.
29. DeFronzo RA, Humphrey RL, Wright JR, et al. Acute renal failure in multiple myeloma. *Medicine (Baltimore)*. 1975;54:209-223.
30. Crittenden DR, Ackerman GL. Hyperuricemic acute renal failure in disseminated carcinoma. *Arch Intern Med*. 1977;137:97-99.
31. Molina JM, Belenfant X, Doco-Lecompte T, et al. Sulfadiazine-induced crystalluria in AIDS patients with toxoplasma encephalitis. *AIDS*. 1991;5:587-589.
32. Goldschmidt H, Lannert H, Bommer J, et al. Multiple myeloma and renal failure. *Nephrol Dial Transplant*. 2000;15:301-304.
33. Waugh DA, Ibels LS. Multiple myeloma presenting as recurrent obstructive uropathy. *Aust N Z J Med*. 1980;10:555-558.
34. Johnson CM, Wilson DM, O'Fallon WM, et al. Renal stone epidemiology: a 25-year study in Rochester, Minnesota. *Kidney Int*. 1979;16:624-631.
35. Stamatelou KK, Francis ME, Jones CA, et al. Time trends in reported prevalence of kidney stones in the United States: 1976-1994. *Kidney Int*. 2003;63:1817-1823.
36. DeFrances CJ, Lucas CA, Buie VC, et al. 2006 National Hospital Discharge Survey. *Natl Health Stat Report*. 2008(5):1-20.
37. Eknoyan G, Qunibi WY, Grissom RT, et al. Renal papillary necrosis: an update. *Medicine (Baltimore)*. 1982;61:55-73.
38. Pham PT, Pham PC, Wilkinson AH, et al. Renal abnormalities in sickle cell disease. *Kidney Int*. 2000;57:1-8.
39. Desport E, Bridoux F, Ayache RA, et al. Papillary necrosis following segmental renal infarction: an unusual cause of early renal allograft dysfunction. *Nephrol Dial Transplant*. 2005;20:830-833.
40. Jameson RM, Heal MR. The surgical management of acute renal papillary necrosis. *Br J Surg*. 1973;60:428-430.
41. Amos AM, Figlesthaler WM, Cookson MS. Bilateral ureteritis cystica with unilateral ureteropelvic junction obstruction. *Tech Urol*. 1999;5:108-112.
42. de Groat WC, Yoshimura N. Pharmacology of the lower urinary tract. *Annu Rev Pharmacol Toxicol*. 2001;41:691-721.
43. Wein AJ. Lower urinary tract dysfunction in neurologic injury and disease. In: Wein AJ, Kavoussi LR, Novick AC, et al, eds. *Campbell-Walsh urology*. 9th ed. Philadelphia: Saunders; 2007:2011-2045.
44. Novicki DE, Willscher MK. Case profile: anticholinergic-induced hydronephrosis. *Urology*. 1979;13:324-325.
45. Murdock MI, Olsson CA, Sax DS, et al. Effects of levodopa on the bladder outlet. *J Urol*. 1975;113:803-805.
46. Crew JP, Donat R, Roskell D, et al. Bilateral ureteric obstruction secondary to the prolonged use of tiaprofenic acid. *Br J Clin Pract*. 1997;51:59-60.
47. Hadas-Halpern I, Farkas A, Patlas M, et al. Sonographic diagnosis of ureteral tumors. *J Ultrasound Med*. 1999;18:639-645.
48. Bolling T, Willich N, Ernst I. Late effects of abdominal irradiation in children: a review of the literature. *Anticancer Res*. 2010;30:227-231.
49. Magrina JF. Therapy for urologic complications secondary to irradiation of gynecologic malignancies. *Eur J Gynaecol Oncol*. 1993;14:265-273.
50. MacGregor GA, Jones NF, Barraclough MA, et al. Ureteric stricture with analgesic nephropathy. *Br Med J*. 1973;2:271-272.
51. Neal PM. Schistosomiasis—an unusual cause of ureteral obstruction: a case history and perspective. *Clin Med Res*. 2004;2:216-227.
52. Christensen WI. Genitourinary tuberculosis: review of 102 cases. *Medicine (Baltimore)*. 1974;53:377-390.
53. Scerpella EG, Alhalel R. An unusual cause of acute renal failure: bilateral ureteral obstruction due to *Candida tropicalis* fungus balls. *Clin Infect Dis*. 1994;18:440-442.
54. Murao F. Ultrasonic evaluation of hydronephrosis during pregnancy and puerperium. *Gynecol Obstet Invest*. 1993;35:94-98.
55. Klein EA. Urologic problems of pregnancy. *Obstet Gynecol Surv*. 1984;39:605-615.
56. Roy C, Saussine C, Lebras Y, et al. Assessment of painful ureterohydronephrosis during pregnancy by MR urography. *Eur Radiol*. 1996;6:334-338.
57. Jarrard DJ, Gerber GS, Lyon ES. Management of acute ureteral obstruction in pregnancy utilizing ultrasound-guided placement of ureteral stents. *Urology*. 1993;42:263-267.
58. Kouba E, Wallen EM, Pruthi RS. Management of ureteral obstruction due to advanced malignancy: optimizing therapeutic and palliative outcomes. *J Urol*. 2008;180:444-450.
59. Gomes CM, Rovner ES, Banner MP, et al. Simultaneous upper and lower urinary tract obstruction associated with severe genital prolapse: diagnosis and evaluation with magnetic resonance imaging. *Int Urogynecol J Pelvic Floor Dysfunct*. 2001;12:144-146.
60. Pais VM, Strandhoy JW, Assimos DG. Pathophysiology of urinary tract obstruction. In: Wein AJ, Kavoussi LR, Novick AC, et al, eds. *Campbell-Walsh urology*. 9th ed. Philadelphia: Saunders; 2007:1195-1226.
61. Deprest J, Marchal G, Brosens I. Obstructive uropathy secondary to endometriosis. *N Engl J Med*. 1997;337:1174-1175.
62. Nasu K, Narahara H, Hayata T, et al. Ureteral obstruction caused by endometriosis. *Gynecol Obstet Invest*. 1995;40:215-216.
63. Dowling RA, Corriere Jr JN, Sandler CM. Iatrogenic ureteral injury. *J Urol*. 1986;135:912-915.
64. Fitzpatrick JM. The natural history of benign prostatic hyperplasia. *BJU Int*. 2006;97(suppl 2):3-6.
65. Burnett AL, Wein AJ. Benign prostatic hyperplasia in primary care: what you need to know. *J Urol*. 2006;175:S19-S24.
66. Alam AM, Sugimura K, Okizuka H, et al. Comparison of MR imaging and urodynamic findings in benign prostatic hyperplasia. *Radiat Med*. 2000;18:123-128.

67. Marks LS, Gallo DA. Ureteral obstruction in the patient with prostatic carcinoma. *Br J Urol.* 1972;44:411-416.
68. Rotariu P, Yohannes P, Alexianu M, et al. Management of malignant extrinsic compression of the ureter by simultaneous placement of two ipsilateral ureteral stents. *J Endourol.* 2001;15:979-983.
69. Batata MA, Whitmore WF, Hilaris BS, et al. Primary carcinoma of the ureter: a prognostic study. *Cancer.* 1975;35:1626-1632.
70. Ben-Ami H, Lavy A, Behar DM, et al. Left hydronephrosis caused by Crohn disease successfully treated conservatively. *Am J Med Sci.* 2000;320:286-287.
71. Schofield PF, Staff WG, Moore T. Ureteral involvement in regional ileitis (Crohn's disease). *J Urol.* 1968;99:412-416.
72. Shield DE, Lytton B, Weiss RM, et al. Urologic complications of inflammatory bowel disease. *J Urol.* 1976;115:701-706.
73. Cook GT. Appendiceal abscess causing urinary obstruction. *J Urol.* 1969;101:212-215.
74. Bissada NK, Redman JF. Ureteral complications in diverticulitis of the colon. *J Urol.* 1974;112:454-456.
75. Knobel B, Rosman P, Gewurtz G. Bilateral hydronephrosis due to fecaloma in an elderly woman. *J Clin Gastroenterol.* 2000;30:311-313.
76. Kiviat MD, Miller EV, Ansell JS. Pseudocysts of the pancreas presenting as renal mass lesions. *Br J Urol.* 1971;43:257-262.
77. Gibson GE, Tiernan E, Cronin CC, et al. Reversible bilateral ureteric obstruction due to a pancreatic pseudocyst. *Gut.* 1993;34:1267-1268.
78. Morehouse HT, Thornhill BA, Alterman DD. Right ureteral obstruction associated with pancreatitis. *Urol Radiol.* 1985;7:150-152.
79. Loughlin K, Kearney G, Helfrich W, et al. Ureteral obstruction secondary to perianeurysmal fibrosis. *Urology.* 1984;24:332-336.
80. Schapira HE, Mitty HA. Right ovarian vein septic thrombophlebitis causing ureteral obstruction. *J Urol.* 1974;112:451-453.
81. Weisman MH, McDonald EC, Wilson CB. Studies of the pathogenesis of interstitial cystitis, obstructive uropathy, and intestinal malabsorption in a patient with systemic lupus erythematosus. *Am J Med.* 1981;70:875-881.
82. Lie JT. Retroperitoneal polyarteritis nodosa presenting as ureteral obstruction. *J Rheumatol.* 1992;19:1628-1631.
83. Plaisier EM, Mougenot B, Khayat R, et al. Ureteral stenosis in Wegener's granulomatosis. *Nephrol Dial Transplant.* 1997;12:1759-1761.
84. Kher KK, Sheth KJ, Makker SP. Stenosing ureteritis in Henoch-Schönlein purpura. *J Urol.* 1983;129:1040-1042.
85. Pfister C, Liard-Zmuda A, Dacher J, et al. Total bilateral ureteral replacement for stenosing ureteritis in Henoch-Schönlein purpura. *Eur Urol.* 2000;38:96-99.
86. Marzano A, Trapani A, Leone N, et al. Treatment of idiopathic retroperitoneal fibrosis using cyclosporin. *Ann Rheum Dis.* 2001;60:427-428.
87. Vaglio A, Salvarani C, Buzio C. Retroperitoneal fibrosis. *Lancet.* 2006;367:241-251.
88. Chung SY, Stein RJ, Landsittel D, et al. 15-year experience with the management of extrinsic ureteral obstruction with indwelling ureteral stents. *J Urol.* 2004;172:592-595.
89. Goldman SM, Fishman EK, Rosenshein NB, et al. Excretory urography and computed tomography in the initial evaluation of patients with cervical cancer: are both examinations necessary? *AJR Am J Roentgenol.* 1984;143:991-996.
90. Jones CR, Woodhouse CR, Hendry WF. Urological problems following treatment of carcinoma of the cervix. *Br J Urol.* 1984;56:609-613.
91. Blum MD, Bahnson RR, Carter MF. Urologic manifestations of von Recklinghausen neurofibromatosis. *Urology.* 1985;26:209-217.
92. David HS, Lavengood Jr RW. Bilateral Wilms' tumor. Treatment, management, and review of the literature. *Urology.* 1974;3:71-78.
93. Schoenfeld RH, Belville WD, Buck AS, et al. Unilateral ureteral obstruction secondary to sarcoidosis. *Urology.* 1985;25:57-59.
94. Bloomberg SD, Neu HC, Ehrlich RM, et al. Chronic granulomatous disease of childhood with renal involvement. *Urology.* 1974;4:193-197.
95. Maeda H, Shichiri Y, Kinoshita H, et al. Urinary undiversion for pelvic actinomycosis: a long-term follow up. *Int J Urol.* 1999;6:111-113.
96. de Feiter PW, Soeters PB. Gastrointestinal actinomycosis: an unusual presentation with obstructive uropathy: report of a case and review of the literature. *Dis Colon Rectum.* 2001;44:1521-1525.
97. Emir L, Karabulut A, Balci U, et al. An unusual cause of urinary retention: a primary retrovesical echinococcal cyst. *Urology.* 2000;56:856.
98. Mark IR, Mansoor A, Derias N, et al. Retroperitoneal malacoplakia: an unusual cause of ureteric obstruction. *Br J Urol.* 1995;76:520-521.
99. Casserly LF, Reddy SM, Rennke HG, et al. Reversible bilateral hydronephrosis without obstruction in hepatitis B–associated polyarteritis nodosa. *Am J Kidney Dis.* 1999;34:e11.
100. Talreja D, Opfell RW. Ureteral metastasis in carcinoma of the breast. *West J Med.* 1980;133:252-254.
101. Roth JA, Diamond DA. Prenatal hydronephrosis. *Curr Opin Pediatr.* 2001;13:138-141.
102. Kessler RM, Quevedo H, Lankau CA, et al. Obstructive vs. nonobstructive dilatation of the renal collecting system in children: distinction with duplex sonography. *AJR Am J Roentgenol.* 1993;160:353-357.
103. Vaidyanathan S, Singh G, Soni BM, et al. Silent hydronephrosis/pyonephrosis due to upper urinary tract calculi in spinal cord injury patients. *Spinal Cord.* 2000;38:661-668.
104. Lementowska T, Nogrady MB, Nearing TN. Intermittent hydronephrosis: a case report demonstrated with overhydration during urography. *J Can Assoc Radiol.* 1970;21:102-104.
105. Tebyani N, Candela J, Patel H, et al. Ureteropelvic junction obstruction presenting as early satiety and weight loss. *J Endourol.* 1999;13:445-446.
106. Chute CG, Panser LA, Girman CJ, et al. The prevalence of prostatism: a population-based survey of urinary symptoms. *J Urol.* 1993;150:85-89.
107. Akcay A, Altun B, Usalan C, et al. Cyclical acute renal failure due to bilateral ureteral endometriosis. *Clin Nephrol.* 1999;52:179-182.
108. Shimada K, Katsumi T, Fujita H. Appendiceal granuloma causing bilateral hydronephrosis and macroscopic haematuria. *Br J Urol.* 1976;48:418.
109. Whiting JC, Stanisic TH, Drach GW. Congenital ureteral valves: report of 2 patients, including one with a solitary kidney and associated hypertension. *J Urol.* 1983;129:1222-1224.
110. Decramer S, Wittke S, Mischak H, et al. Predicting the clinical outcome of congenital unilateral ureteropelvic junction obstruction in newborn by urinary proteome analysis. *Nat Med.* 2006;12:398-400.
111. Shokeir AA. The diagnosis of upper urinary tract obstruction. *BJU Int.* 1999;83:893-900.
112. Noble VE, Brown DF. Renal ultrasound. *Emerg Med Clin North Am.* 2004;22:641-659.
113. Garcia-Pena BM, Keller MS, Schwartz DS, et al. The ultrasonographic differentiation of obstructive versus nonobstructive hydronephrosis in children: a multivariate scoring system. *J Urol.* 1997;158:560-565.
114. Gottlieb RH, Weinberg EP, Rubens DJ, et al. Renal sonography: can it be used more selectively in the setting of an elevated serum creatinine level?. *Am J Kidney Dis.* 1997;29:362-367.
115. Talner LB. Urinary obstruction. In: Pollack HM, ed. *Clinical urology: an atlas and textbook of urological imaging.* Philadelphia: Saunders; 1990:pp 1535-1628.
116. Dorio PJ, Pozniak MA, Lee Jr FT, et al. Non–contrast-enhanced helical computed tomography for the evaluation of patients with acute flank pain. *WMJ.* 1999;98:30-34.
117. Lalli AF. Retroperitoneal fibrosis and inapparent obstructive uropathy. *Radiology.* 1977;122:339-342.
118. Amis Jr ES, Cronan JJ, Pfister RC, et al. Ultrasonic inaccuracies in diagnosing renal obstruction. *Urology.* 1982;19:101-105.
119. Liatsikos EN, Karnabatidis D, Katsanos K, et al. Ureteral metal stents: 10-year experience with malignant ureteral obstruction treatment. *J Urol.* 2009;182:2613-2617.
120. Cronan JJ, Amis ES, Scola FH, et al. Renal obstruction in patients with ileal loops: US evaluation. *Radiology.* 1986;158:647-648.
121. Cronan JJ, Amis Jr ES, Yoder IC, et al. Peripelvic cysts: an impostor of sonographic hydronephrosis. *J Ultrasound Med.* 1982;1:229-236.
122. Charasse C, Camus C, Darnault P, et al. Acute nondilated anuric obstructive nephropathy on echography: difficult diagnosis in the intensive care unit. *Intensive Care Med.* 1991;17:387-391.
123. Garrett WJ, Grunwald G, Robinson DE. Prenatal diagnosis of fetal polycystic kidney by ultrasound. *Aust N Z J Obstet Gynaecol.* 1970;10:7-9.
124. Brown T, Mandell J, Lebowitz RL. Neonatal hydronephrosis in the era of sonography. *Am J Roentgenol.* 1987;148:959-963.
125. Tublin ME, Bude RO, Platt JF. The resistive index in renal Doppler sonography: where do we stand? *AJR Am J Roentgenol.* 2003;180:885-892:(review).
126. Shokeir AA, Nijman RJ, el-Azab M, et al. Partial ureteral obstruction: effect of intravenous normal saline and furosemide upon the renal resistive index. *J Urol.* 1997;157:1074-1077.
127. Reddy PP, Mandell J. Prenatal diagnosis. Therapeutic implications. *Urol Clin North Am.* 1998;25:171-180.
128. Kaefer M, Peters CA, Retik AB, et al. Increased renal echogenicity: a sonographic sign for differentiating between obstructive and nonobstructive etiologies of in utero bladder distension. *J Urol.* 1997;158:1026-1029.
129. Woodward M, Frank D. Postnatal management of antenatal hydronephrosis. *BJU Int.* 2002;89:149-156.
130. Feldman DM, DeCambre M, Kong E, et al. Evaluation and follow-up of fetal hydronephrosis. *J Ultrasound Med.* 2001;20:1065-1069.
131. Little MA, Stafford Johnson DB, O'Callaghan JP, et al. The diagnostic yield of intravenous urography. *Nephrol Dial Transplant.* 2000;15:200-204.
132. Parfrey PS, Griffiths SM, Barrett BJ, et al. Contrast material–induced renal failure in patients with diabetes mellitus, renal insufficiency, or both. A prospective controlled study. *N Engl J Med.* 1989;320:143-149.
133. Dalla Palma L. What is left of i.v. urography? *Eur Radiol.* 2001;11:931-939.
134. Sheth S, Fishman EK. Multi-detector row CT of the kidneys and urinary tract: techniques and applications in the diagnosis of benign diseases. *Radiographics.* 2004;24:e20.

135. Grenier N, Hauger O, Cimpean A, et al. Update of renal imaging. *Semin Nucl Med.* 2006;36:3-15.

136. Smith RC, Rosenfield AT, Choe KA, et al. Acute flank pain: comparison of non–contrast-enhanced CT and intravenous urography. *Radiology.* 1995;194:789-794.

137. Boridy IC, Kawashima A, Goldman SM, et al. Acute ureterolithiasis: nonenhanced helical CT findings of perinephric edema for prediction of degree of ureteral obstruction. *Radiology.* 1999;213:663-667.

138. Lacey NA, Massouh H. Use of helical CT in assessment of crossing vessels in pelviureteric junction obstruction. *Clin Radiol.* 2000;55:212-216.

139. Testa HJ. Nuclear medicine. In: O'Reilly PH, George NJR, Weiss RM, eds. *Diagnostic techniques in urology.* Philadelphia: Saunders; 1990:99-118.

140. O'Reilly P, Aurell M, Britton K, et al. Consensus on diuresis renography for investigating the dilated upper urinary tract. Radionuclides in Nephrourology Group. Consensus Committee on Diuresis Renography. *J Nucl Med.* 1996;37:1872-1876.

141. O'Reilly PH, Testa HJ, Lawson RS, et al. Diuresis renography in equivocal urinary tract obstruction in dilated ureters. *Br J Urol.* 1978;50:76-80.

142. O'Reilly PH, Lawson RS, Shields RA, et al. Idiopathic hydronephrosis—the diuresis renogram: a new non-invasive method of assessing equivocal pelviureteral junction obstruction. *J Urol.* 1979;121:153-155.

143. Conway JJ. "Well-tempered" diuresis renography: its historical development, physiological and technical pitfalls, and standardized technique protocol. *Semin Nucl Med.* 1992;22:74-84.

144. Taylor A, Manatunga A, Garcia EV. Decision support systems in diuresis renography. *Semin Nucl Med.* 2008;38:67-81.

145. Frøkiaer J, Eskild-Jensen A, Dissing TH. Antenatally detected hydronephrosis: the nuclear medicine techniques. In: Prigent A, Piepsz A, eds. *Functional imaging in nephrourology.* London: Taylor & Francis; 2005.

146. Grenier N, Basseau F, Ries M, et al. Functional MRI of the kidney. *Abdom Imaging.* 2003;28:164-175.

147. Kawashima A, Glockner JF, King Jr BF. CT urography and MR urography. *Radiol Clin North Am.* 2003;41:945-961.

148. Little SB, Jones RA, Grattan-Smith JD. Evaluation of UPJ obstruction before and after pyeloplasty using MR urography. *Pediatr Radiol.* 2008;38(suppl 1):S106-S124.

149. Prasad PV. Functional MRI of the kidney: tools for translational studies of pathophysiology of renal disease. *Am J Physiol Renal Physiol.* 2006;290:F958-F974.

150. Pedersen M, Dissing TH, Morkenborg J, et al. Validation of quantitative BOLD MRI measurements in kidney: application to unilateral ureteral obstruction. *Kidney Int.* 2005;67:2305-2312.

151. Thomsen HS, Marckmann P, Logager VB. Update on nephrogenic systemic fibrosis. *Magn Reson Imaging Clin N Am.* 2008;16:551-560:vii.

152. Whitaker RH. Perfusion pressure flow studies. In: O'Reilly PH, George NJR, Weiss RM, eds. *Diagnostic techniques in urology.* Philadelphia: Saunders; 1990:135-141.

153. Lupton EW, George NJ. The Whitaker test: 35 years on. *BJU Int.* 2010;105:94-100.

154. Streem SB, Perminger GM. Surgical management of calculous diseases. In: Gillenwater JY, Grayhack JT, Howards SS, et al, eds. *Adult and pediatric urology.* Philadelphia: Lippincott Williams & Wilkins; 2002:pp 393-448.

155. Alivizatos G, Skolarikos A. Is there still a role for open surgery in the management of renal stones?. *Curr Opin Urol.* 2006;16:106-111.

156. Dal Canton A, Stanziale R, Corradi A, et al. Effects of acute ureteral obstruction on glomerular hemodynamics in the rat kidney. *Kidney Int.* 1977;12:403-411.

157. Ichikawa I. Evidence for altered glomerular hemodynamics during acute nephron obstruction. *Am J Physiol.* 1982;242:F580-F585.

158. Gaudio KM, Siegel NJ, Hayslett JP, et al. Renal perfusion and intratubular pressure during ureteral occlusion in the rat. *Am J Physiol.* 1980;238:F205-F209.

159. Navar LG, Baer PG. Renal autoregulatory and glomerular filtration responses to gradated ureteral obstruction. *Nephron.* 1970;7:301-316.

160. Francisco LL, Hoversten LG, DiBona GF. Renal nerves in the compensatory adaptation to ureteral occlusion. *Am J Physiol.* 1980;238:F229-F234.

161. Wright FS, Briggs JP. Feedback control of glomerular blood flow, pressure, and filtration rate. *Physiol Rev.* 1979;59:958-1006.

162. Schramm LP, Carlson DE. Inhibition of renal vasoconstriction by elevated ureteral pressure. *Am J Physiol.* 1975;228:1126-1133.

163. Allen JT, Vaughan Jr ED, Gillenwater JY. The effect of indomethacin on renal blood flow and ureteral pressure in unilateral ureteral obstruction in awake dogs. *Invest Urol.* 1978;15:324-327.

164. Harris RH, Gill JM. Changes in glomerular filtration rate during complete ureteral obstruction in rats. *Kidney Int.* 1981;19:603-608.

165. Moody TE, Vaughan Jr ED, Gillenwater JY. Relationship between renal blood flow and ureteral pressure during 18 hours of total unilateral ureteral occlusion. *Invest Urol.* 1975;13:246-251.

166. Harris RH, Yarger WE. Renal function after release of unilateral ureteral obstruction in rats. *Am J Physiol.* 1974;227:806-815.

167. Dal Canton A, Corradi A, Stanziale R, et al. Glomerular hemodynamics before and after release of 24-hour bilateral ureteral obstruction. *Kidney Int.* 1980;17:491-496.

168. Dal Canton A, Corradi A, Stanziale R, et al. Effects of 24-hour unilateral ureteral obstruction on glomerular hemodynamics in rat kidney. *Kidney Int.* 1979;15:457-462.

169. Tanner GA. Effects of kidney tubule obstruction glomerular function in rats. *Am J Physiol.* 1979;237(5):F379-F385.

170. Yarger WE, Aynedjian HS, Bank N. A micropuncture study of postobstructive diuresis in the rat. *J Clin Invest.* 1972;51:625-637.

171. Wahlberg J, Stenberg A, Wilson DR, et al. Tubuloglomerular feedback and interstitial pressure in obstructive nephropathy. *Kidney Int.* 1984;26:294-301.

172. Yarger WE, Schocken DD, Harris RH. Obstructive nephropathy in the rat: possible roles for the renin-angiotensin system, prostaglandins, and thromboxanes in postobstructive renal function. *J Clin Invest.* 1980;65:400-412.

173. Vaughan Jr ED, Sweet RC, Gillenwater JY. Peripheral renin and blood pressure changes following complete unilateral ureteral occlusion. *J Urol.* 1970;104:89-92.

174. Moody TE, Vaughan Jr ED, Wyker AT, et al. The role of intrarenal angiotensin II in the hemodynamic response to unilateral obstructive uropathy. *Invest Urol.* 1977;14:390-397.

175. Jensen AM, Li C, Praetorius HA, et al. Angiotensin II mediates downregulation of aquaporin water channels and key renal sodium transporters in response to urinary tract obstruction. *Am J Physiol Renal Physiol.* 2006;291:F1021-F1032.

176. Topcu SO, Pedersen M, Norregaard R, et al. Candesartan prevents long-term impairment of renal function in response to neonatal partial unilateral ureteral obstruction. *Am J Physiol Renal Physiol.* 2007;292:F736-F748.

177. Morrison AR, Benabe JE. Prostaglandins in vascular tone in experimental obstructive nephropathy. *Kidney Int.* 1981;19:786-790.

178. Klotman PE, Smith SR, Volpp BD, et al. Thromboxane synthetase inhibition improves function of hydronephrotic rat kidneys. *Am J Physiol.* 1986;250:F282-F287.

179. Ichikawa I, Purkerson ML, Yates J, et al. Dietary protein intake conditions the degree of renal vasoconstriction in acute renal failure caused by ureteral obstruction. *Am J Physiol.* 1985;249:F54-F61.

180. Yanagisawa H, Morrissey J, Morrison AR, et al. Eicosanoid production by isolated glomeruli of rats with unilateral ureteral obstruction. *Kidney Int.* 1990;37:1528-1535.

181. Folkert VW, Schlondorff D. Altered prostaglandin synthesis by glomeruli from rats with unilateral ureteral ligation. *Am J Physiol.* 1981;241:F289-F299.

182. Schreiner GF, Harris KP, Purkerson ML, et al. Immunological aspects of acute ureteral obstruction: immune cell infiltrate in the kidney. *Kidney Int.* 1988;34:487-493.

183. Harris KP, Schreiner GF, Klahr S. Effect of leukocyte depletion on the function of the postobstructed kidney in the rat. *Kidney Int.* 1989;36:210-215.

184. Reyes AA, Martin D, Settle S, et al. EDRF role in renal function and blood pressure of normal rats and rats with obstructive uropathy. *Kidney Int.* 1992;41:403-413.

185. Harris RH, Yarger WE. The pathogenesis of post-obstructive diuresis. *J Clin Invest.* 1975;56:880-887.

186. Brenner BM, Ballermann BJ, Gunning ME, et al. Diverse biological actions of atrial natriuretic peptide. *Physiol Rev.* 1990;70:665-699.

187. Harris RH, Yarger WE. Urine-reinfusion natriuresis: evidence for potent natriuretic factors in rat urine. *Kidney Int.* 1977;11:93-105.

188. Bhangdia DK, Gulmi FA, Chou SY, et al. Alterations of renal hemodynamics in unilateral ureteral obstruction mediated by activation of endothelin receptor subtypes. *J Urol.* 2003;170:2057-2062.

189. Moridaira K, Yanagisawa H, Nodera M, et al. Enhanced expression of vsmNOS mRNA in glomeruli from rats with unilateral ureteral obstruction. *Kidney Int.* 2000;57:1502-1511.

190. Bander SJ, Buerkert J, Martin D, et al. Long-term effects of 24-hr unilateral ureteral obstruction on renal function in the rat. *Kidney Int.* 1985;28:614-620.

191. Kerr Jr WS. Effect of complete ureteral obstruction for one week on kidney function. *J Appl Physiol.* 1954;6:762-772.

192. Provoost AP, Molenaar JC. Renal function during and after a temporary complete unilateral ureter obstruction in rats. *Invest Urol.* 1981;18:242-246.

193. Wilson DR. Micropuncture study of chronic obstructive nephropathy before and after release of obstruction. *Kidney International.* 1972;2:119-130.

194. Shi Y, Pedersen M, Li C, et al. Early release of neonatal ureteral obstruction preserves renal function. *Am J Physiol Renal Physiol.* 2004;286:F1087-F1099.

195. Sonnenberg H, Wilson DR. The role of the medullary collecting duct in postobstructive diuresis. *J Clin Invest.* 1976;57:1564-1574.

196. Buerkert J, Martin D, Head M, et al. Deep nephron function after release of acute unilateral ureteral obstruction in the young rat. *J Clin Invest.* 1978;62:1228-1239.

197. Hanley MJ, Davidson K. Isolated nephron segments from rabbit models of obstructive nephropathy. *J Clin Invest.* 1982;69:165-174.

198. Hwang SJ, Haas M, Harris Jr HW, et al. Transport defects of rabbit medullary thick ascending limb cells in obstructive nephropathy. *J Clin Invest.* 1993;91:21-28.

199. Miyata Y, Muto S, Ebata S, et al. Sodium and potassium transport properties of the cortical collecting duct following unilateral ureteral obstruction. *J Am Soc Nephrol.* 1992;3:815A.

200. Campbell HT, Bello Reuss E, Klahr S. Hydraulic water permeability and transepithelial voltage in the isolated perfused rabbit cortical collecting tubule following acute unilateral ureteral obstruction. *J Clin Invest.* 1985;75:219-225.

201. Hwang SJ, Harris Jr HW, Otuechere G, et al. Transport defects of rabbit inner medullary collecting duct cells in obstructive nephropathy. *Am J Physiol.* 1993;264:F808-F815.

202. Nagle RB, Bulger RE, Cutler RE, et al. Unilateral obstructive nephropathy in the rabbit. I. Early morphologic, physiologic, and histochemical changes. *Lab Invest.* 1973;28:456-467.

203. McDougal WS, Rhodes RS, Persky L. A histochemical and morphologic study of postobstructive diuresis in the rat. *J Urol.* 1976;14:169-176.

204. Wilson DR. The influence of volume expansion on renal function after relief of chronic unilateral ureteral obstruction. *Kidney Int.* 1974;5: 402-410.

205. Li C, Wang W, Kwon TH, et al. Altered expression of major renal Na transporters in rats with unilateral ureteral obstruction. *Am J Physiol Renal Physiol.* 2003;284:F155-F166.

206. Hwang SJ, Hu G, Charness ME, et al. Regulation of Na/K-ATPase expression in obstructive uropathy. *Clin Res.* 1993;41:141A.

207. Li C, Wang W, Norregaard R, et al. Altered expression of epithelial sodium channel in rats with bilateral or unilateral ureteral obstruction. *Am J Physiol Renal Physiol.* 2007;293:F333-F341.

208. Li C, Wang W, Knepper MA, et al. Downregulation of renal aquaporins in response to unilateral ureteral obstruction. *Am J Physiol Renal Physiol.* 2003;284:F1066-F1079.

209. Hegarty NJ, Watson RW, Young LS, et al. Cytoprotective effects of nitrates in a cellular model of hydronephrosis. *Kidney Int.* 2002;62:70-77.

210. Zeidel ML. Hormonal regulation of inner medullary collecting duct sodium transport. *Am J Physiol.* 1993;265:F159-F173.

211. Grossman EB, Hebert SC. Modulation of Na-K-ATPase activity in the mouse medullary thick ascending limb of Henle. Effects of mineralocorticoids and sodium. *J Clin Invest.* 1988;81:885-892.

212. Petty KJ, Kokko JP, Marver D. Secondary effect of aldosterone on Na-KATPase activity in the rabbit cortical collecting tubule. *J Clin Invest.* 1981;68:1514-1521.

213. Rokaw MD, Sarac E, Lechman E, et al. Chronic regulation of transepithelial Na⁺ transport by the rate of apical Na⁺ entry. *Am J Physiol.* 1996;270:C600-C607.

214. Lebowitz J, An B, Edinger RS, et al. Effect of altered Na⁺ entry on expression of apical and basolateral transport proteins in A6 epithelia. *Am J Physiol Renal Physiol.* 2003;285:F524-F531.

215. Okegawa T, Jonas PE, DeSchryver K, et al. Metabolic and cellular alterations underlying the exaggerated renal prostaglandin and thromboxane synthesis in ureter obstruction in rabbits. Inflammatory response involving fibroblasts and mononuclear cells. *J Clin Invest.* 1983;71:81-90.

216. Norregaard R, Jensen BL, Li C, et al. COX-2 inhibition prevents downregulation of key renal water and sodium transport proteins in response to bilateral ureteral obstruction. *Am J Physiol Renal Physiol.* 2005;289:F322-F333.

217. Lear S, Silva P, Kelley VE, et al. Prostaglandin E₂ inhibits oxygen consumption in rabbit medullary thick ascending limb. *Am J Physiol.* 1990;258:F1372-F1378.

218. Jabs K, Zeidel ML, Silva P. Prostaglandin E₂ inhibits Na⁺-K⁺-ATPase activity in the inner medullary collecting duct. *Am J Physiol.* 1989;257: F424-F430.

219. Stokes JB, Kokko JP. Inhibition of sodium transport by prostaglandin E₂ across the isolated, perfused rabbit collecting tubule. *J Clin Invest.* 1977;59:1099-1104.

220. Norregaard R, Jensen BL, Topcu SO, et al. COX-2 activity transiently contributes to increased water and NaCl excretion in the polyuric phase after release of ureteral obstruction. *Am J Physiol Renal Physiol.* 2007;292:F1322-F1333.

221. Purkerson ML, Blaine EH, Stokes TJ, et al. Role of atrial peptide in the natriuresis and diuresis that follows relief of obstruction in rat. *Am J Physiol.* 1989;256:F583-F589.

222. Purkerson ML, Klahr S. Prior inhibition of vasoconstrictors normalizes GFR in postobstructed kidneys. *Kidney Int.* 1989;35:1306-1314.

223. Frøkiaer J, Marples D, Knepper MA, et al. Bilateral ureteral obstruction downregulates expression of vasopressin-sensitive AQP-2 water channel in rat kidney. *Am J Physiol.* 1996;270:F657-F668.

224. Li C, Wang W, Kwon TH, et al. Downregulation of AQP1, -2, and -3 after ureteral obstruction is associated with a long-term urine-concentrating defect. *Am J Physiol Renal Physiol.* 2001;281:F163-F171.

225. Zeidel ML, Strange K, Emma F, et al. Mechanisms and regulation of water transport in the kidney. *Semin Nephrol.* 1993;13:155-167.

226. Brown D. Cell biology of vasopressin action. In: Taal MW, Chertow GM, Marsden PA, et al. (Eds.). *Brenner and Rector's the kidney.* 9th ed. Philadelphia: Elsevier; 2012.

227. Nielsen S, Frøkiaer J, Marples D, et al. Aquaporins in the kidney: from molecules to medicine. *Physiol Rev.* 2002;82:205-244.

228. Frøkiaer J, Christensen BM, Marples D, et al. Downregulation of aquaporin-2 parallels changes in renal water excretion in unilateral ureteral obstruction. *Am J Physiol.* 1997;273:F213-F223.

229. Harris Jr HW, Strange K, Zeidel ML. Current understanding of the cellular biology and molecular structure of the antidiuretic hormone-stimulated water transport pathway. *J Clin Invest.* 1991;88:1-8.

230. Jensen AM, Bae EH, Fenton RA, et al. Angiotensin II regulates V₂ receptor and pAQP2 during ureteral obstruction. *Am J Physiol Renal Physiol.* 2009;296:F127-F134.

231. Nadler SP, Zimpelmann JA, Hebert RL. PGE₂ inhibits water permeability at a post-cAMP site in rat terminal inner medullary collecting duct. *Am J Physiol.* 1992;262:F229-F235.

232. Cheng X, Zhang H, Lee HL, et al. Cyclooxygenase-2 inhibitor preserves medullary aquaporin-2 expression and prevents polyuria after ureteral obstruction. *J Urol.* 2004;172:2387-2390.

233. Ribeiro C, Suki WN. Acidification in the medullary collecting duct following ureteral obstruction. *Kidney Int.* 1986;29:1167-1171.

234. Laski ME, Kurtzman NA. Site of the acidification defect in the perfused postobstructed collecting tubule. *Miner Electrolyte Metab.* 1989;15:195-200.

235. Wang G, Li C, Kim SW, et al. Ureter obstruction alters expression of renal acid-base transport proteins in rat kidney. *Am J Physiol Renal Physiol.* 2008;295:F497-F506.

236. Wang G, Topcu SO, Ring T, et al. Age-dependent renal expression of acid-base transporters in neonatal ureter obstruction. *Pediatr Nephrol.* 2009;24:1487-1500.

237. Purcell H, Bastani B, Harris KP, et al. Cellular distribution of H(+)-ATPase following acute unilateral ureteral obstruction in rats. *Am J Physiol.* 1991;261:F365-F376.

238. Blondin J, Purkerson ML, Rolf D, et al. Renal function and metabolism after relief of unilateral ureteral obstruction. *Proc Soc Exp Biol Med.* 1975;150:71-76.

239. Klahr S, Schwab SJ, Stokes TJ. Metabolic adaptations of the nephron in renal disease. *Kidney Int.* 1986;29:80-89.

240. Buerkert J, Head M, Klahr S. Effects of acute bilateral ureteral obstruction on deep nephron and terminal collecting duct function in the young rat. *J Clin Invest.* 1977;59:1055-1065.

241. McDougal WS, Wright FS. Defect in proximal and distal sodium transport in post-obstructive diuresis. *Kidney Int.* 1972;2:304-317.

242. Buerkert J, Martin D, Head M. Effect of acute ureteral obstruction on terminal collecting duct function in the weanling rat. *Am J Physiol.* 1979;236:F260-F267.

243. Thirakomen K, Kozlov N, Arruda JA, et al. Renal hydrogen ion secretion after release of unilateral ureteral obstruction. *Am J Physiol.* 1976;231:1233-1239.

244. Beck N. Phosphaturia after release of bilateral ureteral obstruction in rats. *Am J Physiol.* 1979;237:F14-F19.

245. Li C, Wang W, Kwon TH, et al. Altered expression of major renal Na transporters in rats with bilateral ureteral obstruction and release of obstruction. *Am J Physiol Renal Physiol.* 2003;285:F889-F901.

246. Purkerson ML, Rolf DB, Chase LR, et al. Tubular reabsorption of phosphate after release of complete ureteral obstruction in the rat. *Kidney Int.* 1974;5:326-336.

247. Purkerson ML, Rolf DB, Chase LR, et al. Tubular reabsorption of phospate after release of complete ureteral obstruction in the rat. *Kidney Int.* 1974;5:326-336.

248. Stecker Jr JF, Vaughan Jr ED, Gillenwater JY. Alteration in renal metabolism occurring in ureteral obstruction in vivo. *Surg Gynecol Obstet.* 1971;133:846-848.

249. Nito H, Descoeudres C, Kurokawa K, et al. Effect of unilateral obstruction on renal cell metabolism and function. *J Lab Clin Med.* 1978;91:60-71.

250. Storch S, Saggi S, Megyesi J, et al. Ureteral obstruction decreases renal prepro-epidermal growth factor and Tamm-Horsfall expression. *Kidney Int.* 1992;42:89-94.

251. Sawczuk IS, Hoke G, Olsson CA, et al. Gene expression in response to acute unilateral ureteral obstruction. *Kidney Int.* 1989;35:1315-1319.

252. Docherty NG, O'Sullivan OE, Healy DA, et al. Evidence that inhibition of tubular cell apoptosis protects against renal damage and development of fibrosis following ureteric obstruction. *Am J Physiol Renal Physiol.* 2006;290:F4-F13.

253. Ma LJ, Yang H, Gaspert A, et al. Transforming growth factor-beta–dependent and -independent pathways of induction of tubulointerstitial fibrosis in beta6(–/–) mice. *Am J Pathol.* 2003;163:1261-1273.

254. Sato M, Muragaki Y, Saika S, et al. Targeted disruption of TGF-beta1/Smad3 signaling protects against renal tubulointerstitial fibrosis induced by unilateral ureteral obstruction. *J Clin Invest.* 2003;112:1486-1494.

255. Matsuo S, Lopez-Guisa JM, Cai X, et al. Multifunctionality of PAI-1 in fibrogenesis: evidence from obstructive nephropathy in PAI-1-overexpressing mice. *Kidney Int.* 2005;67:2221-2238.

256. Misseri R, Meldrum DR, Dinarello CA, et al. TNF-alpha mediates obstruction-induced renal tubular cell apoptosis and proapoptotic signaling. *Am J Physiol Renal Physiol.* 2005;288:F406-F411.

257. Ito K, Chen J, El CM, et al. Renal damage progresses despite improvement of renal function after relief of unilateral ureteral obstruction in adult rats. *Am J Physiol Renal Physiol.* 2004;287:F1283-F1293.

258. Grande MT, Lopez-Novoa JM. Fibroblast activation and myofibroblast generation in obstructive nephropathy. *Nat Rev Nephrol.* 2009;5:319-328.

259. Rohatgi R, Flores D. Intratubular hydrodynamic forces influence tubulointerstitial fibrosis in the kidney. *Curr Opin Nephrol Hypertens.* 2010;19:65-71.

260. Broadbelt NV, Stahl PJ, Chen J, et al. Early upregulation of iNOS mRNA expression and increase in NO metabolites in pressurized renal epithelial cells. *Am J Physiol Renal Physiol.* 2007;293:F1877-F1888.

261. Broadbelt NV, Chen J, Silver RB, et al. Pressure activates epidermal growth factor receptor leading to the induction of iNOS via NFkappaB and STAT3 in human proximal tubule cells. *Am J Physiol Renal Physiol.* 2009;297:F114-F124.

262. Quinlan MR, Docherty NG, Watson RW, et al. Exploring mechanisms involved in renal tubular sensing of mechanical stretch following ureteric obstruction. *Am J Physiol Renal Physiol.* 2008;295:F1-F11.

263. Yokoi H, Mukoyama M, Sugawara A, et al. Role of connective tissue growth factor in fibronectin expression and tubulointerstitial fibrosis. *Am J Physiol Renal Physiol.* 2002;282:F933-F942.

264. Lenda DM, Kikawada E, Stanley ER, et al. Reduced macrophage recruitment, proliferation, and activation in colony-stimulating factor-1–deficient mice results in decreased tubular apoptosis during renal inflammation. *J Immunol.* 2003;170:3254-3262.

265. Anders HJ, Vielhauer V, Frink M, et al. A chemokine receptor CCR-1 antagonist reduces renal fibrosis after unilateral ureter ligation. *J Clin Invest.* 2002;109:251-259.

266. Gao X, Mae H, Ayabe N, et al. Hepatocyte growth factor gene therapy retards the progression of chronic obstructive nephropathy. *Kidney Int.* 2002;62:1238-1248.

267. Morrissey JJ, Ishidoya S, McCracken R, et al. Nitric oxide generation ameliorates the tubulointerstitial fibrosis of obstructive nephropathy. *J Am Soc Nephrol.* 1996;7:2202-2212.

268. Felsen D, Dardashti K, Ostad M, et al. Inducible nitric oxide synthase promotes pathophysiological consequences of experimental bladder outlet obstruction. *J Urol.* 2003;169:1569-1572.

269. Li C, Shi Y, Wang W, et al. alpha-MSH prevents impairment in renal function and dysregulation of AQPs and Na-K-ATPase in rats with bilateral ureteral obstruction. *Am J Physiol Renal Physiol.* 2006;290:F384-F396.

270. Park SH, Choi MJ, Song IK, et al. Erythropoietin decreases renal fibrosis in mice with ureteral obstruction: role of inhibiting TGF-beta–induced epithelial-to-mesenchymal transition. *J Am Soc Nephrol.* 2007;18:1497-1507.

271. Chevalier RL. Perinatal obstructive nephropathy. *Semin Perinatol.* 2004;28:124-131.

272. Chevalier RL. Pathogenesis of renal injury in obstructive uropathy. *Curr Opin Pediatr.* 2006;18:153-160.

273. Silverstein DM, Travis BR, Thornhill BA, et al. Altered expression of immune modulator and structural genes in neonatal unilateral ureteral obstruction. *Kidney Int.* 2003;64:25-35.

274. Lange-Sperando B, Schimpgen K, Rodenbeck B, et al. Distinct roles of Mac-1 and its counter-receptors in neonatal obstructive nephropathy. *Kidney Int.* 2006;69:81-88.

275. Agarwal SK, Fisk NM. In utero therapy for lower urinary tract obstruction. *Prenat Diagn.* 2001;21:970-976.

276. Edouga D, Hugueny B, Gasser B, et al. Recovery after relief of fetal urinary obstruction: morphological, functional and molecular aspects. *Am J Physiol Renal Physiol.* 2001;281:F26-F37.

277. Bunduki V, Saldanha LB, Sadek L, et al. Fetal renal biopsies in obstructive uropathy: feasibility and clinical correlations—preliminary results. *Prenat Diagn.* 1998;18:101-109.

278. Freedman AL, Johnson MP, Smith CA, et al. Long-term outcome in children after antenatal intervention for obstructive uropathies. *Lancet.* 1999;354:374-377.

279. Chevalier RL. Obstructive nephropathy: towards biomarker discovery and gene therapy. *Nat Clin Pract Nephrol.* 2006;2:157-168.

280. Hsu THS, Streem SB, Nakada SY. Management of upper urinary tract obstruction. In: Wein AJ, Kavoussi LR, Novick AC, et al, eds. *Campbell-Walsh urology.* 9th ed. Philadelphia: Saunders; 2007:1227-1273.

281. Auge BK, Preminger GM. Ureteral stents and their use in endourology. *Curr Opin Urol.* 2002;12:217-222.

282. Moe OW. Kidney stones: pathophysiology and medical management. *Lancet.* 2006;367:333-344.

283. Lepor H, Lowe FC. Evaluation and nonsurgical management of benign prostatic hyperplasia. In: Walsh PC, Retik AB, Vaughan ED, et al, eds. *Campbell's urology.* 9th ed. Philadelphia: Saunders; 2002:1337-1378.

284. Wyndaele JJ. Intermittent catheterization: which is the optimal technique? *Spinal Cord.* 2002;40:432-437.

285. Jezernik S, Craggs M, Grill WM, et al. Electrical stimulation for the treatment of bladder dysfunction: current status and future possibilities. *Neurol Res.* 2002;24:413-430.

286. Streem SB, Franke JJ, Smith AJ. Management of upper urinary tract obstruction. In: Walsh PC, Retik AB, Vaughan ED, et al, eds. *Campell's urology.* 8th ed. Philadelphia: Saunders; 2002:463-512.

287. Gillenwater JY, Howards SS, Grayhack JT. *Adult and pediatric urology.* Philadelphia: Lippincott Williams & Wilkins; 2002.

288. Gulmi FA, Felsen D, Vaughan Jr ED. Pathophysiology of urinary tract obstruction. In: Walsh PC, Retik AB, Vaughan ED, et al, eds. *Campbell's urology.* 8th ed. Philadelphia: Saunders; 2002:411-462.

289. Lewis HY, Pierce JM. Return of function after relief of complete ureteral obstruction of 69 days' duration. *J Urol.* 1962;88:377-379.

290. Shapiro SR, Bennett AH. Recovery of renal function after prolonged unilateral ureteral obstruction. *J Urol.* 1976;115:136-140.

291. Moridaira K, Morrissey J, Fitzgerald M, et al. ACE inhibition increases expression of the ETB receptor in kidneys of mice with unilateral obstruction. *Am J Physiol Renal Physiol.* 2003;284:F209-F217.

Diabetic Nephropathy

Hans-Henrik Parving, Michael Mauer, Paola Fioretto,
Peter Rossing, and Eberhard Ritz

Persistent albuminuria (>300 mg/24 hr or 200 µg/min) is the hallmark of diabetic nephropathy, which can be diagnosed clinically if the following additional criteria are fulfilled: presence of diabetic retinopathy and absence of clinical or laboratory evidence of other kidney or renal tract disease. This clinical definition of diabetic nephropathy is valid in both type 1 diabetes and type 2 diabetes.[1]

During the last decades several longitudinal studies have shown that raised urinary albumin excretion (based on a single measurement) that is below the level of clinical albuminuria (by reagent strip), so-called microalbuminuria, strongly predicts the development of diabetic nephropathy in both type 1 and type 2 diabetes.[2-4] Microalbuminuria is defined as urinary albumin excretion of more than 30 mg/24 hours (20 µg/min) and less than or equal to 300 mg/24 hr (200 µg/min), irrespective of how the urine is collected.

Nephropathy is a major cause of illness and death in diabetes. Indeed, the excess mortality of diabetes occurs mainly in proteinuric diabetic patients and results not only from end-stage renal disease (ESRD) but also from cardiovascular disease, with the latter being particularly common in type 2

diabetic patients.[5-7] Diabetic nephropathy is the single most common cause of ESRD in Europe, Japan, and the United States, with diabetic patients accounting for 25% to 45% of all patients enrolled in ESRD programs.

Pathology of the Kidney in Diabetes

This section outlines the renal pathology evident in type 1 diabetes, followed by a comparison of the similarities and differences in renal pathology in type 2 diabetes. When its features are taken together, diabetic nephropathology in type 1 diabetes is unique to this disease (Table 38-1)[8-10] Thickening of the glomerular basement membrane (GBM) is the first change that can be quantitated (Figure 38-1*A* and *C*).[11] Thickening of tubular basement membranes (TBMs) parallels this GBM thickening (Figure 38-2).[12,13]

Afferent and efferent glomerular arteriolar hyalinosis can also be detected within 3 to 5 years after onset of diabetes or following transplantation of a normal kidney into the diabetic patient.[14] This can eventuate in the total replacement

TABLE 38-1 Pathology of Diabetic Nephropathy in Patients with Type 1 Diabetes and Proteinuria		
ALWAYS PRESENT	**OFTEN OR USUALLY PRESENT**	**SOMETIMES PRESENT**
Glomerular basement membrane thickening*	Kimmelstiel-Wilson nodules (nodular glomerulosclerosis)*; global glomerular sclerosis; focal-segmental glomerulosclerosis, atubular glomeruli	Hyaline "exudative" lesions (subendothelial)†
Tubular basement membrane thickening*	Foci of tubular atrophy	Capsular drops†
Mesangial expansion with predominance of increased mesangial matrix (diffuse glomerulosclerosis)*	Afferent and efferent arteriolar hyalinosis*	Atherosclerosis
Interstitial expansion with predominance of increased extracellular matrix material		Glomerular microaneurysms
Increased glomerular basement membrane, tubular basement membrane, and Bowman's capsule staining for albumin and immunoglobulin G*		

*In combination, diagnostic of diabetic nephropathy.
†Highly characteristic of diabetic nephropathy.

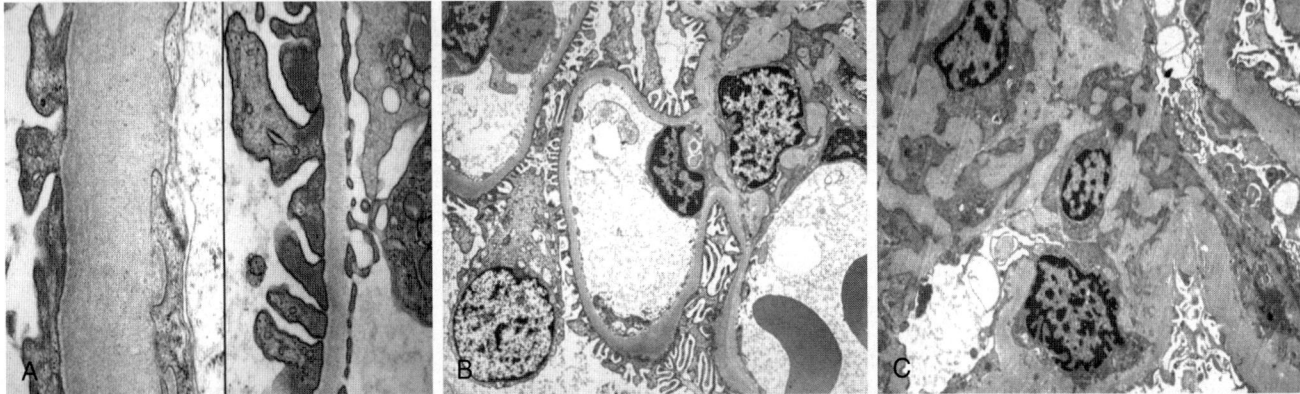

FIGURE 38-1 Electron photomicrographs of (**A**) normal glomerular basement membrane (GBM) on the *left* compared with thickened GBM from a proteinuric type 1 diabetic patient on the *right*, (**B**) normal glomerular capillary loops and mesangial zone, and (**C**) thickened glomerular basement membrane (GBM), mesangial expansion (predominantly with mesangial matrix), and capillary luminal narrowing in a proteinuric type 1 diabetic patient.

of the smooth muscle cells of these small vessels by waxy, homogeneous, translucent-appearing material that is positive for the periodic acid–Schiff reaction (Figure 38-3*A* and *B*) and consists of immunoglobulins, complement, fibrinogen, albumin, and other plasma proteins.[15,16] Arteriolar hyalinosis, glomerular capillary subendothelial hyaline (hyaline caps), and capsular drops along the parietal surface of Bowman's capsule (Figure 38-3*C*) make up the so-called exudative lesions of diabetic nephropathy.

Progressive increases in the fraction of glomerular afferent and efferent arterioles occupied by extracellular matrix (ECM) and in medial thickness have also been reported in young patients with type 1 diabetes mellitus.[17] Increases in the fraction of the volume of the glomerulus occupied by the mesangium, or Vv(Mes/glom), can be documented as early as 4 to 5 years after the onset of type 1 diabetes.[11] In many cases it may take 15 or more years to manifest.[18] This may be because the relationship of mesangial expansion to diabetes duration is nonlinear, with slow development earlier and more rapid development later in the disease.[18] This mesangial expansion is due, in major part, to absolute and relative increases in mesangial matrix, with a lesser contribution from fractional increases in mesangial cell volume (Figure 38-1*C* and 38-4).[19]

The first change in the volume fraction of cortex that is interstitium, or Vv(Int/cortex), is a decrease in this parameter,[20] perhaps due to the expansion of the tubular compartment of the cortex. In contrast to the mesangial expansion,

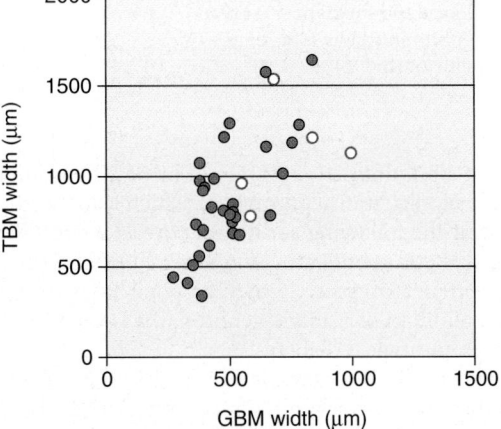

FIGURE 38-2 Relationship of proximal tubular basement membrane (TBM) width and glomerular basement membrane (GBM) width in 35 type 1 diabetic patients, 25 of whom were normoalbuminuric ($r = 0.64$; $P < 0.001$). The hypertensive patients are represented by the *white circles*. (From Brito PL, Fioretto P, Drummond K, et al. Proximal tubular basement membrane width in insulin-dependent diabetes mellitus. *Kidney Int* 53[3]: 754-761, 1998.)

initial interstitial expansion is primarily due to an increase in the cellular component of this renal compartment.[21] An increase in interstitial ECM fibrillar collagen is a relatively late finding in this disease, measurable only in patients with

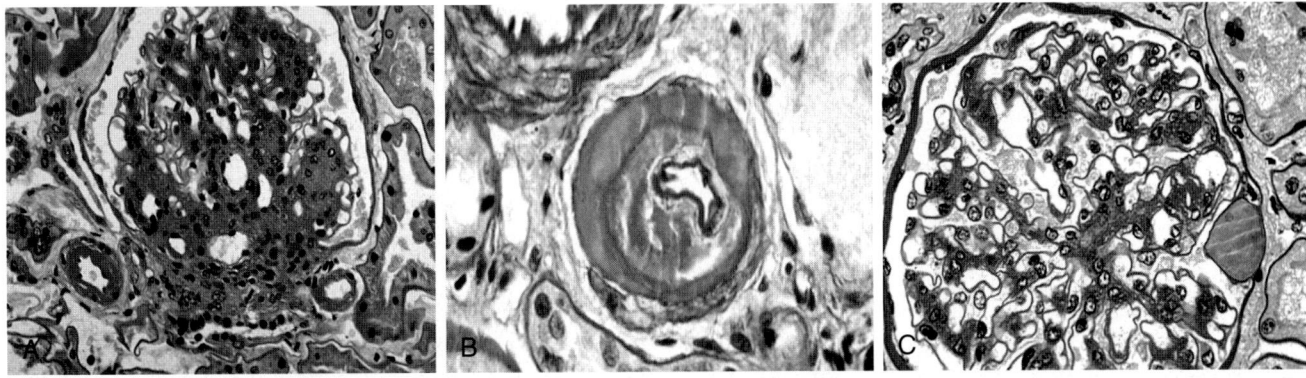

FIGURE 38-3 Light photomicrographs of (**A**) afferent and efferent arteriolar hyalinosis in a glomerulus from a type 1 diabetic patient, which shows diffuse and nodular mesangial expansion (periodic acid–Schiff [PAS] stain); (**B**) glomerular arteriole showing almost complete replacement of the smooth muscle wall by hyaline material and luminal narrowing (PAS stain); and (**C**) glomerulus with minimal mesangial expansion and a capsular drop at the 3 o'clock position.

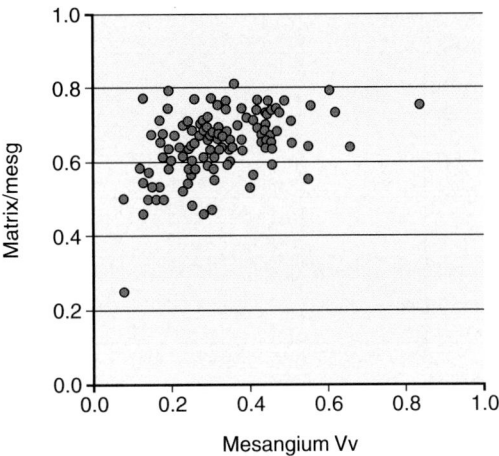

FIGURE 38-4 Mesangial matrix expressed as a fraction of the total mesangium (matrix/mesg) plotted against mesangial fractional volume (mesangium Vv) in patients with long-standing type 1 diabetes. The normal value for matrix/mesg is approximately 0.5. Note that most diabetic patients have elevated values of matrix/mesg (i.e., values above 0.24) whether or not there is an increase in mesangium Vv. (From Steffes MW, Bilous RW, Sutherland DE, et al. Cell and matrix components of the glomerular mesangium in type 1 diabetes. *Diabetes* 41[6]:679-684, 1992.)

an already established decline in glomerular filtration rate (GFR).[21] Abnormalities of the glomerulotubular junction with focal adhesions and obstruction of the proximal tubular takeoff from the glomerulus detachment of the tubule from the glomerulus (atubular glomerulus) (Figure 38-5*A* through *D*) are also late disease manifestations largely restricted to patients with overt proteinuria (Figure 38-6).[21]

These various lesions of diabetic nephropathy can progress at varying rates within and between type 1 diabetic patients,[22,23] and, as discussed later, this is even more the case in patients with type 2 diabetes. For example, GBM width and Vv(Mes/glom) are not highly correlated with one another; some patients have relatively marked GBM thickening without much mesangial expansion and others have the converse (Figure 38-7).[22] Marked renal extracellular basement membrane accumulation resulting in extreme mesangial expansion and GBM thickening are present in the vast majority of type 1 diabetic patients who develop overt diabetic nephropathy manifesting as proteinuria, hypertension, and declining GFR[22,23] (also see later). Ultimately, focal and

global glomerulosclerosis, tubular atrophy, interstitial expansion and fibrosis, and glomerulotubular junction abnormalities are evident when rates of functional loss are marked.[21]

The diffuse and generalized process of mesangial expansion has been termed *diffuse diabetic glomerulosclerosis* (Figure 38-8*A* through *C*). Nodular glomerulosclerosis (Kimmelstiel-Wilson nodular lesions) represents areas of marked mesangial expansion appearing as large round fibrillar mesangial zones with palisading of mesangial nuclei around the periphery of the nodule, often with extreme compression of the adjacent glomerular capillaries (Figure 38-9*C*). This is typically a focal and segmental change likely resulting from glomerular capillary wall detachment from a mesangial anchoring point with consequent microaneurysm formation (Figure 38-9*A*)[24] and subsequent filling of the increased capillary space with mesangial matrix material (Figure 38-9*B*).

Approximately 50% of type 1 diabetic patients with proteinuria have at least a few glomeruli with nodular lesions. Typically, this occurs in patients with moderate to severe diffuse diabetic glomerulosclerosis. However, there are some patients who have occasional nodular lesions and little diffuse mesangial expansion, which suggests that these two forms of diabetic mesangial change may, at least in part, have a different pathogenesis. As mentioned earlier, most (about two thirds) of the mesangial expansion in diabetes is due to increased mesangial matrix and one third is due to mesangial cell expansion. Thus, the mesangial matrix fraction of mesangium, as opposed to the mesangial cellular fraction, is increased in diabetic patients, often even in those in whom Vv(Mes/glom) is still within the normal range (see Figure 38-4).[18] The relative contribution of increased cell number versus cell size to the cellular component of mesangial expansion is currently unknown.

Clinical diabetic nephropathy is primarily the consequence of ECM accumulation, which must result from an imbalance in renal ECM dynamics whereby over many years the rate of ECM production exceeds the rate of removal. The accumulation of mesangial, GBM, and TBM ECM materials represents the accumulation of the intrinsic ECM components of these structures, including types IV and VI collagen, laminin, and fibronectin, and perhaps additional ECM components not yet identified. However, not all renal ECM components change in parallel. Thus, α3- and α4-chains of type IV collagen increase in density in the GBM of patients with diabetic renal lesions, whereas α1 and α2 type

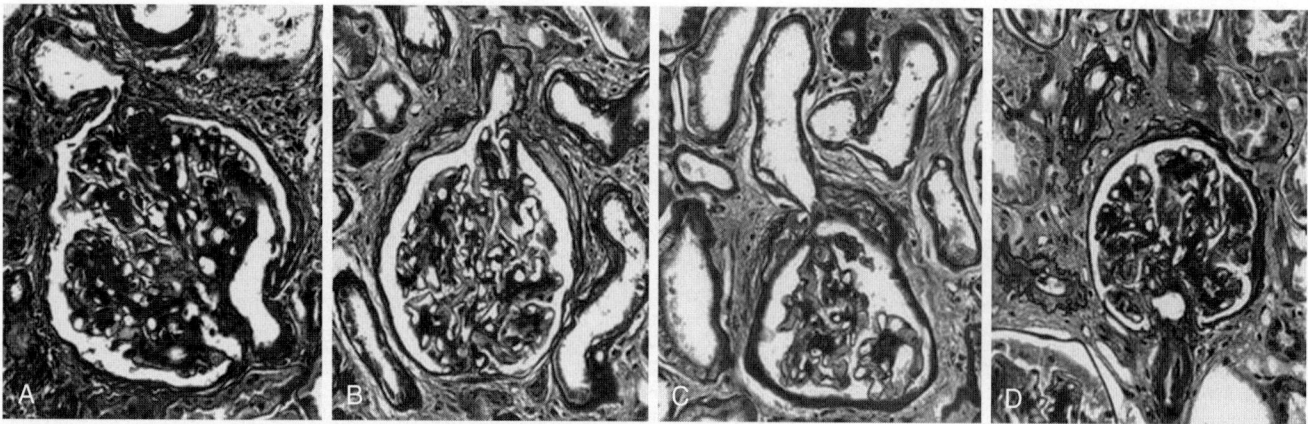

FIGURE 38-5 Glomerulotubular junction (GTJ) abnormalities (GTJA). **A,** Glomerulus attached to a short atrophic tubule (SAT). **B,** Glomerulus attached to a long atrophic tubule (LAT). **C,** Glomerulus attached to an atrophic tubule with no observable opening (ATNO) and a tip lesion. **D,** Atubular glomerulus (AG). (From Najafian B, Crosson JT, Kim Y, et al: Glomerulotubular junction abnormalities are associated with proteinuria in type 1 diabetes, *J Am Soc Nephrol* 17:S53-S60, 2006.)

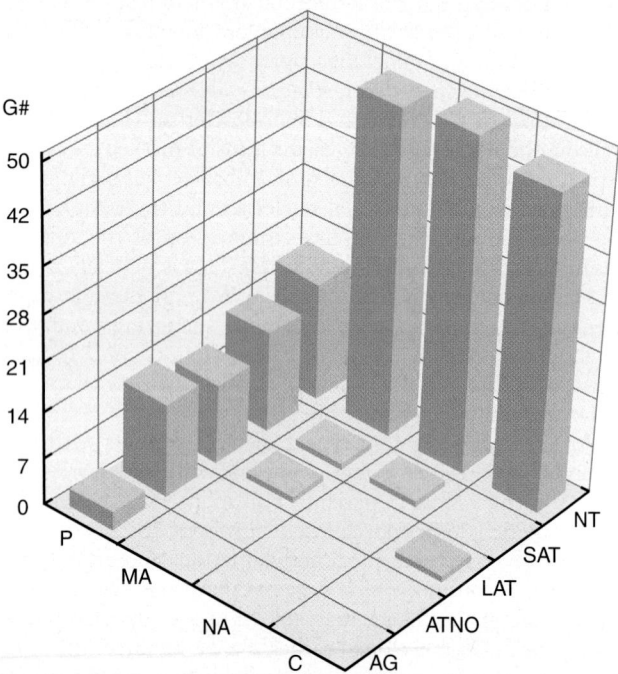

FIGURE 38-6 Frequency of glomerulotubular junction abnormalities (GTJA) in normoalbuminuric (NA), microalbuminuric (MA), and proteinuric (P) patients and control subjects (C). G#, Number of glomeruli; NT, normal tubules. (From Najafian B, Crosson JT, Kim Y, et al: Glomerulotubular junction abnormalities are associated with proteinuria in type 1 diabetes, *J Am Soc Nephrol* 17:S53-S60, 2006.)

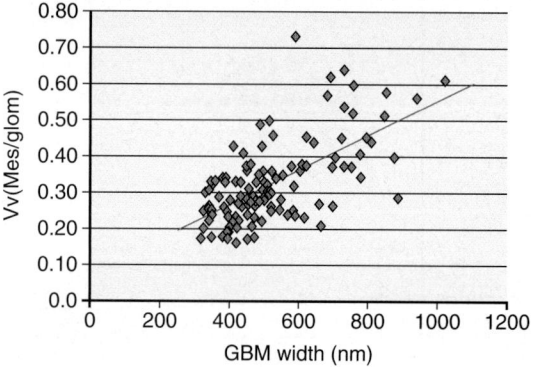

FIGURE 38-7 Relationship between glomerular basement membrane (GBM) width and mesangial fractional volume [Vv(Mes/glom)] in 123 patients with long-standing type 1 diabetes, of whom 88 were normoalbuminuric, 17 were microalbuminuric, and 18 were proteinuric ($r = 0.58$; $P < 0.001$).

IV collagen chains and type IV collagen decrease in density in the mesangium and in the subendothelial space.[25,26] However, the absolute amount of these ECM components per glomerulus is increased due to the marked absolute increase in mesangial matrix material.

The glomerular expression of "scar" collagen is very late in the evolution of diabetic glomerulopathy, occurring primarily in association with global glomerulosclerosis. As the disease progresses toward renal insufficiency, more glomeruli become totally sclerosed or have capillary closure within incompletely scarred glomeruli due to massive mesangial expansion (see Figure 38-9D). However, an increased fraction of glomeruli may become globally sclerosed in diabetic

patients when other glomeruli do not show marked mesangial changes.[27]

Hørlyck and colleagues[28] found that the distribution pattern of scarred glomeruli in type 1 diabetic patients was more often in the plane vertical to the capsule of the kidney than chance would dictate. This finding suggests that glomerular scarring results, at least in part, from obstruction of medium-sized renal arteries.[28] In fact, patients with increased numbers of globally sclerosed glomeruli have more severe arteriolar hyalinosis lesions.[27] In general, global glomerular sclerosis and mesangial expansion are correlated in type 1 diabetic patients,[27] but this may be less often the case in type 2 diabetes (see later).

Podocyte number and/or numerical density (number/volume) are reportedly reduced in both type 1 and 2 diabetes.[29-32] These changes may be associated with albuminuria and disease progression. Podocyte detachment from GBM may be an early phenomenon in type 1 diabetes, appears to worsen with increasing albuminuria, and could be responsible for podocyte loss.[33] However, the experimental techniques used currently to quantify podocyte number are problematic and unstandardized, and more work is needed.

When research renal biopsies were performed in patients with diabetes of at least 10 years' duration who were selected

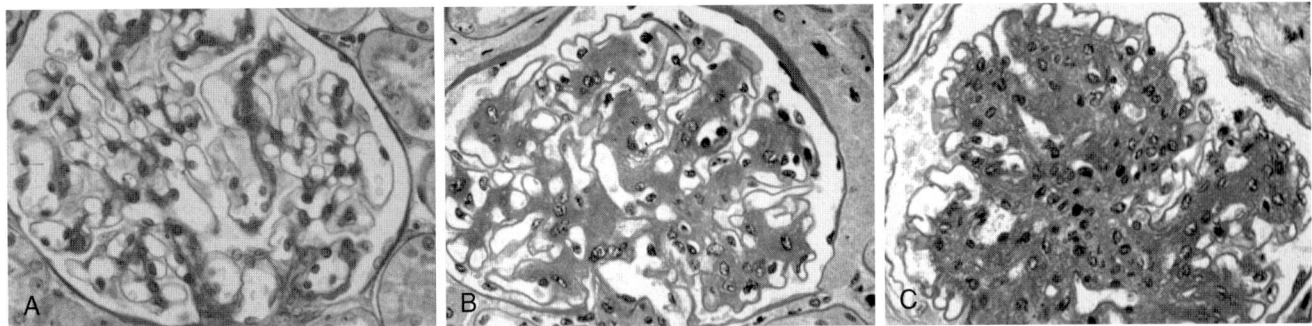

FIGURE 38-8 Light photomicrographs (periodic acid–Schiff stain) of (**A**) a normal glomerulus, (**B**) a glomerulus from a normoalbuminuric type 1 diabetic patient with glomerular basement membrane (GBM) thickening and moderate mesangial expansion, and (**C**) a glomerulus from a type 1 diabetic patient with overt diabetic nephropathy and severe diffuse mesangial expansion.

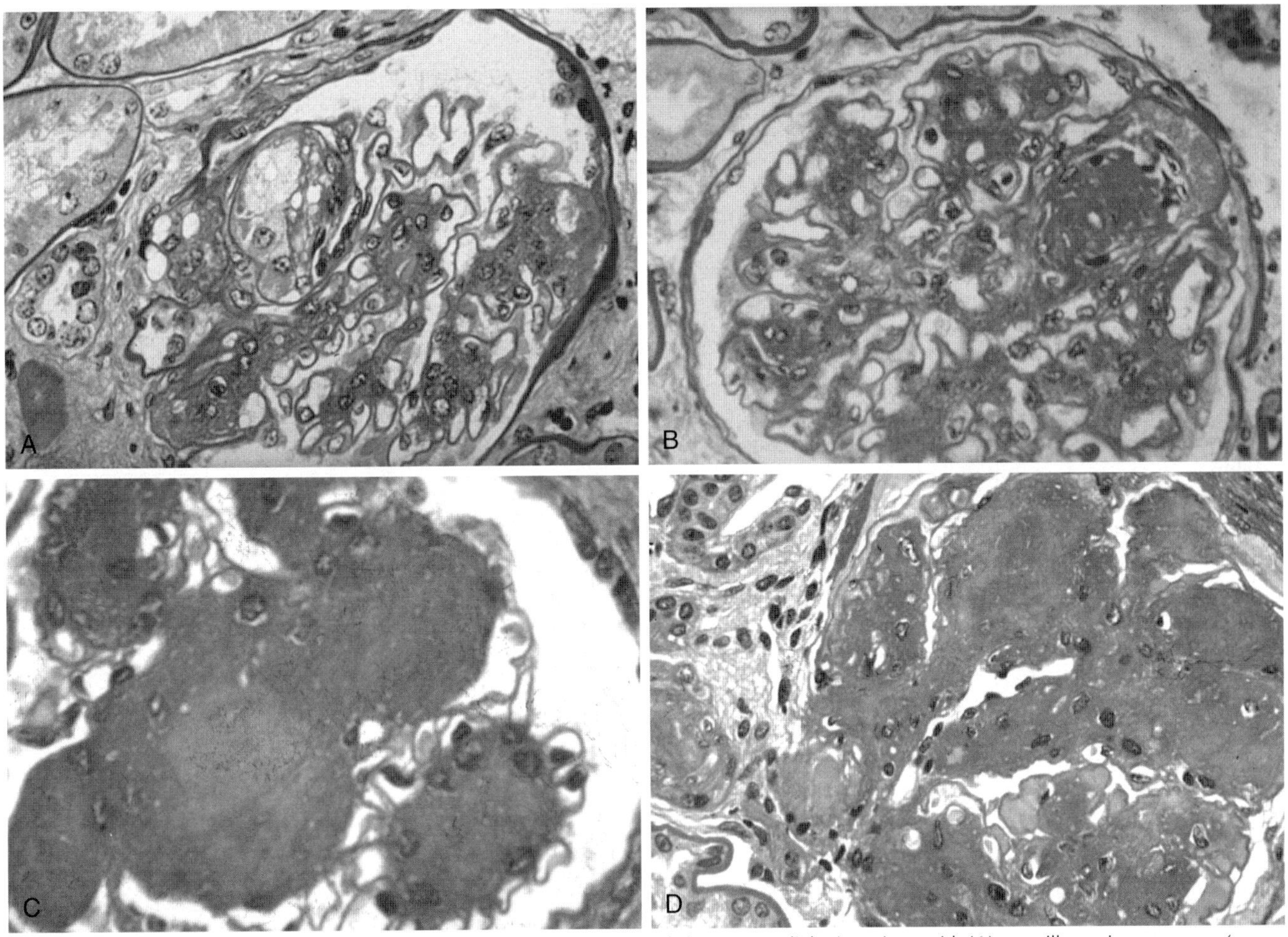

FIGURE 38-9 Light photomicrographs (periodic acid–Schiff stain) of glomeruli from type 1 diabetic patients with (**A**) a capillary microaneurysm (mesangiolysis) at the 11 o'clock position, (**B**) nodule formation within a capillary microaneurysm, (**C**) nodular glomerulosclerosis (Kimmelstiel-Wilson nodules), and (**D**) end-stage diabetic glomerular changes with nearly complete capillary closure.

using no other criteria, significant but only imprecise relationships were found between renal pathology and duration of diabetes.[22] This is consistent with the marked variability in both glycemia and in susceptibility to diabetic nephropathy, with some patients in renal failure after 15 years of diabetes and others without complications despite having had type 1 diabetes for many decades.

Renal extracellular membranes, including GBM, TBM, and Bowman's capsule, demonstrate increased intensity of immunofluorescent linear staining for plasma proteins, especially albumin and immunoglobulin G (IgG).[15] Because these changes are seen in all diabetic patients and appear unrelated to disease risk, their only clinical importance is that they should not be confused with other entities, such as anti-GBM antibody disorders. Immunohistochemical studies have also revealed decreased nephrin expression in association with decreased nephrin messenger RNA expression in podocytes of albuminuric diabetic patients,[34-36] which opens up interesting research avenues for study of these associations[32] and diabetic nephropathy pathogenesis.

Structural-Functional Relationships in Type 1 Diabetic Nephropathy

Mesangial expansion is the major lesion of diabetic nephropathy leading to renal dysfunction in type 1 diabetes patients.[22] Mesangial expansion out of proportion to increases in glomerular volume—that is, increased Vv(Mes/glom)—is strongly correlated with decreased peripheral GBM filtration surface density, or Sv(PGBM/glom) (Figure 38-10),[22] and filtration surface per glomerulus is strongly correlated with GFR in type 1 diabetes.[37] Vv(Mes/glom) is also closely related to urinary albumin excretion rate (AER)[22,23] (Figure 38-11A) and is a strong concomitant of hypertension.[22] Thus, all of the clinical manifestations of diabetic nephropathy are associated with mesangial expansion and the consequent restriction of the filtration surface.

Although GBM width is also directly correlated with blood pressure and AER (Figure 38-12A) and inversely correlated with GFR, the relationships are somewhat weaker than those seen with Vv(Mes/glom).[22,23] However, Vv(Mes/glom) and GBM width, together, explain nearly 60% of AER variability in type 1 diabetic patients over the full range of proteinuria with AERs ranging from normoalbuminuria to proteinuria.[23]

As noted earlier, decreased glomerular podocyte number and detachment has been related to glomerular permeability alterations in diabetes. In addition, changes in podocyte shape, including increases in foot process width and decreases in filtration slit-length density, correlate with AER increases in type 1 and type 2 diabetic patients.[30,32,38,39] Heparin sulfate proteoglycans, presumed to represent an epithelial cell product important in glomerular charge–based permselectivity, are decreased in density in the lamina rara externa in proportion to the increase in AER in type 1 diabetic patients.[40] Whether the addition of podocyte cell structural variables would reduce the residual unexplained variability in AER or GFR in diabetic nephropathy (see later) has not yet been tested. If true, this would support the idea that podocyte

alterations contribute to proteinuria and renal insufficiency. Moreover, confirmation that reduced podocyte number predicts diabetic nephropathy development or progression[41] would add further credence to the importance of this cell in this disease.

The total peripheral capillary filtration surface is directly correlated with GFR across the spectrum from hyperfiltration to renal insufficiency.[38,42] Nonetheless, as already noted, diabetic glomerulopathy structural parameters, examined in linear regression models, explain only a minority of GFR variability in type 1 diabetic patients.[23] Percent global sclerosis[27] and interstitial expansion[9] are also linearly correlated with the clinical manifestations of diabetic nephropathy and are, to some extent, independent predictors of renal dysfunction and hypertension in type 1 diabetes. In fact, some have argued that renal dysfunction in diabetes is primarily consequent to interstitial rather than glomerular lesions.[43,44] However, the conclusion that the interstitium is more closely related to renal dysfunction in diabetes than glomerular changes has been derived from studies in which most, if not all, patients already have elevated serum creatinine

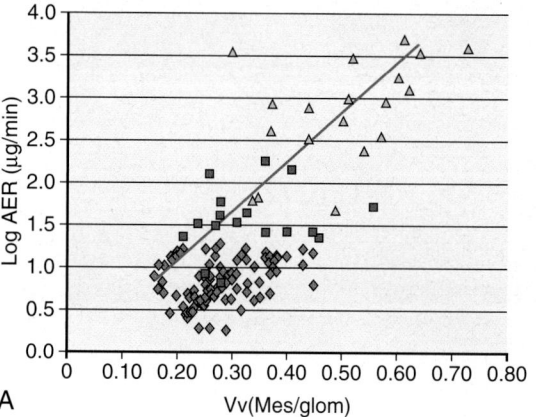

A

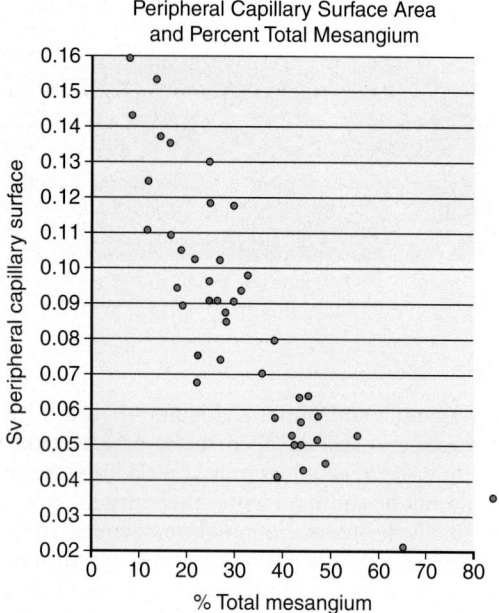

FIGURE 38-10 Relationship of mesangial fractional volume (% Total Mesangium) and filtration surface density [Sv(Peripheral Capillary/Surface)] in type 1 diabetic patients.

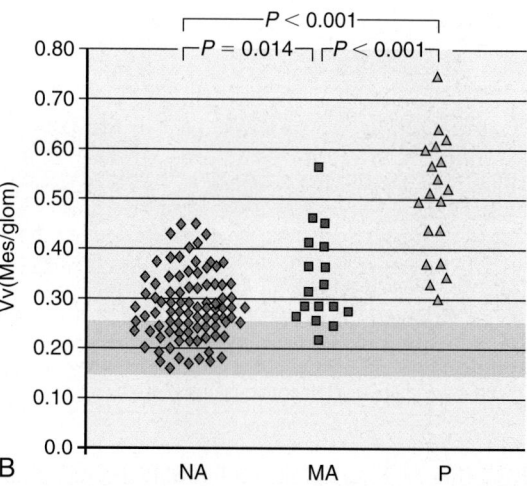

B

FIGURE 38-11 A, Correlation between mesangial fractional volume [Vv(Mes/glom)] and albumin excretion rate (AER) in 124 patients with type 1 diabetes ($r = 0.75$; $P < 0.001$). ◆, Normoalbuminuric patients; □, microalbuminuric patients; △, proteinuric patients. **B,** Vv(Mes/glom) in 88 normoalbuminuric (NA), 17 microalbuminuric (MA), and 19 proteinuric (P) patients with type 1 diabetes. The *shaded area* represents the mean ± 2 standard deviation units in a group of 76 age-matched normal control subjects. The means for all groups are significantly different from the mean for control subjects. (From Caramori ML, Kim Y, Huang C, et al. Cellular basis of diabetic nephropathy: 1. Study design and renal structural-functional relationships in patients with long-standing type 1 diabetes. *Diabetes* 51[2]:506-513, 2002.)

values and in which the interstitium is carefully measured but the glomerular structure is only subjectively estimated.[43,44]

In fact, throughout most of the natural history of diabetic nephropathy, glomerular parameters are more important determinants of renal dysfunction, whereas interstitial changes may become a stronger determinant of the rate of progression from established renal insufficiency to terminal uremia.[45] Furthermore, as mentioned earlier, in the first decade of diabetes, Vv(Int/cortex) is decreased, whereas Vv(Mes/glom) and GBM width are already increased. Moreover, early interstitial expansion in type 1 diabetes is mainly due to expansion of the cellular component of this compartment, and increased interstitial fibrillar collagen is seen in patients whose GFR is already reduced.[20] These and other findings suggest that the interstitial and glomerular changes of diabetes have somewhat different pathogenetic mechanisms and that advancing interstitial fibrosis generally follows the glomerular processes in type 1 diabetes.

Through much of the natural history of diabetic nephropathy, lesions develop in complete clinical silence, and when microalbuminuria and proteinuria initially manifest, lesions are often far advanced and loss of GFR may then progress relatively rapidly toward ESRD. This typical clinical story is best mirrored by nonlinear analyses of structural-functional relationships.[21] When piecewise regression models were used, glomerular structural variables alone [Vv(Mes/glom), GBM width, and total filtration surface per glomerulus] explained 95% of variability in AER ranging from normoalbuminuria to proteinuria; this leaves little room for improvement in predictive models by adding nonglomerular structural variables to the parameters. These same glomerular structures, however, explained only 78% of GFR variability. With the addition of indices of glomerulotubular junction abnormalities and Vv(Int/cortex), this increased to 92%.[21]

In summary, most of the AER and GFR changes in type 1 diabetes are explained by diabetic glomerulopathy changes. These structural-functional relationships are largely driven by more advanced lesions, however; structural changes are highly variable (from virtually none to moderately severe) in patients without functional abnormalities. Predictive tools for the first decade of type 1 diabetes are needed.

Microalbuminuria and Renal Structure

As discussed elsewhere in this chapter, persistent microalbuminuria is a predictor of the development of clinical nephropathy, whereas the absence of microalbuminuria in patients with long-standing type 1 diabetes indicates a lower nephropathy risk. Proteinuria in type 1 diabetes of 10 or more years' duration is typically associated with advanced diabetic glomerular pathology.[22,23] One might reason that microalbuminuria is therefore associated with underlying renal structural changes that are predictive of the ultimate progression of this pathology. However, the relationship of renal structural changes to these low levels of albuminuria (i.e., normoalbuminuria or microalbuminuria) is complex and incompletely understood.

As a group, normoalbuminuric patients who have had type 1 diabetes for a mean of 20 years have increased GBM width and Vv(Mes/glom).[23,46] The structural parameters within this group vary from within the normal range to advanced abnormalities that overlap those of patients with microalbuminuria and proteinuria (Figure 38-11B and 38-12B).[23,46] Patients with microalbuminuric AERs (20 to 200 µg/min) have, on average, even greater GBM and mesangial expansion, with almost no values in the normal range, but these values overlap with those of normoalbuminuric and proteinuric patients (see Figures 38-11B and 38-12B).[23,46]

The incidence of hypertension and reduced GFR is greater in patients with microalbuminuria.[23,46] Thus, microalbuminuria is a marker of more advanced lesions as well as other functional disturbances.[23,46] Studies suggest that greater GBM width in baseline biopsy specimens of normoalbuminuric patients is predictive of later clinical progression to microalbuminuria.[46] Further, microalbuminuric patients with greater GBM width are more likely to progress to proteinuria.[47,48] Some normoalbuminuric patients with long-standing type 1 diabetes, particularly females with retinopathy or hypertension, have reduced GFR, and this is associated with worse diabetic glomerulopathy lesions.[49,50] Thus, increased AER is not always the initial clinical indicator of diabetic nephropathy, and GFR measurements may be indicated in normoalbuminuric female patients with the aforementioned characteristics.[50]

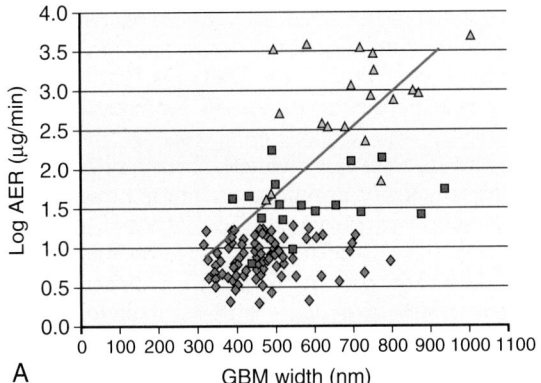

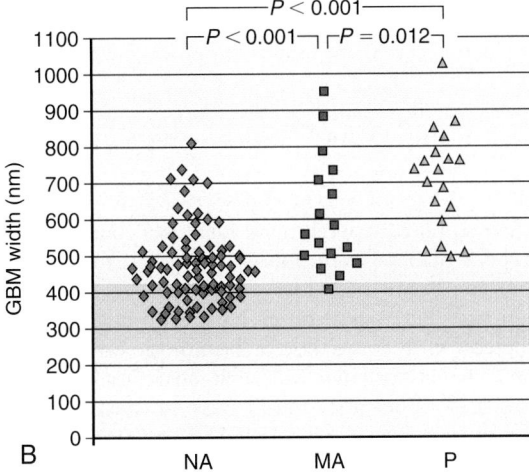

FIGURE 38-12 **A,** Correlation between glomerular basement membrane (GBM) width and albumin excretion rate (AER) in 124 patients with type 1 diabetes (*r* = 0.62; *P* < 0.001). ◆, Normoalbuminuric patients; □, microalbuminuric patients; △, proteinuric patients. **B,** GBM width in 88 normoalbuminuric (NA), 17 microalbuminuric (MA), and 19 proteinuric (P) patients with type 1 diabetes. The *shaded area* represents the mean ± 2 standard deviation units in a group of 76 age-matched normal control subjects. The means for all groups are significantly different from the mean for control subjects. (From Caramori ML, Kim Y, Huang C, et al. Cellular basis of diabetic nephropathy: 1. Study design and renal structural-functional relationships in patients with long-standing type 1 diabetes. *Diabetes* 51[2]:506-513, 2002.)

Risk Factors for Nephropathy Intrinsic to the Kidney

In nondiabetic members of identical twin pairs discordant for type 1 diabetes glomerular structure is within the normal range.[12] In every pair studied, the diabetic twin had higher values for GBM and TBM width and Vv(Mes/glom) than the nondiabetic twin. Several discordant diabetic twins had values for GBM width and Vv(Mes/glom) that were within the range of normal and had "lesions" only in comparison with their nondiabetic twin,[12] whereas others had more severe lesions. Thus, given sufficient duration, probably all type 1 diabetic patients have structural changes that are similar in direction, but the rate at which these lesions develop varies markedly among individuals.

There is a growing body of information, discussed elsewhere in this chapter, which supports the view that not only is glycemia as a risk factor, but genetic variables also confer susceptibility or resistance to diabetic nephropathy. This is also suggested by the marked variability in the rate of development of kidney lesions of diabetic nephropathy in transplanted kidneys, despite the fact that the recipients all had ESRD secondary to diabetic nephropathy.[51] This variability, only partially explained by glycemic control, argues for genetically determined renal tissue responses as important in determining nephropathy clinical outcomes.[51]

Glomerular volume and number could be structural determinants of nephropathy risk. Mean glomerular volumes were higher in patients developing diabetic nephropathy after 25 years of type 1 diabetes compared with a group developing nephropathy after only 15 years.[52] These studies suggest that as mesangial expansion develops, glomerular volume increases, and argue that patients unable to respond to mesangial expansion with glomerular enlargement will more quickly develop overt nephropathy than those whose glomeruli enlarge to provide compensatory preservation of glomerular filtration surface.

The number of glomeruli per kidney can vary markedly among nondiabetic individuals and among diabetic patients,[53] and it has been suggested that fewer glomeruli per kidney could be a risk factor for diabetic nephropathy.[54] However, studies of transplant recipients with type 1 diabetes indicate that having a single kidney does not result in accelerated lesion development compared with having two kidneys.[55] Diabetic patients with advanced renal failure have reduced numbers of glomeruli, but this likely results from resorption of sclerotic glomeruli.[53] If reduced glomerular number were a risk factor, it would be predicted that proteinuric patients without advanced renal failure would have fewer glomeruli, but this was not the case.[53] Although probably not important in the initiation phase of diabetic nephropathology, reduced glomerular number could be associated with more rapid progression to ESRD once advanced lesions and overt diabetic nephropathy have developed.

Comparisons of Nephropathy in Type 1 and Type 2 Diabetes

Renal pathology and structural-functional relationships have been less well studied in type 2 diabetic patients, despite the fact that 80% or more of diabetic patients with ESRD have type 2 diabetes. Proteinuric white Danish patients with type 2 diabetes were reported to have structural changes similar to those of proteinuric patients with type 1 diabetes, and the severity of these changes was strongly correlated with the subsequent rate of decline of GFR.[56] However, the study reporting these findings also noted that some proteinuric patients with type 2 diabetes had little or no diabetic glomerulopathy.[56]

A study of 52 type 2 diabetic patients from northern Italy who underwent biopsy for clinical indications described greater heterogeneity in renal structure, with one third having nondiabetic renal diseases.[57] In a Danish study, three fourths of proteinuric type 2 diabetic patients had diabetic nephropathology,[58] but one fourth had a variety of nondiabetic glomerulopathies, including "minimal lesions," glomerulonephritis, mixed diabetic and glomerulonephritic changes, and chronic glomerulonephritis. All patients with proteinuria and diabetic retinopathy had diabetic nephropathy; only 40% of patients without retinopathy had diabetic nephropathy.[58]

It is very likely that these high incidences of diagnoses other than or in addition to diabetic nephropathy represent a significant selection bias, since many patients in these studies had clinical indications for kidney biopsy, many because of atypical clinical presentations or findings. In fact, the likelihood of finding nondiabetic renal disease among type 2 diabetic patients is highly influenced by a center's clinical indications for renal biopsy in type 2 diabetic patients.[59]

When renal biopsies are performed for research and not for diagnostic purposes, definable renal diseases other than those secondary to diabetes are distinctly uncommon.[59] However, marked heterogeneity in renal structure is present in type 2 diabetic patients with increased AER.[60] Indeed, only a minority of patients have histopathologic patterns resembling those typically present in patients with type 1 diabetes (the typical pattern is 30% of patients with microalbuminuria[60] and 50% of those with proteinuria; P. Fioretto, personal observations). The remainder have either minimal renal abnormalities or tubulointerstitial, vascular, and global glomerulosclerotic changes, which are disproportionally severe relative to the diabetic glomerulopathy lesions (atypical pattern, about 40% of patients with microalbuminuria and proteinuria).[60]

Structural-Functional Relationships in Type 2 Diabetic Nephropathy

Renal structural-functional relationships in Japanese patients with type 2 diabetes were initially reported to be similar to those in type 1 patients.[61] However, a more recent study indicated greater heterogeneity in Japanese patients with type 2 diabetes, with some microalbuminuric and proteinuric patients having normal glomerular structural parameters.[62] Østerby and colleagues found less advanced glomerular changes in type 2 than type 1 diabetic patients with similar AERs.[56] However, the type 1 patients had lower GFR levels than type 2 patients with similar AERs.[56] These findings could reflect much larger glomerular volumes in the type 2 patients, with associated preservation of filtration surface. In fact, GFR and filtration surface per glomerulus were correlated in these patients.[56] Also, the proteinuria in these type 2 patients was, at least in part, unexplained.

Vv(Mes/glom) increased progressively from early to long-term diabetes, with clinical findings ranging from normoalbuminuria, to microalbuminuria, to clinical nephropathy[30] in

Pima Indian patients with type 2 diabetes. Global glomerular sclerosis correlated inversely with GFR in these patients.[30] The authors of this study also suggested, as noted earlier, that glomerular podocyte loss was related to proteinuria in these patients, although this was not seen in microalbuminuric patients (see earlier).

The imprecise correlation between glomerular structure and renal function in patients with type 2 versus type 1 diabetes may be related to the more complex patterns of renal injury seen in type 2 diabetic patients (see earlier).[61] These considerations are relevant to prognosis, in that the patients with more typical diabetic glomerulopathy morphometric findings of mesangial expansion on electron microscopy were more likely to have progressive loss of GFR over the next 4 years of follow-up.[63] This was confirmed in a study of proteinuric Danish patients with type 2 diabetes in which those whose biopsy specimens showed changes of diabetic glomerulopathy on light microscopy experienced much more rapid decline in GFR over a median of 7.7 years of follow-up.[58]

In summary, it appears that in patients with type 2 diabetes renal structural changes are more heterogeneous and diabetic glomerulopathy lesions are less severe than in type 1 patients with similar urine albumin levels. Approximately 40% of the patients show atypical renal injury patterns, and these patterns are associated with higher body mass index and less diabetic retinopathy.[61]

Further cross-sectional and longitudinal studies in type 2 diabetic patients are required before these complexities can be better understood. It is possible that the atypical manifestations of renal injury in type 2 diabetes could be related to the pathogenesis of type 2 diabetes per se. Obesity, hypertension, increased plasma triglyceride levels, decreased high-density lipoprotein cholesterol concentrations, and accelerated atherosclerosis accompany hyperglycemia in many type 2 diabetic patients (metabolic syndrome). Renal dysfunction in these patients could be the consequence of hypertensive nephrosclerosis, hyperlipidemic renal vascular atherosclerosis, renal hypoperfusion due to congestive heart failure, or the synergistic effects of these multiple risk factors for renal disease, which could clinically simulate nephropathy in type 2 diabetes.

The increased risk of clinical renal disease in distinct populations, such as African American, American Indian, or Hispanic patients, could represent variability in the renal consequence of one or more of these pathogenetic influences. For example, there are differences in the renal structural consequences of hypertension in African American compared with white patients.[64]

Other Renal Disorders in Diabetic Patients

It has been reported that renal disorders such as minimal change nephrotic syndrome[65] and membranous nephropathy[66] occur with greater frequency in patients with type 1 diabetes than in nondiabetic persons. In fact, when biopsies are performed for research purposes only and not for clinical indications, fewer than 1% of patients with type 1 diabetes for 10 or more years and fewer than 4% of those with proteinuria and long duration of diabetes will be found to have conditions other than, or in addition to, diabetic nephropathy (M. Mauer, personal observations). As already discussed, proteinuric type 2 diabetic patients without retinopathy may

have a high incidence of atypical renal biopsy findings or other diseases. Proteinuric patients with type 1 diabetes of less than 10 years' duration and type 2 diabetic patients without retinopathy should be thoroughly evaluated for other renal diseases, and renal biopsy for diagnosis and prognosis should be strongly considered.

Reversibility of Diabetic Nephropathy Lesions

Mesangial expansion present after 7 months of diabetes reversed within 2 months after normoglycemia was induced by islet transplantation in rats with streptozotocin-induced diabetes.[67] It was thus disappointing that no improvement in diabetic nephropathy lesions in their native kidneys was found after 5 years of normoglycemia following successful pancreatic transplantation[68] in type 1 patients with a diabetes duration of approximately 20 years. After 10 years of normoglycemia, however, these same patients showed marked reversal of diabetic glomerulopathy lesions. Thus, GBM and TBM width were reduced at 10 years compared with the baseline and 5-year values, with several patients having measures at 10 years that had returned to the normal range (Figure 38-13*A* and *B*).[69] Similar results were obtained for Vv(Mes/glom), primarily due to a marked decrease in mesangial matrix fractional volume (Figure 38-13*C* and *D*). Remarkable glomerular architectural remodeling was seen by light microscopy, including the complete disappearance of Kimmelstiel-Wilson nodular lesions (Figure 38-14).[69]

The reason for the long delay in this reversal process is not understood and could include epigenetic memory of the diabetic state, the slow process of replacement of glycated by nonglycated ECM, or other, as yet undetermined processes. Regardless of the mechanism, relevant renal or circulating cells must be able to recognize the abnormal ECM environment and to initiate and sustain a state of imbalance in which the rate of ECM removal exceeds that of ECM production. This is clearly not the normal situation, because throughout adult life GBM width and mesangial matrix remain quite constant, consistent with balanced ECM production and removal.[70]

More recently, remodeling and healing in the tubulointerstitium has also been demonstrated in these same patients.[71] These studies demonstrated reduction in total cortical interstitial collagen and underscore the remarkable potential for healing of kidney tissue that has been damaged by long-standing diabetes.[71] Blockade of the renin-angiotensin system (RAS) for 5 years did not lead to regression nor to slowing of the progression of diabetic glomerulopathy lesions in young patients with type 1 diabetes and normoalbuminuria.[72] Whether healing can be induced by treatments other than cure of the diabetic state is currently unknown.

Epidemiology of Microalbuminuria and Diabetic Nephropathy

Prevalence and Incidence

Table 38-2 displays the prevalence, incidence, and cumulative incidence of abnormally elevated urinary albumin excretion in type 1 and type 2 diabetes. The overall prevalence of microalbuminuria and macroalbuminuria is around 30% to

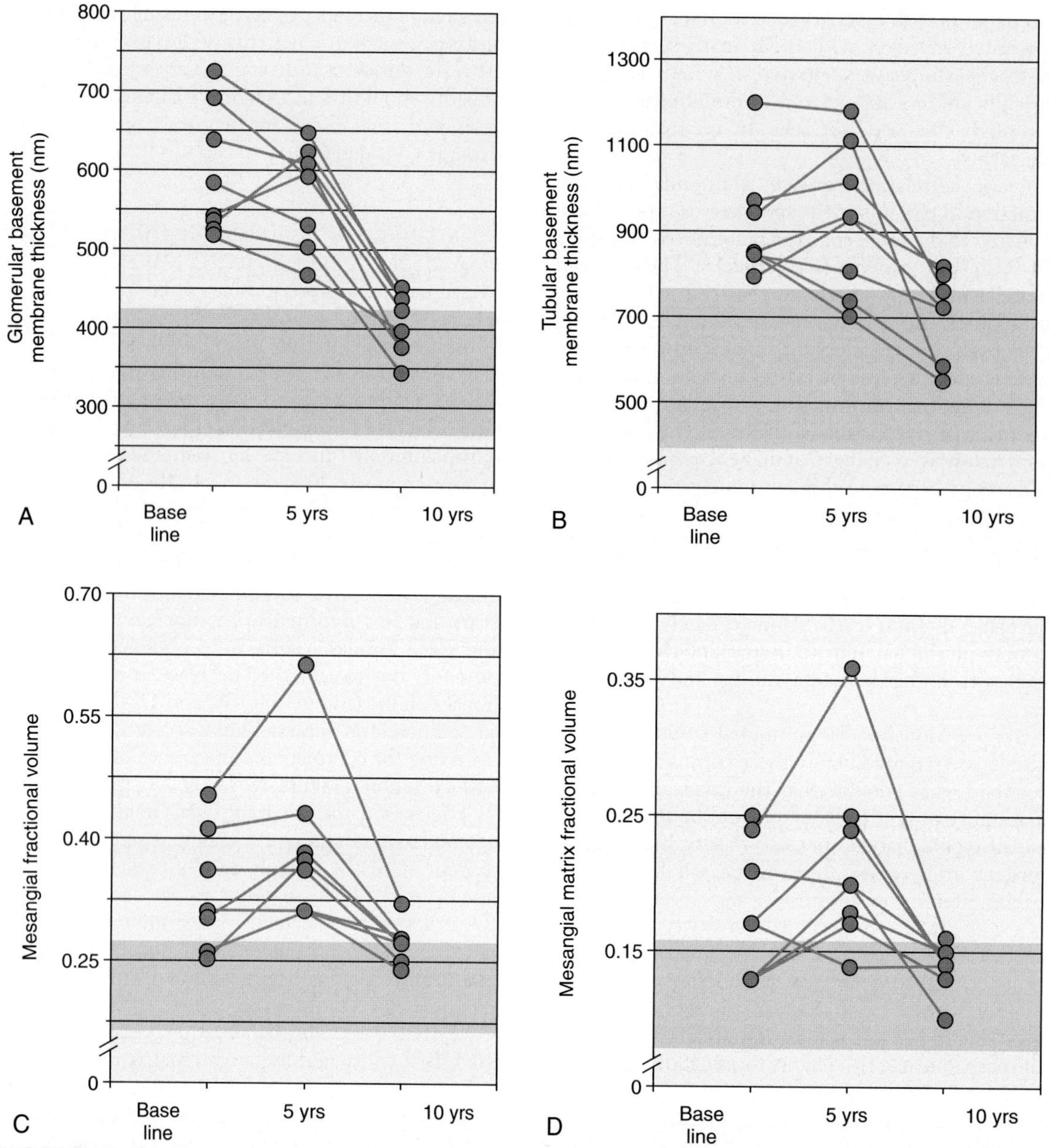

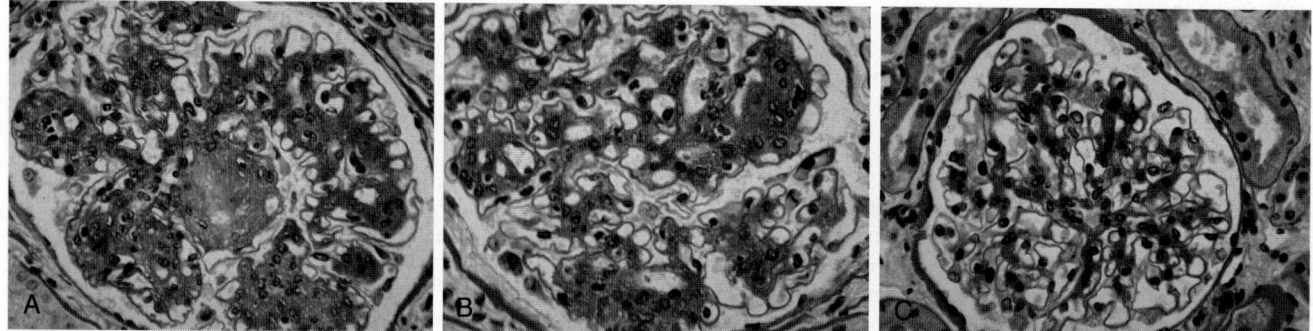

FIGURE 38-13 Thickness of the glomerular basement membrane (GBM), thickness of the tubular basement membrane (TBM), mesangial fractional volume, and mesangial-matrix fractional volume at baseline and 5 and 10 years after pancreas transplantation. The *shaded area* represents the normal ranges obtained in the 66 age- and sex-matched normal control subjects (means ± 2 standard deviation units). Data for individual patients are connected by lines. (From Fioretto P, Steffes MW, Sutherland DER, et al. Reversal of lesions of diabetic nephropathy after pancreas transplantation. *N Engl J Med* 339:69-75, 1998.)

FIGURE 38-14 Light photomicrographs (periodic acid–Schiff stain) of renal biopsy specimens obtained before and after pancreas transplantation from a 33-year-old woman with type 1 diabetes of 17 years' duration at the time of transplantation. **A,** Typical glomerulus from the baseline biopsy specimen, which is characterized by diffuse and nodular (Kimmelstiel-Wilson) diabetic glomerulopathy. **B,** Typical glomerulus 5 years after transplantation with persistence of the diffuse and nodular lesions. **C,** Typical glomerulus 10 years after transplantation, with marked resolution of diffuse and nodular mesangial lesions and more open glomerular capillary lumina. (From Fioretto P, Steffes MW, Sutherland DER, et al. Reversal of lesions of diabetic nephropathy after pancreas transplantation. *N Engl J Med* 339:69-75, 1998.)

<table>
TABLE 38-2 Prevalence, Incidence, and Cumulative Incidence of Microalbuminuria and Nephropathy in Diabetes
</table>

| | CLINIC BASED | | POPULATION BASED |
	TYPE 1	TYPE 2	TYPE 2
Prevalence of microalbuminuria (%)[76,82,525,526]	13 (9-20)	25 (13-27)	20 (17-21)
Prevalence of macroalbuminuria (%)[2,76,525]	15 (8-22)	14 (5-48)	16 (9-46)
Incidence of macroalbuminuria (%/yr)[6]	1.2 (0-3)	1.5 (1-2)	—
Cumulative incidence of macroalbuminuria (%/25 yr)[2,6,74,527]	31 (22-34)	28 (25-31)	—

Median and range are indicated.

TABLE 38-3 Risk Factors and Markers for Development of Diabetic Nephropathy in Patients with Type 1 and Type 2 Diabetes

	TYPE 1	TYPE 2
Normoalbuminuria above median[137,138,528]	+	+
Microalbuminuria[77,80,149,529,530]	+	+
Sex[5,76]	M>F	M>F
Familial clustering[531-534]	+	+
Predisposition to arterial hypertension[168-170]	+/−	+
Increased sodium-lithium countertransport[168,169,535-540]	+/−	−
Ethnic group[73,541]	+	+
Onset of type 1 diabetes before age 20 yr[5,77]	+	?
Poor glycemic control[3,4,133,530,542]	+	+
Hyperfiltration[132-134,136]	+/−	+/−
Increased prorenin level[355,543-545]	+	?
Smoking[184,546]	+	+
High cholesterol level[137,138,547]	+	+
Retinopathy[56,137,138,174,548]	+	+
Use of oral contraceptives[549]	+	?
Inflammation[120,550,551]	+	+
Increased adiponectin level[552]	+	+
Nocturnal hypertension[553]	+	+
Increased uric acid level[143]	+	?
Increased mannose-binding lectin level[551]	+	?
Tubular damage[554]	+	?
Obesity[230]	?	+

+, Risk factor/marker; −, not a risk factor/marker; ?, no relevant information; *IDDM*, insulin-dependent diabetes mellitus.

35% in both types of diabetes. However, the range in prevalence of diabetic nephropathy is much wider in type 2 diabetic patients. Clearly the inability to define the onset of disease in type 2 diabetes is a confounding issue. However, ethnic differences are also a major influence. The highest prevalence, exceeding 50%, is found in Native Americans followed by Asians, Mexican-Americans, black Americans, and European white patients.[73] It should be stressed that a good agreement has been documented between the results of clinic- and population-based studies.

The cumulative incidence of persistent proteinuria in patients whose type 1 diabetes was diagnosed before 1942 was about 40% to 50% after diabetes of 25 to 30 years' duration, but it declined to 15% to 30% in patients receiving a diagnosis of type 1 diabetes after 1953.[2,74] This so-called calendar effect unfortunately has not been seen in white European patients with type 2 diabetes. The reason for the declining cumulative incidence of proteinuria in type 1 diabetic patients is unknown, but improved diabetes care and control,[75] in addition to a decline in the prevalence of smoking and a general decline in nondiabetic glomerulopathies, have been suggested as factors.

Diabetic nephropathy rarely develops in patients with type 1 diabetes before 10 years after diagnosis, whereas approximately 3% of patients with newly diagnosed type 2 diabetes already have overt nephropathy.[76] The incidence peak (3% per year) is usually found in those who have had diabetes for 10 to 20 years; thereafter a progressive decline in incidence takes place. Thus, the risk of developing diabetic nephropathy is reduced for a normoalbuminuric patient who has had diabetes for longer than 30 years.[77] This changing pattern of risk indicates that the magnitude of exposure to diabetes is not sufficient to explain the development of diabetic nephropathy and suggests that only a subset of patients are susceptible to kidney complications.

Microalbuminuria as a Predictor of Nephropathy

The subpopulation of patients with type 1 diabetes who are at risk for nephropathy may now be identified fairly accurately by the detection of microalbuminuria.[3] Several longitudinal studies have shown that microalbuminuria strongly predicts the development of diabetic nephropathy in type 1 diabetic patients with a predictive power of 80%.[78,79] It has

been suggested that 58% of microalbuminuric patients revert to normoalbuminuria,[80] but in contrast to treatment-induced regression, long-lasting spontaneous normalization is seen in only 16% of microalbuminuric patients with type 1 diabetes.[4]

Type 1 diabetic patients with microalbuminuria have a median risk ratio of 21 for developing diabetic nephropathy, whereas the risk ratio for developing diabetic nephropathy ranges from 4.4 to 21 (median = 8.5) in type 2 diabetic patients with microalbuminuria.[81] In addition to microalbuminuria, several other risk factors or markers for development of diabetic nephropathy have been documented or suggested, as discussed in detail later (Table 38-3).

Prognosis of Microalbuminuria

Microalbuminuria is a strong predictor of total and cardiovascular mortality and cardiovascular morbidity in diabetic patients, as confirmed in recent meta-analyses.[82,83] Similarly, microalbuminuria predicts coronary and peripheral vascular disease and death from cardiovascular disease in the general nondiabetic population.[83-85] Microalbuminuria and proteinuria were also linked to stroke in recent meta-analysis.[86]

The mechanisms linking microalbuminuria to death from cardiovascular disease are poorly understood. Microalbuminuria has been proposed to be a marker of widespread endothelial dysfunction, which might predispose to enhanced penetrations of atherogenic lipoprotein particles into the arterial wall,[87] as well as a marker of established cardiovascular disease.[88] In addition, microalbuminuria is associated with an excess of both well-accepted Framingham and nontraditional cardiovascular risk factors.[88] Raised blood pressure, dyslipoproteinemia, increased platelet aggregability, endothelial dysfunction, insulin resistance, and hyperinsulinemia have all been demonstrated in microalbuminuric diabetic patients, as previously reviewed.[3,78,82]

Autonomic neuropathy, which is also associated with microalbuminuria, predicts death (often sudden) from cardiovascular disease in diabetic patients.[89-91] Surprisingly, the prevalence of coronary heart disease based on a Minnesota-coded electrocardiogram is not increased in microalbuminuric patients with type 2 diabetes.[76] Echocardiographic studies have revealed impaired diastolic function and cardiac hypertrophy in microalbuminuric patients with type 1 and type 2 diabetes.[92-94] Left ventricular hypertrophy predisposes the individual to ischemic heart disease, ventricular arrhythmia, heart failure, and sudden death.[95] Recently, it has been demonstrated that a high level of N-terminal pro–brain natriuretic peptide is a major risk marker for cardiovascular disease in type 2 diabetic patients with microalbuminuria.[96]

Prognosis of Diabetic Nephropathy

In a cohort of 1030 patients in whom type 1 diabetes was diagnosed between 1933 and 1952, patients who did not develop proteinuria had a low and constant relative mortality, whereas patients with proteinuria had a 40 times higher relative mortality on average.[5] Type 1 diabetic patients with proteinuria showed the characteristic bell-shaped relationship between diabetes duration/age and relative mortality, with a maximal relative mortality of 110 in females and 80 in males in the age interval of 34 to 38 years.

Several other studies have confirmed the poor prognosis for type 1 diabetic patients with diabetic nephropathy, as reviewed by Borch-Johnsen.[5] In three early studies that described the natural course of diabetic nephropathy in patients with type 1 diabetes, the cumulative death rate 10 years after onset of nephropathy ranged from 50% to 77% as reviewed by Parving.[78,79] The 50% figure represents a minimal value because the study included only death due to ESRD. The overall decrease in relative mortality from 1933 to 1972 was 40% and is partly explained by the decrease in the cumulative incidence of proteinuria.

Unfortunately this calendar effect is not seen in proteinuric type 2 diabetic patients, and subsequently no improved prognosis has been reported.[6] However, the prognostic importance of proteinuria in type 2 diabetic patients is considerably less than in type 1 diabetes. Proteinuria confers a 3.5 times higher risk of death, and the concomitant presence of arterial hypertension increases this relative risk to 7 in Pima Indians with type 2 diabetes.[97] Among European patients with type 2 diabetes, those with proteinuria have a fourfold excess of premature death compared with patients without proteinuria.[98] The cumulative death rate 10 years after onset of abnormally elevated urinary albumin excretion in European patients with type 2 diabetes was 70% compared with 45% in normoalbuminuric type 2 diabetic patients.[99] It is important to realize

that among patients with type 2 diabetes approximately 90% of the proteinuric patients will die from cardiovascular or nonrenal causes before developing ESRD. Thus the 10% who develop ESRD are "survivors," and improvement in cardiovascular prognosis will subsequently increase the number of patients developing ESRD.

ESRD is the major cause of mortality, accounting for 59% to 66% of all deaths, in type 1 diabetic patients with nephropathy.[5] The cumulative incidence of ESRD 10 years after onset of persistent proteinuria in type 1 diabetic patients is 50%, compared with 3% to 11% in proteinuric European patients with type 2 diabetes and 65% in proteinuric Pima Indians with type 2 diabetes. However, renal insufficiency was defined as a serum creatinine level of 2.0 mg/dL or more in the Pima study.

Recent data suggest that the increase in ESRD due to diabetic nephropathy has been levelling off in several countries, including the United States.[100,101] In addition, the survival of diabetic patients with ESRD has also been improved.[102] Ninety-seven percent of the excess mortality associated with type 2 diabetes in the Pima population is found in patients with proteinuria: 16% of deaths were ascribed to ESRD, whereas 22% were due to cardiovascular disease.[97] Cardiovascular disease is also a major cause of death (15% to 25%) in type 1 diabetic patients with nephropathy, despite the relatively low age at death.[5] Borch-Johnsen and Kreiner[103] studied a cohort of 2890 patients with type 1 diabetes and demonstrated that the relative mortality from cardiovascular disease was 37 times higher in proteinuric type 1 diabetic patients than in the general population.

Abnormalities related to well-established cardiovascular risk factors cannot alone account for this finding. Data from the RENAAL (Reduction of Endpoints in NIDDM with the Angiotensin II Antagonist Losartan) study by Parving and colleagues have shown that type 2 diabetic patients with diabetic retinopathy have a poor prognosis.[104] Several studies have shown abnormally raised levels of serum apolipoprotein (a) to be an independent risk factor for premature ischemic heart disease in nondiabetic subjects. However, studies in type 1 and type 2 diabetic patients with diabetic nephropathy have yielded conflicting results.[105-108]

Most studies have demonstrated that a familial predisposition to cardiovascular disease is present in type 1 diabetic patients with diabetic nephropathy.[109-111] Increased left ventricular hypertrophy, an established cardiovascular disease risk factor, and a decrease in diastolic function occur early in the course of diabetic nephropathy.[91,112,113] Left ventricular hypertrophy is a well-established risk factor for cardiovascular disease. Recently, it has been demonstrated that cardiac autonomic neuropathy predicts cardiovascular morbidity and mortality in type 1 diabetic patients with diabetic nephropathy.[90,91] Increased plasma homocysteine concentration is also a cardiovascular disease risk factor and predicts mortality in type 2 diabetic patients with albuminuria.[114]

It has been demonstrated that increased urinary albumin excretion, endothelial dysfunction, and chronic inflammation are interrelated processes that develop in parallel, progress with time, and are strongly and independently associated with risk of death in type 2 diabetes.[115] Early multifactorial intervention to target glycemia, block the RAS, reduce blood pressure, correct dyslipidemia, improve coagulation (aspirin), and address lifestyle factors is therefore important and has been demonstrated to reduce development of microvascular and macrovascular complications and mortality by approximately 50%, as discussed later.[116]

Tarnow and colleagues[117,118] have demonstrated that an elevated level of circulating N-terminal pro–brain natriuretic peptide is a new independent predictor of the excess overall and cardiovascular mortality in type 1 and type 2 diabetic patients with proteinuria but without symptoms of heart failure. In addition, several new circulating biomarkers of cardiovascular risk in diabetic nephropathy have been identified, such as asymmetric dimethylarginine,[119] mannose-binding lectin,[120] osteoprotegerin,[121] connective tissue growth factor,[122] and adiponectin.[123] Finally, it should be reiterated that reduced kidney function is a major cardiovascular risk factor.[124,125]

Clinical Course and Pathophysiology

A preclinical phase of diabetic nephropathy consisting of a normoalbuminuric and a microalbuminuric stage and a clinical phase characterized by albuminuria are well documented in both type 1 and type 2 diabetic patients.

Normoalbuminuria

Approximately one third of type 1 diabetic patients have a GFR above the upper normal range for age-matched healthy nondiabetic subjects.[126] The degree of hyperfiltration is less in type 2 diabetic patients,[127,128] and hyperfiltration is even reported to be lacking by some studies.[129] The GFR elevation is particularly pronounced in patients with newly diagnosed diabetes and during other intervals with poor metabolic control. Intensified insulin treatment and control to near-normal blood glucose levels reduce GFR toward normal levels after a period of days to weeks in both type 1 and type 2 diabetic patients.[127] Additional metabolites, vasoactive hormones, and increased kidney and glomerular size have been suggested as mediators of hyperfiltration in diabetes, as reviewed by Mogensen.[126]

Four factors regulate GFR. First, the glomerular plasma flow influences the mean ultrafiltration pressure and thereby GFR. Enhanced renal plasma flow has been demonstrated in type 1 and type 2 diabetic patients with elevated GFR.[127] Second, GFR is also regulated by the systemic oncotic pressure, which is reported to be normal in diabetes as calculated from plasma protein concentrations. The third determinant of GFR is glomerular transcapillary hydraulic pressure difference, which cannot be measured in humans. However, the demonstrated increase in filtration fraction is compatible with enhanced transglomerular hydraulic pressure difference. The last determinant of GFR is the glomerular ultrafiltration coefficient, K_f, which is determined by the product of the hydraulic conductance of the glomerular capillary and the glomerular capillary surface area available for filtration. Total glomerular capillary surface area is clearly increased at the onset of human diabetes. Studies of rats with experimentally induced diabetes treated with insulin have revealed hyperfiltration, hyperperfusion, enhanced glomerular capillary hydraulic pressure, reduced proximal tubular pressure, unchanged systemic oncotic pressure, and unchanged or slightly elevated K_f.[130]

Several studies suggest that insulin-like growth factor-1 plays a major role in the initiation of renal and glomerular growth in diabetic animals, as reviewed by Flyvbjerg.[131] Longitudinal studies suggest that hyperfiltration is a risk factor for subsequent increase in urinary albumin excretion and development of diabetic nephropathy in type 1 diabetic patients,[132,133] but conflicting results have also been reported.[134] A recent meta-analysis, based on 10 cohort studies following 780 patients, found a hazard ratio of 2.71 (95% confidence interval [CI] = 1.20 to 6.11) for progression to microalbuminuria in patients with hyperfiltration. These authors also found evidence of heterogeneity.[135]

The prognostic significance of hyperfiltration in type 2 diabetic patients is still debated.[136] Six prospective cohort studies following normoalbuminuric type 1 and type 2 diabetic patients for 4 to 10 years revealed that slight elevation of urinary albumin excretion that remained within the normal range, poor glycemic control, hyperfiltration, elevated arterial blood pressure, retinopathy, and smoking contribute to the development of persistent microalbuminuria and overt diabetic nephropathy.[133,137-141] Because several of these risk factors are modifiable, intervention is feasible, as discussed later. It has been suggested that uric acid level is related to hypertension, metabolic syndrome, and renal disease.[142] Recently, elevated serum uric acid was found to be a predictor of the development of diabetic nephropathy in type 1 diabetic patients.[143]

Microalbuminuria

In 1969, Keen and colleagues[144] demonstrated elevated urinary albumin excretion in patients with newly diagnosed type 2 diabetes. This abnormal but subclinical AER has been termed *microalbuminuria*, and it can be normalized by improving glycemic control. In addition to hyperglycemia, many other factors can induce microalbuminuria in diabetic patients, such as hypertension, massive obesity, heavy exercise, various acute or chronic illnesses, and cardiac failure.[145,146]

The day-to-day variation in urinary AER is high, 30% to 50%. Consequently more than one urine sample is needed to determine whether an individual patient has persistent microalbuminuria. Urinary albumin excretion within the microalbuminuric range (30 mg to 300 mg/24 hr) in at least two out of three consecutive nonketotic sterile urine samples is the generally accepted definition of persistent microalbuminuria. For convenience it has been recommended to use early morning spot urine samples for screening and monitoring. Urinary albumin/creatinine ratio is measured, and microalbuminuria is defined as 30 to 300 mg/g creatinine (× 0.1131 for mg/mmol).[147]

Persistent microalbuminuria has not been detected in children with type 1 diabetes younger than 12 years of age and, in general, is exceptional in the first 5 years of diabetes.[148] The annual rate of increase in urinary albumin excretion is about 20% in both type 2 diabetic patients[149] and type 1 diabetic patients with persistent microalbuminuria.[150]

The excretion of albumin in the urine is determined by the amount filtered across the glomerular capillary barrier and the amount reabsorbed by the tubular cells. A normal urinary β_2-microglobulin excretion rate in microalbuminuria suggests that albumin derives from enhanced glomerular leakage rather than from reduced tubular reabsorption of protein.

The transglomerular passage of macromolecules is governed by the size- and charge-selective properties of the glomerular capillary membrane and hemodynamic forces operating across the capillary wall. Alterations in glomerular pressure and flow influence both the diffusive and the convective driving forces for transglomerular passage of proteins. Studies using renal clearance of endogenous plasma proteins or dextrans have not detected a simple size-selective defect.[151-153] Determination of IgG/IgG4 ratio suggests that loss of glomerular charge selectivity precedes or accompanies the formation of new glomerular macromolecular pathways in the development of diabetic nephropathy.[151] Reduction in the negatively charged moieties of the glomerular capillary wall, particularly sialic acid and heparan sulfate, has been suggested.[88] Not all studies have confirmed these findings.[40,154]

Long-term diabetes in spontaneously hypertensive rats is associated with a reduction in both messenger RNA and protein expression of nephrin within the kidney.[155] As discussed earlier, changes in podocyte number and morphology have been implicated in the pathogenesis of proteinuria and progression of diabetic kidney disease.[30,156-158] Filtration fraction is presumed to reflect the glomerular hydraulic pressure, and microalbuminuric type 1 diabetic patients have elevated filtration both at rest and during exercise compared with normal controls.

A close correlation between filtration fraction and urinary albumin excretion has been shown as well. The demonstration that microalbuminuria diminishes promptly with acute reduction in arterial blood pressure argues that reversible hemodynamic factors play an important role in the pathogenesis of microalbuminuria. Imanishi and colleagues[159] have demonstrated that glomerular hypertension is present in type 2 diabetic patients with early nephropathy and is closely correlated with increased urinary albumin excretion. In addition, it should be mentioned that increased pressure has been demonstrated in the nail fold capillaries of microalbuminuric type 1 diabetic patients.[160]

GFR measured using the single-injection chromium 51–radiolabeled ethylenediaminetetraacetic acid (^{51}Cr-EDTA) plasma clearance method or the renal clearance of inulin is normal or slightly elevated in type 1 diabetic patients with microalbuminuria. Prospective studies have demonstrated that GFR remains stable at normal or supranormal levels for at least 5 years if clinical nephropathy does not develop.[161] Nephromegaly is still present and is even more pronounced in microalbuminuric than in normoalbuminuric type 1 diabetic patients.[162] In microalbuminuric type 2 patients GFR declines at rates approximating 3 to 4 mL/min/yr.[163]

Changes in tubular function take place early in diabetes and are related to the degree of glycemic control. The proximal tubular reabsorption of fluid, sodium, and glucose is enhanced.[164] This process could diminish distal sodium delivery and thereby modify tubuloglomerular feedback signals, which would result in enhancement of GFR. A direct effect of insulin in increasing distal sodium reabsorption has also been demonstrated.[164,165] The consequences of these alterations in tubular transport for overall kidney function are unknown.

Several studies have demonstrated blood pressure elevation in children and adults with type 1 diabetes and microalbuminuria.[78,79] The prevalence of arterial hypertension (Seventh Report of the Joint National Committee on Prevention, Detection, Evaluation, and Treatment of High Blood Pressure criterion of ≥140/90 mm Hg) in adult patients with type 1 diabetes increases with urine albumin level, and prevalence rates are 42%, 52%, and 79% in individuals with normoalbuminuria, microalbuminuria, and macroalbuminuria, respectively.[166] The prevalence of hypertension in those with type 2 diabetes (mean age 60 years) was higher: 71%, 90%, and 93% in the normoalbuminuria, microalbuminuria, and macroalbuminuric group, respectively.[76,166]

A genetic predisposition to hypertension in type 1 diabetic patients who develop diabetic nephropathy has been suggested,[167] but other studies did not confirm the concept.[168,169] Recently the original finding has been confirmed by conducting 24-hour blood pressure monitoring in a large group of parents of type 1 diabetic patients, both with and without diabetic nephropathy.[170] The cumulative incidence of hypertension was found to be higher among parents of proteinuric patients, with a shift toward younger age at onset of hypertension in this parental group. However, the difference in prevalence of parental hypertension was not evident when office blood pressure measurements were used.

Several studies have reported that sodium and water retention play a dominant role in the initiation and maintenance of systemic hypertension in patients with microalbuminuria and diabetic nephropathy, whereas the contribution of the renin-angiotensin-aldosterone system (RAAS) is smaller.[171]

Diabetic Nephropathy

Diabetic nephropathy is a clinical syndrome characterized by persistent albuminuria (>300 mg/24 hr, or 300 mg/g creatinine), a relentless decline in GFR, raised arterial blood pressure, and enhanced cardiovascular morbidity and mortality.[78,79] Although albuminuria is the first sign, peripheral edema is often the first symptom of diabetic nephropathy. Fluid retention is frequently observed early in the course of this kidney disease; that is, at a stage characterized by well-preserved renal function and only a modest reduction in serum albumin level. A recent study suggests that capillary hypertension, increased capillary surface area, and reduced capillary reflection coefficient for plasma proteins contribute to the edema formation, whereas the washdown of subcutaneous interstitial protein tends to prevent progressive edema formation in diabetic nephropathy.[172,173]

Most studies dealing with the natural history of diabetic nephropathy have demonstrated a relentless, often linear rate of decline in GFR. Importantly, this rate of decline is highly variable across individuals, ranging from 2 to 20 mL/min/yr, with a mean approximating 12 mL/min/yr.[3,78,79] Type 2 diabetic patients who have nephropathy display the same degree of loss in filtration function and in variability of GFR.[174,175]

Morphologic studies in both type 1 and type 2 diabetic patients have demonstrated a close inverse correlation between the degree of glomerular and tubulointerstitial lesions, on the one hand, and the GFR level, on the other, as discussed in detail previously. Myers and colleagues[176,177] have demonstrated a reduction in the number of restrictive pores leading to loss of ultrafiltration capacity (K_f) and impairment of glomerular barrier size selectivity resulting in progressive albuminuria and IgG-uria in diabetic nephropathy. Furthermore, the extent to which ultrafiltration capacity is impaired appears to be related to the magnitude of the defect in the barrier size selectivity. A defect in the glomerular barrier size selectivity has also been demonstrated in type 2 diabetic patients with diabetic nephropathy.[178] The reduction in renal plasma flow is proportional to the reduction in GFR (filtration fraction unchanged), and the impact on GFR is partially offset by the diminished systemic colloid osmotic pressure.

Several putative promoters of progression in kidney dysfunction have been studied in patients with type 1 diabetes[179-183] and type 2 diabetes[174,184,185] who have nephropathy (Figure 38-15). A close correlation between blood pressure and the rate of decline in GFR has been documented in type 1 and type 2 diabetic patients.[45,181,183,184,186-188] This suggests that systemic blood pressure accelerates the progression of diabetic nephropathy. Previously, the adverse impact of systemic hypertension on renal function and structure was thought to be mediated through vasoconstriction and arteriolar nephrosclerosis.[189] However, evidence from rat models shows that systemic hypertension is transmitted to the single glomerulus, which results in increases in glomerular hydrostatic pressure in such a way as to lead to hyperperfusion and increased capillary pressure.[190] Intraglomerular hypertension has also been documented directly in rats with streptozotocin-induced diabetess[190] and has been estimated to prevail in human diabetic patients, particularly those whose diabetes is complicated by kidney disease.[159]

Impaired or abolished renal autoregulation of GFR and renal plasma flow as demonstrated in type 1 and type 2 diabetic patients with nephropathy increases vulnerability to hypertension or ischemic injury of glomerular capillaries.[191] Defective autoregulation of GFR has been demonstrated in rats with streptozotocin-induced diabetes during hyperglycemia.[192] In contrast, studies in humans with type 2 diabetes revealed no impact of glycemic control on GFR autoregulation.[193]

Several components of the RAAS are elevated and are considered to contribute to the progression of diabetic nephropathy.[194] Accordingly, blocking the RAAS has been demonstrated to be renoprotective (see later). Experimental studies suggested that succinate, formed by the tricarboxylic acid cycle, provides a direct link between high glucose and renin release in the kidney through the G protein–coupled receptor for succinate, GPR91, which functions as a detector of cell metabolism.[195]

Initially focus was on the damaging effect of angiotensin II. Recently a kidney biopsy study revealed increased angiotensin converting enzyme (ACE) activity and reduced expression of ACE2 in patients with diabetic nephropathy compared with controls and patients with nondiabetic kidney disease.[196]

Aldosterone represents another component of the RAAS that should be considered important in the pathophysiology of diabetic nephropathy. Aldosterone is a hormone that, in addition to regulating electrolyte and fluid homeostasis, has widespread actions through genomic and nongenomic effects both in the kidney and in tissues not originally considered target tissue for aldosterone, such as the vasculature, central nervous system, and heart.[197,198] This includes upregulation of the prosclerotic growth factors plasminogen activator inhibitor-1 and transforming growth factor-β_1, as well as promotion of macrophage infiltration, which consequently leads to renal fibrosis.[199,200]

A longitudinal observational study involving a heterogeneous group of type 1 and type 2 diabetic patients with microalbuminuria demonstrated that systolic blood pressure, hyperangiotensinemia, and hyperaldosteronemia acted as independent predictors of more rapidly declining kidney function (measured as 1/Cr, reciprocal creatinine slope).[201] Increasing levels of aldosterone during long-term treatment with the angiotensin II receptor antagonist losartan were demonstrated to be associated with faster decline in GFR.[202]

Originally, Remuzzi and Bertani[203] suggested that proteinuria itself may contribute to renal damage. Type 1 diabetic patients with diabetic nephropathy and nephrotic-range proteinuria (>3 g/24 hr) had the worst prognosis. Several observational studies and treatment trials have confirmed and extended the aforementioned findings to include also subnephrotic-range proteinuria.[45,97,186,204]

For many years it was believed that once albuminuria had become persistent, glycemic control had lost its beneficial impact on kidney function and structure, and consequently the concept of a "point of no return" was advocated by many investigators, as reviewed by Parving.[78] This misconception was based on investigations involving a limited number of patients and studies that used inappropriate methods for monitoring kidney function (serum creatinine level) and glycemic control (random blood glucose level). Several more recent studies encompassing large numbers of type 1 diabetic patients have documented the important impact of glycemic control on the progression of diabetic nephropathy.[186,188,204] In contrast, most of the studies involving proteinuric patients with type 2 diabetes have failed to demonstrate any significant impact,[173,174,205] with two exceptions.[184,206]

Nearly all studies in type 1 and type 2 diabetic patients have demonstrated a correlation between serum cholesterol concentration and progression of diabetic nephropathy, at least in univariate analyses, but some have failed to demonstrate cholesterol level as an independent risk factor in multiple regression analysis.[173,174,181,183,184,186-188] Dietary protein restriction retards the progression of renal disease in virtually every experimental animal model tested.[189] Surprisingly, all major observational studies in type 1 and type 2 diabetic patients with diabetic nephropathy have failed to demonstrate an impact of dietary protein intake on the rate of decline in GFR.[173-175,186-188] Some, but not all, studies suggest that smoking may act as a progression promoter in both type 1 and type 2 diabetic patients with proteinuria.[207,208] However, larger, long-term studies have not been able to confirm these initial findings[184,209]

Several gene variants have been investigated as risk factors for diabetic nephropathy. One of the most intensively studied is the insertion/deletion (I/D) polymorphism of the ACE

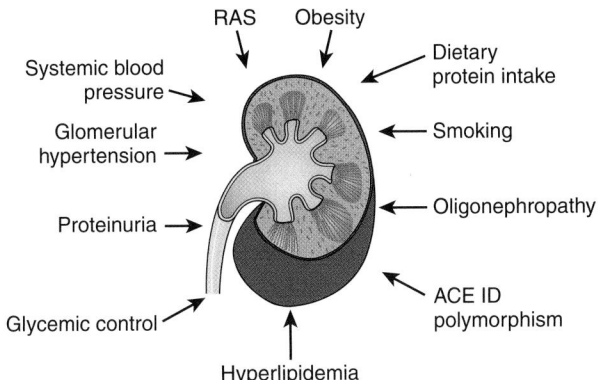

FIGURE 38-15 Putative promoters of progression of diabetic nephropathy.

gene (*ACE*/ID), which is strongly associated with the level of circulating ACE and increased risk of coronary heart disease in nondiabetic and diabetic patients.[210,211] The I/D polymorphism represents a common allelic variant in the sequence of the human *ACE* gene that reflects the insertion (I genotype) or deletion (D genotype) of a 282-nucleotide repetitive element within a downstream intron of the gene. The plasma ACE level in DD homozygous individuals is about twice that of II homozygous individuals, with ID heterozygous individuals having intermediate levels.[212]

Yoshida and colleagues[213] followed 168 proteinuric type 2 diabetic patients for 10 years. Analysis of the clinical course of individuals with the three *ACE* genotypes revealed that the majority (95%) of the patients with the DD genotype progressed to ESRD within 10 years. Moreover the DD genotype appeared be associated with increase mortality once dialysis was initiated. Three observational studies have confirmed that the D allele has a deleterious effect on kidney function.[214-216] Finally, more severe diabetic glomerulopathy lesions have been documented during both the development and the progression of renal disease in type 2 diabetic patients with the D allele.[217] Furthermore, microalbuminuric type 1 diabetic patients carrying the D allele show increased progression of diabetic glomerulopathy, based on the findings in renal biopsy specimens obtained at baseline and after 26 to 48 months of follow-up.[218]

In a large, double-blind, placebo-controlled randomized study (RENAAL) examining the renoprotective effects of losartan administered along with conventional blood pressure–lowering drugs in proteinuric type 2 diabetic patients, Parving and colleagues demonstrated that the presence of the D allele of the *ACE* gene had a harmful impact in terms of the likelihood of reaching the composite endpoint of a doubling of baseline creatinine concentration, ESRD, or death.[219] The impact was more pronounced in the white and the Asian patient group than the black and Hispanic group. The beneficial effects of losartan were greatest in the ACE/DD group and intermediate in the ID group for nearly all endpoints, a trend which suggests a quantitative interaction between treatment and ACE genotype in progression of renal disease. Such interaction was most significant for reduction of risk of reaching the ESRD endpoint.[219]

Parving and colleagues showed an accelerated initial and sustained loss of GFR during ACE inhibitor treatment of albuminuric type 1 patients homozygous for the DD polymorphism of the *ACE* gene.[220] The DD genotype independently influenced the sustained rate of decline in GFR—in other words, it acted as a progression promoter. Three other studies have demonstrated that the D allele is a risk factor for an accelerated course of diabetic nephropathy in patients with type 1 diabetes.[221-223]

A potential contribution from other candidate genes in relation to the RAS has also been suggested.[223] Recently genome-wide association studies have been performed in the search for genes linked to diabetic nephropathy, and although some areas of the genome have attracted attention, no major susceptibility genes have been identified so far.[224-226] For example, genetic heterogeneity in or near the *MHY9* gene on chromosome 19 explains an important component of the susceptibility of those with African ancestry to nondiabetic chronic kidney disease (CKD). This genetic variant does not predict diabetic nephropathy risk.

A common feature in severe CKD is anemia. Anemia seems to occur at an earlier stage in diabetic nephropathy than in other kidney diseases, so that anemia is a frequent finding in patients with diabetic nephropathy and moderately reduced renal function.[227] Furthermore, the degree of anemia has been found to be an independent risk factor associated with the decline in GFR[184] or development of ESRD[185] in type 2 diabetic patients with diabetic nephropathy. Importantly, the Trial to Reduce Cardiovascular Events with Aranesp Therapy (TREAT) has revealed that correction of anemia with erythropoiesis-stimulating agents, specifically darbepoetin, did not improve the prognosis of CKD in iron-replete diabetic patients with mild anemia and modest impairments of GFR.[228]

Obesity is an increasing problem in the general and diabetic population. Several studies have indicated that severe obesity (body mass index [BMI] of >40 kg/m^2) enhances ESRD risk sevenfold.[229] Even a BMI higher than 25 kg/m^2 was found to increase ESRD risk.[229] This effect is independent of the effects of hypertension and diabetes, the prevalence of which is increased in individuals with obesity. An effect of obesity on renal hemodynamics leading to increased glomerular pressure and hyperfiltration has been suggested as the mechanism.[230]

As discussed in Chapter 48, pregnancy in women with diabetic nephropathy is accompanied by an increase in complications such as hypertension and proteinuria and by increases in premature birth and fetal loss. The impact of pregnancy on the long-term course of renal function in women with diabetic nephropathy has not been clarified until recently. A study by Rossing and colleagues suggests that pregnancy has no adverse long-term impact on kidney function and survival in type 1 diabetic patients with diabetic nephropathy who have well-preserved kidney function (serum creatinine concentration of <100 μmol/L at the start of pregnancy).[222]

Nondiabetic glomerulopathy is very seldom seen in proteinuric type 1 diabetic patients, although this condition is common in proteinuric type 2 diabetic patients without retinopathy.[231] A prevalence of biopsy specimens with normal glomerular structure or nondiabetic kidney diseases of approximately 30% was demonstrated. Furthermore, a more rapid decline in GFR and a progressive rise in albuminuria in type 2 diabetic patients with diabetic glomerulopathy compared with type 2 diabetic patients without diabetic glomerulopathy has been demonstrated.[58,232]

Systemic blood pressure elevation to a hypertensive level is an early and frequent phenomenon in diabetic nephropathy.[76,78,79] Furthermore, nocturnal blood pressure elevation ("nondipping") occurs more frequently in type 1 and type 2 diabetic patients with nephropathy.[233,234] Exaggerated blood pressure response to exercise has also been reported in patients with long-standing type 1 diabetes who have microangiopathy. Finally, the increase in glomerular pressure consequent to nephron adaption may be accentuated with concomitant diabetes, as suggested in animal studies.[235]

Recently several new biomarkers associated with renal and cardiovascular outcome has been identified, as discussed later. Connective tissue growth factor (CTGF) has been recognized as a key factor in ECM production and other profibrotic activity mediated by transforming growth factor-β$_1$. CTGF is induced in renal cells by elevated glucose levels and is upregulated in diabetic nephropathy. Elevated levels were found to be independently associated with faster decline in GFR and development of ESRD in type 1 diabetic patients with diabetic nephropathy.[122]

Osteoprotegerin is a 120-kDa secretory glycoprotein belonging to the tumor necrosis factor receptor superfamily. It was first discovered in bone but is also present in the arterial wall. Osteoprotegerin may be involved in the development of vascular calcification. In cross-sectional studies osteoprotegerin level was elevated in type 1 and type 2 diabetic patients with microvascular and macrovascular complications.[236,237] A prospective study demonstrated that elevated levels of osteoprotegerin predict increased all-cause and cardiovascular mortality as well as enhanced decline in GFR in type 1 diabetic patients with nephropathy.[121]

Adiponectin is secreted by adipocytes and has been shown to possess antiinflammatory, antiatherogenic, and cardioprotective properties in type 2 diabetic patients. Paradoxically, in type 1 diabetic patients elevated levels were found in patients with diabetic nephropathy, and these increased levels were associated with an enhanced rate of decline in GFR and development of ESRD.[123] Experimental studies suggest that adiponectin affects podocytes and thereby could link obesity and kidney disease.[238] Urinary proteomic profiles characteristic of diabetic nephropathy have been identified.[239] These changes are partly normalized during renoprotective intervention.[240]

Extrarenal Complications in Diabetic Nephropathy

Diabetic retinopathy is present in virtually all type 1 diabetic patients with nephropathy, whereas only 50% to 60% of proteinuric type 2 diabetic patients have retinopathy.[76] Absence of retinopathy should prompt further investigation for nondiabetic glomerulopathies.[1] Blindness due to severe proliferative retinopathy or maculopathy is approximately five times more frequent in type 1 and type 2 diabetic patients with nephropathy than in normoalbuminuric patients.[76] Macroangiopathies (e.g., stroke, carotid artery stenosis, coronary heart disease, and peripheral vascular disease) are two to five times more common in patients with diabetic nephropathy.[76] Peripheral neuropathy is present in almost all patients with advanced nephropathy. Foot ulcers with sepsis leading to amputation occur frequently (>25% of cases), probably due to a combination of neural and arterial disease. Autonomic neuropathy may be asymptomatic and manifest simply as abnormal cardiovascular reflexes, or it may result in debilitating symptoms. Nearly all patients with nephropathy have grossly abnormal results on autonomic function tests.[90]

Treatment

The major therapeutic interventions that have been investigated include control of blood glucose to near-normal levels, antihypertensive treatment, lipid-lowering therapy, and restriction of dietary proteins. The impact of these four treatment modalities on progression from normoalbuminuria to microalbuminuria (primary prevention), microalbuminuria to diabetic nephropathy (secondary prevention), and diabetic nephropathy to ESRD is described and discussed.

Glycemic Control

Primary Prevention

Strict metabolic control achieved by insulin treatment or islet cell transplantation normalizes hyperfiltration, hyperperfusion, and glomerular capillary hypertension, and reduces the rate of increase in urinary albumin excretion in experimental diabetic animals.[78] The treatment also mitigates the development of diabetic glomerulopathy, although the glomerular enlargement remains unaffected. Risk factors for progression from normoalbuminuria to microalbuminuria and macroalbuminuria have been identified (see Table 38-3).

Short-term blood glucose control to near-normal levels in normoalbuminuric type 1 diabetic patients reduces GFR, renal plasma flow, urinary AER, and observed increases in kidney size. Increased kidney size is associated with an exaggerated renal response to amino acid infusion, and studies suggest that both abnormalities can be corrected by 3 weeks of intensified insulin treatment.[241]

A meta-analysis of long-term intensive blood glucose control (8 to 60 months) documented a beneficial effect on the progression from normoalbuminuria to microalbuminuria in type 1 diabetic patients.[242] The odds ratio for progressing from normoalbuminuria to microalbuminuria ranged from 0.22 to 0.40 in the intensified treatment groups. A worsening of diabetic retinopathy was observed during the initial months of intensive therapy, but in the longer term the rate of deterioration was slower than it was in the type 1 diabetic patients receiving conventional treatment.[243] Side effects are a major concern with intensive therapy, and the frequency of severe hypoglycemia and diabetic ketoacidosis was greater in several studies.[242]

In the Diabetes Control and Complications Trial (DCCT),[244] intensive therapy reduced the occurrence of microalbuminuria by 39% (95% CI = 21% to 52%), and that of albuminuria by 54% (95% CI = 19% to 74%), when the primary and secondary prevention cohorts were combined for analysis. Despite this, however, 16% in the primary prevention cohort and 26% in the secondary prevention cohort developed microalbuminuria during the 9 years of intensive treatment. This clearly documents the need for additional treatment modalities to reduce the burden of diabetic nephropathy.

In Japanese type 2 diabetic patients a beneficial impact of strict glycemic control on progression of normoalbuminuria to microalbuminuria and macroalbuminuria was demonstrated in a small study with a design similar to that of the DCCT.[245] Results of this study have been confirmed and extended by data from the UK Prospective Diabetes Study (UKPDS) documenting a progressive beneficial effect of intensive metabolic control on the development of microalbuminuria and overt proteinuria,[246] and a 10-year poststudy follow-up demonstrated a long-lasting beneficial effect.[247] The beneficial effect was recently confirmed in the Action in Diabetes and Vascular Disease: Preterax and Diamicron Modified-Release Controlled Evaluation (ADVANCE) study, in which 11,140 patients with type 2 diabetes were followed for a median of 5 years and a 21% reduction (95%

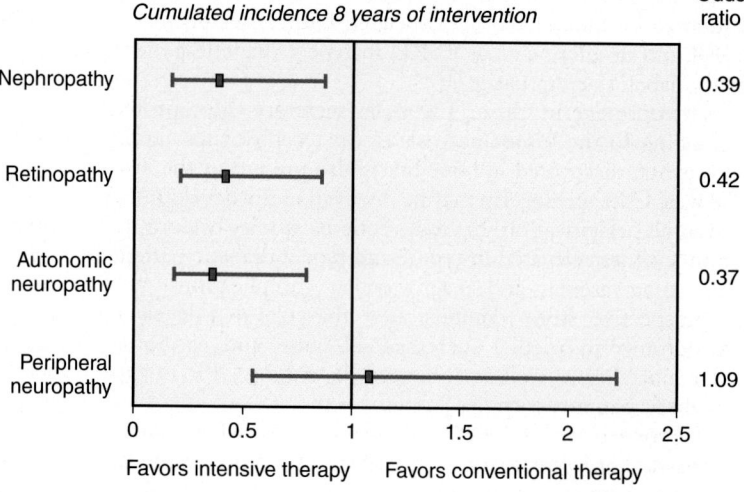

FIGURE 38-16 Odds ratio for progression of microvascular complications in microalbuminuric type 2 diabetic patients receiving multifactorial intensive therapy compared with similar patients receiving standard therapy in the STENO-2 trial (N = 160). (From Gaede P, Vedel P, Larsen N, et al: Multifactorial intervention and cardiovascular disease in patients with type 2 diabetes, *N Engl J Med* 348[5]:383-393, 2003.)

CI = 7% to 34%) in development of nephropathy was seen in patients randomly assigned to strict glycemic control.[248] The same trend was seen in the smaller Veterans Affair Diabetes Trial, but the values did not reach statistical significance.[249]

Secondary Prevention

Several modifiable risk factors for progression from microalbuminuria to overt diabetic nephropathy (including level of urinary albumin excretion, hemoglobin A_{1C} [HbA_{1C}] level, smoking, blood pressure, and serum cholesterol concentration) have been identified in clinical trials and observational studies of type 1 and type 2 diabetic patients.[3,4,149,250-253]

Data regarding the renal impact of intensive diabetic treatment versus conventional diabetic treatment on progression or regression of microalbuminuria in type 1 diabetic patients have been conflicting, as reviewed by Parving.[78] These disappointing results might be due partly to the relatively short length of follow-up, since the UKPDS with 15 years of follow-up documented a progressive beneficial effect with time on the development of proteinuria and a twofold increase in plasma creatinine level.[246] Furthermore, pancreatic transplantation was found to reverse glomerulopathy in patients with type 1 diabetes and normoalbuminuria (N = 3) or microalbuminuria (N = 4), but reversal required more than 5 years of normoglycemia.[69] It has been demonstrated that intensified multifactorial intervention (pharmacologic therapy targeting hyperglycemia, hypertension, dyslipidemia, and microalbuminuria) in patients with type 2 diabetes and microalbuminuria substantially slows progression to overt nephropathy, retinopathy, and autonomic neuropathy[89,254] (Figure 38-16). Furthermore, a follow-up study demonstrated that the rate of development of ESRD was significantly reduced by the intensive multifactorial intervention after 13 years (Figure 38-17).[255]

Nephropathy

The impact of improved metabolic control on progression of kidney function in type 1 diabetic patients with nephropathy has been disappointing. Studies have not found the rate of

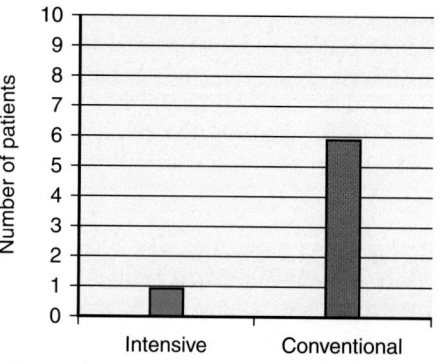

FIGURE 38-17 Development of end-stage renal disease (ESRD) in microalbuminuric type 2 diabetic patients in the STENO-2 trial (N = 160). One patient in the intensive treatment group had progression to ESRD compared with 6 patients in the conventional treatment group (P = 0.04). (Adapted from Gaede P, Lund-Andersen H, Parving H-H, et al: Effect of a multifactorial intervention on mortality in type 2 diabetes, *N Engl J Med* 358[6]:580-591, 2008.)

decline in GFR and the rise in proteinuria and systemic blood pressure to be affected by improved glycemic control. However, it should be stressed that none of the trials was randomized and the number of patients included was small. In contrast, most major prospective observational studies have indicated an important role for glycemic control in the progression of diabetic nephropathy, as discussed earlier.[78,186,188,204]

Blood Pressure Control

Primary Prevention

Originally, Zatz and colleagues[256] showed that prevention of glomerular capillary hypertension in normotensive insulin-treated rats with streptozotocin-induced diabetes effectively protects against the subsequent development of proteinuria and focal and segmental glomerular structural lesions. Other studies confirmed the beneficial effect of ACE inhibition in uninephrectomized rats made diabetic by streptozotocin. Anderson and colleagues[257,258] have demonstrated that antihypertensive therapy slows the development of diabetic glomerulopathy but found that ACE inhibitors provide better long-term protection than triple therapy with reserpine, hydralazine, and hydrochlorothiazide or a calcium channel blocker (nifedipine).

Recent observations are consistent with the concept that glomerular hypertension is a major factor in the pathogenesis of experimental diabetic glomerulopathy and indicate that a lowering of systemic blood pressure without concomitant reduction of glomerular capillary pressure may be insufficient to prevent glomerular injury.[257-259] Reduction of systemic blood pressure by ACE inhibitors or conventional antihypertensive treatment affords significant renoprotection in spontaneously hypertensive rats with streptozotocin-induced diabetes.[260] No specific added benefit of ACE inhibition was observed in this hypertensive model in contrast to the aforementioned normotensive models.

Three randomized placebo-controlled trials in normotensive type 1 and type 2 diabetic patients with normal AER have suggested a beneficial effect of ACE inhibitors on the development of microalbuminuria.[261-263] In contrast to these three studies, which were carried out as placebo-controlled trials, subsequent studies compared the effect of ACE inhibitors versus a long-acting dihydropyridine calcium antagonist[264,265] or versus a β-blocker[266] in hypertensive type 2 diabetic patients with normoalbuminuria. All three of the latter studies reported a similar beneficial renoprotective effect of blood pressure reduction with and without ACE inhibition. Furthermore, the UKPDS study reported that by 6 years a smaller proportion of patients in the group in whom blood pressure was tightly controlled had developed microalbuminuria, and the tight-control group had a 29% reduction in risk for microalbuminuria ($P < 0.009$), with a nonsignificant 39% reduction in the risk for proteinuria ($P = 0.061$).[266]

Aggressive blood pressure control in normotensive (blood pressure of <160/90 mm Hg) type 2 diabetic patients has recently been demonstrated to have beneficial effects on albuminuria, retinopathy, and incidence of stroke.[267] The results were the same whether enalapril or nisoldipine was used as the initial blood pressure–lowering drug.

The Renin Angiotensin System Study (RASS), compared the effect of ACE inhibition, angiotensin II receptor blockade, and placebo on the primary renal structural endpoint of mesangial volume fraction in type 1 diabetic patients who were normotensive (blood pressure of <135/85 mm Hg) and normoalbuminuric (median AER of 5 μg/min). This 5-year randomized controlled trial did not find any benefit of RAS blockade on the progression of nephropathy as measured in terms of the primary endpoint and other secondary renal structural parameters.[72] Also, RAS blockade did not prevent an increase in AER.[72] In contrast, the odds for progression of retinopathy were significantly reduced by 65% to 70% with the RAS blocking agents compared with placebo.

Originally, the EUCLID study group[268] demonstrated a significant beneficial effect of ACE inhibition on progression of diabetic retinopathy and development of proliferative retinopathy in type 1 diabetic patients. The DIRECT study evaluated the effect of angiotensin II receptor blockade with candesartan versus placebo on the development or progression of retinopathy in a randomized controlled trial lasting 5 years involving 3326 patients with type 1 diabetes and 1905 patients with type 2 diabetes.[269,270] Most patients were normotensive, and all had normoalbuminuria (median urinary

AER of 5.0 μg/min). Development of microalbuminuria was also evaluated.[271] In type 1 diabetic patients the incidence of retinopathy was reduced by candesartan treatment but progression was not affected, whereas significant regression of retinopathy was seen in type 2 diabetic patients. The DIRECT study did not show any significant effect on the incidence of microalbuminuria.[271]

The Bergamo Nephrologic Diabetes Complications Trial (BENEDICT) demonstrated that use of an ACE inhibitor, alone or in combination with a calcium channel blocker, decreases the incidence of microalbuminuria in hypertensive type 2 diabetic patients with normoalbuminuria. The effect of the calcium channel block verapamil alone was similar to that of placebo.[272] In the recent ADVANCE study, which included type 2 diabetic patients with or without hypertension, the fixed combination of perindopril and the diuretic indapamide also reduced blood pressure, and the development of new-onset microalbuminuria was reduced by 21% (95% CI = 14% to 27%).[273]

In the ONTARGET study, 25,620 patients with atherosclerotic disease or diabetes (38% with diabetes) who had end-organ damage were randomly assigned to treatment with an ACE inhibitor, angiotensin II receptor blocker (ARB), or both and were followed for a median of 56 months. The mean urinary albumin/creatinine ratio was 7.2 mg/g, and the sustained rate of decline in GFR was less than 1 mL/min/yr. Although the combination treatment reduced the increase in urinary AER, the number of events for the composite primary outcome of doubling of serum creatinine level, need for dialysis, or death was similar for telmisartan ($N = 1147$ [13.4%]) and ramipril ($N = 1150$ [13.5%]; hazard ratio [HR] = 1.00; 95% CI = 0.92 to 1.09), but was increased with combination therapy ($N = 1233$ [14.5%]; HR = 1.09; CI = 1.01 to 1.18; $P = 0.037$).[274] It is important to stress that the ONTARGET study did not include important numbers of patients with overt diabetic nephropathy. Therefore, the therapeutic risk or benefit for RAS combination therapy in patients with diabetic nephropathy could not be addressed by this study.

Patients intolerant of ACE inhibition ($N = 5927$) but otherwise similar to those in the ONTARGET study were randomly assigned to receive a placebo or an ARB in the TRANSCEND study. Albuminuria increased less in patients receiving the ARB than in those receiving the placebo (32% [CI = 23% to 41%] vs. 63% [CI = 52% to 76%]). Very few patients (<2%) reached the prespecified renal endpoints, which were identical to those of the ONTARGET study, and no difference was seen between treatment groups with regard to these endpoints.[275]

In conclusion, RAS blockade has been effective in reducing the frequency of development of microalbuminuria in hypertensive normoalbuminuric patients, whereas the effect has not been significant in normotensive patients. Possibly the intrarenal RAS is not enhanced in normotensive patients in contrast to hypertensive patients. However, the studies have used variable endpoints: intermittent or persistent microalbuminuria. The studies have furthermore enrolled patients with very low levels of urinary albumin excretion. The use of ACE inhibitors or other antihypertensive agents for primary prevention of nephropathy in normotensive normoalbuminuric patients is not recommended in guidelines.[147]

Secondary Prevention

A meta-analysis of 12 trials encompassing 698 type 1 diabetic patients with microalbuminuria who were followed for at least 1 year revealed that treatment with ACE inhibitors reduced the risk of progression to macroalbuminuria compared with placebo (odds ratio = 0.38; 95% CI = 0.25 to 0.57).[276] The rate of regression to normoalbuminuria was three times higher than in the patients receiving placebo. At 2 years, the urinary AER was 50% lower in patients taking ACE inhibitors than in those receiving placebo. Furthermore, it has been shown that the beneficial effect of ACE inhibitors in preventing progression from microalbuminuria to overt nephropathy is long-lasting (8 years), and more importantly, it is associated with preservation of normal GFR.[277] Recent data from a 3-year double-blind randomized study found that long-acting dihydropyridine calcium antagonists are as effective as ACE inhibitors in delaying the occurrence of macroalbuminuria in normotensive patients with type 1 diabetes with persistent microalbuminuria.[278] Finally, agents blocking the effect of the RAS have a beneficial impact on glomerular structural changes in type 1 and type 2 diabetic patients with early diabetic glomerulopathy.[279-281]

Borch-Johnsen and colleagues[150] analyzed the cost versus benefit of screening and antihypertensive treatment of early renal disease indicated by microalbuminuria in type 1 diabetic patients. The authors concluded that screening and intervention programs are likely to have lifesaving effects and lead to considerable economic savings.

The impact of ACE inhibition in microalbuminuric type 2 diabetic patients has also been evaluated. A randomized study[282] was conducted in which diabetic patients with microalbuminuria were treated with perindopril or nifedipine for 12 months. Both treatments significantly reduced mean arterial blood pressure and urinary AER. Unfortunately, the study enrolled a heterogeneous group of hypertensive and normotensive patients with either type 1 or type 2 diabetes.

Ravid and colleagues[149] conducted a double-blind randomized study of 94 normotensive microalbuminuric type 2 diabetic patients who received enalapril or placebo for 5 years. In the actively treated group kidney function remained stable and only 12% of the patients developed diabetic nephropathy, whereas in the group receiving placebo kidney function declined by 13% and 42% of the patients developed nephropathy. These data have been confirmed in other studues.[252,253,267,283]

Antihypertensive treatment has a renoprotective effect in hypertensive patients with type 2 diabetes and microalbuminuria.[254,263-266,284-289] Evidence has been conflicting regarding the existence of a specific renoprotective effect—that is, a beneficial effect on kidney function beyond the hypotensive effect—of agents that block the RAS in patients with type 2 diabetes and microalbuminuria.[254,263-266,284-289] The inconclusive nature of the previous evidence may have been due, in part, to the small size of the patient groups studied and the short duration of antihypertensive treatment in most trials. An exception is the long-lasting UKPDS, which suggested the equivalence of a β-blocker and an ACE inhibitor.[266]

To address this issue, Parving and colleagues evaluated the renoprotective effect of the angiotensin II receptor antagonist irbesartan in hypertensive patients with type 2 diabetes and microalbuminuria in a study known as the IRMA 2 trial.[290] A total of 590 hypertensive patients with type 2 diabetes and microalbuminuria were enrolled in this multinational, randomized, double-blind, placebo-controlled study of irbesartan at a dosage of either 150 mg daily or 300 mg daily and were followed for 2 years. The primary outcome was the time to the onset of diabetic nephropathy, defined by persistent albuminuria in overnight specimens, with a urinary AER that was greater than 200 μg/min and at least 30% higher than the baseline level. The baseline characteristics in the three subject groups (placebo, irbesartan at 150 mg daily, and irbesartan at 300 mg daily) were similar.

Ten of the 194 patients in the 300-mg group (5.2%) and 19 patients of the 195 patients in the 150-mg group (9.7%) reached the primary endpoint, compared with 30 of the 201 patients receiving the placebo (14.9%) (HR = 0.30, 95% CI = 0.14 to 0.61, $P < 0.001$; and HR = 0.61, 95% CI = 0.34 to 1.08, $P = 0.08$, for the two irbesartan groups, respectively) (Figure 38-18). The average blood pressure during the course of the study was 144/83 mm Hg in the placebo group, 143/83 mm Hg in the 150-mg group, and 141/83 mm Hg in the 300-mg group ($P = 0.004$ for the comparison of systolic blood pressure between the placebo group and the combined irbesartan groups). Serious adverse events were less frequent among the patients treated with irbesartan ($P = 0.02$).

The IRMA 2 study demonstrated that irbesartan is renoprotective independent of its blood pressure–lowering effect in patients with type 2 diabetes and microalbuminuria. In a substudy of IRMA 2, irbesartan was found to be renoprotective independent of its beneficial effect in lowering 24-hour blood pressure.[291] Another substudy showed a persistent reduction of microalbuminuria after withdrawal of all antihypertensive treatment, which suggests that the dosage of 300-mg irbesartan daily confers long-term renoprotection.[292] In addition, irbesartan treatment diminished inflammatory markers such as highly sensitive C-reactive protein, fibrinogen, and interleukin-6 compared with placebo. The changes in interleukin-6 were associated with the changes in albumin excretion.[293] Remission to normoalbuminuria was more common in the irbesartan-treated patients than in those treated with placebo.[294] The importance of this finding is a slower decrease in GFR, as also demonstrated in the STENO-2 study.[163] Another study has demonstrated an enhanced renoprotective effect of ultrahigh dosages of irbesartan (900 mg daily) in patients with type 2 diabetes and microalbuminuria.[295] Finally, the cost effectiveness of early irbesartan treatment versus placebo in addition to standard conventional blood pressure–lowering treatment has been demonstrated.[296] The beneficial effect of RAS blockade in microalbuminuric patients has also been shown in the INNOVATION study in an Asian population.[297]

Cardiovascular morbidity is a major burden in patients with type 2 diabetes. The STENO-2 study, which enrolled patients with type 2 diabetes and microalbuminuria, evaluated the effect on cardiovascular and microvascular diseases of an intensified, targeted, multifactorial intervention comprising behavior modification and polypharmacologic therapy aimed at several modifiable risk factors (hyperglycemia, hypertension, dyslipidemia, and microalbuminuria), along with secondary prevention of cardiovascular disease with aspirin. This approach was compared with a conventional intervention addressing multiple risk factors.[89] Patients receiving intensive therapy had a

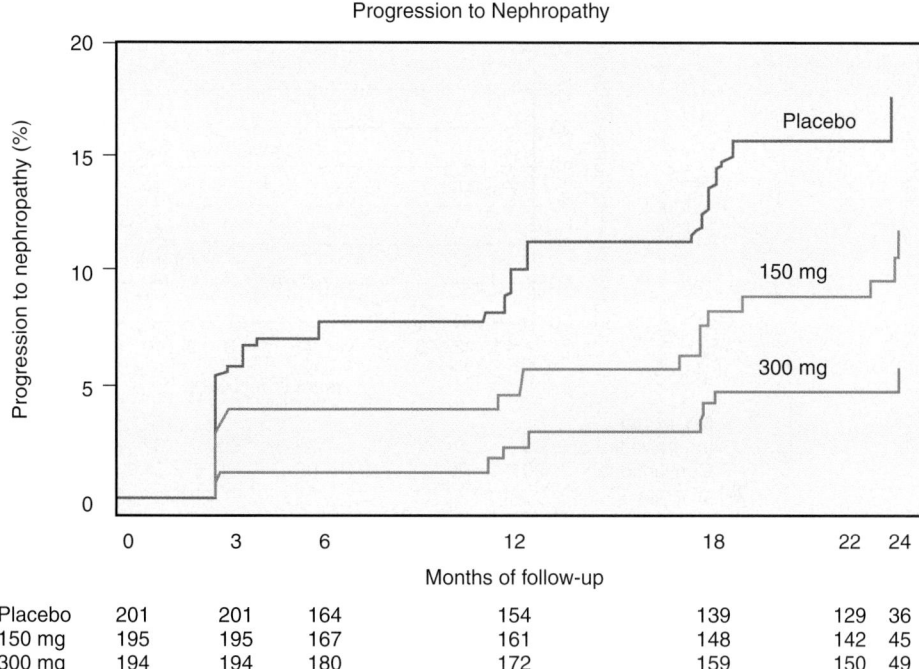

Progression to Nephropathy

	0	3	6	12	18	22	24
Placebo	201	201	164	154	139	129	36
150 mg	195	195	167	161	148	142	45
300 mg	194	194	180	172	159	150	49

FIGURE 38-18 Probability of progression to diabetic nephropathy during treatment with irbesartan 150 mg daily, irbesartan 300 mg daily, or placebo in hypertensive type 2 diabetic patients with persistent microalbuminuria. The difference between placebo and irbesartan 150 mg daily was not significant ($P = 0.08$ by log-rank test), but the difference between placebo and irbesartan 300 mg daily was significant ($P < 0.001$ by log-rank test).

significantly lower risk of cardiovascular disease (HR = 0.47; 95% CI = 0.24 to 0.73), nephropathy (HR = 0.39; 95% CI = 0.17 to 0.87), retinopathy (HR = 0.42; 95% CI = 0.21 to 0.86), and autonomic neuropathy (HR = 0.37; 95% CI = 0.18 to 0.79). In conclusion, a target-driven, long-term, intensified intervention aimed at multiple risk factors in patients with type 2 diabetes and microalbuminuria reduces the risk of cardiovascular and microvascular events by about 50%.

In a poststudy follow-up, after an additional 5 years the effects were maintained, and as mentioned earlier the incidence of ESRD was significantly reduced in the intensively treated group. Even more important, mortality was reduced in the intensively treated group (HR = 0.54; 95% CI = 0.32 to 0.89), which corresponded to an absolute risk reduction of 20%[116] (Figure 38-19). The cost effectiveness of treatment was assessed after 8 years, and intensive therapy was found to be more cost effective than conventional treatment. On the assumption that patients in both arms are treated in a primary care setting, intensive therapy is both cost saving and lifesaving.[298]

In 1995 a consensus report on the detection, prevention, and treatment of diabetic nephropathy with special reference to microalbuminuria was published.[299] Improved blood glucose control (HbA_{1C} below 7.5% to 8%) and treatment with an ACE inhibitor is recommended. Recently an audit of the implementation of this strategy in clinical practice demonstrated that the beneficial outcome found the initial short-term randomized clinical trials could be confirmed and maintained for 10 years.[300] The American Diabetes Association now states the following: "In patients with hypertension and any degree of albuminuria ACE inhibitors have been shown to delay the progression of nephropathy. In patients with type 2 diabetes, hypertension and microalbuminuria, both ACE inhibitors and ARBs have been shown to delay the progression to macroalbuminuria. In patients with type 2 diabetes, hypertension,

macroalbuminuria and renal insufficiency (serum creatinine >1.5 mg/dl), ARBs have been shown to delay the progression of nephropathy".[147]

Nephropathy

From a clinical point of view the ability to predict the long-term effect on kidney function of a recently initiated treatment modality (e.g., antihypertensive therapy) would be of great value, because this could allow for early identification of patients in need of an intensified or alternative therapeutic regimen. In two prospective studies dealing with conventional antihypertensive treatment and ACE inhibition, Rossing and colleagues found that the initial reduction in albuminuria (surrogate endpoint) predicted a beneficial long-term treatment effect on rate of decline in GFR (principal endpoint) in diabetic nephropathy.[301,302] These findings have been confirmed and extended.[188,303] Furthermore, similar findings have been demonstrated in nondiabetic nephropathies.[304,305]

The antiproteinuric effect of ACE inhibition in patients with diabetic nephropathy varies considerably. Individual differences in the RAS may influence this variation. Therefore, the potential role of an I/D polymorphism of the ACE gene on this early antiproteinuric responsiveness was tested in an observational follow-up study of young type 1 diabetic patients with hypertension and diabetic nephropathy.[306] The data showed that type 1 diabetic patients with the II homozygous genotype are particularly likely to benefit from commonly advocated renoprotective treatment.

The EUCLID Study Group[261] demonstrated that urinary AER during lisinopril treatment was 57% lower in the II group, 19% lower in the ID group, and 19% higher in the DD group compared with the placebo group. Furthermore, the polymorphism of the *ACE* gene predicts therapeutic efficacy of ACE inhibitor against progression of nephropathy in type 2 diabetic patients.[216] All previous observational

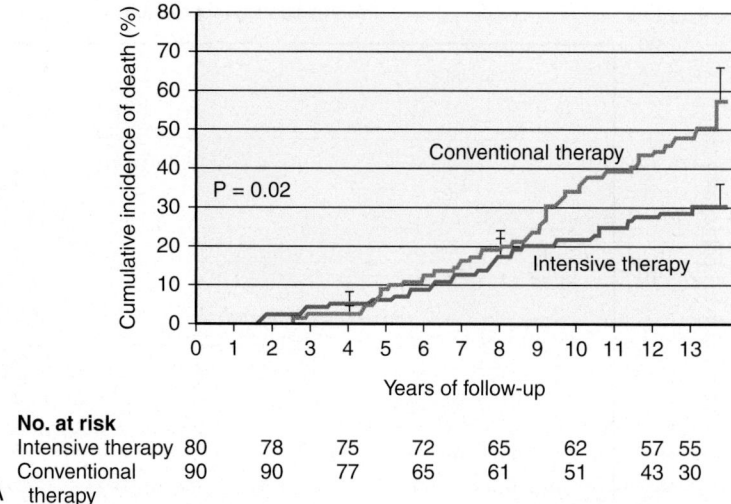

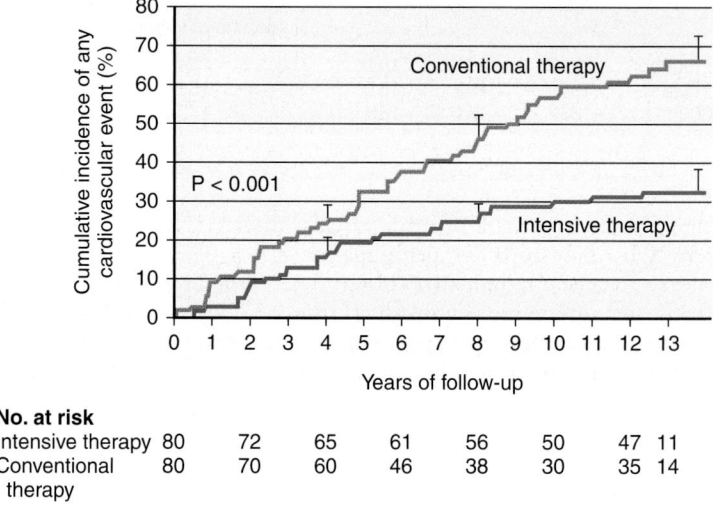

FIGURE 38-19 Kaplan-Meier estimates of the risk of death from any cause and from cardiovascular causes, and the number of cardiovascular events, for microalbuminuric type 2 diabetic patients treated with intensive therapy and for those treated with conventional therapy. **A,** Cumulative incidence of death from any cause (the study's primary endpoint) during the 13.3-year study period. **B,** Cumulative incidence of a secondary composite endpoint of cardiovascular events, including death from cardiovascular causes, nonfatal stroke, nonfatal myocardial infarction, coronary-artery bypass grafting (CABG), percutaneous coronary intervention (PCI), revascularization for peripheral atherosclerotic artery disease, and amputation. **C,** Number of events for each component of the composite endpoint. In **A** and **B,** the *bars* represent standard errors. (From Gaede P, Lund-Andersen H, Parving H-H, et al: Effect of a multifactorial intervention on mortality in type 2 diabetes, *N Engl J Med* 358[6]:580-591, 2008.)

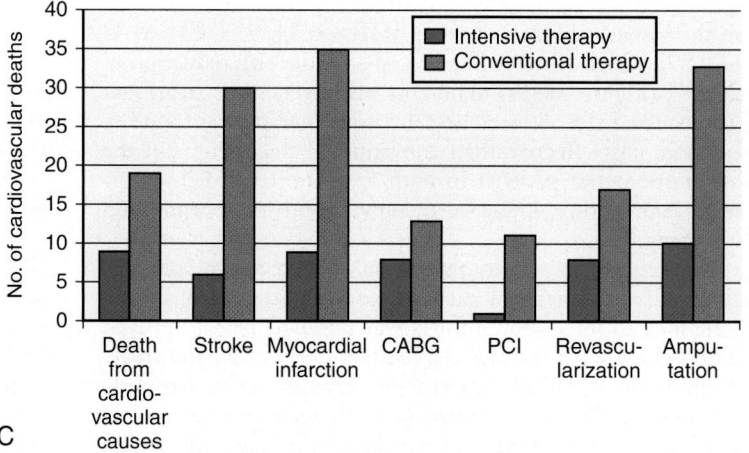

studies in patients with diabetic and nondiabetic nephropathies have demonstrated that the deletion polymorphism of the *ACE* gene, particularly the DD genotype, is a risk factor for an accelerated loss of kidney function.[214,215,220,221,307-312] Furthermore, the *ACE* deletion polymorphism reduces the long-term beneficial effect of ACE inhibition on progression of diabetic and nondiabetic kidney disease.[220,310] These

findings may suggest that the DD genotype patient should be offered more aggressive ACE inhibition or treatment with ARBs or dual blockade of the RAS. Further study of appropriate therapy in patients with the DD genotype is warranted.

In an attempt to overcome this interaction between ACE inhibitor therapy and *ACE* deletion polymorphism, two studies evaluated the short- and long-term renoprotective effect of losartan in type 1 diabetic patients with diabetic nephropathy who were homozygous for either the insertion or the deletion allele.[313,314] The data suggest that this ARB offers similar short- and long-term renoprotective and blood pressure–lowering effects in albuminuric hypertensive type 1 diabetic patients with the *ACE II* and DD genotypes. Also, data from the RENAAL study mentioned earlier indicate that proteinuric type 2 diabetic patients with the D allele of the *ACE* gene have an unfavorable renal prognosis that can be mitigated and even improved by treatment with losartan.[315]

Another example of pharmacogenetic interaction is the relationship between losartan and *CYP2C9* of the cytochrome P450 superfamily, which encodes an enzyme that metabolizes losartan and forms the active metabolite E-3174 that is responsible for the antihypertensive effect. The *CYP2C9*3* polymorphism could modulate the blood pressure–lowering response to optimal monotherapeutic losartan treatment in hypertensive type 1 diabetic patients with diabetic nephropathy.[316] This illustrates the future potential of individualized therapy based on pharmacogenomic profiling.

Head-to-head comparisons of ACE inhibitors and ARBs suggest that these drugs have similar ability to reduce albuminuria and blood pressure in diabetic patients with elevated urinary albumin excretion.[317-319] These results indicate that the reduction in albuminuria and blood pressure induced by ACE inhibition is primarily caused by interference with the RAS. Because reduction of proteinuria is a prerequisite for successful long-term renoprotection, one study investigated whether individual patient factors are determinants of antiproteinuric efficacy.[320] The results suggested that patients responding favorably to one class of antiproteinuric drugs also respond favorably to other classes of available drugs.

Dose-escalation studies of different ARBs have demonstrated that the optimal renoprotective dosage is 100 mg daily for losartan, 16 mg daily for candesartan,[321,322] 900 mg daily for irbesartan,[295] and 320 to 640 mg daily for valsartan.[323] In the SMART study, which included patients with urine protein levels of more than 1 g, of which 54% had diabetes, 128 mg of candesartan had a higher antiproteinuric effect than 16 mg of candesartan.[324] Unfortunately, less information is available about the optimal renoprotective dosage of the various ACE inhibitors. At least for lisinopril, 40 mg daily seems to be the optimal dose.[325]

A comparison of the antiproteinuric effect of the ARBs telmisartan and losartan in diabetic nephropathy suggested that telmisartan was more effective.[326] Short-term studies indicate that the combination of ACE inhibition and angiotensin II receptor blockade may offer additional renal and cardiovascular protection in diabetic patients with elevated AER.[327-333] In a meta-analysis it was concluded that the combination reduced albuminuria approximately 25% more than monotherapy.[334] In accordance with this finding, animal studies suggest that low-dose dual blockade of RAS achieves more important reduction in kidney tissue angiotensin II activity than high doses of captopril or losartan.[335] In addition, it should be mentioned that ARBs reduce blood pressure without adversely altering the ability to autoregulate GFR in diabetic patients.[336] Long-term data in diabetic nephropathy are lacking. The COOPERATE trial found a beneficial effect of combined treatment with an ACE inhibitor and ARB on the endpoint of doubling of creatinine concentration or ESRD in patients with nondiabetic renal disease,[337] but subsequent

analysis of the data has identified concerns about this data set.[338] The IMPROVE trial (*N* = 414) in microalbuminuric hypertensive subjects, the majority with diabetes, randomly assigned patients to ACE inhibition or dual blockade and did not find any difference between monotherapy and dual therapy.[339]

As discussed earlier, the ONTARGET study of patients with low renal risk who had a mean urinary albumin/creatinine ratio of 7.2 mg/g and a sustained decline in GFR of less than 1 mL/min/yr, but high cardiovascular risk, demonstrated a beneficial effect of dual blockade with telmisartan and ramipril on urinary AER within the normal range, but an increase in the composite primary endpoint of doubling of creatinine level, need for dialysis, or death.[274]

Based on the results of the ONTARGET study dealing with renal outcome,[274] Messerli[340] concluded that albuminuria, at least at very low levels, can no longer be regarded as a valid surrogate endpoint in renal disease and argued that compelling evidence in favor of dual RAS blockade was lacking. A meticulous analysis of the study findings led to a completely different conclusion, however: the ONTARGET study, which investigated RAS blockade in a population at low risk for progressive kidney disease and applied insufficiently measured renal endpoints, confounded by death and the need for acute dialysis, has resulted in inconclusive evidence and misinterpretation of the role of dual RAS blockade and the importance of albuminuria as a valid endpoint for renal disease.[341] Furthermore, a Lancet editorial on the ONTARGET study stated, "One needs to interpret the ONTARGET findings in the context of the cohort studied and how renal endpoint data were collected." Data collection on kidney function was argued to be scant. Specifically, urine albumin excretion was not assessed annually, and the need for dialysis was established arbitrarily with no predetermined protocol and the data were assessed post hoc. A robust prospective trial of patients with advanced proteinuric CKD is still needed to answer the question of the efficacy of combination therapy to block the RAS in reducing the progression of CKD.[342]

In recent years it has become clear that aldosterone should be considered a hormone with widespread unfavorable effects on the vasculature, the heart, and the kidneys.[200,343-345] It has been demonstrated that elevated plasma aldosterone level during long-term treatment with losartan is associated with an enhanced decline in GFR in type 1 diabetic patients with diabetic nephropathy.[202] Consequently, aldosterone blockade could be considered in patients with suboptimal renoprotection during conventional RAS blockade.

Short-term studies in type 1 and type 2 proteinuric diabetic patients have demonstrated that spironolactone safely adds to the renal and cardiovascular protective benefits of treatment with maximally recommended dosages of ACE inhibitors or ARBs by reducing albuminuria and blood pressure.[346-348] This selective aldosterone blocker eplerenone has also been demonstrated to reduce proteinuria by 48% when added to an ACE inhibitor in type 2 diabetic patients with albuminuria (urine protein level of >50 mg/g).[349]

Recently aliskiren, the first oral direct renin inhibitor, has been developed for treatment of hypertension, which makes it feasible to block the RAS at the first rate-limiting step in the RAAS cascade, and without an increase in plasma renin activity. In transgenic (mRen-2)27 rats the ACE inhibitor perindopril was compared with aliskiren. The drugs had similar effects on albuminuria and glomerular structural changes, but the amount of interstitial fibrosis was attenuated to a greater extent with aliskiren.[350] Another study of aliskiren[351] using the same rat model demonstrated reduced expression of the (pro)renin receptor, which was described by Nguyen and colleagues[352] in 2002 and has been suggested to be important for the development of renal and cardiac fibrosis.[353,354] Prorenin level has been demonstrated to predict diabetic microvascular complications,[355,356] but whether aliskiren has specific protective effects remains to be established.

In type 2 diabetic patients with albuminuria a significant reduction in urinary AER was seen after 2 to 4 days of treatment with aliskiren 300 mg daily, with a maximal reduction of 44% after 28 days. Systolic blood pressure was significantly lowered after 7 days with no further reduction after 28 days.[357] Another study of type 2 diabetic patients with elevated albumin excretion demonstrated a similar antiproteinuric effect of aliskiren and the ARB irbesartan, but an additional antiproteinuric effect was seen when the agents were combined.[358] Increasing the aliskiren dosage to 600 mg daily did not significantly increase the antiproteinuric effect.[359]

The renoprotective effect of adding a renin inhibitor to optimal renoprotective treatment with losartan 100 mg was demonstrated in the AVOID study in which patients receiving optimal standard therapy were randomly assigned to receive aliskiren or placebo for 6 months. The study included 599 patients with type 2 diabetes. After 6 months a reduction in albuminuria of 20% (95% CI = 9% to 30%) was seen in the aliskiren-treated patients compared with those receiving only standard therapy. Side effects were few; in particular, hyperkalemia was not more frequent in the intervention group.[360] The long-term effect of combined therapy with aliskiren plus conventional antihypertensive treatment on cardiovascular and renal morbidity and mortality in type 2 diabetic patients will be evaluated in the Aliskiren Trial in Type 2 Diabetes Using Cardio-Renal Endpoints (ALTITUDE) study, which aims to recruit 8600 patients and plans a 4-year follow-up.[361]

Initiation of antihypertensive treatment usually induces an initial drop in GFR that is three to five times higher per unit of time than that during the sustained treatment period.[362] This phenomenon occurs with conventional antihypertensive treatment with β-blockers and diuretics, and when ACE inhibitors are used. Whether this initial phenomenon is reversible (hemodynamic effect) or irreversible (structural damage) with prolonged antihypertensive treatment has recently been investigated in type 1 diabetic patients with diabetic nephropathy. The results support the hypothesis that the faster initial decline in GFR is due to a functional (hemodynamic) effect of antihypertensive treatment that does not attenuate over time, whereas the subsequent slower decline reflects the beneficial effect on progression of nephropathy.[362] A similar effect has been demonstrated in nondiabetic glomerulopathies.[363] In contrast, results of another study suggest that the faster initial decline in GFR after initiation of antihypertensive therapy in hypertensive type 2 diabetic patients with diabetic nephropathy is due to an irreversible effect.[364]

In 1982, Mogensen described a beneficial effect of long-term antihypertensive treatment in five hypertensive men with type 1 diabetes and nephropathy.[365] A prospective study initiated in 1976 demonstrated that early and aggressive antihypertensive treatment reduces albuminuria and the rate of decline in GFR in young men and women with type 1 diabetes and nephropathy.[366-368] Figure 38-20 shows the mean values for arterial blood pressure, GFR, and albuminuria in nine patients undergoing long-term treatment (>9 years) with metoprolol, furosemide, and hydralazine.[368] Note that the data are consistent with a time-dependent renoprotective effect of antihypertensive treatment that in the long term might lead to regression of the disease (ΔGFR ≤1 mL/min/yr), at least in some patients. The same progressive benefit in ΔGFR with time has also been demonstrated in patients with nondiabetic renal diseases.[369]

Regression of kidney disease (ΔGFR ≤1 mL/min/yr) has been documented in a sizable fraction (22%) of type 1 diabetic patients receiving aggressive antihypertensive therapy for diabetic nephropathy.[370] Remission of proteinuria for at least 1 year (urine protein excretion of ≤1 g/24 hr) has been described in patients with type 1 diabetes participating in the captopril collaborative study.[371] Eight of 108 patients experienced remission during long-term follow-up.[371] These findings were confirmed and extended in a long-term prospective observational study of 321 patients with type 1 diabetes and nephropathy.[372] The remission group, not surprisingly, is characterized by slow progression of diabetic nephropathy and an improved cardiovascular risk profile. More importantly, the prospective study suggests that remission of nephrotic-range albuminuria in type 1 and type 2 diabetic patients, induced by aggressive antihypertensive treatment with and without the use of ACE inhibitors, is associated with a slower progression in diabetic nephropathy and a substantially improved survival.[373,374]

In 1992, Björck and colleagues suggested that the use of ACE inhibitors in patients with diabetic nephropathy confers renoprotection; that is, it has a beneficial effect on renal function and structure above and beyond that expected from the blood-pressure–lowering effect alone.[375] Their investigation was a prospective, open, randomized study lasting for 2.2 years involving patients with type 1 diabetes.

In 1993, the Captopril Collaborative Study Group demonstrated a significant reduction (48%; 95% CI = 16% to 69%) in the risk of a doubling of serum creatinine concentrations in patients with type 1 diabetes and nephropathy who received captopril.[376] In comparison, the placebo-treated patients received conventional antihypertensive therapy, excluding calcium channel blockers. Long-term treatment (4 years) with an ACE inhibitor or a long-acting dihydropyridine calcium channel antagonist was observed to have similar beneficial effects on progression of diabetic nephropathy in hypertensive patients with type 1 diabetes.[377] Thus, it was initially demonstrated that pharmacologic interruption of the RAS slows the progression of renal disease in patients with type 1 diabetes, but similar data were not available for patients with type 2 diabetes, as reviewed by Parving.[78]

Against this background, two large multinational double-blind, randomized, placebo-controlled trials of ARBs—the RENAAL study and the Irbesartan Diabetic Nephropathy Trial (IDNT)—were carried out in comparable populations of hypertensive patients with type 2 diabetes, proteinuria, and elevated serum creatinine levels.[378,379] In both trials, the primary outcome was the composite of a doubling of the baseline serum creatinine concentration, ESRD, or death. A comparison of the benefits obtained in the RENAAL and IDNT studies is shown in Table 38-4. Side effects were low, and fewer than 2% of the patients had to stop taking an ARB because

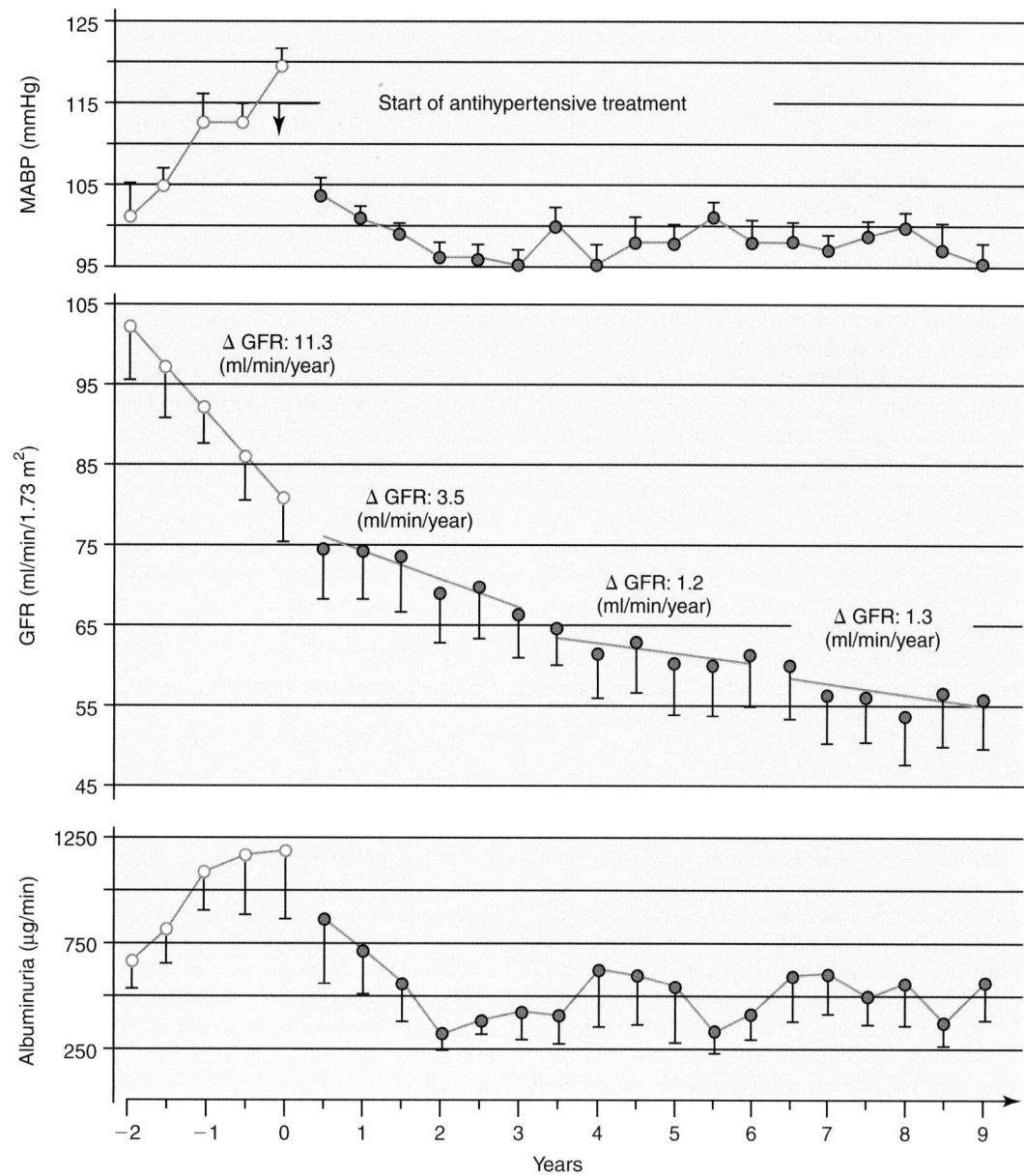

The Effect of Antihypertensive Treatment Upon Kidney
Function in 9 Type 1 Diabetic Patients with Diabetic Nephropathy

FIGURE 38-20 Average course of mean arterial blood pressure, glomerular filtration rate (GFR), and urine albumin level before (○) and during (●) long-term effective antihypertensive treatment in nine type 1 diabetic patients with diabetic nephropathy. (From Parving H-H, Rossing P, Hommel E, et al: Angiotensin converting enzyme inhibition in diabetic nephropathy: ten years experience, *Am J Kidney Dis* 26:99-107, 1995.)

TABLE 38-4 RENAAL and IDNT Results: Comparison of Primary Composite Endpoints and Components

	RISK REDUCTION IN % (95% CI)			
ENDPOINT	LOSARTAN VS. PLACEBO[378]	IRBESARTAN VS. PLACEBO[379]	IRBESARTAN VS. AMLODIPINE[379]	AMLODIPINE VS. PLACEBO[379]
DsCr, ESRD, death	16 (2 to 28)	20 (3 to 34)	23 (7 to 37)	−4 (14 to −25)
DsCr	25 (8 to 39)	33 (13 to 48)	37 (19 to 52)	−6 (16 to −35)
ESRD	28 (11 to 42)	23 (−3 to 43)	23 (−3 to 43)	0 (−32 to 24)
Death	−2 (−27 to 19)	8 (−31 to 23)	−4 (23 to −40)	12 (−19 to 34)
ESRD or death	20 (5 to 32)	—	—	—

CI, Confidence interval; DsCr, doubling of serum creatinine level; ESRD, end-stage renal disease; IDNT, Irbesartan Diabetic Nephropathy Trial; RENAAL, Reduction of End Points in NIDDM with the Angiotensin II Antagonist Losartan study.

of severe hyperkalemia. The number of sudden deaths was not significantly different in the various treatment groups. Taken together, the results of these two landmark studies lead to the following conclusion: "Losartan and irbesartan conferred significant renal benefits in patients with type 2 diabetes and nephropathy. This protection is independent of the reduction in blood pressure it causes. The ARB's are generally safe and well tolerated."[147]

A meta-analysis of the IRMA study[290] and the two aforementioned ARB trials[378,379] revealed a significant reduction (15%) in the risk of cardiovascular events in the experimental groups compared with the control groups.[380] Based on these three outcome trials of ARBs, the American Diabetes Association now states, "In patients with type 2 diabetes, hypertension, macroalbuminuria and renal insufficiency (serum creatinine >1.5 mg/dl), ARBs have been shown to delay the progression of nephropathy."[147]

Early studies describing the prognosis for overt diabetic nephropathy observed a median patient survival time of 5 to 7 years after the onset of persistent proteinuria. End-stage renal failure was the primary cause of death in 66% of patients. When deaths attributed only to ESRD were considered, the median survival time was 10 years. All this was before patients were offered antihypertensive therapy.[78] Long-term antihypertensive therapy was evaluated prospectively in 45 type 1 diabetic patients who developed overt diabetic nephropathy between 1974 and 1978. The cumulative death rate was 18% at 10 years after the onset of diabetic nephropathy, and the median survival time was more than 16 years.[381,382]

Rossing and colleagues went on to examine whether antihypertensive therapy also improved survival in an unselected cohort of 263 patients with diabetic nephropathy who were followed for up to 20 years, and observed a median survival time of 13.9 years; only 35% of patients died because of ESRD (serum creatinine level of >500 μmol/L).[383] Fortunately, survival continues to improve, and a more recent study showed a median survival time of 21 years after the onset of diabetic nephropathy[384] (Figure 38-21).

The first information regarding the effect of antihypertensive treatment on progression of nephropathy to come from a randomized, double-blind, placebo-controlled trial was presented by the Collaborative Study Group of Angiotensin Converting Enzyme Inhibition, which examined the use of captopril in type 1 diabetic patients with diabetic nephropathy.[376] In this study, which lasted on average 2.7 years, the risk of death or progression to dialysis or transplantation was reduced by 61% (95% CI = 26% to 80%; $P = 0.002$) in the subgroup of 102 captopril-treated patients with a baseline serum creatinine concentration of more than 133 μmol/L and by 46% (95% CI = 22% to 76%; $P = 0.14$) in the 307 patients with a baseline serum creatinine concentration below 133 μmol/L, compared with placebo-treated patients. An economic analysis of the use of captopril in patients with diabetic nephropathy revealed that ACE inhibition will provide significant savings in health care costs.[385]

In conclusion, the prognosis for diabetic nephropathy in type 1 diabetic patients has improved during the past decade, largely because of effective antihypertensive treatment with conventional drugs (β-blockers, diuretics) and ACE inhibitors. Unfortunately, scant information on this important issue is available for type 2 diabetic patients with diabetic nephropathy, but the IDNT and RENAAL studies demonstrated that there is a need for further improvement in prognosis for these patients.[378,379]

Lipid-Lowering Therapy

In albuminuric patients with diabetes the risk of cardiovascular disease is enhanced. Consequently these patients should be treated with statins according to current guidelines for patients at high risk.[386] The renoprotective effect of 3-hydroxy-3-methylglutaryl–coenzyme A reductase inhibitors in patients with type 1 or type 2 diabetes who have microalbuminuria or macroalbuminuria appears to be highly variable.[124] However, all nine studies examining this effect were of short duration, enrolled a small number of patients, and evaluated only a surrogate endpoint, namely urinary albumin excretion. Large, long-term, double-blind, randomized trials with hard endpoints (e.g., doubling of serum creatinine level and/or ESRD) are urgently needed.

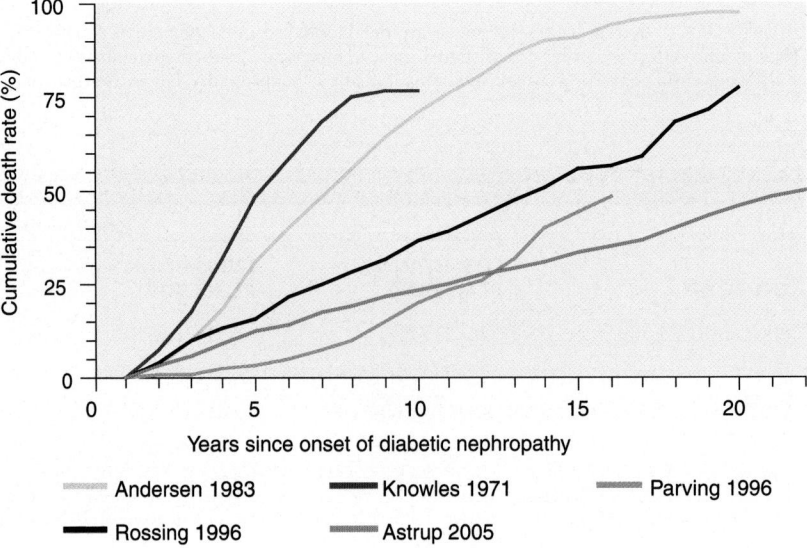

FIGURE 38-21 Cumulative rate of death from the onset of diabetic nephropathy in type 1 diabetic patients during the natural history of diabetic nephropathy (*red line*, N = 45 [Knowles[523]]; *yellow line*, N = 360 [Andersen et al.[524]]) compared with the rate for patients who received effective antihypertensive treatment (*orange line*, N = 45 [Parving et al.[382]]; *black line*, N = 263 [Rossing et al.[383]]; *green line*, n = 199 (Astrup et al.[384]]).

In a recent meta-analysis examining the effect of statins on renal function a small positive effect on urinary albumin excretion and renal function was suggested. This effect was observed mainly in patients with cardiovascular disease and not in patients with renal disease.[387] The effect of fenofibrate on macrovascular and microvascular outcome was evaluated in the FIELD study, which included 9795 type 2 diabetic patients.[388] The study also evaluated the effect on urinary albumin excretion. There was no effect on progression of urinary albumin excretion alone, but when data were combined for a slightly improved regression from microalbuminuria to normoalbuminuria and a reduced progression of albuminuria it was observed that 2.6% more patients treated with fenofibrate showed no progression or a regression of albuminuria. This result was significantly different from that for the placebo group ($P = 0.002$).

Dietary Protein Restriction

Short-term studies in type 1 diabetic patients with normoalbuminuria, microalbuminuria, or macroalbuminuria have shown that low-protein diet (0.6 to 0.8 g/kg/day) reduces urinary albumin excretion and hyperfiltration independently of changes in glucose control and blood pressure.[389,390] Longer-term trials in type 1 patients with diabetic nephropathy suggest that protein restriction reduces the progression of kidney function,[391,392] but this interpretation has been challenged.[393,394] Pedrini and colleagues[395] performed a meta-analysis and concluded that dietary protein restriction effectively slows the progression of diabetic renal disease, but their conclusion has been disputed.[396,397] A 4-year prospective, randomized, controlled trial with concealed randomization compared the effects of a low-protein diet with a usual-protein diet in 82 type 1 diabetic patients with progressive diabetic nephropathy. The endpoint of ESRD or death occurred in 27% of patients consuming a usual-protein diet compared with 10% consuming a low-protein diet (log-rank test, $P = 0.04$).[398] The relative risk of ESRD or death was 0.23 (95% CI = 0.07 to 0.72) for patients assigned to a low-protein diet after an adjustment for the presence of cardiovascular disease at baseline. Currently a dietary protein intake of 0.8 g/kg body weight per day is recommended in the Kidney Disease Outcomes Quality Initiative guidelines for patients with diabetes and chronic renal disease stages 1 through 4.[386]

New Treatment Options

New options are needed to treat diabetic nephropathy despite the success of the aforementioned treatment modalities. A number of new options are suggested by experimental and clinical studies (Table 38-5). Vitamin D (1,25-dihydroxyvitamin D_3) or activation of the vitamin D receptor with vitamin D analogs has recently been suggested to play a role in the development of diabetic nephropathy. In addition, vitamin D is a negative regulator of the RAS.[399] In experimental studies the combination of an ARB and a vitamin D analog was more effective than either agent alone in preventing renal injury.[400] In three short-term studies evaluating the safety of the vitamin D analog paricalcitol in patients with CKD, an antiproteinuric effect was observed.[401] In a small pilot trial a 46% reduction in albuminuria was seen after 1 month of treatment with paricalcitol.[402] This therapy is currently being evaluated in type 2 diabetic patients with microalbuminuria or macroalbuminuria in the Selective Vitamin D Receptor Activator for Albuminuria Lowering (VITAL) study.[403]

Soludexide, a glycosaminoglycan mixture of heparin sulfate and dermatan sulfate, was found to reduce albuminuria in a pilot study[404] but subsequently failed to reduce albuminuria in microalbuminuric or macroalbuminuric type 2 diabetic patients.

Tranilast is an antifibrotic agent that has been shown to suppress collagen synthesis in experimental models. Small studies in human patients found reduced albuminuria and type IV collagen excretion with tranilast treatment.[405] Analogs are now being developed due to concerns about potential adverse effects related to tranilast use.

End-Stage Renal Disease in Diabetic Patients

Epidemiology

Diabetic nephropathy has become the leading cause of ESRD in most Western countries.[406] In the 2005 report of the U.S. Renal Data System (http://www.usrds.org) diabetes was reported as a comorbid condition in 44.8% of incident ESRD patients in the United States (4.3%, type 1 diabetes; 40.5%, type 2 diabetes). In 2006 the number of incident ESRD patients with diabetes was 159 patients per million (45% of all ESRD patients). This number represents a 50% increase compared with more than a decade earlier, but this trend is currently plateauing.

TABLE 38-5 Potential New Treatment Modalities for Diabetic Nephropathy

Tested in Humans*

Vitamin D receptor stimulation[401,402]

Sulodexide[404]

Tranilast[405]

Protein kinase C inhibition[555]

Advanced glycation end product cross-link breakers[556]

Pyridoxamine[557]

Growth hormone inhibition (L. Tarnow, personal communication, September 2009)

Benfothiamine[558]

Pentoxifylline (MCP-1 inhibition?)[559]

Thiozolidinediones[560]

Endothelin antagonist[561]

Connective tissue growth factor inhibition[562]

Allopurinol, antioxidants (not tested)

Tested in Experimental Models

Tissue transglutaminase inhibition[563]

Monocyte chemoattractant CC chemokine ligand (MCP-1)[564]

Uric acid lowering (allopurinol)[565]

*Most of the studies are preliminary, enrolling small numbers of patients and measuring surrogate endpoints.
MCP-1, Monocyte chemoattractant protein-1.

In Europe the proportion of diabetic individuals varies considerably among countries.[407] An average of 117 diabetic patients per million population per year develop ESRD. It is an encouraging observation that recently the incidence of type 2 diabetic patients entering hemodialysis has plateaued in some European countries.[100] The 5-year survival of patients with type 2 diabetes receiving dialysis treatment was 20% in Europe,[408] but is considerably higher in Japan.

Registry figures tend to underestimate the renal burden of diabetes. One study found that diabetes as a comorbid condition was present in no fewer than 48.9% of patients admitted for renal replacement therapy; 90% of these had type 2 diabetes.[409] Clinical features of classic Kimmelstiel-Wilson disease (large kidneys, heavy proteinuria) were found only in 60%, however. Thirteen percent had an atypical presentation consistent with ischemic nephropathy (i.e., shrunken kidneys with no major proteinuria), and 27% had known primary renal disease (e.g., polycystic disease, analgesic nephropathy, primary or secondary glomerulonephritis) with superimposed diabetes. At the time of admission diabetes had not been diagnosed in 11% of these patients. Although many factors may account for this, it has been argued that because patients often lose weight with advanced CKD secondary to anorexia, self-correction of hyperglycemia occurs. Patients with diabetic nephropathy may completely lose hyperglycemia after weight loss in the preterminal stage and regain weight following refeeding on dialysis. Therefore, new-onset diabetes developing while patients are receiving dialysis may represent changes in dietary caloric intake as appetite improves with improvement in the uremic diathesis.[410]

A diabetic patient with ESRD has several options for renal replacement therapy:

1. Transplantation (kidney only, pancreas plus kidney simultaneously, pancreas after kidney)
2. Hemodialysis
3. Continuous ambulatory peritoneal dialysis (CAPD).

There is consensus that today medical rehabilitation and survival are best after transplantation,[411] particularly after transplantation of pancreas plus kidney.[412] The results of CAPD and hemodialysis are inferior to transplantation, but are comparable for CAPD and hemodialysis.

Management of the Patient with Advanced Renal Failure

The diabetic patient with advanced renal failure, or more correctly CKD, has a much higher burden of microvascular and macrovascular complications (Table 38-6) than the diabetic patient without proteinuria or in the earliest stages of diabetic nephropathy. The morbidity of diabetic patients with CKD is usually more severe than that of the average patient seen in the diabetes outpatient clinic. Consequently, even when such patients are asymptomatic, they must be monitored at regular intervals for timely detection of complications (ophthalmologic examination at half-yearly intervals, cardiac and angiologic status yearly, foot inspection at each visit)

The physician in charge of the care of a diabetic patient with impaired renal function has to face a spectrum of therapeutic challenges. These are listed in Table 38-7. The most vexing clinical problems are related to coronary heart disease and autonomic polyneuropathy.

TABLE 38-6 Complications of Diabetic Nephropathy

Microvascular Complications

Retinopathy
Polyneuropathy, including autonomic neuropathy (gastroparesis, diarrhea or obstipation, detrusor paresis, painless myocardial ischemia, erectile dysfunction, supine hypertension/orthostatic hypotension)

Macrovascular Complications

Coronary heart disease, left ventricular hypertrophy, congestive heart failure
Cerebrovascular complications (stroke)
Peripheral artery occlusive disease

Mixed Complications

Diabetic foot (neuropathic, vascular)

TABLE 38-7 Frequent Therapeutic Challenges in the Diabetic Patient with Renal Failure

Hypertension (blood pressure amplitude, circadian rhythm)
Hypervolemia
Glycemic control (prolongation of insulin half-life, accumulation of oral hypoglycemic agents)
Malnutrition
Bacterial infections (diabetic foot)
Timely creation of vascular access

Hypertension

At any given level of GFR, blood pressure tends to be higher in diabetic than in nondiabetic patients with CKD. Because of their beneficial effect on cardiovascular complications[413] and progression of CKD,[290,376,378,379] ACE inhibitors or ARBs are obligatory unless there are temporary or persistent absolute or relative contraindications, for example, an acute major increase in serum creatinine concentration (e.g., renal artery stenosis, hypovolemia) or hyperkalemia resistant to corrective maneuvers (such as loop diuretics, dietary potassium restriction, omission of β-blockers, or correction of metabolic acidosis).

Because of their marked propensity to retain salt, patients with diabetic nephropathy have a tendency to develop hypervolemia and edema.[414] Therefore, dietary salt restriction and the use of loop diuretics are usually indicated. At least as monotherapy, thiazides are no longer sufficient once GFR falls below 30 to 50 mL/min. When the creatinine concentration is elevated, multidrug antihypertensive therapy and dietary salt restriction are indicated.

To normalize blood pressure it is necessary to administer, on average, three to five antihypertensive agents. In these patients, hypertension is also characterized by a high blood pressure amplitude (as a result of increased aortic stiffness) and by an attenuated nighttime decrease in blood pressure (nondipping), which in itself is a potent risk predictor of cardiovascular events and accelerated progression to CKD.[415,416]

Glucose Control

Insulin resistance develops in the early stages of CKD as a result of accumulation of a (hypothetical) circulating factor thought to interfere with the action of insulin. This causes progressive impairment of glucose tolerance and hyperglycemia. Insulin resistance is improved after the start of dialysis.

On the other hand, the biologic half-life of insulin is prolonged and renal gluconeogenesis is impaired, which causes a tendency to develop hypoglycemic episodes.

This risk is further compounded by anorexia and—apart from the impaired clearance of insulin—also by the accumulation of many insulin secretagogues or their metabolites,[417] specifically most sulfonylurea compounds (with the exception of gliquidone or glimepiride). Glinides and glitazones do not accumulate. Metformin should not be given in CKD, although this guideline statement has been disputed. For details on dosing contraindications and pharmacokinetics, refer to the 2009 report of Haneda and Morikawa.[417]

As a result of the aforementioned opposing influences, glycemia is difficult to predict. Therefore close monitoring of plasma glucose concentrations is advisable. There is an increasing trend in patients with advanced CKD to use short-acting insulin more liberally, particularly during intercurrent illness (infections, surgery), especially given that insulin treatment also reduces catabolism and malnutrition.

Malnutrition

Patients are often severely catabolic and are predisposed to develop malnutrition, particularly during periods of intercurrent illness and fasting, but also from ill-advised recommendation of protein-restricted diets without attention to the potential risk of concomitant reduction of energy intake in such anorectic patients. Malnutrition is a potent independent predictor of mortality,[418] and its presence justifies an early start of renal replacement treatment. Anorectic obese patients with type 2 diabetes and advanced CKD often undergo massive weight loss leading to normalization of fasting and even postloading glycemia. The diagnosis of Kimmelstiel-Wilson disease then requires documentation of retinopathy or renal biopsy.

Wasting with low muscle mass is an important dilemma for treating physicians. The severity of renal failure may be underappreciated because, for any given level of GFR, serum creatinine concentrations can be spuriously low in such patients. This contributes to errors in dosing of drugs, which accumulate in renal failure, and may also cause a belated start of renal replacement therapy. In advanced CKD, (i.e., GFR of <60 mL/min/1.73 m^2), it is advisable to estimate GFR (eGFR) using the Modification of Diet in Renal Disease equation.[419] Importantly, some investigators[420] argue that eGFR is imprecise in diabetic patients with a GFR of over 60 mL/min/1.73 m^2. An alternative is measurement of cystatin C concentration.

Acute and "Acute-on-Chronic" Renal Failure

Diabetic patients with diabetic nephropathy who have multiple morbid conditions are particularly prone to develop superimposed acute renal failure (new nomenclature: acute kidney injury [AKI]).[421] In one series, 27% of patients with AKI had diabetes.[409] The most common causes of AKI were emergency cardiologic interventions involving the administration of radiocontrast agents, septicemia, low cardiac output, and shock. Prevention of radiocontrast-induced AKI necessitates adequate preparation of the patient with saline as well as temporary interruption of diuretic treatment.[422] The high susceptibility of the kidney to ischemic injury, at least in experimental diabetes, may be a contributory factor.[423] Not infrequently, AKI necessitates hemodialysis and carries a high risk of leading to irreversible chronic renal failure. This mode of presentation as irreversible acute renal failure has a particularly poor prognosis.[424] Even when the patient recover from AKI the risk of developing delayed CKD is high.[425]

Vascular Access

Timely creation of vascular access is of overriding importance. It should be considered when the eGFR is approximately 20 to 25 mL/min. Although venous runoff problems are not unusual (due to venous occlusion from prior injections, infusions, or infections as well as hypoplasia of veins, particularly in elderly female diabetic patients), inadequate arterial inflow is increasingly recognized as the major cause of fistula malfunction.[426] If distal arteries are severely sclerotic, anastomosis at a more proximal level may be necessary. Use of native vessels is clearly the first choice and results of grafts are definitely inferior. It is often necessary to create an upper arm native arteriovenous fistula[427-429] or use more sophisticated approaches.[430] Arteriosclerosis of arm arteries not only jeopardizes fistula flow but also predisposes to the steal phenomenon with the potential for neurovascular compromise and the risk of finger gangrene or Volkmann's ischemic contracture.[431]

Anemia

Anemia is more frequent and more severe at any given level of GFR in diabetic patients with renal failure than in nondiabetic patients.[432] The major cause of anemia is an inappropriate response of the plasma erythropoietin (EPO) concentration to anemia. Inhibition of the RAS may be an additional factor. In patients whose serum creatinine concentration is still normal, the EPO concentration predicts the future rate of loss of GFR.[433] Interestingly, a single nucleotide polymorphism in the EPO gene promoter is associated with a higher risk of nephropathy and retinopathy.[434]

There had been some concern that correction of anemia by EPO administration may accelerate the rate of loss of GFR, but this has not been confirmed.[435] There is no controlled evidence concerning the effect of reversal of anemia by EPO on diabetic end-organ damage. Although EPO is a retinal proangiogenic factor in diabetes,[436] uncontrolled observations show some improvement of diabetic retinopathy after EPO therapy,[437] in line with experimental observations showing a protective role for EPO in retinal ischemia[438] and diabetic polyneuropathy.[439] The recent TREAT study in type 2 diabetic patients with CKD found no significant survival benefit from EPO therapy, at least beyond guideline recommendations, and noted an increased risk of strokes.[439a]

Initiation of Renal Replacement Therapy

Many, but not all, nephrologists are of the opinion that renal replacement therapy should be started earlier in diabetic than in nondiabetic patients, that is, at an eGFR of approximately 15 mL/min. An even earlier start may be justified when hypervolemia and blood pressure become uncontrollable, when the patient is anorectic and cachectic, and when the patient vomits as the combined result of uremia and gastroparesis.

Hemodialysis

In recent years survival of diabetic patients receiving hemodialysis has tended to improve.[407] Astonishingly high survival rates—for example, 50% at 5 years for diabetic patients undergoing dialysis—have been reported in East Asia. To a large extent the differences between countries may reflect the frequency of cardiovascular death in the background populations.

INTRADIALYTIC AND INTERDIALYTIC BLOOD PRESSURE

Diabetic patients receiving dialysis tend to be more hypertensive than nondiabetic patients receiving dialysis. Blood pressure is exquisitely volume dependent in diabetic patients. The problem is compounded by the fact that patients are predisposed to intradialytic hypotension, so that it is difficult to reach the target "dry weight" by ultrafiltration. Although reduced dietary salt intake, long slow dialysis, nocturnal hemodialysis, and added ultrafiltration may permit control of hypertension without medication, antihypertensive agents are required in virtually all patients.

The main causes of intradialytic hypotension are, on the one hand, disturbed counterregulation (autonomous polyneuropathy) and, on the other hand, disturbed left ventricular compliance so that cardiac output decreases abruptly when left ventricular filling pressure is reduced by ultrafiltration.[440] One or more of the following approaches are useful to avoid intradialytic hypotension: long dialysis sessions, omission of antihypertensive agents immediately before dialysis sessions, and controlled ultrafiltration. If none of these methods works, however, alternative treatment modalities such as hemofiltration, nocturnal hemodialysis, and CAPD should be considered.

Intradialytic hypotension increases the risk of cardiac death by a factor of three.[441] It also predisposes to myocardial ischemia, arrhythmia, deterioration of maculopathy, and (particularly in the elderly) nonthrombotic mesenteric infarction. Elevated pulse pressure and impaired elasticity as well as calcification of central arteries are major predictors of death and of cardiovascular events in nonuremic patients. They are also significant predictors of death in nondiabetic patients but, for uncertain reasons, not in diabetic patients on hemodialysis.[442]

CARDIOVASCULAR PROBLEMS

The survival of diabetic patients receiving hemodialysis (and CAPD) is inferior to that of nondiabetic patients because of the high rate of cardiovascular death in diabetic hemodialysis patients. Stack and Bloembergen[443] examined the prevalence of congestive heart failure in a national random sample of patients entering renal replacement programs and noted that the prevalence of congestive heart failure was significantly higher in diabetic than in nondiabetic patients, with the difference between these two groups even exceeding the difference observed between sexes.

Diabetic patients are at a greater risk of acquiring cardiovascular disease in the predialytic phase. The odds ratio for development of new cardiovascular disease was 5.35 for diabetic patients with established kidney disease who were not yet receiving dialysis.[444] This explains the high prevalence of cardiovascular complications when diabetic patients enter

dialysis programs. The rate of onset of ischemic heart disease is strikingly and significantly higher in diabetic patients than in nondiabetic patients on hemodialysis.[443-445]

When coronary complications supervene, the prognosis is also worse for diabetic patients than for nondiabetic patients. If myocardial infarction occurs, the short-term and long-term survival is poor in all hemodialysis patients, but it is poorest in diabetic patients on hemodialysis, with a mortality of 62.3% in diabetic patients versus 55.4% in nondiabetic patients after 1 year and 93.3% versus 86.9% after 5 years.[446] Diabetic patients are also more prone to develop sudden cardiac death during dialysis sessions[447] and more likely to die from sudden death in the interdialytic interval.

In diabetic patients receiving dialysis coronary calcification is more pronounced and complex triple-vessel lesions are more frequent, but the high mortality rate is not fully explained by the severity of stenosing coronary lesions. The impact of ischemic heart disease is presumably amplified by further cardiac abnormalities such as congestive heart failure, left ventricular hypertrophy, and disturbed sympathetic innervations.[448,449] Fibrosis of the heart and microvessel disease with diminished coronary reserve and deranged cardiomyocyte metabolism with reduced ischemia tolerance may also contribute.[450] Such functional abnormalities, particularly insufficient nitric oxide–dependent vasodilator reserve and perturbed sympathetic innervation, have been documented even in the earliest stages of diabetes[451] and are especially frequent in diabetic patients receiving dialysis.

Therapeutic challenges include prevention in the asymptomatic patient and intervention in the symptomatic patient. With respect to prevention, unfortunately, little evidence-based information is available. But it is sensible to reduce afterload (by controlling blood pressure) and preload (by reducing hypervolemia). Despite the evidence of benefit from statin therapy in diabetic patients without renal failure,[452] the 4D study (Die Deutsche Diabetes Dialyse Studie) found no reduction of the composite cardiac endpoint with atorvastatin therapy in type 2 diabetic patients receiving dialysis.[453]

Diabetic patients with renal failure are characterized by the development of premature and more pronounced anemia. No controlled data are available regarding which target hemoglobin value is protective. In view of the outcome of the TREAT study, it is prudent to follow the guidelines strictly.[439a]

There is limited controlled evidence for the efficacy of ACE inhibitors in diabetic patients undergoing dialysis. One controlled study in patients on hemodialysis treated with fosinopril showed no significant beneficial effect on outcome,[454] but based on pathophysiologic reasoning the administration of ACE inhibitors or ARBs appears to be logical. In view of the importance of disturbed sympathetic innervation,[455] it is surprising that β-blockers are only sparingly administered to diabetic patients undergoing dialysis, although β-blockers were shown to lead to better survival in observational studies[456] and carvedilol therapy resulted in substantially better survival in heart failure patients receiving dialysis in a controlled interventional study.[457] It has been recommended to use the metabolically more advantageous β-blockers in this situation.[458]

In a very small series of diabetic patients with symptomatic coronary heart disease, active intervention—percutaneous transluminal coronary angioplasty (PTCA) or coronary artery bypass graft (CABG)—was superior to medical treatment alone.[459] In another series only 15% of the surgically managed patients had experienced a cardiovascular endpoint after 8.4 months of follow-up compared with 77% of the medically managed group.[460] Because patients often fail to complain of pain, and because screening tests such as exercise electrocardiography and thallium scintigraphy are notoriously poor predictors, one should resort directly to coronary angiography if there is any suspicion of coronary heart disease. The use of gadolinium-enhanced magnetic resonance imaging is contraindicated at that stage of renal function.[461]

No dogmatic statements concerning the type of intervention are possible in the absence of controlled prospective evidence. Retrospective interventional studies[460,462,463] have consistently shown more adverse outcomes in diabetic than in nondiabetic patients treated with either CABG or PTCA. After PTCA, the coronary reocclusion rate had been devastating in the past, in some series reaching 70% at 1 year even in nondiabetic hemodialysis patients. Results have improved considerably in recent years. More recent series suggest markedly better outcomes after PTCA plus stenting than after PTCA alone.[464] However, the frequency of diffuse three-vessel disease with heavy calcification in diabetic patients receiving dialysis remains a major problem.[465] A recent retrospective analysis of data for diabetic patients undergoing dialysis suggested that CABG using internal mammary artery grafts, rather than CABG using venous grafts, yielded superior outcome compared with PTCA with or without stenting.[463]

In view of the fact that renal failure per se aggravates insulin resistance[466] and that in uremia insulin-mediated glucose uptake of the heart is reduced,[467] normalization of blood glucose levels by insulin and glucose infusion is presumably important in uremic patients with diabetes and ischemic heart disease.

GLYCEMIC CONTROL

Dialysis partially reverses insulin resistance, so that insulin requirements often become less than before dialysis. Upon institution of hemodialysis even patients with type 1 diabetes may occasionally lose their need for insulin, at least transiently. In other patients, however, insulin requirements increase, presumably because anorexia is reversed so that appetite and food consumption increase. It is conventional to use dialysates that contain glucose, usually about 200 mg/mL. This allows insulin to be administered at the usual times of day, reduces the risk of hyperglycemic or hypoglycemic episodes, and causes fewer hypotensive episodes.[468]

Adequate control of glycemia is important, because hyperglycemia causes thirst and high fluid intake, as well as an osmotic shift of water and potassium from the intracellular to the extracellular space. This leads to circulatory congestion and hyperkalemia. Diabetic patients with poor glucose control are also more susceptible to infection. Observational studies suggest that good glycemic control in patients entering dialysis programs[469] as well as patients already receiving dialysis[470] reduces overall and cardiovascular mortality.

As an indicator for monitoring glycemic control glycated albumin[471] is theoretically superior to HbA_{1C}, but this test is not routinely available. HbA_{1C} level may be falsely low because of shortened erythrocyte half-life or EPO use, and in some assays is confounded by carbamylation of hemoglobin. Recent studies suggest that survival of diabetic hemodialysis patients is optimal at an HbA_{1C} value of 7.3%,[472] but

given the risks and many interfering factors this goal must be approached with prudence.

MALNUTRITION

Because of anorexia and prolonged habituation to dietary restriction, in diabetic patients on hemodialysis the dietary intake of energy (recommended to be 30 to 35 kcal/kg/day) and protein (recommended to be 1.3 g/kg/day) often falls short of the target. Malnutrition is a potent predictor of death. It is of concern that indications of malnutrition and microinflammation are more commonly found in diabetic patients than in nondiabetic patients receiving hemodialysis.[473] Surprisingly, conventional indicators of malnutrition were not predictive of survival in diabetic hemodialysis patients.[474]

RETINOPATHY

In the distant past the visual prognosis for diabetic dialysis patients was extremely poor, and a high proportion of patients were blind after several months. Despite the use of heparin (which in the past had been accused of being a culprit) de novo amaurosis in patients on hemodialysis has become very rare.

AMPUTATION

At the start of hemodialysis 16% of diabetic patients have undergone amputation, most frequently above-the-ankle amputation.[475] The distinction between neuropathic and vascular foot lesions is crucial to improve outcomes, because the treatment of the two conditions is quite different,[475,476] and major amputation can be prevented by making the right diagnosis.[477] The presence of diabetic foot lesions is the most powerful predictor of survival in diabetic dialysis patients, possibly as a result of the associated microinflammatory state.[476]

Peritoneal Dialysis

Peritoneal dialysis (PD) is not the most common treatment modality, at least in the United States. According to the U.S. Renal Data System, as of 2003, some 41,940 incident diabetic patients were treated with hemodialysis, 2808 were treated with PD, and 367 underwent renal transplantation. The proportion of diabetic patients treated with PD varies greatly among countries, which illustrates that selection of treatment modality not only is based on medical considerations, but also is strongly influenced by logistics and reimbursement policies.

There are very good a priori reasons to offer CAPD treatment to diabetic patients with ESRD at the outset. For example, forearm vessels are often sclerosed, so that it is not possible to create a fistula. The alternative of hemodialysis via intravenous catheters (instead of arteriovenous fistulas or grafts) yields unsatisfactory long-term results, because blood flow is low and the risk of infection is high. Long-term dialysis via catheter was identified as one major predictor of poor survival of patients receiving hemodialysis.[478]

There are additional reasons for offering PD to the diabetic patient, at least as the initial mode of renal replacement therapy. According to Heaf and colleagues, during the first 2 years survival is better for patients treated with PD than for those treated with hemodialysis, and this was also true for diabetic patients,[479] except for the very elderly.[480] A survival advantage is no longer demonstrable beyond the second year (presumably because by then residual renal function has decayed). Moreover, PD provides slow and sustained ultrafiltration without rapid fluctuations of fluid volumes and electrolyte concentrations, facilitating blood pressure control and prevention of heart failure.

An interesting concept has been proposed by van Biesen and colleagues.[481] Patients who started treatment with PD and were transferred to hemodialysis after residual renal function had decayed had better long-term survival than patients who started treatment with hemodialysis and remained on hemodialysis throughout. As a potential explanation it has been proposed that an early start on CAPD prevents the organ damage that accumulates in the terminal stage of uremia. Survival of patients who remained on CAPD for more than 48 months was inferior to that of patients on hemodialysis, presumably because CAPD is no longer sufficiently effective when residual renal function is gone, at least in heavier patients. It is also relevant that CAPD treatment presents no surgical contraindications to renal transplantation.

Although protein is lost across the peritoneal membrane, the main nutritional problem in PD is gain of glucose and calories, because high glucose concentrations in the dialysate are necessary for osmotic removal of excess body fluid. This leads to weight gain and obesity. Daily glucose absorption is 100 to 150 g, and the CAPD patient is exposed to 3 to 7 tons of fluid containing 50 to 175 kg of glucose per year.

The use of glucose-containing fluids causes another problem. Heat sterilization of glucose under acid conditions creates highly reactive glucose degradation products such as methylglyoxal, glyoxal, formaldehyde, 3-deoxyglucosone, and 3,4-dideoxyglucosone-3-ene.[482] Glucose degradation products are cytotoxic and cause formation of advanced glycation end products (AGEs). Even in nondiabetic patients on CAPD, deposits of AGEs are found in the peritoneal membrane. AGEs trigger fibrogenesis and neoangiogenesis, presumably by interaction with RAGE, one of the receptors for AGEs.[483] The products also enter the systemic circulation, most likely contributing to systemic microinflammation.[484] These findings have led many to apply the term *local diabetes mellitus.*[485] Heat sterilization of two-compartment bags circumvents the generation of toxic glucose degradation products. In prospective studies, CAPD fluid produced using this technique of sterilization was much less toxic than conventional CAPD fluid despite the high glucose concentration.[486]

Transplantation

Kidney Transplantation

There is consensus that medical rehabilitation of the diabetic patient with uremia is best after transplantation.[411] Survival of a diabetic patient with a kidney graft is worse than that of a nondiabetic patient with a kidney graft. Nevertheless, because survival of a diabetic patient is so much poorer on dialysis, the percent gain in life expectancy of a diabetic patient with a graft compared with a diabetic patient receiving dialysis who is on the waiting list, is much greater than that of a nondiabetic patient.

Wolfe and colleagues calculated an adjusted relative risk of death in transplant recipients compared with patients on the waiting list. The adjusted relative risk was 0.27 in patients with diabetes and 0.39 in patients with glomerulonephritis.[411]

Unfortunately the perioperative risk is higher in diabetic than in nondiabetic patients. Nevertheless, in diabetic patients the predicted survival after transplantation is substantially higher than the survival on dialysis (i.e., on the waiting list).

Currently patients with type 1 diabetes constitute the majority of diabetic patients receiving a transplant. Graft and patient survival were found to be acceptable in carefully selected type 2 diabetic patients without macrovascular complications who received kidney grafts,[487] but transplantation of kidneys into type 2 diabetic patients violates current transplant criteria of the Eurotransplant International Foundation.

Diabetic patients must be subjected to rigorous pretransplantation evaluation, which in most centers includes routine coronary angiography. Patients should also undergo Doppler ultrasonography of pelvic arteries and, if necessary, angiography to avoid attachment of a renal allograft to an iliac artery with compromised arterial flow and the attendant risk of ischemia of an extremity and amputation. Preemptive transplantation (i.e., transplantation before initiation of dialysis) provides some modest long-term benefit.[488]

Combined Kidney-Pancreas Transplantation

After the seminal double transplantation by Lillehei[493] in Minneapolis, the results of simultaneous pancreas and kidney transplantation (SPK) remained disappointing for a long time. The breakthrough[412] came with the introduction of calcineurin inhibitors and low-steroid protocols. The current regimens usually include initial induction therapy (antithymocyte globulin, alemtuzumab or interleukin-2 receptor antagonists) and mycophenolate mofetil, tacrolimus, and steroids. This regimen reduced acute rejections after combined kidney-pancreas transplantation from 30% to 18%.[489] The bladder drainage of the exocrine pancreas secretion has been abandoned and enteric drainage has been substituted. Efforts to anastomose the pancreatic graft vein to the portal vein have been abandoned.

There are three transplantation strategies:
1. Kidney only
2. Simultaneous pancreas plus kidney
3. Pancreas after kidney

Reversal of established microvascular complications after SPK, at least in the short term, is minor with the important exception of improvement in autonomic polyneuropathy[490] and some improvement in nerve conduction.[491] SPK is associated with superior quality of life, better metabolic control, and improved survival.[412] It has recently been shown that excessive cardiovascular risk is also reduced by pancreas transplantation, but approximately 10 years are required for the difference to show up.[492] This is analogous to the time span necessary for reversal of glomerular lesions in the kidney[69]—presumably another example of "metabolic" or "epigenetic" memory.

Survival of patients undergoing SPK was equal to and later surpassed that of patients undergoing isolated cadaver-donor and even live-donor kidney transplantation. Beyond the tenth year the hazard ratio was 0.55 for pancreas plus kidney transplantation compared with live-donor kidney transplantation alone.

There is an increasing tendency for early or even preemptive SPK.[493] Because graft outcome is progressively more adverse with increasing time spent on hemodialysis,[494] this strategy may make sense. In the United States, diabetic patients younger than 55 years of age are usually considered for SPK when GFR has become less than 40 mL/min, whereas in Europe the criteria are more conservative, requiring a GFR of less than 20 mL/min.[495] An alternative strategy must be considered in the diabetic patient who has a live kidney donor: in a first step the living-donor kidney can be transplanted and subsequently, once stable renal function is achieved (GFR ≥50 mL/min), a cadaver-donor pancreas can be transplanted. The outcomes are quite satisfactory.[496]

Oral glucose tolerance normalizes after SPK unless the pancreatic graft is damaged by ischemia or by subclinical rejection related to HLA-DR mismatch.[497] Most investigators find either normalization of insulin sensitivity[498] or some impairment of insulin-stimulated nonoxidative glucose metabolism,[499,500] possibly related to insulin delivery into the systemic circulation (as opposed to physiologic delivery into the portal circulation). Impressive normalization of lipoprotein lipase activity and of the lipid spectrum have also been reported consistent with reduced atherogenic risk.[501]

An interesting issue is whether graft rejection affects kidney and pancreatic grafts in parallel. Although this is most frequently the case (which permits use of renal function as a surrogate marker of rejection in the pancreas), it is by no means obligatory. Pancreatic biopsies are increasingly used. Pancreatic graft biopsy findings are also able to distinguish graft pancreatitis from immune injury to the graft. Pancreatic grafts are usually lost because of alloimmunity reactions, but in rare cases graft loss resulting from destruction by autoimmune mechanisms has been described.[502]

Recurrence of autoimmune inflammation (insulitis) in the recipient with lymphocytic infiltration and selective loss of insulin-producing β-cells (while glucagon, somatostatin, and pancreatic polypeptide–secreting cells were spared) was often seen in the pioneering era when segmental pancreatic grafts were exchanged between monozygotic twins. Today this has become rare, presumably because immunosuppression keeps autoimmunity under control. Rejection of the pancreas responds poorly to steroid therapy. Its treatment should always include administration of T cell antibodies.

Islet Cell Transplantation

Sophisticated procedures such as transplantation of stem cells or precursor cells, transplantation of encapsulated islet cells, islet xenotransplantation, and insulin gene therapy are still beyond the horizon. Only islet cell transplantation has been tested so far. The initial enthusiasm raised by the Edmonton protocol[503] waned after the long-term results were not confirmed by a multicenter study, which possibly reflected single-site expertise or the effect of the heavy immunosuppression regimens.[504] Therefore this approach currently has been largely abandoned.

Diabetes in Nondiabetic Solid Organ Graft Recipients

An increasingly serious problem of solid organ transplantation, including renal transplantation, is the de novo appearance of diabetes in graft recipients who had no diabetes at the time of transplantation. This was seen in 17.4% of recipients in Spain[505] and in up to 21% of recipients in the United States at 10 years.[506] De novo diabetes is presumably the result of several factors. One possible cause is the diabetogenic action of steroids and calcineurin inhibitors, particularly tacrolimus. The unmasking of diabetes after rapid weight gain in previously anorectic individuals, as discussed earlier, also contributes.

Predictors of de novo diabetes are a family history of diabetes, older age, African American ethnicity, obesity, hepatitis C, and treatment with tacrolimus.[505,507] The DIRECT study found a significantly lower incidence of new-onset diabetes and impaired fasting glucose level in patients treated with cyclosporine (26.0%) than in those receiving tacrolimus (33.6%).[508] Reduction of the steroid dosage improves glycemic control, but complete withdrawal provides no metabolic benefit compared with 5 mg/day prednisolone and increases the risk of graft rejection.[509,510] Complications include increased cardiovascular events[511] and even delayed graft loss from allograft diabetic nephropathy.[512]

Bladder Dysfunction

Bladder dysfunction as a sequela of autonomic diabetic polyneuropathy is frequent in diabetic patients. In males this is often combined with erectile dysfunction.[513] Disabling symptoms are rare, however. Bladder dysfunction is frequently associated with other features of autonomic polyneuropathy, such as postural hypotension, gastroparesis, constipation, and nocturnal diarrhea.

Urinary Tract Infection

For a long time it has been controversial whether the frequency of bacteriuria is higher in diabetic patients, but there has never been any doubt that symptomatic urinary tract infections (UTIs) are more severe and more aggressive. A higher prevalence of UTI, usually asymptomatic, was initially found by Vejlsgaard[514] in female diabetic patients (18.8% vs. 7.9% in controls), but not in males with diabetes. The results of prospective studies remained controversial. A more recent prospective study in diabetic and nondiabetic women showed that the incidence of UTIs as well as asymptomatic bacteriuria was twice as high in diabetic than in nondiabetic women.[515] UTIs may also pose problems after renal transplantation.[516] The spectrum of bacterial isolates as well as the resistance rates to antibiotics did not differ between diabetic and nondiabetic individuals.[517]

Symptomatic UTIs definitely run a more aggressive course in diabetic patients. By multivariate analysis diabetes and poor glycemic control are independent factors associated with upper urinary tract involvement.[518] UTIs in diabetic patients may also lead to complications, such as prostatic abscess, emphysematous cystitis and pyelonephritis,[519] intrarenal abscess formation, renal carbuncle,[119] and penile necrosis (Fournier's disease).[520] Renal papillary necrosis was common in the past but has virtually disappeared according to one autopsy series.[521] Extrarenal bacterial metastases (e.g., endophthalmitis,[522] spondylitis, endocarditis, iliopsoas abscess formation) are common in patients with UTI and septicemia, particularly UTI caused by methicillin-resistant staphylococci.

The reasons for the possibly higher frequency and the definitely higher severity of UTIs in diabetic patients are not known, but may include more favorable conditions for bacterial growth (glucosuria), defective neutrophil function, increased adherence to uroepithelial cells, and impaired bladder evacuation (detrusor paresis).

As to the management of UTI, no clear benefits of antibiotic therapy have been demonstrated for treatment of asymptomatic bacteriuria in diabetic patients. Community-acquired symptomatic lower UTI may be managed with trimethoprim, trimethoprim-sulfamethoxazole, or gyrase inhibitors. For nosocomially acquired UTI, sensitivity testing and sensitivity-directed antibiotic intervention are necessary. Invasive candiduria can be managed with amphotericin by irrigation or systemic administration of fungicidal agents.

References

1. Parving H-H, Gall M-A, Skøtt P, et al. Prevalence and causes of albuminuria in non–insulin-dependent diabetic patients. *Kidney Int*. 1992;41:758-762.
2. Rossing P. The changing epidemiology of diabetic microangiopathy in type 1 diabetes. *Diabetologia*. 2005;48(8):1439-1444.
3. Rossing P. Prediction, progression and prevention of diabetic nephropathy. The Minkowski Lecture 2005. *Diabetologia*. 2006;49(1):11-19.
4. Hovind P, Tarnow L, Rossing P, et al. Predictors for the development of microalbuminuria and macroalbuminuria in patients with type 1 diabetes: inception cohort study. *BMJ*. 2004;328(7448):1105.
5. Borch-Johnsen K. The prognosis of insulin-dependent diabetes mellitus. An epidemiological approach. *Dan Med Bull*. 1989;39:336-349.
6. Ballard DJ, Humphrey LL, Melton III LJ, et al. Epidemiology of persistent proteinuria in type II diabetes mellitus. Population-based study in Rochester, Minnesota. *Diabetes*. 1988;37:405-412.
7. Gall M-A, Borch-Johnsen K, Hougaard P, et al. Albuminuria and poor glycemic control predicts mortality in NIDDM. *Diabetes*. 1995;44:1303-1309.
8. Fioretto P, Mauer M. Histopathology of diabetic nephropathy. *Semin Nephrol*. 2007;27(2):195-207.
9. Fioretto P, Caramori ML, Mauer M. The kidney in diabetes: dynamic pathways of injury and repair. The Camillo Golgi Lecture 2007. *Diabetologia*. 2008;51(8):1347-1355.
10. Lane PH, Steffes MW, Fioretto P, et al. Renal interstitial expansion in insulin-dependent diabetes mellitus. *Kidney Int*. 1993;43(3):661-667.
11. Østerby R. Early phases in the development of diabetic glomerulopathy. A quantitative electron microscopic study. *Acta Med Scand*. 1975;574(suppl):1-80.
12. Steffes MW, Sutherland DER, Goetz FC, et al. Studies of kidney and muscle biopsy specimens from identical twins discordant for type I diabetes mellitus. *N Engl J Med*. 1985;312:1282-1287.
13. Brito PL, Fioretto P, Drummond K, et al. Proximal tubular basement membrane width in insulin-dependent diabetes mellitus. *Kidney Int*. 1998;53:754-761.
14. Mauer SM, Barbosa J, Vernier RL, et al. Development of diabetic vascular lesions in normal kidneys transplanted into patients with diabetes mellitus. *N Engl J Med*. 1976;295:916-920.
15. Mauer SM, Miller K, Goetz FC, et al. Immunopathology of renal extracellular membranes in kidneys transplanted into patients with diabetes mellitus. *Diabetes*. 1976;25(8):709-712.
16. Østerby R, Hartmann A, Bangstad HJ. Structural changes in renal arterioles in type I diabetic patients. *Diabetologia*. 2002;45(4):542-549.
17. Drummond KN, Kramer MS, Suissa S, et al. Effects of duration and age at onset of type 1 diabetes on preclinical manifestations of nephropathy. *Diabetes*. 2003;52(7):1818-1824.
18. Steffes MW, Bilous RW, Sutherland DER, et al. Cell and matrix components of the glomerular mesangium in type 1 diabetes. *Diabetes*. 1992;41:679-684.
19. Drummond K, Mauer M. The early natural history of nephropathy in type 1 diabetes: II. Early renal structural changes in type 1 diabetes. *Diabetes*. 2002;51(5):1580-1587.
20. Katz A, Caramori ML, Sisson-Ross S, et al. An increase in the cell component of the cortical interstitium antedates interstitial fibrosis in type 1 diabetic patients. *Kidney Int*. 2002;61(6):2058-2066.
21. Najafian B, Crosson JT, Kim Y, et al. Glomerulotubular junction abnormalities are associated with proteinuria in type 1 diabetes. *J Am Soc Nephrol*. 2006;17(4 suppl 2):S53-S60.
22. Mauer SM, Steffes MW, Ellis EN, et al. Structural-functional relationships in diabetic nephropathy. *J Clin Invest*. 1984;74:1143-1155.
23. Caramori ML, Kim Y, Huang C, et al. Cellular basis of diabetic nephropathy: 1. Study design and renal structural-functional relationships in patients with long-standing type 1 diabetes. *Diabetes*. 2002;51(2):506-513.
24. Saito Y, Kida H, Takeda S, et al. Mesangiolysis in diabetic glomeruli: its role in the formation of nodular lesions. *Kidney Int*. 1988;34:389-396.
25. Zhu D, Kim Y, Steffes MW, et al. Glomerular distribution of type IV collagen in diabetes by high resolution quantitative immunochemistry. *Kidney Int*. 1994;45:425-433.
26. Moriya T, Groppoli TJ, Kim Y, et al. Quantitative immunoelectron microscopy of type VI collagen in glomeruli in type I diabetic patients. *Kidney Int*. 2001;59(1):317-323.
27. Harris RD, Steffes MW, Bilous RW, et al. Global glomerular sclerosis and glomerular arteriolar hyalinosis in insulin dependent diabetes. *Kidney Int*. 1991;40:107-114.
28. Hørlyck A, Gundersen HJG, Østerby R. The cortical distribution pattern of diabetic glomerulopathy. *Diabetologia*. 1986;29:146-150.
29. White KE, Bilous RW, Marshall SM, et al. Podocyte number in normotensive type 1 diabetic patients with albuminuria. *Diabetes*. 2002;51(10):3083-3089.
30. Pagtalunan ME, Miller PL, Jumping-Eagle S. Podocyte loss and progressive glomerular injury in type II diabetes. *J Clin Invest*. 1996;99:342-348.
31. White KE, Bilous RW. Structural alterations to the podocyte are related to proteinuria in type 2 diabetic patients. *Nephrol Dial Transplant*. 2004;19(6):1437-1440.
32. Dalla VM, Masiero A, Roiter AM, et al. Is podocyte injury relevant in diabetic nephropathy? Studies in patients with type 2 diabetes. *Diabetes*. 2003;52(4):1031-1035.
33. Toyoda M, Najafian B, Kim Y, et al. Podocyte detachment and reduced glomerular capillary endothelial fenestration in human type 1 diabetic nephropathy. *Diabetes*. 2007;56(8):2155-2160.
34. Langham RG, Kelly DJ, Cox AJ, et al. Proteinuria and the expression of the podocyte slit diaphragm protein, nephrin, in diabetic nephropathy: effects of angiotensin converting enzyme inhibition. *Diabetologia*. 2002;45(11):1572-1576.
35. Toyoda M, Suzuki D, Umezono T, et al. Expression of human nephrin mRNA in diabetic nephropathy. *Nephrol Dial Transplant*. 2004;19(2):380-385.
36. Benigni A, Gagliardini E, Tomasoni S, et al. Selective impairment of gene expression and assembly of nephrin in human diabetic nephropathy. *Kidney Int*. 2004;65(6):2193-2200.
37. Ellis EN, Steffes MW, Goetz FC, et al. Glomerular filtration surface in type 1 diabetes mellitus. *Kidney Int*. 1986;29:889-894.
38. Ellis EN, Steffes MW, Chavers BM, et al. Observations of glomerular epithelial cell structure in patients with type 1 diabetes mellitus. *Kidney Int*. 1987;32:736-741.
39. Bjørn SF, Bangstad H-J, Hanssen KF. Glomerular epithelial foot processes and filtration slits in IDDM diabetic patients. *Diabetologia*. 1995;38:1197-1204.
40. Vernier RL, Steffes MW, Sisson-Ross S, et al. Heparan sulfate proteoglycan in the glomerular basement membrane in type 1 diabetes mellitus. *Kidney Int*. 1992;41:1070-1080.
41. Meyer TW, Bennett PH, Nelson RG. Podocyte number predicts long-term urinary albumin excretion in Pima Indians with type II diabetes and microalbuminuria. *Diabetologia*. 1999;42(11):1341-1344.
42. Hirose K, Tsuchida H, Østerby R, et al. A strong correlation between glomerular filtration rate and filtration surface in diabetic kidney hyperfunction. *Lab Invest*. 1980;43:434-437.
43. Thomsen OF, Andersen AR, Christiansen JS, et al. Renal changes in long-term type 1 (insulin-dependent) diabetic patients with and without clinical nephropathy: a light microscopic, morphometric study of autopsy material. *Diabetologia*. 1984;26(5):361-365.
44. Bohle A, Wehrmann M, Bogenschutz O, et al. The pathogenesis of chronic renal failure in diabetic nephropathy. Investigation of 488 cases of diabetic glomerulosclerosis. *Pathol Res Pract*. 1991;187(2-3):251-259.
45. Taft JL, Nolan CJ, Yeung SP, et al. Clinical and histological correlations of decline in renal function in diabetic patients with proteinuria. *Diabetes*. 1994;43:1046-1051.
46. Fioretto P, Steffes MW, Mauer SM. Glomerular structure in nonproteinuric IDDM patients with various levels of albuminuria. *Diabetes*. 1994;43:1358-1364.
47. Steinke JM, Sinaiko AR, Kramer MS, et al. The early natural history of nephropathy in type 1 diabetes: III. Predictors of 5-year urinary albumin excretion rate patterns in initially normoalbuminuric patients. *Diabetes*. 2005;54(7):2164-2171.
48. Bangstad HJ, Østerby R, Hartmann A, et al. Severity of glomerulopathy predicts long-term urinary albumin excretion rate in patients with type 1 diabetes and microalbuminuria. *Diabetes Care*. 1999;22(2):314-319.

49. Caramori ML, Fioretto P, Mauer M. Low glomerular filtration rate in normoalbuminuric type 1 diabetic patients: an indicator of more advanced glomerular lesions. *Diabetes.* 2003;52(4):1036-1040.

50. Caramori ML, Fioretto P, Mauer M. Enhancing the predictive value of urinary albumin for diabetic nephropathy. *J Am Soc Nephrol.* 2006;17(2):339-352.

51. Mauer SM, Goetz FC, McHugh LE, et al. Long-term study of normal kidneys transplanted into patients with type I diabetes. *Diabetes.* 1989;38:516-523.

52. Bilous RW, Mauer SM, Sutherland DER, et al. Mean glomerular volume and rate of development of diabetic nephropathy. *Diabetes.* 1989;38:1142-1147.

53. Bendtsen TF, Nyengaard JR. The number of glomeruli in type 1 (insulin-dependent. and type 2 (non–insulin-dependent) diabetic patients. *Diabetologia.* 1992;35:844-850.

54. Brenner BM, Garcia DL, Anderson S. Glomeruli and blood pressure. Less of one, more the other? *Am J Hypertens.* 1988;1:335-347.

55. Chang S, Caramori ML, Moriya R, et al. Having one kidney does not accelerate the rate of development of diabetic nephropathy lesions in type 1 diabetic patients. *Diabetes.* 2008;57(6):1707-1711.

56. Østerby R, Gall M-A, Schmitz A, et al. Glomerular structure and function in proteinuric type 2 (non–insulin-dependent) diabetic patients. *Diabetologia.* 1993;36:1064-1070.

57. Gambara V, Mecca G, Remuzzi G, et al. Heterogeneous nature of renal lesions in type II diabetes. *J Am Soc Nephrol.* 1993;3:1458-1466.

58. Christensen PK, Larsen S, Horn T, et al. Renal function and structure in albuminuric type 2 diabetic patients without retinopathy. *Nephrol Dial Transplant.* 2001;16(12):2337-2347.

59. Mazzucco G, Bertani T, Fortunato M, et al. Different patterns of renal damage in type 2 diabetes mellitus: a multicentric study on 393 biopsies. *Am J Kidney Dis.* 2002;39(4):713-720.

60. Fioretto P, Mauer SM, Brocco E, et al. Patterns of renal injury in NIDDM patients with microalbuminuria. *Diabetologia.* 1996;39:1569-1576.

61. Hayashi H, Karasawa R, Inn H, et al. An electron microscopic study of glomeruli in Japanese patients with non–insulin dependent diabetes mellitus. *Kidney Int.* 1992;41:749-757.

62. Moriya T, Moriya R, Yajima Y, et al. Urinary albumin as an indicator of diabetic nephropathy lesions in Japanese type 2 diabetic patients. *Nephron.* 2002;91(2):292-299.

63. Nosadini R, Velussi M, Brocco E, et al. Course of renal function in type 2 diabetic patients with abnormalities of albumin excretion rate. *Diabetes.* 2000;49(3):476-484.

64. Marcantoni C, Ma LJ, Federspiel C, et al. Hypertensive nephrosclerosis in African Americans versus Caucasians. *Kidney Int.* 2002;62(1):172-180.

65. Urizar RE, Schwartz A, Top Jr F, et al. The nephrotic syndrome in children with diabetes mellitus of recent onset. *N Engl J Med.* 1969;281(4):173-181.

66. Cavallo T, Pinto JA, Rajaraman S. Immune complex disease complicating diabetic glomerulosclerosis. *Am J Nephrol.* 1984;4(6):347-354.

67. Mauer SM, Steffes MW, Sutherland DER, et al. Studies of the rate of regression of the glomerular lesions in diabetic rats treated with pancreatic islet transplantation. *Diabetes.* 1974;24:280-285.

68. Fioretto P, Mauer SM, Bilous RW, et al. Effects of pancreas transplantation of glomerular structure in insulin-dependent diabetic patients with their own kidneys. *Lancet.* 1993;342:1193-1196.

69. Fioretto P, Steffes MW, Sutherland DER, et al. Reversal of lesions of diabetic nephropathy after pancreas transplantation. *N Engl J Med.* 1998;339:69-75.

70. Steffes MW, Barbosa J, Basgen JM, et al. Quantitative glomerular morphology of the normal human kidney. *Lab Invest.* 1983;49(1):82-86.

71. Fioretto P, Sutherland DE, Najafian B, et al. Remodeling of renal interstitial and tubular lesions in pancreas transplant recipients. *Kidney Int.* 2006;69(5):907-912.

72. Mauer M, Zinman B, Gardiner R, et al. Renal and retinal effects of enalapril and losartan in type 1 diabetes. *N Engl J Med.* 2009;361(1):40-51.

73. Parving H-H, Lewis JB, Ravid M, et al. Prevalence and risk factors for microalbuminuria in a referred cohort of type II diabetic patients: A global perspective. *Kidney Int.* 2006;69(11):2057-2063.

74. Hovind P, Tarnow L, Rossing K, et al. Decreasing incidence of severe diabetic microangiopathy in type 1 diabetes. *Diabetes Care.* 2003;26(4):1258-1264.

75. Bojestig M, Arnqvist HJ, Hermansson G, et al. Declining incidence of nephropathy in insulin-dependent diabetes mellitus. *N Engl J Med.* 1994;330:15-18.

76. Gall M-A, Rossing P, Skøtt P, et al. Prevalence of micro- and macroalbuminuria, arterial hypertension, retinopathy and large vessel disease in European type 2 (non–insulin-dependent) diabetic patients. *Diabetologia.* 1991;34:655-661.

77. Rossing P, Hougaard P, Parving H-H. Progression of microalbuminuria in type 1 diabetes: ten-year prospective observational study. *Kidney Int.* 2005;68(4):1446-1450.

78. Parving H-H. Renoprotection in diabetes: genetic and non-genetic risk factors and treatment. *Diabetologia.* 1998;41:745-759.

79. Parving H-H. Diabetic nephropathy: prevention and treatment. *Kidney Int.* 2001;60(5):2041-2055.

80. Perkins BA, Ficociello LH, Silva KH, et al. Regression of microalbuminuria in type 1 diabetes. *N Engl J Med.* 2003;348(23):2285-2293.

81. Parving H-H, Chaturvedi N, Viberti G, et al. Does microalbuminuria predict diabetic nephropathy? *Diabetes Care.* 2002;25(2):406-407.

82. Dinneen SF, Gerstein HC. The association of microalbuminuria and mortality in non–insulin-dependent diabetes mellitus. *Arch Intern Med.* 1997;157:1413-1418.

83. Perkovic V, Verdon C, Ninomiya T, et al. The relationship between proteinuria and coronary risk: a systematic review and meta-analysis. *PLoS Med.* 2008;5(10):e207.

84. Damsgaard EM, Frøland A, Jørgensen OD, et al. Microalbuminuria as predictor of increased mortality in elderly people. *BMJ.* 1990;300:297-300.

85. Deckert T, Yokoyama H, Mathiesen ER, et al. Cohort study of predictive value of urinary albumin excretion for atherosclerotic vascular disease in patients with insulin dependent diabetes. *BMJ.* 1996;312:871-874.

86. Ninomiya T, Perkovic V, Verdon C, et al. Proteinuria and stroke: a meta-analysis of cohort studies. *Am J Kidney Dis.* 2009;53(3):417-425.

87. Deckert T, Feldt-Rasmussen B, Borch-Johnsen K, et al. Albuminuria reflects widespread vascular damage. The Steno hypothesis. *Diabetologia.* 1989;32:219-226.

88. Winocour PH. Microalbuminuria. *Bmj.* 1992;304:1196-1197.

89. Gaede P, Vedel P, Larsen N, et al. Multifactorial intervention and cardiovascular disease in patients with type 2 diabetes. *N Engl J Med.* 2003;348(5):383-393.

90. Astrup AS, Tarnow L, Rossing P, et al. Cardiac autonomic neuropathy predicts cardiovascular morbidity and mortality in type 1 diabetic patients with diabetic nephropathy. *Diabetes Care.* 2006;29(2):334-339.

91. Giunti S, Bruno G, Veglio M, et al. Electrocardiographic left ventricular hypertrophy in type 1 diabetes: prevalence and relation to coronary heart disease and cardiovascular risk factors: the Eurodiab IDDM Complications Study. *Diabetes Care.* 2005;28(9):2255-2257.

92. Sato A, Tarnow L, Nielsen FS, et al. Left ventricular hypertrophy in normoalbuminuric type 2 diabetic patients not taking antihypertensive treatment. *QJM.* 2005;98(12):879-884.

93. Sampson MJ, Chambers JB, Sprigings DC, et al. Abnormal diastolic function in patients with type 1 diabetes and early nephropathy. *Br Heart J.* 1990;64:266-271.

94. Nielsen FS, Ali S, Rossing P, et al. Left ventricular hypertrophy in non–insulin dependent diabetic patients with and without diabetic nephropathy. *Diabet Med.* 1997;14:538-546.

95. Frolich E, Apstein C, Chobanian AV, et al. The heart in hypertension. *N Engl J Med.* 1992;327(14):998-1008.

96. Gaede P, Hildebrandt P, Hess G, et al. Plasma N-terminal pro-brain natriuretic peptide as a major risk marker for cardiovascular disease in patients with type 2 diabetes and microalbuminuria. *Diabetologia.* 2005;48(1):156-163.

97. Nelson RG, Pettitt DJ, Carraher MJ, et al. Effect of proteinuria on mortality in NIDDM. *Diabetes.* 1988;37:1499-1504.

98. Morrish NJ, Stevens LK, Head J, et al. A prospective study of mortality among middle-aged diabetic patients (the London cohort of the WHO Multinational Study of Vascular Disease in Diabetics). II: Associated risk factors. *Diabetologia.* 1990;33:542-548.

99. Schmitz A. The kidney in non–insulin-dependent diabetes. *Acta Diabetol.* 1992;29:47-69.

100. Sorensen VR, Hansen PM, Heaf J, et al. Stabilized incidence of diabetic patients referred for renal replacement therapy in Denmark. *Kidney Int.* 2006;70(1):187-191.

101. National Institute of Diabetes and Digestive and Kidney Diseases. *United States Renal Data System: USRDS 2008 annual data report.* Bethesda, MD: National Institutes of Health; 2009.

102. Sorensen VR, Mathiesen ER, Heaf J, et al. Improved survival rate in patients with diabetes and end-stage renal disease in Denmark. *Diabetologia.* 2007;50(5):922-929.

103. Borch-Johnsen K, Kreiner S. Proteinuria: value as predictor of cardiovascular mortality in insulin dependent diabetes mellitus. *BMJ.* 1987;294:1651-1654.

104. Parving H-H, Mogensen CE, Thomas MC, et al. Poor prognosis in proteinuric type 2 diabetic patients with retinopathy: insights from the RENAAL study. *QJM.* 2005;98(2):119-126.

105. Kapelrud H, Bangstad H-J, Dahl-Jørgensen K, et al. Serum Lp(a) lipoprotein concentrations in insulin dependent diabetic patients with microalbuminuria. *BMJ.* 1991;303:675-678.

106. Gall M-A, Rossing P, Hommel E, et al. Apolipoprotein(a) in insulin-dependent diabetic patients with and without diabetic nephropathy. *Scand J Clin Lab Invest.* 1992;52:513-521.

107. Nielsen FS, Voldsgaard AI, Gall M-A, et al. Apolipoprotein(a) and cardiovascular disease in type 2 (non–insulin-dependent) diabetic patients with and without diabetic nephropathy. *Diabetologia*. 1993;36:438-444.

108. Tarnow L, Rossing P, Nielsen FS, et al. Increased plasma apolipoprotein(a) levels in IDDM patients with diabetic nephropathy. *Diabetes Care*. 1996;19(12):1382-1387.

109. de Cosmo S, Bacci S, Piras GP, et al. High prevalence of risk factors for cardiovascular disease in parents of IDDM patients with albuminuria. *Diabetologia*. 1997;40:1191-1196.

110. Tarnow L, Rossing P, Nielsen FS, et al. Cardiovascular morbidity and early mortality cluster in parents of type 1 diabetic patients with diabetic nephropathy. *Diabetes Care*. 2000;23:30-33.

111. Earle K, Walker J, Hill C, et al. Familial clustering of cardiovascular disease in patients with insulin-dependent diabetes and nephropathy. *N Engl J Med*. 1992;326:673-677.

112. Sato A, Tarnow L, Parving H-H. Prevalence of left ventricular hypertrophy in type 1 diabetic patients with diabetic nephropathy. *Diabetologia*. 1999;42:76-80.

113. Boner G, Cooper ME, McCarroll K, et al. Adverse effects of left ventricular hypertrophy in the reduction of endpoints in NIDDM with the angiotensin II antagonist losartan (RENAAL) study. *Diabetologia*. 2005;48(10):1980-1987.

114. Stehouwer CD, Gall MA, Hougaard P, et al. Plasma homocysteine concentration predicts mortality in non–insulin-dependent diabetic patients with and without albuminuria. *Kidney Int*. 1999;55(1):308-314.

115. Stehouwer CD, Gall MA, Twisk JW, et al. Increased urinary albumin excretion, endothelial dysfunction, and chronic low-grade inflammation in type 2 diabetes: progressive, interrelated, and independently associated with risk of death. *Diabetes*. 2002;51:1157-1165.

116. Gaede P, Lund-Andersen H, Parving H-H, et al. Effect of a multifactorial intervention on mortality in type 2 diabetes. *N Engl J Med*. 2008;358(6):580-591.

117. Tarnow L, Hildebrandt P, Hansen BV, et al. Plasma N-terminal pro-brain natriuretic peptide as an independent predictor of mortality in diabetic nephropathy. *Diabetologia*. 2005;48(1):149-155.

118. Tarnow L, Gall M-A, Hansen BV, et al. Plasma N-terminal pro-B-type natriuretic peptide and mortality in type 2 diabetes. *Diabetologia*. 2006;49:2256-2262.

119. Tarnow L, Hovind P, Teerlink T, et al. Elevated plasma asymmetric dimethylarginine as a marker of cardiovascular morbidity in early diabetic nephropathy in type 1 diabetes. *Diabetes Care*. 2004;27(3):765-769.

120. Hansen TK, Tarnow L, Thiel S, et al. Association between mannose-binding lectin and vascular complications in type 1 diabetes. *Diabetes*. 2004;53(6):1570-1576.

121. Jorsal A, Tarnow L, Flyvbjerg A, et al. Plasma osteoprotegerin levels predict cardiovascular and all-cause mortality and deterioration of kidney function in type 1 diabetic patients with nephropathy. *Diabetologia*. 2008;51(11):2100-2107.

122. Nguyen TQ, Tarnow L, Jorsal A, et al. Plasma connective tissue growth factor is an independent predictor of end-stage renal disease and mortality in type 1 diabetic nephropathy. *Diabetes Care*. 2008;31(6):1177-1182.

123. Jorsal A, Tarnow L, Frystyk J, et al. Serum adiponectin predicts all-cause mortality and end stage renal disease in patients with type I diabetes and diabetic nephropathy. *Kidney Int*. 2008;74(5):649-654.

124. Sarnak MJ, Levey AS, Schoolwerth AC, et al. Kidney disease as a risk factor for development of cardiovascular disease: a statement from the American Heart Association Councils on Kidney in Cardiovascular Disease, High Blood Pressure Research, Clinical Cardiology, and Epidemiology and Prevention. *Circulation*. 2003;108(17):2154-2169.

125. Go AS, Chertow GM, Fan D, et al. Chronic kidney disease and the risks of death, cardiovascular events, and hospitalization. *N Engl J Med*. 2004;351(13):1296-1305.

126. Mogensen CE. Glomerular hyperfiltration in human diabetes. *Diabetes Care*. 1994;17:770-775.

127. Myers BD, Nelson RG, Williams GW, et al. Glomerular function in Pima Indians with noninsulin-dependent diabetes mellitus of recent onset. *J Clin Invest*. 1991;88:524-530.

128. Vora JP, Dolben J, Dean JD, et al. Renal hemodynamics in newly presenting non–insulin dependent diabetes mellitus. *Kidney Int*. 1992;41:829-835.

129. Schmitz A, Christensen T, Jensen FT. Glomerular filtration rate and kidney volume in normoalbuminuric non–insulin-dependent diabetics—lack of glomerular hyperfiltration and renal hypertrophy in uncomplicated NIDDM. *Scand J Clin Lab Invest*. 1989;49:103-108.

130. Hostetter TH, Troy JL, Brenner BM. Glomerular hemodynamics in experimental diabetes mellitus. *Kidney Int*. 1981;19:410-415.

131. Flyvbjerg A. The role of insulin-like growth factor I in initial renal hypertrophy in experimental diabetes. In: Flyvbjerg A, Ørskov H, Alberti KGMM, eds. *Growth hormone and insulin-like growth factor I in human and experimental diabetes*. New York: John Wiley & Sons; 1993:pp 271-306.

132. Rudberg S, Persson B, Dahlquist G. Increased glomerular filtration rate as a predictor of diabetic nephropathy—an 8-year prospective study. *Kidney Int*. 1992;41:822-828.

133. Rossing P, Hougaard P, Parving H-H. Risk factors for development of incipient and overt diabetic nephropathy in type 1 diabetic patients. *Diabetes Care*. 2002;25:859-864.

134. Jones SL, Wiseman MJ, Viberti GC. Glomerular hyperfiltration as a risk factor for diabetic nephropathy: five year report of a prospective study. *Diabetologia*. 1991;34:59-60.

135. Magee GM, Bilous RW, Cardwell CR, et al. Is hyperfiltration associated with the future risk of developing diabetic nephropathy? A meta-analysis. *Diabetologia*. 2009;52(4):691-697.

136. Vedel P, Obel J, Nielsen FS, et al. Glomerular hyperfiltration in microalbuminuric NIDDM patients. *Diabetologia*. 1996;39:1584-1589.

137. Microalbuminuria Collaborative Study Group UK. Risk factors for development of microalbuminuria in insulin dependent diabetic patients: a cohort study. *BMJ*. 1993;306:1235-1239.

138. Gall M-A, Hougaard P, Borch-Johnsen K, et al. Risk factors for development of incipient and overt diabetic nephropathy in patients with non–insulin dependent diabetes mellitus: prospective, observational study. *BMJ*. 1997;314:783-788.

139. Microalbuminuria Collaborative Study Group UK. Predictors of the development of microalbuminuria in patients with type 1 diabetes mellitus: a seven year prospective study. *Diabet Med*. 1999;16:918-925.

140. Royal College of Physicians of Edinburgh Diabetes Register Group. Near normal urinary albumin concentrations predict progression to diabetic nephropathy in type 1 diabetes. *Diabet Med*. 2000;17:782-791.

141. Schultz CJ, Neil H, Dalton R, et al. Risk of nephropathy can be detected before the onset of microalbuminuria during the early years after diagnosis of type 1 diabetes. *Diabetes Care*. 2000;23:1811-1815.

142. Feig DI, Kang DH, Johnson RJ. Uric acid and cardiovascular risk. *N Engl J Med*. 2008;359(17):1811-1821.

143. Hovind P, Rossing P, Tarnow L, et al. Serum uric acid as a predictor for development of diabetic nephropathy in type 1 diabetes: an inception cohort study. *Diabetes*. 2009;58(7):1668-1671.

144. Keen H, Chlouverakis C, Fuller JH, et al. The concomitants of raised blood sugar: studies in newly-detected hyperglycaemics. II. Urinary albumin excretion, blood pressure and their relation to blood sugar levels. *Guys Hosp Rep*. 1969;118:247-254.

145. Mogensen CE, Vestbo E, Poulsen PL, et al. Microalbuminuria and potential confounders. *Diabetes Care*. 1995;18(4):572-581.

146. Parving H-H. Microalbuminuria in essential hypertension and diabetes mellitus. *J Hypertens*. 1996;14(2):S89-S94.

147. American Diabetes Association. Standards of medical care in diabetes—2009. *Diabetes Care*. 2009;32(suppl 1):S13-S61.

148. Viberti GC, Walker JD, Pinto J, et al. Diabetic nephropathy. In: Alberti KGMM, DeFronzo RA, Keen H, eds. *International textbook of diabetes mellitus*. New York: John Wiley & Sons; 1992:1267-1328.

149. Ravid M, Savin H, Jutrin I, et al. Long-term stabilizing effect of angiotensin-converting enzyme inhibition on plasma creatinine and on proteinuria in normotensive type II diabetic patients. *Ann Intern Med*. 1993;118:577-581.

150. Borch-Johnsen K, Wenzel H, Viberti GC, et al. Is screening and intervention for microalbuminuria worthwhile in patients with insulin dependent diabetes. *BMJ*. 1993;306:1722-1725.

151. Deckert T, Kofoed-Enevoldsen A, Vidal P, et al. Size- and charge-selectivity of glomerular filtration in type 1 (insulin-dependent) diabetic patients with and without albuminuria. *Diabetologia*. 1993;36:244-251.

152. Scandling JD, Myers BD. Glomerular size-selectivity and microalbuminuria in early diabetic glomerular disease. *Kidney Int*. 1992;41:840-846.

153. Pietravalle P, Morano S, Christina G, et al. Charge selectivity of proteinuria in type 1 diabetes explored by Ig subclass clearance. *Diabetes*. 1991;40:1685-1690.

154. van den Born J, van Kraats AA, Bakker MAH, et al. Reduction of heparan sulphate–associated anionic sites in the glomerular basement of rats with streptozotocin-induced diabetic nephropathy. *Diabetologia*. 1995;38:1169-1175.

155. Bonnet F, Cooper ME, Kawachi H, et al. Irbesartan normalises the deficiency in glomerular nephrin expression in a model of diabetes and hypertension. *Diabetologia*. 2001;44(7):874-877.

156. Mifsud SA, Allen TJ, Bertram JF, et al. Podocyte foot process broadening in experimental diabetic nephropathy: amelioration with renin-angiotensin blockade. *Diabetologia*. 2001;44(7):878-882.

157. Nakamura T, Ushiyama C, Suzuki S, et al. Urinary excretion of podocytes in patients with diabetic nephropathy. *Nephrol Dial Transplant*. 2000;15(9):1379-1383.

158. Steffes MW, Schmidt D, McCrery R, et al. Glomerular cell number in normal subjects and in type 1 diabetic patients. *Kidney Int*. 2001;59(6):2104-2113.

159. Imanishi M, Yoshioka K, Konishi Y, et al. Glomerular hypertension as one cause of albuminuria in type II diabetic patients. *Diabetologia.* 1999;42:999-1005.
160. Sandeman DD, Shore AC, Tooke JE. Relation of skin capillary pressure in patients with insulin-dependent diabetes mellitus to complications and metabolic control. *N Engl J Med.* 1992;327:760-764.
161. Mathiesen ER, Feldt-Rasmussen B, Hommel E, et al. Stable glomerular filtration rate in normotensive IDDM patients with stable microalbuminuria. *Diabetes Care.* 1997;20(3):286-289.
162. Lawson ML, Sochett EB, Chait PG, et al. Effect of puberty on markers of glomerular hypertrophy and hypertension in IDDM. *Diabetes.* 1996;45:51-55.
163. Gaede P, Tarnow L, Vedel P, et al. Remission to normoalbuminuria during multifactorial treatment preserves kidney function in patients with type 2 diabetes and microalbuminuria. *Nephrol Dial Transplant.* 2004;19(11):2784-2788.
164. Skøtt P. Lithium clearance in the evaluation of segmental renal tubular reabsorption of sodium and water in diabetes mellitus. *Dan Med Bull.* 1993;41:23-37.
165. DeFronzo RA. The effect of insulin on renal sodium metabolism. *Diabetologia.* 1981;21:165-171.
166. Tarnow L, Rossing P, Gall M-A, et al. Prevalence of arterial hypertension in diabetic patients before and after the JNC-V. *Diabetes Care.* 1994;17(11):1247-1251.
167. Viberti GC, Keen H, Wiseman MJ. Raised arterial pressure in parents of proteinuric insulin-dependent diabetics. *BMJ.* 1987;295:515-517.
168. Walker JD, Tariq T, Viberti GC. Sodium-lithium countertransport activity in red cells of patients with insulin-dependent diabetes and nephropathy and their parents. *BMJ.* 1990;301:635-638.
169. Jensen JS, Mathiesen ER, Nørgaard K, et al. Increased blood pressure and erythrocyte sodium-lithium countertransport activity are not inherited in diabetic nephropathy. *Diabetologia.* 1990;33:619-624.
170. Fagerudd JA, Tarnow L, Jacobsen P, et al. Predisposition to essential hypertension and development of diabetic nephropathy in IDDM patients. *Diabetes.* 1998;47:439-444.
171. Parving H-H. Arterial hypertension in diabetes mellitus. In: Alberti KGMM, DeFronzo RA, Keen H, eds. *International textbook of diabetes mellitus.* New York: John Wiley & Sons; 1992:1521-1534.
172. Hommel E, Mathiesen ER, Aukland K, et al. Pathophysiological aspects of edema formation in diabetic nephropathy. *Kidney Int.* 1990;38:1187-1192.
173. Ritz E, Stefanski A. Diabetic nephropathy in type II diabetes. *Am J Kidney Diseases.* 1996;27:167-194.
174. Gall M-A, Nielsen FS, Smidt UM, et al. The course of kidney function in type 2 (non–insulin-dependent) diabetic patients with diabetic nephropathy. *Diabetologia.* 1993;36:1071-1078.
175. Nelson RG, Bennett PH, Beck GJ, et al. Development and progression of renal disease in Pima Indians with non–insulin-dependent diabetes mellitus. *N Engl J Med.* 1996;335:1636-1642.
176. Myers BD, Nelson RG, Williams GW, et al. Glomerular function in Pima Indians with noninsulin-dependent diabetes mellitus of recent onset. *J Clin Invest.* 1991;88:524-530.
177. Andersen S, Blouch K, Bialek J, et al. Glomerular permselectivity in early stages of overt diabetic nephropathy. *Kidney Int.* 2000;58(5):2129-2137.
178. Gall M-A, Rossing P, Kofoed-Enevoldsen A, et al. Glomerular size- and charge-selectivity in type 2 (non–insulin-dependent) diabetic patients with diabetic nephropathy. *Diabetologia.* 1993;37:195-201.
179. Rossing P, Hommel E, Smidt UM, et al. Impact of arterial blood pressure and albuminuria on the progression of diabetic nephropathy in IDDM patients. *Diabetes.* 1993;42:715-719.
180. Parving H-H. Impact of blood pressure and antihypertensive treatment on incipient and overt nephropathy, retinopathy, and endothelial permeability in diabetes mellitus. *Diabetes Care.* 1991;14:260-269.
181. Rossing P. Promotion, prediction, and prevention of progression of diabetic nephropathy in type 1 diabetes mellitus. *Diabet Med.* 1998;15(11):900-919.
182. Jacobsen P, Rossing K, Tarnow L, et al. Progression of diabetic nephropathy in normotensive type 1 diabetic patients. *Kidney Int.* 1999;56(71):S101-S105.
183. Hovind P, Rossing P, Tarnow L, et al. Progression of diabetic nephropathy. *Kidney Int.* 2001;59:702-709.
184. Rossing K, Christensen PK, Hovind P, et al. Progression of nephropathy in type 2 diabetic patients. *Kidney Int.* 2004;66(4):1596-1605.
185. Keane WF, Brenner BM, de Zeeuw D, et al. The risk of developing end-stage renal disease in patients with type 2 diabetes and nephropathy: the RENAAL study. *Kidney Int.* 2003;63(4):1499-1507.
186. Yokoyama H, Tomonaga O, Hirayama M, et al. Predictors of the progression of diabetic nephropathy and the beneficial effect of angiotensin-converting enzyme inhibitors in NIDDM patients. *Diabetologia.* 1997;40:405-411.
187. Krolewski AS, Warram JH, Christlieb AR. Hypercholesterolemia—a determinant of renal function loss and deaths in IDDM patients with nephropathy. *Kidney Int.* 1994;45(suppl 45):S125-S131.
188. Breyer JA, Bain P, Evans JK, et al. Predictors of the progression of renal insufficiency in patients with insulin-dependent diabetes and overt diabetic nephropathy. *Kidney Int.* 1996;50:1651-1658.
189. Jacobson HR. Chronic renal failure: pathophysiology. *Lancet.* 1991;338:419-423.
190. Hostetter TH, Rennke HG, Brenner BM. The case for intrarenal hypertension in the initiation and progression of diabetic and other glomerulopathies. *Am J Med.* 1982;72:375-380.
191. Christensen PK, Hansen HP, Parving H-H. Impaired autoregulation of GFR in hypertensive non–insulin dependent diabetic patients. *Kidney Int.* 1997;52:1369-1374.
192. Hayashi K, Epstein M, Loutzenhiser R, et al. Impaired myogenic responsiveness of the afferent arteriole in streptozotocin-induced diabetic rats: role of eicosanoid derangements. *J Am Soc Nephrol.* 1992;2:1578-1586.
193. Christensen PK, Lund S, Parving H-H. The impact of glycaemic control on autoregulation of glomerular filtration rate in patients with non–insulin dependent diabetes. *Scand J Clin Lab Invest.* 2001;61:43-50.
194. Gurley SB, Coffman TM. The renin-angiotensin system and diabetic nephropathy. *Semin Nephrol.* 2007;27(2):144-152.
195. Toma I, Kang JJ, Sipos A, et al. Succinate receptor GPR91 provides a direct link between high glucose levels and renin release in murine and rabbit kidney. *J Clin Invest.* 2008;118(7):2526-2534.
196. Reich HN, Oudit GY, Penninger JM, et al. Decreased glomerular and tubular expression of ACE2 in patients with type 2 diabetes and kidney disease. *Kidney Int.* 2008;74(12):1610-1616.
197. Stier Jr CT, Rocha R, Chander PN. Effect of aldosterone and MR blockade on the brain and the kidney. *Heart Fail Rev.* 2005;10(1):53-62.
198. Epstein M, Calhoun DA. The role of aldosterone in resistant hypertension: implications for pathogenesis and therapy. *Curr Hypertens Rep.* 2007;9(2):98-105.
199. Fujisawa G, Okada K, Muto S, et al. Spironolactone prevents early renal injury in streptozotocin-induced diabetic rats. *Kidney Int.* 2004;66(4):1493-1502.
200. Ritz E, Tomaschitz A. Aldosterone, a vasculotoxic agent—novel functions for an old hormone. *Nephrol Dial Transplant.* 2009;24(8):2302-2305.
201. Walker WG. Hypertension-related renal injury: a major contributor to end-stage renal disease. *Am J Kidney Dis.* 1993;22(1):164-173.
202. Schjoedt KJ, Andersen S, Rossing P, et al. Aldosterone escape during blockade of the renin-angiotensin-aldosterone system in diabetic nephropathy is associated with enhanced decline in glomerular filtration rate. *Diabetologia.* 2004;47(11):1936-1939.
203. Remuzzi G, Bertani T. Is glomerulosclerosis a consequence of altered glomerular permeability to macromolecules? *Kidney Int.* 1990;38:384-394.
204. Parving H-H, Rossing P, Hommel E, et al. Angiotensin converting enzyme inhibition in diabetic nephropathy: ten years experience. *Am J Kidney Diseases.* 1995;26:99-107.
205. Biesenbach G, Janko O, Zazgornik J. Similar rate of progression in the predialysis phase in type I and type II diabetes mellitus. *Nephrol Dial Transplant.* 1994;9:1097-1102.
206. Wu M-S, Yu C-C, Yang C-W, et al. Poor pre-dialysis glycaemic control is a predictor of mortality in type II diabetic patients on maintenance haemodialysis. *Nephrol Dial Transplant.* 1997;12:2105-2110.
207. Orth SR, Ritz E, Schrier RW. The renal risk of smoking. *Kidney Int.* 1997;51:1669-1677.
208. Sawicki PT, Didjurgeit U, Mühlhauser I, et al. Smoking is associated with progression of diabetic nephropathy. *Diabetes Care.* 1994;17:126-131.
209. Hovind P, Rossing P, Tarnow L, et al. Smoking and progression of diabetic nephropathy in type 1 diabetes. *Diabetologia.* 2002;45:A361:abstract.
210. Cambien F, Poirier O, Lecerf L, et al. Deletion polymorphism in the gene for angiotensin-converting enzyme is a potent risk factor for myocardial infarction. *Nature.* 1992;359-60:641-644.
211. Tarnow L, Cambien F, Rossing P, et al. Insertion/deletion polymorphism in the angiotensin-I-converting enzyme gene is associated with coronary heart disease in IDDM patients with diabetic nephropathy. *Diabetologia.* 1995;38:798-803.
212. Rigat B, Hubert C, Corvol P, et al. PCR detection of the insertion/deletion polymorphism of the human angiotensin converting enzyme gene (DCP 1) (dipeptidyl-carboxy peptidase 1). *Nucleic Acids Res.* 1992;20:1433-1433.
213. Yoshida H, Kuriyama S, Atsumi Y, et al. Angiotensin I converting enzyme gene polymorphism in non–insulin dependent diabetes mellitus. *Kidney Int.* 1996;50:657-664.
214. Schmidt S, Strojek K, Grzeszczak W, et al. Excess of DD homozygotes in haemodialysed patients with type II diabetes. *Nephrol Dial Transplant.* 1997;12:427-429.
215. Schmidt S, Ritz E. Angiotensin I converting enzyme gene polymorphism and diabetic nephropathy in type II diabetes. *Nephrol Dial Transplant.* 1997;12(2):37-41.
216. So WY, Ma RC, Ozaki R, et al. Angiotensin-converting enzyme (ACE) inhibition in type 2, diabetic patients—interaction with ACE insertion/deletion polymorphism. *Kidney Int.* 2006;69:1438-1443.

217. Solini A, Dalla VM, Saller A, et al. The angiotensin-converting enzyme DD genotype is associated with glomerulopathy lesions in type 2 diabetes. *Diabetes.* 2002;51(1):251-255.
218. Rudberg S, Rasmussen LM, Bangstad H-J, et al. Influence of insertion/deletion polymorphism in the ACE-I gene on the progression of diabetic glomerulopathy in type 1 diabetic patients with microalbuminuria. *Diabetes Care.* 2000;23(4):544-548.
219. Parving H-H, de Zeeuw D, Cooper ME, et al. ACE gene polymorphism and losartan treatment in type 2 diabetic patients with nephropathy. *J Am Soc Nephrol.* 2008;19(4):771-779.
220. Parving H-H, Jacobsen P, Tarnow L, et al. Effect of deletion polymorphism of angiotensin converting enzyme gene on progression of diabetic nephropathy during inhibition of angiotensin converting enzyme: observational follow-up study. *BMJ.* 1996;313:591-594.
221. Marre M, Jeunemaitre X, Gallois Y, et al. Contribution of genetic polymorphism in the renin-angiotensin system to the development of renal complications in insulin-dependent diabetes. *J Clin Invest.* 1997;99(7):1585-1595.
222. Rossing K, Jacobsen P, Hommel E, et al. Pregnancy and progression of diabetic nephropathy. *Diabetologia.* 2002;45:36-41.
223. Jacobsen P, Tarnow L, Carstensen B, et al. Genetic variation in the renin-angiotensin system and progression of diabetic nephropathy. *J Am Soc Nephrol.* 2003;14:2843-2850.
224. Pezzolesi MG, Poznik GD, Mychaleckyj JC, et al. Genome-wide association scan for diabetic nephropathy susceptibility genes in type 1 diabetes. *Diabetes.* 2009;58(6):1403-1410.
225. Rogus JJ, Poznik GD, Pezzolesi MG, et al. High-density single nucleotide polymorphism genome-wide linkage scan for susceptibility genes for diabetic nephropathy in type 1 diabetes: discordant sibpair approach. *Diabetes.* 2008;57(9):2519-2526.
226. Schelling JR, Abboud HE, Nicholas SB, et al. Genome-wide scan for estimated glomerular filtration rate in multi-ethnic diabetic populations: the Family Investigation of Nephropathy and Diabetes (FIND). *Diabetes.* 2008;57(1):235-243.
227. Thomas MC, Cooper ME, Rossing K, et al. Anaemia in diabetes: is there a rationale to TREAT? *Diabetologia.* 2006;49(6):1151-1157.
228. Pfeffer MA, Burdmann EA, Chen CY, et al. Baseline characteristics in the Trial to Reduce Cardiovascular Events with Aranesp Therapy (TREAT). *Am J Kidney Dis.* 2009;54(1):59-69.
229. Hsu CY, McCulloch CE, Iribarren C, et al. Body mass index and risk for end-stage renal disease. *Ann Intern Med.* 2006;144(1):21-28.
230. Krikken JA, Bakker SJ, Navis GJ. Role of renal haemodynamics in the renal risks of overweight. *Nephrol Dial Transplant.* 2009;24(6):1708-1711.
231. Christensen PK, Larsen S, Horn T, et al. The causes of albuminuria in patients with type 2 diabetes without diabetic retinopathy. *Kidney Int.* 2000;58:1719-1731.
232. Christensen PK, Gall MA, Parving H-H. Course of glomerular filtration rate in albuminuric type 2 diabetic patients with or without diabetic glomerulopathy. *Diabetes Care.* 2000;23(suppl 2):B14-B20.
233. Nielsen FS, Rossing P, Bang LE, et al. On the mechanisms of blunted nocturnal decline in arterial blood pressure in NIDDM patients with diabetic nephropathy. *Diabetes.* 1995;44:783-789.
234. Torffvit O, Agardh C-D. Day and night variation in ambulatory blood pressure in type 1 diabetes mellitus with nephropathy and autonomic neuropathy. *J Intern Med.* 1993;233:131-137.
235. Hostetter TH. Pathogenesis of diabetic glomerulopathy: hemodynamic considerations. *Semin Nephrol.* 1990;10:219-227.
236. Rasmussen LM, Tarnow L, Hansen TK, et al. Plasma osteoprotegerin levels are associated with glycaemic status, systolic blood pressure, kidney function and cardiovascular morbidity in type 1 diabetic patients. *Eur J Endocrinol.* 2006;154(1):75-81.
237. Knudsen ST, Foss CH, Poulsen PL, et al. Increased plasma concentrations of osteoprotegerin in type 2 diabetic patients with microvascular complications. *Eur J Endocrinol.* 2003;149(1):39-42.
238. Sharma K, Ramachandrarao S, Qiu G, et al. Adiponectin regulates albuminuria and podocyte function in mice. *J Clin Invest.* 2008;118(5):1645-1656.
239. Rossing K, Mischak H, Dakna M, et al. Urinary proteomics in diabetes and CKD. *J Am Soc Nephrol.* 2008;19(7):1283-1290.
240. Rossing K, Mischak H, Parving H-H, et al. Impact of diabetic nephropathy and angiotensin II receptor blockade on urinary polypeptide patterns. *Kidney Int.* 2005;68(1):193-205.
241. Tuttle KR, Bruton JL, Perusek M, et al. Effect of strict glycemic control on renal hemodynamic response to amino acid infusion. *N Engl J Med.* 1991;324:1626-1632.
242. Wang PH, Lau J, Chalmers TC. Meta-analysis of effects of intensive blood-glucose control on late complications of type I diabetes. *Lancet.* 1993;341:1306-1309.
243. Brinchmann-Hansen O, Dahl-Jørgensen K, Hanssen KF, et al. The response of diabetic retinopathy to 41 months of multiple insulin injections, insulin pumps, and conventional insulin therapy. *Arch Ophthalmol.* 1988;106:1242-1246.
244. The Diabetes Control and Complications Trial Research Group. Effect of intensive therapy on the development and progression of diabetic nephropathy in the Diabetes Control And Complications Trial. *Kidney Int.* 1995;47:1703-1720.
245. Ohkubo Y, Kishikawa H, Araki E, et al. Intensive insulin therapy prevents the progression of diabetic microvascular complications in Japanese patients with non–insulin-dependent diabetes mellitus: a randomized prospective 6-year study. *Diabetes Res Clin Pract.* 1995;28:103-117.
246. UK Prospective Diabetes Study (UKPDS) Group. Intensive blood-glucose control with sulphonylureas or insulin compared with conventional treatment and risk of complications in patients with type 2 diabetes (UKPDS 33). *Lancet.* 1998;352:837-853.
247. Holman RR, Paul SK, Bethel MA, et al. Ten-year follow-up of intensive glucose control in type 2 diabetes. *N Engl J Med.* 2008;359(15):1577-1589.
248. ADVANCE Collaborative Group, Patel A, MacMahon S, et al. Intensive blood glucose control and vascular outcomes in patients with type 2 diabetes. *N Engl J Med.* 2008;358(24):2560-2572.
249. Duckworth W, Abraira C, Moritz T, et al. Glucose control and vascular complications in veterans with type 2 diabetes. *N Engl J Med.* 2009;360(2):129-139.
250. The Microalbuminuria Captopril Study Group. Captopril reduces the risk of nephropathy in IDDM patients with microalbuminuria. *Diabetologia.* 1996;39:587-593.
251. Ravid M, Lang R, Rachmani R, et al. Long-term renoprotective effect of angiotensin-converting enzyme inhibition in non–insulin-dependent diabetes mellitus. *Arch Intern Med.* 1996;156:286-289.
252. Sano T, Kawamura T, Matsumae H, et al. Effects of long-term enalapril treatment on persistent microalbuminuria in well-controlled hypertensive and normotensive NIDDM patients. *Diabetes Care.* 1994;7:420-424.
253. Ahmad J, Siddiqui MA, Ahmad H. Effective postponement of diabetic nephropathy with enalapril in normotensive type 2 diabetic patients with microalbuminuria. *Diabetes Care.* 1997;20(10):1576-1581.
254. Gaede P, Vedel P, Parving H-H, et al. Intensified multifactorial intervention in patients with type 2 diabetes mellitus and microalbuminuria: the Steno type 2 randomised study. *Lancet.* 1999;353:617-622.
255. Gaede P, Lund-Andersen H, Parving H-H, et al. Effect of a multifactorial intervention on mortality in type 2 diabetes. *N Engl J Med.* 2008;358(6):580-591.
256. Zatz R, Dunn BR, Meyer TW, et al. Prevention of diabetic glomerulopathy by pharmacological amelioration of glomerular capillary hypertension. *J Clin Invest.* 1986;77:1925-1930.
257. Anderson S, Rennke HG, Garcia DL, et al. Short and long term effects of antihypertensive therapy in the diabetic rat. *Kidney Int.* 1989;36:526-536.
258. Anderson S, Rennke HG, Brenner BM. Nifedipine versus fosinopril in uninephrectomized diabetic rats. *Kidney Int.* 1992;41:891-897.
259. Flyihara CK, Padilha RM, Zatz R. Glomerular abnormalities in long-term experimental diabetes. *Diabetes.* 1992;41:286-293.
260. Cooper ME, Allen TJ, O'Brien RC, et al. Nephropathy in model combining genetic hypertension with experimental diabetes. *Diabetes.* 1990;39:1575-1579.
261. The EUCLID. Study Group. Randomised placebo-controlled trial of lisinopril in normotensive patients with insulin-dependent diabetes and normoalbuminuria or microalbuminuria. *Lancet.* 1997;349:1787-1792.
262. Ravid M, Brosh D, Levi Z, et al. Use of enalapril to attenuate decline in renal function in normotensive, normoalbuminuric patients with type 2 diabetes mellitus. *Ann Intern Med.* 1998;128:982-988.
263. Heart Outcomes Prevention Evaluation (HOPE) Study Investigators. Effects of ramipril on cardiovascular and microvascular outcomes in people with diabetes mellitus: results of the HOPE study and MICRO-HOPE substudy. *Lancet.* 2000;355:253-259.
264. Tatti P, Pahor M, Byington RP, et al. Outcome results of the fosinopril versus amlodipine cardiovascular events randomized trial (FACET) in patients with hypertension and NIDDM. *Diabetes Care.* 1998;21(4):597-603.
265. Estacio RO, Jeffers BW, Gifford N, et al. Effect of blood pressure control on diabetic microvascular complications in patients with hypertension and type 2 diabetes. *Diabetes Care.* 2000;23(suppl 2):B54-B64.
266. UK Prospective Diabetes Study (UKPDS) Group. Efficacy of atenolol and captopril in reducing risk of macrovascular and microvascular complications in type 2 diabetes: UKPDS 39. UK Prospective Diabetes Study Group. *BMJ.* 1998;317(7160):713-720.
267. Schrier RW, Estacio RO, Esler A, et al. Effects of aggressive blood pressure control in normotensive type 2 diabetic patients on albuminuria, retinopathy and strokes. *Kidney Int.* 2002;61(3):1086-1097.

268. Chaturvedi N, Sjolie A-K, Stephenson JM, et al. Effect of lisinopril on progression of retinopathy in normotensive people with type 1 diabetes. *Lancet.* 1998;351:28-31.

269. Chaturvedi N, Porta M, Klein R, et al. Effect of candesartan on prevention (DIRECT-Prevent 1) and progression (DIRECT-Protect 1) of retinopathy in type 1 diabetes: randomised, placebo-controlled trials. *Lancet.* 2008;372(9647):1394-1402.

270. Sjolie AK, Klein R, Porta M, et al. Effect of candesartan on progression and regression of retinopathy in type 2 diabetes (DIRECT-Protect 2): a randomised placebo-controlled trial. *Lancet.* 2008;372(9647):1385-1393.

271. Bilous R, Chaturvedi N, Sjolie AK, et al. Effect of candesartan on microalbuminuria and albumin excretion rate in diabetes: three randomized trials. *Ann Intern Med.* 2009;151(1):11-14.

272. Ruggenenti P, Fassi A, Ilieva AP, et al. Preventing microalbuminuria in type 2 diabetes. *N Engl J Med.* 2004;351(19):1941-1951.

273. Patel A, ADVANCE Collaborative Group, MacMahon S, et al. Effects of a fixed combination of perindopril and indapamide on macrovascular and microvascular outcomes in patients with type 2 diabetes mellitus (the ADVANCE trial): a randomised controlled trial. *Lancet.* 2007;370(9590):829-840.

274. Mann JF, Schmieder RE, McQueen M, et al. Renal outcomes with telmisartan, ramipril, or both, in people at high vascular risk (the ONTARGET study): a multicentre, randomised, double-blind, controlled trial. *Lancet.* 2008;372(9638):547-553.

275. Mann JF, Schmieder RE, Dyal L, et al. Effect of telmisartan on renal outcomes: a randomized trial. *Ann Intern Med.* 2009;151(1):1-2.

276. The ACE. Inhibitors in Diabetic Nephropathy Trialist Group. Should all type 1 diabetic microalbuminuric patients receive ACE inhibitors? A meta-regression analysis. *Ann Intern Med.* 2001;134:370-379.

277. Mathiesen ER, Hommel E, Hansen HP, et al. Randomised controlled trial of long term efficacy of captopril on preservation of kidney function in normotensive patients with insulin dependent diabetes and microalbuminuria. *BMJ.* 1999;319:24-25.

278. Crepaldi G, Carta Q, Deferrari G, et al. Effects of lisinopril and nifedipine on the progression of overt albuminuria in IDDM patients with incipient nephropathy and normal blood pressure. *Diabetes Care.* 1998;21(1):104-110.

279. Rudberg S, Osterby R, Bangstad HJ, et al. Effect of angiotensin converting enzyme inhibitor or beta blocker on glomerular structural changes in young microalbuminuric patients with type I (insulin-dependent) diabetes mellitus. *Diabetologia.* 1999;42(5):589-595.

280. Osterby R, Bangstad HJ, Rudberg S. Follow-up study of glomerular dimensions and cortical interstitium in microalbuminuric type 1 diabetic patients with or without antihypertensive treatment. *Nephrol Dial Transplant.* 2000;15(10):1609-1616.

281. Cordonnier DJ, Pinel N, Barro C, et al. Expansion of cortical interstitium is limited by converting enzyme inhibition in type 2 diabetic patients with glomerulosclerosis. *J Am Soc Nephrol.* 1999;10:1253-1263.

282. Melbourne Diabetic Nephropathy Study Group. Comparison between perindopril and nifedipine in hypertensive and normotensive diabetic patients with microalbuminuria. *BMJ.* 1991;302:210-216.

283. Chan JCN, Cockram CS, Nicholls MG, et al. Comparison of enalapril and nifedipine in treating non–insulin dependent diabetics associated with hypertension: one year analysis. *BMJ.* 1992;305:981-985.

284. Lacourciere Y, Nadeau A, Poirier L. Captopril or conventional therapy in hypertensive type II diabetics. Three-year analysis. *Hypertension.* 1993;21(6 pt 1):786-794.

285. Lebovitz HE, Wiegmann TB, Cnaan A, et al. Renal protective effects of enalapril in hypertensive NIDDM: role of baseline albuminuria. *Kidney Int Suppl.* 1994;45(suppl 45):S150-S155.

286. Trevisan R, Tiengo A. Effect of low-dose ramipril on microalbuminuria in normotensive or mild hypertensive non–insulin-dependent diabetic patients. North-East Italy Microalbuminuria Study Group. *Am J Hypertens.* 1995;8(9):876-883.

287. Agardh C-D, Garcia-Puig J, Charbonnel B, et al. Greater reduction of urinary albumin excretion in hypertensive type II diabetic patients with incipient nephropathy by lisinopril than by nifedipine. *J Hum Hypertens.* 1996;10:185-192.

288. Chan JC, Ko GT, Leung DH, et al. Long-term effects of angiotensin-converting enzyme inhibition and metabolic control in hypertensive type 2 diabetic patients. *Kidney Int.* 2000;57(2):590-600.

289. Viberti G, Wheeldon NM. Microalbuminuria reduction with valsartan in patients with type 2 diabetes mellitus: a blood pressure–independent effect. *Circulation.* 2002;106(6):672-678.

290. Parving H-H, Lehnert H, Bröchner-Mortensen J, et al. The effect of irbesartan on the development of diabetic nephropathy in patients with type 2 diabetes. *N Engl J Med.* 2001;345:870-878.

291. Rossing K, Christensen PK, Andersen S, et al. Comparative effects of irbesartan on ambulatory and office blood pressure: a substudy of ambulatory blood pressure from the Irbesartan in Patients with Type 2 Diabetes and Microalbuminuria Study. *Diabetes Care.* 2003;26(3):569-574.

292. Andersen S, Brochner-Mortensen J, Parving H-H, Kidney function after withdrawal of long-term antihypertensive treatment in patients with type 2 diabetes and microalbuminuria. *Diabetes Care.* 2003;26(12):3296-3302.

293. Persson F, Rossing P, Hovind P, et al. Irbesartan treatment reduces biomarkers of inflammatory activity in patients with type 2 diabetes and microalbuminuria: an IRMA 2 substudy. *Diabetes.* 2006;55(12):3550-3555.

294. Parving H-H, Lehnert H, Brochner-Mortensen J, et al. The effect of irbesartan on the development of diabetic nephropathy in patients with type 2 diabetes. *N Engl J Med.* 2001;345(12):870-878.

295. Rossing K, Schjoedt KJ, Jensen BR, et al. Enhanced renoprotective effects of ultrahigh doses of irbesartan in patients with type 2 diabetes and microalbuminuria. *Kidney Int.* 2005;68(3):1190-1198.

296. Palmer AJ, Annemans L, Roze S, et al. Cost-effectiveness of early irbesartan treatment versus control (standard antihypertensive medications excluding ACE inhibitors, other angiotensin-2 receptor antagonists, and dihydropyridine calcium channel blockers) or late irbesartan treatment in patients with type 2 diabetes, hypertension, and renal disease. *Diabetes Care.* 2004;27(8):1897-1903.

297. Makino H, Haneda M, Babazono T, et al. Prevention of transition from incipient to overt nephropathy with telmisartan in patients with type 2 diabetes. *Diabetes Care.* 2007;30(6):1577-1578.

298. Gaede P, Valentine WJ, Palmer AJ, et al. Cost-effectiveness of intensified versus conventional multifactorial intervention in type 2 diabetes: results and projections from the Steno-2 study. *Diabetes Care.* 2008;31(8):1510-1515.

299. Mogensen CE, Keane WF, Bennett PH, et al. Prevention of diabetic renal disease with special reference to microalbuminuria. *Lancet.* 1995;346:1080-1084.

300. Schjoedt KJ, Hansen HP, Tarnow L, et al. Long-term prevention of diabetic nephropathy: an audit. *Diabetologia.* 2008;51(6):956-961.

301. Rossing P, Hommel E, Smidt UM, et al. Reduction in albuminuria predicts a beneficial effect on diminishing the progression of human diabetic nephropathy during antihypertensive treatment. *Diabetologia.* 1994;37:511-516.

302. Rossing P, Hommel E, Smidt UM, et al. Reduction in albuminuria predicts diminished progression in diabetic nephropathy. *Kidney Int.* 1994;45(suppl 45):S145-S149.

303. de Zeeuw D, Remuzzi G, Parving H-H, et al. Proteinuria, a target for renoprotection in patients with type 2 diabetic nephropathy: lessons from RENAAL. *Kidney Int.* 2004;65(6):2309-2320.

304. Apperloo AJ, de Zeeuw D, de Jong PE. Short-term antiproteinuric response to antihypertensive treatment predicts long-term GFR decline in patients with non-diabetic renal disease. *Kidney Int.* 1994;45(suppl 45):S174-S178.

305. Peterson JC, Adler S, Burkart JM, et al. Blood pressure control, proteinuria, and the progression of renal disease. The Modification of Diet in Renal Disease study. *Ann Intern Med.* 1995;123:754-762.

306. Jacobsen P, Rossing K, Rossing P, et al. Angiotensin converting enzyme gene polymorphism and ACE inhibition in diabetic nephropathy. *Kidney Int.* 1998;53:1002-1006.

307. Vlemming LJ, van der Pijl JW, Lemkes HHPJ, et al. The DD genotype of the ACE gene polymorphism is associated with progression of diabetic nephropathy to end stage renal failure in IDDM. *Clin Nephrol.* 1999;51(3):133-140.

308. Thomas SM, Alaveras A, Margaglione M, et al. Metabolic and genetic predictors of progression of diabetic kidney disease (DKD). *Diabet Med.* 1997;14(1):S17:(abstract).

309. Jacobsen P, Tarnow L, Hovind P, et al. Genetic variation in the renin-angiotensin system and progression of diabetic nephropathy in type 1 diabetic patients. *J Am Soc Nephrol.* 2002;13:247A:(abstract).

310. Harden PN, Geddes C, Rowe PA, et al. Polymorphisms in angiotensin-converting-enzyme gene and progression of IgA nephropathy. *Lancet.* 1995;345:1540-1542.

311. van Essen GG, Rensma PL, de Zeeuw D, et al. Association between angiotensin-converting-enzyme gene polymorphism and failure of renoprotective therapy. *Lancet.* 1996;347:94-95.

312. Fava S, Azzopardi J, Ellard S, et al. ACE gene polymorphism as a prognostic indicator in patients with type 2 diabetes and established renal disease. *Diabetes Care.* 2001;24(12):2115-2120.

313. Andersen S, Tarnow L, Cambien F, et al. Renoprotective effects of losartan in diabetic nephropathy: interaction with ACE insertion/deletion genotype?. *Kidney Int.* 2002;62(1):192-198.

314. Andersen S, Tarnow L, Cambien F, et al. Long-term renoprotective effects of losartan in diabetic nephropathy: interaction with ACE insertion/deletion genotype? *Diabetes Care.* 2003;26:1501-1506.

315. Parving H-H, de Zeeuw D, Cooper ME, et al. ACE gene polymorphism and losartan treatment in type 2 diabetic patients with nephropathy. *J Am Soc Nephrol.* 2008;19(4):771-779.

316. Lajer M, Tarnow L, Andersen S, et al. CYP2C9 variant modifies blood pressure–lowering response to losartan in type 1 diabetic patients with nephropathy. *Diabet Med.* 2007;24(3):323-325.

317. Muirhead N, Feagan BF, Mahon J, et al. The effects of valsartan and captopril on reducing microalbuminuria in patients with type 2 diabetes mellitus: a placebo-controlled trial. *Curr Ther Res.* 2002;60(12):650:(abstract).

318. Andersen S, Tarnow L, Rossing P, et al. Renoprotective effects of angiotensin II receptor blockade in type 1 diabetic patients with diabetic nephropathy. *Kidney Int.* 2000;57:601-606.

319. Lacourciere Y, Belanger A, Godin C, et al. Long-term comparison of losartan and enalapril on kidney function in hypertensive type 2 diabetics with early nephropathy. *Kidney Int.* 2000;58(2):762-769.

320. Bos H, Andersen S, Rossing P, et al. Role of patient factors in therapy resistance to antiproteinuric intervention in nondiabetic and diabetic nephropathy. *Kidney Int.* 2000;57(suppl 75):S32-S37.

321. Andersen S, Rossing P, Juhl TR, et al. Optimal dose of losartan for renoprotection in diabetic nephropathy. *Nephrol Dial Transplant.* 2002;17(8):1413-1418.

322. Rossing K, Christensen PK, Hansen BV, et al. Optimal dose of candesartan for renoprotection in type 2 diabetic patients with nephropathy: a double-blind randomized crossover study. *Diabetes Care.* 2003;26:150-155.

323. Hollenberg NK, Parving H-H, Viberti G, et al. Albuminuria response to very high-dose valsartan in type 2 diabetes mellitus. *J Hypertens.* 2007;25(9):1921-1926.

324. Burgess E, Muirhead N, Rene de CP, et al. Supramaximal dose of candesartan in proteinuric renal disease. *J Am Soc Nephrol.* 2009;20(4):893-900.

325. Schjoedt KJ, Astrup AS, Persson F, et al. Optimal dose of lisinopril for renoprotection in type 1 diabetic patients with diabetic nephropathy: a randomised crossover trial. *Diabetologia.* 2009;52(1):46-49.

326. Bakris G, Burgess E, Weir M, et al. Telmisartan is more effective than losartan in reducing proteinuria in patients with diabetic nephropathy. *Kidney Int.* 2008;74(3):364-369.

327. Mogensen CE, Neldam S, Tikkanen I, et al. Randomised controlled trial of dual blockade of renin-angiotensin system in patients with hypertension, microalbuminuria, and non–insulin dependent diabetes: the Candesartan And Lisinopril Microalbuminuria (CALM) study. *BMJ.* 2000;321(7274):1440-1444.

328. Jacobsen P, Andersen S, Rossing K, et al. Dual blockade of the renin-angiotensin system in type 1 patients with diabetic nephropathy. *Nephrol Dial Transplant.* 2002;17(6):1019-1024.

329. Rossing K, Christensen PK, Jensen BR, et al. Dual blockade of the renin-angiotensin system in diabetic nephropathy: a randomized double-blind crossover study. *Diabetes Care.* 2002;25(1):95-100.

330. Hilgers KF, Mann JF. ACE inhibitors versus AT(1) receptor antagonists in patients with chronic renal disease. *J Am Soc Nephrol.* 2002;13(4):1100-1108.

331. Jacobsen P, Andersen S, Jensen BR, et al. Additive effect of ACE-inhibition and angiotensin II receptor blockade in type I diabetic patients with diabetic nephropathy. *J Am Soc Nephrol.* 2003;14(4):992-999.

332. Jacobsen P, Andersen S, Rossing K, et al. Dual blockade of the renin-angiotensin system versus maximal recommended dose of ACE inhibition in diabetic nephropathy. *Kidney Int.* 2003;63(5):1874-1880.

333. Rossing K, Jacobsen P, Pietraszek L, et al. Renoprotective effects of adding angiotensin II receptor blocker to maximal recommended doses of ACE-inhibitor in diabetic nephropathy. A randomized double-blind cross-over trial. *Diabetes Care.* 2003;26(8):2268-2274.

334. Kunz R, Friedrich C, Wolbers M, et al. Meta-analysis: effect of monotherapy and combination therapy with inhibitors of the renin angiotensin system on proteinuria in renal disease. *Ann Intern Med.* 2008;148:30-48.

335. Komine N, Khang S, Wead LM, et al. Effect of combining an ACE inhibitor and an angiotensin II receptor blocker on plasma and kidney tissue angiotensin II levels. *Am J Kidney Dis.* 2002;39(1):159-164.

336. Christensen PK, Lund S, Parving H-H. Autoregulated glomerular filtration rate during candesartan treatment in hypertensive type 2 diabetic patients. *Kidney Int.* 2001;60(4):1435-1442.

337. Nakao N, Yoshimura A, Morita H, et al. Combination therapy of angiotensin-II receptor blocker and angiotensin-converting enzyme inhibitor in non-diabetic renal disease: a randomized, controlled trial in Japan (COOPERATE). *Lancet.* 2003;361:117-124.

338. Kunz R, Wolbers M, Glass T, et al. The COOPERATE trial: a letter of concern. *Lancet.* 2008;371(9624):1575-1576.

339. Bakris GL, Ruilope L, Locatelli F, et al. Treatment of microalbuminuria in hypertensive subjects with elevated cardiovascular risk: results of the IMPROVE trial. *Kidney Int.* 2007;72(7):879-885.

340. Messerli FH. The sudden demise of dual renin-angiotensin system blockade or the soft science of the surrogate end point. *J Am Coll Cardiol.* 2009;53(6):468-470.

341. Parving HH, Brenner BM, McMurray JJ, et al. Dual renin-angiotensin system blockade and kidney disease. *J Am Coll Cardiol.* 2009;54(3):278-279.

342. Sarafidis PA, Bakris GL. Renin-angiotensin blockade and kidney disease. *Lancet.* 2008;372(9638):511-512.

343. Epstein M. Aldosterone and the hypertensive kidney: its emerging role as a mediator of progressive renal dysfunction: a paradigm shift. *J Hypertens.* 2001;19(5):829-842.

344. Epstein M. Aldosterone as a determinant of cardiovascular and renal dysfunction. *J R Soc Med.* 2001;94(8):378-383.

345. Becker GJ, Hewitson TD, Chrysostomou A. Aldosterone in clinical nephrology—old hormone, new questions. *Nephrol Dial Transplant.* 2009;24(8):2316-2321.

346. Rossing K, Schjoedt KJ, Smidt UM, et al. Beneficial effects of adding spironolactone to recommended antihypertensive treatment in diabetic nephropathy: a randomized, double-masked, cross-over study. *Diabetes Care.* 2005;28(9):2106-2112.

347. Schjoedt KJ, Rossing K, Juhl TR, et al. Beneficial impact of spironolactone in diabetic nephropathy. *Kidney Int.* 2005;68(6):2829-2836.

348. Schjoedt KJ, Rossing K, Juhl TR, et al. Beneficial impact of spironolactone on nephrotic range albuminuria in diabetic nephropathy. *Kidney Int.* 2006;70(3):536-542.

349. Epstein M, Williams GH, Weinberger M, et al. Selective aldosterone blockade with eplerenone reduces albuminuria in patients with type 2 diabetes. *Clin J Am Soc Nephrol.* 2006;1(5):940-951.

350. Kelly DJ, Zhang Y, Moe G, et al. Aliskiren, a novel renin inhibitor, is renoprotective in a model of advanced diabetic nephropathy in rats. *Diabetologia.* 2007;50(11):2398-2404.

351. Feldman DL, Jin L, Xuan H, et al. Effects of aliskiren on blood pressure, albuminuria, and (pro)renin receptor expression in diabetic TG(mRen-2)27 rats. *Hypertension.* 2008;52(1):130-136.

352. Nguyen G, Delarue F, Burckle C, et al. Pivotal role of the renin/prorenin receptor in angiotensin II production and cellular responses to renin. *J Clin Invest.* 2002;109(11):1417-1427.

353. Ichihara A, Kaneshiro Y, Suzuki F. Prorenin receptor blockers: effects on cardiovascular complications of diabetes and hypertension. *Expert Opin Investig Drugs.* 2006;15(10):1137-1139.

354. Ichihara A, Suzuki F, Nakagawa T, et al. Prorenin receptor blockade inhibits development of glomerulosclerosis in diabetic angiotensin II type 1a receptor–deficient mice. *J Am Soc Nephrol.* 2006;17(7):1950-1961.

355. Wilson DM, Luetscher JA. Plasma prorenin activity and complications in children with insulin-dependent diabetes mellitus. *N Engl J Med.* 1990;323:1101-1106.

356. Luetscher JA, Kraemer FB. Microalbuminuria and increased plasma prorenin. Prevalence in diabetics followed up for four years. *Arch Intern Med.* 1988;148:937-941.

357. Persson F, Rossing P, Schjoedt KJ, et al. Time course of the antiproteinuric and antihypertensive effects of direct renin inhibition in type 2 diabetes. *Kidney Int.* 2008;73(12):1419-1425.

358. Persson F, Rossing P, Reinhard H, et al. Renal effects of aliskiren compared to and in combination with irbesartan in patients with type 2 diabetes, hypertension and albuminuria. *Diabetes Care.* 2009;32(10):1873-1879.

359. Persson F, Rossing P, Reinhard H, et al. Optimal antiproteinuric dose of the direct renin inhibitor aliskiren in type 2 diabetes: a randomized crossover trial. *Diabetes.* 2009;58(S1):A147:(abstract).

360. Parving H-H, Persson F, Lewis JB, et al. Aliskiren combined with losartan in type 2 diabetes and nephropathy. *N Engl J Med.* 2008;358(23):2433-2446.

361. Parving HH, Brenner BM, McMurray JJ, et al. Aliskiren Trial in Type 2 Diabetes Using Cardio-Renal Endpoints (ALTITUDE): rationale and study design. *Nephrol Dial Transplant.* 2009;24(5):1663-1671.

362. Hansen HP, Nielsen FS, Rossing P, et al. Kidney function after withdrawal of long-term antihypertensive treatment in diabetic nephropathy. *Kidney Int.* 1997;52(63):S49-S53.

363. Apperloo AJ, de Zeeuw D, de Jong PE. A short-term antihypertensive treatment-induced fall in glomerular filtration rate predicts long-term stability of renal function. *Kidney Int.* 1997;51:793-797.

364. Hansen HP, Rossing P, Tarnow L, et al. Increased glomerular filtration rate after withdrawal of long-term antihypertensive treatment in diabetic nephropathy. *Kidney Int.* 1995;47:1726-1731.

365. Mogensen CE. Long-term antihypertensive treatment inhibiting progression of diabetic nephropathy. *BMJ.* 1982;285:685-688.

366. Parving H-H, Andersen AR, Smidt UM, et al. Early aggressive antihypertensive treatment reduces rate of decline in kidney function in diabetic nephropathy. *Lancet.* 1983;1(8335):1175-1179.

367. Parving H-H, Andersen AR, Smidt UM, et al. Effect of antihypertensive treatment on kidney function in diabetic nephropathy. *BMJ.* 1987;294:1443-1447.

368. Parving H-H, Smidt UM, Hommel E, et al. Effective antihypertensive treatment postpones renal insufficiency in diabetic nephropathy. *Am J Kidney Dis.* 1993;22:188-195.

369. Ruggenenti P, Perna A, Gheradi G, et al. Renal function and requirement for dialysis in chronic nephropathy patients on long-term ramipril: REIN follow-up trial. *Lancet.* 1998;352:1252-1256.

370. Hovind P, Rossing P, Tarnow L, et al. Remission and regression in the nephropathy of type 1 diabetes when blood pressure is controlled aggressively. *Kidney Int.* 2001;60(1):277-283.

371. Wilmer WA, Hebert LA, Lewis EJ, et al. Remission of nephrotic syndrome in type 1 diabetes: long-term follow-up of patients in the captopril study. *Am J Kidney Dis.* 1999;34(2):308-314.

372. Hovind P, Rossing P, Tarnow L, et al. Remission of nephrotic-range albuminuria in type 1 diabetic patients. *Diabetes Care.* 2000;24(11):1972-1977.

373. Hovind P, Tarnow L, Rossing P, et al. Improved survival in patients obtaining remission of nephrotic range albuminuria in diabetic nephropathy. *Kidney Int.* 2004;66(3):1180-1186.

374. Rossing K, Christensen PK, Hovind P, et al. Remission of nephrotic range albuminuria reduces risk of end-stage renal disease and improves survival in type 2 diabetic patients. *Diabetologia.* 2005;48(11):2241-2247.

375. Björck S, Mulec H, Johnsen S, et al. Renal protective effect of enalapril in diabetic nephropathy. *BMJ.* 1992;304:339-343.

376. Lewis E, Hunsicker L, Bain R, et al. The effect of angiotensin-converting-enzyme inhibition on diabetic nephropathy. *N Engl J Med.* 1993;329:1456-1462.

377. Tarnow L, Rossing P, Jensen C, et al. Long-term renoprotective effect of nisoldipine and lisinopril in type 1 diabetic patients with diabetic nephropathy. *Diabetes Care.* 2000;23:1725-1730.

378. Brenner BM, Cooper ME, de Zeeuw D, et al. Effects of losartan on renal and cardiovascular outcomes in patients with type 2 diabetes and nephropathy. *N Engl J Med.* 2001;345:861-869.

379. Lewis EJ, Hunsicker LG, Clarke WR, et al. Renoprotective effect of the angiotensin-receptor antagonist irbesartan in patients with nephropathy due to type 2 diabetes. *N Engl J Med.* 2001;345(12):851-860.

380. Pourdjabbar A, Lapointe N, Rouleau JL. Angiotensin receptor blockers: powerful evidence with cardiovascular outcomes? *Can J Cardiol.* 2002;18(suppl A):7A-14A.

381. Parving H-H, Hommel E. Prognosis in diabetic nephropathy. *BMJ.* 1989;299:230-233.

382. Parving H-H, Jacobsen P, Rossing K, et al. Benefits of long-term antihypertensive treatment on prognosis in diabetic nephropathy. *Kidney Int.* 1996;49:1778-1782.

383. Rossing P, Hougaard P, Borch-Johnsen K, et al. Predictors of mortality in insulin dependent diabetes: 10 year follow-up study. *BMJ.* 1996;313:779-784.

384. Astrup AS, Tarnow L, Rossing P, et al. Improved prognosis in type 1 diabetic patients with nephropathy: a prospective follow-up study. *Kidney Int.* 2005;68(3):1250-1257.

385. Rodby RA, Firth LM, Lewis E. the Collaborative Study Group. An economic analysis of captopril in the treatment of diabetic nephropathy. *Diabetes Care.* 1996;19(10):1051-1061.

386. KDOQI Clinical Practice Guidelines and Clinical Practice Recommendations for Diabetes and Chronic Kidney Disease. *Am J Kidney Dis.* 2007;49(2 suppl 2):S12-S154.

387. Strippoli GF, Navaneethan SD, Johnson DW, et al. Effects of statins in patients with chronic kidney disease: meta-analysis and meta-regression of randomised controlled trials. *BMJ.* 2008;336(7645):645-651.

388. Keech A, Simes RJ, Barter P, et al. Effects of long-term fenofibrate therapy on cardiovascular events in 9795 people with type 2 diabetes mellitus (the FIELD study): randomised controlled trial. *Lancet.* 2005;366(9500):1849-1861.

389. Dullaart PF, Beusekamp BJ, Meijer S, et al. Long-term effects of protein-restricted diet on albuminuria and renal function in IDDM patients without clinical nephropathy and hypertension. *Diabetes Care.* 1993;16(2):483-492.

390. Hansen HP, Christensen PK, Tauber-Lassen E, et al. Low-protein diet and kidney function in insulin-dependent diabetic patients with diabetic nephropathy. *Kidney Int.* 1999;55(2):621-628.

391. Walker JD, Bending JJ, Dodds RA, et al. Restriction of dietary protein and progression of renal failure in diabetic nephropathy. *Lancet.* 1989;2(8677):1411-1415.

392. Zeller KR, Whittaker E, Sullivan L, et al. Effect of restricting dietary protein on the progression of renal failure in patients with insulin-dependent diabetes mellitus. *N Engl J Med.* 1991;324:78-84.

393. Parving H-H. Low-protein diet and progression of renal disease in diabetic nephropathy. *Lancet.* 1990;335:411.

394. Parving H-H. Protein restriction and renal failure in diabetes mellitus. *N Engl J Med.* 1991;324:1743-1744.

395. Pedrini MT, Levey AS, Lau J, et al. The effect of dietary protein restriction on the progression of diabetic and nondiabetic renal diseases: meta-analysis. *Ann Intern Med.* 1996;124:627-632.

396. Parving H-H. Effects of dietary protein on renal disease. *Ann Intern Med.* 1997;126(4):330-331.

397. Shah N, Horwitz RI, Cancato J. Effects of dietary protein on renal disease. *Ann Intern Med.* 1997;126(4):331.

398. Hansen HP, Tauber-Lassen E, Jensen BR, et al. Effect of dietary protein restriction on prognosis in patients with diabetic nephropathy. *Kidney Int.* 2002;62(1):220-228.

399. Li YC, Kong J, Wei M, et al. 1,25-Dihydroxyvitamin D(3) is a negative endocrine regulator of the renin-angiotensin system. *J Clin Invest.* 2002;110(2):229-238.

400. Zhang Z, Zhang Y, Ning G, et al. Combination therapy with AT1 blocker and vitamin D analog markedly ameliorates diabetic nephropathy: blockade of compensatory renin increase. *Proc Natl Acad Sci U S A.* 2008;105(41):15896 15901.

401. Agarwal R, Acharya M, Tian J, et al. Antiproteinuric effect of oral paricalcitol in chronic kidney disease. *Kidney Int.* 2005;68(6):2823-2828.

402. Alborzi P, Patel NA, Peterson C, et al. Paricalcitol reduces albuminuria and inflammation in chronic kidney disease: a randomized double-blind pilot trial. *Hypertension.* 2008;52(2):249-255.

403. Lambers Heerspink HJ, Agarwal R, Coyne DW, et al. The Selective Vitamin D Receptor Activator for Albuminuria Lowering (VITAL) Study: study design and baseline characteristics. *Am J Nephrol.* 2009;30(3):280-286.

404. Heerspink HL, Greene T, Lewis JB, et al. Effects of sulodexide in patients with type 2 diabetes and persistent albuminuria. *Nephrol Dial Transplant.* 2008;23(6):1946-1954.

405. Soma J, Sato K, Saito H, et al. Effect of tranilast in early-stage diabetic nephropathy. *Nephrol Dial Transplant.* 2006;21(10):2795-2799.

406. Ritz E, Rychlik I, Locatelli F, et al. End-stage renal failure in type 2 diabetes: a medical catastrophe of worldwide dimensions. *Am J Kidney Dis.* 1999;34(5):795-808.

407. Van Dijk PC, Jager KJ, Stengel B, et al. Renal replacement therapy for diabetic end-stage renal disease: data from 10 registries in Europe (1991-2000). *Kidney Int.* 2005;67(4):1489-1499.

408. Stengel B, Billon S, Van Dijk PC, et al. Trends in the incidence of renal replacement therapy for end-stage renal disease in Europe, 1990-1999. *Nephrol Dial Transplant.* 2003;18(9):1824-1833.

409. Schwenger V, Mussig C, Hergesell O, et al. Incidence and clinical characteristics of renal insufficiency in diabetic patients. *Dtsch Med Wochenschr.* 2001;126(47):1322-1326.

410. Kalantar-Zadeh K, Derose SF, Nicholas S, et al. Burnt-out diabetes: impact of chronic kidney disease progression on the natural course of diabetes mellitus. *J Ren Nutr.* 2009;19(1):33-37.

411. Wolfe RA, Ashby VB, Milford EL, et al. Comparison of mortality in all patients on dialysis, patients on dialysis awaiting transplantation, and recipients of a first cadaveric transplant. *N Engl J Med.* 1999;341(23):1725-1730.

412. Becker BN, Brazy PC, Becker YT, et al. Simultaneous pancreas-kidney transplantation reduces excess mortality in type 1 diabetic patients with end-stage renal disease. *Kidney Int.* 2000;57:2129-2135.

413. Yusuf S, Sleight P, Pogue J, et al. Effects of an angiotensin-converting-enzyme inhibitor, ramipril, on cardiovascular events in high-risk patients. The Heart Outcomes Prevention Evaluation Study Investigators. *N Engl J Med.* 2000;342(3):145-153.

414. Feldstein CA. Salt intake, hypertension and diabetes mellitus. *J Hum Hypertens.* 2002;16(suppl 1):S48-S51.

415. Nakano S, Ogihara M, Tamura C, et al. Reversed circadian blood pressure rhythm independently predicts endstage renal failure in non-insulin-dependent diabetes mellitus subjects. *J Diabetes Complications.* 1999;13(4):224-231.

416. Sturrock ND, George E, Pound N, et al. Non-dipping circadian blood pressure and renal impairment are associated with increased mortality in diabetes mellitus. *Diabet Med.* 2000;17(5):360-364.

417. Haneda M, Morikawa A. Which hypoglycaemic agents to use in type 2 diabetic subjects with CKD and how? *Nephrol Dial Transplant.* 2009;24(2):338-341.

418. Flanigan MJ, Frankenfield DL, Prowant BF, et al. Nutritional markers during peritoneal dialysis: data from the 1998 Peritoneal Dialysis Core Indicators Study. *Perit Dial Int.* 2001;21(4):345-354.

419. Levey AS, Stevens LA, Schmid CH, et al. A new equation to estimate glomerular filtration rate. *Ann Intern Med.* 2009;150(9):604-612.

420. Rossing P, Rossing K, Gaede P, et al. Monitoring kidney function in type 2 diabetic patients with incipient and overt diabetic nephropathy. *Diabetes Care.* 2006;29(5):1024-1030.

421. Bellomo R, Ronco C, Kellum JA, et al. Acute renal failure—definition, outcome measures, animal models, fluid therapy and information technology needs: the Second International Consensus Conference of the Acute Dialysis Quality Initiative (ADQI) Group. *Crit Care.* 2004;8(4):R204-R212.

422. Mueller C, Buerkle G, Buettner HJ, et al. Prevention of contrast media–associated nephropathy: randomized comparison of 2 hydration regimens in 1620 patients undergoing coronary angioplasty. *Arch Intern Med.* 2002;162(3):329-336.

423. Melin J, Hellberg O, Larsson E, et al. Protective effect of insulin on ischemic renal injury in diabetes mellitus. *Kidney Int.* 2002;61(4):1383-1392.

424. Chantrel F, Enache I, Bouiller M, et al. Abysmal prognosis of patients with type 2 diabetes entering dialysis. *Nephrol Dial Transplant.* 1999;14(1):129-136.

425. Liangos O, Wald R, O'Bell JW, et al. Epidemiology and outcomes of acute renal failure in hospitalized patients: a national survey. *Clin J Am Soc Nephrol.* 2006;1(1):43-51.

426. Konner K, Nonnast-Daniel B, Ritz E. The arteriovenous fistula. *J Am Soc Nephrol.* 2003;14(6):1669-1680.

427. Konner K. Primary vascular access in diabetic patients: an audit. *Nephrol Dial Transplant.* 2000;15(9):1317-1325.

428. Dixon BS, Novak L, Fangman J. Hemodialysis vascular access survival: upper-arm native arteriovenous fistula. *Am J Kidney Dis.* 2002;39(1):92-101.

429. Revanur VK, Jardine AG, Hamilton DH, et al. Outcome for arterio-venous fistula at the elbow for haemodialysis. *Clin Transplant.* 2000;14(4 pt 1):318-322.

430. Gefen JY, Fox D, Giangola G, et al. The transposed forearm loop arteriovenous fistula: a valuable option for primary hemodialysis access in diabetic patients. *Ann Vasc Surg.* 2002;16(1):89-94.

431. Yeager RA, Moneta GL, Edwards JM, et al. Relationship of hemodialysis access to finger gangrene in patients with end-stage renal disease. *J Vasc Surg.* 2002;36(2):245-249.

432. Ritz E, Haxsen V. Diabetic nephropathy and anaemia. *Eur J Clin Invest.* 2005;35(suppl 3):66-74.

433. Inomata S, Itoh M, Imai H, et al. Serum levels of erythropoietin as a novel marker reflecting the severity of diabetic nephropathy. *Nephron.* 1997;75(4):426-430.

434. Tong Z, Yang Z, Patel S, et al. Promoter polymorphism of the erythropoietin gene in severe diabetic eye and kidney complications. *Proc Natl Acad Sci U S A.* 2008;105(19):6998-7003.

435. Ritz E, Laville M, Bilous RW, et al. Target level for hemoglobin correction in patients with diabetes and CKD: primary results of the Anemia Correction in Diabetes (ACORD) Study. *Am J Kidney Dis.* 2007;49(2):194-207.

436. Watanabe D, Suzuma K, Matsui S, et al. Erythropoietin as a retinal angiogenic factor in proliferative diabetic retinopathy. *N Engl J Med.* 2005;353(8):782-792.

437. Sinclair SH, Delvecchio C, Levin A. Treatment of anemia in the diabetic patient with retinopathy and kidney disease. *Am J Ophthalmol.* 2003;135(5):740-743.

438. Junk AK, Mammis A, Savitz SI, et al. Erythropoietin administration protects retinal neurons from acute ischemia-reperfusion injury. *Proc Natl Acad Sci U S A.* 2002;99(16):10659-10664.

439. Lipton SA. Erythropoietin for neurologic protection and diabetic neuropathy. *N Engl J Med.* 2004;350(24):2516-2517.

439a. Pfeffer MA, Burdmann EA, Chen CY, et al. A trial of darbepoetin alfa in type 2 diabetes and chronic kidney disease. *N Engl J Med.* 2009;361(21):2019-2032.

440. Daugirdas JT. Pathophysiology of dialysis hypotension: an update. *Am J Kidney Dis.* 2001;38(4 suppl 4):S11-S17.

441. Koch M, Thomas B, Tschöpe W, et al. Survival and predictors of death in dialysed diabetic patients. *Diabetologia.* 1993;36:1113-1117.

442. Tozawa M, Iseki K, Iseki C, et al. Pulse pressure and risk of total mortality and cardiovascular events in patients on chronic hemodialysis. *Kidney Int.* 2002;61(2):717-726.

443. Stack AG, Bloembergen WE. A cross-sectional study of the prevalence and clinical correlates of congestive heart failure among incident U.S. dialysis patients. *Am J Kidney Dis.* 2001;38(5):992-1000.

444. Levin A, Djurdjev O, Barrett B, et al. Cardiovascular disease in patients with chronic kidney disease: getting to the heart of the matter. *Am J Kidney Dis.* 2001;38(6):1398-1407.

445. Foley RN, Culleton BF, Parfrey PS, et al. Cardiac disease in diabetic end-stage renal disease. *Diabetologia.* 1997;40:1307-1312.

446. Herzog CA, Ma JZ, Collins AJ. Poor long-term survival after acute myocardial infarction among patients on long-term dialysis. *N Engl J Med.* 1998;339(12):799-805.

447. Karnik JA, Young BS, Lew NL, et al. Cardiac arrest and sudden death in dialysis units. *Kidney Int.* 2001;60(1):350-357.

448. Giordano M, Manzella D, Paolisso G, et al. Differences in heart rate variability parameters during the post-dialytic period in type II diabetic and non-diabetic ESRD patients. *Nephrol Dial Transplant.* 2001;16(3):566-573.

449. Hathaway DK, Abell T, Cardoso S, et al. Improvement in autonomic and gastric function following pancreas-kidney versus kidney-alone transplantation and the correlation with quality of life. *Transplantation.* 1994;57:816-822.

450. Amann K, Ritz E. Microvascular disease—the Cinderella of uraemic heart disease. *Nephrol Dial Transplant.* 2000;15(10):1493-1503.

451. Standl E, Schnell O. A new look at the heart in diabetes mellitus: from ailing to failing. *Diabetologia.* 2000;43(12):1455-1469.

452. Colhoun HM, Betteridge DJ, Durrington PN, et al. Primary prevention of cardiovascular disease with atorvastatin in type 2 diabetes in the Collaborative Atorvastatin Diabetes Study (CARDS): multicentre randomised placebo-controlled trial. *Lancet.* 2004;364(9435):685-696.

453. Wanner C, Krane V, Marz W, et al. Atorvastatin in patients with type 2 diabetes mellitus undergoing hemodialysis. *N Engl J Med.* 2005;353(3):238-248.

454. Zannad F, Kessler M, Lehert P, et al. Prevention of cardiovascular events in end-stage renal disease: results of a randomized trial of fosinopril and implications for future studies. *Kidney Int.* 2006;70(7):1318-1324.

455. Zuanetti G, Maggioni AP, Keane W, et al. Nephrologists neglect administration of betablockers to dialysed diabetic patients. *Nephrol Dial Transplant.* 1997;12:2497-2500.

456. Goodkin DA, Mapes DL, Held PJ. The dialysis outcomes and practice patterns study (DOPPS): how can we improve the care of hemodialysis patients? *Semin Dial.* 2001;14(3):157-159.

457. Cice G, Ferrara L, D'Andrea A, et al. Carvedilol increases two-year survival in dialysis patients with dilated cardiomyopathy: a prospective, placebo-controlled trial. *J Am Coll Cardiol.* 2003;41(9):1438-1444.

458. Bakris GL, Hart P, Ritz E. Beta blockers in the management of chronic kidney disease. *Kidney Int.* 2006;70(11):1905-1913.

459. Manske CL, Wang Y, Rector T, et al. Coronary revascularization in insulin-dependent diabetic patients with chronic renal failure. *Lancet.* 1992;340:998-1002.

460. Matzkies FK, Reinecke H, Regetmeier A, et al. Long-term outcome after percutaneous transluminal coronary angioplasty in patients with chronic renal failure with and without diabetic nephropathy. *Nephron.* 2001;89(1):10-14.

461. Broome ME, Knafl K. Back to the future: building on the past. *J Pediatr Nurs.* 1994;9(3):208-210.

462. Hosoda Y, Yamamoto T, Takazawa K, et al. Coronary artery bypass grafting in patients on chronic hemodialysis: surgical outcome in diabetic nephropathy versus nondiabetic nephropathy patients. *Ann Thorac Surg.* 2001;71(2):543-548.

463. Herzog CA, Ma JZ, Collins AJ. Comparative survival of dialysis patients in the United States after coronary angioplasty, coronary artery stenting, and coronary artery bypass surgery and impact of diabetes. *Circulation.* 2002;106(17):2207-2211.

464. Le Feuvre C, Dambrin G, Helft G, et al. Clinical outcome following coronary angioplasty in dialysis patients: a case-control study in the era of coronary stenting. *Heart.* 2001;85(5):556-560.

465. Hatada K, Sugiura T, Nakamura S, et al. Coronary artery diameter and left ventricular function in patients on maintenance hemodialysis treatment: comparison between diabetic and nondiabetic patients. *Nephron.* 1998;80(3):269-273.

466. Becker B, Kronenberg F, Kielstein JT, et al. Rexnal insulin resistance syndrome, adiponectin and cardiovascular events in patients with kidney disease: the mild and moderate kidney disease study. *J Am Soc Nephrol.* 2005;16(4):1091-1098.

467. Ritz E, Koch M. Morbidity and mortality due to hypertension in patients with renal failure. *Am J Kidney Dis.* 1993;21(5 suppl 2):113-118.

468. Simic-Ogrizovic S, Backus G, Mayer A, et al. The influence of different glucose concentrations in haemodialysis solutions on metabolism and blood pressure stability in diabetic patients. *Int J Artif Organs.* 2001;24(12):863-869.

469. Wu MS, Yu CC, Yang CW, et al. Poor pre-dialysis glycaemic control is a predictor of mortality in type II diabetic patients on maintenance haemodialysis. *Nephrol Dial Transplant.* 1997;12(10):2105-2110.

470. Morioka T, Emoto M, Tabata T, et al. Glycemic control is a predictor of survival for diabetic patients on hemodialysis. *Diabetes Care.* 2001;24(5):909-913.

471. Inaba M, Okuno S, Kumeda Y, et al. Glycated albumin is a better glycemic indicator than glycated hemoglobin values in hemodialysis patients with diabetes: effect of anemia and erythropoietin injection. *J Am Soc Nephrol.* 2007;18(3):896-903.

472. Hayashino Y, Fukuhara S, Akiba T, et al. Diabetes, glycaemic control and mortality risk in patients on haemodialysis: the Japan Dialysis Outcomes and Practice Pattern Study. *Diabetologia.* 2007;50(6):1170-1177.

473. Suliman ME, Stenvinkel P, Heimburger O, et al. Plasma sulfur amino acids in relation to cardiovascular disease, nutritional status, and diabetes mellitus in patients with chronic renal failure at start of dialysis therapy. *Am J Kidney Dis.* 2002;40(3):480-488.

474. Cano NJ, Roth H, Aparicio M, et al. Malnutrition in hemodialysis diabetic patients: evaluation and prognostic influence. *Kidney Int.* 2002;62(2):593-601.

475. Schomig M, Ritz E, Standl E, et al. The diabetic foot in the dialyzed patient. *J Am Soc Nephrol.* 2000;11(6):1153-1159.

476. Koch M, Trapp R, Kulas W, et al. Critical limb ischaemia as a main cause of death in patients with end-stage renal disease: a single-centre study. *Nephrol Dial Transplant.* 2004;19(10):2547-2552.

477. Sheahan MG, Hamdan AD, Veraldi JR, et al. Lower extremity minor amputations: the roles of diabetes mellitus and timing of revascularization. *J Vasc Surg.* 2005;42(3):476-480.

478. Sehgal AR, Leon JB, Siminoff LA, et al. Improving the quality of hemodialysis treatment: a community-based randomized controlled trial to overcome patient-specific barriers. *JAMA*. 2002;287(15):1961-1967.

479. Heaf JG, Lokkegaard H, Madsen M. Initial survival advantage of peritoneal dialysis relative to haemodialysis. *Nephrol Dial Transplant*. 2002;17(1):112-117.

480. Winkelmayer WC, Glynn RJ, Mittleman MA, et al. Comparing mortality of elderly patients on hemodialysis versus peritoneal dialysis: a propensity score approach. *J Am Soc Nephrol*. 2002;13(9):2353-2362.

481. Van Biesen W, Vanholder RC, Veys N, et al. An evaluation of an integrative care approach for end-stage renal disease patients. *J Am Soc Nephrol*. 2000;11(1):116-125.

482. Linden T, Cohen A, Deppisch R, et al. 3,4-Dideoxyglucosone-3-ene (3,4-DGE): a cytotoxic glucose degradation product in fluids for peritoneal dialysis. *Kidney Int*. 2002;62(2):697-703.

483. Schwenger V, Morath C, Salava A, et al. Damage to the peritoneal membrane by glucose degradation products is mediated by the receptor for advanced glycation end-products. *J Am Soc Nephrol*. 2006;17(1):199-207.

484. Zeier M, Schwenger V, Deppisch R, et al. Glucose degradation products in PD fluids: do they disappear from the peritoneal cavity and enter the systemic circulation? *Kidney Int*. 2003;63(1):298-305.

485. Wieslander AP. Cytotoxicity of peritoneal dialysis fluid—is it related to glucose breakdown products? *Nephrol Dial Transplant*. 1996;11(6):958-959.

486. Rippe B, Simonsen O, Heimburger O, et al. Long-term clinical effects of a peritoneal dialysis fluid with less glucose degradation products. *Kidney Int*. 2001;59(1):348-357.

487. Mieghem AV, Fonck C, Coosemans W, et al. Outcome of cadaver kidney transplantation in 23 patients with type 2 diabetes mellitus. *Nephrol Dial Transplant*. 2001;16(8):1686-1691.

488. Becker BN, Rush SH, Dykstra DM, et al. Preemptive transplantation for patients with diabetes-related kidney disease. *Arch Intern Med*. 2006;166(1):44-48.

489. Cohen DJ, St Martin L, Christensen LL, et al. Kidney and pancreas transplantation in the United States, 1995-2004. *Am J Transplant*. 2006;6(5 pt 2):1153-1169.

490. Tyden G, Bolinder J, Solders G, et al. Improved survival in patients with insulin-dependent diabetes mellitus and end-stage diabetic nephropathy 10 years after combined pancreas and kidney transplantation. *Transplantation*. 1999;67(5):645-648.

491. Solders G, Tydén G, Tibell A, et al. Improvement in nerve conduction 8 years after combined pancreatic and renal transplantation. *Transplant Proc*. 1995;27:3091.

492. Morath C, Zeier M, Dohler B, et al. Metabolic control improves long-term renal allograft and patient survival in type 1 diabetes. *J Am Soc Nephrol*. 2008;19(8):1557-1563.

493. Kelly WD, Lillehei RC, Merkel FK, et al. Allotransplantation of the pancreas and duodenum along with the kidney in diabetic nephropathy. *Surgery*. 1967;61:827-837.

494. Mange KC, Joffe MM, Feldman HI. Effect of the use or nonuse of long-term dialysis on the subsequent survival of renal transplants from living donors. *N Engl J Med*. 2001;344(10):726-731.

495. Kahl A, Bechstein WO, Frei U. Trends and perspectives in pancreas and simultaneous pancreas and kidney transplantation. *Curr Opin Urol*. 2001;11(2):165-174.

496. Hariharan S, Pirsch JD, Lu CY, et al. Pancreas after kidney transplantation. *J Am Soc Nephrol*. 2002;13(4):1109-1118.

497. Pfeffer F, Nauck MA, Benz S, et al. Determinants of a normal (versus impaired) oral glucose tolerance after combined pancreas-kidney transplantation in IDDM patients. *Diabetologia*. 1996;39:462-468.

498. Cottrell DA. Normalization of insulin sensitivity and glucose homeostasis in type I diabetic pancreas transplant recipients: a 48-month cross-sectional study—a clinical research study. *J Clin Endocrinol Metab*. 1996;81:3513-3519.

499. Christiansen E, Vestergaard H, Tibell A, et al. Impaired insulin-stimulated nonoxidative glucose metabolism in pancreas-kidney transplant recipients. Dose-response effects of insulin on glucose turnover. *Diabetes*. 1996;45:1267-1275.

500. Rooney DP, Robertson RP. Hepatic insulin resistance after pancreas transplantation in type I diabetes. *Diabetes*. 1996;45:134-138.

501. Foger B, Konigsrainer A, Palos G, et al. Effects of pancreas transplantation on distribution and composition of plasma lipoproteins. *Metabolism*. 1996;45:856-861.

502. Tyden G, Reinholt FP, Sundkvist G, et al. Recurrence of autoimmune diabetes mellitus in recipients of cadaveric pancreatic grafts. *N Engl J Med*. 1996;335(12):860-863.

503. Shapiro AM, Lakey JR, Ryan EA, et al. Islet transplantation in seven patients with type 1 diabetes mellitus using a glucocorticoid-free immunosuppressive regimen. *N Engl J Med*. 2000;343(4):230-238.

504. Senior PA, Zeman M, Paty BW, et al. Changes in renal function after clinical islet transplantation: four-year observational study. *Am J Transplant*. 2007;7(1):91-98.

505. Martinez-Castelao A, Hernandez MD, Pascual J, et al. Detection and treatment of post kidney transplant hyperglycemia: a Spanish multicenter cross-sectional study. *Transplant Proc*. 2005;37(9):3813-3816.

506. Cosio FG, Pesavento TE, Osei K, et al. Post-transplant diabetes mellitus: increasing incidence in renal allograft recipients transplanted in recent years. *Kidney Int*. 2001;59(2):732-737.

507. Araki M, Flechner SM, Ismail HR, et al. Posttransplant diabetes mellitus in kidney transplant recipients receiving calcineurin or mTOR inhibitor drugs. *Transplantation*. 2006;81(3):335-341.

508. Vincenti F, Friman S, Scheuermann E, et al. Results of an international, randomized trial comparing glucose metabolism disorders and outcome with cyclosporine versus tacrolimus. *Am J Transplant*. 2007;7(6):1506-1514.

509. Midtvedt K, Hjelmesaeth J, Hartmann A, et al. Insulin resistance after renal transplantation: the effect of steroid dose reduction and withdrawal. *J Am Soc Nephrol*. 2004;15(12):3233-3239.

510. Kasiske BL, Chakkera HA, Louis TA, et al. A meta-analysis of immunosuppression withdrawal trials in renal transplantation. *J Am Soc Nephrol*. 2000;11(10):1910-1917.

511. Cosio FG, Kudva Y, van der Velde M, et al. New onset hyperglycemia and diabetes are associated with increased cardiovascular risk after kidney transplantation. *Kidney Int*. 2005;67(6):2415-2421.

512. Salifu MO, Nicastri AD, Markell MS, et al. Allograft diabetic nephropathy may progress to end-stage renal disease. *Pediatr Transplant*. 2004;8(4):351-356.

513. Fedele D. Therapy insight: sexual and bladder dysfunction associated with diabetes mellitus. *Nat Clin Pract Urol*. 2005;2(6):282-290.

514. Vejlsgaard R. Studies on urinary infection in diabetics. II. Significant bacteriuria in relation to long-term diabetic manifestations. *Acta Med Scand*. 1966;179(2):183-188.

515. Boyko EJ, Fihn SD, Scholes D, et al. Risk of urinary tract infection and asymptomatic bacteriuria among diabetic and nondiabetic postmenopausal women. *Am J Epidemiol*. 2005;161(6):557-564.

516. Tolkoff-Rubin NE, Rubin RH. The infectious disease problems of the diabetic renal transplant recipient. *Infect Dis Clin North Am*. 1995;9(1):117-130.

517. Bonadio M, Costarelli S, Morelli G, et al. The influence of diabetes mellitus on the spectrum of uropathogens and the antimicrobial resistance in elderly adult patients with urinary tract infection. *BMC Infect Dis*. 2006;6:54.

518. Tseng CC, Wu JJ, Liu HL, et al. Roles of host and bacterial virulence factors in the development of upper urinary tract infection caused by *Escherichia coli*. *Am J Kidney Dis*. 2002;39(4):744-752.

519. Perlemoine C, Neau D, Ragnaud JM, et al. Emphysematous cystitis. *Diabetes Metab*. 2004;30(4):377-379.

520. Jeong HJ, Park SC, Seo IY, et al. Prognostic factors in Fournier gangrene. *Int J Urol*. 2005;12(12):1041-1044.

521. Waldherr R, Ilkenhans C, Ritz E. How frequent is glomerulonephritis in diabetes mellitus type II? *Clin Nephrol*. 1992;37:271-273.

522. Walmsley RS, David DB, Allan RN, et al. Bilateral endogenous *Escherichia coli* endophthalmitis: a devastating complication in an insulin-dependent diabetic. *Postgrad Med J*. 1996;72:361-363.

523. Knowles HCJ. Long term juvenile diabetes treated with unmeasured diet. *Trans Assoc Am Physicians*. 1971;84:95-101.

524. Andersen AR, Christiansen JS, Andersen JK, et al. Diabetic nephropathy in type 1 (insulin-dependent) diabetes: an epidemiological study. *Diabetologia*. 1983;25:496-501.

525. Bruno G, Cavallo-Perin P, Bargero G, et al. Prevalence and risk factors for micro- and macroalbuminuria in an Italian population-based cohort of NIDDM subjects. *Diabetes Care*. 1996;19(1):43-47.

526. Mogensen CE, Poulsen PL. Epidemiology of microalbuminuria in diabetes and in the background population. *Curr Opin Nephrol Hypertens*. 1996;3:248-256.

527. Kofoed-Enevoldsen A, Borch-Johnsen K, Kreiner S, et al. Declining incidence of persistent proteinuria in type 1 (insulin-dependent) diabetic patients in Denmark. *Diabetes*. 1987;36:205-209.

528. Mathiesen ER, Rønn B, Jensen T, et al. Relationship between blood pressure and urinary albumin excretion in development of microalbuminuria. *Diabetes*. 1990;39:245-249.

529. Nelson RG, Knowler WC, Pettitt DJ, et al. Assessing risk of overt nephropathy in diabetic patients from albumin excretion in untimed urine specimens. *Arch Intern Med*. 1991;151:1761-1765.

530. Rudberg S, Dahlquist G. Determinants of progression of microalbuminuria in adolescents with IDDM. *Diabetes Care*. 1996;19(4):369-371.

531. Borch-Johnsen K, Nørgaard K, Hommel E, et al. Is diabetic nephropathy an inherited complication? *Kidney Int*. 1992;41:719-722.

532. Pettitt DJ, Saad MF, Bennett PH, et al. Familial predisposition to renal disease in two generations of Pima Indians with type 2 (non–insulin-dependent) diabetes mellitus. *Diabetologia*. 1990;33:438-443.

533. Ditscherlein G. *Nierenveränderungen bei Diabetikern*. Jena, Germany: VEB Gustav Fischer; 1969.

534. Faronato PP, Maioli M, Tonolo G, et al. Clustering of albumin excretion rate abnormalities in Caucasian patients with NIDDM. *Diabetologia.* 1997;40:816-823.

535. Gall M-A, Rossing P, Jensen JS, et al. Red cell Na/Li countertransport in non–insulin-dependent diabetics with diabetic nephropathy. *Kidney Int.* 1991;39:135-140.

536. Elving LD, Wetzels JFM, de Nobel E, et al. Erythrocyte sodium-lithium countertransport is not different in type 1 (insulin-dependent) diabetic patients with and without diabetic nephropathy. *Diabetologia.* 1991;34: 126-128.

537. Carr S, Mbanya J-C, Thomas T, et al. Increase in glomerular filtration rate in patients with insulin-dependent diabetes and elevated erythrocyte sodium-lithium countertransport. *N Engl J Med.* 1990;322:500-505.

538. Ng LL, Davies JE, Siczkowski M, et al. Abnormal Na⁺/H⁺ antiporter phenotype and turnover of immortalized lymphoblasts from type 1 diabetic patients with nephropathy. *J Clin Invest.* 1994;93:2750-2757.

539. Koren W, Koldanov R, Pronin VS, et al. Enhanced erythrocyte Na⁺/H⁺ exchange predicts diabetic nephropathy in patients with IDDM. *Diabetologia.* 1998;41:201-205.

540. Monciotti CG, Semplicini A, Morocutti A, et al. Elevated sodium-lithium countertransport activity in erythrocytes is predictive of the development of microalbuminuria in IDDM. *Diabetologia.* 1997;40:654-661.

541. Cowie CC, Port FK, Wolfe RA, et al. Disparities in incidence of diabetic end-stage renal disease according to race and type of diabetes. *N Engl J Med.* 1989;321:1074-1079.

542. Krolewski M, Eggers PW, Warram JH. Magnitude of end-stage renal disease in IDDM: a 35 year follow-up study. *Kidney Int.* 1996;50:2041-2046.

543. Franken AAM, Derkx FHM, Man in't Veld AJ, et al. High plasma prorenin in diabetes mellitus and its correlation with some complications. *J Clin Endocrinol Metab.* 1990;71:1008-1015.

544. Daneman D, Crompton CH, Balfe JA, et al. Plasma prorenin as an early marker of nephropathy in diabetic (IDDM) adolescents. *Kidney Int.* 1994;46:1154-1159.

545. Allen TJ, Cooper ME, Gilbert RE, et al. Serum total renin is increased before microalbuminuria in diabetes. *Kidney Int.* 1996;50:902-907.

546. Chase HP, Garg SK, Marshall G, et al. Cigarette smoking increases the risk of albuminuria among subjects with type 1 diabetes. *JAMA.* 1991;265: 614-617.

547. Ravid M, Neumann L, Lishner M. Plasma lipids and the progression of nephropathy in diabetes mellitus type II: effect of ACE inhibitors. *Kidney Int.* 1995;47:907-910.

548. Stephenson J, Fuller JH, Viberti GC, et al. the EURODIAB IDDM Complications Study Group. Blood pressure, retinopathy and urinary albumin excretion in IDDM. *Diabetologia.* 1995;38(5):599-603.

549. Ahmed SB, Hovind P, Parving H-H, et al. Oral contraceptives, angiotensin-dependent renal vasoconstriction, and risk of diabetic nephropathy. *Diabetes Care.* 2005;28(8):1988-1994.

550. Schram MT, Chaturvedi N, Schalkwijk CG, et al. Markers of inflammation are cross-sectionally associated with microvascular complications and cardiovascular disease in type 1 diabetes—the EURODIAB Prospective Complications Study. *Diabetologia.* 2005;48(2):370-378.

551. Hovind P, Hansen TK, Tarnow L, et al. Mannose-binding lectin as a predictor of microalbuminuria in type 1 diabetes: an inception cohort study. *Diabetes.* 2005;54(5):1523-1527.

552. Frystyk J, Tarnow L, Hansen TK, et al. Increased serum adiponectin levels in type 1 diabetic patients with microvascular complications. *Diabetologia.* 2005;48(9):1911-1918.

553. Lurbe E, Redon J, Kesani A, et al. Increase in nocturnal blood pressure and progression to microalbuminuria in type 1 diabetes. *N Engl J Med.* 2002;347(11):797-805.

554. Vaidya VS, Niewczas MA, Ficociello LH, et al. Regression of microalbuminuria in type 1 diabetes is associated with lower levels of urinary tubular injury biomarkers, kidney injury molecule-1, and N-acetyl-β-D-glucosaminidase. *Kidney Int.* 2011;79(4):464-470.

555. Tuttle KR, Bakris GL, Toto RD, et al. The effect of ruboxistaurin on nephropathy in type 2 diabetes. *Diabetes Care.* 2005;28(11):2686-2690.

556. Sourris KC, Forbes JM, Cooper ME. Therapeutic interruption of advanced glycation in diabetic nephropathy: do all roads lead to Rome? *Ann NY Acad Sci.* 2008;1126:101-106.

557. Williams ME, Bolton WK, Khalifah RG, et al. Effects of pyridoxamine in combined phase 2 studies of patients with type 1 and type 2 diabetes and overt nephropathy. *Am J Nephrol.* 2007;27(6):605-614.

558. Rabbani N, Alam SS, Riaz S, et al. High-dose thiamine therapy for patients with type 2 diabetes and microalbuminuria: a randomised, double-blind placebo-controlled pilot study. *Diabetologia.* 2009;52(2):208-212.

559. Navarro JF, Mora C, Muros M, et al. Additive antiproteinuric effect of pentoxifylline in patients with type 2 diabetes under angiotensin II receptor blockade: a short-term, randomized, controlled trial. *J Am Soc Nephrol.* 2005;16(7):2119-2126.

560. Bakris GL, Ruilope LM, McMorn SO, et al. Rosiglitazone reduces microalbuminuria and blood pressure independently of glycemia in type 2 diabetes patients with microalbuminuria. *J Hypertens.* 2006;24(10):2047-2055.

561. Wenzel RR, Littke T, Kuranoff S, et al. Avosentan reduces albumin excretion in diabetics with macroalbuminuria. *J Am Soc Nephrol.* 2009;20(3):655-664.

562. Adler SG. Dose escalation phase 1 study of FG 3019 anti CTGF monoclonal antibody in subjects with type 1/2 diabetes mellitus and microalbuminuria. *J Am Soc Nephrol.* 2006;17:157A:(abstract).

563. Huang L, Haylor JL, Hau Z, et al. Transglutaminase inhibition ameliorates experimental diabetic nephropathy. *Kidney Int.* 2009;76(4):383-394.

564. Ninichuk V, Clauss S, Kulkarni O, et al. Late onset of Ccl2 blockade with the Spiegelmer mNOX-E36-3′PEG prevents glomerulosclerosis and improves glomerular filtration rate in db/db mice. *Am J Pathol.* 2008;172(3):628-637.

565. Kosugi T, Nakayama T, Heinig M, et al. Effect of lowering uric acid on renal disease in the type 2 diabetic db/db mice. *Am J Physiol Renal Physiol.* 2009;297(2):F481-F488.

Index

Note: Page numbers followed by *f* indicate figures; those followed by *t* indicate tables.

Congestive heart failure *(Continued)*
  hypervolemia and
    alterations in glomerular hemodynamics in, 498–499, 499f
    effector mechanism abnormalities in, 498–499
    enhanced tubular sodium reabsorption in, 473f, 499
    neurohumoral mediators of, 499
    sensing mechanism abnormalities in, 496–498
  hyponatremia in, 572–573
  neuropeptide Y in, 508
  nitric oxide in, 505–506
  pathophysiology of, 521–523
  peroxisome proliferator–activated receptor τ agonists and, 508
  prostaglandins in, 506–507
  renal artery stenosis and, 1766
  renin-angiotensin-aldosterone system in, 499–501, 508t
  right ventricular, 1898
  sympathetic nervous system in, 501–502
  treatment of, 521–523
    beta-blockade in, 521
    endothelin antagonists in, 521–522
    natriuretic peptides in, 522
    neutral endopeptidase inhibitors in, 522
    nitric oxide donors in, 521
    renin-angiotensin-aldosterone system inhibition in, 521
    vasopeptidase inhibitors in, 522
    vasopressin receptor antagonists in, 522–523
  urotensin in, 507
  vasoconstrictor/antinatriuretic systems in, 499–503
  vasodilatory/natriuretic systems in, 503–508
  vasopressin in, 502
Congo red stain, 1010–1011
Conivaptan, 1889–1890
  for hyponatremia, 583–584
Connecting tubule
  in acid-base homeostasis in, 302
  bicarbonate reabsorption in, 302
  chloride transport in, 182–183, 182f
  potassium transport in, 67, 188–189
  sodium chloride transport in, 183–186
  sodium reabsorption in, 1879, 1880f
  sodium transport in, 181–186, 181f
  structure and function of, 66–67, 66f, 177–178, 328–329
Connective tissue disease, mixed, glomerular manifestations of, 1208–1209
Connective tissue growth factor, 1426–1427
  in renal fibrosis, 1033
Connexins, 49
  in blood pressure homeostasis, 1690
Conn's syndrome, 218
Consanguinity, genetic disorders and, 2752–2760
Continuous ambulatory peritoneal dialysis, 2356, 2356f. *See also* Peritoneal dialysis.
  for diabetic nephropathy, 1442
  in Near and Middle East, 2759–2760
Continuous positive airway pressure (CPAP)
  for sleep apnea, 2150
Continuous renal replacement therapy, 2387–2390, 2388f, 2388t. *See also* Dialysis; Extracorporeal therapy; Hemofiltration; Renal replacement therapy.
  for acute kidney injury, 1084–1085
  alternatives to, 2389–2390
  in children, 2607
    for acute kidney injury, 2607, 2687–2691
    anticoagulation for, 2688
    complications of, 2690
    drug dosing during, 2689
    equipment for, 2687–2688
    membrane reactions in, 2690
    modes of, 2688
      selection of, 2690
    nutrition in, 2689–2690
    outcomes in, 2690–2691
    prescription for, 2689
    solutions for, 2688
    vascular access for, 2687
  for cirrhosis, 525–526
  drug therapy in, 2267
  indications for, 2387–2388
  initiation of, timing of, 2388t, 2389

Continuous renal replacement therapy *(Continued)*
  intensity of, 2389
  outcome in, 2388–2389, 2388f, 2388t
  for poisoning, 2416. *See also* Poisoning, extracorporeal therapy for.
    vs. sustained low-efficiency dialysis, 2416
  for sepsis, 2389
  vs. intermittent hemodialysis, 2388–2389, 2388f
Continuous venovenous hemofiltration, for theophylline poisoning, 2428–2429
Contralateral ratio, in aldosteronism diagnosis, 1711
Contrast media
  gadolinium chelate, nephrogenic systemic fibrosis and, 940–942, 941f
  iodinated, 932–933
    "allergic" reactions to, 932–933
    renal injury from, 933, 1049–1050, 1776
      in allograft recipient, 2534
Convection, in hemodialysis, 2301–2302, 2302f, 2304
Coomassie blue method, 2624
Copeptin, 544
Copper metabolism, in Wilson's disease, 1593
Copper sulfate poisoning, 2771, 2772t, 2776
Copy number variants, 1555–1556
COQ2 gene, in focal segmental glomerulosclerosis, 1114t
Cori cycle, 149, 626
Cornell criterion, in electrocardiography, 1727
Coronary angiography, in renovascular disease, 1753f
Coronary artery calcifications. *See also* Calcifications, vascular.
  in pediatric chronic kidney disease, 2668–2669, 2668f
Coronary artery disease. *See also* Atherosclerosis.
  beta blockers for, 1840
Cortex
  anatomy of, 31, 32f
  bilateral necrosis of, in pregnancy, 1811
  blood flow in, 104
    measurement of, 104
  circulation in, 95–101
    peritubular capillary dynamics and, 97–101
  COX-2 in, 425–427, 426f
  hemodynamic parameters in, 440
  lymphatics of, 83, 83f
Cortical calcifications, 955
Cortical collecting duct. *See* Collecting duct(s), cortical.
Cortical interstitium, 80–82, 80f
  in nephrogenesis, 6
Corticosteroids. *See also* Glucocorticoid(s); *specific steroid.*
  for acute interstitial nephritis, 1343
  adverse effects of, 1285–1286
  angiotensin II inhibition with, for IgA nephropathy, 1149–1150
  for anorexia, in peritoneal dialysis, 2362
  anti-inflammatory, in regulation of COX gene expression, 424
  for childhood polyarteritis nodosa, 2659
  for Churg-Strauss syndrome, 1220
  fetal exposure to, nephrogenesis and, 798
  for focal segmental glomerulosclerosis, 1118–1119
  for glomerular disease, 1284–1286
  for Henoch-Schönlein purpura, 2658–2659
  for hypercalcemia, in children, 2600t
  for hypercalcemia of malignancy, 1541
  for idiopathic nephrotic syndrome, 2641–2642
  for IgA nephropathy, 1149
  immunosuppression with
    maintenance, 2518t, 2522
    in pregnant patient, 1816, 1817t
  indications for, 1284–1285
  for membranous glomerulopathy, 1127–1128
  for minimal change glomerulopathy, 1110, 1110t
  posttransplant, hypertension and, 1720
  in regulation of COX gene expression, 424
  resistance to, minimal change glomerulopathy and, 1110–1111
  for scleroderma, 1316t
  toxicity of, 2696t
Cortisol
  in primary hyperaldosteronism, 1710
    adrenal vein sampling and, 1711
    fludrocortisone suppression test and, 1710
    intravenous saline loading and, 1710
  synthesis of, 203, 204f

Corynebacterium urealyticum infection, 1367–1369. *See also* Urinary tract infections (UTIs).
Costimulatory molecules, in immune response to allografts, 2480–2482, 2481f
Costimulatory signal blockers, immunosuppression with, 2521–2522
Cosyntropin, in adrenal vein catheterization, 1711
Cough, ACE inhibitor–related, 1829
Countercurrent multiplication hypothesis, 334–335, 334f
Coupled plasma filtration adsorption, 2389, 2390t
COX. *See under* Cyclooxygenase (COX).
CPAP, for sleep apnea, 2150
CPR, ethical aspects of, 2829
Cramps, in hemodialysis, 2335
Cranberry, for cystitis, 1364
CREATE trial, of erythropoiesis-stimulating agents, 2103–2104
Creatinine, 2002f, 2004
  in bicarbonate generation, 308
  serum
    atherosclerotic renal artery stenosis and, 1769–1770
      management of, 1778
      surgery in, 1784–1785, 1784f
    captopril renography and, 1772
    as GFR biomarker, 1021, 2263
    in GFR estimation, 870t, 871–874
    heart failure and, diuretic therapy in, 1898
    in hypovolemia diagnosis, 493
  toxic metabolites of, 2002f, 2004
  turnover of, in uremia, 2173
  urinary, excretion of, age-related differences in, 883, 883f
Creatinine clearance
  in children, 2623–2624
  in GFR estimation, 872–873
    in children, 2624
  in peritoneal dialysis, 2357–2358, 2358t
  residual function and, 2263
Creatinine-ethylenediaminetetraacetic acid (Cr-EDTA), in GFR estimation, 876–877
Creatol, 2004
Crescendo angina, renal artery stenosis and, 1766
Crescentic glomerulonephritis
  categorization of, 1153–1155, 1153f–1154f, 1154t–1155t
  immune complex-mediated, 1155–1156
    electron microscopy of, 1156
    epidemiology of, 1155
    immunofluorescence microscopy of, 1155–1156
    light microscopy of, 1155
    pathogenesis of, 1156
    pathology of, 1155–1156
    treatment of, 1156
  nomenclature in, 1153
  pauci-immune, 1161–1168
    clinical features of, 1164–1165
    electron microscopy of, 1162–1163
    epidemiology of, 1161
    immunofluorescence microscopy of, 1162
    laboratory findings in, 1165–1166
    light microscopy of, 1155t, 1158t, 1161–1162, 1162f
    natural history of, 1164–1165
    pathogenesis of, 1163–1164
    pathology of, 1161–1163
    treatment of, 1166–1168
P-Cresol, 2002f, 2005
Critical care nephrology, 2378
  acid-base disorders in, 2380t–2381t, 2381–2383
  acute kidney injury and, 2380–2381, 2380t
    in Africa, 2737
  blood purification methods in, 2389–2390, 2390t
  cardiorenal syndromes in, 2383–2387. *See also* Cardiorenal syndromes.
  continuous renal replacement therapy in, 2387–2390
  as core component, 2379
  intensivists in, 2379–2380
  multiorgan support therapy in, 2390
  origins of, 2379
  practice of, 2379–2380
  scope of, 2379–2380, 2379t–2380t
Critical illness, hypocalcemia in, 703
Critical Path Initiative (FDA), 1036

Delta values, comparison of, in acid-base disorders, 607–608

Demeclocycline, for hyponatremia, 583

Dementia. *See also* Cognitive impairment.
  age-related, 2148, 2148f
  Alzheimer's, 2147–2149
  delirium and, 2149
  depression and, 2149
  dialysis, 2147
  epidemiology of, 2147–2148
  evaluation of, 2149
  hypertension and, 1679
  management of, 2149
  risk factors for, 2148
  urinary tract infections and, 1367
  vascular, 2147–2149

Demographic factors, 742. *See also* Gender; Race/
  ethnicity; Socioeconomic status.
  in hypertension, 1670

Demyelination, osmotic, 902
  diuretics and, 1903

Dendritic cell(s), interstitial, 1982–1983

Dendroaspis natriuretic peptide (DNP), 396–397
  structure and synthesis of, 398

Dengue fever
  in Far East, 2789
  in Latin America, 2720–2721

Dense deposit disease, 1134–1136
  clinical features of, 1136
  epidemiology of, 1134
  pathogenesis of, 1135–1136
  pathology of, 1134–1135, 1135f
  treatment of, 1136

Dentin matrix protein, 1599, 1599t
  in autosomal recessive hypophosphatemic rickets, 1600

Dent's disease, 243–244, 1476t–1478t, 1587–1588
  nephrolithiasis in, 2654

Denys-Drash syndrome, 23–24, 1579–1580

Deoxyribonucleic acid (DNA), complementary. *See* Complementary DNA (cDNA).

Depigmentation, 2157f, 2158

Depleting agents, immunosuppression with, 2519–2520

Depression
  dementia and, 2149
  in end-stage kidney disease, 2297

Dermatitis
  arteriovenous shunt, 2163
  diuretic-related, 1907

Desamino d-arginine-8 vasopressin (dDVP), 354
  for diabetes insipidus, 357

Deserpidine, in single-pill combination therapy, 1859t

Desmopressin
  for diabetes insipidus, 564t, 565–567
  for nephrogenic diabetes insipidus, in children, 2578
  for uremic bleeding, 2106, 2107f

Desmopressin test, for nephrogenic diabetes insipidus, 901, 2577, 2627

Developmental abnormalities. *See also* Cognitive impairment; Congenital anomalies.
  in chronic kidney disease, 2665–2666
  in pediatric renal transplant recipients, 2713

DEXA, in nutritional assessment, 2327

Dexamethasone, for scleroderma, 1316t

Dextran 70, for thrombotic microangiopathy, 1302t

DGoodpasture's syndrome, 1224–1226, 1225f–1226f.
  See also Anti–glomerular basement membrane disease.

Diabetes insipidus, 357–358, 1614–1619
  AVP-AVPR2-AQP shuttle pathway in, 1614–1615
  central, 553–557
    autosomal dominant form of, 553–554, 554f
    case study of, 902–903, 903t
    diagnosis of, 2578t
    etiology of, 553–555, 554f
    insufficient vasopressin causing, 552, 552t
    partial, 902–903, 902f, 903t
    pathophysiology of, 357, 555–557, 555f–556f
      triphasic response in, 555–556
    treatment of, 566–567
  clinical manifestations of, 561
  differential diagnosis of, 561–564, 562f, 563t
  dipsogenic, 552, 560
  diuretics in, 1902
  evaluation of, 900–901, 901f
  familial neurohypophyseal, 1614

Diabetes insipidus *(Continued)*
  gestational, 552, 1794
    etiology of, 558
    pathophysiology of, 558
    treatment of, 567
  nephrogenic, 552, 558–560
    acquired, 372–375
    aquaporin-2 in, 357–358, 372
    in children, 2648–2649
    congenital, 372, 1615–1618, 2576–2578, 2578t, 2648–2649
      carrier detection for, 1619
      clinical presentation of, 1615–1618, 2577
      diagnosis of, 1619, 2577, 2578t
      history in, 1615–1618, 2577
      mutations in, 1617–1618, 2576–2577
      pathogenesis of, 1615–1618, 2576–2577
      perinatal testing for, 1619
      prevention of complications in, 1619, 2578
      treatment of, 1619, 2578
    etiology of, 558–560, 559f
    knockout mice for, 348
    lithium-induced, 357, 372–373, 375f
    pathophysiology of, 357–358, 560
    treatment of, 567–568
      potential strategies in, 370–371
      V_2R agonists in, 357–358
      V_2R mutations in, 357–358
    vasopressin in, 1615
  pathogenesis of, 1614–1615
  pathophysiology of, 900, 901f
  polyuria in, 900–902, 901f
  treatment of, 564–568, 564t

Diabetes mellitus
  ACE inhibitors in, 1828
  acquired perforating dermatosis in, 2158, 2158f
  acute kidney injury in, 738–739, 739f
  calcineurin inhibitor–induced, 1290
  in chronic kidney disease, 2069
    randomized controlled dietary trials in, 2190–2191
  COX metabolites in, 445–446
  diuretic-related, 1905, 1906f
  hypomagnesemia in, 706
  microalbuminuria in
    clinical course and pathophysiology of, 1423–1424
    epidemiology of, 1419–1421
    as predictor of nephropathy, 1411, 1421, 1421t
    prevalence and incidence of, 1419–1421, 1421t
    prognosis of, 1421–1422
    renal structure and, 1416f–1417f, 1417
  in nondiabetic solid organ graft recipients, 1443
  in peritoneal dialysis, 2364–2365
  pheochromocytoma and, 1701
  posttransplant
    in children, 2710
    treatment of, 2544
  in renal cyst and diabetes syndrome, 2631
  renal transplantation in, 2549
  renin-angiotensin system and, 392–393
  treatment of
    drug dosing in, 2286–2287
    end-stage kidney disease in, 731
    osmotic diuresis in, 905–906
    pyelonephritis in, 1364–1365
    stroke risk in, 2140, 2140t, 2143–2144
    uric acid stones in, 1492–1493, 1492f
  type 1
    renal pathology in, 1411–1419, 1412f, 1412t, 1415f
    vs. nephropathy, 1418
  type 2
    high birth weight and, 792–793
    obesity and, 2209
    structural-functional relationships in, 1418–1419
    vs. nephropathy, 1418

Diabetic glomerulosclerosis, diffuse, 1413, 1415f

Diabetic ketoacidosis, 628
  evaluation of, 922–924
  hypophosphatemia in, 717, 2601

Diabetic nephropathy, 1411
  in Africa, 2740
  bladder dysfunction in, 1443
  clinical course of, 1424–1427, 1425f
  complications in
    extrarenal, 1427
    microvascular and macrovascular, 1438t

Diabetic nephropathy *(Continued)*
  endothelin system in, 395–396
  with end-stage kidney disease, 731, 768, 1437–1442
    epidemiology of, 1437–1438
    management of, 1438–1442, 1438t
      acute-on-chronic renal failure and, 1439
      anemia and, 1439
      blood pressure control in, 1438
      glucose control in, 1438–1439
      hemodialysis in, 1440–1441
      malnutrition and, 1439
      peritoneal dialysis in, 1441–1442
      renal replacement therapy in, 1439–1440
      vascular access in, 1439
  epidemiology of, 1419–1421
  in Far East, 2792–2793
  genetic analysis in, 1562–1565
    candidate gene approach in, 1562–1563
    familial aggregation studies in, 1562
    future of, 1565
    genome-wide association studies in, 1564–1565
    linkage analysis in, 1563–1564
    positional cloning in, 1564
    resources for, 1562
  genetic factors in, 1555, 1562–1565
  in Indian subcontinent, 2778
  kallikrein-kinin system in, 407–408
  in Latin America, 2727–2729
  microalbuminuria as predictor of, 1411, 1421, 1421t
  in Near and Middle East, 2748–2749, 2751
  nephrotic syndrome and, 850–851
  in New Zealand, 2814, 2816
  in Pacific Islands, 2817
  pathology of, 1411–1419, 1412f, 1412t, 1415f
  pathophysiology of, 1424–1427, 1425f
  persistent albuminuria in, 1411
  posttransplant, 2536
  pregnancy and, 1813–1814
  prevalence and incidence of, 1419–1421, 1421t
  prognosis of, 1422–1423
  progression of, gender and, 745
  randomized controlled dietary trials in, 2190–2191
  reversibility of, 1419, 1420f
  risk factors for, 1418, 1421t
  risk scores for, 775t
  structural-functional relationships in, 1415f–1417f, 1416–1417
    in type 2 diabetes, 1418–1419
  treatment of, 1427–1437
    ACE inhibitors in, 2215–2216, 2215f
    blood pressure control in, 1428–1436, 1431f–1432f, 1435f–1436f, 1435t
    dietary protein restriction in, 1437
    glycemic control in, 1427–1428, 1428f
    lipid-lowering therapy in, 1436–1437
    new therapy options in, 1437, 1437t
  transplantation in, 1442–1443
    islet cell, 1443
    kidney, 1442
    kidney-pancreas, 1442–1443
  in type 1 vs. type 2 diabetes, 1418
  urinary tract infection and, 1443–1444

Dialysance, 2304

Dialysate. *See* Hemodialysis, dialysate in.

Dialysate clearance, 2414

Dialysate pump, 2310–2311

Dialysis. *See also* Hemodialysis; Peritoneal dialysis; Renal replacement therapy.
  in Africa, 2737, 2740–2741, 2740f
  amyloidosis and, 2162–2163
  asymmetric dimethylarginine and, 1717
  atherosclerosis and, 2142
  in Australia, 2805–2808, 2805f–2806f, 2806t
  brain edema in, 2147
  calciphylaxis in, 2158–2159
  in children, 2680
    for acute kidney injury, 2606, 2684–2691
    for chronic kidney disease, 2681
    hemodialysis in, 2681–2683
    indications for, 2681
    peritoneal dialysis in, 2683–2684
    vascular access for, 2681–2684
  cognitive impairment in, 2147
  daily, 2258
  drug clearance in, 2258